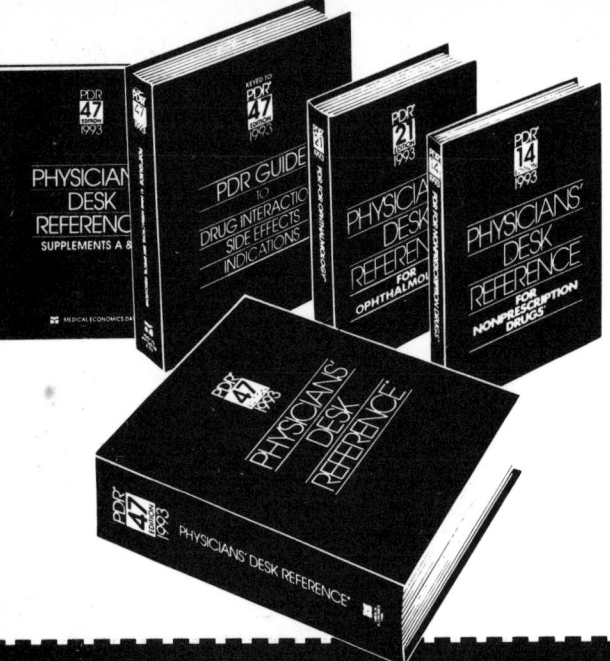

MEDICAL ECONOMICS

Today's top source of definitive medical

Medical Economics Data has long been the most respected, most trusted publisher of essential medical information in the country. Thousands of professionals regularly rely on its vital publications in their day-to-day work.

For more than 45 years, PHYSICIANS' DESK REFERENCE® has been universally recognized as the "last word" on prescription medicines and their effects. Medical Economics Data has proudly continued that tradition of providing the finest reference resources for the entire healthcare industry in all its publications. Every edition is guaranteed to be:

COMPREHENSIVE — Complete coverage of all the essential details assures you of getting all the facts.

AUTHORITATIVE — FDA-approved information gives you the confidence of always getting the official data you need.

UP-TO-DATE — Since current medical news is so critical, Medical Economics Data prides itself on its cutting-edge information network which gets the latest facts almost instantaneously.

EASY-TO-USE — Organized and indexed for quick, easy access, all publications are ready for fast reference.

SEE OTHER SIDE FOR PRODUCT DESCRIPTIONS

COMPLETE YOUR 1993 PDR® LIBRARY NOW!

519975

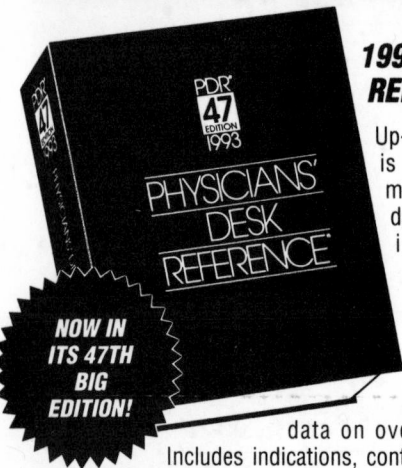
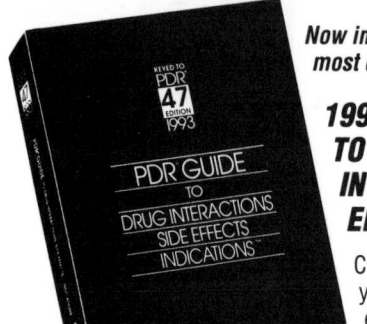
PHYSICIANS' CHANGE OF ADDRESS NOTIFICATION

NO POSTAGE NECESSARY IF MAILED IN THE UNITED STATES

BUSINESS REPLY MAIL
FIRST CLASS MAIL   PERMIT NO. 648   OAK BROOK, IL

POSTAGE WILL BE PAID BY ADDRESSEE

PHYSICIANS' DESK REFERENCE®
Professional Relations Department
P.O. Box 3309
OAK BROOK IL 60522-9879

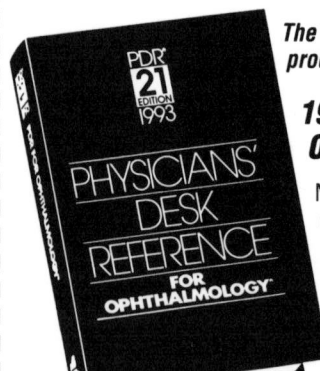

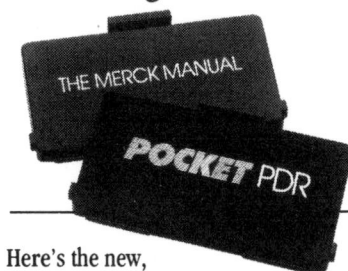

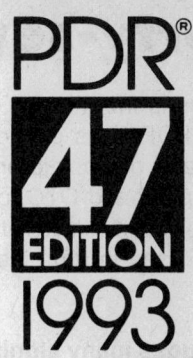

PDR 47 EDITION 1993

PHYSICIANS' DESK REFERENCE®

Product Manager
DANIEL B. ZURICH

Sales Manager
CHARLIE J. MEITNER

Account Managers
CHAD E. ALCORN
JAMES R. PANTALEO
MICHAEL S. SARAJIAN
JOANNE C. TERZIDES

Commercial Sales Manager
ROBIN B. BARTLETT

Direct Marketing Manager
ROBERT W. CHAPMAN

Manager, Professional Data
MUKESH MEHTA, R. Ph.

Index Editor
ADELE L. DOWD

Director of Production
MARJORIE A. DUFFY

Assistant Director of Production
CARRIE WILLIAMS

Production Manager
KIMBERLY V. HILLER

Format Editor
MILDRED M. SCHUMACHER

Production Coordinator
ELIZABETH A. KARST

Art Associate
JOAN K. AKERLIND

Medical Consultant
LOUIS V. NAPOLITANO, MD

Officers of Medical Economics Data, a division of Medical Economics Company Inc: **President and Chief Executive Officer**, Norman R. Snesil; **Executive Vice President**, Mark L. Weinstein; **Senior Vice President and Chief Financial Officer**, J. Crispin Ashworth; **Senior Vice President of Business Development**, Stephen J. Sorkenn; **Vice President of Product Management**, Curtis B. Allen; **Vice President of Sales and Marketing**, Thomas F. Rice; **Vice President of Operations**, John R. Ware; **Vice President of Information Systems and Services**, Edward J. Zecchini

ISBN 1-56363-015-X

Foreword to the Forty-seventh Edition

Excellence in prescribing information for physicians is the mission of the PHYSICIANS' DESK REFERENCE®. This edition represents the 47th consecutive year the PDR® has provided the most complete and fully cross-referenced labeling information available on pharmaceutical and diagnostic products. Included in this reference is full product information for most pharmaceuticals, both prescription and OTC, product overviews for selected drugs and accurate photographs of many products for their easy identification. Information is also provided on active and inactive ingredients, educational materials, pregnancy categories used in drug labeling, poison control centers, and procedures for reporting drug and vaccine adverse events.

The 1993 PHYSICIANS' DESK REFERENCE includes many significant improvements such as addition of generic names to the Product Name Index (Pink Section) so that this single index covers both brand and generic names, and addition of page numbers to Product Identification photographs for easy look-up in the Product Information section.

PHYSICIANS' DESK REFERENCE is published annually by Medical Economics Data with the cooperation of the manufacturers whose products appear in the Product Identification (Gray Section), the Product Information (White Section), and the Diagnostic Product Information (Green Section). Intended primarily for physicians, the purpose of PDR is to provide essential information on major pharmaceutical and diagnostic products. In addition to this volume, the complete library of PDR publications includes: PDR GUIDE TO DRUG INTERACTIONS / SIDE EFFECTS / INDICATIONS™, PDR FOR NONPRESCRIPTION DRUGS®, and PDR FOR OPHTHALMOLOGY®. The PHYSICIANS' DESK REFERENCE database is also available on highly powerful electronic platforms: Pocket PDR®—a handheld device, PDR Drug Interactions and Side Effects diskettes™, and PDR Library on CD-ROM™ for personal computers. For additional information on these databases please see the endsheets in this volume. The complete text computer tape version, PDR Direct Access™, is also available.

This edition of PHYSICIANS' DESK REFERENCE includes the latest available information on nearly 3000 products. During the year as important new or revised information about these products becomes available to us, it is published in a PDR Supplement. Retain the Supplement with this PDR and before prescribing or administering any product described in PHYSICIANS' DESK REFERENCE, consult the latest Supplement to determine if new information about the product has been published.

Under the federal Food, Drug & Cosmetic (FD&C) Act, a drug approved for marketing may be labeled, promoted, and advertised by the manufacturer only for those uses for which the drug's safety and effectiveness have been established. The Code of Federal Regulations 201.100(d)(1) pertaining to labeling for prescription products require that for PDR content, "indications, effects, dosages, routes, methods, and frequency and duration of administration and any relevant warnings, hazards, contraindications, side effects, and precautions" must be the *same in language and emphasis*" as the approved labeling for the products. FDA regards the words *same in language and emphasis"* as requiring VERBATIM use of the approved labeling providing such information. Furthermore, information in the approved labeling that is emphasized by the use of type set in a box or in capitals, bold face, or italics must also be given the same emphasis in PDR.

The FDA has also announced that the FD&C Act "does not, however, limit the manner in which a physician may use an approved drug. Once a product has been approved for marketing, a physician may prescribe it for uses or in treatment regimens or patient populations that are not included in approved labeling." Thus the FDA states also that "accepted medical practice" often includes drug use that is not reflected in approved drug labeling. For products which do not have official package circulars, the publisher has emphasized to manufacturers the necessity of describing such products comprehensively so that physicians would have access to all information essential for intelligent and informed prescribing. Additional information on any product may be obtained through the manufacturer.

The function of the publisher is the compilation, organization, and distribution of this information. Each product description has been prepared by the manufacturer, and edited and approved by the manufacturer's medical department, medical director, and/or medical consultant. In organizing and presenting the material in PHYSICIANS' DESK REFERENCE, the publisher does not warrant or guarantee any of the products described herein or perform any independent analysis in connection with any of the product information contained herein. PHYSICIANS' DESK REFERENCE does not assume, and expressly disclaims, any obligation to obtain and include information other than that provided to it by the manufacturer. It should also be understood that the publisher is not advocating the use of any product described herein. Manufacturers suggest headings under which products should appear in the Product Category Index (Blue Section) and the Generic and Chemical Name Index (Yellow Section).

PDR Customer Service is available at 1-800-232-7379 or Fax 201-573-4956.

Contents

SECTION 1
Manufacturers' Index

The manufacturers appearing in this index (white pages) have provided information concerning their pharmaceutical products in either the Product Information or Diagnostic Product Information Section. It is through their patronage that PHYSICIANS' DESK REFERENCE® is made available to you. Included in this index are the names and addresses of these manufacturers, individuals or departments to whom you may address inquiries, a partial list of products as well as emergency telephone numbers wherever available.

The symbol ♦ indicates the product is shown in the Product Identification Section.

The symbol ᴅ indicates the product is described in PDR FOR NONPRESCRIPTION DRUGS®.

Italic page number indicates a brief listing.

ABANA PHARMACEUTICALS, INC. 403, 502
1 Chase Corporate Drive, Suite 260
Birmingham, AL 35244
Address inquiries to:
Customer Service (205) 988-4588
FAX (205) 988-3294
For Medical Emergencies Contact:
(205) 988-4588
FAX (205) 988-3294
Products Described
♦ Nasabid Capsules 403, *502*
♦ Norcet Capsules 403, *502*
♦ Obe-Nix Capsules 403, *502*
♦ Vanex Forte Caplets 403, *502*
♦ Vanex-HD Liquid 403, *502*
Other Products Available
Endagen-HD Liquid
Otocain Drops
Vanex Expectorant Liquid
Vanex-LA Tablets

ABBOTT LABORATORIES 403, 502
Pharmaceutical Products Division
Medical Information:
(800) 441-4987
Customer Service/To Place Orders:
(800) 255-5162
Physician Services: (800) 222-6885
Hospital Products Division
Medical Information
(708) 937-3806
Customer Service/To Place Orders:
(800) 222-6883
Products Described
♦ Abbokinase 403, 503
♦ Abbokinase Open-Cath 403, 504
Abbo-Pac *502*
♦ Biaxin Tablets 403, 505
Butesin Picrate Ointment 507
Calcidrine Syrup 508
Calcijex Calcitriol Injection 508
♦ Cartrol Tablets 403, 509
♦ Cefol Filmtab 403, 511
♦ Cylert Chewable Tablets 403, 511
♦ Cylert Tablets 403, 511
Dayalets Filmtab .... ᴅ
Dayalets Plus Iron Filmtab .... ᴅ
♦ Depakene Capsules & Syrup .. 403, 512
♦ Depakote Sprinkle Capsules 403, 514
♦ Depakote Tablets 403, 514
♦ Desoxyn Gradumet Tablets 403, 516
Dical-D Tablets & Wafers 517
♦ E.E.S. 400 Filmtab 403, 522
E.E.S. Granules 522
E.E.S. 200 Liquid 522
E.E.S. 400 Liquid 522
♦ Enduron Tablets 403, 517
♦ Enduronyl Forte Tablets 403, 518

♦ Enduronyl Tablets 403, 518
♦ EryPed Drops and Chewable
   Tablets 403, 520
♦ EryPed 200 & EryPed 400
   Granules 403, 520
♦ Ery-Tab Tablets 403, 521
♦ Erythrocin Stearate Filmtab 403, 524
♦ Erythromycin Base Filmtab 403, 525
♦ Erythromycin Delayed-Release
   Capsules, USP 403, 526
♦ Fero-Folic-500 Filmtab 403, 528
♦ Fero-Grad-500 Filmtab 403, 528
Fero-Gradumet Filmtab 528
H-BIG 528
Harmonyl Tablets 529
♦ Hytrin Tablets 403, 529
Iberet Filmtab 531
♦ Iberet-500 Filmtab 403, 531
Iberet-500 Liquid 531
♦ Iberet-Folic-500 Filmtab 403, 528
Iberet-Liquid 531
♦ K-Lor Powder Packets 403, 531
♦ K-Tab Filmtab 403, 532
♦ Nembutal Sodium Capsules 403, 534
Nembutal Sodium Solution 536
Nembutal Sodium
   Suppositories 538
Norisodrine with Calcium
   Iodide Syrup *540*
♦ Ogen Tablets 403, 540
♦ Ogen Vaginal Cream 403, 540
♦ Optilets-500 Filmtab 403
♦ Optilets-M-500 Filmtab 403
♦ Oretic Tablets 403, 543
Oreticyl Forte Tablets 544
Oreticyl Tablets 544
♦ PCE Dispertab Tablets 403, 547
Panhematin 546
♦ Paradione Capsules 403, 546
♦ Peganone Tablets 403, 549
Phenurone Tablets 550
♦ Placidyl Capsules 404, 551
♦ ProSom Tablets 404, 552
Quelidrine Syrup 553
Surbex .... ᴅ
Surbex with C .... ᴅ
Surbex-750 with Iron Filmtab 404
Surbex-750 with Zinc Filmtab 404
Surbex-T Filmtab 404
♦ Tranxene T-TAB Tablets 404, 554
♦ Tranxene-SD Half Strength
   Tablets 404, 554
♦ Tranxene-SD Tablets 404, 554
♦ Tridione Capsules 404, 555
♦ Tridione Dulcet Tablets 404, 555
Tridione Solution 555
Tronothane Hydrochloride
   Cream 556

Other Products Available
0.25% Acetic Acid Irrigation, USP
   (Aqualite)
Sterile A-hydroCort
5% Alcohol & 5% Dextrose Injection
Sterile A-methaPred
Amidate (Etomidate Injection) Ampul,
   Abboject
Aminophylline 250 mg, 10 mL, Ampul
   & Vial
Aminophylline 500 mg, 20 mL, Ampul
   & Vial
Aminosyn 3.5% M
Aminosyn 5%
Aminosyn 7%
Aminosyn II 7%
Aminosyn 7% TPN Kit
Aminosyn 7% with Electrolytes
Aminosyn 7% with Electrolytes TPN Kit
Aminosyn 8.5%
Aminosyn II 8.5%
Aminosyn 8.5% TPN Kit
Aminosyn 8.5% with Electrolytes
Aminosyn 10%
Aminosyn II 10%
Aminosyn 10% TPN Kit
Aminosyn with Dextrose, Nutrimix Dual
   Chamber
Aminosyn II in Dextrose, Nutrimix
   Dual Chamber
Aminosyn-HBC 7%
Aminosyn-PF 7% and 10%
Ammonium Chloride
Anticoagulant Citrate Phosphate
   Dextrose Solution, USP
Atropine 0.1 mg/mL, 5 mL, Abboject
   Syringe
Atropine 0.1 mg/mL, 10 mL, Abboject
   Syringe
Balanced Salt Solution
Bretylium Tosylate in 5% Dextrose
   Injection (2 mg/mL and 4 mg/mL)
Bupivacaine Hydrochloride Injection,
   USP, 0.25%, 0.5%, 0.75%, Ampul,
   Abboject Syringe
Calcium Acetate 0.5 mEq/mL Injection
Calcium Chloride 10%, Abboject
Calcium Glucepate Injection Ampul &
   Abboject
Cecon Solution
Cenolate Ampules
Chromium 10 mL (4 mg/mL)
Colchicine Tablets
Copper 10 mL (4 mg/mL)
Cysteine Hydrochloride Injection
Dehydrated Alcohol Injection, USP
6% Dextran 75 w/v & 5% Dextrose
   Injection
6% Dextran 75 w/v & 0.9% Sodium
   Chloride Injection

2.5% Dextrose & ½ Str Lactated
   Ringer's Injection
5% Dextrose & Lactated Ringer's
   Injection
5% Dextrose & Ringer's Injection
2.5% Dextrose & 0.45% Sodium
   Chloride Injection, USP
5% Dextrose & 0.225% Sodium
   Chloride Injection, USP
5% Dextrose & 0.3% Sodium Chloride
   Injection, USP
5% Dextrose & 0.45% Sodium
   Chloride Injection, USP
5% Dextrose & 0.9% Sodium Chloride
   Injection, USP
10% Dextrose & 0.9% Sodium
   Chloride Injection, USP
2.5% Dextrose Injection, USP
5% Dextrose Injection, USP
5% Dextrose Injection, USP
   (ADD-Vantage)
5% Dextrose Injection, USP (Partial fill)
5% Dextrose & 0.15% Pot Chl
   Injection (20 mEq)
5% Dextrose & 0.224% Pot Chl
   Injection (30 mEq)
5% Dextrose & 0.3% Pot Chl Injection
   (40 mEq)
5% Dextrose & 0.225% Sodium
   Chloride with 0.075% Potassium
   Chloride Injection (10 mEq)
5% Dextrose & 0.225% Sodium
   Chloride with 0.15% Potassium
   Chloride Injection (20 mEq)
5% Dextrose & 0.225% Sodium
   Chloride with 0.224% Potassium
   Chloride Injection (30 mEq)
5% Dextrose & 0.225% Sodium
   Chloride with 0.3% Potassium
   Chloride Injection (40 mEq)
5% Dextrose & 0.3% Sodium Chloride
   with 0.075% Potassium Chloride
   Injection (10 mEq)
5% Dextrose & 0.3% Sodium Chloride
   with 0.15% Potassium Chloride
   Injection (20 mEq)
5% Dextrose & 0.3% Sodium Chloride
   with 0.224% Potassium Chloride
   Injection (30 mEq)
5% Dextrose & 0.45% Sodium
   Chloride with 0.075% Potassium
   Chloride Injection (10 mEq)
5% Dextrose & 0.45% Sodium
   Chloride with 0.15% Potassium
   Chloride Injection (20 mEq)

5% Dextrose & 0.45% Sodium
Chloride with 0.224% Potassium
Chloride Injection (30 mEq)
5% Dextrose & 0.45% Sodium
Chloride with 0.3% Potassium
Chloride Injection (40 mEq)
10% Dextrose Injection, USP
20% Dextrose Injection, USP
30% Dextrose Injection, USP
40% Dextrose Injection, USP
50% Dextrose Injection, USP
60% Dextrose Injection, USP
70% Dextrose Injection, USP
Dopamine Hydrochloride in 5%
Dextrose Injection (800, 1600, 3200
mcg/mL)
Empty Evacuated Container
Endrate Solution, Ampoules
Ephedrine Sulfate, Injection
Epinephrine 1:10,000, 10 ml., Abboject
Erythrocin ADD-Vantage Kits
Erythrocin-I.V.
Erythrocin Lactobionate-I.V.
Erythrocin Piggyback
Fentanyl Injection, Ampul, Vial
Gentamicin Premix ADD-Vantage
Products
Gentamicin Sulfate in 0.9% Sodium
Chloride Injection (0.8, 0.9, 1.0, 1.2,
1.4 mg/mL)
1.5% Glycine Irrigation/Aqualite
1.5% Glycine Irrigation, USP
(Flex & Aqualite)
Glycopyrrolate Injection
Heparin Sodium in 5% Dextrose
Injection (50 & 100 Units/mL)
Heparin Sodium in 0.45% Sodium
Chloride Injection (50 & 100
Units/mL)
Hydroxyzine HCl Injection, Abbojects,
Ampuls, Vials, Syringes
Inpersol & 1.5% Dextrose
Inpersol & 2.5% Dextrose
Inpersol & 4.25% Dextrose
Inpersol-LM with 1.5% Dextrose
Inpersol-LM with 2.5% Dextrose
Inpersol-LM with 4.25% Dextrose
Isoproterenol HCl 1:5,000 5 mL,
Universal Add Syringe
Isoproterenol HCl 1:5,000 10 mL,
Universal Add Syringe
Isoproterenol HCl 1:50,000, 10 mL,
Abboject
10% LMD w/v and 5% Dextrose
Injection
10% LMD w/v and 0.9% Sodium
Chloride Injection
LTA Kit, Preattached
LTA II Kit
LTA Pediatric Kit
Lactated Ringers for Irrigation (Flex)
Lactated Ringer's Injection, USP
Lidocaine HCl Injection, 0.2% in 5%
Dextrose
Lidocaine HCl Injection, 0.4% in 5%
Dextrose
Lidocaine HCl Injection, 0.8% in 5%
Dextrose
Lidocaine HCl Injection, USP, 1%,
mL, Abboject
Lidocaine HCl Injection, USP, 1%, 5
mL, Sterile Pack Abboject
Lidocaine HCl Injection, USP, 2%, 5
mL, Abboject
Lidocaine HCl Injection, USP, 2%, 5
mL, Sterile Pack Abboject
Lidocaine HCl Injection, USP, 20%, 5
mL, 1 gram-Pintop, U.A.S.
Lidocaine HCl Injection, USP, 20%, 10
mL, 2 gram-Pintop, U.A.S.
Lidocaine HCl Injection, USP, 5% with
7.5% Dextrose
Liposyn II 10% and 20%
Magnesium Sulfate 12.5%, 8 mL,
Pintop
Magnesium Sulfate 50% w/v Ampoules,
Vials & Abboject
Mammol Ointment
Manganese 10 mL (1 mg/mL)
5% Mannitol Injection, USP
10% Mannitol Injection, USP
15% Mannitol Injection, USP
20% Mannitol Injection, USP
25% Mannitol Injection, USP
Meperidine HCl Injection (10 mg/mL,
PCA Vials)
Metronidazole Injection, USP (5 mg/mL)
Morphine Sulfate Injection, USP
(1 & 5 mg/mL, PCA Vials)
Nalbuphine Hydrochloride Injection, USP
Nembutal Elixir
Neut Abbo-Vial & Pintop
Nitropress
Normosol-M 900 CAL
Normosol-M & 5% Dextrose Injection
Normosol-R
Normosol-R pH 7.4
Normosol-R & 5% Dextrose Injection
Penthrane
Pentothal (Sterile Powder)
Pentothal (Thiopental Sodium for
Injection)
Pentothal Kit
Pentothal RTM Syringe
Pentothal Rectal Suspension in Syringe
Phenobarbital Sodium Ampoules
Physisol Irrigation (Aqualite)

Plegisol
Potassium Acetate 40 mEq Vial, Pintop
& Fliptop
Potassium Chloride Injection Ampoules
& Vials, Pintop & Universal Additive
Syringe
Potassium Chloride 20 mEq. in D-5 W
in Abbo-Vac
Potassium Phosphate 15 mM Vial,
Pintop & Fliptop
Potassium Phosphate 45 mM Vial
Procainamide Hydrochloride Injection,
USP
Procaine Hydrochloride Injection 1% &
2% Vial
Quelicin (Succinylcholine Chloride
Injection) Ampul & Vial, Pintop
Ringer's Injection, USP
Ringer's Irrigation, USP (Aqualite)
Selsun Suspension
Sodium Acetate 40 mEq, 100 mEq and
200 mEq Vials
5% Sodium Bicarbonate Injection, USP
4.2% Sodium Bicarbonate Injection, 10
mEq in 10 mL Abboject (Neonatal)
7.5% Sodium Bicarbonate Injection,
44.6 mEq in 50 mL ampul or
Abboject
8.4% Sodium Bicarbonate Injection, 50
mEq in 50 mL Abboject or Fliptop
Vial
8.4% Sodium Bicarbonate Injection,
10 mEq in 10 mL Abboject
(Pediatric)
0.45% Sodium Chloride Injection, USP
5% Sodium Chloride
0.9% Sodium Chloride Injection
0.9% Sodium Chloride Injection, USP
(ADD-Vantage)
0.9% Sodium Chloride Injection,
USP (Partial Fill)
0.9% Sodium Chloride Irrigation, USP
(Flex and Aqualite)
0.45% Sodium Chloride Irrigation, USP
(Aqualite)
Sodium Lactate Injection, USP, 1/6
Molar
Sodium Phosphate 45 mg/15 mL
Sorbitol-Mannitol Irrigation (Flex &
Aqualite)
Sterile Urea
TPN Electrolytes
Tham-E
Tham Solution
Theophylline in 5% Dextrose Injection
(0.4, 0.8, 1.6, 2, 4 mg/mL)
Tubocurarine Chloride Injection, USP
Ureaphil
Urologic G Irrigation (Aqualite)
Vercyte Tablets
Water for Injection, Ampoules, Vial
Water for Injection Bacteriostatic 30 mL
Fliptop
Water for Injection, Sterile, USP
Water, for Irrigation, Sterile, USP (Flex
and Aqualite)
Water for Respiratory Therapy, Sterile
(Flex)
Zinc 10 mL (1 mg/1 mL)

ADAMS LABORATORIES, INC.   **556**
14801 Sovereign Road
Fort Worth, TX 76155-2645
Address inquiries to:
John Q. Adams   (817) 545-7791
FAX (817) 354-7820
For Medical Emergencies Contact:
John Q. Adams   (817) 545-7791
FAX (817) 354-7820
Products Described
Airet Solution for Inhalation 556
Atrohist Plus Tablets 557
Atrohist Sprinkle Capsules 557
Deconsal Sprinkle Capsules 558
Deconsal II Tablets 558
Humibid DM Sprinkle
Capsules 559
Humibid DM Tablets 559
Humibid L.A. Tablets 559
Humibid Sprinkle Capsules 559

ADRIA LABORATORIES   **560**
Division of Erbamont Inc.
Administrative Offices:
7001 Post Road
Dublin, OH 43017
Mailing Address:
P. O. Box 16529
Columbus, OH 43216-6529
Address inquiries to:
Medical Department
(614) 764-8100
Products Described
Adriamycin PFS 560
Adriamycin RDF 561
Evac-Q-Kwik ....■□
Idamycin for Injection 563
Neosar 565
Other Products Available
Adrucil
Amphocin
Axotal
Chymex
Folex PFS
Ilopan Choline Tablets
Ilopan Injection (Ampules)
Ilopan Stat-pak (disposable syringe)
Ilozyme Tablets
K-Lease 10 mEq Capsules

Kaochlor 10% Liquid
Kaochlor S-F 10% Liquid
Kaon-Cl Tablets
Kaon-Cl 10 Tablets
Kaon Elixir
Magan Tablets
Modane Bulk
Modane Plus Tablets
Modane Soft Capsules
Modane Tablets
Nitrol Ointment
Nitrol Ointment Appli-Kit
Octamide PFS
Tympagesic Otic Solution
Vincasar PFS
Xylo-Pfan

ADVANCED NUTRITIONAL   **567**
TECHNOLOGY, INC.
1111 Jefferson Avenue
P.O. Box 3225
Elizabeth, NJ 07207-3225
Address inquiries to:
Wayne L. Phillips   (908) 354-2740
(908) 354-2741
Products Described
Alpha E Softgels 567
Biotene Softgel 567
Crangel 567
Formula 3/6/9 567
Lactrol Enzyme Softgels 567
Laxagel 567
Liqui-Cal/Mag 567
Liqui-Cal Softgels 567
N'Odor Softgels 567
Nutr-E-Sol Liquid 567
Nutr-E-Sol Softgels 567
Pediavit Multivitamin Liquid
with Minerals 567
PhosChol Concentrate 567
PhosChol Forte 567
PhosChol 565 Softgels 567
PhosChol 900 Softgels 567
SuperEPA 1200 Softgels 568
SuperEPA 2000 568
UltraVim 568
XL-1 Multivitamin Liquid with
Iron 568

AKORN, INC.   **568**
100 Akorn Drive
Abita Springs, LA 70420
Address inquiries to:
Dave Hanak
Director of Marketing
(800) 535-7155
(504) 893-9300
Manufacturing Facility
Taylor Pharmacal Co.
150 S. Wyckles Road
Decatur, IL 62522   (217) 428-1100

Please consult PDR FOR
OPHTHALMOLOGY

ALCON LABORATORIES, INC.   **568**
Alcon Laboratories, Inc.
And its affiliates Inc.
Corporate Headquarters
P.O. Box 6600
6201 South Freeway
Fort Worth, TX 76134
Address inquiries to:
Sales Services   (817) 293-0450
Products Described
Betoptic Sterile Ophthalmic
Solution 568
Betoptic S Sterile Ophthalmic
Suspension 569
Ciloxan Ophthalmic Solution 570
Eye-Stream Eye Irrigating
Solution 571
Naphcon-A Ophthalmic
Solution 571
Tears Naturale II Lubricant
Eye Drops 572
Tears Naturale Free 572
TobraDex Ophthalmic
Suspension and Ointment 572
Tobrex Ophthalmic Ointment
and Solution 573
Other Products Available
A-OK Ophthalmic Knife
Alcon Surgical System
(Irrigation/Aspiration Kits;
Phacoemulsification Kits)
BSS Irrigation Solution (15mL, 30mL,
250mL, 500mL)
BSS Plus Irrigation Solution (30mL,
500mL)
BSS and BSS Plus Irrigation Solution
Administration Set
Cetamide Ointment
Cetapred Ointment
Cryophake Sterile, Disposable
Cryoextractor
Cyclogyl Ophthalmic Solution
Cyclomydril Ophthalmic Solution
Cystitomes & Cannulas
Duratears Naturale Lubricant Eye
Ointment
Enuclene Ophthalmic Solution
Epinal Ophthalmic Solution
Eye Pak Surgical Drape
Eye Stream Eye Irrigating Solution
Fluorescite Injection
Gonioscopic Prism Solution
I-Knife Ophthalmic Knife

Intraocular Lenses
Iopidine Ophthalmic Solution
Ismotic Solution
Maxidex Ointment
Maxitrol Ointment
Microphake Sterile Disposable
Cryoextractor
Microsponge Miniature Surgical Sponge
Miostat Intraocular Solution
Natacyn Ophthalmic Suspension
Optemp Sterile Disposable Cautery
Osmoglyn Oral Osmotic Agent
PTG, Alcon Applanation
Pneumatonograph
Pilopine HS Gel
Post-Operative Kits
Procedure Packs
Steri-Units Sterile Ophthalmic Units for
Single Use Only
Zolyse Ophthalmic Solution

ALCON (PUERTO RICO) INC.
P.O. Box 3000
Humacao, Puerto Rico 00661
Address inquiries to:
Medical Department
P.O. Box 6380
Fort Worth, TX 76115
(817) 293-0450

Products Available
Adsorbocarpine
Adsorbonac
Adsorbotear
Alcaine
Econopred
Econopred Plus
Glaucon
Isopto Atropine
Isopto Carbachol
Isopto Carpine
Isopto Cetamide
Isopto Cetapred
Isopto Homatropine
Isopto Hyoscine
Maxidex Suspension
Maxitrol Suspension
Mydfrin 2.5%
Mydrapred
Mydriacyl
Naphcon
Naphcon Forte
Zincfrin

ALLEN & HANBURYS   **404, 574**
Division of Glaxo Inc.
Five Moore Drive
Research Triangle Park
North Carolina 27709
(919) 248-2100
Address inquiries to:
Medical Services Department
(919) 248-2100
For Medical Emergencies Contact:
(919) 248-2100
Products Described
◆ Beclovent Inhalation Aerosol
and Refill 404, 574
◆ Beconase AQ Nasal Spray 404, 575
◆ Beconase Inhalation Aerosol &
Refill 404, 575
◆ Ceftin Tablets 404, 577
◆ Trandate Injection 404, 578
◆ Trandate Tablets 404, 578
◆ Ventolin Inhalation Aerosol
and Refill 404, 582
◆ Ventolin Inhalation Solution 404, 582
◆ Ventolin Nebules Inhalation
Solution 404, 582
◆ Ventolin Rotacaps for
Inhalation 404, 582
◆ Ventolin Syrup 404, 582
◆ Ventolin Tablets 404, 582

ALLERGAN HERBERT   **585**
Skin Care Division of Allergan,
Inc.
2525 Dupont Drive
P.O. Box 19534
Irvine, CA 92713-9534
(714) 752-4500
Products Described
Aeroseb-Dex Topical Aerosol
Spray 585
Aeroseb-HC Topical Aerosol
Spray 585
AquaTar Therapeutic Tar Gel ....■□
Bluboro Powder Astringent
Soaking Solution ....■□
Danex Dandruff Shampoo ....■□
Elimite (permethrin) 5%
Cream 585
Erygel Topical Gel 585
Erymax Topical Solution 585
Exsel Shampoo/Lotion 585
Fluonid Topical Solution 586
Fluoroplex Topical Solution &
Cream 1% 586
Gris-PEG Tablets, 125 mg &
250 mg 586
Maxiflor Cream 587
Maxiflor Ointment 587
Naftin Cream 1% 587
Naftin Gel 1% 588
Penecort Cream 1% 588

Manufacturers' Index 5

For Medical Emergency Contact:
(203) 853-0123
FAX (203) 852-9349
Products Described
Soothe & Clean Personal
Cleansing Foam 699
Other Products Available
Calamatum Lotion
Calamatum Spray
Gentlax B Granules
Gentlax S Tablets
Saratoga Ointment

BOCK PHARMACAL COMPANY 700
P.O. Box 8519
St. Louis, MO 63126-0519
(314) 343-0994
Products Described
Broncholate CS *700*
Broncholate Softgels *700*
Broncholate Syrup *700*
Emetrol Solution - Cherry *700*
Emetrol Solution - Lemon-Mint *700*
Hemaspan Caplets *700*
Histussin HC *700*
Poly-Histine CS *700*
Poly-Histine DM Syrup *700*
Poly-Histine Elixir *700*
Poly-Histine-D Capsules *700*
Poly-Histine-D Elixir *700*
Poly-Histine-D Ped Caps *700*
Prenate 90 Tablets *700*
Zephrex Tablets *700*
Zephrex LA Tablets *700*

BOEHRINGER INGELHEIM PHARMACEUTICALS, INC. 405, 700
A subsidiary of Boehringer Ingelheim Corporation
900 Ridgebury Road
P.O. Box 368
Ridgefield, CT 06877-0368
Address inquiries to:
Medical Services Dept.
(203) 798-9988
Products Described
◆ Alupent Inhalation Aerosol 405, 700
◆ Alupent Inhalation Solution 405, 700
Alupent Syrup 700
Alupent Tablets 700
◆ Atrovent Inhalation Aerosol 405, 702
◆ Catapres Tablets 405, 703
◆ Catapres-TTS 405, 704
◆ Combipres Tablets 405, 705
◆ Mexitil Capsules 405, 707
◆ Persantine Tablets 405, 710
◆ Prelu-2 Capsules 405, 710
◆ Respbid Tablets 405, 711
Serentil Ampuls 713
Serentil Concentrate 713
◆ Serentil Tablets 405, 713

BOOTS LABORATORIES 405, 715
a division of Boots Pharmaceuticals, Inc.
Suite 200
300 Tri-State International Center
Lincolnshire, IL 60069
Address inquiries to:
Medical Services Department
(708) 405-7400
FAX (708) 405-7505
For Medical Emergencies Contact:
Medical Services Department
Outside Illinois (800) 356-2225
Inside Illinois (708) 451-3797
FAX (708) 405-7505
Products Described
◆ E-Mycin Tablets 405, 715
IBU (Ibuprofen Tablets, USP) 716
◆ SSD RP Cream 405, 718
Other Products Available
Allopurinol Tablets

BOOTS PHARMACEUTICALS, INC. 405, 719
Suite 200
300 Tri-State International Center
Lincolnshire, IL 60069
Address inquiries to:
Medical Services Department
(708) 405-7400
FAX (708) 405-7505
For Medical Emergencies Contact:
Medical Services Department
Outside IL (800) 356-2225
Inside IL (708) 451-3797
FAX (708) 405-7505
Products Described
◆ Ru-Tuss DE Tablets 405, 720
◆ Ru-Tuss II Capsules 405, 719
Ru-Tuss with Hydrocodone 720
◆ Ru-Tuss Tablets 405, 719
◆ SSD Cream 406, 721
◆ SSD AF Cream 406, 721
◆ Synthroid Injection 406, 721
◆ Synthroid Tablets 405, 721
◆ Travase Ointment 406, 723
Other Products Available
Choloxin
Chymodiactin (chymopapain for injection)
Lopurin Tablets
Rufen Tablets
Ru-Tuss Expectorant
Ru-Tuss Liquid
Twin K Liquid
ZORprin Tablets

BRAINTREE LABORATORIES, INC. 406, 724
P.O. Box 361
Braintree, MA 02184
Address inquiries to:
Mr. Harry P. Keegan, President
(617) 843-2202
For Medical Emergencies Contact:
Geoffrey E. Clark, M.D.
(617) 843-2202
Products Described
◆ GoLYTELY 406, 724
◆ NuLYTELY 406, 724
◆ PhosLo Tablets 406, 725

BRISTOL LABORATORIES
See BRISTOL-MYERS SQUIBB COMPANY

BRISTOL-MYERS ONCOLOGY DIVISION
See BRISTOL-MYERS SQUIBB COMPANY

BRISTOL-MYERS PRODUCTS
See BRISTOL-MYERS SQUIBB COMPANY

BRISTOL-MYERS SQUIBB COMPANY

APOTHECON 611
A Bristol-Myers Squibb Company
General Offices
P.O. Box 4500
Princeton, NJ 08543-4500
Address inquiries to:
Bristol-Myers Squibb Drug Information Dept.
P.O. Box 4500
Princeton, NJ 08543-4500
(800) 321-1335

Adverse Drug Experience and Product Defects Reporting During Business Hours Only Call (609) 243-6991

Orders for Apothecon Products may be placed by:
1. Calling toll-free between 8:30 AM - 6:00 PM EST
(800) 631-5244
2. Mailing your purchase orders to:
Apothecon
Attn: Customer Service Dept.
P.O. Box 5250
Princeton, NJ 08543-5250
3. Orders may be telefaxed to Our Customer Service Dept. using the FAX number:
(800) 523-2965
For listing of standard, purified, and human insulins, see NOVO NORDISK PHARMACEUTICALS INC.
Products Described
Amikin Injectable 612
Ampicillin Sodium Injection USP *611*
Atenolol Tablets USP *611*
Betapen-VK Tablets and Oral Solution 624
Cefanex Capsules *611*
Cefazolin Sodium Injection USP *611*
Cephalexin Capsules and for Oral Suspension USP *611*
Cloxacillin Sodium Capsules USP *611*
Colace 614
Dicloxacillin Sodium Capsules USP *611*
Doxycycline Hyclate Capsules & Tablets USP *611*
Dynapen Capsules *611*
Florinef Acetate Tablets *611*
Fungizone Intravenous *614*
K-Lyte/Cl 50 Effervescent Tablets *615*
K-Lyte/Cl Tablets *615*
K-Lyte & K-Lyte DS Effervescent Tablets *615*
Kantrex Capsules *611*
Klotrix Tablets *615*
Mucomyst and Mucomyst-10 .... *615*
Mycostatin Oral Tablets *611*
Naldecon CX Adult Liquid .... ▣
Naldecon DX Adult Liquid .... ▣
Naldecon DX Children's Syrup .... ▣
Naldecon DX Pediatric Drops .... ▣
Naldecon EX Children's Syrup .... ▣
Naldecon EX Pediatric Drops .... ▣
Naldecon Senior DX .... ▣
Naldecon Senior EX .... ▣
Naldecon Syrup, Tablets, Pediatric Drops and Pediatric Syrup *616*
Naturetin-5 Tablets and Naturetin-10 Tablets *611*
Niacin Tablets USP *611*
Peri-Colace 616
Polycillin Capsules, Oral Suspension, and Pediatric Drops *611*
Polymox Capsules, for Oral Suspension and Pediatric Drops 616
Principen Capsules and for Oral Suspension *611*
Principen with Probenecid Capsules *611*
Prolixin Decanoate 617
Prolixin Elixir 617
Prolixin Enanthate 617
Prolixin Injection 617
Prolixin Oral Concentrate 617
Prolixin Tablets 617
Pronestyl Capsules and Tablets *611*
Pronestyl-SR Tablets *611*
Prostaphlin Capsules and for Oral Solution *611*
Quibron Capsules 620
Quibron-300 Capsules 620
Quibron-T Tablets 620
Quibron-T/SR Tablets 620
Raudixin Tablets *611*
Rauzide Tablets *611*
Saluron Tablets *611*
Salutensin/Salutensin-Demi Tablets *611*
Stadol Injection *623*
Sumycin Tablets, Capsules and Syrup *623*
Tegopen Capsules & Oral Suspension *611*
Theragran Liquid .... ▣
Theragran Stress Formula .... ▣
Theragran Tablets .... ▣
Theragran-M Tablets .... ▣
Trimox Capsules and for Oral Suspension 616
Veetids Tablets and for Oral Suspension 624
Velosef Capsules and for Oral Suspension *625*
Other Products Available
B Complex Vitamin Tablets
Cefadyl for Injection and in ADD-Vantage Vials
Cod Liver Oil Capsules
Cod Liver Oil Plain & Mint Flavored
Crysticillin '300' AS
Fungizone Cream, Lotion and Ointment
Fungizone for Tissue Culture
Glycerin Suppositories
Heparin Sodium Injection USP
Kantrex Injection
Kantrex Pediatric Injection
Kenacort Diacetate Syrup
Kenacort Tablets
Kenalog in Orabase
Mineral Oil
Mycostatin Oral Suspension
Nafcil Injection and in ADD-Vantage Vials
Nafcillin Sodium for Injection USP
Neostigmine Methylsulfate Injection USP
Nitrazine Paper
Nydrazid Injection
Ophthaine Solution
Oxacillin Capsules USP
Oxacillin for Injection USP
Penicillin G Potassium for Injection USP
Penicillin G Sodium for Injection USP
Polycillin-N Injection and in ADD-Vantage Vials
Polycillin-PRB Oral Suspension
Pronestyl Injection
Prostaphlin for Injection
Rubramin PC (Cyanocobalamin Injection USP)
SMZ-TMP Oral Solution
SMZ-TMP Tablets
Spec-T Sore Throat Anesthetic Lozenges
Spec-T Sore Throat/Cough Suppressant Lozenges
Spec-T Sore Throat/Decongestant Lozenges
Staphcillin Injection and Staphcillin Piggyback
Sucostrin High Potency
Sucostrin Injection
Suppositories, Glycerin, USP
Tobramycin Sulfate Injection USP
Tubocurarine Chloride Injection USP
Vesprin Injection
Zolicef Injection

BRISTOL LABORATORIES 406, 726
A Bristol-Myers Squibb Company
P.O. Box 4500
Princeton, NJ 08543-4500
(609) 897-2000
Address medical inquiries to:
Bristol-Myers Squibb Drug Information Department
P.O. Box 4500
Princeton, NJ 08543-4500
(800) 321-1335
Adverse Drug Experience and Product Defects Reporting During Business Hours Only Call (609) 252-3737
Orders may be placed by calling the following toll free number:
Continental US/Alaska/Hawaii
(800) 631-5244
Mail orders and all inquiries should be sent to:
Bristol Laboratories
Attn: Customer Service
P.O. Box 5250
Princeton, NJ 08543-5250
Products Described
◆ Cefzil Tablets and Oral Suspension 406, 726
◆ Corgard Tablets 406, 728
Corzide Tablets 729
◆ Questran Light 406, 733
◆ Questran Powder 406, 732
◆ Videx Tablets, Powder for Oral Solution, & Pediatric Powder for Oral Solution 406, 734

BRISTOL-MYERS ONCOLOGY DIVISION 406, 740
A Bristol-Myers Squibb Company
P.O. Box 4500
Princeton, NJ 08543-4500
(609) 897-2000
Address medical inquiries to:
Scientific Information Section
Medical Department
Adverse Drug Experience and Product Defects Reporting During Business Hours Only Call (609) 897-2126
Orders may be placed by calling the following toll free number:
Continental US (800) 631-5244
Alaska-Hawaii (800) 631-5244
Mail orders and all inquiries should be sent to:
Bristol-Myers Oncology Division
Attn: Customer Service
P.O. Box 5250
Princeton, NJ 08543-5250
Products Described
BiCNU 740
Blenoxane 742
CeeNU 743
◆ Cytoxan for Injection 406, 744
◆ Cytoxan Tablets 406, 744
◆ IFEX 406, 745
Lysodren 747
◆ Megace Tablets 406, 748
◆ Mesnex Injection 406, 749
◆ Mutamycin 406, 749
Mycostatin Pastilles 751
◆ Paraplatin for Injection 406, 751
Platinol 754
◆ Platinol-AQ Injection 406, 756
Teslac Tablets 757
◆ VePesid Capsules and Injection 406, 758

BRISTOL-MYERS PRODUCTS 406, 760
A Bristol-Myers Squibb Company
345 Park Avenue
New York, NY 10154
Address Product Inquiries to:
Products Division
Consumer Affairs Department
U.S. Highway 202/206 North
Somerville, NJ 08876-1279
Address Medical Inquiries about Non-prescription Drug Products to:
Department of Medical Services
1350 Liberty Avenue
Hillside, NJ 07205
In Emergencies Call:
(800) 468-7746
Products Described
Alpha Keri Moisture Rich Body Oil .... ▣
Alpha Keri Moisture Rich Cleansing Bar .... ▣
◆ Arthritis Strength Bufferin Analgesic Caplets 406, 761
◆ Extra Strength Bufferin Analgesic Tablets 406, 761
◆ Bufferin Analgesic Tablets and Caplets 406, 760
◆ Bufferin AF Nite Time Analgesic/Sleeping Aid Caplets 406, 761
◆ Allergy-Sinus Comtrex Multi-Symptom Allergy Sinus Formula Tablets & Caplets 406, 762
Cough Formula Comtrex 763
◆ Comtrex Multi-Symptom Cold Reliever Tablets/Caplets/Liqui-Gels/Liquid 406, 761
◆ Day & Night Comtrex 406, 763
◆ Non-Drowsy Comtrex 406, 764
Congespirin For Children Aspirin Free Chewable Cold Tablets 764
◆ Aspirin Free Excedrin Analgesic Caplets 406, 765
◆ Excedrin Extra-Strength Analgesic Tablets & Caplets 406, 765
Excedrin P.M. Analgesic/Sleeping Aid Tablets, Caplets and Liquid 765
Sinus Excedrin Analgesic, Decongestant Tablets & Caplets 766
4-Way Cold Tablets 767
4-Way Fast Acting Nasal Spray - New Formula 767
4-Way Fast Acting Nasal Spray - Original Formula (regular & mentholated) & Metered Spray Pump (regular) 767
4-Way Long Lasting Nasal Spray & Metered Spray Pump 767
Keri Lotion-Original Formula .... ▣
Keri Lotion-Silky Smooth Formula .... ▣
Keri Lotion-Silky Smooth Fragrance-Free Formula .... ▣

(◆ Shown in Product Identification Section) *Italic Page Number* Indicates Brief Listing (▣ Described in PDR For Nonprescription Drugs)

Multitest CMI Skin Test Antigens for Cellular Hypersensitivity 919, *2664*
ProHIBiT Haemophilus b Conjugate Vaccine (Diphtheria Toxoid Conjugate) 919
Rabies Immune Globulin (Human), Imogam Rabies Vaccine *918*
Rabies Vaccine Human Diploid Cell, Imovax Rabies *918*
Rabies Vaccine Human Diploid Cell, Imovax Rabies I.D. *918*
Skin Test Antigens for Cellular Hypersensitivity, Multitest CMI 919, *2664*
TheraCys BCG Live (Intravesical) 921
Tuberculin, Mono-Vacc Test (O.T.) *2664*

Other Products Available

Diphtheria Antitoxin USP
Diphtheria & Tetanus Toxoids Adsorbed USP (For Pediatric Use) (DT)
MSTA (Mumps Skin Test Antigen USP)
Menomune A/C/Y/W-135 (Meningococcal Polysaccharide Vaccine, Groups A,C,Y,W-135 Combined)
Tetanus Toxoid USP
Tetanus Toxoid Adsorbed USP
Tetanus & Diphtheria Toxoids Adsorbed For Adult Use USP (Td)
Tubersol (Tuberculin Purified Protein Derivative [Mantoux])
YF-VAX (Yellow Fever Vaccine)

CONVATEC
See BRISTOL-MYERS SQUIBB COMPANY

CURATEK PHARMACEUTICALS 926
1965 Pratt Boulevard
Elk Grove Village, IL 60007

Address inquiries to:
Professional Services Department
(708) 806-7680

For Medical Emergencies Contact:
Robert J. Borgman, Ph.D
(708) 806-7680

Products Described
MetroGel 926
MetroGel-Vaginal Gel 927

DANIELS PHARMACEUTICALS, INC. 408, 928
2517 25th Avenue North
St. Petersburg, FL 33713-3918

Address inquiries to:
(800) 237-7427

Products Described
Levothyroxine Sodium for Injection *929*
◆ Levoxine Tablets 408, 928
Tussigon Tablets *929*

DARTMOUTH PHARMACEUTICALS, INC. 929
19 Whaler's Way
North Dartmouth, MA 02747-1058

Address inquiries to:
(508) 636-5553

For Medical Emergency Contact:
Michael J. Greco (508) 636-5553

Products Described
Touro A&H Capsules *929*
Touro LA Caplets *929*
Zartan Capsules *929*

Other Products Available
Touro DM
Touro EXP

DAYTON LABORATORIES, INC. 408, 929
3307 N.W. 74 Avenue
Miami, FL 33122

Address inquiries to:
3307 N.W. 74 Avenue
Miami, FL 33122
(305) 594-0988
Toll Free (800) 446-0255

For Medical Emergencies Contact:
Rey Farinas (305) 594-0988

Products Described
◆ Dayto Himbin Tablets and Liquid 408, 929
◆ Flatulex Tablets 408, 930

Other Products Available
Almebex Plus B-12
Dayto Anase Tablets
Dayto Sulf Vaginal Cream
Enzymax Tablets
Flatulex Drops
Periavit Liquid
Veniphlex Tablets

DELMONT LABORATORIES, INC. 930
P.O. Box 269
Swarthmore, PA 19081

Address inquiries to:
(800) 562-5541
(215) 543-3365
FAX (215) 543-6298

Products Described
Staphage Lysate (SPL) 930

DERMAIDE RESEARCH CORPORATION 931
P.O. Box 562
Palos Heights, IL 60463

Address inquiries to:
P.O. Box 562
Palos Heights, IL 60463
(800) 344-ALOE

For Medical Emergencies Contact:
(800) 344-ALOE

Products Described
Dermaide Aloe Cream 931

DERMIK LABORATORIES, INC. 931
500 Arcola Road, P.O. Box 1200
Collegeville, PA 19426-0107

Distribution Centers
Oak Forest, IL 60452
P.O. Box 230 (312) 687-7440
Sparks, NV 89431
655 Spice Islands Drive
Suite 101 (702) 353-4100
Tucker, GA 30084
4660 Hammermill Road
(404) 496-8484

Products Described
Anthra-Derm Ointment 1%, ½%, ¼%, 1/10% *931*
5 Benzagel (5% benzoyl peroxide) & 10 Benzagel (10% benzoyl peroxide), Acne Gels, Microgel Formula *931*
Benzamycin Topical Gel 931
Florone Cream 0.05% 932
Florone E Emollient Cream 0.05% 932
Florone Ointment 0.05% 932
Hytone Cream 1%, 2 ½% 933
Hytone Lotion 1%, 2 ½% 933
Hytone Ointment 1%, 2 ½% 933
Psorcon Ointment 0.05% 933
Sulfacet-R Acne Lotion 934
Vanoxide-HC Acne Lotion *935*
Vytone Cream 1% *935*
Zetar Emulsion *935*

Other Products Available
Anthra-Derm Ointment 1%, ½%, ¼%, 1/10%
Benzagel (5% benzoyl peroxide) & 10 Benzagel (10% benzoyl peroxide), Acne Gels, Microgel Formula
Loroxide Acne Lotion
Shepard's Cream Lotion
Shepard's Skin Cream
Vanoxide Acne Lotion
Vanoxide-HC Acne Lotion
Vytone Cream 1%
Zetar Emulsion
Zetar Shampoo

DEY LABORATORIES, INC. 935
2751 Napa Valley Corporate Drive
Napa, CA 94558

Address inquiries to:
Susan Lopuszynski (800) 755-5560
FAX (707) 224-3235

For Medical Emergencies Contact:
John Siebert (707) 224-3200
FAX (707) 224-3235

Products Described
Albuterol Sulfate Inhalation Solution *935*
Dey-Pak *935*
Dey-Vial *935*
Dey-Wash Skin Wound Cleanser *935*
Isoetharine Inhalation Solution, Sulfite-Free, USP *935*
Metaproterenol Sulfate Inhalation Solution, USP *935*
Mucosil Acetylcysteine Solution *935*
Nebu-Sol Metered-Dose Dispenser *935*
Purified Water, USP *935*
Racepinephrine Inhalation Solution, Sulfite-Free *935*
Sodium Chloride Solutions *935*

DISTA PRODUCTS COMPANY 408, 935
Division of Eli Lilly and Company

For Medical Information, Write:
Lilly Research Laboratories
Lilly Corporate Center
Indianapolis, IN 46285
(317) 276-3714

For Other Inquiries:
Dista Products Company
Lilly Corporate Center
Indianapolis, IN 46285
(317) 276-4000

Regional Sales Offices
Atlanta, GA 30328
North Park Town Center
Building 500, Suite 710
1100 Abernathy Road, NE
(404) 551-5380
Chicago, IL 60631
Suite 810, O'Hare Plaza
8725 West Higgins Road
(312) 693-8360
Pasadena, CA 91101
811 Mutual Savings Building
301 East Colorado Blvd.
(818) 792-3197
Stamford, CT 06902
300 First Stamford Place
(203) 357-1422

Products Described
Ilosone Liquid, Oral Suspensions 936
◆ Ilosone Pulvules & Tablets 408, 936
Ilotycin Gluceptate, IV, Vials 938
Ilotycin Ophthalmic Ointment 937
◆ Keflex Pulvules, Oral Suspension & Pediatric Drops 408, 939
◆ Keftab Tablets 408, 940
◆ Nalfon 200 Pulvules & Nalfon Tablets 408
◆ Prozac Pulvules & Liquid, Oral Solution 409, 943

Other Products Available
Becotin-T Tablets
Cinobac Pulvules
Co-Pyronil 2 Pulvules
Cordran Ointment & Lotion
Cordran SP Cream
Cordran Tape
Cordran-N Cream
Keflet Tablets
Mi-Cebrin Tablets
Mi-Cebrin T Tablets

DORSEY LABORATORIES
See SANDOZ PHARMACEUTICALS/CONSUMER DIVISION

DORSEY PHARMACEUTICALS 946
See SANDOZ PHARMACEUTICALS CORPORATION, DORSEY DIVISION

DU PONT MULTI-SOURCE PRODUCTS 946
1000 Stewart Avenue
Garden City, NY 11530
(800) 626-8584

For Pharmaceutical Product-Related Inquiries write:
Professional Services
P.O. Box 80026
Wilmington, DE 19880-0026
Business Hours:
8:00 AM to 4:30 PM Eastern Time
Telephone: (302) 992-4240

For Adverse Experience Reporting
Business Hours Only
(302) 992-4240

For Medical Emergency Information Only
After hours or on weekends call:
(302) 996-3240

Products Described
Bretylol Injection 946
Calciparine Injection 948
Intropin Injection 949
Moban Tablets and Concentrate 950
Narcan Injection 952
Nubain Injection 953
Numorphan Injection 954
Numorphan Suppositories 954
Symmetrel Capsules and Syrup 955
Trexan Tablets 956
Tridil Ampuls and Vials 958
Zydone Capsules 960

Other Products Available
Acetylcysteine Solution 10%, 20%
Amoxicillin Capsules 250, 500 mg
Amoxicillin Suspension 125 mg/5 mL, 250 mg/5 mL
Droperidol Injection 2.5 mg/mL
Methyldopate HCl Injection 50 mg/mL
Metoclopramide Injection 5 mg/mL

DU PONT PHARMACEUTICALS 409, 961
Wilmington, DE 19880-0026
Corporate Telephone Number
(302) 992-5000

For Pharmaceutical Product-Related Inquiries Write:
Professional Services
P.O. Box 80026
Wilmington, DE 19880-0026
Business Hours:
8:00 AM to 4:30 PM Eastern Time
Telephone: (302) 992-4240
FAX (302) 992-7771

For Adverse Experience Reporting
Business Hours Only
(302) 992-4240

For Medical Emergency Information Only
After hours or on weekends call:
(302) 996-3240

Products Described
Brevibloc Injection 961
◆ Coumadin Tablets 409, 963
◆ Ethmozine Tablets 409, 965
Hespan Injection 967
Hycodan Tablets and Syrup 968
Hycomine Compound Tablets 970
Hycomine Pediatric Syrup 969
Hycomine Syrup 969
Hycotuss Expectorant Syrup 971
Pentaspan Injection 972
◆ Percocet Tablets 409, 973
◆ Percodan Tablets 409, 974
◆ Percodan-Demi Tablets 409, 974
◆ Sinemet Tablets 409, 974
◆ Sinemet CR Tablets 409, 976

DURA PHARMACEUTICALS, INC 978
San Diego, CA 92121-1203

Address inquiries to:
Same as above (619) 457-2553

For Medical Emergencies Contact:
Medical Affairs Department
(619) 457-2553

For Product Information call
(619) 457-2553

Products Described
D.A. Chewable Tablets *978*
Dura-Gest Capsules *978*
Dura-Tap/PD Capsules *978*
Dura-Vent/A Capsules *978*
Dura-Vent/DA Tablets *978*
Dura-Vent Tablets *978*
Fenesin Tablets *979*
Tornalate Inhalation Solution, 0.2% 979
Tornalate Metered Dose Inhaler 980

DURAMED PHARMACEUTICALS, INC. 981
5040 Lester Road
Cincinnati, OH 45213

Address inquiries to:
Karen Coates (513) 731-9900

For Medical Emergencies Contact:
Charles F. Hicks (800) 543-8338

Products Described
Amantadine Capsules *981*
Aspirin 15gr Delayed Release Tablets *981*
Aspirin 800 mg. Tablets *981*
Benztropine Mesylate Tablets *981*
Iodur DM Liquid *981*
Iodur with Codeine Liquid *981*
Isoniazid Tablets *981*
Methylprednisolone Tablets *981*
Metoclopramide Tablets *981*
Phenylpropanolamine HCl and Guaifenesin Long Acting Tablets *981*
Salsalate Tablets *981*
Tricosal Tablets *981*

Other Products Available
Duradrin Capsules
Duratex Capsules
Iodur Elixir & Tablets
Triotann Liquid
Triotann Tablets
Triotann-S Pediatric Suspension

EASTMAN KODAK COMPANY, DENTAL PRODUCTS 981
Health Sciences Division
343 State Street
Rochester, NY 14650

Address inquiries to:
Kodak Information Center, Dental Products
(800) 242-2424, Ext. 50

Products Described
Carbocaine Hydrochloride 3% Injection 981
Carbocaine Hydrochloride 2% with Neo-Cobefrin 981
Marcaine Hydrochloride 0.5% with Epinephrine 1:200,000 (as bitartrate) 983

Other Products Available
Ravocaine Hydrochloride 0.4% and Novocain 2% with Levophed 1:30,000
Ravocaine Hydrochloride 0.4% and Novocain 2% with Neo-Cobefrin 1:20,000

ELDER PHARMACEUTICALS, INC.
ICN Plaza
3300 Hyland Avenue
Costa Mesa, CA 92626
See ICN PHARMACEUTICALS, INC.

ELKINS-SINN, INC. 984
2 Esterbrook Lane
Cherry Hill, NJ 08003-4099

Address inquiries to:
Professional Service

For General Information Call:
(215) 688-4400

For Medical Emergency Information:
Day or night call (215) 688-4400

Products Described
Amikacin Sulfate Injection, USP 985
Aminocaproic Acid Injection *984*
Aminophylline Injection (Preservative-Free) *984*
Atropine Sulfate Injection *984*
Bretylium Tosylate Injection (Preservative-Free) *984*
Chlorpromazine Hydrochloride Injection *984*
Clindamycin Phosphate Injection *984*
Codeine Phosphate Injection *984*
Cyanocobalamin (Vit. B_{12}) Injection *984*
Cyclophosphamide for Injection (Preservative-Free) *984*
Dexamethasone Sodium Phosphate Injection *984*
Dextrose Injection *984*
Diazepam Injection *984*
Digoxin Injection *984*
Diphenhydramine Hydrochloride Injection *984*

Beesix Injectable
Biamine Injectable
Brompheniramine Maleate Injection
Cebocap Capsules
Cetane Timed Capsules
Choron "10" Injectable Pak
Conex DA Tablet
Conex Liquid
Conex Lozenges
Conex Plus Tablets
Conex with Codeine Liquid
Cyomin Injectable
Dalalone Injectable
Dalalone L.A. Injectable
Dehist Capsules
depAndro "100" & "200" Injectable
depAndrogyn Injectable
depGynogen Injectable
depMedalone "40" Injectable
depMedalone "80" Injectable
Disotate Injectable
Dommanate Injectable
Duradyne DHC Tablets
Duradyne Tablets
G.B.S. Tablets
Gesterol "50" Injectable
Gesterol L.A. "250" Injectable
Gynogen L.A. "10", "20" & "40" Injectable
Iodo-Niacin Tablets
Levothroid Injectables
Lidocaine 1% & 2% Injectable
Livroben Injectable
Lorcet Plus
Metra Tablets
N.B.P. Ointment
Neoquess Tablets
Niac Capsules
Paral Liquid
Pedameth Capsules
Pedameth Liquid
Predalone "50" Injectable
Predalone T.B.A. Injectable
Q.Y.S.
Queltuss Tablets
Rogenic Injectable
Rogenic Tablets
Solu-Eze Solvent
Triamcinolone Diacetate Injectable
Triamonide "40" Injectable
Verazinc Capsules

FUJISAWA PHARMACEUTICAL COMPANY 1035
Division of Fujisawa USA, Inc.
Parkway North Center
3 Parkway North
Deerfield, IL 60015-2548
Address inquiries to:
Medical and Scientific Information
(800) 727-7003
For Medical Emergencies Contact:
Medical and Scientific Information
(800) 727-7003
Products Described
Adenocard Injection ... 1035
Aristocort Suspension (Forte Parenteral) ... 1036
Aristocort Suspension (Intralesional) ... 1036
Aristocort Tablets ... *1036*
Aristocort A Topical Cream ... 1039
Aristocort A Topical Ointment ... 1039
Aristospan Suspension (Intra-articular) ... 1040
Aristospan Suspension (Intralesional) ... 1040
Cefizox for Intramuscular or Intravenous Use ... 1041
Cyclocort Topical Cream 0.1% ... 1043
Cyclocort Topical Lotion 0.1% ... 1043
Cyclocort Topical Ointment 0.1% ... 1043
Elase Ointment ... 1044
Elase Vials ... 1044
Elase-Chloromycetin Ointment ... 1044
Ganite Injection ... 1045
Grivate Tablets & Suspension ... 1047
NebuPent for Inhalation Solution ... 1048
Pentam 300 Injection ... 1049

GALDERMA LABORATORIES, INC. 1050
3000 Altamesa Blvd., Suite 300
Fort Worth, TX 76133
(817) 551-8664
Products Described
Benzac 5 & 10 Gel ... 1050
Benzac AC 2½%, 5%, and 10% Water-Base Gel ... 1050
Benzac AC Wash 2½%, 5%, 10% Water-Base Cleanser ... 1050
Benzac W Wash 5 & 10 Water-Base Cleanser ... 1050
Benzac W 2½, 5 & 10 Water-Base Gel ... 1050
Cetaphil Skin Cleanser ... 1051
DesOwen Cream, Ointment and Lotion ... 1051
Ionil Plus Shampoo ... 1051
Ionil T Plus Shampoo ... 1052
Nutracort Cream & Lotion ... 1052
Nutraderm Cream & Lotion ... 1052
Nutraderm 30 Lotion ... 1053

GALENPHARMA, INC.
See GENDERM CORPORATION

GATE PHARMACEUTICALS 409, 1053
Division of Lemmon Company
P.O. Box 904
Sellersville, PA 18960
Toll Free (800) 292-GATE
(215) 723-5544
Products Described
◆ Adipex-P Tablets and Capsules ... 409, 1053
◆ Orap Tablets ... 409, 1053

GEBAUER COMPANY 1056
9410 St. Catherine Avenue
Cleveland, OH 44104
Address inquiries to:
(800) 321-9348
OH (216) 271-5252
For Medical Emergencies Contact:
(800) 321-9348
OH (216) 271-5252
After Hours Emergency call:
Chemtrec (800) 424-9300
Products Described
Ethyl Chloride, U.S.P. ... 1056
Fluori-Methane ... 1056
Fluro-Ethyl ... 1056
Other Products Available
Dr. Caldwell's Senna Laxative
Gebauer's "114"
Salivart

GEIGY PHARMACEUTICALS 409, 1057
Division of CIBA-GEIGY Corporation
Ardsley, NY 10502
Address inquiries to:
Medical Services Department
556 Morris Avenue
Summit, NJ 07901
(908) 277-5000
Warehouse Offices and Shipping Branches
Eastern
14 Henderson Drive
West Caldwell, NJ 07006
(201) 882-4700
Central
900 Corporate Grove Drive
Buffalo Grove, IL 60089
Buffalo Grove (708) 520-7770
Western
12850 Moore Street
P.O. Box 6300
Cerritos, CA 90701
(310) 404-2651
Products Described
◆ Brethaire Inhaler ... 409, 1057
Brethancer Inhaler ... 1059
◆ Brethine Ampuls ... 409, 1060
◆ Brethine Tablets ... 409, 1059
◆ Constant-T Tablets ... 410, 1061
◆ Lamprene Capsules ... 410, 1062
◆ Lioresal Tablets ... 410, 1063
Lopressor Ampuls ... 1064
◆ Lopressor HCT Tablets ... 410, 1066
◆ Lopressor Tablets ... 410, 1064
Otrivin Nasal Spray and Nasal Drops ... 1069
Otrivin Pediatric Nasal Drops ... 1069
◆ PBZ Tablets ... 410, 1070
◆ PBZ-SR Tablets ... 410, 1069
Tofranil Ampuls ... 1070
◆ Tofranil Tablets ... 410, 1071
◆ Tofranil-PM Capsules ... 410, 1073
◆ Voltaren Tablets ... 410, 1074

GENDERM CORPORATION 1077
600 Knightsbridge Parkway
Lincolnshire, IL 60069
Address inquiries to:
Medical Services Department
(708) 634-7373
Products Described
Occlusal ... 1077
Occlusal-HP ... 1077
Pentrax Anti-dandruff Shampoo ... 1077
PrameGel ... 1077
SalAc ... 1077
Zostrix ... 1077
Zostrix-HP Topical Analgesic Cream ... 1077
Other Products Available
A-Fil
Maxafil
Meted Shampoo
Ovide Lotion
Packer's Pine Tar Shampoo
Packer's Pine Tar Soap
Step 2
Texacort Topical Solution 1%
Texacort Topical Solution 2.5%

GENENTECH, INC. 410, 1078
460 Point San Bruno Blvd.
South San Francisco, CA 94080
(415) 225-1000
For Medical Information, 24 Hours a Day
Call: Medical Information and Drug Experience Dept.
(800) 821-8590
(415) 225-1000
Or write:
Medical Information and Drug Experience Dept.
Genentech, Inc.
460 Point San Bruno Blvd.
South San Francisco, CA 94080
Field Office
100 Tri-County Parkway
Suite 402
Springdale, OH 45246
Steve Aselage, Director of Field Sales
(513) 771-3317
FAX (513) 771-3760
Products Described
◆ Actimmune ... 410, 1078
◆ Activase ... 410, 1079
◆ Protropin ... 410, 1082

GENEVA MARSAM 1083
2555 West Midway Boulevard
P.O. Box 446
Broomfield, CO 80038-0446
Address inquiries to:
Customer Service Department
(800) 525-8747
(303) 466-2400
FAX (303) 469-6467
Products Described
Sterile Ampicillin Sodium, USP ... *1083*
Sterile Cefazolin Sodium, USP ... *1083*
Nafcillin Sodium for Injection, USP ... *1083*
Neostigmine Methylsulfate Injection ... *1083*
Oxacillin Sodium For Injection, USP ... *1083*
Tobramycin Sulfate Injection, USP ... *1083*

GENEVA PHARMACEUTICALS, INC. 1083
2555 West Midway Blvd.
P.O. Box 446
Broomfield, CO 80038-0446
Address inquiries to:
Customer Service Department
(800) 525-8747
(303) 466-2400
FAX (303) 469-6467
Products Described
Acetaminophen/Codeine Phosphate Tablets ... *1083*
Allopurinol Tablets ... *1083*
Aminophylline Tablets ... *1083*
Amitriptyline HCl Tablets ... *1083*
Amoxapine Tablets ... *1083*
Aspirin and Codeine Phosphate Tablets ... *1083*
Atenolol Tablets ... *1083*
Butalbital Compound Tablets ... *1083*
Carisoprodol Tablets ... *1083*
Chlorpheniramine Maleate Extended Release Capsules ... *1083*
Chlorpheniramine Maleate Tablets ... *1083*
Chlorpromazine Oral Concentrate ... *1083*
Chlorpromazine HCl Tablets ... *1083*
Chlorpropamide Tablets ... *1083*
Chlorthalidone Tablets ... *1083*
Chlorzoxazone Tablets ... *1083*
Clonidine HCl Tablets ... *1083*
Cyclobenzaprine HCl Tablets ... *1083*
Desipramine HCl Tablets ... *1083*
Diazepam Tablets ... *1083*
Diphenhydramine HCl Capsules ... *1083*
Dipyridamole Tablets ... *1083*
Disopyramide Phosphate Capsules ... *1083*
Doxepin HCl Capsules ... *1083*
Fenoprofen Calcium Capsules ... *1083*
Fluphenazine HCl Tablets ... *1083*
Furosemide Tablets ... *1083*
Haloperidol Tablets ... *1083*
Hydroxyzine HCl Tablets ... *1083*
Hydroxyzine Pamoate Capsules ... 1083
Imipramine HCl Tablets ... *1083*
Indomethacin Capsules ... *1083*
Isosorbide Dinitrate Tablets ... *1083*
Isoxsuprine HCl Tablets ... *1083*
Lorazepam Tablets ... *1083*
Meclizine HCl Tablets ... *1083*
Meclofenamate Sodium Capsules ... *1083*
Meprobamate Tablets ... *1083*
Methocarbamol Tablets ... *1083*
Methyclothiazide Tablets ... *1083*
Methyldopa/Hydrochlorothiazide Tablets ... *1083*
Methyldopa Tablets ... *1083*
Metronidazole Tablets ... *1083*
Nitroglycerin S.R. Capsules ... *1083*
Oxazepam Capsules ... *1083*
Papaverine HCl S.R. Capsules ... *1083*
Perphenazine Tablets ... *1083*
Perphenazine/Amitriptyline HCl Tablets ... *1083*
Prednisolone Tablets ... *1083*
Prednisone Tablets ... *1083*
Procainamide HCl Extended-Release Tablets ... *1083*
Propoxyphene HCl/Acetaminophen Tablets ... *1083*
Propoxyphene HCl/Aspirin & Caffeine Capsules ... *1083*
Propoxyphene HCl Capsules ... *1083*
Propoxyphene Napsylate/Acetaminophen Tablets ... *1083*
Propranolol HCl Tablets ... *1083*
Propranolol HCl/Hydrochlorothiazide Tablets ... *1083*
Quinidine Gluconate E.R. Tablets ... *1083*
Quinidine Sulfate Tablets ... *1083*
Salsalate Tablets ... *1083*
Spironolactone/Hydrochlorothiazide Tablets ... *1083*
Spironolactone Tablets ... *1083*
Sulfisoxazole Tablets ... *1083*
Sulindac Tablets ... *1083*
Temazepam Capsules ... *1083*
Thioridazine HCl Tablets ... *1083*
Thiothixene Capsules ... *1083*
Timolol Maleate Tablets ... *1083*
Tolazamide Tablets ... *1083*
Tolmetin Sodium ... *1083*
Trazodone HCl Tablets ... *1083*
Triamterene/Hydrochlorothiazide Tablets ... *1083*
Trifluoperazine HCl Tablets and Concentrate ... *1083*
Verapamil HCl Tablets ... *1083*
Other Products Available
Clinoxide Capsules
Decongestant S.R. Tablets
Disobrom Tablets
Ercaf Tablets
Lonox Tablets
Quifile
Resaid S.R. Capsules
T.E.H.
Tamine S.R. Tablets

GENZYME CORPORATION 410, 1084
One Kendall Square
Cambridge, MA 02139
Address inquiries to:
Clinical Services (800) 745-4447
FAX (617) 252-7600
For Medical Emergencies Contact:
(800) 745-4447
Products Described
◆ Ceredase Injection ... 410, 1084

GLAXO DERMATOLOGY 410, 1085
Division of Glaxo Inc.
Five Moore Drive
Research Triangle Park
North Carolina 27709
(919) 248-2100
Address inquiries to:
Medical Services Department
For Medical Emergencies Contact:
(919) 248-2100
Products Described
◆ Aclovate Cream ... 410, 1085
◆ Aclovate Ointment ... 410, 1085
◆ Cutivate Cream ... 410, 1086
◆ Cutivate Ointment ... 410, 1086
◆ Emgel 2% Topical Gel ... 410, 1087
◆ Oxistat Cream ... 410, 1088
◆ Temovate Cream ... 410, 1088
◆ Temovate Ointment ... 410, 1088
◆ Temovate Scalp Application ... 410, 1088

GLAXO PHARMACEUTICALS 410, 1089
Division of Glaxo Inc.
Five Moore Drive
Research Triangle Park
North Carolina 27709
(919) 248-2100
Address inquiries to:
Medical Services Department
(919) 248-2100
For Medical Emergencies Contact:
(919) 248-2100
Products Described
◆ Ceptaz ... 411, 1089
◆ Fortaz ... 410,411, 1092
◆ Zantac Injection and Zantac Injection Premixed ... 411, 1096
◆ Zantac Syrup ... 411, 1097
◆ Zantac 150 & 300 Tablets ... 411, 1097
◆ Zinacef ... 411, 1099

GLENWOOD, INC. 411, 1102
83 North Summit Street
Tenafly, NJ 07670
Address inquiries to:
Professional Services Dept. 1A
(201) 569-0050
Products Described
Bichloracetic Acid Kahlenberg ... 1102
Calphosan ... 1102
Myotonachol ... *1102*
◆ Potaba ... 411, 1102
Primer Unna Boot ... 1103
Yodoxin ... 1103

GORDON LABORATORIES, INC. 1104
State and Parkview Roads
Upper Darby, PA 19082
Address inquiries to:
David Dercher (215) 789-3055
FAX (215) 789-4635
For Medical Emergencies Contact:
David Dercher (215) 789-3055
FAX (215) 789-4635
Products Described
Gordochom Solution ... 1104
Other Products Available
Abscents Deodorizing Powder
Aloe Grandé Creme & Lotion
Bromi-Lotion
Bromi-Talc
Bromi-Talc Plus

Emollia-Creme & Lotion
Formadon
Forma-Ray
Gordofilm
Gordogesic Creme
Gordon's Vite A Creme & Lotion
Gordon's Vite E Cream
Gordon's Urea 22%
Gordon's Urea 40%
Gormel Creme & Lotion
Mecholyl Ointment
Mono-Chlor
Oxyzal Wet Dressing
Pyrogallic Acid
Salacid 25%, 60%
Silver Nitrate Solutions 10%, 25%, 50%
Sodium Hydroxide 10%
Sorbidon Hydrate
Tri-Chlor

GRAY PHARMACEUTICAL CO. 1104
Affiliate, The Purdue Frederick Company
100 Connecticut Avenue
Norwalk, CT 06850-3590
Address inquiries to:
Medical Department
(203) 853-0123
Products Described
Senna X-Prep Bowel Evacuant Liquid 1104
Other Products Available
X-Prep Kit 1
X-Prep Kit 2

GUARDIAN LABORATORIES 1104
A Division of United-Guardian, Inc.
230 Marcus Boulevard
Hauppauge, NY 11788
P.O. Box 2500
Smithtown, NY 11787
(516) 273-0900
(800) 645-5566
Address inquiries to:
Director of Medical Research
Products Described
Clorpactin WCS-90 1104
Lubraseptic Jelly 1104
Renacidin Irrigation *1104*
Other Products Available
Clorpactin XCB
pHos-pHaid Tablets
Renacidin Powder

GYNEX PHARMACEUTICALS, INC. 1105
1175 Corporate Woods Parkway
Vernon Hills, IL 60061
Address inquiries to:
(708) 913-1144
For Medical Emergency Contact
(708) 913-1144
For Ordering Information:
(800) 424-9639
Products Described
Delatestryl Injection *1105*

GYNOPHARMA INC. 411, 1105
50 Division Street
Somerville, NJ 08876
Address inquiries to:
(908) 725-3100
For Medical Information Contact:
(908) 725-3100
Products Described
◆ ParaGard T380A Intrauterine Copper Contraceptive 411, 1105

HAUCK PHARMACEUTICALS
See ROBERTS PHARMACEUTICAL CORPORATION

HEALTH MAINTENANCE PROGRAMS, INC. 1110
7 Westchester Plaza
Elmsford, NY 10523
Address inquiries to:
(800) 362-8673
Products Described
Calcium Health Packs *1110*
Carotene-E Forté Capsules *1111*
Carotene Health Packs *1111*
Endurance Packs *1111*
For Two Capsules *1111*
Glutathione Health Packs *1111*
Glutathione-Forté Capsules *1111*
Glutathione-500 .... *1111*
Performance Packs *1111*
Pure-E Capsules and Liquid *1111*
Superkids Chewable Tablets *1111*

DOW B. HICKAM, INC. 1112
P.O. Box 2006
Sugar Land, TX 77487-2006
Address inquiries to:
Professional Service Dept.
(713) 240-1000
Products Described
Granulex 1112
Other Products Available
Biobrane Temporary Wound Dressing
Proderm Topical Dressing
Sorbsan Topical Wound Dressing
Sulfamylon Cream (mafenide acetate cream)
Unifiber

HIGH CHEMICAL COMPANY 1112
1760 N. Howard St.
Philadelphia, PA 19122
Address inquiries to:
Professional Service Dept.
(215) 634-2224
Products Described
Sarapin 1112
Other Products Available
Amo-Derm
Klorlyptus
Mus-L-Tone

HOECHST-ROUSSEL PHARMACEUTICALS INC. 411, 1112
Route 202-206, P.O. Box 2500
Somerville, NJ 00876-1258
Address medical inquiries to:
Scientific Services Dept.
(8:30AM-5:00PM EST)
(800) 445-4774
Customer Service (800) 451-4455
For medical emergency information only, after hours and on weekends, call:
(201) 231-2000
Products Described
◆ A/T/S Topical Gel and Topical Solution 411, 1114
◆ Altace Capsules 411, 1112
Claforan Sterile Injection 1115
◆ DiaBeta 411, 1117
◆ Lasix Oral Solution 411, 1119
◆ Lasix Tablets and Injection 411, 412,
◆ Loprox Cream 1% and Lotion 1% 412, 1121
Prokine for I.V. Infusion 1121
◆ Topicort Cream 412, 1124
◆ Topicort Gel 412, 1124
◆ Topicort LP 412, 1124
◆ Topicort Ointment 412, 1124
◆ Trental 412, 1125
Other Products Available
Doxinate
Doxinate Solution
Duadacin
Festal II Digestive Aid

HOFFMANN-LA ROCHE INC.
See ROCHE DERMATOLOGICS, ROCHE LABORATORIES & ROCHE PRODUCTS INC.
Contact numbers of other operating units:
Drug Abuse Policy Initiative
Branchburg, NJ (908) 253-7560

Roche Biomedical Laboratories, Inc.
Drugs of Abuse
Research Triangle Park, NC
(800) 872-5727

Roche Biomedical Laboratories, Inc.:
Birmingham, AL (800) 621-8037
Burlington, NC (800) 334-5161
Dublin, OH (800) 282-7300
Raritan, NJ (800) 631-5250

Roche Diagnostic Systems, Inc.
Roche Response Center
Montclair, NJ (800) 526-1247

Roche Professional Service Centers, Inc.
(Home Health Care/Infusion Therapy)
Paramus, NJ (201) 261-5151
(800) 888-7442

HYLAND DIVISION
See BAXTER HEALTHCARE CORPORATION

HYNSON, WESTCOTT & DUNNING PRODUCTS
See BECTON DICKINSON MICROBIOLOGY SYSTEMS

ICI PHARMA 412, 1126
A business unit of ICI Americas Inc.
Wilmington, DE 19897 USA
Address Pharmaceutical product-related inquiries to:
Yvonne Graham, Manager
Professional Services
(302) 886-2231
For Medical Emergencies Contact:
After Hours or On Weekends, call
(302) 886-3000
Products Described
◆ Nolvadex Tablets 412, 1126
◆ Sorbitrate Chewable Tablets 412, 1128
◆ Sorbitrate Oral Tablets 412, 1128
◆ Sorbitrate Sublingual Tablets 412, 1128
◆ Sorbitrate Sustained Action Tablets 412, 1128
◆ Tenoretic Tablets 412, 1129
◆ Tenormin Tablets and I.V. Injection 412, 1132
◆ Zoladex 412, 1134

ICN PHARMACEUTICALS, INC. 412, 1136
ICN Plaza
3300 Hyland Avenue
Costa Mesa, CA 92626
Address inquiries to:
Professional Service Dept.
(800) 556-1937
In CA (800) 331-2331
(714) 545-0100
Products Described
Android-10 Tablets 1136
Android-25 Tablets 1136
Benoquin Cream 20% 1137
Eldecort Cream 1.0% 1137
Eldecort Cream 2.5% 1137
Eldopaque Forte 4% Cream 1138
Eldoquin Forte 4% Cream 1138
Fluonex Cream 1139
Fototar Cream .... ⊡
Kato Potassium Supplement 1140
Mestinon Injectable 1140
Mestinon Syrup 1141
Mestinon Tablets 1141
Mestinon Timespan Tablets 1141
Oxsoralen Lotion 1% 1141
◆ Oxsoralen-Ultra Capsule 412, 1142
Prostigmin Injectable 1145
Prostigmin Tablets 1146
Psorion Cream 0.05% 1147
Solaquin Forte 4% Cream 1147
Solaquin Forte 4% Gel 1148
Tensilon Injectable 1148
◆ Testred Capsules 412, 1149
◆ Trisoralen Tablets 412, 1151
Virazole 1151
Other Products Available
Eldopaque 2% Cream
Eldoquin 2% Cream
Eldoquin 2% Lotion
Precef
RVP Ointment
RVPaba Lip Stick
RVPaque Ointment
Solaquin 2% Cream
Vitadye Lotion

IMMUNEX CORPORATION 1152
51 University Street
Seattle, WA 98101
Address inquiries to:
Professional Services
(800) 334-6273
(206) 587-0430
FAX (800) 441-6303
FAX (206) 343-8926
For Medical Emergencies Contact:
Professional Services
(800) 334-6273
(206) 587-0430
FAX (800) 441-6303
FAX (206) 343-8926
Products Described
Hydrea Capsules 1152
Leukine for IV Infusion 1153
Rubex Injection *1156*

IMMUNO-U.S., INC. 1156
1200 Parkdale Road
Rochester, MI 48307-1744
Address inquiries to:
Telephone: (313) 652-7872
Telex: 4320100
Telefax: (313) 652-0670
Products Described
Albumin (Human) 5% *1156*
Albumin (Human) 25% *1156*
Feiba VH Immuno *1156*
Iveegam *1156*

INTERNATIONAL ETHICAL LABS. 412, 1156
1021 Avenue Americo Miranda
Reparto Metropolitano
Rio Piedras, PR 00921
Address inquiries to:
Mr. Sammy Diaz, President
(809) 765-3510
(809) 763-8414
FAX (809) 767-1110
Products Described
◆ Biocef Capsules and Oral Suspension 412, *1156*
Bio-Tab Tablets *1156*
◆ Despec Capsules 412, *1156*
Despec Liquid *1156*
Mio-Rel Injectable *1156*
Molixin Capsules *1156*
Molixin O/S *1156*
Neuroforte-R Vial *1156*
Neuroforte-Six Monovial *1156*
Remular-S and Remular-500 .... *1156*
◆ Tencon Capsules 412, *1156*

INWOOD LABORATORIES 409, 1157
Subsidiary of Forest Laboratories
300 Prospect Street
Inwood, NY 11696
Address inquiries to:
(718) 471-8000
Products Described
Carbamazepine Tablets *1157*
Indomethacin E.R. Capsules *1157*
Isosorbide Dinitrate E.R. Tablets *1157*
Propranolol Hydrochloride E.R. Capsules *1157*
◆ Theochron E.R. Tablets 409, *1157*

ION LABORATORIES, INC. 1157
7431 Pebble Drive
Fort Worth, TX 76118
Address inquiries to:
Ralph E. Brown (817) 589-7257
FAX (817) 590-0973
For Medical Emergencies Contact:
Ralph E. Brown (817) 589-7257
FAX (817) 590-0973
Products Described
Rescon Capsules *1157*
Rescon-DM Liquid *1157*
Rescon-ED Capsules *1157*
Rescon-GG Liquid *1157*
Rescon JR Capsules *1157*
Rescon Liquid *1157*
Sinupan Capsules *1157*
Other Products Available
Liquibid Tablets
Rexigen Forte Capsules
Zantryl Capsules

JACOBUS PHARMACEUTICAL CO., INC. 1157
37 Cleveland Lane
P.O. Box 5290
Princeton, NJ 08540
Address inquiries to:
Professional Services
(609) 921-7447
For Medical Emergencies Contact:
Medical Department
(609) 921-7447
FAX (609) 799-1176
Products Described
Dapsone USP 1157

JAMOL LABORATORIES INC. 1158
13 Ackerman Avenue
Emerson, NJ 07630
Address inquiries to:
(201) 262-6363
Products Described
Ponaris Nasal Mucosal Emollient 1158

JANSSEN PHARMACEUTICA INC. 412, 1158
1125 Trenton-Harbourton Road
P.O. Box 200
Titusville, NJ 08560-0200
Address inquiries to:
Professional Services
(800) 253-3682
(609) 730-2000
FAX (609) 730-3044
After 5PM EST or on weekends:
(800) 253-3682
Holidays: Routine: (800) 253-3682
Emergencies: (908) 524-0400
Products Described
◆ Alfenta Injection 412, 1158
◆ Duragesic Transdermal System 412, 1160
◆ Ergamisol Tablets 412, 1164
◆ Hismanal Tablets 412, 1165
◆ Imodium Capsules 412, 1166
◆ Inapsine Injection 412, 1167
◆ Innovar Injection 412, 1168
◆ Monistat I.V. 412, 1170
◆ Nizoral 2% Cream 412, 1171
◆ Nizoral 2% Shampoo 412, 1171
◆ Nizoral Tablets 412, 1172
◆ Sublimaze Injection 412, 1173
◆ Sufenta Injection 413, 1174
◆ Vermox Chewable Tablets 412, 1177

JOHNSON & JOHNSON MEDICAL, INC. 1177
P.O. Box 130
Arlington, TX 76004-0130
(800) 433-5009
Products Described
INSTAT Collagen Absorbable Hemostat 1177
SURGICEL Absorbable Hemostat 1178
SURGICEL NU-KNIT Absorbable Hemostat 1178
THROMBOGEN Topical Thrombin, USP 1179
THROMBOGEN Topical Thrombin, USP, Spray Kit 1179
THROMBOGEN Topical Thrombin, USP, Transfer Needle 1179

JOHNSON & JOHNSON • MERCK CONSUMER PHARMACEUTICALS CO. 413, 1180
Camp Hill Road
Ft. Washington, PA 19034
Address inquiries to:
Consumer Affairs Department
Fort Washington, PA 19034
(215) 233-7000
For Medical Emergencies Contact:
(215) 233-7000
Products Described
◆ ALternaGEL Liquid 413, 1180
◆ Dialose Tablets 413, 1180
◆ Dialose Plus Tablets 413, 1181
◆ Effer-Syllium Natural Fiber Bulking Agent 413, 1181
◆ Ferancee Chewable Tablets 413, 1181
◆ Ferancee-HP Tablets 413, 1181
◆ Mylanta Gas Tablets - 40 mg 413, 1183
◆ Mylanta Gas Tablets 413, 1183
◆ Maximum Strength Mylanta Gas Tablets 413, 1183
◆ Mylanta Gelcaps Antacid 413, 1182
◆ Mylanta Liquid 413, 1181
◆ Mylanta Tablets 413, 1181
◆ Mylanta Double Strength Liquid 413, 1182
◆ Mylanta Double Strength Tablets 413, 1182
◆ Mylicon Drops 413, 1183
◆ The Stuart Formula Tablets 413, 1183
◆ Stuartinic Tablets 413, 1183

JOHNSON & JOHNSON PROFESSIONAL DIAGNOSTICS INC.
See ORTHO DIAGNOSTIC SYSTEMS INC.

KABI PHARMACIA 413, 1184
800 Centennial Avenue
P.O. Box 1327
Piscataway, NJ 08855-1327
(908) 457-8000
(800) 526-3619
(908) 457-8283 (Telefax)
Products Described
◆ Azulfidine Tablets and EN-tabs ... 413, 1184
Cyklokapron Tablets and Injection ... 1185
◆ Dipentum Capsules ... 413, 1186
◆ Emcyt Capsules ... 413, 1187
Hyskon Hysteroscopy Fluid ... 1188
Kabikinase (Streptokinase) ... *1189*
Macrodex ... *1189*
Rheomacrodex ... *1189*

KENWOOD LABORATORIES 1189
a division of BRADLEY PHARMACEUTICALS, INC.
383 Route 46 West
Fairfield, NJ 07004-2402
Address inquiries to:
(201) 882-1505
Products Described
Apatate Liquid/Tablets ... *1189*
Apatate Liquid with Fluoride ... *1189*
Duadacin Cold & Allergy Capsules ... *1189*
Glutofac Caplets ... *1189*
ILX B_{12} Caplets Crystalline ... *1189*
ILX B_{12} Elixir Crystalline and ILX B_{12} Sugar Free Elixir ... *1189*
ILX Elixir ... *1189*
Ircon Tablets ... *1189*
Ircon-FA Tablets ... *1189*
Kenwood Therapeutic Liquid ... *1189*
Neoloid Emulsified Castor Oil ... *1189*
Nitroglyn Extended Release Capsules ... *1189*
Tyzine Nasal Solution/Nasal Spray/Pediatric Nasal Drops ... *1189*

KEY PHARMACEUTICALS, INC. 413, 1190
Galloping Hill Road
Kenilworth, NJ 07033
(908) 298-4000
Address inquiries to:
Professional Services Department
9:00 AM to 5:00 PM EST:
(800) 526-4099
After regular hours and on weekends:
(908) 298-4000
Products Described
◆ K-Dur Microburst Release System (potassium chloride, USP) E.R. Tablets .. 413, 1190
◆ Nitro-Dur (nitroglycerin) Transdermal Infusion System ... 413, 1191
◆ Theo-Dur Sprinkle Sustained Action Capsules ... 413, 1195
◆ Theo-Dur Extended-Release Tablets ... 413, 1192
◆ Trinalin Repetabs Tablets ... 413, 1197
Other Products Available
Guanidine Hydrochloride Tablets

KNOLL PHARMACEUTICALS 413, 1198
A Unit of BASF K&F Corporation
30 North Jefferson Road
Whippany, NJ 07981
General Number (201) 887-8300
Customer Service (800) 526-0710
Medical Information
(800) 526-0221
NJ (201) 428-8250
Products Described
Akineton Injection ... 1198
◆ Akineton Tablets ... 413, 1198
◆ Collagenase Santyl Ointment .. 414, 1199
Dilaudid Cough Syrup ... 1200
Dilaudid Hydrochloride Ampules ... 1199
Dilaudid Injection ... 1199
Dilaudid Multiple Dose Vials (Sterile Solution) ... 1199
Dilaudid Powder ... 1199
Dilaudid Rectal Suppositories ... 1199
◆ Dilaudid Tablets ... 413, 1199
◆ Dilaudid-HP Injection ... 413, 1201
◆ Isoptin Ampules ... 413
◆ Isoptin for Intravenous Injection ... 414, 1203
◆ Isoptin Oral Tablets ... 414, 1205
◆ Isoptin SR Sustained Release Tablets ... 414, 1207
◆ Quadrinal Tablets ... 414, 1210
◆ Rythmol Tablets ... 414, 1211
◆ Vicodin Tablets ... 414, 1214
◆ Vicodin ES Tablets ... 414, 1215
Other Products Available
Codeine Sulfate Tablets

KRAMER LABORATORIES INC. 1217
8778 S.W. 8th Street
Miami, FL 33174
Address inquiries to:
8778 S.W. 8th Street
Miami, FL 33174 (800) 824-4894
For Medical Emergencies Contact:
Professional Director
(800) 824-4894
Products Described
Charcoal Plus Tablets ... 1217
Fungi-Nail Tincture ... 1217
Yohimex Tablets ... 1217

KREMERS URBAN COMPANY 1217
See SCHWARZ PHARMA

LACTAID, INC. 414, 1217
Pleasantville, NJ 08232
Address inquiries to:
Alan E. Kligerman (609) 645-5100
Products Described
◆ Lactaid Caplets ... 414, 1217
◆ Lactaid Drops ... 414, 1217

LASER, INC. 1218
2000 N. Main Street,
P.O. Box 905
Crown Point, IN 46307
Address inquiries to:
Donald A. Laser (219) 663-1165
Products Described
Dallergy Capsules, Tablets, Syrup ... *1218*
Dallergy-JR Capsules ... *1218*
Donatussin DC Syrup ... *1218*
Donatussin Drops ... *1218*
Lactocal-F Tablets ... *1218*
Respaire-SR Capsules 60, 120 ... *1218*
Theostat 80 Syrup ... *1218*
Other Products Available
Dallergy-D Capsules
Dallergy-D Syrup
Donatussin Syrup
Fumatinic Capsules
Fumerin Tablets
Kie Syrup

LEDERLE LABORATORIES 414, 1218, 2666
Division of American Cyanamid Company
One Cyanamid Plaza
Wayne, NJ 07470
LEDERLE PARENTERALS, INC.
Carolina, Puerto Rico 00630
LEDERLE PIPERACILLIN, INC.
Carolina, Puerto Rico 00630
PRAXIS BIOLOGICS, INC.
Rochester, NY 14623
A Subsidiary of American Cyanamid Company
Address medical/pharmacy inquiries on marketed products only to:
Professional Services Department
Lederle Laboratories
Pearl River, NY 10965
During business hours (8 AM to 4:30 PM E.S.T.):
(914) 735-2815
All other inquiries and after hours emergencies:
(914) 732-5000
Distribution Centers
ATLANTA
Contact EASTERN (Philadelphia) Distribution Center
CHICAGO
Bulk Address
1100 E. Business Center Drive
Mt. Prospect, IL 60056
Mail Address
P.O. Box 7614
Mt. Prospect, IL 60056-7614
(800) 533-3753
(708) 827-8871
DALLAS
Bulk Address
7611 Carpenter Freeway
Dallas, TX 75247
Mail Address
P.O. Box 655731
Dallas, TX 75265 (800) 533-3753
(214) 631-2130
LOS ANGELES
Bulk Address
2300 S. Eastern Avenue
Los Angeles, CA 90040
Mail Address
T.A. Box 2202
Los Angeles, CA 90051
(800) 533-3753
(213) 726-1016
EASTERN (Philadelphia)
Bulk Address
202 Precision Drive
Horsham, PA 19044
Mail Address
P.O. Box 993
Horsham, PA 19044
(800) 533-3753
(215) 672-5400
Products Described
◆ Acel-Imune Diphtheria and Tetanus Toxoids and Pertussis Vaccine Adsorbed 414, 1219
◆ Achromycin V Capsules ... 414, 1222
Achromycin 3% Ointment ... *1223*
Achromycin Ophthalmic Ointment 1% (See PDR For Ophthalmology) ... *1223*
◆ Achromycin Ophthalmic Suspension 1% (See PDR For Ophthalmology) ... 414, *1222*
Albuterol Sulfate Tablets ... *1218*
◆ Amicar Syrup, Tablets, and Injection ... 414, 1223
Amoxicillin Capsules, Oral Suspension ... *1218*
Ampicillin Trihydrate Capsules, Oral Suspension ... *1218*
◆ Artane Elixir ... 414, 1224
◆ Artane Sequels ... 414, 1224
◆ Artane Tablets ... 414, 1224
◆ Asendin Tablets ... 414, 1225
Atenolol Tablets ... *1218*
Aureomycin Ophthalmic Ointment 1.0% ... *1218*
Benztropine Mesylate Tablets ... *1218*
◆ Caltrate 600 Tablets ... 414, 1226
◆ Caltrate 600 + Iron & Vitamin D ... 414, 1227
◆ Caltrate 600 + Vitamin D ... 414, 1226
Centrum ... ▣
Centrum, Jr. (Children's Chewable) + Extra C ... ▣
Centrum, Jr. (Children's Chewable) + Extra Calcium ... ▣
Centrum, Jr. (Children's Chewable) + Iron ... ▣
Centrum Liquid ... ▣
Centrum Silver ... ▣
Cephalexin Tablets, Oral Suspension ... *1218*
Cephradine Capsules ... *1218*
Clindamycin Phosphate Injection ... *1218*
Clonidine HCl Tablets ... *1218*
Clorazepate Dipotassium Capsules, Tablets ... *1218*
Cloxacillin Sodium Capsules ... *1218*
◆ Declomycin Tablets ... 414, 1227
Diamox Parenteral ... 1228
◆ Diamox Sequels (Sustained Release) ... 414, 1229
◆ Diamox Tablets ... 414, 1228
Diazepam Injection, Tablets ... *1218*
Dicloxacillin Sodium Capsules ... *1218*
Diphtheria & Tetanus Toxoids, Adsorbed Purogenated ... 1230
Dipyridamole Tablets ... *1218*
Disopyramide Phosphate Capsules ... *1218*
Docusate Sodium Capsules ... *1218*
Docusate Sodium with Casanthranol Capsules ... *1218*
Doxepin HCl Capsules ... *1218*
Doxycycline Hyclate Capsules, Tablets ... *1218*
Erythromycin Estolate Oral Suspension ... *1218*
Erythromycin Ethylsuccinate Oral Suspension ... *1218*
Sterile Erythromycin Lactobionate for Injection ... *1218*
Erythromycin Ethylsuccinate/ Sulfisoxazole Acetyl Oral Suspension ... *1218*
Fenoprofen Calcium Tablets ... *1218*
◆ Ferro-Sequels ... 414, 1231
Ferrous Gluconate Iron Supplement Tablets ... *1218*
◆ FiberCon Tablets ... 414, 1231
◆ Filibon F.A. Prenatal Vitamin Tablets ... 414, 1232
◆ Filibon Forte Tablets ... 414, 1232
◆ Filibon Prenatal Vitamin Tablets ... 414, 1232
Flu-Imune Influenza Virus Vaccine ... 1232
Folic Acid Tablets ... *1218*
Furosemide Tablets ... *1218*
Gevrabon Liquid ... ▣
Gevral T Tablets ... ▣
◆ HibTITER ... 414, 1234
Hydralazine HCl Tablets ... *1218*
Hydrochlorothiazide Tablets ... *1218*
◆ Hydromox Tablets ... 414, 1237
Incremin with Iron Syrup ... ▣
Indomethacin Capsules ... *1218*
Ledercillin VK Oral Solution, Tablets ... *1218*
◆ Leucovorin Calcium for Injection ... 415, 1238
◆ Leucovorin Calcium Tablets ... 414, 1240
◆ LEVO-T Tablets ... 415
◆ Loxitane C Oral Concentrate ... 415, 1241
◆ Loxitane Capsules ... 415, 1241
◆ Loxitane IM ... 415, 1241
◆ Materna Tablets ... 415, 1243
◆ Maxzide Tablets ... 415, 1243
◆ Maxzide-25 MG Tablets ... 415, 1243
Methocarbamol Tablets ... *1218*
◆ Methotrexate Sodium Tablets, for Injection and LPF Injection ... 415, 1245
Methyldopa & Hydrochlorothiazide Tablets ... *1218*
Methyldopa Tablets ... *1218*
Metoclopramide Tablets ... *1218*
Metronidazole Tablets ... *1218*
◆ Minocin Intravenous ... 415, 1250
◆ Minocin Oral Suspension ... 415, 1252
◆ Minocin Pellet-Filled Capsules 415, 1251
◆ Minocycline Hydrochloride Tablets ... 415
◆ Myambutol Tablets ... 415, 1254
◆ Neptazane Tablets ... 415, 1255
◆ Nilstat for Preparation of Oral Suspension ... 415
◆ Nilstat Oral Suspension ... 415
Nitroglycerin S.R. Capsules ... *1218*
◆ Novantrone for Injection Concentrate ... 415, 1256
Occucoat (See PDR For Ophthalmology) ... *1258*
Ocuvite (See PDR For Ophthalmology) ... ▣
◆ Orimune Poliovirus Vaccine Live Oral Trivalent ... 415, 1258
◆ PPD Tine Test ... 416, 2666
◆ Pipracil ... 415, 1259
◆ Pnu-Imune 23 Pneumococcal Vaccine Polyvalent ... 415, 1262
Prazosin HCl Capsules ... *1218*
Procainamide HCl SR Tablets ... *1218*
Propranolol Hydrochloride Tablets ... *1218*
Propylthiouracil Tablets ... *1218*
◆ Prostep (nicotine transdermal system) ... 415, 1264
◆ Pyrazinamide Tablets ... 415, 1267
Quinidine Sulfate Tablets ... *1218*
◆ Rheumatrex Methotrexate Dose Pack ... 415, 1268
Stresstabs ... ▣
Stresstabs + Iron, Advanced Formula ... ▣
Stresstabs + Zinc ... ▣
Sulfamethoxazole & Trimethoprim Pediatric Suspension, Tablets ... *1218*
Sulfasalazine Tablets ... *1218*
Sulindac Tablets ... *1218*
◆ Suprax Powder for Oral Suspension ... 416, 1268
◆ Suprax Tablets ... 416, 1268
Tetanus & Diphtheria Toxoids, Adsorbed Purogenated ... 1270
Tetanus Toxoid, Adsorbed Purogenated ... 1272
◆ Thiotepa For Injection ... 415, 1274
Tobramycin Sulfate Injection ... *1218*
Trazodone HCl Tablets ... *1218*
◆ Tri-Immunol Diphtheria & Tetanus Toxoids & Pertussis Vaccine, Adsorbed ... 415, 1274
◆ Tuberculin, Old, Tine Test ... 416, 2667
Vancoled ... *1218*
Verapamil HCl Tablets ... *1218*
◆ Verelan Capsules ... 416, 1277
Zincon Dandruff Shampoo ... ▣
Other Products Available
Folvite Parenteral & Tablets
Pronemia Capsules
TriHEMIC 600 Tablets

LEMMON COMPANY 1279
Post Office Box 904
Sellersville, PA 18960
Address inquiries to:
Toll Free (800) 545-8800
See GATE PHARMACEUTICALS
Products Not Described
Other Products Available
Acetaminophen and Codeine Phosphate Tablets
Albuterol Sulfate Syrup and Tablets
Amantadine HCl Capsules
Amoxicillin Capsules
Betamethasone Dipropionate Cream, Lotion and Ointment
Beta-Val (Betamethasone Valerate) Cream, Lotion & Ointment
Carbamazepine Tablets
Cefazolin Sodium, Sterile
Cephalexin Capsules & Suspension
Chlorzoxazone Tablets
Clemastine Fumarate Tablets
Cotrim Tablets, D.S. Tablets and Pediatric Suspension
Desipramine HCl Tablets
Doxycycline Hyclate Capsules and Tablets
Epitol Tablets
Fluocinonide Gel, Ointment, Topical Solution and Cream (Emulsified Base)
Haloperidol Oral Solution
Ibuprofen Tablets
Indomethacin Extended Release Capsules
Loperamide HCl Capsules
Megestrol Acetate Tablets
Metronidazole Tablets
Myco-Triacet II (Nystatin and Triamcinolone Acetonide) Cream and Ointment
Neothylline (Dyphylline) Tablets
Neothylline GG (Dyphylline and Guaifenesin) Tablets
Nifedipine Capsules
Nystatin Cream, Oral Tablets and Oral Suspension
Otocort Sterile Ear Solution and Suspension
Perphenazine Tablets
Propacet-100 Tablets
Propoxyphene Compound 65 mg Capsules (CIV)
Propoxyphene HCl Capsules 65 mg (CIV)
Propoxyphene Napsylate and Acetaminophen Tablets
Propranolol HCl Extended Release Capsules
Statobex (Phendimetrazine Tartrate) Tablets
Sulfamethoxazole and Trimethoprim Tablets and Pediatric Suspension

(◆ Shown in Product Identification Section) *Italic Page Number* Indicates Brief Listing (▣ Described in PDR For Nonprescription Drugs)

Sulfanilamide Vaginal Cream
Sulindac Tablets
Theochron (Theophylline Anhydrous) (A trademark of Inwood Laboratories) Extended Release Tablets
Trazodone HCl Tablets
Triacet (Triamcinolone Acetonide) Cream

LIFESCAN INC. 2668
a Johnson & Johnson Company
1000 Gibraltar Drive
Milpitas, CA 95035-6312
For the name of your local representative, call toll-free
In the US: (800) 227-8862
In Canada: (800) 663-5521
Products Described
One Touch II Blood Glucose Monitoring System 2668

ELI LILLY AND COMPANY 416, 1279, 2668
For Medical Information, Write
Lilly Research Laboratories
Lilly Corporate Center
Indianapolis, IN 46285
(317) 276-3714
For Other Inquiries
Lilly Corporate Center
Indianapolis, IN 46285
(317) 276-2000

Lilly Regional Sales Offices
Atlanta, GA 30328
North Park Town Center
Bldg. 500, Suite 710
1100 Abernathy Road, NE
(404) 551-5360
Chicago, IL 60631
Suite 810, O'Hare Plaza
8725 West Higgins Road
(312) 693-8740
Dallas, TX 75248
15301 Dallas Parkway
Suite 960, Box 66
(214) 960-7637
Pasadena, CA 91101
811 Mutual Savings Building
301 East Colorado Blvd.
(818) 792-5121
Stamford, CT 06902
300 First Stamford Place
(203) 357-1422
Products Described
◆ Axid Pulvules 416, 1280
Brevital Sodium Vials 1282
Capastat Sulfate Vials 1283
◆ Ceclor Pulvules & Suspension 416, 1284
Colchicine Ampoules 1286
Crystodigin Tablets 1287
◆ Darvocet-N 50 Tablets 416, 1288
◆ Darvocet-N 100 Tablets 416, 1288
◆ Darvon Compound-65 Pulvules 416, 1290
◆ Darvon Pulvules 416, 1290
◆ Darvon-N Suspension & Tablets 416, 1288
Diethylstilbestrol Tablets 1291
Dobutrex Solution Vials 1293
Dolophine Hydrochloride Ampoules & Vials 1294
Dolophine Hydrochloride Tablets 1295
Ergotrate Maleate Ampoules 1297
Glucagon for Injection Vials and Emergency Kit 1297
Heparin Sodium Vials 1298
Humatrope Vials 1300
Humulin 50/50, 100 Units 1301
Humulin 70/30, 100 Units 1302
Humulin BR, 100 Units 1304
Humulin L, 100 Units 1304
Humulin N, 100 Units 1305
Humulin R, 100 Units 1307
Humulin U, 100 Units 1307
◆ Identi-Code 416
Identi-Dose *1279*
Iletin I 1308
Lente, 100 Units 1308
NPH, 100 Units 1308
Regular, 100 Units 1308
Semilente, 100 Units 1308
Ultralente, 100 Units 1308
Iletin II 1310
Beef Lente, 100 Units 1310
Beef NPH, 100 Units 1310
Beef Regular, 100 Units 1310
Pork Lente, 100 Units 1310
Pork NPH, 100 Units 1310
Pork Regular, 100 Units 1311
Pork Regular (Concentrated), 500 Units 1312
Kefurox Vials, Faspak & ADD-Vantage 1312
Kefzol Vials, Faspak & ADD-Vantage 1315
◆ Lorabid Suspension and Pulvules 416, 1317
Mandol Vials, Faspak & ADD-Vantage 1320
◆ Methadone Hydrochloride Diskets 416, 1322
Metubine Iodide Vials 1323
Nebcin Vials, Hyporets & ADD-Vantage 1324
Oncovin Solution Vials & Hyporets 1327
Papaverine Hydrochloride Vials and Ampoules 1328
◆ Permax Tablets 416, 1329
Phenobarbital Elixir and Tablets 1331
Protamine Sulfate Ampoules & Vials 1333
Reverse-numbered Package *1279*
Seconal Sodium Pulvules 1334
Seromycin Pulvules 1336
Tapazole Tablets 1337
Tazidime Vials, Faspak & ADD-Vantage 1338
Tes-Tape 2668
Vancocin HCl, Oral Solution & Pulvules 1342
Vancocin HCl, Vials & ADD-Vantage 1341
Velban Vials 1343
Other Products Available
Amytal Sodium Vials
Atropine Sulfate Vials
Aventyl HCl Liquid & Pulvules
Calcium Carbonate Tablets, Aromatic
Capsules, Empty Gelatin
Cevalin Ampoules
Cocaine Hydrochloride Solvets
Codeine Phosphate Soluble Tablets
Codeine Sulfate Tablets & Soluble Tablets
Cyanide Antidote Package
Deltalin Gelseals
Dymelor Tablets
Ephedrine Sulfate Ampoules
Keflin, Neutral, Vials, & ADD-Vantage
Morphine Sulfate Vials & Soluble Tablets
Opium (Deodorized) Tincture
Quinidine Gluconate Vials
Silver Nitrate Wax Ampoules
Sodium Bicarbonate Tablets
Sodium Chloride Vials & Tablets
Tubocurarine Chloride Vials
Tuinal Pulvules
V-Cillin K Oral Solution
Vitamin D, Gelseals

LOTUS BIOCHEMICAL CORPORATION 416, 1346
Kirk Building, Main Street
P. O. Box 126
Bland, VA 24315
Address inquiries to:
Jay Kirk
(703) 688-4711
FAX (703) 688-4178
For Medical Emergency Contact:
(800) 521-7468, Ext. 419
FAX (703) 688-3021
Products Described
◆ Adapin Capsules 416, 1346
Other Products Available
Proferdex Iron Dextran Injection USP

LUNSCO, INC. 1346
Route 2, Box 62
Pulaski, VA 24301
Address inquiries to:
(703) 980-4358
For Medical Emergencies Contact:
(703) 980-4358
Products Described
Dytuss *1346*
Fetrin Capsules *1346*
Hyco-Pap Capsules *1347*
Pacaps Capsules *1347*
Protid Tablets *1347*

MDR FITNESS CORPORATION 1347
Medical Doctors' Research
5207 NW 163rd Street
Miami, FL 33014
Address inquiries to:
(800) MDR-TABS
Products Described
MDR Fitness Tabs for Men and Women 1347

MGI PHARMA, INC. 1347
Suite 300-E, Opus Center
9900 Bren Road East
Minneapolis, MN 55343-9667
Address inquiries to:
Medical Affairs (800) 562-5580
FAX (612) 935-0468
For Medical Emergencies Contact:
Medical Affairs (800) 562-5580
FAX (612) 935-0468
Products Described
Didronel I.V. Infusion 1347
Oratect Gel 1348

3M PHARMACEUTICALS 416, 1349
275-3W-01 3M Center
St. Paul, MN 55144-1000
For Medical Information:
Write:
Medical Services Department
3M Pharmaceuticals
275-3W-01 3M Center
St. Paul, MN 55144-1000
Call (612) 736-4930
(Outside 612 Area) (800) 328-0255
For Medical Emergencies:
Call: (612) 736-4930 (all hours)
Customer Service and other services:
Call: (800) 423-5197
(Outside of CA) (800) 423-5146
(CA Residents) (818) 341-1300
Pharmacy Returns:
(800) 447-4537
Products Described
Alu-Cap Capsules 1349
Alu-Tab Tablets 1349
Calcium Disodium Versenate Injection 1349
◆ Disalcid Capsules 416, 1351
◆ Disalcid Tablets 416, 1351
Duo-Medihaler Aerosol *1352*
◆ Maxair Inhaler 416, 1352
Medihaler-Epi Aerosol *1353*
Medihaler-Iso Aerosol *1353*
◆ Minitran Transdermal Delivery System 416, 1353
◆ Norflex Injection 416, 1354
◆ Norflex Sustained-Release Tablets 416, 1354
◆ Norgesic Forte Tablets 416, 1355
◆ Norgesic Tablets 416, 1355
◆ Tambocor Tablets 416, 1355
Theolair Liquid 1358
◆ Theolair Tablets 416, 1358
◆ Theolair-SR Tablets 416, 1360
Urex Tablets 1362

MACSIL, INC. 1362
1326 Frankford Avenue
Philadelphia, PA 19125
(215) 739-7300
Products Described
Balmex Baby Powder ..... ▣
Balmex Emollient Lotion ..... ▣
Balmex Ointment ..... ▣

MARION MERRELL DOW INC. 416, 1362
9300 Ward Parkway
Mail: P.O. Box 8480
Kansas City, MO 64114-0480

MARION MERRELL DOW INC.
PRESCRIPTION PRODUCTS DIVISION
9300 Ward Parkway
Mail: P.O. Box 8480
Kansas City, MO 64114-0480

MARION MERRELL DOW INC.
CONSUMER PRODUCTS DIVISION
10123 Alliance Road
Mail: P.O. Box 429553
Cincinnati, OH 45242-9553
Address inquiries for products labeled with a (+) to:
Professional Information Department
Business hours only (9:00 AM to 4:30 PM EST)
(800) 552-3656
For medical emergency information after hours or on weekends only for products labeled with a (+):
(513) 948-9111
Address inquiries for products labeled with an (*) to:
Product Surveillance Department
P.O. Box 9627
Kansas City, MO 64134
(816) 966-5666
For medical emergency information after hours or on weekends only for products labeled with an (*):
(816) 966-5000
Products Described
AVC Cream (+) 1362
AVC Suppositories (+) 1362
◆ Bentyl 10 mg Capsules (+) 416, 1363
Bentyl Injection (+) 1363
Bentyl Syrup (+) 1363
◆ Bentyl 20 mg Tablets (+) 416, 1363
◆ Bricanyl Injection (+) 416, 1364
◆ Bricanyl Tablets (+) 416, 1365
◆ Cantil Tablets (+) 417, 1366
◆ Carafate Tablets (*) 416, 1367
◆ Cardizem CD Capsules-180 mg, 240 mg and 300 mg(*) 417, 1368
◆ Cardizem SR Capsules-60 mg, 90 mg and 120 mg (*) 417, 1372
◆ Cardizem Injectable (*) 416, 1370
◆ Cardizem Tablets-30 mg, 60 mg, 90 mg and 120 mg (*) 417, 1374
Cēpacol Anesthetic Lozenges (Troches) (+) ..... ▣
Cēpacol/Cēpacol Mouthwash/Gargle (+) ..... ▣
Cēpacol Throat Lozenges (+) ..... ▣
CĒPASTAT Cherry Flavor Sore Throat Lozenges (+) ..... ▣
CĒPASTAT Lozenges (+) ..... ▣
◆ Cephulac Syrup (+) 417, 1376
◆ Chronulac Syrup (+) 417, 1376
◆ Clomid Tablets (+) 417, *1377*
Debrox Drops (*) ..... ▣
Ditropan Syrup (*) 1377
◆ Ditropan Tablets (*) 417, 1377
Gaviscon Antacid Tablets (*) ..... ▣
Gaviscon Extra Strength Relief Formula Antacid Tablets (*) ..... ▣
Gaviscon Extra Strength Relief Formula Liquid Antacid (*) ..... ▣
Gaviscon Liquid Antacid (*) ..... ▣
Gly-Oxide Liquid (*) ..... ▣
◆ Hiprex Tablets (+) 417, 1378
◆ Lorelco Tablets (+) 417, 1378
◆ Nicoderm Nicotine Transdermal System(+) 417, 1380
◆ Nicorette (+) 417, 1384
Nitro-Bid IV (*) 1387
Nitro-Bid Ointment (*) 1388
◆ Norpramin Tablets (+) 417, 1389
◆ Novafed A Capsules (+) 417, 1390
◆ Novafed Capsules (+) 417, 1391
◆ Novahistine DH (+) 417, 1391
Novahistine DMX (+) ..... ▣
Novahistine Elixir (+) ..... ▣
◆ Novahistine Expectorant (+) .. 417, 1392
Os-Cal 250+D Tablets (*) ..... ▣
Os-Cal 500 Chewable Tablets (*) ..... ▣
Os-Cal 500 Tablets (*) ..... ▣
Os-Cal 500+D Tablets (*) ..... ▣
Os-Cal Fortified Tablets (*) ..... ▣
Os-Cal Plus Tablets (*) ..... ▣
◆ Pavabid Capsules (*) 417, 1392
◆ Quinamm Tablets (+) 417, 1393
◆ Rifadin Capsules (+) 417, 1394
Rifadin I.V. (+) 1394
◆ Rifamate Capsules (+) 417, 1396
◆ Seldane Tablets (+) 417, 1397
◆ Seldane-D Extended-Release Tablets 417, 1399
◆ Silvadene Cream 1% 417, 1400
Singlet Tablets (+) ..... ▣
◆ TACE 12 mg Capsules (+) 417, 1401
◆ TACE 25 mg Capsules (+) 417, 1401
◆ Tenuate Dospan Controlled-release Tablets (+) 417, 1403
◆ Tenuate Immediate-release Tablets (+) 417, 1403
Throat Discs Throat Lozenges (+) ..... ▣
Other Products Available
Accurbron
DV Cream
Metahydrin
Metatensin

MARLYN HEALTH CARE 1404
14851 North Scottsdale Road
Scottsdale, AZ 85254
(602) 991-0200
Address inquiries to:
Services Department
14851 North Scottsdale Road
Scottsdale, AZ 85254
Toll Free (800) 4- MARLYN
In AZ call (602) 991-0200
Products Described
Hep-Forte Capsules 1404
Marlyn Formula 50 Capsules 1404
Marlyn Formula 50 Mega Forte Capsules 1404
Pro-Hepatone Capsules 1405
Other Products Available
Daily Nutritional Paks
Care-4
Pro-Formance
Soft Stress
Liver Plus
Marlyn PMS
Marlyn Daily Multi Vitamin-Mineral Supplements
4-Beauty
4-Hair
4-Nails
Family Vita Health
Hi-Vita
Kiddy Bees (children vitamins)
Marbec Tablets
Osteo-Fem
Pro-Skin
Vitamin E 1000 IU
Wobenzyme

MASON PHARMACEUTICALS, INC. 417, 1405
4425 Jamboree
Newport Beach, CA 92660
(714) 851-6860
Products Described
◆ Damason-P 417, 1405
◆ DuoCet 417, *1406*

MAYRAND PHARMACEUTICALS, INC. 1407
P.O. Box 8869
4 Dundas Circle
Greensboro, NC 27419
(919) 292-5347
Products Described
Anatuss DM Syrup *1407*
Anatuss DM Tablets *1407*
Anatuss LA Tablets 1407
Antiox Capsules *1407*
Eldercaps *1407*
Eldertonic 1407
May-Vita Elixir 1407
Nu-Iron 150 Caps 1407
Nu-Iron V Tablets *1408*
Nu-Iron Elixir 1407
Nu-Iron Plus Elixir *1408*
Sedapap Tablets 50 mg/650 mg 1408

Bugs Bunny Complete Children's Chewable Vitamins + Minerals with Iron and Calcium (Sugar Free) ◘
Bugs Bunny With Extra C Children's Chewable Vitamins (Sugar Free) ◘
Bugs Bunny Plus Iron Children's Chewable Vitamins (Sugar Free) ◘
Domeboro Astringent Solution Effervescent Tablets ◘
Domeboro Astringent Solution Powder Packets ◘
Flintstones Children's Chewable Vitamins ◘
Flintstones Children's Chewable Vitamins With Extra C ◘
Flintstones Children's Chewable Vitamins Plus Iron ◘
Flintstones Complete With Calcium, Iron & Minerals Children's Chewable Vitamins ◘
Miles Nervine Nighttime Sleep-Aid ◘
Mycelex OTC Cream Antifungal **1630**
Mycelex OTC Solution Antifungal **1630**
Mycelex-7 Vaginal Cream and Inserts **1630**
One-A-Day Essential Vitamins with Beta Carotene ◘
One-A-Day Maximum Formula Vitamins and Minerals with Beta Carotene ◘
One-A-Day Plus Extra C Vitamins with Beta Carotene ◘
One-A-Day Stressgard Formula Vitamins ◘
One-A-Day Women's Formula Multivitamins with Calcium, Extra Iron, Zinc and Beta Carotene ◘

MILES INC. PHARMACEUTICAL DIVISION **420, 1631**
400 Morgan Lane
West Haven, CT 06516
Address Inquiries to:
Director, Medical Services
(800) 468-0894
(203) 937-2000
Products Described
◆ Adalat Capsules (10 mg and 20 mg) **420, 1631**
◆ Biltricide Tablets **420, 1633**
Cipro I.V. **1636**
Cipro I.V. Pharmacy Bulk Package **1639**
◆ Cipro Tablets **420, 1633**
DTIC-Dome **1641**
◆ Lithane Tablets **420, 1642**
Mezlin **1643**
Mezlin Pharmacy Bulk Package **1646**
Mithracin **1649**
◆ Mycelex Troches **420, 1650**
Mycelex-G 1% Vaginal Cream **1651**
◆ Mycelex-G 500 mg Vaginal Tablets **420, 1652**
◆ Niclocide Chewable Tablets **420, 1652**
◆ Nimotop Capsules **420, 1653**
Otic Domeboro Solution **1655**
Otic Tridesilon Solution 0.05% **1658**
◆ Stilphostrol Tablets and Ampuls **420, 1655**
Tridesilon Cream 0.05% **1656**
Tridesilon Ointment 0.05% **1657**
Other Products Available
Cort-Dome High Potency Suppositories
Cort-Dome ½%, and 1% Creme
Dome-Paste Bandage (Unna's Boot)
Mycelex Twin Pack

MILES INC., PHARMACEUTICAL DIVISION ALLERGY PRODUCTS **1658**
400 Morgan Lane
West Haven, CT 06516
Products Described
Ana-Kit Anaphylaxis Emergency Treatment Kit **1658**

MILES INC. PHARMACEUTICAL DIVISION Biological Products **420, 1660**
400 Morgan Lane
West Haven, CT 06516
Products Described
◆ Gamimune N Immune Globulin Intravenous (Human) **420, 1662**
Hyperab Rabies Immune Globulin (Human) **1663**
HyperHep Hepatitis B Immune Globulin (Human) **1665**
Hyper-Tet Tetanus Immune Globulin (Human) **1666**
HypRho-D Rh_o-D Immune Globulin (Human) **1668**
HypRho-D Mini-Dose Rh_o-D Immune Globulin (Human) **1667**
Koāte-HP Antihemophilic Factor (Human) **1669**
Konyne 80 Factor IX Complex **1660**
Plague Vaccine **1670**
Prolastin Alpha$_1$-Proteinase Inhibitor (Human) **1672**
Thrombate III Antithrombin III **1673**
Other Products Available
Plasbumin-5 Albumin (Human) 5%
Plasbumin-25 Albumin (Human) 25%
Plasmanate Plasma Protein Fraction (Human) 5%

MILEX PRODUCTS, INC. **1675**
5915 Northwest Highway
Chicago, IL 60631 (312) 631-6484
Shipping Offices
Milex Western
Post Office Box 46305
Los Angeles, CA 90046
(213) 651-4301

Milex Puerto Rico
GPO Box 554
San Juan, PR 00936
(809) 764-8602

Milex Hawaii
Box 6337
Honolulu, HI 96818
(808) 422-9581

Milex Southeastern
Post Office Drawer 4647
Clearwater, FL 34618
(813) 461-1949

Milex Southern
Post Office Drawer "M"
Weatherford, TX 76086
(817) 599-7604

Milex Carolinas
Post Office Box 23060
Charlotte, NC 28212
(704) 545-4567
Products Described
Amino-Cerv **1675**
Pro-Ception **1675**

MISSION PHARMACAL COMPANY **1675**
1325 E. Durango
San Antonio, TX 78210
Address inquiries to:
Professional Service Dept.
(512) 533-7118
Post Office Box 1676
San Antonio, TX 78296
Products Described
Calcet *1675*
Calcet Plus *1675*
Calcibind *1676*
Citracal *1675*
Citracal Caplets + D *1675*
Citracal Liquitab **1675**
Compete *1675*
Ferralet *1676*
Fosfree *1676*
Iromin-G *1676*
Lithostat *1676*
Medilax *1676*
Mission Prenatal *1676*
Mission Prenatal F.A. *1676*
Mission Prenatal H.P. *1676*
Mission Prenatal RX *1676*
Mission Surgical Supplement *1676*
Prulet *1676*
Supac *1676*
Therabid *1676*
Thera-Gesic **1676**
Thiola Tablets *1676*
Urocit-K *1676*

MURO PHARMACEUTICAL, INC. **1677**
890 East Street
Tewksbury, MA 01876-9987
Address inquiries to:
Professional Service Dept.
1-(800) 225-0974
(617) 851-5981
Products Described
Bromfed Capsules (Timed Release) **1677**
Bromfed Syrup ◘
Bromfed Tablets **1677**
Bromfed-DM Cough Syrup *1677*
Bromfed-PD Capsules (Timed Release) **1677**
Guaifed Capsules (Timed Release) **1677**
Guaifed-PD Capsules (Timed Release) **1677**
Guaifed Syrup ◘
Guaitab Tablets ◘
IoTuss Liquid *1678*
IoTuss-DM Liquid *1678*
Liquid Pred Syrup *1678*
Prelone Syrup *1678*
Salinex Nasal Mist and Drops ◘

MYLAN PHARMACEUTICALS INC. **1678**
781 Chestnut Ridge Road
P.O. Box 4310
Morgantown, WV 26505-4310
(304) 599-2595
Direct medical inquiries to:
Pharmacy Affairs Department
(800) 82-MYLAN
Direct orders to:
Sales Department (800) 82-MYLAN
Products Described
Albuterol Sulfate Tablets *1678*
Allopurinol Tablets *1678*
Amiloride Hydrochloride and Hydrochlorothiazide Tablets *1678*
Amitriptyline Hydrochloride Tablets *1678*
Amoxicillin Trihydrate Capsules & for Oral Suspension *1678*
Ampicillin Trihydrate Capsules & for Oral Suspension *1678*
Atenolol Tablets *1678*
Chlordiazepoxide & Amitriptyline Hydrochloride Tablets *1678*
Chlorothiazide Tablets *1678*
Chlorpropamide Tablets *1678*
Chlorthalidone Tablets *1678*
Clonidine Hydrochloride Tablets *1678*
Clonidine Hydrochloride & Chlorthalidone Tablets *1678*
Clorazepate Dipotassium Tablets *1678*
Cyclobenzaprine Hydrochloride Tablets *1678*
Cyproheptadine Hydrochloride Tablets *1678*
Diazepam Tablets *1678*
Diltiazem Hydrochloride Hydrochloride Tablets *1678*
Diphenoxylate Hydrochloride & Atropine Sulfate Tablets *1678*
Doxepin Hydrochloride Capsules *1678*
Doxycycline Hyclate Capsules & Tablets *1678*
Erythromycin Ethylsuccinate Tablets *1678*
Erythromycin Stearate Tablets *1678*
Fenoprofen Calcium Tablets *1678*
Fluphenazine Hydrochloride Tablets *1678*
Flurazepam Hydrochloride Capsules *1678*
Furosemide Tablets *1678*
Haloperidol Tablets *1678*
Ibuprofen Tablets *1678*
Indomethacin Capsules *1678*
Loperamide Hydrochloride Capsules *1678*
Lorazepam Tablets *1678*
Maprotiline Hydrochloride Tablets *1678*
Meclofenamate Sodium Capsules *1678*
Methotrexate Tablets *1678*
Methyclothiazide Tablets *1678*
Methyldopa Tablets *1678*
Methyldopa & Hydrochlorothiazide Tablets *1678*
Nitroglycerin Transdermal System Patches *1678*
Penicillin V Postassium Tablets *1678*
Perphenazine & Amitriptyline Hydrochloride Tablets *1678*
Prazosin Hydrochloride Capsules *1678*
Probenecid Tablets *1678*
Propoxyphene Hydrochloride & Acetaminophen Tablets *1678*
Propoxyphene Napsylate & Acetaminophen Tablets *1678*
Propranolol Hydrochloride Tablets *1678*
Propranolol Hydrochloride & Hydrochlorothiazide Tablets *1678*
Reserpine & Chlorothiazide Tablets *1678*
Spironolactone Tablets *1678*
Spironolactone & Hydrochlorothiazide Tablets *1678*
Temazepam Capsules *1678*
Tetracycline Hydrochloride Capsules *1678*
Thioridazine Hydrochloride Tablets *1678*
Thiothixene Capsules *1678*
Timolol Maleate Tablets *1678*
Tolazamide Tablets *1678*
Tolbutamide Tablets *1678*
Verapamil Tablets *1678*

NATURE'S BOUNTY, INC. **420, 1680**
90 Orville Drive
Bohemia, NY 11716
Address inquiries to:
Professional Services Dept.
(516) 567-9500
(800) 645-5412
FAX (516) 563-1623
Products Described
◆ Ener-B Vitamin B_{12} Nasal Gel Dietary Supplement **420, 1680**
Other Products Available
ABC to Z
Acidophilus
B-6 50 mg., 100 mg., 200 mg.
B-12 and B-12 Sublingual Tablets
B-50 Tablets
B-100 Tablets-Ultra B Complex
B-Complex + C (Long Acting) Tablets
Beta-Carotene Capsules
Bounty Bears (Children's Chewables)
C-500 mg., C-1000 mg., C-1500 mg. & Time Release Formulas
E-Oil
Garlic Oil 15 gr. & 77 gr.
KLB6 Capsules
Lecithin 1200 mg. Capsules
l-Lysine 500 mg. Tablets and 1000 mg. Tablets
M-KYA
Niacin 50 mg., 100 mg. and 250 mg.
Oat Bran 850 mg.
Oystercal 500 and Oystercal 500+D
Ultra Vita-Time Tablets
Vitamin A 10,000 I.U. & 25,000 I.U.
Vitamin E (Natural d-alpha tocopheryl)
Water Pill (Natural Diuretic)
Zinc 10 mg., 25 mg., 50 mg. Tablets

NEUTROGENA DERMATOLOGICS **420, 1680**
5760 West 96th Street
Los Angeles, CA 90045
Address inquiries to:
Mitchell S. Wortzman , Ph.D.
(310) 642-1150
FAX (310) 337-5530
For Medical Emergencies Contact:
Mitchell S. Wortzman, Ph.D.
(310) 642-1150
FAX (310) 337-5557
Products Described
Neutrogena Cleansing Wash ◘
◆ Neutrogena Melanex Topical Solution **421, 1680**
Neutrogena Moisture ◘
Neutrogena Moisture SPF 15 Untinted ◘
Neutrogena Moisture SPF 15 with Sheer Tint ◘
Neutrogena Norwegian Formula Emulsion ◘
Neutrogena Norwegian Formula Hand Cream ◘
Neutrogena Sunblock SPF 15 ◘
Neutrogena T/Derm Tar Emollient ◘
Neutrogena T/Gel Therapeutic Shampoo ◘
Neutrogena T/Sal Therapeutic Shampoo ◘
Other Products Available
Melanex Topical Solution, Neutrogena (see Neutrogena Melanex Topical Solution)
Neutrogena Acne Mask
Neutrogena Antiseptic
Neutrogena Cleansing Bar for Acne-prone Skin
Neutrogena Cleansing Bar for Dry Skin
Neutrogena Cleansing Bar for Dry Skin fragrance-free
Neutrogena Cleansing Bar for Oily Skin
Neutrogena Cleansing Bar Original Formula
Neutrogena Cleansing Bar Original Formula fragrance-free
Neutrogena Lip Moisturizer
Neutrogena Rainbath
Neutrogena Shampoo
Neutrogena Sunblock SPF 30
Neutrogena T/Gel Therapeutic Conditioner
Neutrogena Vehicle/N
Neutrogena Vehicle/N Mild

NICHÉ PHARMACEUTICALS, INC. **1680**
300 Trophy Club Drive
#400
Roanoke, TX 76262
Address inquiries to:
Steve F. Brandon (817) 491-2770
FAX (817) 491-3533
For Medical Emergency Contact:
Gerald L. Beckloff, M.D.
(817) 491-2770
FAX (817) 491-3533
Products Described
MagTab SR Caplets **1680**

NORDISK-USA
See NOVO NORDISK PHARMACEUTICALS INC.

NORTHAMPTON MEDICAL, INC. **1681**
3039 Amwiler Road, Suite 122
Atlanta, GA 30360
Address inquiries to:
Professional Services Department
(404) 416-8889
FAX (404) 416-0633
For Medical Emergency Contact:
Medical Department (404) 416-8889
FAX (404) 416-0633
Products Described
Femcet Capsules *1681*
Ferrocon Caplets *1681*
NutraVescent *1681*
PDRx .25 *1681*
Precare Caplets *1681*

NORWICH EATON PHARMACEUTICALS, INC.
See PROCTER & GAMBLE PHARMACEUTICALS, INC.

NOVO NORDISK PHARMACEUTICALS INC. **1681**
Suite 200
100 Overlook Center
Princeton, NJ 08540-7810
Address inquiries to:
Professional Services
(609) 987-5800

For Medical Emergencies Contact:
Professional Services
(609) 987-5800
Products Described
Insulatard NPH ... 1682
Insulatard NPH Human ... 1684
Lente Insulin ... 1681
Lente Purified Pork Insulin ... 1682
Mixtard 70/30 ... 1682
Mixtard Human 70/30 ... 1684
NPH Insulin ... 1681
NPH Purified Pork Isophane Insulin ... 1682
Novolin L ... 1683
Novolin N ... 1684
Novolin N PenFill Cartridges ... 1685
Novolin 70/30 ... 1682
Novolin 70/30 PenFill Cartridges ... 1685
Novolin 70/30 Prefilled ... 1685
Novolin R ... 1684
Novolin R PenFill Cartridges ... 1684
NovoPen (Insulin Delivery Device) ... 1686
PenNeedle Disposable Needle ... 1686
Regular Insulin ... 1681
Regular Purified Pork Insulin ... 1682
Semilente Insulin ... 1681
Ultralente Insulin ... 1681
Velosulin ... 1682
Velosulin Human ... 1684

NOVOPHARM, INC. **1686**
165 East Commerce Drive
Suites 100-101-200
Schaumburg, IL 60173-5326
Address inquiries to:
Robert J. Gunter, President
(800) 635-5067
FAX (708) 882-4232
Products Described
Amoxicillin Capsules USP and Oral Suspension ... *1686*
Cephalexin Capsules USP and Oral Suspension ... *1686*
Clofibrate Capsules USP ... *1686*
Indomethacin Capsules ... *1686*
Loperamide Hydrochloride Capsules USP ... *1686*
Methyldopa Tablets USP ... *1686*
Methyldopa and Hydrochlorothiazide Tablets USP ... *1686*
Nifedipine Capsules USP ... *1686*
Tolmetin Sodium Capsules USP ... *1686*

NUTRIPHARM LABORATORIES, INC. **1686**
8 Bartles Corner Road, Suite 101
Flemington, NJ 08822
Address inquiries to:
S. Rao Kolli, Ph.D. (908) 806-8954
FAX (908) 806-8934
For Medical Emergencies Contact:
S. Rao Kolli, Ph.D. (908) 806-8954
FAX: (908) 806-8934
Products Described
Isocom Capsules ... 1686
Other Products Available
Aclophen Long Acting Tablets
Carbiset Tablets
Carbiset-TR Tablets
Klerist-D Capsules (Long-Acting)
Klerist-D Tablets
Tricom Caplets

OCLASSEN PHARMACEUTICALS, INC. **420, 1687**
100 Pelican Way
San Rafael, CA 94901
Address inquiries to:
Marketing Department
(800) 288-4508
For Medical Emergencies Contact:
Director, Clinical Operations
(800) 288-4508
Products Described
◆ Condylox ... 420, 1687
◆ Monodox Capsules ... 420, 1688

ORGANON INC. **420, 1689**
375 Mount Pleasant Ave.
West Orange, NJ 07052
(201) 325-4500
Products Described
Arduan ... *1689*
BCG Vaccine, USP (Tice) ... 1689
◆ Calderol Capsules ... 420, *1692*
Cortrosyn ... *1692*
◆ Cotazym ... 420, 1692
◆ Cotazym-S ... 420, *1693*
Deca-Durabolin ... *1693*
Durabolin ... *1693*
Hexadrol Elixir ... *1693*
Hexadrol Phosphate Injection ... *1693*
◆ Hexadrol Tablets ... 420, *1693*
Hydrocortisone USP ... *1693*
◆ Jenest-28 Tablets ... 421, 1693
Liquaemin Sodium ... *1698*
Norcuron ... 1698
Pavulon ... *1700*
Pregnyl ... 1700
Regonol ... *1701*
Reversol ... *1701*
Succinylcholine Chloride ... *1701*
Tice BCG, USP ... 1689

◆ Wigraine Tablets & Suppositories ... 421, 1701
◆ Zymase Capsules ... 421, 1702

ORTHO BIOTECH (Distributor) **421, 1702**
P.O. Box 300
Raritan, NJ 08869-0602
Products Described
Orthoclone OKT3 Sterile Solution ... 1702
◆ Procrit for Injection ... 421, 1703

ORTHO DIAGNOSTIC SYSTEMS INC. **1707**
Route 202
Raritan, NJ 08869
Address inquiries to:
Customer Service Division
(800) 322-6374
Products Described
MICRhoGAM $Rh_o(D)$ Immune Globulin (Human) ... 1707
RhoGAM $Rh_o(D)$ Immune Globulin (Human) ... 1707

ORTHO PHARMACEUTICAL CORPORATION **421, 1708**
Route 202, P. O. Box 300
Raritan, NJ 08869-0602
For medical inquiries contact:
(800) 682-6532
For Medical Emergency Contact:
(908) 218-7325
Products Described
Aci-Jel Therapeutic Vaginal Jelly ... 1708
◆ All-Flex Arcing Spring Diaphragm (See Ortho Diaphragm Kit) ... 421, 1719
Conceptrol Contraceptive Gel, Single Use Applicators ... ▣
Conceptrol Contraceptive Inserts ... ▣
Delfen Contraceptive Foam ... ▣
◆ Floxin I.V. ... 421, 1708
◆ Floxin Tablets ... 421, 1712
Gynol II Extra Strength Contraceptive Jelly ... ▣
Gynol II Original Formula Contraceptive Jelly ... ▣
Lippes Loop Intrauterine Double-S ... 1715
Lutrepulse for Injection ... 1716
◆ Micronor Tablets ... 421, 1723
◆ Modicon 21 Tablets ... 421, 1723
Modicon 28 Tablets ... 1723
◆ Monistat Dual-Pak ... 421, 1718
◆ Monistat 3 Vaginal Suppositories ... 421, 1718
◆ Ortho Diaphragm Kit/All-Flex Arcing Spring ... 421
Ortho Diaphragm Kit-Coil Spring ... 1719
Ortho Dienestrol Cream ... 1720
Ortho-Gynol Contraceptive Jelly ... ▣
◆ Ortho-Novum 1/35□21 Tablets ... 421, 1723
Ortho-Novum 1/35□28 Tablets ... 1723
◆ Ortho-Novum 1/50□21 Tablets ... 421, 1723
Ortho-Novum 1/50□28 Tablets ... 1723
◆ Ortho-Novum 7/7/7 □21 Tablets ... 421, 1723
Ortho-Novum 7/7/7 □28 Tablets ... 1723
◆ Ortho-Novum 10/11□21 Tablets ... 421, 1723
Ortho-Novum 10/11□28 Tablets ... 1723
Ortho-White Diaphragm Kit-Flat Spring ... 1719
◆ Protostat Tablets ... 421, 1730
Sultrin Triple Sulfa Cream ... 1731
Sultrin Triple Sulfa Vaginal Tablets ... 1731
◆ Terazol 3 Vaginal Cream ... 421, 1732
◆ Terazol 3 Vaginal Suppositories ... 421, 1733
◆ Terazol 7 Vaginal Cream ... 421, 1733

ORTHO PHARMACEUTICAL CORPORATION, DERMATOLOGICAL DIVISION **421, 1734**
Route 202, P.O. Box 300
Raritan, NJ 08869-0602
(908) 218-6000
Address inquiries to:
Dermatological Medical Information
(800) 426-7762
Medical Information (800) 682-6532
Products Described
◆ Erycette (erythromycin 2%) Topical Solution ... 421, 1734
◆ Grifulvin V (griseofulvin microsize tablets), (griseofulvin oral suspension) ... 421, 1734
◆ Meclan (meclocycline sulfosalicylate) Cream ... 421, 1735
◆ Monistat-Derm (miconazole nitrate) Cream ... 421, 1735
◆ Persa-Gel (benzoyl peroxide) .. 421, 1736
◆ Persa-Gel W (benzoyl peroxide) ... 421, 1736
◆ Retin-A (tretinoin) Cream/Gel/Liquid ... 421, 1736
◆ Spectazole (econazole nitrate) Cream ... 421, 1737

PADDOCK LABORATORIES, INC. **1737**
3101 Louisiana Avenue North
Minneapolis, MN 55427
(800) 328-5113
Address inquiries to:
Medical Department
Products Described
Actidose with Sorbitol ... *1737*
Actidose-Aqua ... *1737*
Erythra-Derm (formerly ETS-2%) ... *1737*
Glutose (Oral Glucose Gel) ... *1737*
Glutose Tablets ... *1737*
Nystatin, USP for Extemporaneous Preparation of Oral Suspension ... 1737
Other Products Available
Acetaminophen Tablets 325 mg
Albuterol Sulfate, USP
Aluminium Paste
5-Aminosalicylic Acid Powder
Aquabase
Ascorbic Acid Tablets 500 mg
Aspirin Suppositories 125 mg, 300 mg, 600 mg
Aspirin Tablets 325 mg
Aspirin Tablets, Enteric-Coated 325 mg, 650 mg
Bacitracin Powder, USP
Benzoin Compound Tincture, USP
Betamethasone Valerate Powder, USP
Bisacodyl Suppositories 10 mg
Bisacodyl Tablets 5 mg
Castor Oil, USP
Clindamycin Phosphate Powder, USP
Colistin Sulfate Powder, USP
Dermabase
Dexamethasone Acetate Powder USP
Dexamethasone Sodium Phosphate Powder, USP, Micronized
Docusate Calcium Capsules 240 mg
Docusate Sodium Capsules 100 mg, 250 mg
Docusate Sodium Capsules w/Casanthranol Capsules 100 mg/30 mg
Emulsoil (Self-Emulsifying Castor Oil)
Erythromycin Powder, USP
Fattibase
Ferrous Gluconate Tablets
Ferrous Sulfate Tablets
Folic Acid Tablets
Gentamicin Sulfate Powder, USP
Glutol
Green Soap Tincture, USP
Hydrocortisone Acetate Powder, USP
Hydrocortisone Acetate Suppositories 25 mg
Hydrocortisone Powder, USP
Hydrocream Base
Ipecac Syrup, USP
Liqua-Gel
Liquaderm-A
Methyltestosterone Powder, USP
Milk of Magnesia, USP
Morphine Sulfate Suppositories 5 mg, 10 mg, 20 mg, 30 mg
Neomycin Sulfate Powder, USP
Nystatin Powder, USP
Ora-Plus
Ora-Sweet
Ora-Sweet SF
Podocon-25
Podophyllum Resin, USP
Polybase
Polymyxin B Sulfate Powder, USP
Prednisolone Acetate Powder, USP
Prednisone Powder, USP
Progesterone Injectable, USP
Progesterone Powder, USP, Micronized
Progesterone Powder, USP, Wettable, Microcrystalline
Retinoic Acid, USP
Schamberg Lotion
Sebacide
Sorbitol Solution, 70%
Suspendol-S
Testosterone Crystalline Injectable
Testosterone Powder, USP
Testosterone Propionate Injectable
Testosterone Propionate Powder, USP
Triamcinolone Acetonide Powder, USP
Trimethobenzamide Suppositories 100 mg, 200 mg
Vehicle-A (See Liquaderm-A)
Vehicle-S (See Suspendol-S)
Zincate Capsules 220 mg

PALISADES PHARMACEUTICALS, INC. **422, 1738**
219 County Road
Tenafly, NJ 07670
Address inquiries to:
President (201) 569-8502
(800) 237-9083
For Medical Emergencies Contact:
President (201) 569-8502
(800) 237-9083
Products Described
PALS Internal Deodorant ... *1738*
Pod-Ben-25 ... *1738*
◆ Scleromate ... 422, 1738
Verr-Canth ... *1738*
◆ Yocon ... 422, 1739

PAR PHARMACEUTICAL, INC. **1739**
One Ram Ridge Road
Spring Valley, NY 10977
Address inquiries to:
Customer Services
Toll Free (800) 828-9393
In NY (914) 425-7100
Products Described
Allopurinol Tablets ... *1739*
Amiloride HCl Tablets ... *1739*
Amiloride HCl and Hydrochlorothiazide Tablets ... *1739*
Amitriptyline Hydrochloride Tablets ... *1739*
Benztropine Mesylate Tablets ... *1739*
Carisoprodol and Aspirin Tablets ... *1739*
Chlordiazepoxide and Amitriptyline HCl Tablets ... *1739*
Chlorpropamide Tablets ... *1739*
Chlorzoxazone Tablets ... *1739*
Clonidine HCl and Chlorthalidone Tablets ... *1739*
Clonidine HCl Tablets ... *1739*
Cyproheptadine HCl Tablets ... *1739*
Dexamethasone Tablets ... *1739*
Diazepam Tablets ... *1739*
Disulfiram Tablets ... *1739*
Doxepin HCl Capsules ... *1739*
Doxycycline Hyclate Capsules ... *1739*
Fenoprofen Calcium Capsules & Tablets ... *1739*
Fluphenazine HCl Tablets ... *1739*
Flurazepam HCl Capsules ... *1739*
Haloperidol Tablets ... *1739*
Hydralazine HCl Tablets ... *1739*
Hydra-Zide (Hydralazine HCl and Hydrochlorothiazide) Capsules ... *1739*
Hydroflumethiazide Tablets ... *1739*
Hydroxyzine HCl Tablets ... *1739*
Ibuprofen Tablets ... *1739*
Imipramine HCl Tablets ... *1739*
Indomethacin Capsules ... *1739*
Isosorbide Dinitrate Tablets ... *1739*
Lorazepam Tablets ... *1739*
Meclizine HCl Tablets ... *1739*
Megestrol Acetate Tablets ... *1739*
Metaproterenol Sulfate Inhalation Solution ... *1739*
Metaproterenol Sulfate Tablets ... *1739*
Methocarbamol and Aspirin Tablets ... *1739*
Methocarbomol Tablets ... *1739*
Methyclothiazide Tablets ... *1739*
Methyldopa and Chlorothiazide Tablets ... *1739*
Methyldopa and Hydrochlorothiazide Tablets ... *1739*
Methyldopa Tablets ... *1739*
Methylprednisolone Tablets ... *1739*
Metoclopramide Tablets ... *1739*
Metronidazole Compressed Tablets ... *1739*
Metronidazole Film Coated Tablets ... *1739*
Minoxidil Tablets ... *1739*
Nystatin Tablets ... *1739*
Par-Glycerol Elixir ... *1739*
Par-Glycerol-DM Liquid ... *1739*
Par-Glycerol-C (C-V) Liquid ... *1739*
Perphenazine and Amitriptyline Tablets ... *1739*
Propantheline Bromide Tablets ... *1739*
Propranolol HCl Tablets ... *1739*
Reserpine and Hydroflumethiazide Tablets ... *1739*
Salsalate Tablets ... *1739*
Silver Sulfadiazine Cream ... *1739*
Sulfinpyrazone Capsules & Tablets ... *1739*
Temazepam Capsules ... *1739*
Thioridazine HCl Tablets ... *1739*
Tolazamide Tablets ... *1739*
Trichlormethiazide Tablets ... *1739*
Valproic Acid Capsules ... *1739*

PARKE-DAVIS **422, 1740, 2668**
Division of Warner-Lambert Company
201 Tabor Rd
Morris Plains, NJ
(201) 540-2000
During working hours:
Product Medical Information
(800) 223-0432
FAX (201) 540-2248
After hours or on weekends:
(201) 540-2000 540-6089
Regional Sales Offices
Atlanta, GA 30328
5901 Peachtree Dunwoody Road
(404) 396-4080
Baltimore (Cockeysville), MD 21030
311 International Circle
(410) 584-7810
Chicago (Schaumburg), IL. 60173
1750 East Golf Road
(708) 240-1740
Cincinnati, OH 45242
4445 Lake Forest Drive
(513) 563-6658

(◆ Shown in Product Identification Section) *Italic Page Number* Indicates Brief Listing **(▣ Described in PDR For Nonprescription Drugs)**

Betadine Shampoo
Betadine Skin Cleanser Foam
Betadine Solution Swab Aid
Betadine Solution Swabsticks
Betadine Surgi-Prep Sponge-Brush
Betadine Viscous Formula Antiseptic Gauze Pad
Betadine Whirlpool Concentrate
Phyllocontin
Senokot Suppositories
Senokot Tablets Unit Strip Pack

R&D LABORATORIES, INC. **1895**
4204 Glencoe Avenue
Marina del Rey, CA 90292
Address inquiries to:
Rhoda Makoff, PhD
(310) 305-8053
For Medical Emergencies Contact:
Dwight Makoff, M.D.
(310) 652-9162
Products Described
Calci-Chew Tablets **1895**
Calci-Mix Capsules **1895**
Nephro-Calci Tablets **1895**
Nephro-Derm Cream *1895*
Nephro-Fer Tablets **1895**
Nephro-Fer Rx **1895**
Nephro-Vite Tablets *1895*
Nephro-Vite Rx **1895**
Other Products Available
d-Biotin
L-Carnitine

RECKITT & COLMAN PHARMACEUTICALS, INC. **424, 1895**
1901 Huguenot Road
Richmond, VA 23235
Address inquiries to:
Professional Services
(804) 379-1090
FAX (804) 379-1215
For Medical Emergency Contact:
Medical Department
(804) 379-1090
FAX (804) 379-1215
Branch Offices
Distribution Center
3 Boulden Circle
New Castle, DE 19720
(302) 328-4578
FAX (302) 323-3222
Products Described
◆ Buprenex Injectable **424, 1895**

REED & CARNRICK **424, 1897**
Division of Block Drug Company, Inc.
257 Cornelison Avenue
Jersey City, NJ 07302-9988
Address inquiries to:
R & C Professional Services
(201) 434-4000, Ext. 1821
FAX (201) 434-3032
For Medical Emergency Contact
R & C Professional Services
(201) 434-4000, Ext. 1821
FAX (201) 434-3032
Products Described
◆ Colyte and Colyte Flavored **424, 1897**
◆ Cortifoam **424, 1897**
◆ Dilatrate-SR **424, 1898**
◆ Epifoam **424, 1899**
◆ Kwell Cream **424, 1900**
◆ Kwell Lotion **424, 1901**
◆ Kwell Shampoo **424, 1902**
◆ Levatol **424, 1903**
Phazyme Drops .... ◘
Phazyme-125 Softgels Maximum Strength .... ◘
Phazyme Tablets .... ◘
Phazyme-95 Tablets .... ◘
◆ ProctoCream-HC **424, 1905**
◆ Proctofoam-HC **424, 1906**
ProctoFoam-NS (Non-Steroid) .... ◘
R&C Lice Treatment Kit .... ◘
R&C Shampoo .... ◘
R & C Spray .... ◘
Other Products Available
Ethamolin (ethanolamine oleate) Injection 5%
Proxigel
Trichotine Liquid, Vaginal Douche
Trichotine Powder, Vaginal Douche

REGENCY MEDICAL RESEARCH, LTD. **1906**
2401 South 24th Street
Phoenix, AZ 85034
Address inquiries to:
Marketing Director
(602) 244-8899
Products Described
Medi-Mist Intra-Oral Spray Dietary Supplements **1906**
Medi-Mist Intra-Oral Spray Dietary Supplements **1906**
Multiple
Nico-free
Nutra-Lean
Stress
Vitamin A
Vitamin B-12
Vitamin C, E+ Zinc
Other Products Available
Medi-Mist Spray Supplements
Aerobic
Anti-cholesterol
Anti-oxidant
Circuflex
Menopausal
Pre-natal

REID-ROWELL
See SOLVAY PHARMACEUTICALS.

RESEARCH INDUSTRIES CORPORATION **1907**
Pharmaceutical Division
6864 South 300 West
Midvale, UT 84047
Address inquiries to:
R. D. Hibbert (801) 562-0200
FAX (801) 562-1122
For Medical Emergencies Contact:
R. D. Hibbert (801) 562-0200
FAX (801) 562-1122
Products Described
Rimso-50 .... **1907**

REXAR PHARMACAL CORPORATION **424, 1907**
396 Rockaway Avenue
Valley Stream, NY 11581
Products Described
◆ Dextroamphetamine Sulfate Tablets **424,** *1907*
◆ Obetrol Tablets **424,** *1907*
Oby-Trim Capsules *1907*
Rexatal Tablets *1907*
X-Trozine Capsules and Tablets *1907*
X-Trozine L.A. Capsules *1907*

RHÔNE-POULENC RORER PHARMACEUTICALS INC. **424, 1908**
500 Arcola Road
Collegeville, PA 19426-2911
(215) 454-8000
For Medical Emergencies/ Product Information Contact:
Medical Affairs
Weekdays 8:15 a.m. to 4:45 p.m.
Eastern Time (215) 454-8110
(215) 454-8000
Other times: (919) 967-8090
For Reports of Adverse Drug Experience Contact:
Drug Product Safety
Weekdays 8:15 a.m. to 4:45 p.m.
Eastern Time (215) 454-8110
Other times: (919) 967-8090
For Quality Assurance Questions Contact:
John Chiles
Technical Complaint Coordinator
(215) 454-3129
For Regulatory Affairs Questions Contact:
Margaret Masters
Associate Director, Regulatory Control
(215) 454-3881
Ron Panner
Director, Regulatory Affairs
(215) 454-3026
Products Described
Acthar *1908*
◆ Azmacort Oral Inhaler **424, 1908**
Barotrast *1908*
◆ Calcimar Injection, Synthetic **424, 1910**
Calel-D *1908*
Clysodrast *1908*
◆ DDAVP Injection **424, 1911**
◆ DDAVP Nasal Spray **424, 1912**
◆ DDAVP Rhinal Tube **424, 1912**
◆ Demi-Regroton Tablets **425,** *1908*
Dialume Capsules *1908*
◆ Dilacor XR Extended-release Capsules **424, 1914**
Esophotrast Cream *1908*
HP Acthar Gel *1908*
◆ Hygroton Tablets **424,** *1908*
◆ Lozol Tablets **424, 1916**
◆ Nasacort Nasal Inhaler **425, 1917**
Nicobid **1919**
Nicolar Tablets **1919**
◆ Nitrolingual Spray **425, 1920**
Oratrast *1908*
Parathar *1908*
Parepectolin Suspension *1908*
◆ Penetrex Tablets **425, 1921**
◆ Regroton Tablets **425,** *1908*
◆ Slo-bid Gyrocaps **425, 1923**
Slo-Phyllin GG Capsules *1908*
Slo-Phyllin GG Syrup *1908*
◆ Slo-Phyllin Gyrocaps **425,** *1908*
Slo-Phyllin 80 Syrup *1908*
◆ Slo-Phyllin Tablets **425,** *1908*
Thyrar Tablets *1908*
Thytropar *1908*
Tussar-2 .... *1908*
Tussar DM *1908*
Tussar SF *1908*

RHÔNE-POULENC RORER PHARMACEUTICALS INC. **1926**
CONSUMER PHARMACEUTICAL PRODUCTS
a division of Rhone-Poulenc Rorer
Former Address: 500 Virginia Drive
Fort Washington, PA 19034
New Address: 500 Arcola Road
Collegeville, PA 19426-2911
(215) 454-8000
For Medical Emergencies/ Product Information Contact:
Drug Product Safety
And Product Information
(215) 454-8870
For Regulatory Affairs Questions Contact:
Margaret Masters
Associate Director,
Regulatory Affairs
(215) 454-3881
Products Described
Ascriptin A/D Caplets **1926**
Regular Strength Ascriptin Tablets **1926**
Maalox Suspension and Tablets .... ◘
Maalox HRF Suspension Antacid **1926**
Maalox Plus Tablets **1926**
Extra Strength Maalox Plus Suspension/Tablets **1927**
Maalox TC Suspension Antacid **1928**
Extra Strength Maalox Plus Tablets **1927**
Perdiem Fiber Granules **1928**
Perdiem Granules **1928**

RICHARDSON-VICKS INC **1929**
A Procter & Gamble Company
P.O. Box 5516
Cincinnati, OH 45201
(Also see Procter & Gamble and Procter & Gamble Pharmaceuticals, Inc.)
Address inquiries to:
Arnold P. Austin (800) 358-8707
For medical emergencies and to report adverse reactions:
Call collect (513) 751-2823
Products Described
Children's Chloraseptic Lozenges .... ◘
Children's Chloraseptic Spray .... ◘
Chloraseptic Liquid, Cherry, Menthol or Cool Mint .... ◘
Chloraseptic Lozenges, Cherry, Cool Mint or Menthol .... ◘
Oil of Olay Daily UV Protectant SPF 15 Beauty Fluid-Regular & Fragrance Free (Olay Co. Inc.) .... ◘
Oil of Olay Daily UV Protectant SPF 15 Moisture Replenishing Cream-Regular & Fragrance Free (Olay Co. Inc.) .... ◘
Oil of Olay Foaming Face Wash (Olay Co. Inc.) .... ◘
Percogesic Analgesic Tablets .... ◘
Vicks Children's Cough Syrup .... ◘
Vicks Children's NyQuil Nighttime Cold/Cough Medicine .... ◘
Vicks Children's NyQuil Nighttime Head Cold & Allergy Medicine .... ◘
Vicks Cough Silencers .... ◘
Extra Strength Vicks Cough Drops .... ◘
Vicks DayQuil .... ◘
Vicks DayQuil LiquiCaps .... ◘
Vicks Formula 44 Cough Control Discs .... ◘
Vicks Formula 44 Cough Medicine .... ◘
Vicks Formula 44D Cough & Decongestant Cough Medicine .... ◘
Vicks Formula 44E Cough & Expectorant Medicine .... ◘
Vicks Formula 44M Multi-Symptom Cough & Cold Medicine .... ◘
Vicks Inhaler .... ◘
Vicks NyQuil LiquiCaps Nighttime Cold/Flu Medicine .... ◘
Vicks NyQuil Nighttime Cold/Flu Medicine-Regular & Cherry Flavor .... ◘
Vicks Pediatric Formula 44 Cough Medicine .... ◘
Vicks Pediatric Formula 44d Cough & Decongestant Medicine .... ◘
Vicks Pediatric Formula 44e Cough & Expectorant Medicine .... ◘
Vicks Pediatric Formula 44m Multi-Symptom Cough & Cold Medicine .... ◘
Vicks Sinex Decongestant Nasal Spray .... ◘
Vicks Sinex Long-Acting Decongestant Nasal Spray .... ◘
Vicks Vaporub .... ◘
Vicks Vaposteam .... ◘
Vicks Vatronol Nose Drops .... ◘

RICHWOOD PHARMACEUTICAL COMPANY, INC. **1930**
7902 Tanner's Gate Drive
P.O. Box 6497
Florence, KY 41022
Address inquiries to:
(606) 282-2100
FAX (606) 282-2103
Products Described
Acuprin Adult Low Dose Aspirin *1930*
Anema Trinsic Hematinic Concentrate Capsules **1930**
HydroStat *1930*
MS/S Suppositories **1930**
Verin Constant Release Rate Aspirin *1930*

RIKER LABORATORIES, INC.
See 3M PHARMACEUTICALS

ROBERTS PHARMACEUTICAL CORPORATION **425, 1930**
Meridian Center III
6G Industrial Way West
Eatontown, NJ 07724 U.S.A.
Address inquiries to:
Customer Service (908) 389-1182
(800) 828-2088
FAX: (908) 389-1014
TLX: (910) 250-1110
For Medical Inquiries Contact:
(800) 992-9306
Somogard/Anagrelide Inquiries:
(800) 752-4255
Products Described
Cevi-Fer Capsules (sustained release) **1930**
◆ Cheracol Cough Syrup **425, 1931**
Cheracol-D Cough Formula .... ◘
Cheracol Nasal Spray Pump .... ◘
Cheracol Plus Cough/Cold .... ◘
Cheracol Sore Throat Spray .... ◘
Chlorafed H.S. Timecelles **1931**
Chlorafed Liquid *1931*
Chlorafed Timecelles **1931**
Citrocarbonate Antacid .... ◘
Clocream Skin Cream .... ◘
◆ Dopar Capsules **425, 1932**
◆ Duvoid Tablets **425, 1932**
Entuss Expectorant **1933**
Entuss Tablets **1933**
Entuss-D Jr. Liquid *1934*
Entuss-D Liquid *1934*
Entuss-D Tablets *1934*
◆ Furacin Soluble Dressing **425, 1934**
Furacin Topical Cream **1934**
Furacin Topical Solution 0.2% **1935**
◆ Furoxone Liquid **425, 1935**
◆ Furoxone Tablets **425, 1935**
Haltran Tablets .... ◘
Kasof Capsules .... ◘
Orthoxicol Cough/Cold Syrup .... ◘
P-A-C (Revised Formula) Analgesic Tablets .... ◘
Pyrroxate Capsules & Tablets .... ◘
Romycin Topical Solution **1936**
Sigtab Tablets .... ◘
Sinufed Timecelles **1937**
Sinumist-SR Capsulets *1937*
Supprelin Injection **1937**
◆ Topicycline for Topical Solution **425, 1938**
Zymacap Capsules .... ◘
Other Products Available
Alkets Tablets
Calcium Lactate Tablets, USP
Cheracol Sinus 12-hour Tablets
Cheracol Sore Throat Discs
Clocort Cream
Clomycin Antibiotic Ointment
D-Vert Capsules
Diostate D Tablets
Dolacet Capsules
Gastrosed Drops
Gastrosed Tablets
Histor-D Timecelles
Lipomul Oral Liquid
Niacels Capsules
Orexin Tablets
Probec-T Tablets
Super D Perles
Tencet Capsules

A. H. ROBINS COMPANY, INC. **425, 1939**
P.O. Box 26609
Richmond, VA 23261-6609
Telephone (804) 257-2000
For Medical Emergency Information day or night call:
(215) 688-4400
Products Described
Dimetane-DC Cough Syrup **1939**
Dimetane-DX Cough Syrup **1940**
◆ Donnatal Capsules **425, 1940**
Donnatal Elixir **1940**
◆ Donnatal Extentabs **425, 1941**
◆ Donnatal Tablets **425, 1940**
◆ Donnazyme Tablets **425, 1941**
◆ Dopram Injectable **425, 1942**
◆ Entozyme Tablets **425, 1943**
◆ Exna Tablets **425, 1944**
◆ Micro-K Extencaps **425, 1944**
◆ Micro-K 10 Extencaps **425, 1944**
Micro-K LS Packets **1946**
◆ Phenaphen Caplets **425**
◆ Phenaphen with Codeine Capsules **425, 1947**
◆ Phenaphen-650 with Codeine Tablets **425, 1948**
◆ Pondimin Tablets **425, 1949**
◆ Quinidex Extentabs **425, 1950**
◆ Reglan Injectable **425, 1951**
Reglan Syrup **1951**
◆ Reglan Tablets **425, 1951**
◆ Robaxin Injectable **425, 1953**
◆ Robaxin Tablets **425, 1954**
◆ Robaxin-750 Tablets **425, 1954**
◆ Robaxisal Tablets **425, 1954**

(◆ Shown in Product Identification Section) *Italic Page Number* Indicates Brief Listing (◘ Described in PDR For Nonprescription Drugs)

A. H. ROBINS CONSUMER 1959
PRODUCTS DIVISION
1405 Cummings Drive
Richmond, VA 23230
Address inquiries to:
Consumer Affairs Department
1405 Cummings Drive
Richmond, VA 23230
(804) 257-2790
For Medical Emergencies Contact:
Consumer Affairs Department
Day (804) 257-2790
Evening (804) 257-2000
Products Described

E. C. ROBINS COMPANY, INC. 1959
E. C. Robins/William P. Poythress
3911 Deep Rock Road, P.O. Box
71600
Richmond, VA 23255
Address inquiries to:
Professional Services Department
(804) 527-1950
FAX (804) 527-1959
For Medical Emergency Contact:
Professional Services Department
(804) 527-1950
FAX (804) 527-1959
Products Described

ROCHE DERMATOLOGICS 425, 1960
a division of Hoffmann-La Roche Inc.
Nutley, NJ 07110
**For Medical Information or
To Report Adverse Events**
Write: Professional Services/
 Dermatology Division or
Call: (800) 526-6367 (Teleprompt 2,3)
 or (201) 812-2000
 (8:30 AM to 5:00 PM EST)

For Medical Emergencies
(24-hour service)
Call: (800) 526-6367 (Teleprompt 1)
Other Operating Units
See: Hoffmann-La Roche Inc.
Products Described

ROCHE LABORATORIES 425, 1965
a division of Hoffmann-La Roche Inc.
Nutley, NJ 07110 (201) 235-5000
For Medical Information
Write: Professional Services Department
 For: Medical Emergency Information
 (24-hour service)
 Product Information
 Or Reporting Adverse Events
 Call (800) 526-6367
Branch Warehouse
Belvidere, NJ 07823-0200
 200 Roche Drive (201) 475-5337
 Outside NJ (800) 526-0625
Other Operating Units
See: Hoffmann-La Roche Inc.
Products Described

ROCHE PRODUCTS INC. 425, 2016
Manati, Puerto Rico 00674
Address inquiries to:
Roche Laboratories
(800) 526-6367
Products Described

ROERIG DIVISION 426, 2029
Pfizer Incorporated
235 East 42nd Street
New York, NY 10017
Address inquiries to:
Medical Department
(212) 573-2187
Distribution Center
Hoffman Estates, IL 60196
2400 W. Central Road
(708) 765-9500
Customer Service: (800) 533-4535
Products Described

**RORER CONSUMER
PHARMACEUTICALS**
See RHÔNE-POULENC RORER
PHARMACEUTICALS INC., CONSUMER
PHARMACEUTICAL PRODUCTS.

RORER PHARMACEUTICALS
See RHÔNE-POULENC RORER
PHARMACEUTICALS INC.

ROSS LABORATORIES 2061
Div. Abbott Laboratories
Columbus, OH 43216
Address inquiries to:
Henry S. Sauls, M.D., Vice President,
Medical Affairs (614) 624-7677
Products Described

ROXANE LABORATORIES, 427, 2074
INC.
1809 Wilson Road
Columbus, OH 43228
Address inquiries to:
Professional Services Department
P.O. 16532
Columbus, OH 43216-6532
(Toll Free) (800) 848-0120
(614) 276-4000

RUSS PHARMACEUTICALS, INC.
See WHITBY PHARMACEUTICALS, INC.

RYSTAN COMPANY, INC.   2085
47 Center Avenue
P.O. Box 214
Little Falls, NJ 07424-0214
Address inquiries to:
Professional Service Dept.
                (201) 256-3737

SANDOZ NUTRITION   2086
CORPORATION
Clinical Products Division
5320 West Twenty-Third Street
Minneapolis, MN 55416
Address inquiries to:
Account Services
                (800) 821-3559
          FAX (612) 593-2087

SANDOZ PHARMACEUTICALS/   2088
CONSUMER DIVISION
Division of Sandoz Pharmaceutical Corp.
59 Route 10
East Hanover, NJ 07936

Address Medical Inquiries to:
Medical Department
Sandoz Pharmaceuticals
East Hanover, NJ 07936
               (201) 503-7500
Other Inquiries to:
               (201) 503-7500
       FAX (201) 503-8265

SANDOZ   427, 2090
PHARMACEUTICALS
CORPORATION
DORSEY DIVISION
SANDOZ DIVISION
Route 10, East Hanover, NJ 07936
Address inquiries to:
William F. Westlin, M.D.
               (201) 503-7500

SANOFI WINTHROP   428, 2134, 2670
PHARMACEUTICALS
90 Park Avenue
New York, NY 10016
               (212) 907-2000
Product Information Services
               (800) 446-6267
Customer Relations/Orders
     East Coast-(800) 223-1062
     West Coast-(800) 223-5511

Hypaque Meglumine 30%
Hypaque Meglumine 60%
Hypaque Sodium Oral Powder
Hypaque Sodium Oral Solution
Hypaque Sodium 25%
Hypaque Sodium 50% Injection
Hypaque-Cysto 30%
Hypaque-Cysto 30% Pediatric
Hypaque-76 Injection
Hytakerol Capsules
Luminal Sodium Injection
Modrastane Capsules
Morphine Sulfate Carpuject
Mytelase Chloride Caplets
Phenytoin Sodium Injection Carpuject
Pontocaine Cream
Pontocaine Ointment
Pontocaine Hydrochloride Eye Ointment
Pontocaine Hydrochloride Topical Solution
Pontocaine 0.2% with Dextrose 6%
Pontocaine 0.3% with Dextrose 6%
Primaquine Phosphate Tablets
Procainamide Hydrochloride Carpuject
Prochlorperazine Edisylate Injection Carpuject
Sal-Pak 2 Convenience Package
Sodium Chloride Injection
Sodium Chloride Injection Carpuject
Telepaque Tablets
Trimethobenzamide Hydrochloride Carpuject
Verapamil Hydrochloride Carpuject
Vitamins
Vitamin D, USP
Drisdol 50,000 Unit Capsules
Drisdol in Propylene Glycol

SAVAGE LABORATORIES 428, 2172, 2678
a division of Altana Inc.
60 Baylis Road
Melville, NY 11747
Address inquiries to:
Customer Service (800) 231-0206
For Medical Emergencies Contact:
H.H. Albrecht, M.D.
(516) 454-9071
Products Described
Alphatrex Cream, Ointment & Lotion ... 2172
Betatrex Cream, Ointment & Lotion ... 2172
◆ Brexin L.A. Capsules ... 428, 2173
◆ Chromagen Capsules ... 428, 2173
Dilor Elixir ... *2174*
◆ Dilor Injectable ... 428, *2174*
◆ Dilor-200 Tablets ... 428, 2174
◆ Dilor-400 Tablets ... 428, 2174
◆ Dilor-G Tablets & Liquid ... 428, 2174
◆ Doctar Gel ... 428, 2175
Ethiodol ... 2175, *2678*
◆ Mytrex Cream & Ointment ... 428, 2175
◆ Mytrex Foilpac ... 428
Trysul Vaginal Cream ... 2176
Other Products Available
Nystex Cream & Ointment
Nystex Oral Suspension
Theo-Sav

SCHEIN PHARMACEUTICAL, INC. 428, 2176
1800 Northern Boulevard
Roslyn, NY 11576
Address inquires to:
Customer Service (800) 537-2980
FAX (516) 686-3010
For Medical Emergency Contact:
Dr. Herbert Carlin (800) 548-6236
FAX (914) 225-1763
Branch Office
620 North 51st Avenue
Phoenix, AZ 85043 (800) 524-1843
FAX (602) 269-7468
Products Described
◆ InFeD Iron Dextran Injection ... 428, 2176
Other Products Available
Dexamethasone Acetate Suspension, Sterile
Dicyclomine Injection
Dimenhydrinate Injection
Doxapram Injection
Meperidine Hydrochloride Injection (Preservative Free)
Methylprednisolone Sodium Acetate Suspension, Sterile
Neomycin and Polymyxin B Sulfates and Hydrocortisone Otic Solution
Neomycin and Polymyxin B Sulfates and Hydrocortisone Otic Suspension
Neomycin and Polymyxin B Sulfates Solution for Irrigation
Primidone Tablets
Triamcinolone Acetonide Suspension, Sterile
Triamcinolone Diacetate Suspension, Sterile
Trihexyphenidyl Hydrochloride Tablets

SCHERING CORPORATION 428, 2177
Galloping Hill Road
Kenilworth, NJ 07033
(908) 298-4000
Address inquiries to:
Professional Services Department
9:00 AM to 5:00 PM EST:
(800) 526-4099
After regular hours and on weekends:
(908) 298-4000
Branch Offices
Southeast Branch
5884 Peachtree Rd., N.E.
Chamblee, GA 30341
(404) 457-6315
Midwest Branch
7500 N. Natchez Ave.
Niles, IL 60648 (708) 647-9363
Southwest Branch
1921 Gateway Dr.
Irving, TX 75062 (214) 714-2200
West Coast Branch
14775 Wicks Blvd.
San Leandro, CA 94577
(510) 357-3125
Products Described
Celestone Soluspan Suspension ... 2178
Diprolene AF Cream ... 2180
Diprolene Gel 0.05% ... 2180
Diprolene Lotion 0.05% ... 2180
Diprolene Ointment 0.05% ... 2180
Elocon Cream 0.1% ... 2181
Elocon Lotion 0.1% ... 2181
Elocon Ointment 0.1% ... 2181
◆ Etrafon Forte Tablets (4-25) ... 428, 2182
◆ Etrafon 2-10 Tablets (2-10) ... 428, 2182
◆ Etrafon Tablets (2-25) ... 428, 2182
◆ Etrafon-A Tablets (4-10) ... 428, 2182
◆ Eulexin Capsules ... 428, 2185
◆ Fulvicin P/G Tablets ... 428, 2186
◆ Fulvicin P/G 165 & 330 Tablets ... 428, 2187
Garamycin Cream 0.1% ... *2187*
Garamycin Injectable ... 2187
Garamycin Intrathecal Injection ... 2192
Garamycin Ointment 0.1% ... *2187*
Garamycin Ophthalmic Ointment—Sterile ... *2187*
Garamycin Ophthalmic Solution—Sterile ... *2187*
Garamycin Pediatric Injectable ... 2190
Hyperstat I.V. Injection ... 2193
InspirEase ... *2194*
Intron A ... 2194
Lotrimin Cream 1% ... 2201
Lotrimin Lotion 1% ... 2201
Lotrimin Solution 1% ... 2201
Lotrisone Cream ... 2202
Netromycin Injection 100 mg/ml ... 2203
◆ Normodyne Injection ... 428, 2206
◆ Normodyne Tablets ... 428, 2208
◆ Proventil Inhalation Aerosol ... 428, 2211
◆ Proventil Repetabs Tablets ... 428, 2215
Proventil Solution for Inhalation 0.5% ... 2212
Proventil Solution for Inhalation 0.083% ... 2213
Proventil Syrup ... 2214
◆ Proventil Tablets ... 428, 2215
Sodium Sulamyd Ophthalmic Ointment 10%-Sterile ... 2216
Sodium Sulamyd Ophthalmic Solution 10%-Sterile ... 2216
Sodium Sulamyd Ophthalmic Solution 30%-Sterile ... 2216
Solganal Suspension ... 2216
Trilafon Concentrate ... 2218
Trilafon Injection ... 2218
◆ Trilafon Tablets ... 428, 2218
◆ Vancenase AQ Nasal Spray 0.042% ... 428, 2221
◆ Vancenase PocketHaler Nasal Inhaler ... 429, 2220
◆ Vanceril Inhaler ... 428, 2222
Other Products Available
Celestone Phosphate Injection
Celestone Syrup
Celestone Tablets
Chlor-Trimeton Injection
Diprosone Cream 0.05%
Diprosone Lotion 0.05%
Diprosone Ointment 0.05%
Diprosone Topical Aerosol 0.1%
Estinyl Tablets
Fulvicin-U/F Tablets
Meticorten Tablets
Metimyd Ophthalmic Ointment—Sterile
Metimyd Ophthalmic Suspension—Sterile
Miradon Tablets
Naqua Tablets
Optimine Tablets
Optimyd Ophthalmic Solution
Oreton Methyl Buccal Tablets
Oreton Methyl Tablets
Otobiotic Otic Solution
Paxipam Tablets
Permitil Oral Concentrate
Permitil Tablets
Polaramine Expectorant
Polarmine Repetabs Tablets
Polaramine Syrup
Polaramine Tablets
Sebizon Lotion
Theovent Long-Acting Capsules
Valisone Cream 0.1%
Valisone Lotion 0.1%
Valisone Ointment 0.1%
Valisone Reduced Strength Cream 0.1%

SCHERING-PLOUGH HEALTHCARE PRODUCTS 429, 2224
110 Allen Road
Liberty Corner, NJ 07938
Address inquiries to:
Public Relations (908) 604-1969
For Medical Emergencies Contact:
Clinical Department
(901) 320-2998
Products Described
◆ Gyne-Lotrimin Vaginal Cream Antifungal ... 429, 2224
◆ Gyne-Lotrimin Vaginal Inserts ... 429, 2224

SCHIAPPARELLI SEARLE 429, 2224
Box 5110
Chicago, IL 60680-5110
Customer Service/Order Entry
(800) 323-1603
Address medical inquiries to:
G.D. Searle & Co.
Medical & Scientific Information Department
4901 Searle Parkway
Skokie, IL 60077
For Medical Emergencies Contact:
Outside IL
(800) 323-4204 (business hours)
(708) 982-7000 (at other times)
Within IL
(708) 982-7000
Products Described
Banthīne ... *2224*
Cyclobenzaprine Hydrochloride Tablets USP ... *2224*
◆ Flagyl I.V. ... 429, 2224
◆ Flagyl I.V. RTU ... 429, 2224
Haloperidol Oral Solution USP ... *2224*
Lactulose Syrup USP ... *2224*
◆ Norethin 1/35E-21 ... 429, 2226
◆ Norethin 1/35E-28 ... 429, 2226
◆ Norethin 1/50M-21 ... 429, 2226
◆ Norethin 1/50M-28 ... 429, 2226
◆ Piroxicam Capsules USP ... 429, 2235
Pro-Banthīne Tablets ... 2236

SCHWARZ PHARMA 429, 2237
Kremers Urban Company
P.O. Box 2038
5600 W. County Line Road
Milwaukee, WI 53201
Address inquiries to:
Technical Services Department
(414) 354-4300
(800) 558-5114
For Medical Emergencies Contact:
Technical Services Department
(414) 354-4300
(800) 558-5114
Products Described
Calciferol Drops ... *2237*
Calciferol in Oil Injection ... *2237*
Calciferol Tablets ... *2237*
◆ Deponit NTG Transdermal Delivery System ... 429, 2237
◆ Fedahist Gyrocaps ... 429, 2238
Fedahist Timecaps ... 2238
Kutapressin Injection ... 2239
◆ Kutrase Capsules ... 429, 2240
◆ Ku-Zyme Capsules ... 429, 2240
◆ Ku-Zyme HP Capsules ... 429, 2241
Levsin Drops ... 2241
Levsin Elixir ... 2241
Levsin Injection ... 2241
◆ Levsin Tablets ... 429, 2241
◆ Levsin/SL Tablets ... 429, 2241
◆ Levsinex Timecaps ... 429, 2241
Pre-Pen ... 2242
Other Products Available
Chardonna-2 Tablets
Fedahist Decongestant Syrup
Fedahist Expectorant Pediatric Drops
Fedahist Expectorant Syrup
Fedahist Tablets
Gemnisyn Tablets
Kudrox Suspension
Lactrase Capsules
Levsin with Phenobarbital Drops
Levsin with Phenobarbital Tablets
Milkinol

G.D. SEARLE & CO. 429, 2243
Box 5110
Chicago, IL 60680-5110
Customer Service/Order Entry
(800) 323-1603
Address medical inquiries to:
G.D. Searle & Co.
Medical & Scientific Information Department
4901 Searle Parkway
Skokie, IL 60077
For Medical Emergencies Contact:
Outside IL
(800) 323-4204 (business hours)
(708) 982-7000 (at other times)
Within IL
(708) 982-7000
Products Described
◆ Aldactazide ... 429, 2243
◆ Aldactone ... 429, 2245
◆ Calan SR Caplets ... 429, 2249
◆ Calan Tablets ... 429, 2246
◆ Cytotec ... 429, 2251
◆ Demulen 1/35-21 ... 429, 2253
◆ Demulen 1/35-28 ... 429, 2253
◆ Demulen 1/50-21 ... 429, 2253
◆ Demulen 1/50-28 ... 429, 2253
◆ Flagyl Tablets ... 429, 2259
◆ Kerlone Tablets ... 429, 2261
Lomotil Liquid ... 2264
◆ Lomotil Tablets ... 429, 2264
◆ Maxaquin Tablets ... 429, 2265
◆ Nitrodisc ... 429, 2268
◆ Norpace Capsules ... 429, 2270
◆ Norpace CR Capsules ... 429, 2270

SERES LABORATORIES, INC. 2272
3331 Industrial Drive
Box 470
Santa Rosa, CA 95402
Address inquiries to:
Kathryn M. MacLeod, Ph.D.
(707) 526-4526
Products Described
Cantharone ... *2272*
Cantharone Plus ... *2272*
Night Cast Regular (Medicated Acne Mask-lotion) ... *2272*
Night Cast Special (Medicated Acne Mask-lotion) ... *2272*

SERONO LABORATORIES, INC. 2272, 2678
100 Longwater Circle
Norwell, MA 02061
Address inquiries to:
Drug Information and Surveillance Group
(800) 283-8088
(617) 982-9000
For Medical Emergencies Contact:
(800) 283-8088
(617) 982-9000
Products Described
Geref (sermorelin acetate for injection) ... 2678
Metrodin (urofollitropin for injection) ... 2272
Pergonal (menotropins for injection, USP) ... 2274
Profasi (chorionic gonadotropin for injection, USP) ... 2276
Serophene (clomiphene citrate tablets, USP) ... 2277

SIGMA-TAU PHARMACEUTICALS, INC. 2278
200 Orchard Ridge Drive
Gaithersburg MD 20878
Address inquiries to:
(301) 948-1041
Products Described
Carnitor ... 2278

SMITHKLINE BEECHAM CONSUMER BRANDS 429, 2279
Unit of SmithKline Beecham Inc.
P.O. Box 1467
Pittsburgh, PA 15230
Address inquiries to:
Professional Services Dept.
800-BEECHAM
PA Residents: 800-242-1718
Products Described
◆ A-200 Lice Control Spray and Kit ... 429, 2279
◆ A-200, Pediculicide Shampoo Concentrate ... 429, 2279
Contac Continuous Action Decongestant/Antihistamine Capsules ... ◘
Contac Cough Formula ... ◘
Contac Cough & Sore Throat Formula ... ◘
Contac Jr. Non-Drowsy Cold Liquid ... ◘
Contac Maximum Strength Continuous Action Decongestant/Antihistamine Caplets ... ◘
Contac Severe Cold and Flu Formula Caplets ... ◘
Contac Severe Cold & Flu Nighttime Cold Medicine ... ◘
Contac Sinus Caplets Maximum Strength Non-Drowsy Formula ... ◘
Contac Sinus Tablets Maximum Strength Non-Drowsy Formula ... ◘
Ecotrin Enteric Coated Aspirin Maximum Strength Tablets and Caplets ... 2280
Ecotrin Enteric Coated Aspirin Regular Strength Tablets and Caplets ... 2280
Feosol Capsules ... 2281
Feosol Elixir ... 2281
Feosol Tablets ... 2281
Massengill Disposable Douche ... 2282
Massengill Fragrance-Free Soft Cloth Towelette ... 2282
Massengill Liquid Concentrate ... 2282
Massengill Medicated Disposable Douche ... 2282
Massengill Medicated Liquid Concentrate ... 2282
Massengill Medicated Soft Cloth Towelettes ... 2282
Massengill Powder ... 2282
Nature's Remedy Mineral Oil Enema ... ◘
Nature's Remedy Natural Vegetable Laxative ... ◘
Nature's Remedy Regular Enema ... ◘
Oxy Facial Scrub ... ◘

(◆ Shown in Product Identification Section) *Italic Page Number* Indicates Brief Listing (◘ Described in PDR For Nonprescription Drugs)

Other Products Available

Benzathine Penicillin G (see Bicillin)
CVC Heparin Flush Kits
Codeine Phosphate Injection
Cyanocobalamin Injection
Dicloxacillin Sodium Monohydrate (see
Pathocil)
Digoxin Injection
Dimenhydrinate Injection
Diphenhydramine HCl Injection
Diphtheria & Tetanus Toxoids Adsorbed,
Pediatric
Epinephrine Injection (1:1000)
Estrogenic Substance (estrone) In
Aqueous Suspension
Fluor-I-Strip Applicators
Fluor-I-Strip A.T. Applicators
Heparin Flush Kits
Hydromorphone HCl Injection
Largon Injection
Meperidine HCl Injection
Meperidine HCl Tablets, Redipak
Morphine Sulfate Injection
Naloxone HCl Injection
Ophthalgan
Opium & Belladonna Rectal
Suppositories
Pentobarbital Sodium Injection
Phenobarbital Sodium Injection
Prochlorperazine Edisylate Injection
Redipak Unit Dose Medications (Strip
Pack and/or Individually Wrapped)
Products:
Ativan Tablets, 0.5 mg
Ativan Tablets, 1 mg
Ativan Tablets, 2 mg
Isordil Sublingual Tablets, 2.5 mg
Isordil Sublingual Tablets, 5 mg
Isordil 5 Titradose Tablets, 5 mg
Isordil 10 Titradose Tablets, 10 mg
Isordil 20 Titradose Tablets, 20 mg
Isordil 30 Titradose Tablets, 30 mg
Isordil 40 Titradose Tablets, 40 mg
Meperidine HCl Tablets
Pen•Vee K Tablets, 250 mg
Pen•Vee K Tablets, 500 mg
Phenergan Tablets, 25 mg
Sectral Capsules, 200 mg
Serax Capsules, 10 mg
Serax Capsules, 15 mg
Serax Capsules, 30 mg
Surmontil Capsules, 50 mg
Wygesic Tablets
Wytensin Tablets, 4 mg
Redipak (Respiratory Therapy Unit)
Products:
Sodium Chloride 0.9%
RediTemp-C, Disposable Cold Pack
Saline Solution (see Sodium Chloride
Injection)
Secobarbital Sodium Injection
Sodium Chloride Injection, Bacteriostatic
Sodium Chloride Solution, 0.9%
Sonacide
Sparine Injection
Testuria
Thiamine Hydrochloride Injection
Vitamin B₁₂ Injection
Wyamine Sulfate Injection
Wydase, Stabilized Solution

YOUNG PHARMACEUTICALS INC. 2660
1840 Berlin Turnpike
Wethersfield, CT 06109
Address inquiries to:
Professional Services Department
Toll-free (800) 874-9686
(203) 529-7919

Products Described
BlemErase Acne Masking
Lotion 2660
CuraStain Dermatologic Stain
Reducing Spray 2660
PharmaCreme Emollient
Topical Vehicle 2660

Instructions For Using The Product Name Index

This new, easy-to-use index helps the healthcare professional rapidly locate information on specific pharmaceuticals by either product or generic/chemical name. The index is sorted alphabetically with product name and generic/chemical names intermixed.

Entries appearing under the product name include the manufacturers' name and page numbers where information on this product can be located in the PDR®.

Generic/chemical name headings are followed by products listed in the PDR that include this active ingredient. **Products shown under the generic/chemical name heading are sorted alphabetically— first by products that are fully described in the PDR, followed by the products not fully described in the PDR.**

Products listed with bold page numbers are fully described in the PDR, others are partially described.

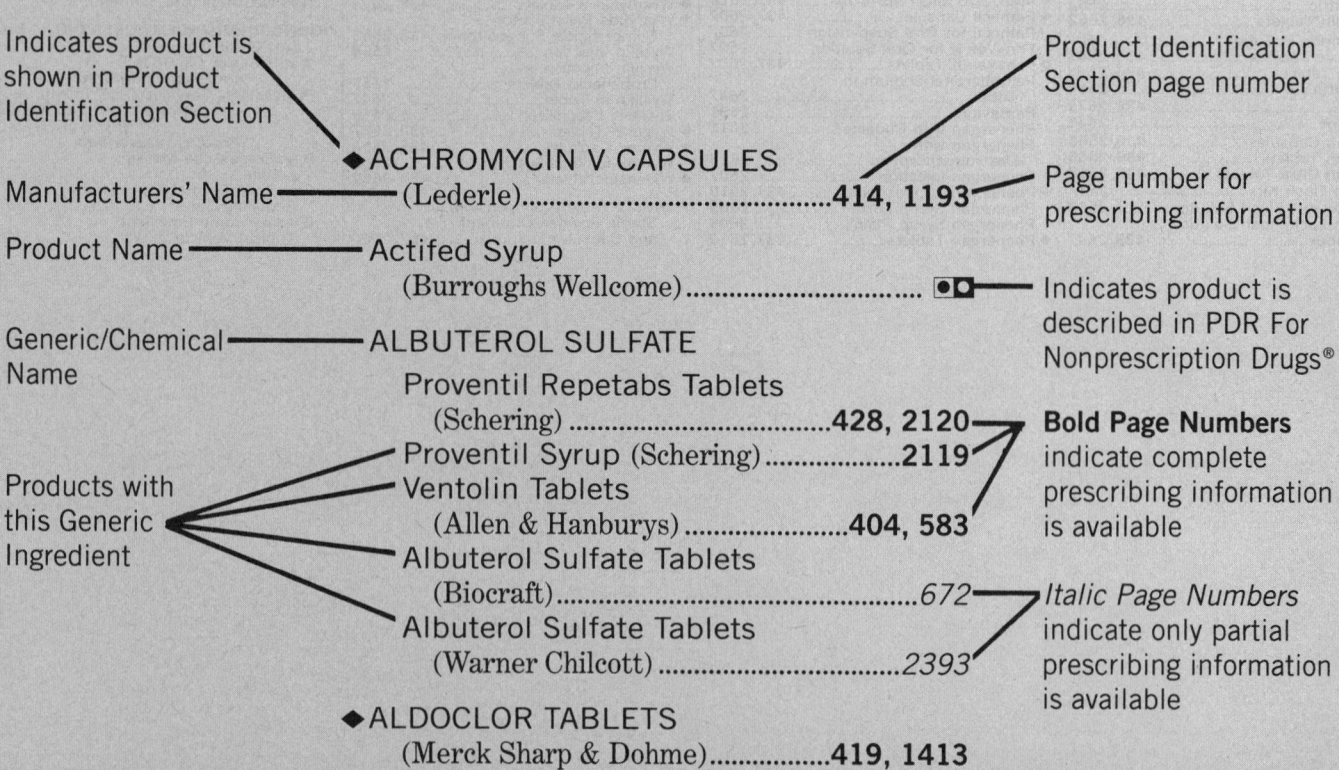

(Sample Page)

SECTION 2

Product Name Index

In response to requests, this section has been re-designed to provide both product and generic/chemical names in the same index. Accordingly, **you will find complete instructions for use on the facing page**.

Here are key features:

- Fully described products have **bold page numbers**.
- Brief listings have *italic page numbers*.
- The symbol ◆ indicates the product is shown in the Product Identification Section.
- The symbol ▣ indicates the product is described in the PDR FOR NONPRESCRIPTION DRUGS®.

(◆ Shown in Product Identification Section)   *Italic Page Number* Indicates Brief Listing   (▣ Described in PDR For Nonprescription Drugs)

Fioricet Tablets (Sandoz Pharmaceuticals)............... **427, 2100**
Fioricet with Codeine Capsules (Sandoz Pharmaceuticals)............... **2101**
Fiorinal Capsules (Sandoz Pharmaceuticals)............... **427, 2102**
Fiorinal with Codeine Capsules (Sandoz Pharmaceuticals)............... **427, 2103**
Fiorinal Tablets (Sandoz Pharmaceuticals)............... **427, 2102**
No Doz Fast Acting Alertness Aid Tablets (Bristol-Myers Products).......... **767**
No Doz Maximum Strength Caplets (Bristol-Myers Products)............... **768**
Norgesic Forte Tablets (3M Pharmaceuticals)............ **416, 1355**
Norgesic Tablets (3M Pharmaceuticals)............ **416, 1355**
Synalgos-DC Capsules (Wyeth-Ayerst)............ **438, 2639**
Wigraine Tablets & Suppositories (Organon).. **421, 1701**
Esgic Tablets & Capsules (Forest Pharmaceuticals)....*409, 1030*
Femcet Capsules (Northampton Medical)............... *1681*
Gelpirin Tablets (Alra Laboratories)............... *594*
Medigesic Capsules/Tablets (U.S. Pharmaceutical)............ *2430*
PC-CAP Propoxyphene Hydrochloride Compound, USP (Alra Laboratories)............... *594*
Pacaps Capsules (Lunsco)..... *1347*
Propoxyphene HCl/Aspirin & Caffeine Capsules (Geneva)............... *1083*
Repan Tablets and Capsules (Everett)............... *996*
◆ CALAN SR CAPLETS (Searle)....**429, 2249**
◆ CALAN TABLETS (Searle)...... **429, 2246**
Calcet (Mission)............... *1675*
Calcet Plus (Mission)............... *1675*
Calcibind (Mission)............... *1676*
CALCI-CHEW TABLETS (R&D Laboratories)............... **1895**
CALCIDRINE SYRUP (Abbott).... **508**

CALCIFEDIOL
Calderol Capsules (Organon).. *420, 1692*

CALCIFEROL
Calciferol Drops (Schwarz Pharma)............... *2237*
Calciferol in Oil Injection (Schwarz Pharma)............... *2237*
Calciferol Tablets (Schwarz Pharma)............... *2237*

CALCIJEX CALCITRIOL INJECTION (Abbott)............... 508

◆ CALCIMAR INJECTION, SYNTHETIC (Rhone-Poulenc Rorer Pharmaceuticals Inc.)....... **424, 1910**
CALCI-MIX CAPSULES (R&D Laboratories)............... **1895**
CALCIPARINE INJECTION (Du Pont Multi-Source Products)............... **948**

CALCITONIN-SALMON
Calcimar Injection, Synthetic (Rhone-Poulenc Rorer Pharmaceuticals Inc.).. **424, 1910**
Miacalcin Injection (Sandoz Pharmaceuticals)............ **427, 2112**

CALCITONIN, SYNTHETIC
Cibacalcin Double-chambered Syringes (CIBA Pharmaceutical)............... **889**

CALCITRIOL
Calcijex Calcitriol Injection (Abbott)............... **508**
Rocaltrol Capsules (Roche Laboratories)............ **426, 2002**

CALCIUM ACETATE
Pedi-Boro Soak Paks (Pedinol)............... *1826*
PhosLo Tablets (Braintree).... **406, 725**

CALCIUM CARBONATE
Ascriptin A/D Caplets (Rhone-Poulenc Rorer Consumer)............... *1926*

Regular Strength Ascriptin Tablets (Rhone-Poulenc Rorer Consumer)............... *1926*
Calci-Chew Tablets (R&D Laboratories)............... **1895**
Calci-Mix Capsules (R&D Laboratories)............... **1895**
Caltrate 600 Tablets (Lederle)............... **414, 1226**
Caltrate 600 + Iron & Vitamin D (Lederle)....... **414, 1227**
Caltrate 600 + Vitamin D (Lederle)............... **414, 1226**
Gerimed Tablets (Fielding)............... **1000**
Materna Tablets (Lederle)...... **415, 1243**
Mylanta Gelcaps Antacid (J&J•Merck Consumer).......... **413, 1182**
Natalins Rx (Mead Johnson Laboratories)............... **419, 1440**
Natalins Tablets (Mead Johnson Laboratories)............ **419, 1440**
Nephro-Calci Tablets (R&D Laboratories)............... **1895**
Pramet FA (Ross)............... **2065**
Pramilet FA (Ross)............... **2065**
Tylenol, Extra Strength, Headache Plus Pain Reliever Caplets (McNeil Consumer)............... **418, 1415**
Zenate Tablets (Solvay)...... **432, 2351**
Calcet (Mission)............... *1675*
Calcet Plus (Mission)............... *1675*
Calcium Carbonate Tablets & Oral Suspension (Roxane)............... *2074*
Calcium Health Packs (Health Maintenance)............... *1110*
Calel-D (Rhone-Poulenc Rorer Pharmaceuticals Inc.)............... *1908*
Endurance Packs (Health Maintenance)............... *1111*
For Two Capsules (Health Maintenance)............... *1111*
Liqui-Cal Softgels (Advanced Nutritional)............... *567*
Liquid Cal-600 Capsules (Carlson)............... *855*
Mission Prenatal (Mission)............... *1676*
Mission Prenatal H.P. (Mission)............... *1676*
Nu-Iron V Tablets (Mayrand Pharmaceuticals)............... *1408*
Prenate 90 Tablets (Bock)....... *700*
Total Formula-2 (multivitamin/multimineral) (Vitaline)............... *2492*

CALCIUM CASEINATE
Promote High Protein Liquid Nutrition (Ross)...... *2066*

CALCIUM CHLORIDE
Calcium Chloride 10% Injection, USP (Astra)............... *635*

CALCIUM CITRATE
Citracal Liquitab (Mission)....... *1675*
Citracal (Mission)............... *1675*
Citracal Caplets + D (Mission)............... *1675*
Liqui-Cal/Mag (Advanced Nutritional)............... *567*
NutraVescent (Northampton Medical)............... *1681*
Total Formula-2 (multivitamin/multiminera-l) (Vitaline)............... *2492*

CALCIUM DISODIUM EDETATE
Calcium Disodium Versenate Injection (3M Pharmaceuticals)............... **1349**

CALCIUM GLUBIONATE
Neo-Calglucon Syrup (Sandoz Pharmaceuticals)......... **2114**

CALCIUM GLUCONATE
Calcet (Mission)............... *1675*
Calcium Gluconate Tablets (Roxane)............... *2074*
Mission Prenatal (Mission)....... *1676*
Mission Prenatal H.P. (Mission)............... *1676*

CALCIUM GLYCEROPHOSPHATE
Calphosan (Glenwood)............... **1102**

Calcium Health Packs (Health Maintenance)............... *1110*

CALCIUM IODIDE
Calcidrine Syrup (Abbott)............... **508**
Norisodrine with Calcium Iodide Syrup (Abbott)............... *540*

CALCIUM LACTATE
Calphosan (Glenwood)............... **1102**
Calcet (Mission)............... *1675*

Cal-Lactate (calcium lactate) Caplets (Vitaline)...... *2492*
Mission Prenatal (Mission)............... *1676*
Mission Prenatal H.P. (Mission)............... *1676*

CALCIUM PANTOTHENATE
Mega-B (Arco)............... **625**
Natalins Rx (Mead Johnson Laboratories)............ **419, 1440**
Natalins Tablets (Mead Johnson Laboratories)............ **419, 1440**
Vicon Forte Capsules (Whitby)............ **435, 2529**
Calcium Health Packs (Health Maintenance)............... *1110*
Eldercaps (Mayrand Pharmaceuticals)............... *1407*
Endurance Packs (Health Maintenance)............... *1111*

CALCIUM PHOSPHATE, DIBASIC
Dical-D Tablets & Wafers (Abbott)............... **517**
Gerimed Tablets (Fielding)............... **1000**

CALCIUM PHOSPHATE, TRIBASIC
Posture 600 mg (Whitehall)...... **2534**
Posture-D 600 mg (Whitehall)............... **2534**

CALCIUM POLYCARBOPHIL
FiberCon Tablets (Lederle)...... **414, 1231**

CALCIUM SODIUM ALGINATE FIBER
Kaltostat Wound Dressing (Calgon Vestal)............... **854**

Caldecort Anti-Itch Hydrocortisone Cream (Fisons Consumer Health)............... ▣
Caldecort Anti-Itch Hydrocortisone Spray (Fisons Consumer Health)............... ▣
Caldecort Light Creme (Fisons Consumer Health)............... ▣
◆ Calderol Capsules (Organon)...... **420, 1692**
Caldesene Medicated Ointment (Fisons Consumer Health)............... ▣
Caldesene Medicated Powder (Fisons Consumer Health)............... ▣
Calel-D (Rhone-Poulenc Rorer Pharmaceuticals Inc.)............... *1908*
Cal-Lactate (calcium lactate) Caplets (Vitaline)............... *2492*
CALPHOSAN (Glenwood)............... **1102**
◆ CALTRATE 600 TABLETS (Lederle)............... **414, 1226**
◆ CALTRATE 600 + IRON & VITAMIN D (Lederle)............... **414, 1227**
◆ CALTRATE 600 + VITAMIN D (Lederle)............... **414, 1226**
Cama Arthritis Pain Reliever (Sandoz Consumer)............... ▣

CAMPHOR
Pazo Hemorrhoid Ointment & Suppositories (Bristol-Myers Products)............... **768**
Nephro-Derm Cream (R&D Laboratories)............... *1895*
Panalgesic Gold Liniment (E. C. Robins)............... *1959*

CANTHARIDIN
Cantharone (Seres)............... *2272*
Cantharone Plus (Seres)............... *2272*
Verr-Canth (Palisades Pharmaceuticals)............... *1738*

◆ CANTIL TABLETS (Marion Merrell Dow)............ **417, 1366**
CAPASTAT SULFATE (Lilly).... **1283**
◆ Capital and Codeine Suspension (Carnrick)............*407, 858*
CAPITROL SHAMPOO (Westwood-Squibb)............... **2511**
◆ CAPOTEN (Princeton)............ **423, 1858**
◆ CAPOTEN (Squibb)............ **432, 2356**
◆ CAPOZIDE (Squibb)............ **432, 2359**

CAPREOMYCIN SULFATE
Capastat Sulfate (Lilly)............... **1283**

CAPSAICIN
Zostrix (GenDerm)............... **1077**
Zostrix-HP Topical Analgesic Cream (GenDerm)............... **1077**

CAPTOPRIL
Capoten (Princeton)............ **423, 1858**
Capoten (Squibb)............ **432, 2356**
Capozide (Squibb)............ **432, 2359**
◆ CARAFATE TABLETS (Marion Merrell Dow)............ **416, 1367**

CARAMIPHEN EDISYLATE
Tuss-Ornade Liquid (SmithKline Beecham Pharmaceuticals)............... **2337**
Tuss-Ornade Spansule Capsules (SmithKline Beecham Pharmaceuticals).... **431, 2337**

CARBAMAZEPINE
Atretol Tablets (Athena Neurosciences)............... **666**
Tegretol Chewable Tablets (Basel)............... **405, 679**
Tegretol Suspension (Basel)............... **679**
Tegretol Tablets (Basel)....... **405, 679**
Carbamazepine Tablets (Taro Pharmaceuticals)............... *2425*
Carbamazepine Chewable Tablets, USP (Warner Chilcott)............... *2507*
Carbamazepine Tablets (Inwood)............... *1157*

CARBENICILLIN INDANYL SODIUM
Geocillin Tablets (Roerig)........ **427, 2040**

CARBETAPENTANE TANNATE
Rynatuss Pediatric Suspension (Wallace)............ **435, 2503**
Rynatuss Tablets (Wallace).... **435, 2503**

CARBIDOPA
Sinemet Tablets (Du Pont Pharmaceuticals)............ **409, 974**
Sinemet CR Tablets (Du Pont Pharmaceuticals)............ **409, 976**

CARBINOXAMINE MALEATE
Rondec Oral Drops (Ross)............ **2066**
Rondec Syrup (Ross)............... **2066**
Rondec Tablet (Ross)............... **2066**
Rondec-DM Oral Drops (Ross)............... **2067**
Rondec-DM Syrup (Ross)............... **2067**
Rondec-TR Tablet (Ross)............ **2066**
Tussafed Drops & Syrup (Everett)............... *996*

CARBOCAINE HYDROCHLORIDE 3% INJECTION (Eastman Kodak)............ 981
CARBOCAINE HYDROCHLORIDE INJECTION (Sanofi Winthrop Pharmaceuticals)............ 2137
CARBOCAINE HYDROCHLORIDE 2% WITH NEO-COBEFRIN (Eastman Kodak)............ 981

CARBOHYDRATES
SMA Lo-Iron Infant Formula, Concentrated, Ready-To-Feed & Powder (Wyeth-Ayerst)............ **437, 2637**

CARBOLIC ACID
(see under PHENOL)

CARBOPLATIN
Paraplatin for Injection (Bristol-Myers Oncology).......... **406, 751**

CARBOXYMETHYLCELLULOSE SODIUM
Glandosane Synthetic Saliva (Tsumura Medical)............... **2425**

◆ CARDENE CAPSULES (Syntex). **433, 2393**
◆ CARDENE SR CAPSULES (Syntex)............... **433, 2395**
◆ CARDILATE ORAL/SUBLINGUAL TABLETS (Burroughs Wellcome)............... **407, 773**
◆ CARDIOQUIN TABLETS (Purdue Frederick)............ **424, 1882**
◆ CARDIZEM CD CAPSULES-180 MG, 240 MG AND 300 MG (Marion Merrell Dow)............ **417, 1368**
◆ CARDIZEM SR CAPSULES-60 MG, 90 MG AND 120 MG (Marion Merrell Dow)............ **417, 1372**
◆ CARDIZEM INJECTABLE (Marion Merrell Dow)............ **416, 1370**
◆ CARDIZEM TABLETS-30 MG, 60 MG, 90 MG AND 120 MG (Marion Merrell Dow)............ **417, 1374**
◆ CARDURA TABLETS (Roerig)....**427, 2031**

CARISOPRODOL
Soma Compound w/Codeine Tablets (Wallace)............ **435, 2505**
Soma Compound Tablets (Wallace)............ **435, 2504**
Soma Tablets (Wallace)............ **435, 2503**
Carisoprodol Tablets (Geneva)............... *1083*

Limbitrol Tablets (Roche Products)..................426, 2022
Menrium Tablets (Roche Products)..................426, 2023
Chlordiazepoxide & Amitriptyline Hydrochloride Tablets (Mylan).......................1678
Chlordiazepoxide and Amitriptyline HCl Tablets (Par).............................1739

CHLORDIAZEPOXIDE HYDROCHLORIDE
Librax Capsules (Roche Products)..................426, 2018
Librium Capsules (Roche Products)..................426, 2020
Librium Injectable (Roche Products)..........................2021

Chlordiazepoxide & Amitriptyline Hydrochloride Tablets (Mylan).......................1678
Chlordiazepoxide and Amitriptyline HCl Tablets (Par)............................1739

CHLORESIUM OINTMENT (Rystan)...........................2085

CHLORESIUM SOLUTION (Rystan)...........................2085

CHLORHEXIDINE GLUCONATE
Hibiclens Antimicrobial Skin Cleanser (Stuart)...............432, 2374
Hibistat Germicidal Hand Rinse (Stuart)..................432, 2375
Hibistat Towelette (Stuart)...432, 2375
Peridex (Procter & Gamble)...........1867

CHLORMEZANONE
Trancopal Caplets (Sanofi Winthrop Pharmaceuticals)............2170

CHLOROETHANE
Ethyl Chloride, U.S.P. (Gebauer)..........................1056

CHLOROMYCETIN CREAM, 1% (Parke-Davis)...................1748

CHLOROMYCETIN HYDROCORTISONE OPHTHALMIC (Parke-Davis)...........1748

◆ **CHLOROMYCETIN KAPSEALS** (Parke-Davis)..................422, 1749

CHLOROMYCETIN OPHTHALMIC OINTMENT, 1% (Parke-Davis)...................1750

CHLOROMYCETIN OPHTHALMIC SOLUTION (Parke-Davis).......................1750

CHLOROMYCETIN OTIC (Parke-Davis).......................1751

CHLOROMYCETIN PALMITATE (Parke-Davis).......1751

CHLOROMYCETIN SODIUM SUCCINATE (Parke-Davis)..............1752

CHLOROPHYLL PREPARATIONS
Chloresium Ointment (Rystan)...........................2085
Chloresium Solution (Rystan).........2085
Derifil Tablets (Rystan)...............2086
Panafil Ointment (Rystan)..............2086
Prophyllin Wet Dressing Powder and Ointment (Rystan)...........................2086

CHLOROPHYLLIN COPPER COMPLEX
Chloresium Ointment (Rystan)...........................2085
Chloresium Solution (Rystan).........2085
Derifil Tablets (Rystan)...............2086
Panafil Ointment (Rystan)..............2086
N'Odor Softgels (Advanced Nutritional)........................567
PALS Internal Deodorant (Palisades Pharmaceuticals)........1738
Prophyllin Wet Dressing Powder and Ointment (Rystan)...........................2086

CHLOROPROCAINE HYDROCHLORIDE
Nesacaine Injections (Astra).......650
Nesacaine-MPF Injection (Astra)...........................650

CHLOROQUINE HYDROCHLORIDE
Aralen Hydrochloride Injection (Sanofi Winthrop Pharmaceuticals)...................2134

CHLOROQUINE PHOSPHATE
Aralen Phosphate Tablets (Sanofi Winthrop Pharmaceuticals).............428, 2135
Chloroquine Phosphate Tablets (Biocraft)................698

CHLOROTHIAZIDE
Aldoclor Tablets (Merck & Co., Inc.)...................419, 1464
Diupres Tablets (Merck & Co., Inc.)...................419, 1512
Diuril Oral Suspension (Merck & Co., Inc.)..............1515
Diuril Tablets (Merck & Co., Inc.)...................419, 1515
Chlorothiazide Tablets (Mylan).......................1678
Methyldopa and Chlorothiazide Tablets (Par).............................1739
Reserpine & Chlorothiazide Tablets (Mylan).................1678

CHLOROTHIAZIDE SODIUM
Diuril Sodium Intravenous (Merck & Co., Inc.)...............1514

CHLOROTRIANISENE
TACE 12 mg Capsules (Marion Merrell Dow)...........417, 1401
TACE 25 mg Capsules (Marion Merrell Dow)...........417, 1401

CHLOROXINE
Capitrol Shampoo (Westwood-Squibb)..............2511

CHLOROXYLENOL
BAZA Cream, Occlusive Skin Protectant (Sween)..............2388
Fungoid Creme (Pedinol)............1825
Fungoid HC Creme (Pedinol)........1825
Fungoid Solution (Pedinol)..........1825
Fungoid Tincture (Pedinol)..........1825
Gordochom Solution (Gordon)........................1104
Micro-Guard Cream, Antiseptic, Antifungal Skin Cream (Sween).................2389
Micro-Guard Powder, Antifungal Powder (Sween).........2389
Ony-Clear Nail Spray (Pedinol)..........................1826
Pedi-Pro Foot Powder (Pedinol)..........................1826
Sween Prep, Protective Skin Barrier (Sween)..................2390

CHLORPHENIRAMINE MALEATE
Ana-Kit Anaphylaxis Emergency Treatment Kit (Miles Allergy)..................1658
Atrohist Plus Tablets (Adams)............................557
Brexin L.A. Capsules (Savage)......................428, 2173
Cerose-DM (Wyeth-Ayerst)...........2555
Chlorafed H.S. Timecelles (Roberts)........................1931
Chlorafed Timecelles (Roberts)........................1931
Comhist LA Capsules (Procter & Gamble Pharmaceuticals)..................1869
Allergy-Sinus Comtrex Multi-Symptom Allergy Sinus Formula Tablets & Caplets (Bristol-Myers Products)................406, 762
Comtrex Multi-Symptom Cold Reliever Tablets/Caplets/Liqui-Gels-/Liquid (Bristol-Myers Products)................406, 761
Day & Night Comtrex (Bristol-Myers Products)...406, 763
Deconamine SR Capsules (Berlex)....................405, 686
Deconamine Syrup (Berlex).............686
Deconamine Tablets (Berlex)...405, 686
Dristan Cold & Flu (Whitehall)................435, 2532
Dristan Cold Nasal Decongestant/ Antihistamine/ Analgesic Coated Tablets (Whitehall) 435, 2532
Extendryl Chewable Tablets (Fleming)..........................1023
Extendryl Sr. & Jr. T.D. Capsules (Fleming)..............1023
Extendryl Syrup (Fleming)............1023
4-Way Cold Tablets (Bristol-Myers Products)...........767
Fedahist Gyrocaps (Schwarz Pharma)....................429, 2238
Fedahist Timecaps (Schwarz Pharma)........................2238
Hycomine Compound Tablets (Du Pont Pharmaceuticals).................970
Kronofed-A Kronocaps (Ferndale)........................997

Kronofed-A-Jr. Kronocaps (Ferndale)........................997
Nolamine Timed-Release Tablets (Carnrick)..........407, 860
Novafed A Capsules (Marion Merrell Dow)..........417, 1390
Novahistine DH (Marion Merrell Dow)..........417, 1391
Ornade Spansule Capsules (SmithKline Beecham Pharmaceuticals)...........431, 2310
PediaCare Cold-Allergy Chewables (McNeil Consumer)..................417, 1410
PediaCare Cough-Cold Liquid (McNeil Consumer)...417, 1410
PediaCare Night Rest Cough-Cold Liquid (McNeil Consumer)..........417, 1410
PediaCare 6-12 Cough-Cold Chewable Tablets (McNeil Consumer)..................417, 1410
Quelidrine Syrup (Abbott)............553
Ru-Tuss II Capsules (Boots Pharmaceuticals)...........405, 719
Ru-Tuss Tablets (Boots Pharmaceuticals)...........405, 719
Sinulin Tablets (Carnrick)........407, 863
Teldrin Timed-Release Allergy Capsules, 12 mg. (SmithKline Beecham Consumer Brands)...............2283
Tylenol Allergy Sinus Medication Caplets and Gelcaps, Maximum Strength (McNeil Consumer)...................418, 1421
Children's Tylenol Cold Liquid Formula and Chewable Tablets (McNeil Consumer)...................418, 1417
Children's Tylenol Cold Plus Cough Liquid Formula (McNeil Consumer).............1417
Tylenol Cold & Flu Hot Medication, Packets (McNeil Consumer)..................418, 1418
Tylenol Cold Medication Caplets and Tablets (McNeil Consumer)..................418, 1418
Tylenol Cold Medication, Effervescent Tablets (McNeil Consumer)..................418, 1417
Chlorafed Liquid (Roberts)..............1931
Chlorpheniramine Maleate Extended Release Capsules (Geneva)...............1083
Chlorpheniramine Maleate Tablets (Geneva)................1083
Chlorpheniramine Maleate Tablets (Roxane)...................2074
Codimal-L.A. Capsules (Central Pharmaceuticals)....408, 868
Codimal-L.A. HALF Capsules (Central Pharmaceuticals)...........408, 868
D.A. Chewable Tablets (Dura)..............................978
Dallergy Capsules, Tablets, Syrup (Laser)...................1218
Donatussin Drops (Laser)..............1218
Duadacin Cold & Allergy Capsules (Kenwood)..............1189
Dura-Tap/PD Capsules (Dura)..............................978
Dura-Vent/A Capsules (Dura)..............................978
Dura-Vent/DA Tablets (Dura)..............................978
Endal-HD (UAD Laboratories)...........2427
Gelpirin CCF Tablets (Alra Laboratories)....................594
Histussin HC (Bock)....................700
Naldecon Syrup, Tablets, Pediatric Drops and Pediatric Syrup (Apothecon)......................616
P-V-Tussin Syrup (Solvay)..............2349
Pediacof Cough Syrup (Sanofi Winthrop Pharmaceuticals)................2162
Protid Tablets (Lunsco)................1347
Rescon Capsules (Ion Laboratories)...................1157
Rescon-DM Liquid (Ion Laboratories)...................1157
Rescon-ED Capsules (Ion Laboratories)...................1157
Rescon JR Capsules (Ion Laboratories)...................1157
Rescon Liquid (Ion Laboratories)...................1157
Tussar DM (Rhone-Poulenc Rorer Pharmaceuticals Inc.)....1908
Vanex Forte Caplets (Abana)...403, 502
Vanex-HD Liquid (Abana)......403, 502

CHLORPHENIRAMINE POLISTIREX
Tussionex Pennkinetic Extended-Release Suspension (Fisons Pharmaceuticals)...............1017

CHLORPHENIRAMINE TANNATE
Rynatan Tablets (Wallace)...435, 2502
Rynatan-S Pediatric Suspension (Wallace)......435, 2502
Rynatuss Pediatric Suspension (Wallace)......435, 2503
Rynatuss Tablets (Wallace)....435, 2503
R-Tannate Tablets and Pediatric Suspension (Warner Chilcott)................2507

CHLORPROMAZINE
Thorazine Suppositories (SmithKline Beecham Pharmaceuticals)...........431, 2327

CHLORPROMAZINE HYDROCHLORIDE
Thorazine Ampuls (SmithKline Beecham Pharmaceuticals)...........431, 2327
Thorazine Concentrate (SmithKline Beecham Pharmaceuticals)...........431, 2327
Thorazine Multi-dose Vials (SmithKline Beecham Pharmaceuticals)...........431, 2327
Thorazine Spansule Capsules (SmithKline Beecham Pharmaceuticals)...431, 2327
Thorazine Syrup (SmithKline Beecham Pharmaceuticals)...431, 2327
Thorazine Tablets (SmithKline Beecham Pharmaceuticals)...........431, 2327
Chlorpromazine Oral Concentrate (Geneva)..........1083
Chlorpromazine Hydrochloride Injection (Elkins-Sinn).................984
Chlorpromazine HCl Tablets (Geneva)........................1083

CHLORPROPAMIDE
Diabinese (Pfizer Labs Division)..................423, 1831
Chlorpropamide Tablets (Geneva)........................1083
Chlorpropamide Tablets (Mylan).......................1678
Chlorpropamide Tablets (Par).............................1739

CHLORPROTHIXENE
Taractan Tablets (Roche Laboratories)....................2010

CHLORPROTHIXENE HYDROCHLORIDE
Taractan Concentrate (Roche Laboratories).............2010
Taractan Injectable (Roche Laboratories).............2010

CHLORPROTHIXENE LACTATE
Taractan Concentrate (Roche Laboratories).............2010

CHLORTETRACYCLINE HYDROCHLORIDE
Aureomycin Ophthalmic Ointment 1.0% (Lederle)............1218

CHLORTHALIDONE
Combipres Tablets (Boehringer Ingelheim)............405, 705
Tenoretic Tablets (ICI Pharma)....................412, 1129
Chlorthalidone Tablets (Geneva)........................1083
Chlorthalidone Tablets (Mylan).......................1678
Clonidine HCl and Chlorthalidone Tablets (Par).............................1739
Clonidine Hydrochloride & Chlorthalidone Tablets (Mylan).......................1678
Demi-Regroton Tablets (Rhone-Poulenc Rorer Pharmaceuticals Inc.).........425, 1908
Hygroton Tablets (Rhone-Poulenc Rorer Pharmaceuticals Inc.).........424, 1908
Regroton Tablets (Rhone-Poulenc Rorer Pharmaceuticals Inc.).........425, 1908

CHLORZOXAZONE
Paraflex Caplets (McNeil Pharmaceutical)................1427
Parafon Forte DSC Caplets (McNeil Pharmaceutical)........418, 1428
Chlorzoxazone Tablets (Geneva)........................1083

Dilaudid-HP Injection (Knoll).. 413, 1201
Hydromorphone HCl Injection (Astra)... *648*
Hydromorphone Hydrochloride Injection (Elkins-Sinn)... *984*
Hydromorphone Hydrochloride in Tubex (Wyeth-Ayerst)... *2647*
Hydromorphone Hydrochloride Tablets (Roxane)... *2074*
HydroStat (Richwood)... *1930*

◆HYDROMOX TABLETS (Lederle)... 414, 1237

◆HYDROPRES TABLETS (Merck & Co., Inc.)... 419, 1536

HYDROQUINONE
Eldopaque Forte 4% Cream (ICN Pharmaceuticals)... 1138
Eldoquin Forte 4% Cream (ICN Pharmaceuticals)... 1138
Neutrogena Melanex Topical Solution (Neutrogena)... 421, 1680
Solaquin Forte 4% Cream (ICN Pharmaceuticals)... 1147
Solaquin Forte 4% Gel (ICN Pharmaceuticals)... 1148

HydroStat (Richwood)... *1930*

HYDROXYCHLOROQUINE SULFATE
Plaquenil Sulfate Tablets (Sanofi Winthrop Pharmaceuticals)... 428, 2163

HYDROXYPROPYL CELLULOSE
Lacrisert Sterile Ophthalmic Insert (Merck & Co., Inc.)... 1544

HYDROXYPROPYL METHYLCELLULOSE
Tears Naturale II Lubricant Eye Drops (Alcon Laboratories)... 572
Tears Naturale Free (Alcon Laboratories)... 572
Occucoat (See PDR For Ophthalmology) (Lederle)... *1258*

HYDROXYUREA
Hydrea Capsules (Immunex)... 1152

HYDROXYZINE HYDROCHLORIDE
Atarax Tablets & Syrup (Roerig)... 426, 2030
Marax Tablets & DF Syrup (Roerig)... 427, 2042
Vistaril Intramuscular Solution (Roerig)... 2058
Hydroxyzine Syrup (Warner Chilcott)... *2507*
Hydroxyzine HCl Tablets (Par)... *1739*
Hydroxyzine HCl Tablets (Geneva)... *1083*
Hydroxyzine Hydrochloride Injection (Elkins-Sinn)... *984*

HYDROXYZINE PAMOATE
Hydroxyzine Pamoate Capsules (Geneva)... 1083
Vistaril Capsules (Pfizer Labs Division)... 423, 1844
Vistaril Oral Suspension (Pfizer Labs Division)... 1844

◆Hygroton Tablets (Rhone-Poulenc Rorer Pharmaceuticals Inc.)... *424, 1908*

HYLOREL TABLETS (Fisons Pharmaceuticals)... 1003

HYOSCINE HYDROBROMIDE (see under SCOPOLAMINE HYDROBROMIDE)

HYOSCYAMINE
Cystospaz (Webcon)... 2509
Urised Tablets (Webcon)... 2510

HYOSCYAMINE HYDROBROMIDE
Pyridium Plus (Parke-Davis).... 423, 1818

HYOSCYAMINE SULFATE
Arco-Lase Plus (Arco)... 625
Atrohist Plus Tablets (Adams)... 557
Cystospaz-M (Webcon)... 2509
Donnatal Capsules (Robins Company)... 425, 1940
Donnatal Elixir (Robins Company)... 1940
Donnatal Extentabs (Robins Company)... 425, 1941
Donnatal Tablets (Robins Company)... 425, 1940
Kutrase Capsules (Schwarz Pharma)... 429, 2240
Levsin Drops (Schwarz Pharma)... 2241
Levsin Elixir (Schwarz Pharma)... 2241
Levsin Injection (Schwarz Pharma)... 2241
Levsin Tablets (Schwarz Pharma)... 429, 2241
Levsin/SL Tablets (Schwarz Pharma)... 429, 2241
Levsinex Timecaps (Schwarz Pharma)... 429, 2241
Ru-Tuss Tablets (Boots Pharmaceuticals)... 405, 719
Anaspaz Tablets (Ascher)... *632*
Rexatal Tablets (Rexar)... *1907*

HYPERAB RABIES IMMUNE GLOBULIN (HUMAN) (Miles Biological)... 1663
HYPERHEP HEPATITIS B IMMUNE GLOBULIN (HUMAN) (Miles Biological)... 1665
HYPERSTAT I.V. INJECTION (Schering)... 2193
HYPER-TET TETANUS IMMUNE GLOBULIN (HUMAN) (Miles Biological)... 1666
HYPRHO-D RH_o-D IMMUNE GLOBULIN (HUMAN) (Miles Biological)... 1668
HYPRHO-D MINI-DOSE RH_o-D IMMUNE GLOBULIN (HUMAN) (Miles Biological)... 1667
HYSKON HYSTEROSCOPY FLUID (Kabi Pharmacia)... 1188
HYTONE CREAM 1%, 2 ½% (Dermik)... 933
HYTONE LOTION 1%, 2 ½% (Dermik)... 933
HYTONE OINTMENT 1%, 2 ½% (Dermik)... 933
◆HYTRIN TABLETS (Abbott)... 403, 529

I

IBU-TAB OTC Tablets, Ibuprofen Tablets, USP (Alra Laboratories)... *594*
IBU (IBUPROFEN TABLETS, USP) (Boots Laboratories)... 716
ILX B_{12} Caplets Crystalline (Kenwood)... *1189*
ILX B_{12} Elixir Crystalline and ILX B_{12} Sugar Free Elixir (Kenwood)... *1189*
ILX Elixir (Kenwood)... *1189*
INH TABLETS (CIBA Pharmaceutical)... 898
IBERET (Abbott)... 531
◆IBERET-500 FILMTAB (Abbott).... 403, 531
IBERET-500 LIQUID (Abbott)... 531
◆IBERET-FOLIC-500 (Abbott)... 403, 528
IBERET-LIQUID (Abbott)... 531

IBUPROFEN
Advil Cold & Sinus Caplets (formerly CoAdvil) (Whitehall)... 435, 2530
Advil Ibuprofen Tablets and Caplets (Whitehall)... 435, 2529
Children's Advil Suspension (Wyeth-Ayerst)... 436, 2537
Dristan Sinus Caplets (Whitehall)... 436, 2533
IBU (Ibuprofen Tablets, USP) (Boots Laboratories)... 716
Motrin Tablets (Upjohn)... 434, 2466
Nuprin Ibuprofen/Analgesic Tablets & Caplets (Bristol-Myers Products)... 406, 768
Pedia-Profen Suspension (McNeil Consumer)... 417, 1411
IBU-TAB OTC Tablets, Ibuprofen Tablets, USP (Alra Laboratories)... *594*
Ibuprofen Tablets (Mylan)... *1678*
Ibuprofen Tablets (Par)... *1739*
Ibuprofen Tablets (Warner Chilcott)... *2507*
IBU-TAB Rx Tablets, Ibuprofen Tablets, USP (Alra Laboratories)... *594*

IDAMYCIN FOR INJECTION (Adria)... 563

IDARUBICIN HYDROCHLORIDE
Idamycin for Injection (Adria)... 563

◆Identi-Code (Lilly)... *416*
Identi-Dose (Lilly)... *1279*
◆IFEX (Bristol-Myers Oncology)... 406, 745

IFOSFAMIDE
IFEX (Bristol-Myers Oncology)... 406, 745

ILETIN I (Lilly)... 1308
ILETIN I, LENTE (Lilly)... 1308
ILETIN I NPH (Lilly)... 1308
ILETIN I, REGULAR (Lilly)... 1308
ILETIN I, SEMILENTE (Lilly)... 1308
ILETIN I, ULTRALENTE (Lilly)... 1308
ILETIN II (Lilly)... 1310
LENTE ILETIN II, BEEF (Lilly)... 1310
NPH ILETIN II, BEEF (Lilly)... 1310
REGULAR ILETIN II, BEEF (Lilly)... 1310
LENTE ILETIN II, PORK (Lilly)... 1310
NPH ILETIN II, PORK (Lilly)... 1310
REGULAR ILETIN II, PORK, 100 UNITS (Lilly)... 1311
REGULAR ILETIN II (CONCENTRATED), PORK, 500 UNITS (Lilly)... 1312
ILOSONE LIQUID, ORAL SUSPENSIONS (Dista)... 936
◆ILOSONE PULVULES & TABLETS (Dista)... 408, 936
ILOTYCIN GLUCEPTATE (Dista)... 938
ILOTYCIN OPHTHALMIC OINTMENT (Dista)... 937
IMFERON (Fisons Pharmaceuticals)... 1005

IMIPENEM-CILASTATIN SODIUM
Primaxin I.M. (Merck & Co., Inc.)... 1585
Primaxin IV (Merck & Co., Inc.)... 1587

IMIPRAMINE HYDROCHLORIDE
Tofranil Ampuls (Geigy)... 1070
Tofranil Tablets (Geigy)... 410, 1071
Imipramine Hydrochloride Tablets (Biocraft)... *698*
Imipramine HCl Tablets (Geneva)... *1083*
Imipramine HCl Tablets (Par)... *1739*
Imipramine Hydrochloride Tablets (Roxane)... *2074*

IMIPRAMINE PAMOATE
Tofranil-PM Capsules (Geigy) 410, 1073

IMMUNE GLOBULIN (HUMAN)
Gamimune N Immune Globulin Intravenous (Human) (Miles Biological).. 420, 1662
Gammagard, Immune Globulin, Intravenous (Human) (Baxter Healthcare)... 681
HypRho-D Rh_o-D Immune Globulin (Human) (Miles Biological)... 1668
HypRho-D Mini-Dose Rh_o-D Immune Globulin (Human) (Miles Biological)... 1667
MICRhoGAM (Ortho Diagnostic Systems)... 1707
Polygam, Immune Globulin Intravenous (Human) (American Red Cross)... 601
RhoGAM (Ortho Diagnostic Systems)... 1707
Sandoglobulin I.V. (Sandoz Pharmaceuticals)... 427, 2122
Iveegam (Immuno-U.S.)... *1156*
Venoglobulin-I (Alpha Therapeutic)... *593*
Venoglobulin-S 5% Solution Solvent Detergent Treated, Immune Globulin Intravenous (Human) (Alpha Therapeutic)... *593*

◆IMODIUM A-D CAPLETS AND LIQUID (McNeil Consumer)... 417, 1410
◆IMODIUM CAPSULES (Janssen).. 412, 1166
Imogam Rabies Immune Globulin (Human) (Connaught)... *918*
Imovax Rabies I.D. (Connaught)... *918*
Imovax Rabies Vaccine (Merieux) (Connaught)... *918*
IMPREGON CONCENTRATE (Fleming)... 1023
IMURAN INJECTION (Burroughs Wellcome)... 785
◆IMURAN TABLETS (Burroughs Wellcome)... 407, 785
◆INAPSINE INJECTION (Janssen)... 412, 1167
Incremin with Iron Syrup (Lederle)... ▣

INDAPAMIDE
Lozol Tablets (Rhone-Poulenc Rorer Pharmaceuticals Inc.).. 424, 1916

◆INDERAL INJECTABLE (Wyeth-Ayerst)... 436, 2571
◆INDERAL TABLETS (Wyeth-Ayerst)... 436, 2571
◆INDERAL LA LONG ACTING CAPSULES (Wyeth-Ayerst)... 436, 2573
◆INDERIDE TABLETS (Wyeth-Ayerst)... 436, 2575
◆INDERIDE LA LONG ACTING CAPSULES (Wyeth-Ayerst)... 436, 2576
◆INDOCIN CAPSULES (Merck & Co., Inc.)... 419, 1538
INDOCIN I.V. (Merck & Co., Inc.)... 1541
INDOCIN ORAL SUSPENSION (Merck & Co., Inc.)... 1538
◆INDOCIN SR CAPSULES (Merck & Co., Inc.)... 419, 1538
◆INDOCIN SUPPOSITORIES (Merck & Co., Inc.)... 419, 1538

INDOMETHACIN
Indocin Capsules (Merck & Co., Inc.)... 419, 1538
Indocin Oral Suspension (Merck & Co., Inc.)... 1538
Indocin SR Capsules (Merck & Co., Inc.)... 419, 1538
Indocin Suppositories (Merck & Co., Inc.)... 419, 1538
Indomethacin Capsules (Lederle)... *1218*
Indomethacin Capsules (Mylan)... *1678*
Indomethacin Capsules (Novopharm)... *1686*
Indomethacin Capsules (Par)... *1739*
Indomethacin Capsules (Geneva)... *1083*
Indomethacin Capsules and Extended-Release Capsules, USP (Warner Chilcott)... *2507*
Indomethacin E.R. Capsules (Inwood)... *1157*

INDOMETHACIN SODIUM TRIHYDRATE
Indocin I.V. (Merck & Co., Inc.)... 1541

◆INFED IRON DEXTRAN INJECTION (Schein Pharmaceutical)... 428, 2176

INFLUENZA VIRUS VACCINE
Flu-Imune Influenza Virus Vaccine (Lederle)... 1232
Fluogen (Parke-Davis)... *1776*
Influenza Virus Vaccine, Trivalent, Types A & B (chromatographed and filter-purified subviron antigen) 1992-93 Formula (Wyeth-Ayerst)... *2578*
Influenza Virus Vaccine, Trivalent, Types A & B, 1992-93 Formula, in Tubex (Wyeth-Ayerst)... *2647*

INFUMORPH 200 AND INFUMORPH 500 STERILE SOLUTIONS (Elkins-Sinn)... 989
◆INNOVAR INJECTION (Janssen)... 412, 1168
INOCOR LACTATE INJECTION (Sanofi Winthrop Pharmaceuticals)... 2143

INOSITOL
Amino-Cerv (Milex)... 1675
Mega-B (Arco)... 625
Megadose (Arco)... *625*

InspirEase (Schering)... *2194*
INSTAT COLLAGEN ABSORBABLE HEMOSTAT (Johnson & Johnson Medical)... 1177
INSULATARD NPH (Novo Nordisk)... 1682
INSULATARD NPH HUMAN (Novo Nordisk)... 1684

INSULIN, HUMAN ISOPHANE SUSPENSION
Novolin N (Novo Nordisk)... 1684

INSULIN, HUMAN NPH
Humulin N, 100 Units (Lilly)... 1305

(◆ Shown in Product Identification Section)   *Italic Page Number* Indicates Brief Listing   (▣ Described in PDR For Nonprescription Drugs)

(♦ **Shown in Product Identification Section**)   *Italic Page Number* Indicates Brief Listing   (▣ **Described in PDR For Nonprescription Drugs**)

SECTION 3
Product Category Index

Products described in the Product Information (White) or Diagnostic Product Information (Green) Sections are listed according to their classifications. The headings and sub-headings have been determined by the Publisher with the cooperation of the individual manufacturers. In cases where there were differences of opinion or where the manufacturer had no opinion, the Publisher made the final decision. A QUICK-REFERENCE INDEX of headings and sub-headings can be found below.

Product Category Quick-Reference

A
AIDS CHEMOTHERAPEUTIC AGENTS
AIDS RELATED COMPLEX (ARC) THERAPEUTIC AGENTS
ALCOHOL ABUSE REDUCTION PREPARATIONS
ALLERGENS
AMINO ACID PREPARATIONS
ANALGESICS
  ACETAMINOPHEN & COMBINATIONS
  ACETAMINOPHEN WITH ANTACIDS
  ASPIRIN
  ASPIRIN COMBINATIONS
  ASPIRIN WITH ANTACIDS
  ASPIRIN WITH CODEINE
  NSAIDS
  NARCOTIC AGONIST-ANTAGONIST
  NARCOTICS, SYNTHETICS & COMBINATIONS
  NEURALEPTANALGESIA
  NON-NARCOTIC AGONIST-ANTAGONIST
  OTHER SALICYLATES & COMBINATIONS
  TOPICAL-ANALGESIC
  TOPICAL-ANTINEURALGIA
  TOPICAL-COUNTERIRRITANT
  OTHER
ANESTHETICS
  CAUDAL
  EPIDURAL
  INHALATION
  INJECTABLE
  LOCAL
  RECTAL
  RETROBULBAR
  SPINAL
  TOPICAL
  TOPICAL MUCOSAL
ANORECTAL PRODUCTS
  CREAMS, FOAMS, LOTIONS, OINTMENTS
  SUPPOSITORIES
  OTHER
ANTACIDS & ANTIFLATULENTS
  ALUMINUM ANTACIDS
  ANTACID/ANTIFLATULENT COMBINATIONS
  ANTIFLATULENTS
  CALCIUM ANTACIDS
  COMBINATION ANTACIDS
  MAGALDRATE ANTACIDS
  MAGNESIUM ANTACIDS
ANTIBIOTICS, SYSTEMIC
  (see also ANTI-INFECTIVES,
  MISCELLANEOUS SYSTEMIC;
  ANTIPARASITICS; QUINOLONES, SYSTEMIC;
  SULFONAMIDES & COMBINATIONS,
  SYSTEMIC; URINARY ANTI-INFECTIVES &
  ANALGESIC COMBINATIONS)
  AMINOGLYCOSIDES & COMBINATIONS
  CEPHALOSPORINS
    1ST GENERATION
    2ND GENERATION
    3RD GENERATION
  MACROLIDES
    ERYTHROMYCINS
    OTHER
  MONOBACTAMS
  PENICILLINS
  TETRACYCLINES
  MISCELLANEOUS ANTIBIOTICS
ANTICOAGULANT ANTAGONIST
ANTICOAGULANTS
ANTIDOTES
  ANTICHOLINESTERASE
  BENZODIAZEPINE ANTAGONIST
  DIGOXIN
  NARCOTIC ANTAGONIST
  METAL POISONING
ANTIHISTAMINES

ANTI-INFECTIVES, MISCELLANEOUS SYSTEMIC
ANTI-INFLAMMATORY AGENTS
  NON-STEROIDALS
  SALICYLATES
  STEROIDS & COMBINATIONS
  OTHER
ANTINEOPLASTICS
  ADJUNCT
  ANDROGEN INHIBITOR
  ANTIBIOTIC DERIVATIVES
  ANTIESTROGEN
  ANTIMETABOLITES
  CYTOTOXIC AGENTS
  HORMONES
  IMMUNOMODULATORS
  NITROGEN MUSTARD DERIVATIVES
  STEROIDS & COMBINATIONS
  OTHER
ANTIOXIDANTS
ANTIPARASITICS
  ARTHROPODS
    LICE
    SCABIES
  HELMINTHS
    ASCARIS (ROUNDWORM)
    ENTEROBIUS (PINWORM)
    HOOKWORM
    STRONGYLOIDS (THREADWORM)
    TAENIA (TAPEWORM)
    TREMATODES (SCHISTOSOMES)
    TRICHURIS (WHIPWORM)
  PROTOZOA
    AMEBAS, EXTRAINTESTINAL
    AMEBAS, INTESTINAL
    GIARDIAS
    MALARIA
    TOXOPLASMA
    TRICHOMONAS
ANTIPYRETICS
ANTISEPTICS
ANTISPASMODICS & ANTICHOLINERGICS
  GASTROINTESTINAL
  OTHER
ANTIVIRALS, SYSTEMIC
APPETITE SUPPRESSANTS
  AMPHETAMINES
  NON-AMPHETAMINES
ARTHRITIS MEDICATIONS
  GOLD COMPOUNDS
  NSAIDS
  SALICYLATES
  STEROIDS
  OTHERS

B
BABY PRODUCTS
BIOLOGICAL RESPONSE MODIFIERS
BIOLOGICALS
  ALPHA₁-ANTITRYPSIN
  ANTIGENS
  ANTISERUM
  RH₀ (D) IMMUNE GLOBULIN (HUMAN)
  SERUM
  TOXOIDS
  VACCINES
  VACCINES (LIVE)
  OTHER
BLOOD & BLOOD COMPONENTS
BONE METABOLISM REGULATOR
  HETEROTOPIC OSSIFICATION AGENT
  HYPERCALCEMIC AGENT
  PAGETIC AGENT
BOWEL EVACUANTS

C
CALCIUM PREPARATIONS
  CALCIUM REGULATOR
  CALCIUM SUPPLEMENTS
  CALCIUM SUPPLEMENTS WITH VITAMINS
CARDIOVASCULAR AGENTS
  ADRENERGIC BLOCKERS, PERIPHERAL & COMBINATIONS
  ADRENERGIC STIMULANTS, CENTRAL & COMBINATIONS
  ALPHA/BETA ADRENERGIC BLOCKERS
  ANGIOTENSIN CONVERTING ENZYME INHIBITORS
  ANGIOTENSIN CONVERTING ENZYME INHIBITORS WITH DIURETICS
  ANTIARRHYTHMICS
    GROUP I
    GROUP II
    GROUP III
    GROUP IV
    MISCELLANEOUS ANTIARRHYTHMICS
  BETA BLOCKERS
  BETA BLOCKERS WITH DIURETICS
  CALCIUM CHANNEL BLOCKERS
  DIURETICS
    CARBONIC ANHYDRASE INHIBITORS
    COMBINATION DIURETICS
    LOOP DIURETICS
    POTASSIUM-SPARING DIURETICS
    THIAZIDES & RELATED DIURETICS
  HYPERTENSIVE EMERGENCY AGENTS
  INOTROPIC AGENTS
  PATENT DUCTUS ARTERIOSUS THERAPY
  RAUWOLFIA DERIVATIVES & COMBINATIONS
  VASODILATORS, CEREBRAL
  VASODILATORS, CORONARY
  VASODILATORS, PERIPHERAL & COMBINATIONS
  VASOPRESSORS
  MISCELLANEOUS CARDIOVASCULAR AGENTS
CATECHOLAMINE SYNTHESIS INHIBITOR
CENTRAL NERVOUS SYSTEM STIMULANTS
CEREBRAL METABOLIC ENHANCER
CERUMENOLYTICS
CHOLINESTERASE INHIBITOR
COLD & COUGH PREPARATIONS
  ANTIHISTAMINES & COMBINATIONS
  ANTITUSSIVES & COMBINATIONS
  ANTITUSSIVES & COMBINATIONS WITH NARCOTICS
  DECONGESTANTS
    DECONGESTANTS, EXPECTORANTS & COMBINATIONS
    ORAL & COMBINATIONS
    TOPICAL
  EXPECTORANTS & COMBINATIONS
  OTHER
COLONY STIMULATING FACTORS
  GRANULOCYTE (G-CSF)
  GRANULOCYTE MACROPHAGE (GM-CSF)
CONTRACEPTIVES
  DEVICES
  DEVICES, COPPER CONTAINING
  IMPLANTS
  ORAL
COSMETICS
CYTOPROTECTIVE AGENTS

D
DENTAL PREPARATIONS
  OTHER
DEODORANTS
  INTERNAL
  ORAL
  TOPICAL
DERMATOLOGICALS
  ABRADANT
  ACNE PREPARATIONS

ANALGESIC
ANTIBACTERIALS
ANTIBACTERIALS, ANTIFUNGALS & COMBINATIONS
ANTIBIOTICS
ANTI-INFLAMMATORY AGENTS
ANTIPERSPIRANTS
BARRIER
BURN RELIEF
CLEANSING AGENTS
COAL TAR
CONDITIONING RINSES
DANDRUFF MEDICATIONS
DEODORANTS
DEPIGMENTING AGENT
DERMATITIS HERPETIFORMIS
DERMATITIS RELIEF
DETERGENTS
DIAPER RASH RELIEF
DRYING AGENT
EMOLLIENTS
EPIDERMAL & CELLULAR GROWTH
FUNGICIDES
GENERAL
HERPES TREATMENT
INSECT BITES & STINGS
KERATOLYTICS
MOISTURIZERS
NAIL ENHANCER
PHOTOSENSITIZER
POISON IVY, OAK OR SUMAC
POWDERS
PRURITUS MEDICATIONS
PSORIASIS AGENTS
SCABICIDES
SEBORRHEA TREATMENT
SHAMPOOS
SHAVE CREAM
SKIN BLEACHES
SKIN PROTECTANT
STEROIDS & COMBINATIONS
SUNBURN PREPARATIONS
SUNSCREENS
WART REMOVERS
WET DRESSINGS
WOUND CLEANSER
WOUND DRESSINGS
OTHER

DETOXIFYING AGENT
DIABETES AGENTS
  INTERMEDIATE ACTING INSULINS
  INTERMEDIATE ACTING INSULINS (PREMIXED)
  INTERMEDIATE AND RAPID ACTING INSULIN COMBINATIONS (PREMIXED)
  LONG ACTING INSULINS
  ORAL
  RAPID ACTING INSULINS
DIAGNOSTICS
  ACTH TEST
  ALLERGY, SKIN TESTS
  ANGIOCARDIOGRAPHY
  ANGIOGRAPHY
  AORTOGRAPHY
  ARTHROGRAPHY
  BLOOD GLUCOSE
  BRONCHIAL AIRWAY HYPERREACTIVITY
  CEREBRAL ANGIOGRAPHY
  CISTERNOGRAPHY-CT
  CT SCAN ENHANCEMENT
  DIABETES TESTS
    BLOOD
  ENDOSCOPIC RETROGRADE PANCREATOGRAPHY (ERP)/ENDOSCOPIC RETROGRADE CHOLANGIOPANCREATOGRAPHY (ERCP)
  EXCRETORY UROGRAPHY
  GASTRIC ACID TEST
  HERNIOGRAPHY
  HYPOTHALAMIC DYSFUNCTION TEST
  HYSTEROSALPINGOGRAPHY

Product Category Index

A

Italic Page Number **Indicates Brief Listing**

MAGNESIUM PREPARATIONS
Beelith Tablets (Beach) ... 405, 682
Magonate Tablets and Liquid (Fleming) ... 1023
Mag-Ox 400 (Blaine) ... 699
MagTab SR Caplets (Niché Pharmaceuticals) ... 1680
Uro-Mag (Blaine) ... 699
POTASSIUM PREPARATIONS
K-Dur (Key Pharmaceuticals) ... 413, 1190
K-Lor Powder Packets (Abbott) 403, 531
K-Norm Extended-Release Capsules (Fisons Pharmaceuticals) ... 1011
K-Tab (Abbott) ... 403, 532
Kato Potassium Supplement (ICN Pharmaceuticals) ... 1140
Klor-Con 8/Klor-Con 10 Tablets (Upsher-Smith) ... 434, 2489
Klorvess Effervescent Granules (Sandoz Pharmaceuticals) ... 2106
Klorvess Effervescent Tablets (Sandoz Pharmaceuticals) ... 2106
Klorvess 10% Liquid (Sandoz Pharmaceuticals) ... 2106
Kolyum Liquid (Fisons Pharmaceuticals) ... 1012
Micro-K Extencaps (Robins Company) ... 425, 1944
Micro-K 10 Extencaps (Robins Company) ... 425, 1944
Micro-K LS Packets (Robins Company) ... 1946
Polycitra-K Crystals (Baker Norton) ... 670
Polycitra-K Oral Solution (Baker Norton) ... 670
Rum-K (Fleming) ... 1023
Slow-K (Summit) ... 433, 2384
Ten-K Controlled-Release Tablets (Summit) ... 433, 2385
OTHER
GoLYTELY (Braintree) ... 406, 724
NuLYTELY (Braintree) ... 406, 724
Uro-Mag (Blaine) ... 699

ENDOMETRIOSIS MANAGEMENT
Danocrine Capsules (Sanofi Winthrop Pharmaceuticals) ... 428, 2141
Synarel Nasal Solution (Syntex) ... 433, 2407

ENURESIS
DDAVP Nasal Spray (Rhone-Poulenc Rorer Pharmaceuticals Inc.) ... 424, 1912
DDAVP Rhinal Tube (Rhone-Poulenc Rorer Pharmaceuticals Inc.) ... 424, 1912
Tofranil Tablets (Geigy) ... 410, 1071

ENZYMES & DIGESTANTS
ADENOSINE DEAMINASE DEFICIENCY
Adagen Injection (Enzon) ... 994
COLLAGENOLYTIC
Collagenase Santyl Ointment (Knoll) ... 414, 1199
DIGESTANTS
Arco-Lase Plus (Arco) ... 625
Arco-Lase (Arco) ... 625
Cotazym (Organon) ... 420, 1692
Creon Capsules (Solvay) ... 432, 2340
Creon 25 Capsules (Solvay) ... 432, 2340
Donnazyme Tablets (Robins Company) ... 425, 1941
Entozyme Tablets (Robins Company) ... 425, 1943
Kutrase Capsules (Schwarz Pharma) ... 429, 2240
Ku-Zyme Capsules (Schwarz Pharma) ... 429, 2240
Ku-Zyme HP Capsules (Schwarz Pharma) ... 429, 2241
Lactaid Caplets (Lactaid) ... 414, 1217
Lactaid Drops (Lactaid) ... 414, 1217
Pancrease Capsules (McNeil Pharmaceutical) ... 418, 1426
Pancrease MT Capsules (McNeil Pharmaceutical) ... 418, 1427
Viokase Powder (Robins Company) ... 1959
Viokase Tablets (Robins Company) ... 425, 1959
Zymase Capsules (Organon) ... 421, 1702
FIBRINOLYTIC & PROTEOLYTIC
Elase Ointment (Fujisawa) ... 1044
Elase Vials (Fujisawa) ... 1044
Elase-Chloromycetin Ointment (Fujisawa) ... 1044
Granulex (Dow Hickam) ... 1112
Panafil Ointment (Rystan) ... 2086
Panafil-White Ointment (Rystan) ... 2086
Travase Ointment (Boots Pharmaceuticals) ... 406, 723
Zymase Capsules (Organon) ... 421, 1702
TOPICAL
Collagenase Santyl Ointment (Knoll) ... 414, 1199
Panafil Ointment (Rystan) ... 2086
Panafil-White Ointment (Rystan) ... 2086
Travase Ointment (Boots Pharmaceuticals) ... 406, 723

EPILEPSY
(see SEIZURE DISORDERS)

ERGOT PREPARATIONS
MIGRAINE PREPARATIONS
Cafergot Suppositories (Sandoz Pharmaceuticals) ... 2092
Cafergot Tablets (Sandoz Pharmaceuticals) ... 427, 2092
Wigraine Tablets & Suppositories (Organon) ... 421, 1701
UTERINE CONTRACTANT
Methergine Injection (Sandoz Pharmaceuticals) ... 2112
Methergine Tablets (Sandoz Pharmaceuticals) ... 2112

ERYTHROPOIESIS ENHANCERS
(see HEMATINICS)

EXPECTORANTS
(see COLD & COUGH PREPARATIONS)

EYEWASHES
(see OPHTHALMIC PREPARATIONS)

F

FERTILITY AGENTS
Metrodin (urofollitropin for injection) (Serono) ... 2272
Parlodel Capsules (Sandoz Pharmaceuticals) ... 427, 2116
Parlodel SnapTabs (Sandoz Pharmaceuticals) ... 427, 2116
Pergonal (menotropins for injection, USP) (Serono) ... 2274
Profasi (chorionic gonadotropin for injection, USP) (Serono) ... 2276
Serophene (clomiphene citrate tablets, USP) (Serono) ... 2277

FEVER BLISTER AIDS
(see HERPES TREATMENT)

FEVER PREPARATIONS
(see ANALGESICS)

FIBER SUPPLEMENTS
Ensure With Fiber (Ross) ... 2062
Glucerna Specialized Nutrition with Fiber for Patients with Abnormal Glucose Tolerance (Ross) ... 2062
Jevity Isotonic Liquid Nutrition with Fiber (Ross) ... 2062

FIBRINOLYTIC AGENTS
Amicar (Lederle) ... 414, 1223
Cyklokapron Tablets and Injection (Kabi Pharmacia) ... 1185

FIBROTICS, SYSTEMIC
Potaba (Glenwood) ... 411, 1102

FLUORESCENT IMMUNOASSAYS
(see THERAPEUTIC DRUG ASSAYS)

FLUORIDE PREPARATIONS
Fluoritab Liquid (Fluoritab) ... 1024
Fluoritab Tablets (Fluoritab) ... 1024
Luride Drops (Colgate-Hoyt/Gel-Kam) ... 913
Luride Lozi-Tabs Tablets (Colgate-Hoyt/Gel-Kam) ... 913
Pediaflor Drops (Ross) ... 2063

FOODS
ALLERGY DIET
Tolerex (Sandoz Nutrition) ... 2086
CARBOHYDRATE
Polycose Glucose Polymers (Ross) ... 2065
COMPLETE THERAPEUTIC
AlitraQ Specialized Elemental Nutrition With Glutamine (Ross) ... 2061
Ensure Liquid Nutrition (Ross) ... 2061
Ensure Plus High Calorie Liquid Nutrition (Ross) ... 2062
Ensure With Fiber (Ross) ... 2062
Nepro Specialized Liquid Nutrition (Ross) ... 2063
Osmolite Isotonic Liquid Nutrition (Ross) ... 2063
Osmolite HN High Nitrogen Isotonic Liquid Nutrition (Ross) ... 2063
PediaSure Liquid Nutrition for Children (Ross) ... 2064
Perative Specialized Liquid Nutrition (Ross) ... *2065*
Pulmocare Specialized Nutrition for Pulmonary Patients (Ross) ... 2066
Tolerex (Sandoz Nutrition) ... 2086
Vital High Nitrogen Nutritionally Complete Partially Hydrolyzed Diet (Ross) ... 2074
Vivonex T.E.N. (Sandoz Nutrition) ... 2087
ENTERAL
AlitraQ Specialized Elemental Nutrition With Glutamine (Ross) ... 2061
Ensure Liquid Nutrition (Ross) ... 2061
Ensure Plus High Calorie Liquid Nutrition (Ross) ... 2062
Ensure With Fiber (Ross) ... 2062
Glucerna Specialized Nutrition with Fiber for Patients with Abnormal Glucose Tolerance (Ross) ... 2062
Jevity Isotonic Liquid Nutrition with Fiber (Ross) ... 2062
Nepro Specialized Liquid Nutrition (Ross) ... 2063
Osmolite Isotonic Liquid Nutrition (Ross) ... 2063
Osmolite HN High Nitrogen Isotonic Liquid Nutrition (Ross) ... 2063
PediaSure Liquid Nutrition for Children (Ross) ... 2064
Perative Specialized Liquid Nutrition (Ross) ... *2065*
Polycose Glucose Polymers (Ross) ... 2065
Promote High Protein Liquid Nutrition (Ross) ... 2066
Pulmocare Specialized Nutrition for Pulmonary Patients (Ross) ... 2066
Tolerex (Sandoz Nutrition) ... 2086
Vital High Nitrogen Nutritionally Complete Partially Hydrolyzed Diet (Ross) ... 2074
Vivonex T.E.N. (Sandoz Nutrition) ... 2087
HIGH CALORIE
Nepro Specialized Liquid Nutrition (Ross) ... 2063
Suplena Specialized Liquid Nutrition (Ross) ... 2069
HIGH FAT
Pulmocare Specialized Nutrition for Pulmonary Patients (Ross) ... 2066
HIGH NITROGEN
AlitraQ Specialized Elemental Nutrition With Glutamine (Ross) ... 2061
Jevity Isotonic Liquid Nutrition with Fiber (Ross) ... 2062
Osmolite HN High Nitrogen Isotonic Liquid Nutrition (Ross) ... 2063
Perative Specialized Liquid Nutrition (Ross) ... *2065*
Promote High Protein Liquid Nutrition (Ross) ... 2066
Pulmocare Specialized Nutrition for Pulmonary Patients (Ross) ... 2066
Vital High Nitrogen Nutritionally Complete Partially Hydrolyzed Diet (Ross) ... 2074
Vivonex T.E.N. (Sandoz Nutrition) ... 2087
INFANT
(see INFANT FORMULAS)
LACTOSE FREE
Ensure Liquid Nutrition (Ross) ... 2061
Ensure Plus High Calorie Liquid Nutrition (Ross) ... 2062
Ensure With Fiber (Ross) ... 2062
Jevity Isotonic Liquid Nutrition with Fiber (Ross) ... 2062
Osmolite Isotonic Liquid Nutrition (Ross) ... 2063
Osmolite HN High Nitrogen Isotonic Liquid Nutrition (Ross) ... 2063
Promote High Protein Liquid Nutrition (Ross) ... 2066
Pulmocare Specialized Nutrition for Pulmonary Patients (Ross) ... 2066
Tolerex (Sandoz Nutrition) ... 2086
Vivonex T.E.N. (Sandoz Nutrition) ... 2087
LOW NITROGEN
Suplena Specialized Liquid Nutrition (Ross) ... 2069
LOW PROTEIN
Suplena Specialized Liquid Nutrition (Ross) ... 2069
LOW RESIDUE
AlitraQ Specialized Elemental Nutrition With Glutamine (Ross) ... 2061
Ensure Liquid Nutrition (Ross) ... 2061
Ensure Plus High Calorie Liquid Nutrition (Ross) ... 2062
Osmolite Isotonic Liquid Nutrition (Ross) ... 2063
Osmolite HN High Nitrogen Isotonic Liquid Nutrition (Ross) ... 2063
Perative Specialized Liquid Nutrition (Ross) ... *2065*
Promote High Protein Liquid Nutrition (Ross) ... 2066
Pulmocare Specialized Nutrition for Pulmonary Patients (Ross) ... 2066
Tolerex (Sandoz Nutrition) ... 2086
Vital High Nitrogen Nutritionally Complete Partially Hydrolyzed Diet (Ross) ... 2074
Vivonex T.E.N. (Sandoz Nutrition) ... 2087
MEDIUM CHAIN TRIGLYCERIDES
Jevity Isotonic Liquid Nutrition with Fiber (Ross) ... 2062
Osmolite Isotonic Liquid Nutrition (Ross) ... 2063
Osmolite HN High Nitrogen Isotonic Liquid Nutrition (Ross) ... 2063
Vital High Nitrogen Nutritionally Complete Partially Hydrolyzed Diet (Ross) ... 2074
METABOLIC DYSFUNCTION
Nepro Specialized Liquid Nutrition (Ross) ... 2063
Ross Metabolic Formula System (Ross) ... *2068*

FORMULAS
(see INFANT FORMULAS)

FUNGAL MEDICATIONS, SYSTEMIC
Ancobon Capsules (Roche Laboratories) ... 425, 1967
Diflucan Injection and Tablets (Roerig) ... 427, 2038
Fulvicin P/G Tablets (Schering) 428, 2186
Fulvicin P/G 165 & 330 Tablets (Schering) ... 428, 2187
Grifulvin V Tablets/Suspension (Ortho Pharmaceutical (Dermatological Div.)) ... 421, 1734
Grisactin Capsules (Wyeth-Ayerst) ... 436, 2566
Grisactin Tablets (Wyeth-Ayerst) ... 436, 2566
Grisactin Ultra Tablets (Wyeth-Ayerst) ... 436, 2567
Gris-PEG Tablets, 125 mg & 250 mg (Allergan Herbert) ... 586
Grivate Tablets & Suspension (Fujisawa) ... 1047
Monistat I.V. (Janssen) ... 412, 1170
Mycelex Troches (Miles Pharmaceutical) ... 420, 1650
Mycostatin Pastilles (Bristol-Myers Oncology) ... 751
Nizoral Tablets (Janssen) ... 412, 1172
Nystatin, USP for Extemporaneous Preparation of Oral Suspension (Paddock) ... 1737

FUNGAL MEDICATIONS, TOPICAL
(see DERMATOLGICALS; OPHTHALMIC PREPARATIONS; VAGINAL PREPARATIONS)

G

GALACTOKINETIC
Syntocinon Nasal Spray (Sandoz Pharmaceuticals) ... 2129

GALACTORRHEA INHIBITOR
Parlodel Capsules (Sandoz Pharmaceuticals) ... 427, 2116
Parlodel SnapTabs (Sandoz Pharmaceuticals) ... 427, 2116

GALLSTONE DISSOLUTION AGENT
Actigall Capsules (Summit) ... 433, 2383

GASTRIC ACID SECRETION INHIBITOR
Cytotec (Searle) ... 429, 2251

GASTRITIS AIDS
(see ANTACIDS)

GASTROINTESTINAL ANTIGRANULOMATOUS DISEASE
Azulfidine Tablets and EN-tabs (Kabi Pharmacia) ... 413, 1184
Dipentum Capsules (Kabi Pharmacia) ... 413, 1186

GASTROINTESTINAL MOTILITY FACTOR
Reglan Injectable (Robins Company) ... 425, 1951
Reglan Syrup (Robins Company) ... 1951
Reglan Tablets (Robins Company) ... 425, 1951

GAUCHER DISEASE
Ceredase Injection (Genzyme) .. 410, 1084

GERMICIDES/MICROBICIDES
(see ANTIBIOTICS & ANTISEPTICS)

GONADOTROPIN INHIBITORS
Danocrine Capsules (Sanofi Winthrop Pharmaceuticals) ... 428, 2141
Synarel Nasal Solution (Syntex) ... 433, 2407

GOUT TREATMENT
(see also ARTHRITIS MEDICATIONS)
Anturane Tablets (CIBA Pharmaceutical) ... 408, 883

UNIT DOSE SYSTEMS

SECTION 4

Generic and Chemical Name Index

In this section the products described in the Product Information (White) and Diagnostic Product Information (Green) Sections are listed under generic and chemical name headings according to the principal ingredient(s). The headings under which products are listed have been determined by the Publisher with the cooperation of the individual manufacturers. **Note: Only fully described products are listed in this index.**

Tylenol Cold Medication Caplets and Tablets (McNeil Consumer) ... 418, 1418
Tylenol Cold Medication No Drowsiness Formula Caplets and Gelcaps (McNeil Consumer) ... 418, 1419
Tylenol Cold Night Time Medication Liquid (McNeil Consumer) ... 418, 1420
Tylenol Cough Medication Liquid, Maximum Strength (McNeil Consumer) ... 418, 1421
Tylenol Cough Medication Liquid with Decongestant, Maximum Strength (McNeil Consumer) ... 418, 1421

DEZOCINE
Dalgan Injection (Astra) ... 636

DIAZEPAM
Valium Injectable (Roche Products) ... 426, 2027
Valium Tablets (Roche Products) ... 426, 2028
Valrelease Capsules (Roche Laboratories) ... 426, 2012

DIAZOXIDE
Hyperstat I.V. Injection (Schering) ... 2193
Proglycem Capsules (Baker Norton) ... 670
Proglycem Suspension (Baker Norton) ... 670

DIBUCAINE
Nupercainal Cream and Ointment (CIBA Pharmaceutical) ... 906

DICHLORALPHENAZONE
Atarin Capsules (Athena Neurosciences) ... 665
Isocom Capsules (Nutripharm) ... 1686
Midrin Capsules (Carnrick) ... 407, 859

DICHLOROACETIC ACID
Bichloracetic Acid Kahlenberg (Glenwood) ... 1102

DICHLORODIFLUOROMETHANE
Fluori-Methane (Gebauer) ... 1056

DICHLOROTETRAFLUOROETHANE
Fluro-Ethyl (Gebauer) ... 1056

DICHLORPHENAMIDE
Daranide Tablets (Merck & Co., Inc.) ... 419, 1496

DICLOFENAC SODIUM
Voltaren Tablets (Geigy) ... 410, 1074

DICYCLOMINE HYDROCHLORIDE
Bentyl 10 mg Capsules (Marion Merrell Dow) ... 416, 1363
Bentyl Injection (Marion Merrell Dow) ... 1363
Bentyl Syrup (Marion Merrell Dow) ... 1363
Bentyl 20 mg Tablets (Marion Merrell Dow) ... 416, 1363

DIDANOSINE
Videx Tablets, Powder for Oral Solution, & Pediatric Powder for Oral Solution (Bristol Laboratories) ... 406, 734

DIENESTROL
Ortho Dienestrol Cream (Ortho Pharmaceutical) ... 1720

DIETHYLPROPION HYDROCHLORIDE
Tenuate Dospan Controlled-release Tablets (Marion Merrell Dow) ... 417, 1403
Tenuate Immediate-release Tablets (Marion Merrell Dow) 417, 1403

DIETHYLSTILBESTROL
Diethylstilbestrol Tablets (Lilly) ... 1291

DIETHYLSTILBESTROL DIPHOSPHATE
Stilphostrol Tablets and Ampuls (Miles Pharmaceutical) ... 420, 1655

DIFENOXIN HYDROCHLORIDE
Motofen Tablets (Carnrick) ... 407, 859

DIFLORASONE DIACETATE
Florone Cream 0.05% (Dermik) ... 932
Florone E Emollient Cream 0.05% (Dermik) ... 932
Florone Ointment 0.05% (Dermik) ... 932
Psorcon Ointment 0.05% (Dermik) ... 933

DIFLUNISAL
Dolobid Tablets (Merck & Co., Inc.) ... 419, 1516

DIGITOXIN
Crystodigin Tablets (Lilly) ... 1287

DIGOXIN
Lanoxicaps (Burroughs Wellcome) ... 407, 788
Lanoxin Elixir Pediatric (Burroughs Wellcome) ... 791
Lanoxin Injection (Burroughs Wellcome) ... 794
Lanoxin Injection Pediatric (Burroughs Wellcome) ... 797
Lanoxin Tablets (Burroughs Wellcome) ... 407, 800

DIGOXIN IMMUNE FAB (OVINE)
Digibind (Burroughs Wellcome) ... 778

DIHYDROCODEINE BITARTRATE
Synalgos-DC Capsules (Wyeth-Ayerst) ... 438, 2639

DIHYDROERGOTAMINE MESYLATE
D.H.E. 45 Injection (Sandoz Pharmaceuticals) ... 2097

DIHYDROTACHYSTEROL
DHT (Dihydrotachysterol) Tablets & Intensol (Roxane) ... 2074

DIIODOHYDROXYQUIN (see IODOQUINOL)

DILTIAZEM HYDROCHLORIDE
Cardizem CD Capsules-180 mg, 240 mg and 300 mg (Marion Merrell Dow) ... 417, 1368
Cardizem SR Capsules-60 mg, 90 mg and 120 mg (Marion Merrell Dow) ... 417, 1372
Cardizem Injectable (Marion Merrell Dow) ... 416, 1370
Cardizem Tablets-30 mg, 60 mg, 90 mg and 120 mg (Marion Merrell Dow) ... 417, 1374
Dilacor XR Extended-release Capsules (Rhone-Poulenc Rorer Pharmaceuticals Inc.) ... 424, 1914

DIMERCAPROL
BAL in Oil Ampules (Becton Dickinson Microbiology) ... 684

DIMETHICONE
Moisturel Cream (Westwood-Squibb) ... 2519
Moisturel Lotion (Westwood-Squibb) ... 2519

DIMETHICONE COPOLYOL
Theraplex HydroLotion (Medicis) ... 1461

DIMETHYL SULFOXIDE
Rimso-50 (Research Industries Corporation) ... 1907

DIOCTYL SODIUM SULFOSUCCINATE (see DOCUSATE SODIUM)

DIOXYBENZONE
Solaquin Forte 4% Gel (ICN Pharmaceuticals) ... 1148
Solbar Plus 15 Cream (Persön & Covey) ... 1828

DIPHENHYDRAMINE CITRATE
Bufferin AF Nite Time Analgesic/Sleeping Aid Caplets (Bristol-Myers Products) ... 406, 761
Excedrin P.M. Analgesic/Sleeping Aid Tablets, Caplets and Liquid (Bristol-Myers Products) ... 765

DIPHENHYDRAMINE HYDROCHLORIDE
Benadryl Capsules (Parke-Davis) ... 422, 1745
Benadryl Kapseals (Parke-Davis) ... 422, 1745
Benadryl Parenteral (Parke-Davis) ... 1746
Benadryl Steri-Vials, Ampoules, and Steri-Dose Syringe (Parke-Davis) ... 1746
Tylenol Cold Night Time Medication Liquid (McNeil Consumer) ... 418, 1420
Tylenol PM, Extra Strength Gelcaps, Caplets and Tablets (McNeil Consumer) ... 418, 1416
Unisom With Pain Relief-Nighttime Sleep Aid and Pain Reliever (Pfizer Consumer Health Care) ... 1829

DIPHENIDOL
Vontrol Tablets (SmithKline Beecham Pharmaceuticals) ... 432, 2338

DIPHENOXYLATE HYDROCHLORIDE
Lomotil Liquid (Searle) ... 2264
Lomotil Tablets (Searle) ... 429, 2264

DIPHTHERIA TOXOID, CONJUGATE
ProHIBiT Haemophilus b Conjugate Vaccine (Diphtheria Toxoid Conjugate) (Connaught) ... 919

DIPHTHERIA & TETANUS TOXOIDS ADSORBED, (FOR PEDIATRIC USE)
Diphtheria & Tetanus Toxoids, Adsorbed Purogenated (Lederle) ... 1230

DIPHTHERIA & TETANUS TOXOIDS W/PERTUSSIS VACCINE COMBINED, ALUMINUM PHOSPHATE ADSORBED
Acel-Imune Diphtheria and Tetanus Toxoids and Pertussis Vaccine Adsorbed (Lederle) ... 414, 1219
Tri-Immunol Diphtheria & Tetanus Toxoids & Pertussis Vaccine, Adsorbed (Lederle) ... 415, 1274

DIPHTHERIA & TETANUS TOXOIDS W/PERTUSSIS VACCINE COMBINED, ALUMINUM POTASSIUM SULFATE ADSORBED
Diphtheria and Tetanus Toxoids and Pertussis Vaccine Adsorbed USP (For Pediatric Use) (Connaught) ... 915

DIPYRIDAMOLE
Persantine Tablets (Boehringer Ingelheim) ... 405, 710

DISOPYRAMIDE PHOSPHATE
Norpace Capsules (Searle) ... 429, 2270
Norpace CR Capsules (Searle) .. 429, 2270

DISULFIRAM
Antabuse Tablets (Wyeth-Ayerst) ... 436, 2540

DIVALPROEX SODIUM
Depakote Sprinkle Capsules (Abbott) ... 403, 514
Depakote Tablets (Abbott) ... 403, 514

DOBUTAMINE HYDROCHLORIDE
Dobutrex Solution (Lilly) ... 1293

DOCUSATE SODIUM
Colace (Apothecon) ... 614
Dialose Tablets (J&J•Merck Consumer) ... 413, 1180
Dialose Plus Tablets (J&J•Merck Consumer) ... 413, 1181
Ferro-Sequels (Lederle) ... 414, 1231
Peri-Colace (Apothecon) ... 616
Senokot-S Tablets (Purdue Frederick) ... 1889

DOPAMINE HYDROCHLORIDE
Intropin Injection (Du Pont Multi-Source Products) ... 949

DOXACURIUM CHLORIDE
Nuromax Injection (Burroughs Wellcome) ... 815

DOXAPRAM HYDROCHLORIDE
Dopram Injectable (Robins Company) ... 425, 1942

DOXAZOSIN MESYLATE
Cardura Tablets (Roerig) ... 427, 2031

DOXEPIN HYDROCHLORIDE
Adapin Capsules (Lotus Biochemical) ... 416, 1346
Sinequan Capsules (Roerig) ... 427, 2048
Sinequan Oral Concentrate (Roerig) ... 2048

DOXORUBICIN HYDROCHLORIDE
Adriamycin PFS (Adria) ... 560
Adriamycin RDF (Adria) ... 561
Doxorubicin Hydrochloride for Injection, USP (Astra) ... 638
Doxorubicin Hydrochloride Injection, USP (Cetus Oncology) ... 873

DOXYCYCLINE HYCLATE
Doryx Capsules (Parke-Davis) ... 422, 1768
Vibramycin Hyclate Capsules (Pfizer Labs Division) ... 423, 1842
Vibramycin Hyclate Intravenous (Roerig) ... 2056
Vibra-Tabs Film Coated Tablets (Pfizer Labs Division) 423, 1842

DOXYCYCLINE MONOHYDRATE
Monodox Capsules (Oclassen) .. 420, 1688
Vibramycin Monohydrate for Oral Suspension (Pfizer Labs Division) ... 1842

DOXYLAMINE SUCCINATE
Unisom Nighttime Sleep Aid (Pfizer Consumer Health Care) ... 1830

DRONABINOL
Marinol (Dronabinol) Capsules (Roxane) ... 427, 2076

DROPERIDOL
Inapsine Injection (Janssen) ... 412, 1167
Innovar Injection (Janssen) ... 412, 1168

DYCLONINE HYDROCHLORIDE
Dyclone 0.5% and 1% Topical Solutions, USP (Astra) ... 642

DYPHYLLINE
Dilor-200 Tablets (Savage) ... 428, 2174
Dilor-400 Tablets (Savage) ... 428, 2174
Dilor-G Tablets & Liquid (Savage) ... 428, 2174
Lufyllin & Lufyllin-400 Tablets (Wallace) ... 435, 2499
Lufyllin-GG Elixir & Tablets (Wallace) ... 435, 2500

E

ECONAZOLE NITRATE
Spectazole Cream (Ortho Pharmaceutical (Dermatological Div.)) ... 421, 1737

EDROPHONIUM CHLORIDE
Enlon-Plus Injection (Anaquest) ... 608
Tensilon Injectable (ICN Pharmaceuticals) ... 1148

ELECTROLYTE SUPPLEMENT
Pedialyte Oral Electrolyte Maintenance Solution (Ross) ... 2063
Rehydralyte Oral Electrolyte Rehydration Solution (Ross) ... 2066

ENALAPRIL MALEATE
Vaseretic Tablets (Merck & Co., Inc.) ... 420, 1615
Vasotec Tablets (Merck & Co., Inc.) ... 420, 1621

ENALAPRILAT
Vasotec I.V. (Merck & Co., Inc.) ... 1618

ENOXACIN
Penetrex Tablets (Rhone-Poulenc Rorer Pharmaceuticals Inc.) ... 425, 1921

ENTSUFON SODIUM
pHisoHex (Sanofi Winthrop Pharmaceuticals) ... 2162

ENZYMES, COLLAGENOLYTIC
Collagenase Santyl Ointment (Knoll) ... 414, 1199

ENZYMES, DEBRIDEMENT
Collagenase Santyl Ointment (Knoll) ... 414, 1199
Panafil Ointment (Rystan) ... 2086
Panafil-White Ointment (Rystan) ... 2086
Travase Ointment (Boots Pharmaceuticals) ... 406, 723

ENZYMES, DIGESTIVE
Arco-Lase Plus (Arco) ... 625
Arco-Lase (Arco) ... 625
Donnazyme Tablets (Robins Company) ... 425, 1941
Entozyme Tablets (Robins Company) ... 425, 1943
Kutrase Capsules (Schwarz Pharma) ... 429, 2240
Ku-Zyme Capsules (Schwarz Pharma) ... 429, 2240
Ku-Zyme HP Capsules (Schwarz Pharma) ... 429, 2241

ENZYMES, FIBRINOLYTIC
Elase Ointment (Fujisawa) ... 1044
Elase Vials (Fujisawa) ... 1044
Elase-Chloromycetin Ointment (Fujisawa) ... 1044

ENZYMES, PROTEOLYTIC
Panafil Ointment (Rystan) ... 2086
Panafil-White Ointment (Rystan) ... 2086
Travase Ointment (Boots Pharmaceuticals) ... 406, 723

EPHEDRINE HYDROCHLORIDE
Primatene Tablets (Whitehall) .. 436, 2535
Quadrinal Tablets (Knoll) ... 414, 1210
Quelidrine Syrup (Abbott) ... 553
Tedral SA Tablets (Parke-Davis) ... 1820

EPHEDRINE SULFATE
Marax Tablets & DF Syrup (Roerig) ... 427, 2042
Pazo Hemorrhoid Ointment & Suppositories (Bristol-Myers Products) ... 768

SECTION 5

Product Identification Section

Designed to help you identify products, this section contains actual size, full-color reproductions selected for inclusion by participating manufacturers. Each Product Identification illustration includes the page number where the product's information first appears in the PRODUCT INFORMATION SECTION (White Section).

Because tablets and capsules, for the most part, are shown here, you should not infer that these are the only dosage forms. Where other dosage forms are available, the product name is preceded by the ▼ symbol. Refer to the product's description in the PRODUCT INFORMATION SECTION or check directly with the manufacturer.

Letters and/or numbers followed by an asterisk (*) accompanying a product photograph designate the manufacturers' identification code.

While every effort has been made to reproduce products faithfully, this section should be considered only as a quick reference identification aid.

INDEX BY MANUFACTURER

This section is made possible through the courtesy of the manufacturers whose products appear on the following pages.

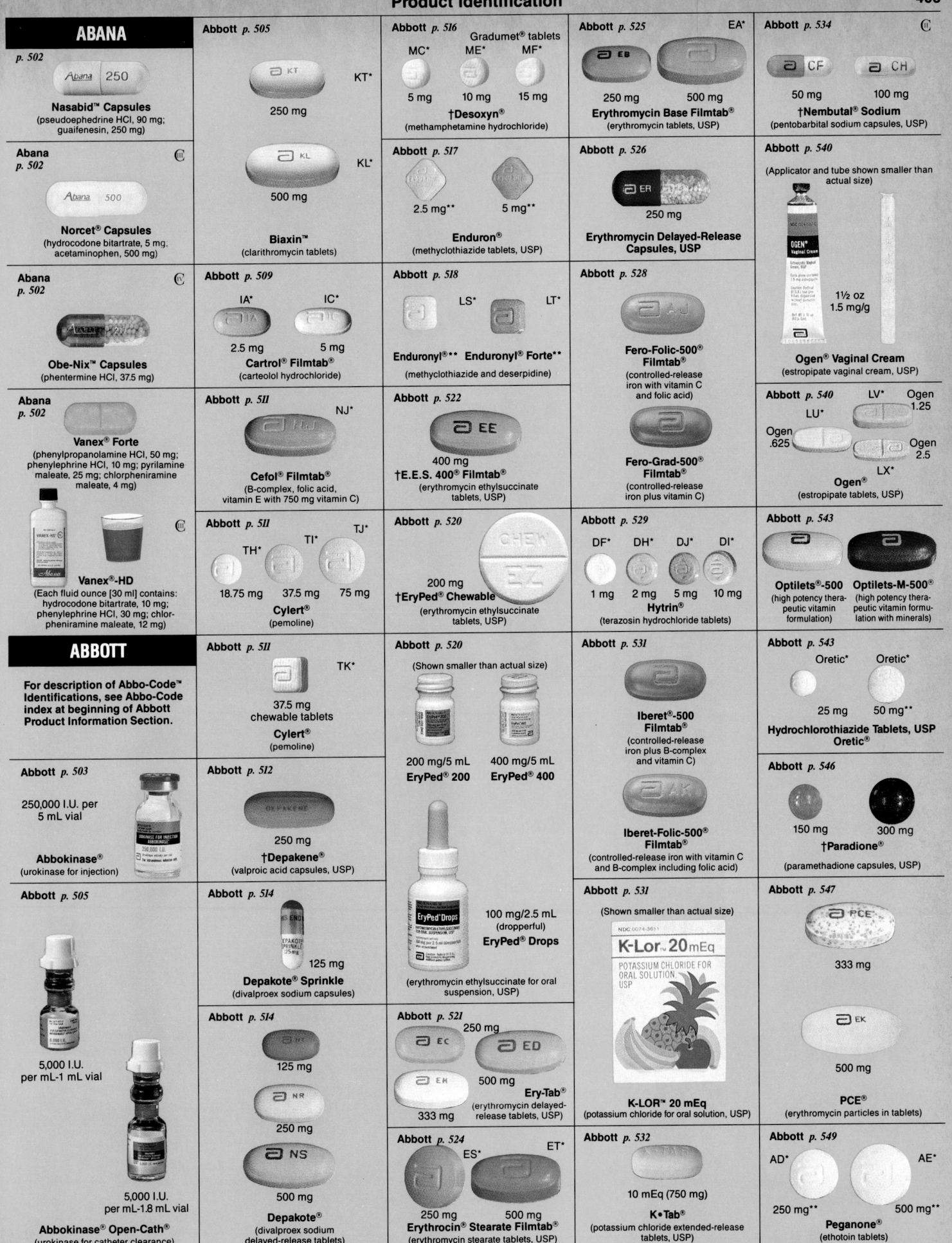

ABANA

p. 502

Nasabid™ Capsules
(pseudoephedrine HCl, 90 mg; guaifenesin, 250 mg)

Abana
p. 502

Norcet® Capsules
(hydrocodone bitartrate, 5 mg, acetaminophen, 500 mg)

Abana
p. 502

Obe-Nix™ Capsules
(phentermine HCl, 37.5 mg)

Abana
p. 502

Vanex® Forte
(phenylpropanolamine HCl, 50 mg; phenylephrine HCl, 10 mg; pyrilamine maleate, 25 mg; chlorpheniramine maleate, 4 mg)

Vanex®-HD
(Each fluid ounce [30 ml] contains: hydrocodone bitartrate, 10 mg; phenylephrine HCl, 30 mg; chlorpheniramine maleate, 12 mg)

ABBOTT

For description of Abbo-Code™ Identifications, see Abbo-Code index at beginning of Abbott Product Information Section.

Abbott p. 503

250,000 I.U. per 5 mL vial

Abbokinase®
(urokinase for injection)

Abbott p. 505

5,000 I.U. per mL-1 mL vial

5,000 I.U. per mL-1.8 mL vial

Abbokinase® Open-Cath®
(urokinase for catheter clearance)

Abbott p. 505

KT*

250 mg

KL*

500 mg

Biaxin™
(clarithromycin tablets)

Abbott p. 509

IA*   IC*

2.5 mg   5 mg

Cartrol® Filmtab®
(carteolol hydrochloride)

Abbott p. 511

NJ*

Cefol® Filmtab®
(B-complex, folic acid, vitamin E with 750 mg vitamin C)

Abbott p. 511

TH*   TI*   TJ*

18.75 mg   37.5 mg   75 mg

Cylert®
(pemoline)

Abbott p. 511

TK*

37.5 mg chewable tablets

Cylert®
(pemoline)

Abbott p. 512

250 mg

†Depakene®
(valproic acid capsules, USP)

Abbott p. 514

125 mg

Depakote® Sprinkle
(divalproex sodium capsules)

Abbott p. 514

125 mg

250 mg

500 mg

Depakote®
(divalproex sodium delayed-release tablets)

Abbott p. 516

MC*   ME*   MF*
Gradumet® tablets

5 mg   10 mg   15 mg

†Desoxyn®
(methamphetamine hydrochloride)

Abbott p. 517

2.5 mg**   5 mg**

Enduron®
(methyclothiazide tablets, USP)

Abbott p. 518

LS*   LT*

Enduronyl®   **Enduronyl® Forte****
(methyclothiazide and deserpidine)

Abbott p. 522

EE

400 mg

†E.E.S. 400® Filmtab®
(erythromycin ethylsuccinate tablets, USP)

Abbott p. 520

200 mg
†EryPed® Chewable
(erythromycin ethylsuccinate tablets, USP)

Abbott p. 520

(Shown smaller than actual size)

200 mg/5 mL   400 mg/5 mL
EryPed® 200   **EryPed® 400**

100 mg/2.5 mL (dropperful)
EryPed® Drops

(erythromycin ethylsuccinate for oral suspension, USP)

Abbott p. 521

250 mg

EC   ED

500 mg

EH
333 mg   **Ery-Tab®**
(erythromycin delayed-release tablets, USP)

Abbott p. 524

ES*   ET*

250 mg   500 mg
Erythrocin® Stearate Filmtab®
(erythromycin stearate tablets, USP)

Abbott p. 525

EA*

EB

250 mg   500 mg
Erythromycin Base Filmtab®
(erythromycin tablets, USP)

Abbott p. 526

ER

250 mg
Erythromycin Delayed-Release Capsules, USP

Abbott p. 528

AJ

Fero-Folic-500® Filmtab®
(controlled-release iron with vitamin C and folic acid)

Fero-Grad-500® Filmtab®
(controlled-release iron plus vitamin C)

Abbott p. 529

DF*   DH*   DJ*   DI*

1 mg   2 mg   5 mg   10 mg

Hytrin®
(terazosin hydrochloride tablets)

Abbott p. 531

Iberet®-500 Filmtab®
(controlled-release iron plus B-complex and vitamin C)

AK

Iberet-Folic-500® Filmtab®
(controlled-release iron with vitamin C and B-complex including folic acid)

Abbott p. 531

(Shown smaller than actual size)

NDC 0074-3611
K-Lor™ 20 mEq
POTASSIUM CHLORIDE FOR ORAL SOLUTION, USP

K-LOR™ 20 mEq
(potassium chloride for oral solution, USP)

Abbott p. 532

10 mEq (750 mg)
K•Tab®
(potassium chloride extended-release tablets, USP)

Abbott p. 534

CF   CH

50 mg   100 mg
†Nembutal® Sodium
(pentobarbital sodium capsules, USP)

Abbott p. 540

(Applicator and tube shown smaller than actual size)

OGEN®
Vaginal Cream

1½ oz
1.5 mg/g

Ogen® Vaginal Cream
(estropipate vaginal cream, USP)

Abbott p. 540

LV*   Ogen 1.25
LU*
Ogen .625

Ogen 2.5

LX*

Ogen®
(estropipate tablets, USP)

Abbott p. 543

Optilets®-500   **Optilets-M-500®**
(high potency thera-peutic vitamin formulation)   (high potency thera-peutic vitamin formu-lation with minerals)

Abbott p. 543

Oretic*   Oretic*

25 mg   50 mg**
Hydrochlorothiazide Tablets, USP Oretic®

Abbott p. 546

150 mg   300 mg
†Paradione®
(paramethadione capsules, USP)

Abbott p. 547

PCE

333 mg

EK

500 mg
PCE®
(erythromycin particles in tablets)

Abbott p. 549

AD*   AE*

250 mg**   500 mg**
Peganone®
(ethotoin tablets)

---

*Abbott Abbo-Code identification letters. Filmtab®—Film-sealed tablets, Abbott. **Grooved tablets.

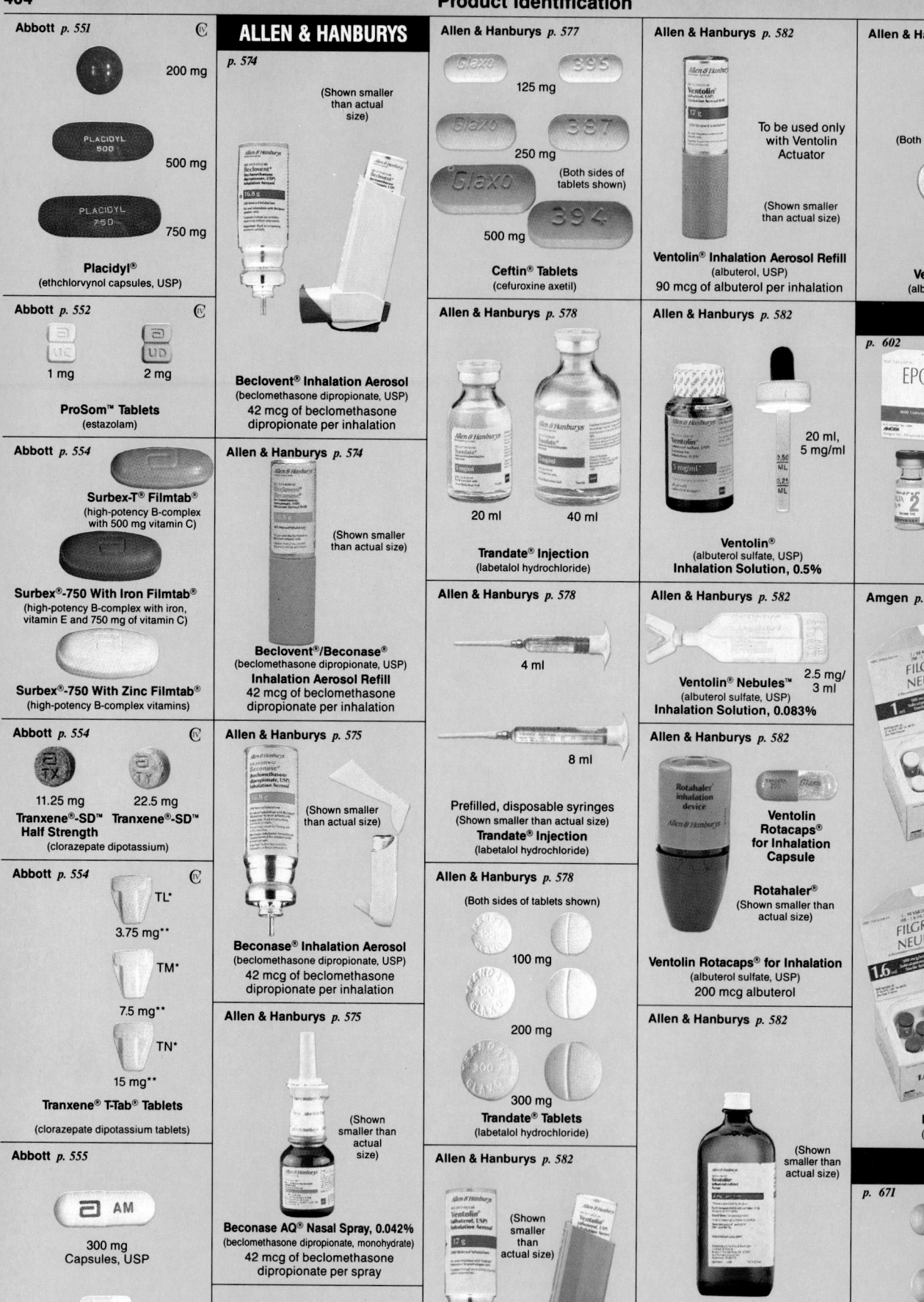

Abbott p. 551

200 mg

PLACIDYL 500 — 500 mg

PLACIDYL 750 — 750 mg

Placidyl®
(ethchlorvynol capsules, USP)

Abbott p. 552

1 mg   2 mg

ProSom™ Tablets
(estazolam)

Abbott p. 554

Surbex-T® Filmtab®
(high-potency B-complex
with 500 mg vitamin C)

Surbex®-750 With Iron Filmtab®
(high-potency B-complex with iron,
vitamin E and 750 mg of vitamin C)

Surbex®-750 With Zinc Filmtab®
(high-potency B-complex vitamins)

Abbott p. 554

11.25 mg   22.5 mg
Tranxene®-SD™   **Tranxene®-SD™**
Half Strength
(clorazepate dipotassium)

Abbott p. 554

TL* — 3.75 mg**

TM* — 7.5 mg**

TN* — 15 mg**

Tranxene® T-Tab® Tablets
(clorazepate dipotassium tablets)

Abbott p. 555

AM

300 mg
Capsules, USP

LE*

150 mg Dulcet®
Tablet, USP

†Tridione®
(trimethadione)

ALLEN & HANBURYS

p. 574

(Shown smaller
than actual
size)

Beclovent® Inhalation Aerosol
(beclomethasone dipropionate, USP)
42 mcg of beclomethasone
dipropionate per inhalation

Allen & Hanburys p. 574

(Shown smaller
than actual size)

Beclovent®/Beconase®
(beclomethasone dipropionate, USP)
Inhalation Aerosol Refill
42 mcg of beclomethasone
dipropionate per inhalation

Allen & Hanburys p. 575

(Shown smaller
than actual size)

Beconase® Inhalation Aerosol
(beclomethasone dipropionate, USP)
42 mcg of beclomethasone
dipropionate per inhalation

Allen & Hanburys p. 575

(Shown
smaller than
actual
size)

Beconase AQ® Nasal Spray, 0.042%
(beclomethasone dipropionate, monohydrate)
42 mcg of beclomethasone
dipropionate per spray

While every effort has been made to
reproduce products faithfully, this
section is to be considered a quick-
reference identification aid. In cases
of suspected overdosage, etc., chemical analysis of the product should
be done.

Allen & Hanburys p. 577

Glaxo / 395 — 125 mg

Glaxo / 387 — 250 mg

(Both sides of
tablets shown)

Glaxo / 394 — 500 mg

Ceftin® Tablets
(cefuroxine axetil)

Allen & Hanburys p. 578

20 ml   40 ml

Trandate® Injection
(labetalol hydrochloride)

Allen & Hanburys p. 578

4 ml

8 ml

Prefilled, disposable syringes
(Shown smaller than actual size)
Trandate® Injection
(labetalol hydrochloride)

Allen & Hanburys p. 578

(Both sides of tablets shown)

100 mg

200 mg

300 mg

Trandate® Tablets
(labetalol hydrochloride)

Allen & Hanburys p. 582

(Shown
smaller
than
actual size)

Ventolin® Inhalation Aerosol
(albuterol, USP)
90 mcg of albuterol per inhalation

Allen & Hanburys p. 582

To be used only
with Ventolin
Actuator

(Shown smaller
than actual size)

Ventolin® Inhalation Aerosol Refill
(albuterol, USP)
90 mcg of albuterol per inhalation

Allen & Hanburys p. 582

20 ml,
5 mg/ml

Ventolin®
(albuterol sulfate, USP)
Inhalation Solution, 0.5%

Allen & Hanburys p. 582

2.5 mg/
3 ml

Ventolin® Nebules™
(albuterol sulfate, USP)
Inhalation Solution, 0.083%

Allen & Hanburys p. 582

Rotahaler
inhalation
device

Ventolin
Rotacaps®
for Inhalation
Capsule

Rotahaler®
(Shown smaller than
actual size)

Ventolin Rotacaps® for Inhalation
(albuterol sulfate, USP)
200 mcg albuterol

Allen & Hanburys p. 582

(Shown
smaller than
actual size)

Ventolin® Syrup
(albuterol sulfate)
2 mg/5 ml

Allen & Hanburys p. 582

2 mg
(Both sides of tablets shown)

4 mg

Ventolin® Tablets
(albuterol sulfate, USP)

AMGEN

p. 602

EPOETIN ALFA
EPOGEN® 3

2   3   4   10

1 mL vials
EPOGEN®
(Epoetin alfa)

Amgen p. 605

FILGRASTIM
NEUPOGEN®
1

1 mL vials

FILGRASTIM
NEUPOGEN®
1.6

1.6 mL vials

NEUPOGEN®
(Filgrastim)

BASEL

p. 671

AFRAN 25 mg — 25 mg. 115*

AFRAN 50 mg — 50 mg. 116*

AFRAN 75 mg — 75 mg. 117*

Anafranil®
(clomipramine
hydrochloride)

---

*Abbott Abbo-Code identification letters. Filmtab®—Film-sealed tablets, Abbott. **Grooved tablets.

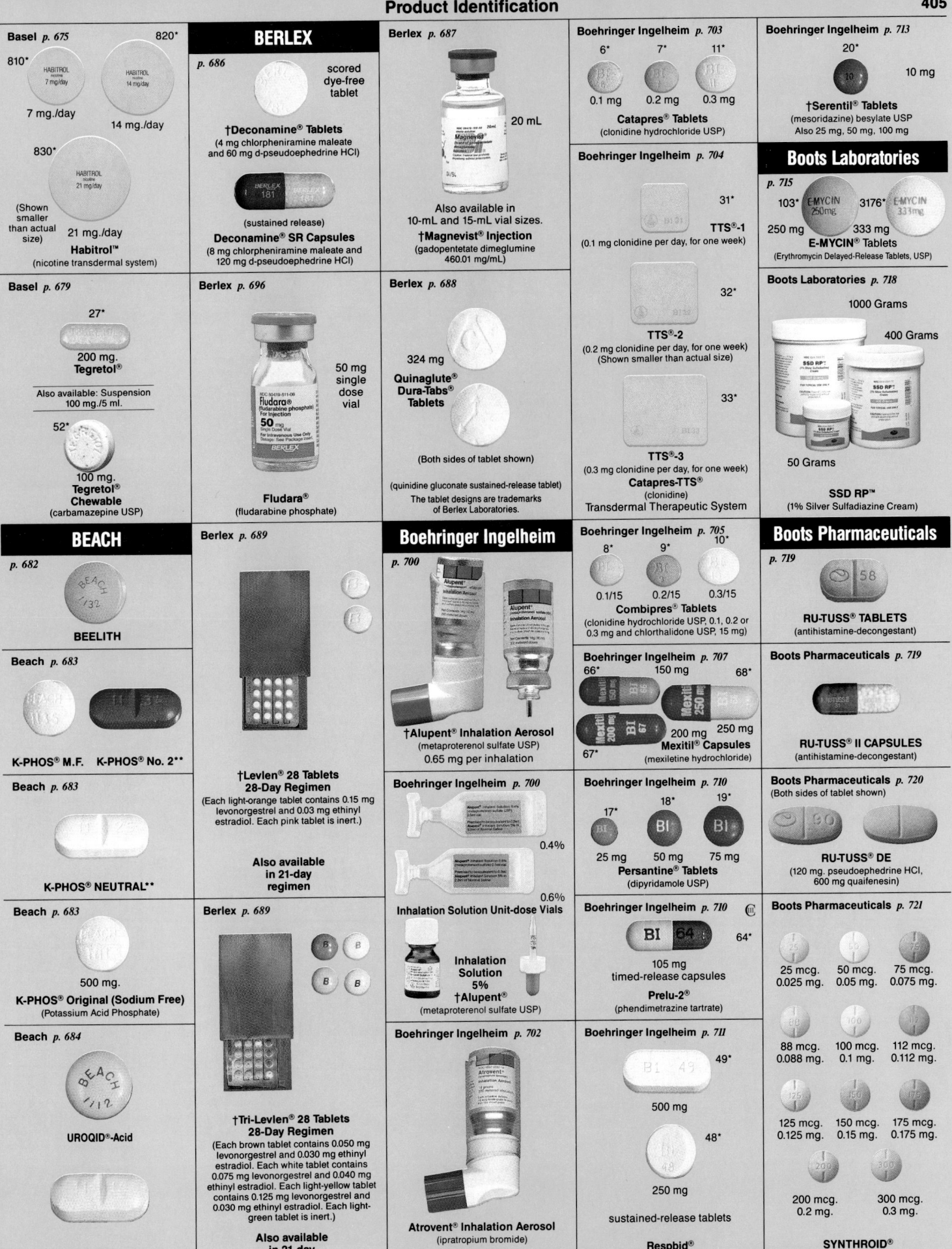

Basel *p. 675* 810* 820*

HABITROL nicotine 7 mg/day

HABITROL nicotine 14 mg/day

7 mg./day

14 mg./day

830*

HABITROL nicotine 21 mg/day

(Shown smaller than actual size) 21 mg./day

Habitrol™
(nicotine transdermal system)

Basel *p. 679* 27*

200 mg.
Tegretol®

Also available: Suspension 100 mg./5 ml.

52*

100 mg.
Tegretol® Chewable
(carbamazepine USP)

BEACH
p. 682

BEACH 132

BEELITH

Beach *p. 683*

BEACH 1135

11 35

K-PHOS® M.F. **K-PHOS® No. 2**

Beach *p. 683*

K-PHOS® NEUTRAL

Beach *p. 683*

500 mg.
K-PHOS® Original (Sodium Free)
(Potassium Acid Phosphate)

Beach *p. 684*

BEACH 112

UROQID®-Acid

UROQID®-Acid No. 2

BERLEX
p. 686

scored dye-free tablet

†Deconamine® Tablets
(4 mg chlorpheniramine maleate and 60 mg d-pseudoephedrine HCl)

BERLEX 181 BERLEX 181

(sustained release)
Deconamine® SR Capsules
(8 mg chlorpheniramine maleate and 120 mg d-pseudoephedrine HCl)

Berlex *p. 696*

fludara (fludarabine phosphate) For Injection 50 mg

50 mg single dose vial

Fludara®
(fludarabine phosphate)

Berlex *p. 689*

B B

B B

†Levlen® 28 Tablets 28-Day Regimen
(Each light-orange tablet contains 0.15 mg levonorgestrel and 0.03 mg ethinyl estradiol. Each pink tablet is inert.)

Also available in 21-day regimen

Berlex *p. 689*

†Tri-Levlen® 28 Tablets 28-Day Regimen
(Each brown tablet contains 0.050 mg levonorgestrel and 0.030 mg ethinyl estradiol. Each white tablet contains 0.075 mg levonorgestrel and 0.040 mg ethinyl estradiol. Each light-yellow tablet contains 0.125 mg levonorgestrel and 0.030 mg ethinyl estradiol. Each light-green tablet is inert.)

Also available in 21-day regimen

Berlex *p. 687*

Magnevist 20 mL

20 mL

Also available in 10-mL and 15-mL vial sizes.
†Magnevist® Injection
(gadopentetate dimeglumine 460.01 mg/mL)

Berlex *p. 688*

324 mg
Quinaglute® Dura-Tabs® Tablets

(Both sides of tablet shown)

(quinidine gluconate sustained-release tablet)
The tablet designs are trademarks of Berlex Laboratories.

Boehringer Ingelheim
p. 700

Alupent Inhalation Aerosol

†Alupent® Inhalation Aerosol
(metaproterenol sulfate USP)
0.65 mg per inhalation

Boehringer Ingelheim *p. 700*

0.4%

0.6%
Inhalation Solution Unit-dose Vials

Inhalation Solution 5%
†Alupent®
(metaproterenol sulfate USP)

Boehringer Ingelheim *p. 702*

Atrovent Inhalation Aerosol

Atrovent® Inhalation Aerosol
(ipratropium bromide)
18 mcg per inhalation

Boehringer Ingelheim *p. 703*

6* 7* 11*

0.1 mg 0.2 mg 0.3 mg

Catapres® Tablets
(clonidine hydrochloride USP)

Boehringer Ingelheim *p. 704*

31*
BI 31
TTS®-1
(0.1 mg clonidine per day, for one week)

32*
TTS®-2
(0.2 mg clonidine per day, for one week)
(Shown smaller than actual size)

33*
BI 33
TTS®-3
(0.3 mg clonidine per day, for one week)
Catapres-TTS®
(clonidine)
Transdermal Therapeutic System

Boehringer Ingelheim *p. 705*

8* 9* 10*

0.1/15 0.2/15 0.3/15

Combipres® Tablets
(clonidine hydrochloride USP, 0.1, 0.2 or 0.3 mg and chlorthalidone USP, 15 mg)

Boehringer Ingelheim *p. 707*

66* 150 mg 68*

Mexitil 150 mg BI Mexitil 250 mg BI

Mexitil 200 mg BI 67

200 mg 250 mg
Mexitil® Capsules
(mexiletine hydrochloride)
67*

Boehringer Ingelheim *p. 710*

17* 18* 19*

BI BI BI

25 mg 50 mg 75 mg
Persantine® Tablets
(dipyridamole USP)

Boehringer Ingelheim *p. 710*

BI 64 64*

105 mg
timed-release capsules
Prelu-2®
(phendimetrazine tartrate)

Boehringer Ingelheim *p. 711*

BI 49 49*

500 mg

BI 48 48*

250 mg

sustained-release tablets
Respbid®
(anhydrous theophylline)

Boehringer Ingelheim *p. 713*

20*
10
10 mg
†Serentil® Tablets
(mesoridazine) besylate USP
Also 25 mg, 50 mg, 100 mg

Boots Laboratories
p. 715

103* E-MYCIN 250 mg 3176* E-MYCIN 333 mg

250 mg 333 mg
E-MYCIN® Tablets
(Erythromycin Delayed-Release Tablets, USP)

Boots Laboratories *p. 718*

1000 Grams

400 Grams

SSD RP SSD RP

SSD RP

50 Grams

SSD RP™
(1% Silver Sulfadiazine Cream)

Boots Pharmaceuticals
p. 719

58

RU-TUSS® TABLETS
(antihistamine-decongestant)

Boots Pharmaceuticals *p. 719*

RU-TUSS® II CAPSULES
(antihistamine-decongestant)

Boots Pharmaceuticals *p. 720*
(Both sides of tablet shown)

90

RU-TUSS® DE
(120 mg. pseudoephedrine HCl, 600 mg quaifenesin)

Boots Pharmaceuticals *p. 721*

25 mcg. 0.025 mg. | 50 mcg. 0.05 mg. | 75 mcg. 0.075 mg.

88 mcg. 0.088 mg. | 100 mcg. 0.1 mg. | 112 mcg. 0.112 mg.

125 mcg. 0.125 mg. | 150 mcg. 0.15 mg. | 175 mcg. 0.175 mg.

200 mcg. 0.2 mg. | 300 mcg. 0.3 mg.

SYNTHROID®
(Levothyroxine Sodium Tablets, USP)

**The name BEACH appears on the reverse side of these tablets.

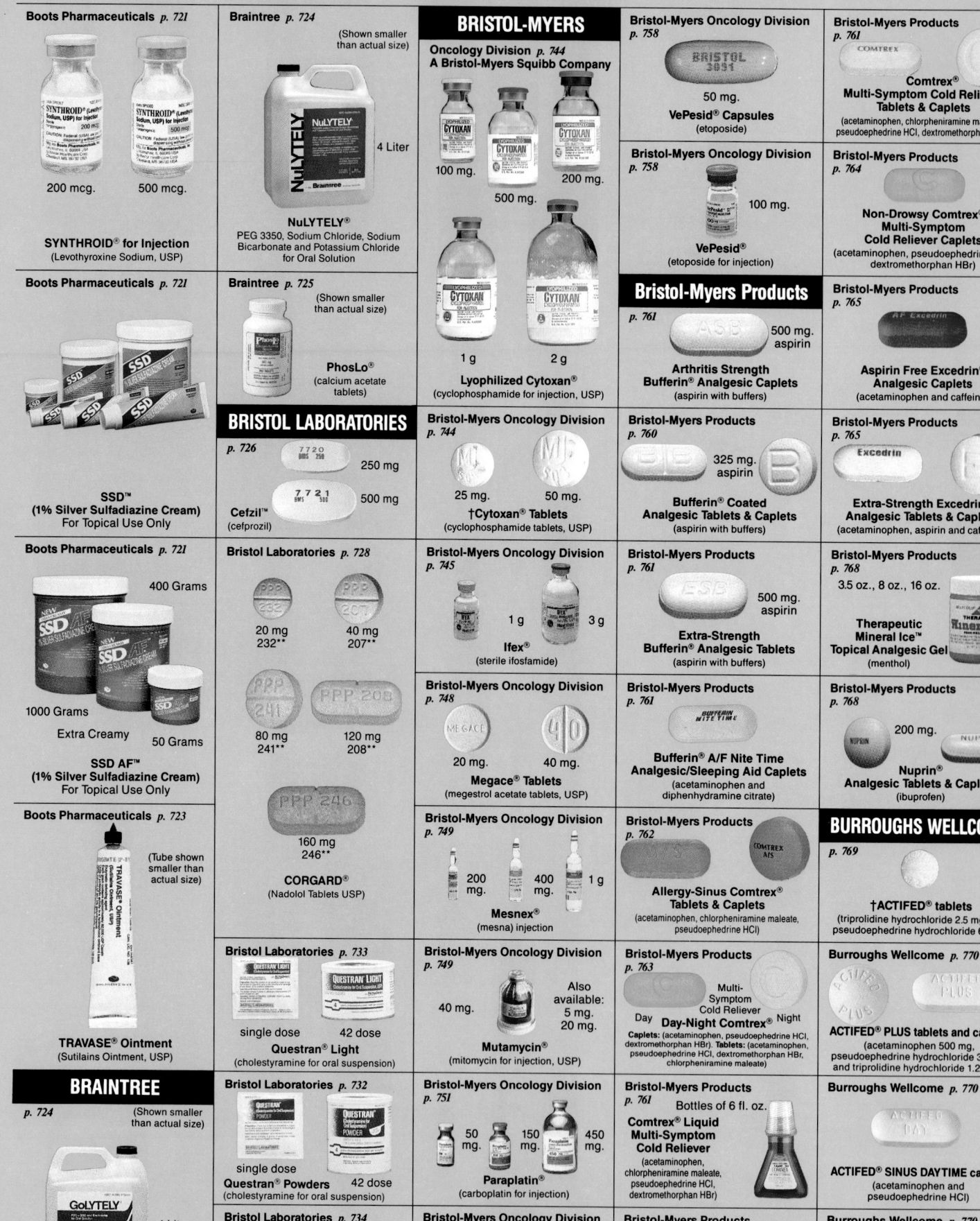

Boots Pharmaceuticals p. 721

200 mcg.   500 mcg.

SYNTHROID® for Injection
(Levothyroxine Sodium, USP)

Boots Pharmaceuticals p. 721

SSD™
(1% Silver Sulfadiazine Cream)
For Topical Use Only

Boots Pharmaceuticals p. 721

400 Grams

1000 Grams

Extra Creamy   50 Grams

SSD AF™
(1% Silver Sulfadiazine Cream)
For Topical Use Only

Boots Pharmaceuticals p. 723

(Tube shown smaller than actual size)

TRAVASE® Ointment
(Sutilains Ointment, USP)

BRAINTREE

p. 724   (Shown smaller than actual size)

GoLYTELY®
PEG-3350 and Electrolytes for Oral Solution

Braintree p. 724

(Shown smaller than actual size)

4 Liter

NuLYTELY®
PEG 3350, Sodium Chloride, Sodium Bicarbonate and Potassium Chloride for Oral Solution

Braintree p. 725

(Shown smaller than actual size)

PhosLo®
(calcium acetate tablets)

BRISTOL LABORATORIES

p. 726

7720 BMS 250   250 mg

7721 BMS 500   500 mg

Cefzil™
(cefprozil)

Bristol Laboratories p. 728

PPP 232   PPP 207

20 mg 232**   40 mg 207**

PPP 241   PPP 208

80 mg 241**   120 mg 208**

PPP 246

160 mg 246**

CORGARD®
(Nadolol Tablets USP)

Bristol Laboratories p. 733

single dose   42 dose
Questran® Light
(cholestyramine for oral suspension)

Bristol Laboratories p. 732

single dose   42 dose
Questran® Powders
(cholestyramine for oral suspension)

Bristol Laboratories p. 734

VIDEX 1   100

100 mg

Videx®
(didanosine)

BRISTOL-MYERS

Oncology Division p. 744
A Bristol-Myers Squibb Company

100 mg.   200 mg.

500 mg.

1 g   2 g

Lyophilized Cytoxan®
(cyclophosphamide for injection, USP)

Bristol-Myers Oncology Division p. 744

25 mg.   50 mg.

†Cytoxan® Tablets
(cyclophosphamide tablets, USP)

Bristol-Myers Oncology Division p. 745

1 g   3 g

Ifex®
(sterile ifosfamide)

Bristol-Myers Oncology Division p. 748

20 mg.   40 mg.

Megace® Tablets
(megestrol acetate tablets, USP)

Bristol-Myers Oncology Division p. 749

200 mg.   400 mg.   1 g

Mesnex®
(mesna) injection

Bristol-Myers Oncology Division p. 749

40 mg.   Also available: 5 mg. 20 mg.

Mutamycin®
(mitomycin for injection, USP)

Bristol-Myers Oncology Division p. 751

50 mg.   150 mg.   450 mg.

Paraplatin®
(carboplatin for injection)

Bristol-Myers Oncology Division p. 756

50 mg.   100 mg.

Platinol®-AQ
(cisplatin injection)

Bristol-Myers Oncology Division p. 758

50 mg.

VePesid® Capsules
(etoposide)

Bristol-Myers Oncology Division p. 758

100 mg.

VePesid®
(etoposide for injection)

Bristol-Myers Products

p. 761

500 mg. aspirin

Arthritis Strength Bufferin® Analgesic Caplets
(aspirin with buffers)

Bristol-Myers Products p. 760

325 mg. aspirin

Bufferin® Coated Analgesic Tablets & Caplets
(aspirin with buffers)

Bristol-Myers Products p. 761

500 mg. aspirin

Extra-Strength Bufferin® Analgesic Tablets
(aspirin with buffers)

Bristol-Myers Products p. 761

Bufferin® A/F Nite Time Analgesic/Sleeping Aid Caplets
(acetaminophen and diphenhydramine citrate)

Bristol-Myers Products p. 762

Allergy-Sinus Comtrex® Tablets & Caplets
(acetaminophen, chlorpheniramine maleate, pseudoephedrine HCl)

Bristol-Myers Products p. 763

Multi-Symptom Cold Reliever
Day **Day-Night Comtrex®** Night
Caplets: (acetaminophen, pseudoephedrine HCl, dextromethorphan HBr). **Tablets:** (acetaminophen, pseudoephedrine HCl, dextromethorphan HBr, chlorpheniramine maleate)

Bristol-Myers Products p. 761

Bottles of 6 fl. oz.

Comtrex® Liquid Multi-Symptom Cold Reliever
(acetaminophen, chlorpheniramine maleate, pseudoephedrine HCl, dextromethorphan HBr)

Bristol-Myers Products p. 761

Liquid Filled Gelatin Capsules

Comtrex® Liqui-Gel Multi-Symptom Cold Reliever
(acetaminophen, chlorpheniramine maleate, phenylpropanolamine HCl, dextromethorphan HBr)

Bristol-Myers Products p. 761

Comtrex® Multi-Symptom Cold Reliever Tablets & Caplets
(acetaminophen, chlorpheniramine maleate, pseudoephedrine HCl, dextromethorphan HBr)

Bristol-Myers Products p. 764

Non-Drowsy Comtrex® Multi-Symptom Cold Reliever Caplets
(acetaminophen, pseudoephedrine HCl, dextromethorphan HBr)

Bristol-Myers Products p. 765

Aspirin Free Excedrin® Analgesic Caplets
(acetaminophen and caffeine)

Bristol-Myers Products p. 765

Extra-Strength Excedrin® Analgesic Tablets & Caplets
(acetaminophen, aspirin and caffeine)

Bristol-Myers Products p. 768

3.5 oz., 8 oz., 16 oz.

Therapeutic Mineral Ice™ Topical Analgesic Gel
(menthol)

Bristol-Myers Products p. 768

200 mg.

Nuprin® Analgesic Tablets & Caplets
(ibuprofen)

BURROUGHS WELLCOME

p. 769

†ACTIFED® tablets
(triprolidine hydrochloride 2.5 mg and pseudoephedrine hydrochloride 60 mg)

Burroughs Wellcome p. 770

ACTIFED® PLUS tablets and caplets
(acetaminophen 500 mg, pseudoephedrine hydrochloride 30 mg, and triprolidine hydrochloride 1.25 mg)

Burroughs Wellcome p. 770

ACTIFED® SINUS DAYTIME caplets
(acetaminophen and pseudoephedrine HCl)

Burroughs Wellcome p. 770

ACTIFED® SINUS NIGHTTIME caplets
(acetaminophen, diphenhydramine HCl, and pseudoephedrine HCl)

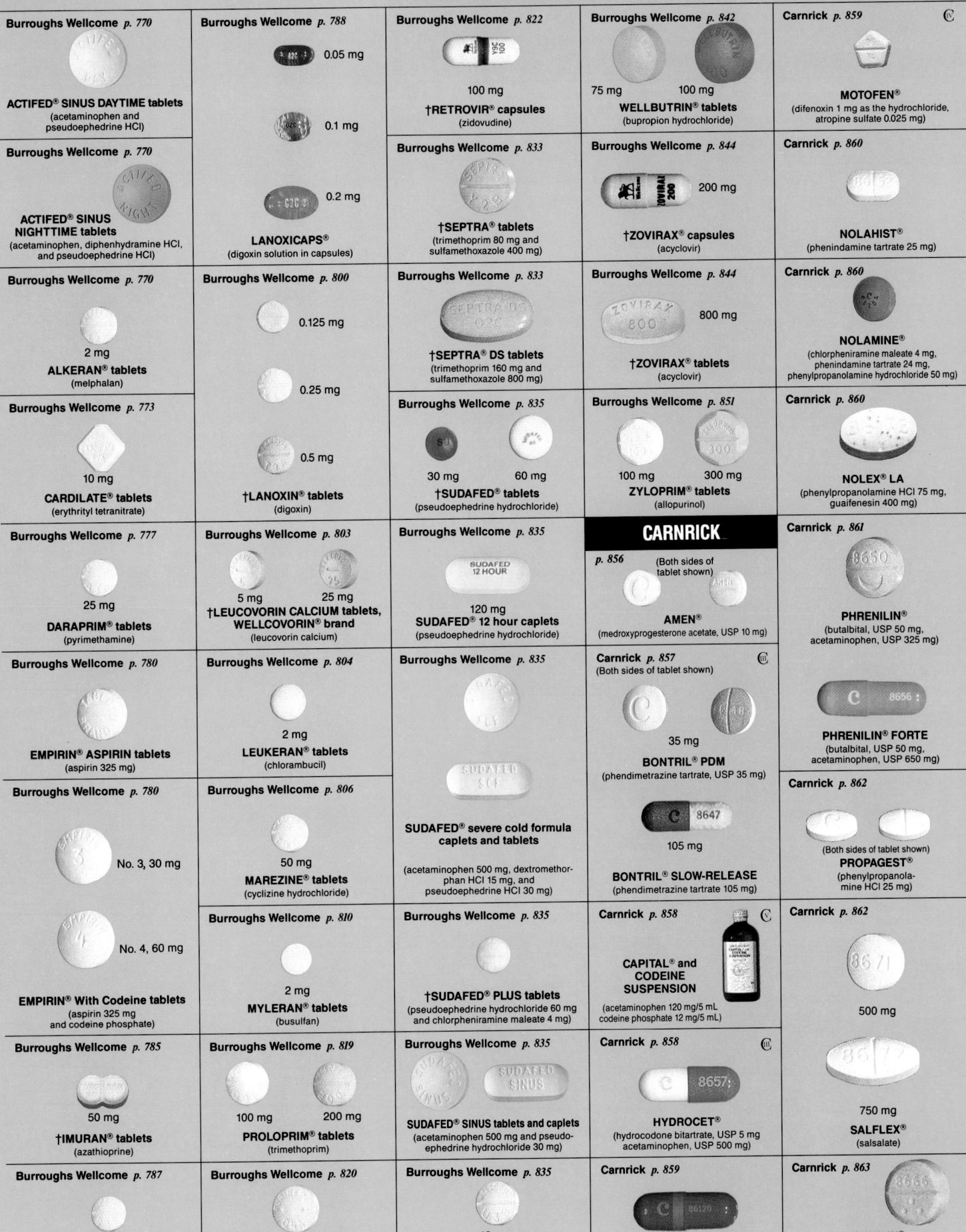

Burroughs Wellcome *p. 770*

ACTIFED® SINUS DAYTIME tablets
(acetaminophen and pseudoephedrine HCl)

Burroughs Wellcome *p. 770*

ACTIFED® SINUS NIGHTTIME tablets
(acetaminophen, diphenhydramine HCl, and pseudoephedrine HCl)

Burroughs Wellcome *p. 770*

2 mg

ALKERAN® tablets
(melphalan)

Burroughs Wellcome *p. 773*

10 mg

CARDILATE® tablets
(erythrityl tetranitrate)

Burroughs Wellcome *p. 777*

25 mg

DARAPRIM® tablets
(pyrimethamine)

Burroughs Wellcome *p. 780*

EMPIRIN® ASPIRIN tablets
(aspirin 325 mg)

Burroughs Wellcome *p. 780*

No. 3, 30 mg

No. 4, 60 mg

EMPIRIN® With Codeine tablets
(aspirin 325 mg and codeine phosphate)

Burroughs Wellcome *p. 785*

50 mg

†IMURAN® tablets
(azathioprine)

Burroughs Wellcome *p. 787*

5 mg

KEMADRIN® tablets
(procyclidine hydrochloride)

Burroughs Wellcome *p. 788*

0.05 mg

0.1 mg

0.2 mg

LANOXICAPS®
(digoxin solution in capsules)

Burroughs Wellcome *p. 800*

0.125 mg

0.25 mg

0.5 mg

†LANOXIN® tablets
(digoxin)

Burroughs Wellcome *p. 803*

5 mg   25 mg

†LEUCOVORIN CALCIUM tablets, WELLCOVORIN® brand
(leucovorin calcium)

Burroughs Wellcome *p. 804*

2 mg

LEUKERAN® tablets
(chlorambucil)

Burroughs Wellcome *p. 806*

50 mg

MAREZINE® tablets
(cyclizine hydrochloride)

Burroughs Wellcome *p. 810*

2 mg

MYLERAN® tablets
(busulfan)

Burroughs Wellcome *p. 819*

100 mg   200 mg

PROLOPRIM® tablets
(trimethoprim)

Burroughs Wellcome *p. 820*

50 mg

PURINETHOL® tablets
(mercaptopurine)

Burroughs Wellcome *p. 822*

100 mg

†RETROVIR® capsules
(zidovudine)

Burroughs Wellcome *p. 833*

†SEPTRA® tablets
(trimethoprim 80 mg and sulfamethoxazole 400 mg)

Burroughs Wellcome *p. 833*

†SEPTRA® DS tablets
(trimethoprim 160 mg and sulfamethoxazole 800 mg)

Burroughs Wellcome *p. 835*

30 mg   60 mg

†SUDAFED® tablets
(pseudoephedrine hydrochloride)

Burroughs Wellcome *p. 835*

120 mg

SUDAFED® 12 hour caplets
(pseudoephedrine hydrochloride)

Burroughs Wellcome *p. 835*

SUDAFED® severe cold formula caplets and tablets

(acetaminophen 500 mg, dextromethorphan HCl 15 mg, and pseudoephedrine HCl 30 mg)

Burroughs Wellcome *p. 835*

†SUDAFED® PLUS tablets
(pseudoephedrine hydrochloride 60 mg and chlorpheniramine maleate 4 mg)

Burroughs Wellcome *p. 835*

SUDAFED® SINUS tablets and caplets
(acetaminophen 500 mg and pseudoephedrine hydrochloride 30 mg)

Burroughs Wellcome *p. 835*

40 mg

THIOGUANINE tablets, TABLOID® brand
(thioguanine)

Burroughs Wellcome *p. 842*

75 mg   100 mg

WELLBUTRIN® tablets
(bupropion hydrochloride)

Burroughs Wellcome *p. 844*

200 mg

†ZOVIRAX® capsules
(acyclovir)

Burroughs Wellcome *p. 844*

800 mg

†ZOVIRAX® tablets
(acyclovir)

Burroughs Wellcome *p. 851*

100 mg   300 mg

ZYLOPRIM® tablets
(allopurinol)

CARNRICK

p. 856   (Both sides of tablet shown)

AMEN®
(medroxyprogesterone acetate, USP 10 mg)

Carnrick *p. 857*
(Both sides of tablet shown)

35 mg

BONTRIL® PDM
(phendimetrazine tartrate, USP 35 mg)

105 mg

BONTRIL® SLOW-RELEASE
(phendimetrazine tartrate 105 mg)

Carnrick *p. 858*

CAPITAL® and CODEINE SUSPENSION

(acetaminophen 120 mg/5 mL codeine phosphate 12 mg/5 mL)

Carnrick *p. 858*

HYDROCET®
(hydrocodone bitartrate, USP 5 mg acetaminophen, USP 500 mg)

Carnrick *p. 859*

MIDRIN®
(isometheptene mucate 65 mg, dichloralphenazone 100 mg, acetaminophen 325 mg)

Carnrick *p. 859*

MOTOFEN®
(difenoxin 1 mg as the hydrochloride, atropine sulfate 0.025 mg)

Carnrick *p. 860*

NOLAHIST®
(phenindamine tartrate 25 mg)

Carnrick *p. 860*

NOLAMINE®
(chlorpheniramine maleate 4 mg, phenindamine tartrate 24 mg, phenylpropanolamine hydrochloride 50 mg)

Carnrick *p. 860*

NOLEX® LA
(phenylpropanolamine HCl 75 mg, guaifenesin 400 mg)

Carnrick *p. 861*

8650

PHRENILIN®
(butalbital, USP 50 mg, acetaminophen, USP 325 mg)

8656

PHRENILIN® FORTE
(butalbital, USP 50 mg, acetaminophen, USP 650 mg)

Carnrick *p. 862*

(Both sides of tablet shown)

PROPAGEST®
(phenylpropanolamine HCl 25 mg)

Carnrick *p. 862*

8671

500 mg

8672

750 mg

SALFLEX®
(salsalate)

Carnrick *p. 863*

SINULIN®
(acetaminophen 650 mg, chlorpheniramine maleate 4 mg, phenylpropanolamine HCl 25 mg)

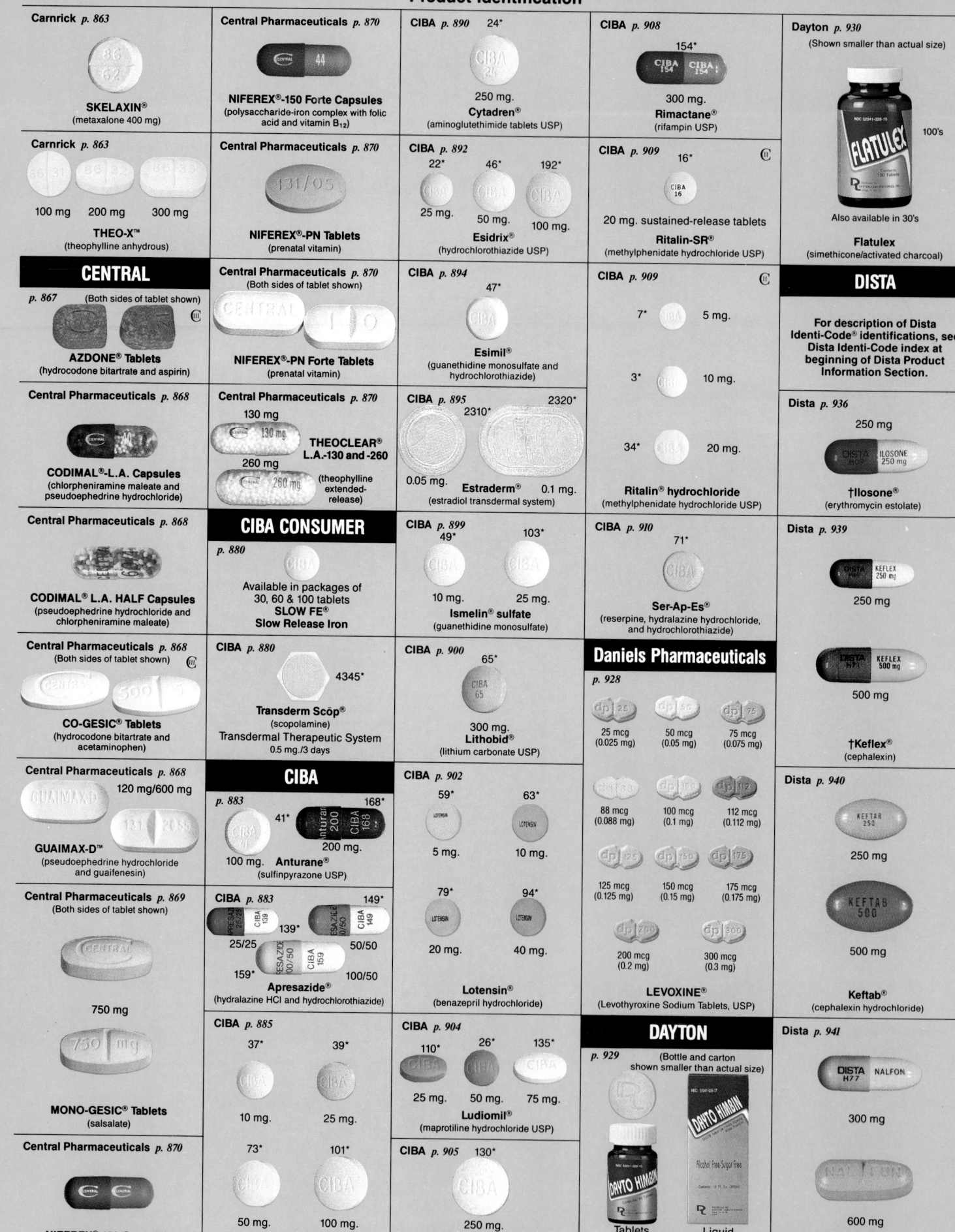

Carnrick p. 863

SKELAXIN®
(metaxalone 400 mg)

Carnrick p. 863

100 mg   200 mg   300 mg

THEO-X™
(theophylline anhydrous)

CENTRAL

p. 867   (Both sides of tablet shown)

AZDONE® Tablets
(hydrocodone bitartrate and aspirin)

Central Pharmaceuticals p. 868

CODIMAL®-L.A. Capsules
(chlorpheniramine maleate and
pseudoephedrine hydrochloride)

Central Pharmaceuticals p. 868

CODIMAL® L.A. HALF Capsules
(pseudoephedrine hydrochloride and
chlorpheniramine maleate)

Central Pharmaceuticals p. 868
(Both sides of tablet shown)

CO-GESIC® Tablets
(hydrocodone bitartrate and
acetaminophen)

Central Pharmaceuticals p. 868

120 mg/600 mg

GUAIMAX-D™
(pseudoephedrine hydrochloride
and guaifenesin)

Central Pharmaceuticals p. 869
(Both sides of tablet shown)

750 mg

MONO-GESIC® Tablets
(salsalate)

Central Pharmaceuticals p. 870

NIFEREX®-150 Capsules
(polysaccharide-iron complex)

Central Pharmaceuticals p. 870

44

NIFEREX®-150 Forte Capsules
(polysaccharide-iron complex with folic
acid and vitamin B_{12})

Central Pharmaceuticals p. 870

131/05

NIFEREX®-PN Tablets
(prenatal vitamin)

Central Pharmaceuticals p. 870
(Both sides of tablet shown)

NIFEREX®-PN Forte Tablets
(prenatal vitamin)

Central Pharmaceuticals p. 870

130 mg

260 mg

THEOCLEAR®
L.A.-130 and -260
(theophylline
extended-
release)

CIBA CONSUMER

p. 880

Available in packages of
30, 60 & 100 tablets
SLOW FE®
Slow Release Iron

CIBA p. 880

4345*

Transderm Scōp®
(scopolamine)
Transdermal Therapeutic System
0.5 mg./3 days

CIBA

p. 883   168*

41*

100 mg.   **Anturane®**
(sulfinpyrazone USP)

200 mg.

CIBA p. 883   149*

139*

25/25   50/50

159*   100/50

Apresazide®
(hydralazine HCl and hydrochlorothiazide)

CIBA p. 885

37*   39*

10 mg.   25 mg.

73*   101*

50 mg.   100 mg.

Apresoline® hydrochloride
(hydralazine hydrochloride USP)

CIBA p. 890   24*

250 mg.

Cytadren®
(aminoglutethimide tablets USP)

CIBA p. 892

22*   46*   192*

25 mg.

50 mg.

100 mg.

Esidrix®
(hydrochlorothiazide USP)

CIBA p. 894

47*

Esimil®
(guanethidine monosulfate and
hydrochlorothiazide)

CIBA p. 895

2310*   2320*

0.05 mg.   **Estraderm®**   0.1 mg.
(estradiol transdermal system)

CIBA p. 899

49*   103*

10 mg.   25 mg.

Ismelin® sulfate
(guanethidine monosulfate)

CIBA p. 900

65*

300 mg.
Lithobid®
(lithium carbonate USP)

CIBA p. 902

59*   63*

5 mg.   10 mg.

79*   94*

20 mg.   40 mg.

Lotensin®
(benazepril hydrochloride)

CIBA p. 904

110*   26*   135*

25 mg.   50 mg.   75 mg.

Ludiomil®
(maprotiline hydrochloride USP)

CIBA p. 905   130*

250 mg.
Metopirone®
(metyrapone USP)

CIBA p. 908

154*

300 mg.
Rimactane®
(rifampin USP)

CIBA p. 909   16*

20 mg. sustained-release tablets
Ritalin-SR®
(methylphenidate hydrochloride USP)

CIBA p. 909

7*   5 mg.

3*   10 mg.

34*   20 mg.

Ritalin® hydrochloride
(methylphenidate hydrochloride USP)

CIBA p. 910

71*

Ser-Ap-Es®
(reserpine, hydralazine hydrochloride,
and hydrochlorothiazide)

Daniels Pharmaceuticals

p. 928

25 mcg   50 mcg   75 mcg
(0.025 mg)   (0.05 mg)   (0.075 mg)

88 mcg   100 mcg   112 mcg
(0.088 mg)   (0.1 mg)   (0.112 mg)

125 mcg   150 mcg   175 mcg
(0.125 mg)   (0.15 mg)   (0.175 mg)

200 mcg   300 mcg
(0.2 mg)   (0.3 mg)

LEVOXINE®
(Levothyroxine Sodium Tablets, USP)

DAYTON

p. 929   (Bottle and carton
shown smaller than actual size)

Tablets   Liquid
Dayto Himbin
(vohimbine HCl, 5.4 mg)

Dayton p. 930
(Shown smaller than actual size)

100's

Also available in 30's

Flatulex
(simethicone/activated charcoal)

DISTA

For description of Dista
Identi-Code® identifications, see
Dista Identi-Code index at
beginning of Dista Product
Information Section.

Dista p. 936

250 mg

†**Ilosone®**
(erythromycin estolate)

Dista p. 939

250 mg

500 mg

†**Keflex®**
(cephalexin)

Dista p. 940

250 mg

500 mg

Keftab®
(cephalexin hydrochloride)

Dista p. 941

300 mg

600 mg

Nalfon®
(fenoprofen calcium)

Dista p. 941

200 mg
Nalfon® 200
(fenoprofen calcium)

Dista p. 943

20 mg
Prozac®
(fluoxetine hydrochloride)

Because tablets and capsules are shown in this section, do not infer that these are the only dosage forms available. Where a product name is preceded by the symbol †, refer to the description in the Product Information (White Section) for other forms.

Du Pont Pharmaceuticals

p. 963

1 mg
pink

2 mg
lavender

2½ mg
green

(Both sides of tablets shown)

5 mg
peach

7½ mg
yellow

10 mg
white

COUMADIN® Tablets
(crystalline warfarin sodium, USP)

Du Pont Pharmaceuticals
p. 965

200 mg

250 mg

300 mg

ETHMOZINE® Tablets
(moricizine hydrochloride)

Du Pont Pharmaceuticals
p. 973

0590-0127

PERCOCET® Tablets
[5 mg oxycodone HCl and 325 mg acetaminophen (USP)/tablet]

(Both sides of tablets shown)

0590-0135

PERCODAN® Tablets
[4.50 mg oxycodone HCl, 0.38 mg oxycodone terephthalate, 325 mg aspirin/tablet]

Du Pont Pharmaceuticals
p. 974

647*

650*

10-100

25-100

654*

25-250

SINEMET® Tablets
(carbidopa-levodopa)

Du Pont Pharmaceuticals
p. 976

521*

Sustained-Release Tablets
SINEMET® CR
(50 mg carbidopa, 200 mg levodopa)

FERRING

p. 1000

NDC 55566-1075-1
SECRETIN-FERRING

NDC 55566-1075-1
SECRETIN-FERRING

75 c.u./vial

Secretin-Ferring
(secretin)

Ferring Laboratories p. 1000

NDC 55566-0981-5 5 x 1 mL Ampul
Relefact® TRH
INJECTION
0.50 mg (500 mcg)/mL

0.5 mg/mL

Relefact® TRH Injection
(protirelin)

FOREST

p. 1024

7g

100 metered inhalations

250 mcg/ per puff

**AEROBID®
Inhaler System**
(flunisolide)

Forest
p. 1024

7g

100 metered inhalations

250 mcg/ per puff

**AEROBID®-M
Inhaler System**
(flunisolide)

Forest
p. 1026

(Aerosol holding chambers for use with metered-dose inhalers)

AeroChamber

AeroChamber

AeroChamber®

**AeroChamber®
With Mask**

Forest
p. 1030

535-12

capsule

Esgic®
(butalbital 50 mg
[Warning: May be habit forming]
acetaminophen 325 mg/caffeine 40 mg)

Ferring Laboratories p. 999

Kit

Pump

0.8 mg

3.2 mg

Lutrepulse® for Injection
(gonadorelin acetate)

Forest
p. 1030

FOREST

678

(Both sides of tablet shown)

Esgic-plus™ Tablet
(butalbital 50 mg
[Warning: May be habit forming]/
acetaminophen 500 mg/caffeine 40 mg)

Forest
p. 1031

25 mcg   50 mcg   75 mcg

100 mcg   125 mcg   150 mcg

175 mcg   200 mcg   300 mcg

Levothroid®
(levothyroxine sodium tablets, USP)

Forest
p. 1035

100 mg

Tessalon® Perles
(benzonatate USP)

Forest
p. 1157

See Product Information under Inwood Laboratories—Subsidiary of Forest Laboratories.

100 mg   200 mg

300 mg

Theochron™
(theophylline anhydrous)

Forest
p. 1028

¼ gr.   ½ gr.   1 gr.   1½ gr.

2 gr.   3 gr.

4 gr.   5 gr.

Armour® Thyroid   (thyroid USP)

Forest
p. 1035

Thyrolar-   Thyrolar-   Thyrolar-
¼   ½   1

Thyrolar-2   Thyrolar-3

Each Thyrolar-1 tablet contains
50 mcg T₄ and 12.5 mcg T₃

Thyrolar®
(liotrix) tablets

GATE

p. 1053

37.5 mg.   (Both sides of tablet shown)
†Adipex-P®
(phentermine hydrochloride)

Gate p. 1053

2 mg.

Orap™
(pimozide)

GEIGY

p. 1057

(Shown smaller than actual size)

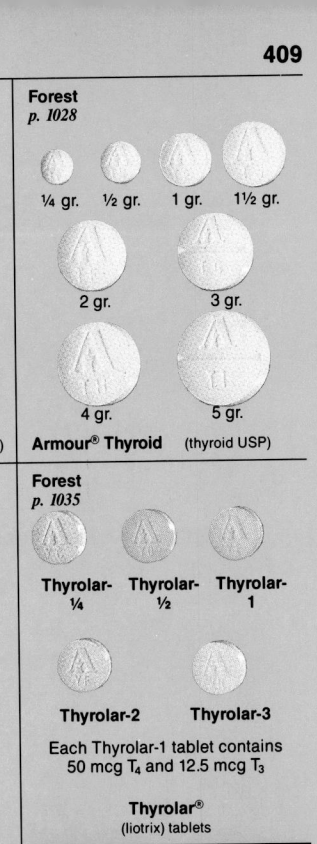

5557*

Brethaire®
(terbutaline sulfate USP
inhalation aerosol)

Geigy p. 1059

7507*

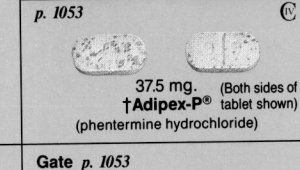

Brethine
terbutaline sulfate USP

1 mg./ml.

Ampul
(Shown smaller than actual size)

72*   105*

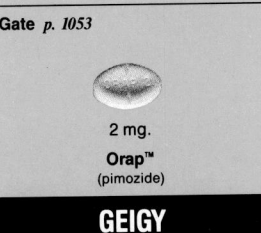

2.5 mg.   5 mg.

Tablets

†Brethine®
(terbutaline sulfate USP)

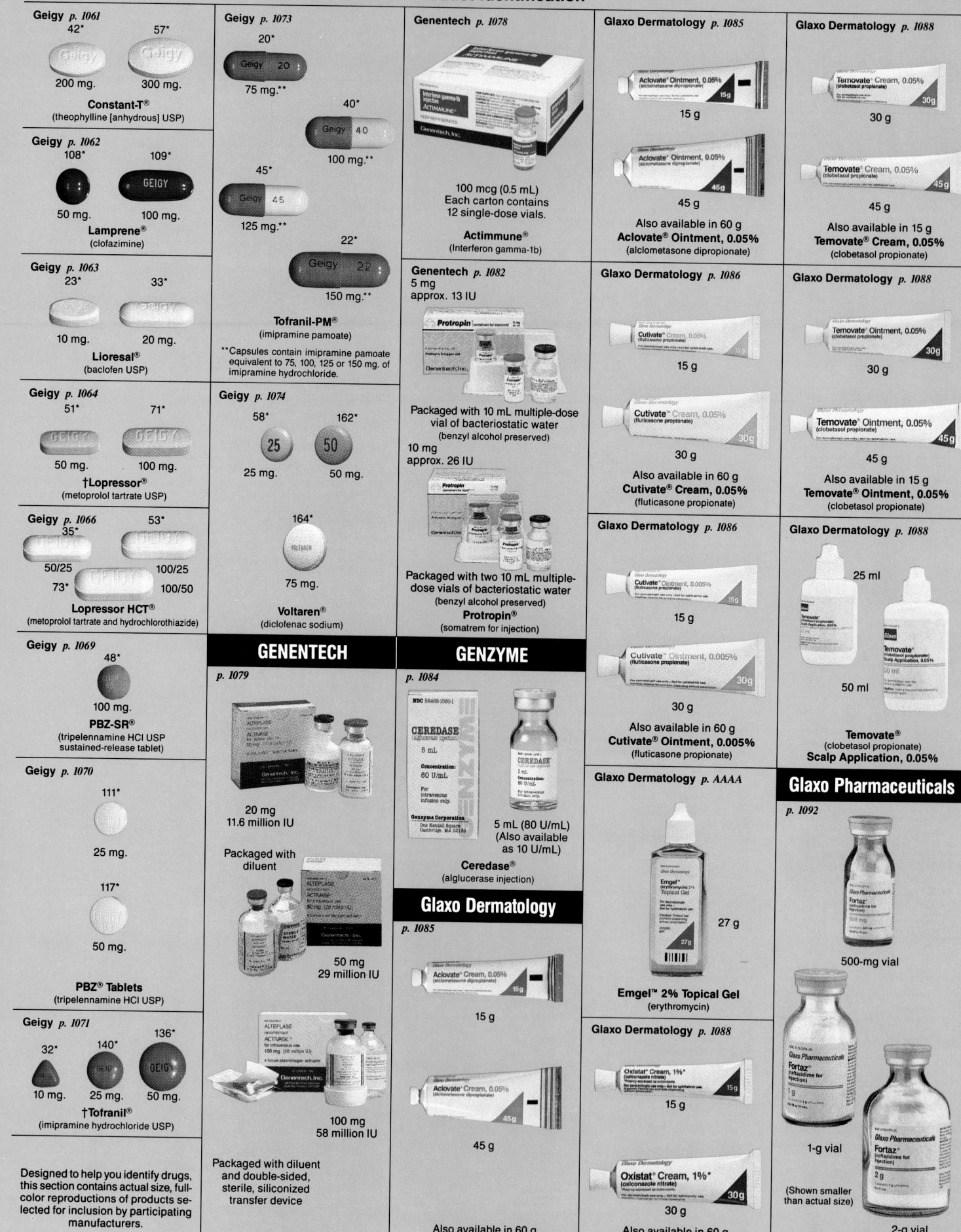

Geigy p. 1061

42* — 200 mg.   57* — 300 mg.

Constant-T®
(theophylline [anhydrous] USP)

Geigy p. 1062

108* — 50 mg.   109* — 100 mg.

Lamprene®
(clofazimine)

Geigy p. 1063

23* — 10 mg.   33* — 20 mg.

Lioresal®
(baclofen USP)

Geigy p. 1064

51* — 50 mg.   71* — 100 mg.

†Lopressor®
(metoprolol tartrate USP)

Geigy p. 1066

35* — 50/25   53* — 100/25   73* — 100/50

Lopressor HCT®
(metoprolol tartrate and hydrochlorothiazide)

Geigy p. 1069

48* — 100 mg.

PBZ-SR®
(tripelennamine HCl USP
sustained-release tablet)

Geigy p. 1070

111* — 25 mg.

117* — 50 mg.

PBZ® Tablets
(tripelennamine HCl USP)

Geigy p. 1071

32* — 10 mg.   140* — 25 mg.   136* — 50 mg.

†Tofranil®
(imipramine hydrochloride USP)

Designed to help you identify drugs, this section contains actual size, full-color reproductions of products selected for inclusion by participating manufacturers.

Geigy p. 1073

20* — 75 mg.**

40* — 100 mg.**

45* — 125 mg.**

22* — 150 mg.**

Tofranil-PM®
(imipramine pamoate)

**Capsules contain imipramine pamoate equivalent to 75, 100, 125 or 150 mg. of imipramine hydrochloride.

Geigy p. 1074

58* — 25 mg.   162* — 50 mg.

164* — 75 mg.

Voltaren®
(diclofenac sodium)

GENENTECH

p. 1079

20 mg
11.6 million IU

Packaged with diluent

50 mg
29 million IU

100 mg
58 million IU

Packaged with diluent and double-sided, sterile, siliconized transfer device

Activase®
(Alteplase, recombinant)

Genentech p. 1078

100 mcg (0.5 mL)
Each carton contains
12 single-dose vials.

Actimmune®
(Interferon gamma-1b)

Genentech p. 1082

5 mg
approx. 13 IU

Packaged with 10 mL multiple-dose vial of bacteriostatic water
(benzyl alcohol preserved)

10 mg
approx. 26 IU

Packaged with two 10 mL multiple-dose vials of bacteriostatic water
(benzyl alcohol preserved)

Protropin®
(somatrem for injection)

GENZYME

p. 1084

NDC 58468-1060-1

CEREDASE
(alglucerase injection)
5 mL

Concentration:
80 U/mL

For intravenous infusion only.

Genzyme Corporation
One Kendall Square
Cambridge, MA 02139

5 mL (80 U/mL)
(Also available as 10 U/mL)

Ceredase®
(alglucerase injection)

Glaxo Dermatology

p. 1085

15 g

Aclovate® Cream, 0.05%
(alclometasone dipropionate)

45 g

Also available in 60 g
Aclovate® Cream, 0.05%
(alclometasone dipropionate)

Glaxo Dermatology p. 1085

15 g

Aclovate® Ointment, 0.05%
(alclometasone dipropionate)

45 g

Also available in 60 g
Aclovate® Ointment, 0.05%
(alclometasone dipropionate)

Glaxo Dermatology p. 1086

15 g

Cutivate™ Cream, 0.05%
(fluticasone propionate)

30 g

Also available in 60 g
Cutivate® Cream, 0.05%
(fluticasone propionate)

Glaxo Dermatology p. 1086

15 g

Cutivate™ Ointment, 0.005%
(fluticasone propionate)

30 g

Also available in 60 g
Cutivate® Ointment, 0.005%
(fluticasone propionate)

Glaxo Dermatology p. AAAA

27 g

Emgel™ 2% Topical Gel
(erythromycin)

Glaxo Dermatology p. 1088

15 g

Oxistat® Cream, 1%*
(oxiconazole nitrate)

30 g

Also available in 60 g
Oxistat® Cream, 1%
(oxiconazole nitrate)

Glaxo Dermatology p. 1088

30 g

Temovate® Cream, 0.05%
(clobetasol propionate)

45 g

Also available in 15 g
Temovate® Cream, 0.05%
(clobetasol propionate)

Glaxo Dermatology p. 1088

30 g

Temovate® Ointment, 0.05%
(clobetasol propionate)

45 g

Also available in 15 g
Temovate® Ointment, 0.05%
(clobetasol propionate)

Glaxo Dermatology p. 1088

25 ml

50 ml

Temovate®
(clobetasol propionate)
Scalp Application, 0.05%

Glaxo Pharmaceuticals

p. 1092

500-mg vial

1-g vial

(Shown smaller than actual size)

2-g vial

Fortaz®
(ceftazidime for injection)

Glaxo Pharmaceuticals p. 1092

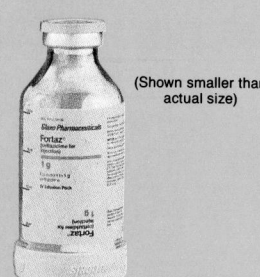

(Shown smaller than actual size)

1-g
IV infusion pack

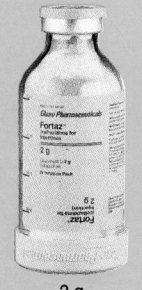

2-g
IV infusion pack

Fortaz®
(ceftazidime for injection)

Glaxo Pharmaceuticals p. 1092

(Shown smaller than actual size)

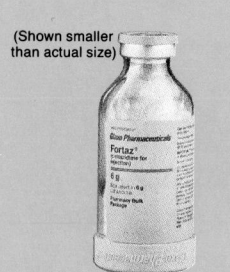

6-g pharmacy bulk package
Fortaz®
(ceftazidime for injection)

Glaxo Pharmaceuticals p. 1092

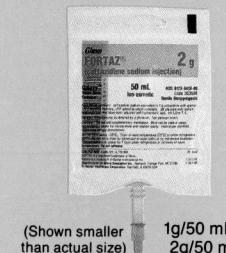

(Shown smaller than actual size)   1g/50 mL &
2g/50 mL

Fortaz®
(ceftazidime sodium injection)

Designed to help you identify drugs, this section contains actual size, full-color reproductions of products selected for inclusion by participating manufacturers.

Important Notice

Before prescribing or administering any product described in PHYSICIANS' DESK REFERENCE always consult the PDR Supplement for possible new or revised information.

Glaxo Pharmaceuticals p. 1089

(Shown smaller than actual size)

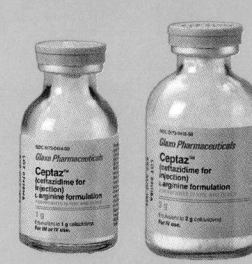

1-g vial   2-g vial

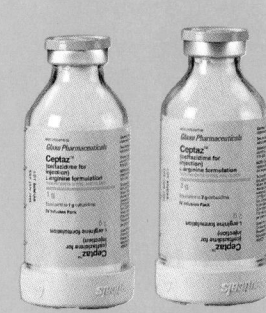

1-g   2-g
infusion pack   infusion pack

Ceptaz™

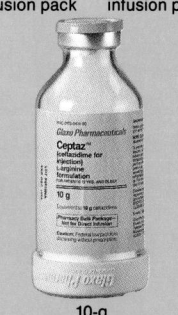

10-g
pharmacy bulk package
Ceptaz™
(ceftazidime for injection)
L-arginine formulation

Glaxo Pharmaceuticals p. 1096

(Shown smaller than actual size)

Available in:
2-mL vial
6-mL vial
40-mL pharmacy
bulk package

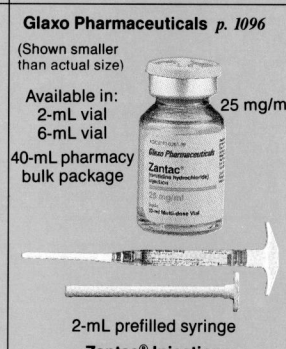   25 mg/mL

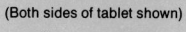

2-mL prefilled syringe
Zantac® Injection
(ranitidine hydrochloride)

Glaxo Pharmaceuticals p. 1097

(Both sides of tablet shown)

150 mg
Zantac® 150 Tablets
(ranitidine hydrochloride)

Glaxo Pharmaceuticals p. 1097

(Both sides of tablet shown)

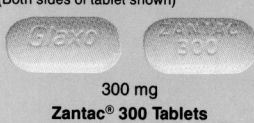

300 mg
Zantac® 300 Tablets
(ranitidine hydrochloride)

Glaxo Pharmaceuticals p. 1096

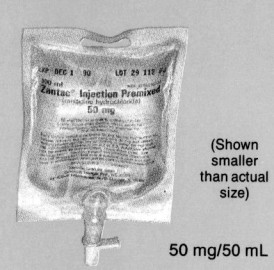

(Shown
smaller
than actual
size)

50 mg/50 mL

Zantac® Injection Premixed
(ranitidine hydrochloride)

Glaxo Pharmaceuticals p. 1097

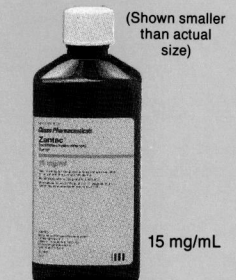

(Shown smaller
than actual
size)

15 mg/mL

Zantac® Syrup
(ranitidine hydrochloride)

Glaxo Pharmaceuticals p. 1099

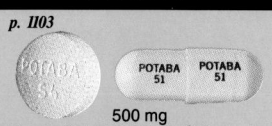

750-mg vial   1.5-g vial

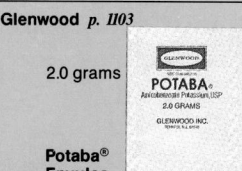

750-mg IV   1.5-g IV
infusion pack   infusion pack

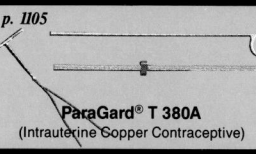

(Shown
smaller
than actual
size)

7.5-g
pharmacy bulk
package

Zinacef®
(sterile cefuroxime sodium)

Glaxo Pharmaceuticals p. 1099

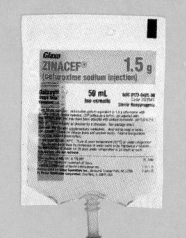

(Shown smaller   750 mg/50 mL &
than actual size)   1.5 g/50 mL

Zinacef®
(cefuroxime sodium injection)

Cerenex Pharmaceuticals
A Division of Glaxo, Inc.
p. 871

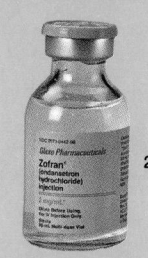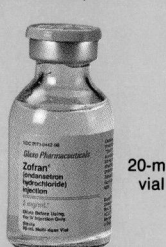   20-mL
vial

(Shown smaller than actual size)

Zofran® Injection
(ondansetron hydrochloride)

GLENWOOD

p. 1103

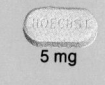   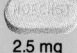

500 mg
Potaba® Tablet   Potaba® Capsule

Glenwood p. 1103

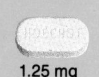

2.0 grams

**Potaba®
Envules**

GYNOPHARMA

p. 1105

ParaGard® T 380A
(Intrauterine Copper Contraceptive)

HOECHST-ROUSSEL

p. 1112

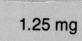

1.25 mg

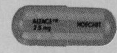

2.5 mg

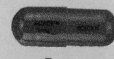

5 mg

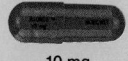

10 mg

ALTACE™ Capsules
(ramipril)

Hoechst-Roussel p. 1114

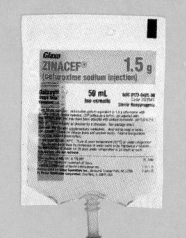

(Shown smaller than actual size)

60 mL
(with applicator)
2% Acne Topical Solution

2% Acne
TOPICAL
SOLUTION
60 mL

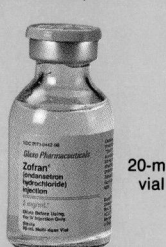

30 g
2% Topical Gel

A/T/S®
(erythromycin)

Hoechst-Roussel p. 1117

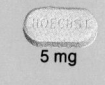

5 mg

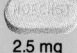

2.5 mg

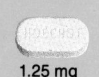

1.25 mg

DIABETA® Tablets
(glyburide)

Hoechst-Roussel p. 1119

60 mL
(with graduated dropper)

Also available,
120 mL
(with graduated
dropper)

**LASIX®
Oral Solution**
(furosemide)

(Lasix Oral Solution shown
smaller than actual size)

Hoechst-Roussel p. 1119

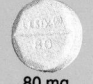

20 mg   40 mg

80 mg

LASIX® Tablets
(furosemide)

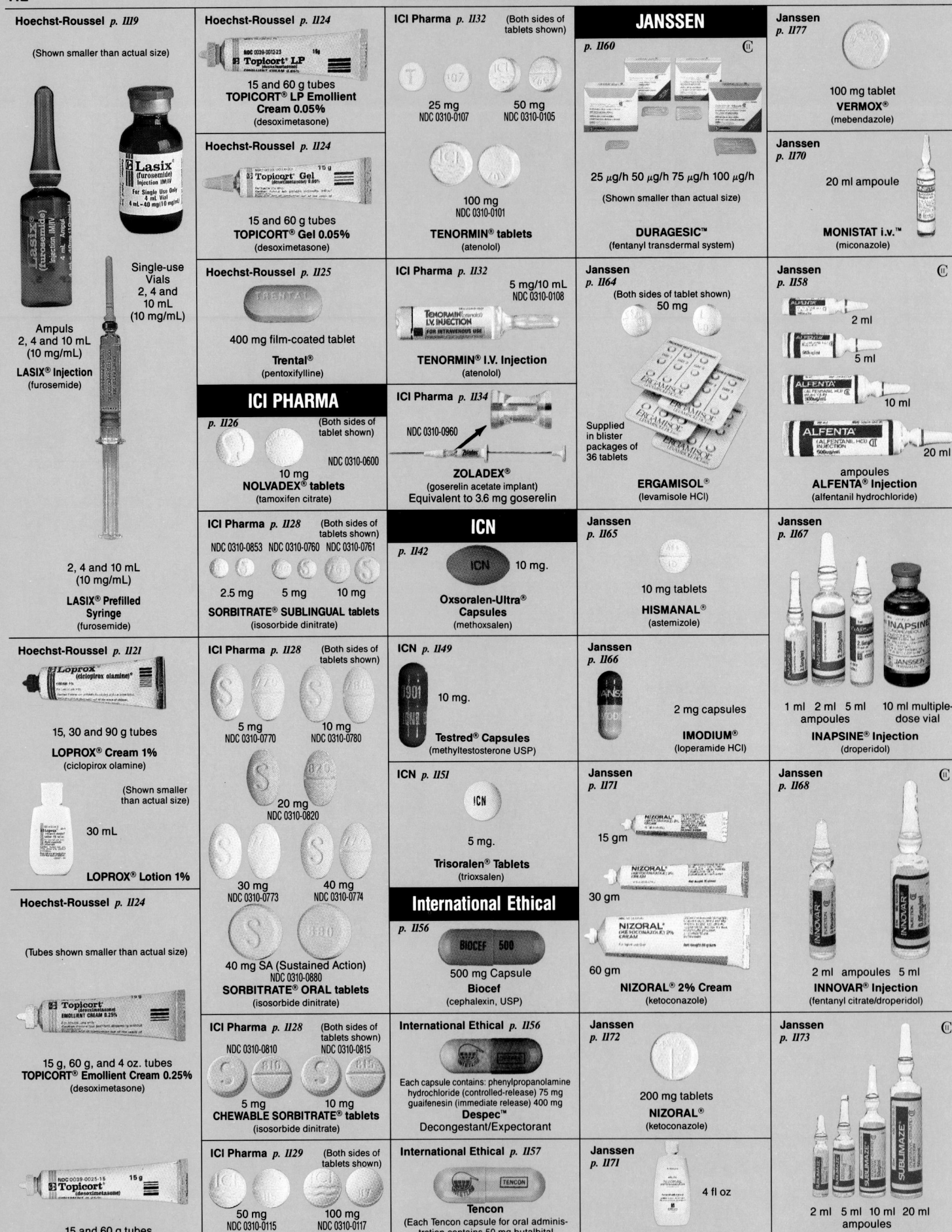

Hoechst-Roussel p. 1119

(Shown smaller than actual size)

Ampuls
2, 4 and 10 mL
(10 mg/mL)

LASIX® Injection
(furosemide)

Single-use
Vials
2, 4 and
10 mL
(10 mg/mL)

2, 4 and 10 mL
(10 mg/mL)

**LASIX® Prefilled
Syringe**
(furosemide)

Hoechst-Roussel p. 1121

15, 30 and 90 g tubes
LOPROX® Cream 1%
(ciclopirox olamine)

(Shown smaller
than actual size)

30 mL

LOPROX® Lotion 1%

Hoechst-Roussel p. 1124

(Tubes shown smaller than actual size)

15 g, 60 g, and 4 oz. tubes
TOPICORT® Emollient Cream 0.25%
(desoximetasone)

15 and 60 g tubes
TOPICORT® Ointment 0.25%
(desoximetasone)

Hoechst-Roussel p. 1124

15 and 60 g tubes
**TOPICORT® LP Emollient
Cream 0.05%**
(desoximetasone)

Hoechst-Roussel p. 1124

15 and 60 g tubes
TOPICORT® Gel 0.05%
(desoximetasone)

Hoechst-Roussel p. 1125

400 mg film-coated tablet
Trental®
(pentoxifylline)

ICI PHARMA

p. 1126   (Both sides of
                  tablet shown)

NDC 0310-0600

10 mg
NOLVADEX® tablets
(tamoxifen citrate)

ICI Pharma p. 1128   (Both sides of
                                tablets shown)

NDC 0310-0853 NDC 0310-0760 NDC 0310-0761

2.5 mg   5 mg   10 mg
SORBITRATE® SUBLINGUAL tablets
(isosorbide dinitrate)

ICI Pharma p. 1128   (Both sides of
                                tablets shown)

5 mg   10 mg
NDC 0310-0770   NDC 0310-0780

20 mg
NDC 0310-0820

30 mg   40 mg
NDC 0310-0773   NDC 0310-0774

40 mg SA (Sustained Action)
NDC 0310-0880
SORBITRATE® ORAL tablets
(isosorbide dinitrate)

ICI Pharma p. 1128   (Both sides of
                                tablets shown)
NDC 0310-0810   NDC 0310-0815

5 mg   10 mg
CHEWABLE SORBITRATE® tablets
(isosorbide dinitrate)

ICI Pharma p. 1129   (Both sides of
                                tablets shown)

50 mg   100 mg
NDC 0310-0115   NDC 0310-0117
TENORETIC® tablets
(atenolol, chlorthalidone, 25 mg)

ICI Pharma p. 1132   (Both sides of
                                tablets shown)

25 mg   50 mg
NDC 0310-0107   NDC 0310-0105

100 mg
NDC 0310-0101
TENORMIN® tablets
(atenolol)

ICI Pharma p. 1132

5 mg/10 mL
NDC 0310-0108

TENORMIN® I.V. Injection
(atenolol)

ICI Pharma p. 1134

NDC 0310-0960

ZOLADEX®
(goserelin acetate implant)
Equivalent to 3.6 mg goserelin

ICN

p. 1142

ICN 10 mg.

**Oxsoralen-Ultra®
Capsules**
(methoxsalen)

ICN p. 1149

10 mg.

Testred® Capsules
(methyltestosterone USP)

ICN p. 1151

ICN

5 mg.

Trisoralen® Tablets
(trioxsalen)

International Ethical

p. 1156

BIOCEF 500

500 mg Capsule
Biocef
(cephalexin, USP)

International Ethical p. 1156

Each capsule contains: phenylpropanolamine
hydrochloride (controlled-release) 75 mg
guaifenesin (immediate release) 400 mg
Despec™
Decongestant/Expectorant

International Ethical p. 1157

TENCON

Tencon
(Each Tencon capsule for oral administration contains 50 mg butalbital
[WARNING: may be habit forming] and
650 mg of acetaminophen)

JANSSEN

p. 1160

25 µg/h 50 µg/h 75 µg/h 100 µg/h

(Shown smaller than actual size)

DURAGESIC™
(fentanyl transdermal system)

Janssen p. 1164

(Both sides of tablet shown)
50 mg

Supplied
in blister
packages of
36 tablets

ERGAMISOL®
(levamisole HCl)

Janssen p. 1165

10 mg tablets
HISMANAL®
(astemizole)

Janssen p. 1166

2 mg capsules
IMODIUM®
(loperamide HCl)

Janssen p. 1171

15 gm

30 gm

60 gm

NIZORAL® 2% Cream
(ketoconazole)

Janssen p. 1172

200 mg tablets
NIZORAL®
(ketoconazole)

Janssen p. 1171

4 fl oz

NIZORAL® 2% Shampoo
(ketoconazole)

Janssen
p. 1177

100 mg tablet
VERMOX®
(mebendazole)

Janssen p. 1170

20 ml ampoule

MONISTAT i.v.™
(miconazole)

Janssen p. 1158

2 ml

5 ml

10 ml

20 ml

ampoules
ALFENTA® Injection
(alfentanil hydrochloride)

Janssen p. 1167

1 ml 2 ml 5 ml   10 ml multiple-
ampoules   dose vial
INAPSINE® Injection
(droperidol)

Janssen p. 1168

2 ml ampoules 5 ml
INNOVAR® Injection
(fentanyl citrate/droperidol)

Janssen p. 1173

2 ml 5 ml 10 ml 20 ml
ampoules
SUBLIMAZE® Injection
(fentanyl citrate)

Janssen
p. 1175

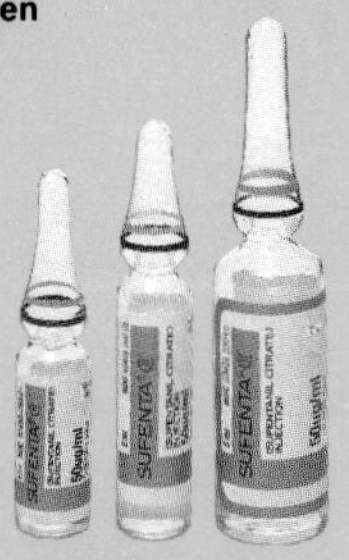

1 ml   2 ml   5 ml
ampoules
SUFENTA® Injection
(sufentanil citrate)

While every effort has been made to reproduce products faithfully, this section is to be considered a quick-reference identification aid. In cases of suspected overdosage, etc., chemical analysis of the product should be done.

J&J-MERCK
p. 1180

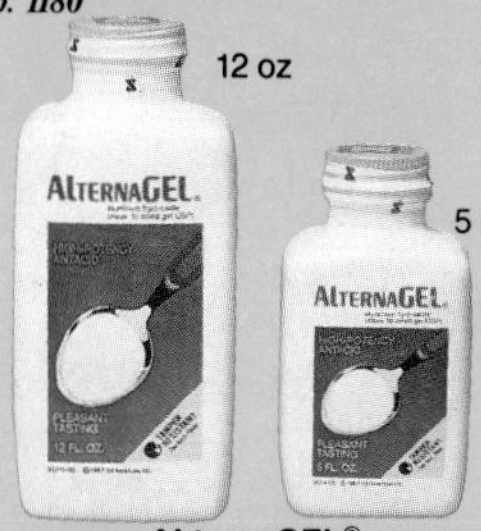

12 oz

5 oz

ALternaGEL®
High Potency Aluminum Hydroxide
Antacid

J&J-Merck
p. 1180

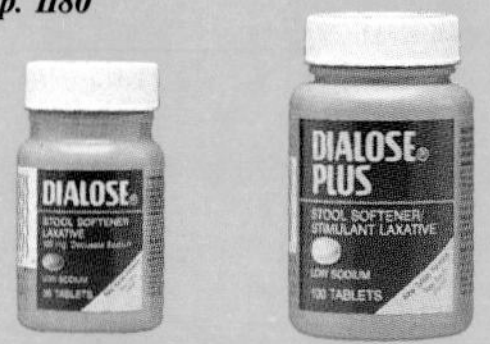

DIALOSE   DIALOSE PLUS

Bottles of 36 & 100 tablets

DIALOSE®   **DIALOSE® PLUS**
(docusate sodium,   (docusate sodium,
100 mg)   100 mg
                     yellow phenolph-
                     thalein, 65 mg)

J&J-Merck
p. 1181

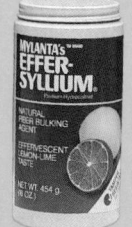

Available in
9 oz and 16 oz
bottles and
convenience
packets, 12's
and 24's

**MYLANTA'S™ BRAND
EFFER-SYLLIUM®**
(psyllium hydrocolloid)
Bulk Laxative containing
Natural Dietary Fiber

J&J-Merck   (layered tablet)
p. 1181

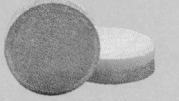

FERANCEE® Chewable Tablets

J&J-Merck
p. 1181

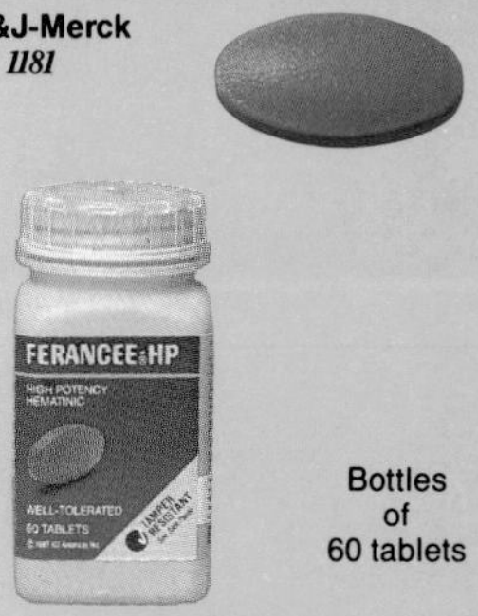

FERANCEE®-HP
High Potency Hematic

J&J-Merck
p. 1183

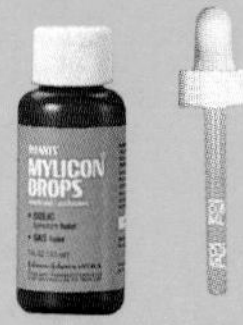

40 mg
per 0.6 mL

Available in
0.5 oz and
1.0 oz bottles
MYLICON® Drops
(simethicone)

J&J-Merck
p. 1183

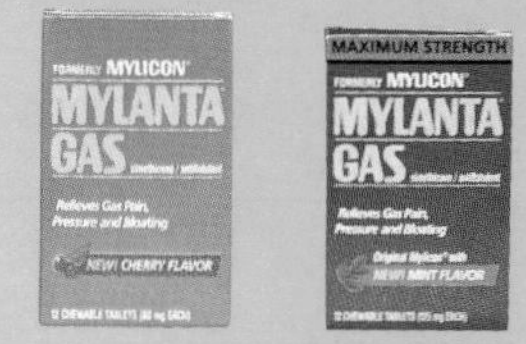

Bottles of 100
12 & 48 tablet
Convenience
Packs

12 & 60
tablet
Convenience
Packs

**MYLANTA®   MAXIMUM
GAS   STRENGTH
             MYLANTA®
             GAS**

(simethicone,   (simethicone,
80 mg)   125 mg)

J&J-Merck
p. 1183

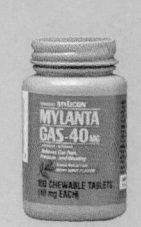

Antiflatulent
Bottles of 100 tablets

MYLANTA® GAS-40 MG
(simethicone, 40 mg)

J&J-Merck
p. 1182

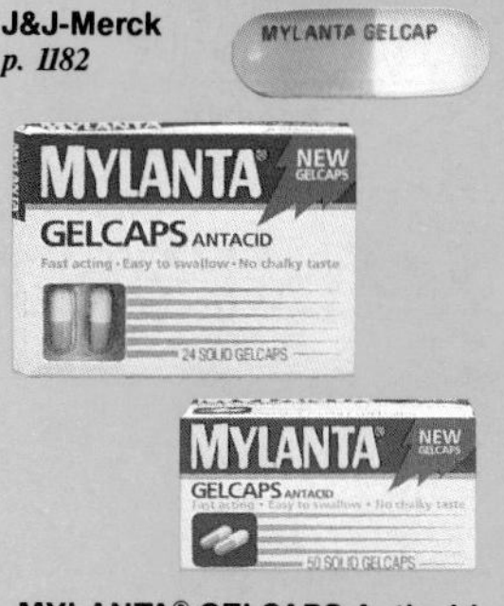

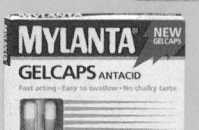

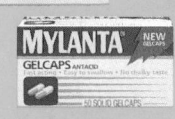

MYLANTA® GELCAPS Antacid
(calcium carbonate 311 mg,
magnesium carbonate 232 mg)

J&J-Merck
p. 1181

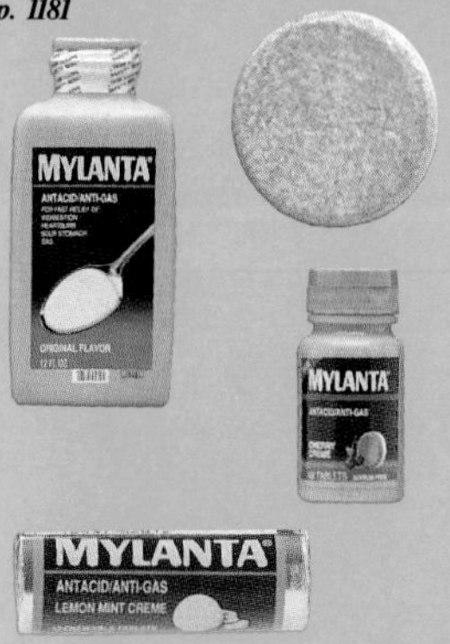

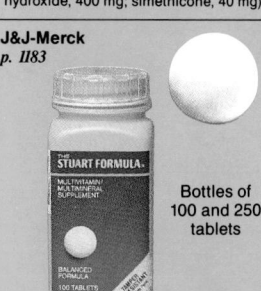

Bottles of 5, 12, 24 oz; tablets
in 48 & 100 count bottles;
12 tablet rollpack

MYLANTA® LIQUID & TABLETS
(aluminum hydroxide 200 mg,
and magnesium hydroxide 200 mg;
simethicone 20 mg)

J&J-Merck
p. 1182

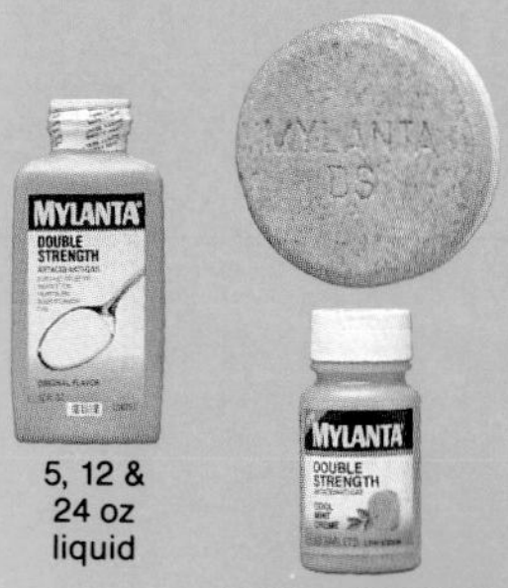

5, 12 &
24 oz
liquid

Bottles of 30 & 60
tablets & 8 tablet
rollpacks

**MYLANTA® DOUBLE STRENGTH
LIQUID & TABLETS**
(aluminum hydroxide, 400 mg; magnesium
hydroxide, 400 mg; simethicone, 40 mg)

J&J-Merck
p. 1183

Bottles of
100 and 250
tablets

STUART FORMULA® TABLETS
Multivitamin/Multimineral Supplement

J&J-Merck
p. 1183

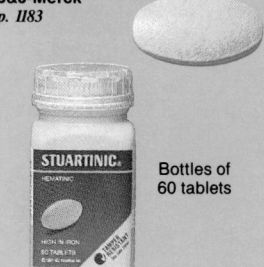

Bottles of
60 tablets

STUARTINIC®
Hematic

KABI PHARMACIA
p. 1184

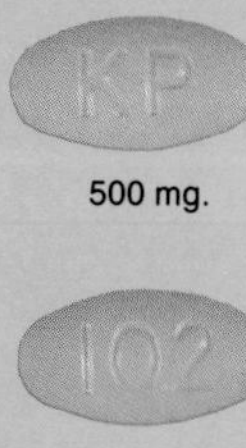

500 mg.

Azulfidine EN-tabs®
(sulfasalazine delayed-release
tablets, USP) Enteric Coated

Kabi Pharmacia
p. 1187

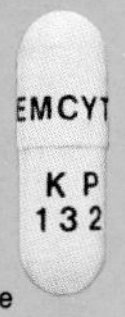

140 mg.

EMCYT
K P
1 3 2

Emcyt®
(estramustine phosphate
sodium/Pharmacia)

Kabi Pharmacia
p. 1186

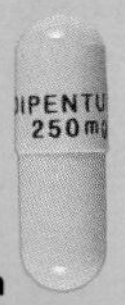

250 mg.

DIPENTU
250 mg

Dipentum
(olsalazine sodium)

Key Pharmaceuticals
p. 1190

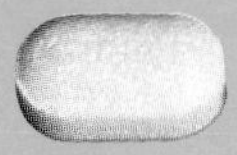

K-Dur® 10

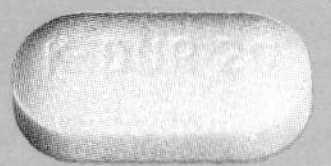

K-Dur® 20

(potassium chloride USP)
Microburst Release System®

Key Pharmaceuticals p. 1191
(Shown smaller than actual size)

0.1 mg/hr   0.2 mg/hr

0.3 mg/hr

                   0.4 mg/hr

                   0.6 mg/hr

Nitro-Dur®
(nitroglycerin)
Transdermal Infusion System

Key Pharmaceuticals p. 1197

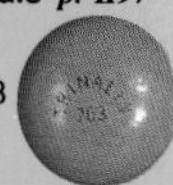

703

**TRINALIN®
Long-Acting
Antihistamine/Decongestant
REPETABS® Tablets**
(azatadine maleate, USP and
pseudoephedrine sulfate, USP)

Key Pharmaceuticals p. 1192

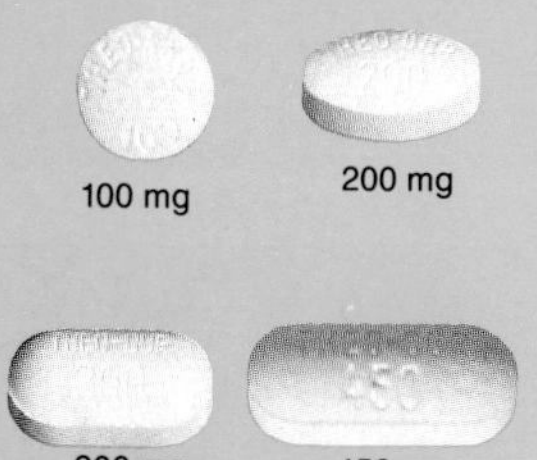

100 mg   200 mg

300 mg   450 mg

Theo-Dur®
(theophylline anhydrous)
Sustained Action Tablets

Key Pharmaceuticals p. 1195

Sustained
Action
Capsules

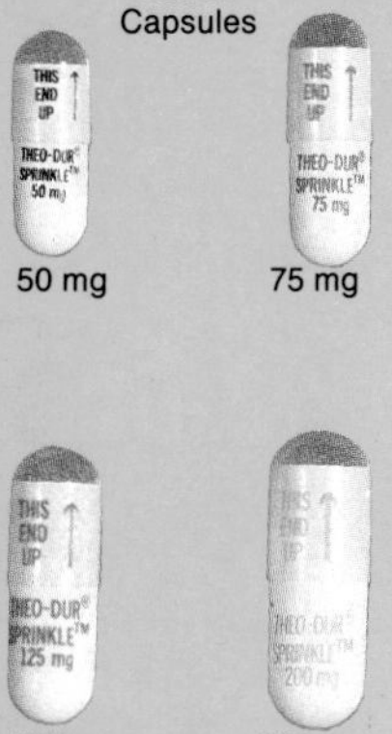

50 mg   75 mg

125 mg   200 mg

Theo-Dur® Sprinkle
(theophylline anhydrous)

KNOLL

p. 1198   (Both sides of tablet shown)

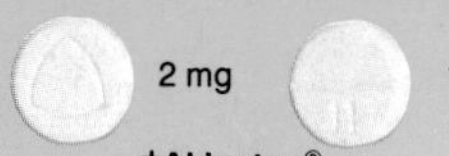

2 mg   11*

†Akineton®
(biperiden HCl)

Knoll p. 1199   (Both sides of tablets shown)

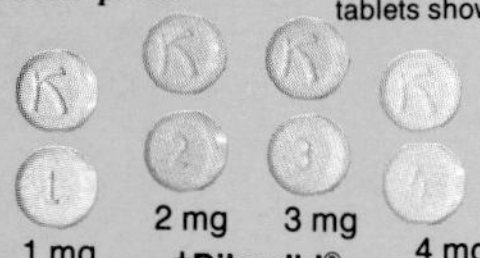

1 mg   2 mg   3 mg   4 mg
†Dilaudid®
(hydromorphone HCl)

Knoll p. 1201

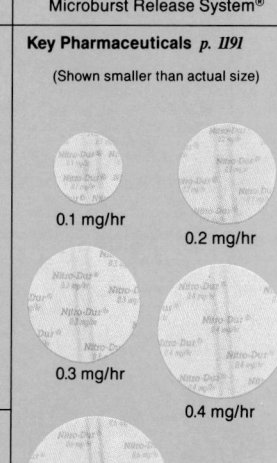

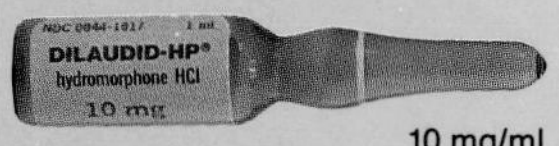

DILAUDID-HP®
hydromorphone HCl
10 mg

10 mg/ml

Dilaudid-HP® Injection
(hydromorphone HCl)

Knoll p. 1203

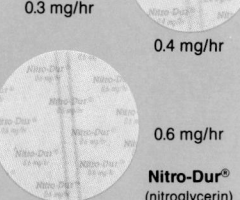

Dilaudid-HP®
hydromorphone HCl
50 mg/5 mL

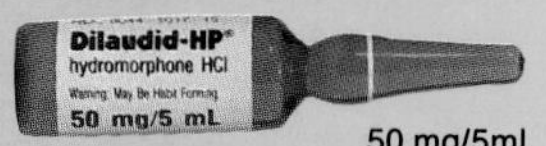

50 mg/5ml

Dilaudid-HP® Injection
(hydromorphone HCl)

Knoll p. 1203

ISOPTIN®
verapamil HCl

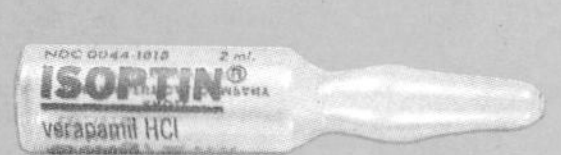

Isoptin® 5 mg/2ml Ampule
(verapamil HCl)

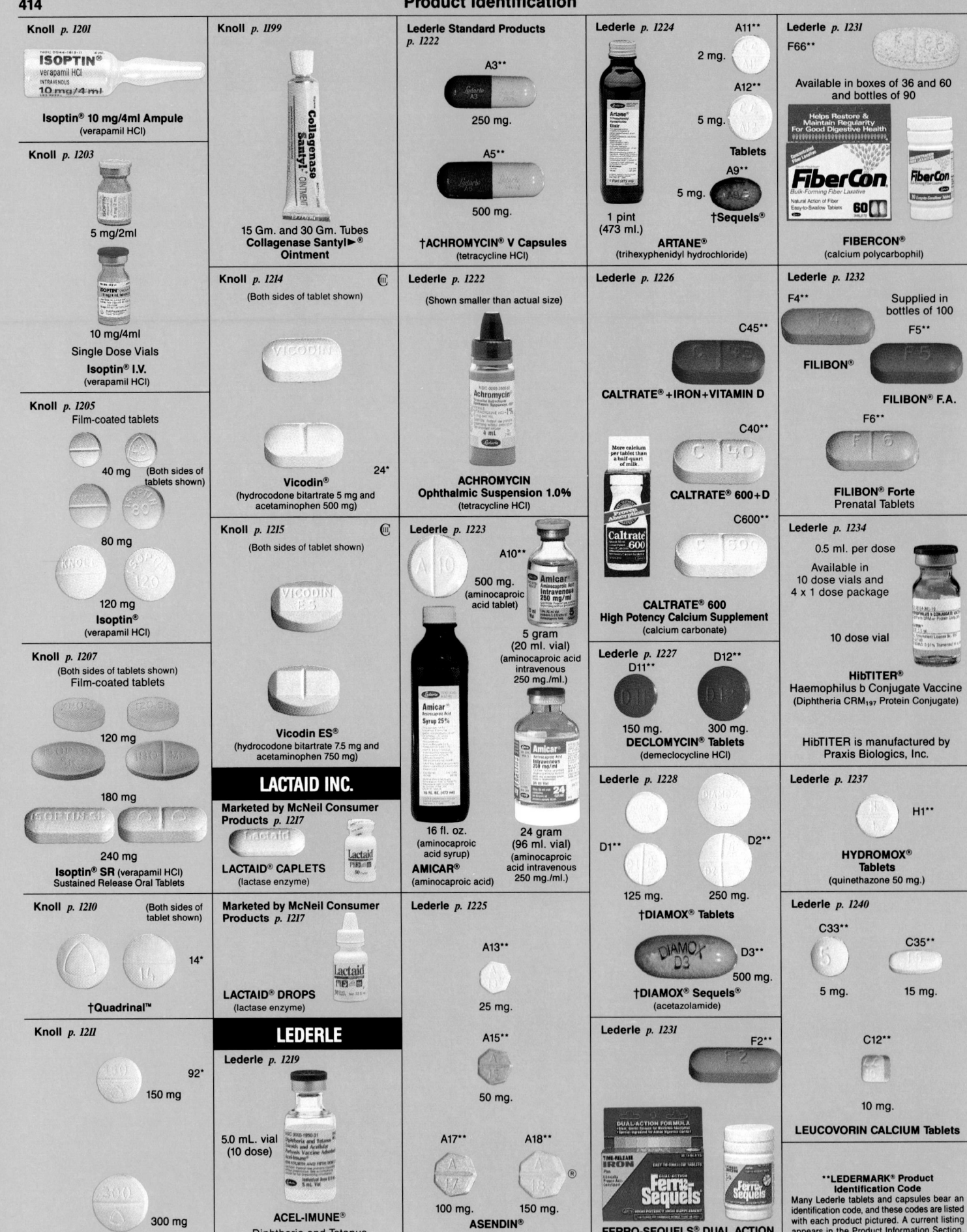

Knoll p. 1201

Isoptin® 10 mg/4ml Ampule
(verapamil HCl)

Knoll p. 1203

5 mg/2ml

10 mg/4ml
Single Dose Vials
Isoptin® I.V.
(verapamil HCl)

Knoll p. 1205
Film-coated tablets

40 mg (Both sides of tablets shown)

80 mg

120 mg
Isoptin®
(verapamil HCl)

Knoll p. 1207
(Both sides of tablets shown)
Film-coated tablets

120 mg

180 mg

240 mg
Isoptin® SR (verapamil HCl)
Sustained Release Oral Tablets

Knoll p. 1210 (Both sides of tablet shown)

14*

†Quadrinal™

Knoll p. 1211

92*

150 mg

300 mg
Rythmol®
(propafenone HCl)

Knoll p. 1199

15 Gm. and 30 Gm. Tubes
Collagenase Santyl►®
Ointment

Knoll p. 1214

(Both sides of tablet shown)

VICODIN

Vicodin® 24*
(hydrocodone bitartrate 5 mg and
acetaminophen 500 mg)

Knoll p. 1215

(Both sides of tablet shown)

VICODIN ES

Vicodin ES®
(hydrocodone bitartrate 7.5 mg and
acetaminophen 750 mg)

LACTAID INC.

**Marketed by McNeil Consumer
Products** p. 1217

LACTAID® CAPLETS
(lactase enzyme)

**Marketed by McNeil Consumer
Products** p. 1217

LACTAID® DROPS
(lactase enzyme)

LEDERLE

Lederle p. 1219

5.0 mL. vial
(10 dose)

ACEL-IMUNE®
Diphtheria and Tetanus
Toxoids and Acellular
Pertussis Vaccine Adsorbed

Lederle Standard Products
p. 1222

A3**
250 mg.

A5**
500 mg.

†ACHROMYCIN® V Capsules
(tetracycline HCl)

Lederle p. 1222

(Shown smaller than actual size)

ACHROMYCIN
Ophthalmic Suspension 1.0%
(tetracycline HCl)

Lederle p. 1223

A10**
500 mg.
(aminocaproic
acid tablet)

A10**

5 gram
(20 ml. vial)
(aminocaproic acid
intravenous
250 mg./ml.)

16 fl. oz.
(aminocaproic
acid syrup)
AMICAR®
(aminocaproic acid)

24 gram
(96 ml. vial)
(aminocaproic
acid intravenous
250 mg./ml.)

Lederle p. 1225

A13**

25 mg.

A15**

50 mg.

A17**   A18**

100 mg.   150 mg.
ASENDIN®
(amoxapine)
®: Unique tablet shape is a trademark
of American Cyanamid Company.

Lederle p. 1224

A11**
2 mg.

A12**
5 mg.
Tablets

A9**
5 mg.
†Sequels®

1 pint
(473 ml.)
ARTANE®
(trihexyphenidyl hydrochloride)

Lederle p. 1226

C45**

CALTRATE® +IRON+VITAMIN D

C40**

CALTRATE® 600+D

C600**

CALTRATE® 600
High Potency Calcium Supplement
(calcium carbonate)

Lederle p. 1227

D11**   D12**

150 mg.   300 mg.
DECLOMYCIN® Tablets
(demeclocycline HCl)

Lederle p. 1228

D1**   D2**

125 mg.   250 mg.
†DIAMOX® Tablets

DIAMOX
D3
D3**
500 mg.
†DIAMOX® Sequels®
(acetazolamide)

Lederle p. 1231

F2**

FERRO-SEQUELS® DUAL ACTION
High Potency Iron Supplement
(ferrous fumarate)

Lederle p. 1231

F66**

Available in boxes of 36 and 60
and bottles of 90

FiberCon

FIBERCON®
(calcium polycarbophil)

Lederle p. 1232

F4**

FILIBON®

F5**

FILIBON® F.A.

F6**

FILIBON® Forte
Prenatal Tablets

Supplied in
bottles of 100

Lederle p. 1234

0.5 ml. per dose
Available in
10 dose vials and
4 x 1 dose package

10 dose vial

HibTITER®
Haemophilus b Conjugate Vaccine
(Diphtheria CRM$_{197}$ Protein Conjugate)

HibTITER is manufactured by
Praxis Biologics, Inc.

Lederle p. 1237

H1**

HYDROMOX®
Tablets
(quinethazone 50 mg.)

Lederle p. 1240

C33**   C35**

5 mg.   15 mg.

C12**

10 mg.
LEUCOVORIN CALCIUM Tablets

****LEDERMARK® Product
Identification Code**
Many Lederle tablets and capsules bear an
identification code, and these codes are listed
with each product pictured. A current listing
appears in the Product Information Section.

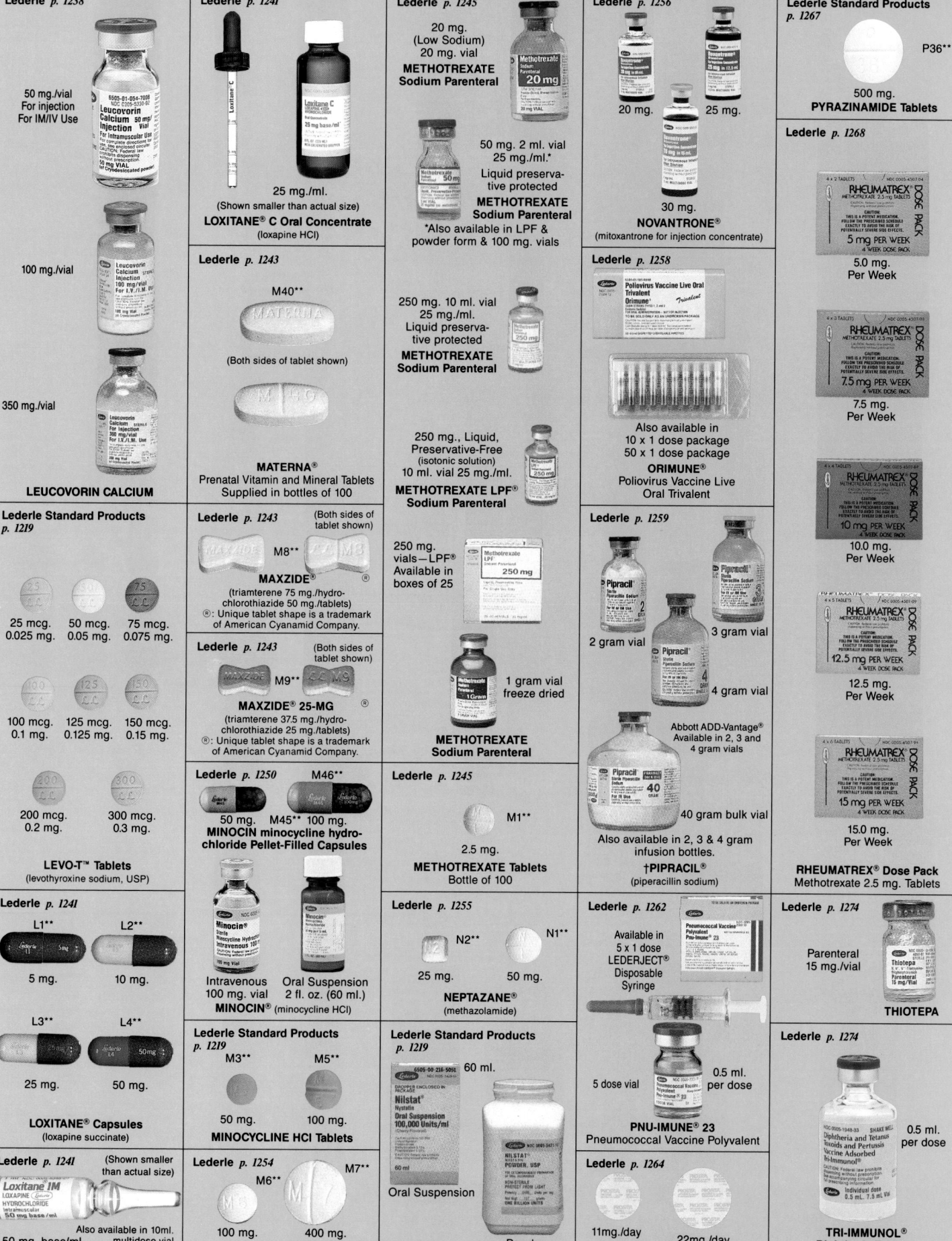

Lederle p. 1238

50 mg./vial
For injection
For IM/IV Use

100 mg./vial

350 mg./vial

LEUCOVORIN CALCIUM

Lederle Standard Products p. 1219

25 mcg.
0.025 mg.

50 mcg.
0.05 mg.

75 mcg.
0.075 mg.

100 mcg.
0.1 mg.

125 mcg.
0.125 mg.

150 mcg.
0.15 mg.

200 mcg.
0.2 mg.

300 mcg.
0.3 mg.

LEVO-T™ Tablets
(levothyroxine sodium, USP)

Lederle p. 1241

L1**
5 mg.

L2**
10 mg.

L3**
25 mg.

L4**
50 mg.

LOXITANE® Capsules
(loxapine succinate)

Lederle p. 1241 (Shown smaller than actual size)

50 mg. base/ml.

Also available in 10ml. multidose vial

†LOXITANE® Intramuscular
(loxapine HCl)

Lederle p. 1241

25 mg./ml.
(Shown smaller than actual size)

LOXITANE® C Oral Concentrate
(loxapine HCl)

Lederle p. 1243

M40**

(Both sides of tablet shown)

MATERNA®
Prenatal Vitamin and Mineral Tablets
Supplied in bottles of 100

Lederle p. 1243 (Both sides of tablet shown)

M8**

MAXZIDE®
(triamterene 75 mg./hydro-
chlorothiazide 50 mg./tablets)
®: Unique tablet shape is a trademark
of American Cyanamid Company.

Lederle p. 1243 (Both sides of tablet shown)

M9**

MAXZIDE® 25-MG
(triamterene 37.5 mg./hydro-
chlorothiazide 25 mg./tablets)
®: Unique tablet shape is a trademark
of American Cyanamid Company.

Lederle p. 1250

50 mg. M45** 100 mg. M46**

**MINOCIN minocycline hydro-
chloride Pellet-Filled Capsules**

Intravenous
100 mg. vial

Oral Suspension
2 fl. oz. (60 ml.)

MINOCIN® (minocycline HCl)

Lederle Standard Products p. 1219

M3**
50 mg.

M5**
100 mg.

MINOCYCLINE HCl Tablets

Lederle p. 1254

M6**
100 mg.

M7**
400 mg.

MYAMBUTOL® Tablets
(ethambutol hydrochloride)

Lederle p. 1245

20 mg.
(Low Sodium)
20 mg. vial

**METHOTREXATE
Sodium Parenteral**

50 mg. 2 ml. vial
25 mg./ml.*
Liquid preserva-
tive protected

**METHOTREXATE
Sodium Parenteral**
*Also available in LPF &
powder form & 100 mg. vials

250 mg. 10 ml. vial
25 mg./ml.
Liquid preserva-
tive protected

**METHOTREXATE
Sodium Parenteral**

250 mg., Liquid,
Preservative-Free
(isotonic solution)
10 ml. vial 25 mg./ml.

**METHOTREXATE LPF®
Sodium Parenteral**

250 mg.
vials—LPF®
Available in
boxes of 25

1 gram vial
freeze dried

**METHOTREXATE
Sodium Parenteral**

Lederle p. 1245

M1**
2.5 mg.

METHOTREXATE Tablets
Bottle of 100

Lederle p. 1255

N2**
25 mg.

N1**
50 mg.

NEPTAZANE®
(methazolamide)

Lederle Standard Products p. 1219

60 ml.

Nilstat®
Nystatin
Oral Suspension
100,000 Units/ml.

Oral Suspension

Powder

NILSTAT®
(nystatin)

Lederle p. 1256

20 mg.

25 mg.

30 mg.

NOVANTRONE®
(mitoxantrone for injection concentrate)

Lederle p. 1258

Poliovirus Vaccine Live Oral Trivalent Orimune®

Also available in
10 x 1 dose package
50 x 1 dose package

ORIMUNE®
Poliovirus Vaccine Live
Oral Trivalent

Lederle p. 1259

2 gram vial

3 gram vial

4 gram vial

Abbott ADD-Vantage®
Available in 2, 3 and
4 gram vials

40 gram bulk vial

Also available in 2, 3 & 4 gram
infusion bottles.

†PIPRACIL®
(piperacillin sodium)

Lederle p. 1262

Available in
5 x 1 dose
LEDERJECT®
Disposable
Syringe

5 dose vial

0.5 ml.
per dose

PNU-IMUNE® 23
Pneumococcal Vaccine Polyvalent

Lederle p. 1264

11mg./day

22mg./day

PROSTEP™
Nicotine Transdermal System

Lederle Standard Products p. 1267

P36**

500 mg.
PYRAZINAMIDE Tablets

Lederle p. 1268

RHEUMATREX®
METHOTREXATE 2.5 mg TABLETS
5 mg PER WEEK
4 WEEK DOSE PACK
5.0 mg.
Per Week

RHEUMATREX®
METHOTREXATE 2.5 mg TABLETS
7.5 mg PER WEEK
4 WEEK DOSE PACK
7.5 mg.
Per Week

RHEUMATREX®
METHOTREXATE 2.5 mg TABLETS
10 mg PER WEEK
4 WEEK DOSE PACK
10.0 mg.
Per Week

RHEUMATREX®
METHOTREXATE 2.5 mg TABLETS
12.5 mg PER WEEK
4 WEEK DOSE PACK
12.5 mg.
Per Week

RHEUMATREX®
METHOTREXATE 2.5 mg TABLETS
15 mg PER WEEK
4 WEEK DOSE PACK
15.0 mg.
Per Week

RHEUMATREX® Dose Pack
Methotrexate 2.5 mg. Tablets

Lederle p. 1274

Parenteral
15 mg./vial

Thiotepa

THIOTEPA

Lederle p. 1274

0.5 ml.
per dose

Diphtheria and Tetanus
Toxoids and Pertussis
Vaccine Adsorbed
Tri-Immunol®

Individual dose
0.5 ml. 7.5 Adsorbed

**TRI-IMMUNOL®
Diphtheria Tetanus
Toxoids and Pertussis
Vaccine Adsorbed**

**Ledermark Product Identification Codes.

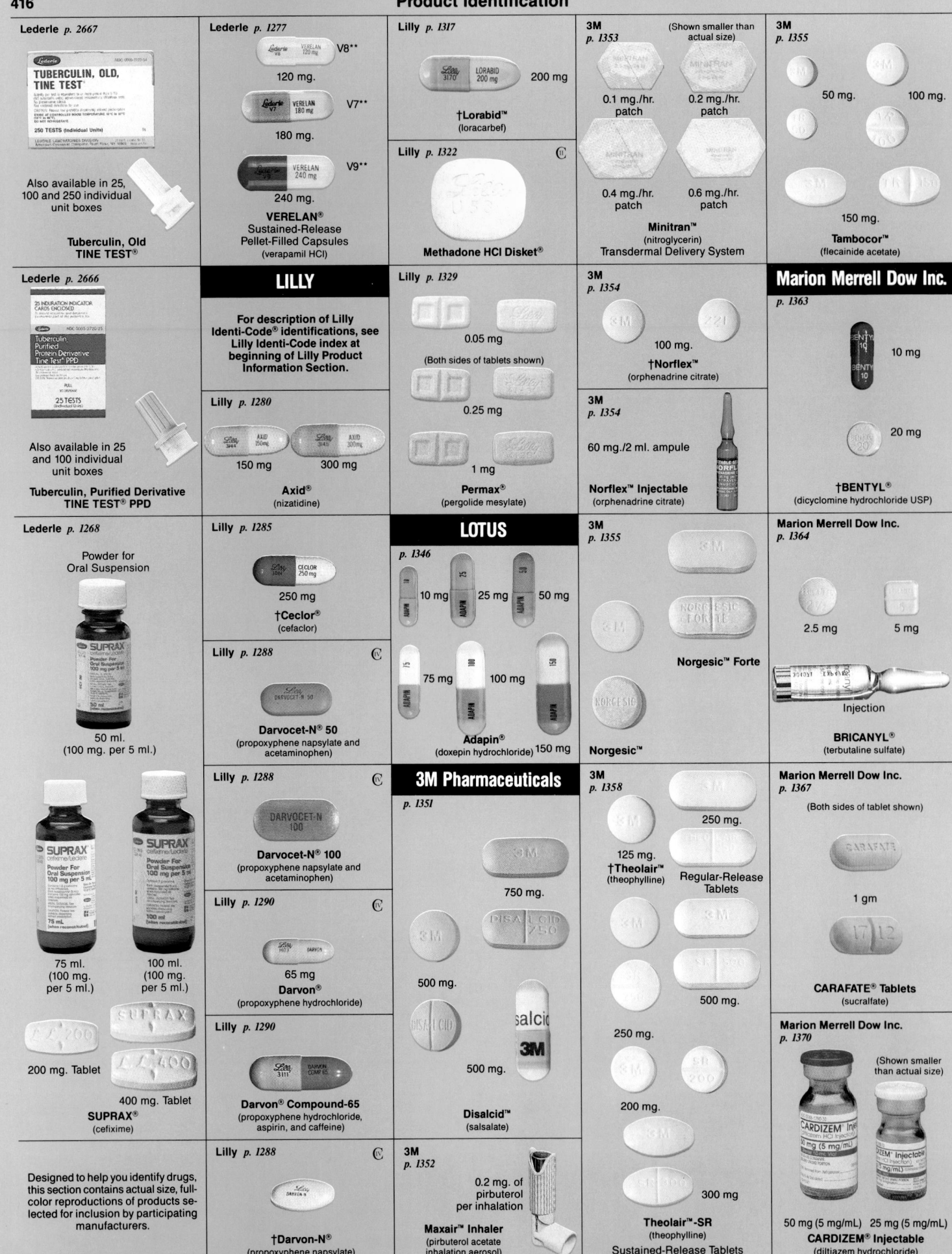

Lederle p. 2667

TUBERCULIN, OLD, TINE TEST

250 TESTS (Individual Units)

Also available in 25, 100 and 250 individual unit boxes

Tuberculin, Old TINE TEST®

Lederle p. 2666

25 INDURATION INDICATOR CARDS ENCLOSED

Tuberculin, Purified Protein Derivative Tine Test® PPD

25 TESTS (Individual Units)

Also available in 25 and 100 individual unit boxes

Tuberculin, Purified Derivative TINE TEST® PPD

Lederle p. 1268

Powder for Oral Suspension

SUPRAX
50 ml. (100 mg. per 5 ml.)

SUPRAX Powder For Oral Suspension 100 mg per 5 ml

75 ml. (100 mg. per 5 ml.)

100 ml. (100 mg. per 5 ml.)

200 mg. Tablet — LL 200

400 mg. Tablet — LL 400

SUPRAX®
(cefixime)

Designed to help you identify drugs, this section contains actual size, full-color reproductions of products selected for inclusion by participating manufacturers.

Lederle p. 1277

Lederle VERELAN V8** 120 mg.
120 mg.

Lederle V7 VERELAN V7**
180 mg.

VERELAN 240 mg V9**
240 mg.

VERELAN®
Sustained-Release Pellet-Filled Capsules
(verapamil HCl)

LILLY

For description of Lilly Identi-Code® identifications, see Lilly Identi-Code index at beginning of Lilly Product Information Section.

Lilly p. 1280

Lilly AXID 150mg   *Lilly* AXID 300mg

150 mg   300 mg

Axid®
(nizatidine)

Lilly p. 1285

Lilly CECLOR 250mg

250 mg

†**Ceclor®**
(cefaclor)

Lilly p. 1288   ⓘⅤ

Lilly DARVOCET-N 50

Darvocet-N® 50
(propoxyphene napsylate and acetaminophen)

Lilly p. 1288   ⓘⅤ

DARVOCET-N 100

Darvocet-N® 100
(propoxyphene napsylate and acetaminophen)

Lilly p. 1290   ⓘⅤ

Lilly DARVON

65 mg

Darvon®
(propoxyphene hydrochloride)

Lilly p. 1290   ⓘⅤ

Lilly DARVON COMP 65

Darvon® Compound-65
(propoxyphene hydrochloride, aspirin, and caffeine)

Lilly p. 1288   ⓘⅤ

Lilly DARVON-N

†**Darvon-N®**
(propoxyphene napsylate)

Lilly p. 1317

Lilly LORABID 200 mg   200 mg

†**Lorabid™**
(loracarbef)

Lilly p. 1322   ©

Methadone HCl Disket®

Lilly p. 1329

0.05 mg

(Both sides of tablets shown)

0.25 mg

1 mg

Permax®
(pergolide mesylate)

LOTUS

p. 1346

10 mg   25 mg   50 mg

75 mg   100 mg   150 mg

Adapin®
(doxepin hydrochloride)

3M Pharmaceuticals

p. 1351

3M
750 mg.

DISALCID 750
3M
500 mg.

DISALCID
500 mg.

salcid
3M

Disalcid™
(salsalate)

3M
p. 1352

0.2 mg. of pirbuterol per inhalation

Maxair™ Inhaler
(pirbuterol acetate inhalation aerosol)

3M
p. 1353

(Shown smaller than actual size)

0.1 mg./hr. patch   0.2 mg./hr. patch

0.4 mg./hr. patch   0.6 mg./hr. patch

Minitran™
(nitroglycerin)
Transdermal Delivery System

3M
p. 1354

100 mg.   221

†**Norflex™**
(orphenadrine citrate)

3M
p. 1354

60 mg./2 ml. ampule

Norflex™ Injectable
(orphenadrine citrate)

3M
p. 1355

3M

NORGESIC FORTE

Norgesic™ Forte

NORGESIC

Norgesic™

3M
p. 1358

3M   250 mg.
125 mg.   Regular-Release Tablets

†**Theolair™**
(theophylline)

3M   3M
SR 300
500 mg.

250 mg.   SR 200

200 mg.

3M

SR 100
300 mg

Theolair™-SR
(theophylline)
Sustained-Release Tablets

3M
p. 1355

3M

50 mg.   100 mg.

3M   TM 150

150 mg.

Tambocor™
(flecainide acetate)

Marion Merrell Dow Inc.

p. 1363

BENTYL 10
10 mg

BENTYL 20
20 mg

†**BENTYL®**
(dicyclomine hydrochloride USP)

Marion Merrell Dow Inc.
p. 1364

2.5 mg   5 mg

Injection

BRICANYL®
(terbutaline sulfate)

Marion Merrell Dow Inc.
p. 1367

(Both sides of tablet shown)

CARAFATE

1 gm

17 12

CARAFATE® Tablets
(sucralfate)

Marion Merrell Dow Inc.
p. 1370

(Shown smaller than actual size)

CARDIZEM Injectable

50 mg (5 mg/mL)   25 mg (5 mg/mL)

CARDIZEM® Injectable
(diltiazem hydrochloride)

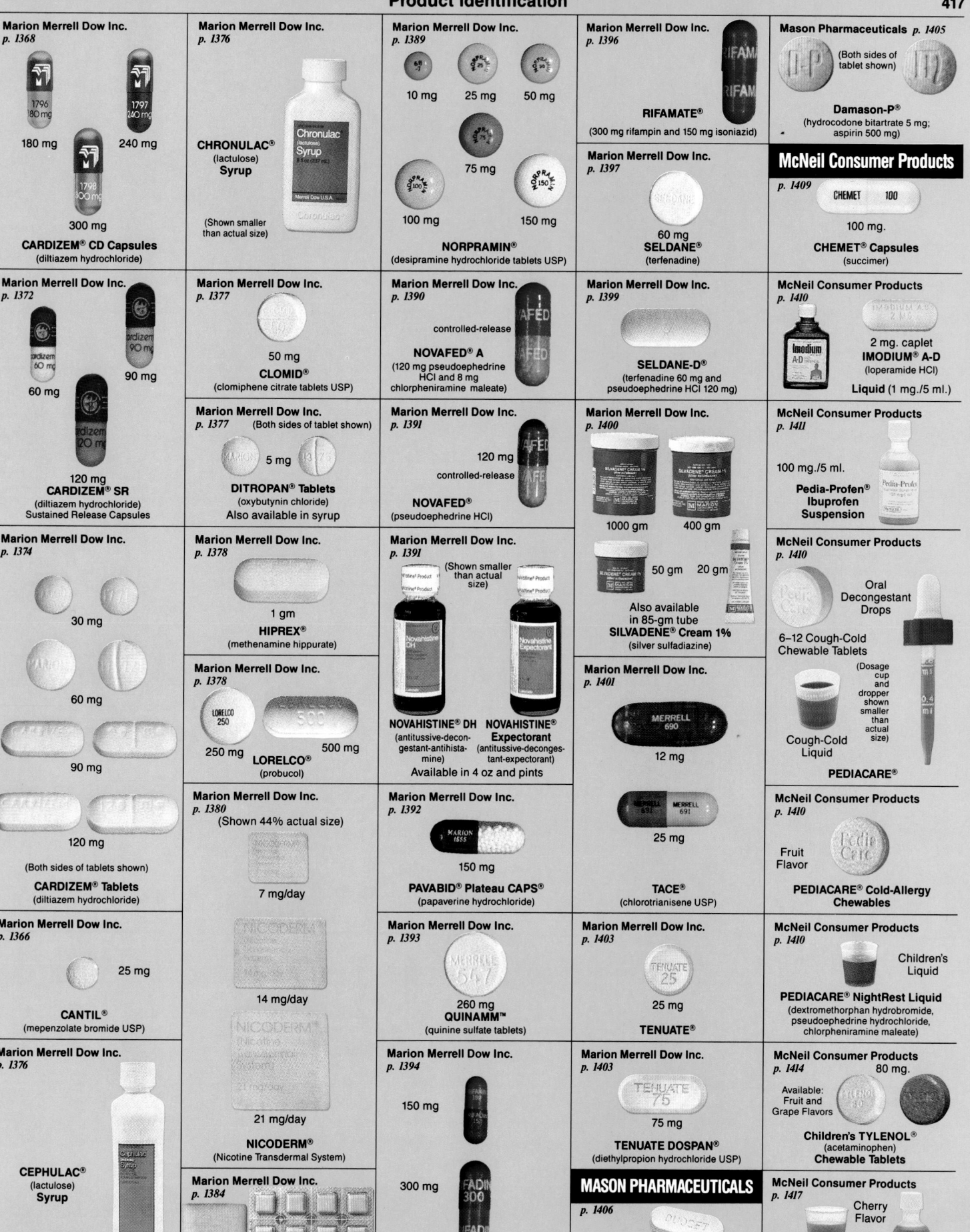

Marion Merrell Dow Inc.
p. 1368

180 mg   240 mg

300 mg

CARDIZEM® CD Capsules
(diltiazem hydrochloride)

Marion Merrell Dow Inc.
p. 1372

60 mg   90 mg

120 mg

CARDIZEM® SR
(diltiazem hydrochloride)
Sustained Release Capsules

Marion Merrell Dow Inc.
p. 1374

30 mg

60 mg

90 mg

120 mg

(Both sides of tablets shown)

CARDIZEM® Tablets
(diltiazem hydrochloride)

Marion Merrell Dow Inc.
p. 1366

25 mg

CANTIL®
(mepenzolate bromide USP)

Marion Merrell Dow Inc.
p. 1376

CEPHULAC®
(lactulose)
Syrup

(Shown smaller
than actual size)

Marion Merrell Dow Inc.
p. 1376

Chronulac
(lactulose)
Syrup

CHRONULAC®
(lactulose)
Syrup

(Shown smaller
than actual size)

Marion Merrell Dow Inc.
p. 1377

50 mg
CLOMID®
(clomiphene citrate tablets USP)

Marion Merrell Dow Inc.
p. 1377 (Both sides of tablet shown)

5 mg
DITROPAN® Tablets
(oxybutynin chloride)
Also available in syrup

Marion Merrell Dow Inc.
p. 1378

1 gm
HIPREX®
(methenamine hippurate)

Marion Merrell Dow Inc.
p. 1378

LORELCO 250

250 mg   500 mg
LORELCO®
(probucol)

Marion Merrell Dow Inc.
p. 1380 (Shown 44% actual size)

7 mg/day

14 mg/day

21 mg/day

NICODERM®
(Nicotine Transdermal System)

Marion Merrell Dow Inc.
p. 1384

2 mg
NICORETTE® (nicotine polacrilex)

Marion Merrell Dow Inc.
p. 1389

10 mg   25 mg   50 mg

75 mg

100 mg   150 mg

NORPRAMIN®
(desipramine hydrochloride tablets USP)

Marion Merrell Dow Inc.
p. 1390

controlled-release
NOVAFED® A
(120 mg pseudoephedrine
HCl and 8 mg
chlorpheniramine maleate)

Marion Merrell Dow Inc.
p. 1391

120 mg
controlled-release
NOVAFED®
(pseudoephedrine HCl)

Marion Merrell Dow Inc.
p. 1391

(Shown smaller
than actual
size)

Novahistine
DH

Novahistine
Expectorant

NOVAHISTINE® DH   **NOVAHISTINE®**
(antitussive-decon-   **Expectorant**
gestant-antihista-   (antitussive-deconges-
mine)   tant-expectorant)

Available in 4 oz and pints

Marion Merrell Dow Inc.
p. 1392

MARION 1855

150 mg
PAVABID® Plateau CAPS®
(papaverine hydrochloride)

Marion Merrell Dow Inc.
p. 1393

MERRELL 547

260 mg
QUINAMM™
(quinine sulfate tablets)

Marion Merrell Dow Inc.
p. 1394

150 mg

300 mg

RIFADIN
300

RIFADIN
300

RIFADIN®
(rifampin)

Marion Merrell Dow Inc.
p. 1396

RIFAMA
RIFAM

RIFAMATE®
(300 mg rifampin and 150 mg isoniazid)

Marion Merrell Dow Inc.
p. 1397

SELDANE

60 mg
SELDANE®
(terfenadine)

Marion Merrell Dow Inc.
p. 1399

SELDANE-D®
(terfenadine 60 mg and
pseudoephedrine HCl 120 mg)

Marion Merrell Dow Inc.
p. 1400

SILVADENE CREAM 1%   SILVADENE CREAM 1%

1000 gm   400 gm

50 gm   20 gm

Also available
in 85-gm tube
SILVADENE® Cream 1%
(silver sulfadiazine)

Marion Merrell Dow Inc.
p. 1401

MERRELL 690

12 mg

MERRELL 691   MERRELL 691

25 mg

TACE®
(chlorotrianisene USP)

Marion Merrell Dow Inc.
p. 1403

TENUATE 25

25 mg
TENUATE®

Marion Merrell Dow Inc.
p. 1403

TENUATE 75

75 mg
TENUATE DOSPAN®
(diethylpropion hydrochloride USP)

MASON PHARMACEUTICALS
p. 1406

DUOCET

DuoCet™
(hydrocodone bitartrate 5 mg;
acetaminophen 500 mg)

Mason Pharmaceuticals *p. 1405*

(Both sides of
tablet shown)

Damason-P®
(hydrocodone bitartrate 5 mg;
aspirin 500 mg)

McNeil Consumer Products
p. 1409

CHEMET   100

100 mg.
CHEMET® Capsules
(succimer)

McNeil Consumer Products
p. 1410

Imodium
A-D

IMODIUM A-D
2 MG

2 mg. caplet
IMODIUM® A-D
(loperamide HCl)
Liquid (1 mg./5 ml.)

McNeil Consumer Products
p. 1411

Pedia-Profen

100 mg./5 ml.
Pedia-Profen
Ibuprofen
Suspension

McNeil Consumer Products
p. 1410

Oral
Decongestant
Drops

6–12 Cough-Cold
Chewable Tablets

(Dosage
cup
and
dropper
shown
smaller
than
actual
size)

Cough-Cold
Liquid

PEDIACARE®

McNeil Consumer Products
p. 1410

Fruit
Flavor

PEDIACARE® Cold-Allergy
Chewables

McNeil Consumer Products
p. 1410

Children's
Liquid

PEDIACARE® NightRest Liquid
(dextromethorphan hydrobromide,
pseudoephedrine hydrochloride,
chlorpheniramine maleate)

McNeil Consumer Products
p. 1414

80 mg.

Available:
Fruit and
Grape Flavors

TYLENOL 80

Children's TYLENOL®
(acetaminophen)
Chewable Tablets

McNeil Consumer Products
p. 1417

Cherry
Flavor

TYLENOL
COLD

Children's
TYLENOL® Cold
Plus Cough

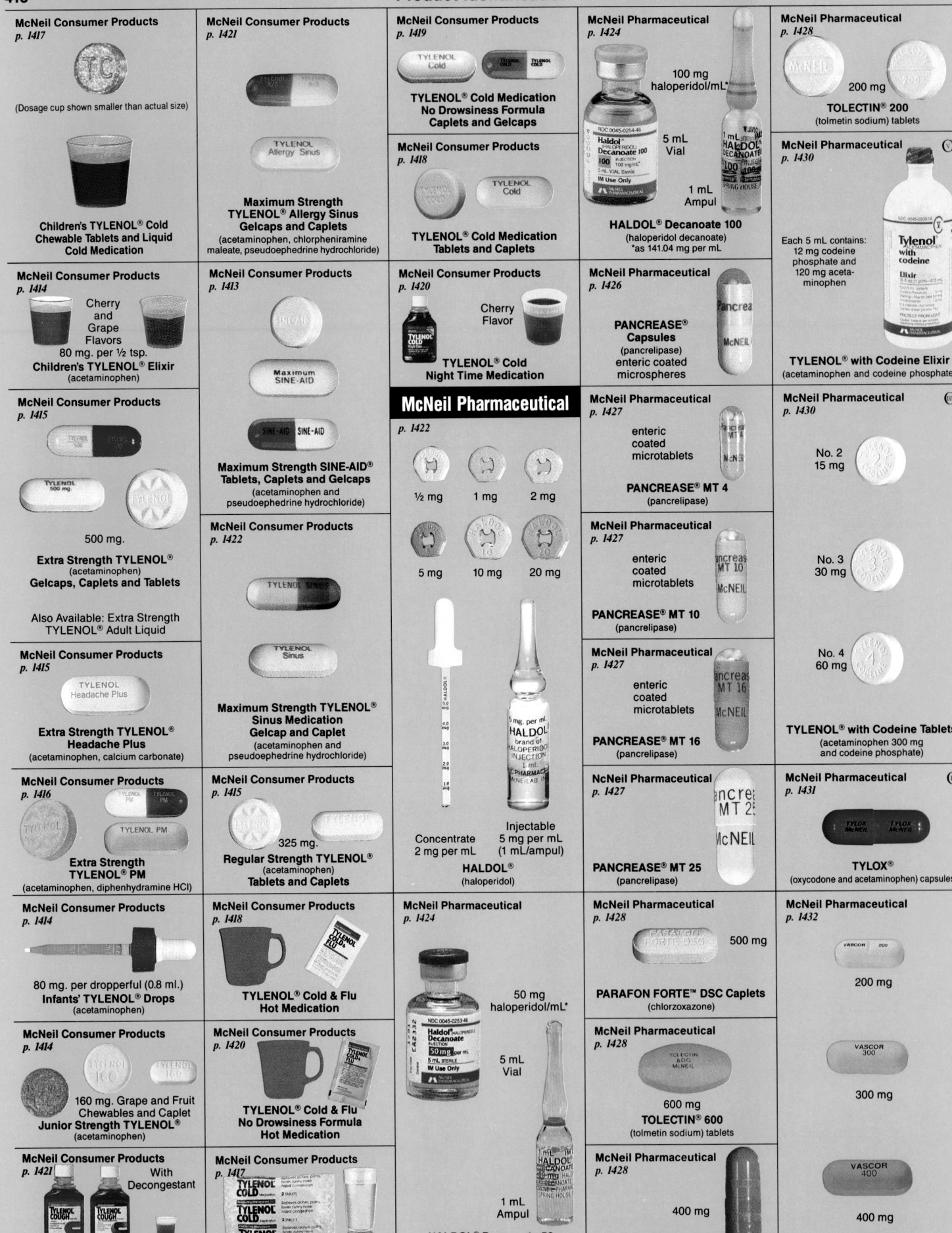

McNeil Consumer Products
p. 1417

(Dosage cup shown smaller than actual size)

**Children's TYLENOL® Cold
Chewable Tablets and Liquid
Cold Medication**

McNeil Consumer Products
p. 1414

Cherry
and
Grape
Flavors
80 mg. per ½ tsp.
Children's TYLENOL® Elixir
(acetaminophen)

McNeil Consumer Products
p. 1415

500 mg.
Extra Strength TYLENOL®
(acetaminophen)
Gelcaps, Caplets and Tablets

Also Available: Extra Strength
TYLENOL® Adult Liquid

McNeil Consumer Products
p. 1415

TYLENOL
Headache Plus

**Extra Strength TYLENOL®
Headache Plus**
(acetaminophen, calcium carbonate)

McNeil Consumer Products
p. 1416

**Extra Strength
TYLENOL® PM**
(acetaminophen, diphenhydramine HCl)

McNeil Consumer Products
p. 1414

80 mg. per dropperful (0.8 ml.)
Infants' TYLENOL® Drops
(acetaminophen)

McNeil Consumer Products
p. 1414

160 mg. Grape and Fruit
Chewables and Caplet
Junior Strength TYLENOL®
(acetaminophen)

McNeil Consumer Products
p. 1421

With
Decongestant

**Maximum Strength
TYLENOL® COUGH**

McNeil Consumer Products
p. 1421

**Maximum Strength
TYLENOL® Allergy Sinus
Gelcaps and Caplets**
(acetaminophen, chlorpheniramine
maleate, pseudoephedrine hydrochloride)

McNeil Consumer Products
p. 1413

Maximum
SINE-AID

**Maximum Strength SINE-AID®
Tablets, Caplets and Gelcaps**
(acetaminophen and
pseudoephedrine hydrochloride)

McNeil Consumer Products
p. 1422

**Maximum Strength TYLENOL®
Sinus Medication
Gelcap and Caplet**
(acetaminophen and
pseudoephedrine hydrochloride)

McNeil Consumer Products
p. 1415

325 mg.
Regular Strength TYLENOL®
(acetaminophen)
Tablets and Caplets

McNeil Consumer Products
p. 1418

**TYLENOL® Cold & Flu
Hot Medication**

McNeil Consumer Products
p. 1420

**TYLENOL® Cold & Flu
No Drowsiness Formula
Hot Medication**

McNeil Consumer Products
p. 1417

**TYLENOL® Cold Medication
Effervescent Formula**

McNeil Consumer Products
p. 1419

**TYLENOL® Cold Medication
No Drowsiness Formula
Caplets and Gelcaps**

McNeil Consumer Products
p. 1418

**TYLENOL® Cold Medication
Tablets and Caplets**

McNeil Consumer Products
p. 1420

Cherry
Flavor

**TYLENOL® Cold
Night Time Medication**

McNeil Pharmaceutical
p. 1422

½ mg　　1 mg　　2 mg

5 mg　　10 mg　　20 mg

Concentrate
2 mg per mL

Injectable
5 mg per mL
(1 mL/ampul)

HALDOL®
(haloperidol)

McNeil Pharmaceutical
p. 1424

50 mg
haloperidol/mL*

5 mL
Vial

1 mL
Ampul

HALDOL® Decanoate 50
(haloperidol decanoate)
*as 70.5 mg haloperidol decanoate

McNeil Pharmaceutical
p. 1424

100 mg
haloperidol/mL*

5 mL
Vial

1 mL
Ampul

HALDOL® Decanoate 100
(haloperidol decanoate)
*as 141.04 mg per mL

McNeil Pharmaceutical
p. 1426

**PANCREASE®
Capsules**
(pancrelipase)
enteric coated
microspheres

McNeil Pharmaceutical
p. 1427

enteric
coated
microtablets

PANCREASE® MT 4
(pancrelipase)

McNeil Pharmaceutical
p. 1427

enteric
coated
microtablets

PANCREASE® MT 10
(pancrelipase)

McNeil Pharmaceutical
p. 1427

enteric
coated
microtablets

PANCREASE® MT 16
(pancrelipase)

NcNeil Pharmaceutical
p. 1427

PANCREASE® MT 25
(pancrelipase)

McNeil Pharmaceutical
p. 1428

500 mg

PARAFON FORTE™ DSC Caplets
(chlorzoxazone)

McNeil Pharmaceutical
p. 1428

600 mg
TOLECTIN® 600
(tolmetin sodium) tablets

McNeil Pharmaceutical
p. 1428

400 mg

TOLECTIN® DS
(tolmetin sodium) capsules

McNeil Pharmaceutical
p. 1428

200 mg
TOLECTIN® 200
(tolmetin sodium) tablets

McNeil Pharmaceutical
p. 1430

Each 5 mL contains:
12 mg codeine
phosphate and
120 mg aceta-
minophen

TYLENOL® with Codeine Elixir
(acetaminophen and codeine phosphate)

McNeil Pharmaceutical
p. 1430

No. 2
15 mg

No. 3
30 mg

No. 4
60 mg

TYLENOL® with Codeine Tablets
(acetaminophen 300 mg
and codeine phosphate)

McNeil Pharmaceutical
p. 1431

TYLOX®
(oxycodone and acetaminophen) capsules

McNeil Pharmaceutical
p. 1432

200 mg

300 mg

400 mg

VASCOR® Tablets
(bepridil hydrochloride)

McNeil Pharmaceutical

p. 1422

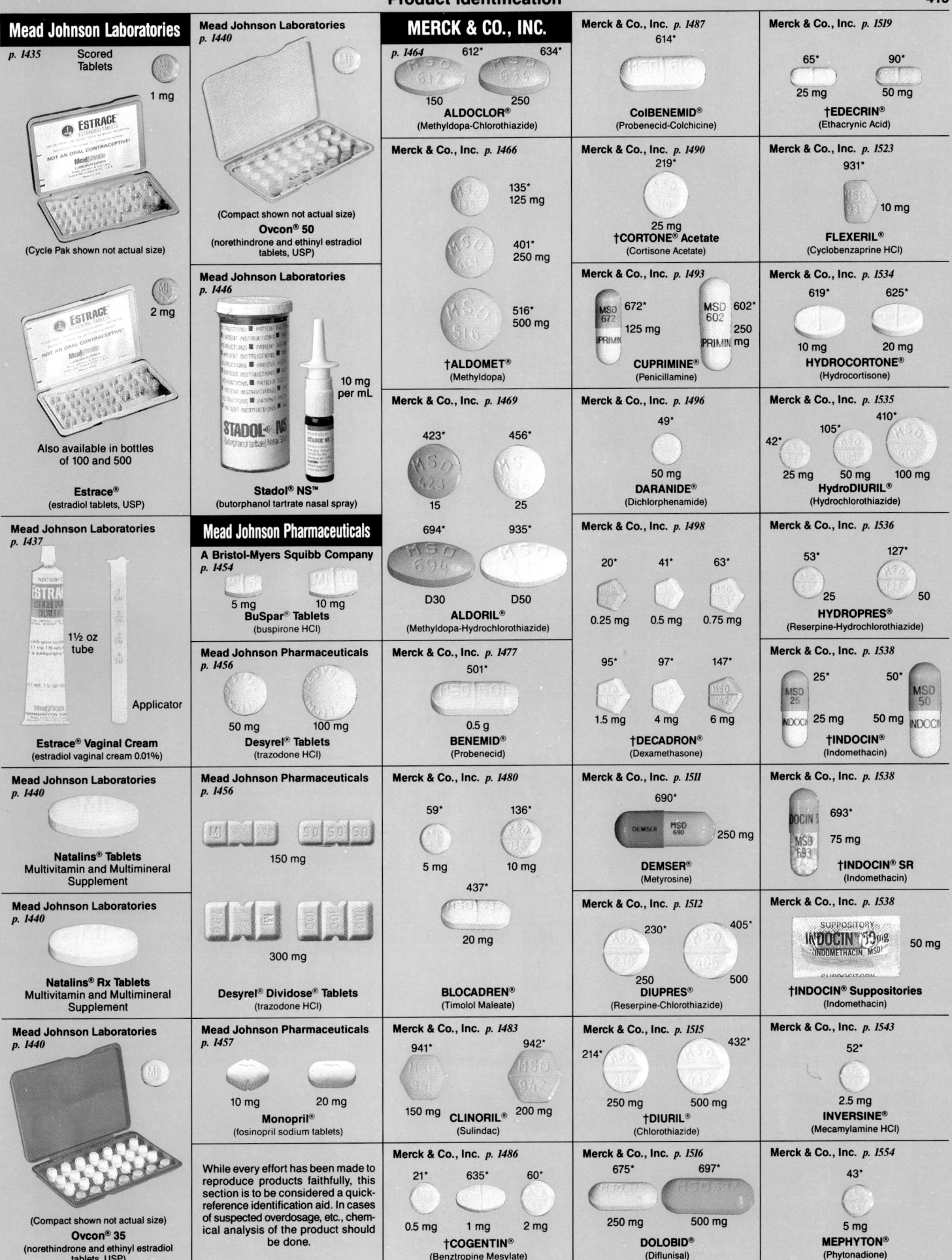

Mead Johnson Laboratories

p. 1435 Scored Tablets

1 mg

(Cycle Pak shown not actual size)

Estrace®
(estradiol tablets, USP)

2 mg

Also available in bottles of 100 and 500

Mead Johnson Laboratories
p. 1437

1½ oz tube

Applicator

Estrace® Vaginal Cream
(estradiol vaginal cream 0.01%)

Mead Johnson Laboratories
p. 1440

Natalins® Tablets
Multivitamin and Multimineral Supplement

Mead Johnson Laboratories
p. 1440

Natalins® Rx Tablets
Multivitamin and Multimineral Supplement

Mead Johnson Laboratories
p. 1440

(Compact shown not actual size)

Ovcon® 35
(norethindrone and ethinyl estradiol tablets, USP)

Mead Johnson Laboratories
p. 1440

(Compact shown not actual size)

Ovcon® 50
(norethindrone and ethinyl estradiol tablets, USP)

Mead Johnson Laboratories
p. 1446

10 mg per mL

Stadol® NS™
(butorphanol tartrate nasal spray)

Mead Johnson Pharmaceuticals

A Bristol-Myers Squibb Company
p. 1454

5 mg   10 mg

BuSpar® Tablets
(buspirone HCl)

Mead Johnson Pharmaceuticals
p. 1456

50 mg   100 mg

Desyrel® Tablets
(trazodone HCl)

Mead Johnson Pharmaceuticals
p. 1456

150 mg

300 mg

Desyrel® Dividose® Tablets
(trazodone HCl)

Mead Johnson Pharmaceuticals
p. 1457

10 mg   20 mg

Monopril®
(fosinopril sodium tablets)

While every effort has been made to reproduce products faithfully, this section is to be considered a quick-reference identification aid. In cases of suspected overdosage, etc., chemical analysis of the product should be done.

MERCK & CO., INC.

p. 1464   612*   634*

150   250
ALDOCLOR®
(Methyldopa-Chlorothiazide)

Merck & Co., Inc. p. 1466

135*
125 mg

401*
250 mg

516*
500 mg

†ALDOMET®
(Methyldopa)

Merck & Co., Inc. p. 1469

423*   456*

15   25

694*   935*

D30   D50

ALDORIL®
(Methyldopa-Hydrochlorothiazide)

Merck & Co., Inc. p. 1477
501*

0.5 g
BENEMID®
(Probenecid)

Merck & Co., Inc. p. 1480

59*   136*

5 mg   10 mg

437*

20 mg
BLOCADREN®
(Timolol Maleate)

Merck & Co., Inc. p. 1483
941*   942*

150 mg   **CLINORIL®**   200 mg
(Sulindac)

Merck & Co., Inc. p. 1486

21*   635*   60*

0.5 mg   1 mg   2 mg
†COGENTIN®
(Benztropine Mesylate)

Merck & Co., Inc. p. 1487
614*

ColBENEMID®
(Probenecid-Colchicine)

Merck & Co., Inc. p. 1490
219*

25 mg
†CORTONE® Acetate
(Cortisone Acetate)

Merck & Co., Inc. p. 1493
672*   602*

125 mg   250 mg
CUPRIMINE®
(Penicillamine)

Merck & Co., Inc. p. 1496
49*

50 mg
DARANIDE®
(Dichlorphenamide)

Merck & Co., Inc. p. 1498

20*   41*   63*

0.25 mg   0.5 mg   0.75 mg

95*   97*   147*

1.5 mg   4 mg   6 mg
†DECADRON®
(Dexamethasone)

Merck & Co., Inc. p. 1511
690*

250 mg
DEMSER®
(Metyrosine)

Merck & Co., Inc. p. 1512

230*   405*

250   500
DIUPRES®
(Reserpine-Chlorothiazide)

Merck & Co., Inc. p. 1515
214*   432*

250 mg   500 mg
†DIURIL®
(Chlorothiazide)

Merck & Co., Inc. p. 1516
675*   697*

250 mg   500 mg
DOLOBID®
(Diflunisal)

Merck & Co., Inc. p. 1519

65*   90*

25 mg   50 mg
†EDECRIN®
(Ethacrynic Acid)

Merck & Co., Inc. p. 1523
931*

10 mg
FLEXERIL®
(Cyclobenzaprine HCl)

Merck & Co., Inc. p. 1534
619*   625*

10 mg   20 mg
HYDROCORTONE®
(Hydrocortisone)

Merck & Co., Inc. p. 1535
42*   105*   410*

25 mg   50 mg   100 mg
HydroDIURIL®
(Hydrochlorothiazide)

Merck & Co., Inc. p. 1536
53*   127*

25   50
HYDROPRES®
(Reserpine-Hydrochlorothiazide)

Merck & Co., Inc. p. 1538
25*   50*

25 mg   50 mg
†INDOCIN®
(Indomethacin)

Merck & Co., Inc. p. 1538
693*

75 mg
†INDOCIN® SR
(Indomethacin)

Merck & Co., Inc. p. 1538

50 mg
†INDOCIN® Suppositories
(Indomethacin)

Merck & Co., Inc. p. 1543
52*

2.5 mg
INVERSINE®
(Mecamylamine HCl)

Merck & Co., Inc. p. 1554
43*

5 mg
MEPHYTON®
(Phytonadione)

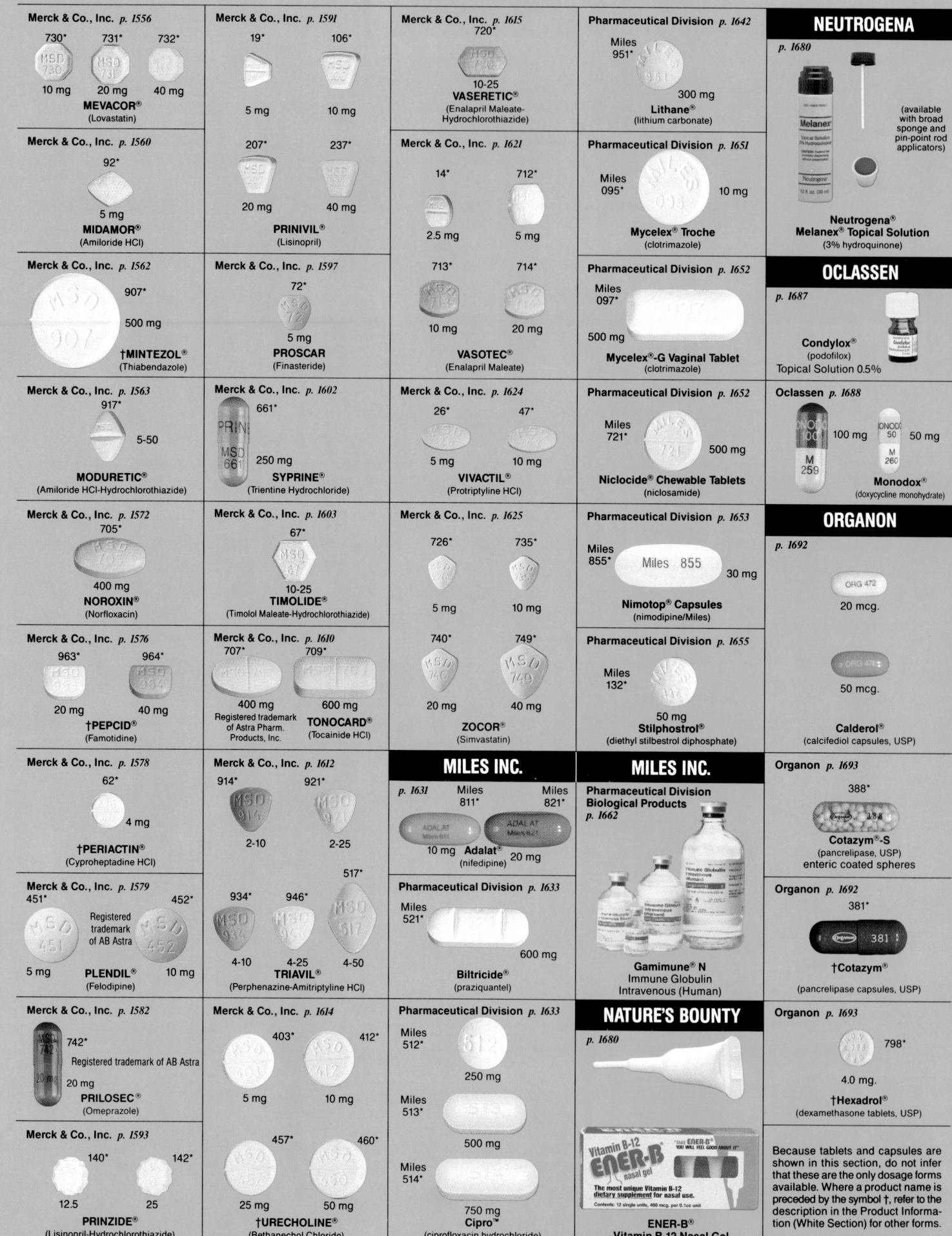

Merck & Co., Inc. *p. 1556*

730*   731*   732*
MSD 730   MSD 731   732
10 mg   20 mg   40 mg
MEVACOR®
(Lovastatin)

Merck & Co., Inc. *p. 1560*

92*
5 mg
MIDAMOR®
(Amiloride HCl)

Merck & Co., Inc. *p. 1562*

907*
500 mg
MSD 907
†MINTEZOL®
(Thiabendazole)

Merck & Co., Inc. *p. 1563*

917*
5-50
MODURETIC®
(Amiloride HCl-Hydrochlorothiazide)

Merck & Co., Inc. *p. 1572*

705*
400 mg
NOROXIN®
(Norfloxacin)

Merck & Co., Inc. *p. 1576*

963*   964*
20 mg   40 mg
†PEPCID®
(Famotidine)

Merck & Co., Inc. *p. 1578*

62*
4 mg
†PERIACTIN®
(Cyproheptadine HCl)

Merck & Co., Inc. *p. 1579*

451*   452*
Registered trademark of AB Astra
MSD 451   MSD 452
5 mg   **PLENDIL®**   10 mg
(Felodipine)

Merck & Co., Inc. *p. 1582*

742*
Registered trademark of AB Astra
20 mg
PRILOSEC®
(Omeprazole)

Merck & Co., Inc. *p. 1593*

140*   142*
12.5   25
PRINZIDE®
(Lisinopril-Hydrochlorothiazide)

Merck & Co., Inc. *p. 1591*

19*   106*
MSD 100
5 mg   10 mg

207*   237*
20 mg   40 mg
PRINIVIL®
(Lisinopril)

Merck & Co., Inc. *p. 1597*

72*
MSD 72
5 mg
PROSCAR
(Finasteride)

Merck & Co., Inc. *p. 1602*

661*
PRIN
MSD 661
250 mg
SYPRINE®
(Trientine Hydrochloride)

Merck & Co., Inc. *p. 1603*

67*
MSD 67
10-25
TIMOLIDE®
(Timolol Maleate-Hydrochlorothiazide)

Merck & Co., Inc. *p. 1610*

707*   709*
400 mg   600 mg
Registered trademark of Astra Pharm. Products, Inc.   **TONOCARD®**
(Tocainide HCl)

Merck & Co., Inc. *p. 1612*

914*   921*
MSD 914   MSD 921
2-10   2-25

  517*
934*   946*   MSD 517
MSD 934   MSD 946
4-10   4-25   4-50
TRIAVIL®
(Perphenazine-Amitriptyline HCl)

Merck & Co., Inc. *p. 1614*

403*   412*
MSD 403   MSD 412
5 mg   10 mg

457*   460*
MSD 457   MSD 460
25 mg   50 mg
†URECHOLINE®
(Bethanechol Chloride)

Merck & Co., Inc. *p. 1615*

720*
MSD 720
10-25
VASERETIC®
(Enalapril Maleate-Hydrochlorothiazide)

Merck & Co., Inc. *p. 1621*

14*   712*
2.5 mg   5 mg

713*   714*
MSD 713   MSD 714
10 mg   20 mg
VASOTEC®
(Enalapril Maleate)

Merck & Co., Inc. *p. 1624*

26*   47*
5 mg   10 mg
VIVACTIL®
(Protriptyline HCl)

Merck & Co., Inc. *p. 1625*

726*   735*
MSD 726   MSD 735
5 mg   10 mg

740*   749*
MSD 740   MSD 749
20 mg   40 mg
ZOCOR®
(Simvastatin)

MILES INC.

p. 1631   Miles 811*   Miles 821*
ADALAT Miles 611   ADALAT Miles 621
10 mg   **Adalat®**   20 mg
(nifedipine)

Pharmaceutical Division *p. 1633*

Miles 521*
600 mg
Biltricide®
(praziquantel)

Pharmaceutical Division *p. 1633*

Miles 512*
512
250 mg

Miles 513*
513
500 mg

Miles 514*
514
750 mg
Cipro™
(ciprofloxacin hydrochloride)

Pharmaceutical Division *p. 1642*

Miles 951*
MILES 951
300 mg
Lithane®
(lithium carbonate)

Pharmaceutical Division *p. 1651*

Miles 095*
MILES 095
10 mg
Mycelex® Troche
(clotrimazole)

Pharmaceutical Division *p. 1652*

Miles 097*
500 mg
Mycelex®-G Vaginal Tablet
(clotrimazole)

Pharmaceutical Division *p. 1652*

Miles 721*
MILES 721
500 mg
Niclocide® Chewable Tablets
(niclosamide)

Pharmaceutical Division *p. 1653*

Miles 855*
Miles 855
30 mg
Nimotop® Capsules
(nimodipine/Miles)

Pharmaceutical Division *p. 1655*

Miles 132*
MILES 132
50 mg
Stilphostrol®
(diethyl stilbestrol diphosphate)

MILES INC.

Pharmaceutical Division
Biological Products
p. 1662

Gamimune® N
Immune Globulin
Intravenous (Human)

NATURE'S BOUNTY

p. 1680

Vitamin B-12
ENER-B
nasal gel
"TAKE ENER-B YOU WILL FEEL GOOD ABOUT IT"
The most unique Vitamin B-12 dietary supplement for nasal use.
Contents: 12 single units, 400 mcg. per 0.1cc unit
ENER-B®
Vitamin B-12 Nasal Gel

NEUTROGENA

p. 1680

Melanex
Topical Solution 3% Hydroquinone
Neutrogena
(available with broad sponge and pin-point rod applicators)
Neutrogena®
Melanex® Topical Solution
(3% hydroquinone)

OCLASSEN

p. 1687

Condylox®
(podofilox)
Topical Solution 0.5%

Oclassen *p. 1688*

ONODOX 100   100 mg   ONODOX 50   50 mg
M 259   M 260
Monodox®
(doxycycline monohydrate)

ORGANON

p. 1692

ORG 472
20 mcg.

ORG 474
50 mcg.
Calderol®
(calcifediol capsules, USP)

Organon *p. 1693*

388*
Cotazym 388
Cotazym®-S
(pancrelipase, USP)
enteric coated spheres

Organon *p. 1692*

381*
Organon 381
†Cotazym®
(pancrelipase capsules, USP)

Organon *p. 1693*

798*
ORGANON 798
4.0 mg.
†Hexadrol®
(dexamethasone tablets, USP)

Because tablets and capsules are shown in this section, do not infer that these are the only dosage forms available. Where a product name is preceded by the symbol †, refer to the description in the Product Information (White Section) for other forms.

Organon *p. 1693*

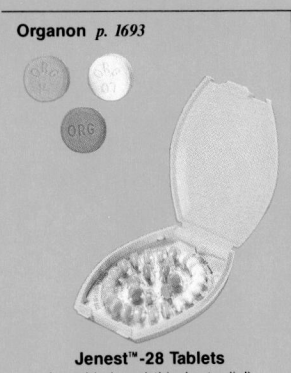

Jenest™-28 Tablets
(norethindrone/ethinyl estradiol)

Organon *p. 1701*

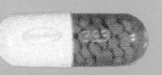

542*

Wigraine®
(ergotamine tartrate and caffeine
tablets, USP)

Organon *p. 1701*

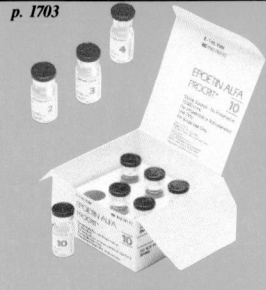

Wigraine®
(ergotamine tartrate and caffeine
suppositories, USP)

Organon *p. 1702*

393*

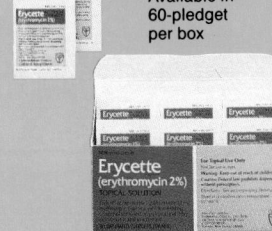

Zymase®
(pancrelipase, USP)
enteric coated spheres

ORTHO BIOTECH

p. 1703

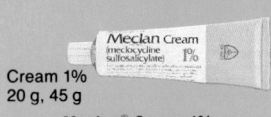

PROCRIT®
(Epoetin alfa)

ORTHO

Ortho Dermatological *p. 1734*

Available in
60-pledget
per box

Erycette® Topical Solution
(erythromycin 2%)

Ortho Dermatological *p. 1735*

Cream 1%
20 g, 45 g

Meclan® Cream 1%
(meclocycline sulfosalicylate)

Ortho Dermatological *p. 1734*

Tablets
available in
250 mg and
500 mg

125 mg/
5 cc oral
suspension

Grifulvin V®
(griseofulvin microsize)
Tablets/Suspension

Ortho Dermatological *p. 1735*

Cream
15 g, 1 oz, 3 oz (85 g)
Monistat-Derm®
(miconazole nitrate 2%)

Ortho Dermatological *p. 1736*

Gel
1.5 oz
and
3 oz

Persa-Gel® 5%
Persa-Gel® 10%
(benzoyl peroxide)

Gel W
1.5 oz
and
3 oz

Persa-Gel® W 5%
Persa-Gel® W 10%
(benzoyl peroxide)

Ortho Dermatological *p. 1737*

Cream 1%
15 g, 30 g, 85 g
Spectazole® (econazole nitrate 1%)

Ortho Dermatological *p. 1736*

Cream 0.025%
20 g, 45 g

Cream 0.05%
20 g, 45 g

Cream 0.1%
20 g, 45 g

Retin-A® (tretinoin)
with Delcap®
Unit Dispensing Cap

Ortho Dermatological *p. 1736*

Liquid 0.05%
28 mL

Retin-A® (tretinoin)

Ortho Dermatological *p. 1736*

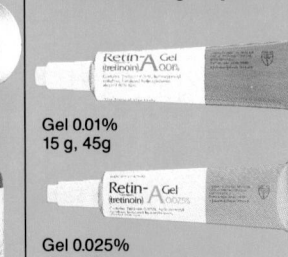

Gel 0.01%
15 g, 45g

Gel 0.025%
15 g, 45 g

Retin-A® (tretinoin)
with Delcap®
Unit Dispensing Cap

ORTHO

p. 1719

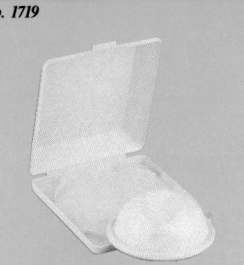

ALL-FLEX
Arcing Spring Diaphragm

Ortho *p. 1708*

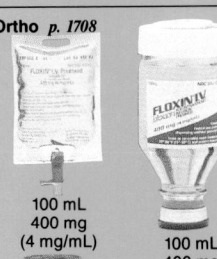

100 mL
400 mg
(4 mg/mL)

100 mL
400 mg
(4 mg/mL)

20 mL
400 mg
(20 mg/mL)

10 mL
400 mg
40 mg/mL)

FLOXIN I.V.
(ofloxacin injection) for
intravenous infusion

Ortho *p. 1712*

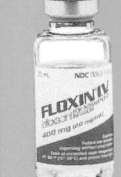

200 mg

300 mg

400 mg

FLOXIN® Tablets
(ofloxacin)

Ortho *p. 1718*

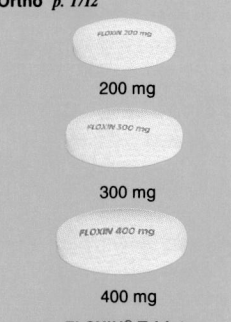

MONISTAT™ 3
Vaginal Suppositories
(200 mg miconazole nitrate)

Ortho *p. 1718*

MONISTAT™ Dual-Pak™
(miconazole nitrate)

Ortho *p. 1723*

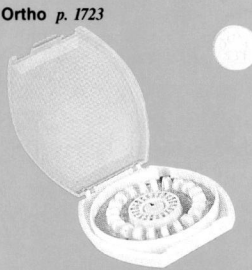

MODICON™ 21 Day Regimen
(0.5 mg of norethindrone with
0.035 mg of ethinyl estradiol)
Also available in 28-day regimen
containing 7 inert green tablets

Ortho *p. 1723*

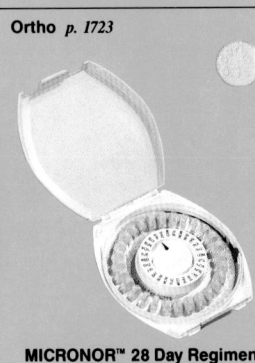

MICRONOR™ 28 Day Regimen
(0.35 mg of norethindrone)

Ortho *p. 1723*

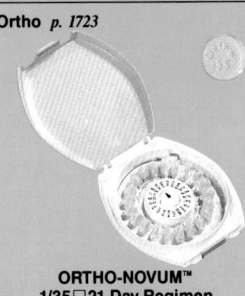

ORTHO-NOVUM™
1/35□21 Day Regimen
(1 mg of norethindrone with
0.035 mg of ethinyl estradiol)
Also available in 28-day regimen
containing 7 inert green tablets

Ortho *p. 1723*

ORTHO-NOVUM™
1/50□21 Day Regimen
(1 mg of norethindrone with
0.05 mg of mestranol)
Also available in 28-day regimen
containing 7 inert green tablets

Ortho *p. 1723*

Ortho
compacts
shown smaller
than actual
size

Also available
in 28-day
regimen
containing 7
inert green
tablets

ORTHO-NOVUM™
7/7/7□21 Day Regimen
(Each white tablet contains
0.5 mg of norethindrone and
0.035 mg of ethinyl estradiol)
(Each light peach tablet contains
0.75 mg of norethindrone and
0.035 mg of ethinyl estradiol)
(Each peach tablet contains
1 mg of norethindrone and
0.035 mg of ethinyl estradiol)

Ortho *p. 1723*

Also
available
in 28-day
regimen con-
taining 7 inert
green tablets

ORTHO-NOVUM™
10/11□21 Day Regimen
(Each white tablet contains 0.5 mg of norethindrone with 0.035 mg of ethinyl estradiol)
(Each peach tablet contains 1 mg of norethindrone with 0.035 mg of ethinyl estradiol)

Ortho *p. 1730*

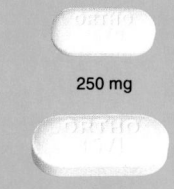

250 mg

500 mg

PROTOSTAT™
(metronidazole)
tablets

Ortho *p. 1732*

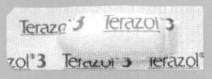

TERAZOL® 3
Vaginal Suppositories
(terconazole)

Ortho *p. 1733*

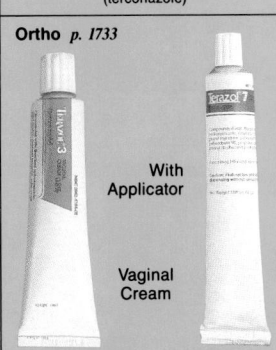

With
Applicator

Vaginal
Cream

TERAZOL® 3   TERAZOL® 7
(terconazole)

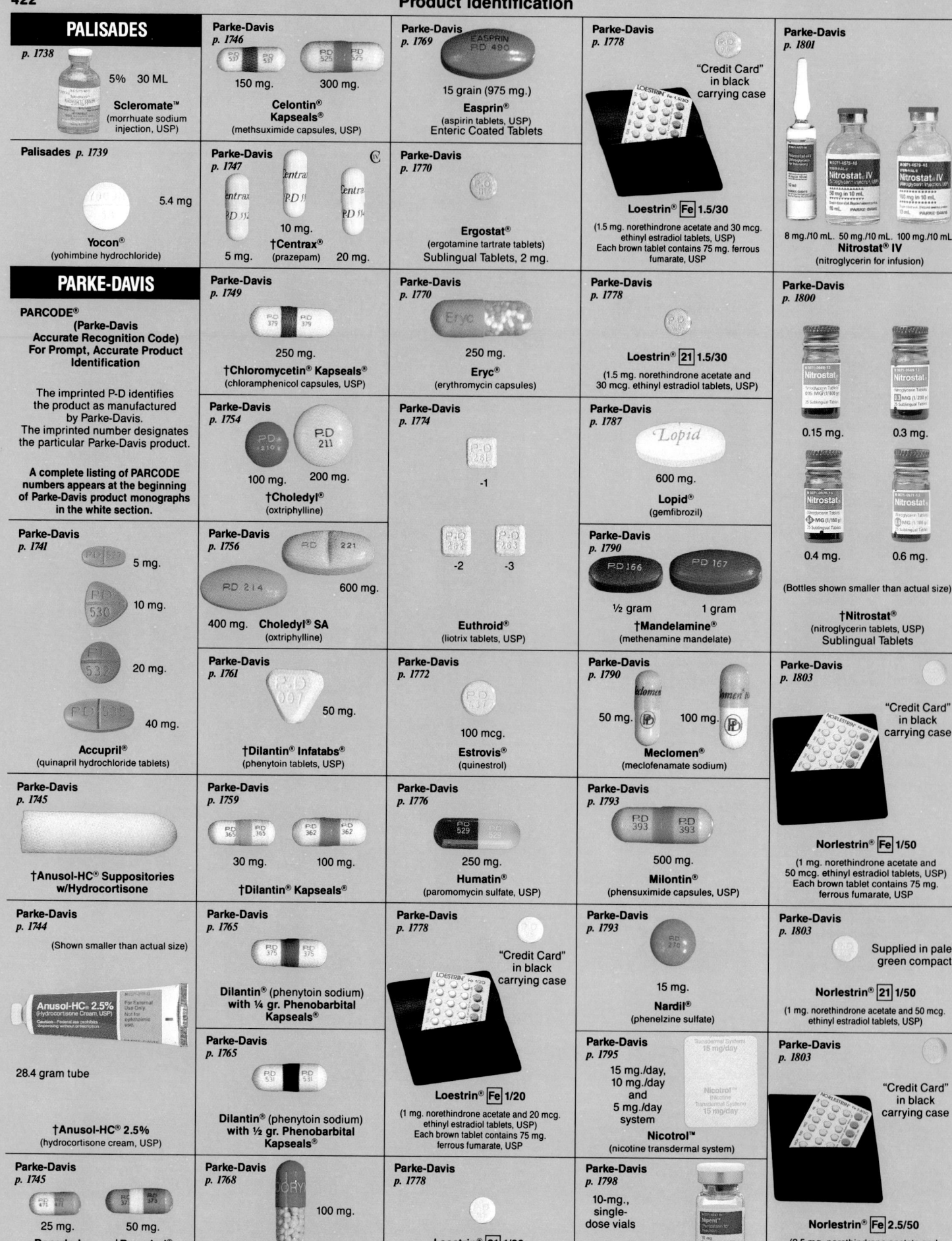

PALISADES

p. 1738

5%   30 ML

Scleromate™
(morrhuate sodium
injection, USP)

Palisades *p. 1739*

5.4 mg.

Yocon®
(yohimbine hydrochloride)

PARKE-DAVIS

PARCODE®
(Parke-Davis
Accurate Recognition Code)
For Prompt, Accurate Product
Identification

The imprinted P-D identifies
the product as manufactured
by Parke-Davis.
The imprinted number designates
the particular Parke-Davis product.

**A complete listing of PARCODE
numbers appears at the beginning
of Parke-Davis product monographs
in the white section.**

Parke-Davis
p. 1741

5 mg.

10 mg.

20 mg.

40 mg.

Accupril®
(quinapril hydrochloride tablets)

Parke-Davis
p. 1745

(Shown smaller than actual size)

†**Anusol-HC® Suppositories
w/Hydrocortisone**

Parke-Davis
p. 1744

(Shown smaller than actual size)

Anusol-HC. 2.5%
(Hydrocortisone Cream, USP)

28.4 gram tube

†**Anusol-HC® 2.5%**
(hydrocortisone cream, USP)

Parke-Davis
p. 1745

25 mg.   50 mg.

**Benadryl
Capsules**   †**Benadryl®
Kapseals®**
(diphenhydramine hydrochloride capsules, USP)

Parke-Davis
p. 1746

150 mg.   300 mg.

**Celontin®
Kapseals®**
(methsuximide capsules, USP)

Parke-Davis
p. 1747

5 mg.   10 mg.   20 mg.

†**Centrax®**
(prazepam)

Parke-Davis
p. 1749

250 mg.

†**Chloromycetin® Kapseals®**
(chloramphenicol capsules, USP)

Parke-Davis
p. 1754

100 mg.   200 mg.

†**Choledyl®**
(oxtriphylline)

Parke-Davis
p. 1756

400 mg.   600 mg.

Choledyl® SA
(oxtriphylline)

Parke-Davis
p. 1761

50 mg.

†**Dilantin® Infatabs®**
(phenytoin tablets, USP)

Parke-Davis
p. 1759

30 mg.   100 mg.

†**Dilantin® Kapseals®**

Parke-Davis
p. 1765

Dilantin® (phenytoin sodium)
with ¼ gr. Phenobarbital
Kapseals®

Parke-Davis
p. 1765

Dilantin® (phenytoin sodium)
with ½ gr. Phenobarbital
Kapseals®

Parke-Davis
p. 1768

100 mg.

Doryx®
(coated doxycycline hyclate pellets)

Parke-Davis
p. 1769

15 grain (975 mg.)

Easprin®
(aspirin tablets, USP)
Enteric Coated Tablets

Parke-Davis
p. 1770

Ergostat®
(ergotamine tartrate tablets)
Sublingual Tablets, 2 mg.

Parke-Davis
p. 1770

250 mg.

Eryc®
(erythromycin capsules)

Parke-Davis
p. 1774

-1

-2   -3

Euthroid®
(liotrix tablets, USP)

Parke-Davis
p. 1772

100 mcg.

Estrovis®
(quinestrol)

Parke-Davis
p. 1776

250 mg.

Humatin®
(paromomycin sulfate, USP)

Parke-Davis
p. 1778

"Credit Card"
in black
carrying case

Loestrin® Fe 1/20
(1 mg. norethindrone acetate and 20 mcg.
ethinyl estradiol tablets, USP)
Each brown tablet contains 75 mg.
ferrous fumarate, USP

Parke-Davis
p. 1778

Loestrin® 21 1/20
(1 mg. norethindrone acetate and
20 mcg. ethinyl estradiol tablets, USP)

Parke-Davis
p. 1778

"Credit Card"
in black
carrying case

Loestrin® Fe 1.5/30
(1.5 mg. norethindrone acetate and 30 mcg.
ethinyl estradiol tablets, USP)
Each brown tablet contains 75 mg. ferrous
fumarate, USP

Parke-Davis
p. 1778

Loestrin® 21 1.5/30
(1.5 mg. norethindrone acetate and
30 mcg. ethinyl estradiol tablets, USP)

Parke-Davis
p. 1787

600 mg.

Lopid®
(gemfibrozil)

Parke-Davis
p. 1790

½ gram   1 gram

†**Mandelamine®**
(methenamine mandelate)

Parke-Davis
p. 1790

50 mg.   100 mg.

Meclomen®
(meclofenamate sodium)

Parke-Davis
p. 1793

500 mg.

Milontin®
(phensuximide capsules, USP)

Parke-Davis
p. 1793

15 mg.

Nardil®
(phenelzine sulfate)

Parke-Davis
p. 1795

15 mg./day,
10 mg./day
and
5 mg./day
system

Nicotrol™
(nicotine transdermal system)

Parke-Davis
p. 1798

10-mg.,
single-
dose vials

Nipent™
(pentostatin for injection)

Parke-Davis
p. 1801

8 mg./10 mL.   50 mg./10 mL.   100 mg./10 mL.

Nitrostat® IV
(nitroglycerin for infusion)

Parke-Davis
p. 1800

0.15 mg.   0.3 mg.

0.4 mg.   0.6 mg.

(Bottles shown smaller than actual size)

†**Nitrostat®**
(nitroglycerin tablets, USP)
Sublingual Tablets

Parke-Davis
p. 1803

"Credit Card"
in black
carrying case

Norlestrin® Fe 1/50
(1 mg. norethindrone acetate and
50 mcg. ethinyl estradiol tablets, USP)
Each brown tablet contains 75 mg.
ferrous fumarate, USP

Parke-Davis
p. 1803

Supplied in pale
green compact

Norlestrin® 21 1/50
(1 mg. norethindrone acetate and 50 mcg.
ethinyl estradiol tablets, USP)

Parke-Davis
p. 1803

"Credit Card"
in black
carrying case

Norlestrin® Fe 2.5/50
(2.5 mg. norethindrone acetate and
50 mcg. ethinyl estradiol tablets, USP)
Each brown tablet contains 75 mg.
ferrous fumarate, USP

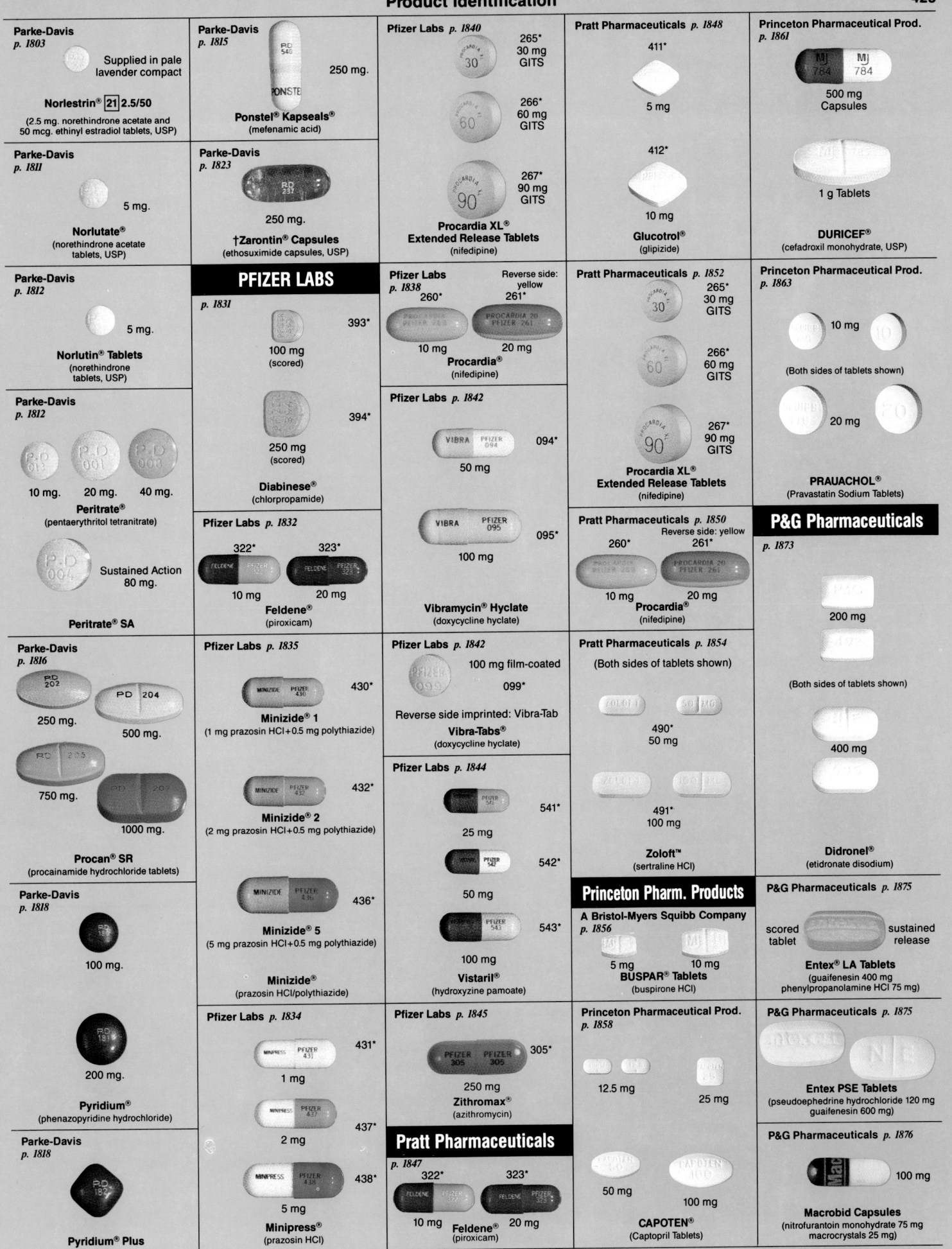

Parke-Davis *p. 1803*

Supplied in pale lavender compact

Norlestrin® 21 2.5/50

(2.5 mg. norethindrone acetate and 50 mcg. ethinyl estradiol tablets, USP)

Parke-Davis *p. 1811*

5 mg.

Norlutate®
(norethindrone acetate tablets, USP)

Parke-Davis *p. 1812*

5 mg.

Norlutin® Tablets
(norethindrone tablets, USP)

Parke-Davis *p. 1812*

10 mg. 20 mg. 40 mg.

Peritrate®
(pentaerythritol tetranitrate)

Sustained Action 80 mg.

Peritrate® SA

Parke-Davis *p. 1816*

250 mg. 500 mg.

750 mg. 1000 mg.

Procan® SR
(procainamide hydrochloride tablets)

Parke-Davis *p. 1818*

100 mg.

200 mg.

Pyridium®
(phenazopyridine hydrochloride)

Parke-Davis *p. 1818*

Pyridium® Plus

Parke-Davis *p. 1815*

250 mg.

Ponstel® Kapseals®
(mefenamic acid)

Parke-Davis *p. 1823*

250 mg.

†Zarontin® Capsules
(ethosuximide capsules, USP)

PFIZER LABS

p. 1831

100 mg (scored) 393*

250 mg (scored) 394*

Diabinese®
(chlorpropamide)

Pfizer Labs *p. 1832*

322* 323*

10 mg 20 mg

Feldene®
(piroxicam)

Pfizer Labs *p. 1835*

430*

Minizide® 1
(1 mg prazosin HCl + 0.5 mg polythiazide)

432*

Minizide® 2
(2 mg prazosin HCl + 0.5 mg polythiazide)

436*

Minizide® 5
(5 mg prazosin HCl + 0.5 mg polythiazide)

Minizide®
(prazosin HCl/polythiazide)

Pfizer Labs *p. 1834*

431*

1 mg

437*

2 mg

438*

5 mg

Minipress®
(prazosin HCl)

Pfizer Labs *p. 1840*

265* 30 mg GITS

266* 60 mg GITS

267* 90 mg GITS

Procardia XL®
Extended Release Tablets

Pfizer Labs *p. 1838*

260* Reverse side: yellow 261*

10 mg 20 mg

Procardia®
(nifedipine)

Pfizer Labs *p. 1842*

094*

50 mg

095*

100 mg

Vibramycin® Hyclate
(doxycycline hyclate)

Pfizer Labs *p. 1842*

100 mg film-coated 099*

Reverse side imprinted: Vibra-Tab

Vibra-Tabs®
(doxycycline hyclate)

Pfizer Labs *p. 1844*

541*

25 mg

542*

50 mg

543*

100 mg

Vistaril®
(hydroxyzine pamoate)

Pfizer Labs *p. 1845*

305*

250 mg

Zithromax®
(azithromycin)

Pratt Pharmaceuticals

p. 1847

322* 323*

10 mg **Feldene®** 20 mg
(piroxicam)

Pratt Pharmaceuticals *p. 1848*

411*

5 mg

412*

10 mg

Glucotrol®
(glipizide)

Pratt Pharmaceuticals *p. 1852*

265* 30 mg GITS

266* 60 mg GITS

267* 90 mg GITS

Procardia XL®
Extended Release Tablets
(nifedipine)

Pratt Pharmaceuticals *p. 1850*

Reverse side: yellow
260* 261*

10 mg 20 mg

Procardia®
(nifedipine)

Pratt Pharmaceuticals *p. 1854*

(Both sides of tablets shown)

490* 50 mg

491* 100 mg

Zoloft™
(sertraline HCl)

Princeton Pharm. Products

A Bristol-Myers Squibb Company
p. 1856

5 mg 10 mg

BUSPAR® Tablets
(buspirone HCl)

Princeton Pharmaceutical Prod.
p. 1858

12.5 mg 25 mg

50 mg 100 mg

CAPOTEN®
(Captopril Tablets)

Princeton Pharmaceutical Prod.
p. 1861

500 mg Capsules

1 g Tablets

DURICEF®
(cefadroxil monohydrate, USP)

Princeton Pharmaceutical Prod.
p. 1863

10 mg

(Both sides of tablets shown)

20 mg

PRAVACHOL®
(Pravastatin Sodium Tablets)

P&G Pharmaceuticals

p. 1873

200 mg

(Both sides of tablets shown)

400 mg

Didronel®
(etidronate disodium)

P&G Pharmaceuticals *p. 1875*

scored tablet sustained release

Entex® LA Tablets
(guaifenesin 400 mg
phenylpropanolamine HCl 75 mg)

P&G Pharmaceuticals *p. 1875*

Entex PSE Tablets
(pseudoephedrine hydrochloride 120 mg
guaifenesin 600 mg)

P&G Pharmaceuticals *p. 1876*

100 mg

Macrobid Capsules
(nitrofurantoin monohydrate 75 mg
macrocrystals 25 mg)

P&G Pharmaceuticals *p. 1877*

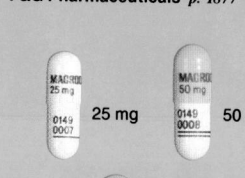

25 mg   50 mg

100 mg

Macrodantin® Capsules
(nitrofurantoin macrocrystals)

PURDUE FREDERICK

p. 1879

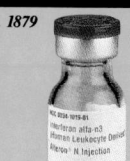

(Shown smaller than actual size)

5 million IU per vial
Contents: 1 ml

**ALFERON® N Injection
Interferon alfa-n3**
(human leukocyte derived)

Purdue Frederick *p. 1882*

(Both sides of tablet shown)

275 mg

Bottles of 100 and 500 tablets
CARDIOQUIN® Tablets
(quinidine polygalacturonate)

Purdue Frederick *p. 1884*

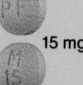 15 mg — Bottles of 100 and 500 tablets and also in unit-dose packaging

(Both sides of tablets shown)

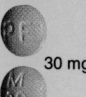 30 mg — Bottles of 50, 100, 250, and 500 tablets and also in unit-dose packaging.

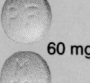 60 mg — Bottles of 100 and 500 tablets and also in unit-dose packaging.

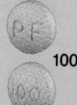 100 mg — Bottles of 100 tablets and also in unit-dose packaging.

MS CONTIN® Tablets
(morphine sulfate controlled-release)

Purdue Frederick *p. 1886*

(Both sides of tablets shown)

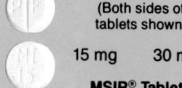

15 mg   30 mg

MSIR® Tablets
(morphine sulfate immediate-release)
Bottles of 50 tablets.

Purdue Frederick *p. 1886*

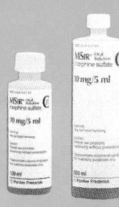

Oral Solution
MSIR Oral Solution (pleasantly flavored) 10 mg/5 ml and 20 mg/5 ml in plastic bottles of 120 ml and 500 ml. Also available in 5 ml unit dose cups.

Oral Solution Concentrate
MSIR Oral Solution Concentrate (unflavored) 20 mg/1 ml in child-resistant plastic bottles of 30 ml and 120 ml with child-resistant dropper.

MSIR® Solutions
(morphine sulfate immediate-release)

Purdue Frederick *p. 1891*

Trilisate Tablets 500 mg and 750 mg available in bottles of 100 and 500 tablets and in unit dose packaging. Trilisate 1000 mg available in bottles of 100 tablets. Trilisate Liquid 500 mg available in bottles of 8 fluid ounces.

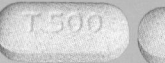

500 mg

(Both sides of tablets shown)

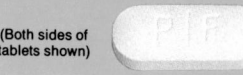

750 mg

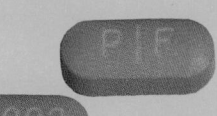

1000 mg

TRILISATE® Tablets
(choline magnesium trisalicylate)

Purdue Frederick *p. 1889*

(Both sides of tablet shown)

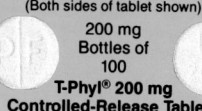

200 mg
Bottles of 100

**T-Phyl® 200 mg
Controlled-Release Tablets**
(theophylline, anhydrous)
(Formerly UNIPHYL® 200 mg tablets)

Purdue Frederick *p. 1892*

(Both sides of tablet shown)

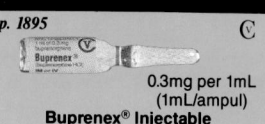

400 mg
Bottles of 100 and 500, and Unit-Dose Packaging

**UNIPHYL® 400 mg
Controlled-Release Tablets**
(theophylline, anhydrous)

RECKITT & COLMAN

p. 1895

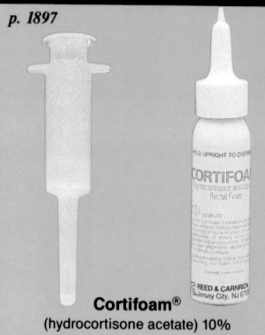

0.3mg per 1mL
(1mL/ampul)
Buprenex® Injectable
(Buprenorphine Hydrochloride)

REED & CARNRICK

p. 1897

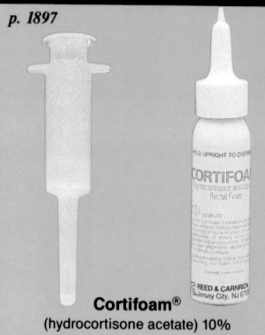

Cortifoam®
(hydrocortisone acetate) 10%

Reed & Carnrick *p. 1897*

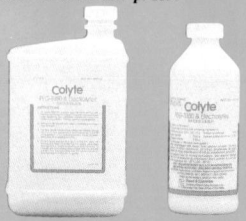

4 liter size   1 gallon size

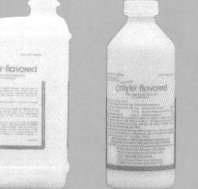

Colyte®/Colyte®-flavored
(PEG-3350 & Electrolytes)
for Oral Solution

Reed & Carnrick *p. 1898*

Sustained Release Capsules

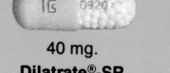

40 mg.
Dilatrate®-SR
(isosorbide dinitrate)

Reed & Carnrick *p. 1899*

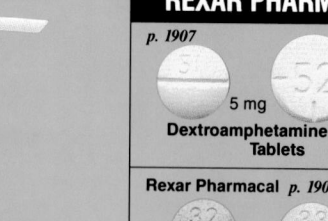

Epifoam®
(hydrocortisone acetate 1% and pramoxine hydrochloride 1%)
topical aerosol

Reed & Carnrick *p. 1900*

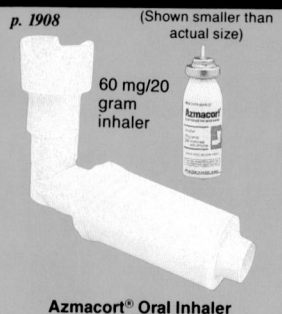

**Kwell®
Cream**
(lindane) 1%

Reed & Carnrick *p. 1901*

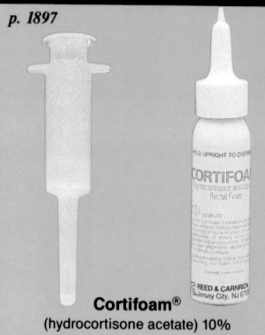

**Kwell®
Lotion**   **Kwell®
Shampoo**
(lindane) 1%

Reed & Carnrick *p. 1903*

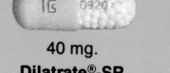

20 mg.
Levatol®
(penbutolol sulfate)

Reed & Carnrick *p. 1905*

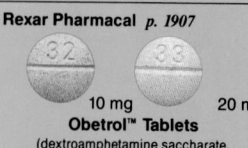

ProctoCream®-HC
(hydrocortisone acetate 1% and pramoxine hydrochloride 1%)

Reed & Carnrick *p. 1906*

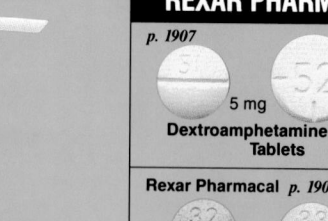

ProctoFoam®-HC
(hydrocortisone acetate 1% and pramoxine hydrochloride 1%)
topical aerosol

REXAR PHARMACAL

p. 1907

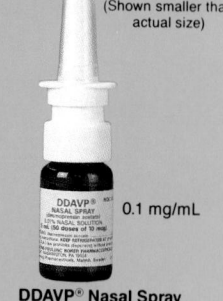

5 mg   10 mg

**Dextroamphetamine Sulfate
Tablets**

Rexar Pharmacal *p. 1907*

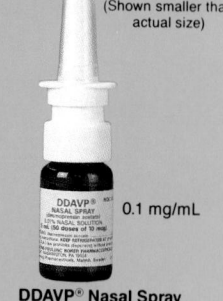

10 mg   20 mg

Obetrol™ Tablets
(dextroamphetamine saccharate, amphetamine aspartate, dextroamphetamine sulfate and amphetamine sulfate)

**Rhône-Poulenc Rorer

p. 1908

(Shown smaller than actual size)

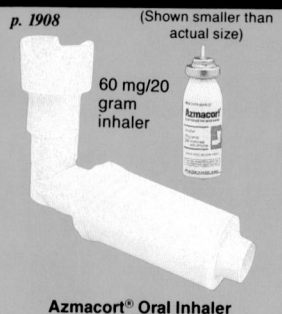

60 mg/20 gram inhaler

Azmacort® Oral Inhaler
(triamcinolone acetonide)

Rhône-Poulenc Rorer
p. 1910

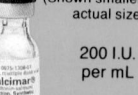

(Shown smaller than actual size)

200 I.U. per mL

Calcimar® Injection, Synthetic
(calcitonin-salmon)

Rhône-Poulenc Rorer
p. 1911

(Shown smaller than actual size)

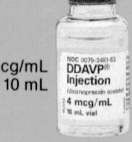

4 mcg/mL
1 mL

4 mcg/mL
10 mL

DDAVP® Injection
(desmopressin acetate)

Rhône-Poulenc Rorer
p. 1912

(Shown smaller than actual size)

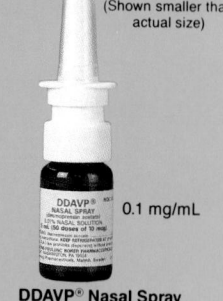

0.1 mg/mL

DDAVP® Nasal Spray
(desmopressin acetate)

Rhône-Poulenc Rorer
p. 1912

(Shown smaller than actual size)

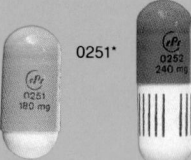

0.1 mg/mL

DDAVP® Rhinal Tube
(desmopressin acetate)

Rhône-Poulenc Rorer
p. 1914

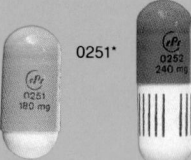

0251*   0252*

180 mg   240 mg

**Dilacor™ XR
Extended-release Capsules**
(diltiazem HCl)

Rhône-Poulenc Rorer
p. 1908

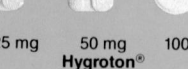

22*   20*   21*

25 mg   50 mg   100 mg

Hygroton®
(chlorthalidone USP)

Rhône-Poulenc Rorer
p. 1916

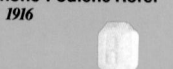

2.5 mg
Lozol®
(indapamide)

**During the next year new Rhône-Poulenc Rorer Identification will appear on the products.

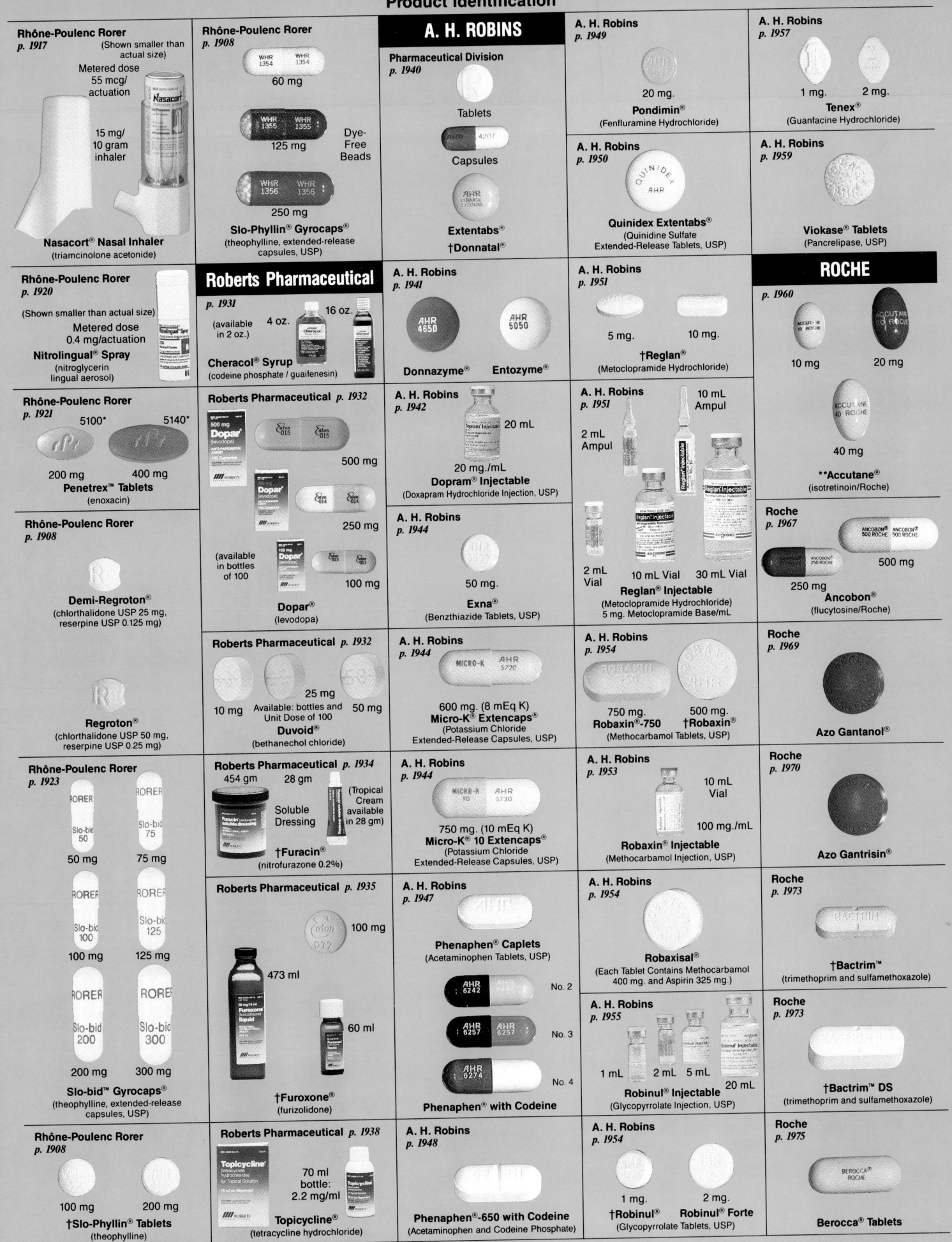

Rhône-Poulenc Rorer
p. 1917 *(Shown smaller than actual size)*

Metered dose
55 mcg/
actuation

15 mg/
10 gram
inhaler

Nasacort® Nasal Inhaler
(triamcinolone acetonide)

Rhône-Poulenc Rorer
p. 1920
(Shown smaller than actual size)

Metered dose
0.4 mg/actuation

Nitrolingual® Spray
(nitroglycerin
lingual aerosol)

Rhône-Poulenc Rorer
p. 1921
5100*   5140*

200 mg   400 mg
Penetrex™ Tablets
(enoxacin)

Rhône-Poulenc Rorer
p. 1908

Demi-Regroton®
(chlorthalidone USP 25 mg,
reserpine USP 0.125 mg)

Regroton®
(chlorthalidone USP 50 mg,
reserpine USP 0.25 mg)

Rhône-Poulenc Rorer
p. 1923

Slo-bid 50 — 50 mg
Slo-bid 75 — 75 mg
Slo-bid 100 — 100 mg
Slo-bid 125 — 125 mg
Slo-bid 200 — 200 mg
Slo-bid 300 — 300 mg

Slo-bid™ Gyrocaps®
(theophylline, extended-release
capsules, USP)

Rhône-Poulenc Rorer
p. 1908

100 mg   200 mg
†Slo-Phyllin® Tablets
(theophylline)

Rhône-Poulenc Rorer
p. 1908

WHR 1354 — 60 mg
WHR 1355 — 125 mg
WHR 1356 — 250 mg

Dye-Free Beads

Slo-Phyllin® Gyrocaps®
(theophylline, extended-release
capsules, USP)

Roberts Pharmaceutical

p. 1931
(available in 2 oz.)   4 oz.   16 oz.

Cheracol® Syrup
(codeine phosphate / guaifenesin)

Roberts Pharmaceutical p. 1932
500 mg

Eaton 015 — 500 mg
Eaton 014 — 250 mg
Eaton 013 — 100 mg

(available in bottles of 100)

Dopar®
(levodopa)

Roberts Pharmaceutical p. 1932
10 mg   25 mg   50 mg

Available: bottles and
Unit Dose of 100
Duvoid®
(bethanechol chloride)

Roberts Pharmaceutical p. 1934
454 gm   28 gm

Soluble Dressing
(Tropical Cream available in 28 gm)

†Furacin®
(nitrofurazone 0.2%)

Roberts Pharmaceutical p. 1935
Eaton 072 — 100 mg

473 ml
†Furoxone®
(furizolidone)

60 ml

Roberts Pharmaceutical p. 1938
70 ml bottle: 2.2 mg/ml

Topicycline®
(tetracycline hydrochloride)

A. H. ROBINS

Pharmaceutical Division
p. 1940

Tablets

AHR 4207 — Capsules

Extentabs®

†Donnatal®

A. H. Robins
p. 1941

AHR 4650 — **Donnazyme®**
AHR 5050 — **Entozyme®**

A. H. Robins
p. 1942
20 mL

20 mg./mL
Dopram® Injectable
(Doxapram Hydrochloride Injection, USP)

A. H. Robins
p. 1944

AHR — 50 mg.
Exna®
(Benzthiazide Tablets, USP)

A. H. Robins
p. 1944

MICRO-K AHR 5720
600 mg. (8 mEq K)
Micro-K® Extencaps®
(Potassium Chloride
Extended-Release Capsules, USP)

A. H. Robins
p. 1944

MICRO-K 10 AHR 5730
750 mg. (10 mEq K)
Micro-K® 10 Extencaps®
(Potassium Chloride
Extended-Release Capsules, USP)

A. H. Robins
p. 1947

AHR — **Phenaphen® Caplets**
(Acetaminophen Tablets, USP)

AHR 6242 — No. 2
AHR 6257 — No. 3
AHR 0274 — No. 4
Phenaphen® with Codeine

A. H. Robins
p. 1948

Phenaphen®-650 with Codeine
(Acetaminophen and Codeine Phosphate)

A. H. Robins
p. 1949

20 mg.
Pondimin®
(Fenfluramine Hydrochloride)

A. H. Robins
p. 1950

QUINIDEX AHR
Quinidex Extentabs®
(Quinidine Sulfate
Extended-Release Tablets, USP)

A. H. Robins
p. 1951

5 mg.   10 mg.
†Reglan®
(Metoclopramide Hydrochloride)

A. H. Robins
p. 1951
2 mL Ampul   10 mL Ampul

2 mL Vial   10 mL Vial   30 mL Vial
Reglan® Injectable
(Metoclopramide Hydrochloride)
5 mg. Metoclopramide Base/mL

A. H. Robins
p. 1954

750 mg.   500 mg.
Robaxin®-750   **†Robaxin®**
(Methocarbamol Tablets, USP)

A. H. Robins
p. 1953
10 mL Vial

100 mg./mL
Robaxin® Injectable
(Methocarbamol Injection, USP)

A. H. Robins
p. 1954

Robaxisal®
(Each Tablet Contains Methocarbamol
400 mg. and Aspirin 325 mg.)

A. H. Robins
p. 1955
1 mL   2 mL   5 mL   20 mL

Robinul® Injectable
(Glycopyrrolate Injection, USP)

A. H. Robins
p. 1954

1 mg.   2 mg.
†Robinul®   Robinul® Forte
(Glycopyrrolate Tablets, USP)

A. H. Robins
p. 1957

1 mg.   2 mg.
Tenex®
(Guanfacine Hydrochloride)

A. H. Robins
p. 1959

Viokase® Tablets
(Pancrelipase, USP)

ROCHE

p. 1960

ACCUTANE 10 ROCHE — 10 mg
ACCUTANE 20 ROCHE — 20 mg
ACCUTANE 40 ROCHE — 40 mg

Accutane®
(isotretinoin/Roche)

Roche
p. 1967

ANCOBON 500 ROCHE — 500 mg
ANCOBON 250 ROCHE — 250 mg
Ancobon®
(flucytosine/Roche)

Roche
p. 1969

Azo Gantanol®

Roche
p. 1970

Azo Gantrisin®

Roche
p. 1973

BACTRIM
†Bactrim™
(trimethoprim and sulfamethoxazole)

Roche
p. 1973

†Bactrim™ DS
(trimethoprim and sulfamethoxazole)

Roche
p. 1975

BEROCCA ROCHE
Berocca® Tablets

---

‡Dalmane, Endep, Librax, Libritabs, Librium, Limbitrol, Menrium, Quarzan and Valium are products of Roche Products Inc., Manati, PR 00701.
**Accutane, Solatene and Tegison are products of Roche Dermatologics, Nutley, NJ 07110.

Roche p. 1975

Berocca® Plus

Roche p. 1976

0.5 mg

1 mg

2 mg

†Bumex®
(bumetanide/Roche)

Roche p. 2016

15 mg

30 mg

‡Dalmane®
(flurazepam HCl/Roche)

Roche p. 2017

10 mg   25 mg

50 mg   75 mg

100 mg   150 mg

‡Endep®
(amitriptyline HCl/Roche)

Roche p. 1977

Fansidar®
(sulfadoxine and pyrimethamine)

Roche p. 1981

500 mg

†Gantanol®
(sulfamethoxazole/Roche)

Roche p. 1982

500 mg

†Gantrisin®
(sulfisoxazole/Roche)

Roche p. 1983

0.375 mg   0.750 mg

Hivid® Tablets
(zalcitabine)

Roche p. 1989

0.5 mg   1 mg   2 mg

Klonopin™
(clonazepam/Roche)

Roche p. 1991

250 mg
Lariam®
(mefloquine hydrochloride)

Roche p. 1992

Larobec®

Roche p. 1992

0.1 Gm Tablet   0.25 Gm Tablet

0.5 Gm Tablet

Larodopa®
(levodopa/Roche)

Roche p. 1993

2 mg

†Levo-Dromoran®
(levorphanol tartrate/Roche)

Roche p. 2018

‡Librax®

Roche p. 2019

5 mg   10 mg   25 mg

‡Libritabs®
(chlordiazepoxide/Roche)

Roche p. 2020

5 mg   10 mg   25 mg

‡†Librium®
(chlordiazepoxide HCl/Roche)

Roche p. 2022

‡Limbitrol®   ‡Limbitrol® DS
(chlordiazepoxide and amitriptyline HCl/Roche)

Roche p. 1993

10 mg
Marplan®
(isocarboxazid/Roche)

Roche p. 1995

50 mg
Matulane®
(procarbazine HCl/Roche)

Roche p. 2023

‡Menrium®   ‡Menrium®   ‡Menrium®
5-2   5-4   10-4

Roche p. 2026

2.5 mg   5 mg

‡Quarzan®
(clidinium bromide/Roche)

Roche p. 2002

0.25 mcg   0.5 mcg

Rocaltrol®
(calcitriol/Roche)

Roche p. 1962

30 mg
****Solatene®**
(beta-carotene/Roche)

Roche p. 2009

5 mg
†Synkayvite®
(menadiol sodium diphosphate/Roche)

Roche p. 1963

10 mg   25 mg

****Tegison®**
(etretinate/Roche)

Roche p. 2011

100 mg
Trimpex®
(trimethoprim/Roche)

Roche p. 2028

2 mg   5 mg   10 mg

‡†Valium®
(diazepam/Roche)

Roche p. 2027

(Shown slightly smaller than actual size)

Scale in mg on both sides of barrel eases visibility during administration.

Prefilled disposable syringe with a 1½" needle to help insure deep administration into muscle.

Tel-E-Ject®
2 ml = 10 mg

†Valium Injectable
(diazepam/Roche)

Roche p. 2012

15 mg
Valrelease™
(diazepam/Roche)

ROERIG DIVISION

p. 2030

210*

12.5 mg.
Antivert®
(meclizine HCl)

Roerig Division p. 2030

211*

25 mg.
Antivert®/25
(meclizine HCl)

Roerig Division p. 2030

214*

50 mg.
Antivert®/50
(meclizine HCl)

Roerig Division p. 2030

10 mg.   25 mg.
560*   561*

50 mg.   100 mg.
562*   563*

†Atarax®
(hydroxyzine hydrochloride)

Designed to help you identify drugs, this section contains actual size, full-color reproductions of products selected for inclusion by participating manufacturers.

Important Notice

Before prescribing or administering any product described in PHYSICIANS' DESK REFERENCE always consult the PDR Supplement for possible new or revised information.

TEL-E-DOSE® ROCHE®

p. 2011

Example:

BUMEX® 0.5 mg
(bumetanide)
ROCHE, NUTLEY, N.J.
LOT 0103
EXP. 12-1-93

Bumex®
(bumetanide/Roche)

Tel-E-Dose is a unit package designed by Roche for convenience in dispensing medications in the hospital and nursing home. Each unit, sealed against contamination and moisture, is clearly identified by product name and strength and carries the control number and expiration date.

Currently available in this package form are the following Roche products: Bactrim™ (80 mg trimethoprim and 400 mg sulfamethoxazole) tablets; Bactrim™ DS (160 mg trimethoprim and 800 mg sulfamethoxazole) tablets; Bumex® (bumetanide) tablets, 0.5 mg, 1 mg, 2 mg; Gantanol® (sulfamethoxazole) tablets, 0.5 Gm; Gantrisin® (sulfisoxazole) tablets, 0.5 Gm; Klonopin® (clonazepam) tablets, 0.5 mg, 1 mg, 2 mg; Larium® (mefloquine hydrochloride) tablets, 250 mg; Librax® (5 mg chlordiazepoxide HCl and 2.5 mg clidinium Br) capsules; Librium® (chlordiazepoxide HCl) capsules, 5 mg, 10 mg, 25 mg; Limbitrol® (5 mg chlordiazepoxide and 12.5 mg amitriptyline HCl) tablets; Limbitrol® DS (10 mg chlordiazepoxide and 25 mg amitriptyline HCl) tablets; Trimpex® (trimethoprim) tablets, 100 mg; and Valium® (diazepam) tablets, 2 mg, 5 mg, 10 mg.

‡Dalmane, Endep, Librax, Libritabs, Librium, Limbitrol, Menrium, Quarzan and Valium are products of Roche Products Inc., Manati, PR 00701.
**Accutane, Solatene and Tegison are products of Roche Dermatologics, Nutley, NJ 07110.

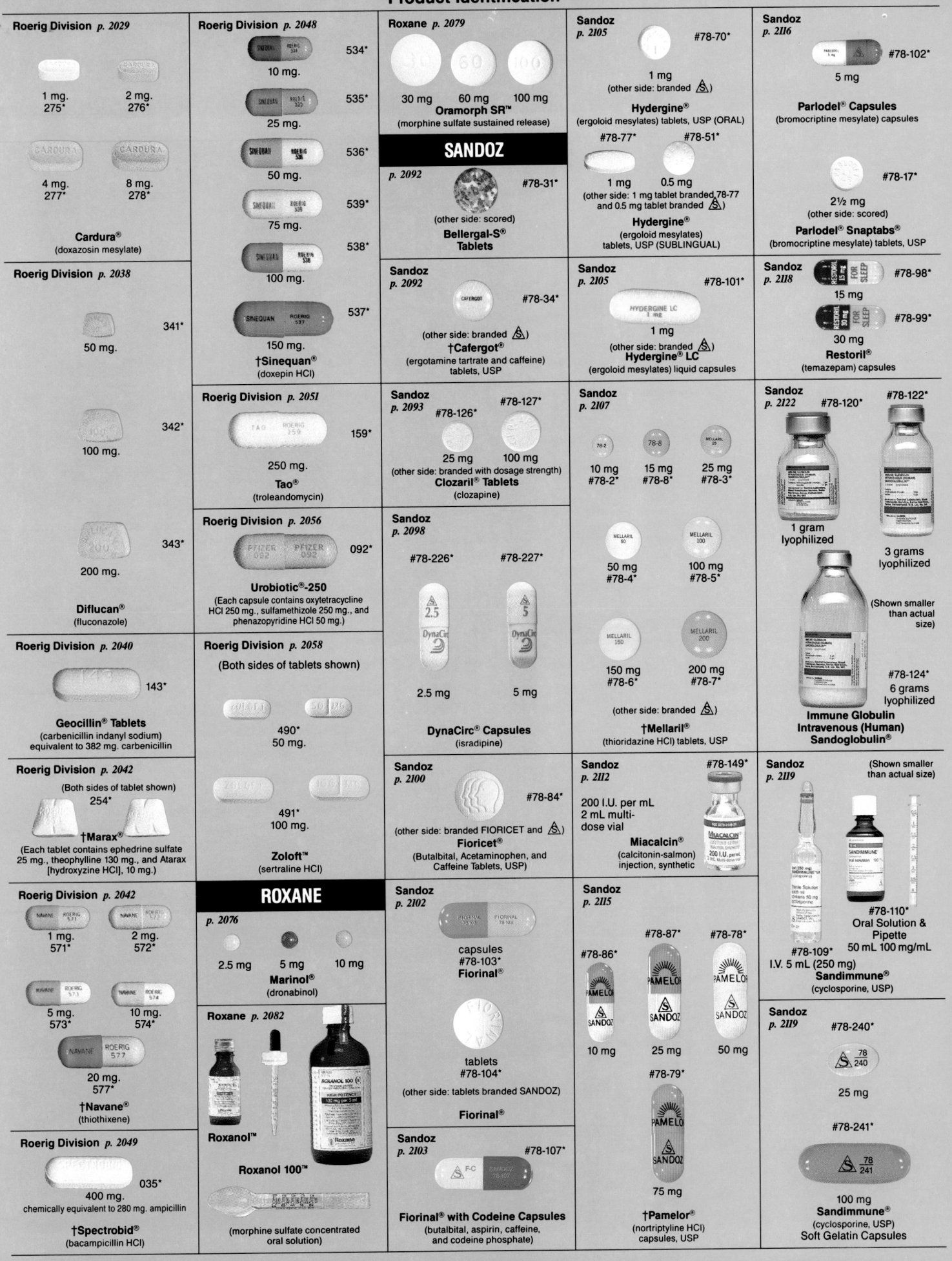

Roerig Division p. 2029

1 mg. 275*
2 mg. 276*
4 mg. 277*
8 mg. 278*

Cardura®
(doxazosin mesylate)

Roerig Division p. 2038

50 mg. 341*
100 mg. 342*
200 mg. 343*

Diflucan®
(fluconazole)

Roerig Division p. 2040

143*

Geocillin® Tablets
(carbenicillin indanyl sodium)
equivalent to 382 mg. carbenicillin

Roerig Division p. 2042

(Both sides of tablet shown)
254*

†Marax®
(Each tablet contains ephedrine sulfate 25 mg., theophylline 130 mg., and Atarax [hydroxyzine HCl], 10 mg.)

Roerig Division p. 2042

1 mg. 571*
2 mg. 572*
5 mg. 573*
10 mg. 574*
20 mg. 577*

†Navane®
(thiothixene)

Roerig Division p. 2049

400 mg. 035*
chemically equivalent to 280 mg. ampicillin

†Spectrobid®
(bacampicillin HCl)

Roerig Division p. 2048

10 mg. 534*
25 mg. 535*
50 mg. 536*
75 mg. 539*
100 mg. 538*
150 mg. 537*

†Sinequan®
(doxepin HCl)

Roerig Division p. 2051

250 mg. 159*

Tao®
(troleandomycin)

Roerig Division p. 2056

092*

Urobiotic®-250
(Each capsule contains oxytetracycline HCl 250 mg., sulfamethizole 250 mg., and phenazopyridine HCl 50 mg.)

Roerig Division p. 2058

(Both sides of tablets shown)

490*
50 mg.

491*
100 mg.

Zoloft™
(sertraline HCl)

ROXANE

p. 2076

2.5 mg   5 mg   10 mg

Marinol®
(dronabinol)

Roxane p. 2082

Roxanol™

Roxanol 100™

(morphine sulfate concentrated oral solution)

Roxane p. 2079

30 mg   60 mg   100 mg

Oramorph SR™
(morphine sulfate sustained release)

SANDOZ

p. 2092

#78-31*

(other side: scored)

Bellergal-S®
Tablets

Sandoz p. 2092

#78-34*

(other side: branded ⓢ)

†Cafergot®
(ergotamine tartrate and caffeine) tablets, USP

Sandoz p. 2093

#78-126*   #78-127*

25 mg   100 mg

(other side: branded with dosage strength)

Clozaril® Tablets
(clozapine)

Sandoz p. 2098

#78-226*   #78-227*

2.5 mg   5 mg

DynaCirc® Capsules
(isradipine)

Sandoz p. 2100

#78-84*

(other side: branded FIORICET and ⓢ)

Fioricet®
(Butalbital, Acetaminophen, and Caffeine Tablets, USP)

Sandoz p. 2102

capsules
#78-103*
Fiorinal®

tablets
#78-104*

(other side: tablets branded SANDOZ)

Fiorinal®

Sandoz p. 2103

#78-107*

Fiorinal® with Codeine Capsules
(butalbital, aspirin, caffeine, and codeine phosphate)

Sandoz p. 2105

#78-70*

1 mg
(other side: branded ⓢ)

Hydergine®
(ergoloid mesylates) tablets, USP (ORAL)

#78-77*   #78-51*

1 mg   0.5 mg
(other side: 1 mg tablet branded 78-77 and 0.5 mg tablet branded ⓢ)

Hydergine®
(ergoloid mesylates)
tablets, USP (SUBLINGUAL)

Sandoz p. 2105

#78-101*

1 mg
(other side: branded ⓢ)

Hydergine® LC
(ergoloid mesylates) liquid capsules

Sandoz p. 2107

10 mg   15 mg   25 mg
#78-2*   #78-8*   #78-3*

50 mg   100 mg
#78-4*   #78-5*

150 mg   200 mg
#78-6*   #78-7*

(other side: branded ⓢ)

†Mellaril®
(thioridazine HCl) tablets, USP

Sandoz p. 2112

#78-149*

200 I.U. per mL
2 mL multi-dose vial

Miacalcin®
(calcitonin-salmon) injection, synthetic

Sandoz p. 2115

#78-86*   #78-87*   #78-78*

10 mg   25 mg   50 mg

#78-79*

75 mg

†Pamelor®
(nortriptyline HCl) capsules, USP

Sandoz p. 2116

#78-102*

5 mg

Parlodel® Capsules
(bromocriptine mesylate) capsules

#78-17*

2½ mg
(other side: scored)

Parlodel® Snaptabs®
(bromocriptine mesylate) tablets, USP

Sandoz p. 2118

#78-98*
15 mg

#78-99*
30 mg

Restoril®
(temazepam) capsules

Sandoz p. 2122

#78-120*   #78-122*

1 gram lyophilized   3 grams lyophilized

(Shown smaller than actual size)

#78-124*
6 grams lyophilized

Immune Globulin Intravenous (Human)
Sandoglobulin®

Sandoz p. 2119

(Shown smaller than actual size)

#78-110*
Oral Solution & Pipette
50 mL 100 mg/mL

#78-109*
I.V. 5 mL (250 mg)

Sandimmune®
(cyclosporine, USP)

Sandoz p. 2119

#78-240*

25 mg

#78-241*

100 mg

Sandimmune®
(cyclosporine, USP)
Soft Gelatin Capsules

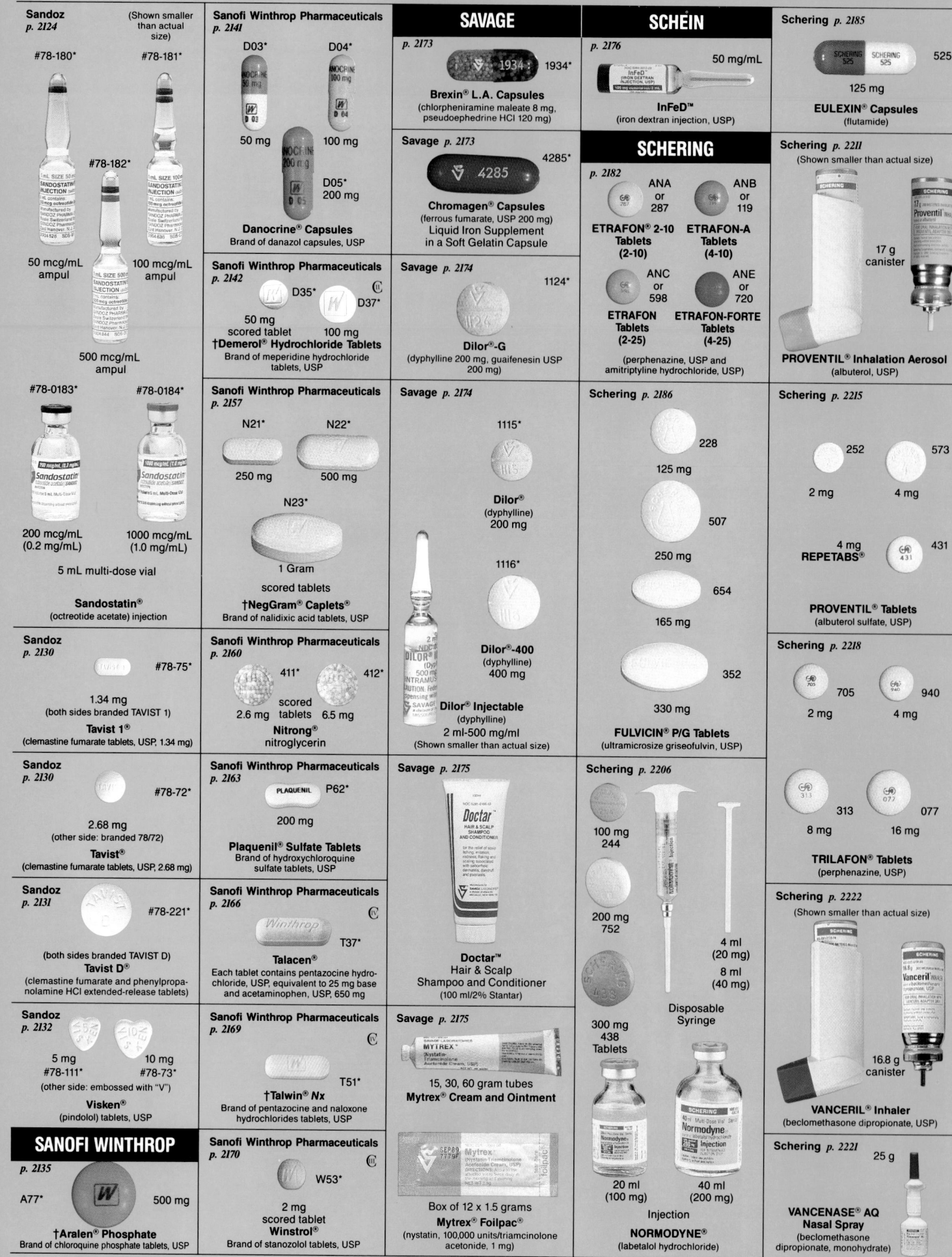

Sandoz p. 2124 (Shown smaller than actual size)

#78-180*

#78-181*

#78-182*

50 mcg/mL ampul

100 mcg/mL ampul

500 mcg/mL ampul

#78-0183*

#78-0184*

200 mcg/mL (0.2 mg/mL)

1000 mcg/mL (1.0 mg/mL)

5 mL multi-dose vial

Sandostatin® (octreotide acetate) injection

Sandoz p. 2130

#78-75*

1.34 mg (both sides branded TAVIST 1)

Tavist 1® (clemastine fumarate tablets, USP, 1.34 mg)

Sandoz p. 2130

#78-72*

2.68 mg (other side: branded 78/72)

Tavist® (clemastine fumarate tablets, USP, 2.68 mg)

Sandoz p. 2131

#78-221*

(both sides branded TAVIST D)

Tavist D® (clemastine fumarate and phenylpropa-nolamine HCl extended-release tablets)

Sandoz p. 2132

5 mg #78-111*

10 mg #78-73*

(other side: embossed with "V")

Visken® (pindolol) tablets, USP

SANOFI WINTHROP

p. 2135

A77*

500 mg

†Aralen® Phosphate Brand of chloroquine phosphate tablets, USP

Sanofi Winthrop Pharmaceuticals p. 2141

D03*

D04*

50 mg

100 mg

D05* 200 mg

Danocrine® Capsules Brand of danazol capsules, USP

Sanofi Winthrop Pharmaceuticals p. 2142

D35*

D37*

50 mg scored tablet

100 mg

†Demerol® Hydrochloride Tablets Brand of meperidine hydrochloride tablets, USP

Sanofi Winthrop Pharmaceuticals p. 2157

N21*

N22*

250 mg

500 mg

N23*

1 Gram scored tablets

†NegGram® Caplets® Brand of nalidixic acid tablets, USP

Sanofi Winthrop Pharmaceuticals p. 2160

411*

412*

scored 2.6 mg tablets 6.5 mg

Nitrong® nitroglycerin

Sanofi Winthrop Pharmaceuticals p. 2163

PLAQUENIL P62*

200 mg

Plaquenil® Sulfate Tablets Brand of hydroxychloroquine sulfate tablets, USP

Sanofi Winthrop Pharmaceuticals p. 2166

Winthrop T37*

Talacen® Each tablet contains pentazocine hydro-chloride, USP, equivalent to 25 mg base and acetaminophen, USP, 650 mg

Sanofi Winthrop Pharmaceuticals p. 2169

T51*

†Talwin® Nx Brand of pentazocine and naloxone hydrochlorides tablets, USP

Sanofi Winthrop Pharmaceuticals p. 2170

W53*

2 mg scored tablet **Winstrol®** Brand of stanozolol tablets, USP

SAVAGE

p. 2173

1934*

Brexin® L.A. Capsules (chlorpheniramine maleate 8 mg, pseudoephedrine HCl 120 mg)

Savage p. 2173

4285*

Chromagen® Capsules (ferrous fumarate, USP 200 mg) Liquid Iron Supplement in a Soft Gelatin Capsule

Savage p. 2174

1124*

Dilor®-G (dyphylline 200 mg, guaifenesin USP 200 mg)

Savage p. 2174

1115*

Dilor® (dyphylline) 200 mg

1116*

Dilor®-400 (dyphylline) 400 mg

Dilor® Injectable (dyphylline) 2 ml-500 mg/ml (Shown smaller than actual size)

Savage p. 2175

Doctar™ Hair & Scalp Shampoo and Conditioner (100 ml/2% Stantar)

Savage p. 2175

15, 30, 60 gram tubes **Mytrex® Cream and Ointment**

Box of 12 x 1.5 grams **Mytrex® Foilpac** (nystatin, 100,000 units/triamcinolone acetonide, 1 mg)

SCHEIN

p. 2176

50 mg/mL

InFeD™ (iron dextran injection, USP)

SCHERING

p. 2182

ANA or 287

ANB or 119

ETRAFON® 2-10 Tablets (2-10)

ETRAFON-A Tablets (4-10)

ANC or 598

ANE or 720

ETRAFON Tablets (2-25)

ETRAFON-FORTE Tablets (4-25)

(perphenazine, USP and amitriptyline hydrochloride, USP)

Schering p. 2186

228 125 mg

507 250 mg

654 165 mg

352 330 mg

FULVICIN® P/G Tablets (ultramicrosize griseofulvin, USP)

Schering p. 2206

100 mg 244

200 mg 752

300 mg 438 Tablets

4 ml (20 mg)

8 ml (40 mg)

Disposable Syringe

20 ml (100 mg)

40 ml (200 mg)

Injection **NORMODYNE®** (labetalol hydrochloride)

Schering p. 2185

525

125 mg

EULEXIN® Capsules (flutamide)

Schering p. 2211 (Shown smaller than actual size)

17 g canister

PROVENTIL® Inhalation Aerosol (albuterol, USP)

Schering p. 2215

252 2 mg

573 4 mg

4 mg **REPETABS®**

431

PROVENTIL® Tablets (albuterol sulfate, USP)

Schering p. 2218

705 2 mg

940 4 mg

313 8 mg

077 16 mg

TRILAFON® Tablets (perphenazine, USP)

Schering p. 2222 (Shown smaller than actual size)

16.8 g canister

VANCERIL® Inhaler (beclomethasone dipropionate, USP)

Schering p. 2221

25 g

VANCENASE® AQ Nasal Spray (beclomethasone dipropionate, monohydrate)

Product Identification

Schering p. 2220

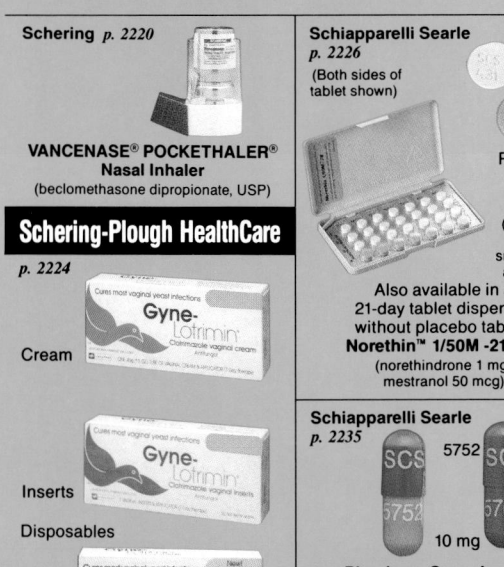

VANCENASE® POCKETHALER®
Nasal Inhaler
(beclomethasone dipropionate, USP)

Schering-Plough HealthCare

p. 2224

Cream

Inserts

Disposables

GYNE-LOTRIMIN®
Clotrimazole Vaginal
Antifungal

Schiapparelli Searle

p. 2224

1804

Sterile lyophilized
powder in
single-dose vials
(equivalent to 500 mg
metronidazole)

(Vial shown smaller
than actual size)

Flagyl® I.V.
(metronidazole HCl)

Schiapparelli Searle
p. 2224

1847

500 mg
metronidazole
in 100-ml
ready-to-use
containers
(5 mg/ml)

(Container is
shown smaller
than actual size)

Flagyl® I.V. RTU®
(metronidazole)

Schiapparelli Searle 221
p. 2226
(Both sides of
tablet shown)

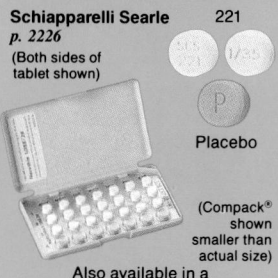

Placebo

(Compack®
shown
smaller than
actual size)

Also available in a
21-day tablet dispenser
without placebo tablets
Norethin™ 1/35E -21, -28
(norethindrone 1 mg,
ethinyl estradiol 35 mcg)

Schiapparelli Searle 431
p. 2226
(Both sides of
tablet shown)

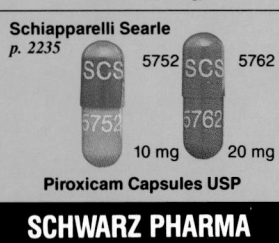

Placebo

(Compack®
shown
smaller than
actual size)

Also available in a
21-day tablet dispenser
without placebo tablets
Norethin™ 1/50M -21, -28
(norethindrone 1 mg,
mestranol 50 mcg)

Schiapparelli Searle
p. 2235

SCS 5752   SCS 5762

10 mg   20 mg

Piroxicam Capsules USP

SCHWARZ PHARMA

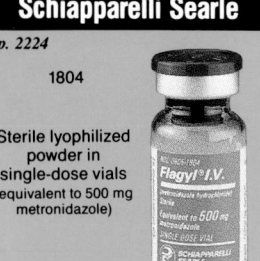

p. 2237

One System

0.2 mg/hr.
(Shown
smaller
than actual
size)

Deponit®
(nitroglycerin transdermal
delivery system)

Schwarz Pharma p. 2238

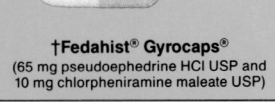   timed release

†Fedahist® Gyrocaps®
(65 mg pseudoephedrine HCl USP and
10 mg chlorpheniramine maleate USP)

Schwarz Pharma p. 2240

KREMERS
URBAN   522

Ku-Zyme®
(amylase, lipase,
protease,
cellulase)

KREMERS
URBAN

Kutrase®
(Ku-Zyme® plus
hyoscyamine sulfate/
phenyltoloxamine
citrate)

Schwarz Pharma p. 2241

KREMERS
URBAN   525

Ku-Zyme® HP
(pancrelipase capsules USP)

Schwarz Pharma p. 2241

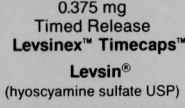

0.125 mg   0.125 mg
Levsin®/SL   **Levsin® Tablets**
Tablets

0.375 mg
Timed Release
Levsinex™ Timecaps™
Levsin®
(hyoscyamine sulfate USP)

G.D. SEARLE & CO.

p. 2243

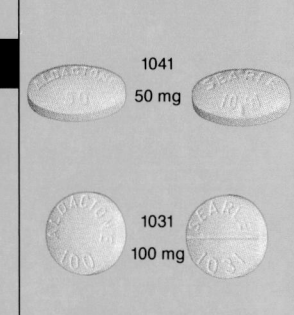

1011
25 mg/25 mg

Both sides of tablets shown

1021

50 mg/50 mg

Aldactazide®
(spironolactone/hydrochlorothiazide)

G.D. Searle & Co. p. 2245

1001
25 mg

1041
50 mg

1031
100 mg

Both sides of tablets shown

Aldactone®
(spironolactone)

G.D. Searle & Co. p. 2246
Both sides of tablets shown

1771
40 mg

1851
80 mg

1861
120 mg

Calan®
(verapamil HCl)

G.D. Searle & Co. p. 2249
Both sides of caplets shown

1901   120 mg

1911   180 mg

1891   240 mg

Calan® SR
(verapamil HCl)
Sustained-Release Oral Caplets

G.D. Searle & Co. p. 2264
Both sides of tablet shown

61

†Lomotil®
(diphenoxylate hydrochloride 2.5 mg/
atropine sulfate 0.025 mg)

G.D. Searle & Co. p. 2251

Both sides of tablets shown

1451
100 mcg

1461
200 mcg

Cytotec®
(misoprostol)

G.D. Searle & Co. p. 2253
Both sides of tablet shown

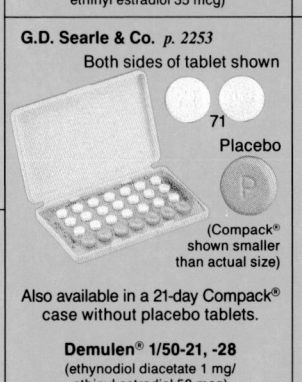

151

Placebo

(Compack®
shown smaller
than actual size)

Also available in a 21-day Compack®
case without placebo tablets.
Demulen® 1/35-21, -28
(ethynodiol diacetate 1 mg/
ethinyl estradiol 35 mcg)

G.D. Searle & Co. p. 2253
Both sides of tablet shown

71

Placebo

(Compack®
shown smaller
than actual size)

Also available in a 21-day Compack®
case without placebo tablets.
Demulen® 1/50-21, -28
(ethynodiol diacetate 1 mg/
ethinyl estradiol 50 mcg)

G.D. Searle & Co. p. 2259

1831
250 mg

Both sides of tablets shown

1821
500 mg

Flagyl®
(metronidazole)

G.D. Searle & Co. p. 2261
Both sides of tablets shown

5101
10 mg

5201
20 mg

Kerlone®
(betaxolol hydrochloride)

G.D. Searle & Co. p. 2265
Both sides of tablet shown

1651

400 mg
Maxaquin®
(lomefloxacin hydrochloride)

G.D. Searle & Co. p. 2268

0.2 mg/hr

(Discs shown
smaller than
actual size)

2058

0.3 mg/hr   0.4 mg/hr

2078   2068

Nitrodisc®
(nitroglycerin transdermal system)

G.D. Searle & Co. p. 2270

2762
NORPACE
150 MG.

2752
NORPACE
100 MG

100 mg   150 mg
Norpace®
(disopyramide phosphate)

G.D. Searle & Co. p. 2270

2732   2742

NORPACE   NORPACE
100 mg   150 mg

SEARLE   SEARLE
2732   2742

100 mg   150 mg

Norpace® CR
(disopyramide phosphate extended-release)

SMITHKLINE BEECHAM

Consumer Brands
p. 2279

Special Comb
Included

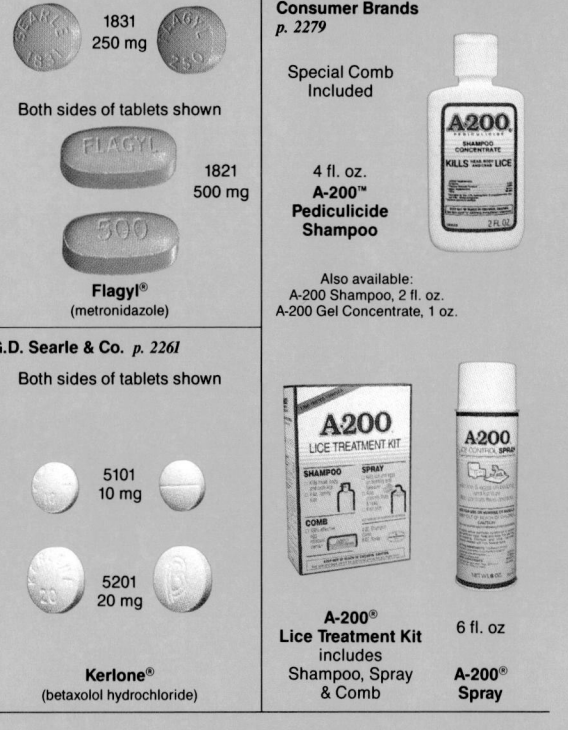

4 fl. oz.
A-200™
Pediculicide
Shampoo

Also available:
A-200 Shampoo, 2 fl. oz.
A-200 Gel Concentrate, 1 oz.

A-200®
Lice Treatment Kit
includes
Shampoo, Spray
& Comb

6 fl. oz

A-200®
Spray

429

SMITHKLINE BEECHAM

Pharmaceuticals *p. 2283*

Available also as oral suspension, pediatric drops and chewable tablets

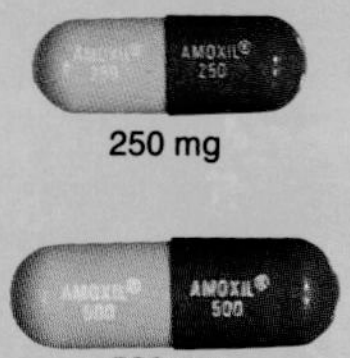

250 mg

500 mg

†AMOXIL® Capsules
(amoxicillin)

SmithKline Beecham
p. 2283

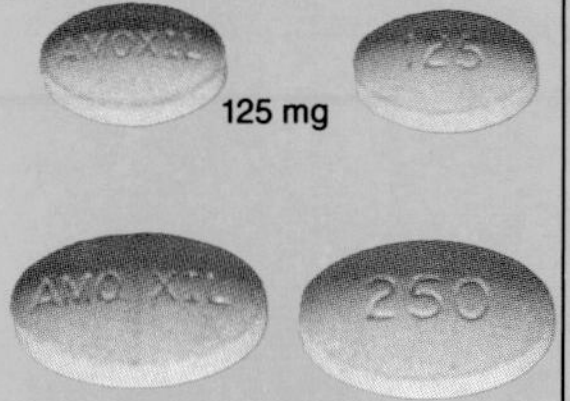

125 mg

250 mg

(Both sides of tablets shown)

†AMOXIL® Chewable Tablets
(amoxicillin)

SmithKline Beecham
p. 2284

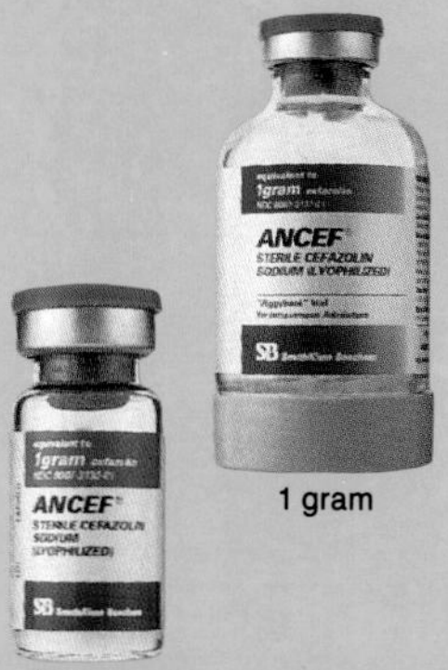

1 gram
Also 500 mg

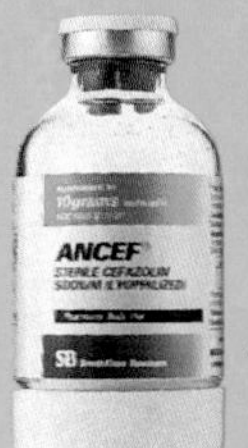

10 grams
Also 5 grams

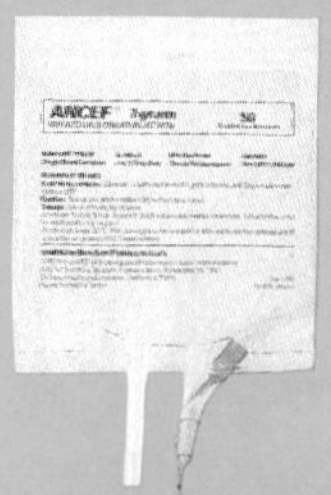

1 gram
Also 500 mg

ANCEF®
(sterile cefazolin sodium and cefazolin sodium injection)

SmithKline Beecham
p. 2289

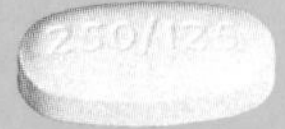

250 mg amoxicillin trihydrate/
125 mg clavulanate potassium

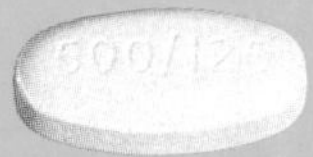

500 mg amoxicillin trihydrate/
125 mg clavulanate potassium

†AUGMENTIN® Tablets
(amoxicillin/clavulanate potassium)

SmithKline Beecham
p. 2289

125 mg amoxicillin trihydrate/
31.25 mg clavulanate potassium

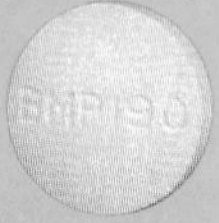

250 mg amoxicillin trihydrate/
62.5 mg clavulanate potassium

†AUGMENTIN® Chewable Tablets

SmithKline Beecham
p. 2287

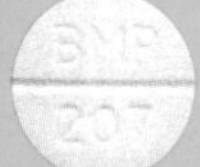

ANEXSIA® 5/500 Tablets
(hydrocodone bitartrate 5 mg and acetaminophen 500 mg)

SmithKline Beecham
p. 2288

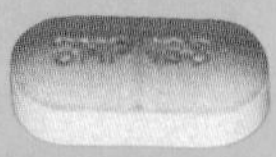

ANEXSIA® 7.5/650 Tablets
(hydrocodone bitartrate 7.5 mg and acetaminophen 650 mg)

SmithKline Beecham
p. 2283

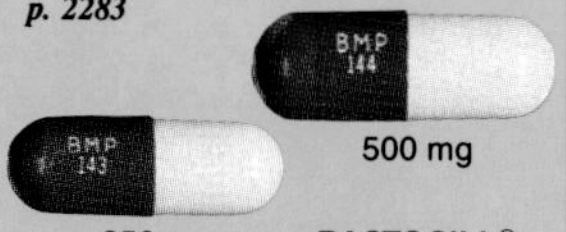

250 mg   500 mg   BACTOCILL®
(oxacillin)

SmithKline Beecham
p. 2283

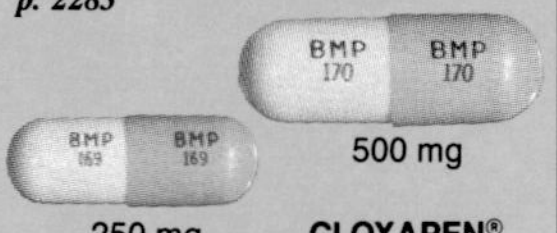

250 mg   500 mg   CLOXAPEN®
(cloxacillin)

SmithKline Beecham
p. 2291

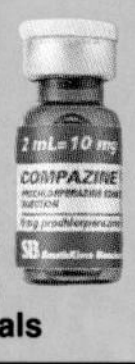

†COMPAZINE®
(prochlorperazine)
2 mL (5 mg/mL) Vials

SmithKline Beecham
p. 2291

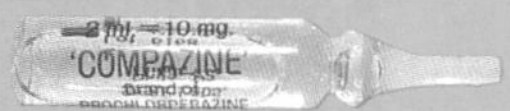

†COMPAZINE®
(prochlorperazine)
2 mL (5 mg/mL) Ampuls

SmithKline Beecham
p. 2291

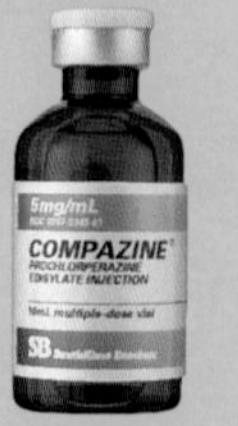

†COMPAZINE®
(prochlorperazine)
10 mL (5 mg/mL)
Multi-dose Vials

SmithKline Beecham
p. 2291   C46

C44
10 mg   15 mg

†COMPAZINE® SPANSULE®
Capsules

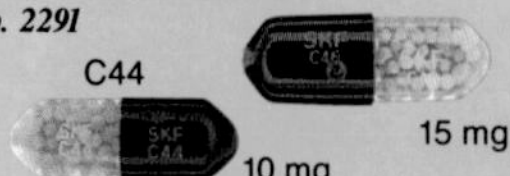

SmithKline Beecham
p. 2291

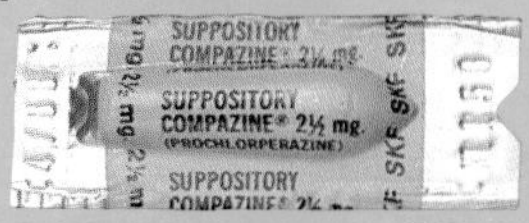

C60
2½ mg

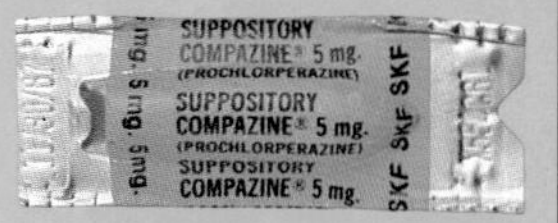

C61
5 mg

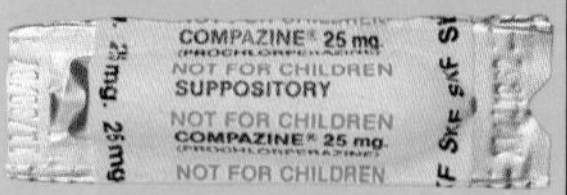

C62
25 mg

†COMPAZINE® Suppositories
(prochlorperazine)

SmithKline Beecham
p. 2291

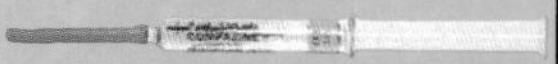

†COMPAZINE®
(prochlorperazine)
2 mL (5 mg/mL)
Prefilled Disposable Syringes

SmithKline Beecham
p. 2291

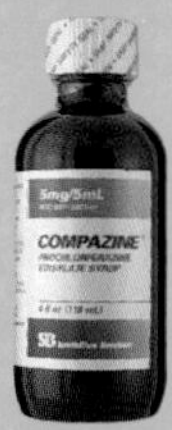

4 fl oz

†COMPAZINE®
(prochlorperazine)
Syrup
(5 mg/5 mL)

SmithKline Beecham
p. 2291   C66
5 mg

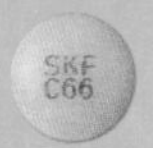

Also 10 mg C67, 25 mg C69
†COMPAZINE® Tablets
(prochlorperazine)

SmithKline Beecham
p. 2293   D14   D16   D17

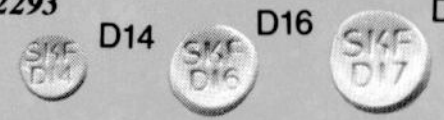

5 mcg   25 mcg   50 mcg
liothyronine as the sodium salt
CYTOMEL® Tablets
(liothyronine sodium)

SmithKline Beecham
p. 2295   E14
15 mg

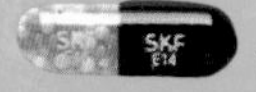

Also 5 mg E12, 10 mg E13
†DEXEDRINE® SPANSULE®
(dextroamphetamine sulfate)
Capsules

SmithKline Beecham
p. 2295   E19

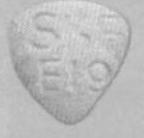

5 mg
†DEXEDRINE® Tablets
(dextroamphetamine sulfate)

SmithKline Beecham
p. 2297   E33

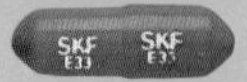

10 mg
DIBENZYLINE® Capsules
(phenoxybenzamine hydrochloride)

SmithKline Beecham
p. 2297   DYAZIDE

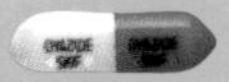

DYAZIDE® Capsules
(25 mg hydrochlorothiazide/
50 mg triamterene)

SmithKline Beecham
p. 2283

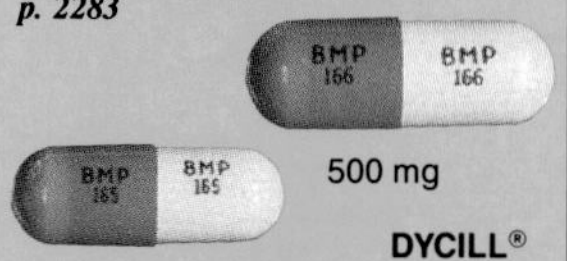

BMP 166

BMP 165   500 mg

250 mg   DYCILL®
(dicloxacillin)

SmithKline Beecham
p. 2300

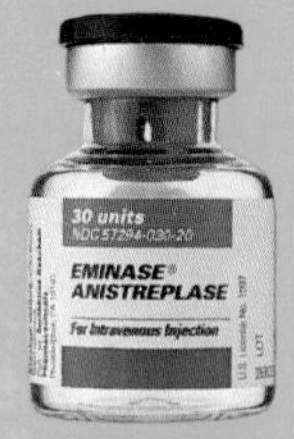

30 units
EMINASE ANISTREPLASE
For Intravenous Injection

30-unit vial
(Shown smaller than actual size)

EMINASE®
(anistreplase)

SmithKline Beecham Biologicals
p. 2302

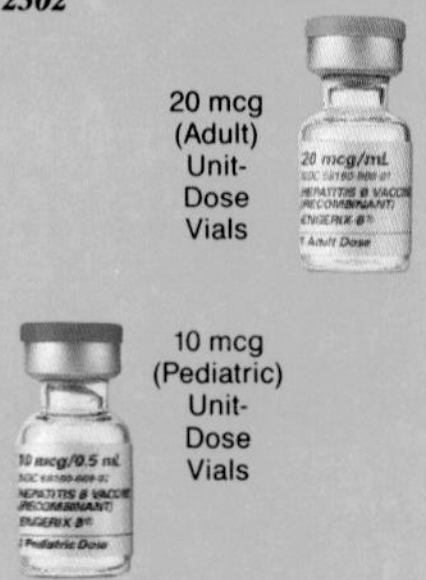

20 mcg
(Adult)
Unit-
Dose
Vials

10 mcg
(Pediatric)
Unit-
Dose
Vials

ENGERIX-B®
(Hepatitis B Vaccine [Recombinant])

SmithKline Beecham
p. 2299

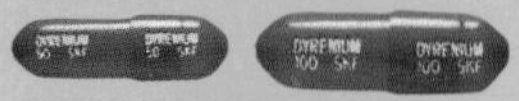

50 mg   100 mg
DYRENIUM® Capsules
(triamterene)

SmithKline Beecham
p. 2304

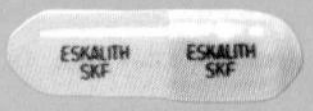

ESKALITH SKF   ESKALITH SKF   ESKALITH

300 mg
ESKALITH® Capsules
(lithium carbonate)

SmithKline Beecham
p. 2304   J09

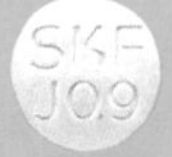

300 mg
ESKALITH® Tablets
(lithium carbonate)

SmithKline Beecham
p. 2304   J10
450 mg

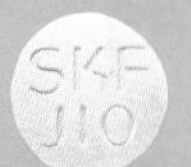

ESKALITH CR®
(lithium carbonate)
Controlled Release Tablets

SmithKline Beecham
p. 2305

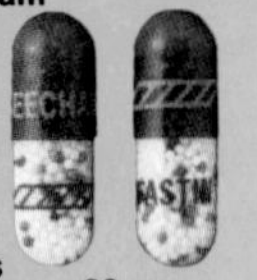

FASTIN® Capsules
(phentermine HCl)   30 mg

SmithKline Beecham
p. 2306

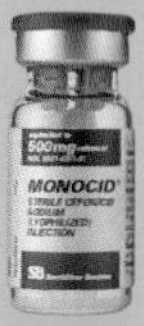

500 mg

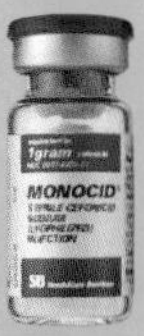

1 gram

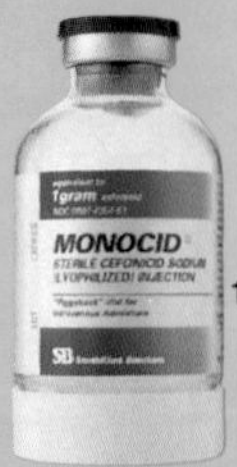

1 gram

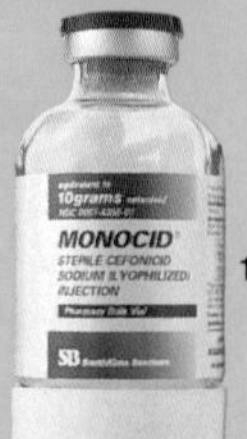

10 grams

MONOCID®
(sterile cefonicid sodium)
(lyophilized)

SmithKline Beecham
p. 2307

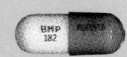

†NUCOFED® Capsules
(20 mg codeine phosphate/
60 mg pseudoephedrine HCl)

SmithKline Beecham
p. 2310

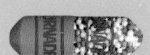

ORNADE

ORNADE® SPANSULE® Capsules

SmithKline Beecham
p. 2311

PARNATE

10 mg

PARNATE® Tablets
(tranylcypromine sulfate)

SmithKline Beecham
p. 2316

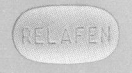

RELAFEN

(Both sides of tablet shown)

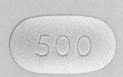

500

500 mg

RELAFEN® Tablets
(nabumetone)

SmithKline Beecham
p. 2318

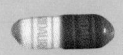

RIDAURA

3 mg

RIDAURA® Capsules
(auranofin)

SmithKline Beecham
p. 2319

2 mg S04
Also 1 mg S03,
5 mg S06,
10 mg S07

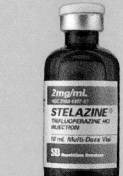

†STELAZINE® Tablets
(trifluoperazine HCl)

SmithKline Beecham
p. 2319

10 mL
(2 mg/mL)
Multi-dose Vials

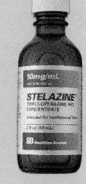

†STELAZINE®
(trifluoperazine HCl)

STELAZINE®
(trifluoperazine hydrochloride)
Concentrate
(10 mg/mL)

SmithKline Beecham
p. 2321

 TAGAMET 200 mg

 TAGAMET 300 mg

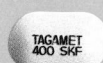 TAGAMET 400 mg

TAGAMET® Tablets
(cimetidine)

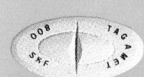 TAGAMET 800 mg

TAGAMET® TILTAB® Tablets
(cimetidine)

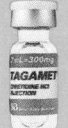 2 mL **Single-dose vials**

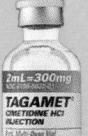 8 mL **Multi-dose vials**

TAGAMET® INJECTION
(cimetidine hydrochloride)
300 mg/2 mL

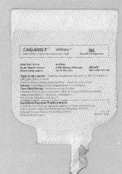 300 mg/50 mL

TAGAMET® INJECTION
(cimetidine hydrochloride)

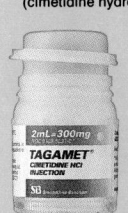 300 mg/2 mL

TAGAMET® INJECTION
(cimetidine hydrochloride in
ADD-Vantage® Vials)

SmithKline Beecham
p. 2321

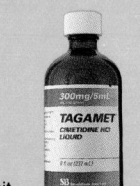 300 mg/5mL TAGAMET

Single-dose unit

8 fl oz

Each 5 mL contains cimetidine
hydrochloride equivalent to
cimetidine, 300 mg
TAGAMET® LIQUID
(cimetidine hydrochloride)

SmithKline Beecham
p. 2324

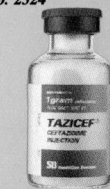 1 gram

2 grams

1 gram
Also 2 grams

6 grams

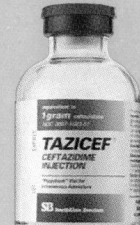

TAZICEF®
(ceftazidime for injection)

SmithKline Beecham
p. 2327

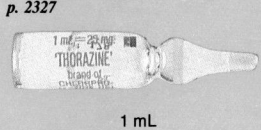 1 mL

2 mL

THORAZINE®
(chlorpromazine hydrochloride)
Ampuls
(25 mg/mL)

SmithKline Beecham
p. 2327

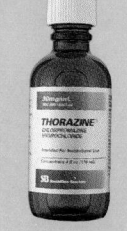

THORAZINE®
(chlorpromazine hydrochloride)
Concentrate
(30 mg/mL)
(100 mg/mL)

SmithKline Beecham
p. 2327

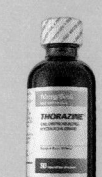

THORAZINE®
(chlorpromazine hydrochloride)
Multi-dose Vials
10 mL (25 mg/mL)

SmithKline Beecham
p. 2327

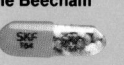 T64 75 mg

Also 30 mg T63, 150 mg T66,
200 mg T67
†THORAZINE® SPANSULE®
(chlorpromazine hydrochloride)
Capsules

SmithKline Beecham
p. 2327

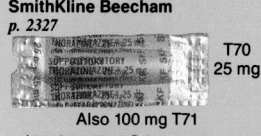 T70 25 mg

Also 100 mg T71
†THORAZINE® Suppositories
(chlorpromazine)

SmithKline Beecham
p. 2327

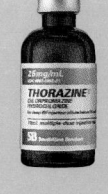

THORAZINE®
(chlorpromazine hydrochloride)
Syrup
(10 mg/5 mL)

SmithKline Beecham
p. 2327

 T74 25 mg

Also 10 mg T73, 50 mg T76,
100 mg T77, 200 mg T79
†THORAZINE® Tablets
(chlorpromazine hydrochloride)

SmithKline Beecham
p. 2330

Also available
in 1 gram

3 grams

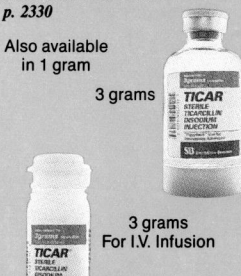

3 grams
For I.V. Infusion

30 grams

Also available
in 20 grams

TICAR®
(sterile ticarcillin disodium)

SmithKline Beecham
p. 2331

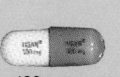 100 mg

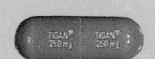 250 mg

†TIGAN® Capsules
(trimethobenzamide HCl)

SmithKline Beecham
p. 2333
(Shown smaller than actual size)

 3.1 gram Vial

 3.1 gram PB

31 gram Pharmacy Bulk Package

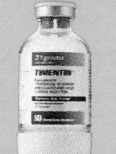

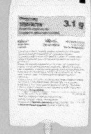 3.1 gram Frozen Bag

3.1 gram
Advantage® Vials

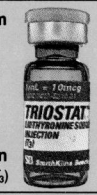

TIMENTIN®
(sterile ticarcillin disodium
and clavulanate potassium)

SmithKline Beecham
p. 2335

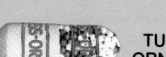

TRIOSTAT™ Injection
(liothyronine sodium) (T₃)

SmithKline Beecham
p. 2337

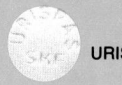 TUSS-ORNADE

**†TUSS-ORNADE®
SPANSULE® Capsules**

SmithKline Beecham
p. 2337

URISPAS

100 mg

URISPAS® Tablets
(flavoxate HCl)

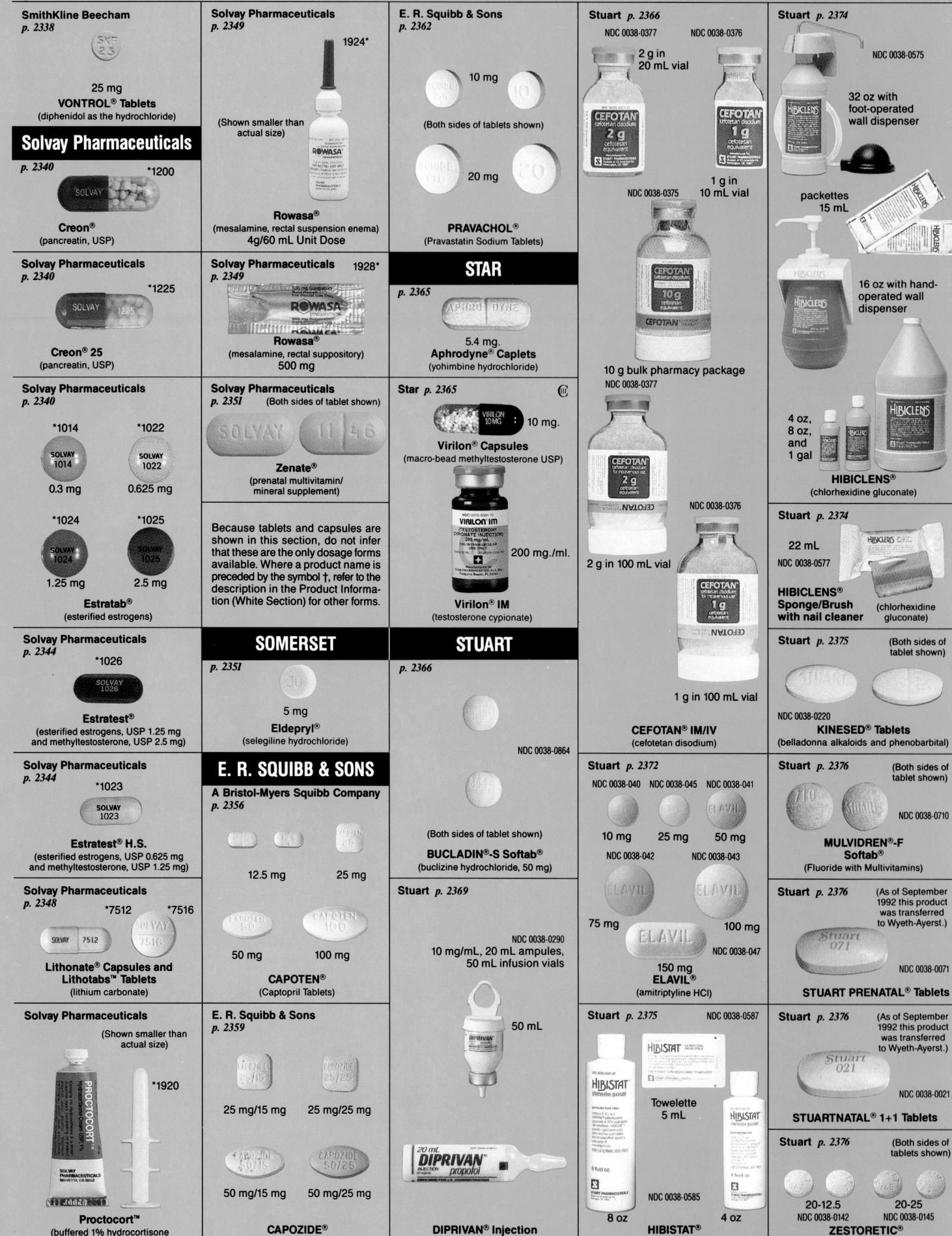

SmithKline Beecham
p. 2338

25 mg
VONTROL® Tablets
(diphenidol as the hydrochloride)

Solvay Pharmaceuticals

p. 2340   *1200

Creon®
(pancreatin, USP)

Solvay Pharmaceuticals
p. 2340   *1225

Creon® 25
(pancreatin, USP)

Solvay Pharmaceuticals
p. 2340

*1014   *1022

0.3 mg   0.625 mg

*1024   *1025

1.25 mg   2.5 mg

Estratab®
(esterified estrogens)

Solvay Pharmaceuticals
p. 2344   *1026

Estratest®
(esterified estrogens, USP 1.25 mg
and methyltestosterone, USP 2.5 mg)

Solvay Pharmaceuticals
p. 2344   *1023

Estratest® H.S.
(esterified estrogens, USP 0.625 mg
and methyltestosterone, USP 1.25 mg)

Solvay Pharmaceuticals
p. 2348   *7512   *7516

**Lithonate® Capsules and
Lithotabs™ Tablets**
(lithium carbonate)

Solvay Pharmaceuticals
(Shown smaller than
actual size)   *1920

Proctocort™
(buffered 1% hydrocortisone
cream, USP, 1%)

Solvay Pharmaceuticals
p. 2349   1924*

(Shown smaller than
actual size)

Rowasa®
(mesalamine, rectal suspension enema)
4g/60 mL Unit Dose

Solvay Pharmaceuticals   1928*
p. 2349

Rowasa®
(mesalamine, rectal suppository)
500 mg

Solvay Pharmaceuticals
p. 2351   (Both sides of tablet shown)

Zenate®
(prenatal multivitamin/
mineral supplement)

Because tablets and capsules are
shown in this section, do not infer
that these are the only dosage forms
available. Where a product name is
preceded by the symbol †, refer to the
description in the Product Information (White Section) for other forms.

SOMERSET

p. 2351

5 mg
Eldepryl®
(selegiline hydrochloride)

E. R. SQUIBB & SONS

A Bristol-Myers Squibb Company
p. 2356

12.5 mg   25 mg

50 mg   100 mg

CAPOTEN®
(Captopril Tablets)

E. R. Squibb & Sons
p. 2359

25 mg/15 mg   25 mg/25 mg

50 mg/15 mg   50 mg/25 mg

CAPOZIDE®
(Captopril-Hydrochlorothiazide Tablets)

E. R. Squibb & Sons
p. 2362

10 mg

(Both sides of tablets shown)

20 mg

PRAVACHOL®
(Pravastatin Sodium Tablets)

STAR

p. 2365

5.4 mg.
Aphrodyne® Caplets
(yohimbine hydrochloride)

Star p. 2365

VIRILON 10 MG   10 mg.
Virilon® Capsules
(macro-bead methyltestosterone USP)

200 mg./ml.

Virilon® IM
(testosterone cypionate)

STUART

p. 2366

NDC 0038-0864

(Both sides of tablet shown)
BUCLADIN®-S Softab®
(buclizine hydrochloride, 50 mg)

Stuart p. 2369

NDC 0038-0290
10 mg/mL, 20 mL ampules,
50 mL infusion vials

50 mL

DIPRIVAN® Injection
(propofol)

Stuart p. 2366
NDC 0038-0377   NDC 0038-0376

2 g in
20 mL vial

1 g in
10 mL vial
NDC 0038-0375

10 g bulk pharmacy package
NDC 0038-0377

NDC 0038-0376

2 g in 100 mL vial

1 g in 100 mL vial
CEFOTAN® IM/IV
(cefotetan disodium)

Stuart p. 2372
NDC 0038-040 NDC 0038-045 NDC 0038-041

10 mg   25 mg   50 mg
NDC 0038-042   NDC 0038-043

75 mg   100 mg
NDC 0038-047

150 mg
ELAVIL®
(amitriptyline HCl)

Stuart p. 2375   NDC 0038-0587

Towelette
5 mL

HIBISTAT

8 oz   4 oz
NDC 0038-0585
HIBISTAT®
(chlorhexidine gluconate)

Stuart p. 2374

NDC 0038-0575

32 oz with
foot-operated
wall dispenser

packettes
15 mL

16 oz with hand-
operated wall
dispenser

4 oz,
8 oz,
and
1 gal

HIBICLENS®
(chlorhexidine gluconate)

Stuart p. 2374

22 mL
NDC 0038-0577

**HIBICLENS®
Sponge/Brush
with nail cleaner**   (chlorhexidine
gluconate)

Stuart p. 2375   (Both sides of
tablet shown)

NDC 0038-0220
KINESED® Tablets
(belladonna alkaloids and phenobarbital)

Stuart p. 2376   (Both sides of
tablet shown)

NDC 0038-0710

**MULVIDREN®-F
Softab®**
(Fluoride with Multivitamins)

Stuart p. 2376   (As of September
1992 this product
was transferred
to Wyeth-Ayerst.)

Stuart
071
NDC 0038-0071

STUART PRENATAL® Tablets

Stuart p. 2376   (As of September
1992 this product
was transferred
to Wyeth-Ayerst.)

Stuart
021
NDC 0038-0021

STUARTNATAL® 1+1 Tablets

Stuart p. 2376   (Both sides of
tablets shown)

20-12.5   20-25
NDC 0038-0142   NDC 0038-0145
ZESTORETIC®
(lisinopril and hydrochlorothiazide)

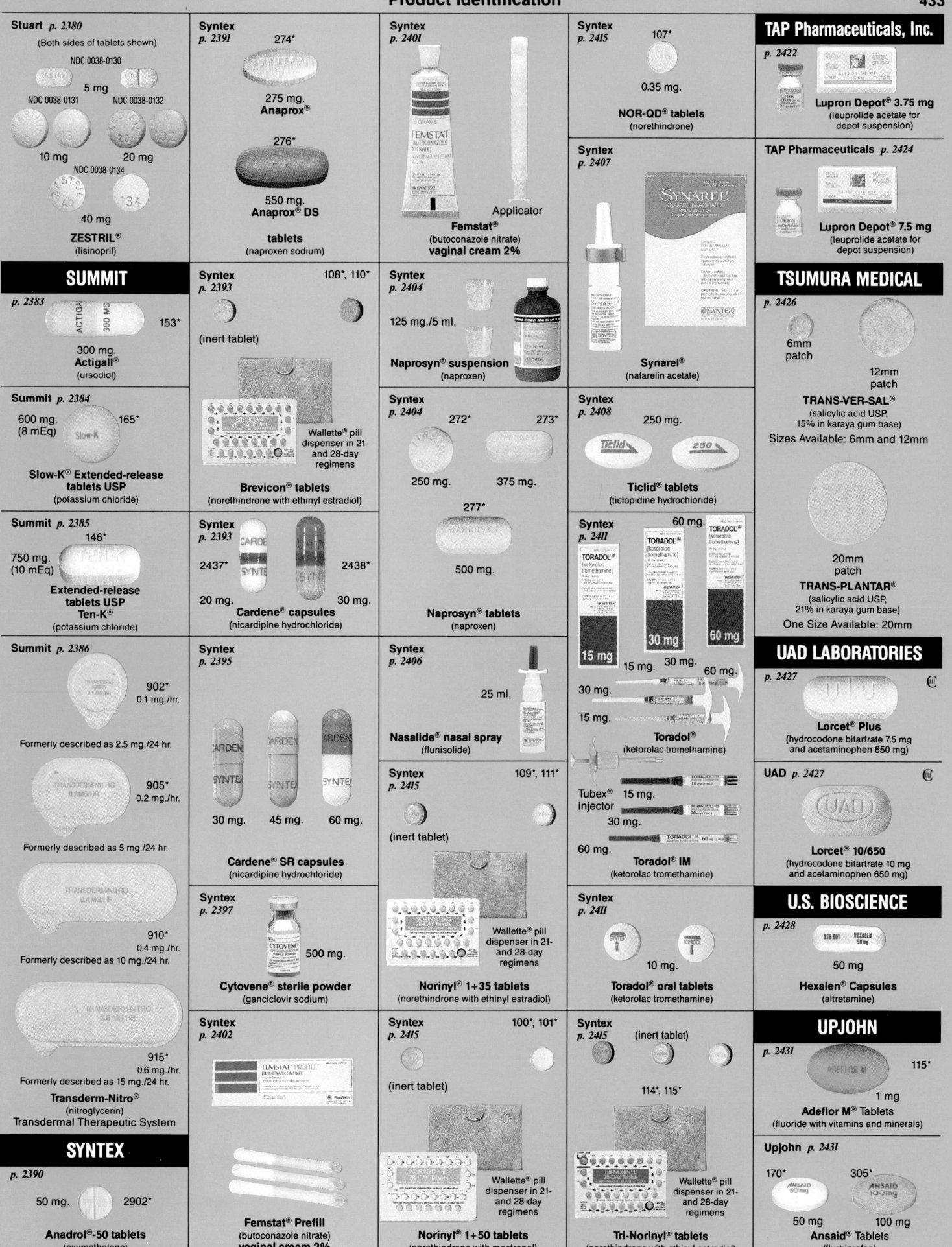

Stuart p. 2380

(Both sides of tablets shown)

NDC 0038-0130

5 mg

NDC 0038-0131   NDC 0038-0132

10 mg   20 mg

NDC 0038-0134

40 mg

ZESTRIL®
(lisinopril)

SUMMIT

p. 2383

153*

300 mg.
Actigall®
(ursodiol)

Summit p. 2384

600 mg.
(8 mEq)   165*

Slow-K® Extended-release tablets USP
(potassium chloride)

Summit p. 2385

146*

750 mg.
(10 mEq)

Extended-release tablets USP Ten-K®
(potassium chloride)

Summit p. 2386

902*
0.1 mg./hr.

Formerly described as 2.5 mg./24 hr.

905*
0.2 mg./hr.

Formerly described as 5 mg./24 hr.

910*
0.4 mg./hr.

Formerly described as 10 mg./24 hr.

915*
0.6 mg./hr.

Formerly described as 15 mg./24 hr.

Transderm-Nitro®
(nitroglycerin)
Transdermal Therapeutic System

SYNTEX

p. 2390

50 mg.   2902*

Anadrol®-50 tablets
(oxymetholone)

Syntex p. 2391

274*

275 mg.
Anaprox®

276*

550 mg.
Anaprox® DS

tablets
(naproxen sodium)

Syntex p. 2393

108*, 110*

(inert tablet)

153*

Wallette® pill dispenser in 21- and 28-day regimens

Brevicon® tablets
(norethindrone with ethinyl estradiol)

Syntex p. 2393

CARDE   SYNTE

2437*   2438*

20 mg.   30 mg.
Cardene® capsules
(nicardipine hydrochloride)

Syntex p. 2395

CARDEN   CARDEN   CARDEN

SYNTEX   SYNTEX   SYNTEX

30 mg.   45 mg.   60 mg.

Cardene® SR capsules
(nicardipine hydrochloride)

Syntex p. 2397

CYTOVENE   500 mg.

Cytovene® sterile powder
(ganciclovir sodium)

Syntex p. 2402

FEMSTAT PREFILL

Femstat® Prefill
(butoconazole nitrate)
vaginal cream 2%

Syntex p. 2401

FEMSTAT   Applicator

Femstat®
(butoconazole nitrate)
vaginal cream 2%

Syntex p. 2404

125 mg./5 ml.

Naprosyn® suspension
(naproxen)

Syntex p. 2404

272*   273*

250 mg.   375 mg.

277*

500 mg.

Naprosyn® tablets
(naproxen)

Syntex p. 2406

25 ml.

Nasalide® nasal spray
(flunisolide)

Syntex p. 2415

109*, 111*

(inert tablet)

Wallette® pill dispenser in 21- and 28-day regimens

Norinyl® 1+35 tablets
(norethindrone with ethinyl estradiol)

Syntex p. 2415

100*, 101*

(inert tablet)

Wallette® pill dispenser in 21- and 28-day regimens

Norinyl® 1+50 tablets
(norethindrone with mestranol)

Syntex p. 2415

107*

0.35 mg.

NOR-QD® tablets
(norethindrone)

Syntex p. 2407

SYNAREL

Synarel®
(nafarelin acetate)

Syntex p. 2408

250 mg.

Ticlid   250

Ticlid® tablets
(ticlopidine hydrochloride)

Syntex p. 2411

60 mg.

TORADOL   TORADOL

TORADOL

15 mg   30 mg   60 mg

15 mg.   30 mg.

30 mg.   60 mg.

15 mg.

Toradol®
(ketorolac tromethamine)

Tubex® injector   15 mg.

30 mg.

60 mg.

Toradol® IM
(ketorolac tromethamine)

Syntex p. 2411

10 mg.

Toradol® oral tablets
(ketorolac tromethamine)

Syntex p. 2415

(inert tablet)

114*, 115*

Wallette® pill dispenser in 21- and 28-day regimens

Tri-Norinyl® tablets
(norethindrone with ethinyl estradiol)

TAP Pharmaceuticals, Inc.

p. 2422

Lupron Depot® 3.75 mg
(leuprolide acetate for depot suspension)

TAP Pharmaceuticals p. 2424

Lupron Depot® 7.5 mg
(leuprolide acetate for depot suspension)

TSUMURA MEDICAL

p. 2426

6mm patch

12mm patch

TRANS-VER-SAL®
(salicylic acid USP, 15% in karaya gum base)

Sizes Available: 6mm and 12mm

20mm patch

TRANS-PLANTAR®
(salicylic acid USP, 21% in karaya gum base)

One Size Available: 20mm

UAD LABORATORIES

p. 2427

Lorcet® Plus
(hydrocodone bitartrate 7.5 mg and acetaminophen 650 mg)

UAD p. 2427

UAD

Lorcet® 10/650
(hydrocodone bitartrate 10 mg and acetaminophen 650 mg)

U.S. BIOSCIENCE

p. 2428

50 mg

Hexalen® Capsules
(altretamine)

UPJOHN

p. 2431

ADEFLOR M   115*

1 mg

Adeflor M® Tablets
(fluoride with vitamins and minerals)

Upjohn p. 2431

170*   305*

50 mg   100 mg

Ansaid® Tablets
(flurbiprofen)

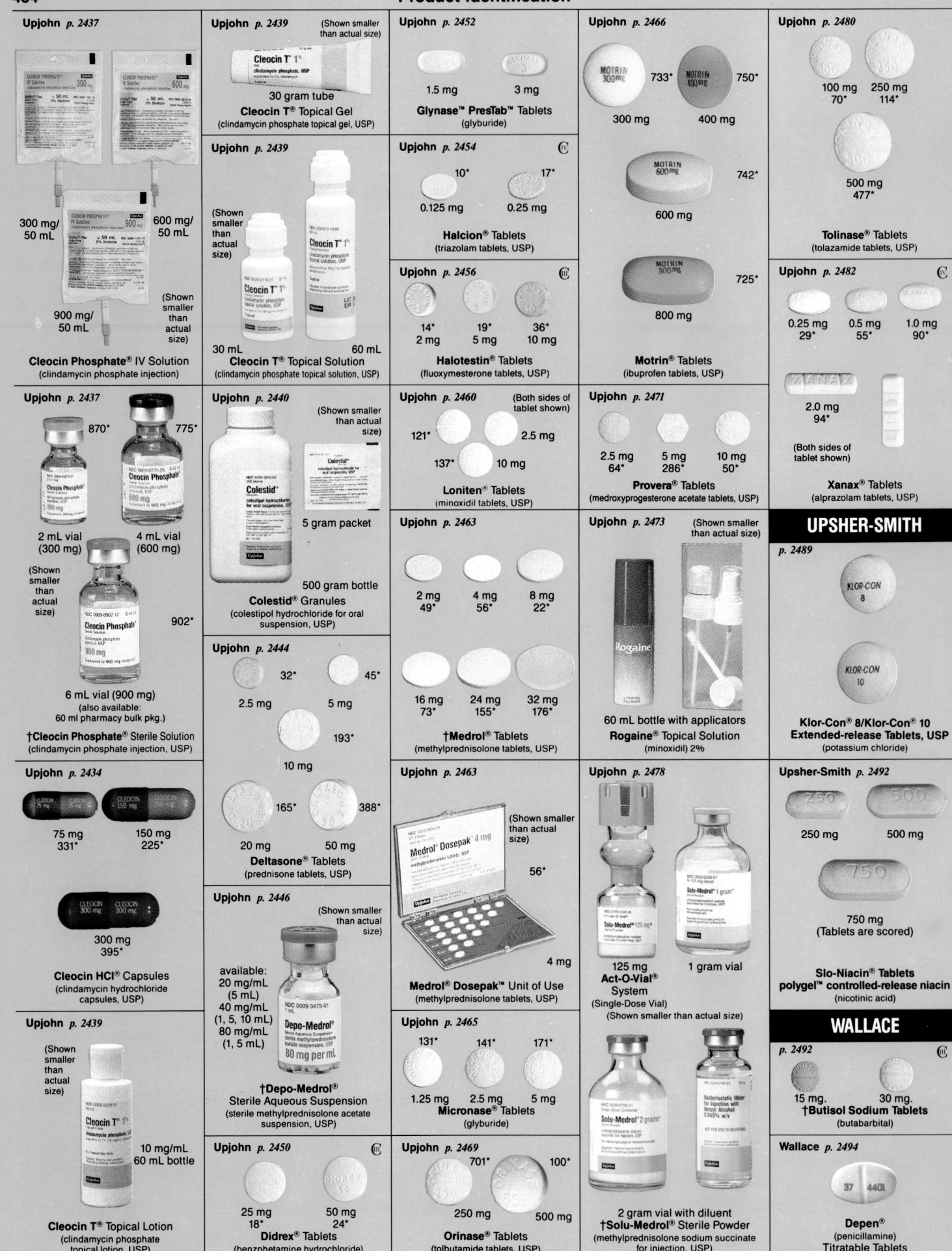

Upjohn *p. 2437*

300 mg/ 50 mL — 600 mg/ 50 mL
900 mg/ 50 mL (Shown smaller than actual size)

Cleocin Phosphate® IV Solution
(clindamycin phosphate injection)

Upjohn *p. 2437*

870* — 775*
2 mL vial (300 mg) — 4 mL vial (600 mg)
(Shown smaller than actual size)
902*
6 mL vial (900 mg)
(also available: 60 ml pharmacy bulk pkg.)

†Cleocin Phosphate® Sterile Solution
(clindamycin phosphate injection, USP)

Upjohn *p. 2434*

75 mg 331* — 150 mg 225*
300 mg 395*

Cleocin HCl® Capsules
(clindamycin hydrochloride capsules, USP)

Upjohn *p. 2439*

(Shown smaller than actual size)
10 mg/mL 60 mL bottle

Cleocin T® Topical Lotion
(clindamycin phosphate topical lotion, USP)

Upjohn *p. 2439* (Shown smaller than actual size)

30 gram tube
Cleocin T® Topical Gel
(clindamycin phosphate topical gel, USP)

Upjohn *p. 2439*

(Shown smaller than actual size)
30 mL — 60 mL
Cleocin T® Topical Solution
(clindamycin phosphate topical solution, USP)

Upjohn *p. 2440*

(Shown smaller than actual size)
5 gram packet
500 gram bottle
Colestid® Granules
(colestipol hydrochloride for oral suspension, USP)

Upjohn *p. 2444*

32* — 45*
2.5 mg — 5 mg
193*
10 mg
165* — 388*
20 mg — 50 mg
Deltasone® Tablets
(prednisone tablets, USP)

Upjohn *p. 2446*

(Shown smaller than actual size)
available:
20 mg/mL (5 mL)
40 mg/mL (1, 5, 10 mL)
80 mg/mL (1, 5 mL)
Depo-Medrol® 80 mg per mL
†Depo-Medrol®
Sterile Aqueous Suspension
(sterile methylprednisolone acetate suspension, USP)

Upjohn *p. 2450*

25 mg 18* — 50 mg 24*
Didrex® Tablets
(benzphetamine hydrochloride)

Upjohn *p. 2452*

1.5 mg — 3 mg
Glynase™ PresTab™ Tablets
(glyburide)

Upjohn *p. 2454*

10* — 17*
0.125 mg — 0.25 mg
Halcion® Tablets
(triazolam tablets, USP)

Upjohn *p. 2456*

14* 2 mg — 19* 5 mg — 36* 10 mg
Halotestin® Tablets
(fluoxymesterone tablets, USP)

Upjohn *p. 2460* (Both sides of tablet shown)

121* — 2.5 mg
137* — 10 mg
Loniten® Tablets
(minoxidil tablets, USP)

Upjohn *p. 2463*

2 mg 49* — 4 mg 56* — 8 mg 22*
16 mg 73* — 24 mg 155* — 32 mg 176*
†Medrol® Tablets
(methylprednisolone tablets, USP)

Upjohn *p. 2463*

(Shown smaller than actual size)
56*
Medrol® Dosepak 4 mg
4 mg
Medrol® Dosepak™ Unit of Use
(methylprednisolone tablets, USP)

Upjohn *p. 2465*

131* — 141* — 171*
1.25 mg — 2.5 mg — 5 mg
Micronase® Tablets
(glyburide)

Upjohn *p. 2469*

701* — 100*
250 mg — 500 mg
Orinase® Tablets
(tolbutamide tablets, USP)

Upjohn *p. 2466*

733* — 750*
300 mg — 400 mg
742*
600 mg
725*
800 mg
Motrin® Tablets
(ibuprofen tablets, USP)

Upjohn *p. 2471*

2.5 mg 64* — 5 mg 286* — 10 mg 50*
Provera® Tablets
(medroxyprogesterone acetate tablets, USP)

Upjohn *p. 2473* (Shown smaller than actual size)

Rogaine
60 mL bottle with applicators
Rogaine® Topical Solution
(minoxidil) 2%

Upjohn *p. 2478*

Solu-Medrol 125 mg — Solu-Medrol 1 gram
125 mg — 1 gram vial
Act-O-Vial®
System
(Single-Dose Vial)
(Shown smaller than actual size)

Solu-Medrol 2 grams — Bacteriostatic Water for Injection with Benzyl Alcohol 0.945% w/v
2 gram vial with diluent
†Solu-Medrol® Sterile Powder
(methylprednisolone sodium succinate for injection, USP)

Upjohn *p. 2480*

100 mg 70* — 250 mg 114*
500 mg 477*
Tolinase® Tablets
(tolazamide tablets, USP)

Upjohn *p. 2482*

0.25 mg 29* — 0.5 mg 55* — 1.0 mg 90*
2.0 mg 94*
(Both sides of tablet shown)
Xanax® Tablets
(alprazolam tablets, USP)

UPSHER-SMITH

p. 2489

KLOR-CON 8
KLOR-CON 10
Klor-Con® 8/Klor-Con® 10
Extended-release Tablets, USP
(potassium chloride)

Upsher-Smith *p. 2492*

250 mg — 500 mg
750 mg
(Tablets are scored)
Slo-Niacin® Tablets
polygel™ controlled-release niacin
(nicotinic acid)

WALLACE

p. 2492

15 mg. — 30 mg.
†Butisol Sodium Tablets
(butabarbital)

Wallace *p. 2494*

37 440L
Depen®
(penicillamine)
Titratable Tablets

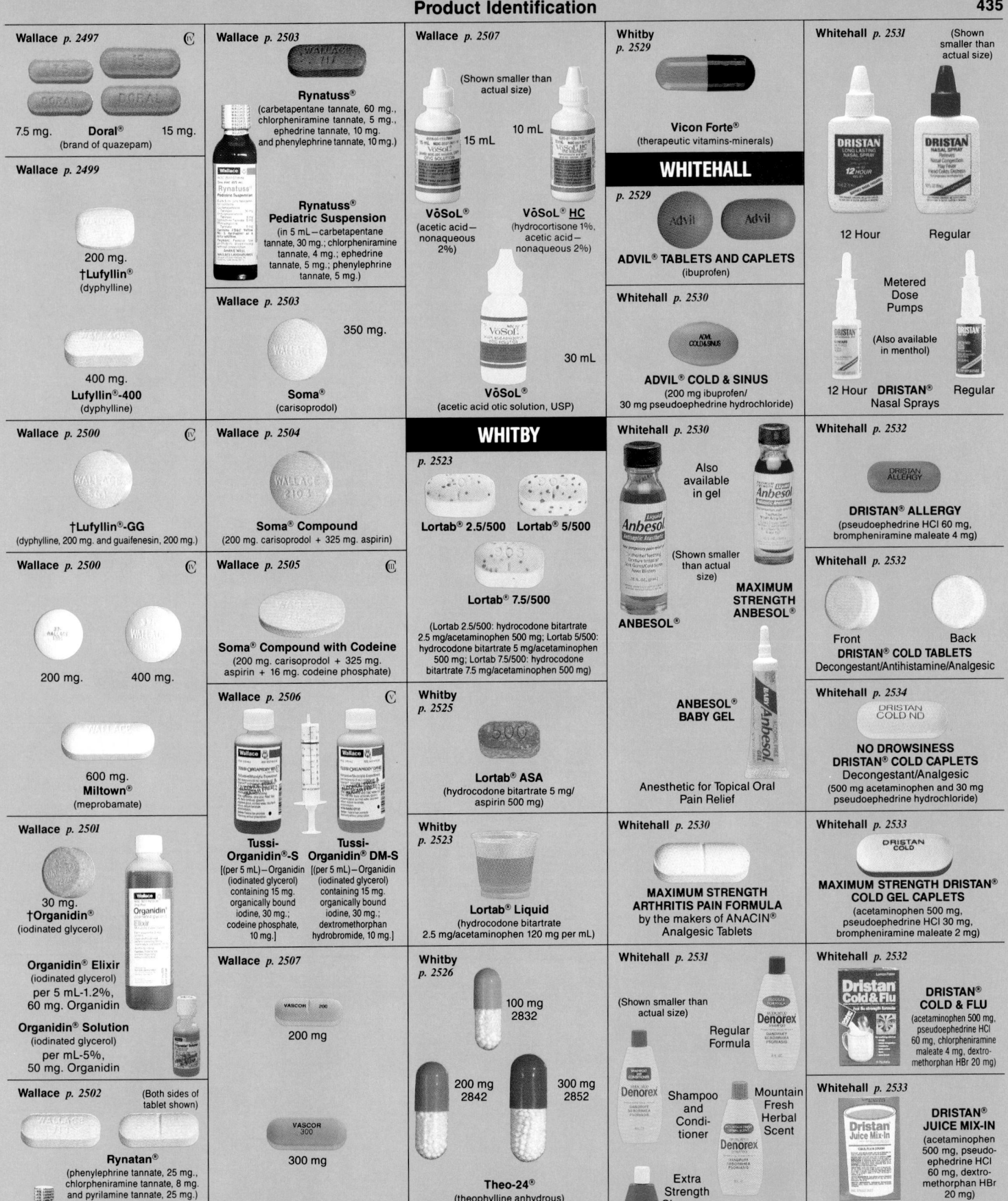

Wallace p. 2497 (IV)

7.5 mg. **Doral®** 15 mg.
(brand of quazepam)

Wallace p. 2499

200 mg.
†**Lufyllin®**
(dyphylline)

400 mg.
Lufyllin®-400
(dyphylline)

Wallace p. 2500 (IV)

†**Lufyllin®-GG**
(dyphylline, 200 mg. and guaifenesin, 200 mg.)

Wallace p. 2500 (IV)

200 mg. 400 mg.

600 mg.
Miltown®
(meprobamate)

Wallace p. 2501

30 mg.
†**Organidin®**
(iodinated glycerol)

Organidin® Elixir
(iodinated glycerol)
per 5 mL-1.2%,
60 mg. Organidin

Organidin® Solution
(iodinated glycerol)
per mL-5%,
50 mg. Organidin

Wallace p. 2502 (Both sides of tablet shown)

Rynatan®
(phenylephrine tannate, 25 mg.,
chlorpheniramine tannate, 8 mg.
and pyrilamine tannate, 25 mg.)

Rynatan®-S*
Pediatric Suspension
(each teaspoonful 5 mL contains: phenylephrine tannate,
5 mg.; chlorpheniramine
tannate, 2 mg.; pyrilamine
tannate, 12.5 mg.)

*Patent Pending
Rynatan®-S is Rynatan Pediatric Suspension either in a 4 fl. oz. unit of use container
with a 10 mL graduated oral syringe (patent
pending) or in a 15 mL sample container.

Wallace p. 2503

Rynatuss®
(carbetapentane tannate, 60 mg.,
chlorpheniramine tannate, 5 mg.,
ephedrine tannate, 10 mg.
and phenylephrine tannate, 10 mg.)

Rynatuss®
Pediatric Suspension
(in 5 mL–carbetapentane
tannate, 30 mg.; chlorpheniramine
tannate, 4 mg.; ephedrine
tannate, 5 mg.; phenylephrine
tannate, 5 mg.)

Wallace p. 2503

350 mg.
Soma®
(carisoprodol)

Wallace p. 2504

Soma® Compound
(200 mg. carisoprodol + 325 mg. aspirin)

Wallace p. 2505 (III)

Soma® Compound with Codeine
(200 mg. carisoprodol + 325 mg.
aspirin + 16 mg. codeine phosphate)

Wallace p. 2506 (IV)

Tussi- **Tussi-**
Organidin®-S **Organidin® DM-S**
[(per 5 mL)–Organidin [(per 5 mL)–Organidin
(iodinated glycerol) (iodinated glycerol)
containing 15 mg. containing 15 mg.
organically bound organically bound
iodine, 30 mg.; iodine, 30 mg.;
codeine phosphate, dextromethorphan
10 mg.] hydrobromide, 10 mg.]

Wallace p. 2507

VASCOR 200
200 mg

VASCOR 300
300 mg

VASCOR 400
400 mg

VASCOR® Tablets
(bepridil hydrochloride)

Wallace p. 2507

(Shown smaller than
actual size)

15 mL 10 mL

VõSoL® **VõSoL® HC**
(acetic acid– (hydrocortisone 1%,
nonaqueous acetic acid–
2%) nonaqueous 2%)

30 mL

VõSoL®
(acetic acid otic solution, USP)

WHITBY

p. 2523

Lortab® 2.5/500 **Lortab® 5/500**

Lortab® 7.5/500

(Lortab 2.5/500: hydrocodone bitartrate
2.5 mg/acetaminophen 500 mg; Lortab 5/500:
hydrocodone bitartrate 5 mg/acetaminophen
500 mg; Lortab 7.5/500: hydrocodone
bitartrate 7.5 mg/acetaminophen 500 mg)

Whitby
p. 2525

Lortab® ASA
(hydrocodone bitartrate 5 mg/
aspirin 500 mg)

Whitby
p. 2523

Lortab® Liquid
(hydrocodone bitartrate
2.5 mg/acetaminophen 120 mg per mL)

Whitby
p. 2526

100 mg
2832

200 mg 300 mg
2842 2852

Theo-24®
(theophylline anhydrous)

Whitby
p. 2528

Trinsicon®
(hematinic concentrate with
intrinsic factor)

Whitby
p. 2529

Vicon Forte®
(therapeutic vitamins-minerals)

WHITEHALL

p. 2529

Advil Advil

ADVIL® TABLETS AND CAPLETS
(ibuprofen)

Whitehall p. 2530

ADVIL
COLD&SINUS

ADVIL® COLD & SINUS
(200 mg ibuprofen/
30 mg pseudoephedrine hydrochloride)

Whitehall p. 2530

Also
available
in gel

Anbesol

(Shown smaller
than actual
size)

MAXIMUM
STRENGTH
ANBESOL®

ANBESOL®

ANBESOL®
BABY GEL

Anesthetic for Topical Oral
Pain Relief

Whitehall p. 2530

MAXIMUM STRENGTH
ARTHRITIS PAIN FORMULA
by the makers of ANACIN®
Analgesic Tablets

Whitehall p. 2531

(Shown smaller than
actual size)

Regular
Formula

Denorex

Denorex
Shampoo
and
Condi-
tioner

Mountain
Fresh
Herbal
Scent

Denorex

Extra
Strength
Shampoo

Extra
Strength
Denorex

Extra
Strength
Shampoo
with
Condi-
tioners

Extra
Strength
Denorex

DENOREX®
Medicated Shampoo

Whitehall p. 2531 (Shown
smaller than
actual size)

DRISTAN
LONG LASTING
NASAL SPRAY
12 HOUR

DRISTAN
NASAL SPRAY

12 Hour Regular

Metered
Dose
Pumps

DRISTAN

(Also available
in menthol)

12 Hour **DRISTAN®** Regular
Nasal Sprays

Whitehall p. 2532

DRISTAN
ALLERGY

DRISTAN® ALLERGY
(pseudoephedrine HCl 60 mg,
brompheniramine maleate 4 mg)

Whitehall p. 2532

Front Back
DRISTAN® COLD TABLETS
Decongestant/Antihistamine/Analgesic

Whitehall p. 2534

DRISTAN
COLD ND

NO DROWSINESS
DRISTAN® COLD CAPLETS
Decongestant/Analgesic
(500 mg acetaminophen and 30 mg
pseudoephedrine hydrochloride)

Whitehall p. 2533

DRISTAN
COLD

MAXIMUM STRENGTH DRISTAN®
COLD GEL CAPLETS
(acetaminophen 500 mg,
pseudoephedrine HCl 30 mg,
brompheniramine maleate 2 mg)

Whitehall p. 2532

Dristan
Cold&Flu

DRISTAN®
COLD & FLU
(acetaminophen 500 mg,
pseudoephedrine HCl
60 mg, chlorpheniramine
maleate 4 mg, dextro-
methorphan HBr 20 mg)

Whitehall p. 2533

Dristan
Juice Mix-In

DRISTAN®
JUICE MIX-IN
(acetaminophen
500 mg, pseudo-
ephedrine HCl
60 mg, dextro-
methorphan HBr
20 mg)

Whitehall p. 2533

Dristan
saline spray

DRISTAN®
SALINE SPRAY
Non-Medicated
Moisturizer

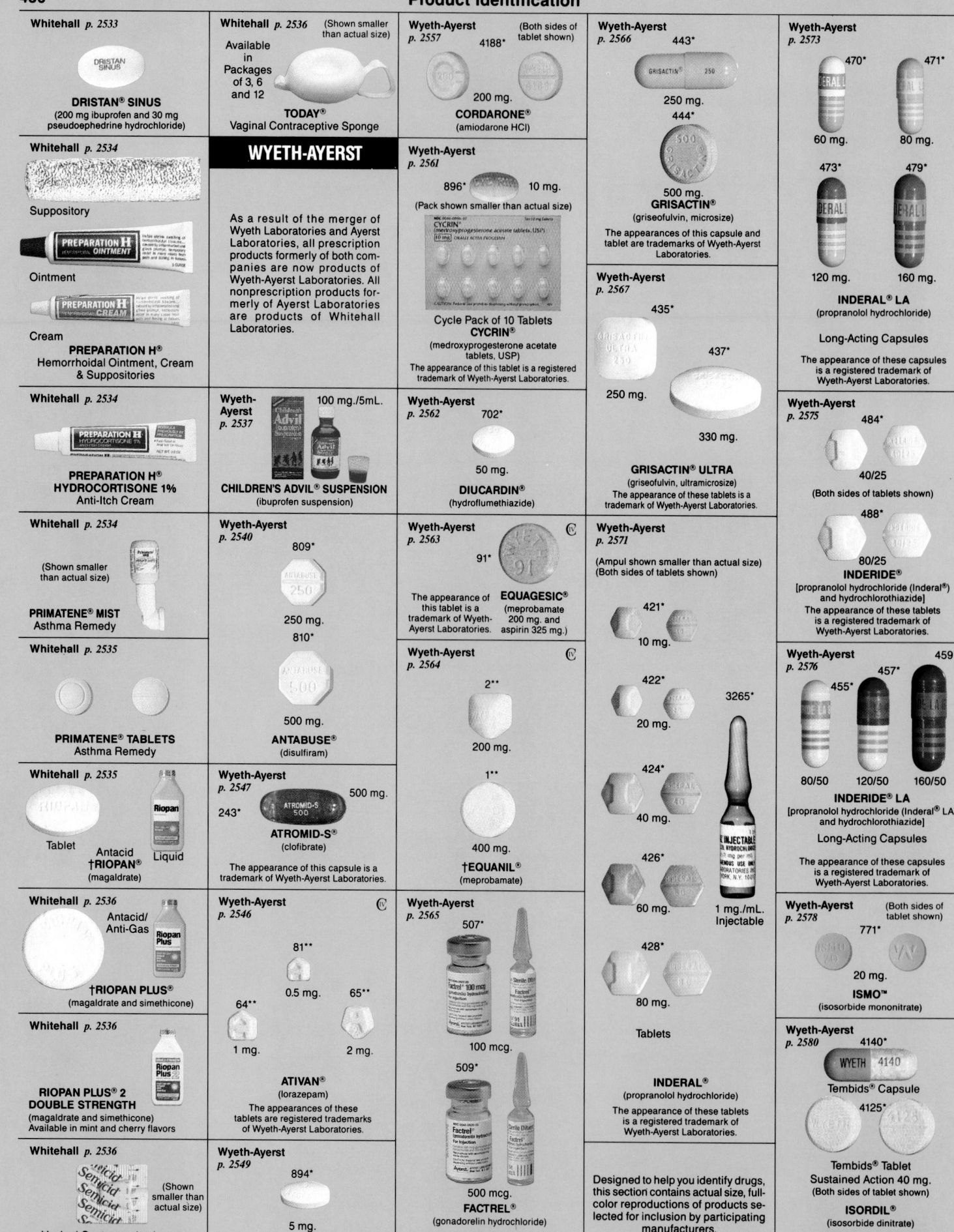

Whitehall *p. 2533*

DRISTAN SINUS

DRISTAN® SINUS
(200 mg ibuprofen and 30 mg
pseudoephedrine hydrochloride)

Whitehall *p. 2534*

Suppository

PREPARATION H OINTMENT

Ointment

PREPARATION H CREAM

Cream

PREPARATION H®
Hemorrhoidal Ointment, Cream
& Suppositories

Whitehall *p. 2534*

PREPARATION H HYDROCORTISONE 1%

PREPARATION H®
HYDROCORTISONE 1%
Anti-Itch Cream

Whitehall *p. 2534*

(Shown smaller
than actual size)

PRIMATENE® MIST
Asthma Remedy

Whitehall *p. 2535*

PRIMATENE® TABLETS
Asthma Remedy

Whitehall *p. 2535*

Tablet   Antacid
†RIOPAN®   Liquid
(magaldrate)

Whitehall *p. 2536*

Antacid/
Anti-Gas

Riopan Plus

†RIOPAN PLUS®
(magaldrate and simethicone)

Whitehall *p. 2536*

Riopan Plus 2

RIOPAN PLUS® 2
DOUBLE STRENGTH
(magaldrate and simethicone)
Available in mint and cherry flavors

Whitehall *p. 2536*

(Shown smaller
than actual size)

Vaginal Contraceptive Inserts

SEMICID®

Whitehall *p. 2536*   (Shown smaller
than actual size)

Available
in
Packages
of 3, 6
and 12

TODAY®
Vaginal Contraceptive Sponge

WYETH-AYERST

As a result of the merger of
Wyeth Laboratories and Ayerst
Laboratories, all prescription
products formerly of both companies are now products of
Wyeth-Ayerst Laboratories. All
nonprescription products formerly of Ayerst Laboratories
are products of Whitehall
Laboratories.

**Wyeth-
Ayerst**
p. 2537

Children's Advil   100 mg./5mL.

CHILDREN'S ADVIL® SUSPENSION
(ibuprofen suspension)

Wyeth-Ayerst
p. 2540

809*
ANTABUSE 250
250 mg.

810*
ANTABUSE 500
500 mg.

ANTABUSE®
(disulfiram)

Wyeth-Ayerst
p. 2547

500 mg.
243*   ATROMID-S 500

ATROMID-S®
(clofibrate)

The appearance of this capsule is a
trademark of Wyeth-Ayerst Laboratories.

Wyeth-Ayerst
p. 2546   Ⓒ

81**
0.5 mg.   65**

64**
1 mg.   2 mg.

ATIVAN®
(lorazepam)
The appearances of these
tablets are registered trademarks
of Wyeth-Ayerst Laboratories.

Wyeth-Ayerst
p. 2549

894*

5 mg.
AYGESTIN®
(norethindrone acetate tablets, USP)

Wyeth-Ayerst   (Both sides of
p. 2557   4188*   tablet shown)

200 mg.
CORDARONE®
(amiodarone HCl)

Wyeth-Ayerst
p. 2561

896*   10 mg.
(Pack shown smaller than actual size)

CYCRIN
medroxyprogesterone acetate tablets, USP
10 mg.

Cycle Pack of 10 Tablets
CYCRIN®
(medroxyprogesterone acetate
tablets, USP)
The appearance of this tablet is a registered
trademark of Wyeth-Ayerst Laboratories.

Wyeth-Ayerst
p. 2562   702*

50 mg.
DIUCARDIN®
(hydroflumethiazide)

Wyeth-Ayerst
p. 2563   Ⓒ

91*

The appearance of
this tablet is a
trademark of Wyeth-
Ayerst Laboratories.

EQUAGESIC®
(meprobamate
200 mg. and
aspirin 325 mg.)

Wyeth-Ayerst
p. 2564   Ⓒ

2**

200 mg.

1**

400 mg.
†EQUANIL®
(meprobamate)

Wyeth-Ayerst
p. 2565

507*

100 mcg.

509*

500 mcg.
FACTREL®
(gonadorelin hydrochloride)
Synthetic Luteinizing Hormone
Releasing Hormone (LH-RH)

Wyeth-Ayerst
p. 2566   443*

GRISACTIN 250
250 mg.

444*
500 GRISACTIN
500 mg.
GRISACTIN®
(griseofulvin, microsize)

The appearances of this capsule and
tablet are trademarks of Wyeth-Ayerst
Laboratories.

Wyeth-Ayerst
p. 2567

435*
GRISACTIN ULTRA 250
250 mg.

437*

330 mg.

GRISACTIN® ULTRA
(griseofulvin, ultramicrosize)
The appearance of these tablets is a
trademark of Wyeth-Ayerst Laboratories.

Wyeth-Ayerst
p. 2571

(Ampul shown smaller than actual size)
(Both sides of tablets shown)

421*
10 mg.

422*
20 mg.

424*
40 mg.

426*
60 mg.

428*
80 mg.

Tablets

3265*

1 mg./mL.
Injectable

INDERAL®
(propranolol hydrochloride)
The appearance of these tablets is a
trademark of Wyeth-Ayerst
Laboratories.

Designed to help you identify drugs,
this section contains actual size, full-
color reproductions of products selected for inclusion by participating
manufacturers.

Wyeth-Ayerst
p. 2573

470*   471*

60 mg.   80 mg.

473*   479*

120 mg.   160 mg.

INDERAL® LA
(propranolol hydrochloride)

Long-Acting Capsules

The appearance of these capsules
is a registered trademark of
Wyeth-Ayerst Laboratories.

Wyeth-Ayerst
p. 2575   484*

40/25
(Both sides of tablets shown)

488*

80/25
INDERIDE®
[propranolol hydrochloride (Inderal®)
and hydrochlorothiazide]
The appearance of these tablets
is a registered trademark of
Wyeth-Ayerst Laboratories.

Wyeth-Ayerst
p. 2576   459*

455*   457*

80/50   120/50   160/50
INDERIDE® LA
[propranolol hydrochloride (Inderal® LA)
and hydrochlorothiazide]

Long-Acting Capsules

The appearance of these capsules
is a registered trademark of
Wyeth-Ayerst Laboratories.

Wyeth-Ayerst   (Both sides of
p. 2578   tablet shown)

771*

20 mg.
ISMO™
(isosorbide mononitrate)

Wyeth-Ayerst
p. 2580   4140*

WYETH 4140
Tembids® Capsule

4125*

Tembids® Tablet
Sustained Action 40 mg.
(Both sides of tablet shown)

ISORDIL®
(isosorbide dinitrate)
The appearances of this
capsule and this tablet are trademarks
of Wyeth-Ayerst Laboratories.

**Product identification number on reverse side of tablet.

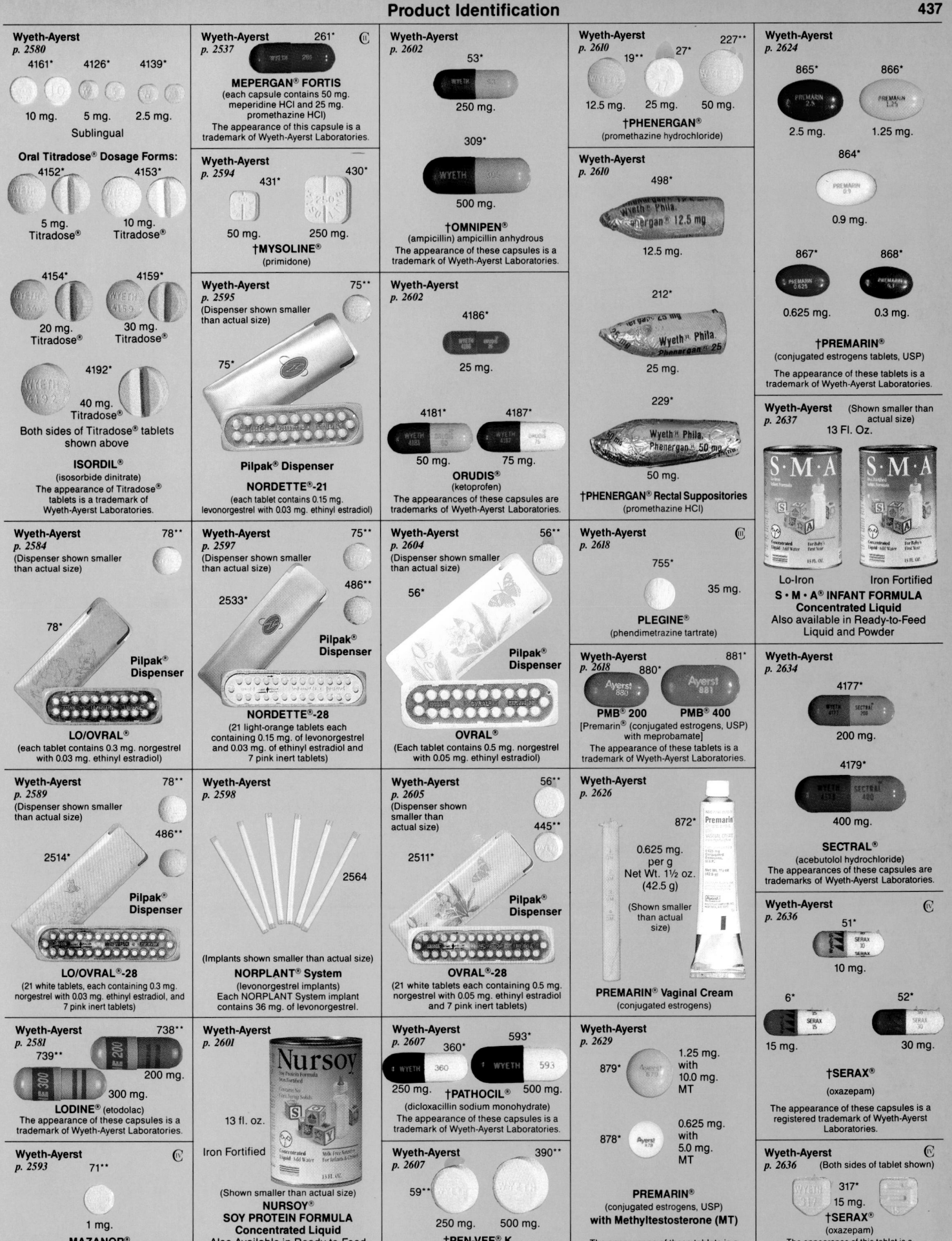

Wyeth-Ayerst
p. 2580

4161*   4126*   4139*

10 mg.   5 mg.   2.5 mg.
Sublingual

Oral Titradose® Dosage Forms:

4152*   4153*

5 mg.   10 mg.
Titradose®   Titradose®

4154*   4159*

20 mg.   30 mg.
Titradose®   Titradose®

4192*

40 mg.
Titradose®

Both sides of Titradose® tablets
shown above

ISORDIL®
(isosorbide dinitrate)
The appearance of Titradose®
tablets is a trademark of
Wyeth-Ayerst Laboratories.

Wyeth-Ayerst   261*   Ⓒ
p. 2537

MEPERGAN® FORTIS
(each capsule contains 50 mg.
meperidine HCl and 25 mg.
promethazine HCl)
The appearance of this capsule is a
trademark of Wyeth-Ayerst Laboratories.

Wyeth-Ayerst
p. 2594

431*   430*

50 mg.   250 mg.

†MYSOLINE®
(primidone)

Wyeth-Ayerst   75**
p. 2595
(Dispenser shown smaller
than actual size)

75*

Pilpak® Dispenser

NORDETTE®-21
(each tablet contains 0.15 mg.
levonorgestrel with 0.03 mg. ethinyl estradiol)

Wyeth-Ayerst
p. 2602

53*

250 mg.

309*

500 mg.

†OMNIPEN®
(ampicillin) ampicillin anhydrous
The appearance of these capsules is a
trademark of Wyeth-Ayerst Laboratories.

Wyeth-Ayerst
p. 2602

4186*

25 mg.

4181*   4187*

50 mg.   75 mg.

ORUDIS®
(ketoprofen)
The appearances of these capsules are
trademarks of Wyeth-Ayerst Laboratories.

Wyeth-Ayerst   227**
p. 2610   19**   27*

12.5 mg.   25 mg.   50 mg.

†PHENERGAN®
(promethazine hydrochloride)

Wyeth-Ayerst
p. 2610

498*

12.5 mg.

212*

25 mg.

229*

50 mg.

†PHENERGAN® Rectal Suppositories
(promethazine HCl)

Wyeth-Ayerst
p. 2624

865*   866*

2.5 mg.   1.25 mg.

864*

0.9 mg.

867*   868*

0.625 mg.   0.3 mg.

†PREMARIN®
(conjugated estrogens tablets, USP)

The appearance of these tablets is a
trademark of Wyeth-Ayerst Laboratories.

Wyeth-Ayerst   (Shown smaller than
p. 2637   actual size)
13 Fl. Oz.

Lo-Iron   Iron Fortified
**S · M · A® INFANT FORMULA
Concentrated Liquid**
Also available in Ready-to-Feed
Liquid and Powder

Wyeth-Ayerst   78**
p. 2584
(Dispenser shown smaller
than actual size)

78*

Pilpak® Dispenser

LO/OVRAL®
(each tablet contains 0.3 mg. norgestrel
with 0.03 mg. ethinyl estradiol)

Wyeth-Ayerst   75**
p. 2597
(Dispenser shown smaller
than actual size)

2533*   486**

**Pilpak®
Dispenser**

NORDETTE®-28
(21 light-orange tablets each
containing 0.15 mg. of levonorgestrel
and 0.03 mg. of ethinyl estradiol and
7 pink inert tablets)

Wyeth-Ayerst   56**
p. 2604
(Dispenser shown smaller
than actual size)

56*

**Pilpak®
Dispenser**

OVRAL®
(Each tablet contains 0.5 mg. norgestrel
with 0.05 mg. ethinyl estradiol)

Wyeth-Ayerst   Ⓒ
p. 2618

755*

35 mg.

PLEGINE®
(phendimetrazine tartrate)

Wyeth-Ayerst   881*
p. 2618   880*

PMB® 200   **PMB® 400**
[Premarin® (conjugated estrogens, USP)
with meprobamate]
The appearance of these tablets is a
trademark of Wyeth-Ayerst Laboratories.

Wyeth-Ayerst
p. 2634

4177*

200 mg.

4179*

400 mg.

SECTRAL®
(acebutolol hydrochloride)
The appearances of these capsules are
trademarks of Wyeth-Ayerst Laboratories.

Wyeth-Ayerst   Ⓒ
p. 2636

51*

10 mg.

Wyeth-Ayerst   78**
p. 2589
(Dispenser shown smaller
than actual size)

2514*   486**

**Pilpak®
Dispenser**

LO/OVRAL®-28
(21 white tablets, each containing 0.3 mg.
norgestrel with 0.03 mg. ethinyl estradiol, and
7 pink inert tablets)

Wyeth-Ayerst
p. 2598

2564

(Implants shown smaller than actual size)

NORPLANT® System
(levonorgestrel implants)
Each NORPLANT System implant
contains 36 mg. of levonorgestrel.

Wyeth-Ayerst   56**
p. 2605
(Dispenser shown
smaller than actual
size)

2511*   445**

**Pilpak®
Dispenser**

OVRAL®-28
(21 white tablets each containing 0.5 mg.
norgestrel with 0.05 mg. ethinyl estradiol
and 7 pink inert tablets)

Wyeth-Ayerst
p. 2626

872*

0.625 mg.
per g
Net Wt. 1½ oz.
(42.5 g)
(Shown smaller
than actual
size)

PREMARIN® Vaginal Cream
(conjugated estrogens)

6*   52*

15 mg.   30 mg.

†SERAX®
(oxazepam)

The appearance of these capsules is a
registered trademark of Wyeth-Ayerst
Laboratories.

Wyeth-Ayerst   Ⓒ
p. 2636   (Both sides of tablet shown)

317*
15 mg.

†SERAX®
(oxazepam)
The appearance of this tablet is a
trademark of Wyeth-Ayerst Laboratories.

Wyeth-Ayerst   738**
p. 2581
739**

200 mg.

300 mg.

LODINE® (etodolac)
The appearance of these capsules is a
trademark of Wyeth-Ayerst Laboratories.

Wyeth-Ayerst   Ⓒ
p. 2593

71**

1 mg.

MAZANOR®
(mazindol)

Wyeth-Ayerst
p. 2601

13 fl. oz.

Iron Fortified

(Shown smaller than actual size)

**NURSOY®
SOY PROTEIN FORMULA
Concentrated Liquid**
Also Available in Ready-to-Feed
Liquid and Powder

Wyeth-Ayerst   593*
p. 2607   360*

250 mg.   500 mg.

†PATHOCIL®
(dicloxacillin sodium monohydrate)
The appearance of these capsules is a
trademark of Wyeth-Ayerst Laboratories.

Wyeth-Ayerst   390**
p. 2607
59**

250 mg.   500 mg.

†PEN-VEE® K
(penicillin V potassium)

Wyeth-Ayerst
p. 2629

879*

1.25 mg.
with
10.0 mg.
MT

878*

0.625 mg.
with
5.0 mg.
MT

PREMARIN®
(conjugated estrogens, USP)
with Methyltestosterone (MT)

The appearance of these tablets is a
trademark of Wyeth-Ayerst Laboratories.

**Product identification number on reverse side of tablet.

Wyeth-Ayerst
p. 2537

29*

28*

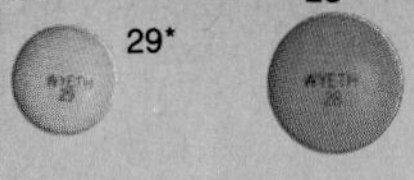

25 mg.

50 mg.

200*

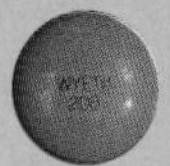

100 mg.

†SPARINE®
(promazine hydrochloride)
The appearance of these tablets is a
trademark of Wyeth-Ayerst Laboratories.

Wyeth-Ayerst
p. 2638

4132*

4133*

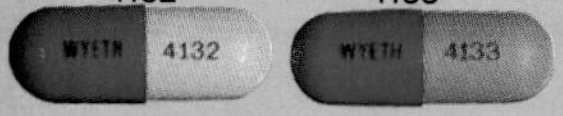

25 mg.

50 mg.

4158*

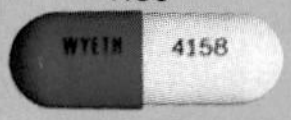

100 mg.

SURMONTIL®
(trimipramine maleate)
The appearances of these capsules
are trademarks of
Wyeth-Ayerst Laboratories.

Wyeth-Ayerst
p. 2639

WYETH 4191

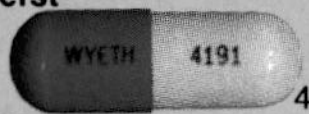

4191*

SYNALGOS®-DC
(each capsule contains 16 mg. drocode
[dihydrocodeine] bitartrate, 356.4 mg.
aspirin, and 30 mg. caffeine)
The appearance of this capsule is a
trademark of Wyeth-Ayerst Laboratories.

Wyeth-Ayerst
p. 2640

786*

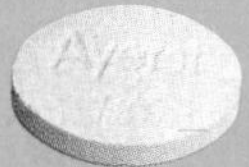

500 mg.
THIOSULFIL® FORTE
(sulfamethizole 500 mg.)

Wyeth-Ayerst
p. 2641

**   **

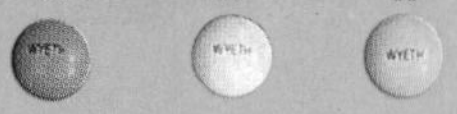

**   **

641

642

643

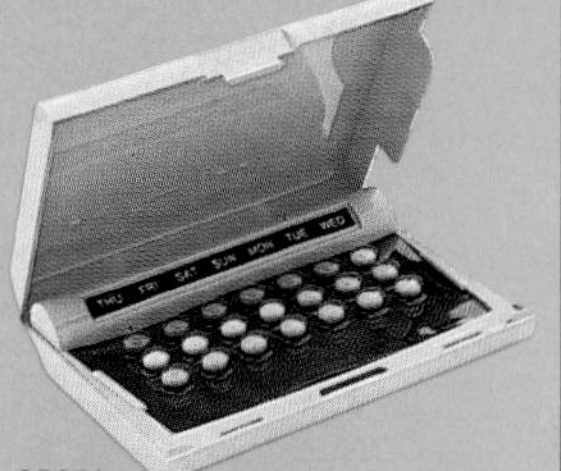

2535*

(Compact shown smaller
than actual size)

TRIPHASIL®-21

(21 tablets containing the following: 6
brown tablets—0.050 mg. levonorgestrel
+ 0.030 mg. ethinyl estradiol; 5 white
tablets—0.075 mg. levonorgestrel +
0.040 mg. ethinyl estradiol; 10 light-
yellow tablets—0.125 mg. levonorgestrel
+ 0.030 mg. ethinyl estradiol)

Wyeth-Ayerst
p. 2646

**   **

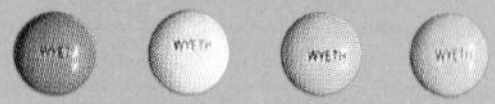

**   **

**   **

**   **

641

642

643

650

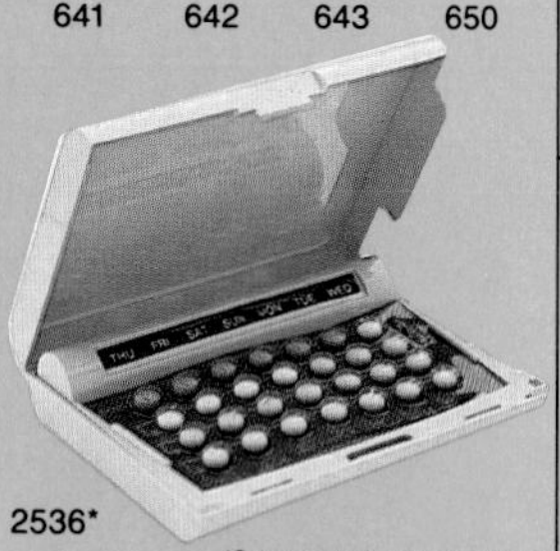

2536*

(Compact shown smaller
than actual size)

TRIPHASIL®-28

(28 tablets containing the following: 6
brown tablets—0.050 mg. levonorgestrel
+ 0.030 mg. ethinyl estradiol; 5 white
tablets—0.075 mg. levonorgestrel +
0.040 mg. ethinyl estradiol; 10 light-
yellow tablets—0.125 mg. levonorgestrel
+ 0.030 mg. ethinyl estradiol;
7 light-green tablets—inert)

Wyeth-Ayerst
p. 2649

57*

WYETH 57

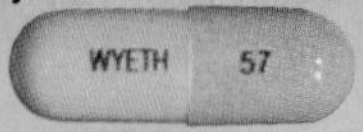

250 mg.
†UNIPEN®
(nafcillin sodium)
The appearance of this capsule is a
trademark of Wyeth-Ayerst Laboratories.

Wyeth-Ayerst
p. 2649

464**

500 mg.
†UNIPEN®
(nafcillin sodium)

Wyeth-Ayerst
p. 2653

576*

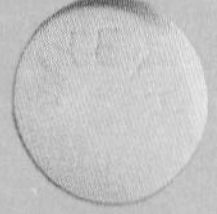

250 mg.

578*

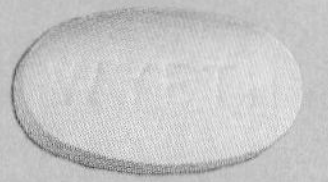

500 mg.
WYAMYCIN® S
(erythromycin stearate)

Wyeth-Ayerst
p. 2653

659*

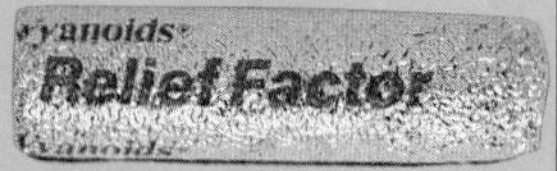

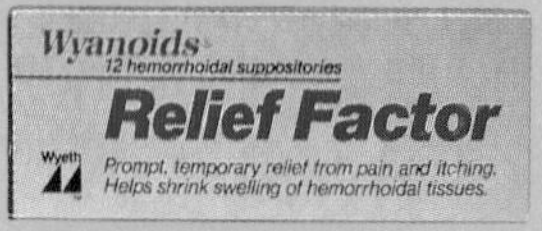

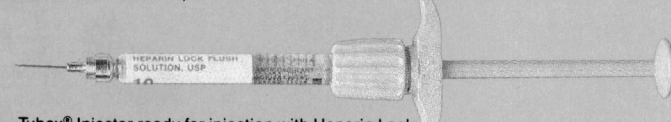

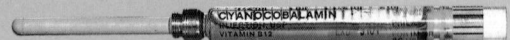

Wyanoids®
12 hemorrhoidal suppositories
Relief Factor
Wyeth
Prompt, temporary relief from pain and itching.
Helps shrink swelling of hemorrhoidal tissues.

(Box shown smaller than actual size)
Box of 24 suppositories
WYANOIDS®
RELIEF FACTOR
Also available in boxes of 12

Wyeth-Ayerst
p. 2657

85**

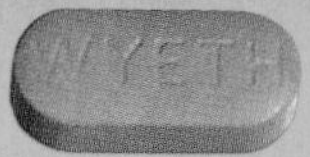

WYGESIC®
(each tablet contains 65 mg. propoxyphene
HCl, USP, and 650 mg. acetaminophen,
USP)

Wyeth-Ayerst
p. 2658

559*

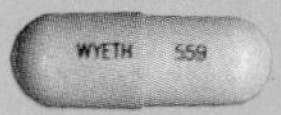

WYETH 559

250 mg.

560*

WYETH 560

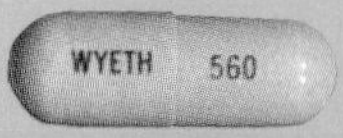

500 mg.

†WYMOX®
(amoxicillin)

Wyeth-Ayerst
p. 2659

73**

74**

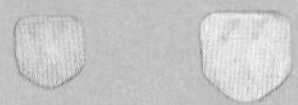

4 mg.

8 mg.

WYTENSIN® (guanabenz acetate)
The appearance of these tablets is a
registered trademark of Wyeth-Ayerst
Laboratories.

Winthrop Pharmaceuticals

Important Notice
Winthrop Pharmaceuticals
products are now distributed
by Sanofi Winthrop
Pharmaceuticals. See page 428
for product identification.

Designed to help you identify drugs,
this section contains actual size, full-
color reproductions of products selected for inclusion by participating
manufacturers.

Wyeth-Ayerst
p. 2647

(Shown smaller than actual size)

HEPARIN LOCK FLUSH
SOLUTION, USP

Tubex® Injector ready for injection with Heparin Lock
Flush Solution, USP, 10 USP units per mL

CYANOCOBALAMIN
INJECTION, USP
VITAMIN B12

Cyanocobalamin Injection, USP (Vitamin B_{12}) 1000 mcg./mL; 1 mL fill in 2 mL size
Tubex® Sterile Cartridge-Needle Unit

TUBEX® CLOSED INJECTION SYSTEM

Examples of Tubex® Sterile Cartridge-Needle Units and the Tubex® Injector, components of the
Tubex Closed Injection System, the most comprehensive line of small-volume unit-dose injectables. For a complete
list of products available, consult TUBEX listing in the Product Information Section.

**Product identification number on reverse side of tablet.

SECTION 6

Product Information Section

This section is made possible through the courtesy of the manufacturers whose products appear on the following pages. The information concerning each product has been prepared, edited and approved by the medical department, medical director, and/or medical counsel of each manufacturer.

Products described in PHYSICIANS' DESK REFERENCE® which have official package circulars must be in full compliance with Food & Drug Administration regulations pertaining to labeling for prescription drugs. These regulations require that for PDR® copy, "indications, effects, dosages, routes, methods, and frequency and duration of administration, and any relevant warnings, hazards, contraindications, side effects, and precautions" must be the "*same in language and emphasis*" as the approved labeling for the product. FDA regards the words "*same language and emphasis*" as requiring VERBATIM use of the approved labeling providing such information. Furthermore, information in the approved labeling that is emphasized by the use of type set in a box or in capitals, bold face, or italics must also be given the same emphasis in PDR. For products which do not have official package circulars, the Publisher has emphasized to manufacturers the necessity of describing such products comprehensively so that physicians would have access to all information essential for intelligent and informed prescribing. In organizing and presenting the material in PHYSICIANS' DESK REFERENCE, the Publisher is providing all the information made available to PDR by manufacturers.

This edition of PHYSICIANS' DESK REFERENCE contains the latest product information available at press-time. During the year, however, new and revised information about the products described herein may be furnished us. This information will be published in the PDR Supplements. Therefore, before prescribing or administering any product described in the following pages, you should first consult the PDR Supplements.

In presenting the following material to the medical profession, the Publisher is not necessarily advocating the use of any product listed.

Abana Pharmaceuticals, Inc.
1 CHASE CORPORATE DRIVE SUITE 260
BIRMINGHAM, AL 35244

NASABID™ Capsules ℞
[nā'za-bĭd]

DESCRIPTION
Each yellow capsule is imprinted in black with the name
Abana and "250" and contains:
Pseudoephedrine HCl .... 90 mg
Guaifenesin .... 250 mg
HOW SUPPLIED
Bottles of 100's (NDC 12463-250-01).
Shown in Product Identification Section, page 403

NORCET® Capsules Ⓒ
[nōr-set']
Hydrocodone Bitartrate and Acetaminophen

DESCRIPTION
Each white capsule is imprinted in blue with the name
Abana and the number "500" and contains:
Hydrocodone Bitartrate* 5mg
*WARNING: May be habit forming
Acetaminophen 500mg
HOW SUPPLIED
Bottles of 100's (NDC 12463-500-01).
Shown in Product Identification Section, page 403

OBE-NIX™ Capsules Ⓒ
[ō-bē-nĭks]
Phentermine Hydrochloride USP, 37.5 mg

DESCRIPTION
Each green and clear capsule is imprinted in white with the
name *Abana* and the number "217" and contains:
Phentermine HCl 37.5mg
HOW SUPPLIED
Bottles of 100's (NDC 12463-217-01).
Shown in Product Identification Section, page 403

VANEX® FORTE ℞
[vān-ĕks' for'tā]
Antihistamine Decongestant
Long-Acting Caplet

DESCRIPTION
Each pink scored caplet is imprinted with an "A" and con-
tains:
Phenylpropanolamine HCl .... 50 mg
Phenylephrine HCl .... 10 mg
Pyrilamine Maleate .... 25 mg
Chlorpheniramine Maleate .... 4 mg
HOW SUPPLIED
Bottles of 100's (NDC 12463-125-01).
Shown in Product Identification Section, page 403

VANEX®-HD Ⓒ
[vān-ĕks]
Hydrocodone Bitartrate, Phenylephrine Hydrochloride, and
Chlorpheniramine Maleate

DESCRIPTION
Each fluid ounce (30ml) contains:
Hydrocodone Bitartrate* .... 10 mg
*WARNING: May be habit forming
Phenylephrine HCl .... 30 mg
Chlorpheniramine Maleate .... 12 mg
HOW SUPPLIED
Bottles of one pint (473ml). (NDC 12463-300-16).
Shown in Product Identification Section, page 403

Products are cross-indexed by
generic and chemical names in the
YELLOW SECTION.

Abbott Laboratories
Pharmaceutical Products Division
NORTH CHICAGO, IL 60064, U.S.A.

ABBO–CODE™ INDEX

The Abbo-Code identification system provides positive identification of a drug and dosage strength. The following Abbott products are imprinted or debossed with an Abbo-Code
designation:

PRODUCT	ABBO-CODE
Biaxin™ Tablets (clarithromycin tablets)	
250 mg	KT
500 mg	KL
Cartrol® (carteolol hydrochloride)	
Filmtab® Tablets	
2.5 mg	IA
5 mg	IC
Cefol® Filmtab® Tablets	
B-complex vitamins with folic	
acid, vitamin E, and vitamin C	NJ
Colchicine Tablets, USP	
0.6 mg	AF
Cylert® Tablets Ⓒ	
(pemoline)	
18.75 mg	TH
37.5 mg	TI
75 mg	TJ
37.5 mg Chewable	TK
Depakene® Capsules	
(valproic acid capsules, USP)	
250 mg	DEPAKENE
Depakote® Sprinkle Capsules (divalproex sodium	
coated particles in capsules)	
125 mg	DEPAKOTE SPRINKLE
Depakote® Tablets (divalproex sodium	
delayed-release tablets)	
125 mg	NT
250 mg	NR
500 mg	NS
Desoxyn® Ⓒ	
(methamphetamine hydrochloride)	
5 mg Tablet	TE
5 mg Gradumet®	MC
10 mg Gradumet	ME
15 mg Gradumet	MF
Dicumarol Tablets, USP	
25 mg	AN
E.E.S. 400® Filmtab® Tablets	
(erythromycin ethylsuccinate tablets, USP)	
400 mg erythromycin activity	EE
EryPed® Chewable Tablets	
(erythromycin ethylsuccinate tablets, USP)	
200 mg erythromycin activity	EZ
Enduron® Tablets	
(methyclothiazide tablets, USP)	
2.5 mg	ENDURON
5 mg	ENDURON
Enduronyl® Tablets	
5 mg methyclothiazide and	
0.25 mg deserpidine	LS
Enduronyl® Forte Tablets	
5 mg methyclothiazide and	
0.5 mg deserpidine	LT
Ery-Tab® Enteric-Coated Tablets	
(erythromycin delayed-release tablets, USP)	
250 mg	EC
333 mg	EH
500 mg	ED
Erythrocin® Stearate Filmtab® Tablets	
(erythromycin stearate tablets, USP)	
250 mg erythromycin activity	ES
500 mg erythromycin activity	ET
Erythromycin Base Filmtab® Tablets	
(erythromycin tablets, USP)	
250 mg	EB
500 mg	EA
Erythromycin Delayed-release Capsules, USP	
250 mg	ER
Fero-Folic-500® Filmtab® Tablets	
controlled-release iron, folic acid, and	
vitamin C	AJ
Harmonyl® Tablets	
(deserpidine tablets)	
0.25 mg	LK
Hytrin® Tablets	
(terazosin hydrochloride tablets)	
1 mg	DF
2 mg	DH
5 mg	DJ
10 mg	DI

PRODUCT	ABBO-CODE
Iberet-Folic-500® Filmtab® Tablets	
controlled-release iron, B-complex	
vitamins with folic acid,	
and vitamin C	AK
Janimine® Filmtab® Tablets	
(imipramine hydrochloride tablets, USP)	
25 mg	NE
50 mg	NL
K ·Tab® Filmtab® Tablets	
(potassium chloride extended-release tablets, USP)	
10 mEq (750 mg)	K-TAB
Nembutal® Sodium Capsules Ⓒ	
(pentobarbital sodium capsules, USP)	
50 mg	CF
100 mg	CH
Ogen® Tablets	
(estropipate tablets, USP)	
0.625 tablet (0.75 mg estropipate)	LU
1.25 tablet (1.5 mg estropipate)	LV
2.5 tablet (3 mg estropipate)	LX
5 tablet (6 mg estropipate)	LY
Oretic® Tablets	
(hydrochlorothiazide tablets, USP)	
25 mg	ORETIC
50 mg	ORETIC
Oreticyl® 25 Tablets	
25 mg hydrochlorothiazide and	
0.125 mg deserpidine	AH
Oreticyl® 50 Tablets	
50 mg hydrochlorothiazide and	
0.125 mg deserpidine	AI
Oreticyl® Forte Tablets	
25 mg hydrochlorothiazide and	
0.25 mg deserpidine	LL
PCE® Dispertab® Tablets	
(erythromycin particles in tablets)	
333 mg	PCE
500 mg	EK
Peganone® Tablets	
(ethotoin tablets, USP)	
250 mg	AD
500 mg	AE
Phenurone® Tablets	
(phenacemide tablets, USP)	
500 mg	I I
Placidyl® Capsules Ⓒ	
(ethchlorvynol capsules, USP)	
500 mg	PLACIDYL 500
750 mg	PLACIDYL 750
ProSom™ Tablets Ⓒ	
(estazolam tablets)	
1 mg	UC
2 mg	UD
Tranxene® T-Tab® Tablets Ⓒ	
(clorazepate dipotassium)	
3.75 mg Tablet	TL
7.5 mg Tablet	TM
15 mg Tablet	TN
Tranxene-SD™ Ⓒ	
Single Dose Tablets	
(clorazepate dipotassium)	
11.25 mg Half Strength	TX
22.5 mg	TY
Tridione® Dulcet® Tablets	
(trimethadione tablets, USP)	
150 mg	LE
Tridione® Capsules	
(trimethadione capsules, USP)	
300 mg	AM
Vercyte® Tablets	
(pipobroman tablets, USP)	
25 mg	AT

ABBO-PAC®
Unit Dose Packages

The Abbo-Pac unit dose system from Abbott Laboratories
offers a wide range of drugs.
Each individual dose is clearly identified by generic name,
Abbott trademark name, strength, NDC identification number, expiration date and lot number. Abbo-Pac unit dose containers are designed to accommodate virtually all hospital
pharmacy storage racks and to provide maximum accessibility and ease of handling.
The following is a list of products which are now available:

PRODUCT	DOSAGE STRENGTH
Biaxin™ Tablets	
(clarithromycin tablets)	250 mg
Biaxin Tablets	500 mg
Depakene® Capsules	
(valproic acid capsules, USP)	250 mg
Depakote® Sprinkle Capsules	
(divalproex sodium coated particles	
in capsules)	125 mg

Depakote® Tablets
(divalproex sodium delayed-release tablets) .... 125 mg
Depakote Tablets .... 250 mg
Depakote Tablets .... 500 mg
Enduron® Tablets
(methyclothiazide tablets, USP) .... 5 mg
Enduronyl® Tablets
(methyclothiazide 5 mg and deserpidine 0.25 mg)
E.E.S. 400® Filmtab
(erythromycin ethylsuccinate tablets, USP) 200 mg
EryPed® Chewable Tablets
(erythromycin ethylsuccinate tablets, USP) .... 200 mg
EryPed® 200 Granules
(erythromycin ethylsuccinate
for oral suspension, USP) .... 200 mg/5 mL
EryPed® 400 Granules
(erythromycin ethylsuccinate
for oral suspension, USP) .... 400 mg/5 mL
Ery-Tab® Enteric-Coated Tablets
(erythromycin delayed-release tablets, USP) ...... 250 mg
Ery-Tab Tablets .... 333 mg
Ery-Tab Tablets .... 500 mg
Erythrocin® Stearate Filmtab
(erythromycin stearate tablets, USP) .... 250 mg
Erythromycin Base Filmtab®
(erythromycin tablets, USP) .... 250 mg
Fero-Grad-500® Filmtab
Controlled-Release Iron plus Vitamin C
Hytrin® Tablets
(terazosin hydrochloride tablets) .... 1 mg
Hytrin Tablets .... 2 mg
Hytrin Tablets .... 5 mg
Hytrin Tablets .... 10 mg
Iberet®-500 Filmtab
Controlled-Release Iron plus B-Complex and Vitamin C
K-Lor™ 20 mEq
(potassium chloride
for oral solution, USP) .... 20 mEq Potassium
20 mEq Chloride/Packet
K-Lor™ 15 mEq .... 15 mEq Potassium
15 mEq Chloride/Packet
K-Tab® Filmtab®
(potassium chloride extended-release
tablets, USP) .... 10 mEq (750 mg)
Nembutal® Sodium Capsules CII
(pentobarbital sodium capsules, USP) .... 100 mg
Oretic® Tablets
(hydrochlorothiazide tablets, USP) .... 25 mg
Oretic® Tablets .... 50 mg
Placidyl® Capsules CIV
(ethchlorvynol capsules, USP) .... 500 mg
ProSom™ Tablets CIV
(estazolam tablets) .... 1 mg
ProSom™ Tablets CIV .... 2 mg
Surbex-T® Filmtab® Tablets
High-Potency B-Complex with Vitamin C
Tranxene® T-Tab® Tablets CIV
(clorazepate dipotassium) .... 3.75 mg
Tranxene® T-Tab® Tablets CIV .... 7.5 mg
Tranxene® T-Tab® Tablets CIV .... 15 mg

ABBOKINASE® ℞

[*ab-bo-kī'nāze*]

(Urokinase For Injection)

ABBOKINASE (urokinase for injection) should be used in hospitals where the recommended diagnostic and monitoring techniques are available. Thrombolytic therapy should be considered in all situations where the benefits to be achieved outweigh the risk of potentially serious hemorrhage. When internal bleeding does occur, it may be more difficult to manage than that which occurs with conventional anticoagulant therapy.

Urokinase treatment should be instituted as soon as possible after onset of pulmonary embolism, preferably no later than seven days after onset. Any delay in instituting lytic therapy to evaluate the effect of heparin decreases the potential for optimal efficacy.[1]

When urokinase is used for treatment of coronary artery thrombosis associated with evolving transmural myocardial infarction, therapy should be instituted within six hours of symptom onset.

DESCRIPTION

Urokinase is an enzyme (protein) produced by the kidney, and found in the urine. There are two forms of urokinase differing in molecular weight but having similar clinical effects. ABBOKINASE (urokinase for injection) is a thrombolytic agent obtained from human kidney cells by tissue culture techniques and is primarily the low molecular weight form. It is supplied as a sterile lyophilized white powder containing mannitol (25 mg/vial), Albumin (Human) (250 mg/vial), and sodium chloride (50 mg/vial).

Thin translucent filaments may occasionally occur in reconstituted ABBOKINASE vials, but do not indicate any decrease in potency of this product. No clinical problems have been associated with these filaments. See "Dosage and Administration" section.

Following reconstitution with 5 mL of Sterile Water for Injection, USP, it is a clear, slightly straw-colored solution; each mL contains 50,000 IU of urokinase activity, 0.5% mannitol, 5% Albumin (Human), and 1% sodium chloride. The pH is adjusted with sodium hydroxide and/or hydrochloric acid prior to lyophilization.

ABBOKINASE is for intravenous and intracoronary infusion only.

CLINICAL PHARMACOLOGY

Urokinase acts on the endogenous fibrinolytic system. It converts plasminogen to the enzyme plasmin. Plasmin degrades fibrin clots as well as fibrinogen and other plasma proteins.

Intravenous infusion of urokinase in doses recommended for lysis of pulmonary embolism is followed by increased fibrinolytic activity. This effect disappears within a few hours after discontinuation, but a decrease in plasma levels of fibrinogen and plasminogen and an increase in the amount of circulating fibrin (ogen) degradation products may persist for 12–24 hours.[2,3] There is a lack of correlation between embolus resolution and changes in coagulation and fibrinolytic assay results.

Information is incomplete about the pharmacokinetic properties in man. Urokinase administered by intravenous infusion is cleared rapidly by the liver. The serum half-life in man is 20 minutes or less. Patients with impaired liver function (e.g., cirrhosis) would be expected to show a prolongation in half-life. Small fractions of an administered dose are excreted in bile and urine.

INDICATIONS AND USAGE

Pulmonary Embolism

ABBOKINASE (urokinase for injection) is indicated in adults:

—For the lysis of acute massive pulmonary emboli, defined as obstruction of blood flow to a lobe or multiple segments.

—For the lysis of pulmonary emboli accompanied by unstable hemodynamics, i.e., failure to maintain blood pressure without supportive measures.

The diagnosis should be confirmed by objective means, such as pulmonary angiography via an upper extremity vein, or non-invasive procedures such as lung scanning.

Angiographic and hemodynamic measurements demonstrate a more rapid improvement with lytic therapy than with heparin therapy.[4–8]

Coronary Artery Thrombosis

ABBOKINASE has been reported to lyse acute thrombi obstructing coronary arteries, associated with evolving transmural myocardial infarction.[9] The majority of patients who received ABBOKINASE by intracoronary infusion within six hours following onset of symptoms showed recanalization of the involved vessel.

IT HAS NOT BEEN ESTABLISHED THAT INTRACORONARY ADMINISTRATION OF ABBOKINASE DURING EVOLVING TRANSMURAL MYOCARDIAL INFARCTION RESULTS IN SALVAGE OF MYOCARDIAL TISSUE, NOR THAT IT REDUCES MORTALITY. THE PATIENTS WHO MIGHT BENEFIT FROM THIS THERAPY CANNOT BE DEFINED.

I.V. Catheter Clearance

ABBOKINASE is indicated for the restoration of patency to intravenous catheters, including central venous catheters, obstructed by clotted blood or fibrin.[10,11] (See separate section at end of insert concerning I.V. catheter clearance for information regarding warnings, precautions, adverse reactions, and dosage and administration.)

CONTRAINDICATIONS

Because thrombolytic therapy increases the risk of bleeding, urokinase is contraindicated in the following situations: (See WARNINGS.)

—Active internal bleeding

—History of cerebrovascular accident

—Recent (within two months) intracranial or intraspinal surgery

—Recent trauma including cardiopulmonary resuscitation

—Intracranial neoplasm, arteriovenous malformation, or aneurysm

—Known bleeding diathesis

—Severe uncontrolled arterial hypertension

WARNINGS

Bleeding

The aim of urokinase is the production of sufficient amounts of plasmin for lysis of intravascular deposits of fibrin; however, fibrin deposits which provide hemostasis, for example, at sites of needle puncture, will also lyse, and bleeding from such sites may occur.

Intramuscular injections and nonessential handling of the patient must be avoided during treatment with urokinase. Venipunctures should be performed carefully and as infrequently as possible.

Should an arterial puncture be necessary (except for intracoronary administration), upper extremity vessels are preferable. Pressure should be applied for at least 30 minutes, a pressure dressing applied, and the puncture site checked frequently for evidence of bleeding.

In the following conditions, the risks of therapy may be increased and should be weighed against the anticipated benefits:

—Recent (within 10 days) major surgery, obstetrical delivery, organ biopsy, previous puncture of non-compressible vessels

—Recent (within 10 days) serious gastrointestinal bleeding

—High likelihood of a left heart thrombus, e.g., mitral stenosis with atrial fibrillation

—Subacute bacterial endocarditis

—Hemostatic defects including those secondary to severe hepatic or renal disease

—Pregnancy

—Cerebrovascular disease

—Diabetic hemorrhagic retinopathy

—Any other condition in which bleeding might constitute a significant hazard or be particularly difficult to manage because of its location

Should serious spontaneous bleeding (not controllable by local pressure) occur, the infusion of urokinase should be terminated immediately, and treatment instituted as described under ADVERSE REACTIONS.

Use of Anticoagulants

Concurrent use of anticoagulants with intravenous administration of ABBOKINASE is not recommended. However, concurrent use of heparin may be required during intracoronary administration of ABBOKINASE. A clinical study[9] with concurrent use of heparin and ABBOKINASE during intracoronary administration has demonstrated no tendency toward increased bleeding that would not be attributable to the procedure or ABBOKINASE alone. Nevertheless, careful monitoring for excessive bleeding is advised.

Arrhythmias

Rapid lysis of coronary thrombi has been reported occasionally to cause atrial or ventricular dysrhythmias as a result of reperfusion requiring immediate treatment. Careful monitoring for arrhythmias should be maintained during and immediately following intracoronary administration of ABBOKINASE.

PRECAUTIONS

Laboratory Tests

Before commencing thrombolytic therapy, obtain a hematocrit, platelet count, and a thrombin time (TT), activated partial thromboplastin time (APTT), or prothrombin time (PT). If heparin has been given, it should be discontinued unless it is to be used in conjunction with ABBOKINASE for intracoronary administration. TT or APTT should be less than twice the normal control value before thrombolytic therapy is started.

During the infusion, coagulation tests and/or measures of fibrinolytic activity may be performed if desired. Results do not, however, reliably predict either efficacy or a risk of bleeding. The clinical response should be observed frequently, and vital signs, i.e., pulse, temperature, respiratory rate and blood pressure, should be checked at least every four hours. The blood pressure should not be taken in the lower extremities to avoid dislodgement of possible deep vein thrombi.

Following the intravenous infusion, *before (re)instituting heparin*, the TT or APTT should be less than twice the upper limits of normal. Following intracoronary infusion of ABBOKINASE, blood coagulation parameters should be determined and heparin therapy continued as appropriate.

Drug Interactions

The interaction of urokinase with other drugs has not been studied. Drugs that alter platelet function should not be used. Common examples are: aspirin, indomethacin and phenylbutazone.

Although a bolus dose of heparin is recommended prior to intracoronary use of urokinase, oral anticoagulants or heparin should not be given concurrently with large doses of urokinase such as those used for pulmonary embolism. Concomitant use of intravenous urokinase and oral anticoagulants or heparin may increase the risk of hemorrhage. (See "WARNINGS" section.)

Carcinogenicity

Adequate data are not available on the long-term potential for carcinogenicity in animals or humans.

Pregnancy

Pregnancy category B. Reproduction studies have been performed in mice and rats at doses up to 1,000 times the human dose and have revealed no evidence of impaired fertility or harm to the fetus due to urokinase. There are, however, no adequate and well-controlled studies in pregnant women. Because animal reproduction studies are not always predic-

Continued on next page

If desired, additional literature on any Abbott product will be provided upon request to Abbott Laboratories.

Abbott Laboratories—Cont.

tive of human response, this drug should be used during pregnancy only if clearly needed.

Nursing Mothers

It is not known whether this drug is excreted in human milk. Because many drugs are excreted in human milk, caution should be exercised when urokinase is administered to a nursing woman.

Pediatric Use

Safety and effectiveness in children have not been established.

ADVERSE REACTIONS

The following adverse reactions have been associated with intravenous therapy but may also occur with intracoronary artery infusion.

Bleeding

The type of bleeding associated with thrombolytic therapy can be placed into two broad categories:

—Superficial or surface bleeding, observed mainly at invaded or disturbed sites (e.g., venous cutdowns, arterial punctures, sites of recent surgical intervention, etc.).

—Internal bleeding, involving, e.g., the gastrointestinal tract, genitourinary tract, vagina, or intramuscular, retroperitoneal, or intracranial sites.

Several fatalities due to intracranial or retroperitoneal hemorrhage have occurred during thrombolytic therapy.

Should serious bleeding occur, urokinase infusion should be discontinued and, if necessary, blood loss and reversal of the bleeding tendency can be effectively managed with whole blood (fresh blood preferable), packed red blood cells and cryoprecipitate or fresh frozen plasma. Dextran should not be used. Although the use of aminocaproic acid (ACA, AMICAR®) in humans as an antidote for urokinase has not been documented, it may be considered in an emergency situation.

Allergic Reactions:

In vitro tests with urokinase, as well as intradermal tests in humans, gave no evidence of induced antibody formation. Relatively mild allergic type reactions, e.g., bronchospasm and skin rash, have been reported. When such reactions occur, they usually respond to conventional therapy. In addition, rare cases of anaphylaxis have been reported.

Miscellaneous:

Fever and chills, including shaking chills (rigors), nausea and/or vomiting, transient hypotension or hypertension, dyspnea, tachycardia, cyanosis, back pain, hypoxemia, and acidosis have been reported together and separately. Rare cases of myocardial infarction have also been reported. A cause and effect relationship has not been established. Aspirin is not recommended for treatment of fever.

DOSAGE AND ADMINISTRATION

ABBOKINASE IS INTENDED FOR INTRAVENOUS AND INTRACORONARY INFUSION ONLY.

A. Pulmonary Embolism:

Preparation

Reconstitute ABBOKINASE (urokinase for injection) by aseptically adding 5 mL of Sterile Water for Injection, USP, to the vial. (It is important that ABBOKINASE be reconstituted *only* with Sterile Water for Injection, USP, *without* preservatives. Bacteriostatic Water for Injection should *not* be used.) Each vial should be visually inspected for discoloration (slightly straw-colored solution) and for the presence of particulate material. Highly colored solutions should not be used. Because ABBOKINASE contains no preservatives, it should not be reconstituted until immediately before using. Any unused portion of the reconstituted material should be discarded.

To minimize formation of filaments, avoid shaking the vial during reconstitution. Roll and tilt the vial to enhance reconstitution. The solution may be terminally filtered, e.g., through a 0.45 micron or smaller cellulose membrane filter. No other medication should be added to this solution.

Reconstituted ABBOKINASE is diluted with 0.9% Sodium Chloride Injection, USP or 5% Dextrose Injection, USP, prior to intravenous infusion. (See Table I, **Dose Preparation-Pulmonary Embolism.**)

Administration

Administer ABBOKINASE (urokinase for injection) by means of a constant infusion pump that is capable of delivering a total volume of 195 mL. The table may be used as an aid in the preparation of ABBOKINASE (urokinase for injection) for administration.

A priming dose of 2,000 IU/lb (4,400 IU/kg) of ABBOKINASE is given as the ABBOKINASE -0.9% Sodium Chloride Injection or 5% Dextrose Injection admixture at a rate of 90 mL/hour over a period of 10 minutes. This is followed by a continuous infusion of 2,000 IU/lb/hr (4,400 IU/kg/hr) of ABBOKINASE at a rate of 15 mL/hour for 12 hours. Since some ABBOKINASE admixture will remain in the tubing at the end of an infusion pump delivery cycle, the following flush procedure should be performed to insure that the total dose of ABBOKINASE is administered. A solution of 0.9%

Sodium Chloride Injection or 5% Dextrose Injection approximately equal in amount to the volume of the tubing in the infusion set should be administered via the pump to flush the ABBOKINASE admixture from the entire length of the infusion set. The pump should be set to administer the flush solution at the continuous infusion rate of 15 mL/hour.

Anticoagulation After Terminating Urokinase Treatment

At the end of urokinase therapy, treatment with heparin by continuous intravenous infusion is recommended to prevent recurrent thrombosis. Heparin treatment, without a loading dose, should not begin until the thrombin time has decreased to *less than twice* the normal control value (approximately 3 to 4 hours after completion of the infusion). See manufacturer's prescribing information for proper use of heparin. This should then be followed by oral anticoagulants in the conventional manner.

B. Lysis of Coronary Artery Thrombi:[9]

Preparation

Reconstitute three (3) 250,000 IU vials of ABBOKINASE by aseptically adding 5 mL of Sterile Water for Injection, USP, to each vial. (It is important that ABBOKINASE be reconstituted *only* with Sterile Water for Injection, USP, *without* preservatives. Bacteriostatic Water for Injection should *not* be used.) Each vial should be visually inspected for discoloration (slightly straw-colored solution) and for the presence of particulate material. Highly colored solutions should not be used. Because ABBOKINASE contains no preservatives, it should not be reconstituted until immediately before using. Any unused portion of the reconstituted material should be discarded.

To minimize formation of filaments, avoid shaking the vial during reconstitution. Roll and tilt the vial to enhance reconstitution. The solution may be terminally filtered, e.g., through a 0.45 micron or smaller cellulose membrane filter. Add the contents of the three (3) reconstituted ABBOKINASE vials to 500 mL of 5% Dextrose Injection, USP. The resulting solution admixture will have a concentration of approximately 1500 IU per mL. No other medication should be added to the solution.

The admixture should be administered immediately as described under Administration. Any solution remaining after administration should be discarded.

NOTE: Adsorption of drug from dilute protein solutions to various materials has been reported in the literature. Therefore, the directions for Preparation and Administration must be followed to assure that significant drug loss does not occur.

Administration

Prior to the infusion of ABBOKINASE, a bolus dose of heparin ranging from 2500 to 10,000 units should be administered intravenously. Prior heparin administration should be considered when calculating the heparin dose for this procedure. Following the bolus dose of heparin, the prepared ABBOKINASE solution should be infused into the occluded artery at a rate of 4 mL per minute (6000 IU per minute) for periods up to 2 hours. In a clinical study, the average total dose of ABBOKINASE utilized for lysis of coronary artery thrombi was 500,000 IU.[9]

To determine response to ABBOKINASE therapy, periodic angiography during the infusion is recommended. It is suggested that the angiography be repeated at approximately 15 minute intervals. ABBOKINASE therapy should be contin-

ued until the artery is maximally opened, usually 15 to 30 minutes after the initial opening. Following the infusion, coagulation parameters should be determined. It is advisable to continue heparin therapy after the artery is opened by ABBOKINASE.

When ABBOKINASE was administered selectively into thrombosed coronary arteries via coronary catheter within 6 hours following onset of symptoms of acute transmural myocardial infarction, 60% of the occlusions were opened.[9]

I.V. CATHETER CLEARANCE

Warnings

Excessive pressure should be avoided when ABBOKINASE is injected into the catheter. Such force could cause rupture of the catheter or expulsion of the clot into the circulation.

Precautions

Catheters may be occluded by substances other than blood products, such as drug precipitate. ABBOKINASE is not effective in such a case, and there is the possibility that the precipitate may be forced into the vascular system.

Adverse Reactions

Although there have been no adverse reactions reported as a result of using ABBOKINASE for the removal of clot obstruction from I.V. catheters, the possibility of reactions should nevertheless be considered.

Dosage and Administration

Preparation: Reconstitute ABBOKINASE (urokinase for injection) by aseptically adding 5 mL of Sterile Water for Injection, USP, to the vial. (It is important that ABBOKINASE be reconstituted *only* with Sterile Water for Injection, USP, *without* preservatives. Bacteriostatic Water for Injection should *not* be used.) Add 1 mL of the reconstituted drug to 9 mL Sterile Water for Injection, USP, to make a final dilution equivalent to 5,000 IU/mL. One mL of this preparation is to be utilized for each catheter clearing procedure. BECAUSE ABBOKINASE CONTAINS NO PRESERVATIVES, IT SHOULD NOT BE RECONSTITUTED UNTIL IMMEDIATELY BEFORE USING.

Administration: NOTE: When the following procedure is used to clear a central venous catheter, the patient should be instructed to exhale and hold his breath any time the catheter is not connected to I.V. tubing or a syringe. This is to prevent air from entering the open catheter.

Aseptically disconnect the I.V. tubing connection at the catheter hub and attach a 10 mL syringe. Determine occlusion of the catheter by *gently* attempting to aspirate blood from the catheter with the 10 mL syringe. If aspiration is not possible, remove the 10 mL syringe and attach a 1 mL tuberculin syringe filled with prepared ABBOKINASE to the catheter. Slowly and gently inject an amount of ABBOKINASE equal to the volume of the catheter. Aseptically remove the tuberculin syringe and connect a 5 mL syringe to the catheter. Wait at least 5 minutes before attempting to aspirate the drug and residual clot with the 5 mL syringe. Repeat aspiration attempts every 5 minutes. If the catheter is not open within 30 minutes, the catheter may be capped allowing ABBOKINASE to remain in the catheter for 30 to 60 minutes before again attempting to aspirate. A second injection of ABBOKINASE may be necessary in resistant cases.

When patency is restored, aspirate 4 to 5 mL of blood to assure removal of all drug and clot residual. Remove the blood-

TABLE I
Dose Preparation-Pulmonary Embolism

Weight (pounds)	Total Dose* Urokinase (IU)	Number Vials ABBOKINASE (urokinase for injection)	Volume of ABBOKINASE After Reconstitution (mL)**	+	Volume of Diluent (mL)	=	Final Volume (mL)
81–90	2,250,000	9	45		150		195
91–100	2,500,000	10	50		145		195
101–110	2,750,000	11	55		140		195
111–120	3,000,000	12	60		135		195
121–130	3,250,000	13	65		130		195
131–140	3,500,000	14	70		125		195
141–150	3,750,000	15	75		120		195
151–160	4,000,000	16	80		115		195
161–170	4,250,000	17	85		110		195
171–180	4,500,000	18	90		105		195
181–190	4,750,000	19	95		100		195
191–200	5,000,000	20	100		95		195
201–210	5,250,000	21	105		90		195
211–220	5,500,000	22	110		85		195
221–230	5,750,000	23	115		80		195
231–240	6,000,000	24	120		75		195
241–250	6,250,000	25	125		70		195

	Priming Dose	Dose for 12-Hour Period
Infusion Rate:	15 mL/10 min***	15 mL/hr for 12 hrs

*Priming dose + dose administered during 12-hour period.
**After addition of 5 mL of Sterile Water for Injection, USP, per vial (See Preparation.)
***Pump rate = 90 mL/hr

filled syringe and replace it with a 10 mL syringe filled with 0.9% Sodium Chloride Injection, USP. The catheter should then be gently irrigated with this solution to assure patency of the catheter. After the catheter has been irrigated, remove the 10 mL syringe and aseptically reconnect sterile I.V. tubing to the catheter hub.

[See table bottom right on preceding page.]

HOW SUPPLIED

ABBOKINASE (urokinase for injection) is supplied as a sterile lyophilized preparation (**NDC** 0074-6109-05). Each vial contains 250,000 IU urokinase activity, 25 mg mannitol, 250 mg Albumin (Human), and 50 mg sodium chloride. Store ABBOKINASE powder at 2° to 8°C.

[See table bottom right on preceding page.]

REFERENCES

1. Sherry S, et al. Thrombolytic therapy in thrombosis: A National Institutes of Health consensus development conference. *Ann Intern Med.* 1980:93:141–144.
2. Bang NU. Physiology and biochemistry of fibrinolysis. In: Bang NU, Beller FK, Deutsch E, Mammen EF, eds. *Thrombosis and Bleeding Disorders.* New York, NY: Academic Press; 1971;292–327.
3. McNicol GP. The fibrinolytic enzyme system. *Postgrad Med J.* August 1973;49 (suppl 5):10–12.
4. Sasahara AA, Hyers TM, Cole CM, et al. The urokinase pulmonary embolism trial. *Circulation.* 1973;47 (suppl 2):1–108.
5. Urokinase pulmonary embolism trial study group: Urokinase-streptokinase embolism trial. *JAMA.* 1974;229:1606–1613.
6. Sasahara AA, Bell WR, Simon TL, et al. The Phase II urokinase-streptokinase pulmonary embolism trial, *Thrombos Diathes Haemorrh* (Stuttg) 1975;33:464–476.
7. Bell WR. Thrombolytic therapy: A comparison between urokinase and streptokinase. *Sem Thromb Hemost.* 1975;2:1–13.
8. Fratantoni JC, Ness P, Simon TL. Thrombolytic therapy: Current status. *N Eng J Med.* 1975;293:1073–1078.
9. Tennant SN, Campbell WB, et al: Intracoronary thrombolysis in acute myocardial infarction: Comparison of the efficacy of urokinase to streptokinase. *Circulation.* 1984;69:756–760.
10. Lawson M, et al. The use of urokinase to restore the patency of occluded central venous catheters. *Am J Intravenous Therapy and Clinical Nutrition.* 1982;9:29–32.
11. Glynn MFX, et al. Therapy for thrombotic occlusion of long-term intravenous alimentation catheters. *Journal of Parenteral and Enteral Nutrition.* 1980;4:387–390.

Ref. 01-2588-R9

Shown in Product Identification Section, page 403

ABBOKINASE® OPEN-CATH® ℞

[ab-bō-kī'nāze open-cath]

(Urokinase for Catheter Clearance)

DESCRIPTION

Urokinase is an enzyme (protein) produced by the kidney, and found in the urine. There are two forms of urokinase differing in molecular weight but having similar clinical effects. Urokinase is a thrombolytic agent obtained from human kidney cells by tissue culture techniques and is primarily the low molecular weight form. It is supplied as a sterile lyophilized white powder. Following reconstitution ABBOKINASE OPEN-CATH solution is clear and essentially colorless.

Each mL of reconstituted ABBOKINASE OPEN-CATH solution contains 5000 IU of urokinase activity, 5 mg gelatin, 15 mg mannitol, 1.7 mg sodium chloride and 4.6 mg monobasic sodium phosphate anhydrous. The pH is adjusted with sodium hydroxide and/or hydrochloric acid prior to lyophilization.

CLINICAL PHARMACOLOGY

Urokinase acts on the endogenous fibrinolytic system. It converts plasminogen to the enzyme plasmin. Plasmin degrades fibrin clots as well as fibrinogen and other plasma proteins.

When used as directed for I.V. catheter clearance, only small amounts of urokinase may reach the circulation; therefore, therapeutic serum levels are not expected to be achieved. Nevertheless, one should be aware of the clinical pharmacology of urokinase.

Intravenous infusion of urokinase in doses recommended for lysis of pulmonary embolism is followed by increased fibrinolytic activity. This effect disappears within a few hours after discontinuation, but a decrease in plasma levels of fibrinogen and plasminogen and an increase in the amount of circulating fibrin (ogen) degradation products may persist for 12–24 hours.[1,2] There is a lack of correlation between embolus resolution and changes in coagulation and fibrinolytic assay results.

Information is incomplete about the pharmacokinetic properties in man. Urokinase administered by intravenous infusion is cleared rapidly by the liver. The serum half-life in man is 20 minutes or less. Patients with impaired liver function (e.g., cirrhosis) would be expected to show a prolongation in half-life. Small fractions of an administered dose are excreted in bile and urine.

INDICATIONS AND USAGE

ABBOKINASE OPEN-CATH (urokinase for catheter clearance) is indicated for the restoration of patency to intravenous catheters, including central venous catheters, obstructed by clotted blood or fibrin.[3,4,5]

CONTRAINDICATIONS

Because thrombolytic therapy increases the risk of bleeding, urokinase is contraindicated in the following situations:

—Active internal bleeding
—History of cerebrovascular accident
—Recent (within two months) intracranial or intraspinal surgery
—Recent trauma including cardiopulmonary resuscitation
—Intracranial neoplasm, arteriovenous malformation, or aneurysm
—Known bleeding diathesis
—Severe uncontrolled arterial hypertension

There have been no reports, however, which would suggest a contraindication for the use of urokinase for I.V. catheter clearance.

WARNINGS

Excessive pressure should be avoided when ABBOKINASE solution is injected into the catheter. Such force could cause rupture of the catheter or expulsion of the clot into the circulation. During attempts to determine catheter occlusion, vigorous suction should not be applied due to possible damage to the vascular wall or collapse of soft-wall catheters. Catheters may be occluded by substances other than fibrin clots, such as drug precipitates. ABBOKINASE solution is not effective in such cases and there is the possibility that the substances may be forced into the vascular system.

PRECAUTIONS

Carcinogenicity: Adequate data is not available on the long-term potential for carcinogenicity in animals or humans.

Pregnancy: Pregnancy category B. Reproduction studies have been performed in mice and rats at doses up to 1,000 times the human therapeutic dose and have revealed no evidence of impaired fertility or harm to the fetus due to urokinase. There are, however, no adequate and well-controlled studies in pregnant women. Because animal reproduction studies are not always predictive of human response, this drug should be used during pregnancy only if clearly needed.

Nursing Mothers: It is not known whether this drug is excreted in human milk. Because many drugs are excreted in human milk, caution should be exercised when urokinase is administered to a nursing woman.

Pediatric Use: Safety and effectiveness in children have not been established.

ADVERSE REACTIONS

The following reactions have been associated with ABBOKINASE (urokinase for injection) in doses recommended for lysis of pulmonary embolism.

Bleeding: The type of bleeding associated with thrombolytic therapy can be placed into two broad categories:

—Superficial or surface bleeding, observed mainly at invaded or disturbed sites (e.g., venous cutdowns, arterial punctures, sites of recent surgical intervention, etc.).
—Internal bleeding, involving, e.g., the gastrointestinal tract, genitourinary tract, vagina, or intramuscular, retroperitoneal, or intracranial sites.

Several fatalities due to intracranial or retroperitoneal hemorrhage have occurred during thrombolytic therapy.

Should serious bleeding occur, urokinase infusion should be discontinued and, if necessary, blood loss and reversal of the bleeding tendency can be effectively managed with whole blood (fresh blood preferable), packed red blood cells and cryoprecipitate or fresh frozen plasma. Dextran and hetastarch should not be used. Although the use of aminocaproic acid (ACA, AMICAR®) in humans as an antidote for urokinase has not been documented, it may be considered in an emergency situation.

Allergic Reactions: *In vitro* tests with urokinase, as well as intradermal tests in humans, gave no evidence of induced antibody formation. Relatively mild allergic type reactions, e.g., bronchospasm and skin rash, have been reported. When such reactions occur, they usually respond to conventional therapy. In addition, rare cases of anaphylaxis have been reported.

Miscellaneous: Fever and chills, including shaking chills (rigors), nausea and/or vomiting, transient hypotension or hypertension, dyspnea, tachycardia, cyanosis, back pain, hypoxemia, and acidosis have been reported together and separately. Rare cases of myocardial infarction have also been reported. A cause and effect relationship has not been established.

Aspirin is not recommended for treatment of fever.

DOSAGE AND ADMINISTRATION

BECAUSE ABBOKINASE OPEN-CATH POWDER CONTAINS NO PRESERVATIVE, RECONSTITUED SOLUTION SHOULD BE USED IMMEDIATELY AFTER RECONSTITUTION. DISCARD ANY UNUSED PORTION.

Preparation of Solution: *Univial:*

1. Remove protective cap. Turn plunger-stopper a quarter turn and press to force diluent into lower chamber.
2. Roll and tilt to effect solution. Use only a clear, colorless solution.
3. Sterilize top of stopper with a suitable germicide.
4. Insert needle through the center of stopper until tip is barely visible. Withdraw dose.

It is recommended that vigorous shaking be avoided during reconstitution; roll and tilt to enhance reconstitution.

Parenteral drug products should be inspected visually for particulate matter and discoloration prior to administration, whenever solution and container permit.

ADMINISTRATION

When the following procedure is used to clear a central venous catheter, the patient should be instructed to exhale and hold his breath any time the catheter is not connected to I.V. tubing or a syringe. This is to prevent air from entering the open catheter.

Aseptically disconnect the I.V. tubing connection at the catheter hub and attach an empty 10 mL syringe. Determine occlusion of the catheter by *gently* attempting to aspirate blood from the catheter with the 10 mL syringe. If aspiration is not possible, remove the 10 mL syringe and attach a syringe filled with an amount of prepared ABBOKINASE OPEN-CATH solution equal to the internal volume of the catheter.

Slowly and gently inject the ABBOKINASE solution into the catheter. Aseptically remove the syringe and connect a 5 mL syringe to the catheter. Wait at least 5 minutes before attempting to aspirate the drug and residual clot with the empty syringe. Repeat aspiration attempts every 5 minutes. If the catheter is not open within 30 minutes, the catheter may be capped allowing ABBOKINASE solution to remain in the catheter for an additional 30 to 60 minutes before again attempting to aspirate. A second injection of ABBOKINASE (urokinase for catheter clearance) may be necessary in resistant cases.

When patency is restored, aspirate 4 to 5 mL of blood to assure removal of all drug and residual clot. Remove the blood-filled syringe and replace it with a 10 mL syringe filled with 0.9% Sodium Chloride Injection, USP. The catheter should then be gently irrigated with this solution to assure patency of the catheter. After the catheter has been irrigated, remove the 10 mL syringe and aseptically reconnect sterile I.V. tubing to the catheter hub.

HOW SUPPLIED

ABBOKINASE OPEN-CATH (urokinase for catheter clearance) is supplied as a sterile lyophilized preparation in single dose Univial® packages of 1 mL (**NDC** 0074-6111-01) and 1.8 mL (**NDC 0074-6145-02). Store powder below 77°F (25°C). Avoid freezing.**

REFERENCES

1. Bang NU. Physiology and biochemistry of fibrinolysis. In: Bang NU, Beller FK, Deutsch E, Mammen EF, eds. *Thrombosis and Bleeding Disorders.* New York, NY: Academic Press; 1971: 292–327.
2. McNicol GP. The fibrinolytic enzyme system. *Postgrad. Med. J.* August 1973; 49 (suppl 5):10–12.
3. Hurtubise, MR, Bottino, JC, Lawson, M, et al. Restoring patency of occluded central venous catheters. *Arch. Surg.* 1980; 115:212–213.
4. Glynn, MFX, et al. Therapy for thrombotic occlusion of long-term intravenous alimentation catheters. *Journal of Parenteral and Enteral Nutrition.* 1980; 4:387–390.
5. Lawson M, Bottino JC, Hurtubise MR, et al. The use of urokinase to restore the patency of occluded central venous catheters. *Am J IV Ther and Clin Nutr.* 1982; 9:29–30,32.

Ref. 01-2589-R5

Shown in Product Identification Section, page 403

BIAXIN (clarithromycin) ℞

Filmtab® Tablets

DESCRIPTION

BIAXIN (clarithromycin) is a semi-synthetic macrolide antibiotic. Chemically, it is 6-0-Methylerythromycin. The molec-

Continued on next page

If desired, additional literature on any Abbott product will be provided upon request to Abbott Laboratories.

Abbott Laboratories—Cont.

ular formula is $C_{38}H_{69}NO_{13}$, and the molecular weight is 747.96. The structural formula is:

Clarithromycin is a white to off-white crystalline powder. It is soluble in acetone, slightly soluble in methanol, ethanol and acetonitrile, and practically insoluble in water.
Each yellow oval film-coated BIAXIN tablet contains 250 mg or 500 mg of clarithromycin for oral administration.

Inactive Ingredients:
250 mg tablet: Cellulosic polymers, croscarmellose sodium, D&C Yellow No. 10, FD&C Blue No. 1, magnesium stearate, povidone, propylene glycol, silicon dioxide, sorbic acid, sorbitan monooleate, pregelatinized starch, stearic acid, talc, titanium dioxide, and vanillin.
500 mg tablet: Cellulosic polymers, croscarmellose sodium, D&C Yellow No. 10, FD&C Blue No. 1, magnesium stearate, povidone, propylene glycol, silicon dioxide, sorbic acid, sorbitan monooleate, stearic acid, talc, titanium dioxide, and vanillin.

CLINICAL PHARMACOLOGY

Clarithromycin is rapidly absorbed from the gastrointestinal tract after oral administration. The absolute bioavailability of 250 mg clarithromycin tablets was approximately 50%. Food slightly delays both the onset of clarithromycin absorption and the formation of the antimicrobially active metabolite, 14-OH clarithromycin, but does not affect the extent of bioavailability. Therefore, BIAXIN tablets may be given without regard to meals.
In fasting healthy human subjects, peak serum concentrations were attained within 2 hours after oral dosing. Steady-state peak serum clarithromycin concentrations were attained in 2 to 3 days and were approximately 1 mcg/mL with a 250 mg dose administered every 12 hours and 2 to 3 mcg/mL with a 500 mg dose administered every 12 hours. The elimination half-life of clarithromycin was about 3 to 4 hours with 250 mg administered every 12 hours but increased to 5 to 7 hours with 500 mg administered every 12 hours. The nonlinearity of clarithromycin pharmacokinetics is slight at the recommended doses of 250 mg and 500 mg administered every 12 hours. With a 250 mg every 12 hours dosing, the principal metabolite, 14-OH clarithromycin, attains a peak steady-state concentration of about 0.6 mcg/mL and has an elimination half-life of 5 to 6 hours. With a 500 mg every 12 hours dosing, the peak steady-state concentrations of 14-OH clarithromycin are slightly higher (up to 1 mcg/mL), and its elimination half-life is about 7 hours. With either dose, the steady-state concentration of this metabolite is generally attained within 2 to 3 days.
After a 250 mg every 12 hours oral dose, approximately 20% of the dose is excreted in the urine as the unchanged parent drug, clarithromycin. After a 500 mg every 12 hours dosing, the urinary excretion of clarithromycin is somewhat greater, approximately 30%. The renal clearance of clarithromycin is, however, relatively independent of the dose size and approximates the normal glomerular filtration rate. The major metabolite found in the urine is 14-OH clarithromycin which accounts for an additional 10% to 15% of the dose with either 250 mg or 500 mg administered every 12 hours.
The steady-state concentrations of clarithromycin in subjects with impaired hepatic function did not differ from those in normal subjects; however, the 14-OH clarithromycin concentrations were lower in the hepatically impaired subjects. The decreased formation of 14-OH clarithromycin was at least partially offset by an increase in renal clearance of clarithromycin in the subjects with impaired hepatic function when compared to healthy subjects.
The pharmacokinetics of clarithromycin were also altered in subjects with impaired renal function. (See PRECAUTIONS and DOSAGE AND ADMINISTRATION.)
Clarithromycin and the 14-OH clarithromycin metabolite distribute readily into body tissues and fluids. There are no data available on cerebrospinal fluid penetration. Because of high intracellular concentrations, tissue concentrations are higher than serum concentrations. Examples from tissue and serum concentrations are presented above.
[See table at top of next column.]

Microbiology:
Clarithromycin exerts its antibacterial action by binding to the 50S ribosomal subunit of susceptible organisms and inhibiting protein synthesis.

CONCENTRATION
(after 250 mg q 12h)

Tissue Type	Tissue (mcg/g)	Serum (mcg/mL)
Tonsil	1.6	0.8
Lung	8.8	1.7

Clarithromycin is active *in vitro* against a variety of aerobic and anaerobic gram-positive and gram-negative organisms. Additionally, the 14-OH clarithromycin metabolite also has clinically significant antimicrobial activity. Against *Haemophilus influenzae*, 14-OH clarithromycin is twice as active as the parent compound.
Clarithromycin has been shown to be active against most strains of the following organisms both *in vitro* and in clinical infections: (See INDICATIONS AND USAGE.)

Gram-positive aerobes
Staphylococcus aureus
Streptococcus pneumoniae
Streptococcus pyogenes
Gram-negative aerobes
Haemophilus influenzae
Moraxella (Branhamella) catarrhalis
Other aerobes
Mycoplasma pneumoniae
Beta-lactamase production should have no effect on clarithromycin activity.
NOTE: Most strains of methicillin-resistant and oxacillin-resistant staphylococci are resistant to clarithromycin.
Clarithromycin has been shown to be active *in vitro* against most strains of the following organisms. The following *in vitro* data are available; however, their clinical significance is unknown.

Gram-positive aerobes
Listeria monocytogenes
Streptococcus agalactiae
Streptococci (Groups C, F, G)
Viridans group streptococci
Gram-negative aerobes
Bordetella pertussis
Campylobacter jejuni
Legionella pneumophila
Neisseria gonorrhoeae
Pasteurella multocida
Other aerobes
Chlamydia trachomatis
Mycobacterium kansasii
Gram-positive anaerobes
Clostridium perfringens
Peptococcus niger
Propionibacterium acnes
Gram-negative anaerobes
Bacteroides melaninogenicus
Susceptibility Tests:
Diffusion Techniques:
Quantitative methods that require measurement of zone diameters give the most precise estimate of the susceptibility of bacteria to antimicrobial agents. One such standard procedure[1] which has been recommended for use with disks to test susceptibility of organisms to clarithromycin, uses the 15-mcg disk. Interpretation involves the correlation of the diameter obtained in the disk test with minumum inhibitory concentration (MIC) for clarithromycin.
Reports from the laboratory giving results of the standard single-disk susceptibility test with a 15-mcg clarithromycin disk should be interpreted according to the following criteria:

Zone Diameter (mm)	Interpretation
≥18	(S) Susceptible
14–17	(I) Intermediate
≤13	(R) Resistant

A report of 'Susceptible' indicates that the pathogen is likely to respond to monotherapy with clarithromycin.
A report of 'Intermediate' indicates that the result be considered equivocal and, if the organism is not fully susceptible to alternative clinically feasible drugs, the test should be repeated. This category provides a buffer zone which prevents small uncontrolled technical factors from causing major discrepancies in interpretations.
However, standardized diffusion methods for routine *in vitro* susceptibility testing, using the 15-mcg clarithromycin disk, do not measure the additive antimicrobial activity of the 14-OH metabolite and thus may underestimate the drug's potential activity against *Haemophilus influenzae*. *Haemophilus influenzae* isolates falling into the 'Intermediate' category often respond to treatment.
A report of 'Resistant' indicates that achievable drug concentrations are unlikely to be inhibitory, and other therapy should be selected.

Standardized procedures require the use of laboratory control organisms. The 15-mcg clarithromycin disk should give the following zone diameters:

Organism	Zone Diameter (mm)
S. aureus ATCC 25923	23–30

Dilution Techniques:
Use a standardized dilution method[2] (broth, agar, microdilution) or equivalent with clarithromycin powder. The MIC values obtained should be interpreted according to the following criteria:

MIC (mcg/mL)	Interpretation
≤2.0	(S) Susceptible
4.0	(I) Intermediate
≥8.0	(R) Resistant

As with standard diffusion techniques, dilution methods require the use of laboratory control organisms. Standard clarithromycin powder should provide the following MIC values:

Organism	MIC (mcg/mL)
S. aureus ATCC 29213	0.06–0.25
E. faecalis ATCC 29212	0.25–1.0

INDICATIONS AND USAGE

BIAXIN (clarithromycin) is indicated for the treatment of mild to moderate infections caused by susceptible strains of the designated microorganisms in the conditions listed below:
Upper Respiratory Tract Infections
  Pharyngitis/Tonsillitis due to *Streptococcus pyogenes*
  Acute maxillary sinusitis due to *Streptococcus pneumoniae*
Lower Respiratory Tract Infections
  Acute bacterial exacerbation of chronic bronchitis due to *Haemophilus influenzae*, *Moraxella catarrhalis*, or *Streptococcus pneumoniae*
  Pneumonia due to *Myocplasma pneumoniae*, or *Streptococcus pneumoniae*
Uncomplicated Skin and Skin Structure Infections due to *Staphylococcus aureus*, or *Streptococcus pyogenes*. Abscesses usually require surgical drainage.

CONTRAINDICATIONS

Clarithromycin is contraindicated in patients with known hypersensitivity to clarithromycin, erythromycin, or any of the macrolide antibiotics.

WARNINGS

CLARITHROMYCIN SHOULD NOT BE USED IN PREGNANT WOMEN EXCEPT IN CLINICAL CIRCUMSTANCES WHERE NO ALTERNATIVE THERAPY IS APPROPRIATE. IF PREGNANCY OCCURS WHILE TAKING THIS DRUG, THE PATIENT SHOULD BE APPRISED OF THE POTENTIAL HAZARD TO THE FETUS. CLARITHROMYCIN HAS DEMONSTRATED ADVERSE EFFECTS ON PREGNANCY OUTCOME AND/OR EMBRYO-FETAL DEVELOPMENT IN MONKEYS, RATS, MICE, AND RABBITS AT DOSES THAT PRODUCED PLASMA LEVELS 2 TO 17 TIMES THE SERUM LEVELS ACHIEVED IN HUMANS TREATED AT THE MAXIMUM RECOMMENDED HUMAN DOSES. (SEE PREGNANCY.)
Pseudomembranous colitis has been reported with nearly all antibacterial agents, including macrolides, and may range in severity from mild to life threatening. Therefore, it is important to consider this diagnosis in patients who present with diarrhea subsequent to the administration of antibacterial agents.
Treatment with antibacterial agents alters the normal flora of the colon and may permit overgrowth of clostridia. Studies indicate that a toxin produced by *Clostridium difficile* is a primary cause of 'antibiotic-associated colitis.'
After the diagnosis of pseudomembranous colitis has been established, therapeutic measures should be initiated. Mild cases of pseudomembranous colitis usually respond to discontinuation of the drug alone. In moderate to severe cases, consideration should be given to management with fluids and electrolytes, protein supplementation, and treatment with an antibacterial drug effective against *Clostridium difficile*.

PRECAUTIONS

General: Clarithromycin is principally excreted via the liver and kidney. Clarithromycin may be administered without dosage adjustment to patients with hepatic impairment and normal renal function. However, in the presence of severe renal impairment with or without coexisting hepatic impairment, decreased dosage or prolonged dosing intervals may be appropriate.
Drug Interactions: Clarithromycin use in patients who are receiving theophylline may be associated with an increase of serum theophylline concentrations. Monitoring of serum theophylline concentrations should be considered for pa-

tients receiving high doses of theophylline or with baseline concentrations in the upper therapeutic range. In two studies in which theophylline was administered with clarithromycin (a theophylline sustained-release formulation was dosed at either 6.5 mg/kg or 12 mg/kg together with 250 mg or 500 mg q 12 h clarithromycin), the steady-state levels of C_{max}, C_{min}, and the area under the serum concentration time curve (AUC) increased about 20%.

Single-dose administration of clarithromycin has been shown to result in increased concentrations of carbamazepine. Blood level monitoring of carbamazepine may be considered.

The following drug interactions have not been reported in clinical trials with clarithromycin; however, they have been observed with erythromycin products:

   Concomitant administration of erythromycin and digoxin has been reported to result in elevated digoxin levels.

   There have been reports of increased anticoagulant effects when erythromycin and oral anticoagulants were used concomitantly.

   Concurrent use of erythromycin and ergotamine or dihydroergotamine has been associated in some patients with acute ergot toxicity characterized by severe peripheral vasospasm and dysesthesia.

   Erythromycin has been reported to decrease the clearance of triazolam and thus may increase the pharmacologic effect of triazolam.

   The use of erythromycin in patients concurrently taking drugs metabolized by the cytochrome P450 system may be associated with elevations in serum levels of these other drugs. There have been reports of interactions of erythromycin with carbamazepine, cyclosporine, hexobarbital, and phenytoin. Serum concentrations of drugs metabolized by the cytochrome P450 system should be monitored closely in patients concurrently receiving erythromycin.

Carcinogenesis, Mutagenesis, Impairment of Fertility: The following *in vitro* mutagenicity tests have been conducted with clarithromycin:

   Salmonella/Mammalian Microsome Test
   Bacterial Induced Mutation Frequency Test
   In vitro Chromosome Aberration Test
   Rat Hepatocyte DNA Synthesis Assay
   Mouse Lymphoma Assay
   Mouse Dominant Lethal Study
   Mouse Micronucleus Test

All tests had negative results except the *In Vitro* Chromosome Aberration Test which was weakly positive in one test and negative in another.

In addition, a Bacterial Reserve-Mutation Test (Ames Test) has been performed on clarithromycin metabolites with negative results.

Fertility and reproduction studies have shown that daily doses of 150–160 mg/kg/day to male and female rats caused no adverse effects on the estrous cycle, fertility, parturition, or number and viability of offspring. Plasma levels in rats after 150 mg/kg/day were 2 times the human serum levels. In the 150 mg/kg/day monkey studies, plasma levels were 3 times the human serum levels. When given orally after the 150 mg/kg/day, clarithromycin was shown to produce embryonic loss in monkeys. This effect has been attributed to marked maternal toxicity of the drug at this high dose.

In rabbits, *in utero* fetal loss occurred at an intravenous dose of 33 mg/sq m, which is 17 times less than the maximum proposed human oral daily dose of 618 mg/sq m.

Long-term studies in animals have not been performed to evaluate carcinogenic potential.

Pregnancy: Teratogenic Effects: Pregnancy Category C. Four teratogenicity studies in rats (three with oral doses and one with intravenous doses up to 160 mg/kg/day administered during the period of major organogenesis) and two in rabbits (at oral doses up to 125 mg/kg/day or intravenous doses of 30 mg/kg/day administered during gestation days 6 to 18) failed to demonstrate any teratogenicity from clarithromycin. Two additional oral studies in a different rat strain at similar doses and similar conditions demonstrated a low incidence of cardiovascular anomalies at doses of 150 mg/kg/day administered during gestation days 6 to 15. Plasma levels after 150 mg/kg/day were 2 times the human serum levels. Four studies in mice revealed a variable incidence of cleft palate following oral doses of 1000 mg/kg/day during gestation days 6 to 15. Cleft palate was also seen at 500 mg/kg/day. The 1000 mg/kg/day exposure resulted in plasma levels 17 times the human serum levels. In monkeys, an oral dose of 70 mg/kg/day produced fetal growth retardation at plasma levels that were 2 times the human serum levels.

There are no adequate and well-controlled studies in pregnant women. Clarithromycin should be used during pregnancy only if the potential benefit justifies the potential risk to the fetus. (SEE WARNINGS.)

Nursing Mothers: It is not known whether clarithromycin is excreted in human milk. Because many drugs are excreted in human milk, caution should be exercised when clarithromycin is administered to a nursing woman. It is known that clarithromycin is excreted in the milk of lactating animals

DOSAGE GUIDELINES

Infection	Dosage (q 12 h)	Normal Duration (days)
Upper respiratory tract	250–500 mg	10–14
Pharyngitis/Tonsillitis	250 mg	10
Acute maxillary sinusitis	500 mg	14
Lower respiratory tract	250–500 mg	7–14
Acute exacerbation of chronic bronchitis due to:		
S. pneumoniae	250 mg	7–14
M. catarrhalis	250 mg	7–14
H. influenzae	500 mg	7–14
Pneumonia due to:		
S. pneumoniae	250 mg	7–14
M. pneumoniae	250 mg	7–14
Uncomplicated skin and skin structure	250 mg	7–14

and that other drugs of this class are excreted in human milk.

Pediatric Use: Safety and effectiveness of clarithromycin in children under 12 years of age have not been established.

Geriatric Use: In a steady-state study in which healthy elderly subjects (age 65 to 81 years old) were given 500 mg every 12 hours, the maximum concentrations of clarithromycin and 14-OH clarithromycin were increased. The AUC was also increased. These changes in pharmacokinetics parallel known age-related decreases in renal function. In clinical trials, elderly patients did not have an increased incidence of adverse events when compared to younger patients. Dosage adjustment should be considered in the elderly patients with severe renal impairment.

ADVERSE REACTIONS

The majority of side effects observed in clinical trials were of a mild and transient nature. Fewer than 3% of patients discontinued therapy because of drug-related side effects.

The most frequently reported events, whether drug-related or not, were diarrhea (3%), nausea (3%), abnormal taste (3%), dyspepsia (2%), abdominal pain/discomfort (2%), and headache (2%). Most of these events were described as mild or moderate in severity. Of the reported adverse events, only 1% were described as severe.

In studies of pneumonia comparing clarithromycin to erythromycin base or erythromycin stearate, there were fewer adverse events involving the digestive system in clarithromycin-treated patients compared to erythromycin-treated patients (13% vs 32%; p < 0.01). Twenty percent of erythromycin-treated patients discontinued therapy due to adverse events compared to 4% of clarithromycin-treated patients.

The following adverse events have been reported with erythromycin products but not in clinical trials of clarithromycin: Rarely, erythromycin has been associated with ventricular arrhythmias, including ventricular tachycardia, and torsades de pointes, in individuals with prolonged QT intervals.

Changes in Laboratory Values: Changes in laboratory values with possible clinical significance were as follows:

Hepatic—Elevated SGPT (ALT) <1%, SGOT (AST) <1%, GGT <1%, alkaline phosphatase <1%, LDH <1%, and total billirubin <1%.

Hematologic—Decreased WBC <1%, and elevated prothrombin time 1%.

Renal—Elevated BUN 4%, and elevated serum creatinine <1%.

DOSAGE AND ADMINISTRATION

BIAXIN (clarithromycin) tablets may be given with or without meals.

[See table above.]

Beta-lactamase production should have no effect on clarithromycin activity.

Clarithromycin may be administered without dosage adjustment in the presence of hepatic impairment if there is normal renal function. However, in the presence of severe renal impairment with or without coexisting hepatic impairment, decreased doses or prolongation of dosing intervals may be appropriate.

HOW SUPPLIED

BIAXIN (clarithromycin) tablets are supplied as yellow oval film-coated tablets in the following strengths and package sizes:

250 mg tablets:
Bottles of 60 ....(NDC 0074-3368-60)
ABBO-PAC® unit dose strip
packages of 100 ....(NDC 0074-3368-11)
500 mg tablets:
Bottles of 60 ....(NDC 0074-2586-60)
ABBO-PAC® unit dose packages
of 100 ....(NDC 0074-2586-11)

Store tablets at controlled room temperature 15° to 30°C (59° to 86°F) in a well-closed container. Protect from light.

ANIMAL PHARMACOLOGY AND TOXICOLOGY

Clarithromycin is rapidly and well-absorbed with dose-linear kinetics, low protein binding, and a high volume of distribution. Plasma half-life ranged from 1–6 hours and was species dependent. High tissue concentrations were achieved, but negligible accumulation was observed. Fecal clearance predominated. Hepatotoxicity occurred in all species tested (i.e., in rats and monkeys at doses 2 times greater than and in dogs at doses comparable to the maximum human daily dose, based on a mg/sq m basis). Renal tubular degeneration (calculated on a mg/sq m basis) occurred in rats at doses 2 times, in monkeys at doses 8 times, and in dogs at doses 12 times greater than the maximum human daily dose. Testicular atrophy (on a mg/sq m basis) occurred in rats at doses 7 times, in dogs at doses 3 times, and in monkeys at doses 8 times greater than the maximum human daily dose. Corneal opacity (on a mg/sq m basis) occurred in dogs at doses 12 times and in monkeys at doses 8 times greater than the maximum human daily dose. Lymphoid depletion (on a mg/sq m basis) occurred in dogs at doses 3 times greater than and in monkeys at doses 2 times greater than the maximum human daily dose. These adverse events were absent during clinical trials.

REFERENCES

1. National Committee for Clinical Laboratory Standards. *Performance Standards for Antimicrobial Disk Susceptibility Tests*—Fourth Edition. Approved Standard NCCLS Document M2-A4, Vol. 10, No. 7, NCCLS, Villanova, PA, 1990.
2. National Committee for Clinical Laboratory Standards. *Methods for Dilution Antimicrobial Susceptibility Tests for Bacteria that Grow Aerobically*—Second Edition. Approved Standard NCCLS Document M7-A2, Vol. 10, No. 8, NCCLS, Villanova, PA, 1990.
Ref. 03-4444-R3
   Shown in Product Identification Section, page 403

BUTESIN® PICRATE Ointment   **OTC**
[*bū'ti-sin pick'rate*]
(butamben picrate)

DESCRIPTION

Butesin Picrate is an anesthetic ointment containing Butesin Picrate (Butamben Picrate), 1%.

Inactive Ingredients: Anhydrous lanolin, ceresin wax, methylparaben, mineral oil, mixed triglycerides, potassium chloride, propylparaben, sodium borate, water, and white wax.

INDICATION

For temporary relief of pain due to minor burns.

WARNING

Certain persons, due to idiosyncrasy, are sensitive to this ointment and may develop a rash following its application. In such cases its use should be discontinued, and the ointment remaining on the skin removed with soap and water.

PRECAUTIONS

Should not be applied repeatedly or to large areas except under a physician's instructions.

Continued on next page

If desired, additional literature on any Abbott product will be provided upon request to Abbott Laboratories.

Abbott Laboratories—Cont.

Butamben Picrate stains cannot be removed. Contact with fabrics and hair should be avoided.

DOSAGE AND ADMINISTRATION

Spread thinly on painful or denuded lesions of the skin, if these are small. Apply a loose bandage to protect the clothing.

HOW SUPPLIED

1 oz tube (**NDC** 0074-4392-01).
Store below 77°F (25°C).

Ref. 09-6440-3/R6

CALCIDRINE® SYRUP ℞ Ⓒ

[*cal'si-drīne*]

DESCRIPTION

Calcidrine is an oral antitussive, expectorant syrup. Each 5 ml (teaspoonful) contains Codeine, USP, 8.4 mg, (Warning—May be habit forming); Calcium Iodide, anhydrous 152 mg. The chemical formula for calcium iodide is CaI_2. Codeine is methylmorphine, a natural alkaloid of opium. The chemical formula for codeine is $C_{18}H_{21}NO_3 \cdot H_2O$.

Inactive Ingredients: Alcohol 6%, FD&C Yellow No. 6, glycerin, liquid glucose, sucrose, water, natural and artificial flavors and other ingredients to form a palatable syrup.

CLINICAL PHARMACOLOGY

The major effects of codeine in man are on the central nervous system. The antitussive effect is produced by depression of the cough reflex. Codeine is rapidly absorbed from the gastrointestinal tract and is metabolized in the liver.

Iodides are readily absorbed from the gastrointestinal tract and are distributed to extracellular fluid as well as gastric and salivary secretions. Iodides are accumulated by the thyroid gland. Excretion occurs mainly through the kidneys.

INDICATIONS AND USAGE

In adults and children as an expectorant, and for symptomatic relief of coughs.

CONTRAINDICATIONS

Calcidrine should not be used in patients with a history of iodism, or with known hypersensitivity to iodides or codeine. Long-term use of iodide-containing preparations is contraindicated during pregnancy.

WARNINGS

Physiological dependence may develop with the use of codeine.

Usage During Pregnancy: Calcidrine Syrup can cause fetal harm when administered to a pregnant woman. Maternal ingestion of large amounts of iodides during pregnancy has been associated with development of fetal goiter and resultant acute respiratory distress of the neonate. If this drug is used during pregnancy, or if the patient becomes pregnant while taking this drug, the patient should be apprised of the potential hazard to the fetus.

Severe and occasionally fatal skin eruptions have been reported rarely in patients receiving prolonged administration of iodides.

PRECAUTIONS

Laboratory Tests: Patients who must receive prolonged iodide therapy should be evaluated periodically for possible depression of thyroid function.

Drug Interactions: The concurrent administration of calcium iodide and lithium carbonate may enhance the hypothyroid and goitrogenic effects of either drug.

Laboratory Test Interactions: Elevated values may be obtained on thyroid function tests or protein-bound iodine tests when iodide-containing compounds have been ingested. False positive results may be obtained if iodides have been ingested prior to guaiac or benzidine testing.

Carcinogenesis: No data is available on long-term carcinogenicity in animals or humans.

Pregnancy: Pregnancy Category D. See "WARNINGS" section.

Nursing Mothers: Iodine is excreted in breast milk. Caution should be exercised when Calcidrine is administered to a nursing woman.

ADVERSE REACTIONS

In decreasing order of severity: severe and sometimes fatal skin eruptions (ioderma) occur rarely after the prolonged use of iodides. Iodism can occur. Symptoms of iodism include metallic taste, acneform skin lesions, mucous membrane irritation, salivary gland swelling, and gastric distress. These side effects subside quickly upon discontinuance of the iodide-containing drug.

Codeine may produce vomiting, nausea, and constipation.

OVERDOSAGE

Symptoms of acute codeine poisoning include respiratory and central nervous system depression, pinpoint pupils and coma. Blood pressure and body temperature may fall.

Acute iodide poisoning is associated with gastrointestinal irritation. Angioedema with laryngeal swelling may develop. Shock may also occur.

Treatment for overdose of Calcidrine is:

a. Establish a patent airway and ventilate if needed. b. Gastric evacuation. c. Treatment for shock. d. General supportive measures including replacement of fluids and electrolytes may be indicated. e. The use of naloxone to antagonize the narcotic depression of the central nervous system should be considered.

DOSAGE AND ADMINISTRATION

Adults and children over ten years of age, usual dose, 1 to 2 teaspoonfuls every 4 hours. Children 6 to 10 years of age, ½ to 1 teaspoonful every 4 hours. Children 2 to 6 years of age, ½ teaspoonful every 4 hours.

HOW SUPPLIED

Orange-colored syrup in pint bottles (**NDC** 0074-5763-16).
Calcidrine must be dispensed in USP tight, light-resistant glass containers.
Store below 86°F (30°C).
Ref. 02-7353-2/R10

CALCIJEX® ℞

CALCITRIOL INJECTION
1 mcg and 2 mcg/mL

DESCRIPTION

Calcijex® (calcitriol injection) is synthetically manufactured calcitriol and is available as a sterile, isotonic, clear, aqueous solution for intravenous injection. Calcijex is available in 1 mL ampuls. Each 1 mL contains calcitriol, 1 or 2 mcg; Polysorbate 20, 4 mg; sodium chloride 1.5 mg; sodium ascorbate 10 mg added; dibasic sodium phosphate, anhydrous 7.6 mg; monobasic sodium phosphate, monohydrate 1.8 mg; edetate disodium, dihydrate 1.1 mg added. pH 7.2 (6.5 to 8.0).

Calcitriol is a colorless, crystalline compound which occurs naturally in humans. It is soluble in organic solvents but relatively insoluble in water. Calcitriol is chemically designated (5Z,7E)-9, 10-secocholesta-5,7,10(19)-triene-1α,3β,25-triol and has the following structural formula:

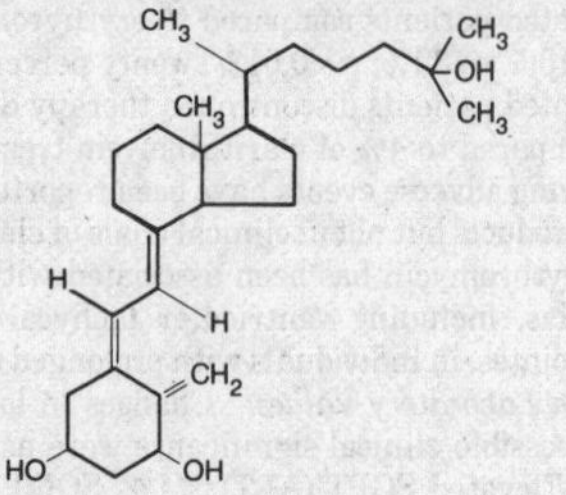

Molecular Formula: $C_{27}H_{44}O_3$

The other names frequently used for calcitriol are 1α, 25-dihydroxycholecalciferol, 1α,25-dihydroxyvitamin D_3, 1,25-DHCC, 1,25$(OH)_2D_3$ and 1,25-diOHC.

CLINICAL PHARMACOLOGY

Calcitriol is the active form of vitamin D_3 (cholecalciferol). The natural or endogenous supply of vitamin D in man mainly depends on ultraviolet light for conversion of 7-dehydrocholesterol to vitamin D_3 in the skin. Vitamin D_3 must be metabolically activated in the liver and the kidney before it is fully active on its target tissues. The initial transformation is catalyzed by a vitamin D_3-25-hydroxylase enzyme present in the liver, and the product of this reaction is 25-$(OH)D_3$ (calcifediol). The latter undergoes hydroxylation in the mitochondria of kidney tissue, and this reaction is activated by the renal 25-hydroxyvitamin D_3-1-α-hydroxylase to produce 1,25-$(OH)_2D_3$ (calcitriol), the active form of vitamin D_3.

The known sites of action of calcitriol are intestine, bone, kidney and parathyroid gland. Calcitriol is the most active known form of vitamin D_3 in stimulating intestinal calcium transport. In acutely uremic rats, calcitriol has been shown to stimulate intestinal calcium absorption. In bone, calcitriol, in conjunction with parathyroid hormone, stimulates resorption of calcium; and in the kidney, calcitriol increases the tubular reabsorption of calcium. In-vitro and in-vivo studies have shown that calcitriol directly suppresses secretion and synthesis of PTH. A vitamin D-resistant state may exist in uremic patients because of the failure of the kidney to adequately convert precursors to the active compound, calcitriol.

Calcitriol when administered by bolus injection is rapidly available in the blood stream. Vitamin D metabolites are known to be transported in blood, bound to specific plasma proteins. The pharmacologic activity of an administered dose of calcitriol is about 3 to 5 days. Two metabolic pathways for calcitriol have been identified, conversion to 1,24,25-$(OH)_3D_3$ and to calcitroic acid.

INDICATIONS AND USAGE

Calcijex® (calcitriol injection) is indicated in the management of hypocalcemia in patients undergoing chronic renal dialysis. It has been shown to significantly reduce elevated parathyroid hormone levels. Reduction of PTH has been shown to result in an improvement in renal osteodystrophy.

CONTRAINDICATIONS

Calcijex® (calcitriol injection) should not be given to patients with hypercalcemia or evidence of vitamin D toxicity.

WARNINGS

Since calcitriol is the most potent metabolite of vitamin D available, vitamin D and its derivatives should be withheld during treatment.

A non-aluminum phosphate-binding compound should be used to control serum phosphorus levels in patients undergoing dialysis.

Overdosage of any form of vitamin D is dangerous (see also OVERDOSAGE). Progressive hypercalcemia due to overdosage of vitamin D and its metabolites may be so severe as to require emergency attention. Chronic hypercalcemia can lead to generalized vascular calcification, nephrocalcinosis and other soft-tissue calcification. The serum calcium times phosphate (Ca × P) product should not be allowed to exceed 70. Radiographic evaluation of suspect anatomical regions may be useful in the early detection of this condition.

PRECAUTIONS

1. **General**
Excessive dosage of Calcijex® (calcitriol injection) induces hypercalcemia and in some instances hypercalciuria; therefore, early in treatment during dosage adjustment, serum calcium and phosphorus should be determined at least twice weekly. Should hypercalcemia develop, the drug should be discontinued immediately.
Calcijex should be given cautiously to patients on digitalis, because hypercalcemia in such patients may precipitate cardiac arrhythmias.
2. **Information for the Patient**
The patient and his or her parents should be informed about adherence to instructions about diet and calcium supplementation and avoidance of the use of unapproved nonprescription drugs, including magnesium-containing antacids. Patients should also be carefully informed about the symptoms of hypercalcemia (see ADVERSE REACTIONS).
3. **Essential Laboratory Tests**
Serum calcium, phosphorus, magnesium and alkaline phosphatase and 24-hour urinary calcium and phosphorus should be determined periodically. During the initial phase of the medication, serum calcium and phosphorus should be determined more frequently (twice weekly).
4. **Drug Interactions**
Magnesium-containing antacid and Calcijex should not be used concomitantly, because such use may lead to the development of hypermagnesemia.
5. **Carcinogenesis, Mutagenesis, Impairment of Fertility**
Long-term studies in animals have not been performed to evaluate the carcinogenic potential of Calcijex (calcitriol injection). There was no evidence of mutagenicity as studied by the Ames Method. No significant effects of calcitriol on fertility were reported using oral Calcitriol.
6. **Use in Pregnancy:** *Pregnancy Category C:*
Calcitriol given orally has been reported to be teratogenic in rabbits when given in doses 4 and 15 times the dose recommended for human use.
All 15 fetuses in 3 litters at these doses showed external and skeletal abnormalities. However, none of the other 23 litters (156 fetuses) showed significant abnormalities compared with controls.
Teratology studies in rats showed no evidence of teratogenic potential. There are no adequate and well-controlled studies in pregnant women. Calcijex should be used during pregnancy only if the potential benefit justifies the potential risk to the fetus.
7. **Nursing Mothers**
It is not known whether this drug is excreted in human milk. Because many drugs are excreted in human milk and because of the potential for serious adverse reactions in nursing infants from calcitriol, a decision should be made whether to discontinue nursing or to discontinue the drug, taking into account the importance of the drug to the mother.
8. **Pediatric Use**
Safety and efficacy of Calcijex in children have not been established.

ADVERSE REACTIONS

Adverse effects of Calcijex® (calcitriol injection) are, in general, similar to those encountered with excessive vitamin

D intake. The early and late signs and symptoms of vitamin D intoxication associated with hypercalcemia include:

1. **Early**
   Weakness, headache, somnolence, nausea, vomiting, dry mouth, constipation, muscle pain, bone pain and metallic taste.
2. **Late**
   Polyuria, polydipsia, anorexia, weight loss, nocturia, conjunctivitis (calcific), pancreatitis, photophobia, rhinorrhea, pruritus, hyperthermia, decreased libido, elevated BUN, albuminuria, hypercholesterolemia, elevated SGOT and SGPT, ectopic calcification, hypertension, cardiac arrhythmias and, rarely, overt psychosis.

Occasional mild pain on injection has been observed.

OVERDOSAGE

Administration of Calcijex® (calcitriol injection) to patients in excess of their requirements can cause hypercalcemia, hypercalciuria and hyperphosphatemia. High intake of calcium and phosphate concomitant with Calcijex may lead to similar abnormalities.

1. **Treatment of Hypercalcemia and Overdosage in Patients on Hemodialysis**
   General treatment of hypercalcemia (greater than 1 mg/dl above the upper limit of normal range) consists of immediate discontinuation of Calcijex therapy, institution of a low calcium diet and withdrawal of calcium supplements. Serum calcium levels should be determined daily until normocalcemia ensues. Hypercalcemia usually resolves in two to seven days. When serum calcium levels have returned to within normal limits, Calcijex therapy may be reinstituted at a dose 0.5 mcg less than prior therapy. Serum calcium levels should be obtained at least twice weekly after all dosage changes.
   Persistent or markedly elevated serum calcium levels may be corrected by dialysis against a calcium-free dialysate.
2. **Treatment of Accidental Overdosage of Calcitriol Injection**
   The treatment of acute accidental overdosage of Calcijex should consist of general supportive measures. Serial serum electrolyte determinations (especially calcium), rate of urinary calcium excretion and assessment of electrocardiographic abnormalities due to hypercalcemia should be obtained. Such monitoring is critical in patients receiving digitalis. Discontinuation of supplemental calcium and low calcium diet are also indicated in accidental overdosage. Due to the relatively short duration of the pharmacological action of calcitriol, further measures are probably unnecessary. Should, however, persistent and markedly elevated serum calcium levels occur, there are a variety of therapeutic alternatives which may be considered, depending on the patients' underlying condition. These include the use of drugs such as phosphates and corticosteroids as well as measures to induce an appropriate forced diuresis. The use of peritoneal dialysis against a calcium-free dialysate has also been reported.

DOSAGE AND ADMINISTRATION

The optimal dose of Calcijex® (calcitriol injection) must be carefully determined for each patient.

The effectiveness of Calcijex therapy is predicated on the assumption that each patient is receiving an adequate and appropriate daily intake of calcium. The RDA for calcium in adults is 800 mg. To ensure that each patient receives an adequate daily intake of calcium, the physician should either prescribe a calcium supplement or instruct the patient in proper dietary measures.

The recommended initial dose of Calcijex is 0.5 mcg (0.01 mcg/kg) administered three times weekly, approximately every other day. Calcijex can be administered as a bolus dose intravenously through the catheter at the end of hemodialysis. If a satisfactory response in the biochemical parameters and clinical manifestations of the disease state is not observed, the dose may be increased by 0.25 to 0.50 mcg at two to four week intervals. During this titration period, serum calcium and phosphorus levels should be obtained at least twice weekly, and if hypercalcemia is noted, the drug should be immediately discontinued until normocalcemia ensues.

Most patients undergoing hemodialysis respond to doses between 0.5 and 3.0 mcg (0.01 to 0.05 mcg/kg) three times per week.

Parenteral drug products should be inspected visually for particulate matter and discoloration prior to administration, whenever solution and container permit.

Discard unused portion.

HOW SUPPLIED

Calcijex® (calcitriol injection) is supplied in 1 mL ampuls containing 1 mcg (List No. 1200) and 2 mcg (List No. 1210).

Protect from light.

Store at controlled room temperature 15° to 30°C (59° to 86°F).

Caution: Federal (USA) law prohibits dispensing without prescription.

©Abbott 1986 06-4630-R5-Rev. Oct, 1990

ABBOTT LABORATORIES, NORTH CHICAGO, IL 60064, USA

CARTROL® ℞

[*kär 'trōl*]

(carteolol hydrochloride)

Filmtab® Tablets

DESCRIPTION

CARTROL (carteolol hydrochloride) is a synthetic, nonselective, beta-adrenergic receptor blocking agent with intrinsic sympathomimetic activity. It is chemically described as 5-[3-[(1,1-dimethylethyl) amino]-2-hydroxypropoxy]-3,4-dihydro-2(1H)-quinolinone monohydrochloride.

Carteolol hydrochloride is a stable, white crystalline powder which is soluble in water and slightly soluble in ethanol. The molecular weight is 328.84 and $C_{16}H_{24}N_2O_3 \cdot HCl$ is the empirical formula.

CARTROL (carteolol hydrochloride) is available as tablets containing either 2.5 mg or 5 mg of carteolol hydrochloride for oral administration.

INACTIVE INGREDIENTS

2.5 mg Tablet: Cellulosic polymers, corn starch, iron oxide, lactose, magnesium stearate, microcrystalline cellulose, polyethylene glycol, propylene glycol, and titanium dioxide.

5 mg Tablet: Cellulosic polymers, corn starch, lactose, magnesium stearate, microcrystalline cellulose, polyethylene glycol, propylene glycol, and titanium dioxide.

CLINICAL PHARMACOLOGY

CARTROL (carteolol hydrochloride) is a long-acting, nonselective, beta-adrenergic receptor blocking agent with intrinsic sympathomimetic activity (ISA) and without significant membrane stabilizing (local anesthetic) activity.

Pharmacodynamics:

Carteolol specifically competes with beta-adrenergic receptor agonists for both $beta_1$-receptors located principally in cardiac muscle and $beta_2$-receptors located in the bronchial and vascular musculature, blocking the chronotropic, inotropic, and vasodilator responses to beta-adrenergic stimulation proportionately. Because of its partial agonist activity, however, carteolol does not reduce resting beta-agonist activity as much as beta-adrenergic blockers lacking this activity. Thus, in clinical trials in man, the decreases in resting pulse rate produced by carteolol (2–5 beats per minute in various studies) were less than those produced by beta-blockers (nadolol and propranolol) without ISA (10–12 beats per minute). There are also equivocal effects on renin secretion, in contrast to beta-blockers without ISA, which inhibit renin secretion.

In controlled clinical trials carteolol, at doses up to 20 mg as monotherapy or in combination with thiazide type diuretics, produced significantly greater reductions in blood pressure than did placebo, with the full effect seen between two and four weeks. The observed differences from placebo ranged from 3.1 to 6.7 mmHg for supine diastolic blood pressure. The antihypertensive effects of carteolol are smaller in black populations but do not seem to be affected by age or sex. Doses of carteolol greater than 10 mg once a day did not produce greater reductions in blood pressure. In fact, doses of 20 mg and above appeared to produce blood pressure reductions less than those produced by 10 mg and below. When carteolol was compared to nadolol and propranolol, although the differences were not statistically significant in relatively small studies, carteolol at doses up to 20 mg produced supine diastolic blood pressure changes consistently 2 mmHg less than that produced by either nadolol or propranolol.

Although the mechanism of the antihypertensive effect of beta-adrenergic blocking agents has not been established, multiple factors are thought to contribute to the lowering of blood pressure, including diminished response to sympathetic nerve outflow from vasomotor centers in the brain, diminished release of renin from the kidneys, and decreased cardiac output. Carteolol does not have a consistent effect on renin and other agents with ISA have been shown to have less effect than other beta-blockers on resting cardiac output (although they cause the usual decrease in exercise cardiac output so that the difference is of uncertain clinical importance), so that the mechanism of its action is particularly uncertain.

Beta-blockade interferes with endogenous adrenergic bronchodilator activity and diminishes the response to exogenous bronchodilators. This is especially important in patients subject to bronchospasm.

Single intravenous doses of carteolol (0.5 mg, 1 mg, 2.5 mg and 5 mg) produced statistically, but not clinically, significant increases from baseline in AV node conduction time and RR and PR intervals.

CARTROL (carteolol hydrochloride) induced no significant alteration in total serum cholesterol and triglycerides.

Following discontinuation of carteolol treatment in man, pharmacologic activity (evaluated by blockade of the tachycardia induced by isoproterenol or postural changes) is present for 2 to 21 days (median 14 days) after the last dose of carteolol. Following administration of recommended doses of CARTROL (carteolol hydrochloride), both beta-blocking and antihypertensive effects persist for at least 24 hours.

Pharmacokinetics and Metabolism:

Following oral administration in man, peak plasma concentrations of carteolol usually occur within one to three hours. Carteolol is well absorbed when administered orally as CARTROL (carteolol hydrochloride) tablets. The presence of food in the gastrointestinal tract somewhat slows the rate of absorption, but the extent of absorption is not appreciably affected. Compared to intravenous administration, the absolute bioavailability of carteolol from CARTROL (carteolol hydrochloride) tablets is approximately 85%.

The plasma half-life of carteolol averages approximately six hours. Steady-state serum levels are achieved within one to two days after initiating therapeutic doses of carteolol in persons with normal renal function. Since approximately 50 to 70% of a carteolol dose is eliminated unchanged by the kidneys, the half-life is increased in patients with impaired renal function. Significant reductions in the rate of carteolol elimination (and prolongations of the half-life) occur in patients as creatinine clearance decreases. Therefore, a reduction in maintenance dose and/or prolongation in dosing interval is appropriate (see DOSAGE and ADMINISTRATION).

Carteolol is 23–30% bound to plasma proteins in humans. The major metabolites of carteolol are 8-hydroxycarteolol and the glucuronic acid conjugates of both carteolol and 8-hydroxycarteolol. In man, 8-hydroxycarteolol is an active metabolite with a half-life of approximately 8 to 12 hours and represents approximately 5% of the administered dose excreted in the urine.

INDICATIONS AND USAGE

CARTROL (carteolol hydrochloride) is indicated in the management of hypertension. It may be used alone or in combination with other antihypertensive agents, especially thiazide diuretics. Preliminary data indicate that carteolol does not have a favorable effect on arrhythmias.

CONTRAINDICATIONS

CARTROL (carteolol hydrochloride) is contraindicated in patients with: 1) bronchial asthma, 2) severe bradycardia, 3) greater than first degree heart block, 4) cardiogenic shock, and 5) clinically evident congestive heart failure (see WARNINGS).

WARNINGS

Congestive Heart Failure:

Sympathetic stimulation may be a vital component supporting circulatory function in patients with congestive heart failure, and impairing that support by beta-blockade may precipitate more severe decompensation. Although CARTROL (carteolol hydrochloride) should be avoided in clinically evident congestive heart failure, it can be used with caution, if necessary, in patients with a history of failure who are well-compensated and are receiving digitalis and diuretics. Beta-adrenergic blocking agents do not abolish the inotropic action of digitalis on heart muscle.

IN PATIENTS WITHOUT A HISTORY OF CONGESTIVE HEART FAILURE, the use of beta-blockers can, in some instances, lead to congestive heart failure. Therefore, at the first sign or symptom of cardiac decompensation, discontinuation of beta-blocker therapy should be considered. The patient should be closely observed and treatment should include a diuretic and/or digitalization as necessary.

Exacerbation of Angina Pectoris Upon Withdrawal:

In patients with angina pectoris, exacerbation of angina and, in some cases, myocardial infarction have been reported following abrupt discontinuation of therapy with some beta-blockers. Therefore such patients should be cautioned against interruption of therapy without a physician's advice. The long persistence of beta-adrenergic blockade following abrupt discontinuation of CARTROL (carteolol hydrochloride), however, might be expected to minimize the possibility of this complication. When discontinuation of CARTROL (carteolol hydrochloride) is planned, dosage should be tapered gradually, as it is with other beta-blockers. If exacerbation of angina occurs when CARTROL (carteolol hydrochloride) therapy is interrupted, it is advisable to reinstitute CARTROL (carteolol hydrochloride) or other beta-blocker therapy, at least temporarily, and to take other measures appropriate for the management of unstable angina pectoris.

PATIENTS WITHOUT CLINICALLY RECOGNIZED ANGINA PECTORIS should be carefully monitored after withdrawal of CARTROL (carteolol hydrochloride) therapy, since coronary artery disease may be unrecognized.

Nonallergic Bronchospasm (e.g., chronic bronchitis, emphysema):

Patients with bronchospastic disease generally should not receive beta-blocker therapy and carteolol is contraindicated in patients with bronchial asthma. If use of CARTROL (carteolol hydrochloride) is essential, it should be administered with caution since it may block bronchodilation produced by

Continued on next page

If desired, additional literature on any Abbott product will be provided upon request to Abbott Laboratories.

Abbott Laboratories—Cont.

endogenous catecholamine stimulation of beta$_2$-receptors or diminish response to therapy with a beta-receptor agonist.

Major Surgery:
The necessity, or desirability, of withdrawal of beta-blocking therapy prior to major surgery is controversial. Because beta-blockade impairs the ability of the heart to respond to reflex stimuli and may increase risks of general anesthesia and surgical procedures resulting in protracted hypotension or low cardiac output, and difficulty in restarting or maintaining a heartbeat, it has been suggested that beta-blocker therapy should be withdrawn several days prior to surgery. It is also recognized, however, that increased sensitivity to catecholamines of patients recently withdrawn from beta-blocker therapy could increase certain risks. Given the persistence of the beta-blocking activity of CARTROL (carteolol hydrochloride), effective withdrawal would take several weeks and would ordinarily be impractical. When beta-blocker therapy is not discontinued, anesthetic agents that depress the myocardium should be avoided. In one study using intravenous carteolol during surgery, recovery from anesthesia was somewhat delayed in three patients who received carteolol near the end of anesthesia, and respiratory arrest occurred in one of these patients immediately following administration of intravenous carteolol.

In the event that CARTROL (carteolol hydrochloride) treatment is not discontinued before surgery, the anesthesiologist should be informed that the patient is receiving CARTROL (carteolol hydrochloride). The effects on the heart of beta-adrenergic blocking agents, such as CARTROL (carteolol hydrochloride), may be reversed by cautious administration of isoproterenol or dobutamine.

Diabetes Mellitus and Hypoglycemia:
Beta-adrenergic blockade may prevent the appearance of premonitory signs and symptoms (e.g., tachycardia and blood pressure changes) of acute hypoglycemia, and it inhibits glycogenolysis, a normal compensatory mechanism for hypoglycemia. This is especially important for patients with labile diabetes mellitus. Beta-blockade also reduces the release of insulin in response to hyperglycemia; therefore, it may be necessary to adjust the dose of antidiabetic agents used to treat hyperglycemia.

Thyrotoxicosis:
Beta-adrenergic blockade may mask certain clinical signs of hyperthyroidism such as tachycardia. Patients suspected of having thyrotoxicosis should be managed carefully to avoid abrupt withdrawal of beta-adrenergic blockade which might precipitate a thyroid storm.

PRECAUTIONS

General:
Impaired Renal Function:
CARTROL (carteolol hydrochloride) should be used with caution in patients with impaired renal function. Patients with impaired renal function clear carteolol at a reduced rate, and dosage should be reduced accordingly (see Dosage and Administration).

Beta-adrenoreceptor blockade can cause reduction in intraocular pressure. Therefore, CARTROL (carteolol hydrochloride) may interfere with glaucoma testing. Withdrawal may lead to a return of increased intraocular pressure.

Information for Patients:
Patients, especially those with evidence of coronary artery insufficiency, should be warned against interruption or discontinuation of CARTROL (carteolol hydrochloride) therapy without the physician's advice. Although cardiac failure rarely occurs in properly selected patients, patients being treated with beta-adrenergic blocking agents should be advised to consult the physician at the first sign or symptom of impending failure (i.e., fatigue with exertion, difficulty breathing, cough or unusually fast heartbeat).

Drug Interactions:
Catecholamine-depleting drugs (e.g., reserpine) may have an additive effect when given with beta-blocking agents. Therefore, patients treated with CARTROL (carteolol hydrochloride) plus a catecholamine-depleting agent must be observed carefully for evidence of hypotension and/or excessive bradycardia, which may produce syncope or postural hypotension.

Risk of Anaphylactic Reaction: While taking beta-blockers, patients with a history of severe anaphylactic reaction to a variety of allergens may be more reactive to repeated challenge, either accidental, diagnostic, or therapeutic. Such patients may be unresponsive to the usual doses of epinephrine used to treat allergic reaction.

Concurrent administration of *general anesthetics* and beta-blocking agents may result in exaggeration of the hypotension induced by general anesthetics (see WARNINGS, Major Surgery).

Blunting of the antihypertensive effect of beta-adrenoreceptor blocking agents by *non-steroidal anti-inflammatory drugs* has been reported. When using these agents concomitantly, patients should be observed carefully to confirm that the desired therapeutic effect has been obtained.

TABLE 1
Adverse Reactions During
Placebo-Controlled Studies

	Placebo (n=448) %	Carteolol (n=761) %
Body as a Whole		
†Asthenia	4.0	7.1*
Abdominal Pain	0.4	1.3
Back Pain	1.6	2.1
Chest Pain	1.8	2.2
Digestive System		
Diarrhea	2.0	2.1
Nausea	1.8	2.1
Metabolic/Nutritional Disorders		
Abnormal Lab Test	1.1	1.2
Peripheral Edema	1.1	1.7
Musculoskeletal System		
Arthralgia	1.1	1.2
Muscle Cramps	0.2	2.6*
Lower Extremity Pain	0.2	1.2
Nervous System		
Insomnia	0.7	1.7
Paresthesia	1.1	2.0
Respiratory System		
Nasal Congestion	0.9	1.1
Pharyngitis	0.9	1.1
Skin and Appendages		
Rash	1.1	1.3

† Includes weakness, tiredness, lassitude and fatigue.
* Statistically significant at p=0.05 level.

Literature reports suggest that *oral calcium antagonists* may be used in combination with beta-adrenergic blocking agents when heart function is normal, but should be avoided in patients with impaired cardiac function. Hypotension, AV conduction disturbances, and left ventricular failure have been reported in some patients receiving beta-adrenergic blocking agents when an oral calcium antagonist was added to the treatment regimen. Hypotension was more likely to occur if the calcium antagonist were a dihydropyridine derivative, e.g., nifedipine, while left ventricular failure and AV conduction disturbances were more likely to occur with either verapamil or diltiazem.

Intravenous calcium antagonists should be used with caution in patients receiving beta-adrenergic blocking agents. The concomitant use of beta-adrenergic blocking agents with digitalis and either diltiazem or verapamil may have additive effects in prolonging AV conduction time.

Concomitant use of oral antidiabetic agents or *insulin* with beta-blocking agents may be associated with hypoglycemia or possibly hyperglycemia. Dosage of the antidiabetic agent should be adjusted accordingly (see WARNINGS, Diabetes Mellitus and Hypoglycemia).

Carcinogenesis, Mutagenesis, Impairment of Fertility:
CARTROL (carteolol hydrochloride) did not produce carcinogenic effects at doses 280 times the maximum recommended human dose (10 mg/70 kg/day) in two-year oral rat and mouse studies.

Tests of mutagenicity, including the Ames Test, recombinant (rec)-assay, *in vivo* cytogenetics and dominant lethal assay demonstrated no evidence for mutagenic potential.

Fertility of male and female rats and male and female mice was unaffected by administration of CARTROL (carteolol hydrochloride) at dosages up to 150 mg/kg/day. This dosage is approximately 1052 times the maximum recommended human dose.

Pregnancy:
Teratogenic Effects: Pregnancy Category C. CARTROL (carteolol hydrochloride) increased resorptions and decreased fetal weights in rabbits and rats at maternally toxic doses approximately 1052 and 5264 times the maximum recommended human dose (10 mg/70 kg/day), respectively. A dose-related increase in wavy ribs was noted in the developing rat fetus when pregnant females received daily doses of approximately 212 times the maximum recommended human dose. No such effects were noted in pregnant mice subjected to up to 1052 times the maximum recommended human dose. There are no adequate and well-controlled studies in pregnant women. CARTROL (carteolol hydrochloride) should be used during pregnancy only if the potential benefit justifies the potential risk to the fetus.

Nursing Mothers:
Studies have not been conducted in lactating humans and, therefore, it is not known whether carteolol is excreted in human milk. Studies in lactating rats indicate that CARTROL (carteolol hydrochloride) is excreted in milk. Because many drugs are excreted in human milk, caution should be exercised when CARTROL (carteolol hydrochloride) is administered to a nursing woman.

Pediatric Use:
Safety and effectiveness in children have not been established.

ADVERSE REACTIONS

The prevalence of adverse reactions has been ascertained from clinical studies conducted primarily in the United States. All adverse experiences (events) reported during these studies were recorded as adverse reactions. The prevalence rates presented below are based on combined data from nineteen placebo-controlled studies of patients with hypertension, angina or dysrhythmias, using once-daily carteolol at doses up to 60 mg. Table 1 summarizes those adverse experiences reported for patients in these studies where the prevalence in the carteolol group is 1% or greater and exceeds the prevalence in the placebo group. Asthenia and muscle cramps were the only symptoms that were significantly more common in patients receiving carteolol than in patients receiving placebo. Patients in clinical trials were carefully selected to exclude those, such as patients with asthma or known bronchospasm, or congestive heart failure, who would be at high risk of experiencing beta-adrenergic blocker adverse effect (See WARNINGS and CONTRAINDICATIONS): [See Table 1 at left.]

The adverse experiences were usually mild or moderate in intensity and transient, but sometimes were serious enough to interrupt treatment. The adverse reactions that were most bothersome, as judged by their being reported as reasons for discontinuation of therapy by at least 0.4% of the carteolol group are shown in Table 2.

TABLE 2
Discontinuations During
Placebo-Controlled Studies

	Placebo (n=448) %	Carteolol (n=761) %
Body as a Whole		
Asthenia	0.2	0.5
Headache	0.7	0.7
Chest Pain	0.2	0.4
Skin and Appendages		
Rash	0.0	0.4
Sweating	0.2	0.4
Digestive System		
Nausea	0.0	0.4
Overall Adverse Reactions	4.2	3.3

Additional adverse reactions have been reported, but these are, in general, not distinguishable from symptoms that might have occurred in the absence of exposure to carteolol. The following additional adverse reactions were reported by at least 1% of 1568 patients who received carteolol in controlled or open, short- or long-term clinical studies, or represent less common, but potentially important, reactions reported in clinical studies or marketing experience (these rare reactions are shown in italics): *Body as a Whole:* fever, infection, injury, malaise, pain, neck pain, shoulder pain; *Cardiovascular System:* angina pectoris, arrhythmia, *heart failure,* palpitations, *second degree heart block,* vasodilation; *Digestive System: acute hepatitis with jaundice,* constipation, dyspepsia, flatulence, gastrointestinal disorder; *Metabolic/Nutritional Disorder:* gout, *Musculoskeletal System:* pain in extremity, joint disorder, arthritis; *Nervous System: abnormal dreams,* anxiety, depression, dizziness, nervousness, somnolence; *Respiratory System:* bronchitis, *bronchospasm,* cold symptoms, cough, dyspnea, flu symptoms, lung disorder, rhinitis, sinusitis, *wheezing; Skin and Appendages:* sweating; *Special Senses:* blurred vision, conjunctivitis, eye disorder, tinnitus; *Urogenital:* impotence, urinary frequency, urinary tract infection.

In studies of patients with hypertension or angina pectoris where carteolol and positive reference beta-adrenergic blocking agents [nadolol (n=82) and propranolol (n=50)] have been compared, the differences in prevalence rates between the carteolol group and the reference agent group were statistically significant (p ≤ 0.05) for the adverse reactions listed in Table 3.

TABLE 3
Adverse Reactions During
Positive-Controlled Studies

	Reference Agents (n=132) %	Carteolol (n=135) %
Body as a Whole		
Chest Pain	5.3	0.7
Cardiovascular System		
Bradycardia	4.5	0.0
Digestive System		
Diarrhea	11.4	4.4
Nervous System		
Somnolence	0.8	7.4
Skin and Appendages		
Sweating	5.3	0.7

POTENTIAL ADVERSE REACTIONS

In addition, other adverse reactions not listed above have been reported with other beta-adrenergic blocking agents and should be considered potential adverse reactions of CARTROL (carteolol hydrochloride).

Body as a Whole:
Fever combined with aching and sore throat.
Cardiovascular System:
Intensification of AV block. (See *CONTRAINDICATIONS.*)
Digestive System:
Mesenteric arterial thrombosis, ischemic colitis.
Hemic/Lymphatic System:
Agranulocytosis, thrombocytopenic and non-thrombocytopenic purpura.
Nervous System:
Reversible mental depression progressing to catatonia; an acute reversible syndrome characterized by disorientation to time and place, short-term memory loss, emotional lability, slightly clouded sensorium, and decreased performance on neuropsychometric testing.
Respiratory System:
Laryngospasm, respiratory distress.
Skin and Appendages:
Erythematous rash, reversible alopecia.
Urogenital System:
Peyronie's disease.
The oculomucocutaneous syndrome associated with the beta-adrenergic blocking agent practolol has not been reported with carteolol.

OVERDOSAGE

No specific information on emergency treatment of overdosage in humans is available. The most common effects expected with overdosage of a beta-adrenergic blocking agent are bradycardia, bronchospasm, congestive heart failure and hypotension.
In case of overdosage, treatment with CARTROL (carteolol hydrochloride) should be discontinued and gastric lavage considered. The patient should be closely observed and vital signs carefully monitored. The prolonged effects of carteolol must be considered when determining the duration of corrective therapy. On the basis of the pharmacologic profile, the following additional measures should be considered as appropriate.
Symptomatic Bradycardia:
Administer atropine. If there is no response to vagal blockade, administer isoproterenol cautiously.
Bronchospasm:
Administer a beta$_2$-stimulating agent such as isoproterenol and/or a theophylline derivative.
Congestive Heart Failure:
Administer diuretics and digitalis glycosides as necessary.
Hypotension:
Administer vasopressors such as intravenous dopamine, epinephrine or norepinephrine bitartrate.

DOSAGE AND ADMINISTRATION

Dosage must be individualized. The initial dose of CARTROL (carteolol hydrochloride) is 2.5 mg given as a single daily oral dose either alone or added to diuretic therapy. If an adequate response is not achieved, the dose can be gradually increased to 5 mg and 10 mg as single daily doses. Increasing the dose above 10 mg per day is unlikely to produce further substantial benefits and, in fact, may decrease the response. The usual maintenance dose of carteolol is 2.5 or 5 mg once daily.
Dosage Adjustment in Renal Impairment:
Carteolol is excreted principally by the kidneys. When administering CARTROL (carteolol hydrochloride) to patients with renal impairment, the dosage regimen should be adjusted individually by the physician. Guidelines for dose interval adjustment are shown below:

Creatinine Clearance (mL/min)	Dosage Interval (hours)
>60	24
20–60	48
<20	72

HOW SUPPLIED

CARTROL (carteolol hydrochloride) is supplied as:
2.5 mg gray tablets:
Bottles of 100 ....(**NDC** 0074-1664-13).
5 mg white tablets:
Bottles of 100 ....(**NDC** 0074-1665-13).
Recommended storage: Store under controlled room temperature, 59°–86°F (15°–30°C).
Ref. 01-2531-R3

Shown in Product Identification Section, page 403

CEFOL® Filmtab® Tablets ℞
[cē'full]
(B-Complex, folic acid, vitamin E with 750 mg vitamin C)

DESCRIPTION

Each oral tablet provides:

Ascorbic Acid (C) (as sodium ascorbate)	750 mg
Niacinamide	100 mg
Calcium Pantothenate	20 mg
Thiamine Mononitrate (B$_1$)	15 mg
Riboflavin (B$_2$)	10 mg
Pyridoxine Hydrochloride (B$_6$)	5 mg
Folic Acid	500 mcg
Cyanocobalamin (B$_{12}$)	6 mcg
Vitamin E (as dl-alpha tocopheryl acetate)	30 IU

Inactive Ingredients: Cellulosic polymers, colloidal silicon dioxide, corn starch, D&C Yellow No. 10, FD&C Blue No. 1, magnesium stearate, microcrystalline cellulose, polyethylene glycol, povidone, titanium dioxide, and vanillin.

CLINICAL PHARMACOLOGY

The vitamin components of Cefol are absorbed by the active transport process. All but Vitamin E are rapidly eliminated and not stored in the body. Vitamin E is stored in body tissues.

INDICATIONS AND USAGE

Indicated in non-pregnant* adults for the treatment of Vitamin C deficiency states with an associated deficient intake or increased need for Vitamin B-Complex, Folic Acid, and Vitamin E.

CONTRAINDICATIONS

Rare hypersensitivity to Folic Acid.

WARNINGS

Folic Acid alone is improper treatment of pernicious anemia and other megaloblastic anemias where Vitamin B$_{12}$ is deficient.

PRECAUTIONS

Folic Acid above 0.1 mg daily may obscure pernicious anemia (hematologic remission may occur while neurological manifestations remain progressive).

ADVERSE REACTIONS

Allergic sensitization has been reported following oral and parenteral administration of Folic Acid.

DOSAGE

Usual adult dose is one tablet daily.

HOW SUPPLIED

Green Filmtab tablets in bottles of 100.
Filmtab—Film-sealed tablets, Abbott.
Store below 77°F (25°C).
Ref. 03-2037-3/R23

*Pregnancy may require greater Folic Acid intake.

Shown in Product Identification Section, page 403

CYLERT® Tablets ℞ Ⓒ
[cī'lert]
(Pemoline)

DESCRIPTION

CYLERT (pemoline) is a central nervous system stimulant. Pemoline is structurally dissimilar to the amphetamines and methylphenidate.
It is an oxazolidine compound and is chemically identified as 2-amino-5-phenyl-2-oxazolin-4-one.
Pemoline is a white, tasteless, odorless powder, relatively insoluble (less than 1 mg/mL) in water, chloroform, ether, acetone, and benzene; its solubility in 95% ethyl alcohol is 2.2 mg/mL.
CYLERT (pemoline) is supplied as tablets containing 18.75 mg, 37.5 mg or 75 mg of pemoline for oral administration. CYLERT is also available as chewable tablets containing 37.5 mg of pemoline.
Inactive Ingredients
18.75 mg tablet: corn starch, gelatin, lactose, magnesium hydroxide, polyethylene glycol and talc.
37.5 mg tablet: corn starch, FD&C Yellow No. 6, gelatin, lactose, magnesium hydroxide, polyethylene glycol and talc.
37.5 mg chewable tablet: corn starch, FD&C Yellow No. 6, magnesium hydroxide, magnesium stearate, mannitol, polyethylene glycol, povidone, talc and artificial flavor.
75 mg tablet: corn starch, gelatin, iron oxide, lactose, magnesium hydroxide, polyethylene glycol and talc.

CLINICAL PHARMACOLOGY

CYLERT (pemoline) has a pharmacological activity similar to that of other known central nervous system stimulants; however, it has minimal sympathomimetic effects. Although studies indicate that pemoline may act in animals through dopaminergic mechanisms, the exact mechanism and site of action of the drug in man is not known.
There is neither specific evidence which clearly establishes the mechanism whereby CYLERT produces its mental and behavioral effects in children, nor conclusive evidence regarding how these effects relate to the condition of the central nervous system.
Pemoline is rapidly absorbed from the gastrointestinal tract. Approximately 50% is bound to plasma proteins. The serum half-life of pemoline is approximately 12 hours. Peak serum levels of the drug occur within 2 to 4 hours after ingestion of a single dose. Multiple dose studies in adults at several dose levels indicate that steady state is reached in approximately 2 to 3 days. In animals given radiolabeled pemoline, the drug was widely and uniformly distributed throughout the tissues, including the brain.
Pemoline is metabolized by the liver. Metabolites of pemoline include pemoline conjugate, pemoline dione, mandelic acid, and unidentified polar compounds. CYLERT is excreted primarily by the kidneys with approximately 50% excreted unchanged and only minor fractions present as metabolites.
CYLERT (pemoline) has a gradual onset of action. Using the recommended schedule of dosage titration, significant clinical benefit may not be evident until the third or fourth week of drug administration.

INDICATIONS AND USAGE

CYLERT (pemoline) is indicated in Attention Deficit Disorder (ADD) with hyperactivity as an integral part of a total treatment program which typically includes other remedial measures (psychological, educational, social) for a stabilizing effect in children with a behavioral syndrome characterized by the following group of developmentally inappropriate symptoms: moderate to severe distractibility, short attention span, hyperactivity, emotional lability, and impulsivity. The diagnosis of this syndrome should not be made with finality when these symptoms are only of comparatively recent origin. Nonlocalizing (soft) neurological signs, learning disability, and abnormal EEG may or may not be present, and a diagnosis of central nervous system dysfunction may or may not be warranted.

CONTRAINDICATIONS

CYLERT (pemoline) is contraindicated in patients with known hypersensitivity or idiosyncrasy to the drug. CYLERT should not be administered to patients with impaired hepatic function. (See "ADVERSE REACTIONS" section.)

WARNINGS

Decrements in the predicted growth (i.e., weight gain and/or height) rate have been reported with the long-term use of stimulants in children. Therefore, patients requiring long-term therapy should be carefully monitored.

PRECAUTIONS

General: Clinical experience suggests that in psychotic children, administration of CYLERT may exacerbate symptoms of behavior disturbance and thought disorder.
CYLERT should be administered with caution to patients with significantly impaired renal function.
Laboratory Tests: Liver function tests should be performed prior to and periodically during therapy with CYLERT. The drug should be discontinued if abnormalities are revealed and confirmed by follow-up tests. (See "ADVERSE REACTIONS" section regarding reports of abnormal liver function tests, hepatitis and jaundice.)
Drug Interactions: The interaction of CYLERT (pemoline) with other drugs has not been studied in humans. Patients who are receiving CYLERT concurrently with other drugs, especially drugs with CNS activity, should be monitored carefully.
Decreased seizure threshold has been reported in patients receiving CYLERT concomitantly with *antiepileptic medications.*
Carcinogenesis: Long-term studies have been conducted in rats with doses as high as 150 mg/kg/day for eighteen months. There was no significant difference in the incidence of any neoplasm between treated and control animals.
Mutagenesis: Data are not available concerning long-term effects on mutagenicity in animals or humans.
Impairment of Fertility: The results of studies in which rats were given 18.75 and 37.5 mg/kg/day indicated that pemoline did not affect fertility in males or females at those doses.
Pregnancy: Teratogenic effects: Pregnancy Category B. Reproduction studies have been performed in rats and rabbits at doses of 18.75 and 37.5 mg/kg/day and have revealed no evidence of impaired fertility or harm to the fetus. There are, however, no adequate and well-controlled studies in pregnant women. Because animal reproduction studies are not always predictive of human response, this drug should be used during pregnancy only if clearly needed.
Nonteratogenic effects: Studies in rats have shown an increased incidence of stillbirths and cannibalization when pemoline was administered at a dose of 37.5 mg/kg/day. Postnatal survival of offspring was reduced at doses of 18.75 and 37.5 mg/kg/day.
Nursing Mothers: It is not known whether this drug is excreted in human milk. Because many drugs are excreted in human milk, caution should be exercised when CYLERT is administered to a nursing woman.
Pediatric Use: Safety and effectiveness in children below the age of 6 years have not been established.
Long-term effects of CYLERT in children have not been established (See "WARNINGS" section).

Continued on next page

Abbott Laboratories—Cont.

CNS stimulants, including pemoline, have been reported to precipitate motor and phonic tics and Tourette's syndrome. Therefore, clinical evaluation for tics and Tourette's syndrome in children and their families should precede use of stimulant medications.

Drug treatment is not indicated in all cases of ADD with hyperactivity and should be considered only in light of complete history and evaluation of the child. The decision to prescribe CYLERT (pemoline) should depend on the physician's assessment of the chronicity and severity of the child's symptoms and their appropriateness for his/her age. Prescription should not depend solely on the presence of one or more of the behavioral characteristics.

ADVERSE REACTIONS

The following are adverse reactions in decreasing order of severity within each category associated with CYLERT:

Hepatic: There have been reports of hepatic dysfunction including elevated liver enzymes, hepatitis and jaundice in patients taking CYLERT. The occurrence of elevated liver enzymes is not rare and these reactions appear to be reversible upon drug discontinuance. Most patients with elevated liver enzymes were asymptomatic. Although no causal relationship has been established, there have been rare reports of hepatic-related fatalities involving patients taking CYLERT.

Hematopoietic: There have been isolated reports of aplastic anemia.

Central Nervous System: The following CNS effects have been reported with the use of CYLERT: convulsive seizures; literature reports indicate that CYLERT may precipitate attacks of Gilles de la Tourette syndrome; hallucinations; dyskinetic movements of the tongue, lips, face and extremities; abnormal oculomotor function including nystagmus and oculogyric crisis; mild depression; dizziness; increased irritability; headache; and drowsiness.

Insomnia is the most frequently reported side effect of CYLERT; it usually occurs early in therapy prior to an optimum therapeutic response. In the majority of cases it is transient in nature or responds to a reduction in dosage.

Gastrointestinal: Anorexia and weight loss may occur during the first weeks of therapy. In the majority of cases it is transient in nature; weight gain usually resumes within three to six months.

Nausea and stomach ache have also been reported.

Genitourinary: A case of elevated acid phosphatase in association with prostatic enlargement has been reported in a 63 year old male who was treated with CYLERT for sleepiness. The acid phosphatase normalized with discontinuation of CYLERT and was again elevated with rechallenge.

Miscellaneous: Suppression of growth has been reported with the long-term use of stimulants in children. (See "WARNINGS" section.) Skin rash has been reported with CYLERT.

Mild adverse reactions appearing early during the course of treatment with CYLERT often remit with continuing therapy. If adverse reactions are of a significant or protracted nature, dosage should be reduced or the drug discontinued.

DRUG ABUSE AND DEPENDENCE

Controlled Substance: CYLERT is subject to control under DEA schedule IV.

Abuse: CYLERT failed to demonstrate a potential for self-administration in primates. However, the pharmacologic similarity of pemoline to other psychostimulants with known dependence liability suggests that psychological and/or physical dependence might also occur with CYLERT. There have been isolated reports of transient psychotic symptoms occurring in adults following the long-term misuse of excessive oral doses of pemoline. CYLERT should be given with caution to emotionally unstable patients who may increase the dosage on their own initiative.

OVERDOSAGE

Signs and symptoms of acute overdosage, resulting principally from overstimulation of the central nervous system and from excessive sympathomimetic effects, may include the following: vomiting, agitation, tremors, hyperreflexia, muscle twitching, convulsions (may be followed by coma), euphoria, confusion, hallucinations, delirium, sweating, flushing, headache, hyperpyrexia, tachycardia, hypertension and mydriasis. Treatment consists of appropriate supportive measures. The patient must be protected against self-injury and against external stimuli that would aggravate overstimulation already present. If signs and symptoms are not too severe and the patient is conscious, gastric contents may be evacuated. Chlorpromazine has been reported in the literature to be useful in decreasing CNS stimulation and sympathomimetic effects.

Efficacy of peritoneal dialysis or extracorporeal hemodialysis for CYLERT overdosage has not been established.

DOSAGE AND ADMINISTRATION

CYLERT (pemoline) is administered as a single oral dose each morning. The recommended starting dose is 37.5 mg/day. This daily dose should be gradually increased by 18.75 mg at one week intervals until the desired clinical response is obtained. The effective daily dose for most patients will range from 56.25 to 75 mg. The maximum recommended daily dose of pemoline is 112.5 mg.

Clinical improvement with CYLERT is gradual. Using the recommended schedule of dosage titration, significant benefit may not be evident until the third or fourth week of drug administration.

Where possible, drug administration should be interrupted occasionally to determine if there is a recurrence of behavioral symptoms sufficient to require continued therapy.

HOW SUPPLIED

CYLERT (pemoline) is supplied as monogrammed, grooved tablets in three dosage strengths:

18.75 mg tablets (white) in bottles of 100 (**NDC** 0074-6025-13);

37.5 mg tablets (orange-colored) in bottles of 100 (**NDC** 0074-6057-13);

75 mg tablets (tan-colored) in bottles of 100 (**NDC** 0074-6073-13).

CYLERT (pemoline) Chewable is supplied as 37.5 mg monogrammed, grooved tablets (orange-colored) in bottles of 100 (**NDC** 0074-6088-13).

Recommended Storage: Store below 86°F (30°C).

Ref. 03-4409-R15

Shown in Product Identification Section, page 403

DAYALETS® Filmtab® OTC

[*dāy 'a-lets*]

Multivitamin Supplement for adults and children 4 or more years of age

DAYALETS® PLUS IRON Filmtab®

Multivitamin Supplement with Iron for adults and children 4 or more years of age

(See PDR For Nonprescription Drugs.)

DEPAKENE® Capsules and Syrup ℞

[*dep 'a-kāne*]

(Valproic Acid)

WARNING

HEPATIC FAILURE RESULTING IN FATALITIES HAS OCCURRED IN PATIENTS RECEIVING VALPROIC ACID. EXPERIENCE HAS INDICATED THAT CHILDREN UNDER THE AGE OF TWO YEARS ARE AT A CONSIDERABLY INCREASED RISK OF DEVELOPING FATAL HEPATOTOXICITY. ESPECIALLY THOSE ON MULTIPLE ANTICONVULSANTS, THOSE WITH CONGENITAL METABOLIC DISORDERS, THOSE WITH SEVERE SEIZURE DISORDERS ACCOMPANIED BY MENTAL RETARDATION, AND THOSE WITH ORGANIC BRAIN DISEASE. WHEN DEPAKENE PRODUCTS ARE USED IN THIS PATIENT GROUP, IT SHOULD BE USED WITH EXTREME CAUTION AND AS A SOLE AGENT. THE BENEFITS OF SEIZURE CONTROL SHOULD BE WEIGHED AGAINST THE RISKS. ABOVE THIS AGE GROUP, EXPERIENCE HAS INDICATED THAT THE INCIDENCE OF FATAL HEPATOTOXICITY DECREASES CONSIDERABLY IN PROGRESSIVELY OLDER PATIENT GROUPS.

THESE INCIDENTS USUALLY HAVE OCCURRED DURING THE FIRST SIX MONTHS OF TREATMENT. SERIOUS OR FATAL HEPATOTOXICITY MAY BE PRECEDED BY NON-SPECIFIC SYMPTOMS SUCH AS LOSS OF SEIZURE CONTROL, MALAISE, WEAKNESS, LETHARGY, FACIAL EDEMA, ANOREXIA, AND VOMITING. PATIENTS SHOULD BE MONITORED CLOSELY FOR APPEARANCE OF THESE SYMPTOMS. LIVER FUNCTION TESTS SHOULD BE PERFORMED PRIOR TO THERAPY AND AT FREQUENT INTERVALS THEREAFTER, ESPECIALLY DURING THE FIRST SIX MONTHS.

DESCRIPTION

DEPAKENE (valproic acid) is a carboxylic acid designated as 2-propylpentanoic acid. It is also known as dipropylacetic acid.

Valproic acid (pKa 4.8) has a molecular weight of 144 and occurs as a colorless liquid with a characteristic odor. It is slightly soluble in water (1.3 mg/mL) and very soluble in organic solvents.

DEPAKENE capsules and syrup are antiepileptics for oral administration. Each soft elastic capsule contains 250 mg valproic acid. The syrup contains the equivalent of 250 mg valproic acid per 5 mL as the sodium salt.

Inactive Ingredients:

250 mg capsules: corn oil, FD&C Yellow No. 6, gelatin, glycerin, iron oxide, methylparaben, propylparaben, and titanium dioxide.

Syrup: FD&C Red No. 40, glycerin, methylparaben, propylparaben, sorbitol, sucrose, water, and natural and artificial flavors.

CLINICAL PHARMACOLOGY

Valproic acid is an antiepileptic agent which dissociates to the valproate ion in the gastrointestinal tract. The mechanism by which valproate exerts its antiepileptic effects has not been established. It has been suggested that its activity is related to increased brain levels of gamma-aminobutyric acid (GABA).

Valproic acid is rapidly absorbed after oral administration. Peak plasma concentrations of valproate ion are observed 1 to 4 hours after a single oral dose of valproic acid. A slight delay in absorption occurs when the drug is administered with meals, but this does not affect the total absorption. Accordingly, administration of oral valproate products with food and substitution among the various DEPAKENE (valproic acid) and DEPAKOTE® (divalproex sodium) products should be without consequence. Nonetheless, any changes in dosage administration, or the addition or discontinuance of concomitant drugs should ordinarily be accompanied by close monitoring of clinical status and valproate plasma concentrations.

The plasma half-life of valproate is typically in the range of 6 to 16 hours. Half-lives in the lower part of the range are usually found in patients taking other antiepileptic drugs capable of enzyme induction.

Valproate is primarily metabolized in the liver. The major metabolic routes are glucuronidation, mitochrondrial beta oxidation, and microsomol oxidation. The major metabolites formed are the glucuronide conjugate, 2-propyl-3-keto-pentanoic acid, and 2-propylhydroxypentanoic acids. Other unsaturated metabolites have been reported. The major route of elimination of these metabolites is in the urine.

Patients on monotherapy will generally have longer half-lives and higher concentrations of valproate at a given dosage than patients receiving polytherapy. This is primarily due to enzyme induction caused by other antiepileptics, which results in enhanced clearance of valproate by glucuronidation and microsomal oxidation. Because of these changes in valproate clearance, monitoring of antiepileptic concentrations should be intensified whenever concomitant antiepileptics are introduced or withdrawn.

The therapeutic range is commonly considered to be 50 to 100 mcg/mL of total valproate, although some patients may be controlled with lower or higher plasma concentrations.

Valproate is highly bound (90%) to plasma proteins in the therapeutic range; however, protein binding is concentration-dependent and decreases at high valproate concentrations. The binding is variable among patients, and may be affected by fatty acids or by highly bound drugs such as salicylate. Some clinicians favor monitoring free valproate concentrations, which may more accurately reflect CNS penetration of valproate. As yet, a consensus on the therapeutic range of free concentrations has not been established; however, monitoring total and free valproate may be informative when there are changes in clinical status, concomitant medication, or valproate dosage.

INDICATIONS AND USAGE

DEPAKENE (valproic acid) is indicated for use as sole and adjunctive therapy in the treatment of simple and complex absence seizures, and adjunctively in patients with multiple seizure types which include absence seizures.

Simple absence is defined as very brief clouding of the sensorium or loss of consciousness accompanied by certain generalized epileptic discharges without other detectable clinical signs. Complex absence is the term used when other signs are also present.

SEE WARNINGS FOR STATEMENT REGARDING FATAL HEPATIC DYSFUNCTION.

CONTRAINDICATIONS

VALPROIC ACID SHOULD NOT BE ADMINISTERED TO PATIENTS WITH HEPATIC DISEASE OR SIGNIFICANT DYSFUNCTION.

Valproic acid is contraindicated in patients with known hypersensitivity to the drug.

WARNINGS

Hepatic failure resulting in fatalities has occurred in patients receiving valproic acid. These incidents usually have occurred during the first six months of treatment. Serious or fatal hepatotoxicity may be preceded by nonspecific symptoms such as loss of seizure control, malaise, weakness, lethargy, facial edema, anorexia and vomiting. Patients should be monitored closely for appearance of these symptoms. Liver function tests should be performed prior to therapy and at frequent intervals thereafter, especially during the first six months. However, physicians should not rely totally on

serum biochemistry since these tests may not be abnormal in all instances, but should also consider the results of careful interim medical history and physical examination. Caution should be observed when administering DEPAKENE (valproic acid) to patients with a prior history of hepatic disease. Patients on multiple anticonvulsants, children, those with congenital metabolic disorders, those with severe seizure disorders accompanied by mental retardation, and those with organic brain disease may be at particular risk. Experience has indicated that children under the age of two years are at considerably increased risk of developing fatal hepatotoxicity, especially those with the aforementioned conditions. When DEPAKENE products are used in this patient group, it should be used with extreme caution and as a sole agent. The benefits of seizure control should be weighed against the risks. Above this age group, experience has indicated that the incidence of fatal hepatotoxicity decreases considerably in progressively older patient groups.

The drug should be discontinued immediately in the presence of significant hepatic dysfunction, suspected or apparent. In some cases, hepatic dysfunction has progressed in spite of discontinuation of drug.

The frequency of adverse effects (particularly elevated liver enzymes) may be dose-related. The benefit of improved seizure control which may accompany the higher doses should be weighed against the possibility of a greater incidence of adverse effects.

Usage in Pregnancy: ACCORDING TO PUBLISHED AND UNPUBLISHED REPORTS, VALPROIC ACID MAY PRODUCE TERATOGENIC EFFECTS IN THE OFFSPRING OF HUMAN FEMALES RECEIVING THE DRUG DURING PREGNANCY.

THERE ARE MULTIPLE REPORTS IN THE CLINICAL LITERATURE WHICH INDICATE THAT THE USE OF ANTIEPILEPTIC DRUGS DURING PREGNANCY RESULTS IN AN INCREASED INCIDENCE OF BIRTH DEFECTS IN THE OFFSPRING. ALTHOUGH DATA ARE MORE EXTENSIVE WITH RESPECT TO TRIMETHADIONE, PARAMETHADIONE, PHENYTOIN, AND PHENOBARBITAL, REPORTS INDICATE A POSSIBLE SIMILAR ASSOCIATION WITH THE USE OF OTHER ANTIEPILEPTIC DRUGS. THEREFORE, ANTIEPILEPTIC DRUGS SHOULD BE ADMINISTERED TO WOMEN OF CHILDBEARING POTENTIAL ONLY IF THEY ARE CLEARLY SHOWN TO BE ESSENTIAL IN THE MANAGEMENT OT THEIR SEIZURES.

THE INCIDENCE OF NEURAL TUBE DEFECTS IN THE FETUS MAY BE INCREASED IN MOTHERS RECEIVING VALPROATE DURING THE FIRST TRIMESTER OF PREGNANCY. THE CENTERS FOR DISEASE CONTROL (CDC) HAS ESTIMATED THE RISK OF VALPROIC ACID EXPOSED WOMEN HAVING CHILDREN WITH SPINA BIFIDA TO BE APPROXIMATELY 1 to 2%.[1] OTHER CONGENITAL ANOMALIES (EG, CRANIOFACIAL DEFECTS, CARDIOVASCULAR MALFORMATIONS AND ANOMALIES INVOLVING VARIOUS BODY SYSTEMS), COMPATIBLE AND INCOMPATIBLE WITH LIFE, HAVE BEEN REPORTED. SUFFICIENT DATA TO DETERMINE THE INCIDENCE OF THESE CONGENITAL ANOMALIES IS NOT AVAILABLE.

THE HIGHER INCIDENCE OF CONGENITAL ANOMALIES IN ANTIEPILEPTIC DRUG-TREATED WOMEN WITH SEIZURE DISORDERS CANNOT BE REGARDED AS A CAUSE AND EFFECT RELATIONSHIP. THERE ARE INTRINISIC METHODOLOGIC PROBLEMS IN OBTAINING ADEQUATE DATA ON DRUG TERATOGENICITY IN HUMANS; GENETIC FACTORS OR THE EPILEPTIC CONDITION ITSELF, MAY BE MORE IMPORTANT THAN DRUG THERAPY IN CONTRIBUTING TO CONGENITAL ANOMALIES.

PATIENTS TAKING VALPROATE MAY DEVELOP CLOTTING ABNORMALITIES. A PATIENT WHO HAD LOW FIBROGEN WHEN TAKING MULTIPLE ANTICONVULSANTS INCLUDING VALPROATE GAVE BIRTH TO AN INFANT WITH AFIBRINOGENEMIA WHO SUBSEQUENTLY DIED OF HEMORRHAGE. IF VALPROATE IS USED IN PREGNANCY, THE CLOTTING PARAMETERS SHOULD BE MONITORED CAREFULLY.

HEPATIC FAILURE, RESULTING IN THE DEATH OF A NEWBORN AND OF AN INFANT, HAVE BEEN REPORTED FOLLOWING THE USE OF VALPROATE DURING PREGNANCY.

ANIMAL STUDIES ALSO HAVE DEMONSTRATED VALPROATE INDUCED TERATOGENICITY. Studies in rats and human females demonstrated placental transfer of the drug. Doses greater than 65 mg/kg/day given to pregnant rats and mice produced skeletal abnormalities in the offspring, primarily involving ribs and vertebrae; doses greater than 150 mg/kg/day given to pregnant rabbits produced fetal resorptions and (primarily) soft-tissue abnormalities in the offspring. In rats a dose-related delay in the onset of parturition was noted. Postnatal growth and survival of the progeny were adversely affected, particularly when drug administration spanned the entire gestation and early lactation period.

Antiepileptic drugs should not be discontinued in patients in whom the drug is administered to prevent major seizures because of the strong possibility of precipitating status epilepticus with attendant hypoxia and threat to life. In individual cases where the severity and frequency of the seizure disorder are such that the removal of medication does not pose a serious threat to the patient, discontinuation of the drug may be considered prior to and during pregnancy, although it cannot be said with any confidence that even minor seizures do not pose some hazard to the developing embryo or fetus.

The prescribing physician will wish to weigh these considerations in treating or counseling epileptic women of childbearing potential.

Tests to detect neural tube and other defects using current accepted procedures should be considered a part of routine prenatal care in childbearing women receiving valproate.

PRECAUTIONS

Hepatic Dysfunction: See BOXED WARNING, CONTRAINDICATIONS, AND WARNINGS.

General: Because of reports of thrombocytopenia, inhibition of the secondary phase of platelet aggregation, and abnormal coagulation parameters (eg, low fibrinogen), platelet counts and coagulation tests are recommended before initiating therapy and at periodic intervals. It is recommended that patients receiving DEPAKENE (valproic acid) be monitored for platelet count and coagulation parameters prior to planned surgery. Evidence of hemorrhage, bruising, or a disorder of hemostasis/coagulation is an indication for reduction of the dosage or withdrawal of therapy.

Hyperammonemia with or without lethargy or coma has been reported and may be present in the absence of abnormal liver function tests. Asymptomatic elevations of ammonia are more common and when present require more frequent monitoring. If clinically significant symptoms occur, DEPAKENE therapy should be modified or discontinued.

Since valproate may interact with concurrently administered antiepileptic drugs, periodic plasma concentration determinations of concomitant antiepileptic drugs are recommended during the early course of therapy (see DRUG INTERACTIONS).

Valproate is partially eliminated in the urine as a keto-metabolite which may lead to a false interpretation of the urine ketone test.

There have been reports of altered thyroid function tests associated with valproate. The clinical significance of these is unknown.

Information for Patients: Since DEPAKENE products may produce CNS depression, especially when combined with CNS depressants (eg, alcohol), patients should be advised not to engage in hazardous activities, such as driving an automobile or operating dangerous machinery, until it is known that they do not become drowsy from the drug.

Drug Interactions: Valproate may potentiate the action of CNS depressants (ie, alcohol, benzodiazepines, etc).

The concomitant administration of valproate with drugs that exhibit extensive protein binding (eg, aspirin, carbamazepine, dicumarol, and phenytoin) may result in alteration of serum drug concentrations.

There is evidence that valproate can cause an increase in serum phenobarbital concentrations by impairment of nonrenal clearance. This phenomenon can result in severe CNS depression. The combination of valproate and phenobarbital has also been reported to produce CNS depression without significant elevations of barbiturate or valproate serum concentrations. All patients receiving concomitant barbiturate therapy should be closely monitored for neurological toxicity. Serum barbiturate concentrations should be obtained, if possible, and the barbiturate dosage decreased, if appropriate.

Primidone is metabolized into a barbiturate and, therefore, may also be involved in a similar or identical interaction.

There have been reports of breakthrough seizures occurring with the combination of valproate and phenytoin. Most reports have noted a decrease in total plasma phenytoin concentration. However, increases in total phenytoin serum concentration have been reported. An initial fall with subsequent increase in total phenytoin concentrations has also been reported. In addition, a decrease in total serum phenytoin with an increase in the free vs. protein bound phenytoin concentrations has been reported. The dosage of phenytoin should be adjusted as required by the clinical situation.

The concomitant use of valproic acid and clonazepam may induce absence status in patients with a history of absence type seizures.

There is inconclusive evidence regarding the effects of valproate on serum ethosuximide concentrations. Patients receiving valproate and ethosuximide, especially along with other anticonvulsants, should be monitored for alterations in serum concentrations of both drugs.

Caution is recommended when valproate is used with drugs affecting coagulation (eg, aspirin, warfarin). See ADVERSE REACTIONS.

Evidence suggests that there is an association between the use of certain antiepileptics and failure of oral contraceptives. One explanation for this interaction is that enzyme-inducing antiepileptics effectively lower plasma concentrations of the relevant steroid hormones, resulting in unimpaired ovulation. However, other mechanisms, not related to enzyme induction may contribute to the failure of oral contraceptives. While valproate is not a significant enzyme inducer, and, therefore, would not be expected to decrease concentrations of steroid hormones, clinical data about the interaction of valproate with oral contraceptives is minimal.[2]

Carcinogenesis: Valproic acid was administered to Sprague Dawley rats and ICR (HA/ICR) mice at doses of 0, 80 and 170 mg/kg/day for two years. A variety of neoplasms were observed in both species. The chief findings were a statistically significant increase in the incidence of subcutaneous fibrosarcomas in high dose male rats receiving valproic acid and a statistically significant dose-related trend for benign pulmonary adenomas in male mice receiving valproic acid. The significance of these findings for man is unknown.

Mutagenesis: Studies of valproate have been performed using bacterial and mammalian systems. These studies have provided no evidence of a mutagenic potential for valproate.

Fertility: Chronic toxicity studies in juvenile and adult rats and dogs demonstrated reduced spermatogenesis and testicular atrophy at doses greater than 200 mg/kg/day in rats and greater than 90 mg/kg/day in dogs. Segment I fertility studies in rats have shown doses up to 350 mg/kg/day for 60 days to have no effect on fertility. THE EFFECT OF VALPROATE ON TESTICULAR DEVELOPMENT AND ON SPERM PRODUCTION AND FERTILITY IN HUMANS IS UNKNOWN.

Pregnancy: Pregnancy Category D: See WARNINGS.

Nursing Mothers: Valproate is excreted in breast milk. Concentrations in breast milk have been reported to be 1–10% of serum concentrations. It is not known what effect this would have on a nursing infant. Caution should be exercised when valproic acid is administered to a nursing woman.

ADVERSE REACTIONS

Since DEPAKENE (valproic acid) has usually been used with other antiepileptic drugs, it is not possible, in most cases, to determine whether the following adverse reactions can be ascribed to valproic acid alone, or the combination of drugs.

Gastrointestinal: The most commonly reported side effects at the initiation of therapy are nausea, vomiting, and indigestion. These effects are usually transient and rarely require discontinuation of therapy. Diarrhea, abdominal cramps, and constipation have been reported. Both anorexia with some weight loss and increased appetite with weight gain have also been reported. Some patients experiencing gastrointestinal side effects may benefit by converting therapy from DEPAKENE (valproic acid) to Depakote® (divalproex sodium).[3]

CNS Effects: Sedative effects have occurred in patients receiving valproate alone but occur most often in patients receiving combination therapy. Sedation usually abates upon reduction of other antiepileptic medication. Tremor (may be dose-related), hallucinations, ataxia, headache, nystagmus, diplopia, asterixis, "spots before eyes", dysarthria, dizziness, and incoordination. Rare cases of coma have been noted in patients receiving valproic acid alone or in conjunction with phenobarbital. In rare instances encephalopathy with fever has developed shortly after the introduction of valproate monotherapy without evidence of hepatic dysfunction or inappropriate plasma levels; all patients recovered after the drug was withdrawn.

Dermatologic: Transient hair loss, skin rash, photosensitivity, generalized pruritus, erythema multiforme, and Stevens-Johnson syndrome. A case of fatal epidermal necrolysis has been reported in a 6 month old infant taking valproate and several other concomitant medications.

Psychiatric: Emotional upset, depression, psychosis, aggression, hyperactivity and behavioral deterioration.

Musculoskeletal: Weakness.

Hematologic: Thrombocytopenia and inhibition of the secondary phase of platelet aggregation may be reflected in altered bleeding time, petechiae, bruising, hematoma formation and frank hemorrhage (see PRECAUTIONS—*General* and *Drug Interactions*). Relative lymphocytosis, macrocytosis, hypofibrinogenemia, leukopenia, eosinophilia, anemia including macrocytic with or without folate deficiency, bone marrow suppression, and acute intermittent porphyria.

Hepatic: Minor elevations of transaminases (eg, SGOT and SGPT) and LDH are frequent and appear to be dose-related. Occasionally, laboratory test results include increases in serum bilirubin and abnormal changes in other liver function tests. These results may reflect potentially serious hepatotoxicity. (See WARNINGS).

Continued on next page

Abbott Laboratories—Cont.

Weight (kg)	Weight (lb)	Total Daily Dose (mg)	Number of Capsules or Teaspoonfuls of Syrup Dose 1	Dose 2	Dose 3
10—24.9	22— 54.9	250	0	0	1
25—39.9	55— 87.9	500	1	0	1
40—59.9	88—131.9	750	1	1	1
60—74.9	132—164.9	1,000	1	1	2
75—89.9	165—197.9	1,250	2	1	2

Endocrine: Irregular menses, secondary amenorrhea, breast enlargement, galactorrhea, and parotid gland swelling. Abnormal thyroid function tests (see PRECAUTIONS).
Pancreatic: Acute pancreatitis including fatalities.
Metabolic: Hyperammonemia (see PRECAUTIONS), hyponatremia, and inappropriate ADH secretion.
Decreased carnitine concentrations have been reported although the clinical relevance is undetermined.
Hyperglycinemia has occurred and was associated with a fatal outcome in a patient with preexistent nonketotic hyperglycinemia.
Genitourinary: Enuresis.
Special Senses: Hearing loss, either reversible or irreversible, has been reported; however, a cause and effect relationship has not been established.
Other: Edema of the extremities, lupus erythematous, and fever.

OVERDOSAGE

Overdosage with valproate may result in somnolence, heart block, and deep coma. Fatalities have been reported.
Since valproic acid is absorbed very rapidly, the benefit of gastric lavage or emesis will vary with the time since ingestion. General supportive measures should be applied with particular attention to the maintenance of adequate urinary output.
Naloxone has been reported to reverse the CNS depressant effects of valproate overdosage. Because naloxone could theoretically also reverse the antiepileptic effects of valproate, it should be used with caution.

DOSAGE AND ADMINISTRATION

DEPAKENE (valproic acid) is administered orally. The recommended initial dose is 15 mg/kg/day, increasing at one week intervals by 5 to 10 mg/kg/day, until seizures are controlled or side effects preclude further increases. The maximum recommended dosage is 60 mg/kg/day. If the total daily dose exceeds 250 mg, it should be given in a divided regimen.
The following table is a guide for the initial daily dose of DEPAKENE (valproic acid) (15 mg/kg/day):
[See table
The frequency of adverse effects (particularly elevated liver enzymes) may be dose-related. The benefit of improved seizure control with higher doses should be weighed against the possibility of a greater incidence of adverse reactions.
A good correlation has not been established between daily dose, serum concentration and therapeutic effect. However, therapeutic valproate serum concentrations for most patients will range from 50 to 100 mcg/mL. Some patients may be controlled with lower or higher serum concentrations (see CLINICAL PHARMACOLOGY).
As the DEPAKENE dosage is titrated upward, blood concentrations of phenobarbital and/or phenytoin may be affected. (See PRECAUTIONS).
Patients who experience G.I. irritation may benefit from administration of the drug with food or by slowly building up the dose from an initial low level.
THE CAPSULES SHOULD BE SWALLOWED WITHOUT CHEWING TO AVOID LOCAL IRRITATION OF THE MOUTH AND THROAT.

HOW SUPPLIED

DEPAKENE (valproic acid) is available as orange-colored soft gelatin capsules of 250 mg valproic acid in bottles of 100 capsules (**NDC** 0074-5681-13), in ABBO-PAC® unit dose packages of 100 capsules (**NDC** 0074-5681-11), and as a red syrup containing the equivalent of 250 mg valproic acid per 5 mL as the sodium salt in bottles of 16 ounces (**NDC** 0074-5682-16).
Recommended Storage:
Store capsules at 59–77°F (15–25°C).
Store syrup below 86°F (30°C).

REFERENCES

1. Centers for Disease Control, valproate: a new cause of birth defects—report from Italy and follow-up from France, *Morbidity and Mortality Weekly Report.* 1983;32(33):438–439.
2. Mattson RH, et al. Use of oral contraceptives by women with epilepsy. *JAMA.* 1986;256(2):238–240.
3. Wilder BJ, et al. Gastrointestinal tolerance of divalproex sodium. *Neurology.* 1983;33:808–811.
4. Wilder BJ, et al. Twice-daily dosing of valproate with divalproex. *Clin Pharmacol Ther.* 1983;34(4):501–504.
5. Hurst DL. Expanded therapeutic range of valproate. *Pediatr Neurol.* 1987;3:342–344.

Caution—Federal (USA) Law prohibits dispensing without prescription.
Ref. 01-2591-R21
Shown in Product Identification Section, page 403

DEPAKOTE® Sprinkle Capsules ℞
DIVALPROEX SODIUM
COATED PARTICLES IN CAPSULES

DEPAKOTE® Tablets ℞
DIVALPROEX SODIUM
DELAYED-RELEASE TABLETS

WARNING
HEPATIC FAILURE RESULTING IN FATALITIES HAS OCCURRED IN PATIENTS RECEIVING VALPROIC ACID AND ITS DERIVATIVES. EXPERIENCE HAS INDICATED THAT CHILDREN UNDER THE AGE OF TWO YEARS ARE AT A CONSIDERABLY INCREASED RISK OF DEVELOPING FATAL HEPATOTOXICITY, ESPECIALLY THOSE ON MULTIPLE ANTICONVULSANTS, THOSE WITH CONGENITAL METABOLIC DISORDERS, THOSE WITH SEVERE SEIZURE DISORDERS ACCOMPANIED BY MENTAL RETARDATION, AND THOSE WITH ORGANIC BRAIN DISEASE. WHEN DEPAKOTE IS USED IN THIS PATIENT GROUP, IT SHOULD BE USED WITH EXTREME CAUTION AND AS A SOLE AGENT. THE BENEFITS OF SEIZURE CONTROL SHOULD BE WEIGHED AGAINST THE RISKS. ABOVE THIS AGE GROUP, EXPERIENCE HAS INDICATED THAT THE INCIDENCE OF FATAL HEPATOTOXICITY DECREASES CONSIDERABLY IN PROGRESSIVELY OLDER PATIENT GROUPS.
THESE INCIDENTS USUALLY HAVE OCCURRED DURING THE FIRST SIX MONTHS OF TREATMENT. SERIOUS OR FATAL HEPATOTOXICITY MAY BE PRECEDED BY NON-SPECIFIC SYMPTOMS SUCH AS LOSS OF SEIZURE CONTROL, MALAISE, WEAKNESS, LETHARGY, FACIAL EDEMA, ANOREXIA, AND VOMITING. PATIENTS SHOULD BE MONITORED CLOSELY FOR APPEARANCE OF THESE SYMPTOMS. LIVER FUNCTION TESTS SHOULD BE PERFORMED PRIOR TO THERAPY AND AT FREQUENT INTERVALS THEREAFTER, ESPECIALLY DURING THE FIRST SIX MONTHS.

DESCRIPTION

Divalproex sodium is a stable co-ordination compound comprised of sodium valproate and valproic acid in a 1:1 molar relationship and formed during the partial neutralization of valproic acid with 0.5 equivalent of sodium hydroxide. Chemically it is designated as sodium hydrogen bis (2-propylpentanoate).
Divalproex sodium occurs as a white powder with a characteristic odor.
DEPAKOTE tablets and Sprinkle capsules are antiepileptics for oral administration. DEPAKOTE Sprinkle capsules contain specially coated particles of divalproex sodium equivalent to 125 mg of valproic acid in a hard gelatin capsule. DEPAKOTE tablets are supplied in three dosage strengths containing divalproex sodium equivalent to 125 mg, 250 mg, or 500 mg of valproic acid.
Inactive Ingredients
125 mg Sprinkle capsules: cellulosic polymers, D&C Red No. 28, FD&C Blue No. 1, gelatin, iron oxide, magnesium stearate, silica gel, titanium dioxide, and triethyl citrate.
DEPAKOTE tablets: cellulosic polymers, diacetylated monoglycerides, povidone, pregelatinized starch (contains corn starch) silica gel, talc, titanium dioxide, and vanillin.
In addition, individual tablets contain:
125 mg tablets: FD&C Blue No. 1 and FD&C Red No. 40.
250 mg tablets: FD&C Yellow No. 6 and iron oxide.
500 mg tablets: D&C Red No. 30, FD&C Blue No. 2, and iron oxide.

CLINICAL PHARMACOLOGY

Divalproex sodium is an antiepileptic agent which dissociates to the valproate ion in the gastrointestinal tract. The mechanism by which valproate exerts its antiepileptic effects has not been established. It has been suggested that its activity is related to increased brain levels of gamma-aminobutyric acid (GABA).
Equivalent oral doses of DEPAKOTE (divalproex sodium) products and DEPAKENE (valproic acid) capsules deliver equivalent quantities of valproate ion systemically. However, the rate of valproate ion absorption may vary with the conditions of use (eg, fasting or postprandial) and the method of administration (eg, whether the contents of the capsule are sprinkled on food or the capsule is taken intact).
When subjects are in a fasting state, peak plasma concentrations of valproate ion are observed approximately 3 to 4 hours following administration of all DEPAKOTE products.
Experiments indicate that feeding can influence the rate of systemic absorption of valproate. In studies in which the contents of DEPAKOTE (divalproex sodium) Sprinkle capsules were sprinkled on applesauce, feeding was found to delay the time to peak plasma concentration by approximately 1.5 hours.
Compared to DEPAKOTE tablets, however, DEPAKOTE Sprinkle capsules (in the fasting state) exhibit a slower rate of absorption, resulting in lower peak plasma concentrations (ie, fluctuations between minimum and maximum plasma valproate concentrations are attentuated).
While absorption rate from the GI tract and fluctuation in valproate plasma concentrations vary with dosing regimen and formulation, the efficacy of valproate in chronic use is not affected. Experience employing dosing regimens from once-a-day to four-times-a-day, as well as studies in primate epilepsy models involving constant rate infusion, indicate that total daily systemic bioavailability (extent of absorption) is the primary determinant of seizure control and that differences in the ratios of plasma peak to trough concentrations between valproate formulations are inconsequential from a practical clinical standpoint.
Accordingly, coadministration of oral valproate products with food and substitution among the various DEPAKOTE and DEPAKENE formulations should cause no clinical problems (see DOSAGE AND ADMINISTRATION). Nonetheless, any changes in dosage administration, or the addition or discontinuance of concomitant drugs should ordinarily be accompanied by close monitoring of clinical status and valproate plasma concentrations.
The plasma half-life of valproate is typically in the range of 6 to 16 hours. Half-lives in the lower part of the range are usually found in patients taking other antiepileptic drugs capable of enzyme induction.
Valproate is primarily metabolized in the liver. The major metabolic routes are glucuronidation, mitochondrial beta oxidation, and microsomal oxidation. The major metabolites formed are the glucuronide conjugate, 2-propyl-3-keto-pentanoic acid, and 2-propylhydroxypentanoic acids. Other unsaturated metabolites have been reported. The major route of elimination of these metabolites is in the urine.
Patients on monotherapy will generally have longer half-lives and higher concentrations of valproate at a given dosage than patients receiving polytherapy. This is primarily due to enzyme induction caused by other antiepileptics, which results in enhanced clearance of valproate by glucuronidation and microsomal oxidation. Because of these changes in valproate clearance, monitoring of antiepileptic concentrations should be intensified whenever concomitant antiepileptics are introduced or withdrawn.
The therapeutic range is commonly considered to be 50 to 100 mcg/ml of total valproate, although some patients may be controlled with lower or higher plasma concentrations.[5]
Valproate is highly bound (90%) to plasma proteins in the therapeutic range; however, protein binding is concentration-dependent and decreases at high valproate concentrations. The binding is variable among patients and may be affected by fatty acids or by highly bound drugs such as salicylate. Some clinicians favor monitoring free valproate concentrations, which may more accurately reflect CNS penetration of valproate. As yet, a consensus on the therapeutic range of free concentrations has not been established; however, monitoring total and free valproate may be informative when there are changes in clinical status, concomitant medication, or valproate dosage.

INDICATIONS AND USAGE

DEPAKOTE (divalproex sodium) is indicated for use as sole and adjunctive therapy in the treatment of simple and complex absence seizures, and adjunctively in patients with multiple seizure types that include absence seizures.
Simple absence is defined as very brief clouding of the sensorium or loss of consciousness accompanied by certain generalized epileptic discharges without other detectable clinical signs. Complex absence is the term used when other signs are also present.
SEE WARNINGS FOR STATEMENT REGARDING FATAL HEPATIC DYSFUNCTION.

CONTRAINDICATIONS

DIVALPROEX SODIUM SHOULD NOT BE ADMINISTERED TO PATIENTS WITH HEPATIC DISEASE OR SIGNIFICANT DYSFUNCTION.

Divalproex sodium is contraindicated in patients with known hypersensitivity to the drug.

WARNINGS

Hepatic failure resulting in fatalities has occurred in patients receiving valproic acid. These incidents usually have occurred during the first six months of treatment. Serious or fatal hepatotoxicity may be preceded by nonspecific symptoms such as loss of seizure control, malaise, weakness, lethargy, facial edema, anorexia, and vomiting. Patients should be monitored closely for appearance of these symptoms. Liver function tests should be performed prior to therapy and at frequent intervals thereafter, especially during the first six months. However, physicians should not rely totally on serum biochemistry since these tests may not be abnormal in all instances, but should also consider the results of careful interim medical history and physical examination. Caution should be observed when administering DEPAKOTE products to patients with a prior history of hepatic disease. Patients on multiple anticonvulsants, children, those with congenital metabolic disorders, those with severe seizure disorders accompanied by mental retardation, and those with organic brain disease may be at particular risk. Experience has indicated that children under the age of two years are at considerably increased risk of developing fatal hepatotoxicity, especially those with the aforementioned conditions. When DEPAKOTE is used in this patient group, it should be used with extreme caution and as a sole agent. The benefits of seizure control should be weighed against the risks. Above this age group, experience has indicated that the incidence of fatal hepatotoxicity decreases considerably in progressively older patient groups.

The drug should be discontinued immediately in the presence of significant hepatic dysfunction, suspected or apparent. In some cases, hepatic dysfunction has progressed in spite of discontinuation of drug.

The frequency of adverse effects (particularly elevated liver enzymes) may be dose-related. The benefit of improved seizure control which may accompany the higher doses should therefore be weighed against the possibility of a greater incidence of adverse effects.

Usage in Pregnancy: ACCORDING TO PUBLISHED AND UNPUBLISHED REPORTS, VALPROIC ACID MAY PRODUCE TERATOGENIC EFFECTS IN THE OFFSPRING OF HUMAN FEMALES RECEIVING THE DRUG DURING PREGNANCY.

THERE ARE MULTIPLE REPORTS IN THE CLINICAL LITERATURE WHICH INDICATE THAT THE USE OF ANTIEPILEPTIC DRUGS DURING PREGNANCY RESULTS IN AN INCREASED INCIDENCE OF BIRTH DEFECTS IN THE OFFSPRING. ALTHOUGH DATA ARE MORE EXTENSIVE WITH RESPECT TO TRIMETHADIONE, PARAMETHADIONE, PHENYTOIN, AND PHENOBARBITAL, REPORTS INDICATE A POSSIBLE SIMILAR ASSOCIATION WITH THE USE OF OTHER ANTIEPILEPTIC DRUGS. THEREFORE, ANTIEPILEPTIC DRUGS SHOULD BE ADMINISTERED TO WOMEN OF CHILDBEARING POTENTIAL ONLY IF THEY ARE CLEARLY SHOWN TO BE ESSENTIAL IN THE MANAGEMENT OF THEIR SEIZURES.

THE INCIDENCE OF NEURAL TUBE DEFECTS IN THE FETUS MAY BE INCREASED IN MOTHERS RECEIVING VALPROATE DURING THE FIRST TRIMESTER OF PREGNANCY. THE CENTERS FOR DISEASE CONTROL (CDC) HAS ESTIMATED THE RISK OF VALPROIC ACID EXPOSED WOMEN HAVING CHILDREN WITH SPINA BIFIDA TO BE APPROXIMATELY 1 to 2%.[1]

OTHER CONGENITAL ANOMALIES (EG, CRANIOFACIAL DEFECTS, CARDIOVASCULAR MALFORMATIONS AND ANOMALIES INVOLVING VARIOUS BODY SYSTEMS), COMPATIBLE AND INCOMPATIBLE WITH LIFE, HAVE BEEN REPORTED. SUFFICIENT DATA TO DETERMINE THE INCIDENCE OF THESE CONGENITAL ANOMALIES IS NOT AVAILABLE.

THE HIGHER INCIDENCE OF CONGENITAL ANOMALIES IN ANTIEPILEPTIC DRUG-TREATED WOMEN WITH SEIZURE DISORDERS CANNOT BE REGARDED AS A CAUSE AND EFFECT RELATIONSHIP. THERE ARE INTRINSIC METHODOLOGIC PROBLEMS IN OBTAINING ADEQUATE DATA ON DRUG TERATOGENICITY IN HUMANS; GENETIC FACTORS OR THE EPILEPTIC CONDITION ITSELF, MAY BE MORE IMPORTANT THAN DRUG THERAPY IN CONTRIBUTING TO CONGENITAL ANOMALIES.

PATIENTS TAKING VALPROATE MAY DEVELOP CLOTTING ABNORMALITIES. A PATIENT WHO HAD LOW FIBRINOGEN WHEN TAKING MULTIPLE ANTICONVULSANTS INCLUDING VALPROATE GAVE BIRTH TO AN INFANT WITH AFIBRINOGENEMIA WHO SUBSEQUENTLY DIED OF HEMORRHAGE. IF VALPROATE IS USED IN PREGNANCY, THE CLOTTING PARAMETERS SHOULD BE MONITORED CAREFULLY.

HEPATIC FAILURE, RESULTING IN THE DEATH OF A NEWBORN AND OF AN INFANT, HAVE BEEN REPORTED FOLLOWING THE USE OF VALPROATE DURING PREGNANCY.

ANIMAL STUDIES ALSO HAVE DEMONSTRATED VALPROATE INDUCED TERATOGENICITY. Studies in rats and human females demonstrated placental transfer of the drug. Doses greater than 65 mg/kg/day given to pregnant rats and mice produced skeletal abnormalities in the offspring, primarily involving ribs and vertebrae; doses greater than 150 mg/kg/day given to pregnant rabbits produced fetal resorptions and (primarily) soft-tissue abnormalities in the offspring. In rats a dose-related delay in the onset of parturition was noted. Postnatal growth and survival of the progeny were adversely affected, particularly when drug administration spanned the entire gestation and early lactation period.

Antiepileptic drugs should not be discontinued in patients in whom the drug is administered to prevent major seizures because of the strong possibility of precipitating status epilepticus with attendant hypoxia and threat to life. In individual cases where the severity and frequency of the seizure disorder are such that the removal of medication does not pose a serious threat to the patient, discontinuation of the drug may be considered prior to and during pregnancy, although it cannot be said with any confidence that even minor seizures do not pose some hazard to the developing embryo or fetus.

The prescribing physician will wish to weigh these considerations in treating or counseling epileptic women of childbearing potential.

Tests to detect neural tube and other defects using current accepted procedures should be considered a part of routine prenatal care in childbearing women receiving valproate.

PRECAUTIONS

Hepatic Dysfunction: See BOXED WARNING, CONTRAINDICATIONS AND WARNINGS.

General: Because of reports of thrombocytopenia, inhibition of the secondary phase of platelet aggregation, and abnormal coagulation parameters (eg. low fibrinogen), platelet counts and coagulation tests are recommended before initiating therapy and at periodic intervals. It is recommended that patients receiving DEPAKOTE (divalproex sodium) be monitored for platelet count and coagulation parameters prior to planned surgery. Evidence of hemorrhage, bruising, or a disorder of hemostasis/coagulation is an indication for reduction of the dosage or withdrawal of therapy.

Hyperammonemia with or without lethargy or coma has been reported and may be present in the absence of abnormal liver function tests. Asympatomatic elevations of ammonia are more common and when present require more frequent monitoring. If clinically significant symptoms occur, DEPAKOTE therapy should be modified or discontinued.

Since valproate may interact with concurrently administered antiepileptic drugs, periodic plasma concentration determinations of concomitant antiepileptic drugs are recommended during the early course of therapy. (See DRUG INTERACTIONS).

Valproate is partially eliminated in the urine as a keto-metabolite which may lead to a false interpretation of the urine ketone test.

There have been reports of altered thyroid function tests associated with valproate. The clinical significance of these is unknown.

Information for Patients: Since DEPAKOTE products may produce CNS depression, especially when combined CNS depressants (eg, alcohol), patients should be advised not to engage in hazardous activities, such as driving an automobile or operating dangerous machinery, until it is known that they do not become drowsy from the drug.

The specially coated particles in DEPAKOTE Sprinkle capsules have been observed in the stool, but this occurrence has not been associated with clinically significant effects.

Drug Interactions: Valproate may potentiate the action of CNS depressants (ie, alcohol, benzodiazepines, etc).

The concomitant administration of valproate with drugs that exhibit extensive protein binding (eg, aspirin, carbamazepine, dicumarol, and phenytoin) may result in alteration of serum drug concentrations.

There is evidence that valproate can cause an increase in serum phenobarbital concentrations by impairment of nonrenal clearance. This pnenomenon can result in severe CNS depression. The combination of valproate and phenobarbital has also beeen reported to produce CNS depression without significant elevations of barbiturate or valproate serum concentrations. All patients receiving concomitant barbiturate therapy should be closely monitored for neurological toxicity. Serum barbiturate levels should be obtained, if possible, and the barbiturate dosage decreased, if appropriate.

Primidone is metabolized to a barbiturate and, therefore, may also be involved in a similar or identical interaction.

There have been reports of breakthrough seizures occurring with the combination of valproate and phenytoin. Most reports have noted a decrease in total plasma phenytoin concentration. However, increases in total phenytoin serum concentration have been reported. An initial fall with subsequent increase in total phenytoin concentrations has also been reported. In addition, a decrease in total serum phenytoin with an increase in the free vs. protein bound phenytoin concentrations has been reported. The dosage of phenytoin should be adjusted as required by the clinical situation.

The concomitant use of valproic acid and clonazepam may induce absence status in patients with a history of absence type seizures.

There is inconclusive evidence regarding the effect of valproate on serum ethosuximide concentrations. Patients receiving valproate and ethosuximide, especially along with other anticonvulsants, should be monitored for alterations in serum concentrations of both drugs.

Caution is recommended when valproate is used with drugs affecting coagulation, (eg, aspirin, warfarin). See ADVERSE REACTIONS.

Evidence suggests that there is an association between the use of certain antiepileptics and failure of oral contraceptives. One explanation for this interaction is that enzyme-inducing antiepileptics effectively lower plasma concentrations of the relevant steroid hormones, resulting in unimpaired ovulation. However, other mechanisms, not related to enzyme induction, may contribute to the failure of oral contraceptives. While valproate is not a significant enzyme inducer, and, therefore, would not be expected to decrease concentrations of steroid hormones, clinical data about the interaction of valproate with oral contraceptives is minimal.[2]

Carcinogenesis: Valproic acid was administered to Sprague Dawley rats and ICR (HA /ICR) mice at doses of 0, 80, and 170 mg/kg/day for two years. A variety of neoplasms were observed in both species. The chief findings were a statistically significant increase in the incidence of subcutaneous fibrosarcomas in high dose male rats receiving valproic acid and a statistically significant dose-related trend for benign pulmonary adenomas in male mice receiving valproic acid. The significance of these findings for humans is unknown.

Mutagenesis: Studies of valproate have been performed using bacterial and mammalian systems. These studies have provided no evidence of a mutagenic potential for valproate.

Fertility: Chronic toxicity studies in juvenile and adult rats and dogs demonstrated reduced spermatogenesis and testicular atrophy at doses greater than 200 mg/kg/day in rats and greater than 90 mg/kg/day in dogs. Segment I fertility studies in rats have shown doses up to 350 mg/kg/day for 60 days to have no effect on fertility. THE EFFECT OF VALPROATE ON TESTICULAR DEVELOPMENT AND ON SPERM PRODUCTION AND FERTILITY IN HUMANS IS UNKNOWN.

Pregnancy: Pregnancy Category D: See WARNINGS.

Nursing Mothers: Valproate is excreted in breast milk. Concentrations in breast milk have been reported to be 1–10% of serum concentrations. It is not known what effect this would have on a nursing infant. Caution should be exercised when divalproex sodium is administered to a nursing woman.

ADVERSE REACTIONS

Since divalproex sodium has usually been used with other antiepileptic drugs, it is not possible, in most cases, to determine whether the following adverse reactions can be ascribed to divalproex sodium alone, or the combination of drugs.

Gastrointestinal: The most commonly reported side effects at the initiation of therapy are nausea, vomiting and indigestion. These effects are usually transient and rarely require discontinuation of therapy. Diarrhea, abdominal cramps, and constipation have been reported. Both anorexia with some weight loss and increased appetite with weight gain have also been reported. The administration of delayed-release divalproex sodium may result in reduction of gastrointestinal side effects in some patients.[3]

CNS Effects: Sedative effects have occurred in patients receiving valproate alone but occur most often in patients receiving combination therapy. Sedation usually abates upon reduction of other antiepileptic medication. Tremor (may be dose-related), hallucinations, ataxia, headache, nystagmus, diplopia, asterixis, "spots before eyes", dysarthria, dizziness, and incoordination. Rare cases of coma have occurred in patients receiving valproate alone or in conjunction with phenobarbital. In rare instances encephalopathy with fever has developed shortly after the introduction of valproate monotherapy without evidence of hepatic dysfunction or inappropriate plasma levels; all patients recovered after the drug was withdrawn.

Dermatologic: Transient hair loss, skin rash, photosensitivity, generalized pruritus, erythema multiforme, and Stevens-Johnson syndrome. A case of fatal epidermal necrolysis has been reported in a 6 month old infant taking valproate and several other concomitant medications.

Psychiatric: Emotional upset, depression, psychosis, aggression, hyperactivity and behavioral deterioration.

Continued on next page

If desired, additional literature on any Abbott product will be provided upon request to Abbott Laboratories.

Abbott Laboratories—Cont.

Musculoskeletal: Weakness.
Hematologic: Thrombocytopenia and inhibition of the secondary phase of platelet aggregation may be reflected in altered bleeding time, petechiae, bruising, hematoma formation, and frank hemorrhage (see PRECAUTIONS—*General* and *Drug Interactions*). Relative lymphocytosis, macrocytosis, hypofibrinogenemia, leukopenia, eosinophilia, anemia including macrocytic with or without folate deficiency, bone marrow suppression, and acute intermittent porphyria.
Hepatic: Minor elevations of transaminases (eg, SGOT and SGPT) and LDH are frequent and appear to be dose-related. Occasionally, laboratory test results include increases in serum bilirubin and abnormal changes in other liver function tests. These results may reflect potentially serious hepatotoxicity (see WARNINGS).
Endocrine: Irregular menses and secondary amenorrhea, breast enlargement, galactorrhea and parotid gland swelling. Abnormal thyroid function tests (see PRECAUTIONS), hyponatremia, and inappropriate ADH secretion.
Decreased carnitine concentrations have been reported although the clinical relevance is undetermined.
Pancreatic: Acute pancreatitis including fatalities.
Metabolic: Hyperammonemia (see PRECAUTIONS), hyponatremia, and inappropriate ADH secretion.
Decreased carnitine concentrations have been reported although the clinical relevance is undetermined.
Hyperglycinemia has occurred and was associated with a fatal outcome in a patient with preexistent nonketotic hyperglycinemia.
Genitourinary: Enuresis.
Special Senses: Hearing loss, either reversible or irreversible, has been reported; however, a cause and effect relationship has not been established.
Other: Edema of the extremities, lupus erythematosus, and fever.

OVERDOSAGE

Overdosage with valproate may result in somnolence, heart block, and deep coma. Fatalities have been reported.
The benefit of gastric lavage or emesis will vary with the time since ingestion. General supportive measures should be applied with particular attention to the maintenance of adequate urinary output.
Naloxone has been reported to reverse the CNS depressant effects of valproate overdosage. Because naloxone could theoretically also reverse the antiepileptic effects of valproate, it should be used with caution.

DOSAGE AND ADMINISTRATION

DEPAKOTE tablets and Sprinkle capsules are administered orally. The recommended initial dose is 15 mg/kg/day, increasing at one week intervals by 5 to 10 mg/kg/day until seizures are controlled or side effects preclude further increases. The maximum recommended dosage is 60 mg/kg/day. If the total daily dose exceeds 250 mg, it should be given in a divided regimen.
Administration of Sprinkle Capsule: DEPAKOTE Sprinkle capsules may be swallowed whole or may be administered by carefully opening the capsule and sprinkling the entire contents on a small amount (teaspoonful) of soft food such as applesauce or pudding. The drug/food mixture should be swallowed immediately (avoid chewing) and not stored for future use. Each capsule is oversized to allow ease of opening.
Conversion from DEPAKENE to DEPAKOTE: In patients previously receiving DEPAKENE (valproic acid) therapy, DEPAKOTE products should be initiated at the same daily dose and dosing schedule. After the patient is stabilized on a DEPAKOTE product, a dosing schedule of two or three times a day may be elected in selected patients.[4]
DEPAKOTE products provide equal extents of absorption, although they may not produce identical trough and peak valproate concentrations. DEPAKOTE tablets produce slightly higher peak concentrations than DEPAKOTE Sprinkle capsules. Such differences in the maximum and minimum valproate plasma concentrations are unlikely to be of clinical significance; however, changes in dosage administration of valproate or concomitant medications should be accompanied by increased monitoring of plasma concentrations of valproate and other medications, as well as the patient's clinical status.
The frequency of adverse effects (particularly elevated liver enzymes) may be dose-related. The benefit of improved seizure control with higher doses should be weighed against the possibility of a greater incidence of adverse reactions.
A good correlation has not been established between daily dose, serum concentration and therapeutic effect. However, therapeutic valproate serum concentrations for most patients will range from 50 to 100 mcg/ml. Some patients may be controlled with lower or higher serum concentrations (see CLINICAL PHARMACOLOGY).
As the DEPAKOTE dosage is titrated upward, blood concentrations of phenobarbital and/or phenytoin may be affected. (See PRECAUTIONS).
Patients who experience G. I. irritation may benefit from administration of the drug with food or by slowly building up the dose from an initial low level.

HOW SUPPLIED

DEPAKOTE Sprinkle capsules (divalproex sodium coated particles in capsules), 125 mg, are white opaque and blue, and are supplied in bottles of 100 (**NDC** 0074-6114-13) and Abbo-Pac® unit dose packages of 100 (**NDC** 0074-6114-11).
Recommended Storage: Store capsules below 77°F (25°C).
DEPAKOTE tablets (divalproex sodium delayed-release tablets) are supplied as:
125 mg salmon pink-colored tablets:
Bottles of 100 ....(**NDC** 0074-6212-13)
Abbo-Pac® unit dose packages of
100 ....(**NDC** 0074-6212-11)
250 mg peach-colored tablets:
Bottles of 100 ....(**NDC** 0074-6214-13)
Bottles of 500 ....(**NDC** 0074-6214-53)
Abbo-Pac® unit dose packages of
100 ....(**NDC** 0074-6214-11)
500 mg lavender-colored tablets:
Bottles of 100 ....(**NDC** 0074-6215-13)
Bottles of 500 ....(**NDC** 0074-6215-53)
Abbo-Pac® unit dose packages of
100 ....(**NDC** 0074-6215-11)
Recommended Storage: Store tablets below 86°F (30°C).

REFERENCES

1. Centers for Disease Control, valproate: a new cause of birth defects—report from Italy and follow-up from France. *Morbidity and Mortality Weekly Report.* 1983; 32(33); 438–439.
2. Mattson RH, et al. Use of oral contraceptives by women with epilepsy. *JAMA.* 1986; 256(2): 238–240.
3. Wilder, BJ, et al. Gastrointestinal tolerance of divalproex sodium. *Neurology.* 1983; 33: 808–811.
4. Wilder BJ, et al. Twice-daily dosing of valproate with divalproex, *Clin Pharmacol Ther.* 1983; 34(4): 501–504.
5. Hurst DL. Expanded therapeutic range of valproate. *Pediatr Neurol.* 1987; 3:342–344.

Caution—Federal (USA) Law prohibits dispensing without prescription.
Ref. 01-2596-R19
Shown in Product Identification Section, page 403

DESOXYN® ℞ Ⓒ
(methamphetamine hydrochloride)
Gradumet® Tablets

METHAMPHETAMINE HAS A HIGH POTENTIAL FOR ABUSE. IT SHOULD THUS BE TRIED ONLY IN WEIGHT REDUCTION PROGRAMS FOR PATIENTS IN WHOM ALTERNATIVE THERAPY HAS BEEN INEFFECTIVE. ADMINISTRATION OF METHAMPHETAMINE FOR PROLONGED PERIODS OF TIME IN OBESITY MAY LEAD TO DRUG DEPENDENCE AND MUST BE AVOIDED. PARTICULAR ATTENTION SHOULD BE PAID TO THE POSSIBILITY OF SUBJECTS OBTAINING METHAMPHETAMINE FOR NON-THERAPEUTIC USE OR DISTRIBUTION TO OTHERS, AND THE DRUG SHOULD BE PRESCRIBED OR DISPENSED SPARINGLY.

DESCRIPTION

Methamphetamine hydrochloride, chemically known as (S)-N, α-dimethylbenzeneethanamine hydrochloride, is a member of the amphetamine group of sympathomimetic amines.
DESOXYN Gradumet sustained-release tablets are available containing 5 mg, 10 mg or 15 mg of methamphetamine hydrochloride for oral administration. The Gradumet is an inert, porous, plastic matrix, which is impregnated with methamphetamine hydrochloride. The drug is leached slowly from the Gradumet as it passes through the gastrointestinal tract. The expended matrix is not absorbed and is excreted in the stool.
Inactive Ingredients: 5 mg Gradumet tablet: magnesium stearate, methyl acrylate-methyl methacrylate copolymer, povidone and talc.
10 mg Gradumet tablet: FD&C Yellow No. 6 (Sunset Yellow), magnesium stearate, methyl acrylate-methyl methacrylate copolymer, povidone and talc.
15 mg Gradumet tablet: FD&C Yellow No. 5 (tartrazine), magnesium stearate, methyl acrylate-methyl methacrylate copolymer, povidone and talc.

CLINICAL PHARMACOLOGY

Methamphetamine is a sympathomimetic amine with CNS stimulant activity. Peripheral actions include elevation of systolic and diastolic blood pressures and weak bronchodilator and respiratory stimulant action. Drugs of this class used in obesity are commonly known as "anorectics" or "anorexigenics." It has not been established, however, that the action of such drugs in treating obesity is primarily one of appetite suppression. Other central nervous system actions, or metabolic effects, may be involved, for example.
Adult obese subjects instructed in dietary management and treated with "anorectic" drugs, lose more weight on the average than those treated with placebo and diet, as determined in relatively short-term clinical trials.
The magnitude of increased weight loss of drug-treated patients over placebo-treated patients is only a fraction of a pound a week. The rate of weight loss is greatest in the first weeks of therapy for both drug and placebo subjects and tends to decrease in succeeding weeks. The origins of the increased weight loss due to the various possible drug effects are not established. The amount of weight loss associated with the use of an "anorectic" drug varies from trial to trial, and the increased weight loss appears to be related in part to variables other than the drug prescribed, such as the physician-investigator, the population treated, and the diet prescribed. Studies do not permit conclusions as to the relative importance of the drug and non-drug factors on weight loss.
The natural history of obesity is measured in years, whereas the studies cited are restricted to a few weeks duration; thus, the total impact of drug-induced weight loss over that of diet alone must be considered clinically limited.
The mechanism of action involved in producing the beneficial behavioral changes seen in hyperkinetic children receiving methamphetamine is unknown.
In humans, methamphetamine is rapidly absorbed from the gastrointestinal tract. The primary site of metabolism is in the liver by aromatic hydroxylation, N-dealkylation and deamination. At least seven metabolites have been identified in the urine. The biological half-life has been reported in the range of 4 to 5 hours. Excretion occurs primarily in the urine and is dependent on urine pH. Alkaline urine will significantly increase the drug half-life. Approximately 62% of an oral dose is eliminated in the urine within the first 24 hours with about one-third as intact drug and the remainder as metabolites.

INDICATIONS AND USAGE

Attention Deficit Disorder with Hyperactivity—DESOXYN Gradumet tablets are indicated as an integral part of a total treatment program which typically includes other remedial measures (psychological, educational, social) for a stabilizing effect in children over 6 years of age with a behavioral syndrome characterized by the following group of developmentally inappropriate symptoms: moderate to severe distractibility, short attention span, hyperactivity, emotional lability, and impulsivity. The diagnosis of this syndrome should not be made with finality when these symptoms are only of comparatively recent origin. Nonlocalizing (soft) neurological signs, learning disability, and abnormal EEG may or may not be present, and a diagnosis of central nervous system dysfunction may or may not be warranted.
Exogenous Obesity—as a short-term (i.e., a few weeks) adjunct in a regimen of weight reduction based on caloric restriction, for patients in whom obesity is refractory to alternative therapy, e.g., repeated diets, group programs, and other drugs. The limited usefulness of DESOXYN Gradumet tablets (see "Clinical Pharmacology" section) should be weighed against possible risks inherent in use of the drug, such as those described below.

CONTRAINDICATIONS

DESOXYN Gradumet tablets are contraindicated during or within 14 days following the administration of monoamine oxidase inhibitors; hypertensive crises may result. It is also contraindicated in patients with glaucoma, advanced arteriosclerosis, symptomatic cardiovascular disease, moderate to severe hypertension, hyperthyroidism or known hypersensitivity or idiosyncrasy to sympathomimetic amines. Methamphetamine should not be given to patients who are in an agitated state or who have a history of drug abuse.

WARNINGS

Tolerance to the anorectic effect usually develops within a few weeks. When this occurs, the recommended dose should not be exceeded in an attempt to increase the effect; rather, the drug should be discontinued (see "Drug Abuse and Dependence" section).
Decrements in the predicted growth (i.e., weight gain and/or height) rate have been reported with the long-term use of stimulants in children. Therefore, patients requiring long-term therapy should be carefully monitored.
Usage in Nursing Mothers: Amphetamines are excreted in human milk. Mothers taking amphetamines should be advised to refrain from nursing.

PRECAUTIONS

General: DESOXYN (methamphetamine hydrochloride) Gradumet tablets should be used with caution in patients with even mild hypertension.
Methamphetamine should not be used to combat fatigue or to replace rest in normal persons.
Prescribing and dispensing of methamphetamine should be limited to the smallest amount that is feasible at one time in order to minimize the possibility of overdosage.

The 15 mg dosage strength of DESOXYN Gradumet tablets contains FD&C Yellow No. 5 (tartrazine) which may cause allergic-type reactions (including bronchial asthma) in certain susceptible individuals. Although the overall incidence of FD&C Yellow No. 5 (tartrazine) sensitivity in the general population is low, it is frequently seen in patients who also have aspirin hypersensitivity.

Information for Patients: The patient should be informed that methamphetamine may impair the ability to engage in potentially hazardous activities, such as, operating machinery or driving a motor vehicle.

The patient should be cautioned not to increase dosage, except on advice of the physician.

Drug Interactions: Insulin requirements in diabetes mellitus may be altered in association with the use of methamphetamine and concomitant dietary regimen.

Methamphetamine may decrease the hypotensive effect of *guanethidine.*

DESOXYN should not be used concurrently with *monoamine oxidase inhibitors* (see "Contraindications" section).

Concurrent administration of *tricyclic antidepressants* and indirect-acting sympathomimetic amines such as amphetamines, should be closely supervised and dosage carefully adjusted.

Phenothiazines are reported in the literature to antagonize the CNS stimulant action of the amphetamines.

Drug/Laboratory Test Interactions: Literature reports suggest that amphetamines may be associated with significant elevation of plasma corticosteroids. This should be considered if determination of plasma corticosteroid levels is desired in a person receiving amphetamines.

Carcinogensis, Mutagenesis, Impairment of Fertility: Data are not available on long-term potential for carcinogenicity, mutagenicity, or impairment of fertility.

Pregnancy: Teratogenic effects: Pregnancy Category C. Methamphetamine has been shown to have teratogenic and embryocidal effects in mammals given high multiples of the human dose. There are no adequate and well-controlled studies in pregnant women. DESOXYN Gradumet tablets should not be used during pregnancy unless the potential benefit justifies the potential risk to the fetus.

Nonteratogenic effects: Infants born to mothers dependent on amphetamines have an increased risk of premature delivery and low birth weight. Also, these infants may experience symptoms of withdrawal as demonstrated by dysphoria, including agitation and significant lassitude.

Nursing Mothers: See "Warnings" section.

Pediatric Use: Safety and effectiveness for use as an anorectic agent in children below the age of 12 years have not been established.

Long-term effects of methamphetamine in children have not been established (see "Warnings" section).

Drug treatment is not indicated in all cases of the behavioral syndrome characterized by moderate to severe distractibility, short attention span, hyperactivity, emotional lability and impulsivity. It should be considered only in light of the complete history and evaluation of the child. The decision to prescribe DESOXYN Gradumet tablets should depend on the physician's assessment of the chronicity and severity of the child's symptoms and their appropriateness for his/her age. Prescription should not depend solely on the presence of one or more of the behavioral characteristics.

When these symptoms are associated with acute stress reaction, treatment with DESOXYN Gradumet tablets is usually not indicated.

Clinical experience suggests that in psychotic children, administration of DESOXYN Gradumet tablets may exacerbate symptoms of behavior disturbance and thought disorder.

Amphetamines have been reported to exacerbate motor and phonic tics and Tourette's syndrome. Therefore, clinical evaluation for tics and Tourette's syndrome in children and their families should precede use of stimulant medications.

ADVERSE REACTIONS

The following are adverse reactions in decreasing order of severity within each category that have been reported:

Cardiovascular: Elevation of blood pressure, tachycardia and palpitation.

Central Nervous System: Psychotic episodes have been rarely reported at recommended doses. Dizziness, dysphoria, overstimulation, euphoria, insomnia, tremor, restlessness and headache. Exacerbation of motor and phonic tics and Tourette's syndrome.

Gastrointestinal: Diarrhea, constipation, dryness of mouth, unpleasant taste and other gastrointestinal disturbances.

Hypersensitivity: Urticaria.

Endocrine: Impotence and changes in libido.

Miscellaneous: Suppression of growth has been reported with the long-term use of stimulants in children (see "Warnings" section).

DRUG ABUSE AND DEPENDENCE

Controlled Substance: DESOXYN Gradumet tablets are subject to control under DEA schedule II.

Abuse: Methamphetamine has been extensively abused. Tolerance, extreme psychological dependence, and severe social disability have occurred. There are reports of patients who have increased the dosage to many times that recommended. Abrupt cessation following prolonged high dosage administration results in extreme fatigue and mental depression; changes are also noted on the sleep EEG. Manifestations of chronic intoxication with methamphetamine include severe dermatoses, marked insomnia, irritability, hyperactivity, and personality changes. The most severe manifestation of chronic intoxication is psychosis, often clinically indistinguishable from schizophrenia.

OVERDOSAGE

Manifestations of acute overdosage with methamphetamine include restlessness, tremor, hyperreflexia, rapid respiration, confusion, assaultiveness, hallucinations, panic states, hyperpyrexia, and rhabdomyolysis. Fatigue and depression usually follow the central stimulation. Cardiovascular effects include arrhythmias, hypertension or hypotension, and circulatory collapse. Gastrointestinal symptoms include nausea, vomiting, diarrhea, and abdominal cramps. Fatal poisoning usually terminates in convulsions and coma.

Management of acute methamphetamine intoxication is largely symptomatic and includes gastric evacuation and sedation with a barbiturate. Experience with hemodialysis or peritoneal dialysis is inadequate to permit recommendations in this regard.

Acidification of urine increases methamphetamine excretion. Intravenous phentolamine (Regitine®) has been suggested for possible acute, severe hypertension, if this complicates methamphetamine overdosage. Usually a gradual drop in blood pressure will result when sufficient sedation has been achieved. Chlorpromazine has been reported to be useful in decreasing CNS stimulation and sympathomimetic effects.

Since the Gradumet tablet releases methamphetamine gradually, therapy should be directed at reversing the effects of the ingested drug and at supporting the patient until symptoms subside. Saline cathartics are useful for hastening the evacuation of the tablets that have not already released medication.

DOSAGE AND ADMINISTRATION

DESOXYN Gradumet tablets are given orally.

Methamphetamine should be administered at the lowest effective dosage, and dosage should be individually adjusted. Late evening medication should be avoided because of the resulting insomnia.

Attention Deficit Disorder with Hyperactivity:

For treatment of children 6 years or older with a behavioral syndrome characterized by moderate to severe distractibility, short attention span, hyperactivity, emotional lability and impulsivity: an initial dose of 5 mg DESOXYN once or twice a day is recommended. Daily dosage may be raised in increments of 5 mg at weekly intervals until optimum clinical response is achieved. The usual effective dose is 20 to 25 mg daily. The total daily dose may be given once daily using the Gradumet tablet. The Gradumet form should not be utilized for initiation of dosage nor until the titrated daily dosage is equal to or greater than the dosage provided in a Gradumet tablet.

Where possible, drug administration should be interrupted occasionally to determine if there is a recurrence of behavioral symptoms sufficient to require continued therapy.

For obesity: one Gradumet tablet, 10 or 15 mg, once a day in the morning. Treatment should not exceed a few weeks in duration. Methamphetamine is not recommended for use as an anorectic agent in children under 12 years of age.

HOW SUPPLIED

DESOXYN (methamphetamine hydrochloride) Gradumet tablets are supplied as follows:

5 mg, white, in bottles of 100 (**NDC** 0074-6941-04); 10 mg, orange, in bottles of 100 (**NDC** 0074-6948-08); and 15 mg, yellow, in bottles of 100 (**NDC** 0074-6959-07).

Recommended Storage: Store below 86°F (30°C).

Ref. 03-4426-R2

Shown in Product Identification Section, page 403

DICAL-D® TABLETS—WAFERS OTC

[dī'cal-d]

(Dibasic Calcium Phosphate with Vitamin D)

DESCRIPTION

Tablets

Daily dosage (three tablets) provides:

Vitamin D	399 IU (10 mcg)	99% USRDA*
Calcium	0.35 g	35% USRDA
Phosphorus	0.27 g	27% USRDA

*% U.S. Recommended Daily Allowance for adults and children 4 or more years of age.

Each tablet contains:

Dibasic Calcium Phosphate, hydrous (as anhydrous form)	500 mg
Cholecalciferol	3.33 mcg (133 IU)

Microcrystalline cellulose, sodium starch glycolate, corn starch, hydrogenated vegetable oil wax, magnesium stearate and talc added.

Calcium to phosphorous ratio 1.3 to 1.

Wafers

Daily dosage (two wafers) provides:

Vitamin D	400 IU (10 mcg)	100% USRDA
Calcium	0.464 g	46% USRDA
Phosphorus	0.36 g	36% USRDA

Each wafer contains:

Cholecalciferol	5 mcg (200 IU)
Dibasic Calcium Phosphate, hydrous	1 g

Added dextrose, sucrose, talc, stearic acid, mineral oil, salt, and natural and artificial flavorings.

Calcium to phosphorus ratio 1.29 to 1.

INDICATIONS

For those individuals who must restrict their intake of dairy products.

DOSAGE AND ADMINISTRATION

Usual dose for adults and children 4 years and older:

Tablets—1 tablet 3 times daily with meals, or as directed by the physician or dentist.

Wafers—Chew 1 wafer twice daily with meals, or as directed by the physician or dentist.

HOW SUPPLIED

Dical-D Tablets in bottles of 100 (**NDC** 0074-3741-13) and 500 (**NDC** 0074-3741-53).

Dical-D Wafers in box of 51 (**NDC** 0074-3589-01).

Recommended storage: Store below 77°F (25°C).

Ref. 03-1924-2/R4 and 09-6484-5/R10

ENDURON® ℞

[en'de-ron]

(methyclothiazide tablets, USP)

DESCRIPTION

Methyclothiazide is a member of the benzothiadiazine (thiazide) class of drugs. It is an analogue of hydrochlorothiazide and occurs as a white to practically white crystalline powder which is basically odorless. Methyclothiazide is very slightly soluble in water and chloroform, and slightly soluble in alcohol. Chemically, methyclothiazide is represented as 6-chloro-3-(chloromethyl)-3, 4-dihydro-2-methyl-2H-1,2,4-benzothiadiazine-7-sulfonamide 1,1-dioxide.

Clinically, ENDURON (methyclothiazide) is an oral diuretic-antihypertensive agent. ENDURON tablets are available in two dosage strengths containing 2.5 mg and 5 mg of methyclothiazide.

Inactive Ingredients:

2.5 mg tablets: corn starch, FD&C Yellow No. 6, lactose, magnesium stearate and talc.

5 mg tablets: corn starch, D&C Red No. 36, lactose, magnesium stearate and talc.

CLINICAL PHARMACOLOGY

The diuretic and saluretic effects of methyclothiazide result from a drug-induced inhibition of the renal tubular reabsorption of electrolytes. The excretion of sodium and chloride is greatly enhanced. Potassium excretion is also enhanced to a variable degree, as it is with the other thiazides. Although urinary excretion of bicarbonate is increased slightly, there is usually no significant change in urinary pH. Methyclothiazide has a per mg natriuretic activity approximately 100 times that of the prototype thiazide, chlorothiazide. At maximal therapeutic dosages, all thiazides are approximately equal in their diuretic/natriuretic effects.

There is significant natriuresis and diuresis within two hours after administration of a single dose of methyclothiazide. These effects reach a peak in about six hours and persist for 24 hours following oral administration of a single dose.

Like other benzothiadiazines, methylclothiazide also has antihypertensive properties, and may be used for this purpose either alone or to enhance the antihypertensive action of other drugs. The mechanism by which the benzothiadiazines, including methyclothiazide, produce a reduction of elevated blood pressure is not known. However, sodium depletion appears to be involved.

Methyclothiazide is rapidly absorbed and slowly eliminated by the kidneys as intact drug but primarily as an inactive metabolite. Additional information on the pharmacokinetics is not known at this time.

Continued on next page

Abbott Laboratories—Cont.

INDICATIONS AND USAGE

ENDURON (methyclothiazide) is indicated in the management of hypertension either as the sole therapeutic agent or to enhance the effect of other antihypertensive drugs in the more severe forms of hypertension.

ENDURON tablets are indicated as adjunctive therapy in edema associated with congestive heart failure, hepatic cirrhosis, and corticosteroid and estrogen therapy.

ENDURON tablets have also been found useful in edema due to various forms of renal dysfunction such as the nephrotic syndrome, acute glomerulonephritis, and chronic renal failure.

Usage in Pregnancy: The routine use of diuretics in an otherwise healthy pregnant woman is inappropriate and exposes mother and fetus to unnecessary hazard. Diuretics do not prevent development of toxemia of pregnancy, and there is no satisfactory evidence that they are useful in the treatment of developed toxemia.

Edema during pregnancy may arise from pathological causes or from the physiological and mechanical consequences of pregnancy. Thiazides are indicated in pregnancy when edema is due to pathological causes, just as they are in the absence of pregnancy (see PRECAUTIONS—Pregnancy). Dependent edema in pregnancy, resulting from restriction of venous return by the expanded uterus, is properly treated through elevation of the lower extremities and use of support hose; use of diuretics to lower intravascular volume in this case is illogical and unnecessary. There is hypervolemia during normal pregnancy that is harmful to neither the fetus nor the mother (in the absence of cardiovascular disease), but that is associated with edema, including generalized edema, in the majority of pregnant women. If this edema produces discomfort, increased recumbency will often provide relief. In rare instances, this edema may cause extreme discomfort that is not relieved by rest. In these cases, a short course of diuretics may provide relief and may be appropriate.

CONTRAINDICATIONS

Methyclothiazide is contraindicated in patients with anuria and in patients with a history of hypersensitivity to this compound or other sulfonamide-derived drugs.

WARNINGS

Methyclothiazide shares with other thiazides the propensity to deplete potassium reserves to an unpredictable degree.

There have been isolated reports that certain non-edematous individuals developed severe fluid and electrolyte derangements after only brief exposure to normal doses of thiazide and non-thiazide diuretics.

Thiazides should be used with caution in patients with renal disease or significant impairment of renal function, since azotemia may be precipitated and cumulative drug effects may occur.

Thiazides should be used with caution in patients with impaired hepatic function or progressive liver disease, since minor alterations of fluid and electrolyte balance may precipitate hepatic coma.

Sensitivity reactions may occur in patients with a history of allergy or bronchial asthma.

The possibility of exacerbation or activation of systemic lupus erythematosus has been reported.

Hyperuricemia may occur or frank gout may be precipitated in certain patients receiving thiazide therapy.

PRECAUTIONS

Laboratory Tests: Initial and periodic determinations of serum electrolytes should be performed at appropriate intervals for the purpose of detecting possible electrolyte imbalances such as hyponatremia, hypochloremic alkalosis, and hypokalemia. Serum and urine electrolyte determinations are particularly important when a patient is vomiting excessively or receiving parenteral fluids.

General: All patients should be observed for clinical signs of electrolyte imbalances such as dryness of mouth, thirst, weakness, lethargy, drowsiness, restlessness, muscle pains or cramps, muscular fatigue, hypotension, oliguria, tachycardia, and gastrointestinal disturbances such as nausea and vomiting.

Hypokalemia may develop, especially with brisk diuresis, when severe cirrhosis is present, during concomitant use of corticosteroids or ACTH, or after prolonged therapy.

Interference with adequate oral electrolyte intake will also contribute to hypokalemia. Hypokalemia may be avoided or treated by use of potassium supplements or foods with a high potassium content.

Any chloride deficit is generally mild and usually does not require specific treatment except under extraordinary circumstances (as in liver disease or renal disease). Dilutional hyponatremia may occur in edematous patients in hot weather; appropriate therapy is water restriction rather than administration of salt, except in rare instances when the hyponatremia is life threatening. In actual salt depletion, appropriate replacement is the therapy of choice.

Latent diabetes mellitus may become manifest during thiazide administration.

The antihypertensive effects of the drug may be enhanced in the postsympathectomy patient.

If progressive renal impairment becomes evident as indicated by a rising nonprotein nitrogen or blood urea nitrogen, a careful reappraisal of therapy is necessary with consideration given to withholding or discontinuing diuretic therapy.

Thiazides may decrease urinary calcium excretion. Thiazides may cause intermittent and slight elevation of serum calcium in the absence of known disorders of calcium metabolism. Marked hypercalcemia may be evidence of hidden hyperparathyroidism. Thiazides should be discontinued before carrying out tests for parathyroid function.

Thiazides may cause increased concentrations of total serum cholesterol, total triglycerides, and low-density lipoproteins in some patients. Use thiazides with caution in patients with moderate or high cholesterol concentrations and in patients with elevated triglyceride levels.

Information for Patients: Patients should inform their doctor if they have: 1) had an allergic reaction to methyclothiazide or other diuretics 2) asthma 3) kidney disease 4) liver disease 5) gout 6) systemic lupus erythematosus, or 7) been taking other drugs such as cortisone, digitalis, lithium carbonate, or drugs for diabetes.

The physician should inform patients of possible side effects and caution the patient to report any of the following symptoms of electrolyte imbalance; dryness of mouth, thirst, weakness, tiredness, drowsiness, restlessness, muscle pains or cramps, nausea, vomiting or increased heart rate.

The physician should advise the patient to take this medication every day as directed. Physicians should also caution patients that drinking alcohol can increase the chance of dizziness.

Drug Interactions: Hypokalemia can sensitize or exaggerate the response of the heart to the toxic effects of *digitalis* (e.g., increased ventricular irritability).

Hypokalemia may develop during concomitant use of *steroids* or *ACTH.*

Insulin requirements in diabetic patients may be increased, decreased, or unchanged.

Thiazides may decrease arterial responsiveness to *norepinephrine.* This diminution is not sufficient to preclude effectiveness of the pressor agent for therapeutic use.

Thiazide drugs may increase the responsiveness to *tubocurarine.*

Lithium renal clearance is reduced by thiazides, increasing the risk of lithium toxicity.

Thiazides may add to or potentiate the action of *other antihypertensive drugs.* Potentiation occurs with ganglionic or peripheral adrenergic blocking drugs.

Drug/Laboratory Test Interactions: Thiazides may decrease serum PBI levels without signs of thyroid disturbance.

Thiazides should be discontinued before carrying out tests for parathyroid function.

Carcinogenesis, Mutagenesis, Impairment of Fertility: No data are available concerning the potential for carcinogenicity or mutagenicity in animals or humans. Methyclothiazide did not impair fertility in rats receiving up to 4 mg/kg/day (at least 20 times the maximum recommended human dose of 10 mg, assuming patient weight equal to or greater than 50 kg).

Pregnancy—Teratogenic Effects: Pregnancy Category B. Reproduction studies performed in rats and rabbits at doses up to 4 mg/kg/day have revealed no evidence of harm to the fetus due to methyclothiazide. There are, however, no adequate and well-controlled studies in pregnant women. Because animal reproduction studies are not always predictive of human response, this drug should be used during pregnancy only if clearly needed.

Nonteratogenic Effects: Thiazides cross the placental barrier and appear in cord blood. The use of thiazides in pregnant women requires that the anticipated benefit be weighed against possible hazards to the fetus. These hazards include fetal or neonatal jaundice, thrombocytopenia and possible other adverse reactions that have occurred in the adult.

Nursing Mothers: Thiazides are excreted in breast milk. Because of the potential for serious adverse reactions in nursing infants, a decision should be made whether to discontinue nursing or to discontinue the drug taking into account the importance of the drug to the mother.

Pediatric Use: Safety and effectiveness in children have not been established.

ADVERSE REACTIONS

Adverse reactions are usually reversible upon reduction of dosage or discontinuation of ENDURON tablets. Whenever adverse reactions are moderate or severe, it may be necessary to discontinue the drug.

The following adverse reactions have been observed, but there has not been enough systematic collection of data to support an estimate of their frequency. Consequently the reactions are categorized by organ system and are listed in decreasing order of severity and not frequency.

Body as a Whole: Headache, cramping, weakness.

Cardiovascular System: Orthostatic hypotension (may be potentiated by alcohol, barbiturates, or narcotics).

Digestive System: Pancreatitis, jaundice (intrahepatic cholestatic), sialadenitis, vomiting, diarrhea, nausea, gastric irritation, constipation, anorexia.

Hemic and Lymphatic System: Aplastic anemia, hemolytic anemia, agranulocytosis, leukopenia, thrombocytopenia.

Hypersensitivity Reactions: Anaphylactic reactions, necrotizing angiitis (vasculitis, cutaneous vasculitis), Stevens-Johnson syndrome, respiratory distress including pneumonitis and pulmonary edema, fever, purpura, urticaria, rash, photosensitivity.

Metabolic and Nutritional Disorders: Hyperglycemia, hyperuricemia, electrolyte imbalance (see PRECAUTIONS section), hypercalcemia.

Nervous System: Vertigo, dizziness, paresthesias, muscle spasm, restlessness.

Special Senses: Transient blurred vision, xanthopsia.

Urogenital System: Glycosuria.

OVERDOSAGE

Symptoms of overdosage include electrolyte imbalance and signs of potassium deficiency such as confusion, dizziness, muscular weakness, and gastrointestinal disturbances. General supportive measures including replacement of fluids and electrolytes may be indicated in treatment of overdosage.

DOSAGE AND ADMINISTRATION

ENDURON (methyclothiazide) is administered orally. Therapy should be individualized according to patient response. This therapy should be titrated to gain maximal therapeutic response as well as the minimal dose possible to maintain that therapeutic response.

For edematous conditions: The usual adult dose ranges from 2.5 to 10 mg once daily. Maximum effective single dose is 10 mg; larger single doses do not accomplish greater diuresis, and are not recommended.

For the treatment of hypertension: The usual adult dose ranges from 2.5 to 5 mg once daily.

If control of blood pressure is not satisfactory after 8 to 12 weeks of therapy with 5 mg once daily, another antihypertensive drug should be added. Increasing the dosage of methylclothiazide will usually not result in further lowering of blood pressure.

Methyclothiazide may be either employed alone for mild to moderate hypertension or concurrently with other antihypertensive drugs in the management of more severe forms of hypertension. Combined therapy may provide adequate control of hypertension with lower dosage of the component drugs and fewer or less severe side effects. An enhanced response frequently follows its concurrent administration with Harmonyl® (deserpidine) so that dosage of both drugs may be reduced.

When other antihypertensive agents are to be added to the regimen, this should be accomplished gradually. Ganglionic blocking agents should be given at only half the usual dose since their effect is potentiated by pretreatment with ENDURON tablets.

HOW SUPPLIED

ENDURON (methyclothiazide tablets, USP) is provided in two dosage sizes as monogrammed, grooved, square-shaped tablets:

2.5 mg, orange-colored:
- bottles of 100 (**NDC** 0074-6827-01),
- bottles of 1000 (**NDC** 0074-6827-02).

5 mg, salmon-colored:
- bottles of 100 (**NDC** 0074-6812-01),
- bottles of 1000 (**NDC** 0074-6812-02),
- bottles of 5000 (**NDC** 0074-6812-03),
- Abbo-Pac® unit dose packages of 100 (**NDC** 0074-6812-10).

Dispense in a USP tight container.

Recommended storage: Store below 86°F (30°C).

Ref. 03-4404-R9

Shown in Product Identification Section, page 403

ENDURONYL® Tablets ℞
[en-du 're-nil]
(methyclothiazide and deserpidine)

Oral thiazide-rauwolfia therapy for hypertension.

WARNING

This fixed combination drug is not indicated for initial therapy of hypertension. Hypertension requires therapy titrated to the individual patient. If the fixed combination represents the dosage so determined, its use may be more convenient in patient management. The treatment of hypertension is not static, but must be reevaluated as conditions in each patient warrant.

DESCRIPTION

ENDURONYL is an orally-administered combination of Enduron® (methyclothiazide) and Harmonyl® (deserpidine). Methyclothiazide is an oral diuretic-antihypertensive of the benzothiadiazine (thiazide) class. Deserpidine is a purified rauwolfia alkaloid, chemically identified as 11-desmethoxyreserpine, which produces antihypertensive effects.

Inactive Ingredients:

Enduronyl tablets: corn starch, D&C Yellow No. 10, FD&C Yellow No. 6, lactose, magnesium stearate and talc.

Enduronyl Forte tablets: corn starch, iron oxide, lactose, magnesium stearate and talc.

ACTIONS

The combined antihypertensive actions of methyclothiazide and deserpidine result in a total clinical antihypertensive effect which is greater than can ordinarily be achieved by either drug given individually.

The diuretic and saluretic effects of methyclothiazide result from a drug-induced inhibition of the renal tubular reabsorption of electrolytes. The excretion of sodium and chloride is greatly enhanced. Potassium excretion is also enhanced to a variable degree, as it is with the other thiazides. Although urinary excretion of bicarbonate is increased slightly, there is usually no significant change in urinary pH. Methyclothiazide has a per mg natriuretic activity approximately 100 times that of the prototype thiazide, chlorothiazide. At maximal therapeutic dosages, all thiazides are approximately equal in their diuretic/natriuretic effects.

There is significant natriuresis and diuresis within two hours after administration of a single dose of methyclothiazide. These effects reach a peak in about six hours and persist for 24 hours following oral administration of a single dose.

Like other benzothiadiazines, methyclothiazide also has antihypertensive properties, and may be used for this purpose either alone or to enhance the antihypertensive action of other drugs. The mechanism by which the benzothiadiazines, including methyclothiazide, produce a reduction of elevated blood pressure is not known. However, sodium depletion appears to be involved.

Methyclothiazide is rapidly absorbed and slowly eliminated by the kidney as both intact drug and as a metabolite showing no diuretic activity in a rat model.

The pharmacologic actions of Harmonyl (deserpidine) are essentially the same as those of other active rauwolfia alkaloids. Deserpidine probably produces its antihypertensive effects through depletion of tissue stores of catecholamines (epinephrine and norepinephrine) from peripheral sites. The antihypertensive effect is often accompanied by bradycardia. There is no significant alteration in cardiac output or renal blood flow. The carotid sinus reflex is inhibited, but postural hypotension is rarely seen with the use of conventional doses of Harmonyl alone.

Deserpidine, like other rauwolfia alkaloids, is characterized by slow onset of action and sustained effect which may persist following withdrawal of the drug.

INDICATIONS

ENDURONYL (methyclothiazide and deserpidine) is indicated in the treatment of mild to moderately severe hypertension (see boxed warning). In many cases ENDURONYL alone produces an adequate reduction of blood pressure. In resistant or unusually severe cases ENDURONYL also may be supplemented by more potent antihypertensive agents. When administered with ENDURONYL, more potent agents can be given at reduced dosage to minimize undesirable side effects.

CONTRAINDICATIONS

Methyclothiazide is contraindicated in patients with renal decompensation and in those who are hypersensitive to this or other sulfonamide-derived drugs.

Deserpidine is contraindicated in patients with known hypersensitivity, history of mental depression especially with suicidal tendencies, active peptic ulcer, and ulcerative colitis. It is also contraindicated in patients receiving electroconvulsive therapy.

WARNINGS

Methyclothiazide

Methyclothiazide shares with other thiazides the propensity to deplete potassium reserves to an unpredictable degree.

Thiazides should be used with caution in patients with renal disease or significant impairment of renal function, since azotemia may be precipitated and cumulative drug effects may occur.

Thiazides should be used with caution in patients with impaired hepatic function or progressive liver disease, since minor alterations of fluid and electrolyte balance may precipitate hepatic coma.

Thiazides may be additive or potentiative of the action of other antihypertensive drugs. Potentiation occurs with ganglionic or peripheral adrenergic blocking drugs.

Sensitivity reactions may occur in patients with a history of allergy or bronchial asthma.

The possibility of exacerbation or activation of systemic lupus erythematosus has been reported.

Deserpidine

Deserpidine differs slightly in chemical structure from reserpine, however, its actions, indications, cautions and adverse reactions are common to the class of rauwolfia alkaloids. Reserpine may cause mental depression. Recognition of depression may be difficult because this condition may often be disguised by somatic complaints (Masked Depression). The drug should be discontinued at first signs of depression such as despondency, early morning insomnia, loss of appetite, impotence, or self-deprecation. Drug-induced depression may persist for several months after drug withdrawal and may be severe enough to result in suicide.

Usage in Pregnancy and Lactation:

Methyclothiazide

Thiazides cross the placental barrier and appear in cord blood. The use of thiazides in pregnant women requires that the anticipated benefit be weighed against possible hazards to the fetus. These hazards include fetal or neonatal jaundice, thrombocytopenia, and possible other adverse reactions that have occurred in the adult.

Thiazides appear in breast milk. If use of the drug is deemed essential, the patient should stop nursing.

Deserpidine

The safety of deserpidine for use during pregnancy or lactation has not been established; therefore, it should be used in pregnant women or in women of childbearing potential only when in the judgment of the physician its use is deemed essential to the welfare of the patient. Increased respiratory secretions, nasal congestion, cyanosis, and anorexia may occur in infants born to rauwolfia alkaloid-treated mothers, since these preparations are known to cross the placental barrier to enter the fetal circulation and appear in cord blood. They also are secreted by nursing mothers into breast milk.

Reproductive and teratology studies in rats reduced the mating index and neonatal survival indices; the no-effect dosage has not been established.

PRECAUTIONS

Periodic determinations of serum electrolytes should be performed at appropriate intervals for the purpose of detecting possible electrolyte imbalances such as hyponatremia, hypochloremic alkalosis, and hypokalemia. Serum and urine electrolyte determinations are particularly important when a patient is vomiting excessively or receiving parenteral fluids. All patients should be observed for other clinical signs of electrolyte imbalances such as dryness of mouth, thirst, weakness, lethargy, drowsiness, restlessness, muscle pains or cramps, muscular fatigue, hypotension, oliguria, tachycardia, and gastrointestinal disturbances such as nausea and vomiting.

Hypokalemia may develop with thiazides as with any other potent diuretic, especially when brisk diuresis occurs, severe cirrhosis is present, or when corticosteroids or ACTH are given concomitantly. Interference with the adequate oral intake of electrolytes will also contribute to the possible development of hypokalemia. Potassium depletion, even of a mild degree, resulting from thiazide use, may sensitize a patient to the effects of cardiac glycosides such as digitalis.

Any chloride deficit is generally mild and usually does not require specific treatment except under extraordinary circumstances (as in liver disease or renal disease). Dilutional hyponatremia may occur in edematous patients in hot weather; appropriate therapy is water restriction rather than administration of salt, except in rare instances when the hyponatremia is life threatening.

In actual salt depletion, appropriate replacement is the therapy of choice.

Hyperuricemia may occur or frank gout may be precipitated in certain patients receiving thiazide therapy.

Insulin requirements in diabetic patients may be increased, decreased, or unchanged. Latent diabetes mellitus may become manifest during thiazide administration.

Thiazide drugs may increase the responsiveness to tubocurarine.

The antihypertensive effects of the drug may be enhanced in the postsympathectomy patient.

Thiazides may decrease arterial responsiveness to norepinephrine. This diminution is not sufficient to preclude effectiveness of the pressor agent for therapeutic use.

If progressive renal impairment becomes evident as indicated by a rising nonprotein nitrogen or blood urea nitrogen, a careful reappraisal of therapy is necessary with consideration given to withholding or discontinuing diuretic therapy.

Thiazides may decrease serum PBI levels without signs of thyroid disturbance.

Thiazides have been reported, on rare occasions, to have elevated serum calcium to hypercalcemic levels. The serum calcium levels have returned to normal when the medication has been stopped. This phenomenon may be related to the ability of the thiazide diuretics to lower the amount of calcium excreted in the urine.

Because rauwolfia preparations increase gastrointestinal motility and secretion, this drug should be used cautiously in patients with a history of peptic ulcer, ulcerative colitis, or gallstones, where biliary colic may be precipitated.

Caution should be exercised when treating hypertensive patients with renal insufficiency since they adjust poorly to lowered blood pressure levels.

Use deserpidine cautiously with digitalis and quinidine since cardiac arrhythmias have occurred with rauwolfia preparations.

Preoperative withdrawal of deserpidine does not assure that circulatory instability will not occur. It is important that the anesthesiologist be aware of the patient's drug intake and consider this in the overall management, since hypotension has occurred in patients receiving rauwolfia preparations. Anticholinergic and/or adrenergic drugs (metaraminol, norepinephrine) have been employed to treat adverse vagocirculatory effects.

Animal tumorigenicity: There are no studies demonstrating that deserpidine is an animal tumorigen, although it is a prolactin stimulator and structurally related to reserpine. Rodent studies with reserpine, however, have shown that reserpine is an animal tumorigen, causing an increased incidence of mammary fibroadenomas in female mice, malignant tumors of the seminal vesicles in male mice, and malignant adrenal medullary tumors in male rats. These findings arose in 2 year studies in which the drug was administered in the feed at concentrations of 5 to 10 ppm—about 100 to 300 times the usual human dose. The breast neoplasms are thought to be related to reserpine's prolactin-elevating effect. Several other prolactin-elevating drugs have also been associated with an increased incidence of mammary neoplasia in rodents.

The extent to which these findings indicate a risk to humans is uncertain. Tissue culture experiments show that about one-third of human breast tumors are prolactin-dependent *in vitro,* a factor of considerable importance if the use of the drug is contemplated in a patient with previously detected breast cancer. The possibility of an increased risk of breast cancer in reserpine users has been studied extensively; however, no firm conclusion has emerged. Although a few epidemiologic studies have suggested a slightly increased risk (less than twofold in all studies except one) in women who have used reserpine, other studies of generally similar design have not confirmed this. Epidemiologic studies conducted using other drugs (neuroleptic agents) that, like reserpine, increase prolactin levels and, therefore, would be considered rodent mammary carcinogens, have not shown an association between chronic administration of the drug and human mammary tumorigenesis. While long-term clinical observation has not suggested such an association, the available evidence is considered too limited to be conclusive at this time. An association of reserpine intake with pheochromocytoma or tumors of the seminal vesicles has not been explored.

ADVERSE REACTIONS

Methyclothiazide

Gastrointestinal System Reactions: Anorexia, gastric irritation, nausea, vomiting, cramping, diarrhea, constipation, jaundice (intrahepatic cholestatic jaundice), pancreatitis.

Central Nervous System Reactions: Dizziness, vertigo, paresthesias, headache, xanthopsia.

Hematologic Reactions: Leukopenia, agranulocytosis, thrombocytopenia, aplastic anemia.

Dermatologic — Hypersensitivity Reactions: Purpura, photosensitivity, rash, urticaria, necrotizing angiitis (vasculitis) (cutaneous vasculitis).

Cardiovascular Reaction: Orthostatic hypotension may occur and may be aggravated by alcohol, barbiturates, or narcotics.

Other: Hyperglycemia, glycosuria, hypercalcemia, hyperuricemia, muscle spasm, weakness, restlessness.

There have been isolated reports that certain nonedematous individuals developed severe fluid and electrolyte derangements after only brief exposure to normal doses of thiazide and non-thiazide diuretics. The condition is usually manifested as severe dilutional hyponatremia, hypokalemia, and hypochloremia. It has been reported to be due to inappropriately increased ADH secretion and appears to be idiosyncratic. Potassium replacement is apparently the most important therapy in the treatment of this syndrome along with removal of the offending drug.

Whenever adverse reactions are severe, treatment should be discontinued.

Deserpidine

The following adverse reactions have been reported with rauwolfia preparations. These reactions are usually reversible and disappear when the drug is discontinued.

Gastrointestinal: Including hypersecretion, anorexia, diarrhea, nausea, and vomiting.

Cardiovascular: Including angina-like symptoms, arrhythmias (particularly when used concurrently with digitalis or quinidine), and bradycardia.

Continued on next page

Abbott Laboratories—Cont.

Central Nervous System: Including drowsiness, depression, nervousness, paradoxical anxiety, nightmares, extrapyramidal tract symptoms, CNS sensitization manifested by dull sensorium, and deafness.
Dermatologic—Hypersensitivity: Including pruritus, rash, and asthma in asthmatic patients.
Ophthalmologic: Including glaucoma, uveitis, optic atrophy, and conjunctival injection.
Hematologic: Thrombocytopenic purpura.
Miscellaneous: Nasal congestion, weight gain, impotence or decreased libido, dysuria, dyspnea, muscular aches, dryness of mouth, dizziness, and headache.

DOSAGE AND ADMINISTRATION

Dosage should be determined by individual titration of ingredients (see boxed warning). Dosage of both components should be carefully adjusted to the needs of the individual patient. Since at least ten days to two weeks may elapse before the full effects of the drugs become manifest, the dosage of the drugs should not be adjusted more frequently.
Two tablet strengths, ENDURONYL (methyclothiazide 5 mg, deserpidine 0.25 mg) and ENDURONYL FORTE (methyclothiazide 5 mg, deserpidine 0.5 mg), each grooved, are provided to permit considerable latitude in meeting the dosage requirements of individual patients.*
The following table will help in determining which dose of ENDURONYL or ENDURONYL FORTE best represents the equivalent of the titrated dose.

Daily Dosage of ENDURONYL	methyclothiazide	deserpidine
½ tablet	2.5 mg	0.125 mg
1 tablet	5.0 mg	0.250 mg
1½ tablet	7.5 mg	0.375 mg
2 tablets	10.0 mg	0.500 mg

Daily Dosage of ENDURONYL FORTE	methyclothiazide	deserpidine
½ tablet	2.5 mg	0.250 mg
1 tablet	5.0 mg	0.500 mg
1½ tablet	7.5 mg	0.750 mg
2 tablets	10.0 mg	1.000 mg

The appropriate dose of ENDURONYL is administered orally, once daily. The usual adult dosage is one lower-strength ENDURONYL tablet daily.
There is no contraindication to combining the administration of ENDURONYL with other antihypertensive agents. When other antihypertensive agents are to be added to the regimen, this should be accomplished gradually. Ganglionic blocking agents should be given at only half the usual dose since their effect is potentiated by pretreatment with ENDURONYL.

OVERDOSAGE

Symptoms of thiazide overdosage include electrolyte imbalance and signs of potassium deficiency such as confusion, dizziness, muscular weakness, and gastrointestinal disturbances. General supportive measures including replacement of fluids and electrolytes may be indicated in treatment of overdosage.
An overdosage of deserpidine is characterized by flushing of the skin, conjunctival injection, and pupillary constriction. Sedation ranging from drowsiness to coma may occur. Hypotension, hypothermia, central respiratory depression and bradycardia may develop in cases of severe overdosage. Treatment consists of the careful evacuation of stomach contents followed by the usual procedures for the symptomatic management of CNS depressant overdosage. If severe hypotension occurs it should be treated with a direct acting vasopressor such as norepinephrine bitartrate injection.

HOW SUPPLIED

ENDURONYL (methyclothiazide and deserpidine) is supplied as monogrammed, grooved, square-shaped tablets in the following dosage sizes and quantities:
ENDURONYL (5 mg of methyclothiazide and 0.25 mg of deserpidine) yellow tablets in bottles of 100 (**NDC** 0074-6838-01) and 1000 (**NDC** 0074-6838-02). Also available in ABBO-PAC® unit dose packages, 100 tablets (**NDC** 0074-6838-06), in strips of 10 tablets.
ENDURONYL FORTE (5 mg of methyclothiazide and 0.5 mg of deserpidine) gray-colored tablets in bottles of 100 (**NDC** 0074-6854-01) and 1000 (**NDC** 0074-6854-02).

*Each component is separately available as ENDURON (methyclothiazide) and HARMONYL (deserpidine).
Recommended Storage: Store below 86°F (30°C).
Ref. 03-4405-R10
Shown in Product Identification Section, page 403

ERYPED® ℞
[*erē 'ped*]
(erythromycin ethylsuccinate)

DESCRIPTION

Erythromycin is produced by a strain of *Streptomyces erythraeus* and belongs to the macrolide group of antibiotics. It is basic and readily forms salts with acids. The base, the stearate salt, and the esters are poorly soluble in water. Erythromycin ethylsuccinate is an ester of erythromycin suitable for oral administration.
EryPed 200 and EryPed Drops (erythromycin ethylsuccinate for oral suspension) when reconstituted with water, forms a suspension containing erythromycin ethylsuccinate equivalent to 200 mg erythromycin per 5 mL (teaspoonful) or 100 mg per 2.5 mL (dropperful) with an appealing fruit flavor.
EryPed 400 when reconstituted with water, forms a suspension containing erythromycin ethylsuccinate equivalent to 400 mg of erythromycin per 5 mL (teaspoonful) with an appealing banana flavor. After mixing, EryPed must be stored below 77°F (25°C) and used within 35 days; refrigeration is not required.
Fruit-flavored EryPed Chewable tablets are easily ingested and are particularly acceptable for the administration of antibiotic medication to young children who are unable to swallow regular tablets or in whom persuasion of a pleasant taste insures cooperation. Each chewable tablet contains the equivalent of 200 mg of erythromycin activity and is scored for division into half-dose (100 mg) portions.
These products are intended primarily for pediatric use but can also be used in adults.
Inactive Ingredients: EryPed 200, EryPed 400 and EryPed Drops: Caramel, polysorbate, sodium citrate, sucrose, xanthan gum and artificial flavors.
EryPed Chewable Tablets: Citric acid, confectioner's sugar (contains corn starch), magnesium aluminum silicate, magnesium stearate, sodium carboxymethyl cellulose, sodium citrate and artificial flavor.

ACTIONS

Microbiology: Biochemical tests demonstrate that erythromycin inhibits protein synthesis of the pathogen without directly affecting nucleic acid synthesis. Antagonism has been demonstrated between clindamycin and erythromycin.
NOTE: Many strains of *Hemophilus influenzae* are resistant to erythromycin alone, but are susceptible to erythromycin and sulfonamides together. Staphylococci resistant to erythromycin may emerge during a course of erythromycin therapy. Culture and susceptibility testing should be performed.
Disc Susceptibility Tests: Quantitative methods that require measurement of zone diameters give the most precise estimates of antibiotic susceptibility. One recommended procedure (21 CFR section 460.1) uses erythromycin class discs for testing susceptibility; interpretations correlate zone diameters of this disc test with MIC values for erythromycin. With this procedure, a report from the laboratory of "susceptible" indicates that the infecting organism is likely to respond to therapy. A report of "resistant" indicates, that the infective organism is not likely to respond to therapy. A report of "intermediate susceptibility" suggests that the organism would be susceptible if higher doses were used.
Clinical Pharmacology: Erythromycin binds to the 50 S ribosomal subunits of susceptible bacteria and suppresses protein synthesis.
Orally administered erythromycin ethylsuccinate suspension is readily and reliably absorbed under both fasting and nonfasting conditions.
Erythromycin diffuses readily into most body fluids. Only low concentrations are normally achieved in the spinal fluid, but passage of the drug across the blood-brain barrier increases in meningitis. In the presence of normal hepatic function, erythromycin is concentrated in the liver and excreted in the bile; the effect of hepatic dysfunction on excretion of erythromycin by the liver into the bile is not known. Less than 5 percent of the orally administered dose of erythromycin is excreted in active form in the urine.
Erythromycin crosses the placental barrier and is excreted in breast milk.

INDICATIONS

Streptococcus pyogenes (Group A beta-hemolytic streptococcus): Upper and lower respiratory tract, skin, and soft tissue infections of mild to moderate severity.
Injectable benzathine penicillin G is considered by the American Heart Association to be the drug of choice in the treatment and prevention of streptococcal pharyngitis and in long-term prophylaxis of rheumatic fever.
When oral medication is preferred for treatment of the above conditions, penicillin G, V, or erythromycin are alternate drugs of choice.
When oral medication is given, the importance of strict adherence by the patient to the prescribed dosage regimen must be stressed. A therapeutic dose should be administered for at least 10 days.
Alpha-hemolytic streptococci (viridans group): Although no controlled clinical efficacy trials have been conducted, oral erythromycin has been suggested by the American Heart Association and American Dental Association for use in a regimen for prophylaxis against bacterial endocarditis in patients hypersensitive to penicillin who have congenital heart disease, or rheumatic or other acquired valvular heart disease when they undergo dental procedures and surgical procedures of the upper respiratory tract.[1] Erythromycin is not suitable prior to genitourinary or gastrointestinal tract surgery. NOTE: When selecting antibiotics for the prevention of bacterial endocarditis the physician or dentist should read the full joint statement of the American Heart Association and the American Dental Association.[1]
Staphylococcus aureus: Acute infections of skin and soft tissue of mild to moderate severity. Resistant organisms may emerge during treatment.
Streptococcus pneumoniae (Diplococcus pneumoniae): Upper respiratory tract infections (e.g., otitis media, pharyngitis) and lower respiratory tract infections (e.g., pneumonia) of mild to moderate degree.
Mycoplasma pneumoniae (Eaton agent, PPLO): For respiratory infections due to this organism.
Hemophilus influenzae: For upper respiratory tract infections of mild to moderate severity when used concomitantly with adequate doses of sulfonamides. (See sulfonamide labeling for appropriate prescribing information). The concomitant use of the sulfonamides is necessary since not all strains of *Hemophilus influenzae* are susceptible to erythromycin at the concentrations of the antibiotic achieved with usual therapeutic doses.
Chlamydia trachomatis: For the treatment of urethritis in adult males due to *Chlamydia trachomatis.*
Ureaplasma urealyticum: For the treatment of urethritis in adult males due to *Ureaplasma urealyticum.*
Treponema pallidum: Erythromycin is an alternate choice of treatment for primary syphilis in patients allergic to the penicillins. In treatment of primary syphilis, spinal fluid examinations should be done before treatment and as part of follow-up after therapy.
Corynebacterium diphtheriae: As an adjunct to antitoxin, to prevent establishment of carriers, and to eradicate the organism in carriers.
Corynebacterium minutissimum: For the treatment of erythrasma.
Entamoeba histolytica: In the treatment of intestinal amebiasis only. Extraenteric amebiasis requires treatment with other agents.
Listeria monocytogenes: Infections due to this organism.
Bordetella pertussis: Erythromycin is effective in eliminating the organism from the nasopharynx of infected individuals, rendering them non-infectious. Some clinical studies suggest that erythromycin may be helpful in the prophylaxis of pertussis in exposed susceptible individuals.
Legionnaires' Disease: Although no controlled clinical efficacy studies have been conducted, *in vitro* and limited preliminary clinical data suggest that erythromycin may be effective in treating Legionnaires' Disease.

CONTRAINDICATIONS

Erythromycin is contraindicated in patients with known hypersensitivity to this antibiotic.

WARNINGS

There have been reports of hepatic dysfunction with or without jaundice, occurring in patients receiving oral erythromycin products.

PRECAUTIONS

General: Erythromycin is principally excreted by the liver. Caution should be exercised when erythromycin is administered to patients with impaired hepatic function. (See "Clinical Pharmacology" and "Warnings" sections).
Prolonged or repeated use of erythromycin may result in an overgrowth of nonsusceptible bacteria or fungi. If superinfection occurs, erythromycin should be discontinued and appropriate therapy instituted.
When indicated, incision and drainage or other surgical procedures should be performed in conjunction with antibiotic therapy.
Laboratory Tests: Erythromycin interferes with the fluorometric determination of urinary catecholamines.
Drug Interactions: Erythromycin use in patients who are receiving high doses of theophylline may be associated with an increase in serum theophylline levels and potential theophylline toxicity. In case of theophylline toxicity and/or elevated serum theophylline levels, the dose of theophylline should be reduced while the patient is receiving concomitant erythromycin therapy.
Concomitant administration of erythromycin and digoxin has been reported to result in elevated digoxin serum levels.
There have been reports of increased anticoagulant effects when erythromycin and oral anticoagulants were used concomitantly.
Concurrent use of erythromycin and ergotamine or dihydroergotamine has been associated in some patients with acute

ergot toxicity characterized by severe peripheral vasospasm and dysesthesia.

Erythromycin has been reported to decrease the clearance of triazolam and thus may increase the pharmacologic effect of triazolam.

The use of erythromycin in patients concurrently taking drugs metabolized by the cytochrome P450 system may be associated with elevations in serum erythromycin with carbamazepine, cyclosporine, hexobarbital and phenytoin. Serum concentrations of drugs metabolized by the cytochrome P450 system should be monitored closely in patients concurrently receiving erythromycin.

Troleandomycin significantly alters the metabolism of terfenadine when taken concomitantly; therefore, observe caution when erythromycin and terfenadine are used concurrently.

Patients receiving concomitant lovastatin and erythromycin should be carefully monitored; cases of rhabdomyolysis have been reported in seriously ill patients.

Carcinogenesis, Mutagenesis, Impairment of Fertility: Long-term (2-year) oral studies conducted in rats with erythromycin base did not provide evidence of tumorigenicity. Mutagenicity studies have not been conducted. There was no apparent effect on male or female fertility in rats fed erythromycin (base) at levels up to 0.25 percent of diet.

Pregnancy: Pregnancy Category B: There is no evidence of teratogenicity or any other adverse effect on reproduction in female rats fed erythromycin base (up to 0.25 percent of diet) prior to and during mating, during gestation, and through weaning of two successive litters. There are, however, no adequate and well-controlled studies in pregnant women. Because animal reproduction studies are not always predictive of human response, this drug should be used during pregnancy only if clearly needed. Erythromycin has been reported to cross the placental barrier in humans, but fetal plasma levels are generally low.

Labor and Delivery: The effect of erythromycin on labor and delivery is unknown.

Nursing Mothers: Erythromycin is excreted in breast milk, therefore, caution should be exercised when erythromycin is administered to a nursing woman.

Pediatric Use: See "Indications and Usage" and "Dosage and Administration" sections.

ADVERSE REACTIONS

The most frequent side effects of oral erythromycin preparations are gastrointestinal and are dose-related. They include nausea, vomiting, abdominal pain, diarrhea and anorexia. Symptoms of hepatic dysfunction and/or abnormal liver function test results may occur (see "Warnings" section). Pseudomembranous colitis has been rarely reported in association with erythromycin therapy.

There have been isolated reports of transient central nervous system side effects including confusion, hallucinations, seizures, and vertigo; however, a cause and effect relationship has not been established.

Occasional case reports of cardiac arrhythmias such as ventricular tachycardia have been documented in patients receiving erythromycin therapy. There have been isolated reports of other cardiovascular symptoms such as chest pain, dizziness, and palpitations; however, a cause and effect relationship has not been established.

Allergic reactions ranging from urticaria and mild skin eruptions to anaphylaxis have occurred.

There have been isolated reports of reversible hearing loss occurring chiefly in patients with renal insufficiency and in patients receiving high doses of erythromycin.

OVERDOSAGE

In case of overdosage, erythromycin should be discontinued. Overdosage should be handled with the prompt elimination of unabsorbed drug and all other appropriate measures. Erythromycin is not removed by peritoneal dialysis or hemodialysis.

DOSAGE AND ADMINISTRATION

EryPed (erythromycin ethylsuccinate) oral suspensions and chewable tablets may be administered without regard to meals.

Children: Age, weight, and severity of the infection are important factors in determining the proper dosage. In mild to moderate infections the usual dosage of erythromycin ethylsuccinate for children is 30 to 50 mg/kg/day in equally divided doses every six hours. For more severe infections this dosage may be doubled. If twice-a-day dosage is desired, one-half of the total daily dose may be given every 12 hours. Doses may also be given three times daily by administering one-third of the total daily dose every 8 hours.

The following dosage schedule is suggested for mild to moderate infections:

Body Weight	Total Daily Dose
Under 10 lbs	30-50 mg/kg/day 15-25 mg/lb/day
10 to 15 lbs	200 mg
16 to 25 lbs	400 mg
26 to 50 lbs	800 mg
51 to 100 lbs	1200 mg
over 100 lbs	1600 mg

Adults: 400 mg erythromycin ethylsuccinate every 6 hours is the usual dose. Dosage may be increased up to 4 g per day according to the severity of the infection. If twice-a-day dosage is desired, one-half of the total daily dose may be given every 12 hours. Doses may also be given three times daily by administering one-third of the total daily dose every 8 hours. For adult dosage calculation, use a ratio of 400 mg of erythromycin activity as the ethylsuccinate to 250 mg of erythromycin activity as the stearate, base or estolate.

In the treatment of streptococcal infections, a therapeutic dosage of erythromycin ethylsuccinate should be administered for at least 10 days. In continuous prophylaxis against recurrences of streptococcal infections in persons with a history of rheumatic heart disease, the usual dosage is 400 mg twice a day.

For prophylaxis against bacterial endocarditis[1] in patients with congenital heart disease, or rheumatic or other acquired valvular heart disease when undergoing dental procedures or surgical procedures of the upper respiratory tract, give 1.6 g (20 mg/kg for children) orally 1 ½ to 2 hours before the procedure, and then, 800 mg (10 mg/kg for children) orally every 6 hours for 8 doses.

For treatment of urethritis due to *C. trachomatis* or *U. urealyticum:* 800 mg three times a day for 7 days.

For treatment of primary syphilis: Adults: 48 to 64 g given in divided doses over a period of 10 to 15 days.

For intestinal amebiasis: Adults: 400 mg four times daily for 10 to 14 days. Children: 30 to 50 mg/kg/day in divided doses for 10 to 14 days.

For use in pertussis: Although optimal dosage and duration have not been established, doses of erythromycin utilized in reported clinical studies were 40 to 50 mg/kg/day, given in divided doses for 5 to 14 days.

For treatment of Legionnaires' Disease: Although optimal doses have not been established, doses utilized in reported clinical data were 1.6 to 4 g daily in divided doses.

HOW SUPPLIED

EryPed 200 (erythromycin ethylsuccinate for oral suspension, USP) is supplied in bottles of 100 mL (**NDC** 0074-6302-13), 200 mL (**NDC** 0074-6302-53), and 5 mL unit dose in ABBO-PAC® packages (**NDC** 0074-6302-05). Each 5 mL (teaspoonful) of reconstituted suspension contains activity equivalent to 200 mg erythromycin.

EryPed 400 (erythromycin ethylsuccinate for oral suspension, USP) is supplied in bottles of 60 mL (**NDC** 0074-6305-60). 100 mL (**NDC** 0074-6305-13), 200 mL (**NDC** 0074-6305-53), and 5 mL unit dose in ABBO-PAC packages (**NDC** 0074-6305-05). Each 5 mL (teaspoonful) of reconstituted suspension contains activity equivalent to 400 mg erythromycin.

EryPed Drops (erythromycin ethylsuccinate for oral suspension) is supplied in 50 mL bottles (**NDC** 0074-6303-50). Each 2.5 mL dropperful (½ teaspoonful of reconstituted suspension contains activity equivalent to 100 mg of erythromycin.

Recommended Storage: Before mixing, store EryPed granules below 86°F (30°C).

After reconstitution, EryPed must be stored below 77°F (25°C) and used within 35 days; refrigeration not required. EryPed Chewable (erythromycin ethylsuccinate tablets, USP) are fruit-flavored wafers containing activity equivalent to 200 mg of erythromycin and are available in packages of 40 (**NDC** 0074-6314-40). Each wafer is individually sealed in a blister package.

Recommended Storage: Store EryPed Chewable below 86°F (30°C).

Reference: 1. American Heart Association. 1977. Prevention of bacterial endocarditis. Circulation 56:139A-143A. Ref. 01-2573-R5

Shown in Product Identification Section, page 403

ERY-TAB® ℞
[êrē'tab]
(erythromycin delayed-release tablets, USP)
Enteric-Coated

DESCRIPTION

Erythromycin is produced by a strain of *Streptomyces erythraeus* and belongs to the macrolide group of antibiotics. It is basic and readily forms salts with acids. The base is white to off-white crystals or powder slightly soluble in water, soluble in alcohol, in chloroform, and in ether. ERY-TAB (erythromycin delayed-release tablets) is specially enteric-coated to protect the contents from the inactivating effects of gastric acidity and to permit efficient absorption of the antibiotic in the small intestine.

ERY-TAB is available in three dosage strengths containing either 250 mg, 333 mg, or 500 mg of erythromycin as the free base.

Inactive Ingredients: 250 mg tablet: cellulosic polymers, corn starch, diacetylated monoglycerides, D&C red no. 30, iron oxide, magnesium hydroxide, magnesium stearate, sodium starch glycolate, titanium dioxide and vanillin.

333 mg tablet: cellulosic polymers, diacetylated monoglycerides, FD&C blue no. 1, magnesium stearate, microcrystalline cellulose, povidone, sodium citrate, soybean derivatives, talc, titanium dioxide and vanillin.

500 mg tablet: cellulosic polymers, diacetylated monoglycerides, FD&C red no. 40, iron oxide, magnesium stearate, microcrystalline cellulose, povidone, sodium citrate, soybean derivatives, talc, titanium dioxide and vanillin.

ACTIONS

The mode of action of erythromycin is inhibition of protein synthesis without affecting nucleic acid synthesis. Resistance to erythromycin of some strains of *Hemophilus influenzae* and staphylococci has been demonstrated. Culture and susceptibility testing should be done. If the Kirby-Bauer method of disc susceptibility is used, a 15 mcg erythromycin disc should give a zone diameter of at least 18 mm when tested against an erythromycin susceptible organism. Bioavailability data are available from Abbott Laboratories, Dept. 355.

ERY-TAB is well absorbed and may be given without regard to meals.

After absorption, erythromycin diffuses readily into most body fluids. In the absence of meningeal inflammation, low concentrations are normally achieved in the spinal fluid but passage of the drug across the blood-brain barrier increases in meningitis. In the presence of normal hepatic function, erythromycin is concentrated in the liver and excreted in the bile; the effect of hepatic dysfunction on excretion of erythromycin by the liver into the bile is not known. After oral administration, less than 5 percent of the activity of the administered dose can be recovered in the urine.

Erythromycin crosses the placental barrier but fetal plasma levels are low.

INDICATIONS

Streptococcus pyogenes (Group A beta-hemolytic streptococcus): For upper and lower respiratory tract, skin, and soft tissue infections of mild to moderate severity.

Injectable benzathine penicillin G is considered by the American Heart Association to be the drug of choice in the treatment and prevention of streptococcal pharyngitis and in long-term prophylaxis of rheumatic fever.

When oral medication is preferred for treatment of the above conditions, penicillin G, V, or erythromycin are alternate drugs of choice.

When oral medication is given, the importance of strict adherence by the patient to the prescribed dosage regimen must be stressed. A therapeutic dose should be administered for at least 10 days.

Alpha-hemolytic streptococci (viridans group): Although no controlled clinical efficacy trials have been conducted, oral erythromycin has been suggested by the American Heart Association and American Dental Association for use in a regimen for prophylaxis against bacterial endocarditis in patients hypersensitive to penicillin who have congenital heart disease, or rheumatic or other acquired valvular heart disease when they undergo dental procedures and surgical procedures of the upper respiratory tract.[1] Erythromycin is not suitable prior to genitourinary or gastrointestinal tract surgery. NOTE: When selecting antibiotics for the prevention of bacterial endocarditis the physician or dentist should read the full joint statement of the American Heart Association and the American Dental Association.[1]

Staphylococcus aureus: For acute infections of skin and soft tissue of mild to moderate severity. Resistant organisms may emerge during treatment.

Streptococcus pneumoniae (Diplococcus pneumoniae): For upper respiratory tract infections (e.g., otitis media, pharyngitis) and lower respiratory tract infections (e.g., pneumonia) of mild to moderate degree.

Mycoplasma pneumoniae (Eaton agent, PPLO): For respiratory infections due to this organism.

Hemophilus influenzae: For upper respiratory tract infections of mild to moderate severity when used concomitantly with adequate doses of sulfonamides. Not all strains of this organism are susceptible at the erythromycin concentrations ordinarily achieved (see appropriate sulfonamide labeling for prescribing information).

Continued on next page

If desired, additional literature on any Abbott product will be provided upon request to Abbott Laboratories.

Abbott Laboratories—Cont.

Chlamydia trachomatis: Erythromycin is indicated for treatment of the following infections caused by *Chlamydia trachomatis:* conjunctivitis of the newborn, pneumonia of infancy and urogenital infections during pregnancy. When tetracyclines are contraindicated or not tolerated, erythromycin is indicated for the treatment of uncomplicated urethral, endocervical, or rectal infections in adults due to *Chlamydia trachomatis.*[2]

Treponema pallidum: Erythromycin is an alternate choice of treatment for primary syphilis in patients allergic to the penicillins. In treatment of primary syphilis, spinal fluid examinations should be done before treatment and as part of follow-up after therapy.

Corynebacterium diphtheriae and C. minutissimum: As an adjunct to antitoxin, to prevent establishment of carriers, and to eradicate the organism in carriers.

In the treatment of erythrasma.

Entamoeba histolytica: In the treatment of intestinal amebiasis only. Extra-enteric amebiasis requires treatment with other agents.

Listeria monocytogenes: Infections due to this organism.

Neisseria gonorrhoeae: Erythrocin® Lactobionate-I.V. (erythromycin lactobionate for injection, USP) in conjunction with erythromycin base orally, as an alternative drug in treatment of acute pelvic inflammatory disease caused by *N. gonorrhoeae* in female patients with a history of sensitivity to penicillin. Before treatment of gonorrhea, patients who are suspected of also having syphilis should have a microscopic examination for *T. pallidum* (by immunofluorescence or darkfield) before receiving erythromycin, and monthly serologic tests for a minimum of 4 months.

Bordetella pertussis: Erythromycin is effective in eliminating the organism from the nasopharynx of infected individuals, rendering them non-infectious. Some clinical studies suggest that erythromycin may be helpful in the prophylaxis of pertussis in exposed susceptible individuals.

Legionnaires' Disease: Although no controlled clinical efficacy studies have been conducted, *in vitro* and limited preliminary clinical data suggest that erythromycin can be effective in treating Legionnaires' Disease.

CONTRAINDICATIONS
Erythromycin is contraindicated in patients with known hypersensitivity to this antibiotic.

WARNINGS
There have been reports of hepatic dysfunction with or without jaundice, occurring in patients receiving oral erythromycin products.

PRECAUTIONS
General: Erythromycin is principally excreted by the liver. Caution should be exercised when erythromycin is administered to patients with impaired hepatic function. (See "Clinical Pharmacology" and "Warnings" sections).

Prolonged or repeated use of erythromycin may result in an overgrowth of nonsusceptible bacteria or fungi. If superinfection occurs, erythromycin should be discontinued and appropriate therapy instituted.

When indicated, incision and drainage or other surgical procedures should be performed in conjunction with antibiotic therapy.

Laboratory Tests: Erythromycin interferes with the fluorometric determination of urinary catecholamines.

Drug Interactions: Erythromycin use in patients who are receiving high doses of theophylline may be associated with an increase in serum theophylline levels and potential theophylline toxicity. In case of theophylline toxicity and/or elevated serum theophylline levels, the dose of theophylline should be reduced while the patient is receiving concomitant erythromycin therapy.

Concomitant administration of erythromycin and digoxin has been reported to result in elevated digoxin serum levels.

There have been reports of increased anticoagulant effects when erythromycin and oral anticoagulants were used concomitantly.

Concurrent use of erythromycin and ergotamine or dihydroergotamine has been associated in some patients with acute ergot toxicity characterized by severe peripheral vasospasm and dysesthesia.

Erythromycin has been reported to decrease the clearance of triazolam and thus may increase the pharmacologic effect of triazolam.

The use of erythromycin in patients concurrently taking drugs metabolized by the cytochrome P450 system may be associated with elevations in serum erythromycin with carbamazepine, cyclosporine, hexobarbital and phenytoin. Serum concentrations of drugs metabolized by the cytochrome P450 system should be monitored closely in patients concurrently receiving erythromycin.

Troleandomycin significantly alters the metabolism of terfenadine when taken concomitantly; therefore, observe caution when erythromycin and terfenadine are used concurrently.

Patients receiving concomitant lovastatin and erythromycin should be carefully monitored; cases of rhabdomyolysis have been reported in seriously ill patients.

Carcinogenesis, Mutagenesis, Impairment of Fertility: Long-term (2-year) oral studies conducted in rats with erythromycin base did not provide evidence of tumorigenicity. Mutagenicity studies have not been conducted. There was no apparent effect on male or female fertility in rats fed erythromycin (base) at levels up to 0.25 percent of diet.

Pregnancy: Pregnancy Category B: There is no evidence of teratogenicity or any other adverse effect on reproduction in female rats fed erythromycin base (up to 0.25 percent of diet) prior to and during mating, during gestation, and through weaning of two successive litters. There are, however, no adequate and well-controlled studies in pregnant women. Because animal reproduction studies are not always predictive of human response, this drug should be used during pregnancy only if clearly needed. Erythromycin has been reported to cross the placental barrier in humans, but fetal plasma levels are generally low.

Labor and Delivery: The effect of erythromycin on labor and delivery is unknown.

Nursing Mothers: Erythromycin is excreted in breast milk, therefore, caution should be exercised when erythromycin is administered to a nursing woman.

Pediatric Use: See "Indications and Usage" and "Dosage and Administration" sections.

ADVERSE REACTIONS
The most frequent side effects of oral erythromycin preparations are gastrointestinal and are dose-related. They include nausea, vomiting, abdominal pain, diarrhea and anorexia. Symptoms of hepatic dysfunction and/or abnormal liver function test results may occur (see "Warnings" section). Pseudomembranous colitis has been rarely reported in association with erythromycin therapy.

There have been isolated reports of transient central nervous system side effects including confusion, hallucinations, seizures, and vertigo; however, a cause and effect relationship has not been established.

Occasional case reports of cardiac arrhythmias such as ventricular tachycardia have been documented in patients receiving erythromycin therapy. There have been isolated reports of other cardiovascular symptoms such as chest pain, dizziness, and palpitations; however, a cause and effect relationship has not been established.

Allergic reactions ranging from urticaria and mild skin eruptions to anaphylaxis have occurred.

There have been isolated reports of reversible hearing loss occurring chiefly in patients with renal insufficiency and in patients receiving high doses of erythromycin.

OVERDOSAGE
In case of overdosage, erythromycin should be discontinued. Overdosage should be handled with the prompt elimination of unabsorbed drug and all other appropriate measures. Erythromycin is not removed by peritoneal dialysis or hemodialysis.

DOSAGE AND ADMINISTRATION
ERY-TAB (erythromycin delayed-release tablets) is well absorbed and may be given without regard to meals.

Adults: The usual dose is 250 mg four times daily in equally spaced doses. The 333 mg tablet is recommended if dosage is desired every 8 hours. If twice-a-day dosage is desired, the recommended dose is 500 mg every 12 hours.

Dosage may be increased up to 4 or more grams per day according to the severity of the infection. Twice-a-day dosing is not recommended when doses larger than 1 gram daily are administered.

Children: Age, weight, and severity of the infection are important factors in determining the proper dosage. 30 to 50 mg/kg/day, in divided doses, is the usual dose. For more severe infections, this dose may be doubled.

In the treatment of streptococcal infections, a therapeutic dosage of erythromycin should be administered for at least 10 days. In continuous prophylaxis of streptococcal infections in persons with a history of rheumatic heart disease, the dose is 250 mg twice a day.

For prophylaxis against bacterial endocarditis[1] in patients with congenital heart disease, or rheumatic or other acquired valvular heart disease when undergoing dental procedures or surgical procedures of the upper respiratory tract, give 1 g (20 mg/kg for children) orally 1½ to 2 hours before the procedure, and then, 500 mg (10 mg/kg in children) orally every 6 hours for 8 doses.

For conjunctivitis of the newborn caused by *Chlamydia trachomatis:* Oral erythromycin suspension 50 mg/kg/day in 4 divided doses for at least 2 weeks.[2]

For pneumonia of infancy caused by *Chlamydia trachomatis:* Although the optimal duration of therapy has not been established, the recommended therapy is oral erythromycin suspension 50 mg/kg/day in 4 divided doses for at least 3 weeks.[2]

For urogenital infections during pregnancy due to *Chlamydia trachomatis:* Although the optimal dose and duration of therapy have not been established, the suggested treatment is erythromycin 500 mg, by mouth, 4 times a day for at least 7 days. For women who cannot tolerate this regimen, a decreased dose of 250 mg, by mouth, 4 times a day should be used for at least 14 days.[2]

For adults with uncomplicated urethral, endocervical, or rectal infections caused by *Chlamydia trachomatis* in whom tetracyclines are contraindicated or not tolerated: 500 mg, by mouth, 4 times a day for at least 7 days.[2]

For treatment of primary syphilis: 30 to 40 grams given in divided doses over a period of 10 to 15 days.

For treatment of acute pelvic inflammatory disease caused by *N. gonorrhoeae:* After initial treatment with Erythrocin® Lactobionate-I.V. (erythromycin lactobionate for injection, USP) 500 mg every 6 hours for 3 days, the oral dosage recommendation is 250 mg every 6 hours for 7 days.

For dysenteric amebiasis: 250 mg four times daily for 10 to 14 days, for adults; 30 to 50 mg/kg/day in divided doses for 10 to 14 days, for children.

For use in pertussis: Although optimal dosage and duration have not been established, doses of erythromycin utilized in reported clinical studies were 40 to 50 mg/kg/day, given in divided doses for 5 to 14 days.

For treatment of Legionnaires' Disease: Although optimal doses have not been established, doses utilized in reported clinical data were 1 to 4 grams erythromycin base daily in divided doses.

HOW SUPPLIED
ERY-TAB (erythromycin delayed-release tablets, USP), 250 mg, is supplied as pink tablets in bottles of 100 (NDC 0074-6304-13), bottles of 500 (NDC 0074-6304-53), and Abbo-Pac® unit dose packages of 100 (NDC 0074-6304-11).

ERY-TAB, 333 mg, is supplied as white tablets in bottles of 100 (NDC 0074-6320-13), bottles of 500 (NDC 0074-6320-53), and Abbo-Pac® unit dose packages of 100 (NDC 0074-6320-11).

ERY-TAB, 500 mg, is supplied as pink tablets in bottles of 100 (NDC 0074-6321-13) and Abbo-Pac® unit dose packages of 100 (NDC 0074-6321-11).

Recommended Storage: Store below 86°F (30°C).

REFERENCES
1. American Heart Association. 1977. Prevention of bacterial endocarditis. Circulation 56:139A-143A.
2. CDC Sexually Transmitted Diseases Treatment Guidelines 1982.

333 mg and 500 mg tablets—U.S. Pat. No. 4,340,582.
Ref. 01-2526-R6

Shown in Product Identification Section, page 403

E.E.S.®   ℞
[ē-ē-s]
(erythromycin ethylsuccinate)

DESCRIPTION
Erythromycin is produced by a strain of *Streptomyces erythraeus* and belongs to the macrolide group of antibiotics. It is basic and readily forms salts with acids. The base, the stearate salt, and the esters are poorly soluble in water. Erythromycin ethylsuccinate is an ester of erythromycin suitable for oral administration.

The granules are intended for reconstitution with water. When reconstituted, they are palatable cherry-flavored suspensions.

The pleasant tasting, fruit-flavored liquids are supplied ready for oral administration.

Granules and ready-made suspensions are intended primarily for pediatric use but can also be used in adults.

The Filmtab® tablets are intended primarily for adults or older children.

Inactive Ingredients: E.E.S. 200 Liquid: FD&C Red No. 40, methylparaben, polysorbate 60, propylparaben, sodium citrate, sucrose, water, xanthan gum and natural and artificial flavors.

E.E.S. 400 Liquid: D&C Yellow No. 10, FD&C Yellow No. 6, methylparaben, polysorbate 60, propylparaben, sodium citrate, sucrose, water, xanthan gum and natural and artificial flavors.

E.E.S. Granules: Citric acid, FD&C Red No. 3, magnesium aluminum silicate, sodium carboxymethyl cellulose, sodium citrate, sucrose and artificial flavor.

E.E.S. 400 Filmtab Tablets: Cellulosic polymers, confectioner's sugar (contains corn starch), corn starch, D&C Red No. 30, D&C Yellow No. 10, FD&C Red No. 40, magnesium stearate, polacrilin potassium, polyethylene glycol, propylene glycol, sodium citrate, sorbic acid, sorbitan monooleate, titanium dioxide and vitamin E.

ACTIONS
Microbiology: Biochemical tests demonstrate that erythromycin inhibits protein synthesis of the pathogen without directly affecting nucleic acid synthesis. Antagonism has been demonstrated between clindamycin and erythromycin. NOTE: Many strains of *Hemophilus influenzae* are resistant to erythromycin alone, but are susceptible to erythromycin

and sulfonamides together. Staphylococci resistant to erythromycin may emerge during a course of erythromycin therapy. Culture and susceptibility testing should be performed.

Disc Susceptibility Tests: Quantitative methods that require measurement of zone diameters give the most precise estimates of antibiotic susceptibility. One recommended procedure (21 CFR section 460.1) uses erythromycin class discs for testing susceptibility; interpretations correlate zone diameters of this disc test with MIC values for erythromycin. With this procedure, a report from the laboratory of "susceptible" indicates that the infecting organism is likely to respond to therapy. A report of "resistant" indicates that the infective organism is not likely to respond to therapy. A report of "intermediate susceptibility" suggests that the organism would be susceptible if higher doses were used.

Clinical Pharmacology: Erythromycin binds to the 50 S ribosomal subunits of susceptible bacteria and suppresses protein synthesis.

Orally administered erythromycin ethylsuccinate suspensions and Filmtab tablets are readily and reliably absorbed. Comparable serum levels of erythromycin are achieved in the fasting and nonfasting states.

Erythromycin diffuses readily into most body fluids. Only low concentrations are normally achieved in the spinal fluid, but passage of the drug across the blood-brain barrier increases in meningitis. In the presence of normal hepatic function, erythromycin is concentrated in the liver and excreted in the bile; the effect of hepatic dysfunction on excretion of erythromycin by the liver into the bile is not known. Less than 5 percent of the orally administered dose of erythromycin is excreted in active form in the urine.

Erythromycin crosses the placental barrier and is excreted in breast milk.

INDICATIONS

Streptococcus pyogenes (Group A beta-hemolytic streptococcus): Upper and lower respiratory tract, skin, and soft tissue infections of mild to moderate severity.

Injectable benzathine penicillin G is considered by the American Heart Association to be the drug of choice in the treatment and prevention of streptococcal pharyngitis and in long-term prophylaxis of rheumatic fever.

When oral medication is preferred for treatment of the above conditions, penicillin G, V, or erythromycin are alternate drugs of choice.

When oral medication is given, the importance of strict adherence by the patient to the prescribed dosage regimen must be stressed. A therapeutic dose should be administered for at least 10 days.

Alpha-hemolytic streptococci (viridans group): Although no controlled clinical efficacy trials have been conducted, oral erythromycin has been suggested by the American Heart Association and American Dental Association for use in a regimen for prophylaxis against bacterial endocarditis in patients hypersensitive to penicillin who have congenital heart disease, or rheumatic or other acquired valvular heart disease when they undergo dental procedures and surgical procedures of the upper respiratory tract.[1] Erythromycin is not suitable prior to genitourinary or gastrointestinal tract surgery. NOTE: When selecting antibiotics for the prevention of bacterial endocarditis the physician or dentist should read the full joint statement of the American Heart Association and the American Dental Association.[1]

Staphylococcus aureus: Acute infections of skin and soft tissue of mild to moderate severity. Resistant organisms may emerge during treatment.

Streptococcus pneumoniae (Diplococcus pneumoniae): Upper respiratory tract infections (e.g., otitis media, pharyngitis) and lower respiratory tract infections (e.g., pneumonia) of mild to moderate degree.

Mycoplasma pneumoniae (Eaton agent, PPLO): For respiratory infections due to this organism.

Hemophilus influenzae: For upper respiratory tract infections of mild to moderate severity when used concomitantly with adequate doses of sulfonamides. (See sulfonamide labeling for appropriate prescribing information). The concomitant use of the sulfonamides is necessary since not all strains of *Hemophilus influenzae* are susceptible to erythromycin at the concentrations of the antibiotic achieved with usual therapeutic doses.

Chlamydia trachomatis: For the treatment of urethritis in adult males due to *Chlamydia trachomatis.*

Ureaplasma urealyticum: For the treatment of urethritis in adult males due to *Ureaplasma urealyticum.*

Treponema pallidum: Erythromycin is an alternate choice of treatment for primary syphilis in patients allergic to the penicillins. In treatment of primary syphilis, spinal fluid examinations should be done before treatment and as part of follow-up after therapy.

Corynebacterium diphtheriae: As an adjunct to antitoxin, to prevent establishment of carriers, and to eradicate the organism in carriers.

Corynebacterium minutissimum: For the treatment of erythrasma.

Entamoeba histolytica: In the treatment of intestinal amebiasis only. Extraenteric amebiasis requires treatment with other agents.

Listeria monocytogenes: Infections due to this organism.

Bordetella pertussis: Erythromycin is effective in eliminating the organism from the nasopharynx of infected individuals, rendering them non-infectious. Some clinical studies suggest that erythromycin may be helpful in the prophylaxis of pertussis in exposed susceptible individuals.

Legionnaires' Disease: Although no controlled clinical efficacy studies have been conducted, *in vitro* and limited preliminary clinical data suggest that erythromycin may be effective in treating Legionnaires' Disease.

CONTRAINDICATIONS

Erythromycin is contraindicated in patients with known hypersensitivity to this antibiotic.

WARNINGS

There have been reports of hepatic dysfunction with or without jaundice, occurring in patients receiving oral erythromycin products.

PRECAUTIONS

General: Erythromycin is principally excreted by the liver. Caution should be exercised when erythromycin is administered to patients with impaired hepatic function. (See "Clinical Pharmacology" and "Warnings" sections).

Prolonged or repeated use of erythromycin may result in an overgrowth of nonsusceptible bacteria or fungi. If superinfection occurs, erythromycin should be discontinued and appropriate therapy instituted.

When indicated, incision and drainage or other surgical procedures should be performed in conjunction with antibiotic therapy.

Laboratory Tests: Erythromycin interferes with the fluorometric determination of urinary catecholamines.

Drug Interactions: Erythromycin use in patients who are receiving high doses of theophylline may be associated with an increase in serum theophylline levels and potential theophylline toxicity. In case of theophylline toxicity and/or elevated serum theophylline levels, the dose of theophylline should be reduced while the patient is receiving concomitant erythromycin therapy.

Concomitant administration of erythromycin and digoxin has been reported to result in elevated digoxin serum levels. There have been reports of increased anticoagulant effects when erythromycin and oral anticoagulants were used concomitantly.

Concurrent use of erythromycin and ergotamine or dihydroergotamine has been associated in some patients with acute ergot toxicity characterized by severe peripheral vasospasm and dysesthesia.

Erythromycin has been reported to decrease the clearance of triazolam and thus may increase the pharmacologic effect of triazolam.

The use of erythromycin in patients concurrently taking drugs metabolized by the cytochrome P450 system may be associated with elevations in serum erythromycin with carbamazepine, cyclosporine, hexobarbital and phenytoin. Serum concentrations of drugs metabolized by the cytochrome P450 system should be monitored closely in patients concurrently receiving erythromycin.

Troleandomycin significantly alters the metabolism of terfenadine when taken concomitantly; therefore, observe caution when erythromycin and terfenadine are used concurrently.

Patients receiving concomitant lovastatin and erythromycin should be carefully monitored; cases of rhabdomyolysis have been reported in seriously ill patients.

Carcinogenesis, Mutagenesis, Impairment of Fertility: Long-term (2-year) oral studies conducted in rats with erythromycin base did not provide evidence of tumorigenicity. Mutagenicity studies have not been conducted. There was no apparent effect on male or female fertility in rats fed erythromycin (base) at levels up to 0.25 percent of diet.

Pregnancy: Pregnancy Category B: There is no evidence of teratogenicity or any other adverse effect on reproduction in female rats fed erythromycin base (up to 0.25 percent of diet) prior to and during mating, during gestation, and through weaning of two successive litters. There are, however, no adequate and well-controlled studies in pregnant women. Because animal reproduction studies are not always predictive of human response, this drug should be used during pregnancy only if clearly needed. Erythromycin has been reported to cross the placental barrier in humans, but fetal plasma levels are generally low.

Labor and Delivery: The effect of erythromycin on labor and delivery is unknown.

Nursing Mothers: Erythromycin is excreted in breast milk; therefore, caution should be exercised when erythromycin is administered to a nursing woman.

Pediatric Use: See "Indications and Usage" and "Dosage and Administration" sections.

ADVERSE REACTIONS

The most frequent side effects of oral erythromycin preparations are gastrointestinal and are dose-related. They include nausea, vomiting, abdominal pain, diarrhea and anorexia. Symptoms of hepatic dysfunction and/or abnormal liver function test results may occur (see "Warnings" section). Pseudomembranous colitis has been rarely reported in association with erythromycin therapy.

There have been isolated reports of transient central nervous system side effects including confusion, hallucinations, seizures, and vertigo; however, a cause and effect relationship has not been established.

Occasional case reports of cardiac arrhythmias such as ventricular tachycardia have been documented in patients receiving erythromycin therapy. There have been isolated reports of other cardiovascular symptoms such as chest pain, dizziness, and palpitations; however, a cause and effect relationship has not been established.

Allergic reactions ranging from urticaria and mild skin eruptions to anaphylaxis have occurred.

There have been isolated reports of reversible hearing loss occurring chiefly in patients with renal insufficiency and in patients receiving high doses of erythromycin.

OVERDOSAGE

In case of overdosage, erythromycin should be discontinued. Overdosage should be handled with the prompt elimination of unabsorbed drug and all other appropriate measures. Erythromycin is not removed by peritoneal dialysis or hemodialysis.

DOSAGE AND ADMINISTRATION

Erythromycin ethylsuccinate suspensions and Filmtab tablets may be administered without regard to meals.

Children: Age, weight, and severity of the infection are important factors in determining the proper dosage. In mild to moderate infections the usual dosage of erythromycin ethylsuccinate for children is 30 to 50 mg/kg/day in equally divided doses every 6 hours. For more severe infections this dosage may be doubled. If twice-a-day dosage is desired, one-half of the total daily dose may be given every 12 hours. Doses may also be given three times daily by administering one-third of the total daily dose every 8 hours.

The following dosage schedule is suggested for mild to moderate infections:

Body Weight	Total Daily Dose
Under 10 lbs	30–50 mg/kg/day 15–25 mg/lb/day
10 to 15 lbs	200 mg
16 to 25 lbs	400 mg
26 to 50 lbs	800 mg
51 to 100 lbs	1200 mg
over 100 lbs	1600 mg

Adults: 400 mg erythromycin ethylsuccinate every 6 hours is the usual dose. Dosage may be increased up to 4 g per day according to the severity of the infection. If twice-a-day dosage is desired, one-half of the total daily dose may be given every 12 hours. Doses may also be given three times daily by administering one-third of the total daily dose every 8 hours. For adult dosage calculation, use a ratio of 400 mg of erythromycin activity as the ethylsuccinate to 250 mg of erythromycin activity as the stearate, base or estolate.

In the treatment of streptococcal infections, a therapeutic dosage of erythromycin ethylsuccinate should be administered for at least 10 days. In continuous prophylaxis against recurrences of streptococcal infections in persons with a history of rheumatic heart disease, the usual dosage is 400 mg twice a day.

For prophylaxis against bacterial endocarditis[1] in patients with congenital heart disease, or rheumatic or other acquired valvular heart disease when undergoing dental procedures or surgical procedures of the upper respiratory tract, give 1.6 g (20 mg/kg for children) orally 1½ to 2 hours before the procedure, and then, 800 mg (10 mg/kg for children) orally every 6 hours for 8 doses.

For treatment of urethritis due to *C. trachomatis* or *U. urealyticum:* 800 mg three times a day for 7 days.

For treatment of primary syphilis: Adults: 48 to 64 g given in divided doses over a period of 10 to 15 days.

For intestinal amebiasis: Adults: 400 mg four times daily for 10 to 14 days. Children: 30 to 50 mg/kg/day in divided doses for 10 to 14 days.

Continued on next page

Abbott Laboratories—Cont.

For use in pertussis: Although optimal dosage and duration have not been established, doses of erythromycin utilized in reported clinical studies were 40 to 50 mg/kg/day, given in divided doses for 5 to 14 days.

For treatment of Legionnaires' Disease: Although optimal doses have not been established, doses utilized in reported clinical data were those recommended above (1.6 to 4 g daily in divided doses).

HOW SUPPLIED

E.E.S. 200 Liquid (erythromycin ethylsuccinate oral suspension, USP) is supplied in 1 pint bottles (**NDC** 0074-6306-16) and in packages of six 100-mL bottles (**NDC** 0074-6306-13). Each 5-mL teaspoonful of fruit-flavored suspension contains activity equivalent to 200 mg of erythromycin.

E.E.S. 400® Liquid (erythromycin ethylsuccinate oral suspension, USP) is supplied in 1 pint bottles (**NDC** 0074-6373-16) and in packages of six 100-mL bottles (**NDC** 0074-6373-13). Each 5-mL teaspoonful of orange, fruit-flavored suspension contains activity equivalent to 400 mg of erythromycin. Both liquid products require refrigeration to preserve taste until dispensed. Refrigeration by patient is not required if used within 14 days.

E.E.S. Granules (erythromycin ethylsuccinate for oral suspension, USP) is supplied in 100-mL (**NDC** 0074-6369-02) and 200-mL (**NDC** 0074-6369-10) size bottles. Each 5-mL teaspoonful of reconstituted cherry-flavored suspension contains activity equivalent to 200 mg of erythromycin.

E.E.S. 400 Filmtab tablets (erythromycin ethylsuccinate tablets, USP) 400 mg, are available in bottles of 100 (**NDC** 0074-5729-13), 500 (**NDC** 0074-5729-53) and 1000 (**NDC** 0074-5729-19) and in Abbo-Pac® unit dose strip packages of 100 (**NDC** 0074-5729-11). Tablets are pink in color.

Recommended Storage: Store tablets and granules (prior to mixing) below 86°F (30°C)

REFERENCE

1. American Heart Association. 1977. Prevention of bacterial endocarditis. Circulation 56: 139A-143A.

Filmtab—Film-sealed tablets, Abbott.
Ref. 01-2562-R17
Shown in Product Identification Section, page 403

ERYTHROCIN® STEARATE   ℞
[e-ry'thrō-sin]
(erythromycin stearate tablets, USP)
Filmtab® Tablets

DESCRIPTION

Erythromycin is produced by a strain of *Streptomyces erythraeus* and belongs to the macrolide group of antibiotics. It is basic and readily forms salts with acids. The base, the stearate salt, and the esters are poorly soluble in water, and are suitable for oral administration.

Erythrocin Stearate Filmtab tablets contain the stearate salt of the antibiotic in a unique film coating.

Inactive Ingredients: 250 mg tablet: Cellulosic polymers, corn starch, D&C Red No. 7, polacrilin potassium, polyethylene glycol, povidone, propylene glycol, sodium carboxymethylcellulose, sodium citrate, sorbic acid, sorbitan monooleate and titanium dioxide.

500 mg tablet: Cellulosic polymers, corn starch, FD&C Red No. 3, magnesium hydroxide, polacrilin potassium, povidone, propylene glycol, sorbitan monooleate, titanium dioxide and vanillin.

ACTIONS

Microbiology: Biochemical tests demonstrate that erythromycin inhibits protein synthesis of the pathogen without directly affecting nucleic acid synthesis. Antagonism has been demonstrated between clindamycin and erythromycin. NOTE: Many strains of *Hemophilus influenzae* are resistant to erythromycin alone, but are susceptible to erythromycin and sulfonamides together. Staphylococci resistant to erythromycin may emerge during a course of erythromycin therapy. Culture and susceptibility testing should be performed.

Disc Susceptibility Tests: Quantitative methods that require measurement of zone diameters give the most precise estimates of antibiotic susceptibility. One recommended procedure (21 CFR section 460.1) uses erythromycin class discs for testing susceptibility; interpretations correlate zone diameters of this disc test with MIC values for erythromycin. With this procedure, a report from the laboratory of "susceptible" indicates that the infecting organism is likely to respond to therapy. A report of "resistant" indicates that the infective organism is not likely to respond to therapy. A report of "intermediate susceptibility" suggests that the organism would be susceptible if higher doses were used.

Clinical Pharmacology: Erythromycin binds to the 50 S ribosomal subunits of susceptible bacteria and suppresses protein synthesis.

Orally administered Erythrocin Stearate tablets are readily and reliably absorbed. Optimal serum levels of erythromycin are reached when the drug is taken in the fasting state or immediately before meals.

Erythromycin diffuses readily into most body fluids. Only low concentrations are normally achieved in the spinal fluid, but passage of the drug across the blood-brain barrier increases in meningitis. In the presence of normal hepatic function, erythromycin is concentrated in the liver and excreted in the bile; the effect of hepatic dysfunction on excretion of erythromycin by the liver into the bile is not known. Less than 5 percent of the orally administered dose of erythromycin is excreted in active form in the urine.

Erythromycin crosses the placental barrier and is excreted in breast milk.

INDICATIONS

Streptococcus pyogenes (Group A beta-hemolytic streptococcus): Upper and lower respiratory tract, skin, and soft tissue infections of mild to moderate severity.

Injectable benzathine penicillin G is considered by the American Heart Association to be the drug of choice in the treatment and prevention of streptococcal pharyngitis and in long-term prophylaxis of rheumatic fever.

When oral medication is preferred for treatment of the above conditions, penicillin G, V, or erythromycin are alternate drugs of choice.

When oral medication is given, the importance of strict adherence by the patient to the prescribed dosage regimen must be stressed. A therapeutic dose should be administered for at least 10 days.

Alpha-hemolytic streptococci (viridans group):
Although no controlled clinical efficacy trials have been conducted, oral erythromycin has been suggested by the American Heart Association and American Dental Association for use in a regimen for prophylaxis against bacterial endocarditis in patients hypersensitive to penicillin who have congenital heart disease, or rheumatic or other acquired valvular heart disease when they undergo dental procedures and surgical procedures of the upper respiratory tract.[1] Erythromycin is not suitable prior to genitourinary or gastrointestinal tract surgery. NOTE: When selecting antibiotics for the prevention of bacterial endocarditis the physician or dentist should read the full joint statement of the American Heart Association and the American Dental Association.[1]

Staphylococcus aureus: Acute infections of skin and soft tissue of mild to moderate severity. Resistant organisms may emerge during treatment.

Streptococcus pneumoniae (Diplococcus pneumoniae): Upper respiratory tract infections (e.g., otitis media, pharyngitis) and lower respiratory tract infections (e.g., pneumonia) of mild to moderate degree.

Mycoplasma pneumoniae (Eaton agent, PPLO): For respiratory infections due to this organism.

Hemophilus influenzae: For upper respiratory tract infections of mild to moderate severity when used concomitantly with adequate doses of sulfonamides. (See sulfonamide labeling for appropriate prescribing information). The concomitant use of the sulfonamides is necessary since not all strains of *Hemophilus influenzae* are susceptible to erythromycin at the concentrations of the antibiotic achieved with usual therapeutic doses.

Chlamydia trachomatis: Erythromycin is indicated for treatment of the following infections caused by *Chlamydia trachomatis:* conjunctivitis of the newborn, pneumonia of infancy and urogenital infections during pregnancy. When tetracyclines are contraindicated or not tolerated, erythromycin is indicated for the treatment of uncomplicated urethral, endocervical, or rectal infections in adults due to *Chlamydia trachomatis.*[2]

Treponema pallidum: Erythromycin is an alternate choice of treatment for primary syphilis in patients allergic to the penicillins. In treatment of primary syphilis, spinal fluid examinations should be done before treatment and as part of follow-up after therapy.

Corynebacterium diphtheriae: As an adjunct to antitoxin, to prevent establishment of carriers, and to eradicate the organism in carriers.

Corynebacterium minutissimum: For the treatment of erythrasma.

Entamoeba histolytica: In the treatment of intestinal amebiasis only. Extra-enteric amebiasis requires treatment with other agents.

Listeria monocytogenes: Infections due to this organism.

Neisseria gonorrhoeae: Erythrocin Lactobionate-I.V. (erythromycin lactobionate for injection) in conjunction with erythromycin stearate orally, as an alternative drug in treatment of acute pelvic inflammatory disease caused by *N. gonorrhoeae* in female patients with a history of sensitivity to penicillin. Before treatment of gonorrhea, patients who are suspected of also having syphilis should have a microscopic examination for *T. pallidum* (by immunofluorescence or darkfield) before receiving erythromycin, and monthly serologic tests for a minimum of 4 months.

Bordetella pertussis: Erythromycin is effective in eliminating the organism from the nasopharynx of infected individuals,

rendering them non-infectious. Some clinical studies suggest that erythromycin may be helpful in the prophylaxis of pertussis in exposed susceptible individuals.

Legionnaires' Disease: Although no controlled clinical efficacy studies have been conducted, *in vitro* and limited preliminary clinical data suggest that erythromycin may be effective in treating Legionnaires' Disease.

CONTRAINDICATIONS

Erythromycin is contraindicated in patients with known hypersensitivity to this antibiotic.

WARNINGS

There have been reports of hepatic dysfunction with or without jaundice, occurring in patients receiving oral erythromycin products.

PRECAUTIONS

General: Erythromycin is principally excreted by the liver. Caution should be exercised when erythromycin is administered to patients with impaired hepatic function. (See "Clinical Pharmacology" and "Warnings" sections).

Prolonged or repeated use of erythromycin may result in an overgrowth of nonsusceptible bacteria or fungi. If superinfection occurs, erythromycin should be discontinued and appropriate therapy instituted.

When indicated, incision and drainage or other surgical procedures should be performed in conjunction with antibiotic therapy.

Laboratory Tests: Erythromycin interferes with the fluorometric determination of urinary catecholamines.

Drug Interactions: Erythromycin use in patients who are receiving high doses of theophylline may be associated with an increase in serum theophylline levels and potential theophylline toxicity. In case of theophylline toxicity and/or elevated serum theophylline levels, the dose of theophylline should be reduced while the patient is receiving concomitant erythromycin therapy.

Concomitant administration of erythromycin and digoxin has been reported to result in elevated digoxin serum levels.

There have been reports of increased anticoagulant effects when erythromycin and oral anticoagulants were used concomitantly.

Concurrent use of erythromycin and ergotamine or dihydroergotamine has been associated in some patients with acute ergot toxicity characterized by severe peripheral vasospasm and dysesthesia.

Erythromycin has been reported to decrease the clearance of triazolam and thus may increase the pharmacologic effect of triazolam.

The use of erythromycin in patients concurrently taking drugs metabolized by the cytochrome P450 system may be associated with elevations in serum erythromycin with carbamazepine, cyclosporine, hexobarbital and phenytoin. Serum concentrations of drugs metabolized by the cytochrome P450 system should be monitored closely in patients concurrently receiving erythromycin.

Troleandomycin significantly alters the metabolism of terfenadine when taken concomitantly; therefore, observe caution when erythromycin and terfenadine are used concurrently.

Patients receiving concomitant lovastatin and erythromycin should be carefully monitored; cases of rhabdomyolysis have been reported in seriously ill patients.

Carcinogenesis, Mutagenesis, Impairment of Fertility: Long-term (2-year) oral studies conducted in rats with erythromycin base did not provide evidence of tumorigenicity. Mutagenicity studies have not been conducted. There was no apparent effect on male or female fertility in rats fed erythromycin (base) at levels up to 0.25 percent of diet.

Pregnancy: Pregnancy Category B: There is no evidence of teratogenicity or any other adverse effect on reproduction in female rats fed erythromycin base (up to 0.25 percent of diet) prior to and during mating, during gestation, and through weaning of two successive litters. There are, however, no adequate and well-controlled studies in pregnant women. Because animal reproduction studies are not always predictive of human response, this drug should be used during pregnancy only if clearly needed. Erythromycin has been reported to cross the placental barrier in humans, but fetal plasma levels are generally low.

Labor and Delivery: The effect of erythromycin on labor and delivery is unknown.

Nursing Mothers: Erythromycin is excreted in breast milk, therefore, caution should be exercised when erythromycin is administered to a nursing woman.

Pediatric Use: See "Indications and Usage" and "Dosage and Administration" sections.

ADVERSE REACTIONS

The most frequent side effects of oral erythromycin preparations are gastrointestinal and are dose-related. They include nausea, vomiting, abdominal pain, diarrhea and anorexia. Symptoms of hepatic dysfunction and/or abnormal liver function test results may occur (see "Warnings" section). Pseudomembranous colitis has been rarely reported in association with erythromycin therapy.

There have been isolated reports of transient central nervous system side effects including confusion, hallucinations, seizures, and vertigo; however, a cause and effect relationship has not been established.

Occasional case reports of cardiac arrhythmias such as ventricular tachycardia have been documented in patients receiving erythromycin therapy. There have been isolated reports of other cardiovascular symptoms such as chest pain, dizziness, and palpitations; however, a cause and effect relationship has not been established.

Allergic reactions ranging from urticaria and mild skin eruptions to anaphylaxis have occurred.

There have been isolated reports of reversible hearing loss occurring chiefly in patients with renal insufficiency and in patients receiving high doses of erythromycin.

OVERDOSAGE

In case of overdosage, erythromycin should be discontinued. Overdosage should be handled with the prompt elimination of unabsorbed drug and all other appropriate measures. Erythromycin is not removed by peritoneal dialysis or hemodialysis.

DOSAGE AND ADMINISTRATION

Optimal serum levels of erythromycin are reached when ERYTHROCIN STEARATE (erythromycin stearate) is taken in the fasting state or immediately before meals.

Adults: The usual dosage is 250 mg every 6 hours; or 500 mg every 12 hours, taken in the fasting state or immediately before meals. Up to 4 g per day may be administered, depending upon the severity of the infection.

Children: Age, weight, and severity of the infection are important factors in determining the proper dosage. For the treatment of mild to moderate infections, the usual dosage is 30 to 50 mg/kg/day in 3 or 4 divided doses. When dosage is desired on a twice-a-day schedule, one-half of the total daily dose may be taken every 12 hours in the fasting state or immediately before meals. For the treatment of more severe infections the total daily dose may be doubled.

In the treatment of streptococcal infections, a therapeutic dosage of erythromycin should be administered for at least 10 days. In continuous prophylaxis of streptococcal infections in persons with a history of rheumatic heart disease, the dose is 250 mg twice a day.

For prophylaxis against bacterial endocarditis[1] in patients with congenital heart disease, or rheumatic or other acquired valvular heart disease when undergoing dental procedures or surgical procedures of the upper respiratory tract, give 1 g (20 mg/kg for children) orally 1½ to 2 hours before the procedure, and then, 500 mg (10 mg/kg for children) orally every 6 hours for 8 doses.

For conjunctivitis of the newborn caused by *Chlamydia trachomatis:* Oral erythromycin suspension 50 mg/kg/day in 4 divided doses for at least 2 weeks.[2]

For pneumonia of infancy caused by *Chlamydia trachomatis:* Although the optimal duration of therapy has not been established, the recommended therapy is oral erythromycin suspension 50 mg/kg/day in 4 divided doses for at least 3 weeks.[2]

For urogenital infections during pregnancy due to *Chlamydia trachomatis:* Although the optimal dose and duration of therapy have not been established, the suggested treatment is erythromycin 500 mg, by mouth, 4 times a day on an empty stomach for at least 7 days. For women who cannot tolerate this regimen, a decreased dose of 250 mg, by mouth, 4 times a day should be used for at least 14 days.[2]

For adults with uncomplicated urethral, endocervical, or rectal infections caused by *Chlamydia trachomatis* in whom tetracyclines are contraindicated or not tolerated: 500 mg, by mouth, 4 times a day for at least 7 days.[2]

For treatment of primary syphilis: 30 to 40 g given in divided doses over a period of 10 to 15 days.

For treatment of acute pelvic inflammatory disease caused by *N. gonorrhoeae:* 500 mg Erythrocin Lactobionate-I.V. (erythromycin lactobionate for injection) every 6 hours for 3 days, followed by 250 mg ERYTHROCIN STEARATE every 6 hours for 7 days.

For intestinal amebiasis: Adults: 250 mg four times daily for 10 to 14 days. Children: 30 to 50 mg/kg/day in divided doses for 10 to 14 days.

For use in pertussis: Although optimal dosage and duration have not been established, doses of erythromycin utilized in reported clinical studies were 40 to 50 mg/kg/day, given in divided doses for 5 to 14 days.

For treatment of Legionnaires' Disease: Although optimal doses have not been established, doses utilized in reported clinical data were 1 to 4 g daily in divided doses.

HOW SUPPLIED

ERYTHROCIN STEARATE Filmtab Tablets (erythromycin stearate tablets, USP) are supplied as:

ERYTHROCIN STEARATE Filmtab, 250 mg

Bottles of 100 ....(NDC 0074-6346-20)
Bottles of 500 ....(NDC 0074-6346-53)
Bottles of 1000 ....(NDC 0074-6346-19)
ABBO-PAC® unit dose strip packages of
100 tablets ....(NDC 0074-6346-38)

ERYTHROCIN STEARATE Filmtab, 500 mg

Bottles of 100 ....(NDC 0074-6316-13)
Recommended storage: Store below 86°F (30°C).

REFERENCES

1. American Heart Association. 1977. Prevention of bacterial endocarditis. Circulation 56: 139A-143A.
2. CDC Sexually Transmitted Diseases Treatment Guidelines 1982.

FILMTAB—Film-sealed tablets, Abbott
Ref. 01-2538-R13

Shown in Product Identification Section, page 403

ERYTHROMYCIN BASE FILMTAB®   ℞
[e-ri-thrō-mī'sin]
(erythromycin tablets, USP)

DESCRIPTION

Erythromycin is produced by a strain of *Streptomyces erythraeus* and belongs to the macrolide group of antibiotics. It is basic and readily forms salts with acids. The base, the stearate salt, and the esters are poorly soluble in water, and are suitable for oral administration.

ERYTHROMYCIN BASE FILMTAB tablets contain erythromycin, USP, in a unique, nonenteric film coating.

Inactive Ingredients: 250 mg tablet: Cellulosic polymers, corn starch, D&C Red No. 30, iron oxide, magnesium hydroxide, magnesium stearate, polyethylene glycol, propylene glycol, sodium starch glycolate, sorbic acid, sorbitan monooleate and titanium dioxide.

500 mg tablet: Cellulosic polymers, corn starch, D&C Red No. 30, magnesium hydroxide, magnesium stearate, microcrystalline cellulose, polyethylene glycol, propylene glycol, sodium starch glycolate, sorbic acid, sorbitan monooleate and titanium dioxide.

ACTIONS

Microbiology: Biochemical tests demonstrate that erythromycin inhibits protein synthesis of the pathogen without directly affecting nucleic acid synthesis. Antagonism has been demonstrated between clindamycin and erythromycin. NOTE: Many strains of *Hemophilus influenzae* are resistant to erythromycin alone, but are susceptible to erythromycin and sulfonamides together. Staphylococci resistant to erythromycin may emerge during a course of erythromycin therapy. Culture and susceptibility testing should be performed.

Disc Susceptibility Tests: Quantitative methods that require measurement of zone diameters give the most precise estimates of antibiotic susceptibility. One recommended procedure (21 CFR section 460.1) uses erythromycin class discs for testing susceptibility; interpretations correlate zone diameters of this disc test with MIC values for erythromycin. With this procedure, a report from the laboratory of "susceptible" indicates that the infecting organism is likely to respond to therapy. A report of "resistant" indicates that the infective organism is not likely to respond to therapy. A report of "intermediate susceptibility" suggests that the organism would be susceptible if higher doses were used.

Clinical Pharmacology: Erythromycin binds to the 50 S ribosomal subunits of susceptible bacteria and suppresses protein synthesis.

Orally administered erythromycin is readily absorbed by most patients, especially on an empty stomach, but patient variation is observed. Due to its formulation and nonenteric coating, this erythromycin tablet gives reliable blood levels in the average subject; however, the levels may vary with the individual.

Erythromycin diffuses readily into most body fluids. Only low concentrations are normally achieved in the spinal fluid, but passage of the drug across the blood-brain barrier increases in meningitis. In the presence of normal hepatic function, erythromycin is concentrated in the liver and excreted in the bile; the effect of hepatic dysfunction on excretion of erythromycin by the liver into the bile is not known. Less than 5 percent of the orally administered dose of erythromycin is excreted in active form in the urine.

Erythromycin crosses the placental barrier and is excreted in breast milk.

INDICATIONS

Streptococcus pyogenes (Group A beta-hemolytic streptococcus): Upper and lower respiratory tract, skin, and soft tissue infections of mild to moderate severity.

Injectable benzathine penicillin G is considered by the American Heart Association to be the drug of choice in the treatment and prevention of streptococcal pharyngitis and in long-term prophylaxis of rheumatic fever.

When oral medication is preferred for treatment of the above conditions, penicillin G, V, or erythromycin are alternate drugs of choice.

When oral medication is given, the importance of strict adherence by the patient to the prescribed dosage regimen must be stressed. A therapeutic dose should be administered for at least 10 days.

Alpha-hemolytic streptococci (viridans group): Although no controlled clinical efficacy trials have been conducted, oral erythromycin has been suggested by the American Heart Association and American Dental Association for use in a regimen for prophylaxis against bacterial endocarditis in patients hypersensitive to penicillin who have congenital heart disease, or rheumatic or other acquired valvular heart disease when they undergo dental procedures and surgical procedures of the upper respiratory tract.[1] Erythromycin is not suitable prior to genitourinary or gastrointestinal tract surgery. NOTE: When selecting antibiotics for the prevention of bacterial endocarditis the physician or dentist should read the full joint statement of the American Heart Association and the American Dental Association.[1]

Staphylococcus aureus: Acute infections of skin and soft tissue of mild to moderate severity. Resistant organisms may emerge during treatment.

Streptococcus pneumoniae (Diplococcus pneumoniae): Upper respiratory tract infections (e.g., otitis media, pharyngitis) and lower respiratory tract infections (e.g., pneumonia) of mild to moderate degree.

Mycoplasma pneumoniae (Eaton agent, PPLO): For respiratory infections due to this organism.

Hemophilus influenzae: For upper respiratory tract infections of mild to moderate severity when used concomitantly with adequate doses of sulfonamides. (See sulfonamide labeling for appropriate prescribing information). The concomitant use of the sulfonamides is necessary since not all strains of *Hemophilus influenzae* are susceptible to erythromycin at the concentrations of the antibiotic achieved with usual therapeutic doses.

Chlamydia trachomatis: Erythromycin is indicated for treatment of the following infections caused by *Chlamydia trachomatis:* conjunctivitis of the newborn, pneumonia of infancy and urogenital infections during pregnancy. When tetracyclines are contraindicated or not tolerated, erythromycin is indicated for the treatment of uncomplicated urethral, endocervical, or rectal infections in adults due to *Chlamydia trachomatis.*[2]

Treponema pallidum: Erythromycin is an alternate choice of treatment for primary syphilis in patients allergic to the penicillins. In treatment of primary syphilis, spinal fluid examinations should be done before treatment and as part of follow-up after therapy.

Corynebacterium diphtheriae: As an adjunct to antitoxin, to prevent establishment of carriers, and to eradicate the organism in carriers.

Corynebacterium minutissimum: For the treatment of erythrasma.

Entamoeba histolytica: In the treatment of intestinal amebiasis only. Extra-enteric amebiasis requires treatment with other agents.

Listeria monocytogenes: Infections due to this organism.

Neisseria gonorrhoeae: Erythrocin® Lactobionate-I.V. (erythromycin lactobionate for injection) in conjunction with erythromycin base orally, as an alternative drug in treatment of acute pelvic inflammatory disease caused by *N. gonorrhoeae* in female patients with a history of sensitivity to penicillin. Before treatment of gonorrhea, patients who are suspected of also having syphilis should have a microscopic examination for *T. pallidum* (by immunofluorescence or darkfield) before receiving erythromycin, and monthly serologic tests for a minimum of 4 months.

Bordetella pertussis: Erythromycin is effective in eliminating the organism from the nasopharynx of infected individuals, rendering them non-infectious. Some clinical studies suggest that erythromycin may be helpful in the prophylaxis of pertussis in exposed susceptible individuals.

Legionnaires' Disease: Although no controlled clinical efficacy studies have been conducted, *in vitro* and limited preliminary clinical data suggest that erythromycin may be effective in treating Legionnaires' Disease.

CONTRAINDICATIONS

Erythromycin is contraindicated in patients with known hypersensitivity to this antibiotic.

WARNINGS

There have been reports of hepatic dysfunction with or without jaundice, occurring in patients receiving oral erythromycin products.

PRECAUTIONS

General: Erythromycin is principally excreted by the liver. Caution should be exercised when erythromycin is administered to patients with impaired hepatic function. (See "Clinical Pharmacology" and "Warnings" sections).

Prolonged or repeated use of erythromycin may result in an overgrowth of nonsusceptible bacteria or fungi. If superinfection occurs, erythromycin should be discontinued and appropriate therapy instituted.

Continued on next page

Abbott Laboratories—Cont.

When indicated, incision and drainage or other surgical procedures should be performed in conjunction with antibiotic therapy.

Laboratory Tests: Erythromycin interferes with the fluorometric determination of urinary catecholamines.

Drug Interactions: Erythromycin use in patients who are receiving high doses of theophylline may be associated with an increase in serum theophylline levels and potential theophylline toxicity. In case of theophylline toxicity and/or elevated serum theophylline levels, the dose of theophylline should be reduced while the patient is receiving concomitant erythromycin therapy.

Concomitant administration of erythromycin and digoxin has been reported to result in elevated digoxin serum levels. There have been reports of increased anticoagulant effects when erythromycin and oral anticoagulants were used concomitantly.

Concurrent use of erythromycin and ergotamine or dihydroergotamine has been associated in some patients with acute ergot toxicity characterized by severe peripheral vasospasm and dysethesia.

Erythromycin has been reported to decrease the clearance of triazolam and thus may increase the pharmacologic effect of triazolam.

The use of erythromycin in patients concurrently taking drugs metabolized by the cytochrome P450 system may be associated with elevations in serum erythromycin with carbamazepine, cyclosporine, hexobarbital and phenytoin. Serum concentrations of drugs metabolized by the cytochrome P450 system should be monitored closely in patients concurrently receiving erythromycin.

Troleandomycin significantly alters the metabolism of terfenadine when taken concomitantly; therefore, observe caution when erythromycin and terfenadine are used concurrently.

Patients receiving concomitant lovastatin and erythromycin should be carefully monitored; cases or rhabdomyolysis have been reported in seriously ill patients.

Carcinogenesis, Mutagenesis, Impairment of Fertility: Long-term (2-year) oral studies conducted in rats with erythromycin base did not provide evidence of tumorigenicity. Mutagenicity studies have not been conducted. There was no apparent effect on male or female fertility in rats fed erythromycin (base) at levels up to 0.25 percent of diet.

Pregnancy: Pregnancy Category B: There is no evidence of teratogenicity or any other adverse effect on reproduction in female rats fed erythromycin base (up to 0.25 percent of diet) prior to and during mating, during gestation, and through weaning of two successive litters. There are, however, no adequate and well-controlled studies in pregnant women. Because animal reproduction studies are not always predictive of human response, this drug should be used during pregnancy only if clearly needed. Erythromycin has been reported to cross the placental barrier in humans, but fetal plasma levels are generally low.

Labor and Delivery: The effect of erythromycin on labor and delivery is unknown.

Nursing Mothers: Erythromycin is excreted in breast milk, therefore, caution should be exercised when erythromycin is administered to a nursing woman.

Pediatric Use: See "Indications and Usage" and "Dosage and Administration" sections.

ADVERSE REACTIONS

The most frequent side effects of oral erythromycin preparations are gastrointestinal and are dose-related. They include nausea, vomiting, abdominal pain, diarrhea and anorexia. Symptoms of hepatic dysfunction and/or abnormal liver function test results may occur (see "Warnings" section). Pseudomembranous colitis has been rarely reported in association with erythromycin therapy.

There have been isolated reports of transient central nervous system side effects including confusion, hallucinations, seizures, and vertigo; however, a cause and effect relationship has not been established.

Occasional case reports of cardiac arrhythmias such as ventricular tachycardia have been documented in patients receiving erythromycin therapy. There have been isolated reports of other cardiovascular symptoms such as chest pain, dizziness, and palpitations; however a cause and effect relationship has not been established.

Allergic reactions ranging from urticaria and mild skin eruptions to anaphylaxis have occurred.

There have been isolated reports of reversible hearing loss occurring chiefly in patients with renal insufficiency and in patients receiving high doses of erythromycin.

OVERDOSAGE

In case of overdosage, erythromycin should be discontinued. Overdosage should be handled with the prompt elimination of unabsorbed drug and all other appropriate measures. Erythromycin is not removed by peritoneal dialysis or hemodialysis.

DOSAGE AND ADMINISTRATION

Optimum blood levels are obtained when doses are given on an empty stomach.

Adults: 250 mg every 6 hours is the usual dose; or 500 mg every 12 hours one hour before meals. Dosage may be increased up to 4 g per day according to the severity of the infection.

Children: Age, weight, and severity of the infection are important factors in determining the proper dosage. 30 to 50 mg/kg/day, in divided doses, is the usual dose. For more severe infections this dose may be doubled. If dosage is desired on a twice-a-day schedule, one-half of the total daily dose may be given every 12 hours, one hour before meals.

For treatment of streptococcal infections: a therapeutic dosage should be administered for at least 10 days. In continuous prophylaxis of streptococcal infections in persons with rheumatic heart disease history, the dose is 250 mg twice a day.

For prophylaxis against bacterial endocarditis[1] in patients with congenital heart disease, or rheumatic or other acquired valvular heart disease when undergoing dental procedures or surgical procedures of the upper respiratory tract, give 1 g (20 mg/kg for children) orally 1½ to 2 hours before the procedure, and then, 500 mg (10 mg/kg for children) orally every 6 hours for 8 doses.

For conjunctivitis of the newborn caused by *Chlamydia trachomatis:* Oral erythromycin suspension 50 mg/kg/day in 4 divided doses for at least 2 weeks.[2]

For pneumonia of infancy caused by *Chlamydia trachomatis:* Although the optimal duration of therapy has not been established, the recommended therapy is oral erythromycin suspension 50 mg/kg/day in 4 divided doses for at least 3 weeks.[2]

For urogenital infections during pregnancy due to *Chlamydia trachomatis:* Although the optimal dose and duration of therapy have not been established, the suggested treatment is erythromycin 500 mg, by mouth, 4 times a day on an empty stomach for at least 7 days. For women who cannot tolerate this regimen, a decreased dose of 250 mg, by mouth 4 times a day should be used for at least 14 days.[2]

For adults with uncomplicated urethral, endocervical, or rectal infections caused by *Chlamydia trachomatis* in whom tetracyclines are contraindicated or not tolerated: 500 mg, by mouth, 4 times a day for at least 7 days.[2]

For treatment of primary syphilis: 30 to 40 g given in divided doses over a period of 10 to 15 days.

For treatment of acute pelvic inflammatory disease caused by *N. gonorrhoeae:* 500 mg Erythrocin® Lactobionate-I.V. (erythromycin lactobionate for injection) every 6 hours for 3 days, followed by 250 mg erythromycin base every 6 hours for 7 days.

For intestinal amebiasis: Adults: 250 mg four times daily for 10 to 14 days. Children: 30 to 50 mg/kg/day in divided doses for 10 to 14 days.

For use in pertussis: Although optimal dosage and duration have not been established, doses of erythromycin utilized in reported clinical studies were 40 to 50 mg/kg/day, given in divided doses for 5 to 14 days.

For treatment of Legionnaires' Disease: Although optimal doses have not been established, doses utilized in reported clinical data were 1 to 4 g daily in divided doses.

HOW SUPPLIED

ERYTHROMYCIN BASE FILMTAB tablets (erythromycin tablets, USP) are supplied as pink capsule-shaped tablets in two dosage strengths:

250 mg tablets:

Bottles of 100 ....(NDC 0074-6326-13)
Bottles of 500 ....(NDC 0074-6326-53)
ABBO-PAC® unit dose strip packages of
100 tablets..(NDC 0074-6326-11)
500 mg tablets:
Bottles of 100 ....(NDC 0074-6227-13)
Recommended storage: Store below 86°F (30°C).

REFERENCES

1. American Heart Association. 1977. Prevention of bacterial endocarditis. Circulation. 56: 139A-143A.
2. CDC Sexually Transmitted Diseases Treatment Guidelines 1982.

FILMTAB—Film-sealed tablets, Abbott.
Ref. 01-2541-R3
Shown in Product Identification Section, page 403

ERYTHROMYCIN DELAYED-RELEASE CAPSULES, USP   ℞

DESCRIPTION

Erythromycin Delayed-Release Capsules contain enteric-coated pellets of erythromycin base for oral administration. Erythromycin is produced by a strain of *Streptomyces erythraeus* and belongs to the macrolide group of antibiotics. It is basic and readily forms salts with acids, but it is the base which is microbiologically active. Each Erythromycin Delayed-Release Capsule contains 250 milligrams of erythromycin base.

Inactive Ingredients: Cellulosic polymers, citrate ester, D&C Red No. 30, D&C Yellow No. 10, magnesium stearate and povidone. The capsule shell contains FD&C Blue No. 1, FD&C Red No. 3, gelatin, and titanium dioxide.

Erythromycin base is (3R*, 4S*, 5S*, 6R*, 7R*, 9R*, 11R*, 12R*, 13S*, 14R*)-4-[(2,6-Dideoxy-3-C-methyl-3-0-methyl-α-L-*ribo*-hexopyranosyl)oxy]-14-ethyl-7,12,13-trihydroxy-3, 5, 7, 9, 11, 13-hexamethyl-6-[[3, 4, 6-trideoxy-3-(dimethyl-amino)-β-D-*xylo*-hexopyranosyl]oxy]oxacyclotetradecane-2,10-dione.

CLINICAL PHARMACOLOGY

Orally administered erythromycin base and its salts are readily absorbed in the microbiologically active form. Interindividual variations in the absorption of erythromycin are, however, observed, and some patients do not achieve acceptable serum levels. Erythromycin is largely bound to plasma proteins, and the freely dissociating bound fraction after administration of erythromycin base represents 90% of the total erythromycin absorbed. After absorption, erythromycin diffuses readily into most body fluids. In the absence of meningeal inflammation, low concentrations are normally achieved in the spinal fluid, but the passage of the drug across the blood-brain barrier increases in meningitis. Erythromycin is excreted in breast milk. The drug crosses the placental barrier but plasma levels are low.

In the presence of normal hepatic function, erythromycin is concentrated in the liver and is excreted in the bile; the effect of hepatic dysfunction in biliary excretion of erythromycin is not known. After oral administration, less than 5% of the administered dose can be recovered in the active form in the urine.

The enteric coating of pellets in Erythromycin Delayed-Release Capsules protects the erythromycin base from inactivation by gastric acidity. Because of their small size and enteric coating, the pellets readily pass intact from the stomach to the small intestine and dissolve efficiently to allow absorption of erythromycin in a uniform manner. After administration of a single dose of a 250 mg Erythromycin Delayed-Release Capsule, peak serum levels in the range of 1.13 to 1.68 mcg/mL are attained in approximately 3 hours and decline to 0.30-0.42 mcg/mL in 6 hours. Optimal conditions for stability in the presence of gastric secretion and for complete absorption are attained when Erythromycin Delayed-Release Capsules are taken on an empty stomach.

Microbiology

Erythromycin acts by inhibition of protein synthesis by binding 50 S ribosomal subunits of susceptible organisms. It does not affect nucleic acid synthesis. Antagonism has been demonstrated between clindamycin and erythromycin. Resistance to erythromycin of many strains of *Haemophilus influenzae* and some strains of staphylococci has been demonstrated. Specimens should be obtained for culture and susceptibility testing.

Erythromycin is usually active against the following organisms *in vitro* and in clinical infections:

Streptococcus pyogenes
Alpha-hemolytic streptococci (viridans group)
Staphylococcus aureus (Resistant organisms may emerge during treatment.)
Streptococcus pneumoniae
Mycoplasma pneumoniae (Eaton's Agent)
Haemophilus influenzae (Many strains are resistant to erythromycin alone, but are susceptible to erythromycin and sulfonamides together.)
Treponema pallidum
Corynebacterium diphtheriae
Corynebacterium minutissimum
Entamoeba histolytica
Listeria monocytogenes
Neisseria gonorrhoeae
Bordetella pertussis
Legionella pneumophila (agent of Legionnaires' disease)

Susceptibility Testing

Quantitative methods that require measurement of zone diameters give the most precise estimates of antibiotic susceptibility. One such standardized single-disc procedure has been recommended for use with discs to test susceptibility to erythromycin.[1] Interpretation involves correlation of the zone diameters obtained in the disc test with minimal inhibitory concentration (MIC) values for erythromycin.

Reports from the laboratory giving results of the standardized single-disc susceptibility test using a 15 mcg erythromycin disc should be interpreted according to the following criteria:

Susceptible organisms produce zones of 18 mm or greater, indicating that the tested organism is likely to respond to therapy.

Resistant organisms produce zones of 13 mm or less, indicating that other therapy should be selected.

Organisms of intermediate susceptibility produce zones of 14 to 17 mm. The "intermediate" category provides a "buffer zone" which should prevent small, uncontrolled technical

factors from causing major discrepancies in interpretations; thus, when a zone diameter falls within the "intermediate" range, the results may be considered equivocal. If alternative drugs are not available, confirmation by dilution tests may be indicated.

A bacterial isolate may be considered susceptible if the MIC value[2] (minimal inhibitory concentration) for erythromycin is not more than 2 mcg/mL. Organisms are considered resistant if the MIC is 8 mcg/mL or higher.

INDICATIONS AND USAGE

Erythromycin Delayed-Release Capsules are indicated in adults and children for treatment of the following conditions:

Upper respiratory tract infections of mild to moderate degree caused by *Streptococcus pyogenes* (Group A beta-hemolytic streptococci); *Streptococcus pneumoniae (Diplococcus pneumoniae); Haemophilus influenzae* (when used concomitantly with adequate doses of sulfonamides, since many strains of *H. influenzae* are not susceptible to the erythromycin concentrations ordinarily achieved). (See appropriate sulfonamide labeling for prescribing information.)

Lower respiratory tract infections of mild to moderate severity caused by *Streptococcus pyogenes* (Group A beta-hemolytic streptococci); *Streptococcus pneumoniae (Diplococcus pneumoniae).*

Respiratory tract infections due to *Mycoplasma pneumoniae* (Eaton's agent).

Pertussis (whooping cough) caused by *Bordetella pertussis.* Erythromycin is effective in eliminating the organism from the nasopharynx of infected individuals, rendering them noninfectious. Some clinical studies suggest that erythromycin may be helpful in the prophylaxis of pertussis in exposed susceptible individuals.

Diphtheria—As an adjunct to antitoxin in infections due to *Corynebacterium diphtheriae,* to prevent establishment of carriers and to eradicate the organism in carriers.

Erythrasma—In the treatment of infections due to *Corynebacterium minutissimum.*

Intestinal amebiasis caused by *Entamoeba histolytica* (oral erythromycins only). Extraenteric amebiasis requires treatment with other agents.

Infections due to *Listeria monocytogenes.*

Skin and soft tissue infections of mild to moderate severity caused by *Streptococcus pyogenes* and *Staphylococcus aureus* (resistant staphylococci may emerge during treatment).

Primary syphilis caused by *Treponema pallidum.* Erythromycin (oral forms only) is an alternate choice of treatment for primary syphilis in patients allergic to the penicillins. In treatment of primary syphilis, spinal fluid should be examined before treatment and as part of the follow-up after therapy. The use of erythromycin for the treatment of *in utero* syphilis is not recommended. (See "CLINICAL PHARMACOLOGY" section.)

Erythromycins are indicated for treatment of the following infections caused by *Chlamydia trachomatis:* conjunctivitis of the newborn, pneumonia of infancy, and urogenital infections during pregnancy. When tetracyclines are contraindicated or not tolerated, erythromycin is indicated for the treatment of uncomplicated urethral, endocervical, or rectal infections in adults due to *Chlamydia trachomatis.*[3]

Legionnaires' disease caused by *Legionella pneumophila.* Although no controlled clinical efficacy studies have been conducted, *in vitro* and limited preliminary clinical data suggest that erythromycin may be effective in treating Legionnaires' disease.

Therapy with erythromycin should be monitored by bacteriological studies and by clinical response. (See "CLINICAL PHARMACOLOGY—Microbiology" section.)

Injectable benzathine penicillin G is considered by the American Heart Association to be the drug of choice in the treatment and prevention of streptococcal pharyngitis and in long-term prophylaxis of rheumatic fever. When oral medication is preferred for treatment of the above conditions, penicillin G, V or erythromycin are alternate drugs of choice.

Although no controlled clinical efficacy trials have been conducted, erythromycin has been suggested by the American Heart Association and the American Dental Association for use in a regimen for prophylaxis against bacterial endocarditis in patients allergic to penicillin who have congenital and/or rheumatic or other acquired valvular heart disease when they undergo dental procedures and surgical procedures of the upper respiratory tract.[3] (Erythromycin is not suitable prior to genitourinary surgery where the organisms likely to lead to bacteremia are gram-negative bacilli or the enterococcal group of streptococci.)

NOTE: When selecting antibiotics for the prevention of bacterial endocarditis the physician or dentist should read the full joint 1984 statement of the American Heart Association and the American Dental Association.[3]

CONTRAINDICATION

Erythromycin is contraindicated in patients with known hypersensitivity to this antibiotic.

WARNINGS

There have been a few reports of hepatic dysfunction, with or without jaundice, occurring in patients receiving oral erythromycin products.

PRECAUTIONS

General: Erythromycin is principally excreted by the liver. Caution should be exercised when erythromycin is administered to patients with impaired hepatic function. (See "Clinical Pharmacology" and "Warnings" sections).

Prolonged or repeated use of erythromycin may result in an overgrowth of nonsusceptible bacteria or fungi. If superinfection occurs, erythromycin should be discontinued and appropriate therapy instituted.

When indicated, incision and drainage or other surgical procedures should be performed in conjunction with antibiotic therapy.

Laboratory Tests: Erythromycin interferes with the fluorometric determination of urinary catecholamines.

Drug Interactions: Erythromycin use in patients who are receiving high doses of theophylline may be associated with an increase in serum theophylline levels and potential theophylline toxicity. In case of theophylline toxicity and/or elevated serum theophylline levels, the dose of theophylline should be reduced while the patient is receiving concomitant erythromycin therapy.

Concomitant administration of erythromycin and digoxin has been reported to result in elevated digoxin serum levels.

There have been reports of increased anticoagulant effects when erythromycin and oral anticoagulants were used concomitantly.

Concurrent use of erythromycin and ergotamine or dihydroergotamine has been associated in some patients with acute ergot toxicity characterized by severe peripheral vasospasm and dysesthesia.

Erythromycin has been reported to decrease the clearance of triazolam and thus may increase the pharmacologic effect of triazolam.

The use of erythromycin in patients concurrently taking drugs metabolized by the cytochrome P450 system may be associated with elevations in serum erythromycin with carbamazepine, cyclosporine, hexobarbital and phenytoin. Serum concentrations of drugs metabolized by the cytochrome P450 system should be monitored closely in patients concurrently receiving erythromycin.

Troleandomycin significantly alters the metabolism of terfenadine when taken concomitantly; therefore, observe caution when erythromycin and terfenadine are used concurrently.

Patients receiving concomitant lovastatin and erythromycin should be carefully monitored; cases or rhabdomyolysis have been reported in seriously ill patients.

Carcinogenesis, Mutagenesis, Impairment of Fertility: Long-term (2-year) oral studies conducted in rats with erythromycin base did not provide evidence of tumorigenicity. Mutagenicity studies have not been conducted. There was no apparent effect on male or female fertility in rats fed erythromycin (base) at levels up to 0.25 percent of diet.

Pregnancy: Pregnancy Category B: There is no evidence of teratogenicity or any other adverse effect on reproduction in female rats fed erythromycin base (up to 0.25 percent of diet) prior to and during mating, during gestation, and through weaning of two successive litters. There are, however, no adequate and well-controlled studies in pregnant women. Because animal reproduction studies are not always predictive of human response, this drug should be used during pregnancy only if clearly needed. Erythromycin has been reported to cross the placental barrier in humans, but fetal plasma levels are generally low.

Labor and Delivery: The effect of erythromycin on labor and delivery is unknown.

Nursing Mothers: Erythromycin is excreted in breast milk, therefore, caution should be exercised when erythromycin is administered to a nursing woman.

Pediatric Use: See "Indications and Usage" and "Dosage and Administration" sections.

ADVERSE REACTIONS

The most frequent side effects of oral erythromycin preparations are gastrointestinal and are dose-related. They include nausea, vomiting, abdominal pain, diarrhea and anorexia. Symptoms of hepatic dysfunction and/or abnormal liver function test results may occur (see "Warnings" section). Pseudomembranous colitis has been rarely reported in association with erythromycin therapy.

There have been isolated reports of transient central nervous system side effects including confusion, hallucinations, seizures, and vertigo; however, a cause and effect relationship has not been established.

Occasional case reports of cardiac arrhythmias such as ventricular tachycardia have been documented in patients receiving erythromycin therapy. There have been isolated reports of other cardiovascular symptoms such as chest pain, dizziness, and palpitations; however a cause and effect relationship has not been established.

Allergic reactions ranging from urticaria and mild skin eruptions to anaphylaxis have occurred.

There have been isolated reports of reversible hearing loss occurring chiefly in patients with renal insufficiency and in patients receiving high doses of erythromycin.

OVERDOSAGE

In case of overdosage, erythromycin should be discontinued. Overdosage should be handled with the prompt elimination of unabsorbed drug and all other appropriate measures. Erythromycin is not removed by peritoneal dialysis or hemodialysis.

DOSAGE AND ADMINISTRATION

Administration of a dose of Erythromycin Delayed-Release Capsules in the presence of food lowers the blood levels of systemically available erythromycin. Although the blood levels obtained upon administration of enteric-coated erythromycin products in the presence of food are still above minimum inhibitory concentrations (MICs) of most organisms for which erythromycin is indicated, optimum blood levels are obtained on a fasting stomach (administration at least ½ hour and preferably two hours before or after a meal).

Adults: The usual dose is 250 mg every 6 hours taken one hour before meals. If twice-a-day dosage is desired, the recommended dose is 500 mg every 12 hours. Dosage may be increased up to 4 grams per day, according to the severity of infection. Twice-a-day dosing is not recommended when doses larger than 1 gram daily are administered.

Children: Age, weight, and severity of the infection are important factors in determining the proper dosage. The usual dosage is 30 to 50 mg/kg/day, in divided doses. For the treatment of more severe infections this dosage may be doubled.

Streptococcal infections: A therapeutic dosage of oral erythromycin should be administered for at least 10 days. For continuous prophylaxis against recurrences of streptococcal infections in persons with a history of rheumatic heart disease, the dose is 250 mg twice a day.

For the prevention of bacterial endocarditis in penicillin-allergic patients with valvular heart disease who are to undergo dental procedures or surgical procedures of the upper respiratory tract, the adult dose is 1 gram orally (20 mg/kg for children) one hour prior to the procedure and then 500 mg (10 mg/kg for children) orally 6 hours later.[3] (See "INDICATIONS AND USAGE" section.)

Primary syphilis: 30 to 40 g given in divided doses over a period of 10 to 15 days.

Intestinal amebiasis: 250 mg every 6 hours for 10 to 14 days for adults; 30 to 50 mg/kg/day in divided doses for 10 to 14 days for children.

Legionnaires' disease: Although optimal doses have not been established, doses utilized in reported clinical data were those recommended above (1 to 4 g daily in divided doses).

Urogenital infections during pregnancy due to *Chlamydia trachomatis:* Although the optimal dose and duration of therapy have not been established, the suggested treatment is 500 mg by mouth four times a day on an empty stomach for at least 7 days. For women who cannot tolerate this regimen, a decreased dose of 250 mg by mouth four times a day should be used for at least 14 days.[4]

For adults with uncomplicated urethral, endocervical, or rectal infections caused by *Chlamydia trachomatis,* when tetracycline is contrainidicated or not tolerated, 500 mg of erythromycin by mouth four times a day for at least 7 days.[4]

Pertussis: Although optimum dosage and duration of therapy have not been established, doses of erythromycin utilized in reported clinical studies were 40 to 50 mg/kg/day, given in divided doses for 5 to 14 days.

HOW SUPPLIED

Erythromycin Delayed-Release Capsules, USP, are clear and opaque maroon capsules with pink and yellow particles containing 250 mg of erythromycin supplied in bottles of 100 (**NDC** 0074-6301-13) and 500 (**NDC** 0074-6301-53).

Storage Conditions: Protect from moisture and excessive heat. **Store below 86°F (30°C).**

REFERENCES

1. Approved Standard ASM-2 "Performance Standards for Antimicrobial Disc Susceptibility Test." National Committee for Clinical Laboratory Standards, 771 East Lancaster Avenue, Villanova, PA 19085.
2. Ericson, H.M., Sherris, J.C.: "Antibiotic Sensitivity Testing Report of an International Collaborative Study." *Acta Pathologica et Microbiologica Scandinavica,* Section B, Supp. 217, 1971.
3. American Heart Assoc. and American Dental Assoc. "Prevention of Bacterial Endocarditis," *Circulation:* Vol. 70, No. 6, December, 1984, 1123A-1127A.

Continued on next page

Abbott Laboratories—Cont.

4. CDC Sexually Transmitted Diseases Treatment Guidelines 1982.

Ref. 01-2563-R4

Shown in Product Identification Section, page 403

FERO–FOLIC–500® Filmtab® Tablets ℞
[*fe 'ro fo-lic*]
Controlled-Release Iron with Folic Acid and Vitamin C

IBERET–FOLIC–500® Filmtab® Tablets ℞
Controlled-Release Iron with Vitamin C, and B-Complex, including Folic Acid

DESCRIPTION

FERO-FOLIC-500 Filmtab is a hematinic for oral administration containing 525 mg of ferrous sulfate (equivalent to 105 mg of elemental iron) in a unique controlled-release vehicle, the Gradumet®. In addition, this product contains 800 mcg of folic acid and 500 mg of ascorbic acid present as sodium ascorbate.

Inactive Ingredients: Castor oil, cellulosic polymers, D&C Red No. 30, magnesium stearate, methyl acrylate-methyl methacrylate copolymer, pregelatinized starch (contains corn starch), polyethylene glycol, povidone, propylene glycol, talc, titanium dioxide and vanillin.

IBERET-FOLIC-500 is an Abbott hematinic containing iron in the Gradumet® controlled-release vehicle; vitamin C for enhancement of iron absorption; and the B-Complex vitamins including folic acid. The IBERET-FOLIC-500 Filmtab is for oral use.

Each Filmtab tablet provides:

*Ferrous Sulfate (equivalent to 105 mg of elemental iron)	525 mg
Ascorbic Acid (present as sodium ascorbate) (C)	500 mg
Niacinamide	30 mg
Calcium Pantothenate	10 mg
Thiamine Mononitrate (B_1)	6 mg
Riboflavin (B_2)	6 mg
Pyridoxine Hydrochloride (B_6)	5 mg
Folic Acid	800 mcg
Cyanocobalamin (B_{12})	25 mcg

*In controlled-release form (Gradumet)

Inactive Ingredients: Castor oil, cellulosic polymers, corn starch, D&C Red No. 7, FD&C Blue No. 1, FD&C Blue No. 2, magnesium stearate, methyl acrylate-methyl methacrylate copolymer, polyethylene glycol, povidone, propylene glycol, stearic acid, talc, titanium dioxide and vanillin.

Controlled-release of iron from the Gradumet protects against gastric side effects. The Gradumet is an inert, porous, plastic matrix which is impregnated with ferrous sulfate. Iron is leached from the Gradumet as it passes through the gastrointestinal tract, and the expended matrix is excreted harmlessly in the stool. Controlled-release iron is particularly helpful in patients who have demonstrated intolerance to oral iron preparations.

CLINICAL PHARMACOLOGY

Oral iron is absorbed most efficiently when it is administered between meals. Conventional iron preparations, however, frequently cause gastric irritation when taken on an empty stomach. Studies with iron in the Gradumet have indicated that relatively little of the iron is released in the stomach, gastric intolerance is seldom encountered, and hematologic response ranks with that obtained from plain ferrous sulfate.

Iron is found in the body principally as hemoglobin. Storage in the form of ferritin occurs in the liver, spleen, and bone marrow. Concentrations of plasma iron and the total iron-binding capacity of plasma vary greatly in different physiological conditions and disease states.

Large amounts of ascorbic acid administered orally with ferrous sulfate have been shown to enhance iron absorption. Apparently this is due to the ability of ascorbic acid to prevent the oxidation of ferrous iron to the less effectively absorbed ferric form.

Folic acid and iron are absorbed in the proximal small intestine, particularly the duodenum. Folic acid is absorbed maximally and rapidly at this site, and iron is absorbed in a descending gradient from the duodenum distally.

After absorption folic acid is rapidly converted into its metabolically active forms. Approximately two-thirds is bound to plasma protein. Half of the folic acid stored in the body is found in the liver. Folic acid is also concentrated in spinal fluid.

Except for the folates ingested in liver, yeast, and egg yolk, the percentage of absorption of food folates averages about 10%.

The B-complex vitamins in IBERET-FOLIC-500 are absorbed by the active transport process. B-complex vitamins are rapidly eliminated and therefore are not stored in the body.

Calcium pantothenate is absorbed readily from the gastrointestinal tract and distributed to all body tissues.

INDICATIONS AND USAGE

FERO-FOLIC-500 is indicated for the treatment of iron deficiency and prevention of concomitant folic acid deficiency in non-pregnant adults. FERO-FOLIC-500 is also indicated in pregnancy for the prevention and treatment of iron deficiency and to supply a maintenance dosage of folic acid.

IBERET-FOLIC-500 is indicated in non-pregnant adults for the treatment of iron deficiency and prevention of concomitant folic acid deficiency where there is an associated deficient intake or increased need for the B-complex vitamins. IBERET-FOLIC-500 is also indicated in pregnancy for the prevention and treatment of iron deficiency where there is a concomitant deficient intake or increased need for the B-complex vitamins (including folic acid).

CONTRAINDICATIONS

FERO-FOLIC-500 and IBERET-FOLIC-500 are contraindicated in patients with pernicious anemia.

FERO-FOLIC-500 and IBERET-FOLIC-500 are also contraindicated in the rare instance of hypersensitivity to folic acid.

WARNINGS

Folic acid alone is improper therapy in the treatment of pernicious anemia and other megaloblastic anemias where vitamin B_{12} is deficient.

PRECAUTIONS

Where anemia exists, its nature should be established and underlying causes determined.

FERO-FOLIC-500 and IBERET-FOLIC-500 contain 800 mcg of folic acid per tablet. Folic acid especially in doses above 0.1 mg daily may obscure pernicious anemia, in that hematologic remission may occur while neurological manifestations remain progresssive. Concomitant parenteral therapy with vitamin B_{12} may be necessary in patients with deficiency of vitamin B_{12}. Pernicious anemia is rare in women of childbearing age, and the likelihood of its occurrence along with pregnancy is reduced by the impairment of fertility associated with vitamin B_{12} deficiency.

Like other oral iron preparations, FERO-FOLIC-500 and IBERET-FOLIC-500 should be stored out of the reach of children to guard against accidental iron poisoning (see Overdosage).

Laboratory Tests: In older patients and those with conditions tending to lead to vitamin B_{12} depletion, serum B_{12} levels should be regularly assessed during treatment with FERO-FOLIC-500 or IBERET-FOLIC-500.

Drug Interactions: Absorption of iron is inhibited by *magnesium trisilicate* and *antacids containing carbonates.* Ferrous sulfate may interfere with the absorption of *tetracyclines.*

The antiparkinsonism effects of *levodopa* may be reversed by pyridoxine.

Iron absorption is inhibited by the ingestion of eggs or milk.

Carcinogenesis: Adequate data are not available on long-term potential for carcinogenesis in animals or humans.

Pregnancy: Pregnancy Category A. Studies in pregnant women have not shown that FERO-FOLIC-500 or IBERET-FOLIC-500 increase the risk of fetal abnormalities if administered during pregnancy. If either of these drugs is used during pregnancy, the possibility of fetal harm appears remote. Because studies cannot rule out the possibility of harm, however, FERO-FOLIC-500 or IBERET-FOLIC-500 should be used during pregnancy only if clearly needed.

Nursing Mothers: Folic acid, ascorbic acid, and B-complex vitamins are excreted in breast milk.

ADVERSE REACTIONS

The likelihood of gastric intolerance to iron in the controlled-release Gradumet vehicle is remote. If such should occur, the tablet may be taken after a meal. Allergic sensitization has been reported following both oral and parenteral administration of folic acid.

OVERDOSAGE

Signs of serious toxicity may be delayed because the iron is in a controlled-release dose form. Increased capillary permeability, reduced plasma volume, increased cardiac output, and sudden cardiovascular collapse may occur in acute iron intoxication. In overdosage, efforts should be made to hasten the elimination of the Gradumet tablets ingested. An emetic should be administered as soon as possible, followed by gastric lavage if indicated. Immediately following emesis, a large dose of a saline cathartic should be used to speed passage through the intestinal tract. X-ray examination may then be considered to determine the position and number of Gradumet tablets remaining in the gastrointestinal tract.

DOSAGE AND ADMINISTRATION

FERO-FOLIC-500 is administered orally and may be taken on an empty stomach.

Adults: For treatment of iron deficiency and prevention of folic acid deficiency, the recommended dose is one tablet daily.

Pregnant Adults: For prevention and treatment of iron deficiency and to supply a maintenance dosage of folic acid, the recommended dose is one tablet daily.

IBERET-FOLIC-500 is administered orally and may be taken on an empty stomach.

Adults: For the treatment of iron deficiency and prevention of concomitant folic acid deficiency where there is an associated deficient intake or increased need for the B-complex vitamins, the recommended dose is one tablet daily.

Pregnant Adults: For the prevention and treatment of iron deficiency where there is a concomitant deficient intake or increased need for the B-complex vitamins including folic acid, the recommended dose is one tablet daily.

HOW SUPPLIED

FERO-FOLIC-500 is supplied as red Filmtab tablets in bottles of 100 (**NDC** 0074-7079-13) and 500 (**NDC** 0074-7079-53).

IBERET-FOLIC-500 is supplied as red Filmtab tablets in bottles of 60 (**NDC** 0074-7125-60).

Recommended storage: Store below 77°F (25°C).

Ref. 03-4410-R9

Shown in Product Identification Section, page 403

FERO–GRAD–500® Filmtab® tablets OTC
[*fe 'ro-grad*]
IRON plus Vitamin C
Well-tolerated once-daily hematinic with controlled-release iron.

FERO-GRADUMET® Filmtab® tablets
Hematinic supplying controlled-release iron

DESCRIPTION

Each Fero-Gradumet and Fero-Grad-500 tablet contains the equivalent of 105 mg of elemental iron (525 mg of ferrous sulfate) in a unique controlled-release vehicle, the Gradumet®. In addition, each Fero-Grad-500 tablet contains 500 mg of vitamin C (as sodium ascorbate) to improve iron absorption.

Inactive Ingredients: Fero-Grad-500: Cellulosic polymers, D&C Red No. 7, FD&C Blue No. 1, magnesium stearate, methyl acrylate-methyl methacrylate copolymer, polyethylene glycol, povidone, pregelatinized starch (contains corn starch), propylene glycol, talc, titanium dioxide and vanillin.

Fero-Gradumet: Castor oil, cellulosic polymers, FD&C Red No. 40, FD&C Yellow No. 6, magnesium stearate, methyl acrylate-methyl methacrylate copolymer, polyethylene glycol, povidone, propylene glycol, talc, titanium dioxide and vanillin.

INDICATIONS

Fero-Grad-500: For the treatment of iron deficiency or iron deficiency anemia. Fero-Gradumet: For the prevention and treatment of iron deficiency.

PRECAUTIONS

Like other oral iron preparations Fero-Gradumet and Fero-Grad-500 should be stored out of the reach of children.

DOSAGE AND ADMINISTRATION

Fero-Grad-500: Usual adult dose, including pregnant females: One tablet daily, or as directed by the physician.

Fero-Gradumet: Usual adult dose: Prevention: One tablet daily; Treatment: One tablet twice daily, or as directed by the physician. Pregnant females: Prevention: One tablet daily, or as directed by physician.

HOW SUPPLIED

Fero-Gradumet is supplied as red tablets in bottles of 100 (**NDC** 0074-6852-02); Fero-Grad-500 is supplied as red tablets in bottles of 100 (**NDC** 0074-7238-01) and 500 (**NDC** 0074-7238-02), and in Abbo-Pac unit dose strip packages of 100 tablets (**NDC** 0074-7238-11). Keep tightly closed. The ingredients of these products are listed in one or more of the Medicare designated compendia.

Recommended storage: Store below 77°F (25°C).

Ref. 03-1972-8/R32 and 03-1954-8/R28

Shown in Product Identification Section, page 403

H-BIG® ℞
(Hepatitis B Immune Globulin [Human])

½ ml syringe	(**NDC** 0074-8399-11)
1 ml vial	(**NDC** 0074-8399-01)
4 ml vial	(**NDC** 0074-8399-04)
5 ml vial	(**NDC** 0074-8399-05)

HARMONYL® Tablets   ℞
[har'mō-nil]
(deserpidine)

DESCRIPTION
Harmonyl (deserpidine) is a purified rauwolfia alkaloid chemically identified as 11-desmethoxyreserpine.
Inactive Ingredients: Corn starch, D&C Red No. 36, lactose, magnesium stearate, stearic acid and talc.

ACTIONS
The pharmacologic actions of HARMONYL (deserpidine) are essentially the same as those of other active rauwolfia alkaloids. Deserpidine probably produces its antihypertensive effects through depletion of tissue stores of catecholamines (epinephrine and norepinephrine) from peripheral sites. By contrast, its sedative and tranquilizing properties are thought to be related to depletion of 5-hydroxytryptamine from the brain.
The antihypertensive effect is often accompanied by bradycardia. There is no significant alteration in cardiac output or renal blood flow. The carotid sinus reflex is inhibited, but postural hypotension is rarely seen with the use of conventional doses of HARMONYL alone.
Deserpidine, like other rauwolfia alkaloids, is characterized by slow onset of action and sustained effect which may persist following withdrawal of the drug.

INDICATIONS
HARMONYL (deserpidine) is indicated for the treatment of mild essential hypertension. It is also useful as adjunctive therapy with other antihypertensive agents in the more severe forms of hypertension.
The drug is also indicated for the relief of symptoms in agitated psychotic states, e.g., schizophrenia—primarily in those individuals unable to tolerate phenothiazine derivatives or those who also require antihypertensive medication.

CONTRAINDICATIONS
HARMONYL (deserpidine) is contraindicated in patients with known hypersensitivity, history of mental depression especially with suicidal tendencies, active peptic ulcer, and ulcerative colitis. It is also contraindicated in patients receiving electroconvulsive therapy.

WARNINGS
HARMONYL (deserpidine) differs slightly in chemical structure from reserpine, however, its actions, indications, cautions and adverse reactions are common to the class of rauwolfia alkaloids. Reserpine may cause mental depression. Recognition of depression may be difficult because this condition may often be disguised by somatic complaints (Masked Depression). The drug should be discontinued at first signs of depression such as despondency, early morning insomnia, loss of appetite, impotence, or self-deprecation. Drug-induced depression may persist for several months after drug withdrawal and may be severe enough to result in suicide.
Usage in Pregnancy and Lactation
The safety of deserpidine for use during pregnancy or lactation has not been established; therefore, it should be used in pregnant women or in women of childbearing potential only when, in the judgment of the physician, its use is deemed essential to the welfare of the patient. Increased respiratory secretions, nasal congestion, cyanosis, and anorexia may occur in infants born to rauwolfia alkaloid-treated mothers since these preparations are known to cross the placental barrier to enter the fetal circulation and appear in cord blood. They also are secreted by nursing mothers into breast milk.
Reproductive and teratology studies in rats reduced the mating index and neonatal survival indices; the no-effect dosage has not been established.

PRECAUTIONS
Because rauwolfia preparations increase gastrointestinal motility and secretion, this drug should be used cautiously in patients with a history of peptic ulcer, ulcerative colitis, or gallstones, where biliary colic may be precipitated.
Caution should be exercised when treating hypertensive patients with renal insufficiency since they adjust poorly to lowered blood pressure levels.
Use HARMONYL (deserpidine) cautiously with digitalis and quinidine since cardiac arrhythmias have occurred with rauwolfia preparations.
Preoperative withdrawal of deserpidine does not assure that circulatory instability will not occur. It is important that the anesthesiologist be aware of the patient's drug intake and consider this in the overall management, since hypotension has occurred in patients receiving rauwolfia preparations. Anticholinergic and/or adrenergic drugs (metaraminol, norepinephrine) have been employed to treat adverse vagocirculatory effects.
Animal tumorigenicity: There are no studies demonstrating that deserpidine is an animal tumorigen, although it is a prolactin stimulator and structurally related to reserpine. Rodent studies with reserpine, however, have shown that reserpine is an animal tumorigen, causing an increased inci-

dence of mammary fibroadenomas in female mice, malignant tumors of the seminal vesicles in male mice, and malignant adrenal medullary tumors in male rats. These findings arose in 2 year studies in which the drug was administered in the feed at concentrations of 5 and 10 ppm—about 100 to 300 times the usual human dose. The breast neoplasms are thought to be related to reserpine's prolactin-elevating effect. Several other prolactin-elevating drugs have also been associated with an increased incidence of mammary neoplasia in rodents.
The extent to which these findings indicate a risk to humans is uncertain. Tissue culture experiments show that about one-third of human breast tumors are prolactin-dependent *in vitro,* a factor of considerable importance if the use of the drug is contemplated in a patient with previously detected breast cancer. The possibility of an increased risk of breast cancer in reserpine users has been studied extensively; however, no firm conclusion has emerged. Although a few epidemiologic studies have suggested a slightly increased risk (less than twofold in all studies except one) in women who have used reserpine, other studies of generally similar design have not confirmed this. Epidemiologic studies conducted using other drugs (neuroleptic agents) that, like reserpine, increase prolactin levels and, therefore, would be considered rodent mammary carcinogens, have not shown an association between chronic administration of the drug and human mammary tumorigenesis. While long-term clinical observation has not suggested such an association, the available evidence is considered too limited to be conclusive at this time. An association of reserpine intake with pheochromocytoma or tumors of the seminal vesicles has not been explored.

ADVERSE REACTIONS
The following adverse reactions have been reported with rauwolfia preparations. These reactions are usually reversible and disappear when the drug is discontinued.
Gastrointestinal: Including hypersecretion, anorexia, diarrhea, nausea, and vomiting.
Cardiovascular: Including angina-like symptoms, arrhythmias (particularly when used concurrently with digitalis or quinidine), and bradycardia.
Central Nervous System: Including drowsiness, depression, nervousness, paradoxical anxiety, nightmares, extrapyramidal tract symptoms, CNS sensitization manifested by dull sensorium, and deafness.
Dermatologic-Hypersensitivity: Including pruritus, rash, and asthma in asthmatic patients.
Ophthalmologic: Including glaucoma, uveitis, optic atrophy, and conjunctival injection.
Hematologic: Thrombocytopenic purpura.
Miscellaneous: Nasal congestion, weight gain, impotence or decreased libido, dysuria, dyspnea, muscular aches, dryness of mouth, dizziness, and headache.
Water retention with edema in patients with hypertensive vascular disease may occur rarely, but the condition generally clears with cessation of therapy or with the administration of a diuretic agent.

DOSAGE AND ADMINISTRATION
HARMONYL (deserpidine) is administered orally. For the management of mild essential hypertension in the average patient not receiving other antihypertensive agents, the usual initial adult dose is 0.75 to 1 mg daily. Because 10 to 14 days are required to produce the full effects of the drug, adjustments in dosage should not be made more frequently. If the therapeutic response is not adequate, it is generally advisable to add another antihypertensive agent to the regimen. For maintenance, dosage should be reduced. A single daily dose of 0.25 mg of deserpidine may suffice for some patients.
Concomitant use of deserpidine with ganglionic blocking agents, guanethidine, veratrum, hydralazine, methyldopa, chlorthalidone, or thiazides necessitates careful titration of dosage with each agent.
For psychiatric disorders: The average initial oral dose is 0.5 mg daily with a range of 0.125 to 1 mg. Adjust dosage upward or downward according to the patient's response.

OVERDOSAGE
An overdosage of deserpidine is characterized by flushing of the skin, conjunctival injection, and pupillary constriction. Sedation ranging from drowsiness to coma may occur. Hypotension, hypothermia, central respiratory depression and bradycardia may develop in cases of severe overdosage. Treatment consists of the careful evacuation of stomach contents followed by the usual procedures for the symptomatic management of CNS depressant overdosage. If severe hypotension occurs, it should be treated with a direct acting vasopressor such as Levophed® (norepinephrine bitartrate injection, USP).

HOW SUPPLIED
HARMONYL (deserpidine tablets) grooved, salmon-pink, 0.25 mg tablets are supplied in bottles of 100 (**NDC** 0074-6906-07).
Ref. 01-2471-R4

HYTRIN®   ℞
[hī'trin]
(terazosin hydrochloride)

DESCRIPTION
HYTRIN (terazosin hydrochloride), an alpha-1-selective adrenoceptor blocking agent, is a quinazoline derivative represented by the following chemical name and structural formula: (RS)-Piperazine, 1-(4-amino-6,7-dimethoxy-2-quinazolinyl)-4-[(tetrahydro-2-furanyl)carbonyl]-, monohydrochloride, dihydrate.
Terazosin hydrochloride is a white, crystalline substance, freely soluble in water and isotonic saline and has a molecular weight of 459.93. HYTRIN tablets (terazosin hydrochloride tablets) for oral ingestion are supplied in four dosage strengths containing terazosin hydrochloride equivalent to 1 mg, 2 mg, 5 mg, or 10 mg of terazosin.
Inactive Ingredients:
1 mg tablet: corn starch, lactose, magnesium stearate, povidone and talc.
2 mg tablet: corn starch, FD&C Yellow No. 6, lactose, magnesium stearate, povidone and talc.
5 mg tablet: corn starch, iron oxide, lactose, magnesium stearate, povidone and talc.
10 mg tablet: corn starch, D&C Yellow No. 10, FD&C Blue No. 2, lactose, magnesium stearate, povidone and talc.

CLINICAL PHARMACOLOGY
Pharmacodynamics:
In animals, terazosin causes a decrease in blood pressure by decreasing total peripheral vascular resistance. The vasodilatory hypotensive action of terazosin appears to be produced mainly by blockade of alpha-1-adrenoceptors. Terazosin decreases blood pressure gradually within 15 minutes following oral administration.
Clinical studies of terazosin in man used once daily (the great majority) and twice daily regimens with total doses usually in the range of 5–20 mg/day, in patients with mild (about 77%, diastolic pressure 95–105 mmHg) or moderate (23%, diastolic pressure 105–115 mmHg) hypertension. Because terazosin, like all alpha antagonists, can cause unusually large falls in blood pressure after the first dose or first few doses, the initial dose was 1 mg in virtually all studies, with subsequent titration to a specified fixed dose or titration to some specified blood pressure end point (usually a supine diastolic pressure of 90 mmHg).
Blood pressure responses were measured at the end of the dosing interval (usually 24 hours) and effects were shown to persist throughout the interval, with the usual supine responses 5–10 mmHg systolic and 3.5–8 mmHg diastolic greater than placebo. The responses in the standing position tended to be somewhat larger, by 1–3 mmHg, although this was not true in all studies. The magnitude of the blood pressure responses was similar to prazosin and less than hydrochlorothiazide (in a single study). In measurements 24 hours after dosing, heart rate was unchanged.
Limited measurements of peak response (2–3 hours after dosing) during chronic terazosin administration indicate that it is greater than about twice the trough (24 hour) response, suggesting some attenuation of response at 24 hours, presumably due to a fall in blood terazosin concentrations at the end of the dose interval. This explanation is not established with certainty, however, and is not consistent with the similarity of blood pressure response to once daily and twice daily dosing and with the absence of an observed dose-response relationship over a range of 5–20 mg, i.e., if blood concentrations had fallen to the point of providing less than full effect at 24 hours, a shorter dosing interval or larger dose should have led to increased response. Further dose response and dose duration studies are being carried out. Blood pressure should be measured at the end of the dose interval; if response is not satisfactory, patients may be tried on a larger dose or twice daily dosing regimen. The latter should also be considered if possibly blood pressure-related side effects, such as dizziness, palpitations, or orthostatic complaints, are seen within a few hours after dosing.
The greater blood pressure effect associated with peak plasma concentrations (first few hours after dosing) appears somewhat more position-dependent (greater in the erect position) than the effect of terazosin at 24 hours and in the erect position there is also a 6–10 beat per minute increase in heart rate in the first few hours after dosing. During the first 3 hours after dosing 12.5% of patients had a systolic pressure fall of 30 mmHg or more from supine to standing, or standing systolic pressure below 90 mmHg with a fall of at least 20 mmHg, compared to 4% of a placebo group.
There was a tendency for patients to gain weight during terazosin therapy. In placebo-controlled monotherapy trials, male and female patients receiving terazosin gained a mean

Continued on next page

Abbott Laboratories—Cont.

of 1.7 and 2.2 pounds respectively, compared to losses of 0.2 and 1.2 pounds respectively, in the placebo group. Both differences were statistically significant.

During controlled clinical studies, patients receiving terazosin monotherapy had a small but statistically significant decrease (a 3% fall) compared to placebo in total cholesterol and the combined low-density and very-low-density lipoprotein fractions. No significant changes were observed in high-density lipoprotein fraction and triglycerides compared to placebo.

Analysis of clinical laboratory data following administration of terazosin suggested the possibility of hemodilution based on decreases in hematocrit, hemoglobin, white blood cells, total protein and albumin. Decreases in hematocrit and total protein have been observed with alpha-blockade and are attributed to hemodilution.

Pharmacokinetics:

Relative to solution, terazosin hydrochloride administered as HYTRIN tablets is essentially completely absorbed in man. Food had little or no effect on the bioavailability of terazosin. Terazosin has been shown to undergo minimal hepatic first-pass metabolism and nearly all of the circulating dose is in the form of parent drug. The plasma levels peak about one hour after dosing, and then decline with a half-life of approximately 12 hours. The drug is highly bound to plasma proteins and binding is constant over the clinically observed concentration range. Approximately 10% of an orally administered dose is excreted as parent drug in the urine and approximately 20% is excreted in the feces. The remainder is eliminated as metabolites. Overall, approximately 40% of the administered dose is excreted in the urine and approximately 60% in the feces. The disposition of the compound in animals is qualitatively similar to that in man.

INDICATIONS AND USAGE

HYTRIN (terazosin hydrochloride) is indicated for the treatment of hypertension. It can be used alone or in combination with other antihypertensive agents such as diuretics or beta-adrenergic blocking agents.

CONTRAINDICATIONS

Clinical studies and available literature do not suggest any contraindication to the use of HYTRIN.

WARNINGS

Syncope and "First-dose" Effect:
Terazosin, like other alpha-adrenergic blocking agents, can cause marked hypotension, especially postural hypotension, and syncope in association with the first dose or first few doses of therapy. A similar effect can be anticipated if therapy is interrupted for more than a few doses. Syncope has also been reported with other alpha-adrenergic blocking agents in association with rapid dosage increases or the introduction of another antihypertensive drug. Syncope is believed to be due to an excessive postural hypotensive effect, although occasionally the syncopal episode has been preceded by a bout of severe supraventricular tachycardia with heart rates of 120–160 beats per minute.
To decrease the likelihood of syncope or excessive hypotension, treatment should always be initiated with a 1 mg dose of terazosin, given at bedtime. The 2 mg, 5 mg and 10 mg tablets are not indicated as initial therapy. Dosage should then be increased slowly, according to recommendations in the Dosage and Administration section and additional antihypertensive agents should be added with caution. The patient should be cautioned to avoid situations where injury could result should syncope occur during initiation of therapy.
In early investigational studies, where increasing single doses up to 7.5 mg were given at 3 day intervals, tolerance to the first dose phenomenon did not necessarily develop and the "first dose" effect could be observed at all doses. Syncopal episodes occurred in 3 of the 14 subjects given terazosin at doses of 2.5, 5 and 7.5 mg, which are higher than the recommended initial dose; in addition, severe orthostatic hypotension (blood pressure falling to 50/0 mmHg) was seen in two others and dizziness, tachycardia, and lightheadedness occurred in most subjects. These adverse effects all occurred within 90 minutes of dosing.
In multiple dose clinical trials involving nearly 2000 patients, syncope was reported in about 1% of patients, in no case severe or prolonged, and was not necessarily associated with early doses.
If syncope occurs, the patient should be placed in a recumbent position and treated supportively as necessary. There is evidence that the orthostatic effect of terazosin is greater, even in chronic use, shortly after dosing.

PRECAUTIONS

General:
Orthostatic Hypotension
While syncope is the most severe orthostatic effect of terazosin (see Warnings), other symptoms of lowered blood pressure, such as dizziness, lightheadedness and palpita-

tions, are more common, occurring in some 28% of patients in clinical trials. Patients with occupations in which such events represent potential problems should be treated with particular caution.
Information for Patients:
Patients should be made aware of the possibility of syncopal and orthostatic symptoms, especially at the initiation of therapy, and to avoid driving or hazardous tasks for 12 hours after the first dose, after a dosage increase, and after interruption of therapy when treatment is resumed. They should be cautioned to avoid situations where injury could result should syncope occur during initiation of terazosin therapy. They should also be advised of the need to sit or lie down when symptoms of lowered blood pressure occur, although these symptoms are not always orthostatic, and to be careful when rising from a sitting or lying position. If dizziness, lightheadedness, or palpitations are bothersome they should be reported to the physician, so that dose adjustment can be considered.
Patients should also be told that drowsiness or somnolence can occur with terazosin, requiring caution in people who must drive or operate heavy machinery.
Laboratory Tests:
Small but statistically significant decreases in hematocrit, hemoglobin, white blood cells, total protein and albumin were observed in controlled clinical trials. The magnitude of the decreases did not worsen with time. These laboratory findings suggested the possibility of hemodilution.
Drug Interactions:
In controlled trials, terazosin has been added to diuretics, and several beta-adrenergic blockers; no unexpected interactions were observed. Terazosin has also been used in patients on a variety of concomitant therapies; while these were not formal interaction studies, no interactions were observed. Terazosin has been used concomitantly in at least 50 patients on the following drugs or drug classes: 1) analgesic/anti-inflammatory (e.g., acetaminophen, aspirin, codeine, ibuprofen, indomethacin); 2) antibiotics (e.g., erythromycin, trimethoprim and sulfamethoxazole); 3) anticholinergic/sympathomimetics (e.g., phenylephrine hydrochloride, phenylpropanolamine hydrochloride, pseudoephedrine hydrochloride); 4) antigout (e.g., allopurinol); 5) antihistamines (e.g., chlorpheniramine); 6) cardiovascular agents (e.g., atenolol, hydrochlorothiazide, methyclothiazide, propranolol); 7) corticosteroids; 8) gastrointestinal agents (e.g., antacids); 9) hypoglycemics; 10) sedatives and tranquilizers (e.g., diazepam).
Carcinogenesis, Mutagenesis, Impairment of Fertility:
HYTRIN was devoid of mutagenic potential when evaluated *in vivo* and *in vitro* (the Ames test, *in vivo* cytogenetics, the dominant lethal test in mice, *in vivo* Chinese hamster chromosome aberration test and V79 forward mutation assay). HYTRIN, administered in the feed to rats at doses of 8, 40, and 250 mg/kg/day for two years, was associated with a statistically significant increase in benign adrenal medullary tumors of male rats exposed to the 250 mg/kg dose. This dose is 695 times the maximum recommended human dose of 20 mg/55 kg patient. Female rats were unaffected. HYTRIN was not oncogenic in mice when administered in feed for 2 years at a maximum tolerated dose of 32 mg/kg/day.
The absence of mutagenicity in a battery of tests, of tumorigenicity of any cell type in the mouse carcinogenicity assay, of increased total tumor incidence in either species, and of proliferative adrenal lesions in female rats, suggests a male rat species-specific event. Numerous other diverse pharmaceutical and chemical compounds have also been associated with benign adrenal medullary tumors in male rats without supporting evidence for carcinogenicity in man.
The effect of HYTRIN on fertility was assessed in a standard fertility/reproductive performance study in which male and female rats were administered oral doses of 8, 30 and 120 mg/kg/day. Four of 20 male rats given 30 mg/kg and five of 19 male rats given 120 mg/kg failed to sire a litter. Testicular weights and morphology were unaffected by treatment. Vaginal smears at 30 and 120 mg/kg/day, however, appeared to contain less sperm than smears from control matings and good correlation was reported between sperm count and subsequent pregnancy.
Oral administration of HYTRIN for one or two years elicited a statistically significant increase in the incidence of testicular atrophy in rats exposed to 40 and 250 mg/kg/day, but not in rats exposed to 8 mg/kg/day (> 20 times the maximum recommended human dose). Testicular atrophy was also observed in dogs dosed with 300 mg/kg/day (> 800 times the maximum recommended human dose) for three months but not after one year when dosed with 20 mg/kg/day. This lesion has also been seen with Minipress®, another (marketed) selective-alpha-1 blocking agent.
Pregnancy:
Teratogenic effects: Pregnancy Category C. HYTRIN was not teratogenic in either rats or rabbits when administered at oral doses up to 1330 and 165 times, respectively, the maximum recommended human dose. Fetal resorptions occurred in rats dosed with 480 mg/kg/day, approximately 1330 times the maximum recommended human dose. Increased fetal resorptions, decreased fetal weight and an increased number

of supernumerary ribs were observed in offspring of rabbits dosed with 165 times the maximum recommended human dose. These findings (in both species) were most likely secondary to maternal toxicity. There are no adequate and well-controlled studies in pregnant women and the safety of terazosin in pregnancy has not been established. HYTRIN is not recommended during pregnancy unless the potential benefit justifies the potential risk to the mother and fetus. Nonteratogenic effects: In a peri- and post-natal development study in rats, significantly more pups died in the group dosed at 120 mg/kg/day (> 300 times the maximum recommended human dose) than in the control group during the three-week post-partum period.
Nursing Mothers:
It is not known whether terazosin is excreted in breast milk. Because many drugs are excreted in breast milk, caution should be exercised when terazosin is administered to a nursing woman.
Pediatric Use:
Safety and effectiveness in children have not been determined.

ADVERSE REACTIONS

The prevalence of adverse reactions has been ascertained from clinical studies conducted primarily in the United States. All adverse experiences (events) reported during these studies were recorded as adverse reactions. The prevalence rates presented below are based on combined data from fourteen placebo-controlled studies involving once-a-day administration of terazosin as monotherapy or in combination with other antihypertensive agents, at doses ranging from 1 to 40 mg. Table 1 summarizes those adverse experiences reported for patients in these studies where the prevalence rate in the terazosin group was at least 5%, where the prevalence rate for the terazosin group was at least 2% and was greater than the prevalence rate for the placebo group, or where the reaction is of particular interest. Asthenia, blurred vision, dizziness, nasal congestion, nausea, peripheral edema, palpitations and somnolence were the only symptoms that were significantly (p < 0.05) more common in patients receiving terazosin than in patients receiving placebo. Similar adverse reaction rates were observed in placebo-controlled monotherapy trials.

TABLE 1
ADVERSE REACTIONS DURING
PLACEBO-CONTROLLED STUDIES

	Terazosin (N=859)	Placebo (N=506)
BODY AS A WHOLE		
†Asthenia	11.3%*	4.3%
Back Pain	2.4%	1.2%
Headache	16.2%	15.8%
CARDIOVASCULAR SYSTEM		
Palpitations	4.3%*	1.2%
Postural Hypotension	1.3%	0.4%
Tachycardia	1.9%	1.2%
DIGESTIVE SYSTEM		
Nausea	4.4%*	1.4%
METABOLIC/NUTRITIONAL DISORDERS		
Edema	0.9%	0.6%
Peripheral Edema	5.5%*	2.4%
Weight Gain	0.5%	0.2%
MUSCULOSKELETAL SYSTEM		
Pain-Extremities	3.5%	3.0%
NERVOUS SYSTEM		
Depression	0.3%	0.2%
Dizziness	19.3%*	7.5%
Libido Decreased	0.6%	0.2%
Nervousness	2.3%	1.8%
Paresthesia	2.9%	1.4%
Somnolence	5.4%*	2.6%
RESPIRATORY SYSTEM		
Dyspnea	3.1%	2.4%
Nasal Congestion	5.9%*	3.4%
Sinusitis	2.6%	1.4%
SPECIAL SENSES		
Blurred Vision	1.6%*	0.0%
UROGENITAL SYSTEM		
Impotence	1.2%	1.4%

† Includes weakness, tiredness, lassitude, and fatigue.
* Statistically significant at p=0.05 level.

The adverse reactions were usually mild or moderate in intensity but sometimes were serious enough to interrupt treatment. The adverse reactions that were most bothersome, as judged by their being reported as reasons for discon-

tinuation of therapy by at least 0.5% of the terazosin group and being reported more often than in the placebo group are shown in Table 2.

TABLE 2
DISCONTINUATIONS DURING
PLACEBO-CONTROLLED STUDIES

	Terazosin (N=859)	Placebo (N=506)
BODY AS A WHOLE		
Asthenia	1.6%	0.0%
Headache	1.3%	1.0%
CARDIOVASCULAR SYSTEM		
Palpitations	1.4%	0.2%
Postural Hypotension	0.5%	0.0%
Syncope	0.5%	0.2%
Tachycardia	0.6%	0.0%
DIGESTIVE SYSTEM		
Nausea	0.8%	0.0%
METABOLIC/NUTRITIONAL DISORDERS		
Peripheral Edema	0.6%	0.0%
NERVOUS SYSTEM		
Dizziness	3.1%	0.4%
Paresthesia	0.8%	0.2%
Somnolence	0.6%	0.2%
RESPIRATORY SYSTEM		
Dyspnea	0.9%	0.6%
Nasal Congestion	0.6%	0.0%
SPECIAL SENSES		
Blurred Vision	0.6%	0.0%

Additional adverse reactions have been reported, but these are, in general, not distinguishable from symptoms that might have occurred in the absence of exposure to terazosin. The following additional adverse reactions were reported by at least 1% of 1987 patients who received terazosin in controlled or open, short- or long-term clinical studies or have been reported during marketing experience: *Body as a Whole:* chest pain, facial edema, fever, abdominal pain, neck pain, shoulder pain; *Cardiovascular System:* arrhythmia, vasodilation; *Digestive System:* constipation, diarrhea, dry mouth, dyspepsia, flatulence, vomiting; *Metabolic/Nutritional Disorders:* gout; *Musculoskeletal System:* arthralgia, arthritis, joint disorder, myalgia; *Nervous System:* anxiety, insomnia; *Respiratory System:* bronchitis, cold symptoms, epistaxis, flu symptoms, increased cough, pharyngitis, rhinitis; *Skin and Appendages:* pruritus, rash, sweating; *Special Senses:* abnormal vision, conjunctivitis, tinnitus; *Urogenital System:* urinary frequency, urinary incontinence primarily reported in postmenopausal women, urinary tract infection.

OVERDOSAGE

Should overdosage of HYTRIN lead to hypotension, support of the cardiovascular system is of first importance. Restoration of blood pressure and normalization of heart rate may be accomplished by keeping the patient in the supine position. If this measure is inadequate, shock should first be treated with volume expanders. If necessary, vasopressors should then be used and renal function should be monitored and supported as needed. Laboratory data indicate that HYTRIN is highly protein bound; therefore, dialysis may not be of benefit.

DOSAGE AND ADMINISTRATION

The dose of HYTRIN and the dose interval (12 or 24 hours) should be adjusted according to the patient's individual blood pressure response. The following is a guide to its administration:

Initial Dose:

1 mg at bedtime is the starting dose for all patients, and this dose should not be exceeded. This initial dosing regimen should be strictly observed to minimize the potential for severe hypotensive effects.

Subsequent Doses:

The dose may be slowly increased to achieve the desired blood pressure response. The usual recommended dose range is 1 mg to 5 mg administered once a day; however, some patients may benefit from doses as high as 20 mg per day. Doses over 20 mg do not appear to provide further blood pressure effect and doses over 40 mg have not been studied. Blood pressure should be monitored at the end of the dosing interval to be sure control is maintained throughout the interval. It may also be helpful to measure blood pressure 2–3 hours after dosing to see if the maximum and minimum responses are similar, and to evaluate symptoms such as dizziness or palpitations which can result from excessive hypotensive response. If response is substantially diminished at 24 hours an increased dose or use of a twice daily regimen can be considered. If terazosin administration is discontinued for several days or longer, therapy should be reinstituted using the initial dosing regimen. In clinical trials, except for the initial dose, the dose was given in the morning.

Use With Other Drugs:

Caution should be observed when terazosin is administered concomitantly with other antihypertensive agents (e.g., calcium antagonists) to avoid the possibility of significant hypotension. When adding a diuretic or other antihypertensive agent, dosage reduction and retitration may be necessary.

HOW SUPPLIED

HYTRIN tablets (terazosin hydrochloride tablets) are available in four dosage strengths:

1 mg, white:
Bottles of 100 ....(NDC 0074-3322-13)
Abbo-Pac® unit dose strip packages of
100 tablets ....(NDC 0074-3322-11).
2 mg, orange:
Bottles of 100 ....(NDC 0074-3323-13)
Abbo-Pac® unit dose strip packages of
100 tablets ....(NDC 0074-3323-11).
5 mg, tan:
Bottles of 100 ....(NDC 0074-3324-13)
Abbo-Pac® unit dose strip packages of
100 tablets ....(NDC 0074-3324-11).
10 mg, green:
Bottles of 100 ....(NDC 0074-3325-13)
Abbo-Pac® unit dose strip packages of
100 tablets ....(NDC 0074-3325-11)
Recommended storage: Store below 86°F (30°C).
Ref. 03-4401-R6

Shown in Product Identification Section, page 403

IBERET®-500 Filmtab® tablets OTC

[ĭ'be-ret]
IRON plus B-complex and Vitamin C
Well-tolerated once-daily hematinic with controlled-release iron.
IBERET® Filmtab® tablets
Hematinic Supplying Controlled-Release Iron, Vitamin C and Vitamin B-Complex

DESCRIPTION

Each Iberet-500 and Iberet Filmtab tablet contains 525 mg of ferrous sulfate (equivalent to 105 mg elemental iron) in the Gradumet® controlled-release vehicle. To enhance iron absorption, 500 mg of vitamin C has been added to each Iberet-500 Filmtab.
Each Iberet-500 Filmtab tablet contains:

Ferrous Sulfate..525 mg
(equivalent to 105 mg of elemental iron)
Vitamin C (as Sodium Ascorbate)................................500 mg
Niacinamide..30 mg
Calcium Pantothenate..10 mg
Vitamin B$_1$ (Thiamine Mononitrate).............................6 mg
Vitamin B$_2$ (Riboflavin)...6 mg
Vitamin B$_6$ (Pyridoxine Hydrochloride).......................5 mg
Vitamin B$_{12}$ (Cyanocobalamin)..............................25 mcg
The formulation of Iberet differs from Iberet-500 only in that it contains a lesser amount of vitamin C, 150 mg per Filmtab tablet.

Inactive Ingredients:

Iberet Filmtab: Castor oil, cellulosic polymers, corn starch, FD&C Red No. 40, FD&C Yellow No. 6, iron oxide, magnesium stearate, methyl acrylate-methyl methacrylate copolymer, polyethylene glycol, povidone, propylene glycol, stearic acid, talc, titanium dioxide and vanillin.
Iberet-500 Filmtab: Castor oil, cellulosic polymers, corn starch, FD&C Red No. 40, FD&C Yellow No. 6, magnesium stearate, methyl acrylate-methyl methacrylate copolymer, polyethylene glycol, povidone, propylene glycol, stearic acid, talc, titanium dioxide and vanillin.

INDICATIONS

Iberet-500: For the treatment of iron deficiency or iron deficiency anemia when there is also a deficient intake or increased need for B-complex vitamins. Iberet: For conditions in which iron deficiency and vitamin C deficiency occur concomitantly with deficient intake or increased need for the B-complex vitamins.

PRECAUTIONS

Like other oral iron preparations, Iberet-500 and Iberet should be stored out of the reach of children.

DOSAGE AND ADMINISTRATION

Iberet-500 and Iberet; Usual Adult Dose, including pregnant females: One tablet daily, or as directed by the physician.

HOW SUPPLIED

Iberet-500 is supplied as red, oval shaped tablets in bottles of 60 (NDC 0074-7235-01) and 500 (NDC 0074-7235-03), and in Abbo-Pac® unit dose packages of 100 (NDC 0074-7235-11); Iberet is supplied as red, round tablets in bottles of 60 (NDC 0074-6863-01). Keep tightly closed.

Recommended storage: Store below 77°F (25°C).
Ref. 03-1929-9/R25 and 03-1932-4/R32
Iberet-500 shown in Product Identification Section, page 403

IBERET–FOLIC–500® ℞

Controlled-Release Iron with Vitamin C, and B-Complex, including Folic Acid
Filmtab® Tablets

See combined listing under Fero-Folic-500.
Shown in Product Identification Section, page 403

IBERET®-500 LIQUID OTC

[ĭ'bĕ-rĕt]
Hematinic Supplying Iron, Vitamin C and Vitamin B-Complex
IBERET®-LIQUID
Hematinic Supplying Iron, Vitamin C and Vitamin B-Complex

DESCRIPTION

Iberet-500 Liquid and Iberet-Liquid are hematinic preparations of ferrous sulfate, B-complex vitamins and ascorbic acid. Each teaspoonful (5 ml) of Iberet-500 Liquid provides:
Elemental Iron (as Ferrous Sulfate) .... 26.25 mg
Vitamin C (Ascorbic Acid) .... 125 mg
Niacinamide .... 7.5 mg
Dexpanthenol .... 2.5 mg
VitaminB$_1$ (Thiamine Hydrochloride) .... 1.5 mg
Vitamin B$_2$ (Riboflavin) .... 1.5 mg
Vitamin B$_6$ (Pyridoxine Hydrochloride) .... 1.25 mg
Vitamin B$_{12}$ (Cyanocobalamin) .... 6.25 mcg
In a citrus-flavored vehicle.
Iberet-Liquid has a raspberry-mint flavored vehicle; Iberet-Liquid has a smaller amount of ascorbic acid: 37.5 mg per teaspoonful. Riboflavin 5' phosphate sodium is the source of riboflavin in Iberet Liquid.

INACTIVE INGREDIENTS

Iberet-Liquid: Alcohol 1%, methylparaben, propylparaben, sorbitol, water and natural and artificial flavors.
Iberet-500 Liquid: Glycerin, methylparaben, propylene glycol, propylparaben, sodium bicarbonate, sorbitol, sucrose, water and artificial flavor.

INDICATIONS

Iberet-500 Liquid: For conditions in which iron deficiency occurs concomitantly with deficient intake or increased need for the B-complex vitamins. Iberet-Liquid: For conditions in which iron deficiency and vitamin C deficiency occur concomitantly with deficient intake or increased need for the B-complex vitamins.

PRECAUTIONS

Iberet-500 Liquid and Iberet-Liquid should be stored out of the reach of children.

DOSAGE AND ADMINISTRATION

Iberet-500 Liquid: Usual dosage; Adults, including pregnant females and children 4 years of age and older—2 teaspoonfuls (10 ml) twice daily, after meals; Children 1–3 years of age—1 teaspoonful (5 ml) twice daily, after meals. Otherwise as directed by the physician. Iberet-Liquid: Usual dosage: Adults including pregnant females and children 4 years of age and older—2 teaspoonfuls (10 ml) three times daily, after meals; Children 1–3 years of age—1 teaspoonful (5 ml) three times daily, after meals. Otherwise as directed by the physician.

HOW SUPPLIED

Iberet-500 Liquid (NDC 0074-8422-02) and Iberet-Liquid (NDC 0074-7173-01) are supplied in 8 fl oz bottles. Protect from temperatures above 77°F (25°C). Dispense in amber bottle only.
Ref. 07-8120-4/R18 and 07-8119-4/R21

K–LOR™ Powder ℞

[k'lor]
(potassium chloride for oral solution, USP)

DESCRIPTION

Natural fruit-flavored K-Lor (potassium chloride for oral solution, USP) is an oral potassium supplement offered in individual packets as a powder for reconstitution. Each packet of K-Lor 20 mEq powder contains potassium 20 mEq and chloride 20 mEq provided by potassium chloride 1.5 g.

Continued on next page

If desired, additional literature on any Abbott product will be provided upon request to Abbott Laboratories.

Abbott Laboratories—Cont.

Each packet of K-Lor 15 mEq powder contains potassium 15 mEq and chloride 15 mEq provided by potassium chloride 1.125 g.

K-Lor powder is an electrolyte replenisher. The chemical name is potassium chloride, and the structural formula is KCl. Potassium chloride, USP, occurs as a white, granular powder or as colorless crystals. It is odorless and has a saline taste. Its solutions are neutral to litmus. It is freely soluble in water and insoluble in alcohol.

Inactive Ingredients: FD&C Yellow No. 6, maltodextrin (contains corn derivative), malic acid, saccharin, silica gel and natural flavoring.

CLINICAL PHARMACOLOGY

Potassium ion is the principal intracellular cation of most body tissues. Potassium ions participate in a number of essential physiological processes including the maintenance of intracellular tonicity, the transmission of nerve impulses, the contraction of cardiac, skeletal and smooth muscle, and the maintenance of normal renal function.

The intracellular concentration of potassium is approximately 150 to 160 mEq per liter. The normal adult plasma concentration is 3.5 to 5 mEq per liter. An active ion transport system maintains this gradient across the plasma membrane.

Potassium is a normal dietary constituent and under steady state conditions the amount of potassium absorbed from the gastrointestinal tract is equal to the amount excreted in the urine. The usual dietary intake of potassium is 50 to 100 mEq per day.

Potassium depletion will occur whenever the rate of potassium loss through renal excretion and/or loss from the gastrointestinal tract exceeds the rate of potassium intake. Such depletion usually develops as a consequence of therapy with diuretics, primary or secondary hyperaldosteronism, diabetic ketoacidosis, or inadequate replacement of potassium in patients on prolonged parenteral nutrition. Depletion can develop rapidly with severe diarrhea, especially if associated with vomiting. Potassium depletion due to these causes is usually accompanied by a concomitant loss of chloride and is manifested by hypokalemia and metabolic alkalosis. Potassium depletion may produce weakness, fatigue, disturbances of cardiac rhythm (primarily ectopic beats), prominent U-waves in the electrocardiogram, and, in advanced cases, flaccid paralysis and/or impaired ability to concentrate urine.

If potassium depletion associated with metabolic alkalosis cannot be managed by correcting the fundamental cause of the deficiency, e.g., where the patient requires long term diuretic therapy, supplemental potassium in the form of high potassium food or potassium chloride may restore normal potassium levels.

In rare circumstances, (e.g., patients with renal tubular acidosis) potassium depletion may be associated with metabolic acidosis and hyperchloremia. In such patients potassium replacement should be accomplished with potassium salts other than the chloride, such as potassium bicarbonate, potassium citrate, potassium acetate, or potassium gluconate.

INDICATIONS AND USAGE

1. For the treatment of patients with hypokalemia with or without metabolic alkalosis, in digitalis intoxication, and in patients with hypokalemic familial periodic paralysis. If hypokalemia is the result of diuretic therapy, consideration should be given to the use of a lower dose of diuretic, which may be sufficient without leading to hypokalemia.
2. For the prevention of hypokalemia in patients who would be at particular risk if hypokalemia were to develop, e.g., digitalized patients or patients with significant cardiac arrhythmias.

The use of potassium salts in patients receiving diuretics for uncomplicated essential hypertension is often unnecessary when such patients have a normal dietary pattern, and when low doses of the diuretic are used. Serum potassium should be checked periodically, however, and, if hypokalemia occurs, dietary supplementation with potassium-containing foods may be adequate to control milder cases. In more severe cases, and if dose adjustment of the diuretic is ineffective or unwarranted, supplementation with potassium salts may be indicated.

CONTRAINDICATIONS

Potassium supplements are contraindicated in patients with hyperkalemia since a further increase in serum potassium concentration in such patients can produce cardiac arrest. Hyperkalemia may complicate any of the following conditions: chronic renal failure, systemic acidosis such as diabetic acidosis, acute dehydration, extensive tissue breakdown as in severe burns, adrenal insufficiency, or the administration of a potassium-sparing diuretic, e.g., spironolactone, triamterene, or amiloride (see OVERDOSAGE).

K-Lor (potassium chloride for oral solution) is contraindicated in patients with known hypersensitivity to any ingredient in this product.

WARNINGS

Hyperkalemia: (See OVERDOSAGE): In patients with impaired mechanisms for excreting potassium, the administration of potassium salts can produce hyperkalemia and cardiac arrest. This occurs most commonly in patients given potassium intravenously, but may also occur in patients given potassium orally. Potentially fatal hyperkalemia can develop rapidly and can be asymptomatic. The use of potassium salts in patients with chronic renal disease, or any other condition which impairs potassium excretion, requires particularly careful monitoring of the serum potassium concentration and appropriate dosage adjustment.

Interaction with Potassium-Sparing Diuretics: Hypokalemia should not be treated by the concomitant administration of potassium salts and a potassium-sparing diuretic, e.g., spironolactone, triamterene or amiloride, since the simultaneous administration of these agents can produce severe hyperkalemia.

Interaction with Angiotensin Converting Enzyme Inhibitors: Angiotensin converting enzyme (ACE) inhibitors (e.g., captopril, enalapril) will produce some potassium retention by inhibiting aldosterone production. Potassium supplements should be given to patients receiving ACE inhibitors only with close monitoring.

Metabolic Acidosis: Hypokalemia in patients with metabolic acidosis should be treated with an alkalinizing potassium salt such as potassium bicarbonate, potassium citrate, potassium acetate or potassium gluconate.

PRECAUTIONS

General: The diagnosis of potassium depletion is ordinarily made by demonstrating hypokalemia in a patient with a clinical history suggesting some cause for potassium depletion. In interpreting the serum potassium level, the physician should bear in mind that acute alkalosis *per se* can produce hypokalemia in the absence of a deficit in total body potassium, while acute acidosis *per se* can increase the serum potassium concentration to within the normal range even in the presence of a reduced total body potassium. The treatment of potassium depletion, particularly in the presence of cardiac disease, renal disease, or acidosis, requires careful attention to acid-base balance and appropriate monitoring of serum electrolytes, the electrocardiogram, and the clinical status of the patient.

Information for Patients: Physicians should consider reminding the patient of the following:

To dilute each packet of powder in ½ glassful of water or other liquid and take each dose after a meal.

To take this medicine following the frequency and amount prescribed by the physician. This is especially important if the patient is also taking diuretics and/or digitalis preparations.

Laboratory Tests: When blood is drawn for analysis of plasma potassium it is important to recognize that artifactual elevations can occur after improper venipuncture technique or as a result of *in vitro* hemolysis of the sample.

Drug Interactions: Potassium-sparing diuretics, angiotensin converting enzyme inhibitors (see WARNINGS).

Carcinogenesis, Mutagenesis, Impairment of Fertility: Carcinogenicity, mutagenicity and fertility studies in animals have not been performed. Potassium is a normal dietary constituent.

Pregnancy Category C: Animal reproduction studies have not been conducted with K-Lor powder. It is unlikely that potassium supplementation that does not lead to hyperkalemia would have an adverse effect on the fetus or would affect reproductive capacity.

Nursing Mothers: The normal potassium ion content of human milk is about 13 mEq per liter. Since oral potassium becomes part of the body potassium pool, as long as body potassium is not excessive, the contribution of potassium chloride supplementation should have little or no effect on the level in human milk.

Pediatric Use: Safety and effectiveness in children have not been established.

ADVERSE REACTIONS

One of the most severe adverse effects is hyperkalemia (see CONTRAINDICATIONS, WARNINGS and OVERDOSAGE).

The most common adverse reactions to oral potassium salts are nausea, vomiting, flatulence, abdominal pain/discomfort, and diarrhea. These symptoms are due to irritation of the gastrointestinal tract and are best managed by diluting the preparation further, taking the dose with meals, or reducing the amount taken at one time.

Skin rash has been reported rarely.

OVERDOSAGE

The administration of oral potassium salts to persons with normal excretory mechanisms for potassium rarely causes serious hyperkalemia. However, if excretory mechanisms are impaired or if intravenous administration is too rapid, potentially fatal hyperkalemia can result (see CONTRAINDICATIONS and WARNINGS). It is important to recognize that hyperkalemia is usually asymptomatic and may be manifested only by an increased serum potassium concentra-

tion (6.5–8 mEq/L) and characteristic electrocardiographic changes (peaking of T-waves, loss of P-waves, depression of S-T segments, and prolongation of the QT intervals). Late manifestations include muscle paralysis and cardiovascular collapse from cardiac arrest (9–12 mEq/L).

Treatment measures for hyperkalemia include the following:

1. Elimination of foods and medications containing potassium and of any agents with potassium-sparing properties;
2. Intravenous administration of 300 to 500 ml/hr of 10% dextrose solution containing 10–20 units of crystalline insulin per 1,000 ml;
3. Correction of acidosis, if present, with intravenous sodium bicarbonate;
4. Use of exchange resins, hemodialysis, or peritoneal dialysis.

In treating hyperkalemia, it should be recalled that in patients who have been stabilized on digitalis, lowering the serum potassium concentration too rapidly can produce digitalis toxicity.

DOSAGE AND ADMINISTRATION

The usual dietary potassium intake by the average adult is 50 to 100 mEq per day. Potassium depletion sufficient to cause hypokalemia usually requires the loss of 200 or more mEq of potassium from the total body store.

Dosage must be adjusted to the individual needs of each patient. The dose for the prevention of hypokalemia is typically in the range of 20 mEq per day. Doses of 40–100 mEq per day or more are used for the treatment of potassium depletion. Dosage should be divided if more than 20 mEq per day is given such that no more than 20 mEq is given in a single dose. The dose should be taken after a meal.

K-Lor 20 mEq powder provides 20 mEq and K-Lor 15 mEq powder provides 15 mEq of potassium chloride.

Each 20 mEq (one K-Lor mEq packet) of potassium should be dissolved in at least 4 oz (approximately ½ glassful) cold water or juice. Each 15 mEq (One K-Lor 15 mEq packet) of potassium should be dissolved in at least 3 oz (approximately ½ glassful) cold water or juice. These preparations, like other potassium supplements, must be properly diluted to avoid the possibility of gastrointestinal irritation.

HOW SUPPLIED

K-Lor 20 mEq (potassium chloride for oral solution, USP) is supplied in cartons of 30 packets (NDC 0074-3611-01), and cartons of 100 packets (NDC 0074-3611-02). Each packet contains potassium, 20 mEq, and chloride, 20 mEq, provided by potassium chloride, 1.5 g.

K-Lor 15 mEq (potassium chloride for oral solution, USP) is supplied in cartons of 100 packets (NDC 0074-3633-11). Each packet contains potassium, 15 mEq, and chloride, 15 mEq, provided by potassium chloride, 1.125 g.

Recommended storage: Store below 86°F (30°C).

Caution: Federal law prohibits dispensing without prescription.

TM—Trademark

Ref. 09-6691-5/R24

Shown in Product Identification Section, page 403

K•Tab®   ℞

[k 'tăb]

(Potassium Chloride Extended-Release Tablets, USP)

DESCRIPTION

K-TAB (potassium chloride extended-release tablets) is a solid oral dosage form of potassium chloride containing 750 mg of potassium chloride, USP, equivalent to 10 mEq of potassium in a film-coated (not enteric-coated), wax matrix tablet. This formulation is intended to slow the release of potassium so that the likelihood of a high localized concentration of potassium chloride within the gastrointestinal tract is reduced. The expended inert, porous, wax/polymer matrix is not absorbed and may be excreted intact in the stool.

K-TAB tablets are an electrolyte replenisher. The chemical name is potassium chloride, and the structural formula is KCl. Potassium chloride, USP, occurs as a white, granular powder or as colorless crystals. It is odorless and has a saline taste. Its solutions are neutral to litmus. It is freely soluble in water and insoluble in alcohol.

Inactive Ingredients

Castor oil, cellulosic polymers, colloidal silicon dioxide, D&C Yellow No. 10, magnesium stearate, paraffin, polyvinyl acetate, titanium dioxide, vanillin and vitamin E.

CLINICAL PHARMACOLOGY

Potassium ion is the principal intracellular cation of most body tissues. Potassium ions participate in a number of essential physiological processes including the maintenance of intracellular tonicity, the transmission of nerve impulses, the contraction of cardiac, skeletal, and smooth muscle, and the maintenance of normal renal function.

The intracellular concentration of potassium is approximately 150 to 160 mEq per liter. The normal adult plasma

concentration is 3.5 to 5 mEq per liter. An active ion transport system maintains this gradient across the plasma membrane.

Potassium is a normal dietary constituent and under steady state conditions the amount of potassium absorbed from the gastrointestinal tract is equal to the amount excreted in the urine. The usual dietary intake of potassium is 50 to 100 mEq per day.

Potassium depletion will occur whenever the rate of potassium loss through renal excretion and/or loss from the gastrointestinal tract exceeds the rate of potassium intake. Such depletion usually develops as a consequence of therapy with diuretics, primary or secondary hyperaldosteronism, diabetic ketoacidosis, or inadequate replacement of potassium in patients on prolonged parenteral nutrition. Depletion can develop rapidly with severe diarrhea, expecially if associated with vomiting. Potassium depletion due to these causes is usually accompanied by a concomitant loss of chloride and is manifested by hypokalemia and metabolic alkalosis. Potassium depletion may produce weakness, fatigue, disturbances of cardiac rhythm (primarily ectopic beats), prominent U-waves in the electrocardiogram, and in advanced cases, flaccid paralysis and/or impaired ability to concentrate urine.

If potassium depletion associated with metabolic alkalosis cannot be managed by correcting the fundamental causes of the deficiency, e.g., where the patient requires long term diuretic therapy, supplemental potassium in the form of high potassium food or potassium chloride may restore normal levels.

In rare circumstances, (e.g., patients with renal tubular acidosis) potassium depletion may be associated with metabolic acidosis and hyperchloremia. In such patients potassium replacement should be accomplished with potassium salts other than the chloride, such as potassium bicarbonate, potassium citrate, potassium acetate, or potassium gluconate.

INDICATIONS AND USAGE

BECAUSE OF REPORTS OF INTESTINAL AND GASTRIC ULCERATION AND BLEEDING WITH CONTROLLED-RELEASE POTASSIUM CHLORIDE PREPARATIONS, THESE DRUGS SHOULD BE RESERVED FOR THOSE PATIENTS WHO CANNOT TOLERATE OR REFUSE TO TAKE LIQUID OR EFFERVESCENT POTASSIUM PREPARATIONS, OR FOR PATIENTS WITH WHOM THERE IS A PROBLEM OF COMPLIANCE WITH THESE PREPARATIONS.

1. For the treatment of patients with hypokalemia with or without metabolic alkalosis, in digitalis intoxication, and in patients with hypokalemic familial periodic paralysis. If hypokalemia is the result of diuretic therapy, consideration should be given to the use of a lower dose of diuretic, which may be sufficient without leading to hypokalemia.
2. For the prevention of hypokalemia in patients who would be at particular risk if hypokalemia were to develop, e.g., digitalized patients or patients with significant cardiac arrhythmias.

The use of potassium salts in patients receiving diuretics for uncomplicated essential hypertension is often unnecessary when such patients have a normal dietary pattern, and when low doses of the diuretic are used. Serum potassium should be checked periodically, however, and, if hypokalemia occurs, dietary supplementation with potassium-containing foods may be adequate to control milder cases. In more severe cases, and if dose adjustment of the diuretic is ineffective or unwarranted, supplementation with potassium salts may be indicated.

CONTRAINDICATIONS

Potassium supplements are contraindicated in patients with hyperkalemia since a further increase in serum potassium concentration in such patients can produce cardiac arrest. Hyperkalemia may complicate any of the following conditions: chronic renal failure, systemic acidosis such as diabetic acidosis, acute dehydration, extensive tissue breakdown as in severe burns, adrenal insufficiency, or the administration of potassium-sparing diuretic, e.g., spironolactone, triamterene, or amiloride, (see OVERDOSAGE).

K-TAB tablets are contraindicated in patients with known hypersensitivity to any ingredient in this product.

Controlled-release formulations of potassium chloride have produced esophageal ulceration in certain cardiac patients with esophageal compression due to an enlarged left atrium. Potassium supplementation, when indicated in such patients, should be given as a liquid preparation.

All solid dosage forms of potassium supplements are contraindicated in any patient in whom there is structural, pathological, e.g., diabetic gastroparesis, or pharmacologic (use of anticholinergic agents or other agents with anticholinergic properties at sufficient doses to exert anticholinergic effects) cause for arrest or delay in tablet passage through the gastrointestinal tract.

WARNINGS

Hyperkalemia (see OVERDOSAGE)

In patients with impaired mechanisms for excreting potassium, the administration of potassium salts can produce hyperkalemia and cardiac arrest. This occurs most commonly in patients given potassium intravenously, but may also occur in patients given potassium orally. Potentially fatal hyperkalemia can develop rapidly and can be asymptomatic. The use of potassium salts in patients with chronic renal disease, or any other condition which impairs potassium excretion, requires particularly careful monitoring of the serum potassium concentration and appropriate dosage adjustment.

Interaction with Potassium-Sparing Diuretics

Hypokalemia should not be treated by the concomitant administration of potassium salts and a potassium-sparing diuretic e.g., spironolactone, triamterene, or amiloride, since the simultaneous administration of these agents can produce severe hyperkalemia.

Interaction with Angiotensin Converting Enzyme Inhibitors

Angiotensin converting enzyme (ACE) inhibitors (e.g., captopril, enalapril) will produce some potassium retention by inhibiting aldosterone production. Potassium supplements should be given to patients receiving ACE inhibitors only with close monitoring.

Gastrointestinal Lesions

Solid oral dosage forms of potassium chloride can produce ulcerative and/or stenotic lesions of the gastrointestinal tract. Based on spontaneous adverse reaction reports, enteric-coated preparations of potassium chloride are associated with an increased frequency of small bowel lesions (40-50 per 100,000 patient years) compared to sustained-release wax matrix formulations (less than one per 100,000 patient years). Because of the lack of extensive marketing experience with microencapsulated products, a comparison between such products and wax matrix or enteric-coated products is not available. K-TAB tablets consist of a wax matrix formulated to provide a controlled rate of release of potassium chloride and thus to minimize the possibility of a high local concentration of potassium near the gastrointestinal wall.

Prospective trials have been conducted in normal human volunteers in which the upper gastrointestinal tract was evaluated by endoscopic inspection before and after one week of solid oral potassium chloride therapy. The ability of this model to predict events occuring in usual clinical practice is unknown. Trials which approximated usual clinical practice did not reveal any clear differences between the wax matrix and microencapsulated dosage forms. In contrast, there was a higher incidence of gastric and duodenal lesions in subjects receiving a high dose of a wax matrix controlled-release formulation under conditions which did not resemble usual or recommended clinical practice, i.e., 96 mEq per day in divided doses of potassium chloride administered to fasted patients in the presence of an anticholinergic drug to delay gastric emptying. The upper gastrointestinal lesions observed by endoscopy were asymptomatic and were not accompanied by evidence of bleeding (hemoccult testing). The relevance of these findings to the usual conditions, i.e., non-fasting, no anticholinergic agent, and smaller doses, under which controlled-release potassium chloride products are used is uncertain. Epidemiologic studies have not identified an elevated risk, compared to microencapsulated products, for upper gastrointestinal lesions in patients receiving wax matrix formulations. K-TAB tablets should be discontinued immediately and the possibility of ulceration, obstruction or perforation considered if severe vomiting, abdominal pain, distention, or gastrointestinal bleeding occurs.

Metabolic Acidosis

Hypokalemia in patients with metabolic acidosis should be treated with an alkalinizing potassium salt such as potassium bicarbonate, potassium citrate, potassium acetate, or potassium gluconate.

PRECAUTIONS

General: The diagnosis of potassium depletion is ordinarily made by demonstrating hypokalemia in a patient with a clinical history suggesting some cause for potassium depletion. In interpreting the serum potassium level, the physician should bear in mind that acute alkalosis *per se* can produce hypokalemia in the absence of a deficit in total body potassium, while acute acidosis *per se* can increase the serum potassium concentration to within the normal range even in the presence of a reduced total body potassium. The treatment of potassium depletion, particularly in the presence of cardiac disease, renal disease, or acidosis, requires careful attention to acid-base balance and appropriate monitoring of serum electrolytes, the electrocardiogram, and the clinical status of the patient.

Information for Patients: Physicians should consider reminding the patient of the following:

To take each dose with meals and with a full glass of water or other liquid.

To take this medicine following the frequency and amount prescribed by the physician. This is especially important if the patient is also taking diuretics and/or digitalis preparations.

To check with the physician if there is trouble swallowing tablets or if the tablets seem to stick in the throat.

To check with the physician at once if tarry stools or other evidence of gastrointestinal bleeding is noticed.

To take each dose without crushing, chewing or sucking the tablets.

Laboratory Tests: When blood is drawn for analysis of plasma potassium it is important to recognize that artifactual elevations can occur after improper venipuncture technique or as a result of *in vitro* hemolysis of the sample.

Drug Interactions: Potassium-sparing diuretics, angiotensin converting enzyme inhibitors (see WARNINGS).

Carcinogenesis, Mutagenesis, Impairment of Fertility: Carcinogenicity, mutagenicity and fertility studies in animals have not been performed. Potassium is a normal dietary constituent.

Pregnancy Category C: Animal reproduction studies have not been conducted with K-TAB tablets. It is unlikely that potassium supplementation that does not lead to hyperkalemia would have an adverse effect on the fetus or would affect reproductive capacity.

Nursing Mothers: The normal potassium ion content of human milk is about 13 mEq per liter. Since oral potassium becomes part of the body potassium pool, as long as body potassium is not excessive, the contribution of potassium chloride supplementation should have little or no effect on the level in human milk.

Pediatric Use: Safety and effectiveness in children have not been established.

ADVERSE REACTIONS

One of the most severe adverse effects is hyperkalemia (see CONTRAINDICATIONS, WARNINGS, and OVERDOSAGE). There also have been reports of upper and lower gastrointestinal conditions including obstruction, bleeding, ulceration, and perforation (see CONTRAINDICATIONS and WARNINGS).

The most common adverse reactions to oral potassium salts are nausea, vomiting, flatulence, abdominal pain/discomfort, and diarrhea. These symptoms are due to irritation of the gastrointestinal tract and are best managed by taking the dose with meals, or reducing the amount taken at one time.

Skin rash has been reported rarely.

OVERDOSAGE

The administration of oral potassium salts to persons with normal excretory mechanisms for potassium rarely causes serious hyperkalemia. However, if excretory mechanisms are impaired or if intravenous administration is too rapid, potentially fatal hyperkalemia can result (see CONTRAINDICATIONS and WARNINGS). It is important to recognize that hyperkalemia is usually asymptomatic and may be manifested only by an increased serum potassium concentration (6.5-8.0 mEq/L) and characteristic electrocardiographic changes (peaking of T-waves, loss of P-waves, depression of S-T segments, and prolongation of QT intervals). Late manifestations include muscle paralysis and cardiovascular collapse from cardiac arrest. (9-12 mEq/L).

Treatment measures for hyperkalemia include the following:

1. Elimination of foods and medications containing potassium and of any agents with potassium-sparing properties;
2. Intravenous administration of 300 to 500 mL/hr of 10% dextrose solution containing 10-20 units of crystalline insulin per 1,000 mL;
3. Correction of acidosis, if present, with intravenous sodium bicarbonate;
4. Use of exchange resins, hemodialysis, or peritoneal dialysis.

In treating hyperkalemia, it should be recalled that in patients who have been stabilized on digitalis, lowering the serum potassium concentration too rapidly can produce digitalis toxicity.

DOSAGE AND ADMINISTRATION

The usual dietary potassium intake by the average adult is 50 to 100 mEq per day. Potassium depletion sufficient to cause hypokalemia usually requires the loss of 200 or more mEq of potassium from the total body store.

Dosage must be adjusted to the individual needs of each patient.The dose for the prevention of hypokalemia is typically in the range of 20 mEq per day. Doses of 40-100 mEq per day or more are used for the treatment of potassium depletion. Dosage should be divided if more than 20 mEq per day is given such that no more than 20 mEq is given in a single dose.

K-TAB tablets provide 10 mEq of potassium chloride.

K-TAB tablets should be taken with meals and with a glass of water or other liquid. This product should not be taken on an empty stomach because of its potential for gastric irritation (see WARNINGS).

Continued on next page

Abbott Laboratories—Cont.

NOTE: K-TAB tablets are to be swallowed whole without crushing, chewing or sucking the tablets.

HOW SUPPLIED

K-TAB (potassium chloride extended-release tablets, USP) contains 750 mg of potassium chloride (equivalent to 10 mEq). K-TAB tablets are provided as yellow, ovaloid, extended-release Filmtab® tablets in bottles of 100 (**NDC** 0074-7804-13), 1000 (**NDC** 0074-7804-19) and 5000 (**NDC** 0074-7804-59) and in ABBO-PAC® unit dose packages of 100 (**NDC** 0074-7804-11).

Recommended Storage: Store below 86°F (30°C).

Filmtab—Film-sealed tablets, Abbott
Ref. 03-4415-R14

Shown in Product Identification Section, page 403

NEMBUTAL® SODIUM CAPSULES ℞ Ⓒ

[*nĕm-bū-tal sō-dī-um*]
(pentobarbital sodium capsules, USP)

WARNING: MAY BE HABIT FORMING

DESCRIPTION

The barbiturates are nonselective central nervous system depressants which are primarily used as sedative hypnotics. The barbiturates and their sodium salts are subject to control under the Federal Controlled Substances Act (See "Drug Abuse and Dependence" section).

Barbiturates are substituted pyrimidine derivatives in which the basic structure common to these drugs is barbituric acid, a substance which has no central nervous system (CNS) activity. CNS activity is obtained by substituting alkyl, alkenyl, or aryl groups on the pyrimidine ring. Nembutal (pentobarbital sodium) is chemically represented by sodium 5-ethyl-5-(1-methylbutyl) barbiturate.

The sodium salt of pentobarbital occurs as a white, slightly bitter powder which is freely soluble in water and alcohol but practically insoluble in benzene and ether. Nembutal Sodium capsules for oral administration contain either 50 mg or 100 mg of pentobarbital sodium.

Inactive Ingredients: 50 mg Capsule: FD&C Blue No. 1, FD&C Red No. 3, FD&C Yellow No. 6, gelatin, lactose, magnesium stearate, polacrilin potassium and potassium chloride.

100 mg Capsule: colloidal silicon dioxide, corn starch, FD&C Blue No. 1, FD&C Red No. 3, FD&C Yellow No. 5 (tartrazine), FD&C Yellow No. 6, gelatin, magnesium stearate and potassium chloride.

CLINICAL PHARMACOLOGY

Barbiturates are capable of producing all levels of CNS mood alteration from excitation to mild sedation, to hypnosis, and deep coma. Overdosage can produce death. In high enough therapeutic doses, barbiturates induce anesthesia.

Barbiturates depress the sensory cortex, decrease motor activity, alter cerebellar function, and produce drowsiness, sedation, and hypnosis.

Barbiturate-induced sleep differs from physiological sleep. Sleep laboratory studies have demonstrated that barbiturates reduce the amount of time spent in the rapid eye movement (REM) phase of sleep or dreaming stage. Also, Stages III and IV sleep are decreased. Following abrupt cessation of barbiturates used regularly, patients may experience markedly increased dreaming, nightmares, and/or insomnia. Therefore, withdrawal of a single therapeutic dose over 5 or 6 days has been recommended to lessen the REM rebound and disturbed sleep which contribute to drug withdrawal syndrome (for example, decrease the dose from 3 to 2 doses a day for 1 week).

In studies, secobarbital sodium and pentobarbital sodium have been found to lose most of their effectiveness for both inducing and maintaining sleep by the end of 2 weeks of continued drug administration at fixed doses. The short-, intermediate-, and, to a lesser degree, long-acting barbiturates have been widely prescribed for treating insomnia. Although the clinical literature abounds with claims that the short-acting barbiturates are superior for producing sleep while the intermediate-acting compounds are more effective in maintaining sleep, controlled studies have failed to demonstrate these differential effects. Therefore, as sleep medications, the barbiturates are of limited value beyond short-term use.

Barbiturates have little analgesic action at subanesthetic doses. Rather, in subanesthetic doses these drugs may increase the reaction to painful stimuli. All barbiturates exhibit anticonvulsant activity in anesthetic doses. However, of the drugs in this class, only phenobarbital, mephobarbital, and metharbital have been clinically demonstrated to be effective as oral anticonvulsants in subhypnotic doses.

Barbiturates are respiratory depressants. The degree of respiratory depression is dependent upon dose. With hypnotic doses, respiratory depression produced by barbiturates is similar to that which occurs during physiologic sleep with slight decrease in blood pressure and heart rate.

Studies in laboratory animals have shown that barbiturates cause reduction in the tone and contractility of the uterus, ureters, and urinary bladder. However, concentrations of the drugs required to produce this effect in humans are not reached with sedative-hypnotic doses.

Barbiturates do not impair normal hepatic function, but have been shown to induce liver microsomal enzymes, thus increasing and/or altering the metabolism of barbiturates and other drugs. (See "Precautions—*Drug Interactions*" section).

Pharmacokinetics: Barbiturates are absorbed in varying degrees following oral, rectal, or parenteral administration. The salts are more rapidly absorbed than are the acids. The rate of absorption is increased if the sodium salt is ingested as a dilute solution or taken on an empty stomach.

The onset of action for oral or rectal administration varies from 20 to 60 minutes.

Duration of action, which is related to the rate at which the barbiturates are redistributed throughout the body, varies among persons and in the same person from time to time. In Table 1, the barbiturates are classified according to their duration of action. This classification should not be used to predict the exact duration of effect, but the grouping of drugs should be used as a guide in the selection of barbiturates.

No studies have demonstrated that the different routes of administration are equivalent with respect to bioavailability.

[See Table 1 below.]

Barbiturates are weak acids that are absorbed and rapidly distributed to all tissues and fluids with high concentrations in the brain, liver, and kidneys. Lipid solubility of the barbiturates is the dominant factor in their distribution within the body. The more lipid soluble the barbiturate, the more rapidly it penetrates all tissues of the body. Barbiturates are bound to plasma and tissue proteins to a varying degree with the degree of binding increasing directly as a function of lipid solubility.

Phenobarbital has the lowest lipid solubility, lowest plasma binding, lowest brain protein binding, the longest delay in onset of activity, and the longest duration of action. At the opposite extreme is secobarbital which has the highest lipid solubility, plasma protein binding, brain protein binding, the shortest delay in onset of activity, and the shortest duration of action. Butabarbital is classified as an intermediate barbiturate.

The plasma half-life for pentobarbital in adults is 15 to 50 hours and appears to be dose dependent.

Barbiturates are metabolized primarily by the hepatic microsomal enzyme system, and the metabolic products are excreted in the urine, and less commonly, in the feces. Approximately 25 to 50 percent of a dose of aprobarbital or phenobarbital is eliminated unchanged in the urine, whereas the amount of other barbiturates excreted unchanged in the urine is negligible. The excretion of unmetabolized barbiturate is one feature that distinguishes the long-acting category from those belonging to other categories which are almost entirely metabolized. The inactive metabolites of the barbiturates are excreted as conjugates of glucuronic acid.

INDICATIONS AND USAGE

Oral:

a. Sedatives.
b. Hypnotics, for the short-term treatment of insomnia, since they appear to lose their effectiveness for sleep induction and sleep maintenance after 2 weeks (See "Clinical Pharmacology" section).
c. Preanesthetics.

Table 1.—*Classification, Onset, and Duration of Action of Commonly used Barbiturates Taken Orally*

Classification	Onset of action	Duration of action
Long-acting Phenobarbital.	1 hour or longer	10 to 12 hours
Intermediate Amobarbital Butabarbital.	¾ to 1 hour	6 to 8 hours
Short-acting Pentobarbital Secobarbital.	10 to 15 minutes	3 to 4 hours

CONTRAINDICATIONS

Barbiturates are contraindicated in patients with known barbiturate sensitivity. Barbiturates are also contraindicated in patients with a history of manifest or latent porphyria.

WARNINGS

1. *Habit forming:* Barbiturates may be habit forming. Tolerance, psychological and physical dependence may occur with continued use. (See "Drug Abuse and Dependence" and "Pharmacokinetics" sections). Patients who have psychological dependence on barbiturates may increase the dosage or decrease the dosage interval without consulting a physician and may subsequently develop a physical dependence on barbiturates. To minimize the possibility of overdosage or the development of dependence, the prescribing and dispensing of sedative-hypnotic barbiturates should be limited to the amount required for the interval until the next appointment. Abrupt cessation after prolonged use in the dependent person may result in withdrawal symptoms, including delirium, convulsions, and possibly death. Barbiturates should be withdrawn gradually from any patient known to be taking excessive dosage over long periods of time. (See "Drug Abuse and Dependence" section).
2. *Acute or chronic pain:* Caution should be exercised when barbiturates are administered to patients with acute or chronic pain, because paradoxical excitement could be induced or important symptoms could be masked. However, the use of barbiturates as sedatives in the postoperative surgical period and as adjuncts to cancer chemotherapy is well established.
3. *Use in pregnancy:* Barbiturates can cause fetal damage when administered to a pregnant woman. Retrospective, case-controlled studies have suggested a connection between the maternal consumption of barbiturates and a higher than expected incidence of fetal abnormalities. Following oral or parenteral administration, barbiturates readily cross the placental barrier and are distributed throughout fetal tissues with highest concentrations found in the placenta, fetal liver, and brain.
   Withdrawal symptoms occur in infants born to mothers who receive barbiturates throughout the last trimester of pregnancy. (See "Drug Abuse and Dependence" section). If this drug is used during pregnancy, or if the patient becomes pregnant while taking this drug, the patient should be apprised of the potential hazard to the fetus.
4. *Synergistic effects:* The concomitant use of alcohol or other CNS depressants may produce additive CNS depressant effects.

PRECAUTIONS

General: Barbiturates may be habit forming. Tolerance and psychological and physical dependence may occur with continuing use. (See "Drug Abuse and Dependence" section). Barbiturates should be administered with caution, if at all, to patients who are mentally depressed, have suicidal tendencies, or a history of drug abuse.

Elderly or debilitated patients may react to barbiturates with marked excitement, depression, and confusion. In some persons, barbiturates repeatedly produce excitement rather than depression.

In patients with hepatic damage, barbiturates should be administered with caution and initially in reduced doses. Barbiturates should not be administered to patients showing the premonitory signs of hepatic coma.

The 100 mg dosage strength of Nembutal Sodium capsules contains FD&C Yellow No. 5 (tartrazine) which may cause allergic-type reactions (including bronchial asthma) in certain susceptible individuals. Although the overall incidence of FD&C Yellow No. 5 (tartrazine) sensitivity in the general population is low, it is frequently seen in patients who also have aspirin hypersensitivity.

Information for the patient: Practitioners should give the following information and instructions to patients receiving barbiturates.

1. The use of barbiturates carries with it an associated risk of psychological and/or physical dependence. The patient should be warned against increasing the dose of the drug without consulting a physician.
2. Barbiturates may impair mental and/or physical abilities required for the performance of potentially hazardous tasks (e.g., driving, operating machinery, etc.).
3. Alcohol should not be consumed while taking barbiturates. Concurrent use of the barbiturates with other CNS depressants (e.g., alcohol, narcotics, tranquilizers, and antihistamines) may result in additional CNS depressant effects.

Laboratory tests: Prolonged therapy with barbiturates should be accompanied by periodic laboratory evaluation of organ systems, including hematopoietic, renal, and hepatic systems. (See "Precautions—*General*" and "Adverse Reactions" sections).

Drug interactions: Most reports of clinically significant drug interactions occurring with the barbiturates have involved phenobarbital. However, the application of these data

to other barbiturates appears valid and warrants serial blood level determinations of the relevant drugs when there are multiple therapies.

1. *Anticoagulants:* Phenobarbital lowers the plasma levels of dicumarol (name previously used: bishydroxycoumarin) and causes a decrease in anticoagulant activity as measured by the prothrombin time. Barbiturates can induce hepatic microsomal enzymes resulting in increased metabolism and decreased anticoagulant response of oral anticoagulants (e.g., warfarin, acenocoumarol, dicumarol, and phenprocoumon). Patients stabilized on anticoagulant therapy may require dosage adjustments if barbiturates are added to or withdrawn from their dosage regimen.

2. *Corticosteroids:* Barbiturates appear to enhance the metabolism of exogenous corticosteroids probably through the induction of hepatic microsomal enzymes. Patients stabilized on corticosteroid therapy may require dosage adjustments if barbiturates are added to or withdrawn from their dosage regimen.

3. *Griseofulvin:* Phenobarbital appears to interfere with the absorption of orally administered griseofulvin, thus decreasing its blood level. The effect of the resultant decreased blood levels of griseofulvin on therapeutic response has not been established. However, it would be preferable to avoid concomitant administration of these drugs.

4. *Doxycycline:* Phenobarbital has been shown to shorten the half-life of doxycycline for as long as 2 weeks after barbiturate therapy is discontinued.
This mechanism is probably through the induction of hepatic microsomal enzymes that metabolize the antibiotic. If phenobarbital and doxycycline are administered concurrently, the clinical response to doxycycline should be monitored closely.

5. *Phenytoin, sodium valproate, valproic acid:* The effect of barbiturates on the metabolism of phenytoin appears to be variable. Some investigators report an accelerating effect, while others report no effect. Because the effect of barbiturates on the metabolism of phenytoin is not predictable, phenytoin and barbiturate blood levels should be monitored more frequently if these drugs are given concurrently. Sodium valproate and valproic acid appear to decrease barbiturate metabolism; therefore, barbiturate blood levels should be monitored and appropriate dosage adjustments made as indicated.

6. *Central nervous system depressants:* The concomitant use of other central nervous system depressants including other sedatives or hypnotics, antihistamines, tranquilizers, or alcohol, may produce additive depressant effects.

7. *Monoamine oxidase inhibitors (MAOI):* MAOI prolong the effects of barbiturates probably because metabolism of the barbiturate is inhibited.

8. *Estradiol, estrone, progesterone and other steroidal hormones:* Pretreatment with or concurrent administration of phenobarbital may decrease the effect of estradiol by increasing its metabolism. There have been reports of patients treated with antiepileptic drugs (e.g., phenobarbital) who became pregnant while taking oral contraceptives. An alternate contraceptive method might be suggested to women taking phenobarbital.

Carcinogenesis: 1. Animal data. Phenobarbital sodium is carcinogenic in mice and rats after lifetime administration. In mice, it produced benign and malignant liver cell tumors. In rats, benign liver cell tumors were observed very late in life.

2. Human Data. In a 29-year epidemiological study of 9,136 patients who were treated on an anticonvulsant protocol that included phenobarbital, results indicated a higher than normal incidence of hepatic carcinoma. Previously, some of these patients were treated with thorotrast, a drug that is known to produce hepatic carcinomas. Thus, this study did not provide sufficient evidence that phenobarbital sodium is carcinogenic in humans.

Data from one retrospective study of 235 children in which the types of barbiturates are not identified suggested an association between exposure to barbiturates prenatally and an increased incidence of brain tumor. (Gold, E., et al., "Increased Risk of Brain Tumors in Children Exposed to Barbiturates," Journal of National Cancer Institute, 61:1031–1034, 1978).

Pregnancy: 1. *Teratogenic effects.* Pregnancy Category D—See "Warnings—Use in Pregnancy" section.

2. *Nonteratogenic effects.* Reports of infants suffering from long-term barbiturate exposure in utero included the acute withdrawal syndrome of seizures and hyperirritability from birth to a delayed onset of up to 14 days. (See "Drug Abuse and Dependence" section).

Labor and delivery: Hypnotic doses of these barbiturates do not appear to significantly impair uterine activity during labor. Full anesthetic doses of barbiturates decrease the force and frequency of uterine contractions. Administration of sedative-hypnotic barbiturates to the mother during labor may result in respiratory depression in the newborn. Premature infants are particularly susceptible to the depressant effects of barbiturates. If barbiturates are used during labor and delivery, resuscitation equipment should be available.

Table 2.—*Concentration of Barbiturate in the Blood Versus Degree of CNS Depression*
Blood barbiturate level in ppm (μg/ml)

Barbiturate	Onset/ duration	Degree of depression in nontolerant persons*				
		1	2	3	4	5
Pentobarbital	Fast/short	≤2	0.5 to 3	10 to 15	12 to 25	15 to 40
Secobarbital	Fast/short	≤2	0.5 to 5	10 to 15	15 to 25	15 to 40
Amobarbital	Intermediate/ intermediate	≤3	2 to 10	30 to 40	30 to 60	40 to 80
Butabarbital	Intermediate/ intermediate	≤5	3 to 25	40 to 60	50 to 80	60 to 100
Phenobarbital	Slow/long	≤10	5 to 40	50 to 80	70 to 120	100 to 200

* Categories of degree of depression in nontolerant persons.
1. Under the influence and appreciably impaired for purposes of driving a motor vehicle or performing tasks requiring alertness and unimpaired judgment and reaction time.
2. Sedated, therapeutic range, calm, relaxed, and easily aroused.
3. Comatose, difficult to arouse, significant depression of respiration.
4. Compatible with death in aged or ill persons or in presence of obstructed airway, other toxic agents, or exposure to cold.
5. Usual lethal level, the upper end of the range includes those who received some supportive treatment.

Data are currently not available to evaluate the effect of these barbiturates when forceps delivery or other intervention is necessary. Also, data are not available to determine the effect of these barbiturates on the later growth, development, and functional maturation of the child.

Nursing mothers: Caution should be exercised when a barbiturate is administered to a nursing woman since small amounts of barbiturates are excreted in the milk.

ADVERSE REACTIONS

The following adverse reactions and their incidence were compiled from surveillance of thousands of hospitalized patients. Because such patients may be less aware of certain of the milder adverse effects of barbiturates, the incidence of these reactions may be somewhat higher in fully ambulatory patients.

More than 1 in 100 patients. The most common adverse reaction estimated to occur at a rate of 1 to 3 patients per 100 is:
Nervous System: Somnolence.
Less than 1 in 100 patients. Adverse reactions estimated to occur at a rate of less than 1 in 100 patients listed below, grouped by organ system, and by decreasing order of occurrence are:
Nervous system: Agitation, confusion, hyperkinesia, ataxia, CNS depression, nightmares, nervousness, psychiatric disturbance, hallucinations, insomnia, anxiety, dizziness, thinking abnormality.
Respiratory system: Hypoventilation, apnea.
Cardiovascular system: Bradycardia, hypotension, syncope.
Digestive system: Nausea, vomiting, constipation.
Other reported reactions: Headache, injection site reactions, hypersensitivity reactions (angioedema, skin rashes, exfoliative dermatitis), fever, liver damage, megaloblastic anemia following chronic phenobarbital use.

DRUG ABUSE AND DEPENDENCE

Pentobarbital sodium capsules are subject to control by the Federal Controlled Substances Act under DEA schedule II. Barbiturates may be habit forming. Tolerance, psychological dependence, and physical dependence may occur especially following prolonged use of high doses of barbiturates. Daily administration in excess of 400 mg of pentobarbital or secobarbital for approximately 90 days is likely to produce some degree of physical dependence. A dosage of from 600 to 800 mg taken for at least 35 days is sufficient to produce withdrawal seizures. The average daily dose for the barbiturate addict is usually about 1.5 grams. As tolerance to barbiturates develops, the amount needed to maintain the same level of intoxication increases; tolerance to a fatal dosage, however, does not increase more than two-fold. As this occurs, the margin between an intoxicating dosage and fatal dosage becomes smaller.

Symptoms of acute intoxication with barbiturates include unsteady gait, slurred speech, and sustained nystagmus. Mental signs of chronic intoxication include confusion, poor judgment, irritability, insomnia, and somatic complaints. Symptoms of barbiturate dependence are similar to those of chronic alcoholism. If an individual appears to be intoxicated with alcohol to a degree that is radically disproportionate to the amount of alcohol in his or her blood the use of barbiturates should be suspected. The lethal dose of a barbiturate is far less if alcohol is also ingested.

The symptoms of barbiturate withdrawal can be severe and may cause death. Minor withdrawal symptoms may appear 8 to 12 hours after the last dose of a barbiturate. These symptoms usually appear in the following order: anxiety, muscle twitching, tremor of hands and fingers, progressive weakness, dizziness, distortion in visual perception, nausea, vomiting, insomnia, and orthostatic hypotension. Major withdrawal symptoms (convulsions and delirium) may occur within 16 hours and last up to 5 days after abrupt cessation of these drugs. Intensity of withdrawal symptoms gradually declines over a period of approximately 15 days. Individuals

susceptible to barbiturate abuse and dependence include alcoholics and opiate abusers, as well as other sedative-hypnotic and amphetamine abusers.

Drug dependence to barbiturates arises from repeated administration of a barbiturate or agent with barbiturate-like effect on a continuous basis, generally in amounts exceeding therapeutic dose levels. The characteristics of drug dependence to barbiturates include: (a) a strong desire or need to continue taking the drug; (b) a tendency to increase the dose; (c) a psychic dependence on the effects of the drug related to subjective and individual appreciation of those effects; and (d) a physical dependence on the effects of the drug requiring its presence for maintenance of homeostasis and resulting in a definite, characteristic, and self-limited abstinence syndrome when the drug is withdrawn.

Treatment of barbiturate dependence consists of cautious and gradual withdrawal of the drug. Barbiturate-dependent patients can be withdrawn by using a number of different withdrawal regimens. In all cases withdrawal takes an extended period of time. One method involves substituting a 30 mg dose of phenobarbital for each 100 to 200 mg dose of barbiturate that the patient has been taking. The total daily amount of phenobarbital is then administered in 3 to 4 divided doses, not to exceed 600 mg daily. Should signs of withdrawal occur on the first day of treatment, a loading dose of 100 to 200 mg of phenobarbital may be administered IM in addition to the oral dose. After stabilization on phenobarbital, the total daily dose is decreased by 30 mg a day as long as withdrawal is proceeding smoothly. A modification of this regimen involves initiating treatment at the patient's regular dosage level and decreasing the daily dosage by 10 percent if tolerated by the patient.

Infants physically dependent on barbiturates may be given phenobarbital 3 to 10 mg/kg/day. After withdrawal symptoms (hyperactivity, disturbed sleep, tremors, hyperreflexia) are relieved, the dosage of phenobarbital should be gradually decreased and completely withdrawn over a 2 week period.

OVERDOSAGE

The toxic dose of barbiturates varies considerably. In general, an oral dose of 1 g of most barbiturates produces serious poisoning in an adult. Death commonly occurs after 2 to 10 g of ingested barbiturate. Barbiturate intoxication may be confused with alcoholism, bromide intoxication, and with various neurological disorders.

Acute overdosage with barbiturates is manifested by CNS and respiratory depression which may progress to Cheyne-Stokes respiration, areflexia, constriction of the pupils to a slight degree (though in severe poisoning they may show paralytic dilation), oliguria, tachycardia, hypotension, lowered body temperature, and coma. Typical shock syndrome (apnea, circulatory collapse, respiratory arrest, and death) may occur.

In extreme overdose, all electrical activity in the brain may cease, in which case a "flat" EEG normally equated with clinical death cannot be accepted. This effect is fully reversible unless hypoxic damage occurs. Consideration should be given to the possibility of barbiturate intoxication even in situations that appear to involve trauma.

Complications such as pneumonia, pulmonary edema, cardiac arrhythmias, congestive heart failure, and renal failure may occur. Uremia may increase CNS sensitivity to barbiturates. Differential diagnosis should include hypoglycemia, head trauma, cerebrovascular accidents, convulsive states, and diabetic coma. Blood levels from acute overdosage for some barbiturates are listed in Table 2. [See table above.]

Continued on next page

If desired, additional literature on any Abbott product will be provided upon request to Abbott Laboratories.

Abbott Laboratories—Cont.

Treatment of overdosage is mainly supportive and consists of the following:

1. Maintenance of an adequate airway, with assisted respiration and oxygen administration as necessary.
2. Monitoring of vital signs and fluid balance.
3. If the patient is conscious and has not lost the gag reflex, emesis may be induced with ipecac. Care should be taken to prevent pulmonary aspiration of vomitus. After completion of vomiting, 30 g activated charcoal in a glass of water may be administered.
4. If emesis is contraindicated, gastric lavage may be performed with a cuffed endotracheal tube in place with the patient in the face down position. Activated charcoal may be left in the emptied stomach and a saline cathartic administered.
5. Fluid therapy and other standard treatment for shock, if needed.
6. If renal function is normal, forced diuresis may aid in the elimination of the barbiturate. Alkalinization of the urine increases renal excretion of some barbiturates, especially phenobarbital, also aprobarbital, and mephobarbital (which is metabolized to phenobarbital).
7. Although not recommended as a routine procedure, hemodialysis may be used in severe barbiturate intoxications or if the patient is anuric or in shock.
8. Patient should be rolled from side to side every 30 minutes.
9. Antibiotics should be given if pneumonia is suspected.
10. Appropriate nursing care to prevent hypostatic pneumonia, decubiti, aspiration, and other complications of patients with altered states of consciousness.

DOSAGE AND ADMINISTRATION

Adults: The usual hypnotic dose consists of 100 mg at bedtime.

Children: The preoperative dose is 2 to 6 mg/kg/24 hours (maximum 100 mg), depending on age, weight, and the desired degree of sedation.

The proper hypnotic dose for children must be judged on the basis of individual age and weight.

Dosages of barbiturates must be individualized with full knowledge of their particular characteristics and recommended rate of administration. Factors of consideration are the patient's age, weight, and condition.

Special patient population: Dosage should be reduced in the elderly or debilitated because these patients may be more sensitive to barbiturates. Dosage should be reduced for patients with impaired renal function or hepatic disease.

HOW SUPPLIED

NEMBUTAL Sodium Capsules (pentobarbital sodium capsules, USP) are supplied as follows:

50 mg transparent and orange-colored capsules in bottles of 100 (**NDC** 0074-3150-11);

100 mg yellow capsules in bottles of 100 (**NDC** 0074-3114-01), 500 (**NDC** 0074-3114-02) and in the Abbo-Pac® unit dose packages of 100 (**NDC** 0074-3114-21).

Recommended Storage: Store below 86°F (30°C).

Ref. 03-4433-R10

Shown in Product Identification Section, page 403

NEMBUTAL® SODIUM SOLUTION ℞ Ⓒ II

[nem ʹ-bū-tal]

(pentobarbital sodium injection, USP)

Ampuls—Vials

WARNING: MAY BE HABIT FORMING. DO NOT USE IF MATERIAL HAS PRECIPITATED.

DESCRIPTION

The barbiturates are nonselective central nervous system depressants which are primarily used as sedative hypnotics and also anticonvulsants in subhypnotic doses. The barbiturates and their sodium salts are subject to control under the Federal Controlled Substances Act (See "Drug Abuse and Dependence" section).

The sodium salts of amobarbital, pentobarbital, phenobarbital, and secobarbital are available as sterile parenteral solutions.

Barbiturates are substituted pyrimidine derivatives in which the basic structure common to these drugs is barbituric acid, a substance which has no central nervous system (CNS) activity. CNS activity is obtained by substituting alkyl, alkenyl, or aryl groups on the pyrimidine ring.

NEMBUTAL Sodium Solution (pentobarbital sodium injection) is a sterile solution for intravenous or intramuscular injection. Each ml contains pentobarbital sodium 50 mg, in a vehicle of propylene glycol, 40%, alcohol, 10% and water for injection, to volume. The pH is adjusted to approximately 9.5 with hydrochloric acid and/or sodium hydroxide.

NEMBUTAL Sodium is a short-acting barbiturate, chemically designated as sodium 5-ethyl-5-(1-methylbutyl) barbiturate. The sodium salt occurs as a white, slightly bitter powder which is freely soluble in water and alcohol but practically insoluble in benzene and ether.

CLINICAL PHARMACOLOGY

Barbiturates are capable of producing all levels of CNS mood alteration from excitation to mild sedation, to hypnosis, and deep coma. Overdosage can produce death. In high enough therapeutic doses, barbiturates induce anesthesia.

Barbiturates depress the sensory cortex, decrease motor activity, alter cerebellar function, and produce drowsiness, sedation, and hypnosis.

Barbiturate-induced sleep differs from physiological sleep. Sleep laboratory studies have demonstrated that barbiturates reduce the amount of time spent in the rapid eye movement (REM) phase of sleep or dreaming stage. Also, Stages III and IV sleep are decreased. Following abrupt cessation of barbiturates used regularly, patients may experience markedly increased dreaming, nightmares, and/or insomnia. Therefore, withdrawal of a single therapeutic dose over 5 or 6 days has been recommended to lessen the REM rebound and disturbed sleep which contribute to drug withdrawal syndrome (for example, decrease the dose from 3 to 2 doses a day for 1 week).

In studies, secobarbital sodium and pentobarbital sodium have been found to lose most of their effectiveness for both inducing and maintaining sleep by the end of 2 weeks of continued drug administration at fixed doses. The short-, intermediate-, and, to a lesser degree, long-acting barbiturates have been widely prescribed for treating insomnia. Although the clinical literature abounds with claims that the short-acting barbiturates are superior for producing sleep while the intermediate-acting compounds are more effective in maintaining sleep, controlled studies have failed to demonstrate these differential effects. Therefore, as sleep medications, the barbiturates are of limited value beyond short-term use.

Barbiturates have little analgesic action at subanesthetic doses. Rather, in subanesthetic doses these drugs may increase the reaction to painful stimuli. All barbiturates exhibit anticonvulsant activity in anesthetic doses. However, of the drugs in this class, only phenobarbital, mephobarbital, and metharbital have been clinically demonstrated to be effective as oral anticonvulsants in subhypnotic doses.

Barbiturates are respiratory depressants. The degree of respiratory depression is dependent upon dose. With hypnotic doses, respiratory depression produced by barbiturates is similar to that which occurs during physiologic sleep with slight decrease in blood pressure and heart rate.

Studies in laboratory animals have shown that barbiturates cause reduction in the tone and contractility of the uterus, ureters, and urinary bladder. However, concentration of the drugs required to produce this effect in humans are not reached with sedative-hypnotic doses.

Barbiturates do not impair normal hepatic function, but have been shown to induce liver microsomal enzymes, thus increasing and/or altering the metabolism of barbiturates and other drugs. (See "Precautions—*Drug Interactions*" section).

Pharmacokinetics: Barbiturates are absorbed in varying degrees following oral, rectal, or parenteral administration. The salts are more rapidly absorbed than are the acids.

The onset of action for oral or rectal administration varies from 20 to 60 minutes. For IM administration, the onset of action is slightly faster. Following IV administration, the onset of action ranges from almost immediately for pentobarbital sodium to 5 minutes for phenobarbital sodium. Maximal CNS depression may not occur until 15 minutes or more after IV administration for phenobarbital sodium.

Duration of action, which is related to the rate at which the barbiturates are redistributed throughout the body, varies among persons and in the same person from time to time.

No studies have demonstrated that the different routes of administration are equivalent with respect to bioavailability.

Barbiturates are weak acids that are absorbed and rapidly distributed to all tissues and fluids with high concentration in the brain, liver, and kidneys. Lipid solubility of the barbiturates is the dominant factor in their distribution within the body. The more lipid soluble the barbiturate, the more rapidly it penetrates all tissues of the body. Barbiturates are bound to plasma and tissue proteins to a varying degree with the degree of binding increasing directly as a function of lipid solubility.

Phenobarbital has the lowest lipid solubility, lowest plasma binding, lowest brain protein binding, the longest delay in onset of activity, and the longest duration of action. At the opposite extreme is secobarbital which has the highest lipid solubility, plasma protein binding, brain protein binding, the shortest delay in onset of activity, and the shortest duration of action. Butabarbital is classified as an intermediate barbiturate.

The plasma half-life for pentobarbital in adults is 15 to 50 hours and appears to be dose dependent.

Barbiturates are metabolized primarily by the hepatic microsomal enzyme system, and the metabolic products are excreted in the urine, and less commonly, in the feces. Approximately 25 to 50 percent of a dose of aprobarbital or phenobarbital is eliminated unchanged in the urine, whereas the amount of other barbiturates excreted unchanged in the urine is negligible. The excretion of unmetabolized barbiturate is one feature that distinguishes the long-acting category from those belonging to other categories which are almost entirely metabolized. The inactive metabolites of the barbiturates are excreted as conjugates of glucuronic acid.

INDICATIONS AND USAGE

Parenteral:

a. Sedatives.

b. Hypnotics, for the short-term treatment of insomnia, since they appear to lose their effectiveness for sleep induction and sleep maintenance after 2 weeks (See "Clinical Pharmacology" section).

c. Preanesthetics.

d. Anticonvulsant, in anesthetic doses, in the emergency control of certain acute convulsive episodes, e.g., those associated with status epilepticus, cholera, eclampsia, meningitis, tetanus, and toxic reactions to strychnine or local anesthetics.

CONTRAINDICATIONS

Barbiturates are contraindicated in patients with known barbiturate sensitivity. Barbiturates are also contraindicated in patients with a history of manifest or latent porphyria.

WARNINGS

1. *Habit forming:* Barbiturates may be habit forming. Tolerance, psychological and physical dependence may occur with continued use. (See "Drug Abuse and Dependence" and "Pharmacokinetics" sections). Patients who have psychological dependence on barbiturates may increase the dosage or decrease the dosage interval without consulting a physician and may subsequently develop a physical dependence on barbiturates. To minimize the possibility of overdosage or the development of dependence, the prescribing and dispensing of sedative-hypnotic barbiturates should be limited to the amount required for the interval until the next appointment. Abrupt cessation after prolonged use in the dependent person may result in withdrawal symptoms, including delirium, convulsions, and possibly death. Barbiturates should be withdrawn gradually from any patient known to be taking excessive dosage over long periods of time. (See "Drug Abuse and Dependence" section).
2. *IV administration:* Too rapid administration may cause respiratory depression, apnea, laryngospasm, or vasodilation with fall in blood pressure.
3. *Acute or chronic pain:* Caution should be exercised when barbiturates are administered to patients with acute or chronic pain, because paradoxical excitement could be induced or important symptoms could be masked. However, the use of barbiturates as sedatives in the postoperative surgical period and as adjuncts to cancer chemotherapy is well established.
4. *Use in pregnancy:* Barbiturates can cause fetal damage when administered to a pregnant woman. Retrospective, case-controlled studies have suggested a connection between the maternal consumption of barbiturates and a higher than expected incidence of fetal abnormalities. Following oral or parenteral administration, barbiturates readily cross the placental barrier and are distributed throughout fetal tissues with highest concentrations found in the placenta, fetal liver, and brain. Fetal blood levels approach maternal blood levels following parenteral administration.

   Withdrawal symptoms occur in infants born to mothers who receive barbiturates throughout the last trimester of pregnancy. (See "Drug Abuse and Dependence" section). If this drug is used during pregnancy, or if the patient becomes pregnant while taking this drug, the patient should be apprised of the potential hazard to the fetus.
5. *Synergistic effects:* The concomitant use of alcohol or other CNS depressants may produce additive CNS depressant effects.

PRECAUTIONS

General: Barbiturates may be habit forming. Tolerance and psychological and physical dependence may occur with continuing use. (See "Drug Abuse and Dependence" section). Barbiturates should be administered with caution, if at all, to patients who are mentally depressed, have suicidal tendencies, or a history of drug abuse.

Elderly or debilitated patients may react to barbiturates with marked excitement, depression, and confusion. In some persons, barbiturates repeatedly produce excitement rather than depression.

In patients with hepatic damage, barbiturates should be administered with caution and initially in reduced doses. Barbiturates should not be administered to patients showing the premonitory signs of hepatic coma.

Parenteral solutions of barbiturates are highly alkaline. Therefore, extreme care should be taken to avoid perivascular extravasation or intra-arterial injection. Extravascular injection may cause local tissue damage with subsequent necrosis; consequences of intra-arterial injection may vary from transient pain to gangrene of the limb. Any complaint of pain in the limb warrants stopping the injection.

Information for the patient: Practitioners should give the following information and instructions to patients receiving barbiturates.

1. The use of barbiturates carries with it an associated risk of psychological and/or physical dependence. The patient should be warned against increasing the dose of the drug without consulting a physician.
2. Barbiturates may impair mental and/or physical abilities required for the performance of potentially hazardous tasks (e.g., driving, operating machinery, etc.).
3. Alcohol should not be consumed while taking barbiturates. Concurrent use of the barbiturates with other CNS depressants (e.g., alcohol, narcotics, tranquilizers, and antihistamines) may result in additional CNS depressant effects.

Laboratory tests: Prolonged therapy with barbiturates should be accompanied by periodic laboratory evaluation of organ systems, including hematopoietic, renal, and hepatic systems. (See "Precautions-*General*" and "Adverse Reactions" sections).

Drug interactions: Most reports of clinically significant drug interactions occurring with the barbiturates have involved phenobarbital. However, the application of these data to other barbiturates appears valid and warrants serial blood level determinations of the relevant drugs when there are multiple therapies.

1. *Anticoagulants:* Phenobarbital lowers the plasma levels of dicumarol (name previously used: bishydroxycoumarin) and causes a decrease in anticoagulant activity as measured by the prothrombin time. Barbiturates can induce hepatic microsomal enzymes resulting in increased metabolism and decreased anticoagulant response of oral anticoagulants (e.g., warfarin, acenocoumarol, dicumarol, and phenprocoumon). Patients stabilized on anticoagulant therapy may require dosage adjustments if barbiturates are added to or withdrawn from their dosage regimen.
2. *Corticosteroids:* Barbiturates appear to enhance the metabolism of exogenous corticosteroids probably through the induction of hepatic microsomol enzymes. Patients stabilized on corticosteroid therapy may require dosage adjustments if barbiturates are added to or withdrawn from their dosage regimen.
3. *Griseofulvin:* Phenobarbital appears to interfere with the absorption of orally administered griseofulvin, thus decreasing its blood level. The effect of the resultant decreased blood levels of griseofulvin on therapeutic response has not been established. However, it would be preferable to avoid concomitant administration of these drugs.
4. *Doxycycline:* Phenobarbital has been shown to shorten the half-life of doxycycline for as long as 2 weeks after barbiturate therapy is discontinued.
This mechanism is probably through the induction of hepatic microsomal enzymes that metabolize the antibiotic. If phenobarbital and doxycycline are administered concurrently, the clinical response to doxycycline should be monitored closely.
5. *Phenytoin, sodium valproate, valproic acid:* The effect of barbiturates on the metabolism of phenytoin appears to be variable. Some investigators report an accelerating effect, while others report no effect. Because the effect of barbiturates on the metabolism of phenytoin is not predictable, phenytoin and barbiturate blood levels should be monitored more frequently if these drugs are given concurrently. Sodium valproate and valproic acid appear to decrease barbiturate metabolism; therefore, barbiturate blood levels should be monitored and appropriate dosage adjustments made as indicated.
6. *Central nervous system depressants:* The concomitant use of other central nervous system depressants, including other sedatives or hypnotics, antihistamines, tranquilizers, or alcohol, may produce additive depressant effects.
7. *Monoamine oxidase inhibitors (MAOI):* MAOI prolong the effects of barbiturates probably because metabolism of the barbiturate is inhibited.
8. *Estradiol, estrone, progesterone and other steroidal hormones:* Pretreatment with or concurrent administration of phenobarbital may decrease the effect of estradiol by increasing its metabolism. There have been reports of patients treated with antiepileptic drugs (e.g., phenobarbital) who became pregnant while taking oral contraceptives. An alternate contraceptive method might be suggested to women taking phenobarbital.

Carcinogenesis:
1. Animal data. Phenobarbital sodium is carcinogenic in mice and rats after lifetime administration. In mice, it produced benign and malignant liver cell tumors. In rats, benign liver cell tumors were obsserved very late in life.
2. Human data. In a 29-year epidemiological study of 9,136 patients who were treated on an anticonvulsant protocol that included phenobarbital, results indicated a higher than normal incidence of hepatic carcinoma. Previously, some of these patients were treated with thorotrast, a drug that is known to produce hepatic carcinomas. Thus, this study did not provide sufficient evidence that phenobarbital sodium is carcinogenic in humans.

Data from one retrospective study of 235 children in which the types of barbiturates are not identified suggested an association between exposure to barbiturates prenatally and an increased incidence of brain tumor. (Gold, E., et al., "Increased Risk of Brain Tumors in Children Exposed to Barbiturates," *Journal of National Cancer Institute*, 61:1031–1034, 1978).

Pregnancy: 1. *Teratogenic effects.* Pregnancy Category D—See "Warnings—Use in Pregnancy" section.

2. *Nonteratogenic effects.* Reports of infants suffering from long-term barbiturate exposure in utero included the acute withdrawal syndrome of seizures and hyperirritability from birth to a delayed onset of up to 14 days. (See "Drug Abuse and Dependence" section).

Labor and delivery: Hypnotic doses of these barbiturates do not appear to significantly impair uterine activity during labor. Full anesthetic doses of barbiturates decrease the force and frequency of uterine contractions. Administration of sedative-hypnotic barbiturates to the mother during labor may result in respiratory depression in the newborn. Premature infants are particularly susceptible to the depressant effects of barbiturates. If barbiturates are used during labor and delivery, resuscitation equipment should be available. Data are currently not available to evaluate the effect of these barbiturates when forceps delivery or other intervention is necessary. Also, data are not available to determine the effect of these barbiturates on the later growth, development, and functional maturation of the child.

Nursing mothers: Caution should be exercised when a barbiturate is administered to a nursing woman since small amounts of barbiturates are excreted in the milk.

ADVERSE REACTIONS

The following adverse reactions and their incidence were compiled from surveillance of thousands of hospitalized patients. Because such patients may be less aware of certain of the milder adverse effects of barbiturates, the incidence of these reactions may be somewhat higher in fully ambulatory patients.

More than 1 in 100 patients. The most common adverse reaction estimated to occur at a rate of 1 to 3 patients per 100 is: *Nervous System:* Somnolence.

Less than 1 in 100 patients. Adverse reactions estimated to occur at a rate of less than 1 in 100 patients listed below, grouped by organ system, and by decreasing order of occurrence are:

Nervous system: Agitation, confusion, hyperkinesia, ataxia, CNS depression, nightmares, nervousness, psychiatric disturbance, hallucinations, insomnia, anxiety, dizziness, thinking abnormality.

Respiratory system: Hypoventilation, apnea.

Cardiovascular system: Bradycardia, hypotension, syncope.

Digestive system: Nausea, vomiting, constipation.

Other reported reactions: Headache, injection site reactions, hypersensitivity reactions (angioedema, skin rashes, exfoliative dermatitis), fever, liver damage, megaloblastic anemia following chronic phenobarbital use.

DRUG ABUSE AND DEPENDENCE

Pentobarbital sodium injection is subject to control by the Federal Controlled Substances Act under DEA schedule II. Barbiturates may be habit forming. Tolerance, psychological dependence, and physical dependence may occur especially following prolonged use of high doses of barbiturates. Daily administration in excess of 400 mg of pentobarbital or secobarbital for approximately 90 days is likely to produce some degree of physical dependence. A dosage of from 600 to 800 mg taken for at least 35 days is sufficient to produce withdrawal seizures. The average daily dose for the barbiturate addict is usually about 1.5 g. As tolerance to barbiturates develops, the amount needed to maintain the same level of intoxication increases; tolerance to a fatal dosage, however, does not increase more than two-fold. As this occurs, the margin between an intoxicating dosage and fatal dosage becomes smaller.

Symptoms of acute intoxication with barbiturates include unsteady gait, slurred speech, and sustained nystagmus. Mental signs of chronic intoxication include confusion, poor judgment, irritability, insomnia, and somatic complaints. Symptoms of barbiturate dependence are similar to those of chronic alcoholism. If an individual appears to be intoxicated with alcohol to a degree that is radically disproportionate to the amount of alcohol in his or her blood the use of barbitu-

rates should be suspected. The lethal dose of a barbiturate is far less if alcohol is also ingested.

The symptoms of barbiturate withdrawal can be severe and may cause death. Minor withdrawal symptoms may appear 8 to 12 hours after the last dose of a barbiturate. These symptoms usually appear in the following order: anxiety, muscle twitching, tremor of hands and fingers, progressive weakness, dizziness, distortion in visual perception, nausea, vomiting, insomnia, and orthostatic hypotension. Major withdrawal symptoms (convulsions and delirium) may occur within 16 hours and last up to 5 days after abrupt cessation of these drugs. Intensity of withdrawal symptoms gradually declines over a period of approximately 15 days. Individuals susceptible to barbiturate abuse and dependence include alcoholics and opiate abusers, as well as other sedative-hypnotic and amphetamine abusers.

Drug dependence to barbiturates arises from repeated administration of a barbiturate or agent with barbiturate-like effect on a continuous basis, generally in amounts exceeding therapeutic dose levels. The characteristics of drug dependence to barbiturates include: (a) a strong desire or need to continue taking the drug; (b) a tendency to increase the dose; (c) a psychic dependence on the effects of the drug related to subjective and individual appreciation of those effects; and (d) a physical dependence on the effects of the drug requiring its presence for maintenance of homeostasis and resulting in a definite, characteristic, and self-limited abstinence syndrome when the drug is withdrawn.

Treatment of barbiturate dependence consists of cautious and gradual withdrawal of the drug. Barbiturate-dependent patients can be withdrawn by using a number of different withdrawal regimens. In all cases withdrawal takes an extended period of time. One method involves substituting a 30 mg dose of phenobarbital for each 100 to 200 mg dose of barbiturate that the patient has been taking. The total daily amount of phenobarbital is then administered in 3 to 4 divided doses, not to exceed 600 mg daily. Should signs of withdrawal occur on the first day of treatment, a loading dose of 100 to 200 mg of phenobarbital may be administered IM in addition to the oral dose. After stabilization on phenobarbital, the total daily dose is decreased by 30 mg a day as long as withdrawal is proceeding smoothly. A modification of this regimen involves initiating treatment at the patient's regular dosage level and decreasing the daily dosage by 10 percent if tolerated by the patient.

Infants physically dependent on barbiturates may be given phenobarbital 3 to 10 mg/kg/day. After withdrawal symptoms (hyperactivity, disturbed sleep, tremors, hyperreflexia) are relieved, the dosage of phenobarbital should be gradually decreased and completely withdrawn over a 2-week period.

OVERDOSAGE

The toxic dose of barbiturates varies considerably. In general, an oral dose of 1 g of most barbiturates produces serious poisoning in an adult. Death commonly occurs after 2 to 10 g of ingested barbiturate. Barbiturate intoxication may be confused with alcoholism, bromide intoxication, and with various neurological disorders.

Acute overdosage with barbiturates is manifested by CNS and respiratory depression which may progress to Cheyne-Stokes respiration, areflexia, constriction of the pupils to a slight degree (though in severe poisoning they may show paralytic dilation), oliguria, tachycardia, hypotension, lowered body temperature, and coma. Typical shock syndrome (apnea, circulatory collapse, respiratory arrest, and death) may occur.

In extreme overdose, all electrical activity in the brain may cease, in which case a "flat" EEG normally equated with clinical death cannot be accepted. This effect is fully reversible unless hypoxic damage occurs. Consideration should be given to the possibility of barbiturate intoxication even in situations that appear to involve trauma.

Complications such as pneumonia, pulmonary edema, cardiac arrhythmias, congestive heart failure, and renal failure may occur. Uremia may increase CNS sensitivity to barbiturates. Differential diagnosis should include hypoglycemia, head trauma, cerebrovascular accidents, convulsive states, and diabetic coma. Blood levels from acute overdosage for some barbiturates are listed in Table 2. [See Table 2 in Nembutal Capsules prescribing information.]

Treatment of overdosage is mainly supportive and consists of the following:
1. Maintenance of an adequate airway, with assisted respiration and oxygen administration as necessary.
2. Monitoring of vital signs and fluid balance.
3. Fluid therapy and other standard treatment for shock, if needed.
4. If renal function is normal, forced diuresis may aid in the elimination of the barbiturate. Alkalinization of the urine increases renal excretion of some barbitu-

Continued on next page

Abbott Laboratories—Cont.

rates, especially phenobarbital, also aprobarbital, and mephobarbital (which is metabolized to phenobarbital).

5. Although not recommended as a routine procedure, hemodialysis may be used in severe barbiturate intoxications or if the patient is anuric or in shock.
6. Patient should be rolled from side to side every 30 minutes.
7. Antibiotics should be given if pneumonia is suspected.
8. Appropriate nursing care to prevent hypostatic pneumonia, decubiti, aspiration, and other complications of patients with altered states of consciousness.

DOSAGE AND ADMINISTRATION

Dosages of barbiturates must be individualized with full knowledge of their particular characteristics and recommended rate of administration. Factors of consideration are the patient's age, weight, and condition. Parenteral routes should be used only when oral administration is impossible or impractical.

Intramuscular Administration: IM injection of the sodium salts of barbiturates should be made deeply into a large muscle, and a volume of 5 ml should not be exceeded at any one site because of possible tissue irritation. After IM injection of a hypnotic dose, the patient's vital signs should be monitored. The usual adult dosage of NEMBUTAL Sodium Solution is 150 to 200 mg as a single IM injection; the recommended pediatric dosage ranges from 2 to 6 mg/kg as a single IM injection not to exceed 100 mg.

Intravenous Administration: NEMBUTAL Sodium Solution should not be admixed with any other medication or solution. IV injection is restricted to conditions in which other routes are not feasible, either because the patient is unconscious (as in cerebral hemorrhage, eclampsia, or status epilepticus), or because the patient resists (as in delirium), or because prompt action is imperative. Slow IV injection is essential and patients should be carefully observed during administration. This requires that blood pressure, respiration, and cardiac function be maintained, vital signs be recorded, and equipment for resuscitation and artificial ventilation be available. The rate of IV injection should not exceed 50 mg/min for pentobarbital sodium.

There is no average intravenous dose of NEMBUTAL Sodium Solution (pentobarbital sodium injection) that can be relied on to produce similar effects in different patients. The possibility of overdose and respiratory depression is remote when the drug is injected slowly in fractional doses.

A commonly used initial dose for the 70 kg adult is 100 mg. Proportional reduction in dosage should be made for pediatric or debilitated patients. At least one minute is necessary to determine the full effect of intravenous pentobarbital. If necessary, additional small increments of the drug may be given up to a total of from 200 to 500 mg for normal adults.

Anticonvulsant use: In convulsive states, dosage of NEMBUTAL Sodium Solution should be kept to a minimum to avoid compounding the depression which may follow convulsions. The injection must be made slowly with due regard to the time required for the drug to penetrate the blood-brain barrier.

Special patient population: Dosage should be reduced in the elderly or debilitated because these patients may be more sensitive to barbiturates. Dosage should be reduced for patients with impaired renal function or hepatic disease.

Inspection: Parenteral drug products should be inspected visually for particulate matter and discoloration prior to administration, whenever solution containers permit. Solutions for injection showing evidence of precipitation should not be used.

HOW SUPPLIED

NEMBUTAL Sodium Solution (pentobarbital sodium injection, USP) is available in the following sizes:

2-ml ampul, 100 mg, in boxes of 25 (**NDC** 0074-6899-04); 20-ml multiple-dose vial, 1 g per vial (**NDC** 0074-3778-04); and 50-ml multiple-dose vial, 2.5 g per vial (**NDC** 0074-3778-05).

Each ml contains:

Pentobarbital Sodium,
derivative of barbituric acid .... 50 mg
Warning—May be habit forming.
Propylene glycol .... 40% v/v
Alcohol 10%
Water for Injection .... qs
(pH adjusted to approximately 9.5 with hydrochloric acid and/or sodium hydroxide.)

Exposure of pharmaceutical products to heat should be minimized. Avoid excessive heat. Protect from freezing. It is recommended that the product be stored at room temperature—86°F (30°C); however, brief exposure up to 104°F (40°C) does not adversely affect the product.

Ref. 01-2577-R5

NEMBUTAL® SODIUM SUPPOSITORIES ℞ Ⓒ

[*nĕm-bū 'tal*]

(pentobarbital sodium suppositories)

WARNING: MAY BE HABIT FORMING

DESCRIPTION

The barbiturates are nonselective central nervous system depressants which are primarily used as sedative hypnotics. The barbiturates and their sodium salts are subject to control under the Federal Controlled Substances Act (See "Drug Abuse and Dependence" section).

Barbiturates are substituted pyrimidine derivatives in which the basic structure common to these drugs is barbituric acid, a substance which has no central nervous system (CNS) activity. CNS activity is obtained by substituting alkyl, alkenyl, or aryl groups on the pyrimidine ring. Nembutal (pentobarbital sodium) is chemically represented by sodium 5-ethyl-5-(1-methylbutyl) barbiturate.

The sodium salt of pentobarbital occurs as a white, slightly bitter powder which is freely soluble in water and alcohol but practically insoluble in benzene and ether. Each rectal suppository contains either 30 mg, 60 mg, 120 mg, or 200 mg of pentobarbital sodium.

Inactive Ingredients: Semi-synthetic glycerides.

CLINICAL PHARMACOLOGY

Barbiturates are capable of producing all levels of CNS mood alteration from excitation to mild sedation, to hypnosis, and deep coma. Overdosage can produce death. In high enough therapeutic doses, barbiturates induce anesthesia.

Barbiturates depress the sensory cortex, decrease motor activity, alter cerebellar function, and produce drowsiness, sedation, and hypnosis.

Barbiturate-induced sleep differs from physiological sleep. Sleep laboratory studies have demonstrated that barbiturates reduce the amount of time spent in the rapid eye movement (REM) phase of sleep or dreaming stage. Also, Stages III and IV sleep are decreased. Following abrupt cessation of barbiturates used regularly, patients may experience markedly increased dreaming, nightmares, and/or insomnia. Therefore, withdrawal of a single therapeutic dose over 5 or 6 days has been recommended to lessen the REM rebound and disturbed sleep which contribute to drug withdrawal syndrome (for example, decrease the dose from 3 to 2 doses a day for 1 week).

In studies, secobarbital sodium and pentobarbital sodium have been found to lose most of their effectiveness for both inducing and maintaining sleep by the end of 2 weeks of continued drug administration at fixed doses. The short-, intermediate-, and, to a lesser degree, long-acting barbiturates have been widely prescribed for treating insomnia. Although the clinical literature abounds with claims that the short-acting barbiturates are superior for producing sleep while the intermediate-acting compounds are more effective in maintaining sleep, controlled studies have failed to demonstrate these differential effects. Therefore, as sleep medications, the barbiturates are of limited value beyond short-term use.

Barbiturates have little analgesic action at subanesthetic doses. Rather, in subanesthetic doses these drugs may increase the reaction to painful stimuli. All barbiturates exhibit anticonvulsant activity in anesthetic doses. However, of the drugs in this class, only phenobarbital, mephobarbital, and metharbital have been clinically demonstrated to be effective as oral anticonvulsants in subhypnotic doses.

Barbiturates are respiratory depressants. The degree of respiratory depression is dependent upon dose. With hypnotic doses, respiratory depression produced by barbiturates is similar to that which occurs during physiologic sleep with slight decrease in blood pressure and heart rate.

Studies in laboratory animals have shown that barbiturates cause reduction in the tone and contractility of the uterus, ureters, and urinary bladder. However, concentrations of the drugs required to produce this effect in humans are not reached with sedative-hypnotic doses.

Barbiturates do not impair normal hepatic function, but have been shown to induce liver microsomal enzymes, thus increasing and/or altering the metabolism of barbiturates and other drugs. (See "Precautions—*Drug Interactions*" section).

Pharmacokinetics: Barbiturates are absorbed in varying degrees following oral, rectal, or parenteral administration. The onset of action for oral or rectal administration varies from 20 to 60 minutes.

Duration of action, which is related to the rate at which the barbiturates are redistributed throughout the body, varies among persons and in the same person from time to time.

No studies have demonstrated that the different routes of administration are equivalent with respect to bioavailability.

Barbiturates are weak acids that are absorbed and rapidly distributed to all tissues and fluids with high concentrations in the brain, liver, and kidneys. Lipid solubility of the barbiturates is the dominant factor in their distribution within the body. The more lipid soluble the barbiturate, the more rapidly it penetrates all tissues of the body. Barbiturates are bound to plasma and tissue proteins to a varying degree with the degree of binding increasing directly as a function of lipid solubility.

Phenobarbital has the lowest lipid solubility, lowest plasma binding, lowest brain protein binding, the longest delay in onset of activity, and the longest duration of action. At the opposite extreme is secobarbital which has the highest lipid solubility, plasma protein binding, brain protein binding, the shortest delay in onset of activity, and the shortest duration of action. Butabarbital is classsified as an intermediate barbiturate.

The plasma half-life for phentobarbital in adults is 15 to 50 hours and appears to be dose dependent.

Barbiturates are metabolized primarily by the hepatic microsomal enzyme system, and the metabolic products are excreted in the urine, and less commonly, in the feces. Approximately 25 to 50 percent of a dose of aprobarbital or phenobarbital is eliminated unchanged in the urine, whereas the amount of other barbiturates excreted unchanged in the urine is negligible. The excretion of unmetabolized barbiturate is one feature that distinguishes the long-acting category from those belonging to other categories which are almost entirely metabolized. The inactive metabolites of the barbiturates are excreted as conjugates of glucuronic acid.

INDICATIONS AND USAGE

Rectal: Barbiturates administered rectally are absorbed from the colon and are used when oral or parenteral administration may be undesirable.

1. Sedative.
2. Hypnotic, for the short-term treatment of insomnia, since they appear to lose their effectiveness for sleep induction and sleep maintenance after 2 weeks (See "Clinical Pharmacology" section).

CONTRAINDICATIONS

Barbiturates are contraindicated in patients with known barbiturate sensitivity. Barbiturates are also contraindicated in patients with a history of manifest or latent porphyria.

WARNINGS

1. *Habit forming:* Barbiturates may be habit forming. Tolerance, psychological and physical dependence may occur with continued use. (See "Drug Abuse and Dependence" and "Pharmacokinetics" sections). Patients who have psychological dependence on barbiturates may increase the dosage or decrease the dosage interval without consulting a physician and may subsequently develop a physical dependence on barbiturates. To minimize the possibility of overdosage or the development of dependence, the prescribing and dispensing of sedative-hypnotic barbiturates should be limited to the amount required for the interval until the next appointment. Abrupt cessation after prolonged use in the dependent person may result in withdrawal symptoms, including delirium, convulsions, and possibly death. Barbiturates should be withdrawn gradually from any patient known to be taking excessive dosage over long periods of time. (See "Drug Abuse and Dependence" section).

2. *Acute or chronic pain:* Caution should be exercised when barbiturates are administered to patients with acute or chronic pain, because paradoxical excitement could be induced or important symptoms could be masked. However, the use of barbiturates as sedatives in the postoperative surgical period and as adjuncts to cancer chemotherapy is well established.

3. *Use in pregnancy:* Barbiturates can cause fetal damage when administered to a pregnant woman. Retrospective, case-controlled studies have suggested a connection between the maternal consumption of barbiturates and a higher than expected incidence of fetal abnormalities. Following oral or parenteral administration, barbiturates readily cross the placental barrier and are distributed throughout fetal tissues with highest concentrations found in the placenta, fetal liver, and brain. It is presumed that this effect will also be seen following rectal administration.

Withdrawal symptoms occur in infants born to mothers who receive barbiturates throughout the last trimester of pregnancy. (See "Drug Abuse and Dependence" section). If this drug is used during pregnancy, or if the patient becomes pregnant while taking this drug, the patient should be apprised of the potential hazard to the fetus.

4. *Synergistic effects:* The concomitant use of alcohol or other CNS depressants may produce additive CNS depressant effects.

PRECAUTIONS

General: Barbiturates may be habit forming. Tolerance and psychological and physical dependence may occur with continuing use. (See "Drug Abuse and Dependence" section). Barbiturates should be administered with caution, if at all, to patients who are mentally depressed, have suicidal tendencies, or a history of drug abuse.

Elderly or debilitated patients may react to barbiturates with marked excitement, depression, and confusion. In some

persons, barbiturates repeatedly produce excitement rather than depression.

In patients with hepatic damage, barbiturates should be administered with caution and initially in reduced doses. Barbiturates should not be administered to patients showing the premonitory signs of hepatic coma.

Information for the patient: Practitioners should give the following information and instructions to patients receiving barbiturates.

1. The use of barbiturates carries with it an associated risk of psychological and/or physical dependence. The patient should be warned against increasing the dose of the drug without consulting a physician.
2. Barbiturates may impair mental and/or physical abilities required for the performance of potentially hazardous tasks (e.g., driving, operating machinery, etc.)
3. Alcohol should not be consumed while taking barbiturates. Concurrent use of the barbiturates with other CNS depressants (e.g., alcohol, narcotics, tranquilizers, and antihistamines) may result in additional CNS depressant effects.

Laboratory tests: Prolonged therapy with barbiturates should be accompanied by periodic laboratory evaluation of organ systems, including hematopoietic, renal, and hepatic systems. (See "Precautions — *General*" and "Adverse Reactions" sections).

Drug interactions: Most reports of clinically significant drug interactions occurring with the barbiturates have involved phenobarbital. However, the application of these data to other barbiturates appears valid and warrants serial blood level determinations of the relevant drugs when there are multiple therapies.

1. *Anticoagulants:* Phenobarbital lowers the plasma levels of dicumarol (name previously used: bishydroxycoumarin) and causes a decrease in anticoagulant activity as measured by the prothrombin time. Barbiturates can induce hepatic microsomal enzymes resulting in increased metabolism and decreased anticoagulant response of oral anticoagulants (e.g., warfarin, acenocoumarol, dicumarol, and phenprocoumon). Patients stabilized on anticoagulant therapy may require dosage adjustments if barbiturates are added to or withdrawn from their dosage regimen.
2. *Corticosteroids:* Barbiturates appear to enhance the metabolism of exogenous corticosteroids probably through the induction of hepatic microsomal enzymes. Patients stabilized on corticosteroid therapy may require dosage adjustments if barbiturates are added to or withdrawn from their dosage regimen.
3. *Griseofulvin:* Phenobarbital appears to interfere with the absorption of orally administered griseofulvin, thus decreasing its blood level. The effect of the resultant decreased blood levels of griseofulvin on therapeutic response has not been established. However, it would be preferable to avoid concomitant administration of these drugs.
4. *Doxycycline:* Phenobarbital has been shown to shorten the half-life of doxycycline for as long as 2 weeks after barbiturate therapy is discontinued. This mechanism is probably through the induction of hepatic microsomal enzymes that metabolize the antibiotic. If phenobarbital and doxycycline are administered concurrently, the clinical response to doxycycline should be monitored closely.
5. *Phenytoin, sodium valproate, valproic acid:* The effect of barbiturates on the metabolism of phenytoin appears to be variable. Some investigators report an accelerating effect, while others report no effect. Because the effect of barbiturates on the metabolism of phenytoin is not predictable, phenytoin and barbiturate blood levels should be monitored more frequently if these drugs are given concurrently. Sodium valproate and valproic acid appear to decrease barbiturate metabolism; therefore, barbiturate blood levels should be monitored and appropriate dosage adjustments made as indicated.
6. *Central nervous system depressants:* The concomitant use of other central nervous system depressants, including other sedatives or hypnotics, antihistamines, tranquilizers, or alcohol, may produce additive depressant effects.
7. *Monoamine oxidase inhibitors (MAOI):* MAOI prolong the effects of barbiturates probably because metabolism of the barbiturate is inhibited.
8. *Estradiol, estrone, progesterone and other steroidal hormones:* Pretreatment with or concurrent administration of phenobarbital may decrease the effect of estradiol by increasing its metabolism. There have been reports of patients treated with antiepileptic drugs (e.g., phenobarbital) who became pregnant while taking oral contraceptives. An alternate contraceptive method might be suggested to women taking phenobarbital.

Carcinogenesis:

1. Animal data. Phenobarbital sodium is carcinogenic in mice and rats after lifetime administration. In mice, it produced benign and malignant liver cell tumors. In rats, benign liver cell tumors were observed very late in life.
2. Human data. In a 29-year epidemiological study of 9,136 patients who were treated on an anticonvulsant protocol that included phenobarbital, results indicated a higher than normal incidence of hepatic carcinoma. Previously, some of these patients were treated with thorotrast, a drug that is known to produce hepatic carcinomas. Thus, this study did not provide sufficient evidence that phenobarbital sodium is carcinogenic in humans.

Data from one retrospective study of 235 children in which the types of barbiturates are not identified suggested an association between exposure to barbiturates prenatally and an increased incidence of brain tumor. (Gold, E., et al., "Increased Risk of Brain Tumors in Children Exposed to Barbiturates," Journal of National Cancer Institute, 61:1031–1034, 1978).

Pregnancy: 1. Teratogenic effects. Pregnancy Category D — See "Warnings — Use in Pregnancy" section.

2. *Nonteratogenic effects.* Reports of infants suffering from long-term barbiturate exposure in utero included the acute withdrawal syndrome of seizures and hyperirritability from birth to a delayed onset of up to 14 days. (See "Drug Abuse and Dependence" section).

Labor and delivery: Hypnotic doses of these barbiturates do not appear to significantly impair uterine activity during labor. Full anesthetic doses of barbiturates decrease the force and frequency of uterine contractions. Administration of sedative-hypnotic barbiturates to the mother during labor may result in respiratory depression in the newborn. Premature infants are particularly susceptible to the depressant effects of barbiturates. If barbiturates are used during labor and delivery, resuscitation equipment should be available. Data are currently not available to evaluate the effect of these barbiturates when forceps delivery or other intervention is necessary. Also, data are not available to determine the effect of these barbiturates on the later growth, development, and functional maturation of the child.

Nursing mothers: Caution should be exercised when a barbiturate is administered to a nursing woman since small amounts of barbiturates are excreted in the milk.

Table 1.—*Concentration of Barbiturate in the Blood Versus Degree of CNS Depression*

Blood barbiturate level in ppm (μg/ml)

Barbiturate	Onset/ duration	Degree of depression in nontolerant persons* 1	2	3	4	5
Pentobarbital	Fast/short	≤2	0.5 to 3	10 to 15	12 to 25	15 to 40
Secobarbital	Fast/short	≤2	0.5 to 5	10 to 15	15 to 25	15 to 40
Amobarbital	Intermediate/ intermediate	≤3	2 to 10	30 to 40	30 to 60	40 to 80
Butabarbital	Intermediate/ intermediate	≤5	3 to 25	40 to 60	50 to 80	60 to 100
Phenobarbital	Slow/long	≤10	5 to 40	50 to 80	70 to 120	100 to 200

*Categories of degree of depression in nontolerant persons:
1. Under the influence and appreciably impaired for purposes of driving a motor vehicle or performing tasks requiring alertness and unimpaired judgment and reaction time.
2. Sedated, therapeutic range, calm, relaxed, and easily aroused.
3. Comatose, difficult to arouse, significant depression of respiration.
4. Compatible with death in aged or ill persons or in presence of obstructed airway, other toxic agents, or exposure to cold.
5. Usual lethal level, the upper end of the range includes those who received some supportive treatment.

ADVERSE REACTIONS

The following adverse reactions and their incidence were compiled from surveillance of thousands of hospitalized patients. Because such patients may be less aware of certain of the milder adverse effects of barbiturates, the incidence of these reactions may be somewhat higher in fully ambulatory patients.

More than 1 in 100 patients. The most common adverse reaction estimated to occur at a rate of 1 to 3 patients per 100 is:
Nervous System: Somnolence.

Less than 1 in 100 patients. Adverse reactions estimated to occur at a rate of less than 1 in 100 patients listed below, grouped by organ system, and by decreasing order of occurrence are:

Nervous system: Agitation, confusion, hyperkinesia, ataxia, CNS depression, nightmares, nervousness, psychiatric disturbance, hallucinations, insomnia, anxiety, dizziness, thinking abnormality.
Respiratory system: Hypoventilation, apnea.
Cardiovascular system: Bradycardia, hypotension, syncope.
Digestive system: Nausea, vomiting, constipation.
Other reported reactions: Headache, injection site reactions, hypersensitivity reactions (angioedema, skin rashes, exfoliative dermatitis), fever, liver damage, megaloblastic anemia following chronic phenobarbital use.

DRUG ABUSE AND DEPENDENCE

Pentobarbital sodium suppositories are subject to control by the Federal Controlled Substances Act under DEA schedule III.

Barbiturates may be habit forming. Tolerance, psychological dependence, and physical dependence may occur especially following prolonged use of high doses of barbiturates. Daily administration in excess of 400 mg of pentobarbital or secobarbital for approximately 90 days is likely to produce some degree of physical dependence. A dosage of from 600 to 800 mg taken for at least 35 days is sufficient to produce withdrawal seizures. The average daily dose for the barbiturate addict is usually about 1.5 grams. As tolerance to barbiturates develops, the amount needed to maintain the same level of intoxication increases; tolerance to a fatal dosage, however, does not increase more than two-fold. As this occurs, the margin between an intoxicating dosage and fatal dosage becomes smaller.

Symptoms of acute intoxication with barbiturates include unsteady gait, slurred speech, and sustained nystagmus. Mental signs of chronic intoxication include confusion, poor judgment, irritability, insomnia, and somatic complaints. Symptoms of barbiturate dependence are similar to those of chronic alcoholism. If an individual appears to be intoxicated with alcohol to a degree that is radically disproportionate to the amount of alcohol in his or her blood the use of barbiturates should be suspected. The lethal dose of a barbiturate is far less if alcohol is also ingested.

The symptoms of barbiturate withdrawal can be severe and may cause death. Minor withdrawal symptoms may appear 8 to 12 hours after the last dose of a barbiturate. These symptoms usually appear in the following order: anxiety, muscle twitching, tremor of hands and fingers, progressive weakness, dizziness, distortion in visual perception, nausea, vomiting, insomnia, and orthostatic hypotension. Major withdrawal symptoms (convulsions and delirium) may occur within 16 hours and last up to 5 days after abrupt cessation of these drugs. Intensity of withdrawal symptoms gradually declines over a period of approximately 15 days. Individuals susceptible to barbiturate abuse and dependence include alcoholics and opiate abusers, as well as other sedative-hypnotic and amphetamine abusers.

Drug dependence to barbiturates arises from repeated administration of a barbiturate or agent with barbiturate-like effect on a continuous basis, generally in amounts exceeding therapeutic dose levels. The characteristics of drug dependence to barbiturates include: (a) a strong desire or need to continue taking the drug; (b) a tendency to increase the dose; (c) a psychic dependence on the effects of the drug related to subjective and individual appreciation of those effects; and (d) a physical dependence on the effects of the drug requiring its presence for maintenance of homeostasis and resulting in a definite, characteristic, and self-limited abstinence syndrome when the drug is withdrawn.

Treatment of barbiturate dependence consists of cautious and gradual withdrawal of the drug. Barbiturate-dependent patients can be withdrawn by using a number of different withdrawal regimens. In all cases withdrawal takes an extended period of time. One method involves substituting a 30 mg dose of phenobarbital for each 100 to 200 mg dose of barbiturate that the patient has been taking. The total daily amount of phenobarbital is then administered in 3 to 4 divided doses, not to exceed 600 mg daily. Should signs of withdrawal occur on the first day of treatment, a loading dose of 100 to 200 mg of phenobarbital may be administered IM in addition to the oral dose. After stabilization on phenobarbital, the total daily dose is decreased by 30 mg a day as long as withdrawal is proceeding smoothly. A modification of this regimen involves initiating treatment at the patient's regu-

Continued on next page

Abbott Laboratories—Cont.

lar dosage level and decreasing the daily dosage by 10 percent if tolerated by the patient.
Infants physically dependent on barbiturates may be given phenobarbital 3 to 10 mg/kg/day. After withdrawal symptoms (hyperactivity, disturbed sleep, tremors, hyperreflexia) are relieved, the dosage of phenobarbital should be gradually decreased and completely withdrawn over a 2 week period.

OVERDOSAGE

The toxic dose of barbiturates varies considerably. In general, an oral dose of 1 g of most barbiturates produces serious poisoning in an adult. Death commonly occurs after 2 to 10 g of ingested barbiturate. Barbiturate intoxication may be confused with alcoholism, bromide intoxication, and with various neurological disorders.
Acute overdosage with barbiturates is manifested by CNS and respiratory depression which may progress to Cheyne-Stokes respiration, areflexia, constriction of the pupils to a slight degree (though in severe poisoning they may show paralytic dilation), oliguria, tachycardia, hypotension, lowered body temperature, and coma. Typical shock syndrome (apnea, circulatory collapse, respiratory arrest, and death) may occur.
In extreme overdose, all electrical activity in the brain may cease, in which case a "flat" EEG normally equated with clinical death cannot be accepted. This effect is fully reversible unless hypoxic damage occurs. Consideration should be given to the possibility of barbiturate intoxication even in situations that appear to involve trauma.
Complications such as pneumonia, pulmonary edema, cardiac arrhythmias, congestive heart failure, and renal failure may occur. Uremia may increase CNS sensitivity to barbiturates. Differential diagnosis should include hypoglycemia, head trauma, cerebrovascular accidents, convulsive states, and diabetic coma. Blood levels from acute overdosage for some barbiturates are listed in Table 1.
[See table at top of preceding page.]
Treatment of overdosage is mainly supportive and consists of the following:

1. Maintenance of an adequate airway, with assisted respiration and oxygen administration as necessary.
2. Monitoring of vital signs and fluid balance.
3. Fluid therapy and other standard treatment for shock, if needed.
4. If renal function is normal, forced diuresis may aid in the elimination of the barbiturate. Alkalinization of the urine increases renal excretion of some barbiturates, especially phenobarbital, also aprobarbital, and mephobarbital (which is metabolized to phenobarbital).
5. Although not recommended as a routine procedure, hemodialysis may be used in severe barbiturate intoxications or if the patient is anuric or in shock.
6. Patient should be rolled from side to side every 30 minutes.
7. Antibiotics should be given if pneumonia is suspected.
8. Appropriate nursing care to prevent hypostatic pneumonia, decubiti, aspiration, and other complications of patients with altered states of consciousness.

DOSAGE AND ADMINISTRATION

Typical hypnotic doses for adults and children are given below. These are intended only as a guide, and administration should be adjusted to the individual needs of each patient. For sedation, in children 5–14 years and in adults, reduce dose appropriately.
Adults (average to above average weight)— one 120 mg or one 200 mg suppository.
Children —

12–14 years (80–110 lbs)	one 60 mg or one 120 mg suppository
5–12 years (40–80 lbs)	one 60 mg suppository
1–4 years (20–40 lbs)	one 30 mg or one 60 mg suppository
2 months–1 year (10–20 lbs)	one 30 mg suppository

Suppositories should not be divided.
Dosages of barbiturates must be individualized with full knowledge of their particular characteristics and recommended rate of administration. Factors of consideration are the patient's age, weight, and condition.
Special patient population: Dosage should be reduced in the elderly or debilitated because these patients may be more sensitive to barbiturates. Dosage should be reduced for patients with impaired renal function or hepatic disease.

HOW SUPPLIED

NEMBUTAL Sodium Suppositories (pentobarbital sodium suppositories) are available as suppositories containing pentobarbital sodium in the amount of 30 mg (**NDC** 0074-3272-01); 60 mg (**NDC** 0074-3148-01); 120 mg (**NDC** 0074-3145-01) and 200 mg (**NDC** 0074-3164-01). Supplied in boxes of 12 suppositories.
Store in a refrigerator (36°–46°F).
Ref. 01-2578-R12

NORISODRINE® WITH CALCIUM IODIDE SYRUP ℞

[*nō-rī 'sō-drēen*]
(isoproterenol sulfate and calcium iodide)

HOW SUPPLIED

Each teaspoonful of NORISODRINE WITH CALCIUM IODIDE SYRUP contains 3 mg of isoproterenol sulfate and 150 mg of anhydrous calcium iodide. Norisodrine with Calcium Iodide Syrup is supplied in pint (**NDC** 0074-6953-01) bottles.
Inactive Ingredients: Alcohol 6%, ascorbic acid, caramel coloring, glycerin, liquid glucose, sucrose, water, and artificial flavors forming a palatable, aromatic syrup.
Store below 77°F (25°C).
Ref. 07-8118-5/R34

OGEN® ℞

[*ō 'jên*]
(estropipate tablets, USP)
(estropipate vaginal cream, USP)

WARNING

1. ESTROGENS HAVE BEEN REPORTED TO INCREASE THE RISK OF ENDOMETRIAL CARCINOMA.
Three independent case control studies have shown an increased risk of endometrial cancer in postmenopausal women exposed to exogenous estrogens for prolonged periods.[1–3] This risk was independent of the other known risk factors for endometrial cancer. These studies are further supported by the finding that incidence rates of endometrial cancer have increased sharply since 1969 in eight different areas of the United States with population-based cancer reporting systems, an increase which may be related to the rapidly expanding use of estrogens during the last decade.[4]
The three case control studies reported that the risk of endometrial cancer in estrogen users was about 4.5 to 13.9 times greater than in nonusers. The risk appears to depend on both duration of treatment[1] and on estrogen dose.[3] In view of these findings, when estrogens are used for the treatment of menopausal symptoms, the lowest dose that will control symptoms should be utilized and medication should be discontinued as soon as possible. When prolonged treatment is medically indicated, the patient should be reassessed on at least a semiannual basis to determine the need for continued therapy. Although the evidence must be considered preliminary, one study suggests that cyclic administration of low doses of estrogen may carry less risk than continuous administration;[3] it therefore appears prudent to utilize such a regimen.
Close clinical surveillance of all women taking estrogens is important. In all cases of undiagnosed persistent or recurring abnormal vaginal bleeding, adequate diagnostic measures should be undertaken to rule out malignancy.
There is no evidence at present that "natural" estrogens are more or less hazardous than "synthetic" estrogens at equiestrogenic doses.
2. OGEN SHOULD NOT BE USED DURING PREGNANCY.
According to some investigators, the use of female sex hormones, both estrogens and progestogens, during early pregnancy may seriously damage the offspring. Studies have reported that females exposed in utero to diethylstilbestrol, a non-steroidal estrogen, have an increased risk of developing in later life a form of vaginal or cervical cancer that is ordinarily extremely rare.[5,6] In one of these studies, this risk was estimated as not greater than 4 per 1000 exposures.[7] Furthermore, there are reports that a high percentage of such exposed women (from 30 to 90 percent) have been found to have vaginal adenosis,[8–12] epithelial changes of the vagina and cervix. Although these reported changes are histologically benign, the investigators have not determined whether they are precursors of adenocarcinoma.
Several reports suggest an association between intrauterine exposure to female sex hormones and congenital anomalies in the offspring, including heart defects and limb reduction defects.[13–16] One case control study[16] estimated a 4.7 fold increased risk of limb reduction defects in infants exposed in utero to sex hormones (oral contraceptives, hormone withdrawal tests for pregnancy, or attempted treatment for threatened abortion). Some of these exposures were very short and involved only a few days of treatment. The data suggest that the risk of limb reduction defects in exposed fetuses is somewhat less than 1 per 1000.
In the past, female sex hormones have been used during pregnancy in an attempt to treat threatened or habitual abortion. OGEN has not been studied for these uses, and therefore should not be used during pregnancy. There is no evidence from well controlled studies that progestogens are effective for these uses.
If OGEN (estropipate) is used during pregnancy, or if the patient becomes pregnant while taking the tablets or using the vaginal cream, she should be apprised of the potential risks to the fetus, and the question of continuation of the pregnancy should be addressed.

DESCRIPTION

OGEN (estropipate), (formerly piperazine estrone sulfate), is a natural estrogenic substance prepared from purified crystalline estrone, solubilized as the sulfate and stabilized with piperazine. It is appreciably soluble in water and has almost no odor or taste. The amount of piperazine in OGEN is not sufficient to exert a pharmacological action. Its addition ensures solubility, stability, and uniform potency of the estrone sulfate. Chemically estropipate is represented by estra-1,3,5(10) -trien-17-one, 3-(sulfooxy)-, compound with piperazine (1:1).
OGEN is available as tablets for oral administration containing either 0.75 mg (OGEN .625), 1.5 mg (OGEN 1.25), 3 mg (OGEN 2.5) or 6 mg (OGEN 5) estropipate.
Each gram of Ogen Vaginal Cream contains 1.5 mg estropipate.
Inactive Ingredients: OGEN .625 tablet: Corn starch, D&C Yellow No. 10, FD&C Yellow No. 6, hydroxypropyl cellulose, lactose, methylparaben, piperazine, propylparaben, stearic acid and talc.
OGEN 1.25 tablet: Corn starch, FD&C Yellow No. 6, hydroxypropyl cellulose, lactose, methylparaben, piperazine, propylparaben, stearic acid and talc.
OGEN 2.5 tablet: Corn starch, FD&C Blue No. 2, hydroxypropyl cellulose, lactose, methylparaben, piperazine, propylparaben, stearic acid and talc.
OGEN 5 tablet: Corn starch, D&C Yellow No. 10, FD&C Blue No. 2, hydroxypropyl cellulose, lactose, methylparaben, piperazine, propylparaben, stearic acid and talc.
The base of OGEN Vaginal Cream is composed of the following ingredients: glycerin, mineral oil, glyceryl monostearate, polyethylene glycol ether complex of higher fatty alcohols, cetyl alcohol, anhydrous lanolin, sodium biphosphate, cis-N-(3-chloroallyl) hexaminium chloride, propylparaben, methylparaben, piperazine hexahydrate, citric acid and water.

CLINICAL PHARMACOLOGY

Estrogens are important in the development and maintenance of the female reproductive system and secondary sex characteristics. They promote growth and development of the vagina, uterus, and fallopian tubes, and enlargement of the breasts. Indirectly, they contribute to the shaping of the skeleton, maintenance of tone and elasticity of urogenital structures, changes in the epiphyses of the long bones that allow for the pubertal growth spurt and its termination, growth of axillary and pubic hair, and pigmentation of the nipples and genitals. Along with other hormones such as progesterone, estrogens are intricately involved in the process of menstruation. Estrogens also affect the release of pituitary gonadotropins.
OGEN (estropipate) owes its therapeutic action to estrone, one of the three principal estrogenic steroid hormones of man: estradiol, estrone, and estriol. Estradiol is rapidly hydrolyzed in the body to estrone, which in turn may be hydrated to the less active estriol. These transformations occur readily, mainly in the liver, where there is also free interconversion between estrone and estradiol.
A depletion of endogenous estrogens occurs postmenopausally as a result of a decline in ovarian function, and may cause symptomatic vulvovaginal atrophy. The signs and symptoms of these atrophic changes in the vaginal and vulval epithelia may be alleviated by the topical application of an estrogenic hormone such as OGEN.
Gastrointestinal absorption of orally administered estrogens is usually prompt and complete. OGEN Vaginal Cream may be absorbed transmucosally and may produce systemic estrogenic effects. Inactivation of estrogens in the body occurs mainly in the liver. During cyclic passage through the liver, estrogens are degraded to less active estrogenic compounds and conjugated with sulfuric and glucuronic acids. Estrone is 50–80% bound to protein as it circulates in the blood, primarily as a conjugate with sulfate.

INDICATIONS AND USAGE

The cyclic administration (See "DOSAGE AND ADMINISTRATION" section) of OGEN Tablets is indicated for the treatment of estrogen deficiency associated with:

1. Moderate to severe *vasomotor* symptoms of menopause. (There is no evidence that estrogens are effective for nervous symptoms or depression which might occur during menopause, and they should not be used to treat these conditions.)

2. Atrophic vaginitis.

3. Kraurosis vulvae.

4. Female hypogonadism.

5. Female castration.

6. Primary ovarian failure.

The cyclic administration of OGEN Vaginal Cream is indicated for the treatment of atrophic vaginitis or kraurosis vulvae. (See "DOSAGE AND ADMINISTRATION" section.)

OGEN (ESTROPIPATE) HAS NOT BEEN TESTED FOR EFFICACY FOR ANY PURPOSE DURING PREGNANCY. SINCE ITS EFFECT UPON THE FETUS IS UNKNOWN, IT CANNOT BE RECOMMENDED FOR ANY CONDITION DURING PREGNANCY (SEE BOXED WARNING).

Concomitant Progestin Use: The lowest effective dose appropriate for the specific indication should be utilized. Studies of the addition of a progestin for seven or more days of a cycle of estrogen administration have reported a lowered incidence of endometrial hyperplasia. Morphological and biochemical studies of endometrium suggest that 10 to 13 days of progestin are needed to provide maximal maturation of the endometrium and to eliminate any hyperplastic changes. Whether this will provide protection from endometrial carcinoma has not been clearly established. There are possible additional risks which may be associated with the inclusion of progestin in estrogen replacement regimens. (See "PRECAUTIONS" section.) The choice of progestin and dosage may be important in minimizing these adverse effects.

CONTRAINDICATIONS

OGEN should not be used in women with any of the following conditions:

1. Known or suspected cancer of the breast.

2. Known or suspected estrogen-dependent neoplasia.

3. OGEN may cause fetal harm when administered to a pregnant woman. OGEN is contraindicated in women who are or may become pregnant (See Boxed Warning).

4. Undiagnosed abnormal genital bleeding.

5. Active thrombophlebitis or thromboembolic disorders.

6. A past history of thrombophlebitis, thrombosis, or thromboembolic disorders associated with previous estrogen use.

OGEN Vaginal Cream is contraindicated in patient's hypersensitive to its ingredients.

WARNINGS

1. *Induction of malignant neoplasms.* Long-term continuous administration of natural and synthetic estrogens in certain animal species has been reported by some investigators to increase the frequency of carcinomas of the breast, cervix, vagina, and liver. There is now evidence that estrogens increase the risk of carcinoma of the endometrium in humans. (See Boxed Warning).

At the present time there is no conclusive evidence that estrogens given to postmenopausal women increase the risk of cancer of the breast.[17,40,41] There are, however, a few retrospective studies which suggest a small but statistically significant increase in the risk factor for breast cancer among these women.[18,42–44] Therefore, caution should be exercised when administering estrogens to women with a strong family history of breast cancer or who have breast nodules, fibrocystic disease, or abnormal mammograms. Careful breast examinations should be performed periodically.

2. *Gallbladder disease.* A recent study has reported a 2 to 3-fold increase in the risk of surgically confirmed gallbladder disease in women receiving postmenopausal estrogens,[17] similar to the 2-fold increase previously noted in users of oral contraceptives.[19,22] In the case of oral contraceptives, the increased risk appeared after two years of use.[22]

3. *Effects similar to those caused by estrogen-progestogen oral contraceptives.* There are several serious adverse effects of oral contraceptives, most of which have not, up to now, been documented as consequences of postmenopausal estrogen therapy. This may reflect the comparatively low doses of estrogen used in postmenopausal women. It would be expected that the larger doses of estrogen used to treat postpartum breast engorgement would be more likely to result in these adverse effects, and, in fact, it has been shown that there is an increased risk of thrombosis in women receiving estrogens for postpartum breast engorgement.[20,21]

a. *Thromboembolic disease.* It is now well established that users of oral contraceptives have an increased risk of various thromboembolic and thrombotic vascular diseases, such as thrombophlebitis, pulmonary embolism, stroke, and myocardial infarction.[22–29] Cases of retinal thrombosis, mesenteric thrombosis, and optic neuritis have been reported in oral contraceptive users. There is evidence that the risk of several of these adverse reactions is related to the dose of the drug.[30,31] An increased risk of post-surgery thromboembolic complications has also been reported in users of oral contraceptives.[32,33] If feasible, estrogen should be discontinued at least 4 weeks before surgery of the type associated with an

increased risk of thromboembolism; it should also be discontinued during periods of prolonged immobilization.

While an increased rate of thromboembolic and thrombotic disease in postmenopausal users of estrogens has not been found[17,34] this does not rule out the possibility that such an increase may be present or that subgroups of women who have underlying risk factors or who are receiving relatively large doses of estrogens may have increased risk. Therefore estrogens should not be used in persons with active thrombophlebitis or thromboembolic disorders, and they should not be used in persons with a history of such disorders in association with estrogen use. They should be used with caution in patients with cerebral vascular or coronary artery disease and only for those in whom estrogens are clearly needed. Large doses of estrogen (5 mg conjugated estrogens per day), comparable to those used to treat cancer of the prostate and breast, have been shown in a large prospective clinical trial in men[35] to increase the risk of nonfatal myocardial infarction, pulmonary embolism and thrombophlebitis. When estrogen doses of this size are used, any of the thromboembolic and thrombotic adverse effects associated with oral contraceptive use should be considered a clear risk.

b. *Hepatic adenoma.* Benign hepatic adenomas appear to be associated with the use of oral contraceptives.[36–38] Although benign, and rare, these may rupture and cause death through intraabdominal hemorrhage. Such lesions have not yet been reported in association with other estrogen or progestogen preparations but should be considered in estrogen users having abdominal pain and tenderness, abdominal mass, or hypovolemic shock. Hepatocellular carcinoma has also been reported in women taking estrogen-containing oral contraceptives.[37] The relationship of this malignancy to these drugs is not known at this time.

c. *Elevated blood pressure.* Increased blood pressure is not uncommon in women using oral contraceptives. There is now a report that this may occur with use of estrogens in the menopause[39] and blood pressure should be monitored with estrogen use, especially if high doses are used.

d. *Glucose tolerance.* A worsening of glucose tolerance has been observed in a significant percentage of patients on estrogen-containing oral contraceptives. For this reason, diabetic patients should be carefully observed while receiving estrogen.

4. *Hypercalcemia.* Administration of estrogens may lead to severe hypercalcemia in patients with breast cancer and bone metastases. If this occurs, the drug should be stopped and appropriate measures taken to reduce the serum calcium level.

PRECAUTIONS

A. General Precautions.

1. A complete medical and family history should be taken prior to the initiation of any estrogen therapy. The pretreatment and periodic physical examinations should include special reference to blood pressure, breasts, abdomen, and pelvic organs, and should include a Papanicolau smear. As a general rule, estrogen should not be prescribed for longer than one year without another physical examination being performed.

2. Diagnostic measures should be taken to rule out gonorrhea or neoplasia before prescribing OGEN Vaginal Cream. Trichomonal, monilial, or bacterial infection should be treated by appropriate anti-microbial therapy.

3. Fluid retention—Estrogens may cause some degree of fluid retention. Therefore, patients with conditions such as epilepsy, migraine, and cardiac or renal dysfunction, which might be influenced by this factor, require careful observation.

4. Certain patients may develop undesirable manifestations of excessive estrogenic stimulation, such as abnormal or excessive uterine bleeding, mastodynia, etc.

5. Oral contraceptives appear to be associated with an increased incidence of mental depression.[22] Although it is not clear whether this is due to the estrogenic or progestogenic component of the contraceptive, patients with a history of depression should be carefully observed.

6. Preexisting uterine leiomyomata may increase in size during estrogen use.

7. The pathologist should be advised of the patient's use of estrogen therapy when relevant specimens are submitted.

8. Patients with a past history of jaundice during pregnancy have an increased risk of recurrence of jaundice while receiving estrogen-containing oral contraceptive therapy. If jaundice develops in any patient receiving estrogen, the medication should be discontinued while the cause is investigated.

9. Estrogens may be poorly metabolized in patients with impaired liver function and they should be administered with caution in such patients.

10. Because estrogens influence the metabolism of calcium and phosphorus, they should be used with caution in patients with metabolic bone diseases that are associated with hypercalcemia or in patients with renal insufficiency.

11. Concomitant Progestin Use: The lowest effective dose appropriate for the specific indication should be utilized. Studies of the addition of a progestin for seven or more days

of a cycle of estrogen administration have reported a lowered incidence of endometrial hyperplasia. Morphological and biochemical studies of endometrium suggest that 10 to 13 days of progestin are needed to provide maximal maturation of the endometrium and to eliminate any hyperplastic changes. Whether this will provide protection from endometrial carcinoma has not been clearly established. There are possible additional risks which may be associated with the inclusion of progestin in estrogen replacement regimens. The potential risks may include adverse effects on carbohydrate and lipid metabolism. The choice of progestin and dosage may be important in minimizing these adverse effects.

B. Information for the Patient. See text of Patient Package Insert which appears after PHYSICIAN REFERENCES.

C. Drug Interactions. The concomitant use of any drugs which can induce hepatic microsomal enzymes with estrogens may produce estrogen levels which are lower than would be expected from the dose of estrogen administered. The use of *broad spectrum antibiotics* which profoundly effect intestinal flora may influence the oral absorption of steroidal compounds including the estrogens.

Diabetics receiving *insulin* may have increased insulin requirements when receiving estrogens.

Laboratory Test Interference. Certain endocrine and liver function tests may be affected by estrogen-containing oral contraceptives. The following similar changes may be expected with larger doses of estrogen:

a. Increased sulfobromophthalein retention.

b. Increased prothrombin and factors VII, VIII, IX, and X; decreased antithrombin 3; increased norepinephrine-induced platelet aggregability.

c. Increased thyroid binding globulin (TBG) leading to increased circulating total thyroid hormone, as measured by PBI, T4 by column, or T4 by radioimmunoassay. Free T3 resin uptake is decreased, reflecting the elevated TBG; free T4 concentration is unaltered.

d. Abnormal glucose tolerance test results.

e. Decreased pregnanediol excretion.

f. Reduced response to metyrapone test.

g. Reduced serum folate concentration.

h. Increased serum triglyceride and phospholipid concentration.

D. Carcinogenesis. Studies have shown an increased risk of endometrial cancer in postmenopausal women exposed to exogenous estrogens for prolonged periods (see Boxed Warning). At the present time there is no conclusive evidence that estrogens given to postmenopausal women increase the risk of cancer of the breast.[17,40,41] There are, however, a few retrospective studies which suggest a small but statistically significant increase in the risk factor for breast cancer among these women.[18,42–44] (See "WARNINGS" section.)

E. Pregnancy. Pregnancy Category X. See "CONTRAINDICATIONS" section and Boxed Warning.

F. Nursing Mothers. Estrogens have been reported to be excreted in human breast milk. Caution should be excercised when OGEN (estropipate) is administered to a nursing woman.

G. Pediatric Use. Because of the effects of estrogens on epiphyseal closure, they should be used judiciously in young patients in whom bone growth is not complete.

ADVERSE REACTIONS

Hypersensitivity reactions, systemic effects such as breast tenderness, and rarely, withdrawal bleeding, have occurred with the use of topical estrogens. Local irritation (especially when prior inflammation is present) has occurred at initiation of therapy.

(See Warnings regarding reports of possible induction of neoplasia, unknown effects upon the fetus, increased incidence of gallbladder disease, and adverse effects similar to those of oral contraceptives, including thromboembolism.) The following additional adverse reactions in decreasing order of severity within each category have been reported with estrogenic therapy, including oral contraceptives:

1. *Genitourinary system.*

Increase in size of uterine fibromyomata.

Vaginal candidiasis.

Cystitis-like syndrome.

Dysmenorrhea.

Amenorrhea during and after treatment.

Change in cervical eversion and in degree of cervical secretion.

Breakthrough bleeding, spotting, change in menstrual flow.

Premenstrual-like syndrome.

2. *Breast.*

Tenderness, enlargement, secretion.

3. *Gastrointestinal.*

Cholestatic jaundice.

Vomiting, nausea.

Abdominal cramps, bloating.

Continued on next page

Abbott Laboratories—Cont.

4. *Skin.*
Hemorrhagic eruption.
Erythema nodosum.
Erythema multiforme.
Hirsutism.
Chloasma or melasma which may persist when drug is discontinued.
Loss of scalp hair.
5. *Eyes.*
Steepening of corneal curvature.
Intolerance to contact lenses.
6. *CNS.*
Chorea.
Mental depression.
Migraine, dizziness, headache.
7. *Miscellaneous.*
Aggravation of porphyria.
Edema.
Reduced carbohydrate tolerance.
Increase or decrease in weight.
Changes in libido.

OVERDOSAGE

Numerous reports of ingestion of large doses of estrogen-containing oral contraceptives by young children indicate that serious ill effects do not occur. Overdosage of estrogen may cause nausea and withdrawal bleeding may occur in females.

DOSAGE AND ADMINISTRATION

OGEN (estropipate) Tablets:
1. *Given cyclically for short-term use:*
For treatment of moderate to severe *vasomotor* symptoms, atrophic vaginitis, or kraurosis vulvae associated with the menopause.
The lowest dose that will control symptoms should be chosen and medication should be discontinued as promptly as possible.
Administration should be cyclic (e.g., 3 weeks on and 1 week off).
Attempts to discontinue or taper medication should be made at 3 to 6 month intervals.
Usual dosage ranges:
Vasomotor symptoms—One OGEN .625 (estropipate) Tablet to one OGEN 5 Tablet per day. The lowest dose that will control symptoms should be chosen. If the patient has not menstruated within the last two months or more, cyclic administration is started arbitrarily. If the patient is menstruating, cyclic administration is started on day 5 of bleeding.
Atrophic vaginitis and kraurosis vulvae—One OGEN .625 Tablet to one OGEN 5 Tablet daily, depending upon the tissue response of the individual patient. The lowest dose that will control symptoms should be chosen. Administer cyclically.
2. *Given cyclically:*
Female hypogonadism; female castration; primary ovarian failure.
Usual dosage ranges:
Female hypogonadism—A daily dose of one OGEN 1.25 Tablet to three OGEN 2.5 Tablets may be given for the first three weeks of a theoretical cycle, followed by a rest period of eight to ten days. The lowest dose that will control symptoms should be chosen. If bleeding does not occur by the end of this period, the same dosage schedule is repeated. The number of courses of estrogen therapy necessary to produce bleeding may vary depending on the responsiveness of the endometrium. If satisfactory withdrawal bleeding does not occur, an oral progestogen may be given in addition to estrogen during the third week of the cycle.
Female castration and primary ovarian failure—A daily dose of one OGEN 1.25 Tablet to three OGEN 2.5 Tablets may be given for the first three weeks of a theoretical cycle, followed by a rest period of eight to ten days. Adjust dosage upward or downward according to severity of symptoms and response of the patient. For maintenance, adjust dosage to lowest level that will provide effective control.
Treated patients with an intact uterus should be monitored closely for signs of endometrial cancer and appropriate diagnostic measures should be taken to rule out malignancy in the event of persistent or recurring abnormal vaginal bleeding.
OGEN (estropipate) Vaginal Cream:
To be administered cyclically for short-term use only:
For treatment of atrophic vaginitis or kraurosis vulvae.
The lowest dose that will control symptoms should be chosen and medication should be discontinued as promptly as possible.
Administration should be cyclic (e.g., three weeks on and one week off).
Attempts to discontinue or taper medication should be made at three to six-month intervals.
Treated patients with an intact uterus should be monitored closely for signs of endometrial cancer and appropriate diagnostic measures should be taken to rule out malignancy in the event of persistent or recurring abnormal vaginal bleeding.
Usual dosage: Intravaginally, 2 to 4 grams of OGEN Vaginal Cream daily, depending upon the severity of the condition.
The following instructions for use are intended for the patient and are printed on the carton label for OGEN Vaginal Cream (estropipate).
1. Remove cap from tube.
2. Make sure plunger of applicator is all the way into the barrel.
3. Screw nozzle end of applicator onto the tube.
4. Squeeze tube to force sufficient cream into applicator so that number on plunger indicating prescribed dose is level with top of barrel.
5. Unscrew applicator from tube and replace cap on tube.
6. To deliver medication, insert end of applicator into vagina and push plunger all the way down.
Between uses, pull plunger out of barrel and wash applicator in warm, soapy water. DO NOT PUT APPLICATOR IN HOT OR BOILING WATER.

HOW SUPPLIED

OGEN (estropipate tablets, USP) is supplied as OGEN .625 (0.75 mg estropipate), yellow tablets, **NDC** 0074-3943-04; OGEN 1.25 (1.5 mg estropipate), peach-colored tablets, **NDC** 0074-3946-04; OGEN 2.5 (3 mg estropipate), blue tablets, **NDC** 0074-3951-04; and OGEN 5 (6 mg estropipate), light green tablets, **NDC** 0074-3958-13. Tablets of all four dosage levels are standardized to provide uniform estrone activity and are grooved (Divide-Tab®) to provide dosage flexibility. All tablet sizes of OGEN are available in bottles of 100.
Store tablets below 77°F (25°C).
OGEN (estropipate vaginal cream, USP), 1.5 mg estropipate per gram, is available in packages containing a 1½ oz (42.5 Gm) tube with one plastic applicator calibrated at 1, 2, 3, and 4 Gm levels. (**NDC** 0074-2467-42).

PHYSICIAN REFERENCES

[1]Ziel, H. K., Finkel, W. D., "Increased Risk of Endometrial Carcinoma Among Users of Conjugated Estrogens", *New England Journal of Medicine,* 293:1167–1170, 1975.
[2]Smith, D. C., Prentic, R., Thompson, D. J., et al., "Association of Exogenous Estrogen and Endometrial Carcinoma," *New England Journal of Medicine,* 293:1164–1167, 1975.
[3]Mack, T. M., Pike, M. C., Henderson, B. E., et al., "Estrogens and Endometrial Cancer in a Retirement Community," *New England Journal of Medicine,* 294:1262–1267, 1976.
[4]Weiss, N. S., Szekely, D. R., Austin, D. F., "Increasing Incidence of Endometrial Cancer in the United States," *New England Journal of Medicine,* 294:1259–1262, 1976.
[5]Herbst, A. L., Ulfelder, H., Poskanzer, D. C., "Adenocarcinoma of Vagina," *New England Journal of Medicine,* 284:878–881, 1971.
[6]Greenwald, P., Barlow, J., Nasca, P., et al., "Vaginal Cancer after Maternal Treatment with Synthetic Estrogens," *New England Journal of Medicine,* 285:390–392, 1971.
[7]Lanier, A., Noller, K., Decker, D., et al., "Cancer and Stilbestrol. A Follow-up of 1719 Persons Exposed to Estrogens In Utero and Born 1943–1959," *Mayo Clinic Proceedings,* 48:793–799, 1973.
[8]Herbst, A., Kurman, R., Scully, R., "Vaginal and Cervical Abnormalities After Exposure to Stilbestrol In Utero" *Obstetrics and Gynecology,* 40:287–298, 1972.
[9]Herbst, A., Robboy, S., Madonald, G., et al., "The Effects of Local Progesterone on Stilbestrol-Associated Vaginal Adenosis," *American Journal of Obstetrics and Gynecology,* 118:607–615, 1974.
[10]Herbst, A., Poskanzer, D., Robboy, S., et al., "Prenatal Exposure to Stilbestrol, A Prospective Comparison of Exposed Female Offspring with Unexposed Controls," *New England Journal of Medicine,* 292:334–339, 1975.
[11]Stafl, A., Mattingly, R., Foley, D., et al., "Clinical Diagnosis of Vaginal Adenosis," *Obstetrics and Gynecology,* 43:118–128, 1974.
[12]Sherman, A. I., Goldrath, M., Berlin, A., et al., "Cervical-Vaginal Adenosis After *In Utero* Exposure to Synthetic Estrogens," *Obstetrics and Gynecology,* 44:531–545, 1974.
[13]Gal, I., Kirman, B., Stern, J., "Hormone Pregnancy Tests and Congenital Malformation," *Nature,* 216:83, 1967.
[14]Levy, E. P., Cohen, A., Fraser, F. C., "Hormone Treatment During Pregnancy and Congenital Heart Defects," *Lancet* 1:611, 1973.
[15]Nora, J., Nora, A., "Birth Defects and Oral Contraceptives," *Lancet,* 1:941–942, 1973.
[16]Janerich, D. T., Piper, J. M., Clebatis, D. M., "Oral Contraceptives and Congenital Limb-Reduction Defects," *New England Journal of Medicine,* 291:697–700, 1974.
[17]Boston Collaborative Drug Surveillance Program "Surgically Confirmed Gall Bladder Disease, Venous Thromboembolism and Breast Tumors in Relation to Post-Menopausal Estrogen Therapy," *New England Journal of Medicine,* 290:15–19, 1974.
[18]Brinton, L. A., Hoover, R. N., Szklo, M., et al., "Menopausal Estrogen Use and Risk of Breast Cancer," *Cancer,* 47(10): 2517–2522, 1981.
[19]Boston Collaborative Drug Surveillance Program, "Oral Contraceptives and Venous Thromboembolic Disease, Surgically Confirmed Gall Bladder Disease and Breast Tumors," *Lancet* 1:1399–1404, 1973.
[20]Daniel, D. G., Campbell, H., Turnbull, A. C., "Puerperal Thromboembolism and Suppression of Lactation," *Lancet,* 2:287–289, 1967.
[21]Bailar, J. C., "Thromboembolism and Oestrogen Therapy," *Lancet,* 2:560, 1967.
[22]Royal College of General Practitioners, "Oral Contraception and Thromboembolic Disease," *Journal of the Royal College of General Practitioners,* 13:267–279, 1967.
[23]Inman, W. H. W., Vessey, M. P., "Investigation of Deaths from Pulmonary, Coronary, and Cerebral Thrombosis and Embolism in Women of Child-Bearing Age," *British Medical Journal,* 2:193–199, 1968.
[24]Vessey, M. P., Doll, R., "Investigation of Relation Between Use of Oral Contraceptives and Thromboembolic Disease. A Further Report," *British Medical Journal,* 2:651–657, 1969.
[25]Sartwell, P. E., Masi, A. T., Arthes, F. G., et al., "Thromboembolism and Oral Contraceptives: An Epidemiological Case Control Study," *American Journal of Epidemiology,* 90:365–380, 1969.
[26]Collaborative Group for the Study of Stroke in Young Women, "Oral Contraception and Increased Risk of Cerebral Ischemia or Thrombosis," *New England Journal of Medicine,* 288:871–878, 1973.
[27]Collaborative Group for the Study of Stroke in Young Women, "Oral Contraceptives and Stroke in Young Women: Associated Risk Factors," *Journal of the American Medical Association,* 231:718–722, 1975.
[28]Mann, J. I., Inman, W. H. W., "Oral Contraceptives and Death from Myocardial Infarction," *British Medical Journal,* 2:245–248, 1975.
[29]Mann, J. I., Vessey, M. P., Thorogood, M., et al., "Myocardial Infarction in Young Women with Special Reference to Oral Contraceptive Practice," *British Medical Journal,* 2:241–245, 1975.
[30]Inman, W. H. W., Vessey, M. P., Westerholm, B., et al., "Thromboembolic Disease and the Steroidal Content of Oral Contraceptives," *British Medical Journal,* 2:203–209, 1970.
[31]Stolley, P. D., Tonascia, J. A., Tockman, M. S., et al., "Thrombosis with Low-Estrogen Oral Contraceptives," *American Journal of Epidemiology,* 102:197–208, 1975.
[32]Vessey, M. P., Doll, R., Fairbairn, A. S., et al., "Post-Operative Thromboembolism and the Use of the Oral Contraceptives," *British Medical Journal,* 3:123–126, 1970.
[33]Greene, G. R., Sartwell, P. E., "Oral Contraceptive Use in Patients with Thromboembolism Following Surgery, Trauma or Infection," *American Journal of Public Health,* 62:680–685, 1972.
[34]Rosenberg, L., Armstrong, M. B., Jick, H., "Myocardial Infarction and Estrogen Therapy in Postmenopausal Women," *New England Journal of Medicine,* 294:1256–1259, 1976.
[35]Coronary Drug Project Research Group, "The Coronary Drug Project: Initial Findings Leading to Modifications of Its Research Protocol," *Journal of the American Medical Association,* 214:1303–1313, 1970.
[36]Baum, J., Holtz, F., Bookstein, J. J., et al., "Possible Association Between Benign Hepatomas and Oral Contraceptives," *Lancet,* 2:926–928, 1973.
[37]Mays, E. T., Christopherson, W. M., Mahr, M. M., et al., "Hepatic Changes in Young Women Ingesting Contraceptive Steroids, Hepatic Hemorrhage and Primary Hepatic Tumors," *Journal of the American Medical Association,* 235:730–782, 1976.
[38]Edmondson, H. A., Henderson, B., Benton, B., "Liver Cell Adenomas Associated with the Use of Oral Contraceptives," *New England Journal of Medicine,* 294:470–472, 1976.
[39]Pfeffer, R. I., Van Den Noort, S., "Estrogen Use and Stroke Risk in Postmenopausal Women," *American Journal of Epidemiology,* 103:445–456, 1976.
[40]Gambrell, R. D., Massey, F. M., Castaneda, T. A., et al., "Estrogen Therapy and Breast Cancer in Postmenopausal Women," *Journal of the American Geriatrics Society,* 28(6): 251–257, 1980.
[41]Kelsey, J. L., Fischer, D. B., Holford, T. R., et al., "Exogenous Estrogens and Other Factors in the Epidemiology of Breast Cancer," *Journal of the National Cancer Institute,* 57(2):327–333, 1981.
[42]Ross, R. K., Paganini-Hill, A., Gerkins, V., et al., "A Case-Control Study of Menopausal Estrogen Therapy and Breast Cancer," *Journal of the American Medical Association,* 243(16):1635–1639, 1980.
[43]Hoover, R., Glass, A., Finkle, W. D., et al., "Conjugated Estrogens and Breast Cancer Risk in Women," *Journal of the National Cancer Institute,* 67(4):815–820, 1981.
[44]Lawson, D. H., Jick, H., Hunter, J. R., et al., "Exogenous Estrogens and Breast Cancer," *American Journal of Epidemiology,* 114(5):710, 1981.

INFORMATION FOR PATIENTS
OGEN®
(estropipate tablets and vaginal cream, USP)

Estrogen cream is used for the local treatment of certain symptoms of estrogen deficiency: the soreness and itching of the vagina and vulva caused by drying and thinning (atrophy) of these tissues.

The discussion that follows is about estrogens that are taken internally for the treatment of symptoms of estrogen deficiency. Some or all of the information below on the systemic use of estrogens may also apply to the estrogen cream.

WHAT YOU SHOULD KNOW ABOUT ESTROGENS: Estrogens are female hormones produced by the ovaries. The ovaries make several different kinds of estrogens. In addition, scientists have been able to make a variety of synthetic estrogens. As far as we know, all these estrogens have similar properties and therefore much the same usefulness, side effects, and risks. This leaflet is intended to help you understand what estrogens are used for, the risks involved in their use, and how to use them as safely as possible.

This leaflet includes the most important information about estrogens, but not all the information. If you want to know more, you can ask your doctor or pharmacist to let you read the package insert prepared for the doctor.

Uses of Estrogen: Estrogens are prescribed by doctors for a number of purposes, including:

1. To provide estrogen during a period of adjustment when a woman's ovaries no longer produce it, in order to prevent certain uncomfortable symptoms of estrogen deficiency. (All women normally stop producing estrogens, generally between the ages of 45 and 55; this is called the menopause.)

2. To prevent symptoms of estrogen deficiency when a woman's ovaries have been removed surgically before the natural menopause.

3. To prevent pregnancy. (Estrogens are given along with a progestogen, another female hormone; these combinations are called oral contraceptives or birth control pills. Patient labeling is available to women taking oral contraceptives and they will not be discussed in this leaflet.)

THERE IS NO PROPER USE OF OGEN (ESTROPIPATE) IN A PREGNANT WOMAN.

Estrogens in the Menopause: In the natural course of their lives, all women eventually experience a decrease in estrogen production. This usually occurs between ages 45 and 55 but may occur earlier or later. Sometimes the ovaries may need to be removed before natural menopause by an operation, producing a "surgical menopause."

When the amount of estrogen in the blood begins to decrease, many women may develop typical symptoms: Feelings of warmth in the face, neck, and chest or sudden intense episodes of heat and sweating throughout the body (called "hot flashes" or "hot flushes"). These symptoms are sometimes very uncomfortable. A few women eventually develop changes in the vagina (called "atrophic vaginitis") which cause discomfort, especially during and after intercourse. Estrogens can be prescribed to treat these symptoms of the menopause. It is estimated that considerably more than half of all women undergoing the menopause have only mild symptoms or no symptoms at all and therefore do not need estrogens. Other women may need estrogens for a few months, while their bodies adjust to lower estrogen levels. Sometimes the need will be for periods longer than six months. In an attempt to avoid over-stimulation of the uterus (womb), estrogens are usually given cyclically during each month of use, that is three weeks of pills followed by one week without pills.

Sometimes women experience nervous symptoms or depression during menopause. There is no evidence that estrogens are effective for such symptoms and they should not be used to treat them, although other treatment may be needed.

You may have heard that taking estrogens for long periods (years) after the menopause will keep your skin soft and supple and keep you feeling young. There is no evidence that this is so, however, and such long-term treatment carries important risks.

The Dangers of Estrogens: 1. *Cancer of the uterus.* If estrogens are used in the postmenopausal period for more than a year, there is an increased risk of *endometrial cancer* (cancer of the uterus). Women taking estrogens have roughly 5 to 10 times as great a chance of getting this cancer as women who take no estrogens. To put this another way, while a postmenopausal woman not taking estrogens has 1 chance in 1,000 each year of getting cancer of the uterus, a woman taking estrogens has 5 to 10 chances in 1,000 each year. For this reason *it is important to take estrogens only when you really need them.*

The risk of this cancer is greater the longer estrogens are used and also seems to be greater when larger doses are taken. For this reason *it is important to take the lowest dose of estrogen that will control symptoms and to take it only as long as it is needed.* If estrogens are needed for longer periods of time, your doctor will want to reevaluate your need for estrogens at least every six months.

Women using estrogens should report any irregular vaginal bleeding to their doctors; such bleeding may be of no importance, but it can be an early warning of cancer of the uterus.

If you have undiagnosed vaginal bleeding, you should not use estrogens until a diagnosis is made and you are certain there is no cancer of the uterus.

If you have had your uterus completely removed (total hysterectomy), there is no danger of developing cancer of the uterus.

2. *Other possible cancers.* Estrogens can cause development of other tumors in animals, such as tumors of the breast, cervix, vagina, or liver, when given for a long time. At present there is no good evidence that women using estrogen in the menopause have an increased risk of such tumors, but there is no way yet to be sure they do not; and one study raises the possibility that use of estrogens in the menopause may increase the risk of breast cancer many years later. This is a further reason to use estrogens only when clearly needed. While you are taking estrogens, it is important that you go to your doctor at least once a year for a physical examination. Also, if members of your family have had breast cancer or if you have breast nodules or abnormal mammograms (breast x-rays), your doctor may wish to carry out more frequent examinations of your breasts.

3. *Gallbladder disease.* Women who use estrogens after menopause are more likely to develop gallbladder disease needing surgery than women who do not use estrogens. Birth control pills have a similar effect.

4. *Abnormal blood clotting.* Oral contraceptives increase the risk of blood clotting in various parts of the body. This can result in a stroke (if the clot is in the brain), a heart attack (clot in a blood vessel of the heart), or a pulmonary embolus (a clot which forms in the legs or pelvis, then breaks off and travels to the lungs). Any of these can be fatal.

At this time use of estrogens in the menopause is not known to cause such blood clotting, but this has not been fully studied and there could still prove to be such a risk. It is recommended that if you have had clotting in the legs or lungs or a heart attack or stroke while you were using estrogens or birth control pills, you should not use estrogens. If you have had a stroke or heart attack or if you have angina pectoris, estrogens should be used with great caution and only if clearly needed (for example, if you have severe symptoms of the menopause).

Special Warning About Pregnancy: You should not receive OGEN (estropipate) if you are pregnant. Some scientists have reported that if estrogens are used during pregnancy, there may be a greater than usual chance that the developing baby will be born with a birth defect, although the risk remains small. In addition, other scientists have reported that there is an association between another estrogen-type product (diethylstilbestrol) and appearance of a particular cancer of the vagina or cervix (adenocarcinoma) in young women whose mothers took that drug in pregnancy. Every effort should be made to avoid exposure to OGEN in pregnancy. If exposure occurs, see your doctor.

Other Effects of Estrogens: In addition to the serious known risks of estrogens described above estrogens have the following side effects and potential risks:

1. *Nausea and vomiting.* The most common side effect of estrogen therapy is nausea. Vomiting is less common.

2. *Effects on breasts.* Estrogens may cause breast tenderness or enlargement and may cause the breasts to secrete a liquid. These effects are not dangerous.

3. *Effects on the uterus.* Estrogens may cause benign fibroid tumors of the uterus to get larger.

Some women will have menstrual bleeding when estrogens are stopped. But if the bleeding occurs on days you are still taking estrogens you should report this to your doctor.

4. *Effects on liver.* Women taking oral contraceptives develop on rare occasions a tumor of the liver which can rupture and bleed into the abdomen. So far, these tumors have not been reported in women using estrogens in the menopause, but you should report any swelling or unusual pain or tenderness in the abdomen to your doctor immediately.

Women with a past history of jaundice (yellowing of the skin and white parts of the eyes) may get jaundice again during estrogen use. If this occurs, stop taking estrogens and see your doctor.

5. *Other effects.* Estrogens may cause excess fluid to be retained in the body. This may make some conditions worse, such as epilepsy, migraine, heart disease, or kidney disease.

SUMMARY

Estrogens have important uses, but they have serious risks as well. You must decide, with your doctor, whether the risks are acceptable to you in view of the benefits of treatment. You should not use OGEN (estropipate) if you have cancer of the breast or uterus, are pregnant, have undiagnosed abnormal vaginal bleeding, clotting in the legs or lungs, or have had a stroke, heart attack or angina, or clotting in the legs or lungs in the past while you were taking estrogens.

You can use estrogens as safely as possible by understanding that your doctor will require regular physical examinations while you are taking them and will try to discontinue the drug as soon as possible and use the smallest dose possible. Be alert for signs of trouble including:

1. Abnormal bleeding from the vagina.
2. Pains in the calves or chest or sudden shortness of breath, or coughing blood (indicating possible clots in the legs, heart or lungs).
3. Severe headache, dizziness, faintness, or changes in vision (indicating possible developing clots in the brain or eye).
4. Breast lumps (you should ask your doctor how to examine your own breasts).
5. Jaundice (yellowing of the skin).
6. Mental depression.

Based on his or her assessment of your medical needs, your doctor has prescribed this drug for you. Do not give the drug to anyone else.

Ref. 03-4380-R14 and 01-2305-R5

Shown in Product Identification Section, page 403

OPTILETS®-500   OTC
[ōp'ti-lets]
High potency multivitamin for use in treatment of multivitamin deficiency.

OPTILETS-M-500®
High potency multivitamin for use in treatment of multivitamin deficiency. Mineral supplementation added.

(See PDR For Nonprescription Drugs.)
Shown in Product Identification Section, page 403

ORETIC®   ℞
[ō-re'tic]
(hydrochlorothiazide tablets, USP)

DESCRIPTION

ORETIC (hydrochlorothiazide) is a member of the benzothiadiazine (thiazide) family of drugs. It is closely related to chlorothiazide. Clinically, hydrochlorothiazide is an orally active diuretic-antihypertensive agent.

Inactive Ingredients:

25 and 50 mg tablets: corn starch, lactose, magnesium stearate and talc.

ACTIONS

The diuretic and saluretic effects of hydrochlorothiazide result from a drug-induced inhibition of the renal tubular reabsorption of electrolytes. The excretion of sodium and chloride is greatly enhanced. Potassium excretion is also enhanced to a variable degree, as it is with the other thiazides. Although urinary excretion of bicarbonate is increased slightly, there is usually no significant change in urinary pH. Hydrochlorothiazide has a per mg natriuretic activity approximately 10 times that of the prototype thiazide, chlorothiazide. At maximal therapeutic dosages, all thiazides are approximately equal in their diuretic/natriuretic effects. There is significant natriuresis and diuresis within two hours after administration of a single oral dose of hydrochlorothiazide. These effects reach a peak in about 6 hours and persist for about 12 hours following oral administration of a single dose.

Like other benzothiadiazines, hydrochlorothiazide also has antihypertensive properties, and may be used for this purpose either alone or to enhance the antihypertensive action of other drugs. The mechanism by which the benzothiadiazines, including hydrochlorothiazide, produce a reduction of elevated blood pressure is not known. However, sodium depletion appears to be involved.

Hydrochlorothiazide is readily absorbed from the gastrointestinal tract and is excreted unchanged by the kidneys.

INDICATIONS

ORETIC (hydrochlorothiazide) is indicated in the management of hypertension either as the sole therapeutic agent or to enhance the effect of other antihypertensive drugs in the more severe forms of hypertension.

ORETIC tablets are indicated as adjunctive therapy in edema associated with congestive heart failure, hepatic cirrhosis, and corticosteroid and estrogen therapy.

ORETIC tablets have also been found useful in edema due to various forms of renal dysfunction such as the nephrotic syndrome, acute glomerulonephritis and chronic renal failure.

Usage in Pregnancy: The routine use of diuretics in an otherwise healthy pregnant woman is inappropriate and exposes mother and fetus to unnecessary hazard. Diuretics do not prevent development of toxemia of pregnancy, and there

Continued on next page

Abbott Laboratories—Cont.

is no satisfactory evidence that they are useful in the treatment of developed toxemia.

Edema during pregnancy may arise from pathological causes or from the physiological and mechanical consequences of pregnancy. Thiazides are indicated in pregnancy when edema is due to pathological causes, just as they are in the absence of pregnancy (see WARNINGS). Dependent edema in pregnancy, resulting from restriction of venous return by the expanded uterus, is properly treated through elevation of the lower extremities and use of support hose; use of diuretics to lower intravascular volume in this case is illogical and unnecessary. There is hypervolemia during normal pregnancy which is harmful to neither the fetus nor the mother (in the absence of cardiovascular disease), but which is associated with edema, including generalized edema, in the majority of pregnant women. If this edema produces discomfort, increased recumbency will often provide relief. In rare instances, this edema may cause extreme discomfort which is not relieved by rest. In these cases, a short course of diuretics may provide relief and may be appropriate.

CONTRAINDICATIONS

Renal decompensation.
Hypersensitivity to this or other sulfonamide-derived drugs.

WARNINGS

Hydrochlorothiazide shares with other thiazides the propensity to deplete potassium reserves to an unpredictable degree.

Thiazides should be used with caution in patients with renal disease or significant impairment of renal function, since azotemia may be precipitated and cumulative drug effects may occur.

Thiazides should be used with caution in patients with impaired hepatic function or progressive liver disease, since minor alterations of fluid and electrolyte balance may precipitate hepatic coma.

Thiazides may be additive or potentiative of the action of other antihypertensive drugs. Potentiation occurs with ganglionic or peripheral adrenergic blocking drugs.

Sensitivity reactions may occur in patients with a history of allergy or bronchial asthma.

The possibility of exacerbation or activation of systemic lupus erythematosus has been reported.

Usage in Pregnancy: Thiazides cross the placental barrier and appear in cord blood. The use of thiazides in pregnant women requires that the anticipated benefit be weighed against possible hazards to the fetus. These hazards include fetal or neonatal jaundice, thrombocytopenia, and possible other adverse reactions that have occurred in the adult.

Nursing Mothers: Thiazides appear in breast milk. If use of the drug is deemed essential, the patient should stop nursing.

PRECAUTIONS

Periodic determinations of serum electrolytes should be performed at appropriate intervals for the purpose of detecting possible electrolyte imbalances such as hyponatremia, hypochloremic alkalosis, and hypokalemia. Serum and urine electrolyte determinations are particularly important when a patient is vomiting excessively or receiving parenteral fluids. All patients should be observed for other clinical signs of electrolyte imbalances such as dryness of mouth, thirst, weakness, lethargy, drowsiness, restlessness, muscle pains or cramps, muscular fatigue, hypotension, oliguria, tachycardia, and gastrointestinal disturbances such as nausea and vomiting.

Hypokalemia may develop with thiazides as with any other potent diuretic, especially when brisk diuresis occurs, severe cirrhosis is present, or when corticosteroids or ACTH are given concomitantly. Interference with the adequate oral intake of electrolytes will also contribute to the possible development of hypokalemia. Potassium depletion, even of a mild degree, resulting from thiazide use, may sensitize a patient to the effects of cardiac glycosides such as digitalis. Any chloride deficit is generally mild and usually does not require specific treatment except under extraordinary circumstances (as in liver disease or renal disease). Dilutional hyponatremia may occur in edematous patients in hot weather; appropriate therapy is water restriction rather than administration of salt, except in rare instances when the hyponatremia is life threatening.

In actual salt depletion, appropriate replacement is the therapy of choice.

Hyperuricemia may occur or frank gout may be precipitated in certain patients receiving thiazide therapy.

Insulin requirements in diabetic patients may be increased, decreased, or unchanged. Latent diabetes mellitus may become manifest during thiazide administration.

Thiazide drugs may increase the responsiveness to tubocurarine.

The antihypertensive effects of the drug may be enhanced in the postsympathectomy patient.

Thiazides may decrease arterial responsiveness to norepinephrine. This diminution is not sufficient to preclude effectiveness of the pressor agent for therapeutic use.

If progressive renal impairment becomes evident as indicated by a rising-nonprotein nitrogen or blood urea nitrogen, a careful reappraisal of therapy is necessary with consideration given to withholding or discontinuing diuretic therapy. Thiazides may decrease serum PBI levels without signs of thyroid disturbance.

Thiazides have been reported, on rare occasions, to have elevated serum calcium to hypercalcemic levels. The serum calcium levels have returned to normal when the medication has been stopped. This phenomenon may be related to the ability of the thiazide diuretics to lower the amount of calcium excreted in the urine.

ADVERSE REACTIONS

Gastrointestinal system reactions: Anorexia, gastric irritation, nausea, vomiting, cramping, diarrhea, constipation, jaundice (intrahepatic cholestatic jaundice), pancreatitis.

Central nervous system reactions: Dizziness, vertigo, paresthesias, headache, xanthopsia.

Hematologic reactions: Leukopenia, agranulocytosis, thrombocytopenia, aplastic anemia.

Dermatologic — hypersensitivity reactions: Purpura, photosensitivity, rash, urticaria, necrotizing angiitis (vasculitis) (cutaneous vasculitis).

Cardiovascular reaction: Orthostatic hypotension may occur and may be aggravated by alcohol, barbiturates, or narcotics.

Other: Hyperglycemia, glycosuria, hypercalcemia, hyperuricemia, muscle spasm, weakness, restlessness, respiratory distress including pneumonitis and pulmonary edema.

There have been isolated reports that certain nonedematous individuals developed severe fluid and electrolyte derangements after only brief exposure to normal doses of thiazide and non-thiazide diuretics. The condition is usually manifested as severe dilutional hyponatremia, hypokalemia, and hypochloremia. It has been reported to be due to inappropriately increased ADH secretion and appears to be idiosyncratic. Potassium replacement is apparently the most important therapy in the treatment of this syndrome along with removal of the offending drug.

Whenever adverse reactions are severe, treatment should be discontinued.

DOSAGE AND ADMINISTRATION

Oretic (hydrochlorothiazide) is administered orally. Therapy should be individualized according to patient response. This therapy should be titrated to gain maximal therapeutic response as well as the minimal dose possible to maintain that therapeutic response.

For the management of edema the adult dosage ranges from 25 to 200 mg daily and may be given in single or divided doses. Usually 75 to 100 mg will produce the desired diuretic effect.

For the management of hypertension the usual initial adult dosage is 25 to 50 mg two times daily. The dosage may be increased if necessary to a maximum of 100 mg twice daily. When therapy is prolonged or large doses are used, particular attention should be given to the patient's electrolyte status. Supplemental potassium may be required.

In the treatment of hypertension hydrochlorothiazide may be either employed alone or concurrently with other antihypertensive drugs. Combined therapy may provide adequate control of hypertension with lower dosage of the component drugs and fewer or less severe side effects. An enhanced response frequently follows its concurrent administration with Harmonyl® (deserpidine) so that dosage of both drugs may be reduced.

For treatment of moderately severe or severe hypertension, supplemental use of other more potent antihypertensive agents such as pargyline hydrochloride may be indicated. When other antihypertensive agents are to be added to the regimen, this should be accomplished gradually. Additional potent antihypertensive agents should be given at only half the usual dose since their effect is potentiated by pretreatment with Oretic.

OVERDOSAGE

Symptoms of overdosage include electrolyte imbalance and signs of potassium deficiency such as confusion, dizziness, muscular weakness, and gastrointestinal disturbances. General supportive measures including replacement of fluids and electrolytes may be indicated in treatment of overdosage.

HOW SUPPLIED

Oretic (hydrochlorothiazide tablets, USP) is provided in two dosage sizes as white tablets:

    25 mg tablets:
    bottles of 100 (**NDC** 0074-6978-01),
    bottles of 1000 (**NDC** 0074-6978-02),
    Abbo-Pac® unit dose packages, 100 tablets (**NDC** 0074-6978-05).

    50 mg tablets:
    bottles of 100 (**NDC** 0074-6985-01),
    bottles of 1000 (**NDC** 0074-6985-02),
    Abbo-Pac® unit dose packages, 100 tablets (**NDC** 0074-6985-06).

Recommended Storage: Store below 86°F (30°C).
Ref. 01-2527-R7
Shown in Product Identification Section, page 403

ORETICYL®   ℞

[ō-re'ti-sill]
(hydrochlorothiazide and deserpidine tablets)

Oral thiazide-rauwolfia therapy for hypertension.

> ### WARNING
>
> This fixed combination drug is not indicated for initial therapy of hypertension. Hypertension requires therapy titrated to the individual patient. If the fixed combination represents the dosage so determined, its use may be more convenient in patient management. The treatment of hypertension is not static, but must be reevaluated as conditions in each patient warrant.

DESCRIPTION

Oreticyl tablets are an orally administered combination of Oretic® (hydrochlorothiazide) and Harmonyl® (deserpidine). Hydrochlorothiazide is a diuretic-antihypertensive agent of the benzothiadiazine (thiazide) class. Deserpidine is a purified rauwolfia alkaloid, chemically identified as 11-desmethoxyreserpine, which produces antihypertensive effects.

Inactive Ingredients:
Oreticyl 25 and Oreticyl 50 tablets: corn starch, lactose, magnesium stearate, red ferric oxide and talc.
Oreticyl Forte tablets: corn starch, iron oxide, lactose, magnesium stearate and talc.

ACTIONS

The combined antihypertensive actions of hydrochlorothiazide and deserpidine result in a total clinical antihypertensive effect which is greater than can ordinarily be achieved by either drug given individually.

The diuretic and saluretic effects of hydrochlorothiazide result from a drug-induced inhibition of the renal tubular reabsorption of electrolytes. The excretion of sodium and chloride is greatly enhanced. Potassium excretion is also enhanced to a variable degree, as it is with the other thiazides. Although urinary excretion of bicarbonate is increased slightly, there is usually no significant change in urinary pH. Hydrochlorothiazide has a per mg natriuretic activity approximately 10 times that of the prototype thiazide, chlorothiazide. At maximal therapeutic dosages, all thiazides are approximately equal in their diuretic/natriuretic effects.

There is significant natriuresis and diuresis within two hours after administration of a single oral dose of hydrochlorothiazide. These effects reach a peak in about 6 hours and persist for about 12 hours following oral administration of a single dose.

Like other benzothiadiazines, hydrochlorothiazide also has antihypertensive properties, and may be used for this purpose either alone or to enhance the antihypertensive action of other drugs. The mechanism by which the benzothiadiazines, including hydrochlorothiazide, produce a reduction of elevated blood pressure is not known. However, sodium depletion appears to be involved.

Hydrochlorothiazide is readily absorbed from the gastrointestinal tract and is excreted unchanged by the kidneys.

The pharmacologic actions of Harmonyl (deserpidine) are essentially the same as those of other active rauwolfia alkaloids. Deserpidine probably produces its antihypertensive effects through depletion of tissue stores of catecholamines (epinephrine and norepinephrine) from peripheral sites. The antihypertensive effect is often accompanied by bradycardia. There is no significant alteration in cardiac output or renal blood flow. The carotid sinus reflex is inhibited, but postural hypotension is rarely seen with the use of conventional doses of Harmonyl alone.

Deserpidine, like other rauwolfia alkaloids, is characterized by slow onset of action and sustained effect which may persist following withdrawal of the drug.

INDICATIONS

Oreticyl (hydrochlorothiazide and deserpidine) is indicated in the treatment of patients with mild to moderately severe hypertension (see boxed warning). It may be used alone for this purpose or added to other antihypertensive agents for the management of more severe hypertension. When administered with Oreticyl tablets, more potent agents can be given at reduced dosage to minimize undesirable side effects.

CONTRAINDICATIONS

Hydrochlorothiazide is contraindicated in patients with renal decompensation and in those who are hypersensitive to this or other sulfonamide-derived drugs.

Deserpidine is contraindicated in patients with known hypersensitivity, history of mental depression especially with suicidal tendencies, active peptic ulcer, and ulcerative colitis. It is also contraindicated in patients receiving electroconvulsive therapy.

WARNINGS

Hydrochlorothiazide

Hydrochlorothiazide shares with other thiazides the propensity to deplete potassium reserves to an unpredictable degree.

Thiazides should be used with caution in patients with renal disease or significant impairment of renal function, since azotemia may be precipitated and cumulative drug effects may occur.

Thiazides should be used with caution in patients with impaired hepatic function or progressive liver disease, since minor alterations of fluid and electrolyte balance may precipitate hepatic coma.

Thiazides may be additive or potentiative of the action of other antihypertensive drugs. Potentiation occurs with ganglionic or peripheral adrenergic blocking drugs.

Sensitivity reactions may occur in patients with a history of allergy or bronchial asthma.

The possibility of exacerbation or activation of systemic lupus erythematosus has been reported.

Deserpidine

Deserpidine differs slightly in chemical structure from reserpine, however, its actions, indications, cautions and adverse reactions are common to the class of rauwolfia alkaloids. Reserpine may cause mental depression. Recognition of depression may be difficult because this condition may often be disguised by somatic complaints (Masked Depression). The drug should be discontinued at first signs of depression such as despondency, early morning insomnia, loss of appetite, impotence, or self-deprecation. Drug-induced depression may persist for several months after drug withdrawal and may be severe enough to result in suicide.

Usage in Pregnancy and Lactation:

Hydrochlorothiazide

Thiazides cross the placental barrier and appear in cord blood. The use of thiazides in pregnant women requires that the anticipated benefit be weighed against possible hazards to the fetus. These hazards include fetal or neonatal jaundice, thrombocytopenia, and possible other adverse reactions that have occurred in the adult.

Thiazides appear in breast milk. If use of the drug is deemed essential, the patient should stop nursing.

Deserpidine

The safety of deserpidine for use during pregnancy or lactation has not been established; therefore, it should be used in pregnant women or in women of childbearing potential only when in the judgment of the physician its use is deemed essential to the welfare of the patient. Increased respiratory secretions, nasal congestion, cyanosis, and anorexia may occur in infants born to rauwolfia alkaloid-treated mothers, since these preparations are known to cross the placental barrier to enter the fetal circulation and appear in cord blood. They also are secreted by nursing mothers into breast milk.

Reproductive and teratology studies in rats reduced the mating index and neonatal survival indices. The no-effect dosage has not been established.

PRECAUTIONS

Periodic determinations of serum electrolytes should be performed at appropriate intervals for the purpose of detecting possible electrolyte imbalances such as hyponatremia, hypochloremic alkalosis, and hypokalemia. Serum and urine electrolyte determinations are particularly important when a patient is vomiting excessively or receiving parenteral fluids. All patients should be observed for other clinical signs of electrolyte imbalances such as dryness of mouth, thirst, weakness, lethargy, drowsiness, restlessness, muscle pains or cramps, muscular fatigue, hypotension, oliguria, tachycardia, and gastrointestinal disturbances such as nausea and vomiting.

Hypokalemia may develop with thiazides as with any other potent diuretic, especially when brisk diuresis occurs, severe cirrhosis is present, or when corticosteroids or ACTH are given concomitantly. Interference with the adequate oral intake of electrolytes will also contribute to the possible development of hypokalemia. Potassium depletion, even of a mild degree, resulting from thiazide use, may sensitize a patient to the effects of cardiac glycosides such as digitalis. Any chloride deficit is generally mild and usually does not require specific treatment except under extraordinary circumstances (as in liver disease or renal disease). Dilutional hyponatremia may occur in edematous patients in hot weather; appropriate therapy is water restriction rather than administration of salt, except in rare instances when the hyponatremia is life threatening.

In actual salt depletion, appropriate replacement is the therapy of choice.

Hyperuricemia may occur or frank gout may be precipitated in certain patients receiving thiazide therapy.

Insulin requirements in diabetic patients may be increased, decreased, or unchanged. Latent diabetes mellitus may become manifest during thiazide administration.

Thiazide drugs may increase the responsiveness to tubocurarine.

The antihypertensive effects of the drug may be enhanced in the postsympathectomy patient.

Thiazides may decrease arterial responsiveness to norepinephrine. This diminution is not sufficient to preclude effectiveness of the pressor agent for therapeutic use.

If progressive renal impairment becomes evident as indicated by a rising-nonprotein nitrogen or blood urea nitrogen, a careful reappraisal of therapy is necessary with consideration given to withholding or discontinuing diuretic therapy. Thiazides may decrease serum protein bound iodine levels without signs of thyroid disturbance.

Thiazides have been reported, on rare occasions, to have elevated serum calcium to hypercalcemic levels. The serum calcium levels have returned to normal when the medication has been stopped. This phenomenon may be related to the ability of the thiazide diuretics to lower the amount of calcium excreted in the urine.

Because rauwolfia preparations increase gastrointestinal motility and secretion, this drug should be used cautiously in patients with a history of peptic ulcer, ulcerative colitis, or gallstones, where biliary colic may be precipitated.

Caution should be exercised when treating hypertensive patients with renal insufficiency since they adjust poorly to lowered blood pressure levels.

Use deserpidine cautiously with digitalis and quinidine since cardiac arrhythmias have occurred with rauwolfia preparations.

Preoperative withdrawal of deserpidine does not assure that circulatory instability will not occur. It is important that the anesthesiologist be aware of the patient's drug intake and consider this in the overall management, since hypotension has occurred in patients receiving rauwolfia preparations. Anticholinergic and/or adrenergic drugs (metaraminol, norepinephrine) have been employed to treat adverse vagocirculatory effects.

Animal tumorigenicity: There are no studies demonstrating that deserpidine is an animal tumorigen, although it is a prolactin stimulator and structurally related to reserpine. Rodent studies with reserpine, however, have shown that reserpine is an animal tumorigen, causing an increased incidence of mammary fibroadenomas in female mice, malignant tumors of the seminal vesicles in male mice, and malignant adrenal medullary tumors in male rats. These findings arose in 2 year studies in which the drug was administered in the feed at concentrations of 5 and 10 ppm—about 100 to 300 times the usual human dose. The breast neoplasms are thought to be related to reserpine's prolactin-elevating effect. Several other prolactin-elevating drugs have also been associated with an increased incidence of mammary neoplasia in rodents.

The extent to which these findings indicate a risk to humans is uncertain. Tissue culture experiments show that about one-third of human breast tumors are prolactin-dependent *in vitro*, a factor of considerable importance if the use of the drug is contemplated in a patient with previously detected breast cancer. The possibility of an increased risk of breast cancer in reserpine users has been studied extensively; however, no firm conclusion has emerged. Although a few epidemiologic studies have suggested a slightly increased risk (less than twofold in all studies except one) in women who have used reserpine, other studies of generally similar design have not confirmed this. Epidemiologic studies conducted using other drugs (neuroleptic agents) that, like reserpine, increase prolactin levels and, therefore, would be considered rodent mammary carcinogens, have not shown an association between chronic administration of the drug and human mammary tumorigenesis. While long-term clinical observation has not suggested such an association, the available evidence is considered too limited to be conclusive at this time. An association of reserpine intake with pheochromocytoma or tumors of the seminal vesicles has not been explored.

ADVERSE REACTIONS

Hydrochlorothiazide

Gastrointestinal System Reactions: Anorexia, gastric irritation, nausea, vomiting, cramping, diarrhea, constipation, jaundice (intrahepatic cholestatic jaundice), pancreatitis.

Central Nervous System Reactions: Dizziness, vertigo, paresthesias, headache, xanthopsia.

Hematologic Reactions: Leukopenia, agranulocytosis, thrombocytopenia, aplastic anemia.

Dermatologic — Hypersensitivity Reactions: Purpura, photosensitivity, rash, urticaria, necrotizing angitis (vasculitis) (cutaneous vasculitis).

Cardiovascular Reaction: Orthostatic hypotension may occur and may be aggravated by alcohol, barbiturates, or narcotics.

Other: Hyperglycemia, glycosuria, hypercalcemia, hyperuricemia, muscle spasm, weakness, restlessness, respiratory distress including pnemonitis and pulmonary edema.

There have been isolated reports that certain nonedematous individuals developed severe fluid and electrolyte derangements after only brief exposure to normal doses of thiazide and non-thiazide diuretics. The condition is usually manifested as severe dilutional hyponatremia, hypokalemia, and hypochloremia. It has been reported to be due to inappropriately increased ADH secretion and appears to be idiosyncratic. Potassium replacement is apparently the most important therapy in the treatment of this syndrome along with the removal of the offending drug.

Whenever adverse reactions are severe, treatment should be discontinued.

Deserpidine

The following adverse reactions have been reported with rauwolfia preparations. These reactions are usually reversible and disappear when the drug is discontinued.

Gastrointestinal: Including hypersecretion, anorexia, diarrhea, nausea, and vomiting.

Cardiovascular: Including angina-like symptoms, arrhythmias (particularly when used concurrently with digitalis or quinidine), and bradycardia.

Central Nervous System: Including drowsiness, depression, nervousness, paradoxical anxiety, nightmares, extrapyramidal tract symptoms, CNS sensitization manifested by dull sensorium, and deafness.

Dermatologic—Hypersensitivity: Including pruritus, rash, and asthma in asthmatic patients.

Ophthalmologic: Including glaucoma, uveitis, optic atrophy, and conjunctival injection.

Hematologic: Thrombocytopenic purpura.

Miscellaneous: Nasal congestion, weight gain, impotence or decreased libido, dysuria, dyspnea, muscular aches, dryness of mouth, dizziness and headache.

DOSAGE AND ADMINISTRATION

Dosage should be determined by individual titration of ingredients (see boxed warning). Dosage of both components should be carefully adjusted to the needs of the individual patient. Since at least 10 days to 2 weeks may elapse before the full effects of the drugs become manifest, the dosage should not be adjusted more frequently.

Three tablet strengths, ORETICYL 25 (hydrochlorothiazide 25 mg, deserpidine 0.125 mg); ORETICYL 50 (hydrochlorothiazide 50 mg, deserpidine 0.125 mg); and ORETICYL FORTE (hydrochlorothiazide 25 mg, deserpidine 0.25 mg), all grooved, are provided to permit considerable latitude in meeting the dosage requirements of individual patients.

The table below will help in determining which dose of ORETICYL 25, ORETICYL 50, or ORETICYL FORTE best represents the equivalent of the titrated dose.

ORETICYL 25	hydro-chlorothiazide	deserpidine
1 tablet bid	25.0 mg bid	0.125 mg bid
1½ tablets bid	37.5 mg bid	0.188 mg bid
2 tablets bid	50.0 mg bid	0.250 mg bid
ORETICYL 50	hydro-chlorothiazide	deserpidine
1 tablet bid	50 mg bid	0.125 mg bid
1½ tablets bid	75 mg bid	0.188 mg bid
2 tablets bid	100 mg bid	0.250 mg bid
ORETICYL FORTE	hydro-chlorothiazide	deserpidine
1 tablet bid	25.0 mg bid	0.250 mg bid
1½ tablets bid	37.5 mg bid	0.375 mg bid
2 tablets bid	50.0 mg bid	0.500 mg bid

The usual adult dosage is one ORETICYL 50 tablet two times daily.

When other antihypertensive agents are to be added to the regimen, this should be accomplished gradually. Ganglionic blocking agents should be given at only half the usual dose since their effect is potentiated by pretreatment with ORETICYL (hydrochlorothiazide and deserpidine).

OVERDOSAGE

Symptoms of thiazide overdosage include electrolyte imbalance and signs of potassium deficiency such as confusion, dizziness, muscular weakness, and gastrointestinal disturbances. General supportive measures including replacement of fluids and electrolytes may be indicated in treatment of overdosage.

An overdosage of deserpidine is characterized by flushing of the skin, conjunctival injection, and pupillary constriction. Sedation ranging from drowsiness to coma may occur. Hypo-

Continued on next page

Abbott Laboratories—Cont.

tension, hypothermia, central respiratory depression and bradycardia may develop in cases of severe overdosage. Treatment consists of the careful evacuation of stomach contents followed by the usual procedures for the symptomatic management of CNS depressant overdosage. If severe hypotension occurs it should be treated with a direct acting vasopressor such as norepinephrine bitartrate injection.

HOW SUPPLIED

ORETICYL (hydrochlorothiazide and deserpidine) is supplied as grooved tablets in the following dosage sizes:
Rose-colored ORETICYL 25, contains hydrochlorothiazide 25 mg, deserpidine 0.125 mg, in bottles of 100 (**NDC** 0074-6922-01).
Rose-colored ORETICYL 50, contains hydrochlorothiazide 50 mg, deserpidine 0.125 mg, in bottles of 100 (**NDC** 0074-6931-01).
Gray-colored ORETICYL FORTE, contains hydrochlorothiazide 25 mg, deserpidine 0.25 mg, in bottles of 100 (**NDC** 0074-6927-01).
Recommended Storage: Store below 86°F (30°C).
Ref. 01-2555-R9

PANHEMATIN® ℞

[pan-hē'ma-tin]
(hemin for injection)
For I.V. Use Only

> PANHEMATIN (hemin for injection) should only be used by physicians experienced in the management of porphyrias in hospitals where the recommended clinical and laboratory diagnostic and monitoring techniques are available.
> PANHEMATIN therapy should be considered after an appropriate period of alternate therapy (i.e., 400 g glucose/day for 1 to 2 days). (See "WARNINGS", "PRECAUTIONS" and "DOSAGE AND ADMINISTRATION" sections.)

DESCRIPTION

PANHEMATIN (hemin for injection) is an enzyme inhibitor derived from processed red blood cells. Hemin for injection was known previously as hematin. The term hematin has been used to describe the chemical reaction product of hemin and sodium carbonate solution. Hemin is an iron containing metalloporphyrin. Chemically hemin is represented as chloro [7,12-diethenyl-3,8,13,17-tetramethyl-21H,23H-porphine-2,18-dipropanoato (2-)-N^{21},N^{22}, N^{23}, N^{24}] iron.
PANHEMATIN is a sterile, lyophilized powder suitable for intravenous administration after reconstitution. Each dispensing vial of PANHEMATIN contains the equivalent of 313 mg hemin, 215 mg sodium carbonate and 300 mg of sorbitol. The pH may have been adjusted with hydrochloric acid; the product contains no preservatives. When mixed as directed with Sterile Water for Injection, USP, each 43 mL provides the equivalent of approximately 301 mg hematin (7 mg/mL).

CLINICAL PHARMACOLOGY

Heme acts to limit the hepatic and/or marrow synthesis of porphyrin. This action is likely due to the inhibition of delta-aminolevulinic acid synthetase, the enzyme which limits the rate of the porphyrin/heme biosynthetic pathway. The exact mechanism by which hematin produces symptomatic improvement in patients with acute episodes of the hepatic porphyrias has not been elucidated.[1,9]
Following intravenous administration of hematin in non-jaundiced human patients, an increase in fecal urobilinogen can be observed which is roughly proportional to the amount of hematin administered. This suggests an enterohepatic pathway as at least one route of elimination. Bilirubin metabolites are also excreted in the urine following hematin injections.[2]
PANHEMATIN (hemin for injection) therapy for the acute porphyrias is not curative. After discontinuation of PANHEMATIN treatment, symptoms generally return although in some cases remission is prolonged. Some neurological symptoms have improved weeks to months after therapy although little or no response was noted at the time of treatment.
Other aspects of human pharmacokinetics have not been defined.

INDICATIONS AND USAGE

PANHEMATIN (hemin for injection) is indicated for the amelioration of recurrent attacks of acute intermittent porphyria temporarily related to the menstrual cycle in susceptible women.
Manifestations such as pain, hypertension, tachycardia, abnormal mental status and mild to progressive neurologic signs may be controlled in selected patients with this disorder.
Similar findings have been reported in other patients with acute intermittent porphyria, porphyria variegata and hereditary coproporphyria. PANHEMATIN is not indicated in porphyria cutanea tarda.

CONTRAINDICATIONS

Hemin for injection is contraindicated in patients with known hypersensitivity to this drug.

WARNINGS

PANHEMATIN (hemin for injection) therapy is intended to limit the rate of porphyria/heme biosynthesis possibly by inhibiting the enzyme delta-aminolevulinic acid synthetase. For this reason, drugs such as estrogens, barbituric acid derivatives and steroid metabolites which increase the activity of delta-aminolevulinic acid synthetase should be avoided.
Also, because PANHEMATIN has exhibited transient, mild anticoagulant effects during clinical studies, concurrent anticoagulant therapy should be avoided.[9] The extent and duration of the hypocoagulable state induced by PANHEMATIN has not been established.

PRECAUTIONS

General: Clinical benefit from PANHEMATIN depends on prompt administration. Attacks of porphyria may progress to a point where irreversible neuronal damage has occurred. PANHEMATIN therapy is intended to prevent an attack from reaching the critical stage of neuronal degeneration. PANHEMATIN is not effective in repairing neuronal damage.[9]
Recommended dosage guidelines should be strictly followed. Reversible renal shutdown has been observed in a case where an excessive hematin dose (12.2 mg/kg) was administered in a single infusion. Oliguria and increased nitrogen retention occurred although the patient remained asymptomatic.[4] No worsening of renal function has been seen with administration of recommended dosages of hematin.[9]
A large arm vein or a central venous catheter should be utilized for the administration of hemin for injection to avoid the possibility of phlebitis.
Since reconstituted PANHEMATIN is not transparent, any undissolved particulate matter is difficult to see when inspected visually. Therefore, terminal filtration through a sterile 0.45 micron or smaller filter is recommended.
Tests for Diagnosis and Monitoring of Therapy: Before PANHEMATIN therapy is begun, the presence of acute porphyria must be diagnosed using the following criteria:[9]
a. Presence of clinical symptoms.
b. Positive Watson-Schwartz or Hoesch test. (A negative Watson-Schwartz or Hoesch test indicates a porphyric attack is highly unlikely. When in doubt quantitative measures of delta-aminolevulinic acid and porphobilinogen in serum or urine may aid in diagnosis.)
Urinary concentrations of the following compounds may be *monitored* during PANHEMATIN therapy. Drug effect will be demonstrated by a decrease in one or more of the following compounds:[3–6] ALA—delta-aminolevulinic acid, UPG—uroporphyrinogen, PBG—porphobilinogen or coproporphyrin.
Carcinogenesis, Mutagenesis, Impairment of Fertility: No data are available on potential for carcinogenicity, mutagenicity or impairment of fertility in animals or humans.
Pregnancy: Teratogenic effects: Pregnancy Category C. Animal reproduction studies have not been conducted with hematin. It is also not known whether hematin can cause fetal harm when administered to a pregnant woman or can affect reproduction capacity. For this reason hemin for injection should not be given to a pregnant woman unless the expected benefits are sufficiently important to the health and welfare of the patient to outweigh the unknown hazard to the fetus.
Nursing Mothers: It is not known whether this drug is excreted in human milk. Because many drugs are excreted in human milk, caution should be exercised when hemin for injection is administered to a nursing woman.
Pediatric Use: Safety and effectiveness in children have not been established.

ADVERSE REACTIONS

Reversible renal shutdown has occurred with administration of excessive doses (See "PRECAUTIONS" section).
Phlebitis with or without leucocytosis and with or without mild pyrexia has occurred after administration of hematin through small arm veins.
There has been one report in the literature[8] of coagulopathy occurring in a patient receiving hematin therapy. This patient exhibited prolonged prothrombin time and partial thromboplastin time, thrombocytopenia, mild hypofibrinogenemia, mild elevation of fibrin split products and a 10% fall in hematocrit.

OVERDOSAGE

Reversible renal shutdown has been observed in a case where an excessive hematin dose (12.2 mg/kg) was administered in a single infusion. Treatment of this case consisted of ethacrynic acid and mannitol.[7]

DOSAGE AND ADMINISTRATION

Before administering hemin for injection, an appropriate period of alternate therapy (i.e., 400 g glucose/day for 1 to 2 days) must be considered. If improvement is unsatisfactory for the treatment of acute attacks of porphyria, an intravenous infusion of PANHEMATIN containing a dose of 1 to 4 mg/kg/day of hematin should be given over a period of 10 to 15 minutes for 3 to 14 days based on the clinical signs. In more severe cases this dose may be repeated no earlier than every 12 hours. No more than 6 mg/kg of hematin should be given in any 24-hour period.
After reconstitution each mL of PANHEMATIN contains the equivalent of approximately 7 mg of hematin. The drug may be administered directly from the vial.

Dosage Calculation Table

1 mg hematin equivalent	= 0.14 mL PANHEMATIN
2 mg hematin equivalent	= 0.28 mL PANHEMATIN
3 mg hematin equivalent	= 0.42 mL PANHEMATIN
4 mg hematin equivalent	= 0.56 mL PANHEMATIN

Since reconstituted PANHEMATIN is not transparent, any undissolved particulate matter is difficult to see when inspected visually. Therefore, terminal filtration through a sterile 0.45 micron or smaller filter is recommended.
Preparation of Solution: Reconstitute PANHEMATIN by aseptically adding 43 mL of Sterile Water for Injection, USP, to the dispensing vial. Immediately after adding diluent, the product should be shaken well for a period of 2 to 3 minutes to aid dissolution. **NOTE: Because PANHEMATIN contains no preservative and because PANHEMATIN undergoes rapid chemical decomposition in solution, it should not be reconstituted until immediately before use. After the first withdrawal from the vial, any solution remaining must be discarded.**
No drug or chemical agent should be added to a PANHEMATIN fluid admixture unless its effect on the chemical and physical stability has first been determined.

HOW SUPPLIED

PANHEMATIN (hemin for injection) is supplied as a sterile, lyophilized black powder in single dose dispensing vials (**NDC** 0074-2000-43). When mixed as directed with Sterile Water for Injection, USP, each 43 mL provides the equivalent of approximately 301 mg hematin (7 mg/mL). Store lyophilized powder in refrigerator (2–8°C) until time of use.

REFERENCES

1. Bickers, D., Treatment of the Porphyrias: Mechanisms of Action, *J Invest Dermatol* 77(1):107–113, 1981.
2. Watson, C. J., Hematin and Porphyria, editorial, *N Engl J Med* 293(12):605–607, September 18, 1975.
3. Lamon, J. M., Hematin Therapy for Acute Porphyria, *Medicine* 58(3):252–269, 1979.
4. Dhar, G. J., et al., Effects of Hematin in Hepatic Porphyria, *Ann Intern Med* 83:20–30, 1975.
5. Watson, C. J., et al., Use of Hematin in the Acute Attack of the "Inducible" Hepatic Porphyrias, *Adv Intern Med* 23:265–286, 1978.
6. McColl, K. E., et al., Treatment with Haematin in Acute Hepatic Porphyria, *Q J Med*, New Series L (198):161–174, Spring, 1981.
7. Dhar, G. J., et al., Transitory Renal Failure Following Rapid Administration of a Relatively Large Amount of Hematin in a Patient with Acute Intermittent Porphyria in Clinical Remission, *Acta Med Scand* 203:437–443, 1978.
8. Morris, D. L., et al., Coagulopathy Associated with Hematin Treatment for Acute Intermittent Porphyria, *Ann Intern Med* 95:700–701, 1981.
9. Pierach, C. A., Hematin Therapy for the Porphyric Attack, *Semin Liver Dis* 2(2):125–131, May, 1982.
Ref. 01-2388-R4

PARADIONE® ℞

[pă-rā-dī'own]
(paramethadione)
Capsules

> BECAUSE OF ITS POTENTIAL TO PRODUCE FETAL MALFORMATIONS AND SERIOUS SIDE EFFECTS, PARADIONE (paramethadione) SHOULD ONLY BE UTILIZED WHEN OTHER LESS TOXIC DRUGS HAVE BEEN FOUND INEFFECTIVE IN CONTROLLING ABSENCE (PETIT MAL) SEIZURES.

DESCRIPTION

PARADIONE (paramethadione) is an antiepileptic agent. An oxazolidinedione compound, it is chemically identified as 5-Ethyl-3,5-dimethyl-2,4-oxazolidinedione. PARADIONE is a synthetic, oily, slightly water-soluble liquid. It is supplied in capsule form for oral use only. The capsules are available in two dosage strengths. One strength contains 150 mg the other 300 mg of paramethadione per capsule.

Inactive Ingredients: 150 mg capsule: FD&C Yellow No. 6, gelatin, glycerin, methylparaben, olive oil ethyl ester and propylparaben.
300 mg capsule: FD&C Blue No. 1, FD&C Yellow No. 5 (tartrazine), FD&C Yellow No. 6, gelatin, glycerin, methylparaben, olive oil ethyl ester and propylparaben.

CLINICAL PHARMACOLOGY

PARADIONE has been shown to prevent pentylenetetrazol-induced and thujone-induced seizures in experimental animals; the drug has a less marked effect on seizures induced by picrotoxin, procaine, cocaine, or strychnine. Unlike the hydantoins and antiepileptic barbiturates, PARADIONE does not modify the maximal seizure pattern in patients undergoing electroconvulsive therapy. PARADIONE has a sedative effect that may increase to the point of ataxia when excessive doses are used. A toxic dose of the drug in animals (approximately 1 g/kg) produced sleep, unconsciousness, and respiratory depression.
Paramethadione is rapidly absorbed from the gastrointestinal tract. It is demethylated by liver microsomes to an active N-demethylated metabolite, and is excreted slowly in this form by the kidney; almost no unmetabolized PARADIONE is excreted.

INDICATIONS AND USAGE

PARADIONE (paramethadione) is indicated for the control of absence (petit mal) seizures that are refractory to treatment with other drugs.

CONTRAINDICATIONS

PARADIONE is contraindicated in patients with a known hypersensitivity to the drug.

WARNINGS

PARADIONE may cause serious side effects. Strict medical supervision of the patient is mandatory, especially during the initial year of therapy.
USAGE DURING PREGNANCY: THERE ARE MULTIPLE REPORTS IN THE CLINICAL LITERATURE WHICH INDICATE THAT THE USE OF ANTIEPILEPTIC DRUGS DURING PREGNANCY RESULTS IN AN INCREASED INCIDENCE OF BIRTH DEFECTS IN THE OFFSPRING. DATA ARE MORE EXTENSIVE WITH RESPECT TO TRIMETHADIONE, PARAMETHADIONE, PHENYTOIN AND PHENOBARBITAL THAN WITH OTHER ANTIEPILEPTIC DRUGS.
THEREFORE, ANTIEPILEPTIC DRUGS SUCH AS PARADIONE (PARAMETHADIONE) SHOULD BE ADMINISTERED TO WOMEN OF CHILDBEARING POTENTIAL ONLY IF THEY ARE CLEARLY SHOWN TO BE ESSENTIAL IN THE MANAGEMENT OF THEIR SEIZURES. EFFECTIVE MEANS OF CONTRACEPTION SHOULD ACCOMPANY THE USE OF PARADIONE IN SUCH PATIENTS. IF A PATIENT BECOMES PREGNANT WHILE TAKING PARADIONE, TERMINATION OF THE PREGNANCY SHOULD BE CONSIDERED. A PATIENT WHO REQUIRES THERAPY WITH PARADIONE AND WHO WISHES TO BECOME PREGNANT SHOULD BE ADVISED OF THE RISKS.
REPORTS HAVE SUGGESTED THAT THE MATERNAL INGESTION OF ANTIEPILEPTIC DRUGS, PARTICULARLY BARBITURATES, IS ASSOCIATED WITH A NEONATAL COAGULATION DEFECT THAT MAY CAUSE BLEEDING DURING THE EARLY (USUALLY WITHIN 24 HOURS OF BIRTH) NEONATAL PERIOD. THE POSSIBILITY OF THE OCCURRENCE OF THIS DEFECT WITH THE USE OF PARADIONE SHOULD BE KEPT IN MIND. THE DEFECT IS CHARACTERIZED BY DECREASED LEVELS OF VITAMIN K-DEPENDENT CLOTTING FACTORS, AND PROLONGATION OF EITHER THE PROTHROMBIN TIME OR THE PARTIAL THROMBOPLASTIN TIME, OR BOTH. IT HAS BEEN SUGGESTED THAT PROPHYLACTIC VITAMIN K BE GIVEN TO THE MOTHER ONE MONTH PRIOR TO, AND DURING DELIVERY, AND TO THE INFANT, INTRAVENOUSLY, IMMEDIATELY AFTER BIRTH.

PRECAUTIONS

General: Abrupt discontinuation of PARADIONE may precipitate absence (petit mal) status. PARADIONE (paramethadione) should always be withdrawn gradually unless serious adverse effects dictate otherwise. In the latter case, another antiepileptic may be substituted to protect the patient.
PARADIONE (paramethadione) should be withdrawn promptly if skin rash appears, because of the grave possibility of the occurrence of exfoliative dermatitis or severe forms of erythema multiforme. Even a minor acneiform or morbilliform rash should be allowed to clear completely before treatment with PARADIONE is resumed; reinstitute therapy cautiously.
PARADIONE should ordinarily not be used in patients with severe blood dyscrasias.
Hepatitis has been associated rarely with the use of oxazolidinediones. Jaundice or other signs of liver dysfunction are an indication for withdrawal of PARADIONE. PARADIONE should ordinarily not be used in patients with severe hepatic impairment.
Fatal nephrosis has been reported with the use of oxazolidinediones. Persistent or increasing albuminuria, or the development of any other significant renal abnormality, is an indication for withdrawal of the drug. PARADIONE should ordinarily not be used in patients with severe renal dysfunction.
Hemeralopia has occurred with the use of oxazolidinedione compounds; this appears to be an effect of the drugs on the neural layers of the retina, and usually can be reversed by a reduction in dosage. Scotomata are an indication for withdrawal of the drug. Caution should be observed when treating patients who have diseases of the retina or optic nerve.
Manifestations of systemic lupus erythematosus have been associated with the use of the oxazolidinediones, as they have with the use of certain other antiepileptics. Lymphadenopathies simulating malignant lymphoma have also occurred. Lupus-like manifestations or lymph node enlargement are indications for withdrawal of PARADIONE. Signs and symptoms may disappear after discontinuation of therapy, and specific treatment may be unnecessary.
A myasthenia gravis-like syndrome has been associated with the chronic use of the oxazolidinediones. Symptoms suggestive of this condition are indications for withdrawal of PARADIONE.
The 300 mg capsule of PARADIONE contains FD&C Yellow No. 5 (tartrazine) which may cause allergic-type reactions (including bronchial asthma) in certain susceptible individuals. Although the overall incidence of FD&C Yellow No. 5 (tartrazine) sensitivity in the general population is low, it is frequently seen in patients who also have aspirin hypersensitivity.
Information for Patients: Patients should be advised to report immediately such signs and symptoms as sore throat, fever, malaise, easy-bruising, petechiae, or epistaxis, or others that may be indicative of an infection or bleeding tendency.
Laboratory Tests: A complete blood count should be done prior to initiating therapy with PARADIONE, and at monthly intervals thereafter. A marked depression of the blood count is an indication for withdrawal of the drug. If no abnormality appears within 12 months, the interval between blood counts may be extended. A moderate degree of neutropenia with or without a corresponding drop in the leukocyte count is not uncommon. Therapy need not be withdrawn unless the neutrophil count is 2500 or less; more frequent blood examinations should be done when the count is less than 3,000. Other blood dyscrasias, including leukopenia, eosinophilia, thrombocytopenia, pancytopenia, agranulocytosis, hypoplastic anemia, and fatal aplastic anemia, have occurred with the use of oxazolidinediones.
Liver function tests should be done prior to initiating therapy with PARADIONE, and at monthly intervals thereafter.
A urinalysis should be done prior to initiating therapy with PARADIONE and at monthly intervals thereafter.
Drug Interactions: Drugs known to cause toxic effects similar to those of the oxazolidinediones should be avoided or used only with extreme caution during therapy with PARADIONE.
Carcinogenesis: No data are available on long-term potential for carcinogenicity in animals or humans.
Pregnancy: Pregnancy Category D. See "Warnings" section.
Nursing Mothers: It is not known whether this drug is excreted in human milk. Because many drugs are excreted in human milk and because of the potential for serious adverse reactions in nursing infants from PARADIONE, a decision should be made whether to discontinue nursing or to discontinue the drug, taking into account the importance of the drug to the mother.

ADVERSE REACTIONS

The following side effects, in decreasing order of severity, have been associated with the use of oxazolidinedione compounds. Although not all of them have been reported with the use of PARADIONE, the possibility of their occurrence should be kept in mind when the drug is prescribed.
Renal: Fatal nephrosis has occurred. Albuminuria.
Hematologic: Fatal aplastic anemia, hypoplastic anemia, pancytopenia, agranulocytosis, leukopenia, neutropenia, thrombocytopenia, eosinophilia, retinal and petechial hemorrhages, vaginal bleeding, epistaxis, and bleeding gums.
Hepatic: Hepatitis has been reported rarely.
Dermatologic: Acneiform or morbilliform skin rash that may progress to severe forms of erythema multiforme or to exfoliative dermatitis. Hair loss.
CNS/Neurologic: A myasthenia gravis-like syndrome has been reported. Precipitation of tonic-clonic (grand mal) seizures, vertigo, personality changes, increased irritability, drowsiness, headache, parasthesias, fatigue, malaise, and insomnia.
Drowsiness usually subsides with continued therapy. If it persists, a reduction in dosage is indicated.
Ophthalmologic: Diplopia, hemeralopia, and photophobia.
Cardiovascular: Changes in blood pressure.
Gastrointestinal: Vomiting, abdominal pain, gastric distress, nausea, anorexia, weight loss, and hiccups.
Other: Lupus erythematosus, and lymphadenopathies simulating malignant lymphoma, have been reported. Pruritus associated with lymphadenopathy and hepatosplenomegaly has occurred in hypersensitive individuals.

OVERDOSAGE

Symptoms of acute PARADIONE overdosage include drowsiness, nausea, dizziness, ataxia, visual disturbances. Coma may follow massive overdosage.
Gastric evacuation, either by induced emesis, or by lavage, or both, should be done immediately. General supportive care, including frequent monitoring of the vital signs and close observation of the patient, are required.
It has been reported that alkalinization of the urine may be expected to increase the excretion of the N-demethylated metabolite of PARADIONE.
A blood count and a careful evaluation of hepatic and renal function should be done following recovery.

DOSAGE AND ADMINISTRATION

PARADIONE is administered orally.
Usual Adult Dosage: 0.9–2.4 g daily in 3 or 4 equally divided doses (i.e., 300–600 mg 3 or 4 times daily).
Initially, give 0.9 g daily; increase this dose by 300 mg at weekly intervals until therapeutic results are seen or until toxic symptoms appear.
Maintenance dosage should be the least amount of drug required to maintain control.
Children's Dosage: Usually 0.3–0.9 g daily in 3 or 4 equally divided doses.

HOW SUPPLIED

PARADIONE Capsules (paramethadione capsules, USP) are round capsules supplied as 150 mg (orange color) (**NDC** 0074-3976-01), and 300 mg (green color) (**NDC** 0074-3838-01) in bottles of 100.
Recommended Storage: 59°–77°F (15°–25°C).
Ref. 01-2594-R10

Shown in Product Identification Section, page 403

PCE® ℞
(erythromycin particles in tablets)
Dispertab® Tablets

DESCRIPTION

PCE (erythromycin particles in tablets) is an antibacterial product containing specially coated erythromycin base particles for oral administration. The coating protects the antibiotic from the inactivating effects of gastric acidity and permits efficient absorption of the antibiotic in the small intestine. PCE is available in two strengths containing either 333 mg or 500 mg of erythromycin base. PCE 500 mg tablets contain no synthetic dyes or artificial colors.
Inactive Ingredients:
PCE 333 mg tablets: Cellulosic polymers, citrate ester, colloidal silicon dioxide, D&C Red No. 30, hydrogenated vegetable oil wax, lactose, magnesium stearate, microcrystalline cellulose, povidone, propylene glycol, sodium starch glycolate, stearic acid and vanillin.
PCE 500 mg tablets: Cellulosic polymers, citrate ester, colloidal silicon dioxide, crospovidone, hydrogenated vegetable oil wax, iron oxide, microcrystalline cellulose, polyethylene glycol, povidone, propylene glycol, stearic acid, talc, titanium dioxide and vanillin.
Erythromycin is produced by a strain of *Streptomyces erythraeus* and belongs to the macrolide group of antibiotics. It is basic and readily forms salts with acids. Erythromycin is a white to off-white powder, slightly soluble in water, and soluble in alcohol, chloroform, and ether. Erythromycin is known chemically as (3R*,4S*,5S*,6R*,7R*,9R*,11R*,12R*,13S*,14R*)-4-[(2,6-Dideoxy-3-C-methyl-3-O-methyl-α-L-*ribo*-hexopyranosyl)oxy]-14-ethyl-7,12,13-trihydroxy-3,5,7,9,11,-13-hexamethyl-6-[[3,4,6-trideoxy-3-(dimethylamino)-β-D-*xylo*-hexopyranosyl]oxy]oxacyclotetradecane-2,10-dione.
The structural formula is:

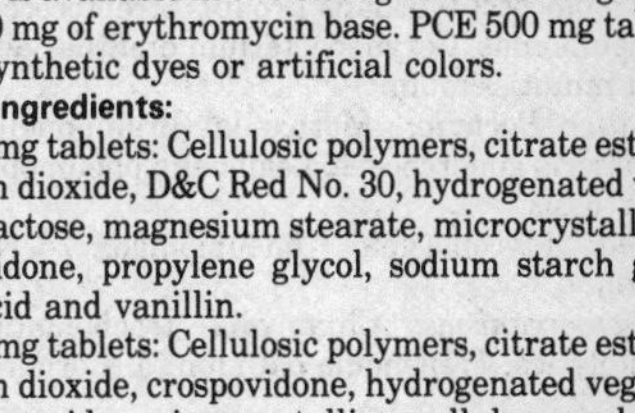

Continued on next page

Abbott Laboratories—Cont.

CLINICAL PHARMACOLOGY

Orally administered erythromycin base and its salts are readily absorbed in the microbiologically active form. Interindividual variations in the absorption of erythromycin are, however, observed, and some patients do not achieve optimal serum levels. Erythromycin is largely bound to plasma proteins. After absorption, erythromycin diffuses readily into most body fluids. In the absence of meningeal inflammation, low concentrations are normally achieved in the spinal fluid but the passage of the drug across the blood-brain barrier increases in meningitis. Erythromycin crosses the placental barrier and is excreted in breast milk. Erythromycin is not removed by peritoneal dialysis or hemodialysis. In the presence of normal hepatic function, erythromycin is concentrated in the liver and is excreted in the bile; the effect of hepatic dysfunction on biliary excretion of erythromycin is not known. After oral administration, less than 5% of the administered dose can be recovered in the active form in the urine.

The erythromycin particles in PCE tablets are coated with a polymer whose dissolution is pH dependent. This coating allows for minimal release of erythromycin in acidic environments, e.g. stomach. This delivery system is designed for optimal drug release and absorption in the small intestine. In multiple-dose, steady-state studies, PCE tablets have demonstrated rapid and generally adequate drug delivery in both fasting and nonfasting conditions. However, the presence of food results in lower blood levels, and optimal blood levels are obtained when PCE tablets are given in the fasting state (at least $\frac{1}{2}$ hour and preferably 2 hours before meals). Bioavailability data are available from Abbott Laboratories, Dept. 355.

Microbiology:

Erythromycin acts by inhibition of protein synthesis by binding 50 S ribosomal subunits of susceptible organisms. It does not affect nucleic acid synthesis. Antagonism has been demonstrated *in vitro* between erythromycin and clindamycin, lincomycin, and chloramphenicol.

Many strains of *Haemophilus influenzae* are resistant to erythromycin alone, but are susceptible to erythromycin and sulfonamides together.

Staphylococci resistant to erythromycin may emerge during a course of erythromycin therapy. Culture and susceptibility testing should be performed.

Erythromycin is usually active against the following organisms *in vitro* (prior to use, refer to "Indications and Usage" section):

Gram-positive Bacteria: Staphylococcus aureus (resistant organisms may emerge during treatment), Streptococcus pyogenes (Group A beta-hemolytic streptococci), Alpha-hemolytic streptococci (viridans group), Streptococcus (diplococcus) pneumoniae, Corynebacterium diphtheriae, Corynebacterium minutissimum.

Gram-negative Bacteria: Moraxella (Branhamella) catarrhalis, Neisseria gonorrhoeae, Legionella pneumophila, Bordetella pertussis.

Mycoplasma: Mycoplasma pneumoniae, Ureaplasma urealyticum.

Other Microorganisms: Chlamydia trachomatis, Entamoeba histolytica, Treponema pallidum, Listeria monocytogenes.

Susceptibility Testing:

Quantitative methods that require measurement of zone diameters give the most precise estimates of antibiotic susceptibility. One such standardized single-disc procedure has been recommended for use with discs to test susceptibility to erythromycin.[1] Interpretation involves correlation of the zone diameters obtained in the disc test with minimal inhibitory concentration (MIC) values for erythromycin.

Reports from the laboratory giving results of the standardized single-disc susceptibility test using a 15 mcg erythromycin disc should be interpreted according to the following criteria:

Susceptible organisms produce zones of 18 mm or greater, indicating that the tested organism is likely to respond to therapy.

Resistant organisms produce zones of 13 mm or less, indicating that other therapy should be selected.

Organisms of intermediate susceptibility produce zones of 14 to 17 mm. The "intermediate" category provides a "buffer zone" which should prevent small, uncontrolled technical factors from causing major discrepancies in interpretations; thus, when a zone diameter falls within the "intermediate" range, the results may be considered equivocal. If alternative drugs are not available, confirmation by dilution tests may be indicated.

Standardized procedures require the use of control organisms. The 15 mcg erythromycin disc should give zone diameters between 22 and 30 mm for the *S. aureus* ATCC 25923 control strain.

A bacterial isolate may be considered susceptible if the MIC value[2] for erythromycin is not more than 2 mcg/mL. Organisms are considered resistant if the MIC is 8 mcg/mL or higher. The MIC of erythromycin for *S. aureus* ATCC 29213 control strain should be between 0.12 and 0.5 mcg/mL.

INDICATIONS AND USAGE

PCE tablets are indicated in the treatment of infections caused by susceptible strains of the designated microorganisms in the diseases listed below:

Upper respiratory tract infections of mild to moderate degree caused by *Streptococcus pyogenes* (Group A beta-hemolytic streptococci); *Streptococcus pneumoniae* (*Diplococcus pneumoniae*); *Haemophilus influenzae* (when used concomitantly with adequate doses of sulfonamides, since many strains of *H. influenzae* are not susceptible to the erythromycin concentrations ordinarily achieved). (See appropriate sulfonamide labeling for prescribing information.)

Lower respiratory tract infections of mild to moderate severity caused by *Streptococcus pyogenes* (Group A beta-hemolytic streptococci); *Streptococcus pneumoniae* (*Diplococcus pneumoniae*).

Respiratory tract infections due to *Mycoplasma pneumoniae.*

Skin and skin structure infections of mild to moderate severity caused by *Streptococcus pyogenes* and *Staphylococcus aureus* (resistant staphylococci may emerge during treatment).

Pertussis (whooping cough) caused by *Bordetella pertussis.* Erythromycin is effective in eliminating the organism from the nasopharynx of infected individuals, rendering them noninfectious. Some clinical studies suggest that erythromycin may be helpful in the prophylaxis of pertussis in exposed susceptible individuals.

Diphtheria—As an adjunct to antitoxin in infections due to *Corynebacterium diphtheriae,* to prevent establishment of carriers and to eradicate the organism in carriers.

Erythrasma—In the treatment of infections due to *Corynebacterium minutissimum.*

Intestinal amebiasis caused by *Entamoeba histolytica* (oral erythromycins only). Extraenteric amebiasis requires treatment with other agents.

Acute pelvic inflammatory disease caused by *Neisseria gonorrhoeae:* Erythrocin® Lactobionate-I.V. (erythromycin lactobionate for injection, USP) followed by erythromycin base orally, as an alternative drug in treatment of acute pelvic inflammatory disease caused by *N. gonorrhoeae* in female patients with a history of sensitivity to penicillin. Before treatment of gonorrhea, patients who are suspected of also having syphilis should have a microscopic examination for *T. pallidum* (by immunofluorescence or darkfield) before receiving erythromycin and monthly serologic tests for a minimum of 4 months thereafter.

Erythromycins are indicated for treatment of the following infections caused by *Chlamydia trachomatis:* conjunctivitis of the newborn, pneumonia of infancy, and urogenital infections during pregnancy. When tetracyclines are contraindicated or not tolerated, erythromycin is indicated for the treatment of uncomplicated urethral, endocervical, or rectal infections in adults due to *Chlamydia trachomatis.*[3]

When tetracyclines are contraindicated or not tolerated, erythromycin is indicated for the treatment of nongonococcal urethritis caused by *Ureaplasma urealyticum.*[3]

Primary syphilis caused by *Treponema pallidum.* Erythromycin (oral forms only) is an alternative choice of treatment for primary syphilis in patients allergic to the penicillins. In treatment of primary syphilis, spinal fluid should be examined before treatment and as part of the follow-up after therapy.

Legionnaires' Disease caused by *Legionella pneumophila.* Although no controlled clinical efficacy studies have been conducted, *in vitro* and limited preliminary clinical data suggest that erythromycin may be effective in treating Legionnaires' Disease.

Prevention of Initial Attacks of Rheumatic Fever—Penicillin is considered by the American Heart Association to be the drug of choice in the prevention of initial attacks of rheumatic fever (treatment of Group A beta-hemolytic streptococcal infections of the upper respiratory tract e.g., tonsillitis, or pharyngitis).[4] Erythromycin is indicated for the treatment of penicillin-allergic patients. The therapeutic dose should be administered for ten days.

Prevention of Recurrent Attacks of Rheumatic Fever—Penicillin or sulfonamides are considered by the American Heart Association to be the drugs of choice in the prevention of recurrent attacks of rheumatic fever. In patients who are allergic to penicillin and sulfonamides, oral erythromycin is recommended by the American Heart Association in the long-term prophylaxis of streptococcal pharyngitis (for the prevention of recurrent attacks of rheumatic fever).[4]

Prevention of Bacterial Endocarditis—Although no controlled clinical efficacy trials have been conducted, oral erythromycin has been recommended by the American Heart Association for prevention of bacterial endocarditis in penicillin-allergic patients with most congenital cardiac malformations, rheumatic or other acquired valvular dysfunction, idiopathic hypertrophic subaortic stenosis (IHSS), previous history of bacterial endocarditis and mitral valve prolapse with insufficiency when they undergo dental procedures and surgical procedures of the upper respiratory tract.[5]

CONTRAINDICATIONS

Erythromycin is contraindicated in patients with known hypersensitivity to this antibiotic.

WARNINGS

There have been reports of hepatic dysfunction with or without jaundice, occurring in patients receiving oral erythromycin products.

PRECAUTIONS

General: Erythromycin is principally excreted by the liver. Caution should be exercised when erythromycin is administered to patients with impaired hepatic function. (See "Clinical Pharmacology" and "Warnings" sections).

Prolonged or repeated use of erythromycin may result in an overgrowth of nonsusceptible bacteria or fungi. If superinfection occurs, erythromycin should be discontinued and appropriate therapy instituted.

When indicated, incision and drainage or other surgical procedures should be performed in conjunction with antibiotic therapy.

Laboratory Tests: Erythromycin interferes with the fluorometric determination of urinary catecholamines.

Drug Interactions: Erythromycin use in patients who are receiving high doses of theophylline may be associated with an increase of serum theophylline levels and potential theophylline toxicity. In case of theophylline toxicity and/or elevated serum theophylline levels, the dose of theophylline should be reduced while the patient is receiving concomitant erythromycin therapy.

Concomitant administration of erythromycin and digoxin has been reported to result in elevated digoxin serum levels.

There have been reports of increased anticoagulant effects when erythromycin and oral anticoagulants were used concomitantly.

Concurrent use of erythromycin and ergotamine or dihydroergotamine has been associated in some patients with acute ergot toxicity characterized by severe peripheral vasospasm and dysesthesia.

Erythromycin has been reported to decrease the clearance of triazolam and thus may increase the pharmacologic effect of triazolam.

The use of erythromycin in patients concurrently taking drugs metabolized by the cytochrome P450 system may be associated with elevations in serum erythromycin with carbamazepine, cyclosporine, hexobarbital and phenytoin. Serum concentrations of drugs metabolized by the cytochrome P450 system should be monitored closely in patients concurrently receiving erythromycin.

Troleandomycin significantly alters the metabolism of terfenadine when taken concomitantly; therefore, observe caution when erythromycin and terfenadine are used concurrently.

Patients receiving concomitant lovastatin and erythromycin should be carefully monitored; cases of rhabdomyolysis have been reported in seriously ill patients.

Carcinogenesis, Mutagenesis, Impairment of Fertility: Long-term (2-year) oral studies conducted in rats with erythromycin base did not provide evidence of tumorigenicity. Mutagenicity studies have not been conducted. There was no apparent effect on male or female fertility in rats fed erythromycin (base) at levels up to 0.25 percent of diet.

Pregnancy: Pregnancy Category B: There is no evidence of teratogenicity or any other adverse effect on reproduction in female rats fed erythromycin base (up to 0.25 percent of diet) prior to and during mating, during gestation, and through weaning of two successive litters. There are, however, no adequate and well-controlled studies in pregnant women. Because animal reproduction studies are not always predictive of human response, this drug should be used during pregnancy only if clearly needed. Erythromycin has been reported to cross the placental barrier in humans, but fetal plasma levels are generally low.

Labor and Delivery: The effect of erythromycin on labor and delivery is unknown.

Nursing Mothers: Erythromycin is excreted in breast milk, therefore, caution should be exercised when erythromycin is administered to a nursing woman.

Pediatric Use: See "Indications and Usage" and "Dosage and Administration" sections.

ADVERSE REACTIONS

The most frequent side effects of oral erythromycin preparations are gastrointestinal and are dose-related. They include nausea, vomiting, abdominal pain, diarrhea and anorexia. Symptoms of hepatic dysfunction and/or abnormal liver function test results may occur (See "Warnings" section).

Pseudomembranous colitis has been rarely reported in association with erythromycin therapy.

There have been isolated reports of transient central nervous system side effects including confusion, hallucinations, seizures, and vertigo; however, a cause and effect relationship has not been established.

Occasional case reports of cardiac arrhythmias such as ventricular tachycardia have been documented in patients receiving erythromycin therapy. There have been isolated reports of other cardiovascular symptoms such as chest pain, dizziness, and palpitations; however, a cause and effect relationship has not been established.
Allergic reactions ranging from urticaria and mild skin eruptions to anaphylaxis have occurred.
There have been isolated reports of reversible hearing loss occurring chiefly in patients with renal insufficiency and in patients receiving high doses of erythromycin.

OVERDOSAGE

In case of overdosage, erythromycin should be discontinued. Overdosage should be handled with the prompt elimination of unabsorbed drug and all other appropriate measures.
Erythromycin is not removed by peritoneal dialysis or hemodialysis.

DOSAGE AND ADMINISTRATION

In most patients, PCE tablets are well absorbed and may be dosed orally without regard to meals. However, optimal blood levels are obtained when either PCE 333 mg or PCE 500 mg tablets are given in the fasting state (at least ½ hour and preferably 2 hours before meals).
Adults: The usual dosage of PCE is one 333 mg tablet every 8 hours or one 500 mg tablet every 12 hours. Dosage may be increased up to 4 g per day according to the severity of the infection. However, twice-a-day dosing is not recommended when doses larger than 1 g daily are administered.
Children: Age, weight, and severity of the infection are important factors in determining the proper dosage. The usual dosage is 30 to 50 mg/kg/day, in equally divided doses. For more severe infections this dosage may be doubled but should not exceed 4 g per day.
In the treatment of Group A beta-hemolytic streptococcal infections of the upper respiratory tract (e.g., tonsillitis or pharyngitis), the therapeutic dosage of erythromycin should be administered for ten days. The American Heart Association suggests a dosage of 250 mg of erythromycin orally, twice a day in long-term prophylaxis of streptococcal upper respiratory tract infections for the prevention of recurring attacks of rheumatic fever in patients allergic to penicillin and sulfonamides.[4]
In prophylaxis against bacterial endocarditis (see "Indications and Usage" section) the oral regimen for penicillin allergic patients is erythromycin 1 gram, 1 hour before the procedure followed by 500 mg six hours later.[5]
Conjunctivitis of the newborn caused by *Chlamydia trachomatis:* Oral erythromycin suspension 50 mg/kg/day in 4 divided doses for at least 2 weeks.[3]
Pneumonia of infancy caused by *Chlamydia trachomatis:* Although the optimal duration of therapy has not been established, the recommended therapy is oral erythromycin suspension 50 mg/kg/day in 4 divided doses for at least 3 weeks.[3]
Urogenital infections during pregnancy due to *Chlamydia trachomatis:* Although the optimal dose and duration of therapy have not been established, the suggested treatment is 500 mg of erythromycin by mouth four times a day or two erythromycin 333 mg tablets orally every 8 hours on an empty stomach for at least 7 days. For women who cannot tolerate this regimen, a decreased dose of one erythromycin 500 mg tablet orally every 12 hours, one 333 mg tablet orally every 8 hours or 250 mg by mouth four times a day should be used for at least 14 days.[3,6]
For adults with uncomplicated urethral, endocervical, or rectal infections caused by *Chlamydia trachomatis,* when tetracycline is contraindicated or not tolerated: 500 mg of erythromycin by mouth four times a day or two 333 mg tablets orally every 8 hours for at least 7 days.[3,6]
For patients with nongonococcal urethritis caused by *Ureaplasma urealyticum* when tetracycline is contraindicated or not tolerated: 500 mg of erythromycin by mouth four times a day or two 333 mg tablets orally every 8 hours for at least seven days.[3,6]
Primary syphilis: 30 to 40 g given in divided doses over a period of 10 to 15 days.
Acute pelvic inflammatory disease caused by *N. gonorrhoeae:* 500 mg Erythrocin Lactobionate-I.V. (erythromycin lactobionate for injection, USP) every 6 hours for 3 days, followed by 500 mg of erythromycin base orally, every 12 hours or 333 mg of erythromycin base orally every 8 hours for 7 days.
Intestinal amebiasis: Adults: 500 mg every 12 hours, 333 mg every 8 hours or 250 mg every 6 hours for 10 to 14 days. Children: 30 to 50 mg/kg/day in divided doses for 10 to 14 days.
Pertussis: Although optimal dosage and duration have not been established, doses of erythromycin utilized in reported clinical studies were 40 to 50 mg/kg/day, given in divided doses for 5 to 14 days.
Legionnaires' Disease: Although optimal dosage has not been established, doses utilized in reported clinical data were 1 to 4 g daily in divided doses.

HOW SUPPLIED

PCE (erythromycin particles in tablets) is supplied as unscored, ovaloid, Dispertab® tablets in the following strengths and packages.
333 mg, pink-speckled white (imprinted with ᗣ and PCE):
Bottles of 60 ....(**NDC** 0074-6290-60);
Bottles of 500 ....(**NDC** 0074-6290-53).
500 mg, white (imprinted with ᗣ and EK):
Bottles of 100 ....(**NDC** 0074-3389-13).
Recommended Storage: Store below 86°F (30°C).

REFERENCES

1. National Committee for Clinical Laboratory Standards, Approved Standard: *Performance Standards for Antimicrobial Disk Susceptibility Tests,* 3rd Edition, Vol. 4(16):M2–A3, Villanova, PA, December 1984.
2. Ericson, H.M., Sherris, J.C., Antibiotic Sensitivity Testing: Report of an International Collaborative Study, *Acta Pathologica et Microbiologica Scandinavica* Section B Suppl. 217:1–90, 1971.
3. CDC Sexually Transmitted Diseases Treatment Guidelines 1985.
4. Committee on Rheumatic Fever and Infective Endocarditis of the Council on Cardiovascular Disease of the Young: Prevention of Rheumatic Fever, *Circulation* 70(6):1118A–1122A, December 1984.
5. Committee on Rheumatic Fever and Infective Endocarditis of the Council on Cardiovascular Disease of the Young: Prevention of Bacterial Endocarditis, *Circulation* 70(6):1123A–1127A, December 1984.
6. Data on file, Abbott Laboratories.

Ref. 01-2546-R3

Shown in Product Identification Section, page 403

PEGANONE® ℞

[*pĕg'ă-noon*]
(ethotoin tablets, USP)

DESCRIPTION

PEGANONE (ethotoin tablets, USP) is an oral antiepileptic of the hydantoin series and is chemically identified as 3-ethyl-5-phenyl-2, 4-imidazolidinedione. PEGANONE tablets are available in two dosage strengths of 250 mg and 500 mg respectively.
Inactive Ingredients: 250 mg and 500 mg tablets: Acacia, lactose, sodium carboxymethylcellulose, stearic acid and talc.

CLINICAL PHARMACOLOGY

PEGANONE (ethotoin tablets, USP) exerts an antiepileptic effect without causing general central nervous system depression. The mechanism of action is probably very similar to that of phenytoin. The latter drug appears to stabilize rather than to raise the normal seizure threshold, and to prevent the spread of seizure activity rather than to abolish the primary focus of seizure discharges.
In laboratory animals, the drug was found effective against electroshock convulsions, and to a lesser extent, against complex partial (psychomotor) and pentylenetetrazol-induced seizures.
In mice, the duration of antiepileptic activity was prolonged by hepatic injury but not by bilateral nephrectomy; the drug is apparently biotransformed by the liver.
Ethotoin is fairly rapidly absorbed; the extent of oral absorption is not known. The drug exhibits saturable metabolism with respect to the formation of N-deethyl and p-hydroxyl-ethotoin, the major metabolites. Where plasma concentrations are below about 8 mcg/mL, the elimination half-life of ethotoin is in the range of 3 to 9 hours. A study comparing single doses of 500 mg, 1000 mg, and 1500 mg of PEGANONE (ethotoin tablets, USP) demonstrated that ethotoin, and to a lesser extent 5-phenylhydantoin, a major metabolite, exhibits substantial nonlinear kinetics. The degree of nonlinearity with multiple dosing may be increased over that seen after a single dose, given the likelihood of plasma accumulation based on a reported elimination half-life of 6 to 9 hours and a dosing interval of 4 to 6 hours. Experience suggests that therapeutic plasma concentrations fall in the range of 15 to 50 mcg/mL; however, this range is not as extensively documented as those quoted for other antiepileptics.

INDICATIONS AND USAGE

PEGANONE (ethotoin tablets, USP) is indicated for the control of tonic-clonic (grand mal) and complex partial (psychomotor) seizures.

CONTRAINDICATIONS

PEGANONE (ethotoin tablets, USP) is contraindicated in patients with hepatic abnormalities or hematologic disorders.

WARNINGS

USAGE DURING PREGNANCY— THERE ARE MULTIPLE REPORTS IN THE CLINICAL LITERATURE WHICH INDICATE THAT THE USE OF ANTIEPILEPTIC DRUGS DURING PREGNANCY RESULTS IN AN INCREASED INCIDENCE OF BIRTH DEFECTS IN THE OFFSPRING. ALTHOUGH DATA ARE MORE EXTENSIVE WITH RESPECT TO TRIMETHADIONE, PARAMETHADIONE, PHENYTOIN, AND PHENOBARBITAL, REPORTS INDICATE A POSSIBLE SIMILAR ASSOCIATION WITH THE USE OF OTHER ANTIEPILEPTIC DRUGS. THEREFORE, ANTIEPILEPTIC DRUGS SHOULD BE ADMINISTERED TO WOMEN OF CHILDBEARING POTENTIAL ONLY IF THEY ARE CLEARLY SHOWN TO BE ESSENTIAL IN THE MANAGEMENT OF THEIR SEIZURES.
ANTIEPILEPTIC DRUGS SHOULD NOT BE DISCONTINUED IN PATIENTS IN WHOM THE DRUG IS ADMINISTERED TO PREVENT MAJOR SEIZURES BECAUSE OF THE STRONG POSSIBILITY OF PRECIPITATING STATUS EPILEPTICUS WITH ATTENDANT HYPOXIA AND RISK TO BOTH MOTHER AND THE UNBORN CHILD. CONSIDERATION SHOULD, HOWEVER, BE GIVEN TO DISCONTINUATION OF ANTIEPILEPTICS PRIOR TO AND DURING PREGNANCY WHEN THE NATURE, FREQUENCY AND SEVERITY OF THE SEIZURES DO NOT POSE A SERIOUS THREAT TO THE PATIENT. IT IS NOT, HOWEVER, KNOWN WHETHER EVEN MINOR SEIZURES CONSTITUTE SOME RISK TO THE DEVELOPING EMBRYO OR FETUS.
REPORTS HAVE SUGGESTED THAT THE MATERNAL INGESTION OF ANTIEPILEPTIC DRUGS, PARTICULARLY BARBITURATES, IS ASSOCIATED WITH A NEONATAL COAGULATION DEFECT THAT MAY CAUSE BLEEDING DURING THE EARLY (USUALLY WITHIN 24 HOURS OF BIRTH) NEONATAL PERIOD. THE POSSIBILITY OF THE OCCURRENCE OF THIS DEFECT WITH THE USE OF PEGANONE SHOULD BE KEPT IN MIND. THE DEFECT IS CHARACTERIZED BY DECREASED LEVELS OF VITAMIN K-DEPENDENT CLOTTING FACTORS, AND PROLONGATION OF EITHER THE PROTHROMBIN TIME OR THE PARTIAL THROMBOPLASTIN TIME, OR BOTH. IT HAS BEEN SUGGESTED THAT VITAMIN K BE GIVEN PROPHYLACTICALLY TO THE MOTHER ONE MONTH PRIOR TO, AND DURING DELIVERY, AND TO THE INFANT, INTRAVENOUSLY, IMMEDIATELY AFTER BIRTH.
THE PHYSICIAN SHOULD WEIGH THESE CONSIDERATIONS IN TREATMENT AND COUNSELING OF EPILEPTIC WOMEN OF CHILDBEARING POTENTIAL.

PRECAUTIONS

General: Blood dyscrasias have been reported in patients receiving PEGANONE. Although the etiologic role of PEGANONE has not been definitely established, physicians should be alert for general malaise, sore throat and other symptoms indicative of possible blood dyscrasia.
There is some evidence suggesting that hydantoin-like compounds may interfere with folic acid metabolism, precipitating a megaloblastic anemia. If this should occur during gestation, folic acid therapy should be considered.
Information for Patients: Patients should be advised to report immediately such signs and symptoms as sore throat, fever, malaise, easy bruising, petechiae, epistaxis, or others that may be indicative of an infection or bleeding tendency.
Laboratory Tests: Liver function tests should be performed if clinical evidence suggests the possibility of hepatic dysfunction. Signs of liver damage are indication for withdrawal of the drug.
It is recommended that blood counts and urinalyses be performed when therapy is begun and at monthly intervals for several months thereafter. As in patients receiving other hydantoin compounds and other antiepileptic drugs, blood dyscrasias have been reported in patients receiving PEGANONE (ethotoin tablets, USP). Marked depression of the blood count is indication for withdrawal of the drug.
Drug Interactions: PEGANONE used in combination with other drugs known to adversely affect the hematopoietic system should be avoided if possible.
Considerable caution should be exercised if PEGANONE is administered concurrently with *Phenurone (phenacemide)* since paranoid symptoms have been reported during therapy with this combination.
A two-way interaction between the hydantoin antiepileptic, *phenytoin,* and the *coumarin anticoagulants* has been suggested. Presumably, phenytoin acts as a stimulator of coumarin metabolism and has been reported to cause decreased serum levels of the coumarin anticoagulants and increased prothrombin-proconvertin concentrations. Conversely, the coumarin anticoagulants have been reported to increase the serum levels and prolong the serum half-life of phenytoin by inhibiting its metabolism. Although there is no documentation of such, a similar interaction between ethotoin and the coumarin anticoagulants may occur. Caution is therefore advised when administering PEGANONE to patients receiving coumarin anticoagulants.

Continued on next page

If desired, additional literature on any Abbott product will be provided upon request to Abbott Laboratories.

Abbott Laboratories—Cont.

Carcinogenesis: No data are available on long-term potential for carcinogenicity in animals or humans.

Pregnancy: Pregnancy Category C. See "Warnings" section.

Nursing Mothers: Ethotoin is excreted in breast milk. Because of the potential for serious adverse reactions in nursing infants from ethotoin, a decision should be made whether to discontinue nursing or to discontinue the drug, taking into account the importance of the drug to the mother.

ADVERSE REACTIONS

Adverse reactions associated with PEGANONE, in decreasing order of severity, are:

Isolated cases of lymphadenopathy and systemic lupus erythematosus have been reported in patients taking hydantoin compounds, and lymphadenopathy has occurred with PEGANONE. Withdrawal of therapy has resulted in remission of the clinical and pathological findings. Therefore, if a lymphoma-like syndrome develops, the drug should be withdrawn and the patient should be closely observed for regression of signs and symptoms before treatment is resumed.

Ataxia and gum hypertrophy have occurred only rarely—usually only in patients receiving an additional hydantoin derivative. It is of interest to note that ataxia and gum hypertrophy have subsided in patients receiving other hydantoins when PEGANONE was given as a substitute antiepileptic.

Occasionally, vomiting or nausea after ingestion of PEGANONE has been reported, but if the drug is administered after meals, the incidence of gastric distress is reduced. Other side effects have included chest pain, nystagmus, diplopia, fever, dizziness, diarrhea, headache, insomnia, fatigue, numbness and skin rash.

OVERDOSAGE

Symptoms of acute overdosage include drowsiness, visual disturbance, nausea and ataxia. Coma is possible at very high dosage.

Treatment should be begun by inducing emesis; gastric lavage may be considered as an alternative. General supportive measures will be necessary. A careful evaluation of blood-forming organs should be made following recovery.

DOSAGE AND ADMINISTRATION

PEGANONE (ethotoin tablets, USP) is administered orally in 4 to 6 divided doses daily. The drug should be taken after food, and doses should be spaced as evenly as practicable. Initial dosage should be conservative. For adults, the initial daily dose should be 1 g or less, with subsequent gradual dosage increases over a period of several days. The optimum dosage must be determined on the basis of individual response. The usual adult maintenance dose is 2 to 3 g daily. Less than 2 g daily has been found ineffective in most adults.

Pediatric dosage depends upon the age and weight of the patient. The initial dose should not exceed 750 mg daily. The usual maintenance dose in children ranges from 500 mg to 1 g daily, although occasionally 2 or (rarely) 3 g daily may be necessary.

If a patient is receiving another antiepileptic drug, it should not be discontinued when PEGANONE therapy is begun. The dosage of the other drug should be reduced gradually as that of PEGANONE is increased. PEGANONE may eventually replace the other drug or the optimal dosage of both antiepileptics may be established.

PEGANONE is compatible with all commonly employed antiepileptic medications with the possible exception of Phenurone® (phenacemide). In tonic-clonic (grand mal) seizures, use of the drug with phenobarbital may be beneficial. PEGANONE may be used in combination with drugs such as Tridione® (trimethadione) or Paradione® (paramethadione), as an adjunct in those patients with absence (petit mal) associated with tonic-clonic (grand mal).

HOW SUPPLIED

PEGANONE (ethotoin tablets, USP) grooved, white tablets are supplied in two dosage strengths: 250 mg, bottles of 100 (NDC 0074-6902-01); 500 mg, bottles of 100 (NDC 0074-6905-04).

Recommended Storage: Store below 77°F (25°C)

This product is listed in N.D., a Medicare designated compendium.

Ref. 01-2537-R9

Shown in Product Identification Section, page 403

PHENURONE®   ℞
[fĕn 'ū-rōne]
(phenacemide tablets, USP)

DESCRIPTION

PHENURONE (phenacemide) is a valuable antiepileptic drug for use in selected patients with epilepsy. Since therapy with PHENURONE involves certain risks, *physicians should thoroughly familiarize themselves with the undesirable side effects which may occur and the precautions to be observed.* PHENU-

RONE (phenacemide) is a substituted acetylurea derivative. Chemically PHENURONE is identified as N-(aminocarbonyl)-benzeneacetamide. PHENURONE tablets contain 500 mg phenacemide for oral administration.

Inactive Ingredients: Corn starch, lactose and talc.

CLINICAL PHARMACOLOGY

In experimental animals, PHENURONE in doses well below those causing neurological signs, elevates the threshold for minimal electroshock convulsions and abolishes the tonic phase of maximal electroshock seizures. The drug prevents or modifies seizures induced by pentylenetetrazol or other convulsants. In comparative tests, PHENURONE was found to be equal or more effective than other commonly used antiepileptics against complex partial (psychomotor) seizures which were induced in mice by low frequency stimulation of the cerebral cortex. Studies in mice have shown that PHENURONE exerts a synergistic antiepileptic effect with mephenytoin, phenobarbital, or trimethadione.

Given orally to laboratory animals, PHENURONE has a low acute toxicity. In mice, slight ataxia appears at 400 mg/kg and light sleep occurs at 800 mg/kg. In high doses the drug causes marked ataxia and coma, the fatal dose being in the range of 3 to 5 g/kg for mice, rats, and cats.

PHENURONE is metabolized by the liver, however, further definition of human pharmacokinetics has not been determined.

INDICATIONS AND USAGE

PHENURONE (phenacemide) is indicated for the control of severe epilepsy, particularly mixed forms of complex partial (psychomotor) seizures, refractory to other drugs.

CONTRAINDICATIONS

PHENURONE should not be administered unless other available antiepileptics have been found to be ineffective in satisfactorily controlling seizures.

WARNINGS

PHENURONE (phenacemide) can produce serious side effects as well as direct organ toxicity. As a consequence its use entails the assumption of certain risks which must be weighed against the benefit to the patient. *Ordinarily PHENURONE should not be administered unless other available antiepileptics have been found to be ineffective in controlling seizures.* Death attributable to liver damage during therapy with PHENURONE has been reported. PHENURONE should be used with caution in patients with a history of previous liver dysfunction. If jaundice or other signs of hepatitis appear, the drug should be discontinued.

Aplastic anemia has occurred in association with PHENURONE therapy and death from this condition has been reported. PHENURONE should ordinarily not be used in patients with severe blood dyscrasias. Marked depression of the blood count is an indication for withdrawal of the drug.

Usage During Pregnancy: PHENURONE can cause fetal harm when administered to a pregnant woman. There are multiple reports in the clinical literature which indicate that the use of antiepileptic drugs during pregnancy results in an increased incidence of birth defects in the offspring. Reports have also suggested that the maternal ingestion of antiepileptic drugs, particularly barbiturates, is associated with a neonatal coagulation defect that may cause bleeding during the early (usually within 24 hours of birth) neonatal period. The possibility of the occurrence of this defect with the use of PHENURONE should be kept in mind. The defect is characterized by decreased levels of vitamin K-dependent clotting factors, and prolongation of either the prothrombin time or the partial thromboplastin time, or both. It has been suggested that vitamin K be given prophylactically to the mother one month prior to and during delivery, and to the infant, intravenously, immediately after birth. If this drug is used during pregnancy, or if the patient becomes pregnant while taking this drug, the patient should be apprised of the potential hazard to the fetus.

PRECAUTIONS

General: Extreme caution must be exercised in treating patients who previously have shown personality disorders. It may be advisable to hospitalize such patients during the first week of treatment. Personality changes, including attempts at suicide and the occurrence of psychoses requiring hospitalization, have been reported during therapy with PHENURONE (phenacemide). Severe or exacerbated personality changes are an indication for withdrawal of the drug.

PHENURONE (phenacemide) should be used with caution in patients with a history of previous liver dysfunction. PHENURONE should be administered with caution to patients with a history of allergy, particularly in association with the administration of other antiepileptics. The drug should be discontinued at the first sign of a skin rash or other allergic manifestation.

Information for Patients: The patient and his family should be aware of the possibility of personality changes so the family can watch for changes in the behavior of the patient such as decreased interest in surroundings, depression, or aggressiveness.

The patient should be told to report immediately any symptoms indicative of a developing blood dyscrasia such as malaise, sore throat, or fever.

Laboratory Tests: Liver function tests should be performed before and during therapy. Death attributable to liver damage during therapy with PHENURONE has been reported. If jaundice or other signs of hepatitis appear, the drug should be discontinued.

Complete blood counts should be made before instituting PHENURONE, and at monthly intervals thereafter. If no abnormality appears within 12 months, the interval between blood counts may be extended. Blood changes have been reported with leukopenia (leukocyte count of 4,000 or less per cubic millimeter of blood) as the most commonly observed effect. However, aplastic anemia has occurred in association with PHENURONE therapy, and death from this condition has been reported. *The total number of each cellular element per cubic millimeter is a better index of possible blood dyscrasia than the percentage of cells.* Marked depression of the blood count is an indication for withdrawal of the drug.

Similarly, as nephritis has occasionally occurred in patients on PHENURONE, the urine should be examined at regular intervals. Abnormal urinary findings are an indication for discontinuance of therapy.

Drug Interactions: Extreme caution is essential if PHENURONE is administered with any other antiepileptic which is known to cause similar toxic effects.

Considerable caution should be exercised if PHENURONE (phenacemide) is administered concurrently with *Peganone (ethotoin)* since paranoid symptoms have been reported during therapy with this combination.

Carcinogenesis: No data are available on long-term potential for carcinogenicity in animals or humans.

Pregnancy: Pregnancy Category D. See "Warnings" section.

Nursing Mothers: It is not known whether this drug is excreted in human milk. Because many drugs are excreted in human milk and because of the potential for serious adverse reactions in nursing infants from PHENURONE, a decision should be made whether to discontinue nursing or to discontinue the drug, taking into account the importance of the drug to the mother.

Pediatric Use: Safety and effectiveness in children below the age of 5 years have not been established.

ADVERSE REACTIONS

The following adverse effects associated with PHENURONE are listed by decreasing order of frequency based on data from one large clinical study.[1]

Psychiatric: Psychic changes (17 in 100 patients).

Gastrointestinal: Gastrointestinal disturbances (8 in 100 patients), including anorexia (5 in 100 patients) and weight loss (less than 1 in 100 patients).

Dermatologic: Skin rash (5 in 100 patients). Stevens-Johnson Syndrome with epidermal necrolysis has been reported in one non-fatal case.

CNS: Drowsiness (4 in 100 patients), headache (2 in 100 patients), insomnia (1 in 100 patients), dizziness and paresthesias (less than 1 in 100 patients).

Hematopoietic: Blood dyscrasias (primarily leukopenia), including fatal aplastic anemia (2 in 100 patients).

Hepatic: Hepatitis, including fatalities (2 in 100 patients).

Renal: Abnormal urinary findings, including a rise in serum creatinine[2], and nephritis (1 in 100 patients or less).

Other: Fatigue, fever, muscle pain and palpitation (less than 1 in 100 patients).

OVERDOSAGE

Symptoms of acute overdosage include excitement or mania, followed by drowsiness, ataxia and coma. In one case of acute overdosage, dizziness was followed by coma which lasted nearly 24 hours. Treatment should be started by inducing emesis; gastric lavage may be considered as an alternative or adjunct. General supportive measures will be necessary. A careful evaluation of liver and kidney function, mental state, and the blood-forming organs should be made following recovery.

DOSAGE AND ADMINISTRATION

PHENURONE is administered orally.

Since PHENURONE may produce serious toxic effects, it is strongly recommended that the dosage be held to the minimum amount necessary to achieve an adequate therapeutic effect.

For adults the usual starting dose is 1.5 g daily, administered in three divided doses of 500 mg each. After the first week, if seizures are not controlled and the drug is well tolerated, an additional 500 mg tablet may be taken upon arising. In the third week, if necessary, the dosage may be further increased by another 500 mg at bedtime. Satisfactory results have been noted in some patients on an initial dose of 250 mg three times per day. The effective total daily dose for adults usually ranges from 2 to 3 g, although some patients have required as much as 5 g daily.

For the pediatric patient from 5 to 10 years of age, approximately one-half the adult dose is recommended. It should be given at the same intervals as for adults.

PHENURONE may be administered alone or in conjunction with other antiepileptics. However, extreme caution must be exercised if other antiepileptics cause toxic effects similar to PHENURONE.
When PHENURONE is to replace other antiepileptic medication, the latter should be withdrawn gradually as the dosage of PHENURONE is increased to maintain seizure control.

HOW SUPPLIED

PHENURONE (Phenacemide Tablets, USP), grooved, white, 500 mg are supplied in bottles of 100 (**NDC** 0074-3971-05).

REFERENCES

1. Tyler, M. W., King, E. Q.: Phenacemide in Treatment of Epilepsy. JAMA 147: 17–21 (1951).
2. Richards, R.K., Bjornsson, T. D., Waterbury, L. D.: Rise in Serum and Urine Creatinine After Phenacemide. Clin. Pharmacol. Ther. 23: 430–437 (1978).
Ref. 01-2503-R10

PLACIDYL® ℞ Ⓒ

[pla 'ci-dil]
(ethchlorvynol capsules, USP)
Oral hypnotic

DESCRIPTION

PLACIDYL (ethchlorvynol) is a tertiary carbinol. It is chemically designated as 1-chloro-3-ethyl-1-penten-4-yn-3-ol. Ethchlorvynol occurs as a liquid which is immiscible with water and miscible with most organic solvents. PLACIDYL is an oral hypnotic available in capsule form containing either 200 mg, 500 mg or 750 mg of ethchlorvynol.
Inactive Ingredients: 200 mg capsule: FD&C Red No. 40, gelatin, glycerin, methylparaben, polyethylene glycol, propylparaben, sorbitol and titanium dioxide.
500 mg capsule: FD&C Red No. 40, gelatin, glycerin, iron oxide, methylparaben, polyethylene glycol, propylparaben, sorbitol and titanium dioxide.
750 mg capsule: FD&C Blue No. 1, FD&C Yellow No. 5 (tartrazine), FD&C Yellow No. 6, gelatin, glycerin, iron oxide, methylparaben, polyethylene glycol, propylparaben, sorbitol and titanium dioxide.

CLINICAL PHARMACOLOGY

The usual hypnotic dose of PLACIDYL induces sleep within 15 minutes to one hour. The duration of the hypnotic effect is about five hours. The mechanism of action is unknown.
PLACIDYL is rapidly absorbed from the gastrointestinal tract with peak plasma concentrations usually occurring within two hours after a single oral fasting dose. Plasma concentrations required for hypnotic effects are unknown. The plasma half-life ($t_{1/2}$, β) of the parent compound is approximately ten to twenty hours. Studies with ^{14}C-PLACIDYL have demonstrated that within 24 hours, 33% of a single 500 mg dose is excreted in the urine mostly as metabolites. The major plasma and urinary metabolite is the secondary alcohol of PLACIDYL. The free and conjugated forms of this metabolite in the urine account for about 40% of the dose. Other minor metabolites have been identified as the primary alcohol and a secondary alcohol with an altered acetylene group. Studies with ^{14}C-PLACIDYL in animals indicate that the parent compound and its metabolites undergo extensive enterohepatic recirculation.
Distribution studies indicate that there is extensive tissue localization of ethchlorvynol, particularly in adipose tissue. Ethchlorvynol and/or its metabolites have also been detected in liver, kidneys, spleen, brain, bile and cerebrospinal fluid.

INDICATIONS AND USAGE

PLACIDYL is indicated as short-term hypnotic therapy for periods up to one week in duration for the management of insomnia. If retreatment becomes necessary, after drug-free intervals of one or more weeks, it should only be undertaken upon further evaluation of the patient.

CONTRAINDICATIONS

PLACIDYL is contraindicated in patients with known hypersensitivity to the drug and in patients with porphyria.

WARNINGS

PLACIDYL SHOULD BE ADMINISTERED WITH CAUTION TO MENTALLY DEPRESSED PATIENTS WITH OR WITHOUT SUICIDAL TENDENCIES. IT SHOULD ALSO BE ADMINISTERED WITH CAUTION TO THOSE WHO HAVE A PSYCHOLOGICAL POTENTIAL FOR DRUG DEPENDENCE. THE LEAST AMOUNT OF DRUG THAT IS FEASIBLE SHOULD BE PRESCRIBED FOR THESE PATIENTS.
Psychological and Physical Dependence: PROLONGED USE OF PLACIDYL MAY RESULT IN TOLERANCE AND PSYCHOLOGICAL AND PHYSICAL DEPENDENCE. PROLONGED ADMINISTRATION OF THE DRUG IS NOT RECOMMENDED. (See "Drug Abuse and Dependence" section.)

PRECAUTIONS

General: Elderly or debilitated patients should receive the smallest effective amount of PLACIDYL (ethchlorvynol).
Caution should be exercised when treating patients with impaired hepatic or renal function.
Patients who exhibit unpredictable behavior, or paradoxical restlessness or excitement in response to barbiturates or alcohol may react in this manner to PLACIDYL.
PLACIDYL should not be used for the management of insomnia in the presence of pain unless insomnia persists after pain is controlled with analgesics.
The 750 mg dosage strength of PLACIDYL contains FD&C Yellow No. 5 (tartrazine) which may cause allergic-type reactions (including bronchial asthma) in certain susceptible individuals. Although the overall incidence of FD&C Yellow No. 5 (tartrazine) sensitivity in the general population is low, it is frequently seen in patients who also have aspirin hypersensitivity.
Information for Patients: The use of ethchlorvynol carries with it an associated risk of psychological and/or physical dependence. The patient should be warned against increasing the dose of the drug without consulting a physician.
Patients should be advised that, for the duration of the effect of PLACIDYL, mental and/or physical abilities required for the performance of potentially hazardous tasks such as the operation of dangerous machinery including motor vehicles, may be impaired.
Patients should be cautioned to avoid the concomitant use of PLACIDYL with alcohol, barbiturates, other CNS depressants, or MAO inhibitors.
Drug Interactions: The concomitant use of PLACIDYL with alcohol, barbiturates, other CNS depressants, or MAO inhibitors may produce exaggerated depressant effects.
Ethchlorvynol may cause a decreased prothrombin time response to coumarin anticoagulants; therefore, the dosage of these drugs may require adjustment when therapy with ethchlorvynol is initiated and after it is discontinued.
Transient delirium has been reported with the concomitant use of PLACIDYL and amitriptyline; therefore, PLACIDYL should be administered with caution to patients receiving tricyclic antidepressants.
Carcinogenesis: A study in mice receiving oral doses of PLACIDYL up to 7 times the maximum human daily dose for 22 to 24 months produced equivocal results. When compared to controls, a statistically significant increase in total lung tumors was found in female mice given the high dose of PLACIDYL. However, the 48% incidence is not substantially higher than the high value (39%) reported for the historical laboratory controls.
No evidence of carcinogenic potential was observed in rats given PLACIDYL at 5 to 15 times the maximum human daily dose for up to 2 years.
Usage During Pregnancy: 1. Teratogenic—Pregnancy Category C. Ethchlorvynol has been associated with a higher percentage of stillbirths and a lower survival rate of progeny among rats given 40 mg/kg/day. There are no adequate and well-controlled studies in pregnant women. Therefore, ethchlorvynol is not recommended for use during the first and second trimesters of pregnancy. Ethchlorvynol should be used during pregnancy only if the potential benefit justifies the potential risk to the fetus.
2. Non-teratogenic—Clinical experience has indicated that ethchlorvynol taken during the third trimester of pregnancy may produce CNS depression and transient withdrawal symptoms in the newborn. These symptoms resemble congenital narcotic withdrawal symptoms (See "Drug Abuse and Dependence" section).
Nursing Mothers: It is not known whether this drug is excreted in breast milk. Because many drugs are excreted in human milk and because of the potential for serious adverse reactions in nursing infants from PLACIDYL, a decision should be made whether to discontinue nursing or to discontinue the drug, taking into account the importance of the drug to the mother.
Pediatric Use: PLACIDYL is not recommended for use in children since its safety and effectiveness in the pediatric age group has not been determined.

ADVERSE REACTIONS

Adverse effects in decreasing order of severity within each of the following categories are:
Hypersensitivity: cholestatic jaundice, urticaria and rash.
Hematologic: thrombocytopenia—one case of fatal immune thrombocytopenia due to ethchlorvynol has been reported.
Gastrointestinal: vomiting, gastric upset, nausea and aftertaste.
Neurologic: dizziness and facial numbness.
Miscellaneous: blurred vision, hypotension and mild "hangover".
The following idiosyncratic responses have been reported occasionally: syncope without marked hypotension, profound muscular weakness, hysteria, marked excitement, prolonged hypnosis and mild stimulation.
Transient ataxia and giddiness have occurred in patients in whom absorption of the drug is especially rapid. These effects can sometimes be controlled by giving PLACIDYL with food.
(See "Drug Abuse and Dependence" section for the signs and symptoms of chronic intoxication).

DRUG ABUSE AND DEPENDENCE

PLACIDYL is subject to control by the Federal Controlled Substances Act under DEA schedule IV.
Abuse: Pulmonary edema of rapid onset has resulted from the I.V. abuse of PLACIDYL (ethchlorvynol).
Dependence: Signs and symptoms of intoxication have been reported with the prolonged use of doses as low as 1 g/day. Signs and symptoms of chronic intoxication may include incoordination, tremors, ataxia, confusion, slurred speech, hyperreflexia, diplopia, and generalized muscle weakness. Toxic amblyopia, scotoma, nystagmus, and peripheral neuropathy have also been reported with prolonged use of ethchlorvynol; these symptoms are usually reversible.
Severe withdrawal symptoms similar to those seen during barbiturate and alcohol withdrawal have been reported following abrupt discontinuance of prolonged use of PLACIDYL. These symptoms may appear as late as nine days after sudden withdrawal of the drug. Signs and symptoms of PLACIDYL withdrawal may include convulsions, delirium, hallucinations, schizoid reaction, perceptual distortions, memory loss, ataxia, insomnia, slurring of speech, unusual anxiety, irritability, agitation, and tremors. Other signs and symptoms may include anorexia, nausea, vomiting, weakness, dizziness, sweating, muscle twitching, and weight loss.
Management of a patient who manifests withdrawal symptoms from PLACIDYL involves readministration of the drug to approximately the same level of chronic intoxication which existed before the abrupt discontinuance. (Phenobarbital may be substituted for PLACIDYL.) A gradual, stepwise reduction of dosage may then be made over a period of days or weeks. A phenothiazine compound may be used in addition to this regimen for those patients who exhibit psychotic symptoms during the withdrawal period. The patient undergoing withdrawal from PLACIDYL must be hospitalized or closely observed, and given general supportive care as indicated.
In one report an infant born to a mother who received 500 mg PLACIDYL at bedtime daily throughout the third trimester, exhibited withdrawal symptoms on the second day of life. The symptoms included episodic jitteriness, hyperactivity, restlessness, irritability, disturbed sleep and hunger. The neonate responded to a single oral dose of phenobarbital (3 mg/kg). The withdrawal symptoms gradually decreased and completely disappeared by the tenth day of life.

OVERDOSAGE

Acute intoxication is characterized by prolonged deep coma, severe respiratory depression, hypothermia, hypotension, and relative bradycardia. Nystagmus and pancytopenia resulting from acute PLACIDYL overdose have been reported. Although death has occurred following the ingestion of 6 g of PLACIDYL, there have been reports of patients who have survived overdoses of 50 g and more with intensive care. Fatal blood concentrations usually range from 20 to 50 μg/mL.[1] Because large amounts of ethchlorvynol are taken up by adipose tissue, the blood concentration is an unreliable indicator of the magnitude of overdose.
Management of acute PLACIDYL intoxication is similar to that of acute barbiturate intoxication.[2] Gastric evacuation should be performed immediately. (In the unconscious patient, gastric lavage should be preceded by tracheal intubation with a cuffed tube.) Supportive care (assisted ventilation, frequent and careful monitoring of vital signs, control of blood pressure) is essential. Emphasis should be placed on pulmonary care and monitoring of blood gases. Hemoperfusion utilizing the Amberlite column technique has been reported in the literature to be the most effective method in the management of acute PLACIDYL overdose.[3] In addition, hemodialysis and peritoneal dialysis have each been reported to be of some value. (Aqueous and oil dialysates have been used. Forced diuresis with maintenance of a high urinary output has also been reported of some value.)
(See "Drug Abuse and Dependence" section for the signs and symptoms of chronic intoxication.)

DOSAGE AND ADMINISTRATION

The usual adult hypnotic dose of PLACIDYL (ethchlorvynol) is 500 mg taken orally at bedtime. A dose of 750 mg may be required for patients whose sleep response to a 500 mg capsule is inadequate, or for patients being changed from barbiturates or other nonbarbiturate hypnotics. Up to 1000 mg may be given as a single bedtime dose when insomnia is unusually severe. A single supplemental dose of 200 mg may be given to reinstitute sleep in patients who may awaken after the original bedtime dose of 500 or 750 mg.

Continued on next page

If desired, additional literature on any Abbott product will be provided upon request to Abbott Laboratories.

Abbott Laboratories—Cont.

For patients whose insomnia is characterized only by untimely awakening during the early morning hours, a single dose of 200 mg taken upon awakening may be adequate for relief.

The smallest effective dose of PLACIDYL should be given to elderly or debilitated patients.

PLACIDYL should not be prescribed for periods exceeding one week. (See "Drug Abuse and Dependence" section.)

HOW SUPPLIED

PLACIDYL (ethchlorvynol capsules, USP) is supplied as:
200 mg red capsules:
Bottles of 100 ....(NDC 0074-6661-08).
500 mg red capsules:
Bottles of 100 ....(NDC 0074-6685-15).
ABBO-PAC® unit dose strip
packages of 100 ....(NDC 0074-6685-10).
750 mg green capsules:
Bottles of 100 ....(NDC 0074-6630-01).
Recommended storage: 59°–77° F (15°–25° C).

REFERENCES

1. AMA Dept. of Drugs. *AMA Drug Evaluations*, Massachusetts: Publishing Sciences Group, Inc., 1980.
2. Khantzian, E. J., McKenna, G. J., Acute Toxic and Withdrawal Reactions Associated with Drug Abuse, *Annals of Internal Medicine*, 90:361–372, 1979.
3. Lynn, R.I., et al., Resin Hemoperfusion for Treatment of Ethchlorvynol Overdose, *Annals of Internal Medicine*, 91:549–553, 1979.
Ref. 01-2542-R10

Shown in Product Identification Section, page 404

PROSOM™   ℞ ℭ
[prō'som]
(estazolam tablets)

DESCRIPTION

ProSom (estazolam), a triazolobenzodiazepine derivative, is an oral hypnotic agent. Estazolam occurs as a fine, white, odorless powder that is soluble in alcohol and practically insoluble in water. The chemical name for estazolam is 8-chloro-6-phenyl-4H-s-triazolo [4,3-α][1,4] benzodiazepine. The empirical formula is $C_{16}H_{11}ClN_4$.

ProSom tablets are scored and contain either 1 mg or 2 mg of estazolam.

Inactive Ingredients: 1 mg tablets: corn starch, lactose, and stearic acid.

2 mg tablets: corn starch, iron oxide, lactose, and stearic acid.

CLINICAL PHARMACOLOGY

Pharmacokinetics: ProSom tablets have been found to be equivalent in absorption to an orally administered solution of estazolam. Independent of concentration, estazolam in plasma is 93% protein bound.

In healthy subjects who received up to three times the recommended dose of ProSom, peak estazolam plasma concentrations occurred within two hours after dosing (range 0.5 to 6.0 hours) and were proportional to the administered dose, suggesting linear pharmacokinetics over the dosage range tested.

The range of estimates for the mean elimination half-life of estazolam varied from 10 to 24 hours. The clearance of benzodiazepines is accelerated in smokers compared to nonsmokers, and there is evidence that this occurs with estazolam. This decrease in half-life, presumably due to enzyme induction by smoking, is consistent with other drugs with similar hepatic clearance characteristics. In all subjects and at all doses, the mean elimination half-life appeared to be independent of the dose.

In a small study (N=8) using various doses in older subjects (59 to 68 years), peak estazolam concentrations were found to be similar to those observed in younger subjects with a mean elimination half-life of 18.4 hours (range 13.5 to 34.6 hours). Estazolam is extensively metabolized, and the metabolites are excreted primarily in the urine. Less than 5% of a 2 mg dose of estazolam is excreted unchanged in the urine, with only 4% of the dose appearing in the feces. 4'-hydroxy estazolam is the major metabolite in plasma, with concentrations approaching 12% of those of the parent eight hours after administration. While it and the lesser metabolite, 1-oxo-estazolam, have some pharmacologic activity, their low potencies and low concentrations preclude any significant contribution to the hypnotic effect of ProSom.

Postulated relationship between elimination rate of benzodiazepine hypnotics and their profile of common untoward effects: The type and duration of hypnotic effects and the profile of unwanted effects during administration of benzodiazepine drugs may be influenced by the biologic half-life of administered drug and any active metabolites formed. If half-lives are long, drug or metabolites may accumulate during periods of nightly administration and may be associated

with impairments of cognitive and/or motor performance during waking hours; the possibility of interaction with other psychoactive drugs or alcohol will be increased. In contrast, if half-lives are short, drug and metabolites will be cleared before the next dose is ingested, and carry-over effects related to excessive sedation or CNS depression should be minimal or absent. However, during nightly use for an extended period, pharmacodynamic tolerance or adaptation to some effects of benzodiazepine hypnotics may develop. If the drug has a short elimination half-life, it is possible that a relative deficiency of the drug or its active metabolites (ie, in relationship to the receptor site) may occur at some point in the interval between each night's use. This sequence of events may account for two clinical findings reported to occur after several weeks of nightly use of rapidly eliminated benzodiazepine hypnotics, namely, increased wakefulness during the last third of the night and increased daytime anxiety in selected patients.

Controlled Trials Supporting Efficacy: In three 7-night, double-blind, parallel-group trials comparing estazolam 1 mg and/or 2 mg with placebo in adult outpatients with chronic insomnia, estazolam 2 mg was consistently superior to placebo in subjective measures of sleep induction (latency) and sleep maintenance (duration, number of awakenings, depth and quality of sleep); estazolam 1 mg was similarly superior to placebo on all measures of sleep maintenance, however, it significantly improved sleep induction in only one of two studies. In a similarly designed trial comparing estazolam 0.5 mg and 1 mg with placebo in geriatric outpatients with chronic insomnia, only the 1 mg estazolam dose was consistently superior to placebo in sleep induction (latency) and in only one measure of sleep maintenance (ie, duration of sleep).

In a single-night, double-blind, parallel-group trial comparing estazolam 2 mg and placebo in patients admitted for elective surgery and requiring sleep medications, estazolam was superior to placebo in subjective measures of sleep induction and maintenance.

In a 12-week, double-blind, parallel-group trial including a comparison of estazolam 2 mg and placebo in adult outpatients with chronic insomnia, estazolam was superior to placebo in subjective measures of sleep induction (latency) and maintenance, (duration, number of awakenings, total wake time during sleep) at week 2, but produced consistent improvement over 12 weeks only for sleep duration and total wake time during sleep. Following withdrawal at week 12, rebound insomnia was seen at the first withdrawal week, but there was no difference between drug and placebo by the second withdrawal week in all parameters except latency, for which normalization did not occur until the fourth withdrawal week.

Adult outpatients with chronic insomnia were evaluated in a sleep laboratory trial comparing four doses of estazolam (0.25, 0.50, 1.0 and 2.0 mg) and placebo, each administered for 2 nights in a crossover design. The higher estazolam doses were superior to placebo in most EEG measures of sleep induction and maintenance, especially at the 2 mg dose, but only for sleep duration in subjective measures of sleep.

INDICATIONS AND USAGE

ProSom (estazolam) is indicated for the short-term management of insomnia characterized by difficulty in falling asleep, frequent nocturnal awakenings, and/or early morning awakenings. Both outpatient studies and a sleep laboratory study have shown that ProSom administered at bedtime improved sleep induction and sleep maintenance (see CLINICAL PHARMACOLOGY).

Because insomnia is often transient and intermittent, the prolonged administration of ProSom is generally neither necessary nor recommended. Since insomnia may be a symptom of several other disorders, the possibility that the complaint may be related to a condition for which there is a more specific treatment should be considered.

There is evidence to support the ability of ProSom to enhance the duration and quality of sleep for intervals up to 12 weeks (see CLINICAL PHARMACOLOGY).

CONTRAINDICATIONS

Benzodiazepines may cause fetal damage when administered during pregnancy. An increased risk of congenital malformations associated with the use of diazepam and chlordiazepoxide during the first trimester of pregnancy has been suggested in several studies. Transplacental distribution has resulted in neonatal CNS depression and also withdrawal phenomena following the ingestion of therapeutic doses of a benzodiazepine hypnotic during the last weeks of pregnancy. ProSom is contraindicated in pregnant women. If there is a likelihood of the patient becoming pregnant while receiving ProSom she should be warned of the potential risk to the fetus and instructed to discontinue the drug prior to becoming pregnant. The possibility that a woman of childbearing potential is pregnant at the time of institution of therapy should be considered.

WARNINGS

ProSom, like other benzodiazepines, has CNS depressant effects. For this reason, patients should be cautioned against engaging in hazardous occupations requiring complete mental alertness, such as operating machinery or driving a motor vehicle, after ingesting the drug, including potential impairment of the performance of such activities that may occur the day following ingestion of ProSom. Patients should also be cautioned about possible combined effects with alcohol and other CNS depressant drugs.

As with all benzodiazepines, amnesia, paradoxical reactions (eg, excitement, agitation, etc.), and other adverse behavioral effects may occur unpredictably.

There have been reports of withdrawal signs and symptoms of the type associated with withdrawal from CNS depressant drugs following the rapid decrease or the abrupt discontinuation of benzodiazepines (see DRUG ABUSE AND DEPENDENCE).

PRECAUTIONS

General: Impaired motor and/or cognitive performance attributable to the accumulation of benzodiazepines and their active metabolites following several days of repeated use at their recommended doses is a concern in certain vulnerable patients (eg, those especially sensitive to the effects of benzodiazepines or those with a reduced capacity to metabolize and eliminate them) (see DOSAGE AND ADMINISTRATION).

Elderly or debilitated patients and those with impaired renal or hepatic function should be cautioned about these risks and advised to monitor themselves for signs of excessive sedation or impaired conditions.

ProSom appears to cause dose-related respiratory depression that is ordinarily not clinically relevant at recommended doses in patients with normal respiratory function. However, patients with compromised respiratory function may be at risk and should be monitored appropriately. As a class, benzodiazepines have the capacity to depress respiratory drive; there are insufficient data available, however, to characterize their relative potency in depressing respiratory drive at clinically recommended doses.

As with other benzodiazepines, ProSom should be administered with caution to patients exhibiting signs or symptoms of depression. Suicidal tendencies may be present in such patients and protective measures may be required. Intentional overdosage is more common in this group of patients; therefore, the least amount of drug that is feasible should be prescribed for the patient at any one time.

Information for Patients: To assure the safe and effective use of ProSom, the following information and instructions should be given to patients:

1. Inform your physician about any alcohol consumption and medicine you are taking now, including drugs you may buy without a prescription. Alcohol should not be used during treatment with hypnotics.
2. Inform your physician if you are planning to become pregnant, if you are pregnant, or if you become pregnant while you are taking this medicine.
3. You should not take this medicine if you are nursing, as the drug may be excreted in breast milk.
4. Until you experience the way this medicine affects you, do not drive a car, operate potentially dangerous machinery, or engage in hazardous occupations requiring complete mental alertness after taking this medicine.
5. Since benzodiazepines may produce psychological and physical dependence, you should not increase the dose before consulting your physician. In addition, since the abrupt discontinuation of ProSom may be associated with temporary sleep disturbances, you should consult your physician before abruptly discontinuing doses of 2 mg per night or more.

Laboratory Tests: Laboratory tests are not ordinarily required in otherwise healthy patients. When treatment with ProSom is protracted, periodic blood counts, urinalyses, and blood chemistry analyses are advisable.

Drug Interactions: If ProSom is given concomitantly with other drugs acting on the central nervous system, careful consideration should be given to the pharmacology of all agents. The action of the benzodiazepines may be potentiated by anticonvulsants, antihistamines, alcohol, barbiturates, monoamine oxidase inhibitors, narcotics, phenothiazines, psychotropic medications, or other drugs that produce CNS depression. Smokers have an increased clearance of benzodiazepines as compared to nonsmokers; this was seen in studies with estazolam (see CLINICAL PHARMACOLOGY).

Carcinogenesis, Mutagenesis, Impairment of Fertility: Two-year carcinogenicity studies were conducted in mice and rats at dietary doses of 0.8, 3, and 10 mg/kg/day and 0.5, 2, and 10 mg/kg/day, respectively. Evidence of tumorigenicity was not observed in either study. Incidence of hyperplastic liver nodules increased in female mice given the mid- and high-dose levels. The significance of such modules in mice is not known at this time.

In vitro and *in vivo* mutagenicity tests including the Ames test, DNA repair in *B. subtilis*, *in vivo* cytogenetics in mice and rats, and the dominant lethal test in mice did not show a mutagenic potential for estazolam.

Fertility in male and female rats was not affected by doses up to 30 times the usual recommended human dose.

Pregnancy:

1. Teratogenic Effects: Pregnancy Category X (see CONTRA-INDICATIONS).
2. Nonteratogenic Effects: The child born of a mother taking benzodiazepines may be at some risk for withdrawal symptoms during the postnatal period. Neonatal flaccidity has been reported in an infant born of a mother who received benzodiazepines during pregnancy.

Labor and Delivery: ProSom has no established use in labor or delivery.

Nursing Mothers: Human studies have not been conducted; however, studies in lactating rats indicate that estazolam and/or its metabolites are secreted in the milk. The use of ProSom in nursing mothers is not recommended.

Pediatric Use: Safety and effectiveness in children below the age of 18 have not been established.

Geriatric Use: Approximately 18% of individuals participating in the premarketing clinical trials of ProSom were 60 years of age or older. Overall, the adverse event profile did not differ substantively from that observed in younger individuals. Care should be exercised when prescribing benzodiazepines to small or debilitated elderly patients (see DOSAGE AND ADMINISTRATION).

ADVERSE REACTIONS

Commonly Observed: The most commonly observed adverse events associated with the use of ProSom, not seen at an equivalent incidence among placebo-treated patients were somnolence, hypokinesia, dizziness, and abnormal coordination.

Associated with Discontinuation of Treatment: Approximately 3% of 1277 patients who received ProSom in US premarketing clinical trials discontinued treatment because of an adverse clinical event. The only event commonly associated with discontinuation, accounting for 1.3% of the total, was somnolence.

Incidence in Controlled Clinical Trials: Table 1 enumerates adverse events that occurred at an incidence of 1% or greater among patients with insomnia who received ProSom in 7-night, placebo-controlled trials. Events reported by investigators were classified into standard dictionary (COSTART) terms to establish event frequencies. Event frequencies reported were not corrected for the occurrence of these events at baseline. The frequencies were obtained from data pooled across six studies: ProSom, N = 685; placebo, N = 433. The prescriber should be aware that these figures cannot be used to predict the incidence of side effects in the course of usual medical practice in which patient characteristics and other factors differ from those that prevailed in these six clinical trials. Similarly, the cited frequencies cannot be compared with figures obtained from other clinical investigators involving related drug products and uses, since each group of drug trials was conducted under a different set of conditions. However, the cited figures provide the physician with a basis of estimating the relative contribution of drug and nondrug factors to the incidence of side effects in the population studied.

ProSom™ Table 1
INCIDENCE OF ADVERSE EXPERIENCES IN PLACEBO-CONTROLLED CLINICAL TRIALS
(Percentage of Patients Reporting)

Body System/ Adverse Event*	ProSom (N=685)	Placebo (N=433)
Body as a Whole		
Headache	16	27
Asthenia	11	8
Malaise	5	5
Lower extremity pain	3	2
Back pain	2	2
Body pain	2	2
Abdominal pain	1	2
Chest pain	1	1
Digestive System		
Nausea	4	5
Dyspepsia	2	2
Musculoskeletal System		
Stiffness	1	—
Nervous System		
Somnolence	42	27
Hypokinesia	8	4
Nervousness	8	11
Dizziness	7	3
Coordination abnormal	4	1
Hangover	3	2
Confusion	2	—
Depression	2	3
Dream abnormal	2	2
Thinking abnormal	2	1
Respiratory System		
Cold symptoms	3	5
Pharyngitis	1	2
Skin and Appendages		
Pruritus	1	—

*Events reported by at least 1% of ProSom patients.

Other Adverse Events: During clinical trials conducted by Abbott, some of which were not placebo-controlled, ProSom was administered to approximately 1300 patients. Untoward events associated with this exposure were recorded by clinical investigators using terminology of their own choosing. To provide a meaningful estimate of the proportion of individuals experiencing adverse events, similar types of untoward events must be grouped into a smaller number of standardized event categories. In the tabulations that follow, a standard COSTART dictionary terminology has been used to classify reported adverse events. The frequencies presented, therefore, represent the proportion of the 1277 individuals exposed to ProSom who experienced an event of the type cited on at least one occasion while receiving ProSom. All reported events are included except those already listed in the previous table, those COSTART terms too general to be informative, and those events where a drug cause was remote. Events are further classified within body system categories and enumerated in order of decreasing frequency using the following definitions: frequent adverse events are defined as those occurring on one or more occasions in at least 1/100 patients; infrequent adverse events are those occurring in 1/100 to 1/1000 patients; rare events are those occurring in less than 1/1000 patients. It is important to emphasize that, although the events reported did occur during treatment with ProSom, they were not necessarily caused by it.

Body as a Whole —Infrequent: allergic reaction, chills, fever, neck pain, upper extremity pain; Rare: edema, jaw pain, swollen breast.

Cardiovascular System —Infrequent: flushing, palpitation; Rare: arrhythmia, syncope.

Digestive System —Frequent: constipation, dry mouth; Infrequent: decreased appetite, flatulence, gastritis, increased appetite, vomiting; Rare: enterocolitis, melena, ulceration of the mouth.

Endocrine System —Rare: thyroid nodule.

Hematologic and Lymphatic System —Rare: leukopenia, purpura, swollen lymph nodes.

Metabolic/Nutritional Disorders —Infrequent: thirst; Rare: increased SGOT, weight gain, weight loss.

Musculoskeletal System —Infrequent: arthritis, muscle spasm, myalgia; Rare: arthralgia.

Nervous System —Frequent: anxiety; Infrequent: agitation, amnesia, apathy, emotional lability, euphoria, hostility, paresthesia, seizure, sleep disorder, stupor, twitch; Rare: ataxia, circumoral paresthesia, decreased libido, decreased reflexes, hallucinations, neuritis, nystagmus, tremor.

Minor changes in EEG patterns, usually low-voltage fast activity, have been observed in patients during ProSom therapy or withdrawal and are of no known clinical significance.

Respiratory System —Infrequent: asthma, cough, dyspnea, rhinitis, sinusitis; Rare: epistaxis, hyperventilation, laryngitis.

Skin and Appendages —Infrequent: rash, sweating, urticaria; Rare: acne, dry skin.

Special Senses —Infrequent: abnormal vision, ear pain, eye irritation, eye pain, eye swelling, perverse taste, photophobia, tinnitus; Rare: decreased hearing, diplopia, scotomata.

Urogenital System —Infrequent: frequent urination, menstrual cramps, urinary hesitancy, urinary urgency, vaginal discharge/itching; Rare: hematuria, nocturia, oliguria, penile discharge, urinary incontinence.

Postintroduction Reports —Voluntary reports of non-US postmarketing experience with estazolam have included rare occurrences of photosensitivity and agranulocytosis. Because of the uncontrolled nature of these spontaneous reports, a causal relationship to estazolam treatment has not been determined.

DRUG ABUSE AND DEPENDENCE

Controlled Substance: ProSom tablets are a controlled substance in Schedule IV.

Abuse and Dependence: Withdrawal symptoms similar to those noted with sedatives/hypnotics and alcohol have occurred following the abrupt discontinuation of drugs in the benzodiazepine class. The symptoms can range from mild dysphoria and insomnia to a major syndrome that may include abdominal and muscle cramps, vomiting, sweating, tremors, and convulsions.

Although withdrawal symptoms are more commonly noted after the discontinuation of higher than therapeutic doses of benzodiazepines, a proportion of patients taking benzodiazepines chronically at therapeutic doses may become physically dependent on them. Available data, however, cannot provide a reliable estimate of the incidence of dependency or the relationship of the dependency to dose and duration of treatment. There is some evidence to suggest that gradual reduction of dosage will attenuate or eliminate some withdrawal phenomena. In most instances, withdrawal phenomena are relatively mild and transient; however, life-threatening events (eg, seizures, delirium, etc.) have been reported. Gradual withdrawal is the preferred course for any patient taking benzodiazepines for a prolonged period. Patients with a history of seizures, regardless of their concomitant antisei-

zure drug therapy, should not be withdrawn abruptly from benzodiazepines.

Individuals with a history of addiction to or abuse of drugs or alcohol should be under careful surveillance when receiving benzodiazepines because of the risk of habituation and dependence to such patients.

OVERDOSAGE

As with other benzodiazepines, experience with ProSom indicates that manifestations of overdosage include somnolence, respiratory depression, confusion, impaired coordination, slurred speech, and ultimately, coma. Patients have recovered from overdosage as high as 40 mg. As in the management of intentional overdose with any drug, the possibility should be considered that multiple agents may have been taken.

Gastric evacuation, either by the induction of emesis, lavage, or both, should be performed immediately. Maintenance of adequate ventilation is essential. General supportive care, including frequent monitoring of the vital signs and close observation of the patient, is indicated. Fluids should be administered intravenously to maintain blood pressure and encourage diuresis. The value of dialysis in treatment of benzodiazepine overdose has not been determined. The physician may wish to consider contacting a Poison Control Center for up-to-date information on the management of hypnotic drug product overdose.

DOSAGE AND ADMINISTRATION

The recommended initial dose for adults is 1 mg at bedtime; however, some patients may need a 2 mg dose. In healthy elderly patients, 1 mg is also the appropriate starting dose, but increases should be initiated with particular care. In small or debilitated older patients, a starting dose of 0.5 mg, while only marginally effective in the overall elderly population, should be considered.

HOW SUPPLIED

ProSom tablets are scored tablets supplied as:
ProSom Tablets 1 mg (white)
Bottles of 100 ....(NDC 0074-3735-13)
ABBO-PAC® unit dose strip
packages of 100 tablets..........................(NDC 0074-3735-11)
ProSom Tablets 2 mg (coral-colored)
Bottles of 100 ....(NDC 0074-3736-13)
ABBO-PAC® unit dose strip
packages of 100 tablets..........................(NDC 0074-3736-11)
Recommended Storage: Store below 86°F (30°C).
Ref. 01-2567-R3

Shown in Product Identification Section, page 404

QUELIDRINE® SYRUP   OTC
[quel 'i-drēen]
(non-narcotic, antihistaminic cough suppressant)

COMPOSITION

Each teaspoonful (5 ml) contains:

Dextromethorphan Hydrobromide	10 mg
Chlorpheniramine Maleate	2 mg
Ephedrine Hydrochloride	5 mg
Phenylephrine Hydrochloride	5 mg
Ammonium Chloride	40 mg
Ipecac Fluidextract	0.005 ml

INACTIVE INGREDIENTS

Alcohol 2%, D&C Red No. 33, glycerin, liquid glucose, magnesium carbonate, methylparaben, propylparaben, sucrose, tolu balsam tincture, water, artificial flavors and other ingredients forming a palatable, aromatic syrup.

ACTION AND INDICATIONS

Quelidrine is designed as an aid in the management of cough associated with acute or subacute simple respiratory infections. Quelidrine provides a wide range of therapeutic action against the cough complex—without the risk of addiction or the production of undue central depression.

WARNINGS

As with any drug, if you are pregnant or nursing a baby, seek the advice of a health professional before using this product. Keep this and all medicines out of the reach of children.

PRECAUTIONS

Quelidrine should be administered with caution to patients with hypertension, serious organic heart disease, angina pectoris, diabetes, thyroid disease, or to persons receiving digitalis. When cough persists or accompanies a high fever, the underlying cause and need for other medication should be reevaluated.

Continued on next page

If desired, additional literature on any Abbott product will be provided upon request to Abbott Laboratories.

Abbott Laboratories—Cont.

SIDE EFFECTS

Quelidrine is safe for patients of all ages, but professional supervision of dosage for young patients is essential. Side effects are infrequent. Drowsiness, nausea, vomiting, nervousness, palpitation, blurred vision and insomnia may occur in susceptible patients. Constipation is seldom a problem. If side effects are encountered, dosage should be reduced or medication withdrawn.

DOSAGE AND ADMINISTRATION

Adults —1 teaspoonful, one to four times daily. Children 6 years of age or older, ½ teaspoonful, one to four times daily. Children 2 to 6 years old, ¼ teaspoonful one to four times daily. Under 2, as directed by physician. Quelidrine may be diluted with Syrup, NF in order to facilitate pediatric administration.

HOW SUPPLIED

Quelidrine Syrup is supplied in bottles of 4 fluid ounces (NDC 0074-6883-04), with or without a prescription.
Store below 77°F (25°C).
Ref. 07-8117-4/R22

SURBEX® OTC
[sir'bex]
Vitamin B-Complex
SURBEX® with C
Vitamin B-Complex with Vitamin C

(See PDR For Nonprescription Drugs.)

SURBEX–T® OTC
[sir'bex-t]
High-Potency Vitamin B-Complex with 500 mg of Vitamin C

(See PDR For Nonprescription Drugs.)
Shown in Product Identification Section, page 404

SURBEX®–750 with IRON OTC
[sir'bex ī-ron]
High-potency B-complex with iron, vitamin E and 750 mg vitamin C

(See PDR For Nonprescription Drugs.)
Shown in Product Identification Section, page 404

SURBEX®–750 with ZINC OTC
[sir'bex zinc]
High-potency B-complex with zinc, vitamin E and 750 mg vitamin C

(See PDR For Nonprescription Drugs.)
Shown in Product Identification Section, page 404

TRANXENE® ℞ ℂ
[tran'zēen]
(clorazepate dipotassium)
T-TAB® Tablets
TRANXENE®-SD™
& TRANXENE®-SD™ HALF STRENGTH
(clorazepate dipotassium)
Tablets

DESCRIPTION

Chemically, TRANXENE is a benzodiazepine. The empirical formula is $C_{16}H_{11}ClK_2N_2O_4$; the molecular weight is 408.92. The compound occurs as a fine, light yellow, practically odorless powder. It is insoluble in the common organic solvents, but very soluble in water. Aqueous solutions are unstable, clear, light yellow, and alkaline.
TRANXENE T-TAB tablets contain either 3.75 mg, 7.5 mg or 15 mg of clorazepate dipotassium for oral administration. TRANXENE- SD and TRANXENE-SD HALF STRENGTH tablets contain 22.5 mg and 11.25 mg of clorazepate dipotassium respectively. TRANXENE-SD and TRANXENE-SD HALF STRENGTH tablets gradually release clorazepate and are designed for once-a-day administration in patients already stabilized on TRANXENE T-TAB tablets.
Inactive ingredients for TRANXENE T-TAB® Tablets: Colloidal silicon dioxide, FD&C Blue No. 2 (3.75 mg only), FD&C Yellow No. 6 (7.5 mg only), FD&C Red No. 3 (15 mg only), magnesium oxide, magnesium stearate, microcrystalline cellulose, potassium carbonate, potassium chloride, and talc.
Inactive ingredients for TRANXENE-SD and TRANXENE-SD HALF STRENGTH Tablets: Castor oil wax, FD&C Blue No. 2 (SD Half Strength, 11.25 mg only), iron oxide (SD, 22.5 mg only), lactose, magnesium oxide, magnesium stearate, potassium carbonate, potassium chloride, and talc.

ACTIONS

Pharmacologically, clorazepate dipotassium has the characteristics of the benzodiazepines. It has depressant effects on the central nervous system. The primary metabolite, nordiazepam, quickly appears in the blood stream. The serum half-life is about 2 days. The drug is metabolized in the liver and excreted primarily in the urine. (See ANIMAL AND CLINICAL PHARMACOLOGY section).

INDICATIONS

TRANXENE is indicated for the management of anxiety disorders or for the short-term relief of the symptoms of anxiety. Anxiety or tension associated with the stress of everyday life usually does not require treatment with an anxiolytic.
TRANXENE is indicated as adjunctive therapy in the management of partial seizures.
The effectiveness of TRANXENE in long-term management of anxiety, that is, more than 4 months, has not been assessed by systematic clinical studies. Long-term studies in epileptic patients, however, have shown continued therapeutic activity. The physician should reassess periodically the usefulness of the drug for the individual patient.
TRANXENE is indicated for the symptomatic relief of acute alcohol withdrawal.

CONTRAINDICATIONS

TRANXENE is contraindicated in patients with a known hypersensitivity to the drug, and in those with acute narrow angle glaucoma.

WARNINGS

TRANXENE is not recommended for use in depressive neuroses or in psychotic reactions.
Patients on TRANXENE should be cautioned against engaging in hazardous occupations requiring mental alertness, such as operating dangerous machinery including motor vehicles. Since TRANXENE has a central nervous system depressant effect, patients should be advised against the simultaneous use of other CNS-depressant drugs, and cautioned that the effects of alcohol may be increased.
Because of the lack of sufficient clinical experience, TRANXENE is not recommended for use in patients less than 9 years of age.
Physical and Psychological Dependence: Withdrawal symptoms (similar in character to those noted with barbiturates and alcohol) have occurred following abrupt discontinuance of clorazepate. Symptoms of nervousness, insomnia, irritability, diarrhea, muscle aches, hallucinations, tremor, and memory impairment have followed abrupt withdrawal after long-term use of high dosage. Withdrawal symptoms have also been reported following abrupt discontinuance of benzodiazepines taken continuously at therapeutic levels for several months.
Caution should be observed in patients who are considered to have a psychological potential for drug dependence.
Evidence of drug dependence has been observed in dogs and rabbits which was characterized by convulsive seizures when the drug was abruptly withdrawn or the dose was reduced; the syndrome in dogs could be abolished by administration of clorazepate.
Usage in Pregnancy: **An increased risk of congenital malformations associated with the use of minor tranquilizers (chlordiazepoxide, diazepam, and meprobamate) during the first trimester of pregnancy has been suggested in several studies. TRANXENE, a benzodiazepine derivative, has not been studied adequately to determine whether it, too, may be associated with an increased risk of fetal abnormality. Because use of these drugs is rarely a matter of urgency, their use during this period should almost always be avoided. The possibility that a woman of childbearing potential may be pregnant at the time of institution of therapy should be considered. Patients should be advised that if they become pregnant during therapy or intend to become pregnant they should communicate with their physician about the desirability of discontinuing the drug.**
Usage during Lactation: TRANXENE should not be given to nursing mothers since it has been reported that nordiazepam is excreted in human breast milk.

PRECAUTIONS

In those patients in which a degree of depression accompanies the anxiety, suicidal tendencies may be present and protective measures may be required. The least amount of drug that is feasible should be available to the patient.
Patients on TRANXENE for prolonged periods should have blood counts and liver function tests periodically. The usual precautions in treating patients with impaired renal or hepatic function should also be observed.
In elderly or debilitated patients, the initial dose should be small, and increments should be made gradually, in accordance with the response of the patient, to preclude ataxia or excessive sedation.

ADVERSE REACTIONS

The side effect most frequently reported was drowsiness. Less commonly reported (in descending order of occurrence) were: dizziness, various gastrointestinal complaints, nervousness, blurred vision, dry mouth, headache, and mental confusion. Other side effects included insomnia, transient skin rashes, fatigue, ataxia, genitourinary complaints, irritability, diplopia, depression, tremor, and slurred speech.
There have been reports of abnormal liver and kidney function tests and of decrease in hematocrit.
Decrease in systolic blood pressure has been observed.

DOSAGE AND ADMINISTRATION

For the symptomatic relief of anxiety: TRANXENE (clorazepate dipotassium) T-TAB® tablets are administered orally in divided doses. The usual daily dose is 30 mg. The dose should be adjusted gradually within the range of 15 to 60 mg daily in accordance with the response of the patient. In elderly or debilitated patients it is advisable to initiate treatment at a daily dose of 7.5 to 15 mg.
TRANXENE may also be administered in a single dose daily at bedtime; the recommended initial dose is 15 mg. After the initial dose, the response of the patient may require adjustment of subsequent dosage. Lower doses may be indicated in the elderly patient. Drowsiness may occur at the initiation of treatment and with dosage increment.
TRANXENE-SD (22.5 mg tablet) may be administered as a single dose every 24 hours. This tablet is intended as an alternate dosage form for the convenience of patients stabilized on a dose of 7.5 mg tablets three times a day. TRANXENE-SD should not be used to initiate therapy.
TRANXENE-SD HALF STRENGTH (11.25 mg tablet) may be administered as a single dose every 24 hours. This tablet is intended as an alternate dosage form for the convenience of patients stabilized on a dose of 3.75 mg tablets three times a day. TRANXENE-SD HALF STRENGTH should not be used to initiate therapy.
For the symptomatic relief of acute alcohol withdrawal: The following dosage schedule is recommended:

1st 24 hours (Day 1)	30 mg Tranxene, initially; followed by 30 to 60 mg in divided doses
2nd 24 hours (Day 2)	45 to 90 mg in divided doses
3rd 24 hours (Day 3)	22.5 to 45 mg in divided doses
Day 4	15 to 30 mg in divided doses

Thereafter, gradually reduce the daily dose to 7.5 to 15 mg. Discontinue drug therapy as soon as patient's condition is stable.
The maximum recommended total daily dose is 90 mg. Avoid excessive reductions in the total amount of drug administered on successive days.
As an Adjunct to Antiepileptic Drugs:
In order to minimize drowsiness, the recommended initial dosages and dosage increments should not be exceeded.
Adults: The maximum recommended initial dose in patients over 12 years old is 7.5 mg three times a day. Dosage should be increased by no more than 7.5 mg every week and should not exceed 90 mg/day.
Children (9-12 years): The maximum recommended initial dose is 7.5 mg two times a day. Dosage should be increased by no more than 7.5 mg every week and should not exceed 60 mg/day.

DRUG INTERACTIONS

If TRANXENE is to be combined with other drugs acting on the central nervous system, careful consideration should be given to the pharmacology of the agents to be employed. Animal experience indicates that TRANXENE prolongs the sleeping time after hexobarbital or after ethyl alcohol, increases the inhibitory effects of chlorpromazine, but does not exhibit monoamine oxidase inhibition. Clinical studies have shown increased sedation with concurrent hypnotic medications. The actions of the benzodiazepines may be potentiated by barbiturates, narcotics, phenothiazines, monoamine oxidase inhibitors or other antidepressants.
If TRANXENE is used to treat anxiety associated with somatic disease states, careful attention must be paid to possible drug interaction with concomitant medication.
In bioavailability studies with normal subjects, the concurrent administration of antacids at therapeutic levels did not significantly influence the bioavailability of TRANXENE.

MANAGEMENT OF OVERDOSAGE

Overdosage is usually manifested by varying degrees of CNS depression ranging from slight sedation to coma. As in the management of overdosage with any drug, it should be borne in mind that multiple agents may have been taken.

There are no specific antidotes for the benzodiazepines. The treatment of overdosage should consist of the general measures employed in the management of overdosage of any CNS depressant. Gastric evacuation either by the induction of emesis, lavage, or both, should be performed immediately. General supportive care, including frequent monitoring of the vital signs and close observation of the patient, is indicated. Hypotension, though rarely reported, may occur with large overdoses. In such cases the use of agents such as Levophed® Bitartrate (norepinephrine bitartrate injection, USP) or Aramine® Injection (metaraminol bitartrate injection, USP) should be considered.

While reports indicate that individuals have survived overdoses of TRANXENE as high as 450 to 675 mg, these doses are not necessarily an accurate indication of the amount of drug absorbed since the time interval between ingestion and the institution of treatment was not always known. Sedation in varying degrees was the most common physiological manifestation of TRANXENE overdosage. Deep coma when it occurred was usually associated with the ingestion of other drugs in addition to TRANXENE.

ANIMAL AND CLINICAL PHARMACOLOGY

Studies in rats and monkeys have shown a substantial difference between doses producing tranquilizing, sedative and toxic effects. In rats, conditioned avoidance response was inhibited at an oral dose of 10 mg/kg; sedation was induced at 32 mg/kg; the LD_{50} was 1320 mg/kg. In monkeys aggressive behavior was reduced at an oral dose of 0.25 mg/kg; sedation (ataxia) was induced at 7.5 mg/kg; the LD_{50} could not be determined because of the emetic effect of large doses, but the LD_{50} exceeds 1600 mg/kg.

Twenty-four dogs were given TRANXENE orally in a 22-month toxicity study; doses up to 75 mg/kg were given. Drug-related changes occurred in the liver; weight was increased and cholestasis with minimal hepatocellular damage was found, but lobular architecture remained well preserved.

Eighteen rhesus monkeys were given oral doses of TRANXENE from 3 to 36 mg/kg daily for 52 weeks. All treated animals remained similar to control animals. Although total leucocyte count remained within normal limits it tended to fall in the female animals on the highest doses.

Examination of all organs revealed no alterations attributable to TRANXENE. There was no damage to liver function or structure.

Reproduction Studies: Standard fertility, reproduction, and teratology studies were conducted in rats and rabbits. Oral doses in rats up to 150 mg/kg and in rabbits up to 15 mg/kg produced no abnormalities in the fetuses. TRANXENE (clorazepate dipotassium) did not alter the fertility indices or reproductive capacity of adult animals. As expected, the sedative effect of high doses interfered with care of the young by their mothers (*see Usage in Pregnancy*).

Clinical Pharmacology: Studies in healthy men have shown that TRANXENE has depressant effects on the central nervous system. Prolonged administration of single daily doses as high as 120 mg was without toxic effects. Abrupt cessation of high doses was followed in some patients by nervousness, insomnia, irritability, diarrhea, muscle aches, or memory impairment.

Absorption —Excretion: After oral administration of TRANXENE, there is essentially no circulating parent drug. Nordiazepam, its primary metabolite, quickly appears in the blood stream. In 2 volunteers given 15 mg (50 μC) of ^{14}C-TRANXENE, about 80% was recovered in the urine and feces within 10 days. Excretion was primarily in the urine with about 1% excreted per day on day 10.

HOW SUPPLIED

TRANXENE (clorazepate dipotassium) is supplied as:

3.75 mg blue-colored, scored T-TAB® tablets:
Bottles of 100 ....(**NDC** 0074-4389-13).
Bottles of 500 ....(**NDC** 0074-4389-53).
ABBO-PAC® unit dose packages:
100 ....(**NDC** 0074-4389-11).

7.5 mg peach-colored, scored T-TAB® tablets:
Bottles of 100 ....(**NDC** 0074-4390-13).
Bottles of 500 ....(**NDC** 0074-4390-53).
ABBO-PAC® unit dose packages:
100 ....(**NDC** 0074-4390-11).

15 mg lavender-colored, scored T-TAB® tablets:
Bottles of 100 ....(**NDC** 0074-4391-13).
Bottles of 500 ....(**NDC** 0074-4391-53).
ABBO-PAC® unit dose packages:
100 ....(**NDC** 0074-4391-11).

T-TAB, tablet appearance and shape are registered trademarks of Abbott Laboratories.
U.S. Design Patent No. D–300,879

TRANXENE®-SD™ 22.5 mg tan-colored, single dose tablets:
Bottles of 100 ....(**NDC** 0074-2997-13).

TRANXENE®-SD™ HALF STRENGTH 11.25 mg blue-colored, single dose tablets:
Bottles of 100 ....(**NDC** 0074-2699-13).

Recommended storage: Store below 77°F (25°C).
Ref. 03-4400-R12

Shown in Product Identification Section, page 404

TRIDIONE® ℞

[*try'dē-own*]
(trimethadione, USP)
Tablets, Capsules, and Oral Solution

> BECAUSE OF ITS POTENTIAL TO PRODUCE FETAL MALFORMATIONS AND SERIOUS SIDE EFFECTS, TRIDIONE (trimethadione) SHOULD ONLY BE UTILIZED WHEN OTHER LESS TOXIC DRUGS HAVE BEEN FOUND INEFFECTIVE IN CONTROLLING PETIT MAL SEIZURES.

DESCRIPTION

TRIDIONE (trimethadione) is an antiepileptic agent. An oxazolidinedione compound, it is chemically identified as 3,5,5-trimethyloxozolidine-2,4-dione.

TRIDIONE is a synthetic, water-soluble, white, crystalline powder. It is supplied in capsular, tablet, and liquid forms for oral use only.

Inactive Ingredients: 300 mg Capsule: Corn starch, FD&C Blue No. 1, FD&C Red No. 3, FD&C Yellow No. 6, gelatin, titanium dioxide and artificial flavor.

150 mg Dulcet Tablet: Corn starch, lactose, magnesium stearate, magnesium trisilicate, sucrose and natural/synthetic flavor.

Solution: FD&C Yellow No. 6, methylparaben, sucrose, water and natural/synthetic flavors.

CLINICAL PHARMACOLOGY

TRIDIONE has been shown to prevent pentylenetetrazol-induced and thujone-induced seizures in experimental animals; the drug has a less marked effect on seizures induced by picrotoxin, procaine, cocaine, or strychnine. Unlike the hydantoins and antiepileptic barbiturates, TRIDIONE does not modify the maximal seizure pattern in patients undergoing electroconvulsive therapy.

TRIDIONE has a sedative effect that may increase to the point of ataxia when excessive doses are used. A toxic dose of the drug in animals (approximately 2 g/kg) produced sleep, unconsciousness, and respiratory depression.

Trimethadione is rapidly absorbed from the gastrointestinal tract. It is demethylated by liver microsomes to the active metabolite, dimethadione.

Approximately 3% of a daily dose of TRIDIONE is recovered in the urine as unchanged drug. The majority of trimethadione is excreted slowly by the kidney in the form of dimethadione.

INDICATIONS

TRIDIONE (trimethadione) is indicated for the control of petit mal seizures that are refractory to treatment with other drugs.

CONTRAINDICATIONS

TRIDIONE is contraindicated in patients with a known hypersensitivity to the drug.

WARNINGS

TRIDIONE may cause serious side effects. Strict medical supervision of the patient is mandatory, especially during the initial year of therapy.

TRIDIONE (trimethadione) should be withdrawn promptly if skin rash appears, because of the grave possibility of the occurrence of exfoliative dermatitis or severe forms of erythema multiforme. Even a minor acneiform or morbilliform rash should be allowed to clear completely before treatment with TRIDIONE is resumed; reinstitute therapy cautiously.

A complete blood count should be done prior to intiating therapy with TRIDIONE, and at monthly intervals thereafter. A marked depression of the blood count is an indication for withdrawal of the drug. If no abnormality appears within 12 months, the interval between blood counts may be extended. A moderate degree of neutropenia with or without a corresponding drop in the leukocyte count is not uncommon. Therapy need not be withdrawn unless the neutrophil count is 2500 or less; more frequent blood examinations should be done when the count is less than 3,000. Other blood dyscrasias, including leukopenia, eosinophilia, thrombocytopenia, pancytopenia, agranulocytosis, hypoplastic anemia, and fatal aplastic anemia, have occurred. Patients should be advised to report immediately such signs and symptoms as sore throat, fever, malaise, easy bruising, petechiae, or epistaxis, or others that may be indicative of an infection or bleeding tendency. TRIDIONE should ordinarily not be used in patients with severe blood dyscrasias.

Liver function tests should be done prior to initiating therapy with TRIDIONE, and at monthly intervals thereafter. Hepatitis has been reported rarely. Jaundice or other signs of liver dysfunction are an indication for withdrawal of the drug. TRIDIONE should ordinarily not be used in patients with severe hepatic impairment.

A urinalysis should be done prior to initiating therapy with TRIDIONE and at monthly intervals thereafter. Fatal nephrosis has been reported. Persistent or increasing albuminuria, or the development of any other significant renal abnormality, is an indication for withdrawal of the drug. TRIDIONE should ordinarily not be used in patients with severe renal dysfunction.

Hemeralopia has occurred; this appears to be an effect of TRIDIONE on the neural layers of the retina, and usually can be reversed by a reduction in dosage. Scotomata are an indication for withdrawal of the drug. Caution should be observed when treating patients who have diseases of the retina or optic nerve.

Manifestations of systemic lupus erythematosus have been associated with the use of TRIDIONE, as they have with the use of certain other anticonvulsants. Lymphadenopathies simulating malignant lymphoma have occurred. Lupus-like manifestations or lymph node enlargement are indications for withdrawal of the drug. Signs and symptoms may disappear after discontinuation of therapy, and specific treatment may be unnecessary.

A myasthenia gravis-like syndrome has been associated with the chronic use of trimethadione. Symptoms suggestive of this condition are indications for withdrawal of the drug.

Drugs known to cause toxic effects similar to those of TRIDIONE should be avoided or used only with extreme caution during therapy with TRIDIONE.

USAGE DURING PREGNANCY AND LACTATION:

THERE ARE MULTIPLE REPORTS IN THE CLINICAL LITERATURE WHICH INDICATE THAT THE USE OF ANTICONVULSANT DRUGS DURING PREGNANCY RESULTS IN AN INCREASED INCIDENCE OF BIRTH DEFECTS IN THE OFFSPRING. DATA ARE MORE EXTENSIVE WITH RESPECT TO TRIMETHADIONE, PARAMETHADIONE, PHENYTOIN AND PHENOBARBITAL THAN WITH OTHER ANTICONVULSANT DRUGS. THEREFORE, ANTICONVULSANT DRUGS SUCH AS TRIDIONE (TRIMETHADIONE) SHOULD BE ADMINISTERED TO WOMEN OF CHILDBEARING POTENTIAL ONLY IF THEY ARE CLEARLY SHOWN TO BE ESSENTIAL IN THE MANAGEMENT OF THEIR SEIZURES. EFFECTIVE MEANS OF CONTRACEPTION SHOULD ACCOMPANY THE USE OF TRIDIONE IN SUCH PATIENTS. IF A PATIENT BECOMES PREGNANT WHILE TAKING TRIDIONE, TERMINATION OF THE PREGNANCY SHOULD BE CONSIDERED. A PATIENT WHO REQUIRES THERAPY WITH TRIDIONE AND WHO WISHES TO BECOME PREGNANT SHOULD BE ADVISED OF THE RISKS.

REPORTS HAVE SUGGESTED THAT THE MATERNAL INGESTION OF ANTICONVULSANT DRUGS, PARTICULARLY BARBITURATES, IS ASSOCIATED WITH A NEONATAL COAGULATION DEFECT THAT MAY CAUSE BLEEDING DURING THE EARLY (USUALLY WITHIN 24 HOURS OF BIRTH) NEONATAL PERIOD. THE POSSIBILITY OF THE OCCURRENCE OF THIS DEFECT WITH THE USE OF TRIDIONE SHOULD BE KEPT IN MIND. THE DEFECT IS CHARACTERIZED BY DECREASED LEVELS OF VITAMIN K-DEPENDENT CLOTTING FACTORS, AND PROLONGATION OF EITHER THE PROTHROMBIN TIME OR THE PARTIAL THROMBOPLASTIN TIME, OR BOTH. IT HAS BEEN SUGGESTED THAT PROPHYLACTIC VITAMIN K BE GIVEN TO THE MOTHER ONE MONTH PRIOR TO, AND DURING DELIVERY, AND TO THE INFANT, INTRAVENOUSLY, IMMEDIATELY AFTER BIRTH.

THE SAFETY OF TRIDIONE FOR USE DURING LACTATION HAS NOT BEEN ESTABLISHED.

PRECAUTIONS

Abrupt discontinuation of TRIDIONE may precipitate petit mal status. TRIDIONE should always be withdrawn gradually unless serious adverse effects dictate otherwise. In the latter case, another anticonvulsant may be substituted to protect the patient.

Usage during Pregnancy and Lactation:
See WARNINGS.

ADVERSE REACTIONS

The following side effects, some of them serious, have been associated with the use of TRIDIONE.

Gastrointestinal: nausea, vomiting, abdominal pain, gastric distress.

CNS/Neurologic: drowsiness, fatigue, malaise, insomnia, vertigo, headache, paresthesias, precipitation of grand mal seizures, increased irritability, personality changes.

Drowsiness usually subsides with continued therapy. If it persists, a reduction in dosage is indicated.

Hematologic: bleeding gums, epistaxis, retinal and petechial hemorrhages, vaginal bleeding; neutropenia, leukopenia, eosinophilia, thrombocytopenia, pancytopenia, agranulocytosis, hypoplastic anemia, and fatal aplastic anemia.

Dermatologic: acneiform or morbilliform skin rash that may progress to exfoliative dermatitis or to severe forms of erythema multiforme.

Continued on next page

If desired, additional literature on any Abbott product will be provided upon request to Abbott Laboratories.

Abbott Laboratories—Cont.

Other: hiccups, anorexia, weight loss, hair loss, changes in blood pressure, albuminuria, hemeralopia, photophobia, diplopia.
Fatal nephrosis has occurred.
Hepatitis has been reported rarely.
Lupus erythematosus, and lymphadenopathies simulating malignant lymphoma, have been reported.
Pruritus associated with lymphadenopathy and hepatosplenomegaly has occurred in hypersensitive individuals.
A myasthenia gravis-like syndrome has been reported.

OVERDOSAGE

Symptoms of acute TRIDIONE overdosage include drowsiness, nausea, dizziness, ataxia, visual disturbances. Coma may follow massive overdosage.
Gastric evacuation, either by induced emesis, or by lavage, or both, should be done immediately. General supportive care, including frequent monitoring of the vital signs and close observation of the patient, are required.
Alkalinization of the urine has been reported to enhance the renal excretion of dimethadione, the active metabolite of TRIDIONE.
A blood count and a careful evaluation of hepatic and renal function should be done following recovery.

DOSAGE AND ADMINISTRATION

TRIDIONE is administered orally.
Usual Adult Dosage: 0.9–2.4 g daily in 3 or 4 equally divided doses (i.e. 300–600 mg 3 or 4 times daily).
Initially, give 0.9 g daily; increase this dose by 300 mg at weekly intervals until therapeutic results are seen or until toxic symptoms appear.
Maintenance dosage should be the least amount of drug required to maintain control.
Children's Dosage: Usually 0.3–0.9 g daily in 3 or 4 equally divided doses.

HOW SUPPLIED

TRIDIONE Capsules (trimethadione capsules, USP), 300 mg (white) are supplied in bottles of 100 (**NDC** 0074-3709-01).
Recommended storage: Store capsules below 77°F (25°C).
TRIDIONE Dulcet® Tablets (trimethadione tablets, USP), 150 mg (white) chewable tablets are supplied in bottles of 100 (**NDC** 0074-3753-01).
Recommended storage: Store Dulcet tablets in refrigerator (2°–8°C) to minimize crystallization. However some crystallization not harmful to product may occur. Keep tightly closed.
TRIDIONE Solution (trimethadione oral solution, USP), 1.2 g per fluid ounce (40 mg per mL), is supplied in pint bottles (**NDC** 0074-3721-01).
Recommended storage: Store solution below 86°F (30°C).

®Dulcet—Sweetened tablets, Abbott.
Ref. 01-2592-R8
Shown in Product Identification Section, page 404

TRONOTHANE® HYDROCHLORIDE OTC

[*tro'nō-thāne hy-drō-clō'rīde*]
(pramoxine hydrochloride)
Cream

DESCRIPTION

Tronothane Hydrochloride (pramoxine hydrochloride) is a surface anesthetic agent, chemically unrelated to the benzoate esters of the "caine" type. It is chemically designated as 4-n-butoxyphenyl gammamorpholinopropyl ether hydrochloride.

INDICATIONS

Tronothane Hydrochloride is indicated for temporary relief of pain and itching due to minor burns, sunburn, minor cuts, abrasions, insect bites, minor skin irritations, hemorrhoids and other anorectal disorders.

CONTRAINDICATIONS

Tronothane Hydrochloride is not suitable for and should not be injected into the tissues. It should not be used for bronchoscopy or gastroscopy, or in patients who are hypersensitive to the drug.

WARNINGS

Tronothane Hydrochloride is not intended for prolonged use. Do not apply to large areas of the body. Do not use in the eyes or nose.
If condition worsens, or persists for 7 days, consult physician.
If bleeding or increased pain occurs when using the product in the rectum, consult physician promptly.
For topical use in children under 2 years or anorectal use in children under 12 years, use only as directed by physician.
Keep out of reach of children.

ADVERSE REACTIONS

Local skin reactions, e.g. stinging and burning. Discontinue use if redness, irritation, swelling or pain occur.

DOSAGE AND ADMINISTRATION

Topical—Adults and children 2 years of age or older: Apply to affected area 3 to 4 times daily, or as directed by a physician.
Anorectal—When practical, wash the area with soap and warm water, and rinse off all soap before application. Adults and children 12 years of age or older: Apply up to 5 times daily, especially morning, night and after bowel movements, or as directed by a physician.
External—Apply liberally to affected area.
Intrarectal—Remove cap from tube and attach clean applicator. Squeeze tube to fill and lubricate applicator. Remove cap from applicator. Gently insert applicator into rectum and squeeze tube. Thoroughly cleanse applicator with soap and warm water after use. Replace applicator cap.

HOW SUPPLIED

Tronothane Hydrochloride 1% Cream (pramoxine hydrochloride cream, USP), pramoxine hydrochloride 1% in a water miscible base containing cetyl alcohol, cetyl esters wax, glycerin, sodium lauryl sulfate, methylparaben, and propylparaben, is supplied in a 1-oz tube with rectal applicator (**NDC** 0074-6645-01).
Store at 59°–86°F (15°–30°C).
These products are listed in USP, a Medicare designated compendium.
Ref. 09-6486-3/R4

If desired, additional literature on any Abbott Product will be provided upon request to Abbott Laboratories.

Adams Laboratories, Inc.

14801 SOVEREIGN ROAD
FORT WORTH, TEXAS 76155-2645

AIRET™ ℞

Albuterol Sulfate Inhalation
Solution 0.083%
(*Potency expressed as albuterol)

DESCRIPTION

Albuterol Sulfate Inhalation Solution is a relatively selective beta$_2$-adrenergic bronchodilator (see **CLINICAL PHARMACOLOGY** section below). Albuterol sulfate has the chemical name α^1-[(*tert*-butylamino)methyl]-4-hydroxy-*m*-xylene-α,α'-diol sulfate (2:1) (salt).
Albuterol sulfate has a molecular weight of 576.7 and the molecular formula $(C_{13}H_{21}NO_3)_2 \cdot H_2SO_4$. Albuterol sulfate is a white or practically white powder, freely soluble in water and slightly soluble in alcohol.
The World Health Organization recommended name for albuterol base is salbutamol. Albuterol Sulfate Inhalation Solution is available in an 0.083% solution requiring no dilution prior to administration.
Each mL of Albuterol Sulfate Inhalation Solution (0.083%) contains 0.83 mg of albuterol (as 1 mg of albuterol sulfate) in an isotonic aqueous solution containing sodium chloride, edetate disodium, sodium citrate, and hydrochloric acid used to adjust the pH between 3 and 5. Albuterol Sulfate Inhalation Solution (0.083%) contains no sulfiting agents. It is supplied in 3 mL unit dose vials.
Albuterol Sulfate Inhalation Solution is a clear, colorless to light yellow solution.

CLINICAL PHARMACOLOGY

The prime action of beta-adrenergic drugs is to stimulate adenyl cyclase, the enzyme which catalyzes the formation of cyclic-3′,5′-adenosine monophosphate (cyclic AMP) from adenosine triphosphate (ATP). The cyclic AMP thus formed mediates the cellular responses. *In vitro* studies and *in vivo* pharmacologic studies have demonstrated that albuterol has a preferential effect on beta$_2$-adrenergic receptors compared with isoproterenol. While it is recognized that beta$_2$-adrenergic receptors are the predominant receptors in bronchial smooth muscle, recent data indicate that 10 to 50% of the beta receptors in the human heart may be beta$_2$ receptors. The precise function of these receptors, however, is not yet established.
Albuterol has been shown in most controlled clinical trials to have more effect on the respiratory tract in the form of bronchial smooth muscle relaxation than isoproterenol at comparable doses while producing fewer cardiovascular effects. Controlled clinical studies and other clinical experience have shown that inhaled albuterol, like other beta-adrenergic agonist drugs, can produce a significant cardiovascular effect in some patients, as measured by pulse rate, blood pressure, symptoms, and/or ECG changes.
Albuterol is longer acting than isoproterenol in most patients by any route of administration because it is not a substrate for the cellular uptake processes for catecholamines nor for catechol-*O*-methyl transferase.
Studies in asthmatic patients have shown that less than 20% of a single albuterol dose was absorbed following the IPPB or nebulizer administration; the remaining amount was recovered from the nebulizer and apparatus and expired air. Most of the absorbed dose was recovered in the urine 24 hours after drug administration. There was a significant dose-related response in FEV, and peak flow rate (PFR). It has been demonstrated that following oral administration of 4 mg albuterol, the elimination half-life was five to six hours.
Animal studies show that albuterol does not pass the blood-brain barrier. Recent studies in laboratory animals (minipigs, rodents, and dogs) recorded the occurrence of cardiac arrhythmias and sudden death (with histologic evidence of myocardial necrosis) when beta-agonists and methylxanthines were administered concurrently. This significance of these findings when applied to humans is currently unknown.
In controlled clinical trials, most patients exhibited an onset of improvement in pulmonary function within 5 minutes as determined by FEV_1. FEV_1 measurements also showed that the maximum average improvement in pulmonary function usually occurred at approximately 1 hour following inhalation of 2.5 mg of albuterol by compressor-nebulizer, and remained close to peak for 2 hours. Clinically significant improvement in pulmonary function (defined as maintenance of a 15% or more increase in FEV_1 over baseline values) continued for 3 to 4 hours in most patients and in some patients continued up to 6 hours.
In repetitive dose studies, continued effectiveness was demonstrated throughout the three-month period of treatment in some patients.

INDICATIONS AND USAGE

Albuterol Sulfate Inhalation Solution is indicated for the relief of bronchospasm in patients with reversible obstructive airway disease and acute attacks of bronchospasm.

CONTRAINDICATIONS

Albuterol Sulfate Inhalation Solution is contraindicated in patients with a history of hypersensitivity to any of its components.

WARNINGS

As with other inhaled beta-adrenergic agonists, Albuterol Sulfate Inhalation Solution can produce paradoxical bronchospasm, which can be life threatening. If it occurs, the preparation should be discontinued immediately and alternative therapy instituted.
Fatalities have been reported in association with excessive use of inhaled sympathomimetic drugs and with the home use of sympathomimetic nebulizers. It is, therefore, essential that the physician instruct the patient in the need for further evaluation if his/her asthma becomes worse. In individual patients, any beta$_2$-adrenergic agonist, including albuterol solution for inhalation, may have a clinically significant cardiac effect.
Immediate hypersensitivity reactions may occur after administration of albuterol as demonstrated by rare cases of urticaria, angioedema, rash, bronchospasm, and oropharyngeal edema.

PRECAUTIONS

General

Albuterol, as with all sympathomimetic amines, should be used with caution in patients with cardiovascular disorders, especially coronary insufficiency, cardiac arrhythmias and hypertension. In patients with convulsive disorders, hyperthyroidism or diabetes mellitus and in patients who are unusually responsive to sympathomimetic amines.
Large doses of intravenous albuterol have been reported to aggravate preexisting diabetes mellitus and ketoacidosis. Additionally, beta-agonists, including albuterol, when given intravenously, may cause a decrease in serum potassium, possibly through intracellular shunting. The decrease is usually transient, not requiring supplementation. The relevance of these observations to the use of Albuterol Sulfate Inhalation Solution is unknown.
Information for Patients: The action of Albuterol Sulfate Inhalation Solution may last up to six hours and therefore it should not be used more frequently than recommended. Do not increase the dose or frequency of medication without medical consultation. If symptoms get worse, medical consultation should be sought promptly. While taking Albuterol Sulfate Inhalation Solution, other anti-asthma medicines should not be used unless prescribed.

Drug Interactions

Other sympathomimetic aerosol bronchodilators or epinephrine should not be used concomitantly with albuterol.
Albuterol should be administered with extreme caution to patients being treated with monoamine oxidase inhibitors or tricyclic antidepressants, since the action of albuterol on the vascular system may be potentiated.

Beta-receptor blocking agents and albuterol inhibit the effect of each other.

Carcinogenesis, Mutagenesis, and Impairment of Fertility

Albuterol sulfate, like other agents in its class, caused a significant dose-related increase in the incidence of benign leiomyomas of the mesovarium in a 2-year study in the rat, at oral doses corresponding to 10, 50 and 250 times the maximum human nebulizer dose. In another study, this effect was blocked by the coadministration of propranolol. The relevance of these findings to humans is not known. An 18-month study in mice and a lifetime study in hamsters revealed no evidence of tumorigenicity. Studies with albuterol revealed no evidence of mutagenesis. Reproduction studies in rats revealed no evidence of impaired fertility.

Teratogenic Effects—Pregnancy Category C: Albuterol has been shown to be teratogenic in mice when given subcutaneously in doses corresponding to the human nebulization dose. There are no adequate and well-controlled studies in pregnant women. Albuterol should be used during pregnancy only if the potential benefit justifies the potential risk to the fetus. A reproduction study in CD-1 mice with albuterol (0.025, 0.25 and 2.5 mg/kg subcutaneously, corresponding to 0.1, 1, and 12.5 times the maximum human nebulization dose, respectively) showed cleft palate formation in 5 of 111 (4.5%) of fetuses at 0.25 mg/kg and in 10 of 108 (9.3%) of fetuses at 2.5 mg/kg. None were observed at 0.025 mg/kg. Cleft palate also occurred in 22 of 72 (30.5%) fetuses treated with 2.5 mg/kg isoproterenol (positive control). A reproduction study in Stride Dutch rabbits revealed cranioschisis in 7 of 19 (37%) of fetuses at 50 mg/kg, corresponding to 250 times the maximum human nebulization dose.

Labor and Delivery

Oral albuterol has been shown to delay preterm labor in some reports. There are presently no well controlled studies which demonstrate that it will stop preterm labor at term. Therefore, cautious use of Albuterol Sulfate Inhalation Solution is required in pregnant patients when given for relief of bronchospasm so as to avoid interference with uterine contractibility.

Nursing Mothers

It is not known whether this drug is excreted in human milk. Because of the potential for tumorigenicity shown for albuterol in some animal studies, a decision should be made whether to discontinue nursing or to discontinue the drug, taking into accord the importance of the drug to the mother.

Pediatric Use

Safety and effectiveness of albuterol solution for inhalation in children below the age of 12 years have not been established.

ADVERSE REACTION

The results of clinical trials with Albuterol Sulfate Inhalation Solution in 135 patients showed the following side effects which were considered probably or possibly drug related:

Central Nervous System: tremors (20%), dizziness (7%), nervousness (4%), headache (3%), insomnia (1%).
Gastrointestinal: nausea (4%), dyspepsia (1%).
Ear, Nose and Throat: pharyngitis (<1%), nasal congestion (1%).
Cardiovascular: tachycardia (1%), hypertension (1%).
Respiratory: bronchospasm (8%), cough (4%), bronchitis (4%), wheezing (1%).

No clinically relevant laboratory abnormalities related to Albuterol Sulfate Inhalation Solution administration were determined in these studies.

In comparing the adverse reactions reported for patients treated with Albuterol Sulfate Inhalation Solution with those of patients treated with isoproterenol during clinical trials of three months, the following moderate to severe reactions as judged by the investigators, were reported. This table does not include mild reactions. [See table above.]

Rare cases of urticaria, angioedema, rash, bronchospasm and oropharyngeal edema have been reported after the use of inhaled albuterol.

OVERDOSAGE

Manifestations of overdosage may include anginal pain, hypertension, hypokalemia, and exaggeration of the pharmacological effects listed in **ADVERSE REACTIONS.**

The oral LD_{50} in rats and mice was greater than 2,000 mg/kg. The inhalational LD_{50} could not be determined.

There is insufficient evidence to determine if dialysis is beneficial for overdosage of albuterol.

DOSAGE AND ADMINISTRATION

The ususal dosage for adults and children 12 years and older is 2.5 mg of albuterol administered 3 or 4 times daily by nebulization. More frequent administration or high doses is not recommended. To administer 2.5 mg of albuterol, use the entire contents of one unit-dose vial (3 mL of 0.083% nebulizer solution) by nebulization. The flow rate is regulated to suit the particular nebulizer so that the Albuterol Sulfate Inhalation Solution will be delivered over approximately 5 to 15 minutes. (A 2.5 mg dose of albuterol is also equal to 0.5 mL of a 0.5% solution.)

Percent Incidence of Moderate to Severe Adverse Reactions

Reaction	*Albuterol* N=65	*Isoproterenol* N=65
Central Nervous System		
Tremors	10.7%	13.8%
Headache	3.1%	1.5%
Insomnia	3.1%	1.5%
Cardiovascular		
Hypertension	3.1%	3.1%
Arrhythmias	0%	3.0%
**Palpitation	0%	22.0%
Respiratory		
*Bronchospasm	15.4%	18%
Cough	3.1%	5%
Bronchitis	1.5%	5%
Wheeze	1.5%	1.5%
Sputum Increase	1.5%	1.5%
Dyspnea	1.5%	1.5%
Gastrointestinal		
Nausea	3.1%	0%
Dyspepsia	1.5%	0%
Systemic		
Malaise	1.5%	0%

*In most cases of bronchospasm, this term was generally used to describe exacerbations in the underlying pulmonary disease.

**The finding of no arrhythmias and no palpitations after albuterol administration in this clinical study should not be interpreted as indicating that these adverse effects can not occur after the administration of inhaled albuterol.

The use of Albuterol Sulfate Inhalation Solution can be continued as medically indicated to control recurring bouts of bronchospasm. During treatment, most patients gain optimum benefit from regular use of the nebulizer solution.

If a previously effective dosage regimen fails to provide the usual relief, medical advice should be sought immediately, as this is often a sign of seriously worsening asthma which would require reassessment of therapy.

HOW SUPPLIED

AIRET™ Albuterol Sulfate Inhalation Solution 0.083% 3 mL vials. Equivalent to 0.5 mL albuterol (as the sulfate) 0.5% (2.5 mg albuterol) diluted to 3 mL. Supplied in cartons as listed below.

NDC 53014-075-25
Twenty-five vials per carton.
NDC 53014-075-60
Sixty vials per carton.

Storage: Store between 2° and 25°C (36° and 77°F).

CAUTION

Federal law prohibits dispensing without prescription.

Distributed by:
Adams®
LABORATORIES, INC.
FORT WORTH, TEXAS 76155-2645
03-272-00
754/492 April 1992

ATROHIST® PLUS Tablets ℞

DESCRIPTION

Each yellow, scored Atrohist PLUS Tablet provides: 25 mg phenylephrine hydrochloride, 50 mg phenylpropanolamine hydrochloride, 8 mg chlorpheniramine maleate, 0.19 mg hyoscyamine sulfate, 0.04 mg atropine sulfate and 0.01 mg scopolamine hydrobromide in a sustained-release formulation. Atrohist PLUS Tablets are intended for oral administration. Atrohist PLUS Tablets are a antihistaminic, nasal decongestant and anti-secretory preparation. Inactive ingredients: Lactose, Stearic Acid, Sterotex, PVP Povidone, Magnesium Stearate, Silicon Dioxide, Ethyl Cellulose, D & C Yellow #10 Lake.

INDICATIONS AND USAGE

Atrohist PLUS Tablets provide relief of the symptoms resulting from irritation of sinus, nasal and upper respiratory tract tissues. Phenylephrine and phenylpropanolamine combine to exert a vasoconstrictive and decongestive action while chlorpheniramine maleate decreases the symptoms of watering eyes, post nasal drip and sneezing which may be associated with an allergic-like response. The belladonna alkaloids, hyoscyamine, atropine and scopolamine further augment the anti-secretory activity of Atrohist PLUS Tablets.

CONTRAINDICATIONS

This product is contraindicated in patients with hypersensitivity to antihistamines or sympathomimetics. Atrohist PLUS Tablets are contraindicated in children under 12 years of age and in patients with glaucoma, bronchial asthma and women who are pregnant. Concomitant use of MAO inhibitors is contraindicated.

WARNINGS

Atrohist PLUS Tablets may cause drowsiness. Patients should be warned of possible additive effects caused by taking antihistamines with alcohol, hypnotics or tranquilizers.

PRECAUTIONS

Atrohist PLUS Tablets contain belladonna alkaloids, and must be administered with care to those patients with urinary bladder neck obstruction. Caution should be exercised when Atrohist PLUS Tablets are given to patients with hypertension, cardiac or peripheral vascular disease or hyperthyroidism. Patients should avoid driving a motor vehicle or operating dangerous machinery. (See **WARNINGS.**)

ADVERSE REACTIONS

Hypersensitivity reactions such as rash, urticaria, leukopenia, agranulocytosis, and thrombocytopenia may occur. Large overdoses may cause tachypnea, delirium, fever, stupor, coma and respiratory failure.

Gastrointestinal: nausea, vomiting, diarrhea, constipation, epigastric distress.

Genitourinary System: urinary frequency and dysuria.

Cardiovascular: tightness of the chest, palpitation, tachycardia, hypotension/hypertension.

Central Nervous System: drowsiness, giddiness, faintness, dizziness, headache, incoordination, mydriasis, hyperirritability, nervousness, and insomnia.

Metabolic/Endocrine: lassitude, anorexia.

Miscellaneous: dryness of mucous membranes, xerostomia.

Respiratory: thickening of bronchial secretions.

Special Senses: tinnitus, visual disturbances, blurred vision.

OVERDOSAGE

Since the action of sustained release products may continue for as long as 12 hours, treatment of overdoses directed at reversing the effects of the drug and supporting the patient should be maintained for at least that length of time. In children and infants, antihistamine overdosage may produce convulsions and death.

DOSAGE AND ADMINISTRATION

Adults and children over 12 years of age: One tablet every 12 hours not to exceed 2 tablets in 24 hours. Not recommended for use in children under 12 years of age. Tablets are to be swallowed whole.

HOW SUPPLIED

Bottles of 100 tablets (NDC 53014-024-10). Scored, yellow tablets are embossed with "Adams/024". Store at controlled room temperature between 15° C and 30° C (59° F and 86° F). Dispense in tight, light-resistant containers.

CAUTION: Federal law prohibits dispensing without prescription.

MANUFACTURED BY:
ANABOLIC, INC.
Irvine, California 92714

Adams®
LABORATORIES, INC.
FORT WORTH, TEXAS 76155-2645 244/692

ATROHIST® SPRINKLE Capsules ℞

DESCRIPTION

Each ATROHIST® SPRINKLE Capsule provides 2 mg brompheniramine maleate, 25 mg phenyltoloxamine citrate, and 10 mg phenylephrine hydrochloride in a sustained-release formulation intended for oral administration. The microencapsulated contents of a capsule may be sprinkled on a small amount of soft food immediately prior to ingestion, making the product ideal for children and other patients unable to swallow capsules or tablets. Capsules are oversized to facilitate opening but may also be swallowed whole.

ATROHIST® SPRINKLE Capsules have antihistaminic and nasal decongestant effects. Chemically, brompheniramine maleate is 2-[p-bromo-α-[2-(dimethylamino) ethyl]benzyl]pyridine maleate; phenyltoloxamine citrate is N,N-dimethyl-2(alpha phenyl-ortho-toloxy)-ethylamine; and phenylephrine hydrochloride is (R)-3-hydroxy-α-[(methylamino)methyl]benzenemethanol hydrochloride.

CLINICAL PHARMACOLOGY

Brompheniramine maleate and phenyltoloxamine citrate are antihistamines which act on H_1 receptors as antagonists and interfere with the action of histamine, primarily in capillaries surrounding mucous tissues and sensory nerves of nasal and adjacent areas. Both drugs are rapidly and almost completely absorbed from the gastrointestinal tract and distributed throughout the body, including the central nervous system (CNS). Little, if any, of the drugs is excreted unchanged in the urine; most is apparently metabolized by the liver and excreted as degradation products within 24 hours.

Alkylamine-type antihistamines such as brompheniramine maleate are among the most potent H_1 blockers and are gen-

Continued on next page

Adams Laboratories—Cont.

erally effective in relatively low doses. Although brompheniramine is not so prone as other types of antihistamines to cause drowsiness, a significant proportion of patients do experience this effect. CNS stimulation is more common with alkylamines. Ethanolamine-type antihistamines such as phenyltoloxamine citrate are potent and effective H_1 blockers that possess significant antimuscarinic activity and have a pronounced tendency to induce sedation.

Phenylephrine hydrochloride effects its vasoconstrictor activity by releasing noradrenaline from sympathetic nerve endings, and from direct stimulation of α-adrenoreceptors in blood vessels. Following oral administration, constriction of blood vessels in the nasal mucosa helps relieve nasal congestion. In therapeutic doses the drug causes little, if any, central nervous system stimulation.

INDICATIONS AND USAGE

ATROHIST® SPRINKLE Capsules are indicated for symptomatic relief of seasonal and perennial allergic rhinitis, vasomotor rhinitis, and eustachian tube congestion. The product is particularly suitable for use in children and other patients unable to swallow tablets or capsules.

CONTRAINDICATIONS

This product is contraindicated in patients with hypersensitivity to antihistamines or sympathomimetic amines, and in patients receiving monoamine oxidase (MAO) inhibitor therapy (see **Drug Interactions** section).

Patients known to be hypersensitive to other sympathomimetic amines may exhibit cross sensitivity to phenylephrine. Phenylephrine is contraindicated in patients with severe hypertension or severe coronary artery disease. Patient idiosyncrasy to adrenergic agents may be manifested by insomnia, dizziness, weakness, tremors or arrhythmias.

WARNINGS

Antihistamines should be used with considerable caution in patients with: narrow angle glaucoma; stenosing peptic ulcer; pyloroduodenal obstruction; symptomatic prostatic hypertrophy; bladder neck obstruction.

Sympathomimetic amines should be used with caution in patients with hypertension, ischemic heart disease, diabetes mellitus, increased intraocular pressure, hyperthyroidism, or prostatic hypertropy. Sympathomimetics may produce central nervous system stimulation with convulsions or cardiovascular collapse with accompanying hypotension. **Do not exceed recommended dosage.**

Hypertensive crises can occur with concurrent use of phenylephrine and monoamine oxidase (MAO) inhibitors, indomethacin or with beta-blockers and methyldopa. If a hypertensive crisis occurs, these drugs should be discontinued immediately and therapy to lower blood pressure should be instituted. Fever should be managed by means of external cooling.

PRECAUTIONS

General: Antihistamines have an atropine-like action and therefore should be used with caution in patients with a history of bronchial asthma, increased intraocular pressure, hyperthyroidism, cardiovascular disease and hypertension. Phenylephrine should be used with caution in patients with diabetes, hypertension, cardiovascular disease and hyperreactivity to ephedrine.

Information for Patients: Antihistamines may impair mental and physical abilities required for the performance of potentially hazardous tasks, such as driving a vehicle or operating machinery. Patients should be warned accordingly. Capsules may be swallowed whole or the entire contents sprinkled on a small amount of soft food (jam etc.) immediately prior to ingestion. Capsule contents should not be subdivided. Capsule contents should not be crushed or chewed.

Pediatric Use: This product is not recommended for use in children under 2 years of age. In infants and children, antihistamines in **overdosage** may cause hallucinations, convulsions or death. As in adults, antihistamines may diminish mental alertness in children. In the young child particularly, they may produce excitation.

Use in Elderly: The elderly (60 years and older) are more likely to experience adverse reactions to sympathomimetics. Overdosage of sympathomimetics in this age group may cause hallucinations, convulsions, CNS depression, and death.

Drug Interactions: MAO inhibitors and tricyclic antidepressants may prolong and intensify the anticholinergic (drying) effects of antihistamines. Beta-adrenergic blockers and MAO inhibitors may potentiate the pressor effect of phenylephrine (see **WARNINGS**). Concurrent use of digitalis glycosides may increase the possibility of cardiac arrhythmias. Sympathomimetics may reduce the hypotensive effects of guanethidine, mecamylamine, methyldopa, reserpine and veratrum alkaloids. Concurrent use of tricyclic antidepressants may antagonize the effects of phenylephrine. Concomitant use of antihistamines with alcohol, tricyclic antidepressants, barbiturates and other CNS depressants may have an additive effect.

Carcinogenesis, Mutagenesis, Impairment of Fertility: No data are available on the long-term potential of the components of this product for carcinogenesis, mutagenesis, or impairment of fertility in animals or humans.

Pregnancy: Category C: Animal reproduction studies have not been conducted with the components of this product. It is also not known whether these drugs can cause fetal harm when administered to a pregnant woman or can affect reproduction capacity. Accordingly, this product should be given to a pregnant woman only if clearly needed.

Nursing Mothers: Use of this product by nursing mothers is not recommended because of the higher than usual risk for infants from sympathomimetic amines.

ADVERSE REACTIONS

Hyper-reactive individuals may display ephedrine-like reactions such as tachycardia, palpitations, headache, dizziness, or nausea. Sympathomimetics have been associated with certain untoward reactions including fear, anxiety, nervousness, restlessness, tremor, weakness, pallor, respiratory difficulty, dysuria, insomnia, hallucinations, convulsions, CNS depression, arrhythmias, and cardiovascular collapse with hypotension.

Possible side effects of antihistamines are drowsiness, dry mouth, anorexia, nausea, vomiting, headache and nervousness, blurring of vision, polyuria, heartburn, dysuria and very rarely, dermatitis.

OVERDOSAGE

Since ATROHIST® SPRINKLE Capsules contain pharmacologically different compounds, treatment of overdosage should be based upon the symptomatology of the patient as it relates to the individual ingredients. A detailed description of the symptoms which are likely to appear after ingestion of an excess of the individal components follows:

Manifestations of antihistamine overdosage may vary from CNS depression (sedation, apnea, cardiovascular collapse) to stimulation (insomnia, hallucinations, tremors or convulsions). Other signs and symptoms may be dizziness, tinnitus, ataxia, blurred vision, and hypotension. Stimulation is particularly likely in children, as are atropine-like signs and symptoms (dry-mouth; fixed, dilated pupils; flushing; hyperthermia and gastrointestinal symptoms).

Overdosage with phenylephrine may manifest itself as excessive CNS stimulation resulting in excitment, tremor, restlessness and insomnia. Other effects may include tachycardia, hypertension, pallor, mydriasis, hyperglycemia and urinary retention. Severe overdosage may cause tachypnea or hyperpnea, hallucination, convulsions or delirium, but in some individuals there may be CNS depression with somnolence, stupor or respiratory depression. Arrhythmias (including ventricular fibrillation) may lead to hypotension and circulatory collapse. Severe hypokalemia can occur, probably due to a compartmental shift rather than a depletion of potassium.

The LD_{50} of phenylephrine (single oral dose) has been reported to be 120 mg/kg in the mouse and 350 mg/kg in the rat. The toxic and lethal concentrations in human biologic fluids are not known. No information is available regarding the LD_{50} of brompheniramine maleate and phenyltoloxamine citrate, and their toxic and lethal concentrations in human biologic fluids are not known. Cases of fatal overdosage with antihistamines have been reported in the literature.

In the event of overdosage, emergency treatment should be started immediately. Since the action of sustained release products may continue for as long as 12 hours, treatment of overdosage should be directed toward reducing further absorption and supporting the patient for at least that length of time. Gastric emptying (Syrup of Ipecac) and/or lavage is recommended as soon as possible after ingestion, even if the patient has vomited spontaneously. Either isotonic or half-isotonic saline may be used for lavage. Administration of an activated charcoal slurry is benefical after lavage and/or emesis if less than 4 hours have passed since ingestion. Saline cathartics, such as Milk of Magnesia, are useful for hastening the evacuation of unreleased medication.

Adrenergic receptor blocking agents are antidotes to phenylephrine. In practice, the most useful is the beta-blocker propranolol which is indicated when there are signs of cardiac toxicity. Theoretically, phenylephrine is dialyzable but procedures have not been clinically established.

In severe cases of overdosage, it is essential to monitor both the heart (by electrocardiograph) and plasma electrolytes, and to give intravenous potassium as indicated. Vasopressors may be used to treat hypotension. Excessive CNS stimulation may be counteracted with parenteral diazepam. Stimulants should not be used. Hyperpyrexia, especially in children, may require treatment with tepid water sponge baths or a hyperthermic blanket. Apnea is treated with ventilatory support.

DOSAGE AND ADMINISTRATION

Adults and children over 12 years of age: Three capsules every 12 hours not to exceed 6 capsules in 24 hours. **Children 6 to 12 years:** One or two capsules every 12 hours not to exceed 4 capsules in 24 hours. **Children 2 to 6 years:** One capsule every 12 hours not to exceed 2 capsules in 24 hours. Capsules may be swallowed whole or the entire contents sprinkled on a small amount of soft food immediately prior to ingestion. **Subdividing the contents of a capsule is not recommended.**

HOW SUPPLIED

Bottles of 100 capsules (NDC 53014-022-10). White beads in a yellow and clear capsule imprinted with "Adams/022." Store at controlled room temperature between 15° C and 30° C (59° F and 86° F). Dispense in tight, light-resistant containers.

CAUTION: Federal law prohibits dispensing without prescription.

DECONSAL® II Tablets ℞
PSEUDOEPHEDRINE HCl/GUAIFENESIN

DECONSAL® SPRINKLE Capsules ℞
PHENYLEPHRINE HCl/GUAIFENESIN

DESCRIPTION

DECONSAL® II Tablets: Each scored, dark blue tablet provides 60 mg pseudoephedrine hydrochloride and 600 mg guaifenesin in a sustained-release formulation intended for oral administration. Inactive ingredients: stearic acid, dibasic calcium phosphate, FD & C Blue #1 Lake, sodium lauryl sulfate, ethyl cellulose, magnesium stearate.

DECONSAL® SPRINKLE Capsules: Each blue and clear capsule provides 300 mg guaifenesin and 10 mg phenylephrine hydrochloride in a sustained-release formulation intended for oral administration. The microencapsulated contents of a capsule may be sprinkled on a small amount of soft food immediately prior to ingestion, making the product ideal for children and other patients unable to swallow capsules or tablets. Capsules are oversized to facilitate opening but may also be swallowed whole.

Pseudoephedrine hydrochloride and phenylephrine hydrochloride are orally effective nasal decongestants. Chemically, pseudoephedrine hydrochloride is [S-(R*, R*)]-α-[1-(methylamino)ethyl]benzenemethanol hydrochloride, and phenylephrine hydrochloride is (R)-3-hydroxy-α-[(methylamino)methyl]benzenemethanol hydrochloride. Guaifenesin is an expectorant. Chemically, it is 3-(2 methoxyphenoxy)-1,2-propanediol.

CLINICAL PHARMACOLOGY

Pseudephedrine hydrochloride and phenylephrine hydrochloride are orally active sympathomimetic amines which exerts a decongestant action on the nasal mucosa.

Pseudoephedrine hydrochloride acts by vasoconstriction which results in reduction of tissue hyperemia, edema, nasal congestion, and an increase in nasal airway patency. The vasoconstriction action of pseudoephedrine is similar to that of ephedrine. In the usual dose it has minimal vasopressor effects. Pseudoephedrine is rapidly and almost completely absorbed from the gastrointestinal tract. It has a plasma half-life of 6 to 8 hours. Acidic urine is associated with faster elimination of the drug. The drug is distributed to body tissues and fluids, including the fetal tissue, breast milk and the central nervous system (CNS). Approximately 50% to 75% of the administered dose is excreted unchanged in the urine; the remainder is apparently metabolized in the liver to inactive compounds by N-demethylation, parahydroxylation, and oxidative deamination.

Phenylephrine hydrochloride effects its vasoconstrictor activity by releasing noradrenaline from sympathetic nerve endings, and from direct stimulation of α-adrenoreceptors in blood vessels. Following oral administration, constriction of blood vessels in the nasal mucosa helps relieve nasal congestion. In therapeutic doses the drug causes little, if any, central nervous system stimulation.

Guaifenesin is an expectorant which increases respiratory tract fluid secretions and helps to loosen phlegm and bronchial secretions. By reducing the viscosity of secretions, guaifenesin increases the efficiency of the cough reflex and of ciliary action in removing accumulated secretions from the trachea and bronchi. Guaifenesin is readily absorbed from the gastrointestinal tract and is rapidly metabolized and excreted in the urine. Guaifenesin has a plasma half-life of one hour. The major urinary metabolite is β-(2-methoxyphenoxy) lactic acid.

INDICATIONS AND USAGE

DECONSAL® II Tablets and Deconsal® SPRINKLE Capsules are indicated for the temporary relief of nasal congestion and cough associated with respiratory tract infections and related conditions such as sinusitis, pharyngitis, bronchitis, and asthma, when these conditions are complicated by tenacious mucus and/or mucus plugs and congestion. The products are effective in productive as well as non-productive cough, but are of particular value in dry, non-productive cough which tends to injure the mucous membrane of the air passages.

CONTRAINDICATIONS

These products are contraindicated in patients with hypersensitivity to guaifenesin or hypersensitivity or idiosyncrasy to sympathomimetic amines which may be manifested by insomnia, dizziness, weakness, tremor, or arrhythmias.

Patients known to be hypersensitive to other sympathomimetic amines may exhibit cross sensitivity with pseudoephedrine and phenylephrine. Sympathomimetic amines are contraindicated in patients with severe hypertension, severe coronary artery disease, and patients on monoamine oxidase (MAO) inhibitor therapy (see **Drug Interactions** section).

WARNINGS

Sympathomimetic amines should be used with caution in patients with hypertension, ischemic heart disease, diabetes mellitus, increased intraocular pressure, hyperthyroidism, or prostatic hypertrophy. Sympathomimetics may produce central nervous stimulation with convulsions or cardiovascular collapse with accompanying hypotension. **Do not exceed recommended dosage.**

Hypertensive crises can occur with concurrent use of pseudoephedrine or phenylephrine and monoamine oxidase (MAO) inhibitors, indomethacin, or with beta-blockers and methyldopa. If a hypertensive crisis occurs, these drugs should be discontinued immediately and therapy to lower blood pressure should be instituted. Fever should be managed by means of external cooling.

PRECAUTIONS

General: Use with caution in patients with diabetes, hypertension, cardiovascular disease, or hyperreactivity to ephedrine.

Before prescribing medication to suppress or modify cough, it is important to ascertain that the underlying cause of cough is identified, that modification of cough does not increase the risk of clinical or physiologic complications, and that appropriate therapy for the primary disease is instituted.

Information for Patients: Patients should be instructed to check with physician if symptoms do not improve within 5 days or if fever is present.

Pediatric Use: These products are not recommended for use in children under 2 years of age.

Use in Elderly: The elderly (60 years and older) are more likely to experience adverse reactions to sympathomimetics. Overdosage of sympathomimetics in this age group may cause hallucinations, convulsions, CNS depression, and death.

Drug Interactions: Beta-adrenergic blockers and MAO inhibitors may potentiate the pressor effects of pseudoephedrine and phenylephrine (see **WARNINGS**). Concurrent use of digitalis glycosides may increase the possibility of cardiac arrhythmias. Sympathomimetics may reduce the hypotensive effects of guanethidine, mecamylamine, methyldopa, reserpine, and veratrum alkaloids. Concurrent use of tricyclic antidepressants may antagonize the effects of pseudoephedrine and phenylephrine.

Drug/Laboratory Test Interactions: Guaifenesin may increase renal clearance for urate and therby lower serum uric acid levels. Guaifenesin may produce an increase in urinary 5-hydroxyindoleacetic acid and may therefore interfere with the interpretation of this test for the diagnosis of carcinoid syndrome. It may also falsely elevate the VMA test for catechols. Administration of this drug should be discontinued 48 hours prior to the collection of urine specimens for such tests.

Carcinogenesis, Mutagenesis, Impairment of Fertility: No data are available on the long-term potential of the components of these products for carcinogenesis, mutagenesis, or impairment of fertility in animals or humans.

Pregnancy: Category C: Animal reproduction studies have not been conducted with the components of these products. It is also not known whether these drugs can cause fetal harm when administered to a pregnant woman or can affect reproduction capacity. Accordingly, these products should be given to a pregnant woman only if clearly needed.

Nursing Mothers: Pseudoephedrine is excreted in breast milk. Use of these products by nursing mothers is not recommended because of the higher than usual risk for infants from sympathomimetic amines.

ADVERSE REACTIONS

Hyperreactive individuals may display ephedrine-like reactions such as tachycardia, palpitations, headache, dizziness, or nausea. Sympathomimetics have been associated with certain untoward reactions including fear, anxiety, nervousness, restlessness, tremor, weakness, pallor, respiratory difficulty, dysuria, insomnia, hallucinations, convulsions, CNS depression, arrhythmias, and cardiovascular collapse with hypotension. No serious side effects have been reported with the use of guaifenesin.

OVERDOSAGE

Since DECONSAL® II Tablets and Deconsal® SPRINKLE Capsules contain two pharmacologically different compounds, treatment of overdosage should be based upon the symptomatology of the patient as it relates to the individual ingredients. Treatment of acute overdosage would probably be based upon treating the patient for pseudoephedrine or phenylephrine toxicity which may manifest itself as excessive CNS stimulation resulting in excitement, tremor, restlessness, and insomnia. Other effets may include tachycardia, hypertension, pallor, mydriasis, hyperglycemia and urinary retention. Severe overdosage may cause tachypnea or hyperpnea, hallucinations, convulsions, or delirium, but in some individuals there may be CNS depression. Arrhythmias (including ventricular fibrillation) may lead to hypotension and circulatory collapse. Severe hypokalemia can occur, probably due to a compartmental shift rather than a depletion of potassium. Overdosage with guaifenesin is unlikely to produce toxic effects since its toxicity is much lower than that of pseudoephedrine.

The LD_{50} of pseudoephedrine (single oral dose) has been reported to be 726 mg/kg in the mouse, 2206 mg/kg in the rat, and 1177 mg/kg in the rabbit. The toxic and lethal concentrations in human biologic fluids are not known. Urinary excretion increases with acidification and decreases with alkalinization of the urine. There are few published reports of toxicity due to pseudoephedrine and no case of fatal overdosage has been reported. The LD_{50} of phenylephrine (single oral dose) has been reported to be 120 mg/kg in the mouse and 350 mg/kg in the rat. The toxic and lethal concentrations in human biologic fluids are not known. Guaifenesin, when administered by stomach tube to test animals in doses up to 5 grams/kg, produced no signs of toxicity.

Since the action of sustained-release products may continue for as long as 12 hours, treatment of overdosage should be directed toward reducing further absorption and supporting the patient for at least that length of time. Gastric emptying (Syrup of Ipecac) and/or lavage is recommended as soon as possible after ingestion, even if the patient has vomited spontaneously. Either isotonic or half-isotonic saline may be used for lavage. Administration of an activated charcoal slurry is beneficial after lavage and/or emesis if less than 4 hours have passed since ingestion. Saline cathartics, such as Milk of Magnesia, are useful for hastening the evacuation of unreleased medication.

Adrenergic receptor blocking agents are antidotes to pseudoephedrine and phenylephrine. In practice, the most useful is the beta-blocker propranolol which is indicated when there are signs of cardiac toxicity. Theoretically, pseudoephedrine and phenylephrine are dialyzable but procedures have not been clinically established.

In severe cases of overdosage, it is essential to monitor both the heart (by electrocardiograph) and plasma electrolytes, and to give intravenous potassium as indicated. Vasopressors may be used to treat hypotension. Excessive CNS stimulation may be counteracted with parenteral diazepam. Stimulants should not be used.

DOSAGE AND ADMINISTRATION

DECONSAL® II Tablets: Adults and children over 12 years of age: One or two tablets every 12 hours not to exceed 4 tablets in 24 hours. **Children 6 to 12 years:** One tablet every 12 hours not to exceed 2 tablets in 24 hours. **Children 2 to 6 years:** ½ tablet every 12 hours not to exceed 1 tablet in 24 hours.

DECONSAL® SPRINKLE Capsules: Adults and children over 12 years of age: Two to three capsules every 12 hours not to exceed six capsules in 24 hours. **Children 6 to 12 years:** One to two capsules every 12 hours not to exceed four capsules in 24 hours. **Children 2 to 6 years:** One capsule every 12 hours not to exceed two capsules in 24 hours.

HOW SUPPLIED

DECONSAL® II Tablets: Bottles of 100 (NDC 53014-017-10) and 500 (NDC 53014-017-50) tablets. Scored, dark blue tablets are embossed with "Adams/017".

DECONSAL® SPRINKLE Capsules: Bottles of 100 capsules (NDC 53014-019-10). White beads in a blue and clear capsule imprinted with "Adams/019".

Caution: Federal law prohibits dispensing without prescription.

5/89

HUMIBID® L.A. Tablets ℞
GUAIFENESIN

HUMIBID® SPRINKLE Capsules
GUAIFENESIN

HUMIBID® DM Tablets
GUAIFENESIN/DEXTROMETHORPHAN HYDROBROMIDE

HUMIBID® DM SPRINKLE Capsules
GUAIFENESIN/DEXTROMETHORPHAN HYDROBROMIDE

DESCRIPTION

HUMIBID® L.A. Tablets: Each light green, scored, sustained-release tablet provides 600 mg guaifenesin. Inactive ingredients: dibasic calcium phosphate, ethyl cellulose, FD & C Blue #1 Lake, D & C Yellow #10 Lake, magnesium stearate, sodium lauryl sulfate, stearic acid.

HUMIBID® SPRINKLE Capsules: Each green and clear capsule provides 300 mg guaifenesin in a sustained-release formulation intended for oral administration. The microencapsulated contents of a capsule may be sprinkled on a small amount of soft food immediately prior to ingestion, making the product ideal for children and other patients unable to swallow capsules or tablets. Capsules are oversized to facilitate opening but may also be swallowed whole.

HUMIBID® DM Tablets: Each dark green, scored, sustained-release tablet provides 600 mg guaifenesin and 30 mg dextromethorphan hydrobromide. Inactive ingredients: stearic acid, dibasic calcium phosphate, FD & C Blue #1 Lake, D & C Yellow #10 Lake, sodium lauryl sulfate, ethyl cellulose, magnesium stearate.

HUMIBID® DM SPRINKLE Capsules: Each dark green and clear capsule provides 15 mg dextromethorphan HBr and 300 mg guaifenesin in a sustained-release formulation intended for oral administration. The microencapsulated contents of a capsule may be sprinkled on a small amount of soft food immediately prior to ingestion, making the product ideal for children and other patients unable to swallow capsules or tablets. Capsules are oversized to facilitate opening but may also be swallowed whole.

Chemically, guaifenesin is 3-(2-methoxyphenoxy)-1, 2-propanediol. Dextromethorphan is a salt of the methyl ether of the dextrorotatory isomer of levorphanol, a narcotic analgesic. Chemically, it is 3-methoxy-17-methyl-(9α, 13α, 14α)-morphinan hydrobromide monohydrate.

CLINICAL PHARMACOLOGY

Guaifenesin is an expectorant which increases respiratory tract fluid secretions and helps to loosen phlegm and bronchial secretions. By reducing the viscosity of secretions, guaifenesin increases the efficiency of the cough reflex and of ciliary action in removing accumulated secretions from the trachea and bronchi. Guaifenesin is readily absorbed from the gastrointestinal tract and is rapidly metabolized and excreted in the urine. Guaifenesin has a plasma half-life of one hour. The major urinary metabolite is β-(2-methoxyphenoxy) lactic acid.

Dextromethorphan is an antitussive agent which, unlike the isomeric levorphanol, has no analgesic or addictive properties. The drug acts centrally and elevates the threshold for coughing. It is about equal to codeine in depressing the cough reflex. In therapeutic dosage, dextromethorphan does not inhibit ciliary activity. Dextromethorphan is rapidly absorbed from the gastrointestinal tract, metabolized by the liver and excreted primarily in the urine.

INDICATIONS AND USAGE

HUMIBID® L.A. Tablets and HUMIBID® SPRINKLE Capsules are indicated for the temporary relief of coughs associated with respiratory tract infections and related conditions such as sinusitis, pharyngitis and bronchitis, and asthma, when these conditions are complicated by tenacious mucus and/or mucus plugs and congestion.

HUMIBID® DM Tablets and HUMIBID® DM SPRINKLE Capsules are indicated for the temporary relief of coughs associated with upper respiratory tract infections and related conditions such as sinusitis, pharyngitis and bronchitis, particularly when these conditions are complicated by tenacious mucus and/or mucus plugs and congestion.

HUMIBID® L.A. Tablets, HUMIBID® SPRINKLE Capsules, HUMIBID® DM Tablets and HUMIBID® SPRINKLE Capsules are effective in productive as well as non-productive cough, but are of particular value in dry, non-productive cough which tends to injure the mucous membrane of the air passages.

CONTRAINDICATIONS

These products are contraindicated in patients with hypersensitivity to guaifenesin or dextromethorphan.

HUMIBID® DM Tablets and HUMIBID® DM SPRINKLE Capsules should not be used in patients receiving monoamine oxidase (MAO) inhibitor therapy.

PRECAUTIONS

General: Before prescribing medication to suppress or modify cough, it is important that the underlying cause of cough is identified, that modification of cough does not increase the risk of clinical or physiological complications, and that appropriate therapy for the primary disease is instituted.

Dextromethorphan should be used with caution in sedated or debilitated patients, and in patients to be confined to the supine position.

Information for Patients: HUMIBID® SPRINKLE Capsules and HUMIBID® DM SPRINKLE Capsules may be swallowed whole or the entire contents sprinkled on a small amount of soft food (jam, etc.) immediately prior to ingestion. Capsule contents should not be subdivided, nor should they be crushed or chewed.

Drug/Laboratory Test Interactions: Guaifenesin may increase renal clearance for urate and thereby lower serum uric acid levels. Guaifenesin may produce an increase in urinary 5-hydroxyindoleacetic acid and may therefore inter-

Continued on next page

Adams Laboratories—Cont.

fere with the interpretation of this test for the diagnosis of carcinoid syndrome. It may also falsely elevate the VMA test for catechols. Administration of these products should be discontinued 48 hours prior to the collection of urine specimens for such tests.

Carcinogenesis, Mutagenesis, Impairment of Fertility: No data are available on the long-term potential of guaifenesin or of dextromethorphan for carcinogenesis, mutagenesis, or impairment of fertility in animals or humans.

Pregnancy: Category C: Animal reproduction studies have not been conducted with guaifenesin or with dextromethorphan. It is also not known whether these drugs can cause fetal harm when administered to a pregnant woman or can affect reproduction capacity. Therefore, these products should be given to a pregnant woman only if clearly needed.

Nursing Mothers: It is not known whether guaifenesin or dextromethorphan is excreted in human milk. Because many drugs are excreted in human milk, caution should be exercised when these products are administered to a nursing woman and a decision should be made whether to discontinue nursing or to discontinue the drug, taking into account the importance of the drug to the mother.

ADVERSE REACTIONS

No serious side effects from guaifenesin or dextromethorphan have been reported.

OVERDOSAGE

Overdosage with guaifenesin is unlikely to produce toxic effects since its toxicity is low. Guaifenesin, when administered by stomach tube to test animals in doses up to 5 grams/kg, produced no signs of toxicity. In severe cases of overdosage, treatment should be aimed at reducing further absorption of the drug. Gastric emptying (Syrup of Ipecac) and/or lavage is recommended as soon as possible after ingestion.

Overdosage with dextromethorphan may produce central excitement and mental confusion. Very high doses may produce respiratory depression. One case of toxic psychosis (hyperactivity, marked visual and auditory hallucinations) after ingestion of a single 300 mg dose of dextromethorphan has been reported.

DOSAGE AND ADMINISTRATION

HUMIBID® L.A. and HUMIBID® DM Tablets: Adults and children over 12 years of age: One or two tablets every 12 hours not to exceed 4 tablets in 24 hours . **Children 6 to 12 years:** One tablet every 12 hours not to exceed 2 tablets in 24 hours. **Children 2 to 6 years:** ½ tablet every 12 hours not to exceed 1 tablet in 24 hours.

HUMIBID® SPRINKLE Capsules: Adults and children over 12 years of age: Two to four capsules every 12 hours not to exceed 8 capsules in 24 hours. **Children 6 to 12 years:** Two capsules every 12 hours not to exceed 4 capsules in 24 hours. **Children 2 to 6 years:** One capsule every 12 hours not to exceed 2 capsules in 24 hours.

HUMIBID® DM SPRINKLE Capsules: Adults and children over 12 years of age: Two to four capsules every 12 hours not to exceed 8 capsules in 24 hours. **Children 6 to 12 years:** One to two capsules every 12 hours not to exceed 4 capsules in 24 hours. **Children 2 to 6 years:** One capsule every 12 hours not to exceed 2 capsules in 24 hours.

HOW SUPPLIED

HUMIBID® L.A. Tablets: Bottles of 100 tablets (NDC 53014-012-10) and 500 tablets (NDC 53014-012-50). Light green, scored tablets are embossed with "Adams/012".

HUMIBID® SPRINKLE Capsules: Bottles of 100 capsules (NDC 53014-018-10). White beads in a green and clear capsule imprinted with "Adams/018".

HUMIBID® DM Tablets: Bottles of 100 tablets (NDC 53014-030-10). Dark green, scored tablets are embossed with "Adams/030."

HUMIBID® DM SPRINKLE Capsules: Bottles of 100 capsules (NDC 53014-034-10). White beads in a dark green and clear capsule imprinted with "Adams/034".

Store at controlled room temperature between 15° C and 30° C (59° F and 86° F). Dispense in tight containers.

CAUTION: Federal law prohibits dispensing without prescription.

6/92

Adria Laboratories
Division of Erbamont Inc.
7001 POST ROAD
DUBLIN, OH 43017

PRODUCT IDENTIFICATION CODES

To provide quick and positive identification of Adria Laboratories products, we have imprinted the product identification number on one side of all tablets and capsules. The other side of the tablet displays the name "ADRIA".

In order that you may quickly identify a product by its code number, we have compiled above a numerical list of code numbers of prescription products with their corresponding product names:

[See table above].

PRODUCT IDENTIFICATION CODE	PRODUCT INDEX
130	Axotal® (butalbital, USP, 50 mg and aspirin, USP, 650 mg. Warning: May be habit forming)
200	Ilozyme® (pancrelipase, USP) Tablets
231	Ilopan-Choline® Tablets (dexpanthenol 50 mg./choline bitartrate 25 mg)
Kaon-CL 10	Kaon-CL® 10 (potassium chloride) Controlled Release Tablets, 750 mg. (10 mEq)
307	Kaon-CL® (potassium chloride) Controlled Release Tablets, 500 mg (6.7 mEq)
308	K-Lease® 10 mEq (potassium chloride extended-release capsules, USP) 750 mg
412	Magan® (magnesium salicylate) Tablets, 545 mg.

ADRIAMYCIN PFS™ ℞

[adrēē'ah-mī-cĭn]
(Doxorubicin Hydrochloride, USP)
Injection
FOR INTRAVENOUS USE ONLY

WARNINGS

1. Severe local tissue necrosis will occur if there is extravasation during administration (See Dosage and Administration). ADRIAMYCIN PFS must not be given by the intramuscular or subcutaneous route.
2. Serious irreversible myocardial toxicity with delayed congestive failure often unresponsive to any cardiac supportive therapy may be encountered as total dosage approaches 550 mg/m². This toxicity may occur at lower cumulative doses in patients with prior mediastinal irradiation or on concurrent cyclophosphamide therapy.
3. Dosage should be reduced in patients with impaired hepatic function.
4. Severe myelosuppression may occur.
5. ADRIAMYCIN PFS should be administered only under the supervision of a physician who is experienced in the use of cancer chemotherapeutic agents.

DESCRIPTION

Doxorubicin is a cytotoxic anthracycline antibiotic isolated from cultures of *Streptomyces peucetius* var. *caesius.* Doxorubicin consists of a naphthacenequinone nucleus linked through a glycosidic bond at ring atom 7 to an amino sugar, daunosamine.

Doxorubicin binds to nucleic acids, presumably by specific intercalation of the planar anthracycline nucleus with the DNA double helix. The anthracycline ring is lipophilic but the saturated end of the ring system contains abundant hydroxyl groups adjacent to the amino sugar, producing a hydrophilic center. The molecule is amphoteric, containing acidic functions in the ring phenolic groups and a basic function in the sugar amino group. It binds to cell membranes as well as plasma proteins.

ADRIAMYCIN PFS (doxorubicin hydrochloride, USP) Injection is a parenteral, isotonic, solution containing no preservative, available in 5 mL (10 mg), 10 mL (20 mg), and 25 mL (50 mg) single dose vials and 100 mL (200 mg) multidose vial. Each mL contains doxorubicin hydrochloride and the following inactive ingredients: sodium chloride 0.9% and water for injection q.s. Hydrochloric acid is used to adjust pH to a target pH of 3.0.

CLINICAL PHARMACOLOGY

Though not completely elucidated, the mechanism of action of doxorubicin is related to its ability to bind DNA and inhibit nucleic acid synthesis. Cell culture studies have demonstrated rapid cell penetration and perinucleolar chromatin binding, rapid inhibition of mitotic activity and nucleic acid synthesis, mutagenesis and chromosomal aberrations. Animal studies have shown activity in a spectrum of experimental tumors, immunosuppression, carcinogenic properties in rodents, induction of a variety of toxic effects, including delayed and progressive cardiac toxicity, myelosuppression in all species and atrophy to testes in rats and dogs.

Pharmacokinetic studies show the intravenous administration of normal or radiolabeled doxorubicin is followed by rapid plasma clearance and significant tissue binding. Urinary excretion, as determined by fluorimetric methods, accounts for approximately 4–5% of the administered dose in five days. Biliary excretion represents the major excretion route, 40–50% of the administered dose being recovered in the bile or the feces in seven days. Impairment of liver function results in slower excretion, and consequently, increased retention and accumulation in plasma and tissues. Doxorubicin does not cross the blood brain barrier.

INDICATIONS AND USAGE

ADRIAMYCIN® (Doxorubicin HCl, USP) for injection has been used successfully to produce regression in disseminated neoplastic conditions such as acute lymphoblastic leukemia, acute myeloblastic leukemia, Wilms' tumor, neuroblastoma, soft tissue and bone sarcomas, breast carcinoma, ovarian carcinoma, transitional cell bladder carcinoma, thyroid carcinoma, lymphomas of both Hodgkin and non-Hodgkin types, bronchogenic carcinoma in which the small cell histologic type is the most responsive compared to other cell types and gastric carcinoma.

A number of other solid tumors have also shown some responsiveness but in numbers too limited to justify specific recommendation. Studies to date have shown malignant melanoma, kidney carcinoma, large bowel carcinoma, brain tumors and metastases to the central nervous system not to be significantly responsive to ADRIAMYCIN therapy.

CONTRAINDICATIONS

ADRIAMYCIN therapy should not be started in patients who have marked myelosuppression induced by previous treatment with other antitumor agents or by radiotherapy. Conclusive data are not available on pre-existing heart disease as a co-factor of increased risk of ADRIAMYCIN induced cardiac toxicity. Preliminary data suggest that in such cases cardiac toxicity may occur at doses lower than the recommended cumulative limit. It is therefore not recommended to start ADRIAMYCIN in such cases. ADRIAMYCIN treatment is contraindicated in patients who received previous treatment with complete cumulative doses of ADRIAMYCIN and/or daunorubicin.

WARNINGS

Special attention must be given to the cardiac toxicity exhibited by ADRIAMYCIN. Although uncommon, acute left ventricular failure has occurred, particularly in patients who have received total dosage of the drug exceeding the currently recommended limit of 550 mg/m². This limit appears to be lower (400 mg/m²) in patients who received radiotherapy to the mediastinal area or concomitant therapy with other potentially cardiotoxic agents such as cyclophosphamide. The total dose of ADRIAMYCIN administered to the individual patient should also take into account a previous or concomitant therapy with related compounds such as daunorubicin. Congestive heart failure and/or cardiomyopathy may be encountered several weeks after discontinuation of ADRIAMYCIN therapy.

Cardiac failure is often not favorably affected by presently known medical or physical therapy for cardiac support. Early clinical diagnosis of drug induced heart failure appears to be essential for successful treatment with digitalis, diuretics, low salt diet and bed rest. Severe cardiac toxicity may occur precipitously without antecedent EKG changes. A baseline EKG and EKGs performed prior to each dose or course after 300 mg/m² cumulative dose has been given is suggested. Transient EKG changes consisting of T-wave flattening, S-T depression and arrhythmias lasting for up to two weeks after a dose or course of ADRIAMYCIN are presently not considered indications for suspension of ADRIAMYCIN therapy. ADRIAMYCIN cardiomyopathy has been reported to be associated with a persistent reduction in the voltage of the QRS wave, a prolongation of the systolic time interval and a reduction of the ejection fraction as determined by echocardiography or radionuclide angiography. None of these tests have yet been confirmed to consistently identify those individual patients that are approaching their maximally tolerated cumulative dose of ADRIAMYCIN. If test results indicate change in cardiac function associated with ADRIAMYCIN the benefit of continued therapy must be carefully evaluated against the risk of producing irreversible cardiac damage.

Acute life-threatening arrhythmias have been reported to occur during or within a few hours after ADRIAMYCIN administration.

There is a high incidence of bone marrow depression, primarily of leukocytes, requiring careful hematologic monitoring. With the recommended dosage schedule, leukopenia is usually transient, reaching its nadir at 10–14 days after treat-

ment with recovery usually occurring by the 21st day. White blood cell counts as low as 1000 mm^3 are to be expected during treatment with appropriate doses of ADRIAMYCIN. Red blood cell and platelet levels should also be monitored since they may also be depressed. Hematologic toxicity may require dose reduction or suspension or delay of ADRIAMYCIN therapy. Persistent severe myelosuppression may result in superinfection or hemorrhage.

ADRIAMYCIN may potentiate the toxicity of other anticancer therapies. Exacerbation of cyclophosphamide induced hemorrhagic cystitis and enhancement of the hepatotoxicity of 6-mercaptopurine have been reported. Radiation induced toxicity to the myocardium, mucosae, skin and liver have been reported to be increased by the administration of ADRIAMYCIN.

Toxicity to recommended doses of ADRIAMYCIN is enhanced by hepatic impairment, therefore, prior to the individual dosing, evaluation of hepatic function is recommended using conventional clinical laboratory tests such as SGOT, SGPT, alkaline phosphatase and bilirubin. (See Dosage and Administration).

Necrotizing colitis manifested by typhlitis (cecal inflammation), bloody stools and severe and sometimes fatal infections have been associated with a combination of ADRIAMYCIN given by i.v. push daily for 3 days and cytarabine given by continuous infusion daily for 7 or more days.

On intravenous administration of ADRIAMYCIN extravasation may occur with or without an accompanying stinging or burning sensation and even if blood returns well on aspiration of the infusion needle (See Dosage and Administration). If any signs or symptoms of extravasation have occurred the injection or infusion should be immediately terminated and restarted in another vein.

ADRIAMYCIN and related compounds have also been shown to have mutagenic and carcinogenic properties when tested in experimental models.

Usage in Pregnancy—Safe use of ADRIAMYCIN in pregnancy has not been established. ADRIAMYCIN is embryotoxic and teratogenic in rats and embryotoxic and abortifacient in rabbits. Therefore, the benefits to the pregnant patient should be carefully weighed against the potential toxicity to fetus and embryo. The possible adverse effects on fertility in males and females in humans or experimental animals have not been adequately evaluated.

PRECAUTIONS

Initial treatment with ADRIAMYCIN requires close observation of the patient and extensive laboratory monitoring. It is recommended, therefore, that patients be hospitalized at least during the first phase of the treatment.

Like other cytotoxic drugs, ADRIAMYCIN may induce hyperuricemia secondary to rapid lysis of neoplastic cells. The clinician should monitor the patient's blood uric acid level and be prepared to use such supportive and pharmacologic measures as might be necessary to control this problem.

ADRIAMYCIN imparts a red coloration to the urine for 1–2 days after administration and patients should be advised to expect this during active therapy.

ADRIAMYCIN is not an anti-microbial agent.

ADVERSE REACTIONS

Dose limiting toxicities of therapy are myelosuppression and cardiotoxicity (See Warnings). Other reactions reported are:

Cutaneous—Reversible complete alopecia occurs in most cases. Hyperpigmentation of nailbeds and dermal creases, primarily in children, and onycholysis have been reported in a few cases. Recall of skin reaction due to prior radiotherapy has occurred with ADRIAMYCIN administration.

Gastrointestinal—Acute nausea and vomiting occurs frequently and may be severe. This may be alleviated by antiemetic therapy. Mucositis (stomatitis and esophagitis) may occur 5–10 days after administration. The effect may be severe leading to ulceration and represents a site of origin for severe infections. The dose regimen consisting of administration of ADRIAMYCIN on three successive days results in the greater incidence and severity of mucositis. Ulceration and necrosis of the colon, especially the cecum, may occur leading to bleeding or severe infections which can be fatal. This reaction has been reported in patients with acute non-lymphocytic leukemia treated with a 3-day course of ADRIAMYCIN combined with cytarabine. Anorexia and diarrhea have been occasionally reported.

Vascular—Phlebosclerosis has been reported especially when small veins are used or a single vein is used for repeated administration. Facial flushing may occur if the injection is given too rapidly.

Local—Severe cellulitis, vesication and tissue necrosis will occur if ADRIAMYCIN is extravasated during administration. Erythematous streaking along the vein proximal to the site of the injection has been reported (See Dosage and Administration).

Hypersensitivity—Fever, chills and urticaria have been reported occasionally. Anaphylaxis may occur. A case of apparent cross sensitivity to lincomycin has been reported.

Other—Conjunctivitis and lacrimation occur rarely.

OVERDOSAGE

Acute overdosage with ADRIAMYCIN enhances the toxic effects of mucositis, leukopenia and thrombopenia. Treatment of acute overdosage consists of treatment of the severely myelosuppressed patient with hospitalization, antibiotics, platelet and granulocyte transfusions and symptomatic treatment of mucositis. **The 200 mg vial is packaged as a multiple dose vial and caution should be exercised to prevent inadvertent overdosage.**

Chronic overdosage with cumulative doses exceeding 550 mg/m^2 increases the risk of cardiomyopathy and resultant congestive heart failure. Treatment consists of vigorous management of congestive heart failure with digitalis preparations and diuretics. The use of peripheral vasodilators has been recommended.

DOSAGE AND ADMINISTRATION

Care in the administration of ADRIAMYCIN will reduce the chance of perivenous infiltration. It may also decrease the chance of local reactions such as urticaria and erythematous streaking. On intravenous administration of ADRIAMYCIN, extravasation may occur with or without an accompanying stinging or burning sensation and even if blood returns well on aspiration of the infusion needle. If any signs or symptoms of extravasation have occurred, the injection or infusion should be immediately terminated and restarted in another vein. If it is known or suspected that subcutaneous extravasation has occurred, local infiltration with an injectable corticosteroid and flooding the site with normal saline has been reported to lessen the local reaction. Because of the progressive nature of extravasation reactions, the area of injection should be frequently examined and plastic surgery consultation obtained. If ulceration begins, early wide excision of the involved area should be considered.[1]

The most commonly used dosage schedule is 60–75 mg/m^2 as a single intravenous injection administered at 21-day intervals. The lower dose should be given to patients with inadequate marrow reserves due to old age, or prior therapy, or neoplastic marrow infiltration. An alternative dose schedule is weekly doses of 20 mg/m^2 which has been reported to produce a lower incidence of congestive heart failure. Thirty mg/m^2 on each of three successive days repeated every 4 weeks has also been used. ADRIAMYCIN dosage must be reduced if the bilirubin is elevated as follows: serum bilirubin 1.2–3.0 mg/dL—give ½ normal dose, > 3 mg/dL—give ¼ normal dose.

It is recommended that ADRIAMYCIN PFS be slowly administered into the tubing of a freely running intravenous infusion of Sodium Chloride Injection USP or 5% Dextrose Injection USP. The tubing should be attached to a Butterfly® needle inserted preferably into a large vein. If possible, avoid veins over joints or in extremities with compromised venous or lymphatic drainage. The rate of administration is dependent on the size of the vein and the dosage. However the dose should be administered in not less than 3 to 5 minutes. Local erythematous streaking along the vein as well as facial flushing may be indicative of too rapid an administration. A burning or stinging sensation may be indicative of perivenous infiltration and the infusion should be immediately terminated and restarted in another vein. Perivenous infiltration may occur painlessly.

ADRIAMYCIN should not be mixed with heparin or 5-fluorouracil since it has been reported that these drugs are incompatible to the extent that a precipitate may form. Until specific compatibility data are available, it is not recommended that ADRIAMYCIN PFS be mixed with other drugs.

ADRIAMYCIN has been used concurrently with other approved chemotherapeutic agents. Evidence is available that in some types of neoplastic disease combination chemotherapy is superior to single agents. The benefits and risks of such therapy continue to be elucidated.

Handling and Disposal: Skin reactions associated with ADRIAMYCIN have been reported. Caution in the handling of the solution must be exercised and the use of gloves is recommended. If ADRIAMYCIN PFS contacts the skin or mucosae, immediately wash thoroughly with soap and water.

Procedures for proper handling and disposal of anti-cancer drugs should be considered. Several guidelines on this subject have been published.[2–7] There is no general agreement that all of the procedures recommended in the guidelines are necessary or appropriate.

HOW SUPPLIED

ADRIAMYCIN PFS™ (doxorubicin hydrochloride, USP) Injection

Sterile, single use only, contains no preservative

NDC 0013-1136-91 10 mg vial, 2 mg/mL, 5 mL, 10 vial packs.

NDC 0013-1146-91 20 mg vial, 2 mg/mL, 10 mL, 10 vial packs.

NDC 0013-1156-79 50 mg vial, 2 mg/mL, 25 mL, single vial packs.

Store under refrigeration, 2°–8°C (36°–46°F), protect from light and retain in carton until time of use. Discard unused solution.

Sterile, multidose vial, contains no preservative.

NDC 0013-1166-83 200 mg, 2 mg/mL, 100 mL multidose vial, single vial packs.

Store under refrigeration 2°–8°C (36°–46°F), protect from light and retain in carton until time of use.

REFERENCES

1. Rudolph R et al: Skin Ulcers Due to ADRIAMYCIN. Cancer 38: 1087–1094, Sept. 1976.
2. Recommendations for the Safe Handling of Parenteral Antineoplastic Drugs. NIH Publication No. 83-2621. For sale by the Superintendent of Documents, U.S. Government Printing Office, Washington, D.C. 20402.
3. AMA Council Report. Guidelines for Handling Parenteral Antineoplastics. JAMA, March 15, 1985.
4. National Study Commission on Cytotoxic Exposure—Recommendations for Handling Cytotoxic Agents. Available from Louis P. Jeffrey, Sc. D., Director of Pharmacy Services, Rhode Island Hospital, 593 Eddy Street, Providence, Rhode Island 02902.
5. Clinical Oncological Society of Australia: Guidelines and recommendations for safe handling of antineoplastic agents. Med J. Australia 1:426–428, 1983.
6. Jones R., et al. Safe handling of chemotherapeutic agents: A report from the Mount Sinai Medical Center. Ca—A Cancer Journal for Clinicians Sept/Oct, 258–263, 1983.
7. American Society of Hospital Pharmacists technical assistance bulletin on handling cytotoxic drugs in hospitals. Am J Hosp Pharm 42:131–137, 1985.

Manufactured by:
FARMITALIA CARLO ERBA
MILAN, ITALY
Distributed by:
ADRIA LABORATORIES
Division of Erbamont Inc.
COLUMBUS, OHIO 43216.

ADRIAMYCIN RDF™ ℞

[*a 'dreeah-mī "sin*]
(Doxorubicin Hydrochloride, USP)
For Injection
FOR INTRAVENOUS USE ONLY

PRODUCT OVERVIEW

KEY FACTS

ADRIAMYCIN RDF is a cytotoxic agent active against a variety of hematologic malignancies and solid tumors. The active ingredient, doxorubicin hydrochloride, is an anthracycline antibiotic that selectively kills malignant cells and causes tumor regression. ADRIAMYCIN RDF contains a small amount of methylparaben (to enhance dissolution).

MAJOR USES

ADRIAMYCIN RDF is clinically effective against disseminated neoplastic conditions including acute lymphoblastic and myeloblastic leukemia, Wilm's tumor, neuroblastoma, soft tissue and bone sarcomas, breast carcinoma, ovarian carcinoma, transitional cell bladder carcinoma, thyroid carcinoma, Hodgkin's and non-Hodgkin's lymphoma, bronchogenic carcinoma and gastric carcinoma.

SAFETY INFORMATION

ADRIAMYCIN RDF is intended for intravenous use only. Care must be taken to avoid extravasation. Patients must be carefully monitored and doses adjusted to avoid too severe myelosuppression or mucositis. Too large cumulative doses may cause cardiomyopathy leading to congestive heart failure.

PRESCRIBING INFORMATION

ADRIAMYCIN RDF™ ℞

[*a 'dreeah-mī "sin*]
(Doxorubicin Hydrochloride, USP)
For Injection
FOR INTRAVENOUS USE ONLY

WARNINGS

1. Severe local tissue necrosis will occur if there is extravasation during administration (See Dosage and Administration). ADRIAMYCIN RDF must not be given by the intramuscular or subcutaneous route.
2. Serious irreversible myocardial toxicity with delayed congestive failure often unresponsive to any cardiac supportive therapy may be encountered as total dosage approaches 550 mg/m^2. This toxicity may occur at lower cumulative doses in patients with prior mediastinal irradiation or on concurrent cyclophosphamide therapy.
3. Dosage should be reduced in patients with impaired hepatic function.

Continued on next page

Adria Laboratories—Cont.

4. Severe myelosuppression may occur.
5. ADRIAMYCIN RDF should be administered only under the supervision of a physician who is experienced in the use of cancer chemotherapeutic agents.

DESCRIPTION

Doxorubicin is a cytotoxic anthracycline antibiotic isolated from cultures of *Streptomyces peucetius* var. *caesius*. Doxorubicin consists of a naphthacenequinone nucleus linked through a glycosidic bond at ring atom 7 to an amino sugar, daunosamine.

Doxorubicin binds to nucleic acids, presumably by specific intercalation of the planar anthracycline nucleus with the DNA double helix. The anthracycline ring is lipophilic but the saturated end of the ring system contains abundant hydroxyl groups adjacent to the amino sugar, producing a hydrophilic center. The molecule is amphoteric, containing acidic functions in the ring phenolic groups and a basic function in the sugar amino group. It binds to cell membranes as well as plasma proteins. It is supplied in the hydrochloride form as a freeze-dried powder containing lactose and methylparaben (added to enhance dissolution).

CLINICAL PHARMACOLOGY

Though not completely elucidated, the mechanism of action of doxorubicin is related to its ability to bind to DNA and inhibit nucleic acid synthesis. Cell culture studies have demonstrated rapid cell penetration and perinucleolar chromatin binding, rapid inhibition of mitotic activity and nucleic acid synthesis, mutagenesis and chromosomal aberrations.

Animal studies have shown activity in a spectrum of experimental tumors, immunosuppression, carcinogenic properties in rodents, induction of a variety of toxic effects, including delayed and progressive cardiac toxicity, myelosuppression in all species and atrophy to testes in rats and dogs.

Pharmacokinetic studies show the intravenous administration of normal or radiolabeled doxorubicin is followed by rapid plasma clearance and significant tissue binding. Urinary excretion, as determined by fluorimetric methods, accounts for approximately 4–5% of the administered dose in five days. Biliary excretion represents the major excretion route, 40–50% of the administered dose being recovered in the bile or the feces in seven days. Impairment of liver function results in slower excretion, and, consequently, increased retention and accumulation in plasma and tissues. Doxorubicin does not cross the blood brain barrier.

INDICATIONS AND USAGE

ADRIAMYCIN® (Doxorubicin HCl, USP) for Injection has been used successfully to produce regression in disseminated neoplastic conditions such as acute lymphoblastic leukemia, acute myeloblastic leukemia, Wilms' tumor, neuroblastoma, soft tissue and bone sarcomas, breast carcinoma, ovarian carcinoma, transitional cell bladder carcinoma, thyroid carcinoma, lymphomas of both Hodgkin and non-Hodgkin types, bronchogenic carcinoma in which the small cell histologic type is the most responsive compared to other cell types and gastric carcinoma.

A number of other solid tumors have also shown some responsiveness but in numbers too limited to justify specific recommendation. Studies to date have shown malignant melanoma, kidney carcinoma, large bowel carcinoma, brain tumors and metastases to the central nervous system not to be significantly responsive to ADRIAMYCIN therapy.

CONTRAINDICATIONS

ADRIAMYCIN therapy should not be started in patients who have marked myelosuppression induced by previous treatment with other antitumor agents or by radiotherapy. Conclusive data are not available on pre-existing heart disease as a co-factor of increased risk of ADRIAMYCIN induced cardiac toxicity. Preliminary data suggest that in such cases cardiac toxicity may occur at doses lower than the recommended cumulative limit. It is therefore not recommended to start ADRIAMYCIN in such cases. ADRIAMYCIN treatment is contraindicated in patients who received previous treatment with complete cumulative doses of ADRIAMYCIN and/or daunorubicin.

WARNINGS

Special attention must be given to the cardiac toxicity exhibited by ADRIAMYCIN. Although uncommon, acute left ventricular failure has occurred, particularly in patients who have received total dosage of the drug exceeding the currently recommended limit of 550 mg/m^2. This limit appears to be lower (400 mg/m^2) in patients who received radiotherapy to the mediastinal area or concomitant therapy with other potentially cardiotoxic agents such as cyclophosphamide. The total dose of ADRIAMYCIN administered to the individual patient should also take into account a previous or concomitant therapy with related compounds such as daunorubicin. Congestive heart failure and/or cardiomyopathy may be encountered several weeks after discontinuation of ADRIAMYCIN therapy.

Cardiac failure is often not favorably affected by presently known medical or physical therapy for cardiac support. Early clinical diagnosis of drug induced heart failure appears to be essential for successful treatment with digitalis, diuretics, low salt diet and bed rest. Severe cardiac toxicity may occur precipitously without antecedent EKG changes. A baseline EKG and EKGs performed prior to each dose or course after 300 mg/m^2 cumulative dose has been given is suggested. Transient EKG changes consisting of T-wave flattening, S-T depression and arrhythmias lasting for up to two weeks after a dose or course of ADRIAMYCIN are presently not considered indications for suspension of ADRIAMYCIN therapy. ADRIAMYCIN cardiomyopathy has been reported to be associated with a persistent reduction in the voltage of the QRS wave, a prolongation of the systolic time interval and a reduction of the ejection fraction as determined by echocardiography or radionuclide angiography. None of these tests have yet been confirmed to consistently identify those individual patients that are approaching their maximally tolerated cumulative dose of ADRIAMYCIN. If test results indicate change in cardiac function associated with ADRIAMYCIN the benefit of continued therapy must be carefully evaluated against the risk of producing irreversible cardiac damage.

Acute life-threatening arrhythmias have been reported to occur during or within a few hours after ADRIAMYCIN administration.

There is a high incidence of bone marrow depression, primarily of leukocytes, requiring careful hematologic monitoring. With the recommended dosage schedule, leukopenia is usually transient, reaching its nadir at 10–14 days after treatment with recovery usually occurring by the 21st day. White blood cell counts as low as 1000 mm^3 are to be expected during treatment with appropriate doses of ADRIAMYCIN. Red blood cell and platelet levels should also be monitored since they may also be depressed. Hematologic toxicity may require dose reduction or suspension or delay of ADRIAMYCIN therapy. Persistent severe myelosuppression may result in superinfection or hemorrhage.

ADRIAMYCIN may potentiate the toxicity of other anticancer therapies. Exacerbation of cyclophosphamide induced hemorrhagic cystitis and enhancement of the hepatotoxicity of 6-mercaptopurine have been reported. Radiation induced toxicity to the myocardium, mucosae, skin and liver have been reported to be increased by the administration of ADRIAMYCIN.

Toxicity to recommended doses of ADRIAMYCIN is enhanced by hepatic impairment, therefore, prior to the individual dosing, evaluation of hepatic function is recommended using conventional clinical laboratory tests, such as SGOT, SGPT, alkaline phosphatase and bilirubin. (See Dosage and Administration).

Necrotizing colitis manifested by typhlitis (cecal inflammation), bloody stools and severe and sometimes fatal infections has been associated with a combination of ADRIAMYCIN given by i.v. push daily for 3 days and cytarabine given by continuous infusion daily for 7 or more days.

On intravenous administration of ADRIAMYCIN extravasation may occur with or without an accompanying stinging or burning sensation and even if blood returns well on aspiration of the infusion needle (See Dosage and Administration). If any signs or symptoms of extravasation have occurred the injection or infusion should be immediately terminated and restarted in another vein.

ADRIAMYCIN and related compounds have also been shown to have mutagenic and carcinogenic properties when tested in experimental models.

Usage in Pregnancy—Safe use of ADRIAMYCIN in pregnancy has not been established. ADRIAMYCIN is embryotoxic and teratogenic in rats and embryotoxic and abortifacient in rabbits. Therefore, the benefits to the pregnant patient should be carefully weighed against the potential toxicity to fetus and embryo. The possible adverse effects on fertility in males and females in humans or experimental animals have not been adequately evaluated.

PRECAUTIONS

Initial treatment with ADRIAMYCIN requires close observation of the patient and extensive laboratory monitoring. It is recommended, therefore, that patients be hospitalized at least during the first phase of the treatment.

Like other cytotoxic drugs, ADRIAMYCIN may induce hyperuricemia secondary to rapid lysis of neoplastic cells. The clinician should monitor the patient's blood uric acid level and be prepared to use such supportive and pharmacologic measures as might be necessary to control this problem.

ADRIAMYCIN imparts a red coloration to the urine for 1-2 days after administration and patients should be advised to expect this during active therapy.

ADRIAMYCIN is not an anti-microbial agent.

ADVERSE REACTIONS

Dose limiting toxicities of therapy are myelosuppression and cardiotoxicity (See Warnings). Other reactions reported are:

Cutaneous—Reversible complete alopecia occurs in most cases. Hyperpigmentation of nailbeds and dermal creases, primarily in children, and onycholysis have been reported in a few cases. Recall of skin reaction due to prior radiotherapy has occurred with ADRIAMYCIN administration.

Gastrointestinal—Acute nausea and vomiting occurs frequently and may be severe. This may be alleviated by antiemetic therapy. Mucositis (stomatitis and esophagitis) may occur 5–10 days after administration. The effect may be severe leading to ulceration and represents a site of origin for severe infections. The dose regimen consisting of administration of ADRIAMYCIN on three successive days results in the greater incidence and severity of mucositis. Ulceration and necrosis of the colon, especially the cecum, may occur leading to bleeding or severe infections which can be fatal. This reaction has been reported in patients with acute non-lymphocytic leukemia treated with a 3-day course of ADRIAMYCIN combined with cytarabine. Anorexia and diarrhea have been occasionally reported.

Vascular—Phlebosclerosis has been reported especially when small veins are used or a single vein is used for repeated administration. Facial flushing may occur if the injection is given too rapidly.

Local—Severe cellulitis, vesication and tissue necrosis will occur if ADRIAMYCIN is extravasated during administration. Erythematous streaking along the vein proximal to the site of the injection has been reported (See Dosage and Administration).

Hypersensitivity—Fever, chills and urticaria have been reported occasionally. Anaphylaxis may occur. A case of apparent cross sensitivity to lincomycin has been reported.

Other—Conjunctivitis and lacrimation occur rarely.

OVERDOSAGE

Acute overdosage with ADRIAMYCIN enhances the toxic effects of mucositis, leukopenia and thrombopenia. Treatment of acute overdosage consists of treatment of the severely myelosuppressed patient with hospitalization, antibiotics, platelet and granulocyte transfusions and symptomatic treatment of mucositis. **The 150 mg vial is packaged as a multiple dose vial and caution should be exercised to prevent inadvertent overdosage.**

Chronic overdosage with cumulative doses exceeding 550 mg/m^2 increases the risk of cardiomyopathy and resultant congestive heart failure. Treatment consists of vigorous management of congestive heart failure with digitalis preparations and diuretics. The use of peripheral vasodilators has been recommended.

DOSAGE AND ADMINISTRATION

Care in the administration of ADRIAMYCIN will reduce the chance of perivenous infiltration. It may also decrease the chance of local reactions such as urticaria and erythematous streaking. On intravenous administration of ADRIAMYCIN, extravasation may occur with or without accompanying stinging or burning sensation and even if blood returns well on aspiration of the infusion needle. If any signs or symptoms of extravasation have occurred, the injection or infusion should be immediately terminated and restarted in another vein. If it is known or suspected that subcutaneous extravasation has occurred, local infiltration with an injectable corticosteroid and flooding the site with normal saline has been reported to lessen the local reaction. Because of the progressive nature of extravasation reactions, the area of injection should be frequently examined and plastic surgery consultation obtained. If ulceration begins, early wide excision of the involved area should be considered.[1]

The most commonly used dosage schedule is 60–75 mg/m^2 as a single intravenous injection administered at 21-day intervals. The lower dose should be given to patients with inadequate marrow reserves due to old age, or prior therapy, or neoplastic marrow infiltration. An alternative dose schedule is weekly doses of 20 mg/m^2 which has been reported to produce a lower incidence of congestive heart failure. Thirty mg/m^2 on each of three successive days repeated every 4 weeks has also been used. ADRIAMYCIN dosage must be reduced if the bilirubin is elevated as follows: Serum Bilirubin 1.2–3.0 mg/dL-give ½ normal dose, > 3 mg/dL—give ¼ normal dose.

Preparation of Solution: ADRIAMYCIN RDF 10 mg, 20 mg, 50 mg, and 150 mg vials should be reconstituted with 5 mL, 10 mL, 25 mL, and 75 mL respectively, of Sodium Chloride Injection, USP (0.9%) to give a final concentration of 2 mg/mL of doxorubicin hydrochloride. An appropriate volume of air should be withdrawn from the vial during reconstitution to avoid excessive pressure build-up. Bacteriostatic diluents are not recommended.

After adding the diluent, the vial should be shaken and the contents allowed to dissolve. The reconstituted solution is stable for 7 days at room temperature and under normal room light (100 foot-candles) and 15 days under refrigeration (2°-8°C). It should be protected from exposure to sunlight. Discard any unused solution from the 10 mg, 20 mg and 50 mg single dose vials. Unused solutions of the multiple dose vial remaining beyond the recommended storage times should be discarded.

It is recommended that ADRIAMYCIN be slowly administered into the tubing of a freely running intravenous infusion of Sodium Chloride Injection, USP or 5% Dextrose Injection, USP. The tubing should be attached to a Butterfly® needle inserted preferably into a large vein. If possible, avoid veins over joints or in extremities with compromised venous or lymphatic drainage. The rate of administration is dependent on the size of the vein and the dosage. However, the dose should be administered in not less than 3 to 5 minutes. Local erythematous streaking along the vein as well as facial flushing may be indicative of too rapid an administration. A burning or stinging sensation may be indicative of perivenous infiltration and the infusion should be immediately terminated and restarted in another vein. Perivenous infiltration may occur painlessly.

ADRIAMYCIN should not be mixed with heparin or 5-fluorouracil since it has been reported that these drugs are incompatible to the extent that a precipitate may form. Until specific compatibility data are available, it is not recommended that ADRIAMYCIN be mixed with other drugs.

ADRIAMYCIN has been used concurrently with other approved chemotherapeutic agents. Evidence is available that in some types of neoplastic disease combination chemotherapy is superior to single agents. The benefits and risks of such therapy continue to be elucidated.

Handling and Disposal: Skin reactions associated with ADRIAMYCIN have been reported. Caution in handling and preparation of the powder and solution must be exercised and the use of gloves is recommended. If ADRIAMYCIN powder or solution contacts the skin or mucosae, immediately wash thoroughly with soap and water.

Procedures for proper handling and disposal of anti-cancer drugs should be considered. Several guidelines on this subject have been published.[2–7] There is no general agreement that all of the procedures recommended in the guidelines are necessary or appropriate.

HOW SUPPLIED

ADRIAMYCIN RDF™ (DOXORUBICIN HYDROCHLORIDE, USP) FOR INJECTION is available as follows:

10 mg—Each single dose vial contains 10 mg of doxorubicin HCl, USP, 50 mg of lactose, N.F. and 1 mg of methylparaben, N.F. (added to enhance dissolution) as a sterile red-orange lyophilized powder. Packaged and supplied in 10-vial packs NDC 0013-1086-91.

20 mg—Each single dose vial contains 20 mg of doxorubicin HCl,USP, 100 mg of lactose, N.F. and 2 mg of methylparaben, N.F. (added to enhance dissolution) as a sterile red-orange lyophilized powder. Packaged and supplied in 10-vial packs NDC 0013-1096-91.

50 mg—Each single dose vial contains 50 mg of doxorubicin HCl, USP, 250 mg of lactose, N.F. and 5 mg of methylparaben, N.F. (added to enhance dissolution) as a sterile red-orange lyophilized powder. Packaged and supplied in a single vial pack NDC 0013-1106-79.

Protect from exposure to sunlight and discard any unused solution.

150 mg—Each multi-dose vial contains 150 mg of doxorubicin HCl, USP, 750 mg of lactose, N.F. and 15 mg of methylparaben, N.F. (added to enhance dissolution) as a sterile red-orange lyophilized powder. Packaged and supplied in a single vial pack. NDC 0013-1116-83.

Protect from exposure to sunlight and discard any solution remaining beyond the recommended reconstitution storage times.

REFERENCES

1. Rudolph R et al: Skin Ulcers Due to ADRIAMYCIN. Cancer 38: 1087–1094, Sept. 1976.
2. Recommendations for the Safe Handling of Parenteral Antineoplastic Drugs. NIH Publication No. 83-2621. For sale by the Superintendent of Documents, U.S. Government Printing Office, Washington, D.C. 20402.
3. AMA Council Report. Guidelines for Handling Parenteral Antineoplastics. JAMA, March 15, 1985.
4. National Study Commission on Cytotoxic Exposure—Recommendations for Handling Cytotoxic Agents. Available from Louis P. Jeffrey, Sc. D., Director of Pharmacy Services, Rhode Island Hospital, 593 Eddy Street, Providence, Rhode Island 02902.
5. Clinical Oncological Society of Australia: Guidelines and recommendations for safe handling of antineoplastic agents. Med J Australia 1:426–428 1983.
6. Jones RB, et al. Safe handling of chemotherapeutic agents: A report from the Mount Sinai Medical Center. CA—A Cancer Journal for Clinicians Sept/Oct, 258–263 1983.
7. American Society of Hospital Pharmacists technical assistance bulletin on handling cytotoxic drugs in hospitals. Am J Hosp Pharm 42:131–137, 1985.

Distributed by:
ADRIA LABORATORIES
Division of Erbamont Inc.
COLUMBUS, OHIO 43216.

Manufactured by:
FARMITALIA CARLO ERBA
MILAN, ITALY

IDAMYCIN® ℞

[*eye-dă-mī-sĭn*]
(Idarubicin Hydrochloride for Injection)
For Intravaneous Use Only

WARNINGS

1. IDAMYCIN should be given slowly into a freely flowing intravenous infusion. It must *never* be given intramuscularly or subcutaneously. Severe local tissue necrosis can occur if there is extravasation during administration.
2. As in the case with other anthracyclines the use of IDAMYCIN can cause myocardial toxicity leading to congestive heart failure. Cardiac toxicity is more common in patients who have received prior anthracyclines or who have pre-existing cardiac disease.
3. As is usual with antileukemic agents, severe myelosuppression occurs when IDAMYCIN is used at effective therapeutic doses.
4. It is recommended that IDAMYCIN be administered only under the supervision of a physician who is experienced in leukemia chemotherapy and in facilities with laboratory and supportive resources adequate to monitor drug tolerance and protect and maintain a patient compromised by drug toxicity. The physician and institution must be capable of responding rapidly and completely to severe hemorrhagic conditions and/or overwhelming infection.
5. Dosage should be reduced in patients with impaired hepatic or renal function. (See DOSAGE AND ADMINISTRATION).

DESCRIPTION

IDAMYCIN® (idarubicin hydrochloride for injection) is a sterile, synthetic antineoplastic anthracycline for intravenous use. Chemically, idarubicin hydrochloride is 5,12-Naphthacenedione, 9-acetyl-7-{(3-amino-2,3,6-trideoxy-α-L-*lyxo*-hexopyranosyl)oxy}-7,8,9,10-tetrahydro-6, 9, 11-trihydroxy-hydrochloride, (7S-*cis*). The structural formula is as follows:

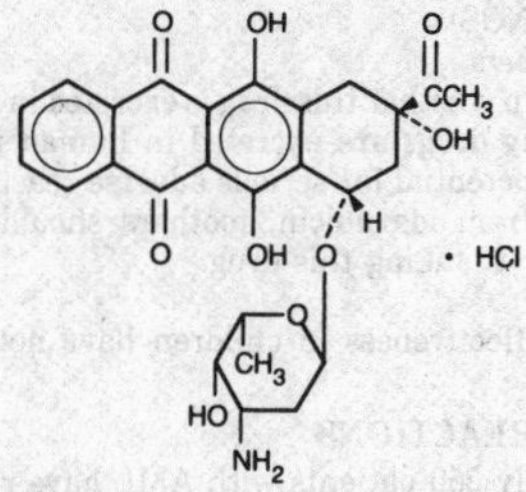

$C_{26}H_{27}NO_9 \cdot HCl$ M.W. 533.96

IDAMYCIN, a sterile parenteral, is available in 5 mg and 10 mg single use only vials.

Each 5 mg vial contains 5 mg idarubicin hydrochloride and 50 mg of Lactose NF(hydrous) as an orange-red, lyophilized powder.

Each 10 mg vial contains 10 mg idarubicin hydrochloride and 100 mg of Lactose NF(hydrous) as an orange-red, lyophilized powder.

CLINICAL PHARMACOLOGY

IDAMYCIN is a DNA-intercalating analog of daunorubicin which has an inhibitory effect on nucleic acid synthesis and interacts with the enzyme topoisomerase II. The absence of a methoxy group at position 4 of the anthracycline structure gives the compound a high lipophilicity which results in an increased rate of cellular uptake compared with other anthracyclines.

Pharmacokinetic studies have been performed in adult leukemia patients with normal renal and hepatic function following intravenous administration of 10-12 mg/m^2 of IDAMYCIN daily for 3 to 4 days, as a single agent or combined with cytarabine (Ara-C). The plasma concentrations of IDAMYCIN are best described by a two or three compartment open model. The disposition profile shows a rapid distributive phase with a very high volume of distribution presumably reflecting extensive issue binding. The plasma clearance is twice the expected hepatic plasma flow indicating extensive extrahepatic metabolism. The drug is eliminated predominately by biliary and to a lesser extent by renal excretion, mostly in the form of the primary metabolite, 13-dihydroidarubicin (idarubicinol).

The elimination rate of IDAMYCIN from plasma is slow with an estimated mean terminal half-life of 22 hours (range: 4 to 46 hours) when used as a single agent and 20 hours (range: 7 to 38 hours) when used in combination with cytarabine. The elimination of idarubicinol is considerably slower than that of the parent drug with an estimated mean terminal half-life that exceeds 45 hours; hence its plasma levels are sustained for a period greater than 8 days. As idarubicinol has cytotoxic activity it presumably contributes to the effects of IDAMYCIN.

The extent of drug and metabolite accumulation predicted in leukemia patients for Day 2 and 3 of dosing, based on the mean plasma levels and half-life obtained after the first dose, is 1.7-and 2.3-fold, respectively, and suggests no change in kinetics following a daily × 3 regimen.

The pharmacokinetics if IDAMYCIN have not been evaluated in leukemia patients with hepatic impairment. It is expected that in patients with moderate or severe hepatic dysfunction, the metabolism of IDAMYCIN may be impaired and lead to higher systemic drug levels.

Studies of cellular (nucleated blood and bone marrow cells) drug concentrations in leukemia patients have shown that peak cellular idarubicin concentrations are reached a few minutes after injection. Idarubicin and idarubicinol concentrations in nucleated blood and bone marrow cells are more than a hundred times the plasma concentrations. Idarubicin disappearance rates in plasma and cells were comparable with a terminal half-life of about 15 hours. The terminal half-life of idarubicinol in cells was about 72 hours.

Protein binding was studied *in vitro* by equilibrium dialysis at concentrations of idarubicin and idarubicinol similar to the maximum plasma level obtained in the pharmacokinetic studies. The percentages of idarubicin and idarubicinol bound to human plasma proteins averaged 97% and 94%, respectively. The binding is concentration independent.

IDAMYCIN studies in pediatric leukemia patients, at doses of 4.2 to 13.3 mg/m^2/day × 3, suggest dose independent kinetics. There is no difference between the half-lives of the drug following daily × 3 or weekly × 3 administration.

Cerebrospinal fluid (CSF) levels of idarubicin and its active metabolite, idarubicinol, were measured in pediatric leukemia patients treated intravenously. Idarubicin was detected in 2 of 21 CSF samples (0.14 and 1.57 ng/mL), while idarubicinol was detected in 20 of these 21 CSF samples obtained 18-30 hours after dosing (mean = 0.51 ng/mL, range 0.22 − 1.05 ng/mL). The clinical relevance of these findings is currently being evaluated.

CLINICAL STUDIES

Four prospective randomized studies, three U.S. and one Italian, have been conducted to compare the efficacy and safety of idarubicin (IDR) to that of daunorubicin (DNR), each in combination with cytarabine (Ara-C) as induction therapy in previously untreated adult patients with acute myeloid leukemia (AML). These data are summarized in the following table and demonstrate significantly greater complete remission rates for the IDR regimen in two of the three U.S. studies and significantly longer overall survival for the IDR regimen in two of the three U.S. studies.

[See table on next page.]

There is no consensus regarding optional regimens to be used for consolidation; however, the following consolidation regimens were used in U.S. controlled trials. Patients received the same anthracycline for consolidation as was used for induction.

Studies 1 and 3 utilized 2 courses of consolidation therapy consisting of idarubicin 12 or 13 mg/m^2 daily for 2 days, respectively (or DNR 50 or 45 mg/m^2 daily for 2 days), and Ara-C, either 25 mg/m^2 daily by IV bolus followed by 200 mg/m^2 daily by continuous infusion for 4 days (Study 1), or 100 mg/m^2 daily for 5 days by continuous infusion (Study 3). A rest period of 4 to 6 weeks is recommended prior to initiation of consolidation and between the courses. Hematologic recovery is mandatory prior to initiation of each consolidation course.

Study 2 utilized 3 consolidation courses, administered at intervals of 21 days or upon hematologic recovery. Each course consisted of idarubicin 15 mg/m^2 IV for 1 dose (or DNR 50 mg/m^2 IV for 1 dose), Ara-C 100 mg/m^2 every 12 hours for 10 doses and 6-thioguanine 100 mg/m^2 po for 10 doses. If severe myelosuppression occurred, subsequent courses were given with 25% reduction in the doses of all drugs. In addition, this study included 4 courses of maintenance therapy (2 days of the same anthracycline as was used in induction and 5 days of Ara-C).

Toxicities and duration of aplasia were similar during induction on the 2 arms in the U.S. studies except for an increase in mucositis on the IDR arm in one study. During consolidation, duration of aplasia on the IDR arm was longer in all three studies and mucositis was more frequent in two studies. During consolidation, transfusion requirements were higher on the IDR arm in the two studies in which they were tabulated, and patients on the IDR arm in Study 3 spent more days on IV antibiotics (Study 3 used a higher dose of IDAMYCIN).

Continued on next page

Adria Laboratories—Cont.

The benefit of consolidation and maintenance therapy in prolonging the duration of remission and survival is not proven.
Intensive maintenance with IDAMYCIN is not recommended in view of the considerable toxicity (including deaths in remission) experienced by patients during the maintenance phase of Study 2.
A higher induction death rate was noted in patients on the IDR arm in the Italian trial. Since this was not noted in patients of similar age in the U.S. trials, one may speculate that it was due to a difference in the level of supportive care.

INDICATIONS AND USAGE

IDAMYCIN in combination with other approved antileukemic drugs is indicated for the treatment of acute myeloid leukemia (AML) in adults. This includes French-American-British (FAB) classifications M1 through M7.

WARNINGS

IDAMYCIN is intended for administration under the supervision of a physician who is experienced in leukemia chemotherapy.
IDAMYCIN is a potent bone marrow suppressant. IDAMYCIN should not be given to patients with pre-existing bone marrow suppression induced by previous drug therapy or radiotherapy unless the benefit warrants the risk.
Severe myelosuppression will occur in all patients given a therapeutic dose of this agent for induction, consolidation or maintenance. Careful hematologic monitoring is required. Deaths due to infection and/or bleeding have been reported during the period of severe myelosuppression. Facilities with laboratory and supportive resources adequate to monitor drug tolerability and protect and maintain a patient compromised by drug toxicity should be available. It must be possible to treat rapidly and completely a severe hemorrhagic condition and/or a severe infection.
Pre-existing heart disease and previous therapy with anthracyclines at high cumulative doses or other potentially cardiotoxic agents are co-factors for increased risk of idarubicin-induced cardiac toxicity and the benefit to risk ratio of idarubicin therapy in such patients should be weighed before starting treatment with IDAMYCIN.
Myocardial toxicity as manifested by potentially fatal congestive heart failure, acute life-threatening arrhythmias or other cardiomyopathies may occur following therapy with IDAMYCIN. Appropriate therapeutic measures for the management of congestive heart failure and/or arrhythmias are indicated.
Cardiac function should be carefully monitored during treatment in order to minimize the risk of cardiac toxicity of the type described for other anthracycline compounds. The risk of such myocardial toxicity may be higher following concomitant or previous radiation to the mediastinal-pericardial area or in patients with anemia, bone marrow depression, infections, leukemic pericarditis and/or myocarditis. While there are no reliable means for predicting congestive heart failure, cardiomyopathy induced by anthracyclines is usually associated with a decrease of the left ventricular ejection fraction (LVEF) from pretreatment baseline values.
Since hepatic and/or renal function impairment can affect the disposition of IDAMYCIN, liver and kidney function should be evaluated with conventional clinical laboratory tests (using serum bilirubin and serum creatinine as indicators) prior to and during treatment. In a number of Phase III clinical trials, treatment was not given if bilirubin and/or creatinine serum levels exceeded 2 mg%. However, in one Phase III trial, patients with bilirubin levels between 2.6 and 5 mg% received the anthracycline with a 50% reduction in dose. Dose reduction of IDAMYCIN should be considered if the bilirubin and/or creatinine levels are above normal range. (See DOSAGE AND ADMINISTRATION).
Pregnancy Category D—Idarubicin was embryotoxic and teratogenic in the rat at a dose of 1.2 mg/m^2/day or one tenth the human dose, which was nontoxic to dams. Idarubicin was embryotoxic but not teratogenic in the rabbit even at a dose of 2.4 mg/m^2/day or two tenths the human dose, which was toxic to dams. There is no conclusive information about idarubicin adversely affecting human fertility or causing teratogenesis.
There are no adequate and well-controlled studies in pregnant women. If IDAMYCIN is to be used during pregnancy, or if the patient becomes pregnant during therapy, the patient should be apprised of the potential hazard to the fetus. Women of childbearing potential should be advised to avoid pregnancy.

PRECAUTIONS

General
Therapy with IDAMYCIN requires close observation of the patient and careful laboratory monitoring. Hyperuricemia secondary to rapid lysis of leukemic cells may be induced. Appropriate measures must be taken to prevent hyperuricemia and to control any systemic infection before beginning therapy.
Extravasation of IDAMYCIN can cause severe local tissue necrosis. Extravasation may occur with or without an accompanying stinging or burning sensation even if blood returns well on aspiration of the infusion needle. If signs or symptoms of extravasation occur the injection or infusion should be terminated immediately and restarted in another vein. (See DOSAGE AND ADMINISTRATION).
Laboratory Tests
Frequent complete blood counts and monitoring of hepatic and renal function tests are recommended.
Carcinogenesis, Mutagenesis, Impairment of Fertility
Formal long-term carcinogenicity studies have not been conducted with IDAMYCIN. IDAMYCIN and related compounds have been shown to have mutagenic and carcinogenic properties when tested in experimental models (including bacterial systems, mammalian cells in culture and female Sprague-Dawley rats).
In male dogs given 1.8 mg/m^2/day or more idarubicin (3 times/wk for 13 weeks), testicular atrophy was observed with inhibition of spermiogenesis and sperm maturation, and few or no mature sperm. Effects were not readily reversible after an eight week recovery period.
Pregnancy Category D
(*See* WARNINGS).
Nursing Mothers
It is not known whether this drug is excreted in human milk. Because many drugs are excreted in human milk and because of the potential for serious adverse reactions in nursing infants from idarubicin, mothers should discontinue nursing prior to taking this drug.
Pediatric Use
Safety and effectiveness in children have not been established.

ADVERSE REACTIONS

Approximately 550 patients with AML have received IDAMYCIN in combination with Ara-C in controlled clinical trials worldwide. In addition, over 550 patients with acute leukemia have been treated in uncontrolled trials utilizing IDAMYCIN as a single agent or in combination. The table below lists the adverse experiences reported in U.S. Study 2 (see CLINICAL STUDIES) and is representative of the experiences in other studies. These adverse experiences constitute all reported or observed experiences, including those not considered to be drug related. Patients undergoing induction therapy for AML are seriously ill due to their disease, are receiving multiple transfusions, and concomitant medications including potentially toxic antibiotics and antifungal agents. The contribution of the study drug to the adverse experience profile is difficult to establish.

Induction Phase	Percentage of Patients	
	IDR	DNR
Adverse Experiences	(N=110)	(N=118)
Infection	95%	97%
Nausea & Vomiting	82%	80%
Hair Loss	77%	72%
Abdominal Cramps/ Diarrhea	73%	68%
Hemorrhage	63%	65%
Mucositis	50%	55%
Dermatologic	46%	40%
Mental Status	41%	34%
Pulmonary-Clinical	39%	39%
Fever (not elsewhere classified)	26%	28%
Headache	20%	24%
Cardiac-Clinical	16%	24%
Neurologic-Peripheral Nerves	7%	9%
Pulmonary Allergy	2%	4%
Seizure	4%	5%
Cerebellar	4%	4%

The duration of aplasia and incidence of mucositis were greater on the IDR arm than the DNR arm, especially during consolidation in some U.S. controlled trials (see CLINICAL STUDIES).
The following information reflects experience based on U.S. controlled clinical trials.
Myelosuppression
Severe myelosuppression is the major toxicity associated with IDAMYCIN therapy, but this effect of the drug is required in order to eradicate the leukemic clone. During the period of myelosuppression, patients are at risk of developing infection and bleeding which may be life-threatening or fatal.
Gastrointestinal
Nausea and/or vomiting, mucositis, abdominal pain and diarrhea were reported frequently, but were severe (equivalent to WHO Grade 4) in less than 5% of patients. Severe enterocolitis with perforation has been reported rarely. The risk of perforation may be increased by instrumental intervention. The possibility of perforation should be considered in patients who develop severe abdominal pain and appropriate steps for diagnosis and management should be taken.
Dermatologic
Alopecia was reported frequently and dermatologic reactions including generalized rash, urticaria and a bullous erythrodermatous rash of the palms and soles have occurred. The dermatologic reactions were usually attributed to concomitant antibiotic therapy. Local reactions including hives at the injection site have been reported.
Hepatic and Renal
Changes in hepatic and renal function tests have been observed. These changes were usually transient and occurred in the setting of sepsis and while patients were receiving potentially hepatotoxic and nephrotoxic antibiotics and antifungal agents. Severe changes in renal function (equivalent to WHO Grade 4) occurred in no more than 1% of patients, while severe changes in hepatic function (equivalent to WHO Grade 4) occurred in less than 5% of patients.
Cardiac
Congestive heart failure (frequently attributed to fluid overload), serious arrhythmias including atrial fibrillation, chest pain, myocardial infarction and asymptomatic declines in LVEF have been reported in patients undergoing induction therapy for AML. Myocardial insufficiency and arrhythmias were usually reversible and occurred in the setting of sepsis, anemia and aggressive intravenous fluid administration. The events were reported more frequently in patients over age 60 years and in those with pe-existing cardiac disease.

OVERDOSAGE

There is no known antidote to IDAMYCIN. Two cases of fatal overdosage in patients receiving therapy for AML have been reported. The doses were 135 mg/m^2 over 3 days and 45 mg/m^2 of idarubicin and 90 mg/m^2 of daunorubicin over a three day period.
It is anticipated that overdosage with idarubicin will result in severe and prolonged myelosuppression and possibly in increased severity of gastrointestinal toxicity. Adequate supportive care including platelet transfusions, antibiotics and symptomatic treatment of mucositis is required. The effect of acute overdose on cardiac function is not fully known, but severe arrhythmia occurred in 1 of the 2 patients exposed. It is anticipated that very high doses of idarubicin may cause acute cardiac toxicity and may be associated with a higher incidence of delayed cardiac failure.
Disposition studies with idarubicin in patients undergoing dialysis have not been carried out. The profound multicompartment behavior, extensive extravascular distribution and tissue binding, coupled with the low unbound fraction available in the plasma pool make it unlikely that therapeutic

	Induction[A] Regimen Dose in mg/m^2 Daily × 3 Days		Complete Remission Rate, All Pts Randomized		Median Survival (Days) All Pts Randomized	
	IDR	DNR	IDR	DNR	IDR	DNR
U.S. (IND Studies)						
1. MSKCC* (Age ≤ 60 years)	12[b]	50[b]	51/65+ (78%)	38/65 (58%)	508+	435
2. SEG** (Age ≥ 15 years)	12[c]	45[c]	76/111+ (69%)	65/119 (55%)	328	277
3. U.S. Multicenter (Age ≥ 18 years)	13[c]	45[c]	68/101 (67%)	66/113 (58%)	393+	281
Foreign (non-IND study)						
GIMEMA*** (Age ≥ 55 years)	12[c]	45[c]	49/124 (40%)	49/125 (39%)	87	169

* Memorial Sloan Kettering Cancer Center
** Southeastern Cancer Study Group
*** Gruppo Italiano Malattie Emetologiche Maligne dell Adulto
+ Overall $p < 0.05$, unadjusted for prognostic factors or multiple endpoints.
[a] Patients who had persistent leukemia after the first induction course received a second course.
[b] Ara-C 25 mg/m^2 bolus IV followed by 200 mg/m^2 daily × 5 days by continuous infusion.
[c] Ara-C 100 mg/m^2 daily × 7 days by continuous infusion.

efficacy or toxicity would be altered by conventional peritoneal or hemodialysis.

DOSAGE AND ADMINISTRATION (See WARNINGS.)

For induction therapy in adult patients with AML the following dose schedule is recommended:

IDAMYCIN 12 mg/m² daily for 3 days by slow (10 to 15 min) intravenous injection in combination with Ara-C. The Ara-C may be given as 100 mg/m² daily by continuous infusion for 7 days or as Ara-C 25 mg/m² intravenous bolus followed by Ara-C 200 mg/m² daily for 5 days continuous infusion. In patients with unequivocal evidence of leukemia after the first induction course, a second course may be administered. Administration of the second course should be delayed in patients who experience severe mucositis, until recovery from this toxicity has occurred, and a dose reduction of 25% is recommended. In patients with hepatic and/or renal impairment, a dose reduction of IDAMYCIN should be considered. IDAMYCIN should not be administered if the bilirubin level exceeds 5 mg%. (See WARNINGS).

The benefit of consolidation in prolonging the duration of remissions and survival is not proven. There is no consensus regarding optional regimens to be used for consolidation. (See CLINICAL STUDIES for doses used in U.S. clinical studies).

Preparation of Solution

Caution in handling of the powder and preparation of the solution must be exercised as skin reactions associated with IDAMYCIN may occur. Skin accidently exposed to IDAMYCIN should be washed thoroughly with soap and water and if the eyes are involved, standard irrigation techniques should be used immediately. The use of goggles, gloves, and protective gowns is recommended during preparation and administration of the drug.

IDAMYCIN 5 mg and 10 mg vials should be reconstituted with 5 mL and 10 mL, respectively, of Sodium Chloride Injection USP (0.9%) to give a final concentration of 1 mg/mL of idarubicin hydrochloride. Bacteriostatic diluents are not recommended.

The vial contents are under a negative pressure to minimize aerosol formation during reconstitution; therefore, particular care should be taken when the needle is inserted. Inhalation of any aerosol produced during reconstitution must be avoided.

Reconstituted solutions are physically and chemically stable for at least 168 hours (7 days) under refrigeration (2°–8°C, 36°–46°F) and 72 hours (3 days) at controlled room temperature, (15°–30°C, 59°–86°F). Discard unused solutions in an appropriate manner (see *Handling and Disposal*).

Care in the administration of IDAMYCIN will reduce the chance of perivenous infiltration. It may also decrease the chance of local reactions such as urticaria and erythematous streaking. During intravenous administration of IDAMYCIN extravasation may occur with or without an accompanying stinging or burning sensation even if blood returns well on aspiration of the influsion needle. If any signs or symptoms of extravasation have occurred, the injection or infusion should be immediately terminated and restarted in another vein. If it is known or suspected that subcutaneous extravasation has occurred it is recommended that intermittent ice packs (½ hour immediately, then ½ hour 4 times per day for 3 days) be placed over the area of extravasation and that the affected extremity be elevated. Because of the progressive nature of extravasation reactions, the area of injection should be frequently examined and plastic surgery consultation obtained early if there is any sign of a local reaction such as pain, erythema, edema or vesication. If ulceration begins or there is severe persistent pain at the site of extravasation, early wide excision of the involved area should be considered.[1]

IDAMYCIN should be administered slowly (over 10 to 15 minutes) into the tubing of a freely running intravenous infusion of Sodium Chloride Injection USP (0.9%) or 5% Dextrose Injection USP. The tubing should be attached to a Butterfly needle or other suitable device and inserted preferably into a large vein.

Incompatibility

Unless specific compatability data are available, IDAMYCIN should not be mixed with other drugs. Precipitation occurs with heparin. Prolonged contact with any solution of an alkaline pH will result in degradation of the drug.

Parenteral drug products should be inspected visually for particulate matter and discoloration prior to administration whenever solution and containers permit.

Handling and Disposal—Procedures for handling and disposal of anticancer drugs should be considered. Several guidelines on this subject have been published.[2–8] There is no general agreement that all of the procedures recommended in the guidelines are necessary or appropriate.

HOW SUPPLIED

IDAMYCIN® (idarubicin hydrochloride for injection)

NDC 0013-2506-94 5 mg single dose vial. Available in 5 vial packs.

NDC 0013-2516-86 10 mg single dose vial. Available in single vials.

Store at controlled room temperature, 15°–30°C (59°–86°F), and protect from light.

CAUTION: Federal law prohibits dispensing without prescription.

Manufactured by:
FARMITALIA CARLO ERBA
MILAN, ITALY
For:
ADRIA LABORATORIES
Division of Erbamont Inc.
COLUMBUS, OHIO 43216

REFERENCES

1. Rudolph R, Larson DL: Etiology and Treatment of Chemotherapeutic Agent Extravasation Injuries: A Review. J. Clin Oncol 5: 1116–1126, 1987.
2. Recommendations for the Safe Handling of Parenteral Antineoplastic Drugs. NIH Publication No. 83-2621, US Government Printing Office, Washington, DC 20402.
3. Council on Scientific Affairs: Guidelines for Handling Parenteral Antineoplastics. JAMA 1985; 253:1590.
4. National Study Commission on Cytotoxic Agents. Available from Louis P. Jeffrey, ScD., Director of Pharmacy Services, Rhode Island Hospital, 593 Eddy Street, Providence, Rhode Island 02902.
5. Clinical Oncological Society of Australia: Guidelines and Recommendations for Safe Handling of Antineoplastic Agents. Med J Aust 1983; 1:426.
6. Jones RB, et al.: Safe Handling of Chemotherapeutic Agents: A Report from the Mount Sinai Medical Center. CA 33:258; Sept/Oct 1983.
7. American Society of Hospital Pharmacists: Technical Assistance Bulletin on Handling Cytotoxic Drugs in Hospitals. Am J Hosp Pharm 1990; 47:1033–1049.
8. OSHA Work-Practice Guidelines for Personnel Dealing with Cytotoxic (Antineoplastic) Drugs. Am J Hosp Pharm 1986; 43:1193–1204.

052001290–1 December 7, 1990

NEOSAR® ℞

[nē'ō-săr]

(cyclophosphamide for injection, USP)

DESCRIPTION

NEOSAR® (Cyclophosphamide for Injection, USP) is supplied as a sterile powder for parenteral use containing 45 mg sodium chloride per 100 mg cyclophosphamide (anhydrous). Cyclophosphamide is a synthetic antineoplastic drug chemically related to the nitrogen mustards. Cyclophosphamide is a white crystalline powder with the molecular formula $C_7H_{15}Cl_2N_2O_2P \cdot H_2O$ and a molecular weight of 279.1. The chemical name for cyclophosphamide is 2-[bis(2-chloroethyl) amino]tetrahydro-2H-1,3,2-oxazaphosphorine 2-oxide monohydrate. Cyclophosphamide is soluble in water, saline, or ethanol.

CLINICAL PHARMACOLOGY

NEOSAR is biotransformed principally in the liver to active alkylating metabolites by a mixed function microsomal oxidase system. These metabolites interfere with the growth of susceptible rapidly proliferating malignant cells. The mechanism of action is thought to involve cross-linking of tumor cell DNA.

Cyclophosphamide is well absorbed after oral administration with a bioavailability greater than 75%. The unchanged drug has an elimination half-life of 3 to 12 hours. It is eliminated primarily in the form of metabolites, but from 5 to 25% of the dose is excreted in urine as unchanged drug. Several cytotoxic and noncytotoxic metabolites have been identified in urine and in plasma. Concentrations of metabolites reach a maximum in plasma 2 to 3 hours after an intravenous dose. Plasma protein binding of unchanged drug is low but some metabolites are bound to an extent greater than 60%. It has not been demonstrated that any single metabolite is responsible for either the therapeutic or toxic effects of cyclophosphamide. Although elevated levels of metabolites of cyclophosphamide have been observed in patients with renal failure, increased clinical toxicity in such patients has not been demonstrated.

INDICATIONS AND USAGE

Malignant Diseases

NEOSAR, although effective alone in susceptible malignancies, is more frequently used concurrently or sequentially with other antineoplastic drugs. The following malignancies are often susceptible to NEOSAR treatment:

1. Malignant lymphomas (Stages III and IV of the Ann Arbor staging system), Hodgkin's disease, lymphocytic lymphoma (nodular or diffuse), mixed-cell type lymphoma, histiocytic lymphoma, Burkitt's lymphoma.
2. Multiple myeloma.
3. Leukemias: Chronic lymphocytic leukemia, chronic granulocytic leukemia (it is usually ineffective in acute blast crisis), acute myelogenous and monocytic leukemia, acute lymphoblastic (stem cell) leukemia in children (NEOSAR given during remission is effective in prolonging its duration).
4. Cutaneous T-cell lymphoma (Mycosis fungoides-advanced disease).
5. Neuroblastoma (disseminated disease).
6. Adenocarcinoma of the ovary.
7. Retinoblastoma.
8. Carcinoma of the breast.

Non-Malignant Disease: Biopsy Proven "Minimal Change" Nephrotic Syndrome in Children

Cyclophosphamide is useful in carefully selected cases of biopsy proven "minimal change" nephrotic syndrome in children but should not be used as primary therapy. In children whose disease fails to respond adequately to appropriate adrenocorticosteroid therapy or in whom the adrenocorticosteroid therapy produces or threatens to produce intolerable side effects, cyclophosphamide may induce a remission. Cyclophosphamide is not indicated for the nephrotic syndrome in adults or for any other renal disease.

CONTRAINDICATIONS

Continued use of cyclophosphamide is contraindicated in patients with severely depressed bone marrow function. See WARNINGS and PRECAUTIONS sections.

WARNINGS

Carcinogenesis, Mutagenesis, Impairment of Fertility

Second malignancies have developed in some patients treated with cyclophosphamide used alone or in association with other antineoplastic drugs and/or modalities. Most frequently, they have been urinary bladder, myeloproliferative, or lymphoproliferative malignancies. Second malignancies most frequently were detected in patients treated for primary myeloproliferative or lymphoproliferative malignancies or nonmalignant disease in which immune processes are believed to be involved pathologically. In some cases, the second malignancy developed several years after cyclophosphamide treatment had been discontinued. Urinary bladder malignancies generally have occurred in patients who previously had hemorrhagic cystitis. One case of carcinoma of the renal pelvis was reported in a patient receiving long-term cyclophosphamide therapy for cerebral vasculitis. The possibility of cyclophosphamide-induced malignancy should be considered in any benefit-to-risk assessment for use of the drug.

Cyclophosphamide can cause fetal harm when administered to a pregnant woman and such abnormalities have been reported following cyclophosphamide therapy in pregnant women. Abnormalities were found in two infants and a six-month old fetus born to women treated with cyclophosphamide. Ectrodactylia was found in two of the three cases. Normal infants have also been born to women treated with cyclophosphamide during pregnancy, including the first trimester. If this drug is used during pregnancy, or if the patient becomes pregnant while taking (receiving) this drug, the patient should be apprised of the potential hazard to the fetus. Women of childbearing potential should be advised to avoid becoming pregnant.

Cyclophosphamide interferes with oogenesis and spermatogenesis. It may cause sterility in both sexes. Development of sterility appears to depend on the dose of cyclophosphamide, duration of therapy, and the state of gonadal function at the time of treatment. Cyclophosphamide-induced sterility may be irreversible in some patients.

Amenorrhea associated with decreased estrogen and increased gonadotropin secretion develops in a significant proportion of women treated with cyclophosphamide. Affected patients generally resume regular menses within a few months after cessation of therapy. Girls treated with cyclophosphamide during prepubescence generally develop secondary sexual characteristics normally and have regular menses. Ovarian fibrosis with apparently complete loss of germ cells after prolonged cyclophosphamide treatment in late prepubescence has been reported. Girls treated with cyclophosphamide during prepubescence subsequently have conceived.

Men treated with cyclophosphamide may develop oligospermia or azoospermia associated with increased gonadotropin but normal testosterone secretion. Sexual potency and libido are unimpaired in these patients. Boys treated with cyclophosphamide during prepubescence develop secondary sexual characteristics normally, but may have oligospermia or azoospermia and increased gonadotropin secretion. Some degree of testicular atrophy may occur. Cyclophosphamide-induced azoospermia is reversible in some patients, though the reversibility may not occur for several years after cessation of therapy. Men temporarily rendered sterile by cyclophosphamide have subsequently fathered normal children.

Urinary System

Hemorrhagic cystitis may develop in patients treated with cyclophosphamide. Rarely, this condition can be severe and even fatal. Fibrosis of the urinary bladder, sometimes extensive, also may develop with or without accompanying cystitis. Atypical urinary bladder epithelial cells may appear in

Continued on next page

Adria Laboratories—Cont.

the urine. These adverse effects appear to depend on the dose of cyclophosphamide and the duration of therapy. Such bladder injury is thought to be due to cyclophosphamide metabolites excreted in the urine. Forced fluid intake helps to assure an ample output of urine, necessitates frequent voiding, and reduces the time the drug remains in the bladder. This helps to prevent cystitis. Hematuria usually resolves in a few days after cyclophosphamide treatment is stopped, but it may persist. Medical and/or surgical supportive treatment may be required, rarely, to treat protracted cases of severe hemorrhagic cystitis. It is usually necessary to discontinue cyclophosphamide therapy in instances of severe hemorrhagic cystitis.

Cardiac Toxicity

Although a few instances of cardiac dysfunction have been reported following use of recommended doses of cyclophosphamide, no causal relationship has been established. Cardiotoxicity has been observed in some patients receiving high doses of cyclophosphamide ranging from 120 to 270 mg/kg administered over a period of a few days, usually as a portion of an intensive antineoplastic multi-drug regimen or in conjunction with transplantation procedures. In a few instances with high doses of cyclophosphamide, severe, and sometimes fatal, congestive heart failure has occurred within a few days after the first cyclophosphamide dose. Histopathologic examination has primarily shown hemorrhagic myocarditis. Hemopericardium has occurred secondary to hemorrhagic myocarditis and myocardial necrosis. Pericarditis has been reported independent of any hemopericardiums.

No residual cardiac abnormalities, as evidenced by electrocardiogram or echocardiogram appear to be present in patients surviving episodes of apparent cardiac toxicity associated with high doses of cyclophosphamide.

Cyclophosphamide has been reported to potentiate doxorubicin-induced cardiotoxicity.

Infections

Treatment with cyclophosphamide may cause significant suppression of immune responses. Serious, sometimes fatal, infections may develop in severely immunosuppressed patients. Cyclophosphamide treatment may not be indicated or should be interrupted or the dose reduced in patients who have or who develop viral, bacterial, fungal, protozoan, or helminthic infections.

Other

Rare instances of anaphylactic reaction including one death have been reported. One instance of possible cross-sensitivity with other alkylating agents has been reported.

PRECAUTIONS

General

Special attention to the possible development of toxicity should be exercised in patients being treated with cyclophosphamide if any of the following conditions are present.
1. Leukopenia
2. Thrombocytopenia
3. Tumor cell infiltration of bone marrow
4. Previous X-ray therapy
5. Previous therapy with other cytotoxic agents
6. Impaired hepatic function
7. Impaired renal function

Laboratory Tests

During treatment, the patient's hematologic profile (particularly neutrophils and platelets) should be monitored regularly to determine the degree of hematopoietic suppression. Urine should also be examined regularly for red cells which may precede hemorrhagic cystitis.

Drug Interactions

The rate of metabolism and the leukopenic activity of cyclophosphamide reportedly are increased by chronic administration of high doses of phenobarbital.

The physician should be alert for possible combined drug actions, desirable or undesirable, involving cyclophosphamide even though cyclophosphamide has been used successfully concurrently with other drugs, including other cytotoxic drugs.

Cyclophosphamide treatment, which causes a marked and persistent inhibition of cholinesterase activity, potentiates the effect of succinylcholine chloride.

If a patient has been treated with cyclophosphamide within 10 days of general anesthesia, the anesthesiologist should be alerted.

Adrenalectomy

Since cyclophosphamide has been reported to be more toxic in adrenalectomized dogs, adjustment of the doses of both replacement steroids and cyclophosphamide may be necessary for the adrenalectomized patient.

Wound Healing

Cyclophosphamide may interfere with normal wound healing.

Carcinogenesis, Mutagenesis, Impairment of Fertility

See WARNINGS section for information on carcinogenesis, mutagenesis, and impairment of fertility.

Pregnancy

Pregnancy Category D—See WARNINGS section.

Nursing Mothers

Cyclophosphamide is excreted in breast milk. Because of the potential for serious adverse reactions and the potential for tumorigenicity shown for cyclophosphamide in humans, a decision should be made whether to discontinue nursing or to discontinue the drug, taking into account the importance of the drug to the mother.

ADVERSE REACTIONS

Information on adverse reactions associated with the use of NEOSAR is arranged according to body system affected or type of reaction. The adverse reactions are listed in order of decreasing incidence. The most serious adverse reactions are described in the WARNINGS section.

Reproductive System

See WARNINGS section for information on impairment of fertility.

Digestive System

Nausea and vomiting commonly occur with cyclophosphamide therapy. Anorexia and, less frequently, abdominal discomfort or pain and diarrhea may occur. There are isolated reports of hemorrhagic colitis, oral mucosal ulceration and jaundice occurring during therapy. These adverse drug effects generally remit when cyclophosphamide treatment is stopped.

Skin and Its Structures

Alopecia occurs commonly in patients treated with cyclophosphamide. The hair can be expected to grow back after treatment with the drug or even during continued drug treatment, though it may be different in texture or color. Skin rash occurs occasionally in patients receiving the drug. Pigmentation of the skin and changes in nails can occur.

Hematopoietic System

Leukopenia occurs in patients treated with cylcophosphamide, is related to the dose of the drug, and can be used as a dosage guide. Leukopenia of less than 2000 cells/mm^3 develops commonly in patients treated with an intial loading dose of the drug, and less frequently in patients maintained on smaller doses. The degree of neutropenia is particularly important because it correlates with a reduction in resistance to infections.

Thrombocytopenia or anemia develop occasionally in patients treated with cyclophosphamide. These hematologic effects usually can be reversed by reducing the drug dose or by interrupting treatment. Recovery from leukopenia usually begins in 7 to 10 days after cessation of therapy.

Urinary System

See WARNINGS section for information on cystitis and urinary bladder fibrosis.

Hemorrhagic ureteritis and renal tubular necrosis have been reported to occur in patients treated with cyclophasphamide. Such lesions usually resolve following cessation of therapy.

Infections

See WARNINGS section for information on reduced host resistance to infections.

Carcinogenesis

See WARNINGS section for information on carcinogenesis.

Respiratory System

Interstitial pulmonary fibrosis has been reported in patients receiving high doses of cyclophosphamide over a prolonged period.

Other

Rare instances of anaphylactic reaction including one death have been reported. One instance of possible cross-sensitivity with other alkylating agents has been reported.

OVERDOSAGE

No specific antidote for cyclophosphamide is known. Overdosage should be managed with supportive measures, including appropriate treatment for any concurrent infection, myelosuppression, or cardiac toxicity should it occur.

DOSAGE AND ADMINISTRATION

Adults and Children

When used as the only oncolytic drug therapy, the initial course of NEOSAR for patients with no hematologic deficiency usually consists of 40 to 50 mg/kg given intravenously in divided doses over a period of 2 to 5 days. Other intravenous regimens include 10 to 15 mg/kg given every 7 to 10 days or 3 to 5 mg/kg twice weekly.

Many other regimens of intravenous NEOSAR have been reported. Dosages must be adjusted in accord with evidence of antitumor activity and/or leukopenia. The total leukocyte count is a good, objective guide for regulating dosage. Transient decreases in the total white blood cell count to 2000 cells/mm^3(following short courses) or more persistent reduction of 3000 cells/mm^3(with continuing therapy) are tolerated without serious risk of infection if there is no marked granulocytopenia.

When NEOSAR is included in combined cytotoxic regimens, it may be necessary to reduce the dose of NEOSAR as well as that of the other drugs.

NEOSAR and its metabolites are dialyzable although there are probably quantitative differences depending upon the

dialysis system being used. Patients with compromised renal function may show some measurable changes in pharmacokinetic parameters of NEOSAR metabolism, but there is no consistent evidence indicating a need for NEOSAR dosage modification in patients with renal function impairment.

Treatment of Nonmalignant Diseases

Biopsy Proven "Minimal Change" Nephrotic Syndrome in Children

An oral dose of 2.5 to 3 mg/kg daily for a period of 60 to 90 days is recommended. In males, the incidence of oligospermia and azoospermia increases if the duration of cyclophosphamide treatment exceeds 60 days. Treatment beyond 90 days increases the probability of sterility. Adrenocorticosteroid therapy may be tapered and discontinued during the course of cyclophosphamide therapy. See PRECAUTIONS section concerning hematologic monitoring.

Preparation and Handling of Solutions

Parenteral drug products should be inspected visually for particulate matter and discoloration prior to administration, whenever solution and container permit.

NEOSAR for Injection should be prepared for parenteral use by adding Bacteriostatic Water for Injection, USP, (paraben preserved only) or Sterile Water for Injection, USP to the vial and shaking to dissolve. Use the quantity of diluent shown below to reconstitute the product.

Dosage Strength	Quantity of Diluent
100 mg	5 mL
200 mg	10 mL
500 mg	25 mL
1g	50 mL
2g	100 mL

Solutions of NEOSAR may be injected intravenously, intramuscularly, intraperitoneally, or intrapleurally or they may be infused intravenously in the following:

Dextrose Injection, USP (5% dextrose)
Dextrose and Sodium Chloride Injection, USP (5% dextrose and 0.9% sodium chloride)
5% Dextrose and Ringer's Injection
Lactated Ringer's Injection, USP
Sodium Chloride Injection, USP (0.45% sodium chloride)
Sodium Lactate Injection, USP ($\frac{1}{6}$ molar sodium lactate)

Reconstituted NEOSAR is chemically and physically stable for 24 hours at room temperature or for six days in the refrigerator; it does not contain any antimicrobial preservative and thus care must be taken to assure the sterility of prepared solutions.

NEOSAR prepared by adding Bacteriostatic Water for Injection, USP (paraben preserved only) should be used within 24 hours if stored at room temperature or within 6 days if stored under refrigeration.

If NEOSAR is not prepared by adding Bacteriostatic Water for Injection, USP (paraben preserved only), it is recommended that the solution be used promptly (preferably within six hours).

The osmolarities of solutions of NEOSAR for Injection and normal saline are compared in the following table:

	mOsm/L
NEOSAR	352
Normal saline	287

Extemporaneous liquid preparations of NEOSAR for oral administration may be prepared by dissolving NEOSAR in Aromatic Elixir, N.F. Such preparations should be stored under refrigeration in glass containers and used within 14 days.

Handling and Disposal

Procedures for proper handling and disposal of anticancer drugs should be considered. Several guidelines on this subject have been published.[1–7] There is no general agreement that all the procedures recommended in the guidelines are necessary or appropriate.

HOW SUPPLIED

NEOSAR® (Cyclophosphamide for Injection, USP) contains 45 mg sodium chloride per 100 mg cyclophosphamide (anhydrous) and is available in the following single dose vials:
NDC 0013-5606-93   100 mg vials (yellow cap), cartons of 12
NDC 0013-5616-93   200 mg vials (blue cap), cartons of 12
NDC 0013-5626-93   500 mg vials (red cap), cartons of 12
NDC 0013-5636-70   1 gram vials (gray cap), cartons of 6
NDC 0013-5646-70   2 gram vials (violet cap), cartons of 6
Storage at temperatures not exceeding 25°C (77°F) is recommended. It will withstand brief exposure to temperatures up to 30°C (86°F), but is to be protected from temperatures above 30°C (86°F).

Caution: Federal law prohibits dispensing without prescription.

Manufactured by:
ASTA Pharma AG
BIELEFELD, GERMANY

For:
ADRIA LABORATORIES
Division of Erbamont Inc.
COLUMBUS, OHIO 43216

REFERENCES

1. Recommendations for the Safe Handling of Parenteral Antineoplastic Drugs. NIH Publication No. 83-2621. For sale by the Superintendent of Documents, U.S. Government Printing Office, Washington, D.C. 20402.
2. AMA Council Report. Guidelines for Handling Parenteral Antineoplastics, JAMA, March 15, 1985.
3. National Study Commission on Cytotoxic Exposure—Recommendations for Handling Cytotoxic Agents. Available from Louis P. Jeffrey, ScD, Director of Pharmacy Services, Rhode Island Hospital, 593 Eddy Street, Providence, Rhode Island 02902.
4. Clinical Oncological Society of Australia. Guidelines and recommendations for safe handling of antineoplastic agents. Med J Australia 1:426–428 1983.
5. Jones R.B., et al: Safe handling of chemotherapeutic agents: A report from the Mount Sinai Medical Center, CA-A Cancer Journal for Clinicians Sept./Oct., 258–263 1983.
6. American Society of Hospital Pharmacists technical assistance bulletin on handling cytotoxic drugs in hospitals. Am J Hosp Pharm 42:131–137, 1985.
7. OSHA Work-Practice Guidelines for Personnel Dealing with Cytotoxic (Antineoplastic) Drugs, AM J Hosp Pharm 1986;43:1193–1204.

Advanced Nutritional Technology, Inc.
1111 JEFFERSON AVENUE
P.O. BOX 3225
ELIZABETH, NJ 07207-3225

ALPHA E Softgels   OTC
Natural Vitamin E as D-Alpha Tocopherol

100's	NDC #10888-1167-4
250's	NDC #10888-1167-9

BIOTENE Softgel   OTC
Natural Beta Carotene derived from Sea Algae.

30's	NDC #10888-4128-1
60's	NDC #10888-4128-3
100's	NDC #10888-4128-5

CRANGEL®   OTC
Each three softgels contain 3000 mg of cranberry powder and essential fatty acids.

HOW SUPPLIED
Bottles of 60's	NDC #10888-5319-2
Bottles of 90's	NDC #10888-5319-1

FORMULA 3/6/9   OTC
Each softgel contains all essential fatty acids.

HOW SUPPLIED
Bottles of 30's	NDC #10888-5317-1
Bottles of 60's	NDC #10888-5317-3

LACTROL ENZYME   OTC
Each softgel contains 125 mg of lactase enzyme.

HOW SUPPLIED
125 mg 100's	NDC #10888-5305-1
125 mg 250's	NDC #10888-5305-3

LAXAGEL®   OTC
Each softgel contains senna useful as a stimulant laxative for short time relief of constipation.

HOW SUPPLIED
Bottles of 50's	NDC #10888-3070-1
Bottles of 100 's	NDC #10888-3070-3

LIQUI–CAL®   OTC
Two softgels provide 1200 mg of calcium from calcium carbonate.

HOW SUPPLIED
600 mg 60's	NDC #10888-5304-6

LIQUI-CAL/MAG   OTC
Each softgel contains calcium from calcium citrate and magnesium.

HOW SUPPLIED
Bottles of 60's	NDC #10888-5318-1

N'ODOR®   OTC
Each softgel contains 50 mg of chlorophyllin copper complex effective for urinary & fecal odor control.

HOW SUPPLIED
50 mg 120's	NDC #10888-1010-5

NUTR-E-SOL™ Liquid   OTC
Pleasant-tasting water-soluble Vitamin E designed for fat mal-absorbers in diseases such as: Cystic Fibrosis, Crohn's Disease, Short Bowel Syndrome and Biliary Cirrhosis.

8 oz	NDC #10888-35000-2
16 oz	NDC #10888-35000-3

NUTR-E-SOL™ Softgels   OTC
Water-soluble Vitamin E designed for fat mal-absorbers in diseases such as: Cystic Fibrosis, Crohn's Disease, Short Bowel Syndrome and Biliary Cirrhosis.

400 IU 30's	NDC #10888-5238-1
200 IU 30's	NDC #10888-5329-1
200 IU 100's	NDC #10888-5329-5

PEDIAVIT Children's Multivitamin Liquid   OTC
with Minerals
Pleasant tasting 100% RDA vitamins with iron and zinc for children.

HOW SUPPLIED
Bottles of 8 oz	NDC #10888-8630-1

PHOSCHOL®   OTC
[fos'kol]
Phosphatidylcholine (highly purified lecithin)
Softgels and Concentrate

DESCRIPTION
PhosChol 900 contains 900 mg of pure phosphatidylcholine in each softgel.
PhosChol 565 contains 565 mg of pure phosphatidylcholine in each softgel.
PhosChol Concentrate contains 3000 mg of pure phosphatidylcholine in each teaspoonful.

ACTION & USES
Choline circulating in the blood after PC ingestion is taken up into all cells of the body. The brain has a unique way of ensuring that its nerve cells will receive adequate supplies of circulating choline.
A special protein molecule within the brain's capillaries traps the circulating choline, and then transports it across the blood-brain barrier, into the brain. Once in the brain, choline is incorporated into the brain's own PC, which is an essential and major part of neuronal membranes. Circulating choline transported into the brain has an additional very important function for a special group of nerve cells that make a biochemical, acetylcholine, which is released into synapses as a neurotransmitter. It provides the essential precursor used to synthesize acetylcholine. Moreover, when nerve cells are active, firing frequently and releasing large quantities of acetylcholine, their ability to make adequate amounts of the neurotransmitter requires that they receive adequate amounts of choline from the blood stream. In the absence of adequate choline, the ability of nerve cells to transmit messages to other cells across synapses is impaired and neuronal cell membranes can be depleted of PC causing cell damage. In contrast, when supplemental choline is provided, these messages can be amplified and membrane structure maintained.
PhosChol® brand of highly purified lecithin has been carefully developed to contain the highest concentration of phosphatidylcholine commercially available and can provide for the highest blood choline levels.

Figure 1.
LEVELS OF CHOLINE IN HUMAN PLASMA AFTER THE ADMINISTRATION OF 3, 6, 9, AND 18 GRAM DOSES OF LECITHIN AS PHOSCHOL

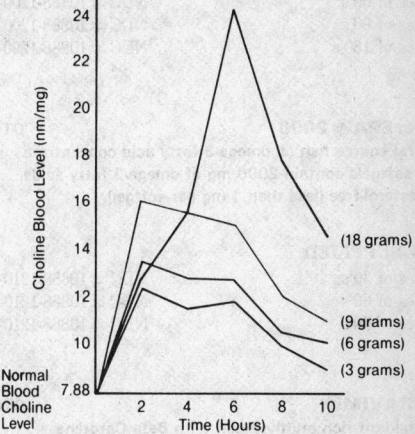

(One 9-gram dose at baseline, one 9-gram dose at 4 hours)

DOSAGE AND ADMINISTRATION
PhosChol® nutritional supplements may be recommended for two purposes:
To guard against low blood choline levels, and to restore blood choline levels in patients suffering from selected brain disorders. Amounts of PC sufficient to increase blood choline levels would help support normal cellular membrane composition and repair; they would also provide sufficient precursor choline for the maintenance of acetylcholine biosynthesis. Taken according to these schedules, dietary supplements of PC are an aid to good health, and protect against low choline stores.
To increase blood choline by 50%, patients should take 3 grams of PhosChol before meals by noon. To double blood choline levels, patients should take 9 grams of PhosChol before meals by noon. If ingestion before meals causes intestinal distress, it is recommended that PhosChol be taken either with meals or immediately thereafter.

ADVERSE REACTIONS
No major side effects have been reported in connection with consumption of large quantities of phosphatidylcholine or commercially available (less pure) lecithin.
Minor side effects may be seen such as increased salivation, nausea and upset stomach.

HOW SUPPLIED
Two dosage strengths as clear, amber colored, one-piece sealed softgels.
PhosChol 900 contains 900 mg of pure phosphatidylcholine in each softgel and is available in bottles of 100 and 300 softgels. Ten softgels a day provide 9 grams of phosphatidylcholine.
100's NDC #10888-9000-1
300's NDC #10888-9000-5
PhosChol 565 contains 565 mg of pure phosphatidylcholine and is available in bottles of 100 and 300 softgels. Sixteen softgels per day provide 9 grams of phosphatidylcholine.
100's NDC #10888-5650-1
300's NDC #10888-5650-5
One dosage strength as a liquid concentrate.
PhosChol Concentrate contains 3000 mg of pure phosphatidylcholine in each teaspoonful and is available in 4 oz., 8 oz., and 16 oz. bottles. Three teaspoonsful a day provide 9 grams of phosphatidylcholine.
4 oz NDC #10888-0121-4
8 oz NDC #10888-0121-1
16 oz NDC #10888-0121-2

PHOSCHOL® FORTE   OTC
Each softgel contains phosphatidylcholine enriched with B vitamins.

HOW SUPPLIED
Bottles of 30's	NDC #10888-5314-1
Bottles of 60's	NDC #10888-5314-3

Continued on next page

Advanced Nutritional—Cont.

SuperEPA® 1200 OTC
Natural source fish oil omega-3 fatty acid concentrate
Two softgels contain 1200 mg of omega-3 fatty acids.
Cholesterol-free (less than 1 mg per softgel)

HOW SUPPLIED
Bottles of 60's   NDC #10888-1200-3
Bottles of 90's   NDC #10888-1200-5
Bottles of 180's   NDC #10888-1200-7

SuperEPA® 2000 OTC
Natural source fish oil omega-3 fatty acid concentrate
Two softgels contain 2000 mg of omega-3 fatty acids.
Cholesterol-free (less than 1 mg per softgel).

HOW SUPPLIED
Bottles of 30's   NDC #10888-1210-3
Bottles of 60's   NDC #10888-1210-6
Bottles of 90's   NDC #10888-1210-9

ULTRAVIM® OTC
Antioxidant rich multivitamin with Beta Carotene

HOW SUPPLIED
Bottles of 30's   NDC #10888-5313-1
Bottles of 60's   NDC #10888-5313-3

XL-1 Multivitamin Liquid with Iron OTC
Pleasant tasting multivitamin liquid for adults.

HOW SUPPLIED
Bottles of 8 oz   NDC #10888-8710-1

Akorn, Inc.
100 AKORN DRIVE
ABITA SPRINGS, LA 70420

OPHTHALMIC PRODUCTS

For information on Akorn ophthalmic pharmaceutical products, consult the PDR For Ophthalmology. For literature, sample material or service items, please contact Akorn, Inc. directly.

Alcon Laboratories, Inc.
and its affiliates
CORPORATE HEADQUARTERS:
PO BOX 6600
6201 SOUTH FREEWAY
FORT WORTH, TX 76134

OPHTHALMIC PRODUCTS

For information on Alcon ophthalmic products, consult the PDR For Ophthalmology. See a complete listing of products in the Manufacturers' Index section of this book. For information, literature, samples or service items contact Alcon Sales Services.

BETOPTIC® ℞
(betaxolol hydrochloride)
0.5% as base
Sterile Ophthalmic Solution

DESCRIPTION
BETOPTIC® Sterile Ophthalmic Solution contains betaxolol hydrochloride, a cardioselective beta-adrenergic receptor blocking agent, in a sterile isotonic solution. Betaxolol hydrochloride is a white, crystalline powder, soluble in water, with a molecular weight of 343.89. The chemical structure is presented above.   [See next column.]

FEV$_1$ —Percent Change from Baseline[1]			
	Means		
	Betaxolol 1.0%[a]	Timolol 0.5%	Placebo
Baseline	1.6	1.4	1.4
60 Minutes	2.3	−25.7*	5.8
120 Minutes	1.6	−27.4*	7.5
240 Minutes	−6.4	−26.9*	6.9
Isoproterenol[b]	36.1	−12.4*	42.8

[1] Schoene, R. B., et al., Am. J. Ophthal. 97:86, 1984.
[a] Twice the clinical concentration.
[b] Inhaled at 240 minutes; measurement at 270 minutes.
* Timolol statistically different from betaxolol and placebo (p < 0.05).

(CH$_3$)$_2$CHNHCH$_2$CHCH$_2$O—⟨⟩—CH$_2$CH$_2$OCH$_2$—◁ •HCl
OH

Empirical Formula:
C$_{18}$H$_{29}$NO$_3$·HCl
Chemical Name
(±)-1-[p-[2-(Cyclopropylmethoxy)ethyl]phenoxy]-3-(isopropylamino)-2-propanol hydrochloride.
Each mL of BETOPTIC Ophthalmic Solution (0.5%) contains: Active: 5.6 mg betaxolol hydrochloride equivalent to betaxolol base 5 mg. Preservative: Benzalkonium Chloride 0.01%. Inactive: Edetate Disodium, Sodium Chloride, Hydrochloric Acid and/or Sodium Hydroxide (to adjust pH), and Purified Water.

CLINICAL PHARMACOLOGY
Betaxolol HCl, a cardioselective (beta-1-adrenergic) receptor blocking agent, does not have significant membrane-stabilizing (local anesthetic) activity and is devoid of intrinsic sympathomimetic action. Orally administered beta-adrenergic blocking agents reduce cardiac output in healthy subjects and patients with heart disease. In patients with severe impairment of myocardial function, beta-adrenergic receptor antagonists may inhibit the sympathetic stimulatory effect necessary to maintain adequate cardiac function.
When instilled in the eye, BETOPTIC Ophthalmic Solution has the action of reducing elevated as well as normal intraocular pressure, whether or not accompanied by glaucoma. Ophthalmic betaxolol has minimal effect on pulmonary and cardiovascular parameters.
Ophthalmic betaxolol (one drop in each eye) was compared to timolol and placebo in a three-way crossover study challenging nine patients with reactive airway disease who were selected on the basis of having at least a 15% reduction in the forced expiratory volume in one second (FEV$_1$) after administration of ophthalmic timolol. Betaxolol HCl had no significant effect on pulmonary function as measured by FEV$_1$, Forced Vital Capacity (FVC) and FEV$_1$/VC. Additionally, the action of isoproterenol, a beta stimulant, administered at the end of the study was not inhibited by ophthalmic betaxolol. In contrast, ophthalmic timolol significantly decreased these pulmonary functions.
[See table above.]
No evidence of cardiovascular beta-adrenergic blockade during exercise was observed with betaxolol in a double-masked, three-way crossover study in 24 normal subjects comparing ophthalmic betaxolol, timolol and placebo for effect on blood pressure and heart rate. Mean arterial blood pressure was not affected by any treatment; however, ophthalmic timolol produced a significant decrease in the mean heart rate. [See table below.]

Clinical Studies: Optic nerve head damage and visual field loss are the result of a sustained elevated intraocular pressure and poor ocular perfusion. BETOPTIC Ophthalmic Solution has the action of reducing elevated as well as normal intraocular pressure, and the mechanism of ocular hypotensive action appears to be a reduction of aqueous production as demonstrated by tonography and aqueous fluorophotometry. The onset of action with BETOPTIC Ophthalmic Solution can generally be noted within 30 minutes and the maximal effect can usually be detected 2 hours after topical administration. A single dose provides a 12-hour reduction in intraocular pressure. Clinical observation of glaucoma patients treated with BETOPTIC Ophthalmic Solution for up to three years shows that the intraocular pressure lowering effect is well maintained.
Clinical studies show that topical BETOPTIC Ophthalmic Solution reduces mean intraocular pressure 25% from baseline. In trials using 22 mmHg as a generally accepted index of intraocular pressure control, BETOPTIC Ophthalmic Solution was effective in more than 94% of the population studied, of which 73% were treated with the beta blocker alone. In controlled, double-masked studies, the magnitude and duration of the ocular hypotensive effect of BETOPTIC Ophthalmic Solution and ophthalmic timolol solution were clinically equivalent.
BETOPTIC Ophthalmic Solution has also been used successfully in glaucoma patients who have undergone a laser trabeculoplasty and have needed additional long-term ocular hypotensive therapy.
BETOPTIC Ophthalmic Solution has been well tolerated in glaucoma patients wearing hard or soft contact lenses and in aphakic patients.
BETOPTIC Ophthalmic Solution does not produce miosis or accommodative spasm which are frequently seen with miotic agents. The blurred vision and night blindness often associated with standard miotic therapy are not associated with BETOPTIC Ophthalmic Solution. Thus, patients with central lenticular opacities avoid the visual impairment caused by a constricted pupil.

INDICATIONS AND USAGE
BETOPTIC® Ophthalmic Solution has been shown to be effective in lowering intraocular pressure and is indicated in the treatment of ocular hypertension and chronic open-angle glaucoma. It may be used alone or in combination with other anti-glaucoma drugs.

Mean Heart Rates[1]			
	TREATMENT		
Bruce Stress Exercise Test			
Minutes	Betaxolol 1%[a]	Timolol 0.5%	Placebo
0	79.2	79.3	81.2
2	130.2	126.0	130.4
4	133.4	128.0*	134.3
6	136.4	129.2*	137.9
8	139.8	131.8*	139.4
10	140.8	131.8*	141.3

[1] Atkins, J. M., et al., Am. J. Oph. 99:173–175, Feb., 1985.
[a] Twice the clinical concentration.
* Mean pulse rate significantly lower for timolol than betaxolol or placebo (p < 0.05).

In clinical studies BETOPTIC® was safely used to lower intraocular pressure in 47 patients with both glaucoma and reactive airway disease who were followed for a mean period of 15 months. However, caution should be used in treating patients with severe reactive airway disease or a history of asthma.

CONTRAINDICATIONS

Hypersensitivity to any component of this product. BETOPTIC Ophthalmic Solution is contraindicated in patients with sinus bradycardia, greater than a first degree atrioventricular block, cardiogenic shock, or patients with overt cardiac failure.

WARNING

Topically applied beta-adrenergic blocking agents may be absorbed systemically. The same adverse reactions found with systemic administration of beta-adrenergic blocking agents may occur with topical administration. For example, severe respiratory reactions and cardiac reactions, including death due to bronchospasm in patients with asthma, and rarely death in association with cardiac failure, have been reported with topical application of beta-adrenergic blocking agents.

BETOPTIC Ophthalmic Solution has been shown to have a minor effect on heart rate and blood pressure in clinical studies. Caution should be used in treating patients with a history of cardiac failure or heart block. Treatment with BETOPTIC Ophthalmic Solution should be discontinued at the first signs of cardiac failure.

PRECAUTIONS

General: Information for Patients. Do not touch dropper tip to any surface as this may contaminate the solution.

Diabetes Mellitus. Beta-adrenergic blocking agents should be administered with caution in patients subject to spontaneous hypoglycemia or to diabetic patients (especially those with labile diabetes) who are receiving insulin or oral hypoglycemic agents. Beta-adrenergic receptor blocking agents may mask the signs and symptoms of acute hypoglycemia.

Thyrotoxicosis. Beta-adrenergic blocking agents may mask certain clinical signs (e.g., tachycardia) of hyperthyroidism. Patients suspected of developing thyrotoxicosis should be managed carefully to avoid abrupt withdrawal of beta-adrenergic blocking agents, which might precipitate a thyroid storm.

Muscle Weakness. Beta-adrenergic blockade has been reported to potentiate muscle weakness consistent with certain myasthenic symptoms (e.g., diplopia, ptosis, and generalized weakness).

Major Surgery. Consideration should be given to the gradual withdrawal of beta-adrenergic blocking agents prior to general anesthesia because of the reduced ability of the heart to respond to beta-adrenergically mediated sympathetic reflex stimuli.

Pulmonary: Caution should be exercised in the treatment of glaucoma patients with excessive restriction of pulmonary function. There have been reports of asthmatic attacks and pulmonary distress during betaxolol treatment. Although rechallenges of some such patients with ophthalmic betaxolol have not adversely affected pulmonary function test results, the possibility of adverse pulmonary effects in patients sensitive to beta blockers cannot be ruled out.

Risk from Anaphylactic Reaction: While taking beta-blockers, patients with a history of atopy or a history of severe anaphylactic reaction to a variety of allergens may be more reactive to repeated accidental, diagnostic, or therapeutic challenge with such allergens. Such patients may be unresponsive to the usual doses of epinephrine used to treat anaphylactic reactions.

Drug Interactions: Patients who are receiving a beta-adrenergic blocking agent orally and BETOPTIC Ophthalmic Solution should be observed for a potential additive effect either on the intraocular pressure or on the known systemic effects of beta blockade.

Close observation of the patient is recommended when a beta-blocker is administered to patients receiving catecholamine-depleting drugs such as reserpine, because of possible additive effects and the production of hypotension and/or bradycardia.

Betaxolol is an adrenergic blocking agent; therefore, caution should be exercised in patients using concomitant adrenergic psychotropic drugs.

Ocular: In patients with angle-closure glaucoma, the immediate treatment objective is to re-open the angle by constriction of the pupil with a miotic agent. Betaxolol has little or no effect on the pupil. When BETOPTIC Ophthalmic Solution is used to reduce elevated intraocular pressure in angle-closure glaucoma, it should be used with a miotic and not alone.

Carcinogenesis, Mutagenesis, Impairment of Fertility: Lifetime studies with betaxolol HCl have been completed in mice at oral doses of 6, 20 or 60 mg/kg/day and in rats at 3, 12 or 48 mg/kg/day; betaxolol HCl demonstrated no carcinogenic effect. Higher dose levels were not tested.

In a variety of *in vitro* and *in vivo* bacterial and mammalian cell assays, betaxolol HCl was nonmutagenic.

Pregnancy: Pregnancy Category C: Reproduction, teratology, and peri- and postnatal studies have been conducted with orally administered betaxolol HCl in rats and rabbits. There was evidence of drug related postimplantation loss in rabbits and rats at dose levels above 12 mg/kg and 128 mg/kg, respectively. Betaxolol HCl was not shown to be teratogenic, however, and there were no other adverse effects on reproduction at subtoxic dose levels. There are no adequate and well-controlled studies in pregnant women. BETOPTIC Ophthalmic Solution should be used during pregnancy only if the potential benefit justifies the potential risk to the fetus.

Nursing Mothers: It is not known whether betaxolol HCl is excreted in human milk. Because many drugs are excreted in human milk, caution should be exercised when BETOPTIC Ophthalmic Solution is administered to nursing women.

Pediatric Use: Safety and effectiveness in children have not been established.

ADVERSE REACTIONS

The following adverse reactions have been reported in clinical trials with BETOPTIC Ophthalmic Solution.

Ocular: Discomfort of short duration was experienced by one in four patients, but none discontinued therapy; occasional tearing has been reported. Rare instances of decreased corneal sensitivity, erythema, itching sensation, corneal punctate staining, keratitis, anisocoria, edema, and photophobia have been reported.

Additional medical events reported with other formulations of betaxolol include blurred vision, foreign body sensation, dryness of the eyes, inflammation, discharge, ocular pain, decreased acuity, and crusty lashes.

Systemic: Systemic reactions following administration of BETOPTIC Ophthalmic Solution 0.5% or BETOPTIC S Ophthalmic Suspension 0.25% have been rarely reported. These include:

Cardiovascular: Bradycardia, heart block and congestive failure.

Pulmonary: Pulmonary distress characterized by dyspnea, bronchospasm, thickened bronchial secretions, asthma and respiratory failure.

Central Nervous System: Insomnia, dizziness, vertigo, headaches, depression, lethargy, and increase in signs and symptoms of myasthenia gravis.

Other: Hives, toxic epidermal necrolysis, hair loss and glossitis.

OVERDOSAGE

No information is available on overdosage of humans. The oral LD_{50} of the drug ranged from 350–920 mg/kg in mice and 860–1050 mg/kg in rats. The symptoms which might be expected with an overdose of a systemically administered beta-1-adrenergic receptor blocker agent are bradycardia, hypotension and acute cardiac failure. A topical overdose of BETOPTIC Ophthalmic Solution may be flushed from the eye(s) with warm tap water.

DOSAGE AND ADMINISTRATION

The recommended dose is one to two drops of BETOPTIC Ophthalmic Solution in the affected eye(s) twice daily. In some patients, the intraocular pressure lowering responses to BETOPTIC Ophthalmic Solution may require a few weeks to stabilize. As with any new medication, careful monitoring of patients is advised.

If the intraocular pressure of the patient is not adequately controlled on this regimen, concomitant therapy with pilocarpine and other miotics, and/or epinephrine and/or carbonic anhydrase inhibitors can be instituted.

HOW SUPPLIED

BETOPTIC Ophthalmic Solution is a sterile, isotonic, aqueous solution of betaxolol hydrochloride. Supplied as follows: 2.5, 5, 10 and 15 mL in plastic ophthalmic DROP-TAINER® dispensers.

2.5 mL: **NDC** 0065-0245-20	10 mL: **NDC** 0065-0245-10
5 mL: **NDC** 0065-0245-05	15 mL: **NDC** 0065-0245-15

STORAGE

Store at room temperature.

CAUTION

Federal (USA) law prohibits dispensing without prescription.

U.S. Patent Nos. 4,252,984; 4,311,708; 4,342,783

BETOPTIC® S ℞

(betaxolol HCl)
0.25% as base
Sterile Ophthalmic Suspension

DESCRIPTION

BETOPTIC S Ophthalmic Suspension 0.25% contains betaxolol hydrochloride, a cardioselective beta-adrenergic receptor blocking agent, in a sterile resin suspension formulation. Betaxolol hydrochloride is a white, crystalline powder, with a molecular weight of 343.89. The chemical structure is presented below:

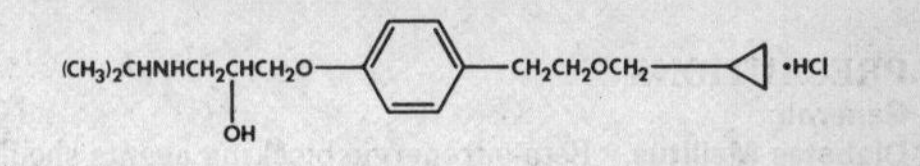

Empirical Formula:
$C_{18}H_{29}NO_3 \cdot HCl$

Chemical Name:
(±)-1-[p-[2-(cyclopropylmethoxy)ethyl]phenoxy]-3-(isopropylamino)-2-propanol hydrochloride.

Each mL of BETOPTIC S Ophthalmic Suspension contains: Active: betaxolol HCl 2.8 mg equivalent to 2.5 mg of betaxolol base. Preservative: benzalkonium chloride 0.01%. Inactive: Mannitol, Poly(Styrene-Divinyl Benzene) sulfonic acid, Carbomer 934P, edetate disodium, hydrochloric acid or sodium hydroxide (to adjust pH) and purified water.

CLINICAL PHARMACOLOGY

Betaxolol HCl, a cardioselective (beta-1-adrenergic) receptor blocking agent, does not have significant membrane-stabilizing (local anesthetic) activity and is devoid of intrinsic sympathomimetic action. Orally administered beta-adrenergic blocking agents reduce cardiac output in healthy subjects and patients with heart disease. In patients with severe impairment of myocardial function, beta-adrenergic receptor antagonists may inhibit the sympathetic stimulatory effect necessary to maintain adequate cardiac function.

When instilled in the eye, BETOPTIC S Ophthalmic Suspension 0.25% has the action of reducing elevated intraocular pressure, whether or not accompanied by glaucoma. Ophthalmic betaxolol has minimal effect on pulmonary and cardiovascular parameters.

Elevated IOP presents a major risk factor in glaucomatous field loss. The higher the level of IOP, the greater the likelihood of optic nerve damage and visual field loss. Betaxolol has the action of reducing elevated as well as normal intraocular pressure and the mechanism of ocular hypotensive action appears to be a reduction of aqueous production as demonstrated by tonography and aqueous fluorophotometry. The onset of action with betaxolol can generally be noted within 30 minutes and the maximal effect can usually be detected 2 hours after topical administration. A single dose provides a 12-hour reduction in intraocular pressure.

In controlled, double-masked studies, the magnitude and duration of the ocular hypotensive effect of BETOPTIC S Ophthalmic Suspension 0.25% and BETOPTIC Ophthalmic Solution 0.5% were clinically equivalent. BETOPTIC S Suspension was significantly more comfortable than BETOPTIC Solution.

Ophthalmic betaxolol solution at 1% (one drop in each eye) was compared to placebo in a crossover study challenging nine patients with reactive airway disease. Betaxolol HCl had no significant effect on pulmonary function as measured by FEV_1, Forced Vital Capacity (FVC), FEV_1/FVC and was not significantly different from placebo. The action of isoproterenol, a beta stimulant, administered at the end of the study was not inhibited by ophthalmic betaxolol.

No evidence of cardiovascular beta adrenergic-blockade during exercise was observed with betaxolol in a double-masked, crossover study in 24 normal subjects comparing ophthalmic betaxolol and placebo for effects on blood pressure and heart rate.

INDICATIONS AND USAGE

BETOPTIC S Ophthalmic Suspension 0.25% has been shown to be effective in lowering intraocular pressure and may be used in patients with chronic open-angle glaucoma and ocular hypertension. It may be used alone or in combination with other intraocular pressure lowering medications.

CONTRAINDICATIONS

Hypersensitivity to any component of this product. BETOPTIC S Ophthalmic Suspension 0.25% is contraindicated in patients with sinus bradycardia, greater than a first degree atrioventricular block, cardiogenic shock, or patients with overt cardiac failure.

WARNING

Topically applied beta-adrenergic blocking agents may be absorbed systemically. The same adverse reactions found with systemic administration of beta-adrenergic blocking agents may occur with topical administration. For example, severe respiratory reactions and cardiac reactions, including death due to bronchospasm in patients with asthma, and rarely death in association with cardiac failure, have been reported with topical application of beta-adrenergic blocking agents.

BETOPTIC S Ophthalmic Suspension 0.25% has been shown to have a minor effect on heart rate and blood pressure in clinical studies. Caution should be used in treating patients with a history of cardiac failure or heart block. Treatment with BETOPTIC S Ophthalmic Suspension 0.25% should be discontinued at the first signs of cardiac failure.

Continued on next page

Alcon Laboratories—Cont.

PRECAUTIONS

General:

Diabetes Mellitus. Beta-adrenergic blocking agents should be administered with caution in patients subject to spontaneous hypoglycemia or to diabetic patients (especially those with labile diabetes) who are receiving insulin or oral hypoglycemic agents. Beta-adrenergic receptor blocking agents may mask the signs and symptoms of acute hypoglycemia.

Thyrotoxicosis. Beta-adrenergic blocking agents may mask certain clinical signs (e.g., tachycardia) of hyperthyroidism. Patients suspected of developing thyrotoxicosis should be managed carefully to avoid abrupt withdrawal of beta-adrenergic blocking agents, which might precipitate a thyroid storm.

Muscle Weakness. Beta-adrenergic blockade has been reported to potentiate muscle weakness consistent with certain myasthenic symptoms (e.g., diplopia, ptosis and generalized weakness).

Major Surgery. Consideration should be given to the gradual withdrawal of beta-adrenergic blocking agents prior to general anesthesia because of the reduced ability of the heart to respond to beta-adrenergically mediated sympathetic reflex stimuli.

Pulmonary. Caution should be exercised in the treatment of glaucoma patients with excessive restriction of pulmonary function. There have been reports of asthmatic attacks and pulmonary distress during betaxolol treatment. Although rechallenges of some such patients with ophthalmic betaxolol has not adversely affected pulmonary function test results, the possibility of adverse pulmonary effects in patients sensitive to beta blockers cannot be ruled out.

Information for Patients: Do not touch dropper tip to any surface, as this may contaminate the contents. Do not use with contact lenses in eyes.

Drug Interactions: Patients who are receiving a beta-adrenergic blocking agent orally and BETOPTIC S Ophthalmic Suspension 0.25% should be observed for a potential additive effect either on the intraocular pressure or on the known systemic effects of beta blockade.

Close observation of the patient is recommended when a beta blocker is administered to patients receiving catecholamine-depleting drugs such as reserpine, because of possible additive effects and the production of hypotension and/or bradycardia.

Betaxolol is an adrenergic blocking agent; therefore, caution should be exercised in patients using concomitant adrenergic psychotropic drugs.

Risk from anaphylactic reaction: While taking beta-blockers, patients with a history of atopy or a history of severe anaphylactic reaction to a variety of allergens may be more reactive to repeated accidental, diagnostic, or therapeutic challenge with such allergens. Such patients may be unresponsive to the usual doses of epinephrine used to treat anaphylactic reactions.

Ocular: In patients with angle-closure glaucoma, the immediate treatment objective is to reopen the angle by constriction of the pupil with a miotic agent. Betaxolol has little or no effect on the pupil. When BETOPTIC S Ophthalmic Suspension 0.25% is used to reduce elevated intraocular pressure in angle-closure glaucoma, it should be used with a miotic and not alone.

Carcinogenesis, Mutagenesis, Impairment of Fertility: Lifetime studies with betaxolol HCl have been completed in mice at oral doses of 6, 20 or 60 mg/kg/day and in rats at 3, 12 or 48 mg/kg/day; betaxolol HCl demonstrated no carcinogenic effect. Higher dose levels were not tested.

In a variety of *in vitro* and *in vivo* bacterial and mammalian cell assays, betaxolol HCl was nonmutagenic.

Pregnancy:

Pregnancy Category C. Reproduction, teratology, and peri- and postnatal studies have been conducted with orally administered betaxolol HCl in rats and rabbits. There was evidence of drug related postimplantation loss in rabbits and rats at dose levels above 12 mg/kg and 128 mg/kg, respectively. Betaxolol HCl was not shown to be teratogenic, however, and there were no other adverse effects on reproduction at subtoxic dose levels. There are no adequate and well-controlled studies in pregnant women. BETOPTIC S should be used during pregnancy only if the potential benefit justifies the potential risk to the fetus.

Nursing Mothers: It is not known whether betaxolol HCl is excreted in human milk. Because many drugs are excreted in human milk, caution should be exercised when BETOPTIC S Ophthalmic Suspension 0.25% is administered to nursing women.

Pediatric Use: Safety and effectiveness in children have not been established.

ADVERSE REACTIONS

Ocular: In clinical trials, the most frequent event associated with the use of BETOPTIC S Ophthalmic Suspension 0.25% has been transient ocular discomfort. The following other conditions have been reported in small numbers of patients: blurred vision, corneal punctate keratitis, foreign body sensation, photophobia, tearing, itching, dryness of eyes, erythema, inflammation, discharge, ocular pain, decreased visual acuity and crusty lashes.

Additional medical events reported with other formulations of betaxolol include allergic reactions, decreased corneal sensitivity, edema and anisocoria.

Systemic: Systemic reactions following administration of BETOPTIC S Ophthalmic Suspension 0.25% or BETOPTIC Ophthalmic Solution 0.5% have been rarely reported. These include:

Cardiovascular: Bradycardia, heart block and congestive failure.

Pulmonary: Pulmonary distress characterized by dyspnea, bronchospasm, thickened bronchial secretions, asthma and respiratory failure.

Central Nervous System: Insomnia, dizziness, vertigo, headaches, depression, lethargy, and increase in signs and symptoms of myasthenia gravis.

Other: Hives, toxic epidermal necrolysis, hair loss, and glossitis.

OVERDOSAGE

No information is available on overdosage of humans. The oral LD50 of the drug ranged from 350–920 mg/kg in mice and 860–1050 mg/kg in rats. The symptoms which might be expected with an overdose of a systemically administered beta-1-adrenergic receptor blocking agent are bradycardia, hypotension and acute cardiac failure.

A topical overdose of BETOPTIC S Ophthalmic Suspension 0.25% may be flushed from the eye(s) with warm tap water.

DOSAGE AND ADMINISTRATION

The recommended dose is one to two drops of BETOPTIC S Ophthalmic Suspension 0.25% in the affected eye(s) twice daily. In some patients, the intraocular pressure lowering responses to BETOPTIC S may require a few weeks to stabilize. As with any new medication, careful monitoring of patients is advised.

If the intraocular pressure of the patient is not adequately controlled on this regimen, concomitant therapy with pilocarpine and other miotics, and/or epinephrine and/or carbonic anhydrase inhibitors can be instituted.

HOW SUPPLIED

BETOPTIC S Ophthalmic Suspension 0.25% is supplied as follows: 2.5, 5, 10 and 15 mL in plastic ophthalmic DROP-TAINER® dispensers.

2.5 mL:	**NDC** 0065-0246-20
5.0 mL:	**NDC** 0065-0246-05
10 mL:	**NDC** 0065-0246-10
15.0 mL:	**NDC** 0065-0246-15

STORAGE

Store upright at room temperature. Shake well before using.

CAUTION

Federal (USA) Law Prohibits Dispensing Without a Prescription.

U.S. Patents Nos. 4,252,984; 4,311,708; 4,342,783; 4,911,920

CILOXAN™ ℞

(Ciprofloxacin HCl)
0.3% as base
Sterile Ophthalmic Solution

DESCRIPTION

CILOXAN™ (Ciprofloxacin HCl) Ophthalmic Solution is a synthetic, sterile, multiple dose, antimicrobial for topical ophthalmic use. Ciprofloxacin is a fluoroquinolone antibacterial active against a broad spectrum of gram-positive and gram-negative ocular pathogens. It is available as the monohydrochloride monohydrate salt of 1-cyclopropyl-6-fluoro-1,4-dihydro-4-oxo-7- (1-piperazinyl)-3-quinoline-carboxylic acid. It is a faint to light yellow crystalline powder with a molecular weight of 385.8. Its empirical formula is $C_{17}H_{18}FN_3O_3 \cdot HCl \cdot H_2O$ and its chemical structure is as follows:

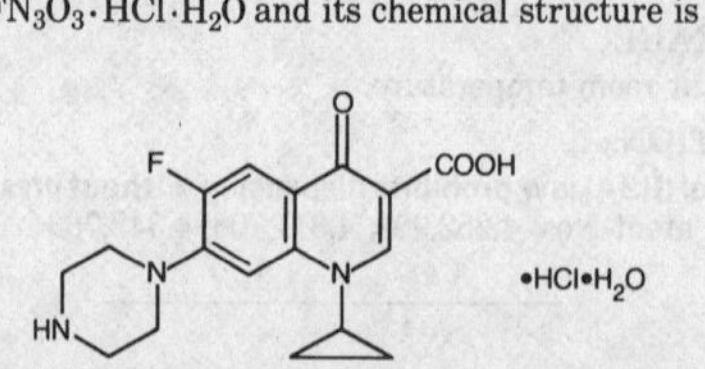

Ciprofloxacin differs from other quinolones in that it has a fluorine atom at the 6-position, a piperazine moiety at the 7-position, and a cyclopropyl ring at the 1-position.

Each mL of CILOXAN Ophthalmic Solution contains: Active: Ciprofloxacin HCl 3.5 mg equivalent to 3 mg base. Preservative: Benzalkonium Chloride 0.006%. Inactive: Sodium Acetate, Acetic Acid, Mannitol 4.6%, Edetate Disodium 0.05%, Hydrochloric Acid and/or Sodium Hydroxide (to adjust pH) and Purified Water. The pH is approximately 4.5 and the osmolality is approximately 300 mOsm.

CLINICAL PHARMACOLOGY

Systemic Absorption: A systemic absorbtion study was performed in which CILOXAN Ophthalmic Solution was administered in each eye every two hours while awake for two days followed by every four hours while awake for an additional 5 days. The maximum reported plasma concentration of ciprofloxacin was less than 5 ng/mL. The mean concentration was usually less than 2.5 ng/mL.

Microbiology: Ciprofloxacin has *in vitro* activity against a wide range of gram-negative and gram-positive organisms. The bactericidal action of ciprofloxacin results from interference with the enzyme DNA gyrase which is needed for the synthesis of bacterial DNA.

Ciprofloxacin has been shown to be active against most strains of the following organisms both *in vitro* and in clinical infections. (See *Indications and Usage* section).

Gram-Positive:
Staphylococcus aureus (including methicillin-susceptible and methicillin-resistant strains)
Staphylococcus epidermidis
Streptococcus pneumoniae
Streptococcus (Viridans Group)

Gram-Negative:
Pseudomonas aeruginosa
Serratia marcescens

Ciprofloxacin has been shown to be active *in vitro* against most strains of the following organisms, however, *the clinical significance of these data is unknown:*

Gram-Positive:
Enterococcus faecalis (Many strains are only moderately susceptible)
Staphylococcus haemolyticus
Staphylococcus hominis
Staphylococcus saprophyticus
Streptococcus pyogenes

Gram-Negative:
Acinetobacter calcoaceticus subsp. anitratus
Aeromonas caviae
Aeromonas hydrophila
Brucella melitensis
Campylobacter coli
Campylobacter jujuni
Citrobacter diversus
Citrobacter freundii
Edwardsiella tarda
Enterobacter aerogenes
Enterobacter cloacae
Escherichia coli
Haemophilus ducreyi
Haemophilus influenzae
Haemophilus parainfluenzae
Klebsiella pneumoniae
Klebsiella oxytoca
Legionella pneumophila
Moraxella (Branhamella) catarrhalis
Morganella morganii
Neisseria gonorrhoeae
Neisseria meningitidis
Pasteurella multocida
Proteus mirabilis
Proteus vulgaris
Providencia rettgeri
Providencia stuartii
Salmonella enteritidis
Salmonella typhi
Shigella sonneii
Shigella flexneri
Vibrio cholerae
Vibrio parahaemolyticus
Vibrio vulnificus
Yersinia enterocolitica

Other Organisms: *Chlamydia trachomatis* (only moderately susceptible) and *Mycobacterium tuberculosis* (only moderately susceptible).

Most strains of *Pseudomonas cepacia* and some strains of *Pseudomonas maltophilia* are resistant to ciprofloxacin as are most anaerobic bacteria, including *Bacteroides fragilis* and *Clostridium difficile.*

The minimal bactericidal concentration (MBC) generally does not exceed the minimal inhibitory concentration (MIC) by more than a factor of 2. Resistance to ciprofloxacin *in vitro* usually develops slowly (multiple-step mutation).

Ciprofloxacin does not cross-react with other antimicrobial agents such as beta-lactams or aminoglycosides; therefore, organisms resistant to these drugs may be susceptible to ciprofloxacin.

Clinical Studies:

Following therapy with CILOXAN Ophthalmic Solution, 76% of the patients with corneal ulcers and positive bacterial cultures were clinically cured and complete re-epithelialization occurred in about 92% of the ulcers.

In 3 and 7 day multicenter clinical trials, 52% of the patients with conjunctivitis and positive conjunctival cultures were clinically cured and 70–80% had all causative pathogens eradicated by the end of treatment.

INDICATIONS AND USAGE

CILOXAN Ophthalmic Solution is indicated for the treatment of infections caused by susceptible strains of the designated microorganisms in the conditions listed below:

Corneal Ulcers:	*Pseudomonas aeruginosa*
	Serratia marcescens*
	Staphylococcus aureus
	Staphylococcus epidermidis
	Streptococcus pneumoniae
	Streptococcus (Viridans Group)*
Conjunctivitis:	*Staphylococcus aureus*
	Staphylococcus epidermidis
	Streptococcus pneumoniae*

*Efficacy for this organism was studied in fewer than 10 infections.

CONTRAINDICATIONS

A history of hypersensitivity to ciprofloxacin or any other component of the medication is a contraindication to its use. A history of hypersensitivity to other quinolones may also contraindicate the use of ciprofloxacin.

WARNINGS

NOT FOR INJECTION INTO THE EYE.

Serious and occasionally fatal hypersensitivity (anaphylactic) reactions, some following the first dose, have been reported in patients receiving systemic quinolone therapy. Some reactions were accompanied by cardiovascular collapse, loss of consciousness, tingling, pharyngeal or facial edema, dyspnea, urticaria, and itching. Only a few patients had a history of hypersensitivity reactions. Serious anaphylactic reactions require immediate emergency treatment with epinephrine and other resuscitation measures, including oxygen, intravenous fluids, intravenous antihistamines, corticosteroids, pressor amines and airway management, as clinically indicated.

PRECAUTIONS

General: As with other antibacterial preparations, prolonged use of ciprofloxacin may result in overgrowth of nonsusceptible organisms, including fungi. If superinfection occurs, appropriate therapy should be initiated. Whenever clinical judgment dictates, the patient should be examined with the aid of magnification, such as slit lamp biomicroscopy and, where appropriate, fluorescein staining.

Ciprofloxacin should be discontinued at the first appearance of a skin rash or any other sign of hypersensitivity reaction. In clinical studies of patients with bacterial corneal ulcer, a white crystalline precipitate located in the superficial portion of the corneal defect was observed in 35 (16.6%) of 210 patients. The onset of the precipitate was within 24 hours to 7 days after starting therapy. In one patient, the precipitate was immediately irrigated out upon its appearance. In 17 patients, resolution of the precipitate was seen in 1 to 8 days (seven within the first 24–72 hours); in five patients, resolution was noted in 10–13 days. In nine patients, exact resolution days were unavailable; however, at follow-up examinations, 18–44 days after onset of the event, complete resolution of the precipitate was noted. In three patients, outcome information was unavailable. The precipitate did not preclude continued use of ciprofloxacin, nor did it adversely affect the clinical course of the ulcer or visual outcome. (SEE ADVERSE REACTIONS).

Drug Interactions: Specific drug interaction studies have not been conducted with ophthalmic ciprofloxacin. However, the systemic administration of some quinolones has been shown to elevate plasma concentrations of theophylline, interfere with the metabolism of caffeine, enhance the effects of the oral anticoagulant, warfarin, and its derivatives and have been associated with transient elevations in serum creatinine in patients receiving cyclosporine concomitantly.

Carcinogenesis, Mutagenesis, Impairment of Fertility: Eight *in vitro* mutagenicity tests have been conducted with ciprofloxacin and the test results are listed below:

Salmonella/Microsome Test (Negative)
E. coli DNA Repair Assay (Negative)
Mouse Lymphoma Cell Forward Mutation Assay (Positive)
Chinese Hamster V$_{79}$ Cell HGPRT Test (Negative)
Syrian Hamster Embryo Cell Transformation Assay (Negative)
Saccharomyces cerevisiae Point Mutation Assay (Negative)
Saccharomyces cerevisiae Mitotic Crossover and Gene Conversion Assay (Negative)
Rat Hepatocyte DNA Repair Assay (Positive)

Thus, two of the eight tests were positive, but the results of the following three *in vivo* test systems gave negative results:

Rat Hepatocyte DNA Repair Assay
Micronucleus Test (Mice)
Dominant Lethal Test (Mice)

Long term carcinogenicity studies in mice and rats have been completed. After daily oral dosing for up to two years, there is no evidence that ciprofloxacin had any carcinogenic or tumorigenic effects in these species.

Pregnancy—Pregnancy Category C: Reproduction studies have been performed in rats and mice at doses up to six times the usual daily human oral dose and have revealed no evidence of impaired fertility or harm to the fetus due to ciprofloxacin. In rabbits, as with most antimicrobial agents, ciprofloxacin (30 and 100 mg/kg orally) produced gastrointestinal disturbances resulting in maternal weight loss and an increased incidence of abortion. No teratogenicity was observed at either dose. After intravenous administration, at doses up to 20 mg/kg, no maternal toxicity was produced and no embryotoxicity or teratogenicity was observed. There are no adequate and well controlled studies in pregnant women. CILOXAN Ophthalmic Solution should be used during pregnancy only if the potential benefit justifies the potential risk to the fetus.

Nursing Mothers: It is not known whether topically applied ciprofloxacin is excreted in human milk; however, it is known that orally administered ciprofloxacin is excreted in the milk of lactating rats and oral ciprofloxacin has been reported in human breast milk after a single 500 mg dose. Caution should be exercised when CILOXAN Ophthalmic Solution is administered to a nursing mother.

Pediatric Use: Safety and effectiveness in children below the age of 12 have not been established.

Although ciprofloxacin and other quinolones cause arthropathy in immature animals after oral administration, topical ocular administration of ciprofloxacin to immature animals did not cause any arthropathy and there is no evidence that the ophthalmic dosage form has any effect on the weight bearing joints.

ADVERSE REACTIONS

The most frequently reported drug related adverse reaction was local burning or discomfort. In corneal ulcer studies with frequent administration of the drug, white crystalline precipitates were seen in approximately 17% of patients (SEE PRECAUTIONS). Other reactions occurring in less than 10% of patients included lid margin crusting, crystals/scales, foreign body sensation, itching, conjunctival hyperemia and a bad taste following instillation. Additional events occurring in less than 1% of patients included corneal staining, keratopathy/keratitis, allergic reactions, lid edema, tearing, photophobia, corneal infiltrates, nausea and decreased vision.

OVERDOSAGE

A topical overdose of CILOXAN Ophthalmic Solution may be flushed from the eye(s) with warm tap water.

DOSAGE AND ADMINISTRATION

The recommended dosage regimen for the treatment of **corneal ulcers** is: Two drops into the affected eye every 15 minutes for the first six hours and then two drops into the affected eye every 30 minutes for the remainder of the first day. On the second day, instill two drops in the affected eye hourly. On the third through the fourteenth day, place two drops in the affected eye every four hours. Treatment may be continued after 14 days if corneal re-epithelialization has not occurred.

The recommended dosage regimen for the treatment of **bacterial conjunctivitis** is: One or two drops instilled into the conjunctival sac(s) every two hours while awake for two days and one or two drops every four hours while awake for the next five days.

HOW SUPPLIED

As a sterile ophthalmic solution: 2.5 mL and 5 mL in plastic DROP-TAINER® dispensers.

2.5 mL—NDC 0065-0656-25
5 mL —NDC 0065-0656-05

STORAGE

Store at 2° to 30°C (36° to 86°F). Protect from light.

ANIMAL PHARMACOLOGY

Ciprofloxacin and related drugs have been shown to cause arthropathy in immature animals of most species tested following oral administration. However, a one-month topical ocular study using immature Beagle dogs did not demonstrate any articular lesions.

CAUTION

Federal (USA) law prohibits dispensing without prescription.

U.S. Patent No. 4,670,444

EYE-STREAM®   OTC
Sterile Eye Irrigating Solution

EYE-STREAM® is a sterile and stable irrigating solution that is specially designed and packaged for use in the eye(s). Formulated as a buffered salt solution, it closely approximates normal human tear fluid.

INGREDIENTS

Each mL contains: **Tonicity Agents:** Sodium Chloride 0.64%, Potassium Chloride 0.075%, Calcium Chloride Dihydrate 0.048%, Magnesium Chloride Hexahydrate 0.03%. **Buffering Agents:** Sodium Acetate Trihydrate 0.39%, Sodium Citrate Dihydrate 0.17%. **pH Adjusters:** Sodium Hydroxide and/or Hydrochloric Acid. **Preservative:** Benzalkonium Chloride 0.013%. **Purified Water.** The pH of the solution is in the physiologic range.

INDICATIONS

> ### FDA APPROVED USES
> For irrigating the eye to help relieve irritation, discomfort and burning by removing loose foreign material, air pollutants (smog or pollen), or chlorinated water.

WARNINGS

If you experience eye pain, changes in vision, continued redness or irritation of the eye, or if the condition worsens or persists, consult a doctor. Obtain immediate medical treatment for all open wounds in or near the eyes. If solution changes color or becomes cloudy, do not use. To avoid contamination, do not touch tip of container to any surface. Replace cap after using. Keep this and all drugs out of the reach of children. In case of accidental ingestion, seek professional assistance or contact a Poison Control Center immediately. Not to be used as a saline solution for rinsing and soaking soft contact lenses. Not for injection or intraocular surgery.

DIRECTIONS

Flush the affected eye as needed, controlling the rate of flow of solution by pressure on the bottle.

HOW SUPPLIED

In 1 fluid ounce and 4 fluid ounce plastic squeeze bottles.
1 fl. oz: NDC 0065-0530-01
4 fl. oz.: NDC 0065-0530-04

STORAGE

Store at 46°–80°F.

NAPHCON-A®   ℞
(naphazoline hydrochloride and pheniramine maleate)
Sterile Ophthalmic Solution

DESCRIPTION

NAPHCON-A® (naphazoline hydrochloride, pheniramine maleate) is a combination of an antihistamine and a decongestant prepared as a sterile topical ophthalmic solution. The active ingredients are represented by the chemical structures:

Established name:
Naphazoline Hydrochloride
Chemical name:
1H-Imidazole, 4, 5-dihydro- 2-(1- naphthalenylmethyl)-, monohydrochloride.

Established name:
Pheniramine Maleate
Chemical name:
N,N-Dimethyl -y -phenyl -2- pyridine-propanamine, (Z)- Butenedioic acid.

Each mL contains: Active: Naphazoline Hydrochloride 0.025%, Pheniramine Maleate 0.3%. Preservative: Benzalkonium Chloride 0.01%. Inactive: Boric Acid, Sodium Borate, Edetate Disodium, Sodium Chloride, Sodium Hydroxide and/or Hydrochloric Acid (to adjust pH), and Purified Water.

CLINICAL PHARMACOLOGY

NAPHCON-A® combines the effects of the antihistamine, pheniramine maleate, and the decongestant, naphazoline.

> **INDICATIONS AND USAGE:** Based on a review of a related combination of drugs by the National Academy of Sciences—National Research Council and/or other information, FDA has classified the indications as follows: "Possibly" effective: For relief of ocular irritation and/or congestion or for the treatment of allergic or

Continued on next page

Alcon Laboratories—Cont.

inflammatory ocular conditions. Final classification of the less-than-effective indication requires further investigation.

CONTRAINDICATIONS

Hypersensitivity to one or more of the components of this preparation.

Do not use in the presence of narrow angle glaucoma or in patients predisposed to narrow angle glaucoma.

WARNINGS

Patients under MAO inhibitors may experience a severe hypertensive crisis if given a sympathomimetic drug such as Naphazoline HCl. Use in infants and children may result in CNS depression leading to coma and marked reduction in body temperature.

PRECAUTIONS

General

For topical eye use only—not for injection. This preparation should be used with caution in patients with severe cardiovascular disease including cardiac arrhythmias, patients with poorly controlled hypertension, patients with diabetes, especially those with a tendency toward diabetic ketoacidosis.

Information For Patients: To prevent contaminating the dropper tip and solution, care should be taken not to touch the eyelids or surrounding area with the dropper tip of the bottle.

Carcinogenesis, Mutagenesis, Impairment of Fertility: There have been no long-term studies done using naphazoline hydrochloride and/or pheniramine maleate in animals to evaluate carcinogenic potential.

Pregnancy: Pregnancy Category C. Animal reproduction studies have not been conducted with naphazoline hydrochloride and/or pheniramine maleate. It is also not known whether naphazoline hydrochloride and/or pheniramine maleate can cause fetal harm when administered to a pregnant woman or can affect reproduction capacity. NAPHCON-A® Ophthalmic Solution should be given to a pregnant woman only if clearly needed.

Nursing Mothers: It is not known whether these drugs are excreted in human milk. Because many drugs are excreted in human milk, caution should be exercised when NAPHCON-A Ophthalmic Solution is administered to a nursing woman.

ADVERSE REACTIONS

The following adverse reactions may occur: Pupillary dilation, increase in intraocular pressure, systemic effects due to absorption (i.e., hypertension, cardiac irregularities, hyperglycemia). Drowsiness may be experienced by some patients.

DOSAGE AND ADMINISTRATION

One or two drops instilled in each eye every 3 to 4 hours or less frequently, as required to relieve symptoms.

HOW SUPPLIED

In 15mL plastic DROP-TAINER® Dispenser.
NDC 0998-0080-15

STORAGE

Store at 36° to 80°F. Keep bottle tightly closed when not in use. Protect from light and excessive heat.

CAUTION

Federal (USA) law prohibits dispensing without prescription.

TEARS NATURALE® II   OTC
Lubricant Eye Drops
TEARS NATURALE® FREE
Lubricant Eye Drops

DESCRIPTION

TEARS NATURALE II is the only lubricant eye drop preserved with safe, nonsensitizing POLYQUAD 0.001%. *In vitro* studies have shown that POLYQUAD substantially avoids the damaging effects of epithelial cell toxicity possible with other tear substitute preservatives and allows epithelial cell growth. POLYQUAD has been shown to be 99% reaction-free in normal subjects and 97% reaction-free in subjects known to be preservative sensitive. TEARS NATURALE FREE is a preservative-free version of TEARS NATURALE II.

With their unique mucin like polymeric formulation, and with their natural pH, low viscosity, and isotonicity, TEARS NATURALE II and TEARS NATURALE FREE provide dry eye patients with comfort and prompt relief of dry eye symptoms.

Sterile-For Topical Eye Use Only

INGREDIENTS

TEARS NATURALE II: each mL contains:
Active: DUASORB®, a water soluble polymeric system containing Dextran 70 0.1% and Hydroxypropyl Methylcellulose 2910 0.3%.
Preservative: POLYQUAD®* (Polyquaternium-1) 0.001%.
Inactive: Sodium Borate, Potassium Chloride, Sodium Chloride, Purified Water. May contain Hydrochloric Acid and/or Sodium Hydroxide to adjust pH.
TEARS NATURALE FREE: each mL contains:
Active: DUASORB, a water soluble polymeric system containing Dextran 70 0.1% and Hydroxypropyl Methylcellulose 2910 0.3%.
Inactive: Sodium Borate, Potassium Chloride, Sodium Chloride, Purified Water. May contain Hydrochloric Acid and/or Sodium Hydroxide to adjust pH.

INDICATIONS

For the temporary relief of burning and irritation due to dryness of the eye and for use as a protectant against further irritation. For temporary relief of discomfort due to minor irritations of the eye or to exposure to wind or sun.

WARNINGS

If you experience eye pain, changes in vision, continued redness or irritation of the eye, or if the condition worsens or persists for more than 72 hours, discontinue use and consult a doctor.

If solution changes color or becomes cloudy, do not use.
To avoid contamination, do not touch tip of container to any surface. TEARS NATURALE II: Replace cap after using. TEARS NATURALE FREE: Do not reuse. Once opened, discard. Keep this and all drugs out of the reach of children. In case of accidental ingestion, seek professional assistance or contact a Poison Control Center immediately.

DIRECTIONS

TEARS NATURALE II: Instill 1 or 2 drops in the affected eye(s) as needed. TEARS NATURALE FREE: Completely twist off tab: do not pull. Instill 1 or 2 drops in the affected eye(s) as needed.

HOW SUPPLIED

TEARS NATURALE II Lubricant Eye Drops are supplied in 15 mL and 30 mL plastic DROP-TAINER® bottles.
15 mL NDC 0065-0418-15
30 mL NDC 0065-0418-30
TEARS NATURALE FREE Lubricant Eye Drops are supplied in boxes of 24 0.02 fl. oz. single-use containers.
NDC 0065-0416-24

STORAGE

Store at room temperature.
* U.S. Patent No. 3,931,319 and others.

TOBRADEX®   ℞
(Tobramycin and Dexamethasone)
Sterile Ophthalmic Suspension and Ointment

DESCRIPTION

TOBRADEX® (Tobramycin and Dexamethasone) Ophthalmic Suspension and Ointment are sterile, multiple dose antibiotic and steroid combinations for topical ophthalmic use. The chemical structures for tobramycin and dexamethasone are presented below:

Tobramycin   Empirical Formula: $C_{18}H_{37}N_5O_9$

Chemical name:
O-3-Amino-3-deoxy-α-D-glucopyranosyl-$(1 \rightarrow 4)$-O-[2,6-diamino-2,3,6-trideoxy-α-D-*ribo*-hexopyranosyl-$(1 \rightarrow 6)$]-2-deoxy-L-streptamine

Dexamethasone   Empirical Formula: $C_{22}H_{29}FO_5$

Chemical Name:
9-Fluoro-11β,17,21-trihydroxy-16α-methylpregna-1,4-diene-3,20-dione

Each mL of TOBRADEX® Suspension contains: Active: Tobramycin 0.3% (3 mg) and Dexamethasone 0.1% (1 mg). Preservative: Benzalkonium Chloride 0.01%. Inactive: Tyloxapol, Edetate Disodium, Sodium Chloride, Hydroxyethyl Cellulose, Sodium Sulfate, Sulfuric Acid and/or Sodium Hydroxide (to adjust pH) and Purified Water.

Each gram of TOBRADEX® Ointment contains: Active: Tobramycin 0.3% (3 mg) and Dexamethasone 0.1% (1 mg). Preservative: Chlorobutanol 0.5%. Inactive: Mineral Oil and White Petrolatum.

CLINICAL PHARMACOLOGY

Corticoids suppress the inflammatory response to a variety of agents and they probably delay or slow healing. Since corticoids may inhibit the body's defense mechanism against infection, a concomitant antimicrobial drug may be used when this inhibition is considered to be clinically significant. Dexamethasone is a potent corticoid.

The antibiotic component in the combination (tobramycin) is included to provide action against susceptible organisms. *In vitro* studies have demonstrated that tobramycin is active against susceptible strains of the following microorganisms: Staphylococci, including *S. aureus* and *S. epidermidis* (coagulase-positive and coagulase-negative), including penicillin-resistant strains.

Streptococci, including some of the Group A beta-hemolytic species, some nonhemolytic species, and some *Streptococcus pneumoniae*.

Pseudomonas aeruginosa, Escherichia coli, Klebsiella pneumoniae, Enterobacter aerogenes, Proteus mirabilis, Morganella morganii, most *Proteus vulgaris* strains, *Haemophilus influenzae* and *H. aegyptius, Moraxella lacunata*, and *Acinetobacter calcoaceticus* and some *Neisseria* species.

Bacterial susceptibility studies demonstrate that in some cases microorganisms resistant to gentamicin remain susceptible to tobramycin. A significant bacterial population resistant to tobramycin has not yet emerged; however, bacterial resistance may develop upon prolonged use.

No data are available on the extent of systemic absorption from TOBRADEX® Ophthalmic Suspension or Ointment; however, it is known that some systemic absorption can occur with ocularly applied drugs. If the maximum dose of TOBRADEX Ophthalmic Suspension is given for the first 48 hours (two drops in each eye every 2 hours) and complete systemic absorption occurs, which is highly unlikely, the daily dose of dexamethasone would be 2.4 mg. The usual physiologic replacement dose is 0.75 mg daily. If TOBRADEX Ophthalmic Suspension is given after the first 48 hours as two drops in each eye every 4 hours, the administered dose of dexamethasone would be 1.2 mg daily. For TOBRADEX Ophthalmic Ointment the administered dose for both eyes four times daily would be 0.4 mg of dexamethasone daily.

INDICATIONS AND USAGE

TOBRADEX® Ophthalmic Suspension and Ointment are indicated for steroid-responsive inflammatory ocular conditions for which a corticosteroid is indicated and where superficial bacterial ocular infection or a risk of bacterial ocular infection exists.

Ocular steroids are indicated in inflammatory conditions of the palpebral and bulbar conjunctiva, cornea and anterior segment of the globe where the inherent risk of steroid use in certain infective conjunctivitides is accepted to obtain a diminution in edema and inflammation. They are also indicated in chronic anterior uveitis and corneal injury from chemical, radiation or thermal burns, or penetration of foreign bodies. The use of a combination drug with an anti-infective component is indicated where the risk of superficial ocular infection is high or where there is an expectation that potentially dangerous numbers of bacteria will be present in the eye. The particular anti-infective drug in this product is active against the following common bacterial eye pathogens: Staphylococci, including *S. aureus* and *S. epidermidis* (coagulase-positive and coagulase-negative), including penicillin-resistant strains.

Streptococci, including some of the Group A beta-hemolytic species, some nonhemolytic species, and some *Streptococcus pneumoniae*.

Pseudomonas aeruginosa, Escherichia coli, Klebsiella pneumoniae, Enterobacter aerogenes, Proteus mirabilis, Morganella morganii, most *Proteus vulgaris* strains, *Haemophilus influenzae* and *H. aegyptius, Moraxella lacunata*, and *Acinetobacter calcoaceticus* and some *Neisseria* species.

CONTRAINDICATIONS

Epithelial herpes simplex keratitis (dendritic keratitis), vaccinia, varicella, and many other viral diseases of the cornea and conjunctiva. Mycobacterial infection of the eye. Fungal diseases of ocular structures. Hypersensitivity to a component of the medication.

The use of this combination is always contraindicated after uncomplicated removal of a corneal foreign body.

WARNINGS

NOT FOR INJECTION INTO THE EYE. Sensitivity to topically applied aminoglycosides may occur in some patients. If a sensitivity reaction does occur, discontinue use. Prolonged use of steroids may result in glaucoma, with damage to the optic nerve, defects in visual acuity and fields of vision, and posterior subcapsular cataract formation. Intraocular pressure should be routinely monitored even though it may be difficult in children and uncooperative patients. Prolonged use may suppress the host response and thus increase the hazard of secondary ocular infections. In those diseases causing thinning of the cornea or sclera, perforations have been known to occur with the use of topical steroids. In acute purulent conditions of the eye, steroids may mask infection or enhance existing infection.

PRECAUTIONS

General. The possibility of fungal infections of the cornea should be considered after long-term steroid dosing. As with other antibiotic preparations, prolonged use may result in overgrowth of nonsusceptible organisms, including fungi. If superinfection occurs, appropriate therapy should be initiated. When multiple prescriptions are required, or whenever clinical judgement dictates, the patient should be examined with the aid of magnification, such as slit lamp biomicroscopy and, where appropriate, fluorescein staining.
Information for Patients: Do not touch dropper or tube tip to any surface as this may contaminate the contents.
Carcinogenesis, Mutagenesis, Impairment of Fertility. No studies have been conducted to evaluate the carcinogenic or mutagenic potential. No impairment of fertility was noted in studies of subcutaneous tobramycin in rats at doses of 50 and 100 mg/kg/day.
Pregnancy Category C. Corticosteroids have been found to be teratogenic in animal studies. Ocular administration of 0.1% dexamethasone resulted in 15.6% and 32.3% incidence of fetal anomalies in two groups of pregnant rabbits. Fetal growth retardation and increased mortality rates have been observed in rats with chronic dexamethasone therapy. Reproduction studies have been performed in rats and rabbits with tobramycin at doses up to 100 mg/kg/day parenterally and have revealed no evidence of impaired fertility or harm to the fetus. There are no adequate and well-controlled studies in pregnant women. TOBRADEX® Ophthalmic Suspension and Ointment should be used during pregnancy only if the potential benefit justifies the potential risk to the fetus.
Nursing Mothers. It is not known whether this drug is excreted in human milk. Because many drugs are excreted in human milk, a decision should be considered to discontinue nursing temporarily while using TOBRADEX Ophthalmic Suspension or Ointment.
Pediatric Use. Safety and effectiveness in children have not been established.

ADVERSE REACTIONS

Adverse reactions have occurred with steroid/anti-infective combination drugs which can be attributed to the steroid component, the anti-infective component, or the combination. Exact incidence figures are not available. The most frequent adverse reactions to topical ocular tobramycin (TOBREX®) are hypersensitivity and localized ocular toxicity, including lid itching and swelling, and conjunctival erythema. These reactions occur in less than 4% of patients. Similar reactions may occur with the topical use of other aminoglycoside antibiotics. Other adverse reactions have not been reported; however, if topical ocular tobramycin is administered concomitantly with systemic aminoglycoside antibiotics, care should be taken to monitor the total serum concentration. The reactions due to the steroid component are: elevation of intraocular pressure (IOP) with possible development of glaucoma, and infrequent optic nerve damage; posterior subcapsular cataract formation; and delayed wound healing.
Secondary Infection. The development of secondary infection has occurred after use of combinations containing steroids and antimicrobials. Fungal infections of the cornea are particularly prone to develop coincidentally with long-term applications of steroids. The possibility of fungal invasion must be considered in any persistent corneal ulceration where steroid treatment has been used. Secondary bacterial ocular infection following suppression of host responses also occurs.

DOSAGE AND ADMINISTRATION

Suspension: One or two drops instilled into the conjunctival sac(s) every four to six hours. During the initial 24 to 48 hours, the dosage may be increased to one or two drops every two (2) hours. Frequency should be decreased gradually as warranted by improvement in clinical signs. Care should be taken not to discontinue therapy prematurely. **Ointment:** Apply a small amount (approximately ½ inch ribbon) into the conjunctival sac(s) up to three or four times daily. TOBRADEX Ophthalmic Ointment may be used at bedtime in conjunction with TOBRADEX Ophthalmic Suspension

used during the day. Not more than 20 mL or 8 g should be prescribed initially and the prescription should not be refilled without further evaluation as outlined in PRECAUTIONS above.

HOW SUPPLIED

Sterile ophthalmic suspension in 2.5 mL (NDC 0065-0647-25) and 5 mL (NDC 0065-0647-05) DROP-TAINER® dispensers. Sterile ophthalmic ointment in 3.5 g ophthalmic tube (NDC 0065-0648-35).

STORAGE

Store 46° to 80°F (8° to 27°C).
Store suspension upright and shake well before using.

CAUTION

Federal (USA) law prohibits dispensing without prescription.
Patent Pending.

TOBREX® ℞
(tobramycin 0.3%)
Ophthalmic Solution and Ointment

DESCRIPTION

TOBREX® (tobramycin 0.3%) is a sterile topical ophthalmic antibiotic formulation prepared specifically for topical therapy of external ophthalmic infections. This product is supplied in solution and ointment forms.
Each mL of TOBREX Ophthalmic solution contains: Active: Tobramycin 0.3% (3 mg). Preservative: Benzalkonium Chloride 0.01%. Inactive: Boric Acid, Sodium Sulfate, Sodium Chloride, Tyloxapol, Sodium Hydroxide and/or Sulfuric Acid (to adjust pH), and Purified Water.
Each gram of TOBREX Ophthalmic ointment contains: Active: Tobramycin 0.3% (3 mg). Preservative: Chlorobutanol 0.5%. Inactive: Mineral Oil and White Petrolatum.
The chemical structure of tobramycin is:

Chemical name:
0-{3-amino-3-deoxy-α-D-gluco-pyranosyl-(1→4)}-0-{2,6-diamino-2,3,6-trideoxy-α-D-ribohexo-pyranosyl-(1→6)}-2-deoxystreptamine.
Tobramycin is a water-soluble aminoglycoside antibiotic active against a wide variety of gram-negative and grampositive ophthalmic pathogens.

CLINICAL PHARMACOLOGY

In Vitro Data: In vitro studies have demonstrated tobramycin is active against susceptible strains of the following microorganisms:
Staphylococci, including *S. aureus* and *S. epidermidis* (coagulase-positive and coagulase-negative), including penicillinresistant strains.
Streptococci, including some of the Group A-betahemolytic species, some nonhemolytic species, and some *Streptococcus pneumoniae*.
Pseudomonas aeruginosa, Escherichia coli, Klebsiella pneumoniae, Enterobacter aerogenes, Proteus mirabilis, Morganella morganii, most *Proteus vulgaris* strains, *Haemophilus influenzae* and *H. aegyptius, Moraxella lacunata*, and *Acinetobacter calcoaceticus* and some *Neisseria* species. Bacterial susceptibility studies demonstrate that in some cases, microorganisms resistant to gentamicin retain susceptibility to tobramycin. A significant bacterial population resistant to tobramycin has not yet emerged; however, bacterial resistance may develop upon prolonged use.

INDICATIONS AND USAGE

TOBREX® is a topical antibiotic indicated in the treatment of external infections of the eye and its adnexa caused by susceptible bacteria. Appropriate monitoring of bacterial response to topical antibiotic therapy should accompany the use of TOBREX.
Clinical studies have shown tobramycin to be safe and effective for use in children.

CONTRAINDICATIONS

TOBREX Ophthalmic Solution and Ointment are contraindicated in patients with known hypersensitivity to any of their components.

WARNINGS

NOT FOR INJECTION INTO THE EYE. Do not touch tube or dropper tip to any surface, as this may contaminate the

contents. Sensitivity to topically applied aminoglycosides may occur in some patients. If a sensitivity reaction to TOBREX® occurs, discontinue use.

PRECAUTIONS

As with other antibiotic preparations, prolonged use may result in overgrowth of nonsusceptible organisms, including fungi. If superinfection occurs, appropriate therapy should be initiated. Ophthalmic ointments may retard corneal wound healing.
Pregnancy Category B. Reproduction studies in three types of animals at doses up to thirty-three times the normal human systemic dose have revealed no evidence of impaired fertility or harm to the fetus due to tobramycin. There are, however, no adequate and well-controlled studies in pregnant women. Because animal studies are not always predictive of human response, this drug should be used during pregnancy only if clearly needed.
Nursing Mothers: Because of the potential for adverse reactions in nursing infants from TOBREX, a decision should be made whether to discontinue nursing the infant or discontinue the drug, taking into account the importance of the drug to the mother.

ADVERSE REACTIONS

The most frequent adverse reactions to TOBREX Ophthalmic Solution and Ointment are hypersensitivity and localized ocular toxicity, including lid itching and swelling, and conjunctival erythema. These reactions occur in less than three of 100 patients treated with TOBREX. Similar reactions may occur with the topical use of other aminoglycoside antibiotics. Other adverse reactions have not been reported from TOBREX therapy; however, if topical ocular tobramycin is administered concomitantly with systemic aminoglycoside antibiotics, care should be taken to monitor the total serum concentration.
In clinical trials, TOBREX Ophthalmic Ointment produced significantly fewer adverse reactions (3.7%) than did GARAMYCIN® Ophthalmic Ointment (10.6%).

OVERDOSAGE

Clinically apparent signs and symptoms of an overdose of TOBREX Ophthalmic Solution or Ointment (punctate keratitis, erythema, increased lacrimation, edema and lid itching) may be similar to adverse reaction effects seen in some patients.

DOSAGE AND ADMINISTRATION

Solution: In mild to moderate disease, instill one or two drops into the affected eye(s) every four hours. In severe infections, instill two drops into the eye(s) hourly until improvement, following which treatment should be reduced prior to discontinuation.
Ointment: In mild to moderate disease, apply a half-inch ribbon into the affected eye(s) two or three times per day. In severe infections, instill a half-inch ribbon into the affected eye(s) every three to four hours until improvement, following which treatment should be reduced prior to discontinuation.
How to Apply TOBREX® Ointment
1. Tilt your head back.
2. Place a finger on your cheek just under your eye and gently pull down until a "V" pocket is formed between your eyeball and your lower lid.
3. Place a small amount (about ½ inch) of TOBREX in the "V" pocket. Do not let the tip of the tube touch your eye.
4. Look downward before closing your eye.
TOBREX Ointment may be used in conjunction with TOBREX Solution.

HOW SUPPLIED

5 mL Sterile solution in Drop-Tainer® dispenser (NDC 0998-0643-05), containing tobramycin 0.3% (3 mg/mL) and 3.5 g Sterile ointment in ophthalmic tube (NDC 0065-0644-35), containing tobramycin 0.3% (3 mg/g).

STORAGE

Store at 8°-27°C (46°-80°F).

CAUTION

Federal (USA) law prohibits dispensing without prescription.

Products are cross-indexed by
generic and chemical names
in the
YELLOW SECTION.

Allen & Hanburys
Division of Glaxo Inc.
FIVE MOORE DRIVE
RESEARCH TRIANGLE PARK, NC 27709

BECLOVENT® Inhalation Aerosol ℞
[*be'klō-vent"*]
(beclomethasone dipropionate, USP)
For Oral Inhalation Only

DESCRIPTION

Beclomethasone dipropionate, USP, the active component of Beclovent® Inhalation Aerosol, is an anti-inflammatory steroid having the chemical name 9-chloro-11β, 17, 21-trihydroxy-16β-methylpregna-1, 4-diene-3, 20-dione 17, 21-dipropionate.

Beclovent Inhalation Aerosol is a metered-dose aerosol unit containing a microcrystalline suspension of beclomethasone dipropionate-trichloromonofluoromethane clathrate in a mixture of propellants (trichloromonofluoromethane and dichlorodifluoromethane) with oleic acid. Each canister contains beclomethasone dipropionate–trichloromonofluoromethane clathrate having a molecular proportion of beclomethasone dipropionate to trichloromonofluoromethane between 3:1 and 3:2. Each actuation delivers from the mouthpiece a quantity of clathrate equivalent to 42 mcg of beclomethasone dipropionate, USP. The contents of one canister provide at least 200 oral inhalations.

CLINICAL PHARMACOLOGY

Beclomethasone 17, 21-dipropionate is a diester of beclomethasone, a synthetic halogenated corticosteroid. Animal studies show that beclomethasone dipropionate has potent anti-inflammatory activity. When beclomethasone dipropionate was administered systemically to mice, the anti-inflammatory activity was accompanied by other features typical of glucocorticoid action, including thymic involution, liver glycogen deposition, and pituitary-adrenal suppression. However, after systemic administration of beclomethasone dipropionate to rats, the anti-inflammatory action was associated with little or no effect on other tests of glucocorticoid activity.

Beclomethasone dipropionate is sparingly soluble and is poorly mobilized from subcutaneous or intramuscular injection sites. However, systemic absorption occurs after all routes of administration. When given to animals in the form of an aerosolized suspension of the trichloromonofluoromethane clathrate, the drug is deposited in the mouth and nasal passages, the trachea and principal bronchi, and the lung; a considerable portion of the drug is also swallowed. Absorption occurs rapidly from all respiratory and gastrointestinal tissues, as indicated by the rapid clearance of radioactively labeled drug from local tissues and appearance of tracer in the circulation. There is no evidence of tissue storage of beclomethasone dipropionate or its metabolites. Lung slices can metabolize beclomethasone dipropionate rapidly to beclomethasone 17-monopropionate and more slowly to free beclomethasone (which has very weak anti-inflammatory activity). However, irrespective of the route of administration (injection, oral, or aerosol), the principal route of excretion of the drug and its metabolites is the feces. Less than 10% of the drug and its metabolites is excreted in the urine. In humans, 12%–15% of an orally administered dose of beclomethasone dipropionate was excreted in the urine as both conjugated and free metabolites of the drug.

The mechanisms responsible for the anti-inflammatory action of beclomethasone dipropionate are unknown. The precise mechanism of the aerosolized drug's action in the lung is also unknown.

INDICATIONS AND USAGE

Beclovent® (beclomethasone dipropionate) Inhalation Aerosol is indicated only for patients who require chronic treatment with corticosteroids for control of the symptoms of bronchial asthma. Such patients would include those already receiving systemic corticosteroids, and selected patients who are inadequately controlled on a nonsteroid regimen and in whom steroid therapy has been withheld because of concern over potential adverse effects.

Beclovent Inhalation Aerosol is NOT indicated:

1. For relief of asthma that can be controlled by bronchodilators and other nonsteroid medications.
2. In patients who require systemic corticosteroid treatment infrequently.
3. In the treatment of nonasthmatic bronchitis.

CONTRAINDICATIONS

Beclovent® (beclomethasone dipropionate) Inhalation Aerosol is contraindicated in the primary treatment of status asthmaticus or other acute episodes of asthma where intensive measures are required.

Hypersensitivity to any of the ingredients of this preparation contraindicates its use.

WARNINGS

> Particular care is needed in patients who are transferred from systemically active corticosteroids to Beclovent® (beclomethasone dipropionate) Inhalation Aerosol because deaths due to adrenal insufficiency have occurred in asthmatic patients during and after transfer from systemic corticosteroids to aerosol beclomethasone dipropionate. After withdrawal from systemic corticosteroids, a number of months are required for recovery of hypothalamic-pituitary-adrenal (HPA) function. During this period of HPA suppression, patients may exhibit signs and symptoms of adrenal insufficiency when exposed to trauma, surgery, or infections, particularly gastroenteritis. Although Beclovent Inhalation Aerosol may provide control of asthmatic symptoms during these episodes, it does NOT provide the systemic steroid that is necessary for coping with these emergencies.
>
> During periods of stress or a severe asthmatic attack, patients who have been withdrawn from systemic corticosteroids should be instructed to resume systemic steroids (in large doses) immediately and to contact their physician for further instruction. These patients should also be instructed to carry a warning card indicating that they may need supplementary systemic steroids during periods of stress or a severe asthma attack. To assess the risk of adrenal insufficiency in emergency situations, routine tests of adrenal cortical function, including measurement of early morning resting cortisol levels, should be performed periodically in all patients. An early morning resting cortisol level may be accepted as normal only if it falls at or near the normal mean level.

Children who are on immunosuppressant drugs are more susceptible to infections than healthy children. Chickenpox and measles, for example, can have a more serious or even fatal course in children on immunosuppressant corticosteroids. In such children, or in adults who have not had these diseases, particular care should be taken to avoid exposure. If exposed, therapy with varicella zoster immune globulin (VZIG) or pooled intravenous immunoglobulin (IVIG), as appropriate, may be indicated. If chickenpox develops, treatment with antiviral agents may be considered.

Localized infections with *Candida albicans* or *Aspergillus niger* have occurred frequently in the mouth and pharynx and occasionally in the larynx. Positive cultures for oral *Candida* may be present in up to 75% of patients. Although the frequency of clinically apparent infection is considerably lower, these infections may require treatment with appropriate antifungal therapy or discontinuation of treatment with Beclovent Inhalation Aerosol.

Beclovent Inhalation Aerosol is not to be regarded as a bronchodilator and is not indicated for rapid relief of bronchospasm.

Patients should be instructed to contact their physician immediately when episodes of asthma that are not responsive to bronchodilators occur during the course of treatment with Beclovent Inhalation Aerosol. During such episodes, patients may require therapy with systemic corticosteroids.

There is no evidence that control of asthma can be achieved by the administration of Beclovent Inhalation Aerosol in amounts greater than the recommended doses.

Transfer of patients from systemic steroid therapy to Beclovent Inhalation Aerosol may unmask allergic conditions previously suppressed by the systemic steroid therapy, e.g., rhinitis, conjunctivitis, and eczema.

PRECAUTIONS

During withdrawal from oral steroids, some patients may experience symptoms of systemically active steroid withdrawal, e.g., joint and/or muscular pain, lassitude, and depression, despite maintenance or even improvement of respiratory function (see DOSAGE AND ADMINISTRATION).

In responsive patients, beclomethasone dipropionate may permit control of asthmatic symptoms without suppression of HPA function, as discussed below (see CLINICAL STUDIES). Since beclomethasone dipropionate is absorbed into the circulation and can be systemically active, the beneficial effects of Beclovent® (beclomethasone dipropionate) Inhalation Aerosol in minimizing or preventing HPA dysfunction may be expected only when recommended dosages are not exceeded.

The long-term effects of beclomethasone dipropionate in human subjects are still unknown. In particular, the local effects of the agent on developmental or immunologic processes in the mouth, pharynx, trachea, and lung are unknown. There is also no information about the possible long-term systemic effects of the agent.

The potential effects of Beclovent Inhalation Aerosol on acute, recurrent, or chronic pulmonary infections, including active or quiescent tuberculosis, are not known. Similarly, the potential effects of long-term administration of the drug on lung or other tissues are unknown.

Pulmonary infiltrates with eosinophilia may occur in patients on Beclovent Inhalation Aerosol therapy. Although it is possible that in some patients this state may become manifest because of systemic steroid withdrawal when inhalational steroids are administered, a causative role for beclomethasone dipropionate and/or its vehicle cannot be ruled out.

Information for Patients: Patients who are on immunosuppressant doses of corticosteroids should be warned to avoid exposure to chickenpox or measles and, if exposed, to obtain medical advice.

Pregnancy: ***Teratogenic Effects:*** Glucocorticoids are known teratogens in rodent species and beclomethasone dipropionate is no exception.

Teratology studies were done in rats, mice, and rabbits treated with subcutaneous beclomethasone dipropionate. Beclomethasone dipropionate was found to produce fetal resorption, cleft palate, agnathia, microstomia, absence of tongue, delayed ossification, and partial agenesis of the thymus. Well-controlled trials relating to fetal risk in humans are not available. Glucocorticoids are secreted in human milk. It is not known whether beclomethasone dipropionate would be secreted in human milk, but it is safe to assume that it is likely. The use of beclomethasone dipropionate in pregnant women, nursing mothers, or women of childbearing potential requires that the possible benefits of the drug be weighed against the potential hazards to the mother, embryo, or fetus. Infants born of mothers who have received substantial doses of corticosteroids during pregnancy should be carefully observed for hypoadrenalism.

ADVERSE REACTIONS

Deaths due to adrenal insufficiency have occurred in asthmatic patients during and after transfer from systemic corticosteroids to aerosol beclomethasone dipropionate (see WARNINGS).

Suppression of HPA function (reduction of early morning plasma cortisol levels) has been reported in adult patients who received 1,600-mcg daily doses of Beclovent® (beclomethasone dipropionate) Inhalation Aerosol for 1 month. A few patients on Beclovent Inhalation Aerosol have complained of hoarseness or dry mouth.

Rare cases of immediate and delayed hypersensitivity reactions, including urticaria, angioedema, rash, and bronchospasm, have been reported after the use of beclomethasone oral or intranasal inhalers.

DOSAGE AND ADMINISTRATION

Adults and Children 12 Years of Age and Older: The usual recommended dosage is two inhalations (84 mcg) given three or four times a day. Alternatively, four inhalations (168 mcg) given twice daily have been shown to be effective in some patients. In patients with severe asthma, it is advisable to start with 12–16 inhalations a day and adjust the dosage downward according to the response of the patient. The maximal daily intake should not exceed 20 inhalations, 840 mcg (0.84 mg), in adults.

Children 6–12 Years of Age: The usual recommended dosage is one or two inhalations (42–84 mcg) given three or four times a day according to the response of the patient. Alternatively, four inhalations (168 mcg) given twice daily have been shown to be effective in some patients. The maximal daily intake should not exceed 10 inhalations, 420 mcg (0.42 mg), in children 6–12 years of age. Insufficient clinical data exist with respect to the administration of Beclovent® (beclomethasone dipropionate) Inhalation Aerosol in children below the age of 6.

Rinsing the mouth after inhalation is advised.

Patients receiving bronchodilators by inhalation should be advised to use the bronchodilator before Beclovent Inhalation Aerosol in order to enhance penetration of beclomethasone dipropionate into the bronchial tree. After use of an aerosol bronchodilator, several minutes should elapse before use of the Beclovent Inhalation Aerosol to reduce the potential toxicity from the inhaled fluorocarbon propellants in the two aerosols.

Different considerations must be given to the following groups of patients in order to obtain the full therapeutic benefit of Beclovent Inhalation Aerosol.

Patients Not Receiving Systemic Steroids: The use of Beclovent Inhalation Aerosol is straightforward in patients who are inadequately controlled with nonsteroid medications but in whom systemic steroid therapy has been withheld because of concern over potential adverse reactions. In patients who respond to Beclovent Inhalation Aerosol, an improvement in pulmonary function is usually apparent within 1–4 weeks after the start of Beclovent Inhalation Aerosol.

Patients Receiving Systemic Steroids: In those patients dependent on systemic steroids, transfer to Beclovent Inhalation Aerosol and subsequent management may be more difficult because recovery from impaired adrenal function is usually slow. Such suppression has been known to last for up to 12 months. Clinical studies, however, have demonstrated that Beclovent Inhalation Aerosol may be effective in the management of these asthmatic patients and may permit

replacement or significant reduction in the dosage of systemic corticosteroids.
The patient's asthma should be reasonably stable before treatment with Beclovent Inhalation Aerosol is started. Initially, the aerosol should be used concurrently with the patient's usual maintenance dose of systemic steroid. After approximately 1 week, gradual withdrawal of the systemic steroid is started by reducing the daily or alternate-daily dose. The next reduction is made after an interval of 1 or 2 weeks, depending on the response of the patient. Generally, these decrements should not exceed 2.5 mg of prednisone or its equivalent. A slow rate of withdrawal cannot be overemphasized. During withdrawal some patients may experience symptoms of systemically active steroid withdrawal, e.g., joint and/or muscular pain, lassitude, and depression, despite maintenance or even improvement of respiratory function. Such patients should be encouraged to continue with the inhaler but should be watched carefully for objective signs of adrenal insufficiency such as hypotension and weight loss. If evidence of adrenal insufficiency occurs, the systemic steroid dose should be boosted temporarily and thereafter further withdrawal should continue more slowly. During periods of stress or a severe asthma attack, transfer patients will require supplementary treatment with systemic steroids. Exacerbations of asthma that occur during the course of treatment with Beclovent Inhalation Aerosol should be treated with a short course of systemic steroid that is gradually tapered as these symptoms subside. There is no evidence that control of asthma can be achieved by administration of Beclovent Inhalation Aerosol in amounts greater than the recommended doses.

Directions for Use: Illustrated Patient's Instructions for Use accompany each package of Beclovent Inhalation Aerosol.

CONTENTS UNDER PRESSURE. Do not puncture. Do not use or store near heat or open flame. Exposure to temperatures above 120°F may cause bursting. Never throw container into fire or incinerator. Keep out of reach of children.

HOW SUPPLIED

Beclovent® (beclomethasone dipropionate) Inhalation Aerosol is supplied in a 16.8-g canister containing 200 metered inhalations with oral adapter and patient's instructions (NDC 0173-0312-88). Also available is a 16.8-g refill canister only with patient's instructions (NDC 0173-0360-98).

Store between 2° and 30°C (36° and 86°F). As with most inhaled medications in aerosol canisters, the therapeutic effect of this medication may decrease when the canister is cold. Shake well before using.

ANIMAL PHARMACOLOGY AND TOXICOLOGY

Studies in a number of animal species, including rats, rabbits, and dogs, have shown no unusual toxicity during acute experiments. However, the effects of beclomethasone dipropionate in producing signs of glucocorticoid excess during chronic administration by various routes were dose related.

CLINICAL STUDIES

The effects of beclomethasone dipropionate on HPA function have been evaluated in adult volunteers. There was no suppression of early morning plasma cortisol concentrations when beclomethasone dipropionate was administered in a dose of 1,000 mcg per day for 1 month as an aerosol or for 3 days by intramuscular injection. However, partial suppression of plasma cortisol concentration was observed when beclomethasone dipropionate was administered in doses of 2,000 mcg per day either intramuscularly or by aerosol. Immediate suppression of plasma cortisol concentrations was observed after single doses of 4,000 mcg of beclomethasone dipropionate.
In one study the effects of beclomethasone dipropionate on HPA function were examined in patients with asthma. There was no change in basal early morning plasma cortisol concentrations or in the cortisol responses to tetracosactrin (ACTH 1:24) stimulation after daily administration of 400, 800, or 1,200 mcg of beclomethasone dipropionate for 28 days. After daily administration of 1,600 mcg each day for 28 days, there was slight reduction in basal cortisol concentrations and a statistically significant ($p<.01$) reduction in plasma cortisol responses to tetracosactrin stimulation. The effects of a more prolonged period of beclomethasone dipropionate administration on HPA function have not been evaluated. However, a number of investigators have noted that when systemic corticosteroid therapy in asthmatic subjects can be replaced with recommended doses of beclomethasone dipropionate, there is gradual recovery of endogenous cortisol concentrations to the normal range. There is still no documented evidence of recovery from other adverse systemic corticosteroid-induced reactions during prolonged therapy of patients with beclomethasone dipropionate.
Clinical experience has shown that some patients with bronchial asthma who require corticosteroid therapy for control of symptoms can be partially or completely withdrawn from systemic corticosteroids if therapy with beclomethasone dipropionate aerosol is substituted. Beclomethasone dipropionate aerosol is not effective for all patients with bronchial asthma or at all stages of the disease in a given patient.
The early clinical experience has revealed several new problems that may be associated with the use of beclomethasone dipropionate by inhalation for treatment of patients with bronchial asthma.

1. There is a risk of adrenal insufficiency when patients are transferred from systemic corticosteroids to aerosol beclomethasone dipropionate. Although the aerosol may provide adequate control of asthma during the transfer period, it does not provide the systemic steroid that is needed during acute stress situations. Deaths due to adrenal insufficiency have occurred in asthmatic patients during and after transfer from systemic corticosteroids to aerosol beclomethasone dipropionate (see WARNINGS).
2. Transfer of patients from systemic steroid therapy to beclomethasone dipropionate aerosol may unmask allergic conditions that were previously controlled by the systemic steroid therapy, e.g., rhinitis, conjunctivitis, and eczema.
3. Localized infections with *Candida albicans* or *Aspergillus niger* have occurred frequently in the mouth and pharynx and occasionally in the larynx. It has been reported that up to 75% of the patients who receive prolonged treatment with beclomethasone dipropionate have positive oral cultures for *Candida albicans*. The incidence of clinically apparent infection is considerably lower but may require therapy with appropriate antifungal agents or discontinuation of treatment with beclomethasone dipropionate aerosol.

The long-term effects of beclomethasone dipropionate in human subjects are still unknown. In particular, the local effects of the agent on developmental or immunologic processes in the mouth, pharynx, trachea, and lung are unknown. There is also no information about the possible long-term systemic effects of the agent. The possible relevance of the data in animal studies to results in human subjects cannot be evaluated.

Shown in Product Identification Section, page 404

BECONASE® Inhalation Aerosol ℞
[*be'kō-nāz''*]
(beclomethasone dipropionate, USP)
For Nasal Inhalation Only

BECONASE AQ® Nasal Spray, 0.042%*
[*be'kō-nāz''AQ*]
(beclomethasone dipropionate, monohydrate)
***Calculated on the dried basis.** **SHAKE WELL**
For Intranasal Use Only **BEFORE USE.**

DESCRIPTION

Beconase® Inhalation Aerosol:
Beclomethasone dipropionate, USP, the active component of Beconase Inhalation Aerosol, is an anti-inflammatory steroid having the chemical name 9-chloro-11β,17,21-trihydroxy-16β-methylpregna-1, 4-diene-3, 20-dione 17,21-dipropionate.
Beclomethasone dipropionate is a white to creamy-white, odorless powder with a molecular weight of 521.25. It is very slightly soluble in water, very soluble in chloroform, and freely soluble in acetone and in alcohol.
Beconase Inhalation Aerosol is a metered-dose aerosol unit containing a microcrystalline suspension of beclomethasone dipropionate-trichloromonofluoromethane clathrate in a mixture of propellants (trichloromonofluoromethane and dichlorodifluoromethane) with oleic acid. Each canister contains beclomethasone dipropionate-trichloromonofluoromethane clathrate having a molecular proportion of beclomethasone dipropionate to trichloromonofluoromethane between 3:1 and 3:2. Each actuation delivers from the nasal adapter a quantity of clathrate equivalent to 42 mcg of beclomethasone dipropionate, USP. The contents of one canister provide at least 200 metered doses.

Beconase AQ® Nasal Spray:
Beclomethasone dipropionate, monohydrate, the active component of Beconase AQ Nasal Spray, is an anti-inflammatory steroid having the chemical name 9-chloro-11β, 17,21-trihydroxy- 16β-methylpregna-1,4-diene-3,20-dione 17,21-dipropionate, monohydrate.
Beclomethasone dipropionate, monohydrate is a white to creamy-white, odorless powder with a molecular weight of 539.06. It is very slightly soluble in water, very soluble in chloroform, and freely soluble in acetone and in alcohol.
Beconase AQ Nasal Spray is a metered-dose, manual pump spray unit containing a microcrystalline suspension of beclomethasone dipropionate, monohydrate equivalent to 0.042% w/w beclomethasone dipropionate, calculated on the dried basis, in an aqueous medium containing microcrystalline cellulose, carboxymethylcellulose sodium, dextrose, benzalkonium chloride, polysorbate 80, and 0.25% v/w phenylethyl alcohol. Hydrochloric acid may be added to adjust pH. The pH is between 4.5 and 7.0.
After initial priming (three to four actuations), each actuation of the pump delivers from the nasal adapter 100 mg of suspension containing beclomethasone dipropionate, monohydrate equivalent to 42 mcg of beclomethasone dipropionate. Each bottle of Beconase AQ Nasal Spray will provide at least 200 metered doses.

CLINICAL PHARMACOLOGY

Beclomethasone 17,21-dipropionate is a diester of beclomethasone, a synthetic halogenated corticosteroid. Animal studies show that beclomethasone dipropionate has potent glucocorticoid and weak mineralocorticoid activity.
The mechanisms responsible for the anti-inflammatory action of beclomethasone dipropionate are unknown. The precise mechanism of the aerosolized drug's action in the nose is also unknown. Biopsies of nasal mucosa obtained during clinical studies showed no histopathologic changes when beclomethasone dipropionate was administered intranasally.
The effects of beclomethasone dipropionate on hypothalamic-pituitary-adrenal (HPA) function have been evaluated in adult volunteers by other routes of administration. Studies with beclomethasone dipropionate by the intranasal route may demonstrate that there is more or that there is less absorption by this route of administration. There was no suppression of early morning plasma cortisol concentrations when beclomethasone dipropionate was administered in a dose of 1,000 mcg per day for 1 month as an oral aerosol or for 3 days by intramuscular injection. However, partial suppression of plasma cortisol concentrations was observed when beclomethasone dipropionate was administered in doses of 2,000 mcg per day either by oral aerosol or intramuscular injection. Immediate suppression of plasma cortisol concentrations was observed after single doses of 4,000 mcg of beclomethasone dipropionate. Suppression of HPA function (reduction of early morning plasma cortisol levels) has been reported in adult patients who received 1,600-mcg daily doses of oral beclomethasone dipropionate for 1 month. In clinical studies using beclomethasone dipropionate aerosol intranasally, there was no evidence of adrenal insufficiency. The effect of Beconase AQ® (beclomethasone dipropionate, monohydrate) Nasal Spray on HPA function was not evaluated but would not be expected to differ from intranasal beclomethasone dipropionate aerosol.
In one study in asthmatic children, the administration of inhaled beclomethasone at recommended daily doses for at least 1 year was associated with a reduction in nocturnal cortisol secretion. The clinical significance of this finding is not clear. It reinforces other evidence, however, that topical beclomethasone may be absorbed in amounts that can have systemic effects and that physicians should be alert for evidence of systemic effects, especially in chronically treated patients (see PRECAUTIONS).
Beclomethasone dipropionate is sparingly soluble. When given by nasal inhalation in the form of an aqueous or aerosolized suspension, the drug is deposited primarily in the nasal passages. A portion of the drug is swallowed. Absorption occurs rapidly from all respiratory and gastrointestinal tissues. There is no evidence of tissue storage of beclomethasone dipropionate or its metabolites. *In vitro* studies have shown that tissue other than the liver (lung slices) can rapidly metabolize beclomethasone dipropionate to beclomethasone 17-monopropionate and more slowly to free beclomethasone (which has very weak anti-inflammatory activity). However, irrespective of the route of entry, the principal route of excretion of the drug and its metabolites is the feces. In humans, 12%–15% of an orally administered dose of beclomethasone dipropionate is excreted in the urine as both conjugated and free metabolites of the drug.
Studies have shown that the degree of binding to plasma proteins is 87%.

INDICATIONS AND USAGE

Beconase® (beclomethasone dipropionate) Inhalation Aerosol is indicated for the relief of the symptoms of seasonal or perennial rhinitis in those cases poorly responsive to conventional treatment. **Beconase AQ® (beclomethasone dipropionate, monohydrate) Nasal Spray** is indicated for the relief of the symptoms of seasonal or perennial allergic and nonallergic (vasomotor) rhinitis.
Both preparations are also indicated for the prevention of recurrence of nasal polyps following surgical removal.
Clinical studies with Beconase Inhalation Aerosol in patients with seasonal or perennial rhinitis have shown that improvement is usually apparent within a few days. Results from two clinical trials have shown that significant symptomatic relief was obtained with Beconase AQ Nasal Spray within 3 days. With either preparation, however, symptomatic relief may not occur in some patients for as long as 2 weeks. Although systemic effects are minimal at recommended doses, Beconase Inhalation Aerosol and Beconase AQ Nasal Spray should not be continued beyond 3 weeks in the absence of significant symptomatic improvement. Both preparations should not be used in the presence of untreated localized infection involving the nasal mucosa.
Clinical studies have shown that treatment of the symptoms associated with nasal polyps may have to be continued for several weeks or more before a therapeutic result can be

Continued on next page

Allen & Hanburys—Cont.

fully assessed. Recurrence of symptoms due to polyps can occur after stopping treatment, depending on the severity of the disease.

CONTRAINDICATIONS

Hypersensitivity to any of the ingredients of either preparation contraindicates its use.

WARNINGS

The replacement of a systemic corticosteroid with Beconase® (beclomethasone dipropionate) Inhalation Aerosol or Beconase AQ® (beclomethasone dipropionate, monohydrate) Nasal Spray can be accompanied by signs of adrenal insufficiency.

Careful attention must be given when patients previously treated for prolonged periods with systemic corticosteroids are transferred to Beconase Inhalation Aerosol or Beconase AQ Nasal Spray. This is particularly important in those patients who have associated asthma or other clinical conditions where too rapid a decrease in systemic corticosteroids may cause a severe exacerbation of their symptoms. Studies have shown that the combined administration of alternate-day prednisone systemic treatment and orally inhaled beclomethasone increases the likelihood of HPA suppression compared with a therapeutic dose of either one alone. Therefore, Beconase Inhalation Aerosol and Beconase AQ Nasal Spray treatment should be used with caution in patients already on alternate-day prednisone regimens for any disease.

If recommended doses of intranasal beclomethasone are exceeded or if individuals are particularly sensitive or predisposed by virtue of recent systemic steroid therapy, symptoms of hypercorticism may occur, including very rare cases of menstrual irregularities, acneiform lesions, and cushingoid features. If such changes occur, Beconase Inhalation Aerosol and Beconase AQ Nasal Spray should be discontinued slowly consistent with accepted procedures for discontinuing oral steroid therapy.

Children who are on immunosuppressant drugs are more susceptible to infections than healthy children. Chickenpox and measles, for example, can have a more serious or even fatal course in children on immunosuppressant corticosteroids. In such children, or in adults who have not had these diseases, particular care should be taken to avoid exposure. If exposed, therapy with varicella zoster immune globulin (VZIG) or pooled intravenous immunoglobulin (IVIG), as appropriate, may be indicated. If chickenpox develops, treatment with antiviral agents may be considered.

PRECAUTIONS

General: During withdrawal from oral steroids, some patients may experience symptoms of withdrawal, e.g., joint and/or muscular pain, lassitude, and depression.

In clinical studies with beclomethasone dipropionate administered intranasally, the development of localized infections of the nose and pharynx with *Candida albicans* has occurred only rarely. When such an infection develops, it may require treatment with appropriate local therapy or discontinuation of treatment with Beconase® (beclomethasone dipropionate) Inhalation Aerosol or Beconase AQ® (beclomethasone dipropionate, monohydrate) Nasal Spray.

Beclomethasone dipropionate is absorbed into the circulation. Use of excessive doses of Beconase Inhalation Aerosol or Beconase AQ Nasal Spray may suppress HPA function. Beconase Inhalation Aerosol and Beconase AQ Nasal Spray should be used with caution, if at all, in patients with active or quiescent tuberculous infections of the respiratory tract; untreated fungal, bacterial, or systemic viral infections; or ocular herpes simplex.

For either preparation to be effective in the treatment of nasal polyps, the aerosol or spray must be able to enter the nose. Therefore, treatment of nasal polyps with these preparations should be considered adjunctive therapy to surgical removal and/or the use of other medications that will permit effective penetration of these preparations into the nose. Nasal polyps may recur after any form of treatment.

As with any long-term treatment, patients using Beconase Inhalation Aerosol or Beconase AQ Nasal Spray over several months or longer should be examined periodically for possible changes in the nasal mucosa.

Because of the inhibitory effect of corticosteroids on wound healing, patients who have experienced recent nasal septum ulcers, nasal surgery, or trauma should not use a nasal corticosteroid until healing has occurred.

Although systemic effects have been minimal with recommended doses, this potential increases with excessive doses. Therefore, larger than recommended doses of Beconase Inhalation Aerosol and Beconase AQ Nasal Spray should be avoided.

Beconase Inhalation Aerosol: Rare instances of nasal septum perforation have been spontaneously reported.

Rare instances of increased intraocular pressure have been reported following the intranasal application of aerosolized corticosteroids.

Beconase AQ Nasal Spray: Rarely, immediate hypersensitivity reactions may occur after the intranasal administration of beclomethasone.

Extremely rare instances of wheezing, nasal septum perforation, and increased intraocular pressure have been reported following the intranasal application of aerosolized corticosteroids. Although these have not been observed in clinical trials with Beconase AQ Nasal Spray, vigilance should be maintained.

If persistent nasopharyngeal irritation occurs, it may be an indication for stopping Beconase AQ Nasal Spray.

Information for Patients: Patients being treated with Beconase Inhalation Aerosol or Beconase AQ Nasal Spray should receive the following information and instructions. This information is intended to aid in the safe and effective use of this medication. It is not a disclosure of all possible adverse or intended effects. Patients should use these preparations at regular intervals since their effectiveness depends on their regular use. The patient should take the medication as directed. It is not acutely effective, and the prescribed dosage should not be increased. Instead, nasal vasoconstrictors or oral antihistamines may be needed until the effects of Beconase Inhalation Aerosol or Beconase AQ Nasal Spray are fully manifested. One to 2 weeks may pass before full relief is obtained. The patient should contact the physician if symptoms do not improve, or if the condition worsens, or if sneezing or nasal irritation occurs. For the proper use of either unit and to attain maximum improvement, the patient should read and follow carefully the patient's instructions section of the package insert.

Patients who are on immunosuppressant doses of corticosteroids should be warned to avoid exposure to chickenpox or measles and, if exposed, to obtain medical advice.

Carcinogenesis, Mutagenesis, Impairment of Fertility: Treatment of rats for a total of 95 weeks, 13 weeks by inhalation and 82 weeks by the oral route, resulted in no evidence of carcinogenic activity. Mutagenic studies have not been performed.

Impairment of fertility, as evidenced by inhibition of the estrous cycle in dogs, was observed following treatment by the oral route. No inhibition of the estrous cycle in dogs was seen following treatment with beclomethasone dipropionate by the inhalation route.

Pregnancy: *Teratogenic Effects: Pregnancy Category C:* Like other corticoids, parenteral (subcutaneous) beclomethasone dipropionate has been shown to be teratogenic and embryocidal in the mouse and rabbit when given in doses approximately 10 times the human dose. In these studies, beclomethasone was found to produce fetal resorption, cleft palate, agnathia, microstomia, absence of tongue, delayed ossification, and agenesis of the thymus. No teratogenic or embryocidal effects have been seen in the rat when beclomethasone dipropionate was administered by inhalation at 10 times the human dose or orally at 1,000 times the human dose. There are no adequate and well-controlled studies in pregnant women. Beclomethasone dipropionate should be used during pregnancy only if the potential benefit justifies the potential risk to the fetus.

Nonteratogenic Effects: Hypoadrenalism may occur in infants born of mothers receiving corticosteroids during pregnancy. Such infants should be carefully observed.

Nursing Mothers: It is not known whether beclomethasone dipropionate is excreted in human milk. Because other corticosteroids are excreted in human milk, caution should be exercised when Beconase Inhalation Aerosol or Beconase AQ Nasal Spray is administered to a nursing woman.

Pediatric Use: Safety and effectiveness in children below 6 years of age have not been established.

ADVERSE REACTIONS

In general, side effects in clinical studies with both preparations have been primarily associated with irritation of the nasal mucous membranes.

Rare cases of immediate and delayed hypersensitivity reactions, including urticaria, angioedema, rash, and bronchospasm, have been reported following the oral and intranasal inhalation and administration of beclomethasone.

Beconase® (beclomethasone dipropionate) Inhalation Aerosol: Adverse reactions reported in controlled clinical trials and long-term open studies in patients treated with Beconase Inhalation Aerosol are described below.

Sensations of irritation and burning in the nose (11 per 100 patients) following the use of Beconase Inhalation Aerosol have been reported. Also, occasional sneezing attacks (10 per 100 adult patients) have occurred immediately following the use of the intranasal inhaler. This symptom may be more common in children. Rhinorrhea may occur occasionally (1 per 100 patients).

Localized infections of the nose and pharynx with *Candida albicans* have occurred rarely (see PRECAUTIONS).

Transient episodes of epistaxis have been reported in 2 per 100 patients.

Rare cases of ulceration of the nasal mucosa and instances of nasal septum perforation have been spontaneously reported (see PRECAUTIONS).

Rare instances of increased intraocular pressure have been reported following the intranasal application of aerosolized corticosteroids (see PRECAUTIONS).

Systemic corticosteroid side effects were not reported during controlled clinical trials. If recommended doses are exceeded, however, or if individuals are particularly sensitive, symptoms of hypercorticism, i.e., Cushing's syndrome, could occur.

Beconase AQ® (beclomethasone dipropionate, monohydrate) Nasal Spray: Adverse reactions reported in controlled clinical trials and open studies in patients treated with Beconase AQ Nasal Spray are described below.

Mild nasopharyngeal irritation following the use of beclomethasone aqueous nasal spray has been reported in up to 24% of patients treated, including occasional sneezing attacks (about 4%) occurring immediately following use of the spray. In patients experiencing these symptoms, none had to discontinue treatment. The incidence of transient irritation and sneezing was approximately the same in the group of patients who received placebo in these studies, implying that these complaints may be related to vehicle components of the formulation.

Fewer than 5 per 100 patients reported headache, nausea, or lightheadedness following the use of Beconase AQ Nasal Spray. Fewer than 3 per 100 patients reported nasal stuffiness, nosebleeds, rhinorrhea, or tearing eyes.

Extremely rare instances of wheezing, nasal septum perforation, and increased intraocular pressure have been reported following the intranasal administration of aerosolized corticosteroids (see PRECAUTIONS).

OVERDOSAGE

When used at excessive doses, systemic corticosteroid effects such as hypercorticism and adrenal suppression may appear. If such changes occur, the dosage of Beconase® (beclomethasone dipropionate) Inhalation Aerosol should be decreased, and Beconase AQ® (beclomethasone dipropionate, monohydrate) Nasal Spray should be discontinued slowly consistent with accepted procedures for discontinuing oral steroid therapy. The oral LD_{50} of beclomethasone dipropionate is greater than 1 g/kg in rodents. One canister of Beconase Inhalation Aerosol contains 8.4 mg of beclomethasone dipropionate, and one bottle of Beconase AQ Nasal Spray contains beclomethasone dipropionate, monohydrate equivalent to 10.5 mg of beclomethasone dipropionate; therefore, acute overdosage is unlikely.

DOSAGE AND ADMINISTRATION

Beconase® (beclomethasone dipropionate) Inhalation Aerosol: *Adults and Children 12 Years of Age and Older:* The usual dosage is one inhalation (42 mcg) in each nostril two to four times a day (total dose, 168–336 mcg per day). Patients can often be maintained on a maximum dose of one inhalation in each nostril three times a day (252 mcg per day). *Children 6–12 Years of Age:* The usual dosage is one inhalation in each nostril three times a day (252 mcg per day). Beconase Inhalation Aerosol is *not* recommended for children below 6 years of age since safety and efficacy studies have not been conducted in this age-group.

CONTENTS UNDER PRESSURE. Do not puncture. Do not use or store near heat or open flame. Exposure to temperatures above 120°F may cause bursting. Never throw container into fire or incinerator. Keep out of reach of children.

Beconase AQ® (beclomethasone dipropionate, monohydrate) Nasal Spray: *Adults and Children 6 Years of Age and Older:* The usual dosage is one or two inhalations (42–84 mcg) in each nostril twice a day (total dose, 168–336 mcg per day).

Beconase AQ Nasal Spray is *not* recommended for children below 6 years of age.

In patients who respond to Beconase Inhalation Aerosol and to Beconase AQ Nasal Spray, an improvement of the symptoms of seasonal or perennial rhinitis usually becomes apparent within a few days after the start of therapy. However, symptomatic relief may not occur in some patients for as long as 2 weeks. Beconase Inhalation Aerosol and Beconase AQ Nasal Spray should not be continued beyond 3 weeks in the absence of significant symptomatic improvement.

The therapeutic effects of corticosteroids, unlike those of decongestants, are not immediate. This should be explained to the patient using either preparation in advance in order to ensure cooperation and continuation of treatment with the prescribed dosage regimen.

In the presence of excessive nasal mucous secretion or edema of the nasal mucosa, the drug may fail to reach the site of intended action. In such cases it is advisable to use a nasal vasoconstrictor during the first 2–3 days of Beconase Inhalation Aerosol or Beconase AQ Nasal Spray therapy.

Directions for Use: Illustrated patient's instructions for use accompany each package of Beconase Inhalation Aerosol and Beconase AQ Nasal Spray.

HOW SUPPLIED

Beconase® (beclomethasone dipropionate) Inhalation Aerosol is supplied in a 16.8-g canister containing 200 metered

doses with beige compact actuator and patient's instructions (NDC 0173-0336-02). Also available is a 16.8-g refill canister only with patient's instructions (NDC 0173-0360-98).
Store between 2° and 30°C (36° and 86°F). As with most inhaled medications in aerosol canisters, the therapeutic effect of this medication may decrease when the canister is cold. Shake well before using.
Beconase AQ® (beclomethasone dipropionate, monohydrate) Nasal Spray, 0.042%* is supplied in an amber glass bottle fitted with a metering atomizing pump and nasal adapter in a box of one (NDC 0173-0388-79) with patient's instructions for use. Each bottle contains 25 g of suspension.
Store between 15° and 30°C (59° and 86°F).

*Calculated on the dried basis.

Shown in Product Identification Section, page 404

CEFTIN® Tablets ℞
[*sef'tin*]
(cefuroxime axetil)

DESCRIPTION

Ceftin® (cefuroxime axetil) Tablets contain a semisynthetic, broad-spectrum cephalosporin antibiotic for oral administration. Cefuroxime axetil is the 1-(acetyloxy) ethyl ester of cefuroxime (Zinacef®, Glaxo), which in turn is chemically designated as (6R,7R)-3-carbamoyloxymethyl-7- [Z-2-methoxyimino-2- (fur-2-yl)acetamido] ceph-3-em-4-carboxylate. Cefuroxime axetil is in the amorphous form.
Each Ceftin Tablet contains the equivalent of 125, 250, or 500 mg of cefuroxime. Each tablet also contains the inactive ingredients colloidal silicon dioxide, croscarmellose sodium, FD&C Blue No. 1 (250- and 500-mg tablets only), hydrogenated vegetable oil, hydroxypropyl methylcellulose, methylparaben, microcrystalline cellulose, propylene glycol, propylparaben, sodium benzoate (125-mg tablets only), sodium lauryl sulfate, and titanium dioxide.

CLINICAL PHARMACOLOGY

After oral administration, cefuroxime axetil is absorbed from the gastrointestinal tract and rapidly hydrolyzed by nonspecific esterases in the intestinal mucosa and blood to release cefuroxime into the circulation. Cefuroxime is subsequently distributed throughout the extracellular fluids. The axetil moiety is metabolized to acetaldehyde and acetic acid. Cefuroxime is excreted unchanged in the urine.
Serum cefuroxime concentrations and urinary excretion data are shown in the table below.

Bioavailability of Cefuroxime Administered as Cefuroxime Axetil

Dose* (Cefuroxime Equivalent)	Serum Cefuroxime Concentration† (mcg/mL)		12-h Urinary Excretion† (% of dose)
	Peak	6 h	
125 mg	2.1	0.3	52
250 mg	4.1	0.7	51
500 mg	7.0	2.2	48
1,000 mg	13.6	3.4	43

*Administered immediately after a meal.
†Mean values of 12 normal volunteers. Peak concentrations occurred around 2 hours after the dose.

While cefuroxime axetil can be taken after food or on an empty stomach, absorption is greater when taken after food (absolute bioavailability of 52% compared with 37%). Peak serum cefuroxime concentrations after a 500-mg dose are also greater when taken with food (mean = 7.0 mcg/mL) compared with the fasting state (mean = 4.9 mcg/mL). Despite this difference in absorption, the clinical and bacteriologic responses of patients were independent of food intake at the time of dosing in two studies where this was assessed.
Approximately 50% of serum cefuroxime is bound to protein. The half-life of cefuroxime after oral administration of Ceftin® (cefuroxime axetil) Tablets is 1.2 hours. Concomitant administration of probenecid increases the area under the serum concentration versus time curve by 50%. Peak serum cefuroxime concentration after a 1.5-g single dose is greater when taken with 1 g of probenecid (mean = 14.8 mcg/mL) than without probenecid (mean = 12.2 mcg/mL). Concomitant probenecid also increases the time for which serum cefuroxime concentrations exceed 0.25 mcg/mL from 10.7 hours to 14.0 hours.
Pharmacokinetic studies of cefuroxime axetil in elderly patients indicate that a dosage adjustment based on age is not necessary. Since cefuroxime is renally eliminated, however, the serum half-life is increased in elderly patients with declining renal function associated with normal aging. In a study of twenty elderly patients (mean age=83.9 years) having a mean creatinine clearance of 34.9 mL per minute, the mean serum elimination half-life was 3.5 hours.

Microbiology: The *in vivo* bactericidal activity of cefuroxime axetil is due to cefuroxime. Cefuroxime has bactericidal activity against a wide range of common pathogens, including many beta-lactamase-producing strains.
Cefuroxime is highly stable to bacterial beta-lactamases, especially plasmid-mediated enzymes that are commonly found in Enterobacteriaceae. The bactericidal action of cefuroxime results from inhibition of cell-wall synthesis by binding to essential target proteins.
Cefuroxime has been shown to be active against most strains of the following organisms both *in vitro* and in clinical infections (see INDICATIONS AND USAGE):
Gram-positive: *Staphylococcus aureus, Streptococcus pneumoniae, and Streptococcus pyogenes.*
NOTE: Certain strains of enterococci, e.g., *Enterococcus faecalis* (formerly *Streptococcus faecalis*), are resistant to cefuroxime. Methicillin-resistant staphylococci are resistant to cefuroxime.
Gram-negative: *Moraxella (Branhamella) catarrhalis, Escherichia coli, Haemophilus influenzae, Haemophilus parainfluenzae, Klebsiella pneumoniae,* and *Neisseria gonorrhoeae* (non–penicillinase-producing strains).
NOTE: *Pseudomonas* spp. and *Campylobacter* spp., *Acinetobacter calcoaceticus,* and most strains of *Serratia* spp. and *Proteus vulgaris* are resistant to most first- and second-generation cephalosporins. Some strains of *Morganella morganii, Enterobacter cloacae, and Citrobacter* spp. have been shown by *in vitro* tests to be resistant to cefuroxime and other cephalosporins.
Cefuroxime has been shown to be active *in vitro* against the following micoorganisms; however, the clinical significance of these findings is unknown.
Gram-positive: *Staphylococcus epidermidis, Staphylococcus saprophyticus,* and *Streptococcus agalactiae.*
Gram-negative: *Citrobacter* spp., *Enterobacter* spp., *Klebsiella* spp., *Morganella morganii, Neisseria gonorrhoeae* (including penicillinase- and non–penicillinase-producing strains), *Proteus inconstans, Proteus mirabilis, Providencia rettgeri, Salmonella* spp., *and Shigella* spp.
Anaerobes: *Bacteroides* spp., *Clostridium* spp., *Fusobacterium* spp., *Peptococcus* spp., *Peptostreptococcus* spp., and *Propionibacterium* spp.
NOTE: Most strains of *Clostridium difficile* and *Bacteroides fragilis* are resistant to cefuroxime.
Susceptibility Tests: *Diffusion Techniques:* Quantitative methods that require measurement of zone diameters give the most precise estimate of antibiotic susceptibility. One such standard procedure[1] that has been recommended for use with disks to test susceptibility of organisms to cefuroxime uses the 30-mcg cefuroxime disk. Interpretation involves the correlation of the diameters obtained in the disk test with the minimum inhibitory concentration (MIC) for cefuroxime.
Reports from the laboratory giving results of the standard single-disk susceptibility test with a 30-mcg cefuroxime disk should be interpreted according to the following criteria:

Zone diameter (mm)	Interpretation
≥ 23	(S) Susceptible
15–22	(MS) Moderately Susceptible
≤ 14	(R) Resistant

A report of "Susceptible" indicates that the pathogen is likely to be inhibited by generally achievable blood levels. A report of "Moderately Susceptible" suggests that the organism would be susceptible if high dosage is used or if the infection is confined to tissues and fluids in which high antibiotic levels are attained. A report of "Resistant" indicates that achievable concentrations of the antibiotic are unlikely to be inhibitory and other therapy should be selected.
Standardized procedures require the use of laboratory control organisms. The 30-mcg cefuroxime disk should give the following zone diameters:

Organism	Zone Diameter (mm)
Staphylococcus aureus ATCC 25923	27–35
Escherichia coli ATCC 25922	20–26

Dilution Techniques: Use a standardized dilution method[2] (broth, agar, microdilution) or equivalent with cefuroxime powder. The MIC values obtained should be interpreted according to the following criteria:

MIC (mcg/mL)	Interpretation
≤ 4	(S) Susceptible
8–16	(MS) Moderately Susceptible
≥ 32	(R) Resistant

As with standard diffusion techniques, dilution methods require the use of laboratory control organisms. Standard cefuroxime powder should provide the following MIC values:

Organism	MIC (mcg/mL)
Staphylococcus aureus ATCC 29213	0.5–2
Escherichia coli ATCC 25922	2–8

INDICATIONS AND USAGE

Ceftin® (cefuroxime axetil) Tablets are indicated for the treatment of patients with infections caused by susceptible strains of the designated organisms in the following diseases:

1. **Pharyngitis and Tonsillitis** caused by *Streptococcus pyogenes.* (Penicillin is the usual drug of choice in the treatment and prevention of streptococcal infections, including the prophylaxis of rheumatic fever. Ceftin Tablets are generally effective in the eradication of streptococci from the oropharynx.Ceftin Tablets are not indicated for the prophylaxis of subsequent rheumatic fever because data to support such use are not yet available.)
2. **Otitis Media** caused by *Streptococcus pneumoniae, Haemophilus influenzae* (ampicillin-susceptible and ampicillin-resistant strains), *Moraxella (Branhamella) catarrhalis* and *Streptococcus pyogenes.*
3. **Lower Respiratory Tract Infections** (bronchitis) caused by *Streptococcus pneumoniae, Haemophilus influenzae* (ampicillin-susceptible strains), and *Haemophilus parainfluenzae* (ampicillin-susceptible strains).
4. **Urinary Tract Infections** caused by *Escherichia coli* and *Klebsiella pneumoniae* in the absence of urological complications.
5. **Skin and Skin Structure Infections** caused by *Staphylococcus aureus* and *Streptococcus pyogenes.*
6. **Uncomplicated Gonorrhea** (urethral and endocervical) caused by non–penicillinase-producing strains of *Neisseria gonorrhoeae.*

Bacteriologic studies to determine the causative organism and its susceptibility to cefuroxime should be performed. Therapy may be started while awaiting the results of these studies. Once these results become available, antibiotic treatment should be adjusted accordingly.

CONTRAINDICATIONS

Ceftin® (cefuroxime axetil) Tablets are contraindicated in patients with known allergy to the cephalosporin group of antibiotics.

WARNINGS

BEFORE THERAPY WITH CEFTIN® (CEFUROXIME AXETIL) TABLETS IS INSTITUTED, CAREFUL INQUIRY SHOULD BE MADE TO DETERMINE WHETHER THE PATIENT HAS HAD PREVIOUS HYPERSENSITIVITY REACTIONS TO CEPHALOSPORINS, PENICILLINS, OR OTHER DRUGS. IF THIS PRODUCT IS TO BE GIVEN TO PENICILLIN-SENSITIVE PATIENTS, CAUTION SHOULD BE EXERCISED BECAUSE CROSS-HYPERSENSITIVITY AMONG BETA-LACTAM ANTIBIOTICS HAS BEEN CLEARLY DOCUMENTED AND MAY OCCUR IN UP TO 10% OF PATIENTS WITH A HISTORY OF PENICILLIN ALLERGY. ANTIBIOTICS SHOULD BE ADMINISTERED WITH CAUTION TO ANY PATIENT WHO HAS DEMONSTRATED SOME FORM OF ALLERGY, PARTICULARLY TO DRUGS. IF AN ALLERGIC REACTION TO CEFTIN TABLETS OCCURS, DISCONTINUE THE DRUG. SERIOUS ACUTE HYPERSENSITIVITY REACTIONS MAY REQUIRE TREATMENT WITH EPINEPHRINE AND OTHER EMERGENCY MEASURES, INCLUDING OXYGEN, INTRAVENOUS FLUIDS, INTRAVENOUS ANTIHISTAMINES, CORTICOSTEROIDS, PRESSOR AMINES, AND AIRWAY MANAGEMENT, AS CLINICALLY INDICATED.
Pseudomembranous colitis has been reported with nearly all antibacterial agents, including cefuroxime, and may range from mild to life-threatening. Therefore, it is important to consider this diagnosis in patients who present with diarrhea subsequent to the administration of antibacterial agents.
Treatment with broad-spectrum antibiotics alters normal flora of the colon and may permit overgrowth of clostridia. Studies indicate that a toxin produced by *Clostridium difficile* is one primary cause of antibiotic-associated colitis. Cholestyramine and colestipol resins have been shown to bind the toxin *in vitro.*
Mild cases of colitis may respond to drug discontinuation alone. Moderate to severe cases should be managed with fluid, electrolyte, and protein supplementation as indicated. Elderly patients may be susceptible to fluid losses and should be treated aggressively.
When the colitis is not relieved by drug discontinuation or when it is severe, metronidazole and oral vancomycin have been shown to be beneficial. Oral vancomycin is the treatment of choice for antibiotic-associated pseudomembranous colitis produced by *Clostridium difficile.* Other causes of colitis should also be considered.

PRECAUTIONS

General: If an allergic reaction to Ceftin® (cefuroxime axetil) Tablets occurs, the drug should be discontinued, and, if necessary, the patient should be treated with appropriate agents, e.g., antihistamines, pressor amines, or corticosteroids.
As with other antibiotics, prolonged use of Ceftin Tablets may result in overgrowth of nonsusceptible organisms. If superinfection occurs during therapy, appropriate measures should be taken.
Broad-spectrum antibiotics should be prescribed with caution for individuals with a history of colitis.
Information for Patients: (Pediatric) Ceftin is only available in tablet form. During clinical trials, the tablet was well tolerated by children who could swallow the tablet whole. Chil-

Continued on next page

Allen & Hanburys—Cont.

dren who cannot swallow the tablet whole may have the tablet crushed and mixed with food (e.g., applesauce, ice cream). However, it should be noted that the crushed tablet has a strong, persistent, bitter taste. Discontinuation of therapy due to the taste and/or problems of administering this drug occurred in 13% of children (range, 2%–28% across centers). Thus, the physician and parent should ascertain, preferably while still in the physician's office, that the child can ingest Ceftin Tablets reliably. If not, alternative therapy should be considered.

Geriatric Use: In clinical trials involving 1,349 adult patients treated with Ceftin, 241 (17.9%) patients were 65 years of age or older. No overall differences in effectiveness were observed between elderly patients and younger patients, although the rate of drug-related adverse reactions was significantly lower in elderly (9.6%) than in younger (14.6%) patients. No clinically important differences in laboratory results were observed between elderly patients and younger patients treated with Ceftin.

Drug/Laboratory Test Interactions: A false-positive reaction for glucose in the urine may occur with copper reduction tests (Benedict's or Fehling's solution or with Clinitest® tablets), but not with enzyme-based tests for glycosuria (e.g., Clinistix®, Tes-Tape®). As a false-negative result may occur in the ferricyanide test, it is recommended that either the glucose oxidase or hexokinase method be used to determine blood plasma glucose levels in patients receiving Ceftin Tablets.

Cefuroxime does not interfere with the assay of serum and urine creatinine by the alkaline picrate method.

Carcinogenesis, Mutagenesis, Impairment of Fertility: Although no long-term studies in animals have been performed to evaluate carcinogenic potential, no mutagenic potential of cefuroxime was found in standard laboratory tests.

Reproductive studies revealed no impairment of fertility in animals.

Pregnancy: ***Pregnancy Category B:*** Reproduction studies have been performed in rats and mice at doses up to 50–160 times the human dose and have revealed no evidence of impaired fertility or harm to the fetus due to cefuroxime axetil. There are, however, no adequate and well-controlled studies in pregnant women. Because animal reproduction studies are not always predictive of human response, this drug should be used during pregnancy only if clearly needed.

Nursing Mothers: Since cefuroxime is excreted in human milk, consideration should be given to discontinuing nursing temporarily during treatment with Ceftin Tablets.

Pediatric Use: See DOSAGE AND ADMINISTRATION.

ADVERSE REACTIONS

The adverse reactions to Ceftin® (cefuroxime axetil) Tablets are similar to reactions to other orally administered cephalosporins. Ceftin Tablets were usually well tolerated in controlled clinical trials. Pediatric patients taking crushed tablets during clinical trials complained of the bitter taste of Ceftin Tablets (see ADVERSE REACTIONS: Gastrointestinal and PRECAUTIONS: Information for Patients: (Pediatric)). The majority of adverse events were mild, reversible in nature, and did not require discontinuation of the drug. The incidence of gastrointestinal adverse events increased with the higher recommended doses. Twenty-five (25) patients have received Ceftin Tablets 500 mg twice a day for 1–2.5 months with no increase in frequency or severity of adverse events.

The following adverse reactions have been reported in clinical trials using dosage regimens of 125–500 mg twice a day.

Gastrointestinal: Nausea occurred in 2.4% of patients. Vomiting occurred in 2.0% of patients. Diarrhea occurred in 3.5% of patients. Loose stools occurred in 1.3% of patients. Onset of pseudomembranous colitis symptoms may occur during or after antibiotic treatment (see WARNINGS).

Crushed tablets have a bitter taste. In pediatric clinical studies conducted with crushed tablets, complaints due to taste ranged from 0/8 (0%) in one center to 47/71 (66%) in another center.

Hypersensitivity: Rash (0.6% of patients), pruritus (0.3% of patients), and urticaria (0.2% of patients) have been observed. One case of severe bronchospasm has been reported among the approximately 1,600 patients treated with Ceftin Tablets. Of the patients treated with Ceftin Tablets who reported a history of delayed hypersensitivity to a penicillin and not a cephalosporin, 2.9% of patients experienced a delayed hypersensitivity reaction to Ceftin Tablets.

Hypersensitivity reactions including Stevens-Johnson syndrome, erythema multiforme, toxic epidermal necrolysis, drug fever, serum sickness-like reactions, and anaphylaxis have been reported.

Central Nervous System: Headache occurred in less than 0.7% of patients, and dizziness occurred in less than 0.2% of patients.

Vaginitis, including vaginal candidiasis, occurred in 1.9% of female patients.

Clinical Laboratory Tests: Transient elevations in AST (SGOT, 2.0% of patients), ALT (SGPT, 1.6% of patients), and LDH (1.0% of patients) have been observed. Eosinophilia (1.1% of patients) and positive Coombs' test (0.4% of patients) have been reported.

Adverse Reactions Following a Single Oral 1-g Dose for the Treatment of Gonorrhea: The incidence of drug-related adverse experiences in patients treated for gonorrhea who received a single 1-g dose of cefuroxime axetil was 16%. The most common adverse experiences were diarrhea (4.8%), nausea (4.6%), vomiting (2.5%), abdominal pain (1.2%), and dizziness (1.2%).

In addition to the adverse reactions listed above that have been observed in patients treated with Ceftin Tablets, the following adverse reactions and altered laboratory tests have been reported for cephalosporin class antibiotics:

Adverse Reactions: Renal dysfunction, toxic nephropathy, hepatic dysfunction including cholestasis, abdominal pain, superinfection, aplastic anemia, hemolytic anemia, hemorrhage, and pain and/or phlebitis at the injection site.

Several cephalosporins have been implicated in triggering seizures, particularly in patients with renal impairment when the dosage was not reduced. If seizures associated with drug therapy should occur, the drug should be discontinued. Anticonvulsant therapy can be given if clinically indicated.

Altered Laboratory Tests: Increased prothrombin time, increased BUN, increased creatinine, false-positive test for urinary glucose, increased alkaline phosphatase, neutropenia, thrombocytopenia, leukopenia, elevated bilirubin, pancytopenia, and agranulocytosis.

OVERDOSAGE

Overdosage of cephalosporins can cause cerebral irritation leading to convulsions. Serum levels of cefuroxime can be reduced by hemodialysis and peritoneal dialysis.

DOSAGE AND ADMINISTRATION

Ceftin® (cefuroxime axetil) Tablets may be given orally without regard to meals. However, absorption is enhanced when Ceftin Tablets are administered with food.

Adults and Children 12 Years of Age and Older: The recommended dosage is 250 mg twice a day. For more severe infections or infections caused by less susceptible organisms, the dosage may be increased to 500 mg twice a day.

For uncomplicated urinary tract infections, the usual recommended dosage is 125 mg twice a day. Dosage may be increased to 250 mg twice a day for some patients with urinary tract infections.

Geriatric Use: In clinical trials involving patients 65 years of age and older, no overall differences in effectiveness were observed between elderly patients and younger patients, although the rate of drug-related adverse reactions was significantly lower in elderly (9.6%) than in younger (14.6%) patients (see PRECAUTIONS: Geriatric Use). Therefore, no adjustment of the usual adult dose is necessary.

Treatment of Gonorrhea: A single oral 1-g dose is recommended for treating uncomplicated urethral and endocervical gonorrhea.

Infants and Children Up to 12 Years of Age: The recommended dosage for children is 125 mg twice a day. For children with otitis media, the recommended dosage is 125 mg twice a day for children less than 2 years of age and 250 mg twice a day for children 2 years of age and older.

Ceftin Tablets administered as a crushed tablet have a strong, persistent, bitter taste. Alternative therapy should be considered for children who cannot swallow tablets (see PRECAUTIONS: Information for Patients: (Pediatric)).

In the treatment of infections due to *Streptococcus pyogenes*, a therapeutic dosage of Ceftin Tablets should be administered for at least 10 days.

HOW SUPPLIED

Ceftin® (cefuroxime axetil) Tablets, 125 mg, are white, capsule-shaped, film-coated tablets engraved with "395" on one side and "GLAXO" on the other in bottles of 20 (NDC 0173-0395-00) and 60 (NDC 0173-0395-01) and unit dose packs of 100 (NDC 0173-0395-02).

Ceftin Tablets, 250 mg, are light blue, capsule-shaped, film-coated tablets engraved with "387" on one side and "GLAXO" on the other in bottles of 20 (NDC 0173-0387-00) and 60 (NDC 0173-0387-42) and unit dose packs of 100 (NDC 0173-0387-01).

Ceftin Tablets, 500 mg, are dark blue, capsule-shaped, film-coated tablets engraved with "394" on one side and "GLAXO" on the other in bottles of 20 (NDC 0173-0394-00) and 60 (NDC 0173-0394-42) and unit dose packs of 50 (NDC 0173-0394-01).

Store between 15° and 30°C (59° and 86°F). Replace cap securely after each opening. Protect unit dose packs from excessive moisture.

REFERENCES

1. National Committee for Clinical Laboratory Standards. *Performance Standards for Antimicrobial Disk Susceptibility Tests.* 4th ed. Aproved Standard NCCLS Document M2-A4, Vol. 10, No. 7. Villanova, Pa: NCCLS; 1990.
2. National Committee for Clinical Laboratory Standards. *Methods for Dilution Antimicrobial Susceptibility Tests for Bacteria That Grow Aerobically.* 2nd ed. Approved Standard NCCLS Document M7-A2, Vol. 10, No. 8. Villanova, Pa: NCCLS; 1990.

Shown in Product Identification Section, page 404

TRANDATE® Tablets ℞
[tran 'dāt]
(labetalol hydrochloride)

TRANDATE® Injection
[tran 'dāt]
(labetalol hydrochloride)

DESCRIPTION

Trandate® (labetalol HCl) Tablets and Injection are adrenergic receptor blocking agents that have both selective $alpha_1$-adrenergic and nonselective beta-adrenergic receptor blocking actions in a single substance.

Labetalol HCl is a racemate chemically designated as 2-hydroxy-5-[1-hydroxy-2-[(1-methyl-3-phenylpropyl)amino] ethyl]benzamide monohydrochloride. Labetalol HCl has the empirical formula $C_{19}H_{24}N_2O_3 \cdot HCl$ and a molecular weight of 364.9. It has two asymmetric centers and therefore exists as a molecular complex of two diastereoisomeric pairs.

Labetalol HCl is a white or off-white crystalline powder, soluble in water.

Trandate Tablets contain 100, 200, or 300 mg of labetalol HCl and are taken orally. The tablets also contain the inactive ingredients corn starch, FD&C Yellow No. 6 (100- and 300-mg tablets only), hydroxypropyl methylcellulose, lactose, magnesium stearate, methylparaben, pregelatinized corn starch, propylparaben, sodium benzoate (200-mg tablet only), talc (100-mg tablet only), and titanium dioxide.

Trandate® (labetalol HCl) Injection is a clear, colorless to light yellow, aqueous, sterile, isotonic solution for intravenous (IV) injection. It has a pH range of 3–4. Each milliliter contains 5 mg of labetalol HCl, 45 mg of anhydrous dextrose, 0.1 mg of edetate disodium; 0.8 mg of methylparaben and 0.1 mg of propylparaben as preservatives; and citric acid monohydrate and sodium hydroxide, as necessary, to bring the solution into the pH range.

CLINICAL PHARMACOLOGY

Labetalol HCl combines both selective, competitive, $alpha_1$-adrenergic blocking and nonselective, competitive, beta-adrenergic blocking activity in a single substance. In man, the ratios of alpha- to beta-blockade have been estimated to be approximately 1:3 and 1:7 following oral and IV administration, respectively. $Beta_2$-agonist activity has been demonstrated in animals with minimal $beta_1$-agonist (ISA) activity detected. In animals, at doses greater than those required for alpha- or beta-adrenergic blockade, a membrane stabilizing effect has been demonstrated.

Pharmacodynamics: The capacity of labetalol HCl to block alpha receptors in man has been demonstrated by attenuation of the pressor effect of phenylephrine and by a significant reduction of the pressor response caused by immersing the hand in ice-cold water ("cold-pressor test"). Labetalol HCl's $beta_1$-receptor blockade in man was demonstrated by a small decrease in the resting heart rate, attenuation of tachycardia produced by isoproterenol or exercise, and by attenuation of the reflex tachycardia to the hypotension produced by amyl nitrite. $Beta_2$-receptor blockade was demonstrated by inhibition of the isoproterenol-induced fall in diastolic blood pressure. Both the alpha- and beta-blocking actions of orally administered labetalol HCl contribute to a decrease in blood pressure in hypertensive patients. Labetalol HCl consistently, in dose-related fashion, blunted increases in exercise-induced blood pressure and heart rate, and in their double product. The pulmonary circulation during exercise was not affected by labetalol HCl dosing.

Single oral doses of labetalol HCl administered in patients with coronary artery disease had no significant effect on sinus rate, intraventricular conduction, or QRS duration. The atrioventricular (A-V) conduction time was modestly prolonged in two of seven patients. In another study, IV labetalol HCl slightly prolonged A-V nodal conduction time and atrial effective refractory period with only small changes in heart rate. The effects on A-V nodal refractoriness were inconsistent.

Labetalol HCl produces dose-related falls in blood pressure without reflex tachycardia and without significant reduction in heart rate, presumably through a mixture of its alpha- and beta-blocking effects. Hemodynamic effects are variable, with small, nonsignificant changes in cardiac output seen in some studies, but not others, and small decreases in total peripheral resistance. Elevated plasma renins are reduced. Doses of labetalol HCl that controlled hypertension did not affect renal function in mildly to severely hypertensive patients with normal renal function.

Due to the alpha$_1$-receptor blocking activity of labetalol HCl, blood pressure is lowered more in the standing than in the supine position, and symptoms of postural hypotension (2%), including rare instances of syncope, can occur. Following oral administration, when postural hypotension has occurred, it has been transient and is uncommon when the recommended starting dose and titration increments are closely followed (see **DOSAGE AND ADMINISTRATION**). Symptomatic postural hypotension is most likely to occur 2–4 hours after a dose, especially following the use of large initial doses or upon large changes in dose.

During dosing with IV labetalol HCl, the contribution of the postural component should be considered when positioning the patient for treatment, and the patient should not be allowed to move to an erect position unmonitored until his ability to do so is established.

The peak effects of single oral doses of labetalol HCl occur within 2–4 hours. The duration of effect depends upon dose, lasting at least 8 hours following single oral doses of 100 mg and more than 12 hours following single oral doses of 300 mg. The maximum, steady-state blood pressure response upon oral, twice-a-day dosing occurs within 24–72 hours.

The antihypertensive effect of labetalol has a linear correlation with the logarithm of labetalol plasma concentration, and there is also a linear correlation between the reduction in exercise-induced tachycardia occurring at 2 hours after oral administration of labetalol HCl and the logarithm of the plasma concentration.

About 70% of the maximum beta-blocking effect is present for 5 hours after the administration of a single oral dose of 400 mg with suggestion that about 40% remains at 8 hours.

The antianginal efficacy of labetalol HCl has not been studied. In 37 patients with hypertension and coronary artery disease, labetalol HCl did not increase the incidence or severity of angina attacks.

In a clinical pharmacologic study in severe hypertensives, an initial 0.25-mg/kg injection of labetalol HCl administered to patients in the supine position decreased blood pressure by an average of 11/7 mmHg. Additional injections of 0.5 mg/kg at 15-minute intervals up to a total cumulative dose of 1.75 mg/kg of labetalol HCl caused further dose-related decreases in blood pressure. Some patients required cumulative doses of up to 3.25 mg/kg. The maximal effect of each dose level occurred within 5 minutes. Following discontinuation of IV treatment with labetalol HCl, the blood pressure rose gradually and progressively, approaching pretreatment baseline values within an average of 16–18 hours in the majority of patients.

Similar results were obtained in the treatment of patients with severe hypertension who required urgent blood pressure reduction with an initial dose of 20 mg (which corresponds to 0.25 mg/kg for an 80-kg patient) followed by additional doses of either 40 or 80 mg at 10-minute intervals to achieve the desired effect, or up to a cumulative dose of 300 mg.

Labetalol HCl administered as a continuous IV infusion, with a mean dose of 136 mg (27–300 mg) over a period of 2–3 hours (mean of 2 hours and 39 minutes), lowered the blood pressure by an average of 60/35 mmHg.

Exacerbation of angina and, in some cases, myocardial infarction and ventricular dysrhythmias have been reported after abrupt discontinuation of therapy with beta-adrenergic blocking agents in patients with coronary artery disease. Abrupt withdrawal of these agents in patients without coronary artery disease has resulted in transient symptoms, including tremulousness, sweating, palpitation, headache, and malaise. Several mechanisms have been proposed to explain these phenomena, among them increased sensitivity to catecholamines because of increased numbers of beta receptors.

Although beta-adrenergic receptor blockade is useful in the treatment of angina and hypertension, there are also situations in which sympathetic stimulation is vital. For example, in patients with severely damaged hearts, adequate ventricular function may depend on sympathetic drive. Beta-adrenergic blockade may worsen A-V block by preventing the necessary facilitating effects of sympathetic activity on conduction. Beta$_2$-adrenergic blockade results in passive bronchial constriction by interfering with endogenous adrenergic bronchodilator activity in patients subject to bronchospasm, and it may also interfere with exogenous bronchodilators in such patients.

Pharmacokinetics and Metabolism: Labetalol HCl is completely absorbed from the gastrointestinal tract with peak plasma levels occurring 1–2 hours after oral administration. The relative bioavailability of labetalol HCl tablets compared to an oral solution is 100%. The absolute bioavailability (fraction of drug reaching systemic circulation) of labetalol when compared to an IV infusion is 25%; this is due to extensive "first-pass" metabolism. Despite "first-pass" metabolism, there is a linear relationship between oral doses of 100–3,000 mg and peak plasma levels. The absolute bioavailability of labetalol is increased when administered with food. The plasma half-life of labetalol following oral administration is about 6–8 hours. Steady-state plasma levels of labetalol during repetitive dosing are reached by about the third day of dosing. Following IV infusion of labetalol, the elimination half-life is about 5.5 hours and the total body clearance is approximately 33 mL/min/kg. In patients with decreased hepatic or renal function, the elimination half-life of labetalol is not altered; however, the relative bioavailability in hepatically impaired patients is increased due to decreased "first-pass" metabolism.

The metabolism of labetalol is mainly through conjugation to glucuronide metabolites. These metabolites are present in plasma and are excreted in the urine and, via the bile, into the feces. Approximately 55%–60% of a dose appears in the urine as conjugates or unchanged labetalol within the first 24 hours of dosing.

Labetalol has been shown to cross the placental barrier in humans. Only negligible amounts of the drug crossed the blood-brain barrier in animal studies. Labetalol is approximately 50% protein bound. Neither hemodialysis nor peritoneal dialysis removes a significant amount of labetalol HCl from the general circulation (<1%).

INDICATIONS AND USAGE

Trandate® (labetalol HCl) Tablets are indicated in the management of hypertension. Trandate Tablets may be used alone or in combination with other antihypertensive agents, especially thiazide and loop diuretics.

Trandate® (labetalol HCl) Injection is indicated for control of blood pressure in severe hypertension.

CONTRAINDICATIONS

Trandate® (labetalol HCl) Tablets and Injection are contraindicated in bronchial asthma, overt cardiac failure, greater-than-first-degree heart block, cardiogenic shock, severe bradycardia, other conditions associated with severe and prolonged hypotension, and in patients with a history of hypersensitivity to any component of the product (see **WARNINGS**).

WARNINGS

Hepatic Injury: Severe hepatocellular injury, confirmed by rechallenge in at least one case, occurs rarely with labetalol therapy. The hepatic injury is usually reversible, but hepatic necrosis and death have been reported. Injury has occurred after both short- and long-term treatment and may be slowly progressive despite minimal symptomatology. Appropriate laboratory testing should be done at the first symptom/sign of liver dysfunction (e.g., pruritus, dark urine, persistent anorexia, jaundice, right upper quadrant tenderness, or unexplained "flu-like" symptoms). If the patient has laboratory evidence of liver injury or jaundice, labetalol should be stopped and not restarted.

Cardiac Failure: Sympathetic stimulation is a vital component supporting circulatory function in congestive heart failure. Beta-blockade carries a potential hazard of further depressing myocardial contractility and precipitating more severe failure. Although beta-blockers should be avoided in overt congestive heart failure, if necessary, labetalol HCl can be used with caution in patients with a history of heart failure who are well compensated. Congestive heart failure has been observed in patients receiving labetalol HCl. Labetalol HCl does not abolish the inotropic action of digitalis on heart muscle.

In Patients Without a History of Cardiac Failure: In patients with latent cardiac insufficiency, continued depression of the myocardium with beta-blocking agents over a period of time can, in some cases, lead to cardiac failure. At the first sign or symptom of impending cardiac failure, patients should be fully digitalized and/or be given a diuretic, and the response should be observed closely. If cardiac failure continues despite adequate digitalization and diuretic, Trandate® (labetalol HCl) Tablets and Trandate® (labetalol HCl) Injection therapy should be withdrawn (gradually, if possible).

Exacerbation of Ischemic Heart Disease Following Abrupt Withdrawal: Angina pectoris has not been reported upon labetalol HCl discontinuation. However, hypersensitivity to catecholamines has been observed in patients withdrawn from beta-blocker therapy; exacerbation of angina and, in some cases, myocardial infarction have occurred after *abrupt* discontinuation of such therapy. When discontinuing chronically administered Trandate Tablets, particularly in patients with ischemic heart disease, the dosage should be gradually reduced over a period of 1–2 weeks and the patient should be carefully monitored. If angina markedly worsens or acute coronary insufficiency develops, Trandate Tablets therapy should be reinstituted promptly, at least temporarily, and other measures appropriate for the management of unstable angina should be taken. Patients should be warned against interruption or discontinuation of therapy without the physician's advice. Because coronary artery disease is common and may be unrecognized, it may be prudent not to discontinue Trandate Tablets therapy abruptly in patients being treated for hypertension.

Ischemic Heart Disease: Angina pectoris has not been reported upon labetalol HCl discontinuation. However, following abrupt cessation of therapy with some beta-blocking agents in patients with coronary artery disease, exacerbations of angina pectoris and, in some cases, myocardial infarction have been reported. Therefore, such patients should be cautioned against interruption of therapy without the physician's advice. Even in the absence of overt angina pectoris, when discontinuation of Trandate Injection is planned, the patient should be carefully observed and should be advised to limit physical activity. If angina markedly worsens or acute coronary insufficiency develops, Trandate Injection administration should be reinstituted promptly, at least temporarily, and other measures appropriate for the management of unstable angina should be taken.

Nonallergic Bronchospasm (e.g., Chronic Bronchitis and Emphysema): Patients with bronchospastic disease should, in general, not receive beta-blockers. Trandate Tablets may be used with caution, however, in patients who do not respond to, or cannot tolerate, other antihypertensive agents. It is prudent, if Trandate Tablets are used, to use the smallest effective dose, so that inhibition of endogenous or exogenous beta-agonists is minimized.

Since Trandate Injection at the usual IV therapeutic doses has not been studied in patients with nonallergic bronchospastic disease, it should not be used in such patients.

Pheochromocytoma: Labetalol HCl has been shown to be effective in lowering blood pressure and relieving symptoms in patients with pheochromocytoma; higher than usual IV doses may be required. However, paradoxical hypertensive responses have been reported in a few patients with this tumor; therefore, use caution when administering labetalol HCl to patients with pheochromocytoma.

Diabetes Mellitus and Hypoglycemia: Beta-adrenergic blockade may prevent the appearance of premonitory signs and symptoms (e.g., tachycardia) of acute hypoglycemia. This is especially important with labile diabetics. Beta-blockade also reduces the release of insulin in response to hyperglycemia; it may therefore be necessary to adjust the dose of antidiabetic drugs.

Major Surgery: The necessity or desirability of withdrawing beta-blocking therapy before major surgery is controversial. Protracted severe hypotension and difficulty in restarting or maintaining a heartbeat have been reported with beta-blockers. The effect of labetalol HCl's alpha-adrenergic activity has not been evaluated in this setting.

A synergism between labetalol HCl and halothane anesthesia has been shown (see **PRECAUTIONS**: Drug Interactions).

Rapid Decreases of Blood Presure: Trandate Injection: Caution must be observed when reducing severely elevated blood pressure. Although such findings have not been reported with IV labetalol HCl, a number of adverse reactions, including cerebral infarction, optic nerve infarction, angina, and ischemic changes in the electrocardiogram, have been reported with other agents when severely elevated blood pressure was reduced over time courses of several hours to as long as 1 or 2 days. The desired blood pressure lowering should therefore be achieved over as long a period of time as is compatible with the patient's status.

PRECAUTIONS

General: ***Impaired Hepatic Function:*** Trandate® (labetalol HCl) Tablets and Injection should be used with caution in patients with impaired hepatic function since metabolism of the drug may be diminished.

Hypotension: Symptomatic postural hypotension (incidence, 58%) is likely to occur if patients are tilted or allowed to assume the upright position within 3 hours of receiving Trandate Injection. Therefore, the patient's ability to tolerate an upright position should be established before permitting any ambulation.

Jaundice or Hepatic Dysfunction: (see **WARNINGS**).

Information for Patients: As with all drugs with beta-blocking activity, certain advice to patients being treated with labetalol HCl is warranted. This information is intended to aid in the safe and effective use of this medication. It is not a disclosure of all possible adverse or intended effects. While no incident of the abrupt withdrawal phenomenon (exacerbation of angina pectoris) has been reported with labetalol HCl, dosing with Trandate Tablets should not be interrupted or discontinued without a physician's advice. Patients being treated with Trandate Tablets should consult a physician at any signs or symptoms of impending cardiac failure or hepatic dysfunction (see WARNINGS). Also, transient scalp tingling may occur, usually when treatment with Trandate Tablets is initiated (see **ADVERSE REACTIONS**).

During and immediately following (for up to 3 hours) Trandate Injection, the patient should remain supine. Subsequently, the patient should be advised on how to proceed gradually to become ambulatory and should be observed at the time of first ambulation.

When the patient is started on Trandate Tablets following adequate control of blood pressure with Trandate Injection, appropriate directions for titration of dosage should be provided (see **DOSAGE AND ADMINISTRATION**).

Laboratory Tests: As with any new drug given over prolonged periods, laboratory parameters should be observed over regular intervals. In patients with concomitant ill-

Continued on next page

Allen & Hanburys—Cont.

nesses, such as impaired renal function, appropriate tests should be done to monitor these conditions.

Routine laboratory tests are ordinarily not required before or after IV labetalol HCl.

Drug Interactions: Since Trandate Injection may be administered to patients already being treated with other medications, including other antihypertensive agents, careful monitoring of these patients is necessary to detect and treat promptly any undesired effect from concomitant administration.

In one survey, 2.3% of patients taking labetalol HCl orally in combination with tricyclic antidepressants experienced tremor, as compared to 0.7% reported to occur with labetalol HCl alone. The contribution of each of the treatments to this adverse reaction is unknown, but the possibility of a drug interaction cannot be excluded.

Drugs possessing beta-blocking properties can blunt the bronchodilator effect of beta-receptor agonist drugs in patients with bronchospasm; therefore, doses greater than the normal antiasthmatic dose of beta-agonist bronchodilator drugs may be required.

Cimetidine has been shown to increase the bioavailability of labetalol HCl administered orally. Since this could be explained either by enhanced absorption or by an alteration of hepatic metabolism of labetalol HCl, special care should be used in establishing the dose required for blood pressure control in such patients.

Synergism has been shown between halothane anesthesia and intravenously administered labetalol HCl. During controlled hypotensive anesthesia using labetalol HCl in association with halothane, high concentrations (3% or above) of halothane should not be used because the degree of hypotension will be increased and because of the possibility of a large reduction in cardiac output and an increase in central venous pressure. The anesthesiologist should be informed when a patient is receiving labetalol HCl.

Labetalol HCl blunts the reflex tachycardia produced by nitroglycerin without preventing its hypotensive effect. If labetalol HCl is used with nitroglycerin in patients with angina pectoris, additional antihypertensive effects may occur. Care should be taken if labetalol is used concomitantly with calcium antagonists of the verapamil type.

Risk of Anaphylactic Reaction: While taking beta-blockers, patients with a history of severe anaphylactic reaction to a variety of allergens may be more reactive to repeated challenge, either accidental, diagnostic, or therapeutic. Such patients may be unresponsive to the usual doses of epinephrine used to treat allergic reaction.

Drug/Laboratory Test Interactions: The presence of labetalol metabolites in the urine may result in falsely elevated levels of urinary catecholamines, metanephrine, normetanephrine, and vanillylmandelic acid when measured by fluorimetric or photometric methods. In screening patients suspected of having a pheochromocytoma and being treated

with labetalol HCl, a specific method, such as a high performance liquid chromatographic assay with solid phase extraction (e.g., *J Chromatogr* 385:241,1987) should be employed in determining levels of catecholamines.

Labetalol HCl has also been reported to produce a false-positive test for amphetamine when screening urine for the presence of drugs using the commercially available assay methods Toxi-Lab A® (thin-layer chromatographic assay) and Emit-d.a.u.® (radioenzymatic assay). When patients being treated with labetalol have a positive urine test for amphetamine using these techniques, confirmation should be made by using more specific methods, such as a gas chromatographic-mass spectrometer technique.

Carcinogenesis, Mutagenesis, Impairment of Fertility: Long-term oral dosing studies with labetalol HCl for 18 months in mice and for 2 years in rats showed no evidence of carcinogenesis. Studies with labetalol HCl using dominant lethal assays in rats and mice and exposing microorganisms according to modified Ames tests showed no evidence of mutagenesis.

Pregnancy: *Teratogenic Effects: Pregnancy Category C:* Teratogenic studies were performed with labetalol in rats and rabbits at oral doses up to approximately six and four times the maximum recommended human dose (MRHD), respectively. No reproducible evidence of fetal malformations was observed. Increased fetal resorptions were seen in both species at doses approximating the MRHD. A teratology study performed with labetalol in rabbits at IV doses up to 1.7 times the MRHD revealed no evidence of drug-related harm to the fetus. There are no adequate and well-controlled studies in pregnant women. Labetalol should be used during pregnancy only if the potential benefit justifies the potential risk to the fetus.

Nonteratogenic Effects: Hypotension, bradycardia, hypoglycemia, and respiratory depression have been reported in infants of mothers who were treated with labetalol HCl for hypertension during pregnancy. Oral administration of labetalol to rats during late gestation through weaning at doses of two to four times the MRHD caused a decrease in neonatal survival.

Labor and Delivery: Labetalol HCl given to pregnant women with hypertension did not appear to affect the usual course of labor and delivery.

Nursing Mothers: Small amounts of labetalol (approximately 0.004% of the maternal dose) are excreted in human milk. Caution should be exercised when Trandate is administered to a nursing woman.

Pediatric Use: Safety and effectiveness in children have not been established.

ADVERSE REACTIONS

Trandate® (labetalol HCl) Tablets: Most adverse effects are mild and transient and occur early in the course of treatment. In controlled clinical trials of 3–4 months' duration, discontinuation of Trandate Tablets due to one or more adverse effects was required in 7% of all patients. In these same trials, other agents with solely beta-blocking activity used in the control groups led to discontinuation in 8%–10% of patients, and a centrally acting alpha-agonist led to discontinuation in 30% of patients.

The incidence rates of adverse reactions listed in the following table were derived from multicenter, controlled clinical trials comparing labetalol HCl, placebo, metoprolol, and propranolol over treatment periods of 3 and 4 months. Where the frequency of adverse effects for labetalol HCl and placebo is similar, causal relationship is uncertain. The rates are based on adverse reactions considered probably drug related by the investigator. If all reports are considered, the rates are somewhat higher (e.g., dizziness, 20%; nausea, 14%; fatigue, 11%), but the overall conclusions are unchanged.

[See table below.]

The adverse effects were reported spontaneously and are representative of the incidence of adverse effects that may be observed in a properly selected hypertensive patient population, i.e., a group excluding patients with bronchospastic disease, overt congestive heart failure, or other contraindications to beta-blocker therapy.

The incidence of adverse reactions depends upon the dose of labetalol HCl. The largest experience is with oral labetalol. Clinical trials included studies utilizing daily doses up to 2,400 mg in more severely hypertensive patients. Certain of the side effects increased with increasing dose, as shown in the following table that depicts the entire US therapeutic trials data base for adverse reactions that are clearly or possibly dose related.

[See table above.]

In addition, a number of other less common adverse events have been reported:

Body as a Whole: Fever.

Cardiovascular: Hypotension, and rarely, syncope, bradycardia, heart block.

Central and Peripheral Nervous Systems: Paresthesia, most frequently described as scalp tingling. In most cases, it was mild and transient and usually occurred at the beginning of treatment.

Collagen Disorders: Systemic lupus erythematosus, positive antinuclear factor.

Eyes: Dry eyes.

Immunological System: Antimitochondrial antibodies.

Liver and Biliary System: Hepatic necrosis, hepatitis, cholestatic jaundice, elevated liver function tests.

Musculoskeletal System: Muscle cramps, toxic myopathy.

Respiratory System: Bronchospasm.

Skin and Appendages: Rashes of various types, such as generalized maculopapular, lichenoid, urticarial, bullous lichen planus, psoriasiform, and facial erythema; Peyronie's disease; reversible alopecia.

Urinary System: Difficulty in micturition, including acute urinary bladder retention.

Hypersensitivity: Rare reports of hypersensitivity (e.g., rash, urticaria, pruritus, angioedema, dyspnea) and anaphylactoid reactions.

Following approval for marketing in the United Kingdom, a monitored release survey involving approximately 6,800 patients was conducted for further safety and efficacy evalu-

Labetalol HCl Daily Dose (mg)	200	300	400	600	800	900	1,200	1,600	2,400
Number of patients	522	181	606	608	503	117	411	242	175
Dizziness (%)	2	3	3	3	5	1	9	13	16
Fatigue	2	1	4	4	5	3	7	6	10
Nausea	<1	0	1	2	4	0	7	11	19
Vomiting	0	0	<1	<1	<1	0	1	2	3
Dyspepsia	1	0	2	1	1	0	2	2	4
Paresthesia	2	0	2	2	1	1	2	5	5
Nasal stuffiness	1	1	2	2	2	2	4	5	6
Ejaculation failure	0	2	1	2	3	0	4	3	5
Impotence	1	1	1	1	2	4	3	4	3
Edema	1	0	1	1	1	0	1	2	2

	Labetalol HCl (n=227) %	Placebo (n=98) %	Propranolol (n=84) %	Metoprolol (n=49) %
Body as a whole				
fatigue	5	0	12	12
asthenia	1	1	1	0
headache	2	1	1	2
Gastrointestinal				
nausea	6	1	1	2
vomiting	<1	0	0	0
dyspepsia	3	1	1	0
abdominal pain	0	0	1	2
diarrhea	<1	0	2	0
taste distortion	1	0	0	0
Central and peripheral nervous systems				
dizziness	11	3	4	4
paresthesia	<1	0	0	0
drowsiness	<1	2	2	2
Autonomic nervous system				
nasal stuffiness	3	0	0	0
ejaculation failure	2	0	0	0
impotence	1	0	1	3
increased sweating	<1	0	0	0
Cardiovascular				
edema	1	0	0	0
postural hypotension	1	0	0	0
bradycardia	0	0	5	12
Respiratory				
dyspnea	2	0	1	2
Skin				
rash	1	0	0	0
Special senses				
vision abnormality	1	0	0	0
vertigo	2	1	0	0

ation of this product. Results of this survey indicate that the type, severity, and incidence of adverse effects were comparable to those cited above.

Potential Adverse Effects: In addition, other adverse effects not listed above have been reported with other beta-adrenergic blocking agents.

Central Nervous System: Reversible mental depression progressing to catatonia, an acute reversible syndrome characterized by disorientation for time and place, short-term memory loss, emotional lability, slightly clouded sensorium, and decreased performance on psychometrics.

Cardiovascular: Intensification of A-V block (see CONTRAINDICATIONS).

Allergic: Fever combined with aching and sore throat, laryngospasm, respiratory distress.

Hematologic: Agranulocytosis, thrombocytopenic or non-thrombocytopenic purpura.

Gastrointestinal: Mesenteric artery thrombosis, ischemic colitis.

Trandate® (labetalol HCl) Injection: Trandate Injection is usually well tolerated. Most adverse effects have been mild and transient and, in controlled trials involving 92 patients, did not require labetalol HCl withdrawal. Symptomatic postural hypotension (incidence, 58%) is likely to occur if patients are tilted or allowed to assume the upright position within 3 hours of receiving Trandate Injection. Moderate hypotension occurred in 1 of 100 patients while supine. Increased sweating was noted in 4 of 100 patients, and flushing occurred in 1 of 100 patients.

The following also were reported with Trandate Injection with the incidence per 100 patients as noted:

Cardiovascular System: Ventricular arrhythmia in 1.

Central and Peripheral Nervous Systems: Dizziness in 9, tingling of the scalp/skin in 7, hypoesthesia (numbness) and vertigo in 1 each.

Gastrointestinal System: Nausea in 13, vomiting in 4, dyspepsia and taste distortion in 1 each.

Metabolic Disorders: Transient increases in blood urea nitrogen and serum creatinine levels occurred in 8 of 100 patients; these were associated with drops in blood pressure, generally in patients with prior renal insufficiency.

Psychiatric Disorders: Somnolence/yawning in 3.

Respiratory System: Wheezing in 1.

Skin: Pruritus in 1.

In addition, a number of other less common adverse events have been reported:

Cardiovascular: Hypotension, and rarely, syncope, bradycardia, heart block.

Liver and Biliary System: Hepatic necrosis, hepatitis, cholestatic jaundice, elevated liver function tests.

Hypersensitivity: Rare reports of hypersensitivity (e.g., rash, urticaria, pruritus, angioedema, dyspnea) and anaphylactoid reactions.

The oculomucocutaneous syndrome associated with the beta-blocker practolol has not been reported with labetalol HCl.

Clinical Laboratory Tests: Among patients dosed with Trandate Tablets, there have been reversible increases of serum transaminases in 4% of patients tested and, more rarely, reversible increases in blood urea.

OVERDOSAGE

Overdosage with labetalol HCl causes excessive hypotension that is posture sensitive and, sometimes, excessive bradycardia. Patients should be placed supine and their legs raised if necessary to improve the blood supply to the brain. If overdosage with labetalol HCl follows oral ingestion, gastric lavage or pharmacologically induced emesis (using syrup of ipecac) may be useful for removal of the drug shortly after ingestion. The following additional measures should be employed if necessary: *Excessive bradycardia*—administer atropine or epinephrine. *Cardiac failure*—administer a digitalis glycoside and a diuretic. Dopamine or dobutamine may also be useful. *Hypotension*—administer vasopressors, e.g., norepinephrine. There is pharmacologic evidence that norepinephrine may be the drug of choice. *Bronchospasm*—administer epinephrine and/or an aerosolized beta₂-agonist.

Seizures—administer diazepam.

In severe beta-blocker overdose resulting in hypotension and/or bradycardia, glucagon has been shown to be effective when administered in large doses (5–10 mg rapidly over 30 seconds, followed by continuous infusion of 5 mg per hour that can be reduced as the patient improves).

Neither hemodialysis nor peritoneal dialysis removes a significant amount of labetalol HCl from the general circulation (<1%).

The oral LD_{50} value of labetalol HCl in the mouse is approximately 600 mg/kg and in the rat is greater than 2 g/kg. The IV LD_{50} in these species is 50–60 mg/kg.

DOSAGE AND ADMINISTRATION

Trandate® (labetalol HCl) Tablets: DOSAGE MUST BE INDIVIDUALIZED. The recommended *initial* dosage is 100 mg *twice* daily whether used alone or added to a diuretic regimen. After 2 or 3 days, using standing blood pressure as an indicator, dosage may be titrated in increments of 100 mg b.i.d. every 2 or 3 days. The usual *maintenance* dosage of labetalol HCl is between 200 and 400 mg *twice* daily.

Since the full antihypertensive effect of labetalol HCl is usually seen within the first 1–3 hours of the initial dose or dose increment, the assurance of a lack of an exaggerated hypotensive response can be clinically established in the office setting. The antihypertensive effects of continued dosing can be measured at subsequent visits, approximately 12 hours after a dose, to determine whether further titration is necessary.

Patients with severe hypertension may require from 1,200–2,400 mg per day, with or without thiazide diuretics. Should side effects (principally nausea or dizziness) occur with these doses administered twice daily, the same total daily dose administered three times daily may improve tolerability and facilitate further titration. Titration increments should not exceed 200 mg twice daily.

When a diuretic is added, an additive antihypertensive effect can be expected. In some cases this may necessitate a labetalol HCl dosage adjustment. As with most antihypertensive drugs, optimal dosages of Trandate Tablets are usually lower in patients also receiving a diuretic.

When transferring patients from other antihypertensive drugs, Trandate Tablets should be introduced as recommended and the dosage of the existing therapy progressively decreased.

Trandate® (labetalol HCl) Injection: Trandate Injection is intended for IV use in hospitalized patients. DOSAGE MUST BE INDIVIDUALIZED depending upon the severity of hypertension and the response of the patient during dosing.

Patients should always be kept in a supine position during the period of IV drug administration. A substantial fall in blood pressure on standing should be expected in these patients. The patient's ability to tolerate an upright position should be established before permitting any ambulation, such as using toilet facilities.

Either of two methods of administration of Trandate Injection may be used: a) repeated IV injection, or b) slow continuous infusion.

Repeated Intravenous Injection: Initially, Trandate Injection should be given in a 20-mg dose (which corresponds to 0.25 mg/kg for an 80-kg patient) by slow IV injection over a 2-minute period.

Immediately before the injection and at 5 and 10 minutes after injection, supine blood pressure should be measured to evaluate response. Additional injections of 40 or 80 mg can be given at 10-minute intervals until a desired supine blood pressure is achieved or a total of 300 mg of labetalol HCl has been injected. The maximum effect usually occurs within 5 minutes of each injection.

Slow Continuous Infusion: Trandate Injection is prepared for continuous IV infusion by diluting the vial contents with commonly used IV fluids (see below). Examples of two methods of preparing the infusion solution are:

    Add 40 mL of Trandate Injection to 160 mL of a commonly used IV fluid such that the resultant 200 mL of solution contains 200 mg of labetalol HCl, 1 mg/mL. The diluted solution should be administered at a rate of 2 mL per minute to deliver 2 mg per minute.

    Alternatively, add 40 mL of Trandate Injection to 250 mL of a commonly used IV fluid. The resultant solution will contain 200 mg of labetalol HCl, approximately 2 mg/3 mL. The diluted solution should be administered at a rate of 3 mL per minute to deliver approximately 2 mg per minute.

The rate of infusion of the diluted solution may be adjusted according to the blood pressure response, at the discretion of the physician. To facilitate a desired rate of infusion, the diluted solution can be infused using a controlled administration mechanism, e.g., graduated burette or mechanically driven infusion pump.

Since the half-life of labetalol is 5–8 hours, steady-state blood levels (in the face of a constant rate of infusion) would not be reached during the usual infusion time period. The infusion should be continued until a satisfactory response is obtained and should then be stopped and oral labetalol HCl started (see below). The effective IV dose is usually in the range of 50–200 mg. A total dose of up to 300 mg may be required in some patients.

Blood Pressure Monitoring: The blood pressure should be monitored during and after completion of the infusion or IV injection. Rapid or excessive falls in either systolic or diastolic blood pressure during IV treatment should be avoided. In patients with excessive systolic hypertension, the de-

crease in systolic pressure should be used as an indicator of effectiveness in addition to the response of the diastolic pressure.

Initiation of Dosing with Trandate Tablets After Blood Pressure Control With Trandate Injection: Subsequent oral dosing with Trandate Tablets should begin when it has been established that the supine diastolic blood pressure has begun to rise. The recommended initial dose is 200 mg, followed in 6–12 hours by an additional dose of 200 or 400 mg, depending on the blood pressure response. Thereafter, **inpatient titration with Trandate Tablets** may proceed as follows:

Inpatient Titration Instruction

Regimen	Daily Dose*
200 mg b.i.d.	400 mg
400 mg b.i.d.	800 mg
800 mg b.i.d.	1,600 mg
1,200 mg b.i.d.	2,400 mg

* If needed, the total daily dose may be given in three divided doses.

The dosage of Trandate Tablets used in the hospital may be increased at 1-day intervals to achieve the desired blood pressure reduction.

Compatibility With Commonly Used Intravenous Fluids: Parenteral drug products should be inspected visually for particulate matter and discoloration before administration whenever solution and container permit.

Trandate Injection was tested for compatibility with commonly used IV fluids at final concentrations of 1.25–3.75 mg of labetalol HCl per milliliter of the mixture.

Trandate Injection was found to be compatible with and stable (for 24 hours refrigerated or at room temperature) in mixtures with the following solutions: ringer's injection, USP; lactated ringer's injection, USP; 5% dextrose and ringer's injection; 5% lactated ringer's and 5% dextrose injection; 5% dextrose injection, USP; 0.9% sodium chloride injection, USP; 5% dextrose and 0.2% sodium chloride injection, USP; 2.5% dextrose and 0.45% sodium chloride injection, USP; 5% dextrose and 0.9% sodium chloride injection, USP; and 5% dextrose and 0.33% sodium chloride injection, USP.

Trandate Injection was NOT compatible with 5% sodium bicarbonate injection, USP.

HOW SUPPLIED

Trandate® (labetalol HCl) Tablets, 100 mg, light orange, round, scored, film-coated tablets engraved on one side with "TRANDATE 100 GLAXO," bottles of 100 (NDC 0173-0346-43) and 500 (NDC 0173-0346-44) and unit dose packs of 100 tablets (NDC 0173-0346-47).

Trandate Tablets, 200 mg, white, round, scored, film-coated tablets engraved on one side with "TRANDATE 200 GLAXO," bottles of 100 (NDC 0173-0347-43) and 500 (NDC 0173-0347-44) and unit dose packs of 100 tablets (NDC 0173-0347-47).

Trandate Tablets, 300 mg, peach, round, scored, film-coated tablets engraved on one side with "TRANDATE 300 GLAXO," bottles of 100 (NDC 0173-0348-43) and 500 (NDC 0173-0348-44) and unit dose packs of 100 tablets (NDC 0173-0348-47).

Trandate Tablets should be stored between 2° and 30°C (36° and 86°F). Trandate Tablets in the unit dose boxes should be protected from excessive moisture.

Trandate® (labetalol HCl) Injection, 5 mg/mL, is supplied in 20-mL (100-mg) vials, box of one (NDC 0173-0350-58); 40-mL (200-mg) vials, box of one (NDC 0173-0350-57); 4-mL (20-mg) single-dose, prefilled, disposable syringes, box of one, (NDC 0173-0350-00); and 8-mL (40-mg) single-dose, prefilled, disposable syringes, box of one (NDC 0173-0350-01).

Store between 2° and 30°C (36° and 86°F). Do not freeze. Protect from light.

Note: To ensure patient safety, the needle with the prefilled syringes should be handled with care and should be destroyed and discarded if damaged in any manner. If the cannula is bent, no attempt should be made to straighten it. To prevent needle-stick injuries, needles should not be recapped, purposely bent, or broken by hand.

Shown in Product Identification Section, page 404

Continued on next page

Allen & Hanburys—Cont.

VENTOLIN® Inhalation Aerosol   ℞
[*vent 'ō-lin*]
(albuterol, USP)
Bronchodilator Aerosol
For Oral Inhalation Only

VENTOLIN® Inhalation Solution, 0.5%*   ℞
(albuterol sulfate, USP)
*Potency expressed as albuterol.

VENTOLIN® NEBULES™ Inhalation Solution, 0.083%*
(albuterol sulfate, USP)
*Potency expressed as albuterol.

VENTOLIN ROTACAPS® for Inhalation   ℞
(albuterol sulfate, USP)
For Inhalation Only

VENTOLIN® Syrup   ℞
(albuterol sulfate)

VENTOLIN® Tablets   ℞
(albuterol sulfate, USP)

DESCRIPTION

The active component of **Ventolin®** Inhalation Aerosol is albuterol, USP, racemic (α^1-[*tert* -butylamino)methyl-4-hydroxy-*m* -xylene- α, α' -diol) and a relatively selective beta$_2$-adrenergic bronchodilator.
Albuterol is the official generic name in the United States. The World Health Organization recommended name for the drug is salbutamol. The molecular weight of albuterol is 239.3, and the empirical formula is $C_{13}H_{21}NO_3$. Albuterol is a white to off-white crystalline solid. It is soluble in ethanol, sparingly soluble in water, and very soluble in chloroform.
Ventolin Inhalation Aerosol is a metered-dose aerosol unit for oral inhalation. It contains a microcrystalline (95% $\leq$10 μm) suspension of albuterol in propellants (trichloromonofluoromethane and dichlorodifluoromethane) with oleic acid. Each actuation delivers from the mouthpiece 90 mcg of albuterol. Each canister provides at least 200 inhalations.
The active component of Ventolin® Inhalation Solution, Ventolin® Nebules™ Inhalation Solution, Ventolin Rotacaps® for Inhalation, Ventolin® Syrup, and Ventolin® Tablets is albuterol sulfate, the racemic form of albuterol and a relatively selective beta$_2$-adrenergic bronchodilator with the chemical name α^1-[(*tert* -butylamino)methyl]-4-hydroxy-*m* -xylene- α, α' -diol sulfate (2:1) (salt).
Albuterol sulfate has a molecular weight of 576.7, and the empirical formula is $(C_{13}H_{21}NO_3)_2 \cdot H_2SO_4$. Albuterol sulfate is a white crystalline powder, soluble in water and slightly soluble in ethanol.
The World Health Organization recommended name for albuterol base is salbutamol.
Ventolin Inhalation Solution is in concentrated form. Dilute 0.5 mL of the solution with 2.5 mL of sterile normal saline solution before administration. Each milliliter of Ventolin Inhalation Solution contains 5 mg of albuterol (as 6 mg of albuterol sulfate) in an aqueous solution containing benzalkonium chloride; sulfuric acid is used to adjust the pH to between 3 and 5. Ventolin Inhalation Solution contains no sulfiting agents. Ventolin Inhalation Solution is a clear, colorless to light yellow solution.
Ventolin Nebules Inhalation Solution requires no dilution before administration. Each milliliter of Ventolin Nebules Inhalation Solution contains 0.83 mg of albuterol (as 1 mg of albuterol sulfate) in an isotonic, sterile, aqueous solution containing sodium chloride; sulfuric acid is used to adjust the pH to between 3 and 5. Ventolin Nebules Inhalation Solution contains no sulfiting agents or preservatives. Ventolin Nebules Inhalation Solution is a clear, colorless solution.
Ventolin Rotacaps for Inhalation contain a dry powder presentation of albuterol sulfate intended for oral inhalation only. Each light blue and clear, hard gelatin capsule contains a mixture of 200 mcg of microfine (95% $\leq$10 μm) albuterol (as the sulfate) with 25 mg of lactose. The contents of each capsule are inhaled using a specially designed plastic device for inhaling powder called the Rotahaler®. When turned, this device opens the capsule and facilitates dispersion of the albuterol sulfate into the airstream created when the patient inhales through the mouthpiece. Ventolin Rotacaps for Inhalation are an alternative inhalation form of albuterol to the metered-dose pressurized inhaler.
Ventolin Syrup contains 2 mg of albuterol as 2.4 mg of albuterol sulfate in each teaspoonful (5 mL). Ventolin Syrup also contains the inactive ingredients citric acid, FD&C Yellow No. 6, hydroxypropyl methylcellulose, saccharin sodium, sodium benzoate, sodium citrate, artificial strawberry flavor, and purified water.
Each **Ventolin Tablet** contains 2 or 4 mg of albuterol as 2.4 or 4.8 mg, respectively, of albuterol sulfate. Each tablet also contains the inactive ingredients corn starch, lactose, and magnesium stearate.

CLINICAL PHARMACOLOGY

In vitro studies and *in vivo* pharmacologic studies have demonstrated that albuterol has a preferential effect on beta$_2$-adrenergic receptors compared with isoproterenol. While it is recognized that beta$_2$-adrenergic receptors are the predominant receptors in bronchial smooth muscle, recent data indicate that there is a population of beta$_2$-receptors in the human heart existing in a concentration between 10% and 50%. The precise function of these, however, is not yet established (see WARNINGS).
The pharmacologic effects of beta-adrenergic agonist drugs, including albuterol, are at least in part attributable to stimulation through beta-adrenergic receptors of intracellular adenyl cyclase, the enzyme that catalyzes the conversion of adenosine triphosphate (ATP) to cyclic-3',5'-adenosine monophosphate (cyclic AMP). Increased cyclic AMP levels are associated with relaxation of bronchial smooth muscle and inhibition of release of mediators of immediate hypersensitivity from cells, especially from mast cells.
Albuterol has been shown in most controlled clinical trials to have more effect on the respiratory tract, in the form of bronchial smooth muscle relaxation, than isoproterenol at comparable doses while producing fewer cardiovascular effects. Controlled clinical studies and other clinical experience have shown that inhaled albuterol, like other beta-adrenergic agonist drugs, can produce a significant cardiovascular effect in some patients, as measured by pulse rate, blood pressure, symptoms, and/or electrocardiographic changes. Albuterol is longer acting than isoproterenol in most patients by any route of administration because it is not a substrate for the cellular uptake processes for catecholamines nor for catechol-*O* -methyl transferase.
Because of its gradual absorption from the bronchi, systemic levels of albuterol are low after inhalation of recommended doses. Studies undertaken with four subjects administered tritiated albuterol from a metered-dose aerosol inhaler resulted in maximum plasma concentrations occurring within 2–4 hours. Due to the sensitivity of the assay method, the metabolic rate and half-life of elimination of albuterol in plasma could not be determined. However, urinary excretion provided data indicating that albuterol has an elimination half-life of 3.8 hours. Approximately 72% of the inhaled dose is excreted within 24 hours in the urine, and consists of 28% as unchanged drug and 44% as metabolite.
Studies in asthmatic patients have shown that less than 20% of a single albuterol dose was absorbed following either IPPB (intermittent positive-pressure breathing) or nebulizer administration; the remaining amount was recovered from the nebulizer and apparatus and expired air. Most of the absorbed dose was recovered in the urine 24 hours after drug administration. Following a 3-mg dose of nebulized albuterol, the maximum albuterol plasma levels at 0.5 hours were 2.1 ng/mL (range, 1.4–3.2 ng/mL). There was a significant dose-related response in FEV_1 (forced expiratory volume in 1 second) and peak flow rate. It has been demonstrated that following oral administration of 4 mg of albuterol, the elimination half-life was 5–6 hours.
Albuterol is rapidly absorbed after oral administration of 10 mL of Ventolin® (albuterol sulfate) Syrup (4 mg of albuterol) and of 4-mg Ventolin® (albuterol sulfate) Tablets in normal volunteers. Maximum plasma concentrations of about 18 ng/mL of albuterol are achieved within 2 hours, and the drug is eliminated with a half-life of about 5 hours. In other studies, the analysis of urine samples of patients given 8 mg of tritiated albuterol orally showed that 76% of the dose was excreted over 3 days, with the majority of the dose being excreted within the first 24 hours. Sixty percent of this radioactivity was shown to be the metabolite. Feces collected over this period contained 4% of the administered dose.
Animal studies show that albuterol does not pass the blood-brain barrier.
Recent studies in laboratory animals (minipigs, rodents, and dogs) recorded the occurrence of cardiac arrhythmias and sudden death (with histologic evidence of myocardial necrosis) when beta-agonists and methylxanthines were administered concurrently. The significance of these findings when applied to humans is currently unknown.
The effects of rising doses of albuterol and isoproterenol aerosols were studied in volunteers and asthmatic patients. Results in normal volunteers indicated that albuterol is one half to one quarter as active as isoproterenol in producing increases in heart rate. In asthmatic patients similar cardiovascular differentiation between the two drugs was also seen.
In controlled clinical trials with Ventolin® (albuterol) Inhalation Aerosol involving adults with asthma, the onset of improvement in pulmonary function was within 15 minutes, as determined by both MMEF (maximum midexpiratory flow rate) and FEV_1. MMEF measurements also showed that near maximum improvement in pulmonary function generally occurs within 60–90 minutes following two inhalations of albuterol and that clinically significant improvement generally continues for 3–4 hours in most patients. Some patients showed a therapeutic response (defined as maintain-

ing FEV_1 values 15% or more above baseline) that was still apparent at 6 hours. Continued effectiveness of albuterol was demonstrated over a 13-week period in these same trials. In controlled clinical trials involving children 4–12 years of age, FEV_1 measurements showed that maximum improvement in pulmonary function occurs within 30–60 minutes. The onset of clinically significant ($\geq$15%) improvement in FEV_1 was observed as soon as 5 minutes following 180 mcg of albuterol in 18 of 30 (60%) children in a controlled dose-ranging study. Clinically significant improvement in FEV_1 continued in the majority of patients for 2 hours and in 33%–47% for 4 hours among 56 patients receiving inhalation aerosol in one pediatric study. In a second study among 48 patients receiving inhalation aerosol, clinically significant improvement continued in the majority for up to 1 hour and in 23%–40% for 4 hours. In addition, at least 50% of the patients in both studies achieved an improvement in $FEF_{25\%-75\%}$ (forced expiratory flow rate between 25% and 75% of the forced vital capacity) of at least 20% for 2–5 hours. Continued effectiveness of albuterol was demonstrated over the 12-week study period.
In other clinical studies, two inhalations of albuterol taken approximately 15 minutes before exercise prevented exercise-induced bronchospasm, as demonstrated by the maintenance of FEV_1 within 80% of baseline values in the majority of patients. One of these studies also evaluated the duration of the prophylactic effect to repeated exercise challenges, which was evident at 4 hours in the majority of patients and at 6 hours in approximately one third of the patients.
In controlled clinical trials with Ventolin® (albuterol sulfate) Inhalation Solution, most patients exhibited an onset of improvement in pulmonary function within 5 minutes as determined by FEV_1. FEV_1 measurements also showed that the maximum average improvement in pulmonary function usually occurred at approximately 1 hour following inhalation of 2.5 mg of albuterol by compressor-nebulizer and remained close to peak for 2 hours. Clinically significant improvement in pulmonary function (defined as maintenance of a 15% or more increase in FEV_1 over baseline values) continued for 3–4 hours in most patients, with some patients continuing up to 6 hours. In repetitive dose studies, continued effectiveness was demonstrated throughout the 3-month period of treatment in some patients.
In single, dose-range, crossover trials with Ventolin Rotacaps® (albuterol sulfate) for Inhalation in patients 12 years of age and older, the onset of improvement in pulmonary function was within 5 minutes, as determined by a 15% increase in FEV_1 following administration of either a 200- or 400-mcg dose. Maximum increases in FEV_1 occurred within 60 minutes following inhalation of either dose. The duration of effect (defined as an increase in FEV_1 of 15% or greater in a single-dose study) was 1–2 hours after the 200-mcg dose and 3–4 hours after the 400-mcg dose. In a single-dose study, an increase in $FEF_{25\%-75\%}$ of 20% or greater continued for 3–4 hours after the 200-mcg dose and for 3–6 hours following the 400-mcg dose. A therapeutic response continued for 4 hours in the majority of patients and for 6 hours in 38% of the patients following the 400-mcg dose. Twenty-two percent of the patients receiving the 200-mcg dose had a duration of effect of 8 hours.
In 12-week, double-blind, comparative evaluations in patients 12 years of age and older of one 200-mcg Ventolin Rotacaps for Inhalation capsule versus two inhalations of Ventolin Inhalation Aerosol, the two dosage regimens were found to be equivalent. Based on a 15% or more increase in FEV_1 determinations, both provided a therapeutic response that persisted for 2 or 3 hours in 50% of 231 patients aged 12 years and older. Similar results were found in two controlled, 12-week clinical trials involving 204 children aged 4–11 years. Both formulations produced a therapeutic response (defined as maintenance of mean increase over baseline of at least 15% in FEV_1, or 20% in $FEF_{25\%-75\%}$). Therapeutic improvement of $FEF_{25\%-75\%}$ persisted for 3–5 hours in over 50% of the children throughout the study. Continued effectiveness and safety of Ventolin Rotacaps for Inhalation were demonstrated over the 12-week study periods in both adults and children.
In controlled clinical trials with Ventolin Syrup and Ventolin Tablets in patients with asthma, the onset of improvement in pulmonary function, as measured by MMEF and FEV_1 and by MMEF, respectively, was within 30 minutes, with peak improvement occurring between 2 and 3 hours.
In a controlled clinical trial with Ventolin Syrup involving 55 children, clinically significant improvement (defined as maintenance of mean values over baseline of 15%–20% or more in the FEV_1 and MMEF, respectively) continued to be recorded up to 6 hours. No decrease in the effectiveness was reported in one uncontrolled study of 32 children who took Ventolin Syrup for a 3-month period.
In controlled clinical trials with Ventolin Tablets in which measurements were conducted for 6 hours, clinically significant improvement (defined as maintaining a 15% or more increase in FEV_1 and a 20% or more increase in MMEF over baseline values) was observed in 60% of patients at 4 hours and in 40% at 6 hours. In other single-dose, controlled clini-

cal trials, clinically significant improvement was observed in at least 40% of the patients at 8 hours. No decrease in the effectiveness of Ventolin Tablets has been reported in patients who received long-term treatment with the drug in uncontrolled studies for periods up to 6 months.

INDICATIONS AND USAGE

Ventolin® (albuterol) Inhalation Aerosol is indicated for the prevention and relief of bronchospasm in patients 4 years of age and older with reversible obstructive airway disease and for the prevention of exercise-induced bronchospasm in patients 12 years of age and older. Ventolin Inhalation Aerosol can be used with or without concomitant steroid therapy.

Ventolin® (albuterol sulfate) Inhalation Solution is indicated for the relief of bronchospasm in patients with reversible obstructive airway disease and acute attacks of bronchospasm.

Ventolin® Nebules™ Inhalation Solution is indicated for the relief of bronchospasm in patients with reversible obstructive airway disease and acute attacks of bronchospasm.

Ventolin Rotacaps® (albuterol sulfate) for Inhalation are indicated for the prevention and relief of bronchospasm in patients 4 years of age and older with reversible obstructive airway disease and for the prevention of exercise-induced bronchospasm in patients 12 years of age and older. This formulation is particularly useful in patients who are unable to properly use the pressurized aerosol form of albuterol or who prefer an alternative formulation. Ventolin Rotacaps for Inhalation can be used with or without concomitant steroid therapy.

Ventolin® (albuterol sulfate) Syrup is indicated for the relief of bronchospasm in adults and children 2 years of age and older with reversible obstructive airway disease.

Ventolin® (albuterol sulfate) Tablets are indicated for the relief of bronchospasm in patients with reversible obstructive airway disease.

CONTRAINDICATIONS

The Ventolin® (albuterol/albuterol sulfate) preparations are contraindicated in patients with a history of hypersensitivity to any of the components.

WARNINGS

As with other inhaled beta-adrenergic agonists, Ventolin® (albuterol) Inhalation Aerosol, Ventolin® (albuterol sulfate) Inhalation Solution, Ventolin® Nebules™ (albuterol sulfate) Inhalation Solution, and Ventolin Rotacaps® (albuterol sulfate) for Inhalation can produce paradoxical bronchospasm that can be life-threatening. If it occurs, the preparation should be discontinued immediately and alternative therapy instituted.

Fatalities have been reported in association with excessive use of inhaled sympathomimetic drugs and with the home use of nebulizers. The exact cause of death is unknown, but cardiac arrest following the unexpected development of a severe acute asthmatic crisis and subsequent hypoxia is suspected. It is therefore essential that the physician instruct the patient in the need for further evaluation if his/her asthma becomes worse. In individual patients, any beta₂-adrenergic agonist, including albuterol inhalation solution, may have a clinically significant cardiac effect.

Immediate hypersensitivity reactions may occur after administration of albuterol, as demonstrated by rare cases of urticaria, angioedema, rash, bronchospasm, anaphylaxis, and oropharyngeal edema. Albuterol, like other beta-adrenergic agonists, can produce a significant cardiovascular effect in some patients, as measured by pulse rate, blood pressure, symptoms, and/or electrocardiographic changes.

The contents of Ventolin Inhalation Aerosol are under pressure. Do not puncture. Do not use or store near heat or open flame. Exposure to temperatures above 120°F may cause bursting. Never throw container into fire or incinerator. Keep out of reach of children.

PRECAUTIONS

General: Although no effect on the cardiovascular system is usually seen after the administration of inhaled albuterol at recommended doses, cardiovascular and central nervous system effects seen with all sympathomimetic drugs can occur after use of inhaled albuterol and may require discontinuation of the drug. As with all sympathomimetic amines, albuterol should be used with caution in patients with cardiovascular disorders, especially coronary insufficiency, cardiac arrhythmias, and hypertension; in patients with convulsive disorders, hyperthyroidism, or diabetes mellitus; and in patients who are unusually responsive to sympathomimetic amines. Clinically significant changes in systolic and diastolic blood pressure have been seen in individual patients and could be expected to occur in some patients after use of any beta-adrenergic bronchodilator.

Large doses of intravenous albuterol have been reported to aggravate pre-existing diabetes mellitus and ketoacidosis. As with other beta-agonists, inhaled and intravenous albuterol may produce significant hypokalemia in some patients, possibly through intracellular shunting, which has the potential to produce adverse cardiovascular effects. The decrease is usually transient, not requiring supplementation.

Although there have been no reports concerning the use of Ventolin® (albuterol) Inhalation Aerosol or Ventolin Rotacaps® (albuterol sulfate) for Inhalation during labor and delivery, it has been reported that high doses of albuterol administered intravenously inhibit uterine contractions. Although this effect is extremely unlikely as a consequence of Ventolin Inhalation Aerosol or Ventolin Rotacaps for Inhalation use, it should be kept in mind.

Information for Patients: The action of Ventolin Inhalation Aerosol, Ventolin® (albuterol sulfate) Inhalation Solution, Ventolin® Nebules™ (albuterol sulfate) Inhalation Solution, and Ventolin® (albuterol sulfate) Syrup may last up to 6 hours; the action of Ventolin Rotacaps for Inhalation may last for 6 hours or longer; and the action of Ventolin® (albuterol sulfate) Tablets may last for 8 hours or longer. Therefore, they should not be used more frequently than recommended. Do not increase the dose or frequency of medication without medical consultation. If the recommended dosage does not provide relief of symptoms or symptoms become worse, seek immediate medical attention.

While taking Ventolin Inhalation Aerosol or Ventolin Rotacaps for Inhalation, other inhaled drugs should not be used unless prescribed. While taking Ventolin Inhalation Solution or Ventolin Nebules Inhalation Solution, other antiasthma medicines should not be used unless prescribed. In general, the technique for administering Ventolin Inhalation Aerosol to children is similar to that for adults, since children's smaller ventilatory exchange capacity automatically provides proportionally smaller aerosol intake. Children should use Ventolin Inhalation Aerosol and Ventolin Rotacaps for Inhalation under adult supervision, as instructed by the patient's physician.

See package inserts for Ventolin Inhalation Aerosol, Ventolin Inhalation Solution, Ventolin Nebules Inhalation Solution, and Ventolin Rotacaps for Inhalation for illustrated Patient's Instructions for Use.

Drug Interactions: Other sympathomimetic aerosol bronchodilators or epinephrine should not be used concomitantly with albuterol. If additional adrenergic drugs are to be administered by any route to patients using Ventolin Inhalation Aerosol or Ventolin Rotacaps for Inhalation, they should be used with caution to avoid deleterious cardiovascular effects.

In addition, the concomitant use of Ventolin Syrup or Ventolin Tablets and other oral sympathomimetic agents is not recommended since such combined use may lead to deleterious cardiovascular effects. This recommendation does not preclude the judicious use of an aerosol bronchodilator of the adrenergic stimulant type in patients receiving Ventolin Syrup or Ventolin Tablets. Such concomitant use, however, should be individualized and not given on a routine basis. If regular coadministration is required, then alternative therapy should be considered.

Albuterol should be administered with extreme caution to patients being treated with monoamine oxidase inhibitors or tricyclic antidepressants because the action of albuterol on the vascular system may be potentiated.

Beta-receptor blocking agents and albuterol inhibit the effect of each other.

Carcinogenesis, Mutagenesis, Impairment of Fertility: Albuterol sulfate, like other agents in its class, caused a significant dose-related increase in the incidence of benign leiomyomas of the mesovarium in a 2-year study in the rat at doses corresponding to 93, 463, and 2,315 times, the maximum inhalational dose for a 50-kg human; to 10, 50, and 250 times the maximum nebulization dose for a 50-kg human; to 42, 248, and 1,042 times the maximum inhalational dose for a 50-kg human (Ventolin Rotacaps for Inhalation); to 2, 9, and 46 times the maximum human (child weighing 21 kg) oral dose (syrup); and to 3, 16, and 78 times the maximum oral dose for a 50-kg human (tablets). In another study this effect was blocked by the coadministration of propranolol. The relevance of these findings to humans is not known. An 18-month study in mice (at doses corresponding to 10,417 times the human inhalational dose) and a lifetime study in hamsters (at doses corresponding to 1,042 times the human inhalational dose) revealed no evidence of tumorigenicity. Studies with albuterol revealed no evidence of mutagenesis. Reproduction studies in rats (at doses corresponding to 1,042 times the human inhalational dose) revealed no evidence of impaired fertility.

Pregnancy: *Teratogenic Effects: Pregnancy Category C:* Albuterol has been shown to be teratogenic in mice when given subcutaneously in doses corresponding to 14 times the human aerosol dose; to five times the human inhalational dose (Ventolin Rotacaps for Inhalation); to 0.2 times the maximum human (child weighing 21 kg) oral dose (syrup); to 0.4 times the maximum human oral dose (tablets); and when given in doses corresponding to the human nebulization dose. There are no adequate and well-controlled studies in pregnant women. Albuterol should be used during pregnancy only if the potential benefit justifies the potential risk to the fetus.

A reproduction study in CD-1 mice given albuterol subcutaneously (0.025, 0.25, and 2.5 mg/kg, corresponding to 1.15, 11.5, and 115 times, respectively, the maximum inhalational dose for a 50-kg human; to 0.1, 1, and 12.5 times the maximum human nebulization dose; to 0.52, 5.2, and 52 times, respectively, the maximum inhalational dose for a 50-kg human [Ventolin Rotacaps for Inhalation];and to 0.04, 0.4, and 3.9 times, respectively, the maximum oral dose for a 50-kg human [tablets] showed cleft palate formation in 5 of 111 (4.5%) fetuses at 0.25 mg/kg and in 10 of 108 (9.3%) fetuses at 2.5 mg/kg. None was observed at 0.025 mg/kg. Cleft palate also occurred in 22 of 72 (30.5%) fetuses treated with 2.5 mg/kg isoproterenol (positive control). A reproduction study with oral albuterol in Stride Dutch rabbits revealed cranioschisis in 7 of 19 (37%) fetuses at 50 mg/kg, corresponding to 2,315 times the maximum inhalational dose for a 50-kg human; to 1,042 times the maximum inhalational dose for a 50-kg human (Ventolin Rotacaps for Inhalation); to 250 times the maximum human nebulization dose; to 46 times the maximum human (child weighing 21 kg) oral dose (syrup) of albuterol sulfate; and to 78 times the maximum oral dose for a 50 kg human (tablets).

Labor and Delivery: Oral albuterol has been shown to delay preterm labor in some reports. There are presently no well-controlled studies that demonstrate that it will stop preterm labor or prevent labor at term. Therefore, cautious use of Ventolin Inhalation Solution, Ventolin Nebules Inhalation Solution, Ventolin Rotacaps for Inhalation, Ventolin Syrup, and Ventolin Tablets is required in pregnant patients when given for relief of bronchospasm so as to avoid interference with uterine contractility. Use in such patients should be restricted to those patients in whom the benefits clearly outweigh the risks.

Nursing Mothers: It is not known whether albuterol is excreted in human milk. Because of the potential for tumorigenicity shown for albuterol in some animal studies, a decision should be made whether to discontinue nursing or to discontinue the drug, taking into account the importance of the drug to the mother.

Pediatric Use: Safety and effectiveness have not been established in children below 12 years of age for Ventolin Inhalation Solution and Ventolin Nebules Inhalation Solution; in children below 6 years of age for Ventolin Tablets; in children below 4 years of age for Ventolin Inhalation Aerosol and Ventolin Rotacaps for Inhalation; and in children below 2 years of age for Ventolin Syrup.

ADVERSE REACTIONS

The adverse reactions to albuterol are similar in nature to reactions to other sympathomimetic agents, although the incidence of certain cardiovascular effects is lower with albuterol. Rare cases of urticaria, angioedema, rash, bronchospasm, hoarseness, and oropharyngeal edema have been reported after the use of inhaled albuterol. In addition to the reactions given below by specific dosage form, albuterol, like other sympathomimetic agents, can cause adverse reactions such as angina, vertigo, and CNS stimulation.

Ventolin® (albuterol) Inhalation Aerosol: A 13-week, double-blind study compared albuterol and isoproterenol aerosols in 147 asthmatic patients aged 12 years and older. The results of this study showed that the incidence of cardiovascular effects was: palpitations, fewer than 10 per 100 with albuterol and fewer than 15 per 100 with isoproterenol; tachycardia, 10 per 100 with both albuterol and isoproterenol; and increased blood pressure, fewer than 5 per 100 with both albuterol and isoproterenol. In the same study, both drugs caused tremor or nausea in fewer than 15 patients per 100, and dizziness or heartburn in fewer than 5 per 100 patients. Nervousness occurred in fewer than 10 per 100 patients receiving albuterol and in fewer than 15 per 100 patients receiving isoproterenol.

Twelve-week, double-blind studies involving the use of Ventolin Inhalation Aerosol 180 mcg q.i.d. by 104 asthmatic children aged 4–11 years showed the following side effects:

Central Nervous System: Headache, 3 of 104 patients (3%); nervousness, lightheadedness, agitation, nightmares, hyperactivity, and aggressive behavior, each in 1%.

Gastrointestinal: Nausea and/or vomiting, 6 of 104 (6%); stomachache, 3 of 104 (3%); diarrhea in 1%.

Oropharyngeal: Throat irritation, 6 of 104 (6%); discoloration of teeth in 1%.

Respiratory: Epistaxis, 3 of 104 (3%); coughing, 2 of 104 (2%).

Musculoskeletal: Tremor and muscle cramp, each in 1%.

Ventolin® (albuterol sulfate) Inhalation Solution: The results of clinical trials in 135 patients showed the following side effects that were considered probably or possibly drug related:

Central Nervous System: Tremors (20%), dizziness (7%), nervousness (4%), headache (3%), insomnia (1%).

Gastrointestinal: Nausea (4%), dyspepsia (1%).

Ear, Nose, and Throat: Pharyngitis (<1%), nasal congestion (1%).

Cardiovascular: Tachycardia (1%), hypertension (1%).

Respiratory: Bronchospasm (8%), cough (4%), bronchitis (4%), wheezing (1%).

Continued on next page

Allen & Hanburys—Cont.

No clinically relevant laboratory abnormalities related to Ventolin Inhalation Solution administration were determined in these studies.

In comparing the adverse reactions reported for patients treated with Ventolin Inhalation Solution with those of patients treated with isoproterenol during clinical trials of 3 months, the following moderate to severe reactions, as judged by the investigators, were reported. This table does not include mild reactions.

Percent Incidence of Moderate to Severe Adverse Reactions

Reaction	Albuterol n=65	Isoproterenol n=65
Central nervous system		
Tremor	10.7%	13.8%
Headache	3.1%	1.5%
Insomnia	3.1%	1.5%
Cardiovascular		
Hypertension	3.1%	3.1%
Arrhythmias	0%	3.0%
Palpitation*	0%	22.0%
Respiratory		
Bronchospasm†	15.4%	18.0%
Cough	3.1%	5.0%
Bronchitis	1.5%	5.0%
Wheezing	1.5%	1.5%
Sputum increase	1.5%	1.5%
Dyspnea	1.5%	1.5%
Gastrointestinal		
Nausea	3.1%	0%
Dyspepsia	1.5%	0%
Systemic		
Malaise	1.5%	0%

* The finding of no arrhythmias and no palpitations after albuterol administration in this clinical study should not be interpreted as indicating that these adverse effects cannot occur after the administration of inhaled albuterol.
† In most cases of bronchospasm, this term was generally used to describe exacerbations in the underlying pulmonary disease.

Ventolin Rotacaps® (albuterol sulfate) for Inhalation: Results of clinical trials with Ventolin Rotacaps for Inhalation 200 mcg in 172 patients aged 12 years and older (adults) and 129 patients aged 4–12 years (children) showed the following side effects:

Central Nervous System: **Adults:** Headache, 4 of 172 patients (2%); nervousness, 2 of 172 (1%); dizziness, insomnia, lightheadedness, each in <1%. **Children:** Headache, 6 of 129 (5%), dizziness and hyperactivity, each in <1%.

Gastrointestinal: **Adults:** Burning in stomach in <1%. **Children:** Nausea and/or vomiting in 5 of 129 (4%), stomachache in 2 of 129 (2%), diarrhea in <1%.

Oropharyngeal: **Adults:** Throat irritation in 3 of 172 (2%); dry mouth and voice changes, each in <1%. **Children:** Throat irritation in 3 of 129 (2%), unusual taste in 2 of 129 (2%).

Respiratory: **Adults:** Cough in 8 of 172 (5%), bronchospasm in 2 of 172 (1%). **Children:** Cough and nasal congestion, each in 3 of 129 (2%); hoarseness and epistaxis, each in 2 of 129 (2%).

Musculoskeletal: **Adults:** Tremor in 2 of 172 (1%). **Children:** None reported.

Ventolin® (albuterol sulfate) Syrup: The most frequent adverse reactions to Ventolin Syrup in adults and older children were tremor, 10 of 100 patients, and nervousness and shakiness, each in 9 of 100 patients. Other reported adverse reactions were headache, 4 of 100 patients; dizziness and increased appetite, each in 3 of 100 patients; hyperactivity and excitement, each in 2 of 100 patients; and tachycardia, epistaxis, and sleeplessness, each in 1 of 100 patients. The following adverse effects each occurred in fewer than 1 of 100 patients: muscle spasm, disturbed sleep, epigastric pain, cough, palpitations, stomachache, irritable behavior, dilated pupils, sweating, chest pain, and weakness.

In young children 2–6 years of age, some adverse reactions were noted more frequently than in adults and older children. Excitement was noted in approximately 20% of patients and nervousness in 15%. Hyperkinesia occurred in 4% of patients, with insomnia, tachycardia, and gastrointestinal symptoms in 2% each. Anorexia, emotional lability, pallor, fatigue, and conjunctivitis were seen in 1%.

Ventolin® (albuterol sulfate) Tablets: The most frequent adverse reactions to Ventolin Tablets were nervousness and tremor, with each occurring in approximately 20 of 100 patients. Other reported reactions were headache, 7 of 100 patients; tachycardia and palpitations, 5 of 100 patients; muscle cramps, 3 of 100 patients; and insomnia, nausea, weakness, and dizziness, each in 2 of 100 patients. Drowsiness, flushing, restlessness, irritability, chest discomfort, and diffi-

culty in micturition each occurred in fewer than 1 of 100 patients.

The reactions to Ventolin Syrup and Ventolin Tablets are generally transient in nature, and it is usually not necessary to discontinue treatment. In selected cases, however, dosage may be reduced temporarily; after the reaction has subsided, dosage should be increased in small increments to the optimal dosage.

OVERDOSAGE

The expected symptoms with overdosage are those of excessive beta-stimulation and/or occurrence or exaggeration of any of the symptoms listed under ADVERSE REACTIONS, e.g., seizures, angina, hypertension or hypotension, tachycardia with rates up to 200 beats per minute, arrhythmias, nervousness, headache, tremor, dry mouth, palpitation, nausea, dizziness, fatigue, malaise, and insomnia. Hypokalemia may also occur.

Treatment consists of discontinuation of albuterol together with appropriate symptomatic therapy.

As with all sympathomimetic aerosol medications, cardiac arrest and even death may be associated with abuse of aerosol albuterol.

The oral LD_{50} in male and female rats and mice was greater than 2,000 mg/kg. The inhalational LD_{50} could not be determined.

Dialysis is not appropriate treatment for overdosage of Ventolin® (albuterol) Inhalation Aerosol, Ventolin Rotacaps® (albuterol sulfate) for Inhalation, or Ventolin® (albuterol sulfate) Syrup. The judicious use of a cardioselective beta-receptor blocker, such as metoprolol tartrate, is suggested, bearing in mind the danger of inducing an asthmatic attack. There is insufficient evidence to determine if dialysis is beneficial for overdosage of Ventolin® (albuterol sulfate) Inhalation Solution, Ventolin® Nebules™ (albuterol sulfate) Inhalation Solution, or Ventolin® (albuterol sulfate) Tablets.

DOSAGE AND ADMINISTRATION

Ventolin® (albuterol) Inhalation Aerosol: For treatment of acute episodes of bronchospasm or prevention of asthmatic symptoms, the usual dosage for adults and children 4 years and older is two inhalations repeated every 4–6 hours; in some patients, one inhalation every 4 hours may be sufficient. More frequent administration or a larger number of inhalations are not recommended.

The use of Ventolin Inhalation Aerosol can be continued as medically indicated to control recurring bouts of bronchospasm. During this time most patients gain optimal benefit from regular use of the inhaler. Safe usage for periods extending over several years has been documented.

If a previously effective dosage regimen fails to provide the usual relief, medical advice should be sought immediately as this is often a sign of seriously worsening asthma that would require reassessment of therapy.

Exercise-induced Bronchospasm Prevention: The usual dosage for adults and children 12 years and older is two inhalations 15 minutes before exercise.

For treatment, see above.

Ventolin® (albuterol sulfate) Inhalation Solution: The usual dosage for adults and children 12 years of age and older is 2.5 mg of albuterol administered three to four times daily by nebulization. More frequent administration or higher doses are not recommended. To administer 2.5 mg of albuterol, dilute 0.5 mL of the 0.5% inhalation solution with 2.5 mL of sterile normal saline solution. The flow rate is regulated to suit the particular nebulizer so that Ventolin Inhalation Solution will be delivered over approximately 5–15 minutes.

The use of Ventolin Inhalation Solution can be continued as medically indicated to control recurring bouts of bronchospasm. During this time most patients gain optimal benefit from regular use of the inhalation solution.

If a previously effective dosage regimen fails to provide the usual relief, medical advice should be sought immediately as this is often a sign of seriously worsening asthma that would require reassessment of therapy.

Ventolin® Nebules™ (albuterol sulfate) Inhalation Solution: The usual dosage for adults and children 12 years and older is 2.5 mg of albuterol administered three to four times daily by nebulization. More frequent administration or higher doses are not recommended. To administer 2.5 mg of albuterol, administer the contents of one sterile unit dose Nebule® (3 mL of 0.083% inhalation solution) by nebulization. The flow rate is regulated to suit the particular nebulizer so that Ventolin Nebules Inhalation Solution will be delivered over approximately 5–15 minutes.

The use of Ventolin Nebules Inhalation Solution can be continued as medically indicated to control recurring bouts of bronchospasm. During this time most patients gain optimal benefit from regular use of the inhalation solution.

If a previously effective dosage regimen fails to provide the usual relief, medical advice should be sought immediately as this is often a sign of seriously worsening asthma that would require reassessment of therapy.

Ventolin Rotacaps® (albuterol sulfate) for Inhalation: The usual dosage for adults and children 4 years of age and older is the contents of one 200-mcg capsule inhaled every 4–6 hours using a Rotahaler® inhalation device. In some patients, the contents of two 200-mcg capsules inhaled every 4–6 hours may be required. Larger doses or more frequent administration are not recommended.

The use of Ventolin Rotacaps for Inhalation can be continued as medically indicated to control recurring bouts of bronchospasm. During this time most patients gain optimal benefit from regular use of the Ventolin Rotacaps for Inhalation formulation.

If a previously effective dosage regimen fails to provide the usual relief, medical advice should be sought immediately as this is often a sign of seriously worsening asthma that would require reassessment of therapy.

Exercise-induced Bronchospasm Prevention: The usual dosage of Ventolin Rotacaps for Inhalation for adults and children 12 years of age and older is the contents of one 200-mcg capsule inhaled using a Rotahaler 15 minutes before exercise.

Ventolin® (albuterol sulfate) Syrup: The following dosages of Ventolin Syrup are expressed in terms of albuterol base.
Usual Dosage: The usual starting dosage for adults and children over age 14 is 2 mg (1 teaspoonful) or 4 mg (2 teaspoonfuls) three or four times a day.

The usual starting dosage for children 6–14 years of age is 2 mg (1 teaspoonful) three or four times a day.

For children 2–6 years of age, dosing should be initiated at 0.1 mg/kg of body weight three times a day. This starting dosage should not exceed 2 mg (1 teaspoonful) three times a day.

Dosage Adjustment: For adults and children over age 14, a dosage above 4 mg four times a day should be used *only* when the patient fails to respond. If a favorable response does not occur, the dosage may be cautiously increased stepwise, but not to exceed 8 mg four times a day.

For children 6–14 years of age who fail to respond to the initial starting dosage of 2 mg four times a day, the dosage may be cautiously increased stepwise, but not to exceed 24 mg per day (given in divided doses).

For children 2–6 years of age who do not respond satisfactorily to the initial dosage, the dosage may be increased stepwise to 0.2 mg/kg of body weight three times a day, but not to exceed a maximum of 4 mg (2 teaspoonfuls) given three times a day.

Elderly Patients and Those Sensitive to Beta-adrenergic Stimulators: The initial dosage should be restricted to 2 mg three or four times a day and individually adjusted thereafter.

Ventolin® (albuterol sulfate) Tablets: The following dosages of Ventolin Tablets are expressed in terms of albuterol base.
Usual Dosage: The usual starting dosage for adults and children 12 years of age and older is 2 or 4 mg three or four times a day.

The usual starting dosage for children 6–12 years of age is 2 mg three or four times a day.

Dosage Adjustment: For adults and children 12 years of age and older, a dosage above 4 mg four times a day should be used only when the patient fails to respond. If a favorable response does not occur with the 4-mg initial dosage, it should be cautiously increased stepwise up to a maximum of 8 mg four times a day as tolerated.

For children 6–12 years of age who fail to respond to the initial starting dosage of 2 mg four times a day, the dosage may be cautiously increased stepwise, but not to exceed 24 mg per day (given in divided doses).

Elderly Patients and Those Sensitive to Beta-adrenergic Stimulators: An initial dosage of 2 mg three or four times a day is recommended for elderly patients and for those with a history of unusual sensitivity to beta-adrenergic stimulators. If adequate bronchodilatation is not obtained, dosage may be increased gradually to as much as 8 mg three or four times a day.

The total daily dose should not exceed 32 mg in adults and children 12 years of age and older.

HOW SUPPLIED

Ventolin® (albuterol) Inhalation Aerosol is supplied in 17-g canisters containing 200 metered inhalations in boxes of one. Each actuation delivers 90 mcg of albuterol from the mouthpiece. Each canister is supplied with an oral adapter and patient's instructions (NDC 0173-0321-88). Also available, Ventolin Inhalation Aerosol Refill 17-g canister only with patient's instructions (NDC 0173-0321-98). **Store between 15° and 30°C (59° and 86°F). As with most inhaled medications in aerosol canisters, the therapeutic effect of this medication may decrease when the canister is cold. Shake well before using.**

Ventolin® (albuterol sulfate) Inhalation Solution, 0.5% is supplied in bottles of 20 mL (NDC 0173-0385-58) with accompanying calibrated dropper in boxes of one. **Store between 2° and 25°C (36° and 77°F).**

Ventolin® Nebules™ (albuterol sulfate) Inhalation Solution, 0.083% is supplied in sterile unit dose nebules of 3 mL each in boxes of 25 (NDC 0173-0419-00). **Protect from light.**

Store in a refrigerator between 2° and 8°C (36° and 46°F). Ventolin Nebules Inhalation Solution may be held at room temperature for up to 2 weeks before use. (Nebules must be used within 2 weeks of removal from refrigerator; record date the nebules are removed from the refrigerator in the space provided on the product carton.) Discard if solution becomes discolored. (Note: Ventolin Nebules Inhalation Solution is colorless.)

Ventolin Rotacaps® (albuterol sulfate) for Inhalation, 200 mcg, are light blue and clear, with "VENTOLIN 200" printed on the blue cap and "GLAXO" printed on the clear body. Ventolin Rotacaps for Inhalation are supplied in a unit dose kit containing one unit dose pack of 96 capsules and one Rotahaler® inhalation device (NDC 0173-0389-81) and a hospital unit dose kit containing one unit dose pack of 24 capsules and one Rotahaler inhalation device (NDC 0173-0389-03). **Store between 2° and 30°C (36° and 86°F).**

Ventolin® (albuterol sulfate) Syrup, a clear, orange-yellow liquid with a strawberry flavor, contains 2 mg of albuterol as the sulfate per 5 mL in bottles of 16 fluid ounces (one pint) (NDC 0173-0351-54). **Store between 2° and 30°C (36° and 86°F).**

Ventolin® (albuterol sulfate) Tablets, 2 mg of albuterol as the sulfate, are white, round, compressed tablets impressed with the product name (VENTOLIN) and the number 2 on one side and scored on the other with "GLAXO" impressed on each side of the score in bottles of 100 (NDC 0173-0341-43) and 500 (NDC 0173-0341-44).

Ventolin® Tablets, 4 mg of albuterol as the sulfate, are white, round, compressed tablets impressed with the product name (VENTOLIN) and the number 4 on one side and scored on the other with "GLAXO" impressed on each side of the score in bottles of 100 (NDC 0173-0342-43) and 500 (NDC 0173-0342-44).

Store between 2° and 25°C (36° and 77°F). Replace cap securely after each opening.

Shown in Product Identification Section, page 404

Allergan Herbert
Skin Care Division of Allergan, Inc.
2525 DUPONT DRIVE
P.O. BOX 19534
IRVINE, CA 92713-9534

AEROSEB–DEX® ℞
(dexamethasone) 0.01%
Topical Aerosol Spray

Active Ingredient: dexamethasone 0.01%
Inactive Ingredients: SD Alcohol 40-2 (59%), isopropyl myristate and propellant (butane).
Each 1 second of spray dispenses approximately 0.02 mg of dexamethasone.

HOW SUPPLIED
In a 58 g aerosol with applicator tube.* NDC 0023-0852-90
© 1992 Allergan, Inc.

*U.S. Patent 3,730,182

AEROSEB–HC® ℞
(hydrocortisone) 0.5%
Topical Aerosol Spray

Active Ingredient: hydrocortisone 0.5%
Inactive Ingredients: SD Alcohol 40-2 (58%), isopropyl myristate and propellant (butane).
Each 1 second of spray dispenses approximately 1 mg of hydrocortisone.

HOW SUPPLIED
In a 58 g aerosol with applicator tube.* NDC 0023-0804-90
© 1992 Allergan, Inc.

*U.S. Patent 3,730,182

ELIMITE® ℞
(permethrin) 5% Cream

DESCRIPTION
Elimite® (permethrin) 5% Cream is a topical scabicidal agent for the treatment of infestation with *Sarcoptes scabiei* (scabies). It is available in an off-white vanishing cream base. Each gram contains: *Active Ingredient:* permethrin 50 mg (5%). *Inactive Ingredients:* butylated hydroxytoluene, carbomer 934P, fractionated coconut oil, glycerin, glyceryl monostearate, isopropyl myristate, lanolin alcohols, mineral oil, polyoxyethylene cetylethers, purified water, and sodium hydroxide. Formaldehyde 1 mg (0.1%) is added as a preservative.

The permethrin used is an approximate 1:3 mixture of the *cis* and *trans* isomers of the pyrethroid (±)-3-phenoxybenzyl 3-(2,2-dichlorovinyl)-2,2-dimethylcyclopropane-carboxylate. It is a yellow to light orange-brown, low melting solid or viscous liquid. The molecular weight is 391.29 and the structural formula is:

CLINICAL PHARMACOLOGY
Permethrin, a pyrethroid, is active against a broad range of pests including lice, ticks, fleas, mites, and other arthropods. It acts on the nerve cell membrane to disrupt the sodium channel current by which the polarization of the membrane is regulated. Delayed repolarization and paralysis of the pests are the consequences of this disturbance.

Permethrin is rapidly metabolized by ester hydrolysis to inactive metabolites which are excreted primarily in the urine. Although the amount of permethrin absorbed after a single application of the 5% Cream has not been determined precisely, data from studies with ^{14}C-labeled permethrin and absorption studies of the cream applied to patients with moderate to severe scabies indicate it is 2% or less of the amount applied.

INDICATIONS AND USAGE
Elimite (permethrin) 5% Cream is indicated for the single-application treatment of infestation with *Sarcoptes scabiei* (scabies).

CONTRAINDICATIONS
Elimite is contraindicated in patients with known hypersensitivity to any of its components, to any synthetic pyrethroid or pyrethrin.

WARNINGS
If hypersensitivity to Elimite occurs, discontinue use.

PRECAUTIONS
General: Scabies infestation is often accompanied by pruritus, edema and erythema. Treatment with Elimite may temporarily exacerbate these conditions.
Information for patients: Patients with scabies should be advised that itching, mild burning and/or stinging may occur after application of Elimite. In clinical trials approximately 75% of patients treated with Elimite who continued to manifest pruritus at 2 weeks had cessation by 4 weeks. If irritation persists, they should consult their physician. Elimite may be very mildly irritating to the eyes. Patients should be advised to avoid contact with eyes during application and to flush with water immediately if Elimite gets in the eyes.
Carcinogenesis, mutagenesis, impairment of fertility: Six carcinogenicity bioassays were evaluated with permethrin, three each in rats and mice. No tumorigenicity was seen in the rat studies. However, species-specific increases in pulmonary adenomas, a common benign tumor of mice of high spontaneous background incidence, were seen in the three mouse studies. In one of these studies there was an increased incidence of pulmonary alveolar-cell carcinomas and benign liver adenomas only in female mice when permethrin was given in their food at a concentration of 5000 ppm. Mutagenicity assays, which give useful correlative data for interpreting results from carcinogenicity bioassays in rodents, were negative. Permethrin showed no evidence of mutagenic potential in a battery of *in vitro* and *in vivo* genetic toxicity studies.
Permethrin did not have any adverse effect on reproductive function at a dose of 180 mg/kg/day orally in a three-generation rat study.
Pregnancy: *teratogenic effects:* Pregnancy Category B: Reproduction studies have been performed in mice, rats, and rabbits (200 to 400 mg/kg/day orally) and have revealed no evidence of impaired fertility or harm to the fetus due to permethrin. There are, however, no adequate and well-controlled studies in pregnant women. Because animal reproduction studies are not always predictive of human response, this drug should be used during pregnancy only if clearly needed.
Nursing mothers: It is not known whether this drug is excreted in human milk. Because many drugs are excreted in human milk and because of the evidence for tumorigenic potential of permethrin in animal studies, consideration should be given to discontinuing nursing temporarily or withholding the drug while the mother is nursing.
Pediatric use: Elimite is safe and effective in children two months of age and older. Safety and effectiveness in children less than two months of age have not been established.

ADVERSE REACTIONS
In clinical trials, generally mild and transient burning and stinging followed application with Elimite in 10% of patients and was associated with the severity of infestation. Pruritus

---

was reported in 7% of patients at various times post-application. Erythema, numbness, tingling, and rash were reported in 1 to 2% or less of patients (see PRECAUTIONS: General).

OVERDOSAGE
No instance of accidental ingestion of Elimite has been reported. If ingested, gastric lavage and general supportive measures should be employed.

DOSAGE AND ADMINISTRATION
Adults and children: Thoroughly massage Elimite into the skin from the head to the soles of the feet. Scabies rarely infests the scalp of adults, although the hairline, neck, temple, and forehead may be infested in infants and geriatric patients. Usually 30 grams is sufficient for an average adult. The cream should be removed by washing (shower or bath) after 8 to 14 hours. Infants should be treated on the scalp, temple and forehead. One application is curative.

Patients may experience persistent pruritus after treatment. This is rarely a sign of treatment failure and is not an indication for retreatment.

HOW SUPPLIED
Elimite® (permethrin) 5% (wt./wt.) Cream is supplied in tubes in the following size: 60 g—NDC 0023-7915-60.
Note: Store at 15° to 25°C (59° to 77°F).
Caution: Federal (U.S.A.) law prohibits dispensing without prescription.
Manufactured for:
ALLERGAN Herbert
Skin Care Division of Allergan, Inc.
Irvine, CA 92713, U.S.A.
by Burroughs Wellcome Co.
Research Triangle Park, NC 27709
© 1992 Allergan, Inc.

ERYGEL® ℞
[ār'ē-jel]
(erythromycin) 2%
Topical Gel

Active Ingredient: erythromycin, USP .... 2% (20 mg/g)
Inactive Ingredients: alcohol 92% and hydroxypropyl cellulose

HOW SUPPLIED
Erygel® (erythromycin) 2% Topical Gel is supplied in plastic tubes in the following sizes: 30 g—NDC 0023-4312-30.
60 g—NDC 0023-4312-60.
Note: FLAMMABLE. Keep away from heat and flame. Keep tube tightly closed. Store at room temperature.
© 1992 Allergan, Inc.

ERYMAX® ℞
(Erythromycin Topical Solution USP) 2%

Active Ingredient: erythromycin .... 2% (20 mg/mL)
Inactive Ingredients: SD Alcohol 40-2 (66%), propylene glycol, and citric acid

HOW SUPPLIED
In a 2 fl oz plastic bottle with optional Dab-O-Matic applicator and a 4 fl oz plastic bottle:
2 fl oz (59 mL)—NDC 0023-0540-02
4 fl oz (118 mL)—NDC 0023-0540-04
© 1992 Allergan, Inc.

EXSEL® Lotion/Shampoo ℞
(Selenium sulfide lotion, USP) 2.5%

Active Ingredient: selenium sulfide .... 2.5% (w/v) in aqueous suspension
Inactive Ingredients: edetate disodium; bentonite; sodium dodecylbenzene sulfonate; sodium C14-16 olefin sulfonate; glyceryl ricinoleate; dimethicone copolyol; titanium dioxide; citric acid monohydrate; sodium phosphate monobasic, monohydrate; fragrance; and purified water

HOW SUPPLIED
Exsel is available in a 4 fl oz plastic bottle—NDC 0023-0817-99
© 1992 Allergan, Inc.

Continued on next page

Allergan Herbert—Cont.

FLUONID® ℞
(fluocinolone acetonide) 0.01%
Topical Solution

Active Ingredient: fluocinolone acetonide 0.01%
Inactive Ingredients: propylene glycol and citric acid

HOW SUPPLIED
Topical Solution 0.01%—20 mL and 60 mL plastic squeeze bottles.
   20 mL NDC 0023-0878-20
   60 mL NDC 0023-0878-60
© 1992 Allergan, Inc.

FLUOROPLEX® ℞
(fluorouracil)
1% Topical Cream and
1% Topical Solution

PRODUCT OVERVIEW

KEY FACTS
Effective treatment for multiple Actinic Keratoses sites.
Provides effective treatment for both clinical and subclinical lesions.
Fluoroplex Cream does not contain irritating parabens or propylene glycol.

MAJOR USES
Multiple actinic keratoses.

SAFETY INFORMATION
Contraindicated in persons hypersensitive to fluorouracil or its listed ingredients.
Contraindicated in pregnancy.
Prolonged exposure to sunlight or other forms of ultraviolet irradiation may increase intensity of reaction.
Adequate long-term studies in animals to evaluate carcinogenic potential have not been conducted with fluorouracil.

PRESCRIBING INFORMATION

FLUOROPLEX® ℞
(fluorouracil)
1% Topical Cream and
1% Topical Solution

DESCRIPTION
Fluoroplex (fluorouracil) 1% Topical Cream and 1% Topical Solution are antineoplastic/antimetabolite products for dermatological use. Fluorouracil has the empirical formula $C_4H_3FN_2O_2$ and a molecular weight of 130.08. It is sparingly soluble in water and slightly soluble in alcohol. The pH is approximately 8.5 for Fluoroplex Topical Cream and 9.2 for Fluoroplex Topical Solution.
Chemical Name:
2,4(1*H*, 3*H*)-Pyrimidinedione,5-fluoro-.
Fluoroplex 1% Topical Cream contains:
Active Ingredient: fluorouracil 1.0%
Inactive Ingredients: benzyl alcohol, emulsifying wax, mineral oil, isopropyl myristate, sodium hydroxide and purified water
Fluoroplex 1% Topical Solution contains:
Active Ingredient: fluorouracil 1.0%
Inactive Ingredients: propylene glycol, sodium hydroxide and/or hydrochloric acid to adjust the pH, and purified water
Structural Formula:

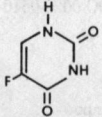

fluorouracil

CLINICAL PHARMACOLOGY
There is evidence that fluorouracil (or its metabolites) blocks the methylation reaction of deoxyuridylic acid to thymidylic acid. In this fashion, fluorouracil interferes with the synthesis of deoxyribonucleic acid (DNA) and to a lesser extent inhibits the formation of ribonucleic acid (RNA).

INDICATIONS AND USAGE
Fluoroplex is indicated for the topical treatment of multiple actinic (solar) keratoses.

CONTRAINDICATIONS
Fluorouracil is contraindicated in women who are or may become pregnant. These products should not be used by patients who are allergic to any of their components.

WARNINGS
There exists the potential for a delayed hypersensitivity reaction to fluorouracil. Patch testing to prove hypersensitivity may be inconclusive.[1]
If an occlusive dressing is used, there may be an increase in the incidence of inflammatory reactions in the adjacent normal skin.
The patient should avoid prolonged exposure to sunlight or other forms of ultraviolet irradiation during treatment with Fluoroplex, as the intensity of the reaction may be increased.

PRECAUTIONS
General: There is a possibility of increased absorption through ulcerated or inflamed skin.
Information for patients: The medication should be applied with care near the eyes, nose and mouth. Excessive reaction in these areas may occur due to irritation from accumulation of drug. If Fluoroplex is applied with the fingers, the hands should be washed immediately afterward.
The reaction to Fluoroplex in treated areas may be unsightly during therapy, and, in some cases, for several weeks following cessation of therapy.
Laboratory Tests: To rule out the presence of a frank neoplasm, a biopsy should be made of those areas failing to respond to treatment or recurring after treatment.
Carcinogenesis, mutagenesis, impairment of fertility: Adequate long-term studies in animals to evaluate carcinogenic potential have not been conducted with fluorouracil. In three *in-vitro* cell transformation assays, fluorouracil produced morphological transformation of cells. Morphological transformation was also produced in one of these *in-vitro* assays by a metabolite of fluorouracil and the transformed cells produced malignant tumors when injected into immunosuppressed syngeneic mice. Fluorouracil has been shown to exert mutagenic activity in the yeast cells. **Bacillus subtilis,** and **Drosophila** assays. In addition, fluorouracil has produced chromosome damage at concentrations of 1.0 and 2.0 mcg/mL in an *in vitro* hamster fibroblast assay and increases in micronuclei formation in the bone marrow of mice at intraperitoneal doses within the human therapeutic dose range of 12–15 mg/kg/day. Patients receiving cumulative doses of 0.24–1.0 g of fluorouracil parenterally have shown an increase in numerical and structural chromosome aberrations in peripheral blood lymphocytes. Fluorouracil has been shown to impair fertility after parenteral administration in rats. In mice, single-dose intravenous and intraperitoneal injections of fluorouracil have been reported to kill differentiated spermatogonia and spermatocytes at a dose of 500 mg/kg and produce abnormalities in spermatids at 50 mg/kg.
Fluorouracil was negative in the dominant lethal mutation assay performed in mice.
Pregnancy: Teratogenic effects: Pregnancy Category X: Fluorouracil may cause fetal harm when administered to a pregnant woman. Fluorouracil administered parenterally has been shown to be teratogenic in mice, rats and hamsters, and embryolethal in monkeys. Fluorouracil is contraindicated in women who are or may become pregnant. If this drug is used during pregnancy, or if the patient becomes pregnant while taking this drug, the patient should be apprised of the potential hazard to the fetus.
Nursing mothers: It is not known whether this drug is excreted in human milk. Because many drugs are excreted in human milk, and because there is some systemic absorption of fluorouracil after topical administration (see **PRECAUTIONS: General**), mothers should not nurse their infants while receiving this drug.
Pediatric use: Safety and effectiveness in children have not been established.

ADVERSE REACTIONS
Pain, pruritus, burning, irritation, inflammation, allergic contact dermatitis and telangiectasia have been reported. Occasionally, hyperpigmentation and scarring have also been reported.

OVERDOSAGE
Ordinarily, overdosage will not cause acute problems. If Fluoroplex accidentally comes in contact with the eye(s), flush the eye(s) with water or normal saline. If Fluoroplex is accidentally ingested, induce emesis and gastric lavage. Administer symptomatic and supportive care as needed.

DOSAGE AND ADMINISTRATION
The patient should be instructed to apply sufficient medication to cover the entire face or other affected areas.
Apply medication twice daily with non-metallic applicator or fingertips and wash hands afterwards. A treatment period of 2–6 weeks is usually required.
Increasing the frequency of application and a longer period of administration with Fluoroplex may be required on areas other than the head and neck.
When Fluoroplex is applied to keratotic skin, a response occurs with the following sequence: erythema, usually followed by scaling, tenderness, erosion, ulceration, necrosis and re-epithelization. When the inflammatory reaction reaches the erosion, ulceration and necrosis stages, the use of

the drug should be terminated. Responses may sometimes occur in areas which appear clinically normal. These may be sites of subclinical actinic (solar) keratosis which the medication is affecting.

HOW SUPPLIED
Fluoroplex® (fluorouracil) 1% Topical Cream is available in 30 g tubes (NDC 0023-0812-30).
Fluoroplex® (fluorouracil) 1% Topical Solution is available in 30 mL plastic dropper bottles (NDC 0023-0810-30).
Note: Avoid freezing. Store at 15°–25°C (59°–77°F) in tight containers.
CAUTION: Federal (U.S.A.) law prohibits dispensing without prescription.

REFERENCE
1. Epstein E. Testing for 5-fluorouracil allergy: patch and intradermal tests. Contact Dermatitis 1984; 10:311.
© 1992 Allergan, Inc.

Gris-PEG® ℞
(griseofulvin ultramicrosize)
Tablets, USP
125 mg; 250 mg

DESCRIPTION
Gris-PEG Tablets contain ultramicrosize crystals of griseofulvin, an antibiotic derived from a species of *Penicillium*. Each Gris-PEG Tablet contains:
Active Ingredient: griseofulvin ultramicrosize ...... 125 mg
Inactive Ingredients: colloidal silicon dioxide, lactose, magnesium stearate; methylcellulose; methylparaben; polyethylene glycol 400 and 8000, polyvinylpolypyrrolidone; povidone; and titanium dioxide, or
Active Ingredient: griseofulvin ultramicrosize .... 250 mg
Inactive Ingredients: colloidal silicon dioxide; magnesium stearate; methylcellulose; methylparaben; polyethylene glycol 400 and 8000; povidone; sodium lauryl sulfate; and titanium dioxide.

ACTION
Microbiology—Griseofulvin is fungistatic with *in vitro* activity against various species of *Microsporum, Epidermophyton* and *Trichophyton.* It has no effect on bacteria or other genera of fungi.
Human Pharmacology—Following oral administration, griseofulvin is deposited in the keratin precursor cells and has a greater affinity for diseased tissue. The drug is tightly bound to the new keratin which becomes highly resistant to fungal invasions.
The efficiency of gastrointestinal absorption of ultramicrocrystalline griseofulvin is approximately one and one-half times that of the conventional microsize griseofulvin. This factor permits the oral intake of two-thirds as much ultramicrocrystalline griseofulvin as the microsize form. However, there is currently no evidence that this lower dose confers any significant clinical differences with regard to safety and/or efficacy.

INDICATIONS
Gris-PEG (griseofulvin ultramicrosize) is indicated for the treatment of the following ringworm infections; tinea corporis (ringworm of the body), tinea pedis (athlete's foot), tinea cruris (ringworm of the groin and thigh), tinea barbae (barber's itch), tinea capitis (ringworm of the scalp), and tinea unguium (onychomycosis, ringworm of the nails), when caused by one or more of the following genera of fungi: *Trichophyton rubrum, Trichophyton tonsurans, Trichophyton mentagrophytes, Trichophyton interdigitalis, Trichophyton verrucosum, Trichophyton megnini, Trichophyton gallinae, Trichophyton crateriform, Trichophyton sulphureum, Trichophyton schoenleini, Microsporum audouini, Microsporum canis, Microsporum gypseum* and *Epidermophyton floccosum.*
Note: Prior to therapy, the type of fungi responsible for the infection should be identified. The use of the drug is not justified in minor or trivial infections which will respond to topical agents alone. Griseofulvin is *not* effective in the following: bacterial infections, candidiasis (moniliasis), histoplasmosis, actinomycosis, sporotrichosis, chromoblastomycosis, coccidioidomycosis, North American blastomycosis, cryptococcosis (torulosis), tinea versicolor and nocardiosis.

CONTRAINDICATIONS
Two cases of conjoined twins have been reported since 1977 in patients taking griseofulvin during the first trimester of pregnancy. Griseofulvin should not be prescribed to pregnant patients. If the patient becomes pregnant while taking this drug, the patient should be apprised of the potential hazard to the fetus.
This drug is contraindicated in patients with porphyria or hepatocellular failure and in individuals with a history of hypersensitivity to griseofulvin.

WARNINGS
Prophylactic Usage—Safety and efficacy of griseofulvin for prophylaxis of fungal infections have not been established.

Animal Toxicology—Chronic feeding of griseofulvin, at levels ranging from 0.5%–2.5% of the diet resulted in the development of liver tumors in several strains of mice, particularly in males. Smaller particle sizes result in an enhanced effect. Lower oral dosage levels have not been tested. Subcutaneous administration of relatively small doses of griseofulvin once a week during the first three weeks of life has also been reported to induce hepatomata in mice. Thyroid tumors, mostly adenomas but some carcinomas, have been reported in male rats receiving griseofulvin at levels of 2.0%, 1.0% and 0.2% of the diet, and in female rats receiving the two higher dose levels. Although studies in other animal species have not yielded evidence of tumorigenicity, these studies were not of adequate design to form a basis for conclusion in this regard. In subacute toxicity studies, orally administered griseofulvin produced hepatocellular necrosis in mice, but this has not been seen in other species. Disturbances in porphyrin metabolism have been reported in griseofulvin-treated laboratory animals. Griseofulvin has been reported to have a colchicine-like effect on mitosis and cocarcinogenicity with methylcholanthrene in cutaneous tumor induction in laboratory animals. *Usage in Pregnancy*—See CONTRAINDICATIONS section. *Animal Reproduction Studies*—It has been reported in the literature that griseofulvin was found to be embryotoxic and teratogenic on oral administration to pregnant rats. Pups with abnormalities have been reported in the litters of a few bitches treated with griseofulvin. Suppression of spermatogenesis has been reported to occur in rats, but investigation in man failed to confirm this.

PRECAUTIONS

Patients on prolonged therapy with any potent medication should be under close observation. Periodic monitoring of organ system function, including renal, hepatic and hematopoietic, should be done. Since griseofulvin is derived from species of *Penicillium*, the possibility of cross-sensitivity with penicillin exists; however, known penicillin-sensitive patients have been treated without difficulty. Since a photosensitivity reaction is occasionally associated with griseofulvin therapy, patients should be warned to avoid exposure to intense natural or artificial sunlight. Lupus erythematosus or lupus-like syndromes have been reported in patients receiving griseofulvin. Griseofulvin decreases the activity of warfarin-type anticoagulants so that patients receiving these drugs concomitantly may require dosage adjustment of the anticoagulant during and after griseofulvin therapy. Barbiturates usually depress griseofulvin activity and concomitant administration may require a dosage adjustment of the antifungal agent. There have been reports in the literature of possible interactions between griseofulvin and oral contraceptives. The effect of alcohol may be potentiated by griseofulvin, producing such effects as tachycardia and flush.

ADVERSE REACTIONS

When adverse reactions occur, they are most commonly of the hypersensitivity type such as skin rashes, urticaria, and rarely, angioneurotic edema, and may necessitate withdrawal of therapy and appropriate countermeasures. Paresthesias of the hands and feet have been reported rarely after extended therapy. Other side effects reported occasionally are oral thrush, nausea, vomiting, epigastric distress, diarrhea, headache, fatigue, dizziness, insomnia, mental confusion, and impairment of performance of routine activities. Proteinuria and leukopenia have been reported rarely. Administration of the drug should be discontinued if granulocytopenia occurs. When rare, serious reactions occur with griseofulvin, they are usually associated with high dosages, long periods of therapy, or both.

DOSAGE AND ADMINISTRATION

Accurate diagnosis of the infecting organism is essential. Identification should be made either by direct microscopic examination of a mounting of infected tissue in a solution of potassium hydroxide or by culture on an appropriate medium. Medication must be continued until the infecting organism is completely eradicated as indicated by appropriate clinical or laboratory examination. Representative treatment periods are tinea capitis, 4 to 6 weeks; tinea corporis, 2 to 4 weeks; tinea pedis, 4 to 8 weeks; tinea unguium—depending on rate of growth—fingernails, at least 4 months; toenails, at least 6 months.
General measures in regard to hygiene should be observed to control sources of infection or reinfection. Concomitant use of appropriate topical agents is usually required, particularly in treatment of tinea pedis. In some forms of athlete's foot, yeasts and bacteria may be involved as well as fungi. Griseofulvin will not eradicate the bacterial or monilial infection.
Adults: Daily administration of 375 mg (as a single dose or in divided doses) will give a satisfactory response in most patients with tinea corporis, tinea cruris, and tinea capitis. For those fungal infections more difficult to eradicate, such as tinea pedis and tinea unguium, a divided dose of 750 mg is recommended.
Children: Approximately 3.3 mg per pound of body weight per day of ultramicrosize griseofulvin is an effective dose for most children. On this basis, the following dosage schedule is suggested: Children weighing 35–60 pounds—125 mg to 187.5 mg daily. Children weighing over 60 pounds—187.5 mg to 375 mg daily. Children 2 years of age and younger—dosage has not been established.
Clinical experience with griseofulvin in children with tinea capitis indicates that a single daily dose is effective. Clinical relapse will occur if the medication is not continued until the infecting organism is eradicated.

HOW SUPPLIED

Gris-PEG® (griseofulvin ultramicrosize) Tablets, 125 mg, white, scored, elliptical-shaped, embossed "Gris-PEG®" on one side and "125" on the other. Gris-PEG® (griseofulvin ultramicrosize) Tablets, 250 mg, white, scored, capsule-shaped, embossed "Gris-PEG" on one side and "250" on the other. The 125 mg strength is available in bottles of 100 and 500 (NDC 0023-0763-04, and NDC 0023-0763-99 respectively). The 250 mg strength is available in bottles of 100, 250 and 500 (NDC 0023-0773-04, NDC 0023-0773-25, and NDC 0023-0773-50 respectively). Both strengths are film-coated.

CAUTION

Federal (U.S.A.) law prohibits dispensing without prescription.

STORAGE

Store Gris-PEG tablets at controlled room temperature 15°–30°C (59°–86°F) in tight, light-resistant containers.
Manufactured for ALLERGAN Herbert
Skin Care Division of Allergan, Inc.
Irvine, CA 92713, U.S.A.
by SANDOZ PHARMACEUTICALS CORPORATION
© 1992 Allergan, Inc.

MAXIFLOR®   ℞
(diflorasone diacetate)
Cream, USP, 0.05%
Ointment, USP, 0.05%

DESCRIPTION

MAXIFLOR Cream Contains:
Active Ingredient: 0.5 mg diflorasone diacetate, USP, in an emulsified and hydrophilic cream base.
Inactive Ingredients: Propylene glycol, stearic acid, polysorbate 60, sorbitan monostearate and monooleate, sorbic acid, citric acid and water. The corticosteroid is formulated as a solution in the vehicle using 15 percent propylene glycol to optimize drug delivery.
MAXIFLOR Ointment Contains:
Active Ingredient: 0.5 mg diflorasone diacetate, USP, in an emollient, occlusive base. *Inactive Ingredients:* Polyoxypropylene 15-stearyl ether, stearic acid, lanolin alcohol and white petrolatum.

HOW SUPPLIED

MAXIFLOR® (diflorasone diacetate) Cream, USP, 0.05% is available in collapsible tubes in the following sizes:
    15 gram NDC 0023-0766-15
    30 gram NDC 0023-0766-30
    60 gram NDC 0023-0766-60
MAXIFLOR® (diflorasone diacetate) Ointment, USP, 0.05% is available in collapsible tubes in the following sizes:
    15 gram NDC 0023-0770-15
    30 gram NDC 0023-0770-30
    60 gram NDC 0023-0770-60
Manufactured for **ALLERGAN Herbert**
Skin Care Division of **Allergan, Inc.**
Irvine, California 92713, USA
by **The Upjohn Company**
Kalamazoo, Michigan 49001
© 1992 Allergan, Inc.

NAFTIN®   ℞
(naftifine hydrochloride) 1%
Cream

DESCRIPTION

Naftin Cream, 1% contains the synthetic, broad-spectrum, antifungal agent naftifine hydrochloride.
Naftin Cream, 1% is for topical use only.
Chemical Name: (E)-N-Cinnamyl-N-methyl-1-naphthalenemethyl-amine hydrochloride. Naftifine hydrochloride has an empirical formula of $C_{21}H_{21}N \cdot HCl$ and a molecular weight of 323.86.
Active Ingredient: Naftifine hydrochloride 1%
Inactive Ingredients: benzyl alcohol, cetyl alcohol, cetyl esters wax, isopropyl myristate, polysorbate 60, purified water, sodium hydroxide, sorbitan monostearate, and stearyl alcohol. Hydrochloric acid may be added to adjust pH.

CLINICAL PHARMACOLOGY

Naftifine hydrochloride is a synthetic allylamine derivative. The following *in vitro* data are available, but their clinical significance is unknown. Naftifine hydrochloride has been shown to exhibit fungicidal activity *in vitro* against a broad spectrum of organisms including *Trichophyton rubrum*, *Trichophyton mentagrophytes*, *Trichophyton tonsurans*, *Epidermophyton floccosum*, *Microsporum canis*, *Microsporum audouini*, and *Microsporum gypseum;* and fungistatic activity against *Candida* species, including *Candida albicans*. Naftin Cream, 1% has only been shown to be clinically effective against the disease entities listed in the INDICATIONS AND USAGE section.
Although the exact mechanism of action against fungi is not known, naftifine hydrochloride appears to interfere with sterol biosynthesis by inhibiting the enzyme squalene 2,3-epoxidase. This inhibition of enzyme activity results in decreased amounts of sterols, especially ergosterol, and a corresponding accumulation of squalene in the cells.
Pharmacokinetics: *In vitro* and *in vivo* bioavailability studies have demonstrated that naftifine penetrates the stratum corneum in sufficient concentration to inhibit the growth of dermatophytes.
Following a single topical application of 1% naftifine cream to the skin of healthy subjects, systemic absorption of naftifine was approximately 6% of the applied dose. Naftifine and/or its metabolites are excreted via the urine and feces with a half-life of approximately two to three days.

INDICATIONS AND USAGE

Naftin Cream, 1% is indicated for the topical application in the treatment of tinea pedis, tinea cruris and tinea corporis caused by the organisms *Tricophyton rubrum*, *Tricophyton mentagrophytes*, and *Epidermophyton floccosum*.

CONTRAINDICATIONS

Naftin Cream, 1% is contraindicated in individuals who have shown hypersensitivity to any of its components.

WARNING

Naftin Cream, 1% is for topical use only and not for ophthalmic use.

PRECAUTIONS

General: Naftin Cream, 1% is for external use only. If irritation or sensitivity develops with the use of Naftin Cream 1%, treatment should be discontinued and appropriate therapy instituted. Diagnosis of the disease should be confirmed either by direct microscopic examination of a mounting of infected tissue in a solution of potassium hydroxide or by culture on an appropriate medium.
Information for patients: The patient should be told to:
1. Avoid the use of occlusive dressings or wrappings unless otherwise directed by the physician.
2. Keep Naftin Cream, 1% away from the eyes, nose, mouth and other mucous membranes.
Carcinogenesis, mutagenesis, impairment of fertility: Long-term animal studies to evaluate the carcinogenic potential of Naftin Cream, 1% have not been performed. *In vitro* and animal studies have not demonstrated any mutagenic effect or effect on fertility.
Pregnancy: Teratogenic Effects: Pregnancy Category B: Reproduction studies have been performed in rats and rabbits (via oral administration) at doses 150 times or more the topical human dose and have revealed no significant evidence of impaired fertility or harm to the fetus due to naftifine. There are, however, no adequate and well-controlled studies in pregnant women. Because animal reproduction studies are not always predictive of human response, this drug should be used during pregnancy only if clearly needed.
Nursing mothers: It is not known whether this drug is excreted in human milk. Because many drugs are excreted in human milk, caution should be exercised when Naftin Cream, 1% is administered to a nursing woman.
Pediatric use: Safety and effectiveness in children have not been established.

ADVERSE REACTIONS

During clinical trials with Naftin Cream 1%, the incidence of adverse reactions was as follows: burning/stinging (6%), dryness (3%), erythema (2%), itching (2%), local irritation (2%).

DOSAGE AND ADMINISTRATION

A sufficient quantity of Naftin Cream, 1% should be gently massaged into the affected and surrounding skin areas once a day. The hands should be washed after application.
If no clinical improvement is seen after four weeks of treatment with Naftin Cream, 1% the patient should be re-evaluated.

HOW SUPPLIED

Naftin® (naftifine hydrochloride) 1% Cream is supplied in collapsible tubes in the following sizes:

Continued on next page

Allergan Herbert—Cont.

15 g-NDC-0023-4126-15
30 g-NDC-0023-4126-30
60 g-NDC-0023-4126-60
Note: Store below 30°C (86°F).
Caution: Federal (U.S.A.) law prohibits dispensing without prescription.
© 1992 Allergan, Inc.

NAFTIN®   ℞
(naftifine hydrochloride) 1%
Gel

DESCRIPTION

Naftin Gel, 1% contains the synthetic, broad-spectrum, antifungal agent naftifine hydrochloride.
Naftin Gel, 1% is for topical use only.
Chemical Name: (E)-N-Cinnamyl-N-methyl-1-naphthalenemethylamine hydrochloride. Naftifine hydrochloride has an empirical formula of $C_{21}H_{21}N \cdot HCl$ and a molecular weight of 323.86.
Contains:
Active Ingredient: Naftifine hydrochloride 1%
Inactive Ingredients: polysorbate 80, carbomer 934P, diisopropanolamine, edetate disodium, alcohol (52% $\%_v$), and purified water.

CLINICAL PHARMACOLOGY

Naftifine hydrochloride is a synthetic allylamine derivative. The following *in vitro* data are available but their clinical significance is unknown. Naftifine hydrochloride has been shown to exhibit fungicidal activity *in vitro* against a broad spectrum of organisms including *Trichophyton rubrum, Trichophyton mentagrophytes, Trichophyton tonsurans, Epidermophyton floccosum,* and *Microsporum canis, Microsporum audouini,* and *Microsporum gypseum;* and fungistatic activity against *Candida* species including *Candida albicans.* Naftin Gel, 1% has only been shown to be clinically effective against the disease entities listed in the INDICATIONS AND USAGE section.
Although the exact mechanism of action against fungi is not known, naftifine hydrochloride appears to interfere with sterol biosynthesis by inhibiting the enzyme squalene 2,3-epoxidase. This inhibition of enzyme activity results in decreased amounts of sterols, especially ergosterol, and a corresponding accumulation of squalene in the cells.
Pharmacokinetics: *In vitro* and *in vivo* bioavailability studies have demonstrated that naftifine penetrates the stratum corneum in sufficient concentration to inhibit the growth of dermatophytes.
Following single topical application of ^{3}H-labeled naftifine gel 1% to the skin of healthy subjects, up to 4.2% of the applied dose was absorbed. Naftifine and/or its metabolites are excreted via the urine and feces with a half-life of approximately two to three days.

INDICATION AND USAGE

Naftin Gel, 1% is indicated for the topical treatment of tinea pedis, tinea cruris and tinea corporis caused by the organisms *Trichophyton rubrum, Trichophyton mentagrophytes, Trichophyton tonsurans** and *Epidermophyton floccosum.**

CONTRAINDICATIONS

Naftin Gel, 1% is contraindicated in individuals who have shown hypersensitivity to any of its components.

WARNINGS

Naftin Gel, 1% is for topical use only and not for ophthalmic use.

PRECAUTIONS

General: Naftin Gel, 1% is for external use only. If irritation or sensitivity develop with the use of Naftin Gel, 1%, treatment should be discontinued and appropriate therapy instituted. Diagnosis of the disease should be confirmed either by direct microscopic examination of a mounting of infected tissue in a solution of potassium hydroxide or by culture on an appropriate medium.
Information for patients:
The patient should be told to:
1. Avoid the use of occlusive dressings or wrappings unless otherwise directed by the physician.
2. Keep Naftin Gel, 1% away from the eyes, nose, mouth and other mucous membranes.
Carcinogenesis, mutagenesis, impairment of fertility: Long-term studies to evaluate the carcinogenic potential of Naftin Gel, 1% have not been performed. *In vitro* and animal studies have not demonstrated any mutagenic effect or effect on fertility.
Pregnancy: Teratogenic Effects: Pregnancy Category B: Reproduction studies have been performed in rats and rab-

*Efficacy for this organism in this organ system was studied in fewer than 10 infections.

---

bits (via oral administration) at doses 150 times or more than the topical human dose and have revealed no evidence of impaired fertility or harm to the fetus due to naftifine. There are, however, no adequate and well-controlled studies in pregnant women. Because animal reproduction studies are not always predictive of human response, this drug should be used during pregnancy only if clearly needed.
Nursing mothers: It is not known whether this drug is excreted in human milk. Because many drugs are excreted in human milk, caution should be exercised when Naftin Gel, 1% is administered to a nursing woman.
Pediatric use: Safety and effectiveness in children have not been established.

ADVERSE REACTIONS

During clinical trials with Naftin Gel, 1%, the incidence of adverse reactions was as follows: burning/stinging (5.0%), itching (1.0%), erythema (0.5%), rash (0.5%), skin tenderness (0.5%).

DOSAGE AND ADMINISTRATION

A sufficient quantity of Naftin Gel, 1% should be gently massaged into the affected and surrounding skin areas twice a day, in the morning and evening. The hands should be washed after application.
If no clinical improvement is seen after four weeks of treatment with Naftin Gel, 1%, the patient should be re-evaluated.

HOW SUPPLIED

Naftin® (naftifine hydrochloride) is supplied in collapsible tubes in the following sizes:
20 g-NDC-0023-4770-20
40 g-NDC-0023-4770-40
60 g-NDC-0023-4770-60
Note: Store at room temperature.
Caution: Federal (U.S.A.) law prohibits dispensing without prescription.
© 1992 Allergan, Inc.

PENECORT®   ℞
(hydrocortisone)
Cream, USP, 1%
Topical Solution 1%

PENECORT Cream contains:
Active Ingredient: hydrocortisone, USP 1%
Inactive Ingredients: benzyl alcohol; petrolatum; stearyl alcohol; propylene glycol; isopropyl myristate; polyoxyl 40 stearate; carbomer 934; sodium lauryl sulfate; edetate disodium; sodium hydroxide to adjust the pH; and purified water.
PENECORT Topical Solution contains:
Active Ingredient: hydrocortisone, USP 1%
Inactive Ingredients: alcohol (57%); propylene glycol; benzyl alcohol; and purified water.

HOW SUPPLIED

PENECORT® (hydrocortisone):
Cream, USP, 1%—30 g collapsible tubes: NDC 0023-0510-30
Topical Solution 1%—30 mL and 60 mL plastic bottles:
30 mL NDC 0023-0889-30; 60 mL NDC 0023-0889-60
© 1992 Allergan, Inc.

TAC™-3   ℞
(sterile triamcinolone acetonide suspension) 3mg/mL
NOT FOR INTRAVENOUS USE
FOR INTRALESIONAL AND INTRADERMAL USE

Each mL of aqueous suspension contains: **Active Ingredient:** triamcinolone acetonide 3 mg. **Inactive Ingredients:** benzyl alcohol 0.9% as preservative; carboxymethylcellulose sodium 7.5 mg; polysorbate 80 0.4 mg; sodium chloride 2 mg; in water for injection q.s. Sodium hydroxide and/or hydrochloric acid may have been used to adjust pH.

HOW SUPPLIED

Multiple dose vials of 5 mL containing triamcinolone acetonide 3 mg/mL.
NDC 0023-0218-05.
Manufactured for ALLERGAN Herbert
Skin Care Division of Allergan, Inc.
Irvine, California 92713, U.S.A.
by
Steris Laboratories, Inc.
Phoenix, AZ 85043
© 1992 Allergan, Inc.

TEMARIL®   ℞
(trimeprazine tartrate)
Tablets 2.5 mg, Syrup 2.5 mg/5mL and
Spansule® capsules 5 mg
(extended-release capsules)

DESCRIPTION

Temaril, available as trimeprazine tartrate, a phenothiazine derivative, is 10-[3-(dimethylamino)-2-methylpropyl]-phenothiazine tartrate.
Trimeprazine tartrate is a white to off-white odorless, crystalline powder readily soluble in water.
Tablets—Each round, gray, coated tablet is imprinted HL and T41 and contains trimeprazine tartrate equivalent to 2.5 mg of trimeprazine. Inactive ingredients consist of acacia, calcium sulfate, FD&C Yellow No. 6, gelatin, iron oxide, mineral oil, starch, stearic acid, sucrose, talc, titanium dioxide and trace amounts of other inactive ingredients.
Syrup—Each 5 mL (one teaspoonful) of clear, red, raspberry/strawberry flavored liquid contains trimeprazine tartrate equivalent to 2.5 mg of trimeprazine, and alcohol, 5.7%. Inactive ingredients consist of citric acid, FD&C Green No. 3, FD&C Red No. 40, flavors, glycerin, saccharin sodium, sodium benzoate, sucrose and water.
Spansule® extended-release capsules— Each 'Spansule' extended-release capsule is so prepared that an initial dose is released promptly and the remaining medication is released gradually over a prolonged period. Each capsule, with opaque gray cap and natural body, is imprinted HL and T50 and contains trimeprazine tartrate equivalent to 5 mg of trimeprazine. Inactive ingredients consist of benzyl alcohol, cetylpyridinium chloride, FD&C Green No. 3, FD&C Red No. 40, FD&C Yellow No. 6, gelatin, glyceryl distearate, glyceryl monostearate, iron oxide, sodium lauryl sulfate, starch, sucrose, titanium dioxide, wax and trace amounts of other inactive ingredients.

ACTIONS

Temaril (trimeprazine tartrate), a phenothiazine, possesses antipruritic and antihistaminic properties with anticholinergic (drying) and sedative side effects.

INDICATIONS

Treatment of pruritic symptoms in urticaria. Relief of pruritic symptoms in a variety of allergic and non-allergic conditions including atopic dermatitis, neurodermatitis, contact dermatitis, pityriasis rosea, poison ivy dermatitis, eczematous dermatitis, pruritus ani and vulvae, and drug rash.

CONTRAINDICATIONS

Temaril (trimeprazine tartrate) is contraindicated: in comatose patients; in patients who have received large amounts of central nervous system depressants (alcohol, barbiturates, narcotics, etc.); in patients with bone marrow depression; in patients who have demonstrated an idiosyncrasy or hypersensitivity to Temaril or other phenothiazines; in newborn or premature children; and in nursing mothers. It should not be used in children who are acutely ill and/or dehydrated, as there is an increased susceptibility to dystonias in such patients.

WARNINGS

Temaril (trimeprazine tartrate) may impair the mental and/or physical ability required for the performance of potentially hazardous tasks, such as driving a vehicle or operating machinery. Similarly, it may impair mental alertness in children. The concomitant use of alcohol or other central nervous system depressants may have an additive effect. Patients should be warned accordingly.
Temaril should be used with extreme caution in patients with:
    Asthmatic attack
    Narrow-angle glaucoma
    Prostatic hypertrophy
    Stenosing peptic ulcer
    Pyloroduodenal obstruction
    Bladder neck obstruction
    Patients receiving monoamine oxidase inhibitors
Usage in Pregnancy: The safe use of Temaril has not been established with respect to the possible adverse effects upon fetal development. Therefore, it should not be used in women of childbearing potential. Jaundice and prolonged extrapyramidal symptoms have been reported in infants whose mothers received phenothiazines during pregnancy.
Usage in Children: Temaril should be used with caution in children who have a history of sleep apnea or a family history of sudden infant death syndrome (SIDS). It should also be used with caution in young children, in whom it may cause excitation.
Overdosage may produce hallucinations, convulsions and sudden death.
Usage in Elderly Patients (60 years or older): Elderly patients are more prone to develop the following side effects from phenothiazines:
    Hypotension
    Syncope
    Toxic confusional states

Extrapyramidal symptoms, especially parkinsonism
Excessive sedation

PRECAUTIONS

Temaril (trimeprazine tartrate) may significantly affect the actions of other drugs. It may increase, prolong or intensify the sedative action of central nervous system depressants such as anesthetics, barbiturates or alcohol. When Temaril is administered concomitantly the dose of a narcotic or barbiturate should be reduced to ¼ or ½ the usual amount. In the patient with pain, receiving treatment with narcotics, excessive amounts of Temaril may lead to restlessness and motor hyperactivity. Temaril can block and even reverse the usual pressor effect of epinephrine.

Temaril should be used cautiously in persons with acute or chronic respiratory impairment, particularly children, as it may suppress the cough reflex.

This drug should be used cautiously in persons with cardiovascular disease, impairment of liver function, or those with a history of ulcer disease.

Since Temaril has a slight antiemetic action, it may obscure signs of intestinal obstruction, brain tumor, or overdosage of toxic drugs.

Phenothiazines have been shown to elevate prolactin levels; the elevation persists during chronic administration. Tissue culture experiments indicate that approximately one-third of human breast cancers are prolactin-dependent in vitro, a factor of potential importance if the prescribing of these drugs is contemplated in a patient with a previously detected breast cancer. Although disturbances such as galactorrhea, amenorrhea, gynecomastia, and impotence have been reported, the clinical significance of elevated serum prolactin levels is unknown for most patients. An increase in mammary neoplasms has been found in rodents after chronic administration of neuroleptic drugs. Neither clinical nor epidemiologic studies conducted to date, however, have shown an association between chronic administration of these drugs and mammary tumorigenesis; the available evidence is considered too limited to be conclusive at this time.

Drugs which lower the seizure threshold, including phenothiazine derivatives, should not be used with metrizamide. As with other phenothiazine derivatives, 'Temaril' should be discontinued at least 48 hours before myelography, should not be resumed for at least 24 hours postprocedure, and should not be used for the control of nausea and vomiting occurring either prior to myelography or postprocedure.

ADVERSE REACTIONS

Temaril (trimeprazine tartrate) may produce adverse reactions attributable to both phenothiazines and antihistamines.

Note: Not all of the following adverse reactions have been reported with Temaril (trimeprazine tartrate); however, pharmacological similarities among the phenothiazine derivatives require that each be considered when Temaril is administered. There have been occasional reports of sudden death in patients receiving phenothiazine derivatives chronically.

C.N.S. Effects: Drowsiness is the most common C.N.S. effect of this drug. Extrapyramidal reactions (opisthotonos, dystonia, akathisia, dyskinesia, parkinsonism) occur, particularly with high doses. (See Overdosage section for management of extrapyramidal symptoms.) Hyperreflexia has been reported in the newborn when a phenothiazine was used during pregnancy. Other reported reactions include dizziness, headache, lassitude, tinnitus, incoordination, fatigue, blurred vision, euphoria, diplopia, nervousness, insomnia, tremors and grand mal seizures, excitation, catatonic-like states, neuritis and hysteria, oculogyric crises, disturbing dreams/nightmares, pseudoschizophrenia, and intensification and prolongation of the action of C.N.S. depressants (opiates, analgesics, antihistamines, barbiturates, alcohol), atropine, heat, organophosphorus insecticides.

Cardiovascular Effects: Postural hypotension is the most common cardiovascular effect of phenothiazines. Reflex tachycardia may be seen. Bradycardia, faintness, dizziness and cardiac arrest have been reported. ECG changes, including blunting of T waves and prolongation of the Q-T interval, may be seen.

Gastrointestinal: Anorexia, nausea, vomiting, epigastric distress, diarrhea, constipation, and dry mouth may occur. Increased appetite and weight gain have also been reported.

Genitourinary: Urinary frequency and dysuria, urinary retention, early menses, induced lactation, gynecomastia, decreased libido, inhibition of ejaculation and false positive pregnancy tests have been reported.

Respiratory: Thickening of bronchial secretions, tightness of the chest, wheezing and nasal stuffiness may occur.

Allergic Reactions: These include urticaria, dermatitis, asthma, laryngeal edema, angioneurotic edema, photosensitivity, lupus erythematosus-like syndrome and anaphylactoid reactions.

Other Reported Reactions: Leukopenia, agranulocytosis, pancytopenia, hemolytic anemia, elevation of plasma cholesterol levels and thrombocytopenic purpura have been reported. Jaundice of the obstructive type has also been re-

ported; it is usually reversible but chronic jaundice has been reported. Erythema, peripheral edema, and stomatitis have been reported. High or prolonged glucose tolerance curves, glycosuria, elevated spinal fluid proteins and reversed epinephrine effects may also occur.

Rare occurrences of neuroleptic malignant syndrome (NMS) have been reported in patients receiving phenothiazines. This syndrome is comprised of the symptom complex of hyperthermia, altered consciousness, muscular rigidity and autonomic dysfunction and is potentially fatal.

Long-Term Therapy Considerations: After prolonged phenothiazine administration at high dosage, pigmentation of the skin has occurred, chiefly in the exposed areas. Ocular changes consist of the appearance of lenticular and corneal opacities, epithelial keratopathies and pigmentary retinopathy. Vision may be impaired.

DOSAGE AND ADMINISTRATION

Tablets and Syrup:
Adults: Usual dosage is 2.5 mg q.i.d.
Children over three years: Usual dosage is 2.5 mg h.s., or t.i.d. if needed.
Children 6 months to 3 years: Usual dosage is 1.25 mg (½ teaspoonful of syrup) h.s., or t.i.d. if needed.
Spansule capsules:
Adults: Usual daily dosage is 1 capsule q12h.
Children over 6 years of age: 1 capsule daily.
This product form is not recommended for children under 6 years of age. Use tablets or syrup for their dosage flexibility. Because some side effects appear to be dose-related, it is important to use the lowest effective dosage.

DRUG INTERACTIONS

MAO inhibitors and thiazide diuretics prolong and intensify the anticholinergic effects of Temaril (trimeprazine tartrate). Combined use of MAO inhibitors and phenothiazines may result in hypertension and extrapyramidal reactions.

Narcotics: The C.N.S. depressant and analgesic effects of narcotics are potentiated by phenothiazines.

The following drugs may result in potentiation of phenothiazine effects:
Oral contraceptives
Progesterone
Reserpine
Nylidrin hydrochloride

MANAGEMENT OF OVERDOSAGE

Signs and symptoms of Temaril (trimeprazine tartrate) overdosage range from mild depression of the central nervous system and cardiovascular system to profound hypotension, respiratory depression and unconsciousness. Stimulation may be evident, especially in children and geriatric patients. Atropine-like signs and symptoms—dry mouth, fixed, dilated pupils, flushing, etc.—as well as gastrointestinal symptoms may occur. The treatment of overdosage is essentially symptomatic and supportive. Early gastric lavage may be beneficial. **Do not administer emetics or attempt to induce vomiting because a dystonic reaction of the head or neck might result in aspiration of vomitus.** Extrapyramidal symptoms may be treated with anti-parkinsonism drugs, barbiturates, or diphenhydramine hydrochloride.

Avoid analeptics, which may cause convulsions. Severe hypotension usually responds to the administration of levarterenol or phenylephrine. EPINEPHRINE SHOULD NOT BE USED, since its use in a patient with partial adrenergic blockade may further lower the blood pressure. Additional measures include oxygen and intravenous fluids. Limited experience with dialysis indicates that it is not helpful.

Special note on 'Spansule' capsules —Since much of the 'Spansule' capsule medication is coated for gradual release, therapy directed at reversing the effects of the ingested drug and at supporting the patient should be continued for as long as overdosage symptoms remain. Saline cathartics are useful for hastening evacuation of pellets that have not already released medication.

HOW SUPPLIED

Tablets—2.5 mg in bottles of 100; Single Unit Packages of 100 (intended for institutional use only).

Syrup—2.5 mg/5 mL (teaspoonful) and alcohol 5.7%, in 4 fl oz bottles.

Spansule capsules—5 mg in bottles of 50; Single Unit Packages of 100 (intended for institutional use only).

CAUTION

Federal (U.S.A.) law prohibits dispensing without prescription.
Manufactured for
ALLERGAN Herbert
Skin Care Division of Allergan, Inc.
By SmithKline Beecham Pharmaceuticals
Philadelphia, PA 19101
© 1992 Allergan, Inc.

Allergan Optical
Allergan Pharmaceuticals
Divisions of Allergan, Inc.
2525 DUPONT DRIVE
P.O. BOX 19534
IRVINE, CA 92713-9534

OPHTHALMIC PRODUCTS

For information on Allergan, Inc., prescription, OTC, ophthalmic and contact lens products, consult the Physicians' Desk Reference For Ophthalmology. Allergan OTC artificial tear preparations also appear in the Physicians' Desk Reference For Nonprescription Drugs. For literature, service items or sample material, contact Allergan directly. See a complete listing of products in the Manufacturers' Index section of this book.

BLEPH®-10   ℞
(sulfacetamide sodium
ophthalmic solution) 10%
BLEPH®-10
(sulfacetamide sodium
ophthalmic ointment) 10%

DESCRIPTION

BLEPH®-10 (sulfacetamide sodium ophthalmic solution and ointment) 10% are topical anti-infective agents for ophthalmic use.
CHEMICAL NAME
N-Sulfanilylacetamide monosodium salt monohydrate.
CONTAINS
Bleph®-10 solution:
Sulfacetamide sodium 10%
with: Liquifilm® (polyvinyl alcohol) 1.4%; benzalkonium chloride (0.005%); sodium thiosulfate; sodium phosphate dibasic; sodium phosphate monobasic; edetate disodium; polysorbate 80; hydrochloric acid and/or sodium hydroxide to adjust the pH; and purified water.
Bleph®-10 ointment:
Sulfacetamide sodium 10%
with: phenylmercuric acetate (0.0008%), white petrolatum, mineral oil, and petrolatum (and) lanolin alcohol.

CLINICAL PHARMACOLOGY

Sulfonamides exert a bacteriostatic effect against a wide range of gram-positive and gram-negative organisms by restricting, through competition with para-aminobenzoic acid, the synthesis of folic acid which bacteria require for growth.

INDICATIONS AND USAGE

BLEPH®-10 is indicated for the treatment of conjunctivitis, corneal ulcer and other superficial ocular infections caused by susceptible microorganisms, and as adjunctive treatment in systemic sulfonamide therapy of trachoma.

CONTRAINDICATIONS

BLEPH®-10 is contraindicated in individuals who have a hypersensitivity to sulfonamide preparations or to any of the ingredients of the preparation.

WARNINGS

Bleph®-10 solution is **FOR TOPICAL EYE USE ONLY—NOT FOR INJECTION.** As with all sulfonamide preparations, severe sensitivity reactions, e.g., Stevens-Johnson syndrome, fever, skin rash, GI disturbances and bone marrow depression have been identified in individuals with no prior history of sulfonamide hypersensitivity. A significant percentage of staphylococcal isolates are completely resistant to sulfa drugs.

PRECAUTIONS

Sulfacetamide preparations are incompatible with silver preparations. Nonsusceptible organisms, including fungi, may proliferate with the use of this preparation. Sulfonamides are inactivated by the aminobenzoic acid present in purulent exudates. Sensitization may occur when a sulfonamide is readministered irrespective of the route of administration, and cross-sensitivity between different sulfonamides may occur. If signs of sensitivity or other untoward reactions occur, discontinue use of the preparation.
Ophthalmic ointments may retard corneal healing.
Do not touch dropper tip to any surface since this may contaminate the contents.

ADVERSE REACTIONS

Sulfacetamide sodium may cause local irritation, stinging and burning. While the irritation may be transient, occasionally, use of the medication has to be discontinued.
Although sensitivity reactions to sulfacetamide sodium are rare, an isolated incident of Stevens-Johnson syndrome was reported in a patient who had experienced a previous bullous

Continued on next page

Allergan—Cont.

drug reaction to an orally administered sulfonamide, and a single instance of local hypersensitivity was reported which progressed to a fatal syndrome resembling systemic lupus erythematosus. The development of secondary infection has occurred after the use of antimicrobials.

DOSAGE AND ADMINISTRATION

Bleph®-10 solution: One to two drops into the lower conjunctival sac every 2 or 3 hours during the day, less often at night.

Bleph®-10 ointment: Apply a small amount of ointment in the conjunctival sac 4 times daily and at bedtime.

HOW SUPPLIED

Bleph®-10 (sulfacetamide sodium ophthalmic solution) 10% is supplied sterile in plastic dropper bottles in the following sizes:

2.5 mL—NDC 11980-011-03
5 mL—NDC 11980-011-05
15 mL—NDC 11980-011-15

BLEPH®-10 (sulfacetamide sodium ophthalmic ointment) 10% is supplied sterile in ophthalmic ointment tubes in the following size:

3.5 g—NDC 0023-0311-04

Note: Store ointment away from heat. Store solution between 8°-25°C (46°-77°F). Protect from light. Do not use if solution is discolored (dark brown).

CAUTION

Federal (U.S.A.) law prohibits dispensing without prescription.

BLEPHAMIDE®   ℞
(sulfacetamide sodium—prednisolone acetate)
LIQUIFILM®
sterile ophthalmic suspension
and
BLEPHAMIDE®
(sulfacetamide sodium—prednisolone acetate)
S.O.P.®
sterile ophthalmic ointment

DESCRIPTION

BLEPHAMIDE® is a topical anti-inflammatory/anti-infective combination product for ophthalmic use.
CHEMICAL NAMES
Sulfacetamide sodium: N-Sulfanilylacetamide monosodium salt monohydrate
Prednisolone acetate: 11β, 17, 21-Trihydroxypregna-1, 4-diene-3, 20-dione 21-acetate
BLEPHAMIDE® LIQUIFILM sterile ophthalmic suspension contains:
sulfacetamide sodium 10.0%
prednisolone acetate
(microfine suspension) 0.2%
with: LIQUIFILM® (polyvinyl alcohol) 1.4%; benzalkonium chloride; polysorbate 80; edetate disodium; sodium phosphate, dibasic; potassium phosphate, monobasic; sodium thiosulfate; hydrochloric acid and/or sodium hydroxide to adjust the pH; and purified water.
BLEPHAMIDE® SOP sterile ophthalmic ointment contains:
sulfacetamide sodium 10.0%
prednisolone acetate 0.2%
(microfine suspension)
with: phenylmercuric acetate (0.0008%), mineral oil, white petrolatum and petrolatum (and) lanolin alcohol.

CLINICAL PHARMACOLOGY

Corticosteroids suppress the inflammatory response to a variety of agents and they probably delay or slow healing. Since corticosteroids may inhibit the body's defense mechanism against infection, a concomitant antimicrobial drug may be used when this inhibition is considered to be clinically significant in a particular case.
The anti-infective component in BLEPHAMIDE® is included to provide action against specific organisms susceptible to it. Sulfacetamide sodium is considered active against the following microorganisms: **Escherichia coli, Staphylococcus aureus, Streptococcus pneumoniae, Streptococcus (viridans group), Pseudomonas** species, **Haemophilus influenzae, Klebsiella** species, and **Enterobacter** species.
When a decision to administer both a corticosteroid and an antimicrobial is made, the administration of such drugs in combination has the advantage of greater patient compliance and convenience, with the added assurance that the appropriate dosage of both drugs is administered. When both types of drugs are in the same formulation, compatibility of ingredients is assured and the correct volume of drug is delivered and retained. The relative potency of corticosteroids depends on the molecular structure, concentration, and release from the vehicle.

INDICATIONS AND USAGE

A steroid/anti-infective combination is indicated for steroid-responsive inflammatory ocular conditions for which a corticosteroid is indicated and where bacterial infection or a risk of bacterial ocular infection exists.
Ocular steroids are indicated in inflammatory conditions of the palpebral and bulbar conjunctiva, cornea, and anterior segment of the globe where the inherent risk of steroid use in certain infective conjunctivitides is accepted to obtain a diminution in edema and inflammation. They are also indicated in chronic anterior uveitis and corneal injury from chemical, radiation, or thermal burns or penetration of foreign bodies. The use of a combination drug with an anti-infective component is indicated where the risk of infection is high or where there is an expectation that potentially dangerous numbers of bacteria will be present in the eye.
The particular anti-infective drug in this product is active against the following common bacterial eye pathogens: **Escherichia coli, Staphylococcus aureus, Streptococcus pneumoniae, Streptococcus (viridans group), Pseudomonas** species, **Haemophilus influenzae, Klebsiella** species, and **Enterobacter** species. This product does not provide adequate coverage against **Neisseria** species and **Serratia marcescens**.

CONTRAINDICATIONS

Epithelial herpes simplex keratitis (dendritic keratitis), vaccinia, varicella, and many other viral diseases of the cornea and conjunctiva. Mycobacterial infection of the eye. Fungal diseases of the ocular structures. Hypersensitivity to a component of the medication. (Hypersensitivity to the antimicrobial component occurs at a higher rate than for other components.)
The use of these combinations is always contraindicated after uncomplicated removal of a corneal foreign body.

WARNINGS

Prolonged use may result in glaucoma, with damage to the optic nerve, defects in visual acuity and fields of vision, and in posterior subcapsular cataract formation. Prolonged use may suppress the host response and thus increase the hazard of secondary ocular infections. In those diseases causing thinning of the cornea or sclera, perforations have been known to occur with the use of topical steroids. In acute purulent conditions of the eye, steroids may mask infection or enhance existing infection. If these products are used for 10 days or longer, intraocular pressure should be routinely monitored even though it may be difficult in children and uncooperative patients.
Employment of a steroid medication in the treatment of herpes simplex requires great caution.
A significant percentage of staphylococcal isolates are completely resistant to sulfa drugs.

PRECAUTIONS

The initial prescription and renewal of the medication order beyond 20 milliliters (BLEPHAMIDE® suspension) or 8 grams (BLEPHAMIDE® ointment) should be made by a physician only after examination of the patient with the aid of magnification, such as slit lamp biomicroscopy and, where appropriate, fluorescein staining.
The possibility of fungal infections of the cornea should be considered after prolonged steroid dosing.
Ophthalmic ointments may retard corneal healing.

ADVERSE REACTIONS

Adverse reactions have occurred with steroid/anti-infective combination drugs which can be attributed to the steroid component, the anti-infective component, or the combination. Exact incidence figures are not available since no denominator of treated patients is available.
Reactions occurring most often from the presence of the anti-infective ingredient are allergic sensitizations. The reactions due to the steroid component in decreasing order of frequency are: elevation of intraocular pressure (IOP) with possible development of glaucoma, and infrequent optic nerve damage; posterior subcapsular cataract formation; and delayed wound healing.
Secondary infection: The development of secondary infection has occurred after use of combinations containing steroids and antimicrobials. Fungal infections of the cornea are particularly prone to develop coincidentally with long-term applications of steroid. The possibility of fungal invasion must be considered in any persistent corneal ulceration where steroid treatment has been used.
Secondary bacterial ocular infection following suppression of host responses also occurs.

DOSAGE AND ADMINISTRATION

BLEPHAMIDE® Suspension: Optimal dosage is 1 drop two to four times daily, depending upon the severity of the condition.
In general, during early or acute stages of blepharitis, BLEPHAMIDE® LIQUIFILM® sterile ophthalmic suspension produces results most rapidly—and most efficiently—with instillation directly into the eye, with the excess spread on the lid (Method I). When the condition is confined to the

lid, however, BLEPHAMIDE® may be applied directly to the site of the lesions (Method II).
METHOD I: In the Eye and On the Lid
1. Wash hands carefully. Tilt head back and drop **1 drop** into the eye.
2. Close the eye and spread the excess medication present after closing the eye on the full length of the upper and lower lids.
3. Do not wipe any of the medication off the lids. It will dry completely in 4 or 5 minutes to a clear film that remains on the lids for several hours—it cannot be seen by others, nor will it interfere with vision.
4. The medication should be washed off the lids once or twice a day. However, it should be reapplied after each washing.
METHOD II: On the Lid
1. Wash hands carefully. With head tilted back and **eye closed**, drop 1 drop onto the lid—preferably at the corner of the eye close to the nose.
2. Spread the medication over the full length of the upper and lower lids.
3. Do not wipe away any medication—it will dry in 4 to 5 minutes to a clear, invisible film which will remain on the lids for several hours.
4. The medication should be washed off the lids once or twice a day. **However, it should be reapplied after each washing.**
Not more than 20 milliliters should be prescribed initially and the prescription should not be refilled without further evaluation as outlined in **Precautions** above.
BLEPHAMIDE® Ointment: A small amount should be applied in the conjunctival sac three or four times daily and once or twice at night. Not more than 8 grams should be prescribed initially and the prescription should not be refilled without further evaluation as outlined in **Precautions** above.

HOW SUPPLIED

BLEPHAMIDE® LIQUIFILM® is supplied in plastic dropper bottles in the following sizes:
2.5 mL—NDC 11980-022-03
5 mL—NDC 11980-022-05
10 mL—NDC 11980-022-10
BLEPHAMIDE® S.O.P.® sterile ophthalmic ointment is supplied in ophthalmic ointment tubes in the following size:
3.5 g—NDC 0023-0313-04
Note: Store ointment away from heat. Protect suspension from freezing. Shake suspension well before using.

CAUTION

Federal (U.S.A.) law prohibits dispensing without prescription.

BOTOX®   ℞
(Botulinum Toxin Type A)

DESCRIPTION

Botox® (Botulinum Toxin Type A) is a sterile, lyophilized form of purified botulinum toxin type A, produced from a culture of the Hall strain of *Clostridium botulinum* grown in a medium containing N-Z amine and yeast extract. It is purified from the culture solution by a series of acid precipitations to a crystalline complex consisting of the active high molecular weight toxin protein and an associated hemagglutinin protein. The crystalline complex is re-dissolved in a solution containing saline and albumin and sterile filtered (0.2 microns) prior to lyophilization. **Botox®** is to be reconstituted with sterile non-preserved saline prior to intramuscular injection.
Each vial of **Botox®** contains 100 units (U) of *Clostridium botulinum* toxin type A, 0.5 milligrams of albumin (human), and 0.9 milligrams of sodium chloride in a sterile, lyophilized form without a preservative. One unit (U) corresponds to the calculated median lethal intraperitoneal dose (LD/50) in mice of the reconstituted **Botox®** injected.

CLINICAL PHARMACOLOGY

Botox® (Botulinum Toxin Type A) blocks neuromuscular conduction by binding to receptor sites on motor nerve terminals, entering the nerve terminals, and inhibiting the release of acetylcholine. When injected intramuscularly at therapeutic doses, **Botox®** produces a localized chemical denervation muscle paralysis. When the muscle is chemically denervated, it atrophies and may develop extrajunctional acetylcholine receptors. There is evidence that the nerve can sprout and reinnervate the muscle, with the weakness thus being reversible.
The paralytic effect on muscles injected with **Botox®** is useful in reducing the excessive, abnormal contractions associated with blepharospasm. When used for the treatment of strabismus, it is postulated that the administration of **Botox®** affects muscle pairs by inducing an atrophic lengthening of the injected muscle and a corresponding shortening of the muscle's antagonist. Following peri-ocular injection of **Botox®**, distant muscles show electrophysiologic changes but no clinical weakness or other clinical change for a period

of several weeks or months, parallel to the duration of local clinical paralysis.[1]

In one study, botulinum toxin was evaluated in 27 patients with essential blepharospasm. Twenty-six of the patients had previously undergone drug treatment utilizing benztropine mesylate, clonazepam and/or baclofen without adequate clinical results. Three of these patients then underwent muscle stripping surgery still without an adequate outcome. One patient of the 27 was previously untreated. Upon using botulinum toxin, 25 of the 27 patients reported improvement within 48 hours. One of the other patients was later controlled with a higher dosage. The remaining patient reported only mild improvement but remained functionally impaired.[2]

In another study, twelve patients with blepharospasm were evaluated in a double-blind, placebo-controlled study. All patients receiving botulinum toxin (n=8) were improved compared with no improvements in the placebo group (n=4). The mean dystonia score improved by 72%, the self-assessment score rating improved by 61%, and a videotape evaluation rating improved by 39%. The effects of the treatment lasted a mean of 12.5 weeks.[3]

One thousand six hundred eighty-four patients with blepharospasm evaluated in an open trial showed clinical improvement lasting an average of 12.5 weeks prior to the need for re-treatment.[4]

Six hundred seventy-seven patients with strabismus treated with one or more injections of **Botox®** were evaluated in an open trial. Fifty-five percent of these patients were improved to an alignment of 10 prism diopters or less when evaluated 6 months or more following injection.[5] These results are consistent with results from additional open label trials which were conducted for this indication.[4]

INDICATIONS AND USAGE

Botox® (Botulinum Toxin Type A) is indicated for the treatment of strabismus and blepharospasm associated with dystonia, including benign essential blepharospasm or VII nerve disorders in patients 12 years of age and above.

The efficacy of **Botox®** in deviations over 50 prism diopters, in restrictive strabismus, in Duane's syndrome with lateral rectus weakness, and in secondary strabismus caused by prior surgical over-recession of the antagonist is doubtful, or multiple injections over time may be required. **Botox®** is ineffective in chronic paralytic strabismus except to reduce antagonist contracture in conjunction with surgical repair.

Presence of antibodies to botulinum toxin type A may reduce the effectiveness of **Botox®** therapy. In clinical studies, reduction in effectiveness due to antibody production has occurred in one patient with blepharospasm receiving 3 doses of **Botox®** over a 6 week period totalling 92 U, and in several patients with torticollis who received multiple doses experimentally, totalling over 300 U in a one-month period. For this reason, the dose of **Botox®** for strabismus and blepharospasm should be kept as low as possible, in any case below 200 U in a one month period.

CONTRAINDICATIONS

Botox® (Botulinum Toxin Type A) is contraindicated in individuals with known hypersensitivity to any ingredient in the formulation.

WARNINGS

The recommended dosages and frequencies of administration for **Botox®** should not be exceeded. There have not been any reported instances of systemic toxicity resulting from accidental injection or oral ingestion of **Botox®**. Should accidental injection or oral ingestion occur, the person should be medically supervised for several days on an office or outpatient basis for signs or symptoms of systemic weakness or muscle paralysis. The entire contents of a vial is below the estimated dose for systemic toxicity in humans weighing 6 kg. or greater.

In the event of overdosage or injection into the wrong muscle, additional information may be obtained by contacting Allergan Pharmaceuticals at (800) 347-5063 from 8:00 a.m. to 4:00 p.m. Pacific Time, or at (714) 724-5954 for a recorded message at other times.

The effect of botulinum toxin may be potentiated by aminoglycoside antibiotics or any other drugs that interfere with neuromuscular transmission. Caution should be exercised when **Botox®** is used in patients taking any of these drugs.[6]

PRECAUTIONS

General: The safe and effective use of **Botox® (Botulinum Toxin Type A)** depends upon proper storage of the product, selection of the correct dose, and proper reconstitution and administration techniques. Physicians administering **Botox®** must understand the relevant neuromuscular and orbital anatomy and any alterations to the anatomy due to prior surgical procedures, and standard electromyographic techniques.

As with all biologic products, epinephrine and other precautions as necessary should be available should an anaphylactic reaction occur.

During the administration of **Botox®** for the treatment of strabismus, retrobulbar hemorrhages sufficient to compromise retinal circulation have occurred from needle penetrations into the orbit. It is recommended that appropriate instruments to decompress the orbit be accessible. Ocular (globe) penetrations by needles have also occurred. An ophthalmoscope to diagnose this condition should be available.

Reduced blinking from **Botox®** injection of the orbicularis muscle can lead to corneal exposure, persistent epithelial defect and corneal ulceration, especially in patients with VII nerve disorders. One case of corneal perforation in an aphakic eye requiring corneal grafting has occurred because of this effect. Careful testing of corneal sensation in eyes previously operated upon, avoidance of injection into the lower lid area to avoid ectropion, and vigorous treatment of any epithelial defect should be employed. This may require protective drops, ointment, therapeutic soft contact lenses, or closure of the eye by patching or other means.

Information for Patients: Patients with blepharospasm may have been extremely sedentary for a long time. Sedentary patients should be cautioned to resume activity slowly and carefully following the administration of **Botox® (Botulinum Toxin Type A)**.

Drug Interactions: The effect of botulinum toxin may be potentiated by aminoglycoside antibiotics or any other drugs that interfere with neuromuscular transmission. Caution should be exercised when **Botox®** is used in patients taking any of these drugs.[6] (See Warnings).

Pregnancy: ***Pregnancy Category C:*** Animal reproduction studies have not been conducted with **Botox® (Botulinum Toxin Type A)**. It is also not known whether **Botox®** can cause fetal harm when administered to a pregnant woman or can affect reproduction capacity. **Botox®** should be administered to pregnant women only if clearly needed.

Carcinogenesis, Mutagenesis, Impairment of Fertility: Long term studies in animals have not been performed to evaluate carcinogenic potential of **Botox®**.

Nursing Mothers: It is not known whether this drug is excreted in human milk. Because many drugs are excreted in human milk, caution should be exercised when **Botox® (Botulinum Toxin Type A)** is administered to a nursing woman.

Pediatric Use: Safety and effectiveness in children below the age of 12 have not been established.

ADVERSE REACTIONS[4]

There have been reports of seven cases of diffuse skin rash and two cases of local swelling of the eyelid skin lasting for several days following eyelid injection.

Strabismus: Inducing paralysis in one or more extraocular muscles may produce spatial disorientation, double vision, or past-pointing. Covering the affected eye may alleviate these symptoms. Extraocular muscles adjacent to the injection site are often affected, causing ptosis or vertical deviation, especially with higher doses of **Botox® (Botulinum Toxin Type A)**. The incidence rates of these side effects in 2058 adults who received 3650 injections for horizontal strabismus are listed below:

Ptosis	15.7%
Vertical deviation	16.9%

The incidence of ptosis was much less after inferior rectus injection (0.9%) and much greater after superior rectus injection (37.7%).

The incidence rates of these side effects persisting for over 6 months in an enlarged series of 5587 injections of horizontal muscles in 3104 patients are listed below:

Ptosis lasting over 180 days	0.3%
Vertical deviation greater than 2 prism diopters lasting over 180 days	2.1%

In these patients, the injection procedure itself caused 9 scleral perforations. A vitreous hemorrhage occurred and later cleared in one case. No retinal detachment or visual loss occurred in any case. Sixteen retrobulbar hemorrhages occurred. Decompression of the orbit after 5 minutes was done to restore retinal circulation in one case. No eye lost vision from retrobulbar hemorrhage. Five eyes had pupillary change consistent with ciliary ganglion damage (Adies pupil).

Blepharospasm: In 1684 patients who received 4258 treatments (involving multiple injections) for blepharospasm, the incidence rates of adverse reactions per treated eye are listed below:

Ptosis	11.0%
Irritation/Tearing (includes dry eye, lagophthalmos, and photophobia)	10.0%

Ectropion, keratitis, diplopia and entropion were reported rarely (incidence less than 1%)

Ecchymosis occurs easily in the soft eyelid tissues. This can be prevented by applying pressure at the injection site immediately after the injection.

In two cases of VII nerve disorder (one case of an aphakic eye) reduced blinking from **Botox® (Botulinum Toxin Type A)** injection of the orbicularis muscle led to serious corneal exposure, persistent epithelial defect and corneal ulceration. Perforation requiring corneal grafting occurred in one case, an aphakic eye. Avoidance of injection into the lower lid area to avoid ectropion may reduce this hazard. Vigorous treatment of any corneal epithelial defect should be employed. This may require protective drops, ointment, therapeutic soft contact lenses, or closure of the eye by patching or other means.

Two patients previously incapacitated by blepharospasm experienced cardiac collapse attributed to over-exertion within three weeks following **Botox®** therapy. Sedentary patients should be cautioned to resume activity slowly and carefully following the administration of **Botox®**.

OVERDOSAGE

In the event of overdosage or injection into the wrong muscle, additional information may be obtained by contacting Allergan Pharmaceuticals at (800) 347-5063 from 8:00 a.m. to 4:00 p.m. Pacific Time, or at (714) 724-5954 for a recorded message at other times.

DOSAGE AND ADMINISTRATION

Strabismus: **Botox® (Botulinum Toxin Type A)** is intended for injection into extraocular muscles utilizing the electrical activity recorded from the tip of the injection needle as a guide to placement within the target muscle. Injection without surgical exposure or electromyographic guidance should not be attempted. Physicians should be familiar with electromyographic technique.

An injection of **Botox®** is prepared by drawing into a sterile 1.0 mL tuberculin syringe an amount of the properly diluted toxin (see Dilution Table) slightly greater than the intended dose. Air bubbles in the syringe barrel are expelled and the syringe is attached to the electromyographic injection needle, preferably a 1½", 27 gauge needle. Injection volume in excess of the intended dose is expelled through the needle into an appropriate waste container to assure patency of the needle and to confirm that there is no syringe-needle leakage. A new, sterile needle and syringe should be used to enter the vial on each occasion for dilution or removal of **Botox®**.

To prepare the eye for **Botox®** injection, it is recommended that several drops of a local anesthetic and an ocular decongestant be given several minutes prior to injection.

Note: The volume of **Botox®** injected for treatment of strabismus should be between 0.05 mL to 0.15 mL per muscle.

Strabismus dosage: The initial listed doses of the diluted **Botox® (Botulinum Toxin Type A)** (see Dilution Table below) typically create paralysis of injected muscles beginning one to two days after injection and increasing in intensity during the first week. The paralysis lasts for 2–6 weeks and gradually resolves over a similar time period. Overcorrections lasting over 6 months have been rare. About one half of patients will require subsequent doses because of inadequate paralytic response of the muscle to the initial dose, or because of mechanical factors such as large deviations or restrictions, or because of the lack of binocular motor fusion to stabilize the alignment.

I. Initial doses in units (abbreviated as U). Use the lower listed doses for treatment of small deviations. Use the larger doses only for large deviations.
   A. For vertical muscles, and for horizontal strabismus of less than 20 prism diopters: 1.25 U to 2.5 U in any one muscle.
   B. For horizontal strabismus of 20 prism diopters to 50 prism diopters: 2.5 U to 5.0 U in any one muscle.
   C. For persistent VI nerve palsy of one month or longer duration: 1.25 U to 2.5 U in the medial rectus muscle.
II. Subsequent doses for residual or recurrent strabismus.
   A. It is recommended that patients be re-examined 7–14 days after each injection to assess the effect of that dose.
   B. Patients experiencing adequate paralysis of the target muscle that require subsequent injections should receive a dose comparable to the initial dose.
   C. Subsequent doses for patients experiencing incomplete paralysis of the target muscle may be increased up to twice the size of the previously administered dose.
   D. Subsequent injections should not be administered until the effects of the previous dose have dissipated as evidenced by substantial function in the injected and adjacent muscles.
   E. The maximum recommended dose as a single injection for any one muscle is 25 U.

Blepharospasm: For blepharospasm, diluted **Botox® (Botulinum Toxin Type A)** (see Dilution Table) is injected using a sterile, 27–30 gauge needle without electromyographic guidance. 1.25 U to 2.5 U (0.05 mL to 0.1 mL volume at each site) injected into the medial and lateral pre-tarsal orbicularis oculi of the upper lid and into the lateral pre-tarsal orbicularis oculi of the lower lid is the initial recommended dose. In general, the initial effect of the injections is seen within three days and reaches a peak at one to two weeks post-treatment. Each treatment lasts approximately three months, following which the procedure can be repeated indefinitely. At repeat treatment sessions, the dose may be increased up to two-fold if the response from the initial treatment is considered insufficient—usually defined as an effect that does not last longer than two months. However there appears to be little benefit obtainable from injecting more than 5.0 Units per site. Some tolerance may be found when **Botox®** is

Continued on next page

Allergan—Cont.

used in treating blepharospasm if treatments are given any more frequently than every three months, and it is rare to have the effect be permanent.
The cumulative dose of **Botox®** in a 30-day period should not exceed 200 U.

DILUTION TECHNIQUE

To reconstitute lyophilized **Botox® (Botulinum Toxin Type A)**, use sterile normal saline **without** a preservative; 0.9% Sodium Chloride Injection is the recommended diluent. Draw up the proper amount of diluent in the appropriate size syringe. Since **Botox®** is denatured by bubbling or similar violent agitation, inject the diluent into the vial gently. Discard the vial if a vacuum does not pull the diluent into the vial. Record the date and time of reconstitution on the space on the label. **Botox®** should be administered within 4 hours after reconstitution.
During this time period, reconstituted **Botox®** should be stored in a refrigerator (2° to 8°C). Reconstituted **Botox®** should be clear, colorless and free of particulate matter. Parenteral drug products should be inspected visually for particulate matter and discoloration prior to administration and whenever the solution and the container permit. The use of one vial for more than one patient is not recommended because the product and diluent do not contain a preservative.
Dilution Table

Diluent Added (0.9% Sodium Chloride Injection)	Resulting dose in Units per 0.1 mL
1.0 mL	10.0 U
2.0 mL	5.0 U
4.0 mL	2.5 U
8.0 mL	1.25 U

Note: These dilutions are calculated for an injection volume of 0.1 mL. A decrease or increase in the **Botox®** dose is also possible by administering a smaller or larger injection volume—from 0.05 mL (50% decrease in dose) to 0.15 mL (50% increase in dose).

HOW SUPPLIED

Each vial contains 100 U of lyophilized *Clostridium botulinum* Toxin type A. NDC 0023-0504-01.

CAUTION

Federal (U.S.A.) law prohibits dispensing without prescription.

STORAGE

Store the lyophilized product in a freezer at or below −5°C. Administer **Botox® (Botulinum Toxin Type A)** within 4 hours after the vial is removed from the freezer and reconstituted. During these four hours, reconstituted **Botox®** should be stored in a refrigerator (2° to 8°C). Reconstituted **Botox®** should be clear, colorless and free of particulate matter.
All vials, including expired vials, or equipment used with the drug should be disposed of carefully as is done with all medical waste.

REFERENCES

1. Sanders D, Massey W, Buckley E. Botulinum toxin for blepharospasm: Single-fiber EMG studies. Neurology 1986; 36:545–547.
2. Arthurs B, Flanders M, Codere F, Gauthier S, Dresner S, Stone L. Treatment of blepharospasm with medication, surgery and type A botulinum toxin. Can J Ophthalmol 1987; 22:24–28.
3. Jankovic J, Orman J. Botulinum A toxin for cranial-cervical dystonia: A double-blind, placebo-controlled study. Neurology 1987; 37:616–623.
4. Data on file, Allergan, Inc.
5. Scott A B. Botulinum toxin treatment of strabismus. American Academy of Ophthalmology, Focal Points 1989: Clinical Modules for Ophthalmologists Vol VII Module12.
6. Wang Y C, Burr D H, Korthals G J, Sugiyama H. Acute toxicity of aminoglycoside antibiotics as an aid in detecting botulism. Appl Environ Microbiol 1984; 48:951–955.

Manufactured by:
Allergan, Inc.
2525 DuPont Drive
Irvine, CA 92715
April 1992

POLYTRIM® OPHTHALMIC SOLUTION Sterile (TRIMETHOPRIM SULFATE AND POLYMYXIN B SULFATE) ℞

DESCRIPTION

Polytrim® Ophthalmic Solution (trimethoprim sulfate and polymyxin B sulfate) is a sterile antimicrobial solution for topical ophthalmic use. Each mL contains trimethoprim sulfate equivalent to 1 mg trimethoprim and polymyxin B sulfate 10,000 units. The vehicle contains benzalkonium chloride 0.004% (added as a preservative) and the inactive ingredients sodium chloride, sodium hydroxide or sulfuric acid (added to adjust pH), and Water for Injection.
Trimethoprim sulfate, 2,4-diamino-5-(3,4,5-trimethoxybenzyl)pyrimidine sulfate (2:1), is a white, odorless, crystalline powder with a molecular weight of 678.72.
Polymyxin B sulfate is the sulfate salt of polymyxin B_1 and B_2 which are produced by the growth of *Bacillus polymyxa* (Prazmowski) Migula (Fam. Bacillaceae). It has a potency of not less than 6,000 polymyxin B units per mg, calculated on an anhydrous basis.

CLINICAL PHARMACOLOGY

Trimethoprim is a synthetic antibacterial drug active against a wide variety of aerobic gram-positive and gram-negative ophthalmic pathogens. Trimethoprim blocks the production of tetrahydrofolic acid from dihydrofolic acid by binding to and reversibly inhibiting the enzyme dihydrofolate reductase. This binding is very much stronger for the bacterial enzyme than for the corresponding mammalian enzyme. For that reason, trimethoprim selectively interferes with bacterial biosynthesis of nucleic acids and proteins.
Polymyxin B, a cyclic lipopeptide antibiotic, is rapidly bactericidal for a variety of gram-negative organisms, especially *Pseudomonas aeruginosa*. It increases the permeability of the bacterial cell membrane by interacting with the phospholipid components of the membrane.
When used topically, trimethoprim and polymyxin B absorption through intact skin and mucous membranes is insignificant.
Blood samples were obtained from 11 human volunteers at 20 minutes, 1 hour and 3 hours following instillation in the eye of 2 drops of ophthalmic solution containing 1 mg trimethoprim and 10,000 units polymyxin B per mL. Peak serum concentrations were approximately 0.03 μg/mL trimethoprim and 1 unit/mL polymyxin B.
Microbiology: *In vitro* studies have demonstrated that the anti-infective components of Polytrim are active against the following bacterial pathogens that are capable of causing external infections of the eye:
Trimethoprim: *Staphylococcus aureus* and *Staphylococcus epidermidis, Streptococcus pyogenes, Streptococcus faecalis, Streptococcus pneumoniae, Haemophilus influenzae, Haemophilus aegyptius, Escherichia coli, Klebsiella pneumoniae, Proteus mirabilis* (indole-negative), *Proteus vulgaris* (indole-positive), *Enterobacter aerogenes*, and *Serratia marcescens.*
Polymyxin B: *Pseudomonas aeruginosa, Escherichia coli, Klebsiella pneumoniae, Enterobacter aerogenes* and *Haemophilus influenzae.*

INDICATIONS AND USAGE

Polytrim Ophthalmic Solution is indicated in the treatment of surface ocular bacterial infections, including acute bacterial conjunctivitis, and blepharoconjunctivitis, caused by susceptible strains of the following microorganisms: *Staphylococcus aureus, Staphylococcus epidermidis, Streptococcus pneumoniae, Streptococcus viridans, Haemophilus influenzae* and *Pseudomonas aeruginosa.**

CONTRAINDICATIONS

Polytrim Ophthalmic Solution is contraindicated in patients with known hypersensitivity to any of its components.

WARNINGS

NOT FOR INJECTION INTO THE EYE. If a sensitivity reaction to Polytrim occurs, discontinue use. Polytrim Ophthalmic Solution is not indicated for the prophylaxis or treatment of ophthalmia neonatorum.

PRECAUTIONS

General: As with other antimicrobial preparations, prolonged use may result in overgrowth of nonsusceptible organisms, including fungi. If superinfection occurs, appropriate therapy should be initiated.
Information for Patients: Avoid contaminating the applicator tip with material from the eye, fingers, or other source. This precaution is necessary if the sterility of the drops is to be maintained.
If redness, irritation, swelling or pain persists or increases, discontinue use immediately and contact your physician.
Carcinogenesis, Mutagenesis, Impairment of Fertility:
Carcinogenesis: Long-term studies in animals to evaluate carcinogenic potential have not been conducted with polymyxin B sulfate or trimethoprim.
Mutagenesis: Trimethoprim was demonstrated to be non-mutagenic in the Ames assay. In studies at two laboratories no chromosomal damage was detected in cultured Chinese hamster ovary cells at concentrations approximately 500 times human plasma levels after oral administration; at concentrations approximately 1000 times human plasma levels after oral administration in these same cells a low level of chromosomal damage was induced at one of the laboratories. Studies to evaluate mutagenic potential have not been conducted with polymyxin B sulfate.

*Efficacy for this organism in this organ system was studied in fewer than 10 infections.

Impairment of Fertility: Polymyxin B sulfate has been reported to impair the motility of equine sperm, but its effects on male or female fertility are unknown.
No adverse effects on fertility or general reproductive performance were observed in rats given trimethoprim in oral dosages as high as 70 mg/kg/day for males and 14 mg/kg/day for females.
Pregnancy: ***Teratogenic Effects:*** Pregnancy Category C. Animal reproduction studies have not been conducted with polymyxin B sulfate. It is not known whether polymyxin B sulfate can cause fetal harm when administered to a pregnant woman or can affect reproduction capacity.
Trimethoprim has been shown to be teratogenic in the rat when given in oral doses 40 times the human dose. In some rabbit studies, the overall increase in fetal loss (dead and resorbed and malformed conceptuses) was associated with oral doses 6 times the human therapeutic dose.
While there are no large well-controlled studies on the use of trimethoprim in pregnant women, Brumfitt and Pursell, in a retrospective study, reported the outcome of 186 pregnancies during which the mother received either placebo or oral trimethoprim in combination with sulfamethoxazole. The incidence of congenital abnormalities was 4.5% (3 of 66) in those who received placebo and 3.3% (4 of 120) in those receiving trimethoprim and sulfamethoxazole. There were no abnormalities in the 10 children whose mothers received the drug during the first trimester. In a separate survey, Brumfitt and Pursell also found no congenital abnormalities in 35 children whose mothers had received oral trimethoprim and sulfamethoxazole at the time of conception or shortly thereafter.
Because trimethoprim may interfere with folic acid metabolism, trimethoprim should be used during pregnancy only if the potential benefit justifies the potential risk to the fetus.
Nonteratogenic Effects: The oral administration of trimethoprim to rats at a dose of 70 mg/kg/day commencing with the last third of gestation and continuing through parturition and lactation caused no deleterious effects on gestation or pup growth and survival.
Pediatric Use: Safety and effectiveness in children below the age of 2 months have not been established (see WARNINGS).

ADVERSE REACTIONS

The most frequent adverse reaction to Polytrim Ophthalmic Solution is local irritation consisting of transient burning or stinging, itching or increased redness on instillation. These reactions occur in less than 4 of 100 patients treated. Polytrim has a low incidence of hypersensitivity reactions (less than 2 of 100 patients treated) consisting of lid edema, itching, increased redness, tearing and/or circumocular rash. Although sensitivity reactions to trimethoprim are rare, an isolated incident of photosensitivity was reported in a patient who received the drug orally.

DOSAGE AND ADMINISTRATION

Adults: In mild to moderate infections, instill one drop in the affected eye(s) every three hours (maximum of 6 doses per day) for a period of 7 to 10 days.
Pediatric Use: Clinical studies have shown Polytrim to be safe and effective for use in children over two months of age. The dosage regimen is the same as for adults.

HOW SUPPLIED

A sterile ophthalmic solution, each mL contains trimethoprim sulfate** equivalent to 1 mg trimethoprim and polymyxin B sulfate 10,000 units in a plastic dropper bottle of 10 mL (NDC 0023-7824-10).
Store at 15°–25°C (59°–77°F) and protect from light.

**Mfd. under U.S. Patent No. 3,956,327.

Distributed by:
ALLERGAN PHARMACEUTICALS
A Division of Allergan, Inc.
Irvine, CA 92713, U.S.A.
Manufactured by:
BURROUGHS WELLCOME CO.
Research Triangle Park, North Carolina 27709

IDENTIFICATION PROBLEM?
Consult PDR's
Product Identification Section
where you'll find over 1700
products pictured actual size
and in full color.

Alpha Therapeutic Corporation
5555 VALLEY BLVD.
LOS ANGELES, CA 90032

ALBUTEIN® 5%   ℞
Albumin (Human), USP, 5% Solution

10 bottles per case.

250mL bottle & IV set	NDC 49669-5211-1
500mL bottle & IV set	NDC 49669-5211-2

ALBUTEIN® 25%   ℞
Albumin (Human), USP, 25% Solution

10 bottles per case.

20mL bottle & IV set	NDC 49669-5213-1
50mL bottle & IV set	NDC 49669-5213-2
100mL bottle & IV set	NDC 49669-5213-3

ALPHANINE®   ℞
Heat-Treated/Solvent Suspension
Coagulation Factor IX (Human)

AlphaNine® Coagulation Factor IX (Human) is available in 500, 1000, and 1500 assay ranges with 10 mL diluent. For intravenous administration only. Each carton and single dose vial is labeled with Factor IX dose contained; carton contains sterile diluent, transfer needle, and microaggregate filter. 12 vials per case.
ASSAY RANGE 0-2000 F IX Units/Vial NDC 49669-3900-1

FLUOSOL®   ℞
20% Intravascular Perfluorochemical Emulsion
Product Information

DESCRIPTION
Fluosol® (20% Intravascular Perfluorochemical Emulsion) is a stable emulsion of perfluorochemicals in Water for Injection. The perfluorochemical phase of the emulsion dissolves oxygen and carbon dioxide. The formulation is a sterile and nonpyrogenic fluid for intracoronary administration only during percutaneous transluminal coronary angioplasty. Fluosol® consists of 3 separate parts which must be mixed prior to use: (1) the Fluosol® emulsion; (2) Solution 1; and (3) Solution 2. The additive solutions serve to adjust pH, ionic strength, and osmotic pressure in the final 20% emulsion, and must be added separately and sequentially prior to administration. The Fluosol® emulsion is supplied as 400 mL volume in a 500 mL flexible plastic container. Solutions 1 and 2 are supplied in glass vials, 30 mL and 70 mL, respectively, as sterile, nonpyrogenic aqueous solutions.

HOW SUPPLIED
Fluosol® consists of 3 components which must be mixed before administration. The components included are:
- Fluosol® Emulsion, 400 mL in
  flexible plastic bag   (NDC 49669-1520-1).
- Solution 1, 30 mL in glass vial   (NDC 49669-1521-1).
- Solution 2, 70 mL in glass vial   (NDC 49669-1522-1).

The additive solutions are supplied in a separate kit which includes accessories for effecting oxygenation. The oxygenation kit includes the following accessories:

CARTRIDGE OXYGENATION KIT
1 95% O_2, 5% CO_2 Cartridge
1 30 mL Solution 1
1 70 mL Solution 2
1 Cartridge-Piercing Device
1 18-Gauge Needle
1 0.2 Micron Filter
1 Protective Immersion Bag
1 Directions For Use
1 FLUOSOL Package Insert

PLASMATEIN® 5%   ℞
Plasma Protein Fraction (Human), USP, 5% Solution

10 bottles per case.

250mL bottle & IV set	NDC 49669-5721-1
500mL bottle & IV set	NDC 49669-5721-2

PROFILATE® OSD   ℞
Solvent Detergent Treated
Antihemophilic Factor (Human), Factor VIII (AHF)

Profilate® OSD Solvent Detergent Treated, Antihemophilic Factor (Human) is available in 250 and 500 assay ranges with 10 mL diluent; and 750, 1000, 1250 and 1500 assay ranges with 25 mL diluent. For intravenous administration only. Each carton and single dose vial is labeled with Factor VIII dose contained; carton contains sterile diluent, transfer needle, and microaggregate filter. Isoagglutinin titre available upon request. 12 vials per case.
ASSAY RANGE   0–649 AHF Units/Vial NDC 49669-4300-1
ASSAY RANGE 650–2000 AHF Units/Vial NDC 49669-4300-2

PROFILNINE® HEAT-TREATED   ℞
Factor IX Complex

Profilnine® Heat-Treated Factor IX Complex is available in 250 and 500 assay ranges with 10 mL diluent, and 750, 1000, 1250 and 1500 assay ranges with 25 mL diluent. For intravenous administration only. Each carton and single dose vial is labeled with Factor IX dose contained; carton contains sterile diluent, transfer needle, and microaggregate filter. NAPTT times available upon request. 12 vials per case.
ASSAY RANGE 0–649 AHF Units/Vial NDC 49669-3700-1
ASSAY RANGE 650–2000 AHF Units/Vial NDC 49669-3700-2

VENOGLOBULIN®–I   ℞
Immune Globulin Intravenous (Human)

Sterile highly purified lyophilized preparation of intact, unmodified immunoglobulin. Supplies broad spectrum of IgG antibodies. Manufacturing process includes cold alcohol fractionation plus purification by PEG fractionation and DEAE Sephadex ion exchange adsorption. For intravenous administration. In 0.5g, 2.5g, 5.0g, and 10.0g vials with sterile diluent and transfer device. 6 vials per case.

0.5g with reconstitution kit	NDC 49669-1600-1
2.5g with reconstitution kit	NDC 49669-1602-1
5.0g with reconstitution kit	NDC 49669-1603-1
10.0g with reconstitution kit and administration set	NDC 49669-1604-1

VENOGLOBULIN®–S 5% Solution   ℞
Immune Globulin Intravenous (Human)
SOLVENT DETERGENT TREATED

Venoglobulin®-S 5% Solution, Solvent Detergent Treated is a sterile, highly purified solution of intact, unmodified human immunoglobulin G intended for intravenous use. IgG is isolated from large pools of human plasma using the Cohn-Oncley cold alcohol fractionation process, followed by polyethylene glycol fractionation and ion exchange chromatography. The manufacturing process includes treatment with a mixture of tri-n-butyl phosphate (TNBP) and polysorbate 80.
The process used to produce Venoglobulin®-S inactivates and/or partitions up to 13 cumulative logs of Human Immunodeficiency Virus Type 1 (HIV-1) based on *in vitro* studies. Additional solvent-detergent treatment further removes greater than 10 logs of HIV-1 and greater than 6 logs of HIV-2 as demonstrated *in vitro*, thereby providing an extra measure of safety.
Venoglobulin®-S contains all IgG antibody activities present in the donor population. The distribution of IgG subclasses corresponds to that of normal human plasma. Gamma globulin is isolated without additional chemical or enzymatic modification and the Fc portion of the molecule is maintained functionally intact. Typically IgG purity exceeds 99%.
The composition of Venoglobulin®-S is as follows:

Component	Quantity/mL
Human immunoglobulin G	50 mg
D-sorbitol	50 mg
Albumin (Human)	<1.3 mg
Polyethylene glycol	<100 mcg
Polysorbate 80	<100 mcg
Tri-n-butyl phosphate	< 10 mcg

This formulation contains no preservatives. The pH of the solution ranges from 5.2 to 5.8. The osmolarity is approximately 300 mOsm/L.

10 vials per case:

50 mL	2.5g IgG	NDC 49669-1612-1
100 mL	5.0g IgG	NDC 49669-1613-1
200 mL	10.0g IgG	NDC 49669-1614-1

All sizes are packaged with a sterile I.V. administration set. Recommended storage at or below 25°C or 77°F. Do not freeze.

EDUCATIONAL MATERIAL

Scientific publications, monographs, product literature, brochures and formulary kits available upon request.

Alra Laboratories, Inc.
3850 CLEARVIEW CT.
GURNEE, IL 60031

ALRAMUCIL INSTANT MIX   OTC
Psyllium Hydrophilic Mucilloid For Oral Suspension, USP
Effervescent and Instant mix, Unit dose packets

Each packet provides:
Psyllium hydrophilic mucilloid .... 3.6 gm.

HOW SUPPLIED
Carton of 30 (NDC 51641-150-03) Regular Flavor
Carton of 30 (NDC 51641-151-03) Orange Flavor

APAP-ELIXIR   OTC
Acetaminophen 160mg/5mL

HOW SUPPLIED
4 fl. oz. bottle (NDC 51641-033-64)
4 fl. oz. bottle in carton (NDC 51641-033-46)

CHOLAC   ℞
[kō'lac]
CONSTILAC   ℞
[kŏn'stil-ac]
Lactulose Syrup, USP

Each 15 mL syrup contains:
10 g lactulose (and less than 1.6 g galactose, less than 1.2 g lactose, 0.1 g or less of fructose); plus water and coloring. Sodium hydroxide used to adjust pH.

HOW SUPPLIED
1 fl. oz. bottle (30 mL) (unit-dose)		
100 bottles/carton		NDC #51641-225-61
8 fl. oz. bottle (240 mL)		NDC #51641-224-68
16 fl oz. bottle (480 mL)		NDC #51641-225-76
32 fl. oz. bottle (960 mL)		NDC #51641-224-82
64 fl. oz. bottle (1920 mL)		NDC #51641-225-94
1 gal. (3785 mL)		NDC #51641-225-97

DMH-SYRUP   OTC
Dimenhydrinate Syrup, USP 12.5mg/4ml

HOW SUPPLIED
4 fl. oz. bottle (NDC 51641-013-64)
4 fl. oz. bottle in carton (NDC 51641-013-46)

DPH-ELIXIR   OTC
Diphenhydramine Elixir, USP 12.5/5mL

HOW SUPPLIED
4 fl. oz. bottle (NDC 51641-030-64)
4 fl. oz. bottle in carton (NDC 51641-030-46)
16 fl. oz. bottle (NDC 51641-030-76)
64 fl. oz. bottle (NDC 51641-030-94)

ERYZOLE Granules for Suspension   ℞
erythromycin ethylsuccinate and sulfisoxazole acetyl
for oral suspension USP

When reconstituted each 5mL of suspension contains:
Erythromycin Ethylsuccinate equivalent to 200mg erythromycin and Sulfisoxazole Acetyl equivalent to 600mg sulfisoxazole.

HOW SUPPLIED
Eryzole suspension is available for teaspoon dosage in bottles of,
100 mL (NDC 51641-111-64)
150 mL (NDC 51641-111-66)
200 mL (NDC 51641-111-68)
in the form of granules to be reconstituted with water.

Continued on next page

Alra Laboratories—Cont.

FERROUS SULFATE DROPS   OTC
Ferrous Sulfate Oral Solution, USP
Each 0.6 mL supplies 15 mg of elemental iron.

HOW SUPPLIED
50 mL bottle (NDC 51641-743-50)

GELPIRIN TABLETS   OTC

Each tablet contains:
Acetaminophen	125 mg.
Aspirin	240 mg.
Caffeine	32 mg.
Along with two buffering agents

HOW SUPPLIED
Bottle of 100 (NDC 51641-711-01)
Bottle of 1000 (NDC 51641-711-10)
Unit dose (NDC 51641-711-11)

GELPIRIN CCF COUGH, COLD AND FEVER TABLETS   OTC

Each tablet contains:
Acetaminophen	325mg
Guaifenesin	25mg
Phenylpropanolamine	12.5mg
Chlorpheniramine Maleate	1mg

HOW SUPPLIED
Bottle of 50 (NDC 51641-721-50)

Gen–XENE®   © R
[jen'zĕn]
Clorazepate Dipotassium Tablets

Gen–XENE Tablets are available in 3.75 mg, 7.5 mg or 15 mg strengths for oral administration.

HOW SUPPLIED
3.75 mg gray, scored tablets debossed with ALRA and GX:
Unit dose packages of 100: NDC 51641-242-11
Bottles of 30 NDC 51641-242-03
Bottles of 100 NDC 51641-242-01
Bottles of 500 NDC 51641-242-05

7.5 mg yellow, scored tablets debossed with ALRA and GT:
Unit dose packages of 100: NDC 51641-243-11
Bottles of 30 NDC 51641-243-03
Bottles of 100 NDC 51641-243-01
Bottles of 500 NDC 51641-243-05

15 mg green, scored tablets debossed with ALRA and GN:
Unit dose packages of 100: NDC 51641-244-11
Bottles of 30 NDC 51641-244-03
Bottles of 100 NDC 51641-244-01
Bottles of 500 NDC 51641-244-05

IBU–TAB
Ibuprofen Tablets, USP

Ibuprofen Tablets are available in 200, 400, 600 and 800 mg strengths for oral administration.

HOW SUPPLIED
IBU-TAB OTC
Ibuprofen Tablets, 200 mg (orange) film-coated, round tablets. Debossed 'ALRA' on one side and 215 on the other.
Bottles of 30   NDC 51641-215-03
Bottles of 60   NDC 51641-215-60
Bottles of 100   NDC 51641-215-01
Bottles of 250   NDC 51641-215-25
IBU-TAB R
Ibuprofen Tablets, 400 mg (orange) film-coated, round tablets. Debossed 'ALRA' on one side and IF 400 on the other.
Bottles of 100   NDC 51641-214-01
Bottles of 500   NDC 51641-214-05
Bottles of 1000   NDC 51641-214-10
Unit-dose packages of 100   NDC 51641-214-11
Ibuprofen Tablets, 600 mg (orange) film-coated, oval tablets. Debossed 'ALRA' on one side and IF 600 on the other.
Bottles of 100   NDC 51641-213-01
Bottles of 500   NDC 51641-213-05
Bottles of 1000   NDC 51641-213-10
Unit-dose packages of 100   NDC 51641-213-11

Ibuprofen Tablets, 800 mg (light peach) film-coated, oval tablets. Debossed 'ALRA' on one side and IF 800 on the other.
Bottles of 100   NDC 51641-212-01
Bottles of 500   NDC 51641-212-05
Bottles of 1000   NDC 51641-212-10
Unit-dose packages of 100   NDC 51641-212-11

K+ 10   R
Potassium Chloride Extended-release Tablets, USP

Each K+ 10 tablet contains:
Potassium Chloride, USP ....10 mEq (750 mg)
[Equivalent to 10 mEq (390 mg) of potassium and 10 mEq (360 mg) of chloride]

HOW SUPPLIED
Bottle of 100 (NDC #51641-177-01)
Bottle of 500 (NDC #51641-177-05)
Bottle of 1000 (NDC #51641-177-10)
Unit dose packages of 100: NDC 51641-177-11

K+ CARE 20 mEq   R
Potassium Chloride For Oral Solution, USP

Each powder packet provides:
Potassium Chloride .... 20 mEq (1.5 gm.)
[Equivalent to 20 mEq (780 mg) of potassium and 20 mEq (720 mg) of chloride]

HOW SUPPLIED
Carton of 30 (NDC 51641-120-03) Orange flavor
Carton of 30 (NDC 51641-140-03) Fruit flavor
Carton of 100 (NDC 51641-120-01) Orange flavor
Carton of 100 (NDC 51641-140-01) Fruit flavor

K+ CARE ET 25 mEq   R
Potassium Bicarbonate Effervescent Tablets For Oral Solution, USP

Each tablet contains .... 25 mEq of Potassium
(From 2.5 Gm. of Potassium Bicarbonate)

HOW SUPPLIED
Carton of 30 (NDC 51641-135-03) Orange flavor
Carton of 30 (NDC 51641-125-03) Lime flavor
Carton of 100 (NDC 51641-135-01) Orange flavor
Carton of 100 (NDC 51641-125-01) Lime flavor

MB-TAB   R
Meprobamate Tablets

HOW SUPPLIED
Each tablet contains:
Meprobamate 200mg
Bottle of 100 (NDC 51641-327-01)
Each tablet contains:
Meprobamate 400mg
Bottle of 100 (NDC 51641-327-01)
Bottle of 1000 (NDC 51641-327-10)

MULTI VITAMIN DROPS   OTC

Each 1.0 mL supplies 100% of U.S. recommended daily allowance of vitamins A,D,E,C, Thiamine, Riboflavin, Niacin, B6 and B12.
HOW SUPPLIED
50 mL bottle (NDC 51641-722-50)

MULTI VITAMIN DROPS WITH FLUORIDE   R

Each 1.0 mL supplies 100% of U.S. recommended daily allowance of vitamins A,D,E,C, Thiamine, Riboflavin, B6 and B12 with Fluoride.
HOW SUPPLIED
With 0.25 mg Fluoride
50 mL bottle (NDC 51641-727-50)
With 0.50 mg Fluoride
50 mL bottle (NDC 51641-730-50)

MULTI VITAMIN DROPS WITH IRON   OTC

Each 1.0 mL supplies 100% of U.S. recommended daily allowance of vitamins A,D,E,C, Thiamine, Riboflavin, B6 and B12 with Iron.

HOW SUPPLIED
50 mL bottle (NDC 51641-723-50)
PC-CAP   R
Propoxyphene HCl Compound, USP

Each capsule contains:
Propoxyphene HCl Compound	65 mg
Aspirin	389 mg
Caffeine	32.4 mg
HOW SUPPLIED
Bottle of 100 (NDC 51641-323-01)
Bottle of 500 (NDC 51641-323-05)
Bottle of 1000 (NDC 51641-323-10)
Unit Dose 100 (NDC 51641-323-11)

PP-CAP   R
Propoxyphene HCl Capsules, USP

Each capsule contains:
Propoxyphene HCl .... 65 mg
HOW SUPPLIED
Bottle of 100 (NDC 51641-321-01)
Bottle of 500 (NDC 51641-321-05)
Bottle of 1000 (NDC 51641-321-10)
Unit dose of 100 (NDC 51641-321-11)

VITAMIN DROPS WITH FLUORIDE   R

Each 1.0 mL supplies 100% of U.S. recommended daily allowance of vitamins A,D, and C with Fluoride.
HOW SUPPLIED
With 0.25 mg Fluoride
50 mL bottle (NDC 51641-724-50)
With 0.50 mg Fluoride
50 mL bottle (NDC 51641-725-50)

Alza Corporation
950 PAGE MILL ROAD
P.O. BOX 10950
PALO ALTO, CA 94303-0802

PROGESTASERT® System   R
[prŏ-jes-ta-sert]

DESCRIPTION
System
The PROGESTASERT system is a white, T-shaped unit constructed of ethylene/vinyl acetate copolymer (EVA) containing titanium dioxide. The 36-mm tubular vertical stem of the T contains a reservoir of 38 mg of progesterone, together with barium sulfate for radiopacity; both are dispersed in medical grade silicone fluid. The 32-mm horizontal cross-arms are solid EVA. Two monofilament blue-black nylon indicator/retrieval threads are fastened to the base of the T stem.
The tip of the shorter indicator thread is 9 cm from the top or leading end of the system and is used to ascertain correct placement at insertion. The long thread extends the length of the inserter, to which it is anchored by a plug that retains the system in the inserter.
Inserter
The inserter is a malleable, curved tube designed to conform to the anatomical configuration of most cervical-uterine cavities. The horizontal arms of the T are positioned outside of the inserter and are folded by an arm-cocker attachment immediately prior to insertion. The inserter does not contain a plunger.
DO NOT REMOVE ANY COMPONENT FROM THE INSERTER BEFORE INSERTION OF THE SYSTEM INTO THE UTERUS.

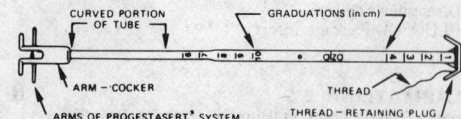

The PROGESTASERT system inserter permits determination of the depth of uterine placement of the PROGESTASERT system. The curvature of the inserter conforms with the usual orientation of the uterus; however, in cases of extreme flexion, the malleable inserter may need to be gently shaped to the desired curvature prior to insertion.
The PROGESTASERT system is packaged sterile within its inserter. Progesterone is released from the system *in situ* at an average rate of 65 μg/day for one year by membrane-controlled diffusion from the reservoir. Inert ingredients of the reservoir or membrane—barium sulfate, silicone fluid, titanium dioxide, or EVA—are not released.

HOW SUPPLIED

Available in cartons containing six packages, each with a sterile system and sterile inserter in a Tyvek polyethylene pouch.

EDUCATIONAL MATERIAL

All educational materials are free.
Booklets—Brochures
A. Patient Information Leaflet
(English and Spanish)
B. Clinical Evidence Brochure
C. Demonstration Kit
Slides—Videos
A. Progestasert® System Insertion Technique
Videocassette
B. Patient Audiocasette Tape
C. Instructional Slide Program

American Dermal Corporation
**51 APPLE TREE LANE
PO BOX 900
PLUMSTEADVILLE, PA 18949-0900**

DRITHOCREME®   ℞
(anthralin) 0.1%, 0.25%, 0.5%, 1.0% (HP)

DESCRIPTION
Drithocreme is a pale yellow topical cream containing 0.1%, 0.25%, 0.5% or 1.0% (HP) anthralin USP in a base of white petrolatum, sodium lauryl sulfate, cetostearyl alcohol, ascorbic acid, salicylic acid, chlorocresol and purified water. The chemical name of anthralin is 1,8-dihydroxy-9-anthrone.
The structural formula:

CLINICAL PHARMACOLOGY
Although the precise mechanism of anthralin's anti-psoriatic action is not fully understood, in vitro evidence suggests that its antimitotic effect results from inhibition of DNA synthesis. Additionally, the chemically reducing properties of anthralin may upset oxidative metabolic processes, providing a further slowing down of epidermal mitosis. Absorption in man has not been finally determined, but in a limited clinical study of Drithocreme, no traces of anthraquinone metabolites were detected in the urine of subjects treated. However, caution is advised in patients with renal disease.

INDICATIONS AND USAGE
An aid in the topical treatment of quiescent or chronic psoriasis. Treatment should be continued until the skin is entirely clear i.e. when there is nothing to feel with the fingers and the texture is normal.

CONTRAINDICATIONS
Do not use Drithocreme on the face, or for acute or actively inflamed psoriatic eruptions. Do not use if sensitive to any of the ingredients.

WARNINGS
Avoid contact with the eyes or mucous membranes. Drithocreme should not normally be applied to intertriginous skin areas and high strengths should not be used on these sites. Discontinue use if a sensitivity reaction occurs or if excessive irritation develops on uninvolved skin areas.

PRECAUTIONS
For external use only. Keep out of the reach of children. To prevent the possibility of staining clothing or bed linen while gaining experience in using Drithocreme, it may be advisable to use protective dressings. To prevent the possibility of discoloration particularly where Drithocreme HP (1.0%) has been used, always rinse the bath/shower with hot water immediately after washing/showering and then use a suitable cleanser to remove any deposit on the surface of the bath or shower. Contact with fabrics, plastics and other materials may cause staining and should be avoided. Always wash hands thoroughly after use. Long-term studies in animals have not been performed to evaluate the carcinogenic potential of the drug. Although anthralin has been found to have tumor-promoting properties on mouse skin, there have been

no reports to suggest carcinogenic effects in humans after many years of clinical use.
As long-term use of topical corticosteroids is known to destabilize psoriasis and withdrawal may also give rise to a 'rebound' phenomenon, an interval of at least one week should be allowed between the discontinuance of such steroids and the commencement of Drithocreme therapy. Petrolatum or a suitably bland emollient may usefully be applied during the intervening period.

PREGNANCY
Pregnancy Category C. Animal reproduction studies have not been conducted with Drithocreme. It is also not known whether Drithocreme can cause fetal harm when administered to a pregnant woman or can affect reproduction capacity. Drithocreme should be given to a pregnant woman only if clearly needed.

NURSING MOTHERS
It is not known whether this drug is excreted in human milk. Because many drugs are excreted in milk and because of the potential for tumorigenicity shown for anthralin in animal studies, a decision should be made whether to discontinue nursing or to discontinue the drug, taking into account the importance of the drug to the mother.

PEDIATRIC USE
Safety and effectiveness in children have not been specifically established.

ADVERSE REACTIONS
Very few instances of contact allergic reactions to anthralin have been reported. However, transient primary irritation of normal skin or uninvolved skin surrounding the treated lesions is more frequently seen and may occasionally be severe. Application of Drithocreme must be restricted to the psoriatic lesions. If the initial treatment produces excessive soreness or if the lesions spread, reduce frequency of application and, in extreme cases, discontinue use and consult physician. Some temporary discoloration of hair and fingernails may arise during the period of treatment but should be minimized by careful application. Drithocreme may stain skin, hair or fabrics. Staining of fabrics may be permanent, so contact should be avoided.

DOSAGE AND ADMINISTRATION
Generally, it is recommended that Drithocreme be applied once a day. Anthralin is known to be a potential skin irritant.The irritant potential of anthralin is directly related to the strength being used and each patient's individual tolerance. Therefore, where the response to anthralin treatment has not previously been established, always commence treatment for at least one week using 0.1% Drithocreme. Increase to the 0.25%, 0.5% or 1.0% (HP) strengths if appropriate. To open the tube, unscrew the cap and invert to pierce membrane. Drithocreme should normally be applied once daily and removed by washing or showering. The optimal period of contact will vary according to the strength used and the patient's response to treatment.
For the Skin: Apply sparingly only to the psoriatic lesions and rub gently and carefully into the skin until absorbed. It is most important to avoid applying an excessive quantity which may cause unnecessary soiling and staining of the clothing and/or bed linen. At the end of each period of treatment, a bath or shower should be taken to remove any surplus cream (which may have become red/brown in color). The margins of the lesions may gradually become stained purple/brown as treatment progresses, but this will disappear after cessation of treatment.
For the Scalp: Comb the hair to remove scalar debris and, after suitably parting, rub the cream well into the lesions. Keep Drithrocreme away from the eyes. Care should be taken to avoid application of the cream to uninvolved scalp margins. Remove any unintended residue which may be deposited behind the ears. At the end of each period of contact, wash the hair and scalp to remove any surplus cream (which may have become red/brown in color).
Keep tightly capped when not in use.
Store in a cool place (46°–59°F)

HOW SUPPLIED
50g tubes
Drithocreme 0.1%   NDC 51201-0029-1
Drithocreme 0.25%   NDC 51201-0028-1
Drithocreme 0.5%   NDC 51201-0027-1
Drithocreme HP 1.0%   NDC 51201-0026-1

CAUTION
Federal law prohibits dispensing without prescription.
Revised 1/90
Distributed by American Dermal Corporation
Plumsteadville, Pa 18949, USA.
Made in UK.

DRITHO–SCALP®   ℞
(anthralin) 0.25%, 0.5%

PRESCRIBING INFORMATION

DESCRIPTION
Dritho-Scalp is a pale yellow topical cream containing 0.25% or 0.5% anthralin USP in a base of white petrolatum, mineral oil, sodium lauryl sulfate, cetostearyl alcohol, ascorbic acid, salicylic acid, chlorocresol and purified water.
The chemical name of anthralin is 1,8-dihydroxy-9-anthrone.
The structural formula:

CLINICAL PHARMACOLOGY
Although the precise mechanism of anthralin's anti-psoriatic action is not fully understood, in vitro evidence suggests that its antimitotic effect results from inhibition of DNA synthesis. Additionally, the chemically reducing properties of anthralin may upset oxidative metabolic processes, providing a further slowing down of epidermal mitosis. Absorption in man has not been finally determined, but in a limited clinical study of anthralin cream, no traces of anthraquinone metabolites were detected in the urine of subjects treated: however, caution is advised in patients with renal disease.

INDICATIONS AND USAGE
An aid in the topical treatment of quiescent or chronic psoriasis of the scalp. Treatment should be continued until the skin is entirely clear i.e. when there is nothing to feel with the fingers and the texture is normal.

CONTRAINDICATIONS
In patients with acute psoriatic eruptions or a history of hypersensitivity to any of the ingredients.

WARNINGS
Avoid contact with the eyes or mucous membranes. Discontinue use if a sensitivity reaction occurs or if excessive irritation develops on uninvolved skin areas.

PRECAUTIONS
For external use only. Keep out of the reach of children. Dritho-Scalp may stain the hair and should be applied sparingly and carefully to psoriasis lesions only. Contact with fabrics, plastics and other materials may cause staining and should be avoided. To prevent the possibility of discoloration, always rinse the bath/shower with hot water immediately after washing/showering and then use a suitable cleanser to remove any deposit on the surface of the bath or shower. Always wash hands thoroughly after use. Long-term studies in animals have not been performed to evaluate the carcinogenic potential of the drug. Although anthralin has been found to have tumor-promoting properties on mouse skin, there have been no reports to suggest carcinogenic effects in humans after many years of clinical use.
As long-term use of topical corticosteroids is known to destabilize psoriasis and withdrawal may also give rise to a 'rebound' phenomenon, an interval of at least one week should be allowed between the discontinuance of such steroids and the commencement of Dritho-Scalp therapy. Petrolatum or a suitably bland emollient may usefully be applied during the intervening period.

PREGNANCY
Pregnancy Category C. Animal reproduction studies have not been conducted with Dritho-Scalp. It is also not known whether Dritho-Scalp can cause fetal harm when administered to a pregnant woman or can affect reproduction capacity. Dritho-Scalp should be given to a pregnant woman only if clearly needed.

NURSING MOTHERS
It is not known whether this drug is excreted in human milk. Because many drugs are excreted in milk and because of the potential for tumorigenicity shown for anthralin in animal studies, a decision should be made whether to discontinue nursing or to discontinue the drug, taking into account the importance of the drug to the mother.

PEDIATRIC USE
Safety and effectiveness in children have not been specifically established.

ADVERSE REACTIONS
Very few instances of contact allergic reactions to anthralin have been reported. However, transient primary irritation of normal skin or uninvolved skin surrounding the treated lesions is more frequently seen and may occasionally be severe. Application of Dritho-Scalp must be restricted to the

Continued on next page

American Dermal—Cont.

psoriatic lesions. If the initial treatment produces excessive soreness or if the lesions spread, reduce frequency of application and, in extreme cases, discontinue use and consult physician. Some temporary discoloration of hair and fingernails may arise during the period of treatment but should be minimized by careful application. Dritho-Scalp may stain skin, hair or fabrics. Staining of fabrics may be permanent, so contact should be avoided.

DOSAGE AND ADMINISTRATION

Before initial use, the tube membrane should be pierced by inverting the white cap, which should then be discarded. The black applicator should then be screwed firmly onto the tube. This applicator includes a black cap which should always be replaced between treatments. Generally, it is recommended that Dritho-Scalp be applied once a day. Anthralin is known to be a potential skin irritant. The irritant potential of anthralin is directly related to the strength being used and each patient's individual tolerance. Therefore, where the response to anthralin treatment has not previously been established, always commence treatment for at least one week using 0.25% Dritho-Scalp. Increase to the 0.5% strength only if appropriate.

Dritho-Scalp should normally be applied once daily and removed by washing or showering. The optimal period of contact will vary according to the strength used and the patient's response to treatment.

Comb the hair to remove scalar debris and, after suitably parting, apply Dritho-Scalp only to the lesions and rub in well, taking care to prevent the cream spreading onto the forehead.

Keep Dritho-Scalp well away from the eyes.

Avoid application of the cream to uninvolved scalp margins. Remove any unintended residue which may be deposited behind the ears. At the end of each period of contact, wash the hair and scalp to remove any surplus cream (which may have become red/brown in color).

Always wash hands thoroughly after use.

Store in a cool place (46°–59°F).

HOW SUPPLIED

50g tube with special applicator
Dritho-Scalp 0.25% NDC 51201-0024-1
Dritho-Scalp 0.5% NDC 51201-0023-1

CAUTION

Federal law prohibits dispensing without prescription.
Revised 1/90
Distributed by American Dermal Corporation
Plumsteadville, Pa 18949, USA.
Made in UK.

VIRANOL® GEL ULTRA ℞
(26% w/w Salicylic Acid)
[*vī'răn"ŏl*]

DESCRIPTION

Viranol Gel Ultra is a topical preparation containing 26% w/w salicylic acid in an evaporative collodion-like gel vehicle composed of camphor, pyroxylin, povidone, ethyl alcohol (2% w/w) and acetone. The pharmacologic activity of Viranol Gel Ultra is generally attributed to the keratolytic action of salicylic acid.

The structural formula of salicylic acid is:

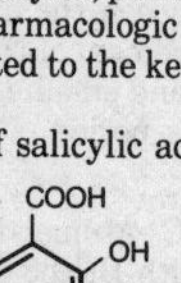

$C_7H_6O_3$ M.Wt. 138.12

CLINICAL PHARMACOLOGY

Although the exact mode of action of salicylic acid in the treatment of warts is not known, its activity appears to be associated with a keratolytic action which results in mechanical removal of epidermal cells infected with wart viruses.

INDICATIONS AND USAGE

Viranol Gel Ultra is indicated for the treatment and removal of common warts and plantar warts.

CONTRAINDICATIONS

This product should not be used by diabetics, patients with poor blood circulation, or patients who are hypersensitive to any of its components. Do not use on moles, birthmarks, unusual warts with hair growing from them, genital warts, or warts on the face.

PRECAUTIONS

Viranol Gel Ultra is for external use only. Do not permit this product to contact eyes or mucous membranes (inside mouth, nose, anus, genitals, or on lips). If contact with eyes or mucous membranes should occur, flush with water for 15 minutes to remove collodion film, and consult a physician.

Viranol Gel Ultra should not be allowed to contact normal skin surrounding the wart. Treatment should be discontinued if excessive irritation occurs.

The product is extremely flammable and should be kept away from fire or flame. Avoid smoking during application and until product has dried. Keep tube tightly capped when not in use. Avoid inhaling vapors. Store at room temperature away from heat. Contact with clothing, fabrics, plastics, wood, metal or other materials may cause damage, and should be avoided. Keep this and all drugs out of the reach of children.

ADVERSE REACTIONS

A localized irritation reaction may occur if Viranol Gel Ultra is applied to the normal skin surrounding the wart. Any irritation will normally be controlled by temporarily discontinuing use of the product and by taking care to apply the medication only to the wart site when treatment is resumed.

DOSAGE AND ADMINISTRATION

To attach special applicator provided before use: Hold the tube upright, cap uppermost, for 30 seconds. With the base of the tube on a firm surface, pierce the tube membrane by unscrewing and inverting the standard cap, which should then be discarded. This procedure should be carried out on a suitable surface, in case of accidental spillage. The accompanying special applicator should then be screwed firmly onto the tube and left in place. This special applicator inlcudes its own cap, which should always be replaced between treatments.

Once daily application.

1. Soak the affected area in warm water for 5 minutes.
2. Dry thoroughly with a clean towel which must not be used by others since the wart virus can be contagious.
3. Remove applicator cap, locate tip of applicator precisely at site of wart and gently squeeze the tube. Apply one or two drops of the gel carefully to the wart and allow to dry over its surface. Take care to avoid spreading onto surrounding normal skin. No adhesive bandage is necessary. Close applicator cap tightly after use.
4. The following day, carefully remove and discard the elastic film formed from the previous application, and then soak the affected area in warm water for 5 minutes. Dry thoroughly, then gently remove any loose tissue by rubbing with the enclosed emery board. Re-apply the gel, again taking care to avoid spreading onto surrounding normal skin.
5. Visible improvement will usually occur during the first one to two weeks of therapy. Maximum resolution may be expected after four to six weeks of drug use.

HOW SUPPLIED

Viranol Gel Ultra is supplied in an 8 g tube with special applicator, NDC 51201-5009-1.

See PRECAUTIONS section for special handling and storage information.

CAUTION

Federal law prohibits dispensing without prescription.
Revised 4/91
American Dermal Corporation, Plumsteadville, PA 18949-0900
Made in UK by Aeropak (Chemical Products) Limited, Great Yarmouth, Norfolk, NR30 3DN UA4/1/1

American Red Cross
Blood Services, Plasma Operations
1730 E. St. N.W.
WASHINGTON, DC 20006-5306

ALBUMIN (HUMAN), USP, ℞
5% SOLUTION

This product is derived from blood collected from volunteer donors by the American Red Cross Blood Services. The cost of processing, testing and packaging was paid by the Red Cross.

DESCRIPTION

Albumin (Human), 5% Solution, contains in each 100 mL, 5 g of albumin prepared from pooled human venous plasma. This product was prepared using the Cohn cold ethanol fractionation process.[1,2] It has been adjusted to physiological pH with sodium bicarbonate and/or sodium hydroxide and has been stablized with 0.004 M sodium caprylate and 0.004 M sodium acetyltryptophanate. The solution contains 145 ± 15 mEq of sodium per liter. Albumin (Human), 5% Solution, contains no preservative and none of the coagulation factors of fresh whole blood or fresh plasma. The transparent or slightly opalescent solution may have a greenish tint or may be pale straw to amber in color.

In addition to sterilization by filtration, this product has been heated for 10 hours at 60°C in the final container. This procedure has been shown to be an effective method of inactivating hepatitis viruses in 25% solutions of albumin even when prepared from plasma known to contain transmissible hepatitis viruses.[3]

The processing of Albumin (Human), 5% Solution, has removed blood group isoagglutinins to permit its administration without regard to the recipient's blood group. Albumin (Human), 5% Solution, must be administered INTRAVENOUSLY.

CLINICAL PHARMACOLOGY

Albumin is a highly soluble, ellipsoidal protein (MW 66,500), accounting for 70-80% of the colloid osmotic pressure of plasma. It is, therefore, important in regulating the volume of circulating blood.[4,5,6] This solution supplies the oncotic equivalent of approximately its volume of normal human plasma. When injected intravenously, 5% albumin will increase the circulating plasma volume by an amount approximately equal to the volume infused. This extra fluid reduces hemoconcentration and decreases blood viscosity. The degree and duration of volume expansion depend upon the initial blood volume. When treating patients with diminished blood volume, the effect of infused albumin may persist for many hours. In individuals with normal blood volumes, the hemodilution lasts for a much shorter time.

Albumin is also a transport protein and binds naturally occurring, therapeutic, and toxic materials in the circulation.[4,5]

Albumin is distributed throughout the extracellular water and more than 60% of the body albumin pool is located in the extravascular fluid compartment. The total body albumin in a 70 kg man is approximately 320 g; it has a circulating life span of 15–20 days, with a turnover of approximately 15 g per day.[5]

The minimum serum albumin level necessary to prevent or reverse peripheral edema is unknown. Although it undoubtedly varies from patient to patient, there is some evidence that it falls near 2.5 g per deciliter. This concentration provides a plasma oncotic pressure of 20 mm Hg (the equivalent of a total protein concentration of 5.2 g/dL).[6,7]

INDICATIONS AND USAGE

1. Hypovolemia (with or without shock)

Hypovolemia is a possible indication for albumin administration. The effectiveness of 5% albumin in reversing hypovolemia depends largely upon its colloid osmotic pressure.

Although crystalloid solutions or colloid-containing plasma substitutes may be used in the emergency treatment of shock, Albumin (Human) has a longer intravascular half-life.[7,8,9]

When the hypovolemia is long-standing and hypoalbuminemia exists in the presence of adequate hydration or edema, 25% albumin is preferable to 5% protein solutions.[4,6]

When the blood volume deficit is the result of hemorrhage, replacement with compatible red blood cells or whole blood should be undertaken as quickly as is possible.

2. Hypoalbuminemia

A. General

Hypoalbuminemia is another possible indication for albumin administration. Hypoalbuminemia may result from one or more of the following:[5]

1. Inadequate production (malnutrition, burns, major injury, congenital analbuminemia, liver disease, infection, malignancy, endocrine disorders).
2. Excessive catabolism (burns, major injury, pancreatitis, thyrotoxicosis, pemphigus, nephrosis).
3. Loss from the body (hemorrhage, excessive renal excretion, burn exudates, exudative enteropathy, exfoliative dermatoses).
4. Redistribution within the body (major surgery, cirrhosis with ascites, various inflammatory conditions).

In almost every instance, treatment of the underlying disorder and emphasis on increased nutritional replacement of amino acids and/or protein will be more likely to restore normal plasma albumin levels than will the transfusion of albumin-containing solutions.[4,6]

Whenever hypoalbuminemia results from excessive protein loss, the effect of albumin administration will be temporary unless the underlying disorder is reversed.

There are occasional patients with hypoproteinemia accompanying major infections or injuries, or severe pancreatitis, for whom reversal of the disorder cannot be accomplished quickly. In these situations, supplementation of nutritional protein intake with amino acid infusions may fail to restore serum albumin to adequate levels, and 5% albumin may be a useful therapeutic adjuvant.

B. Burns

The optimal mix of crystalloid and colloid solutions which should be administered following extensive burns remains the subject of continuing discussion.[4,7] During the initial 24 hours of therapy, large volumes of crystalloids are infused to restore the depleted extracellular fluid volume. Beyond 24 hours, albumin is indicated to replace the protein loss which accompanies any severe burn.[4,6,7]

C. Cirrhosis

When repeated paracenteses are being performed for ascites and the fluid is not being reinfused, supplementary albumin infusion may be needed.[7]

3. Miscellaneous Indications for Albumin (Human), 5% Solution

A. The administration of albumin prior to or during cardiopulmonary bypass surgery has been recommended although there are no clear data indicating its advantages over crystalloid solutions. Which is the most propitious time to infuse albumin is also unclear.[4,7,10]

B. When large volumes of packed red blood cells have been transfused to correct blood loss, 5% albumin may be administered in order to avoid the development of hypoalbuminemia.

Circumstances in Which Albumin Administration Is Usually Not Indicated:

The internal redistribution of plasma albumin which accompanies major surgery only occasionally causes clinical evidence of hypovolemia or insufficient plasma oncotic pressure. Moreover, there is no evidence that this temporary redistribution adversely affects wound healing. Therefore, the administration of 5% albumin to such post-surgical patients is not usually indicated.

The sequestration of protein-rich fluid during the course of acute inflammatory conditions (peritonitis, pancreatitis, cellulitis) rarely causes significant morbidity due to hypovolemia, and treatment with albumin is rarely indicated.

Rarely does a valid reason exist for administering albumin to treat the stabilized hypoproteinemias accompanying chronic cirrhosis, chronic nephrosis, protein-losing enteropathy, malabsorption, or pancreatic insufficiency.[4,6,7] However, when a patient in this category has to cope with a superimposed acute stress (e.g., anesthesia, major injection, etc.) his hemodynamic state, oncotic deficit and fluid balance should be carefully assessed and appropriate measure taken, as indicated by the individual circumstances.[6,7]

There is no valid reason for the use of albumin as an intravenous nutrient.

CONTRAINDICATIONS

The history of an allergic reaction to albumin is a specific contraindication to the use of this product.

WARNINGS

This solution should be administered with great caution to patients with hypertension, cardiac disease, severe pulmonary infection, or severe chronic anemia. For the treatment of patients with hypoalbuminemia accompanied by peripheral edema, 25% albumin solution should be used.

Although the volume administered and the speed of infusion should be adapted to the patient, 5% albumin solution usually can be administered safely to older children and adults at the rate of 100 mL per hour. Patients should always be carefully monitored in order to guard against the possibility of circulatory overload.

DO NOT USE IF TURBID. DO NOT BEGIN ADMINISTRATION MORE THAN 4 HOURS AFTER THE CONTAINER HAS BEEN ENTERED.
DISCARD PARTIALLY USED BOTTLES.

PRECAUTIONS

a) General

The rise in blood pressure following 5% albumin infusion necessitates careful observation of the injured or postoperative patient in order to detect and treat severed blood vessels that may not have bled at the lower blood pressure. The increase in blood volume which follows the administration of 5% albumin may cause a significant fall in hemoglobin concentration and red blood cell transfusion may become appropriate.

b) Laboratory Tests

Although laboratory testing is not necessary in order to monitor the treatment of shock or moderate hypoalbuminemia, when Albumin (Human), 5% Solution, is being administered for treatment of severe hypoproteinemia, periodic measurement of serum albumin levels is advisable.

c) Pregnancy — CATEGORY C

Animal reproduction studies have not been conducted with Albumin (Human), 5% Solution. It is not known if Albumin (Human), 5% Solution, can cause fetal harm when given to a pregnant woman, or can affect reproductive capacity. Albumin (Human), 5% Solution, should be given to a pregnant woman only if clearly needed.

d) Pediatric Use

Safety of this product has been demonstrated in children. Use in children is not associated with special or specific hazards, if dose is appropriate for body weight.

ADVERSE REACTIONS

Untoward reactions to Albumin (Human), 5% Solution, are extremely rare, although nausea, fever chills, or urticaria may occasionally occur. Such symptoms usually disappear when the infusion is slowed or stopped for a short period of time.

DOSAGE AND ADMINISTRATION

Albumin (Human), 5% Solution, must be administered INTRAVENOUSLY. It may be given without dilution, or it may be given in conjunction with, or combined with other parenteral solutions, such as whole blood, plasma, saline, glucose, or sodium lactate.

Hypovolemic Shock

Although the volume of administered 5% albumin and the rate of infusion must be individualized, the initial treatment of acute hypovolemia should be in the range of 500 to 750 mL of 5% albumin (25–37.5 g) for adults or 12 to 20 mL of 5% albumin per kilogram body weight (0.6–1.0 g/kg) for infants and children. The initial dose may be repeated after 15 to 30 minutes, if the response is not adequate.

Hypoproteinemia With or Without Edema

Hypoalbuminemia is usually accompanied by a hidden extravascular albumin deficiency of equal magnitude. This total body albumin deficit must be considered when determining the amount of albumin necessary to reverse the hypoproteinemia. When using the patient's serum albumin concentration to estimate albumin deficit, the body albumin space should be calculated to be 80–100 mL per kilogram body weight.[4,5,7] Daily doses should not exceed 2 g of albumin per kilogram body weight.

When the hypovolemia is long-standing and hypoalbuminemia exists in the presence of adequate hydration or edema, 25% albumin is usually preferable to 5% protein.[4]

Preparation for Administration

1. Remove cap from bottle to expose central portion of rubber stopper.
2. Clean stopper with germicidal solution.
3. Parenteral drug products should be inspected visually for particulate matter and discoloration prior to administration, whenever solution and container permit.

Administration

Follow directions for use printed on the administration set container. Make certain that the administration set contains an adequate filter.

HOW SUPPLIED

Albumin (Human), USP, 5% Solution.

10 bottles per case
250 ml vial w/IV set   NDC 52769-450-25
500 ml vial w/IV set   NDC 52769-450-50

STORAGE

Store Albumin (Human), 5% Solution, at room temperature, not to exceed 30℃ (86℉). Avoid freezing to prevent damage to the bottle. Do not use after expiration date.

REFERENCES

1. Cohn EJ, Strong LE, Hughes WL, *et al:* Preparation and properties of serum and plasma proteins. IV. A system for the separation into fractions of the protein and lipoprotein components of biological tissus and fluids. **J Am Chem Soc** 68:459–475, 1946.
2. Janeway CA: Human serum albumin: Historical review, in **Proceedings of the Workshop on Albumin.** Sgouris JT and René A (eds), Bethesda, MD, DHEW Publication NIH 76–1975, pp 3–21
3. Gerety RJ, Aronson DL: Plasma derivatives and viral hepatitis. **Transfusion** 22:347–351, 1982
4. Finlayson JS: Albumin products. **Sem Thromb Hemostasis** 6:85–120, 1980
5. Peters T Jr: Serum albumin, in **The Plasma Proteins, 2nd Edition, Vol 1.** Putnam FW (ed), New York, Academic Press, 1975, pp 133–181
6. Tullis JL: Albumin 1. Background and use. 2. Guidelines for clinical use. **JAMA** 237:355–360, 460–463, 1977.
7. O'Riordan JP, Aebischer M, Darnborough J, *et al:* The indications for the use of albumin, plasma protein solutions and plasma substitutes. Strasbourg (67006), France. **Council of Europe — Public Health Committee Report,** 1976 Programme. Coordinated Research in Blood Transfusion, 1978
8. Heyl JT, Gibson JG II, Janeway CA: Studies on the plasma proteins. V. The effect of concentrated solutions of human and bovine serum albumin of blood volume after acute blood loss in man. **J Clin Invest** 22:763–773, 1943
9. Shoemaker WC, Hauser CJ: Critique of crystalloid versus colloid therapy in shock and shock lung. **Crit Care Med** 7:117–124, 1979
10. Lowenstein E: Blood conservation in open heart surgery. **Cleve Clin Q** 48:112–125, 1981

Manufactured by:
Baxter Healthcare Corporation
Hyland Division
Glendale, CA 91203 USA
U.S. License No. 140
Distributed by:
American Red Cross
Blood Services
Washington, DC 20006 USA
Revised November 1990

ALBUMIN (HUMAN), USP   ℞
25% Solution

This product is derived from blood collected from volunteer donors by the American Red Cross Blood Services. The cost of processing, testing and packaging was paid by the Red Cross.

DESCRIPTION

Albumin (Human), 25% Solution, contains in each 100 mL, 25 g of albumin prepared from pooled human venous plasma. This product was prepared using the Cohn cold ethanol fractionation process.[1,2] It has been adjusted to physiological pH with sodium bicarbonate and/or sodium hydroxide and has been stabilized with 0.02M sodium caprylate and 0.02M sodium acetyltryptophanate. The solution contains 145 ± 15 mEq of sodium per liter. Albumin (Human), 25% Solution, contains no preservative and none of the coagulation factors of fresh whole blood or fresh plasma. The transparent or slightly opalescent solution may have a greenish tint or may be pale straw to amber in color.

In addition to sterilization by filtration, this product has been heated for 10 hours at 60℃ in the final container. This procedure has been shown to be an effective method of inactivating hepatitis viruses in 25% solutions of albumin even when prepared from plasma known to contain transmissible hepatitis virus.[3]

Albumin (Human), 25% Solution, **must** be administered intravenously.

CLINICAL PHARMACOLOGY

Albumin is a highly soluble, ellipsoidal protein (MW 66,500), accounting for 70 to 80% of the colloid osmotic pressure of plasma. It is, therefore, important in regulating the volume of circulating blood.[4–6] This solution supplies the oncotic equivalent of approximately five times its volume of human plasma. When injected intravenously, 25% albumin will draw approximately 3.5 times its volume of additional fluid into the circulation within 15 minutes, if the recipient is adequately hydrated.[2,7] This extra fluid reduces hemoconcentration and decreases blood viscosity. The degree and duration of volume expansion depend upon the initial blood volume. When treating patients with diminished blood volume, the effect of infused albumin may persist for many hours.

Albumin is also a transport protein and binds naturally occurring, therapeutic, and toxic materials in the circulation.[4,5]

Albumin is distributed throughout the extracellular water and more than 60% of the body albumin pool is located in the extravascular fluid compartment. The total body albumin in a 70 kg man is approximately 320 g; it has a circulating life span of 15 to 20 days, with a turnover of approximately 15 g per day.[5]

The minimum serum albumin level necessary to prevent or reverse peripheral edema is unknown. Although it undoubtedly varies from patient to patient, the range probably falls near 2.5 g per deciliter. This concentration provides a plasma oncotic pressure of 20 mm of mercury (the equivalent of a total protein concentration of 5.2 g/dL).[6]

INDICATIONS AND USAGE

1. Hypovolemia (with or without shock)

Hypovolemia is a possible indication for albumin administration. The effectiveness of 25% albumin in reversing hypovolemia depends largely upon its ability to draw interstitial fluid into the circulation. Thus, it will be maximally effective only if the patient is well hydrated.[2] Generally, except where signs of overhydration and/or edema are present, the treatment of acute blood volume deficit (shock) is best achieved by the administration of 5% plasma protein solution [5% Albumin (Human), 5% Plasma Protein Fraction (Human)][4–7] or, by using 25% albumin with crystalloid solutions in an albumin-to-crystalloid volume ratio of 1:3 or 1:4.

Although crystalloid solutions or colloid-containing plasma substitutes may be used in the emergency treatment of shock, Albumin (Human) has a longer intravascular half-life.[4,8]

When the hypovolemia is long-standing and hypoalbuminemia exists in the presence of adequate hydration or edema, 25% albumin is preferable to 5% protein solutions.[4,5]

When the blood volume deficit is the result of hemorrhage, replacement with compatible red blood cells or whole blood should be undertaken as quickly as is possible.

2. Hypoalbuminemia

A. General

Hypoalbuminemia is another possible indication for albumin administration. Hypoalbuminemia may result from one or more of the following.[5]

1) <u>Inadequate production</u> (malnutrition, burns, major injury, congenital analbuminemia, liver disease, infection, malignancy, endocrine disorders).

Continued on next page

American Red Cross—Cont.

2) <u>Excessive</u> <u>catabolism</u> (burns, major injury, pancreatitis, thyrotoxicosis, pemphigus, nephrosis).

3) <u>Loss</u> <u>from</u> <u>the</u> <u>body</u> (hemorrhage, excessive renal excretion, burn exudates, exudative enteropathy, exfoliative dermatoses).

4) <u>Redistribution</u> <u>within</u> <u>the</u> <u>body</u> (major surgery, cirrhosis with ascites, various inflammatory conditions).

In almost every instance, treatment of the underlying disorder and emphasis on increased nutritional replacement of amino acids and/or protein will be more likely to restore normal plasma albumin levels than will the transfusion of albumin-containing solutions.[4,6,7] Whenever hypoalbuminemia results from excessive protein loss, the effect of albumin administration will be temporary unless the underlying disorder is reversed.

There are occasional patients with hypoproteinemia accompanying major infections or injuries or severe pancreatitis for whom reversal of the disorder cannot be accomplished quickly. In these situations, supplementation of nutritional protein intake with amino acid infusions may fail to restore serum albumin to adequate levels, and 25% albumin may be a useful therapeutic adjuvant.

B. Burns

The optimal mix of crystalloid and colloid solutions which should be administered following extensive burns remains the subject of continuing discussion. During the initial 24 hours of therapy, large volumes of crystalloids are infused to restore the depleted extra-cellular fluid volume. Beyond 24 hours, albumin is generally used to replace the protein loss which accompanies any severe burn.[4,6,7]

C. Adult Respiratory Distress Syndrome (ARDS)

Several factors are usually involved in the development of ARDS.[4,6,9] One of these is a hypoproteinemic state which may be causally related to the interstitial pulmonary edema characteristic of ARDS. Although uncertainty exists concerning the precise indications for albumin infusion in ARDS, when evidence of fluid overload in the lungs is accompanied by hypoalbuminemia, the administration of 25% albumin together with a diuretic may be of therapeutic value.[6]

D. Cirrhosis

When repeated paracenteses are being performed for ascites and the fluid is not being reinfused, supplementary albumin infusion may be needed.[7]

E. Nephrosis

In patients with acute nephrosis who are receiving steroids and/or diuretics, success in treatment of edema may be enhanced by raising plasma oncotic pressure through the administration of the 25% albumin.[4,6]

3. Cardiopulmonary Bypass Surgery

The administration of 25% albumin prior to or during cardiopulmonary bypass surgery has been recommended although there are no clear data indicating its advantages over crystalloid solutions. Which is the most propitious time to infuse albumin is also unclear.[4,6,10]

4. Hemolytic Disease of the Newborn (HDN)

In view of its transport role, 25% albumin may be administered in an attempt to bind and detoxify unconjugated bilirubin circulating in infants with severe HDN, thereby lessening the risk of kernicterus.[4]

Circumstances in Which Albumin Administration Is Usually Not Indicated:

The internal redistribution of plasma albumin which accompanies major surgery only occasionally causes clinical evidence of hypovolemia or insufficient plasma oncotic pressure. Moreover, there is no evidence that this temporary redistribution adversely affects wound healing. Therefore, the administration of 25% albumin to such post-surgical patients is not usually indicated.

The sequestration of protein-rich fluid during the course of acute inflammatory conditions (peritonitis, pancreatitis, cellulitis) rarely causes significant morbidity due to hypovolemia and treatment with albumin is rarely indicated. Rarely does a valid reason exist for administering albumin to treat the stabilized hypoproteinemias accompanying chronic cirrhosis, chronic nephrosis, protein-losing enteropathy, malabsorption, or pancreatic insufficiency.[4,6,7] However, when a patient in this category has to cope with a superimposed acute stress (e.g., anesthesia, major infection, etc.) his hemodynamic state, oncotic deficit and fluid balance should be carefully assessed and appropriate measures taken, as indicated by the individual circumstances.[6]

There is no valid reason for the use of albumin as an intravenous nutrient.

CONTRAINDICATIONS

The history of an allergic reaction to albumin is a specific contraindication to the use of this product.

WARNINGS

This solution should be administered with great caution to patients with hypertension, cardiac disease, severe pulmonary infection, severe chronic anemia or, hypoalbuminemia

with peripheral edema. If patients with hypertension or mild congestive failure are to be infused with concentrated albumin, the 25% solution should be diluted with 5% or 10% glucose solution to reduce the albumin concentration to 10%. This dilute solution can be administered safely at the rate of 100 mL per hour. Patients should always be carefully monitored in order to guard against the possibility of circulatory overload.

DO NOT USE IF TURBID. DO NOT BEGIN ADMINISTRATION MORE THAN FOUR HOURS AFTER THE CONTAINER HAS BEEN ENTERED. DISCARD UNUSED PORTION.

PRECAUTIONS

a. General

The rise in blood pressure following 25% albumin infusion necessitates careful observation of the injured or postoperative patient in order to detect and treat severed blood vessels that may not have bled at the lower blood pressure. The increase in blood volume which follows the administration of 25% albumin may cause a significant fall in hemoglobin concentration and red blood cell transfusion may become appropriate.

Administer 25% albumin slowly (1 mL/min) to patients with normal blood volume.

b. Laboratory Test

Although laboratory testing is not necessary in order to monitor the treatment of shock or moderate hypoalbuminemia, when Albumin (Human), 25% Solution, is being administered for treatment of severe hypoproteinemia, periodic measurement of serum albumin levels is advisable.

c. Pregnancy — Category C

Animal reproduction studies have not been conducted with Albumin (Human), 25% Solution. It is not known if Albumin (Human), 25% Solution can cause fetal harm when given to a pregnant woman, or can affect reproductive capacity. Albumin (Human), 25% Solution, should be given to a pregnant woman only if clearly needed.

d. Pediatric Use

Safety of this product has been demonstrated in children. Use in children is not associated with special or specific hazards, if dose is appropriate for body weight.

ADVERSE REACTIONS

Untoward reactions to Albumin (Human), 25% Solution, are extremely rare, although nausea, fever, chills, or urticaria may occasionally occur. Such symptoms usually disappear when the infusion is slowed or stopped for a short period of time.

DOSAGE AND ADMINISTRATION

Albumin (Human), 25% Solution, must be administered INTRAVENOUSLY. It may be given without dilution, or it may be given in conjunction with, or combined with other parenteral solutions, such as whole blood, plasma, saline, glucose, or sodium lactate. The addition of one volume of albumin solution to four volumes of normal saline or 5% glucose gives a solution approximately isotonic and isosmotic with citrated plasma. Albumin solutions should not be mixed with protein hydrolysates or solutions containing alcohol.

1. Hypovolemic Shock

Although the volume of administered 25% albumin and the speed of infusion must be individualized, the initial treatment of acute hypovolemia should be in the range of 100 to 200 mL of 25% albumin (25 to 50 g) for adults or 2.5 to 5 mL of 25% albumin per kilogram body weight (0.6 to 1.2 g/kg) for children. The initial dose may be repeated after 10 to 30 minutes, if the response is not adequate. For patients with significant plasma volume deficits, albumin replacement is best administered in the form of 5% Albumin (Human).

2. Hypoproteinemia With or Without Edema

Hypoalbuminemia is usually accompanied by a hidden extravascular albumin deficiency of equal magnitude. This total body albumin deficit must be considered when determining the amount of albumin necessary to reverse the hypoproteinemia. When using the patient's serum albumin concentration to estimate albumin deficit, the body albumin space should be calculated to be 80 to 100 mL per kilogram body weight.[4,5,7] Daily doses should not exceed 2 g of albumin per kilogram body weight.

3. Hemolytic Disease of the Newborn

Albumin (Human), 25% Solution, may be administered to jaundiced infants prior to exchange transfusion in a dose of 1 g per kilogram body weight[11] and it may be administered during the procedure.[12]

Preparation for Administration

1. Remove cap from bottle to expose central portion of rubber stopper.
2. Clean stopper with germicidal solution.
3. Parenteral drug products should be inspected visually for particulate matter and discoloration prior to administration, whenever solution and container permit.

Administration

Follow directions for use printed on the administration set container. Make certain that the administration set contains an adequate filter.

HOW SUPPLIED

Albumin (Human), USP, 25% Solution.

10 bottles per case

50 ml vial w/IV set	NDC 52769-451-05
100 ml vial w/IV set	NDC 52769-451-10

STORAGE

Store Albumin (Human), 25% Solution, at room temperature, not to exceed 30°C (86°F). Avoid freezing to prevent damage to the bottle.

REFERENCES

1. Cohn EJ, Strong LE, Hughes WL, *et al:* Preparation and properties of serum and plasma proteins. IV. A system for the separation into fractions of the protein and lipoprotein components of biological tissues and fluids. **J Am Chem Soc 68**: 459–475, 1946
2. Janeway CA: Human serum albumin; Historical review, in **Proceedings of the Workshop on Albumin.** Sgouris JT and René A (eds), Bethesda, MD, DHEW Publication NIH 76-925, 1975, pp 3–21
3. Gellis SS, Neefe JR, Stokes J Jr *et al:* Chemical, clinical and immunological studies on the products of human plasma fractionation. XXXVI. Inactivation of the virus of homologous serum hepatitis in solutions of normal serum albumin by means of heat. **J Clin Invest 27**:239–244, 1948
4. Finlayson JS: Albumin products. **Sem Thromb Hemostas 6**:85–120, 1980
5. Peters T Jr: Serum albumin, in **The Plasma Proteins, 2nd Edition, Vol 1.** Putnam FW (ed), New York, Academic Press, 1975, pp 133–181
6. Tullis JL: Albumin 1. Background and use. 2. Guidelines for clinical use. **JAMA 237**:355–360, 460–463, 1977
7. Silver H: Normal serum albumin and plasma protein fraction in **Blood, Blood Components and Derivatives in Transfusion Therapy: A Technical Workshop.** Washington, DC, American Association of Blood Banks, 1980, pp 89–95
8. Heyl JT, Gibson JG II, Janeway CA: Studies on the plasma proteins. V. The effect of concentrated solutions of human and bovine serum albumin on blood volume after acute blood loss in man. **J Clin Invest 22**:763–773, 1943
9. Shoemaker WC, Hauser CJ: Critque of crystalloid versus colloid therapy in shock and shock lung. **Crit Care Med 7**:117–124, 1979
10. Lowenstein E: Blood conservation in open heart surgery. **Cleve Clin Q 48**:112–125, 1981
11. Wood B, Comley A, Sherwell J: Effect of additional albumin administration during exchange transfusion on plasma albumin-binding capacity. **Arch Dis Child 45**:59–62, 1970
12. Tsao YC, Yu VYH: Albumin in the management of neonatal hyperbilirubinemia. **Arch Dis Child 47**:250–256, 1972

Manufactured by:

Baxter Healthcare Corporation
Hyland Division
Glendale, CA 91203 USA
U.S. License No. 140

Distributed by:

American Red Cross
Blood Services
Washington, DC 20006 USA

4122   Revised November 1990

ANTIHEMOPHILIC FACTOR (HUMAN)   ℞
Method M
Monoclonal Purified

This product is derived from blood collected from volunteer donors by the American Red Cross Blood Services. The cost of processing, testing and packaging was paid by the American Red Cross Blood Services.

DESCRIPTION

Antihemophilic Factor (Human), Method M, is a sterile, nonpyrogenic, dried preparation of antihemophilic factor (Factor VIII, Factor VIII:C, AHF) in concentrated form with a specific activity range of 2 to 15 AHF International Units/mg of total protein. When reconstituted with the appropriate volume of diluent, it contains approximately 12.5 mg/mL Albumin (Human), 1.5 mg/mL polyethylene glycol (3350), 0.055 M histidine and 0.030 M glycine as stabilizing agents. In the absence of the added Albumin (Human), the specific activity is approximately 2,000 AHF International Units/mg of protein. It also contains trace amounts of mouse protein, less than 10 ng/100 AHF activity units. See **CLINICAL PHARMACOLOGY.**

Antihemophilic Factor (Human) is prepared by the Method M process from pooled human plasma by immunoaffinity chromatography utilizing a murine monoclonal antibody to Factor VIII:C, followed by an ion exchange chromatography step for further purification. Method M also includes an organic solvent [tri(n-butyl) phosphate] and detergent (Triton X-100) virus inactivation step designed to reduce the risk of transmission of hepatitis and other viral diseases. However, no procedure has been shown to be totally effective in removing viral infectivity from coagulation factor products.

Each bottle of Antihemophilic Factor (Human) is labeled with the AHF activity expressed in International Units per bottle, which is referenced to the WHO International Standard.

Antihemophilic Factor (Human) is to be administered only intravenously.

CLINICAL PHARMACOLOGY

Antihemophilic factor (AHF) is a protein found in normal plasma which is necessary for clot formation. The administration of Antihemophilic Factor (Human) provides an increase in plasma levels of AHF and can temporarily correct the coagulation defect of patients with hemophilia A (classical hemophilia). The administration of Antihemophilic Factor (Human), Method M, will also correct deficiencies caused by circulating inhibitors when the inhibitor level does not exceed 10 Bethesda Units per mL.

The half-life of Antihemophilic Factor (Human), Method M, administered to Factor VIII deficient patients has been shown to be 14.8 ± 3.0 hours.

Use of an organic solvent [tri(n-butyl) phosphate; TNBP] in the manufacture of Antihemophilic Factor (Human) has little or no effect on AHF activity, while lipid enveloped viruses, such as hepatitis B and human immunodeficiency virus (HIV) are inactivated.[1] Prince, et al, report inactivation of at least 10,000 Chimpanzee Infectious Doses (CID-50) of hepatitis B virus, 10,000 CID-50 of hepatitis non A, non B virus, and 30,000 Tissue Culture Infectious Doses of HIV with TNBP/detergent treatment during manufacture of an Antihemophilic Factor (Human) concentrate.[2]

The effectiveness of the Method M organic solvent/detergent inactivation step in reducing viral infectivity was assessed *in vitro* by using marker viruses. When known quantities of Sindbis virus, Vesicular Stomatitis virus, and Pseudorabies virus were added during manufacture, this step was shown to inactivate 3 to 4 logs of these viruses. The infectivity of HIV seeded into cryoprecipitate was reduced by greater than 4 logs almost instantaneously by the organic solvent/detergent step. In four other experiments, the concentration of both enveloped and non-enveloped viruses were decreased approximately 4 logs during the immunoaffinity chromatography step.

Antihemophilic Factor (Human), Method M, was administered to 11 patients previously untreated with Antihemophilic Factor (Human). They have shown no signs of hepatitis or HIV infection following 3 to 9 months of evaluation. An ongoing study of 25 patients treated with Method M and monitored for 3 to 6 months has demonstrated no evidence of antibody response to mouse protein. More than 1,000 infusions of Antihemophilic Factor (Human), Method M, have been administered during the clinical trials with no significant reactions. Reported events included a single episode each of chest tightness, fuzziness and dizziness and one patient reported an unusual taste after each infusion.

INDICATIONS AND USAGE

The use of Antihemophilic Factor (Human), Method M, is indicated in hemophilia A (classical hemophilia) for the prevention and control of hemorrhagic episodes.

Antihemophilic Factor (Human), Method M, can be of significant therapeutic value in patients with acquired Factor VIII inhibitors not exceeding 10 Bethesda Units per mL.[3] However, in such uses, the dosage should be controlled by frequent laboratory determinations of circulating AHF.

Antihemophilic Factor (Human), Method M, is not indicated in von Willebrand's disease.

CONTRAINDICATIONS

Known hypersensitivity to mouse protein is a contraindication to the use of Antihemophilic Factor (Human), Method M.

WARNINGS

This product is prepared from pooled human plasma which may contain the causative agents of hepatitis and other viral diseases. Prescribed manufacturing procedures utilized at the plasma collection centers, plasma testing laboratories, and the fractionation facilities are designed to reduce the risk of transmitting viral infection. However, the risk of viral infectivity from this product cannot be totally eliminated.

Individuals who receive infusions of blood or plasma products may develop signs and/or symptoms of some viral infections, particularly non A, non B hepatitis. As indicated under **CLINICAL PHARMACOLOGY**, however, a group of such patients treated with Antihemophilic Factor (Human)

did not demonstrate signs or symptoms of non A, non B hepatitis over observation periods ranging from 3 to 9 months.

PRECAUTIONS

General

Identification of the clotting defect as a Factor VIII deficiency is essential before the administration of Antihemophilic Factor (Human) is initiated. No benefit may be expected from this product in treating other deficiencies.

The processing of Antihemophilic Factor (Human), Method M, significantly reduces the presence of blood group specific antibodies in the final product. Nevertheless, when large or frequently repeated doses of product are needed, patients should be monitored by means of hematocrit and direct Coombs tests for signs of progressive anemia.

Formation of Antibodies to Mouse Protein—Although no hypersensitivity reactions have been observed, because Antihemophilic Factor (Human), Method M, contains trace amounts of mouse protein (less than 10 ng/100 AHF activity units), the possibility exists that patients treated with this product may develop hypersensitivity to the mouse proteins. The pulse rate should be determined before and during administration of Antihemophilic Factor (Human).

Should a significant increase occur, reducing the rate of administration or temporarily halting the injection usually allows the symptoms to disappear promptly.

Information for Patients

Patients should be informed of the early signs of hypersensitivity reactions including hives, generalized urticaria, tightness of the chest, wheezing, hypotension, and anaphylaxis, and should be advised to discontinue use of the product and contact their physician if these symptoms occur.

Laboratory Tests

Although dosage can be estimated by the calculations which follow, it is strongly recommended that whenever possible, appropriate laboratory tests be performed on the patient's plasma at suitable intervals to assure that adequate AHF levels have been reached and are maintained.

If the AHF content of the patient's plasma fails to reach expected levels or if bleeding is not controlled after apparently adequate dosage, the presence of inhibitor should be suspected. By appropriate laboratory procedures, the presence of inhibitor can be demonstrated and quantified in terms of AHF units neutralized by each mL of plasma or by the total estimated plasma volume. If the inhibitor is at low levels (i.e., <10 Bethesda Units/mL), after administration of sufficient AHF units to neutralize the inhibitor, additional AHF units will elicit the predicted response.

Pregnancy

Pregnancy Category C. Animal reproduction studies have not been conducted with Antihemophilic Factor (Human). It is not known whether Antihemophilic Factor (Human) can cause fetal harm when administered to pregnant woman or can affect reproduction capacity. Antihemophilic Factor (Human) should be given to a pregnant woman only if clearly needed.

ADVERSE REACTIONS

Allergic reactions may be encountered from the use of Antihemophilic Factor (Human) preparations. See **Information for Patients.**

The protein in greatest concentration in Antihemophilic Factor (Human), Method M, is Albumin (Human). Reactions associated with albumin are extremely rare, although nausea, fever, chills or urticaria have been reported.

DOSAGE AND ADMINISTRATION

Each bottle of Antihemophilic Factor (Human) is labeled with the AHF content expressed in International Units per bottle. This potency assignment is referenced to the World Health Organization International Standard.

The following formulas can be used to calculate the appropriate dose required for a given response (I) or the response to be expected from a given dose (II).

These dosage formulas are presented for reference and as guidelines. The amount of AHF that an individual hemophiliac requires for normal hemostasis varies with circumstances and with the patient. Exact dosage determinations should be based on the medical judgment of the physician regarding circumstances, condition of the patient, degree of Factor VIII deficiency and the level of AHF to be achieved.

I. Units required =
body weight (kg) × 0.4 units/kg × desired AHF increase (% of normal)
Example: 70 kg × 0.4 units/kg × 50 = 1,400 units

II. Expected AHF increase (% of normal) =

$$\frac{\text{units administered}}{\text{body weight (kg)} \times 0.4 \text{ units/kg}}$$

Example: $\dfrac{1{,}400 \text{ units}}{70 \text{ kg} \times 0.4 \text{ units/kg}} = 50\%$

The response factor used in the preceding formulas (0.4 units/kg) was based on the work of Shanbrom and Thelin with adults.[4] Abildgaard, et al, in work with boys 8 months to 14 years of age reported data from which a response factor of 0.5 units/kg can be calculated.[5]

A. Minor hemorrhagic episodes will generally subside with a single infusion if an AHF level of 30% or more is attained.

B. For more serious hemorrhages, an AHF level of 35 to 50% of normal should be obtained for optimum clot formation.

C. In surgery, the initial dose of Antihemophilic Factor (Human), calculated to achieve a level of 80 to 100% of normal, should be given an hour before the procedure. A second dose of Antihemophilic Factor (Human), half the size of the priming dose, should be given five hours after the priming dose. If several units of blood were lost during the operation, a third dose of Antihemophilic Factor (Human) should be given when the patient reaches the recovery room. The AHF level should be maintained at a daily minimum of at least 30% for a healing period of 10 to 14 days.[6]

Other dosage regimens have been proposed, such as that of Hilgartner,[7] which outlines dosage according to various types of bleeding episodes, and Schimpf, et al,[8] which describes continuous maintenance therapy.

Reconstitution: Use Aseptic Technique

1. Bring Antihemophilic Factor (Human), (dry concentrate) and Sterile Water for Injection, USP, (diluent) to room temperature.
2. Remove caps from concentrate and diluent bottles to expose central portion of rubber stoppers.
3. Cleanse stoppers with germicidal solution.
4. Remove protective covering from one end of double-ended needle and insert exposed needle through diluent stopper.
5. Remove protective covering from other end of double-ended needle. Invert diluent bottle over upright Antihemophilic Factor (Human) bottle, then rapidly insert free end of the needle through the Antihemophilic Factor (Human) bottle stopper at its center. The vacuum in the Antihemophilic Factor (Human) bottle will draw in the diluent.
6. Disconnect the two bottles by removing needle from diluent bottle stopper, then remove needle from Antihemophilic Factor (Human) bottle. Swirl gently until all material is dissolved. Be sure that Antihemophilic Factor (Human) is completely dissolved, otherwise active material will be removed by the filter.

Note: Do not refrigerate after reconstitution.

Administration: Use Aseptic Technique

Administer at room temperature.

Antihemophilic Factor (Human) should be administered not more than one hour after reconstitution.

Intravenous Syringe Injection

Parenteral drug products should be inspected for particulate matter and discoloration prior to administration, whenever solution and container permit.

Plastic syringes are recommended for use with this product. The ground glass surface of all-glass syringes tend to stick with solutions of this type.

1. Attach filter needle to a disposable syringe and draw back plunger to admit air into syringe.
2. Insert needle into reconstituted Antihemophilic Factor (Human).
3. Inject air into bottle and then withdraw the reconstituted material into the syringe.
4. Remove and discard the filter needle from the syringe; attach a suitable needle and inject intravenously as instructed under **Rate of Administration.**
5. If a patient is to receive more than one bottle of Antihemophilic Factor (Human), the contents of two bottles may be drawn into the same syringe by drawing up each bottle through a separate unused filter needle. This practice lessens the loss of Antihemophilic Factor (Human). Please note, filter needles are intended to filter the contents of a single bottle of Antihemophilic Factor (Human) only.

Rate of Administration

Preparations of Antihemophilic Factor (Human), Method M, can be administered at a rate of up to 10 mL per minute with no significant reactions.

The pulse rate should be determined before and during administration of Antihemophilic Factor (Human). Should a significant increase occur, reducing the rate of administration or temporarily halting the injection usually allows the symptoms to disappear promptly.

HOW SUPPLIED

Antihemophilic Factor (Human), Method M, is available as single dose bottles. Each bottle is labeled with the potency in International Units, and is packaged together with 10 mL of Sterile Water for Injection, USP, a double-ended needle, and a filter needle.

STORAGE

Antihemophilic Factor (Human), Method M, should be stored under refrigeration (2 to 8°C, 36 to 46°F). Avoid freezing to prevent damage to the diluent bottle.

Continued on next page

American Red Cross—Cont.

REFERENCES

1. Horowitz B, Wiebe ME, Lippin A, et al: Inactivation of viruses in labile blood derivatives: I. Disruption of lipid enveloped viruses by tri(n-butyl)phosphate detergent combinations. **Transfusion** 25:516–522, 1985
2. Prince AM, Horowitz B, Brotman B: Sterilisation of hepatitis and HTLV-III viruses by exposure to tri(n-butyl)-phosphate and sodium cholate. **Lancet** I:706–710, 1986
3. Brinkhous KM, Shanbrom E, Roberts HR, et al: A new high potency glycine-precipitated antihemophilic factor (AHF) concentrate: Treatment of classical hemophilia and hemophilia with inhibitors. **JAMA** 205:613–617, 1968
4. Shanbrom E, Thelin GM: Experimental prophylaxis of severe hemophilia with a Factor VIII concentrate. **JAMA** 208:1853–1856, 1969
5. Abildgaard CF, Simone JV, Corrigan JJ, et al: Treatment of hemophilia with glycine-precipitated Factor VIII. **New Eng J Med** 275:471–475, 1966
6. Kasper CK: Hematologic care, in **Comprehensive Management of Hemophilia**. Boone DC (ed), Philadelphia, F.A. Davis Co., 1976, pp 3–17
7. Hilgartner MW: Factor replacement therapy, in **Hemophilia in the Child and Adult**. Hilgartner MW (ed), New York, Masson Publishing USA, Inc. 1982, pp 63–84
8. Schimpf K, Rothmann P, Zimmermann K: Factor VIII dosis in prophylaxis of hemophilia A; A further controlled study, in **Proc XIth Cong W.F.H.** Kyoto, Japan, Academic Press, 1976, pp 363–366

Manufactured by:
Baxter Healthcare Corporation
Hyland Division
Glendale, CA 91203 USA
U.S. License No. 140
Distributed by:
American Red Cross
Blood Services
Washington, DC 20006 USA
4136
Revised November 1990

PLASMA PROTEIN FRACTION (HUMAN), ℞
USP, 5% SOLUTION

This product is derived from blood collected from volunteer donors by the American Red Cross Blood Services. The cost of processing, testing and packaging was paid by the Red Cross.

DESCRIPTION

Plasma Protein Fraction (Human) is a sterile, nonpyrogenic 5% solution of protein which has been prepared from human venous plasma using the Cohn cold ethanol fractionation method. It has been adjusted to physiological pH by the addition of sodium bicarbonate and/or sodium hydroxide and has been stabilized with 0.004 M sodium acetyltryptophanate and 0.004 M sodium caprylate. The plasma proteins consist of: albumin, not less than 83%; alpha and beta globulins, less than 17%; gamma globulin, less than 1%. Plasma Protein Fraction (Human) contains no preservative nor does it contain any of the coagulation factors of fresh whole blood or plasma. The sodium content of this product is 145 ± 15 mEq/L and the potassium content is not greater than 2 mEq/L. Plasma Protein Fraction (Human) is a transparent or slightly opalescent solution which may vary from pale straw to amber in color.

The method of processing removes isoagglutinins and other antibodies which allows the administration of Plasma Protein Fraction (Human) without regard to the recipient's blood group. Plasma Protein Fraction (Human) is supplied in single dose bottles and must be administered intravenously. This product has been heated for 10 hours at 60℃. This procedure has been shown to be an effective method of inactivating hepatitis virus in albumin solutions even when those solutions were prepared from plasma known to contain transmissible hepatitis virus.[1]

CLINICAL PHARMACOLOGY

The protein in Plasma Protein Fraction (Human) is primarily albumin, which is useful in regulating and increasing circulating blood volume. Administration of Plasma Protein Fraction (Human) will increase blood volume by an amount equal to the volume infused and some of this expansion will last up to 48 hours.[2]

Total body albumin is estimated to be 350 g for a 70 kg man and is distributed throughout the extracellular fluid, with more than 60% located within the extravascular compartment. The half life of albumin is 15 to 20 days and an estimated 5% of this albumin is exchanged between the vascular and extravascular compartments each hour.[3]

The minimum plasma albumin level necessary to prevent or reverse peripheral edema is not known. Some investigators recommend that plasma albumin levels be maintained at approximately 2.5 g/dL. This concentration provides a plasma oncotic pressure value of 20 mm Hg.[4]

INDICATIONS AND USAGE

Plasma Protein Fraction (Human) is indicated for the restoration of circulating blood volume when the infusion rate need not exceed 10 mL/min.

1. Hypovolemia (with or without shock)

Hypovolemia is a possible indication for the use of Plasma Protein Fraction (Human). Although crystalloid solutions or colloid-containing plasma substitutes can be used in emergency treatment of shock, albumin-containing solutions have a prolonged intravascular half-life.[3]

When blood volume deficit is the result of hemorrhage, compatible red blood cells or whole blood should be administered as quickly as possible.

2. Hypoalbuminemia

Hypoalbuminemia is another possible indication for the use of Plasma Protein Fraction (Human).[5]

When albumin deficit is the result of excessive protein loss, the effect of administration of albumin will be temporary unless the underlying disorder is reversed. In most cases, increased nutritional replacement of amino acids and/or protein with concurrent treatment of the underlying disorder will restore normal plasma albumin levels more effectively than administration of albumin solutions. Occasionally, hypoalbuminemia accompanying severe injuries or infections or severe pancreatitis cannot be quickly reversed and nutritional supplements may fail to restore adequate plasma albumin levels. In these cases, Plasma Protein Fraction (Human) may be a useful therapeutic adjuvant.

The internal redistribution of plasma albumin which accompanies major surgery only occasionally causes clinical evidence of hypovolemia or insufficient plasma oncotic pressure. Moreover, there is no evidence that this temporary redistribution adversely affects wound healing. Therefore, the administration of albumin-containing solutions to such post-surgical patients is not usually indicated.

The sequestration of protein-rich fluid during the course of acute inflammatory conditions (peritonitis, pancreatitis, cellulitis) rarely causes significant morbidity due to hypovolemia, and treatment with albumin-containing solutions is rarely indicated.

Rarely does a valid reason exist for administering albumin to treat the stabilized hypoproteinemias accompanying chronic cirrhosis, chronic nephrosis, protein-losing enteropathy, malabsorption, or pancreatic insufficiency.[4,7] However, when a patient in this category has to cope with a superimposed acute stress (e.g., anesthesia, major infection, etc.) his hemodynamic state, oncotic deficit and fluid balance should be carefully assessed and appropriate measures taken, as indicated by the individual circumstances.[4] **There is no valid reason for the use of albumin as an intravenous nutrient.**

3. Burns

The optimal mix of crystalloid and colloid solutions which should be administered following extensive burns has not been definitively elucidated.

In conjunction with appropriate crystalloid therapy, Plasma Protein Fraction (Human) may be useful for treatment of protein deficits after the initial 24 hour period following extensive burns.

CONTRAINDICATIONS

A history of allergic reactions to albumin or to plasma-containing blood products is a specific contraindication to the use of this product.[6]

Plasma Protein Fraction (Human) is contraindicated for use in patients undergoing cardiopulmonary bypass surgery, in severely anemic patients and in patients with cardiac failure.[7]

WARNINGS

This solution should be administered with great caution to patients with hypertension, cardiac disease, severe pulmonary infection, or severe chronic anemia. For treatment of patients with hypoalbuminemia accompanied by peripheral edema, 25% albumin solution should be used.

Patients should always be carefully monitored to guard against the possibility of circulatory overload.

DO NOT USE IF TURBID. DO NOT BEGIN ADMINISTRATION MORE THAN 4 HOURS AFTER THE CONTAINER HAS BEEN ENTERED. Discard partially used bottles.

PRECAUTIONS

The rate of administration should be controlled since infusion faster than 10 mL per minute may result in hypotension.

Blood pressure should be monitored during administration and the infusion should be stopped or slowed if hypotension develops.

When Plasma Protein Fraction (Human) is used following injuries or surgery, the quick rise in blood pressure which follows administration makes it necessary to observe the patient to detect and treat severed blood vessels that may not have bled at a lower blood pressure.

The increase in blood volume which follows the administration of Plasma Protein Fraction (Human) may cause a significant fall in hemoglobin concentration and red blood cell transfusion may become appropriate.

Pregnancy—Category C

Animal reproduction studies have not been conducted with Plasma Protein Fraction (Human). It is not known whether Plasma Protein Fraction (Human) can cause fetal harm when administered to a pregnant woman or can affect reproductive capacity. Plasma Protein Fraction (Human) should be given to a pregnant woman only if clearly needed.

Pediatric Use

The use of Plasma Protein Fraction (Human) in children has not been associated with any special or specific hazards, if the dose is appropriate for the child's body weight.

ADVERSE REACTIONS

Instances of abrupt drop in blood pressure have been observed during rapid administration.[7,8] This symptom may disappear when the infusion is slowed or stopped; however, in some instances vasopressors have been required to restore blood pressure.

The incidence of adverse reactions of Plasma Protein Fraction (Human) is low, although nausea, chills, fever or headache may occur occasionally.[2]

DOSAGE AND ADMINISTRATION

Plasma Protein Fraction (Human) must be administered intravenously. It may be given without dilution, or it may be given in conjunction with or combined with other parenterals such as whole blood, plasma, saline, glucose or sodium lactate. The volume of the total dose and the rate of infusion depend on the patient's condition and response.

Recommended Dosages

1. Hypovolemia

Although the volume of Plasma Protein Fraction (Human) administered must be individualized, the initial dose should be 250 to 500 mL for adults and 12 to 20 mL per kilogram of body weight for infants and children. It may be repeated after 15 to 30 minutes if the response is not adequate.

2. Hypoalbuminemia

Hypoalbuminemia is usually accompanied by a hidden extravascular albumin deficiency of equal magnitude. This total body albumin deficit must be considered when determining the amount of albumin necessary to reverse the hypoalbuminemia. When using the patient's serum albumin concentration to estimate the deficit, the body albumin compartment should be calculated to be 80 to 100 mL per kilogram of body weight.[5,7] Daily doses should not exceed 2 g of albumin per kilogram of body weight.

3. Burns

When Plasma Protein Fraction (Human) is administered after the first 24 hours following burns, the dose should be determined according to the patient's condition and response to treatment.

Preparation for Administration

Parenteral drug products should be inspected visually for particulate matter and discoloration prior to administration, whenever solution and container permit.

1. Remove cap from bottle to expose center portion of rubber stopper.
2. Clean stopper with germicidal solution.
3. Follow directions for use printed on the administration set container.

Make sure that the administration set used contains an adequate filter.

Rate of Administration

The rate of administration should be carefully controlled since infusion rates exceeding 10 mL per minute may result in hypotension.

HOW SUPPLIED

Plasma Protein Fraction (Human), USP, 5% Solution.

10 bottles per case	
250 ml vial w/IV set	NDC 52769-430-25
500 ml vial w/IV set	NDC 52769-430-50

STORAGE

Store Plasma Protein Fraction (Human) at room temperature, not to exceed 30℃ (86°F). Exposure to higher temperatures may cause the formation of particulate matter in the solution. Avoid freezing to prevent damage to the bottle.

REFERENCES

1. Gellis SS, Neefe JR, Stokes J Jr, et al: Chemical, clinical and immunological studies on the products of human plasma fractionation. XXXVI. Inactivation of the virus of homologous serum hepatitis in solutions of normal serum albumin by means of heat. **J Clin Invest** 27:239-244, 1948
2. Bertrand JJ, Feichtmeir TV, Kolomeyer N, et al: Clinical investigations with a heat-treated plasma protein fraction—Plasmanate®. **Vox Sang** 4:384-402, 1959
3. Heyl JT, Gibson JG, Janeway CA, et al: Studies on the plasma proteins. V. The effect of concentrated solutions of

human and bovine serum albumin on blood volume after acute blood loss in man. **J Clin Invest** 22:763-773, 1943

4. Tullis JL: Albumin 1. Background and use. 2. Guidelines for clinical use. **JAMA** 237:355-360, 460-463, 1977

5. Peters T Jr: Serum albumin. In **The Plasma Proteins, 2nd ed.** Putnam FW (ed). New York, Academic Press, vol. 1, pp 133-181, 1975

6. Ring J, Messmer K: Incidence and severity of anaphylactoid reactions to colloid volume substitutes. **Lancet** 1:466-469, 1977

7. Finlayson JS: Albumin Products. **Sem Thromb Hemostas** 6:85-120, 1980

8. Bland JHL, Chir B, Laver MB, *et al:* Vasodilator effect of commercial 5% plasma protein fraction solutions. **JAMA** 224:1721-1724, 1973

Manufactured by:
Baxter Healthcare Corporation
Hyland Division
Glendale, CA 91203 USA
U.S. License No. 140
Distributed by:
American Red Cross
Blood Services
Washington, DC 20006 USA
4124   Revised November 1990

POLYGAM®   ℞
IMMUNE GLOBULIN INTRAVENOUS (HUMAN)

IMMUNE GLOBULIN INTRAVENOUS (HUMAN), POLYGAM®

This product is derived from blood collected from volunteer donors by the American Red Cross Blood Services. The cost of processing, testing, and packaging was paid by the American Red Cross Blood Services.

DESCRIPTION
Immune Globulin Intravenous (Human), Polygam® is a sterile, dried, highly purified preparation of immunoglobulin G (IgG), which is derived from the cold ethanol fractionation process and is further purified using ultrafiltration and ion exchange adsorption. When reconstituted with the appropriate volume of diluent, this preparation contains approximately 50 mg of protein per mL, of which at least 90% is gamma globulin. The reconstituted product contains approximately 0.15 M sodium chloride and has a pH of 6.8 ± 0.4. Stabilizing agents are present in the following maximum amounts: 20 mg/mL glucose, 2 mg/mL polyethylene glycol (PEG), 0.3 M glycine, and 3 mg/mL Albumin (Human). The manufacturing process for Immune Globulin Intravenous (Human), Polygam® isolates IgG without additional chemical or enzymatic modification, and the Fc portion is maintained intact. Immune Globulin Intravenous (Human), Polygam® contains all of the IgG antibody activities which are present in the donor population. On the average, the distribution of IgG subclasses present in this product is the same as is present in normal plasma.[1] Immune Globulin Intravenous (Human), Polygam® contains only trace amounts of IgM and IgA.
Immune Globin Intravenous (Human), Polygam® contains no preservative.
This product has been prepared from large pools of human plasma from which donors found to have elevated alanine aminotransferase (ALT) levels were excluded.

CLINICAL PHARMACOLOGY
Immune Globulin Intravenous (Human), Polygam® contains a broad spectrum of IgG antibodies against bacterial and viral agents that are capable of opsonization and neutralization of microbes and toxins.
Peak levels of IgG are reached immediately after infusion of Immune Globulin Intravenous (Human), Polygam®. It has been shown that IgG is distributed relatively rapidly between plasma and extravascular fluid until approximately half of the total body pool is partitioned in the extravascular space. A rapid initial drop in serum levels is, therefore, to be expected.[2]
As a class, IgG survives longer *in vivo* than other serum proteins.[2,3] Studies show that the half-life of Immune Globulin Intravenous (Human), Polygam® is approximately 24 days. These findings are consistent with reports of a 21-25 day half-life for IgG.[2,3,4] The half-life of IgG can vary considerably from person to person, however. In particular, high concentrations of IgG and hypermetabolism associated with fever and infection have been seen to coincide with a shortened half-life of IgG.[2,3,4,5]

INDICATIONS AND USAGE
Immunodeficiencies
Primary
Immune Globulin Intravenous (Human), Polygam® is indicated for the treatment of primary immunodeficient states such as: congenital agammaglobulinemias, common variable immunodeficiency, Wiskott-Aldrich syndrome, and severe combined immunodeficiencies.[4,5] Immune Globulin Intrave-

nous (Human), Polygam® is especially useful when high levels or rapid elevation of circulating IgG is desired or when intramuscular injections are contraindicated (e.g., small muscle mass).

B-cell Chronic Lympocytic Leukemia
Immune Globulin Intravenous (Human) (IGIV), Polygam® is indicated for prevention of bacterial infections in patients with hypogammaglobulinemia and/or recurrent bacterial infections associated with B-cell Chronic Lymphocytic Leukemia (CLL). In a study of 81 patients, 41 of whom were treated with Immune Globulin Intravenous (Human), Polygam®, bacterial infections were significantly reduced in the treatment group.[6,7] In this study, the placebo group had approximately twice as many bacterial infections as the IGIV group. The median time to first bacterial infection for the IGIV group was greater than 365 days. By contrast, the time to first bacterial infection in the placebo group was 192 days. The number of viral and fungal infections, which were for the most part minor, was not statistically different between the two groups.

Idiopathic Thrombocytopenic Purpura (ITP)
When rapid rise in platelet count is needed to control bleeding or to allow a patient with ITP to undergo surgery, the administration of Immune Globulin Intravenous (Human), Polygam® should be considered. The efficacy of Immune Globulin Intravenous (Human), Polygam® has been demonstrated in a clinical study involving sixteen patients (twelve adults and four children) diagnosed with acute or chronic Idiopathic Thrombocytopenic Purpura (ITP). Each of the sixteen patients (100%) demonstrated an acute, clinically significant rise in platelet count (platelet count greater than 40,000/mm^3) following the administration of Immune Globulin Intravenous (Human), Polygam®.
Ten of the sixteen patients (62%) exhibited a clinically significant rise in platelet count after only one 1g/kg infusion; four patients (25%) exhibited this result after only two 1g/kg infusions; and two patients exhibited this result after more than two 1 g/kg infusions. The rise in platelet count is generally rapid, occurring within 5 days. The rise, however, is transient and should not be considered curative. Platelet rises most often lasted 2 to 3 weeks, with a range of 12 days to 6 months. **It should be noted that childhood ITP may resolve spontaneously without treatment.**

CONTRAINDICATIONS
None known.

WARNINGS
Immune Globulin Intravenous (Human), Polygam® should only be administered intravenously. Other routes of administration have not been evaluated.
Immune Globulin Intravenous (Human), Polygam® contains very low levels of IgA (not more than 10 μg/mL), nonetheless, it should be given with caution to patients with antibodies to IgA or selective IgA deficiencies.[5,8]

PRECAUTIONS
Drug Interactions
Admixtures of Immune Globulin Intravenous (Human), Polygam® with other drugs have not been evaluated. It is recommended that Immune Globulin Intravenous (Human), Polygam® be administered separately from other drugs or medication which the patient may be receiving.
Pregnancy Category C
Animal reproduction studies have not been conducted with Immune Globulin Intravenous (Human), Polygam®. It is also not known whether Immune Globulin Intravenous (Human), Polygam® can cause fetal harm when administered to a pregnant woman or can affect reproduction capacity. Immune Globulin Intravenous (Human), Polygam® should be given to a pregnant woman only if clearly needed.

ADVERSE REACTIONS
In general, adverse reactions to Immune Globulin Intravenous (Human) (IGIV), Polygam® in patients with congenital or acquired immunodeficiencies are similar in kind and frequency. The incidence of untoward reactions in these patients is low, although various minor reactions such as headache, fatigue, chills, backache, leg cramps, lightheadedness, fever, urticaria, flushing, slight elevation of blood pressure, nausea, and vomiting may occasionally occur. The incidence of these reactions directly attributable to the infusion of Immune Globulin Intravenous (Human), Polygam® during the clinical trials of primary immunodeficiencies was about 6%. In the study of patients with B-cell Chronic Lymphocytic Leukemia (CLL), the incidence was about 3%. Slowing or stopping the infusion usually allows the symptoms to disappear promptly.
During the clinical study of this product for treatment of Idiopathic Thrombocytopenic Purpura (ITP), the only side effect reported was headache, which occurred in 12 of 16 patients. Oral antihistamines and analgesics alleviated the headache and were used as pretreatment for those patients requiring additional IGIV therapy. The remaining four patients did not report any side effects and did not require pretreatment.

Immediate anaphylactic and hypersensitivity reactions are a remote possibility. Epinephrine should be available for treatment of any acute anaphylactoid reaction. (See WARNINGS.)

DOSAGE AND ADMINISTRATION
Immunodeficiencies
For patients with primary immunodeficiencies, monthly doses of at least 100 mg/kg are recommended. Initially, patients may receive 200–400 mg/kg. As there are significant differences in the half-life of IgG among patients with primary immunodeficiencies, the frequency and amount of immunoglobulin therapy may vary from patient to patient. The proper amount can be determined by monitoring clinical response. The minimum serum concentration of IgG necessary for protection has not been established.
For patients with hypogammaglobulinemia and/or recurrent bacterial infections due to B-cell Chronic Lymphocytic Leukemia (CLL), a dose of 400 mg/kg every three to four weeks is recommended.
Idiopathic Thrombocytopenic Purpura (ITP)
For patients with acute or chronic Idiopathic Thrombocytopenic Purpura (ITP), a dose of 1 g/kg is recommended. The need for additional doses can be determined by clinical response and platelet count. Up to three doses may be given on alternate days if required.
Rate of Administration
It is recommended that initially a rate of 0.5 mL/kg/Hr be used. If infusion at this rate causes the patient no distress, the administration rate may be gradually increased but should not exceed 4 mL/kg/Hr.
A rate of administration which is too rapid may cause flushing and changes in pulse rate and blood pressure. Slowing or stopping the infusion usually allows the symptoms to disappear promptly.

ADMINISTRATION
Immune Globulin Intravenous (Human), Polygam® should be administered as soon after reconstitution as possible. Administration should begin not more than 2 hours after reconstitution.
The reconstituted material should be at room temperature during administration.
Parenteral drug products should be inspected visually for particulate matter and discoloration prior to administration, whenever solution and container permit.
Follow directions for use printed on the administration set container. Make sure the administration set contains an adequate filter.

STORAGE
Immune Globulin Intravenous (Human), Polygam® is to be stored at a temperature not to exceed 25°C (77°F). Freezing should be avoided to prevent the diluent bottle from breaking.

0.5 g SIZE RECONSTITUTION
Use Aseptic Technic
1. NOTE: RECONSTITUTE IMMEDIATELY BEFORE USE.
2. If refrigerated, warm the Sterile Water for Injection, USP (diluent) and Immune Globulin Intravenous (Human), Polygam® (dried concentrate) to room temperature.
3. Remove caps from concentrate and diluent bottles to expose central portion of rubber stoppers.
4. Cleanse stoppers with germicidal solution.
5. Remove protective covering from one end of double-ended needle and insert exposed needle through diluent stopper.
6. Remove protective covering from the other end of double-ended needle. Invert diluent bottle over upright concentrate bottle, then rapidly insert free end of the needle through the concentrate bottle stopper at its center. The vacuum in the concentrate bottle will draw in the diluent.
7. When diluent transfer is complete, remove empty diluent bottle from needle and then needle from concentrate bottle. Discard needle after single use.
8. Thoroughly wet dried material by tilting or inverting and gently rotating the bottle. DO NOT SHAKE. AVOID FOAMING.
9. Repeat gentle rotation as long as undissolved product is observed.

HOW SUPPLIED
Immune Globulin Intravenous (Human), Polygam® is supplied in 0.5 g single use bottles.

Ten vials per case
0.5 g with reconstitution kit   NDC 52769-470-70

Each bottle of Immune Globulin Intravenous (Human), Polygam® is furnished with a suitable volume of Sterile Water for Injection, USP, a double-ended needle and a filter spike.

2.5 g, 5.0 g, AND 10.0 g SIZES RECONSTITUTION
Use Aseptic Technic
1. NOTE: RECONSTITUTE IMMEDIATELY BEFORE USE.

Continued on next page

American Red Cross—Cont.

2. If refrigerated, warm the Sterile Water for Injection, USP (diluent) and Immune Globulin Intravenous (Human), Polygam® (dried concentrate) to room temperature.
3. Remove caps from concentrate and diluent bottles to expose central portion of rubber stoppers.
4. Cleanse stoppers with germicidal solution.
5. Remove protective covering from the spike at one end of the transfer device (Fig. 1).
6. Place the diluent bottle on a flat surface and, while holding the bottle to prevent slipping, insert the spike of the transfer device perpendicularly through the center of the bottle stopper. Press down firmly so that the transfer device fits snugly against the diluent bottle (Fig. 2). A slight twist at the end of the downward push helps ensure a snug fit.

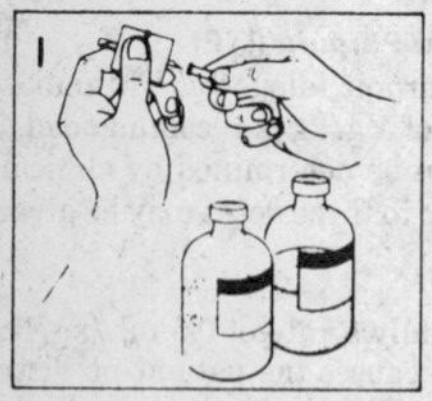

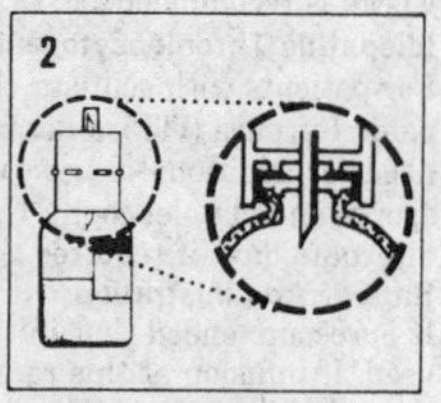

7. Remove the protective covering from the other end of the transfer device. Hold diluent bottle to prevent slipping. Invert concentrate bottle and press firmly onto the transfer device until the concentrate bottle fits snugly against the transfer device.
8. Invert bottle/transfer device assembly (Fig. 3). Diluent will flow into the concentrate bottle. When diluent transfer is complete, remove empty diluent bottle and transfer device from concentrate bottle. Discard transfer device after single use.
9. Thoroughly wet the dried material by tilting or inverting and gently rotating the bottle (Fig. 4). DO NOT SHAKE. AVOID FOAMING.
10. Repeat gentle rotation as long as undissolved product is observed.

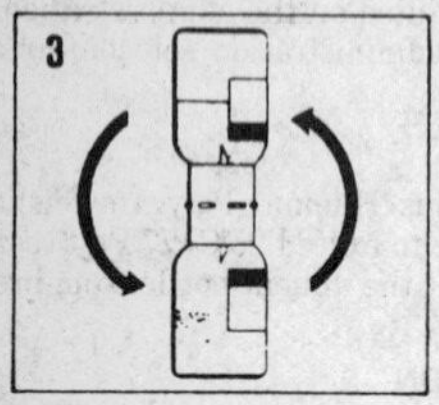

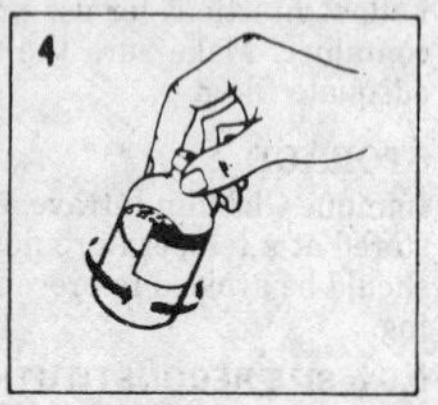

HOW SUPPLIED

Immune Globulin Intravenous (Human), Polygam® is supplied in either 2.5 g, 5.0 g or 10.0 g single use bottles.

Ten vials per case	
5.0 g with reconstitution kit	NDC 52769-470-72
2.5 g with reconstitution kit	NDS 52769-470-75
10.0 g with reconstitution kit	NDC 52769-470-80

Each bottle of Immune Globulin Intravenous (Human), Polygam® is furnished with a suitable volume of Sterile Water for Injection, USP, a transfer device and an administration set which contains an integral airway and a 15 micron filter.

REFERENCES

1. Unpublished data in the files of Baxter Healthcare Corporation
2. Waldman TA, Storber W: Metabolism of immunoglobulins. **Prog Allergy 13**:1–110, 1969
3. Morrell A, Riesen W: Structure, function and catabolism of immunoglobulins in **Immunohemotherapy.** Nydegger UE (ed), London, Academic Press, 1981, pp 17–26
4. Stiehm ER: Standard and special human immune serum globulins as therapeutic agents. **Pediatrics 63**:301–319, 1979
5. Buckley RH: Immunoglobulin replacement therapy: Indications and contraindications for use and variable IgG levels achieved in **Immunoglobulins: Characteristics and Use of Intravenous Preparations.** Alving BM, Finlayson JS (eds), Washington, DC, U.S. Department of Health and Human Services, 1979, pp 3–8
6. Bunch C, Chapel HM, Rai K, *et al:* Intravenous Immune Globulin reduces bacterial infections in Chronic Lymphocytic Leukemia: A controlled, randomized clinical trial. **Blood 70 Suppl 1**:753, 1987
7. Cooperative Group for The Study of Immunoglobulin in Chronic Lymphocytic Leukemia: Intravenous immunoglobulin for the prevention of infection in Chronic Lymphocytic Leukemia: A randomized, controlled clinical trial. **N Eng J Med 314**:902–907, 1988
8. Burks AW, Sampson HA, Buckley RH: Anaphylactic reactions after gammaglobulin administration in patients with hypogammaglobulinemia: Detection of IgE antibodies to IgA. **N Eng J Med 314**:560–564, 1986

BIBLIOGRAPHY

Bussel JB, Kimberly RP, Inman RD, *et al:* Intravenous gammaglobulin treatment of chronic idiopathic thrombocytopenic purpura. **Blood 62**:480–486, 1983

Manufactured by: Baxter Healthcare Corporation
Hyland Division
Glendale, CA 91203 USA
U.S. License No. 140
Distributed by: American Red Cross
Blood Services
Washington, DC 20006 USA
4111 Revised November 1990

Amgen
AMGEN INC.
AMGEN CENTER
THOUSAND OAKS, CA 91320-1789

EPOGEN® ℞
[*'é-pōjen*]
EPOETIN ALFA
For Injection

DESCRIPTION

Erythropoietin is a glycoprotein which stimulates red blood cell production. It is produced in the kidney and stimulates the division and differentiation of committed erythroid progenitors in the bone marrow. EPOGEN® (Epoetin alfa) is the Amgen Inc. trademark for Epoetin alfa which has been selected as the proper name for recombinant human erythropoietin. EPOGEN®, a 165 amino acid glycoprotein manufactured by recombinant DNA technology, has the same biological effects as endogenous erythropoietin.[1] It has a molecular weight of 30,400 daltons and is produced by mammalian cells into which the human erythropoietin gene has been introduced. The product contains the identical amino acid sequence of isolated natural erythropoietin.

EPOGEN® is formulated as a sterile, colorless, preservative-free liquid for intravenous or subcutaneous administration. Each single-use vial contains 2,000, 3,000, 4,000, or 10,000 units of Epoetin alfa formulated in an isotonic sodium chloride/sodium citrate buffered solution (pH 6.9 $\pm$ 0.3) containing Albumin (Human) (2.5 mg), sodium citrate (5.8 mg), sodium chloride (5.8 mg), citric acid (0.06 mg) in Water for Injection, USP.

CLINICAL PHARMACOLOGY

Chronic Renal Failure Patients: Erythropoietin is a glycoprotein which stimulates red blood cell production. Endogenous production of erythropoietin is normally regulated by the level of tissue oxygenation. Hypoxia and anemia generally increase the production of erythropoietin, which in turn stimulates erythropoiesis.[2] In normal subjects, plasma erythropoietin levels range from 0.01 to 0.03 U/mL,[2,3] and increase up to 100- to 1000-fold during hypoxia or anemia.[2,3] In contrast, in patients with chronic renal failure (CRF), production of erythropoietin is impaired, and this erythropoietin deficiency is the primary cause of their anemia.[3,4] Chronic renal failure is the clinical situation in which there is a progressive and usually irreversible decline in kidney function. Such patients may manifest the sequelae of renal dysfunction, including anemia, but do not necessarily require regular dialysis. Patients with end-stage renal disease (ESRD) are those patients with CRF who require regular dialysis or kidney transplantation for survival.

EPOGEN® has been shown to stimulate erythropoiesis in anemic patients with CRF, including both patients on dialysis and those who do not require regular dialysis.[4–13] The first evidence of a response to the three times weekly (T.I.W.) administration of EPOGEN® is an increase in the reticulocyte count within 10 days, followed by increases in the red cell count, hemoglobin, and hematocrit, usually within 2–6 weeks.[4,5] Because of the length of time required for erythropoiesis—several days for erythroid progenitors to mature and be released into the circulation—a clinically significant increase in hematocrit is usually not observed in less than 2 weeks and may require up to 6 weeks in some patients. Once the hematocrit reaches the target range (30–33%), that level can be sustained by EPOGEN® therapy in the absence of iron deficiency and concurrent illnesses.

The rate of hematocrit increase varies between patients and is dependent upon the dose of EPOGEN®, within a therapeutic range of approximately 50–300 U/kg T.I.W.[4]; a greater biologic response is not observed at doses exceeding 300 U/kg T.I.W.[6] Other factors affecting the rate and extent of response include availability of iron stores, the baseline hematocrit, and the presence of concurrent medical problems.

AZT-Treated HIV-Infected Patients: Responsiveness to EPOGEN® in HIV-infected patients is dependent upon the endogenous serum erythropoietin level prior to treatment. Patients with endogenous serum erythropoietin levels $\leq$500 mU/mL, and who are receiving a dose of AZT $\leq$4200 mg/week, may respond to EPOGEN® therapy. Patients with endogenous serum erythropoietin levels >500 mU/mL do not appear to respond to EPOGEN® therapy. In a series of four clinical trials involving 255 patients, sixty to eighty percent of HIV-infected patients treated with Zidovudine (AZT) had endogenous serum erythropoietin levels $\leq$500 mU/mL.

Response to EPOGEN® in AZT-treated HIV-infected patients is manifested by reduced transfusion requirements and increased hematocrit.

Pharmacokinetics: Intravenously administered EPOGEN® is eliminated at a rate consistent with first order kinetics with a circulating half-life ranging from approximately 4 to 13 hours in patients with CRF. Within the therapeutic dose range, detectable levels of plasma erythropoietin are maintained for at least 24 hours.[7] After subcutaneous administration of EPOGEN® to patients with CRF, peak serum levels are achieved within 5–24 hours after administration and decline slowly thereafter. There is no apparent difference in half-life between patients not on dialysis whose serum creatinine levels were greater than 3, and patients maintained on dialysis.

In normal volunteers, the half-life of intravenously administered EPOGEN® is approximately 20% shorter than the half-life in CRF patients. The pharmacokinetics of EPOGEN® have not been studied in HIV-infected patients.

INDICATIONS AND USAGE

Treatment of Anemia of Chronic Renal Failure Patients: EPOGEN® is indicated in the treatment of anemia associated with chronic renal failure, including patients on dialysis (end-stage renal disease) and patients not on dialysis. EPOGEN® is indicated to elevate or maintain the red blood cell level (as manifested by the hematocrit or hemoglobin determinations) and to decrease the need for transfusions in these patients.

EPOGEN® is not intended for patients who require immediate correction of severe anemia. EPOGEN® may obviate the need for maintenance transfusions but is not a substitute for emergency transfusion.

Prior to initiation of therapy, the patient's iron stores, including transferrin saturation and serum ferritin, should be evaluated. Transferrin saturation should be at least 20% and ferritin at least 100 ng/mL. Blood pressure should be adequately controlled prior to initiation of EPOGEN® therapy, and must be closely monitored and controlled during therapy. Non-dialysis patients with symptomatic anemia considered for therapy should have a hematocrit less than 30%. All patients on EPOGEN® therapy should be regularly monitored (see "Laboratory Monitoring" and "Precautions").

EPOGEN® should be administered under the guidance of a qualified physician (see "Dosage and Administration").

Treatment of Anemia in AZT-Treated HIV-Infected Patients: EPOGEN® is indicated for the treatment of anemia related to therapy with Zidovudine (AZT) in HIV-infected patients. EPOGEN® is indicated to elevate or maintain the red blood cell level (as manifested by the hematocrit or hemoglobin determinations) and to decrease the need for transfusions in these patients. EPOGEN® is not indicated for the treatment of anemia in HIV-infected patients due to other factors such as iron or folate deficiencies, hemolysis or gastrointestinal bleeding, which should be managed appropriately.

EPOGEN®, at a dose of 100 U/kg three times per week, is effective in decreasing the transfusion requirement and increasing the red blood cell level of anemic, HIV-infected patients treated with AZT, when the endogenous serum erythropoietin level is $\leq$500 mU/mL and when patients are receiving a dose of AZT $\leq$4200 mg/week.

Clinical Experience: Response to EPOGEN®

Chronic Renal Failure Patients: Response to EPOGEN® was consistent across all studies. In the presence of adequate iron stores (see "Pre-Therapy Iron Evaluation"), the time to reach the target hematocrit is a function of the baseline hematocrit and the rate of hematocrit rise.

The rate of increase in hematocrit is dependent upon the dose of EPOGEN® administered and individual patient variation. In clinical trials at starting doses of 50–150 U/kg T.I.W., patients responded with an average rate of hematocrit rise of:

Starting Dose (T.I.W. IV)	HEMATOCRIT INCREASE Hematocrit Points/Day	Hematocrit Points/2 Weeks
50 U/kg	0.11	1.5
100 U/kg	0.18	2.5
150 U/kg	0.25	3.5

Over this dose range, approximately 95% of all patients responded with a clinically significant increase in hematocrit,

and by the end of approximately two months of therapy virtually all patients were transfusion-independent. Once the target hematocrit was achieved, the maintenance dose was individualized for each patient.

Patients on Dialysis: Thirteen clinical studies were conducted, involving intravenous administration to a total of 1010 anemic patients on dialysis for 986 patient-years of EPOGEN® therapy. In the three largest of these clinical trials, the median maintenance dose necessary to maintain the hematocrit between 30–36% was approximately 75 U/kg (T.I.W.). In the U.S. multicenter Phase III study, approximately 65% of the patients required doses of 100 U/kg T.I.W., or less, to maintain their hematocrit at approximately 35%. Almost 10% of patients required a dose of 25 U/kg, or less, and approximately 10% required a dose of more than 200 U/kg T.I.W. to maintain their hematocrit at this level.

Patients with CRF Not Requiring Dialysis: Four clinical trials were conducted in patients with CRF not on dialysis involving 181 EPOGEN®-treated patients for approximately 67 patient-years of experience. These patients responded to EPOGEN® therapy in a manner similar to that observed in patients on dialysis. Patients with CRF not on dialysis demonstrated a dose-dependent and sustained increase in hematocrit when EPOGEN® was administered by either an intravenous (IV) or subcutaneous (SC) route, with similar rates of rise of hematocrit when EPOGEN® was administered by either route. Moreover, EPOGEN® doses of 75–150 U/kg per week have been shown to maintain hematocrits of 36–38% for up to six months.

Clinical Experience in AZT-Treated HIV-Infected Patients:
EPOGEN® has been studied in four placebo-controlled trials enrolling 297 anemic (hematocrit <30%) HIV-infected (AIDS) patients receiving concomitant therapy with Zidovudine (AZT), (all patients were treated with Epoetin alfa manufactured by Amgen Inc.). In the subgroup of patients (89/125 EPOGEN®, and 88/130 placebo) with prestudy endogenous serum erythropoietin levels ≤500 mU/mL (normal endogenous serum erythropoietin levels are 4–26 mU/mL), EPOGEN® reduced the mean cumulative number of units of blood transfused per patient by approximately 40%, as compared to the placebo group.[14] Among those patients who required transfusions at baseline, 43% of EPOGEN®-treated patients versus 18% of placebo-treated patients were transfusion-independent during the second and third months of therapy. EPOGEN® therapy also resulted in significant increases in hematocrit in comparison to placebo. When examining the results according to the weekly dose of AZT received during Month 3 of therapy, there was a statistically significant (p <0.003) reduction in transfusion requirements in EPOGEN®-treated patients (N=51) compared to placebo-treated patients (N=54) whose mean weekly AZT dose was ≤4200 mg/week.[14] Approximately 17% of the patients with endogenous serum erythropoietin levels ≤500 mU/mL receiving EPOGEN® in doses from 100–200 U/kg three times weekly (T.I.W.) achieved a hematocrit of 38% unrelated to transfusions or to a significant reduction in AZT dose. In the subgroup of patients whose prestudy endogenous serum erythropoietin levels were >500 mU/mL, EPOGEN® therapy did not reduce transfusion requirements or increase hematocrit compared to the corresponding responses in placebo-treated patients.

Responsiveness to EPOGEN® therapy may be blunted by intercurrent infectious/inflammatory episodes and by an increase in AZT dosage. Consequently, the dose of EPOGEN® must be titrated based on these factors to maintain the desired erythropoietic response.

CONTRAINDICATIONS

EPOGEN® is contraindicated in patients with:
1) Uncontrolled hypertension
2) Known hypersensitivity to mammalian cell-derived products
3) Known hypersensitivity to Albumin (Human).

WARNINGS

Chronic Renal Failure Patients

Hypertension: Patients with uncontrolled hypertension should not be treated with EPOGEN®; blood pressure should be controlled adequately before initiation of therapy. Blood pressure may rise during EPOGEN® therapy, often during the early phase of treatment when the hematocrit is increasing.

For patients who respond to EPOGEN® with a rapid increase in hematocrit (e.g., more than 4 points in any two-week period), the dose of EPOGEN® should be reduced because of the possible association of excessive rate of rise of hematocrit with an exacerbation of hypertension.

Seizures: Seizures have occurred in patients with CRF participating in EPOGEN® clinical trials.

In patients on dialysis, there was a higher incidence of seizures during the first 90 days of therapy (occurring in approximately 2.5% of patients), as compared with later timepoints.

Given the potential for an increased risk of seizures during the first 90 days of therapy, blood pressure and the presence of premonitory neurologic symptoms should be monitored closely. Patients should be cautioned to avoid potentially hazardous activities such as driving or operating heavy machinery during this period.

Thrombotic Events: During hemodialysis, patients treated with EPOGEN® may require increased anticoagulation with heparin to prevent clotting of the artificial kidney. Clotting of the vascular access (A-V shunt) has occurred at an annualized rate of about 0.25 events per patient-year on EPOGEN® therapy.

Overall, for patients with CRF (whether on dialysis or not), other thrombotic events (e.g., myocardial infarction, cerebrovascular accident, transient ischemic attack) have occurred at an annualized rate of less than 0.04 events per patient-year of EPOGEN® therapy. Patients with pre-existing vascular disease should be monitored closely.

AZT-Treated HIV-Infected Patients: In contrast to CRF patients, EPOGEN® therapy has not been linked to exacerbation of hypertension, seizures, and thrombotic events in HIV-infected patients.

PRECAUTIONS

Chronic Renal Failure Patients and AZT-Treated HIV-Infected Patients

General: The parenteral administration of any biologic product should be attended by appropriate precautions in case allergic or other untoward reactions occur (see "Contraindications"). While transient rashes have occasionally been observed concurrently with EPOGEN® therapy, no serious allergic or anaphylactic reactions have been reported.

The safety and efficacy of EPOGEN® therapy have not been established in patients with a known history of a seizure disorder or underlying hematologic disease (e.g., sickle cell anemia, myelodysplastic syndromes, or hypercoagulable disorders).

In some female patients, menses have resumed following EPOGEN® therapy; the possibility of potential pregnancy should be discussed and the need for contraception evaluated.

Hematology: Exacerbation of porphyria has been observed rarely in EPOGEN®-treated patients with CRF. However, EPOGEN® has not caused increased urinary excretion of porphyrin metabolites in normal volunteers, even in the presence of a rapid erythropoietic response. Nevertheless, EPOGEN® should be used with caution in patients with known porphyria.

In pre-clinical studies in dogs and rats, but not in monkeys, EPOGEN® therapy was associated with subclinical bone marrow fibrosis. Bone marrow fibrosis is a known complication of CRF in humans and may be related to secondary hyperparathyroidism or unknown factors. The incidence of bone marrow fibrosis was not increased in a study of patients on dialysis who were treated with EPOGEN® for 12–19 months, compared to the incidence of bone marrow fibrosis in a matched group of patients who had not been treated with EPOGEN®.

Hematocrit in CRF patients should be measured twice a week; AZT-treated HIV-infected patients should have hematocrit measured once a week until hematocrit has been stabilized, and measured periodically thereafter.

Delayed or Diminished Response: If the patient fails to respond or to maintain a response, the following etiologies should be considered and evaluated:
1) Iron deficiency: functional iron deficiency may develop with normal ferritin levels but low transferrin saturation (less than 20%), presumably due to the inability to mobilize iron stores rapidly enough to support increased erythropoiesis. Virtually all patients will eventually require supplemental iron therapy.
2) Underlying infectious, inflammatory, or malignant processes.
3) Occult blood loss.
4) Underlying hematologic diseases (i.e., thalassemia, refractory anemia, or other myelodysplastic disorders).
5) Vitamin deficiencies: folic acid or vitamin B12.
6) Hemolysis.
7) Aluminum intoxication.
8) Osteitis fibrosa cystica.

Iron Evaluation: Prior to and during EPOGEN® therapy, the patient's iron stores, including transferrin saturation (serum iron divided by iron binding capacity) and serum ferritin, should be evaluated. Transferrin saturation should be at least 20%, and ferritin should be at least 100 ng/mL. Supplemental iron may be required to increase and maintain transferrin saturation to levels that will adequately support EPOGEN®-stimulated erythropoiesis.

Drug Interaction: No evidence of interaction of EPOGEN® with other drugs was observed in the course of clinical trials.

Carcinogenesis, Mutagenesis, and Impairment of Fertility: Carcinogenic potential of EPOGEN® has not been evaluated. EPOGEN® does not induce bacterial gene mutation (Ames Test), chromosomal aberrations in mammalian cells, micronuclei in mice, or gene mutation at the HGPRT locus. In male and female rats treated intravenously with EPOGEN®, there was a trend for slightly increased fetal wastage at doses of 100 and 500 U/kg.

Pregnancy Category C: EPOGEN® has been shown to have adverse effects in rats when given in doses five times the human dose. There are no adequate and well-controlled studies in pregnant women. EPOGEN® should be used during pregnancy only if potential benefit justifies the potential risk to the fetus.

In studies in female rats, there were decreases in body weight gain, delays in appearance of abdominal hair, delayed eyelid opening, delayed ossification, and decreases in the number of caudal vertebrae in the F1 fetuses of the 500 U/kg group. In female rats treated intravenously, there was a trend for slightly increased fetal wastage at doses of 100 and 500 U/kg. EPOGEN® has not shown any adverse effect at doses as high as 500 U/kg in pregnant rabbits (from day 6 to 18 of gestation).

Nursing Mothers: Postnatal observations of the live offspring (F1 generation) of female rats treated with EPOGEN® during gestation and lactation revealed no effect of EPOGEN® at doses of up to 500 U/kg. There were, however, decreases in body weight gain, delays in appearance of abdominal hair, eyelid opening, and decreases in the number of caudal vertebrae in the F1 fetuses of the 500 U/kg group. There were no EPOGEN®-related effects on the F2 generation fetuses.

It is not known whether EPOGEN® is excreted in human milk. Because many drugs are excreted in human milk, caution should be exercised when EPOGEN® is administered to a nursing woman.

Pediatric Use: The safety and effectiveness of EPOGEN® in children have not been established.

Chronic Renal Failure Patients

Patients with CRF Not Requiring Dialysis: Blood pressure and hematocrit should be monitored no less frequently than for patients maintained on dialysis. Renal function and fluid and electrolyte balance should be closely monitored, as an improved sense of well-being may obscure the need to initiate dialysis in some patients.

Hematology: In order to avoid reaching the target hematocrit too rapidly, or exceeding the target range (hematocrit of 30–33%), the guidelines for dose and frequency of dose adjustments (see "Dosage and Administration") should be followed.

For patients who respond to EPOGEN® with a rapid increase in hematocrit (e.g., more than 4 points in any two-week period), the dose of EPOGEN® should be reduced because of the possible association of excessive rate of rise of hematocrit with an exacerbation of hypertension.

The elevated bleeding time characteristic of CRF decreases toward normal after correction of anemia in EPOGEN®-treated patients. Reduction of bleeding time also occurs after correction of anemia by transfusion.

Sufficient time should be allowed to determine a patient's responsiveness to a dosage of EPOGEN® before adjusting the dose. Because of the time required for erythropoiesis and the red cell half-life, an interval of 2–6 weeks may occur between the time of a dose adjustment (initiation, increase, decrease, or discontinuation) and a significant change in hematocrit.

Laboratory Monitoring: The hematocrit should be determined twice a week until it has stabilized in the target range and the maintenance dose has been established. After any dose adjustment, the hematocrit should also be determined twice weekly for at least 2–6 weeks until it has been determined that the hematocrit has stabilized in response to the dose change. The hematocrit should then be monitored at regular intervals.

A complete blood count with differential and platelet count should be performed regularly. During clinical trials, modest increases were seen in platelets and white blood cell counts. While these changes were statistically significant, they were not clinically significant and the values remained within normal ranges.

In patients with CRF, serum chemistry values [including blood urea nitrogen (BUN), uric acid, creatinine, phosphorus, and potassium] should be monitored regularly. During clinical trials in patients on dialysis, modest increases were seen in BUN, creatinine, phosphorus, and potassium. In some patients with CRF not on dialysis, treated with EPOGEN®, modest increases in serum uric acid and phosphorus were observed. While changes were statistically significant, the values remained within the ranges normally seen in patients with CRF.

Hypertension: Patients with uncontrolled hypertension should not be treated with EPOGEN®; blood pressure should be controlled adequately before initiation of therapy. Blood pressure may rise and episodes of hypertension may increase during EPOGEN® therapy in all CRF patients, whether or not they require dialysis, often during the early phase of treatment when the hematocrit is increasing. To prevent hypertension and its sequelae, particular care needs to be taken in patients treated with EPOGEN® to monitor and aggressively control blood pressure. During the period when hematocrit is increasing, approximately 25% of pa-

Continued on next page

Amgen—Cont.

tients on dialysis may require initiation of, or increases in, antihypertensive therapy. Patients should be advised as to the importance of compliance with antihypertensive therapy and dietary restrictions. For patients who respond to EPOGEN® with a rapid increase in hematocrit (e.g., more than 4 points in any two-week period), the dose of EPOGEN® should be reduced because of the possible association of excessive rate of rise of hematocrit with an exacerbation of hypertension. If blood pressure is difficult to control, the dose of EPOGEN® should be reduced; if clinically indicated, EPOGEN® may be withheld until blood pressure control is re-established.

Seizures: Seizures have occurred in patients with CRF participating in EPOGEN® clinical trials. In patients on dialysis, there was a higher incidence of seizures during the first 90 days of therapy (occurring in approximately 2.5% of patients), as compared with later timepoints.

Given the potential for an increased risk of seizures during the first 90 days of therapy, blood pressure and the presence of premonitory neurologic symptoms should be monitored closely. Patients should be cautioned to avoid potentially hazardous activities such as driving or operating heavy machinery during this period.

Thrombotic Events: During hemodialysis, patients treated with EPOGEN® may require increased anticoagulation with heparin to prevent clotting of the artificial kidney. Clotting of the vascular access has occurred at an annualized rate of about 0.25 events per patient-year on EPOGEN® therapy.

A relationship has not been established with statistical certainty between a rise in hematocrit and the rate of thrombotic events [including thrombosis of vascular access (A-V shunt)] in EPOGEN®-treated patients. Overall, for patients with CRF (whether on dialysis or not), other thrombotic events (e.g., myocardial infarction, cerebrovascular accident, transient ischemic attack) have occurred at an annualized rate of less than 0.04 events per patient-year of EPOGEN® therapy. Patients with pre-existing vascular disease should be monitored closely.

Diet: As the hematocrit increases and patients experience an improved sense of well-being and quality of life, the importance of compliance with dietary and dialysis prescriptions should be reinforced. In particular, hyperkalemia is not uncommon in patients with CRF. In U.S. studies in patients on dialysis, hyperkalemia has occurred at an annualized rate of approximately 0.11 episodes per patient-year of EPOGEN® therapy, often in association with poor compliance to medication, dietary and/or dialysis prescriptions.

Dialysis Management: Therapy with EPOGEN® results in an increase in hematocrit and a decrease in plasma volume which could affect dialysis efficiency. In studies to date, the resulting increase in hematocrit did not appear to adversely affect dialyzer function[9,10] or the efficiency of high-flux hemodialysis.[11] During hemodialysis, patients treated with EPOGEN® may require increased anticoagulation with heparin to prevent clotting of the artificial kidney.

Patients who are marginally dialyzed may require adjustments in their dialysis prescription. As with all patients on dialysis, the serum chemistry values [including blood urea nitrogen (BUN), creatinine, phosphorus, and potassium] in EPOGEN®-treated patients should be monitored regularly to assure the adequacy of the dialysis prescription.

Renal Function: In patients with CRF not on dialysis, renal function and fluid and electrolyte balance should be closely monitored, as an improved sense of well-being may obscure the need to initiate dialysis in some patients. In patients with CRF not on dialysis, placebo-controlled studies of progression of renal dysfunction over periods of greater than one year have not been completed. In shorter-term trials in patients with CRF not on dialysis, changes in creatinine and creatinine clearance were not significantly different in EPOGEN®-treated patients, compared with placebo-treated patients. Analysis of the slope of 1/serum creatinine vs. time plots in these patients indicates no significant change in the slope after the initiation of EPOGEN® therapy.

AZT-Treated HIV-Infected Patients

Hypertension: Exacerbation of hypertension has not been observed in AZT-treated HIV-infected patients treated with EPOGEN®. However, EPOGEN® should be withheld in these patients if pre-existing hypertension is uncontrolled, and should not be started until blood pressure is controlled. In double-blind studies, a single seizure has been experienced by an EPOGEN®-treated patient.[14]

ADVERSE REACTIONS

Chronic Renal Failure Patients

Studies analyzed to date indicate that EPOGEN® is generally well tolerated. The adverse events reported are frequent sequelae of CRF and are not necessarily attributable to EPOGEN® therapy. In double-blind, placebo-controlled studies involving over 300 patients with CRF, the events reported in greater than 5% of EPOGEN®-treated patients during the blinded phase were:

Event	Percent of Patients Reporting Event: EPOGEN®-Treated Patients (n=200)	Placebo-Treated Patients (n=135)
Hypertension	24%	19%
Headache	16%	12%
Arthralgias	11%	6%
Nausea	11%	9%
Edema	9%	10%
Fatigue	9%	14%
Diarrhea	9%	6%
Vomiting	8%	5%
Chest Pain	7%	9%
Skin Reaction (Administration Site)	7%	12%
Asthenia	7%	12%
Dizziness	7%	13%
Clotted Access	7%	2%

Significant adverse events of concern in patients with CRF treated in double-blinded, placebo-controlled trials occurred in the following percent of patients during the blinded phase of the studies:

Seizure	1.1%	1.1%
CVA/TIA	0.4%	0.6%
MI	0.4%	1.1%
Death	0	1.7%

In the U.S. EPOGEN® studies in patients on dialysis (over 567 patients) the incidence (number of events per patient-year) of the most frequently reported adverse events were: hypertension (0.75), headache (0.40), tachycardia (0.31), nausea/vomiting (0.26), clotted vascular access (0.25), shortness of breath (0.14), hyperkalemia (0.11), and diarrhea (0.11). Other reported events occurred at a rate of less than 0.10 events per patient per year.

Events reported to have occurred within several hours of administration of EPOGEN® were rare, mild and transient, and included flu-like symptoms such as arthralgias and myalgias.

In all studies analyzed to date, EPOGEN® administration was generally well tolerated, irrespective of the route of administration.

Allergic Reactions: There have been no reports of serious allergic reactions or anaphylaxis associated with EPOGEN® administration. Skin rashes and urticaria have been observed rarely and when reported have been mild and transient in nature. There has been no evidence for development of antibodies to erythropoietin in patients tested to date, including those receiving intravenous EPOGEN® for over two years. Nevertheless, if an anaphylactoid reaction occurs, EPOGEN® should be immediately discontinued and appropriate therapy initiated.

Seizures: The relationship, if any, of EPOGEN® therapy to seizures is uncertain. The baseline incidence of seizures in the untreated dialysis population is difficult to determine; it appears to be in the range of 5–10% per patient-year.[15–17] There have been 47 seizures in 1010 patients on dialysis, treated with EPOGEN® with an exposure of 986 patient-years for a rate of approximately 0.048 events per patient-year. However, there appeared to be a higher rate of seizures during the first 90 days of therapy (occurring in approximately 2.5% of patients), when compared to subsequent 90-day time periods. While the relationship between seizures and the rate of rise of hematocrit is uncertain, it is recommended that the dose of EPOGEN® be decreased if the hematocrit increase exceeds 4 points in any two-week period.

Hypertension: Up to 80% of patients with CRF have a history of hypertension.[18] Blood pressure may rise during EPOGEN® therapy in CRF patients whether or not maintained on dialysis; during the early phase of treatment when hematocrit is increasing, approximately 25% of patients on dialysis may require initiation or increases in antihypertensive therapy. Hypertensive encephalopathy and seizures have been observed in patients with CRF treated with EPOGEN®. Increases in blood pressure may be associated with the rate of increase in hematocrit. It is recommended that the dose of EPOGEN® be decreased if the hematocrit increase exceeds 4 points in any two-week period.

Increases in blood pressure have been reported in clinical trials, often during the first 90 days of therapy. When data from all patients in the U.S. Phase III multicenter trial were analyzed, there was an apparent trend of more reports of hypertensive adverse events in patients on dialysis with a faster rate of rise of hematocrit (greater than 4 hematocrit points in any two-week period). However, in a double-blind, placebo-controlled trial, hypertensive adverse events were not reported at an increased rate in the EPOGEN®-treated group (150 U/kg T.I.W.) relative to the placebo group. There do not appear to be any direct pressor effects of EPOGEN®. Special care should be taken to closely monitor and control blood pressure in EPOGEN®-treated patients.

Thrombotic Events: During hemodialysis, patients treated with EPOGEN® may require increased anticoagulation with heparin to prevent clotting of the artificial kidney. Clotting of the vascular access has occurred at an annualized rate of about 0.25 events per patient-year on EPOGEN® therapy.

A relationship has not been established with statistical certainty between a rise in hematocrit and the rate of thrombotic events [including thrombosis of vascular access (A-V shunt)] in EPOGEN®-treated patients. Overall, for patients with CRF (whether on dialysis or not), other thrombotic events (e.g., myocardial infarction, cerebrovascular accident, transient ischemic attack) have occurred at an annualized rate of less than 0.04 events per patient-year of EPOGEN® therapy. Patients with pre-existing vascular disease should be monitored closely.

AZT-Treated HIV-Infected Patients

Adverse events reported in clinical trials with EPOGEN® in AZT-treated HIV-infected patients were consistent with the progression of HIV infection. In double-blind, placebo-controlled studies of 3-months duration involving approximately 300 AZT-treated HIV-infected patients, adverse events with an incidence of ≥10% in either EPOGEN®-treated patients or placebo-treated patients were:

Event	Percent of Patients Reporting Event: EPOGEN®-Treated Patients (n=144)	Placebo-Treated Patients (n=153)
Pyrexia	38%	29%
Fatigue	25%	31%
Headache	19%	14%
Cough	18%	14%
Diarrhea	16%	18%
Rash	16%	8%
Congestion, Respiratory	15%	10%
Nausea	15%	12%
Shortness of Breath	14%	13%
Asthenia	11%	14%
Skin Reaction, Medication Site	10%	7%
Dizziness	9%	10%

There were no statistically significant differences between treatment groups in the incidence of the above events.

In the 297 patients studied, EPOGEN® was not associated with significant increases in opportunistic infections or mortality.[14] In 71 patients from this group treated with EPOGEN® at 150 U/kg T.I.W., serum p24 antigen levels did not appear to increase.[14] Preliminary data showed no enhancement of HIV replication in infected cell lines in vitro.[14]

Peripheral white blood cell and platelet counts are unchanged following EPOGEN® therapy.

Allergic Reactions: Two AZT-treated HIV-infected patients had urticarial reactions within 48 hours of their first exposure to study medication. One patient was treated with EPOGEN® and one was treated with placebo (EPOGEN® vehicle alone). Both patients had positive immediate skin tests against their study medication with a negative saline control. The basis for this apparent pre-existing hypersensitivity to components of the EPOGEN® formulation is unknown, but may be related to HIV-induced immunosuppression or prior exposure to blood products.

Seizures: In double-blind and open-label trials of EPOGEN® in AZT-treated HIV-infected patients, ten patients have experienced seizures.[14] In general, these seizures appear to be related to underlying pathology such as meningitis or cerebral neoplasms, not EPOGEN® therapy.

OVERDOSAGE

The maximum amount of EPOGEN® that can be safely administered in single or multiple doses has not been determined. Doses of up to 1500 U/kg T.I.W. for three to four weeks have been administered without any direct toxic effects of EPOGEN® itself.[6]

Therapy with EPOGEN® can result in polycythemia if the hematocrit is not carefully monitored and the dose appropriately adjusted. If the target range is exceeded, EPOGEN® may be temporarily withheld until the hematocrit returns to the target range; EPOGEN® therapy may then be resumed using a lower dose (see "Dosage and Administration"). If polycythemia is of concern, phlebotomy may be indicated to decrease the hematocrit.

DOSAGE AND ADMINISTRATION

Chronic Renal Failure Patients

Starting doses of EPOGEN® over the range of 50–100 U/kg three times weekly (T.I.W.) have been shown to be safe and effective in increasing hematocrit and eliminating transfusion dependency in patients with CRF (see "Clinical Experience"). The dose of EPOGEN® should be reduced when the hematocrit reaches the target range of 30–33% or increases by more than 4 points in any two-week period. The dosage of EPOGEN® must be individualized to maintain the hemato-

crit within the target range. Dose changes should generally be in the range of 25 U/kg, T.I.W. The table below provides general therapeutic guidelines.

Starting Dose:	50–100 U/kg T.I.W.; IV: Dialysis Patients IV or SC: Non-Dialysis CRF Patients
Reduce Dose When:	1) Target range is reached, or 2) Hematocrit increases > 4 points in any 2-week period
Increase Dose if:	Hematocrit does not increase by 5–6 points after 8 weeks of therapy, and hematocrit is below target range
Maintenance Dose:	Individually titrate
Target Hematocrit Range:	30–33% (max. 36%)

In patients on dialysis, EPOGEN® usually has been administered as an IV bolus T.I.W. While the administration of EPOGEN® is independent of the dialysis procedure, EPOGEN® may be administered into the venous line at the end of the dialysis procedure to obviate the need for additional venous access. In patients with CRF not on dialysis, EPOGEN® may be given either as an intravenous or subcutaneous injection.

During therapy, hematological parameters should be monitored regularly (see "Laboratory Monitoring").

Pre-Therapy Iron Evaluation: Prior to and during EPOGEN® therapy, the patient's iron stores, including transferrin saturation (serum iron divided by iron binding capacity) and serum ferritin, should be evaluated. Transferrin saturation should be at least 20%, and ferritin should be at least 100 ng/mL. Supplemental iron may be required to increase and maintain transferrin saturation to levels that will adequately support EPOGEN®-stimulated erythropoiesis.

Dose Adjustment:
- When the hematocrit reaches 30–33%, the dosage should be decreased by approximately 25 U/kg T.I.W., to avoid exceeding the target range. Once the hematocrit is within the target range, the maintenance dose must be individualized for each patient (see "Maintenance Dose").
- At any time, if the hematocrit increases by more than 4 points in a two-week period, the dose should be immediately decreased. After the dose reduction, the hematocrit should be monitored twice weekly for 2–6 weeks, and further dose adjustments should be made as outlined in "Maintenance Dose."
- As the hematocrit approaches, or if it exceeds 36%, EPOGEN® should be temporarily withheld until the hematocrit decreases to the target range of 30–33%; the dose should be reduced by approximately 25 U/kg T.I.W. upon re-initiation of therapy.
- If a hematocrit increase of 5–6 points is not achieved after an eight-week period and iron stores are adequate (see "Delayed or Diminished Response"), the dose of EPOGEN® may be increased in increments of 25 U/kg T.I.W. Further increases of 25 U/kg T.I.W. may be made at 4- to 6-week intervals until the desired response is attained.

Maintenance Dose: The maintenance dose must be individualized for each patient. As the hematocrit approaches, or if it exceeds, 36%, EPOGEN® should be temporarily withheld until the hematocrit is 33% or less. Upon re-initiation of therapy, the dose should be reduced by approximately 25 U/kg T.I.W., or doses omitted, and an appropriate time interval (i.e., 2–6 weeks) allowed for stabilization of response. If the hematocrit remains below, or falls below, the target range, iron stores should be re-evaluated. If the transferrin saturation is less than 20%, supplemental iron should be administered. If the transferrin saturation is greater than 20%, the dose of EPOGEN® may be increased by 25 U/kg T.I.W. Such dose increases should not be made more frequently than once a month, unless clinically indicated, as the response time of the hematocrit to a dose increase can be 2–6 weeks. Hematocrit should be measured twice weekly for 2–6 weeks following dose increases.

In the U.S. Phase III multicenter trial in patients on hemodialysis, the median maintenance dose was 75 U/kg T.I.W., with approximately 65% of the patients requiring doses of 100 U/kg T.I.W., or less, to maintain their hematocrit within the range of 32–38% (maintenance doses ranged from 12.5 to 525 U/kg T.I.W.). Almost 10% of the patients required a dose of 25 U/kg, or less, and approximately 10% of the patients required more than 200 U/kg T.I.W. to maintain their hematocrit in this range.

In patients with CRF not on dialysis, the maintenance dose must also be individualized. EPOGEN® doses of 75–150 U/kg per week have been shown to maintain hematocrits of 36–38% for up to six months.

Delayed or Diminished Response: Over 95% of patients with CRF responded with clinically significant increases in hematocrit, and virtually all patients were transfusion-independent within approximately two months of initiation of EPOGEN® therapy.

If a patient fails to respond or maintain a response, other etiologies should be considered and evaluated as clinically indicated. See "Precautions" section for discussion of delayed or diminished response.

AZT-Treated HIV-Infected Patients

Prior to beginning EPOGEN®, it is recommended that the endogenous serum erythropoietin level be determined (prior to transfusion). Available evidence suggests that patients receiving AZT with endogenous serum erythropoietin levels > 500 mU/mL are unlikely to respond to therapy with EPOGEN®.

Starting Dose: For patients with serum erythropoietin levels ≤ 500 mU/mL who are receiving a dose of AZT ≤ 4200 mg/week, the recommended starting dose of EPOGEN® is 100 U/kg as an intravenous or subcutaneous injection three times weekly (T.I.W.) for 8 weeks.

Increase Dose: During the dose adjustment phase of therapy, the hematocrit should be monitored weekly. If the response is not satisfactory in terms of reducing transfusion requirements or increasing hematocrit after 8 weeks of therapy, the dose of EPOGEN® can be increased by 50–100 U/kg T.I.W. Response should be evaluated every 4–8 weeks thereafter and the dose adjusted accordingly by 50–100 U/kg increments T.I.W. If patients have not responded satisfactorily to an EPOGEN® dose of 300 U/kg T.I.W., it is unlikely that they will respond to higher doses of EPOGEN®.

Maintenance Dose: After attainment of the desired response (i.e., reduced transfusion requirements or increased hematocrit), the dose of EPOGEN® should be titrated to maintain the response based on factors such as variations in AZT dose and the presence of intercurrent infectious or inflammatory episodes. If the hematocrit exceeds 40%, the dose should be discontinued until the hematocrit drops to 36%. The dose should be reduced by 25% when treatment is resumed and then titrated to maintain the desired hematocrit.

PREPARATION AND ADMINISTRATION OF EPOGEN®

1. DO NOT SHAKE. Shaking may denature the glycoprotein, rendering it biologically inactive.
2. Parenteral drug products should be inspected visually for particulate matter and discoloration prior to administration. Do not use any vials exhibiting particulate matter or discoloration.
3. Using aseptic techniques, attach a sterile needle to a sterile syringe. Remove the flip top from the vial containing EPOGEN®, and wipe the septum with a disinfectant. Insert the needle into the vial, and withdraw into the syringe an appropriate volume of solution.
4. Use only one dose per vial; do not re-enter the vial. Discard unused portions. Contains no preservative.
5. Do not administer in conjunction with other drug solutions.

HOW SUPPLIED

EPOGEN® is available in vials containing 2,000 (NDC 55513-126-01), 3,000 (NDC 55513-267-01), 4,000 (NDC 55513-148-01), or 10,000 (NDC 55513-144-01) units of Epoetin alfa in 1.0 mL of a sterile, preservative-free solution. Each dosage form is supplied in boxes containing 10 single-use vials.

STORAGE

Store at 2° to 8°C (36° to 46°F). Do not freeze or shake.

REFERENCES

1. Egrie JC, Strickland TW, Lane J, et al., (1986). "Characterization and biological effects of recombinant human erythropoietin." *Immunobiol.* 72: 213–224.
2. Graber SE and Krantz SB, (1978). "Erythropoietin and the Control of Red Cell Production." *Ann. Rev. Med.* 29: 51–66.
3. Eschbach JW and Adamson JW, (1985). "Anemia of End-Stage Renal Disease (ESRD)." *Kidney Intl.* 28: 1–5.
4. Eschbach JW, Egrie JC, Downing MR, Browne JK, and Adamson JW, (1987). "Correction of the Anemia of End-Stage Renal Disease with Recombinant Human Erythropoietin." *NEJM* 316: 73–78.
5. Eschbach JW, Adamson JW, and Cooperative Multicenter r-HuEPO Trial Group, (1988). "Correction of the Anemia of Hemodialysis (HD) Patients with Recombinant Human Erythropoietin (r-HuEPO): Results of a Multicenter Study." *Kidney Intl.* 33: 189.
6. Eschbach JW, Egrie JC, Downing MR, Browne JK, Adamson JW, (1989). "The Use of Recombinant Human Erythropoietin (r-HuEPO): Effect in End-Stage Renal Disease (ESRD)." *Prevention of Chronic Uremia* (Friedman, Beyer, DeSanto, Giordano, eds.), Field and Wood Inc., Philadelphia, PA, pp 148–155.
7. Egrie JC, Eschbach JW, McGuire T, and Adamson JW, (1988). "Pharmacokinetics of Recombinant Human Erythropoietin (r-HuEPO) Administered to Hemodialysis (HD) Patients." *Kidney Intl.* 33: 262.
8. Lundin AP, Delano BG, Stein R, Quinn RM, and Friedman EA, (1988). "Recombinant Human Erythropoietin (r-HuEPO) Treatment Enhances Exercise Tolerance in Hemodialysis Patients." *Kidney Intl.* 33: 200.
9. Paganini E, Garcia J, Ellis P, Bodnar D, and Magnussen M, (1988). "Clinical Sequelae of Correction of Anemia with Recombinant Human Erythropoietin (r-HuEPO);

Urea Kinetics, Dialyzer Function and Reuse." *Am. J. Kid. Dis.* 11: 16.
10. Delano BG, Lundin AP, Golansky R, Quinn RM, Rao TKS, and Friedman EA, (1988). "Dialyzer Urea and Creatinine Clearances Not Significantly Changed in r-HuEPO Treated Maintenance Hemodialysis (MD) Patients." *Kidney Intl.* 33: 219.
11. Stivelman J, Van Wyck D, and Ogden D, (1988). "Use of Recombinant Erythropoietin (r-HuEPO) with High Flux Dialysis (HFD) Does Not Worsen Azotemia or Shorten Access Survival." *Kidney Intl.* 33: 239.
12. Lim VS, DeGowin RL, Zavala D, Kirchner PT, Abels R, Perry P, and Fangman J, (1989). "Recombinant Human Erythropoietin Treatment in Pre-Dialysis Patients: A Double-Blind Placebo-Controlled Trial." *Ann. Int. Med.* 110: 108–114.
13. Stone WJ, Graber SE, Krantz SB, et al., (1988). "Treatment of the anemia of pre-dialysis patients with recombinant human erythropoietin: a randomized, placebo-controlled trial." *Am. J. Med. Sci.* 296: 171–179.
14. Data on file, Ortho Biologics, Inc.
15. Raskin NH and Fishman RA, (1976). "Neurologic Disorders in Renal Failure (First of Two Parts)." *NEJM* 294: 143–148.
16. Raskin NH and Fishman RA, (1976). "Neurologic Disorders in Renal Failure (Second of Two Parts)." *NEJM* 294: 204–210.
17. Messing RO and Simon RP, (1986). "Seizures as a Manifestation of Systemic Disease." *Neurologic Clinics* 4: 563–584.
18. Kerr DN, (1979). "Chronic Renal Failure." *Cecil Textbook of Medicine,* (Beeson PB, McDermott W, Wyngaarden JB, eds.), W.B. Saunders, Philadelphia, PA, pp 1351–1367.

Manufactured by:
Amgen Inc.
Amgen Center
Thousand Oaks, California 91320-1789
Issue Date: 1/23/91
Shown in Product Identification Section, page 404

NEUPOGEN®   ℞
(Filgrastim)

DESCRIPTION

Filgrastim is a human granulocyte colony stimulating factor (G-CSF), produced by recombinant DNA technology. G-CSF regulates the production of neutrophils within the bone marrow; endogenous G-CSF is a glycoprotein produced by monocytes, fibroblasts, and endothelial cells.[1–5] G-CSF is a colony stimulating factor which has been shown to have minimal direct in vivo or in vitro effects on the production of other hematopoietic cell types.[5,6] NEUPOGEN® is the Amgen Inc. trademark for Filgrastim, which has been selected as the name for recombinant methionyl human granulocyte colony stimulating factor (r-metHuG-CSF).

NEUPOGEN® (Filgrastim) is a 175 amino acid protein manufactured by recombinant DNA technology.[7] NEUPOGEN® is produced by Escherichia coli (E. coli) bacteria into which has been inserted the human granulocyte colony stimulating factor gene. NEUPOGEN® has a molecular weight of 18,800 daltons. The protein has an amino acid sequence that is identical to the natural sequence predicted from human DNA sequence analysis, except for the addition of an N-terminal methionine necessary for expression in E. coli. Because NEUPOGEN® is produced in E. coli, the product is non-glycosylated and thus differs from G-CSF isolated from a human cell.

NEUPOGEN® is a sterile, clear, colorless, preservative-free liquid for parenteral administration. Each single-use vial of NEUPOGEN® contains 300 mcg/mL of Filgrastim at a specific activity of $1.0 \pm 0.6 \times 10^8$ U/mg, (as measured by a cell mitogenesis assay). The product is formulated in a 10 mM sodium acetate buffer at pH 4.0, containing 5% mannitol and 0.004% Tween® 80. The quantitative composition (per mL) of NEUPOGEN® is:

Filgrastim	300 mcg
Acetate	0.59 mg
Mannitol	50.0 mg
Tween® 80	0.004%
Sodium	0.035 mg
Water for Injection USP q.s. ad	1.0 mL

Manufacture is initiated at Amgen Inc. from a master seed lot of E. coli containing the gene for r-metHuG-CSF. The E. coli are grown and the product is purified by conventional means. Prior to final purification, r-metHuG-CSF is allowed to oxidize to its native state and its final purity is achieved by sequential passage over a series of chromatography columns. The product is then formulated in an acetate buffer with mannitol and Tween® 80.

Continued on next page

Amgen—Cont.

Filling and packaging operations for NEUPOGEN® are performed by an outside, FDA-approved contractor.

CLINICAL PHARMACOLOGY

Colony Stimulating Factors

Colony stimulating factors are glycoproteins which act on hematopoietic cells by binding to specific cell surface receptors and stimulating proliferation, differentiation commitment, and some end-cell functional activation.

Endogenous G-CSF is a lineage-specific colony stimulating factor with selectivity for the neutrophil lineage. G-CSF is not species specific and has been shown to primarily affect neutrophil progenitor proliferation,[8,9] differentiation,[8,10] and selected end-cell functional activation (including enhanced phagocytic ability,[11] priming of the cellular metabolism associated with respiratory burst,[12] antibody dependent killing,[13] and the increased expression of some functions associated with cell surface antigens[14]).

Pre-clinical Experience

Filgrastim was administered to monkeys, dogs, hamsters, rats, and mice as part of a comprehensive pre-clinical toxicology program which included both single-dose acute, repeated-dose subacute, and chronic studies. Single-dose administration of Filgrastim by the oral, intravenous, subcutaneous, or intraperitoneal routes resulted in no significant toxicity in mice, rats, hamsters, or monkeys. Although no deaths were observed in mice, rats, or monkeys at dose levels up to 3450 mcg/kg and in hamsters using single doses up to approximately 860 mcg/kg, deaths were observed in a subchronic (13 week) study in monkeys. In this study, evidence of neurological symptoms was seen in monkeys treated with doses of Filgrastim greater than 1150 mcg/kg/day for up to 18 days. Deaths were seen in 5 of the 8 treated animals and were associated with 15- to 28-fold increases in peripheral leukocyte counts, and neutrophil-infiltrated hemorrhagic foci were seen in both the cerebrum and cerebellum. In contrast, no monkeys died following 13 weeks of daily intravenous administration of Filgrastim at a dose level of 115 mcg/kg.

In subacute, repeated-dose studies, changes observed were attributable to the expected pharmacological actions of Filgrastim (i.e., dose-dependent increases in white cell counts, increased circulating segmented neutrophils, and increased myeloid:erythroid ratio in bone marrow). In all species, histopathologic examination of the liver and spleen revealed evidence of ongoing extramedullary granulopoiesis; increased spleen weights were seen in all species and appeared to be dose-related. A dose-dependent increase in serum alkaline phosphatase was observed in rats, and may reflect increased activity of osteoblasts and osteoclasts. Changes in serum chemistry values were reversible following discontinuation of treatment.

In rats treated at doses of 1150 mcg/kg/day for four weeks (5 of 32 animals) and for 13 weeks at doses of 100 mcg/kg/day (4 of 32 animals) and 500 mcg/kg/day (6 of 32 animals) articular swelling of the hind legs was observed. Some degree of hind leg dysfunction was also observed; however, symptoms reversed following cessation of dosing. In rats, osteoclasis and osteoanagenesis were found in the femur, humerus, coccyx and hind legs (where they were accompanied by synovitis) after intravenous treatment for four weeks (115 to 1150 mcg/kg/day), and in the sternum after intravenous treatment for 13 weeks (115 to 575 mcg/kg/day). These effects reversed to normal within 4 to 5 weeks following cessation of treatment.

Pharmacologic Effects of NEUPOGEN®

In Phase I studies involving 96 patients with various nonmyeloid malignancies, NEUPOGEN® administration resulted in a dose-dependent increase in circulating neutrophil counts over the dose range of 1–70 mcg/kg/day.[15–17] This increase in neutrophil counts was observed whether NEUPOGEN® was administered intravenously (1–70 mcg/kg twice daily),[15] subcutaneously (1–3 mcg/kg once daily),[17] or by continuous subcutaneous infusion (3–11 mcg/kg/day).[16] With discontinuation of NEUPOGEN® therapy, neutrophil counts returned to baseline, in most cases within four days. Isolated neutrophils displayed normal phagocytic (measured by zymosan-stimulated chemoluminescence) and chemotactic [measured by migration under agarose using N-formyl-methionyl-leucyl-phenylalanine (fMLP) as the chemotaxin] activity in vitro.

The absolute monocyte count was reported to increase in a dose-dependent manner in most patients receiving NEUPOGEN®, however, the percentage of monocytes in the differential count remained within the normal range. In all studies to date, absolute counts of both eosinophils and basophils did not change and were within the normal range following administration of NEUPOGEN®. Increases in lymphocyte counts following NEUPOGEN® administration have been reported in some normal subjects and cancer patients.

White blood cell differentials obtained during clinical trials have demonstrated a shift towards earlier granulocyte progenitor cells (left shift), including the appearance of promyelocytes and myeloblasts, usually during neutrophil recovery following the chemotherapy-induced nadir. In addition, Dohle bodies, increased granulocyte granulation, as well as hypersegmented neutrophils have been observed. Such changes were transient, and were not associated with clinical sequelae nor were they necessarily associated with infection.

Pharmacokinetics

Absorption and clearance of NEUPOGEN® follows first-order pharmacokinetic modeling without apparent concentration dependence. A positive linear correlation occurred between the parenteral dose and both the serum concentration and area under the concentration-time curves. Continuous intravenous infusion of 20 mcg/kg of NEUPOGEN® over 24 hours resulted in mean and median serum concentrations of approximately 48 and 56 ng/mL, respectively. Subcutaneous administration of 3.45 mcg/kg and 11.5 mcg/kg resulted in maximum serum concentrations and 4 and 49 ng/mL, respectively, within 2 to 8 hours. The volume of distribution averaged 150 mL/kg in both normal subjects and cancer patients. The elimination half-life, in both normal subjects and cancer patients, was approximately 3.5 hours. Clearance rates of NEUPOGEN® were approximately 0.5–0.7 mL/min/kg. Single parenteral doses or daily intravenous doses, over a 14 day period, resulted in comparable half-lives. The half-lives were similar for intravenous administration (231 minutes, following doses of 34.5 mcg/kg) and for subcutaneous administration (210 minutes, following NEUPOGEN® doses of 3.45 mcg/kg). Continuous 24-hour intravenous infusions at 20 mcg/kg over an 11 to 20 day period produced steady state serum concentrations of NEUPOGEN® with no evidence of drug accumulation over the time period investigated.

INDICATIONS AND USAGE

NEUPOGEN® is indicated to decrease the incidence of infection, as manifested by febrile neutropenia, in patients with non-myeloid malignancies receiving myelosuppressive anti-cancer drugs associated with a significant incidence of severe neutropenia with fever (see CLINICAL EXPERIENCE). A complete blood count and platelet count should be obtained prior to chemotherapy, and twice per week (see LABORATORY MONITORING) during NEUPOGEN® therapy to avoid leukocytosis and to monitor the neutrophil count. In Phase III clinical studies, NEUPOGEN® therapy was discontinued when the absolute neutrophil count (ANC) was $\geq$10,000/mm^3 after the expected chemotherapy-induced nadir.

Clinical Experience: Response to NEUPOGEN®

NEUPOGEN® has been shown to be safe and effective in accelerating the recovery of neutrophil counts following a variety of chemotherapy regimens. In a Phase III clinical trial in small cell lung cancer, patients received subcutaneous administration of NEUPOGEN® (4 to 8 mcg/kg/day, days 4–17) or placebo. In this study, the benefits of NEUPOGEN® therapy where shown to be prevention of infection as manifested by febrile neutropenia, decreased hospitalization, and decreased intravenous antibiotic usage. No difference in survival or disease progression was demonstrated.

In the Phase III, randomized, double-blind, placebo-controlled trial conducted in patients with small cell lung cancer, patients were randomized to receive NEUPOGEN® (n=99) or placebo (n=111) starting on day 4, after receiving standard dose chemotherapy with cyclophosphomide, doxorubicin, and etoposide. A total of 210 patients were evaluated for efficacy and 207 evaluated for safety. Treatment with NEUPOGEN® resulted in a clinically and statistically significant reduction in the incidence of infection, as manifested by febrile neutropenia; the incidence of at least one infection over all cycles of chemotherapy was 76% (84/111) for placebo-treated patients, versus 40% (40/99) for NEUPOGEN®-treated patients ($p<0.001$). The following secondary analyses were also performed. The requirements for in-patient hospitalization and antibiotic use were also significantly decreased during the first cycle of chemotherapy; incidence of hospitalization was 69% (77/111) for placebo-treated patients in cycle one, versus 52% (51/99) for NEUPOGEN®-treated patients ($p=0.032$). The incidence of intravenous antibiotic usage was 60% (67/111) for placebo-treated patients in cycle one, versus 38% (38/99) for NEUPOGEN®-treated patients ($p=0.003$). The incidence, severity, and duration of severe neutropenia (ANC <500/mm^3) following chemotherapy were all significantly reduced. The incidence of severe neutropenia in cycle one was 84% (83/99) for patients receiving NEUPOGEN® versus 96% (106/110) for patients receiving placebo ($p = 0.004$). Over all cycles, patients randomized to NEUPOGEN® had a 57% (286/500 cycles) rate of severe neutropenia versus 77% (416/543 cycles) for patients randomized to placebo. The median duration of severe neutropenia in cycle one was reduced from 6 days (range 0–10 days) for patients receiving placebo to 2 days (range 0–9 days) for patients receiving NEUPOGEN® ($p < 0.001$). The mean duration of neutropenia in cycle one was 5.64 ± 2.27 for patients receiving placebo versus 2.44 ± 1.90 for patients receiving NEUPOGEN®. Over all cycles, the median duration of neutropenia was 3 days for patients randomized to placebo versus 1 day for patients randomized to NEUPOGEN®. The median severity of neutropenia (as measured by ANC nadir) was 72/mm^3 (range 0/mm^3–7912/mm^3) in cycle one for patients receiving NEUPOGEN® versus 38/mm^3 (range 0/mm^3–9520/mm^3) for patients receiving placebo ($p = 0.012$). The mean severity of neutropenia in cycle one was 496/mm^3$\pm$1382/mm^3 for patients receiving NEUPOGEN® versus 204/mm^3$\pm$953/mm^3 for patients receiving placebo. Over all cycles, the ANC nadir for patients randomized to NEUPOGEN® was 403/mm^3, versus 161/mm^3 for patients randomized to placebo. Administration of NEUPOGEN® resulted in an earlier ANC nadir following chemotherapy than was experienced by patients receiving placebo (day 10 versus day 12). NEUPOGEN® was well tolerated when given subcutaneously daily at doses of 4–8 mcg/kg for up to 14 consecutive days following each cycle of chemotherapy (see ADVERSE REACTIONS).

Several other Phase I/II studies, which did not directly measure the incidence of infection, but which did measure increases in neutrophils, support the efficacy of NEUPOGEN®. The regimens are presented to provide some background on the clinical experience with NEUPOGEN®. No claim regarding the safety or efficacy of the chemotherapy regimens is made. The effects of NEUPOGEN® on tumor growth or on the antitumor activity of the chemotherapy were not assessed. The doses of NEUPOGEN® used in these studies are considerably greater than those found to be effective in the Phase III study described above. Such Phase I/II studies are summarized in the following table.

[See table on next page.]

CONTRAINDICATIONS

NEUPOGEN® is contraindicated in patients with known hypersensitivity to E. coli-derived proteins.

WARNINGS

In cancer patients who have received NEUPOGEN® to date, no serious adverse reactions that would limit the use of the product have been reported.

PRECAUTIONS

General

Simultaneous Use with Chemotherapy

The safety and efficacy of NEUPOGEN® given simultaneously with cytotoxic chemotherapy have not been established. Because of the potential sensitivity of rapidly dividing myeloid cells to cytotoxic chemotherapy, do not use NEUPOGEN® in the period 24 hours before to 24 hour after the administration of cytotoxic chemotherapy (see DOSAGE AND ADMINISTRATION).

The efficacy of NEUPOGEN® has not been evaluated in patients receiving chemotherapy associated with delayed myelosuppression (e.g., nitrosoureas) or with mitomycin C or with myelosuppressive doses of anti-metabolites such as 5-fluorouracil or cytosine arabinoside.

Growth Factor Potential

NEUPOGEN® is a growth factor that primarily stimulates neutrophils. However, the possibility that NEUPOGEN® can act as a growth factor for any tumor type, particularly myeloid malignancies, cannot be excluded. Therefore, because of the possibility of tumor growth, precaution should be exercised in using this drug in any malignancy with myeloid characteristics.

Leukocytosis

White blood cell counts of 100,000/mm^3 or greater were observed in approximately 2% of patients receiving NEUPOGEN® at doses above 5 mcg/kg/day. There were no reports of adverse events associated with this degree of leukocytosis. In order to avoid the potential complications of excessive leukocytosis, a complete blood count (CBC) is recommended twice per week during NEUPOGEN® therapy (see LABORATORY MONITORING).

Premature Discontinuation of NEUPOGEN® Therapy

A transient increase in neutrophil counts is typically seen 1 to 2 days after initiation of NEUPOGEN® therapy. However, for a sustained therapeutic response, NEUPOGEN® therapy should be continued until the post nadir ANC reaches 10,000/mm^3. Therefore, the premature discontinuation of NEUPOGEN® therapy, prior to the time of recovery from the expected neutrophil nadir, is generally not recommended (see DOSAGE AND ADMINISTRATION).

Chronic Administration

The safety and efficacy of chronic administration of NEUPOGEN® (Filgrastim) have not been established. Preliminary investigational studies with NEUPOGEN® have been conducted in 224 patients with severe chronic neutropenia, 13 of whom have been treated for up to three years. In these patients, subclinical splenomegaly (detected by CT or MRI scanning) was the most frequently observed adverse effect, occurring in approximately one third of patients receiving chronic administration of NEUPOGEN®; 3% of patients were noted to have clinical splenomegaly. Less frequently observed adverse events included exacerbation of some preexisting skin disorders (e.g., psoriasis), alopecia, hematuria/proteinuria, thrombocytopenia (platelets less than 50,000/mm^3) and osteoporosis.

Type of Malignancy	Regimen	Chemotherapy Dose	Number of Pts.	Trial Phase	NEUPOGEN® Daily Dose[a]
Small Cell Lung Cancer	Cyclophosphamide Doxorubicin Etoposide	1 g/m²/day 50 mg/m²/day 120 mg/m²/day x3 q 21 days	210	III	4–8 mcg/kg SC days 4–17
Small Cell Lung Cancer[17]	Ifosfamide Doxorubicin Etoposide Mesna	5 g/m²/day 50 mg/m²/day 120 mg/m²/day x3 8 g/m²/day q 21 days	12	I/II	5.75–46 mcg/kg IV days 4–17
Urothelial Cancer[18]	Methotrexate Vinblastine Doxorubicin Cisplatin	30 mg/m²day x2 3 mg/m²/day x2 30 mg/m²/day 70 mg/m²/day q 28 days	40	I/II	3.45–69 mcg/kg IV days 4–11
Various Non-Myeloid Malignancies[19]	Cyclophosphamide Etoposide Cisplatin	2.5 g/m²/day x2 500 mg/m²/day x3 50 mg/m²/day x3 q 28 days	18	I/II	23–69 mcg/kg[b] IV days 8–28
Breast/ Ovarian[20]	Doxorubicin[c]	75 mg/m²	21	II	11.5 mcg/kg days 2–9 IV
		100 mg/m²			5.75 mcg/kg days 10–12 IV
		125 mg/m² 150 mg/m² q 14 days			
Neuroblastoma	Cyclophosphamide	150 mg/m² x7	12	II	5.45–17.25 mcg/kg SC days 6–19
	Doxorubicin Cisplatin	35 mg/m² 90 mg/m² q 28 days (cycles 1,3,5)[d]			

[a] NEUPOGEN® doses were those that accelerated neutrophil production. Doses which provided no additional acceleration beyond that achieved at the next lower dose are not reported.
[b] Lowest dose(s) tested in the study.
[c] Patients received doxorubicin at either 75, 100, 125 or 150 mg/m².
[d] Cycles 2,6 = cyclophosphamide 150 mg/m² × 7 and etoposide 280 mg/m² × 3
Cycle 4 = cisplatin 90 mg/m² × 1 and etoposide 280 mg/m² × 3

Other
In studies of NEUPOGEN® administration following chemotherapy, most reported side effects were consistent with those usually seen as a result of cytotoxic chemotherapy (see ADVERSE REACTIONS). Because of the potential of receiving higher doses of chemotherapy (i.e., full doses on the prescribed schedule), the patient may be at greater risk of thrombocytopenia, anemia, and non-hematologic consequences of increased chemotherapy doses (please refer to the prescribing information of the specific chemotherapy agents used). Regular monitoring of the hematocrit and platelet count is recommended. Furthermore, care should be exercised in the administration of NEUPOGEN® in conjunction with other drugs known to lower the platelet count. In septic patients receiving NEUPOGEN®, the physician should be alert to the theoretical possibility of adult respiratory distress syndrome, due to the possible influx of neutrophils at the site of inflammation. Cardiac events (myocardial infarctions, arrhythmias) have been reported in 11 of 375 cancer patients receiving NEUPOGEN® in clinical studies; the relationship to NEUPOGEN® therapy is unknown. However, patients with pre-existing cardiac conditions receiving NEUPOGEN® should be monitored closely.

Information for Patients
In those situations in which the physician determines that the patient can safely and effectively self-administer NEUPOGEN®, the patient should be instructed as to the proper dosage and administration. Patients should be referred to the full "Information for Patients" section attached; it is not a disclosure of all, or possible, intended effects. The most common adverse experience occurring with NEUPOGEN® therapy is bone pain. If home use is prescribed, patients should be thoroughly instructed in the importance of proper disposal and cautioned against the reuse of needles, syringes, or drug product. A puncture-resistant container for the disposal of used syringes and needles should be available to the patient. The full container should be disposed of according to the directions provided by the physician.

Laboratory Monitoring
A CBC and platelet count should be obtained prior to chemotherapy, and at regular intervals (twice per week) during NEUPOGEN® therapy. Following cytotoxic chemotherapy, the neutrophil nadir occurred earlier during cycles when NEUPOGEN® was administered, and white blood cell differentials demonstrated a left shift, including the appearance of promyelocytes and myeloblasts. In addition, the duration of severe neutropenia was reduced, and was followed by an accelerated recovery in the neutrophil counts. Therefore, regular monitoring of white blood cell counts, particularly at the time of the recovery from the post chemotherapy nadir, is recommended in order to avoid excessive leukocytosis.

Drug Interaction
No evidence of interaction of NEUPOGEN® with other drugs was observed in the course of clinical trials.

Carcinogensis, Mutagenesis, Impairment of Fertility
The carcinogenic potential of NEUPOGEN® has not been studied. NEUPOGEN® failed to induce bacterial gene mutations in either the presence or absence of a drug metabolizing enzyme system. NEUPOGEN® had no observed effect on the fertility of male or female rats, or on gestation at doses up to 500 mcg/kg.

Pregnancy Category C
NEUPOGEN® has been shown to have adverse effects in pregnant rabbits when given in doses 2 to 10 times the human dose. There are no adequate and well controlled studies in pregnant women. NEUPOGEN® should be used during pregnancy only if the potential benefit justifies the potential risk to the fetus.
In rabbits, increased abortion and embryolethality were observed in animals treated with NEUPOGEN® at 80 mcg/kg/day. NEUPOGEN® administered to pregnant rabbits at doses of 100 mcg/kg/day during the period of organogenesis was associated with increased fetal resorption, genitourinary bleeding, developmental abnormalities, and decreased body weight, live births, and food consumption. External abnormalities were not observed in the fetuses of dams treated at 100 mcg/kg/day. Reproductive studies in pregnant rats have shown that NEUPOGEN® was not associated with lethal, teratogenic, or behavioral effects on fetuses when administered by daily intravenous injection during the period of organogensis at dose levels up to 575 mcg/kg/day.
In Segment III studies in rats, offspring of dams treated at > 20 mcg/kg/day exhibited a delay in external differentiation (detachment of auricles and descent of testes) and slight growth retardation, possibly due to lower body weight of females during rearing and nursing. Offspring of dams treated at 100 mcg/kg/day exhibited decreased body weights at birth, and a slightly reduced four day survival rate.

Nursing Mothers
It is not known whether NEUPOGEN® is excreted in human milk. Because many drugs are excreted in human milk, caution should be exercised if NEUPOGEN® is administered to a nursing woman.

Pediatric Use
Although efficacy of NEUPOGEN® has not been demonstrated in a pediatric population, safety data indicate that NEUPOGEN® does not exhibit any greater toxicity in children than in adults. NEUPOGEN® has been used to treat 128 pediatric severe chronic neutropenia patients; such patients ranged in age from 3 months to 18 years and were treated with NEUPOGEN® at 0.6–120 mcg/kg/day for up to three years. Such doses were well tolerated, and the overall pattern of adverse events in children and adults appeared to be similar. While subclinical increases in spleen size detected by imaging studies (CT or MRI) were reported more often in children than in adults, the clinical significance of these radiographic findings relative to normal growth and development is not known. No hematologic abnormalities were noted which were unique to children treated with NEUPOGEN®. In addition, 12 pediatric patients with neuroblastoma have received up to six cycles of cyclophosphamide, cisplatin, doxorubicin, and etoposide chemotherapy concurrently with NEUPOGEN®; in this population, NEUPOGEN® was well tolerated. There was one report of palpable splenomegaly associated with NEUPOGEN® therapy, however, the only consistently reported adverse event was musculoskeletal pain, which is no different from the experience in the adult population.

ADVERSE REACTIONS
In clinical trials involving over 350 patients receiving NEUPOGEN® following cytotoxic chemotherapy, most adverse experiences were the sequelae of the underlying malignancy or cytotoxic chemotherapy. In all Phase II and III trials, medullary bone pain, reported in 24% of patients, was the only consistently observed adverse reaction attributed to NEUPOGEN® therapy. This bone pain was generally reported to be of mild-to-moderate severity, and could be controlled in most patients with non-narcotic analgesics; infrequently, bone pain was severe enough to require narcotic analgesics. Bone pain was reported more frequently in patients treated with higher doses (20–100 mcg/kg/day) administered intravenously, and less frequently in patients treated with lower subcutaneous doses of NEUPOGEN® (3–10 mcg/kg/day).
In the randomized, double-blind, placebo-controlled trial of NEUPOGEN® therapy following combination chemotherapy in patients (n = 207) with small cell lung cancer, the following adverse events were reported during blinded cycles of study medication (placebo or NEUPOGEN® at 4 to 8 mcg/kg/day). Events are reported as exposure adjusted since patients remained on double-blind NEUPOGEN® a median of three cycles versus one cycle for placebo.

| | % of Blinded Cycles with Events | |
Event	NEUPOGEN® N = 384 patient cycles	Placebo N = 257 patient cycles
Nausea/Vomiting	57	64
Skeletal Pain	22	11
Alopecia	18	27
Diarrhea	14	23
Neutropenic Fever	13	35
Mucositis	12	20
Fever	12	11
Fatigue	11	16
Anorexia	9	11
Dyspnea	9	11
Headache	7	9
Cough	6	8
Skin Rash	6	9
Chest Pain	5	6
Generalized Weakness	4	7
Sore Throat	4	9
Stomatitis	5	10
Constipation	5	10
Pain (Unspecified)	2	7

In this study, there were no serious, life-threatening, or fatal adverse reactions attributed to NEUPOGEN® therapy. Specifically, there were no reports of flu-like symptoms, pleuritis, pericarditis, or other major systemic reactions to NEUPOGEN®.
Spontaneously reversible elevations in uric acid, lactate dehydrogenase, and alkaline phosphatase occurred in 27% to 58% of 98 patients receiving blinded NEUPOGEN® therapy following cytotoxic chemotherapy; increases were generally mild to moderate. Transient decreases in blood pressure (< 90/60 mmHg), which did not require clinical treatment,

Continued on next page

Amgen—Cont.

were reported in 7 to 176 patients in Phase III clinical studies following administration of NEUPOGEN®.

No evidence of interaction of NEUPOGEN® with other drugs was observed in the course of clinical trials (see PRECAUTIONS—SIMULTANEOUS USE WITH CHEMOTHERAPY). To date, there have been no reported allergic reactions or anaphylaxis attributed to NEUPOGEN® administration in over 500 patients treated with NEUPOGEN® for a variety of conditions. In this group of patients, including 33 who have received NEUPOGEN® daily for almost two years, there has been no evidence of the development of antibodies to NEUPOGEN® or of a blunted or diminished response over time.

OVERDOSAGE

The maximum tolerated dose of NEUPOGEN® has not been determined. Twenty-seven patients have been treated at NEUPOGEN® doses of $\geq$ 69 mcg/kg/day. Of those, six patients have been treated at 115 mcg/kg/day with no toxic effects attributable to NEUPOGEN®. Efficacy has been demonstrated using much lower doses. (Doses of 4 to 8 mcg/kg/day showed efficacy in the Phase III study.) Doses of NEUPOGEN® which increase the ANC beyond 10,000/mm^3 may not result in any additional clinical benefit.

In NEUPOGEN® clinical trials, white blood cell counts >100,000/mm^3 have been reported in less than 5% of patients, but were not associated with any reported adverse clinical effects.

It is recommended, to avoid the potential risks of excessive leukocytosis, that NEUPOGEN® therapy should be discontinued if the ANC count surpasses 10,000/mm^3 after the ANC nadir has occurred.

Discontinuation of NEUPOGEN® therapy usually results in a 50% decrease in circulating neutrophils within 1 to 2 days, with a return to pretreatment levels in 1 to 7 days.

DOSAGE AND ADMINISTRATION

The recommended starting dose of NEUPOGEN® is 5 mcg/kg/day, administered subcutaneously or intravenously as a single daily injection. No data are currently available regarding NEUPOGEN'S® stability or compatibility with infusion equipment or diluted in intravenous solutions. A CBC and platelet count should be obtained before instituting NEUPOGEN® therapy, and monitored twice weekly during therapy. Doses may be increased in increments of 5 mcg/kg for each chemotherapy cycle, according to the duration and severity of the ANC nadir.

NEUPOGEN® should be administered no earlier than 24 hours after the administration of cytotoxic chemotherapy. NEUPOGEN® should not be administered in the period 24 hours before the administration of chemotherapy (see PRECAUTIONS). NEUPOGEN® should be administered daily for up to two weeks, until the ANC has reached 10,000/mm^3 following the expected chemotherapy-induced neutrophil nadir. The duration of NEUPOGEN® therapy needed to attenuate chemotherapy-induced neutropenia may be dependent on the myelosuppressive potential of the chemotherapy regimen employed. NEUPOGEN® therapy should be discontinued if the ANC surpasses 10,000/mm^3 after the expected chemotherapy-induced neutrophil nadir (see PRECAUTIONS). In Phase III trials, efficacy was observed at doses of 4 to 8 mcg/kg/day.

Injectable solution: Each 1 mL of NEUPOGEN® contains 300 mcg of Filgrastim in a preservative-free solution containing 0.59 mg acetate, 50 mg mannitol, 0.004% Tween® 80, 0.035 mg sodium, and 1 mL water for injection, USP, pH 4.0. Each 1.6 mL of NEUPOGEN® contains 480 mcg of Filgrastim in a preservative-free solution containing 0.94 mg acetate, 80 mg mannitol, 0.004% Tween® 80, 0.056 mg sodium, and 1.6 mL water for injection, USP, pH 4.0.

NEUPOGEN® should be stored in the refrigerator at 2–8 degrees Centigrade (39–46 degrees Fahrenheit). Do not freeze. Avoid shaking. Prior to injection, NEUPOGEN® may be allowed to reach room temperature for a maximum of 6 hours. Any vial left at room temperature for greater than 6 hours should be discarded.

Parenteral drug products should be inspected visually for particulate matter and discoloration prior to administration, whenever solution and container permit; if particulates or discoloration are observed, the container should not be used.

HOW SUPPLIED

NEUPOGEN®: Use only one dose per vial; do not re-enter the vial. Discard unused portions. Do not save unused drug for later administration.

Single-dose, preservative-free vials containing 300 mcg (1 mL) of Filgrastim (300 mcg/mL). Boxes of 10 (NDC 55513-347-10).

Single-dose, preservative-free vials containing 480 mcg (1.6 mL) of Filgrastim (300 mcg/mL). Boxes of 10 (NDC 55513-348-10).

NEUPOGEN® should be stored at 2–8 degrees Centigrade (36–46 degrees Fahrenheit). Do not freeze. Avoid shaking.

REFERENCES

1. Zsebo KM, Yuschenkoff VN, Schiffer S, et al. Vascular endothelial cells and granulopoiesis: Interleukin-1 stimulates release of G-CSF and GM-CSF. Blood 71:99–103 (1988).
2. Souza LM, Boone TC, Gabrilove J, et al. Recombinant human granulocyte colony-stimulating factor: effects on normal and leukemic myeloid cells. Science 232:61–65 (1986).
3. Koeffler HP, Gasson J, Raynard J, Souza LM, Shepard M, and Munker R. Recombinant human TNF stimulates production of granulocyte colony-stimulating factor. Blood 70:55–59 (1987).
4. Seelentag WK, Mermod JJ, Montesano R, and Vassalli P. Additive effects of interleukin 1 and tumor necrosis factor-alpha on the accumulation of three granulocyte and macrophage colony-stimulating factor mRNAs in human endothelial cells. EMBO J. 6:2261–2265 (1987).
5. Metcalf D. The Haemopoietic colony stimulating factors. Elsevier Sci. Pub. Chp. 13:55–92 (1984).
6. Burgess AW and Metcalf D. Characterization of a serum factor stimulating the differentiation of myelomonocytic leukemic cells. Int. J. Cancer 26:647–654 (1980).
7. Zsebo KM, Cohen AM, Murdock DC, Boone TC, Inque H, Chazin VR, Hines D, and Souza LM. Recombinant human granulocyte colony-stimulating factor: Molecular and biological characterization. Immunobiol. 172:175–184 (1986).
8. Welte K, Bonilla MA, Gillio AP, et al. Recombinant human G-CSF: Effects on hematopoiesis in normal and cyclophosphamide treated primates. J. Exp. Med. 165:941–948 (1987).
9. Duhrsen U, Villefal JL, Boyd J, et al. Effects of recombinant human granulocyte colony-stimulating factor on hematopoietic progenitor cells in cancer patients. Blood 72:2074–2081 (1988).
10. Souza LM, Boone TC, Gabrilove K, et al. Recombinant human granulocyte colony-stimulating factor: Effects on normal and leukemic myeloid cells. Science 232:61–65 (1986).
11. Weisbart RH, Kacena A, Schuh A, Golde DW. GM-CSF induces human neutrophil IgA-mediated phagocytosis by an IgA Fc receptor activation mechanism. Nature 332:647–648 (1988).
12. Kitagawa S, Yuo A, Souza LM, Saito M, Miura Y, Takaku F. Recombinant human granulocyte colony-stimulating factor enhances superoxide release in human granulocytes stimulated by chemotactic peptide. Biochem. Biophys. Res. Commun. 144:1143 (1987).
13. Glaspy JA, Baldwin GC, Robertson PA, et al. Therapy for neutropenia in hairy cell leukemia with recombinant human granulocyte colony-stimulating factor. Ann. Int. Med. 109:789–795 (1988).
14. You A, Kitagawa S, Ohsaka A, et al. Recombinant human granulocyte colony-stimulating factor as an activator of human granulocytes: potentiation of responses triggered by receptor-mediated agonists and stimulation of C3bi receptor expression and adherence. Blood 74:2144–2149 (1989).
15. Gabrilove JL, Jakubowski A, Fain K, et al. Phase I study of granulocyte colony-stimulating factor in patients with transitional cell carcinoma of the urothelium. J. Clin. Invest. 82:1454–1461 (1988).
16. Morstyn G, Souza L, Keech J, et al. Effect of granulocyte colony-stimulating factor on neutropenia induced by cytotoxic chemotherapy. Lancet March 26:667–672 (1988).
17. Bronchud MH, Scarffe JH, Thatcher N, et al. Phase I/II study of recombinant human granulocyte colony-stimulating factor in patients receiving intensive chemotherapy for small cell lung cancer. Br. J. Cancer 56:809–813 (1987).
18. Gabrilove JL, Jakubowski A, Scher H, et al. Effect of granulocyte colony-stimulating factor on neutropenia and associated morbidity due to chemotherapy for transitional cell carcinoma of the urothelium. N. Engl. J. Med. 318:1414–1422 (1988).
19. Neidhart J, Mangalik A, Kohler W, et al. Granulocyte colony-stimulating factor stimulates recovery of granulocytes in patients receiving dose-intensive chemotherapy without bone-marrow transplantation. J. Clin. Oncol. 7:1685–1691 (1981).
20. Bronchud MH, Howell A, Crowther D, et al. The use of granulocyte colony-stimulating factor to increase the intensity of treatment with doxorubicin in patients with advanced breast and ovarian cancer. Br. J. Cancer 60:121–128 (1989).

Manufactured by:
Amgen Inc.
Amgen Center
Thousand Oaks, California 91320-1789
Issue Date 2/21/91

Shown in Product Identification Section, page 404

Anaquest Inc
110 ALLEN ROAD
BOX 804
LIBERTY CORNER, NJ 07938-0804

ENLON®   ℞
[ĕn 'lon]
(edrophonium chloride injection, USP)

DESCRIPTION

Enlon is a short and rapid-acting cholinergic drug. Chemically, edrophonium chloride is ethyl(m-hydroxyphenyl) dimethylammonium chloride and its structural formula is:

Each mL contains, in a sterile solution, 10 mg edrophonium chloride compounded with 0.45% phenol as a preservative, and 0.2% sodium sulfite as an antioxidant, buffered with sodium citrate and citric acid and pH adjusted to approximately 5.4.
Enlon is intended for IV and IM use.

HOW SUPPLIED

ENLON (edrophonium chloride injection, USP):
NDC 10019-873-15   15 mL vials

ENLON-PLUS®
(edrophonium chloride, USP and atropine sulfate, USP) Injection

DESCRIPTION

Enlon-Plus (edrophonium chloride, USP and atropine sulfate, USP) Injection, for intravenous use, is a sterile, nonpyrogenic, nondepolarizing neuromuscular relaxant antagonist. Enlon-Plus is a combination drug containing a rapid acting acetylcholinesterase inhibitor, edrophonium chloride, and an anticholinergic, atropine sulfate. Chemically, edrophonium chloride is ethyl (m-hydroxyphenyl) dimethylammonium chloride; its structural formula is:

Molecular Formula: $C_{10}H_{16}ClNO$
Molecular Weight: 201.70

Table of Pharmacokinetic Values for Edrophonium Chloride

Population	T1/2β hr ± S.D.	VD L/kg ± S.D.	Cl mL/kg/min ± S.D.	N	Ref.
Adults	1.8 ± 0.6	1.1 ± 0.2	9.6 ± 2.7	10	3
Anephric Patients*†	3.4 ± 1.0	0.68 ± 0.13	2.7 ± 1.4	6	4
Infants (3 wks–11 mos)	1.2 ± 0.5	1.2 ± 0.2	1.78 ± 1.2	4	5
Children (1–6 yr)	1.6 ± 0.5	1.2 ± 0.7	14.2 ± 7.3	4	5
Adults	‡0.9 ± 0.3	1.1 ± 0.6	13.3 ± 5	5	6
Elderly* (over 75 yr)	‡1.4 ± 0.3	0.5 ± 0.1	5.1 ± 1	5	6

T½β = Elimination half-life
VD = Volume of distribution
Cl = Clearance
* No adjustments of edrophonium dosage are required because elimination of non-depolarizing muscle relaxants is similarly decreased.
† Values for anephric patients were calculated using a non-compartmental model.
‡ From a study using a different, less sensitive HPLC method and fitting C vs T data to a biexponential curve.

Chemically, atropine sulfate is:
endo-(±)-alpha-(hydroxymethyl)-8-methyl-8-azbicyclo [3.2.1] oct-3-yl benzeneacetate sulfate (2:1) monohydrate. Its structural formula is:

Molecular Formula: $(C_{17}H_{23}NO_3)_2 \cdot H_2SO_4 \cdot H_2O$
Molecular Weight: 694.84
Enlon-Plus contains in each mL of sterile solution:
5 mL Ampuls: 10 mg edrophonium chloride and 0.14 mg atropine sulfate compounded with 2.0 mg sodium sulfite as a preservative and buffered with sodium citrate and citric acid. The pH is adjusted in the range of 4.4–4.6.
15 mL Multidose Vials: 10 mg edrophonium chloride and 0.14 mg atropine sulfate compounded with 2.0 mg sodium sulfite and 4.5 mg phenol as a preservative and buffered with sodium citrate and citric acid. The pH is adjusted in the range of 4.4–4.6.

CLINICAL PHARMACOLOGY

Pharmacodynamics
Enlon-Plus (edrophonium chloride, USP and atropine sulfate, USP) Injection is a combination of an anticholinesterase agent, which antagonizes the action of nondepolarizing neuromuscular blocking drugs, and a parasympatholytic (anticholinergic) drug, which prevents the muscarinic effects caused by inhibition of acetylcholine breakdown by the anticholinesterase. Edrophonium chloride antagonizes the effect of nondepolarizing neuromuscular blocking agents primarily by inhibiting or inactivating acetylcholinesterase. By inactivating the acetylcholinesterase enzyme, acetylcholine is not hydrolyzed as rapidly by acetylcholinesterase and is thereby allowed to accumulate. The greater quantity of acetylcholine reaching the sites of nicotinic cholinergic postjunctional receptors improves transmission of impulses across the myoneural junction. The concomitant, unavoidable accumulation of acetylcholine at the sites of muscarinic cholinergic transmission occurring at the parasympathetic, postganglionic receptors of the autonomic nervous system, may cause **bradycardia, bronchoconstriction, increased secretions,** and other parasympathomimetic side effects. The magnitude of these muscarinic side effects can be expected to vary from patient to patient depending upon the amount of vagal nerve activity present. Atropine sulfate counteracts these side effects.

Intravenous edrophonium chloride in doses of 0.5 to 1.0 mg/kg promptly antagonizes the effects of nondepolarizing muscle relaxants reaching the maximum antagonism within 1.2 minutes. A plateau of maximal antagonism is sustained for 70 minutes.[1] Intravenous atropine sulfate has an immediate effect on heart rate which reaches a peak in 2 to 16 minutes and lasts 170 minutes after an average 0.02 mg/kg dose.

Pharmacokinetics
Edrophonium chloride
Edrophonium chloride given intravenously shows first order elimination in a two compartment open pharmacokinetic model.[3] Onset of reversal of muscle relaxant induced depression in twitch tension occurs within three minutes. Edrophonium is primarily renally excreted with 67% of the dose appearing in the urine.[4] Hepatic metabolism and biliary excretion, have also been demonstrated in animals.[4,8] While infants and children have been shown to have a reduced plasma half-life and an increased clearance of edrophonium, doses in children are not significantly different from adults on a mg/kg basis although they are more variable in effect. Conversely, elderly subjects (>75 years old) have a prolonged plasma half-life and a reduced clearance. Studies have shown that in spite of these changes the onset and duration of action is unchanged in these patients.
[See table above.]

Atropine sulfate
Atropine sulfate given intravenously shows first order elimination in a two compartment open model.[7] Approximately 57% of a dose of atropine appears in the urine as unchanged drug. Tropine is the primary hepatic metabolite of atropine and it accounts for approximately 30% of the dose[2], Atropine is only 14 ± 9% bound to plasma proteins.[7] Atropine clearance in children under 2 years old and in the elderly is decreased in relation to normal healthy adult males.
[See table below.]

INDICATIONS AND USAGE
Enlon-Plus (edrophonium chloride, USP and atropine sulfate, USP) Injection is recommended as a reversal agent or antagonist of nondepolarizing neuromuscular blocking agents. It is not effective against depolarizing neuromuscular blocking agents. It is also useful if used adjunctively in the treatment of respiratory depression caused by curare overdosage.
The appropriateness of the specific fixed ratio of edrophonium and atropine contained in Enlon-Plus has not been evaluated in myasthenia gravis. Therefore, Enlon-Plus is not recommended for use in the differential diagnosis of this condition.

CONTRAINDICATIONS
Enlon-Plus (edrophonium chloride, USP and atropine sulfate, USP) Injection is not to be used in patients with known hypersensitivity to either of the components, or in patients with intestinal or urinary obstruction of mechanical type.

Atropine sulfate is contraindicated in the presence of acute glaucoma, adhesions (synchiae) between the iris and lens of the eye, and pyloric stenosis.

WARNINGS
Enlon-Plus (edophonium chloride, USP and atropine sulfate, USP) Injection should be used with caution in patients with bronchial asthma or cardiac arrhythmias. Cardiac arrest has been reported to occur in digitalized patients as well as in jaundiced subjects receiving cholinesterase inhibitors. In patients with cardiovascular disease, given anesthesia with narcotic and nitrous oxide without a potent inhalational agent, there is increased risk for clinically significant bradycardia. In patients receiving beta-adrenergic blocking agents there is increased risk for excessive bradycardia from unopposed parasympathetic vagal tone. Such patients should receive atropine sulfate alone prior to Enlon-Plus. Isolated instances of respiratory arrest have also been reported following the administration of edrophonium chloride. Additional atropine sulfate (1 mg) should be available for immediate use to counteract severe cholinergic reaction which may occur in hypersensitive individuals when Enlon-Plus is used.
Enlon-Plus contains sodium sulfite, a sulfite that may cause allergic-type reactions including anaphylactic symptoms and life-threatening or less severe asthmatic episodes in certain susceptible people. The overall prevalence of sulfite sensitivity in the general population is unknown and probably low. Sulfite sensitivity is seen more frequently in asthmatic than in nonasthmatic people.
There is a potential for tissue irritation by extravascular injection.

PRECAUTIONS
General: As with any antagonist of nondepolarizing muscle relaxants, adequate recovery of voluntary respiration and neuromuscular transmission must be obtained prior to the discontinuation of respiratory assistance. Should a patient develop "anticholinesterase insensitivity" for brief or prolonged periods, the patient should be carefully monitored and the dosage of anticholinesterase drugs reduced or withheld until the patient again becomes sensitive to them. Use with caution in patients with prostatic hypertrophy and in debilitated patients with chronic lung disease.
When used in therapeutic doses, atropine can cause dryness of the mouth. This effect is additive when the product is administered with other drugs that can cause dryness of the mouth.
Since atropine sulfate slows gastric emptying and gastrointestinal motility, it may interfere with the absorption of other medications. The effect of atropine on dryness of the mouth may be increased if it is given with other drugs that have anticholinergic action (tricyclic antidepressants, antipsychotics, some antihistamines, and antiparkinsonism drugs).

Drug Interactions: Enlon-Plus (edrophonium chloride, USP and atropine sulfate, USP) Injection should not be administered prior to the administration of any nondepolarizing muscle relaxants. It should be administered with caution to patients with symptoms of myasthenic weakness who are also on anticholinesterase drugs. Anticholinesterase overdosage (cholinergic crisis) symptoms may mimic underdosage (myasthenic weakness), so the use of this drug may worsen the condition of these patients (see OVERDOSAGE section for treatment).
Narcotic analgesics, except when combined with potent inhaled anesthetics, appear to potentiate the effect of edrophonium on the sinus node and conduction system, increasing both the frequency and duration of bradycardia. In patients with cardiovascular disease given anesthesia with narcotic and nitrous oxide without a potent inhalational agent, there is increased risk for clinically significant bradycardia. In patients receiving beta-adrenergic blocking agents there is increased risk for excessive bradycardia from unopposed parasympathetic vagal tone. Such patients should receive atropine sulfate alone prior to Enlon-Plus.
Compared to muscle relaxants with some vagolytic activity, muscle relaxants with no vagolytic effects, i.e. vecuronium, may be associated with a slightly higher incidence of vagotonic effects such as bradycardia and first-degree heart block when reversed with Enlon-Plus.

Pregnancy Category C: Animal reproduction studies have not been conducted with Enlon-Plus. It is also not known whether Enlon-Plus can cause fetal harm when administered to a pregnant woman or can affect reproduction capacity. Enlon-Plus should be used during pregnancy only if the potential benefit justifies the potential risk to the fetus.

Table of Pharmacokinetic Values for Atropine Sulfate

Population	T1/2β hr ± S.D.	VD L/kg ± S.D.	Cl mL/kg/min ± S.D.	N	Ref.
Adults	3.0 ± 0.9	1.6 ± 0.4	6.8 ± 2.9	8	7
Children (0.08–10 yrs)	4.8 ± 3.5	2.2 ± 1.5	6.4 ± 3.9	13	7
Elderly (65–75 yrs)	10.0 ± 7.3	1.8 ± 1.2	2.9 ± 1.9	10	7

T1/2β = Elimination half-life
VD = Volume of distribution
Cl = Clearance
* No dose adjustment required because the cardiovascular effect of atropine is diminished in the elderly.

Continued on next page

Anaquest—Cont.

Labor and Delivery: The effect of Enlon-Plus on the mother and fetus, on the duration of labor or delivery, in the possibility that a forceps delivery or other intervention or resuscitation of the newborn will be necessary, is not known. The effect of the combination drug on the later growth, development and functional maturation of the child is also unknown.
Nursing Mothers: The safety of Enlon-Plus during lactation in humans has not been established.
Pediatric Use: Safety and effectiveness in children have not been established. Pediatric patients may have increased vagal tone. The effect of fixed ratios of edrophonium and atropine on heart rate in such patients has not been evaluated.

ADVERSE REACTIONS

Cardiovascular: Arrhythmias Frequency >10%: junctional rhythm, bradycardia, tachycardia:
Frequency 3–10%: first and second degree A-V block, P Wave changes, atrial premature contractions.
Frequency 1–3%: third degree A-V block, ventricular premature contractions;
Frequency less than 1%: 3 second R-R interval.
Of the patients who experienced any arrhythmias, 85% had the onset within two minutes, 74% no longer had any arrhythmias after 10 minutes. Arrhythmias related to increased vagal tone, bradycardia, second and third degree heart block respond to treatment with 0.2–0.4 mg of atropine I.V. (Bigeminy or ventricular ectopy may be treated with lidocaine 50 mg I.V.).
Adverse experiences reported for anticholinesterase agents such as edrophonium chloride, but not observed in the 235 patients studied with Enlon-Plus (edrophonium chloride, USP and atropine sulfate, USP) Injection;
Cardiovascular: Nonspecific EKG changes, fall in cardiac output leading to hypotension;
Respiratory: Increased tracheobronchial secretions, laryngospasm, bronchiolar constriction and respiratory muscle paralysis;
Neurologic: Convulsions, dysarthria, dysphonia, and dysphagia;
Gastrointestinal: Nausea, vomiting, increased peristalsis, increased gastric and intestinal secretions, diarrhea, abdominal cramps;
Musculoskeletal: Weakness and fasciculations;
Miscellaneous: Increased urinary frequency, diaphoresis, increased lacrimation, pupillary constriction, diplopia, and conjunctival hyperemia.
Untoward reactions to atropine sulfate generally are dose-related. Individual tolerance varies greatly but systemic doses of 0.5 to 10 mg are likely to produce the following effects, which were not observed in the 235 patients treated with Enlon-Plus:
Neurologic: Speech disturbances and restlessness with asthenia;
Dermatologic: Flushed, dry skin, formation of a scarlatiniform rash;
Miscellaneous: Dryness of the nose and mouth, thirst, blurred vision, photophobia, slight mydriasis. Atropine may produce fever through inhibition of heat loss by evaporation.

OVERDOSAGE

Muscarinic symptoms (nausea, vomiting, diarrhea, sweating, increased bronchial and salivary secretions and bradycardia) may appear with overdosage (cholinergic crisis) of Enlon-Plus (edrophonium chloride, USP and atropine sulfate, USP) Injection, but may be managed by the use of additional atropine sulfate. Obstruction of the airway by bronchial secretions can arise and may be managed with suction (especially if tracheostomy has been performed).
Should edrophonium chloride overdosage occur:
1. Maintain respiratory exchange.
2. Monitor cardiac function.
Appropriate measures should be taken if convulsions occur or shock is present.
Principal manifestations of overdosage (poisoning) with atropine sulfate are delirium, tachycardia and fever. In the treatment of atropine poisoning, respiratory assistance and symptomatic support are indicated. Death is usually due to paralysis of the medullary centers.
In the clinical studies performed with Enlon-Plus (edrophonium chloride, USP and atropine sulfate, USP) Injection, there were no reported overdoses and therefore no clinical information is available regarding overdosing with Enlon-Plus.

DOSAGE AND ADMINISTRATION

Dosages of Enlon-Plus (edrophonium chloride, USP and atropine sulfate, USP) Injection range from 0.05–0.1 mL/kg given slowly over 45 seconds to 1 minute at a point of at least 5% recovery of twitch response to neuromuscular stimulation (95% block). The dosage delivered is 0.5–1.0 mg/kg of edrophonium chloride and 0.007–0.014 mg/kg of atropine sulfate. A total dosage of 1.0 mg/kg of edrophonium chloride should rarely be exceeded. Response should be monitored carefully and assisted or controlled ventilation secured. Satisfactory reversal permits adequate voluntary respiration and neuromuscular transmission (as tested with a peripheral nerve stimulator). Recurarization has not been reported after satisfactory reversal has been attained.
Parenteral drug products should be inspected visually for particulate matter and discoloration prior to administration.

HOW SUPPLIED

Enlon-Plus (edrophonium chloride, USP and atropine sulfate, USP) Injection should be stored between 15°–26°C (59°–78°F).
NDC 10019–195–05 5 mL ampuls, boxes of 10
NDC 10019–195–15 15 mL multidose vials
Caution: Federal (USA) law prohibits dispensing without prescription.

REFERENCES

1. Cronnelly R, Morris RB, Miller RD; Edrophonium: Duration of action and atropine requirement in humans during halothane anesthesia. Anesthesiology 1982;57:261–266.
2. Hinderling PH, Gundert-Remy U, Schmidlin O, Heinzel G: Integrated pharmacokinetics and pharmacodynamics of atropine in healthy humans. I: Pharmacokinetics; II: Pharmacodynamics. J Pharmaceutical Sci 1985;74:I–703–710; II–711–717.
3. Morris RB, Cronnelly R, Miller RD, Stanski DR, Fahey MR; Pharmacokinetics of edrophonium and neostigmine when antagonizing d-tubocurarine neuromuscular blockade in man. Anesthesiology 1981;54:399–402.
4. Morris RB, Cronnelly R, Miller RD, Stanski DR, Fahey MR: Pharmacokinetics of edrophonium in anephric and renal transplant patients. Br J Anaesth 1981;53:1311–1313.
5. Fisher DM, Cronnelly R, Sharma M, Miller RD; Clinical pharmacology of edrophonium in infants and children. Anesthesiology 1984; 61;428–433.
6. Silverberg PA, Matteo RS, Ornstein E, Young WL, Diaz J: Pharmacokinetics and pharmacodynamics of edrophonium in the elderly. Anesth Analg 1986;65:S142.
7. Virtanen R, Kanto J, Iisalo E, Iisalo EU, Salo M, Sjovall S: Pharmacokinetic studies on atropine with special reference to age. Acta Anaesthesiol Scand 1982;26:297–300.
8. Back DJ, Calvey TN; Excretion of ^{14}C-edrophonium and its metabolites in bile: role of the liver cell and the peribiliary vascular plexus. Br J Pharmacol, 1972; 44:534.

Mfd. for: Anaquest Inc, Liberty Corner, NJ 07938
A Subsidiary of BOC Health Care Inc
By: Taylor Pharmacal Co., Decatur, IL 62525
400–288 A-0528 11-91

ETHRANE® ℞

[ĕ'thrān]
(enflurane, USP)
Liquid For Inhalation

CAUTION: Federal Law Prohibits Dispensing without Prescription.

DESCRIPTION

ETHRANE (enflurane, USP), a nonflammable liquid administered by vaporizing, is a general inhalation anesthetic drug. It is 2-chloro-1,1,2-trifluoroethyl difluoromethyl ether (CHF_2OCF_2CHFCl). The boiling point is 56.5°C at 760 mm Hg, and the vapor pressure (in mm Hg) is 175 at 20°C, 218 at 25°C, and 345 at 36°C. Vapor pressures can be calculated using the equation:

$$\log_{10}P_{vap} = A + \frac{B}{T} \qquad A = 7.967,\quad B = -1678.4,\quad T = {}^{\circ}C + 273.16\ (\text{Kelvin})$$

The specific gravity (25°/25°C) is 1.517. The refractive index at 20°C is 1.3026–1.3030. The blood/gas coefficient is 1.91 at 37°C and the oil/gas coefficient is 98.5 at 37°C.
Enflurane is a clear, colorless, stable liquid whose purity exceeds 99.9% (area percent by gas chromatography). No stabilizers are added as these have been found, through controlled laboratory tests, to be unnecessary even in the presence of ultraviolet light. Enflurane is stable to strong base and does not decompose in contact with soda lime and does not react with aluminum, tin, brass, iron or copper. The partition coefficients of enflurane at 25°C are 74 in conductive rubber and 120 in polyvinyl chloride.

HOW SUPPLIED

ETHRANE (enflurane, USP) is packaged in 125 and 250 mL amber-colored bottles.
125 mL—NDC 10019-350-50
250 mL—NDC 10019-350-60
Storage: Store at room temperature 15–30°C (59–86°F). Enflurane contains no additives and has been demonstrated to be stable at room temperature for periods in excess of five years.

A-0408 Rev 5-87

FORANE® ℞

[for'ān]
(isoflurane, USP)
Liquid for Inhalation

CAUTION: Federal Law Prohibits Dispensing without Prescription.

DESCRIPTION

FORANE (isoflurane, USP) a nonflammable liquid administered by vaporizing, is a general inhalation anesthetic drug. It is 1-chloro-2,2,2-trifluoroethyl difluoromethyl ether, and its structural formula is:

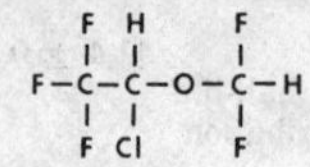

Some physical constants are:

Molecular weight	184.5
Boiling point at 760 mm Hg	48.5°C (uncorr.)
Refractive index n^{20}_D	1.2990–1.3005
Specific gravity 25°/25°C	1.496
Vapor pressure in mm Hg** 20°C	238
25°C	295
30°C	367
35°C	450

** Equation for vapor pressure calculation:

$$\log_{10}P_{vap} = A + \frac{B}{T} \quad \text{where: } A = 8.056,\quad B = -1664.58,\quad T = {}^{\circ}C + 273.16\ (\text{Kelvin})$$

Partition coefficients at 37°C	
Water/gas	0.61
Blood/gas	1.43
Oil/gas	90.8
Partition coefficients at 25°C—rubber and plastic	
Conductive rubber/gas	62.0
Butyl rubber/gas	75.0
Polyvinyl chloride/gas	110.0
Polyethylene/gas	~2.0
Polyurethane/gas	~1.4
Polyolefin/gas	~1.1
Butyl acetate/gas	~2.5
Purity by gas chromatography	>99.9%
Lower limit of flammability in oxygen or nitrous oxide at 9 joules/sec. and 23°C	None
Lower limit of flammability in oxygen or nitrous oxide at 900 joules/sec. and 23°C	Greater than useful concentration in anesthesia.

Isoflurane is a clear, colorless, stable liquid containing no additives or chemical stabilizers. Isoflurane has a mildly pungent, musty, ethereal odor. Samples stored in indirect sunlight in clear, colorless glass for five years, as well as samples directly exposed for 30 hours to a 2 amp, 115 volt, 60 cycle long wave U.V. light were unchanged in composition as determined by gas chromatography. Isoflurane in one normal sodium methoxide-methanol solution, a strong base, for over six months consumed essentially no alkali, indicative of strong base stability. Isoflurane does not decompose in the presence of soda lime, and does not attack aluminum, tin, brass, iron or copper.

CLINICAL PHARMACOLOGY

FORANE (isoflurane, USP) is an inhalation anesthetic. The MAC (minimum alveolar concentration) in man is as follows:

Age	100% Oxygen	70% N_2O
26 ± 4	1.28	0.56
44 ± 7	1.15	0.50
64 ± 5	1.05	0.37

Induction of and recovery from isoflurane anesthesia are rapid. Isoflurane has a mild pungency which limits the rate of induction, although excessive salivation or tracheobronchial secretions do not appear to be stimulated. Pharyngeal and laryngeal reflexes are readily obtunded. The level of anesthesia may be changed rapidly with isoflurane. Isoflurane is a profound respiratory depressant. RESPIRATION MUST BE MONITORED CLOSELY AND SUPPORTED WHEN NECESSARY. As anesthetic dose is increased, tidal volume decreases and respiratory rate is unchanged. This depression is partially reversed by surgical stimulation, even at deeper levels of anesthesia. Isoflurane evokes a sigh response reminiscent of that seen with diethyl ether and enflurane, although the frequency is less than with enflurane.
Blood pressure decreases with induction of anesthesia but returns toward normal with surgical stimulation. Progressive increases in depth of anesthesia produce corresponding decreases in blood pressure. Nitrous oxide diminishes the inspiratory concentration of isoflurane required to reach a desired level of anesthesia and may reduce the arterial hypotension seen with isoflurane alone. Heart rhythm is remarkably stable. With controlled ventilation and normal $PaCO_2$, cardiac output is maintained despite increasing depth of anesthesia primarily through an increase in heart rate

which compensates for a reduction in stroke volume. The hypercapnia which attends spontaneous ventilation during isoflurane anesthesia further increases heart rate and raises cardiac output above awake levels. Isoflurane does not sensitize the myocardium to exogenously administered epinephrine in the dog. Limited data indicate that subcutaneous injection of 0.25 mg of epinephrine (50 mL of 1:200,000 solution) does not produce an increase in ventricular arrhythmias in patients anesthetized with isoflurane.

Muscle relaxation is often adequate for intra-abdominal operations at normal levels of anesthesia. Complete muscle paralysis can be attained with small doses of muscle relaxants. ALL COMMONLY USED MUSCLE RELAXANTS ARE MARKEDLY POTENTIATED WITH ISOFLURANE, THE EFFECT BEING MOST PROFOUND WITH THE NONDEPOLARIZING TYPE. Neostigmine reverses the effect of nondepolarizing muscle relaxants in the presence of isoflurane. All commonly used muscle relaxants are compatible with isoflurane.

Isoflurane can produce coronary vasodilation at the arteriolar level in selected animal models[1,2]; the drug is probably also a coronary dilator in humans. Isoflurane, like some other coronary arteriolar dilators, has been shown to divert blood from collateral dependent myocardium to normally perfused areas in an animal model ("coronary steal")[3]. Clinical studies to date evaluating myocardial ischemia, infarction and death as outcome parameters have not established that the coronary arteriolar dilation property of isoflurane is associated with coronary steal or myocardial ischemia in patients with coronary artery disease[4,5,6,7].

Pharmacokinetics: Isoflurane undergoes minimal biotransformation in man. In the postanesthesia period, only 0.17% of the isoflurane taken up can be recovered as urinary metabolites.

INDICATIONS AND USAGE

FORANE (isoflurane, USP) may be used for induction and maintenance of general anesthesia. Adequate data have not been developed to establish its application in obstetrical anesthesia.

CONTRAINDICATIONS

Known sensitivity to FORANE (isoflurane, USP) or to other halogenated agents.

Known or suspected genetic susceptibility to malignant hyperthermia.

WARNINGS

Since levels of anesthesia may be altered easily and rapidly, only vaporizers producing predictable concentrations should be used. Hypotension and respiratory depression increase as anesthesia is deepened.

Increased blood loss comparable to that seen with halothane has been observed in patients undergoing abortions.

FORANE (isoflurane, USP) markedly increases cerebral blood flow at deeper levels of anesthesia. There may be a transient rise in cerebral spinal fluid pressure which is fully reversible with hyperventilation.

PRECAUTIONS

General: As with any potent general anesthetic, FORANE (isoflurane, USP) should only be administered in an adequately equipped anesthetizing environment by those who are familiar with the pharmacology of the drug and qualified by training and experience to manage the anesthetized patient.

Regardless of the anesthetics employed, maintenance of normal hemodynamics is important to the avoidance of myocardial ischemia in patients with coronary artery disease[4,5,6,7].

Information to Patients: Isoflurane, as well as other general anesthetics, may cause a slight decrease in intellectual function for 2 or 3 days following anesthesia. As with other anesthetics, small changes in moods and symptoms may persist for up to 6 days after administration.

Laboratory Tests: Transient increases in BSP retention, blood glucose and serum creatinine with decrease in BUN, serum cholesterol and alkaline phosphatase have been observed.

Drug Interactions: Isoflurane potentiates the muscle relaxant effect of all muscle relaxants, most notably nondepolarizing muscle relaxants, and MAC (minimum alveolar concentration) is reduced by concomitant administration of N_2O. See CLINICAL PHARMACOLOGY.

Carcinogenesis: Swiss ICR mice were given isoflurane to determine whether such exposure might induce neoplasia. Isoflurane was given at $\frac{1}{2}$, $\frac{1}{8}$ and $\frac{1}{32}$ MAC for four in-utero exposures and for 24 exposures to the pups during the first nine weeks of life. The mice were killed at 15 months of age. The incidence of tumors in these mice was the same as in untreated control mice which were given the same background gases, but not the anesthetic.

Pregnancy Category C: Isoflurane has been shown to have a possible anesthetic-related fetotoxic effect in mice when given in doses 6 times the human dose. There are no adequate and well-controlled studies in pregnant women. Isoflurane should be used during pregnancy only if the potential benefit justifies the potential risk to the fetus.

Nursing Mothers: It is not known whether this drug is excreted in human milk. Because many drugs are excreted in human milk, caution should be exercised when isoflurane is administered to a nursing woman.

Malignant Hyperthermia: In susceptible individuals, isoflurane anesthesia may trigger a skeletal muscle hypermetabolic state leading to high oxygen demand and the clinical syndrome known as malignant hyperthermia. The syndrome includes nonspecific features such as muscle rigidity, tachycardia, tachypnea, cyanosis, arrhythmias, and unstable blood pressure. (It should also be noted that many of these nonspecific signs may appear with light anesthesia, acute hypoxia, etc.) An increase in overall metabolism may be reflected in an elevated temperature (which may rise rapidly early or late in the case, but usually is not the first sign of augmented metabolism) and an increased usage of the CO_2 absorption system (hot canister). PaO_2 and pH may decrease, and hyperkalemia and a base deficit may appear. Treatment includes discontinuance of triggering agents (e.g., isoflurane), administration of intravenous dantrolene sodium, and application of supportive therapy. Such therapy includes vigorous efforts to restore body temperature to normal, respiratory and circulatory support as indicated, and management of electrolyte-fluid-acid-base derangements. (Consult prescribing information for dantrolene sodium intravenous for additional information on patient management.) Renal failure may appear later, and urine flow should be sustained if possible.

ADVERSE REACTION

Adverse reactions encountered in the administration of FORANE (isoflurane, USP) are in general dose dependent extensions of pharmacophysiologic effects and include respiratory depression, hypotension and arrhythmias.

Shivering, nausea, vomiting and ileus have been observed in the postoperative period.

As with all other general anesthetics, transient elevations in white blood count have been observed even in the absence of surgical stress.

See PRECAUTIONS for information regarding malignant hyperthermia.

OVERDOSAGE

In the event of overdosage, or what may appear to be overdosage, the following action should be taken:

Stop drug administration, establish a clear airway and initiate assisted or controlled ventilation with pure oxygen.

DOSAGE AND ADMINISTRATION

Premedication: Premedication should be selected according to the need of the individual patient, taking into account that secretions are weakly stimulated by FORANE (isoflurane, USP) and the heart rate tends to be increased. The use of anticholinergic drugs is a matter of choice.

Inspired Concentration: The concentration of isoflurane being delivered from a vaporizer during anesthesia should be known. This may be accomplished by using:

a) vaporizers calibrated specifically for isoflurane;
b) vaporizers from which delivered flows can be calculated, such as vaporizers delivering a saturated vapor which is then diluted. The delivered concentration from such a vaporizer may be calculated using the formula:

$$\%\ \text{isoflurane} = \frac{100\ P_V F_V}{F_T\,(P_A - P_V)}$$

where: P_A = Pressure of atmosphere
P_V = Vapor pressure of isoflurane
F_V = Flow of gas through vaporizer (mL/min)
F_T = Total gas flow (mL/min)

Isoflurane contains no stabilizer. Nothing in the agent alters calibration or operation of these vaporizers.

Induction: Induction with isoflurane in oxygen or in combination with oxygen-nitrous oxide mixtures may produce coughing, breath holding, or laryngospasm. These difficulties may be avoided by the use of a hypnotic dose of an ultra-short-acting barbiturate. Inspired concentrations of 1.5 to 3.0% isoflurane usually produce surgical anesthesia in 7 to 10 minutes.

Maintenance: Surgical levels of anesthesia may be sustained with a 1.0 to 2.5% concentration when nitrous oxide is used concomitantly. An additional 0.5 to 1.0% may be required when isoflurane is given using oxygen alone. If added relaxation is required, supplemental doses of muscle relaxants may be used.

The level of blood pressure during maintenance is an inverse function of isoflurane concentration in the absence of other complicating problems. Excessive decreases may be due to depth of anesthesia and in such instances may be corrected by lightening anesthesia.

HOW SUPPLIED

FORANE (isoflurane, USP), NDC 10019-360-40, is packaged in 100 mL amber-colored bottles.

Storage: Store at room temperature 15–30°C (59–86°F). Isoflurane contains no additives and has been demonstrated to be stable at room temperature for periods in excess of five years.

REFERENCES

1. JC Sill, et al. *Anesthesiology* 66:273–279, 1987.
2. RF Hickey, et al. *Anesthesiology* 68:21–30, 1988.
3. CW Buffington, et al. *Anesthesiology* 66:280–292, 1987.
4. S Reiz, et al. *Anesthesiology* 59:91–97, 1983.
5. S Slogoff and AS Keats. *Anesthesiology* 70:179–188, 1989.
6. KJ Tuman, et al. *Anesthesiology* 70:189–198, 1989.
7. DT Mangano, Editorial Views. *Anesthesiology* 70:175–178, 1989.

A-0491 Rev 2-90

EDUCATIONAL MATERIAL

Educational Resources

Anaquest offers a wide range of educational materials free of charge to physicians, nurse-anesthetists and hospital pharmacists. They are available from Anaquest representatives, by writing to: Anaquest Inc, 110 Allen Road, Box 804, Liberty Corner, NJ 07938-0804, or by calling "(800) ANA-DRUG".

Apothecon

A Bristol-Myers Squibb Company
P.O. BOX 4500
PRINCETON, NJ 08540-4500

For listing of standard, purified, and human insulins, see Novo Nordisk Pharmaceuticals Inc.

UNILOG®
(Tablet and Capsule Identification Code)
ALPHABETICAL INDEX

Unilog Number	Product
5040	**Atenolol Tablets** 50 mg
5240	**Atenolol Tablets** 100 mg
BL V1	**Betapen Tablets** (Penicillin V Potassium Tablets USP) 250 mg
BL V2	**Betapen Tablets** (Penicillin V Potassium Tablets USP) 500 mg
7375	**Cefanex Capsules** (Cephalexin Capsules USP) 250 mg
7376	**Cefanex Capsules** (Cephalexin Capsules USP) 500 mg
181	**Cephalexin Capsules USP** 250 mg
239	**Cephalexin Capsules USP** 500 mg
W028	**Cloxacillin Sodium Capsules USP** 250 mg
W038	**Cloxacillin Sodium Capsules USP** 500 mg
W048	**Dicloxacillin Sodium Capsules USP** 250 mg
W058	**Dicloxacillin Sodium Capsules USP** 500 mg
940	**Doxycycline Hyclate Capsules USP** 100 mg
674	**Doxycycline Hyclate Capsules USP** 50 mg
812	**Doxycycline Hyclate Tablets USP** 100 mg
7892	**Dynapen Capsules** (Dicloxacillin Sodium Capsules USP) 125 mg
7893	**Dynapen Capsules** (Dicloxacillin Sodium Capsules USP) 250 mg
7658	**Dynapen Capsules** (Dicloxacillin Sodium Capsules USP) 500 mg
429	**Florinef Tablets** Fludrocortisone Acetate Tablets USP) 0.1 mg
3506	**Kantrex Capsules** (Kanamycin Sulfate Capsules) 500 mg
BL 770	**Klotrix Tablets** (Potassium Chloride Tablets) 10 mEq
580	**Mycostatin Oral Tablets** (Nystatin Tablets USP) 500,000 u.
BL NI	**Naldecon Tablets**
606	**Naturetin Tablets** (Bendroflumethazide Tablets USP) 5 mg
618	**Naturetin Tablets** (Bendroflumethazide Tablets USP) 10 mg
611	**Niacin Tablets USP** 50 mg
612	**Niacin Tablets USP** 100 mg
537	**Niacin Tablets USP** 500 mg
7992	**Polycillin Capsules** (Ampicillin Capsules USP) 250 mg
7993	**Polycillin Capsules** (Ampicillin Capsules USP) 500 mg
7278	**Polymox Capsules** (Amoxacillin Capsules USP) 250 mg
7279	**Polymox Capsules** (Amoxacillin Capsules USP) 500 mg

Continued on next page

Apothecon—Cont.

7992	**Principen Capsules**	(Ampicillin Capsules USP) 250 mg
7993	**Principen Capsules**	(Ampicillin Capsules USP) 500 mg
1616	**Principen with Probenecid**	(Ampicillin with Probenecid Capsules)
863	**Prolixin Tablets**	(Fluphenazine Hydrochloride Tablets USP) 1 mg
864	**Prolixin Tablets**	(Fluphenazine Hydrochloride Tablets USP) 2.5 mg
877	**Prolixin Tablets**	(Fluphenazine Hydrochloride Tablets USP) 5 mg
956	**Prolixin Tablets**	(Fluphenazine Hydrochloride Tablets USP) 10 mg
758	**Pronestyl Capsules**	(Procainamide Hydrochloride Capsules USP) 250 mg
756	**Pronestyl Capsules**	(Procainamide Hydrochloride Capsules USP) 375 mg
757	**Pronestyl Capsules**	(Procainamide Hydrochloride Capsules USP) 500 mg
431	**Pronestyl Tablets**	(Procainamide Hydrochloride Tablets USP) 250 mg
434	**Pronestyl Tablets**	(Procainamide Hydrochloride Tablets USP) 375 mg
438	**Pronestyl Tablets**	(Procainamide Hydrochloride Tablets USP) 500 mg
775	**Pronestyl-SR Tablets**	(Procainamide Hydrochloride Tablets) 500 mg
7977	**Prostaphlin Capsules**	(Oxacillin Sodium Capsules USP) 250 mg
7982	**Prostaphlin Capsules**	(Oxacillin Sodium Capsules USP) 500 mg
576	**Quibron Capsules**	(Theophylline with Guiafenesin Capsules) 150 mg-90 mg
512	**Quibron-T Tablets**	(Theophylline Tablets USP)
519	**Quibron-T/SR Tablets**	(Theophylline Tablets Sustained Release)
713	**Raudixin Tablets**	(Rauwolfia Serpentina Tablets USP) 50 mg
776	**Raudixin Tablets**	(Rauwolfia Serpentina Tablets USP) 100 mg
769	**Rauzide Tablets**	(Rauwolfia Serpentina with Bendroflumethazide Tablets) 50 mg - 4 mg
BL S2	**Saluron Tablets**	(Hydroflumethiazide Tablets) 50 mg
BL S1	**Salutensin Tablets**	(Hydroflumethiazide with Reserpine Tablets) 50 mg - 0.125 mg
BL S3	**Salutensin-Demi Tablets**	(Hydroflumethiazide with Reserpine Tablets) 25 mg -0.125 mg
138	**SMZ/TMP Tablets**	(Sulfamethoxazole and Trimethoprim Tablets USP) 400 mg - 80 mg
171	**SMZ/TMP Tablets**	(Sulfamethoxazole and Trimethoprim Tablets USP) 800 mg - 160 mg
655	**Sumycin Capsules**	(Tetracycline Hydrochloride Capsules USP) 250 mg
763	**Sumycin Capsules**	(Tetracycline Hydrochloride Capsules USP) 500 mg
663	**Sumycin Tablets**	(Tetracycline Hydrochloride Tablets USP) 250 mg
603	**Sumycin Tablets**	(Tetracycline Hydrochloride Tablets USP) 500 mg
7936	**Tegopen Capsules**	(Cloxacillin Sodium Capsules USP) 250 mg
7496	**Tegopen Capsules**	(Cloxacillin Sodium Capsules USP) 500 mg
7278	**Trimox Capsules**	(Amoxicillin Capsules USP) 250 mg
7279	**Trimox Capsules**	(Amoxicillin Capsules USP) 500 mg
113	**Velosef '250' Capsules**	(Cephradine Capsules USP) 250 mg
114	**Velosef '500' Capsules**	(Cephradine Capsules USP) 500 mg

AMIKIN® ℞

[ah-mi'kin]

(amikacin sulfate) Injectable, 500 mg vial NSN
6505-01-033-0058 (M & VA)
Injectable, 1 g vial NSN 6505-01-056-1950 (M & VA)

WARNINGS

Patients treated with parenteral aminoglycosides should be under close clinical observation because of the potential ototoxicity and nephrotoxicity associated with their use. Safety for treatment periods which are longer than 14 days has not been established.

Neurotoxicity, manifested as vestibular and permanent bilateral auditory ototoxicity, can occur in patients with preexisting renal damage and in patients with normal renal function treated at higher doses and/or for periods longer than those recommended. The risk of aminoglycoside-induced ototoxicity is greater in patients with renal damage. High frequency deafness usually occurs first and can be detected only by audiometric testing. Vertigo may occur and may be evidence of vestibular injury. Other manifestations of neurotoxicity may include numbness, skin tingling, muscle twitching and convulsions. The risk of hearing loss due to aminoglycosides increases with the degree of exposure to either high peak or high trough serum concentrations. Patients developing cochlear damage may not have symptoms during therapy to warn them of developing eighth-nerve toxicity, and total or partial irreversible bilateral deafness may occur after the drug has been discontinued. Aminoglycoside-induced ototoxicity is usually irreversible.

Aminoglycosides are potentially nephrotoxic. The risk of nephrotoxicity is greater in patients with impaired renal function and in those who receive high doses or prolonged therapy.

Neuromuscular blockade and respiratory paralysis have been reported following parenteral injection, topical instillation (as in orthopedic and abdominal irrigation or in local treatment of empyema), and following oral use of aminoglycosides. The possibility of these phenomena should be considered if aminoglycosides are administered by any route, especially in patients receiving anesthetics, neuromuscular blocking agents such as tubocurarine, succinylcholine, decamethonium, or in patients receiving massive transfusions of citrate-anticoagulated blood. If blockage occurs, calcium salts may reverse these phenomena, but mechanical respiratory assistance may be necessary.

Renal and eighth-nerve function should be closely monitored especially in patients with known or suspected renal impairment at the onset of therapy and also in those whose renal function is initially normal but who develop signs of renal dysfunction during therapy. Serum concentrations of amikacin should be monitored when feasible to assure adequate levels and to avoid potentially toxic levels and prolonged peak concentrations above 35 µg per mL. Urine should be examined for decreased specific gravity, increased excretion of proteins, and the presence of cells or casts. Blood urea nitrogen, serum creatinine, or creatinine clearance should be measured periodically. Serial audiograms should be obtained where feasible in patients old enough to be tested, particularly high risk patients. Evidence of ototoxicity (dizziness, vertigo, tinnitus, roaring in the ears, and hearing loss) or nephrotoxicity requires discontinuation of the drug or dosage adjustment.

Concurrent and/or sequential systemic, oral or topical use of other neurotoxic or nephrotoxic products, particularly bacitracin, cisplatin, amphotericin B, cephaloridine, paromomycin, viomycin, polymyxin B, colistin, vancomycin, or other aminoglycosides should be avoided. Other factors that may increase risk of toxicity are advanced age and dehydration.

The concurrent use of AMIKIN with potent diuretics (ethacrynic acid, or furosemide) should be avoided since diuretics by themselves may cause ototoxicity. In addition, when administered intravenously, diuretics may enhance aminoglycoside toxicity by altering antibiotic concentrations in serum and tissue.

DESCRIPTION

Amikacin sulfate is a semisynthetic aminoglycoside antibiotic derived from kanamycin. It is $C_{22}H_{43}N_5O_{13} \cdot 2H_2SO_4$. D-Streptamine, 0-3-amino-3-deoxy-α-D-glucopyranosyl-(1 → 6)-0-[6-amino-6-deoxy-α-D-glucopyranosyl-(1 → 4)]-N¹-(4-amino-2-hydroxyl-1-oxobutyl)-2-deoxy-, (S)-, sulfate (1:2) (salt).

[See chemical structure at top of next column.]

The dosage form is supplied as a sterile, colorless to light straw colored solution. The 100 mg per 2 mL vial contains, in addition to amikacin sulfate, 0.13% sodium bisulfite and 0.5% sodium citrate with pH adjusted to 4.5 with sulfuric

acid. The 500 mg per 2 mL vial and the 1 gram per 4 mL vial contain 0.66% sodium bisulfite and 2.5% sodium citrate with pH adjusted to 4.5 with sulfuric acid.
Vial headspace contains nitrogen.

CLINICAL PHARMACOLOGY

Intramuscular Administration—AMIKIN is rapidly absorbed after intramuscular administration. In normal adult volunteers, average peak serum concentrations of about 12, 16, and 21 µg/mL are obtained 1 hour after intramuscular administration of 250-mg (3.7mg/kg), 375-mg (5 mg/kg), 500-mg (7.5 mg/kg), single doses, respectively. At 10 hours, serum levels are about 0.3 µg/mL, 1.2 µg/mL, and 2.1 µg/mL, respectively.

Tolerance studies in normal volunteers reveal that amikacin is well tolerated locally following repeated intramuscular dosing, and when given at maximally recommended doses, no ototoxicity or nephrotoxicity has been reported. There is no evidence of drug accumulation with repeated dosing for 10 days when administered according to recommended doses.

With normal renal function, about 91.9% of an intramuscular dose is excreted unchanged in the urine in the first 8 hours, and 98.2% within 24 hours. Mean urine concentrations for 6 hours are 563 µg/mL following a 250-mg dose, 697 µg/mL following a 375-mg dose, and 832 µg/mL following a 500-mg dose.

Preliminary intramuscular studies in newborns of different weights (less than 1.5 kg, 1.5 to 2.0 kg, over 2.0 kg) at a dose of 7.5 mg/kg revealed that, like other aminoglycosides, serum half-life values were correlated inversely with postnatal age and renal clearances of amikacin. The volume of distribution indicates that amikacin, like other aminoglycosides, remains primarily in the extracellular fluid space of neonates. Repeated dosing every 12 hours in all the above groups did not demonstrate accumulation after 5 days.

Intravenous Administration—Single doses of 500 mg (7.5 mg/kg) administered to normal adults as an infusion over a period of 30 minutes produced a mean peak serum concentration of 38 µg/mL at the end of the infusion, and levels of 24 µg/mL, 18 µg/mL, and 0.75 µg/mL at 30 minutes, 1 hour and 10 hours postinfusion, respectively. Eighty-four percent of the administered dose was excreted in the urine in 9 hours and about 94% within 24 hours.

Repeat infusions of 7.5 mg/kg every 12 hours in normal adults were well tolerated and caused no drug accumulation.

General—Pharmacokinetic studies in normal adult subjects reveal the mean serum half-life to be slightly over 2 hours with a mean total apparent volume of distribution of 24 liters (28% of the body weight). By the ultrafiltration technique, reports of serum protein binding range from 0% to 11%. The mean serum clearance rate is about 100 mL/min and the renal clearance rate is 94 mL/min in subjects with normal renal function.

Amikacin is excreted primarily by glomerular filtration. Patients with impaired renal function or diminished glomerular filtration pressure excrete the drug much more slowly (effectively prolonging the serum half-life). Therefore, renal function should be monitored carefully and dosage adjusted accordingly (see suggested dosage schedule under "Dosage and Administration").

Following administration at the recommended dose, therapeutic levels are found in bone, heart, gallbladder, and lung tissue in addition to significant concentrations in urine, bile, sputum, bronchial secretions, interstitial, pleural and synovial fluids.

Spinal fluid levels in normal infants are approximately 10% to 20% of the serum concentrations and may reach 50% when the meninges are inflamed. AMIKIN has been demonstrated to cross the placental barrier and yield significant concentrations in amniotic fluid. The peak fetal serum concentration is about 16% of the peak maternal serum concentration and maternal and fetal serum half-life values are about 2 and 3.7 hours, respectively.

Microbiology

Gram-negative—Amikacin is active in vitro against **Pseudomonas** species, **Escherichia coli**, **Proteus** species (indole-positive and indole-negative), **Providencia** species, **Klebsiella-Enterobacter-Serratia** species, **Acinetobacter** (formerly **Mima-Herellea**) species, and **Citrobacter freundii**.

When strains of the above organisms are found to be resistant to other aminoglycosides, including gentamicin, tobramycin and kanamycin, many are susceptible to amikacin in vitro.

Gram-positive—Amikacin is active in vitro against penicillinase and nonpenicillinase-producing **Staphylococcus** species including methicillin-resistant strains. However, aminoglycosides in general have a low order of activity against other Gram-positive organisms; viz, **Streptococcus pyogenes**, enterococci, and **Streptococcus pneumoniae** (formerly **Diplococcus pneumoniae**).

Amikacin resists degradation by most aminoglycoside inactivating enzymes known to affect gentamicin, tobramycin, and kanamycin.

In vitro studies have shown that AMIKIN combined with a beta-lactam antibiotic acts synergistically against many clinically significant gram-negative organisms.

Disc Susceptibility Tests—Quantitative methods that require measurement of zone diameters give the most precise estimates of antibiotic susceptibility. One such procedure* has been recommended for use with discs to test susceptibility to amikacin. Interpretation involves correlation of the diameters obtained in the disc test with MIC values for amikacin. When the causative organism is tested by the Kirby-Bauer method of disc susceptibility, a 30-µg amikacin disc should give a zone of 17 mm or greater to indicate susceptibility. Zone sizes of 14 mm or less indicate resistance. Zone sizes of 15 to 16 mm indicate intermediate susceptibility. With this procedure, a report from the laboratory of "susceptible" indicates that the infecting organism is likely to respond to therapy. A report of "resistant" indicates that the infecting organism is not likely to respond to therapy. A report of "intermediate susceptibility" suggests that the organism would be susceptible if the infection is confined to tissues and fluids (eg, urine) in which high antibiotic levels are attained.

INDICATIONS AND USAGE

AMIKIN is indicated in the short-term treatment of serious infections due to susceptible strains of Gram-negative bacteria, including **Pseudomonas** species, **Escherichia coli**, species of indole-positive and indole-negative **Proteus, Providencia** species, **Klebsiella-Enterobacter-Serratia** species, and **Acinetobacter (Mima-Herellea)** species.

Clinical studies have shown AMIKIN to be effective in bacterial septicemia (including neonatal sepsis); in serious infections of the respiratory tract, bones and joints, central nervous system (including meningitis) and skin and soft tissue; intra-abdominal infections (including peritonitis); and in burns and postoperative infections (including postvascular surgery). Clinical studies have shown AMIKIN also to be effective in serious complicated and recurrent urinary tract infections due to these organisms. Aminoglycosides, including AMIKIN injectable, are not indicated in uncomplicated initial episodes of urinary tract infections unless the causative organisms are not susceptible to antibiotics having less potential toxicity.

Bacteriologic studies should be performed to identify causative organisms and their susceptibilities to amikacin. AMIKIN may be considered as initial therapy in suspected Gram-negative infections and therapy may be instituted before obtaining the results of susceptibility testing. Clinical trials demonstrated that AMIKIN was effective in infections caused by gentamicin and/or tobramycin-resistant strains of Gram-negative organisms, particularly **Proteus rettgeri, Providencia stuartii, Serratia marcescens,** and **Pseudomonas aeruginosa.** The decision to continue therapy with the drug should be based on results of the susceptibility tests, the severity of the infection, the response of the patient and the important additional considerations contained in the "WARNINGS" box above.

AMIKIN has also been shown to be effective in staphylococcal infections and may be considered as initial therapy under certain conditions in the treatment of known or suspected staphylococcal disease such as, severe infections where the causative organism may be either a Gram-negative bacterium or a staphylococcus, infections due to susceptible strains of staphylococci in patients allergic to other antibiotics, and in mixed staphylococcal/Gram-negative infections. In certain severe infections such as neonatal sepsis, concomitant therapy with a penicillin-type drug may be indicated because of the possibility of infections due to Gram-positive organisms such as streptococci or pneumococci.

CONTRAINDICATIONS

A history of hypersensitivity to amikacin is a contraindication for its use. A history of hypersensitivity or serious toxic reactions to aminoglycosides may contraindicate the use of any other aminoglycoside because of the known cross-sensitivities of patients to drugs in this class.

WARNINGS

See "Warnings" box above.

Aminoglycosides can cause fetal harm when administered to a pregnant woman. Aminoglycosides cross the placenta and there have been several reports of total irreversible, bilateral congenital deafness in children whose mothers received streptomycin during pregnancy. Although serious side effects to the fetus or newborns have not been reported in the treatment of pregnant women with other aminoglycosides, the potential for harm exists. Reproduction studies of amika-

cin have been performed in rats and mice and revealed no evidence of impaired fertility or harm to the fetus due to amikacin. There are no well controlled studies in pregnant women, but investigational experience does not include any positive evidence of adverse effects to the fetus. If this drug is used during pregnancy, or if the patient becomes pregnant while taking this drug, the patient should be apprised of the potential hazard to the fetus.

Contains sodium bisulfite, a sulfite that may cause allergic-type reactions including anaphylactic symptoms and life-threatening or less severe asthmatic episodes in certain susceptible people. The overall prevalence of sulfite sensitivity in the general population is unknown and probably low. Sulfite sensitivity is seen more frequently in asthmatic than nonasthmatic people.

PRECAUTIONS

Aminoglycosides are quickly and almost totally absorbed when they are applied topically, except to the urinary bladder, in association with surgical procedures. Irreversible deafness, renal failure, and death due to neuromuscular blockade have been reported following irrigation of both small and large surgical fields with an aminoglycoside preparation.

AMIKIN is potentially nephrotoxic, ototoxic and neurotoxic. The concurrent or serial use of other ototoxic or nephrotoxic agents should be avoided either systemically or topically because of the potential for additive effects. Increased nephrotoxicity has been reported following concomitant parenteral administration of aminoglycoside antibiotics and cephalosporins. Concomitant cephalosporins may spuriously elevate creatinine determinations.

Since AMIKIN is present in high concentrations in the renal excretory system, patients should be well hydrated to minimize chemical irritation of the renal tubules. Kidney function should be assessed by the usual methods prior to starting therapy and daily during the course of treatment.

If signs of renal irritation appear (casts, white or red cells, or albumin), hydration should be increased. A reduction in dosage (see "Dosage and Administration") may be desirable if other evidence of renal dysfunction occurs such as decreased creatinine clearance; decreased urine specific gravity; increased BUN, creatinine, or oliguria. If azotemia increases or if a progressive decrease in urinary output occurs, treatment should be stopped.

Note: When patients are well hydrated and kidney function is normal the risk of nephrotoxic reactions with amikacin is low if the dosage recomendations (see "Dosage and Administration") are not exceeded.

Elderly patients may have reduced renal function which may not be evident in routine screening tests such as BUN or serum creatinine. A creatinine clearance determination may be more useful. Monitoring of renal function during treatment with aminoglycosides is particularly important.

Aminoglycosides should be used with caution in patients with muscular disorders such as myasthenia gravis or parkinsonism since these drugs may aggravate muscle weakness because of their potential curare-like effect on the neuromuscular junction.

In vitro mixing of aminoglycosides with beta-lactam antibiotics (penicillin or cephalosporins) may result in a significant mutual inactivation. A reduction in serum half-life or serum level may occur when an aminoglycoside or penicillin-type drug is administered by separate routes. Inactivation of the aminoglycoside is clinically significant only in patients with severely impaired renal function. Inactivation may continue in specimens of body fluids collected for assay, resulting in inaccurate aminoglycoside readings. Such specimens should be properly handled (assayed promptly, frozen, or treated with beta-lactamase).

Cross-allergenicity among aminoglycosides has been demonstrated.

As with other antibiotics, the use of amikacin may result in overgrowth of nonsusceptible organisms. If this occurs, appropriate therapy should be instituted.

Aminoglycosides should not be given concurrently with potent diuretics (See "Warnings" box).

Carcinogenesis, Mutagenesis, Impairment of Fertility—Long term studies in animals to evaluate carcinogenic potential have not been performed, and mutagenicity has not been studied. AMIKIN administered subcutaneously to rats at doses up to 4 times the human daily dose did not impair male or female fertility.

Pregnancy—Category D (See "Warnings" section).

Nursing Mothers—It is not known whether AMIKIN is excreted in human milk. Because many drugs are excreted in human milk and because of the potential for serious adverse reactions in nursing infants from AMIKIN, a decision should be made whether to discontinue nursing or to discontinue the drug, taking into account the importance of the drug to the mother.

PEDIATRIC USE—Aminoglycosides should be used with caution in premature and neonatal infants because of the renal immaturity of these patients and the resulting prolongation of serum half-life of these drugs.

ADVERSE REACTIONS

All aminoglycosides have the potential to induce auditory, vestibular, and renal toxicity and neuromuscular blockade (see "Warnings" box). They occur more frequently in patients with present or past history of renal impairment, of treatment with other ototoxic or nephrotoxic drugs, and in patients treated for longer periods and/or with higher doses than recommended.

Neurotoxicity-Ototoxicity—Toxic effects on the eighth cranial nerve can result in hearing loss, loss of balance, or both. Amikacin primarily affects auditory function. Cochlear damage includes high frequency deafness and usually occurs before clinical hearing loss can be detected.

Neurotoxicity-Neuromuscular Blockage—Acute muscular paralysis and apnea can occur following treatment with aminoglycoside drugs.

Nephrotoxicity—Elevation of serum creatinine, albuminuria, presence of red and white cells, casts, azotemia, and oliguria have been reported. Renal function changes are usually reversible when the drug is discontinued.

Other—In addition to those described above, other adverse reactions which have been reported on rare occasions are skin rash, drug fever, headache, paresthesia, tremor, nausea and vomiting, eosinophilia, arthralgia, anemia, and hypotension.

Overdosage—In the event of overdosage or toxic reaction, peritoneal dialysis or hemodialysis will aid in the removal of amikacin from the blood. In the newborn infant, exchange transfusion may also be considered.

DOSAGE AND ADMINISTRATION

The patient's pretreatment body weight should be obtained for calculation of correct dosage. AMIKIN may be given intramuscularly or intravenously.

The status of renal function should be estimated by measurement of the serum creatinine concentration or calculation of the endogenous creatinine clearance rate. The blood urea nitrogen (BUN) is much less reliable for this purpose. Reassessment of renal function should be made periodically during therapy.

Whenever possible, amikacin concentrations in serum should be measured to assure adequate but not excessive levels. It is desirable to measure both peak and trough serum

DOSAGE GUIDELINES				
ADULTS AND CHILDREN WITH NORMAL RENAL FUNCTION				
Patient Weight		**Dosage**		
lbs.	kg	7.5 mg/kg q. 12h	OR	5mg/kg q. 8h
99	45	337.5 mg		225 mg
110	50	375 mg		250 mg
121	55	412.5 mg		275 mg
132	60	450 mg		300 mg
143	65	487.5 mg		325 mg
154	70	525 mg		350 mg
165	75	562.6 mg		375 mg
176	80	600 mg		400 mg
187	85	637.5 mg		425 mg
198	90	675 mg		450 mg
209	95	712.5 mg		475 mg
220	100	750 mg		500 mg

Available as: 100 mg/2 mL vial, 500 mg/2 mL vial, 1g/4 mL vial, 500 mg/2 mL Disposable Syringe

Continued on next page

Apothecon—Cont.

concentrations intermittently during therapy. Peak concentrations (30 to 90 minutes after injection) above 35 μg per mL and trough concentrations (just prior to the next dose) above 10 μg per mL should be avoided. Dosage should be adjusted as indicated.

Intramuscular Administration for Patients with Normal Renal Function—The recommended dosage for adults, children and older infants (see "Warnings" box) with normal renal function is 15 mg/kg/day divided into 2 or 3 equal doses administered at equally-divided intervals, ie, 7.5 mg/kg q.12h or 5 mg/kg q.8h. Treatment of patients in the heavier weight classes should not exceed 1.5 g/day.

When amikacin is indicated in newborns (see "Warnings" box), it is recommended that a loading dose of 10 mg/kg be administered initially to be followed with 7.5 mg/kg every 12 hours.

The usual duration of treatment is 7 to 10 days. It is desirable to limit the duration of treatment to short term whenever feasible. The total daily dose by all routes of administration should not exceed 15 mg/kg/day. In difficult and complicated infections where treatment beyond 10 days is considered, the use of AMIKIN should be reevaluated. If continued, amikacin serum levels, and renal, auditory, and vestibular functions should be monitored. At the recommended dosage level, uncomplicated infections due to amikacin-sensitive organisms should respond in 24 to 48 hours. If definite clinical response does not occur within 3 to 5 days, therapy should be stopped and the antibiotic susceptibility pattern of the invading organism should be rechecked. Failure of the infection to respond may be due to resistance of the organism or to the presence of septic foci requiring surgical drainage.

When AMIKIN is indicated in uncomplicated urinary tract infections, a dose of 250 mg twice daily may be used.

[See table on preceding page.]

Intramuscular Administration for Patients with Impaired Renal Function—Whenever possible, serum amikacin concentrations should be monitored by appropriate assay procedures. Doses may be adjusted in patients with impaired renal function either by administering normal doses at prolonged intervals or by administering reduced doses at a fixed interval.

Both methods are based on the patient's creatinine clearance or serum creatinine values since these have been found to correlate with aminoglycoside half-lives in patients with diminished renal function. These dosage schedules must be used in conjunction with careful clinical and laboratory observations of the patient and should be modified as necessary. Neither method should be used when dialysis is being performed.

Normal Dosage at Prolonged Intervals—If the creatinine clearance rate is not available and the patient's condition is stable, a dosage interval in hours for the normal dose can be calculated by multiplying the patient's serum creatinine by 9; eg, if the serum creatinine concentration is 2 mg/100 mL, the recommended single dose (7.5 mg/kg) should be administered every 18 hours.

Reduced Dosage at Fixed Time Intervals—When renal function is impaired and it is desirable to administer AMIKIN at a fixed time interval, dosage must be reduced. In these patients, serum AMIKIN concentrations should be measured to assure accurate administration of AMIKIN and to avoid concentrations above 35 μg/mL. If serum assay determinations are not available and the patient's condition is stable, serum creatinine and creatinine clearance values are the most readily available indicators of the degree of renal impairment to use as a guide for dosage.

First, initiate therapy by administering a normal dose, 7.5 mg/kg, as a loading dose. This loading dose is the same as the normally recommended dose which would be calculated for a patient with a normal renal function as described above.

To determine the size of maintenance doses administered every 12 hours, the loading dose should be reduced in proportion to the reduction in the patient's creatinine clearance rate:

$$\text{Maintenance Dose Every 12 hours} = \frac{\text{observed CC in mL/min}}{\text{normal CC in mL/min}} \times \text{calculated loading dose in mg}$$

(CC—creatinine clearance rate)

An alternate rough guide for determining reduced dosage at 12-hour intervals (for patients whose steady state serum creatinine values are known) is to divide the normally recommended dose by the patient's serum creatinine.

The above dosage schedules are not intended to be rigid recommendations but are provided as guides to dosage when the measurement of amikacin serum levels is not feasible.

Intravenous Administration—The individual dose, the total daily dose, and the total cumulative dose of AMIKIN are identical to the dose recommended for intramuscular administration. The solution for intravenous use is prepared by adding the contents of a 0.5 gram vial to 100 to 200 mL of sterile diluent such as Normal Saline or 5% Dextrose in Water or any other compatible solutions listed below.

The solution is administered to adults over a 30 to 60 minute period. The total daily dose should not exceed 15 mg/kg/day and may be divided into either 2 or 3 equally-divided doses at equally-divided intervals.

In pediatric patients the amount of fluid used will depend on the amount ordered for the patient. It should be a sufficient amount to infuse the amikacin over a 30 to 60 minute period. Infants should receive a 1- to 2-hour infusion.

Stability in IV Fluids—AMIKIN is stable for 24 hours at room temperature at concentrations of 0.25 and 5.0 mg/mL in the following solutions:

5% Dextrose Injection, USP
5% Dextrose and 0.2% Sodium Chloride Injection, USP
5% Dextrose and 0.45% Sodium Chloride Injection, USP
0.9% Sodium Chloride Injection, USP
Lactated Ringer's Injection, USP
Normosol®M in 5% Dextrose Injection, USP (or Plasma-Lyte 56 Injection in 5% Dextrose in Water)
Normosol®R in 5% Dextrose Injection, USP (or Plasma-Lyte 148 Injection in 5% Dextrose in Water)

In the above solutions with AMIKIN concentrations of 0.25 and 5.0 mg/mL, solutions aged for 60 days at 4°C and then stored at 25°C had utility times of 24 hours.

At the same concentrations, solutions frozen and aged for 30 days at −15°C, thawed, and stored at 25°C had utility times of 24 hours.

Parenteral drug products should be inspected visually for particulate matter and discoloration prior to administration whenever the solution and container permit.

Aminoglycosides administered by any of the above routes should not be physically premixed with other drugs but should be administered separately.

Because of the potential toxicity of aminoglycosides, "fixed dosage" recommendations which are not based upon body weight are not advised. Rather, it is essential to calculate the dosage to fit the needs of each patient.

HOW SUPPLIED

AMIKIN is supplied as a colorless solution which requires no refrigeration. It is stable at room temperature for at least 2 years. At times the solution may become a very pale yellow; this does not indicate a decrease in potency.

AMIKIN (amikacin sulfate injection)
NDC 0015-3015-20—100 mg per 2 mL
NDC 0015-3020-20—500 mg per 2 mL
NDC 0015-3020-21—Disposable Syringe (500 mg per 2 mL)
NDC 0015-3023-20—1 gram per 4 mL

U.S. Patent Nos. 3,781,268, 4,424,343

*Bauer, A. W., Kirby, W. M. M., Sherris, J. C., and Turck, M.: Antibiotic Testing by a Standardized Single Disc Method, Am. J. Clin. Pathol. 45:493, 1966; Standardized Disc Susceptibility Test, FEDERAL REGISTER, 37:20527–29, 1972.

COLACE® OTC

[*kō'lās*]
docusate sodium, Apothecon
capsules • syrup • liquid (drops)
30 mL bottle NSN 6505-00-045-7786 (M)

PRODUCT OVERVIEW

KEY FACTS

Colace is a stool softener. This surface-active agent helps keep stools soft for easy, natural passage. Colace is not a laxative, thus, not habit forming. It is available in three forms: capsules, 50 mg and 100 mg; syrup, 20 mg/5 mL; liquid drops, 1% solution, 10 mg/mL.

MAJOR USES

Colace is useful in constipation due to hard stools in painful anorectal conditions, in cardiac and other conditions in which maximum ease of passage is desirable to avoid difficult or painful defecation, and when peristaltic stimulants are contraindicated.

SAFETY INFORMATION

There are no known contraindications to Colace. The incidence of side effects—none of a serious nature—is exceedingly small. As with any drug, if you are pregnant or nursing a baby, seek the advice of a health professional before using this product.

PRESCRIBING INFORMATION

COLACE®

[*kō' lās*]
docusate sodium, Apothecon
capsules • syrup • liquid (drops)

DESCRIPTION

Colace (docusate sodium) is a stool softener.

Colace Capsules, 50 mg, contain the following inactive ingredients: citric acid, D&C Red No. 33, FD&C Red No. 40, nonporcine gelatin, edible ink, polyethylene glycol, propylene glycol, and purified water.

Colace Capsules, 100 mg, contain the following inactive ingredients: citric acid, D&C Red No. 33, FD&C Red No. 40, FD&C Yellow No. 6, nonporcine gelatin, edible ink, polyethylene glycol, propylene glycol, titanium dioxide, and purified water.

Colace Liquid, 1%, contains the following inactive ingredients: citric acid, D&C Red No. 33, methylparaben, poloxamer, polyethylene glycol, propylene glycol, propylparaben, sodium citrate, vanillin, and purified water.

Colace Syrup, 20 mg/5 mL, contains the following inactive ingredients: alcohol (not more than 1%), citric acid, D&C Red No. 33, FD&C Red No. 40, flavor (natural), menthol, methylparaben, peppermint oil, poloxamer, polyethylene glycol, propylparaben, sodium citrate, sucrose, and purified water.

ACTIONS AND USES

Colace, a surface-active agent, helps to keep stools soft for easy, natural passage and is not a laxative, thus not habit forming. Useful in constipation due to hard stools, in painful anorectal conditions, in cardiac and other conditions in which maximum ease of passage is desirable to avoid difficult or painful defecation, and when peristaltic stimulants are contraindicated. *Note:* When peristaltic stimulation is needed due to inadequate bowel motility, see Peri-Colace® (laxative and stool softener).

CONTRAINDICATIONS

There are no known contraindications to Colace.

WARNING

As with any drug, if you are pregnant or nursing a baby, seek the advice of a health professional before using this product.

SIDE EFFECTS

The incidence of side effects—none of a serious nature—is exceedingly small. Bitter taste, throat irritation, and nausea (primarily associated with the use of the syrup and liquid) are the main side effects reported. Rash has occurred.

ADMINISTRATION AND DOSAGE

Orally —Suggested daily Dosage: *Adults and older children:* 50 to 200 mg. *Children 6 to 12:* 40 to 120 mg. *Children 3 to 6:* 20 to 60 mg. *Infants and children under 3:* 10 to 40 mg. The higher doses are recommended for initial therapy. Dosage should be adjusted to individual response. The effect on stools is usually apparent 1 to 3 days after the first dose. Give Colace liquid in half a glass of milk or fruit juice or in infant formula, to mask bitter taste. *In enemas* —Add 50 to 100 mg Colace (5 to 10 mL Colace liquid) to a retention or flushing enema.

HOW SUPPLIED

Colace® capsules, 50 mg
NDC 0087-0713-01 Bottles of 30
NDC 0087-0713-02 Bottles of 60
NDC 0087-0713-03 Bottles of 250
NDC 0087-0713-05 Bottles of 1000
NDC 0087-0713-07 Cartons of 100 single unit packs

Colace® capsules, 100 mg
NDC 0087-0714-01 Bottles of 30
NDC 0087-0714-02 Bottles of 60
NDC 0087-0714-03 Bottles of 250
NDC 0087-0714-05 Bottles of 1000
NDC 0087-0714-07 Cartons of 100 single unit packs

Note: Colace capsules should be stored at controlled room temperature (59°–86°F or 15°–30°C)

Colace® liquid, 1% solution; 10 mg/mL (with calibrated dropper)
NDC 0087-0717-04 Bottles of 16 fl oz
NDC 0087-0717-02 Bottles of 30 mL.
6505-00-045-7786 (Bottle of 30 mL) Defense

Colace® syrup, 20 mg/5-mL teaspoon; contains not more than 1% alcohol
NDC 0087-0720-01 Bottles of 8 fl oz
NDC 0087-0720-02 Bottles of 16 fl oz

FUNGIZONE® INTRAVENOUS ℞

[*fun'ji-zōn*]
Amphotericin B For Injection USP

DESCRIPTION

FUNGIZONE Intravenous (Amphotericin B for Injection) contains amphotericin B, an antifungal polyene antibiotic obtained from a strain of *Streptomyces nodosus.* Amphotericin B is designated chemically as [1R-(1R*, 3S*,5R*,6R*,9R*, 11R*, 15S*, 16R*, 17R*,18S*, 19E, 21E, 23E,25E,27E, 29E, 31E,33R*,35S*,36R*,37S*)] -33- [(3-Amino-3, 6-dideoxy-β-D-mannopyranosyl) -oxy]- 1,3,5,6,9,11,17,37 -octahydroxy-15,16, 18-trimethyl-13-oxo-14, 39-dioxabicyclo[33.3.1] nonatriaconta-19,21,23,25,27,29,31-heptaene-36-carboxylic acid.

	K-LYTE	K-LYTE DS	K-LYTE/CL	K-LYTE/CL 50
Potassium Chloride	—	—	1.5 g	2.24 g
Potassium Bicarbonate	2.5 g	2.5 g	0.5 g	2.0 g
Potassium Citrate	—	2.7 g	—	—
L-lysine Monohydrochloride	—	—	0.91 g	3.65 g
Citric Acid	2.1 g	2.1 g	0.55 g	1.0 g

Each vial contains a sterile, nonpyrogenic, lyophilized cake (which may partially reduce to powder following manufacture) providing 50 mg amphotericin B and 41 mg sodium desoxycholate with 20.2 mg sodium phosphates as a buffer. Crystalline amphotericin B is insoluble in water; therefore, the antibiotic is solubilized by the addition of sodium desoxycholate to form a mixture which provides a colloidal dispersion for intravenous infusion following reconstitution.

At the time of manufacture the air in the vial is replaced by nitrogen.

HOW SUPPLIED
FUNGIZONE Intravenous (Amphotericin B for Injection USP)
Available as single vials providing 50 mg amphotericin B as a yellow to orange lyophilized cake (which may partially reduce to powder following manufacture). NDC 0003-0437-30.

Storage
Prior to reconstitution FUNGIZONE Intravenous should be stored in the refrigerator, protected against exposure to light. The concentrate (5 mg amphotericin B per mL after reconstitution with 10 mL Sterile Water for Injection USP) may be stored in the dark, at room temperature for 24 hours, or at refrigerator temperatures for one week with minimal loss of potency and clarity. Any unused material should then be discarded. Solutions prepared for intravenous infusion (0.1 mg or less amphotericin B per mL) should be used promptly after preparation and should be protected from light during administration.

K–LYTE®
[k' lĭt]
Effervescent Tablets   ℞

Each tablet in solution provides 25 mEq (978 mg) potassium as bicarbonate and citrate.

K–LYTE® DS
Effervescent Tablets   ℞
Each tablet in solution provides 50 mEq (1955 mg) potassium as bicarbonate and citrate.

K–LYTE/CL®
Effervescent Tablets   ℞
Each tablet in solution provides the equivalent of 25 mEq (1865 mg) potassium chloride.

K–LYTE/CL® 50
Effervescent Tablets   ℞
Each tablet in solution provides the equivalent of 50 mEq (3730 mg) potassium chloride.

DESCRIPTION
[See table above.]
Inactive Ingredients: All of the K-LYTE line of effervescent tablets contain docusate sodium, natural and/or artificial flavors, light mineral oil, saccharin and talc.
K-LYTE and K-LYTE DS lime tablets, and K-LYTE/Cl and K-LYTE/Cl 50 citrus tablets have D&C Yellow No. 10. K-LYTE and K-LYTE DS orange tablets and K-LYTE/Cl and K-LYTE/Cl 50 fruit punch tablets have FD&C Yellow No. 6. K-LYTE orange and lime tablets have dextrose, and K-LYTE DS orange and lime tablets have lactose.
Note: This listing of inactive ingredients is a voluntary action of Pharmaceutical Manufacturers Association members.

HOW SUPPLIED
K-LYTE® Effervescent Tablets. Each tablet in solution provides 25 mEq (978 mg) potassium.
NDC 0087-0760-01 Lime flavor, Boxes of 30
NDC 0087-0760-43 Lime flavor, Boxes of 100
NDC 0087-0760-02 Lime flavor, Boxes of 250
NDC 0087-0761-01 Orange flavor, Boxes of 30
NDC 0087-0761-43 Orange flavor, Boxes of 100
NDC 0087-0761-02 Orange flavor, Boxes of 250
K-LYTE® DS Effervescent Tablets. Each tablet provides 50 mEq (1955 mg) potassium.

NDC 0087-0772-41 Lime flavor, Boxes of 30
NDC 0087-0772-42 Lime flavor, Boxes of 100
NDC 0087-0771-41 Orange flavor, Boxes of 30
NDC 0087-0771-42 Orange flavor, Boxes of 100
K-LYTE/CL® Effervescent Tablets. Each tablet in solution provides the equivalent of 25 mEq (1865 mg) potassium chloride.
NDC 0087-0766-41 Citrus flavor, Boxes of 30
NDC 0087-0766-43 Citrus flavor, Boxes of 100
NDC 0087-0766-42 Citrus flavor, Boxes of 250
NDC 0087-0767-41 Fruit Punch flavor, Boxes of 30
NDC 0087-0767-43 Fruit Punch flavor, Boxes of 100
NDC 0087-0767-42 Fruit Punch flavor, Boxes of 250
K-LYTE/CL® 50 mEq Effervescent Tablets. Each tablet in solution provides the equivalent of 50 mEq (3730 mg) potassium chloride.
NDC 0087-0757-41 Fruit Punch flavor, Boxes of 30
NDC 0087-0757-42 Fruit Punch flavor, Boxes of 100
NDC 0087-0758-41 Citrus flavor, Boxes of 30
NDC 0087-0758-42 Citrus flavor, Boxes of 100
Store Below 86°F (30°C).
U.S. Patent No. 3,970,750

KLOTRIX®   ℞
[klō'trix]
(potassium chloride)
Slow-Release Tablets 10 mEq (750 mg)

DESCRIPTION
KLOTRIX is a solid, oral dosage form of potassium chloride containing 750 mg of potassium chloride, USP (equivalent to 10 mEq of potassium) in a film-coated wax-matrix tablet. This formulation is intended to provide a controlled release of potassium from the matrix to minimize the likelihood of producing high, localized concentrations of potassium within the gastrointestinal tract.
KLOTRIX is an electrolyte replenisher. The chemical name is potassium chloride, and the structural formula is KCl. Potassium chloride, USP, occurs as a white, granular powder or as colorless crystals. It is odorless and has a saline taste. Its solutions are neutral to litmus. It is freely soluble in water and insoluble in alcohol.
This product contains the following inactive ingredients: ethylcellulose, FD&C Yellow No. 6 (aluminum lake), glycerin, hydroxypropyl methylcellulose 2910, edible ink, magnesium stearate, povidone, colloidal silicon dioxide, stearic acid, and titanium dioxide.

HOW SUPPLIED
Tablets (light orange, film-coated) each containing 750 mg potassium chloride (equivalent to 10 mEq each potassium and chloride).

NDC 0087-0770-41   Bottles of 100
NDC 0087-0770-42   Bottles of 1000
NDC 0087-0770-43   Cartons of 100
     individually wrapped tablets
U.S. Patent No. 4,140,756
Do not store at temperatures above 86°F (30°C).

MUCOMYST®   ℞
(ACETYLCYSTEINE)

DESCRIPTION
MUCOMYST brand of acetylcysteine is for inhalation (mucolytic agent) or oral administration (acetaminophen antidote), and available as sterile, unpreserved solutions (not for injection). These solutions contain 20% (MUCOMYST) or 10% (MUCOMYST-10) acetylcysteine, with disodium edetate in purified water. Sodium hydroxide is added to adjust pH to 7. Acetylcysteine is the N-acetyl derivative of the naturally-occurring amino acid, cysteine. The compound is a white crystalline powder with the molecular formula $C_5H_9NO_3S$, a molecular weight of 163.2, and a chemical name of N-acetyl-L-cysteine. Acetylcysteine has the following structural formula:

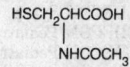

$$HSCH_2CHCOOH$$
$$|$$
$$NHCOCH_3$$

This product contains the following inactive ingredients: disodium edetate, sodium hydroxide, and purified water.

HOW SUPPLIED
MUCOMYST® 20% acetylcysteine solution (200 mg acetylcysteine per mL).[1] Sterile, not for injection.
NDC 0087-0570-03   Cartons of three 10 mL vials, 1 plastic dropper
NDC 0087-0570-09   Cartons of three 30 mL vials.
NDC 0087-0570-07   Cartons of twelve 4 mL vials.
MUCOMYST®-10 10% acetylcysteine solution (100 mg acetylcysteine per mL).[1] Sterile, not for injection.
NDC 0087-0572-01   Cartons of three 10 mL vials, 1 plastic dropper
NDC 0087-0572-02   Cartons of three 30 mL vials.
NDC 0087-0572-03   Cartons of twelve 4 mL vials.
[1] For inhalation (mucolytic agent) or oral administration (acetaminophen antidote).

STORAGE REQUIREMENTS
Store unopened vials at controlled room temperature, 59° to 86°F (15° to 30°C).

REFERENCES
A bibliography on MUCOMYST will be supplied on request by specific subject.

NALDECON®   ℞
[nal'dĕ-côn]
Tablets, Syrup, Pediatric Drops
and Pediatric Syrup
For Oral Use Only
Pediatric Syrup, 16 oz bottle NSN 6505-01-094-1974 (M)

DESCRIPTION
NALDECON is a preparation containing:
(1) phenylpropanolamine hydrochloride
    Benzenemethanol, α-(1-aminoethyl)-hydrochloride

	For immediate action	For delayed action	Total contents
Each sustained-action tablet contains:			
Phenylpropanolamine hydrochloride	20.0 mg	20.0 mg	40.0 mg
Phenylephrine hydrochloride	5.0 mg	5.0 mg	10.0 mg
Phenyltoloxamine citrate	7.5 mg	7.5 mg	15.0 mg
Chlorpheniramine maleate	2.5 mg	2.5 mg	5.0 mg
Each teaspoonful (5 mL) of syrup contains:			
Phenylpropanolamine hydrochloride			20.0 mg
Phenylephrine hydrochloride			5.0 mg
Phenyltoloxamine citrate			7.5 mg
Chlorpheniramine maleate			2.5 mg

	Pediatric Syrup each 5 mL contains:	Pediatric Drops each 1 mL contains:
Each pediatric formulation contains the following ingredients:		
Phenylpropanolamine hydrochloride	5.0 mg	5.0 mg
Phenylephrine hydrochloride	1.25 mg	1.25 mg
Phenyltoloxamine citrate	2.0 mg	2.0 mg
Chlorpheniramine maleate	0.5 mg	0.5 mg

Continued on next page

Apothecon—Cont.

(2) phenylephrine hydrochloride
1-m-hydroxy-α-[(methylamino)methyl]benzyl alcohol hydrochloride

(3) phenyltoloxamine citrate
N,N- dimethyl-2(alpha phenyl -ortho- toloxy)-ethylamine citrate

(4) chlorpheniramine maleate
2-[p-chloro-α-[2-(dimethylamino)ethyl]benzyl]pyridine maleate

Inactive ingredients in NALDECON tablets are: acacia, FD&C Red No. 3, gelatin, lactose, magnesium stearate, polyethylene glycol 8000, starch, sucrose, carnauba wax, and white wax.
Inactive ingredients in NALDECON syrup, pediatric syrup, and pediatric drops are D&C Red No. 33, D&C Yellow No. 10, natural and artificial flavor, glycerin, povidone, purified water, sodium benzoate and sorbitol.
[See table on preceding page.]

HOW SUPPLIED
NDC 0015-5600—NALDECON Tablets
NDC 0015-5601—NALDECON Syrup
NDC 0015-5615—NALDECON Pediatric Drops
NDC 0015-5616—NALDECON Pediatric Syrup
For information on package sizes available, refer to the current price schedule.
BRISTOL, NALDECON and the distinctive speckled tablets are trademarks.

PERI-COLACE® capsules • syrup OTC
[*peri-kō 'lās*]
(casanthranol and docusate sodium)

PRODUCT OVERVIEW

KEY FACTS
Peri-Colace is a combination of the mild stimulant laxative casanthranol and the stool softener Colace® (docusate sodium). This product provides gentle peristaltic stimulation and helps to keep stools soft for easier passage. It is available in two forms: capsules and syrup.

MAJOR USES
Peri-Colace is useful in the management of chronic or temporary constipation.

SAFETY INFORMATION
Do not use Peri-Colace when abdominal pain, nausea, or vomiting are present. Frequent or prolonged use of this preparation may result in dependence on laxatives.
As with any drug, if you are pregnant or nursing a baby, seek the advice of a health professional before using this product.

PRESCRIBING INFORMATION

PERI-COLACE® capsules • syrup
[*peri-kō 'las*]
(casanthranol and docusate sodium)

DESCRIPTION
Peri-Colace is a combination of the mild stimulant laxative casanthranol and the stool-softener Colace (docusate sodium). Each capsule contains 30 mg of casanthranol and 100 mg of Colace; the syrup contains 30 mg of casanthranol and 60 mg of Colace per 15-mL tablespoon (10 mg of casanthranol and 20 mg of Colace per 5-mL teaspoon) and 10% alcohol.
Peri-Colace Capsules contain the following inactive ingredients: D&C Red No. 33, FD&C Red No. 40, nonporcine gelatin, edible ink, polyethylene glycol, propylene glycol, titanium dioxide, and purified water.
Peri-Colace Syrup contains the following inactive ingredients: alcohol (10% v/v), citric acid, flavors, methyl salicylate, methylparaben, poloxamer, polyethylene glycol, propylparaben, sodium citrate, sorbitol solution, sucrose, and purified water.

ACTION AND USES
Peri-Colace provides gentle peristaltic stimulation and helps to keep stools soft for easier passage. Bowel movement is induced gently—usually overnight or in 8 to 12 hours. Nausea, griping, abnormally loose stools, and constipation rebound are minimized. Useful in management of chronic or temporary constipation.
Note: To prevent hard stools when laxative stimulation is not needed or undesirable, see Colace (stool softener).

WARNINGS
Do not use when abdominal pain, nausea, or vomiting are present. Frequent or prolonged use of this preparation may result in dependence on laxatives.
As with any drug, if you are pregnant or nursing a baby, seek the advice of a health professional before using this product.

SIDE EFFECTS
The incidence of side effects—none of a serious nature—is exceedingly small. Nausea, abdominal cramping or discomfort, diarrhea, and rash are the main side effects reported.

ADMINISTRATION AND DOSAGE
Adults —1 or 2 capsules, or 1 or 2 tablespoons syrup at bedtime, or as indicated. In severe cases, dosage may be increased to 2 capsules or 2 tablespoons twice daily, or 3 capsules at bedtime. *Children* —1 to 3 teaspoons of syrup at bedtime, or as indicated.

OVERDOSAGE
In addition to symptomatic treatment, gastric lavage, if timely, is recommended in cases of large overdosage.

HOW SUPPLIED
Peri-Colace® Capsules
NDC 0087-0715-01 Bottles of 30
NDC 0087-0715-02 Bottles of 60
NDC 0087-0715-03 Bottles of 250
NDC 0087-0715-05 Bottles of 1000
NDC 0087-0715-07 Cartons of 100 single unit packs
Note: Peri-Colace capsules should be stored at controlled room temperatures (59°-86°F or 15°- 30°C).
Peri-Colace® Syrup
NDC 0087-0721-01 Bottles of 8 fl oz
NDC 0087-0721-02 Bottles of 16 fl oz

POLYMOX® ℞
TRIMOX®
(Amoxicillin, USP)
CAPSULES
250 mg and 500 mg
FOR ORAL SUSPENSION
125 mg per 5 mL, 250 mg per 5 mL
PEDIATRIC DROPS
50 mg per mL

DESCRIPTION
POLYMOX and TRIMOX (amoxicillin, USP), [2S- [2α,5α, 6β (S*)]]-6- [[amino(4-hydroxyphenyl)-acetyl]amino]-3,3-dimethyl-7-oxo-4-thia-1-azabicyclo[3.2.0] heptane-2-carboxylic acid trihydrate, is a semisynthetic penicillin, an analogue of ampicillin. It is an antibacterial agent with a broad spectrum of bactericidal activity against Gram-positive organisms and many Gram-negative pathogens. It has the following chemical structure:

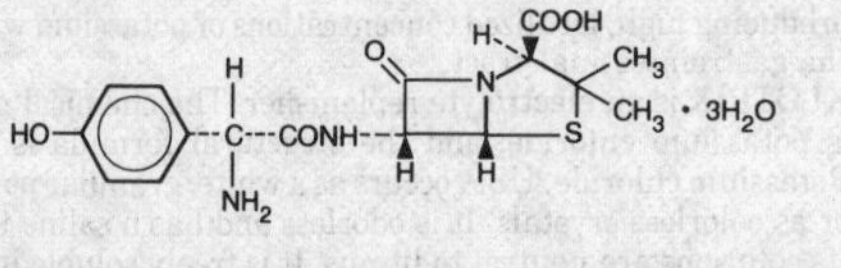

The empirical formula is $C_{16}H_{19}N_3O_5S \cdot 3H_2O$, and the molecular weight is 419.45.
The capsules contain amoxicillin trihydrate equivalent to 250 mg or 500 mg of amoxicillin, respectively. Each 5 mL of reconstituted oral suspension contains amoxicillin trihydrate equivalent to 125 mg or 250 mg of amoxicillin, respectively. Each 1 mL of the reconstituted pediatric drops contains amoxicillin trihydrate equivalent to 50 mg of amoxicillin.
Inactive ingredient in POLYMOX capsules is: magnesium stearate. Inactive ingredients in POLYMOX for oral suspension and pediatric drops are: acacia, Atmos 300, DC antifoam AF emulsion, FD&C Red No. 40, lecithin, natural & artificial flavorings, silicon dioxide colloidal, sodium benzoate, sodium citrate, and sucrose.
Inactive ingredient in TRIMOX capsules is: magnesium stearate. Inactive ingredients in TRIMOX for oral suspension are: acacia, Atmos 300, DC antifoam AF emulsion, FD&C Red No. 40, lecithin, natural & artificial flavorings, silicon dioxide colloidal, sodium benzoate, sodium citrate, and sucrose.

CLINICAL PHARMACOLOGY
POLYMOX and TRIMOX are stable in the presence of gastric acid and is well absorbed from the gastrointestinal tract and may be given with no regard to food. It diffuses readily into most body tissues and fluids, with the exception of brain and spinal fluid, except when meninges are inflamed. The half-life of amoxicillin is 61.3 minutes. Most of the amoxicillin is excreted unchanged in the urine; its excretion can be delayed by concurrent administration of probenecid. Amoxicillin is not highly protein-bound. In blood serum, amoxicillin is approximately 20% protein-bound as compared to 60% for penicillin G.
Orally administered doses of 250 mg and 500 mg amoxicillin capsules result in average peak blood levels one to two hours after administration in the range of 3.5 to 5.0 μg/mL and 5.5 to 7.5 μg/mL, respectively.
Orally administered doses of amoxicillin suspension, 125 mg/5 mL and 250 mg/5 mL, result in average peak blood levels one to two hours after administration in the range of 1.5 to 3.0 μg/mL and 3.5 to 5.0 μg/mL, respectively.
Detectable serum levels are observed up to 8 hours after an orally administered dose of amoxicillin. Approximately 60 percent of an orally administered dose of amoxicillin is excreted in the urine within six to eight hours.
Microbiology: POLYMOX and TRIMOX are similar to ampicillin in its bactericidal action against susceptible organisms during the stage of active multiplication. It acts through the inhibition of biosynthesis of cell wall mucopeptides. While **in vitro** studies have demonstrated the susceptibility of most strains of the following organisms, clinical efficacy for infections other than those included in the **INDICATIONS AND USAGE** section has not been documented.
In vitro studies have demonstrated the susceptibility of most strains of the following Gram-positive bacteria: alpha and beta-hemolytic streptococci, **Diplococcus pneumoniae,** non-penicillinase-producing staphylococci, and **Streptococcus faecalis.** It is active **in vitro** against many strains of **Haemophilus influenzae, Neisseria gonorrhoeae, Escherichia coli,** and **Proteus mirabilis.** Because it does not resist destruction by penicillinase, it is **not** effective against penicillinase-producing bacteria, particularly resistant staphylococci. All strains of Pseudomonas and most strains of Klebsiella and Enterobacter are resistant.
Susceptibility Tests: Susceptibility tests should be performed according to the standards set forth by the National Committee for Clinical Laboratory Standards for the susceptibility testing for ampicillin class antibiotics. A full description of the methods may be found in "Performance Standards for Antimicrobial Disk Susceptibility Tests", 3rd Edition, National Committee for Clinical Laboratory Standards, Vol. 4, No. 16.

INDICATIONS AND USAGE
POLYMOX and TRIMOX (amoxicillin, USP) are indicated in the treatment of infections caused by susceptible strains of the designated organisms in the conditions listed below:
Venereal Disease: Amoxicillin is indicated for the treatment of uncomplicated infections (urethral, endocervical or rectal) due to **N. gonorrhoeae** in males and females.
Upper Respiratory Tract Infections caused by nonpenicillinase-producing staphylococci, **Streptococci sp.,** and **H. influenzae.** Amoxicillin is indicated for treating otitis media caused by **H. influenzae.**
Urinary Tract Infections caused by **E. coli, Proteus mirabilis,** and **Streptococcus faecalis.**
Skin and Skin Structure Infections caused by nonpenicillinase-producing **Staphylococcus sp.** and **Escherichia coli.**
Therapy may be instituted prior to obtaining results from bacteriological and susceptibility studies to determine the causative organisms and their susceptibility to amoxicillin. Indicated surgical procedures should be performed.

CONTRAINDICATIONS
A history of a previous hypersensitivity reaction to any of the penicillins is a contraindication.

WARNINGS
Serious and occasionally fatal hypersensitivity (anaphylactoid) reactions have been reported in patients on penicillin therapy. Although anaphylaxis is more frequent following parenteral therapy, it has occurred in patients on oral penicillins. These reactions are more apt to occur in individuals with a history of penicillin hypersensitivity and/or a history of sensitivity to multiple allergens.
There have been well documented reports of individuals with a history of penicillin hypersensitivity reactions who have experienced severe hypersensitivity reactions when treated with a cephalosporin. Before initiating therapy with any penicillin, careful inquiry should be made concerning previous hypersensitivity reactions to penicillins, cephalosporins, and other allergens. If an allergic reaction occurs, POLYMOX should be discontinued and the appropriate therapy instituted.
SERIOUS ANAPHYLACTOID REACTIONS REQUIRE IMMEDIATE EMERGENCY TREATMENT WITH EPINEPHRINE. OXYGEN, INTRAVENOUS STEROIDS, AND AIRWAY MANAGEMENT, INCLUDING INTUBATION, SHOULD ALSO BE ADMINISTERED AS INDICATED.

PRECAUTIONS
General: The possibility of superinfections with mycotic organisms or bacterial pathogens should be kept in mind during therapy. In such cases, discontinue the drug and substitute appropriate treatment.
Laboratory Tests: As with any potent drug, periodic assessment of organ system function, including renal, hepatic, and hematopoietic should be made during prolonged therapy.
Cases of gonorrhea with a suspected lesion of syphilis should have darkfield examinations before receiving amoxicillin, and monthly serological tests for a minimum of four months.

Carcinogenesis, Mutagenesis, and Impairment of Fertility: Long-term studies in animals have not been performed with these drugs.

Pregnancy Category B: Reproduction studies have been performed in mice and rats at doses up to ten (10) times the human dose and have revealed no evidence of impaired fertility or harm to the fetus due to amoxicillin. There are, however, no adequate and well-controlled studies in pregnant women. Because animal reproduction studies are not always predictive of human response, this drug should be used during pregnancy only if clearly needed.

Labor and Delivery: Oral ampicillin-class antibiotics are poorly absorbed during labor. Studies in guinea pigs showed that intravenous administration of ampicillin slightly decreased the uterine tone and frequency of contractions, but moderately increased the height and duration of contractions. However, it is not known whether use of these drugs in humans during labor or delivery has immediate or delayed adverse effects on the fetus, prolongs the duration of labor, or increases the likelihood that forceps delivery or other obstetrical intervention or resuscitation of the newborn will be necessary.

Nursing Mothers: POLYMOX is excreted in human milk in very small amounts. Therefore caution should be exercised when amoxicillin is administered to a nursing woman.

Pediatric Use: Guidelines for administration of POLYMOX to pediatric patients are presented in **DOSAGE AND ADMINISTRATION.**

ADVERSE REACTIONS

As with other penicillins, it may be expected that untoward reactions will be essentially limited to sensitivity phenomena. They are more likely to occur in individuals who have previously demonstrated hypersensitivity to penicillins and in those with a history of allergy, asthma, hay fever, or urticaria.

The following adverse reactions have been reported as associated with the use of penicillin:

GASTROINTESTINAL: Glossitis, stomatitis, black "hairy" tongue, nausea, vomiting, and diarrhea. (These reactions are usually associated with oral dosage forms.)

HYPERSENSITIVITY REACTIONS: Skin rashes and urticaria have been reported frequently. A few cases of exfoliative dermatitis and erythema multiforme have been reported. Anaphylaxis is the most serious reaction experienced and has usually been associated with the parenteral dosage form.

NOTE: Urticaria, other skin rashes, and serum sickness-like reactions may be controlled with antihistamines and, if necessary, systemic corticosteroids. Whenever such reactions occur, penicillin should be discontinued unless, in the opinion of the physician, the condition being treated is life threatening and amenable only to penicillin therapy. Serious anaphylactic reactions require the immediate use of epinephrine, oxygen, and intravenous steroids.

LIVER: A moderate rise in serum glutamic oxaloacetic transaminase (SGOT) has been noted, particularly in infants, but the significance of this finding is unknown.

HEMIC AND LYMPHATIC SYSTEMS: Anemia, thrombocytopenia, thrombocytopenic purpura, eosinophilia, leukopenia, and agranulocytosis have been reported during therapy with the penicillins. These reactions are usually reversible on discontinuation of therapy and are believed to be hypersensitivity phenomena.

OVERDOSAGE

In case of overdosage, discontinue medication, treat symptomatically and institute supportive measures as required. Amoxicillin can be removed from circulation by hemodialysis.

DOSAGE AND ADMINISTRATION

Infections of the ear, nose, and throat due to streptococci, pneumococci, nonpenicillinase-producing staphylococci, and **H. influenzae:**

Infections of the genitourinary tract due to **E. coli, Proteus mirabilis,** and **Streptococcus faecalis;**

Infections of the skin and soft tissues due to streptococci, susceptible staphylococci, and **E. coli:**

Usage Dosage: Adults—250 mg every 8 hours.

Children—20 mg/kg/day in divided doses every 8 hours. Children weighing 20 kg or more should be dosed according to the adult recommendations.

In severe infections or those caused by less susceptible organisms: 500 mg every 8 hours for adults, and 40 mg/kg/day in divided doses every 8 hours for children may be needed.

Infections of the lower respiratory tract, due to streptococci, pneumococci, nonpenicillinase-producing staphylococci, and **H. influenzae:**

Usual Dosage: Adults—500 mg every 8 hours.

Children—40 mg/kg/day in divided doses every 8 hours. Children weighing 20 kg or more should be dosed according to the adult recommendations.

Larger doses may be required for stubborn or severe infections.

The children's dosage is intended for individuals whose weight will not cause a dosage to be calculated greater than that recommended for adults.

Gonorrhea, acute uncomplicated ano-genital and urethral infections due to **N. gonorrhoeae:** (males and females) 3 grams as a single oral dose.

Cases of gonorrhea with a suspected lesion of syphilis should have darkfield examinations before receiving amoxicillin, and monthly serological tests for a minimum of four months. It should be recognized that in the treatment of chronic urinary tract infections, frequent bacteriological and clinical appraisals are necessary. Smaller doses than those recommended above should not be used. Even higher doses may be needed at times. In stubborn infections, therapy may be required for several weeks. It may be necessary to continue clinical and/or bacteriological followup for several months after cessation of therapy. Except for gonorrhea, treatment should be continued for a minimum of 48 to 72 hours beyond the time that the patient becomes asymptomatic or evidence of bacterial eradication has been obtained. It is recommended that there be at least 10-days treatment for any infection caused by hemolytic streptococci to prevent the occurrence of acute rheumatic fever or glomerulonephritis.

Dosage and Administration of Pediatric Drops: Usual dosage for all indications except infections of the lower respiratory tract:

    Under 6 kg (13 lbs): 0.5 mL every 8 hours

    6 to 8 kg (13 to 18 lbs): 1 mL every 8 hours

Infections of the lower respiratory tract:

    Under 6 kg (13 lbs): 1 mL every 8 hours

    6 to 8 kg (13 to 18 lbs): 2 mL every 8 hours

Children weighing more than 8 kg (18 lbs) should receive the appropriate dose of the Oral Suspension 125 mg or 250 mg/5 mL.

After reconstitution, the required amount of suspension should be placed directly on the child's tongue for swallowing. Alternate means of administration are to add the required amount of suspension to formula, milk, fruit juice, water, ginger ale, or cold drinks. These preparations should then be taken immediately. To be certain the child is receiving full dosage, such preparations should be consumed in entirety.

DIRECTIONS FOR DISPENSING ORAL SUSPENSION AND PEDIATRIC DROPS

Prepare these formulations at the time of dispensing. For ease in preparation, add water to the bottle in two portions and shake well after each addition. Add the total amount of water as directed on the labeling of the package being dispensed.

The reconstituted formulation is stable for 14 days at either room temperature or refrigeration.

HOW SUPPLIED

POLYMOX (amoxicillin Capsules, USP). Each capsule contains amoxicillin trihydrate equivalent to 250 or 500 mg amoxicillin.

250 mg Capsules

NDC 0015-7278-60 Bottles of 100 NDC 0015-7278-80 Bottle of 500

NDC 0015-7278-66 Carton of 100 Unit Doses

500 mg Capsules

NDC 0015-7279-50 Bottle of 50

NDC 0015-7279-60 Bottle of 100

NDC 0015-7279-80 Bottle of 500

NDC 0015-7279-66 Carton of 100 Unit Doses

POLYMOX (amoxicillin for Oral Suspension, USP). Each 5 mL of reconstituted suspension contains amoxicillin trihydrate equivalent to 125 or 250 mg amoxicillin.

125 mg/5 mL

NDC 0015-7276-35 80 mL Bottle

NDC 0015-7276-41 100 mL Bottle

NDC 0015-7276-50 150 mL Bottle

NDC 0015-7276-79 Carton of 25 Unit Doses (5 mL)

250 mg/5 mL

NDC 0015-7277-35 80 mL Bottle

NDC 0015-7277-41 100 mL Bottle

NDC 0015-7277-50 150 mL Bottle

NDC 0015-7277-79 Carton of 25 Unit Doses (5 mL)

POLYMOX (amoxicillin for Oral Suspension, USP). Each mL of reconstituted pediatric drops contains amoxicillin trihydrate equivalent to 50 mg amoxicillin.

NDC 0015-7277-16 15 mL Bottle

TRIMOX (amoxicillin Capsules, USP). Each capsule contains amoxicillin trihydrate equivalent to 250 or 500 mg amoxicillin.

250 mg Capsules

NDC 0003-0101-50 Bottle of 100

NDC 0003-0101-60 Bottle of 500

NDC 0003-0101-51 Carton of 100 Unit Doses

500 mg Capsules

NDC 0003-0109-45 Bottle of 50

NDC 0003-0109-60 Bottle of 500

NDC 0003-0109-51 Carton of 100 Unit Doses

TRIMOX (amoxicillin for Oral Suspension, USP). Each 5 mL of reconstituted suspension contains amoxicillin trihydrate equivalent to 125 or 250 mg amoxicillin.

125 mg/5 mL

NDC 0003-1737-30 80 mL Bottle

NDC 0003-1737-40 100 mL Bottle

NDC 0003-1737-45 150 mL Bottle

NDC 0003-1737-25 Carton of 25 Unit Doses (5 mL)

250 mg/5 mL

NDC 0003-1738-30 80 mL Bottle

NDC 0003-1738-40 100 mL Bottle

NDC 0003-1738-45 150 mL Bottle

NDC 0003-1738-25 Carton of 25 Unit Doses (5 mL)

PROLIXIN® INJECTION ℞
Fluphenazine Hydrochloride Injection USP
FOR INTRAMUSCULAR USE ONLY

PROLIXIN® ORAL CONCENTRATE ℞
Fluphenazine Hydrochloride Oral Solution USP

PROLIXIN® TABLETS ℞
Fluphenazine Hydrochloride Tablets USP

PROLIXIN® ELIXIR ℞
Fluphenazine Hydrochloride Elixir USP

PROLIXIN DECANOATE® ℞
Fluphenazine Decanoate Injection USP

PROLIXIN ENANTHATE® ℞
Fluphenazine Enanthate Injection USP

DESCRIPTION

PROLIXIN is a trifluoromethyl phenothiazine derivative intended for the management of schizophrenia. PROLIXIN Injection (Fluphenazine Hydrochloride Injection) is available in multiple dose vials providing 2.5 mg fluphenazine hydrochloride per mL. The preparation also includes sodium chloride for isotonicity, sodium hydroxide or hydrochloric acid to adjust the pH to 4.8–5.2, and 0.1% methylparaben and 0.01% propylparaben as preservatives. At the time of manufacture, the air in the vials is replaced by nitrogen.

PROLIXIN Oral Concentrate (Fluphenazine Hydrochloride Oral Solution) contains 5 mg fluphenazine hydrochloride per mL. Inactive ingredients: alcohol 14%, glycerin, purified water, and sodium benzoate.

PROLIXIN Tablets (Fluphenazine Hydrochloride Tablets) contain 1, 2.5, 5, and 10 mg fluphenazine hydrochloride per tablet. Inactive ingredients: acacia; carnauba wax for 1 and 2.5 mg only; castor oil; colorants [D&C Yellow No. 10 for 5 and 10 mg only; FD&C Blue No. 1 for 5 and 10 mg only; FD&C Blue No. 2 for 2.5 mg only; FD&C Red No. 3 for 1 and 10 mg only; and FD&C Yellow No. 5 (tartrazine) for 2.5, 5, and 10 mg only]; corn starch; ethylcellulose; gelatin; lactose; magnesium carbonate; magnesium stearate; pharmaceutical glaze; polyethylene glycol for 1 and 2.5 mg only; povidone for 1 and 2.5 mg only; precipitated calcium carbonate; sodium benzoate for 1, 2.5, and 5 mg only; sucrose; synthetic iron oxide; talc; titanium dioxide; white wax for 1 and 2.5 mg only; and other ingredients.

PROLIXIN Elixir (Fluphenazine Hydrochloride Elixir) contains 0.5 mg fluphenazine hydrochloride per mL. Inactive ingredients: alcohol [14% (v/v)], colorant (FD&C Yellow No. 6), flavors, glycerin, polysorbate 40, purified water, sodium benzoate, and sucrose.

PROLIXIN DECANOATE is the decanoate ester of a trifluoromethyl phenothiazine derivative. It is a highly potent behavior modifier with a markedly extended duration of effect. PROLIXIN DECANOATE is available for intramuscular or subcutaneous administration, providing 25 mg fluphenazine decanoate per mL in a sesame oil vehicle with 1.2% (w/v) benzyl alcohol as a preservative. At the time of manufacture, the air in the vials is replaced by nitrogen.

PROLIXIN ENANTHATE (Fluphenazine Enanthate Injection) is an esterified trifluoromethyl phenothiazine derivative, chemically designated as 2-[4-[3-[2-(Trifluoromethyl)-phenothiazin-10-yl]propyl]-1-piperazinyl]ethyl heptanoate. It is a highly potent behavior modifier with a markedly extended duration of effect. PROLIXIN ENANTHATE is available for intramuscular or subcutaneous administration, providing 25 mg fluphenazine enanthate per mL in a sesame oil vehicle with 1.5% (w/v) benzyl alcohol as a preservative. At the time of manufacture, the air in the vials is replaced by nitrogen.

CLINICAL PHARMACOLOGY

PROLIXIN has activity at all levels of the central nervous system as well as on multiple organ systems. The mechanism whereby its therapeutic action is exerted is unknown.

The basic effects of fluphenazine decanoate appear to be no different from those of fluphenazine hydrochloride, with the exception of duration of action. The esterification of fluphenazine markedly prolongs the drug's duration of effect without unduly attenuating its beneficial action.

The basic effects of fluphenazine enanthate appear to be no different from those of fluphenazine hydrochloride, with the exception of duration of action. The esterification of fluphenazine markedly prolongs the drug's duration of effect with-

Continued on next page

Apothecon—Cont.

out unduly attenuating its beneficial action. The onset of action generally appears between 24 to 72 hours after injection, and the effects of the drug on psychotic symptoms become significant within 48 to 96 hours. Amelioration of symptoms then continues for one to three weeks or longer, with an average duration of effect of about two weeks.

Fluphenazine differs from other phenothiazine derivatives in several respects: it is more potent on a milligram basis, it has less potentiating effect on central nervous system depressants and anesthetics than do some of the phenothiazines and appears to be less sedating, and it is less likely than some of the older phenothiazines to produce hypotension (nevertheless, appropriate cautions should be observed—see sections on PRECAUTIONS and ADVERSE REACTIONS).

INDICATIONS AND USAGE

PROLIXIN is indicated in the management of manifestations of psychotic disorders.

Prolixin Decanoate (Fluphenazine Decanoate Injection) is a long-acting parenteral antipsychotic drug intended for use in the management of patients requiring prolonged parenteral neuroleptic therapy (e.g., chronic schizophrenics).

Prolixin Enanthate is a long-acting parenteral antipsychotic drug intended for use in the management of patients requiring prolonged parenteral neuroleptic therapy (e.g., chronic schizophrenics).

PROLIXIN has not been shown effective in the management of behavorial complications in patients with mental retardation.

CONTRAINDICATIONS

Phenothiazines are contraindicated in patients with suspected or established subcortical brain damage, in patients receiving large doses of hypnotics, and in comatose or severely depressed states. The presence of blood dyscrasia or liver damage precludes the use of fluphenazine decanoate, enanthate, or hydrochloride. PROLIXIN is contraindicated in patients who have shown hypersensitivity to fluphenazine; cross-sensitivity to phenothiazine derivatives may occur.

Fluphenazine decanoate and fluphenazine enanthate are not intended for use in children under 12 years of age.

WARNINGS

Tardive Dyskinesia

Tardive dyskinesia, a syndrome consisting of potentially irreversible, involuntary, dyskinetic movements may develop in patients treated with neuroleptic (antipsychotic) drugs. Although the prevalence of the syndrome appears to be highest among the elderly, especially elderly women, it is impossible to rely upon prevalence estimates to predict, at the inception of neuroleptic treatment, which patients are likely to develop the syndrome. Whether neuroleptic drug products differ in their potential to cause tardive dyskinesia is unknown.

Both the risk of developing the syndrome and the likelihood that it will become irreversible are believed to increase as the duration of treatment and the total cumulative dose of neuroleptic drugs administered to the patient increase. However, the syndrome can develop, although much less commonly, after relatively brief treatment periods at low doses. There is no known treatment for established cases of tardive dyskinesia, although the syndrome may remit, partially or completely, if neuroleptic treatment is withdrawn. Neuroleptic treatment, itself, however, may suppress (or partially suppress) the signs and symptoms of the syndrome and thereby may possibly mask the underlying disease process. The effect that symptomatic suppression has upon the long-term course of the syndrome is unknown.

Given these considerations, neuroleptics should be prescribed in a manner that is most likely to minimize the occurrence of tardive dyskinesia. Chronic neuroleptic treatment should generally be reserved for patients who suffer from a chronic illness that, 1) is known to respond to neuroleptic drugs, and, 2) for whom alternative, equally effective, but potentially less harmful treatments are *not* available or appropriate. In patients who do require chronic treatment, the smallest dose and the shortest duration of treatment producing a satisfactory clinical response should be sought. The need for continued treatment should be reassessed periodically.

If signs and symptoms of tardive dyskinesia appear in a patient on neuroleptics, drug discontinuation should be considered. However, some patients may require treatment despite the presence of the syndrome.

(For further information about the description of tardive dyskinesia and its clinical detection, please refer to the sections on PRECAUTIONS, Information for Patients and ADVERSE REACTIONS, Tardive Dyskinesia.)

Neuroleptic Malignant Syndrome (NMS)

A potentially fatal symptom complex sometimes referred to as Neuroleptic Malignant Syndrome (NMS) has been reported in association with antipsychotic drugs. Clinical manifestations of NMS are hyperpyrexia, muscle rigidity,

altered mental status and evidence of autonomic instability (irregular pulse or blood pressure, tachycardia, diaphoresis, and cardiac dysrhythmias).

The diagnostic evaluation of patients with this syndrome is complicated. In arriving at a diagnosis, it is important to identify cases where the clinical presentation includes both serious medical illness (e.g., pneumonia, systemic infection, etc.) and untreated or inadequately treated extrapyramidal signs and symptoms (EPS). Other important considerations in the differential diagnosis include central anticholinergic toxicity, heat stroke, drug fever and primary central nervous system (CNS) pathology.

The management of NMS should include: 1) immediate discontinuation of antipsychotic drugs and other drugs not essential to concurrent therapy; 2) intensive symptomatic treatment and medical monitoring; and 3) treatment of any concomitant serious medical problems for which specific treatments are available. There is no general agreement about specific pharmacological treatment regimens for uncomplicated NMS.

If a patient requires antipsychotic drug treatment after recovery from NMS, the potential reintroduction of drug therapy should be carefully considered. The patient should be carefully monitored, since recurrences of NMS have been reported.

The use of this drug may impair the mental and physical abilities required for driving a car or operating heavy machinery.

Physicians should be alert to the possibility that severe adverse reactions may occur which require immediate medical attention.

Potentiation of the effects of alcohol may occur with the use of this drug.

Since there is no adequate experience in children who have received this drug, safety and efficacy in children have not been established.

Usage in Pregnancy

The safety for the use of this drug during pregnancy has not been established; therefore, the possible hazards should be weighed against the potential benefits when administering this drug to pregnant patients.

PRECAUTIONS

General

Because of the possibility of cross-sensitivity, fluphenazine should be used cautiously in patients who have developed cholestatic jaundice, dermatoses or other allergic reactions to phenothiazine derivatives.

PROLIXIN Tablets (Fluphenazine Hydrochloride Tablets) 2.5, 5, and 10 mg contain FD&C Yellow No. 5 (tartrazine) which may cause allergic-type reactions (including bronchial asthma) in certain susceptible individuals. Although the overall incidence of FD&C Yellow No. 5 (tartrazine) sensitivity in the general population is low, it is frequently seen in patients who also have aspirin hypersensitivity.

Psychotic patients on large doses of a phenothiazine drug who are undergoing surgery should be watched carefully for possible hypotensive phenomena. Moreover, it should be remembered that reduced amounts of anesthetics or central nervous system depressants may be necessary.

The effects of atropine may be potentiated in some patients receiving fluphenazine because of added anticholinergic effects.

Fluphenazine should be used cautiously in patients exposed to extreme heat or phosphorus insecticides; in patients with a history of convulsive disorders, since grand mal convulsions have been known to occur; and in patients with special medical disorders, such as mitral insufficiency or other cardiovascular diseases and pheochromocytoma.

The possibility of liver damage, pigmentary retinopathy, lenticular and corneal deposits, and development of irreversible dyskinesia should be remembered when patients are on prolonged therapy.

Neuroleptic drugs elevate prolactin levels; the elevation persists during chronic administration. Tissue culture experiments indicate that approximately one-third of human breast cancers are prolactin dependent *in vitro*, a factor of potential importance if the prescription of these drugs is contemplated in a patient with a previously detected breast cancer. Although disturbances such as galactorrhea, amenorrhea, gynecomastia, and impotence have been reported, the clinical significance of elevated serum prolactin levels is unknown for most patients. An increase in mammary neoplasms has been found in rodents after chronic administration of neuroleptic drugs. Neither clinical studies nor epidemiologic studies conducted to date, however, have shown an association between chronic administration of these drugs and mammary tumorigenesis; the available evidence is considered too limited to be conclusive at this time.

Information for Patients

Given the likelihood that some patients exposed chronically to neuroleptics will develop tardive dyskinesia, it is advised that all patients in whom chronic use is contemplated be given, if possible, full information about this risk. The decision to inform patients and/or their guardians must obvi-

ously take into account the clinical circumstances and the competency of the patient to understand the information provided.

Abrupt Withdrawal

In general, phenothiazines do not produce psychic dependence; however, gastritis, nausea and vomiting, dizziness, and tremulousness have been reported following abrupt cessation of high dose therapy. Reports suggest that these symptoms can be reduced if concomitant antiparkinsonian agents are continued for several weeks after the phenothiazine is withdrawn.

Outside state hospitals or other psychiatric institutions, fluphenazine decanoate or enanthate should be administered under the direction of a physician experienced in the clinical use of psychotropic drugs, particularly phenothiazine derivatives.

Facilities should be available for periodic checking of hepatic function, renal function and the blood picture. Renal function of patients on long-term therapy should be monitored; if BUN (blood urea nitrogen) becomes abnormal, treatment should be discontinued.

As with any phenothiazine, the physician should be alert to the possible development of "silent pneumonias" in patients under treatment with fluphenazine.

ADVERSE REACTIONS

Central Nervous System: The side effects most frequently reported with phenothiazine compounds are extrapyramidal symptoms including pseudoparkinsonism, dystonia, dyskinesia, akathisia, oculogyric crises, opisthotonos, and hyperreflexia. Muscle rigidity sometimes accompanied by hyperthermia has been reported following use of fluphenazine decanoate. Most often these extrapyramidal symptoms are reversible; however, they may be persistent (see below). The frequency of such reactions is related in part to chemical structure: one can expect a higher incidence with fluphenazine decanoate or enanthate than with less potent piperazine derivatives or with straight-chain phenothiazines such as chlorpromazine. With any given phenothiazine derivative, the incidence and severity of such reactions depend more on individual patient sensitivity than on other factors, but dosage level and patient age are also determinants.

Extrapyramidal reactions may be alarming, and the patient should be forewarned and reassured. These reactions can usually be controlled by administration of antiparkinsonian drugs such as Benztropine Mesylate or intravenous Caffeine and Sodium Benzoate Injection, and by subsequent reductions in dosage.

Tardive Dyskinesia: See WARNINGS. The syndrome is characterized by involuntary choreoathetoid movements which variously involve the tongue, face, mouth, lips, or jaw (e.g., protrusion of the tongue, puffing of cheeks, puckering of the mouth, chewing movements), trunk and extremities. The severity of the syndrome and the degree of impairment produced vary widely.

The syndrome may become clinically recognizable either during treatment, upon dosage reduction, or upon withdrawal of treatment. Early detection of tardive dyskinesia is important. To increase the likelihood of detecting the syndrome at the earliest possible time, the dosage of neuroleptic drug should be reduced periodically (if clinically possible) and the patient observed for signs of the disorder. This maneuver is critical, since neuroleptic drugs may mask the signs of the syndrome.

Other CNS Effects: Occurrences of neuroleptic malignant syndrome (NMS) have been reported in patients on neuroleptic therapy (see WARNINGS, Neuroleptic Malignant Syndrome). Leukocytosis, elevated CPK, liver function abnormalities, and acute renal failure may also occur with NMS. Drowsiness or lethargy, if they occur, may necessitate a reduction in dosage; the induction of a catatonic-like state has been known to occur with dosages of fluphenazine far in excess of the recommended amounts. As with other phenothiazine compounds, reactivation or aggravation of psychotic processes may be encountered.

Phenothiazine derivatives have been known to cause, in some patients, restlessness, excitement, or bizarre dreams.

Autonomic Nervous System: Hypertension and fluctuations in blood pressure have been reported with fluphenazine. Hypotension has rarely presented a problem with fluphenazine. However, patients with pheochromocytoma, cerebral vascular or renal insufficiency, or a severe cardiac reserve deficiency (such as mitral insufficiency) appear to be particularly prone to hypotensive reactions with phenothiazine compounds, and should therefore be observed closely when the drug is administered. If severe hypotension should occur, supportive measures including the use of intravenous vasopressor drugs should be instituted immediately. Levarterenol Bitartrate Injection is the most suitable drug for this purpose; *epinephrine should not be used* since phenothiazine derivatives have been found to reverse its action, resulting in a further lowering of blood pressure.

Autonomic reactions including nausea and loss of appetite, salivation, polyuria, perspiration, dry mouth, headache, and

constipation may occur. Autonomic effects can usually be controlled by reducing or temporarily discontinuing dosage. In some patients, phenothiazine derivatives have caused blurred vision, glaucoma, bladder paralysis, fecal impaction, paralytic ileus, tachycardia, or nasal congestion.

Metabolic and Endocrine: Weight change, peripheral edema, abnormal lactation, gynecomastia, menstrual irregularities, false results on pregnancy tests, impotency in men and increased libido in women have all been known to occur in some patients on phenothiazine therapy.

Allergic Reactions: Skin disorders such as itching, erythema, urticaria, seborrhea, photosensitivity, eczema and even exfoliative dermatitis have been reported with phenothiazine derivatives. The possibility of anaphylactoid reactions occurring in some patients should be borne in mind.

Hematologic: Routine blood counts are advisable during therapy since blood dyscrasias including leukopenia, agranulocytosis, thrombocytopenic or nonthrombocytopenic purpura, eosinophilia, and pancytopenia have been observed with phenothiazine derivatives. Furthermore, if any soreness of the mouth, gums, or throat, or any symptoms of upper respiratory infection occur and confirmatory leukocyte count indicates cellular depression, therapy should be discontinued and other appropriate measures instituted immediately.

Hepatic: Liver damage as manifested by cholestatic jaundice may be encountered, particularly during the first months of therapy; treatment should be discontinued if this occurs. An increase in cephalin flocculation, sometimes accompanied by alterations in other liver function tests, has been reported in patients receiving fluphenazine who have had no clinical evidence of liver damage.

Others: Sudden, unexpected and unexplained deaths have been reported in hospitalized psychotic patients receiving phenothiazines. Previous brain damage or seizures may be predisposing factors; high doses should be avoided in known seizure patients. Several patients have shown sudden flare-ups of psychotic behavior patterns shortly before death. Autopsy findings have usually revealed acute fulminating pneumonia or pneumonitis, aspiration of gastric contents, or intramyocardial lesions.

Although this is not a general feature of fluphenazine, potentiation of central nervous system depressants (opiates, analgesics, antihistamines, barbiturates, alcohol) may occur.

The following adverse reactions have also occurred with phenothiazine derivatives: systemic lupus erythematosus-like syndrome, hypotension severe enough to cause fatal cardiac arrest, altered electrocardiographic and electroencephalographic tracings, altered cerebrospinal fluid proteins, cerebral edema, asthma, laryngeal edema and angioneurotic edema; with long-term use—skin pigmentation, and lenticular and corneal opacities.

Injections of fluphenazine decanoate or enanthate are extremely well tolerated, local tissue reactions occurring only rarely.

DOSAGE AND ADMINISTRATION

Prolixin Injection

The average well-tolerated starting dose for adult psychotic patients is 1.25 mg (0.5 mL) intramuscularly. Depending on the severity and duration of symptoms, initial total daily dosage may range from 2.5 to 10.0 mg and should be divided and given at six- to eight-hour intervals.

The smallest amount that will produce the desired results must be carefully determined for each individual, since optimal dosage levels of this potent drug vary from patient to patient. In general, the parenteral dose for fluphenazine has been found to be approximately $\frac{1}{3}$ to $\frac{1}{2}$ the oral dose. Treatment may be instituted with a *low initial dosage,* which may be increased, if necessary, until the desired clinical effects are achieved. Dosages exceeding 10.0 mg daily should be used with caution.

When symptoms are controlled, oral maintenance therapy can generally be instituted, often with single daily doses. Continued treatment, by the oral route if possible, is needed to achieve maximum therapeutic benefits; further adjustments in dosage may be necessary during the course of therapy to meet the patient's requirements.

Prolixin Oral Concentrate

Depending on the severity and duration of symptoms, total daily dosage for *adult* psychotic patients may range initially from 2.5 to 10.0 mg and should be divided and given at six- to eight-hour intervals.

The smallest amount that will produce the desired results must be carefully determined for each individual, since optimal dosage levels of this potent drug vary from patient to patient. In general, the oral dose has been found to be approximately two to three times the parenteral dose of fluphenazine. Treatment is best instituted with a *low initial dosage,* which may be increased, if necessary, until the desired clinical effects are achieved. Therapeutic effect is often achieved with doses under 20 mg daily. Patients remaining severely disturbed or inadequately controlled may require

upward titration of dosage. Daily doses up to 40 mg may be necessary; controlled clinical studies have not been performed to demonstrate safety of prolonged administration of such doses.

When symptoms are controlled, dosage can generally be reduced gradually to daily maintenance doses of 1.0 or 5.0 mg, often given as a single daily dose. Continued treatment is needed to achieve maximum therapeutic benefits; further adjustments in dosage may be necessary during the course of therapy to meet the patient's requirements.

For psychotic patients who have been stabilized on a fixed daily dosage of orally administered PROLIXIN (fluphenazine hydrochloride) dosage forms, conversion to the long-acting injectable PROLIXIN DECANOATE may be indicated [see package insert for PROLIXIN DECANOATE (Fluphenazine Decanoate Injection) for conversion information]. For *geriatric* patients, the suggested starting dose is 1.0 to 2.5 mg daily, adjusted according to the response of the patient. When the Oral Concentrate dosage form is to be used, the desired dose (measured by calibrated device only) should be added to at least 60 mL (2 fl oz) of a suitable diluent *just prior to administration* to insure palatability and stability. Suggested diluents include tomato or fruit juice, milk, and uncaffeinated soft drinks. The Oral Concentrate should not be mixed with beverages containing caffeine (coffee, cola), tannics (tea), or pectinates (apple juice) because of potential incompatibility.

PROLIXIN Injection (Fluphenazine Hydrochloride Injection USP) is useful when psychotic patients are unable or unwilling to take oral therapy.

Prolixin Tablets and Elixir

PROLIXIN Elixir should be inspected prior to use. Upon standing a slight wispy precipitate or globular material may develop due to the flavoring oils separating from the solution (potency is not affected). Gentle shaking redisperses the oils and the solution becomes clear. Solutions that do not clarify should not be used.

Depending on the severity and duration of symptoms, total daily dosage for *adult* psychotic patients may range initially from 2.5 to 10.0 mg and should be divided and given at six- to eight-hour intervals.

The smallest amount that will produce the desired results must be carefully determined for each individual, since optimal dosage levels of this potent drug vary from patient to patient. In general, the oral dose has been found to be approximately two to three times the parenteral dose of fluphenazine. Treatment is best instituted with a *low initial dosage,* which may be increased, if necessary, until the desired clinical effects are achieved. Therapeutic effect is often achieved with doses under 20 mg daily. Patients remaining severely disturbed or inadequately controlled may require upward titration of dosage. Daily doses up to 40 mg may be necessary; controlled clinical studies have not been performed to demonstrate safety of prolonged administration of such doses.

When symptoms are controlled, dosage can generally be reduced gradually to daily maintenance doses of 1.0 or 5.0 mg, often given as a single daily dose. Continued treatment is needed to achieve maximum therapeutic benefits; further adjustments in dosage may be necessary during the course of therapy to meet the patient's requirements.

For psychotic patients who have been stabilized on a fixed daily dosage of orally administered PROLIXIN (fluphenazine hydrochloride) dosage forms, conversion to the long-acting injectable PROLIXIN DECANOATE may be indicated [see package insert for PROLIXIN DECANOATE (Fluphenazine Decanoate Injection) for conversion information]. For *geriatric* patients, the suggested starting dose is 1.0 to 2.5 mg daily, adjusted according to the response of the patient. PROLIXIN Injection (Fluphenazine Hydrochloride Injection USP) is useful when psychotic patients are unable or unwilling to take oral therapy.

Prolixin Decanoate

Parenteral drug products should be inspected visually for particulate matter and discoloration prior to administration, whenever solution and container permit.

PROLIXIN DECANOATE (Fluphenazine Decanoate Injection) may be given intramuscularly or subcutaneously. A dry syringe and needle of at least 21 gauge should be used. Use of a wet needle or syringe may cause the solution to become cloudy.

To begin therapy with PROLIXIN DECANOATE the following regimens are suggested:

For *most patients,* a dose of 12.5 to 25 mg (0.5 to 1 mL) may be given to initiate therapy. The onset of action generally appears between 24 and 72 hours after injection and the effects of the drug on psychotic symptoms become significant within 48 to 96 hours. Subsequent injections and the dosage interval are determined in accordance with the patient's response. When administered as maintenance therapy, a single injection may be effective in controlling schizophrenic symptoms up to four weeks or longer. The response to a single dose has been found to last as long as six weeks in a few patients on maintenance therapy.

It may be advisable that patients who have no history of taking phenothiazines should be treated initially with a shorter-

acting form of fluphenazine (see HOW SUPPLIED section for the availability of the shorter-acting fluphenazine hydrochloride dosage forms) before administering the decanoate to determine the patient's response to fluphenazine and to establish appropriate dosage. For psychotic patients who have been stabilized on a fixed daily dosage of PROLIXIN Tablets (Fluphenazine Hydrochloride Tablets USP), PROLIXIN Elixir (Fluphenazine Hydrochloride Elixir USP), or PROLIXIN Oral Concentrate (Fluphenazine Hydrochloride Oral Solution), conversion of therapy from these short-acting oral forms to the long-acting injectable PROLIXIN DECANOATE may be indicated.

Appropriate dosage of PROLIXIN DECANOATE (Fluphenazine Decanoate Injection) should be individualized for each patient and responses carefully monitored. No precise formula can be given to convert to use of PROLIXIN DECANOATE; however, a controlled multicentered study,* in patients receiving oral doses from 5 to 60 mg fluphenazine hydrochloride daily, showed that 20 mg fluphenazine hydrochloride daily was equivalent to 25 mg (1 mL) PROLIXIN DECANOATE every three weeks. This represents an approximate conversion ratio of 0.5 mL (12.5 mg) of decanoate every three weeks for every 10 mg of fluphenazine hydrochloride daily.

Once conversion to PROLIXIN DECANOATE is made, careful clinical monitoring of the patient and appropriate dosage adjustment should be made at the time of each injection.

Severely agitated patients may be treated initially with a rapid-acting phenothiazine compound such as PROLIXIN Injection (Fluphenazine Hydrochloride Injection USP—see package insert accompanying that product for complete information). When acute symptoms have subsided, 25 mg (1 mL) of PROLIXIN DECANOATE may be administered; subsequent dosage is adjusted as necessary.

"Poor risk" patients (those with known hypersensitivity to phenothiazines, or with disorders that predispose to undue reactions): Therapy may be initiated cautiously with oral or parenteral fluphenazine hydrochloride (see package inserts accompanying these products for complete information). When the pharmacologic effects and an appropriate dosage are apparent, an equivalent dose of PROLIXIN DECANOATE may be administered. Subsequent dosage adjustments are made in accordance with the response of the patient.

The optimal amount of the drug and the frequency of administration must be determined for each patient, since dosage requirements have been found to vary with clinical circumstances as well as with individual response to the drug.

Dosage should not exceed 100 mg. If doses greater than 50 mg are deemed necessary, the next dose and succeeding doses should be increased cautiously in increments of 12.5 mg.

Prolixin Enanthate

PROLIXIN ENANTHATE (Fluphenazine Enanthate Injection USP) may be given intramuscularly or subcutaneously. A dry syringe and needle of at least 21 gauge should be used. Use of a wet needle or syringe may cause the solution to become cloudy.

To begin therapy with PROLIXIN ENANTHATE the following regimens are suggested:

For most patients a dose of 25 mg (1 mL) every two weeks should prove to be adequate, and therapy may be started on that basis. Subsequent adjustments in the amount and the dosage interval may be made, if necessary, in accordance with the patient's response.

It may be advisable that patients who have no history of taking phenothiazines should be treated initially with a shorter-acting form of fluphenazine before administering the enanthate to determine the patient's response to fluphenazine and to establish appropriate dosage. Since the dosage comparability of the shorter-acting forms of fluphenazine to the longer-acting enanthate is not known, special caution should be exercised when switching from the shorter-acting forms to the enanthate.

Severely agitated patients may be treated initially with a rapid-acting phenothiazine compound such as PROLIXIN Injection (Fluphenazine Hydrochloride Injection USP—see package insert accompanying that product for complete information). When acute symptoms have subsided, 25 mg (1 mL) of PROLIXIN ENANTHATE may be administered; subsequent dosage is adjusted as necessary.

"Poor risk" patients (those with known hypersensitivity to phenothiazines, or with disorders that predispose to undue reactions): Therapy may be initiated cautiously with oral or parenteral fluphenazine hydrochloride. (See package inserts accompanying these products for complete information.) When the pharmacologic effects and an appropriate dosage are apparent, an equivalent dose of PROLIXIN

---

*The Initiation of Long-Term Pharmacotherapy in Schizophrenia: Dosage and Side Effect Comparisons Between Oral and Depot Fluphenazine; N.R. Schooler; Pharmakopsych. 9:159–169, 1976.

Continued on next page

Apothecon—Cont.

ENANTHATE may be administered. Subsequent dosage adjustments are made in accordance with the response of the patient.

The optimal amount of the drug and the frequency of administration must be determined for each patient, since dosage requirements have been found to vary with clinical circumstances as well as with individual response to the drug. Although in a large series of patients the optimal dose was usually 25 mg every two weeks, the amount required ranged from 12.5 to 100 mg (0.5 to 4 mL). The interval between doses ranged from one to three weeks in most instances. The response to a single dose was found to last as long as six weeks in a few patients on maintenance therapy.

Dosage should not exceed 100 mg. If doses greater than 50 mg are deemed necessary, the next dose and succeeding doses should be increased cautiously in increments of 12.5 mg.

HOW SUPPLIED

PROLIXIN Injection (Fluphenazine Hydrochloride Injection USP) is available in multiple dose vials as a sterile aqueous solution providing 2.5 mg fluphenazine hydrochloride per mL. The drug is also available for oral administration as sugar-coated tablets, a flavored elixir, and an oral solution concentrate.

Storage

Solutions should be protected from exposure to light. Parenteral solutions may vary in color from essentially colorless to light amber. If a solution has become any darker than light amber or is discolored in any other way it should not be used. Store at room temperature; avoid freezing.

PROLIXIN Oral Concentrate (Fluphenazine Hydrochloride Oral Solution USP): 120 mL bottle with a 1 mL safety-cap dropper calibrated at 0.1 mL and in 0.2 mL increments. 5 mg fluphenazine hydrochloride per mL. NDC 0003-0801-10.

PROLIXIN (fluphenazine hydrochloride) is also available as a sterile aqueous solution for intramuscular use, plus tablets and elixir for oral administration. See specific package insert for complete information.

Storage

Store at room temperature; avoid freezing. Protect from light. Keep tightly closed.

PROLIXIN Tablets

(Fluphenazine Hydrochloride Tablets USP)

1 mg: bottles of 50 (NDC 0003-0863-40), 100 (NDC 0003-0863-50), and 500 (NDC 0003-0863-70)

2.5 mg: bottles of 50 (NDC 0003-0864-40), 100 (NDC 0003-0864-50), and 500 (NDC 0003-0864-70)

5 mg: bottles of 50 (NDC 0003-0877-40), 100 (NDC 0003-0877-50), and 500 (NDC 0003-0877-70)

10 mg: bottles of 50 (NDC 0003-0956-40), 100 (NDC 0003-0956-50), and 500 (NDC 0003-0956-70)

Unimatic® single dose

(tablets individually sealed) packages

1 mg:	100 (NDC 0003-0863-55)
2.5 mg:	100 (NDC 0003-0864-52)
5 mg:	100 (NDC 0003-0877-52)
10 mg:	100 (NDC 0003-0956-52)

Identification Numbers on Tablets: 1 mg, **863**; 2.5 mg, **864**; 5 mg, **877**; 10 mg, **956**.

PROLIXIN Elixir

(Fluphenazine Hydrochloride Elixir USP) 0.5 mg/mL (2.5 mg per 5 mL teaspoonful)

60 ml bottle with calibrated dropper: NDC 0003-0820-30

473 ml bottle: NDC 0003-0820-50

PROLIXIN (fluphenazine hydrochloride) is also available as an oral solution concentrate and a sterile aqueous solution for intramuscular use. See specific package inserts for complete information.

Storage

Store tablets and elixir at room temperature. Protect from light. Keep tightly closed.

Tablets: Avoid excessive heat.

Elixir: Avoid freezing.

PROLIXIN DECANOATE (Fluphenazine Decanoate Injection) is available in Unimatic® single dose preassembled syringes, and vials, providing 25 mg fluphenazine decanoate per mL.

PROLIXIN ENANTHATE (Fluphenazine Enanthate Injection USP) is available in vials providing 25 mg fluphenazine enanthate per mL.

Storage

Store at room temperature; avoid freezing and excessive heat. Protect from light.

QUIBRON®   ℞

[kwi'bron]

(Theophylline-Guaifenesin)

QUIBRON®-300   ℞

(Theophylline-Guaifenesin)

QUIBRON®-T   ℞

(theophylline tablets, USP)

DIVIDOSE® TABLETS

IMMEDIATE RELEASE BRONCHODILATOR

QUIBRON®-T/SR   ℞

(Theophylline Anhydrous)

DIVIDOSE® TABLETS

SUSTAINED RELEASE BRONCHODILATOR

DESCRIPTION

QUIBRON®-T TABLETS
DIVIDOSE® TABLETS
IMMEDIATE RELEASE BRONCHODILATOR

Theophylline is a bronchodilator structurally classified as a xanthine derivative. It occurs as a white, odorless, crystalline powder having a bitter taste. Theophylline anhydrous has the chemical name, 1H-purine-2,6-dione,3,7-dihydro-1,3-dimethyl-, and is represented by the following structural formula:

$$\text{(structural formula of theophylline)}$$

QUIBRON-T tablets provide 300 mg of anhydrous theophylline as an oral bronchodilator in an immediate release formulation combined with the convenience of the unique DIVIDOSE® tablet design. With functional trisects and bisects, QUIBRON-T tablets can be conveniently and accurately divided into 100, 150, and 200 mg segments to provide a variety of dosing increments, as required.

	QUIBRON-T tablets	
	One-third tablet	= 100 mg
	One-half tablet	= 150 mg
	Two-thirds tablet	= 200 mg
	One tablet	= 300 mg

This product contains the following inactive ingredients: microcrystalline cellulose, yellow ferric oxide, hydroxypropyl methylcellulose 2910, lactose, magnesium stearate, colloidal silicon dioxide, and sodium starch glycolate.

QUIBRON® AND QUIBRON®-300

Guaifenesin is an expectorant classified as a guaiacol compound. It occurs as a white to slightly yellow crystalline powder with a bitter, aromatic taste. Guaifenesin has the chemical name, 3-(o-Methoxyphenoxy)-1,2-propanediol, and is represented by the following structural formula:

$$\text{(structural formula of guaifenesin)}$$

QUIBRON is available as soft gelatin capsules intended for oral administration, containing 150 mg of theophylline anhydrous and 90 mg of guaifenesin. QUIBRON-300 is available as soft gelatin capsules intended for oral administration, containing 300 mg of theophylline anhydrous and 180 mg of guaifenesin. These products contain the following inactive ingredients: D&C Yellow No. 10, non-porcine gelatin, glycerin, edible ink, polyethylene glycol, and titanium dioxide.

QUIBRON®-T/SR DIVIDOSE® TABLETS
SUSTAINED RELEASE BRONCHODILATOR

QUIBRON-T/SR tablets provide 300 mg of anhydrous theophylline as an oral bronchodilator in a sustained release formulation combined with the convenience of the unique Dividose® tablet design. With functional trisects and bisects, QUIBRON-T/SR tablets can be conveniently and accurately divided into 100, 150, and 200 mg segments to provide a variety of dosing increments, as required.

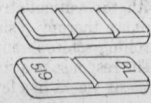

	QUIBRON-T/SR tablets	
	One-third tablet	= 100 mg
	One-half tablet	= 150 mg
	Two-thirds tablet	= 200 mg
	One tablet	= 300 mg

This product contains the following inactive ingredient: magnesium stearate.

CLINICAL PHARMACOLOGY

QUIBRON, QUIBRON-300, QUIBRON-T

Theophylline

Mode of Action

Theophylline directly relaxes the smooth muscle of the bronchial airways and pulmonary blood vessels, thus acting mainly as a bronchodilator and smooth muscle relaxant. It has also been demonstrated that aminophylline has a potent effect on diaphragmatic contractility in normal persons and may then be capable of reducing fatigability and thereby improve contractility in patients with chronic obstructive airways disease. The exact mode of action remains unsettled. Although theophylline does cause inhibition of phosphodiesterase with a resultant increase in intracellular cyclic AMP, other agents similarly inhibit the enzyme producing a rise of cyclic AMP but are unassociated with any demonstrable bronchodilation. Other mechanisms proposed include an effect on translocation of intracellular calcium; prostaglandin antagonism; stimulation of catecholamines endogenously; inhibition of cyclic guanosine monophosphate metabolism and adenosine receptor antagonism. None of these mechanisms has been proved, however.

In vitro, theophylline has been shown to act synergistically with β-agonists and there are now available data which do demonstrate an additive effect *in vivo* with combined use.

Pharmacokinetics

The half-life of theophylline is influenced by a number of known variables. It may be prolonged in chronic alcoholics, particularly those with liver disease (cirrhosis or alcoholic liver disease), in patients with congestive heart failure, and in those patients taking certain other drugs (see PRECAUTIONS, Drug Interactions). Newborns and neonates have extremely slow clearance rates compared to older infants and children, ie, those over 1 year. Older children have rapid clearance rates while most nonsmoking adults have clearance rates between these two extremes. In premature neonates the decreased clearance is related to oxidative pathways that have yet to be established.

Theophylline Elimination Characteristics
Half-Life (in hours)

	Range	Mean
Children	1–9	3.7
Adults	3–15	7.7

In cigarette smokers (1 to 2 packs/day) the mean half-life is 4 to 5 hours, much shorter than in nonsmokers. The increase in clearance associated with smoking is presumably due to stimulation of the hepatic metabolic pathway by components of cigarette smoke. The duration of this effect after cessation of smoking is unknown but may require 6 months to 2 years before the rate approaches that of the nonsmoker.

QUIBRON AND QUIBRON-300

Guaifenesin

Mode of Action

Guaifenesin increases respiratory tract secretions, possibly by stimulating the goblet cells.

Pharmacokinetics

Guaifenesin appears to be well absorbed, but its pharmacokinetics have not been well studied.

QUIBRON-T/SR

Pharmacokinetics

Theophylline excretion, principally as inactive metabolites, occurs primarily via the kidney. The half-life of theophylline varies among individuals with a wide range having been documented. Theophylline half-life is shorter in cigarette smokers. Half-life is prolonged in alcoholism, reduced hepatic or renal function, congestive heart failure and in patients receiving macrolide antibiotics (troleandomycin and erythromycin) or cimetidine. High fever for prolonged periods may decrease theophylline elimination. Older adults (over age 55) and patients with chronic obstructive pulmonary disease, with or without cor pulmonale, may have much slower clearance rates. For such patients, the theophylline half-life may exceed 24 hours. The theophylline half-life is generally shorter in children.

It appears that between 3 months and 2 years of cessation of smoking may be necessary for elimination of the effect of smoking on theophylline pharmacokinetics.

Representative Theophylline Serum Half-lives
Half-life (hours)

	Mean	Range
Adults		
non-smokers	8.7	6.1–12.8
smokers	5.5	4.0–7.7
congestive heart failure	22.9	3.1–82.0
Children (6–16 years)	3.7	1.4–7.9

Therapeutic serum theophylline levels are usually 10–20 μg/mL.

Binding to plasma proteins is not extensive and theophylline is not preferentially taken up by any particular organ.

Theophylline-containing products may increase the plasma levels of free fatty acids and the urinary levels of epinephrine and norepinephrine.

Apparently no development of tolerance occurs with chronic use of theophylline.

In a single-dose study of QUIBRON-T/SR, a 300 mg dose in 12 fasted normal male subjects gave a mean peak plasma level of 5.26 ± 1.04 (S.D.) μg/mL at 6.25 ± 1.10 (S.D.) hours.

In a multi-dose, steady state study of 16 adult patients with a mean age of 39.0 years, the patients were dose-titrated to a therapeutically effective level without toxicity. Doses were administered once every 12 hours and ranged from 7.8 mg/kg/24 hours to 18.6 mg/kg/24 hours with a mean dose of 10.0 ± 2.8 (S.D.) mg/kg/24 hours. No food-fasting conditions were imposed in the study. A mean C_{max} of 13.9 ± 3.2 (S.D.) μg/mL, a mean C_{min} of 7.7 ± 2.0 (S.D.) μg/mL, and a mean percent fluctuation of 87.1 ± 49.6 (S.D.) resulted from the study.

In a multi-dose, steady state study of 15 patients with a mean age of 14.4 years, the patients were dose-titrated to a therapeutically effective level without toxicity. Doses were administered once every 12 hours and ranged from 9.1 mg/kg/24 hours to 22.6 mg/kg/24 hours with a mean dose of 13.3 ± 3.9 (S.D.) mg/kg/24 hours. No food-fasting conditions were imposed in the study. A mean C_{max} of 13.8 ± 3.9 (S.D.) μg/mL, a mean C_{min} of 8.0 ± 2.5 (S.D.) μg/mL, and a mean percent fluctuation of 85.4 ± 57.7 (S.D.) resulted from the study.

INDICATIONS AND USAGE

QUIBRON Capsules, QUIBRON-300 Capsules, QUIBRON-T tablets, and QUIBRON-T/SR tablets are indicated for relief and/or prevention of symptoms from asthma and reversible bronchospasm associated with chronic bronchitis and emphysema.

CONTRAINDICATIONS

QUIBRON Capsules, QUIBRON-300 Capsules, QUIBRON-T tablets, and QUIBRON-T/SR tablets are contraindicated in individuals who have shown hypersensitivity to their components. QUIBRON, QUIBRON-300, and QUIBRON-T are also contraindicated in patients with active peptic ulcer disease, and in individuals with underlying seizure disorders (unless receiving appropriate anticonvulsant medication). QUIBRON-T/SR tablets are also contraindicated in individuals who have shown hypersensitivity to xanthine derivatives.

WARNINGS

Excessive doses may be associated with toxicity, although increasing the dose of theophylline may enhance response. The likelihood of serious toxicity increases significantly when the serum theophylline concentration exceeds 20 μg/mL. Therefore, determination of serum theophylline levels is recommended to assure maximal benefit without excessive risk.

Serum levels above 20 μg/mL are rarely found after appropriate administration of the recommended doses. However, in individuals in whom theophylline plasma clearance is reduced *for any reason*, even conventional doses may result in increased serum levels and potential toxicity. Reduced theophylline clearance has been documented in the following readily identifiable groups: 1) patients with impaired liver function; 2) patients over 55 years of age, particularly males and those with chronic lung disease; 3) those with cardiac failure from any cause; 4) patients with sustained high fever; 5) neonates and infants under 1 year of age; and 6) those patients taking certain drugs (see PRECAUTIONS, Drug Interactions). Frequently, such patients have markedly prolonged theophylline serum levels following discontinuation of the drug. Decreased clearance of theophylline may be associated with either influenza immunization or active influenza infection. Reduction of dosage and laboratory monitoring is especially appropriate in the above individuals.

Serious side effects such as ventricular arrhythmias, convulsions or even death may appear as the first sign of toxicity without any previous warning. Less serious signs of theophylline toxicity (ie, nausea and restlessness) may occur frequently when initiating therapy, but are usually transient; when such signs are persistent during maintenance therapy, they are often associated with serum concentrations above 20 μg/mL. Stated differently: *serious toxicity is not reliably preceded by less severe side effects.* A serum concentration measurement is the only reliable method of predicting potentially life-threatening toxicity.

Many patients who have serum levels >20 μg/mL exhibit tachycardia due to their underlying disease process so that the cause/effect relationship to elevated serum theophylline concentrations may not be appreciated.

Theophylline products may cause dysrhythmia or worsen arrhythmias and any significant change in rate and/or rhythm warrants monitoring and further investigation.

Studies in laboratory animals (minipigs, rodents, and dogs) recorded the occurrence of cardiac arrhythmias and sudden death (with histologic evidence of myocardial necrosis) when β-agonists and methylxanthines were administered concurrently. The significance of these findings when applied to humans is currently unknown.

Status asthmaticus should be considered a medical emergency and is defined as that degree of bronchospasm which is not rapidly responsive to usual doses of conventional bronchodilators. Optimal therapy for such patients frequently requires both *additional medication*, parenterally administered, and *close monitoring*, preferably in an intensive care setting.

Although increasing the dose of theophylline may bring about relief, such treatment may be associated with toxicity. The likelihood of the development of such toxicity increases significantly when the serum theophylline concentration exceeds 20 μg/mL. Therefore, determination of serum theophylline levels is recommended to assure maximal benefit without excessive risk.

PRECAUTIONS

QUIBRON, QUIBRON-300, and QUIBRON-T

General

On the average, theophylline half-life is shorter in cigarette and marijuana smokers than in nonsmokers, but smokers can have half-lives as long as nonsmokers. Theophylline should not be administered concurrently with other xanthines. Use with caution in patients with hypoxemia, hypertension, or those with history of peptic ulcer. Theophylline may occasionally act as a local irritant to G.I. tract although gastrointestinal symptoms are more commonly centrally mediated and associated with serum drug concentrations over 20 μg/mL.

Information for Patients

The importance of taking only the prescribed dose and time interval between doses should be reinforced.

Laboratory Tests

Serum levels should be monitored periodically to determine the theophylline level associated with observed clinical response and as the method of predicting toxicity. For such measurements, the serum sample should be obtained at the time of peak concentration, 1 to 2 hours after administration for immediate release products. It is important that the patient will not have missed or taken additional doses during the previous 48 hours and that dosing intervals will have been reasonably equally spaced. DOSAGE ADJUSTMENT BASED ON SERUM THEOPHYLLINE MEASUREMENTS WHEN THESE INSTRUCTIONS HAVE NOT BEEN FOLLOWED MAY RESULT IN RECOMMENDATIONS THAT PRESENT RISK OF TOXICITY TO THE PATIENT.

Drug Interactions

Toxic synergism with ephedrine has been documented and may occur with other sympathomimetic bronchodilators. In addition, the following drug interactions have been demonstrated:

Theophylline with:	
Allopurinol (high dose)	Increased serum theophylline levels
Cimetidine	Increased serum theophylline levels
Ciprofloxacin	Increased serum theophylline levels
Erythromycin, Troleandomycin	Increased serum theophylline levels
Lithium Carbonate	Increased renal excretion of lithium
Oral Contraceptives	Increased serum theophylline levels
Phenytoin	Decreased theophylline and phenytoin serum levels
Propranolol	Increased serum theophylline levels
Rifampin	Decreased serum theophylline levels

Drug-Laboratory Test Interactions

Currently available analytical methods, including high pressure liquid chromatography and immunoassay techniques, for measuring serum theophylline levels are specific. Metabolites and other drugs generally do not affect the results. Other new analytic methods are also now in use. The physician should be aware of the laboratory method used and whether other drugs will interfere with the assay for theophylline.

Carcinogenesis, Mutagenesis, and Impairment of Fertility

Long-term carcinogenicity studies have not been performed with theophylline.

Chromosome-breaking activity was detected in human cell cultures at concentrations of theophylline up to 50 times the therapeutic serum concentration in humans. Theophylline was not mutagenic in the dominant lethal assay in male mice given theophylline intraperitoneally in doses up to 30 times the maximum daily human oral dose.

Studies to determine the effect on fertility have not been performed with theophylline.

Pregnancy

Category C—Animal reproduction studies have not been conducted with theophylline. It is also not known whether theophylline can cause fetal harm when administered to a pregnant woman or can affect reproduction capacity. Xanthines should be given to a pregnant woman only if clearly needed.

Nursing Mothers

Theophylline is distributed into breast milk and may cause irritability or other signs of toxicity in nursing infants. Because of the potential for serious adverse reactions in nursing infants from theophylline, a decision should be made whether to discontinue nursing or to discontinue the drug, taking into account the importance of the drug to the mother.

Pediatric Use

Safety and effectiveness of QUIBRON, QUIBRON-300 and QUIBRON-T/SR in children under 6 years of age have not been established.

Safety and effectiveness of theophylline immediate-release products in children under 1 year of age have not been established. Because of the potential difficulty of drug administration (eg, tablet swallowability) and the inability to provide small and precise incremental doses, it is recommended that a liquid theophylline preparation be used for children under 6 years of age.

QUIBRON T/SR

General

QUIBRON-T/SR tablets should not be chewed or crushed.

Use with caution in neonates, the elderly (especially males), and in patients with severe cardiac disease, hypertension, acute myocardial injury, congestive heart failure, cor pulmonale, severe hypoxemia, hyperthyroidism, hepatic impairment, history of peptic ulcer or alcoholism.

Concurrent administration with certain antibiotics (see DRUG INTERACTIONS section) may result in increased serum theophylline levels.

A decrease in serum half-life is seen in smokers (see Clinical Pharmacology/Pharmacokinetics).

Particular caution should be used in administering theophylline to patients in congestive heart failure. Reduced theophylline clearance in these patients may cause theophylline blood levels to persist long after discontinuing the drug.

Theophylline should not be administered concurrently with other xanthine medications.

Use theophylline cautiously in patients with a history of peptic ulcer. Theophylline may occasionally act as a local irritant to the GI tract, although gastrointestinal symptoms are more commonly centrally mediated and associated with serum drug concentrations over 20 μg/mL.

Sustained release theophylline is not useful in status asthmaticus.

Information for Patients

Patients should be instructed carefully on how to divide QUIBRON-T/SR tablets along the appropriate tablet score.

The physician should reinforce the importance of taking only the prescribed dose and observing the correct time interval between doses.

The patient should alert the physician if symptoms occur repeatedly, especially near the end of a dosing interval.

Drug Interactions

Drug—Drug: Toxic synergism with ephedrine has been documented and may occur with some other sympathomimetic bronchodilators. In addition, the following drug interactions have been demonstrated:

Drug	Effect
Theophylline with lithium carbonate	Increased renal excretion of lithium
Theophylline with propranolol	Mutual antagonism of therapeutic effects
Theophylline with cimetidine	Increased serum theophylline levels
Theophylline with troleandomycin or erythromycin	Increased serum theophylline levels

Drug—Food: QUIBRON-T/SR has not been adequately studied to determine whether its bioavailability is altered when it is given with food.

Available data suggests that drug administration at the time of food ingestion may influence the absorption characteristics of some or all theophylline controlled-release products, resulting in serum values different from those found after administration in the fasting state.

A drug-food effect, if any, would likely have its greatest clinical significance when high theophylline serum levels are being maintained and/or when large single doses (>13 mg/kg or 900 mg) of a controlled-release theophylline product are given. The influence of type and amount of food on performance of controlled-release theophylline products is under study at this time.

Drug-Laboratory Test Interactions:

Spectrophotometric determination of theophylline is affected by coffee, tea, cola beverages, chocolate, and acetaminophen, which contribute to falsely high values.

Carcinogenesis, Mutagenesis, and Impairment of Fertility

Long-term animal studies have not been performed to evaluate the carcinogenic potential, mutagenic potential, or the effect on fertility of xanthine compounds.

Continued on next page

Apothecon—Cont.

Usage in Pregnancy
Teratogenic Effects
Pregnancy Category C. Animal reproduction studies have not been conducted with QUIBRON-T/SR tablets. It is also not known whether QUIBRON-T/SR tablets can cause fetal harm when administered to a pregnant woman or can affect reproduction capacity. QUIBRON-T/SR tablets should be given to a pregnant woman only if clearly indicated.

Nonteratogenic Effects
It is not known whether use of this drug during labor or delivery has immediate or delayed adverse effects on the fetus, or whether it prolongs the duration of labor or increases the possibility of forceps delivery or other obstetrical intervention.

Nursing Mothers
Theophylline has been reported to be excreted in human milk and to have caused irritability in a nursing infant. Because of the potential for serious adverse reactions, a decision should be made whether to discontinue nursing or to discontinue QUIBRON-T/SR tablets, taking into account the importance of this drug to the mother.

ADVERSE REACTIONS
QUIBRON, QUIBRON-300, and QUIBRON-T
The following adverse reactions have been observed, but there has not been enough systematic collection of data to support an estimate of their frequency. The most consistent adverse reactions are usually due to overdosage.
1. *Gastrointestinal:* nausea, vomiting, epigastric pain, hematemesis, diarrhea.
2. *Central nervous system:* headaches, irritability, restlessness, insomnia, reflex hyperexcitability, muscle twitching, clonic and tonic generalized convulsions.
3. *Cardiovascular:* palpitation, tachycardia, extrasystoles, flushing, hypotension, circulatory failure, ventricular arrhythmias.
4. *Respiratory:* tachypnea.
5. *Renal:* potentiation of diuresis.
6. *Others:* alopecia, hyperglycemia, inappropriate ADH syndrome, rash.

QUIBRON T/SR
The frequency of adverse reactions is related to serum theophylline levels and is usually not a problem at levels below 20 μg/mL. The most consistent adverse reactions are usually due to overdosage and, while not all have been reported with QUIBRON-T and/or with QUIBRON-T/SR tablets, the following reactions may be considered when theophylline is administered. Central nervous system: clonic and tonic generalized convulsions, muscle twitching, reflex hyperexcitability, headaches, insomnia, restlessness, and irritability. Cardiovascular: circulatory failure, ventricular arrhythmias, hypotension, extrasystoles, tachycardia, palpitation, and flushing. Gastrointestinal: hematemesis, vomiting, diarrhea, epigastric pain, and nausea. Renal: increased excretion of renal tubular cells and red blood cells, albuminuria, and diuresis. Respiratory: tachypnea. Other: hyperglycemia and inappropriate ADH syndrome, and rash.

OVERDOSAGE
Symptoms (QUIBRON-T/SR)
Nervousness, agitation, headache, insomnia, nausea, vomiting, tachycardia, extrasystoles, hyperreflexia, fasciculations and clonic and tonic convulsions. Children may be particularly prone to restlessness and hyperactivity that can proceed to convulsions.

Management: It is suggested that the management principles (consistent with the clinical status of the patient when first seen) outlined below be instituted and that simultaneous contact with a Regional Poison Control Center be established. In this way both updated information and individualization regarding required therapy may be provided.
1. When potential oral overdose is established and seizure has not occurred:
  a) If patient is alert and seen within the early hours after ingestion, induction of emesis may be of value. Gastric lavage has been demonstrated to be of no value in influencing outcome in patients who present more than 1 hour after ingestion.
  b) Administer a cathartic. Sorbitol solution is reported to be of value. This is particularly important if a sustained release preparation has been taken.
  c) Administer repeated doses of activated charcoal and monitor theophylline serum levels. Monitor vital signs, maintain blood pressure, and provide adequate hydration.
  d) Prophylactic administration of phenobarbital has been shown to increase the seizure threshold in laboratory animals, and administration of this drug can be considered.
2. If patient presents with a seizure:
  a) Establish an airway.
  b) Administer oxygen.
  c) Treat the seizure with intravenous diazepam, 0.1 to 0.3 mg/kg, up to 10 mg. If seizures cannot be controlled, the use of general anesthesia should be considered.

  d) Monitor vital signs, maintain blood pressure, and provide adequate hydration.
3. If postseizure coma is present:
  a) Maintain airway and oxygenation.
  b) If a result of oral medication, follow above recommendations to prevent absorption of the drug, but intubation and lavage will have to be performed instead of inducing emesis, and the cathartic and charcoal will need to be introduced via a large bore gastric lavage tube.
  c) Continue to provide full supportive care and adequate hydration until the drug is metabolized. In general, drug metabolism is sufficiently rapid so as not to warrant dialysis. If repeated oral activated charcoal is ineffective (as noted by stable or rising serum levels) charcoal hemoperfusion may be indicated.

General
The oral LD_{50} of theophylline in mice is 350 mg/kg. In humans, adverse reactions often occur when serum theophylline levels exceed 20 μg/mL. Information on physiological variables which influence excretion of theophylline can be found under the heading "Clinical Pharmacology."

DOSAGE AND ADMINISTRATION
QUIBRON, QUIBRON-300, and QUIBRON-T
Effective use of theophylline, (ie, the concentration of drug in the serum associated with optimal benefit and minimal risk of toxicity) is considered to occur when the theophylline concentration is maintained from 10 to 20 μg/mL. The early studies from which these levels were derived were carried out in patients immediately or shortly after recovery from acute exacerbations of their disease (some hospitalized with status asthmaticus).

Although the 20 μg/mL level remains appropriate as a critical value (above which toxicity is more likely to occur) for safety purposes, additional data are now available which indicate that the serum theophylline concentrations required to produce maximum physiologic benefit may, in fact, fluctuate with the degree of bronchospasm present and are variable. Therefore, the physician should individualize the range appropriate to the patient's requirements, based on both symptomatic response and improvement in pulmonary function. It should be stressed that serum theophylline concentrations maintained at the upper level of the 10 to 20 μg/mL range may be associated with potential toxicity when factors known to reduce theophylline clearance are operative. (See WARNINGS).

If it is not possible to obtain serum level determinations, restriction of the daily dose (in otherwise healthy adults) to not greater than 13 mg/kg/day, to a maximum of 900 mg, in divided doses will result in relatively few patients exceeding serum levels of 20 μg/mL and the resultant greater risk of toxicity.

Caution should be exercised for younger children who cannot complain of minor side effects. Older adults, those with cor pulmonale, congestive heart failure, and/or liver disease may have unusually low dosage requirements and thus may experience toxicity at the maximal dosage recommended below.

Theophylline does not distribute into fatty tissue. Dosage should be calculated on the basis of lean (ideal) body weight where mg/kg doses are presented.

Frequency of Dosing: When immediate-release products with rapid absorption are used, dosing to maintain serum levels generally requires administration every 6 hours. This is particularly true in children, but dosing intervals up to 8 hours may be satisfactory in adults since they eliminate the drug at a slower rate. Some children, and adults requiring higher-than-average doses (those having rapid rates of clearance, eg, half-lives of under 6 hours), may benefit and be more effectively controlled during chronic therapy when given products with sustained-release characteristics since these provide longer dosing intervals and/or less fluctuation in serum concentration between dosing.

Dosage guidelines are approximations only and the wide range of theophylline clearance between individuals (particularly those with concomitant disease) makes indiscriminate usage hazardous.

Dosage Guidelines
I. Acute symptoms of bronchospasm requiring rapid attainment of theophylline serum levels for bronchodilation.
NOTE: Status asthmaticus should be considered a medical emergency and is defined as that degree of bronchospasm which is not rapidly responsive to usual doses of conventional bronchodilators. Optimal therapy for such patients frequently requires both *additional medication*, parenterally administered, and *close monitoring*, preferably in an intensive care setting. [See table at top of next column.]
The loading dose for theophylline is based on the principle that each 0.5 mg/kg of theophylline administered as a loading dose will result in a 1.0 μg/mL increase in serum theophylline concentration. Ideally, the loading dose should be deferred if a serum theophylline concentration can be obtained rapidly.
If this is not possible, the clinician must exercise judgment in selecting a dose based on the potential for benefit and risk. When there is sufficient respiratory distress to warrant a

A. Patients not currently receiving theophylline products.

	Theophylline Dosage Oral	
	Loading	Maintenance:
Children age: 6* to under 9 years	5 mg/kg	4 mg/kg q 6 hours
Children age: 9 to under 16 years; and smokers	5 mg/kg	3 mg/kg q 6 hours
Otherwise healthy nonsmoking adults	5 mg/kg	3 mg/kg q 8 hours
Older patients and patients with cor pulmonale	5 mg/kg	2 mg/kg q 8 hours
Patients with congestive heart failure	5 mg/kg	1–2 mg/kg q 12 hours

* 1 for QUIBRON-T

B. Patients currently receiving theophylline products.
Determine, where possible, the time, amount, dosage form, and route of administration of the last dose the patient received.

small risk, then 2.5 mg/kg of theophylline administered in rapidly-absorbed form is likely to increase serum concentration by approximately 5 μg/mL. If the patient is not experiencing theophylline toxicity, this is unlikely to result in dangerous adverse effects.
Subsequent to the decision regarding use of a loading dose for this group of patients, the maintenance dosage recommendations are the same as those described above.
II. Chronic Therapy
Theophylline is a treatment for the management of reversible bronchospasm (asthma, chronic bronchitis and emphysema) to prevent symptoms and maintain patent airways. A dosage form which allows small incremental doses is desirable for initiating therapy. A liquid preparation should be considered for children to permit greater ease of and more accurate dosage adjustment. Slow clinical titration is generally preferred to assure acceptance and safety of the medication, and to allow the patient to develop tolerance to transient caffeine-like side effects.
Initial Dose: 16 mg/kg/24 hours or 400 mg/24 hours (whichever is less) of theophylline in divided doses at 6- or 8-hour intervals.
Increasing Dose: The above dosage may be increased in approximately 25% increments at 3-day intervals so long as the drug is tolerated; until clinical response is satisfactory or the maximum dose as indicated in Section III (below) is reached. The serum concentration may be checked at these intervals, but at a minimum, should be determined at the end of this adjustment period.
It is important that no patient be maintained on any dosage that is not tolerated. When instructing patients to increase dosage according to the schedule above, they should be told not to take a subsequent dose if apparent side effects occur and to resume therapy at a lower dose once adverse effects have disappeared.
III. Maximum Dose of Theophylline Where the Serum Concentration is Not Measured
WARNING: DO NOT ATTEMPT TO MAINTAIN ANY DOSE THAT IS NOT TOLERATED.
Not to exceed the following: (or 900 mg, whichever is less)
Age 6*-under 9 years   24 mg/kg/day
Age 9-under 12 years   20 mg/kg/day
Age 12-under 16 years   18 mg/kg/day
Age 16 years and older   13 mg/kg/day

* 1 for QUIBRON-T

IV. Measurement of Serum Theophylline Concentrations During Chronic Therapy:
If the above maximum doses are to be maintained or exceeded, serum theophylline measurement is essential. (See PRECAUTIONS, Laboratory Tests, for guidance).
V. Final Adjustment of Dosage:
Dosage adjustment after serum theophylline measurement

If serum theophylline is:	Directions:
Within desired range	Maintain dosage if tolerated.
Too high 20 to 25 μg/mL	Decrease doses by about 10% and recheck serum level after 3 days
25 to 30 μg/mL	Skip the next dose and decrease subsequent doses by about 25%. Recheck serum level after 3 days.
Over 30 μg/mL	Skip next 2 doses and decrease subsequent doses by 50%. Recheck serum level after 3 days.
Too low	Increase dosage by 25% at 3-day intervals until either the desired serum concentration and/or clinical response is achieved. The total daily dose may need to be administered at more frequent intervals if symptoms occur repeatedly

at the end of a dosing interval.

The serum concentration may be rechecked at appropriate intervals, but at least at the end of any adjustment period. When the patient's condition is otherwise clinically stable and none of the recognized factors which alter elimination are present, measurement of serum levels need be repeated only every 6 to 12 months.

DOSAGE OF THEOPHYLLINE TO PROVIDE mg ANHYDROUS THEOPHYLLINE/kg BODY WEIGHT*/DOSE

Body Weight*		Approximate Dose in mg		
Lbs.	kg	3 mg/kg	4 mg/kg	5 mg/kg
40	18	54	72	90
60	27	81	108	135
70	32	96	128	160
80	36	108	144	180
90	41	123	164	205
100	45	135	180	225
120	55	165	220	275
140	64	192		320
160	73	219		365
180	82	246		410
200	91	273		455
220	100	300		500

*For obese patients, use lean (ie, ideal) body weight.

QUIBRON T/SR

General
QUIBRON-T/SR has not been adequately studied for its bioavailability when administered with food (see PRECAUTIONS, DRUG-FOOD INTERACTIONS).

Therapeutic serum levels associated with optimal likelihood for benefit and minimal risk of toxicity are considered to be between 10 μg/mL and 20 μg/mL. Levels above 20 μg/mL may produce toxic effects and, in a small number of patients, toxicity even be seen with serum levels between 15–20 μg/mL, particularly during initiation of therapy. Because of the variable rates of theophylline elimination among patients, the dose necessary to achieve the desired serum level of 10–20 μg theophylline per mL varies from patient to patient. Therefore, it is essential that not only must dosage be individualized, but titration and monitoring of serum levels be utilized where available. When serum concentrations cannot be obtained, restriction of dosage to amounts and intervals recommended in the guidelines listed below becomes essential.

Since theophylline does not distribute into fatty tissue, dosage should be calculated on the basis of ideal body weight.

Acute Symptoms
QUIBRON-T/SR is not intended for use in status asthmaticus or with patients experiencing an acute episode of bronchospasm (associated with asthma, chronic bronchitis, or emphysema). Such patients require rapid relief of symptoms and should be treated with an immediate-release or intravenous theophylline preparation (or other bronchodilators) and not with controlled-release products.

Chronic Therapy
It is recommended that the appropriate dosage be established using an immediate-release preparation. Slow clinical titration is generally preferred to help assure acceptance of the medication, and to allow the patient to develop tolerance to transient caffeine-like side effects. For children under 25 kg, proper dosage should be established with a liquid preparation to permit titration in small increments. Then, the patient can usually be switched to QUIBRON-T/SR, giving one-half of the daily dose at 12-hour intervals. However, certain patients, such as the young, smokers, and some non-smoking adults, are likely to metabolize theophylline rapidly and require dosing at 8-hour intervals. Such patients can generally be identified as having trough serum concentrations lower than desired or repeatedly exhibiting symptoms near the end of the dosage interval.

The average initial adult and children's (over 25 kg) dose is two-thirds (200 mg) of a QUIBRON-T/SR tablet q.12 h.

If the desired response is not achieved with the recommended initial dose, and there are no adverse reactions, the dose may be cautiously adjusted upward in increments of no more than 25% at 3 day intervals until the following MAXIMUM DOSE WITHOUT MEASUREMENT OF SERUM CONCENTRATION or, in the case of adults, a maximum of 900 mg in any 24 hour period (whichever is less) is attained. Following each adjustment, if the clinical response is satisfactory, that dosage level should be maintained.

[See table at top of next column.]

Do not attempt to maintain any dosage that is not tolerated. If doses higher than those contained in the above MAXIMUM DOSE WITHOUT MEASUREMENT OF SERUM CONCENTRATION are necessary, it is recommended that the theophylline levels be monitored. For therapeutic levels, draw blood sample when last dose peaks (4–5 hours after dosing). It is important that the patient has missed no doses during the

previous 72 hours and that dosing intervals have been reasonably typical with no doses added during that period of

MAXIMUM DOSE WITHOUT MEASUREMENT OF SERUM CONCENTRATION

	mg per kg Body Weight* per day
Children (under 9)	24
Children (9–12)	20
Adolescents (12–16)	18
Adults	13 (or 900 mg, whichever is less)

*Use ideal body weight for obese patients.

time. DOSE ADJUSTMENT BASED ON SERUM THEOPHYLLINE MEASUREMENTS MADE WHEN THESE INSTRUCTIONS HAVE NOT BEEN FOLLOWED, MAY RESULT IN RECOMMENDATIONS THAT PRESENT RISK OF TOXICITY TO THE PATIENT.
[See table below.]

Caution should be exercised for younger children who cannot complain of minor side effects. Older adults, those with cor pulmonale, congestive heart failure, and/or liver disease may have unusually low dosage requirements and thus may experience toxicity at the maximal dosage recommended above.

It is important that no patient be maintained on any dosage that is not tolerated. In instructing patients to increase dosage according to the schedule above, they should be instructed not to take a subsequent dose if apparent side effects occur and to resume therapy at a lower dose once adverse effects have disappeared.

HOW SUPPLIED
QUIBRON® Capsules: One-piece, opaque yellow, soft gelatin capsules printed with the "Bristol" logo and "516" containing 150 mg anhydrous theophylline and 90 mg guaifenesin.

NDC 0087-0516-01	Bottles of 100
NDC 0087-0516-02	Bottles of 1000
NDC 0087-0516-03	Unit Dose 100's

QUIBRON®-300 Capsules: One-piece, half opaque white/half opaque yellow, soft gelatin capsules with the "Bristol" logo and "515" containing 300 mg anhydrous theophylline and 180 mg guaifenesin.

NDC 0087-0515-41	Bottles of 100

Store below 30°C (86°F). Protect from freezing.
Dispense in a tight container as defined in the USP.
QUIBRON®-T Tablets: Ivory, in the Dividose® tablet design with debossed "BL" logo and "512" on one side containing 300 mg anhydrous theophylline.

NDC 0087-0512-41	Bottles of 100
NDC 0087-0512-44	Bottles of 500

Store below 86°F (30°C).
QUIBRON-T/SR tablets (white, in the Dividose® tablet design) containing 300 mg anhydrous theophylline.

NDC-0087-0519-41	Bottles of 100
NDC 0087-0519-44	Bottles of 500

Patent Nos. 4,465,660, 4,547,358, 4,215,104
Store below 86°F (30°C).

STADOL®　　℞
[stā'dŏl]
(butorphanol tartrate, USP)

DESCRIPTION
Stadol (butorphanol tartrate, USP), sterile, parenteral, narcotic analgesic agent with agonist-antagonist activity, is a member of the phenanthrene series. The chemical name is levo-N- cyclobutylmethyl-6, 10aβ-dihydroxy-1,2,3,9,10, 10a-hexahydro- (4H) - 10, 4a-iminoethanophenanthrene tartrate. It is a white crystalline substance soluble in aqueous solu-

tion. The dose is expressed as the salt. One milligram of tartrate salt is equivalent to 0.68 milligram of base. In addition to Stadol (butorphanol tartrate, USP), each mL contains 3.3 mg citric acid, 6.4 mg sodium citrate and 6.4 mg sodium chloride.
The structural formula is:

The molecular weight is 477.56 and the molecular formula is $C_{21}H_{29}NO_2 \cdot C_4H_6O_6$

SUPPLY
Stadol (butorphanol tartrate, USP) Injection for IM or IV use is available as follows:
NDC 0015-5644-20—2 mg per mL, 2-mL vial
NDC 0015-5645-20—1 mg per mL, 1-mL vial
NDC 0015-5646-20—2 mg per mL, 1-mL vial
NDC 0015-5648-20—2 mg per mL, 10-mL multi-dose vial
U.S. Patent Nos. 3,819,635, 4,139,534
For information on package sizes available, refer to the current price schedule.

SUMYCIN® '250' TABLETS　　℞
[sū"mī'sin]
SUMYCIN® '500' TABLETS　　℞
Tetracycline Hydrochloride Tablets USP
SUMYCIN® '250' CAPSULES　　℞
SUMYCIN® '500' CAPSULES　　℞
Tetracycline Hydrochloride Capsules USP
SUMYCIN® SYRUP　　℞
Tetracycline Oral Suspension USP

DESCRIPTION
SUMYCIN '250' and SUMYCIN '500' Tablets (Tetracycline Hydrochloride Tablets) are available for oral administration as FILMLOK®* tablets providing 250 mg and 500 mg tetracycline hydrochloride, respectively. Inactive ingredients: microcrystalline cellulose, colorant (D&C Red No. 30), lactose, magnesium stearate, povidone, pregelatinized starch, stearic acid, and other ingredients.

SUMYCIN '250' and SUMYCIN '500' Capsules (Tetracycline Hydrochloride Capsules) contain 250 mg and 500 mg crystalline tetracycline hydrochloride, respectively. Inactive ingredients: colorants (FD&C Blue No. 1 and Red No. 3), gelatin, lactose, magnesium stearate, mineral oil, and titanium dioxide.

SUMYCIN Syrup (Tetracycline Oral Suspension) is a suspension containing, in each 5 mL teaspoonful, tetracycline equivalent to 125 mg tetracycline hydrochloride. Inactive ingredients: citric acid, colorant (D&C Yellow No. 10), flavor, potassium citrate, potassium metaphosphate, purified water, saccharin sodium, sodium benzoate, sodium citrate, sodium metabisulfite, sorbitol solution, sucrose, and tragacanth.

HOW SUPPLIED
*SUMYCIN '250' and *SUMYCIN '500' Tablets (Tetracycline Hydrochloride Tablets USP) are available for oral administration as tablets containing 250 mg and 500 mg tetracycline hydrochloride, respectively.
*SUMYCIN '250' and *SUMYCIN '500' Capsules (Tetracycline Hydrochloride Capsules USP) are available for oral administration as capsules containing 250 mg and 500 mg tetracycline hydrochloride, respectively.

*FILMLOK is a Squibb trademark for veneer-coated tablets.

If serum theophylline level is:		Directions:
Within normal limits	10 to 20 μg/mL	Maintain dosage if tolerated. Recheck serum theophylline concentration at 6- to 12-month intervals.*
Too high	20 to 25 μg/mL	Decrease doses by about 10%. Recheck serum theophylline concentration at 6- to 12-month intervals.*
	25 to 30 μg/mL	Skip next dose and decrease subsequent doses by about 25%.
	Over 30 μg/mL	Skip next 2 doses and decrease subsequent doses by 50%. Recheck serum theophylline.
Too low	7.5 to 10 μg/mL	Increase dose by about 25%. Recheck serum theophylline concentration at 6- to 12-month intervals.**
	5 to 7.5 μg/mL	Increase dose by about 25% to the nearest dose increment and recheck serum theophylline for guidance in further dosage adjustment (another increase will probably be needed, but this provides a safety check).

* Finer adjustments may be needed for some patients.
** Dividing the daily dosage into 3 doses administered at 8 hour intervals may be indicated if symptoms occur repeatedly at the end of a dosing interval.
From the Journal of Respiratory Diseases 2(7): 16, 1981.

Continued on next page

Apothecon—Cont.

SUMYCIN Syrup (Tetracycline Oral Suspension USP) is available as a fruit-flavored suspension containing, in each 5 mL teaspoonful, tetracycline equivalent to 125 mg tetracycline hydrochloride.

Storage

Store the tablets and capsules at room temperature; avoid excessive heat. Store the syrup below 30° C (86° F); avoid freezing; protect from light; keep tightly closed.

THERAGRAN® LIQUID OTC

[*ther'ah-gran"*]

(High Potency Vitamin Supplement)

(See PDR For Nonprescription Drugs.)

THERAGRAN® TABLETS OTC

[*ther'ah-gran"*]

(High Potency Multivitamin Formula)

ADVANCED FORMULA

(See PDR For Nonprescription Drugs.)

THERAGRAN-M® TABLETS OTC

[*ther'ah-gran"em*]

(High Potency Multivitamin Formula with Minerals)

ADVANCED FORMULA

(See PDR For Nonprescription Drugs.)

THERAGRAN® STRESS FORMULA OTC

(High Potency Multivitamin Formula with Iron and Biotin)

(See PDR For Nonprescription Drugs.)

VEETIDS® ℞

BETAPEN-VK®

Penicillin V Potassium Tablets, USP

500 mg (800,000 units) and

Oral Solution

DESCRIPTION

VEETIDS and BETAPEN-VK, the potassium salt of penicillin V, monopotassium [2S-(2α, 5α, 6β)]-3,3-dimethyl-7-oxo-6-[(phenoxyacetyl) amino]-4-thia-1-azabicyclo[3.2.0] heptane-2-carboxylate, is an antibacterial agent having the following chemical structure:

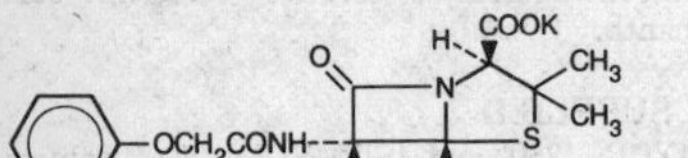

The empirical formula is $C_{16}H_{17}KN_2O_5S$ and the molecular weight is 388.48.

The oral solutions contain 125 mg or 250 mg of penicillin V activity, respectively, in each 5 mL (1 teaspoonful). The tablets each contain 250 mg or 500 mg of penicillin V activity, respectively.

Inactive ingredients in VEETIDS tablets are: carnauba wax, ethyl cellulose, lactose, magnesium stearate, methanol, methyl cellulose, opaspray white, polyethylene glycol, starch, and white wax. Inactive ingredients in VEETIDS oral solution are: acacia, citric acid, DL-menthol, FD&C Red No. 40, natural and artificial flavorings, sodium benzoate, sodium citrate, sodium saccharin, sucrose, and thymol.

CLINICAL PHARMACOLOGY

Penicillin V has the distinct advantage over penicillin G in resistance to inactivation by gastric acid. It may be given with meals; however, blood levels are slightly higher when the drug is given on an empty stomach. Average blood levels are two to five times higher than the levels following the same dose of oral penicillin G and also show much less individual variation.

Once absorbed, penicillin V is about 80% bound to serum protein. Tissue levels are highest in the kidney, with lesser amount in the liver, skin, and intestines. Small amounts are found in all other body tissues and the cerebrospinal fluid. The drug is excreted as rapidly as it is absorbed in individuals with normal renal function; however, recovery of the drug from the urine indicates that only about 25% of the dose is absorbed. In neonates, young infants, and individuals with impaired renal function, excretion is considerably delayed.

Microbiology

Penicillin V exerts a bactericidal action against penicillin-susceptible microorganisms during the stage of active multiplication. It acts through the inhibition of biosynthesis of cell wall mucopeptide. It is not active against the penicillinase-producing bacteria, which include many strains of staphylococci. While **in vitro** studies have demonstrated the susceptibility of most strains of the following organisms, clinical efficacy for infections other than those included in the **INDICATIONS AND USAGE** section has not been documented. The drug exerts high **in vitro** activity against staphylococci (except penicillinase-producing strains), streptococci (Groups A, C, G, H, L, and M), and pneumococci. Other organisms susceptible in **vitro** to penicillin V are **Corynebacterium diphtheriae, Bacillus anthracis,** Clostridia, **Actinomyces bovis, Streptobacillus moniliformis, Listeria monocytogenes,** Leptospira, and **Neisseria gonorrhoeae. Treponema pallidum** is extremely susceptible.

INDICATIONS AND USAGE

VEETIDS and BETAPEN-VK are indicated in the treatment of infections caused by susceptible strains of the designated organisms in the conditions listed below:

Skin and Soft Tissue Infections caused by penicillin G-susceptible staphylococci and **Streptococcal sp.** (mild erysipelas and scarlet fever).

Respiratory Tract Infections caused by **Streptococcus sp.** (Groups A, C, G, H, L, and M) including pneumococcal infections (**Strep. pneumoniae**). Fusospirochetosis (Vincent's gingivitis and pharyngitis) of the oropharynx usually respond to therapy with oral penicillin.

Note: Necessary dental care should be accomplished in infections involving gum tissue.

Prophylaxis for Recurrent Rheumatic Fever may be indicated for oral penicillins. Although no controlled clinical efficacy studies have been conducted, penicillin V has been suggested by the American Heart Association and the American Dental Association for use as part of a parenteral-oral regimen and as an alternative oral regimen for prophylaxis against bacterial endocarditis in patients with congenital heart disease or rheumatic or other acquired valvular heart disease when they undergo dental procedures and surgical procedures of the respiratory tract.[1] Since it may happen that **alpha**-hemolytic streptococci, relatively resistant to penicillin, may be found when patients are receiving continuous oral penicillin for secondary prevention of rheumatic fever, prophylactic agents other than penicillin may be chosen for these patients and prescribed in addition to their continuous rheumatic fever prophylactic regimen. Oral penicillin should not be used as adjunctive prophylaxis for genitourinary instrumentation or surgery, lower intestinal tract surgery, sigmoidoscopy, and childbirth.

Note: When selecting antibiotics for the prevention of bacterial endocarditis the physician or dentist should read the full joint statement of the American Heart Association and the American Dental Association.[1]

Note: Severe pneumonia, empyema, bacteremia, pericarditis, meningitis, and arthritis should not be treated with oral penicillins during the acute stage.

CONTRAINDICATIONS

A previous hypersensitivity reaction to any penicillin is a contraindication.

WARNINGS

Serious and occasionally fatal hypersensitivity (anaphylactoid) reactions have been reported in patients on penicillin therapy. Although anaphylaxis is more frequent following parenteral therapy, it has occurred in patients on oral penicillins. These reactions are more apt to occur in individuals with a history of penicillin hypersensitivity and/or a history of sensitivity to multiple allergens. There have been well documented reports of individuals with a history of penicillin hypersensitivity reactions who experienced severe hypersensitivity reactions when treated with cephalosporins. Before initiating therapy with any penicillin, careful inquiry should be made concerning previous hypersensitivity reactions to penicillins, cephalosporins, and other allergens. If an allergic reaction occurs, the drug should be discontinued and the appropriate therapy instituted.

SERIOUS ANAPHYLACTOID REACTIONS REQUIRE IMMEDIATE EMERGENCY TREATMENT WITH EPINEPHRINE. OXYGEN, INTRAVENOUS STEROIDS, AND AIRWAY MANAGEMENT, INCLUDING INTUBATION, SHOULD ALSO BE ADMINISTERED AS INDICATED.

PRECAUTIONS

General: Penicillins should be used with caution in individuals with a history of significant allergies and/or asthma.

The oral route of administration should not be relied upon in patients with severe illness, or with nausea, vomiting, gastric dilatation, cardiospasm, or intestinal hypermotility.

Occasional patients will not absorb therapeutic amounts of orally administered penicillin.

Prolonged use of antibiotics may promote the overgrowth of nonsusceptible organisms, including fungi. Should superinfection occur, appropriate measures should be taken.

In streptococcal infections, therapy must be sufficient to eliminate the organism (10 days minimum); otherwise the sequelae of streptococcal disease may occur.

Laboratory Tests: In streptoccoal infections, cultures should be taken following completion of treatment to determine whether streptococci have been eradicated.

Carcinogenesis, Mutagenesis, and Impairment of Fertility: No long-term animal studies have been conducted with these drugs.

Pregnancy Category B: Reproduction studies performed in the mouse, rat, and rabbit have revealed no evidence of impaired fertility or harm to the fetus due to penicillin V. Human experience with the penicillins during pregnancy has not shown any positive evidence of adverse effects on the fetus. There are, however, no adequate and well-controlled studies in pregnant women showing conclusively that harmful effects of these drugs on the fetus can be excluded. Because animal reproduction studies are not always predictive of human response, penicillin should be used during pregnancy only if clearly needed.

Nursing Mothers: Penicillins are excreted in milk. Caution should be exercised when penicillins are administered to a nursing woman.

Pediatric Use: Because of incompletely developed renal function in newborns, penicillin elimination may be delayed. Guidelines for administration of this drug to children are presented under DOSAGE AND ADMINISTRATION.

ADVERSE REACTIONS

Althougih the incidence of reactions to oral penicillins has been reported with much less frequency than following parenteral therapy, it should be remembered that all degrees of hypersensitivity, including fatal anaphylaxis, have been reported with oral penicillin.

The most common reactions to oral penicillin are nausea, vomiting, epigastric distress, diarrhea, and black hairy tongue. The hypersensitivity reactions reported are skin eruptions (maculopapular) to exfoliative dermatitis), urticaria and other serum sickness reactions, laryngeal edema, and anaphylaxis. Fever and eosinophilia may frequently be the only reaction observed. Hemolytic anemia, leukopenia, thrombocytopenia, neuropathy, and nephropathy are infrequent reactions and usually associated with high doses of parenteral penicillin.

OVERDOSAGE

In case of overdosage, discontinue medication, treat symptomatically and institute supportive measures as required.

DOSAGE AND ADMINISTRATION

The dosage of VEETIDS and BETAPEN-VK should be determined according to the susceptibility of the causative organism and the severity of infection, and adjusted to the clinical response of the patient.

The usual dosage recommendations for adults and children 12 years and over are as follows:

Streptococcal Infections—mild to moderately severe—of the upper respiratory tract and including scarlet fever and erysipelas: 125 to 250 mg (200,000 to 400,000 units) every 6 to 8 hours for 10 days.

Pneumococcal Infections—mild to moderately severe—of the respiratory tract, including otitis media: 250 mg (400,000 units) every 6 hours until the patient has been afebrile for at least 2 days.

Staphylococcal Infections—mild infections of skin and soft tissue (culture and susceptibility tests should be performed): 250 mg (400,000 units) every 6 to 8 hours.

Fusospirochetosis (Vincent's infection) of the oropharynx —mild to moderately severe infections: 250 mg (400,000 units) every 6 to 8 hours.

For the prevention of recurrence following rheumatic fever and/or chorea: 125 mg (200,000 units) twice daily on a continuing basis. For prophylaxis against bacterial endocarditis[1] in patients with congenital heart disease or rheumatic or other acquired valvular heart disease when undergoing dental procedures or surgical procedures of the upper respiratory tract, 1 of 2 regimens may be selected:

(1) For the oral regimen, give 2 grams of penicillin V (1 gram for children under 60 lbs) ½ to 1 hour before the procedure, and then 500 mg (250 mg for children under 60 lbs) every 6 hours for 8 doses; or

(2) For the combined parenteral-oral regimen, give 1 million units of aqueous crystalline penicillin G (30,000 units/kg in children) intramuscularly mixed with 600,000 units procaine penicillin G (600,000 units for children) ½ to 1 hour before the procedure, and then oral penicillin V, 500 mg for adults or 250 mg for children less than 60 lbs, every 6 hours for 8 doses. Doses for children should not exceed recommendations for adults for a single dose or for a 24-hour period.

DIRECTIONS FOR DISPENSING ORAL SOLUTIONS

Prepare this formulation at the time of dispensing. For ease in preparation, add water to the bottle in two portions and shake well after each addition. Add the total amount of water as directed on the labeling of the package being dispensed. The reconstituted solutions are stable for 14 days under refrigeration.

HOW SUPPLIED

VEETIDS (penicillin V potassium for Oral Solution, USP). Each 5 mL of reconstituted solution contains penicillin V potassium equivalent to 125 or 250 mg penicillin V.

NDC 0003-0681-44   125 mg/5 mL, bottle of 100 mL
NDC 0003-0681-54   125 mg/5 mL, bottle of 200 mL
NDC 0003-0682-44   250 mg/5 mL, bottle of 100 mL
NDC 0003-0682-54   250 mg/5 mL, bottle of 200 mL

VEETIDS (penicillin V potassium Tablets, USP) Film-Coated. Each tablet contains penicillin V potassium equivalent to 250 or 500 mg penicillin V.

NDC 0003-0115-50   250 mg, bottle of 100
NDC 0003-0115-75   250 mg, bottle of 1000
NDC 0003-0116-50   500 mg, bottle of 100
NDC 0003-0116-75   500 mg, bottle of 1000

REFERENCE

1. American Heart Association, 1977. Prevention of bacterial endocarditis. Circulation. 56:139A-143A.

BETAPEN-VK (penicillin V potassium for Oral Solution, USP). Each 5 mL of reconstituted solution contains penicillin V potassium equivalent to 125 or 250 mg penicillin V.

NDC 0015-7506-40   125 mg/5 mL, bottle of 100 mL
NDC 0015-7506-64   126 mg/5 mL, bottle of 200 mL
NDC 0015-7507-40   250 mg/5 mL, bottle of 100 mL
NDC 0015-7507-64   250 mg/5 mL, bottle of 200 mL

BETAPEN-VK (penicillin V potassium Tablets, USP) Film-Coated. Each tablet contains penicillin V potassium equivalent to 250 or 500 mg penicillin V.

NDC 0015-7508-60   250 mg, bottle of 100
NDC 0015-7508-90   250 mg, bottle of 1000
NDC 0015-7509-60   500 mg, bottle of 100
NDC 0015-7509-80   500 mg, bottle of 500

REFERENCE

1. American Heart Association, 1977. Prevention of bacterial endocarditis. Circulation. 56:139A-143A.

VELOSEF® '250' CAPSULES   ℞
[vel 'ō-sef]
VELOSEF® '500' CAPSULES   ℞
Cephradine Capsules USP
VELOSEF® '125' FOR ORAL SUSPENSION   ℞
VELOSEF® '250' FOR ORAL SUSPENSION   ℞
Cephradine for Oral Suspension USP

DESCRIPTION

VELOSEF (Cephradine, Squibb) is a semisynthetic cephalosporin antibiotic; oral dosage forms include capsules containing 250 mg and 500 mg cephradine and cephradine for oral suspension containing, after constitution, 125 mg and 250 mg per 5 mL dose.

Cephradine is designated chemically as (6R,7R)-7-[(R)-2-amino-2-(1,4-cyclohexadien-1-yl) acetamido]-3-methyl-8-oxo-5-thia-1-azabicyclo[4.2.0]oct-2-ene-2-carboxylic acid.

Inactive ingredients: VELOSEF Capsules—colorants (D&C Red No. 33 and Yellow No. 10; FD&C Blue No. 1, and, for '250' only, Red No. 3), gelatin, lactose, magnesium stearate, talc, and titanium dioxide. VELOSEF for Oral Suspension—citric acid, colorants (FD&C Red No. 40 for '250' only; FD&C Yellow No. 6 for '125' only), flavors, guar gum, methylcellulose, sodium citrate, and sucrose.

HOW SUPPLIED

VELOSEF Capsules (Cephradine Capsules USP)

*VELOSEF '250' 250 mg/capsule: bottles of 24 (NDC 0003-0113-24) and 100 (NDC 0003-0113-50) and 100 Unimatic® unit-dose packs (NDC 0003-0113-52). Capsule identification no. 113.

*VELOSEF '500' 500 mg/capsule: bottles of 24 (NDC 0003-0114-26) and 100 (NDC 0003-0114-50) and 100 Unimatic unit-dose packs (NDC 0003-0114-52). Capsule identification no. 114.

VELOSEF for Oral Suspension (Cephradine for Oral Suspension USP)

VELOSEF '125' When constituted as directed on the container label, a pleasant fruit-flavored suspension containing 125 mg per 5 mL, in bottle sizes for preparation of 100 mL (NDC 0003-1193-50) and 200 mL (NDC 0003-1193-80). 125 mg/bottle: packs of 100 Unimatic unit-dose bottles (NDC 0003-1193-20).

VELOSEF '250' When constituted as directed on the container label, a pleasant fruit-flavored suspension containing 250 mg per 5 mL, in bottle sizes for preparation of 100 mL (NDC 0003-1194-50) and 200 mL (NDC 0003-1194-80). 250 mg/bottle: packs of 100 Unimatic unit-dose bottles (NDC 0003-1194-20).

Storage

VELOSEF Capsules—Keep tightly closed. Do not store above 86°F.

VELOSEF for Oral Suspension— Prior to constitution, store at room temperature; avoid excessive heat. After constitution, when stored at room temperature, discard unused portion after seven days; when stored in refrigerator, discard unused portion after 14 days. Keep tightly closed.

Arco Pharmaceuticals, Inc.
105 ORVILLE DRIVE
BOHEMIA, NY 11716

ARCO-LASE®   OTC
(broad pH spectrum digestant)

COMPOSITION

Each soft, mint flavored tablet contains Trizyme*, 38 mg., and Lipase, 25 mg.
*Contains the following standardized enzymes: amylolytic 30 mg.; proteolytic 6 mg.; cellulolytic 2 mg.

ACTION AND USES

Indicated for most gastrointestinal disorders due to poor digestion. Flatulence, gas and bloating, dyspepsia, distention, fullness, heartburn, or in any condition where normal digestion is impaired by digestive insufficiencies. Arcolase provides the highest standardized enzymatic activity, plus the protective action of the widest pH range. Thus it is effective throughout the entire G.I. tract. Requiring no enteric coating, there is assurance of a positive breakdown of its factors. This is advantageous, because quite often patients with digestive disorders cannot digest their food properly, let alone hard, or enteric coated capsules or tablets.

SIDE EFFECTS
None.

ADMINISTRATION AND DOSAGE

One tablet with or immediately following meals. Tablet may be swallowed or chewed.

SUPPLIED

Bottles of 50's. NDC 275-4040.

ARCO-LASE® PLUS   ℞

COMPOSITION

Same as Arco-Lase, plus the addition of Hyoscyamine sulfate 0.10 mg., atropine sulfate 0.02 mg. and phenobarbital ⅛ gr. (Warning: may be habit forming.)

ACTION AND USES

Gastrointestinal disturbances, such as cramps, bloating, spasms, diarrhea, nausea, vomiting and peptic ulcer. The enzymes correct the digestive insufficiencies.

The antispasmodic and phenobarbital contribute to the symptomatic relief of hypermotility and nervous tension, which usually accompanies functional disturbances of the bowel.

ADMINISTRATION AND DOSAGE

One tablet following meals.

SIDE EFFECTS

May cause rapid pulse, dryness of mouth and blurred vision.

CONTRAINDICATIONS

This product is contraindicated in the presence of glaucoma or prostatic hypertrophy.

SUPPLIED

Bottles of 50's. NDC 275-45-45.

LITERATURE AVAILABLE

Yes.

MEGA-B®   OTC
(super potency vitamin B complex, sugar & starch free)

COMPOSITION

Each Mega-B Tablet contains the following Mega Vitamins:

B_1 (Thiamine Mononitrate)	100 mg.
B_2 (Riboflavin)	100 mg.
B_6 (Pyridoxine Hydrochloride)	100 mg.
B_{12} (Cyanocobalamin)	100 mcg.
Choline Bitartrate	100 mg.
Inositol	100 mg.
Niacinamide	100 mg.
Folic Acid	100 mcg.
Pantothenic Acid	100 mg.
d-Biotin	100 mcg.
Para-Aminobenzoic Acid (PABA)	100 mg.

In a base of yeast to provide the identified and unidentified B-Complex Factors.

ADVANTAGES

Each Mega-B capsule-shaped tablet provides the highest vitamin B complex available in a single dose.
Mega-B was designed for those patients who require truly Mega vitamin potencies with the convenience of minimum dosage.

INDICATIONS

Mega-B is indicated in conditions characterized by depletions or increased demand of the water-soluble B-complex vitamins. It may be useful in the nutritional management of patients during prolonged convalescence associated with major surgery. It is also indicated for stress conditions, as an adjunct to antibiotics and diuretic therapy, pre and post operative cases, liver conditions, gastrointestinal disorders interfering with intake or absorption of water-soluble vitamins, prolonged or wasting diseases, diabetes, burns, fractures, severe infections, and some psychological disorders.

WARNING

NOT INTENDED FOR TREATMENT OF PERNICIOUS ANEMIA, OR OTHER PRIMARY OR SECONDARY ANEMIAS.

DOSAGE

Usual dosage is one Mega-B tablet daily, or varied, depending on clinical needs.

SUPPLIED

Yellow capsule shaped tablets in bottles of 30, 100 and 500.

MEGADOSE™   OTC
(multiple mega-vitamin formula with minerals, sugar and starch free)

COMPOSITION

Vitamin A	25,000 USP Units
Vitamin D	1,000 USP Units
Vitamin C w/Rose Hips	250 mg.
Vitamin E	100 IU
Folic Acid	400 mcg.
Vitamin B_1	80 mg.
Vitamin B_2	80 mg.
Niacinamide	80 mg.
Vitamin B_6	80 mg.
Vitamin B_{12}	80 mcg.
Biotin	80 mcg.
Pantothenic Acid	80 mg.
Choline Bitartrate	80 mg.
Inositol	80 mg.
Para-Aminobenzoic Acid	80 mg.
Rutin	30 mg.
Citrus Bioflavonoids	30 mg.
Betaine Hydrochloride	30 mg.
Glutamic Acid	30 mg.
Hesperidin Complex	5 mg.
Iodine (from Kelp)	0.15 mg.
Calcium Gluconate*	50 mg.
Zinc Gluconate*	25 mg.
Potassium Gluconate*	10 mg.
Ferrous Gluconate*	10 mg.
Magnesium Gluconate*	7 mg.
Manganese Gluconate*	6 mg.
Copper Gluconate*	0.5 mg.

*Natural mineral chelates in a base containing natural ingredients.

DOSAGE

One tablet daily.

SUPPLIED

Capsule shaped tablets in bottles of 30, 100 and 250.

Armour Pharmaceutical Company
500 ARCOLA ROAD
P.O. BOX 1200
COLLEGEVILLE, PA 19426-0107

PLASMA DERIVATIVE PRODUCTS

ALBUMINAR®-5 ℞
[*al-byōō'mĭn-är*]
Albumin
(Human) U.S.P. 5%

DESCRIPTION
Albumin (Human) 5%, ALBUMINAR®-5 is a sterile solution of albumin obtained from large pools of adult human venous plasma by low temperature controlled fractionation according to the Cohn process. It is pasteurized at 60°C for 10 hours and stabilized with 0.004M sodium acetyltryptophanate and 0.004M sodium caprylate.
Each 50 mL bottle of 5% solution contains 2.5 grams of albumin in normal saline. Each 250 mL bottle of 5% solution contains 12.5 grams of albumin in normal saline. Each 500 mL bottle of 5% solution contains 25 grams of albumin in normal saline. Each 1000 mL bottle of 5% solution contains 50 grams of albumin in normal saline. The 5% solution is osmotically equivalent with citrated plasma. The pH of the solution is adjusted to 6.9 ± 0.5 with sodium bicarbonate, sodium hydroxide or acetic acid. Approximate concentrations of significant electrolytes per liter are: Sodium—130–160 mEq; and Potassium—n.m.t. 1 mEq. The solution contains no preservative. This product has been prepared in accordance with the requirements established by the Food and Drug Administration and is in compliance with the standards of the United States Pharmacopeia.

CLINICAL PHARMACOLOGY
Albumin (Human) 5%, ALBUMINAR®-5, being active osmotically, is useful in regulating the volume of circulating blood. It is a valuable therapeutic aid for the treatment of conditions that will be benefited by its marked osmotic effect. When the circulating blood volume has been depleted, the hemodilution following albumin administration persists for many hours. In individuals with normal blood volume, it usually lasts only a few hours.
Albumin, unlike whole blood or plasma, is considered free of the danger of viral hepatitis. It is convenient to use since no crossmatching is required and the absence of cellular elements removes the danger of sensitization with repeated infusions.

INDICATIONS
Shock—Albumin 5% is indicated in the emergency treatment of shock due to burns, trauma, operations and infections, in the treatment of severe injuries, and in other similar conditions where the restoration of blood volume is urgent. The primary function is maintenance of colloid osmotic pressure. If there has been considerable loss of red blood cells, transfusion with whole blood is indicated.
Burns—Albumin 5% is indicated in conjunction with adequate infusions of crystalloid to counteract hemoconcentration and the loss of protein, electrolytes and water that usually follow severe burns.
Hypoproteinemia—Albumin (Human) 5%, ALBUMINAR®-5 may be used in acutely hypoproteinemic patients, provided sodium restriction is not a problem.

CONTRAINDICATIONS
Albumin (Human) 5%, ALBUMINAR®-5 is contraindicated in patients with severe anemia or cardiac failure.

WARNING
Do not use if the solution is turbid, or if there is a sediment in the bottle. Since the product contains no antimicrobial preservative, do not begin administration more than 4 hours after the container has been entered. Destroy unused portions to prevent the possibility of subsequent use of a solution that may have become contaminated.

PRECAUTIONS
Administration of large quantities of albumin should be supplemented with or replaced by whole blood to combat the relative anemia which would follow such use. The quick response of blood pressure, which may follow the rapid administration of albumin, necessitates careful observation of the injured patient to detect bleeding points which failed to bleed at lower blood pressure. Albumin (Human) 5%, ALBUMINAR®-5 should be administered with caution to patients with low cardiac reserve or with no albumin deficiency because a rapid increase in plasma volume may cause circulatory embarrassment of pulmonary edema.

ADVERSE REACTIONS
The incidence of untoward reactions to Albumin (Human) 5% is low although nausea, vomiting, increased salivation and febrile reactions occasionally may occur. Urticaria has been reported following administration of albumin.

DOSAGE AND ADMINISTRATION
Albumin (Human) 5%, ALBUMINAR®-5 is given intravenously without further dilution. This concentration is approximately isotonic and iso-osmotic with citrated plasma. Albumin in this concentration provides additional fluid for plasma volume expansion. Therefore, when it is administered to patients with normal blood volume, the rate of infusion should be slow enough to prevent too rapid expansion of plasma volume.
In the treatment of shock in an adult patient an initial dose of 500 mL of the 5% albumin solution is given as rapidly as tolerated. If response within 30 minutes is inadequate, an additional 500 mL of 5% albumin solution may be given. The 50 mL dosage form would be appropriate for pediatric use. Therapy should be guided by the clinical response, blood pressure and an assessment of relative anemia. If more than 1000 mL are given, or if hemorrhage has occurred, the administration of Whole Blood (Human) or Red Blood Cells (Human) may be desirable.
In severe burns, immediate therapy usually includes large volumes of crystalloid with lesser amounts of 5% albumin solution to maintain an adequate plasma volume. After the first 24 hours, the ratio of albumin to crystalloid may be increased to establish and maintain a plasma albumin level of about 2.5 g/100mL or a total serum protein level of about 5.2 g/100mL. However, an optimal regimen for the use of colloids, electrolytes and water after severe burns has not been established.
The infusion of Albumin (Human) as a nutrient in the treatment of chronic hypoproteinemia is not recommended. In acute hypoproteinemia 5% albumin may be used in replacing the protein lost in hypoproteinemic conditions. However, if edema is present or if large amounts of albumin are lost, Albumin (Human) 25% is preferred because of the greater amount of protein in the concentrated solution.

HOW SUPPLIED
Albumin (Human) 5%, ALBUMINAR®-5 is supplied in:
NDC 0053-7670-06 50 mL bottles containing 2.5 grams of albumin,
NDC 0053-7670-01 250 mL bottles containing 12.5 grams of albumin,
NDC 0053-7670-02 500 mL bottles containing 25.0 grams of albumin,
NDC 0053-7670-03 1000 mL bottles containing 50.0 grams of albumin.
Store at controlled room temperature—between 15°–30°C (59°–86°F).
CAUTION: FEDERAL (U.S.A.) LAW PROHIBITS DISPENSING WITHOUT PRESCRIPTION.

REFERENCES
1. Finlayson, J.S.: Albumin Products. Seminars in Thrombosis and Hemostasis 6:85–120, 1980.
2. Tullis, J.L.: Albumin. JAMA 237: 355–360 and 460–463, 1977.
Revised: July, 1990

ALBUMINAR®-25 ℞
[*ăl-byōō'mĭn-är*"]
Albumin
(Human) U.S.P. 25%

DESCRIPTION
Albumin (Human) 25%, ALBUMINAR®-25 is a sterile aqueous solution of albumin obtained from large pools of adult human plasma by low termperature controlled fractionation according to the Cohn process. It is stabilized with 0.02M sodium acetyltryptophanate and 0.02M sodium caprylate and pasteurized at 60°C for 10 hours.
Albumin (Human) 25%, ALBUMINAR®-25 is a solution containing in each 100 mL, 25 grams of serum albumin, osmotically equivalent to 500 mL of normal human plasma. The pH of the solution is adjusted with sodium bicarbonate, sodium hydroxide, or acetic acid. Approximate concentrations of significant electrolytes per liter are: sodium—130–160 mEq; and potassium—n.m.t. 1mEq. The solution contains no preservative. This product has been prepared in accordance with the requirements established by the Food and Drug Administration and is in compliance with the standards of the United States Pharmacopeia.
Albumin (Human) 25%, ALBUMINAR®-25 is to be administered by the intravenous route.

CLINICAL PHARMACOLOGY
ALBUMINAR®-25 is active osmotically and is therefore important in regulating the volume of circulating blood. When injected intravenously, 50 mL of 25% albumin draws approximately 175 mL of additional fluid into the circulation within 15 minutes, except in the presence of marked dehydration. This extra fluid reduces hemoconcentration and blood viscosity. The degree of volume expansion is dependent on the initial blood volume. When the circulating blood volume has been depleted, the hemodilution following albumin administration persists for many hours. In individuals with normal blood volume, it usually lasts only a few hours.
Albumin, unlike whole blood or plasma, is considered free of the danger of homologous serum hepatitis. Albumin (Human) 25%, ALBUMINAR®-25 may be given in conjunction with other parenteral fluids—such as saline, glucose or sodium lactate. It is convenient to use since no crossmatching is required and the absence of cellular elements removes the danger of sensitization with repeated infusions.

INDICATIONS AND USAGE
Shock—Albumin is indicated in the emergency treatment of shock and in other similar conditions where the restoration of blood volume is urgent. If there has been considerable loss of red blood cells, transfusion with whole blood is indicated.
Burns—Albumin or Albumin in either normal saline or glucose is indicated to prevent marked hemoconcentration and to maintain appropriate electrolyte balance.
Hypoproteinemia with or without edema—Albumin is indicated in those clinical situations usually associated with a low concentration of plasma protein and a resulting decreased circulating blood volume. Although diuresis may occur soon after albumin administration has been instituted, best results are obtained if albumin is continued until the normal serum protein level is regained.

CONTRAINDICATIONS
Albumin (Human) 25%, ALBUMINAR®-25 may be contraindicated in patients with severe anemia or cardiac failure.

WARNING
Do not use if the solution is turbid. Since this product contains no antimicrobial preservative, do not begin administration more than 4 hours after the container has been entered.

PRECAUTIONS
General
If dehydration is present additional fluids must accompany or follow the administration of albumin. Administration of large quantities of albumin should be supplemented with or replaced by whole blood to combat the relative anemia which would follow such use. The quick response of blood pressure which may follow the rapid administration of concentrated albumin necessitates careful observation of the injured patient to detect bleeding points which failed to bleed at lower blood pressure. Albumin (Human) 25% should be administered with caution to patients with low cardiac reserve or with no albumin deficiency because a rapid increase in plasma volume may cause circulatory embarrassment or pulmonary edema. In cases of hypertension, a slower rate of administration is desired—200 mL of albumin solution may be mixed with 300 mL of 10% glucose solution and administered at a rate of 10 grams of albumin (100 mL) per hour.
Pregnancy Category C
Animal reproduction studies have not been conducted with Albumin (Human) 25%, ALBUMINAR®-25. It is also not known whether ALBUMINAR®-25 can cause fetal harm when administered to a pregnant woman or can affect reproduction capacity. ALBUMINAR®-25 should be given to a pregnant woman only if clearly needed.

ADVERSE REACTIONS
The incidence of untoward reactions to Albumin (Human) 25% is low although nausea, vomiting, increased salivation and febrile reactions occasionally may occur.

DOSAGE AND ADMINISTRATION
Albumin (Human) 25%, ALBUMINAR®-25 may be given intravenously without dilution or it may be diluted with normal saline or 5% glucose before administration. Two hundred mL per liter gives a solution which is approximately isotonic and ios-osmotic with citrated plasma.
When undiluted albumin solution is administered in patients with normal blood volume, the rate of infusion should be slow enough (1 mL per minute) to prevent too rapid expansion of plasma volume.
In the treatment of shock the amount of albumin and duration of therapy must be based on the responsiveness of the patient as indicated by blood pressure, degree of pulmonary congestion, and hematocrit. The initial dose may be followed by additional albumin within 15–30 minutes if the response is deemed inadequate. If there is continued loss of protein, it also may be desirable to give whole blood and/or other blood fractions.
In the treatment of burns an optimal regimen involving use of albumin, crystalloids, electrolytes and water has not been established. Suggested therapy during the first 24 hours includes administration of large volumes of crystalloid solution to maintain an adequate plasma volume. Continuation of therapy beyond 24 hours usually requires more albumin and less crystalloid solution to prevent marked hemoconcentration and maintain electrolyte balance.

Duration of treatment varies depending upon the extent of protein loss through renal excretion, denuded areas of skin and decreased albumin synthesis. Attempts to raise the albumin level above 4.0 g/100 mL may only result in an increased rate of catabolism.

In the treatment of hypoproteinemia, 200 to 300 mL of 25% albumin may be required to reduce edema and to bring serum protein values to normal. Since such patients usually have approximately normal blood volume, doses of more than 100 mL of 25% albumin should not be given faster than 100 mL in 30 to 45 minutes to avoid circulatory embarrassment. If slower administration is desired, 200 mL of 25% albumin may be mixed with 300 mL of 10% glucose solution and administered by continuous drip at a rate of 100 mL of this glucose solution an hour.

Parenteral drug products should be inspected visually for particulate matter and discoloration prior to administration, whenever solution and container permit.

HOW SUPPLIED

Albumin (Human), ALBUMINAR®-25 is supplied as a 25% solution in:

NDC 0053-7680-01 20 mL vials containing 5.0 grams of albumin

NDC 0053-7680-02 50 mL vials containing 12.5 grams of albumin

NDC 0053-7680-03 100 mL vials containing 25.0 grams of albumin

Store at controlled room temperature—
between 15°–30°C (59°–86°F).
Caution: Federal (U.S.A.) law prohibits
dispensing without prescription

Revised—October, 1990

GAMMAR® ℞
[găm 'är]
**Immune Globulin
(Human) U.S.P.**

DESCRIPTION

Immune Globulin (Human) (IG)—GAMMAR® is a sterile solution of immunoglobulin, primarily immunoglobulin G (IgG), containing $16.5 \pm 1.5\%$ protein. It is prepared by cold alcohol fractionation of pooled plasma. Immune Globulin (Human)—GAMMAR® contains the mercurial preservative, thimerosal, at a concentration of 100 mg per liter and is stabilized with 0.3 M glycine. The pH of the solution has been adjusted to 6.8 ± 0.4 with sodium bicarbonate. The product is intended for the intramuscular route of administration.

CLINICAL PHARMACOLOGY

Peak blood levels of immunoglobulin G are obtained approximately 2 days after intramuscular injection of IG (1). The half-life of IgG in the circulation of individuals with normal IgG levels is 23 days (2).

Passive immunization with IG modifies hepatitis A, prevents or modifies measles, and provides replacement therapy in persons with hypo- or agammaglobulinemia. IG is not standardized with respect to antibody titers against hepatitis B surface antigen (HBsAg) and should not be used for prophylaxis of viral hepatitis type B. Prophylactic treatment to prevent hepatitis B can best be accomplished with the use of Hepatitis B Immune Globulin, often in combination with Hepatitis B Vaccine (10).

IG may be of benefit in women who have been exposed to rubella in the first trimester of pregnancy and who would not consider a therapeutic abortion (4). IG may also be considered for use in immunocompromised patients for passive immunization against varicella if Varicella-Zoster Immune Globulin (Human) is not available (7).

IG is not indicated for routine prophylaxis or treatment of rubella, poliomyelitis, mumps or varicella. It is not indicated for allergy or asthma in patients who have normal levels of immunoglobulin (8).

INDICATIONS AND USAGE

Hepatitis A—The prophylactic value of IG is greatest when given before or soon after exposure to hepatitis A. IG is not indicated in persons with clinical manifestations of hepatitis A or in those exposed more than 2 weeks previously.

Measles (Rubeola)—IG should be given to prevent or modify measles in a susceptible person exposed less than 6 days previously (5). (A susceptible person is one who has not been vaccinated and has not had measles previously.) IG may be especially indicated for susceptible household contacts of measles patients, particularly contacts under one year of age, for whom the risk of complications is highest (5). IG and measles vaccine should not be given at the same time (5). If a child is older than 12 months and has received IG, he should be given measles vaccine about 3 months later, when the measles antibody titer will have disappeared.

If a susceptible child exposed to measles is immunocompromised, IG should be given immediately (9). Children who are immunocompromised should not receive measles vaccine or any other live viral vaccine.

Immunoglobulin Deficiency—In patients with immunoglobulin deficiencies, IG may prevent serious infection. However, IG may not prevent chronic infections of the external secretory tissues such as the respiratory and gastrointestinal tract.

Prophylactic therapy, especially against infections due to encapsulated bacteria, is effective in Bruton-type, sex-linked congenital agammaglobulinemia, agammaglobulinemia and severe combined immunodeficiency.

Varicella—Passive immunization against varicella in immunosuppressed patients is best accomplished by use of Varicella-Zoster Immune Globulin (Human) (VZIG). If VZIG is unavailable, IG, promptly given, may also modify varicella (7).

Rubella—The routine use of IG for prophylaxis of rubella in early pregnancy is of dubious value and cannot be justified (4). Some studies suggest that the use of IG in exposed susceptible women can lessen the likelihood of infection and fetal damage. IG may benefit those women who will not consider a therapeutic abortion (4).

CONTRAINDICATIONS

IG should not be given to persons with isolated immunoglobulin A (IgA) deficiency. Such persons have the potential for developing antibodies to IgA and could have anaphylactic reactions to subsequent administration of blood products that contain IgA (6).

IG should not be administered to patients who have severe thrombocytopenia or any coagulation disorder that would contraindicate intramuscular injections.

WARNINGS

IG should be given with caution to patients with a history of prior systemic allergic reactions following the administration of human immunoglobulin preparations (6).

IG is for intramuscular injection only.

PRECAUTIONS

General—IG should not be administered intravenously because of the potential for serious reactions. Injections should be made intramuscularly, and care should be taken to draw back on the plunger of the syringe before injection in order to be certain that the needle is not in a blood vessel.

Although systemic reactions to intramuscularly administered immunoglobulin preparations are rare, epinephrine should be available for treatment of acute allergic symptoms.

Laboratory Tests—None are required.

Drug Interactions—Antibodies in the globulin preparation may interfere with the response to live viral vaccines such as measles, mumps, and rubella. Therefore, use of such vaccines should be deferred until approximately three months after IG administration.

No interactions with other products are known.

Pregnancy Category C—Animal reproduction studies have not been performed with Immune Globulin (Human) U.S.P. —GAMMAR®. It is also not known whether GAMMAR® can cause fetal harm when administered to a pregnant woman or can affect reproduction capacity. GAMMAR® should be given to a pregnant woman only if clearly needed.

Pediatric Use—See DOSAGE AND ADMINISTRATION section.

ADVERSE REACTIONS

Local pain and tenderness at the injection site, urticaria, and angioedema may occur. Anaphylactic reactions, although rare, have been reported following the injection of human immune globulin preparations (6). Anaphylaxis is more likely to occur if IG is given intravenously; therefore IG must be administered only intramuscularly.

DOSAGE AND ADMINISTRATION

Dosage

Hepatitis A—IG in a dose of 0.01 mL/lb (0.02 mL/kg) is recommended for household and institutional hepatitis A contacts.

The following doses of IG are recommended for persons who plan to travel in areas where hepatitis A is common (3):

Length of Stay	Dose Volume
Less than 3 months	0.02 mL/kg
3 months or longer	0.06 mL/kg (repeat every 4–6 months)

Measles (Rubeola)—IG should be given in a dose of 0.11 mL/lb (0.25 mL/kg) to prevent or modify measles in a susceptible person exposed less than 6 days previously (5).

If a susceptible child who is also immunocompromised is exposed, IG in a dose of 0.5 mL/kg (maximum 15 mL) should be given immediately (9).

Immunoglobulin Deficiency—IG may prevent serious infection in patients with immunoglobulin deficiencies if circulating IgG levels of approximately 200 mg/100 mL plasma are maintained. The recommended dosage is 0.66 mL/kg (at least 100 mg/kg) given every 3 to 4 weeks (8). A double dose is given at onset of therapy: some patients may require more frequent injections.

Varicella—If Varicella-Zoster immune Globulin (Human) is unavailable, IG at a dose of 0.6 to 1.2 mL/kg given promptly, is the recommended dose (7).

Rubella—The recommended dose of 0.55 mL/kg IG may benefit women who will not consider a therapeutic abortion (4).

Administration

IG is administered intramuscularly (see PRECAUTIONS), preferably in the gluteal region. Doses over 10 mL should be divided and injected into several muscle sites to reduce local pain and discomfort.

Parenteral drug products should be inspected visually for particulate matter and discoloration prior to administration whenever solution and container permit.

HOW SUPPLIED

Immune Globulin (Human)—GAMMAR® is available in 2 mL (NDC 0053-7595-01) and 10 mL (NDC 0053-7595-02) vials. Vials should be stored at 2°–8°C (36°–46°F). Do not freeze. Do not use after expiration date.

Caution: Federal (U.S.A.) law prohibits dispensing without prescription.

REFERENCES

1. Smith, GN, Mollison, D, Griffiths, B, and Mollison, PL; Uptake of IgG after intramuscular and subcutaneous injection. Lancet i:1208–1212, 1972.
2. Waldmann, TA, Strober, W, and Blaese, RM: Variations in the metabolism of immunoglobulins measured by turnover rates, in Immunoglobulins. Biologic Aspects and Clinical Uses. Edited by Ezio Merler, National Academy of Sciences, Washington, D.C., 1970, pp. 33–51.
3. Morbidity and Mortality Weekly Report, September 4, 1981 (Vol. 30, No. 34).
4. Report of the Committee on Infectious Diseases, American Academy of Pediatrics, 1982, Red Book p. 231.
5. Morbidity and Mortality Weekly Report, May 7, 1982 (Vol. 31, No. 17).
6. Fudenberg, HH: Sensitization to immunoglobulins and hazards of gamma globulin therapy, in Immunoglobulins. Biologic Aspects and Clinical Uses. Edited by Ezio Merler, National Academy of Sciences, Washington, D.C., 1970, pp. 211–220.
7. Gershon, AA, Pelmelli, S, Karpatkin,, M, Smithwick, E, and Steinberg, S: Antibody to varicella-zoster virus after passive immunization against chickenpox. J. Clin. Microbiol. 8:733–735, 1978.
8. Report of the Committee on Infectious Diseases, American Academy of Pediatrics, 1982, Red Book pp. 34–36.
9. Report of the Committee on Infectious Diseases, American Academy of Pediatrics, 1982, Red Book pp. 134–135.
10. Morbidity and Mortality Weekly Report, June 1, 1984 (Vol. 33, No. 21).

Revised: October, 1990

IMMUNE GLOBULIN
INTRAVENOUS
(HUMAN)
GAMMAR® I.V.
LYOPHILIZED ℞

DESCRIPTION

Immune Globulin Intravenous (Human), Gammar® I.V., is a sterile, lyophilized preparation of intact, unmodified, immunoglobulin, primarily IgG, stabilized with Albumin (Human) and Sucrose. The distribution of IgG sub-classes is similar to that present in normal human plasma. It is prepared by cold alcohol fractionation of pooled plasma and is not chemically altered or enzymatically degraded. When reconstituted with the appropriate volume of Sterile Water for Injection USP, Gammar® I.V. contains 5% IgG, 3% Albumin (Human), 5% sucrose, and 0.5% sodium chloride. The pH of the solution has been adjusted to 6.8 ± 0.4 with citric acid and/or sodium carbonate. Gammar® I.V. contains no preservative. This product is intended for intravenous administration.

CLINICAL PHARMACOLOGY

Immune Globulin Intravenous (Human), Gammar® I.V. provides a broad range of antibodies, capable of opsonization and neutralization of microbes and toxins, against bacterial and viral antigens for prevention or attenuation of infectious diseases. The half-life of Gammar® I.V., as reflected in circulating IgG levels, is approximately three weeks, although individual variations have occurred.

Gammar® I.V. is a native, non-chemically modified IgG fractionated from pooled human donor plasma. The distribution of IgG sub-classes (IgG_1, IgG_2, IgG_3, IgG_4) is similar to that present in Cohn Fraction II. Since the IgG concentrate is prepared from a large pool of at least 1000 donors, it represents the expected diversity of antibodies in that population. The processing steps used in the manufacture of this product

Continued on next page

Armour—Cont.

have been shown capable of eliminating at least 6.75 logs of added HIV.

Albumin (Human) and sucrose are added to the formulation in order to provide adequate stabilization of the IgG molecules and the reconstituted product. Because sucrose, when given intravenously, is excreted unchanged in the urine, Gammar® I.V. may be given to diabetics without compensatory changes in insulin dosage regimen.

INDICATIONS AND USAGE

Gammar® I.V. is indicated for patients with primary defective antibody synthesis such as agammaglobulinemia or hypogammaglobulinemia, who are at increased risk of infection. When high levels or rapid elevation of circulating gamma globulins are desired, intravenous administration is more desirable than intramuscular therapy.

CONTRAINDICATIONS

Gammar® I.V. is contraindicated in individuals with a history of anaphylactic or severe systemic response to immune globulin intramuscular or intravenous preparations.

Gammar® I.V. should not be given to persons with isolated immunoglobulin A (IgA) deficiency. Such persons have the potential for developing antibodies to IgA and could have anaphylactic reactions to subsequent administration of blood products that contain IgA.

WARNINGS

If anaphylactic or severe anaphylactoid reactions occur, discontinue infusion immediately. Epinephrine should be available for the treatment of any acute anaphylactoid reactions.

Patients with agammaglobulinemia or extreme hypogammaglobulinemia who have not received immunoglobulin therapy within the preceding 8 weeks may be at risk of developing inflammatory reactions upon the infusion of human immunoglobulins. These reactions are manifested by a rise in temperature, chills, nausea and vomiting, and appear to be related to the rate of infusion.

Infusion rates and the patient's clinical state should be monitored closely during infusion. (See administration section under DOSAGE AND ADMINISTRATION.)

PRECAUTIONS

General—Epinephrine should be available for treatment of acute allergic reactions.

Pregnancy Category C—Animal reproduction studies have not been performed with Immune Globulin Intravenous (Human), Gammar® I.V. It is also not known whether Gammar® I.V. can cause fetal harm when administered to a pregnant woman or can affect reproduction capacity. Gammar® I.V. should be given to a pregnant woman only if clearly needed.

Drug Interactions—Admixtures of Immune Globulin Intravenous (Human), Gammar® I.V. with other drugs have not been evaluated. It is recommended that Gammar® I.V. be administered by a separate infusion line without mixing with other drugs or medication which the patient may be receiving.

Pediatric Use—See "Dosage and Administration" section.

ADVERSE REACTIONS

Adverse reactions which may occur include headache, backache, myalgia, pyrexia, hypotension, chills, flushing and nausea, usually beginning within one hour of the start of the infusion. Symptoms subside in most cases within 30 minutes. The incidence of adverse reactions reported for a twelve month multi-center, repeated administration crossover study was shown to be 16% for Gammar® I.V. and 11% for another manufacturer's Immune Globulin Intravenous (Human). Data from this clinical evaluation indicated that the numbers of patients experiencing adverse reactions to each preparation were comparable, and that similar reactions were involved regardless of preparation.

True anaphylactic reactions may occur in patients with a history of prior systemic allergic reactions or seizure following administration of human immunoglobulin preparations. Very rarely an anaphylactoid reaction may occur in patients with no prior history of severe allergic reactions to human immunoglobulin preparations. Patients previously sensitized to certain antigens, most commonly IgA, may be at risk of immediate anaphylactoid and hypersensitivity reactions. Epinephrine should be available for the treatment of any acute anaphylactoid reaction. (See WARNINGS and CONTRAINDICATIONS.)

Infusion rates and clinical state should be monitored closely during infusion. If adverse reaction occurs, the infusion rate should be reduced or the infusion stopped until the symptoms have subsided. (See DOSAGE AND ADMINISTRATION.)

DOSAGE AND ADMINISTRATION

The usual dose of Immune Globulin Intravenous (Human) is directed toward restoration of the immune deficient patient's circulating IgG level to near-normal levels. Use of 100–200 mg/kg body weight every three to four weeks is recommended. An initial loading dose of at least 200 mg/kg at more frequent intervals, proceeding to 100–200 mg/kg at three week intervals once a therapeutic plasma level has been established can be used. However, treatment must be individualized for each patient due to variation among patients in catabolic rate of IgG.

Reconstitution

Directions must be followed exactly.

1) Bring diluent and lyophilized product vials to room temperature prior to reconstitution.
2) Remove plastic flip-off caps from both vials.
3) Treat rubber stoppers with antiseptic solution and allow to dry.
4) Insert plastic piercing pin of the transfer spike into the upright diluent vial first.
5) Remove the needle cover, invert the diluent vial with the attached transfer spike and insert metal needle into the upright product vial.
6) The vacuum in the product vial will pull the diluent into the product vial. As soon as all diluent has been transferred the transfer spike will automatically admit filtered air to the product. An additional venting of the product vial after diluent addition is not necessary. Withdraw and discard transfer spike.
7) Do not shake product vial. Solubilize the product by gently swirling it in an upright position. Avoid the formation of foam.
8) Examine solution. Any small particles will dissolve with gentle swirling of vial. The solution should be clear and ready to administer in less than 20 minutes.
9) Product contains no preservative. Use within 3 hours of reconstitution.

Administration

Immune Globulin Intravenous (Human), Gammar® I.V. is to be administered by intravenous infusion. The infusion should begin at a rate of 0.01 mL/kg/minute, increasing to 0.02 mL/kg/minute after 15 to 30 minutes. Most patients tolerate a gradual increase to 0.03–0.06 mL/kg/minute. For the average 70 kg person this is equivalent to 2 to 4 mL/minute. If adverse reactions develop, slowing the infusion rate will usually eliminate the reaction. Discard any unused solution.

Parenteral drug products should be inspected visually for particulate matter and discoloration prior to administration whenever solution and container permit.

HOW SUPPLIED

Immune Globulin Intravenous (Human), Gammar® I.V., is supplied in single dose vials, with diluent and sterile, vented transfer spike for reconstitution.

The following dosage forms are available:

Product	Diluent
NDC 0053-7490-01 1.0 g immune globulin/vial	20 mL
NDC 0053-7490-02 2.5 g immune globulin/vial	50 mL
NDC 0053-7490-05 5.0 g immune globulin/vial	100 mL

STORAGE

When stored at temperatures not exceeding 30°C (86°F), Gammar® I.V. is stable for the period indicated by the expiration date on its label. Avoid freezing which may damage container for diluent.

CAUTION: Federal (U.S.A.) law prohibits dispensing without prescription.

References

Fudenberg, H.H. "Sensitization to immunoglobulins and hazards of gamma globulin therapy" in *Immunoglobulins, Biologic Aspects and Clinical Uses.* Edited by Ezio Merler. National Academy of Sciences, Washington, D.C., (1970), pp. 211–220.

Steele, R.W., Augustine, R.A., Tannenbaum, A.S., and Marmer, D.J. "Intravenous Immune Globulin for Hypogammaglobulinemia: A Comparison of Opsonizing Capacity in Recipient Sera." *Clin. Immunol. Immunopathol* 34 (1985), pp. 275–283.

Martindale. *The Extra Pharmacopoeia* 27th ed. Edited by A. Wade. London: The Pharmaceutical Press (1979) p. 65.

Polley, M.J., Fischetti, V.A., and Landaburu, P.H. "Native Intravenous IgG Exhibits Greater Biological Activity than Modified IgG" from the XX Cong. Int. Soc. of Hematology (1984).

Issued: January, 1991

GAMULIN® Rh ℞

[*găm'yōō-lĭn"*]

Rh_o(D) Immune Globulin (Human)

Rh_o(D) Immune Globulin (Human) Gamulin® Rh, is a sterile immunoglobulin solution containing Rh_o(D) antibodies for intramuscular use only. It is obtained by alcohol fractionation of plasma from human blood donors, concentrated and standardized to give a total globulin content of 11.5± 1.5 percent. All lots are assayed for Rh_o(D) antibody content by serological method (anti-globulin titer). The Rh_o(D) antibody level in each vial or syringe of Gamulin® Rh is equal to or greater than that of the Office of Biologics Research and Review Reference Rh_o(D) Immune Globulin (Human). This dose has been shown to effectively inhibit the immunizing potential of up to 15 mL of Rh-positive packed red blood cells.[1] The final product contains 0.3 molar glycine as a stabilizer and 0.01% thimerosal (mercury derivative) as a preservative.

CLINICAL PHARMACOLOGY

Gamulin® Rh effectively suppresses the immune response on non-sensitized Rh_o(D) negative individuals who receive Rh_o(D) positive blood as the result of a fetomaternal hemorrhage or a transfusion accident. The administration of Rh_o(D) antibody to an Rh_o(D) negative mother or to the Rh negative recipient of Rh positive red cells suppresses the antibody response and the formation of anti-Rh_o(D). Clinical studies indicated that the administration of Rh_o(D) immune globulin within 72 hours of a full term delivery of an Rh_o(D) positive infant to an Rh_o(D) negative mother reduces the incidence of Rh isoimmunization from 12–13% to 1–2%.[13] Data have been reported to indicate that 1.5 to 1.8% of Rh_o(D) negative mothers, carrying Rh_o(D) positive fetuses, who are given Rh immune globulin postpartum may be immunized to Rh during the latter part of their pregnancies or after delivery.[14] Bowman reported that the incidence of immunization can be further reduced from approximately 1.6% to less than 0.1% by administering Rh_o(D) immune globulin in two doses to Rh negative primagravida or multigravida patients, one antepartum at 28 weeks gestation and another following delivery.[11]

INDICATIONS AND USAGE

Full Term Delivery. Rh_o(D) Immune Globulin (Human) Gamulin® Rh is used to prevent sensitization to the Rh_o(D) factor and thus to prevent hemolytic disease of the newborn (Erythroblastosis fetalis) in a pregnancy that follows the injection of Gamulin® Rh. It effectively suppresses the immune response of non-sensitized Rh-negative mothers after delivery of an Rh-positive infant.[1–4]

Criteria for an Rh-incompatible pregnancy requiring administration of Rh_o(D) Immune Globulin (Human) Gamulin® Rh are:

1. The mother must be Rh_o(D) negative.
2. The mother should not have been previously sensitized to the Rh_o(D) factor.
3. The infant must be Rh_o(D) positive and direct antiglobulin negative.

Other Obstetric Conditions. Gamulin® Rh should be administered to all non-sensitized Rh-negative women after spontaneous or induced abortions, after ruptured tubal pregnancies, amniocentesis, and other abdominal trauma, or any occurrence of transplacental hemorrhage unless the blood type of the fetus has been determined to be Rh_o(D) negative.[1–3]

If Rh_o(D) Immune Globulin (Human) Gamulin® Rh is administered antepartum, it is essential that the mother receive another dose of Gamulin® Rh after the delivery of an Rh_o(D) positive infant.

NOTE: In a case of abortion or ectopic pregnancy when Rh typing of the fetus is not possible, the fetus must be assumed to be Rh_o(D) positive. In such an instance, the patient should be considered a candidate for administration of Rh_o(D) Immune Globulin (Human) Gamulin® Rh.

If the father can be determined to be Rh_o(D) negative, Gamulin® Rh need not be given.

Gamulin® Rh should be given within 72 hours following an Rh-incompatible delivery, miscarriage or abortion.

Transfusions. Gamulin® Rh can be used to prevent Rh_o(D) sensitization in Rh_o(D) negative patients accidentally transfused with Rh_o(D) positive RBC or blood components containing RBC.[6–7]

It should be administered within 72 hours following an Rh-incompatible transfusion.

CONTRAINDICATIONS

None known.

WARNINGS

Gamulin® Rh must not be given to the Rh_o(D) positive postpartum infant. Do not give intravenously.

PRECAUTIONS

General. Before administering Gamulin® Rh, it is desirable that all diagnostic laboratory criteria be met, as outlined in the Preadministration Laboratory Procedures section below. Babies born of women given Rh immune globulin antepartum may have a weakly positive antiglobulin test at birth. Passively acquired anti-Rh_o(D) may be detected in maternal serum if antibody screening tests are performed subsequent to antepartum of postpartum administration of Gamulin® Rh.

Pregnancy Category C. Animal reproduction studies have not been conducted with Rh_o(D) Immune Globulin (Human) Gamulin® Rh. It is also not known whether Gamulin® Rh can cause fetal harm when administered to a pregnant woman or can affect reproduction capacity. Gamulin® Rh

should be given to a pregnant woman only if clearly needed. However, use of Rh antibody during the third trimester in full doses of antibody has been reported to produce no evidence of hemolysis in the infant.[12]

The presence of passively administered Rh antibody in the maternal blood sample can, however, affect the interpretation of laboratory tests to identify the patient as a candidate for $Rh_o(D)$ Immune Globulin (Human) Gamulin® Rh. A large fetomaternal hemorrhage late in pregnancy or following delivery may cause a weak, mixed field positive D^U test result. If there is any doubt about the mother's Rh type, she should be given $Rh_o(D)$ Immune Globulin (Human) Gamulin® Rh. A screening test for fetal red blood cells may help in such cases. If more than 15 mL of $Rh_o(D)$ positive fetal red blood cells are present in the mother's circulation, more than a single dose of $Rh_o(D)$ Immune Globulin (Human) Gamulin® Rh is required. Failure to recognize this may result in the administration of inadequate dose. In case of doubt as to the patient's Rh group or immune status, Gamulin® Rh should be administered.

ADVERSE REACTIONS

Since Gamulin® Rh is an $Rh_o(D)$ immune globulin derived from homologous human serum proteins, allergic reactions are not expected but the possibility cannot be ruled out. Such reactions have been reported following extensive use of immune serum globulin in hypogammaglobulinemic patients.[9]

On occasion a patient has shown a systemic reaction manifested by a low-grade fever but, generally, reactions have been mild, infrequent and confined to the site of injection.

$Rh_o(D)$ negative patients inadvertently transfused with $Rh_o(D)$ positive blood have received from 15 to 33 vials of Gamulin® Rh with no adverse reaction other than soreness at the injection site. A 1°F temperature elevation in one patient which could have been due to the underlying illness has been reported.

DOSAGE AND ADMINISTRATION

Preadministration Laboratory Procedure

Infant. Immediately postpartum determine the infant's blood group ABO, $Rh_o(D)$) and perform a direct antiglobulin test. Umbilical cord, venous or capillary blood may be used.

Mother. Confirm that the mother is $Rh_o(D)$ negative.

Dosage

Postpartum prophylaxis, miscarriage, abortion, or ectopic pregnancy: One vial or syringe of $Rh_o(D)$ Immune Globulin (Human) Gamulin® Rh is sufficient to prevent maternal sensitization to the Rh factor if the fetal packed red blood cell volume, which entered the mother's blood due to fetomaternal hemorrhage is less than 15 mL (30 mL of whole blood).[1,2,9]

When the fetomaternal hemorrhage exceeds 15 mL of packed cells or 30 mL of whole blood, more than one vial or syringe of Gamulin® Rh should be administered.

Antepartum Prophylaxis. The contents of one vial or syringe of Gamulin® Rh injected intramuscularly at 28 weeks gestation and the contents of one vial or syringe within 72 hours after an Rh incompatible delivery is highly effective in preventing Rh isoimmunization during pregnancy.[11]

To determine the number of vials or syringes required, the volume of packed fetal red blood cells must be determined by an approved laboratory assay, such as the Kleihauer-Betke Acid Elution Technic or the Clayton Modification.[13] The volume of fetomaternal hemorrhage divided by two gives the volume of packed fetal red blood cells in the maternal blood. The number of vials or syringes of Gamulin® Rh to be administered is determined by dividing the volume (mL) of packed red blood cells by 15.

Transfusion Accidents. The number of vials or syringes of $Rh_o(D)$ Immune Globulin (Human) Gamulin® Rh to be administered is dependent on the volume of packed red cells or whole blood transfused. The method to determine the number of vials or syringes of Gamulin® Rh required to prevent sensitization is outlined below. If the dose calculation results in a fraction, administered the next whole number of vials or syringes of Gamulin® Rh.

Procedure:

a. Multiply the volume (in mL) of Rh-positive whole blood administered by the hematocrit of the donor unit. This value equals the volume of packed red blood cells transfused.
b. Divide the volume (in mL) of packed red blood cells by 15 to obtain the number of vials or syringes of Gamulin® Rh to be administered.

Administration

Single vial or syringe dose. Inject intramuscularly the entire contents of the vial or syringe of $Rh_o(D)$ Immune Globulin (Human) Gamulin® Rh.

Multiple vial or syringe dose. The contents of the total number of vials or syringes may be injected as a divided dose at different injection sites at the same time or the total dosage may be divided and injected at intervals provided the total dosage to be given is injected within 72 hours postpartum or after as transfusion accident.

This product should be administered within 72 hours after Rh-incompatible delivery or transfusion.

Do not inject intravenously.

Parenteral drug products should be inspected visually for particulate matter and discoloration prior to administration, whenever solution and container permit.

The following information should be included in the patient's records:

1. Patient's complete identification.
2. Patient's ABO and Rh group, and date determined.
3. Result of test for prior Rh sensitization.
4. Infant's ABO and Rh group, when known, and result of direct antiglobulin tests in the case of transfusion accident, the ABO and Rh groups of the donor tested and the volume transfused.
5. Notification of patient concerning nature of medication, date and reason for giving it.
6. Lot number of $Rh_o(D)$ Immune Globulin (Human) Gamulin® Rh and date and location of injection and the number of vials or syringes injected.
7. Adequate documentation, if medication is refused by the patient.

CAUTION—Federal (U.S.A.) law prohibits dispensing without prescription.

HOW SUPPLIED

Individual vial packages (NDC 0053-7590-01) containing:
1. One single dose vial of Gamulin® Rh.
2. Patient identification card.
3. Directions for use.
4. Patient information brochure.
5. Laboratory control form.

Cartons of 10 vials in plastic pouches (NDC 0053-7590-06) containing:
1. 10 single dose vials of Gamulin® Rh.
2. 10 patient identification cards.
3. 10 sets of directions for use.
4. 10 patient information brochures.
5. 10 laboratory control forms.

Cartons of 25 vials (NDC 0053-7590-03) containing:
1. 25 single dose vials of Gamulin® Rh.
2. 25 patient identification cards.
3. 10 sets of directions for use.
4. 25 patient information brochures.

Cartons of 6 syringes (NDC 0053-7590-02) containing:
1. 6 single dose syringes of Gamulin® Rh.
2. 6 patient identification cards.
3. 6 sets of directions for use.
4. 6 patient information brochures.
5. 6 laboratory control forms

STORAGE

Keep refrigerated at 2° to 8°C (36° to 46°F). Do not freeze.

REFERENCES

1. $Rh_o(D)$ Immune Globulin (Human). *The Medical Letter on Drugs and Therapeutics* 16:3–4, 1974.
2. Public Health Services Advisory Committee on Immunization Practices. *MMWR* 21:15 (April 21), 1972.
3. Prevention of Rh sensitization. WHO Technical Report Series No. 468, 1971.
4. Eich F G. Tripodi D. Screening and quantitating fetal maternal hemorrhages. *Amer J Clin Path* 61:192–198, 1974.
5. Bowman J M. Chown B. Prevention of Rh immunization after massive Rh-positive transfusion. *Can Med J* 99:385–388, 1968.
6. Keith L. Anti-Rh therapy after transfusion. *J Reprod Med* 8:293–198, 1972.
7. Pollack W. *et al.* Studies of Rh prophylaxis. II. Rh immune prophylaxis after transfusion with Rh-positive blood. *Transfusion* 11:340–344, 1971.
8. Henny C S. Ellis E F. Antibody production to aggregated human γ G-globulin in acquired hypogammaglobulinema. *New England J Med* 278:1144–46, 1968.
9. Walker R H. Fetomaternal hemorrhage. A summary. *American Association of Blood Banks —Technical Workshop.* Chicago: September 12, 1971, pp 17–29.
10. Chalos M K. Detection of fetomaternal hemorrhage. *American Association of Blood Banks —Technical Workshop.* Chicago: September 12, 1971, pp 12–16.
11. Bowman J M. Pollock J M. Antenatal prophylaxis of Rh isoimmunization: 28 weeks'-gestation service program. *Can Med J* 118:627–630, 1978.
12. Zipursky A. and Israels L G. The paibogenesis and prevention of Rh immunization. *Can Med J* 97:1245, 1967.
13. Pollack W. Rh hemolytic disease of the newborn, its cause, and prevention. *Reprod Immunol,* Alan R. Liss, New York, 1981.
14. Bowman J M. *et al.* Rh isoimmunization during pregnancy: antenatal prophylaxis. *Canad Med Assoc J* 118(6):623–627, 1971

REVISED: October, 1990

HUMATE-P™ ℞

[*hyōō'māt*]

Antihemophilic Factor (Human), Pasteurized

Humate-P™, Antihemophilic Factor (Human), Pasteurized, is supplied in single dose vials (I.U. activity is stated on label of each vial) with sterile diluent and needles for reconstitution and withdrawal. Manufactured by Behringwerke AG, Marburg/Lahn West Germany and distributed by Armour Pharmaceutical Company.

MINI-GAMULIN™ Rh ℞

[*mĭ-nē"găm'yoo-lĭn*]

Rh_o (D) Immune Globulin (Human)

REDUCED DOSE—FOR USE FOLLOWING SPONTANEOUS OR INDUCED ABORTION UP TO 12 WEEKS' GESTATION

DESCRIPTION

$Rh_o(D)$ Immune Globulin (Human) Mini-Gamulin™ Rh is a sterile immune globulin solution containing $Rh_o(D)$ antibodies for single dose intramuscular injection. Mini-Gamulin™ Rh is obtained by alcohol fractionation of plasma from human blood donors, concentrated and standardized to give total protein content of 11.5±1.5 percent.

Mini-Gamulin™ Rh contains one-sixth the quantity of $Rh_o(D)$ antibody contained in a standard dose of $Rh_o(D)$ Immune Globulin (Human). The contents of one vial or syringe of Mini-Gamulin™ Rh will suppress the immunizing potential of 5 mL of whole blood or 2.5 mL of packed red blood cells. The final product contains 0.3 molar glycine as a stabilizer and 0.01% thimerosal (mercury derivative) as a preservative.

CLINICAL PHARMACOLOGY

$Rh_o(D)$ Immune Globulin (Human) prevents the formation of anti-$Rh_o(D)$ antibodies in nonsensitized $Rh_o(D)$ negative individuals who receive $Rh_o(D)$ positive red blood cells. Although the precise mechanism of action is not fully understood, passively administered $Rh_o(D)$ antibody binds circulating antigen, thus preventing stimulation of antigen-sensitive cells and the resulting production of anti-$Rh_o(D)$.

In order to prevent sensitization, $Rh_o(D)$ Immune Globulin (Human) must be administered after each exposure to $Rh_o(D)$ positive red blood cells.

ADMINISTRATION AND USAGE

Rh sensitization may occur in nonsensitized $Rh_o(D)$ negative women following transplacental hemorrhage resulting from spontaneous or induced abortions.[1–3] Sensitization occurs more frequently in women undergoing induced abortions than in those aborting spontaneously.[4]

$Rh_o(D)$ Immune Globulin, at the dosage level contained in one vial or syringe of Mini-Gamulin™ Rh, prevents the formation of anti-$Rh_o(D)$ antibodies in nonsensitized $Rh_o(D)$ negative women who receive $Rh_o(D)$ positive blood during transplacental hemorrhage resulting from spontaneous or induced abortion up to 12 weeks' gestation.[5–7]

For spontaneous or induced abortions occurring after 12 weeks' gestation, an appropriate dose of standard $Rh_o(D)$ Immune Globulin (Gamulin® Rh) sufficient to suppress the immunizing potential of 15 mL of Rh-positive packed red blood cells, should be given.

NOTE: Mini-Gamulin™ Rh prophylaxis is not indicated if the fetus or father can be determined to be Rh negative. If Rh typing of the fetus is not possible, the fetus must be assumed to be $Rh_o(D)$ positive and the patient should be considered a candidate for treatment.

Mini-Gamulin™ Rh should be administered promptly following spontaneous or induced abortion. If prompt administration is not possible, Mini-Gamulin™ Rh should be given within 72 hours following termination of the pregnancy. However, if Mini-Gamulin™ Rh is not given within this time period, administration of the product should still be considered.

CONTRAINDICATIONS

None known.

WARNINGS

Do not inject intravenously.

PRECAUTIONS

General. Mini-Gamulin™ Rh should be administered intramuscularly. It must not be administered intravenously.

A separate, sterile syringe and needle should be used for each individual patient to avoid transmission of hepatitis B and other infectious agents from one person to another.

The possibility of a hypersensitivity reaction is very remote but should be borne in mind. Epinephrine should be available for immediate use should a hypersensitivity reaction occur.

Continued on next page

Armour—Cont.

Pregnancy—Category C. Animal reproduction studies have not been conducted with Rh_0(D) Immune Globulin (Human) Mini-Gamulin™ Rh. It is also not known whether Mini-Gamulin™ Rh can cause fetal harm when administered to a pregnant woman or can affect reproduction capacity. Mini-Gamulin™ should be given to a pregnant woman only if clearly needed.

ADVERSE REACTIONS

Reactions following intramuscular injection of Mini- Gamulin™ Rh, as with any immune globulin preparation, are infrequent, usually mild in nature, and confined to the site of injection. An occasional patient may react more strongly with localized tenderness, erythema, or low-grade fever. Rh_0(D) Immune Globulin and other immune globulins rarely cause systemic reactions or induce sensitization upon repeated injections.

DOSAGE AND ADMINISTRATION

Do not inject intravenously.

The contents of one vial or syringe of Mini-Gamulin™ Rh provides protection from Rh immunization for women with transplacental hemorrhage resulting from spontaneous or induced abortion up to 12 weeks' gestation.

Inject intramuscularly the entire contents of vial or syringe. Mini-Gamulin™ Rh should be administered promptly following spontaneous or induced abortion. If prompt administration is not possible, Mini-Gamulin™ Rh should be given within 72 hours following termination of the pregnancy.

Parenteral drug products should be inspected visually for particulate matter and discoloration prior to administration, whenever solution and container permit.

HOW SUPPLIED

Individual vial packages (NDC 0053-7591-02) containing:
1. One single dose vial of Mini-Gamulin™ Rh.
2. Patient identification card.
3. Directions for use.
4. Patient information brochure.
5. Laboratory control form.

Cartons of 10 vials in plasting pouches (NDC 0053-7591-06) containing:
1. 10 single dose vials of Mini-Gamulin™ Rh.
2. 10 patient identification cards.
3. 10 sets of directions for use.
4. 10 patient information brochures.
5. 10 laboratory control forms.

Cartons of 25 vials (NDC 0053-7591-03) containing:
1. 25 single dose vials of Mini-Gamulin™ Rh.
2. 25 patient identification cards.
3. 10 sets of directions for use.
4. 25 patient information brochures.

Cartons of 6 syringes of (NDC 0053-7591-04) containing:
1. 6 single dose syringes of Mini-Gamulin™ Rh.
2. 6 patient identification cards.
3. 6 sets of directions for use.
4. 6 patient information brochures
5. 6 laboratory control forms.

STORAGE

Store at a temperature between 2°-8°C (36°-46°F). Do not freeze.

REFERENCES

1. Queenan JT, et al: Role of induced abortion in *Rhesus* immunization. *Lancet* 1:815–817, 1971.
2. Parmley TH, et al: Transplacental hemorrhage in patients subjected to therapeutic abortion. *Am J Obstet Gynecol* 106:540–542, 1970.
3. Grimes DA, et al: Rh immunoglobulin utilization after spontaneous and induced abortion. *Obstet Gynecol* 50:261:263,1977.
4. American College of Obstetricians and Gynecologists: Current use of Rh_o immune globulin and detection of antibodies. *Technical Bulletin* 35, 1976.
5. World Health Organization: Prevention of Rh sensitization. *Technical Report Series* 468, 1971.
6. Scott JR: Report on Rh immune globulin therapy. *Cont Ob Gyn* 8:27–30, 1976.
7. Keith L, Bozorgi N: Small dose anti-Rh therapy after first trimester abortion. *Intern J Gynecol Obstet* 15:235–237, 1977.

Revised: October, 1990

MONOCLATE-P® Factor VIII:C, Pasteurized ℞

[*mŏn 'ō-clāte "*]

Monoclonal Antibody Purified
Antihemophilic Factor (Human)

DESCRIPTION

Antihemophilic Factor (Human), MONOCLATE-P®, Factor VIII:C Pastuerized is a sterile, stable, lyophilized concentrate of Factor VIII:C with reduced amounts of vWf:Ag and purified of extraneous plasma-derived protein by use of affinity chromatography. A murine monoclonal antibody to vWf:Ag is used as an affinity ligand to first isolate the Factor VIII Complex. Factor VIII:C is then dissociated from vWf:Ag, recovered, formulated and provided as a sterile lyophilized powder.[1,2,3] The concentrate as formulated contains Albumin (Human) as a stabilizer, resulting in a concentrate with a specific activity between 5 and 10 units/mg of total protein. In the absence of this added Albumin (Human) stabilizer, specific activity has been determined to exceed 3000 units/mg of protein.[4] MONOCLATE-P® has been prepared from pooled human plasma and is intended for use in therapy of classical hemophilia (Hemophilia A).

The concentrate has been pasteurized by heating at 60°C for 10 hours in aqueous solution form during its manufacture in order to further reduce the risk of viral transmission.[5] However, no procedure has been shown to be totally effective in removing viral infectivity from coagulant factor concentrates. (See CLINICAL PHARMACOLOGY and WARNINGS)

MONOCLATE-P® is a highly purified preparation of Factor VIII:C. When stored as directed, it will maintain its labeled potency for the period indicated on the container and package labels.[8,9]

Upon reconstitution, a clear, colorless solution is obtained, containing 50 to 150 times as much Factor VIII:C as does an equal volume of plasma.

Each vial contains the labeled amount of antihemophilic factor (AHF) activity as expressed in terms of International Units of antihemophilic activity. One unit of antihemophilic activity is equivalent to that quantity of AHF present in one mL of normal human plasma. When reconstituted as recommended, the resulting solution contains approximately 300 to 450 millimoles of sodium ions per liter and has 2 to 3 times the tonicity of saline. It contains approximately 2–5 millimoles of calcium ions per liter, contributed as calcium chloride, approximately 1 to 2% Albumin (Human), 0.8% mannitol, and 1.2 mM histidine. The pH is adjusted with hydrochloric acid and/or sodium hydroxide. MONOCLATE-P® also contains trace amounts (less than 50 ng per 100 AHF activity units) of mouse protein (see CLINICAL PHARMACOLOGY).

MONOCLATE-P® is to be administered only intravenously.

CLINICAL PHARMACOLOGY

Factor VIII:C is the coagulant portion of the Factor VIII complex circulating in plasma. It is noncovalently associated with the von Willebrand protein responsible for von Willebrand factor activity. These two proteins have distinct biochemical and immunological properties and are under separate genetic control. Factor VIII:C acts as a cofactor for Factor IX to activate Factor X in the intrinsic pathway of blood coagulation.[6] Hemophilia A, an hereditary disorder of blood coagulation due to decreased levels of Factor VIII:C, results in profuse bleeding into joints, muscles or internal organs as a result of a trauma. Antihemophilic Factor (Human), MONOCLATE-P®, Factor VIII:C Pasteurized provides an increase in plasma levels of AHF, thereby enabling temporary correction of Hemophilia A bleeding.

Clinical evaluation of MONOCLATE-P®, Factor VIII:C Pasteurized concentrate for its half-life characteristics in hemophilic patients showed it to be comparable to other commercially available Antihemophilic Factor (Human) concentrates. The mean half-life obtained from six patients was 17.5 hours with a mean recovery of 1.9 Units/dl rise/U/kg.

The pasteurization process used in the manufacture of this concentrate has demonstrated *in vitro* inactivation of human immunodeficiency virus (HIV) and several model viruses. In two separate studies, HIV was reduced by $\geq 7.0\ \log_{10}$ to an undetectable level and by 10.5 $\log_{10}$, respectively. In addition to HIV, studies were also performed using three lipid containing model viruses and one non-lipid, encapsulated model virus. Vesicular stomatitis (VSV) was reduced by ≥ 6.79 $\log_{10}$ to undetectable, Sindbis was reduced by $\geq 6.48\ \log_{10}$ to undetectable and Vaccinia was reduced by $\geq 5.36\ \log_{10}$ to detectable. Murine encephalomyocarditis (EMC), a non-lipid, encapsulated model virus, was reduced by $\geq 7.1\ \log_{10}$ to undetectable.

Evidence of the capability of the purification and preparative steps used in the production of Antihemophilic Factor (Human), MONOCLATE-P®, Factor VIII:C Pasteurized to reduce viral bioburden was obtained in studies involving the addition of known quantities of virus to cryoprecipitate. These studies were conducted using an earlier form of the concentrate which had not undergone liquid pasteurization (Antihemophilic Factor (Human), MONOCLATE®, Factor VIII:C, Heat-Treated). These studies provide evidence of the viral removal potential of the purification and preparative steps of the manufacturing process (exclusive of heat treatment) which are common to both concentrates. In one study, the viruses used were human immunodeficiency virus (HIV), sindbis virus, vesicular stomatitis virus (VSV) and pseudorabies virus (PsRV). A comparison of the cumulative mean reductions for all viruses tested with the individual values obtained in each experiment indicates that the combined effects of the manufacturing steps, which purify the Factor VIII:C and prepare the concentrate in a final sterile container as a lyophilized powder, contribute viral reduction capabilities of approximately 5 to 6 logs. In a separate study, aluminum hydroxide treatment followed by antibody affinity chromatography reduced vaccinia virus infectivity by 4.81 logs. These studies indicate that the purification and preparative steps of the manufacturing process are capable of providing a non-specific, viral reduction of approximately 5 to 6 logs, independent of the pasteurization process.

MONOCLATE-P® contains trace amounts of mouse protein[7] (less than 50 ng per 100 AHF activity units). In a study using an earlier form of the concentrate which had not undergone pasteurization (MONOCLATE®), a number of patients seronegative for anti-HIV-1 were monitored to determine whether they would develop antibody or experience adverse reactions as a result of repeated exposure. These patients were treated on multiple occasions. Pre-study serum measurements of 27 patients for human anti-mouse IgG showed that, prior to treatment, 6 of them had either detectable antibody to mouse proteins or cross-reactive proteins. These patients continued to demonstrate similar or lower antibody levels during the study. Of the remaining 21 patients, 6 were shown to have low antibody levels on one or more occasions. In no case was observance of low antibody level associated with an anamnestic response or with any clinical adverse reaction. Patients were observed for time periods ranging from 2 to 30 months.

INDICATIONS AND USAGE

Antihemophilic Factor (Human), MONOCLATE-P®, Factor VIII:C Pasteurized is indicated for treatment of classical hemophilia (Hemophilia A). Affected individuals frequently require therapy following minor accidents. Surgery, when required in such individuals, must be preceded by temporary corrections of the clotting abnormality. Presurgical correction of severe AHF deficiency can be accomplished with a small volume of MONOCLATE-P®.

MONOCLATE-P® is not effective in controlling the bleeding of patients with von Willebrand's disease.

CONTRAINDICATIONS

Known hypersensitivity to mouse protein is a contraindication to Antihemophilic Factor (Human), MONOCLATE-P®, Factor VIII:C Pasteurized.

WARNINGS

This product is prepared from pooled human plasma which may contain the causative agents of hepatitis and other viral diseases. Prescribed manufacturing procedures utilized at the plasma collection centers, plasma testing laboratories, and the fractionation facilities are designed to reduce the risk of transmitting viral infection. However, the risk of viral infectivity from this product cannot be totally eliminated. Accordingly, the benefits and risks of treatment with this concentrate should be carefully assessed prior to use. Individuals who receive infusions of blood or plasma products may develop signs and/or symptoms of some viral infections, particularly nonA, nonB hepatitis.

PRECAUTIONS

General

Most Antihemophilic Factor (Human) concentrates contain naturally occurring blood group specific antibodies. However, the processing of MONOCLATE-P® significantly reduces the presence of blood group specific antibodies in the final product. Nevertheless, when large or frequently repeated doses of product are needed, patients should be monitored by means of hematocrit and direct Coombs tests for signs of progressive anemia.

Formation of Antibodies to Mouse Protein—Although no hypersensitivity reactions have been observed, because MONOCLATE-P® contains trace amounts of mouse protein (less than 50 ng per 100 AHF activity units), the possibility exists that patients treated with MONOCLATE-P® may develop hypersensitivity to the mouse proteins.

Information for Patients

Patients should be informed of the early signs of hypersensitivity reactions including hives, generalized urticaria, tightness of the chest, wheezing, hypotension, and anaphylaxis, and should be advised to discontinue use of the concentrate and contact their physician if these symptoms occur.

Pregnancy Category C

Animal reproduction studies have not been conducted with Antihemophilic Factor (Human), MONOCLATE-P®, Factor VIII:C Pasteurized. It is also not known whether MONOCLATE-P® can cause fetal harm when administered to a pregnant woman or can affect reproduction capacity. MONOCLATE-P® should be given to a pregnant woman only if clearly needed.

ADVERSE REACTIONS

Products of this type are known to cause allergic reactions, mild chills, nausea or stinging at the infusion site.

DOSAGE AND ADMINISTRATION

Antihemophilic Factor (Human), MONOCLATE-P®, Factor VIII:C Pasteurized is for intravenous administration only.

As a general rule 1 unit of AHF activity per kg will increase the circulating AHF level by 2%.[10] The following formula provides a guide for dosage calculations:

Number of AHF I.U. Required	=	Body weight (in kg)	×	desired Factor VIII increase (% normal)	×	0.5^{10}

Although dosage must be individualized according to the needs of the patient (weight, severity of hemorrhage, presence of inhibitors), the following general dosages are suggested.[11]

1. MILD HEMORRHAGES—Minor hemorrhagic episodes will generally subside with a single infusion if a level of 30% or more is attained.
2. MODERATE HEMORRHAGE AND MINOR SURGERY—For more serious hemorrhages and minor surgical procedures, the patient's Factor VIII level should be raised to 30–50% of normal, which usually requires an initial dose of 15–25 I.U. per kg. If further therapy is required a maintenance dose is 10–15 I.U. per kg every 8–12 hours.
3. SEVERE HEMORRHAGE—In hemorrhages near vital organs (neck, throat, subperitoneal) it may be desirable to raise the Factor VIII level to 80–100% of normal which can be achieved with an initial dose of 40–50 I.U. per kg and a maintenance dose of 20–25 I.U. per kg every 8–12 hours.
4. MAJOR SURGERY—For surgical procedures a dose of AHF sufficient to achieve a level 80–100% of normal should be given an hour prior to surgery. A second dose, half the size of the priming dose, should be given five hours after the first dose. Factor VIII levels should be maintained at a daily minimum of at least 30% for a period of 10–14 days postoperatively. Close laboratory control to maintain AHF plasma levels deemed appropriate to maintain hemostasis is recommended.

Reconstitution

1. Warm both the diluent and Antihemophilic Factor (Human), MONOCLATE-P®, Factor VIII:C Pasteurized in unopened vials to room temperature [not above 37℃ (98°F)].
2. Remove the caps from both vials to expose the central portions of the rubber stoppers.
3. Treat the surface of the rubber stoppers with antiseptic solution and allow them to dry.
4. Using aseptic technique, insert one end of the double-end needle into the rubber stopper of the diluent vial. Invert the diluent vial and insert the other end of the double-end needle into the rubber stopper of the MONOCLATE-P® vial. Direct the diluent, which will be drawn in by vacuum, over the entire surface of the MONOCLATE-P® cake. (In order to assure transfer of all the diluent, adjust the position of the tip of the needle in the diluent vial to the inside edge of the diluent stopper.) Rotate the vial to ensure complete wetting of the cake during the transfer process.
5. Remove the diluent vial to release the vacuum, <u>then remove the double-end needle</u>, from the MONOCLATE-P® vial.
6. Gently swirl the vial until the powder is dissolved and the solution is ready for administration. The concentrate routinely and easily reconstitutes within one minute. To assure sterility, MONOCLATE-P® should be administered within three hours after reconstitution.
7. Parenteral drug preparations should be inspected visually for particulate matter and discoloration prior to administration, whenever solution and container permit.

Administration

Intravenous Injection

Plastic disposable syringes are recommended with Antihemophilic Factor (Human), MONOCLATE-P®, Factor VIII:C Pasteurized solution. The ground glass surface of all-glass syringes tend to stick with solutions of this type. Please note, this concentrate is supplied with a SELF-VENTING filter spike.

1. Using aseptic technique, attach the vented filter spike to a sterile disposable syringe.
   CAUTION: DO NOT INJECT AIR INTO THE MONOCLATE-P® VIAL. The self-venting feature of the vented filter spike precludes the need to inject air in order to facilitate withdrawal of the reconstituted solution. The injection of air could cause partial product loss through the vent filter.
   CAUTION: The use of other, non-vented filter needles or spikes without the proper procedure may result in an air lock and prevent the complete transfer of the concentrate.
2. Insert the vented filter spike into the stopper of the MONOCLATE-P® vial, invert the vial, and position the filter spike so that the orifice is at the inside edge of the stopper.
3. Withdraw the reconstituted solution into the syringe.
4. Discard the filter spike. Perform venipuncture using the enclosed winged needle with microbore tubing. Attach the syringe to the luer end of the tubing.
   CAUTION: Use of other winged needles without microbore tubing, although compatible with the concentrate,

will result in a larger retention of solution within the winged infusion set.

5. Administer solution intravenously at a rate (approximately 2 mL/minute) comfortable to the patient.

STORAGE

When stored at refrigerator temperature, 2°–8℃ (36°–46°F). Antihemophilic Factor (Human), MONOCLATE-P®, Factor VIII:C Pasteurized, is stable for the period indicated by the expiration date on its label. Within this period, MONOCLATE-P® may be stored at room temperature not to exceed 30℃ (86°F), for up to 6 months.
Avoid freezing which may damage container for the diluent.

HOW SUPPLIED

MONOCLATE-P® is supplied in a single dose vial with diluent, double-ended needle for reconstitution, vented filter spike for withdrawal, winged infusion set and alcohol swabs. I.U. activity is stated on the label of each vial.

CAUTION: FEDERAL (U.S.A.) LAW PROHIBITS DISPENSING WITHOUT PRESCRIPTION.

REFERENCES

1. W. Terry, A. Schreiber, C. Tarr, M. Hrinda, W. Curry, and F. Feldman, "Human Factor VIII:C Produced Using Monoclonal Antibodies." in *Research in Clinic and Laboratory*, Vol. XVI, (#1), 202 (1986) from the XVIIth International Congress of the World Federation of Hemophilia.
2. A.B. Schreiber, "The Preclinical Characterization of Monoclate Factor VIII C Antihemophilic Factor Human," *Semin Hematol* 25 (2 Suppl. 1), 1988, pp. 27–32.
3. E. Berntorp and I.M. Nilsson, "Biochemical Properties of Human Factor VIII C Monoclate Purified Using Monoclonal Antibody to VWF," *Thromb Res* O (Suppl.7), 1987, p. 60, from the Satellite Symposia of the XIth International Congress on Thrombosis and Haemostasis, Brussel, Belguim, July 11, 1987.
4. S. Chandra, C.C. Huang, R.L. Weeks, K. Beatty and F. Feldman, "Purity of a Factor VIII:C Preparation (Monoclate) Manufactured by Monoclonal Immunoaffinity Chromatography Technique," from the XVIII International Congress of the World Federation of Hemophilia, May 1988.
5. B. Spire, D. Dormont, F. Barre-Sinousii, L. Montagnier, and J.C. Chermann, "Inactivation of Lumphadenopathy Associated Virus by Heat, Gamma Rays, and Ultraviolet Light," *Lancet*, Jan. 26, 1985, p.188.
6. L.W. Hoyer, "The Factor VIII Complex: Structure and Function," *Blood* 58 (1981), p.1.
7. F. Feldman, S. Chandra, R. Kleszynski, C.C. Huang and R.L. Weeks, "Measurement of Murine Protein Levels in Monoclonal Antibody Purified Coagulation Factor," from the XVIII International Congress of the World Federation of Hemophilia, May 1988.
8. F. Feldman, R. Kleszynski, L. Ho, R. Kling, S. Chandra and C.C. Huang, "Validation of Coagulation Test Methods for Evaluation of Monoclate (Factor VIII:C) Potencies," from the XVIII International Congress of the World Federation of Hemophilia, May 1988.
9. S. Chandra, C.C. Huang, L. Ho, R. Kling, R.L. Weeks and F. Feldman, "Studies on the Stability of Factor VIII:C (Monoclate) in Lyophilized and Solution Form," from the XVIII International Congress of the World Federation of Hemophilia, May 1988.
10. C.F. Abilgaard, J.V. Simone, J.J. Corrigan, et al., "Treatment of Hemophilia with Glycine—Precipitated Factor VIII," *New Eng J Med*, 275 (1966), p.471.
11. C.K. Kasper, "Hematologic Care," *Comprehensive Management of Hemophilia*, ed. Boone, D.C., Philadelphia, F.A. Davis Co., (1976) pp. 2–20.

BIBLIOGRAPHY

Hershman, R.J., Naconti, S.B., and Shulman, N.R., "Prophylactic Treatment of Factor VIII Deficiency." *Blood* 35 (1970), p. 189.
Kasper, C. K., Dietrich, S. I. and Rapaport, S.K. "Hemophilia Prophylaxis in Factor VIII Concentrate." *Arch. Int. Med.* 125 (1970), p. 1004.
Biggs, R., ed. "The Treatment of Hemophilia A and B and von Willebrands Disease." Oxford: Blackwell, 1978.
Fulcher, C.A., Zimmerman, T.S., "Characterization of the Human Factor VIII Procoagulant Protein With a Heterologous Precipitating Antibody." *Proc. Natl. Acad. Sci.* 79 (1982), pp. 1648–1652.
Levine, P.H., "Factor VIII C Purified from Plasma Via Monoclonal Antibodies Human Studies." *Semin Hematol* 25 (2 Suppl. 1), 1988, pp. 38–41.
Revised: May 1992

PLASMA–PLEX®   ℞

[plăz′ma-plĕks]
Plasma Protein Fraction (Human) U.S.P.
5% Solution Heat-Treated

DESCRIPTION

Plasma Protein Fraction (Human) 5%—Plasma-Plex® is a sterile solution of protein consisting of Albumin and Globulin derived from Human venous plasma that was non-reactive when tested for hepatitis B surface antigen (HBsAg) by FDA required test. Each 100 ml contains 5.0 g selected plasma proteins. The plasma proteins, as determined by electrophoresis are at least 83% Albumin and no more than 17% Globulins; no more than 1% of the proteins are Gamma Globulins. The solution is iso-osmotic with normal human plasma. Approximate concentrations of significant electrolytes are: Sodium 130–160 mEq per liter; and Potassium not more than 2mEq per liter.
Plasma-Plex® is stabilized with 0.004 molar Sodium Acetyltryptophanate and 0.004 molar Sodium Caprylate, and contains no preservative. It is heat treated at 60℃ for 10 hours. This product has been prepared in accordance with the requirements established by the Food and Drug Administration and is in compliance with the standards of the United States Pharmacopeia.
Plasma Protein Fraction (Human) 5%—Plasma-Plex® is to be administered by the intravenous route.

CLINICAL PHARMACOLOGY

Plasma Protein Fraction (Human) is effective in the maintenance of a normal blood volume but has not been proved effective in the maintenance of oncotic pressure. When the circulating blood volume has been depleted, the hemodilution following albumin administration persists for many hours. In individuals with normal blood volume, it usually lasts only a few hours.
Unlike whole blood plasma, Plasma Protein Fraction (Human) 5%—Plasma-Plex® is considered free of the danger of homologous serum hepatitis. No cross-matching is required and the absence of cellular elements removes the risk of sensitization with repeated infusions.

INDICATIONS AND USAGE

Shock: Plasma-Plex® is indicated in the emergency treatment of shock due to burns, trauma, surgery, infections, in the treatment of injuries of such severity that shock, although not immediately present, is likely to ensue, and in other similar conditions where the restoration of blood volume is urgent. It supplies additional fluid for adequate plasma volume expansion in dehydrated patients. Blood transfusion may be indicated if there has been considerable loss of red blood cells.
Burns: Plasma-Plex® is indicated to prevent marked hemoconcentration and to maintain appropriate electrolyte balance.
Hypoproteinemia: Plasma Protein Fraction (Human) 5%—Plasma-Plex® may be used in hypoproteinemic patients, providing sodium restriction is not a problem. If sodium restriction is imperative, the use of 25% Normal Serum Albumin (Human) is recommended.

CONTRAINDICATIONS

Plasma-Plex® may be contraindicated in patients with severe anemia or cardiac failure. Do not use in patients on cardiopulmonary bypass.

WARNINGS

Do not use if the solution is turbid, or if there is a sediment in the bottle. Since the product contains no preservative, do not begin administration more than 4 hours after opening the bottle. Unused portions should be discarded.

PRECAUTIONS

General

Administration of large quantities of Plasma-Plex® should be supplemented with or replaced by whole blood to combat the relative anemia which would follow such use. Rapid infusion (greater than 10 ml/minute) may produce hypotension. Blood pressure should be monitored during use and infusion slowed or ceased if sudden hypotension occurs.
When used to reverse shock or hypotension, careful observation of the patient is necessary to detect bleeding points which failed to bleed at lower pressure.
Dehydrated patients require administration of additional fluids to replace fluid withdrawn from tissues by osmotic action of Plasma-Plex®.
Administer with caution to patients with low cardiac reserve or with no albumin deficiency because a rapid increase in plasma volume may cause circulatory embarrassment or pulmonary edema.

Continued on next page

Armour—Cont.

This product cannot be used for correction of defects of the coagulation mechanism. Administration should be by intravenous route only.

Pregnancy Category C
Animal reproduction studies have not been conducted with Plasma Protein Fraction (Human) 5%—Plasma-Plex.® It is also not known whether Plasma-Plex® can cause fetal harm when administered to a pregnant woman or can affect reproduction capacity. Plasma-Plex® should be given to a pregnant woman only if clearly needed.

ADVERSE REACTIONS
Incidence of untoward reactions is low. Nausea may occur, but should be evaluated with respect to the nature of the present illness. Hypotension, particularly following rapid infusion or intraarterial administration to patients on cardiopulmonary bypass.

DOSAGE AND ADMINISTRATION
Plasma Protein Fraction (Human) 5%—Plasma-Plex® is given intravenously without further dilution. This concentration is iso-osmotic with normal human plasma. When it is administered to patients with normal blood volume, the rate of infusion should be slow enough (1 mL per minute) to present too rapid expansion of plasma volume.

Treatment of Shock: Dosage is based almost entirely on the nature of the individual case and the response to therapy. The usual minimum effective dose if 250–500 ml.
The rate of administration for the emergency treatment of shock in adults in dependent on the response to therapy and the flow should be adjusted as the patient improves. Administration rates of 10 ml per minute should not be exceeded.
In infants and small children, Plasma-Plex® has been found to be very useful in the initial therapy of shock due to dehydration and infection. A dose of 15 ml per pound of body weight infused intravenously at a rate up to 5 to 10 ml per minute for the treatment of acute shock states in infants is desirable. As with any plasma expander the rate should be adjusted or slowed according to the clinical response and rising blood pressure.

Treatment of Burns: The dosage is dependent on the extent and severity of the burn. An optimal regimen for use of Plasma Protein Fraction (Human), crystalloids, electrolytes and water in the treatment of burns has not been established.

Treatment of Hypoproteinemia: The adult dose of Plasma Protein Fraction (Human) 5%—Plasma-Plex® is 1000 to 1500 ml daily to yield 50 to 75 g of plasma protein. Since blood volume in these patients may be normal, doses of more than 500 ml should not be given faster than 500 ml in 30 to 45 minutes to avoid circulatory embarrassment. If slower administration is desired, 1000 ml may be given by continuous drip at a rate of 100 ml per hour. If sodium restriction is imperative, 25% Normal Serum Albumin (Human) is recommended.
Parenteral drug products should be inspected visually for particulate matter and discoloration prior to administration whenever solution and container permit.

HOW SUPPLIED
Plasma Protein Fraction (Human) 5%—Plasma-Plex® is supplied as a 5% solution in:
NDC 0053-7753-03 50 ml bottles containing 2.5 g of selected plasma proteins.
NDC 0053-7753-01 250 ml bottles containing 12.5 g of selected plasma proteins.
NDC 0053-7753-02 500 ml bottles containing 25.0 g of selected plasma proteins.
Store at controlled room temperature—between 15°–30°C (59°–86°F). Do not allow to freeze.
Caution: Federal (U.S.A.) law prohibits dispensing without prescription.

BIBLIOGRAPHY
1. Bertrand, J.J.; Feichtmeir, T.V.; Kolomeyer, N.; Beatty, J.O.; Murphy, P.L.; Waldschmidt, W.D.; and McLean, E.B.; Clinical Investigations with a Heat-Treated Plasma Protein Fraction, Vox. Sang. 4:385–402, 1959.
2. Cock, T.C.; Binger, D.C.; and Dennis, J.L.; A New Plasma Substitute for Pediatric Therapy, Calif. Med. 89:257, 1958.
3. Hink, J.H. Jr.; Hidalgo, J.; Seeberg, V.P.; and Johnson, F.F.; Preparation and Properties of a Heat-Treated Human Plasma Protein Fraction, Vox Sanguinis 2:174, 1957.
4. Bland, J.H.; Laver, M.B.; and Lowenstein, E.; Vasodilator Effect of Commercial 5% Plasma Protein Fraction Solutions, JAMA 224:172114 1724, 1973.
Revised August, 1990

EDUCATIONAL MATERIAL

Gamulin
"Confidence Factor" booklets
—in Rh negative women
—in a matter of choice
—in antepartum prophylaxis
—in prenatal diagnostic testing
The above literature is available to physicians, pharmacists and patients.
Monograph Series—"The Prevention of Rh Isoimmunization"
#1— Amniocentesis and Rh Isoimmunization
#2— Antenatal Rh Immune Globulin Use in an Uneventful Pregnancy
#3— Management of the High-Risk Pregnancy
#4— Massive Transplacental Hemorrhage, the Laboratory and the Blood Bank
Film—"Hemolytic disease of the newborn"
The Monograph Series and film are available to physicians and pharmacists—contact Armour Corporate Headquarters.

Monoclate-P® Factor VIII:C
Question and Answer Booklet
Patient Infusion Video
Available to physicians and pharmacists—contact Armour Corporate Headquarters.

B.F. Ascher & Company, Inc.
15501 WEST 109TH STREET
LENEXA, KS 66219-1308

ANASPAZ® Tablets ℞
[*an 'ah-spāz*]

(l-hyoscyamine sulfate) ....0.125 mg

HOW SUPPLIED
Light yellow, compressed, scored tablets with the Ascher logo on one side and the NDC 225/295 on the other.
Bottles of 100—NDC 0225-0295-15
Bottles of 500—NDC 0225-0295-20

AYR® Saline Nasal Mist and Drops OTC
(See PDR For Nonprescription Drugs.)

ITCH–X® Gel OTC
(See PDR For Nonprescription Drugs.)

KWELCOF® Liquid Ⓒ℞
[*kwel 'cof*]

Each teaspoonful (5 ml) contains:
Hydrocodone bitartrate ....5 mg
        (WARNING: May be habit-forming)
Guaifenesin ....100 mg

HOW SUPPLIED
Clear, fruit-flavored liquid which is alcohol-free, dye-free, sugar-free and corn products-free.
1 pint bottles—NDC 0225-0420-45

MOBIGESIC® Analgesic Tablets OTC
(See PDR For Nonprescription Drugs.)

MOBISYL® Analgesic Creme OTC
(See PDR For Nonprescription Drugs.)

PEN•KERA® Creme OTC
(See PDR For Nonprescription Drugs.)

UNILAX® Softgel Capsules OTC
(See PDR For Nonprescription Drugs.)

Astra Pharmaceutical Products, Inc.
50 OTIS STREET
WESTBORO, MA 01581-4500

AQUASOL A® ℞
water-miscible
Vitamin A Capsules, USP
equivalent to
15 mg retinol
50,000 USP Units
vitamin A per capsule
7.5 mg retinol
25,000 USP Units
vitamin A per capsule

DESCRIPTION
Aquasol A (water-miscible vitamin A) capsules provide 15 mg retinol (50,000 USP Units) or 7.5 mg retinol (25,000 USP Units) in the form of vitamin A alcohol, a light yellow to amber oil. One USP Unit is equivalent to the biological activity of 0.3 mcg of retinol or 0.6 mcg of beta-carotene. One molecule of beta-carotene yields two molecules of retinol, which is known as provitamin A.
Vitamin A, one of the fat-soluble vitamins, includes vitamin A itself as well as its precursors, alpha-, beta-, and gamma-carotene and cryptoxanthin. Of the precursors, beta-carotene predominates in nature and is the most active; on splitting, it forms two molecules of vitamin A, whereas the other precursors form only one molecule of vitamin A.
The structural formula of retinol ($C_{20}H_{30}O$) is:

Ordinarily fat-soluble, the vitamin A in this product has been water solubilized by special processing* to enable better absorption and utilization particularly in conditions in which absorption or utilization of fats and fat-soluble substances is impaired. The capsules also contain ethyl vanillin, FD&C Red #40, gelatin, glycerin, methylparaben, polysorbate 80, and propylparaben.

CLINICAL PHARMACOLOGY
Retinol combines with opsin, the rod pigment in the retina, to form rhodopsin, which is necessary for visual adaptation to darkness.
Vitamin A prevents retardation of growth and preserves the integrity of the epithelial cells.
Vitamin A deficiency is characterized by nyctalopia, keratomalacia, keratinization and drying of the skin, lowered resistance to infection, retardation of growth, thickening of bone, diminished production of cortical steroids, and fetal malformations. Vitamin A absorption requires bile salts, pancreatic lipase, and dietary fat. The vitamin is stored (primarily as the palmitate) in the Kupffer cells of the liver. The minimum daily requirement is approximately 20 units of vitamin A or 40 units of beta-carotene per kg of body weight. The daily Recommended Dietary Allowance (RDA) established by the National Academy of Sciences for selected categories of population are as follows: children 4–10 years of age, 2500–3000 units; adult males, 5000 units; adult females, 4000 units; pregnant women, 5000 units; lactating women, 6000 units.
The fat-soluble vitamins (A, D, E and K) are absorbed by complex processes that parallel the absorption of fat. Thus, any condition that causes malabsorption of fat (e.g., celiac disease, tropical sprue, regional enteritis) may result in deficiency of one or all of these vitamins. Fat-soluble vitamins affect permeability or transport in various cell membranes and act as oxidation-reduction agents, coenzymes, or enzyme inhibitors. They are stored principally in the liver and excreted in the feces. Because these vitamins are metabolized very slowly, overdosage may produce toxic effects. Dietary fat is necessary for effective absorption of carotene, and protein is required for absorption of retinols. Protein and, possibly, zinc may be required to mobilize vitamin A reserves in the liver.
Vitamin A is more rapidly absorbed than carotene. Absorption of vitamin A from an aqueous vehicle is appreciably greater than when the drug is given in an oily solution. Carotene is converted to vitamin A in the intestinal wall and in the liver. Vitamin A itself is found only in animal sources; it occurs in high concentrations in the liver of the cod, hali-

---
* Oil-soluble vitamin A alcohol, water solubilized with polysorbate 80.

but, tuna, and shark. It is also prepared synthetically. Carotene is found only in plants.

INDICATIONS AND USAGE

Aquasol A (water-miscible vitamin A) capsules are effective for the treatment of vitamin A deficiency. Unlike fat-soluble vitamin A products, **Aquasol A** capsules are not contraindicated in the malabsorption syndrome, because of the water-solubilizing process.

CONTRAINDICATIONS

Hypervitaminosis A. Sensitivity to any of the ingredients of this preparation.

WARNINGS

Avoid overdosage. Keep out of the reach of children.
Use in Pregnancy; Aquasol A capsules may cause fetal harm when administered to a pregnant woman. Safety of amounts exceeding 6000 units of vitamin A daily during pregnancy has not been established at this time. Therefore, use of **Aquasol A** capsules is contraindicated during pregnancy.
Animal reproduction studies with vitamin A, either alone or combined with other retinoid compounds, have shown fetal abnormalities. Therefore, total intake of vitamin A and other therapeutic retinoids should be considered. Fetal abnormalities in animal reproduction studies have been associated with overdosage in several species. Malformations of the central nervous system, eye, palate, and genitourinary tract have been recorded.
In women of childbearing age, the possibility of pregnancy should be excluded before use of **Aquasol A** capsules. **Aquasol A** is contraindicated in women who are or may become pregnant. If this drug is used during pregnancy, or if the patient becomes pregnant while taking this drug, the patient should be apprised of the potential hazard to the fetus.

PRECAUTIONS

General: Protect from light. Vitamin A ingested in fortified foods, dietary supplements, and other concomitantly taken drugs should be evaluated. Prolonged daily administration of more than 25,000 units should be conducted under close supervision. Blood level assays are not a direct measure of liver storage. Liver storage should be adequate before discontinuing therapy. Single vitamin A deficiency is rare. Multiple vitamin deficiency is expected in any dietary deficiency.
Drug Interactions: Women receiving oral contraceptives have shown a significant increase in plasma vitamin A levels.
Usage in Pregnancy:
Pregnancy Category X:
See WARNINGS.
Nursing Mothers: Human milk supplies sufficient vitamin A for infants unless the maternal diet is grossly inadequate.

ADVERSE REACTIONS

See OVERDOSAGE section.

OVERDOSAGE

The following amounts have been found to be toxic. Toxicity manifestations depend on the age, dose, and duration of administration.
Acute toxicity—Results from a single dose of 25,000 units per kg of body weight; e.g., 350,000 units for an infant and over 2 million units for an adult.
Chronic toxicity—Produced by 4000 units per kg of body weight administered for 6 to 15 months.
Infants 3 to 6 months of age can experience chronic toxicity from 18,500 units (water dispersed) per day for 1 to 3 months.
Adults: 1 million units daily for three days, or 50,000 units daily for longer than 18 months, or 500,000 units daily for two months.
Hypervitaminosis A Syndrome:
1. *General manifestations:*
Fatigue, malaise, lethargy, abdominal discomfort, anorexia, and vomiting.
2. *Specific manifestations:*
a. Skeletal: Slow growth, hard tender cortical thickening over the radius and tibia, migratory arthralgia, and premature closure of the epiphysis.
b. Central Nervous System: Irritability, headache, and increased intracranial pressure as manifested by bulging fontanels, papilledema, and exophthalmos.
c. Dermatologic: Fissures of the lips, drying and cracking of the skin, alopecia, scaling, massive desquamation, and increased pigmentation.
d. Systemic: Hypomenorrhea, hepatosplenomegaly, jaundice, leukopenia, vitamin A plasma level over 1200 units.
The treatment of hypervitaminosis A consists of immediate withdrawal of the vitamin along with symptomatic and supportive treatment.

DOSAGE AND ADMINISTRATION

For adults and children over eight years of age:
1. Severe deficiency with xerophthalmia: 500,000 units daily for three days, followed by 50,000 units daily for two weeks.
2. Severe deficiency: 100,000 units daily for three days followed by 50,000 units daily for two weeks.

3. Follow-up therapy: 10,000 to 20,000 units daily for two months.

HOW SUPPLIED

Aquasol A capsules (water-miscible vitamin A) are available as:
NDC 0186-4301-00; 15 mg retinol (50,000 USP Units), Bottles of 100.
NDC 0186-4291-00; 7.5 mg retinol (25,000 USP units), Bottles of 100.
These products are dark red, soft gelatin capsules.
These products are manufactured for Astra Pharmaceutical Products, Inc., by R.P. Scherer Corp., Clearwater, FL 33518. Store at controlled room temperature, 15°–30°C (59°–86°F). Protect from light. Dispense in a tight, light-resistant container as defined in the USP.
Caution: Federal law prohibits dispensing without prescription.
021678R00   Iss. 6/91

AQUASOL A®   ℞
Parenteral
water-miscible
vitamin A Palmitate
50,000 USP Units
(15 mg retinol)/mL

with 0.5% chlorobutanol as preservative; 12% polysorbate 80, 0.1% citric acid, 0.03% butylated hydroxyanisole, 0.03% butylated hydroxytoluene; and sodium hydroxide to adjust pH.

THIS IS A STERILE PRODUCT FOR INTRAMUSCULAR INJECTION

DESCRIPTION

AQUASOL A PARENTERAL (water-miscible vitamin A) provides 50,000 USP Units of vitamin A per mL as retinol ($C_{20}H_{30}O$) in the form of vitamin A palmitate, a light yellow to amber oil. The structural formula of retinol is:

$$\text{structural formula of retinol}$$

Ordinarily oil-soluble, the vitamin A in this product has been water solubilized by special processing* and is available in a water solution for intramuscular injection.
One USP Unit is equivalent to one international unit (IU) and to 0.3 mcg of retinol or 0.6 mcg of beta-carotene.

CLINICAL PHARMACOLOGY

Beta-carotene, retinol, and retinal have effective and reliable vitamin A activity. Retinal and retinol are in chemical equilibrium in the body and have equivalent antixerophthalmic activity. Retinal combines with the rod pigment, opsin, in the retina to form rhodopsin, necessary for visual dark adaptation. Vitamin A prevents retardation of growth and preserves the epithelial cells' integrity. Normal adult liver storage is sufficient to satisfy two years' requirements of vitamin A.
Vitamin A is readily absorbed from the gastrointestinal tract, where the biosynthesis of vitamin A from beta-carotene takes place. Vitamin A absorption requires bile salts, pancreatic lipase, and dietary fat. It is transported in the blood to the liver by the chylomicron fraction of the lymph. Vitamin A is stored in Kupffer cells of the liver mainly as the palmitate. Normal serum vitamin A is 80–300 Units per 100 mL (plasma range is 30–70μg per dl) and for carotenoids 270–753 Units per 100 mL. The normal adult liver contains approximately 100 to 300 micrograms per gram, mostly as retinol palmitate.

INDICATIONS

Vitamin A injection is effective for the treatment of vitamin A deficiency.
The parenteral administration is indicated when the oral administration is not feasible as in anorexia, nausea, vomiting, pre- and post- operative conditions, or it is not available as in the "Malabsorption Syndrome" with accompanying steatorrhea.

CONTRAINDICATIONS

The intravenous administration. Hypervitaminosis A. Sensitivity to any of the ingredients in this preparation.
Use in Pregnancy: Safety of amounts exceeding 6,000 Units of vitamin A daily during pregnancy has not been established at this time. The use of vitamin A in excess of the recommended dietary allowance may cause fetal harm when

*Oil-soluble vitamin A water solubilized with polysorbate 80.

administered to a pregnant woman. Animal reproduction studies have shown fetal abnormalities associated with overdosage in several species. Malformations of the central nervous system, the eye, the palate, and the urogenital tract are recorded. Vitamin A in excess of the recommended dietary allowance is contraindicated in women who are or may become pregnant. If vitamin A is used during pregnancy, or if the patient becomes pregnant while taking vitamin A, the patient should be apprised of the potential hazard to the fetus.

WARNINGS

Avoid overdosage. Keep out of the reach of children.

PRECAUTIONS

General: Protect from light. Prolonged daily dose administration over 25,000 Units vitamin A should be under close supervision. Blood level assays are not a direct measure of liver storage. Liver storage should be adequate before discontinuing therapy. Single vitamin A deficiency is rare. Multiple vitamin deficiency is expected in any dietary deficiency.
Drug Interactions: Women on oral contraceptives have shown a significant increase in plasma vitamin A levels.
Carcinogenesis: There are no studies that show that administration of vitamin A will cause or prevent cancer.
Pregnancy Category X:
See CONTRAINDICATIONS section.
Nursing Mothers: The U.S. Recommended Daily Allowance (RDA) of vitamin A (5,000 Units) is recommended for nursing mothers.

ADVERSE REACTIONS

See OVERDOSAGE section. Anaphylactic shock and death have been reported using the intravenous route. Allergic reactions have been reported rarely with administration of Aquasol A Parenteral including one case of an anaphylactoid type reaction.

OVERDOSAGE

The following amounts have been found to be toxic orally. Toxicity manifestations depend on the age, dosage, size and duration of administration.
Acute toxicity—single dose (25,000 Units/kg body weight)
Infant: 350,000 Units
Adult: Over 2 million Units
Chronic toxicity   (4,000 Units/kg body weight for 6 to 15 months)
Infants 3 to 6 months old: 18,500 Units (water dispersed)/ day for one to three months.
Adult: 1 million Units daily for three days; 50,000 Units daily for longer than 18 months; 500,000 Units daily for two months.
Hypervitaminosis A Syndrome:
1. *General manifestations:*
Fatigue, malaise, lethargy, abdominal discomfort, anorexia, and vomiting.
2. *Specific manifestations:*
a. Skeletal: Slow growth, hard tender cortical thickening over the radius and tibia, migratory arthralgia and premature closure of the epiphysis.
b. Central Nervous System: Irritability, headache, and increased intracranial pressure as manifested by bulging fontanels, papilledema, and exophthalmos.
c. Dermatologic: Fissures of the lips, drying and cracking of the skin, alopecia, scaling, massive desquamation, and increased pigmentation.
d. Systemic: Hypomenorrhea, hepatosplenomegaly, jaundice, leukopenia, vitamin A plasma level over 1,200 Units/100 mL.
The treatment of hypervitaminosis A consists of immediate withdrawal of the vitamin along with symptomatic and supportive treatment.

DOSAGE AND ADMINISTRATION

For intramuscular use.
I.   Adults
      100,000 Units daily for three days followed by 50,000 daily for two weeks.
II.   Children 1 to 8 years old
      17,500 to 35,000 Units daily for 10 days.
III. Infants
      7,500 to 15,000 Units daily for 10 days.
Follow-up therapy with an oral therapeutic multi-vitamin preparation, containing 10,000 to 20,000 Units vitamin A for persons over 8 years old and 5,000 to 10,000 Units for infants and children, is recommended daily for two months. In malabsorption, the parenteral route must be used for an equivalent preparation.
Poor dietary habits should be corrected and an abundant and well-balanced dietary intake should be prescribed.

HOW SUPPLIED

Aquasol A Parenteral (water-miscible vitamin A Palmitate) is available as: NDC 0186-4239-62; 50,000 USP Units (15 mg retinol/mL); 2 mL single-dose vial, box of 10.

Continued on next page

Astra—Cont.

Caution: Federal law prohibits dispensing without prescription.
Manufactured by:
Armour Pharmaceutical Company
Kankakee, IL 60901
021677R00 Iss. 6/91

ASTRAMORPH/PF™ Ⓒ

[ăs'-trā-mŏrf"]
(morphine sulfate injection, USP) Preservative-Free

DESCRIPTION

Morphine is the most important alkaloid of opium and is a phenanthrene derivative . It is available as the sulfate, having the following structural formula:

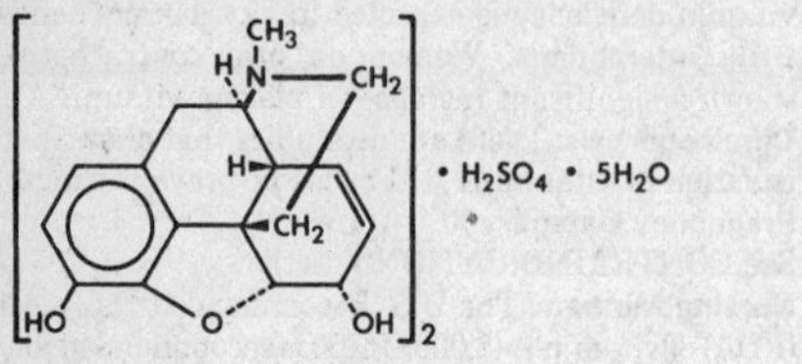

7,8-Didehydro-4,5-epoxy-17-methyl-(5α,6α)-morphinan-3,6-diol sulfate (2:1)(salt), pentahydrate

Preservative-free ASTRAMORPH/PF (Morphine Sulfate Injection, USP) is a sterile, pyrogen-free, isobaric solution free of antioxidants, preservatives or other potentially neurotoxic additives, and is intended for intravenous, epidural or intrathecal administration as a narcotic analgesic. Each milliliter contains morphine sulfate 0.5 mg or 1 mg (Warning: May Be Habit Forming) and sodium chloride 9 mg in Water for Injection. pH may be adjusted with hydrochloric acid to 2.5–6.5. Containers are sealed under nitrogen. Each container is intended for SINGLE USE ONLY. Discard any unused portion. DO NOT AUTOCLAVE.

CLINICAL PHARMACOLOGY

Morphine exerts its primary effects on the central nervous system and organs containing smooth muscle. Pharmacologic effects include analgesia, drowsiness, alteration in mood (euphoria), reduction in body temperature (at low doses), dose-related depression of respiration, interference with adrenocortical response to stress (at high doses), reduction in peripheral resistance with little or no effect on cardiac index and miosis.

Morphine, as other opioids, acts as an agonist interacting with stereo-specific and saturable binding sites/receptors in the brain, spinal cord and other tissues. These sites have been classified as μ receptors and are widely distributed throughout the central nervous system being present in highest concentration in the limbic system (frontal and temporal cortex, amygdala and hippocampus), thalamus, striatum, hypothalamus, midbrain and laminae I, II, IV and V of the dorsal horn in the spinal cord. It has been postulated that exogenously administered morphine exerts its analgesic effect, in part, by altering the central release of neurotransmitter from afferent nerves sensitive to noxious stimuli. Peripheral threshold or responsiveness to noxious stimuli is unaffected leaving monosynaptic reflexes such as the patellar or the Achilles tendon reflex intact.

Autonomic reflexes are not affected by epidural or intrathecal morphine, however morphine exerts spasmogenic effects on the gastrointestinal tract that result in decreased peristaltic activity.

Central nervous system effects of intravenously administered morphine sulfate are influenced by ability to cross the blood-brain barrier.

The delay in the onset of analgesia following epidural or intrathecal injection may be attributed to its relatively poor lipid solubility (i.e., an oil/water partition coefficient of 1.42), and its slow access to the receptor sites. The hydrophilic character of morphine may also explain its retention in the CNS and its slow release into the systemic circulation, resulting in a prolonged effect.

Nausea and vomiting may be prominent and are thought to be the result of central stimulation of the chemoreceptor trigger zone. Histamine release is common; allergic manifestations of urticaria and, rarely, anaphylaxis may occur. Bronchoconstriction may occur either as an idiosyncratic reaction or from large dosages.

Approximately one-third of intravenous morphine is bound to plasma proteins. Free morphine is rapidly redistributed in parenchymatous tissues. The major metabolic pathway is through conjugation with glucuronic acid in the liver. Elimination half-life is approximately 1.5 to 2 hours in healthy volunteers. For intravenously administered morphine, 90% is excreted in the urine within 24 hours and traces are detectable in urine up to 48 hours. About 7–10% of administered morphine eventually appears in the feces as conjugated morphine.

Peak serum levels following epidural or intrathecal administration of ASTRAMORPH/PF are reached within 30 minutes in most subjects and decline to very low levels during the next 2 to 4 hours. The onset of action occurs in 15 to 60 minutes following epidural administration or intrathecal administration; analgesia may last up to 24 hours. Due to this extended duration of action, sustained pain relief can be provided with lower daily doses (by these two routes) than are usually required with intravenous or intramuscular morphine administration.

INDICATIONS AND USAGE

Preservative-free ASTRAMORPH/PF is a systemic narcotic analgesic for administration by the intravenous, epidural or intrathecal routes. It is used for the management of pain not responsive to non-narcotic analgesics. Morphine sulfate, administered epidurally or intrathecally, provides pain relief for extended periods without attendant loss of motor, sensory or sympathetic function.

CONTRAINDICATIONS

ASTRAMORPH/PF is contraindicated in those medical conditions which would preclude the administration of opioids by the intravenous route—allergy to morphine or other opiates, acute bronchial asthma, upper airway obstruction.

Administration of morphine by the epidural or intrathecal route is contraindicated in the presence of infection at the injection site, anticoagulant therapy, bleeding diathesis, parenterally administered corticosteroids within a two week period or other concomitant drug therapy or medical condition which would contraindicate the technique of epidural or intrathecal analgesia.

WARNINGS

ASTRAMORPH/PF administration should be limited to use by those familiar with the management of respiratory depression, and in the case of epidural or intrathecal administration, familiar with the techniques and patient management problems associated with epidural or intrathecal drug administration. Because epidural administration has been associated with lessened potential for immediate or late adverse effects than intrathecal administration, the epidural route should be used whenever possible. Rapid intravenous administration may result in chest wall rigidity.

FACILITES WHERE ASTRAMORPH/PF IS ADMINISTERED MUST BE EQUIPPED WITH RESUSCITATIVE EQUIPMENT, OXYGEN, NALOXONE INJECTION, AND OTHER RESUSCITATIVE DRUGS. WHEN THE EPIDURAL OR INTRATHECAL ROUTE OF ADMINISTRATION IS EMPLOYED, PATIENTS MUST BE OBSERVED IN A FULLY EQUIPPED AND STAFFED ENVIRONMENT FOR AT LEAST 24 HOURS.

SEVERE RESPIRATORY DEPRESSION UP TO 24 HOURS FOLLOWING EPIDURAL OR INTRATHECAL ADMINISTRATION HAS BEEN REPORTED.

Morphine sulfate may be habit forming. (**See Drug Abuse and Dependence section**).

PRECAUTIONS

General

Preservative-free ASTRAMORPH/PF (Morphine Sulfate Injection, USP) should be administered with extreme caution in aged or debilitated patients, in the presence of increased intracranial/intraocular pressure and in patients with head injury. Pupillary changes (miosis) may obscure the course of intracranial pathology. Care is urged in patients who have a decreased respiratory reserve (e.g., emphysema, severe obesity, kyphoscoliosis).

Seizures may result from high doses. Patients with known seizure disorders should be carefully observed for evidence of morphine-induced seizure activity.

It is recommended that administration of ASTRAMORPH/PF by the epidural or intrathecal routes be limited to the lumbar area. Intrathecal use has been associated with a higher incidence of respiratory depression than epidural use.

Smooth muscle hypertonicity may result in biliary colic, difficulty in urination and possible urinary retention requiring catheterization. Consideration should be given to risks inherent in urethral catheterization, e.g., sepsis, when epidural or intrathecal administration is considered, especially in the perioperative period.

Elimination half-life may be prolonged in patients with reduced metabolic rates and with hepatic or renal dysfunction. Hence, care should be exercised in administering morphine in these conditions, particularly with repeated dosing.

Patients with reduced circulating blood volume, impaired myocardial function or on sympatholytic drugs should be observed carefully for orthostatic hypotension, particularly in transport.

Patients with chronic obstructive pulmonary disease and patients with acute asthmatic attack may develop acute respiratory failure with administration of morphine. Use in these patients should be reserved for those whose conditions require endotracheal intubation and respiratory support or control of ventilation.

Drug Interactions

Depressant effects of morphine are potentiated by either concomitant administration or in the presence of other CNS depressants such as alcohol, sedatives, antihistaminics or psychotropic drugs (e.g., MAO inhibitors, phenothiazines, butyrophenones and tricyclic antidepressants). Premedication or intra-anesthetic use of neuroleptics with morphine may increase the risk of respiratory depression.

Carcinogenesis, Mutagenesis, Impairment of Fertility

Studies of morphine sulfate in animals to evaluate the carcinogenic and mutagenic potential or the effect on fertility have not been conducted.

Pregnancy

Teratogenic effects—Pregnancy Category C

Animal reproduction studies have not been conducted with morphine sulfate. It is also not known whether morphine sulfate can cause fetal harm when administered to a pregnant woman or can affect reproduction capacity. Morphine sulfate should be given to a pregnant woman only if clearly needed.

Nonteratogenic effects

Infants born from mothers who have been taking morphine chronically may exhibit withdrawal symptoms.

Labor and Delivery

Intravenous morphine readily passes into the fetal circulation and may result in respiratory depression in the neonate. Naloxone and resuscitative equipment should be available for reversal of narcotic-induced respiratory depression in the neonate. In addition, intravenous morphine may reduce the strength, duration and frequency of uterine contraction resulting in prolonged labor.

Epidurally and intrathecally administered morphine readily passes into the fetal circulation and may result in respiratory depression of the neonate. Controlled clinical studies have shown that *epidural* administration has little or no effect on the relief of labor pain.

However, studies have suggested that in most cases 0.2 to 1 mg of morphine *intrathecally* provides adequate pain relief with little effect on the duration of first stage labor. The second stage labor, though, may be prolonged if the parturient is not encouraged to bear down. A continuous intravenous infusion of naloxone, 0.6 mg/hr, for 24 hours after intrathecal injection may be employed to reduce the incidence of potential side effects.

Nursing Mothers

Morphine is excreted in maternal milk. Effect on the nursing infant is not known.

Pediatric Use

Safety and effectiveness in children have not been established.

ADVERSE REACTIONS

The most serious side effect is respiratory depression. Because of delay in maximum CNS effect with intravenously administered drug (30 min), rapid administration may result in overdosing. Bolus administration by the epidural or intrathecal route may result in early respiratory depression due to direct venous redistribution of morphine to the respiratory centers in the brain. Late (up to 24 hours) onset of acute respiratory depression has been reported with administration by the epidural or intrathecal route and is believed to be the result of rostral spread. Reports of respiratory depression following intrathecal administration have been more frequent, but the dosage used in most of these cases has been considerably higher than that recommended. This depression may be severe and could require intervention (see Warnings and Overdosage sections). Even without clinical evidence of ventilatory inadequacy, a diminished CO_2 ventilation response may be noted for up to 22 hours following epidural or intrathecal administration.

While low doses of intravenously administered morphine have little effect on cardiovascular stability, high doses are excitatory, resulting from sympathetic hyperactivity and increase in circulating catecholamines. Excitation of the central nervous system resulting in convulsions may accompany high doses of morphine given intravenously. Dysphoric reactions may occur and toxic psychoses have been reported.

Epidural or intrathecal administration is accompanied by a high incidence of pruritus which is dose related but not confined to site of administration. Nausea and vomiting are frequently seen in patients following morphine administration. Urinary retention which may persist for 10–20 hours following single epidural or intrathecal administration has been reported in approximately 90% of males. Incidence is somewhat lower in females. Patients may require catheterization (see Precautions). Pruritus, nausea/vomiting and urinary retention frequently can be alleviated by the intravenous administration of low doses of naloxone (0.2 mg).

Tolerance and dependence to chronically administered morphine, by whatever route, is known to occur (**see Drug Abuse and Dependence section**).

Miscellaneous side effects include constipation, headache, anxiety, depression of cough reflex, interference with thermal regulation and oliguria. Evidence of histamine release such as urticaria, wheals and/or local tissue irritation may occur.

In general, side effects are amenable to reversal by narcotic antagonists. **NALOXONE HYDROCHLORIDE INJECTION AND RESUSCITATIVE EQUIPMENT SHOULD BE IMMEDIATELY AVAILABLE FOR ADMINISTRATION IN CASE OF LIFE THREATENING OR INTOLERABLE SIDE EFFECTS.**

DRUG ABUSE AND DEPENDENCE

Controlled Substance
Morphine sulfate injection is a Schedule II substance under the Drug Enforcement Administration classification.

Abuse
Morphine has recognized abuse and dependence potential.

Dependence
Cerebral and spinal receptors may develop tolerance/dependence independently, as a function of local dosage. Care must be taken to avert withdrawal in those patients who have been maintained on parenteral/oral narcotics when epidural or intrathecal administration is considered. Withdrawal may occur following chronic epidural or intrathecal administration, as well as the development of tolerance to morphine by these routes. (**See nonteratogenic effects under Pregnancy**).

OVERDOSAGE

Overdosage is characterized by respiratory depression with or without concomitant CNS depression. Since respiratory arrest may result either through direct depression of the respiratory center or as the result of hypoxia, primary attention should be given to the establishment of adequate respiratory exchange through provision of a patent airway and institution of assisted or controlled ventilation. The narcotic antagonist, naloxone hydrochloride, is a specific antidote. Naloxone hydrochloride (see package insert for full prescribing information) should be administered intravenously, simultaneously with respiratory resuscitation. *As the duration of effect of naloxone is considerably shorter than that of epidural or intrathecal morphine, repeated administration may be necessary.* Patients should be closely observed for evidence of renarcotization.

Note: Respiratory depression may be delayed in onset up to 24 hours following epidural or intrathecal administration. In painful conditions, reversal of narcotic effect may result in acute onset of pain and release of catecholamines. Careful administration of naloxone may permit reversal of side effects without affecting analgesia. Parenteral administration of narcotics in patients receiving epidural or intrathecal morphine may result in overdosage.

DOSAGE AND ADMINISTRATION

Preservative-free ASTRAMORPH/PF (Morphine Sulfate Injection, USP) is intended for intravenous, epidural or intrathecal administration.

Intravenous Administration
Dosage
The initial dose of morphine should be 2 mg to 10 mg/70 kg of body weight. Patients under the age of 18; no information available.

Epidural Administration
ASTRAMORPH/PF SHOULD BE ADMINISTERED EPIDURALLY ONLY BY PHYSICIANS EXPERIENCED IN THE TECHNIQUES OF EPIDURAL ADMINISTRATION AND WHO ARE THOROUGHLY FAMILIAR WITH THE LABELING. IT SHOULD BE ADMINISTERED ONLY IN SETTINGS WHERE ADEQUATE PATIENT MONITORING IS POSSIBLE. RESUSCITATIVE EQUIPMENT AND A SPECIFIC ANTAGONIST (NALOXONE HYDROCHLORIDE INJECTION) SHOULD BE IMMEDIATELY AVAILABLE FOR THE MANAGEMENT OF RESPIRATORY DEPRESSION AS WELL AS COMPLICATIONS WHICH MIGHT RESULT FROM INADVERTENT INTRATHECAL OR INTRAVASCULAR INJECTION. (NOTE: INTRATHECAL DOSAGE IS USUALLY ¹⁄₁₀ THAT OF EPIDURAL DOSAGE). PATIENT MONITORING SHOULD BE CONTINUED FOR AT LEAST 24 HOURS AFTER EACH DOSE, SINCE DELAYED RESPIRATORY DEPRESSION MAY OCCUR.

Proper placement of a needle or catheter in the epidural space should be verified before ASTRAMORPH/PF is injected. Acceptable techniques for verifying proper placement include: a) aspiration to check for absence of blood or cerebrospinal fluid, or b) administration of 5 mL (3 mL in obstetric patients) of 1.5% UNPRESERVED Lidocaine and Epinephrine (1:200,000) Injection and then observe the patient for lack of tachycardia (this indicates that vascular injection has *not* been made) and lack of sudden onset of segmental anesthesia (this indicates that intrathecal injection has *not* been made).

Epidural Adult Dosage
Initial injection of 5 mg in the lumbar region may provide satisfactory pain relief for up to 24 hours. If adequate pain relief is not achieved within one hour, careful administration of incremental doses of 1 to 2 mg at intervals sufficient to assess effectiveness may be given. No more than 10 mg/24 hr should be administered.

Thoracic administration has been shown to dramatically increase the incidence of early and late respiratory depression even at doses of 1 to 2 mg.

For continuous infusion an initial dose of 2 to 4 mg/24 hours is recommended. Further doses of 1 to 2 mg may be given if pain relief is not achieved initially.

Aged or debilitated patients-Administer with extreme caution (**see Precautions section**). Doses of less than 5 mg may provide satisfactory pain relief for up to 24 hours.

Epidural Pediatric Use
No information on use in pediatric patients is available.

Intrathecal Administration

> **NOTE: INTRATHECAL DOSAGE IS USUALLY ¹⁄₁₀ THAT OF EPIDURAL DOSAGE**

ASTRAMORPH/PF SHOULD BE ADMINISTERED INTRATHECALLY ONLY BY PHYSICIANS EXPERIENCED IN THE TECHNIQUES OF INTRATHECAL ADMINISTRATION AND WHO ARE THOROUGHLY FAMILIAR WITH THE LABELING. IT SHOULD BE ADMINISTERED ONLY IN SETTINGS WHERE ADEQUATE PATIENT MONITORING IS POSSIBLE. RESUSCITATIVE EQUIPMENT AND A SPECIFIC ANTAGONIST (NALOXONE HYDROCHLORIDE INJECTION) SHOULD BE IMMEDIATELY AVAILABLE FOR THE MANAGEMENT OF RESPIRATORY DEPRESSION AS WELL AS COMPLICATIONS WHICH MIGHT RESULT FROM INADVERTENT INTRAVASCULAR INJECTION. PATIENT MONITORING SHOULD BE CONTINUED FOR AT LEAST 24 HOURS AFTER EACH DOSE, SINCE DELAYED RESPIRATORY DEPRESSION MAY OCCUR. RESPIRATORY DEPRESSION (BOTH EARLY AND LATE ONSET) HAS OCCURRED MORE FREQUENTLY FOLLOWING INTRATHECAL ADMINISTRATION.

Intrathecal Adult Dosage
A single injection of 0.2 to 1 mg may provide satisfactory pain relief for up to 24 hours. (CAUTION: THIS IS ONLY 0.4 TO 2 ML OF THE 0.5 MG/ML POTENCY OR 0.2 to 1 ML OF THE 1 MG/ML POTENCY OF ASTRAMORPH/PF). DO NOT INJECT INTRATHECALLY MORE THAN 2 ML OF THE 0.5 MG/ML POTENCY OR 1 ML OF THE 1 MG/ML POTENCY. USE IN THE LUMBAR AREA ONLY IS RECOMMENDED. Repeated intrathecal injections of ASTRAMORPH/PF are not recommended. A constant intravenous infusion of naloxone hydrochloride, 0.6 mg/hr, for 24 hours after intrathecal injection may be used to reduce the incidence of potential side effects.

Aged or debilitated patients-Administer with extreme caution (**see Precautions section**). A lower dosage is usually satisfactory.

Repeat Dosage
If pain recurs, alternative routes of administraion should be considered, since experience with repeated doses of morphine by the intrathecal route is limited.

Intrathecal Pediatric Use
No information on use in pediatric patients is available. Parenteral drug products should be inspected for particulate matter and discoloration prior to administration, whenever solution and container permit.

HOW SUPPLIED

The following strengths and container types of ASTRAMORPH/PF are available:

(0.5 mg/mL)
NDC 0186-1159-03	2 mL (1 mg) Ampule, Boxes of 10
NDC 0186-1150-02	10 mL (5 mg) Ampule, Boxes of 5
NDC 0186-1152-12	10 mL (5 mg) Single Dose Vial, Astra E-Z OFF™ vial closure Boxes of 5

(1 mg/mL)
NDC 0186-1160-03	2 mL (2 mg) Ampule, Boxes of 10
NDC 0186-1151-02	10 mL (10 mg) Ampule, Boxes of 5
NDC 0186-1153-12	10 mL (10 mg) Single Dose Vial, Astra E-Z OFF™ vial closure Boxes of 5

Storage
Protect from light. Store in carton at controlled room temperature, 15° to 30° C (59°F to 86°F) until ready to use. ASTRAMORPH/PF contains no preservative. **DISCARD ANY UNUSED PORTION. DO NOT AUTOCLAVE.** Do not use the Injection if darker than pale yellow or if discolored in any other way, or if it contains a precipitate.
Caution: Federal law prohibits dispensing without prescription.
021865R03   10/89 (3)

ATROPINE SULFATE   ℞
[*ā'trow-peen*]
Injection, USP
0.1 mg/mL
Adult Strength

(For details of indications, dosage and administration, precautions, and adverse reactions, see circular in package.)

HOW SUPPLIED
Prefilled syringes equipped with 21 g ¹⁵⁄₁₆″ needle:
5 mL (0.5 mg) NDC 0186-0648-01
10 mL (1 mg) NDC 0186-0649-01
Solution should be stored at controlled room temperature 15°–30°C (59°–86°F)
021880R02   9/91 (2)

BRETYLIUM TOSYLATE INJECTION   ℞
For Intramuscular or Intravenous Use

For details of indications, dosage and administration, precautions, and adverse reactions, see circular in package.

HOW SUPPLIED
NDC 0186-1131-04 10 mL single dose vials, box of 1
NDC 0186-0663-01 10 mL syringes, 21 g ¹⁵⁄₁₆″ needle, box of 1
Each unit contains 500 mg bretylium tosylate in Water for Injection, USP. The pH is adjusted, when necessary with hydrochloric acid and/or sodium hydroxide. Sterile, non-pyrogenic.
021810R01   4/90 (1)

10% CALCIUM CHLORIDE   ℞
[*cal'cium chlor'ide*]
Injection, USP
1 gram (100 mg/mL)
27.3 mg (1.4 mEq) Ca++/mL
2.04 mOsm/mL (calc.)
A Hypertonic Solution for Intravenous Injection

Caution: This solution must not be injected intramuscularly or subcutaneously.

(For details of indications, dosage and administration, precautions, and adverse reactions, see circular in package.)

HOW SUPPLIED
10% Calcium Chloride Injection, USP is supplied as follows:
NDC 0186-1166-04 10 mL single dose vials in packages of 25.
NDC 0186-0651-01 10 mL prefilled syringes with 21 g ¹⁵⁄₁₆″ needle.
The solution should be stored at controlled room temperature 15°–30°C (59°–86°F).
021710R00   7/88

CLINDAMYCIN PHOSPHATE INJECTION, USP   ℞
[*klin"dah-mī'sin*]
Sterile Solution
For Intramuscular and Intravenous Use

> **WARNING**
> Clindamycin therapy has been associated with severe colitis which may end fatally. Therefore, it should be reserved for serious infections where less toxic antimicrobial agents are inappropriate, as described in the INDICATIONS and USAGE Section. It should not be used in patients with nonbacterial infections, such as most upper respiratory tract infections. Studies indicate a toxin(s) produced by *Clostridia* is one primary cause of antibiotic-associated colitis. Cholestyramine and colestipol resins have been shown to bind the toxin *in vitro.* See WARNINGS section. The colitis is usually characterized by severe, persistent diarrhea and severe abdominal cramps and may be associated with the passage of blood and mucus. Endoscopic examination may reveal pseudomembranous colitis. Stool culture for *Clostridium difficile* and stool assay for *C. difficile* toxin may be helpful diagnostically.
> When significant diarrhea occurs, the drug should be discontinued or, if necessary, continued only with close observation of the patient. Large bowel endoscopy has been recommended.
> Antiperistaltic agents such as opiates and diphenoxylate with atropine may prolong and/or worsen the condition. Vancomycin has been found to be effective in the treatment of antibiotic associated pseudomembranous colitis produced by *Clostridium difficile.* The usual adult dose is 500 milligrams to 2 grams of vancomycin orally per day in three to four divided doses administered for 7 to 10 days. Cholestyramine or colestipol resins bind vancomycin *in vitro.* If both a resin and vancomycin are to be administered concurrently, it may be advisable to separate the time of administration of each drug.

Continued on next page

Astra—Cont.

Diarrhea, colitis, and pseudomembranous colitis have been observed to begin up to several weeks following cessation of therapy with clindamycin.

(For details of indications, dosage and administration, precautions, and adverse reactions, see circular in package.)

HOW SUPPLIED
Each mL of Clindamycin Phosphate Injection, USP contains clindamycin phosphate equivalent to 150 mg clindamycin; 0.5 mg disodium edetate; 9.45 mg benzyl alcohol added as preservative. When necessary, pH is adjusted with sodium hydroxide and/or hydrochloric acid. Clindamycin Phosphate Injection, USP is available in the following packages:

2 mL vials	NDC 0186-1450-04 Boxes of 25
4 mL vials	NDC 0186-1451-04 Boxes of 25
6 mL vials	NDC 0186-1452-04 Boxes of 25
Also available in:	
60 mL Pharmacy Bulk Package	NDC 0186-1453-01 Box of 1

Store at controlled room temperature 15°–30°C (59°–86°F).
Caution: Federal law prohibits dispensing without prescription.
021666R01　　　　　　　　　　　　　　　　7/90 (1)

COCAINE HYDROCHLORIDE　　　Ⓒ
Topical Solution

DESCRIPTION
Each mL contains
Cocaine Hydrochloride .... 40 mg or 100 mg
(**Warning:**　May be habit forming.) An aqueous solution.

NOT FOR INJECTION OR OPHTHALMIC USE

NOTE (for Glass Bottle): Do not steam autoclave.
Cocaine Hydrochloride USP is a crystalline, granular, or powder substance having a saline, slightly bitter taste that numbs tongue and lips. Cocaine Hydrochloride is a local anesthetic.

CLINICAL PHARMACOLOGY
Cocaine blocks the initiation or conduction of the nerve impulse following local application, thereby effecting local anesthetic action.
Cocaine is absorbed from all sites of application, including mucous membranes and the gastrointestinal mucosa. Cocaine is degraded by plasma esterases, with the half-life in the plasma being approximately one hour.

INDICATIONS AND USAGE
Cocaine Hydrochloride Topical Solution is indicated for the introduction of local (topical) anesthesia of accessible mucous membranes of the oral, laryngeal and nasal cavities.

CONTRAINDICATIONS
Cocaine Hydrochloride is contraindicated in patients with a known history of hypersensitivity to the drug or to the components of the topical solution.

WARNINGS
RESUSCITATIVE EQUIPMENT AND DRUGS SHOULD BE IMMEDIATELY AVAILABLE WHEN ANY LOCAL ANESTHETIC IS USED.
Carcinogenesis, Mutagenesis
Long-term studies to determine the carcinogenic and mutagenic potential of cocaine are not available.
Pregnancy: Teratogenic Effects —Pregnancy Category C
Animal reproduction studies have not been conducted with cocaine. It is also not known whether cocaine can cause fetal harm when administered to a pregnant woman or can affect reproduction capacity. Cocaine should be given to a pregnant woman only if needed.

PRECAUTIONS
General
The safety and effectiveness of Cocaine Hydrochloride Topical Solution depends on proper dosage, correct technique, adequate precautions, and readiness for emergencies. Standard textbooks should be consulted for specific techniques and precautions for various anesthetic procedures.
The lowest dosage that results in effective anesthesia should be used to avoid high plasma levels and serious adverse effects. Debilitated, elderly patients, acutely ill patients, and children should be given reduced doses commensurate with their age and physical status.
Cocaine Hydrochloride Topical Solution should be used with caution in patients with severely traumatized mucosa and sepsis in the region of the proposed application. Use with caution in persons with known drug sensitivities.

ADVERSE REACTIONS
Adverse reactions may be due to high plasma levels as a result of excessive and rapid absorption of the drug. Reactions are systemic in nature and involve the central nervous system and/or the cardiovascular system. A small number of reactions may result from hypersensitivity, idiosyncrasy or diminished tolerance on the part of the patient.
CNS reactions are excitatory and/or depressant and may be characterized by nervousness, restlessness, and excitement. Tremors and eventually clonictonic convulsions may result. Emesis may occur. Central stimulation is followed by depression, with death resulting from respiratory failure.
Small doses of cocaine slow the heart rate, but after moderate doses, the rate is increased due to central sympathetic stimulation.
Cocaine is pyrogenic, augmenting heat production in stimulating muscular activity and causing vasoconstriction which decreases heat loss. Cocaine is known to interfere with the uptake of norepinephrine by adrenergic nerve terminals, producing sensitization to catecholamines, causing vasoconstriction and mydriasis.
Cocaine causes sloughing of the corneal epithelium, causing clouding, pitting, and occasionally ulceration of the cornea. The drug is not meant for ophthalmic use.

OVERDOSAGE
The fatal dose of cocaine has been approximated at 1.2 g, although severe toxic effects have been reported from doses as low as 20 mg.
Symptoms
The symptoms of cocaine poisoning are referable to the CNS, namely the patient becomes excited, restless, garrulous, anxious, and confused. Enhanced reflexes, headache, rapid pulse, irregular respiration, chills, rise in body temperature, mydriasis, exothalmos, nausea, vomiting and abdominal pain are noticed. In severe overdoses, delirium. Cheyne-Stoke respiration, convulsions, unconsciousness, and death from respiratory arrest result. Acute poisoning by cocaine is rapid in developing.
Treatment
The specific treatment of acute cocaine poisoning is the intravenous administration of a short-acting barbiturate or diazepam. Artificial respiration may be necessary. It is important to limit absorption of the drug. If entrance of the drug into circulation can be checked, and respiratory exchange maintained, the prognosis is favorable since cocaine is eliminated fairly rapidly.

DOSAGE AND ADMINISTRATION
The dosage varies and depends upon the area to be anesthetized, vascularity of the tissues, individual tolerance, and the technique of anesthesia. The lowest dosage needed to provide effective anesthesia should be administered. Dosages should be reduced for children and for elderly and debilitated patients. Cocaine Hydrochloride Topical Solution can be administered by means of cotton applicators or packs, instilled into a cavity, or as a spray.

HOW SUPPLIED
4% Cocaine Hydrochloride Topical Solution

NDC 0186-1790-78	4 mL Unit Dose Bottle Box of 1
NDC 0186-1791-13	10 mL Multiple Dose Bottle Box of 1

10% Cocaine Hydrochloride Topical Solution

NDC 0186-1792-78	4 mL Unit Dose Bottle Box of 1
NDC 0186-1793-13	10 mL Multiple Dose Bottle Box of 1

Store at controlled room temperature: 15°–30°C (59°–86°F)
Caution: Federal law prohibits dispensing without prescription.
021661R01　　　　　　　　　　　　　　　　4/90

DALGAN®　　　　　　　　　　　　　　　　℞
(dezocine)
Injection

DESCRIPTION
Dalgan (dezocine) is a synthetic opioid agonist-antagonist parenteral analgesic of the amino-tetralin series. The chemical name is (-)-[5R-(5α,11α,13S*)]-13-amino-　5,6,7, 8,9,10,11,12-octahydro-5-methyl-5,11　-methanobenzocyclodecen-3-ol. The structural formula is:

The molecular weight of the base is 245.4, and the molecular formula is $C_{16}H_{23}NO$. The n-octanol: water partition coefficient of dezocine is 1.7.
Dalgan is available in three concentrations: 5, 10, and 15 mg of dezocine per mL for intravenous or intramuscular administration. Each mL of the 5 mg strength contains 0.15 mg sodium metabisulfite and 7.236 mg lactic acid. Each mL of the 10 mg strength contains 0.15 mg sodium metabisulfite and 9.406 mg lactic acid. Each mL of the 15 mg strength contains 0.075 mg sodium metabisulfite and 11.578 mg lactic acid. Each mL of all three strengths contains 0.3 mL propylene glycol as a preservative and Water for Injection. The pH of Dalgan solutions is adjusted to 4.0 with sodium hydroxide.

CLINICAL PHARMACOLOGY
PHARMACODYNAMICS
Dalgan (dezocine) is a strong opioid analgesic. Its analgesic potency, onset, and duration of action in the relief of postoperative pain are comparable to morphine. Pain relief in patients with postoperative pain is clinically evident when steady-state serum levels exceed 5 to 9 ng/mL. The side effects listed under **Adverse Reactions** were observed in patients whose average peak levels were less than 45 ng/mL. Peak analgesic effect lags peak serum levels by 20 to 60 minutes.
Table of Estimated Pharmacodynamic Parameters
Following Intramuscular Doses of Dalgan

C(50)est1	5 to 9 ng/mL
C(toxic)est2	45 ng/mL

1. Estimated concentration required to obtain 50% decreases in pain intensity scores in post-operative pain.
2. Estimated concentration above which side effects may be more frequent.

PHARMACOKINETICS　　(see Table [below] and Graph [next page.])
Dalgan (dezocine) is completely and rapidly absorbed following intramuscular injection in normal volunteers with an average peak serum concentration of 19 ng/mL (range 10 to 38 ng/mL) occurring between 10 and 90 minutes after a 10 mg intramuscular injection. Following a 10 mg intravenous infusion over 5 minutes, the average terminal half-life of dezocine is 2.4 hr (range 1.2 to 7.4 hr). The average volume of distribution (Vss) is 10.1 L/kg (range 4.7 to 20.1 L/kg), and the average total body clearance is 3.3 L/hr/kg (range 1.7 to 7.2 L/hr/kg). There is evidence of nonlinear (dose-dependent) pharmacokinetics at doses above 10 mg: in a study where 5, 10, and 20 mg intravenous doses of dezocine were given (N = 12), dose-proportional serum levels were observed after 5 and 10 mg injections, but the area under the serum concentration-time curve for the 20 mg dose was about 25% greater, and the total body clearance was about 20% lower, when compared to the 5 and 10 mg doses. The pharmacokinetics of dezocine following chronic administration (steady-state pharmacokinetics) have not been experimentally determined, but predicted serum levels for 5 and 15 mg intramuscular doses given every 4 hr are presented in the graph.
Approximately two-thirds of a Dalgan dose is recovered in the urine with about 1% being excreted as unchanged dezocine and the remainder as the glucuronide conjugate. Protein binding of dezocine has not been studied.

Mean (range) Pharmacokinetic Parameters of Dezocine In Normal Volunteers

	Dose		
	5 mg (N=12)	10 mg (N=36)	20 mg (N=12)
IV			
Clearance (L/hr/kg)	3.52 (2.1–6.2)	3.33 (1.7–7.2)	2.76 (1.7–4.1)
Vss (L/kg)	10.7 (6.4–15.5)	10.1 (4.7–20.1)	8.8 (5.8–13.5)
t1/2 (hr)	1.7 (0.6–4.4)	2.4 (1.2–7.4)	2.4 (1.4–5.2)
IM		(N = 24)	
Bioavailability		100%	
Cmax1 (ng/mL)		10–38	
tmax2 (min)		10–90	

1. Peak plasma concentration.
2. Time-to-peak plasma concentration.

Hepatic insufficiency did not alter total body clearance in one study of 7 patients with cirrhosis. The volume of distribution and consequently the half-life, however, were increased by 30–50% relative to normal volunteers following a 10 mg intravenous dose. It is not known whether the free concentration of dezocine is altered in cirrhotic patients.
The effect of renal insufficiency on dezocine kinetics (urinary elimination) has not been studied. Because the primary elimination of dezocine is through the urine as a glucuronide, however, use in patients with renal dysfunction should be done cautiously with reduced doses.

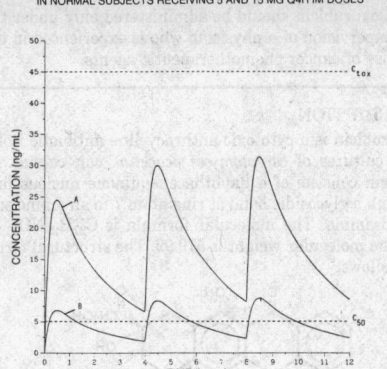

SIMULATED MEAN SERUM CONCENTRATIONS OF DEZOCINE IN NORMAL SUBJECTS RECEIVING 5 AND 15 MG Q4H IM DOSES

A = Dalgan 15 mg q4h
B = Dalgan 5 mg q4h
C_{tox} = Estimated concentration above which side effects may be more frequent
C_{50} = Estimated concentration required to obtain 50% decreases in pain intensity scores in postoperative pain

NARCOTIC ANTAGONIST ACTIVITY
Dalgan is a mixed opioid agonist-antagonist analgesic. Its opioid antagonist activity is less than that of nalorphine but greater than that of pentazocine when measured by antagonism of morphine-induced narcosis in rats.

EFFECT ON RESPIRATION
Dalgan and morphine produce a similar degree of respiratory depression when given in the usual analgesic doses. The effect is dose dependent and may be reversed by naloxone. As the dose of Dalgan is increased, there appears to be an upper limit to the magnitude of the respiratory depression produced by the drug in both animals and healthy human volunteers. Dalgan, like other mixed agonist-antagonist analgesics, may offer increased safety over pure agonist drugs such as morphine.

CARDIOVASCULAR EFFECTS
Dalgan has not been found to be associated with clinically important adverse effects on cardiac performance. Dalgan has been administered to patients as a 4-minute intravenous infusion at approximately 10 times the usual recommended intravenous dose without causing significant changes in mean systemic artery pressure, mean pulmonary artery pressure, pulmonary capillary wedge pressure, cardiac output, stroke index, and left ventricular stroke work index.

CLINICAL TRIALS
Postoperative Analgesia
The analgesic efficacy of Dalgan was investigated in randomized controlled clinical trials in postoperative general surgical pain (orthopedic, gynecologic, and abdominal). The studies were primarily double-blind, single-dose, parallel trials in which Dalgan in intravenous (IV) doses of 2.5 to 10 mg (85 to 160 patients per treatment group) or intramuscular (IM) doses of 5 to 20 mg (39 to 221 patients per treatment group) was compared to 5 to 10 mg of morphine or 1 mg of IV butorphanol in patients with moderate-to-severe pain at baseline. The onset of analgesic action was similar to Dalgan, morphine, and butorphanol, occurring within 15 minutes of IV and 30 minutes of IM administration of the drug. Dalgan in 10 mg IM doses produced analgesia similar to that produced by 10 mg of IM morphine, while 5 mg of Dalgan IV was equivalent to 1 mg of IV butorphanol.
The peak analgesic effect and duration of analgesia were comparable for both routes of administration. The time by which approximately half of the patients remedicated was dose related and independent of the route of administration. Half of the patients remedicated within 2 hours after 5 mg of Dalgan or 1 mg of butorphanol IV, 3 hours after 10 mg of Dalgan or morphine IM, and 4 hours after 15 mg of Dalgan IM.
Another measure of the effect of Dalgan was the number of patients who did not require remedication during the six hours of the trial. The percentage of patients who did not request additional medication during the trial was 21% after a single dose of 15 mg of Dalgan, 15% after 10 mg of Dalgan or morphine, and 4% after placebo.
Pain relief was proportional to the dose of Dalgan for single doses less than 20 mg. In one study with 39 to 42 patients per treatment group, comparing single doses of 20 or 10 mg of IM Dalgan with 10 mg of IM morphine, the patients receiving 20 mg of Dalgan did not obtain as much pain relief as that provided by 15 mg of the drug in other studies (the patients who received 10 mg of Dalgan or morphine in this study did obtain analgesia comparable to that seen in other trials). These results suggest that the maximally effective dose of Dalgan

in postoperative pain may be 15 mg due to Dalgan's mixed agonist-antagonist pharmacology.
Use In Chronic Pain States
Data on the use of Dalgan in chronic pain has been gathered in trials of burn patients (n = 16) and cancer pain (n = 88). The daily dose of Dalgan for most patients with chronic pain has ranged between 20 and 60 mg per day, although doses as large as 90 to 140 mg per day have been used in 15 patients. Dalgan has not been adequately studied in the management of chronic pain. It is not recommended for use in patients who may have developed significant tolerance to opioid drugs from long-term use because of the risk of precipitating acute withdrawal symptoms.

INDICATIONS
Dalgan is indicated for the management of pain when the use of an opioid analgesic is appropriate (see "Clinical Trials").

CONTRAINDICATIONS
Dalgan should not be administered to patients who have been shown to be hypersensitive to it.

WARNINGS
Contains sodium metabisulfite, a sulfite that may cause allergic-type reactions including anaphylactic symptoms and life-threatening or less severe asthmatic episodes in certain susceptible people. The overall prevalence of sulfite sensitivity in the general population is unknown and probably low. Sulfite sensitivity is seen more frequently in asthmatic than in nonasthmatic people.
PATIENTS PHYSICALLY DEPENDENT ON NARCOTICS
Because of its opioid antagonist properties, Dalgan is not recommended for patients who are physically dependent on narcotics. Patients who have recently taken substantial amounts of narcotics may experience withdrawal symptoms. Because of the difficulty in assessing dependence in patients who have previously received substantial amounts of narcotic medication, caution should be used in the administration of Dalgan to such patients. To avoid precipitating an acute narcotic abstinence reaction, a sufficient period of withdrawal from opioids should be allowed before Dalgan is administered.

PRECAUTIONS
DALGAN IS A STRONG OPIOID ANALGESIC AND, LIKE ALL SUCH DRUGS, IT SHOULD BE ADMINISTERED IN CLINICAL SETTINGS WHERE RESPIRATORY DEPRESSION WILL BE PROMPTLY RECOGNIZED AND APPROPRIATELY MANAGED.
RESPIRATORY DEPRESSION INDUCED BY DALGAN CAN BE REVERSED WITH NALOXONE.
HEAD INJURY AND INCREASED INTRACRANIAL PRESSURE
Although there is no clinical experience in patients with head injury, the possible respiratory-depressant effect and the potential of strong analgesics to elevate cerebrospinal-fluid pressure (resulting from vasodilatation following CO_2 retention) may be markedly exaggerated in the presence of head injury, intracranial lesions, or a preexisting increase in intracranial pressure. Furthermore, strong analgesics can produce effects that may obscure the clinical course of patients with head injuries. In such patients, Dalgan should be used only when essential and with extreme caution.
USE IN CHRONIC OBSTRUCTIVE PULMONARY DISEASE
Because strong opioids cause some respiratory depression, they should be administered only with caution and in low doses to patients with preexisting respiratory depression (e.g., from other medication, uremia, or severe infection), severely limited respiratory reserve, bronchial asthma, obstructive respiratory conditions, or cyanosis. Respiratory depression induced by Dalgan can be reversed by naloxone.
USE IN HEPATIC OR RENAL DISEASE
Dezocine undergoes extensive hepatic metabolism and renal excretion of the glucuronide metabolite (see "Clinical Pharmacology"). Administration to patients with hepatic or renal dysfunction should be cautious using reduced doses.
USE IN BILIARY SURGERY
Although there is no evidence that Dalgan alters the tonic pressure within the common bile duct, therapeutic doses of other opioid analgesics can significantly increase pressure within the common bile duct. Therefore, Dalgan should be used with caution in such settings.
USE WITH OTHER CENTRAL NERVOUS SYSTEM DEPRESSANTS
Opioid analgesics, general anesthetics, sedatives, tranquilizers, hypnotics, or other CNS depressants (including alcohol) administered concomitantly with Dalgan may have an additive effect. When such combined therapy is contemplated, the dose of one or both agents should be reduced.
USE IN DRUG OR ALCOHOL DEPENDENCE
Use of Dalgan in combination with alcohol and/or other CNS depressant drugs will result in increased risk to the patient. Dalgan should be used with caution in individuals with active drug or alcohol addiction who are not in a medically controlled environment. Self-administration of any strong

opioid may increase the relapse rate in populations recovering from addiction in abstinence-based recovery programs.
USE IN AMBULATORY PATIENTS
Strong opioid analgesics impair the mental or physical abilities required for the performance of potentially dangerous tasks such as driving a car or operating machinery. Patients who have been given Dalgan should not drive or operate dangerous machinery until the effects of the drug are no longer present.
PREGNANCY CATEGORY C
In reproductive studies, dezocine was shown to cause a dose-related suppression of body weight and food consumption of the parenteral generation in rats receiving either intravenous or intramuscular doses. Pup body weight was suppressed in a dose-related fashion. Teratology studies conducted in mice, rats, and rabbits revealed no evidence of teratogenic effects. There are no adequate and well-controlled studies in pregnant women. Dalgan should be used during pregnancy only if the potential benefit justifies the potential risk to the fetus.
LABOR AND DELIVERY
Safety to the mother and fetus after Dalgan administration during labor is unknown. The drug should be used in labor and delivery only when the physician deems its use essential to the welfare of the mother and infant.
NURSING MOTHERS
The use of Dalgan in mothers nursing infants is not recommended, since it is not known whether this drug is excreted in breast milk.
PEDIATRIC USE
Safety and efficacy in patients under the age of 18 years have not been established.
USE IN THE AGED
Like all strong, mixed opioid agonist-antagonist analgesics, Dalgan has the ability to depress respiration and reduce ventilatory drive to a clinically significant extent. It also has the potential to alter mental status or induce delirium in elderly patients. Dalgan has not undergone sufficient clinical testing in the geriatric population to assess its relative risk compared to other opioid analgesics, but the initial dose of all drugs of this class should be reduced in the geriatric patient and subsequent doses individualized.

ADVERSE REACTIONS
A total of 2192 patients have received Dalgan on an acute or chronic basis in the initial clinical trials of the drug. In nearly all cases, the type of incidence of side effects were those expected of a strong analgesic, and no unforeseen or unusual toxicity was reported. There is, as yet, limited information on the use of Dalgan for periods longer than 48 to 72 hours, but there was no evidence of hepatic, hematologic, or renal toxicity in 73 patients who received the drug for periods of time longer than 7 days.
The occurrence of adverse effects with Dalgan is based on data obtained from patients treated in both controlled and uncontrolled clinical trials. The adverse effects are listed below by frequency of occurrence within the body system affected.
The frequencies shown reflect the actual frequency of each adverse effect in patients who received Dalgan. There has been no attempt to correct for a placebo effect or to subtract the frequencies reported by placebo-treated patients in controlled trials.
The following adverse reactions were reported at a frequency of 1% or greater:
REACTIONS
Gastrointestinal System: Nausea*, vomiting*.
Nervous System: Sedation*, dizziness/vertigo.
Skin: Injection-site reactions*.
(Reactions occurring with a frequency of 1 to <3% are unmarked, while reactions occurring with a frequency of 3 to 9% are marked with an asterisk.*)
The following adverse reactions were reported with a frequency of less than 1% and are probably causally related to the administration of Dalgan:
Body as a whole: Sweating, chills, flushing, low hemoglobin, edema.
Cardiovascular system: Hypotension, heart or pulse irregularity, hypertension, chest pain, pallor, thrombophlebitis.
Gastrointestinal system: Dry mouth, constipation, diarrhea, abdominal pain/distress/disorder.
Musculoskeletal system: Cramps/aching/pain.
Nervous system: Anxiety, confusion, crying, delusions, sleep disturbance, headache, delirium, depression.
Respiratory system: Respiratory depression, respiratory symptoms, atelectasis.
Skin: Pruritus, rash, erythema.
Special senses: Diplopia, slurred speech, blurred vision.
Urogenital system: Urinary frequency, hesitancy, and retention.
The following adverse effects have been reported in less than 1% of the 2192 patients studied, and the association between these events and Dalgan administration is unknown. They

Continued on next page

Astra—Cont.

are being listed to serve as alerting information for the physician.

Gastrointestinal: Increased alkaline phosphatase and SGOT.

Respiratory system: Hiccups.

Special senses: Congestion in ears, tinnitus.

There is no information available from postmarketing experience with the drug.

DRUG ABUSE AND DEPENDENCE

Dezocine has substituted for morphine in abuse-liability testing in animals. It has been identified as a narcotic in abuse-liability testing in experienced drug abusers, but has shown no evidence of abuse in clinical use during drug development. Mixed opioid agonist-antagonists of this type are generally recognized as having less potential for abuse than pure agonists such as morphine or meperidine, but all such drugs have abuse potential in certain individuals, especially those individuals with a prior history of opioid drug abuse or dependence.

Dezocine has a limited capacity to induce physical dependence in animal testing. Increasing tolerance to Dalgan or physical dependence on the drug were not seen in clinical trials.

OVERDOSAGE

CLINICAL PRESENTATION

Although there have been no incidents of overdosage with Dalgan during clinical trials, and thus no human experience with the drug, overdosage with Dalgan is possible. Based on the preclinical pharmacology of dezocine, overdosage will produce acute respiratory depression, cardiovascular compromise, and delirium. The largest dose of Dalgan which has been given to nontolerant healthy volunteers without toxicity has been 30 mg/70 kg.

TREATMENT

The pharmacologic treatment of suspected Dalgan overdosage is intravenously administered naloxone. The respiratory and cardiac status of the patient should be evaluated constantly and appropriate supportive measures instituted, such as oxygen, intravenous fluids, vasopressors, and assisted or controlled respiration.

DOSAGE AND ADMINISTRATION

INTRAMUSCULAR

Although the recommended single dose for an adult is 5 to 20 mg, the majority of patients in clinical trials received an initial dose of 10 mg. Dosage should be adjusted according to the patient's weight, age, severity of pain, physical status, and other medications that the patient may be receiving. Dalgan may be repeated every 3 to 6 hours as necessary. The recommended maximum single dose is 20 mg, with a probable upper limit of 120 mg a day based on preclinical pharmacology of the drug. There is insufficient information regarding the risk of chronic use of Dalgan to establish limits for the maximum recommended duration of treatment with the drug.

INTRAVENOUS

The recommended range for intravenous administration of Dalgan is 2.5 to 10 mg repeated every 2 to 4 hours, with most patients in clinical trials receiving an initial intravenous dose of 5 mg.

SUBCUTANEOUS

Dalgan is not recommended for subcutaneous administration. Repeated injection of Dalgan at a single site has been associated with subcutaneous inflammation, vascular irritation, and venous thrombosis in animals. The significance of this finding for patients is unknown, although injection-site reactions occurred in 4% of patients treated with Dalgan in clinical trials.

CHILDREN AND ADOLESCENTS

Dalgan is not recommended for patients under 18 years of age.

HOW SUPPLIED

Dalgan® (dezocine) Injection (a clear, colorless to slightly yellow solution) is available in the following dosage strengths:

Single-Dose Vials

2 mL (1 mL Fill), 5 mg/mL,   Box of 1, NDC 0186-1520-13
2 mL (1 mL Fill), 10 mg/ml,   Box of 1, NDC 0186-1521-13
2 mL (1 mL Fill), 15 mg/mL,   Box of 1, NDC 0186-1523-13

Multiple-Dose Vials

10 mL, 10 mg/mL,   Box of 1, NDC 0186-1522-12
2 mL (1 mL Fill), 5 mg/mL,   Box of 10, NDC 0186-1529-23
2 mL (1 mL Fill), 10 mg/mL,   Box of 10, NDC 0186-1524-23
2 mL (1 mL Fill), 15 mg/mL,   Box of 10, NDC 0186-1525-23

For intramuscular or intravenous injection.

SAFETY AND HANDLING INSTRUCTIONS

Dalgan is supplied in sealed dosage forms and at low concentrations which pose no known risk to health-care workers. Accidental dermal exposure to Dalgan should be treated by rinsing the affected area with fresh water.

Dalgan should be stored at room temperature and protected from light. As with all parenteral products, Dalgan should be inspected visually for particulate matter and discoloration prior to administration, whenever solution and container permit. Do not use if the solution contains a precipitate. Dalgan, like other mixed agonist-antagonist opioid analgesics, has low abuse potential in patient populations. However, strong mixed agonist-antagonist drugs have reportedly been associated with abuse and dependence in health-care providers and others with ready access to such drugs. Dalgan should be handled accordingly.

Manufactured by:
Wyeth Laboratories Inc.
Philadelphia, PA 19101
Manufactured for:
Astra Pharmaceutical Products, Inc.
Westboro, MA 01581
021665R02   7/90 (2)

50% DEXTROSE   ℞

[dex'trose]
Injection, USP
Concentrated Dextrose
For Intravenous
Administration

NOTE: This solution is hypertonic—see Warnings and Precautions

(For details of indications, dosage and administration, precautions, and adverse reactions, see circular in package.)

HOW SUPPLIED

Dextrose Injection USP, 50% is supplied as follows:
50 mL Prefilled Syringe with 19 g $^{15}/_{16}''$ needle, NDC 0186-0654-01
The solution should be stored at controlled room temperature 15°–30° (59°–86°F).
021857R03   Rev. 5/88 (3)

DOPAMINE HCl Injection, USP   ℞

[dó-pa-mean]

(For details of indications, dosage and administration, precautions, and adverse reactions, see circular in package.)

HOW SUPPLIED

Dopamine HCl 200 mg is supplied in the following forms:
   Single Dose Vial—5 ml (40 mg/ml) NDC 0186-1010-13
   Additive Syringe—5 ml (40 mg/ml) NDC 0186-0638-01
Dopamine HCl 400 mg is supplied in the following forms:
   Single Dose Vial—5 ml (80 mg/ml) NDC 0186-1012-13
   Additive Syringe —5 ml (80 mg/ml) NDC 0186-0641-01
           —10 ml (40 mg/ml) NDC 0186-0639-01
Dopamine HCl 800 mg is supplied in the following forms:
   Single Dose Vial—5 ml (160 mg/ml) NDC 0186-1014-13
   Additive Syringe—5 ml (160 mg/ml) NDC 0186-0642-01
Packages are color coded according to the total dosage content; 200 mg coded blue/white, 400 mg coded green/white and 800 mg coded yellow/white.
Store at controlled room temperature 15°–30°C (59°–86°F). Protect from light.
Avoid contact with alkalies (including sodium bicarbonate), oxidizing agents, or iron salts.
NOTE: Do not use the Injection if it is darker than slightly yellow or discolored in any way.
021861R05   Rev. 8/89 (5)

DOXORUBICIN HYDROCHLORIDE FOR   ℞
INJECTION, USP

[dox-ō-rūbe'-ih-sin]
FOR INTRAVENOUS USE ONLY

WARNINGS

1. Severe local tissue necrosis will occur if there is extravastion during administration (See DOSAGE AND ADMINISTRATION). Doxorubicin must not be given by the intramuscular or subcutaneous route.
2. Serious irreversible myocardial toxicity with delayed congestive failure often unresponsive to any cardiac supportive therapy may be encountered as total dosage approaches 550 mg/m². This toxicity may occur at lower cumulative doses in patients with prior mediastinal irradiation or on concurrent cyclophosphamide therapy.
3. Dosage should be reduced in patients with impaired hepatic function.

---

4. Severe myelosuppression may occur.
5. Doxorubicin should be administered only under the supervision of a physician who is experienced in the use of cancer chemotherapeutic agents.

DESCRIPTION

Doxorubicin is a cytotoxic anthracycline antibiotic isolated from cultures of *Streptomyces peucetius* var. *caesius.* Doxorubicin consists of a naphthacenequinone nucleus linked through a glycosidic bond at ring atom 7 to an amino sugar, daunosamine. The molecular formula is $C_{27}H_{29}NO_{11} \cdot HCl$ and the molecular weight is 579.99. The structural formula is a follows:

Doxorubicin binds to nucleic acids, presumably by specific intercalation of the planar anthracycline nucleus with the DNA double helix. The anthracycline ring is lipophilic but the saturated end of the ring system contains abundant hydroxyl groups adjacent to the amino sugar, producing a hydrophilic center. The molecule is amphoteric, containing acidic functions in the ring phenolic groups and a basic function in the sugar amino group. It binds to cell membranes as well as plasma proteins. Doxorubicin Hydrochloride for Injection, USP is for intravenous use only. It is available in 10 mg, 20 mg, and 50 mg single dose vials as a lyophilized, sterile powder with added lactose (anhydrous), 50 mg, 100 mg, and 250 mg respectively.

CLINICAL PHARMACOLOGY

Though not completely elucidated, the mechanism of action of doxorubicin is related to its ability to bind to DNA and inhibit nucleic acid synthesis. Cell culture studies have demonstrated rapid cell penetration and perinucleolar chromatin binding, rapid inhibition of mitotic activity and nucleic acid synthesis, mutagenesis and chromosomal aberrations. Animal studies have shown activity in a spectrum of experimental tumors, immunosuppression, carcinogenic properties in rodents, induction of a variety of toxic effects, including delayed and progressive cardiac toxicity, myelosuppression in all species and atrophy to testes in rats and dogs. Pharmacokinetic studies show the intravenous administration of normal or radiolabeled doxorubicin is followed by rapid plasma clearance and significant tissue binding. Urinary excretion, as determined by fluorimetric methods, accounts for approximately 4 to 5% of the administered dose in five days. Biliary excretion, represents the major excretion route, 40 to 50% of the administered dose being recovered in the bile or feces in seven days. Impairment of liver function results in slower excretion and consequently, increased retention and accumulation in plasma and tissues. Doxorubicin does not cross the blood brain barrier.

INDICATIONS AND USAGE

Doxorubicin Hydrochloride for Injection has been used successfully to produce regression in disseminated neoplastic conditions such as acute lymphoblastic leukemia, acute myeloblastic leukemia, Wilms' tumor, neuroblastoma, soft tissue and bone sarcomas, breast carcinoma, ovarian carcinoma, transitional cell bladder carcinoma, thyroid carcinoma, lymphomas of both Hodgkin and non-Hodgkin types, bronchogenic carcinoma in which the small cell histologic type is the most responsive compared to other cell types and gastric carcinoma.

A number of other solid tumors have also shown some responsiveness but in numbers too limited to justify specific recommendation. Studies to date have shown malignant melanoma, kidney carcinoma, large bowel carcinoma, brain tumors and metastases to the central nervous system not to be significantly responsive to doxorubicin therapy.

CONTRAINDICATIONS

Doxorubicin therapy should not be started in patients who have marked myelosuppression induced by previous treatment with other antitumor agents or by radiotherapy. Conclusive data are not available on pre-existing heart disease as a co-factor of increased risk of doxorubicin-induced cardiac toxicity. Preliminary data suggest that in such cases cardiac toxicity may occur at doses lower than the recommended cumulative limit. It is therefore not recommended to start doxorubicin in such cases. Doxorubicin treatment is contraindicated in patients who received previous treatment with complete cumulative doses of doxorubicin and/or daunorubicin.

WARNINGS

Special attention must be given to the cardiac toxicity exhibited by doxorubicin. Although uncommon, acute left ventricular failure has occurred, particularly in patients who have received total dosage of the drug exceeding the currently recommended limit of 550 mg/m^2. The limit appears to be lower (400 mg/m^2) in patients who received radiotherapy to the mediastinal area or concomitant therapy with other potentially cardiotoxic agents such as cyclophosphamide. The total dose of doxorubicin administered to the individual patient should also take into account previous or concomitant therapy with related compounds such as daunorubicin. Congestive heart failure and/or cardiomyopathy may be encountered several weeks after discontinuation of doxorubicin therapy.

Cardiac failure is often not favorably affected by presently known medical or physical therapy for cardiac support. Early clinical diagnosis of drug-induced heart failure appears to be essential for successful treatment with digitalis, diuretics, low salt diet and bed rest. Severe cardiac toxicity may occur precipitously without antecedent EKG changes. A baseline EKG and EKGs performed prior to each dose or course after 300 mg/m^2 cumulative dose has been given is suggested. Transient EKG changes consisting of T-wave flattening, S-T depression and arrhythmias lasting for up to two weeks after a dose or course of doxorubicin are presently not considered indications for suspension of doxorubicin therapy. Doxorubicin cardiomyopathy has been reported to be associated with a persistent reduction in the voltage of the QRS wave, a prolongation of the systolic time interval and a reduction of the ejection fraction as determined by echocardiography or radionuclide angiography. None of these tests have yet been confirmed to consistently identify those individual patients that are approaching their maximally tolerated cumulative dose of doxorubicin. If test results indicate change in cardiac function associated with doxorubicin, the benefit of continued therapy must be carefully evaluated against the risk of producing irreversible cardiac damage.

Acute life-threatening arrhythmias have been reported to occur during or within a few hours after doxorubicin hydrochloride administration.

There is a high incidence of bone marrow depression, primarily of leukocytes, requiring careful hematologic monitoring. With the recommended dosage schedule. leukopenia is usually transient, reaching its nadir at 10 to 14 days after treatment with recovery usually occurring by the 21st day. White blood cell counts as low as 1000/mm^3 are to be expected during treatment with appropriate doses of doxorubicin. Red blood cell and platelet levels should also be monitored since they may also be depressed. Hematologic toxicity may require dose reduction or suspension or delay of doxorubicin therapy. Persistent severe myelosuppression may result in superinfection or hemorrhage.

Doxorubicin may potentiate the toxicity of other anticancer therapies. Exacerbation of cyclophosphamide induced hemorrhagic cystitis and enhancement of the hepatotoxicity of 6-mercaptopurine have been reported. Radiation-induced toxicity to the myocardium, mucosae, skin and liver have been reported to be increased by the administration of doxorubicin.

Toxicity to recommended doses of doxorubicin hydrochloride is enhanced by hepatic impairment, therefore, prior to the individual dosing, evaluation of hepatic function is recommended using conventional clinical laboratory tests, such as SGOT, SGPT, alkaline phosphatase and bilirubin. (See DOSAGE AND ADMINISTRATION.)

Necrotizing colitis manifested by typhlitis (cecal inflammation), bloody stools and severe and sometimes fatal infections have been associated with a combination of doxorubicin hydrochloride given by IV push daily for 3 days and cytarabine given by continuous infusion daily for 7 or more days.

On intravenous administration of doxorubicin extravasation may occur with or without an accompanying stinging or burning sensation and even if blood returns well on aspiration of the infusion needle (See DOSAGE AND ADMINISTRATION). If any signs or symptoms of extravasation have occurred the injection or infusion should be immediately terminated and restarted in another vein.

Doxorubicin and related compounds have also been shown to have mutagenic and carcinogenic properties when tested in experimental models.

Usage in Pregnancy—Safe use of doxorubicin in pregnancy has not been established. Doxorubicin is embryotoxic and teratogenic in rats and embryotoxic and abortifacient in rabbits. Therefore, the benefits to the pregnant patient should be carefully weighed against the potential toxicity to fetus and embryo. The possible adverse effects on fertility in males and females in humans or experimental animals have not been adequately evaluated.

PRECAUTIONS

Initial treatment with doxorubicin requires close observation of the patient and extensive laboratory monitoring. It is recommended, therefore, that patients be hospitalized at least during the first phase of the treatment.

Like other cytotoxic drugs, doxorubicin may induce hyperuricemia secondary to rapid lysis of neoplastic cells. The clinician should monitor the patient's blood uric acid level and be prepared to use such supportive and pharmacologic measures as might be necessary to control this problem.

Doxorubicin imparts a red coloration to the urine 1 to 2 days after administration and patients should be advised to expect this during active therapy.

Doxorubicin is not an anti-microbial agent.

ADVERSE REACTIONS

Dose limiting toxicities of therapy are myelosuppression and cardiotoxicity (see WARNINGS). Other reactions reported are:

Cutaneous—Reversible complete alopecia occurs in most cases. Hyperpigmentation of nailbeds and dermal creases, primarily in children, and onycholysis have been reported in a few cases. Recall of skin reaction due to prior radiotherapy has occurred with doxorubicin administration.

Gastrointestinal—Acute nausea and vomiting occurs frequently and may be severe. This may be alleviated by antiemetic therapy. Mucositis (stomatitis and esophagitis) may occur 5 to 10 days after administration. The effect may be severe leading to ulceration and represents a site of origin for severe infections. The dosage regimen consisting of administration of doxorubicin on three successive days results in the greater incidence and severity of mucositis. Ulceration and necrosis of the colon, especially the cecum, may occur leading to bleeding or severe infections which can be fatal. This reaction has been reported in patients with acute nonlymphocytic leukemia treated with a 3-day course of doxorubicin combined with cytarabine. Anorexia and diarrhea have been occasionally reported.

Vascular—Phlebosclerosis has been reported especially when small veins are used or a single vein is used for repeated administration. Facial flushing may occur if the injection is given too rapidly.

Local—Severe cellulitis, vesication and tissue necrosis will occur if doxorubicin is extravasated during administration. Erythematous streaking along the vein proximal to the site of the injection has been reported. (See DOSAGE AND ADMINISTRATION.)

Hypersensitivity—Fever, chills and urticaria have been reported occasionally. Anaphylaxis may occur. A case of apparent cross sensitivity to lincomycin has been reported.

Other—Conjunctivitis and lacrimation occur rarely.

OVERDOSAGE

Acute overdosage of doxorubicin enhances the toxic effects of mucositis, leukopenia and thrombopenia. Treatment of acute overdosage consists of treatment of the severely myelosuppressed patient with hospitalization, antibiotics, platelet and granulocyte transfusions and symptomatic treatment of mucositis.

Chronic overdosage with cumulative doses exceeding 550 mg/m^2 increases the risk of cardiomyopathy and resultant congestive heart failure. Treatment consists of vigorous management of congestive heart failure with digitalis preparations and diuretics. The use of peripheral vasodilators has been recommended.

DOSAGE AND ADMINISTRATION

Care in the administration of doxorubicin hydrochloride will reduce the chance of perivenous infiltration. It may also decrease the chance of local reactions such as urticaria and erythematous streaking. On intravenous administration of doxorubicin, extravasation may occur with or without an accompanying stinging or burning sensation and even if blood returns well on aspiration of the infusion needle. If any signs or symptoms of extravasation have occurred, the injection or infusion should be immediately terminated and restarted in another vein. If it is known or suspected that subcutaneous extravasation has occurred, local infiltration with an injectable corticosteroid and flooding the site with normal saline has been reported to lessen the local reaction. Because of the progressive nature of extravasation reactions, the area of injection should be frequently examined and plastic surgery consultation obtained. If ulceration begins, early wide excision of the involved area should be considered[1].

The most commonly used dosage schedule is 60 to 75 mg/m^2 as a single intravenous injection administered at 21 day intervals. The lower dose should be given to patients with inadequate marrow reserves due to old age, or prior therapy, or neoplastic marrow infiltration. An alternative dosage schedule is weekly doses of 20 mg/m^2 which has been reported to produce a lower incidence of congestive heart failure. Thirty (30) mg/m^2 on each of three successive days repeated every four weeks has also been used. Doxorubicin dosage must be reduced if the bilirubin is elevated as follows: Serum Bilirubin 1.2 to 3.0 mg/dl—give ½ normal dose, > 3 mg/dl—give ¼ normal dose.

Preparation of Solution: Doxorubicin Hydrochloride for Injection, USP 10 mg, 20 mg and 50 mg vials should be reconstituted with 5 mL, 10 mL and 25 mL, respectively of Sodium Chloride Injection, USP (0.9%) to give a final concentration of 2 mg/mL of doxorubicin hydrochloride. An appropriate volume of air should be withdrawn from the vial during reconstitution to avoid excessive pressure build-up. Bacteriostatic diluents are not recommended.

After adding the diluent, the vial should be shaken and the contents allowed to dissolve. The reconstituted solution is stable for 24 hours at room temperature and 48 hours under refrigeration, 2°–8°C (36°–46°F). It should be protected from exposure to sunlight. Discard any unused solution.

It is recommended that doxorubicin be slowly administered into the tubing of a freely running intravenous infusion of Sodium Chloride Injection, USP or 5% Dextrose Injection, USP. The tubing should be attached to a Butterfly® needle inserted preferably into a large vein. If possible, avoid veins over joints or in extremities with compromised venous or lymphatic drainage. The rate of administration is dependent on the size of the vein and the dosage. However, the dose should be administered in not less than 3 to 5 minutes. Local erythematous streaking along the vein as well as facial flushing may be indicative of too rapid an administration. A burning or stinging sensation may be indicative of perivenous infiltration and the infusion should be immediately terminated and restarted in another vein. Perivenous infiltration may occur painlessly.

Doxorubicin should not be mixed with heparin or fluorouricil since it has been reported that these drugs are incompatible to the extent that a precipitate may form. Until specific compatibility data are available, it is not recommended that doxorubicin be mixed with other drugs.

Doxorubicin has been used concurrently with other approved chemotherapeutic agents. Evidence is available that in some types of neoplastic disease combination chemotherapy is superior to single agents. The benefits and risks of such therapy continue to be elucidated.

Parenteral drug products should be inspected visually for particulate matter and discoloration prior to administration, whenever solution and container permit.

Handling and Disposal: Skin reactions associated with doxorubicin have been reported. Caution in the handling and preparation of the powder and solution must be exercised and the use of gloves is recommended. If doxorubicin powder or solution contacts the skin or mucosae, immediately wash thoroughly with soap and water.

Procedures for proper handling and disposal of anti-cancer drugs should be considered. Several guidelines on this subject have been published.[2–8] There is no general agreement that all of the procedures recommended in the guidelines are necessary or appropriate.

HOW SUPPLIED

Doxorubicin Hydrochloride for Injection, USP, is available as follows

10 mg	NDC 0186-1530-13 Box of 5 (for USA)
20 mg	NDC 0186-1575-12 Box of 5
50 mg	NDC 0186-1531-01 Box of 1

Store the dry powder at controlled room temperature 15°–30°C (59°–86°F). Protect from exposure to sunlight. Retain in carton until time of use. The reconstituted solution is stable for 24 hours at room temperature and 48 hours under refrigeration 2°–8°C (36°–46°F).

REFERENCES

1. Rudolph R, et al: Skin Ulcers Due to ADRIAMYCIN. *Cancer* 38; 1087–1094, Sept. 1976.
2. Recommendations for the Safe Handling of Parenteral Antineoplastic Drugs. NIH Publication No. 83-2621. For sale by the Superintendent of Documents, U.S. Government Printing Office, Washington, D.C. 20402.
3. AMA Council Report. Guidelines for Handling Parenteral Antineoplastics. *JAMA*. March 15, 1985.
4. National Study Commission on Cytotoxic Exposure—Recommendations for Handling Cytotoxic Agents. Available from Louis P. Jeffrey, Sc.D., chairman, National Study Commission on Cytotoxic Exposure, Massachusetts College of Pharmacy and Allied Health Services, 179 Longwood Avenue, Boston, Massachusetts, 02115.
5. Clinical Oncological Society of Australia: Guidelines and recommendations for Safe Handling of Antineoplastic agents. *Med J Australia* 1:426–428, 1983.
6. Jones RB, et al: Safe Handling of Chemotherapeutic Agents: A Report from the Mount Sinai Medical Center. *CA-A Cancer Journal for Clinicians*. Sept./Oct., 258–263, 1983.
7. American Society of Hospital Pharmacists Technical Assistance Bulletin on Handling Cytotoxic and Hazardous Drugs. *Am J Hosp Pharm*. 47: 1033–1049, 1990.
8. OSHA Work-Practice Guidelines for Personnel Dealing with Cytotoxic (Antineoplastic) Drugs. *Am J Hosp Pharm*. 43: 1193–1204, 1986.

Manufactured by:
BRISTOL-MYERS SQUIBB
Princeton, N.J. 08540
021642R00 ISS. 2/92

Continued on next page

Astra—Cont.

DROPERIDOL INJECTION, USP ℞
FOR INTRAVENOUS OR INTRAMUSCULAR USE ONLY

(For details of indications, dosage and administration, precautions, and adverse reactions, see circular in package.)

HOW SUPPLIED

Droperidol injection is available as:

Ampules, 2.5 mg/mL

2 mL, (5 mg/2 mL),	box of 10	NDC 0186-1220-03
5 mL, (12.5 mg/5 mL),	box of 10	NDC 0186-1221-03
Single Dose Vials, 2.5 mg/mL		
2 mL, (5 mg/2 mL),	box of 10	NDC 0186-1226-13
5 mL, (12.5 mg/5 mL),	box of 10	NDC 0186-1227-13
Multiple Dose Vials, 2.5 mg/mL		
10 mL,	box of 1	NDC 0186-1224-12

PROTECT FROM LIGHT, STORE AT CONTROLLED ROOM TEMPERATURE 15°–30°C (59°–86°F).

021879R02 9/88 (2)

DURANEST® ℞
[dur'a-nest]
(etidocaine hydrochloride)
Injections for infiltration and nerve block

DESCRIPTION

Duranest (etidocaine HCl) Injections are sterile aqueous solutions that contain a local anesthetic agent and are administered parenterally by injection. See INDICATIONS AND USAGE for specific uses. The specific quantitative composition of each available solution is shown in Table 1. Duranest Injections contain etidocaine HCl, which is chemically designated as butanamide, N-(2,6-dimethylphenyl)-2-(ethylpropylamine)-, monohydrochloride and has the following structural formula:

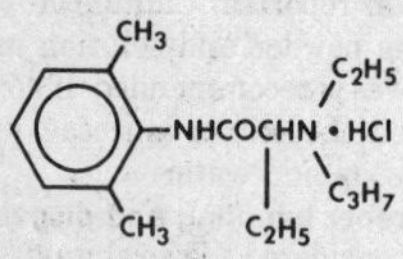

Epinephrine is (-)-3, 4-Dihydroxy-α-[(methylamino) methyl] benzyl alcohol and has the following structural formula:

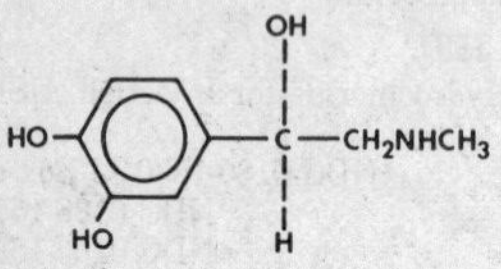

The pKa of etidocaine (7.74) is similar to that of lidocaine (7.86). However, etidocaine possesses a greater degree of lipid solubility and protein binding capacity than does lidocaine. Duranest Injections are sterile and, except for the 1.5% concentration, are available with or without epinephrine 1:200,000. Single dose containers of Duranest Injection without epinephrine may be reautoclaved if necessary.

See Table 1. Composition of available solutions.

CLINICAL PHARMACOLOGY

Mechanism of action: Etidocaine stabilizes the neuronal membrane by inhibiting the ionic fluxes required for the initiation and conduction of impulses, thereby effecting local anesthetic action.

Onset and duration of action: *In vivo* animal studies have shown that etidocaine has a rapid onset (3–5 minutes) and a prolonged duration of action (5–10 hours). Based on comparative clinical studies of lidocaine and etidocaine, the anesthetic properties of etidocaine in man may be characterized as follows: Initial onset of sensory analgesia and motor blockade is rapid (usually 3–5 minutes) and similar to that produced by lidocaine. Duration of sensory analgesia is 1.5 to 2 times longer than that of lidocaine by the peridural route. The difference in analgesic duration between etidocaine and lidocaine may be even greater following peripheral nerve blockade than following central neural block. Duration of analgesia in excess of 9 hours is not infrequent when etidocaine is used for peripheral nerve blocks such as brachial plexus blockade. Etidocaine produces a profound degree of motor blockade and abdominal muscle relaxation when used for peridural analgesia.

Hemodynamics: Excessive blood levels may cause changes in cardiac output, total peripheral resistance and mean arterial pressure. With central neural blockade these changes may be attributable to block of autonomic fibers, a direct depressant effect on the local anesthetic agent on various components of the cardiosvascular system, and/or the beta-adrenergic receptor stimulating action of epinephrine when present. The net effect is normally a modest hypotension when the recommended dosages are not exceeded.

Pharmacokinetics and metabolism: Information derived from diverse formulations, concentrations and usages reveals that etidocaine is completely absorbed following parenteral administration, its rate of absorption depending, for example, upon such factors as the site of administration and the presence or absence of a vasconstrictor agent. Except for intravenous administration, the highest blood levels are obtained following intercostal nerve block and the lowest after subcutaneous administration.

The plasma binding of etidocaine is dependent on drug concentration, and the fraction bound decreases with increasing concentration. At 0.5–1.0 μg/mL, 95% is bound to plasma protein.

Etidocaine crosses the blood-brain barrier and placental barriers, presumably by passive diffusion.

Etidocaine is metabolized rapidly by the liver, and metabolites and unchanged drug are excreted by the kidney. Biotransformation includes oxidative N-dealkylation, ring hydroxylation, cleavage of the amide linkage, and conjugation. To date, approximately 20 metabolites of etidocaine have been found in the urine. The percent of dose excreted as unchanged drug is less than 10%.

The mean elimination half-life of etidocaine following a bolus intravenous injection is about 2.5 hours. Because of the rapid rate at which etidocaine is metabolized, any condition that affects liver function may alter etidocaine kinetics. Renal dysfunction may not affect etidocaine kinetics but may increase the accumulation of metabolites.

Factors such as acidosis and the concomitant use of CNS stimulants and depressants affect the CNS levels of etidocaine required to produce overt systemic effects. In the rhesus monkey arterial blood levels of 4.5 μg/mL have been shown to be threshold for convulsive activity.

INDICATIONS AND USAGE

Duranest (etidocaine HCl) Solutions are indicated for infiltration anesthesia, peripheral nerve blocks (e.g., brachial plexus, intercostal, retrobulbar, ulnar, inferior alveolar), and central neural block (i.e., lumbar or caudal epidural blocks).

CONTRAINDICATIONS

Etidocaine is contraindicated in patients with a known history of hypersensitivity to local anesthetics of the amide type.

WARNINGS

DURANEST INJECTIONS FOR INFILTRATION AND NERVE BLOCK SHOULD BE EMPLOYED ONLY BY CLINICIANS WHO ARE WELL VERSED IN DIAGNOSIS AND MANAGEMENT OF DOSE-RELATED TOXICITY AND OTHER ACUTE EMERGENCIES THAT MIGHT ARISE FROM THE BLOCK TO BE EMPLOYED AND THEN ONLY AFTER ENSURING THE *IMMEDIATE* AVAILABILITY OF OXYGEN, OTHER RESUSCITATIVE DRUGS, CARDIOPULMONARY EQUIPMENT, AND THE PERSONNEL NEEDED FOR PROPER MANAGEMENT OF TOXIC REACTIONS AND RELATED EMERGENCIES (See also ADVERSE REACTIONS and PRECAUTIONS). DELAY IN PROPER MANAGEMENT OF DOSE-RELATED TOXICITY, UNDERVENTILATION FROM ANY CAUSE AND/OR ALTERED SENSITIVITY MAY LEAD TO THE DEVELOPMENT OF ACIDOSIS, CARDIAC ARREST AND, POSSIBLY, DEATH.

To avoid intravascular injection, aspiration should be performed before the local anesthetic solution is injected. The needle must be repositioned until no return of blood can be elicited by aspiration. Note, however, that the absence of blood in the syringe does not guarantee that intravascular injection has been avoided.

Local anesthetic solutions containing antimicrobial preservatives (e.g., methylparaben) should not be used for epidural anesthesia because the safety of these agents has not been established with regard to intrathecal injection, either intentional or accidental.

Vasopressor agents administered for the treatment of hypotension related to caudal or other epidural blocks should not be used in the presence of ergot-type oxytocic drugs, since severe persistent hypertension and even rupture of cerebral blood vessels may occur.

Duranest with epinephrine solutions contain sodium metabisulfite, a sulfite that may cause allergic-type reactions including anaphylactic symptoms and life-threatening or less severe asthmatic episodes in certain susceptible people. The overall prevalence of sulfite sensitivity in the general population is unknown and probably low. Sulfite sensitivity is seen more frequently in asthmatic than in nonasthmatic people.

PRECAUTIONS

General: The safety and effectiveness of etidocaine depend on proper dosage, correct technique, adequate precautions, and readiness for emergencies. Standard textbooks should be consulted for specific techniques and precautions for various regional anesthetic procedures. Resuscitative equipment, oxygen, and other resuscitative drugs should be available for immediate use (See WARNINGS and ADVERSE REACTIONS.) The lowest dosage that results in effective anesthesia should be used to avoid high plasma levels and serious adverse effects. Syringe aspirations should also be performed before and during each supplemental injection when using indwelling catheter techniques. During the administration of epidural anesthesia, it is recommended that a test dose be administered initially and that the patient be monitored for central nervous system toxicity and cardiovascular toxicity, as well as for signs of unintended intrathecal administration, before proceeding. When clinical conditions permit, consideration should be given to employing local anesthetic solutions that contain epinephrine for the test dose because circulatory changes compatible with epinephrine may also serve as a warning sign of unintended intravascular injection. An intravascular injection is still possible even if aspirations for blood are negative. Repeated doses of etidocaine may cause significant increases in blood levels with each repeated dose because of slow accumulation of the drug or its metabolites. Tolerance to elevated blood levels varies with the status of the patient. Debilitated, elderly patients, acutely ill patients, and children should be given reduced doses commensurate with their age and physical condition. Etidocaine should also be used with caution in patients with severe shock or heart block.

Lumbar and caudal epidural anesthesia should be used with extreme caution in persons with the following conditions: existing neurological disease, spinal deformities, septicemia and severe hypertension.

Local anesthetic solutions containing a vasoconstrictor should be used cautiously and in carefully circumscribed quantities in areas of the body supplied by end arteries or having otherwise compromised blood supply. Patients with peripheral vascular disease and those with hypertensive vascular disease may exhibit exaggerated vasoconstrictor response. Ischemic injury or necrosis may result. Preparations containing a vasoconstrictor should be used with caution in patients during or following the administration of potent general anesthetic agents, since cardiac arrhythmias may occur under such conditions.

Careful and constant monitoring of cardiovascular and respiratory (adequacy of ventilation) vital signs and the patient's state of consciousness should be accomplished after each local anesthetic injection. It should be kept in mind at such times that restlessness, anxiety, tinnitus, dizziness, blurred vision, tremors, depression or drowsiness may be early warning signs of central nervous system toxicity.

Since amide-type local anesthetics are metabolized by the liver, Duranest Injections should be used with caution in patients with hepatic disease.

Patients with severe hepatic disease, because of their inability to metabolize local anesthetics normally, are a greater risk of developing toxic plasma concentrations. Duranest Injection should also be used with caution in patients with impaired cardiovascular function since they may be less able to compensate for functional changes associated with the prolongation of A-V conduction produced by these drugs.

Many drugs used during the conduct of anesthesia are considered potential triggering agents for familial malignant hyperthermia. Since it is not known whether amide-type local anesthetics may trigger this reaction and since the need for supplemental general anesthesia cannot be pre-

Table 1. Composition of Available Solutions

Product Identification			Formula		
Duranest (etidocaine HCl) Concentration %	Epinephrine Dilution (as the bitartrate)	pH	Sodium chloride (mg/mL)	Single Dose Vials/ Dental Cartridge Sodium metabisulfite (mg/mL)	Citric acid (mg/mL)
1.0	None	4.0–5.0	7.1	None	—
1.0	1:200,000	3.0–4.5	7.1	0.5	0.2
1.5	1:200,000	3.0–4.5	6.2	0.5	0.2

NOTE: pH of all solutions adjusted with sodium hydroxide or hydrochloric acid. Duranest dental cartridges are only available as 1.5% solution with epinephrine 1:200,000. Filled under nitrogen.

dicted in advance, it is suggested that a standard protocol for the management of malignant hyperthermia should be available. Early unexplained signs of tachycardia, tachypnea, labile blood pressure and metabolic acidosis may precede temperature elevation. Successful outcome is dependent on early diagnosis, prompt discontinuance of the suspect triggering agent(s) and institution of treatment, including oxygen therapy, indicated supportive measures and dantrolene (consult dantrolene sodium intravenous package insert before using).

Etidocaine should be used with caution in persons with known drug sensitivities. Patients allergic to para-amino-benzoic acid derivatives (procaine, tetracaine, benzocaine, etc.) have not shown cross sensitivity to etidocaine.

Use in the Head and Neck Area: Small doses of local anesthetics injected into the head and neck area, including retrobulbar, dental and stellate ganglion blocks, may produce adverse reactions similar to systemic toxicity seen with unintentional intravascular injections of larger doses. The injection procedures require the utmost care. Confusion, convulsions, respiratory depression and/or respiratory arrest, and cardiovascular stimulation or depression have been reported. These reactions may be due to intra-arterial injection of the local anesthetic with retrograde flow to the cerebral circulation. They may also be due to puncture of the dural sheath of the optic nerve during retrobulbar block with diffusion of any local anesthetic along the subdural space to the midbrain. Patients receiving these blocks should have their circulation and respiration monitored and be constantly observed. Resuscitative equipment and personnel for treating adverse reactions should be immediately available. Dosage recommendations should not be exceeded. (See DOSAGE AND ADMINISTRATION.)

Use in Ophthalmic Surgery: When local anesthetic injections are employed for retrobulbar block, lack of corneal sensation should not be relied upon to determine whether or not the patient is ready for surgery. This is because complete lack of corneal sensation usually precedes clinically acceptable external ocular muscle akinesia.

Use in Dentistry: Because of the long duration of anesthesia, when Duranest 1.5% with epinephrine is used for dental injections, patients should be cautioned about the possibility of inadvertent trauma to tongue, lips and buccal mucosa and advised not to chew solid foods or test the anesthetized area by biting or probing.

Information for Patients: When appropriate, patients should be informed in advance that they may experience temporary loss of sensation and motor activity, usually in the lower half of the body, following proper administration of epidural anesthesia.

Clinically significant drug interactions: The administration of local anesthetic solutions containing epinephrine or norepinephrine to patients receiving monoamine oxidase inhibitors, tricyclic antidepressants or phenothiazines may produce severe, prolonged hypotension or hypertension. Concurrent use of these agents should generally be avoided. In situations when concurrent therapy is necessary, careful patient monitoring is essential.

Concurrent administration of vasopressor drugs (for the treatment of hypotension related to epidural blocks) and ergot-type oxytocic drugs may cause severe, persistent hypertension or cerebrovascular accidents.

Drug Laboratory test interactions: The intramuscular injection of etidocaine may result in an increase in creatine phosphokinase levels. Thus, the use of this enzyme determination, without isoenzyme separation, as a diagnostic test for the presence of acute myocardial infarction may be compromised by the intramuscular injection of etidocaine.

Carcinogenesis, mutagenesis, impairment of fertility: Studies of etidocaine in animals to evaluate the carcinogenic and mutagenic potential have not been conducted. Studies in rats at 1.7 times the maximum recommended human dose have revealed no impairment of fertility.

Use in Pregnancy: Teratogenic Effects. Pregnancy Category B. Reproduction studies have been performed in rats and rabbits at doses up to 1.7 times the human dose and have revealed no evidence of harm to the fetus caused by etidocaine. There are, however, no adequate and well-controlled studies in pregnant women. Animal reproduction studies are not always predictive of human response. General consideration should be given to this fact before administering etidocaine to women of childbearing potential, especially during early pregnancy when maximum organogenesis takes place.

Labor and delivery: Local anesthetics rapidly cross the placenta and when used for epidural, paracervical, pudendal or caudal block anesthesia, can cause varying degrees of maternal, fetal and neonatal toxicity. (See CLINICAL PHARMACOLOGY—Pharmacokinetics). The incidence and degree of toxicity depend upon the procedure performed, the type and amount of drug used, and the technique of drug administration. Adverse reactions in the parturient, fetus and neonate involve alterations of the central nervous system, peripheral vascular tone and cardiac function.

Maternal hypotension has resulted from regional anesthesia. Local anesthetics produce vasodilation by blocking sympathetic nerves. Elevating the patient's legs and positioning

her on her left side will help prevent decreases in blood pressure. The fetal heart rate also should be monitored continuously and electronic fetal monitoring is highly advisable. Epidural anesthesia may alter the forces of parturition through changes in uterine contractility or maternal expulsive efforts. Because Duranest Injection may produce profound motor block, it is not recommended for epidural anesthesia in normal delivery. Duranest Injection is, however, recommended for epidural anesthesia when caesarian section is to be performed.

The use of some local anesthetic drug products during labor and delivery may be followed by diminished muscle strength and tone for the first day or two of life. The long-term significance of these observations is unknown.

Fetal bradycardia may occur in 20 to 30 percent of patients receiving paracervical nerve block anesthesia with the amide-type local anesthetics and may be associated with fetal acidosis. Fetal heart rate should always be monitored during paracervical anesthesia. The physician should weigh the possible advantages against risks when considering paracervical block in prematurity, toxemia of pregnancy, and fetal distress. Careful adherence to recommended dosage is of the utmost importance in obstetrical paracervical block. Failure to achieve adequate analgesia with recommended doses should arouse suspicion of intravascular or fetal intracranial injection. Cases compatible with unintended fetal intracranial injection of local anesthetic solution have been reported following intended paracervical or pudendal block or both. Babies so affected present with unexplained neonatal depression at birth, which correlates with high local anesthetic serum levels, and often manifest seizures within six hours. Prompt use of supportive measures combined with forced urinary excretion of the local anesthetic has been used successfully to manage this complication. Case reports of maternal convulsions and cardiovascular collapse following use of some local anesthetics for paracervical block in early pregnancy (as anesthesia for elective abortion) suggest that systemic absorption under these circumstances may be rapid. There are inadequate data in support of safe and effective use of etidocaine for obstetrical or non-obstetrical paracervical block, therefore, such use is not recommended.

Nursing mothers: It is not known whether this drug is excreted in human milk. Because many drugs are excreted in human milk, caution should be exercised when etidocaine is administered to a nursing woman.

Pediatric use: No information is currently available on appropriate pediatric doses.

ADVERSE REACTIONS

Systemic: Adverse experiences following the administration of etidocaine are similar in nature to those observed with other amide local anesthetic agents. These adverse experiences are, in general, dose-related and may result from high plasma levels caused by excessive dosage, rapid absorption or unintended intravascular injection, or may result from a hypersensitivity, idiosyncrasy or diminished tolerance on the part of the patient. Serious adverse experiences are generally systemic in nature. The following types are those most commonly reported:

Central nervous system: CNS manifestations are excitatory and/or depressant and may be characterized by lightheadedness, nervousness, apprehension, euphoria, confusion, dizziness, drowsiness, tinnitus, blurred or double vision, vomiting, sensations of heat, cold or numbness, twitching, tremors, convulsions, unconsciousness, respiratory depression and arrest. The excitatory manifestations may be very brief or may not occur at all, in which case the first manifestation of toxicity may be drowsiness merging into unconsciousness and respiratory arrest.

Drowsiness following the administration of etidocaine is usually an early sign of a high blood level of the drug and may occur as a consequence of rapid absorption.

Cardiovascular system: Cardiovascular manifestations are usually depressant and are characterized by bradycardia, hypotension, and cardiovascular collapse, which may lead to cardiac arrest.

Allergic: Allergic reactions are characterized by cutaneous lesions, urticaria, edema or anaphylactoid reactions. Allergic reactions may occur as a result of sensitivity either to local anesthetic agents or to the methylparaben used as a preservative in multiple dose vials. The detection of sensitivity by skin testing is of doubtful value.

Neurologic: The incidences of adverse reactions associated with the use of local anesthetics may be related to the total dose of local anesthetic administered and are also dependent upon the particular drug used, the route of administration and the physical status of the patient.

In the practice of caudal or lumbar epidural block, occasional unintentional penetration of the subarachnoid space by the catheter may occur. Subsequent adverse effects may depend partially on the amount of drug administered subdurally. These may include spinal block of varying magnitude (including total spinal block), hypotension secondary to spinal block, loss of bladder and bowel control, and loss of perineal sensation and sexual function. Persistent motor, sensory and/or autonomic (sphincter control) deficit of some lower

spinal segments with slow recovery (several months) or incomplete recovery have been reported in rare instances when caudal or lumbar epidural block has been attempted. Backache and headache have also been noted following use of these anesthetic procedures.

OVERDOSAGE

Acute emergencies from local anesthetics are generally related to high plasma levels encountered during therapeutic use of local anesthetics or to unintended subarachnoid injection of local anesthetic solution (see ADVERSE REACTIONS, WARNINGS, and PRECAUTIONS).

Management of local anesthetic emergencies: The first consideration is prevention, best accomplished by careful and constant monitoring of cardiovascular and respiratory vital signs and the patient's state of consciousness after each local anesthetic injection. At the first sign of change, oxygen should be administered.

The first step in the management of convulsions, as well as underventilation or apnea due to unintentional subarachnoid injection of drug solution, consists of immediate attention to the maintenance of a patent airway and assisted or controlled ventilation with oxygen and a delivery system capable of permitting immediate positive airway pressure by mask. Immediately after the institution of these ventilatory measures, the adequacy of the circulation should be evaluated, keeping in mind that drugs used to treat convulsions sometimes depress the circulation when administered intravenously. Should convulsions persist despite adequate respiratory support, and if the status of the circulation permits, small increments of an ultra-short acting barbiturate (such as thiopental or thiamylal) or a benzodiazepine (such as diazepam) may be administered intravenously. The clinician should be familiar, prior to use of local anesthetics, with these anticonvulsant drugs. Supportive treatment of circulatory depression may require administration of intravenous fluids and, when appropriate, a vasopressor as directed by the clinical situation (e.g., ephedrine).

If not treated immediately, both convulsions and cardiovascular depression can result in hypoxia, acidosis, bradycardia, arrhythmias and cardiac arrest. Underventilation or apnea due to unintentional subarachnoid injection of local anesthetic solution may produce these same signs and also lead to cardiac arrest if ventilatory support is not instituted. If cardiac arrest should occur, standard cardiopulmonary resuscitative measures should be instituted.

Endotracheal intubation, employing drugs and techniques familiar to the clinician, may be indicated, after initial administration of oxygen by mask, if difficulty is encountered in the maintenance of a patent airway or if prolonged ventilatory support (assisted or controlled) is indicated.

Dialysis is of negligible value in the treatment of acute overdosage with etidocaine.

The intravenous LD_{50} of etidocaine HCl in female mice is 7.6 (6.6–8.5) mg/kg and the subcutaneous LD_{50} is 112 (96–166) mg/kg.

DOSAGE AND ADMINISTRATION

As with all local anesthetic agents, the dose of Duranest (etidocaine HCl) Injection to be employed will depend upon the area to be anesthetized, the vascularity of the tissues, the number of neuronal segments to be blocked, the type of regional anesthetic technique, and the physical condition and tolerance of the individual patient.

The maximum dose to be employed as a single injection should be determined on the basis of the status of the patient and the type of regional anesthetic technique to be performed. Although single injections of 450 mg have been employed for regional anesthesia without adverse effects, at present it is strongly recommended that the maximal dose as a single injection should not exceed 400 mg (approximately 8.0 mg/kg or 3.6 mg/lb based on a 50 kg person) with epinephrine 1:200,000 and 300 mg (approximately 6 mg/kg and 2.7 mg/lb based on a 50 kg person) without epinephrine. Because etidocaine has been shown to disappear quite rapidly from blood, toxicity is influenced by rapidity of administration, and therefore slow injection in vascular areas is highly recommended. Incremental doses of Duranest Injection may be repeated at 2–3 hour intervals.

Caudal and lumbar epidural block: As a precaution against the adverse experiences sometimes observed following unintentional penetration of the subarachnoid space, a test dose of 2–5 mL should be administered at least 5 minutes prior to injecting the total volume required for a lumbar or caudal epidural block. The test dose should be repeated if the patient is moved in a manner that may have displaced the catheter. Epinephrine, if contained in the test dose (10–15μg have been suggested), may serve as a warning of unintentional intravascular injection. If injected into a blood vessel this amount of epinephrine is likely to produce a transient "epinephrine response" within 45 seconds, consisting of an increase in heart rate and systolic blood pressure, circumoral pallor, palpitations and nervousness in the unsedated patient. The sedated patient may exhibit only a pulse rate in-

Continued on next page

Astra—Cont.

crease of 20 or more beats per minute for 15 or more seconds. Patients on beta-blockers may not manifest changes in heart rate, but blood pressure monitoring can detect an evanescent rise in systolic blood pressure. Adequate time should be allowed for onset of anesthesia after administration of each test dose. The rapid injection of a large volume of Duranest Injection through the catheter should be avoided, and when feasible fractional doses should be administered.

In the event of the known injection of a large volume of local anesthetic solution into the subarchnoid space after suitable resuscitation and if the catheter is in place, consider attempting the recovery of drug by draining a moderate amount of cerebrospinal fluid (such as 10 mL) through the epidural catheter.

Use in Dentistry: When used for local anesthesia in dental procedures the dosage of Duranest (etidocaine HCl) Injection depends on the physical status of the patient, the area of the oral cavity to be anesthetized, the vascularity of the oral tissues, and the technique of anesthesia. The least volume of solution that results in effective local anesthesia should be administered. For specific techniques and procedures of local anesthesia in the oral cavity, refer to standard textbooks. Dosage requirements should be determined on an individual basis. In maxillary infiltration and/or inferior alveolar nerve block, initial dosages of 1.0–5.0 mL (½–2½ cartridges) of Duranest Injection 1.5% with epinephrine 1:200,000 are usually effective.

Aspiration is recommended since it reduces the possibility of intravascular injection, thereby keeping the incidence of side effects and anesthetic failures to a minimum.

The following dosage recommendations are intended as guides for the use of Duranest Injection in the average adult patient. As indicated previously, the dosage should be reduced for elderly or debilitated patients or patients with severe renal disease.

NOTE:

Parenteral drug products should be inspected visually for particulate matter and discoloration prior to administration whenever the solution and container permit. The Injection is not to be used if its color is pinkish or darker than slightly yellow or if it contains a precipitate.

[See Table 2 below.]

HOW SUPPLIED

[See second table below.]
Store at controlled room temperature 15°–30°C (59°–86°F).
021842R08   Rev. 3/91 (8)

DYCLONE® 0.5% and 1%   ℞
Topical Solutions, USP
[*dié-clone*]
(dyclonine HCl)

DESCRIPTION

Dyclone (dyclonine HCl) 0.5% and 1% Topical Solutions contain a local anesthetic agent and are administered topically. See INDICATIONS for specific uses.

Dyclone 0.5% and 1% Topical Solutions contain dyclonine HCl, which is chemically designated as 4'-butoxy-3-piperidinopropiophenone HCl. Dyclonine HCl is a white crystalline powder that is sparingly soluble in water and has the following structural formula:

$$CH_2CH_2C(=O){-}\langle\text{benzene ring}\rangle{-}OCH_2CH_2CH_2CH_3 \cdot HCl$$

COMPOSITIONS OF DYCLONE 0.5% AND 1% TOPICAL SOLUTIONS

Each mL of Dyclone 0.5% Solution contains dyclonine HCl, 5 mg.

Each mL of Dyclone 1% Solution contains dyclonine HCl, 10 mg.

Both solutions also contain chlorbutanol hydrous and sodium chloride, and the pH is adjusted to 3.0–5.0 by means of hydrochloric acid.

CLINICAL PHARMACOLOGY

Dyclone Topical Solutions effect surface anesthesia when applied topically to mucous membranes. Effective anesthesia varies with different patients, but usually occurs from 2 to 10 minutes after application and persists for approximately 30 minutes.

INDICATIONS AND USAGE

Dyclone Topical Solutions are indicated for anesthetizing accessible mucous membranes (e.g., the mouth, pharynx, larynx, trachea, esophagus, and urethra) prior to various endoscopic procedures.

Dyclone 0.5% Topical Solution may also be used to block the gag reflex, to relieve the pain of oral ulcers or stomatitis and to relieve pain associated with ano-genital lesions.

CONTRAINDICATIONS

Dyclonine is contraindicated in patients known to be hypersensitive (allergic) to the local anesthetic or to other components of Dyclone Topical Solutions.

WARNINGS

IN ORDER TO MANAGE POSSIBLE ADVERSE REACTIONS, RESUSCITATIVE EQUIPMENT, OXYGEN AND OTHER RESUSCITATIVE DRUGS SHOULD BE IMMEDIATELY AVAILABLE WHENEVER LOCAL ANESTHETIC AGENTS, SUCH AS DYCLONINE, ARE ADMINISTERED TO MUCOUS MEMBRANES.

Dyclone Topical Solutions should not be injected into tissue or used in the eyes because of highly irritant properties.

Dyclone Topical Solutions should be used with extreme caution in the presence of sepsis or severely traumatized mucosa in the area of application since under such conditions there is the potential for rapid systemic absorption.

PRECAUTIONS

General: The safety and effectiveness of dyclonine depend on proper dosage, correct technique, adequate precautions, and readiness for emergencies (See WARNINGS and AD-

VERSE REACTIONS). The lowest dosage that results in effective anesthesia should be used to avoid high plasma levels and serious adverse effects. Repeated doses of dyclonine may cause significant increases in blood levels with each repeated dose because of slow accumulation of the drug or its metabolites. Tolerance to elevated blood levels varies with the status of the patient. Debilitated, elderly patients, acutely ill patients, and children should be given reduced doses commensurate with their age, weight and physical condition. Dyclonine should also be used with caution in patients with severe shock or heart block.

Dyclone Topical Solutions should be used with caution in persons with known drug sensitivities.

Information for Patients: When topical anesthetics are used in the mouth or throat, the patient should be aware that the production of topical anesthesia may impair swallowing and thus enhance the danger of aspiration. For this reason, food should not be ingested for 60 minutes following use of local anesthetic preparations in the mouth or throat area. This is particularly important in children because of their frequency of eating.

Numbness of the tongue or buccal mucosa may increase the danger of biting trauma. When Dyclone 0.5% Topical Solution is used to relieve the pain of oral ulcers or stomatitis which interferes with eating, patients should be warned about the risk of biting trauma before they accept this treatment; caution should be exercised in selecting food and eating. Following other uses in the mouth and throat area, food and/or chewing gum should not be used while the area is anesthetized.

Drug/Laboratory Test Interactions: Dyclone Topical Solutions should not be used in cystoscopic procedures following intravenous pyelography because an iodine precipitate occurs which interferes with visualization.

Carcinogenesis, mutagenesis, impairment of fertility: Studies of dyclonine in animals to evaluate the carcinogenic and mutagenic potential or the effect on fertility have not been conducted.

Use in Pregnancy: Teratogenic Effects:
Pregnancy Category C. Animal reproduction studies have not been conducted with dyclonine. It is also not known whether dyclonine can cause fetal harm when administered to a pregnant woman or can affect reproduction capacity. General consideration should be given to this fact before administering dyclonine to women of childbearing potential, especially during early pregnancy when maximum organogenesis takes place.

Nursing Mothers: It is not known whether this drug is excreted in human milk. Because many drugs are excreted in human milk, caution should be exercised when dyclonine is administered to a nursing woman.

Pediatric Use: Safety and effectiveness in children under the age of 12 have not been established.

ADVERSE REACTIONS

Adverse experiences following the administration of dyclonine are similar in nature to those observed with other local anesthetic agents. These adverse experiences are, in general, dose-related and may result from high plasma levels caused by excessive dosage or rapid absorption, or may result from a hypersensitivity, idiosyncrasy or diminished tolerance on the part of the patient. Serious adverse experiences are generally systemic in nature. The following types are those most commonly reported:

Central nervous system: CNS manifestations are excitatory and/or depressant and may be characterized by lightheadedness, nervousness, apprehension, euphoria, confusion, dizziness, drowsiness, tinnitus, blurred or double vision, vomiting, sensations of heat, cold or numbness, twitching, tremors, convulsions, unconsciousness, repiratory depression and arrest. The excitatory manifestations may be very brief or may not occur at all, in which case the first manifestation of toxicity may be drowsiness merging into unconsciousness and respiratory arrest.

Drowsiness following the administration of dyclonine is usually an early sign of a high blood level of the drug and may occur as a consequence of rapid absorption.

Cardiovascular system: Cardiovascular manifestations are usually depressant and are characterized by bradycardia, hypotension, and cardiovascular collapse, which may lead to cardiac arrest.

Allergic: Allergic reactions are characterized by cutaneous lesions, urticaria, edema or anaphylactoid reactions. Allergic reactions may occur as a result of sensitivity either to the local anesthetic agent or to the other ingredients used in this formulation. Allergic reactions, if they occur, should be managed by conventional means. The detection of sensitivity by skin testing is of doubtful value. Local reactions include irritation, stinging, urethritis with and without bleeding.

OVERDOSAGE

Acute emergencies from local anesthetics are generally related to high plasma levels encountered during therapeutic use of local anesthetics. (See ADVERSE REACTIONS, WARNINGS, and PRECAUTIONS).

Table 2. Dosage Recommendations

PROCEDURE	Duranest HCl with epinephrine 1:200,000			PROCEDURE	Duranest HCl with epinephrine 1:200,000		
	Conc. (%)	Vol. (mL)	Total Dose (mg)		Conc. (%)	Vol. (mL)	Total Dose (mg)
Peripheral Nerve Block	1.0	5–40	50–400	Caudal	1.0	10–30	100–300
				Retrobulbar	1.0 or 1.5	2–4	20–60
Central Neural Block				Maxillary Infiltration and/or Inferior Alveolar			
Lumbar Peridural				Nerve Block	1.5	1–5	15–75
Intraabdominal or Pelvic Surgery	1.0	10–30	100–300				
Lower Limb Surgery or Caesarean Section	or 1.5	10–20	150–300				

Dosage Form and Volume	Duranest Injection Concentration	Epinephrine Dilution (as the bitartrate)	pH	NDC Number
Single Dose Vials 30 mL	1.0%	None	4.0–5.0	0186-0820-01
	1.0%	1:200,000	3.0–4.5	0186-0825-01
20 mL	1.5%	1:200,000	3.0–4.5	0186-0836-03
Dental Cartridge 1.8 mL	1.5%	1:200,000	3.0–4.5	0186-0840-14

Management of local anesthetic emergencies: The first consideration is prevention, best accomplished by careful and constant monitoring of cardiovascular and respiratory vital signs and the patient's state of consciousness after each local anesthetic administration.

The first step in the management of convulsions consists of immediate attention to the maintenance of a patent airway and assisted or controlled ventilation with oxygen and a delivery system capable of permitting immediate positive airway pressure by mask. Immediately after the institution of these ventilatory measures, the adequacy of the circulation should be evaluated, keeping in mind that drugs used to treat convulsions sometimes depress the circulation when administered intravenously. Should convulsions persist despite adequate respiratory support, and if the status of the circulation permits, small increments of an ultra-short acting barbiturate (such as thiopental or thiamylal) or a benzodiazepine (such as diazepam) may be administered intravenously. The clinician should be familiar, prior to use of local anesthetics, with these anticonvulsant drugs. Supportive treatment of circulatory depression may require administration of intravenous fluids and, when appropriate, a vasopressor as directed by the clinical situation (e.g., ephedrine).

If not treated immediately, both convulsions and cardiovascular depression can result in hypoxia, acidosis, bradycardia, arrhythmias and cardiac arrest. If cardiac arrest should occur, standard cardiopulmonary resuscitative measures should be instituted.

The mean lethal dose (LD$_{50}$) of dyclonine HCl administered orally to female rats is 176 mg/kg and 90 mg/kg in female mice. Intraperitoneally the LD$_{50}$ in female rats is 31 mg/kg and 43 mg/kg in female mice.

DOSAGE AND ADMINISTRATION

As with all local anesthetics, the dosage varies and depends upon the area to be anesthetized, vascularity of the tissues, individual tolerance and the technique of anesthesia. The lowest dosage needed to provide effective anesthesia should be administered.

A maximum dose of 30 mL of 1% Dyclone Topical Solution (300 mg of dyclonine HCl) may be used, although satisfactory anesthesia is usually produced within the range of 4 to 20 mL. For specific techniques and procedures refer to standard textbooks.

Although as much as 300 mg of dyclonine HCl (as a 1% solution) have been tolerated, this dosage as a 0.5% solution has not been administered primarily because satisfactory anesthesia in endoscopic procedures can usually be produced by lesser amounts. For specific techniques for endoscopic procedures refer to standard textbooks.

PROCTOLOGY

Apply pledgets of cotton or sponges moistened with the Dyclone 0.5% Solution to postoperative wounds for the relief of discomfort and pain.

GYNECOLOGY

Apply Dyclone 0.5% Solution as wet compresses or as a spray to relieve the discomfort of episiotomy or perineorrhaphy wounds.

ONCOLOGY-RADIOLOGY

Apply Dyclone 0.5% Solution as a rinse or swab to inflamed or ulcerated mucous membrane of the mouth caused by antineoplastic chemotherapy or radiation therapy. In lesions of the esophagus, 5–15 mL of the anesthetic may be swallowed to relieve pain and allow more comfortable deglutition.

OTORHINOLARYNGOLOGY

To suppress the gag reflex and to facilitate examination of the posterior pharynx or larynx, apply Dyclone 0.5% Solution as a spray or gargle.

Dyclone 0.5% Solution may be applied as a rinse or swab to relieve the discomfort of aphthous stomatitis, herpetic stomatitis, or other painful oral lesions.

DENTISTRY

Dyclone 0.5% Topical Solution is useful to suppress the gag reflex in the positioning of x-ray films, making prosthetic impressions, and doing surgical procedures in the molar areas. It is also useful as a preinjection mucous membrane anesthetic or applied to the gums prior to scaling (prophylaxis). The anesthetic can be applied as a mouthwash or gargle and the excess spit out.

HOW SUPPLIED

Sterile, in one fluid ounce bottles, DYCLONE 0.5% TOPICAL SOLUTION (NDC 0186-3001-01) and DYCLONE 1% TOPICAL SOLUTION (NDC 0186-3002-01). Keep tightly closed. Store at controlled room temperature: 15°–30°C (59°–86°F). Avoid excessive heat (temperatures above 40°C (104°F). Subject to damage by freezing.

021859R02   Rev. 8/89 (2)

EPINEPHRINE   ℞
[*ep-ē-nef'-rin*]
Injection, USP
1:10,000 (0.1 mg/mL)
Adult Strength

(For details of indications, dosage and administration, precautions, and adverse reactions, see circular in package.)

HOW SUPPLIED

Epinephrine Injection USP, 1:10,000, is supplied in 10 mL prefilled syringes with a 21 g $^{15}/_{16}$″ needle. (NDC 0186-0653-01). The solution should be stored at controlled room temperature 15°–30°C (59°–86°F) and should be protected from light by storage in the original carton until use.

021883R03   Rev. 7/91 (3)

FENTANYL CITRATE* and DROPERIDOL   Ⓒ ℞
INJECTION
*WARNING (May be habit forming)
For INTRAVENOUS OR INTRAMUSCULAR USE ONLY

> The two components of Fentanyl Citrate and Droperidol Injection, fentanyl citrate and droperidol, have different pharmacologic actions. Before administering Fentanyl Citrate and Droperidol Injection, the user should become familiar with the special properties of each drug, particularly the widely differing durations of action.

(For details of indication, dosage and administration, precautions, and adverse reactions, see circular in package.)

HOW SUPPLIED

Each mL of Fentanyl Citrate and Droperidol Injection contains fentanyl citrate (WARNING: May be habit forming) equivalent to 0.05 mg (50 mcg) of fentanyl base, droperidol 2.5 mg and lactic acid to adjust pH and is available in the following dosage forms:
Ampules
NDC 0186-1230-03, 2 mL ampule in packages of 10
NDC 0186-1231-03, 5 mL ampule in packages of 10
Vials
NDC 0186-1232-13, 2 mL single dose vial in packages of 10
NDC 0186-1233-13, 5 mL single dose vial in packages of 10
(FOR INTRAVENOUS USE BY HOSPITAL PERSONNEL SPECIFICALLY TRAINED IN THE USE OF OPIOID ANALGESICS.)
PROTECT FROM LIGHT. STORE AT CONTROLLED ROOM TEMPERATURE 15°–30°C (59°–86°F).
021881R01   5/89(1)

FOSCAVIR®   ℞
[*fos-ka-vēer*]
(foscarnet sodium) Injection

> RENAL IMPAIRMENT IS THE MAJOR TOXICITY OF FOSCAVIR, AND OCCURS TO SOME DEGREE IN MOST PATIENTS, CONSEQUENTLY, CONTINUAL ASSESSMENT OF A PATIENT'S RISK AND FREQUENT MONITORING OF SERUM CREATININE WITH DOSE ADJUSTMENT FOR CHANGES IN RENAL FUNCTION ARE IMPERATIVE.
> FOSCAVIR HAS BEEN SHOWN TO CAUSE ALTERATIONS IN PLASMA MINERALS AND ELECTROLYTES THAT HAVE LED TO SEIZURES. THEREFORE, PATIENTS MUST BE MONITORED FREQUENTLY FOR SUCH CHANGES AND THEIR POTENTIAL SEQUELAE.

DESCRIPTION

FOSCAVIR is the brand name for foscarnet sodium. The chemical name of foscarnet sodium is phosphonoformic acid, trisodium salt. Foscarnet sodium is a white, crystalline powder containing 6 equivalents of water of hydration with an empirical formula of $Na_3CO_5P \cdot 6\ H_2O$ and a molecular weight of 300.1. The structural formula is:

$$3\ Na+ \left[O - P - C \right] \cdot 6\ H_2O$$

FOSCAVIR has the potential to chelate divalent metal ions, such as calcium and magnesium, to form stable coordination compounds. FOSCAVIR INJECTION is a sterile, isotonic aqueous solution for intravenous administration only. The solution is clear and colorless. Each milliliter of FOSCAVIR contains 24 mg of foscarnet sodium hexahydrate in Water for Injection, USP. Hydrochloric acid and/or sodium hydrox-

---

ide may have been added to adjust the pH of the solution to 7.4. FOSCAVIR INJECTION contains no preservatives.

CLINICAL PHARMACOLOGY
Microbiology:
FOSCAVIR is an organic analogue of inorganic pyrophosphate that inhibits replication of all known herpesviruses *in vitro* including cytomegalovirus (CMV), herpes simplex virus types 1 and 2 (HSV-1, HSV-2), human herpesvirus 6 (HHV-6), Epstein-Barr virus (EBV), and varicella-zoster virus (VZV).

FOSCAVIR exerts its antiviral activity by a selective inhibition at the pyrophosphate binding site on virus-specific DNA polymerases and reverse transcriptases at concentrations that do not affect cellular DNA polymerases. FOSCAVIR does not require activation (phosphorylation) by thymidine kinase or other kinases, and therefore is active *in vitro* against HSV mutants deficient in thymidine kinase (TK). CMV strains resistant to ganciclovir may be sensitive to FOSCAVIR. No controlled trials have been completed involving FOSCAVIR treatment of patients with CMV resistant to ganciclovir.

The quantitative relationship between the *in vitro* susceptibility of human cytomegalovirus (CMV) to FOSCAVIR and clinical response to therapy has not been clearly established in man and virus sensitivity testing has not been standardized. Sensitivity test results, expressed as the concentration of drug required to inhibit by 50% the growth of virus in cell culture (IC$_{50}$), vary greatly depending on the assay method used, cell type employed and the laboratory performing the test. A number of sensitive viruses and their IC$_{50}$ values are listed below.

TABLE 1

FOSCARNET Inhibition of virus multplication in cell culture

Virus	IC$_{50}$(μM)
CMV	50–800*
HSV-1, HSV-2	10–130
VZV	48–90
EBV	<500**
HHV-6	<67***
Ganciclovir resistant CMV	190
HSV-TK minus mutant	67
HSV-DNA polymerase mutants	5–443

* Mean = 269 μM
** 97% of viral antigen synthesis inhibited at 500 μM
*** IC$_{100}$ = 67 μM

Clinical isolates of CMV taken from patients show different sensitivities to FOSCAVIR *in vitro*. Statistically significant decreases in positive CMV cultures from blood and urine have been demonstrated in two studies (FOS-03 and ACTG-015/915) of patients treated with FOSCAVIR. Although median time to progression of CMV retinitis was reduced in patients treated with the drug, reductions in positive blood or urine cultures have not been shown to correlate with clinical efficacy in individual patients.

TABLE 2
BLOOD AND URINE CULTURE RESULTS FROM CMV RETINITIS PATIENTS*

Blood	+CMV	−CMV
Baseline	27	34
End of Induction**	1	60

Urine	+CMV	−CMV
Baseline	52	6
End of Induction**	21	37

*A combined total of 77 patients were treated with FOSCAVIR in two clinical trials (FOS-03 and ACTG-015/915). Not all patients had blood or urine cultures done and some patients had results from both cultures.
**(60 mg/kg FOSCAVIR TID for 2–3 weeks).

If no clinical response to FOSCAVIR is observed, viral isolates should be tested for sensitivity to foscarnet as naturally resistant mutants may emerge under selective pressure both *in vitro* and *in vivo*. The latent state of any of the human herpesviruses is not known to be sensitive to FOSCAVIR and viral reactivation of CMV occurs after FOSCAVIR therapy is terminated.

Pharmacokinetics:
Protein Binding:
In vitro studies have shown that 14–17% of foscarnet is bound to plasma protein at plasma drug concentrations of 1–1000 μM.

Continued on next page

Astra—Cont.

Plasma Concentrations:
The pharmacokinetics of FOSCAVIR infusions have been determined when administered as an intermittent infusion during induction therapy in AIDS patients with CMV retinitis. Observed plasma foscarnet concentrations in two studies (FOS-01 and ACTG-015 respectively) are summarized in the following table:

[See table below.]

Clearance:
Mean (±SD) plasma clearances were 130 ± 44 and 178 ± 48 mL/min in two studies in which FOSCAVIR was given by intermittent infusion (ACTG-015 and FOS-01 respectively), and 152 ± 59 and 214 ± 25 mL/min/1.73 m^2 in two studies using continuous infusion. Approximately 80–90% of IV FOSCAVIR is excreted unchanged in the urine of patients with normal renal function. Urinary excretion data suggest that both tubular secretion and glomerular filtration account for urinary elimination of foscarnet. In one study, plasma clearance was less than creatinine clearance, suggesting that FOSCAVIR may also undergo tubular reabsorption. In three studies, decreases in plasma clearance of FOSCAVIR were proportional to decreases in creatinine clearance.

Half-life:
Two studies (FOS-01 and ACTG-015) in patients with initially normal renal function who were treated with intermittant infusions of FOSCAVIR showed average drug plasma half-lives of about three hours determined on days 1 or 3 of therapy. This may be an underestimate of the effective half-life of FOSCAVIR due to the limited duration of the observation period. The plasma half-life of FOSCAVIR increases with the severity of renal impairment. Half-lives of 2–8 hours have been reported in patients having estimated or measured 24-hour creatinine clearances of 44–90 mL/min. Careful monitoring of renal function and dose adjustment in patients on FOSCAVIR is imperative (see WARNINGS and DOSAGE AND ADMINISTRATION).
Following the continuous infusion of FOSCAVIR for 72 hours in six HIV+ patients, plasma half-lives of 0.45 ± 0.32 and 3.3 ± 1.3 hours were determined. A terminal half-life (λ_3) of 18 ± 2.8 hours was estimated from the urinary excretion of foscarnet over 48 hours after stopping the infusion. When FOSCAVIR was administered as a continuous infusion to 13 patients with HIV infection for 8 to 21 days, plasma half-lives of 1.4 ± 0.6 and 6.8 ± 5.0 hours were determined. A terminal half-life of 87.5 ± 41.8 hours was estimated from the urinary excretion of foscarnet over six days after the last infusion; however, the renal function of these patients at the time of discontinuing the FOSCAVIR infusion was not known.
Measurements of urinary excretion are required to detect the longer terminal half-life assumed to represent release of foscarnet from bone. In animal studies (mice), 40% of an intravenous dose of FOSCAVIR is deposited in bone in young animals and 7% in adults. Postmortem data on several patients in European clinical trials provide evidence that foscarnet does accumulate in bone in humans; however, the extent to which this occurs has not been determined.

Volume of Distribution:
Mean volumes of distribution at steady state range from 0.3–0.6 L/kg.

Cerebrospinal Fluid:
Variable penetration of FOSCAVIR into cerebrospinal fluid has been observed. Intermittent infusion of 50 mg/kg of FOSCAVIR every 8 hours for 28 days in 9 patients produced foscarnet CSF levels 3 hours after the end of the infusion of 150–260 μM or 39–103% of plasma levels. In another 4 patients, the CSF concentrations of foscarnet were 35–69% of the plasma drug level after a dose of 230 mg/kg/day by continuous infusion for 2–13 days; however, the CSF:plasma ratio was only 13% in one patient while receiving a continuous infusion of FOSCAVIR at a rate of 274 mg/kg/day. Disease-related defects in the blood-brain barrier may be responsible for the variations seen.

Pharmacodynamics:
A pharmacodynamic analysis of patient data from one U.S. clinical trial (FOS-01) revealed a relationship between cumulative exposure to foscarnet (product of plasma foscarnet concentration *x* time) and changes in renal function (serum creatinine) during induction. All patients had their doses adjusted according to the recommended FOSCAVIR dosing nomogram. Seventeen of 24 patients (72%) showed evidence of renal impairment (> 20% suppression from baseline estimated creatinine clearance) during induction. This occurred in 3 patients on days 5–6, in 11 patients on days 7–14 and in 3 patients after day 14. Eleven patients had at least 40% suppression from baseline estimated creatinine clearance and six patients had more than 50% suppression, demonstrating that patients vary in their degree of sensitivity to FOSCAVIR-induced renal impairment. No specific factors were identified that predicted patients at higher risk. No relationship was found between a patient's initial creatinine clearance or initial drug clearance and renal impairment. Thus initial renal function may not be predictive of a patient's potential for renal impairment induced by FOSCAVIR.

CLINICAL TRIALS
Controlled clinical trials of FOSCAVIR have been conducted in the treatment of CMV retinitis. In most studies, treatment was begun with an induction dosage regimen of 60 mg/kg every 8 hours for the first 2–3 weeks, followed by a once-daily maintenance regimen at doses ranging from 60–120 mg/kg. No studies of FOSCAVIR as a treatment for other manifestations of CMV disease (i.e., viremia, pneumonitis, or gastroenteritis) have been conducted.
A prospective, randomized, masked, controlled clinical trial (FOS-03) was conducted in 24 patients with AIDS and CMV retinitis. All diagnoses and determinations of retinitis progression were made from retinal photographs by ophthalmologists who were masked to the patient's treatment assignment. Patients received induction treatment of FOSCAVIR, 60 mg/kg every 8 hours for 3 weeks, followed by maintenance treatment with 90 mg/kg/day until retinitis progression (appearance of a new lesion or advancement of the border of a posterior lesion greater than 750 microns in diameter). The 13 patients randomized to treatment with FOSCAVIR had a significant delay in progression of CMV retinitis compared to untreated controls. Median times to retinitis progression from study entry were 93 days (range 21– > 364) and 22 days (range 7–42), respectively, p < 0.001.
In another prospective clinical trial of CMV retinitis in patients with AIDS (ACTG-915), 33 patients were treated with two to three weeks of FOSCAVIR induction (60 mg/kg TID) and then randomized to two maintenance dose groups, 90 mg/kg/day and 120 mg/kg/day. Median times from study entry to retinitis progression were 96 (range 14– > 176) days and 140 (range 16– > 233) days, respectively (FDA analysis). This difference was not statistically significant. The same criteria for retinitis progression were used as described above for FOS-03.

INDICATIONS
FOSCAVIR is indicated for the treatment of CMV retinitis in patients with acquired immunodeficiency syndrome (AIDS). SAFETY AND EFFICACY OF FOSCAVIR HAVE NOT BEEN ESTABLISHED FOR TREATMENT OF OTHER CMV INFECTIONS (e.g., PNEUMONITIS, GASTROENTERITIS); CONGENITAL OR NEONATAL CMV DISEASE; OR NON-IMMUNOCOMPROMISED INDIVIDUALS.
The diagnosis of CMV retinitis should be made by indirect ophthalmoscopy. Other conditions in the differential diagnosis of CMV retinitis include candidiasis, toxoplasmosis and other diseases producing a similar retinal pattern, any of which may produce a retinal appearance similar to CMV. For this reason it is essential that the diagnosis of CMV retinitis be established by an ophthalmologist familiar with the retinal presentation of these conditions. The diagnosis of CMV retinitis may be supported by culture of CMV from urine, blood, throat, or other sites, but a negative CMV culture does not rule out CMV retinitis.

CONTRAINDICATIONS
FOSCAVIR is contraindicated in patients with clinically significant hypersensitivity to foscarnet sodium.

WARNINGS
Renal Impairment
THE MAJOR TOXICITY OF FOSCAVIR IS RENAL IMPAIRMENT, WHICH OCCURS TO SOME DEGREE IN MOST PATIENTS. Approximately 33% of 189 patients with AIDS and CMV retinitis who received intravenous FOSCAVIR in clinical studies developed significant impairment of renal function, manifested by a rise in serum creatinine concentration to 2.0 mg/dL or greater. FOSCAVIR must therefore be used with caution in all patients, especially those with a history of impairment of renal function. Patients vary in their sensitivity to nephrotoxicity induced by FOSCAVIR and initial renal function may not be predictive of the potential for drug induced renal impairment (see Pharmacodynamics). FOSCAVIR has not been studied in patients with baseline serum creatinine levels greater than 2.8 mg/dL or measured 24-hour creatinine clearances < 50 mL/min.
Analysis of data in one clinical trial (FOS-01) demonstrated renal impairment is most likely to become clinically evident, as assessed by increasing serum creatinine, during the second week of induction therapy at 60 mg/kg TID (see Pharmacodynamics). Renal impairment, however, may occur at any time in any patient during FOSCAVIR treatment and renal function should therefore be monitored especially carefully (see PATIENT MONITORING).
Elevations in serum creatinine are usually, but not uniformly, reversible following discontinuation or dose adjustment of FOSCAVIR. In the U.S. studies, recovery of renal function after FOSCAVIR-induced impairment usually occurred within one week of drug discontinuation. However, of 35 patients in the U.S. controlled clinical studies who experienced grade II renal impairment (serum creatinine 2–3 times the upper limit of normal), two died with renal failure within four weeks of stopping FOSCAVIR, and three others died with renal insufficiency still present less than four weeks after the drug cessation.
BECAUSE OF FOSCAVIR'S POTENTIAL TO CAUSE RENAL IMPAIRMENT, DOSE ADJUSTMENT FOR DECREASED BASELINE RENAL FUNCTION AND ANY CHANGE IN RENAL FUNCTION DURING TREATMENT IS NECESSARY. In addition, it may be beneficial for adequate hydration to be established (e.g. by inducing diuresis) prior to and during FOSCAVIR administration.

Mineral and Electrolyte Imbalances:
FOSCAVIR has been associated with changes in serum electrolytes including hypocalcemia (15%), hypophosphatemia (8%) and hyperphosphatemia (6%), hypomagnesemia (15%), and hypokalemia (16%). Administration of FOSCAVIR has been shown to be associated with a transient, dose-related decrease in ionized serum calcium, which may not be reflected in total serum calcium. This effect most likely is re-

TABLE 3

Mean ±SD Dose mg/kg* (Infusion Time)	Day of Sampling	Mean Plasma Concentration (μM) CMAX**[range]	CMIN***[range]
FOS-01			
57±6 q 8 hr (1 hour)	1	573 [213–1305]	78 [< 33–139]
47±12 q 8 hr (1 hour)	14 or 15	579 [246–922]	110 [< 33–148]
ACTG-015			
55±6 q 8 hr (2 hours)	3	445 [306–720]	88 [< 33–162]
57 ±7 q 8 hr (2 hours)	14 or 15	517 [348–789]	105 [43–205]

* Planned dose = 60 mg/kg q8hr in both studies.
** Observed Maximum Concentration:
FOS-01:
Day 1 (N = 14): Observed 0.9–2.0 hr after start of infusion.
Day 14/15 (N = 10); Observed 0.8–1.3 hr after start of infusion.
ACTG-015:
Day 3 (N = 12): Observed 1.8–2.4 hr after start of infusion.
Day 14/15 (N = 12): Observed 1.7–2.6 hr after start of infusion.
*** Observed Minimum Concentration:
FOS-01:
Day 1 (N = 13): Observed 4–8 hr after start of infusion.
(Mean represents 5/13 observations, 8/13 < 33 μM)
Day 14/15 (N = 10): Observed 6.3–8 hr after start of infusion.
(Mean represents 9/10 observations, 1/10 < 33 μM)
ACTG-015:
Day 3 (N = 12): Observed 7.8–8.1 hr after start of infusion.
(Mean represents 9/12 observations, 3/12 < 33 μM)
Day 14/15 (N = 12): Observed 6.4–8.7 hr after start of infusion.
(Means represents 12/12 observations)

lated to foscarnet's chelation of divalent metal ions such as calcium. Therefore, patients should be advised to report symptoms of low ionized calcium such as perioral tingling, numbness in the extremities and paresthesias. Physicians should be prepared to treat these as well as severe manifestations of electrolyte abnormalities such as tetany and seizures. The rate of FOSCAVIR infusion may affect the transient decrease in ionized calcium. Slowing the rate may decrease or prevent symptoms.

Transient changes in calcium or other electrolytes (including magnesium, potassium or phosphate) may also contribute to a patient's risk for cardiac disturbances and seizures (see below). Therefore, particular caution is advised in patients with altered calcium or other electrolyte levels before treatment, especially those with neurologic or cardiac abnormalities and those receiving other drugs known to influence minerals and electrolytes (see PATIENT MONITORING and Drug Interactions).

Neurotoxicity and Seizures:
FOSCAVIR treatment has been associated with seizures in 18/189 (10%) of AIDS patients in five controlled studies. Three patients were not taking FOSCAVIR at the time of seizure. In most cases (15/18), the patients had an active CNS condition (e.g., toxoplasmosis, HIV encephalopathy) or a history of CNS diseases. The rate of seizures did not increase with duration of treatment. These cases were associated with overdose of FOSCAVIR (see OVERDOSAGE).

A logistic regression analysis was performed comparing the 18 patients in these five studies who had seizures with the 161 who did not. Statistically significant ($p < 0.05$) risk factors associated with seizures were low baseline absolute neutrophil count (ANC), impaired baseline renal function, and low total serum calcium. Several cases of seizures were associated with death. However, occurrence of seizures did not always necessitate discontinuation of FOSCAVIR; ten of fifteen patients with seizures that occurred while receiving the drug continued or resumed FOSCAVIR following treatment of their underlying disease, electrolyte disturbances, and/or dose decreases. If factors predisposing a patient to seizures are present, electrolytes, including calcium and magnesium, must be monitored especially carefully (see PATIENT MONITORING).

PRECAUTIONS
General:
In controlled clinical studies with FOSCAVIR, the maximum single dose administered was 120 mg/kg by intravenous infusion over 2 hours. It is likely that larger doses, or more rapid infusions, would result in increased toxicity. Care must be taken to infuse solutions containing FOSCAVIR only into veins with adequate blood flow to permit rapid dilution and distribution, and avoid local irritation (see DOSAGE AND ADMINISTRATION). Local irritation and ulcerations of penile epithelium have been reported in male patients receiving FOSCAVIR, possibly related to the presence of drug in urine. One case of vulvovaginal ulcerations in a female receiving FOSCAVIR has been reported. Adequate hydration with close attention to personal hygiene may minimize the occurrence of such events.

Hemopoietic System:
Anemia has been reported in 33% of patients receiving FOSCAVIR in controlled studies. This anemia was usually manageable with transfusions and required discontinuation of FOSCAVIR in less than 1% (1/189) of patients in the studies. Granulocytopenia has been reported in 17% of patients receiving FOSCAVIR in controlled studies; however, only 1% (2/189) were terminated from these studies because of neutropenia.

Information for Patients:
Patients should be advised that FOSCAVIR is not a cure for CMV retinitis, and that they may continue to experience progression of retinitis during or following treatment. They should be advised to have regular ophthalmologic examinations. They should be informed that the major toxicities of foscarnet are renal impairment, electrolyte disturbances, and seizures, and that dose modifications and possibly discontinuation may be required. The importance of close monitoring while on therapy must be emphasized. Patients should be advised of the importance of perioral tingling, numbness in the extremities or paresthesias during or after infusion as possible symptoms of electrolyte abnormalities. Should such symptoms occur, the infusion of FOSCAVIR should be stopped, appropriate laboratory samples for assessment of electrolyte concentrations obtained, and a physician consulted before resuming treatment. The rate of infusion must be no more than 1 mg/kg/minute. The potential for renal impairment may be minimized by accompanying FOSCAVIR administration with hydration adequate to establish and maintain a diuresis during dosing.

Drug Interactions:
Coadministration of FOSCAVIR with other drugs could theroretically alter its antiviral activity, toxicity, or pharmacokinetics.

A possible drug interaction of FOSCAVIR and intravenous pentamidine has been described. Concomitant treatment of four patients in the United Kingdom with FOSCAVIR and intravenous pentamidine may have caused hypocalcemia; one patient died with severe hypocalcemia. Toxicity associated with concomitant use of aerosolized pentamidine has not been reported.

The elimination of foscarnet may be impaired by drugs that inhibit renal tubular secretion; however, no studies have been conducted to determine whether this occurs. Nonetheless because of foscarnet's tendency to cause renal impairment, the use of FOSCAVIR should be avoided in combination with potentially nephrotoxic drugs such as aminoglycosides, amphotericin B and intravenous pentamidine (see above) unless the potential benefits outweigh the risks to the patient.

Since FOSCAVIR decreases serum levels of ionized calcium, concurrent treatment with other drugs known to influence serum calcium levels should be used with particular caution. FOSCAVIR was used concomitantly with zidovudine in approximately one-third of patients in the U.S. studies. Although the combination was generally well tolerated, additive effects on anemia may have occurred. In one study of 24 patients (FOS-03), anemia was reported as an adverse event in 60% (3/5) patients receiving FOSCAVIR only, 88% (7/8) of patients receiving both zidovudine and FOSCAVIR, 29% (2/7) of patients receiving only zidovudine and 25% (1/4) of patients receiving neither drug. However, no evidence of increased myelosuppression was seen with FOSCAVIR in combination with zidovudine.

Carcinogenesis, Mutagenesis, Impairment of Fertility:
Carcinogenicity studies were conducted in rats and mice at oral doses of 500 mg/kg/day and 250 mg/kg/day. Oral bioavailability in unfasted rodents is <20%. No evidence of oncogenicity was reported at plasma drug levels equal to $\frac{1}{3}$ and $\frac{1}{5}$, respectively, of those in humans (at the maximum recommended human daily dose) as measured by the area-under-the-time/concentration curve (AUC).

FOSCAVIR showed genotoxic effects in the BALB/3T3 *in vitro* transformation assay at concentrations greater than 0.5 mcg/mL and an increased frequency of chromosome aberrations in the sister chromatid exchange assay at 1000 mcg/mL. A high dose of foscarnet (350 mg/kg) caused an increase in micronucleated polychromatic erythrocytes *in vivo* in mice at doses that produced exposures (Area Under Curve) comparable to that anticipated clinically.

Pregnancy: Teratogenic Effect:
Pregnancy, Category C:
FOSCAVIR did not adversely affect fertility and general reproductive performance in rats. The results of peri- and post-natal studies in rats were also negative. However, these studies used exposures that are inadequate to define the potential for impairment of fertility at human drug exposure levels.

Daily subcutaneous doses up to 75 mg/kg administered to female rats prior to and during mating, during gestation, and 21 days post-partum caused a slight increase (<5%) in the number of skeletal anomalies compared with the control group. Daily subcutaneous doses up to 75 mg/kg administered to rabbits and 150 mg/kg administered to rats during gestation caused an increase in the frequency of skeletal anomalies/variations.

On the basis of estimated drug exposure (as measured by AUC), the 150 mg/kg dose in rats and 75 mg/kg dose in rabbits were approximately one-eighth (rat) and one-third (rabbit) the estimated maximal daily human exposure. These studies are inadequate to define the potential teratogenicity at levels to which women will be exposed. There are no adequate and well controlled studies in pregnant women. Because animal reproductive studies are not always predictive of human response, FOSCAVIR should be used during pregnancy only if clearly needed.

Nursing Mothers:
It is not known whether FOSCAVIR is excreted in human milk; however, in lactating rats administered 75 mg/kg, FOSCAVIR was excreted in maternal milk at concentrations three times higher than peak maternal blood concentrations. Because many drugs are excreted in human milk, caution should be exercised if FOSCAVIR is administered to a nursing woman.

Pediatric Use:
The safety and effectiveness of FOSCAVIR in children have not been studied. FOSCAVIR is deposited in teeth and bone and deposition is greater in young and growing animals. FOSCAVIR has been demonstrated to adversely affect development of tooth enamel in mice and rats. The effects of this deposition on skeletal development have not been studied. Since deposition in human bone also occurs, it is likely that it does so to a greater degree in developing bone in children. Administration to children should be undertaken only after careful evaluation and only if the potential benefits for treatment outweigh the risks.

Use in the Elderly:
No studies of the efficacy or safety of FOSCAVIR in persons over age 65 have been conducted. Since these individuals frequently have reduced glomerular filtration, particular attention should be paid to assessing renal function before and during FOSCAVIR administration (see DOSAGE AND ADMINISTRATION).

ADVERSE REACTIONS
In five controlled U.S. clinical trials in which 189 patients with AIDS and CMV retinitis were treated with FOSCAVIR, the most frequently reported events were the following: fever 65% (123/189), nausea 47% (88/189), anemia 33% (63/189), diarrhea 30% (57/189), abnormal renal function including acute renal failure, decreased creatinine clearance and increased serum creatinine 27% (51/189), vomiting 26% (50, 189), headache 26% (49/189), and seizure 10% (18/189) (see WARNINGS and PRECAUTIONS). These incidence figures were calculated without reference to drug relationship or severity.

From the same controlled studies, adverse events categorized by investigator as "severe" were death (14%), abnormal renal function (14%), marrow suppression (10%), anemia (9%), and seizures (7%). Although death was specifically attributed to FOSCAVIR in only one case, other complications of foscarnet (i.e., renal impairment, electrolyte abnormalities, and seizures) may have contributed to patient deaths (see WARNINGS and PRECAUTIONS).

The types and incidences of adverse events reported worldwide with FOSCAVIR have not been different from, or greater in frequency, than those observed in the U.S. trials. From the five U.S. controlled clinical trials of FOSCAVIR, the following list of adverse events has been compiled regardless of casual relationship to FOSCAVIR. Evaluation of these reports was difficult because of the diverse manifestations of the underlying disease and because most patients received numerous concomitant medications.

Incidence 5% or Greater
Body as a Whole: fever, fatigue, rigors, asthenia, malaise, pain, infection, sepsis, death
Central and Peripheral Nervous System: headache, paresthesia, dizziness, involuntary muscle contractions, hypoesthesia, neuropathy, seizures including grand mal seizures (see WARNINGS)
Gastrointestinal System: anorexia, nausea, diarrhea, vomiting, abdominal pain
Hematologic: anemia, granulocytopenia, leukopenia (see PRECAUTIONS)
Metabolic and Nutritional: mineral and electrolyte imbalances (see WARNINGS) including hypokalemia, hypocalcemia, hypomagnesemia, hypophosphatemia, hyperphosphatemia
Psychiatric: depression, confusion, anxiety
Respiratory System: coughing, dyspnea
Skin and Appendages: rash, increased sweating
Urinary: alterations in renal function including increased serum creatinine, decreased creatinine clearance, and abnormal renal function (see WARNINGS)
Special Senses: vision abnormalities

Incidence between 1% and 5%
Application Site: injection site pain, injection site inflammation
Body as a Whole: back pain, chest pain, edema, influenza-like symptoms, bacterial infections, moniliasis, fungal infections, abscess
Cardiovascular: hypertension, palpitations, ECG abnormalities including sinus tachycardia, first degree AV block and non-specific ST-T segment changes, hypotension, flushing, cerebrovascular disorder (see WARNINGS)
Central and Peripheral Nervous System: tremor, ataxia, dementia, stupor, generalized spasms, sensory disturbances, meningitis, aphasia, abnormal coordination, leg cramps, EEG abnormalities (see WARNINGS)
Gastrointestinal: constipation, dysphagia, dyspepsia, rectal hemorrhage, dry mouth, melena, flatulence, ulcerative stomatitis, pancreatitis
Hematologic: thrombocytopenia, platelet abnormalities, thrombosis, white blood cell abnormalities, lymphadenopathy
Liver and Biliary: abnormal A-G ratio, abnormal hepatic function, increased SGPT, increased SGOT
Metabolic and Nutritional: hyponatremia, decreased weight, increased alkaline phosphatase, increased LDH, increased BUN, acidosis, cachexia, thirst, hypercalcemia (see WARNINGS)
Musculo-Skeletal: arthralgia, myalgia
Neoplasms: lymphoma-like disorder, sarcoma
Psychiatric: insomnia, somnolence, nervousness, amnesia, agitation, aggressive reaction, hallucination
Respiratory System: pneumonia, sinusitis, pharyngitis, rhinitis, respiratory disorders, respiratory insufficiency, pulmonary infiltration, stridor, pneumothorax, hemoptysis, bronchospasm
Skin and Appendages: pruritus, skin ulceration, seborrhea, erythematous rash, maculo-papular rash, skin discoloration
Special Senses: taste perversions, eye abnormalities, eye pain, conjunctivitis
Urinary System: albuminuria, dysuria, polyuria, urethral disorder, urinary retention, urinary tract infections, acute renal failure, nocturia, facial edema

Continued on next page

Astra—Cont.

Incidence less than 1%

Body as a Whole: hypothermia, leg edema, peripheral edema, syncope, ascites, substernal chest pain, abnormal crying, malignant hyperpyrexia, herpes simplex, viral infection, toxoplasmosis

Cardiovascular: cardiomyopathy, cardiac failure, cardiac arrest, bradycardia, extrasystole, arrhythmias, atrial arrhythmias, atrial fibrillation, phlebitis, superficial thrombophlebitis of the arm, mesenteric vein thrombophlebitis

Central and Peripheral Nervous System: vertigo, coma, encephalopathy, abnormal gait, hyperesthesia, hypertonia, visual field defects, dyskinesia, extrapyramidal disorders, hemiparesis, hyperkinesia, vocal cord paralysis, paralysis, paraplegia, speech disorders, tetany, hyporeflexia, neuralgia, neuritis, peripheral neuropathy, hyperreflexia, cerebral edema, nystagmus

Endocrine: antidiuretic hormone disorders, decreased gonadotropins, gynecomastia

Gastrointestinal System: enteritis, enterocolitis, glossitis, proctitis, stomatitis, tenesmus, increased amylase, pseudomembranous colitis, gastroenteritis, oral leukoplakia, oral hemorrhage, rectal disorders, colitis, duodenal ulcer, hematemesis, paralytic ileus, esophageal ulceration, ulcerative proctitis, tongue ulceration

Hematologic: pulmonary embolism, coagulation disorders, decreased coagulation factors, epistaxis, decreased prothrombin, hypochromic anemia, pancytopenia, hemolysis, leukocytosis, cervical lymphadenopathy, lymphopenia

Special Senses: deafness, earache, tinnitus, otitis

Liver and Biliary System: cholecystitis, cholelithiasis, hepatitis, cholestatic hepatitis, hepatosplenomegaly, jaundice

Metabolic and Nutritional: dehydration, glycosuria, increased creatine phosphokinase, diabetes mellitus, abnormal glucose tolerance, hypervolemia, hypochloremia, periorbital edema, hypoproteinemia

Musculo-Skeletal System: arthrosis, synovitis, torticollis

Neoplasms: malignant lymphoma, skin hypertrophy

Psychiatric: impaired concentration, emotional lability, psychosis, suicide attempt, delirium, personality disorders, sleep disorders

Reproductive: perineal pain in women, penile inflammation

Respiratory System: bronchitis, laryngitis, respiratory depression, abnormal chest x-ray, pleural effusion, lobar pneumonia, pulmonary hemorrhage, pneumonitis

Skin and Appendages: acne, alopecia, dermatitis, anal pruritis, genital pruritis, aggravated psoriasis, psoriaform rash, skin disorders, dry skin, urticaria, verruca

Urinary System: hematuria, glomerulonephritis, micturition disorders, micturition frequency, toxic nephropathy, nephrosis, urinary incontinence, renal tubular disorders, pyelonephritis, urethral irritation, uremia

Special Senses: diplopia, blindness, retinal detachment, mydriasis, photophobia

OVERDOSAGE

In controlled clinical trials performed in the United States, overdosage with FOSCAVIR was reported in 10 patients. All 10 patients experienced adverse events and all except one made a complete recovery. One patient died after receiving a total daily dose of 12.5 g for three days instead of the intended 10.9 g. The patient suffered a grand mal seizure and become comatose. Three days later the patient expired with the cause of death listed as respiratory/cardiac arrest. The other nine patients received doses ranging from 1.14 times to 8 times their recommended doses with an average of 4 times their recommended doses. Overall, three patients had seizures, three patients had renal function impairment, four patients had paresthesis either in limbs or periorally, and five patients had documented electrolyte disturbances primarily involving calcium and phosphate.

There is no specific antidote for FOSCAVIR overdose. Hemodialysis and hydration may be of benefit in reducing drug plasma levels in patients who receive an overdosage of FOSCAVIR, but these have not been evaluated in a clinical trial setting. The patient should be observed for signs and symptoms of renal impairment and electrolyte imbalance. Medical treatment should be instituted if clinically warranted.

DOSAGE AND ADMINISTRATION

CAUTION—DO NOT ADMINISTER FOSCAVIR BY RAPID OR BOLUS INTRAVENOUS INJECTION. THE TOXICITY OF FOSCAVIR MAY BE INCREASED AS A RESULT OF EXCESSIVE PLASMA LEVELS. CARE SHOULD BE TAKEN TO AVOID UNINTENTIONAL OVERDOSE BY CAREFULLY CONTROLLING THE RATE OF INFUSION. THEREFORE, AN INFUSION PUMP MUST BE USED. IN SPITE OF THE USE OF AN INFUSION PUMP, OVERDOSES HAVE OCCURRED.

ADMINISTRATION

FOSCAVIR is administered by controlled intravenous infusion, either by using a central venous line or by using a peripheral vein. The standard 24 mg/mL solution may be used without dilution when using a central venous catheter for infusion. When a peripheral vein catheter is used, the 24 mg/mL soluton must be diluted to 12 mg/mL with 5% dextrose in water or with a normal saline solution prior to administration to avoid local irritation of peripheral veins. Since the dose of FOSCAVIR is calculated on the basis of body weight, it may be desirable to remove and discard any unneeded quantity from the bottle before starting with the infusion to avoid overdosage. Dilutions and/or removals of excess quantities should be accomplished under aseptic conditions. Solutions thus prepared should be used within 24 hours of first entry into a sealed bottle.

Other drugs and supplements can be administered to a patient receiving FOSCAVIR. However, care must be taken to ensure that FOSCAVIR is only administered with normal saline or 5% dextrose solution and that no other drug or supplement is administered concurrently via the same catheter. Foscarnet has been reported to be chemically incompatible with 30% dextrose, amphotericin B, and solutions containing calcium such as Ringer's lactate and TPN. Physical incompatibility with other IV drugs has also been reported including acyclovir sodium, ganciclovir, trimetrexate glucuronate, pentamidine isethionate, vancomycin, trimethoprim/sulfamethoxazole, diazepam, midazolam, digoxin, phenytoin, leucovorin, and prochlorperazine. Because of foscarnet's chelating properties, a precipitate can potentially occur when divalent cations are administered concurrently in the same catheter.

Parenteral drug products must be inspected visually for particulate matter and discoloration prior to administration whenever the soluton and container permit. Solutions that are discolored or contain particulate matter should not be used.

DOSAGE

THE RECOMMENDED DOSAGE, FREQUENCY, OR INFUSION RATES SHOULD NOT BE EXCEEDED. ALL DOSES MUST BE INDIVIDUALIZED FOR PATIENTS' RENAL FUNCTION.

Induction Treatment:

The recommended initial dose of FOSCAVIR for patients with normal renal function is 60 mg/kg, adjusted for individual patients' renal function, given intravenously at a constant rate over a minimum of one hour every 8 hours for 2–3 weeks depending on clinical response. An infusion pump must be used to control the rate of infusion. Adequate hydration is recommended to establish a diuresis, both prior to and during treatment to minimize renal toxicity (see WARNINGS), provided there are no clinical contraindications.

Maintenance Treatment:

Following induction treatment the recommended maintenance dose of FOSCAVIR is 90 mg/kg/day to 120 mg/kg/day (individualized for renal function) given as an intravenous infusion over 2 hours. Because the superiority of the 120 mg/kg/day has not been established in controlled trials, and given the likely relationship of higher plasma foscarnet levels to toxicity, it is recommended that most patients be started on maintenance treatment with a dose of 90 mg/kg/day. Escalation to 120 mg/kg/day may be considered should early reinduction be required because of retinitis progression. Some patients who show excellent tolerance to FOSCAVIR may benefit from initiation of maintenance treatment at 120 mg/kg/day earlier in their treatment. An infusion pump must be used to control the rate of infusion with all doses. Again, hydration to establish diuresis both prior to and during treatment is recommended to minimize renal toxicity, provided there are no clinical contraindications (see WARNINGS).

Patients who experience progression of retinitis while receiving FOSCAVIR maintenance therapy may be retreated with the induction and maintenance regimens given above.

Use in Patients with Abnormal Renal Function:

FOSCAVIR should be used with caution in patients with abnormal renal function because reduced plasma clearance of foscarnet will result in elevated plasma levels (see CLINICAL PHARMACOLOGY). In addition, FOSCAVIR has the potential to further impair renal function (see WARNINGS). FOSCAVIR has not been specifically studied in patients with creatinine clearances <50 mL/min or serum creatinines >2.8 mg/dL. Renal function must be monitored carefully at baseline and during induction and maintenance therapy with appropriate dose adjustments for FOSCAVIR as outlined below (see Dose Adjustment and PATIENT MONITORING). During FOSCAVIR therapy if creatinine clearance falls below the limits of the dosing nomograms (0.4 mL/min/kg), FOSCAVIR should be discontinued and the patient monitored daily until resolution of renal impairment is ensured.

Dose Adjustment:

FOSCAVIR dosing must be individualized according to the patient's renal function status. Refer to TABLE 4 below for recommended doses and adjust the dose as indicated.

To use this dosing guide, actual 24-hour creatinine clearance (mL/min) must be divided by body weight (kg), or the estimated creatinine clearance in mL/min/kg can be calculated from serum creatinine (mg/dL) using the following formula (modified Cockcroft and Gault equation):

For males:

$$\frac{140 - \text{age}}{\text{serum creatinine} \times 72} \quad (\times\ 0.85 \text{ for females})$$

TABLE 4
FOSCAVIR DOSING GUIDE
Induction

CrCl mL/min/kg	Equivalent to 60 mg/kg Dose Q8H
≥1.6	60
1.5	57
1.4	53
1.3	49
1.2	46
1.1	42
1.0	39
0.9	35
0.8	32
0.7	28
0.6	25
0.5	21
0.4	18

Maintenance

CrCl (mL/min/kg)	Equivalent to 90 mg/kg Dose Q24H	Equivalent to 120 mg/kg Dose Q24H
≥1.4	90	120
1.2–1.4	78	104
1.0–1.2	75	100
0.8–1.0	71	94
0.6–0.8	63	84
0.4–0.6	57	76

PATIENT MONITORING

The majority of patients will experience some decrease in renal function due to FOSCAVIR administration. Therefore, it is recommended that creatinine clearance, either measured or estimated using the modified Cockcroft and Gault equation based on serum creatinine, be determined at baseline, 2–3 times per week during induction therapy and at least once every one to two weeks during maintenance therapy, with FOSCAVIR dose adjusted accordingly (see Dose Adjustment). More frequent monitoring may be required for some patients. It is also recommended that a 24-hour creatinine clearance be determined at baseline and periodically thereafter to ensure correct dosing (assuming verification of an adequate collection using creatinine index). FOSCAVIR should be discontinued if creatinine clearance drops below 0.4 mL/min/kg.

Due to FOSCAVIR's propensity to chelate divalent metal ions and alter levels of serum electrolytes, patients must be monitored closely for such changes. It is recommended that a schedule similar to that recommended for serum creatinine (see above) be used to monitor serum calcium, magnesium, potassium and phosphorus. Particular caution is advised in patients with decreased total serum calcium or other electrolyte levels before treatment, as well as patients with neurologic or cardiac abnormalities, and in patients receiving other drugs known to influence serum calcium levels. Any clinically significant metabolic changes should be corrected. Also patients who experience mild (e.g., perioral numbness or paresthesias) or severe (e.g., seizures) symptoms of electrolyte abnormalities should have serum electrolyte and mineral levels assessed as close in time to the event as possible.

Careful monitoring and appropriate management of electrolytes, calcium, magnesium and creatinine are of particular importance in patients with conditions that may predispose them to seizures (see WARNINGS).

HOW SUPPLIED

FOSCAVIR (foscarnet sodium) INJECTION, 24 mg/mL for intravenous infusion, is supplied in glass bottles as follows:

NDC 0186-1906-01 500 mL bottles, cases of 12
NDC 0186-1905-01 250 mL bottles, cases of 12

FOSCAVIR INJECTION should be stored at controlled room temperature 15°–30°C (59°–86°F), and should be protected from excessive heat (above 40°C) and from freezing. FOSCAVIR INJECTION should be used only if the bottle and seal are intact, a vacuum is present, and the solution is clear and colorless.

Caution: Federal law prohibits dispensing without prescription.

Manufactured by:
Abbott Laboratories
North Chicago, IL 60064
Manufactured for:
ASTRA®
Astra Pharmaceutical Products, Inc.
Westborough, MA 01581
21662ROO Iss. 9/91

FUROSEMIDE INJECTION, USP

℞

[fū"rō'sĕ-mīde]
10 mg/mL

PROTECT FROM LIGHT ● DO NOT USE IF THE SOLUTION IS DISCOLORED ● STORE AT CONTROLLED ROOM TEMPERATURE

WARNING: Furosemide is a potent diuretic which, if given in excessive amounts, can lead to a profound diuresis with water and electrolyte depletion. Therefore, careful medical supervision is required, and the individual dose and the dosage schedule have to be adjusted to each patient's needs. (See under "DOSAGE AND ADMINISTRATION")

(For details of indications, dosage, and administration, precautions, and adverse reactions, see circular in package.)

HOW SUPPLIED

Furosemide injection, USP, 10 mg/mL is supplied in the following forms:

Single Dose Vials:
2 mL (20 mg), 25 per package, NDC 0186-1114-13
4 mL (40 mg), 25 per package, NDC 0186-1115-13
8 mL (80 mg), 25 per package, NDC 0186-1116-12
10 mL (100 mg), 25 per package, NDC 0186-1117-12
Prefilled Syringes:
4 mL (40 mg), NDC 0186-0635-01
10 mL (100 mg), NDC 0186-0636-01
Syringes supplied with 21 gauge × $^{15}/_{16}$" needle.
All solutions should be stored at controlled room temperature 15°–30°C (59°–86°F) and should be protected from light. Do not use if the solution is discolored. .
021877R07   3/92 (7)

HEMOPAD®

℞

[hē'mō-pǎd]
Absorbable Collagen Hemostat

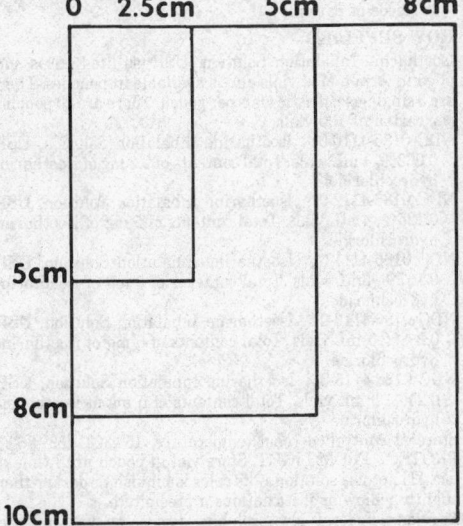

DESCRIPTION

HEMOPAD® Absorbable Collagen Hemostat is a purified bovine collagen. The material, prepared as a textured pad, is sterile, nonpyrogenic, and absorbable. Hemostatic activity, which is an inherent property of collagen, is largely dependent on the basic helical structure of this protein. The helical structure of native collagen is preserved during the manufacture of HEMOPAD Hemostat. When collagen comes into contact with blood, platelets aggregate on the collagen and release coagulation factors which, together with plasma factors result in the formation of fibrin, and finally in the formation of a clot.

INDICATIONS

HEMOPAD is indicated in surgical procedures (other than in neurological, urological and ophthalmological surgery) for use as an adjunct to hemostasis when control of bleeding by ligature or other conventional methods is ineffective or impractical.

CONTRAINDICATIONS

HEMOPAD is contraindicated in the closure of skin incisions as it may interfere with the healing of skin edges. This interference is due to simple mechanical interposition of dry collagen and not due to any intrinsic interference with wound healing.

HEMOPAD is contraindicated on bone surfaces to which prosthetic materials are to be attached with methylmethacrylate adhesives. It has been reported with another absorb-

able collagen hemostat, that by filling porosities of cancellous bone, collagen may reduce the bonding strength of methylmethacrylate.

WARNINGS

HEMOPAD is inactivated by autoclaving. It should not be resterilized. As with any foreign substance, use in contaminated wounds may enhance infection.

HEMOPAD should not be used in instances of pumping arterial hemorrhage.

HEMOPAD should not be used where blood or other fluids have pooled or in cases where the point of hemorrhage is submerged. HEMOPAD will not act as a tampon or plug in a bleeding site nor will it close off an area of blood collecting behind a tampon.

Only the amount of HEMOPAD necessary to provide hemostasis should be used. The long-term effects of leaving HEMOPAD *in situ* are unknown. Opened, unused HEMOPAD should be discarded because it cannot be resterilized.

PRECAUTIONS

As with other hemostatic agents, it is not recommended that HEMOPAD be left in an infected nor contaminated space, nor is it recommended for use in persons known to be sensitive to material of bovine origin. When placed into cavities or closed spaces, care should be exercised to avoid overpacking HEMOPAD as it may absorb fluid and expand and press against neighboring structures.

Safety of this product has not been established in children and pregnant women: therefore, HEMOPAD should only be used when benefit to risk clearly warrants its use.

HEMOPAD is not intended to be used to treat systemic coagulation disorders.

ADVERSE REACTIONS

HEMOPAD is a collagen product. Although several types of post-operative complications were observed in HEMOPAD treated patients, none were attributed to HEMOPAD by the investigator. Adverse reactions reported for other collagen hemostats include hematoma, potentiation of infection, wound dehiscence, inflammation and edema. Other reported adverse reactions that may be related to the use of collagen hemostats include adhesion formation, allergic reaction, foreign body reaction and subgaleal seroma (in a single case). The use of microfibrillar collagen in dental extraction sockets has been reported to increase the incidence of alveolalgia. The possibility that all of the above reactions may occur with HEMOPAD cannot be excluded.

ADMINISTRATION

HEMOPAD is applied directly to the bleeding surface with pressure. HEMOPAD can be cut to size. The amount needed and the period of time necessary to apply pressure will vary with the type and amount of bleeding to be controlled. Hemostasis time depends upon the type of surgery and degree of pretreatment bleeding. It usually occurred between 2 to 6 minutes with HEMOPAD.

HEMOPAD maintains its integrity in the presence of blood and is not dispersed when wet. It is easily removed from the site following hemostatsis. It is most effective when used dry. HEMOPAD may be left *in situ* whenever necessary. However, the surgeon, at his discretion, should remove any excess of HEMOPAD prior to wound closure. Animal implant studies have demonstrated that absorption and tissue reaction to HEMOPAD are similar to those observed with another absorbable collagen hemostatic agent.

CLINICAL STUDIES

The safety, effectiveness and handling characteristics of HEMOPAD Collagen Absorbable Hemostat were evaluated in a variety of surgical procedures. The average time to hemostasis for HEMOPAD was 4.4 minutes. Passive Hemagglutination Assay (PHA) and Enzyme-Linked Immunoabsorbent Assay (ELISA) methods have been used to evaluate the immunological potential for HEMOPAD to produce antibodies in animals. These assays revealed little if any elevation of antibody titers in HEMOPAD treated animals while in animals treated with a collagen control hemostat, mild elevation of antibodies occurred. The handling properties of HEMOPAD were judged superior to those of the collagen control hemostat.

HOW SUPPLIED

HEMOPAD is supplied in a nonwoven form in peelable plastic pouches in the following sizes:
2.5cm × 5cm IN BOXES OF 10
                                PRODUCT No. 0166-2001-00
5cm × 8cm IN BOXES OF 10
                                PRODUCT No. 0186-2002-00
8cm × 10cm IN BOXES OF 10
                                PRODUCT No. 0186-2003-00
The sterility of the product is guaranteed unless the individual envelope is damaged or opened.

CAUTION: Federal (U.S.A.) law restricts this device to sale, distribution, and use by or on the order of a physician.

HEMOPAD is manufactured by DATASCOPE CORP.
021873 R00   Rev. 12/87

HEMOTENE™

℞

[hē'mō-tēēn]

DESCRIPTION

HEMOTENE™ Absorbable Collagen Hemostat is a purified bovine collagen. The material is sterile, non pyrogenic, and absorbable. Hemostatic activity, which is an inherent property of collagen, is largely dependent on the basic helical structure of this protein. The helical structure of native collagen is preserved during the manufacture of HEMOTENE Hemostat. When collagen comes into contact with blood, platelets aggregate on the collagen and release coagulation factors which, together with the plasma factors result in the formulation of fibrin, and finally in the formation of a clot.

INDICATIONS

HEMOTENE is indicated in surgical procedures (other than in neurological, urological and ophthalmological surgery) for use as an adjunct to hemostasis when control of bleeding by ligature or other conventional method is ineffective or impractical.

CONTRAINDICATIONS

HEMOTENE is contraindicated in the closure of skin incisions as it may interfere with the healing of skin edges. This interference is due to simple mechanical interposition of dry collagen and not due to any intrinsic interference with wound healing.

HEMOTENE is contraindicated on bone surfaces to which prosthetic materials are to be attached with methylmethacrylate adhesives. It has been reported with another absorbable collagen hemostat, that by filling porosities of cancellous bone, collagen may reduce the bonding strength of methylmethacrylate.

WARNINGS

HEMOTENE is inactivated by autoclaving. It should not be resterilized. As with any foreign substance, use in contaminated wounds may enhance infection.

HEMOTENE should not be used in instances of pumping arterial hemorrhage.

HEMOTENE should not be used where blood or other fluids have pooled or in cases where the point of hemorrhage is submerged. HEMOTENE will not act as a tampon or plug in a bleeding site nor will it close off an area of blood collecting behind a tampon.

Only the amount of HEMOTENE necessary to provide hemostasis should be used. The long-term effects of leaving HEMOTENE *in-situ* are unknown. Opened, unused HEMOTENE should be discarded because it cannot be resterilized.

PRECAUTIONS

As with other hemostatic agents, it is not recommended that HEMOTENE be left in an infected or contaminated space, nor is it recommended for use in persons known to be sensitive to material of bovine origin. When placed into cavities or closed spaces, care should be exercised to avoid overpacking HEMOTENE as it may absorb fluid and expand and press against neighboring structures.

Safety of this product has not been established in children and pregnant women: therefore, HEMOTENE should only be used when benefit to risk clearly warrants its use.

HEMOTENE is not intended to be used to treat systemic coagulation disorders.

HEMOTENE may fragment when manipulated under water or saline producing small particles which can pass through filters commonly used on blood salvaging apparatus. This same fragmentation may also take place during surgery in applying the fibrillar material to the bleeding site. If a blood salvaging apparatus is used in such a case, these collagen fragments may pass through the filter in the apparatus and subsequently into the blood stream of the patient when the salvaged blood is returned. This may result in the formation of intravascular thrombi. Therefore, HEMOTENE should not be used in areas where use of a blood salvaging device is contemplated.

ADVERSE REACTIONS

HEMOTENE is a collagen product. Adverse reactions reported for other collagen hemostats include hematoma, potentiation of infection, wound dehiscence, inflammation and edema. Other reported adverse reactions that may be related to the use of collagen hemostats include adhesion formation, allergic reaction, foreign body reaction and subgaleal seroma (in a single case). The use of microfibrillar collagen in dental extraction sockets has been reported to increase the incidence of alveolalgia. The possibility that all of the above reactions may occur with HEMOTENE cannot be excluded.

Continued on next page

Astra—Cont.

ADMINISTRATION

HEMOTENE can be shaped by hand or instrument to the needs of the surgical site and is applied directly to the bleeding surface with pressure. The amount needed and the period of time necessary to apply pressure will vary with the type and amount of bleeding to be controlled. Hemostasis time depends upon the type of surgery and degree of pretreatment bleeding. It usually occurs between 2 to 6 minutes with HEMOTENE.

HEMOTENE may be left *in-situ* whenever necessary. However, the surgeon, at his discretion may remove any excess HEMOTENE prior to wound closure.

HOW SUPPLIED

HEMOTENE is supplied in a non-compressed form in plastic containers in the following size: 1 gram in boxes of 5, Product No. 0186-2005-02.

The sterility of the product is guaranteed unless the individual container is damaged or opened.

CAUTION

Federal (U.S.A.) law restricts this device to sale, distribution, and use by or on the order of a physician.

Hemotene is manufactured by Datascope Corp.
for
Astra Pharmaceutical Products, Inc.
Westborough, MA 01581
021602R00   Iss. 7/91

HYDROMORPHONE HCL INJECTION   Ⓒ

(For details of indications, dosages and administration, precautions, and adverse reactions, see circular in package.)

HOW SUPPLIED

2 mg/mL—20 mL multiple dose vials—NDC 0186-1309-01
Storage: Store at 59°–86°F (15°–30°C). Protect from light.
021888R01   11/91 (1)

ISOETHARINE INHALATION   ℞
Solution, USP
Arm a Med®
**0.062%, 0.125%, 0.167%,
0.2%, and 0.25%**

DESCRIPTION

Isoetharine Inhalation Solution, USP (sulfite-free) is a sterile solution for oral inhalation packaged in plastic vials for single use. Each vial contains isoetharine hydrochloride 0.062%, 0.125%, 0.167%, 0.2% or 0.25% in a sterile aqueous solution containing water for injection, sodium chloride, absorbic acid, etetate disodium and hydrochloric acid. The solution is filled under nitrogen. The solution is for use in aerosol bronchodilator therapy employing oxygen aerosolization or intermittent positive pressure breathing (IPPB). Isoetharine hydrochloride is a sympathomimetic amine and is chemically 3,4-dihydroxy-α-[1-(isopropylamino)propyl] benzyl alcohol hydrochloride, with the following structural formula:

$C_{13}H_{21}NO_3 \cdot HCl$ M.W.275.77

CLINICAL PHARMACOLOGY

Isoetharine is a sympathomimetic amine with preferential affinity for $Beta_2$ adrenergic receptor sites of bronchial and certain arteriolar musculature and a lower order of affinity for $Beta_1$ adrenergic receptors. Its activity in symptomatic relief of bronchospasm is rapid and of relatively long duration. By relieving bronchospasm, isoetharine helps give prompt relief and significantly increases FVC, FEV_1, and FEF 25%–75%.

Recent studies in laboratory animals (minipigs, rodents and dogs) recorded the occurrence of cardiac arrhythmias and sudden death (with histologic evidence of myocardial necrosis) when beta agonists and methylxanthines were administered concurrently. The significance of these findings when applied to human usage is currently unknown.

INDICATIONS AND USAGE

Isoetharine hydrochloride is indicated for use as a bronchodilator for bronchial asthma and for reversible bronchospasm that may occur in association with bronchitis and emphysema.

CONTRAINDICATIONS

Isoetharine inhalation solution should not be administered to patients who are hypersensitive to any of its components.

WARNINGS

Not for injection.

Excessive use of an adrenergic aerosol should be discouraged as it may lose its effectiveness. Occasional patients have been reported to develop severe paradoxical airway resistance with repeated excessive use of an aerosol adrenergic inhalation preparation. The cause of this refractory state is unknown. It is advisable that in such instances the use of the aerosol adrenergic be discontinued immediately and alternative therapy instituted, since in the reported cases the patients did not respond to other forms of therapy until the drug was withdrawn. Cardiac arrest has been noted in several instances.

Isoetharine should not be administered along with epinephrine or other sympathomimetic amines, since these drugs are direct cardiac stimulants and may cause excessive tachycardia. They may, however, be alternated if desired.

PRECAUTIONS

General: Dosage must be carefully adjusted in patients with hyperthyroidism, hypertension, acute coronary disease, cardiac asthma, limited cardiac reserve and in individuals sensitive to sympathomimetic amines since overdosage may result in tachycardia, palpitations, nausea, headache or epinephrine-like side effects.

Drug Interactions: Isoetharine should not be administered along with epinephrine or other sympathomimetic amines, since these drugs are direct cardiac stimulants and may cause excessive tachycardia. They may, however, be alternated if desired.

Carcinogenesis, Mutagenesis, Impairment of Fertility: Chronic toxicity studies up to twelve months in dogs with doses up to 20 mg/kg/day (equivalent to approximately 200 times the human dose based on a 70 kg individual) and chronic toxicity studies in rats with the doses up to 45 mg/kg/day (equivalent to approximately 450 times the human dose, based on a 70 kg individual) revealed no evidence of carcinogenicity due to isoetharine.

Pregnancy—Category C: Animal reproduction studies have not been conducted with isoetharine hydrochloride. It is also not known whether isoetharine hydrochloride can cause fetal harm when administered to a pregnant woman or can affect reproduction capacity, although there is no evidence of such harm or effects. Isoetharine hydrochloride should be given to a pregnant woman only if in the physician's judgment the potential benefit to the pregnant woman outweighs the risk to the fetus.

Nursing Mothers: It is not known whether this drug is excreted in human milk. Because many drugs are excreted in human milk, caution should be exercised when isoetharine hydrochloride is administered to a nursing woman.

Pediatric Use: The safety and efficacy of this product in children under the age of 12 have not been established.

ADVERSE REACTIONS

Although isoetharine hydrochloride is relatively free of toxic side effects, too frequent use may cause the following effects, as is the case with other sympathomimetic amines:

CNS Effects: headache, anxiety, tension, restlessness, insomnia, weakness, dizziness, excitement.

Cardiovascular Effects: tachycardia, palpitations, changes in blood pressure.

Gastrointestinal Effects: nausea.

Other: tremor, weakness.

OVERDOSAGE

Overdosage of isoetharine hydrochloride may produce signs and symptoms typical of excessive sympathomimetic effects, including tachycardia, palpitations, nausea, headache, blood pressure changes, anxiety, restlessness, insomnia, tremor, weakness, dizziness, and excitation. Excessive use of adrenergic aerosols may result in loss of effectiveness or severe paradoxical airway resistance. Cardiac arrest has been noted in several instances. In all cases of overdosage, the drug should be discontinued immediately and vital functions supported until the patient is stabilized. It is not known whether isoetharine hydrochloride is dialyzable.

The single dose amount of drug that may be toxic or life threatening is highly variable according to patient characteristics and drug history. The acute oral LD_{50} in mice is 1630 mg/kg of pure drug (isoetharine HCl).

DOSAGE AND ADMINISTRATION

Isoetharine hydrochloride is for oral inhalation only and can be administered by oxygen aerosolization or intermittent positive pressure breathing devices (IPPB). Usually, treatment need not be repeated more than every four hours, although in severe cases more frequent administration may be necessary.

Method of Administration	Usual Dose (1% Solution)*	Range
Oxygen aerosolization**	0.5 mL	0.25 to 0.5 mL
IPPB†	0.5 mL	0.25 to 1 mL

* The doses given are for the 1% solution which must be suitably diluted prior to administration. Below are the dose equivalents for the entire prediluted and ready-to-use product line:

Product Strength (%)	Volume (mL)	Equivalent to mL of Isoetharine HCl 1%
0.062%	4 mL	0.25 mL
0.125%	4 mL	0.5 mL
0.167%	3 mL	0.5 mL
0.2%	2.5 mL	0.5 mL
0.25%	2 mL	0.5 mL

** Administered with oxygen flow adjusted to 4 to 6 liters/minute over a period of 15 to 20 minutes.

† Usually an inspiratory flow rate of 15 liters/minute at a cycling pressure of 15 cm H_2O is recommended. It may be necessary, according to patient and type of IPPB apparatus, to adjust flow rate to 6 to 30 liters per minute, cycling pressure to 10–15 cm H_2O and further dilution according to needs of patient.

HOW SUPPLIED

Isoetharine Inhalation Solution, USP (sulfite-free) is supplied in Arm-a-Med vials and is available in pouches. There are 5 single-use, plastic vials per pouch. There are 20 pouches per carton of 100 vials.

NDC 0186-4110-01   Isoetharine Inhalation Solution, USP, 0.062%, 4 mL vials. Total contents of 2.5 mg of isoetharine hydrochloride.

NDC 0186-4112-01   Isoetharine Inhalation Solution, USP, 0.125%, 4 mL vials. Total contents of 5 mg of isoetharine hydrochloride.

NDC 0186-4111-01   Isoetharine Inhalation Solution, USP, 0.167%, 3mL vials. Total contents of 5 mg of isoetharine hydrochloride.

NDC 0186-4113-01   Isoetharine Inhalation Solution, USP, 0.2%, 2.5 mL vials. Total contents of 5 mg of isoetharine hydrochloride.

NDC 0186-4115-01   Isoetharine Inhalation Solution, USP, 0.25%, 2 mL vials. Total contents of 5 mg of isoetharine hydrochloride.

Store at controlled room temperature, 15°–30°C (59°–86°F). PROTECT FROM LIGHT. Store vial in pouch until time of use. Do not use solution if its color is pinkish or darker than slightly yellow or if it contains a precipitate.

Caution: Federal law prohibits dispensing without prescription.

Manufactured by:
Armour Pharmaceutical Company
Kankakee, Illinois 60901

021673R02   10/91(2)

MAGNESIUM SULFATE INJECTION, USP   ℞

(For details of indications, dosages and administration, precautions, and adverse reactions, see circular in package.)
[See table below.]

No preservative added. Unused portion of container should be discarded. Use only if solution is clear, and seal intact.
021874R01   2/88

NDC No. 0186-	Magnesium Sulfate Heptahydrate Concentration	Container Type	Fill Volume	Magnesium per mL	Sulfate per mL
1203-04	10%	Vial	20 mL	9.9 mg	38.9 mg
1204-04	10%	Vial	50 mL	9.9 mg	38.9 mg
1209-04	50%	Vial	2 mL	49.3 mg	194.7 mg
1210-04	50%	Vial	10 mL	49.3 mg	194.7 mg
1211-04	50%	Vial	20 mL	49.3 mg	194.7 mg
0684-01	50%	Additive Syringe	5 mL	49.3 mg	194.7 mg
0685-01	50%	Additive Syringe	10 mL	49.3 mg	194.7 mg

MANNITOL Injection, USP, 25% ℞
[man-ĭ-tall]

For details of indications, dosage and administration, precautions, and adverse reactions, see circular in package.

HOW SUPPLIED
Mannitol Injection USP, 25% is a sterile solution supplied in single dose containers as follows:
NDC 0186-1168-04; 50 ml vials, 25 vials per package
NDC 0186-0652-01: 50 ml syringes, 10 syringes per package
CAUTION: Federal law prohibits dispensing without prescription.
Store at controlled room temperature 15°–30°C (59°–86°F).
Note: Crystals may form in mannitol solutions especially if solutions are chilled. See PRECAUTIONS to dissolve the crystals.
021855R01   Rev. 5/86(1)

MEPERIDINE HCI INJECTION, USP Ⓒ ℞

(For details of indications, dosage and administration, precautions, and adverse reactions, see circular in package.)

HOW SUPPLIED
Meperidine Hydrochloride Injection, USP is available as:
Multiple Dose Vials
NDC 0186-1283-01   100 mg/mL,   20 mL vial, box of 1
NDC 0186-1284-01   50 mg/mL,   30 mL vial, box of 1
Store at controlled room temperature 15°–30°C (59°–86°F).
021889R03   Iss. 8/91 (3)

METAPROTERENOL SULFATE ℞
ARM-A-MED®
Inhalation Solution, USP
0.4% and 0.6%

DESCRIPTION
Each vial contains metaproterenol sulfate 0.4% or 0.6% in a sterile aqueous solution containing sodium chloride and edetate disodium. Sulfuric acid and/or sodium hydroxide to adjust pH to 2.8–4.0. The solution is filled under nitrogen. The solution is a bronchodilator to be administered by oral inhalation with the aid of an intermittent positive pressure breathing apparatus (IPPB).
Metaproterenol sulfate is a beta adrenergic stimulator and is chemically 1-(3,5 dihydroxyphenyl)-2-isopropylamino-ethanol sulfate, a white, crystalline, racemic mixture of two optically active isomers. It differs from isoproterenol hydrochloride by having two hydroxyl groups attached at the meta positions on the benezene ring rather than one at the meta and one at the para position.

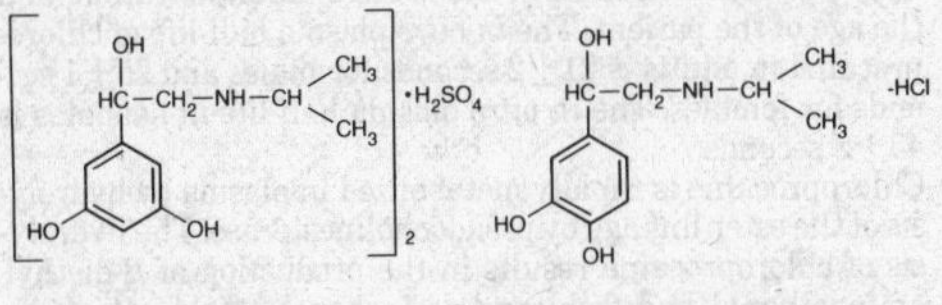

metaproterenol sulfate   isoproterenol hydrochloride

CLINICAL PHARMACOLOGY
Metaproterenol is a potent beta adrenergic stimulator with a rapid onset action. It is postulated that beta adrenergic stimulants produce many of their pharmacological effects by activation of adenyl cyclase, the enzyme which catalyzes the conversion of adenosine triphosphate to cyclic adenosine monophosphate.
Absorption, biotransformation and excretion studies following administration by inhalation have not been performed. Following oral administration in humans, an average of 40% of the drug is absorbed; it is not metabolized by catechol-O-methyltransferase but is excreted primarily as glucuronic acid conjugates.
Recent studies in laboratory animals (minipigs, rodents and dogs) recorded the occurrence of cardiac arrhythmias and sudden death (with histologic evidence of myocardial necrosis) when beta agonists and methylxanthines were administered concurrently. The significance of these findings when applied to humans is currently unknown.

INDICATIONS AND USAGE
Metaproterenol Sulfate Inhalation Solution is indicated as a bronchodilator for bronchial asthma, and for reversible bronchospasm which may occur in association with bronchitis and emphysema.
Following controlled single dose studies by an intermittent positive pressure breathing apparatus (IPPB) and by hand bulb nebulizers, significant improvement (15% or greater increase in FEV_1) occurred within 5 to 30 minutes and persisted for periods varying from 2 to 6 hours.
In these studies, the longer duration of effect occurred in the studies in which the drug was administered by IPPB, i.e., 6 hours versus 2 to 3 hours when administered by hand bulb nebulizer. In these studies the doses used were 0.3 mL by IPPB and 10 inhalations by hand bulb nebulizer.
In controlled repetitive dosing studies by IPPB and by hand bulb nebulizer the onset of effect occurred within 5 to 30 minutes and duration ranged from 4 to 6 hours. In these studies the doses used were 0.3 mL b.i.d. or t.i.d. when given by IPPB, and 10 inhalations q.i.d. (no more often than q4h) when given by hand bulb nebulizer. As in the single-dose studies, effectiveness was measured as a sustained increase in FEV_1 of 15% or greater. In these repetitive dosing studies there was no apparent difference in duration between the two methods of delivery.
During other clinical tolerance studies metaproterenol was administered q.i.d. (by nebulizer) for periods of 60 and 90 days. On specified days before, during, and after these open label trials, patients were referred to a laboratory where the effects of single doses of metaproterenol and isoproterenol on pulmonary function were recorded (in a double blind crossover controlled setting). Both drugs continued to exert significant improvement in function throughout this period of treatment.

CONTRAINDICATIONS
Use in patients with cardiac arrhythmias associated with tachycardia is contraindicated.
Although rare, immediate hypersensitivity reactions can occur. Therefore, Metaproterenol Sulfate Inhalation Solution is contraindicated in patients with a history of hypersensitivity to any of its components.

WARNINGS
Excessive use of adrenergic aerosols is potentially dangerous. Fatalities have been reported following excessive use of metaproterenol, as with other sympathomimetic inhalation preparations, and the exact cause is unknown. Cardiac arrest was noted in several cases.
Paradoxical bronchoconstriction with repeated excessive administration has been reported with other sympathomimetic agents.
Patients should be advised to contact their physicians in the event that they do not respond to their usual dose of sympathomimetic amine aerosol.

PRECAUTIONS
General: Because metaproterenol is a sympathomimetic drug, it should be used with great caution in patients with hypertension, coronary artery disease, congestive heart failure, hyperthyroidism or diabetes, or when there is sensitivity to sympathomimetic amines.
Information for Patients: Extreme care must be exercised with respect to the administration of additional sympathomimetic agents. A sufficient interval of time should elapse prior to administration of another sympathomimetic agent.
Carcinogenesis, Mutagenesis, Impairment of Fertility: Long-term studies in mice and rats to evaluate the oral carcinogenic potential of metaproterenol sulfate have not been completed.
Studies of metaproterenol sulfate have not been conducted to determine mutagenic potential or effect on fertility.
Pregnancy: Teratogenic Effects: Pregnancy Category C. Metaproterenol has been shown to be teratogenic and embryocidal in rabbits when given orally in doses 620 times the human inhalation dose. There are no adequate and well-controlled studies in pregnant women. Metaproterenol sulfate inhalation solution should be used during pregnancy only if the potential benefit justifies the potential risk to the fetus.
Oral reproduction studies in mice, rats and rabbits showed no teratogenic or embryocidal effect at 50 mg/kg corresponding to 310 times the human inhalation dose. Teratogenic effects in the rabbit included skeletal abnormalities and hydrocephalus with bone separation.
Nursing Mothers: It is not known whether this drug is excreted in human milk. Because many drugs are excreted in human milk, caution should be exercised when metaproterenol sulfate is administered to a nursing woman.
Pediatric Use: Safety and effectiveness in children below the age of 12 have not been established.

ADVERSE REACTIONS
Adverse reactions are similar to those noted with other sympathomimetic agents.
The most frequent adverse reactions to metaproterenol sulfate are nervousness and tachycardia which occur in about 1 in 7 patients, tremor which occurs in about 1 in 20 patients and nausea which occurs in about 1 in 50 patients. Less frequent adverse reactions are hypertension, palpitations, vomiting and bad taste occur in approximately 1 in 300 patients.

OVERDOSAGE
The symptoms of overdosage are those of excessive beta adrenergic stimulation listed under ADVERSE REACTIONS. These reactions usually do not require treatment other than reduction of dosage and/or frequency of administration.

DOSAGE AND ADMINISTRATION
Metaproterenol Sulfate Inhalation Solution is administered by oral inhalation using an IPPB device. The usual adult dose is one vial per nebulization treatment. Each 0.4% vial is equivalent to 0.2 mL metaproterenol sulfate 5% solution diluted to 2.5 mL with normal saline. Each 0.6% vial is equivalent to 0.3 mL metaproterenol sulfate 5% solution diluted to 2.5 mL with normal saline.
Usually, treatment need not be repeated more often than every four hours to relieve acute attacks of bronchospasm. As part of a total treatment program in chronic bronchospastic pulmonary diseases, Metaproterenol Sulfate Inhalation Solution may be administered three or four times a day.
As with all medications, the physician should begin therapy with the lowest effective dose and then titrate the dosage according to the individual patient's requirements.
Metaproterenol Sulfate Inhalation Solution, USP is not recommended for use in children under 12 years of age.

HOW SUPPLIED
Metaproterenol Sulfate Inhalation Solution, USP is supplied in Arm-a-Med vials and is available in pouches containing 5 single-use, plastic vials of 2.5 mL each. There are 20 pouches per carton of 100 vials.
NDC 0186-4131-01   0.4% equivalent to 0.2 mL Metaproterenol Sulfate Inhalation Solution, USP 5% diluted to 2.5 mL. Total contents of 10 mg of metaproterenol sulfate.
NDC 0186-4130-01   0.6% equivalent to 0.3 mL Metaproterenol Sulfate Inhalation Solution, USP 5% diluted to 2.5 mL. Total contents of 15 mg of metaproterenol sulfate.
DO NOT STORE ABOVE 25°C (77°F). PROTECT FROM LIGHT. Store vials in pouch until ready for use.
Do not use solution if its color is pinkish or darker than slightly yellow or if it contains a precipitate.
Caution: Federal law prohibits dispensing without prescription.
Manufactured by:
Armour Pharmaceutical Company
Kankakee, Illinois 60901
021674R01   8/91 (1)

METHOTREXATE SODIUM INJECTION, USP ℞

NOTE
See Box "WARNINGS".
(For details of indications, dosages and administration, precautions, and adverse reactions, see circular in package.)

HOW SUPPLIED
Methotrexate Sodium Injection Preservative-Free Solution 25 mg/mL. Single use vials only.
NDC 0186-1420-13   2 mL   (50 mg)
NDC 0186-1421-13   4 mL   (100 mg)
NDC 0186-1422-12   10 mL   (250 mg)
NDC 0186-1423-04   10 mL   (250 mg)
Manufactured by Pharmachemie BV Haarlem, Holland
021894R02   10/88 (2)

MORPHINE SULFATE INJECTION, USP Ⓒ
(morphine sulfate injection, USP)

(For details of indications, dosage and administration, precautions, and adverse reactions, see circular in package.)

HOW SUPPLIED
Morphine Sulfate Injection, USP is available in the following dosage strengths:
8 mg (⅛ gr)/mL, 2 mL (1 mL fill); Ampule
                    NDC 0186-1155-03, Boxes of 25
10 mg (⅙ gr)/mL, 2 mL (1 mL fill); Ampule
                    NDC 0186-1156-03, Boxes of 25
15 mg (¼ gr)/mL, 2 mL (1 mL fill); Ampule
                    NDC 0186-1157-03, Boxes of 25
8 mg (⅛ gr)/mL, 2 mL (1 mL fill); Vial
                    NDC 0186-1138-13, Boxes of 25
10 mg (⅙ gr)/mL, 2 mL (1 mL fill); Vial
                    NDC 0186-1139-13, Boxes of 25
15 mg (¼ gr)/mL, 2 mL (1 mL fill); Vial
                    NDC 0186-1140-13, Boxes of 25
15 mg (¼ gr)/mL, 20 mL Multiple dose vial;
                    NDC 0186-1158-02, Box of 1
Protect from light. Store at controlled room temperature 15°–30°C (59°–86°F).
021869R05   5/91 (5)

Continued on next page

Astra—Cont.

M.V.I.®-12   ℞
Multi-Vitamin Infusion
M.V.I.-12
Multi-Vitamin Infusion
M.V.I.-12 Multi-Dose
PHARMACY BULK PACKAGE
NOT FOR DIRECT INFUSION
Multi-Vitamin Infusion
M.V.I.-12 UNIT VIAL
Multi-Vitamin Infusion
For dilution in intravenous infusions only

(For details of indications, dosage and administration, precautions, and adverse reactions, see circular in package.)

After M.V.I.-12 is diluted in an intravenous infusion, the resulting solution is ready for immediate use. Some of the vitamins in this product, particularly A and D and riboflavin, are light sensitive, and exposure to light should be minimized.
Store at 2°–8°C (36°–46°F).

HOW SUPPLIED
M.V.I.-12—NDC 0186-1199-31 Boxes of 25 and cartons of 100. Each box contains two vials—Vial 1 (5 mL) and Vial 2 (5 mL), both vials to be used for a single dose.
M.V.I.-12 Multi-Dose (PHARMACY BULK PACKAGE) NDC 0186-1199-10 Boxes of 20 vials, 50 mL each (10 Vial 1 and Vial 2). Both solutions to be used for single dose.
M.V.I.-12 UNIT VIAL—NDC 0186-1199-35 Boxes of 25 two-chambered 10 mL vials.
CAUTION: Federal law prohibits dispensing without prescription.
Manufactured by:
Armour Pharmaceutical Company
Kankakee, IL 60901
021675R00   Iss. 6/91

M.V.I.® PEDIATRIC   ℞
Multi-Vitamins for Infusion
For dilution in intravenous infusions only

(For details of indications, dosage and administration, precautions, and adverse reactions, see circular in package.)

DISCARD ANY UNUSED PORTION.
Parenteral drug products should be inspected visually for particulate matter and discoloration prior to administration, whenever solution and container permit.
After M.V.I. Pediatric is reconstituted it should be immediately diluted into the intravenous solution. The resulting solution should be administered immediately. Some of the vitamins in this product, particularly vitamins A and D and riboflavin, are light-sensitive and exposure to light should be minimized.

HOW SUPPLIED
M.V.I Pediatric is available as:
NDC 0186-1839-35, 10 mL Single Dose Vial, Boxes of 25.
NDC 0186-1839-25, 25 mL Single-use, multiple-dose vials (PHARMACY BULK PACKAGE), Boxes of 5.
Store at controlled room temperature, 15°–30°C (59°–86°F).
CAUTION: Federal law prohibits dispensing without prescription.
Manufactured by:
Armour Pharmaceutical Company
Kankakee, IL 60901
021676R00   Iss. 6/91

NALBUPHINE HCl INJECTION   ℞

(For details of indications, dosage and administration, precautions, and adverse reactions, see circular in package.)

HOW SUPPLIED
Nalbuphine HCl Injection for intramuscular, subcutaneous or intravenous use is available in the following dosage forms:

Vials
10 mg/mL, 10 mL vial (box of 1),   NDC 0186-1262-12
20 mg/mL, 10 mL vial (box of 1),   NDC 0186-1266-12
Store at controlled room temperature 15°–30°C (59°–86°F). Protect from light.
021886R04   8/90 (4)

NALOXONE HCl INJECTION, USP   ℞
Narcotic Antagonist

(For details of indications, dosage and administration, precautions, and adverse reactions, see circular in package.)

HOW SUPPLIED
Naloxone HCl Injection for intravenous, intramuscular and subcutaneous administration is available as:
0.02 mg/mL
2 mL vial,   box of 10   NDC 0186-1252-13
0.4 mg/mL
1 mL vial,   box of 10   NDC 0186-1250-13
10 mL vial,   box of 1   NDC 0186-1254-12
1 mg/mL
1 mL vial,   box of 10   NDC 0186-1251-13
5 mL vial,   box of 1   NDC 0186-1253-13
10 mL vial,   box of 1   NDC 0186-1255-12
Store at controlled room temperature 15°–30°C (59°–86°F).
021885R05   8/91 (5)

NEOSTIGMINE METHYLSULFATE   ℞
INJECTION, USP

(For details of indications, dosage and administration, precautions, and adverse reactions, see circular in package.)

HOW SUPPLIED
Neostigmine Methylsulfate Injection, USP is available in the following dosage forms:
1:1000 (1 mg/mL)—NDC 0186-1742-01
10 mL Multiple Dose Vial, box of 5
1:2000 (0.5 mg/mL)—NDC 0186-1741-01
10 mL Multiple Dose Vial, box of 5
021591R02   12/89 (2)

NESACAINE®   ℞
[nes 'a-caine]
(Chloroprocaine HCl) Injection
NESACAINE® MPF
(Chloroprocaine HCl) Injection
for Infiltration and Nerve Block

DESCRIPTION
Nesacaine and Nesacaine-MPF Injections are sterile nonpyrogenic local anesthetics. The active ingredient in Nesacaine and Nesacaine-MPF Injections is chloroprocaine HCl (benzoic acid, 4-amino-2-chloro-2-(diethylamino) ethyl ester, monohydrochloride), which is represented by the following structural formula:

$$NH_2 - \text{C}_6\text{H}_3(\text{Cl}) - COOCH_2CH_2N(C_2H_5)_2 \cdot HCl$$

[See table below.]
The solutions are adjusted to pH 2.7–4.0 by means of sodium hydroxide and/or hydrochloric acid. Filled under nitrogen. Nesacaine and Nesacaine-MPF Injections should not be resterilized by autoclaving.

CLINICAL PHARMACOLOGY
Chloroprocaine, like other local anesthetics, blocks the generation and the conduction of nerve impulses, presumably by increasing the threshold for electrical excitation in the nerve, by slowing the propagation of the nerve impulse and by reducing the rate of rise of the action potential. In general, the progression of anesthesia is related to the diameter, myelination and conduction velocity of affected nerve fibers. Clinically, the order of loss of nerve function is as follows: (1) pain, (2) temperature, (3) touch, (4) proprioception, and (5) skeletal muscle tone.

Systemic absorption of local anesthetics produces effects on the cardiovascular and central nervous systems. At blood concentrations achieved with normal therapeutic doses, changes in cardiac conduction, excitability, refractoriness, contractility, and peripheral vascular resistance are minimal. However, toxic blood concentrations depress cardiac conduction and excitability, which may lead to atrioventricular block and ultimately to cardiac arrest. In addition, with toxic blood concentrations myocardial contractility may be depressed and peripheral vasodilation may occur, leading to decreased cardiac output and arterial blood pressure.
Following systemic absorption, toxic blood concentrations of local anesthetics can produce central nervous system stimulation, depression, or both. Apparent central stimulation may be manifested as restlessness, tremors and shivering, which may progress to convulsions. Depression and coma may occur, possibly progressing ultimately to respiratory arrest.
However, the local anesthetics have a primary depressant effect on the medulla and on higher centers. The depressed stage may occur without a prior stage of central nervous system stimulation.

PHARMACOKINETICS
The rate of systemic absorption of local anesthetic drugs is dependent upon the total dose and concentration of drug administered, the route of administration, the vascularity of the administration site, and the presence or absence of epinephrine in the anesthetic injection. Epinephrine usually reduces the rate of absorption and plasma concentration of local anesthetics and is sometimes added to local anesthetic injections in order to prolong the duration of action.
The onset of action with chloroprocaine is rapid (usually within 6 to 12 minutes), and the duration of anesthesia, depending upon the amount used and the route of administration, may be up to 60 minutes.
Local anesthetics appear to cross the placenta by passive diffusion. However, the rate and degree of diffusion varies considerably among the different drugs as governed by: (1) the degree of plasma protein binding, (2) the degree of ionization, and (3) the degree of lipid solubility. Fetal/maternal ratios of local anesthetics appear to be inversely related to the degree of plasma protein binding, since only the free, unbound drug is available for placental transfer. Thus, drugs with the highest protein binding capacity may have the lowest fetal/maternal ratios. The extent of placental transfer is also determined by the degree of ionization and lipid solubility of the drug. Lipid soluble, nonionized drugs readily enter the fetal blood from the maternal circulation.
Depending upon the route of administration, local anesthetics are distributed to some extent to all body tissues, with high concentrations found in highly perfused organs such as the liver, lungs, heart and brain.
Various pharmacokinetic parameters of the local anesthetics can be significantly altered by the presence of hepatic or renal disease, addition of epinephrine, factors affecting urinary pH, renal blood flow, the route of administration, and the age of the patient. The *in vitro* plasma half-life of chloroprocaine in adults is 21 ± 2 seconds for males and 25 ± 1 seconds for females. The *in vitro* plasma half-life in neonates is 43 ± 2 seconds.
Chloroprocaine is rapidly metabolized in plasma by hydrolysis of the ester linkage by pseudocholinesterase. The hydrolysis of chloroprocaine results in the production of β-diethylaminoethanol and 2-chloro-4-aminobenzoic acid, which inhibits the action of the sulfonamides (SEE PRECAUTIONS). The kidney is the main excretory organ for most local anesthetics and their metabolites. Urinary excretion is affected by urinary perfusion and factors affecting urinary pH.

INDICATIONS AND USAGE
Nesacaine 1% and 2% Injections, in multidose vials with methylparaben as preservative, are indicated for the production of local anesthesia by infiltration and peripheral nerve block. They are not to be used for lumbar or caudal epidural anesthesia.
Nesacaine-MPF 2% and 3% Injections, in single-dose vials without preservative, are indicated for the production of local anesthesia by infiltration, peripheral and central nerve block, including lumbar and caudal epidural blocks.
Nesacaine and Nesacaine-MPF Injections, are not to be used for subarachnoid administration.

CONTRAINDICATIONS
Nesacaine and Nesacaine-MPF Injections are contraindicated in patients hypersensitive (allergic) to drugs of the PABA ester group.
Lumbar and caudal epidural anesthesia should be used with extreme caution in persons with the following conditions: existing neurological disease, spinal deformities, septicemia and severe hypertension.

WARNINGS
LOCAL ANESTHETICS SHOULD ONLY BE EMPLOYED BY CLINICIANS WHO ARE WELL VERSED IN DIAGNOSIS AND MANAGEMENT OF DOSE RELATED TOXICITY

Table 1. Composition of Available Injections

Product Identification	Chloroprocaine HCl	Sodium Chloride	Disodium EDTA dihydrate	Methylparaben
Nesacaine 1%	10	6.7	0.111	1
Nesacaine 2%	20	4.7	0.111	1
Nesacaine-MPF 2%	20	4.7	0.111	—
Nesacaine-MPF 3%	30	3.3	0.111	—

Formula (mg/mL)

AND OTHER ACUTE EMERGENCIES WHICH MIGHT ARISE FROM THE BLOCK TO BE EMPLOYED, AND THEN ONLY AFTER ENSURING THE *IMMEDIATE* AVAILABILITY OF OXYGEN, OTHER RESUSCITATIVE DRUGS, CARDIOPULMONARY RESUSCITATIVE EQUIPMENT, AND THE PERSONNEL RESOURCES NEEDED FOR PROPER MANAGEMENT OF TOXIC REACTIONS AND RELATED EMERGENCIES (See also *ADVERSE REACTIONS and PRECAUTIONS.*) DELAY IN PROPER MANAGEMENT OF DOSE RELATED TOXICITY, UNDERVENTILATION FROM ANY CAUSE AND/OR ALTERED SENSITIVITY MAY LEAD TO THE DEVELOPMENT OF ACIDOSIS, CARDIAC ARREST AND, POSSIBLY, DEATH. NESACAINE (chloroprocaine HCl) INJECTION contains methylparaben and should not be used for lumbar or caudal epidural anesthesia because safety of this antimicrobial preservative has not been established with regard to intrathecal injection, either intentional or unintentional. NESACAINE-MPF Injection contains no preservative; discard unused injection remaining in vial after initial use.

Vasopressors should not be used in the presence of ergot-type oxytocic drugs, since a severe persistent hypertension may occur.

To avoid intravascular injection, aspiration should be performed before the anesthetic solution is injected. The needle must be repositioned until no blood return can be elicited. However, the absence of blood in the syringe does not guarantee that intravascular injection has been avoided.

Mixtures of local anesthetics are sometimes employed to compensate for the slower onset of one drug and the shorter duration of action of the second drug. Experiments in primates suggest that toxicity is probably additive when mixtures of local anesthetics are employed, but some experiments in rodents suggest synergism. Caution regarding toxic equivalence should be exercised when mixtures of local anesthetics are employed.

PRECAUTIONS

General: The safety and effective use of chloroprocaine depend on proper dosage, correct technique, adequate precautions and readiness for emergencies. Resuscitative equipment, oxygen and other resuscitative drugs should be available for immediate use. (See WARNINGS and ADVERSE REACTIONS). The lowest dosage that results in effective anesthesia should be used to avoid high plasma levels and serious adverse effects. Injections should be made slowly, with frequent aspirations before and during the injection to avoid intravascular injection. Syringe aspirations should also be performed before and during each supplemental injection in continuous (intermittent) catheter techniques. During the administration of epidural anesthesia, it is recommended that a test dose be administered (3 mL of 3% or 5 mL of 2% Nesacaine-MPF Injection) initially and that the patient be monitored for central nervous system toxicity and cardiovascular toxicity, as well as for signs of unintended intrathecal administration, before proceeding. When clinical conditions permit, consideration should be given to employing a chloroprocaine solution that contains epinephrine for the test dose because circulatory changes characteristic of epinephrine may also serve as a warning sign of unintended intravascular injection. An intravascular injection is still possible even if aspirations for blood are negative. With the use of continuous catheter techniques, it is recommended that a fraction of each supplemental dose be administered as a test dose in order to verify proper location of the catheter. Injection of repeated doses of local anesthetics may cause significant increases in plasma levels with each repeated dose due to slow accumulation of the drug or its metabolites. Tolerance to elevated blood levels varies with the physical condition of the patient. Debilitated, elderly patients, acutely ill patients, and children should be given reduced doses commensurate with their age and physical status. Local anesthetics should also be used with caution in patients with hypotension or heart block.

Careful and constant monitoring of cardiovascular and respiratory (adequacy of ventilation) vital signs and the patient's state of consciousness should be accomplished after each local anesthetic injection. It should be kept in mind at such times that restlessness, anxiety, tinnitus, dizziness, blurred vision, tremors, depression or drowsiness may be early warning signs of central nervous system toxicity.

Local anesthetic injections containing a vasoconstrictor should be used cautiously and in carefully circumscribed quantities in areas of the body supplied by end arteries or having otherwise compromised blood supply. Patients with peripheral vascular disease and those with hypertensive vascular disease may exhibit exaggerated vasoconstrictor response. Ischemic injury or necrosis may result.

Since ester-type local anesthetics are hydrolyzed by plasma cholinesterase produced by the liver, chloroprocaine should be used cautiously in patients with hepatic disease.

Local anesthetics should also be used with caution in patients with impaired cardiovascular function since they may be less able to compensate for functional changes associated with the prolongation of A-V conduction produced by these drugs.

Use in Ophthalmic Surgery: When local anesthetic injections are employed for retrobulbar block, lack of corneal sensation should not be relied upon to determine whether or not the patient is ready for surgery. This is because complete lack of corneal sensation usually precedes clinically acceptable external ocular muscle akinesia.

INFORMATION FOR PATIENTS

When appropriate, patients should be informed in advance that they may experience temporary loss of sensation and motor activity, usually in the lower half of the body, following proper administration of epidural anesthesia.

CLINICALLY SIGNIFICANT DRUG INTERACTIONS: The administration of local anesthetic solutions containing epinephrine or norepinephrine to patients receiving monoamine oxidase inhibitors, tricyclic antidepressants or phenothiazines may produce severe, prolonged hypotension or hypertension. Concurrent use of these agents should generally be avoided. In situations when concurrent therapy is necessary, careful patient monitoring is essential.

Concurrent administration of vasopressor drugs (for the treatment of hypotension related to obstetric blocks) and ergot-type oxytocic drugs may cause severe, persistent hypertension or cerebrovascular accidents.

The para-aminobenzoic acid metabolite of chloroprocaine inhibits the action of sulfonamides. Therefore, chloroprocaine should not be used in any condition in which a sulfonamide drug is being employed.

CARCINOGENESIS, MUTAGENESIS, AND IMPAIRMENT OF FERTILITY: Long-term studies in animals to evaluate carcinogenic potential and reproduction studies to evaluate mutagenesis or impairment of fertility have not been conducted with chloroprocaine.

PREGNANCY CATEGORY C: Animal reproduction studies have not been conducted with chloroprocaine. It is also not known whether chloroprocaine can cause fetal harm when administered to a pregnant woman or can affect reproduction capacity. Chloroprocaine should be given to a pregnant woman only if clearly needed. This does not preclude the use of chloroprocaine at term for the production of obstetrical anesthesia.

LABOR AND DELIVERY: Local anesthetics rapidly cross the placenta, and when used for epidural, paracervical, pudendal or caudal block anesthesia, can cause varying degrees of maternal, fetal and neonatal toxicity.
(See CLINICAL PHARMACOLOGY and PHARMACOKINETICS.)

The incidence and degree of toxicity depend upon the procedure performed, the type and amount of drug used, and the technique of drug administration. Adverse reactions in the parturient, fetus and neonate involve alterations of the central nervous system, peripheral vascular tone and cardiac function.

Maternal hypotension has resulted from regional anesthesia. Local anesthetics produce vasodilation by blocking sympathetic nerves. Elevating the patient's legs and positioning her on her left side will help prevent decreases in blood pressure. The fetal heart rate also should be monitored continuously, and electronic fetal monitoring is highly advisable. Epidural, paracervical, or pudendal anesthesia may alter the forces of parturition through changes in uterine contractility or maternal expulsive efforts. In one study, paracervical block anesthesia was associated with a decrease in the mean duration of first stage labor and facilitation of cervical dilation. However, epidural anesthesia has also been reported to prolong the second stage of labor by removing the parturient's reflex urge to bear down or by interfering with motor function. The use of obstetrical anesthesia may increase the need for forceps assistance.

The use of some local anesthetic drug products during labor and delivery may be followed by diminished muscle strength and tone for the first day or two of life. The long-term significance of these observations is unknown.

Careful adherence to recommended dosage is of the utmost importance in obstetrical paracervical block. Failure to achieve adequate analgesia with recommended doses should arouse suspicion of intravascular or fetal intracranial injection. Cases compatible with unintended fetal intracranial injection of local anesthetic injection have been reported following intended paracervical or pudendal block or both. Babies so affected present with unexplained neonatal depression at birth which correlates with high local anesthetic serum levels and usually manifest seizures within six hours. Prompt use of supportive measures combined with forced urinary excretion of the local anesthetic has been used successfully to manage this complication.

Case reports of maternal convulsions and cardiovascular collapse following use of some local anesthetics for paracervical block in early pregnancy (as anesthesia for elective abortion) suggest that systemic absorption under these circumstances may be rapid. The recommended maximum dose of each drug should not be exceeded. Injection should be made slowly and with frequent aspiration. Allow a 5-minute interval between sides.

There are no data concerning use of chloroprocaine for obstetrical paracervical block when toxemia of pregnancy is present or when fetal distress or prematurity is anticipated in advance of the block; such use is, therefore, not recommended.

The following information should be considered by clinicians who select chloroprocaine for obstetrical paracervical block anesthesia: 1) Fetal bradycardia (generally a heart rate of less than 120 per minute for more than 2 minutes) has been noted by electronic monitoring in about 5 to 10 percent of the cases (various studies) where initial total doses of 120 mg to 400 mg of chloroprocaine were employed. The incidence of bradycardia, within this dose range, might not be dose related. 2) Fetal acidosis has not been demonstrated by blood gas monitoring around the time of bradycardia or afterwards. These data are limited and generally restricted to nontoxemic cases where fetal distress or prematurity was not anticipated in advance of the block. 3) No intact chloroprocaine and only trace quantities of a hydrolysis product, 2-chloro-4-aminobenzoic acid, have been demonstrated in umbilical cord arterial or venous plasma following properly administered paracervical block with chloroprocaine. 4) The role of drug factors and non-drug factors associated with fetal bradycardia following paracervical block are unexplained at this time.

NURSING MOTHERS: It is not known whether this drug is excreted in human milk. Because many drugs are excreted in human milk, caution should be exercised when chloroprocaine is administered to a nursing woman.

PEDIATRIC USE: Guidlines for the administration of Nesacaine and Nesacaine-MPF Injections to children are presented in DOSAGE AND ADMINISTRATION.

ADVERSE REACTIONS

Systemic: The most commonly encountered acute adverse experiences that demand immediate countermeasures are related to the central nervous system and the cardiovascular system. These adverse experiences are generally dose related and may result from rapid absorption from the injection site, diminished tolerance, or from unintentional intravascular injection of the local anesthetic solution. In addition to systemic dose-related toxicity, unintentional subarachnoid injection of drug during the intended performance of caudal or lumbar epidural block or nerve blocks near the vertebral column (especially in the head and neck region) may result in underventilation or apnea ("Total Spinal"). Factors influencing plasma protein binding, such as acidosis, systemic diseases that alter protein production, or competition of other drugs for protein binding sites, may diminish individual tolerance. Plasma cholinesterase deficiency may also account for diminished tolerance to ester type local anesthetics.

Central Nervous System Reactions: These are characterized by excitation and/or depression. Restlessness, anxiety, dizziness, tinnitus, blurred vision or tremors may occur, possibly proceeding to convulsions. However, excitement may be transient or absent, with depression being the first manifestation of an adverse reaction. This may quickly be followed by drowsiness merging into unconsciousness and respiratory arrest.

The incidence of convulsions associated with the use of local anesthetics varies with the procedure used and the total dose administered. In a survey of studies of epidural anesthesia, overt toxicity progressing to convulsions occurred in approximately 0.1 percent of local anesthetic administrations.

Cardiovascular System Reactions: High doses, or unintended intravascular injection, may lead to high plasma levels and related depression of the myocardium, hypotension, bradycardia, ventricular arrhythmias and, possibly, cardiac arrest.

Allergic: Allergic type reactions are rare and may occur as a result of sensitivity to the local anesthetic or to other formulation ingredients, such as the antimicrobial preservative methylparaben, contained in multiple dose vials. These reactions are characterized by signs such as urticaria, pruritis, erythema, angioneurotic edema (including laryngeal edema), tachycardia, sneezing, nausea, vomiting, dizziness, syncope, excessive sweating, elevated temperature, and possibly, anaphylactoid type symptomatology (including severe hypotension). Cross sensitivity among members of the ester-type local anesthetic group has been reported. The usefulness of screening for sensitivity has not been definitely established.

Neurologic: In the practice of caudal or lumbar epidural block, occasional unintentional penetration of the subarachnoid space by the catheter may occur (see PRECAUTIONS). Subsequent adverse observations may depend partially on the amount of drug administered intrathecally. These observations may include spinal block of varying magnitude (including total spinal block), hypotension secondary to spinal block, loss of bladder, and bowel control, and loss of perineal sensation and sexual function. Arachnoiditis, persistent motor, sensory and/or autonomic (sphincter control) deficit of some lower spinal segments with slow recovery (several

Continued on next page

Astra—Cont.

months) or incomplete recovery have been reported in rare instances. (See DOSAGE AND ADMINISTRATION discussion of *Caudal and Lumbar Epidural Block).* Backache and headache have also been noted following lumbar epidural or caudal block.

OVERDOSAGE

Acute emergencies from local anesthetics are generally related to high plasma levels encountered during therapeutic use of local anesthetics or to unintended subarachnoid injection of local anesthetic solution (see ADVERSE REACTIONS, WARNINGS, and PRECAUTIONS).

In mice, the intravenous LD_{50} of chloroprocaine HCl is 97 mg/kg and the subcutaneous LD_{50} of chloroprocaine HCl is 950 mg/kg.

Management of Local Anesthetic Emergencies: The first consideration is prevention, best accomplished by careful and constant monitoring of cardiovascular and respiratory vital signs and the patient's state of consciousness after each local anesthetic injection. At the first sign of change, oxygen should be administered.

The first step is the management of convulsions, as well as underventilation or apnea due to unintentional subarachnoid injection of drug solution, consists of immediate attention to the maintenance of a patent airway and assisted or controlled ventilation with oxygen and a delivery system capable of permitting immediate positive airway pressure by mask. Immediately after the institution of these ventilatory measures, the adequacy of the circulation should be evaluated, keeping in mind that drugs used to treat convulsions sometimes depress the circulation when administered intravenously. Should convulsions persist despite adequate respiratory support, and if the status of the circulation permits, small increments of an ultra-short acting barbiturate (such as thiopental or thiamylal) or a benzodiazepine (such as diazepam) may be administered intravenously; the clinician should be familiar, prior to the use of local anesthetics, with these anticonvulsant drugs. Supportive treatment of circulatory depression may require administration of intravenous fluids and, when appropriate, a vasopressor dictated by the clinical situation (such as ephedrine to enhance myocardial contractile force).

If not treated immediately, both convulsions and cardiovascular depression can result in hypoxia, acidosis, bradycardia, arrhythmias and cardiac arrest. Underventilation or apnea due to unintentional subarachnoid injection of local anesthetic solution may produce these same signs and also lead to cardiac arrest if ventilatory support is not instituted. If cardiac arrest should occur, standard cardiopulmonary resuscitative measures should be instituted. Recovery has been reported after prolonged resuscitative efforts.

Endotracheal intubation, employing drugs and techniques familiar to the clinician, may be indicated, after initial administration of oxygen by mask, if difficulty is encountered in the maintenance of a patent airway or if prolonged ventilatory support (assisted or controlled) is indicated.

DOSAGE AND ADMINISTRATION

Chloroprocaine may be administered as a single injection or continuously through an indwelling catheter. As with all local anesthetics, the dose administered varies with the anesthetic procedure, the vascularity of the tissues, the depth of anesthesia and degree of muscle relaxation required, the duration of anesthesia desired, and the physical condition of the patient. The smallest dose and concentration required to produce the desired result should be used. Dosage should be reduced for children, elderly and debilitated patients and patients with cardiac and/or liver disease. The maximum single recommended doses of chloroprocaine in adults are: without epinephrine, 11 mg/kg, not to exceed a maximum total dose of 800 mg; with epinephrine (1:200,000), 14 mg/kg, not to exceed a maximum total dose of 1000 mg. For specific techniques and procedures, refer to standard textbooks.

Caudal and Lumbar Epidural Block: In order to guard against adverse experiences sometimes noted following unintended penetration of the subarachnoid space, the following procedure modifications are recommended: 1. Use an adequate test dose (3 mL of Nesacaine-MPF 3% Injection or 5 mL of Nesacaine-MPF 2% Injection) prior to induction of complete block. This test dose should be repeated if the patient is moved in such a fashion as to have displaced the epidural catheter. Allow adequate time for onset of anesthesia following administration of each test dose. 2. Avoid the rapid injection of a large volume of local anesthetic injection through the catheter. Consider fractional doses, when feasible. 3. In the event of the known injection of a large volume of local anesthetic injection into the subarachnoid space, after suitable resuscitation and if the catheter is in place, consider attempting the recovery of drug by draining a moderate amount of cerebrospinal fluid (such as 10 mL) through the epidural catheter.

As a guide for some routine procedures, suggested doses are given below:

1. Infiltration and Peripheral Nerve Block: NESACAINE or NESACAINE-MPF (Chloroprocaine HCl) INJECTION [See table below.]
2. Caudal and Lumbar Epidural Block: NESACAINE-MPF INJECTION. For caudal anesthesia, the initial dose is 15 to 25 mL of a 2% or 3% solution. Repeated doses may be given at 40 to 60 minute intervals.

For lumbar epidural anesthesia, 2 to 2.5 mL per segment of a 2% or 3% solution can be used. The usual total volume of Nesacaine-MPF Injection is from 15 to 25 mL. Repeated doses 2 to 6 mL less than the original dose may be given at 40 to 50 minute intervals.

The above dosages are recommended as a guide for use in the average adult. Maximum dosages of all local anesthetics must be individualized after evaluating the size and physical condition of the patient and the rate of systemic absorption from a particular injection site.

Pediatric Dosage: It is difficult to recommend a maximum dose of any drug for children, since this varies as a function of age and weight. For children over 3 years of age who have a normal lean body mass and normal body development, the maximum dose is determined by the child's age and weight and should not exceed 11 mg/kg (5 mg/lb). For example, in a child of 5 years weighing 50 lbs (23 kg), the dose of chloroprocaine HCl without epinephrine would be 250 mg. Concentrations of 0.5–1.0% are suggested for infiltration and 1.0–1.5% for nerve block. In order to guard against systemic toxicity, the lowest effective concentration and lowest effective dose should be used at all times. Some of the lower concentrations for use in infants and smaller children are not available in pre-packaged containers; it will be necessary to dilute available concentrations with the amount of 0.9% sodium chloride injection necessary to obtain the required final concentration of chloroprocaine solution.

Preparation of Epinephrine Injections—To prepare a 1:200,000 epinephrine-chloroprocaine HCl injection, add 0.15 mL of a 1 to 1000 Epinephrine Injection USP to 30 mL of Nesacaine-MPF Injection.

Chloroprocaine is incompatible with caustic alkalis and their carbonates, soaps, silver salts, iodine and iodides.

Parenteral drug products should be inspected visually for particulate matter and discoloration prior to administration, whenever injection and container permit. As with other anesthetics having a free aromatic amino group, Nesacaine and Nesacaine-MPF Injections are slightly photosensitive and may become discolored after prolonged exposure to light. It is recommended that these vials be stored in the original outer containers, protected from direct sunlight. Discolored injection should not be administered. If exposed to low temperatures, Nesacaine and Nesacaine-MPF Injections may deposit crystals of chloroprocaine HCl which will redissolve with shaking when returned to room temperature. The product should not be used if it contains undissolved (e.g., particulate) material.

HOW SUPPLIED

NESACAINE (Chloroprocaine HCl) INJECTION with preservatives is supplied as follows:

1% solution (NDC 0186-0971-66) in 30 mL multiple dose vials.

2% solution (NDC 0186-0972-66) in 30 mL multiple dose vials.

NESACAINE-MPF (Chloroprocaine HCl) INJECTION without preservatives is supplied as follows:

2% solution (NDC 0186-0993-66) in 30 mL single dose vials.
3% solution (NDC 0186-0994-66) in 30 mL single dose vials.

Keep from freezing. Protect from light. Store at controlled room temperature: 15°–30°C (59°–86°F).

021849R08 Rev. 6/91(8)

Anesthetic Procedure	Solution Concentration %	Volume (mL)	Total Dose (mg)
Mandibular	2	2–3	40–60
Infraorbital	2	0.5–1	10–20
Brachial plexus	2	30–40	600–800
Digital (without epinephrine)	1	3–4	30–40
Pudendal	2	10 each side	400
Paracervical (see also PRECAUTIONS)	1	3 per each of 4 sites	up to 120

PANCURONIUM BROMIDE INJECTION ℞

THIS DRUG SHOULD BE ADMINISTERED BY ADEQUATELY TRAINED INDIVIDUALS FAMILIAR WITH ITS ACTIONS, CHARACTERISTICS, AND HAZARDS.

HOW SUPPLIED

Pancuronium Bromide Injection is packaged in the following forms:

Vials, 1 mg/mL
NDC 0186-1322-12, 10 mL size—boxes of 5, Flip-Off vial closure

Vials, 2 mg/mL
NDC 0186-1331-13, 2 mL size—boxes of 10, Astra E-Z OFF™ vial closure
NDC 0186-1334-03, 2 mL size—boxes of 10, Flip-Off vial closure
NDC 0186-1332-13, 5 mL size—boxes of 10, Astra E-Z OFF™ vial closure
NDC 0186-1335-03, 5 mL size—boxes of 10, Flip-off vial closure

Syringes, 2 mg/mL
NDC 0186-1333-23, 2 mL size—boxes of 10, 22G, 1¼″ needle
NDC 0186-1336-23, 2 mL size—boxes of 10, Luer Hub Only
NDC 0186-0676-01, 5 mL size—box of 1, 21G, 15/16″ needle
NDC 0186-0692-01, 5 mL size—box of 1, Luer Hub Only

STORAGE

Both concentrations of Pancuronium Bromide Injection will maintain full clinical potency for six months if kept at a room temperature of 18° to 22°C (65° to 72°F), or for 18 months when refrigerated at 2° to 8°C (36° to 46°F).

021887R04 12/88 (4)

POLOCAINE® ℞

[pō′-lō-caine″]
(mepivacaine hydrochloride Injection, USP)
THESE SOLUTIONS ARE NOT INTENDED FOR SPINAL ANESTHESIA OR DENTAL USE

(For details of indications, dosages and administration, precautions, and adverse reactions, see circular in package.)

HOW SUPPLIED

1% Single Dose Vial	30 mL (NDC 0186-0412-01)
1% Multiple Dose Vial	50 mL (NDC 0186-0410-01)
1.5% Single Dose Vial	30 mL (NDC 0186-0418-01)
2% Single Dose Vial	20 mL (NDC 0186-0422-01)
2% Multiple Dose Vial	50 mL (NDC 0186-0420-01)

Unused portions of solutions not containing preservatives should be discarded.

021668R00 Issue 1/92

SENSORCAINE® ℞

[sén-sor-caine]
(Bupivacaine HCl Injection, USP)
SENSORCAINE®–MPF (Bupivacaine HCl Injection, USP)
SENSORCAINE® with Epinephrine (Bupivacaine and Epinephrine Injection, USP) 1:200,000 (as bitartrate)
SENSORCAINE®–MPF with Epinephrine (Bupivacaine and Epinephrine Injection, USP) 1:200,000 (as bitartrate)

DESCRIPTION

Sensorcaine® (bupivacaine HCl) injections are sterile isotonic solutions that contain a local anesthetic agent with and without epinephrine (as bitartrate) 1:200,000 and are administered parenterally by injection. See INDICATIONS AND USAGE for specific uses. Solutions of bupivacaine HCl may be autoclaved if they do not contain epinephrine.

Sensorcaine® injections contain bupivacaine HCl which is chemically designated as 2-piperidinecarboxamide, 1-butyl-N-(2,6-dimethylphenyl)-monohydrochloride, monohydrate and has the following structure:

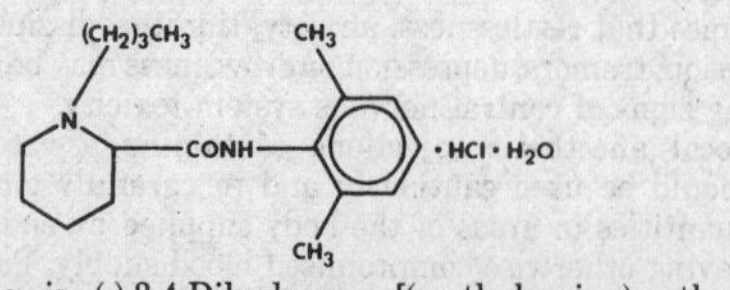

Epinephrine is (-)-3,4-Dihydroxy-α-[(methylamino)methyl] benzyl alcohol. It has the following structural formula: [See chemical structure at top of next column.]

The pKa of bupivacaine (8.1) is similar to that of lidocaine (7.86). However, bupivacaine possesses a greater degree of lipid solubility and is protein bound to a greater extent than lidocaine.

Bupivacaine is related chemically and pharmacologically to the aminoacyl local anesthetics. It is a homologue of mepiva-

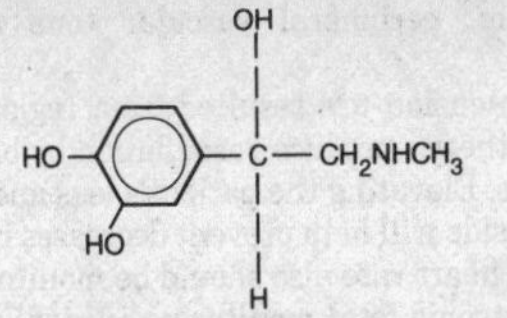

caine and is chemically related to lidocaine. All three of these anesthetics contain an amide linkage between the aromatic nucleus and the amino or piperidine group. They differ in this respect from the procaine-type local anesthetics, which have an ester linkage.

Dosage forms listed as Sensorcaine-MPF indicates single dose solutions that are Methyl Paraben Free (MPF).

Sensorcaine-MPF is a sterile isotonic solution containing sodium chloride. Sensorcaine in multiple dose vials, each mL also contains 1 mg methylparaben as antiseptic preservative. The pH of these solutions is adjusted to between 4.0 and 6.5 with sodium hydroxide and/or hydrochloric acid.

Sensorcaine-MPF with Epinephrine 1:200,000 (as bitartrate) is a sterile isotonic solution containing sodium chloride. Each mL contains bupivacaine hydrochloride and 0.005 mg epinephrine, with 0.5 mg sodium metabisulfite as an antioxidant and 0.2 mg citric acid (anhydrous) as stabilizer. Sensorcaine with Epinephrine 1:200.000 (as bitartrate) in multiple dose vials, each mL also contains 1 mg methylparaben as antiseptic preservative. The pH of this solution is adjusted to between 3.3 to 5.5 with sodium hydroxide and/or hydrochloric acid. Filled under nitrogen.

Note: The user should have an appreciation and awareness of the formulations and their intended uses. (See DOSAGE AND ADMINISTRATION.)

CLINICAL PHARMACOLOGY

Local anesthetics block the generation and the conduction of nerve impulses, presumably by increasing the threshold for electrical excitation in the nerve, by slowing the propagation of the nerve impulse, and by reducing the rate of rise of the action potential. In general, the progression of anesthesia is related to the diameter, myelination and conduction velocity of affected nerve fibers. Clinically, the order of loss of nerve function is as follows: (1) pain, (2) temperature, (3) touch, (4) proprioception, and (5) skeletal muscle tone.

Systemic absorption of local anesthetics produces effects on the cardiovascular and central nervous systems. At blood concentrations achieved with therapeutic doses, changes in cardiac conduction, excitability, refractoriness, contractility, and peripheral vascular resistance are minimal. However, toxic blood concentrations depress cardiac conduction and excitability, which may lead to atrioventricular block, ventricular arrhythmias and to cardiac arrest, sometimes resulting in fatalities. In addition, myocardial contractility is depressed and peripheral vasodilation occurs, leading to decreased cardiac output and arterial blood pressure.

Recent clinical reports and animal research suggest that these cardiovascular changes are more likely to occur after unintended intravascular injection of bupivacaine. Therefore, incremental dosing is necessary.

Following systemic absorption, local anesthetics can produce central nervous system stimulation, depression or both. Apparent central stimulation is usually manifested as restlessness, tremors and shivering, progressing to convulsions, followed by depression and coma, progressing ultimately to respiratory arrest. However, the local anesthetics have a primary depressant effect on the medulla and on higher centers. The depressed stage may occur without a prior excited stage.

Pharmacokinetics: The rate of systemic absorption of local anesthetics is dependent upon the total dose and concentration of drug administered, the route of administration, the vascularity of the administration site, and the presence or absence of epinephrine in the anesthetic solution. A dilute concentration of epinephrine (1:200,000 or 5 μg/mL) usually reduces the rate of absorption and peak plasma concentration of bupivacaine, permitting the use of moderately larger total doses and sometimes prolonging the duration of action.

The onset of action with bupivacaine is rapid and anesthesia is long-lasting. The duration of anesthesia is significantly longer with bupivacaine than with any other commonly used local anesthetic. It has also been noted that there is a period of analgesia that persists after the return of sensation, during which time the need for potent analgesics is reduced.

Local anesthetics are bound to plasma proteins in varying degrees. Generally, the lower the plasma concentration of drug, the higher the percentage of drug bound to plasma proteins.

Local anesthetics appear to cross the placenta by passive diffusion. The rate and degree of diffusion is governed by: (1) the degree of plasma protein binding, (2) the degree of ionization, and (3) the degree of lipid solubility. Fetal/maternal ratios of local anesthetics appear to be inversely related to the degree of plasma protein binding, because only the free, unbound drug is available for placental transfer. Bupivacaine, with a high protein binding capacity (95%), has a low fetal/maternal ratio (0.2–0.4). The extent of placental transfer is also determined by the degree of ionization and lipid solubility of the drug. Lipid soluble, nonionized drugs readily enter the fetal blood from the maternal circulation.

Depending upon the route of administration, local anesthetics are distributed to some extent to all body tissues, with high concentrations found in highly perfused organs such as the liver, lungs, heart and brain.

Pharmacokinetic studies on the plasma profile of bupivacaine after direct intravenous injection suggest a three-compartment open model. The first compartment is represented by the rapid intravascular distribution of the drug. The second compartment represents the equilibration of the drug throughout the highly perfused organs such as the brain, myocardium, lungs, kidneys and liver. The third compartment represents an equilibration of the drug with poorly perfused tissues, such as muscle and fat. The elimination of drug from tissue depends largely upon the ability of binding sites in the circulation to carry it to the liver where it is metabolized.

After injection of Sensorcaine (bupivacaine HCl) injection for caudal, epidural or peripheral nerve block in man, peak levels of bupivacaine in the blood are reached in 30 to 45 minutes, followed by a decline to insignificant levels during the next 3 to 6 hours.

Various pharmacokinetic parameters of the local anesthetics can be significantly altered by the presence of hepatic or renal disease, addition of epinephrine, factors affecting urinary pH, renal blood flow, the route of drug administration, and the age of the patient. The half-life of bupivacaine in adults is 3.5 ± 2.0 hours and in neonates 8.1 hours.

Amide-type local anesthetics such as bupivacaine are metabolized primarily in the liver via conjugation with glucuronic acid.

Patients with hepatic disease, especially those with severe hepatic disease, may be more susceptible to the potential toxicities of the amide-type local anesthetics. The major metabolite of bupivacaine is 2,6-pipecoloxylidine.

The kidney is the main excretory organ for most local anesthetics and their metabolites. Urinary excretion is affected by renal perfusion and factors affecting urinary pH. Only 5% of bupivacaine is excreted unchanged in the urine.

When administered in recommended doses and concentrations, Sensorcaine (bupivacaine HCl) injection does not ordinarily produce irritation or tissue damage and does not cause methemoglobinemia.

INDICATIONS AND USAGE

Sensorcaine (bupivacaine HCl) injection is indicated for the production of local or regional anesthesia or analgesia for surgery, for oral surgery procedures, for diagnostic and therapeutic procedures and for obstetrical procedures. Only the 0.25% and 0.5% concentrations are indicated for obstetrical anesthesia. (See WARNINGS.)

Experience with non-obstetrical surgical procedures in pregnant patients is not sufficient to recommend use of the 0.75% concentration in these patients. Sensorcaine (bupivacaine HCl) injection is not recommended for intravenous regional anesthesia (Bier Block). See WARNINGS.

The routes of administration and indicated Sensorcaine (bupivacaine HCl) concentrations are:

local infiltration	0.25%
peripheral nerve block	0.25%, 0.5%
retrobulbar block	0.75%
sympathetic block	0.25%
lumbar epidural	0.25%, 0.5% and 0.75% (non-obstetrical)
caudal	0.25%, 0.5%
epidural test dose (see PRECAUTIONS)	

(See DOSAGE AND ADMINISTRATION for additional information.) Standard textbooks should be consulted to detemine the accepted procedures and techniques for the administration of Sensorcaine (bupivacaine HCl).

Use only the single-dose ampules and single-dose vials for caudal or epidural anesthesia, the multiple-dose vials contain a preservative and, therefore, should not be used for these procedures.

CONTRAINDICATIONS

Sensorcaine (bupivacaine HCl) injection is contraindicated in obstetrical paracervical block anesthesia. Its use by this technique has resulted in fetal bradycardia and death.

Sensorcaine (bupivacaine HCl) is contraindicated in patients with a known hypersensitivity to it or to any local anesthetic agent of the amide type or to other components of bupivacaine solutions.

WARNINGS

THE 0.75% CONCENTRATION OF SENSORCAINE (BUPIVACAINE HYDROCHLORIDE) INJECTION IS NOT RECOMMENDED FOR OBSTETRICAL ANESTHESIA. THERE HAVE BEEN REPORTS OF CARDIAC ARREST WITH DIFFICULT RESUSCITATION OR DEATH DURING USE OF BUPIVACAINE FOR EPIDURAL ANESTHESIA IN OBSTETRICAL PATIENTS. IN MOST CASES, THIS HAS FOLLOWED USE OF THE 0.75% CONCENTRATION. RESUSCITATION HAS BEEN DIFFICULT OR IMPOSSIBLE DESPITE APPARENTLY ADEQUATE PREPARATION AND APPROPRIATE MANAGEMENT. CARDIAC ARREST HAS OCCURRED AFTER CONVULSIONS RESULTING FROM SYSTEMIC TOXICITY, PRESUMABLY FOLLOWING UNINTENTIONAL INTRAVASCULAR INJECTION. THE 0.75% CONCENTRATION SHOULD BE RESERVED FOR SURGICAL PROCEDURES WHERE A HIGH DEGREE OF MUSCLE RELAXATION AND PROLONGED EFFECT ARE NECESSARY.

LOCAL ANESTHETICS SHOULD ONLY BE EMPLOYED BY CLINICIANS WHO ARE WELL VERSED IN DIAGNOSIS AND MANAGEMENT OF DOSE-RELATED TOXICITY AND OTHER ACUTE EMERGENCIES WHICH MIGHT ARISE FROM THE BLOCK TO BE EMPLOYED, AND THEN ONLY AFTER INSURING THE *IMMEDIATE* AVAILABILITY OF OXYGEN, OTHER RESUSCITATIVE DRUGS, CARDIOPULMONARY RESUSCITATIVE EQUIPMENT, AND THE PERSONNEL RESOURCES NEEDED FOR PROPER MANAGEMENT OF TOXIC REACTIONS AND RELATED EMERGENCIES. (See also ADVERSE REACTIONS, PRECAUTIONS, and OVERDOSAGE.) DELAY IN PROPER MANAGEMENT OF DOSE-RELATED TOXICITY, UNDERVENTILATION FROM ANY CAUSE AND /OR ALTERED SENSITIVITY MAY LEAD TO THE DEVELOPMENT OF ACIDOSIS, CARDIAC ARREST AND, POSSIBLY, DEATH.

Local anesthetic solutions containing antimicrobial preservatives, i.e. those supplied in multiple dose vials, should not be used for epidural or caudal anesthesia because safety has not been established with regard to intrathecal injection, either intentional or unintentional, of such preservatives.

It is essential that aspiration for blood or cerebrospinal fluid (where applicable) be done prior to injecting any local anesthetic, both the original dose and all subsequent doses, to avoid intravascular or subarachnoid injection. However, a negative aspiration does *not* ensure against an intravascular or subarachnoid injection.

Bupivacaine and Epinephrine Injection or other vasopressors should not be used concomitantly with ergot-type oxytocic drugs, because a severe persistent hypertension may occur. Likewise, solutions of bupivacaine containing a vasoconstrictor, such as epinephrine, should be used with extreme caution in patients receiving monoamine oxidase (MAO) inhibitors or antidepressants of the triptyline or imipramine types, because severe prolonged hypertension may result.

Until further experience is gained in children younger than 12 years, administration of bupivacaine in this age group is not recommended.

Reports of cardiac arrest and death have occurred with the use of bupivacaine for intravenous regional anesthesia (Bier Block). Information on safe dosages or techniques of administration of this product are lacking; therefore, bupivacaine is not recommended for use by this technique.

Prior use of chloroprocaine may interfere with subsequent use of bupivacaine. Because of this, and because safety of intercurrent use of bupivacaine and chloroprocaine has not been established, such use is not recommended.

Sensorcaine with epinephrine solutions contain sodium metabisulfite, a sulfite that may cause allergic-type reactions including anaphylactic symptoms and life-threatening or less severe asthmatic episodes in certain susceptible people. The overall prevalence of sulfite sensitivity in the general population is unknown and probably low. Sulfite sensitivity is seen more frequently in asthmatic than in nonasthmatic people.

PRECAUTIONS

General: The safety and effectiveness of local anesthetics depend on proper dosage, correct technique, adequate precautions and readiness for emergencies. Resuscitative equipment, oxygen and other resuscitative drugs should be available for immediate use. (See WARNINGS, ADVERSE REACTIONS, and OVERDOSAGE.) During major regional nerve blocks, the patient should have I.V. fluids running via an indwelling catheter to assure a functioning intravenous pathway. The lowest dosage of local anesthetic that results in effective anesthesia should be used to avoid high plasma levels and serious adverse effects. The rapid injection of a large volume of local anesthetic solution should be avoided and fractional (incremental) doses should be used when feasible.

Epidural Anesthesia: During epidural administration of bupivacaine, concentrated solutions (0.5–0.75%) should be administered in incremental doses of 3 to 5 mL with sufficient time between doses to detect toxic manifestations of unintentional intravascular or intrathecal injection. Syringe aspirations should also be performed before and during each supplemental injection in continuous (intermittent)

Continued on next page

Astra—Cont.

catheter techniques. An intravascular injection is still possible even if aspirations for blood are negative.

During the administration of epidural anesthethesia, it is recommended that a test dose be administered initially and the effects monitored before the full dose is given. When using a "continuous" catheter technique, test doses should be given prior to both the original and all reinforcing doses, because plastic tubing in the epidural space can migrate into a blood vessel or through the dura. When clinical conditions permit, the test dose should contain epinephrine (10 to 15 μg have been suggested) to serve as a warning of unintentional intravascular injection. If injected into a blood vessel, this amount of epinephrine is likely to produce a transient "epinephrine response" within 45 seconds, consisting of an increase in heart rate and systolic blood pressure, circumoral pallor, palpitations and nervousness in the unsedated patient. The sedated patient may exhibit only a pulse rate increase of 20 or more beats per minute for 15 or more seconds. Therefore, following the test dose, the heart rate should be monitored for a heart rate increase. Patients on beta-blockers may not manifest changes in heart rate, but blood pressure monitoring can detect an evanescent rise in systolic blood pressure. The test dose should also contain 10 to 15 mg of Sensorcaine (bupivacaine HCl) injection or an equivalent dose of a short-acting amide anesthetic such as 30 to 40 mg of lidocaine, to detect an unintentional intrathecal administration. This will be manifested within a few minutes by signs of spinal block (e.g. decreased sensation of the buttocks, paresis of the legs, or, in the sedated patient, absent knee jerk). An intravascular or subarachnoid injection is still possible even if results of the test dose are negative. The test dose itself may produce a systemic toxic reaction, high spinal or epinephrine-induced cardiovascular effects.

Injection of repeated doses of local anesthetics may cause significant increases in plasma levels with each repeated dose due to slow accumulation of the drug or its metabolites or to slow metabolic degradation. Tolerance to elevated blood levels varies with the physical condition of the patient. Debilitated, elderly patients, acutely ill patients and children should be given reduced doses commensurate with their age and physical condition. Local anesthetics should also be used with caution in patients with hypotension or heart block.

Careful and constant monitoring of cardiovascular and respiratory vital signs (adequacy of ventilation) and the patient's state of consciousness should be performed after each local anesthetic injection. It should be kept in mind at such times that restlessness, anxiety, incoherent speech, light-headedness, numbness and tingling of the mouth and lips, metallic taste, tinnitus, dizziness, blurred vision, tremors, twitching, depression, or drowsiness may be early warning signs of central nervous system toxicity.

Local anesthetic solutions containing a vasoconstrictor should be used cautiously and in carefully restricted quantities in areas of the body supplied by end arteries or having otherwise compromised blood supply such as digits, nose, external ear, penis, etc. Patients with hypertensive vascular disease may exhibit exaggerated vasoconstrictor response. Ischemic injury or necrosis may result.

Because amide-type local anesthetics such as bupivacaine are metabolized by the liver, these drugs, especially repeat doses, should be used cautiously in patients with hepatic disease. Patients with severe hepatic disease, because of their inability to metabolize local anesthetics normally, are at a greater risk of developing toxic plasma concentrations. Local anesthetics should also be used with caution in patients with impaired cardiovascular function because they may be less able to compensate for functional changes associated with the prolongation of A-V conduction produced by these drugs.

Serious dose-related cardiac arrythmias may occur if preparations containing a vasoconstrictor such as epinephrine are employed in patients during or following the administration of potent inhalation anesthetics. In deciding whether to use these products concurrently in the same patient, the combined action of both agents upon the myocardium, the concentration and volume of vasoconstrictor used, and the time since injection, when applicable, should be taken into account.

Many drugs used during the conduct of anesthesia are considered potential triggering agents for familial malignant hyperthermia. Because it is not known whether amide-type local anesthetics may trigger this reaction and because the need for supplemental general anesthesia cannot be predicted in advance, it is suggested that a standard protocol for management should be available. Early unexplained signs of tachycardia, tachypnea, labile blood pressure and metabolic acidosis may precede temperature elevation. Successful outcome is dependent on early diagnosis, prompt discontinuance of the suspect triggering agent(s) and prompt treatment, including oxygen therapy, dantrolene (consult dantrolene sodium intravenous package insert before using) and other supportive measures.

Use in Head and Neck Area: Small doses of local anesthetics injected into the head and neck area, including retrobulbar, dental and stellate ganglion blocks, may produce adverse reactions similar to systemic toxicity seen with unintentional intravascular injections of larger doses. The injection procedures require the utmost care. Confusion, convulsions, respiratory depression and/or respiratory arrest, and cardiovascular stimulation or depression have been reported. These reactions may be due to intraarterial injection of the local anesthetic with retrograde flow to the cerebral circulation. They also may be due to puncture of the dural sheath of the optic nerve during retrobulbar block with diffusion of any local anesthetic along the subdural space to the midbrain. Patients receiving these blocks should have their circulation and respiration monitored and be constantly observed. Resuscitative equipment and personnel for treating adverse reactions should be immediately available. Dosage recommendations should not be exceeded. (See DOSAGE AND ADMINISTRATION.)

Use in Ophthalmic Surgery: Clinicians who perform retrobulbar blocks should be aware that there have been reports of respiratory arrest following local anesthetic injection. Prior to retrobulbar block, as with all other regional procedures the immediate availability of equipment, drugs, and personnel to manage respiratory arrest or depression, convulsions, and cardiac stimulation or depression should be assured (see also WARNINGS and USE IN HEAD AND NECK AREA, above). As with other anesthetic procedures, patients should be constantly monitored following ophthalmic blocks for signs of these adverse reactions, which may occur following relatively low total doses. A concentration of 0.75% bupvacaine is indicated for retrobulbar block, however this concentration is not indicated for any other peripheral nerve block, including the facial nerve and not indicated for local infiltration, including the conjunctiva (See INDICATIONS and PRECAUTIONS, General). Mixing Sensorcaine (bupivacaine HCl) with other local anesthetics is not recommended because of insufficient data on the clinical use of such mixtures.

When Sensorcaine 0.75% is used for retrobulbar block, complete corneal anesthesia usually precedes onset of clinically acceptable external ocular muscle akinesia. Therefore, presence of akinesia rather than anesthesia alone should determine readiness of the patient for surgery.

Information for Patients: When appropriate, patients should be informed in advance that they may experience temporary loss of sensation and motor activity, usually in the lower half of the body following proper administration of caudal or lumbar epidural anesthesia. Also, when appropriate, the physician should discuss other information including adverse reactions in the Sensorcaine (bupivacaine HCl) package insert.

Clinically Significant Drug Interactions: The administration of local anesthetic solutions containing epinephrine or norepinephrine to patients receiving monoamine oxidase inhibitors or tricyclic antidepressants may produce severe, prolonged hypertension. Concurrent use of these agents should generally be avoided. In situations in which concurrent therapy is necessary, careful patient monitoring is essential.

Concurrent administration of vasopressor drugs and of ergot-type oxytocic drugs may cause severe, persistent hypertension or cerebrovascular accidents.

Phenothiazines and butyrophenones may reduce or reverse the pressor effect of epinephrine.

Carcinogenesis, Mutagenesis, and Impairment of Fertility: Long-term studies in animals of most local anesthetics, including bupivacaine, to evaluate the carcinogenic potential have not been conducted. Mutagenic potential or the effect on fertility have not been determined. There is no evidence from human data that bupivacaine may be carcinogenic or mutagenic or that it impairs fertility.

Pregnancy Category C: Decreased pup survival in rats and embryocidal effect in rabbits have been observed when bupivacaine HCl was administered to these species in doses comparable to nine and five times, respectively, the maximum recommended daily human dose (400 mg). There are no adequate and well-controlled studies in pregnant women of the effect of bupivacaine on the developing fetus. Sensorcaine (bupivacaine HCl) injection should be used during pregnancy only if the potential benefit justifies the potential risk to the fetus. This does not exclude the use of Sensorcaine (bupivacaine HCl) injection (0.25% and 0.5% concentrations) at term for obstetrical anesthesia or analgesia. (See LABOR AND DELIVERY.)

Labor and Delivery: See Box WARNING regarding obstetrical use in 0.75% concentration.

Sensorcaine (bupivacaine HCl) injection is contraindicated in obstetrical paracervical block anesthesia.

Local anesthetics rapidly cross the placenta, and when used for epidural, caudal or pudendal block anesthesia, can cause varying degrees of maternal, fetal and neonatal toxicity. (See Pharmacokinetics in CLINICAL PHARMACOLOGY.) The incidence and degree of toxicity depend upon the procedure performed, the type and amount of drug used, and the technique of drug administration. Adverse reactions in the parturient, fetus and neonate involve alterations of the central nervous system, peripheral vascular tone and cardiac function.

Maternal hypotension has resulted from regional anesthesia. Local anesthetics produce vasodilation by blocking sympathetic nerves. Elevating the patient's legs and positioning her on her left side will help prevent decreases in blood pressure. The fetal heart rate also should be monitored continuously, and electronic fetal monitoring is highly advisable.

Epidural, caudal, or pudendal anesthesia may alter the forces of parturition through changes in uterine contractility or maternal expulsive efforts. Epidural anesthesia has been reported to prolong the second stage of labor by removing the parturient's reflex urge to bear down or by interfering with motor function. The use of obstetrical anesthesia may increase the need for forceps assistance.

The use of some local anesthetic drug products during labor and delivery may be followed by diminished muscle strength and tone for the first day or two of life. This has not been reported with Sensorcaine (bupivacaine HCl) injection.

It is extremely important to avoid aortocaval compression by the gravid uterus during administration of regional block to parturients. To do this, the patient must be maintained in the left lateral decubitus position or a blanket roll or sandbag may be placed beneath the right hip and the gravid uterus displaced to the left.

Nursing Mothers: It is not known whether local anesthetic drugs are excreted in human milk. Because many drugs are excreted in human milk, caution should be exercised when local anesthetics are administered to a nursing mother.

Pediatric Use: Until further experience is gained in children younger than 12 years, administration of Sensorcaine (bupivacaine HCl) injection in this age group is not recommended.

ADVERSE REACTIONS

Reactions to bupivacaine are characteristic of those associated with other amide-type local anesthetics. A major cause of adverse reactions to this group of drugs may be associated with its excessive plasma levels, which may be due to overdosage, unintentional intravascular injection or slow metabolic degradation.

Systemic: The most commonly encountered acute adverse experiences that demand immediate countermeasures are related to the central nervous system and the cardiovascular system. These adverse experiences are generally dose related and due to high plasma levels which may result from overdosage, rapid absorption from the injection site, diminished tolerance or from unintentional intravascular injection of the local anesthetic solution. In addition to systemic dose-related toxicity, unintentional subarachnoid injection of drug during the intended performance of caudal or lumbar epidural block or nerve blocks near the vertebral column (especially in the head and neck region) may result in underventilation or apnea ("Total or High Spinal"). Also, hypotension due to loss of sympathetic tone and respiratory paralysis or underventilation due to cephalad extension of the motor level of anesthesia may occur. This may lead to secondary cardiac arrest if untreated. Factors influencing plasma protein binding, such as acidosis, systemic diseases that alter protein production or competition with other drugs for protein binding sites, may diminish individual tolerance.

Central Nervous System Reactions: These are characterized by excitation and/or depression. Restlessness, anxiety, dizziness, tinnitus, blurred vision or tremors may occur, possibly proceeding to convulsions. However, excitement may be transient or absent, with depression being the first manifestation of an adverse reaction. This may quickly be followed by drowsiness merging into unconsciousness and respiratory arrest. Other central nervous system effects may be nausea, vomiting, chills, and constriction of the pupils.

The incidence of convulsions associated with the use of local anesthetics varies with the procedure used and the total dose administered. In a survey of studies of epidural anesthesia, overt toxicity progressing to convulsions occurred in approximately 0.1 percent of local anesthetic administrations.

Cardiovascular System Reactions: High doses or unintentional intravascular injection may lead to high plasma levels and related depression of the myocardium, decreased cardiac output, heart block, hypotension, bradycardia, ventricular arrhythmias, including ventricular tachycardia and ventricular fibrillation, and cardiac arrest. (See WARNINGS, PRECAUTIONS, and OVERDOSAGE sections.)

Allergic: Allergic type reactions are rare and may occur as a result of sensitivity to the local anesthetic or to other formulation ingredients, such as the antimicrobial preservative methylparaben contained in multiple dose vials or sulfites in epinephrine-containing solutions (see WARNINGS). These reactions are characterized by signs such as urticaria, pruritus, erythema, angioneurotic edema (including laryngeal edema), tachycardia, sneezing, nausea, vomiting, dizziness, syncope, excessive sweating, elevated temperature, and possibly, anaphylactoid symptomatology (including severe hypotension). Cross sensitivity among members of the amide-type local anesthetic group has been reported. The useful-

ness of screening for sensitivity has not been definitely established.

Neurologic: The incidence of adverse neurologic reactions associated with the use of local anesthetics may be related to the total dose of local anesthetic administered and are also dependent upon the particular drug used, the route of administration and the physical status of the patient. Many of these effects may be related to local anesthetic techniques, with or without a contribution from the drug.

In the practice of caudal or lumbar epidural block, occasional unintentional penetration of the subarachnoid space by the catheter or needle may occur. Subsequent adverse effects may depend partially on the amount of drug administered intrathecally and the physiological and physical effects of a dural puncture. A high spinal is characterized by paralysis of the legs, loss of consciousness, respiratory paralysis and bradycardia.

Neurologic effects following unintentional subarachnoid administration during epidural or caudal anesthesia may include spinal block by varying magnitude (including high or total spinal block); hypotension secondary to spinal block; urinary retention; fecal and urinary incontinence; loss of perineal sensation and sexual function; persistent anesthesia, paresthesia, weakness, paralysis of the lower extremities and loss of sphincter control, all of which may have slow, incomplete or no recovery; headache; backache; septic meningitis; meningismus; slowing of labor; increased incidence of forceps delivery; or cranial nerve palsies due to traction on nerves from loss of cerebrospinal fluid.

OVERDOSAGE

Acute emergencies from local anesthetics are generally related to high plasma levels encountered during therapeutic use of local anesthetics or to unintended subarachnoid injection of local anesthetic solution. (See ADVERSE REACTIONS, WARNINGS, and PRECAUTIONS).

Management of Local Anesthetic Emergencies: The first consideration is prevention, best accomplished by careful and constant monitoring of cardiovascular and respiratory vital signs and the patient's state of consciousness after each local anesthetic injection. At the first sign of change, oxygen should be administered.

The first step in the management of systemic toxic reactions, as well as underventilation or apnea due to unintentional subarachnoid injection of drug solution, consists of **immediate** attention to the establishment and maintenance of a patent airway and effective assisted or controlled ventilation with 100% oxygen with a delivery system capable of permitting immediate positive airway pressure by mask. This may prevent convulsions if they have not already occurred.

If necessary, use drugs to control the convulsions. A 50 to 100 mg bolus I.V. injection of succinylcholine will paralyze the patient without depressing the central nervous or cardiovascular systems and facilitate ventilation. A bolus I.V. dose of 5 to 10 mg of diazepam or 50 to 100 mg of thiopental will permit ventilation and counteract central nervous system stimulation, but these drugs also depress the central nervous system, respiratory and cardiac function, add to postictal depression, and may result in apnea. Intravenous barbiturates, anticonvulsant agents, or muscle relaxants should only be administered by those familiar with their use. Immediately after the institution of these ventilatory measures, the adequacy of the circulation should be evaluated. Supportive treatment of circulatory depression may require administration of intravenous fluids, and, when appropriate, a vasopressor dictated by the clinical situation (such as ephedrine or epinephrine to enhance myocardial contractile force).

If difficulty is encountered in the maintenance of a patent airway or if prolonged ventilatory support (assisted or controlled) is indicated, endotracheal intubation, employing drugs and techniques familiar to the clinician, may be indicated after initial administration of oxygen by mask.

Recent clinical data from patients experiencing local anesthetic induced convulsions demonstrated rapid development of hypoxia, hypercarbia and acidosis wih bupivacaine within a minute of the onset of convulsions. These observations suggest the oxygen consumption and carbon dioxide production are greatly increased during local anesthetic convulsions and emphasize the importance of immediate and effective ventilation with oxygen which may avoid cardiac arrest.

If not treated immediately, convulsions with simultaneous hypoxia, hypercarbia and acidosis, plus myocardial depression from the direct effects of the local anesthetic may result in cardiac arrhythmias, bradycardia, asystole, ventricular fibrillation, or cardiac arrest. Respiratory abnormalities, including apnea, may occur. Underventilation or apnea due to unintentional subarachnoid injection of local anesthetic solution may produce these same signs and also lead to cardiac arrest if ventilatory support is not instituted. *If cardiac arrest should occur, a successful outcome may require prolonged resuscitative efforts.*

The supine position is dangerous in pregnant women at term because of aortocaval compression by the gravid uterus. Therefore, during treatment of systemic toxicity, maternal hypotension or fetal bradycardia following regional block, the parturient should be maintained in the left lateral decubitus position if possible, or manual displacement of the uterus off the great vessels be accomplished.

The mean seizure dosage of bupivacaine in rhesus monkeys was found to be 4.4 mg/kg with mean arterial plasma concentration of 4.5 mcg/mL. The intravenous and subcutaneous LD_{50} in mice is 6 to 8 mg/kg and 38 to 54 mg/kg respectively.

TABLE 1. DOSAGE RECOMMENDATIONS—SENSORCAINE (bupivacaine HCl) INJECTIONS

Type of Block	Each Dose conc.(%)	(mL)	(mg)	Motor Block[1]
Local Infiltration	0.25[4]	up to max.	up to max.	—
Epidural	0.75[2,4]	10–20	75–150	Complete
	0.5[4]	10–20	50–100	Moderate to complete
	0.25[4]	10–20	25–50	Partial to moderate
Caudal	0.5[4]	15–30	75–150	Moderate to complete
	0.25[4]	15–30	37.5–75	Moderate
Peripheral Nerves	0.5[4]	5 to max.	25 to max.	Moderate to complete
	0.25[4]	5 to max.	12.5 to max.	Moderate to complete
Retrobulbar[3]	0.75[4]	2–4	15–30	Complete
Sympathetic	0.25	20–50	50–125	—
Epidural[3] Test Dose	0.5 w/epi.	2–3	10–15 (see PRECAUTIONS)	—

[1]With continuous (intermittent) techniques, repeat doses increase the degree of motor block. The first repeat dose of 0.5% may produce complete motor block. Intercostal nerve block with 0.25% may also produce complete motor block for intra-abdominal surgery.
[2]For single-dose use; not for intermittent (catheter) epidural technique. Not for obstetrical anesthesia.
[3]See PRECAUTIONS.
[4]Solutions with or without epinephrine.

DOSAGE AND ADMINISTRATION

The dose of any local anesthetic administered varies with the anesthetic procedure, the area to be anesthetized, the vascularity of the tissues, the number of neuronal segments to be blocked, the depth of anesthesia and degree of muscle relaxation required, the duration of anesthesia desired, individual tolerance, and the physical condition of the patient. The smallest dose and concentration required to produce the desired result should be administered. Dosages of SENSORCAINE should be reduced for young, elderly and debilitated patients and patients with cardiac and/or liver disease. The rapid injection of a large volume of local anesthetic solution should be avoided and fractional (incremental) doses should be used when feasible.

For specific techniques and procedures, refer to standard textbooks.

In recommended doses, SENSORCAINE produces complete sensory block, but the effect on motor function differs among the three concentrations.

0.25%—when used for caudal, epidural, or peripheral nerve block, produces incomplete motor block. Should be used for operations in which muscle relaxation is not important, or when another means of providing muscle relaxation is used concurrently. Onset of action may be slower than with the 0.5% or 0.75% solutions.

0.5%—provides motor blockade for caudal, epidural, or nerve block, but muscle relaxation may be inadequate for operations in which complete muscle relaxation is essential.

0.75%—produces complete motor block. Most useful for epidural block in abdominal operations requiring complete muscle relaxation, and for retrobulbar anesthesia. Not for obstetrical anesthesia.

The duration of anesthesia with SENSORCAINE is such that for most indications, a single dose is sufficient.

Maximum dosage limit must be individualized in each case after evaluating the size and physical status of the patient, as well as the usual rate of systemic absorption from a particular injection site. Most experience to date is with single doses of SENSORCAINE up to 225 mg with epinephrine 1:200,000 and 175 mg without epinephrine, more or less drug may be used depending on individualization of each case. These doses may be repeated up to once every three hours. In clinical studies to date, total daily doses up to 400 mg have been reported. Until further experience is gained, this dose should not be exceeded in 24 hours. The duration of anesthetic effect may be prolonged by the addition of epinephrine.

The dosages in Table 1 have generally proved satisfactory and are recommended as a guide for use in the average adult. These dosages should be reduced for young, elderly or debilitated patients. Until further experience is gained, SENSORCAINE is not recommended for children younger than 12 years. SENSORCAINE is contraindicated for obstetrical paracervical blocks and is not recommended for intravenous regional anesthesia (Bier Block).

Use in Epidural Anesthesia: During epidural administration of SENSORCAINE, 0.5% and 0.75% solutions should be administered in incremental doses of 3 mL to 5 mL, with sufficient time between doses to detect toxic manifestations of unintentional intravascular or intrathecal injection. In obstetrics, only the 0.5% and 0.25% concentrations should be used; incremental doses of 3 mL to 5 mL of the 0.5% solution, not exceeding 50 mg to 100 mg at any dosing interval are recommended. Repeat doses should be preceded by a test dose containing epinephrine if not contraindicated. Use only the single-dose ampules and single-dose vials for caudal or epidural anesthesia; the multiple-dose vials contain a preservative and therefore should not be used for these procedures.

Test dose for Caudal and Lumbar Epidural Blocks: See PRECAUTIONS.

Unused portions of solutions in single dose containers should be discarded, since this product form contains no preservatives.

[See table above.]

NOTE: Parenteral drug products should be inspected visually for particulate matter and discoloration prior to administration whenever the solution and container permit. The injection is not to be used if its color is pinkish or darker than slightly yellow or if it contains a precipitate.

HOW SUPPLIED

SOLUTIONS OF SENSORCAINE (BUPIVACAINE HYDROCHLORIDE) SHOULD NOT BE USED FOR THE PRODUCTION OF SPINAL ANESTHESIA (SUBARACHNOID BLOCK) BECAUSE OF INSUFFICIENT DATA TO SUPPORT SUCH USE.

[See table below.]

Disinfecting agents containing heavy metals, which cause release of respective ions (mercury, zinc, copper, etc.), should

HOW SUPPLIED

Sensorcaine-MPF (methylparaben free) is available in the following forms:

Single Dose Ampules;	
5 mL;	0.5% with epinephrine 1:200,000
30 mL;	0.25%, 0.5% and 0.75% without epinephrine
	0.5% and 0.75% with epinephrine 1:200,000
Single Dose Vials;	
10 mL; with Astra E-Z Off® vial closure	0.25%, 0.5% and 0.75% without epinephrine
	0.25%, 0.5% and 0.75% with epinephrine 1:200,000
30 mL;	0.25% and 0.5% without epinephrine
	0.25%, 0.5% and 0.75% with epinephrine 1:200,000

Sensorcaine is available in the following forms:

Multiple Dose Vials;	
50 mL;	0.25%, and 0.5% without epinephrine
	0.25% and 0.5% with epinephrine 1:200,000

Continued on next page

Astra—Cont.

not be used for skin or mucous membrane disinfection since they have been related to incidents of swelling and edema. When chemical disinfection of the container surface is desired, either isopropyl alcohol (91%) or ethyl alcohol (70%) is recommended. It is recommended that chemical disinfection be accomplished by wiping the ampule or vial stopper thoroughly with cotton or gauze that has been moistened with the recommended alcohol just prior to use.
Solutions should be stored at controlled room temperature 15° to 30°C (59°–86°F).
Solutions containing epinephrine should be protected from light.
021680R00   5/91 (00)

SENSORCAINE®-MPF™ SPINAL   ℞
[sén-sor-caine]
(Bupivacaine in Dextrose Injection USP)
Bupivacaine HCl 0.75% in Dextrose 8.25% Injection
Sterile Hyperbaric Solution for Spinal Anesthesia

(For details of indications, dosages and administration, precautions, and adverse reactions, see circular in package.)
HOW SUPPLIED
NDC 0186-1026-03 2 mL ampule (15 mg bupivacaine HCl with 165 mg dextrose), boxes of 10.
Store at controlled room temperature, between 15° C and 30° C (59° F and 86° F).
021868R02   11/89 (2)

SODIUM BICARBONATE   ℞
[so'-dēum by-car'-bōw-nāte]
Injection, USP

FOR CORRECTION OF METABOLIC ACIDOSIS AND OTHER CONDITIONS REQUIRING SYSTEMIC ALKALINIZATION
(For details of indications, dosage and administration, precautions, and adverse reactions, see circular in package.)

HOW SUPPLIED
Sodium Bicarbonate Injection, USP is supplied in the following dosage forms:
[See table above.]
Solutions should be stored at controlled room temperature 15°–30°C (59°– –86°F).
021701R00   Rev. 6/88

SODIUM CHLORIDE 0.9%,   ℞
SODIUM CHLORIDE 0.45%,
Sterile Water for Inhalation
Arm-A-Vial®

INDICATIONS
For use in respiratory therapy. Contents of these vials are for use in apparatus for intermittent positive pressure-breathing (IPPB) and for tracheal lavage.

WARNING
Not for injection or in preparations to be used for injection.

DOSAGE AND ADMINISTRATION
To verify container integrity squeeze Arm-a-Vial® before use. Twist cap completely off Arm-a-Vial, invert, squeeze prescribed volume in nebulizer cup of IPPB apparatus.
Can also be used for tracheal lavage.
Internal contents sterile.
External surface of vial not sterile.
DISCARD ANY UNUSED PORTION OF THE CONTENTS OF THIS SINGLE DOSE VIAL AS WELL AS ANY UNUSED SOLUTION REMAINING IN THE NEBULIZER CUP.

HOW SUPPLIED
Single dose plastic Arm-a-Vial containing 3 mL or 5 mL solutions.
Sterile water. Non pyrogenic. Available by shelf carton of 100 × 3 mL vials (NDC 0186-4102-01) and 100 × 5 mL vials (NDC 0186-4102-03).
Sodium chloride 0.9% (normal saline-sterile). Non pyrogenic. Available by shelf carton of 100 × 3 mL vials (NDC 0186-4100-01) and 100 × 5 mL vials (NDC 0186-4100-03).
Sodium chloride 0.45% (half-normal saline-sterile). Non pyrogenic. Available by shelf carton of 100 × 3 mL vials (NDC 0186-4101-01) and 100 × 5 mL vials (NDC 0186-4101-03).
Store at controlled room temperature, 15°–30°C (59°–86°F).
021672R00   Iss. 6/91

NDC No. 0186-	Dosage Form	Conc. %	mg/mL (NaHCO₃)	mEq/mL; (Na+)	mEq/mL (HCO₃)	mEq/Container size (mL)	mOsm
0650-01	Syringe	8.4	84	1.0	1.0	50/50	2/mL
0656-01	Syringe (Pediatric)	8.4	84	1.0	1.0	10/10	2/mL
0647-01	Syringe	7.5	75	0.9	0.9	44.6/50	1.79/mL
0646-01	Syringe (Infant)	4.2	42	0.5	0.5	5/10	1/mL
0645-01	Syringe (Infant)	4.2	42	0.5	0.5	2.5/5	1/mL

STREPTASE®   ℞
(streptokinase)

DESCRIPTION
Streptase® (streptokinase) is a sterile, purified preparation of a bacterial protein elaborated by group C β-hemolytic streptococci. It is supplied as a lyophilized white powder containing 25 mg cross-linked gelatin polypeptides, 25 mg sodium L-glutamate, sodium hydroxide to adjust pH, and 100 mg Albumin (Human) per vial as stabilizers. The preparation contains no preservatives and is intended for intravenous and intracoronary administration.

CLINICAL PHARMACOLOGY
Streptase® (streptokinase) acts with plasminogen to produce an "activator complex" that converts plasminogen to the proteolytic enzyme plasmin. The $t_{1/2}$ of the activator complex is about 23 minutes; the complex is inactivated, in part, by antistreptococcal antibodies. The mechanism by which streptokinase is eliminated is unknown; no metabolites of streptokinase have been identified. Plasmin degrades fibrin clots as well as fibrinogen and other plasma proteins. Plasmin is inactivated by circulating inhibitors, such as α-2-plasmin inhibitor or α-2-macroglobulin. These inhibitors are rapidly consumed at high doses of streptokinase.
Intravenous infusion of streptokinase is followed by increased fibrinolytic activity, which decreases plasma fibrinogen levels for 24 to 36 hours. The decrease in plasma fibrinogen is associated with decreases in plasma and blood viscosity and red blood cell aggregation. The hyperfibrinolytic effect disappears within a few hours after discontinuation, but a prolonged thrombin time may persist for up to 24 hours due to the decrease in plasma levels of fibrinogen and an increase in the amount of circulating fibrin(ogen) degradation products (FDP). Depending upon the dosage and duration of infusion of streptokinase, the thrombin time will decrease less than two times the normal control value within 4 hours, and return to normal by 24 hours.
Intravenous administration has been shown to reduce blood pressure and total peripheral resistance with a corresponding reduction in cardiac afterload. These expected responses were not studied with the intracoronary administration of Streptase® (streptokinase). The quantitative benefit has not been evaluated.
Variable amounts of circulating antistreptokinase antibody are present in individuals as a result of recent streptococcal infection. The recommended dosage schedule usually obviates the need for antibody titration.
Two large randomized, placebo-controlled studies conducted with a 60 minute intravenous infusion of 1,500,000 IU of Streptase® (streptokinase) for the treatment of acute myocardial infarction within 6 hours of the onset of symptoms have reported reductions in acute mortality from 20–25%.(1,2)
In the GISSI study, the reduction in mortality was time dependent; there was a 47% reduction in mortality among patients treated within one hour of the onset of chest pain, a 23% reduction among patients treated within three hours, and a 17% reduction among patients treated between three and six hours. There was also a reduction in mortality in patients treated between six and twelve hours from the onset of symptoms, but the reduction was not statistically significant.
One of eight smaller studies using a similar dosing schedule showed statistically significant reduction in mortality. When all of these studies were pooled, the overall decrease in mortality was approximately 23%. Results from pooling several studies using different dosages with long term infusion corroborate these observations.
In addition, studies measuring left ventricular ejection fraction (LVEF) at discharge showed the mean LVEFs were approximately 3–6 percentage points higher in the Streptase® (streptokinase) group when compared to the control group. This difference was statistically significant in some of the studies.(3,4) Furthermore, some studies reported greater improvement in LVEF among patients treated within three hours than in patients treated later. Fewer streptokinase treated patients had very low ejection fractions associated

with congestive heart failure, and the number of patients with clinical symptoms of CHF was reduced.
The rate of reocclusion of the infarct-related vessel has been reported to be approximately 20%. The rate of reocclusion depends on dosage, additional anticoagulant therapy and residual stenosis. When the reinfarctions were evaluated in studies involving 8,800 streptokinase treated patients, the overall rate was 3.8% (range 2–15%). In over 8,500 control patients, the rate of reinfarction was 2.4%.
Streptase® (streptokinase) administered by the intracoronary route has resulted in thrombolysis usually within one hour, and ensuing reperfusion results in limitation of infarct size, improvement of cardiac function, and reduction of mortality.(5,6) LVEF was increased in patients treated with streptokinase when compared to patients treated with conventional therapy. When the initial LVEF was low, the streptokinase-treated patients showed greater improvement than did the controls. Spontaneous reperfusion is known to occur and has been observed with angiography at various time points after infarction. Data from one study show that 73% of the streptokinase-treated patients and 47% of the placebo-allocated patients reperfused during hospitalization.
Studies with thrombolytic therapy for pulmonary embolism show no significant difference in lung perfusion scan between the thrombolysis group and the heparin group at one year follow-up. However, measurements of pulmonary capillary blood volumes and diffusing capacities at two weeks and one year after therapy indicate that a more complete resolution of thrombotic obstruction and normalization of pulmonary physiology was achieved with thrombolytic therapy, thus preventing the long term sequelae of pulmonary hypertension and pulmonary failure.(7)
The long term benefit of Streptase® (streptokinase) therapy for deep vein thrombosis (DVT) has been evaluated venographically.(8) The combined results of five randomized studies show no residual thrombotic material in 60–75% of patients treated with streptokinase versus only 10% of those treated with heparin. Thrombolytic therapy also preserves venous valve function in a majority of cases, thus avoiding the pathologic venous changes that produce the clinical postphlebitic syndrome which occurs in 90% of the DVT patients treated with heparin.
There is a time-related decrease in effectiveness when Streptase® (streptokinase) is used in the management of peripheral arterial thromboembolism. When administered three to ten days after onset of obstruction, rates of clearance of 50–75% were reported.

INDICATIONS AND USAGE
Acute Evolving Transmural Myocardial Infarction
Streptase® (streptokinase) is indicated for use in the management of acute myocardial infarction (AMI) in adults, for the lysis of intracoronary thrombi, for the improvement of ventricular function, for the reduction of the incidence of congestive heart failure associated with AMI, and for the reduction of mortality when administered by either the intravenous or intracoronary route. Earlier administration of streptokinase is correlated with greater clinical benefit. (See **CLINICAL PHARMACOLOGY** section.)
Pulmonary Embolism
Streptase® (streptokinase) is indicated for the lysis of objectively diagnosed (angiography or lung scan) pulmonary emboli, involving obstruction of blood flow to a lobe or multiple segments, with or without unstable hemodynamics.
Deep Vein Thrombosis
Streptase® (streptokinase) is indicated for the lysis of objectively diagnosed (preferably ascending venography), acute, extensive thrombi of the deep veins such as those involving the popliteal and more proximal vessels.
Arterial Thrombosis or Embolism
Streptase® (streptokinase) is indicated for the lysis of acute arterial thrombi and emboli. Streptokinase is not indicated for arterial emboli originating from the left side of the heart due to the risk of new embolic phenomena such as cerebral embolism.
Occlusion of Arteriovenous Cannulae
Streptase® (streptokinase) is indicated as an alternative to surgical revision for clearing totally or partially occluded arteriovenous cannulae when acceptable flow cannot be achieved.

Route	Total Dose	Dosage/Duration
Intravenous infusion	1,500,000 IU	1,500,000 IU within 60 min.
Intracoronary infusion	140,000 IU	20,000 IU by bolus followed by 2,000 IU/min. for 60 min.

CONTRAINDICATIONS

Because thrombolytic therapy increases the risk of bleeding, Streptase® (streptokinase) is contraindicated in the following situations:

- active internal bleeding
- recent (within 2 months) cerebrovascular accident, intracranial or intraspinal surgery (see **WARNINGS**)
- Intracranial neoplasm
- severe uncontrolled hypertension

Streptokinase should not be administered to patients having experienced severe allergic reaction to the product.

WARNINGS

Bleeding

Streptase® (streptokinase) will cause lysis of hemostatic fibrin deposits such as those occuring at sites of needle punctures, and bleeding may occur from such sites. In order to minimize the risk of bleeding during treatment with streptokinase, venipunctures and physicial handling of the patient should be performed carefully and as infrequently as possible, and intramuscular injections must be avoided.

Should arterial puncture be necessary during intravenous therapy, upper extremity vessels are preferable. Pressure should be applied for at least 30 minutes, a pressure dressing applied, and the puncture site checked frequently for evidence of bleeding.

In the following conditions the risks of therapy may be increased and should be weighed against the anticipated benefits.

- Recent (within 10 days) major surgery, obstetrical delivery, organ biopsy, previous puncture of noncompressible vessels.
- Recent (within 10 days) serious gastrointestinal bleeding
- Recent (within 10 days) trauma including cardiopulmonary resuscitation
- Hypertension: systolic BP ≥ 180 mm Hg and/or diastolic BP ≥ 110 mm Hg
- High likelihood of left heart thrombus, e.g., mitral stenosis with artrial fibrillation
- Subacute bacterial endocarditis
- Hemostatic defect including those secondary to severe hepatic or renal disease
- Pregnancy
- Age ≥ 75 years
- Cerebrovascular disease
- Diabetic hemorrhagic retinopathy
- Septic thrombophlebitis or occluded AV cannula at seriously infected site
- Any other condition in which bleeding constitutes a significant hazard or would be particularly difficult to manage because of its location.

Should serious spontaneous bleeding (not controllable by local pressure) occur, the infusion of Streptase® (streptokinase) should be terminated immediately and treatment instituted as described under **ADVERSE REACTIONS.**

Arrhythmias

Rapid lysis of coronary thrombi has been shown to cause reperfusion atrial or ventricular dysrhythmias requiring immediate treatment. Careful monitoring for arrhythmia is recommended during and immediately following administration of Streptase® (streptokinase) for acute myocardial infarction.

Hypotension

Hypotension, sometimes severe, not secondary to bleeding or anaphylaxis has been observed during intravenous Streptase® (streptokinase) infusion in 1% to 10% of patients. Patients should be monitored closely and, should symptomatic or alarming hypotension occur, appropriate treatment should be administered. This treatment may include a decrease in the intravenous streptokinase infusion rate. Smaller hypotensive effects are common and have not required treatment.

Other

Non-cardiogenic pulmonary edema has been reported rarely in patients treated with Streptase® (streptokinase). The risk of this appears greatest in patients who have large myocardial infarctions and are undergoing thrombolytic therapy by the intracoronary route.

Rarely, polyneuropathy has been temporally related to the use of Streptase® (streptokinase).

Should pulmonary embolism or recurrent pulmonary embolism occur during Streptase® (streptokinase) therapy, the originally planned course of treatment should be completed in an attempt to lyse the embolus. While pulmonary embolism may occasionally occur during streptokinase treatment, the incidence is no greater than when patients are treated with heparin alone.

PRECAUTIONS

General

Because of the increased likelihood of resistance, due to anti-streptokinase antibody, Streptase® (streptokinase) may not be effective if administered between five days and twelve months of prior streptokinase or Anistreplase administration or streptococcal infections, such as streptococcal pharyngitis, acute rheumatic fever, or acute glomerulonephritis secondary to a streptococcal infection.

Laboratory Tests

Intravenous or Intracoronary Infusion for Myocardial Infarction.

Intravenous administration of Streptase® (streptokinase) will cause marked decreases in plasminogen and fibrinogen and increases in thrombin time (TT), activated partial thromboplastin time (APTT), and prothrombin time (PT). These changes may also occur in some patients with intracoronary administration of streptokinase.

Intravenous Infusion for Other Indications. Before commencing thrombolytic therapy, it is desirable to obtain an activated partial thromboplastin time (APTT), a prothrombin time (PT), a thrombin time (TT), fibrinogen levels, and a hematocrit and platelet count. If heparin has been given, it should be discontinued and the TT or APTT should be less than twice the normal control value before thrombolytic therapy is started.

During the infusion, decreases in plasminogen and fibrinogen levels and an increase in the level of FDP (the latter two causing a prolongation in the clotting times of coagulation tests) will generally confirm the existence of a lytic state. Therefore, lytic therapy can be confirmed by performing the TT, APTT, PT, or fibrinogen levels approximately 4 hours after initiation of therapy.

If heparin is to be (re)instituted following the Streptase® (streptokinase) infusion, the TT or APTT should be less than twice the normal control value (see manufacturer's prescribing information for proper use of heparin).

Drug Interactions

The interaction of Streptase® (streptokinase) with other drugs has not been well studied.

Use of Anticoagulants and Antiplatelet Agents. Streptase® (streptokinase) alone or in combination with antiplatelet agents and anticoagulants, may cause bleeding complications. Therefore, careful monitoring is advised.

Anticoagulation After Treatment for Myocardial Infarction. Administration of anticoagulant and/or antiplatelet drugs following administration of Streptase® (streptokinase) appears to increase the risk of bleeding (see **ADVERSE REACTIONS**). These agents have been used in an attempt to prevent reocclusion of the target vessel. Use of anticoagulants following administration of streptokinase has not yet been shown to be of unequivocal clinical benefit. Therefore, the use of anticoagulant regimens should be individualized.

Anticoagulation After IV Treatment for Other Indications. Continuous intravenous infusion of heparin, without a loading dose, has been recommended following termination of Streptase® (streptokinase) infusion for treatment of pulmonary embolism or deep vein thrombosis to prevent rethrombosis. The effect of streptokinase on thrombin time (TT) and activated partial thromboplastin time (APTT) will usually diminish with 3 to 4 hours after streptokinase therapy, and heparin therapy without a loading dose can be initiated when the TT or the APTT is less than twice the normal control value.

Pregnancy

Pregnancy Category C. Animal reproduction studies have not been conducted with Streptase® (streptokinase). It is also not known whether streptokinase can cause fetal harm

when administered to a pregnant woman or can affect reproduction capacity. Streptokinase should be given to a pregnant woman only if clearly needed.

Pediatric Use

Safety and effectiveness in children have not been established.

ADVERSE REACTIONS

The following adverse reactions have been associated with intravenous therapy and may also occur with intracoronary artery infusion:

Bleeding

The incidence of bleeding (major or minor) varied widely from study to study depending on dosage, patient population and concomitant therapy.

Minor bleeding can be anticipated mainly at invaded or disturbed sites. If such bleeding occurs, local measures should be taken to control the bleeding.

Severe internal bleeding involving gastrointestinal, genitourinary, retroperitoneal, or intracerebral sites has occurred and has resulted in fatalities. In three studies in which anticoagulation was optional following intravenous administration of Streptase® (streptokinase) for acute myocardial infarction, the incidence of major bleeding ranged from 0.3%–6.2%. In 21 studies in which anticoagulation was compulsory, the incidence of major bleeding ranged from 0–16%. The overall incidence of major bleeding with high-dose intravenous infusion is 1.2%.

Major bleed rates are difficult to determine for other dosages and patient populations because of the different dosing and intervals of infusions. The rates reported appear to be within the ranges reported for intravenous administration in acute myocardial infarction.

Should uncontrollable bleeding occur, streptokinase infusion should be terminated immediately. Slowing the rate of administration of streptokinase will not help correct bleeding and may make it worse. If necessary, bleeding can be reversed and blood loss effectively managed with appropriate replacement therapy. Although the use of aminocaproic acid (ACA, AMICAR®) in humans as an antidote for streptokinase has not been documented, it may be considered in an emergency situation.

Allergic Reactions

Anaphylactic and anaphylactoid reactions have been observed rarely in patients treated intravenously with Streptase® (streptokinase). These ranged in severity from minor breathing difficulty to bronchospasm, periorbital swelling or angioneurotic edema. Other milder allergic effects such as urticaria, itching, flushing, nausea, headache and musculoskeletal pain have also been observed, as have delayed hypersensitivity reactions such as vasculitis and interstitial nephritis. Anaphylactic shock was reported in one study with an incidence rate of 0.1%.

Mild or moderate allergic reactions may be managed with concomitant antihistamine and/or corticosteroid therapy. Severe allergic reactions require immediate discontinuation of Streptase® (streptokinase) with adrenergic, antihistamine, and/or corticosteroid agents administered intravenously as required.

Fever

Although Streptase® (streptokinase) is nonpyrogenic in standard animal tests, recent reports in the literature have noted an incidence of fever ranging from 0 to 21% in patients treated intravenously with streptokinase. Symptomatic treatment is usually sufficient to alleviate discomfort.

DOSAGE AND ADMINISTRATION

Acute Evolving Transmural Myocardial Infarction

Administer streptokinase as soon as possible after onset of symptoms. The greatest benefit in mortality reduction was observed when Streptase® (streptokinase) was administered within one hour; statistically significant benefits were observed up to six hours and some benefit was observed up to 12 hours without statistical significance (See **CLINICAL PHARMACOLOGY.**) [See table above.]

Pulmonary Embolism, Deep Vein Thrombosis, Arterial Thrombosis or Embolism

Streptase® (streptokinase) treatment should be instituted as soon as possible after onset of the thrombotic event, preferably within 7 days. Any delay in instituting lytic therapy to evaluate the effect of heparin therapy decreases the potential for optimal efficacy. Since human exposure to streptococci is common, antibodies to streptokinase are prevalent. Thus, a loading dose of streptokinase sufficient to neutralize these antibodies is required. A dose of 250,000 IU of streptokinase infused into a peripheral vein over 30 minutes has been found appropriate in over 90% of patients. Furthermore, if the thrombin time or any other parameter of lysis after 4 hours of therapy is not significantly different from the normal control level, discontinue streptokinase because excessive resistance is present. [See table at left.]

Arteriovenous Cannulae Occlusion

Before using Streptase® (streptokinase) an attempt should be made to clear the cannula by careful syringe technique,

Indication	Loading Dose	IV Infusion Dosage/Duration
Pulmonary Embolism	250,000 IU/30 min.	100,000 IU/hr for 24 hr (72 hrs if concurrent DVT is suspected).
Deep Vein Thrombosis	250,000 IU/30 min.	100,000 IU/hr for 72 hr
Arterial Thrombosis or Embolism	250,000 IU/30 min.	100,000 IU/hr for 24–72 hr

Continued on next page

Astra—Cont.

using heparinized saline solution. If adequate flow is not reestablished, streptokinase may be employed. Allow the effect of any pretreatment anticoagulants to diminish. Instill 250,000 IU streptokinase in 2 mL of solution into each occluded limb of the cannula slowly. Clamp off cannula limb(s) for 2 hours. Observe the patient closely for possible adverse effects. After treatment, aspirate contents of infused cannula limb(s), flush with saline, reconnect cannula.

Reconstitution and Dilution

The protein nature and lyophilized form of Streptase® (streptokinase) require careful reconstitution and dilution. Slight flocculation (described as thin translucent fibers) of reconstituted streptokinase occurred occasionally during clinical trials but did not interfere with the safe use of the solution. The following reconstitution and dilution procedures are recommended:

1. Slowly add 5 mL Sodium Chloride Injection, USP or Dextrose (5%) Injection, USP to the Streptase® (streptokinase) vial, directing the diluent at the side of the vacuum-packed vial rather than into the drug powder.
2. Roll and tilt the vial gently to reconstitute. **Avoid shaking.** (Shaking may cause foaming.)
3. Withdraw the entire reconstituted contents of the vial; slowly and carefully dilute further to a total volume as recommended in Table I. Avoid shaking and agitation on dilution. (If necessary, total volume may be increased to a maximum of 500 mL in glass or 50 mL in plastic containers, and the infusion pump rate in Table I should be adjusted accordingly.) To facilitate setting the infusion pump rate, a total volume of 45 mL, or a multiple thereof, is recommended.
4. When diluting the 1,500,000 IU infusion bottle (50 mL), slowly add 5 mL Sodium Chloride Injection, USP, or Dextrose (5%) Injection, USP, directing it at the side of the bottle rather than into the drug powder. Roll and tilt the bottle gently to reconstitute. Avoid shaking as it may cause foaming. Add an additional 40 mL of diluent to the bottle, avoiding shaking and agitation (total volume = 45 mL). Administer by infusion pump at the rate indicated in Table I.
5. Parenteral drug products should be inspected visually for particulate matter and discoloration prior to administration. (The albumin (human) may impart a slightly yellow color to the solution.)
6. The reconstituted solution can be filtered through a 0.8 μm or larger pore size filter.
7. Because Streptase® (streptokinase) contains no preservatives, it should be reconstituted immediately before use. The solution may be used for direct intravenous administration within eight hours following reconstitution if stored at 2–8°C (36–46° F).
8. Do not add other medication to the container of Streptase® (streptokinase).

[See table below.]

For Use In Arteriovenous Cannulae

Slowly reconstitute the contents of 250,000 IU Streptase® (streptokinase) vacuum-packed vial with 2 mL Sodium Chloride Injection, USP or Dextrose (5%) Injection, USP.

HOW SUPPLIED

Streptase® (streptokinase) is supplied as a lyophilized white powder in 6.5 mL vials with a color-coded label corresponding to the amount of purified streptokinase in each vial as follows:

green	250,000 IU	NDC 0186-1770-01, box of 1
blue	750,000 IU	NDC 0186-1771-01, box of 1
red	1,500,000 IU	NDC 0186-1773-01, box of 1 (vials) and
		NDC 0186-1774-01, box of 1 (infusion bottle)

Store unopened vials at controlled room temperature (15–30° C or 59–86 ° F). Unused reconstituted drug should be discarded.

REFERENCES

1. GISSI: Effectiveness of intravenous thrombolytic treatment in acute myocardial infarction. Lancet I: 397–402, 1986.
2. ISIS Steering Committee: Intravenous streptokinase given within 0–4 hours of onset of myocardial infarction reduced mortality in ISIS-2. Lancet I: 502, 1987.
3. White, H., Norris, R., Brown, M., et al: Effect of intravenous streptokinase on left ventricular function and early survival after acute myocardial infarction. N Engl J Med 317: 850–5, 1987.
4. The I.S.A.M. Study Group: A prospective trial of intravenous streptokinase in acute myocardial infarction (I.S.A.M.). N Engl J Med 314: 1465–1471, 1986.
5. Anderson, J., Marshall, H., Bray, B., et al: A randomized trial of intracoronary streptokinase in the treatment of acute myocardial infarction. N Engl J Med 308: 1312–18, 1983.
6. Kennedy, J., Ritchie, J., Davis, K., Fritz, J.: Western Washington randomized trial of intracoronary streptokinase in acute myocardial infarction. N Engl J Med 309: 1477–82, 1983.
7. Sharma, G., Burleson, V., Sasahara, A.: Effect of thrombolytic therapy on pulmonary-capillary blood volume in patients with pulmonary embolism. N Engl J Med 303: 842–5, 1980.
8. Arneson, H., Heilo, A., Jakobsen, E., et al: A prospective study of streptokinase and heparin in the treatment of venous thrombosis. Acta Med Scand 203: 457–463, 1978.

Manufactured by
Behringwerke AG
in Marburg/Lahn, Germany
US License No. 97

Distributed by:
ASTRA®
Astra Pharmaceutical Products, Inc.
Westborough, MA 01581

021596RO5 2/92 (5)

TOPROL XL™ TABLETS   ℞
(Metoprolol succinate)
Extended Release Tablets
Tablets: 50 mg, 100 mg, and 200 mg

DESCRIPTION

Toprol XL, metoprolol succinate, is a beta$_1$-selective (cardioselective) adrenoceptor blocking agent for oral administration, available as extended release tablets. Toprol XL has been formulated to provide a controlled and predictable release of metoprolol for once daily administration. The tablets comprise a multiple unit system containing metoprolol succinate in a multitude of controlled release pellets. Each pellet acts as a separate drug delivery unit and is designed to deliver metoprolol continuously over the dosage interval. The tablets contain 47.5 mg, 95 mg and 190 mg of metoprolol succinate equivalent to 50, 100 and 200 mg of metoprolol tartrate, USP, respectively. Its chemical name is (±)-1-(isopropylamino)-3-[p- (2-methoxyethyl) phenoxy]-2-propanol succinate (2:1) (salt). Its structural formula is: [See above.]

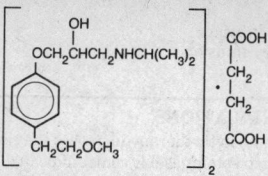

Metoprolol succinate is a white crystalline powder with a molecular weight of 652.8. It is freely soluble in water; soluble in methanol; sparingly soluble in ethanol; slightly soluble in dichloromethane and 2-propanol; practically insoluble in ethyl-acetate, acetone, diethylether and heptane. Inactive ingredients: Silicone dioxide, Cellulose compounds, Acetyltributyl citrate, Maize starch, Lactose powder, Polyvidone, Magnesium stearate, Polyethylene glycol, Titanium dioxide, Paraffin.

CLINICAL PHARMACOLOGY

Metoprolol is a beta$_1$-selective (cardioselective) adrenergic receptor blocking agent. This preferential effect is not absolute, however, and at higher plasma concentrations, metoprolol also inhibits beta$_2$-adrenoreceptors, chiefly located in the bronchial and vascular musculature. Metoprolol has no intrinsic sympathomimetic activity, and membrane-stabilizing activity is detectable only at plasma concentrations much greater than required for beta-blockade. Animal and human experiments indicate that metoprolol slows the sinus rate and decreases AV nodal conduction.

Clinical pharmacology studies have confirmed the beta-blocking activity of metoprolol in man, as shown by (1) reduction in heart rate and cardiac output at rest and upon exercise, (2) reduction of systolic blood pressure upon exercise, (3) inhibition of isoproterenol-induced tachycardia, and (4) reduction of reflex orthostatic tachycardia.

The relative beta$_1$-selectivity of metoprolol has been confirmed by the following: (1) In normal subjects, metoprolol is unable to reverse the beta$_2$-mediated vasodilating effects of epinephrine. This contrasts with the effect of nonselective beta-blockers, which completely reverse the vasodilating effects of epinephrine. (2) In asthmatic patients, metoprolol reduces FEV_1 and FVC significantly less than a nonselective beta-blocker, propranolol, at equivalent beta$_1$-receptor blocking doses.

In five controlled studies in normal healthy subjects, the same daily doses of Toprol XL and immediate release metoprolol were compared in terms of the extent and duration of beta$_1$-blockade produced. Both formulations were given in a dose range equivalent to 100–400 mg of immediate release metoprolol per day. In these studies, Toprol XL was administered once a day and immediate release metoprolol was administered once to four times a day. A sixth controlled study compared the beta$_1$-blocking effects of a 50 mg daily dose of the two formulations. In each study, beta$_1$-blockade was expressed as the percent change from baseline, in exercise heart rate following standardized submaximal exercise tolerance tests at steady state. Toprol XL administered once a day, and immediate release metoprolol administered once to four times a day, provided comparable total beta$_1$-blockade over 24 hours (area under the beta$_1$-blockade versus time curve) in the dose range 100–400 mg. At a dosage of 50 mg once daily, Toprol XL produced significantly higher total beta$_1$-blockade over 24 hours than immediate release metoprolol. For Toprol XL, the percent reduction in exercise heart rate was relatively stable throughout the entire dosage interval and the level of beta$_1$-blockade increased with increasing doses from 50 to 300 mg daily. The effects at peak/trough (i.e. at 24 hours post dosing) were; 14/9, 16/10, 24/14, 27/22 and 27/20% reduction in exercise heart rate for doses of 50, 100, 200, 300 and 400 mg Toprol XL once a day, respectively. In contrast to Toprol XL immediate release metoprolol given at a dose of 50–100 mg once a day, produced a significantly larger peak effect on exercise tachycardia, but the effect was not evident at 24 hours. To match the peak to trough ratio obtained with Toprol XL over the dosing range of 200 to 400 mg, a t.i.d. to q.i.d. divided dosing regimen was required for immediate release metoprolol.

The relationship between plasma metoprolol levels and reduction in exercise heart rate is independent of the pharmaceutical formulation. Using the E_{max} model, the maximal beta$_1$-blocking effect has been estimated to produce a 28.3% reduction in exercise heart rate. Beta$_1$-blocking effects in the range of 30–80% of the maximal effect (corresponding to approximately 8–23% reduction in exercise heart rate) are expected to occur at metoprolol plasma concentrations ranging from 30–540 nmol/L. The concentration-effect curve begins reaching a plateau between 200–300 nmol/L, and higher plasma levels produce little additional beta$_1$-blocking effect. The relative beta$_1$-selectivity of metoprolol diminishes and blockade of beta$_2$-adrenoceptors increases at higher plasma concentrations.

Although beta-adrenergic receptor blockade is useful in the treatment of angina and hypertension, there are situations in which sympathetic stimulation is vital. In patients with

TABLE I
SUGGESTED DILUTIONS AND INFUSION RATES

Dosage	Vial Size (IU)	Total Solution Volume	Infusion Rate
I. Acute Myocardial Infarction			
A. **Intravenous Infusion**	1,500,000	45 mL	Infuse 45 mL within 60 minutes
B. **Intracoronary Infusion**	250,000	125 mL	
1. 20,000 IU bolus			1. Loading dose of 10 mL
2. 2,000 IU/minute for 60 minutes			2. Then 60 mL/hour
II. Pulmonary Embolism, Deep Vein Thrombosis, Arterial Thrombosis or Embolism Intravenous Infusion			
A. 1. 250,000 IU loading dose over 30 minutes	1,500,000	90 mL	1. Infuse 30 mL/hour for 30 minutes
2. 100,000 IU/hour maintenance dose			2. Infuse 6 mL/hour
B. **Same**	1,500,000 infusion bottle	45 mL	1. 15 mL/hour for 30 minutes
			2. Infuse 3 mL/hour

severely damaged hearts, adequate ventricular function may depend on sympathetic drive. In the presence of AV block, beta-blockade may prevent the necessary facilitating effect of sympathetic activity on conduction. Beta$_2$-adrenergic blockade results in passive bronchial constriction by interfering with endogenous adrenergic bronchodilator activity in patients subject to bronchospasm and may also interfere with exogenous bronchodilators in such patients.

Hypertension
The mechanism of the antihypertensive effects of beta-blocking agents has not been elucidated. However, several possible mechanisms have been proposed: (1) competitive antagonism of catecholamines at peripheral (especially cardiac) adrenergic neuron sites, leading to decreased cardiac output; (2) a central effect leading to reduced sympathetic outflow to the periphery; and (3) suppression of renin activity.
In controlled clinical studies, an immediate release dosage form of metoprolol has been shown to be an effective antihypertensive agent when used alone or as concomitant therapy with thiazide-type diuretics at dosages of 100–450 mg daily. Toprol XL, in dosages of 100 to 400 mg once daily, has been shown to possess comparable β_1-blockade as conventional metoprolol tablets administered two to four times daily. In addition, Toprol XL administered at a dose of 50 mg once daily has been shown to lower blood pressure 24-hours post-dosing in placebo controlled studies. In controlled, comparative, clinical studies, immediate release metoprolol appeared comparable as an antihypertensive agent to propranolol, methyldopa, and thiazide-type diuretics, and to be effective both in supine and standing positions. Because of variable plasma levels attained with a given dose and lack of a consistent relationship of antihypertensive activity to drug plasma concentration, selection of proper dosage requires individual titration.

Angina Pectoris
By blocking catecholamine-induced increases in heart rate, in velocity and extent of myocardial contraction, and in blood pressure, metoprolol reduces the oxygen requirements of the heart at any given level of effort, thus making it useful in the long-term management of angina pectoris. However, in patients with heart failure, beta-adrenergic blockade may increase oxygen requirements by increasing left ventricular fiber length and end-diastolic pressure.
In controlled clinical trials, an immediate release formulation of metoprolol has been shown to be an effective antianginal agent, reducing the number of angina attacks and increasing exercise tolerance. The dosage used in these studies ranged from 100 to 400 mg daily. Toprol XL, in dosages of 100 to 400 mg once daily, has been shown to possess comparable β_1-blockade as conventional metoprolol tablets administered two to four times daily.

Pharmacokinetics
In man, absorption of metoprolol is rapid and complete. Plasma levels following oral administration of conventional metoprolol tablets, however, approximate 50% of levels following intravenous administration, indicating about 50% first-pass metabolism. Metoprolol crosses the blood-brain barrier and has been reported in the CSF in a concentration 78% of the simultaneous plasma concentration.
Plasma levels achieved are highly variable after oral administration. Only a small fraction of the drug (about 12%) is bound to human serum albumin. Elimination is mainly by biotransformation in the liver, and the plasma half-life ranges from approximately 3 to 7 hours. Less than 5% of an oral dose of metoprolol is recovered unchanged in the urine; the rest is excreted by the kidneys as metabolites that appear to have no clinical significance. Following intravenous administration of metoprolol, the urinary recovery of unchanged drug is approximately 10%. The systemic availability and half-life of metoprolol in patients with renal failure do not differ to a clinically significant degree from those in normal subjects. Consequently, no reduction in dosage is usually needed in patients with chronic renal failure.
In comparison to conventional metoprolol, the plasma metoprolol levels following administration of Toprol XL are characterized by lower peaks, longer time to peak and significantly lower peak to trough variation. The peak plasma levels following once daily administration of Toprol XL average one-fourth to one-half the peak plasma levels obtained following a corresponding dose of conventional metoprolol, administered once daily or in divided doses. At steady state the average bioavailability of metoprolol following administration of Toprol XL, across the dosage range of 50 to 400 mg once daily, was 77% relative to the corresponding single or divided doses of conventional metoprolol. Nevertheless, over the 24 hour dosing interval, β_1-blockade is comparable and dose-related (see CLINICAL PHARMACOLOGY). The bioavailability of metoprolol shows a dose-related, although not directly proportional increase with dose and is not significantly affected by food following Toprol XL administration.

INDICATIONS AND USAGE
Hypertension
Toprol XL tablets are indicated for the treatment of hypertension. They may be used alone or in combination with other antihypertensive agents.

Angina Pectoris
Toprol XL tablets are indicated in the long-term treatment of angina pectoris.

CONTRAINDICATIONS
Hypertension and Angina
Toprol XL is contraindicated in sinus bradycardia, heart block greater than first degree, cardiogenic shock, and overt cardiac failure (see WARNINGS).

WARNINGS
Hypertension and Angina
Cardiac Failure: Sympathetic stimulation is a vital component supporting circulatory function in congestive heart failure, and beta-blockade carries the potential hazard of further depressing myocardial contractility and precipitating more severe failure. In hypertensive and angina patients who have congestive heart failure controlled by digitalis and diuretics, Toprol XL should be administered cautiously. Both digitalis and Toprol XL slow AV conduction.
In Patients Without a History of Cardiac Failure: Continued depression of the myocardium with beta-blocking agents over a period of time can, in some cases, lead to cardiac failure. At the first sign or symptom of impending cardiac failure, patients should be fully digitalized and/or given a diuretic. The response should be observed closely. If cardiac failure continues, despite adequate digitalization and diuretic therapy, Toprol XL should be withdrawn.
Ischemic Heart Disease: Following abrupt cessation of therapy with certain beta-blocking agents, exacerbations of angina pectoris and, in some cases, myocardial infarction have occurred. When discontinuing chronically administered Toprol XL, particularly in patients with ischemic heart disease, the dosage should be gradually reduced over a period of 1–2 weeks and the patient should be carefully monitored. If angina markedly worsens or acute coronary insufficiency develops, Toprol XL administration should be reinstated promptly, at least temporarily, and other measures appropriate for the management of unstable angina should be taken. Patients should be warned against interruption or discontinuation of therapy without the physician's advice. Because coronary artery disease is common and may be unrecognized, it may be prudent not to discontinue Toprol XL therapy abruptly even in patients treated only for hypertension.
Bronchospastic Diseases: PATIENTS WITH BRONCHOSPASTIC DISEASES SHOULD, IN GENERAL, NOT RECEIVE BETA-BLOCKERS. Because of its relative beta$_1$-selectivity, however, Toprol XL may be used with caution in patients with bronchospastic disease who do not respond to, or cannot tolerate, other antihypertensive treatment. Since beta$_1$-selectivity is not absolute, a beta$_2$-stimulating agent should be administered concomitantly, and the lowest possible dose of Toprol XL should be used (see DOSAGE AND ADMINISTRATION).
Major Surgery: The necessity or desirability of withdrawing beta-blocking therapy prior to major surgery is controversial; the impaired ability of the heart to respond to reflex adrenergic stimuli may augment the risks of general anesthesia and surgical procedures.
Toprol XL like other beta-blockers, is a competitive inhibitor of beta-receptor agonists, and its effects can be reversed by administration of such agents, e.g., dobutamine or isoproterenol. However, such patients may be subject to protracted severe hypotension. Difficulty in restarting and maintaining the heart beat has also been reported with beta-blockers.
Diabetes and Hypoglycemia: Toprol XL should be used with caution in diabetic patients if a beta-blocking agent is required. Beta-blockers may mask tachycardia occurring with hypoglycemia, but other manifestations such as dizziness and sweating may not be significantly affected.
Thyrotoxicosis: Beta-adrenergic blockade may mask certain clinical signs (e.g., tachycardia) of hyperthyroidism. Patients suspected of developing thyrotoxicosis should be managed carefully to avoid abrupt withdrawal of beta-blockade, which might precipitate a thyroid storm.

PRECAUTIONS
General
Toprol XL should be used with caution in patients with impaired hepatic function.
Information for Patients
Patients should be advised to take Toprol XL regularly and continuously, as directed, preferably with or immediately following meals. If a dose should be missed, the patient should take only the next scheduled dose (without doubling it). Patients should not discontinue Toprol XL without consulting the physician.
Patients should be advised (1) to avoid operating automobiles and machinery or engaging in other tasks requiring alertness until the patient's response to therapy with Toprol XL has been determined; (2) to contact the physician if any difficulty in breathing occurs; (3) to inform the physician or dentist before any type of surgery that he or she is taking Toprol XL.

Laboratory Tests
Clinical laboratory findings may include elevated levels of serum transaminase, alkaline phosphatase, and lactate dehydrogenase.
Drug Interactions
Catecholamine-depleting drugs (e.g., reserpine) may have an additive effect when given with beta-blocking agents. Patients treated with Toprol XL plus a catecholamine depletor should therefore be closely observed for evidence of hypotension or marked bradycardia, which may produce vertigo, syncope, or postural hypotension.
Carcinogenesis, Mutagenesis, Impairment of Fertility
Long-term studies in animals have been conducted to evaluate the carcinogenic potential of metoprolol tartrate. In 2-year studies in rats at three oral dosage levels of up to 800 mg/kg/day, there was no increase in the development of spontaneously occurring benign or malignant neoplasms of any type. The only histologic changes that appeared to be drug related were an increased incidence of generally mild focal accumulation of foamy macrophages in pulmonary alveoli and a slight increase in biliary hyperplasia. In a 21-month study in Swiss albino mice at three oral dosage levels of up to 750 mg/kg/day, benign lung tumors (small adenomas) occurred more frequently in female mice receiving the highest dose than in untreated control animals. There was no increase in malignant or total (benign plus malignant) lung tumors, nor in the overall incidence of tumors or malignant tumors. This 21-month study was repeated in CD-1 mice, and no statistically or biologically significant differences were observed between treated and control mice of either sex for any type of tumor.
All mutagenicity tests performed on metoprolol tartrate (a dominant lethal study in mice, chromosome studies in somatic cells, a Salmonella/mammalian-microsome mutagenicity test, and a nucleus anomaly test in somatic interphase nuclei) and metoprolol succinate (a Salmonella/mammalian-microsome mutagenicity test) were negative.
No evidence of impaired fertility due to metoprolol tartrate was observed in a study performed in rats at doses up to 55.5 times the maximum daily human dose of 450 mg.
Pregnancy Category C
Metoprolol tartrate has been shown to increase post-implantation loss and decrease neonatal survival in rats at doses up to 55.5 times the maximum daily human dose of 450 mg. Distribution studies in mice confirm exposure of the fetus when metoprolol tartrate is administered to the pregnant animal. These studies have revealed no evidence of impaired fertility or teratogenicity. There are no adequate and well-controlled studies in pregnant women. Because animal reproduction studies are not always predictive of human response, this drug should be used during pregnancy only if clearly needed.
Nursing Mothers
Metoprolol is excreted in breast milk in very small quantities. An infant consuming 1 liter of breast milk daily would receive a dose of less than 1 mg of the drug. Caution should be exercised when Toprol XL is administered to a nursing woman.
Pediatric Use
Safety and effectiveness in children have not been established.
Risk Of Anaphylactic Reactions
While taking beta-blockers, patients with a history of severe anaphylactic reactions to a variety of allergens may be more reactive to repeated challenge, either accidental, diagnostic or therapeutic. Such patients may be unresponsive to the usual doses of epinephrine used to treat allergic reaction.

ADVERSE REACTIONS
Hypertension and Angina
Most adverse effects have been mild and transient. The following adverse reactions have been reported for metoprolol tartrate.
Central Nervous System: Tiredness and dizziness have occurred in about 10 of 100 patients. Depression has been reported in about 5 of 100 patients. Mental confusion and short-term memory loss have been reported. Headache, somnolence, nightmares, and insomnia have also been reported.
Cardiovascular: Shortness of breath and bradycardia have occurred in approximately 3 of 100 patients. Cold extremities; arterial insufficiency, usually of the Raynaud type; palpitations; congestive heart failure; peripheral edema; syncope; chest pain; and hypotension have been reported in about 1 of 100 patients (see CONTRAINDICATIONS, WARNINGS and PRECAUTIONS).
Respiratory: Wheezing (bronchospasm) and dyspnea have been reported in about 1 of 100 patients (see WARNINGS).
Gastrointestinal: Diarrhea has occurred in about 5 of 100 patients. Nausea, dry mouth, gastric pain, constipation, flatulence, digestive tract disorders and heartburn have been reported in about 1 of 100 patients.
Hypersensitive Reactions: Pruritus or rash have occurred in about 5 of 100 patients. Worsening of psoriasis has also been reported.

Continued on next page

Astra—Cont.

Miscellaneous: Peyronie's disease has been reported in fewer than 1 of 100,000 patients. Musculoskeletal pain, blurred vision, decreased libido and tinnitus have also been reported.

There have been rare reports of reversible alopecia, agranulocytosis, and dry eyes. Discontinuation of the drug should be considered if any such reaction is not otherwise explicable. The oculomucocutaneous syndrome associated with the beta-blocker practolol has not been reported with metoprolol.

Potential Adverse Reactions

A variety of adverse reactions not listed above have been reported with other beta-adrenergic blocking agents and should be considered potential adverse reactions to Toprol XL.

Central Nervous System: Reversible mental depression progressing to catatonia; an acute reversible syndrome characterized by disorientation for time and place, short-term memory loss, emotional lability, slightly clouded sensorium, and decreased performance on neuropsychometrics.

Cardiovascular: Intensification of AV block (see CONTRAINDICATIONS).

Hematologic: Agranulocytosis, nonthrombocytopenic purpura, thrombocytopenic purpura.

Hypersensitive Reactions: Fever combined with aching and sore throat, laryngospasm, and respiratory distress.

OVERDOSAGE

Acute Toxicity

No overdosage has been reported with Toprol XL and no specific overdosage information was obtained with this drug, with the exception of animal toxicology data. However, since Toprol XL (metoprolol succinate salt) contains the same active moiety, metoprolol, as conventional metoprolol tablets (metoprolol tartrate salt), the recommendations on overdosage for metoprolol conventional tablets are applicable to Toprol XL.

Signs and Symptoms

Potential signs and symptoms associated with overdosage with metoprolol are bradycardia, hypotension, bronchospasm, and cardiac failure.

Treatment

There is no specific antidote.

In general, patients with acute or recent myocardial infarction may be more hemodynamically unstable than other patients and should be treated accordingly. On the basis of the pharmacologic actions of metoprolol tartrate, the following general measures should be employed.

Elimination of the Drug: Gastric lavage should be performed.

Bardycardia: Atropine should be administered. If there is no response to vagal blockade, isoproterenol should be administered cautiously.

Hypotension: A vasopressor should be administered, e.g., levarterenol or dopamine.

Branchospasm: A beta$_2$-stimulating agent and/or a theophylline derivative should be administered.

Cardiac Failure: A digitalis glycoside and diuretics should be administered. In shock resulting from inadequate cardiac contractility, administration of dobutamine, isoproterenol or glucagon may be considered.

DOSAGE AND ADMINISTRATION

Toprol XL is an extended release tablet intended for once-a-day administration. When switching from immediate release metoprolol tablet to Toprol XL, the same total daily dose of Toprol XL should be used.

As with immediate release metoprolol, dosages of Toprol XL should be individualized and titration may be needed in some patients.

Hypertension

The usual initial dosage is 50 to 100 mg daily in a single dose, whether used alone or added to a diuretic. The dosage may be increased at weekly (or longer) intervals until optimum blood pressure reduction is achieved. In general, the maximum effect of any given dosage level will be apparent after 1 week of therapy. Dosages above 400 mg per day have not been studied.

Angina Pectoris

The dosage of Toprol XL should be individualized. The usual initial dosage is 100 mg daily, given in a single dose. The dosage may be gradually increased at weekly intervals until optimum clinical response has been obtained or there is a pronounced slowing of the heart rate. Dosages above 400 mg per day have not been studied. If treatment is to be discontinued, the dosage should be reduced gradually over a period of 1–2 weeks (see WARNINGS).

HOW SUPPLIED

<u>Tablets 50 mg:</u>

Contain 47.5 mg of metoprolol succinate equivalent to 50 mg of metoprolol tartrate, USP

Are white, biconvex, round, film-coated

Engraved A/mo on one side and scored on the other

Bottles of 100 NDC 0186-1090-05

<u>Tablets 100 mg:</u>

Contain 95 mg of metoprolol succinate equivalent to 100 mg of metoprolol tartrate, USP

Are white, biconvex, round, film-coated

Engraved A/ms on one side and scored on the other

Bottles of 100 NDC 0186-1092-05

<u>Tablets 200 mg:</u>

Contain 190 mg of metoprolol succinate equivalent to 200 mg of metoprolol tartrate, USP

Are white, biconvex, oval, film-coated

Engraved A/my and scored on one side

Bottles of 100 NDC 0186-1094-05

Store at controlled room temperature 15°-30°C (59°-86°F)

Manufactured by:
Astra Pharmaceutical Production, AB
Södertälje, Sweden
Manufactured for:
ASTRA®
Astra Pharmaceutical Products, Inc.
Westborough, MA 01581
021671ROO Iss. 11/91

XYLOCAINE® (lidocaine hydrochloride) ℞

[zī´lo-caine]

Injections

XYLOCAINE® (lidocaine HCl) with Epinephrine

Injections infiltration and nerve block

DESCRIPTION

Xylocaine (lidocaine HCl) Injections are sterile, non-pyrogenic aqueous solutions that contain a local anesthetic agent with or without epinephrine and are administered parenterally by injection. See INDICATIONS for specific uses.

Xylocaine solutions contain lidocaine HCl, which is chemically designated as acetamide 2-(diethylamino)-N-(2,6-dimethylphenyl)-monohydrochloride and has the molecular wt. 270.8. Its structural formula is:

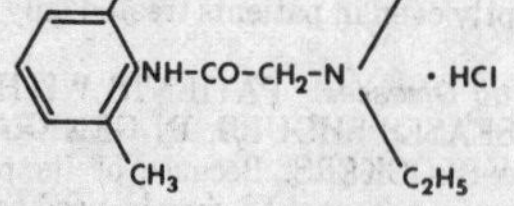

Epinephrine is (−)–3, 4-Dihydroxy-α-[(methylamino) methyl] benzyl alcohol and has the molecular wt. 183.21.

Dosage forms listed as Xylocaine-MPF indicates single dose solutions that are <u>M</u>ethyl <u>P</u>araben <u>F</u>ree (MPF).

<u>Xylocaine</u> <u>MPF</u> is a sterile, non-pyrogenic, isotonic solution containing sodium chloride. <u>Xylocaine</u> in multiple dose vials, each mL also contains 1 mg methylparaben as antiseptic preservative. The pH of these solutions is adjusted to approximately 6.5 (5.0–7.0) with sodium hydroxide and/or hydrochloric acid.

<u>Xylocaine</u> <u>MPF</u> <u>with</u> <u>Epinephrine</u> is a sterile, non-pyrogenic, isotonic solution containing sodium chloride. Each mL contains lidocaine hydrochloride and epinephrine, with 0.5 mg sodium metabisulfite as an antioxidant and 0.2 mg citric acid as a stabilizer. <u>Xylocaine</u> <u>with</u> <u>Epinephrine</u> in multiple dose vials, each mL also contains 1 mg methylparaben as antiseptic preservative. The pH of these solutions is adjusted to approximately 4.5 (3.3–5.5) with sodium hydroxide and/or hydrochloric acid. Filled under nitrogen.

CLINICAL PHARMACOLOGY

Mechanism of action: Lidocaine stabilizes the neuronal membrane by inhibiting the ionic fluxes required for the initiation and conduction of impulses, thereby effecting local anesthetic action.

Hemodynamics: Excessive blood levels may cause changes in cardiac output, total peripheral resistance, and mean arterial pressure. With central neural blockade these changes may be attributable to block of autonomic fibers, a direct depressant effect of the local anesthetic agent on various components of the cardiovascular system and/or the beta-adrenergic receptor stimulating action of epinephrine when present. The net effect is normally a modest hypotension when the recommended dosages are not exceeded.

Pharmacokinetics and metabolism: Information derived from diverse formulations, concentrations and usages reveals that lidocaine is completely absorbed following parenteral administration, its rate of absorption depending, for example, upon various factors such as the site of administration and the presence or absence of a vasoconstrictor agent. Except for intravascular administration, the highest blood levels are obtained following intercoastal nerve block and the lowest after subcutaneous administration.

The plasma binding of lidocaine is dependent on drug concentration, and the fraction bound decreases with increasing concentration. At concentrations of 1 to 4 µg of free base per mL 60 to 80 percent of lidocaine is protein bound. Binding is also dependent on the plasma concentration of the alpha-1-acid glycoprotein.

Lidocaine crosses the blood-brain and placental barriers, presumably by passive diffusion.

Lidocaine is metabolized rapidly by the liver, and metabolites and unchanged drug are excreted by the kidneys. Biotransformation includes oxidative N-dealkylation, ring hydroxylation, cleavage of the amide linkage, and conjugation. N-dealkylation, a major pathway of biotransformation, yields the metabolites monoethylglycinexylidide and glycinexylidide. The pharmacological/toxicological actions of these metabolites are similar to, but less potent than, those of lidocaine. Approximately 90% of lidocaine administered is excreted in the form of various metabolites, and less than 10% is excreted unchanged. The primary metabolite in urine is a conjugate of 4-hydroxy-2, 6-dimethylaniline.

The elimination half-life of lidocaine following an intravenous bolus injection is typically 1.5 to 2.0 hours. Because of the rapid rate at which lidocaine is metabolized, any condition that affects liver function may alter lidocaine kinetics. The half-life may be prolonged two-fold or more in patients with liver dysfunction. Renal dysfunction does not affect lidocaine kinetics but may increase the accumulation of metabolites.

Factors such as acidosis and the use of CNS stimulants and depressants affect the CNS levels of lidocaine required to produce overt systemic effects. Objective adverse manifestations become increasingly apparent with increasing venous plasma levels above 6.0 µg free base per mL. In the rhesus monkey arterial blood levels of 18–21 µg/mL have been shown to be threshold for convulsive activity.

INDICATIONS AND USAGE

Xylocaine (lidocaine HCl) Injections are indicated for production of local or regional anesthesia by infiltration techniques such as percutaneous injection and intravenous regional anesthesia by peripheral nerve block techniques such as brachial plexus and intercostal and by central neural techniques such as lumbar and caudal epidural blocks, when the accepted procedures for these techniques as described in standard textbooks are observed.

CONTRAINDICATIONS

Lidocaine is contraindicated in patients with a known history of hypersensitivity to local anesthetics of the amide type.

WARNINGS

XYLOCAINE INJECTIONS FOR INFILTRATION AND NERVE BLOCK SHOULD BE EMPLOYED ONLY BY CLINICIANS WHO ARE WELL VERSED IN DIAGNOSIS AND MANAGEMENT OF DOSE-RELATED TOXICITY AND OTHER ACUTE EMERGENCIES THAT MIGHT ARISE FROM THE BLOCK TO BE EMPLOYED AND THEN ONLY AFTER ENSURING THE *IMMEDIATE* AVAILABILITY OF OXYGEN. OTHER RESUSCITATIVE DRUGS, CARDIOPULMONARY EQUIPMENT, AND THE PERSONNEL NEEDED FOR PROPER MANAGEMENT OF TOXIC REACTIONS AND RELATED EMERGENCIES (See also ADVERSE REACTIONS and PRECAUTIONS). DELAY IN PROPER MANAGEMENT OF DOSE-RELATED TOXICITY, UNDERVENTILATION FROM ANY CAUSE AND/OR ALTERED SENSITIVITY MAY LEAD TO THE DEVELOPMENT OF ACIDOSIS, CARDIAC ARREST AND, POSSIBLY, DEATH.

To avoid intravascular injection, aspiration should be performed before the local anesthetic solution is injected. The needle must be repositioned until no return of blood can be elicited by aspiration. Note, however, that the absence of blood in the syringe does not guarantee that intravascular injection has been avoided.

Local anesthetic solutions containing antimicrobial preservatives (e.g., methylparaben) should not be used for epidural or spinal anesthesia because the safety of these agents has not been established with regard to intrathecal injection, either intentional or accidental.

Xylocaine with epinephrine solutions contain sodium metabisulfite, a sulfite that may cause allergic-type reactions including anaphylactic symptoms and life-threatening or less severe asthmatic episodes in certain susceptible people. The overall prevalence of sulfite sensitivity in the general population is unknown and probably low. Sulfite sensitivity is seen more frequently in asthmatic than in nonasthmatic people.

PRECAUTIONS

General: The safety and effectiveness of lidocaine depend on proper dosage, correct technique, adequate precautions, and readiness for emergencies. Standard textbooks should be consulted for specific techniques and precautions for various regional anesthetic procedures.

Resuscitative equipment, oxygen, and other resuscitative drugs should be available for immediate use. (See WARNINGS and ADVERSE REACTIONS). The lowest dosage that results in effective anesthesia should be used to avoid high plasma levels and serious adverse effects. Syringe aspira-

tions should also be performed before and during each supplemental injection when using indwelling catheter techniques. During the administration of epidural anesthesia, it is recommended that a test dose be administered initially and that the patient be monitored for central nervous system toxicity and cardiovascular toxicity, as well as for signs of unintended intrathecal administration, before proceeding. When clinical conditions permit, consideration should be given to employing local anesthetic solutions that contain epinephrine for the test dose because circulatory changes compatible with epinephrine may also serve as a warning sign of unintended intravascular injection. An intravascular injection is still possible even if aspirations for blood are negative. Repeated doses of lidocaine may cause significant increases in blood levels with each repeated dose because of slow accumulation of the drug or its metabolites. Tolerance to elevated blood levels varies with the status of the patient. Debilitated, elderly patients, acutely ill patients and children should be given reduced doses commensurate with their age and physical condition. Lidocaine should also be used with caution in patients with severe shock or heart block.

Lumbar and caudal epidural anesthesia should be used with extreme caution in persons with the following conditions: existing neurological disease, spinal deformities, septicemia and severe hypertension.

Local anesthetic solutions containing a vasoconstrictor should be used cautiously and in carefully circumscribed quantities in areas of the body supplied by end arteries or having otherwise compromised blood supply. Patients with peripheral vascular disease and those with hypertensive vascular disease may exhibit exaggerated vasoconstrictor response. Ischemic injury or necrosis may result. Preparations containing a vasoconstrictor should be used with caution in patients during or following the administration of potent general anesthetic agents, since cardiac arrhythmias may occur under such conditions.

Careful and constant monitoring of cardiovascular and respiratory (adequacy of ventilation) vital signs and the patient's state of consciousness should be accomplished after each local anesthetic injection. It should be kept in mind at such times that restlessness, anxiety, tinnitus, dizziness, blurred vision, tremors, depression or drowsiness may be early warning signs of central nervous system toxicity.

Since amide-type local anesthetics are metabolized by the liver, Xylocaine Injection should be used with caution in patients with hepatic disease. Patients with severe hepatic disease, because of their inability to metabolize local anesthetics normally, are at greater risk of developing toxic plasma concentrations. Xylocaine Injection should also be used with caution in patients with impaired cardiovascular function since they may be less able to compensate for functional changes associated with the prolongation of A-V conduction produced by these drugs.

Many drugs used during the conduct of anesthesia are considered potential triggering agents for familial malignant hyperthermia. Since it is not known whether amide-type local anesthetics may trigger this reaction and since the need for supplemental general anesthesia cannot be predicted in advance, it is suggested that a standard protocol for the management of malignant hyperthermia should be available. Early unexplained signs of tachycardia, tachypnea, labile blood pressure and metabolic acidosis may precede temperature elevation. Successful outcome is dependent on early diagnosis, prompt discontinuance of the suspect triggering agent(s) and institution of treatment, including oxygen therapy, indicated supportive measures and dantrolene (consult dantrolene sodium intravenous package insert before using).

Proper tourniquet technique, as described in publications and standard textbooks, is essential in the performance of intravenous regional anesthesia. Solutions containing epinephrine or other vasoconstrictors should not be used for this technique.

Lidocaine should be used with caution in persons with known drug sensitivities. Patients allergic to para-aminobenzoic acid derivatives (procaine, tetracaine, benzocaine, etc.) have not shown cross sensitivity to lidocaine.

Use in the Head and Neck Area: Small doses of local anesthetics injected into the head and neck area, including retrobulbar, dental and stellate ganglion blocks, may produce adverse reactions similar to systemic toxicity seen with unintentional intravascular injections of larger doses. Confusion, convulsions, respiratory depression and/or respiratory arrest, and cardiovascular stimulation or depression have been reported. These reactions may be due to intra-arterial injection of the local anesthetic with retrograde flow to the cerebral circulation. Patients receiving these blocks should have their circulation and respiration monitored and be constantly observed. Resuscitative equipment and personnel for treating adverse reactions should be immediately available. Dosage recommendations should not be exceeded. (See DOSAGE and ADMINISTRATION.)

Information for Patients: When appropriate, patients should be informed in advance that they may experience temporary loss of sensation and motor activity, usually in the lower half of the body, following proper administration of epidural anesthesia.

Clinically significant drug interactions: The administration of local anesthetic solutions containing epinephrine or norepinephrine to patients receiving monamine oxidase inhibitors or tricyclic antidepressants may produce severe, prolonged hypertension.

Phenothiazines and butyrophenones may reduce or reverse the pressor effect of epinephrine.

Concurrent use of these agents should generally be avoided. In situations when concurrent therapy is necessary, careful patient monitoring is essential.

Concurrent administration of vasopressor drugs (for the treatment of hypotension related to obstetric blocks) and ergot-type oxytocic drugs may cause severe, persistent hypertension or cerebrovascular accidents.

Drug Laboratory test interactions: The intramuscular injection of lidocaine may result in an increase in creatine phosphokinase levels. Thus, the use of this enzyme determination without isoenzyme separation, as a diagnostic test for the presence of acute myocardial infarction may be compromised by the intramuscular injection of lidocaine.

Carcinogenesis, mutagenesis, impairment of fertility: Studies of lidocaine in animals to evaluate the carcinogenic and mutagenic potential or the effect on fertility have not been conducted.

Pregnancy: Teratogenic Effects. Pregnancy Category B. Reproduction studies have been performed in rats at doses up to 6.6 times the human dose and have revealed no evidence of harm to the fetus caused by lidocaine. There are, however, no adequate and well-controlled studies in pregnant women. Animal reproduction studies are not always predictive of human response. General consideration should be given to this fact before administering lidocaine to women of childbearing potential, especially during early pregnancy when maximum organogenesis takes place.

Labor and delivery: Local anesthetics rapidly cross the placenta and when used for epidural, paracervical, pudendal or caudal block anesthesia, can cause varying degrees of maternal, fetal, and neonatal toxicity, (See CLINICAL PHARMACOLOGY—Pharmacokinetics). The potential for toxicity depends upon the procedure performed, the type and amount of drug used, and the technique of drug administration. Adverse reactions in the parturient, fetus and neonate involve alterations of the central nervous system peripheral vascular tone and cardiac function.

Maternal hypotension has resulted from regional anesthesia. Local anesthetics produce vasodilation by blocking sympathetic nerves. Elevating the patient's legs and positioning her on her left side will help prevent decreases in blood pressure. The fetal heart rate also should be monitored continuously, and electronic fetal monitoring is highly advisable.

Epidural, spinal, paracervical, or pudendal anesthesia may alter the forces of parturition through changes in uterine contractility or maternal expulsive efforts. In one study paracervical block anesthesia was associated with a decrease in the mean duration of first stage labor and facilitation of cervical dilation. However, spinal and epidural anesthesia have also been reported to prolong the second stage of labor by removing the parturient's reflex urge to bear down or by interfering with motor function. The use of obstetrical anesthesia may increase the need for forceps assistance.

The use of some local anesthetic drug products during labor and delivery may be followed by diminished muscle strength and tone for the first day or two of life. The long term significance of these observations is unknown. Fetal bradycardia may occur in 20 to 30 percent of patients receiving paracervical nerve block anesthesia with the amide-type local anesthetics and may be associated with fetal acidosis. Fetal heart rate should always be monitored during paracervical anesthesia. The physician should weigh the possible advantages against risks when considering paracervical block in prematurity, toxemia of pregnancy, and fetal distress. Careful adherence to recommended dosage is of the utmost importance in obstetrical paracervical block. Failure to achieve adequate analgesia with recommended doses should arouse suspicion of intravascular or fetal intracranial injection. Cases compatible with unintended fetal intracranial injection of local anesthetic solution have been reported following intended paracervical or pudendal block or both. Babies so affected present with unexplained neonatal depression at birth, which correlates with high local anesthetic serum levels, and often manifest seizures within six hours. Prompt use of supportive measures combined with forced urinary excretion of the local anesthetic has been used successfully to manage this complication.

Case reports of maternal convulsions and cardiovascular collapse following use of some local anesthetics for paracervical block in early pregnancy (as anesthesia for elective abortion) suggest that systemic absorption under these circumstances may be rapid. The recommended maximum dose of each drug should not be exceeded. Injection should be made slowly and with frequent aspiration. Allow a 5-minute interval between sides.

Nursing mothers: It is not known whether this drug is excreted in human milk. Because many drugs are excreted in human milk, caution should be exercised when lidocaine is administered to a nursing woman.

Pediatric use: Dosages in children should be reduced, commensurate with age, body weight and physical condition. See DOSAGE AND ADMINISTRATION.

ADVERSE REACTIONS

Systemic: Adverse experiences following the administration of lidocaine are similar in nature to those observed with other amide local anesthetic agents. These adverse experiences are, in general, dose-related and may result from high plasma levels caused by excessive dosage, rapid absorption or inadvertent intravascular injection, or may result from a hypersensitivity, idiosyncrasy or diminished tolerance on the part of the patient. Serious adverse experiences are generally systemic in nature. The following types are those most commonly reported:

Central nervous system: CNS manifestations are excitatory and/or depressant and may be characterized by lightheadedness, nervousness, apprehension, euphoria, confusion, dizziness, drowsiness, tinnitus, blurred or double vision, vomiting, sensations of heat, cold or numbness, twitching, tremors, convulsions, unconsciousness, respiratory depression and arrest. The excitatory manifestations may be very brief or may not occur at all, in which case the first manifestation of toxicity may be drowsiness merging into unconsciousness and respiratory arrest.

Drowsiness following the administration of lidocaine is usually an early sign of a high blood level of the drug and may occur as a consequence of rapid absorption.

Cardiovascular system: Cardiovascular manifestations are usually depressant and are characterized by bradycardia, hypotension, and cardiovascular collapse, which may lead to cardiac arrest.

Allergic: Allergic reactions are characterized by cutaneous lesions, urticaria, edema or anaphylactoid reactions. Allergic reactions may occur as a result of sensitivity either to local anesthetic agents or to the methylparaben used as a preservative in multiple dose vials. Allergic reactions as a result of sensitivity to lidocaine are extremely rare and, if they occur, should be managed by conventional means. The detection of sensitivity by skin testing is of doubtful value.

Neurologic: The incidences of adverse reactions associated with the use of local anesthetics may be related to the total dose of local anesthetic administered and are also dependent upon the particular drug used, the route of administration and the physical status of the patient. In a prospective review of 10,440 patients who received lidocaine for spinal anesthesia, the incidences of adverse reactions were reported to be about 3 percent each for positional headaches, hypotension and backache; 2 percent for shivering; and less than 1 percent each for peripheral nerve symptoms, nausea, respiratory inadequacy and double vision. Many of these observations may be related to local anesthetic techniques, with or without a contribution from the local anesthetic.

In the practice of caudal or lumbar epidural block, occasional unintentional penetration of the subarachnoid space by the catheter may occur. Subsequent adverse effects may depend partially on the amount of drug administered subdurally. These may include spinal block of varying magnitude (including total spinal block), hypotension secondary to spinal block, loss of bladder and bowel control, and loss of perineal sensation and sexual function. Persistent motor, sensory and/or autonomic (sphincter control) deficit of some lower spinal segments with slow recovery (several months) or incomplete recovery have been reported in rare instances when caudal or lumbar epidural block has been attempted. Backache and headache have also been noted following use of these anesthetic procedures.

OVERDOSAGE

Acute emergencies from local anesthetics are generally related to high plasma levels encountered during therapeutic use of local anesthetics or to unintended subarachnoid injection of local anesthetic solution (see ADVERSE REACTIONS, WARNINGS and PRECAUTIONS).

Management of local anesthetic emergencies: The first consideration is prevention, best accomplished by careful and constant monitoring of cardiovascular and respiratory vital signs and the patient's state of consciousness after each local anesthetic injection. At the first sign of change, oxygen should be administered.

The first step in the management of convulsions, as well as underventilation or apnea due to unintended subarachnoid injection of drug solution, consists of immediate attention to the maintenance of a patent airway and assisted or controlled ventilation with oxygen and a delivery system capable of permitting immediate positive airway pressure by mask. Immediately after the institution of these ventilatory measures, the adequacy of the circulation should be evaluated, keeping in mind that drugs used to treat convulsions sometimes depress the circulation when administered intravenously. Should convulsions persist despite adequate repiratory support, and if the status of the circulation per-

Continued on next page

Astra—Cont.

mits, small increments of an ultra-short acting barbiturate (such as thiopental or thiamylal) or a benzodiazepine (such as diazepam) may be administered intravenously. The clinician should be familiar, prior to the use of local anesthetics, with these anticonvulsant drugs. Supportive treatment of circulatory depression may require administration of intravenous fluids and, when appropriate, a vasopressor as directed by the clinical situation (e.g. ephedrine).

If not treated immediately, both convulsions and cardiovascular depression can result in hypoxia, acidosis, bradycardia, arrhythmias and cardiac arrest. Underventilation or apnea due to unintentional subarachnoid injection of local anesthetic solution may produce these same signs and also lead to cardiac arrest if ventilatory support is not instituted. If cardiac arrest should occur standard cardiopulmonary resuscitative measures should be instituted.

Endotracheal intubation, employing drugs and techniques familiar to the clinician, may be indicated, after initial administration of oxygen by mask, if difficulty is encountered in the maintenance of a patent airway or if prolonged ventilatory support (assisted or controlled) is indicated.

Dialysis is of negligible value in the treatment of acute overdosage with lidocaine.

The oral LD_{50} of lidocaine HCl in non-fasted female rats is 459 (346–773) mg/kg (as the salt) and 214 (159–324) mg/kg (as the salt) in fasted female rats.

DOSAGE AND ADMINISTRATION

Table II (Recommended Dosages) summarizes the recommended volumes and concentrations of Xylocaine Injection for various types of anesthetic procedures. The dosages suggested in this table are for normal healthy adults and refer to the use of epinephrine-free solutions. When larger volumes are required only solutions containing epinephrine should be used, except in those cases where vasopressor drugs may be contraindicated.

These recommended doses serve only as a guide to the amount of anesthetic required for most routine procedures. The actual volumes and concentrations to be used depend on a number of factors such as type and extent of surgical procedure, depth of anesthesia and degree of muscular relaxation required, duration of anesthesia required, and the physical condition of the patient. In all cases the lowest concentration and smallest dose that will produce the desired result should be given. Dosages should be reduced for children and for elderly and debilitated patients and patients with cardiac and/or liver disease.

The onset of anesthesia, the duration of anesthesia and the degree of muscular relaxation are proportional to the volume and concentration (i.e. total dose) of local anesthetic used. Thus, an increase in volume and concentration of Xylocaine Injection will decrease the onset of anesthesia, prolong the duration of anesthesia, provide a greater degree of muscular relaxation and increase the segmental spread of anesthesia. However, increasing the volume and concentration of Xylocaine Injection may result in a more profound fall in blood pressure when used in epidural anesthesia. Although the incidence of side effects with lidocaine is quite low, caution should be exercised when employing large volumes and concentrations, since the incidence of side effects is directly proportional to the total dose of local anesthetic agent injected.

For intravenous regional anesthesia, only the 50 mL single dose vial containing Xylocaine (lidocaine HCl) 0.5% Injection should be used.

Epidural Anesthesia

For epidural anesthesia, only the following dosage forms of Xylocaine Injection are recommended:

1% without epinephrine .... 30 mL ampules
       30 mL single dose vials
1% with epinephrine 1:200,000 .... 30 mL ampules
       30 mL single dose vials
1.5% without epinephrine .... 20 mL ampules
       20 mL single dose vials
1.5% with epinephrine 1:200,000 .... 30 mL ampules
       30 mL single dose vials
2% without epinephrine .... 10 mL ampules
       10 mL single dose vials
2% with epinephrine 1:200,000 .... 20 mL ampules
       20 mL single dose vials

Although these solutions are intended specifically for epidural anesthesia, they may also be used for infiltration and peripheral nerve block, provided they are employed as single dose units. These solutions contain no bacteriostatic agent.

In epidural anesthesia, the dosage varies with the number of dermatomes to be anesthetized (generally 2-3 mL of the indicated concentration per dermatome).

Caudal and lumbar epidural block: As a precaution against the adverse experience sometimes observed following unintentional penetration of the subarachnoid space, a test dose such as 2–3 mL of 1.5% lidocaine should be administered at least 5 minutes prior to injecting the total volume required for a lumbar or caudal epidural block. The test dose should be repeated if the patient is moved in a manner that may have displaced the catheter. Epinephrine, if contained in the test dose (10–15 μg have been suggested), may serve as a warning of unintentional intravascular injection. If injected into a blood vessel, this amount of epinephrine is likely to produce a transient "epinephrine response" within 45 seconds, consisting of an increase in heart rate and systolic blood pressure, circumoral pallor, palpitations and nervousness in the unsedated patient. The sedated patient may exhibit only a pulse rate increase of 20 or more beats per minutes for 15 or more seconds. Patients on beta-blockers may not manifest changes in heart rate, but blood pressure monitoring can detect an evanescent rise in systolic blood pressure. Adequate time should be allowed for onset of anesthesia after administration of each test dose. The rapid injection of a large volume of Xylocaine Injection through the catheter should be avoided, and, when feasible, fractional doses should be administered.

In the event of the known injection of a large volume of local anesthetic solution into the subarachnoid space, after suitable resuscitation and if the catheter is in place, consider attempting the recovery of drug by draining a moderate amount of cerebrospinal fluid (such as 10 mL) through the epidural catheter.

MAXIMUM RECOMMENDED DOSAGES

Adults: For normal healthy adults, the individual maximum recommended dose of lidocaine HCl with epinephrine should not exceed 7 mg/kg (3.5 mg/lb) of body weight, and in general it is recommended that the maximum total dose not exceed 500 mg. When used without epinephrine, the maximum individual dose should not exceed 4.5 mg/kg (2 mg per lb) of body weight, and in general it is recommended that the maximum total dose does not exceed 300 mg. For continuous epidural or caudal anesthesia, the maximum recommended dosage should not be administered at intervals of less than 90 minutes. When continuous lumbar or caudal epidural anesthesia is used for non-obstetrical procedures, more drug may be administered if required to produce adequate anesthesia.

The maximum recommended dose per 90 minute period of lidocaine hydrochloride for paracervical block in obstetrical patients and non-obstetrical patients is 200 mg total. One half of the total dose is usually administered to each side. Inject slowly, five minutes between sides. (See also discussion of paracervical block in PRECAUTIONS).

For intravenous regional anesthesia, the dose administered should not exceed 4 mg/kg in adults.

Children: It is difficult to recommend a maximum dose of any drug for children, since this varies as a function of age and weight. For children over 3 years of age who have a normal lean body mass and normal body development, the maximum dose is determined by the child's age and weight. For example, in a child of 5 years weighing 50 lbs., the dose of lidocaine HCl should not exceed 75–100 mg (1.5–2 mg/lb). The use of even more dilute solutions (i.e., 0.25–0.5%) and total dosages not to exceed 3 mg/kg (1.4 mg/lb) are recommended for induction of intravenous regional anesthesia in children.

In order to guard against systemic toxicity, the lowest effective concentration and lowest effective dose should be used at all times. In some cases it will be necessary to dilute available concentrations with 0.9% sodium chloride injection in order to obtain the required final concentration.

NOTE: Parenteral drug products should be inspected visually for particulate matter and discoloration prior to administration whenever the solution and container permit. The injection is not to be used if its color is pinkish or darker than slightly yellow or if it contains a precipitate.

TABLE 1 Recommended Dosages

PROCEDURE	Xylocaine (lidocaine hydrochloride) Injection (without epinephrine)		
	Conc (%)	Vol (mL)	Total Dose (mg)
Infiltration			
Percutaneous	0.5 or 1	1–60	5–300
Intravenous regional	0.5	10–60	50–300
Peripheral Nerve Blocks, e.g.			
Brachial	1.5	15–20	225–300
Dental	2	1–5	20–100
Intercostal	1	3	30
Paravertebral	1	3–5	30–50
Pudendal (each side)	1	10	100
Paracervical			
Obstetrical analgesia (each side)			
	1	10	100
Sympathetic Nerve Blocks, e.g.			
Cervical (stellate ganglion)	1	5	50
Lumbar	1	5–10	50–100
Central Neural Blocks			
Epidural*			
Thoracic	1	20–30	200–300
Lumbar			
Analgesia	1	25–30	250–300
Anesthesia	1.5	15–20	225–300
	2	10–15	200–300
Caudal			
Obstetrical analgesia	1	20–30	200–300
Surgical anesthesia	1.5	15–20	225–300

* Dose determined by number of dermatomes to be anesthetized (2–3 mL/dermatome).

THE ABOVE SUGGESTED CONCENTRATIONS AND VOLUMES SERVE ONLY AS A GUIDE. OTHER VOLUMES AND CONCENTRATIONS MAY BE USED PROVIDED THE TOTAL MAXIMUM RECOMMENDED DOSE IS NOT EXCEEDED.

Sterilization, Storage and Technical Procedures: Disinfecting agents containing heavy metals, which cause release of respective ions (mercury, zinc, copper, etc.) should not be used for skin or mucous membrane disinfection as they have been related to incidents of swelling and edema. When chemical disinfection of multi-dose vials is desired, either isopropyl alcohol (91%) or ethyl alcohol (70%) is recommended. Many commercially available brands of rubbing alcohol, as well as solutions of ethyl alcohol not of U.S.P. grade, contain denaturants which are injurious to rubber and therefore are not to be used.

Dosage forms listed as Xylocaine-MPF indicates single dose solutions that are M̲ethyl P̲araben F̲ree (MPF).

HOW SUPPLIED
[See table at left.]
Protect from light.
021850R13   Rev. 1/92 (13)

HOW SUPPLIED

Xylocaine (lidocaine HCl) Concentration	/Epinephrine Dilution (if present)	Xylocaine—MPF											Xylocaine		
		Ampules (mL)					Single Dose Vials (mL)						Multiple Dose Vials (mL)		
		2	5	10	20	30	2*	5	10	20	30	50	10	20	50
0.5%												X			X
0.5%	/1:200,000											X			
1%		X	X			X	X	X	X		X		X	X	X
1%	/1:100,000												X	X	X
1%	/1:200,000				X			X	X	X		X			
1.5%					X				X	X					
1.5%	/1:200,000			X		X		X	X	X		X			
2%		X		X			X	X	X				X	X	X
2%	/1:100,000												X	X	X
2%	/1:200,000			X			X	X	X						

All solutions should be stored at room temperature, approximately 25°C (77°F).   * = 3 mL vial with 2 mL fill

XYLOCAINE® INJECTION ℞

[$z\bar{\imath}\,'lo\text{-}caine$]
(lidocaine hydrochloride)
FOR VENTRICULAR ARRHYTHMIAS

DESCRIPTION

Xylocaine (lidocaine hydrochloride) Injection is a sterile and non-pyrogenic solution of an antiarrhythmic agent administered intravenously by either direct injection or continuous infusion.

Xylocaine Injections are composed of aqueous solutions of lidocaine hydrochloride. Lidocaine hydrochloride ($C_{14}H_{22}N_2O\cdot HCl$) is chemically designated acetamide, 2-(diethylamino)-N-(2, 6 dimethylphenyl)-, monohydrochloride.
(For details of indications, dosage and administration, precautions, and adverse reactions, see circular in package.)

HOW SUPPLIED

For direct intravenous injection, Xylocaine (lidocaine hydrochloride) Injection without preservatives is supplied in 5 mL, 50 mg and 100 mg prefilled syringes and in 5 mL, 100 mg ampules.

For preparing solutions for intravenous infusions, Xylocaine Injection without sodium chloride or preservatives is supplied in one and two gram additive syringes and in one and two gram single use vials. Vials are available with or without pre-sterilized transfer unit manufactured by the West Company.

Solutions should be stored at controlled room temperature 15°–30°C (59°–86°F).

021834R05 Rev. 5/89 (5)

4% XYLOCAINE®-MPF™ (lidocaine HCl) ℞

[$z\bar{\imath}\,'lo\text{-}caine$]
STERILE SOLUTION
   For transtracheal use,
   retrobulbar injection,
   and for topical application

DESCRIPTION

4% Xylocaine-MPF (lidocaine HCl) Sterile Solution contains a local anesthetic agent and is administered topically or by injection. See INDICATIONS for specific uses.

4% Xylocaine-MPF Sterile Solution contains lidocaine HCl, which is chemically designated as acetamide, 2-(diethylamino)-N-(2,6-dimethylphenyl)-monohydrochloride.

4% Xylocaine-MPF Sterile Solution in 5 mL ampules may be autoclaved repeatedly if necessary.
(For details of indications, dosage and administration, precautions, and adverse reactions, see circular in package.)
Composition of 4% Xylocaine-MPF Sterile Solution
Each mL contains lidocaine HCl, 40.0 mg, and sodium hydroxide and/or hydrochloric acid to adjust pH to 5.0–7.0. A sterile, aqueous solution.

HOW SUPPLIED

4% Xylocaine-MPF (lidocaine HCl) Sterile Solution, 5 mL ampule (NDC 0186-0235-03) and 5 mL prefilled sterile disposable syringe packaged in a presterilized kit containing a laryngotracheal cannula (NDC 0186-0235-72).
Store at controlled room temperature: 15°C–30°C (59°–86°F).
021562R07 Rev. 8/90 (7)

XYLOCAINE® (lidocaine hydrochloride) ℞

[$z\bar{\imath}\,'lo\text{-}caine$]
4% TOPICAL SOLUTION
For topical application

DESCRIPTION

Xylocaine (lidocaine HCl) 4% Topical Solution contains a local anesthetic agent and is administered topically. See INDICATIONS for specific uses.

Xylocaine 4% Topical Solution contains lidocaine HCL, which is chemically designated as acetamide, 2-(diethylamino)-N-(2,6-dimethylphenyl)-, monohydrochloride.

The 50ml screw-cap bottle should not be autoclaved, because the closure employed cannot withstand autoclaving temperatures and pressures. Composition of Xylocaine (lidocaine HCl) 4% Topical Solution: Each ml contains lidocaine HCl, 40mg, methylparaben, and sodium hydroxide and/or hydrochloric acid to adjust pH to 6.0–7.0.
An aqueous solution. NOT FOR INJECTION

HOW SUPPLIED

Xylocaine (lidocaine HCl) 4% Topical Solution 50ml screw-cap bottle, cartoned (NDC 0186-0320-01). NOT FOR INJECTION.
Store at controlled room temperature: 15°-30°C (59°-86°F).
021802R01 7/84

XYLOCAINE®-MPF™ ℞

[$z\bar{\imath}\,'lo\text{-}caine$]
(lidocaine HCl) 1.5% Injection
WITH DEXTROSE 7.5%
   for Spinal Anesthesia
   in Obstetrics

(For details of indications, dosage and administration, precautions, and adverse reactions, see circular in package.)

HOW SUPPLIED

Xylocaine-MPF (lidocaine HCl) 1.5% Injection with Dextrose 7.5% (NDC 0186-0212-03) is supplied in 2 mL ampules in packages of 10. Store at controlled room temperature 15°-30°C (59°-86°F).
021836R06 9/89 (6)

5% XYLOCAINE®-MPF™ ℞

[$z\bar{\imath}\,'lo\text{-}cain$]
(lidocaine hydrochloride) Injection
WITH GLUCOSE 7.5%

(For details of indications, dosage and administration, precautions, and adverse reactions, see circular in package.)

HOW SUPPLIED

Xylocaine-MPF (lidocaine HCl) 5% Injection with Glucose 7.5% (NDC 0186-0225-03) is supplied in 2 mL ampules in packages of 10.
Store at controlled room temperatures 15°-30°C (59°-86°F).
021564R10 8/89 (10)

XYLOCAINE® 2% (lidocaine hydrochloride) ℞

[$z\bar{\imath}\,'lo\text{-}caine$]
JELLY
   A Topical Anesthetic
   for Urological Procedures
   and Lubrication
   of Endotracheal Tubes

DESCRIPTION

Xylocaine (lidocaine HCl) 2% Jelly is a sterile aqueous product that contains a local anesthetic agent and is administered topically. See INDICATIONS for specific uses.

Xylocaine 2% Jelly contains lidocaine HCl which is chemically designated as acetamide, 2-(diethylamino)-N-(2,6-dimethylphenyl)-, monohydrochloride.

Xylocaine 2% Jelly also contains hydroxypropylmethylcellulose, and the resulting mixture maximizes contact with mucosa and provides lubrication for instrumentation.
The unused portion should be discarded after initial use.
Composition of Xylocaine 2% Jelly:
Each mL contains 20 mg of lidocaine HCl. The formulation also contains methylparaben, propylparaben, hydroxypropylmethylcellulose, and sodium hydroxide and/or hydrochloric acid to adjust pH to 6.0–7.0.
(For details of indications, dosage and administration, precautions, and adverse reactions, see circular in package.)

HOW SUPPLIED

Xylocaine (lidocaine HCl) 2% Jelly (NDC 0186-0330-01) is supplied in collapsible tubes that deliver 30 mL. A detachable applicator cone and a key for expressing the contents are included in each package.
Store at controlled room temperature 15°-30°C (59°-86°F).
021838R11 Rev. 6/86 (11)

5% XYLOCAINE®(lidocaine) ℞

[$z\bar{\imath}\,'lo\text{-}caine$]
Ointment
A Water-Soluble Topical Anesthetic Ointment

DESCRIPTION

Xylocaine (lidocaine) 5% Ointment contains a local anesthetic agent and is administered topically. See INDICATIONS for specific uses.

Xylocaine 5% Ointment contains lidocaine, which is chemically designated as acetamide, 2-(diethylamino)-N-(2,6-dimethylphenyl)-.
Composition of Xylocaine 5% Ointment
Each gram of the plain and flavored ointments contains lidocaine, 50 mg, polyethylene glycol 1500, polyethylene glycol 4000, and propylene glycol. The flavored ointment contains sodium saccharin, peppermint oil and spearmint oil.
(For details of indications, dosage and administration, precautions, and adverse reactions, see circular in package.)

HOW SUPPLIED

Xylocaine (lidocaine) 5% Ointment (NDC 0186-0315-21) is available in 35 gm tubes.
Xylocaine (lidocaine) 5% Ointment Flavored for application within the oral cavity, is dispensed in 3.5 gram tubes, 10

---

tubes per carton (NDC 0186-0350-03), and in 35-gram jars (NDC 0186-0350-01).
KEEP CONTAINER TIGHTLY CLOSED AT ALL TIMES WHEN NOT IN USE.
Store at controlled room temperature 15°-30°C (59°-86°F).
021709R12 Rev. 1/88(12)

XYLOCAINE ® (lidocaine) OTC

[$z\bar{\imath}\,'lo\text{-}cain$]
2.5% OINTMENT

(See PDR For Nonprescription Drugs.)

XYLOCAINE® (lidocaine) ℞

[$z\bar{\imath}\,'lo\text{-}caine$]
10% Oral Spray
   Flavored Topical Anesthetic Aerosol
   For Use In The Oral Cavity

WARNING—CONTENTS UNDER PRESSURE

DESCRIPTION

Xylocaine (lidocaine) 10% Oral Spray contains a local anesthetic agent and is administered topically in the oral cavity. See INDICATIONS for specific uses.

Xylocaine 10% Oral Spray contains lidocaine, which is chemically designated as acetamide, 2-(diethylamino)-N-(2,6-dimethylphenyl)-.
Composition of Xylocaine (lidocaine) 10% Oral Spray
Each actuation of the metered dose valve delivers solution containing lidocaine, 10mg, cetylpyridinium chloride, absolute alcohol, saccharin, flavor, and polyethylene glycol.
And as propellants: trichlorofluoromethane/dichlorodifluoromethane (65%/35%).
(For details of indications, dosage and administration, precautions, and adverse reactions, see circular in package.)

HOW SUPPLIED

NDC 0186-0356-01. A 26.8 mL aerosol container provides a total amount of 3.3 g (w/w) of the active ingredient lidocaine. Each actuation of the metered dose valve delivers 10 mg of lidocaine.

Contents under pressure. Do not puncture or incinerate container. Do not expose to heat or store at temperatures above 120°F. Avoid contact with the eyes. Inhalation and swallowing should be avoided.
Keep out of the reach of children.
Use only as directed; intentional misuse by deliberately concentrating and inhaling the contents can be harmful or fatal.
STORE AT CONTROLLED ROOM TEMPERATURE 15°-30°C (59°-86°F).
Manufactured by Armstrong Laboratories, Inc., West Roxbury, MA 02132
A flexible, disposable Cannula, 9035-05, is available in boxes of 50, to provide directed spray for easier access to oropharynx.
021731R07 2/90 (7)

XYLOCAINE® 2% (lidocaine hydrochloride) VISCOUS SOLUTION ℞

[$z\bar{\imath}\,'lo\text{-}caine$]
A Topical Anesthetic
for the Mucous Membranes
of the Mouth and Pharynx

DESCRIPTION

Xylocaine (lidocaine HCl) 2% Viscous Solution contains a local anesthetic agent and is administered topically. Xylocaine 2% Viscous Solution contains lidocaine HCl, which is chemically designated as acetamide, 2-(diethylamino)-N-(2,6-dimethylphenyl)-, monohydrochloride.
The molecular formula of lidocaine is $C_{14}H_{22}N_2O$. The molecular weight is 234.34.
(For details of indications, dosage and administration, precautions, and adverse reactions, see circular in package.)

HOW SUPPLIED

Xylocaine 2% (lidocaine HCl) Viscous Solution is available in 100 mL (NDC 0186-0360-01) and 450 mL (NDC 0186-0360-11) polyethylene squeeze bottles and in unit of use (adult dose) packages of 25 (20 mL) polyethylene bottles (NDC 0186-0361-78).
The solutions should be stored at controlled room temperature 15°-30°C (59°-86°F).
021899R00 Iss. 1/88

Continued on next page

Astra—Cont.

YUTOPAR® ℞

[*yoū 'tow-par*]
(ritodrine hydrochloride)
Injection and Tablets

CAUTION: Federal law prohibits dispensing without prescription.

DESCRIPTION

Yutopar, which contains the betamimetic (beta sympathomimetic amine) ritodrine hydrochloride, is available in two dosage forms. Yutopar for parenteral (intravenous) use is a clear, colorless, sterile, aqueous solution; each milliliter contains either 10 mg. or 15 mg. of ritodrine hydrochloride, 4.35 mg of acetic acid, 2.4 mg of sodium hydroxide, 1 mg of sodium metabisulfite, and 2.4 mg of sodium chloride in Water for injection USP. Hydrochloric acid or additional sodium hydroxide is used to adjust pH. Filled under nitrogen. **FOR INTRAVENOUS USE ONLY. MUST BE DILUTED BEFORE USE. FOR DOSAGE AND ADMINISTRATION INSTRUCTIONS, SEE PRODUCT INFORMATION BELOW. DO NOT USE IF INJECTION IS DISCOLORED OR CONTAINS A PRECIPITATE.**

Each Yutopar tablet contains 10 mg. of ritodine hydrochloride and the following inactive ingredients (in alphabetical order): corn starch, iron oxide yellow synthetic, lactose, magnesium stearate, povidone, and talc.

Ritodrine hydrochloride is a white, odorless crystalline powder, freely soluble in water, with a melting point between 196° and 205°C. The chemical name of ritodrine hydrochloride is erythro-p-hydroxy-α-[1[(p-hydroxyphenethyl)-amino]ethyl]benzyl alcohol hydrochloride and has the chemical structure:

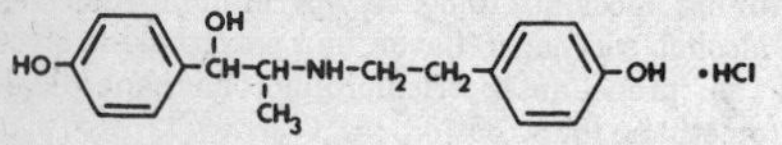

CLINICAL PHARMACOLOGY

Yutopar (ritodrine hydrochloride) is a beta-receptor agonist, which has been shown by *in vitro* and *in vivo* pharmacologic studies in animals to exert a preferential effect on the β_2 adrenergic receptors such as those in the uterine smooth muscle. Stimulation of the β_2 receptors inhibits contractility of the uterine smooth muscle.

In humans, intravenous infusions of 0.05 to 0.30 mg/min. or single oral doses of 10 to 20 mg. decreased the intensity and frequency of uterine contractions. These effects were antagonized by beta-blocking compounds. Intravenous administration induced an immediate dose-related elevation of heart rate with maximum mean increases between 19 and 40 beats per minute. Widening of the pulse pressure was also observed; the average increase in systolic blood pressure was 4.0 mm. Hg, and the average decrease in diastolic pressure was 12.3 mm. Hg. With oral intake, the increase in heart rate was mild and delayed.

During intravenous infusion in humans, transient elevations of blood glucose, insulin, and free fatty acids have been observed. Decreased serum potassium has also been found, but effects on other electrolytes have not been reported.

Serum kinetics in humans (non-pregnant females) of an intravenous infusion of 60 minutes duration were determined by measuring serum ritodrine levels by a radioimmunoassay technique. The distribution half-life was found to be 6 to 9 minutes, and the effective half-life 1.7 to 2.6 hours. In a study of serum kinetics after oral ingestion (male subjects), the decline of serum drug levels could be described in terms of a two-phase decay with an initial half-life of 1.3 hours and a final half-life of 12 hours. With either route of administration, 90% of the excretion was completed within 24 hours after the dose.

Comparison of ritodrine serum levels after intravenous administration with those after oral dosage indicates the oral bioavailability is about 30%. Intravenous infusion at a rate of 0.15 mg./min. for 1 hour yielded maximum serum levels ranging between 32 and 52 ng./mL in a group of 6 non-pregnant female volunteers; maximum serum levels following single and repeated (4 × 10 mg./24 hr.) 10 mg. oral doses ranged between 5 and 15 ng./mL and were obtained within 30 to 60 minutes after ingestion.

Placental transfer was confirmed by measurement of drug concentrations in cord blood showing that ritodrine and its conjugates reach the fetal circulation.

INDICATIONS AND USAGE

Yutopar is indicated for the management of preterm labor in suitable patients.

Administered intravenously, the drug will decrease uterine activity and thus prolong gestation in the majority of such patients. After intravenous Yutopar has arrested the acute episode, oral administration may help to avert relapse. Additional acute episodes may be treated by repeating the intravenous infusion. The incidence of neonatal mortality and respiratory distress syndrome increases when the normal gestation period is shortened.

Since successful inhibition of labor is more likely with early treatment, therapy with Yutopar should be instituted as soon as the diagnosis of preterm labor is established and contraindications ruled out in pregnancies of 20 or more weeks' gestation. The efficacy and safety of Yutopar in advanced labor, that is, when cervical dilatation is more than 4 cm. or effacement is more than 80%, have not been established.

CONTRAINDICATIONS

Yutopar is contraindicated before the 20th week of pregnancy.

Yutopar is also contraindicated in those conditions of the mother or fetus in which continuation of pregnancy is hazardous; specific contraindications include:

1. Antepartum hemorrhage which demands immediate delivery
2. Eclampsia and severe preeclampsia
3. Intrauterine fetal death
4. Chorioamnionitis
5. Maternal cardiac disease
6. Pulmonary hypertension
7. Maternal hyperthyroidism
8. Uncontrolled maternal diabetes mellitus (See PRECAUTIONS.)
9. Pre-existing maternal medical conditions that would be seriously affected by the known pharmacologic properties of a betamimetic drug; such as: hypovolemia, cardiac arrhythmias associated with tachycardia or digitalis intoxication, uncontrolled hypertension, pheochromocytoma, bronchial asthma already treated by betamimetics and/or steroids
10. Known hypersensitivity to any component of the product

WARNINGS

> Maternal pulmonary edema has been reported in patients treated with Yutopar, sometimes after delivery. It has occurred more often when patients were treated concomitantly with corticosteroids. Maternal death from this condition has been reported with or without corticosteroids given concomitantly with drugs of this class.
>
> Patients so treated must be closely monitored in the hospital. The patient's state of hydration should be carefully monitored; fluid overload must be avoided. (See DOSAGE AND ADMINISTRATION.) Intravenous fluid loading may be aggravated by the use of betamimetics with or without corticosteroids and may turn into manifest circulatory overloading with subsequent pulmonary edema. If pulmonary edema develops during administration, the drug should be discontinued. Edema should be managed by conventional means.

Intravenous administration of Yutopar should be supervised by persons having knowledge of the pharmacology of the drug and who are qualified to identify and manage complications of drug administration and pregnancy. Beta-adrenergic drugs increase cardiac output, and even in a normal healthy heart this added myocardial oxygen demand can sometimes lead to myocardial ischemia. Complications may include: myocardial necrosis, which may result in death; arrhythmias, including premature atrial and ventricular contractions, ventricular tachycardia, and bundle branch block; anginal pain, with or without ECG changes. *Because cardiovascular responses are common and more pronounced during intravenous administration of Yutopar, cardiovascular effects, including maternal pulse rate and blood pressure and fetal heart rate, should be closely monitored. Care should be exercised for maternal signs and symptoms of pulmonary edema. A persistent high tachycardia (over 140 beats per minute) may be one of the signs of impending pulmonary edema with drugs of this class. Occult cardiac disease may be unmasked with the use of Yutopar. If the patient complains of chest pain or tightness of chest, the drug should be temporarily discontinued and an ECG should be done as soon as possible.*

The drug should not be administered to patients with mild to moderate preeclampsia, hypertension, or diabetes unless the attending physician considers that the benefits clearly outweigh the risks.

Yutopar Injection contains sodium metabisulfite, a sulfite that may cause serious allergic-type reactions including anaphylactic symptoms and life-threatening or less severe asthmatic episodes in certain susceptible people. The overall prevalence of sulfite sensitivity in the general population is unknown and probably low. Sulfite sensitivity is seen more frequently in asthmatic than in nonasthmatic people.

PRECAUTIONS

When Yutopar is used for the management of preterm labor in a patient with premature rupture of the membranes, the benefits of delaying delivery should be balanced against the potential risks of development of chorioamnionitis.

Among low birth weight infants, approximately 9% may be growth retarded for gestational age. Therefore, Intra-Uterine Growth Retardation (IUGR) should be considered in the differential diagnosis of preterm labor; this is especially important when the gestational age is in doubt. The decision to continue or reinitiate the administration of Yutopar will depend on an assessment of fetal maturity. In addition to clinical parameters, other studies, such as sonography or amniocentesis, may be helpful in establishing the state of fetal maturity if it is in doubt.

Baseline EKG

This should be done to rule out occult maternal heart disease.

Laboratory Tests

Because intravenous administration of Yutopar has been shown to elevate plasma insulin and glucose and to decrease plasma potassium concentrations, monitoring of glucose and electrolyte levels is recommended during protracted infusions. Decrease of plasma potassium concentrations is usually transient, returning to normal within 24 hours. Special attention should be paid to biochemical variables when treating diabetic patients or those receiving potassium-depleting diuretics.

Serial hemograms may be helpful as an index of state of hydration.

Drug Interactions

Corticosteroids used concomitantly may lead to pulmonary edema. (SEE WARNINGS.)

Cardiovascular effects of Yutopar injection (especially cardiac arrhythmia or hypotension) may be potentiated by concomitant use of the following drugs.

1. magnesium sulfate
2. diazoxide
3. meperidine
4. potent general anesthetic agents

Systemic hypertension may be exaggerated in the presence of parasympatholytic agents such as atropine.

The effects of other sympathomimetic amines may be potentiated when concurrently administered and these effects may be additive. A sufficient time interval should elapse prior to administration of another sympathomimetic drug.

With either oral or intravenous administration, 90% of the excretion of Yutopar is completed within 24 hours after the dose.

(See CLINICAL PHARMACOLOGY.)

Beta-adrenergic blocking drugs inhibit the action of Yutopar; coadministration of these drugs should, therefore, be avoided.

With anesthetics used in surgery, the possibility that hypotensive effects may be potentiated should be considered.

Migraine Headache

Transient cerebral ischemia associated with beta sympathomimetic therapy has been reported in two patients with migraine headache.

Carcinogenesis, Mutagenesis, Impairment of Fertility

In rats given oral doses of 1, 10 and 150 mg./kg./day of ritodrine hydrochloride for 82 weeks, benign and malignant tumors were found in the various dosage groups. Since there were no important differences between untreated controls and treated groups and no dose-related trends, it was concluded that there was no evidence of tumorigenicity. The incidence (2–4%) of tumors of the type found in this study is not unusual in this species.

Reproduction studies in rats and rabbits have revealed no evidence of impaired fertility due to ritodrine hydrochloride.

Pregnancy

Teratogenic Effects

(Pregnancy Category B)

Reproduction studies were performed in rats and rabbits. The doses employed intravenously were ⅑ (1 mg./kg.), ⅓ (3 mg./kg.), and 1 (9 mg./kg.) times the maximum human daily intravenous dose (but given to the animals as a bolus rather than by infusion). The oral doses, 10 and 100 mg./kg. represented 5 and 50 times the maximum human daily oral maintenance dose. The results of these studies have revealed no evidence of impaired fertility or harm to the fetus due to ritodrine hydrochloride.

No adverse fetal effects were encountered when single intravenous doses of 1, 3, and 9 mg./kg./day or oral doses of 10 and 100 mg./kg./day were given to rats and rabbits on Days 6 through 15 and 6 through 18 of gestation, respectively. Intravenous doses of 1 and 8 mg./kg./day or oral doses of 10 and 100 mg./kg./day administered to the mother from Day 15 of pregnancy to Day 21 postpartum did not affect perinatal or postnatal development in rats. A slight increase in fetal weight in the rat was observed. Oral administration to both sexes did not impair fertility or reproductive performance. Lethal doses to pregnant rats did not cause immediate fetal demise. There are no adequate and well-controlled studies of Yutopar effects in pregnant women before 20 weeks' gestation; *therefore, this drug should not be used before the 20th week of pregnancy.* Studies of Yutopar administered to pregnant women from the 20th week of gestation have not shown increased risk of fetal abnormalities. Follow-up of selected variables in a small number of children for up to 2 years has not revealed harmful effects on growth, developmental or

functional maturation. Nonetheless, although clinical studies did not demonstrate a risk of permanent adverse fetal effects from Yutopar, the possibility cannot be excluded; therefore, Yutopar should be used only when clearly indicated.

Some studies indicate that infants born before 36 weeks' gestation make up less than 10% of all births but account for as many as 75% of perinatal deaths and one-half of all neurologically handicapped infants. There are data available indicating that infants born at any time prior to full term may manifest a higher incidence of neurologic or other handicaps than occurs in the total population of infants born at or after full term. In delaying or preventing preterm labor, the use of Yutopar should result in an overall increase in neonatal survival. Handicapped infants who might not have otherwise survived may survive.

ADVERSE REACTIONS

The unwanted effects of Yutopar are related to its betamimetic activity and usually are controlled by suitable dosage adjustment.

Effects Associated with Intravenous Administration
Usual effects (80–100% of patients)
Intravenous infusion of Yutopar leads almost invariably to dose-related alterations in maternal and fetal heart rates and in maternal blood pressure. During clinical studies in which the maximum infusion rate was limited to 0.35 mg./min. (one patient received 0.40 mg./min.), the maximum maternal and fetal heart rates averaged, respectively, 130 (range 60 to 180) and 164 (range 130 to 200) beats per minute. The maximum maternal systolic blood pressures averaged 128 mm. Hg (range 96 to 162 mm. Hg), an average increase of 12 mm. Hg from pretreatment levels. The minimum maternal diastolic blood pressures averaged 48 mm. Hg (range 0 to 76 mm. Hg), an average decrease of 23 mm. Hg from pretreatment levels. While the more severe effects were usually managed effectively by dosage adjustments, in less than 1% of patients, persistent maternal tachycardia or decreased diastolic blood pressure required withdrawal of the drug. A persistent high tachycardia (over 140 beats per minute) may be one of the signs of impending pulmonary edema. (See WARNINGS.)

Yutopar infusion is associated with transient elevation of blood glucose and insulin, which decreases toward normal values after 48 to 72 hours despite continued infusion. Elevation of free fatty acids and cAMP has been reported. Reduction of potassium levels should be expected; other biochemical effects have not been reported.

Frequent effects (10–50% of patients)
Intravenous Yutopar, in about one-third of the patients, was associated with palpitation. Tremor, nausea, vomiting, headache, or erythema was observed in 10 to 15% of patients.

Occasional effects (5–10% of patients)
Nervousness, jitteriness, restlessness, emotional upset, or anxiety was reported in 5 to 6% of patients and malaise in similar numbers.

Infrequent effects (1–3% of patients)
Cardiac symptoms including chest pain or tightness (rarely associated with abnormalities of ECG) and arrhythmia were reported in 1 to 2% of patients. (See Warnings.)
Other infrequently reported maternal effects included: anaphylactic shock, rash, heart murmur, epigastric distress, ileus, bloating, constipation, diarrhea, dyspnea, hyperventilation, hemolytic icterus, glycosuria, lactic acidosis, sweating, chills, drowsiness, and weakness. Impaired liver function (i.e., increased transaminase levels and hepatitis) have also been reported infrequently (less than 1%) with the use of ritodrine and other beta sympathomimetics.

Neonatal Effects
Infrequently reported neonatal symptoms include hypoglycemia and ileus. In addition, hypocalcemia and hypotension have been reported in neonates whose mothers were treated with other betamimetic agents.

Effects Associated with Oral Administration
Frequent effects (<50% of patients)
Oral ritodrine in clinical studies was often associated with small increases in maternal heart rate, but little or no effect upon either maternal systolic or diastolic blood pressure or upon fetal heart rate was found.
Oral ritodrine in 10 to 15% of patients was associated with palpitation or tremor. Nausea and jitterness were less frequent (5 to 8%), while rash was observed in some patients (3 to 4%), and arrhythmia was infrequent (about 1%). Impaired liver function (i.e., increased transaminase levels and hepatitis) have also been reported infrequently (less than 1%) with the use of ritodrine and other beta sympathomimetics.

OVERDOSAGE

The symptoms of overdosage are those of excessive beta-adrenergic stimulation including exaggeration of the known pharmacologic effects, the most prominent being tachycardia (maternal and fetal), palpitation, cardiac arrhythmia, hypotension, dyspnea, nervousness, tremor, nausea, and vomiting. If an excess of ritodrine tablets is ingested, gastric lavage or induction of emesis should be carried out followed by administration of activated charcoal. When symptoms of

overdose occur as a result of intravenous administration, ritodrine should be discontinued; an appropriate beta-blocking agent may be used as an antidote. Ritodrine hydrochloride is dialyzable.

Acute intravenous toxicity was studied in rats and rabbits and acute oral toxicity in mice, rats, guinea pigs, and dogs. The LD50 values in the most sensitive of the species used were 64 mg./kg. intravenously in the nonpregnant rabbit and 540 mg./kg. orally in the nonpregnant mouse. The intravenous LD50 value in the pregnant rat was 85 mg./kg. The amount of drug required to produce symptoms of overdose in humans is individually variable. No reports of human mortality due to overdose have been received.

DOSAGE AND ADMINISTRATION

In the management of preterm labor, the initial intravenous treatment should usually be followed by oral administration. The optimum dose of Yutopar is determined by a clinical balance of uterine response and unwanted effects.

Intravenous Therapy
Do not use intravenous Yutopar if the solution is discolored or contains any precipitate or particulate matter. Yutopar injection should be used promptly after preparation, but in no case after 48 hours of preparation.

Method of Administration: To minimize the risks of hypotension, the patient should be maintained in the left lateral position throughout infusion and careful attention given to her state of hydration, but fluid overload must be avoided. For appropriate control and dose titration, a controlled infusion device is recommended to adjust the rate of flow in drops/minute. An IV microdrip chamber (60 drops/mL) can provide a convenient range of infusion rates within the recommended dose range for Yutopar.

Recommended Dilution: 150 mg. ritodrine hydrochloride in 500 mL fluid yielding a final concentration of 0.3 mg/mL*. Ritodrine for intravenous infusion should be diluted with 5% w/v dextrose solution. Because of the increased probability of pulmonary edema, saline diluents such as:
—0.9% w/v sodium chloride solution,
—compound sodium chloride solution (Ringer's solution)
—and Hartmann's solution, should be reserved for cases where dextrose solution is medically undesirable e.g. diabetes mellitus.

Intravenous therapy should be started as soon as possible after diagnosis. The usual initial dose is 0.1 mg./minute (0.33 mL/min., 20 drops/min. using a microdrip chamber at the recommended dilution), to be gradually increased according to the results by 0.05 mg./minute (0.17 mL/min., 10 drops/min. using a microdrip chamber at the recommended dilution) every 10 minutes until the desired result is attained. The effective dosage usually lies between 0.15 and 0.35 mg./minute (0.50 to 1.17 mL/min., 30–70 drops/min. using a microdrip chamber at the recommended dilution). Frequent monitoring of maternal uterine contractions, heart rate, and blood pressure, and of fetal heart rate is required, with dosage individually titrated according to response. If other drugs need to be given intravenously, the use of "piggyback" or other site of intravenous administration permits the continued independent control of the rate of infusion of the Yutopar.

The infusion should generally be continued for at least 12 hours after uterine contractions cease. With the recommended dilution, the maximum volume of fluid that might be administered after 12 hours at the highest dose (0.35 mg./min.) will be approximately 840 mL.
The amount of IV fluids administered and the rate of administration should be monitored to avoid circulatory fluid overload (over-hydration). (See PRECAUTIONS, Laboratory Tests.)

Oral Maintenance
One tablet (10 mg.) may be given approximately 30 minutes before the termination of intravenous therapy. The usual dosage schedule for the first 24 hours of oral administration is 1 tablet (10 mg.) every two hours. Thereafter, the usual maintenance is 1 or 2 tablets (10 to 20 mg.) every four to six hours, the dose depending on uterine activity and unwanted effects. The total daily dose of oral ritodrine should not exceed 120 mg. The treatment may be continued as long as the physician considers it desirable to prolong pregnancy.
Recurrence of unwanted preterm labor may be treated with repeated infusion of Yutopar.

HOW SUPPLIED

NDC 0186-0569-13: 5 mL vial in boxes of 10. Each vial contains 50 mg (10 mg/mL) of ritodrine hydrochloride.
NDC 0186-0599-03: 5 mL ampules in boxes of 10. Each ampule contains 50 mg (10 mg/mL) of ritodrine hydrochloride.
NDC 0186-0597-12: 10 mL vial in box of 1. Each vial contains 150 mg (15 mg/mL) of ritodrine hydrochloride.
NDC 0186-0595-60: 10 mg tablets in bottles of 60. Each round, yellow tablet contains 10 mg ritodrine hydrochloride and is inscribed YUTOPAR on one side and scored on the other.
*In those cases where fluid restriction is medically desirable, a more concentrated solution may be prepared.

NDC 0186-0595-78: 10 mg unit dose tablets in boxes of 100. Each round, yellow tablet contains 10 mg ritodrine hydrochloride and is inscribed YUTOPAR on one side and scored on the other.
NDC 0186-0644-01: 10 mL syringe in box of 1. Each syringe contains 150 mg (15 mg/mL) of ritodrine hydrochloride.
Both the tablet and intravenous dosage forms should be stored at room temperature, preferably below 86°F. (30°C). Protect from excessive heat.
Oral dosage form manufactured by SOLVAY DUPHAR B.V., Holland for
ASTRA®
Astra Pharmaceuticals Products, Inc.
Westborough MA 01581
Yutopar® licensed by Solvay Duphar B. V. Holland
021843R09   Rev. 8/91 (09)

For information on Astra products, write to:
Professional Information Dept.
Astra Pharmaceutical Products, Inc.
50 Otis Street
Westborough Massachusetts 01581-4500

For Emergency Medical Information on any Astra product, call (800) 225-6333.

Athena Neurosciences, Inc.
800F GATEWAY BOULEVARD
SOUTH SAN FRANCISCO, CA 94080

ATARIN™   ℞
Isometheptene Mucate, Dichloralphenazone,
and Acetaminophen
[ă′ter-ĭn]

CAUTION: Federal law prohibits dispensing without prescription.

DESCRIPTION

Each capsule contains Isometheptene Mucate 65 mg., Dichloralphenazone 100 mg., and Acetaminophen 325 mg. Isometheptene Mucate is a white crystalline powder having a characteristic aromatic odor and bitter taste. It is an unsaturated aliphatic amine with sympathomimetic properties. Dichloralphenazone is a white microcrystalline powder, with a slight odor and tastes saline at first, becoming acrid. It is a mild sedative.
Acetaminophen, a non-salicylate, occurs as a white, odorless, crystalline powder possessing a slightly bitter taste.

ACTIONS

Isometheptene Mucate, a sympathomimetic amine, acts by constricting dilated cranial and cerebral arterioles, thus reducing the stimuli that lead to vascular headaches. Dichloralphenazone, a mild sedative, reduces the patient's emotional reaction to the pain of both vascular and tension headaches. Acetaminophen raises the threshold to painful stimuli, thus exerting an analgesic effect against all types of headaches.

INDICATIONS

For relief of vascular and tension headaches.

> Based on a review for this drug (isometheptene mucate), The National Academy of Sciences—National Research Council and/or other information, FDA has classified the other indication as "possibly" effective in the treatment of migraine headache.
> Final classification of the less-than effective indication requires further investigation.

CONTRAINDICATIONS

Atarin™ is contraindicated in glaucoma and/or severe cases of renal disease, hypertension, organic heart disease, hepatic disease and in those patients who are on monoamine-oxidase (MAO) inhibitor therapy.

PRECAUTIONS

Caution should be observed in hypertension, peripheral vascular disease and after recent cardiovascular attacks.

ADVERSE REACTIONS

Transient dizziness and skin rash may appear in hypersensitive patients. This can usually be eliminated by reducing the dose.

DOSAGE AND ADMINISTRATION

FOR RELIEF OF MIGRAINE HEADACHE: The usual adult dose is two capsules at once, followed by one capsule every hour until relieved, up to 5 capsules within a twelve hour period.

Continued on next page

Athena Neurosciences, Inc.—Cont.

FOR RELIEF OF TENSION HEADACHE: The usual adult dose is one or two capsules every four hours up to 8 capsules a day.

HOW SUPPLIED

Bottles of 100 capsules, NDC 59075-576-10, Professional samples in bottles of 5 capsules, NDC 59075-576-01
Manufactured by:
NUTRIPHARM LABORATORIES, INC.
Flemington, NJ 08822
Distributed by
ATHENA NEUROSCIENCES, INC.
South San Francisco, CA 94080

ATRETOL™   ℞
[ă'trĕ-tŏl]
Carbamazepine Tablets, USP 200 mg

> **WARNING**
>
> APLASTIC ANEMIA AND AGRANULOCYTOSIS HAVE BEEN REPORTED IN ASSOCIATION WITH THE USE OF CARBAMAZEPINE. DATA FROM A POPULATION—BASED CASE CONTROL STUDY DEMONSTRATE THAT THE RISK OF DEVELOPING THESE REACTIONS IS 5–8 TIMES GREATER THAN IN THE GENERAL POPULATION. HOWEVER, THE OVERALL RISK OF THESE REACTIONS IN THE UNTREATED GENERAL POPULATION IS LOW, APPROXIMATELY SIX PATIENTS PER ONE MILLION POPULATION PER YEAR FOR AGRANULOCYTOSIS AND TWO PATIENTS PER ONE MILLION POPULATION PER YEAR FOR APLASTIC ANEMIA.
>
> ALTHOUGH REPORTS OF TRANSIENT OR PERSISTENT DECREASED PLATELET OR WHITE BLOOD CELL COUNTS ARE NOT UNCOMMON IN ASSOCIATION WITH THE USE OF CARBAMAZEPINE, DATA ARE NOT AVAILABLE TO ESTIMATE ACCURATELY THEIR INCIDENCE OR OUTCOME. HOWEVER, THE VAST MAJORITY OF THE CASES OF LEUKOPENIA HAVE NOT PROGRESSED TO THE MORE SERIOUS CONDITIONS OF APLASTIC ANEMIA OR AGRANULOCYTOSIS.
>
> BECAUSE OF THE VERY LOW INCIDENCE OF AGRANULOCYTOSIS AND APLASTIC ANEMIA, THE VAST MAJORITY OF MINOR HEMATOLOGIC CHANGES OBSERVED IN MONITORING OF PATIENTS ON CARBAMAZEPINE ARE UNLIKELY TO SIGNAL THE OCCURRENCE OF EITHER ABNORMALITY. NONETHELESS, COMPLETE PRETREATMENT HEMATOLOGICAL TESTING SHOULD BE OBTAINED AS A BASELINE. IF A PATIENT IN THE COURSE OF TREATMENT EXHIBITS LOW OR DECREASED WHITE BLOOD CELL OR PLATELET COUNTS, THE PATIENT SHOULD BE MONITORED CLOSELY. DISCONTINUATION OF THE DRUG SHOULD BE CONSIDERED IF ANY EVIDENCE OF SIGNIFICANT BONE MARROW DEPRESSION DEVELOPS.

Before prescribing Carbamazepine, the physician should be thoroughly familiar with the details of this prescribing information, particularly regarding use with other drugs, especially those which accentuate toxicity potential.

DESCRIPTION

Carbamazepine is an anticonvulsant and specific analgesic for trigeminal neuralgia, available as tablets of 200 mg for oral administration. Its chemical name is 5H-dibenz (b,f)-azepine-5-carboxamide.
Carbamazepine USP is a white to off-white powder, practically insoluble in water and soluble in alcohol and in acetone.
Atretol™ 200 mg tablets contain the inactive ingredients Colloidal Silicon Dioxide, Croscarmellose Sodium, Lactose, Magnesium Stearate, Sodium Starch Glycolate and other ingredients.

CLINICAL PHARMACOLOGY

In controlled clinical trials, carbamazepine has been shown to be effective in the treatment of psychomotor and grand mal seizures, as well as trigeminal neuralgia.
It has demonstrated anticonvulsant properties in rats and mice with electrically and chemically induced seizures. It appears to act by reducing polysynaptic responses and blocking the post-tetanic potentiation. Carbamazepine greatly reduces or abolishes pain induced by stimulation of the intraorbital nerve in cats and rats. It depresses thalamic potential and bulbar and polysynaptic reflexes, including the linguomandibular reflex in cats. Carbamazepine is chemically unrelated to other anticonvulsants or other drugs used to control the pain of trigeminal neuralgia. The mechanism of action remains unknown.

Atretol tablets are adequately absorbed after oral administration at a slower rate than a solution, thus avoiding undesirably high peak concentrations. Carbamazepine in blood is 76% bound to plasma proteins. Plasma levels of carbamazepine are variable and may range from 0.5–25 µg/mL, with no apparent relationship to the daily intake of the drug. Usual adult therapeutic levels are between 4 and 12 µg/mL. Following oral administration, serum levels peak at 4 to 5 hours. The CSF/serum ratio is 0.22 similar to the 22% unbound carbamazepine in serum. Because carbamazepine may induce its own metabolism, the half-life is also variable. Initial half-life values range from 25–65 hours, with 12–17 hours on repeated doses. Carbamazepine is metabolized in the liver. After oral administration of ^{14}C-carbamazepine, 72% of the administered radioactivity was found in the urine and 28% in the feces. This urinary radioactivity was composed largely of hydroxylated and conjugated metabolites, with only 3% of unchanged carbamazepine. Transplacental passage of carbamazepine is rapid (30 to 60 minutes), and the drug is accumulated in fetal tissues, with higher levels found in liver and kidney than in brain and in lungs.

INDICATIONS AND USAGE

Epilepsy: Atretol (Carbamazepine Tablets) is indicated for use as an anticonvulsant drug. Evidence supporting efficacy of carbamazepine as an anticonvulsant was derived from active drug-controlled studies that enrolled patients with the following seizure types:

1. Partial seizures with complex symptomatology (psychomotor, temporal lobe). Patients with these seizures appear to show greater improvement than those with other types.
2. Generalized tonic-clonic seizures (grand mal).
3. Mixed seizure patterns which include the above, or other partial or generalized seizures.

Absence seizures (petit mal) do not appear to be controlled by carbamazepine (see PRECAUTIONS General).

Trigeminal Neuralgia—Atretol is indicated in the treatment of the pain associated with true trigeminal neuralgia.
Beneficial results have also been reported in glossopharyngeal neuralgia.
This drug is not a simple analgesic and should not be used for the relief of trivial aches or pains.

CONTRAINDICATIONS

Carbamazepine should not be used in patients with a history of previous bone marrow depression, hypersensitivity to the drug or known sensitivity to any of the tricyclic compounds, such as amitriptyline, desipramine, imipramine, protriptyline, nortriptyline, etc. Likewise, on theoretical grounds its use with monoamine oxidase inhibitors is not recommended. Before administration of carbamazepine, MAO inhibitors should be discontinued for a minimum of fourteen days, or longer if the clinical situation permits.

WARNINGS

Patients with a history of adverse hematologic reaction to any drug may be particularly at risk.
Severe dermatologic reactions including toxic epidermal necrolysis (Lyell's syndrome) and Stevens-Johnson syndrome, have been reported with carbamazepine. These reactions have been extremely rare. However, a few fatalities have been reported.
Carbamazepine has shown mild anticholinergic activity; therefore, patients with increased intraocular pressure should be closely observed during therapy.
Because of the relationship of the drug to other tricyclic compounds, the possibility of activation of a latent psychosis and, in elderly patients, of confusion or agitation should be borne in mind.

PRECAUTIONS

General—Before initiating therapy, a detailed history and physical examination should be made.
Carbamazepine should be used with caution in patients with a mixed seizure disorder that includes atypical absence seizures, since in these patients carbamazepine has been associated with increased frequency of generalized convulsions (see INDICATIONS AND USAGE).
Therapy should be prescribed only after critical benefit-to-risk appraisal in patients with a history of cardiac, hepatic or renal damage, adverse hematologic reaction to other drugs, or interrupted courses of therapy with carbamazepine.
Information for Patients—Patients should be made aware of the early toxic signs and symptoms of a potential hematologic problem, such as fever, sore throat, ulcers in the mouth, easy bruising, petechial or purpuric hemorrhage, and should be advised to report to the physician immediately if any such signs or symptoms appear.
Since dizziness and drowsiness may occur, patients should be cautioned about the hazards of operating machinery or automobiles or engaging in other potentially dangerous tasks.
Laboratory Tests—Complete pretreatment blood counts, including platelets and possibly reticulocytes and serum iron, should be obtained as a baseline. If a patient in the course of treatment exhibits low or decreased white blood cell or platelet counts, the patient should be monitored closely. Discontinuation of the drug should be considered if any evidence of significant bone marrow depression develops.

Baseline and periodic evaluations of liver function, particularly in patients with a history of liver disease, must be performed during treatment with this drug since liver damage may occur. The drug should be discontinued immediately in cases of aggravated liver dysfunction or active liver disease.
Baseline and periodic eye examinations, including slit-lamp, funduscopy and tonometry, are recommended since many phenothiazines and related drugs have been shown to cause eye changes.
Baseline and periodic complete urinalysis and BUN determinations are recommended for patients treated with this agent because of observed renal dysfunction.
Monitoring of blood levels (see CLINICAL PHARMACOLOGY) has increased the efficacy and safety of anticonvulsants. This monitoring may be particularly useful in cases of dramatic increase in seizure frequency and for verification of compliance. In addition, measurement of drug serum levels may aid in determining the cause of toxicity when more than one medication is being used.
Thyroid function tests have been reported to show decreased values with carbamazepine administered alone.
Hyponatremia has been reported in association with carbamazepine use, either alone or in combination with other drugs.
Drug Interactions—The simultaneous administration of phenobarbital, phenytoin, or primidone, or a combination of two, produces a marked lowering of serum levels of carbamazepine. The effect of valproic acid on carbamazepine blood levels is not clearly established.
The half-lives of phenytoin, warfarin, doxycycline, and theophylline were significantly shortened when administered concurrently with carbamazepine. Haloperidol and valproic acid serum levels may be reduced when the drug is administered with carbamazepine. The doses of these drugs may therefore have to be increased when carbamazepine is added to the therapeutic regimen.
Concomitant administration of carbamazepine with erythromycin, cimetidine, propoxyphene, isoniazid or calcium channel blockers has been reported to result in elevated plasma levels of carbamazepine resulting in toxicity in some cases. Also, concomitant administration of carbamazepine and lithium may increase the risk of neurotoxic side effects.
Alterations of thyroid function have been reported in combination therapy with other anticonvulsant medications.
Breakthrough bleeding has been reported among patients receiving concomitant oral contraceptives and their reliability may be adversely affected.
Carcinogenicity, Mutagenesis, Impairment of Fertility—Carbamazepine, when administered to Sprague-Dawley rats for two years in the diet at doses of 25, 75, and 250 mg/kg/day, resulted in a dose-related increase in the incidence of hepatocellular tumors in females and of benign interstitial cell adenomas in the testes of males.
Carbamazepine must, therefore, be considered to be carcinogenic in Sprague-Dawley rats. Bacterial and mammalian mutagenicity studies using carbamazepine produced negative results. The significance of these findings relative to the use of carbamazepine in humans is, at present, unknown.
Pregnancy Category C—Carbamazepine has been shown to have adverse effects in reproduction studies in rats when given orally in dosages 10–25 times the maximum human daily dosage of 1200 mg. In rat teratology studies, 2 of 135 offspring showed kinked ribs at 250 mg/kg and 4 of 119 offspring at 650 mg/kg showed other anomalies (cleft palate, 1; talipes, 1; anophthalmos, 2). In reproduction studies in rats, nursing offspring demonstrated a lack of weight gain and an unkempt appearance at a maternal dosage level of 2000 mg/kg.
There are no adequate and well-controlled studies in pregnant women. Carbamazepine should be used during pregnancy only if the potential benefit justifies the potential risk to the fetus.
Retrospective case reviews suggest that compared with monotherapy, there may be a higher prevalence of teratogenic effects associated with the use of anticonvulsants in combination therapy. Therefore, monotherapy is recommended for pregnant women.
It is important to note that anticonvulsant drugs should not be discontinued in patients in whom the drug is administered to prevent major seizures because of the strong possibility of precipitating status epilepticus with attendant hypoxia and threat to life. In individual cases where the severity and frequency of the seizure disorder are such that removal of medication does not pose a serious threat to the patient, discontinuation of the drug may be considered prior to and during pregnancy, although it cannot be said with any confidence that even minor seizures do not pose some hazard to the developing embryo or fetus.
Labor and Delivery—The effect of carbamazepine on human labor and delivery is unknown.

Nursing Mothers—During lactation, concentration of carbamazepine in milk is approximately 60% of the maternal plasma concentration.
Because of the potential for serious adverse reactions in nursing infants from carbamazepine, a decision should be made whether to discontinue nursing or to discontinue the drug, taking into account the importance of the drug to the mother.
Pediatric Use—Safety and effectiveness in children below the age of 6 years have not been established.

ADVERSE REACTIONS

If adverse reactions are of such severity that the drug must be discontinued, the physician must be aware that abrupt discontinuation of any anticonvulsant drug in a responsive epileptic patient may lead to seizures or even status epilepticus with its life-threatening hazards.
The most severe adverse reactions have been observed in the hemopoietic system (see boxed WARNING), the skin and the cardiovascular system.
The most frequently observed adverse reactions, particularly during the initial phases of therapy, are dizziness, drowsiness, unsteadiness, nausea, and vomiting. To minimize the possibility of such reactions, therapy should be initiated at the low dosage recommended.
The following additional adverse reactions have been reported:
Hemopoietic System—Aplastic anemia, agranulocytosis, pancytopenia, bone marrow depression, thrombocytopenia, leukopenia, leukocytosis, eosinophilia.
Skin—Pruritic and erythematous rashes, urticaria, toxic epidermal necrolysis (Lyell's syndrome) (see WARNINGS), Stevens-Johnson syndrome (see WARNINGS), photosensitivity reactions, alterations in skin pigmentation, exfoliative dermatitis, erythema multiforme and nodosum, purpura, aggravation of disseminated lupus erythematosus, alopecia, and diaphoresis. In certain cases, discontinuation of therapy may be necessary.
Cardiovascular System—Congestive heart failure, edema, aggravation of hypertension, hypotension, syncope and collapse, aggravation of coronary artery disease, arrhythmias and AV block, primary thrombophlebitis, recurrence of thrombophlebitis, and adenopathy or lymphadenopathy.
Some of these cardiovascular complications have resulted in fatalities. Myocardial infarction has been associated with other tricyclic compounds.
Liver—Abnormalities in liver function tests, cholestatic and hepatocellular jaundice, hepatitis.
Respiratory System—Pulmonary hypersensitivity characterized by fever, dyspnea, pneumonitis or pneumonia.
Genitourinary System—Urinary frequency, acute urinary retention, oliguria with elevated blood pressure, azotemia, renal failure, and impotence. Albuminuria, glycosuria, elevated BUN and microscopic deposits in the urine have also been reported.
Testicular atrophy occurred in rats receiving carbamazepine orally from 4 to 52 weeks at dosage levels of 50 to 400 mg/kg/day. Additionally, rats receiving carbamazepine in the diet for two years at dosage levels of 25, 75, and 250 mg/kg/day had a dose-related incidence of testicular atrophy and aspermatogenesis. In dogs, it produced a brownish discoloration, presumably a metabolite, in the urinary bladder at dosage levels of 50 mg/kg and higher. Relevance of these findings to humans is unknown.
Nervous System—Dizziness, drowsiness, disturbances of coordination, confusion, headache, fatigue, blurred vision, visual hallucinations, transient diplopia, oculomotor disturbances, nystagmus, speech disturbances, abnormal involuntary movements, peripheral neuritis and paresthesias, depression with agitation, talkativeness, tinnitus, and hyperacusis.
There have been reports of associated paralysis and other symptoms of cerebral arterial insufficiency, but the exact relationship of these reactions to the drug has not been established.
Digestive System—Nausea, vomiting, gastric distress and abdominal pain, diarrhea, constipation, anorexia, and dryness of the mouth and pharynx, including glossitis and stomatitis.
Eyes—Scattered, punctate, cortical lens opacities, as well as conjunctivitis have been reported. Although a direct casual relationship has not been established, many phenothiazines and related drugs have been shown to cause eye changes.
Musculoskeletal System—Aching joints and muscles, and leg cramps.
Metabolism—Fever and chills. Inappropriate antidiuretic hormone (ADH) secretion syndrome has been reported. Cases of frank water intoxication, with decreased serum sodium (hyponatremia) and confusion, have been reported in association with carbamazepine use (see PRECAUTIONS, Laboratory Tests).
Other—Isolated cases of a lupus erythematosus-like syndrome have been reported. There have been occasional reports of elevated levels of cholesterol, HDL cholesterol and triglycerides in patients taking anticonvulsants.

DRUG ABUSE AND DEPENDENCE

No evidence of abuse potential has been associated with carbamazepine, nor is there evidence of psychological or physical dependence in humans.

OVERDOSAGE

Acute toxicity—Lowest known lethal dose: adults > 60 g (39-year-old man). Highest known doses survived: adults, 30 g (31-year-old woman); children, 10 g (6-year-old boy), small children 5 g (3-year-old girl).
Oral LD_{50} in animals (mg/kg): mice, 1100–3570; rats, 3850–4025; rabbits, 1500–2680; guinea pigs, 920.
Signs and Symptoms—The first signs and symptoms appear after 1–3 hours. Neuromuscular disturbances are the most prominent. Cardiovascular disorders are generally milder, and severe cardiac complications occur only when very high doses (> 60 g) have been ingested.
Respiration—Irregular breathing, respiratory depression.
Cardiovascular System—Tachycardia, hypertension or hypotension, shock, conduction disorders.
Nervous System and Muscles—Impairment of consciousness ranging in severity to deep coma. Convulsions, especially in small children. Motor restlessness, muscular twitching, tremor, athetoid movements, opisthotonos, ataxia, drowsiness, dizziness, mydriasis, nystagmus, adiadochokinesia, ballism, psychomotor disturbances, dysmetria. Initial hyperreflexia, followed by hyporeflexia.
Gastrointestinal Tract—Nausea, vomiting.
Kidneys and Bladder—Anuria or oliguria, urinary retention.
Laboratory Findings—Isolated instances of overdosage have included leukocytosis, reduced leukocyte count, glycosuria and acetonuria. EEG may show dysrhythmias.
Combined Poisoning—When alcohol, tricyclic antidepressants, barbiturates or hydantoins are taken at the same time, the signs and symptoms of acute poisoning with carbamazepine may be aggravated or modified.
Treatment—The prognosis in cases of severe poisoning is critically dependent upon prompt elimination of the drug, which may be achieved by inducing vomiting, irrigating the stomach and by taking appropriate steps to diminish absorption. If these measures cannot be implemented without risk on the spot, the patient should be transferred at once to a hospital, while ensuring that vital functions are safeguarded. There is no specific antidote.
Elimination of the Drug—Induction of vomiting.
Gastric lavage. Even when more than 4 hours have elapsed following ingestion of the drug, the stomach should be repeatedly irrigated, especially if the patient has also consumed alcohol.
Measures to Reduce Absorption—Activated charcoal, laxatives.
Measures to Accelerate Elimination—Forced diuresis.
Dialysis is indicated only in severe poisoning associated with renal failure. Replacement transfusion is indicated in severe poisoning in small children.
Respiratory Depression—Keep the airways free; resort, if necessary, to endotracheal intubation, artificial respiration, and administration of oxygen.
Hypotension, Shock—Keep the patient's legs raised and administer a plasma expander. If blood pressure fails to rise despite measures taken to increase plasma volume, use of vasoactive substances should be considered.
Convulsions—Diazepam or barbiturates.
Warning—Diazepam or barbiturates may aggravate respiratory depression (especially in children), hypotension, and coma. However, barbiturates should *not* be used if drugs that inhibit monoamine oxidase have also been taken by the patient either in overdosage or in recent therapy (within one week).
Surveillance—Respiration, cardiac function (ECG monitoring), blood pressure, body temperature, pupillary reflexes, and kidney and bladder function should be monitored for several days.
Treatment of Blood Count Abnormalities—If evidence of significant bone marrow depression develops, the following recommendations are suggested: (1) stop the drug, (2) perform daily CBC, platelet and reticulocyte counts, (3) do a bone marrow aspiration and trephine biopsy immediately and repeat with sufficient frequency to monitor recovery.
Specific periodic studies might be helpful as follows: (1) white cell and platelet antibodies, (2) ^{59}Fe-ferrokinetic studies, (3) peripheral blood cell typing, (4) cytogenetic studies on marrow and peripheral blood, (5) bone marrow culture studies for colony-forming units, (6) hemoglobin electrophoresis for A_2 and F hemoglobin, and (7) serum folic acid and B_{12} levels.
A fully developed aplastic anemia will require appropriate, intensive monitoring and therapy, for which specialized consultation should be sought.

DOSAGE AND ADMINISTRATION

Monitoring of blood levels has increased the efficacy and safety of anticonvulsants (see PRECAUTIONS Laboratory Tests). Dosage should be adjusted to the needs of the individual patient. A low initial daily dosage with a gradual increase is advised. As soon as adequate control is achieved, the dosage may be reduced very gradually to the minimum effective level. Tablets should be taken with meals.
Epilepsy (see INDICATIONS AND USAGE).
Adults and children over 12 years of age—Initial: 200 mg b.i.d. Increase at weekly intervals by adding up to 200 mg per day using a t.i.d or q.i.d. regimen until the best response is obtained. Dosage should generally not exceed 1000 mg daily in children 12 to 15 years of age, and 1200 mg daily in patients above 15 years of age. Doses up to 1600 mg daily have been used in adults in rare instances. **Maintenance:** Adjust dosage to the minimum effective level, usually 800–1200 mg daily.
Children 6–12 years of age—Initial: 100 mg b.i.d. Increase at weekly intervals by adding 100 mg per day using a t.i.d. or q.i.d. regimen until the best response is obtained. Dosage should generally not exceed 1000 mg. **Maintenance:** Adjust dosage to the minimum effective level, usually 400–800 mg daily.
Combination Therapy: Atretol may be used alone or with other anticonvulsants. When added to existing anticonvulsant therapy, the drug should be added gradually while the other anticonvulsants are maintained or gradually decreased, except phenytoin, which may have to be increased, (see PRECAUTIONS, Drug Interactions and Pregnancy Category C).
Trigeminal Neuralgia (see INDICATIONS AND USAGE).
Initial: 100 mg b.i.d. on the first day for a total daily dose of 200 mg. This daily dose may be increased by up to 200 mg a day using increments of 100 mg every 12 hours only as needed to achieve freedom from pain. Do not exceed 1200 mg daily. **Maintenance:** Control of pain can be maintained in most patients with 400 mg to 800 mg daily. However, some patients may be maintained on as little as 200 mg daily, while others may require as much as 1200 mg daily. At least once every 3 months throughout the treatment period, attempts should be made to reduce the dose to the minimum effective level or even to discontinue the drug.

HOW SUPPLIED

Atretol™ 200 mg (Carbamazepine Tablets, USP) is available in the following form:
Round, white, single-scored tablets, engraved "A"–"554" and are packaged in bottles of 100.
NDC 59075-554-10 (100's)
Store at controlled room temperature 15°–30°C (59°–86°F).
Protect from light and moisture.
Dispense in a tight, light-resistant container, as defined in the USP/NF.
CAUTION: Federal law prohibits dispensing without prescription.

Rev. 1 8/90

Manufactured by:
TEVA PHARMACEUTICAL IND. LTD.
Jerusalem, 91010, Israel
Distributed by:
ATHENA NEUROSCIENCES, Inc.
South San Francisco, CA 94080

ATROFEN™ ℞

BACLOFEN Tablets, USP
[*ă'trō-fin*]

DESCRIPTION

Baclofen is a muscle relaxant and antispastic.
Its chemical name is 4-amino-3-(4-chlorophenyl) butanoic acid; empirical formula $C_{10}H_{12}ClNO_2$; M.W. 213.66.
Baclofen, USP is a white to off-white, odorless or practically odorless crystalline powder, with a molecular weight of 213.6. It is slightly soluble in water, very slightly soluble in methanol and insoluble in chloroform.
Atrofen™, Baclofen Tablets, USP available as 10 mg and 20 mg strengths for oral administration, contain the following inactive ingredients: anhydrous lactose, colloidal silicon dioxide, hydrous dibasic calcium phosphate, magnesium stearate, microcrystalline cellulose and sodium starch glycolate.

CLINICAL PHARMACOLOGY

The precise mechanism of action of baclofen is not fully known. Baclofen is capable of inhibiting both monosynaptic and polysynaptic reflexes at the spinal level, possibly by hyperpolarization of afferent terminals, although actions at supraspinal sites may also occur and contribute to its clinical effect. Although baclofen is an analog of the putative inhibitory neurotransmitter gamma-aminobutyric acid (GABA), there is no conclusive evidence that actions on GABA systems are involved in the production of its clinical effects. In studies with animals baclofen has been shown to have general CNS depressant properties as indicated by the production of sedation with tolerance, somnolence, ataxia, and respiratory and cardiovascular depression. Baclofen is rapidly and extensively absorbed and eliminated. Absorption may be

Continued on next page

Athena Neurosciences, Inc.—Cont.

dose-dependent, being reduced with increasing doses. Baclofen is excreted primarily by the kidney in unchanged form and there is relatively large intersubject variation in absorption and/or elimination.

INDICATIONS

Atrofen (baclofen) is useful for the alleviation of signs and symptoms of spasticity resulting from multiple sclerosis, particularly for the relief of flexor spasms and concomitant pain, clonus, and muscular rigidity.

Patients should have reversible spasticity so that baclofen treatment will aid in restoring residual functions. Atrofen (baclofen) may also be of some value in patients with spinal cord injuries and other spinal cord diseases.

Atrofen (baclofen) is not indicated in the treatment of skeletal muscle spasm resulting from rheumatic disorders.

The efficacy of baclofen in stroke, cerebral palsy, and Parkinson's disease has not been established and, therefore, it is not recommended for these conditions.

CONTRAINDICATIONS

Hypersensitivity to baclofen.

WARNINGS

a. Abrupt Drug Withdrawal: Hallucinations and seizures have occurred on abrupt withdrawal of baclofen. Therefore, except for serious adverse reactions, the dose should be reduced slowly when the drug is discontinued.

b. Impaired Renal Function: Because baclofen is primarily excreted unchanged through the kidneys, it should be given with caution, and it may be necessary to reduce the dosage.

c. Stroke: Baclofen has not significantly benefited patients with stroke. These patients have also shown poor tolerability to the drug.

d. Pregnancy: Baclofen has been shown to increase the incidence of omphaloceles (ventral hernias) in fetuses of rats given approximately 13 times the maximum dose recommended for human use, at a dose which caused significant reductions in food intake and weight gain in dams. This abnormality was not seen in mice or rabbits. There was also an increased incidence of incomplete sternebral ossification in fetuses of rats given approximately 13 times the maximum recommended human dose, and an increased incidence of unossified phalangeal nuclei of forelimbs and hindlimbs in fetuses of rabbits given approximately 7 times the maximum recommended human dose. In mice, no teratogenic effects were observed, although reductions in mean fetal weight with consequent delays in skeletal ossification were present when dams were given 17 and 34 times the human daily dose. There are no studies in pregnant women. Baclofen should be used during pregnancy only if the benefit clearly justifies the potential risk to the fetus.

PRECAUTIONS

Safe use of baclofen in children under age 12 has not been established, and it is, therefore, not recommended for use in children.

Because of the possiblity of sedation, patients should be cautioned regarding the operation of automobiles or other dangerous machinery, and activities made hazardous by decreased alertness. Patients should also be cautioned that the central nervous system effects of baclofen may be additive to those of alcohol and other CNS depressants. Baclofen should be used with caution where spasticity is utilized to sustain upright posture and balance in locomotion or whenever spasticity is utilized to obtain increased function.

In patients with epilepsy, the clinical state and electroencephalogram should be monitored at regular intervals, since deterioration in seizure control and EEG have been reported occasionally in patients taking baclofen .

It is not known whether this drug is excreted in human milk. As a general rule, nursing should not be undertaken while a patient is on a drug since many drugs are excreted in human milk.

A dose-related increase in incidence of ovarian cysts and a less marked increase in enlarged and/or hemorrhagic adrenal glands was observed in female rats treated chronically with baclofen.

Ovarian cysts have been found by palpation in about 4% of the multiple sclerosis patients that were treated with baclofen for up to one year. In most cases these cysts disappeared spontaneously while patients continued to recieve the drug. Ovarian cysts are estimated to occur spontaneously in approximately 1% to 5% of the normal female population.

ADVERSE REACTIONS

The most common is transient drowsiness (10–63%). In one controlled study of 175 patients, transient drowsiness was observed in 63% of those receiving baclofen compared to 36% of those in the placebo group. Other common adverse reactions are dizziness (5–15%), weakness (5–15%), and fatigue 2–4%).

Other reported:

Neuropsychiatric: Confusion (1–11%), headache (4–8%), insomnia (2–7%); and rarely, euphoria, excitement, depression, hallucinations, paresthesia, muscle pain, tinnitus, slurred speech, coordination disorder, tremor, rigidity, dystonia, ataxia, blurred vision, nystagmus, strabismus, miosis, mydriasis, diplopia, dysarthria, epileptic seizure.

Cardiovascular: Hypotension (0–9%). Rare instances of dyspnea, palpitation, chest pain, sncype.

Gastrointestinal: Nausea (4–12%), constipation (2–6%); and rarely, dry mouth, anorexia, taste disorder, abdominal pain, vomiting, diarrhea, and positive test for occult blood in stool.

Genitourinary: Urinary frequency (2–6%); and rarely, enuresis, urinary retention, dysuria, impotence, inability to ejaculate, nocturia, hematuria.

Other: Instances of rash, pruritus, ankle edema, excessive perspiration, weight gain, nasal congestion.

Some of the CNS and genitourinary symptoms may be related to the underlying disease rather than to drug therapy. The following laboratory tests have been found to be abnormal in a few patients receiving baclofen; increased SGOT, elevated alkaline phosphatase, and elevation of blood sugar.

OVERDOSAGE

Signs and Symptoms: Vomiting, muscular hypotonia, drowsiness, accommodation disorders, coma, respiratory depression, and seizures.

Treatment: In the alert patient, empty the stomach promptly by induced emesis followed by lavage. In the obtunded patient, secure the airway with a cuffed endotracheal tube before beginning lavage (do not induce emesis). Maintain adequate respiratory exchange, do not use respiratory stimulants.

DOSAGE AND ADMINISTRATION

The determination of optimal dosage requires individual titration. Start therapy at a low dosage and increase gradually until optimum effect is achieved (usually between 40–80 mg daily).

The following dosage titration schedule is suggested:

    5 mg t.i.d. for three days
   10 mg t.i.d. for three days
   15 mg t.i.d. for three days
   20 mg t.i.d. for three days

Thereafter additional increases may be necessary but the total daily dose should not exceed a maximum of 80 mg daily (20 mg q.i.d.).

The lowest dose compatible with an optimal response is recommended. If benefits are not evident after a reasonable trial period, patients should be slowly withdrawn from the drug (see **WARNINGS** Abrupt Drug Withdrawal).

HOW SUPPLIED

Available as white, round, flat, scored tablet debossed $^A/_{561}$ on one side and 10 on scored side, containing 10 mg Baclofen, USP packaged in bottles of 50 and 100 tablets; as white, round, flat, scored tablet debossed $^A/_{562}$ on one side and 20 on scored side, containing 20 mg Baclofen, USP packaged in bottles of 100 tablets.

NDC Numbers:

10 mg	**20 mg**
59075-561-05 (50's)	59075-562-10 (100's)
59075-561-10 (100's)	

PHARMACIST: Dispense in a well-closed container as defined in the USP. Use child-resistant closure.

Store at controlled room temperature 15°–30°C (59°–86°F).

CAUTION: Federal law prohibits dispensing without prescription.

MANUFACTURED BY

ZENITH LABORATORIES, INC.

NORTHVALE, NEW JERSEY 07647

Distributed by:

ATHENA NEUROSCIENCES, INC.

South San Francisco, CA 94080

59075
Revised 1/92
A1

IDENTIFICATION PROBLEM?
Consult PDR's
Product Identification Section
where you'll find over 1700
products pictured actual size
and in full color.

Ayerst Laboratories

Division of American Home
  Products Corporation
685 THIRD AVE.
NEW YORK, NY 10017-4071

As a result of a merger of Wyeth Laboratories and Ayerst Laboratories, all prescription products of both companies and all nonprescription products of Wyeth are now products of Wyeth-Ayerst Laboratories.

All of Ayerst's nonprescription products are now products of Whitehall Laboratories.

Baker Norton Pharmaceuticals, Inc.

8800 N. W. 36TH STREET
MIAMI, FL 33178-2404

BICITRA®—Sugar-Free   ℞
[bye "si-trah]
**(Sodium Citrate & Citric Acid
Oral Solution USP)**

DESCRIPTION

BICITRA is a pleasant tasting oral alkalinizing agent and a fast-acting nonparticulate antacid.

BICITRA contains in each tablespoonful (15 mL):

SODIUM CITRATE Dihydrate .... 1500 mg (0.34 Molar)
CITRIC ACID Monohydrate .... 1002 mg (0.32 Molar)

Each mL contains 1 mEq Sodium ion and is equivalent to 1 mEq Bicarbonate (HCO_3).

BICITRA is sugar free and nonalcoholic. BICITRA is the highly palatable, improved SHOHL'S Solution.

CLINICAL PHARMACOLOGY

Sodium Citrate is absorbed and metabolized to sodium bicarbonate, thus acting as a systemic alkalizer. The effects are essentially those of chlorides before absorption and those of bicarbonates subsequently. Oxidation is virtually complete so that less than 5% of the citrate is excreted in the urine unchanged. BICITRA is a useful antacid for effectively buffering gastric acid, offering a maximum buffering capacity due to its equimolar ratio of Sodium Citrate to Citric Acid on a 1:1 basis.

INDICATIONS AND ADVANTAGES

BICITRA is useful for conditions requiring long-term maintenance of an alkaline urine, as in patients where dissolution and control of uric acid and cystine calculi of the urinary tract is indicated, especially when the administration of potassium salts is undesirable or contraindicated. It is highly valuable in preventing uric acid nephropathy when administered to patients with hyperuricosuria due to underlying metabolic defects (e.g. gout), or who are receiving drugs (e.g. cancer chemotherapy or uricosuric agents), resulting in acute or chronic increases in urinary uric acid excretion. BICITRA is also effective for alleviating chronic metabolic acidosis, particularly when caused by conditions which may result from renal insufficiency or renal tubular acidosis, where the administration of Sodium Citrate may be preferable.

BICITRA is concentrated, and when administered after meals and before bedtime, maintains an alkaline pH without the need for a 2 A.M. dose. In the recommended dosage, BICITRA alkalinizes the urine without producing systemic alkalosis.

BICITRA is a fast-acting nonparticulate buffering agent and is useful for raising gastric pH. BICITRA has a rapid onset of action, and is decidedly advantageous over particulate aluminum-magnesium containing antacids as a preanesthesia medication. BICITRA offers these advantages over Shohl's Solution, while supplying equivalent alkalinizing effect and sodium content.

BICITRA is pleasant tasting and highly tolerable, even when administered for long periods.

CONTRAINDICATIONS

Patients on sodium-restricted diets or with severe renal impairment. POLYCITRA-K or POLYCITRA-K CRYSTALS is recommended in those clinical situations where administration of Potassium Citrate is preferred.

PRECAUTIONS

Should be used with caution by patients with low urinary output unless under the supervision of a physician. Patients with renal insufficiency should not ingest BICITRA concurrently with aluminum-based antacids used as phosphate binders. Patients should be directed to dilute adequately with water and preferably to take each dose after meals to avoid saline laxative effect. Sodium salts should be used cautiously in patients with cardiac failure, hypertension, impaired renal function, peripheral and pulmonary edema and

toxemia of pregnancy. Periodic examinations of serum electrolytes, particularly serum bicarbonate level, should be carried out in those patients with renal disease in order to avoid these complications.

ADVERSE REACTIONS

BICITRA is generally well tolerated without any unpleasant side effects when given in recommended doses to patients with normal renal function and urinary output. However, as with any alkalinizing agent, caution must be used in certain patients with abnormal renal mechanisms to avoid development of alkalosis, especially in the presence of hypocalcemia.

DOSAGE AND ADMINISTRATION

BICITRA should be taken diluted in water followed by additional water, if desired.

For Systemic Alkalization: Usual Adult Prescribing Limits: Up to 150 mL daily. Occasional patients may require more or less to achieve the desired alkalinizing effect, and since 1 mEq Sodium and 1 mEq Citrate is supplied per each mL, dosage is easy to regulate. To check urinary pH, HYDRION Paper (pH 6.0-8.0) or NITRAZINE Paper (pH 4.5-7.5) are available and easy to use.

Usual Adult Dose: 10 to 30 mL, diluted in 1 to 3 ounces of water or juice, after meals and at bedtime.

Usual Pediatric Dose: 5 to 10 mL diluted in 1 to 3 ounces of water or juice, after meals and at bedtime.

As a Neutralizing Buffer: 15 mL to 30 mL, taken as a single dose, or diluted, if desired, with 15 mL to 30 mL water, or as directed by physician.

OVERDOSAGE

Overdosage with sodium salts may cause diarrhea, nausea and vomiting, hypernoia, and convulsions.

HOW SUPPLIED

BICITRA—
   16 fl oz. (473 mL) (NDC 11414-207-01);
   4 fl oz (120 mL) (NDC 11414-207-04);
   15 mL Unit-Dose (NDC 11414-207-15);
   30 mL Unit-Dose (NDC 11414-207-30).

DORAL®   Ⓒⁱᵛ
brand of quazepam
   Tablets

Marketed by Wallace Laboratories, Division of Carter-Wallace, Inc. under license from Baker Norton Pharmaceuticals, Inc.

Shown in Product Identification Section, page 435

NEUTRA–PHOS® Powder, Packets & Capsules   OTC
NEUTRA–PHOS®–K Powder, Packets & Capsules OTC
[new "trah foss']
Oral Phosphorus Dietary Supplement

NEUTRA-PHOS and NEUTRA-PHOS-K supply the physiologically important element—PHOSPHORUS—as inorganic orthophosphate, in a well tolerated oral compound. Each contains a chemically balanced combination of readily soluble inorganic phosphates, affording a very high source of elemental Phosphorus. Both products supply equal concentration of elemental Phosphorus.

NEUTRA-PHOS is a stable powder combination of monobasic and dibasic Sodium and Potassium Phosphates.

NEUTRA-PHOS-K is a stable sodium-free powder combination of monobasic and dibasic Potassium Phosphates intended for oral use in low sodium diets.

Both products form an oral solution by reconstitution with water and are neutral (pH 7.3), isotonic, pleasant tasting sources of Phosphorus. There is less than 1 calorie per average dose.

INDICATIONS

NEUTRA-PHOS and NEUTRA-PHOS-K are recommended as oral Phosphorus supplements, particularly if the diet supplies an insufficient quantity of Phosphorus, or if metabolic requirements for Phosphorus are increased. In addition, NEUTRA-PHOS and NEUTRA-PHOS-K are useful in the treatment of children and adults with conditions associated with excessive renal phosphate loss or inadequate gastrointestinal absorption of phosphate. They are also useful as an adjunct supplement in the management of phosphate diabetes.

ADVANTAGES

NEUTRA-PHOS and NEUTRA-PHOS-K, reconstituted to an oral liquid, provide a chemically balanced supply of Phosphorus in a pH neutral solution that shows rapid absorption and utilization from the alimentary tract. These liquid products have the advantage over coated or uncoated tablets, as slowly dissolving tablets may cause local gastrointestinal irritation or inflammation in sensitive individuals. Both products are highly concentrated and thus economically provide inorganic Phosphate. They are especially useful for

long term maintenance of an adequate daily supply of Phosphorus. NEUTRA-PHOS supplies Sodium and Potassium in equimolar proportions—a decided advantage over products which supply a high amount of sodium and a low amount of potassium per dose. NEUTRA-PHOS-K supplies only Potassium and is recommended when a low sodium intake is indicated.

ELECTROLYTES SUPPLIED

75 mL of the reconstituted solution or contents of 1 packet or 1 capsule supplies:

NEUTRA-PHOS

Electrolyte	mg	mEq	mg/mL
Phosphorus	250	14.25	3.33
Phosphate (PO₄)	765	—	10.20
Sodium	164	7.125	2.18
Potassium	278	7.125	3.70

NEUTRA-PHOS-K

Electrolyte	mg	mEq	mg/mL
Phosphorus	250	14.25	3.33
Phosphate (PO₄)	765	—	10.20
Sodium	none	none	none
Potassium	556	14.25	7.41

OSMOLALITY

NEUTRA-PHOS Solution*: 223–236 milliosmols per kg (mOsm/kg)
NEUTRA-PHOS-K Solution*: 240–244 milliosmols per kg (mOsm/kg)
(*reconstituted in water as per label directions. Refer to Packets and Capsules description.)

AVERAGE DIRECTIONS FOR ADULTS AND CHILDREN

4 or more years of age: 75 mL of the oral solution, or contents of 1 packet or capsule, equivalent to 250 mg Phosphorus, taken 4 times a day. (See Packets and Capsules description.)

PEDIATRIC DOSE

Infants and children under 4 years of age: 60 mL of the oral solution, equivalent to 200 mg of Phosphorus, taken 4 times a day.

USUAL DOSE RANGE

75 mL to 600 mL of the oral solution, or contents of 1 to 8 packets or capsules (equivalent from 250 mg to 2 grams of Phosphorus) taken daily in divided doses, after meals and at bedtime.*
75 mL of the reconstituted solution, 1 packet, or 1 capsule, 4 times a day, supplies 1 g Phosphorus. 150 mL of the reconstituted solution, 2 packets, or 2 capsules, 3 times a day, supplies 1.5 g Phosphorus. Phosphorus. (See Packets and Capsules description).*

(*This U.S. R.D.A. for Phosphorus is 0.8 g for children 1 to 10 years; 0.8 g for adults 25 years or older; and 1.2 g for ages 11 to 24, pregnant, or lactating women.)

PRECAUTIONS AND SIDE EFFECTS

Reconstitute powder and contents of packets and capsules as directed before taking. Occasionally some individuals may experience a mild laxative effect for the first day or two when beginning to use NEUTRA-PHOS. If this persists to an unpleasant degree, reduce the daily intake until this effect subsides or, if necessary, discontinue its use. NEUTRA-PHOS-K contains FD&C Yellow #6.

HOW SUPPLIED

NEUTRA-PHOS and NEUTRA-PHOS-K are powder concentrates, to be reconstituted with water or any palatable juice or beverage, and are supplied in multiple bulk dose packages or unit dose packets or unit dose capsules.

MULTIPLE DOSE POWDER CONCENTRATE: For patient convenience, bulk powder concentrates are supplied in a package size sufficient to make 1 gallon (3.785 Liters) and are intended for use while at home. This is the most economical dosage form and is prepared by the patient, who is instructed to dissolve the entire contents of one bottle in one gallon of water or other desirable liquid. This solution is not to be further diluted, but can be chilled, if desired, to increase palatability, and can be stored for up to 60 days. 75 mL of this solution supplies 250 mg Phosphorus (refer to electrolyte chart).

UNIT DOSE PACKETS AND CAPSULES: NEUTRA-PHOS and NEUTRA-PHOS-K are also supplied in premeasured unit dose packets and capsules. The contents of 1 packet or capsule makes 75 mL of an oral suspension equal to the oral solution prepared above. To use, empty the contents of 1 packet or capsule into ⅓ glassful water (approximately 75 mL) and stir well before taking. *NOTE: All active components will dissolve rapidly while the excipients will remain in suspension.* If desired, the contents of 1 or 2 packets or capsules can be mixed into the same amount of water or other liquid, such as juice, depending on dosage requirements. Each

packet or capsule supplies 250 mg Phosphorus (refer to electrolyte chart).

NEUTRA-PHOS POWDER CONCENTRATE (Potassium and Sodium Phosphates for Oral Use)—2¼ oz. (64 g) per bottle. Each bottle reconstitutes to make 1 gallon of solution (Stock No. 201-01).

NEUTRA-PHOS UNIT DOSE PACKETS and
NEUTRA-PHOS UNIT DOSE CAPSULES—Each packet or capsule contains 1.25 g NEUTRA-PHOS POWDER CONCENTRATE and makes 75 mL of oral solution.

NEUTRA-PHOS UNIT DOSE PACKETS are packaged 100 packets per box (Stock No. 201-15).

NEUTRA-PHOS UNIT DOSE CAPSULES are packaged 100 capsules per bottle (Stock No. 202-05).

NEUTRA-PHOS-K POWDER CONCENTRATE (Potassium Phosphates for Oral Use)—2½ oz. (71 g) per bottle. Each bottle reconstitutes to make 1 gallon (Stock No. 203-01).

NEUTRA-PHOS K UNIT DOSE PACKETS and
NEUTRA-PHOS-K UNIT DOSE CAPSULES—Each packet or capsule contains 1.45 g NEUTRA-PHOS-K POWDER CONCENTRATE and makes 75 mL of oral solution.

NEUTRA-PHOS-K UNIT DOSE PACKETS are packaged 100 packets per box (Stock No. 203-25).

NEUTRA-PHOS-K UNIT DOSE CAPSULES are packaged 100 capsules per bottle (Stock No. 204-05).

IS THIS PRODUCT O.T.C.?

Yes.

POLYCITRA® Syrup   ℞
POLYCITRA®–LC–Sugar–Free   ℞
[polly "si-trah]
(Tricitrates Oral Solution USP)

DESCRIPTION

Syrup POLYCITRA and POLYCITRA-LC are pleasant tasting and effective oral alkalinizing agents useful for conditions where long-term maintenance of an alkaline urine is desirable.

Syrup POLYCITRA and POLYCITRA-LC contain in each teaspoonful (5 mL):

POTASSIUM CITRATE Monohydrate .... 550 mg
                              (0.34 Molar)
SODIUM CITRATE Dihydrate .... 500 mg (0.34 Molar)
CITRIC ACID Monohydrate .... 334 mg (0.32 Molar)
Each mL contains 1 mEq Potassium and 1 mEq Sodium and is equivalent to 2 mEq Bicarbonate (HCO₃).

Syrup POLYCITRA is a sugar based solution. POLYCITRA-LC is a sugar free solution. Both products contain identical amounts of active ingredients.

CLINICAL PHARMACOLOGY

Potassium Citrate and Sodium Citrate are absorbed and metabolized to potassium bicarbonate and sodium bicarbonate, thus acting as systemic alkalizers. The effects are essentially those of chlorides before absorption and those of bicarbonates subsequently. Oxidation is virtually complete so that less than 5% of the citrates are excreted in the urine unchanged.

INDICATIONS AND ADVANTAGES

Syrup POLYCITRA and POLYCITRA-LC are effective alkalinizing agents useful for conditions where long-term maintenance of an alkaline urine is desirable, as in patients where dissolution and control of uric acid and cystine calculi of the urinary tract is indicated. They are highly valuable in preventing uric acid nephropathy when administered to patients with hyperuricosuria (e.g. gout), or who are receiving drugs (e.g. cancer chemotherapy or uricosuric agents), resulting in acute or chronic increases in urinary uric acid excretion. They are also effective for alleviating chronic metabolic acidosis, which may result from renal insufficiency or renal tubular acidosis.

Syrup POLYCITRA and POLYCITRA-LC are highly concentrated, and when administered after meals and before bedtime, will maintain an alkaline urine pH without the need for a 2 A.M. dose. In recommended dosage, Syrup POLYCITRA and POLYCITRA-LC alkalinize the urine without producing systemic alkalosis.

CONTRAINDICATIONS

Severe renal impairment with oliguria or azotemia, untreated Addison's disease or severe myocardial damage. POLYCITRA-K or POLYCITRA-K CRYSTALS are recommended when the administration of Potassium Citrate is preferred, such as a sodium-restricted diet. BICITRA is recommended when the administration of Sodium Citrate is preferred, such as a potassium-restricted diet.

PRECAUTIONS AND WARNINGS

Should be used with caution by patients with low urinary output or reduced glomerular filtration rates, unless under the supervision of a physician. Patients with renal insuffi-

Continued on next page

Baker Norton—Cont.

ciency should not ingest POLYCITRA or POLYCITRA-LC concurrently with aluminum-based antacids. Patients should be directed to dilute adequately with water and preferably to take each dose after meals, to minimize the possibility of gastrointestinal injury associated with oral ingestion of potassium salt preparations and to avoid saline laxative effect. Sodium salts should be used cautiously in patients with cardiac failure, hypertension, peripheral and pulmonary edema and toxemia of pregnancy. Concurrent administration of potassium-containing medication, potassium-sparing diuretics, angiotensin converting enzyme (ACE) inhibitors, or cardiac glycosides may lead to toxicity. Periodic examination and determinations of serum electrolytes, particularly serum levels of potassium and bicarbonate, should be carried out in those patients with renal disease in order to avoid these complications. Syrup POLYCITRA contains FD&C Yellow #6.

ADVERSE REACTIONS
Syrup POLYCITRA and POLYCITRA-LC are generally well tolerated without any unpleasant side effects when given in recommended doses to patients with normal renal function and urinary output. However, as with any alkalinizing agent, caution must be used in certain patients with abnormal renal mechanisms to avoid development of hyperkalemia or alkalosis, especially in the presence of hypocalcemia. Potassium intoxication causes listlessness, weakness, mental confusion and tingling of extremities.

DOSAGE AND ADMINISTRATION
Syrup POLYCITRA and POLYCITRA-LC should be taken diluted in water, followed by additional water if desired.
Usual Dosage: Adults: 15 to 30 mL diluted in water, four times a day after meals and at bedtime, or as directed by physician.
Children: 5 to 10 mL diluted in water, four times a day after meals and at bedtime, or as directed by physician.
Usual Dosage Range: 10 to 15 mL diluted with water, four times a day, will usually maintain a urine pH of 6.5-7.4. 15 to 20 mL diluted with water, taken four times a day, will usually maintain a urine pH of 7.0-7.6 throughout most of the 24 hours without unpleasant side effects. To check urinary pH, HYDRION Paper (pH 6.0-8.0) or NITRAZINE Paper (pH 4.5-7.5) are available and easy to use.

OVERDOSAGE
Overdosage with sodium salts may cause diarrhea, nausea and vomiting, hypernoea, and convulsions. Overdosage with potassium salts may cause hyperkalemia and alkalosis, especially in the presence of renal disease.

HOW SUPPLIED
Syrup POLYCITRA—16 fl oz (473 mL) (NDC 11414-205-01)
POLYCITRA-LC—16 fl oz (473 mL) (NDC 11414-208-01)

POLYCITRA®-K Oral Solution   **℞**
POLYCITRA®-K CRYSTALS   **℞**
[polly "si-trah-ka 'y]
(Potassium Citrate and Citric Acid)
Sugar-Free

DESCRIPTION
POLYCITRA-K Oral Solution and POLYCITRA-K CRYSTALS are pleasant tasting and effective oral alkalinizing agents useful for conditions where long- term maintenance of an alkaline urine is desirable.
POLYCITRA-K (Potassium Citrate and Citric Acid Oral Solution USP) contains in each teaspoonful (5 mL):
POTASSIUM CITRATE Monohydrate .... 1100 mg
CITRIC ACID Monohydrate .... 334 mg
Each mL contains 2 mEq Potassium and is equivalent to 2 mEq Bicarbonate (HCO₃).
POLYCITRA-K CRYSTALS (Potassium Citrate and Citric Acid for Oral Solution)—each unit dose packet contains:
POTASSIUM CITRATE Monohydrate .... 3300 mg
CITRIC ACID Monohydrate .... 1002 mg
Each unit dose packet, when reconstituted, supplies the same amount of active ingredients as is contained in 15 mL (one tablespoonful) POLYCITRA-K Oral Solution and provides 30 mEq Potassium and is equivalent to 30 mEq Bicarbonate (HCO₃).

CLINICAL PHARMACOLOGY
Potassium Citrate is absorbed and metabolized to potassium bicarbonate, thus acting as a systemic alkalizer. The effects are essentially those of chlorides before absorption and those of bicarbonates, subsequently. Oxidation is virtually complete so that less than 5% of the citrate is excreted in the urine unchanged.

INDICATIONS AND ADVANTAGES
POLYCITRA-K Oral Solution and POLYCITRA-K CRYSTALS are effective alkalinizing agents useful in those condi-

tions where long-term maintenance of an alkaline urine is desirable, as in patients where dissolution and control of uric acid and cystine calculi of the urinary tract is indicated, especially when the administration of sodium salts is undesirable or contraindicated. They are highly valuable in preventing uric acid nephrophathy when administered to patients with hyperuricosuria (e.g. gout), or who are receiving drugs (e.g. cancer chemotherapy or uricosuric agents), resulting in acute or chronic increases in urinary uric acid excretion. They are also effective for alleviating chronic metabolic acidosis, which may result from renal insufficiency or renal tubular acidosis, where the administration of Potassium Citrate may be preferable. Potassium Citrate has been reported to be effective in controlling mixed calcium oxalate/uric acid calculi.
POLYCITRA-K Oral Solution and POLYCITRA-K CRYSTALS are highly concentrated and when administered after meals and before bedtime, will maintain an alkaline urine pH without the need for a 2 A.M. dose. In recommended dosage, these products alkalinize the urine without producing systemic alkalosis. They are pleasant tasting and tolerable, even when administered over long periods.
POLYCITRA-K is an oral liquid. POLYCITRA-K CRYSTALS, when reconstituted, becomes an oral liquid. Thus, both products provide rapid absorption from the alimentary tract. This is very advantageous compared to the use of tablet dosage forms. (The patient ingests a liquid rather than a slowly dissolving tablet which may cause local irritation or inflammation in sensitive individuals).

CONTRAINDICATIONS
Severe renal impairment with oliguria or azotemia, untreated Addison's disease, adynamia episodica hereditaria, acute dehydration, heat cramps, anuria, severe myocardial damage, and hyperkalemia from any cause.

PRECAUTIONS AND WARNINGS
Should be used with caution by patients with low urinary output unless under the supervision of a physician. As with all liquids containing a high concentration of potassium, patients should be directed to dilute adequately with water or other liquids to minimize the possibility of gastrointestinal injury associated with the oral ingestion of concentrated potassium salt preparations; and preferably, to take each dose after meals to avoid saline laxative effect.
Large doses may cause hyperkalemia and alkalosis, especially in the presence of renal disease. Patients with renal insufficiency or uremia should not ingest POLYCITRA-K concurrently with aluminum-based antacids. Concurrent administration of potassium-containing medication, potassium sparing diuretics, angiotensin converting enzyme (ACE) inhibitors, or cardiac glycosides may lead to toxicity.
Pregnancy: POLYCITRA-K Oral Solution and POLYCITRA-K CRYSTALS are not expected to cause fetal harm when administered in dosages which will not result in hyperkalemia.
Nursing Mothers: Caution should be exercised when administered to a nursing woman.
Pediatric Use: POLYCITRA-K Oral Solution (not POLYCITRA-K CRYSTALS Packets) is recommended for pediatric administration since dosage can be more easily regulated.

ADVERSE REACTIONS
POLYCITRA-K Oral Solution and POLYCITRA-K CRYSTALS are generally well tolerated without any unpleasant side effects when given in recommended doses to patients with normal renal function and urinary output. However, as with any alkalinizing agent, caution must be used in certain patients with abnormal renal mechanisms to avoid development of hyperkalemia or alkalosis. Potassium intoxication causes listlessness, weakness, mental confusion, tingling of extremities, and other symptoms associated with a high concentration of potassium in the serum. Periodic determinations of serum electrolytes should be carried out in those patients with renal disease in order to avoid these complications.

DOSAGE AND ADMINISTRATION
POLYCITRA-K Oral Solution and POLYCITRA-K CRYSTALS should be taken with water or juice according to directions, followed by additional water or juice if desired.
Usual Adult Dose: POLYCITRA-K Oral Solution— 15 mL, diluted with 6 ounces of water or juice, after meals and at bedtime, or as directed by physician.
POLYCITRA-K CRYSTALS—Contents of 1 packet reconstituted with at least 6 ounces of cool water or juice, after meals and at bedtime, or as directed by physician.
Usual Pediatric Dose: POLYCITRA-K Oral Solution—5 to 10 mL, diluted with 6 ounces of water, after meals and at bedtime, or as directed by physician.
(POLYCITRA-K CRYSTALS is not recommended for pediatric use. Dosage can be more easily regulated using POLYCITRA-K Oral Solution.)
Usual Dosage Range: 10 to 15 mL POLYCITRA-K Oral Solution, diluted and taken four times a day, or contents of 1 packet POLYCITRA-K CRYSTALS, reconstituted as di-

rected and taken four times a day, will usually maintain a urinary pH of 6.5 to 7.4.

OVERDOSAGE
The administration of oral potassium salts to persons with normal excretory mechanisms for potassium rarely causes serious hyperkalemia. However, if excretory mechanisms are impaired, hyperkalemia can result (see Contraindications and Warnings). Hyperkalemia, when detected, must be treated immediately because lethal levels can be reached in a few hours.
Treatment of Hyperkalemia: Should hyperkalemia occur, treatment measures include the following: (1) elimination of foods or medications containing potassium. (2) The intravenous administration of 300 to 500 mL/hr of dextrose solution (10 to 25%), containing 10 units of insulin/20 gm dextrose. (3) The use of exchange resins, hemodialysis, or peritoneal dialysis. In treating hyperkalemia, it should be recalled that in patients who have been stabilized on digitalis, too rapid a lowering of the plasma potassium concentration can produce digitalis toxicity.

HOW SUPPLIED
POLYCITRA-K—16 fl oz (473 mL) (NDC 11414-209-01)
POLYCITRA-K CRYSTALS—Unit Dose packets, 100/box (NDC 11414-215-01).

PROGLYCEM®   **℞**
[pro-gli 'sem]
brand of diazoxide
   CAPSULES
   SUSPENSION, USP
   FOR ORAL ADMINISTRATION

DESCRIPTION
Diazoxide is 7-chloro-3-methyl-2H-1,2,4-benzothiadiazine 1,1-diazoxide. It is a white powder practically insoluble to sparingly soluble in water.

CLINICAL PHARMACOLOGY
Diazoxide administered orally produces a prompt dose-related increase in blood glucose level, due primarily to an inhibition of insulin release from the pancreas and also to an extrapancreatic effect. The hyperglycemic effect begins within an hour and generally lasts no more than eight hours in the presence of normal renal function.
PROGLYCEM decreases the excretion of sodium chloride and water resulting in fluid retention which may be clinically significant.
The hypotensive effect of diazoxide on blood pressure is usually not marked with the oral preparation.
Other pharmacologic actions of PROGLYCEM include increased pulse rate, increased serum uric acid levels due to decreased excretion, increased serum levels of free fatty acids, decreased para-aminohippuric acid (PAH) clearance with no appreciable effect on glomerular filtration rate.
PROGLYCEM-induced hyperglycemia is reversed by the administration of insulin or tolbutamide. The inhibition of insulin release by PROGLYCEM is antagonized by alpha-adrenergic blocking agents.
PROGLYCEM is extensively bound (more than 90%) to serum proteins, and is excreted in the kidneys. The plasma half-life 28±8.3 hours. In four children aged four and six years, the plasma half-life varied from 9.5 to 24 hours. The half-life may be prolonged following overdosage, and in patients with impaired renal function.

INDICATIONS AND USAGE
PROGLYCEM (oral diazoxide) is useful in the management of hypoglycemia due to hyperinsulinism associated with the following conditions when surgery or other therapy is unsuccessful.
ADULTS: inoperable islet cell adenoma or carcinoma, or extrapancreatic malignancy.
INFANTS AND CHILDREN: leucine sensitivity, islet cell hyperplasia, nesidioblastosis, extrapancreatic malignancy, islet cell adenoma, or adenomatosis. PROGYLCEM may be used preoperatively as a temporary measure, and postoperatively, if hypoglycemia persists.

CONTRAINDICATIONS
The use of PROGLYCEM for functional hypoglycemia is contraindicated. The drug should not be used in patients hypersensitive to diazoxide or to other thiazides unless the potential benefits outweigh the possible risks.

WARNINGS
Diazoxide may lead to significant fluid retention which in patients with a compromised cardiac reserve, may precipitate congestive heart failure. The fluid retention will respond to conventional therapy with diuretics. It should be noted that concomitantly administered thiazides may potentiate the hyperglycemic and hyperuricemic actions of diazoxide.
Ketoacidosis and nonketotic hyperosmolar coma have been reported in patients treated with recommended doses of

PROGLYCEM usually during intercurrent illness. Prompt recognition and treatment are essential (see OVERDOSAGE), and prolonged surveillance following the acute episode is necessary because of the long drug half-life.

Transient cataracts occur in association with hyperosmolar coma in an infant, and subsided on correction of the hyperosmolarity. Cataracts have been observed in several animals receiving daily doses of intravenous or oral diazoxide.

The development of abnormal facial features in four children treated chronically (> 4 years) with PROGLYCEM for hypoglycemia hyperinsulinism in the same clinic has been reported.

PRECAUTIONS

General: Treatment with PROGLYCEM should be initiated under close clinical supervision, with careful monitoring of blood glucose and clinical response until the patient's condition has stabilized. This usually requires several days. If not effective in two to three weeks, the drug should be discontinued.

Prolonged treatment requires regular monitoring of the urine for sugar and ketones, especially under stress conditions, with prompt reporting of any abnormalities to the physician. Additionally, blood sugar levels should be monitored periodically by the physician to determine the need or dose adjustment.

In some patients, higher blood levels have been observed with the oral suspension than with the capsule formulation of PROGLYCEM. Dosage should be adjusted as necessary in individual patients if changed from one formulation to the other.

The antihypertensive effect of other drugs may be enhanced by PROGLYCEM.

DRUG INTERACTIONS

Since diazoxide is highly bound to serum proteins, it may displace other substances which are also bound to protein, such as bilirubin or coumarin and its derivatives, resulting in higher blood levels of these substances. Concomitant administration of oral diazoxide and diphenylhydantoin may result in a loss of seizure control. The concomitant administration of thiazides or other commonly used diuretics may potentiate the hyperglycemic and other hyperglycemic effects of diazoxide.

Pregnancy Category C: Reproduction studies in rats and rabbits have revealed increased fetal resorptions and delayed parturition, as well as fetal skeletal and cardiac anomalies. The drug has also been demonstrated to cross the placental barrier in animals and to cause degeneration of the fetal pancreatic beta cells. Since there are no adequate data on fetal effects of this drug when given to pregnant women, safety in pregnancy has not been established. When the use of PROGLYCEM is considered, the indications should be limited to those specified for adults and the potential benefits to the mother must be weighed against possible harmful effects to the fetus.

Non-Teratogenic Effects: Diazoxide crosses the placental barrier and appears in cord blood. When given to the mother prior to delivery of the infant, the drug may produce fetal or neonatal hyperbilirubinemia, thrombocytopenia, altered carbohydrate metabolism or possibly other side effects that have occurred in adults. Alopecia and hypertrichosis lanuginosa have occurred in infants whose mothers received oral diazoxide during the last 19 to 60 days of pregnancy.

LABOR AND DELIVERY

Since intravenous administration of the drug during labor may cause cessation of uterine contractions, and administration of oxytocic agents may be required to reinstate labor, caution is advised in administering PROGLYCEM at that time.

ADVERSE REACTIONS

Frequent and Serious: Sodium and fluid retention is most common in young infants and in adults and may precipitate congestive heart failure in patients with compromised cardiac reserve. It usually responds to diuretic therapy. INFREQUENT AND SERIOUS: Diabetic ketoacidosis and hyperosmolar non-ketotic coma may develop very rapidly (see OVERDOSAGE and WARNING).

Other Frequent Adverse Reactions: Hirsutism of the lanugo type, mainly on the forehead, back and limbs subsides on discontinuation of the drug. HYPERGLYCEMIA OR GLYCOSURIA may require reduction in dosage in order to avoid progression towards ketoacidosis or hyperosmolar coma. GASTROINTESTINAL INTOLERANCE may include anorexia, nausea, vomiting, abdominal pain, illeus, diarrhea, transient loss of taste. Tachycardia, palpitations, increased levels of serum uric acid are common. THROMBOCYTOPENIA with or without purpura may require discontinuation of the drug. Neutropenia is transient, is not associated with increased susceptibility to infection, and ordinarily does not require discontinuation of the drug. Skin rash, headache, weakness, and malaise may also occur. Other adverse reactions which have been observed are: CARDIOVASCULAR—hypotension and transient hypertension. Chest pain has been reported rarely. HEMATOLOGIC

—eosinophilia, decreased hemoglobin/hemocrit, excessive bleeding, decreased IgG. HEPATO-RENAL—increased AST, alkaline phosphatase, azotemia, decreased creatinine clearance, reversible nephrotic syndrome, decreased urinary output, hematuria, albuminuria. NEUROLOGIC—anxiety, dizziness, insomnia, polyneuritis, paresthesia, pruritus, extrapyramidal signs. OPHTHALMOLOGIC—transient cataracts, subconjunctival hemorrhage, ring scotoma, blurred vision, diplopia, lacrimation, SKELETAL, INTEGUMENTARY—monilial dermatitis, herpes, advance in bone-age, loss of scalp hair. SYSTEMIC—fever, lymphadenopathy. OTHER—gout, acute pancreatitis, pancreatic necrosis, galactorrhea, enlargement of lump in breast.

OVERDOSAGE

An overdosage of PROGLYCEM causes marked hyperglycemia which may be associated with ketoacidosis. It will respond to prompt insulin administration and restoration of fluid and electrolyte balance. Because of the drug's long half-life (approximately 30 hours), the symptoms of overdosage require prolonged surveillance for periods of up to seven days, until the blood sugar level stabilizes with the normal range. Peritoneal dialysis and hemodialysis have lowered diazoxide blood levels in two patients.

DOSAGE AND ADMINISTRATION

The dosage of PROGLYCEM must be individualized based on the severity of the hypoglycemic condition and the blood glucose level and clinical response of the patient. The dosage should be adjusted until the desired clinical and laboratory effects are produced with the least amount of the drug. Special care should be taken to assure accuracy of dosage in infants and young children.

ADULTS AND CHILDREN: The usual daily dosage is 3 to 8 mg/kg, divided into two or three equal doses every 8 to 12 hours. In certain instances, patients with refractory hypoglycemia may require higher dosages.

INFANTS AND NEWBORNS: The usual daily dosage is 8 to 15 mg/kg, divided into two or three equal doses every 8 to 12 hours.

HOW SUPPLIED

PROGLYCEM Capsules, 50 mg, half opaque orange and half clear capsules, branded in black with BCP 6000, bottle of 100 (NDC#0575-6000-01).

PROGLYCEM Suspension, 50 mg/ml, a chocolate-mint flavored suspension, bottle of 30 ml (NDC #0575-6200-30), with dropper calibrated to deliver 10, 20, 30, 40, and 50 mg diazoxide. **Shake well before each use: Protect from light. Store in carton until contents are used. Store PROGLYCEM Capsules and Suspension between 2° and 30° C (36° and 86° F).**
07/91

Barry Laboratories
**2100 PARK CENTRAL BLVD. NORTH
SUITE 500
POMPANO BEACH, FL 33064**

ALLERGENIC EXTRACTS, DIAGNOSIS AND/OR IMMUNOTHERAPY ℞

COMPOSITION
Fluid allergens are available from the following categories: pollens, foods, dusts, epidermals, insects, fungi (molds & smuts), yeasts, and others.

ACTION AND USES
For diagnosis and immunotherapy.

PRECAUTIONS
Usual precautions used in testing or treating hypersensitive individuals. See product information circulars accompanying each product.

HOW SUPPLIED
Diagnostic materials are available for cutaneous or intracutaneous testing.

Diagnostic Test Sets include a comprehensive selection of perennial and seasonal allergens for each of five botanical zones.

Diagnostic Test Sets available: Multi-Test® , Food and Intradermal.

Immunorex®—Prescription Allergy Treatment Sets—Individualized, four vial treatment sets are prepared from the physician's instructions, based on the patient's skin test reactions and history. RAST based prescriptions and refills of any dilutions are also available.

LITERATURE AVAILABLE
Send for free descriptive literature, report and case history forms.

Basel Pharmaceuticals
**Division of CIBA-GEIGY Corporation
556 MORRIS AVENUE
SUMMIT, NJ 07901**

To provide a convenient and accurate means of identifying Basel Pharmaceuticals' solid dosage form products, a code number has been imprinted on all tablets and capsules. To help you quickly identify a Basel Tablet or Capsule by its code number, a numerical listing of codes (with corresponding product names) and an alphabetical listing of products (with corresponding codes and list numbers) have been compiled below.

Basel Product Identification Number	ALPHABETICAL LISTING	National Drug Code Number
	Anafranil®	
	clomipramine HCl	
115	CAPSULES, 25 mg (ivory/melon yellow)	58887-115-30
116	CAPSULES, 50 mg (ivory/aqua blue)	58887-116-30
117	CAPSULES, 75 mg (ivory/yellow)	58887-117-30
	Tegretol®	
	carbamazepine	
52	TABLETS, 100 mg (round, red-speckled, pink)	58887-052-30
27	TABLETS, 200 mg (capsule-shaped, pink)	58887-027-30

Basel Product Identification Number	NUMERICAL LISTING	
	Tegretol®	
	carbamazepine	
27	TABLETS, 200 mg (capsule-shaped, pink)	
52	TABLETS, 100 mg (round, red-speckled, pink)	
	Anafranil®	
	clomipramine HCl	
115	CAPSULES, 25 mg (ivory/melon yellow)	
116	CAPSULES, 50 mg (ivory/aqua blue)	
117	CAPSULES, 75 mg (ivory/yellow)	

ANAFRANIL® ℞
clomipramine hydrochloride
Capsules

Prescribing Information

DESCRIPTION
Anafranil, clomipramine hydrochloride, is an antiobsessional drug that belongs to the class (dibenzazepine) of pharmacologic agents known as tricyclic antidepressants. Anafranil is available as capsules of 25, 50, and 75 mg for oral administration.

Clomipramine hydrochloride is 3-chloro-5-[3-(dimethylamino)propyl]-10,11-dihydro-5H-dibenz[b,f]azepine monohydrochloride.

Clomipramine hydrochloride is a white to off-white crystalline powder. It is freely soluble in water, in methanol, and in methylene chloride, and insoluble in ethyl ether and in hexane. Its molecular weight is 351.3.

Inactive Ingredients. D&C Red No. 33 (25-mg capsules only), D&C Yellow No. 10, FD&C Blue No. 1 (50-mg capsules only), FD&C Yellow No. 6, gelatin, magnesium stearate, methylparaben, propylparaben, silicon dioxide, sodium lauryl sulfate, starch, and titanium dioxide.

CLINICAL PHARMACOLOGY
Pharmacodynamics
Clomipramine (CMI) is presumed to influence obsessive and compulsive behaviors through its effects on serotonergic neuronal transmission. The actual neurochemical mechanism is unknown, but CMI's capacity to inhibit the reuptake of serotonin (5-HT) is thought to be important.

Pharmacokinetics
Absorption/Bioavailability: CMI from Anafranil capsules is as bioavailable as CMI from a solution. The bioavailability of CMI from capsules is not significantly affected by food.

Continued on next page

The full prescribing information for each Basel product is contained herein and is that in effect as of September 1, 1992.

Basel—Cont.

In a dose proportionality study involving multiple CMI doses, steady-state plasma concentrations (C_{SS}) and area-under-plasma-concentration-time curves (AUC) of CMI and CMI's major active metabolite, desmethylclomipramine (DMI), were not proportional to dose over the ranges evaluated, i.e., between 25–100 mg/day and between 25–150 mg/day, although C_{SS} and AUC are approximately linearly related to dose between 100–150 mg/day. The relationship between dose and CMI/DMI concentrations at higher daily doses has not been systematically assessed, but if there is significant dose dependency at doses above 150 mg/day, there is the potential for dramatically higher C_{SS} and AUC even for patients dosed within the recommended range. This may pose a potential risk to some patients (see WARNINGS and PRECAUTIONS, Drug Interactions).

After a single 50-mg oral dose, maximum plasma concentrations of CMI occur within 2-6 hours (mean, 4.7 hr) and range from 56 ng/ml to 154 ng/ml (mean, 92 ng/ml). After multiple daily doses of 150 mg of Anafranil, steady-state maximum plasma concentrations range from 94 ng/ml to 339 ng/ml (mean, 218 ng/ml) for CMI and from 134 ng/ml to 532 ng/ml (mean, 274 ng/ml) for DMI. No pharmacokinetic information is available for doses ranging from 150 mg/day to 250 mg/day, the maximum recommended daily dose.

Distribution: CMI distributes into cerebrospinal fluid (CSF) and brain and into breast milk. DMI also distributes into CSF, with a mean CSF/plasma ratio of 2.6. The protein binding of CMI is approximately 97%, principally to albumin, and is independent of CMI concentration. The interaction between CMI and other highly protein-bound drugs has not been fully evaluated, but may be important (see PRECAUTIONS, Drug Interactions).

Metabolism: CMI is extensively biotransformed to DMI and other metabolites and their glucuronide conjugates. DMI is pharmacologically active, but its effects on OCD behaviors are unknown. These metabolites are excreted in urine and feces, following biliary elimination. After a 25-mg radiolabeled dose of CMI in two subjects, 60% and 51%, respectively, of the dose were recovered in the urine and 32% and 24%, respectively, in feces. In the same study, the combined urinary recoveries of CMI and DMI were only about 0.8–1.3% of the dose administered. CMI does not induce drug-metabolizing enzymes, as measured by antipyrine half-life.

Elimination: Evidence that the C_{SS} and AUC for CMI and DMI may increase disproportionately with increasing oral doses suggests that the metabolism of CMI and DMI may be capacity limited. This fact must be considered in assessing the estimates of the pharmacokinetic parameters presented below, as these were obtained in individuals exposed to doses of 150 mg. If the pharmacokinetics of CMI and DMI are nonlinear at doses above 150 mg, their elimination half-lives may be considerably lengthened at doses near the upper end of the recommended dosing range (i.e., 200 mg/day to 250 mg/day). Consequently, CMI and DMI may accumulate, and this accumulation may increase the incidence of any dose- or plasma-concentration-dependent adverse reactions, in particular seizures (see WARNINGS).

After a 150-mg dose, the half-life of CMI ranges from 19 hours to 37 hours (mean, 32 hr) and that of DMI ranges from 54 hours to 77 hours (mean, 69 hr). Steady-state levels after multiple dosing are typically reached within 7–14 days for CMI. Plasma concentrations of the metabolite exceed the parent drug on multiple dosing. After multiple dosing with 150 mg/day, the accumulation factor for CMI is approximately 2.5 and for DMI is 4.6. Importantly, it may take two weeks or longer to achieve this extent of accumulation at constant dosing because of the relatively long elimination half-lives of CMI and DMI (see DOSAGE AND ADMINISTRATION). The effects of hepatic and renal impairment on the disposition of Anafranil have not been determined.

Interactions: Coadministration of haloperidol with CMI increases plasma concentrations of CMI. Coadministration of CMI with phenobarbital increases plasma concentrations of phenobarbital (see PRECAUTIONS, Drug Interactions). Younger subjects (18–40 years of age) tolerated CMI better and had significantly lower steady-state plasma concentrations, compared with subjects over 65 years of age. Children under 15 years of age had significantly lower plasma concentration/dose ratios, compared with adults. Plasma concentrations of CMI were significantly lower in smokers than in nonsmokers.

INDICATIONS AND USAGE

Anafranil is indicated for the treatment of obsessions and compulsions in patients with Obsessive-Compulsive Disorder (OCD). The obsessions or compulsions must cause marked distress, be time-consuming, or significantly interfere with social or occupational functioning, in order to meet the DSM-III-R (circa 1989) diagnosis of OCD.

Obsessions are recurrent, persistent ideas, thoughts, images, or impulses that are ego-dystonic. Compulsions are repetitive, purposeful, and intentional behaviors performed in response to an obsession or in a stereotyped fashion, and are recognized by the person as excessive or unreasonable.

The effectiveness of Anafranil for the treatment of OCD was demonstrated in multicenter, placebo-controlled, parallel-group studies, including two 10-week studies in adults and one 8-week study in children and adolescents 10–17 years of age. Patients in all studies had moderate-to-severe OCD (DSM-III), with mean baseline ratings on the Yale-Brown Obsessive Compulsive Scale (YBOCS) ranging from 26 to 28 and a mean baseline rating of 10 on the NIMH Clinical Global Obsessive Compulsive Scale (NIMH-OC). Patients taking CMI experienced a mean reduction of approximately 10 on the YBOCS, representing an average improvement on this scale of 35% to 42% among adults and 37% among children and adolescents. CMI treated patients experienced a 3.5 unit decrement on the NIMH-OC. Patients on placebo showed no important clinical response on either scale. The maximum dose was 250 mg/day for most adults and 3 mg/kg/day (up to 200 mg) for all children and adolescents. The effectiveness of Anafranil for long-term use (i.e., for more than 10 weeks) has not been systematically evaluated in placebo-controlled trials. The physician who elects to use Anafranil for extended periods should periodically reevaluate the long-term usefulness of the drug for the individual patient (see DOSAGE AND ADMINISTRATION).

CONTRAINDICATIONS

Anafranil is contraindicated in patients with a history of hypersensitivity to Anafranil or other tricyclic antidepressants.

Anafranil should not be given in combination, or within 14 days before or after treatment, with a monoamine oxidase (MAO) inhibitor. Hyperpyretic crisis, seizures, coma, and death have been reported in patients receiving such combinations.

Anafranil is contraindicated during the acute recovery period after a myocardial infarction.

WARNINGS

Seizures

During premarket evaluation, seizure was identified as the most significant risk of Anafranil use.

The observed cumulative incidence of seizures among patients exposed to Anafranil at doses up to 300 mg/day was 0.64% at 90 days, 1.12% at 180 days, and 1.45% at 365 days. The cumulative rates correct the crude rate of 0.7% (25 of the 3519 patients) for the variable duration of exposure in clinical trials.

Although dose appears to be a predictor of seizure, there is a confounding of dose and duration of exposure, making it difficult to assess independently the effect of either factor alone. The ability to predict the occurrence of seizures in subjects exposed to doses of CMI greater than 250 mg is limited, given that the plasma concentration of CMI may be dose-dependent and may vary among subjects given the same dose. Nevertheless, prescribers are advised to limit the daily dose to a maximum of 250 mg in adults and 3 mg/kg (or 200 mg) in children and adolescents (see DOSAGE AND ADMINISTRATION).

Caution should be used in administering Anafranil to patients with a history of seizures or other predisposing factors, e.g., brain damage of varying etiology, alcoholism, and concomitant use with other drugs that lower the seizure threshold.

Rare reports of fatalities in association with seizures have been recorded by foreign post-marketing surveillance, but not in U.S. clinical trials. In some of these cases, Anafranil had been administered with other epileptogenic agents; in others, the patients involved had possibly predisposing medical conditions. Thus a causal association between Anafranil treatment and these fatalities has not been established.

Physicians should discuss with patients the risk of taking Anafranil while engaging in activities in which sudden loss of consciousness could result in serious injury to the patient or others, e.g., the operation of complex machinery, driving, swimming, climbing.

PRECAUTIONS

General

Suicide: Since depression is a commonly associated feature of OCD, the risk of suicide must be considered. Prescriptions for Anafranil should be written for the smallest quantity of capsules consistent with good patient management, in order to reduce the risk of overdose.

Cardiovascular Effects: Modest orthostatic decreases in blood pressure and modest tachycardia were each seen in approximately 20% of patients taking Anafranil in clinical trials; but patients were frequently asymptomatic. Among approximately 1400 patients treated with CMI in the premarketing experience who had ECGs, 1.5% developed abnormalities during treatment, compared with 3.1% of patients receiving active control drugs and 0.7% of patients receiving placebo. The most common ECG changes were PVCs, ST-T wave changes, and intraventricular conduction abnormalities. These changes were rarely associated with significant clinical symptoms. Nevertheless, caution is necessary in treating patients with known cardiovascular disease, and gradual dose titration is recommended.

Psychosis, Confusion, And Other Neuropsychiatric Phenomena: Patients treated with Anafranil have been reported to show a variety of neuropsychiatric signs and symptoms including delusions, hallucinations, psychotic episodes, confusion, and paranoia. Because of the uncontrolled nature of many of the studies, it is impossible to provide a precise estimate of the extent of risk imposed by treatment with Anafranil. As with tricyclic antidepressants to which it is closely related, Anafranil may precipitate an acute psychotic episode in patients with unrecognized schizophrenia.

Mania/Hypomania: During premarketing testing of Anafranil in patients with affective disorder, hypomania or mania was precipitated in several patients. Activation of mania or hypomania has also been reported in a small proportion of patients with affective disorder treated with marketed tricyclic antidepressants, which are closely related to Anafranil.

Hepatic Changes: During premarketing testing, Anafranil was occasionally associated with elevations in SGOT and SGPT (pooled incidence of approximately 1% and 3%, respectively) of potential clinical importance (i.e., values greater than 3 times the upper limit of normal). In the vast majority of instances these enzyme increases were not associated with other clinical findings suggestive of hepatic injury; moreover, none were jaundiced. Rare reports of more severe liver injury, some fatal, have been recorded in foreign post-marketing experience. Caution is indicated in treating patients with known liver disease, and periodic monitoring of hepatic enzyme levels is recommended in such patients.

Hematologic Changes: Although no instances of severe hematologic toxicity were seen in the premarketing experience with Anafranil, there have been post-marketing reports of leukopenia, agranulocytosis, thrombocytopenia, anemia, and pancytopenia in association with Anafranil use. As is the case with tricyclic antidepressants to which Anafranil is closely related, leukocyte and differential blood counts should be obtained in patients who develop fever and sore throat during treatment with Anafranil.

Central Nervous System: More than 30 cases of hyperthermia have been recorded by nondomestic post-marketing surveillance systems. Most cases occurred when Anafranil was used in combination with other drugs when Anafranil and a neuroleptic were used concomitantly, the cases were sometimes considered to be examples of a neuroleptic malignant syndrome.

Sexual Dysfunction: The rate of sexual dysfunction in male patients with OCD who were treated with Anafranil in the premarketing experience was markedly increased compared with placebo controls (i.e., 42% experienced ejaculatory failure and 20% experienced impotence, compared with 2.0% and 2.6%, respectively, in the placebo group). Approximately 85% of males with sexual dysfunction chose to continue treatment.

Weight Changes: In controlled studies of OCD, weight gain was reported in 18% of patients receiving Anafranil, compared with 1% of patients receiving placebo. In these studies, 28% of patients receiving Anafranil had a weight gain of at least 7% of their initial body weight, compared with 4% of patients receiving placebo. Several patients had weight gains in excess of 25% of their initial body weight. Conversely, 5% of patients receiving Anafranil and 1% receiving placebo had weight losses of at least 7% of their initial body weight.

Electroconvulsive Therapy: As with closely related tricyclic antidepressants, concurrent administration of Anafranil with electroconvulsive therapy may increase the risks; such treatment should be limited to those patients for whom it is essential, since there is limited clinical experience.

Surgery: Prior to elective surgery with general anesthetics, therapy with Anafranil should be discontinued for as long as is clinically feasible, and the anesthetist should be advised.

Use in Concomitant Illness: As with closely related tricyclic antidepressants, Anafranil should be used with caution in the following:

1. Hyperthyroid patients or patients receiving thyroid medication, because of the possibility of cardiac toxicity.
2. Patients with increased intraocular pressure, a history of narrow-angle glaucoma, or urinary retention, because of the anticholinergic properties of the drug.
3. Patients with tumors of the adrenal medulla (e.g., pheochromocytoma, neuroblastoma) in whom the drug may provoke hypertensive crises.
4. Patients with significantly impaired renal function.

Withdrawal Symptoms: A variety of withdrawal symptoms have been reported in association with abrupt discontinuation of Anafranil, including dizziness, nausea, vomiting, headache, malaise, sleep disturbance, hyperthermia, and irritability. In addition, such patients may experience a worsening of psychiatric status. While the withdrawal effects of Anafranil have not been systematically evaluated in controlled trials, they are well known with closely related tricyclic antidepressants, and it is recommended that the dosage be tapered gradually and the patient monitored

carefully during discontinuation (see DRUG ABUSE AND DEPENDENCE).

Information for Patients
Physicians are advised to discuss the following issues with patients for whom they prescribe Anafranil:
1. The risk of seizure (see WARNINGS);
2. The relatively high incidence of sexual dysfunction among males (see PRECAUTIONS; Sexual Dysfunction);
3. Since Anafranil may impair the mental and/or physical abilities required for the performance of complex tasks, and since Anafranil is associated with a risk of seizures, patients should be cautioned about the performance of complex and hazardous tasks (see WARNINGS);
4. Patients should be cautioned about using alcohol, barbiturates, or other CNS depressants concurrently, since Anafranil may exaggerate their response to these drugs;
5. Patients should notify their physician if they become pregnant or intend to become pregnant during therapy;
6. Patients should notify their physician if they are breast-feeding.

Drug Interactions
The risks of using Anafranil in combination with other drugs have not been systematically evaluated. Given the primary CNS effects of Anafranil, caution is advised in using it concomitantly with other CNS-active drugs (see Information for Patients). Anafranil should *not* be used with MAO inhibitors (see CONTRAINDICATIONS).

Close supervision and careful adjustment of dosage are required when Anafranil is administered with anticholinergic or sympathomimetic drugs.

Several tricyclic antidepressants have been reported to block the pharmacologic effects of guanethidine, clonidine, or similar agents, and such an effect may be anticipated with CMI because of its structural similarity to other tricyclic antidepressants.

The plasma concentration of CMI has been reported to be increased by the concomitant administration of haloperidol; plasma levels of several closely related tricyclic antidepressants have been reported to be increased by the concomitant administration of methylphenidate or hepatic enzyme inhibitors (e.g., cimetidine, fluoxetine) and decreased by the concomitant administration of hepatic enzyme inducers (e.g., barbiturates, phenytoin), and such an effect may be anticipated with CMI as well. Administration of CMI has been reported to increase the plasma levels of phenobarbital, if given concomitantly (see CLINICAL PHARMACOLOGY, Interactions).

Because Anafranil is highly bound to serum protein, the administration of Anafranil to patients taking other drugs that are highly bound to protein (e.g., warfarin, digoxin) may cause an increase in plasma concentrations of these drugs, potentially resulting in adverse effects. Conversely, adverse effects may result from displacement of protein-bound Anafranil by other highly bound drugs (see CLINICAL PHARMACOLOGY, Distribution).

Carcinogenesis, Mutagenesis, Impairment of Fertility
In a 2-year bioassay, no clear evidence of carcinogenicity was found in rats given doses 20 times the maximum daily human dose. Three out of 235 treated rats had a rare tumor (hemangioendothelioma); it is unknown if these neoplasms are compound related.

In reproduction studies, no effects on fertility were found in rats given doses approximately 5 times the maximum daily human dose.

Pregnancy Category C
No teratogenic effects were observed in studies performed in rats and mice at doses up to 20 times the maximum daily human dose. Slight nonspecific fetotoxic effects were seen in the offspring of pregnant mice given doses 10 times the maximum daily human dose. Slight nonspecific embryotoxicity was observed in rats given doses 5–10 times the maximum daily human dose.

There are no adequate or well-controlled studies in pregnant women. Withdrawal symptoms, including jitteriness, tremor, and seizures, have been reported in neonates whose mothers had taken Anafranil until delivery. Anafranil should be used during pregnancy only if the potential benefit justifies the potential risk to the fetus.

Nursing Mothers
Anafranil has been found in human milk. Because of the potential for adverse reactions, a decision should be made whether to discontinue nursing or to discontinue the drug, taking into account the importance of the drug to the mother.

Pediatric Use
In a controlled clinical trial in children and adolescents (10–17 years of age), 46 outpatients received Anafranil for up to 8 weeks. In addition, 150 adolescent patients have received Anafranil in open-label protocols for periods of several months to several years. Of the 196 adolescents studied, 50 were 13 years of age or less and 146 were 14–17 years of age. While the adverse reaction profile in this age group (see ADVERSE REACTIONS) is similar to that in adults, it is unknown what, if any, effects long-term treatment with Anafranil may have on the growth and development of children.

The safety and effectiveness in children below the age of 10 have not been established. Therefore, specific recommendations cannot be made for the use of Anafranil in children under the age of 10.

Use in Elderly
Anafranil has not been systematically studied in older patients; but 152 patients at least 60 years of age participating in U.S. clinical trials received Anafranil for periods of several months to several years. No unusual age-related adverse events have been identified in this elderly population, but these data are insufficient to rule out possible age-related differences, particularly in elderly patients who have concomitant systemic illnesses or who are receiving other drugs concomitantly.

ADVERSE REACTIONS

Commonly Observed
The most commonly observed adverse events associated with the use of Anafranil and not seen at an equivalent incidence among placebo-treated patients were gastrointestinal complaints, including dry mouth, constipation, nausea, dyspepsia, and anorexia; nervous system complaints, including somnolence, tremor, dizziness, nervousness, and myoclonus; genitourinary complaints, including changed libido, ejaculatory failure, impotence, and micturition disorder; and other miscellaneous complaints, including fatigue, sweating, increased appetite, weight gain, and visual changes.

Leading to Discontinuation of Treatment
Approximately 20% of 3616 patients who received Anafranil in U.S. premarketing clinical trials discontinued treatment because of an adverse event. Approximately one-half of the patients who discontinued (9% of the total) had multiple complaints, none of which could be classified as primary. Where a primary reason for discontinuation could be identified, most patients discontinued because of nervous system complaints (5.4%), primarily somnolence. The second-most-frequent reason for discontinuation was digestive system complaints (1.3%), primarily vomiting and nausea.

Incidence in Controlled Clinical Trials
The following table enumerates adverse events that occurred at an incidence of 1% or greater among patients with OCD who received Anafranil in adult or pediatric placebo-controlled clinical trials. The frequencies were obtained from pooled data of clinical trials involving either adults receiving Anafranil (N=322) or placebo (N=319) or children treated with Anafranil (N=46) or placebo (N=44). The prescriber should be aware that these figures cannot be used to predict the incidence of side effects in the course of usual medical practice, in which patient characteristics and other factors differ from those which prevailed in the clinical trials. Similarly, the cited frequencies cannot be compared with figures obtained from other clinical investigations involving different treatments, uses, and investigators. The cited figures, however, provide the physician with a basis for estimating the relative contribution of drug and nondrug factors to the incidence of side effects in the populations studied.
[See tables on next two pages.]

Other Events Observed During the Premarketing Evaluation of Anafranil
During clinical testing in the U.S., multiple doses of Anafranil were administered to approximately 3600 subjects. Untoward events associated with this exposure were recorded by clinical investigators using terminology of their own choosing. Consequently, it is not possible to provide a meaningful estimate of the proportion of individuals experiencing adverse events without first grouping similar types of untoward events into a smaller number of standardized event categories.

In the tabulations that follow, a modified World Health Organization dictionary of terminology has been used to classify reported adverse events. The frequencies presented, therefore, represent the proportion of the 3525 individuals exposed to Anafranil who experienced an event of the type cited on at least one occasion while receiving Anafranil. All events are included except those already listed in the previous table, those reported in terms so general as to be uninformative, and those in which an association with the drug was remote. It is important to emphasize that although the events reported occurred during treatment with Anafranil, they were not necessarily caused by it.

Events are further categorized by body system and listed in order of decreasing frequency according to the following definitions: frequent adverse events are those occurring on one or more occasions in at least 1/100 patients; infrequent adverse events are those occurring in 1/100 to 1/1000 patients; rare events are those occurring in less than 1/1000 patients.

Body as a Whole: Infrequent —general edema, increased susceptibility to infection, malaise. *Rare* —dependent edema, withdrawal syndrome.

Cardiovascular System: Infrequent —abnormal ECG, arrhythmia, bradycardia, cardiac arrest, extrasystoles, pallor. *Rare* —aneurysm, atrial flutter, bundle branch block, cardiac failure, cerebral hemorrhage, heart block, myocardial

infarction, myocardial ischemia, peripheral ischemia, thrombophlebitis, vasospasm, ventricular tachycardia.

Digestive System: Infrequent —abnormal hepatic function, blood in stool, colitis, duodenitis, gastric ulcer, gastritis, gastroesophageal reflux, gingivitis, glossitis, hemorrhoids, hepatitis, increased saliva, irritable bowel syndrome, peptic ulcer, rectal hemorrhage, tongue ulceration, tooth caries. *Rare* —cheilitis, chronic enteritis, discolored feces, gastric dilatation, gingival bleeding, hiccup, intestinal obstruction, oral/pharyngeal edema, paralytic ileus, salivary gland enlargement.

Endocrine System: Infrequent —hypothyroidism. *Rare* —goiter, gynecomastia, hyperthyroidism.

Hemic and Lymphatic System: Infrequent —lymphadenopathy. *Rare* —leukemoid reaction, lymphoma-like disorder, marrow depression.

Metabolic and Nutritional Disorder: Infrequent —dehydration, diabetes mellitus, gout, hypercholesterolemia, hyperglycemia, hyperuricemia, hypokalemia. *Rare* —fat intolerance, glycosuria.

Musculoskeletal System: Infrequent —arthrosis. *Rare* —dystonia, exostosis, lupus erythematosus rash, bruising, myopathy, myositis, polyarteritis nodosa, torticollis.

Nervous System: Frequent —abnormal thinking, vertigo. *Infrequent* —abnormal coordination, abnormal EEG, abnormal gait, apathy, ataxia, coma, convulsions, delirium, delusion, dyskinesia, dysphonia, encephalopathy, euphoria, extrapyramidal disorder, hallucinations, hostility, hyperkinesia, hypnagogic hallucinations, hypokinesia, leg cramps, manic reaction, neuralgia, paranoia, phobic disorder, psychosis, sensory disturbance, somnambulism, stimulation, suicidal ideation, suicide attempt, teeth-grinding. *Rare* —anticholinergic syndrome, aphasia, apraxia, catalepsy, cholinergic syndrome, choreoathetosis, generalized spasm, hemiparesis, hyperesthesia, hyperreflexia, hypoesthesia, illusion, impaired impulse control, indecisiveness, mutism, neuropathy, nystagmus, oculogyric crisis, oculomotor nerve paralysis, schizophrenic reaction, stupor, suicide.

Respiratory System: Infrequent —bronchitis, hyperventilation, increased sputum, pneumonia. *Rare* —cyanosis, hemoptysis, hypoventilation, laryngismus.

Skin and Appendages: Infrequent —alopecia, cellulitis, cyst, eczema, erythematous rash, genital pruritus, maculopapular rash, photosensitivity reaction, psoriasis, pustular rash, skin discoloration. *Rare* —chloasma, folliculitis, hypertrichosis, piloerection, seborrhea, skin hypertrophy, skin ulceration.

Special Senses: Infrequent —abnormal accommodation, deafness, diplopia, earache, eye pain, foreign body sensation, hyperacusis, parosmia, photophobia, scleritis, taste loss. *Rare* —blepharitis, chromatopsia, conjunctival hemorrhage, exophthalmos, glaucoma, keratitis, labyrinth disorder, night blindness, retinal disorder, strabismus, visual field defect.

Urogenital System: Infrequent —endometriosis, epididymitis, hematuria, nocturia, oliguria, ovarian cyst, perineal pain, polyuria, prostatic disorder, renal calculus, renal pain, urethral disorder, urinary incontinence, uterine hemorrhage, vaginal hemorrhage. *Rare* —albuminuria, anorgasmy, breast engorgement, breast fibroadenosis, cervical dysplasia, endometrial hyperplasia, premature ejaculation, pyelonephritis, pyuria, renal cyst, uterine inflammation, vulvar disorder.

DRUG ABUSE AND DEPENDENCE
Anafranil has not been systematically studied in animals or humans for its potential for abuse, tolerance, or physical dependence. While a variety of withdrawal symptoms have been described in association with Anafranil discontinuation (see PRECAUTIONS, Withdrawal Symptoms), there is no evidence for drug-seeking behavior, except for a single report of potential Anafranil abuse by a patient with a history of dependence on codeine, benzodiazepines, and multiple psychoactive drugs. The patient received Anafranil for depression and panic attacks and appeared to become dependent after hospital discharge.

Despite the lack of evidence suggesting an abuse liability for Anafranil in foreign marketing, it is not possible to predict the extent to which Anafranil might be misused or abused once marketed in the U.S. Consequently, physicians should carefully evaluate patients for a history of drug abuse and follow such patients closely.

Continued on next page

The full prescribing information for each Basel product is contained herein and is that in effect as of September 1, 1992.

Basel—Cont.

OVERDOSAGE

Human Experience

In U.S. clinical trials, 2 deaths occurred in 12 reported cases of acute overdosage with Anafranil either alone or in combination with other drugs. One death involved a patient suspected of ingesting a dose of 7000 mg. The second death involved a patient suspected of ingesting a dose of 5750 mg. The 10 nonfatal cases involved doses of up to 5000 mg, accompanied by plasma levels of up to 1010 ng/ml. All 10 patients completely recovered. Among reports from other countries of Anafranil overdose, the lowest dose associated with a fatality was 750 mg. Based upon post-marketing reports in the United Kingdom, CMI's lethality in overdose is considered to be similar to that reported for closely related tricyclic compounds marketed as antidepressants.

Signs and Symptoms

Signs and symptoms vary in severity depending upon factors such as the amount of drug absorbed, the age of the patient, and the time elapsed since drug ingestion. Blood and urine levels of Anafranil may not reflect the severity of poisoning: they have chiefly a qualitative rather than quantitative value, and they are unreliable indicators in the clinical management of the patient. The first signs and symptoms of poisoning with tricyclic antidepressants are generally severe anticholinergic reactions. CNS abnormalities may include drowsiness, stupor, coma, ataxia, restlessness, agitation, delirium, severe perspiration, hyperactive reflexes, muscle rigidity, athetoid and choreiform movements, and convulsions. Cardiac abnormalities may include arrhythmia, tachycardia, ECG evidence of impaired conduction, and signs of congestive heart failure, and in very rare cases, cardiac arrest. Respiratory depression, cyanosis, hypotension, shock, vomiting, hyperpyrexia, mydriasis, oliguria or anuria, and diaphoresis may also be present.

Treatment

The recommended treatment for tricyclic overdose may change periodically. Therefore, it is recommended that the physician contact a poison control center for current information on treatment.

Because CNS involvement, respiratory depression, and cardiac arrhythmia can occur suddenly, hospitalization and close observation may be necessary, even when the amount ingested is thought to be small or the initial degree of intoxication appears slight or moderate. All patients with ECG abnormalities should have continuous cardiac monitoring and be closely observed until well after the cardiac status has returned to normal; relapses may occur after apparent recovery.

In the alert patient, the stomach should be emptied promptly by lavage. In the obtunded patient, the airway should be secured with a cuffed endotracheal tube before beginning lavage (do not induce emesis). Instillation of activated charcoal slurry may help reduce absorption of CMI.

External stimulation should be minimized to reduce the tendency for convulsions. If anticonvulsants are necessary, diazepam and phenytoin may be useful. Adequate respiratory exchange should be maintained, including intubation and artificial respiration, if necessary. Respiratory stimulants should not be used.

In severe hypotension or shock, the patient should be placed in an appropriate position and given a plasma expander, and, if necessary, a vasopressor agent by intravenous drip. The use of corticosteroids in shock is controversial and may be contraindicated in cases of overdosage with tricyclic antidepressants. Digitalis may increase conduction abnormalities and further irritate an already sensitized myocardium. If congestive heart failure necessitates rapid digitalization, particular care must be exercised. Hyperpyrexia should be controlled by whatever external means are available, including ice packs and cooling sponge baths, if necessary. Hemodialysis, peritoneal dialysis, exchange transfusions, and forced diuresis have generally been reported as ineffective because of the rapid fixation of Anafranil in tissues.

The slow intravenous administration of physostigmine salicylate has been used as a last resort to reverse severe CNS anticholinergic manifestations of overdosage with tricyclic antidepressants; however, it should not be used routinely, since it may induce seizures and cholinergic crises.

Body System/ Adverse Event*	Incidence of Treatment-Emergent Adverse Experience in Placebo-Controlled Clinical Trials (Percentage of Patients Reporting Event) Adults		Children and Adolescents	
	Anafranil (N=322)	Placebo (N=319)	Anafranil (N=46)	Placebo (N=44)
Nervous System				
Somnolence	54	16	46	11
Tremor	54	2	33	2
Dizziness	54	14	41	14
Headache	52	41	28	34
Insomnia	25	15	11	7
Libido change	21	3	—	—
Nervousness	18	2	4	2
Myoclonus	13	—	2	—
Increased appetite	11	2	—	2
Paresthesia	9	3	2	2
Memory impairment	9	1	7	2
Anxiety	9	4	2	—
Twitching	7	1	4	5
Impaired concentration	5	2	—	—
Depression	5	1	—	—
Hypertonia	4	1	2	—
Sleep disorder	4	—	9	5
Psychosomatic disorder	3	—	—	—
Yawning	3	—	—	—
Confusion	3	—	2	—
Speech disorder	3	—	—	—
Abnormal dreaming	3	—	—	2
Agitation	3	—	—	—
Migraine	3	—	—	—
Depersonalization	2	—	2	—
Irritability	2	2	2	—
Emotional lability	2	—	—	2
Panic reaction	1	—	2	—
Aggressive reaction	—	—	2	—
Paresis	—	—	2	—
Skin and Appendages				
Increased sweating	29	3	9	—
Rash	8	1	4	2
Pruritis	6	—	2	2
Dermatitis	2	—	—	2
Acne	2	2	—	5
Dry Skin	2	—	—	5
Urticaria	1	—	—	—
Abnormal skin odor	—	—	2	—
Digestive System				
Dry mouth	84	17	63	16
Constipation	47	11	22	9
Nausea	33	14	9	11
Dyspepsia	22	10	13	2
Diarrhea	13	9	7	5
Anorexia	12	—	22	2
Abdominal pain	11	9	13	16
Vomiting	7	2	7	—
Flatulence	6	3	—	2
Tooth disorder	5	—	—	—
Gastrointestinal disorder	2	—	—	2
Dysphagia	2	—	—	—
Esophagitis	1	—	—	—
Eructation	—	—	2	2
Ulcerative stomatitis	—	—	2	—
Body as a Whole				
Fatigue	39	18	35	9
Weight increase	18	1	2	—
Flushing	8	—	7	—
Hot flushes	5	—	2	—
Chest pain	4	4	7	—
Fever	4	—	2	7
Allergy	3	3	7	5
Pain	3	2	4	2
Local edema	2	4	—	—
Chills	2	1	—	—
Weight decrease	—	—	7	—
Otitis media	—	—	4	5
Asthenia	—	—	2	—
Halitosis	—	—	2	—
Cardiovascular System				
Postural hypotension	6	—	4	—
Palpitation	4	2	4	—
Tachycardia	4	—	2	—
Syncope	—	—	2	—
Respiratory System				
Pharyngitis	14	9	—	5
Rhinitis	12	10	7	9
Sinusitis	6	4	2	5
Coughing	6	6	4	5
Bronchospasm	2	—	7	2
Epistaxis	2	—	—	2
Dyspnea	—	—	2	—
Laryngitis	—	1	2	—

Body System/ Adverse Event*	Incidence of Treatment-Emergent Adverse Experience in Placebo-Controlled Clinical Trials (Percentage of Patients Reporting Event)			
	Adults		**Children and Adolescents**	
	Anafranil (N=322)	Placebo (N=319)	Anafranil (N=46)	Placebo (N=44)
Urogenital System				
Male and Female Patients Combined				
Micturition disorder	14	2	4	2
Urinary tract infection	6	1	—	—
Micturition frequency	5	3	—	—
Urinary retention	2	—	7	—
Dysuria	2	2	—	—
Cystitis	2	—	—	—
Female Patients Only	(N=182)	(N=167)	(N=10)	(N=21)
Dysmenorrhea	12	14	10	10
Lactation (nonpuerperal)	4	—	—	—
Menstrual disorder	4	2	—	—
Vaginitis	2	—	—	—
Leukorrhea	2	—	—	—
Breast enlargement	2	—	—	—
Breast pain	1	—	—	—
Amenorrhea	1	—	—	—
Male Patients Only	(N=140)	(N=152)	(N=36)	(N=23)
Ejaculation failure	42	2	6	—
Impotence	20	3	—	—
Special Senses				
Abnormal vision	18	4	7	2
Taste perversion	8	—	4	—
Tinnitus	6	—	4	—
Abnormal lacrimation	3	2	—	—
Mydriasis	2	—	—	—
Conjunctivitis	1	—	—	—
Anisocoria	—	—	2	—
Blepharospasm	—	—	2	—
Ocular allergy	—	—	2	—
Vestibular disorder	—	—	2	2
Musculoskeletal				
Myalgia	13	9	—	—
Back pain	6	6	—	—
Arthralgia	3	5	—	—
Muscle weakness	1	—	2	—
Hemic and Lymphatic				
Purpura	3	—	—	—
Anemia	—	—	2	2
Metabolic and Nutritional				
Thirst	2	2	—	2

*Events reported by at least 1% of Anafranil patients are included.

DOSAGE AND ADMINISTRATION

The treatment regimens described below are based on those used in controlled clinical trials of Anafranil in 520 adults, and 91 children and adolescents with OCD. During initial titration, Anafranil should be given in divided doses with meals to reduce gastrointestinal side effects. The goal of this initial titration phase is to minimize side effects by permitting tolerance to side effects to develop or allowing the patient time to adapt if tolerance does not develop.

Because both CMI and its active metabolite, DMI, have long elimination half-lives, the prescriber should take into consideration the fact that steady-state plasma levels may not be achieved until 2–3 weeks after dosage change (see CLINICAL PHARMACOLOGY). Therefore, after initial titration, it may be appropriate to wait 2–3 weeks between further dosage adjustments.

Initial Treatment/Dose Adjustment (Adults)

Treatment with Anafranil should be initiated at a dosage of 25 mg daily and gradually increased, as tolerated, to approximately 100 mg during the first 2 weeks. During initial titration, Anafranil should be given in divided doses with meals to reduce gastrointestinal side effects. Thereafter, the dosage may be increased gradually over the next several weeks, up to a maximum of 250 mg daily. After titration, the total daily dose may be given once daily at bedtime to minimize daytime sedation.

Initial Treatment/Dose Adjustment (Children and Adolescents)

As with adults, the starting dose is 25 mg daily and should be gradually increased (also given in divided doses with meals to reduce gastrointestinal side effects) during the first 2 weeks, as tolerated, up to a daily maximum of 3 mg/kg or 100 mg, whichever is smaller. Thereafter, the dosage may be increased gradually over the next several weeks up to a daily maximum of 3 mg/kg or 200 mg, whichever is smaller (see PRECAUTIONS, Pediatric Use). As with adults, after titration, the total daily dose may be given once daily at bedtime to minimize daytime sedation.

Maintenance/Continuation Treatment (Adults, Children, and Adolescents)

While there are no systematic studies that answer the question of how long to continue Anafranil, OCD is a chronic condition and it is reasonable to consider continuation for a responding patient. Although the efficacy of Anafranil after 10 weeks has not been documented in controlled trials, patients have been continued in therapy under double-blind conditions for up to 1 year without loss of benefit. However, dosage adjustments should be made to maintain the patient on the lowest effective dosage, and patients should be periodically reassessed to determine the need for treatment. During maintenance, the total daily dose may be given once daily at bedtime.

HOW SUPPLIED

Capsules 25 mg—ivory/melon yellow (imprinted ANAFRANIL 25 mg)

  Bottles of 100 ....NDC 58887-115-30
  Unit Dose (blister pack)
    Box of 100 (strips of 10) ....NDC 58887-115-32

Capsules 50 mg—ivory/aqua blue (imprinted ANAFRANIL 50 mg)

  Bottles of 100 ....NDC 58887-116-30
  Unit Dose (blister pack)
    Box of 100 (strips of 10) ....NDC 58887-116-32

Capsules 75 mg—ivory/yellow (imprinted ANAFRANIL 75 mg)

  Bottles of 100 ....NDC 58887-117-30
  Unit Dose (blister pack)
    Box of 100 (strips of 10) ....NDC 58887-117-32

Samples, when available, are identified by the word *SAMPLE* appearing on each capsule.

Do not store above 86°F (30°C). Protect from moisture.

Dispense in tight container (USP).

ANIMAL TOXICOLOGY

Testicular and lung changes commonly associated with tricyclic compounds have been observed with Anafranil. In 1- and 2-year studies in rats, changes in the testes (atrophy, aspermatogenesis, and calcification) and drug-induced phospholipidosis in the lungs were observed at doses 4 times the maximum daily human dose. Testicular atrophy was also observed in a 1-year oral toxicity study in dogs at 10 times the maximum daily human dose.

Printed in U.S.A.   C91-40 (Rev. 2/92)

BASEL Pharmaceuticals
Division of CIBA-GEIGY Corporation
Summit, New Jersey 07901

Shown in Product Identification Section, page 404

HABITROL™   ℞

(nicotine transdermal system)
Systemic delivery of 21, 14, or 7 mg/day over 24 hours

DESCRIPTION

Habitrol is a transdermal system that provides systemic delivery of nicotine following its application to intact skin for 24 hours.

Nicotine is a tertiary amine composed of a pyridine and a pyrrolidine ring. It is a colorless-to-pale yellow, freely water-soluble, strongly alkaline, oily, volatile, hygroscopic liquid obtained from the tobacco plant. Nicotine has a characteristic pungent odor and turns brown on exposure to air or light. Of its two stereoisomers, S(-)-nicotine is the more active and is the more prevalent form in tobacco. The free alkaloid is absorbed rapidly through the skin and respiratory tract.

Chemical Name: S-3-(1-methyl-2-pyrrolidinyl) pyridine
Molecular Formula: $C_{10}H_{14}N_2$
Molecular Weight: 162.23
Ionization Constants: $pK_{a1}=7.84$, $pK_{a2}=3.04$
Octanol-Water Partition Coefficient: 15.1 at pH 7

Habitrol systems are round, flat, 0.6-mm-thick multi-layer units containing nicotine as the active agent. Proceeding from the visible surface toward the surface attached to the skin are: (1) a tan-colored aluminized backing film; (2) a pressure-sensitive acrylate adhesive; (3) a layer containing a methacrylic acid copolymer solution of nicotine dispersed in a pad of nonwoven viscose and cotton; (4) an adhesive layer similar in composition to (2) above; (5) a protective aluminized release liner which overlays the adhesive layer and must be removed prior to use.

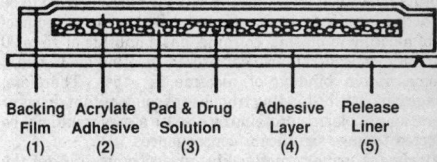

Backing Film (1)	Acrylate Adhesive (2)	Pad & Drug Solution (3)	Adhesive Layer (4)	Release Liner (5)

Nicotine is the active ingredient; other components of the system are pharmacologically inactive.

The amount of nicotine delivered to the patient from each system (29 mcg/cm²-h) is nearly proportional to the surface area. About 60% of the total amount of nicotine remains in the system 24 hours after application. Habitrol systems are labeled as to the dose actually absorbed by the patient. The dose of nicotine absorbed from a Habitrol system represents 98% of the amount released from the system in 24 hours.

Dose Absorbed in 24 hours (mg/day)	System Surface Area (cm²)	Total Nicotine Content (mg)
21	30	52.5
14	20	35.0
7	10	17.5

CLINICAL PHARMACOLOGY

Pharmacologic Action

Nicotine, the chief alkaloid in tobacco products, binds stereoselectively to acetylcholine receptors at the autonomic ganglia, in the adrenal medulla, at neuromuscular junctions, and in the brain. Two types of central nervous system effects are believed to be the basis of nicotine's positively reinforcing properties. A stimulating effect, exerted mainly in the cortex via the locus ceruleus, produces increased alertness and cognitive performance. A "reward" effect via the "pleasure system" in the brain is exerted in the limbic system. At low doses the stimulant effects predominate while at high doses the reward effects predominate. Intermittent intravenous administration of nicotine activates neurohormonal pathways, releasing acetylcholine, norepinephrine, dopamine, serotonin, vasopressin, beta-endorphin, growth hormone, and ACTH.

Pharmacodynamics

The cardiovascular effects of nicotine include peripheral vasoconstriction, tachycardia, and elevated blood pressure.

Continued on next page

The full prescribing information for each Basel product is contained herein and is that in effect as of September 1, 1992.

Basel—Cont.

Acute and chronic tolerance to nicotine develops from smoking tobacco or ingesting nicotine preparations. Acute tolerance (a reduction in response for a given dose) develops rapidly (less than 1 hour), however, not at the same rate for different physiologic effects (skin temperature, heart rate, subjective effects). Withdrawal symptoms, such as cigarette craving, can be reduced in some individuals by plasma nicotine levels lower than those from smoking.

Withdrawal from nicotine in addicted individuals is characterized by craving, nervousness, restlessness, irritability, mood lability, anxiety, drowsiness, sleep disturbances, impaired concentration, increased appetite, minor somatic complaints (headache, myalgia, constipation, fatigue), and weight gain. Nicotine toxicity is characterized by nausea, abdominal pain, vomiting, diarrhea, diaphoresis, flushing, dizziness, disturbed hearing and vision, confusion, weakness, palpitations, altered respirations, and hypotension.

The cardiovascular effects of Habitrol 14 mg/day systems used continuously for 24 hours were compared with smoking every hour druing waking hours, for 10 days. A small increase in blood pressure was detectable on the first day but not after 10 days. Heart rate was increased by 3–7% and stroke volume decreased by 5–12% on the 10th day of application. Habitrol treatment had no significant influence on cutaneous blood flow or skin temperature.

Both smoking and nicotine can increase circulating cortisol and catecholamines, and tolerance does not develop to the catecholamine-releasing effects of nicotine. Changes in the response to a concomitantly administered adrenergic agonist or antagonist should be watched for when nicotine intake is altered during Habitrol therapy and/or smoking cessation (see PRECAUTIONS, Drug Interactions).

Pharmacokinetics

The volume of distribution following IV administration of nicotine is approximately 2 to 3 L/kg and the half-life ranges from 1 to 2 hours. The major eliminating organ is the liver, and average plasma clearance is about 1.2 L/min; the kidney and lung also metabolize nicotine. There is no significant skin metabolism of nicotine. More than 20 metabolites of nicotine have been identified, all of which are believed to be less active than the parent compound. The primary metabolite of nicotine in plasma, cotinine, has a half-life of 15 to 20 hours and concentrations that exceed nicotine by 10-fold. Plasma-protein binding of nicotine is <5%. Therefore, changes in nicotine binding from use of concomitant drugs or alterations of plasma proteins by disease states would not be expected to have significant consequences.

The primary urinary metabolites are cotinine (15% of the dose) and trans-3-hydroxycotinine (45% of the dose). About 10% of nicotine is excreted unchanged in the urine. As much as 30% may be excreted in the urine with high urine flow rates and urine acidification below pH 5.

The pharmacokinetic model which best fits the plasma nicotine concentrations from Habitrol systems is an open, two-compartment disposition model with a skin depot through which nicotine enters the central circulation compartment. The nicotine from the drug matrix is released slowly from the system. Therefore, the decline of plasma nicotine concentrations during the last 12 hours is determined primarily by release of nicotine from the system through the skin.

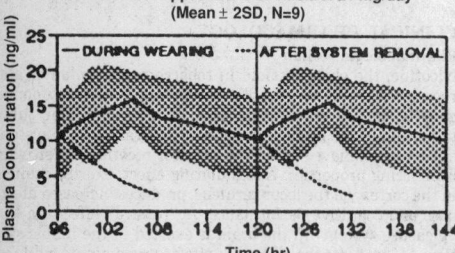

Steady-State Plasma Nicotine Concentrations for Two Consecutive Applications of Habitrol 21 mg/day (Mean ± 2SD, N=9)

Following an initial lag time of 1–2 hours, nicotine concentrations increase to a broad peak between 6 and 12 hours and then decrease gradually. Steady state for nicotine is attained within 2 days of initiating Habitrol treatment and average plasma nicotine concentrations are, on average, 25% higher compared to single dose applications. Upon application of a new system and removal of the old system there is, in some patients, a slight and transient (30–60 min.) increase in nicotine plasma concentration and its variability. Plasma nicotine concentrations are proportional to dose (ie, linear kinetics are observed) for the three dosages of Habitrol systems. Nicotine kinetics are similar for all sites of application on the back, abdomen, or side

Following removal of Habitrol systems, plasma nicotine concentrations decline in an exponential fashion with an apparent mean half-life of 3–4 hours (see dotted line in graph) compared with 1–2 hours for IV administration, due to continued absorption from the skin depot. Most nonsmoking patients will have nondetectable nicotine concentrations in 10 to 12 hours.

Steady-State Nicotine Pharmacokinetic Parameters for Habitrol Systems
(mean, standard deviation, range)

Parameter (units)	14 mg/day (N=9)			21 mg/day (N=9)		
	Mean	SD	Range	Mean	SD	Range
C_{max} (ng/mL)	12	4	6–16	17	3	13–19
C_{avg} (ng/mL)	9	3	5–12	13	2	9–17
C_{min} (ng/mL)	6	2	3–10	9	2	7–14
T_{max} (hrs)	5	3	0– 8	6	3	2– 9

C_{max}: maximum observed plasma concentration
C_{avg}: average plasma concentration
C_{min}: minimum observed plasma concentration
T_{max}: time of maximum plasma concentration

Clinical Studies

The efficacy of Habitrol treatment as an aid to smoking cessation was demonstrated in three placebo-controlled, double-blind trials in otherwise healthy patients smoking at least one pack per day (N=792). In two of these trials, Habitrol therapy was combined with concomitant support and in one trial Habitrol was used without concomitant support. In all three trials, patients were treated for 7 weeks (3 weeks of titration and 4 weeks of maintenance) followed by 3 weeks of weaning. Quitting was defined as total abstinence from smoking as measured by patient diary and verified by expired carbon monoxide. The "quit rates" are the proportions of all persons initially enrolled who abstained after week 3. The two trials in otherwise healthy smokers with concomitant support showed that Habitrol therapy was more effective than placebo after 7 weeks. Quit rates were still significantly different after the additional 3-week weaning period. The quit rates varied approximately 3-fold among clinics for each treatment when Habitrol therapy was used with a concomitant support program. Data from these two studies (N=516) are combined in the Quit Rate table. Greater variability and decreased quit rates were demonstrated in both placebo and Habitrol treatment groups when concomitant support was not employed (N=276, see table [below]).

Patients who used Habitrol treatment in clinical trials had a significant reduction in craving for cigarettes, a major nicotine withdrawal symptom, as compared to placebo-treated patients (see graph). Reduction in craving, as with quit rate, is quite variable. This variability is presumed to be due to inherent differences in patient populations, eg, patient motivation, concomitant illnesses, number of cigarettes smoked per day, number of years smoking, exposure to other smokers, socioeconomic status, etc, as well as differences among the clinics.

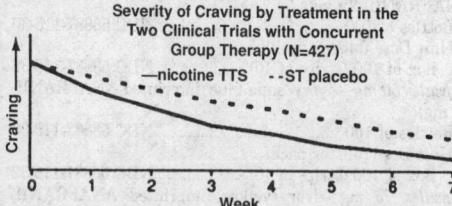

Severity of Craving by Treatment in the Two Clinical Trials with Concurrent Group Therapy (N=427)
—nicotine TTS   - -ST placebo

Patients using Habitrol systems dropped out of the trials less frequently than did patients receiving placebo. Quit rates for the 32 patients over age 60 were comparable to the quit rates for the 369 patients aged 60 and under.

Individualization of Dosage

It is important to make sure that patients read the instructions made available to them and have their questions answered. They should clearly understand the directions for applying and disposing of Habitrol systems. They should be instructed to stop smoking completely when the first system is applied.

The success or failure of smoking cessation depends heavily on the quality, intensity, and frequency of supportive care. Patients are more likely to quit smoking if they are seen frequently and participate in formal smoking cessation programs.

The goal of Habitrol therapy is complete abstinence. Significant health benefits have not been demonstrated for reduction of smoking. If a patient is unable to stop smoking by the fourth week of therapy, treatment should probably be discontinued. Patients who have not stopped smoking after 4 weeks of Habitrol therapy are unlikely to quit on that attempt.

Patients who fail to quit on any attempt may benefit from interventions to improve their chances for success on subsequent attempts. Patients who were unsuccessful should be counseled to determine why they failed. Patients should then probably be given a "therapy holiday" before the next attempt. A new quit attempt should be encouraged when the factors that contributed to failure can be eliminated or reduced, and conditions are more favorable.

Based on the clinical trials, a reasonable approach to assisting patients in their attempt to quit smoking is to assign their initial Habitrol dosage using the recommended dosing schedule (see Dosing Schedule below). The need for dose adjustment should be assessed during the first 2 weeks. Patients should continue the dose selected with counseling and support over the following month. Those who have successfully stopped smoking during that time should be supported during 4 to 8 weeks of weaning, after which treatment should be terminated.

Therapy should generally begin with the Habitrol 21 mg/day dose (see Dosing Schedule below) except if the patient is small (less than 100 lbs), is a light smoker (less than ½ pack of cigarettes per day) or has cardiovascular disease.

Dosing Schedule

	Otherwise Healthy Patients	Other Patients*
Initial/Starting Dose	21 mg/day	14 mg/day
Duration of Treatment	4–8 weeks	4–8 weeks
First Weaning Dose	14 mg/day	7 mg/day
Duration of Treatment	2–4 weeks	2–4 weeks
Second Weaning Dose	7 mg/day	
Duration of Treatment	2–4 weeks	

* small patient (less than 100 lbs)
  or light smoker (less than 10 cigarettes/day)
  or patient with cardiovascular disease

The symptoms of nicotine withdrawal and excess overlap (see Pharmacodynamics and ADVERSE REACTIONS). Since patients using Habitrol treatment may also smoke intermittently, it may be difficult to determine if patients are experiencing nicotine withdrawal or nicotine excess.

The controlled clinical trials using Habitrol therapy suggest that abnormal dreams are more often symptoms of nicotine excess while flatulence, anxiety, and depression are more often symptoms of nicotine withdrawal.

INDICATIONS AND USAGE

Habitrol treatment is indicated as an aid to smoking cessation for the relief of nicotine withdrawal symptoms. Habitrol treatment should be used as a part of a comprehensive behavioral smoking cessation program.

The use of Habitrol systems for longer than 3 months has not been studied.

CONTRAINDICATIONS

Use of Habitrol systems is contraindicated in patients with hypersensitivity or allergy to nicotine or to any of the components of the therapeutic system.

WARNINGS

Nicotine from any source can be toxic and addictive. Smoking causes lung cancer, heart disease, emphysema, and may adversely affect the fetus and the pregnant woman. For any smoker, with or without concomitant disease or pregnancy, the risk of nicotine replacement in a smoking cessation program should be weighed against the hazard of continued smoking while using Habitrol systems, and the likelihood of achieving cessation of smoking without nicotine replacement.

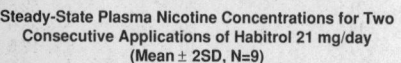

		Quit Rates After Week 3 by Treatment		
Concomitant Support	Treatment	Number of Patients	After 7 Weeks (range)	After Weaning (range)
Yes†	Habitrol	260	19–54%	8–43%
	Placebo*	256	9–30%	8–30%
No††	Habitrol	141	4–28%	4–20%
	Placebo*	135	0–24%	0–22%

*Sub Therapeutic (ST) Placebo systems contained 13% of the nicotine found in the respective-sized active system to allow blinding as to color and odor.
†Two trials with 9 clinics, number of patients per treatment ranged from 22 to 39.
††One trial with 5 clinics, number of patients per treatment ranged from 24 to 40.

Pregnancy Warning
Tobacco smoke, which has been shown to be harmful to the fetus, contains nicotine, hydrogen cyanide, and carbon monoxide. Nicotine has been shown in animal studies to cause fetal harm. It is therefore presumed that Habitrol treatment can cause fetal harm when administered to a pregnant woman. The effect of nicotine delivery by Habitrol systems has not been examined in pregnancy (see PRECAUTIONS, Other Effects). Therefore, pregnant smokers should be encouraged to attempt cessation using educational and behavioral interventions before using pharmacological approaches. If Habitrol therapy is used during pregnancy, or if the patient becomes pregnant while using Habitrol treatment, the patient should be apprised of the potential hazard to the fetus.

Safety Note Concerning Children
The amounts of nicotine that are tolerated by adult smokers can produce symptoms of poisoning and could prove fatal if Habitrol systems are applied or ingested by children or pets. Used 21 mg/day systems contain about 60% (32 mg) of their initial drug content. Therefore, patients should be cautioned to keep both used and unused Habitrol systems out of the reach of children and pets.

May Require a Decrease in Dose at Cessation of Smoking	**Possible Mechanism**
Acetaminophen, caffeine, imipramine, oxazepam, pentazocine, propranolol, theophylline	Deinduction of hepatic emzymes on smoking cessation
Insulin	Increase of subcutaneous insulin absorption with smoking cessation
Adrenergic antagonists (eg, prazosin, labetalol)	Decrease in circulating catecholamines with smoking cessation
May Require an Increase in Dose at Cessation of Smoking	**Possible Mechanism**
Adrenergic agonists (eg, isoproterenol, phenylephrine)	Decrease in circulating catecholamines with smoking cessation

PRECAUTIONS

General
The patient should be urged to stop smoking completely when initiating Habitrol therapy (see DOSAGE AND ADMINISTRATION). Patients should be informed that if they continue to smoke while using Habitrol systems, they may experience adverse effects due to peak nicotine levels higher than those experienced from smoking alone. If there is a clinically significant increase in cardiovascular or other effects attributable to nicotine, the Habitrol dose should be reduced or Habitrol treatment discontinued (see WARNINGS). Physicians should anticipate that concomitant medications may need dosage adjustment (see Drug Interactions).
The use of Habitrol systems beyond 3 months by patients who stop smoking should be discouraged because the chronic consumption of nicotine by any route can be harmful and addicting.

Allergic Reactions: In a 6-week, open-label dermal irritation and sensitization study of Habitrol systems, 22 of 220 patients exhibited definite erythema at 24 hours after application. Upon rechallenge, 3 patients exhibited mild-to-moderate contact allergy. Patients with contact sensitization should be cautioned that a serious reaction could occur from exposure to other nicotine-containing products or smoking. In the efficacy trials, erythema following system removal was typically seen in about 17% of patients, some edema in 4%, and dropouts due to skin reactions occurred in 6% of patients.
Patients should be instructed to promptly discontinue the Habitrol treatment and contact their physicians if they experience severe or persistent local skin reactions at the site of application (eg, severe erythema, pruritus, or edema) or a generalized skin reaction (eg, urticaria, hives, or generalized rash).

Skin Disease: Habitrol systems are usually well tolerated by patients with normal skin, but may be irritating for patients with some skin disorders (atopic or eczematous dermatitis).

Cardiovascular or Peripheral Vascular Diseases: The risks of nicotine replacement in patients with certain cardiovascular and peripheral vascular diseases should be weighed against the benefits of including nicotine replacement in a smoking cessation program for them. Specifically, patients with coronary heart disease (history of myocardial infarction and/or angina pectoris), serious cardiac arrhythmias, or vasospastic diseases (Buerger's disease, Prinzmetal's variant angina) should be carefully screened and evaluated before nicotine replacement is prescribed.
Tachycardia occurring in association with the use of Habitrol treatment was reported occasionally. If serious cardiovascular symptoms occur with Habitrol treatment, it should be discontinued.
Habitrol treatment should generally not be used in patients during the immediate post-myocardial infarction period, patients with serious arrhythmias, and patients with severe or worsening angina pectoris.

Renal or Hepatic Insufficiency: The pharmacokinetics of nicotine have not been studied in the elderly or in patients with renal or hepatic impairment. However, given that nicotine is extensively metabolized and that its total system clearance is dependent on liver blood flow, some influence of hepatic impairment on drug kinetics (reduced clearance) should be anticipated. Only severe renal impairment would be expected to affect the clearance of nicotine or its metabolites from the circulation (see CLINICAL PHARMACOLOGY, Pharmacokinetics).

Endocrine Diseases: Habitrol treatment should be used with caution in patients with hyperthyroidism, pheochromocytoma, or insulin-dependent diabetes since nicotine causes the release of catecholamines by the adrenal medulla.

Peptic Ulcer Disease: Nicotine delays healing in peptic ulcer disease; therefore, Habitrol treatment should be used with caution in patients with active peptic ulcers and only when the benefits of including nicotine replacement in a smoking cessation program outweigh the risks.

Accelerated Hypertension: Nicotine constitutes a risk factor for development of malignant hypertension in patients with accelerated hypertension; therefore, Habitrol treatment should be used with caution in these patients and only when the benefits of including nicotine replacement in a smoking cessation program outweigh the risks.

Information for Patient: A patient instruction sheet is included in the package of Habitrol systems dispensed to the patient. It contains important information and instructions on how to use and dispose of Habitrol systems properly. Patients should be encouraged to ask questions of the physician and pharmacist.
Patients must be advised to keep both used and unused systems out of the reach of children and pets.

Drug Interactions
Smoking cessation, with or without nicotine replacement, may alter the pharmacokinetics of certain concomitant medications.
[See table above.]

Carcinogenesis, Mutagenesis, Impairment of Fertility
Nicotine itself does not appear to be a carcinogen in laboratory animals. However, nicotine and its metabolites increased the incidence of tumors in the cheek pouches of hamsters and forestomach of F344 rats, respectively, when given in combination with tumor-initiators. One study, which could not be replicated, suggested that cotinine, the primary metabolite of nicotine, may cause lymphoreticular sarcoma in the large intestine in rats.
Nicotine and cotinine were not mutagenic in the Ames *Salmonella* test. Nicotine induced repairable DNA damage in an *E. coli* test system. Nicotine was shown to be genotoxic in a test system using Chinese hamster ovary cells. In rats and rabbits, implantation can be delayed or inhibited by a reduction in DNA synthesis that appears to be caused by nicotine. Studies have shown a decrease in litter size in rats treated with nicotine during gestation.

Pregnancy Category D (see WARNINGS)
The harmful effects of cigarette smoking on maternal and fetal health are clearly established. These include low birth weight, an increased risk of spontaneous abortion, and increased perinatal mortality. The specific effects of Habitrol treatment on fetal development are unknown. Therefore, pregnant smokers should be encouraged to attempt cessation using educational and behavioral interventions before using pharmacological approaches.
Spontaneous abortion during nicotine replacement therapy has been reported; as with smoking, nicotine as a contributing factor cannot be excluded.
Habitrol treatment should be used during pregnancy only if the likelihood of smoking cessation justifies the potential risk of use of nicotine replacement by the patient, who may continue to smoke.

Teratogenicity
Animal Studies: Nicotine was shown to produce skeletal abnormalities in the offspring of mice when given doses toxic to the dams (25 mg/kg/day IP or SC).
Human Studies: Nicotine teratogenicity has not been studied in humans except as a component of cigarette smoke (each cigarette smoked delivers about 1 mg of nicotine). It has not been possible to conclude whether cigarette smoking is teratogenic to humans.

Other Effects
Animal Studies: A nicotine bolus (up to 2 mg/kg) to pregnant rhesus monkeys caused acidosis, hypercarbia, and hypotension (fetal and maternal concentrations were about 20 times those achieved after smoking 1 cigarette in 5 minutes). Fetal breathing movements were reduced in the fetal lamb after intraveous injection of 0.25 mg/kg nicotine to the ewe (equivalent to smoking 1 cigarette every 20 seconds for 5 minutes). Uterine blood flow was reduced about 30% after infusion of 0.1 mg/kg/min nicotine for 20 minutes to pregnant rhesus monkeys (equivalent to smoking about six cigarettes every minute for 20 minutes).
Human Experience: Cigarette smoking during pregnancy is associated with an increased risk of spontaneous abortion, low-birth-weight infants and perinatal mortality. Nicotine and carbon monoxide are considered the most likely mediators of these outcomes. The effects of cigarette smoking on fetal cardiovascular parameters have been studied near term. Cigarettes increased fetal aortic blood flow and heart rate and decreased uterine blood flow and fetal breathing movements. Habitrol treatment has not been studied in pregnant humans.

Labor and Delivery
Habitrol systems are not recommended to be left on during labor and delivery. The effects of nicotine on the mother or the fetus during labor are unknown.

Nursing Mothers
Caution should be exercised when Habitrol therapy is administered to nursing women. The safety of Habitrol treatment in nursing infants has not been examined. Nicotine passes freely into breast milk; the milk-to-plasma ratio averages 2.9. Nicotine is absorbed orally. An infant has the ability to clear nicotine by hepatic first-pass clearance; however, the efficiency of removal is probably lowest at birth. The nicotine concentrations in milk can be expected to be lower with Habitrol treatment when used as directed than with cigarette smoking, as maternal plasma nicotine concentrations are generally reduced with nicotine replacement. The risk of exposure of the infant to nicotine from Habitrol systems should be weighed against the risks associated with the infant's exposure to nicotine from continued smoking by the mother (passive smoke exposure and contamination of breast milk with other components of tobacco smoke) and from Habitrol systems alone or in combination with continued smoking.

Pediatric Use
Habitrol systems are not recommended for use in children because the safety and effectiveness of Habitrol treatment in children and adolescents who smoke have not been evaluated.

Geriatric Use
Forty-eight patients over the age of 60 participated in clinical trials of Habitrol therapy. Habitrol therapy appeared to be as effective in this age group as in younger smokers.

ADVERSE REACTIONS

Assessment of adverse events in the 792 patients who participated in controlled clinical trials is complicated by the occurrence of GI and CNS effects of nicotine withdrawal as well as nicotine excess. The actual incidences of both are confounded by concurrent smoking by many of the patients. In the trials, when reporting adverse events, the investigators did not attempt to identify the cause of the symptom.

Topical Adverse Events
The most common adverse event associated with topical nicotine is a short-lived erythema, pruritus, or burning at the application site, which was seen at least once in 35% of patients on Habitrol treatment in the clinical trials. Local erythema after system removal was noted at least once in 17% of patients and local edema in 4%. Erythema generally resolved within 24 hours. Cutaneous hypersensitivity (contact

Continued on next page

The full prescribing information for each Basel product is contained herein and is that in effect as of September 1, 1992.

Basel—Cont.

sensitization) occurred in 2% of patients on Habitrol treatment (see PRECAUTIONS, Allergic Reactions).

Probably Causally Related

The following adverse events were reported more frequently in Habitrol-treated patients than in placebo-treated patients or exhibited a dose response in clinical trials.

Digestive system—Diarrhea*, dyspepsia*.
Mouth/Tooth disorders—Dry mouth.
Musculoskeletal system—Arthralgia*, myalgia*.
Nervous system—Abnormal dreams†, somnolence†.

Frequencies for 21 mg/day system
* Reported in 3% to 9% of patients.
† Reported in 1% to 3% of patients.
Unmarked if reported in <1% of patients.

Causal Relationship Unknown

Adverse events reported in Habitrol- and placebo-treated patients at about the same frequency in clinical trials are listed below. The clinical significance of the association between Habitrol treatment and these events is unknown, but they are reported as alerting information for the clinician.
Body as a whole—Allergy†, back pain†.
Cardiovascular system—Hypertension†
Digestive system—Abdominal pain†, constipation†, nausea†, vomiting.
Nervous system—Dizziness†, concentration impaired†, headache (17%), insomnia*.
Respiratory system—Cough increased†, pharyngitis†, sinusitis†.
Urogenital system—Dysmenorrhea*.

Frequencies for 21 mg/day system
* Reported in 3% to 9% of patients.
† Reported in 1% to 3% of patients.
Unmarked if reported in <1% of patients.

DRUG ABUSE AND DEPENDENCE

Habitrol systems are likely to have a low abuse potential based on differences between it and cigarettes in four characteristics commonly considered important in contributing to abuse: much slower absorption, much smaller fluctuations in blood levels, lower blood levels of nicotine, and less frequent use (ie, once daily).

Dependence on nicotine polacrilex chewing gum replacement therapy has been reported. Such dependence might also occur from transference to Habitrol systems of tobacco-based nicotine dependence. The use of the system beyond 3 months has not been evaluated and should be discouraged.

To minimize the risk of dependence, patients should be encouraged to withdraw gradually from Habitrol treatment after 4 to 8 weeks of usage. Recommended dose reduction is to progressively decrease the dose every 2 to 4 weeks (see DOSAGE AND ADMINISTRATION).

OVERDOSAGE

The effects of applying several Habitrol systems simultaneously or of swallowing unused Habitrol systems are unknown (see WARNINGS, Safety Note Concerning Children).

The oral LD_{50} for nicotine in rodents varies with species but is in excess of 24 mg/kg; death is due to respiratory paralysis. The oral minimum lethal dose of nicotine in dogs is greater than 5 mg/kg. The oral minimum acute lethal dose for nicotine in human adults is reported to be 40 to 60 mg (<1 mg/kg).

Two or three Habitrol 30 cm^2 systems in capsules fed to dogs weighing 8–17 kg were emetic, but did not produce any other significant clinical signs. The administration of these patches corresponds to about 6–17 mg/kg of nicotine.

Signs and symptoms of an overdose of Habitrol systems would be expected to be the same as those of acute nicotine poisoning including: pallor, cold sweat, nausea, salivation, vomiting, abdominal pain, diarrhea, headache, dizziness, disturbed hearing and vision, tremor, mental confusion, and weakness. Prostration, hypotension, and respiratory failure may ensue with large overdoses. Lethal doses produce convulsions quickly and death follows as a result of peripheral or central respiratory paralysis or, less frequently, cardiac failure.

Overdose From Topical Exposure

The Habitrol system should be removed immediately if the patient shows signs of overdosage and the patient should seek immediate medical care. The skin surface may be flushed with water and dried. No soap should be used since it may increase nicotine absorption. Nicotine will continue to be delivered into the bloodstream for several hours (see CLINICAL PHARMACOLOGY, Pharmacokinetics) after removal of the system because of a depot of nicotine in the skin.

Overdose From Ingestion

Persons ingesting Habitrol system should be referred to a health care facility for management. Due to the possibility of nicotine-induced seizures, activated charcoal should be administered. In unconscious patients with a secure airway, instill activated charcoal via nasogastric tube. A saline cathartic or sorbitol added to the first dose of activated charcoal may speed gastrointestinal passage of the system. Repeated doses of activated charcoal should be administered as long as the system remains in the gastrointestinal tract since it will continue to release nicotine for many hours.

Management of Nicotine Poisoning

Other supportive measures include diazepam or barbiturates for seizures, atropine for excessive bronchial secretions or diarrhea, respiratory support for respiratory failure, and vigorous fluid support for hypotension and cardiovascular collapse.

DOSAGE AND ADMINISTRATION

Patients must desire to stop smoking and should be instructed to *stop smoking immediately* as they begin using Habitrol therapy. The patient should read the patient instruction sheet on Habitrol treatment and be encouraged to ask any questions. Treatment should be initiated with Habitrol 21 mg/day or 14 mg/day systems (see CLINICAL PHARMACOLOGY, Individualization of Dosage).

Once the appropriate dosage is selected the patient should begin 4–6 weeks of therapy at that dosage. The patient should stop smoking cigarettes completely during this period. If the patient is unable to stop cigarette smoking within 4 weeks, Habitrol therapy should probably be stopped, since few additional patients in clinical trials were able to quit after this time.

Recommended Dosing Schedule for Healthy Patients[a]
(see Individualization of Dosage)

Dose	Duration
Habitrol 21 mg/day	First 6 Weeks
Habitrol 14 mg/day	Next 2 Weeks[b]
Habitrol 7 mg/day	Last 2 Weeks[c]

[a] Start with Habitrol 14 mg/day for 6 weeks for patients who:
—have coronary artery disease
—weigh less than 100 pounds
—smoke less than ½ a pack of cigarettes/day
Decrease dose to Habitrol 7 mg/day for the final 2–4 weeks.

[b] Patients who have successfully abstained from smoking should have their dose of Habitrol reduced after each 2–4 weeks of treatment until the 7 mg/day dose has been used for 2–4 weeks (see Individualization of Dosage).

[c] The entire course of nicotine substitution and gradual withdrawal should take 8–12 weeks, depending on the size of the initial dose. The use of Habitrol beyond 3 months has not been studied.

The Habitrol system should be applied promptly upon its removal from the protective pouch to prevent evaporative loss of nicotine from the system. Habitrol systems should be used only when the pouch is intact to assure that the product has not been tampered with.

Habitrol systems should be applied only once a day to a non-hairy, clean, and dry skin site on the trunk or upper, outer arm. After 24 hours, the used Habitrol system should be removed and a new system applied to an alternate skin site. Skin sites should not be reused for at least a week. Patients should be cautioned not to continue to use the same system for more than 24 hours.

Safety and Handling

Habitrol systems can be a dermal irritant and can cause contact sensitization. Although exposure of health care workers to nicotine from Habitrol systems should be minimal, care should be taken to avoid unnecessary contact with active systems. If you do handle active systems, wash with water alone, since soap may increase nicotine absorption. Do not touch your eyes.

Disposal

When the used system is removed from the skin, it should be folded over and placed in the protective pouch which contained the new system. The used system should be immediately disposed of in such a way to prevent its access by children or pets. See patient information for further directions for handling and disposal.

Nicotine Delivery Rate *(in vivo)*	Nicotine in System	System Size	Package Size	NDC Number
21 mg/day	52.5 mg	30 cm^2	30 systems	58887-830-26
14 mg/day	35.0 mg	20 cm^2	30 systems	58887-820-26
7 mg/day	17.5 mg	10 cm^2	30 systems	58887-810-26

HOW SUPPLIED

[See table below.]

How to Store

Do not store above 86°F (30°C) because Habitrol systems are sensitive to heat. A slight discoloration of the system is not significant.

Do not store unpouched. Once removed from the protective pouch, Habitrol systems should be applied promptly since nicotine is volatile and the system may lose strength.

The use of this product is covered by U.S. Patent No. 4,597,961.

CAUTION: Federal law prohibits dispensing without prescription.

C92-1 (Rev. 2/92)

BASEL
Pharmaceuticals
Dist. by:
BASEL Pharmaceuticals
Division of CIBA-GEIGY Corporation
Summit, New Jersey 07901

HABITROL™

(nicotine transdermal system)
Patient Instructions

IMPORTANT

YOUR DOCTOR HAS PRESCRIBED THIS DRUG FOR YOUR USE ONLY. DO NOT LET ANYONE ELSE USE IT. KEEP THIS MEDICINE OUT OF THE REACH OF CHILDREN AND PETS. Nicotine can be very toxic and harmful. Small amounts of nicotine can cause serious illness in children. Even used Habitrol patches contain enough nicotine to poison children and pets. Be sure to throw Habitrol patches away out of the reach of children and pets. If a child puts on Habitrol patches or plays with a Habitrol patch that is out of the sealed pouch, take it away from the child and contact a poison control center, or contact a doctor immediately.

Women: Nicotine in any form may cause harm to your unborn baby if you use nicotine while you are pregnant. Do not use Habitrol patches if you are pregnant or nursing unless advised by your doctor. If you become pregnant while using Habitrol patches or if you think you might be pregnant, stop smoking and don't use Habitrol patches until you have talked to your doctor.

This leaflet will provide you with general information about nicotine and specific instruction about how to use Habitrol patches. It is important that you read it carefully and completely before you start using Habitrol patches. Be sure to read the PRECAUTIONS section before using Habitrol patches, because, as with all drugs, Habitrol treatment has side effects. Since this leaflet is only a summary of information, be sure to ask your doctor if you have any questions or want to know more.

INTRODUCTION

IT IS IMPORTANT THAT YOU ARE FIRMLY COMMITTED TO GIVING UP SMOKING.

Habitrol is a skin patch containing nicotine designed to help you quit smoking cigarettes. When you wear a Habitrol patch, it releases nicotine through the skin into your bloodstream while you're wearing it. The nicotine which is in your skin will still be entering your bloodstream for several hours after you take the patch off.

It is the nicotine in cigarettes that causes addiction to smoking. Habitrol therapy replaces some of the nicotine you crave when you are stopping smoking. Habitrol patches may also help relieve other symptoms of nicotine withdrawal that may occur when you stop smoking such as irritability, frustration, anger, anxiety, difficulty in concentration, and restlessness.

There are three doses of Habitrol. Your doctor has chosen the Habitrol system with the correct dose for you and may adjust it during the first week or two. After about 6 weeks, your doctor will give you smaller Habitrol patches approximately every two weeks. The smaller patches give you less nicotine. In time, you will be completely off nicotine.

INFORMATION ABOUT HABITROL PATCHES

How Habitrol Patches Work

Habitrol patches contain nicotine. When you put a Habitrol patch on your skin, nicotine passes from the patch through the skin and into your blood.

How to Apply a Habitrol Patch

Step 1. Choose a non-hairy, clean, dry area of your body or the upper, outer part of your arm. Do not put a Habitrol patch on skin that is very oily, burned, broken out, cut, or irritated in any way.

Step 2. Do not remove the Habitrol patch from its sealed protective pouch until you are ready to use it. Carefully cut open the plastic, child-resistant outer cover, then tear open the pouch. Discard the used patch you take off by folding it in half and putting it into the opened pouch. Throw it away in the trash out of the reach of children and pets (see Step 7).

Step 3. A shiny protective liner covers the sticky side of the Habitrol patch—the side that will be put on

your skin. The liner has a precut slit to help you remove it from the patch. With the silver side facing you, pull the liner away from the Habitrol patch starting at the edge slit. Hold the Habitrol patch at the edge (touch the sticky side as little as possible) and pull off the other piece of the protective liner. Throw away this liner.

Step 4. Immediately apply the sticky side of the Habitrol patch to your skin. Press the Habitrol patch firmly on your skin with the palm of your hand for about 10 seconds. Make sure it sticks well to your skin, expecially around the edges.

Step 5. Wash your hands when you have finished applying the Habitrol patch. Nicotine on your hands could get into your eyes and nose and could cause stinging, redness, or more serious problems.

Step 6. After approximately 24 hours, remove the patch you have been wearing. Choose a *different* place on your skin to apply the next Habitrol patch and repeat Steps 1 to 5. Do not return to a previously used skin site for at least one week. Do not leave on the Habitrol patch for more than 24 hours because it may irritate your skin and because it loses strength after 24 hours.

Step 7. Fold the used Habitrol patch in half with the sticky side together. After you have put on a new Habitrol patch, take its pouch and place the used, folded Habitrol patch inside of it. Throw the pouch in the trash away from children and pets.

When to Apply a Habitrol Patch

If you apply the Habitrol patch at about the same time each day, it will help you to remember when to put on a new Habitrol patch. If you want to change the time when you put on your patch, you can do so. Just remove the Habitrol patch you are wearing and put on a new one. After that, apply the Habitrol patch at the new time each day.

If Your Habitrol Patch Gets Wet

Water will not harm the Habitrol patch you are wearing. You can bathe, swim, use a hot tub, or shower while you are wearing a Habitrol patch.

If Your Habitrol Patch Comes Off

If your Habitrol patch falls off, put on a new one. Remove the Habitrol patch at your regular time to keep your schedule the same, or 24 hours after applying the replacement patch if you wish to change the time each day that you apply a new patch. Before putting on a new patch, make sure you select a non-hairy area which is not irritated and is clean and dry.

Disposing of a Habitrol Patch

Fold the used Habitrol patch in half with the sticky side together. After you put on a new Habitrol patch, take its opened pouch or aluminum foil and place the used folded Habitrol patch inside of it. THROW THE POUCH IN THE TRASH AWAY FROM CHILDREN AND PETS.

Storage Instructions

Keep the Habitrol patch in its protective pouch until you are ready to use it. Do not store your Habitrol patches above 86°F (30°C) because the patch is sensitive to heat. Remember, the inside of your car can reach temperatures much higher than this in the summer.

PRECAUTIONS

What to Ask Your Doctor

Ask your doctor about possible problems with Habitrol therapy. Be sure to tell your doctor if you have had any of the following:

- a recent heart attack (myocardial infarction)
- irregular heart beat (arrhythmia)
- severe or worsening heart pain (angina pectoris)
- allergies to drugs
- rashes from adhesive tape or bandages
- skin diseases
- very high blood pressure
- stomach ulcers
- overactive thyroid
- diabetes requiring insulin
- kidney or liver disease

If You Are Taking Medicines

Habitrol patch use, together with stopping smoking, may change the effect of other medicines. It is important to tell your doctor about all the medicines you are taking.

What to Watch For (Adverse Effects)

You should not smoke while using the Habitrol patch. It is possible to get too much nicotine (an overdose), especially if you use a Habitrol patch and smoke at the same time. Signs of an overdose would include bad headaches, dizziness, upset stomach, drooling, vomiting, diarrhea, cold sweat, blurred vision, difficulty with hearing, mental confusion, and weakness. An overdose might cause you to faint.

If Your Skin Reacts to the Habitrol Patch

When you first put on a Habitrol patch, mild itching, burning, or tingling is normal and should go away within an hour. After you remove a Habitrol patch, the skin under the patch might be somewhat red. Your skin should not stay red for more than a day. If you get a skin rash after using a Habitrol patch, or if the skin under the patch becomes swollen or very red, call your doctor. Do not put on a new patch. You may be allergic to one of the components of the Habitrol patch.

If you do become allergic to the nicotine in the Habitrol patch, you could get sick from using cigarettes or other nicotine-containing products.

What to Do When Problems Occur

IF YOU NOTICE ANY WORRISOME SYMPTOMS OR PROBLEMS, TAKE OFF THE HABITROL PATCH AND CALL YOUR DOCTOR AT ONCE.

C92-2 (Rev. 2/92)

BASEL
Pharmaceuticals
Dist. by:
BASEL Pharmaceuticals
Division of CIBA-GEIGY Corporation
Summit, New Jersey 07901

Shown in Product Identification Section, page 405

TEGRETOL® ℞

carbamazepine USP
Chewable Tablets of 100 mg—red-speckled, pink
Tablets of 200 mg-pink
Suspension of 100 mg/5 ml

Prescribing Information

WARNING

APLASTIC ANEMIA AND AGRANULOCYTOSIS HAVE BEEN REPORTED IN ASSOCIATION WITH THE USE OF TEGRETOL. DATA FROM A POPULATION-BASED CASE CONTROL STUDY DEMONSTRATE THAT THE RISK OF DEVELOPING THESE REACTIONS IS 5–8 TIMES GREATER THAN IN THE GENERAL POPULATION. HOWEVER, THE OVERALL RISK OF THESE REACTIONS IN THE UNTREATED GENERAL POPULATION IS LOW, APPROXIMATELY SIX PATIENTS PER ONE MILLION POPULATION PER YEAR FOR AGRANULOCYTOSIS AND TWO PATIENTS PER ONE MILLION POPULATION PER YEAR FOR APLASTIC ANEMIA.

ALTHOUGH REPORTS OF TRANSIENT OR PERSISTENT DECREASED PLATELET OR WHITE BLOOD CELL COUNTS ARE NOT UNCOMMON IN ASSOCIATION WITH THE USE OF TEGRETOL, DATA ARE NOT AVAILABLE TO ESTIMATE ACCURATELY THEIR INCIDENCE OR OUTCOME. HOWEVER, THE VAST MAJORITY OF THE CASES OF LEUKOPENIA HAVE NOT PROGRESSED TO THE MORE SERIOUS CONDITIONS OF APLASTIC ANEMIA OR AGRANULOCYTOSIS.

BECAUSE OF THE VERY LOW INCIDENCE OF AGRANULOCYTOSIS AND APLASTIC ANEMIA, THE VAST MAJORITY OF MINOR HEMATOLOGIC CHANGES OBSERVED IN MONITORING OF PATIENTS ON TEGRETOL ARE UNLIKELY TO SIGNAL THE OCCURRENCE OF EITHER ABNORMALITY. NONETHELESS, COMPLETE PRETREATMENT HEMATOLOGICAL TESTING SHOULD BE OBTAINED AS A BASELINE. IF A PATIENT IN THE COURSE OF TREATMENT EXHIBITS LOW OR DECREASED WHITE BLOOD CELL OR PLATELET COUNTS, THE PATIENT SHOULD BE MONITORED CLOSELY. DISCONTINUATION OF THE DRUG SHOULD BE CONSIDERED IF ANY EVIDENCE OF SIGNIFICANT BONE MARROW DEPRESSION DEVELOPS.

Before prescribing Tegretol, the physician should be thoroughly familiar with the details of this prescribing information, particularly regarding use with other drugs, especially those which accentuate toxicity potential.

DESCRIPTION

Tegretol, carbamazepine USP, is an anticonvulsant and specific analgesic for trigeminal neuralgia, available for oral administration as chewable tablets of 100 mg, tablets of 200 mg, and as a suspension of 100 mg/5 ml (teaspoon). Its chemical name is *5H*-dibenz[b,f]azepine-5-carboxamide.

Carbamazepine USP is a white to off-white powder, practically insoluble in water and soluble in alcohol and in acetone. Its molecular weight is 236.27.

Inactive Ingredients. Tablets: Colloidal silicon dioxide, FD&C Red No. 3 (chewable tablets only), FD&C Red No. 40 (200-mg tablets only), flavoring (chewable tablets only), gelatin, glycerin, magnesium stearate, sodium starch glycolate (chewable tablets only), starch, stearic acid, and sucrose (chewable tablets only). Suspension: Citric acid, FD&C Yellow No. 6, flavoring, polymer, potassium sorbate, propylene glycol, purified water, sorbitol, sucrose, and xanthan gum.

CLINICAL PHARMACOLOGY

In controlled clinical trials, Tegretol has been shown to be effective in the treatment of psychomotor and grand mal seizures, as well as trigeminal neuralgia.

It has demonstrated anticonvulsant properties in rats and mice with electrically and chemically induced seizures. It appears to act by reducing polysynaptic responses and blocking the post-tetanic potentiation. Tegretol greatly reduces or abolishes pain induced by stimulation of the infraorbital nerve in cats and rats. It depresses thalamic potential and bulbar and polysynaptic reflexes, including the linguomandibular reflex in cats. Tegretol is chemically unrelated to other anticonvulsants or other drugs used to control the pain of trigeminal neuralgia. The mechanism of action remains unknown.

In clinical studies both suspension and conventional tablet delivered equivalent amounts of drug to the systemic circulation. However, the suspension was absorbed somewhat faster than the tablet. Following a b.i.d. dosage regimen, the suspension has higher peak plasma levels and lower trough levels than those obtained from the tablet formulation for the same dosage regimen. On the other hand, following a t.i.d. dosage regimen, Tegretol suspension affords steady-state plasma levels comparable to Tegretol tablets given b.i.d. when administered at the same total mg daily dose. Tegretol chewable tablets may produce higher peak levels than the same dose given as regular tablets. Tegretol in blood is 76% bound to plasma proteins. Plasma levels of Tegretol are variable and may range from 0.5–25 μg/ml, with no apparent relationship to the daily intake of the drug. Usual adult therapeutic levels are between 4 and 12 μg/ml. Following chronic oral administration of suspension, plasma levels peak at approximately 1.5 hours compared to 4 to 5 hours after administration of oral tablets. The CSF/serum ratio is 0.22, similar to the 22% unbound Tegretol in serum. Because Tegretol may induce its own metabolism, the half-life is also variable. Initial half-life values range from 25–65 hours, with 12–17 hours on repeated doses. Tegretol is metabolized in the liver. After oral administration of ^{14}C-carbamazepine, 72% of the administered radioactivity was found in the urine and 28% in the feces. This urinary radioactivity was composed largely of hydroxylated and conjugated metabolites, with only 3% of unchanged Tegretol. Transplacental passage of Tegretol is rapid (30 to 60 minutes), and the drug is accumulated in fetal tissues, with higher levels found in liver and kidney than in brain and lungs.

INDICATIONS AND USAGE

Epilepsy: Tegretol is indicated for use as an anticonvulsant drug. Evidence supporting efficacy of Tegretol as an anticonvulsant was derived from active drug-controlled studies that enrolled patients with the following seizure types:

1. Partial seizures with complex symptomatology (psychomotor, temporal lobe). Patients with these seizures appear to show greater improvement than those with other types.
2. Generalized tonic-clonic seizures (grand mal).
3. Mixed seizure patterns which include the above, or other partial or generalized seizures.

Absence seizures (petit mal) do not appear to be controlled by Tegretol (see PRECAUTIONS, General).

Trigeminal Neuralgia: Tegretol is indicated in the treatment of the pain associated with true trigeminal neuralgia. Beneficial results have also been reported in glossopharyngeal neuralgia.

This drug is not a simple analgesic and should not be used for the relief of trivial aches or pains.

CONTRAINDICATIONS

Tegretol should not be used in patients with a history of previous bone marrow depression, hypersensitivity to the drug, or known sensitivity to any of the tricyclic compounds, such as amitriptyline, desipramine, imipramine, protriptyline, nortriptyline, etc. Likewise, on theoretical grounds its use with monoamine oxidase inhibitors is not recommended. Before administration of Tegretol, MAO inhibitors should be discontinued for a minimum of fourteen days, or longer if the clinical situation permits.

WARNINGS

Patients with a history of adverse hematologic reaction to any drug may be particularly at risk.

Severe dermatologic reactions including toxic epidermal necrolysis (Lyell's syndrome) and Stevens-Johnson syndrome, have been reported with Tegretol. These reactions have been extremely rare. However, a few fatalities have been reported.

Tegretol has shown mild anticholinergic activity; therefore, patients with increased intraocular pressure should be closely observed during therapy.

Because of the relationship of the drug to other tricyclic compounds, the possibility of activation of a latent psychosis and, in elderly patients, of confusion or agitation should be borne in mind.

Continued on next page

The full prescribing information for each Basel product is contained herein and is that in effect as of September 1, 1992.

Basel—Cont.

PRECAUTIONS

General: Before initiating therapy, a detailed history and physical examination should be made.

Tegretol should be used with caution in patients with a mixed seizure disorder that includes atypical absence seizures, since in these patients Tegretol has been associated with increased frequency of generalized convulsions (see INDICATIONS AND USAGE).

Therapy should be prescribed only after critical benefit-to-risk appraisal in patients with a history of cardiac, hepatic or renal damage, adverse hematologic reaction to other drugs, or interrupted courses of therapy with Tegretol.

Since a given dose of Tegretol suspension will produce higher peak levels than the same dose given as the tablet, it is recommended that patients given the suspension be started on lower doses and increased slowly to avoid unwanted side effects (see DOSAGE AND ADMINISTRATION).

Information for Patients: Patients should be made aware of the early toxic signs and symptoms of a potential hematologic problem, such as fever, sore throat, ulcers in the mouth, easy bruising, petechial or purpuric hemorrhage, and should be advised to report to the physician immediately if any such signs or symptoms appear.

Since dizziness and drowsiness may occur, patients should be cautioned about the hazards of operating machinery or automobiles or engaging in other potentially dangerous tasks.

Laboratory Tests: Complete pretreatment blood counts, including platelets and possibly reticulocytes and serum iron, should be obtained as a baseline. If a patient in the course of treatment exhibits low or decreased white blood cell or platelet counts, the patient should be monitored closely. Discontinuation of the drug should be considered if any evidence of significant bone marrow depression develops.

Baseline and periodic evaluations of liver function, particularly in patients with a history of liver disease, must be performed during treatment with this drug since liver damage may occur. The drug should be discontinued immediately in cases of aggravated liver dysfunction or active liver disease.

Baseline and periodic eye examinations, including slit-lamp, funduscopy and tonometry, are recommended since many phenothiazines and related drugs have been shown to cause eye changes.

Baseline and periodic complete urinalysis and BUN determinations are recommended for patients treated with this agent because of observed renal dysfunction.

Monitoring of blood levels (see CLINICAL PHARMACOLOGY) has increased the efficacy and safety of anticonvulsants. This monitoring may be particularly useful in cases of dramatic increase in seizure frequency and for verification of compliance. In addition, measurement of drug serum levels may aid in determining the cause of toxicity when more than one medication is being used.

Thyroid function tests have been reported to show decreased values with Tegretol administered alone.

Hyponatremia has been reported in association with Tegretol use, either alone or in combination with other drugs.

Drug Interactions: The simultaneous administration of phenobarbital, phenytoin, or primidone, or a combination of two, produces a marked lowering of serum levels of Tegretol. The effect of valproic acid on Tegretol blood levels is not clearly established, although an increase in the ratio of active 10, 11-epoxide metabolite to parent compound is a consistent finding.

The half-lives of phenytoin, warfarin, doxycycline, and theophylline were significantly shortened when administered concurrently with Tegretol. Haloperidol and valproic acid serum levels may be reduced when these drugs are administered with Tegretol. The doses of these drugs may therefore have to be increased when Tegretol is added to the therapeutic regimen.

Concomitant administration of Tegretol with erythromycin, cimetidine, propoxyphene, isoniazid, fluoxetine or calcium channel blockers has been reported to result in elevated plasma levels of carbamazepine resulting in toxicity in some cases. Also, concomitant administration of carbamazepine and lithium may increase the risk of neurotoxic side effects.

Alterations of thyroid function have been reported in combination therapy with other anticonvulsant medications.

Breakthrough bleeding has been reported among patients receiving concomitant oral contraceptives and their reliability may be adversely affected.

Carcinogenesis, Mutagenesis, Impairment of Fertility: Carbamazepine, when administered to Sprague-Dawley rats for two years in the diet at doses of 25, 75, and 250 mg/kg/day, resulted in a dose-related increase in the incidence of hepatocellular tumors in females and of benign interstitial cell adenomas in the testes of males.

Carbamazepine must, therefore, be considered to be carcinogenic in Sprague-Dawley rats. Bacterial and mammalian mutagenicity studies using carbamazepine produced negative results. The significance of these findings relative to the use of carbamazepine in humans is, at present, unknown.

Pregnancy Category C: Tegretol has been shown to have adverse effects in reproduction studies in rats when given orally in dosages 10–25 times the maximum human daily dosage of 1200 mg. In rat teratology studies, 2 of 135 offspring showed kinked ribs at 250 mg/kg and 4 of 119 offspring at 650 mg/kg showed other anomalies (cleft palate, 1; talipes, 1; anophthalmos, 2). In reproduction studies in rats, nursing offspring demonstrated a lack of weight gain and an unkempt appearance at a maternal dosage level of 200 mg/kg.

There are no adequate and well-controlled studies in pregnant women. Epidemiological data suggest that there may be an association between the use of carbamazepine during pregnancy and congenital malformations, including spina bifida. Tegretol should be used during pregnancy only if the potential benefit justifies the potential risk to the fetus.

Retrospective case reviews suggest that, compared with monotherapy, there may be a higher prevalence of teratogenic effects associated with the use of anticonvulsants in combination therapy. Therefore, monotherapy is recommended for pregnant women.

It is important to note that anticonvulsant drugs should not be discontinued in patients in whom the drug is administered to prevent major seizures because of the strong possibility of precipitating status epilepticus with attendant hypoxia and threat to life. In individual cases where the severity and frequency of the seizure disorder are such that removal of medication does not pose a serious threat to the patient, discontinuation of the drug may be considered prior to and during pregnancy, although it cannot be said with any confidence that even minor seizures do not pose some hazard to the developing embryo or fetus.

Labor and Delivery: The effect of Tegretol on human labor and delivery is unknown.

Nursing Mothers: During lactation, concentration of Tegretol in milk is approximately 60% of the maternal plasma concentration.

Because of the potential for serious adverse reactions in nursing infants from carbamazepine, a decision should be made whether to discontinue nursing or to discontinue the drug, taking into account the importance of the drug to the mother.

Pediatric Use: Safety and effectiveness in children below the age of 6 years have not been established.

ADVERSE REACTIONS

If adverse reactions are of such severity that the drug must be discontinued, the physician must be aware that abrupt discontinuation of any anticonvulsant drug in a responsive epileptic patient may lead to seizures or even status epilepticus with its life-threatening hazards.

The most severe adverse reactions have been observed in the hemopoietic system (see boxed WARNING), the skin and the cardiovascular system.

The most frequently observed adverse reactions, particularly during the initial phases of therapy, are dizziness, drowsiness, unsteadiness, nausea, and vomiting. To minimize the possibility of such reactions, therapy should be initiated at the low dosage recommended.

The following additional adverse reactions have been reported:

Hemopoietic System: Aplastic anemia, agranulocytosis, pancytopenia, bone marrow depression, thrombocytopenia, leukopenia, leukocytosis, eosinophilia, acute intermittent porphyria.

Skin: Pruritic and erythematous rashes, urticaria, toxic epidermal necrolysis (Lyell's syndrome) (see WARNINGS), Stevens-Johnson syndrome (see WARNINGS), photosensitivity reactions, alterations in skin pigmentation, exfoliative dermatitis, erythema multiforme and nodosum, purpura, aggravation of disseminated lupus erythematosus, alopecia, and diaphoresis. In certain cases, discontinuation of therapy may be necessary. Isolated cases of hirsutism have been reported, but a causal relationship is not clear.

Cardiovascular System: Congestive heart failure, edema, aggravation of hypertension, hypotension, syncope and collapse, aggravation of coronary artery disease, arrhythmias and AV block, primary thrombophlebitis, recurrence of thrombophlebitis, and adenopathy or lymphadenopathy.

Some of these cardiovascular complications have resulted in fatalities. Myocardial infarction has been associated with other tricyclic compounds.

Liver: Abnormalities in liver function tests, cholestatic and hepatocellular jaundice, hepatitis.

Respiratory System: Pulmonary hypersensitivity characterized by fever, dyspnea, pneumonitis or pneumonia.

Genitourinary System: Urinary frequency, acute urinary retention, oliguria with elevated blood pressure, azotemia, renal failure, and impotence. Albuminuria, glycosuria, elevated BUN and microscopic deposits in the urine have also been reported.

Testicular atrophy occurred in rats receiving Tegretol orally from 4 to 52 weeks at dosage levels of 50 to 400 mg/kg/day. Additionally, rats receiving Tegretol in the diet for two years at dosage levels of 25, 75, and 250 mg/kg/day had a dose-related incidence of testicular atrophy and aspermatogenesis. In dogs, it produced a brownish discoloration, presumably a metabolite, in the urinary bladder at dosage levels of 50 mg/kg and higher. Relevance of these findings to humans is unknown.

Nervous System: Dizziness, drowsiness, disturbances of coordination, confusion, headache, fatigue, blurred vision, visual hallucinations, transient diplopia, oculomotor disturbances, nystagmus, speech disturbances, abnormal involuntary movements, peripheral neuritis and paresthesias, depression with agitation, talkativeness, tinnitus, and hyperacusis.

There have been reports of associated paralysis and other symptoms of cerebral arterial insufficiency, but the exact relationship of these reactions to the drug has not been established.

Digestive System: Nausea, vomiting, gastric distress and abdominal pain, diarrhea, constipation, anorexia, and dryness of the mouth and pharynx, including glossitis and stomatitis.

Eyes: Scattered, punctate, cortical lens opacities, as well as conjunctivitis have been reported. Although a direct causal relationship has not been established, many phenothiazines and related drugs have been shown to cause eye changes.

Musculoskeletal System: Aching joints and muscles, and leg cramps.

Metabolism: Fever and chills. Inappropriate antidiuretic hormone (ADH) secretion syndrome has been reported. Cases of frank water intoxication, with decreased serum sodium (hyponatremia) and confusion, have been reported in association with Tegretol use (see PRECAUTIONS, Laboratory Tests).

Other: Isolated cases of a lupus erythematosus-like syndrome have been reported. There have been occasional reports of elevated levels of cholesterol, HDL cholesterol and triglycerides in patients taking anticonvulsants.

A case of aseptic meningitis, accompanied by myoclonus and peripheral eosinophilia, has been reported in a patient taking carbamazepine in combination with other medications. The patient was successfully dechallenged, and the meningitis reappeared upon rechallenge with carbamazepine.

DRUG ABUSE AND DEPENDENCE

No evidence of abuse potential has been associated with Tegretol, nor is there evidence of psychological or physical dependence in humans.

OVERDOSAGE

Acute Toxicity

Lowest known lethal dose: adults, >60 g (39-year-old man). Highest known doses survived: adults, 30 g (31-year-old woman); children, 10 g (6-year-old boy); small children, 5 g (3-year-old girl).

Oral LD_{50} in animals (mg/kg): mice, 1100–3750; rats, 3850–4025; rabbits, 1500–2680; guinea pigs, 920.

Signs and Symptoms

The first signs and symptoms appear after 1–3 hours. Neuromuscular disturbances are the most prominent. Cardiovascular disorders are generally milder, and severe cardiac complications occur only when very high doses (>60 g) have been ingested.

Respiration: Irregular breathing, respiratory depression.

Cardiovascular System: Tachycardia, hypotension or hypertension, shock, conduction disorders.

Nervous System and Muscles: Impairment of consciousness ranging in severity to deep coma. Convulsions, especially in small children. Motor restlessness, muscular twitching, tremor, athetoid movements, opisthotonos, ataxia, drowsiness, dizziness, mydriasis, nystagmus, adiadochokinesia, ballism, psychomotor disturbances, dysmetria. Initial hyperreflexia, followed by hyporeflexia.

Gastrointestinal Tract: Nausea, vomiting.

Kidneys and Bladder: Anuria or oliguria, urinary retention.

Laboratory Findings: Isolated instances of overdosage have included leukocytosis, reduced leukocyte count, glycosuria and acetonuria. EEG may show dysrhythmias.

Combined Poisoning: When alcohol, tricyclic antidepressants, barbiturates or hydantoins are taken at the same time, the signs and symptoms of acute poisoning with Tegretol may be aggravated or modified.

Treatment

The prognosis in cases of severe poisoning is critically dependent upon prompt elimination of the drug, which may be achieved by inducing vomiting, irrigating the stomach, and by taking appropriate steps to diminish absorption. If these measures cannot be implemented without risk on the spot, the patient should be transferred at once to a hospital, while ensuring that vital functions are safeguarded. There is no specific antidote.

Elimination of the Drug: Induction of vomiting.

Gastric lavage. Even when more than 4 hours have elapsed following ingestion of the drug, the stomach should be re-

Indication	Initial Dose		Subsequent Dose		Maximum Dose
	Dosage Information: Tablets and Suspension				
	Tablet	Suspension	Tablet	Suspension	Tablet or Suspension
Epilepsy					
6–12 years of age	100 mg b.i.d. (200 mg/day)	½ teaspoon q.i.d. (200 mg/day)	Add up to 100 mg per day at weekly intervals, t.i.d. or q.i.d.	Add up to 1 teaspoon (100 mg) per day at weekly intervals, t.i.d. or q.i.d.	1000 mg/24 hours
Over 12 years of age	200 mg b.i.d. (400 mg/day)	1 teaspoon q.i.d. (400 mg/day)	Add up to 200 mg per day at weekly intervals, t.i.d. or q.i.d.	Add up to 2 teaspoons (200 mg) per day at weekly intervals, t.i.d. or q.i.d.	1000 mg/24 hours: 12–15 years 1200 mg/24 hours: Over 15 years 1600 mg/24 hours: adults, in rare instances
Trigeminal Neuralgia	100 mg b.i.d. on the first day (200 mg/day)	½ teaspoon q.i.d. (200 mg/day)	Add up to 200 mg per day in increments of 100 mg every 12 hours	Add up to 2 teaspoons (200 mg) per day q.i.d.	1200 mg/24 hours

peatedly irrigated, especially if the patient has also consumed alcohol.

Measures to Reduce Absorption: Activated charcoal, laxatives.

Measures to Accelerate Elimination: Forced diuresis.

Dialysis is indicated only in severe poisoning associated with renal failure. Replacement transfusion is indicated in severe poisoning in small children.

Respiratory Depression: Keep the airways free; resort, if necessary, to endotracheal intubation, artificial respiration, and administration of oxygen.

Hypotension, Shock: Keep the patient's legs raised and administer a plasma expander. If blood pressure fails to rise despite measures taken to increase plasma volume, use of vasoactive substances should be considered.

Convulsions: Diazepam or barbiturates.

Warning: Diazepam or barbiturates may aggravate respiratory depression (especially in children), hypotension, and coma. However, barbiturates should <u>not</u> be used if drugs that inhibit monoamine oxidase have also been taken by the patient either in overdosage or in recent therapy (within one week).

Surveillance: Respiration, cardiac function (ECG monitoring), blood pressure, body temperature, pupillary reflexes, and kidney and bladder function should be monitored for several days.

Treatment of Blood Count Abnormalities: If evidence of significant bone marrow depression develops, the following recommendations are suggested: (1) stop the drug, (2) perform daily CBC, platelet and reticulocyte counts, (3) do a bone marrow aspiration and trephine biopsy immediately and repeat with sufficient frequency to monitor recovery. Special periodic studies might be helpful as follows: (1) white cell and platelet antibodies, (2) [59]Fe—ferrokinetic studies, (3) peripheral blood cell typing, (4) cytogenetic studies on marrow and peripheral blood, (5) bone marrow culture studies for colony-forming units, (6) hemoglobin electrophoresis for A_2 and F hemoglobin, and (7) serum folic acid and B_{12} levels.

A fully developed aplastic anemia will require appropriate, intensive monitoring and therapy, for which specialized consultation should be sought.

DOSAGE AND ADMINISTRATION (see table above)

Monitoring of blood levels has increased the efficacy and safety of anticonvulsants (see PRECAUTIONS, Laboratory Tests). Dosage should be adjusted to the needs of the individual patient. A low initial daily dosage with a gradual increase is advised. As soon as adequate control is achieved, the dosage may be reduced very gradually to the minimum effective level. Medication should be taken with meals.

Since a given dose of Tegretol suspension will produce higher peak levels than the same dose given as the tablet, it is recommended to start with low doses (children 6–12 years: ½ teaspoon q.i.d.) and to increase slowly to avoid unwanted side effects.

Conversion of patients from oral Tegretol tablets to Tegretol suspension: Patients should be converted by administering the same number of mg per day in smaller, more frequent doses (i.e., b.i.d. tablets to t.i.d. suspension).

Epilepsy (see INDICATIONS AND USAGE).

Adults and children over 12 years of age—*Initial:* Either 200 mg b.i.d. for tablets or 1 teaspoon q.i.d. for suspension (400 mg per day). Increase at weekly intervals by adding up to 200 mg per day using a t.i.d. or q.i.d. regimen until the optimal response is obtained. Dosage should generally not exceed 1000 mg daily in children 12 to 15 years of age, and 1200 mg daily in patients above 15 years of age. Doses up to 1600 mg daily have been used in adults in rare instances. *Maintenance:* Adjust dosage to the minimum effective level, usually 800–1200 mg daily.

Children 6–12 years of age—*Initial:* Either 100 mg b.i.d. for tablets or ½ teaspoon q.i.d for suspension (200 mg per day). Increase at weekly intervals by adding up to 100 mg per day using a t.i.d. or q.i.d. regimen until the optimal response is obtained. Dosage generally should not exceed 1000 mg daily. *Maintenance:* Adjust dosage to the minimum effective level, usually 400–800 mg daily.

Combination Therapy: Tegretol may be used alone or with other anticonvulsants. When added to existing anticonvulsant therapy, the drug should be added gradually while the other anticonvulsants are maintained or gradually decreased, except phenytoin, which may have to be increased (see PRECAUTIONS, Drug Interactions and Pregnancy Category C).

Trigeminal Neuralgia (see INDICATIONS AND USAGE).

Initial: On the first day, either 100 mg b.i.d. for tablets or ½ teaspoon q.i.d. for suspension for a total daily dose of 200 mg. This daily dose may be increased by up to 200 mg a day using increments of 100 mg every 12 hours for tablets or 50 mg (½ teaspoon) q.i.d. for suspension, only as needed to achieve freedom from pain. Do not exceed 1200 mg daily. *Maintenance:* Control of pain can be maintained in most patients with 400 mg to 800 mg daily. However, some patients may be maintained on as little as 200 mg daily, while others may require as much as 1200 mg daily. At least once every 3 months throughout the treatment period, attempts should be made to reduce the dose to the minimum effective level or even to discontinue the drug.

HOW SUPPLIED

Chewable Tablets 100 mg—round, red-speckled, pink, single-scored (imprinted Tegretol on one side and 52 twice on the scored side)

    Bottles of 100 .... NDC 58887-052-30
    Unit Dose (blister pack)
    Box of 100 (strips of 10) .... NDC 58887-052-32

Tablets 200 mg—capsule-shaped, pink, single-scored (imprinted Tegretol on one side and 27 twice on the partially scored side)

    Bottles of 100 .... NDC 58887-027-30
    Bottles of 1000 .... NDC 58887-027-40
    Unit Dose (blister pack)
    Box of 100 (strips of 10) .... NDC 58887-027-32

Samples, when available, are identified by the word *SAMPLE* appearing on each tablet.

Protect from moisture. Dispense in tight container (USP).

Suspension 100 mg/5 ml (teaspoon)—yellow-orange, citrus-vanilla flavored

    Bottles of 450 ml ....NDC 58887-019-76

Shake well before using.

Do not store above 86°F.

Dispense in tight, light-resistant container (USP).

[See table above.]

                                   C91-50 (Rev.11/91)

BASEL
Pharmaceuticals
BASEL Pharmaceuticals
Division of CIBA-GEIGY Corporation
Summit, New Jersey 07901

Shown in Product Identification Section, page 405

Baxter Healthcare Corporation
Hyland Division
550 NORTH BRAND BLVD.
GLENDALE, CA 91203

AUTOPLEX® T   R

Anti-Inhibitor Coagulant Complex, Heat Treated

Supplied in 30 mL vials (Hyland Factor VIII correctional activity is stated on label of each vial) with sterile diluent and needles for reconstitution and withdrawal. Heat treated at 60°C for 6 days (144 hours).

BUMINATE® 5%   R
Albumin (Human),
USP, 5% Solution

Supplied as a 5% solution in 250 ml and 500 ml bottles. For use with intravenous administration set.

BUMINATE® 25%   R
Albumin (Human),
USP, 25% Solution

Supplied as a 25% solution in 20 ml, 50 ml, and 100 ml vials. For use with intravenous administration set.

GAMMAGARD®   R
Immune Globulin
Intravenous (Human)

DESCRIPTION

Immune Globulin Intravenous (Human), GAMMAGARD®* is a sterile, dried, highly purified preparation of immunoglobulin G (IgG) which is derived from the cold ethanol fractionation process and is further purified using ultrafiltration and ion exchange adsorption. When reconstituted with the appropriate volume of diluent, this preparation contains approximately 50 mg of protein per mL, of which at least 90% is gamma globulin. The reconstituted product contains approximately 0.15 M sodium chloride and has a pH of 6.8 ± 0.4. Stabilizing agents are present in the following maximum amounts: 20 mg/mL glucose, 2 mg/mL polyethylene glycol (PEG), 0.3 M glycine, and 3 mg/mL Albumin (Human).

The manufacturing process for Immune Globulin Intravenous (Human), Gammagard, isolates IgG without additional chemical or enzymatic modification and the Fc portion is maintained intact. Immune Globulin Intravenous (Human), Gammagard contains all the IgG antibody activities which are present in the donor population. On the average, the distribution of IgG subclasses present in this product is the same as is present in normal plasma.[1] Immune Globulin Intravenous (Human), Gammagard contains only trace amounts of IgM and IgA.

Immune Globulin Intravenous (Human), Gammagard contains no preservative.

This product has been prepared from large pools of human plasma from which donors found to have elevated alanine aminotransferase (ALT) levels were excluded. Each unit of plasma used in the manufacture of this product has been found to be nonreactive for HBsAg by an FDA approved test.

CLINICAL PHARMACOLOGY

Immune Globulin Intravenous (Human), Gammagard contains a broad spectrum of IgG antibodies against bacterial and viral agents that are capable of opsonization and neutralization of microbes and toxins.

Peak levels of IgG are reached immediately after infusion of Immune Globulin Intravenous (Human), Gammagard. It has been shown that IgG is distributed relatively rapidly between plasma and extravascular fluid until approximately half of the total body pool is partitioned in the extravascular space. A rapid initial drop in serum levels is, therefore, to be expected.[2]

As a class, IgG survives longer *in vivo* than other serum proteins.[2,3] Studies show that the half-life of Immune Globulin Intravenous (Human), Gammagard is approximately 24 days. These findings are consistent with reports of a 21 to 25 day half-life for IgG.[2,3,4] The half-life of IgG can vary considerably from person to person, however. In particular, high concentrations of IgG and hypermetabolism associated with fever and infection have been seen to coincide with a shortened half-life of IgG.[2,3,4,5]

INDICATIONS AND USAGE

Immunodeficiencies
Primary

Immune Globulin Intravenous (Human), Gammagard is indicated for the treatment of primary immunodeficient states such as: congenital agammaglobulinemias, common variable immunodeficiency, Wiskott-Aldrich syndrome, and severe combined immunodeficiencies.[4,5] Immune Globulin

*Manufactured under U.S. Patent No. 4,439,421

Continued on next page

Baxter Healthcare—Cont.

Intravenous (Human), Gammagard is especially useful when high levels or rapid elevation of circulating IgG are desired or when intramuscular injections are contraindicated (e.g., small muscle mass).

B-cell Chronic Lymphocytic Leukemia

Immune Globulin Intravenous (Human) (IGIV), Gammagard is indicated for prevention of bacterial infections in patients with hypogammaglobulinemia and/or recurrent bacterial infections associated with B-cell Chronic Lymphocytic Leukemia (CLL). In a study of 81 patients, 41 of whom were treated with Immune Globulin Intravenous (Human), Gammagard, bacterial infections were significantly reduced in the treatment group.[6,7] In this study, the placebo group had approximately twice as many bacterial infections as the IGIV group. The median time to first bacterial infection for the IGIV group was greater than 365 days. By contrast, the time to first bacterial infection in the placebo group was 192 days. The number of viral and fungal infections, which were for the most part minor, was not statistically different between the two groups.

Idiopathic Thrombocytopenic Purpura (ITP)

When a rapid rise in platelet count is needed to control bleeding or to allow a patient with ITP to undergo surgery, the administration of Immune Globulin Intravenous (Human), Gammagard should be considered. The efficacy of Immune Globulin Intravenous (Human), Gammagard has been demonstrated in a clinical study involving sixteen patients (twelve adults and four children) diagnosed with acute or chronic Idiopathic Thrombocytopenic Purpura (ITP). Each of the sixteen patients (100%) demonstrated an acute, clinically significant rise in platelet count (platelet count greater than 40,000/mm³) following the administration of Immune Globulin Intravenous (Human), Gammagard.

Ten of the sixteen patients (62%) exhibited a clinically significant rise in platelet count after only one 1 g/kg infusion; four patients (25%) exhibited this result after only two 1 g/kg infusions; and two patients exhibited this result after more than two 1 g/kg infusions. The rise in platelet count is generally rapid, occurring within 5 days. The rise, however, is transient and should not be considered curative. Platelet rises most often lasted 2 to 3 weeks, with a range of 12 days to 6 months. *It should be noted that childhood ITP may resolve spontaneously without treatment.*

CONTRAINDICATIONS

None known.

WARNINGS

Immune Globulin Intravenous (Human), Gammagard should only be administered intravenously. Other routes of administration have not been evaluated.

Immune Globulin Intravenous (Human), Gammagard contains very low quantities of IgA (not more than 10 μg/mL); nonetheless, it should be given with caution to patients with antibodies to IgA or selective IgA deficiencies.[5,8]

PRECAUTIONS

Drug Interactions

Admixtures of Immune Globulin Intravenous (Human), Gammagard with other drugs have not been evaluated. It is recommended that Immune Globulin Intravenous (Human), Gammagard be administered separately from other drugs or medication which the patient may be receiving.

Pregnancy Category C

Animal reproduction studies have not been conducted with Immune Globulin Intravenous (Human), Gammagard. It is also not known whether Immune Globulin Intravenous (Human), Gammagard can cause fetal harm when administered to a pregnant woman or can affect reproduction capacity. Immune Globulin Intravenous (Human), Gammagard should be given to a pregnant woman only if clearly needed.

ADVERSE REACTIONS

In general, adverse reactions to Immune Globulin Intravenous (Human), IGIV, Gammagard in patients with congenital or acquired immunodeficiencies are similar in kind and frequency. The incidence of untoward reactions in these patients is low, although various minor reactions, such as headache, fatigue, chills, backache, leg cramps, lightheadedness, fever, urticaria, flushing, slight elevation of blood pressure, nausea and vomiting may occasionally occur. The incidence of these reactions directly attributable to the infusion of Immune Globulin Intravenous (Human), Gammagard during the clinical trials of primary immunodeficiencies was about 6%. In the study of patients with B-cell Chronic Lymphocytic Leukemia (CLL), the incidence was about 3%. Slowing or stopping the infusion usually allows the symptoms to disappear promptly.

During the clinical study of this product for treatment of Idiopathic Thrombocytopenic Purpura (ITP), the only side effect reported was headache which occurred in 12 of 16 patients. Oral antihistamines and analgesics alleviated the headache and were used as pretreatment for those patients requiring additional IGIV therapy. The remaining four patients did not report any side effects and did not require pretreatment.

Immediate anaphylactic and hypersensitivity reactions are a remote possibility. Epinephrine should be available for treatment of any acute anaphylactoid reaction. (See *Warnings*.)

DOSAGE AND ADMINISTRATION

Immunodeficiencies

For patients with primary immunodeficiencies, monthly doses of at least 100 mg/kg are recommended. Initially, patients may receive 200–400 mg/kg. As there are significant differences in the half-life of IgG among patients with primary immunodeficiencies, the frequency and amount of immunoglobulin therapy may vary from patient to patient. The proper amount can be determined by monitoring clinical response. The minimum serum concentration of IgG necessary for protection has not been established.

For patients with hypogammaglobulinemia and/or recurrent bacterial infections due to B-cell Chronic Lymphocytic Leukemia (CLL), a dose of 400 mg/kg every three to four weeks is recommended.

Idiopathic Thrombocytopenic Purpura (ITP)

For patients with acute or chronic Idiopathic Thrombocytopenic Purpura (ITP), a dose of 1 g/kg is recommended. The need for additional doses can be determined by clinical response and platelet count. Up to three doses may be given on alternate days if required.

Rate of Administration

It is recommended that initially a rate of 0.5 mL/kg/Hr be used. If infusion at this rate causes the patient no distress, the administration rate may be gradually increased but should not exceed 4 mL/kg/Hr.

A rate of administration which is too rapid may cause flushing and changes in pulse rate and blood pressure. Slowing or stopping the infusion usually allows the symptoms to disappear promptly.

Administration

Immune Globulin Intravenous (Human), Gammagard should be administered as soon after reconstitution as possible. Administration should not begin more than 2 hours after reconstitution.

The reconstituted material should be at room temperature during administration.

Parenteral drug products should be inspected visually for particulate matter and discoloration prior to administration, whenever solution and container permit.

HOW SUPPLIED

Immune Globulin Intravenous (Human), Gammagard is supplied in either 0.5 g, 2.5 g, 5.0 g, or 10.0 g single use bottles. Each bottle of Immune Globulin Intravenous (Human), Gammagard is furnished with a suitable volume of Sterile Water for Injection, USP, and a transfer device. An administration set, which contains an integral airway and a 15 micron filter, is included with the 2.5 g, 5.0 g, and 10.0 g sizes.

STORAGE

Immune Globulin Intravenous (Human), Gammagard is to be stored at a temperature not to exceed 25°C (77°F). Freezing should be avoided to prevent the diluent bottle from breaking.

REFERENCES

1. Unpublished data in the files of Baxter Healthcare Corporation
2. Waldmann TA, Storber W: Metabolism of immunoglobulins. *Prog Allergy 13:* 1–110, 1969
3. Morell A, Riesen W: Structure, function and catabolism of immunoglobulins in *Immunohemotherapy.* Nydegger UE (ed), London, Academic Press, 1981, pp 17–26
4. Stiehm ER: Standard and special human immune serum globulins as therapeutic agents. *Pediatrics 63:* 301–319, 1979
5. Buckley RH: Immunoglobulin replacement therapy: Indications and contraindications for use and variable IgG levels achieved in *Immunoglobulins: Characteristics and Use of Intravenous Preparations.* Alving BM, Finlayson JS (eds), Washington, DC, U.S. Department of Health and Human Services, 1979, pp 3–8
6. Bunch C, Chapel HM, Rai K, et al: Intravenous Immune Globulin reduces bacterial infections in Chronic Lymphocytic Leukemia: A controlled randomized clinical trial, *Blood 70 Suppl 1:* 753, 1987
7. Cooperative Group for The Study Of Immunoglobulin in Chronic Lymphocytic Leukemia: Intravenous immunoglobulin for the prevention of infection in Chronic Lymphocytic Leukemia: A randomized, controlled clinical trial. *N Eng J Med 319:* 902–907, 1988
8. Burks AW, Sampson HA, Buckley RH: Anaphylactic reactions after gammaglobulin administration in patients with hypogammaglobulinemia: Detection of IgE antibodies to IgA. *N Eng J Med 314:* 560–564, 1986

BIBLIOGRAPHY

Bussel JB, Kimberly RP, Inman RD, *et al:* Intravenous gammaglobulin treatment of chronic idiopathic thrombocytopenic purpura. *Blood 62:* 480–486, 1983

Baxter Healthcare Corporation
Hyland Division
Glendale, CA 91203 USA
U.S. License No. 140
G-054   Revised February 1989

HEMOFIL® M   ℞
Antihemophilic Factor (Human)
Method M, Monoclonal Purified

Supplied in single dose bottles. Each bottle is labeled with the potency in international Units, and is packaged together with 10 mL of Sterile Water for Injection, USP, double-ended needle, and a filter needle.

PROPLEX® T   ℞
Factor IX Complex, Heat Treated

Indicated for Factor VII and Factor IX deficiency and Factor VIII inhibitor therapy. Supplied in 30 mL vials (Factor IX and Factor VII content are stated on the label of each vial) with sterile diluent and needles for reconstitution and withdrawal. Heat treated at 60°C for 144 hours (6 days).

PROTENATE® 5%   ℞
Plasma Protein Fraction (Human),
USP, 5% Solution

Supplied as a 5% solution in 250 ml and 500 ml bottles. For use with intravenous administration set.

Beach Pharmaceuticals
Division of BEACH PRODUCTS, INC.
5220 SOUTH MANHATTAN AVE.
TAMPA, FL 33611

BEELITH Tablets   OTC
MAGNESIUM SUPPLEMENT
With PYRIDOXINE HCl
Each tablet supplies 362 mg of
magnesium (31.83 mEq).

DIRECTIONS

As a dietary supplement, take one tablet daily or as directed by a physician. Each tablet yields 362 mg of magnesium and supplies 90% of the Adult U.S. Recommended Daily Allowance (RDA) for magnesium and 1000% of the Adult RDA for vitamin B₆.

Each tablet contains magnesium oxide 600 mg and pyridoxine hydrochloride (Vitamin B₆) 25 mg equivalent to B₆ 20 mg. Also, castor oil, hydroxypropyl methylcellulose, magnesium stearate, microcrystalline cellulose, pharmaceutical glaze, povidone, sodium starch glycolate, D&C Yellow #10, FD&C Yellow #6 (Sunset Yellow), and titanium dioxide.

DRUG INTERACTION PRECAUTIONS

Do not take this product if you are presently taking a prescription antibiotic drug containing any form of tetracycline.

WARNINGS

If you have kidney disease, take only under the supervision of a physician. Excessive dosage may cause laxation. **KEEP OUT OF THE REACH OF CHILDREN.** Do not use if protective printed band around cap is broken or missing.

HOW SUPPLIED

Golden yellow, film coated tablet with the name **BEACH** and the number **1132** printed on each tablet. Packaged in bottles of 100 (NDC 0486-1132-01) tablets.

STORAGE

Keep tightly closed. Store at 15°–30°C (59°–86°F). Protect from light.

R4/90

Shown in Product Identification Section, page 405

CITROLITH TABLETS   ℞

DESCRIPTION

Each white, capsule shaped tablet contains potassium citrate, anhydrous 50 mg and sodium citrate, anhydrous 950 mg.

K–PHOS® M.F.   ℞
K–PHOS® No.2   ℞
Phosphate Urinary Acidifiers

DESCRIPTION

K-PHOS® M.F.: Each tablet contains potassium acid phosphate 155 mg and sodium acid phosphate, anhydrous 350 mg. Each tablet yields approximately 125.6 mg of phosphorus, 44.5 mg of potassium or 1.1 mEq and 67 mg of sodium or 2.9 mEq. **K-PHOS® No.2:** Each tablet contains potassium acid phosphate 305 mg and sodium acid phosphate, anhydrous, 700 mg. Each tablet yields approximately 250 mg of phosphorus, 88 mg of potassium or 2.3 mEq and 134 mg of sodium or 5.8 mEq.

ACTIONS

These products are highly effective urinary acidifiers.

INDICATIONS

For use in patients with elevated urinary pH. These products help keep calcium soluble and reduce odor and rash caused by ammoniacal urine. Also, by acidifying the urine they increase the antibacterial activity of methenamine mandelate and methenamine hippurate.

CONTRAINDICATIONS

These products are contraindicated in patients with infected phosphate stones; in patients with severely impaired renal function (less than 30% of normal) and in the presence of hyperphosphatemia.

PRECAUTIONS

Drug Interactions: Use of antacids containing magnesium, aluminum or calcium in conjunction with phosphate preparations may bind the phosphate and prevent its absorption. Concurrent use of antihypertensives, especially diazoxide, guanethidine, hydralazine, methyldopa or rauwolfia alkaloids; or corticosteroids, especially mineralocorticoids or corticotropin, with sodium phosphate may result in hypernatremia. Potassium-containing medications or potassium-sparing diuretics may cause hyperkalemia when used with potassium phosphates. Patients should have serum potassium level determinations at periodic intervals. Plasma levels of salicylates may be increased since salicylate excretion is decreased in acidified urine; administration of monobasic phosphates to patients stabilized on salicylates may lead to toxic salicylate levels.
General: Contains potassium and sodium and should be used with caution if regulation of these elements is desired. Occasionally, some individuals may experience a mild laxative effect during the first few days of phosphate therapy. If laxation persists to an unpleasant degree, reduce the daily dosage until this effect subsides or, if necessary, discontinue the use of this product. Use of this medication should be carefully considered when the following medical problems exist: Cardiac disease (particularly in digitalized patients), Addison's disease, acute dehydration, extensive tissue breakdown, myotonia congenita, cardiac failure, cirrhosis of the liver or severe hepatic disease, peripheral and pulmonary edema, hypernatremia, hypertension, toxemia of pregnancy, hypoparathyroidism, and acute pancreatitis. Rickets may benefit from phosphate therapy but caution should be observed. High serum phosphate levels increase the risk of extraskeletal calcification.
Information for Patients: Patients with kidney stones may pass old stones when phosphate therapy is started and should be warned of this possibility. Patients should be advised to avoid the use of antacids containing aluminum, magnesium or calcium which may prevent the absorption of phosphate.
Laboratory Tests: Careful monitoring of renal function and serum electrolytes (calcium, phosphorus, potassium, sodium) may be required at periodic intervals. Other tests may be warranted in some patients, depending on conditions.
Carcinogenesis, mutagenesis, impairment of fertility: Long term animal studies to evaluate the carcinogenic, mutagenic, or teratogenic potential of these products have not been performed.
Pregnancy: Pregnancy Category C. Animal reproduction studies have not been conducted with these products. It is also not known whether these products can cause fetal harm when administered to a pregnant woman or can affect reproduction capacity. These products should be given to a pregnant woman only if clearly needed.
Nursing Mothers: It is not known whether these drugs are excreted in human milk. Because many drugs are excreted in human milk, caution should be exercised when these products are administered to a nursing woman.

ADVERSE REACTIONS

Gastrointestinal upset (diarrhea, nausea, stomach pain and vomiting) may occur with phosphate therapy. Also, bone and joint pain (possible phosphate-induced osteomalacia) could occur. The following adverse effects may be observed (primarily from sodium or potassium): headaches; dizziness; mental confusion; seizures; weakness or heaviness of legs; unusual tiredness or weakness; muscle cramps; numbness,

tingling, pain, or weakness of hands or feet; numbness or tingling around lips; fast or irregular heartbeat; shortness of breath or troubled breathing; swelling of feet or lower legs; unusual weight gain; low urine output unusual thirst.

DIRECTIONS

K-PHOS® M.F.: Two tablets four times daily with a full glass of water.
K-PHOS® No.2: One tablet four times daily with a full glass of water. When the urine is difficult to acidify administer one tablet every two hours not to exceed eight tablets in a 24 hour period.

HOW SUPPLIED

K-PHOS® M.F.: White scored tablet with the name **BEACH** and the number **1135** embossed on each tablet. Bottles of 100 (NDC 0486-1135-01) and bottles of 500 (NDC 0486-1135-05) tablets. **K-PHOS® No.2:** Brown capsule shaped tablet with the name **BEACH** and the number **1134** embossed on each tablet. Bottles of 100 (NDC 0486-1134-01) and bottles of 500 (NDC 0486-1134-05) tablets.

CAUTION

Federal law prohibits dispensing without prescription.
Shown in Product Identification Section, page 405

K–PHOS® NEUTRAL   ℞
Supplies 250 mg of phosphorus per tablet.

DESCRIPTION

Each tablet contains 852 mg dibasic sodium phosphate anhydrous, 155 mg monobasic potassium phosphate, and 130 mg monobasic sodium phosphate monohydrate. Each tablet yields approximately 250 mg of phosphorus, 298 mg of sodium (13.0 mEq) and 45 mg of potassium (1.1 mEq).

INDICATIONS

K-PHOS® NEUTRAL increases urinary phosphate and pyrophosphate. As a phosphorus supplement, each tablet supplies 25% of the U.S. Recommended Daily Allowance (U.S.RDA) of phosphorus for adults.

CONTRAINDICATIONS

This product is contraindicated in patients with infected phosphate stones, in patients with severely impaired renal function (less than 30% of normal) and in the presence of hyperphosphatemia.

PRECAUTIONS

General: This product contains potassium and sodium and should be used with caution if regulation of these elements is desired. Occasionally, some individuals may experience a mild laxative effect during the first few days of phosphate therapy. If laxation persists to an unpleasant degree, reduce the daily dosage until this effect subsides or, if necessary, discontinue the use of this product.
Caution should be exercised when prescribing this product in the following conditions: Cardiac disease (particularly in digitalized patients); severe adrenal insufficiency (Addison's disease); acute dehydration; severe renal insufficiency; renal function impairment or chronic renal disease; extensive tissue breakdown (such as severe burns); myotonia congenita; cardiac failure; cirrhosis of the liver or severe hepatic disease; peripheral or pulmonary edema; hypernatremia; hypertension; toxemia of pregnancy; hypoparathyroidism; and acute pancreatitis. Rickets may benefit from phosphate therapy, but caution should be exercised. High serum phosphate may increase the incidence of extra-skeletal calcification.
Information for Patients: Patients with kidney stones may pass old stones when phosphate therapy is started and should be warned of this possibility. Patients should be advised to avoid the use of antacids containing aluminum, magnesium or calcium which may prevent the absorption of phosphate.
Laboratory Tests: Careful monitoring of renal function and serum electrolytes (calcium, phosphorus, potassium, sodium) may be required at periodic intervals during phosphate therapy. Other tests may be warranted in some patients, depending on conditions.
Drug Interactions: The use of antacids containing magnesium, aluminum or calcium in conjunction with phosphate preparations may bind the phosphate and prevent its absorption. Concurrent use of antihypertensives, especially diazoxide, guanethidine, hydralazine, methyldopa, or rauwolfia alkaloids; or corticosteroids, especially mineralocorticoids or corticotropin, with sodium phosphate may result in hypernatremia. Calcium-containing preparations and/or vitamin D may antagonize the effects of phosphates in the treatment of hypercalcemia. Potassium-containing medications or potassium-sparing diuretics may cause hyperkalemia. Patients should have serum potassium level determinations at periodic intervals.
Carcinogenesis, Mutagenesis, Impairment of Fertility: There have been no studies in animals or humans to evaluate the

carcinogenesis, mutagenesis, or impairment of fertility for this product.
Pregnancy: Pregnancy Category C. Animal reproduction studies have not been conducted with this product. It is also not known whether this product can cause fetal harm when administered to a pregnant woman or can affect reproduction capacity. This product should be given to a pregnant woman only if clearly needed.
Nursing Mothers: It is not known whether this drug is excreted in human milk. Because many drugs are excreted in human milk, caution should be exercised when this product is administered to a nursing woman.

ADVERSE REACTIONS

Gastrointestinal upset (diarrhea, nausea, stomach pain, and vomiting) may occur with phosphate therapy. Also, bone and joint pain (possible phosphate-induced osteomalacia) could occur. The following adverse effects may be observed (primarily from sodium or potassium): headaches; dizziness; mental confusion; seizures; weakness or heaviness of legs; unusual tiredness or weakness; muscle cramps; numbness, tingling, pain, or weakness of hands or feet; numbness or tingling around lips; fast or irregular heartbeat; shortness of breath or troubled breathing; swelling of feet or lower legs; unusual weight gain; low urine output; unusual thirst.

DIRECTIONS

Adults: One or two tablets four times a day with a full glass of water.

HOW SUPPLIED

White, film coated, capsule-shaped tablet with the name **BEACH** and number **1125** embossed on each tablet. Bottles of 100 (NDC 0486-1125-01) and 500 (NDC 0486-1125-05) tablets.

CAUTION

Federal law prohibits dispensing without a prescription.
Shown in Product Identification Section, page 405

K–PHOS® ORIGINAL (Sodium Free)   ℞
(Potassium Acid Phosphate)
Urinary Acidifier
Supplies 114 mg of phosphorus per tablet.

DESCRIPTION

Each tablet contains potassium acid phosphate 500 mg. Each tablet yields approximately 114 mg of phosphorus and 144 mg of potassium or 3.7 mEq.

ACTIONS

K-PHOS® ORIGINAL (Sodium Free) is a highly effective urinary acidifier.

INDICATIONS

For use in patients with elevated urinary pH. Helps keep calcium soluble and reduces odor and rash caused by ammoniacal urine. Also, by acidifying the urine, it increases the antibacterial activity of methenamine mandelate and methenamine hippurate.

CONTRAINDICATIONS

This product is contraindicated in patients with infected phosphate stones; in patients with severely impaired renal function (less than 30% of normal) and in the presence of hyperphosphatemia and hyperkalemia.

PRECAUTIONS

General: This product contains potassium and should be used with caution if regulation of this element is desired. Occasionally, some individuals may experience a mild laxative effect during the first few days of phosphate therapy. If laxation persists to an unpleasant degree, reduce the daily dosage until this effect subsides or, if necessary, discontinue the use of this product.
Caution should be exercised when prescribing this product in the following conditions: Cardiac disease (particularly in digitalized patients); severe adrenal insufficiency (Addison's disease); acute dehydration; severe renal insufficiency or chronic renal disease; extensive tissue breakdown (such as severe burns); myotonia congenita; hypoparathyroidism; and acute pancreatitis. Rickets may benefit from phosphate therapy, but caution should be exercised. High serum phosphate levels may increase the incidence of extraskeletal calcification.
Information for Patients: Patients with kidney stones may pass old stones when phosphate therapy is started and should be warned of this possibility. Patients should be advised to avoid the use of antacids containing aluminum, calcium, or magnesium which may prevent the absorption of phosphate. To assure against gastrointestinal injury associated with oral ingestion of concentrated potassium salt preparations, patients should be instructed to dissolve tablets completely in an appropriate amount of water before taking.

Continued on next page

Beach—Cont.

Laboratory Tests: Careful monitoring of renal function and serum electrolytes (calcium, phosphorous, potassium) may be required at periodic intervals during phosphate therapy. Other tests may be warranted in some patients, depending on conditions.

Drug Interactions: The use of antacids containing magnesium, calcium, or aluminum in conjunction with phosphate preparations may bind the phosphate and prevent its absorption. Potassium-containing medications or potassium-sparing diuretics may cause hyperkalemia when used concurrently with potassium salts. Patients should have serum potassium level determinations at periodic intervals. Concurrent use of salicylates may lead to increased serum salicylate levels since excretion of salicylates is reduced in acidified urine. Serum salicylate levels should be closely monitored to avoid toxicity.

Carcincogenesis, Mutagenesis, Impairment of Fertility: There have been no studies in animals or humans to evaluate the carcinogenesis, mutagenesis, or impairment of fertility for this product.

Pregnancy: Pregnancy Category C. Animal reproduction studies have not been conducted with this product. It is also not known whether this product can cause fetal harm when administered to a pregnant woman or can affect reproduction capacity. This product should be given to a pregnant woman only if clearly needed.

Nursing Mothers: It is not known whether this drug is excreted in human milk. Because many drugs are excreted in human milk, caution should be exercised when this product is administered to a nursing woman.

ADVERSE REACTIONS

Gastrointestinal upset (diarrhea, nausea, stomach pain, and vomiting) may occur with the use of potassium phosphates. Also, bone and joint pain (possible phosphate-induced osteomalacia) could occur. The following adverse effects may be observed with potassium administration: irregular heartbeat; dizziness; mental confusion; weakness or heaviness of legs; unusual tiredness; muscle cramps; numbness, tingling, pain, or weakness in hands or feet; numbness or tingling around lips; shortness of breath or troubled breathing.

DIRECTIONS

Two tablets dissolved in 6–8 oz. of water 4 times daily with meals and at bedtime. For best results, let the tablets soak in water for 2 to 5 minutes, or more if necessary, and stir. If any tablet particles remain undissolved, they may be crushed and stirred vigorously to speed dissolution.

HOW SUPPLIED

White scored tablet with the name **BEACH** and the number **1111** embossed on each tablet. Bottles of 100 (NDC 0486-1111-01) and bottles of 500 (NDC 0486-1111-05) tablets.

CAUTION

Federal law prohibits dispensing without prescription.

Shown in Product Identification Section, page 405

UROQID-Acid® Tablets ℞
UROQID-Acid®No. 2 Tablets ℞

DESCRIPTION

Each **UROQID-Acid®** tablet contains methenamine mandelate 350 mg and sodium acid phosphate, monohydrate 200 mg. Each **UROQID-Acid®No. 2** tablet contains methenamine mandelate 500 mg and sodium acid phosphate, monohydrate 500 mg.

CLINICAL PHARMACOLOGY

Methenamine mandelate is rapidly absorbed and excreted in the urine. Formaldehyde is released by acid hydrolysis from methenamine with bactericidal levels rapidly reached at pH 5.0–5.5. Proportionally less formaldehyde is released as urinary pH approaches 6.0 and insufficient quantities are released above this level for therapeutic response. In acid urine, mandelic acid exerts its antibacterial action and also contributes to the acidification of the urine. Mandelic acid is excreted by both glomerular filtration and tubular excretion. In acid urine, there is equally effective antibacterial activity against both gram-positive and gram-negative organisms, since the antibacterial action of mandelic acid and formaldehyde is nonspecific. With Proteus vulgaris and urea splitting strains of Pseudomonas and Aerobacter, results may be discouraging and particular attention is required in monitoring urinary pH and overall management.

INDICATIONS AND USAGE

For the suppression or elimination of bacteriuria associated with chronic and recurrent infections of the urinary tract, including pyelitis, pyelonephritis, cystitis, and infected residual urine accompanying neurogenic bladder. When used as recommended, **UROQID-Acid®** and **UROQID- Acid® No. 2** are particularly suitable for long-term therapy because of their relative safety and because resistance to the nonspecific bactericidal action of formaldehyde does not develop. Pathogens resistant to other antibacterial agents may respond because of the nonspecific effect of formaldehyde formed in an acid urine.

Prophylactic Use Rationale: Urine is a good culture medium for many urinary pathogens. Inoculation by a few organisms (relapse or reinfection) may lead to bacteriuria in susceptible individuals. Thus, the rationale of management in recurring urinary tract infection (bacteriuria) is to change the urine from a growth-supporting to a growth-inhibiting medium. There is a growing body of evidence that long-term administration of methenamine can prevent recurrence of bacteriuria in patients with chronic pyelonephritis.

Therapeutic Use Rationale: Helps to sterilize the urine and, in some situations in which underlying pathologic conditions prevent sterilization by any means, they can help to suppress bacteriuria. As part of the overall management of the urinary tract infection, a thorough diagnostic evaluation should accompany the use of these products.

CONTRAINDICATIONS

UROQID-Acid® and **UROQID-Acid®No. 2** are contraindicated in patients with renal insufficiency, severe hepatic disease, severe dehydration, hyperphosphatemia, and in patients who have exhibited hypersensitivity to any components of these products.

PRECAUTIONS

General: These products should not be used as the sole therapeutic agent in acute parenchymal infections causing systemic symptoms such as chills anf fever.

UROQID-Acid® and **UROQID-Acid®No. 2** contain approximately 33 mg and 83 mg of sodium per tablet, respectively, and should be used with caution in patients on a sodium-restricted diet.

Sodium phosphates should be used with caution in the following conditions: cardiac failure; peripheral or pulmonary edema; hypernatremia; hypertension; toxemia of pregnancy; hypoparathyroidism; and acute pancreatitis. High serum phosphate levels increase the incidence of extraskeletal calcification.

Large doses of methenamine (8 grams daily for 3 to 4 weeks) have caused bladder irritation, painful and frequent micturation, albuminuria and gross hematuria. Dysuria may occur, although usually at higher than recommended doses, and can be controlled by reducing the dosage. These products contain a urinary acidifier and can cause metabolic acidosis. Care should be taken to maintain an acid urinary pH (below 5.5), especially when treating infections due to urea-splitting organisms such as Proteus and strains of Pseudomonas. Drugs and/or foods which produce an alkaline urine should be restricted. Frequent urine pH tests are essential. If acidification of the urine is contraindicated or unattainable, use of these products should be discontinued.

Information for Patients: To assure an acidic pH, patients should be instructed to restrict or avoid most fruits, milk and milk products, and antacids containing sodium carbonate or bicarbonate.

Laboratory Tests: As with all urinary tract infections, the efficacy of therapy should be monitored by repeated urine cultures. During long-term therapy, careful monitoring of renal function, serum phosphorus and sodium may be required at periodic intervals.

Drug Interactions: Formaldehyde and sulfonamides form an insoluble precipitate in acid urine and increase the risk of crystalliuria; therefore, these products should not be used concurrently. Thiazide diuretics, carbonic anhydrase inhibitors, antacids, or urinary alkalinizing agents should not be used concurrently since they may cause the urine to become alkaline and reduce the effectiveness of methenamine by inhibiting its conversion to formaldehyde. Concurrent use of antihypertensives, especially diazoxide, guanethidine, hydralazine, methyldopa, or rauwolfia alkaloids; or corticosteroids, especially mineralocorticoids or corticotropin, with sodium phosphates may result in hypernatremia. Concurrent use of salicylates may lead to increased serum salicylate levels since excretion of salicylates is reduced in acidified urine. Serum salicylate levels should be closely monitored to avoid toxicity.

Laboratory Test Interactions: Formaldehyde interferes with fluorometric procedures for determination of urinary catecholamines and vanilmandelic acid (VMA) causing erroneously high results. Formaldehyde also causes falsely decreased urine estriol levels by reacting with estriol when acid hydrolysis techniques are used; estriol determinations which use enzymatic hydrolysis are unaffected by folmaldehyde. Formaldehyde causes falsely elevated 17-hydroxycorticosteroid levels when the Porter-Silber method is used and falsely decreased 5-hydroxyindoleacetic acid (5HIAA) levels by inhibiting color development when nitrosonaphthol methods are used.

Carcinogenesis, Mutagenesis, Impairment of Fertility: Long-term animal studies to evaluate the carcinogenic, mutagenic, or impairment of fertility potential of these products have not been performed.

Pregnancy: Pregnancy Category C. Animal reproduction studies have not been conducted with these products. It is also not known whether these products can cause fetal harm when administered to a pregnant woman or can affect reproduction capacity. Since methenamine is known to cross the placental barrier, these products should be given to a pregnant woman only if clearly needed.

Nursing Mothers: Methenamine is excreted in breast milk. Caution should be exercised when these products are administered to a nursing woman.

ADVERSE REACTIONS

Gastrointestinal disturbances (nausea, stomach upset), generalized skin rash, dysuria, painful or difficult urination may occur occasionally with the use of methenamine preparations. Microscopic and rarely, gross hematuria have also been reported.

Gastrointestinal upsets (diarrhea, nausea, stomach pain, and vomiting) may occur with the use of sodium phosphates. Also, bone or joint pain (possible phosphate induced osteomalacia) could occur. The following adverse effects may be observed (primarily from sodium or potassium): headaches; dizziness; mental confusion; seizures; weakness or heaviness of legs; unusual tiredness or weakness; muscle cramps; numbness, tingling, pain or weakness of hands or feet; numbness or tingling around lips; fast or irregular heartbeat; shortness of breath or troubled breathing; swelling of feet or lower legs; unusual weight gain; low urine output; unusual thirst.

DIRECTIONS

UROQID-Acid®: Initially, 3 tablets 4 times daily. For maintenance, 1 or 2 tablets 4 times daily. **UROQID-Acid®No. 2:** Initially, 2 tablets 4 times daily. For maintenance, 2 to 4 tablets daily, in divided doses. Give these products with a full glass of water.

HOW SUPPLIED

UROQID-Acid® is a yellow, sugar coated, tablet with the name **BEACH** and the number **1112** printed on each tablet. Packaged in bottles of 100 (NDC 0486-1112-01) tablets. **UROQID-Acid®No. 2** is a yellow, film coated, capsule shaped tablet with the name **BEACH** and the number **1114** embossed on each tablet. Packaged in bottles of 100 (NDC 0486-1114-01) tablets.

CAUTION

Federal law prohibits dispensing without prescription.

Shown in Product Identification Section, page 405

Becton Dickinson Microbiology Systems

Division of Becton Dickinson and Company
P.O. BOX 243
COCKEYSVILLE, MD 21030

BAL IN OIL AMPULES ℞
(Dimercaprol Injection, USP)

DESCRIPTION

Dimercaprol (2,3-dimercapto-1-propanol) is a colorless or almost colorless liquid, having a disagreeable, mercaptan-like odor. Each 1 ml sterile BAL in Oil contains 100 mg Dimercaprol in 200 mg benzyl benzoate and 700 mg peanut oil.

ACTION

Dimercaprol promotes the excretion of arsenic, gold and mercury in cases of poisoning. It is also used in combination with Edetate Calcium Disodium Injection, USP to promote the excretion of lead.

INDICATIONS

BAL in Oil (Dimercaprol Injection, USP) is indicated in the treatment of arsenic, gold and mercury poisoning. It is indicated in acute lead poisoning when used concomitantly with Edetate Calcium Disodium Injection, USP.

Dimercaprol Injection, USP is effective for use in acute poisoning by mercury salts if therapy is begun within one or two hours following ingestion. It is not very effective for chronic mercury poisoning.

Dimercaprol Injection, USP is of questionable value in poisoning caused by other heavy metals such as antimony and bismuth. It should not be used in iron, cadmium, or selenium poisoning because the resulting dimercaprol-metal complexes are more toxic than the metal alone, especially to the kidneys.

CONTRAINDICATIONS

BAL in Oil is contraindicated in most instances of hepatic insufficiency with the exception of postarsenical jaundice. The drug should be discontinued or used only with extreme caution if acute renal insufficiency develops during therapy.

WARNINGS

There may be local pain at the site of the injection. A reaction apparently peculiar to children is fever which may per-

sist during therapy. It occurs in approximately 30% of children. A transient reduction of the percentage of polymorphonuclear leukocytes may also be observed.

PRECAUTIONS

Because the dimercaprol-metal complex breaks down easily in an acid medium, production of an alkaline urine affords protection to the kidney during therapy. Medicinal iron should not be administered to patients under therapy with BAL. Data is not available regarding the use of dimercaprol during pregnancy and it should not be used unless judged by the physician to be necessary in the treatment of life threatening acute poisoning.

ADVERSE REACTIONS

One of the most consistent responses to Dimercaprol Injection, USP is a rise in blood pressure accompanied by tachycardia. This rise is roughly proportional to the dose administered. Doses larger than those recommended may cause other transitory signs and symptoms in approximate order of frequency as follows: (1) nausea and, in some instances, vomiting; (2) headache; (3) a burning sensation in the lips, mouth and throat; (4) a feeling of constriction, even pain, in the throat, chest, or hands; (5) conjunctivitis, lacrimation, blepharal spasm, rhinorrhea, and salivation; (6) tingling of the hands; (7) a burning sensation in the penis; (8) sweating of the forehead, hands and other areas; (9) abdominal pain; and (10) occasional appearance of painful sterile abscesses. Many of the above symptoms are accompanied by a feeling of anxiety, weakness, and unrest and often are relieved by administration of an antihistamine.

DOSAGE AND ADMINISTRATION

By deep intramuscular injection only. For mild arsenic or gold poisoning, 2.5 mg/kg of body weight four times daily for two days, two times on the third day, and once daily thereafter for ten days; for severe arsenic or gold poisoning, 3 mg/kg every four hours for two days, four times on the third day, then twice daily thereafter for ten days. For mercury poisoning, 5 mg/kg initially, followed by 2.5 mg/kg one or two times daily for ten days. For acute lead encephalopathy 4 mg/kg body weight is given alone in the first dose and thereafter at four hour intervals in combination with Edetate Calcium Disodium Injection, USP administered at a separate site. For less severe poisoning the dose can be reduced to 3 mg/kg after the first dose. Treatment is maintained for two to seven days depending on clinical response. Successful treatment depends on beginning injections at the earliest possible moment and on the use of adequate amounts at frequent intervals. Other supportive measures should always be used in conjunction with BAL in Oil therapy.

BAL in Oil should be inspected visually for particulate matter and discoloration prior to administration.

HOW SUPPLIED

3 ml (100 mg/ml, ampules, box of 10 (NDC 0011-8341-09). Store at 15° to 30°C (59° to 85°F).

Beiersdorf Inc.
P.O. BOX 5529
NORWALK, CT 06856-5529

AQUAPHOR®—Original Formula   OTC
Ointment
NDC Numbers—10356-020-01
                10356-020-02

COMPOSITION

Petrolatum, mineral oil, mineral wax and wool wax alcohol.

ACTIONS AND USES

Aquaphor is a stable, neutral, odorless, anhydrous ointment base. Miscible with water or aqueous solutions, Aquaphor will absorb several times its own weight, forming smooth, creamy water-in-oil emulsions. In its pure form, Aquaphor is recommended for use as a topical preparation to help heal severely dry skin. Aquaphor contains no preservatives, fragrances or known irritants.

ADMINISTRATION AND DOSAGES

Use Aquaphor alone or in compounding virtually any ointment using aqueous solutions or in combination with other oil-based substances and all common topical medications. Apply Aquaphor liberally to affected area.

PRECAUTIONS

For external use only. Avoid contact with eyes. Not to be applied over third degree burns, deep or puncture wounds, infections or lacerations. If condition worsens or does not improve within 7 days, patient should consult a doctor.

HOW SUPPLIED

16 oz. jar—List No. 45585
5 lb. jar—List. No. 45586

AQUAPHOR® Antibiotic Formula   OTC
NDC Number—10356-022-01

COMPOSITION

Polymyxin-B Sulfate/Bacitracin Zinc, Petrolatum, Mineral Wax, Mineral Oil, Wood Wax Alcohol.

ACTIONS AND USES

Aquaphor Antibiotic Formula is formulated to help reduce wound healing time and the risk of infection.[1] Recommended for prevention of infection in minor first-aid wounds and for use as a post-operative dressing.

Aquaphor Antibiotic Formula is preservative-free, fragrance-free and hypoallergenic. It is recommended for patients with sensitive skin.

ADMINISTRATION AND DOSAGE

Use Aquaphor Antibiotic Formula whenever a topical antibiotic ointment is needed to help prevent infection in minor cuts, scrapes and burns. Apply Aquaphor Formula liberally to affected area two to three times a day as needed.

PRECAUTIONS

For external use only. Avoid contact with eyes, Not to be applied over third degree burns, deep or puncture wounds, infections or lacerations. If condition worsens or does not improve within seven days, patient should consult a physician.

HOW SUPPLIED

5 oz. tube.
1. Data on file, BDF Inc

AQUAPHOR® Natural Healing Ointment   OTC
NDC Number—10356-021-01

COMPOSITION

Petrolatum, Mineral Oil, Mineral Wax, Wool Wax Alcohol, Eucerite, Panthenol, Bisabolol, Glycerin.

ACTIONS AND USES

Aquaphor Natural Healing Ointment is specially formulated for faster healing of severely dry skin, cracked skin and minor burns. It is recommended for patients suffering from severe skin chapping and from skin disorders that result in severely dry, damaged skin. This formula is also indicated as a follow-up skin treatment for patients undergoing radiation therapy or other drying/burning medical therapies. It is preservative-free, fragrance-free and hypoallergenic, and is clinically proven to reduce wound healing time.[1]

ADMINISTRATION AND DOSAGE

Use Aquaphor Natural Healing Ointment whenever a mild healing agent is needed. Apply liberally to affected areas two to three times a day. In the case of wounds, clean area prior to application.

PRECAUTIONS

For external use only. Avoid contact with the eyes. Not to be applied over third degree burns, deep or puncture wounds, infections or lacerations. If condition worsens or does not improve within seven days, patient should consult a physician.

HOW SUPPLIED

1.75 oz. tube
1. Data on file, BDF Inc

EUCERIN®   OTC
[ū 'sir-in]
Dry Skin Care Cleansing Bar

ACTIVE INGREDIENT

Eucerite®

ACTIONS AND USES

Eucerin® Cleansing Bar has been specially formulated for use on sensitive skin. The formulation contains Eucerite®, a special blend of ingredients that closely resemble the natural oils of the skin, thus providing excellent moisturizing properties. This formulation is fragrance-free and non-comedogenic. Additionally, the pH value of Eucerin Cleansing Bar is neutral so as not to affect the skin's normal acid mantle.

DIRECTIONS

Use during shower, bath, or regular cleansing, or as directed by physician

HOW SUPPLIED

3 ounce bar.
List number 3852

EUCERIN® Creme   OTC
[ū 'sir-in]
Fragrance-Free Moisturizing Formula
NDC Numbers—10356-090-01
                10356-090-05
                10356-090-04
                10356-090-07

COMPOSITION

Water, petrolatum, mineral oil, wool wax alcohol, methylchloroisothiazolinone, methylisothiazolinone.

ACTIONS AND USES

A gentle, non-comedogenic, fragrance-free water-in-oil emulsion. Eucerin can be used as a treatment for dry skin associated with eczema, psoriasis, chapped or chafed skin, sunburn, windburn and itching associated with dryness.

ADMINISTRATION AND DOSAGES

Apply freely to affected areas of the skin as often as necessary or as directed by physician.

PRECAUTIONS

For external use only.

HOW SUPPLIED

16 oz. jar—List Number 0090
8 oz. jar—List Number 3774
4 oz. jar—List Number 3797
2 oz. tube—List Number 3868.

EUCERIN® DAILY FACIAL LOTION   OTC
NDC Number—10356-972-01

COMPOSITION

Active Ingredients: Octyl Methoxycinnamate, micronized Titanium Dioxide, 2-Phenylbenzimidazole-5-Sulfonic Acid, Octyl Salicylate. Other Ingredients: Triple Purified water, Caprylic/capric Triglyceride, Mineral Oil, Octyl Stearate, Cetearyl Alcohol, Glyceryl Stearate, Sodium Hydroxide PEG-40, Castor Oil, Acrylamide/Sodium Acrylate Copolymer, Sodium Cetearyl Sulfate, Wool Wax Alcohol, EDTA, Methylchloroisothiazolinone, Methylisothiazolinone.

ACTIONS AND USES

Eucerin Daily Facial Lotion SPF 20 is fragrance-free, noncomedogenic and non-acnegenic, with a unique chemical-free sun screen (titanium dioxide) to protect skin from UVA and UVB light. It is specially formulated for dry, sensitive skin or for those undergoing therapies which irritate delicate facial skin such as Retin-A® therapy. This light, oil-in-water formula is non-greasy and is easily absorbed into the skin.

ADMINISTRATION AND DOSAGE

Apply Eucerin Daily Facial Lotion twice a day (especially in the morning), or as directed by a physician, to nourish and moisture skin and protect it from harmful UVA and UVB rays.

PRECAUTIONS

For external use only. Avoid contact with eyes.

HOW SUPPLIED

4-oz. bottle.

EUCERIN® Lotion   OTC
[ū 'sir-in]
Dry Skin Care Lotion
NDC Numbers—10356-793-01
                10356-793-04
                10356-793-06

COMPOSITION

Water, Mineral Oil, Isopropyl Myristate, PEG-40 Sorbitan Peroleate, Lanolin Acid Glycerin Ester, Sorbitol, Propylene Glycol, Cetyl Palmitate, Magnesium Sulfate, Aluminum Stearate, Wool Wax Alcohol, BHT, Methylchloroisothiazolinone, Methylisothiazolinone.

ACTIONS AND USES

Eucerin Lotion is a non-comedogenic, fragrance-free, unique water-in-oil formulation that will help to alleviate and soothe excessively dry skin, and provide long-lasting moisturization.

ADMINISTRATION AND DOSAGE

Use daily as preventive care for skin exposed to sun, water, wind, cold or other drying elements.

PRECAUTIONS

For external use only.

Continued on next page

Beiersdorf—Cont.

HOW SUPPLIED

4 fluid oz. plastic bottle—List Number 3771
8 fluid oz. plastic bottle—List Number 3793
16 fluid oz. plastic bottle—List number 3794

EUCERIN® CLEANSING LOTION   OTC
DRY SKIN CARE

COMPOSITION

Water, Sodium Laureth Sulfate, Cocoamphodiacetate, Cocamidopropyl Betaine, Sodium Laureth Sulfate, Glycol Distearate, Cocamide MEA, PEG-7 Glyceryl Cocoate, PEG-5 Lanolate, Citric Acid, PEG-120 Methyl Glucose Dioleate, Lanolin Alcohol, Imidazolidinyl Urea.

ACTIVE INGREDIENT

Eucerite®.

ACTIONS AND USES

Eucerin Cleansing Lotion is formulated for the care of dry, sensitive or irritated skin. Its soap-free formula combines gentle cleansing with unique moisturizing ingredients to both clean skin and protect it against dryness. It contains no fragrances, is non-comedogenic, and leaves no soapy residue.

ADMINISTRATION AND DOSAGE

Wash with water; rinse thoroughly.

PRECAUTIONS

For external use only.

HOW SUPPLIED

8 Fluid oz.—List No. 3962
1 Fluid oz.—List No. 3960

EUCERIN® PLUS   OTC
Moisturizing Lotion
NDC 10356-967-01

COMPOSITION

Water, Mineral Oil, PEG-7, Hydrogenated Castor Oil, Isohexodecane, Sodium Lactate (5%), Urea (5%), Glycerin, Isopropyl Palmitate, Panthenol, Ozokerite, Magnesium Sulfate, Lanolin Alcohol, Bisabolol, Methylchloroisothiazolinone, Methylisothiazolinone

ACTION AND USES

Eucerin Plus in a unique alpha-hydroxy acid moisturizing lotion (5% Sodium Lactate, 5% Urea) that is clinically proven to relieve severely dry, scaly skin conditions.[1] Unlike other alphahydroxy acid moisturizing lotions, Eucerin Plus has low sensitization potential, is fragrance free and non-comedogenic.

ADMINISTRATION AND DOSAGE

Use daily on severely dry, scaly skin.

PRECAUTIONS

Avoid contact with eyes. For external use only. Keep out of reach of children.

HOW SUPPLIED

6 oz bottle—List No. 03967
1. Data on File.

Berlex Laboratories
300 FAIRFIELD ROAD
WAYNE, NJ 07470

DECONAMINE® Tablets   ℞
[dē"con'uh-mēēn]
DECONAMINE® SR Capsules   ℞
DECONAMINE® Syrup   ℞
(chlorpheniramine maleate; d-pseudoephedrine hydrochloride)

DESCRIPTION

Tablets
Each scored, white tablet contains:
  chlorpheniramine maleate ....4 mg
  d-pseudoephedrine hydrochloride ....60 mg
Each DECONAMINE® Tablet also contains the following inactive ingredients: dibasic calcium phosphate, magnesium stearate, microcrystalline cellulose, pregelatinized starch, silica gel, starch (corn), and stearic acid.

SR Capsules
Each sustained-release blue and yellow capsule contains:
  chlorpheniramine maleate ....8 mg
  d-pseudoephedrine hydrochloride ....120 mg
Each DECONAMINE® SR Capsule also contains the following inactive ingredients: coloring agents, gelatin, starch, and sucrose.
Each DECONAMINE® SR Capsule may also contain one or more of the following inactive ingredients: butyl paraben, methyl paraben, propyl paraben, titanium dioxide and other ingredient(s).
  The capsules are designed to provide prolonged release of medication.

Syrup—No alcohol, no dye
Each 5 mL (teaspoonful) clear, colorless to slightly yellow liquid contains:
  chlorpheniramine maleate ....2 mg
  d-pseudoephedrine hydrochloride ....30 mg
  in a grape-flavored, aromatic vehicle
DECONAMINE® Syrup also contains the following inactive ingredients: citric acid, flavoring agent, glycerin, sodium benzoate, sodium chloride, sorbitol, sucrose, and water.

CLINICAL PHARMACOLOGY

Chlorpheniramine maleate antagonizes the physiological action of histamine by acting as an H_1 receptor blocking agent.
Pseudoephedrine is an orally active sympathomimetic amine and exerts a decongestant action on the nasal mucosa. It does this by vasoconstriction, which results in reduction of tissue hyperemia, edema, nasal congestion and an increase in nasal airway patency. The vasoconstrictive action of pseudoephedrine is similar to that of ephedrine. In the usual dose it has minimal vasopressor effects.

INDICATIONS

DECONAMINE® is indicated for the temporary relief of symptoms such as rhinorrhea, sneezing and nasal congestion, due to upper respiratory infections (the common cold), sinusitis or allergic rhinitis; also to help clear nasal passages and shrink swollen membranes, decongest sinus openings and passages, promote sinus drainage and/or relieve sinus pressure.

CONTRAINDICATIONS

Patients with severe hypertension, severe coronary artery disease and patients on MAO inhibitor therapy.
DECONAMINE® medications are also contraindicated in patients sensitive to antihistamines or sympathomimetic agents.

WARNINGS

Chlorpheniramine maleate should be used with extreme caution in patients with narrow angle glaucoma; stenosing peptic ulcer; pyloroduodenal obstruction; symptomatic prostatic hypertrophy; or bladder neck obstruction. Due to its mild atropine-like action, chlorpheniramine maleate should be used cautiously in patients with bronchial asthma, emphysema, chronic pulmonary disease. May cause excitability especially in children.
Sympathomimetic amines should be used with caution in patients with hypertension, ischemic heart disease, diabetes mellitus, increased intraocular pressure, hyperthyroidism and prostatic hypertrophy. Sympathomimetics may produce central nervous system stimulation with convulsions or cardiovascular collapse with accompanying hypotension.
Nervousness, dizziness or sleeplessness may occur at higher doses.

PRECAUTIONS

Information for patients:
Antihistamines may impair mental and physical abilities required for the performance of potentially hazardous tasks, such as driving a vehicle or operating machinery. Patients should also be warned about possible additive effects with alcohol and other central nervous system depressants (hypnotics, sedatives, tranquilizers).
Drug interactions:
Pseudoephedrine-containing drugs should not be given to patients treated with monoamine oxidase (MAO) inhibitors because of the possibility of precipitating a hypertensive crisis. MAO inhibitors also prolong and intensify the anticholinergic effects of antihistamines. Sympathomimetics may reduce the antihypertensive effect of methyldopa, reserpine, veratrum alkaloids and mecamylamine.
Alcohol and other sedative drugs will potentiate the sedative effects of chlorpheniramine.
Care should be taken in administering DECONAMINE® medications concomitantly with other sympathomimetic amines, since their combined effects on the cardiovascular system may be harmful to the patient.
Pregnancy:
Pregnancy Category C: Animal reproduction studies have not been conducted with DECONAMINE® medications. It is also not known whether DECONAMINE® medications can cause fetal harm when administered to a pregnant woman or can affect reproduction capacity. DECONAMINE® medica-

tions should be given to a pregnant woman only if clearly needed.
Nursing Mothers: Due to the possible passage of pseudoephedrine and chlorpheniramine into breast milk, and, because of the higher than usual risk for infants from sympathomimetic amines and antihistamines, the benefit to the mother vs. the potential risk should be considered and a decision should be made whether to discontinue nursing or to discontinue the drug.
Pediatric Use: DECONAMINE® Capsules or Tablets should not be given to children under 12 years of age.

ADVERSE REACTIONS

Chlorpheniramine maleate
Slight to moderate drowsiness may occur and is the most frequent side effect. Other possible side effects of antihistamines in general include:
General: urticaria, drug rash, anaphylactic shock, photosensitivity, excessive perspiration, chills, dryness of mouth, nose and throat;
Cardiovascular: hypotension, headache, palpitation, tachycardia, extrasystoles;
Hematological: hemolytic anemia, thrombocytopenia, agranulocytosis;
CNS: sedation, dizziness, disturbed coordination, fatigue, confusion, restlessness, excitation, nervousness, tremor, irritability, insomnia, euphoria, paresthesia, blurred vision, diplopia, vertigo, tinnitus, hysteria, neuritis, convulsion;
Gastrointestinal: epigastric distress, anorexia, nausea, vomiting, diarrhea, constipation;
Genitourinary: urinary frequency, difficult urination, urinary retention, early menses;
Respiratory: thickening of bronchial secretions, tightness of chest, wheezing and nasal stuffiness.

Pseudoephedrine hydrochloride
Pseudoephedrine may cause mild central nervous system stimulation, especially in those patients who are hypersensitive to sympathomimetic drugs. Nervousness, excitability, restlessness, dizziness, weakness and insomnia may also occur. Headache and drowsiness have also been reported. Large doses may cause lightheadedness, nausea and/or vomiting. Sympathomimetic drugs have also been associated with certain untoward reactions including fear, anxiety, tenseness, restlessness, tremor, weakness, pallor, respiratory difficulty, dysuria, insomnia, hallucination, convulsion, CNS depression, arrhythmias and cardiovascular collapse with hypotension.

OVERDOSAGE

Acute overdosage may produce clinical signs of CNS stimulation and variable cardiovascular effects. Pressor amines should be used with great caution in the presence of pseudoephedrine. Patients with signs of stimulation should be treated conservatively.

DOSAGE AND ADMINISTRATION

Tablets
Adults and children over 12 years, 1 tablet three or four times daily.
Children under 12 years, DECONAMINE® Syrup is recommended.
Syrup
Adults and children over 12 years, 1 to 2 teaspoonfuls (5 to 10 mL) three or four times daily.
Children 6 to 12 years, ½ to 1 teaspoonful (2.5 to 5 mL) three or four times daily, not to exceed 4 teaspoonfuls in 24 hours.
Children 2 to 6 years, ½ teaspoonful (2.5 mL) three or four times daily, not to exceed 2 teaspoonfuls in 24 hours.
Children under 2 years, as directed by physician.
SR Capsules
Adults and children over 12 years, 1 capsule every 12 hours.
Children under 12 years, DECONAMINE® Syrup is recommended.

HOW SUPPLIED

In bottles of:
Tablets
  100 ....NDC 50419-184-10
SR Capsules
  100 ....NDC 50419-181-10
  500 ....NDC 50419-181-50
Syrup
  473 mL ....NDC 50419-185-16
Store at controlled room temperature, between 15°–30°C (59°–86°F). Caution: Federal law prohibits dispensing without prescription.
Manufactured by or for
BERLEX Laboratories, Inc.
Wayne, NJ 07470
Rev. 6/89   60565-3
Shown in Product Identification Section, page 405

MAGNEVIST® ℞
(brand of gadopentetate dimeglumine)
Injection

DESCRIPTION
MAGNEVIST® (brand of gadopentetate dimeglumine) Injection is the N-methylglucamine salt of the gadolinium complex of diethylenetriamine pentaacetic acid, and is an injectable contrast medium for magnetic resonance imaging (MRI). Gadopentetate dimeglumine is to be administered by intravenous injection.
Each mL of MAGNEVIST® Injection contains 469.01 mg gadopentetate dimeglumine, 0.99 mg meglumine, 0.40 mg diethylenetriamine pentaacetic acid and water for injection. MAGNEVIST® Injection contains no antimicrobial preservative.
MAGNEVIST® Injection is provided as a sterile, clear, colorless to slightly yellow aqueous solution.
MAGNEVIST® Injection is a 0.5 mol/L solution of 1-deoxy-1-(methylamino)-D-glucitol dihydrogen [N,N-bis[2-[bis(carboxymethyl)amino]ethyl]glycinato(5-)]gadolinate(2-)(2:1) with a molecular weight of 938 and has the following structural formula:

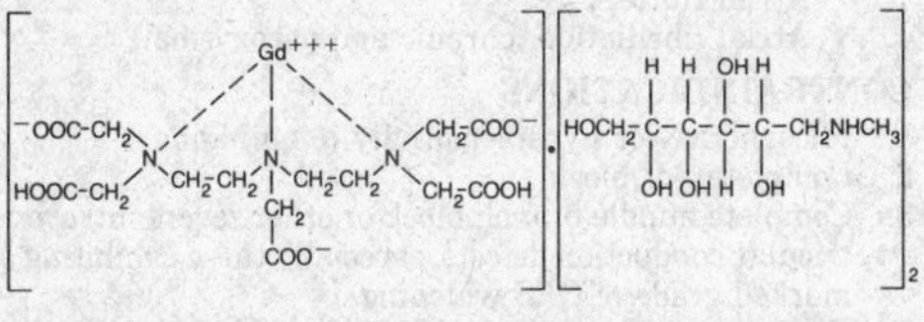

MAGNEVIST® Injection has a pH of 6.5 to 8.0. Pertinent physicochemical data are noted below:

PARAMETER	
Osmolality (mOsmol/kg water) @ 37° C	1,960
Viscosity	
(cP) @ 20° C	4.9
@ 37° C	2.9
Density (g/mL)	1.195

MAGNEVIST® Injection has an osmolality 6.9 times that of plasma (285 mOsmol/kg water) and is hypertonic under conditions of use.

CLINICAL PHARMACOLOGY
The pharmacokinetics of intravenously administered gadopentetate dimeglumine in normal subjects conforms to a two compartment open-model with mean distribution and elimination half-lives (reported as mean ± SD) of about 0.2 ± 0.13 hours and 1.6 ± 0.13 hours, respectively. Upon injection, the meglumine salt is completely dissociated from the gadopentetate dimeglumine complex. Gadopentetate is exclusively eliminated in the urine with 83 ± 14% (mean ± SD) of the dose excreted within 6 hours, and 91 ± 13% (mean ± SD) by 24 hours, post-injection. There was no detectable biotransformation or decomposition of gadopentetate dimeglumine.
The urinary and plasma clearance rates (1.76 ± 0.39 mL/min/kg and 1.94 ± 0.28 mL/min/kg, respectively) of gadopentetate are essentially identical, indicating no alteration in elimination kinetics on passage through the kidneys and that the drug is essentially cleared through the kidney. The volume of distribution (266 ± 43 mL/kg) is equal to that of extracellular water, and clearance is similar to that of substances which are subject to glomerular filtration.
The extent of protein binding and blood cell partitioning of gadopentetate dimeglumine is not known.
Gadopentetate dimeglumine is a paramagnetic agent and, as such, it develops a magnetic moment when placed in a magnetic field. The relatively large magnetic moment produced by the paramagnetic agent results in a relatively large local magnetic field, which can enhance the relaxation rates of water protons in the vicinity of the paramagnetic agent.
In magnetic resonance imaging (MRI), visualization of normal and pathological brain tissue depends in part on variations in the radiofrequency signal intensity that occur with 1) changes in proton density; 2) alteration of the spin-lattice or longitudinal relaxation time (T1); and 3) variation of the spin-spin or transverse relaxation time (T2). When placed in a magnetic field, gadopentetate dimeglumine decreases the T1 and T2 relaxation time in tissues where it accumulates. At usual doses the effect is primarily on the T1 relaxation time.
Gadopentetate dimeglumine does not cross the intact blood-brain barrier and, therefore, does not accumulate in normal brain or in lesions that do not have an abnormal blood-brain barrier, e.g., cysts, mature post-operative scars, etc. However, disruption of the blood-brain barrier or abnormal vascularity allows accumulation of gadopentetate dimeglumine in lesions such as neoplasms, abscesses, subacute infarcts.

INDICATIONS AND USAGE
MAGNEVIST® Injection is indicated for use with magnetic resonance imaging (MRI) in adults and children (2 years of age and older) to provide contrast enhancement in those intracranial lesions with abnormal vascularity or those thought to cause an abnormality in the blood-brain barrier. MAGNEVIST® Injection has been shown to facilitate visualization of intracranial lesions including but not limited to tumors.
MAGNEVIST® Injection is also indicated for use with MRI in adults and children (2 years of age and older) to provide contrast enhancement and facilitate visualization of lesions in the spine and associated tissues. There is, however, only limited clinical experience in children for this indication.

CONTRAINDICATIONS
None known.

WARNINGS
The accepted safety considerations and procedures that are required for magnetic resonance imaging are applicable when MAGNEVIST® Injection is used for contrast enhancement. In addition, deoxygenated sickle erythrocytes have been shown in *in vitro* studies to align perpendicular to a magnetic field which may result in vaso-occlusive complications *in vivo.* The enhancement of magnetic moment by gadopentetate dimeglumine may possibly potentiate sickle erythrocyte alignment. MAGNEVIST® Injection in patients with sickle cell anemia and other hemoglobinopathies has not been studied.
Patients with other hemolytic anemias have not been adequately evaluated following administration of MAGNEVIST® Injection to exclude the possibility of increased hemolysis.
Hypotension may occur in some patients after injection of MAGNEVIST® Injection. In clincial trials two cases were reported and in addition, there was one case of a vasovagal reaction and two cases of pallor with dizziness, sweating and nausea in one and substernal pain and flushing in the other. These were reported within 25 to 85 minutes after injection except for the vasovagal reaction which was described as mild by the patient and occurred after 6-½ hours. In a study in normal volunteers one subject experienced syncope after arising from a sitting position two hours after administration of the drug. Although the relationship of gadopentetate dimeglumine to these events is uncertain, patients should be observed for several hours after drug administration.

PRECAUTIONS
General
Diagnostic procedures that involve the use of contrast agents should be carried out under direction of a physician with the prerequisite training and a thorough knowledge of the procedure to be performed.
In a patient with a history of grand mal seizures, MAGNEVIST® Injection was reported to induce such a seizure.
Since gadopentetate dimeglumine is cleared from the body by glomerular filtration, caution should be exercised in patients with severly impaired renal function.
The possibility of a reaction, including serious, life-threatening, fatal, anaphylactoid or cardiovascular reactions or other idiosyncratic reactions should always be considered (see ADVERSE REACTIONS) especially in those patients with a known clinical hypersensitivity or a history of asthma or other allergic respiratory disorders.
Animal studies suggest that gadopentetate dimeglumine may alter red cell membrane morphology resulting in a slight degree of extravascular (splenic) hemolysis. In clinical trials 15–30% of the patients experienced an asymptomatic transient rise in serum iron. Serum bilirubin levels were slightly elevated in approximately 3.4% of patients. Levels generally returned to baseline within 24 to 48 hours. Hematocrit and red blood cell count were unaffected and liver enzymes were not elevated in these patients. While the effects of gadopentetate dimeglumine on serum iron and bilirubin have not been associated with clinical manifestations, the effect of the drug in patients with hepatic disease is not known and caution is therefore advised.
When MAGNEVIST® Injection is to be injected using plastic disposable syringes, the contrast medium should be drawn into the syringe and used immediately.
If nondisposable equipment is used, scrupulous care should be taken to prevent residual contamination with traces of cleansing agents.
Repeat Procedures: If in the clinical judgment of the physician sequential or repeat examinations are required, a suitable interval of time between administrations should be observed to allow for normal clearance of the drug from the body.
Information for Patients:
Patients receiving MAGNEVIST® Injection should be instructed to:
1. Inform your physician if you are pregnant or breast feeding.
2. Inform your physician if you have anemia or any diseases that affect red blood cells.
3. Inform your physician if you have asthma or other allergic respiratory disorders.

LABORATORY TEST FINDINGS
Transitory changes in serum iron and bilirubin levels have been reported in patients with normal and abnormal liver function (See PRECAUTIONS—General).
CARCINOGENESIS, MUTAGENESIS, AND IMPAIRMENT OF FERTILITY
No animal studies have been performed to evaluate the carcinogenic potential of gadopentetate dimeglumine.
Gadopentetate dimeglumine did not evoke any evidence of mutagenic potential in the Ames test (histidine-dependent *Salmonella typhimurium*) nor in a reverse mutation assay using tryptophan-dependent *Escherichia coli.* Gadopentetate dimeglumine did not induce a positive response in the (C3H 10T½) mouse embryo fibroblast cellular transformation assay, nor did it induce unscheduled DNA repair synthesis in primary cultures of rat hepatocytes at concentrations up to 5000 μg/mL. However, the drug did show some evidence of mutagenic potential *in vivo* in the mouse dominant lethal assay at doses of 6 mmol/kg, but did not show any such potential in the mouse and dog micronucleus tests at intravenous doses of 9 mmol/kg and 2.5 mmol/kg, respectively.
The results of a reproductive study in rats showed that gadopentetate dimeglumine when administered in daily doses of 0.1–2.5 mmol/kg, did not cause a significant change in the pregnancy rate in comparison to a control group. However, suppression of body weight gain and food consumption and a decrease in the mean weights of testis and epididymis occurred in male rats at the 2.5 mmol/kg dose. In female rats a decrease in the number of corpora lutea at the 0.1 mmol/kg dose and the suppression of body weight gain and food consumption at the 2.5 mmol/kg dose were observed.
In a separate experiment, 16 daily intravenous injections were administered to male rats. At a dose of 5 mmol/kg of gadopentetate dimeglumine, spermatogenic cell atrophy was observed. This atrophy was not reversed within a 16-day observation period following the discontinuation of the drug. This effect was not observed at a dose of 2.5 mmol/kg.
PREGNANCY CATEGORY C.
Gadopentetate dimeglumine has been shown to retard development slightly in rats when given in doses 2.5 times the human dose, and in rabbits when given in doses of 7.5 and 12.5 times the human dose. The drug did not exhibit this effect in rabbits when given in doses 2.5 times the human dose. No congenital anomalies were noted in either species. There are no adequate and well-controlled studies in pregnant women. MAGNEVIST® Injection should be used during pregnancy only if the potential benefit justifies the potential risk to the fetus.
NURSING MOTHERS
C^{14} labelled gadopentetate dimeglumine was administered intravenously to lactating rats at a dose of 0.5 mmol/kg. Less than 0.2% of the total dose was transferred to the neonate via the milk during the 24-hour evaluation period. It is not known to what extent MAGNEVIST® Injection is excreted in human milk. Because many drugs are excreted in human milk, caution should be exercised when the drug is administered to a nursing mother and consideration should be given to temporarily discontinuing nursing.
PEDIATRIC USE
Safety and efficacy in children under the age of 2 years have not been established. (See INDICATIONS AND USAGE and DOSAGE AND ADMINISTRATION sections.)

ADVERSE REACTIONS
The most commonly noted adverse experience is headache with an incidence of 8.7%. The majority of headaches are transient and of mild to moderate severity. In 42.3% of the cases it was felt that the headaches were not related to MAGNEVIST® Injection. Injection site coldness/localized coldness is the second most common adverse experience at 4.8%. Nausea occurs in 3.2% of the patients.
Localized pain, vomiting, paresthesia, dizziness and localized warmth occur in less than 2% of the patients.
The following additional adverse events occur in less than 1% of the patients:
Body as a Whole: Injection site symptoms, namely, pain, warmth, burning; localized burning sensation, substernal chest pain, fever, weakness, generalized coldness, localized edema, tiredness, chest tightness, regional lymphangitis, and anaphylactoid reactions (characterized by cardiovascular, respiratory and cutaneous symptoms) rately resulting in death.

Continued on next page

Information on the Berlex products appearing here is based on the labeling in effect on June 1, 1992. Further information for these and other products may be obtained from the Medical Affairs Department, Berlex Laboratories, 300 Fairfield Road, Wayne, New Jersey 07470, (201) 292-3007. Information on oncology products may be obtained from Berlex Laboratories, 15049 San Pablo Avenue, Richmond, California 94804-0016 1-800-888-4112.

Berlex Laboratories—Cont.

Cardiovascular: Hypotension, vasodilation, pallor, non-specific ECG changes, angina pectoris, phlebitis.
Digestive: Gastrointestinal distress, stomach pain, teeth pain, increased salivation.
Nervous System: Agitation, thirst, convulsions (including grand mal).
Respiratory System: Throat irritation, rhinorrhea, sneezing, dyspnea, wheezing, laryngismus, cough.
Skin: Rash, sweating, pruritus, urticaria (hives).
Special Senses: Tinnitus, conjunctivitis, visual field defect, taste abnormality, dry mouth, lacrimation disorder (tearing), eye irritation.
Laboratory: Transient elevation of serum transaminases.
The following other adverse events were reported. A casual relationship has neither been established nor refuted.
Body as a Whole: Back pain, pain, generalized warmth.
Cardiovasular: Hypertension, tachycardia, migraine, syncope, death related to myocardial infarction or other undetermined causes.
Digestive: Constipation, diarrhea.
Nervous System: Anxiety, anorexia, nystagmus, drowsiness, diplopia, stupor.
Skin: facial edema, erythema multiforme, epidermal necrolysis.
Special Senses: Eye pain, ear pain.
Data from foreign studies did not reveal any additional adverse experiences.

OVERDOSAGE

The LD_{50} of intravenously administered gadopentetate dimeglumine injection in mice is 5–12.5 mmol/kg and in rats it is 10–15 mmol/kg. The LD_{50} of intravenously administered MAGNEVIST® Injection in dogs is greater than 6 mmol/kg.
Clinical consequences of overdose with MAGNEVIST® Injection have not been reported.

DOSAGE AND ADMINISTRATION

The recommended dosage of MAGNEVIST® Injection is 0.2 mL/kg (0.1 mmol/kg), administered intravenously, at a rate not to exceed 10 mL per minute. More rapid injection rates may be associated with nausea. The maximum total dose is 20 mL. Any unused portion must be discarded.

DOSAGE CHART

Body Weight (kg)	Dose in mL	Approx. Duration of Injection in Seconds
10	2.0	20
20	4.0	30
30	6.0	40
40	8.0	50
50	10.0	60
60	12.0	70
70	14.0	80
80	16.0	95
90	18.0	110
100	20.0	120

To ensure complete injection of the contrast medium, the injection should be followed by a 5-mL normal saline flush. The imaging procedure should be completed within 1 hour of injection of MAGNEVIST® Injection.
Parenteral products should be inspected visually for particulate matter and discoloration prior to adminstration, whenever solution and container permit.

HOW SUPPLIED

MAGNEVIST® Injection is a clear, colorless to slightly yellow solution containing 469.01 mg/mL of gadopentetate dimeglumine. MAGNEVIST® Injection is supplied in the following sizes:
20 mL single dose vials, rubber stoppered, in individual cartons; Boxes of 20, NDC 50419-188-02.
15 mL single dose vials, rubber stoppered, in individual cartons; Boxes of 20, NDC 50419-188-15.
10 mL single dose vials, rubber stoppered, in individual cartons; Boxes of 20, NDC 50419-188-01.
STORAGE
MAGNEVIST® Injection should be stored at controlled room temperature, between 15°–30°C (59°–86°F) and protected from light. DO NOT FREEZE. Should solidification occur in the vial because of exposure to the cold, MAGNEVIST® Injection should be brought to room temperature before use. If allowed to stand at room temperature for a minimum of 90 minutes, MAGNEVIST® Injection will return to a clear, colorless to slightly yellow solution. Before use, examine the product to assure that all solids are redissolved and that the container and closure have not been damaged.
Caution: Federal Law Prohibits Dispensing Without Prescription.

This product is covered by U.S. Patent No. 4,957,939. The use of this product is covered by U.S. Patent Nos. 4,647,447 and 4,963,344.
Berlex Laboratories
Wayne, New Jersey 07470
USA/Berlex **663 930**/001   60626-1   Revised 8/91
Shown in Product Identification Section, page 405

QUINAGLUTE®   ℞
[kwĭn 'uh-glōōt "]
(quinidine gluconate)
DURA-TABS®
(sustained-release tablets)

DESCRIPTION

Each QUINAGLUTE® (brand of quinidine gluconate) DURA-TABS® (brand of sustained-release tablets) Tablet contains 324 mg quinidine gluconate (equivalent to 202 mg quinidine base) in a tablet matrix specially designed for the sustained-release (8 to 12 hours) of the drug in the gastrointestinal tract. QUINAGLUTE® DURA-TABS® Tablets are to be administered orally.
Quinidine gluconate is the gluconate salt of quinidine [6-methoxy-α-(5-vinyl-2-quinuclidinyl)-4-quinoline-methanol], a dextrorotatory isomer of quinine. Quinidine gluconate is represented by the following structural formula:

Quinidine gluconate contains 62.3% of the anhydrous quinidine alkaloid, whereas quinidine sulfate contains 82.86%. In prescribing QUINAGLUTE® DURA-TABS® Tablets, this factor should be considered.
Therapeutic category: Type I antiarrhythmic.
Each QUINAGLUTE® DURA-TABS® Tablet also contains the following inactive ingredients: confectioner's sugar, magnesium stearate, starch (corn), and other ingredient(s).

CLINICAL PHARMACOLOGY

The antiarrhythmic activity consists of the following basic actions:
1. In arrhythmias due to enhanced automaticity, quinidine decreases the rate of rise of slow diastolic (Phase 4) depolarization, thereby depressing automaticity, particularly in ectopic foci.
2. In addition to the above, quinidine slows depolarization, repolarization and amplitude of the action potential, thus increasing its duration leading to an increase in the refractoriness of atrial and ventricular tissue. Prolongation of the effective refractory period and an increase in conduction time may prevent the reentry phenomenon.
3. Quinidine exerts an indirect anticholinergic effect through blockade of vagal innervation. This anticholinergic effect may facilitate conduction in the atrioventricular junction.
Quinidine absorption from QUINAGLUTE® DURA-TABS® Tablets proceeds at a slower rate than the immediate-release products. In a single-dose pharmacokinetic study conducted in normal volunteers, the time of peak quinidine serum concentration was 1.6 hours for quinidine sulfate tablets and 3.6 hours for QUINAGLUTE® DURA-TABS® Tablets.
The apparent elimination half-life of quinidine ranges from 4 to 10 hours in healthy persons with a usual mean value of 6 to 7 hours. The half-life may be prolonged in elderly persons. From 60% to 80% of the dose is metabolized by the liver. Renal excretion of the intact drug comprises the remainder of the total clearance. Quinidine is approximately 75% bound to serum proteins.
In the past, plasma levels of 1.5 to 5 μg/mL have been reported as therapeutic, based on non-specific assay methodology that quantitates quinidine metabolites as well as intact quinidine. The therapeutic plasma level range using newer, more specific assays has not been definitively established; however, effective reduction of premature ventricular contractions has been reported with blood levels less than 1.0 μg/mL. In general, plasma quinidine levels are lower using specific assays. Clinicians requesting serum quinidine determinations should therefore also ask that the method of analysis be specified.
Due to the wide individual variation in response to quinidine therapy, the usefulness of serum quinidine levels in the planning of optimal quinidine therapy has not been clearly established. A serum quinidine concentration within the reported therapeutic range may not necessarily be the optimal con-

centration for some patients. In the absence of toxicity, such patients may warrant an increase in dose to achieve the desired therapeutic effect. However, for those patients in whom a high blood level has been achieved without significant therapeutic response, increasing the dose to potentially toxic levels is not warranted and consideration should be given to combination or alternate therapy. In all cases, the physician should carefully consider the patient response and evidence of toxicity along with blood levels in determining optimal quinidine therapy.

INDICATIONS AND USAGE

QUINAGLUTE® DURA-TABS® Tablets are indicated in the prevention and/or treatment of:
1. Ventricular arrhythmias
   Premature ventricular contractions
   Ventricular tachycardia (when not associated with complete heartblock)
2. Junctional (nodal) arrhythmias
   AV junctional premature complexes
   Paroxysmal junctional tachycardia
3. Supraventricular (atrial) arrhythmias
   Premature atrial contractions
   Paroxysmal atrial tachycardia
   Atrial flutter
   Atrial fibrillation (chronic and paroxysmal)

CONTRAINDICATIONS

1. Idiosyncrasy or hypersensitivity to quinidine.
2. Complete AV block.
3. Complete bundle branch block or other severe intraventricular conduction defects, especially those exhibiting a marked grade of QRS widening.
4. Digitalis intoxication manifested by AV conduction disorders.
5. Myasthenia gravis.
6. Aberrant impulses and abnormal rhythms due to escape mechanisms.

WARNINGS

1. In the treatment of atrial flutter, reversion to sinus rhythm may be preceded by a progressive reduction in the degree of AV block to a 1:1 ratio resulting in an extremely rapid ventricular rate. This possible hazard may be reduced by digitalization prior to administration of quinidine.
2. Recent reports indicate that plasma concentrations of digoxin increase and may even double when quinidine is administered concurrently. Patients on concomitant therapy should be carefully monitored. Reduction of digoxin dosage may have to be considered.
3. Manifestations of quinidine cardiotoxicity such as excessive prolongation of the QT interval, widening of the QRS complex and ventricular tachyarrhythmias mandate immediate discontinuation of the drug and/or close clinical and electrocardiographic monitoring.
4. In susceptible individuals, such as those with marginally compensated cardiovascular disease, quinidine may produce clinically important depression of cardiac function such as hypotension, bradycardia, or heartblock. Quinidine therapy should be carefully monitored in such individuals.
5. Quinidine should be used with extreme caution in patients with incomplete AV block since complete block and asystole may be produced. Quinidine may cause abnormalities of cardiac rhythm in digitalized patients and therefore should be used with caution in the presence of digitalis intoxication.
6. Quinidine should be used with caution in patients exhibiting renal, cardiac or hepatic insufficiency because of potential accumulation of quinidine in plasma leading to toxicity.
7. Patients taking quinidine occasionally have syncopal episodes, usually resulting from ventricular tachycardia or fibrillation. This syndrome has not been shown to be related to dose or plasma levels. Syncopal episodes frequently terminate spontaneously or in response to treatment, but sometimes are fatal.
8. A few cases of hepatotoxicity, including granulomatous hepatitis, due to quinidine hypersensitivity have been reported in patients taking quinidine. Unexplained fever and/or elevation of hepatic enzymes, particularly in the early stages of therapy, warrant consideration of possible hepatotoxicity. Monitoring liver function during the first 4 to 8 weeks should be considered. Cessation of quinidine in these cases usually results in the disappearance of toxicity.

PRECAUTIONS

General: The precautions to be observed include all those applicable to quinidine. A preliminary test dose of a single tablet of quinidine sulfate may be administered to determine if the patient has an idiosyncrasy to quinidine. Hypersensitivity to quinidine, although rare, should constantly be considered, especially during the first weeks of therapy. Hospitalization for close clinical observation, electrocardiographic monitoring, and possible determination of plasma

quinidine levels is indicated when large doses are used, or with patients who present an increased risk.

Information for Patients: As with all solid oral dosage medications, QUINAGLUTE® DURA-TABS® Tablets should be taken with an adequate amount of fluid, preferably in an upright position, to facilitate swallowing.

Drug Interactions:

Drug	Effect
Quinidine with anti-cholinergic drugs	Additive vagolytic effect
Quinidine with cholinergic drugs	Antagonism of cholinergic effects
Quinidine with carbonic anhydrase inhibitors, sodium bicarbonate, thiazide diuretics	Alkalinization of urine resulting in decreased excretion of quinidine
Quinidine with coumarin anticoagulants	Reduction of clotting factor concentrations
Quinidine with tubocurare, succinylcholine and decamethonium	Potentiation of neuromuscular blockade
Quinidine with phenothiazines and reserpine	Additive cardiac depressive effects
Quinidine with hepatic enzyme-inducing drugs (phenobarbital, phenytoin, rifampin)	Potential for reduction of quinidine plasma levels
Quinidine with cimetidine	Potential for elevation of quinidine plasma levels
Quinidine with digoxin	Increased plasma concentrations of digoxin (See WARNINGS)

Carcinogenesis, Mutagenesis and Impairment of Fertility: Long-term studies in animals have not been performed to evaluate the carcinogenic potential of quinidine. There is currently no evidence of quinidine-induced mutageness or impairment of fertility.

Pregnancy: Teratogenic Effects: Pregnancy Category C. Animal reproduction studies have not been conducted with quinidine. There are no adequate and well-controlled studies in pregnant women. QUINAGLUTE® DURA-TABS® Tablets should be administered to a pregnant woman only if clearly indicated.

Nonteratogenic Effects: Like quinine, quinidine has been reported to have oxytocic properties. The significance of this property in the clinical setting has not been established.

Nursing Mothers: Because of passage of the drug into breast milk, caution should be exercised when QUINAGLUTE® DURA-TABS® Tablets are administered to a nursing woman.

Pediatric Use: There are no adequate and well-controlled studies establishing the safety and effectiveness of QUINAGLUTE® DURA-TABS® Tablets in children.

ADVERSE REACTIONS

Symptoms of cinchonism, ringing in ears, headache, nausea, and/or disturbed vision may appear in sensitive patients after a single dose of the drug.

The most frequently encountered side effects to quinidine are gastrointestinal in nature. These gastrointestinal effects include nausea, vomiting, abdominal pain, diarrhea, and rarely, esophagitis.

Less frequently encountered adverse reactions:

Cardiovascular: Widening of QRS complex, cardiac asystole, ventricular ectopic beats, idioventricular rhythms including ventricular tachycardia and fibrillation, paradoxical tachycardia, arterial embolism and hypotension.

Hematologic: Acute hemolytic anemia, hypoprothrombinemia, thrombocytopenia (purpura), agranulocytosis.

Central Nervous System: Headache, fever, vertigo, apprehension, excitement, confusion, delirium and syncope, disturbed hearing (tinnitus, decreased auditory acuity), disturbed vision (mydriasis, blurred vision, disturbed color perception, reduced vision field, photophobia, diplopia, night blindness, scotomata), optic neuritis.

Dermatologic: Rash, cutaneous flushing with intense pruritus, urticaria. Photosensitivity has also been reported.

Hypersensitivity Reactions: Angioedema, acute asthmatic episode, vascular collapse, respiratory arrest, hepatotoxicity including granulomatous hepatitis (See WARNINGS). Although rare, there have been reports of lupus erythematosus in patients taking quinidine.

OVERDOSAGE

If ingestion of quinidine is recent, gastric lavage, emesis and/or administration of activated charcoal may reduce absorption. Management of overdosage includes symptomatic treatment, ECG and blood pressure monitoring, cardiac pacing if indicated, and acidification of the urine. Artificial respiration and other supportive measures may be required.

IV infusion of ⅙ molar sodium lactate reportedly reduces the cardiotoxic effects of quinidine. Since marked CNS depression may occur even in the presence of convulsions, CNS depressants should not be administered. Hypotension may be treated, if necessary, with metaraminol or norepinephrine after adequate fluid volume replacement. Hemodialysis has been reported to be effective in the treatment of quinidine overdosage in adults and children, but is rarely warranted.

DOSAGE AND ADMINISTRATION

The dosage varies considerably depending upon the general condition and cardiovascular state of the patient. The quantity and frequency of administration of QUINAGLUTE® DURA-TABS® Tablets that will achieve the desired clinical results must be determined for each patient.

The ideal dosage is the minimum amount of total dose and frequency of daily administration that will prevent premature contractions, paroxysmal tachycardias and maintain normal sinus rhythm.

Prevention of premature atrial, nodal or ventricular contractions:

    1 to 2 tablets every 8 or 12 hours.

Maintenance of normal sinus rhythm following conversion of paroxysmal tachycardias:

    2 tablets every 12 hours or 1 ½ to 2 tablets every 8 hours are usually required.

Although most patients may be maintained in normal rhythm on a dosage of 1 QUINAGLUTE® DURA-TABS® Tablet every 8 or 12 hours, other patients may require larger doses or more frequent administration (ie every 6 hours) than the usually recommended schedule. Such increased dosage should be instituted only after careful clinical and laboratory evaluation of the patient, including monitoring of plasma quinidine levels and, if possible, serial electrocardiograms.

QUINAGLUTE® DURA-TABS® Tablets are generally well tolerated. Gastrointestinal disturbances, if they occur, may be minimized by administering the drug with food.

It is frequently desirable to determine if a patient can tolerate maintenance quinidine therapy prior to electrical conversion. Therefore, maintenance therapy may be initiated 2 to 3 days before electrical conversion is attempted. QUINAGLUTE® DURA-TABS® Tablets are well suited for such a program and can be administered at a maintenance dose felt necessary for a given patient as indicated above.

Note: Dosage may be titrated by breaking the tablet in half. Do not crush or chew since sustained-release properties will be lost.

HOW SUPPLIED

White to off-white round tablet imprinted with:

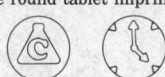

In bottles of:
100 Tablets	....	NDC 50419-101-10
250 Tablets	....	NDC 50419-101-25
		NSN 6505-00-728-2009
500 Tablets	....	NDC 50419-101-50
Unit Dose Boxes		
of 100	....	NDC 50419-101-11

Store at controlled room temperature, between 15° and 30°C (59° and 86°F).

Caution: Federal law prohibits dispensing without prescription.

* Tablet designs are registered trademarks of Berlex Laboratories, Inc.

Revised 4/89   60536-7

Shown in Product Identification Section, page 405

TRI–LEVLEN® 21   ℞
[trī-lĕvlĕn]
Tablets
(levonorgestrel and ethinyl estradiol tablets—triphasic regimen)

TRI–LEVLEN® 28   ℞
[trī-lĕvlĕn]
Tablets
(levonorgestrel and ethinyl estradiol tablets—triphasic regimen)

LEVLEN® 21   ℞
[lĕvlĕn]
Tablets
(levonorgestrel and ethinyl estradiol tablets)

LEVLEN® 28   ℞
[lĕvlĕn]
Tablets
(levonorgestrel and ethinyl estradiol tablets)

DESCRIPTION

TRI-LEVLEN® 21 tablets

Each cycle of TRI-LEVLEN® 21 (Levonorgestrel and Ethinyl Estradiol Tablets—Triphasic Regimen) tablets consists of three different drug phases as follows: Phase 1 comprised of 6 brown tablets, each containing 0.050 mg of levonorgestrel (d(-)-13 beta-ethyl-17-alpha-ethinyl-17-beta-hydroxygon-4-en-3-one), a totally synthetic progestogen, and 0.030 mg of ethinyl estradiol (19-nor-17α-pregna-1,3,5(10)-trien-20-yne-3,17-diol); phase 2 comprised of 5 white tablets, each containing 0.075 mg levonorgestrel and 0.040 mg ethinyl estradiol; and, phase 3 comprised of 10 light-yellow tablets, each containing 0.125 mg levonorgestrel and 0.030 mg ethinyl estradiol. The inactive ingredients present are calcium carbonate, glycerin, iron oxides, lactose, magnesium stearate, methylparaben, polyethylene glycol, povidone, propylparaben, sodium benzoate, starch, sucrose, talc, and titanium dioxide.

TRI-LEVLEN® 28 tablets

Each cycle of TRI-LEVLEN® 28 (Levonorgestrel and Ethinyl Estradiol Tablets—Triphasic Regimen) tablets consists of three different drug phases as follows: Phase 1 comprised of 6 brown tablets, each containing 0.050 mg of levonorgestrel (d(-)-13 beta-ethyl-17-alpha-ethinyl-17-beta-hydroxygon-4-en-3-one), a totally synthetic progestogen, and 0.030 mg of ethinyl estradiol (19-nor-17 α-pregna-1,3,5(10)-trien-20-yne-3, 17-diol); phase 2 comprised of 5 white tablets, each containing 0.075 mg levonorgestrel and 0.040 mg ethinyl estradiol; and phase 3 comprised of 10 light-yellow tablets, each containing 0.125 mg levonorgestrel and 0.030 mg ethinyl estradiol; then followed by 7 light-green inert tablets. The inactive ingredients present are calcium carbonate, cellulose, FD&C Blue 1, glycerin, iron oxides, lactose, magnesium stearate, methylparaben, polyethylene glycol, povidone, propylparaben, sodium benzoate, starch, sucrose, talc, and titanium dioxide.

LEVLEN® 21 tablets:

Each LEVLEN® 21 tablet (Levonorgestrel and Ethinyl Estradiol Tablets) contains 0.15 mg of levonorgestrel (d(-)-13 beta-ethyl-17-alpha-ethinyl-17-beta-hydroxygon-4-en-3-one), a totally synthetic progestogen, and 0.03 mg of ethinyl estradiol (19-nor-17 α-pregna-1,3,5(10)-trien-20-yne-3, 17-diol). The inactive ingredients present are cellulose, FD&C Yellow 6, lactose, magnesium stearate, and polacrillin potassium.

LEVLEN® 28 tablets:

21 light-orange LEVLEN® tablets (Levonorgestrel and Ethinyl Estradiol Tablets), each containing 0.15 mg of levonorgestrel (d(-)-13 beta-ethyl-17-alpha-ethinyl-17-beta-hydroxygon-4-en-3-one), a totally synthetic progestogen, and 0.03 mg of ethinyl estradiol (19-nor-17 α-pregna-1,3,5(10)-trien-20-yne-3, 17-diol), and 7 pink inert tablets. The inactive ingredients present are cellulose, D&C Red 30, FD&C Yellow 6, lactose, magnesium stearate, and polacrillin potassium.

Levonorgestrel   Ethinyl Estradiol

CLINICAL PHARMACOLOGY

Combination oral contraceptives act by suppression of gonadotropins. Although the primary mechanism of this action is inhibition of ovulation, other alterations include changes in the cervical mucus (which increase the difficulty of sperm entry into the uterus) and the endometrium (which reduce the likelihood of implantation).

INDICATIONS AND USAGE

Oral contraceptives are indicated for the prevention of pregnancy in women who elect to use this product as a method of contraception.

Continued on next page

Information on the Berlex products appearing here is based on the labeling in effect on June 1, 1992. Further information for these and other products may be obtained from the Medical Affairs Department, Berlex Laboratories, 300 Fairfield Road, Wayne, New Jersey 07470, (201) 292-3007. Information on oncology products may be obtained from Berlex Laboratories, 15049 San Pablo Avenue, Richmond, California 94804-0016 1-800-888-4112.

Berlex Laboratories—Cont.

Oral contraceptives are highly effective. Table I lists the typical accidental pregnancy rates for users of combination oral contraceptives and other methods of contraception. The efficacy of these contraceptive methods, except sterilization and the IUD, depends upon the reliability with which they are used. Correct and consistent use of methods can result in lower failure rates.

TABLE I: LOWEST EXPECTED AND TYPICAL FAILURE RATES DURING THE FIRST YEAR OF CONTINUOUS USE OF A METHOD

% of Women Experiencing an Accidental Pregnancy in the First Year of Continuous Use

Method	Lowest Expected*	Typical**
(No Contraception)	(89)	(89)
Oral contraceptives		3
combined	0.1	N/A***
progestin only	0.5	N/A***
Diaphragm with spermicidal cream or jelly	3	18
Spermicides alone (foam, creams, jellies and vaginal suppositories)	3	21
Vaginal Sponge		
nulliparous	5	18
multiparous	>8	>28
IUD (medicated)	1	6#
Condom without spermicides	2	12
Periodic abstinence (all methods)	2–10	20
Female sterilization	0.2	0.4
Male sterilization	0.1	0.15

Adapted from J. Trussell and K. Kost, Table II, Studies in Family Planning, *18(5)*, Sept.–Oct. 1987.

* The authors' best guess of the percentage of women expected to experience an accidental pregnancy among couples who initiate a method (not necessarily for the first time) and who use it consistently and correctly during the first year if they do not stop for any other reason.

** This term represents "typical" couples who initiate use of a method (not necessarily for the first time), who experience an accidental pregnancy during the first year if they do not stop use for any other reason.

*** N/A—Data not available.

Combined typical rate for both medicated and non-medicated IUD. The rate for medicated IUD alone is not available.

CONTRAINDICATIONS

Oral contraceptives should not be used in women with any of the following conditions:
  Thrombophlebitis or thromboembolic disorders.
  A past history of deep-vein thrombophlebitis or thrombo-embolic disorders.
  Cerebral-vascular or coronary-artery disease.
  Known or suspected carcinoma of the breast.
  Carcinoma of the endometrium or other known or suspected estrogen-dependent neoplasia.
  Undiagnosed abnormal genital bleeding.
  Cholestatic jaundice of pregnancy or jaundice with prior pill use.
  Hepatic adenomas or carcinomas.
  Known or suspected pregnancy.

WARNINGS

> Cigarette smoking increases the risk of serious cardio-vascular side effects from oral-contraceptive use. This risk increases with age and with heavy smoking (15 or more cigarettes per day) and is quite marked in women over 35 years of age. Women who use oral contraceptives should be strongly advised not to smoke.

The use of oral contraceptives is associated with increased risks of several serious conditions including myocardial infarction, thromboembolism, stroke, hepatic neoplasia, gall-bladder disease, and hypertension, although the risk of serious morbidity or mortality is very small in healthy women without underlying risk factors. The risk of morbidity and mortality increases significantly in the presence of other underlying risk factors such as hypertension, hyper-lipidemias, obesity and diabetes.

Practitioners prescribing oral contraceptives should be familiar with the following information relating to these risks. The information contained in this package insert is based principally on studies carried out in patients who used oral contraceptives with higher formulations of estrogens and

progestogens than those in common use today. The effect of long-term use of the oral contraceptives with lower formulations of both estrogens and progestogens remains to be determined.

Throughout this labeling, epidemiological studies reported are of two types: retrospective or case control studies and prospective or cohort studies. Case control studies provide a measure of the relative risk of disease, namely, a ratio of the incidence of a disease among oral-contraceptive users to that among nonusers. The relative risk does not provide information on the actual clinical occurrence of a disease. Cohort studies provide a measure of attributable risk, which is the difference in the incidence of disease between oral-contraceptive users and nonusers. The attributable risk does provide information about the actual occurrence of a disease in the population. For further information, the reader is referred to a text on epidemiological methods.

1. *Thromboembolic Disorders and Other Vascular Problems*
a. *Myocardial Infarction*
An increased risk of myocardial infarction has been attributed to oral-contraceptive use. This risk is primarily in smokers or women with other underlying risk factors for coronary-artery disease such as hypertension, hypercholesterolemia, morbid obesity, and diabetes. The relative risk of heart attack for current oral-contraceptive users has been estimated to be two to six. The risk is very low under the age of 30.

Smoking in combination with oral-contraceptive use has been shown to contribute substantially to the incidence of myocardial infarctions in women in their mid-thirties or older with smoking accounting for the majority of excess cases. Mortality rates associated with circulatory disease have been shown to increase substantially in smokers over the age of 35 and nonsmokers over the age of 40 (Table II) among women who use oral contraceptives.

TABLE II. (Adapted from P.M. Layde and V. Beral, Lancet, *1* :541–546, 1981.)

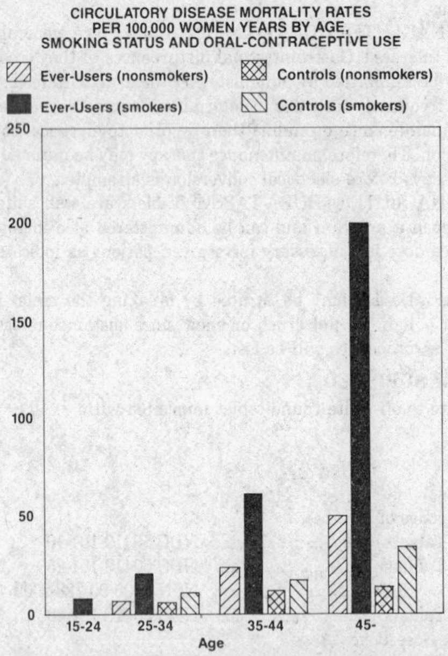

CIRCULATORY DISEASE MORTALITY RATES PER 100,000 WOMEN YEARS BY AGE, SMOKING STATUS AND ORAL-CONTRACEPTIVE USE

Ever-Users (nonsmokers)   Controls (nonsmokers)
Ever-Users (smokers)   Controls (smokers)

Oral contraceptives may compound the effects of well-known risk factors, such as hypertension, diabetes, hyperlipidemias, age and obesity. In particular, some progestogens are known to decrease HDL cholesterol and cause glucose intolerance, while estrogens may create a state of hyperinsulinism. Oral contraceptives have been shown to increase blood pressure among users (see section 9 in "Warnings"). Similar effects on risk factors have been associated with an increased risk of heart disease. Oral contraceptives must be used with caution in women with cardiovascular disease risk factors.
b. *Thromboembolism*
An increased risk of thromboembolic and thrombotic disease associated with the use of oral contraceptives is well established. Case control studies have found the relative risk of users compared to nonusers to be 3 for the first episode of superficial venous thrombosis, 4 to 11 for deep vein thrombosis or pulmonary embolism, and 1.5 to 6 for women with predisposing conditions for venous thromboembolic disease. Cohort studies have shown the relative risk to be somewhat lower, about 3 for new cases and about 4.5 for new cases requiring hospitalization. The risk of thromboembolic disease due to oral contraceptives is not related to length of use and disappears after pill use is stopped.
A two- to four-fold increase in relative risk of postoperative thromboembolic complications has been reported with the use of oral contraceptives. The relative risk of venous throm-

bosis in women who have predisposing conditions is twice that of women without such medical conditions. If feasible, oral contraceptives should be discontinued at least four weeks prior to and for two weeks after elective surgery of a type associated with an increase in risk of thromboembolism and during and following prolonged immobilization. Since the immediate post partum period is also associated with an increased risk of thromboembolism, oral contraceptives should be started no earlier than four to six weeks after delivery in women who elect not to breast-feed, or a midtrimester pregnancy termination.
c. *Cerebrovascular diseases*
Oral contraceptives have been shown to increase both the relative and attributable risks of cerebrovascular events (thrombotic and hemorrhagic strokes), although, in general, the risk is greatest among older (> 35 years), hypertensive women who also smoke. Hypertension was found to be a risk factor for both users and nonusers, for both types of strokes, while smoking interacted to increase the risk for hemorrhagic strokes.
In a large study, the relative risk of thrombotic strokes has been shown to range from 3 for normotensive users to 14 for users with severe hypertension. The relative risk of hemorrhagic stroke is reported to be 1.2 for normotensive users who used oral contraceptives, 2.6 for smokers who did not use oral contraceptives, 7.6 for smokers who used oral contraceptives, 1.8 for normotensive users and 25.7 for users with severe hypertension. The attributable risk is also greater in older women.
d. *Dose-related risk of vascular disease from oral contraceptives*
A positive association has been observed between the amount of estrogen and progestogen in oral contraceptives and the risk of vascular disease. A decline in serum high-density lipoproteins (HDL) has been reported with many progestational agents. A decline in serum high-density lipoproteins has been associated with an increased incidence of ischemic heart disease. Because estrogens increase HDL cholesterol, the net effect of an oral contraceptive depends on a balance achieved between doses of estrogen and progestogen and the nature and absolute amount of progestogen used in the contraceptive. The amount of both hormones should be considered in the choice of an oral contraceptive.
Minimizing exposure to estrogen and progestogen is in keeping with good principles of therapeutics. For any particular estrogen/progestogen combination, the dosage regimen prescribed should be one which contains the least amount of estrogen and progestogen that is compatible with a low failure rate and the needs of the individual patient. New acceptors of oral-contraceptive agents should be started on preparations containing less than 50 mcg of estrogen.
e. *Persistence of risk of vascular disease*
There are two studies which have shown persistence of risk of vascular disease for ever-users of oral contraceptives. In a study in the United States, the risk of developing myocardial infarction after discontinuing oral contraceptives persists for at least 9 years for women 40–49 years who had used oral contraceptives for five or more years, but this increased risk was not demonstrated in other age groups. In another study in Great Britain, the risk of developing cerebrovascular disease persisted for at least 6 years after discontinuation of oral contraceptives, although excess risk was very small. However, both studies were performed with oral contraceptive formulations containing 50 micrograms or higher of estrogens.
2. *Estimates of Mortality from Contraceptive Use*
One study gathered data from a variety of sources which have estimated the mortality rate associated with different methods of contraception at different ages (Table III). These estimates include the combined risk of death associated with contraceptive methods plus the risk attributable to pregnancy in the event of method failure. Each method of contraception has its specific benefits and risks. The study concluded that with the exception of oral-contraceptive users 35 and older who smoke and 40 and older who do not smoke, mortality associated with all methods of birth control is less than that associated with childbirth. The observation of a possible increase in risk of mortality with age for oral-contraceptive users is based on data gathered in the 1970's—but not reported until 1983. However, current clinical practice involves the use of lower estrogen dose formulations combined with careful restriction of oral-contraceptive use to women who do not have the various risk factors listed in this labeling.
Because of these changes in practice and, also, because of some limited new data which suggest that the risk of cardiovascular disease with the use of oral contraceptives may now be less than previously observed, the Fertility and Maternal Health Drugs Advisory Committee was asked to review the topic in 1989. The Committee concluded that although cardiovascular disease risks may be increased with oral-contraceptive use after age 40 in healthy nonsmoking women (even with the newer low-dose formulations), there are greater potential health risks associated with pregnancy in older women and with the alternative surgical and medical procedures which may be necessary if such women do not have

access to effective and acceptable means of contraception. Therefore, the Committee recommended that the benefits of oral-contraceptive use by healthy nonsmoking women over 40 may outweigh the possible risks. Of course, older women, as all women who take oral contraceptives, should take the lowest possible dose formulation that is effective.

[See table at right.]

3. *Carcinoma of the Reproductive Organs*

Numerous epidemiological studies have been performed on the incidence of breast, endometrial, ovarian and cervical cancer in women using oral contraceptives. The overwhelming evidence in the literature suggests that use of oral contraceptives is not associated with an increase in the risk of developing breast cancer, regardless of the age and parity of first use or with most of the marketed brands and doses. The Cancer and Steroid Hormone (CASH) study also showed no latent effect on the risk of breast cancer for at least a decade following long-term use. A few studies have shown a slightly increased relative risk of developing breast cancer, although the methodology of these studies, which included differences in examination of users and nonusers and differences in age at start of use, has been questioned.

Some studies suggest that oral-contraceptive use has been associated with an increase in the risk of cervical intraepithelial neoplasia in some populations of women. However, there continues to be controversy about the extent to which such findings may be due to differences in sexual behavior and other factors.

In spite of many studies of the relationship between oral-contraceptive use and breast and cervical cancers, a cause-and-effect relationship has not been established.

4. *Hepatic Neoplasia*

Benign hepatic adenomas are associated with oral-contraceptive use, although the incidence of benign tumors is rare in the United States. Indirect calculations have estimated the attributable risk to be in the range of 3.3 cases/100,000 for users, a risk that increases after four or more years of use. Rupture of rare, benign, hepatic adenomas may cause death through intra-abdominal hemorrhage.

Studies from Britain have shown an increased risk of developing hepatocellular carcinoma in long-term (>8 years) oral-contraceptive users. However, these cancers are extremely rare in the U.S. and the attributable risk (the excess incidence) of liver cancers in oral-contraceptive users approaches less than one per million users.

5. *Ocular Lesions*

There have been clincial case reports of retinal thrombosis associated with the use of oral contraceptives. Oral contraceptives should be discontinued if there is unexplained partial or complete loss of vision; onset of proptosis or diplopia; papilledema; or retinal vascular lesions. Appropriate diagnostic and therapeutic measures should be undertaken immediately.

6. *Oral-Contraceptive Use Before or During Early Pregnancy*

Extensive epidemiological studies have revealed no increased risk of birth defects in women who have used oral contraceptives prior to pregnancy. Studies also do not suggest a teratogenic effect, particularly insofar as cardiac anomalies and limb-reduction defects are concerned, when taken inadvertently during early pregnancy.

The administration of oral contraceptives to induce withdrawal bleeding should not be used as a test for pregnancy. Oral contraceptives should not be used during pregnancy to treat threatened or habitual abortion.

It is recommended that for any patient who has missed two consecutive periods, pregnancy should be ruled out before continuing oral-contraceptive use. If the patient has not adhered to the prescribed schedule, the possibility of pregnancy should be considered at the time of the first missed period. Oral-contraceptive use should be discontinued if pregnancy is confirmed.

7. *Gallbladder Disease*

Earlier studies have reported an increased lifetime relative risk of gallbladder surgery in users of oral contraceptives and estrogens. More recent studies, however, have shown that the relative risk of developing gallbladder disease among oral-contraceptive users may be minimal. The recent findings of minimal risk may be related to the use of oral-contraceptive formulations containing lower hormonal doses of estrogens and progestogens.

8. *Carbohydrate and Lipid Metabolic Effects*

Oral contraceptives have been shown to cause glucose intolerance in a significant percentage of users. Oral contraceptives containing greater than 75 micrograms of estrogens cause hyperinsulinism, while lower doses of estrogen cause less glucose intolerance. Progestogens increase insulin secretion and create insulin resistance, this effect varying with different progestational agents. However, in the nondiabetic woman, oral contraceptives appear to have no effect on fasting blood glucose. Because of these demonstrated effects, prediabetic and diabetic women should be carefully observed while taking oral contraceptives.

A small proportion of women will have persistent hypertriglyceridemia while on the pill. As discussed earlier (see "Warnings" 1a. and 1d.), changes in serum triglycerides and

TABLE III—ANNUAL NUMBER OF BIRTH-RELATED OR METHOD-RELATED DEATHS ASSOCIATED WITH CONTROL OF FERTILITY PER 100,000 NONSTERILE WOMEN, BY FERTILITY-CONTROL METHOD ACCORDING TO AGE

Method of control and outcome	15–19	20–24	25–29	30–34	35–39	40–44
No fertility—control methods*	7.0	7.4	9.1	14.8	25.7	28.2
Oral contraceptives nonsmoker**	0.3	0.5	0.9	1.9	13.8	31.6
Oral contraceptives smoker**	2.2	3.4	6.6	13.5	51.1	117.2
IUD**	0.8	0.8	1.0	1.0	1.4	1.4
Condom*	1.1	1.6	0.7	0.2	0.3	0.4
Diaphragm/spermicide*	1.9	1.2	1.2	1.3	2.2	2.8
Periodic abstinence*	2.5	1.6	1.6	1.7	2.9	3.6

* Deaths are birth related

** Deaths are method related

Adapted from H.W. Ory, Family Planning Perspectives *15*:57–63, 1983.

lipoprotein levels have been reported in oral-contraceptive users.

9. *Elevated Blood Pressure*

An increase in blood pressure has been reported in women taking oral contraceptives and this increase is more likely in older oral-contraceptive users and with continued use. Data from the Royal College of General Practitioners and subsequent randomized trials have shown that the incidence of hypertension increases with increasing quantities of progestogens.

Women with a history of hypertension or hypertension-related diseases, or renal disease should be encouraged to use another method of contraception. If women with hypertertension elect to use oral contraceptives, they should be monitored closely, and if significant elevation of blood pressure occurs, oral contraceptives should be discontinued. For most women, elevated blood pressure will return to normal after stopping oral contraceptives, and there is no difference in the occurrence of hypertension among ever- and never-users.

10. *Headache*

The onset or exacerbation of migraine or development of headache with a new pattern that is recurrent, persistent, or severe requires discontinuation of oral contraceptives and evaluation of the cause.

11. *Bleeding Irregularities*

Breakthrough bleeding and spotting are sometimes encountered in patients on oral contraceptives, especially during the first three months of use. The type and dose of progestogen may be important. Nonhormonal causes should be considered and adequate diagnostic measures taken to rule out malignancy or pregnancy in the event of breakthrough bleeding, as in the case of any abnormal vaginal bleeding. If pathology has been excluded, time or a change to another formulation may solve the problem. In the event of amenorrhea, pregnancy should be ruled out.

Some women may encounter post-pill amenorrhea or oligomenorrhea, especially when such a condition was preexistent.

PRECAUTIONS

1. PHYSICAL EXAMINATION AND FOLLOW UP

A complete medical history and physical examination should be taken prior to the initiation or reinstitution of oral contraceptives and at least annually during use of oral contraceptives. These physical examinations should include special reference to blood pressure, breasts, abdomen and pelvic organs, including cervical cytology, and relevant laboratory tests. In case of undiagnosed, persistent, or recurrent abnormal vaginal bleeding, appropriate diagnostic measures should be conducted to rule out malignancy. Women with a strong family history of breast cancer or who have breast nodules should be monitored with particular care.

2. LIPID DISORDERS

Women who are being treated for hyperlipidemias should be followed closely if they elect to use oral contraceptives. Some progestogens may elevate LDL levels and may render the control of hyperlipidemias more difficult. (See "Warnings" 1d.)

3. LIVER FUNCTION

If jaundice develops in any woman receiving such drugs, the medication should be discontinued. Steroid hormones may be poorly metabolized in patients with impaired liver function.

4. FLUID RETENTION

Oral contraceptives may cause some degree of fluid retention. They should be prescribed with caution, and only with careful monitoring, in patients with conditions which might be aggravated by fluid retention.

5. EMOTIONAL DISORDERS

Patients becoming significantly depressed while taking oral contraceptives should stop the medication and use an alternate method of contraception in an attempt to determine whether the symptom is drug related. Women with a history of depression should be carefully observed and the drug discontinued if depression recurs to a serious degree.

6. CONTACT LENSES

Contact-lens wearers who develop visual changes or changes in lens tolerance should be assessed by an ophthalmologist.

7. DRUG INTERACTIONS

Reduced efficacy and increased incidence of breakthrough bleeding and menstrual irregularities have been associated with concomitant use of rifampin. A similar assocation, though less marked, has been suggested with barbiturates, phenylbutazone, phenytoin sodium, and possibly with griseofulvin, ampicillin, and tetracyclines.

8. INTERACTIONS WITH LABORATORY TESTS

Certain endocrine- and liver-function tests and blood components may be affected by oral contraceptives:

a. Increased prothrombin and factors VII, VIII, IX, and X; decreased antithrombin 3; increased norepinephrine-induced platelet aggregability.

b. Increased thyroid-binding globulin (TBG) leading to increased circulating total thyroid hormone, as measured by protein-bound iodine (PBI), T4 by column or by radioimmunoassay. Free T3 resin uptake is decreased, reflecting the elevated TBG, free T4 concentration is unaltered.

c. Other binding proteins may be elevated in serum.

d. Sex-binding globulins are increased and result in elevated levels of total circulating sex steroids and corticoids; however, free or biologically active levels remain unchanged.

e. Triglycerides may be increased.

f. Glucose tolerance may be decreased.

g. Serum folate levels may be depressed by oral-contraceptive therapy. This may be of clinical significance if a woman becomes pregnant shortly after discontinuing oral contraceptives.

9. *Carcinogenesis*

See "Warnings" section.

10. *Pregnancy*

Pregnancy Category X. See "Contraindications" and "Warnings" sections.

11. *Nursing Mothers*

Small amounts of oral-contraceptive steroids have been identified in the milk of nursing mothers and a few adverse effects on the child have been reported, including jaundice and breast enlargement. In addition, oral contraceptives given in the postpartum period may interfere with lactation by decreasing the quantity and quality of breast milk. If possible, the nursing mother should be advised not to use oral contraceptives but to use other forms of contraception until she has completely weaned her child.

INFORMATION FOR THE PATIENT

See Patient Labeling Printed Below.

ADVERSE REACTIONS

An increased risk of the following serious adverse reactions has been associated with the use of oral contraceptives (see "Warnings" Section).

Thrombophlebitis	Cerebral thrombosis
Aterial thromboembolism	Hypertension
Pulmonary embolism	Gallbladder disease
Myocardial infarction	Hepatic adenomas or benign liver tumors
Cerebral hemorrhage	

Continued on next page

Information on the Berlex products appearing here is based on the labeling in effect on June 1, 1992. Further information for these and other products may be obtained from the Medical Affairs Department, Berlex Laboratories, 300 Fairfield Road, Wayne, New Jersey 07470, (201) 292-3007. Information on oncology products may be obtained from Berlex Laboratories, 15049 San Pablo Avenue, Richmond, California 94804-0016 1-800-888-4112.

Berlex Laboratories—Cont.

There is evidence of an association between the following conditions and the use of oral contraceptives, although additional confirmatory studies are needed:

- Mesenteric thrombosis
- Retinal thrombosis

The following adverse reactions have been reported in patients receiving oral contraceptives and are believed to be drug related:

- Nausea
- Vomiting
- Gastrointestinal symptoms (such as abdominal cramps and bloating)
- Breakthrough bleeding
- Spotting
- Change in menstrual flow
- Amenorrhea
- Temporary infertility after discontinuation of treatment
- Edema
- Melasma which may persist
- Breast changes: tenderness, enlargement, and secretion
- Change in weight (increase or decrease)
- Change in cervical erosion and cervical secretion
- Diminution in lactation when given immediately postpartum
- Cholestatic jaundice
- Migraine
- Rash (allergic)
- Mental depression
- Reduced tolerance to carbohydrates
- Vaginal candidiasis
- Change in corneal curvature (steepening)
- Intolerance to contact lenses

The following adverse reactions have been reported in users of oral contraceptives and the association has been neither confirmed nor refuted:

Congenital anomalies	Erythema nodosum
Premenstrual syndrome	Hemorrhagic eruption
Cataracts	Vaginitis
Optic neuritis	Porphyria
Changes in appetitie	Impaired renal function
Cystitis-like syndrome	Hemolytic uremic syndrome
Headache	
Nervousness	
Dizziness	Budd-Chiari syndrome
Hirsutism	Acne
Loss of scalp hair	Changes in libido
Erythema multiforme	Colitis
Cerebral-vascular disease with mitral valve prolapse	Sickle-Cell Disease
Lupus-like Syndromes	

OVERDOSAGE

Serious ill effects have not been reported following acute ingestion of large doses of oral contraceptives by young children. Overdosage may cause nausea, and withdrawal bleeding may occur in females.

NONCONTRACEPTIVE HEALTH BENEFITS

The following noncontraceptive health benefits related to the use of oral contraceptives are supported by epidemiological studies which largely utilized oral-contraceptive formulations containing doses exceeding 0.035 mg of ethinyl estradiol or 0.05 mg of mestranol.

Effects on menses:
- increased menstrual cycle regularity
- decreased blood loss and decreased incidence of iron deficiency anemia
- decreased incidence of dysmenorrhea

Effects related to inhibition of ovulation:
- decreased incidence of functional ovarian cysts
- decreased incidence of ectopic pregnancies

Effects from long-term use:
- decreased incidence of fibroadenomas and fibrocystic disease of the breast
- decreased incidence of acute pelvic inflammatory disease
- decreased incidence of endometrial cancer
- decreased incidence of ovarian cancer

DOSAGE AND ADMINISTRATION

TRI-LEVLEN® tablets

To achieve maximum contraceptive effectiveness, TRI-LEVLEN® tablets (Levonorgestrel and Ethinyl Estradiol Tablets—Triphasic Regimen) must be taken exactly as directed and at intervals not exceeding 24 hours.

TRI-LEVLEN® 21 TABLETS (LEVONORGESTREL AND ETHINYL ESTRADIOL TABLETS—TRIPHASIC REGIMEN)

TRI-LEVLEN® 21 tablets are a three-phase preparation. The dosage of TRI-LEVLEN® 21 tablets is **one tablet daily** for 21 consecutive days per menstrual cycle in the following order: 6 brown tablets (phase 1), followed by 5 white tablets (phase 2), and then followed by the last 10 light-yellow tablets (phase 3), according to the prescribed schedule. Tablets are then discontinued for 7 days (three weeks on, one week off).

It is recommended that TRI-LEVLEN® 21 tablets be taken at the same time each day, preferably after the evening meal or at bedtime. During the first cycle of medication, the patient should be instructed to take one TRI-LEVLEN® 21 tablet daily in the order of 6 brown, 5 white and, finally, 10 light-yellow tablets for twenty-one (21) consecutive days, beginning on day one (1) of her menstrual cycle. (The first day of menstruation is day one.) The tablets are then discontinued for one week (7 days). Withdrawal bleeding usually occurs within 3 days following discontinuation of TRI-LEVLEN® 21 Tablets. (If TRI-LEVLEN® 21 tablets are first taken later than the first day of the first menstrual cycle of medication or postpartum, contraceptive reliance should not be placed on TRI-LEVLEN® 21 tablets until after the first 7 consecutive days of administration. The possibility of ovulation and conception prior to initiation of medication should be considered.)

When switching from another oral contraceptive, TRI-LEVLEN® 21 tablets should be started on the first day of bleeding following the last active tablet taken of the previous oral contraceptive.

The patient begins her next and all subsequent 21-day courses of TRI-LEVLEN® 21 tablets on the same day of the week that she began her first course, following the same schedule: 21 days on—7 days off. She begins taking her brown tablets on the 8th day after discontinuance, regardless of whether or not a menstrual period has occurred or is still in progress. Any time the next cycle of TRI-LEVLEN® 21 tablets are started later than the 8th day, the patient should be protected by another means of contraception until she has taken a tablet daily for seven consecutive days.

If spotting or breakthrough bleeding occurs, the patient is instructed to continue on the same regimen. This type of bleeding is usually transient and without significance; however, if the bleeding is persistent or prolonged, the patient is advised to consult her physician. Although the occurrence of pregnancy is highly unlikely if TRI-LEVLEN® 21 tablets are taken according to directions, if withdrawal bleeding does not occur, the possibility of pregnancy must be considered. If the patient has not adhered to the prescribed schedule (missed one or more tablets or started taking them on a day later than she should have), the probability of pregnancy should be considered at the time of the first missed period and appropriate diagnostic measures taken before the medication is resumed. If the patient has adhered to the prescribed regimen and misses two consecutive periods, pregnancy should be ruled out before continuing the contraceptive regimen.

The risk of pregnancy increases with each tablet missed. If the patient misses one tablet, she should be instructed to take it as soon as she remembers, and also to take her next tablet at the regular time, which means that she will be taking two tablets on that day. If she misses two tablets consecutively, she should take the second missed tablet as soon as she remembers, discard the first missed tablet and take her regular tablet for that day at the proper time. Furthermore, she should use an additional method of birth control in addition to taking TRI-LEVLEN® 21 until menses has appeared or pregnancy has been excluded. If breakthrough bleeding occurs following missed tablets, it will usually be transient and of no consequence. If three consecutive tablets are missed, all medication should be discontinued and the remainder of the package discarded. A new package of TRI-LEVLEN® 21 Tablets should be started on the first day of the patient's next bleed after the last tablet was taken. An alternate means of birth control should be prescribed during the days without tablets and continued until the patient has taken a tablet daily for seven consecutive days (six brown and one white).

In the nonlactating mother, TRI-LEVLEN® 21 may be initiated postpartum, for contraception. When the tablets are administered in the postpartum period, an increased risk of thromboembolic disease associated with the postpartum period must be considered (see "Contraindications," "Warnings," and "Precautions" concerning thromboembolic disease). It is to be noted that early resumption of ovulation may occur if Parlodel® (bromocriptine mesylate) has been used for the prevention of lactation.

TRI-LEVLEN® 28 TABLETS (LEVONORGESTREL AND ETHINYL ESTRADIOL TABLETS—TRIPHASIC REGIMEN)

TRI-LEVLEN® 28 tablets are a three-phase preparation plus 7 inert tablets. The dosage of TRI-LEVLEN® 28 tablets is one tablet daily for 28 consecutive days per menstrual cycle in the following order: 6 brown tablets (phase 1), followed by 5 white tablets (phase 2), followed by 10 light-yellow tablets (phase 3), plus 7 light-green inert tablets according to the prescribed schedule.

It is recommended that TRI-LEVLEN® 28 tablets be taken at the same time each day, preferably after the evening meal or at bedtime. During the first cycle of medication, the patient should be instructed to take one TRI-LEVLEN® 28 tablet daily in the order of 6 brown, 5 white, 10 light-yellow tablets, and then 7 light-green inert tablets for twenty-eight (28) consecutive days, beginning on day one (1) of her menstrual cycle. (The first day of menstruation is day one.) Withdrawal bleeding usually occurs within 3 days following the last light-yellow tablet. (If TRI-LEVLEN® 28 tablets are first taken later than the first day of the first menstrual cycle of medication or postpartum, contraceptive reliance should not be placed on TRI-LEVLEN® 28 tablets until after the first 7 consecutive days of administration. The possibility of ovulation and conception prior to initiation of medication should be considered.)

When switching from another oral contraceptive, TRI-LEVLEN® 28 tablets should be started on the first day of bleeding following the last tablet taken of the previous oral contraceptive.

The patient begins her next and all subsequent 28-day courses of TRI-LEVLEN® 28 tablets on the same day of the week that she began her first course, following the same schedule. She begins taking her brown tablets on the next day after ingestion of the last light-green tablet, regardless of whether or not a menstrual period has occurred or is still in progress. Any time a subsequent cycle of TRI-LEVLEN® 28 tablets is started later than the next day, the patient should be protected by another means of contraception until she has taken a tablet daily for seven consecutive days.

If spotting or breakthrough bleeding occurs, the patient is instructed to continue on the same regimen. This type of bleeding is usually transient and without significance; however, if the bleeding is persistent or prolonged, the patient is advised to consult her physician. Although the occurrence of pregnancy is highly unlikely if TRI-LEVLEN® 28 tablets are taken according to directions, if withdrawal bleeding does not occur, the possibility of pregnancy must be considered. If the patient has not adhered to the prescribed schedule (missed one or more tablets or started taking them on a day later than she should have), the probability of pregnancy should be considered at the time of the first missed period and appropriate diagnostic measures taken before the medication is resumed. If the patient has adhered to the prescribed regimen and misses two consecutive periods, pregnancy should be ruled out before continuing the contraceptive regimen.

The risk of pregnancy increases with each active (brown, white, or light-yellow) tablet missed. If the patient misses one active tablet, she should be instructed to take it as soon as she remembers, and also to take her next tablet at the regular time, which means that she will be taking two tablets on that day. If she misses two active tablets consecutively, she should take the second missed tablet as soon as she remembers, discard the first missed tablet and take her regular tablet for that day at the proper time. Furthermore, she should use an additional method of birth control in addition to taking TRI-LEVLEN® 28 until menses has appeared or pregnancy has been excluded. If breakthrough bleeding occurs following missed active tablets, it will usually be transient and of no consequence. If three consecutive active tablets are missed, all medication should be discontinued and the remainder of the package discarded. A new package of TRI-LEVLEN® 28 tablets should be started on the first day of the patient's next bleed after the last tablet was taken. An alternate means of birth control should be prescribed during the days without tablets and continued until the patient has taken a tablet daily for seven consecutive days (six brown, and one white). If the patient misses one or more light-green tablets, she is still protected against pregnancy provided she begins taking brown tablets again on the proper day.

In the nonlactating mother, TRI-LEVLEN® 28 may be initiated postpartum, for contraception. When the tablets are administered in the postpartum period, the increased risk of thromboembolic disease associated with the postpartum period must be considered (see "Contraindications," "Warnings," and "Precautions" concerning thromboembolic disease). It is to be noted that early resumption of ovulation may occur if Parlodel® (bromocriptine mesylate) has been used for the prevention of lactation.

LEVLEN® TABLETS

To achieve maximum contraceptive effectiveness, LEVLEN® 21 tablets and LEVLEN® 28 tablets must be taken exactly as directed and at intervals not exceeding 24 hours.

LEVLEN® 21 TABLETS (LEVONORGESTREL AND ETHINYL ESTRADIOL TABLETS)

The dosage of LEVLEN® 21 is one tablet daily for 21 consecutive days per menstrual cycle according to prescribed schedule. Tablets are then discontinued for 7 days (three weeks on, one week off).

It is recommended that LEVLEN®21 tablets be taken at the same time each day, preferably after the evening meal or at bedtime.

During the first cycle of medication, the patient is instructed to take one LEVLEN® 21 tablet daily for twenty-one consecutive days beginning on day five of her menstrual cycle. (The first day of menstruation is day one.) The tablets are then discontinued for one week (7 days). Withdrawal bleeding

should usually occur within three days following discontinuation of LEVLEN® 21 tablets.
(If LEVLEN® 21 tablets are first taken later than the fifth day of the first menstrual cycle of medication or postpartum, contraceptive reliance should not be placed on LEVLEN® 21 tablets until after the first seven consecutive days of administration. The possibility of ovulation and conception prior to initiation of medication should be considered.)
The patient begins her next and all subsequent 21-day courses of LEVLEN® 21 tablets on the same day of the week that she began her first course, following the same schedule: 21 days on—7 days off. She begins taking her tablets on the 8th day after discontinuance, regardless of whether or not a menstrual period has occurred or is still in progress. Any time a new cycle of LEVLEN® 21 tablets is started later than the 8th day, the patient should be protected by another means of contraception until she has taken a tablet daily for seven consecutive days.
If spotting or breakthrough bleeding occurs, the patient is instructed to continue on the same regimen. This type of bleeding is usually transient and without significance; however, if the bleeding is persistent or prolonged, the patient is advised to consult her physician. Although the occurrence of pregnancy is highly unlikely if LEVLEN® 21 tablets are taken according to directions, if withdrawal bleeding does not occur, the possiblity of pregnancy must be considered. If the patient has not adhered to the prescribed schedule (missed one or more tablets or started taking them on a day later than she should have), the probability of pregnancy should be considered at the time of the first missed period and appropriate diagnostic measures taken before the medication is resumed. If the patient has adhered to the prescribed regimen and misses two consecutive periods, pregnancy should be ruled out before continuing the contraceptive regimen.
The patient should be instructed to take a missed tablet as soon as it is remembered. If two consecutive tablets are missed, they should both be taken as soon as remembered. The next tablet should be taken at the usual time.
Any time the patient misses one or two tablets, she should also use another method of contraception until she has taken a tablet daily for seven consecutive days. If breakthrough bleeding occurs following missed tablets, it will usually be transient and of no consequence. While there is little likelihood of ovulation occurring if only one or two tablets are missed, the possibility of ovulation increases with each successive day that scheduled tablets are missed. If three consecutive tablets are missed, all medication should be discontinued and the remainder of the package discarded. A new tablet cycle should be started on the 8th day after the last tablet was taken and an alternate means of contraception should be prescribed during the seven days without tablets and until the patient has taken a tablet daily for seven consecutive days.
In the nonlactating mother, LEVLEN® 21 may be initiated postpartum, for contraception. When the tablets are administered in the postpartum period, the increased risk of thromboembolic disease associated with the postpartum period must be considered (see "Contraindications," "Warnings," and "Precautions" concerning thromboembolic disease). It is to be noted that early resumption of ovulation may occur if Parlodel® (bromocriptine meslyate) has been used for prevention of lactation.
LEVLEN® 28 TABLETS (LEVONORGESTREL AND ETHINYL ESTRADIOL TABLETS)
The dosage of LEVLEN® 28 tablets is one light-orange tablet daily for 21 consecutive days, followed by one pink inert tablet daily for 7 consecutive days, according to prescribed schedule. It is recommended that tablets be taken at the same time each day, preferably after the evening meal or at bedtime. During the first cycle of medication, the patient is instructed to begin taking LEVLEN® 28 tablets on the first Sunday after the onset of menstruation. If menstruation begins on a Sunday, the first tablet (light-orange) is taken that day. One light-orange tablet should be taken daily for 21 consecutive days, followed by one pink inert tablet daily for 7 consecutive days. Withdrawal bleeding should usually occur within three days following discontinuation of light-orange tablets.
During the first cycle, contraceptive reliance should not be placed on LEVLEN® 28 tablets until a light-orange tablet has been taken daily for 7 consecutive days. The possibility of ovulation and conception prior to initiation of medication should be considered.
The patient begins her next and all subsequent 28-day courses of tablets on the same day of the week (Sunday) on which she began her first course, following the same schedule: 21 days on light-orange tablets—7 days on pink inert tablets. If in any cycle the patient starts tablets later than the proper day, she should protect herself by using another method of birth control until she has taken a light-orange tablet daily for 7 consecutive days.
If spotting or breakthrough bleeding occurs, the patient is instructed to continue on the same regimen. This type of bleeding is usually transient and without significance; however, if the bleeding is persistent or prolonged, the patient is advised to consult her physician. Although the occurrence of pregnancy is highly unlikely if LEVLEN® 28 tablets are taken according to directions, if withdrawal bleeding does not occur, the possiblilty of pregnancy must be considered. If the patient has not adhered to the prescribed schedule (missed one or more tablets or started taking them on a day later than she should have), the probability of pregnancy should be considered at the time of the first missed period and appropriate diagnostic measures taken before the medication is resumed. If the patient has adhered to the prescribed regimen and misses two consecutive periods, pregnancy should be ruled out before continuing the contraceptive regimen.
The patient should be instructed to take a missed light-orange tablet as soon as it is remembered. If two consecutive light-orange tablets are missed, they should both be taken as soon as remembered. The next tablet should be taken at the usual time.
Any time the patient misses one or two light-orange tablets, she should also use another method of contraception until she has taken a light-orange tablet daily for seven consecutive days. If the patient misses one or more pink tablets, she is still protected against pregnancy **provided** she begins taking light-orange tablets again on the proper day.
If breakthrough bleeding occurs following missed light-orange tablets, it will usually be transient and of no consequence. While there is little likelihood of ovulation occurring if only one or two light-orange tablets are missed, the possibility of ovulation increases with each successive day that scheduled light-orange tablets are missed. If three consecutive light-orange LEVLEN® tablets are missed, all medication should be discontinued and the remainder of the 28-day package discarded. A new tablet cycle should be started on the first Sunday following the last missed tablet, and an alternate means of contraception should be prescribed during the days without tablets and until the patient has taken a light-orange tablet daily for 7 consecutive days.
In the nonlactating mother, LEVLEN® 28 may be initiated postpartum, for contraception. When the tablets are administered in the postpartum period, the increased risk of thromboembolic disease associated with the postpartum period must be considered (see "Contraindications," "Warnings," and "Precautions" concerning thromboembolic disease). It is to be noted that early resumption of ovulation may occur if Parlodel® (bromocriptine meslyate) has been used for prevention of lactation.

HOW SUPPLIED

TRI-LEVLEN® 21 tablets (Levonorgestrel and Ethinyl Estradiol Tablets—Triphasic Regimen), are available in packages of 3 and 6 SLIDECASE™ dispensers. Each cycle contains 21 round, coated tablets as follows:
NDC 50419-095, six brown tablets marked "B" on one side and "95" on the other side, each containing 0.050 mg levonorgestrel and 0.030 mg ethinyl estradiol;
NDC 50419-096, five white to off-white tablets marked "B" on one side and "96" on the other side, each containing 0.075 mg levonorgestrel and 0.040 mg ethinyl estradiol; and
NDC 50419-097, ten light-yellow tablets marked "B" on one side and "97" on the other side, each containing 0.125 mg levonorgestrel and 0.030 mg ethinyl estradiol.
In packages of:
3 SLIDECASE™ dispensers ....NDC 50419-430-21
6 SLIDECASE™ dispensers ....NDC 50419-430-06

TRI-LEVLEN® 28 tablets (Levonorgestrel and Ethinyl Estradiol Tablets—Triphasic Regimen), are available in packages of 3 and 6 SLIDECASE™ dispensers. Each cycle contains 28 round, coated tablets as follows:
NDC 50419-095, six brown tablets marked "B" on one side and "95" on the other side, each containing 0.050 mg levonorgestrel and 0.030 mg ethinyl estradiol;
NDC 50419-096, five white to off-white tablets marked "B" on one side and "96" on the other side, each containing 0.075 mg levonorgestrel and 0.040 mg ethinyl estradiol;
NDC 50419-097, ten light-yellow tablets marked "B" on one side and "97" on the other side, each containing 0.125 mg levonorgestrel and 0.030 mg ethinyl estradiol; and
NDC 50419-011, seven light-green inert tablets marked "B" on one side and "11" on the other side.
In packages of:
3 SLIDECASE™ dispensers ....NDC 50419-431-28
6 SLIDECASE™ dispensers ....NDC 50419-431-06

LEVLEN® 21 tablets (Levonorgestrel and Ethinyl Estradiol Tablets), are available in packages of 3 SLIDECASE™ dispensers. Each cycle contains 21 round, tablets as follows:
NDC 50419-021, 21 active, light-orange tablets marked "B" on one side and "21" on the other side, each containing 0.15 mg levonorgestrel and 0.03 mg ethinyl estradiol;
In packages of:
3 SLIDECASE™ dispensers ....NDC 50419-410-21

LEVLEN® 28 tablets (Levonorgestrel and Ethinyl Estradiol Tablets), are available in packages of 3 SLIDECASE™ dispensers. Each cycle contains 28 round tablets as follows:
NDC 50419-021, 21 active, light-orange tablets marked "B" on one side and "21" on the other side, each containing 0.15 mg levonorgestrel and 0.03 mg ethinyl estradiol;
NDC 50419-028, 7 inert pink tablets marked "B" on one side and "28" on the other side.
In packages of:
3 SLIDECASE™ dispensers ....NDC 50419-411-28

References available upon request.

Brief Summary Patient Package Insert

Oral contraceptives, also known as "birth control pills" or "the pill," are taken to prevent pregnancy and when taken correctly, have a failure rate of less than 1.0% per year when used without missing any pills. The typical failure rate of large numbers of pill users is less than 3.0% per year when women who miss pills are included. For most women oral contraceptives are also free of serious or unpleasant side effects. However, forgetting to take pills considerably increases the chances of pregnancy.
For the majority of women, oral contraceptives can be taken safely. But there are some women who are at high risk of developing certain serious diseases that can be life-threatening or may cause temporary or permanent disability or death. The risks associated with taking oral contraceptives increase significantly if you:

- smoke
- have high blood pressure, diabetes, high cholesterol
- have or have had clotting disorders, heart attack, stroke, angina pectoris, cancer of the breast or sex organs, jaundice or malignant or benign liver tumors

You should not take the pill if you suspect you are pregnant or have unexplained vaginal bleeding.

Cigarette smoking increases the risk of serious adverse effects on the heart and blood vessels from oral-contraceptive use. This risk increases with age and with heavy smoking (15 or more cigarettes per day) and is quite marked in women over 35 years of age. Women who use oral contraceptives should not smoke.

Most side effects of the pill are not serious. The most common such effects are nausea, vomiting, bleeding between menstrual periods, weight gain, breast tenderness, and difficulty wearing contact lenses. These side effects, especially nausea, and vomiting, may subside within the first three months of use.
The serious side effects of the pill occur very infrequently, especially if you are in good health and do not smoke. However, you should know that the following medical conditions have been associated with or made worse by the pill:
1. Blood clots in the legs (thrombophlebitis), lungs (pulmonary embolism), stoppage or rupture of a blood vessel in the brain (stroke), blockage of blood vessels in the heart (heart attack and angina pectoris) or other organs of the body. As mentioned above, smoking increases the risk of heart attacks and strokes and subsequent serious medical consequences.
2. Liver tumors, which may rupture and cause severe bleeding. A possible but not definite association has been found with the pill and liver cancer. However, liver cancers are extremely rare. The chance of developing liver cancer from using the pill is thus even rarer.
3. High blood pressure, although blood pressure usually returns to normal when the pill is stopped.
The symptoms associated with these serious side effects are discussed in the detailed leaflet given to you with your supply of pills. Notify your doctor or health-care provider if you notice any unusual physical disturbances while taking the pill. In addition, drugs such as rifampin, as well as some anticonvulsants and some antibiotics may decrease oral contraceptive effectiveness.
Studies to date of women taking the pill have not shown an increase in the incidence of cancer of the breast or cervix. There is, however, insufficient evidence to rule out the possibility that pills may cause such cancers.
Taking the pill provides some important noncontraceptive benefits. These include less painful menstruation, less menstrual blood loss and anemia, fewer pelvic infections, and fewer cancers of the ovary and the lining of the uterus.
Be sure to discuss any medical condition you may have with your health-care provider. Your health-care provider will take a medical and family history before prescribing oral contraceptives and will examine you. You should be reexamined at least once a year while taking oral contraceptives.

Continued on next page

Information on the Berlex products appearing here is based on the labeling in effect on June 1, 1992. Further information for these and other products may be obtained from the Medical Affairs Department, Berlex Laboratories, 300 Fairfield Road, Wayne, New Jersey 07470, (201) 292-3007. Information on oncology products may be obtained from Berlex Laboratories, 15049 San Pablo Avenue, Richmond, California 94804-0016 1-800-888-4112.

Berlex Laboratories—Cont.

The detailed patient information leaflet gives you further information which you should read and discuss with your health-care provider.

DETAILED PATIENT LABELING

INTRODUCTION

Any woman who considers using oral contraceptives (the "birth control pill" or the "pill") should understand the benefits and risks of using this form of birth control. This leaflet will give you much of the information you will need to make this decision and will also help you determine if you are at risk of developing any of the serious side effects of the pill. It will tell you how to use the pill properly so that it will be as effective as possible. However, this leaflet is not a replacement for a careful discussion between you and your health-care provider. You should discuss the information provided in this leaflet with him or her, both when you first start taking the pill and during your revisits. You should also follow your health-care provider's advice with regard to regular check-ups while you are on the pill.

EFFECTIVENESS OF ORAL CONTRACEPTIVES

Oral contraceptives or "birth control pills" or "the pill" are used to prevent pregnancy and are more effective than other nonsurgical methods of birth control. When they are taken correctly, the chance of becoming pregnant is less than 1.0% when used perfectly, without missing pills. Typical failure rates are less than 3.0% per year. The chance of becoming pregnant increases with each missed pill during the menstrual cycle.

In comparison, typical failure rates for other nonsurgical methods of birth control during the first year of use are as follows:

IUD: 6%
Diaphragm with spermicides: 18%
Spermicides alone: 21%
Vaginal sponge: 18 to 30%
Condom alone: 12%
Periodic abstinence: 20%
No method: 89%

WHO SHOULD NOT TAKE ORAL CONTRACEPTIVES

Cigarette smoking increases the risk of serious adverse effects on the heart and blood vessels from oral-contraceptive use. This risk increases with age and with heavy smoking (15 or more cigarettes per day) and is quite marked in women over 35 years of age. Women who use oral contraceptives should not smoke.

Some women should not use the pill. For example, you should not take the pill if you are pregnant or think you may be pregnant. You should also not use the pill if you have had any of the following conditions:

- Heart attack or stroke
- Blood clots in the legs (thrombophlebitis), lungs (pulmonary embolism), or eyes
- Blood clots in the deep veins of your legs
- Known or suspected breast cancer or cancer of the lining of the uterus, cervix or vagina
- Liver tumor (benign or cancerous)

Or, if you have any of the following:

- Chest pain (angina pectoris)
- Unexplained vaginal bleeding (until a diagnosis is reached by your doctor)
- Yellowing of the whites of the eyes or of the skin (jaundice) during pregnancy or during previous use of the pill
- Known or suspected pregnancy

Tell your health-care provider if you have ever had any of these conditions. Your health-care provider can recommend another method of birth control.

OTHER CONSIDERATIONS BEFORE TAKING ORAL CONTRACEPTIVES

Tell your health-care provider if you or any family member has ever had:

- Breast nodules, fibrocystic disease of the breast, an abnormal breast x-ray or mammogram
- Diabetes
- Elevated cholesterol or triglycerides
- High blood pressure
- Migraine or other headaches or epilepsy
- Mental depression
- Gallbladder, heart or kidney disease
- History of scanty or irregular menstrual periods

Women with any of these conditions should be checked often by their health-care provider if they choose to use oral contraceptives. Also, be sure to inform your doctor or health-care provider if you smoke or are on any medications.

RISKS OF TAKING ORAL CONTRACEPTIVES

1. *Risk of developing blood clots*

Blood clots and blockage of blood vessels are the most serious side effects of taking oral contraceptives and can be fatal. In particular, a clot in the legs can cause thrombophlebitis and a clot that travels to the lungs can cause a sudden blocking of the vessel carrying blood to the lungs. Rarely, clots occur in the blood vessels of the eye and may cause blindness, double vision, or impaired vision.

If you take oral contraceptives and need elective surgery, need to stay in bed for a prolonged illness or have recently delivered a baby, you may be at risk of developing blood clots. You should consult your doctor about stopping oral contraceptives three to four weeks before surgery and not taking oral contraceptives for two weeks after surgery or during bed rest. You should also not take oral contraceptives soon after delivery of a baby or a midtrimester pregnancy termination. It is advisable to wait for at least four weeks after delivery if you are not breast-feeding. If you are breast-feeding, you should wait until you have weaned your child before using the pill. (See also the section on Breast-Feeding in "General Precautions".)

2. *Heart attacks and strokes*

Oral contraceptives may increase the tendency to develop strokes (stoppage or rupture of blood vessels in the brain) and angina pectoris and heart attacks (blockage of blood vessels in the heart). Any of these conditions can cause death or serious disability.

Smoking greatly increases the possibility of suffering heart attacks and strokes. Furthermore, smoking and the use of oral contraceptives greatly increase the chances of developing and dying of heart disease.

3. *Gallbladder disease*

Oral-contraceptive users probably have a greater risk than nonusers of having gallbladder disease, although this risk may be related to pills containing high doses of estrogens.

4. *Liver tumors*

In rare cases, oral contraceptives can cause benign but dangerous liver tumors. These benign liver tumors can rupture and cause fatal internal bleeding. In addition, a possible but not definite association has been found with the pill and liver cancers in two studies, in which a few women who developed these very rare cancers were found to have used oral contraceptives for long periods. However, liver cancers are extremely rare. The chance of developing liver cancer from using the pill is thus even rarer.

5. *Cancer of the reproductive organs*

There is, at present, no confirmed evidence that oral contraceptives increase the risk of cancer of the reproductive organs in human studies.

Several studies have found no overall increase in the risk of developing breast cancer. However, women who use oral contraceptives and have a strong family history of breast cancer or who have breast nodules or abnormal mammograms should be closely followed by their doctors.

Some studies have found an increase in the incidence of cancer of the cervix in women who use oral contraceptives. However, this finding may be related to factors other than the use of oral contraceptives.

ESTIMATED RISK OF DEATH FROM A BIRTH-CONTROL METHOD OR PREGNANCY

All methods of birth control and pregnancy are associated with a risk of developing certain diseases which may lead to disability or death. An estimate of the number of deaths associated with different methods of birth control and pregnancy has been calculated and is shown in the following table. [See table below.]

ANNUAL NUMBER OF BIRTH-RELATED OR METHOD-RELATED DEATHS ASSOCIATED WITH CONTROL OF FERTILITY PER 100,000 NONSTERILE WOMEN, BY FERTILITY-CONTROL METHOD ACCORDING TO AGE

Method of control and outcome	15–19	20–24	25–29	30–34	35–39	40–44
No fertility-control methods*	7.0	7.4	9.1	14.8	25.7	28.2
Oral contraceptives nonsmoker**	0.3	0.5	0.9	1.9	13.8	31.6
Oral contraceptives smoker**	2.2	3.4	6.6	13.5	51.1	117.2
IUD**	0.8	0.8	1.0	1.0	1.4	1.4
Condom*	1.1	1.6	0.7	0.2	0.3	0.4
Diaphragm/spermicide*	1.9	1.2	1.2	1.3	2.2	2.8
Periodic abstinence*	2.5	1.6	1.6	1.7	2.9	3.6

* Deaths are birth related
** Deaths are method related

In the table below, the risk of death from any birth-control method is less than the risk of childbirth, except for oral contraceptive users over the age of 35 who smoke and pill users over the age of 40 even if they do not smoke. It can be seen in the table that for women aged 15 to 39, the risk of death was highest with pregnancy (7 to 26 deaths per 100,000 women, depending on age). Among pill users who do not smoke, the risk of death was always lower than that associated with pregnancy for any age group, except for those women over the age of 40 when the risk increases to 32 deaths per 100,000 women, compared to 28 associated with pregnancy at that age. However, for pill users who smoke and are over the age of 35, the estimated number of deaths exceeds those for other methods of birth control. If a woman is over the age of 40 and smokes, her estimated risk of death is four times higher (117/100,000 women) than the estimated risk associated with pregnancy (28/100,000 women) in that age group.

The suggestion that women over 40 who don't smoke should not take oral contraceptives is based on information from older high-dose pills and on less-selective use of pills than is practiced today. An Advisory Committee of the FDA discussed this issue in 1989 and recommended that the benefits of oral-contraceptive use by healthy, nonsmoking women over 40 years of age may outweigh the possible risks. However, all women, especially older women, are cautioned to use the lowest-dose pill that is effective.

WARNING SIGNALS

If any of these adverse effects occur while you are taking oral contraceptives, call your doctor immediately:

- Sharp chest pain, coughing of blood, or sudden shortness of breath (indicating a possible clot in the lung).
- Pain in the calf (indicating a possible clot in the leg).
- Crushing chest pain or heaviness in the chest (indicating a possible heart attack).
- Sudden severe headache or vomiting, dizziness or fainting, disturbances of vision or speech, weakness, or numbness in an arm or leg (indicating a possible stroke).
- Sudden partial or complete loss of vision (indicating a possible clot in the eye).
- Breast lumps (indicating possible breast cancer or fibrocystic disease of the breast; ask your doctor or health-care provider to show you how to examine your breasts).
- Severe pain or tenderness in the stomach area (indicating a possibly ruptured liver tumor).
- Difficulty in sleeping, weakness, lack of energy, fatigue, or change in mood (possibly indicating severe depression).
- Jaundice or a yellowing of the skin or eyeballs, accompanied frequently by fever, fatigue, loss of appetite, dark-colored urine, or light-colored bowel movements (indicating possible liver problems).

SIDE EFFECTS OF ORAL CONTRACEPTIVES

1. *Vaginal bleeding*

Irregular vaginal bleeding or spotting may occur while you are taking the pills. Irregular bleeding may vary from slight staining between menstrual periods to breakthrough bleeding which is a flow much like a regular period. Irregular bleeding occurs most often during the first few months of oral contraceptive use, but may also occur after you have been taking the pill for some time. Such bleeding may be temporary and usually does not indicate any serious problems. It is important to continue taking your pills on schedule. If the bleeding occurs in more than one cycle or lasts for more than a few days, talk to your doctor or health-care provider.

2. *Contact lenses*

If you wear contact lenses and notice a change in vision or an inability to wear your lenses, contact your doctor or health-care provider.

3. *Fluid retention*

Oral contraceptives may cause edema (fluid retention) with swelling of the fingers or ankles and may raise your blood pressure. If you experience fluid retention, contact your doctor or health-care provider.

4. *Melasma*

A spotty darkening of the skin is possible, particularly of the face.

5. *Other side effects*

Other side effects include change in appetite, headache, nervousness, depression, dizziness, loss of scalp hair, rash, and vaginal infections.

If any of these side effects bother you, call your doctor or health-care provider.

GENERAL PRECAUTIONS

1. MISSED PERIODS AND USE OF ORAL CONTRACEPTIVES BEFORE OR DURING EARLY PREGNANCY.

There may be times when you may not menstruate regularly after you have completed taking a cycle of pills. If you have taken your pills regularly and miss one menstrual period, continue taking your pills for the next cycle but be sure to inform your health-care provider before doing so. If you have not taken the pills daily as instructed and missed a menstrual period, or if you missed two consecutive menstrual periods, you may be pregnant. Check with your health-care

provider immediately to determine whether you are pregnant. Do not continue to take oral contraceptives until you are sure you are not pregnant, but continue to use another method of contraception.

There is no conclusive evidence that oral contraceptive use is associated with an increase in birth defects, when taken inadvertently during early pregnancy. Previously, a few studies had reported that oral contraceptives might be associated with birth defects, but these studies have not been confirmed. Nevertheless, oral contraceptives or any other drugs should not be used during pregnancy unless clearly necessary and prescribed by your doctor. You should check with your doctor about risks to your unborn child of any medication taken during pregnancy.

2. WHILE BREAST-FEEDING

If you are breast-feeding, consult your doctor before starting oral contraceptives. Some of the drug will be passed on to the child in the milk. A few adverse effects on the child have been reported, including yellowing of the skin (jaundice) and breast enlargement. In addition, oral contraceptives may decrease the amount and quality of your milk. If possible, do not use oral contraceptives while breast-feeding. You should use another method of contraception since breast-feeding provides only partial protection from becoming pregnant and this partial protection decreases significantly as you breast-feed for longer periods of time. You should consider starting oral contraceptives only after you have weaned your child completely.

3. LABORATORY TESTS

If you are scheduled for any laboratory tests, tell your doctor you are taking birth-control pills. Certain blood tests may be affected by birth-control pills.

4. DRUG INTERACTIONS

Certain drugs may interact with birth control pills to make them less effective in preventing pregnancy or cause an increase in breakthrough bleeding. Such drugs include rifampin, drugs used for epilepsy such as barbiturates (for example, phenobarbital) and phenytoin (Dilantin is one brand of this drug), phenylbutazone (Butazolidin is one brand) and possibly certain antibiotics. You may need to use an additional method of contraception during any cycle in which you take drugs that can make oral contraceptives less effective.

HOW TO TAKE ORAL CONTRACEPTIVES

1. GENERAL INSTRUCTIONS

You must take your pill every day according to the instructions. Oral contraceptives are most effective if taken no more than 24 hours apart. Take your pill at the same time every day so that you are less likely to forget to take it. You will then maintain an effective dose of the oral contraceptive in your body.

If your doctor has scheduled you for surgery, or you need prolonged bed rest, he or she may suggest that you stop taking the pill four weeks before surgery to avoid an increased risk of blood clots. It is also advisable not to start oral contraceptives sooner than four weeks after delivery of a baby or a midtrimester pregnancy termination.

TRI-LEVLEN® 21 TABLETS (LEVONORGESTREL AND ETHINYL ESTRADIOL TABLETS—TRIPHASIC REGIMEN)

TRI-LEVLEN® is a three-phase contraceptive, different from the usual same-dose-every-day combination oral contraceptive.

TRI-LEVLEN® 21 tablets contain 21 active pills divided among 6 brown pills, 5 white pills, and 10 light-yellow pills in each package.

The dosage of TRI-LEVLEN® 21 tablets is ***one pill daily*** for 21 days in a row in your menstrual cycle beginning with the first brown pill, continuing through the white pills and finishing the cycle with the light-yellow pills, ***in that order.*** Pills are then discontinued for 7 days. The basic schedule is 21 days on—7 days off.

In the first month, you should begin taking TRI-LEVLEN® 21 tablets on day one (1) of your menstrual cycle, which is the first day of your menstruation regardless of the amount of bleeding or spotting. (Day 1 is the first day of menstruation, even if it is almost midnight when you start.) Note: During the first month on TRI-LEVLEN® 21 tablets, if you start taking pills later than day 1 of your menstrual cycle, you should protect yourself by also using another method of birth control until you have taken a pill daily for seven days in a row (6 brown pills followed by 1 white pill). Thereafter, if you follow directions carefully, you should obtain the full contraceptive benefit. If you begin taking pills later than the proper day, the possibility of ovulation and pregnancy occurring before or during the taking of the brown pills should be considered.

Take one pill every day until you finish all 21 pills. No pills are then taken for one week (7 days). Your period will usually begin about three days after you take the last light-yellow pill. Don't be alarmed if the amount of bleeding is not the same as before. On the 8th day, start with a brown pill from a new package, even if you still have your period. If, for example, you took TRI-LEVLEN® 21 tablets for the first time on a Tuesday, the 8th day will also be a Tuesday. ***If you have taken the pills as directed,*** you will begin the next cycle on the same day of the week. If you start taking pills later than the 8th day, you should protect yourself by also using another method of birth control until you have taken a pill daily for seven days in a row.

When switching from another oral contraceptive, TRI-LEVLEN® 21 tablets should be started on the first day of bleeding following the last active pill taken of the previous oral contraceptive.

TRI-LEVLEN® 28 TABLETS (LEVONORGESTREL AND ETHINYL ESTRADIOL TABLETS—TRIPHASIC REGIMEN)

TRI-LEVLEN® is a three-phased contraceptive, different from the usual same-dose-every-day combination oral contraceptive.

TRI-LEVLEN® 28 tablets contain 21 active pills divided among 6 brown pills, 5 white pills, and 10 light-yellow pills plus 7 light-green inactive pills per package.

The dosage of TRI-LEVLEN® 28 tablets is one active pill daily for 21 days in a row beginning with the 6 brown pills, followed by the 5 white pills, followed by the 10 light-yellow pills, and then one of the 7 light-green inactive pills daily for the next 7 days. ***In that order,*** for a total of 28 days or 4 weeks. The basic schedule is 21 days on active pills (brown, white, and light-yellow)—7 days on light-green inactive pills. Always take all of the 21 active pills (brown, white, and light-yellow) in each package before taking the light-green pills.

When you start your ***first*** cycle of TRI-LEVLEN® 28 tablets, you should begin taking your pills on the ***first*** day of your next menstrual period, regardless of the day of the week or the amount of the bleeding or spotting. NOTE: During the first month on TRI-LEVLEN® 28 tablets, if you start taking pills later than day 1 of your menstrual cycle, you should protect yourself by also using another method of birth control until you have taken a pill daily for seven days in a row (6 brown pills followed by 1 white pill). Thereafter, if you follow directions carefully you should obtain the full contraceptive benefit. If you begin taking pills later than the proper day, the possibility of ovulation and pregnancy occurring before or during the taking of the brown pills should be considered. Take one pill every day until you finish all 6 brown, 5 white and 10 light-yellow pills in a package followed by all 7 light-green pills. Your period will usually begin about three days after you take the last light-yellow pill, which will be during the time you are taking the light-green pills. Don't be alarmed if the amount of bleeding is not the same as before. The day after you have taken your last light-green pill, begin a new package of pills (first taking the 6 brown, then the 5 white, and then the 10 light-yellow pills one a day just as you did before) so that you will take a pill every day without interruption. ***If you have taken the pills as directed,*** the starting day for each new package will always be the same as in the previous cycle. When switching from another oral contraceptive, TRI-LEVLEN® 28 tablets should be started on the first day of bleeding following the last active pill taken of the previous oral contraceptive.

LEVLEN® 21

The dosage of LEVLEN® 21 tablets is one tablet daily for 21 days in a row per mentstrual cycle. Tablets are then discontinued for 7 days. The basic schedule is 21 days on—7 days off.

During the first month, you should begin taking LEVLEN® 21 on Day 5 of your menstrual cycle whether or not you still have your period. (Day 1 is the first day of menstruation, even if it is almost midnight when you start.) Note: During your first month on LEVLEN® 21, if you start taking tablets later than Day 5 of your menstrual cycle, you should protect yourself by also using another method of birth control until you have taken a tablet daily for seven consecutive days. Thereafter, if you follow directions carefully, you will obtain the full contraceptive benefit. If you begin taking tablets later than the proper day, the possibility of ovulation and pregnancy occurring before beginning medication should be considered. Take one tablet every day until you finish all 21 tablets. No tablets are then taken for one week (7 days) . Your period will usually begin about three days after you take the last tablet. Don't be alarmed if the amount of bleeding is not the same as before. On the 8th day, start a new SLIDECASE™ dispenser, even if you still have your period. If, for example, you took LEVLEN® 21 tablets for the first time on a Tuesday, the 8th day will also be a Tuesday. Thus, you will always begin a new cycle on the same day of the week as long as you do not interrupt your original schedule. If you start taking tablets later than the 8th day, you should protect yourself by also using another method of birth control until you have taken a tablet daily for seven days in a row.

LEVLEN® 28

The dosage of LEVLEN® 28 tablets is one light-orange active tablet daily for 21 consecutive days followed by one pink inactive tablet daily for 7 consecutive days. The basic schedule is 21 days on light-orange active tablets—7 days on pink inactive tablets. Always take all 21 light-orange tablets in each SLIDECASE™ dispenser before taking the pink tablets.

You should begin taking LEVLEN® 28 tablets on the first Sunday after your menstrual period begins, whether or not you are still bleeding. If your period begins on a Sunday, take your first tablet that very same day. Your first light-orange tablet is marked with the word "Start". Note: During your first month on LEVLEN® 28, you should protect yourself by also using another method of birth control until you have taken a light-orange tablet daily for seven consecutive days. Thereafter, if you follow directions carefully, you will obtain the full contraceptive benefit. If you begin taking tablets later than the proper day, the possibility of ovulation and pregnancy occuring before beginning medication should be considered. Take one tablet every day until you finish all 21 light-orange tablets in a SLIDECASE™ dispenser, followed by all seven pink tablets. Your period will usually begin about three days after you take the last light-orange tablet, which will be during the time you are taking the pink tablets. Don't be alarmed if the amount of bleeding is not the same as before. The day after you have taken your last pink tablet, begin a new SLIDECASE™ dispenser of tablets (taking all 21 light-orange tablets first, just as you did before) so that you will take a tablet every day without interruption. The starting day for each new SLIDECASE™ dispenser will always be Sunday. If in any cycle you start tablets later than the proper day, you should also use another method of birth control until you have taken a light-orange tablet daily for 7 days in a row.

Spotting or Breakthrough Bleeding:

Spotting is slight staining between menstrual periods which may not even require a pad. Breakthrough bleeding is a flow much like a regular period, requiring sanitary protection. Spotting is more common than breakthrough bleeding, and both occur more often in the first few cycles than in later cycles. These types of bleeding are usually temporary and without significance. It is important to continue taking your pills on schedule. If the bleeding persists for more than a few days, consult your doctor.

2. IF YOU FORGET TO TAKE YOUR PILL

If you miss only one pill in a cycle, the chance of becoming pregnant is small. Take the missed pill as soon as you realize that you have forgotten it. Since the risk of pregnancy increases with each additional pill you skip, it is very important that you take one pill a day.

TRI-LEVLEN® Tablets

There is a chance of becoming pregnant if you miss one brown, white, or light-yellow pill, and that chance increases with each additional brown, white, or light-yellow pill missed. If you miss any one of these pills, it is important that it be taken as soon as remembered, and also take your next pill at the regular time, which means that you will be taking two pills on that day. If you miss any two of these pills consecutively, it is important that you take the second missed pill as soon as you remember, discard the first missed pill, and take your regular pill that day at the proper time (which means you will be taking two pills on that day). Furthermore, you should use an additional method of birth control for the remainder of the cycle in addition to taking your pills as directed above. If breakthrough bleeding occurs following missed pills, it will usually be temporary and of no consequence. If you miss three or more of any of the brown, white, or light-yellow pills in succession, discontinue the medication and discard the pill card. Then start a new refill card beginning with the first brown pill on the first day of bleeding of your next period. During the days without pills and until you have taken a pill daily for seven consecutive days (six brown and one white), you should also use another means of birth control. If you miss one or more light-green inactive pills (TRI-LEVLEN® 28 tablets only), you are still protected against pregnancy ***provided*** you begin taking your next brown pill on the proper day.

LEVLEN® 21 contains 21 active light-orange tablets per SLIDECASE™ dispenser. LEVLEN® 28 contains 21 active light-orange tablets plus 7 pink inactive tablets per SLIDECASE™ dispenser.

The chance of becoming pregnant is probably quite small if you miss only one light-orange tablet in a cycle. Of course, with each additional one you skip, the chance increases. If you miss one or more pink tablets (LEVLEN® 28), you are still protected against pregnancy as long as you begin taking your next light-orange tablet on the proper day.

It is important to take a missed light-orange tablet as soon as it is remembered. If two consecutive light-orange tablets are

Continued on next page

Information on the Berlex products appearing here is based on the labeling in effect on June 1, 1992. Further information for these and other products may be obtained from the Medical Affairs Department, Berlex Laboratories, 300 Fairfield Road, Wayne, New Jersey 07470, (201) 292-3007. Information on oncology products may be obtained from Berlex Laboratories, 15049 San Pablo Avenue, Richmond, California 94804-0016 1-800-888-4112.

Berlex Laboratories—Cont.

missed they should both be taken as soon as remembered. The next tablet should then be taken at the usual time. Any time you miss one or two light-orange tablets, or begin a new SLIDECASE™ dispenser after the proper starting day, you should also use another method of birth control until you have taken a light-orange tablet daily for seven consecutive days. If breakthrough bleeding occurs following missed tablets, it will usually be temporary and of no consequence. While there is little likelihood of pregnancy occuring if only one or two light-orange tablets are missed, the possibility of pregnancy increases with each successive day that scheduled light-orange tablets are missed.

If you are taking LEVLEN® 21 and forget to take three light-orange tablets in a row, do not take them when you remember. Wait four more days—which makes a whole week without tablets. Then begin a new SLIDECASE™ dispenser on the 8th day after the last tablet was taken. During the seven days without tablets, and until you have taken a light-orange tablet daily for seven consecutive days, you should protect yourself from pregnancy by also using another method of birth control.

If you are taking LEVLEN® 28 and forget to take three light-orange tablets in a row, do not take them when you remember. Stop taking all medication until the first Sunday following the last missed tablet. Then, whether or not you have had your period, and even if you are still bleeding, start a new SLIDECASE™ dispenser. During the days without tablets, and until you have taken a light-orange tablet daily for seven consecutive days, you should protect yourself from pregnancy by also using another method of birth control.

At times there may be no menstrual period after a cycle of pills. Therefore, if you miss one menstrual period but have taken the pills ***exactly as you were supposed to,*** continue as usual into the next cycle. If you have not taken the pills correctly and miss a menstrual period, you may be pregnant and should stop taking oral contraceptives until your doctor determines whether or not you are pregnant. Until you can get to your doctor, use another form of nonhormonal contraception. If two consecutive menstrual periods are missed, you should stop taking pills until it is determined by a physician whether you are pregnant.

If you do become pregnant while using oral contraceptives, the risk to the fetus is small, on the order of no more than one per thousand. You should, however, discuss the risks to the developing child with your doctor.

3. PREGNANCY DUE TO PILL FAILURE

The incidence of pill failure resulting in pregnancy is approximately less than 1.0% if taken every day as directed, but more typical failure rates are less than 3.0%. If failure does occur, the risk to the fetus is minimal.

4. PREGNANCY AFTER STOPPING THE PILL

There may be some delay in becoming pregnant after you stop using oral contraceptives, especially if you had irregular menstrual cycles before you used oral contraceptives. It may be advisable to postpone conception until you begin menstruating regularly once you have stopped taking the pill and desire pregnancy.

There does not appear to be any increase in birth defects in newborn babies when pregnancy occurs soon after stopping the pill.

5. OVERDOSAGE

Serious ill effects have not been reported following ingestion of large doses of oral contraceptives by young children. Overdosage may cause nausea and withdrawal bleeding in females. In case of overdosage, contact your health-care provider or pharmacist.

6. OTHER INFORMATION

Your health-care provider will take a medical and family history before prescribing oral contraceptives and will examine you. You should be reexamined at least once a year. Be sure to inform your health-care provider if there is a family history of any of the conditions listed previously in this leaflet. Be sure to keep all appointments with your health-care provider, because this is a time to determine if there are early signs of side effects of oral-contraceptive use.

Do not use the drug for any condition other than the one for which it was prescribed. This drug has been prescribed specifically for you; do not give it to others who may want birth-control pills.

Health Benefits from Oral Contraceptives

In addition to preventing pregnancy, use of oral contraceptives may provide certain benefits. They are:

- Menstrual cycles may become more regular.
- Blood flow during menstruation may be lighter and less iron may be lost. Therefore, anemia due to iron deficiency is less likely to occur.
- Pain or other symptoms during menstruation may be encountered less frequently.
- Ovarian cycsts may occur less frequently.
- Ectopic (tubal) pregnancy may occur less frequently.
- Noncancerous cysts or lumps in the breast may occur less frequently.
- Acute pelvic inflammatory disease may occur less frequently.
- Oral-contraceptive use may provide some protection against developing two forms of cancer: cancer of the ovaries and cancer of the lining of the uterus.

If you want more information about birth-control pills, ask your doctor or pharmacist. They have a more technical leaflet called the Professional Labeling, which you may wish to read.

Manufactured for
BERLEX Laboratories, Wayne, NJ 07470
Issued May 1991 60627-0
60631-0

Shown in Product Identification Section, page 405

Berlex Laboratories

15049 SAN PABLO AVENUE
RICHMOND, CA 94804-0016

FLUDARA® ℞
(fludarabine phosphate)
FOR INJECTION
FOR INTRAVENOUS USE ONLY

WARNING: FLUDARA FOR INJECTION should be administered under the supervision of a qualified physician experienced in the use of antineoplastic therapy. FLUDARA FOR INJECTION can severely suppress bone marrow function. When used at high doses in dose-ranging studies in patients with acute leukemia, FLUDARA FOR INJECTION was associated with severe neurologic effects, including blindness, coma, and death. This severe central nervous system toxicity occurred in 36% of patients treated with doses approximately four times greater (96 mg/m^2/day for 5–7 days) than the recommended dose. Similar severe central nervous system toxicity has been rarely ($\leq$0.2%) reported in patients treated at doses in the range of the dose recommended for chronic lymphocytic leukemia.
In a clinical investigation using FLUDARA FOR INJECTION in combination with pentostatin (deoxycoformycin) for the treatment of refractory chronic lymphocytic leukemia (CLL), there was an unacceptably high incidence of fatal pulmonary toxicity. Therefore, the use of FLUDARA FOR INJECTION in combination with pentostatin is not recommended.

DESCRIPTION

FLUDARA FOR INJECTION contains fludarabine phosphate, a fluorinated nucleotide analog of the antiviral agent vidarabine, 9-β-D-arabinofuranosyladenine (ara-A) that is relatively resistant to deamination by adenosine deaminase. Each vial of sterile lyophilized solid cake contains 50 mg of the active ingredient fludarabine phosphate, 50 mg of mannitol, and sodium hydroxide to adjust pH to 7.7. The pH range for the final product is 7.2–8.2. Reconstitution with 2 mL of Sterile Water for Injection USP results in a solution containing 25 mg/mL of fludarabine phosphate intended for intravenous administration.

The chemical name for fludarabine phosphate is 9H-Purin-6-amine, 2-fluoro-9-(5-O-phosphono-β-D-arabinofuranosyl). The molecular formula of fludarabine phosphate is $C_{10}H_{13}FN_5O_7P$ (MW 365.2) and the structure is:

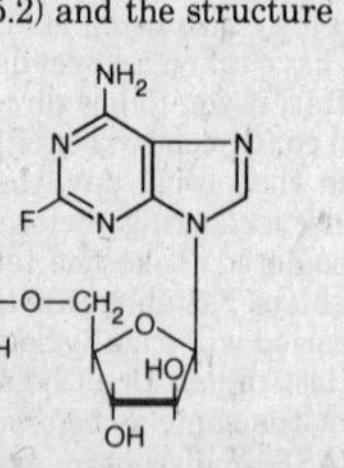

CLINICAL PHARMACOLOGY

Fludarabine phosphate is rapidly dephosphorylated to 2-fluoro-ara-A and then phosphorylated intracellularly by deoxycytidine kinase to the active triphosphate, 2-fluoro-ara-ATP. This metabolite appears to act by inhibiting DNA polymerase alpha, ribonucleotide reductase and DNA primase, thus inhibiting DNA synthesis. The mechanism of action of this antimetabolite is not completely characterized and may be multi-faceted.

Phase I studies in humans have demonstrated that fludarabine phosphate is rapidly converted to the active metabolite, 2-fluoro-ara-A, within minutes after intravenous infusion. Consequently, clinical pharmacology studies have focused on 2-fluoro-ara-A pharmacokinetics. In a study with 4 patients treated with 25 mg/m^2/day for 5 days, the half-life of 2-fluoro-ara-A was approximately 10 hours. The mean total plasma clearance was 8.9 L/hr/m^2 and the mean volume of distribution was 98 L/m^2. Approximately 23% of the dose was excreted in the urine as unchanged 2-fluoro-ara-A. The mean C_{max} after the Day 1 dose was 0.57 mcg/mL and after the Day 5 dose was 0.54 mcg/mL. No information is available on pharmacokinetic parameters, other than C_{max}, following the Day 5 dose of 25 mg/m^2. Total body clearance of 2-fluoro-ara-A has been shown to be inversely correlated with serum creatinine, suggesting renal elimination of the compound.

A correlation was noted between the degree of absolute granulocyte count nadir and increased area under the concentration × time curve (AUC).

Two single-arm open-label studies of FLUDARA FOR INJECTION have been conducted in patients with CLL refractory to at least one prior standard alkylating-agent containing regimen. In a study conducted by M.D. Anderson Cancer Center (MDAH), 48 patients were treated with a dose of 22–40 mg/m^2 daily for 5 days every 28 days. Another study conducted by the Southwest Oncology Group (SWOG) involved 31 patients treated with a dose of 15–25 mg/m^2 daily for 5 days every 28 days. The overall objective response rates were 48% and 32% in the MDAH and SWOG studies, respectively. The complete response rate in both studies was 13%; the partial response rate was 35% in the MDAH study and 19% in the SWOG study. These response rates were obtained using standardized response criteria developed by the National Cancer Institute CLL Working Group[1] and were achieved in heavily pre-treated patients. The ability of FLUDARA FOR INJECTION to induce a significant rate of response in refractory patients suggests minimal cross-resistance with commonly used anti-CLL agents.

The median time to response in the MDAH and SWOG studies was 7 weeks (range of 1 to 68 weeks) and 21 weeks (range of 1 to 53 weeks) respectively. The median duration of disease control was 91 weeks (MDAH) and 65 weeks (SWOG). The median survival of all refractory CLL patients treated with FLUDARA FOR INJECTION was 43 weeks and 52 weeks in the MDAH and SWOG studies, respectively.

Rai stage improved to Stage II or better in 7 of 12 MDAH responders (58%) and in 5 of 7 SWOG responders (71%) who were Stage III or IV at baseline. In the combined studies, mean hemoglobin concentration improved from 9.0 g/dL at baseline to 11.8 g/dL at the time of response, in a subgroup of anemic patients. Similarly, average platelet count improved from 63,500/mm^3 to 103,300/mm^3 at the time of response in a subgroup of patients who were thrombocytopenic at baseline.

INDICATIONS AND USAGE

FLUDARA FOR INJECTION is indicated for the treatment of patients with B-cell chronic lymphocytic leukemia (CLL) who have not responded to or whose disease has progressed during treatment with at least one standard alkylating-agent containing regimen. The safety and effectiveness of FLUDARA FOR INJECTION in previously untreated or non-refractory patients with CLL have not been established.

CONTRAINDICATIONS

FLUDARA FOR INJECTION is contraindicated in those patients who are hypersensitive to this drug or its components.

WARNINGS

(See boxed warning): There are clear dose dependent toxic effects seen with FLUDARA FOR INJECTION. Dose levels approximately 4 times greater (96 mg/m^2/day for 5 to 7 days) than that recommended for CLL (25 mg/m^2/day for 5 days) were associated with a syndrome characterized by delayed blindness, coma and death. Symptoms appeared from 21 to 60 days following the last dose. Thirteen of 36 patients (36%) who received FLUDARA FOR INJECTION at high doses (96 mg/m^2/day for 5 to 7 days) developed this severe neurotoxicity. This syndrome has been reported rarely in patients treated with doses in the range of the recommended CLL dose of 25 mg/m^2/day for 5 days every 28 days. The effect of chronic administration of FLUDARA FOR INJECTION on the central nervous system is unknown, however, patients have received the recommended dose for up to 15 courses of therapy.

Severe bone marrow suppression, notably anemia, thrombocytopenia and neutropenia, has been reported in patients treated with FLUDARA FOR INJECTION. In a Phase I study in solid tumor patients, the median time to nadir counts was 13 days (range, 3–25 days) for granulocytes and 16 days (range, 2–32) for platelets. Most patients had hematologic impairment at baseline either as a result of disease or as a result of prior myelosuppressive therapy. Cumulative myelosuppression may be seen. While chemotherapy-induced myelosuppression is often reversible, administration of FLUDARA FOR INJECTION requires careful hematologic monitoring.

In a clinical investigation using FLUDARA FOR INJECTION in combination with pentostatin (deoxycoformycin) for the treatment of refractory chronic lymphocytic leukemia (CLL), there was an unacceptably high incidence of fatal pulmonary toxicity. Therefore, the use of FLUDARA FOR

INJECTION in combination with pentostatin is not recommended.

Of the 133 CLL patients in the two trials, there were 29 fatalities during study. Approximately 50% of the fatalities were due to infection and 25% due to progressive disease.

Pregnancy Category D: FLUDARA FOR INJECTION may cause fetal harm when administered to a pregnant woman. Fludarabine phosphate was teratogenic in rats and in rabbits. Fludarabine phosphate was administered intravenously at doses of 0, 1, 10 or 30 mg/kg/day to pregnant rats on days 6 to 15 of gestation. At 10 and 30 mg/kg/day in rats, there was an increased incidence of various skeletal malformations. Fludarabine phosphate was administered intravenously at doses of 0, 1, 5 or 8 mg/kg/day to pregnant rabbits on days 6 to 15 of gestation. Dose-related teratogenic effects manifested by external deformities and skeletal malformations were observed in the rabbits at 5 and 8 mg/kg/day. Drug-related deaths or toxic effects on maternal and fetal weights were not observed. There are no adequate and well-controlled studies in pregnant women.

If FLUDARA FOR INJECTION is used during pregnancy, or if the patient becomes pregnant while taking this drug, the patient should be apprised of the potential hazard to the fetus. Women of childbearing potential should be advised to avoid becoming pregnant.

PRECAUTIONS

General: FLUDARA FOR INJECTION is a potent antineoplastic agent with potentially significant toxic side effects. Patients undergoing therapy should be closely observed for signs of hematologic and nonhematologic toxicity. Periodic assessment of peripheral blood counts is recommended to detect the development of anemia, neutropenia and thrombocytopenia.

Tumor lysis syndrome associated with FLUDARA FOR INJECTION treatment has been reported in CLL patients with large tumor burdens. Since FLUDARA FOR INJECTION can induce a response as early as the first week of treatment, precautions should be taken in those patients at risk of developing this complication.

There are inadequate data on dosing of patients with renal insufficiency. FLUDARA FOR INJECTION must be administered cautiously in patients with renal insufficiency. The total body clearance of 2-fluoro-ara-A has been shown to be inversely correlated with serum creatinine, suggesting renal elimination of the compound.

Laboratory Tests: During treatment, the patient's hematologic profile (particularly neutrophils and platelets) should be monitored regularly to determine the degree of hematopoietic suppression.

Drug Interactions: There are no known drug interactions with FLUDARA FOR INJECTION.

Carcinogenesis: No animal carcinogenicity studies with FLUDARA FOR INJECTION have been conducted.

Mutagenesis: Fludarabine phosphate has been shown to be non-mutagenic to several strains of Salmonella typhimurium, including TA-98, TA-100, TA-1535 and TA-1537. In addition, fludarabine phosphate was non-mutagenic to Chinese hamster ovary (CHO) cells at the hypoxanthine-guanine-phosphoribosyltransferase (HGPRT) locus under both activated and non-activated metabolic conditions. Chromosomal aberrations were observed in an in vitro assay using CHO cells under metabolically activated conditions. In addition, fludarabine phosphate was determined to cause increased sister chromatid exchanges using an in vitro sister chromatid exchange (SCE) assay under both metabolically activated and non-activated conditions.

Impairment of Fertility: Studies in mice, rats and dogs have demonstrated dose-related adverse effects on the male reproductive system. Observations consisted of a decrease in mean testicular weights in mice and rats with a trend toward decreased testicular weights in dogs and degeneration and necrosis of spermatogenic epithelium of the testes in mice, rats and dogs. The possible adverse effects on fertility in humans have not been adequately evaluated.

Pregnancy: Pregnancy Category D: (See WARNINGS section).

Nursing Mothers: It is not known whether this drug is excreted in human milk. Because many drugs are excreted in human milk and because of the potential for serious adverse reactions in nursing infants from FLUDARA FOR INJECTION, a decision should be made to discontinue nursing or discontinue the drug, taking into account the importance of the drug for the mother.

Pediatric Use: The safety and effectiveness of FLUDARA FOR INJECTION in children have not been established.

ADVERSE REACTIONS

The most common adverse events include myelosuppression (neutropenia, thrombocytopenia and anemia), fever and chills, infection, and nausea and vomiting. Other commonly reported events include malaise, fatigue, anorexia, and weakness. Serious opportunistic infections have occurred in CLL patients treated with FLUDARA FOR INJECTION. The most frequently reported adverse events and those reactions which are more clearly related to the drug are arranged below according to body system.

Hematopoietic Systems: Hematologic events (neutropenia, thrombocytopenia, and/or anemia) were reported in the majority of CLL patients treated with FLUDARA FOR INJECTION. During FLUDARA FOR INJECTION treatment of 133 patients with CLL, the absolute neutrophil count decreased to less than 500/mm^3 in 59% of patients, hemoglobin decreased from pretreatment values by at least 2 grams percent in 60%, and platelet count decreased from pretreatment values by at least 50% in 55%. Myelosuppression may be severe and cumulative. Bone marrow fibrosis occurred in one CLL patient treated with FLUDARA FOR INJECTION.

Metabolic: Tumor lysis syndrome has been reported in CLL patients treated with FLUDARA FOR INJECTION. This complication may include hyperuricemia, hyperphosphatemia, hypocalcemia, metabolic acidosis, hyperkalemia, hematuria, urate crystalluria, and renal failure. The onset of this syndrome may be heralded by flank pain and hematuria.

Nervous System: (See WARNINGS section) Objective weakness, agitation, confusion, visual disturbances, and coma have occurred in CLL patients treated with FLUDARA FOR INJECTION at the recommended dose. Peripheral neuropathy has been observed in patients treated with FLUDARA FOR INJECTION and one case of wrist-drop was reported.

Pulmonary System: Pneumonia, a frequent manifestation of infection in CLL patients, occurred in 16% and 22% of those treated with FLUDARA FOR INJECTION in the MDAH and SWOG studies, respectively. Pulmonary hypersensitivity reactions to FLUDARA FOR INJECTION characterized by dyspnea, cough and interstitial pulmonary infiltrate have been observed.

Gastrointestinal System: Gastrointestinal disturbances such as nausea and vomiting, anorexia, diarrhea, stomatitis and gastrointestinal bleeding have been reported in patients treated with FLUDARA FOR INJECTION.

Cardiovascular: Edema has been frequently reported. One patient developed a pericardial effusion possibly related to treatment with FLUDARA FOR INJECTION. No other severe cardiovascular events were considered to be drug related.

Skin: Skin toxicity, consisting primarily of skin rashes, has been reported in patients treated with FLUDARA FOR INJECTION.

Data in the following table are derived from the 133 patients with CLL who received FLUDARA FOR INJECTION in the MDAH and SWOG studies.

More than 3000 patients received FLUDARA FOR INJECTION in studies of other leukemias, lymphomas, and other solid tumors. The spectrum of adverse effects reported in these studies was consistent with the data presented above.

OVERDOSAGE

High doses of FLUDARA FOR INJECTION (see Warnings) have been associated with an irreversible central nervous system toxicity characterized by delayed blindness, coma, and death. High doses are also associated with severe thrombocytopenia and neutropenia due to bone marrow suppression. There is no known specific antidote for FLUDARA FOR INJECTION overdosage. Treatment consists of drug discontinuation and supportive therapy.

DOSAGE AND ADMINISTRATION

Usual Dose: The recommended dose of FLUDARA FOR INJECTION is 25 mg/m^2 administered intravenously over a period of approximately 30 minutes daily for five consecutive days. Each 5 day course of treatment should commence every 28 days. Dosage may be decreased or delayed based on evidence of hematologic or nonhematologic toxicity. Physicians should consider delaying or discontinuing the drug if neurotoxicity occurs.

A number of clinical settings may predispose to increased toxicity from FLUDARA FOR INJECTION. These include advanced age, renal insufficiency, and bone marrow impairment. Such patients should be monitored closely for excessive toxicity and the dose modified accordingly.

The optimal duration of treatment has not been clearly established. It is recommended that three additional cycles of FLUDARA FOR INJECTION be administered following the achievement of a maximal response and then the drug should be discontinued. [See table next column.]

Preparation of Solutions: FLUDARA FOR INJECTION should be prepared for parenteral use by aseptically adding Sterile Water for Injection USP. When reconstituted with 2 mL of Sterile Water for Injection, USP, the solid cake should fully dissolve in 15 seconds or less; each mL of the resulting solution will contain 25 mg of fludarabine phosphate, 25 mg of mannitol, and sodium hydroxide to adjust the pH to 7.7. The pH range for the final product is 7.2–8.2. In clinical studies, the product has been diluted in 100 cc or 125 cc of 5% Dextrose Injection USP or 0.9% Sodium Chloride USP. Reconstituted FLUDARA FOR INJECTION contains no antimicrobial preservative and thus should be used within 8 hours of reconstitution. Care must be taken to assure the sterility of prepared solutions. Parenteral drug products should be inspected visually for particulate matter and discoloration prior to administration.

PERCENT OF CLL PATIENTS REPORTING NON-HEMATOLOGIC ADVERSE EVENTS

ADVERSE EVENTS	MDAH (N=101)	SWOG (N=32)
ANY ADVERSE EVENT	88%	91%
BODY AS A WHOLE	72	84
FEVER	60	69
CHILLS	11	19
FATIGUE	10	38
INFECTION	33	44
PAIN	20	22
MALAISE	8	6
DIAPHORESIS	1	13
ALOPECIA	0	3
ANAPHYLAXIS	1	0
HEMORRHAGE	1	0
HYPERGLYCEMIA	1	6
DEHYDRATION	1	0
NEUROLOGICAL	21	69
WEAKNESS	9	65
PARESTHESIA	4	12
HEADACHE	3	0
VISUAL DISTURBANCE	3	15
HEARING LOSS	2	6
SLEEP DISORDER	1	3
DEPRESSION	1	0
CEREBELLAR SYNDROME	1	0
IMPAIRED MENTATION	1	0
PULMONARY	35	69
COUGH	10	44
PNEUMONIA	16	22
DYSPNEA	9	22
SINUSITIS	5	0
PHARYNGITIS	0	9
UPPER RESPIRATORY INFECTION	2	16
ALLERGIC PNEUMONITIS	0	6
EPISTAXIS	1	0
HEMOPTYSIS	1	6
BRONCHITIS	1	0
HYPOXIA	1	0
GASTROINTESTINAL	46	63
NAUSEA/VOMITING	36	31
DIARRHEA	15	13
ANOREXIA	7	34
STOMATITIS	9	0
GI BLEEDING	3	13
ESOPHAGITIS	3	0
MUCOSITIS	2	0
LIVER FAILURE	1	0
ABNORMAL LIVER FUNCTION TEST	1	3
CHOLELITHIASIS	0	3
CONSTIPATION	1	3
DYSPHAGIA	1	0
CUTANEOUS	17	18
RASH	15	15
PRURITUS	1	3
SEBORRHEA	1	0
GENITOURINARY	12	22
DYSURIA	4	3
URINARY INFECTION	2	15
HEMATURIA	2	3
RENAL FAILURE	1	0
ABNORMAL RENAL FUNCTION TEST	1	0
PROTEINURIA	1	0
HESITANCY	0	3
CARDIOVASCULAR	12	38
EDEMA	8	19
ANGINA	0	6
CONGESTIVE HEART FAILURE	0	3
ARRHYTHMIA	0	3
SUPRAVENTRICULAR TACHYCARDIA	0	3
MYOCARDIAL INFARCTION	0	3
DEEP VENOUS THROMBOSIS	1	3
PHLEBITIS	1	3
TRANSIENT ISCHEMIC ATTACK	1	0
ANEURYSM	1	0
CEREBROVASCULAR ACCIDENT	0	3
MUSCULOSKELETAL	7	16
MYALGIA	4	16
OSTEOPOROSIS	2	0
ARTHRALGIA	1	0
TUMOR LYSIS SYNDROME	1	0

Handling and Disposal: Procedures for proper handling and disposal should be considered. Consideration should be given to handling and disposal according to guidelines issued

Continued on next page

Berlex Laboratories—Cont.

for cytotoxic drugs. Several guidelines on this subject have been published.[2-8] There is no general agreement that all of the procedures recommended in the guidelines are necessary or appropriate.

Caution should be exercised in the handling and preparation of FLUDARA FOR INJECTION solution. The use of latex gloves and safety glasses is recommended to avoid exposure in case of breakage of the vial or other accidental spillage. If the solution contacts the skin or mucous membranes, wash thoroughly with soap and water; rinse eyes thoroughly with plain water. Avoid exposure by inhalation or by direct contact of the skin or mucous membranes.

HOW SUPPLIED

FLUDARA FOR INJECTION is supplied as a white, lyophilized solid cake. Each vial contains 50 mg of fludarabine phosphate, 50 mg of mannitol and sodium hydroxide to adjust pH to 7.7. The pH range for the final product is 7.2–8.2. Store under refrigeration, between 2°–8°C (36°–46°F).
FLUDARA FOR INJECTION is supplied in a clear glass single dose vial (6 mL capacity) and packaged in a single dose vial carton in a shelf pack of five.
CAUTION: Federal law prohibits dispensing without prescription.
U.S. Patent Number: 4,357,324
NDC 50419-511-06
Manufactured by: Ben Venue Laboratories, Bedford, OH 44146
Manufactured for: Berlex Laboratories, Alameda, CA 94501
RA 1/3/92

References: 1. Cheson B.D., Bennett J.M., Rai K.R. et al. Guidelines for clinical protocols for chronic lymphocytic leukemia: Recommendations of the National Cancer Institute-Sponsored Working Group. Amer J Hematol 29:152–163, 1988. **2.** Recommendations for the Safe Handling of Parenteral Antineoplastic Drugs. NIH Publication No. 83-2621. For sale by the Superintendent of Documents, U.S. Government Printing Office, Washington, D.C. 20402. **3.** AMA Council Report. Guidelines for Handling Parenteral Antineoplastics, JAMA, 1985; March 15. **4.** National Study Commission on Cytotoxic Exposure—Recommendations for Handling Cytotoxic Agents. Available from Louis P. Jeffrey, Sc.D., Chairman, National Study Commission on Cytotoxic Exposure, Massachusetts College of Pharmacy and Allied Health Sciences, 179 Longwood Avenue, Boston, Massachusetts 02115. **5.** Clinical Oncological Society of Australia: Guidelines and Recommendations for Safe Handling of Antineoplastic Agents, Med. J. Australia 1983;1:426–428. **6.** Jones, R.B. et al. Safe Handling of Chemotherapeutic Agents: A Report from the Mount Sinai Medical Center, Ca—A Cancer Journal for Clinicians 1983; Sept/Oct. 258–263. **7.** American Society of Hospital Pharmacists Technical Assistance Bulletin on Handling Cytotoxic Drugs in Hospitals, Am. J. Hosp. Pharm. 1985;42:131–137. **8.** OSHA Work-Practice Guidelines for Personnel Dealing with Cytotoxic (antineoplastic) Drugs. Am. J. Hosp. Pharm. 1986;43:1193–1204.

Shown in Product Identification Section, page 405

Berna Products Corp.
4216 PONCE DE LEON BLVD.
CORAL GABLES, FL. 33146

TYPHOID VACCINE LIVE ORAL Ty21a   ℞
VIVOTIF BERNA™

DESCRIPTION

Vivotif Berna™ (Typhoid Vaccine Live Oral Ty21a) is a live attenuated vaccine for oral administration. The vaccine contains the attenuated strain Salmonella typhi Ty21a. Vivotif Berna™ Vaccine is manufactured by the Swiss Serum and Vaccine Institute. The vaccine strain is grown under controlled conditions in medium containing a digest of bovine tissues, an acid digest of casein, dextrose and galactose. The bacteria are collected by centrifiguation, mixed with a stabilizer containing lactose and amino acids, and lyophilized. The lyophilized bacteria are filled into gelatin capsules which are coated with organic solution to render them resistant to dissolution in stomach acid. The enteric-coated capsules are then packaged in 4-capsule blisters for distribution.

HOW SUPPLIED

A single foil blister containing 4 doses of vaccine in a single package.
For prescribing information write to:
Customer Service, BERNA PRODUCTS CORP., 4216 Ponce de Leon Blvd., Coral Gables, Fla. 33146, or call 1-800-533-5899.

Beutlich L. P.
7149 N. AUSTIN AVENUE
NILES, IL 60648

CEO–TWO® SUPPOSITORIES   OTC

COMPOSITION

Each adult rectal suppository contains sodium bicarbonate and potassium bitartrate in a water soluble polyethylene glycol base.

ACTIONS

CEO-TWO suppositories are easy to use, effective and predictable. They will not disturb the homeostasis of the bowel. They are gentle and will not irritate the bowel which often would result in a secondary urge to defecate. CEO-TWO will not cause cramping.
CEO-TWO suppositories combine with the natural moisture in the bowel to gently release approximately 175 cc's of carbon dioxide. The slowly released CO_2 distends the rectal ampulla thus stimulating peristalsis. The emollient base allows for easy insertion and lubricates the bowel wall to facilitate passage of feces. Defecation generally occurs within 10 to 30 minutes after insertion of the suppository.

INDICATIONS

CEO-TWO is indicated for the relief of constipation in adolescents through geriatrics. It is used effectively in bowel training and maintenance programs. It will provide predictable results prior to lower endoscopic procedures as well as pre and post operative or pre and post partum bowel emptying. CEO-TWO should be used whenever the last 25 cm of the bowel must be evacuated.

ADMINISTRATION AND DOSAGE

One or two suppositories can be used as needed. Moisten CEO-TWO with warm water before inserting. Patient should retain as long as possible. Dosage can be repeated in 4–6 hours if necessary.

CONTRAINDICATIONS

As with other enemas or laxatives.

WARNINGS

Do not use CEO-TWO when abdominal pain, nausea or vomiting are present unless directed by a physician.

HOW SUPPLIED

In packages of 10, white opaque suppositories. Keep in cool, dry place.
DO NOT REFRIGERATE

HURRICAINE® TOPICAL ANESTHETIC   OTC

COMPOSITION

HURRICAINE contains 20% benzocaine in a flavored, water soluble polyethylene glycol base.

ACTION AND INDICATIONS

HURRICAINE is a topical anesthetic that provides rapid anesthesia in 15 to 30 seconds, short duration of 15 minutes, has virtually no systemic absorption, and tastes good. Hurricaine is used as a lubricant and topical anesthetic to facilitate passage of fiberoptic gastroscopes, laryngoscopes, proctoscopes and sigmoidoscopes. In addition, Hurricaine is effective in suppressing the pharyngeal and tracheal gag reflex during the placement of nasogastric tubes. Hurricaine is used to control pain and discomfort during certain gynecological procedures such as IUD insertion, vaginal speculum placement, LEEP and as a preinjection anesthetic prior to para-cervical blocks. Hurricaine is also effective in controlling various types of pain generally associated with dental procedures.

CONTRAINDICATIONS

Patients with a known hypersensitivity to benzocaine should not use HURRICAINE. True allergic reactions are rare.

ADVERSE REACTIONS

Methemoglobinemia has been reported following the use of benzocaine on extremely rare occasions. Intravenous methylene blue is the specific therapy for this condition.

CAUTIONS

DO NOT USE IN THE EYES.
NOT FOR INJECTION.
KEEP THIS AND ALL DRUGS OUT OF THE REACH OF CHILDREN.

PACKAGING AVAILABLE

Gel
1 oz. Jar Wild Cherry NDC #0283-0871-31
1 oz. Jar Pina Colada NDC #0283-0886-31
1/8 oz. Tube Wild Cherry NDC #0283-0871-12
Liquid
1 fl. oz. Jar Wild Cherry NDC #0283-0569-31
1 fl. oz. Jar Pina Colada NDC #0283-1886-31

1/8 oz. Tube Wild Cherry NDC #0283-0569-12
.25 gm. Packet Wild Cherry NDC #0283-0569-50
.25 gm. Packet Pina Colada NDC #0283-1886-50
Spray
2 oz. Aerosol Wild Cherry NDC #0283-679-02
Spray Kit
2 oz. Aerosol Wild Cherry NDC #0283-183-02 with 200 Disposable Extension Tubes

---

PERIDIN-C®   OTC

COMPOSITION

Each tablet contains Hesperidin Methyl Chalcone 50 mg., Hesperidin Complex 150 mg., Ascorbic Acid 200 mg., F.D. & C. #6.

DOSAGE

1 tablet daily or as directed.

HOW SUPPLIED

In bottles of 100 and 500 orange tablets.

EDUCATIONAL MATERIAL

Samples and literature available upon request.

Biocraft Laboratories, Inc.
18-01 RIVER ROAD
FAIR LAWN, NJ 07410

NDC 0332	PRODUCT	PROD. ID. NO.
	ALBUTEROL SULFATE TABLETS ℞	
2226	2 mg	130
2228	4 mg	131
	AMILORIDE HYDROCHLORIDE AND HYDROCHLOROTHIAZIDE TABLETS ℞	
2205	5 mg/50 mg	52
	AMITRIPTYLINE HYDROCHLORIDE TABLETS ℞	
2120	10 mg	22
2122	25 mg	23
2124	50 mg	24
2126	75 mg	25
2128	100 mg	26
	AMOXICILLIN CAPSULES ℞	
3107	250 mg	01
3109	500 mg	03
	AMOXICILLIN FOR ORAL SUSPENSION ℞	
4150	125 mg/5 mL	
4155	250 mg/5 mL	
	AMPICILLIN CAPSULES ℞	
3111	250 mg	05
3113	500 mg	06
	AMPICILLIN FOR ORAL SUSPENSION ℞	
4129	125 mg/5 mL	
4131	250 mg/5 mL	
	AMPICILLIN-PROBENECID FOR ORAL SUSPENSION ℞	
4140	1 gm Probenecid; 3.5 gm Ampicillin	
	BACLOFEN TABLETS ℞	
2234	10 mg	141
2236	20 mg	142
	CEPHALEXIN CAPSULES ℞	
3145	250 mg	115
3147	500 mg	117
	CEPHALEXIN FOR ORAL SUSPENSION ℞	
4175	125 mg/5 mL	
4177	250 mg/5 mL	
	CEPHALEXIN TABLETS ℞	
2238	250 mg	136
2240	500 mg	137
	CEPHRADINE CAPSULES ℞	
3153	250 mg	112
3155	500 mg	113
	CEPHRADINE FOR ORAL SUSPENSION ℞	
4165	125 mg/5 mL	
4167	250 mg/5 mL	
	CHLOROQUINE PHOSPHATE TABLETS ℞	
2160	250 mg	38
	CINOXACIN CAPSULES ℞	
3181	500 mg	164

	CLINDAMYCIN HYDROCHLORIDE CAPSULES ℞	
3169	75 mg	148
3171	150 mg	149
	CLOXACILLIN SODIUM CAPSULES ℞	
3119	250 mg	28
3121	500 mg	30
	CLOXACILLIN SODIUM FOR ORAL SOLUTION ℞	
4159	125 mg/5 mL	
	DICLOXACILLIN SODIUM CAPSULES ℞	
3123	250 mg	02
3125	500 mg	04
	DISOPYRAMIDE PHOSPHATE CAPSULES ℞	
3127	100 mg	40
3129	150 mg	41
	IMIPRAMINE HYDROCHLORIDE TABLETS ℞	
2111	10 mg	19
2113	25 mg	20
2117	50 mg	21
	METAPROTERENOL SULFATE SYRUP ℞	
6117	10 mg/5 mL	
	METAPROTERENOL SULFATE TABLETS ℞	
2230	10 mg	132
2232	20 mg	133
	METOCLOPRAMIDE SYRUP ℞	
6105	5 mg/5 mL	
	METOCLOPRAMIDE TABLETS ℞	
2203	10 mg	93
	MINOCYCLINE HYDROCHLORIDE CAPSULES ℞	
3165	50 mg	134
3167	100 mg	135
	NEOMYCIN SULFATE TABLETS ℞	
1177	500 mg	18
	NYSTATIN ORAL SUSPENSION ℞	
6109	100,000 units/mL	
	OXACILLIN SODIUM CAPSULES ℞	
3115	250 mg	12
3117	500 mg	14
	OXACILLIN SODIUM FOR ORAL SOLUTION ℞	
4157	250 mg/5 mL	
	PENICILLIN G POTASSIUM TABLETS ℞	
1117	200,000 units	07
1121	250,000 units	09
1123	400,000 units	10
	PENICILLIN V POTASSIUM FOR ORAL SOLUTION ℞	
4125	125 mg/5 mL	
4127	250 mg/5 mL	
	PENICILLIN V POTASSIUM TABLETS ℞	
1171	250 mg ROUND	15
1172	250 mg OVAL	16
1173	500 mg ROUND	17
1174	500 mg OVAL	49
	SULFAMETHOXAZOLE AND TRIMETHOPRIM ORAL SUSPENSION ℞	
6100	200 mg/40 mg per 5 mL	
	SULFAMETHOXAZOLE AND TRIMETHOPRIM TABLETS ℞	
2130	400 mg/80 mg (Single Strength)	32
2132	800 mg/160 mg (Double Strength)	33
	TRIMETHOPRIM TABLETS ℞	
2158	100 mg	34
2159	200 mg	35

Bio-Tech Pharmacal, Inc.
P.O. BOX 1992
FAYETTEVILLE, AR 72702

B-12 RESIN (Sublingual)   OTC

Each tablet contains 1,000 mcg Vit B-12 on Ion Exchange Resin.

BROMASE   OTC
(Proteolytic Enzyme)
(Bromelain)

Each BROMASE capsule contains 500 mg of Bromelain (2400mcu/gm), 15 mg Ascorbic Acid.

C-MAX   OTC

Each gradual release tablet contains Vit C (Mg, Zn, K, Mn Ascorbate) 1,000 mg; Mg (Ascorbate) 40 mg; Zn (Ascorbate) 5 mg; K (Ascorbate) 10 mg; Mn (Ascorbate) 1 mg; Pectin 10 mg.

K-MAG-70   OTC

Each capsule contains: Mg (El) 70 mg (from Mg Aspartate); K (El) 70 mg (from K Aspartate).

MAG-L-100   OTC

Each enteric-coated tablet contains Mg Cl 833 mg.

OB-20 Pre- and Peri-Natal (YEAST FREE)   OTC

Each 2 tablets contain: Vit A (Beta Carotene) 4,000 USP Units; Vit D-3 200 USP Units; Vit E 15 USP Units; Vit C 60 mg; Folic Acid 0.5 mg; Vit B-1 0.86 mg; Vit B-2 1.0 mg; Vit B-3 10.0 mg; Vit B-6 5.0 mg; Vit B-12 (Resin Adsorbate) 4.0 mcg; Biotin 75.0 mcg; Pantothenic Acid 5.0 mg; Calcium (Citrate) 250 mg; Iron (Fe Gluconate) 25.0 mg; Mg (Ascorbate) 75 mg; Zn (Ascorbate) 12.5 mg; Mn (Ascorbate) 2.5 mg; Cr (Chelate) NON-YEAST 12.5 mcg; Se (Chelate) NON-YEAST 12.5 mcg.

P-1000   OTC

Each two (2) capsules contain: Lemon Bioflavonoid Complex 1,000 mg "Testlab 50."

SAM-E.P.A.   OTC

Each softgel contains: Marine Lipid Concentrate 1,000 mg (EPA 300 mg; DHA 200 mg; Total Omega-3 500 mg); Vit E 1 USP Unit.

VITA-MIN   OTC

Hypo-Allergenic YEAST-FREE Highly Bioavailable Vitamin-Mineral Multiple.

Blaine Company, Inc.
1465 JAMIKE LANE
ERLANGER, KY 41018

MAG-OX 400   OTC

DESCRIPTION
Each tablet contains Magnesium Oxide 400 mg. U.S.P. (Heavy), or 241.3 mg. Elemental Magnesium (19.86 mEq.)

INDICATIONS AND USAGE
Hypomagnesemia, magnesium deficiencies and/or magnesium depletion resulting from malnutrition, restricted diet, alcoholism or magnesium depleting drugs. An antacid. For increasing urinary magnesium excretion. Supplemental magnesium during pregnancy.

WARNINGS
Do not take more than 2 tablets in a 24 hour period, or use this maximum dosage for more than 2 weeks, except under the advice and supervision of a physician. Do not use this product except under the advice and supervision of a physician if you have a kidney disease. May have laxative effect. As with any drug, if you are pregnant or nursing a baby, seek professional advice before using this product. Keep this and all medicines out of children's reach.

DOSAGE
Adult dose 1 or 2 tablets daily or as directed by a physician.

HOW SUPPLIED
Bottles of 100 and 1000.

URO-MAG   OTC

DESCRIPTION
Each capsule contains Magnesium Oxide 140 mg. U.S.P. (Heavy), or 84.5 mg. Elemental Magnesium (6.93 mEq.)

INDICATIONS AND USAGE
Hypomagnesemia, magnesium deficiencies and/or magnesium depletion resulting from malnutrition, restricted diet, alcoholism or magnesium depleting drugs. An antacid. For increasing urinary magnesium excretion. Supplemental magnesium during pregnancy.

WARNINGS
Do not take more than 4 capsules in a 24 hour period, or use this maximum dosage for more than 2 weeks, except under

the advice and supervision of a physician. Do not use this product except under the advice and supervision of a physician if you have a kidney disease. May have laxative effect. As with any drug, if you are pregnant or nursing a baby, seek professional advice before using this product. Keep this and all medicines out of children's reach.

DOSAGE
Adult dose 3–4 capsules daily or as directed by a physician.

HOW SUPPLIED
Bottles of 100 and 1000.

EDUCATIONAL MATERIAL

Samples and literature available to physicians upon request.

Blair Laboratories, Inc.
(a division of The Purdue
Frederick Company)
100 CONNECTICUT AVENUE
NORWALK, CT 06850-3590

SOOTHE & CLEAN™   OTC
Personal Cleansing Foam

Distributed by Blair Laboratories, Inc., a division of The Purdue Frederick Company.
ACTION AND USES
SOOTHE & CLEAN is an alcohol-free, lanolin-rich foam that softens and moistens toilet tissue to comfort and clean sensitive areas. Its unique formula gently cleanses personal areas made tender by external hemorrhoids, surgical stitches, or other minor irritations. Use with bathroom tissue to soothe and cleanse anal or outer vaginal areas, SOOTHE & CLEAN removes residue and bacteria that can cause irritation. SOOTHE & CLEAN is convenient, easy to use, and economical—approximately 60 uses per 1.5-oz. canister.
Use of SOOTHE & CLEAN on bathroom tissue is especially appropriate:
● During external hemorrhoid flare-ups.
● When new mothers are tender after childbirth.
● For external cleansing during menstruation.
● When there's irritation from diarrhea.
● Whenever tender rectal or outer vaginal areas need extra gentle, extra soothing cleansing.
● Anytime when bathroom tissue alone is not enough.

DIRECTIONS
Shake well. Dispense small amount (about the size of a cotton ball) onto bathroom tissue and use as a final cleansing step. Use as often as needed, up to a maximum of 6 times per day. For best results hold can upright.

CAUTION
For external use only. In case of rectal bleeding, discontinue use and consult a physician promptly. Keep out of reach of children. In case of accidental ingestion, seek professional assistance or contact a Poison Control Center immediately.

WARNINGS
Contents under pressure. Do not puncture or incinerate. Do not store at temperatures above 120° F.

ACTIVE INGREDIENTS
Glycerin, non-alcoholic witch hazel.

OTHER INGREDIENTS
Water, Polysorbate 80, Cetyl acetate, Acetylated lanolin, Isobutane, Polysorbate 20, Fragrance.

HOW SUPPLIED
1.5 oz. Aerosol Canister.
NDC: 0154-1300-15
Copyright 1991, Blair Laboratories, Inc.

EDUCATIONAL MATERIAL

"A Helpful Guide to Personal Cleansing" booklet (Soothe & Clean)

Products are cross-indexed by
generic and chemical names in the
YELLOW SECTION.

Bock Pharmacal Company
P.O. BOX 8519
ST. LOUIS, MO 63126-0519

BRONCHOLATE® CS   ℃

Each 5 ml cherry flavored red syrup contains:
Codeine Phosphate .... 10.00 mg
  (Warning: May be habit forming)
Ephedrine HCl... 6.25 mg
Guaifenesin .... 100.00 mg

HOW SUPPLIED
Bottles of 16 oz.

BRONCHOLATE® SOFTGELS   ℞

Each orange football shaped softgel contains:
Ephedrine HCl... 12.5 mg
Guaifenesin .... 200.0 mg

HOW SUPPLIED
Bottles of 100

BRONCHOLATE® SYRUP   ℞

Each 5 ml orange flavored syrup contains:
Ephedrine HCl... 6.25 mg
Guaifenesin .... 100.00 mg

HOW SUPPLIED
Bottles of 16 oz.

EMETROL® SOLUTION—CHERRY   OTC

Each teaspoonful (5ml) contains:
  Dextrose (glucose) .... 1.87 g
  Levulose (fructose) .... 1.87 g
  Phosphoric Acid .... 21.5 mg

EMETROL® SOLUTION—LEMON-MINT   OTC

Each teaspoonful (5ml) contains:
  Dextrose (glucose) .... 1.87 g
  Levulose (fructose) .... 1.87 g
  Phosphoric Acid .... 21.5 mg

HEMASPAN®   OTC

Each tan colored caplet embossed bock on one side and HS
bisect 33 on the other contains:
*Elemental Iron .... 110.0 mg
(as Ferrous Fumarate–335 mg)
 Vitamin C .... 200.0 mg
 Docusate Sodium .... 20.0 mg
*In a special base to provide delayed therapeutic action.

HOW SUPPLIED
Bottles of 100.

HISTUSSIN® HC   ℞ Ⓒ

Each 5 ml orange/pineapple flavored syrup contains:
Hydrocodone Bitartrate .... 2.5 mg
  (Warning: May be habit forming.)
Phenylephrine Hydrochloride .... 5.0 mg
Chlorpheniramine Maleate .... 2.0 mg

HOW SUPPLIED
Bottles of 16 oz.

POLY-HISTINE CS®   ℞ ℃

Each 5 ml raspberry/strawberry flavored red syrup con-
tains:
Codeine Phosphate .... 10.0 mg
  (Warning: May be habit forming.)
Phenylpropanolamine HCl .... 12.5 mg
Brompheniramine Maleate .... 2.0 mg

HOW SUPPLIED
Bottles of 16 oz.

POLY-HISTINE ELIXIR®   ℞

Each 5 ml lemon-lime flavored green elixir contains:
Phenyltoloxamine Citrate .... 4.0 mg
Pyrilamine Maleate .... 4.0 mg
Pheniramine Maleate .... 4.0 mg
Alcohol 4%

HOW SUPPLIED
Bottles of 16 oz.

POLY-HISTINE-D® CAPSULES   ℞

Each red-clear timed release capsule* imprinted BOCK
contains:
Phenylpropanolamine HCl .... 50.0 mg
Phenyltoloxamine Citrate .... 16.0 mg
Pyrilamine Maleate .... 16.0 mg
Pheniramine Maleate .... 16.0 mg
*In a special base to provide prolonged therapeutic action.

HOW SUPPLIED
Bottles of 100.

POLY-HISTINE-D® ELIXIR   ℞

Each 5 ml wild cherry flavored red elixir contains:
Phenylpropanolamine HCl .... 12.5 mg
Phenyltoloxamine Citrate .... 4.0 mg
Pyrilamine Maleate .... 4.0 mg
Pheniramine Maleate .... 4.0 mg
Alcohol 4%

HOW SUPPLIED
Bottles of 16 oz.

POLY-HISTINE-D® PED CAPS   ℞

Each clear timed release capsule* imprinted BOCK contains:
Phenylpropanolamine HCl .... 25.0 mg
Phenyltoloxamine Citrate .... 8.0 mg
Pyrilamine Maleate .... 8.0 mg
Pheniramine Maleate .... 8.0 mg
*In a special base to provide prolonged therapeutic action.

HOW SUPPLIED
Bottles of 100.

POLY-HISTINE DM® SYRUP   ℞

Each 5 ml black-raspberry flavored purple syrup contains:
Dextromethorphan HBr .... 10.0 mg
Phenylpropanolamine HCl .... 12.5 mg
Brompheniramine Maleate .... 2.0 mg

HOW SUPPLIED
Bottles of 16 oz.

PRENATE 90®   ℞
Vitamin-Mineral Supplement

Each white film coated tablet embossed BOCK contains:
Elemental Iron .... 90.0 mg*
(as Ferrous Fumarate–270 mg)
Iodine (Potassium Iodide) .... 0.15 mg
Calcium (Calcium Carbonate) .... 250.0 mg
Copper (Cupric Oxide) .... 2.0 mg
Zinc (Zinc Oxide) .... 25.0 mg
Folic Acid .... 1.0 mg
Vitamin A (Acetate) .... 4000.0 I.U.
Vitamin D (Ergocalciferol) .... 400.0 I.U.
Vitamin E (Acetate) .... 30.0 I.U.
Vitamin C (Ascorbic Acid) .... 120.0 mg
Vitamin B₁ (Thiamine Mononitrate) .... 3.0 mg
Vitamin B₂ (Riboflavin) .... 3.4 mg
Vitamin B₆ (Pyridoxine HCl) .... 20.0 mg
Vitamin B₁₂ (Cyanocobalamin) .... 12.0 mcg
Niacinamide .... 20.0 mg
Docusate Sodium .... 50.0 mg
*MICRO IRON (A special base to provide delayed therapeu-
tic action)

HOW SUPPLIED
Bottles of 100.

ZEPHREX® TABLETS   ℞

Each blue film coated tablet embossed BOCK contains:
Pseudoephedrine HCl .... 60.0 mg
Guaifenesin .... 400.0 mg

HOW SUPPLIED
Bottles of 100.

ZEPHREX LA® TABLETS   ℞

Each orange timed release tablet* embossed BOCK contains:
Pseudoephedrine HCl .... 120.0 mg
Guaifenesin .... 600.0 mg
*In a special base to provide prolonged therapeutic action.

HOW SUPPLIED
Bottles of 100.

Boehringer Ingelheim Pharmaceuticals, Inc.
A subsidiary of Boehringer Ingelheim Corporation
900 RIDGEBURY ROAD
POST OFFICE BOX 368
RIDGEFIELD, CT 06877-0368

ALUPENT®   ℞
[al'u-pent]
(metaproterenol sulfate, USP)
Bronchodilator

Tablets 10 mg	BI-CODE 74
Tablets 20 mg	BI-CODE 72
Inhalation Aerosol 10 ml	BI-CODE 70
Syrup 10 mg/5 ml	BI-CODE 73
Inhalation Solution 5%	BI-CODE 71
Inhalation Solution	BI-CODE 69
Unit-dose Vials 0.4% and 0.6%	

DESCRIPTION

Alupent® (metaproterenol sulfate USP) Inhalation Aerosol
is administered by oral inhalation. The Alupent Inhalation
Aerosol containing 150 mg of metaproterenol sulfate as micronized powder is sufficient medication for 200 inhalations.
Each metered dose delivers through the mouthpiece 0.65 mg
of metaproterenol sulfate (each ml contains 15 mg). The inert ingredients are dichlorodifluoromethane, dichlorotetrafluoroethane and trichloromonofluoromethane as propellants, and sorbitan trioleate.
Alupent Inhalation Solution is administered by oral inhalation with the aid of a hand-bulb nebulizer or an intermittent
positive pressure breathing apparatus (IPPB). It contains
Alupent 5% in a pH-adjusted aqueous solution containing
benzalkonium chloride and edetate disodium as preservatives.
Alupent Inhalation Solution Unit-dose Vial is administered
by oral inhalation with the aid of an IPPB. It contains Alupent 0.4% or 0.6% in a sterile pH-adjusted aqueous solution
with edetate disodium and sodium chloride.
Alupent Syrup is administered orally. Each teaspoonful (5
ml) of syrup contains metaproterenol sulfate 10 mg. The
inactive ingredients are edetate disodium, FD&C Red No. 40,
hydroxyethylcellulose, imitation black cherry flavor, methylparaben, propylparaben, saccharin, sorbitol solution.
Alupent Tablets are administered orally. Each tablet contains metaproterenol sulfate 10 mg or 20 mg. The inactive
ingredients are colloidal silicon dioxide, cornstarch, dibasic
calcium phosphate, lactose, magnesium stearate.
Chemically, Alupent is 1-(3,5 dihydroxyphenyl)-2-iso-
propylaminoethanol sulfate, a white crystalline, racemic
mixture of two optically active isomers. It differs from isoproterenol hydrochloride by having two hydroxyl groups
attached at the meta positions on the benzene ring rather
than one at the meta and one at the para position.

Mol. Wt. 520.59
metaproterenol sulfate (Alupent)
$(C_{11}H_{17}NO_3)_2 \cdot H_2SO_4$

CLINICAL PHARMACOLOGY
Alupent® (metaproterenol sulfate USP) is a potent beta-
adrenergic stimulator. Alupent Inhalation Aerosol and Inhalation Solution have a rapid onset of action. It is postu-

lated that beta-adrenergic stimulants produce many of their pharmacological effects by activation of adenyl cyclase, the enzyme that catalyzes the conversion of adenosine triphosphate to cyclic adenosine monophosphate.

Pharmacokinetics: Absorption, biotransformation and excretion studies in humans following administration by inhalation have shown that approximately 3 percent of the actuated dose is absorbed intact through the lungs.

Following oral administration in humans, an average of 40% of the drug is absorbed; it is not metabolized by catechol-O-methyltransferase or sulfatase enzymes in the gut, but is excreted primarily as glucuronic acid conjugates.

When administered orally or by inhalation, Alupent decreases reversible bronchospasm. Pulmonary function tests performed concomitantly usually show improvement following aerosol Alupent administration, e.g., an increase in the one-second forced expiratory volume (FEV_1), an increase in maximum expiratory flow rate, an increase in peak expiratory flow rate, an increase in forced vital capacity, and/or a decrease in airway resistance. The resultant decrease in airway obstruction may relieve the dyspnea associated with bronchospasm.

Controlled single- and multiple-dose studies have been performed with pulmonary function monitoring. The duration of effect of a single dose of Alupent Tablets 20 mg or Alupent Syrup (that is, the period of time during which there is a 15% or greater increase in FEV_1) was up to 4 hours. Four controlled multiple-dose 60-day studies, comparing the effectiveness of Alupent Tablets with ephedrine tablets, have been performed. Because of difficulties in study design, only one study was available which could be analyzed in depth. This study showed a loss of efficacy with time for both Alupent and ephedrine. Therefore, the physician should take this phenomenon into account in evaluating the individual patient's overall management. Further studies are in progress to adequately explain these results.

Controlled single- and multiple-dose studies have been performed with pulmonary function monitoring. The duration of effect of a single dose of two to three inhalations of Alupent Inhalation Aerosol (that is, the period of time during which there is a 20% or greater increase in FEV_1) has varied from 1 to 5 hours.

In repetitive-dosing studies (up to q.i.d.) the duration of effect for a similar dose of Alupent Inhalation Aerosol has ranged from about 1 to 2.5 hours. Present studies are inadequate to explain the divergence in duration of the FEV_1 effect between single- and repetitive-dosing studies, respectively.

Following controlled single dose studies with Alupent Inhalation Solution by an intermittent positive pressure breathing apparatus (IPPB) and by hand-bulb nebulizers, significant improvement (15% or greater increase in FEV_1) occurred within 5 to 30 minutes and persisted for periods varying from 2 to 6 hours.

In these studies, the longer duration of effect occurred in the studies in which the drug was administered by IPPB, i.e., 6 hours, versus 2 to 3 hours when administered by hand-bulb nebulizer. In these studies, the doses used were 0.3 ml by IPPB and 10 inhalations by hand-bulb nebulizer.

In controlled repetitive-dosing studies with Alupent Inhalation Solution by IPPB and by hand-bulb nebulizer the onset of effect occurred within 5 to 30 minutes and duration ranged from 4 to 6 hours. In these studies, the doses used were 0.3 ml b.i.d. or t.i.d. when given by IPPB, and 10 inhalations q.i.d. (no more often than q4h) when given by hand-bulb nebulizer. As in the single dose studies, effectiveness was measured as a sustained increase in FEV_1 of 15% or greater. In these repetitive-dosing studies there was no apparent difference in duration between the two methods of delivery.

Clinical studies were conducted in which the effectiveness of Alupent Inhalation Solution was evaluated by comparison with that of isoproterenol hydrochloride over periods of two to three months. Both drugs continued to produce significant improvement in pulmonary function throughout this period of treatment.

In two well-controlled studies in children 6 to 12 years of age with acute exacerbation of asthma, 70% of patients receiving Alupent Inhalation Solution (0.1 mL to 0.2 mL) showed improvement in pulmonary function as demonstrated by a 15% increase in FEV_1 above baseline.

Recent studies in laboratory animals (minipigs, rodents and dogs) recorded the occurrence of cardiac arrhythmias and sudden death (with histologic evidence of myocardial necrosis) when beta agonists and methylxanthines were administered concurrently. The significance of these findings when applied to humans is currently unknown.

INDICATIONS AND USAGE

Alupent® (metaproterenol sulfate USP) is indicated as a bronchodilator for bronchial asthma and for reversible bronchospasm which may occur in association with bronchitis and emphysema. Alupent Inhalation Solution is additionally indicated for the treatment of acute asthmatic attacks in children age 6 years and older.

CONTRAINDICATIONS

Use in patients with cardiac arrhythmias associated with tachycardia is contraindicated.

Although rare, immediate hypersensitivity reactions can occur. Therefore, Alupent® (metaproterenol sulfate USP) is contraindicated in patients with a history of hypersensitivity to any of its components.

WARNINGS

Excessive use of adrenergic aerosols is potentially dangerous. Fatalities have been reported following excessive use of Alupent® (metaproterenol sulfate USP) as with other sympathomimetic inhalation preparations, and the exact cause is unknown. Cardiac arrest was noted in several cases.

Alupent, like other beta adrenergic agonists, can produce a significant cardiovascular effect in some patients, as measured by pulse rate, blood pressure, symptoms and/or ECG changes. As with other beta adrenergic aerosols, Alupent can produce paradoxical bronchospasm (which can be life threatening). If it occurs, the preparation should be discontinued immediately and alternative therapy instituted.

Alupent® (metaproterenol sulfate USP) should not be used more often than prescribed. Patients should be advised to contact their physician in the event that they do not respond to their usual dose of a sympathomimetic amine aerosol.

PRECAUTIONS

General: Extreme care must be exercised with respect to the administration of additional sympathomimetic agents. Since metaproterenol is a sympathomimetic amine it should be used with caution in patients with cardiovascular disorders, including ischemic heart disease, hypertension or cardiac arrhythmias, in patients with hyperthyroidism or diabetes mellitus, and in patients who are unusually responsive to sympathomimetic amines or who have convulsive disorders. Significant changes in systolic and diastolic blood pressure could be expected to occur in some patients after use of any beta adrenergic bronchodilator.

Physicians should recognize that a single dose of nebulized Alupent® (metaproterenol sulfate USP) in the treatment of acute asthma may alleviate symptoms and improve pulmonary function temporarily but fail to completely abort an attack.

Information for Patients: Extreme care must be exercised with respect to the administration of additional sympathomimetic agents. A sufficient interval of time should elapse prior to administration of another sympathomimetic agent. A single dose of nebulized Alupent in the treatment of an acute attack of asthma may not completely abort an attack.

Drug Interactions: Other beta adrenergic aerosol bronchodilators should not be used concomitantly with Alupent® (metaproterenol sulfate USP) because they may have additive effects. Beta adrenergic agonists should be administered with caution to patients being treated with monoamine oxidase inhibitors or tricyclic antidepressants, since the action of beta adrenergic agonists on the vascular system may be potentiated.

Carcinogenesis/Mutagenesis/Impairment of Fertility: In an 18-month study in mice, Alupent produced an increase in benign ovarian tumors in females at doses corresponding to 320 and 640 times the maximum recommended dose (based on a 50 kg individual). In a two-year study in rats, a non-significant incidence of benign leiomyomata of the mesovarium was noted at 640 times the maximum recommended dose. The relevance of these findings to man is not known. Mutagenic studies with Alupent have not been conducted. Reproduction studies in rats revealed no evidence of impaired fertility.

Pregnancy/Teratogenic Effects *PREGNANCY CATEGORY C:* Alupent has been shown to be teratogenic and embryotoxic in rabbits when given orally in doses 620 times the human inhalation dose and 62 times the human oral dose. There are no adequate and well-controlled studies in pregnant women. Alupent should be used during pregnancy only if the potential benefit justifies the potential risk to the fetus.

Oral reproduction studies in mice, rats and rabbits showed no teratogenic or embryocidal effects at 50 mg/kg corresponding to 310 times the human inhalation dose and 31 times the human oral dose. Teratogenic effects in the rabbit included skeletal abnormalities and hydrocephalus with bone separation.

Nursing Mothers: It is not known whether this drug is excreted in human milk. Because many drugs are excreted in human milk, caution should be exercised when Alupent is administered to a nursing woman.

Pediatric Use: See **DOSAGE AND ADMINISTRATION.**

ADVERSE REACTIONS

Adverse reactions are similar to those noted with other sympathomimetic agents. Adverse reactions such as tachycardia, hypertension, palpitations, nervousness, tremor, nausea and vomiting have been reported.

The most frequent adverse reaction to Alupent® (metaproterenol sulfate USP) administered by metered-dose inhaler among 251 patients in 90-day controlled clinical trials was nervousness. This was reported in 6.8% of patients. Less frequent adverse experiences, occurring in 1–4% of patients were headache, dizziness, palpitations, gastrointestinal distress, tremor, throat irritation, nausea, vomiting, cough and asthma exacerbation. Tachycardia occurred in less than 1% of patients.

Adverse experiences associated with Alupent Inhalation Solution in at least 2% of 120 patients participating in multiple-dose clinical trial of 60- and 90-day duration included nervousness (14.1%; n=17), cough (3.3%; n=4) headache (3.3%; n=4), tachycardia (2.5%; n=3) and tremor (2.5%; n=3).

Alupent Inhalation Solution may be associated with a somewhat higher incidence of eadverse reactions in children. In controlled clinical trials conducted in 160 patients the incidence of adverse reactions observed at the recommended doses was as follows: tachycardia, 16.6%; tremor, 33%; nausea, 14%; vomiting, 7.7%. The corresponding incidence in placebo-treated patients was: tachycardia, 7.6%; tremor, 20%; nausea, 7.7%; vomiting, 2.5%.

In two well-controlled studies in children 6 to 12 years of age with acute exacerbation of asthma, Alupent Inhalation Solution was not efficacious in approximately 30% of patients, where efficacy was defined as a 15% increase in FEV_1 above baseline at two or more time points during the 1-hour testing period. In 8% of patients there was a decrease in FEV_1 of 10% or more from baseline at two or more time points during the testing period. Insufficient information exists to assess the relationship of drug administration to the decline in pulmonary function observed in these patients, but paradoxical bronchospasm is one possibility.

It is important to recognize that adverse reactions from beta agonist bronchodilator solutions for nebulization may occur with the use of a new container of a product in patients who have previously tolerated that same product without adverse effect. There have been reports that indicate that such patients may subsequently tolerate replacement containers of the same product without adverse effect.

OVERDOSAGE

The expected symptoms with overdosage are those of excessive beta-adrenergic stimulation and/or any of the symptoms listed under adverse reactions, e.g. angina, hypertension or hypotension, arrhythmias, nervousness, headache, tremor, dry mouth, palpitation, nausea, dizziness, fatigue, malaise and insomnia.

Treatment consists of discontinuation of metaproterenol together with appropriate symptomatic therapy.

DOSAGE AND ADMINISTRATION

If Alupent® (metaproterenol sulfate USP) is administered before or after other sympathomimetic bronchodilators, caution should be exercised with respect to possible potentiation of adrenergic effects.

Inhalation Aerosol: The usual single dose is two to three inhalations. With repetitive dosing, inhalation should usually not be repeated more often than about every three to four hours. Total dosage per day should not exceed 12 inhalations. Alupent Inhalation Aerosol is not recommended for use in children under 12 years of age.

Inhalation Solution: Usually, treatment need not be repeated more often than every four hours to relieve acute attacks of bronchospasm.

As with all medications, the physician should begin therapy with the lowest effective dose and then titrate the dosage according to the individual patient's requirements.

Inhalation Solution 5%: Alupent Inhalation Solution is administered by oral inhalation with the aid of a hand-bulb nebulizer or an intermittent positive pressure breathing apparatus (IPPB).

Alupent Inhalation Solution may be administered three to four times a day for the treatment of reversible airways dis-

Population	Method of Administration	Usual Single Dose	Range	Dilution
Adult 12 years and older	Hand-bulb nebulizer	10 inhalations	5–15 inhalations	No dilution
	IPPB or nebulizer	0.3 ml	0.2–0.3 ml	Diluted in approx. 2.5 ml saline solution or other diluent
Pediatric 6–12 years	Nebulizer	0.1 ml	0.1–0.2 ml	Diluted in saline solution to a total volume of 3 ml

Continued on next page

Boehringer Ingelheim—Cont.

ease in adults. A single dose of nebulized Alupent in the treatment of an acute attack of asthma may not completely abort an attack. [See table at bottom of preceding page.]

Inhalation Solution 0.4% and 0.6% Unit-dose Vials: Alupent Inhalation Solution Unit-dose Vial is administered by oral inhalation using an IPPB device. The usual adult dose is one vial per nebulization treatment. Each vial of Alupent Inhalation Solution 0.4% is equivalent to 0.2 ml Alupent Inhalation Solution 5% diluted to 2.5 ml with normal saline; each vial of Alupent Inhalation Solution 0.6% is equivalent to 0.3 ml Alupent Inhalation Solution 5% diluted to 2.5 ml with normal saline.

As part of a total treatment program in chronic bronchospastic pulmonary diseases, Alupent Inhalation Solution may be administered three to four times a day.

Alupent Inhalation Solution Unit-dose vial is not recommended for use in children under 12 years of age.

Syrup: *Children:* Aged six to nine years or weight under 60 lbs—one teaspoonful three or four times a day. Children over nine years or weight over 60 lbs—two teaspoonfuls three or four times a day. Experience in children under the age of six is limited to 78 children. Of this number, 40 were treated with Alupent syrup for at least one month. In this group daily doses of approximately 1.3 to 2.6 mg/kg were well tolerated. Adults—two teaspoonfuls three or four times a day.

Tablets: *Adults:* The usual dose is 20 mg three or four times a day. *Children:* Aged six to nine years or weight under 60 lbs—10 mg three or four times a day. Over nine years or weight over 60 lbs—20 mg three or four times a day. Alupent tablets are not recommended for use in children under six years at this time.

HOW SUPPLIED

Inhalation Aerosol: Each 200 inhalations of Alupent® (metaproterenol sulfate USP) Inhalation Aerosol contains 150 mg of metaproterenol sulfate as a micronized powder in inert propellants. Each metered dose delivers through the mouthpiece 0.65 mg metaproterenol sulfate (each ml contains 15 mg). Alupent Inhalation Aerosol with Mouthpiece (NDC 0597-0070-17), net contents 14g (10 mL).The mouthpiece is white with a clear, colorless sleeve and a blue protective cap. Alupent Inhalation Aerosol Refill (NDC 0597-0070-18), net contents 14g (10 mL).

Store between 59°F (15°C) and 77°F (25°C). Avoid excessive humidity.

Inhalation Solution: Alupent Inhalation Solution is supplied as a 5% solution in bottles of 10 ml (NDC 0597-0071-75) or 30 ml (NDC 0597-0071-30) with accompanying calibrated dropper. Plastic cover on dropper should be discarded and not used to retain product. Store between 59°F (15°C) and 77°F (25°C).

Alupent Inhalation Solution Unit-dose Vial is supplied as a 0.4% (NDC 0597-0078-62) or 0.6% (NDC 0597-0069-62) clear colorless or nearly colorless solution containing 2.5 ml with 25 vials per box. Store below 77°F (25°C). Protect from light. Do not use the solution if it is pinkish or darker than slightly yellow or contains a precipitate.

Syrup: Alupent is available as a cherry-flavored syrup, 10 mg per teaspoonful (5 ml) in 16 fl. oz. bottles. Store below 86°F (30°C). Protect from light.

Tablets: Alupent is supplied in two dosage strengths as scored round white tablets in bottles of 100. Tablets of 10 mg coded BI/74. Tablets of 20 mg coded BI/72. *Storage for bottles:* Store below 86°F (30°C). Protect from light. *Storage for blister samples:* Store below 77°F (25°C). Protect from light.

Caution

Federal law prohibits dispensing without prescription.

AL-PI-1/92

Shown in Product Identification Section, page 405

ATROVENT® ℞

[ă 'trō "vĕnt]

(ipratropium bromide)
Inhalation Aerosol
Bronchodilator

<u>PRODUCT</u> <u>OVERVIEW</u>

KEY FACTS

The active ingredient in Atrovent® (ipratropium bromide) Inhalation Aerosol is ipratropium bromide. It is an anticholinergic bronchodilator classified as a synthetic quaternary ammonium compound. The bronchodilating effect of Atrovent is primarily local and site specific. It is not well absorbed systemically, resulting in a low potential for toxicity.

MAJOR USES

Atrovent Inhalation Aerosol has proved to be clinically effective for maintenance treatment of bronchospasm associated with chronic obstructive pulmonary disease, including chronic bronchitis and emphysema.

SAFETY INFORMATION

Atrovent Inhalation Aerosol is contraindicated for patients with a hypersensitivity to atropine or its derivatives. It is not intended for treatment of acute episodes of bronchospasm where rapid response is required.

Before prescribing, please consult full prescribing information below.

<u>PRESCRIBING</u> <u>INFORMATION</u>

ATROVENT® ℞

[ă 'trō"vĕnt]

(ipratropium bromide)
Inhalation Aerosol
Bronchodilator

DESCRIPTION

The active ingredient in Atrovent® (ipratropium bromide) Inhalation Aerosol is ipratropium bromide. It is an anticholinergic bronchodilator chemically described as 8-azoniabicyclo(3.2.1)-octane, 3-(3-hydroxy -1- oxo-2-phenyl propoxy)-8-methyl-8-(1-methylethyl)-, bromide, monohydrate *(endo, syn)-*, (±)-; a synthetic quaternary ammonium compound, chemically related to atropine. It has the following structural formula:

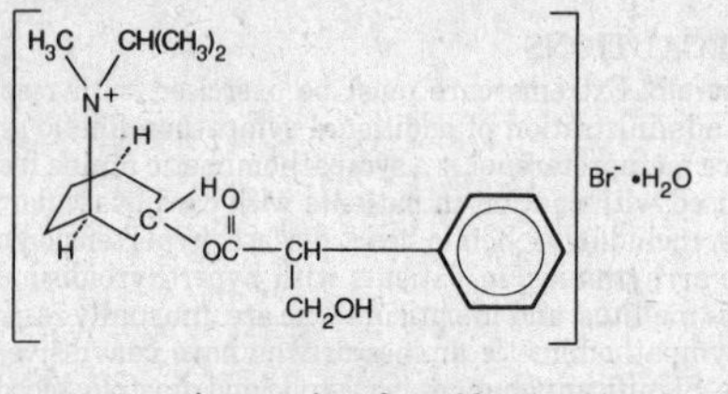

ipratropium bromide
(Atrovent)

$C_{20}H_{30}BrNO_3 \cdot H_2O$ Mol. Wt. 430.4

Ipratropium bromide is a white crystalline substance, freely soluble in water and lower alcohols but insoluble in lipophilic solvents such as ether, chloroform, and fluorocarbons.

Atrovent Inhalation Aerosol is an inhalation aerosol for oral administration. The net weight is 14 grams; it yields 200 inhalations. Each actuation of the valve delivers 18 mcg of ipratropium bromide from the mouthpiece. The inert ingredients are dichlorodifluoromethane, dichlorotetrafluoroethane, and trichloromonofluoromethane as propellants and soya lecithin.

CLINICAL PHARMACOLOGY

Atrovent® (ipratropium bromide) is an anticholinergic (parasympatholytic) agent which, based on animal studies, appears to inhibit vagally mediated reflexes by antagonizing the action of acetylcholine, the transmitter agent released from the vagus nerve. Anticholinergics prevent the increases in intracellular concentration of cyclic guanosine monophosphate (cyclic GMP) which are caused by interaction of acetylcholine with the muscarinic receptor on bronchial smooth muscle.

The bronchodilation following inhalation of Atrovent is primarily a local, site-specific effect, not a systemic one. Much of an inhaled dose is swallowed as shown by fecal excretion studies. Atrovent is not readily absorbed into the systemic circulation either from the surface of the lung or from the gastrointestinal tract as confirmed by blood level and renal excretion studies.

The half-life of elimination is about 2 hours after inhalation or intravenous administration. Autoradiographic studies in rats have shown that Atrovent does not penetrate the blood-brain barrier.

In controlled 90-day studies in patients with bronchospasm associated with chronic obstructive pulmonary disease (chronic bronchitis and emphysema) significant improvements in pulmonary function (FEV_1 and FEF_{25-75}% increases of 15% or more) occurred within 15 minutes, reached a peak in 1–2 hours, and persisted for periods of 3 to 4 hours in the majority of patients and up to 6 hours in some patients. In addition, significant increases in Forced Vital Capacity (FVC) have been demonstrated.

Controlled clinical studies have demonstrated that Atrovent (ipratropium bromide) does not alter either mucociliary clearance or the volume or viscosity of respiratory secretions. In studies without a positive control Atrovent did not alter pupil size, accommodation or visual acuity (See ADVERSE REACTIONS).

Ventilation/perfusion studies have shown no clinically significant effects on pulmonary gas exchange or arterial oxygen tension. Atrovent does not produce clinically significant changes in pulse rate or blood pressure.

INDICATIONS AND USAGE

Atrovent® (ipratropium bromide) is indicated as a bronchodilator for maintenance treatment of bronchospasm associated with chronic obstructive pulmonary disease, including chronic bronchitis and emphysema.

CONTRAINDICATIONS

Hypersensitivity to atropine or its derivatives.

WARNINGS

Atrovent® (ipratropium bromide) is not indicated for the initial treatment of acute episodes of bronchospasm where rapid response is required.

PRECAUTIONS

General: Atrovent® (ipratropium bromide) should be used with caution in patients with narrow-angle glaucoma, prostatic hypertrophy or bladder-neck obstruction.

Information for Patients: Patients should be advised that temporary blurring of vision may result if the aerosol is sprayed into the eyes.

Patients should be reminded that Atrovent is not intended for occasional use, but rather, in order to be maximally effective, must be used consistently as prescribed throughout the course of therapy.

Drug Interactions: Atrovent has been used concomitantly with other drugs, including sympathomimetic bronchodilators, methylxanthines, steroids and cromolyn sodium, commonly used in the treatment of chronic obstructive pulmonary disease, without adverse drug reactions. There are no formal studies fully evaluating the interactive effects of Atrovent and these drugs with respect to effectiveness.

Carcinogenesis, Mutagenesis, Impairment of Fertility: Two-year oral carcinogenicity studies in rats and mice have revealed no carcinogenic potential at doses up to 1,250 times the maximum recommended human daily dose for Atrovent. Results of various mutagenicity studies were negative.

Fertility of male or female rats at oral doses up to approximately 10,000 times the maximum recommended human daily dose was unaffected by Atrovent administration. At doses above 18,000 times the maximum recommended human daily dose, increased resorption and decreased conception rates were observed.

Pregnancy/Teratogenic Effects *PREGNANCY CATEGORY B:* Oral reproduction studies performed in mice, rats and rabbits (at doses approximately 2,000, 200,000 and 26,000 times the maximum recommended human daily dose, respectively) and inhalation reproduction studies in rats and rabbits (at doses approximately 312 and 375 times the maximum recommended human daily dose, respectively) have demonstrated no evidence of teratogenic effects as a result of Atrovent. However, no adequate or well controlled studies have been conducted in pregnant women. Because animal reproduction studies are not always predictive of human response, Atrovent® (ipratropium bromide) should be used during pregnancy only if clearly needed.

Nursing Mothers: It is not known whether Atrovent is excreted in human milk. Although lipid-insoluble quaternary bases pass into breast milk, it is unlikely that Atrovent would reach the infant to an important extent, especially when taken by aerosol. However, because many drugs are excreted in human milk, caution should be exercised when Atrovent is administered to a nursing woman.

Pediatric Use: Safety and effectiveness in children below the age of 12 have not been established.

ADVERSE REACTIONS

Adverse reaction information concerning Atrovent® (ipratropium bromide) is derived from 90 day controlled clinical trials (N = 254), other controlled clinical trials using recommended doses of Atrovent (N = 377) and an uncontrolled study (N = 1924). Additional information is derived from the foreign post-marketing experience and the published literature.

Adverse reactions occurring in greater than one percent of patients in the 90 day controlled clinical trials appear in the following table:

[See table next page.]

Additional adverse reactions reported in less than one percent of the patients considered possibly due to Atrovent include urinary difficulty, fatigue, insomnia and hoarseness.

The large uncontrolled, open-label study included seriously ill patients. About 7% of patients treated discontinued the program because of adverse events.

Of the 2301 patients treated in the large uncontrolled study and in clinical trials other than the 90-day studies, the most common adverse reactions reported were: dryness of the oropharynx, about 5 in 100; cough, exacerbation of symptoms and irritation from aerosol, each about 3 in 100; headache, about 2 in 100; nausea, dizziness, blurred vision/difficulty in accommodation, and drying of secretions, each about 1 in 100. Less frequently reported adverse reactions that were possibly due to Atrovent® (ipratropium bromide) include tachycardia, paresthesias, drowsiness, coordination difficulty, itching, hives, flushing, alopecia, constipation, tremor, mucosal ulcers.

Cases of precipitation or worsening of narrow-angle glaucoma, acute eye pain and hypotension have been reported.

A case of giant urticaria with positive rechallenge has been reported from the foreign marketing experience. (See CONTRAINDICATIONS).

	Percent of Patients	
	Ipratropium bromide	Metaproterenol sulfate
	N = 254	N = 249
Reaction		
Cardiovascular		
Palpitations	1.8	1.6
Central Nervous System		
Nervousness	3.1	6.8
Dizziness	2.4	2.8
Headache	2.4	2.0
Dermatological		
Rash	1.2	0.4
Gastrointestinal		
Nausea	2.8	1.2
Gastrointestinal distress	2.4	2.8
Vomiting	0	1.2
Musculoskeletal		
Tremor	0	2.4
Ophthalmological		
Blurred vision	1.2	0.8
Oro-Otolaryngeal		
Dry mouth	2.4	0.8
Irritation from aerosol	1.6	1.6
Respiratory		
Cough	5.9	1.2
Exacerbation of symptoms	2.4	3.6

OVERDOSAGE

Acute overdosage by inhalation is unlikely since Atrovent® (ipratropium bromide) is not well absorbed systemically after aerosol or oral administration. The oral LD_{50} of Atrovent ranged between 1001 and 2010 mg/kg in mice; between 1667 and more than 4000 mg/kg in rats; and between 400 and 1300 mg/kg in dogs.

DOSAGE AND ADMINISTRATION

The usual starting dose of Atrovent® (ipratropium bromide) is two inhalations (36 mcg) four times a day. Patients may take additional inhalations as required; however, the total number of inhalations should not exceed 12 in 24 hours.

HOW SUPPLIED

Atrovent® (ipratropium bromide) Inhalation Aerosol is supplied as a metered dose inhaler with a white mouthpiece which has a clear, colorless sleeve and a green protective cap. Each 14 gram vial provides sufficient medication for 200 inhalations. NDC 0597-0082-14. Each actuation delivers 18 mcg of ipratropium bromide from the mouthpiece.

Store between 59°F (15°C) and 86°F (30°C). Avoid excessive humidity.

Caution

Federal law prohibits dispensing without prescription.

AT-PI-7/90

Shown in Product Identification Section, page 405

CATAPRES® ℞

[*kah 'tah-pres*]

(clonidine hydrochloride USP)

Oral Antihypertensive

Tablets, 0.1 mg .... BI-CODE 06

Tablets, 0.2 mg .... BI-CODE 07

Tablets, 0.3 mg .... BI-CODE 11

DESCRIPTION

Catapres® (clonidine hydrochloride USP) is a centrally acting antihypertensive agent available as tablets for oral administration in three dosage strengths: 0.1 mg, 0.2 mg and 0.3 mg. The 0.1 mg tablet is equivalent to 0.087 mg of the free base.

The inactive ingredients are colloidal silicon dioxide, corn starch, dibasic calcium phosphate, FD&C Yellow No. 6, gelatin, glycerin, lactose, magnesium stearate, methylparaben, propylparaben. The Catapres 0.1 mg tablet also contains FD&C Blue No. 1 and FD&C Red No. 3.

Clonidine hydrochloride is an imidazoline derivative and exists as a mesomeric compound. The chemical name is 2-(2,6-dichlorophenylamino)-2-imidazoline hydrochloride. The following is the structural formula:

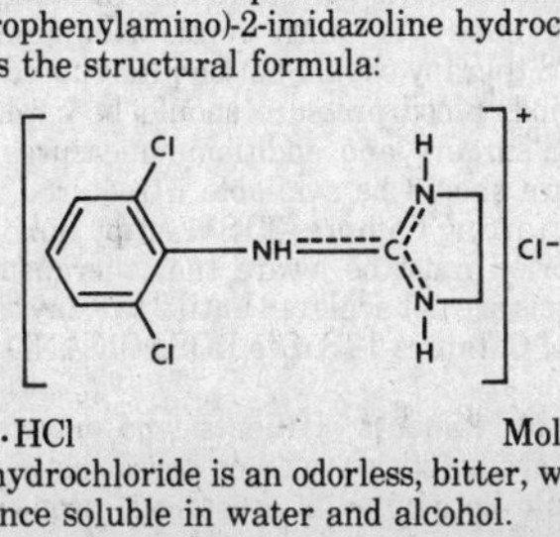

$C_9H_9Cl_2N_3 \cdot HCl$ Mol. Wt. 266.56

Clonidine hydrochloride is an odorless, bitter, white crystalline substance soluble in water and alcohol.

CLINICAL PHARMACOLOGY

Catapres® (clonidine hydrochloride USP) acts relatively rapidly. The patient's blood pressure declines within 30 to 60 minutes after an oral dose, the maximum decrease occurring within 2 to 4 hours. The plasma level of Catapres peaks in approximately 3 to 5 hours and the plasma half-life ranges from 12 to 16 hours. The half-life increases up to 41 hours in patients with severe impairment of renal function. Following oral administration about 40–60% of the absorbed dose is recovered in the urine as unchanged drug in 24 hours. About 50% of the absorbed dose is metabolized in the liver.

Clonidine stimulates alpha-adrenoreceptors in the brain stem, resulting in reduced sympathetic outflow from the central nervous system and a decrease in peripheral resistance, renal vascular resistance, heart rate, and blood pressure. Renal blood flow and glomerular filtration rate remain essentially unchanged. Normal postural reflexes are intact and therefore orthostatic symptoms are mild and infrequent.

Acute studies with clonidine hydrochloride in humans have demonstrated a moderate reduction (15% to 20%) of cardiac output in the supine position with no change in the peripheral resistance; at a 45° tilt there is a smaller reduction in cardiac output and a decrease of peripheral resistance. During long-term therapy, cardiac output tends to return to control values, while peripheral resistance remains decreased. Slowing of the pulse rate has been observed in most patients given clonidine, but the drug does not alter normal hemodynamic response to exercise.

Other studies in patients have provided evidence of a reduction in plasma renin activity and in the excretion of aldosterone and catecholamines, but the exact relationship of these pharmacologic actions to the antihypertensive effect has not been fully elucidated.

Clonidine acutely stimulates growth hormone release in both children and adults, but does not produce a chronic elevation of growth hormone with long-term use.

Tolerance may develop in some patients, necessitating a reevaluation of therapy.

INDICATIONS AND USAGE

Catapres® (clonidine hydrochloride USP) is indicated in the treatment of hypertension. Catapres may be employed alone or concomitantly with other antihypertensive agents.

CONTRAINDICATIONS

None known.

PRECAUTIONS

General In patients who have developed localized contact sensitization to Catapres-TTS® (clonidine), substitution of oral clonidine hydrochloride therapy may be associated with the development of a generalized skin rash.

In patients who develop an allergic reaction from Catapres-TTS® (clonidine) that extends beyond the local patch site (such as generalized skin rash, urticaria, or angioedema), oral clonidine hydrochloride substitution may elicit a similar reaction.

As with all antihypertensive therapy, Catapres® (clonidine hydrochloride USP) should be used with caution in patients with severe coronary insufficiency, recent myocardial infarction, cerebrovascular disease or chronic renal failure.

Withdrawal Patients should be instructed not to discontinue therapy without consulting their physician. Sudden cessation of clonidine treatment has resulted in subjective symptoms such as nervousness, agitation and headache, accompanied or followed by a rapid rise in blood pressure and elevated catecholamine concentrations in the plasma, but such occurrences have usually been associated with previous administration of high oral doses (exceeding 1.2 mg/day) and/or with continuation of concomitant beta-blocker therapy. Rare instances of hypertensive encephalopathy and death have been reported. When discontinuing therapy with Catapres, the physician should reduce the dose gradually over 2 to 4 days to avoid withdrawal symptomatology.

An excessive rise in blood pressure following Catapres discontinuance can be reversed by administration of oral clonidine or by intravenous phentolamine. If therapy is to be discontinued in patients receiving beta-blockers and clonidine concurrently, beta-blockers should be discontinued several days before the gradual withdrawal of Catapres.

Perioperative Use Administration of Catapres should be continued to within four hours of surgery and resumed as soon as possible thereafter. The blood pressure should be carefully monitored and appropriate measures instituted to control it as necessary.

Information for Patients Patients who engage in potentially hazardous activities, such as operating machinery or driving, should be advised of a potential sedative effect of clonidine. Patients should be cautioned against interruption of Catapres therapy without a physician's advice.

Drug Interactions If a patient receiving clonidine hydrochloride is also taking tricyclic antidepressants, the effect of clonidine may be reduced, thus necessitating an increase in dosage. Clonidine hydrochloride may enhance the CNS-depressive effects of alcohol, barbiturates or other sedatives. Amitriptyline in combination with clonidine enhances the manifestation of corneal lesions in rats (see TOXICOLOGY).

Carcinogenesis, Mutagenesis, Impairment of Fertility In a 132-week (fixed concentration) dietary administration study in rats, clonidine hydrochloride administered at 32 to 46 times the maximum recommended daily human dose was unassociated with evidence of carcinogenic potential.

Fertility of male or female rats was unaffected by clonidine hydrochloride doses as high as 150 mcg/kg or about 3 times the maximum recommended daily human dose (MRDHD). Fertility of female rats did, however, appear to be affected (in another experiment) at dose levels of 500 to 2000 mcg/kg or 10 to 40 times the MRDHD.

Usage in Pregnancy/Teratogenic Effects *PREGNANCY CATEGORY C:* Reproduction studies performed in rabbits at doses up to approximately 3 times the maximum recommended daily human dose (MRDHD) of clonidine hydrochloride have revealed no evidence of teratogenic or embryotoxic potential in rabbits. In rats, however, doses as low as ⅓ the MRDHD were associated with increased resorptions in a study in which dams were treated continuously from 2 months prior to mating. Increased resorptions were not associated with treatment at the same or at higher dose levels (up to 3 times the MRDHD) when dams were treated days 6–15 of gestation. Increased resorptions were observed at much higher levels (40 times the MRDHD) in rats and mice treated days 1–14 of gestation (lowest dose employed in that study was 500 mcg/kg). There are, however, no adequate and well-controlled studies in pregnant women. Because animal reproduction studies are not always predictive of human response, this drug should be used during pregnancy only if clearly needed.

Nursing Mothers As clonidine hydrochloride is excreted in human milk, caution should be exercised when Catapres® (clonidine hydrochloride USP) is administered to a nursing woman.

Pediatric Use Safety and effectiveness in children have not been established.

ADVERSE REACTIONS

Most adverse effects are mild and tend to diminish with continued therapy. The most frequent (which appear to be dose-related) are dry mouth, occurring in about 40 of 100 patients; drowsiness, about 33 in 100; dizziness, about 16 in 100; constipation and sedation, each about 10 in 100.

The following less frequent adverse experiences have also been reported in patients receiving Catapres® (clonidine hydrochloride USP), but in many cases patients were receiving concomitant medication and a causal relationship has not been established.

Gastrointestinal Nausea and vomiting, about 5 in 100 patients; anorexia and malaise, each about 1 in 100; mild transient abnormalities in liver function tests, about 1 in 100; rare reports of hepatitis; parotitis, rarely.

Metabolic Weight gain, about 1 in 100 patients; gynecomastia, about 1 in 1000; transient elevation of blood glucose or serum creatine phosphokinase, rarely.

Central Nervous System Nervousness and agitation, about 3 in 100 patients; mental depression, about 1 in 100; headache, about 1 in 100; insomnia, about 5 in 1000. Vivid dreams or nightmares, other behavioral changes, restlessness, anxiety, visual and auditory hallucinations and delirium have been reported.

Cardiovascular Orthostatic symptoms, about 3 in 100 patients; palpitations and tachycardia, bradycardia, each about 5 in 1000. Raynaud's phenomenon, congestive heart failure, and electrocardiographic abnormalities i.e. conduction disturbances and arrhythmias have been reported rarely. Rare cases of sinus bradycardia and atrioventricular block have been reported, both with and without the use of concomitant digitalis.

Dermatological Rash, about 1 in 100 patients; pruritus, about 7 in 1000; hives, angioneurotic edema and urticaria, about 5 in 1000; alopecia, about 2 in 1000.

Genitourinary Decreased sexual activity, impotence and loss of libido, about 3 in 100 patients; nocturia, about 1 in 100; difficulty in micturition, about 2 in 1000; urinary retention, about 1 in 1000.

Other Weakness, about 10 in 100 patients; fatigue, about 4 in 100; discontinuation syndrome, about 1 in 100; muscle or joint pain, about 6 in 1000 and cramps of the lower limbs, about 3 in 1000. Dryness, burning of the eyes, blurred vision, dryness of the nasal mucosa, pallor, weakly positive Coombs' test, increased sensitivity to alcohol and fever have been reported.

OVERDOSAGE

The signs and symptoms of clonidine hydrochloride overdosage include hypotension, bradycardia, lethargy, irritability, weakness, somnolence, diminished or absent reflexes, miosis, vomiting and hypoventilation. With large overdoses, reversible cardiac conduction defects or arrhythmias, apnea, seizures and transient hypertension have been reported. The

Continued on next page

Boehringer Ingelheim—Cont.

oral LD_{50} of clonidine in rats was 465 mg/kg, and in mice 206 mg/kg.

The general treatment of Catapres® (clonidine hydrochloride USP) overdosage may include intravenous fluids as indicated. Bradycardia can be treated with intravenous atropine sulfate and hypotension with dopamine infusion in addition to intravenous fluids. Hypertension, associated with overdosage, has been treated with intravenous furosemide or diazoxide or alpha-blocking agents such as phentolamine. Tolazoline, an alpha-blocker, in intravenous doses of 10 mg at 30-minute intervals, may reverse clonidine's effects if other efforts fail. Routine hemodialysis is of limited benefit, since a maximum of 5% of circulating clonidine is removed.

In a patient who ingested 100 mg clonidine hydrochloride, plasma clonidine levels were 60 ng/ml (one hour), 190 ng/ml (1.5 hours), 370 ng/ml (two hours) and 120 ng/ml (5.5 and 6.5 hours). This patient developed hypertension followed by hypotension, bradycardia, apnea, hallucinations, semicoma, and premature ventricular contractions. The patient fully recovered after intensive treatment.

DOSAGE AND ADMINISTRATION

Adults: The dose of Catapres® (clonidine hydrochloride USP) must be adjusted according to the patient's individual blood pressure response. The following is a general guide to its administration.

Initial Dose 0.1 mg tablet twice daily (morning and bedtime). Elderly patients may benefit from a lower initial dose.

Maintenance Dose Further increments of 0.1 mg per day may be made if necessary until the desired response is achieved. Taking the larger portion of the total daily dose at bedtime may minimize transient adjustment effects of dry mouth and drowsiness. The therapeutic doses most commonly employed have ranged from 0.2 mg to 0.6 mg per day given in divided doses. Studies have indicated that 2.4 mg is the maximum effective daily dose, but doses as high as this have rarely been employed.

Renal Impairment Dosage must be adjusted according to the degree of impairment, and patients should be carefully monitored. Since only a minimal amount of clonidine is removed during routine hemodialysis, there is no need to give supplemental clonidine following dialysis.

HOW SUPPLIED

Catapres® (clonidine hydrochloride USP) is supplied in tablets containing 0.1 mg, 0.2 mg or 0.3 mg of clonidine hydrochloride.

Catapres® 0.1 mg tablets are tan, oval shaped and single scored with the marking BI 6. Available in bottles of 100 (NDC 0597-0006-01) and 1000 (NDC 0597-0006-10) and unit-dose packages of 100 (NDC 0597-0006-61).

Catapres® 0.2 mg tablets are orange, oval shaped and single scored with the marking BI 7. Available in bottles of 100 (NDC 0597-0007-01) and 1000 (NDC 0597-0007-10) and unit-dose packages of 100 (NDC 0597-0007-61).

Catapres® 0.3 mg tablets are peach, oval shaped and single scored with the marking BI 11. Available in bottles of 100 (NDC 0597-0011-01).

Store below 86°F (30°C).

Dispense in tight, light-resistant container.

Caution Federal law prohibits dispensing without prescription.

TOXICOLOGY

In several studies, oral clonidine hydrochloride produced a dose-dependent increase in the incidence and severity of spontaneously occurring retinal degeneration in albino rats treated for 6 months or longer. Tissue distribution studies in dogs and monkeys revealed that clonidine hydrochloride was concentrated in the choroid of the eye. In view of the retinal degeneration observed in rats, eye examinations were performed in 908 patients prior to the start of clonidine hydrochloride therapy, who were then examined periodically thereafter. In 353 of these 908 patients, examinations were performed for periods of 24 months or longer. Except for some dryness of the eyes, no drug-related abnormal ophthalmologic findings were recorded and clonidine hydrochloride did not alter retinal function as shown by specialized tests such as the electroretinogram and macular dazzle. In rats, clonidine hydrochloride in combination with amitriptyline produced corneal lesions within 5 days.

CA-PI-4/88

Shown in Product Identification Section, page 405

CATAPRES-TTS® ℞

(clonidine) **Catapres-TTS®-1**
Transdermal Therapeutic **Catapres-TTS®-2**
System **Catapres-TTS®-3**
(clonidine)

Programmed delivery *in vivo* of 0.1, 0.2 or 0.3 mg clonidine per day, for one week

PRODUCT OVERVIEW

KEY FACTS

Catapres-TTS® (clonidine) delivers a therapeutic dose of the antihypertensive clonidine through an adhesive patch applied to the skin. Each patch delivers clonidine at a constant rate for 7 days, permitting once-a-week dosing.

MAJOR USES

Catapres-TTS has been proven effective in the treatment of hypertension in controlled clinical trials. It may be used alone or with other antihypertensives.

SAFETY INFORMATION

Catapres-TTS is contraindicated in patients with known hypersensitivity to clonidine or any other component of the adhesive layer of the therapeutic system. As with other antihypertensive medications, patients should be instructed not to discontinue therapy without consulting their physician. Before prescribing, please consult full prescribing information below.

PRESCRIBING INFORMATION

CATAPRES-TTS® ℞

(clonidine) **Catapres-TTS®-1**
Transdermal Therapeutic **Catapres-TTS®-2**
System **Catapres-TTS®-3**
(clonidine)

Programmed delivery *in vivo* of 0.1, 0.2 or 0.3 mg clonidine per day, for one week

DESCRIPTION

Catapres-TTS® (clonidine) is a transdermal system providing continuous systemic delivery of clonidine for 7 days at an approximately constant rate. Clonidine is a centrally acting alpha agonist and is an antihypertensive agent. It is an imidazoline derivative whose chemical name is 2, 6-dichloro-N-2-imidazolidinylidenebenzenamine and has the following chemical structure:

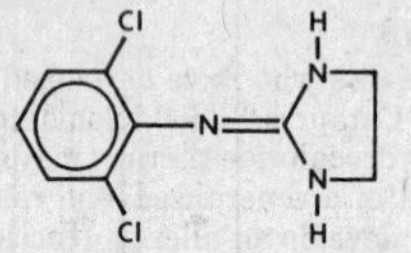

(clonidine)

System Structure and Components Catapres-TTS is a multilayered film, 0.2 mm thick, containing clonidine as the active agent. System area is 3.5, 7.0, or 10.5 cm^2 and the amount of drug released is directly proportional to area. (See Release Rate Concept.) The composition per unit area of all three dosages is identical.

Proceeding from the visible surface towards the surface attached to the skin, are four layers: 1) a backing layer of pigmented polyester film; 2) a drug reservoir of clonidine, mineral oil, polyisobutylene, and colloidal silicon dioxide; 3) a microporous polypropylene membrane that controls the rate of delivery of clonidine from the system to the skin surface; 4) an adhesive formulation of clonidine, mineral oil, polyisobutylene, and colloidal silicon dioxide. Prior to use, a protective peel strip of polyester that covers layer 4 is removed.

Release Rate Concept Catapres-TTS is programmed to release clonidine at an approximately constant rate for 7 days. The energy source for drug release derives from the concentration gradient existing between a saturated solution of drug in the system and the much lower concentration prevailing in the skin. Clonidine flows in the direction of the lower concentration at a constant rate, limited by the rate-controlling membrane, so long as a saturated solution is maintained in the drug reservoir.

Following system application to intact skin, clonidine in the adhesive layer saturates the skin sites below the system. Clonidine from the drug reservoir then begins to flow through the rate-controlling membrane and the adhesive layer of the system into the systemic circulation via the capillaries beneath the skin. Therapeutic plasma clonidine levels are achieved 2 to 3 days after initial application of Catapres-TTS.

The 3.5, 7.0, and 10.5 cm^2 systems respectively deliver 0.1, 0.2, and 0.3 mg clonidine per day. To ensure constant release of drug over 7 days, the total drug content of the system is greater than the total amount of drug delivered. Application of a new system to a fresh skin site at weekly intervals continuously maintains therapeutic plasma concentrations of clonidine. If the Catapres-TTS is removed and not replaced with a new system, therapeutic plasma clonidine levels will persist for about 8 hours and then decline slowly over several days. Over this time period, blood pressure returns gradually to pretreatment levels. If the patient experiences localized skin irritation before completing 7 days of use, the system may be removed and replaced with a new one applied on a fresh skin site.

CLINICAL PHARMACOLOGY

The plasma half-life of clonidine is 12.7 ± 7 hours. Following oral administration, about 40–60% of the absorbed dose is recovered in the urine as unchanged drug in 24 hours. About 50% of the absorbed dose is metabolized in the liver.

Clonidine stimulates alpha-adrenoreceptors in the brain stem, resulting in reduced sympathetic outflow from the central nervous system and a decrease in peripheral resistance, renal vascular resistance, heart rate, and blood pressure. Renal blood flow and glomerular filtration rate remain essentially unchanged. Normal postural reflexes are intact, and therefore orthostatic symptoms are mild and infrequent.

Acute studies with clonidine hydrochloride in humans have demonstrated a moderate reduction (15% to 20%) of cardiac output in the supine position with no change in the peripheral resistance; at a 45° tilt there is a smaller reduction in cardiac output and a decrease of peripheral resistance. During long-term therapy, cardiac output tends to return to control values, while peripheral resistance remains decreased. Slowing of the pulse rate has been observed in most patients given clonidine, but the drug does not alter normal hemodynamic response to exercise.

Other studies in patients have provided evidence of a reduction in plasma renin activity and in the excretion of aldosterone and catecholamines, but the exact relationship of these pharmacologic actions to the antihypertensive effect has not been fully elucidated.

Clonidine acutely stimulates growth hormone release in both children and adults, but does not produce a chronic elevation of growth hormone with long-term use.

Tolerance may develop in some patients, necessitating a reevaluation of therapy.

INDICATIONS FOR USE

Catapres-TTS® (clonidine) is indicated in the treatment of hypertension. It may be employed alone or concomitantly with other antihypertensive agents.

CONTRAINDICATIONS

Catapres-TTS® (clonidine) should not be used in patients with known hypersensitivity to clonidine or to any other component of the adhesive layer of the therapeutic system.

PRECAUTIONS

General In patients who have developed localized contact sensitization to Catapres-TTS® (clonidine), substitution of oral clonidine hydrochloride therapy may be associated with development of a generalized skin rash.

In patients who develop an allergic reaction to Catapres-TTS that extends beyond the local patch site (such as generalized skin rash, urticaria, or angioedema) oral clonidine hydrochloride substitution may elicit a similar reaction.

As with all antihypertensive therapy, Catapres-TTS should be used with caution in patients with severe coronary insufficiency, recent myocardial infarction, cerebrovascular disease, or chronic renal failure.

Transdermal clonidine systems should be removed before attempting defibrillation or cardioversion because of the potential for altered electrical conductivity which may enhance the possibility of arcing, a phenomenon associated with the use of defibrillators.

Withdrawal Patients should be instructed not to discontinue therapy without consulting their physician. Sudden cessation of clonidine treatment has resulted in subjective symptoms such as nervousness, agitation and headache, accompanied or followed by a rapid rise in blood pressure and elevated catecholamine concentrations in the plasma, but such occurrences have usually been associated with previous administration of high oral doses (exceeding 1.2 mg/day) and/or with continuation of concomitant beta-blocker therapy. Rare instances of hypertensive encephalopathy and death have been reported.

An excessive rise in blood pressure following Catapres-TTS discontinuance can be reversed by administration of oral clonidine or by intravenous phentolamine. If therapy is to be discontinued in patients receiving beta-blockers and clonidine concurrently, beta-blockers should be discontinued several days before cessation of Catapres-TTS administration.

Perioperative Use As with oral clonidine therapy, Catapres-TTS therapy should not be interrupted during the surgical period. Blood pressure should be carefully monitored during surgery and additional measures to control blood pressure should be available if required. Physicians considering starting Catapres-TTS therapy during the perioperative period must be aware that therapeutic plasma clonidine levels are not achieved until 2 to 3 days after initial application of Catapres-TTS (See DOSAGE AND ADMINISTRATION).

Information for Patients Patients who engage in potentially hazardous activities, such as operating machinery or driving, should be advised of a potential sedative effect of

clonidine. Patients should be cautioned against interruption of Catapres-TTS therapy without a physician's advice. Patients should be advised that if the system begins to loosen from the skin after application, the adhesive overlay should be applied directly over the system to ensure good adhesion over its 7-day lifetime. Instructions for using the system are provided. Patients who develop moderate or severe erythema and/or localized vesicle formation at the site of application, or a generalized skin rash, should consult their physician promptly about the possible need to remove the patch.

Drug Interactions If a patient receiving clonidine is also taking tricyclic antidepressants, the effect of clonidine may be reduced, thus necessitating an increase in dosage. Clonidine may enhance the CNS-depressive effects of alcohol, barbiturates or other sedatives. Amitriptyline in combination with clonidine enhances the manifestation of corneal lesions in rats. (See TOXICOLOGY section.)

Carcinogenesis, Mutagenesis, Impairment of Fertility In a 132-week (fixed concentration) dietary administration study in rats, Catapres® (clonidine HCl) administered at 32 to 46 times the oral maximum recommended daily human dose (MRDHD) was unassociated with evidence of carcinogenic potential. Results from the Ames test with clonidine hydrochloride revealed no evidence of mutagenesis. Fertility of male or female rats was unaffected by clonidine doses as high as 150 mcg/kg or about 3 times the oral MRDHD. Fertility of female rats did, however, appear to be affected (in another experiment) at the dose levels of 500 to 2000 mcg/kg or 10 to 40 times the oral MRDHD.

Pregnancy/Teratogenic Effects *PREGNANCY CATEGORY C:* Reproduction studies performed in rabbits at doses up to approximately 3 times the oral maximum recommended daily human dose (MRDHD) of Catapres® (clonidine HCl) have revealed no evidence of teratogenic or embryotoxic potential in rabbits. In rats, however, doses as low as 1/3 the oral MRDHD of clonidine were associated with increased resorptions in a study in which dams were treated continuously from 2 months prior to mating. Increased resorptions were not associated with treatment at the same or at higher dose levels (up to 3 times the oral MRDHD) when dams were treated days 6–15 of gestation. Increased resorptions were observed at much higher levels (40 times the oral MRDHD) in rats and mice treated days 1–14 of gestation (lowest dose employed in the study was 500 mcg/kg). There are, however, no adequate and well-controlled studies in pregnant women. Because animal reproduction studies are not always predictive of human response, this drug should be used during pregnancy only if clearly needed.

Nursing Mothers As clonidine is excreted in human milk, caution should be exercised when Catapres-TTS is administered to a nursing woman.

Pediatric Use Safety and effectiveness in children below the age of twelve have not been established.

ADVERSE REACTIONS

Most systemic adverse effects during therapy with Catapres-TTS® (clonidine) have been mild and have tended to diminish with continued therapy. In a 3-month, multiclinic trial of Catapres-TTS in 101 hypertensive patients, the most frequent systemic reactions were dry mouth (25 patients) and drowsiness (12 patients).

Transient localized skin reactions, primarily localized pruritus, occurred in 51 patients. Twenty-six patients experienced localized erythema. This erythema and pruritus were more common in patients utilizing an adhesive overlay for the entire 7-day treatment period. Allergic contact sensitization to Catapres-TTS was observed in 5 patients.

In additional clinical experience contact dermatitis resulting in treatment discontinuation was observed in 128 of 673 patients (about 19 in 100) after a mean duration of treatment of 37 weeks. The incidence in white females was about 34 in 100; in white males about 18 in 100; in black females about 14 in 100; and in black males about 8 in 100.

The following less frequent adverse experiences were also reported in patients involved in the multiclinic trial with Catapres-TTS.

Gastrointestinal Constipation (1 patient); nausea (1); and change in taste (1).

Central Nervous System Fatigue (6 patients); headache (5); lethargy (3); sedation (3); insomnia (2); dizziness (2); and nervousness (1).

Genitourinary Impotence/sexual dysfunction (2 patients).

Dermatological Localized vesiculation (7 patients); hyperpigmentation (5); edema (3); excoriation (3); burning (3); papules (1); throbbing (1); blanching (1); and generalized macular rash (1).

In additional clinical experience involving 3539 patients, less common dermatologic reactions have occurred, where a causal relationship to Catapres-TTS was not established: maculopapular skin rash (10 cases); urticaria (2 cases); angioedema involving the face (2 cases), one of which also involved the tongue.

Oro-otolaryngeal Dry throat (2 patients).

In long experience with oral Catapres® (clonidine HCl), the most common adverse reactions have been dry mouth (about 40%), drowsiness (about 35%) and sedation (about 8%). In addition, the following adverse reactions have been reported less frequently:

Gastrointestinal Nausea and vomiting, about 5 in 100 patients; anorexia and malaise, each about 1 in 100; mild transient abnormalities in liver function tests, about 1 in 100; rare reports of hepatitis; parotitis, rarely.

Metabolic Weight gain, about 1 in 100 patients; gynecomastia, about 1 in 1000; transient elevation of blood glucose or serum creatine phosphokinase, rarely.

Central Nervous System Nervousness and agitation, about 3 in 100 patients; mental depression, about 1 in 100 and insomnia, about 5 in 1000. Vivid dreams or nightmares, other behavioral changes, restlessness, anxiety, visual and auditory hallucinations and delirium have been reported.

Cardiovascular Orthostatic symptoms, about 3 in 100 patients; palpitations and tachycardia, and bradycardia, each about 5 in 1000. Raynaud's phenomenon, congestive heart failure, and electrocardiographic abnormalities (i.e. conduction disturbances and arrhythmias) have been reported rarely. Rare cases of sinus bradycardia and atrioventricular block have been reported, both with and without the use of concomitant digitalis.

Dermatological Rash, about 1 in 100 patients; pruritus, about 7 in 1000; hives, angioneurotic edema and urticaria, about 5 in 1000; alopecia, about 2 in 1000.

Genitourinary Decreased sexual activity, impotence and loss of libido, about 3 in 100 patients; nocturia, about 1 in 100; difficulty in micturition, about 2 in 1000; urinary retention, about 1 in 1000.

Other Weakness, about 10 in 100 patients; fatigue, about 4 in 100; headache, and discontinuation syndrome, each about 1 in 100; muscle or joint pain, about 6 in 1000 and cramps of the lower limbs, about 3 in 1000. Dryness, burning of the eyes, blurred vision, dryness of the nasal mucosa, pallor, weakly positive Coombs' test, increased sensitivity to alcohol and fever have been reported.

OVERDOSAGE

If symptoms of overdosage occur, remove all Catapres-TTS® (clonidine) systems. The signs and symptoms of clonidine overdosage include hypotension, bradycardia, lethargy, irritability, weakness, somnolence, diminished or absent reflexes, miosis, vomiting and hypoventilation. With large overdoses, reversible cardiac conduction defects or arrhythmias, apnea, seizures and transient hypertension have been reported. The oral LD_{50} of clonidine in rats was 465 mg/kg, and in mice 206 mg/kg.

The general treatment of Catapres-TTS overdosage may include intravenous fluids as indicated. Bradycardia can be treated with intravenous atropine sulfate and hypotension with dopamine infusion in addition to intravenous fluids. Hypertension associated with overdosage has been treated with intravenous furosemide or diazoxide or alpha-blocking agents such as phentolamine. Tolazoline, an alpha-blocker, in intravenous doses of 10 mg at 30-minute intervals, may reverse clonidine's effects if other efforts fail. Routine hemodialysis is of limited benefit, since a maximum of 5% of circulating clonidine is removed.

In a patient who ingested 100 mg clonidine hydrochloride, plasma clonidine levels were 60 ng/ml (1 hour), 190 ng/ml (1.5 hours), 370 ng/ml (2 hours) and 120 ng/ml (5.5 and 6.5 hours). This patient developed hypertension followed by hypotension, bradycardia, apnea, hallucinations, semicoma, and premature ventricular contractions. The patient fully recovered after intensive treatment.

DOSAGE AND ADMINISTRATION

Apply Catapres-TTS® (clonidine) to a hairless area of intact skin on the upper arm or torso, once every 7 days. Each new application of Catapres-TTS should be on a different skin site from the previous location. If the system loosens during 7-day wearing, the adhesive overlay should be applied directly over the system to ensure good adhesion.

To initiate therapy, Catapres-TTS dosage should be titrated according to individual therapeutic requirements, starting with Catapres-TTS-1. If after one or two weeks the desired reduction in blood pressure is not achieved, increase the dosage by adding an additional Catapres-TTS-1 or changing to a larger system. An increase in dosage above two Catapres-TTS-3 is usually not associated with additional efficacy.

When substituting Catapres-TTS in patients on prior antihypertensive therapy, physicians should be aware that the antihypertensive effect of Catapres-TTS may not commence until 2 to 3 days after initial application. Therefore, gradual reduction of prior drug dosage is advised. Some or all previous antihypertensive treatment may have to be continued, particularly in patients with more severe forms of hypertension.

	Programmed Delivery Clonidine *in vivo* Per Day Over 1 Week	Clonidine Content	Size	Code
Catapres-TTS®-1 (clonidine)	0.1 mg	2.5 mg	3.5 cm^2	BI-31
Catapres-TTS®-2 (clonidine)	0.2 mg	5.0 mg	7.0 cm^2	BI-32
Catapres-TTS®-3 (clonidine)	0.3 mg	7.5 mg	10.5 cm^2	BI-33

HOW SUPPLIED

Catapres-TTS®-1 (clonidine) and Catapres-TTS®-2 are supplied as 4 pouched systems and 4 adhesive overlays per carton, 3 cartons per shipper (NDC 0597-0031-12 and 0597-0032-12, respectively). Catapres-TTS®-3 is supplied as 4 pouched systems and 4 adhesive overlays per carton (NDC 0597-0033-34).

[See chart above.]

Storage and Handling: Store below 86°F (30°C).

Caution: Federal law prohibits dispensing without prescription.

TOXICOLOGY

In several studies, oral clonidine hydrochloride produced a dose-dependent increase in the incidence and severity of spontaneously occurring retinal degeneration in albino rats treated for six months or longer. Tissue distribution studies in dogs and monkeys revealed that clonidine hydrochloride was concentrated in the choroid of the eye. In view of the retinal degeneration observed in rats, eye examinations were performed in 908 patients prior to the start of clonidine hydrochloride therapy, who were then examined periodically thereafter. In 353 of these 908 patients, examinations were performed for periods of 24 months or longer. Except for some dryness of the eyes, no drug-related abnormal ophthalmologic findings were recorded and clonidine hydrochloride did not alter retinal function as shown by specialized tests such as the electroretinogram and macular dazzle.

In rats, clonidine hydrochloride in combination with amitriptyline produced corneal lesions within 5 days.

CT-PI-7/88

Shown in Product Identification Section, page 405

COMBIPRES® ℞

[*kom'be-pres*]

Each tablet contains:
clonidine hydrochloride USP,
0.1 mg or 0.2 mg or 0.3 mg
and chlorthalidone USP, 15 mg
Oral Antihypertensive

Tablets 0.1	**BI-CODE 08**
Tablets 0.2	**BI-CODE 09**
Tablets 0.3	**BI-CODE 10**

DESCRIPTION

Combipres® is a combination of clonidine hydrochloride (a centrally acting antihypertensive agent) and chlorthalidone (a diuretic). Combipres® is available as tablets for oral administration in three dosage strengths: 0.1/15 mg, 0.2/15 mg and 0.3/15 mg of clonidine hydrochloride/chlorthalidone, respectively.

The inactive ingredients are colloidal silicon dioxide, corn starch, dibasic calcium phosphate, gelatin, glycerin, lactose, magnesium stearate, methylparaben and propylparaben. The Combipres 0.1/15 mg tablet also contains FD&C Red No. 3. The Combipres 0.2/15 mg tablet also contains FD&C Blue No. 1.

Clonidine hydrochloride:

Clonidine hydrochloride is an imidazoline derivative and exists as a mesomeric compound. The chemical name is 2-(2,6-dichlorophenylamino)-2-imidazoline hydrochloride. The following is the structural formula:

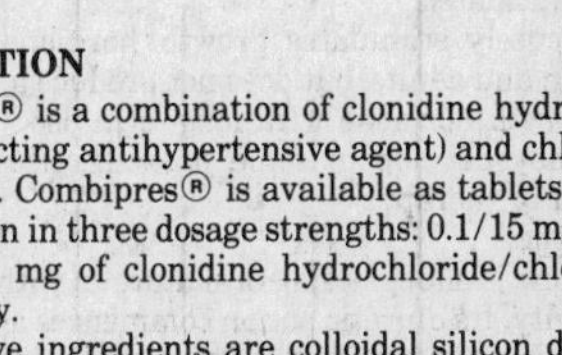

$C_9H_9Cl_2N_3 \cdot HCl$
Mol. Wt. 266.56

Clonidine hydrochloride is an odorless, bitter, white crystalline substance soluble in water and alcohol.

Chlorthalidone

Chlorthalidone is a monosulfamyl diuretic that differs chemically from thiazide diuretics in that a double ring system is incorporated in its structure. It is a racemic mixture of 2-chloro-5-(1- hydroxy-3-oxo-1-isoindolinyl) benzenesulfonamide with the following structural formula: [See top of next page.]

Continued on next page

Boehringer Ingelheim—Cont.

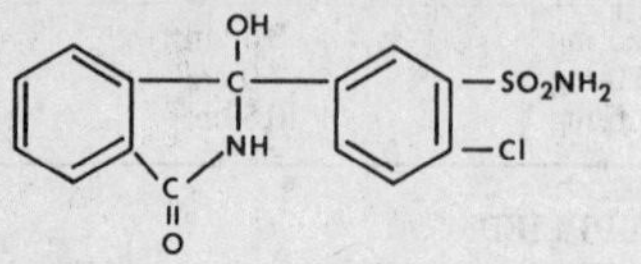

$C_{14}H_{11}Cl\ N_2O_4S$
Mol. Wt. 338.76

Chlorthalidone is practically insoluble in water, in ether and in chloroform; soluble in methanol; slightly soluble in alcohol.

CLINICAL PHARMACOLOGY

Combipres®:
Combipres produces a more pronounced antihypertensive response than occurs after either clonidine hydrochloride or chlorthalidone alone in equivalent doses.

Clonidine hydrochloride:
Clonidine hydrochloride acts relatively rapidly. The patient's blood pressure declines within 30 to 60 minutes after an oral dose, the maximum decrease occurring within 2 to 4 hours. The plasma level of clonidine hydrochloride peaks in approximately 3 to 5 hours and the plasma half-life ranges from 12 to 16 hours. The half-life increases up to 41 hours in patients with severe impairment of renal function. Following oral administration about 40–60% of the absorbed dose is recovered in the urine as unchanged drug in 24 hours. About 50% of the absorbed dose is metabolized in the liver.
Clonidine stimulates alpha-adrenoreceptors in the brain stem, resulting in reduced sympathetic outflow from the central nervous system and a decrease in peripheral resistance, renal vascular resistance, heart rate, and blood pressure. Renal blood flow and glomerular filtration rate remain essentially unchanged. Normal postural reflexes are intact and therefore orthostatic symptoms are mild and infrequent.
Acute studies with clonidine hydrochloride in humans have demonstrated a moderate reduction (15 to 20%) of cardiac output in the supine position with no change in the peripheral resistance; at a 45° tilt there is a smaller reduction in cardiac output and a decrease of peripheral resistance. During long-term therapy, cardiac output tends to return to control values, while peripheral resistance remains decreased. Slowing of the pulse rate has been observed in most patients given clonidine but the drug does not alter normal hemodynamic response to exercise.
Other studies in patients have provided evidence of a reduction in plasma renin activity and in the excretion of aldosterone and catecholamines, but the exact relationship of these pharmacologic actions to the antihypertensive effect has not been fully elucidated.
Clonidine acutely stimulates growth hormone release in both children and adults, but does not produce a chronic elevation of growth hormone with long-term use.
Tolerance may develop in some patients, necessitating a reevaluation of therapy.

Chlorthalidone:
Chlorthalidone is a long-acting oral diuretic with antihypertensive activity. Its diuretic action commences a mean of 2.6 hours after dosing and continues for up to 72 hours. The drug produces diuresis with increased excretion of sodium and chloride. The diuretic effects of chlorthalidone and the benzothiadiazine (thiazide) diuretics appear to arise from similar mechanisms and the maximal effect of chlorthalidone and the thiazides appears to be similar. The site of action appears to be the distal convoluted tubule of the nephron. The diuretic effects of chlorthalidone lead to decreased extracellular fluid volume, plasma volume, cardiac output, total exchangeable sodium, glomerular filtration rate, and renal plasma flow. Although the mechanism of action of chlorthalidone and related drugs is not wholly clear, sodium and water depletion appear to provide a basis for its antihypertensive effect. Like the thiazide diuretics, chlorthalidone produces dose-related reductions in serum potassium levels, elevations in serum uric acid and blood glucose, and it can lead to be decreased sodium and chloride levels.
The mean plasma half-life of chlorthalidone is about 40 to 60 hours. It is eliminated primarily as unchanged drug in the urine. Non-renal routes of elimination have yet to be clarified. In the blood, approximately 75% of the drug is bound to plasma proteins.

INDICATIONS AND USAGE

Combipres® (clonidine hydrochloride USP/chlorthalidone USP) is indicated in the treatment of hypertension. **This fixed combination drug is not indicated for initial therapy of hypertension. Hypertension requires therapy titrated to the individual patient. If the fixed combination represents the dosage so determined, its use may be more convenient in patient management. The treatment of hypertension is not static, but must be reevaluated as conditions in each patient warrant.**

CONTRAINDICATIONS

Anuria. Combipres® is contraindicated in patients with known hypersensitivity to chlorthalidone or other sulfonamide-derived drugs.

WARNINGS

Chlorthalidone should be used with caution in severe renal disease. In patients with renal disease, chlorthalidone or related drugs may precipitate azotemia. Cumulative effects of the drug may develop in patients with impaired renal function. Chlorthalidone should be used with caution in patients with impaired hepatic function or progressive liver disease, because minor alterations of fluid and electrolyte balance may precipitate hepatic coma.
Sensitivity reactions may occur in patients with a history of allergy or bronchial asthma. The possibility of exacerbation or activation of systemic lupus erythematosus has been reported with thiazide diuretics which are structurally related to chlorthalidone. However, systemic lupus erythematosus has not been reported following chlorthalidone administration.

PRECAUTIONS

Clonidine hydrochloride:
General In patients who have developed localized contact sensitization to Catapres-TTS® (clonidine), substitution of oral clonidine hydrochloride therapy may be associated with the development of a generalized skin rash.
In patients who develop an allergic reaction from Catapres-TTS® (clonidine) that extends beyond the local patch site (such as generalized skin rash, urticaria, or angioedema), oral clonidine hydrochloride substitution may elicit a similar reaction.
As with all antihypertensive therapy, clonidine hydrochloride should be used with caution in patients with severe coronary insufficiency, recent myocardial infarction, cerebrovascular disease or chronic renal failure.
Withdrawal Patients should be instructed not to discontinue therapy without consulting their physician. Sudden cessation of clonidine treatment has resulted in subjective symptoms such as nervousness, agitation and headache, accompanied or followed by a rapid rise in blood pressure and elevated catecholamine concentrations in the plasma, but such occurrences have usually been associated with previous administration of high oral doses (exceeding 1.2 mg/day) and/or with continuation of concomitant beta-blocker therapy. Rare instances of hypertensive encephalopathy and death have been reported. When discontinuing therapy with clonidine hydrochloride, the physician should reduce the dose gradually over 2 to 4 days to avoid withdrawal symptomatology.
An excessive rise in blood pressure following clonidine hydrochloride discontinuance can be reversed by administration of oral clonidine or by intravenous phentolamine. If therapy is to be discontinued in patients receiving beta-blockers and clonidine concurrently, beta-blockers should be discontinued several days before the gradual withdrawal of clonidine hydrochloride.
Perioperative Use Administration of clonidine hydrochloride should be continued to within four hours of surgery and resumed as soon as possible thereafter. The blood pressure should be carefully monitored and appropriate measures instituted to control it as necessary.
Information for Patients Patients who engage in potentially hazardous activities, such as operating machinery or driving, should be advised of a potential sedative effect of clonidine. Patients should be cautioned against interruption of clonidine hydrochloride therapy without a physician's advice.
Drug Interactions If a patient receiving clonidine hydrochloride is also taking tricyclic antidepressants, the effect of clonidine may be reduced, thus necessitating an increase in dosage. Clonidine hydrochloride may enhance the CNS-depressive effects of alcohol, barbiturates or other sedatives. Amitriptyline in combination with clonidine enhances the manifestation of corneal lesions in rats (see OCULAR TOXICITY).

OCULAR TOXICITY

In several studies, oral clonidine hydrochloride produced a dose-dependent increase in the incidence and severity of spontaneously occurring retinal degeneration in albino rats treated for six months or longer. Tissue distribution studies in dogs and monkeys revealed that clonidine hydrochloride was concentrated in the choroid of the eye. In view of the retinal degeneration observed in rats, eye examinations were performed in 908 patients prior to the start of clonidine hydrochloride therapy, who were then examined periodically thereafter. In 353 of these 908 patients, examinations were performed for periods of 24 months or longer. Except for some dryness of the eyes, no drug-related abnormal ophthalmologic findings were recorded and clonidine hydrochloride did not alter retinal function as shown by specialized tests such as the electroretinogram and macular dazzle.
In rats, clonidine hydrochloride in combination with amitriptyline produced corneal lesions within 5 days.

Carcinogenesis, Mutagenesis, Impairment of Fertility In a 132-week (fixed concentraiton) dietary administration study in rats, clonidine hydrochloride administered at 32 to 46 times the maximum recommended daily human oral dose was unassociated with evidence of carcinogenic potential.
Fertility of male or female rats was unaffected by clonidine hydrochloride doses as high as 150 mcg/kg or about 3 times the maximum recommended daily human oral dose (MRDHD). Fertility of female rats did, however, appear to be affected (in another experiment) at dose levels of 500 to 2000 mcg/kg or 10 to 40 times the MRDHD.

Usage in Pregnancy
TERATOGENIC EFFECTS Pregnancy Category C. Reproduction studies performed in rabbits at doses up to approximately 3 times the maximum recommended daily human dose (MRDHD) of clonidine hydrochloride have revealed no evidence of teratogenic or embryotoxic potential. In rats however, doses as low as 1/3 the MRDHD were associated with increased resorptions in a study in which dams were treated continuously from 2 months prior to mating. Increased resorptions were not associated with treatment at the same or at higher dose levels (up to 3 times the MRDHD) when dams were treated days 6–15 of gestation. Increased resorptions were observed at much higher levels (40 times the MRDHD) in rats and mice treated days 1–14 of gestation (lowest dose employed in that study was 500 mcg/kg). There are, however, no adequate and well-controlled studies in pregnant women. Because animal reproduction studies are not always predictive of human response, this drug should be used during pregnancy only if clearly needed.
Nursing Mothers As clonidine hydrochloride is excreted in human milk, caution should be exercised when it is administered to a nursing woman.
Pediatric Use Safety and effectiveness in children have not been established.

Chlorthalidone: **General**
Hypokalemia and other electrolyte abnormalities, including hyponatremia and hypochloremic alkalosis, are common in patients receiving chlorthalidone. These abnormalities are dose-related but may occur even at the lowest marketed doses of chlorthalidone. Serum electrolytes should be determined before initiating therapy and at periodic intervals during therapy. Serum and urine electrolyte determinations are particularly important when the patient is vomiting excessively or receiving parenteral fluids. All patients taking chlorthalidone should be observed for clinical signs of electrolyte imbalance, including dryness of mouth, thirst, weakness, lethargy, drowsiness, restlessness, muscle pains or cramps, muscular fatigue, hypotension, oliguria, tachycardia, palpitations and gastrointestinal disturbances, such as nausea and vomiting. Digitalis therapy may exaggerate metabolic effects of hypokalemia especially with reference to myocardial activity.
Any chloride deficit is generally mild and usually does not require specific treatment except under extraordinary circumstances (as in liver disease or renal disease). Dilutional hyponatremia may occur in edematous patients in hot weather: appropriate therapy is water restriction, rather than administration of salt, except in rare instances when the hyponatremia is life-threatening. In cases of actual salt depletion, appropriate replacement is the therapy of choice.
Uric Acid Hyperuricemia may occur or frank gout may be precipitated in certain patients receiving chlorthalidone.
Other Increases in serum glucose may occur and latent diabetes mellitus may become manifest during chlorthalidone therapy (see PRECAUTIONS Drug Interactions). Chlorthalidone and related drugs may decrease serum PBI levels without signs of thyroid disturbance.
Information for Patients Patients should inform their doctor if they have: 1) had an allergic reaction to chlorthalidone or other diuretics or have asthma 2) kidney disease 3) liver disease 4) gout 5) systemic lupus erythematosus, or 6) been taking other drugs such as cortisone, digitalis, lithium carbonate, or drugs for diabetes.
Patients should be cautioned to contact their physician if they experience any of the following symptoms of potassium loss: excess thirst, tiredness, drowsiness, restlessness, muscle pains or cramps, nausea, vomiting or increased heart rate or pulse.
Patients should also be cautioned that taking alcohol can increase the chance of dizziness occurring.
Laboratory Tests Periodic determination of serum electrolytes to detect possible electrolyte imbalance should be performed at appropriate intervals.
All patients receiving chlorthalidone should be observed for clinical signs of fluid or electrolyte imbalance: namely, hyponatremia, hypochloremic alkalosis and hypokalemia. Serum and urine electrolyte determinations are particularly important when the patient is vomiting excessively or receiving parenteral fluids.
Drug Interactions Chlorthalidone may add to or potentiate the action of other antihypertensive drugs. Insulin requirements in diabetic patients may be increased, decreased or unchanged. Higher dosage of oral hypoglycemic agents may be required. Chlorthalidone and related drugs may increase the responsiveness to tubocurarine. Chlorthalidone and re-

lated drugs may decrease arterial responsiveness to norepinephrine. This diminution is not sufficient to preclude effectiveness of the pressor agent for therapeutic use. Lithium renal clearance is reduced by chlorthalidone, increasing the risk of lithium toxicity.

Drug/Laboratory Test Interactions Chlorthalidone and related drugs may decrease serum PBI levels without signs of thyroid disturbance.

Carcinogenesis, Mutagenesis, Impairment of Fertility No information is available.

Usage in Pregnancy

TERATOGENIC EFFECTS Pregnancy Category B. Reproduction studies have been performed in the rat and the rabbit at doses up to 420 times the human dose and have revealed no evidence of harm to the fetus due to chlorthalidone. There are, however, no adequate and well-controlled studies in pregnant women. Because animal reproduction studies are not always predictive of human response, this drug should be used during pregnancy only if clearly needed.

NON-TERATOGENIC EFFECTS Thiazides cross the placental barrier and appear in cord blood. The use of chlorthalidone and related drugs in pregnant women requires that the anticipated benefits of the drug be weighed against possible hazards to the fetus. These hazards include fetal or neonatal jaundice, thrombocytopenia, and possibly other adverse reactions that have occurred in the adult.

Nursing Mothers Thiazides are excreted in human milk. Because of the potential for serious adverse reactions in nursing infants from chlorthalidone, a decision should be made whether to discontinue nursing or to discontinue the drug, taking into account the importance of the drug to the mother.

Pediatric Use Safety and effectiveness in children have not been established.

ADVERSE REACTIONS

Combipres® is generally well tolerated. Most adverse effects are mild and tend to diminish with continued therapy. The most frequent (which appear to be dose-related) are dry mouth, occurring in about 40 to 100 patients; drowsiness, about 33 in 100; dizziness, about 16 in 100; constipation and sedation, each about 10 in 100.

In addition to the reactions listed above, certain less frequent adverse experiences, which are shown below, have also been reported in patients receiving the component drugs of Combipres® but in many cases patients were receiving concomitant medication and a causal relationship has not been established:

Clonidine hydrochloride:

Gastrointestinal Nausea and vomiting, about 5 in 100 patients; anorexia and malaise, each about 1 in 100; mild transient abnormalities in liver function tests, about 1 in 100; rare reports of hepatitis; parotitis, rarely.

Metabolic Weight gain, about 1 in 100 patients; gynecomastia, about 1 in 1000, transient elevation of blood glucose or serum creatine phosphokinase, rarely.

Central Nervous System Nervousness and agitation, about 3 in 100 patients; mental depression, about 1 in 100; headache, about 1 in 100; insomnia, about 5 in 1000. Vivid dreams or nightmares, other behavioral changes, restlessness, anxiety, visual and auditory hallucinations and delirium have been reported.

Cardiovascular Orthostatic symptoms, about 3 in 100 patients; palpitations and tachycardia, and bradycardia, each about 5 in 1000. Raynaud's phenomenon, congestive heart failure, and electrocardiographic abnormalities i.e. conduction disturbances and arrhythmias have been reported rarely. Rare cases of sinus bradycardia and atrioventricular block have been reported, both with and without the use of concomitant digitalis.

Dermatological Rash, about 1 in 100 patients; pruritus, about 7 in 1000; hives, angioneurotic edema and urticaria, about 5 in 1000, alopecia, about 2 in 1000.

Genitourinary Decreased sexual activity, impotence and loss of libido, about 3 in 100 patients; nocturia, about 1 in 100; difficulty in micturition, about 2 in 1000; urinary retention, about 1 in 1000.

Other Weakness, about 10 in 100 patients; fatigue, about 4 in 100; discontinuation syndrome, about 1 in 100; muscle or joint pain, about 6 in 1000 and cramps of the lower limbs, about 3 in 1000. Dryness, burning of the eyes, blurred vision, dryness of the nasal mucosa, pallor, weakly positive Coombs' test, increased sensitivity to alcohol and fever have been reported.

Chlorthalidone:

Gastrointestinal Anorexia, gastric irritation, nausea, vomiting, cramping, diarrhea, constipation, jaundice (intrahepatic cholestatic jaundice), pancreatitis.

Central Nervous System Dizziness, vertigo, paresthesias, headache, xanthopsia.

Hematologic Leukopenia, agranulocytosis, thrombocytopenia, aplastic anemia.

Dermatologic-Hypersensitivity Purpura, photosensitivity, rash, urticaria, necrotizing angiitis (vasculitis) (cutaneous vasculitis), Lyell's syndrome (toxic epidermal necrolysis).

Cardiovascular Orthostatic hypotension may occur and may be aggravated by alcohol, barbiturates or narcotics.

Other adverse reactions Hyperglycemia, glycosuria, hyperuricemia, muscle spasm, weakness, restlessness, impotence. Whenever adverse reactions are moderate or severe, chlorthalidone dosage should be reduced or therapy withdrawn.

OVERDOSAGE

Clonidine hydrochloride:

The signs and symptoms of clonidine hydrochloride overdosage include hypotension, bradycardia, lethargy, irritability, weakness, somnolence, diminished or absent reflexes, miosis, vomiting and hypoventilation. With large overdoses, reversible cardiac conduction defects or arrhythmias, apnea, seizures and transient hypertension have been reported. The oral LD_{50} of clonidine in rats was 465 mg/kg, and in mice 206 mg/kg.

The general treatment of clonidine hydrochloride overdosage may include intravenous fluids as indicated. Bradycardia can be treated with intravenous atropine sulfate and hypotension with dopamine infusion in addition to intravenous fluids. Hypertension, associated with overdosage, has been treated with intravenous furosemide or diazoxide or alpha-blocking agents such as phentolamine. Tolazoline, an alpha-blocker, in intravenous doses of 10 mg at 30-minute intervals, may reverse clonidine's effects if other efforts fail. Routine hemodialysis is of limited benefit, since a maximum of 5% of circulating clonidine is removed.

In a patient who ingested 100 mg clonidine hydrochloride, plasma clonidine levels were 60 ng/ml (one hour), 190 ng/ml (1.5 hours), 370 ng/ml (two hours) and 120 ng/ml (5.5 and 6.5 hours). This patient developed hypertension followed by hypotension, bradycardia, apnea, hallucinations, semicoma, and premature ventricular contractions. The patient fully recovered after intensive treatment.

Chlorthalidone:

Symptoms of acute overdosage include nausea, weakness, dizziness and disturbances of electrolyte balance. The oral LD_{50} of the drug in the mouse and the rat is more than 25,000 mg/kg body weight. The minimum lethal dose (MLD) in humans has not been established. There is no specific antidote but gastric lavage is recommended, followed by supportive treatment. Where necessary, this may include intravenous dextrose-saline with potassium, administered with caution.

DOSAGE AND ADMINISTRATION

The dosage must be determined by individual titration. (See INDICATIONS AND USAGE.)

Chlorthalidone is usually initiated at a dose of 25 mg once daily and may be increased to 50 mg if the response is insufficient after a suitable trial.

Clonidine hydrochloride is usually initiated at a dose of 0.1 mg twice daily. Elderly patients may benefit from a lower initial dose. Further increments of 0.1 mg/day may be made if necessary until the desired response is achieved. The therapeutic doses most commonly employed have ranged from 0.2 to 0.6 mg per day in divided doses.

One Combipres® (clonidine hydrochloride/chlorthalidone) Tablet administered once or twice daily can be used to administer a minimum of 0.1 mg clonidine hydrochloride and 15 mg chlorthalidone to a maximum of 0.6 mg clonidine hydrochloride and 30 mg chlorthalidone.

HOW SUPPLIED

Combipres® 0.1/15 mg (each tablet contains clonidine hydrochloride USP, 0.1 mg + chlorthalidone USP, 15 mg) tablets are pink, oval shaped and single scored with the marking Bl 8. Available in bottles of 100 (NDC 0597-0008-01) and 1000 (NDC 0597-0008-10).

Combipres® 0.2/15 mg (each tablet contains clonidine hydrochloride USP 0.2 mg +chlorthalidone USP, 15 mg) tablets are blue, oval shaped and single scored with the marking Bl 9. Available in bottles of 100 (NDC 0597-0009-01) and 1000 (NDC 0597-0009-10).

Combipres® 0.3/15 mg (each tablet contains clonidine hydrochloride USP, 0.3 mg + chlorthalidone USP, 15 mg) tablets are white, oval shaped and single scored with the marking Bl 10. Available in bottles of 100 (NDC 0597-0010-01).

Store below 86°F (30°C). Avoid excessive humidity.

Dispense in tight, light-resistant container.

Caution: Federal law prohibits dispensing without prescription.

CM-PI-4/91

Shown in Product Identification Section, page 405

MEXITIL® ℞
(mexiletine hydrochloride)
Oral Antiarrhythmic
Capsules of 150 mg, 200 mg and 250 mg

PRODUCT OVERVIEW

KEY FACTS

Mexitil® (mexiletine hydrochloride) is an orally active Class 1B antiarrhythmic agent that is structurally similar to lidocaine. It has no significant negative inotropic effects, nor does it affect QRS or QT intervals.

MAJOR USES

Mexitil has proven to be effective in the suppression of symptomatic ventricular arrhythmias (ventricular tachycardia, couplets and PVCs) in controlled clinical trials and in long-term use.

SAFETY INFORMATION

Mexitil is contraindicated in the presence of cardiogenic shock or pre-existing second- or third-degree AV block (if no pacemaker is present). It is important to optimize response and tolerance for each patient by careful dosage titration. Although serious adverse events have occasionally been reported, the most common adverse reactions to Mexitil are reversible upper GI and CNS effects, which can often be avoided by administration with food and careful dosage titration.

Before prescribing, please consult full prescribing information below.

PRESCRIBING INFORMATION

MEXITIL® ℞
(mexiletine hydrochloride)
Oral Antiarrhythmic
Capsules of 150 mg, 200 mg and 250 mg

DESCRIPTION

Mexitil® (mexiletine hydrochloride) is an orally active antiarrhythmic agent available as 150 mg, 200 mg and 250 mg capsules. 100 mg of mexiletine hydrochloride is equivalent to 83.31 mg of mexiletine base. It is a white to off-white crystalline powder with a slightly bitter taste, freely soluble in water and in alcohol. Mexitil has a pKa of 9.2.

Chemically, Mexitil is 1-methyl-2-(2,6-xylyloxy)-ethylamine hydrochloride and has the following structural formula:

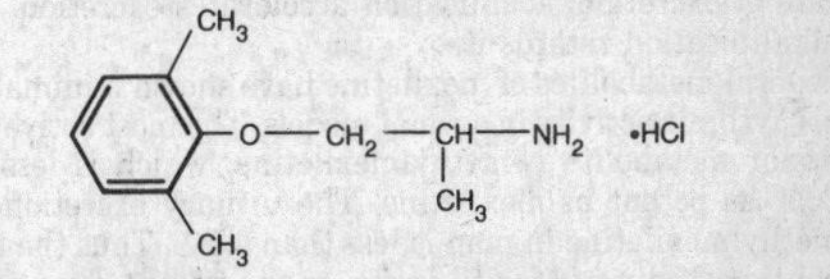

mexiletine hydrochloride (Mexitil)

$C_{11}H_{17}NO \cdot HCl$ Mol. Wt. 215.73

Mexitil Capsules contain the following inactive ingredients: colloidal silicon dioxide, cornstarch, magnesium stearate, titanium dioxide, gelatin, FD&C Red No. 40, D&C Red No. 28, and FD&C Blue No. 1; the Mexitil 150 mg and 250 mg capsules also contain FD&C Yellow No. 10. Mexitil capsules may contain one or more of the following components: sodium lauryl sulfate, sodium propionate, edetate calcium disodium, benzyl alcohol, carboxymethylcellulose sodium, glycerin, butylparaben, propylparaben, methylparaben, pharmaceutical glaze, ethylene glycol monoethyl ether, soya lecithin, dimethylpolysiloxane, refined shellac (food grade) and other inactive ingredients.

CLINICAL PHARMACOLOGY

Mechanism of Action Mexitil® (mexiletine hydrochloride) is a local anesthetic, antiarrhythmic agent, structurally similar to lidocaine, but orally active. In animal studies, Mexitil has been shown to be effective in the suppression of induced ventricular arrhythmias, including those induced by glycoside toxicity and coronary artery ligation. Mexitil, like lidocaine, inhibits the inward sodium current, thus reducing the rate of rise of the action potential, Phase 0. Mexitil decreased the effective refractory period (ERP) in Purkinje fibers. The decrease in ERP was of lesser magnitude than the decrease in action potential duration (APD), with a resulting increase in the ERP/APD ratio.

Electrophysiology in Man Mexiletine is a Class 1B antiarrhythmic compound with electrophysiologic properties in man similar to those of lidocaine, but dissimilar from quinidine, procainamide, and disopyramide.

In patients with normal conduction systems, Mexitil has a minimal effect on cardiac impulse generation and propagation. In clinical trials, no development of second-degree or third-degree AV block was observed. Mexitil did not prolong ventricular depolarization (QRS duration) or repolarization (QT intervals) as measured by electrocardiography. Theoretically, therefore, Mexitil may be useful in the treatment of ventricular arrhythmias associated with a prolonged QT interval.

In patients with pre-existing conduction defects, depression of the sinus rate, prolongation of sinus node recovery time, decreased conduction velocity and increased effective refractory period of the intraventricular conduction system have occasionally been observed.

Continued on next page

Boehringer Ingelheim—Cont.

The antiarrhythmic effect of Mexitil has been established in controlled comparative trials against placebo, quinidine, procainamide and disopyramide. Mexitil, at doses of 200–400 mg q8h, produced a significant reduction of ventricular premature beats, paired beats, and episodes of non-sustained ventricular tachycardia compared to placebo and was similar in effectiveness to the active agents. Among all patients entered into the studies, about 30% in each treatment group had a 70% or greater reduction in PVC count and about 40% failed to complete the three-month studies because of adverse effects. Follow-up of patients from the controlled trials has demonstrated continued effectiveness of Mexitil in long-term use.

Hemodynamics Hemodynamic studies in a limited number of patients, with normal or abnormal myocardial function, following oral administration of Mexitil, have shown small, usually not statistically significant, decreases in cardiac output and increases in systemic vascular resistance, but no significant negative inotropic effect. Blood pressure and pulse rate remain essentially unchanged. Mild depression of myocardial function, similar to that produced by lidocaine, has occasionally been observed following intravenous Mexitil therapy in patients with cardiac disease.

Pharmacokinetics Mexitil is well absorbed (~90%) from the gastrointestinal tract. Unlike lidocaine, its first-pass metabolism is low. Peak blood levels are reached in two to three hours. In normal subjects, the plasma elimination half-life of Mexitil is approximately 10–12 hours. It is 50–60% bound to plasma protein, with a volume of distribution of 5–7 liters/kg. Mexitil is metabolized in the liver. Approximately 10% is excreted unchanged by the kidney. While urinary pH does not normally have much influence on elimination, marked changes in urinary pH influence the rate of excretion: acidification accelerates excretion, while alkalinization retards it.

Several metabolites of mexiletine have shown minimal antiarrhythmic activity in animal models. The most active is the minor metabolite N-methylmexiletine, which is less than 20% as potent as mexiletine. The urinary excretion of N-methylmexiletine in man is less than 0.5%. Thus the therapeutic activity of Mexitil is due to the parent compound.

Hepatic impairment prolongs the elimination half-life of Mexitil. In eight patients with moderate to severe liver disease, the mean half-life was approximately 25 hours.

Consistent with the limited renal elimination of Mexitil, little change in the half-life has been detected in patients with reduced renal function. In eight patients with creatinine clearance less than 10 ml/min, the mean plasma elimination half-life was 15.7 hours; in seven patients with creatinine clearance between 11–40 ml/min, the mean half-life was 13.4 hours.

The absorption rate of Mexitil is reduced in clinical situations such as acute myocardial infarction in which gastric emptying time is increased. Narcotics, atropine and magnesium-aluminum hydroxide have also been reported to slow the absorption of Mexitil. Metoclopramide has been reported to accelerate absorption.

Mexiletine plasma levels of at least 0.5 mcg/ml are generally required for therapeutic response. An increase in the frequency of central nervous system adverse effects has been observed when plasma levels exceed 2.0 mcg/ml. Thus the therapeutic range is approximately 0.5 to 2.0 mcg/ml. Plasma levels within the therapeutic range can be attained with either three times daily or twice daily dosing but peak to trough differences are greater with the latter regimen, creating the possibility of adverse effects at peak and arrhythmic escape at trough. Nevertheless, some patients may be transferred successfully to the twice daily regimen (See DOSAGE AND ADMINISTRATION).

INDICATIONS AND USAGE

Mexitil® is indicated for the treatment of documented ventricular arrhythmias, such as sustained ventricular tachycardia, that, in the judgement of the physician, are life-threatening. Because of the proarrhythmic effects of Mexitil, its use with lesser arrhythmias is generally not recommended. Treatment of patients with asymptomatic ventricular premature contractions should be avoided.

Initiation of Mexitil treatment, as with other antiarrhythmic agents used to treat life-threatening arrhythmias, should be carried out in the hospital.

Antiarrhythmic drugs have not been shown to enhance survival in patients with ventricular arrhythmias.

CONTRAINDICATIONS

Mexitil® (mexiletine hydrochloride) is contraindicated in the presence of cardiogenic shock or pre-existing second- or third-degree AV block (if no pacemaker is present).

WARNINGS

Mortality:

In the National Heart, Lung and Blood Institute's Cardiac Arrhythmia Suppression Trial (CAST), a long-term, multicentered, randomized, double-blind study in patients with asymptomatic non-life-threatening ventricular arrhythmias who had had myocardial infarctions more than six days but less than two years previously, an excessive mortality or non-fatal cardiac arrest rate was seen in patients treated with encainide or flecainide (56/730) compared with that seen in patients assigned to matched placebo-treated groups (22/725). The average duration of treatment with encainide or flecainide in this study was ten months.

The applicability of these results to other populations (e.g., those without recent myocardial infarction) or to other antiarrhythmic drugs is uncertain, but at present it is prudent to consider any antiarrhythmic agent to have a significant risk in patients with structural heart disease.

Acute Liver Injury In postmarketing experience abnormal liver function tests have been reported, some in the first few weeks of therapy with Mexitil® (mexiletine hydrochloride). Most of these have been observed in the setting of congestive heart failure or ischemia and their relationship to Mexitil has not been established.

PRECAUTIONS

General If a ventricular pacemaker is operative, patients with second or third degree heart block may be treated with Mexitil® (mexiletine hydrochloride) if continuously monitored. A limited number of patients (45 of 475 in controlled clinical trials) with pre-existing first degree AV block were treated with Mexitil; none of these patients developed second or third degree AV block. Caution should be exercised when it is used in such patients or in patients with pre-existing sinus node dysfunction or intraventricular conduction abnormalities.

Like other antiarrhythmics Mexitil® (mexiletine hydrochloride) can cause worsening of arrhythmias. This has been uncommon in patients with less serious arrhythmias (frequent premature beats or non-sustained ventricular tachycardia: see ADVERSE REACTIONS), but is of greater concern in patients with life-threatening arrhythmias such as sustained ventricular tachycardia. In patients with such arrhythmias subjected to programmed electrical stimulation or to exercise provocation, 10–15% of patients had exacerbation of the arrhythmia, a rate not greater than that of other agents.

Mexitil should be used with caution in patients with hypotension and severe congestive heart failure because of the potential for aggravating these conditions.

Since Mexitil is metabolized in the liver, and hepatic impairment has been reported to prolong the elimination half-life of Mexitil, patients with liver disease should be followed carefully while receiving Mexitil. The same caution should be observed in patients with hepatic dysfunction secondary to congestive heart failure.

Concurrent drug therapy or dietary regimens which may markedly alter urinary pH should be avoided during Mexitil therapy. The minor fluctuations in urinary pH associated with normal diet do not affect the excretion of Mexitil.

SGOT Elevation and Liver Injury In three-month controlled trials, elevations of SGOT greater than three times the upper limit of normal occurred in about 1% of both mexiletine-treated and control patients. Approximately 2% of patients in the mexiletine compassionate use program had elevations of SGOT greater than or equal to three times the upper limit of normal. These elevations frequently occurred in association with identifiable clinical events and therapeutic measures such as congestive heart failure, acute myocardial infarction, blood transfusions and other medications. These elevations were often asymptomatic and transient, usually not associated with elevated bilirubin levels and usually did not require discontinuation of therapy. Marked elevations of SGOT (>1000 U/L) were seen before death in four patients with end-stage cardiac disease (severe congestive heart failure, cardiogenic shock).

Rare instances of severe liver injury, including hepatic necrosis, have been reported in association with Mexitil treatment. It is recommended that patients in whom an abnormal liver test has occurred, or who have signs or symptoms suggesting liver dysfunction, be carefully evaluated. If persistent or worsening elevation of hepatic enzymes is detected, consideration should be given to discontinuing therapy.

Blood Dyscrasias Among 10,867 patients treated with mexiletine in the compassionate use program, marked leukopenia (neutrophils less than 1000/mm^3) or agranulocytosis were seen in 0.06%, and milder depressions of leukocytes were seen in 0.08%, and thrombocytopenia was observed in 0.16%. Many of these patients were seriously ill and receiving concomitant medications with known hematologic adverse effects. Rechallenge with mexiletine in several cases was negative. Marked leukopenia or agranulocytosis did not occur in any patient receiving Mexitil alone; five of the six cases of agranulocytosis were associated with procainamide (sustained release preparations in four) and one with vinblastine. If significant hematologic changes are observed, the patient should be carefully evaluated, and, if warranted, Mexitil should be discontinued. Blood counts usually return to normal within one month of discontinuation. (See ADVERSE REACTIONS.)

Convulsions (seizures) did not occur in Mexitil controlled clinical trials. In the compassionate use program, convulsions were reported in about 2 of 1000 patients. Twenty-eight percent of these patients discontinued therapy. Convulsions were reported in patients with and without a prior history of seizures. Mexiletine should be used with caution in patients with known seizure disorder.

Drug Interactions In a large compassionate use program Mexitil has been used concurrently with commonly employed antianginal, antihypertensive, and anticoagulant drugs without observed interactions. A variety of antiarrhythmics such as quinidine or propranolol were also added, sometimes with improved control of ventricular ectopy. When phenytoin or other hepatic enzyme inducers such as rifampin and phenobarbital have been taken concurrently with Mexitil, lowered Mexitil plasma levels have been reported. Monitoring of Mexitil plasma levels is recommended during such concurrent use to avoid ineffective therapy.

In a formal study, benzodiazepines were shown not to affect Mexitil plasma concentrations. ECG intervals (PR, QRS and QT) were not affected by concurrent Mexitil and digoxin, diuretics, or propranolol.

Concurrent administration of cimetidine and Mexitil has been reported to increase, decrease, or leave unchanged Mexitil plasma levels; therefore patients should be followed carefully during concurrent therapy.

Mexitil does not alter serum digoxin levels, but magnesium-aluminum hydroxide, when used to treat gastrointestinal symptoms due to Mexitil, has been reported to lower serum digoxin levels.

Concurrent use of Mexitil and theophylline may lead to increased plasma theophylline levels. One controlled study in eight normal subjects showed a 72% mean increase (range 35–136%) in plasma theophylline levels. This increase was observed at the first test point which was the second day after starting Mexitil. Theophylline plasma levels returned to pre-Mexitil values within 48 hours after discontinuing Mexitil. If Mexitil and theophylline are to be used concurrently, theophylline blood levels should be monitored, particularly when the Mexitil dose is changed. An appropriate adjustment in theophylline dose should be considered.

Additionally, in one controlled study in five normal subjects and seven patients, the clearance of caffeine was decreased 50% following the administration of Mexitil.

Carcinogenesis, Mutagenesis and Impairment of Fertility Studies of carcinogenesis in rats (24 months) and mice (18 months) did not demonstrate any tumorigenic potential. Mexitil was found to be non-mutagenic in the Ames test. Mexitil did not impair fertility in the rat.

Pregnancy/Teratogenic Effects

PREGNANCY CATEGORY C

Reproduction studies performed with Mexitil® in rats, mice and rabbits at doses up to four times the maximum human oral dose (24 mg/kg in a 50 kg patient) revealed no evidence of teratogenicity or impaired fertility but did show an increase in fetal resorption. There are no adequate and well-controlled studies in pregnant women; this drug should be used in pregnancy only if the potential benefit justifies the potential risk to the fetus.

Nursing Mothers Mexitil appears in human milk in concentrations similar to those observed in plasma. Therefore, if the use of Mexitil is deemed essential, an alternative method of infant feeding should be considered.

Pediatric Use Safety and effectiveness in children have not been established.

ADVERSE REACTIONS

Mexitil® (mexiletine hydrochloride) commonly produces reversible gastrointestinal and nervous system adverse reactions but is otherwise well tolerated. Mexitil has been evaluated in 483 patients in one-month and three-month controlled studies and in over 10,000 patients in a large compassionate use program. Dosages in the controlled studies ranged from 600–1200 mg/day; some patients (8%) in the compassionate use program were treated with higher daily doses (1600–3200 mg/day). In the three-month controlled trials comparing Mexitil to quinidine, procainamide and disopyramide, the most frequent adverse reactions were upper gastrointestinal distress (41%), lightheadedness (10.5%), tremor (12.6%) and coordination difficulties (10.2%). Similar frequency and incidence were observed in the one-month placebo-controlled trial. Although these reactions were generally not serious, and were dose-related and reversible with a reduction in dosage, by taking the drug with food or antacid or by therapy discontinuation, they led to therapy discontinuation in 40% of patients in the controlled trials. A tabulation of the adverse events reported in the one-month placebo-controlled trial follows:

COMPARATIVE INCIDENCE (%) OF
ADVERSE EVENTS AMONG PATIENTS
TREATED WITH MEXILETINE AND
PLACEBO IN THE 4-WEEK,
DOUBLE-BLIND CROSSOVER TRIAL

	Mexiletine N = 53	Placebo N = 49
Cardiovascular		
Palpitations	7.5	10.2
Chest Pain	7.5	4.1
Increased Ventricular		
Arrhythmias/PVCs	1.9	—
Digestive		
Nausea/Vomiting/Heartburn	39.6	6.1
Central Nervous System		
Dizziness/Lightheadedness	26.4	14.3
Tremor	13.2	—
Nervousness	11.3	6.1
Coordination Difficulties	9.4	—
Changes in Sleep Habits	7.5	16.3
Paresthesias/Numbness	3.8	2.0
Weakness	1.9	4.1
Fatigue	1.9	2.0
Tinnitus	1.9	4.1
Confusion/Clouded Sensorium	1.9	2.0
Other		
Headache	7.5	6.1
Blurred Vision/Visual		
Disturbances	7.5	2.0
Dyspnea/Respiratory	5.7	10.2
Rash	3.8	2.0
Non-specific Edema	3.8	—

A tabulation of adverse reactions occurring in one percent or more of patients in the three-month controlled studies follows: [See table at right.]

Less than 1%: Syncope, edema, hot flashes, hypertension, short-term memory loss, loss of consciousness, other psychological changes, diaphoresis, urinary hesitancy/retention, malaise, impotence/decreased libido, pharyngitis, congestive heart failure.

An additional group of over 10,000 patients has been treated in a program allowing administration of Mexitil® (mexiletine hydrochloride) under compassionate use circumstances. These patients were seriously ill with the large majority on multiple drug therapy. Twenty-four percent of the patients continued in the program for one year or longer. Adverse reactions leading to therapy discontinuation occurred in 15 percent of patients (usually upper gastrointestinal system or nervous system effects). In general, the more common adverse reactions were similar to those in the controlled trials. Less common adverse events possibly related to Mexitil use include:

Cardiovascular System: Syncope and hypotension, each about 6 in 1000; bradycardia, about 4 in 1000; angina/angina-like pain, about 3 in 1000; edema, atrioventricular block/conduction disturbances and hot flashes, each about 2 in 1000; atrial arrhythmias, hypertension and cardiogenic shock, each about 1 in 1000.

Central Nervous System: Short-term memory loss, about 9 in 1000 patients; hallucinations and other psychological changes, each about 3 in 1000; psychosis and convulsions/seizures, each about 2 in 1000; loss of consciousness, about 6 in 10,000.

Digestive: Dysphagia, about 2 in 1000; peptic ulcer, about 8 in 10,000; upper gastrointestinal bleeding, about 7 in 10,000; esophageal ulceration, about 1 in 10,000. Rare cases of severe hepatitis/acute hepatic necrosis.

Skin: Rare cases of exfoliative dermatitis and Stevens-Johnson Syndrome with Mexitil® (mexiletine hydrochloride) treatment have been reported.

Laboratory: Abnormal liver function tests, about 5 in 1000 patients; positive ANA and thrombocytopenia, each about 2 in 1000; leukopenia (including neutropenia and agranulocytosis), about 1 in 1000; myelofibrosis, about 2 in 10,000 patients.

Other: Diaphoresis, about 6 in 1000; altered taste, about 5 in 1000; salivary changes, hair loss and impotence/decreased libido, each about 4 in 1000; malaise, about 3 in 1000; urinary hesitancy/retention, each about 2 in 1000; hiccups, dry skin, laryngeal and pharyngeal changes and changes in oral mucous membranes, each about 1 in 1000; SLE syndrome, about 4 in 10,000.

Hematology: Blood dyscrasias were not seen in the controlled trials but did occur among the 10,867 patients treated with mexiletine in the compassionate use program (see PRECAUTIONS).

Myelofibrosis was reported in two patients in the compassionate use program: one was receiving long-term thiotepa therapy and the other had pretreatment myeloid abnormalities.

In postmarketing experience, there have been isolated, spontaneous reports of pulmonary changes including pulmonary fibrosis during Mexitil therapy with or without other drugs or diseases that are known to produce pulmonary toxicity. A causal relationship to Mexitil therapy has not been estab-

COMPARATIVE INCIDENCE (%) OF ADVERSE EVENTS AMONG PATIENTS TREATED
WITH MEXILETINE OR CONTROL DRUGS IN THE 12-WEEK DOUBLE-BLIND TRIALS

	Mexiletine N = 430	Quinidine N = 262	Procainamide N = 78	Disopyramide N = 69
Cardiovascular				
Palpitations	4.3	4.6	1.3	5.8
Chest Pain	2.6	3.4	1.3	2.9
Angina/Angina-like Pain	1.7	1.9	2.6	2.9
Increased Ventricular				
Arrhythmias/PVCs	1.0	2.7	2.6	—
Digestive				
Nausea/Vomiting/				
Heartburn	39.3	21.4	33.3	14.5
Diarrhea	5.2	33.2	2.6	8.7
Constipation	4.0	—	6.4	11.6
Changes in Appetite	2.6	1.9	—	—
Abdominal Pain/Cramps/				
Discomfort	1.2	1.5	—	1.4
Central Nervous System				
Dizziness/				
Lightheadedness	18.9	14.1	14.1	2.9
Tremor	13.2	2.3	3.8	1.4
Coordination Difficulties	9.7	1.1	1.3	—
Changes in Sleep Habits	7.1	2.7	11.5	8.7
Weakness	5.0	5.3	7.7	2.9
Nervousness	5.0	1.9	6.4	5.8
Fatigue	3.8	5.7	5.1	1.4
Speech Difficulties	2.6	0.4	—	—
Confusion/Clouded				
Sensorium	2.6	—	3.8	—
Paresthesias/Numbness	2.4	2.3	2.6	—
Tinnitus	2.4	1.5	—	—
Depression	2.4	1.1	1.3	1.4
Other				
Blurred Vision/Visual				
Disturbances	5.7	3.1	5.1	7.2
Headache	5.7	6.9	7.7	4.3
Rash	4.2	3.8	10.3	1.4
Dyspnea/Respiratory	3.3	3.1	5.1	2.9
Dry Mouth	2.8	1.9	5.1	14.5
Arthralgia	1.7	2.3	5.1	1.4
Fever	1.2	3.1	2.6	—

lished. In addition, there have been isolated reports of exacerbation of congestive heart failure in patients with pre-existing compromised ventricular function.

OVERDOSAGE

Nine cases of Mexitil® (mexiletine hydrochloride) overdosage have been reported; two were fatal. In one fatality, 4400 mg of the drug was ingested. In the other death, the dose ingested was unknown. There has been a report of non-fatal ingestion of 8000 mg. Symptoms associated with overdosage include nausea, hypotension, sinus bradycardia, paresthesia, seizures, intermittent left bundle branch block and temporary asystole.

There is no specific antidote for Mexitil. Acidification of the urine, which will accelerate the excretion of mexiletine, may be useful. Treatment of overdosage should be supportive, and may include the administration of atropine if hypotension or bradycardia occurs.

DOSAGE AND ADMINISTRATION

The dosage of Mexitil® (mexiletine hydrochloride) must be individualized on the basis of response and tolerance, both of which are dose-related. Administration with food or antacid is recommended. Initiate Mexitil therapy with 200 mg every eight hours when rapid control of arrhythmia is not essential. A minimum of two to three days between dose adjustments is recommended. Dose may be adjusted in 50 or 100 mg increments up or down.

As with any antiarrhythmic drug, clinical and electrocardiographic evaluation (including Holter monitoring if necessary for evaluation) are needed to determine whether the desired antiarrhythmic effect has been obtained and to guide titration and dose adjustment.

Satisfactory control can be achieved in most patients by 200 to 300 mg given every eight hours with food or antacid. If satisfactory response has not been achieved at 300 mg q8h, and the patient tolerates Mexitil well, a dose of 400 mg q8h may be tried. As the severity of CNS side effects increases with total daily dose, the dose should not exceed 1200 mg/day.

In general, patients with renal failure will require the usual doses of Mexitil. Patients with severe liver disease, however, may require lower doses and must be monitored closely. Similarly, marked right-sided congestive heart failure can reduce hepatic metabolism and reduce the needed dose. Plasma level may also be affected by certain concomitant drugs (see PRECAUTIONS: Drug Interactions).

Loading Dose: When rapid control of ventricular arrhythmia is essential, an initial loading dose of 400 mg of Mexitil may be administered, followed by a 200 mg dose in eight hours. Onset of therapeutic effect is usually observed within 30 minutes to two hours.

Q12H Dosage Schedule: Some patients responding to Mex-

itil may be transferred to a 12-hour dosage schedule to improve convenience and compliance. If adequate suppression is achieved on a Mexitil dose of 300 mg or less every eight hours, the same total daily dose may be given in divided doses every 12 hours while carefully monitoring the degree of suppression of ventricular ectopy. This dose may be adjusted up to a maximum of 450 mg every 12 hours to achieve the desired response.

Transferring to Mexitil: The following dosage schedule, based on theoretical considerations rather than experimental data, is suggested for transferring patients from other Class I oral antiarrhythmic agents to Mexitil: Mexitil treatment may be initiated with a 200 mg dose, and titrated to response as described above, 6–12 hours after the last dose of quinidine sulfate, 3–6 hours after the last dose of procainamide, 6–12 hours after the last dose of disopyramide or 8–12 hours after the last dose of tocainide.

In patients in whom withdrawal of the previous antiarrhythmic agent is likely to produce life-threatening arrhythmias, hospitalization of the patient is recommended.

When transferring from lidocaine to Mexitil, the lidocaine infusion should be stopped when the first oral dose of Mexitil is administered. The infusion line should be left open until suppression of the arrhythmia appears to be satisfactorily maintained. Consideration should be given to the similarity of the adverse effects of lidocaine and Mexitil and the possibility that they may be additive.

HOW SUPPLIED

Mexitil® (mexiletine hydrochloride) is supplied in hard gelatin capsules containing 150 mg, 200 mg or 250 mg of mexiletine hydrochloride:

Mexitil® 150 mg capsules are red and caramel with the marking BI 66. Available in bottles of 100 (NDC 0597-0066-01) and individually blister-sealed unit-dose cartons of 100 (NDC 0597-0066-61).

Mexitil® 200 mg capsules are red with the marking BI 67. Available in bottles of 100 (NDC 0597-0067-01) and individually blister-sealed unit-dose cartons of 100 (NDC 0597-0067-61).

Mexitil® 250 mg capsules are red and aqua green with the marking BI 68. Available in bottles of 100 (NDC 0597-0068-01) and individually blister-sealed unit-dose cartons of 100 (NDC 0597-0068-61).

Store below 86°F (30°C).

Caution: Federal law prohibits dispensing without prescription.

ME-PI-6/91

Shown in Product Identification Section, page 405

Continued on next page

Boehringer Ingelheim—Cont.

PERSANTINE® ℞
[*per-san 'tēn*]
(dipyridamole USP)
Tablets of 25 mg ....BI-CODE 17
Tablets of 50 mg ....BI-CODE 18
Tablets of 75 mg ....BI-CODE 19

DESCRIPTION

Persantine® (dipyridamole USP) is a platelet inhibitor chemically described as 2,6-bis-(diethanolamino)-4,8-dipiperidino-pyrimido-(5,4-d) pyrimidine. It has the following structural formula:

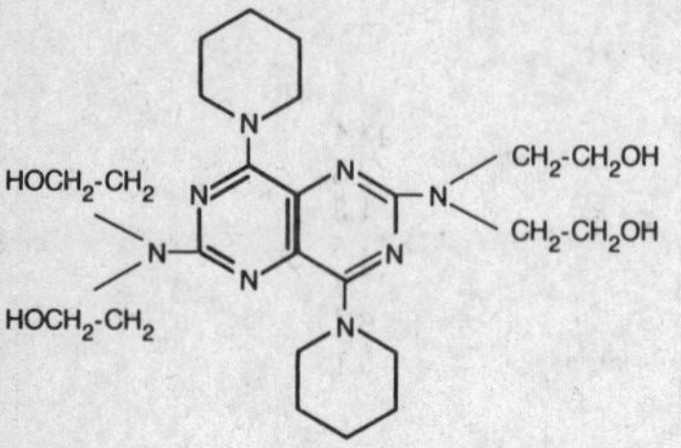

$C_{24}H_{40}N_8O_4$ Mol. Wt. 504.63

Dipyridamole is an odorless yellow crystalline powder, having a bitter taste. It is soluble in dilute acids, methanol and chloroform, and practically insoluble in water.
Persantine tablets for oral administration contain:
Active Ingredient: *TABLETS 25, 50 and 75 mg:* dipyridamole USP 25, 50 and 75 mg respectively.
Inactive Ingredients: *TABLETS 25, 50 and 75 mg:* acacia, carnauba wax, cornstarch, FD&C blue No. 1 aluminum lake, D&C yellow No. 10 aluminum lake, D&C red No. 30 aluminum lake, lactose, magnesium stearate, polyethylene glycol, povidone, shellac, sodium benzoate, sucrose, talc, titanium dioxide, white wax.

CLINICAL PHARMACOLOGY

It is believed that platelet reactivity and interaction with prosthetic cardiac valve surfaces, resulting in abnormally shortened platelet survival time, is a significant factor in thromboembolic complications occurring in connection with prosthetic heart valve replacement.
Persantine® (dipyridamole USP) has been found to lengthen abnormally shortened platelet survival time in a dose-dependent manner.
In three randomized controlled clinical trials involving 854 patients who had undergone surgical placement of a prosthetic heart valve, Persantine, in combination with warfarin, decreased the incidence of postoperative thromboembolic events by 62% to 91% compared to warfarin treatment alone. The incidence of thromboembolic events in patients receiving the combination of Persantine and warfarin ranged from 1.2% to 1.8%. In three additional studies involving 392 patients taking Persantine and coumarin-like anticoagulants, the incidence of thromboembolic events ranged from 2.3% to 6.9%.
In these trials, the coumarin anticoagulant was begun between 24 hours and 4 days postoperatively, and the Persantine was begun between 24 hours and 10 days postoperatively. The length of follow-up in these trials varied from 1 to 2 years.
Persantine does not influence prothrombin time or activity measurements when administered with warfarin.
Mechanism of Action: Persantine is a platelet adhesion inhibitor, although the mechanism of action has not been fully elucidated. The mechanism may relate to inhibition of red blood cell uptake of adenosine, itself an inhibitor of platelet reactivity, phosphodiesterase inhibition leading to increased cyclic-3', 5'-adenosine monophosphate within platelets, and inhibition of thromboxane A_2 formation, which is a potent stimulator of platelet activation.
Hemodynamics: In dogs intraduodenal doses of Persantine of 0.5 to 4.0 mg/kg produced dose-related decreases in systemic and coronary vascular resistance leading to decreases in systemic blood pressure and increases in coronary blood flow. Onset of action was in about 24 minutes and effects persisted for about 3 hours.
Similar effects were observed following IV Persantine in doses ranging from 0.025 to 2.0 mg/kg.
In man the same qualitative hemodynamic effects have been observed. However, acute intravenous administration of Persantine may worsen regional myocardial perfusion distal to partial occlusion of coronary arteries.
Pharmacokinetics and Metabolism: Following an oral dose of Persantine, the average time to peak concentration is about 75 minutes. The decline in plasma concentration following a dose of Persantine fits a two-compartment model. The alpha half-life (the initial decline following peak concentration) is approximately 40 minutes. The beta half-life (the terminal decline in plasma concentration) is approximately 10 hours. Persantine is highly bound to plasma proteins. It is metabolized in the liver where it is conjugated as a glucuronide and excreted with the bile.

INDICATIONS AND USAGE

Persantine® (dipyridamole USP) is indicated as an adjunct to coumarin anticoagulants in the prevention of postoperative thromboembolic complications of cardiac valve replacement.

CONTRAINDICATIONS

None known.

PRECAUTIONS

General: Persantine® (dipyridamole USP) should be used with caution in patients with hypotension since it can produce peripheral vasodilation.
Carcinogenesis, Mutagenesis, Impairment of Fertility: In a 111 week oral study in mice and in a 128-142 week oral study in rats, Persantine produced no significant carcinogenic effects at doses of 8, 25 and 75 mg/kg (1, 3.1 and 9.4 times the maximum recommended daily human dose). Mutagenicity testing with Persantine was negative. Reproduction studies with Persantine revealed no evidence of impaired fertility in rats at dosages up to 60 times the maximum recommended human dose. A significant reduction in number of corpora lutea with consequent reduction in implantations and live fetuses was, however, observed at 155 times the maximum recommended human dose.
Teratogenic Effects: *PREGNANCY CATEGORY B* Reproduction studies have been performed in mice and rats at doses up to 125 mg/kg (15.6 times the maximum recommended daily human dose) and rabbits at doses up to 20 mg/kg and have revealed no evidence of harm to the fetus due to Persantine. There are, however, no adequate and well-controlled studies in pregnant women. Because animal reproduction studies are not always predictive of human response, this drug should be used during pregnancy only if clearly needed.
Nursing Mothers: As dipyridamole is excreted in human milk, caution should be exercised when Persantine is administered to a nursing woman.
Pediatric Use: Safety and effectiveness in children below the age of 12 years have not been established.

ADVERSE REACTIONS

Adverse reactions at therapeutic doses are usually minimal and transient. On long-term use of Persantine® (dipyridamole USP) initial side effects usually disappear. The following reactions were reported in two heart valve replacement trials comparing Persantine and warfarin therapy to either warfarin alone or warfarin and placebo:

	Persantine/ Warfarin (N = 147)	**Placebo/ Warfarin (N = 170)**
Dizziness	13.6%	8.2%
Abdominal distress	6.1%	3.5%
Headache	2.3%	0.0
Rash	2.3%	1.1%

Other reactions from uncontrolled studies include diarrhea, vomiting, flushing and pruritus. In addition, angina pectoris has been reported rarely and there have been rare reports of liver dysfunction. On those uncommon occasions when adverse reactions have been persistent or intolerable, they have ceased on withdrawal of the medication.
When Persantine was administered concomitantly with warfarin, bleeding was no greater in frequency or severity than that observed when warfarin was administered alone.

OVERDOSAGE

Hypotension, if it occurs, is likely to be of short duration, but a vasopressor drug may be used if necessary. The oral LD_{50} in rats is greater than 6,000 mg/kg while in the dogs, the oral LD_{50} is approximately 400 mg/kg. Since Persantine® (dipyridamole USP) is highly protein bound, dialysis is not likely to be of benefit.

DOSAGE AND ADMINISTRATION

Adjunctive Use in Prophylaxis of Thromboembolism after Cardiac Valve Replacement The recommended dose is 75–100 mg four times daily as an adjunct to the usual warfarin therapy. Please note that aspirin is not to be administered concomitantly with coumarin anticoagulants.

HOW SUPPLIED

Persantine® (dipyridamole USP) is available as round, orange, sugar-coated tablets of 25 mg, 50 mg and 75 mg coded BI/17, BI/18 and BI/19 respectively.
They are available in the following package sizes:

25 mg Tablets	
Bottles of 100	(NDC 0597-0017-01)
Bottles of 1000	(NDC 0597-0017-10)
Unit Dose Packages of 100	(NDC 0597-0017-61)
50 mg Tablets	
Bottles of 100	(NDC 0597-0018-01)
Bottles of 1000	(NDC 0597-0018-10)
Unit Dose Packages of 100	(NDC 0597-0018-61)
75 mg Tablets	
Bottles of 100	(NDC 0597-0019-01)
Bottles of 500	(NDC 0597-0019-05)
Unit Dose Packages of 100	(NDC 0597-0019-61)

Store below 86°F (30°C).
Caution: Federal law prohibits dispensing without prescription.

PE-PI-12/90

Shown in Product Identification Section, page 405

PRELU-2® Ⓒⅲ ℞
[*pra 'lu (2)*]
(phendimetrazine tartrate)
Timed Release Capsules BI-CODE 64
105 mg

DESCRIPTION

Chemical name: phendimetrazine tartrate (+) 3, 4 dimethyl-2-phenylmorpholine tartrate. Phendimetrazine tartrate is a white, odorless powder with a bitter taste. It is soluble in water, methanol and ethanol. It has a molecular weight of 341, and has the following molecular structure:

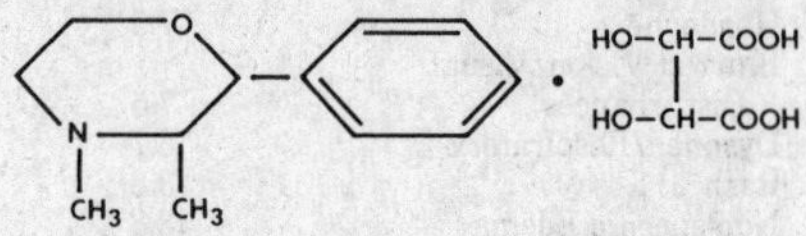

d-3, 4-dimethyl-2-phenylmorpholine tartrate

The capsule is manufactured in a special base which is designed for prolonged release.
Active Ingredient: Each timed-release capsule contains phendimetrazine tartrate 105 mg.
Inactive Ingredients: D&C Red No. 33, D&C Yellow No. 10, FD&C Blue No. 1, FD&C Yellow No. 6, gelatin, povidone, shellac, silica gel, starch, sucrose, talc, titanium dioxide.

CLINICAL PHARMACOLOGY

Phendimetrazine tartrate is a sympathomimetic amine with pharmacologic activity similar to the prototype of drugs of this class used in obesity, the amphetamines. Actions include central nervous system stimulation and elevation of blood pressure. Tachyphylaxis and tolerance have been demonstrated with all drugs of this class in which these phenomena have been looked for.
Drugs of this class used in obesity are commonly known as 'anorectics' or 'anorexigenics.' It has not been established, however, that the action of such drugs in treating obesity is primarily one of appetite suppression. Other central nervous system actions, or metabolic effects, may be involved, for example.
Adult obese subjects instructed in dietary management and treated with 'anorectic' drugs lose more weight on the average than those treated with placebo and diet, as determined in relatively short-term clinical trials.
The magnitude of increased weight loss of drug-treated patients over placebo-treated patients is only a fraction of a pound a week. The rate of weight loss is greatest in the first weeks of therapy for both drug and placebo subjects and tends to decrease in succeeding weeks. The possible origins of the increased weight loss due to the various drug effects are not established. The amount of weight loss associated with the use of an 'anorectic' drug varies from trial to trial, and the increased weight loss appears to be related in part to variables other than the drug prescribed, such as the physician-investigator, the population treated, and the diet prescribed. Studies do not permit conclusions as to the relative importance of the drug and non-drug factors on weight loss.
The natural history of obesity is measured in years, whereas the studies cited are restricted to a few weeks duration; thus, the total impact of drug-induced weight loss over that of diet alone must be considered clinically limited.
The active drug, 105 mg of phendimetrazine tartrate in each capsule of this special timed release dosage form, approximates the action of three 35 mg non-timed doses taken at four-hour intervals.
The major route of elimination is via the kidneys where most of the drug and metabolites are excreted. Some of the drug is metabolized to phenmetrazine and also phendimetrazine-N-oxide.
The average half-life of elimination when studied under controlled conditions is about 3.7 hours for both the timed and non-timed forms. The absorption half-life of the drug from conventional non-timed 35 mg phendimetrazine tablets is appreciably more rapid than the absorption rate of the drug from the timed release formulation.

INDICATIONS AND USAGE

Phendimetrazine tartrate is indicated in the management of exogenous obesity as a short-term adjunct (a few weeks) in a regimen of weight reduction based on caloric restriction. The

limited usefulness of agents of this class (see Clinical Pharmacology) should be measured against possible risk factors inherent in their use such as those described below.

CONTRAINDICATIONS

Advanced arteriosclerosis, symptomatic cardiovascular disease, moderate to severe hypertension, hyperthyroidism, known hypersensitivity, or idiosyncrasy to the sympathomimetic amines, glaucoma.

Agitated states.

Patients with a history of drug abuse.

During or within 14 days following the administration of monoamine oxidase inhibitors (hypertensive crises may result).

WARNINGS

Tolerance to the anorectic effect usually develops within a few weeks. When this occurs, the recommended dose should not be exceeded in an attempt to increase the effect; rather, the drug should be discontinued.

Phendimetrazine tartrate may impair the ability of the patient to engage in potentially hazardous activities such as operating machinery or driving a motor vehicle; the patient should therefore be cautioned accordingly.

DRUG DEPENDENCE

Phendimetrazine tartrate is related chemically and pharmacologically to the amphetamines. Amphetamines and related stimulant drugs have been extensively abused, and the possibility of abuse of phendimetrazine tartrate should be kept in mind when evaluating the desirability of including a drug as part of a weight reduction program. Abuse of amphetamines and related drugs may be associated with intense psychological dependence and severe social dysfunction. There are reports of patients who have increased the dosage to many times that recommended. Abrupt cessation following prolonged high dosage administration results in extreme fatigue and mental depression; changes are also noted on the sleep EEG. Manifestations of chronic intoxication with anorectic drugs include severe dermatoses, marked insomnia, irritability, hyperactivity, and personality changes. The most severe manifestation of chronic intoxication is psychosis, often clinically indistinguishable from schizophrenia.

Usage in Pregnancy: The safety of phendimetrazine tartrate in pregnancy and lactation has not been established. Therefore phendimetrazine tartrate should not be taken by women who are or may become pregnant.

Usage in Children: Phendimetrazine tartrate is not recommended for use in children under 12 years of age.

PRECAUTIONS

Caution is to be exercised in prescribing phendimetrazine tartrate for patients with even mild hypertension.

Insulin requirements in diabetes mellitus may be altered in association with the use of phendimetrazine tartrate and the concomitant dietary regimen.

Phendimetrazine tartrate may decrease the hypotensive effect of guanethidine.

The least amount feasible should be prescribed or dispensed at one time in order to minimize the possibility of overdosage.

ADVERSE REACTIONS

Cardiovascular: Palpitation, tachycardia, elevation of blood pressure.

Central Nervous System: Overstimulation, restlessness, dizziness, insomnia, euphoria, dysphoria, tremor, headache; rarely psychotic episodes at recommended doses.

Gastrointestinal: Dryness of the mouth, unpleasant taste, diarrhea, constipation, other gastrointestinal disturbances.

Allergic: Urticaria.

Endocrine: Impotence, changes in libido.

OVERDOSAGE

Manifestations of acute overdosage with phendimetrazine tartrate include restlessness, tremor, hyperreflexia, rapid respiration, confusion, assaultiveness, hallucinations, panic states.

Fatigue and depression usually follow the central stimulation.

Cardiovascular effects include arrhythmias, hypertension or hypotension and circulatory collapse. Gastrointestinal symptoms include nausea, vomiting, diarrhea, and abdominal cramps. Fatal poisoning usually terminates in convulsions and coma. Management of acute phendimetrazine tartrate intoxication is largely symptomatic and includes lavage and sedation with a barbiturate. Experience with hemodialysis or peritoneal dialysis is inadequate to permit recommendation in this regard. Acidification of the urine increases phendimetrazine tartrate excretion. Intravenous phentolamine (Regitine®*) has been suggested for possible acute, severe hypertension, if this complicates phendimetrazine tartrate overdosage.

*Regitine® (phentolamine mesylate USP) is a registered trademark of CIBA Pharmaceutical Company.

DOSAGE AND ADMINISTRATION

Since this product is a timed release dosage form, limit to one timed release capsule (105 mg phendimetrazine tartrate) in the morning.

Phendimetrazine tartrate is not recommended for use in children under 12 years of age.

HOW SUPPLIED

105 mg capsules (celery and green) in bottles of 100.

Federal law prohibits dispensing without a prescription.

P2-PI-9/85

Shown in Product Identification Section, page 405

RESPBID® ℞

[resp'bid]

(anhydrous theophylline, sustained release)

Tablets

250 mg and 500 mg

Oral Bronchodilator

Prescribing Information

DESCRIPTION

Theophylline is a bronchodilator structurally classified as a xanthine derivative. It occurs as a white, odorless, crystalline powder having a bitter taste. Theophylline anhydrous has the chemical name, 1H-Purine-2, 6-dione, 3,7-dihydro-1,3-dimethyl-, and is represented by the following structural formula:

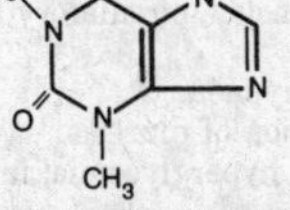

$C_7H_8N_4O_2$ Molecular Weight 180.17

Respbid® (anhydrous theophylline) Tablets contain 250 or 500 mg theophylline anhydrous, in a sustained-release formulation for oral administration. Respbid Tablets also contain: cellulose acetate phthalate, lactose, magnesium stearate.

CLINICAL PHARMACOLOGY

Theophylline directly relaxes the smooth muscle of the bronchial airways and pulmonary blood vessels, thus acting mainly as a bronchodilator and smooth muscle relaxant. It has also been demonstrated that aminophylline has a potent effect on diaphragmatic contractility in normal persons and may then be capable of reducing fatigability and thereby improve contractility in patients with chronic obstructive airways disease. The exact mode of action remains unsettled. Although theophylline does cause inhibition of phosphodiesterase with a resultant increase in intracellular cyclic AMP, other agents similarly inhibit the enzyme producing a rise of cyclic AMP but are unassociated with any demonstrable bronchodilation. Other mechanisms proposed include an effect on translocation of intracellular calcium; prostaglandin antagonism; stimulation of catecholamines endogenously; inhibition of cyclic guanosine monophosphate metabolism and adenosine receptor antagonism. None of these mechanisms has been proved, however.

In vitro, theophylline has been shown to act synergistically with beta agonists and there are now available data which do demonstrate an additive effect *in vivo* with combined use.

Pharmacokinetics: The half-life of theophylline is influenced by a number of known variables. It may be prolonged in chronic alcoholics, particularly those with liver disease (cirrhosis or alcoholic liver disease), in patients with congestive heart failure, and in those patients taking certain other drugs (see PRECAUTIONS, Drug Interactions). Newborns and neonates have extremely slow clearance rates compared to older infants and children, i.e., those over 1 year. Older children have rapid clearance rates while most non-smoking adults have clearance rates between these two extremes. In premature neonates the decreased clearance is related to oxidative pathways that have yet to be established.

Theophylline Elimination Characteristics

	Half-Life (in Hours)	
	Range	Mean
Children	1–9	3.7
Adults	3–15	7.7

In cigarette smokers (1–2 packs/day) the mean half-life is 4–5 hours, much shorter than in non-smokers. The increase in clearance associated with smoking is presumably due to stimulation of the hepatic metabolic pathway by components of cigarette smoke. The duration of this effect after cessation of smoking is unknown but may require 6 months to 2 years before the rate approaches that of the non-smoker.

A single 500 mg dose of Respbid® (anhydrous theophylline) in 8 healthy male subjects fasted for 10 hours predose (overnight) through 4 hours postdose resulted in mean peak theophylline plasma levels of 9.1 ± 3.8 (SD) mcg/ml occurring at 5.0 ± 1.5 hours following dose administration. The extent of theophylline absorption from Respbid® (anhydrous theophylline) was complete in these subjects when compared with that from an immediate-release tablet. In another single dose study, comparable rates and extents of theophylline absorption were seen for the 250 mg Respbid Tablets in 18 healthy male subjects, fasted as above.

In a five-day multiple-dose study, 18 healthy male subjects received 250 mg Respbid Tablets in doses ranging from 375 mg to 625 mg twice daily (mean dose of 11 mg/kg per day). Subjects were allowed to take drug with milk and were permitted their normal daily meals except for fasting from 10 hours before through 4 hours after the morning dose on day 5. Following that dose, mean minimum and maximum plasma theophylline levels were 7.3 ± 2.3 mcg/ml and 10.8 ± 3.1 mcg/ml, respectively. The average percent fluctuation $[(C_{max} - C_{min}/C_{min}) \times 100]$ was 48%. The extent of theophylline absorption from Respbid averaged 94 ± 19% of that from an immediate-release liquid given four times daily.

In other studies: A single 500 mg dose of Respbid was administered to 35 healthy volunteers in both a fasting state and with a high-fat content breakfast. The resultant pharmacokinetic values recorded a delay in the rate of absorption (but not the extent) for the fed group.

In a multiple-dose study involving 12 adolescent patients, the rate and extent of absorption was similar whether the drug was taken immediately after, or two hours after, a low-fat content breakfast (see PRECAUTIONS, Drug/Food Interactions).

INDICATIONS AND USAGE

For relief and/or prevention of symptoms from asthma and reversible bronchospasm associated with chronic bronchitis and emphysema.

CONTRAINDICATIONS

Respbid® (anhydrous theophylline) Tablets are contraindicated in individuals who are hypersensitive to theophylline or any of the tablet components. It is also contraindicated in patients with active peptic ulcer disease, and in individuals with underlying seizure disorders (unless receiving appropriate anti-convulsant therapy).

WARNINGS

Serum levels above 20 mcg/ml are rarely found after appropriate administration of the recommended doses. However, in individuals in whom theophylline plasma clearance is reduced for any reason, even conventional doses may result in increased serum levels and potential toxicity. Reduced theophylline clearance has been documented in the following readily identifiable groups: 1) patients with impaired liver function; 2) patients over 55 years of age, particularly males and those with chronic lung disease; 3) those with cardiac failure from any cause; 4) patients with sustained high fever; 5) neonates and infants under 1 year of age; and 6) those patients taking certain drugs (see PRECAUTIONS, Drug Interactions). Frequently, such patients have markedly prolonged theophylline serum levels following discontinuation of the drug.

Reduction of dosage and laboratory monitoring is especially appropriate in the above individuals.

Serious side effects such as ventricular arrhythmias, convulsions or even death may appear as the first sign of toxicity without any previous warning. Less serious signs of theophylline toxicity (i.e., nausea and restlessness) may occur frequently when initiating therapy, but are usually transient; when such signs are persistent during maintenance therapy; they are often associated with serum concentrations above 20 mcg/ml. Stated differently: serious toxicity is not reliably preceded by less severe side effects. A serum concentration measurement is the only reliable method of predicting potentially life-threatening toxicity.

Many patients who require theophylline exhibit tachycardia due to their underlying disease process so that the cause/effect relationship to elevated serum theophylline concentrations may not be appreciated.

Theophylline products may cause or worsen arrhythmias and any significant change in rate and/or rhythm warrants monitoring and further investigation.

Studies in laboratory animals (minipigs, rodents, and dogs) recorded the occurrence of cardiac arrhythmias and sudden death (with histologic evidence of myocardial necrosis) when beta-agonists and methylxanthines were administered concurrently. The significance of these findings when applied to humans is currently unknown.

PRECAUTIONS

General: On the average, theophylline half-life is shorter in cigarette and marijuana smokers than in non-smokers, but smokers can have half-lives as long as non-smokers. Theophylline should not be administered concurrently with other xanthines. Use with caution in patients with hypoxemia, hypertension, or those with history of peptic ulcer. Theophylline may occasionally act as a local irritant to G.I. tract although gastrointestinal symptoms are more commonly centrally mediated and associated with serum drug concentrations over 20 mcg/ml.

Continued on next page

Boehringer Ingelheim—Cont.

Information for Patients: If nausea, vomiting, restlessness, irregular heartbeat, or convulsions occur, contact a physician immediately.

Take only the amount of drug that has been prescribed. Do not take a larger dose, or take the drug more often, or for a longer time than recommended.

Take this drug consistently with respect to food: either with meals, or fasted (at least two hours pre- or 2 hours post-meals).

Do not take other medicines, especially those for pulmonary disorders, except on the advice of a physician.

Contact your physician if pulmonary symptoms occur repeatedly, especially at the end of a dosing interval.

Avoid drinking large amounts of caffeine-containing beverages, such as coffee, tea, cocoa, or cola, or eating large quantities of chocolate while taking this medicine, since these foods increase the side effects of theophylline.

Respbid® (anhydrous theophylline) Tablets should not be chewed or crushed.

Laboratory Tests: Serum levels should be monitored periodically to determine the theophylline level associated with observed clinical response and as the method of predicting toxicity. For such measurements, the serum sample should be obtained four to six hours after administration of Respbid Tablets. It is important that the patient will not have missed or taken additional doses during the previous 48 hours and that dosing intervals will have been reasonably equally spaced. DOSAGE ADJUSTMENT BASED ON SERUM THEOPHYLLINE MEASUREMENTS WHEN THESE INSTRUCTIONS HAVE NOT BEEN FOLLOWED MAY RESULT IN RECOMMENDATIONS THAT PRESENT RISK OF TOXICITY TO THE PATIENT.

Drug Interactions: *Drug/Drug*—Toxic synergism with ephedrine has been documented and may occur with other sympathomimetic bronchodilators. In addition, the following drug interactions have been demonstrated:

Theophylline with:

Allopurinol (high-dose)	Increased serum theophylline levels
Cimetidine	Increased serum theophylline levels
Erythromycin, Troleandomycin	Increased serum theophylline levels
Lithium carbonate	Increased renal excretion of lithium
Oral Contraceptives	Increased serum theophylline levels
Phenytoin	Decreased theophylline and phenytoin serum levels
Propranolol	Increased serum theophylline levels
Rifampin	Decreased serum theophylline levels

Drug/Food—Administration of a single dose of Respbid immediately after a high-fat content breakfast (8 ounces of whole milk, 2 fried eggs, 2 bacon strips, 2 ounces of hash browns and 2 slices of buttered toast, which equates to approximately 71 grams of fat and 985 calories) to 35 healthy volunteers resulted in plasma concentration levels (for the first 8 hours) of 40–60% of those noted during the fasted state and a delay in the time to peak plasma level (T-max) of 17.1 hours in contrast to the 5.1 hours observed during the fasted state.

However, when Respbid was administered on an every 12 hour schedule for 5 days, no consequential effect on absorption was noted following similar high-fat content breakfast, and the time to peak concentration averaged 5.4 hours. The rate and extent of absorption seen was similar when the drug was taken immediately after, and two hours after, a low-fat content breakfast.

The effect of other types and amounts of food, and the pharmacokinetic profile following an evening meal is not presently known.

Drug-Laboratory Test Interactions: Currently available analytical methods, including high pressure liquid chromatography and immunoassay techniques, for measuring serum theophylline levels are specific. Metabolites and other drugs generally do not affect the results. Other new analytic methods are also now in use. The physician should be aware of the laboratory method used and whether other drugs will interfere with the assay for theophylline.

Carcinogenesis, Mutagenesis, and Impairment of Fertility: Long-term carcinogenicity studies have not been performed with theophylline.

Chromosome-breaking activity was detected in human cell cultures at concentrations of theophylline up to 50 times the therapeutic serum concentration in humans. Theophylline was not mutagenic in the dominant lethal assay in male mice given theophylline intraperitoneally in doses up to 30 times the maximum daily human oral dose.

Studies to determine the effect on fertility have not been performed with theophylline.

Pregnancy: *CATEGORY C*—Animal reproduction studies have not been conducted with theophylline. It is also not known whether theophylline can cause fetal harm when administered to a pregnant woman or can affect reproduction capacity. Xanthines should be given to a pregnant woman only if clearly needed.

Nursing Mothers: Theophylline is distributed into breast milk and may cause irritability or other signs of toxicity in nursing infants. Because of the potential for serious adverse reactions in nursing infants from theophylline, a decision should be made whether to discontinue nursing or to discontinue the drug, taking into account the importance of the drug to the mother.

Pediatric Use: Respbid® (anhydrous theophylline) Tablets are not recommended for administration to children less than six years of age.

ADVERSE REACTIONS

The following adverse reactions have been observed, but there has not been enough systematic collection of data to support an estimate of their frequency. The most consistent adverse reactions are usually due to overdosage.

1. *Gastrointestinal:* nausea, vomiting, epigastric pain, hematemesis, diarrhea.
2. *Central nervous system:* headaches, irritability, restlessness, insomnia, reflex hyperexcitability, muscle twitching, clonic and tonic generalized convulsions.
3. *Cardiovascular:* palpitation, tachycardia, extrasystoles, flushing, hypotension, circulatory failure, ventricular arrhythmias.
4. *Respiratory:* tachypnea.
5. *Renal:* potentiation of diuresis.
6. *Others:* alopecia, hyperglycemia, inappropriate ADH syndrome, rash.

OVERDOSAGE

Management: It is suggested that the management principles (consistent with the clinical status of the patient when first seen) outlined below be instituted and that simultaneous contact with a Regional Poison Control Center be established. In this way both updated information and individualization regarding required therapy may be provided.

1. When potential oral overdose is established and seizure has not occurred:

a) If patient is alert and seen within the early hours after ingestion, induction of emesis may be of value. Gastric lavage has been demonstrated to be of no value in influencing outcome in patients who present more than 1 hour after ingestion.

b) Administer a cathartic. Sorbitol solution is reported to be of value.

c) Administer repeated doses of activated charcoal and monitor theophylline serum levels.

d) Prophylactic administration of phenobarbital has been shown to increase the seizure threshold in laboratory animals, and administration of this drug can be considered.

2. If patient presents with a seizure:

a) Establish an airway.

b) Administer oxygen.

c) Treat the seizure with intravenous diazepam, 0.1 to 0.3 mg/kg up to 10 mg. If seizures cannot be controlled, the use of general anesthesia should be considered.

d) Monitor vital signs, maintain blood pressure and provide adequate hydration.

3. If post-seizure coma is present:

a) Maintain airway and oxygenation.

b) If a result of oral medication, follow above recommendations to prevent absorption of the drug, but intubation and lavage will have to be performed instead of inducing emesis, and the cathartic and charcoal will need to be introduced via a large bore gastric lavage tube.

c) Continue to provide full supportive care and adequate hydration until the drug is metabolized. In general, drug metabolism is sufficiently rapid so as not to warrant dialysis. If repeated oral activated charcoal is ineffective (as noted by stable or rising serum levels) charcoal hemoperfusion may be indicated.

DOSAGE AND ADMINISTRATION

Effective use of theophylline (i.e., the concentration of drug in the serum associated with optimal benefit and minimal risk of toxicity) is considered to occur when the theophylline concentration is maintained from 10 to 20 mcg/ml. The early studies from which these levels were derived were carried out in patients immediately or shortly after recovery from acute exacerbations of their disease (some hospitalized with status asthmaticus).

Although the 20 mcg/ml level remains appropriate as a critical value (above which toxicity is more likely to occur) for safety purposes, additional data are now available which indicate that the serum theophylline concentrations required to produce maximum physiologic benefit may, in fact, fluctuate with the degree of bronchospasm present and are variable. Therefore, the physician should individualize the range appropriate to the patient's requirements, based on both symptomatic response and improvement in pulmonary function. It should be stressed that serum theophylline concentrations maintained at the upper level of the 10 to 20 mcg/ml range may be associated with potential toxicity when factors known to reduce theophylline clearance are operative (see WARNINGS).

If it is not possible to obtain serum level determinations, restriction of the daily dose (in otherwise healthy adults) to not greater than 13 mg/kg/day, to a maximum of 900 mg, in divided doses, will result in relatively few patients exceeding serum levels of 20 mcg/ml and the resultant greater risk of toxicity.

Caution should be exercised for younger children who cannot complain of minor side effects. Older adults, those with cor pulmonale, congestive heart failure, and/or liver diseases may have unusually low dosage requirements and thus may experience toxicity at the maximal dosage recommended below.

Theophylline does not distribute into fatty tissue. Dosage should be calculated on the basis of lean (ideal) body weight where mg/kg doses are presented.

Dosage guidelines are approximations only and the wide range of theophylline clearance between individuals (particularly those with concomitant disease) makes indiscriminate usage hazardous.

Respbid® (anhydrous theophylline) Tablets Should Not Be Chewed or Crushed.

Dosage Guidelines: There is information which shows that taking Respbid consistently after both high-fat and low-fat content breakfasts does not result in a decrease in peak concentration or delay in time to peak concentration that are seen when a single dose of Respbid is taken immediately after a high-fat content breakfast. Therefore, Respbid® (anhydrous theophylline) should be administered consistently with respect to food; either with meals, or fasted (at least 2 hours pre- or 2 hours post-meals). (See PRECAUTIONS, Drug/Food Interactions.)

Status asthmaticus should be considered a medical emergency and is defined as that degree of bronchospasm which is not rapidly responsive to usual doses of conventional bronchodilators. Optimal therapy for such patients frequently requires both additional medication, parenterally administered, and close monitoring, preferably in an intensive care setting.

Acute Symptoms—Respbid Tablets are not intended for patients experiencing an acute episode of bronchospasm (associated with asthma, chronic bronchitis, or emphysema). Such patients require rapid relief of symptoms and should be treated with an immediate release theophylline preparation, an intravenous theophylline preparation or other bronchodilators, and not with controlled-release products.

Chronic Symptoms—Theophylline administration is a treatment for the management of reversible bronchospasm (asthma, chronic bronchitis and emphysema) to prevent symptoms and maintain patent airways. The appropriate dosage of theophylline can be established using an immediate-release preparation. Slow clinical titration is preferred to help assure acceptance and safety of the medication. When appropriate theophylline serum levels have been attained and clinical improvement has been maintained, the patient can usually be switched to Respbid Tablets by dividing the total daily dose of immediate-release theophylline by two and administering the appropriate Respbid Tablet every 12 hours (see conversion chart below). However, certain patients, such as the young, smokers, or some non-smoking adults are likely to metabolize theophylline rapidly and require the total daily dose administered as three equal doses at eight-hour intervals. Such patients can generally be identified as having trough serum levels lower than desired or repeatedly exhibiting symptoms near the end of a dosing interval.

If the established daily dose is:	The q 12 hr regimen is:	
	no. tablets:	strength:
500 mg	1	Respbid 250 mg
1000 mg	1	Respbid 500 mg

Alternatively, therapy can be initiated with Respbid since it is available in dosage strengths which permit titration and adjustment of dosage as noted above. A liquid preparation should be considered for children to permit both greater ease of and more accurate dosage adjustment.

Recommended Doses for Initiating Therapy with Respbid:
Initial Dose—As an initial dose, 16 mg/kg per 24 hours or 400 mg per 24 hours (whichever is less) of Respbid® (anhydrous theophylline) Tablets in divided doses at 8- or 12-hour intervals, as appropriate (see DOSAGE AND ADMINISTRATION).

Increasing Dose—The above dosage may be increased in approximately 25% increments at three-day intervals so long as the drug is tolerated, until clinical response is satisfactory or the maximum dose as indicated in the following section is reached. The serum concentration may be checked at these intervals, but at a minimum, should be determined at the end of this adjustment period.

IT IS IMPORTANT THAT NO PATIENT BE MAINTAINED ON ANY DOSAGE THAT IS NOT TOLERATED. In instruct-

If serum theophylline is:		Directions:
Within desired range		Maintain dosage if tolerated. Recheck serum theophylline concentration at 6- to 12-month intervals.*
Too high	20 to 25 mcg/ml	Decrease doses by about 10% and recheck serum level after 3 days.
	25 to 30 mcg/ml	Skip the next dose and decrease subsequent doses by about 25%. Recheck serum level after 3 days.
	Over 30 mcg/ml	Skip next two doses and decrease subsequent doses by 50%. Recheck serum level after 3 days.
Too low		Increase dosage by 25% at 3 day intervals until either the desired serum concentration and/or clinical response is achieved.* The total daily dose may need to be administered at more frequent intervals if symptoms occur repeatedly at the end of a dosing interval.

The serum concentration may be rechecked at appropriate intervals, but at least at the end of any adjustment period. When the patient's condition is otherwise clinically stable, and none of the recognized factors which alter elimination are present, measurement of serum levels need be repeated only every 6 to 12 months.

*Finer adjustments in dosage may be needed for some patients.

ing patients to increase dosage, they should be instructed not to take a subsequent dose if side effects occur and to resume therapy at a lower dose once adverse effects have disappeared.

Maximum Dose Where the Serum Concentration Is Not Measured:

WARNING: DO NOT ATTEMPT TO MAINTAIN ANY DOSE THAT IS NOT TOLERATED.

Do not exceed the following (or 900 mg, whichever is less):

Age 6 to under 9 years	24 mg/kg/day
Age 9 to under 12 years	20 mg/kg/day
Age 12 to under 16 years	18 mg/kg/day
Age 16 years and older	13 mg/kg/day

Measurement of Serum Theophylline Concentrations During Chronic Therapy If the above maximum doses are to be maintained or exceeded, serum theophylline measurement is essential (see PRECAUTIONS, Laboratory Tests, for guidance).

Dosage Adjustment After Serum Theophylline Measurement: [See table above.]

HOW SUPPLIED

Respbid® brand anhydrous theophylline is supplied as 250 mg white, round, scored sustained release tablets imprinted with "BI 48" (NDC 0597-0048-01) and 500 mg white, capsule-shaped, scored sustained-release tablets imprinted with "BI 49" (NDC 0597-0049-01) in bottles of 100.

STORE AT CONTROLLED ROOM TEMPERATURE 15°–30°C (59°–86°F).

Caution: Federal law prohibits dispensing without prescription.

RE-PI-7/91

Shown in Product Identification Section, page 405

SERENTIL® ℞

[seh-ren 'til]

(mesoridazine besylate USP)

Tablets, 10 mg	**BI-CODE 20**
Tablets, 25 mg	**BI-CODE 21**
Tablets, 50 mg	**BI-CODE 22**
Tablets, 100 mg	**BI-CODE 23**
Concentrate of 25 mg/ml	**BI-CODE 25**
Ampuls of 1 ml (25 mg)	**BI-CODE 27**

Caution: Federal law prohibits dispensing without prescription.

DESCRIPTION

Serentil® (mesoridazine besylate USP), the besylate salt of a metabolite of thioridazine, is a phenothiazine tranquilizer that is effective in the treatment of schizophrenia, organic brain disorders, alcoholism and psychoneuroses.

Serentil is 10-[2(1-methyl-2-piperidyl) ethyl]-2-(methyl-sulfinyl)-phenothiazine [as the besylate].

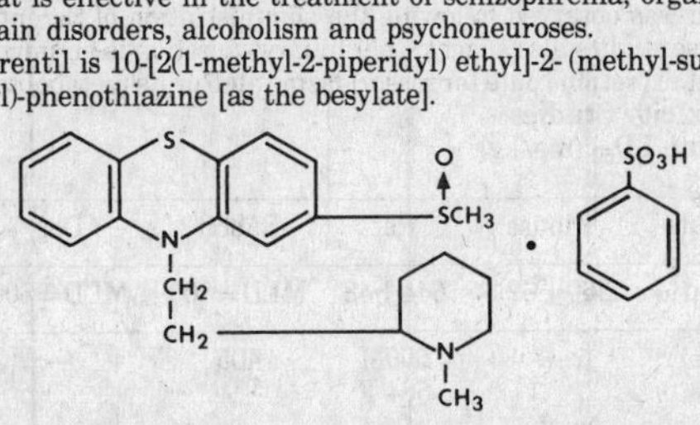

Tablet, 10 mg, for oral administration—Active Ingredient: mesoridazine (as the besylate), 10 mg. Inactive Ingredients: acacia, carnauba wax, colloidal silicon dioxide, FD&C Red No. 40 aluminum lake, lactose, microcrystalline cellulose, povidone, sodium benzoate, starch, stearic acid, sucrose, synthetic black iron oxide, talc, titanium dioxide, and other ingredients.

Tablet, 25 mg, for oral administration—Active Ingredient: mesoridazine (as the besylate), 25 mg. Inactive Ingredients: acacia, carnauba wax, colloidal silicon dioxide, FD&C Red No. 40 aluminum lake, lactose, microcrystalline cellulose, povidone, sodium benzoate, stearic acid, sucrose, synthetic black iron oxide, talc, titanium dioxide, and other ingredients.

Tablet, 50 mg, for oral administration—Active Ingredient: mesoridazine (as the besylate), 50 mg. Inactive Ingredients: acacia, carnauba wax, colloidal silicon dioxide, FD&C Red No. 40 aluminum lake, gelatin, lactose, microcrystalline cellulose, povidone, sodium benzoate, starch, stearic acid, sucrose, synthetic black iron oxide, talc, titanium dioxide, and other ingredients.

Tablet, 100 mg, for oral administration—Active Ingredient: mesoridazine (as the besylate), 100 mg. Inactive Ingredients: acacia, carnauba wax, colloidal silicon dioxide, FD&C Red No. 40 aluminum lake, gelatin, lactose, microcrystalline cellulose, povidone, sodium benzoate, starch, stearic acid, sucrose, synthetic black iron oxide, talc, titanium dioxide, and other ingredients.

Ampuls, 1 ml, for intramuscular administration—Active Ingredient: mesoridazine (as the besylate), 25 mg. Inactive Ingredients: edetate disodium USP, 0.5 mg; sodium chloride USP, 7.2 mg; carbon dioxide gas (bone dry) q.s., water for injection USP, q.s. to 1 ml.

Concentrate, for oral administration—Active Ingredient: mesoridazine (as the besylate), 25 mg per ml. Inactive Ingredients: alcohol, 0.61% by volume; citric acid; FD&C Red No. 40; flavors; methylparaben; propylparaben; purified water; sodium citrate, sorbitol.

ACTIONS

Based upon animal studies, Serentil® (mesoridazine besylate USP), as with other phenothiazines, acts indirectly on reticular formation, whereby neuronal activity into reticular formation is reduced without affecting its intrinsic ability to activate the cerebral cortex. In addition, the phenothiazines exhibit at least part of their activities through depression of hypothalamic centers. Neurochemically, the phenothiazines are thought to exert their effects by a central adrenergic blocking action.

INDICATIONS

In clinical studies Serentil® (mesoridazine besylate USP) has been found useful in the following disease states:

Schizophrenia: Serentil is effective in the treatment of schizophrenia. It substantially reduces the severity of emotional withdrawal, conceptual disorganization, anxiety, tension, hallucinatory behavior, suspiciousness and blunted affect in schizophrenic patients. As with other phenothiazines, patients refractory to previous medication may respond to Serentil.

Behavioral Problems in Mental Deficiency and Chronic Brain Syndrome: The effect of Serentil was found to be excellent or good in the management of hyperactivity and uncooperativeness associated with mental deficiency and chronic brain syndrome.

Alcoholism—Acute and Chronic: Serentil ameliorates anxiety, tension, depression, nausea and vomiting in both acute and chronic alcoholics without producing hepatic dysfunction or hindering the functional recovery of the impaired liver.

Psychoneurotic Manifestations: Serentil reduces the symptoms of anxiety and tension, prevalent symptoms often associated with neurotic components of many disorders, and benefits personality disorders in general.

CONTRAINDICATIONS

As with other phenothiazines, Serentil® (mesoridazine besylate USP) is contraindicated in severe central nervous system depression or comatose states from any cause. Serentil is contraindicated in individuals who have previously shown hypersensitivity to the drug.

WARNINGS

Tardive Dyskinesia: Tardive dyskinesia, a syndrome consisting of potentially irreversible, involuntary, dyskinetic movements may develop in patients treated with neuroleptic (antipsychotic) drugs. Although the prevalence of the syndrome appears to be highest among the elderly, especially elderly women, it is impossible to rely upon prevalence estimates to predict, at the inception of neuroleptic treatment, which patients are likely to develop the syndrome. Whether neuroleptic drug products differ in their potential to cause tardive dyskinesia is unknown.

Both the risk of developing the syndrome and the likelihood that it will become irreversible are believed to increase as the duration of treatment and the total cumulative dose of neuroleptic drugs administered to the patient increase. However, the syndrome can develop, although much less commonly, after relatively brief treatment periods at low doses.

There is no known treatment for established cases of tardive dyskinesia, although the syndrome may remit, partially or completely, if neuroleptic treatment is withdrawn. Neuroleptic treatment, itself, however, may suppress (or partially suppress) the signs and symptoms of the syndrome and thereby may possibly mask the underlying disease process. The effect that symptomatic suppression has upon the long-term course of the syndrome is unknown.

Given these considerations, neuroleptics should be prescribed in a manner that is most likely to minimize the occurrence of tardive dyskinesia. Chronic neuroleptic treatment should generally be reserved for patients who suffer from a chronic illness 1) that is known to respond to neuroleptic drugs, and 2) for which alternative, equally effective but potentially less harmful treatments are *not* available or appropriate. In patients who do require chronic treatment, the smallest dose and the shortest duration of treatment producing a satisfactory clinical response should be sought. The need for continued treatment should be reassessed periodically.

If signs and symptoms of tardive dyskinesia appear in a patient on neuroleptics, drug discontinuation should be considered. However, some patients may require treatment despite the presence of the syndrome.

(For further information about the description of tardive dyskinesia and its clinical detection, please refer to the sections on Information for Patients and Adverse Reactions.)

Neuroleptic Malignant Syndrome (NMS) A potentially fatal symptom complex sometimes referred to as Neuroleptic Malignant Syndrome (NMS) has been reported in association with antipsychotic drugs. Clinical manifestations of NMS are hyperpyrexia, muscle rigidity, altered mental status and evidence of autonomic instability (irregular pulse or blood pressure, tachycardia, diaphoresis, and cardiac dysrhythmias).

The diagnostic evaluation of patients with this syndrome is complicated. In arriving at a diagnosis, it is important to identify cases where the clinical presentation includes both serious medical illness (e.g., pneumonia, systemic infection, etc.) and untreated or inadequately treated extrapyramidal signs and symptoms (EPS). Other important considerations in the differential diagnosis include central anticholinergic toxicity, heat stroke, drug fever and primary central nervous system (CNS) pathology.

The management of NMS should include 1) immediate discontinuation of antipsychotic drugs and other drugs not essential to concurrent therapy, 2) intensive symptomatic treatment and medical monitoring, and 3) treatment of any concomitant serious medical problems for which specific treatments are available. There is no general agreement about specific pharmacological treatment regimens for uncomplicated NMS. If a patient requires antipsychotic drug treatment after recovery from NMS, the potential reintroduction of drug therapy should be carefully considered. The patient should be carefully monitored, since recurrences of NMS have been reported.

Where patients are participating in activities requiring complete mental alertness (e.g., driving), it is advisable to administer the phenothiazines cautiously and to increase the dosage gradually.

Usage in Pregnancy: The safety of this drug in pregnancy has not been established; hence, it should be given only when the anticipated benefits to be derived from treatment exceed the possible risks to mother and fetus.

Usage in Children: The use of Serentil® (mesoridazine besylate USP) in children under 12 years of age is not recommended, because safe conditions for its use have not been established.

Attention should be paid to the fact that phenothiazines are capable of potentiating central nervous system depressants (e.g., anesthetics, opiates, alcohol, etc.) as well as atropine and phosphorus insecticides.

PRECAUTIONS

While ocular changes have not to date been related to Serentil® (mesoridazine besylate USP), one should be aware that such changes have been seen with other drugs of this class.

Because of possible hypotensive effects, reserve parenteral administration for bedfast patients or for acute ambulatory cases, and keep patient lying down for at least one-half hour after injection.

Leukopenia and/or agranulocytosis have been attributed to phenothiazine therapy. A single case of transient granulocytopenia has been associated with Serentil. Since convulsive seizures have been reported, patients receiving anticonvul-

Continued on next page

Boehringer Ingelheim—Cont.

sant medication should be maintained on that regimen while receiving Serentil.

Neuroleptic drugs elevate prolactin levels; the elevation persists during chronic administration. Tissue culture experiments indicate that approximately one-third of human breast cancers are prolactin dependent in vitro, a factor of potential importance if the prescription of these drugs is contemplated in a patient with a previously detected breast cancer. Although disturbances such as galactorrhea, amenorrhea, gynecomastia, and impotence have been reported, the clinical significance of elevated serum prolactin levels is unknown for most patients. An increase in mammary neoplasms has been found in rodents after chronic administration of neuroleptic drugs. Neither clinical studies nor epidemiologic studies conducted to date, however, have shown an association between chronic administration of these drugs and mammary tumorigenesis; the available evidence is considered too limited to be conclusive at this time.

Information for Patients: Given the likelihood that some patients exposed chronically to neuroleptics will develop tardive dyskinesia, it is advised that all patients in whom chronic use is contemplated be given, if possible, full information about this risk.

ADVERSE REACTIONS

Drowsiness and hypotension were the most prevalent side effects encountered. Side effects tended to reach their maximum level of severity early with the exception of a few (rigidity and motoric effects) which occurred later in therapy.

With the exceptions of tremor and rigidity, adverse reactions were generally found among those patients who received relatively high doses early in treatment. Clinical data showed no tendency for the investigators to terminate treatment because of side effects.

Serentil® (mesoridazine besylate USP) has demonstrated a remarkably low incidence of adverse reactions when compared with other phenothiazine compounds.

Central Nervous System: Drowsiness, Parkinson's syndrome, dizziness, weakness, tremor, restlessness, ataxia, dystonia, rigidity, slurring, akathisia, and motoric reactions (opisthotonos) have been reported.

Autonomic Nervous System: Dry mouth, nausea and vomiting, fainting, stuffy nose, photophobia, constipation and blurred vision have occurred in some instances.

Genitourinary System: Inhibition of ejaculation, impotence, enuresis, and incontinence have been reported.

Skin: Itching, rash, hypertrophic papillae of the tongue and angioneurotic edema have been reported.

Cardiovascular System: Hypotension and tachycardia have been reported. EKG changes have occurred in some instances (see Phenothiazine Derivatives: Cardiovascular Effects).

Phenothiazine Derivatives: It should be noted that efficacy, indications and untoward effects have varied with the different phenothiazines. The physician should be aware that the following have occurred with one or more phenothiazines and should be considered whenever one of these drugs is used:

Autonomic Reactions: Miosis, obstipation, anorexia, paralytic ileus.

Cutaneous Reactions: Erythema, exfoliative dermatitis, contact dermatitis.

Blood Dyscrasias: Agranulocytosis, leukopenia, eosinophilia, thrombocytopenia, anemia, aplastic anemia, pancytopenia.

Allergic Reactions: Fever, laryngeal edema, angioneurotic edema, asthma.

Hepatotoxicity: Jaundice, biliary stasis.

Cardiovascular Effects: Changes in the terminal portion of the electrocardiogram, including prolongation of the Q-T interval, lowering and inversion of the T wave and appearance of a wave tentatively identified as a bifid T or a U wave have been observed in some patients receiving the phenothiazine tranquilizers, including Serentil. To date, these appear to be due to altered repolarization and not related to myocardial damage. They appear to be reversible. While there is no evidence at present that these changes are in any way precursors of any significant disturbance of cardiac rhythm, it should be noted that sudden and unexpected deaths apparently due to cardiac arrest have occurred in patients previously showing characteristic electrocardiographic changes while taking the drug. The use of periodic electrocardiograms has been proposed but would appear to be of questionable value as a predictive device.

Hypotension, rarely resulting in cardiac arrest, has been noted.

Extrapyramidal Symptoms: Akathisia, agitation, motor restlessness, dystonic reactions, trismus, torticollis, opisthotonos, oculogyric crises, tremor, muscular rigidity, akinesia.

Tardive Dyskinesia: Chronic use of neuroleptics may be associated with the development of tardive dyskinesia. The salient features of this syndrome are described in the **Warnings** section and below.

The syndrome is characterized by involuntary choreoathetoid movements which variously involve the tongue, face, mouth, lips, or jaw (e.g., protrusion of the tongue, puffing of cheeks, puckering of the mouth, chewing movements), trunk and extremities. The severity of the syndrome and the degree of impairment produced vary widely.

The syndrome may become clinically recognizable either during treatment, upon dosage reduction, or upon withdrawal of treatment. Movements may decrease in intensity and may disappear altogether if further treatment with neuroleptics is withheld. It is generally believed that reversibility is more likely after short- rather than long-term neuroleptic exposure. Consequently, early detection of tardive dyskinesia is important. To increase the likelihood of detecting the syndrome at the earliest possible time, the dosage of neuroleptic drug should be reduced periodically (if clinically possible) and the patient observed for signs of the disorder. This maneuver is critical, for neuroleptic drugs may mask the signs of the syndrome.

Endocrine Disturbances: Menstrual irregularities, altered libido, gynecomastia, lactation, weight gain, edema. False positive pregnancy tests have been reported.

Urinary Disturbances: Retention, incontinence.

Others: Hyperpyrexia. Behavioral effects suggestive of a paradoxical reaction have been reported. These include excitement, bizarre dreams, aggravation of psychoses and toxic confusional states. More recently, a peculiar skin-eye syndrome has been recognized as a side effect following long-term treatment with phenothiazines. This reaction is marked by progressive pigmentation of areas of the skin or conjunctiva and/or accompanied by discoloration of the exposed sclera and cornea. Opacities of the anterior lens and cornea described as irregular or stellate in shape have also been reported. Systemic lupus erythematosus-like syndrome.

OVERDOSAGE

Symptoms of Acute Overdosage

—Drowsiness, confusion, disorientation, agitation, coma, death.

—Dryness of mouth, edema of glottis, laryngeal spasms, nasal congestion, blurred vision, vomiting.

—Hyperpyrexia, dilated pupils, muscle rigidity, hyperactive reflexes, areflexia.

—Stupor, and CNS depression or stimulation with convulsions followed by respiratory depression.

—Cardiac abnormalities, including QRS changes, tachycardia, hypotension, bilateral bundle branch block, ventricular fibrillation, shock, cardiac arrest and congestive heart failure. (See case descriptions below.)

Treatment of Acute Overdosage   No specific antidote is known. The drug is not dialyzable. Treatment should include:

—*General supportive* measures with *emesis* and *gastric lavage.*

—*Respiratory assistance* is apparently the most effective measure when indicated.

—The *administration of barbiturates* for control of convulsions alleviates an increase in the cardiac work load, but should be undertaken with caution to avoid potentiation of respiratory depression.

—*Intramuscular paraldehyde* or *diazepam* provides anticonvulsant activity with less respiratory depression than do the barbiturates; diazepam seems to be preferred.

—The use of *digitalis and/or physostigmine* may be considered in case of serious cardiovascular abnormalities or cardiac failure.

—Due to several cases of severe cardiotoxicity following Serentil® (mesoridazine besylate USP) overdose, *continuous ECG monitoring* of these patients is recommended. Two cases are described below:

Marrs-Simon et al (Cardiotoxic manifestations of mesoridazine overdose. *Ann Emerg Med.* 1988;17:1074-1078) describes the management of a 20-year-old female who experienced severe cardiotoxicity following an overdose of mesoridazine. The paper also describes similar cases from the published literature.

The serum mesoridazine level in a 115-lb patient following ingestion of 4.5 g to 6.0 g of Serentil was 2.5 mcg/mL. She was comatose, hypotensive, convulsing, and had ECG changes. Twenty-four hours later, after hemoperfusion with activated charcoal, the mesoridazine blood levels fell to 1.3 mcg/mL and the patient was normotensive and responsive.

DOSAGE AND ADMINISTRATION

The dosage of Serentil® (mesoridazine besylate USP), as in most medications, should be adjusted to the needs of the individual. The lowest effective dosage should always be used. When maximum response is achieved, dosage may be reduced gradually to a maintenance level.

Schizophrenia: For most patients, regardless of severity, a starting dose of 50 mg t.i.d. is recommended. The usual optimum total daily dose range is 100-400 mg per day.

Behavioral Problems in Mental Deficiency and Chronic Brain Syndrome: For most patients a starting dose of 25 mg t.i.d.

is recommended. The usual optimum total daily dose range is 75-300 mg per day.

Alcoholism: For most patients the usual starting dose is 25 mg b.i.d. The usual optimum total daily dose range is 50-200 mg per day.

Psychoneurotic Manifestations: For most patients the usual starting dose is 10 mg t.i.d. The usual optimum total daily dose range is 30-150 mg per day.

Injectable Form: In those situations in which an intramuscular form of medication is indicated, Serentil injectable is available. For most patients a starting dose of 25 mg is recommended. The dose may be repeated in 30 to 60 minutes, if necessary. The usual optimum total daily dose range is 25-200 mg per day.

HOW SUPPLIED

Tablets: 10 mg, 25 mg, 50 mg, and 100 mg mesoridazine (as the besylate). Bottles of 100.

Ampuls: 1 ml [25 mg mesoridazine (as the besylate)]. Boxes of 20.

Concentrate: Contains 25 mg mesoridazine (as the besylate) per ml; alcohol, USP), 0.61% by volume. Immediate containers: Amber glass bottles of 4 fl oz (118 ml) packaged in cartons of 12 bottles, with an accompanying dropper graduated to deliver 10 mg, 25 mg and 50 mg of mesoridazine (as the besylate).

STORAGE

Tablets: Below 86°F (30°C). **Injection:** Below 86°F (30°C); protect from light. **Oral Solution:** Below 77°F (25°C). Protect from light. Dispense in amber glass bottles only.

The concentrate may be diluted with distilled water, acidified tap water, orange juice or grape juice.

Each dose should be diluted just prior to administration. Preparation and storage of bulk dilutions is not recommended.

Additional information available to physicians.

PHARMACOLOGY

Pharmacological studies in laboratory animals have established that Serentil® (mesoridazine besylate USP) has a spectrum of pharmacodynamic actions typical of a major tranquilizer. In common with other tranquilizers it inhibits spontaneous motor activity in mice, prolongs thiopental and hexobarbital sleeping time in mice and produces spindles and block of arousal reaction in the EEG of rabbits. It is effective in blocking spinal reflexes in the cat and antagonizes d-amphetamine excitation and toxicity in grouped mice. It shows a moderate adrenergic blocking activity in vitro and in vivo and antagonizes 5-hydroxytryptamine in vivo. Intravenously administered, it lowers the blood pressure of anesthetized dogs. It has a weak antiacetylcholine effect in vitro. The most outstanding activity of Serentil is seen in tests developed to investigate antiemotive activity of drugs. Such tests are those in which the rat reacts to acute or chronic stress by increased defecation (emotogenic defecation) or tests in which "emotional mydriasis" is elicited in the mouse by an electric shock. In both of these tests Serentil is effective in reducing emotive reactions. Its ED_{50} in inhibiting emotogenic defecation in the rat is 0.053 mg/kg (subcutaneous administration). Serentil has a potent antiemetic action. The intravenous ED_{50} against apomorphine-induced emesis in the dog is 0.64 mg/kg. Serentil, in common with other phenothiazines, demonstrates antiarrhythmic activity in anesthetized dogs.

Metabolic studies in the dog and rabbit with tritium labeled mesoridazine demonstrate that the compound is well absorbed from the gastrointestinal tract. The biological half-life of Serentil in these studies appears to be somewhere between 24 and 48 hours. Although significant urinary excretion was observed following the administration of Serentil, these studies also suggest that biliary excretion is an important excretion route for mesoridazine and/or its metabolites.

Toxicity Studies

Acute LD_{50} (mg/kg):

Route	Mouse	Rat	Rabbit	Dog
Oral	560±62.5	644±48	MLD=800	MLD=800
I.M.	—	509M 584 F	405	—
I.V.	26±0.08	—	—	—

Chronic toxicity studies were conducted in rats and dogs. Rats were administered Serentil orally seven days per week for a period of 17 months in doses up to 160 mg/kg per day. Dogs were administered Serentil orally seven days per week for a period of 13 months. The daily dosage of the drug was increased during the period of this test such that the "top-dose" group received a daily dose of 120 mg/kg of mesoridazine for the last month of the study.

Untoward effects that occurred upon chronic administration of high dose levels included:

Rats: Reduction of food intake, slowed weight gain, morphological changes in pituitary-supported endocrine organs, and melanin-like pigment deposition in renal tissues.
Dogs: Emesis, muscle tremors, decreased food intake and death associated with aspiration of oral-gastric contents into the respiratory system.
Increased intrauterine resorptions were seen with Serentil in rats at 70 mg/kg and in rabbits at 125 mg/kg but not at 60 and 100 mg/kg, respectively. No drug-related teratology was suggested by these reproductive studies.
Local irritation from the intramuscular injection of Serentil was of the same order of magnitude as with other phenothiazines.

SR-PI-8/91

Shown in Product Identification Section, page 405

Boots Laboratories
a Division of Boots Pharmaceuticals, Inc.
SUITE 200
300 TRI-STATE INTERNATIONAL CENTER
LINCOLNSHIRE, IL 60069-4415

E-MYCIN® ℞
(Erythromycin Delayed-Release)
Tablets, USP
250 mg/333 mg

E-MYCIN® (Erythromycin Delayed-Release) Tablets, USP contain erythromycin as the base.

DESCRIPTION
Erythromycin is produced by a strain of *Streptomyces erythreaus* and belongs to the macrolide group of antibiotics. It is basic and readily forms salts with acids. The base is white to off-white crystal or powder slightly soluble in water, soluble in alcohol, in chloroform, and in ether. The chemical name for erythromycin is (3*R**, 4*S**, 5*S**, 6*R**, 7*R**, 9*R**, 11*R**, 12*R**, 13*S**, 14*R**)-4-[2,6-Dideoxy-3-*C*-methyl-3-*O*-methyl-α-L-*ribo*- hexopyranosyl)-oxy] -14 -ethyl -7, 12, 13-trihydroxy- 3, 5, 7, 9, 11,13-hexamethyl-6-[[3,4,6 -trideoxy-3-(dimethylamino) -β-D-*xylo*-hexopyranosyl] oxy] oxacyclotetradecane-2,10-dione and the molecular weight is 733.94. The structural formula is represented below:

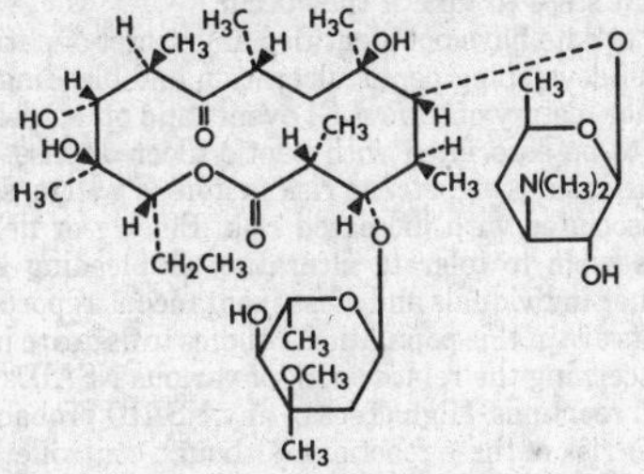

E-MYCIN Tablets, available in 250 mg and 333 mg strengths, are specially coated to protect the contents from the inactivating effects of gastric acidity and to permit efficient absorption of the antibiotic in the small intestine.
Inactive Ingredients: carboxymethylcellulose calcium, carnauba wax, cellulose acetate phthalate, corn starch, hydroxypropyl cellulose, lactose, magnesium stearate, mineral oil, propylene glycol, sorbic acid, sorbitan monooleate, sucrose, talc, titanium dioxide. **250 mg**—FD&C Yellow No. 6.

CLINICAL PHARMACOLOGY
Microbiology: The mode of action of erythromycin is by inhibition of protein synthesis without affecting nucleic acid synthesis. Many strains of *Haemophilus influenzae* are resistant to erythromycin alone, but are susceptible to erythromycin and sulfonamides together.
Erythromycin is usually active against the following organisms *in vitro* (prior to use, refer to **INDICATIONS AND USAGE** section): **Gram-positive Bacteria:** *Staphylococcus aureus* (resistant organisms may emerge during treatment), *Streptococcus pyogenes* (Group A beta-hemolytic streptococci), Alpha-hemolytic streptococci (viridans group), *Streptococcus* (diplococcus) *pneumoniae, Corynebacterium diphtheriae, Corynebacterium minutissimum.*
Gram-negative Bacteria: *Neisseria gonorroeae, Legionella pneumophila* (agent of Legionnaire's Disease), *Bordetella pertussis.*
Mycoplasma: *Mycoplasma pneumoniae* (Eaton's agent), *Ureaplasma urealyticum.*
Other Microorganism: *Chlamydia trachomatis, Entamoeba histolytica, Treponema pallidum, Listeria monocytogenes.*
Antagonism has been demonstrated *in vitro* between clindamycin, lincomycin, chloramphenicol and erythromycin.
Bioavailability data are available from Boots Pharmaceuticals, Inc.
After absorption, erythromycin diffuses readily into most body fluids. Low concentrations are normally achieved in the spinal fluid but passage of the drug across the blood-brain barrier increases in meningitis. In the presence of normal hepatic function, erythromycin is concentrated in the liver and excreted in the bile; the effect of hepatic dysfunction on excretion of erythromycin by the liver into the bile is not known. After oral administration, less than 5 percent of the activity of the administered dose can be recovered in the urine.
Erythromycin crosses the placental barrier but fetal plasma levels are low.
Erythromycin serum levels are not appreciably affected by hemodialysis or peritoneal dialysis.
Susceptibility testing: Culture and susceptibility testing should be done. If the Kirby-Bauer method of disk susceptibility is used, a 15 mcg erythromycin disk should give a zone diameter of at least 18 mm when tested against an erythromycin susceptible organism.

INDICATIONS AND USAGE
E-MYCIN is indicated in the treatment of infections caused by susceptible strains of the designated organisms in the conditions listed below:
Upper respiratory tract infections of mild to moderate severity due to *Streptococcus pyogenes, Streptococcus pneumoniae, and Haemophilius influenzae.* (Since many strains of *H. Influenzae* are not susceptible at the erythromycin concentrations ordinarily achieved, concomitant sulfonamide therapy should be prescribed.)
Lower respiratory tract infections of mild to moderate severity due to *S. pyogenes* and *S. pneumoniae.*
Respiratory infections due to *Mycoplasma pneumoniae* (Eaton's agent, PPLO).
Whooping cough (pertussis) caused by *Bordetella pertussis:* Erythromycin is effective in eliminating the organism from the nasopharynx of infected individuals, rendering them noninfectious. Some clinical studies suggest that erythromycin may be helpful in the prophylaxis of pertussis in exposed susceptible individuals.
Legionnaires' disease due to *Legionella pneumophila:* Although no controlled clinical efficacy studies have been conducted, *in vitro,* preliminary clinical data suggest that erythromycin can be effective in treating Legionnaires' disease.
Infections due to *Chlamydia trachomatis:* Erythromycin is indicated in the treatment of conjunctivitis of the newborn, pneumonia of infancy, and urogenital infections during pregnancy. When tetracyclines are contraindicated or not tolerated, erythromycin is indicated for the treatment of uncomplicated urethral, endocervical or rectal infections in adults due to *C. trachomatis.*
Prophylaxis against bacterial endocarditis due to alpha-hemolytic streptococci (viridans group). Although no controlled clinical efficacy trials have been conducted, or oral erythromycin has been suggested by the American Heart Association and the American Dental Association for use in a regimen for prophylaxis against bacterial endocarditis in patients allergic to penicillin who have congenital heart disease or rheumatic or other acquired valvular heart disease when they undergo dental procedures and surgical procedures of the upper respiratory tract. Erythromycin is not suitable prior to genitourinary or gastrointestinal tract surgery.
Prophylaxis of rheumatic fever: Injectable benzathine penicillin G is considered by the American Heart Association to be the drug of choice in the treatment and prevention of streptococcal pharyngitis and in long-term prophylaxis of rheumatic fever. When oral medication is preferred for treatment of the above conditions, penicillin G, V or erythromycin are alternate choices.
Skin and soft tissue infections of mild to moderate severity due to *S. pyrogenes* and *Staphylococcus aureus* (staphylococci may become resistant during treatment).
Diphtheria due to *Corynebacterium diphtheriae:* Erythromycin may be beneficial as adjunctive therapy with antitoxin and to prevent the establishment of carriers, and to eradicate the organism in carriers.
Erythrasma due to *Corynebacterium minutissium.*
Intestinal amebiasis due to *Entamoiba histolytica:* Extraintestinal amebiasis requires treatment with other agents.
Infections due to *Listeria monocytogenes.*
Syphillis (primary) due to *Treponema pallidum:* Erythromycin is an alternate choice of treatment for patients allergic to the penicillins. Spinal fluid examinations should be done before therapy and as part of the follow-up after therapy.
Acute pelvic inflammatory disease due to *Neisseria gonorrhea:* Erythromycin lactobionate for infection in conjunction with erythromycin base orally is an alternative treatment for patients allergic to penicillin. Before treatment of gonorrhea, patients who are suspected of also having syphillis should have a microscopic examination for *T. pallidum* before receiving erythromycin. Monthly serologic test should be done for a minimum of four months.

CONTRAINDICATIONS
Erythromycin is contraindicated in patients with known hypersensitivity to this antibiotic.

WARNINGS
There have been a few reports of hepatic dysfunction, with or without jaundice, occurring in patients receiving oral erythromycin products.
Rhabdomyolysis with or without renal impairment has been reported in seriously ill patients receiving erythromycin concomitantly with lovastatin. Therefore, patients receiving concomitant lovastatin and erythromycin should be carefully monitored.

PRECAUTIONS
General: Erythromycin is principally excreted by the liver. Caution should be exercised in administering the antibiotic to patients with impaired hepatic function.
When indicated, incision and drainage or other surgical procedures should be performed in conjunction with antibiotic therapy.
During prolonged or repeated therapy, there is a possibility of overgrowth of nonsusceptible bacteria or fungi. If such infections occur, the drug should be discontinued and appropriate therapy instituted.
Laboratory Test: Erythromycin interferes with the fluorometric determination of urinary catecholamines.
Drug Interactions: The use of erythromycin in patients who are receiving high doses of theophylline may be associated with an increase in serum theophylline levels and potential theophylline toxicity.
Erythromycin administration in patients receiving carbamazepine has been reported to cause increased blood levels of carbamazepine with subsequent development of signs of carbamazepine toxicity (ataxia, dizziness, vomiting).
Erythromycin may decrease the clearance of warfarin and thus potentiate the hypoprothrombinemic effect of warfarin.
Erythromycin has been reported to decrease the clearance of triazolam and thus may increase the pharmacologic effect of triazolam.
Erythromycin has been reported to decrease the clearance of cyclosporine causing elevated cyclosporine levels and associated increased serum creatinine. Renal function as well as serum concentration of cyclosporine should be closely monitored when both drugs are administered concomitantly.
An interaction between erythromycin and ergotamine has been reported to increase the vasospasm associated with ergotamine.
Carcinogenesis, mutagenesis, impairment of fertility: Animal studies evaluating carcinogenesis and mutagenesis have not been conducted by Boots Pharmaceuticals, Inc.
Pregnancy category B: Reproduction studies have been performed in rats, mice and rabbits using erythromycin and its various salts and esters, at doses which were several times the usual human dose. No evidence of impaired fertility or harm to the fetus that appeared related to erythromycin was reported in these studies. There are, however, no adequate well controlled studies in pregnant women. Because animal reproduction studies are not always predictive of human response, this drug should be used during pregnancy only if clearly needed.
Labor and delivery: The effect of erythromycin on labor and delivery is unknown.
Nursing mothers: Because erythromycin is excreted in breast milk, caution should be exercised when this drug is administered to a nursing woman.
Pediatric use: See **INDICATIONS AND USAGE** and **DOSAGE AND ADMINISTRATION.**

ADVERSE REACTIONS
The most frequent side effects of erythromycin preparations are gastrointestinal, such as abdominal cramping and discomfort, and are dose related. Nausea, vomiting, and diarrhea occur infrequently with usual oral doses.
Mild allergic reactions such as urticaria and other skin rashes have occurred. Serious allergic reactions, including anaphylaxis, have been reported.
There have been isolated reports of reversible hearing loss occurring chiefly in patients with renal insufficiency and in patients receiving high doses of erythromycin.

DOSAGE AND ADMINISTRATION
E-MYCIN® (Erythromycin Delayed-Release) Tablets, USP are well absorbed and may be given without regard to meals.
Adults: The usual dose is 250 mg four times daily or 333 mg every 8 hours.
If twice a day dosage is desired, the recommended dose is 500 mg every 12 hours.
Dosage may be increased up to 4 or more grams per day according to the severity of the infection. Twice-a-day dosing is not recommended when doses larger than 1 gram daily are administered.
Children: Age, weight, and severity of the infection are important factors in determining the proper dosage. 30 to 50 mg/kg/day, in divided doses, is the usual dose. For more severe infections, this dose may be doubled.
For the treatment of streptococcal infections: A therapeutic dosage of erythromycin should be administered for at

Continued on next page

Boots Laboratories—Cont.

least 10 days. In continuous prophylaxis of streptococcal infections in persons with a history of rheumatic heart disease, the dose is 250 mg twice a day.

For prophylaxis against bacterial endocarditis[1]: In patients with congential heart disease or rheumatic, or other acquired valvular heart disease when undergoing dental procedures or surgical procedures of the upper respiratory tract, give 1.0 gram (20 mg/kg for children) orally 3–4 hours before the procedure and then 500 mg (10 mg/kg for children) orally 6 hours after the first dose.

NOTE: Due to the pharmacokinetic characteristics of E-MYCIN delayed-release tablets, the above indicated timing of the doses differs from the American Heart Association.

For treatment of primary syphillis: 30 to 40 grams given in divided doses over a period of 10 to 15 days.

For treatment of acute pelvic inflammatory disease caused by *N. gonorrhoeae:* After initial treatment with erythromycin lactobionate for injection (500 mg every 6 hours for 3 days), the oral dosage recommendation is 250 mg every 6 hours for 7 days or 333 mg every 8 hours for 7 days.

Urogenital infections during pregnancy due to *Chlamydia trachomatis:* Although the optimal dose and duration of therapy have not been established, the suggested treatment is erythromycin 500 mg, by mouth, four times a day or two 333 mg tablets every eight hours for at least seven days. For women who cannot tolerate this regimen, a decreased dose of 250 mg, by mouth, four times a day or one 333 mg tablet every eight hours should be used for at least 14 days.[2]

For adults with uncomplicated urethral, endocervical, or rectal infections caused by *Chlamydia trachomatis* in whom tetracyclines are contraindicated or not tolerated: 500 mg, by mouth, four times a day or two 333 mg tablets every eight hours for at least seven days.[2]

For dysenteric amebiasis: 250 mg four times daily or 333 mg every 8 hours for 10 to 14 days, for adults; 30 to 50 mg/kg/day in divided doses for 10 to 14 days, for children.

For use in pertussis: Although optimal dosage and duration have not been established, doses of erythromycin utilized in reported clinical studies were 40 to 50 mg/kg/day, given in divided doses for 5 to 14 days.

For treatment of Legionnaires Disease: Although optimal doses have not been established, doses utilized in reported clinical data were those recommended above (1 to 4 grams daily in divided doses).

Preoperative Prophylaxis for Elective Colorectal Surgery: Listed below is an example of a recommended bowel preparation regimen. A proposed surgery time of 8:00 a.m. has been used.

Pre-op Day 3: Minimum residue or clear liquid diet. Bisacodyl, 1 tablet orally at 6:00 p.m.

Pre-op Day 2: Minimum residue or clear liquid diet. Magnesium sulfate, 30 mL, 50% solution (15g) orally at 10:00 a.m., 2:00 p.m. and 6:00 p.m. Enema at 7:00 p.m. and 8:00 p.m.

Pre-op Day 1: Clear liquid diet. Supplemental (IV) fluids as needed. Magnesium sulfate, 30 mL, 50% solution (15g) orally at 10:00 a.m. and 2:00 p.m. Neomycin sulfate (1.0g) and erythromycin base (three 333 mg tablets or four 250 mg tablets) orally at 1:00 p.m., 2:00 p.m. and 11:00 p.m. No enema.

Day of operation: Patient evacuates rectum at 6:30 a.m. for scheduled operation at 8:00 a.m.

HOW SUPPLIED

E-MYCIN® (Erythromycin Delayed-Release) Tablets, USP:

250 mg: round, convex, orange, enteric-coated tablet with "E-MYCIN 250 mg" printed in black on one face.

Bottles of 40	NDC 0524-0207-99
Bottles of 100	NDC 0524-0207-01
Unit Dose Pkg of 100	NDC 0524-0207-21
Bottles of 500	NDC 0524-0207-05

333 mg: round, convex, white, enteric-coated tablet with "E-MYCIN 333 mg" printed in orange on one face.

Bottles 100	NDC 0524-0208-01
Unit Dose Pkg of 100	NDC 0524-0208-21
Bottles of 500	NDC 0524-0208-05

Store at controlled room temperature, 15°–30°C (59°–86°F).

CAUTION

Federal (USA) law prohibits dispensing without prescription.

[1] American Heart Association 1984. Prevention of Bacterial Endocarditis, Circulation 70:1123A–1127A

[2] CDC Sexually Transmitted Diseases Treatment Guidelines 1985.

Manufactured for
Boots Laboratories
a division of
Boots Pharmaceuticals, Inc.
Lincolnshire, Illinois 60069 USA
By
The Upjohn Company
Kalamazoo, Michigan 49001 USA

Rev. 8/27/91

Shown in Product Identification Section, page 405

IBU® ℞

(Ibuprofen Tablets, USP)
400 mg/600 mg/800 mg

DESCRIPTION

IBU (Ibuprofen Tablets, USP) is (±)-2-(*p*-isobutylphenyl) propionic acid. It is a white powder with a melting point of 74–77°C and is very slightly soluble in water (<1 mg/mL) and readily soluble in organic solvents such as ethanol and acetone.

Its structural formula is:

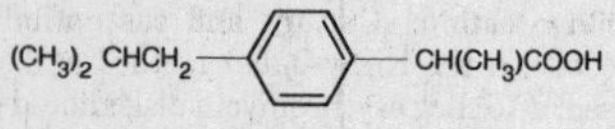
(CH3)2 CHCH2
CH(CH3)COOH

IBU is a nonsteroidal anti-inflammatory agent. It is available in 400, 600 and 800 mg tablets for oral administration.

Inactive Ingredients: 400 mg and 600 mg—colloidal silicon dioxide, hydroxypropyl methylcellulose 2910, Opaspray® M-1-7111-B, pregelatinized starch, starch, stearic acid, talc, 2202C Fine Black Ink or Opacode® Ink S-1-8100HV. **800 mg**—croscarmellose sodium, hydroxypropyl methylcellulose 2910, hydroxpropyl cellulose, lactose, magnesium stearate, propylene glycol, 2202C Fine Black Ink or Opacode® Ink S-1-8100HV.

CLINICAL PHARMACOLOGY

IBU is a nonsteroidal anti-inflammatory agent that possesses analgesic and anti-pyretic activities. Its mode of action, like that of other nonsteroidal anti-inflammatory agents is not completely understood, but may be related to prostaglandin synthetase inhibition.

In clinical studies in patients with rheumatoid arthritis and osteoarthritis, IBU has been shown to be comparable to aspirin in controlling pain and inflammation and to be associated with a statistically significant reduction in the milder gastrointestinal side effects (see **ADVERSE REACTIONS**).

IBU may be well tolerated in some patients who have had gastrointestinal side effects with aspirin, but these patients when treated with IBU should be carefully followed for signs and symptoms of gastrointestinal ulceration and bleeding.

Although it is not definitely known whether ibuprofen causes less peptic ulceration than aspirin, in one study involving 885 patients with rheumatoid arthritis treated for up to one year, there were no reports of gastric ulceration with ibuprofen whereas frank ulceration was reported in 13 patients in the aspirin group (statistically significant $p<001$).

Gastroscopic studies at varying doses show an increased tendency toward gastric irritation at higher doses. However, at comparable doses, gastric irritation is approximately half that seen with aspirin. Studies using ^{51} Cr-tagged red cells indicate that fecal blood loss associated with ibuprofen in doses up to 2400 mg daily did not exceed the normal range, and was significantly less than that seen in aspirin treated patients.

In clinical studies in patients with rheumatoid arthritis, ibuprofen has been shown to be comparable to indomethacin in controlling aforementioned signs and symptoms of disease activity and to be associated with a statistically significant reduction of the milder gastrointestinal (see **ADVERSE REACTIONS**), and CNS side effects.

IBU may be used in combination with gold salts and/or corticosteroids.

Controlled studies have demonstrated that ibuprofen is a more effective analgesic than propoxyphene for the relief of episotomy pain, pain following dental extraction procedures, and for the relief of the symptoms of primary dysmenorrhea.

In patients with primary dysmenorrhea, ibuprofen has been shown to reduce elevated levels of prostaglandin activity in the menstrual fluid and to reduce resting and active intrauterine pressure, as well as the frequency of uterine contractions. The probable mechanism of action is to inhibit prostaglandin synthesis rather than simply to provide analgesia.

Pharmacokinetics: IBU is rapidly absorbed when administered orally. Peak serum ibuprofen levels are generally attained one to two hours after administration. With single doses up to 800 mg, a linear relationship exists between the amount of drug administered and the integrated area under the serum drug concentration vs time curve. Above 800 mg, however, the area under the curve increases less than proportional to increases in dose. There is no evidence of drug accumulation or enzyme induction.

The administration of IBU tablets either under fasting conditions or immediately before meals yields quite similar serum ibuprofen concentration-time profiles. When IBU is administered immediately after a meal, there is a reduction in the rate of absorption but no appreciable decrease in the extent of absorption. The bioavailability of ibuprofen is minimally altered by the presence of food.

A bioavailability study has shown that there was no interference with the absorption of ibuprofen when given in conjunction with an antacid containing both aluminum hydroxide and magnesium hydroxide.

Ibuprofen is rapidly metabolized and eliminated in the urine. The excretion of ibuprofen is virtually complete 24 hours after the last dose. The serum half-life is 18 to 20 hours.

Studies have shown that following ingestion of the drug 45% to 79% of the dose was recovered in the urine within 24 hours as metabolite A (25%),(+)-2-4′-(2 hydroxy-2-methylpropyl)-phenyl propionic acid and metabolite B (37%),(+)-2-4′-(2 carboxypropyl) phenyl propionic acid; the percentages of free and conjugated ibuprofen were approximately 1% and 14% respectively.

INDICATIONS AND USAGE

IBU is indicated for relief of the signs and symptoms of rheumatoid arthritis and osteoarthritis.

IBU is indicated for the relief of mild to moderate pain.

IBU is also indicated for the treatment of primary dysmenorrhea.

Since there have been no controlled trials to demonstrate whether there is any beneficial effect or harmful interaction with the use of IBU in conjunction with aspirin, the combination cannot be recommended (see **Drug Interactions**).

Controlled clinical trials to establish the safety and effectiveness of IBU in children have not been conducted.

CONTRAINDICATIONS

IBU tablets should not be used in patients who have previously exhibited hypersensitivity to it, or in individuals with all or part of the syndrome of nasal polyps, angioedema and bronchospastic reactivity to aspirin or other nonsteroidal anti-inflammatory agents. Anaphylactoid reactions have occurred in such patients.

WARNINGS

Risk of GI Ulceration, Bleeding and Perforation with NSAID Therapy: Serious gastrointestinal toxicity such as bleeding, ulceration, and perforation, can occur at any time, with or without warning symptoms, in patients treated chronically with NSAID therapy. Although minor upper gastrointestinal problems, such as dyspepsia, are common, usually developing early in therapy, physicians should remain alert for ulceration and bleeding in patients treated chronically with NSAIDs even in the absence of previous GI tract symptoms. In patients observed in clinical trials of several months to two years duration, symptomatic upper GI ulcers, gross bleeding or perforation appear to occur in approximately 1% of patients treated for 3–6 months, and in about 2–4% of patients treated for one year. Physicians should inform patients about the signs and/or symptoms of serious GI toxicity and what steps to take if they occur.

Studies to date have not identified any subset of patients not at risk of developing peptic ulceration and bleeding. Except for a prior history of serious GI events and other risk factors known to be associated with peptic ulcer disease, such as alcoholism, smoking, etc. no risk factors (e.g., age, sex) have been associated with increased risk. Elderly or debilitated patients seem to tolerate ulceration or bleeding less well than other individuals and most spontaneous reports of fatal GI events are in this population. Studies to date are inconclusive concerning the relative risk of various NSAIDs in causing such reactions. High doses of any NSAID probably carry a greater risk of these reactions, although controlled clinical trials showing this do not exist in most cases. In considering the use of relatively large doses (within the recommended dosage range), sufficient benefit should be anticipated to offset the potential increased risk of GI toxicity.

PRECAUTIONS

General: Blurred and/or diminished vision, scotomata, and/or changes in color vision have been reported. If a patient develops such complaints while receiving IBU, the drug should be discontinued and the patient should have an ophthalmologic examination which includes central visual fields and color vision testing.

Fluid retention and edema have been reported in association with IBU, therefore, the drug should be used with caution in patients with a history of cardiac decompensation or hypertension.

IBU, like other nonsteroidal anti-inflammatory agents, can inhibit platelet aggregation but the effect is quantitatively less and of shorter duration than that seen with aspirin. Ibuprofen has been shown to prolong bleeding time (but within the normal range), in normal subjects. Because this prolonged bleeding effect may be exaggerated in patients with underlying hemostatic defects, IBU should be used with caution in persons with intrinsic coagulation defects and those on anticoagulant therapy.

Patients on IBU should report to their physicians signs or symptoms of gastrointestinal ulceration or bleeding, blurred vision or other eye symptoms, skin rash, weight gain, or edema.

In order to avoid exacerbation of disease or adrenal insufficiency, patients who have been on prolonged corticosteroid therapy should have their therapy tapered slowly rather than discontinued abruptly when IBU is added to the treatment program.

The antipyretic and anti-inflammatory activity of ibuprofen may reduce fever and inflammation, thus diminishing their utility as diagnostic signs in detecting complications of presumed noninfectious, noninflammatory painful conditions.

Liver Effects: As with other nonsteroidal anti-inflammatory drugs, borderline elevations of one or more liver function tests may occur in up to 15% of patients. These abnormalities may progress, may remain essentially unchanged, or may be transient with continued therapy. The SGPT (ALT) test is probably the most sensitive indicator of liver dysfunction. Meaningful (3 times the upper limit of normal), elevations of SGPT or SGOT (AST) occurred in controlled clinical trials in less than 1% of patients. A patient with symptoms and/or signs suggesting liver dysfunction, or in whom an abnormal liver test has occurred, should be evaluated for evidence of the development of more severe hepatic reactions while on therapy with ibuprofen. Severe hepatic reactions, including jaundice and cases of fatal hepatitis, have been reported with ibuprofen as with other nonsteroidal anti-inflammatory drugs. Although such reactions are rare, if abnormal liver tests persist or worsen, if clinical signs and symptoms consistent with liver disease develop, or if systemic manifestations occur (e.g. eosinophilia, rash, etc), IBU should be discontinued.

Hemoglobin Levels: In cross-study comparisons with doses ranging from 1200 mg to 3200 mg daily for several weeks, a slight dose-response decrease in hemoglobin/hematocrit was noted. This has been observed with other nonsteroidal anti-inflammatory drugs; the mechanism is unknown. However, even with daily doses of 3200 mg, the total decrease in hemoglobin usually does not exceed 1 gram; if there are no signs of bleeding, it is probably not clinically important.

In two postmarketing clinical studies the incidence of a decreased hemoglobin level was greater than previously reported. Decrease in hemoglobin of 1 gram or more was observed in 17.1% of 193 patients on 1600 mg ibuprofen daily (osteoarthritis), and in 22.8% of 189 patients taking 2400 mg of ibuprofen daily (rheumatoid arthritis). Positive stool occult blood tests and elevated serum creatinine levels were also observed in these studies.

Aseptic Meningitis: Aseptic meningitis with fever and coma has been observed on rare occasions in patients on ibuprofen therapy. Although it is probably more likely to occur in patients with systemic lupus erythematosus and related connective tissue diseases, it has been reported in patients who do not have an underlying chronic disease. If signs or symptoms of meningitis develop in a patient on IBU, the possibility of its being related to ibuprofen should be considered.

Renal Effects: As with other nonsteroidal anti-inflammatory drugs, long term administration of ibuprofen to animals has resulted in renal papillary necrosis and other abnormal renal pathology. In humans, there have been reports of acute interstitial nephritis with hematuria, proteinuria, and occasionally nephrotic syndrome.

A second form of renal toxicity has been seen in patients with prerenal conditions leading to a reduction in renal blood flow or blood volume, where the renal prostaglandins have a supportive role in the maintenance of renal perfusion. In these patients administration of a nonsteroidal anti-inflammatory drug may cause a dose dependent reduction in prostaglandin formation and may precipitate overt renal decompensation. Patients at greatest risk of this reaction are those with impaired renal function, heart failure, liver dysfunction, those taking diuretics and the elderly. Discontinuation of nonsteroidal anti-inflammatory drug therapy is typically followed by recovery to the pretreatment state.

Those patients at high risk who chronically take IBU should have renal function monitored if they have signs or symptoms which may be consistent with mild azotemia, such as malaise, fatigue, loss of appetite, etc. Occasional patients may develop some elevation of serum creatinine and BUN levels without signs or symptoms.

Since ibuprofen is elimated primarily by the kidneys, patients with significantly impaired renal function should be closely monitored and a reduction in dosage should be anticipated to avoid drug accumulation. Prospective studies on the safety of ibuprofen in patients with chronic renal failure have not been conducted.

Information for Patients: Ibuprofen, like other drugs of its class, is not free of side effects. The side effects of these drugs can cause discomfort and, rarely, there are more serious side effects, such as gastrointestinal bleeding, which may result in hospitalization and even fatal outcomes.

NSAIDs (Nonsteroidal Anti-Inflammatory Drugs) are often essential agents in the management of arthritis and have a major role in the treatment of pain, but they also may be commonly employed for conditions which are less serious.

Physicians may wish to discuss with their patients the potential risks (see **WARNINGS, PRECAUTIONS, and ADVERSE REACTIONS** sections) and likely benefits of NSAID treatment, particularly when the drugs are used for less serious conditions where treatment without NSAIDs may represent an acceptable alternative to both the patient and physician.

Laboratory Tests: Because serious GI tract ulceration and bleeding can occur without warning symptoms, physicians should follow chronically treated patients for the signs and symptoms of ulceration and bleeding and should inform them of the importance of this follow-up (see **WARNINGS**).

Drug Interactions: ***Coumarin-type anticoagulants:*** Several short-term controlled studies failed to show that ibuprofen significantly affected prothrombin times or a variety of other clotting factors when administered to individuals on coumarin-type anticoagulants. However, because bleeding has been reported when IBU® (Ibuprofen Tablets, USP) and other nonsteroidal anti-inflammatory agents have been administered to patients on coumarin-type anticoagulants, the physician should be cautious when administering IBU to patients on anticoagulants.

Aspirin: Animal studies show that aspirin given with nonsteroidal anti-inflammatory agents, including ibuprofen, yields a net decrease in anti-inflammatory activity with lowered blood levels of the non-aspirin drug. Single dose bioavailability studies in normal volunteers have failed to show an effect of aspirin on ibuprofen blood levels. Correlative clinical studies have not been done.

Methotrexate: Ibuprofen, as well as other nonsteroidal anti-inflammatory drugs, has been reported to competitively inhibit methotrexate accumulation in rabbit kidney slices. This may indicate that ibuprofen could enhance the toxicity of methotrexate. Caution should be used if IBU is administered concomitantly with methotrexate.

H-2 Anatagonists: In studies with human volunteers, coadministration of cimetidine or ranitidine with ibuprofen had no substantive effect on ibuprofen serum concentrations.

Furosemide: Clinical studies, as well as random observations, have shown that ibuprofen can reduce the natriuretic effect of furosemide and thiazides in some patients. This response has been attributed to inhibition of renal prostaglandin synthesis. During concomitant therapy with ibuprofen, the patient should be observed closely for signs of renal failure (see **PRECAUTIONS: Renal Effects**), as well as to assure diuretic efficacy.

Lithium: Ibuprofen produced an elevation of plasma lithium levels and a reduction in renal lithium clearance in a study of eleven normal volunteers. The mean minimum lithium concentration increased 15% and the renal clearance of lithium was decreased by 19% during this period of concomitant drug administration.

This effect has been attributed to inhibition of renal prostaglandin synthesis by ibuprofen. Thus, when ibuprofen and lithium are administered concurrently, subjects should be observed carefully for signs of lithium toxicity. (Read circulars for lithium preparation before use of such concurrent therapy.)

Pregnancy: Reproductive studies conducted in rats and rabbits at doses somewhat less than the maximal clinical dose did not demonstrate evidence of developmental abnormalities. However, animal reproduction studies are not always predictive of human response. As there are no adequate and well-controlled studies in pregnant women, this drug should be used during pregnancy only if clearly needed. Because of the known effects of nonsteroidal anti-inflammatory drugs on the fetal cardiovascular system (closure of ductus arteriosus), use during late pregnancy should be avoided. As with other drugs known to inhibit prostaglandin synthesis, an increased incidence of dystocia and delayed parturition occurred in rats. Administration of IBU is not recommended during pregnancy.

Nursing Mothers: In limited studies, an assay capable of detecting 1 mcg/mL did not demonstrate ibuprofen in the milk of lactating mothers. However, because of the limited nature of the studies and the possible adverse effects of prostaglandin inhibiting drugs on neonates, IBU is not recommended for use in nursing mothers.

ADVERSE REACTIONS

The most frequent type of adverse reaction occurring with ibuprofen is gastrointestinal. In controlled clinical trials, the percentage of patients reporting one or more gastrointestinal complaints ranged from 4% to 16%.

In controlled studies when ibuprofen was compared to aspirin and indomethacin in equally effective doses, the overall incidence of gastrointestinal complaints was about half that seen in either the aspirin-or indomethacin-treated patients.

Adverse reactions observed during controlled clinical trials at an incidence greater than 1% are listed in the following paragraphs. Those reactions listed under the heading. Incidence Greater Than 1% (but less than 3%) Probable Causal Relationship, encompass observations in approximately 3,000 patients. More than 500 of these patients were treated for periods of at least 54 weeks.

Still other reactions occurring less frequently than 1 in 100 were reported in controlled clinical trials and from marketing experience. These reactions have been divided into two categories. Precise Incidence Unknown (but less than 1%) Probable Causal Relationship, lists reactions with ibuprofen therapy where the probability of a causal relationship exists; Precise Incidence Unknown (but less tha 1%) Causal Relationship Unknown, lists reactions with ibuprofen therapy where a causal relationship has not been established.

Reported side effects were higher at doses of 3200 mg/day than at doses of 2400 mg or less per day in clinical trials of patients with rheumatoid arthritis. The increases in incidence were slight and still within the ranges reported in the following paragraphs.

Incidence Greater Than 1%
(but less than 3%)
Probabe Causal Relationship

Gastrointestinal: nausea*, epigastric pain*, heartburn*, diarrhea, abdominal distress, nausea and vomiting, indigestion, constipation, abdominal cramps or pain, fullness of GI tract (bloating and flatulence).
Central Nervous System: dizziness*, headache, nervousness.
Dermatologic: rash* (including maculopapular type), pruritus.
Special Senses: tinnitus.
Metabolic/Endocrine: decreased appetite.
Cardiovascular: edema, fluid retention (generally responds promptly to drug discontinuation) (see **PRECAUTIONS**).

Precise Incidence Unknown
(but less than 1%)
Probable Causal Relationship**

Gastrointestinal: gastric or duodenal ulcer with bleeding and/or perforation, gastrointestinal hemorrhage, pancreatitis, melena, gastritis, hepatitis, jaundice, abnormal liver function tests.
Central Nervous System: depression, insomnia, confusion, emotional lability, somnolence, aseptic meningitis with fever and coma (See **PRECAUTIONS**).
Dermatologic: vesiculobullous eruptions, urticaria, erythema multiforme, Stevens-Johnson syndrome, alopecia.
Special Senses: hearing loss, amblyopia (blurred and/or diminished vision, scotomata and/or changes in color vision) (see **PRECAUTIONS**).
Hematologic: neutropenia, agranulocytosis, aplastic anemia, hemolytic anemia (sometimes Coombs positive), thrombocytopenia with or without purpura, eosinophilia, decrease in hemoglobin and hematocrit (see **PRECAUTIONS**).
Cardiovascular: congestive heart failure in patients with marginal cardiac function, elevated blood pressure, palpitations.
Allergic: syndrome of abdominal pain, fever chills, nausea and vomiting, anaphylaxis, bronchospasm (see **CONTRAINDICATIONS**).
Renal: acute renal failure in patients with pre-existing significantly impaired renal function (see **PRECAUTIONS**), decreased creatinine clearance, polyuria, azotemia, cystitis, hematuria.
Miscellaneous: dry eyes and mouth, gingival ulcer, rhinitis.

Precise Incidence Unknown
(but less than 1%)
Causal Relationship Unknown**

Central Nervous System: paresthesias, hallucinations, dream abnormalities, pseudotumor cerebri.
Dermatologic: toxic epidermal necrolysis, photoallergic skin reactions.
Special Senses: conjunctivitis, diplopia, optic neuritis, cataracts.
Hematologic: bleeding episodes (e.g. epistaxis, menorrhagia).
Metabolic/Endocrine: gynecomastia, hypoglycemic reaction, acidosis.
Cardiovascular: arrhythmias (sinus tachycardia, sinus bradycardia).
Allergic: serum sickness, lupus erythematosus syndrome, Henoch-Schonlein vasculitis, antioedema.
Renal: renal papillary necrosis.

OVERDOSAGE

Approximately $1\frac{1}{2}$ hours after the reported ingestion of from 7 to 10 ibuprofen tablets (400 mg), a 19-month old child weighing 12 kg was seen in the hospital emergency room, apneic and cyanotic, responding only to painful stimuli. This type of stimulus, however, was sufficient to induce respiration. Oxygen and parenteral fluids were given, a greenish-yellow fluid was aspirated from the stomach with no evidence to indicate the presence of ibuprofen. Two hours after ingestion the child's condition seemed stable, she still responded only to painful stimuli and continued to have periods of apnea lasting from 5 to 10 seconds. She was admitted to intensive care and sodium bicarbonate was administered as well as infusions of dextrose and normal saline. By four hours post-ingestion she could be aroused easily, sit by herself and respond to spoken commands. Blood level of ibuprofen was 102.9 mcg/mL approximately $8\frac{1}{2}$ hours after accidental ingestion. At 12 hours she appeared to be completely recovered.

In two other reported cases where children (each weighing approximately 10 kg) accidentally, acutely ingested approxi-

*Reactions occurring in 3% to 9% of patients treated with ibuprofen. (Those reactions occurring in less than 3% of the patients are unmarked.)

**Reactions are classified under "Probable Causal Relationship (PCR)", if there has been one positive rechallenge or if three or more cases occur which might be causally related. Reactions are classified under "Causal Relationship Unknown", if seven or more events have been reported but the criteria for PCR have not been met.

Continued on next page

Boots Laboratories—Cont.

mately 120 mg/kg, there were no signs of acute intoxication or late sequelae. Blood level in one child 90 minutes after ingestion was 700 mcg/mL, about 10 times the peak levels seen in absorption excretion studies.

A 19-year old male who had taken 8,000 mg of ibuprofen over a period of a few hours complained of dizziness, and nystagmus was noted. After hospitalization, parenteral hydration and three days bed rest, he recovered with no reported sequelae.

In cases of acute overdosage, the stomach should be emptied by vomiting or lavage, though little drug will likely be recovered if more than an hour has elapsed since ingestion. Because the drug is acidic and is excreted in the urine, it is theoretically beneficial to administer alkali and induce diuresis. In addition to supportive measures, the use of oral activated charcoal may help reduce the absorption and reabsorption of ibuprofen.

DOSAGE AND ADMINISTRATION

Do not exceed 3200 mg total daily dose. If gastrointestinal complaints occur, administer IBU with meals or milk.

Rheumatoid arthritis and osteoarthritis, including flareups of chronic disease: *Suggested Dosage:* 1200-3200 mg daily (300 mg q.i.d., or 400 mg, 600 mg or 800 mg t.i.d. or q.i.d.). Individual patients may show a better response to 3200 mg daily, as compared with 2400 mg, although in well-controlled clinical trials patients on 3200 mg did not show a better mean response in terms of efficacy. Therefore, when treating patients with 3200 mg/day, the physician should observe sufficient increased clinical benefits to offset potential increased risk.

The dose of ibuprofen should be tailored to each patient and may be lowered or raised from the suggested doses depending on the severity of symptoms either at time of initiating drug therapy or as the patient responds or fails to respond.

In general, patients with rheumatoid arthritis seem to require higher doses of ibuprofen than do patients with osteoarthritis.

The smallest dose of IBU that yields acceptable control should be employed. A linear blood level dose-response relationship exists with single doses up to 800 mg (see **CLINICAL PHARMACOLOGY:** Pharmacokinetics for effects of food on rate of absorption).

The commercial availability of multiple strengths facilitates dosage adjustment.

In chronic conditions, a therapeutic response to IBU therapy is sometimes seen in a few days to a week but most often is observed by two weeks. After a satisfactory response has been achieved, the patient's dose should be reviewed and adjusted as required.

Mild to moderate pain: 400 mg every 4 to 6 hours as necessary for the relief of pain.

In controlled analgesic clinical trials, doses of ibuprofen greater than 400 mg were no more effective than the 400 mg dose.

Dysmenorrhea: For the treatment of dysmenorrhea, beginning with the earliest onset of such pain, IBU should be given in a dose of 400 mg every 4 hours as necessary for the relief of pain.

HOW SUPPLIED

IBU® (Ibuprofen Tablets, USP):

400 mg: elongated, smooth textured, white, film-coated tablet with "IBU 400" printed in black on one face.

Bottles of 100	NDC 0524-0165-01
Bottles of 500	NDC 0524-0165-05

600 mg: elongated, smooth textured, white, film-coated tablet with "IBU 600" printed in black on one face.

Bottles of 100	NDC 0524-0162-01
Bottles of 500	NDC 0524-0162-05
Unit Dose Boxes of 100	NDC 0524-0162-21

800 mg: elongated, smooth textured, white, film-coated tablet with "IBU 800" printed in black on one face.

Bottles of 100	NDC 0524-0173-01
Bottles of 500	NDC 0524-0173-05
Unit Dose Boxes of 100	NDC 0524-0173-21

Store at controlled room temperature 15°-30°C (59°-86°F).

CAUTION: Federal (USA) law prohibits dispensing without prescription.

Boots Laboratories
a division of
Boots Pharmaceuticals, Inc.
Lincolnshire, Illinois 60069 USA

Rev. 12/2/91 6352-04

SSD RP™ ℞
(1% Silver Sulfadiazine) Cream

DESCRIPTION

SSD RP (1% Silver Sulfadiazine) Cream is a topical antibacterial preparation which has as its active antimicrobial ingredient silver sulfadiazine. The active moiety is contained within an opaque, white, water-miscible cream base.

Each 1000 grams of SSD RP Cream contains 10 grams of silver sulfadiazine.

Inactive Ingredients: cetyl alcohol, isopropyl myristate, polyoxyl 40 stearate, propylene glycol, purified water, stearyl alcohol, sodium hydroxide, sorbitan monooleate, white petrolatum; with 0.3% methylparaben, as a preservative.

Silver sulfadiazine has an empirical formula of $C_{10}H_9AgN_4O_2S$, molecular weight of 357.14, and structural formula as shown:

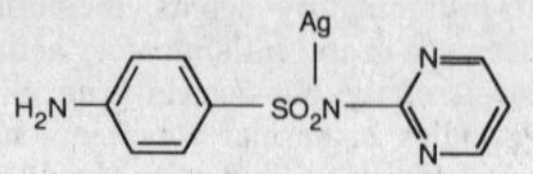

CLINICAL PHARMACOLOGY

Silver sulfadiazine has broad antimicrobial activity. It is bactericidal for many gram-negative and gram-positive bacteria as well as being effective against yeast. Results from *in vitro* testing are listed below.

Sufficient data have been obtained to demonstrate that silver sulfadiazine will inhibit bacteria that are resistant to other antimicrobial agents and that the compound is superior to sulfadiazine.

Studies utilizing radioactive micronized silver sulfadiazine, electron microscopy, and biochemical techniques have revealed that the mechanism of action of silver sulfadiazine on bacteria differs from silver nitrate and sodium sulfadiazine. Silver sulfadiazine acts only on the cell wall to produce its bactericidal effect.

Results of *In Vitro* Testing With
Concentrations of Silver Sulfadiazine
Number of Sensitive Strains/Total Number of
Strains Tested

Genus & Species	50 µg/mL	100 µg/mL
Pseudomonas aeruginosa	130/130	130/130
Pseudomonas maltophilia	7/7	7/7
Enterobacter species	48/50	50/50
Enterobacter cloacae	24/24	24/24
Klebsiella species	53/54	54/54
Escherichia coli	63/63	63/63
Serratia species	27/28	28/28
Proteus mirabilis	53/53	53/53
Morganella morganii	10/10	10/10
Providencia rettgeri	2/2	2/2
Proteus vulgaris	2/2	2/2
Providencia species	1/1	1/1
Citrobacter species	10/10	10/10
Acinetobacter calcoaceticus	10/11	11/11
Staphylococcus aureus	100/101	101/101
Staphylococcus epidermidis	51/51	51/51
β-Hemolytic Streptococcus	4/4	4/4
Enterococcus species	52/53	53/53
Corynebacterium diphtheriae	2/2	2/2
Clostridium perfringens	0/2	2/2
Candida albicans	43/50	50/50

Silver sulfadiazine is not a carbonic anhydrase inhibitor and may be useful in situations where such agents are contraindicated.

INDICATIONS AND USAGE

Silver Sulfadiazine Cream is a topical antimicrobial drug indicated as an adjunct for the prevention and treatment of wound sepsis in patients with second and third degree burns.

CONTRAINDICATIONS

Silver Sulfadiazine Cream is contraindicated in patients who are hypersensitive to silver sulfadiazine or any of the other ingredients in the preparation.

Because sulfonamide therapy is known to increase the possibility of kernicterus, Silver Sulfadiazine Cream should not be used on pregnant women approaching or at term, on premature infants, or on newborn infants during the first 2 months of life.

WARNINGS

There is potential cross-sensitivity between silver sulfadiazine and other sulfonamides. If allergic reactions attributable to treatment with silver sulfadiazine occur, continuation of therapy must be weighed against the potential hazards of the particular allergic reaction.

Fungal proliferation in and below eschar may occur. However, the incidence of clinically reported fungal superinfection is low.

The use of Silver Sulfadiazine Cream in some cases of glucose-6-phosphate dehydrogenase-deficient individuals may be hazardous, as hemolysis may occur.

PRECAUTION

General: If hepatic and renal functions become impaired and elimination of drug decreases, accumulation may occur and discontinuation of Silver Sulfadiazine Cream should be weighed against the therapeutic benefit being achieved.

In considering the use of topical proteolytic enzymes in conjunction with Silver Sulfadiazine Cream, the possibility should be noted that silver may inactivate such enzymes.

Laboratory Tests: In the treatment of burn wounds involving extensive areas of the body, the serum sulfa concentrations may approach adult therapeutic levels (8 to 12 mg%). Therefore, in these patients it would be advisable to monitor serum sulfa concentrations. Renal function should be carefully monitored and the urine should be checked for sulfa crystals.

Absorption of the propylene glycol vehicle has been reported to affect serum osmolality, which may affect the interpretation of laboratory tests.

Carcinogenesis, Mutagenesis, Impairment of Fertility: Long-term dermal toxicity studies of 24 months duration in rats and 18 months in mice with concentrations of silver sulfadiazine three to ten times the concentration in Silver Sulfadiazine Cream revealed no evidence of carcinogenicity.

Pregnancy: Pregnancy category B. A reproductive study has been performed in rabbits at doses up to three to ten times the concentration of silver sulfadiazine in Silver Sulfadiazine Cream and has revealed no evidence of harm to the fetus due to silver sulfadiazine. There are, however, no adequate and well-controlled studies in pregnant women. Because animal reproduction studies are not always predictive of human response, this drug should be used during pregnancy only if clearly justified, especially in pregnant women approaching or at term (see **CONTRAINDICATIONS**).

Nursing Mothers: It is not known whether Silver Sulfadiazine Cream is excreted in human milk. However, sulfonamides are known to be excreted in human milk, and all sulfonamide derivatives are known to increase the possibility of kernicterus. Because of the possibility for serious adverse reactions in nursing infants from sulfonamides, a decision should be made whether to discontinue nursing or to discontinue the drug, taking into account the importance of the drug to the mother.

Pediatric Use: Safety and effectiveness in children have not been established (see **CONTRAINDICATIONS**).

ADVERSE REACTIONS

Several cases of transient leukopenia have been reported in patients receiving silver sulfadiazine therapy. Leukopenia associated with silver sulfadiazine administration is primarily characterized by decreased neutrophil count. Maximal white blood cell depression occurs within two to four days of initiation of therapy. Rebound to normal leukocyte levels follows onset within two to three days. Recovery is not influenced by continuation of silver sulfadiazine therapy. The incidence of leukopenia in various reports averages about 20%. A higher incidence has been seen in patients treated concurrently with cimetidine.

Other infrequently occurring events include skin necrosis, erythema multiforme, skin discoloration, burning sensation, rashes, and interstitial nephritis.

Reduction in bacterial growth after application of topical antibacterial agents has been reported to permit spontaneous healing of deep partial-thickness burns by preventing conversion of the partial thickness to full thickness by sepsis. However, reduction in bacterial colonization has caused delayed separation, in some cases necessitating escharotomy in order to prevent contracture.

Absorption of silver sulfadiazine varies depending upon the percent of body surface area and the extent of the tissue damage. Although few have been reported, it is possible that any adverse reaction associated with sulfonamides may occur. Some of the reactions which have been associated with sulfonamides are as follows: blood dyscrasias, including agranulocytosis, aplastic anemia, thrombocytopenia, leukopenia and hemolytic anemia; dermatologic and allergic reactions, including Stevens-Johnson syndrome and exfoliative dermatitis; gastrointestinal reactions; hepatitis and hepatocellular necrosis; CNS reactions; and toxic nephrosis.

DOSAGE AND ADMINISTRATION

Prompt institution of appropriate regimens for care of the burned patient is of prime importance and includes the control of shock and pain. The burn wounds are then cleansed and debrided and Silver Sulfadiazine Cream is applied under sterile conditions. The burn areas should be covered with Silver Sulfadiazine Cream at all times. The cream should be applied once to twice daily to a thickness of approximately 1/16 inch. Whenever necessary, the cream should be reapplied to any areas from which it has been removed by patient activity. Administration may be accomplished in minimal time because dressings are not required. However, if individual patient requirements make dressings necessary, they may be used.

Reapply immediately after hydrotherapy.

Treatment with Silver Sulfadiazine Cream should be continued until satisfactory healing has occurred or until the burn

site is ready for grafting. The drug should not be withdrawn from the therapeutic regimen while there remains the possibility of infection except if a significant adverse reaction occurs.

HOW SUPPLIED

SSD RP™• (1% Silver Sulfadiazine) **Cream:**

50 gram jar
400 gram jar

•Retail Package
Store at controlled room temperature 15°–30°C (59°–86°F).

CAUTION

Federal (USA) law prohibits dispensing without prescription.

Manufactured by:
Boots Pharmaceuticals, Inc.
Lincolnshire, Illinois 60069 USA

Rev. 12/11/90   7557-01

Shown in Product Identification Section, page 406

Boots Pharmaceuticals, Inc.
SUITE 200
300 TRI-STATE INTERNATIONAL CENTER
LINCOLNSHIRE, IL 60069-4415

PRODUCT INFORMATION WAS PREPARED IN JUNE, 1992. FOR FURTHER INFORMATION ON THESE AND OTHER BOOTS PRODUCTS CONTACT YOUR BOOTS REPRESENTATIVE OR WRITE BOOTS PHARMACEUTICALS, INC., SUITE 200, 300 TRI-STATE INTERNATIONAL CENTER, LINCOLNSHIRE, IL 60069-4415.

RU-TUSS® TABLETS ℞
[roo-tŭs]

DESCRIPTION

Each prolonged action tablet contains:

Phenylephrine Hydrochloride	25 mg
Phenylpropanolamine Hydrochloride	50 mg
Chlorpheniramine Maleate	8 mg
Hyoscyamine Sulfate	0.19 mg
Atropine Sulfate	0.04 mg
Scopolamine Hydrobromide	0.01 mg

Inactive Ingredients: carnauba wax, D&C Yellow No. 10 Lake, ethylcellulose, FD&C Blue No. 1 Lake, magnesium stearate, microcrystalline cellulose, povidone, sodium starch glycolate, starch, sucrose, stearic acid, talc.
RU-TUSS Tablets act continuously for 10 to 12 hours.
RU-TUSS Tablets are an oral antihistaminic, nasal decongestant and anti-secretory preparation.

INDICATIONS AND USAGE

RU-TUSS Tablets provide relief of the symptoms resulting from irritation of sinus, nasal and upper respiratory tract tissues. Phenylephrine and phenylpropanolamine combine to exert a vasoconstrictive and decongestive action while chlorpheniramine maleate decreases the symptoms of watering eyes, post nasal drip and sneezing which may be associated with an allergic-like response. The belladonna alkaloids, hyoscyamine, atropine and scopolamine further augment the anti-secretory activity of RU-TUSS Tablets.

CONTRAINDICATIONS

Hypersensitivity to antihistamines or sympathomimetics. RU-TUSS Tablets are contraindicated in children under 12 years of age and in patients with glaucoma, bronchial asthma and women who are pregnant. Concomitant use of MAO inhibitors is contraindicated.

WARNINGS

RU-TUSS Tablets may cause drowsiness. Patients should be warned of the possible additive effects caused by taking antihistamines with alcohol, hypnotics or tranquilizers.

PRECAUTIONS

RU-TUSS Tablets contain belladonna alkaloids, and must be administered with care to those patients with urinary bladder neck obstruction. Caution should be exercised when RU-TUSS Tablets are given to patients with hypertension, cardiac or peripheral vascular disease or hyperthyroidism. Patients should avoid driving a motor vehicle or operating dangerous machinery (See **WARNINGS**.)

ADVERSE REACTIONS

Hypersensitivity reactions such as rash, urticaria, leukopenia, agranulocytosis, and thrombocytopenia may occur. Large overdoses may cause tachypnea, delirium, fever, stupor, coma and respiratory failure.
Gastrointestinal: nausea, vomiting, diarrhea, constipation, epigastric distress.

Genitourinary System: urinary frequency and dysuria.
Cardiovascular: tightness of the chest, palpitation, tachycardia, hypotension/hypertension.
Central Nervous System: drowsiness, giddiness, faintness, dizziness, headache, incoordination, mydriasis, hyperirritability, nervousness, and insomnia.
Metabolic/Endocrine: lassitude, anorexia.
Miscellaneous: dryness of mucous membranes, xerostomia.
Respiratory: thickening of bronchial secretions.
Special Senses: tinnitus, visual disturbances, blurred vision.

OVERDOSAGE

Since the action of sustained release products may continue for as long as 12 hours, treatment of overdoses directed at reversing the effects of the drug and supporting the patient should be maintained for at least that length of time. In children and infants, antihistamine overdosage may produce convulsions and death.

DOSAGE AND ADMINISTRATION

Adults and children 12 years of age and older, one tablet morning and evening. Not recommended for children under 12 years of age. Tablets are to be swallowed whole.

HOW SUPPLIED

RU-TUSS® Tablets: elongated, light green, scored tablet debossed with BOOTS logo and "58".

Bottles of 100	NDC 0048-0058-01
Bottles of 500	NDC 0048-0058-05

Store at controlled room temperature 15°–30°C (59°–86°F).

CAUTION

Federal (USA) law prohibits dispensing without prescription.

Manufactured for
Boots Pharmaceuticals, Inc.
Lincolnshire, Illinois 60069 USA
By
Vitarine Pharmaceuticals, Inc.
Springfield Gardens, New York 11413 USA
Rev. 1/22/92   8467-02

Shown in Product Identification Section, page 405

RU-TUSS® II CAPSULES ℞
[roo-tŭs]
(Phenylpropanolamine Hydrochloride ... 75 mg
Chlorpheniramine Maleate ... 12 mg)

DESCRIPTION

Each slow-release capsule contains 12 mg of chlorpheniramine maleate and 75 mg of phenylpropanolamine hydrochloride so prepared that an initial dose is released promptly (approximately one-third of the contents) and the remaining medication is released gradually over a prolonged period. White beads are DYE-FREE.
Inactive Ingredients: FD&C Green No. 3, FD&C Yellow No. 10, pharmaceutical glaze, starch, sucrose; in gelatin capsules.
Chlorpheniramine maleate is 2-[p-Chloro-α-[2-(dimethylamino) ethyl] benzyl] pyridine maleate (1:1), an antihistamine.
Phenylpropanolamine hydrochloride is benzenemethanol, α-(1-aminoethyl)-, hydrochloride, (R*, S*), (±), an adrenergic agent.
The structural formulas are as follows:

Chlorpheniramine Maleate
M.W. 390.87

Phenylpropanolamine HCl
M.W. 187.67

CLINICAL PHARMACOLOGY

Chlorpheniramine Maleate: An antihistamine with anticholinergic (drying) and sedative side effects. Antihistamines appear to compete with histamine for cell receptor sites on effector cells. Chlorpheniramine maleate is a member of the alkylamine class of antihistamines which are among the least sedating antihistamines.
Phenylpropanolamine Hydrochloride: The drug may directly stimulate adrenergic receptors but probably indirectly stimulates both alpha (α) and beta (β) adrenergic receptors by releasing norepinephrine from its storage sites. Phenylpropanolamine increases heart rate, force of contraction and

cardiac output, and excitability. It acts on alpha receptors in the mucosa of the respiratory tract, producing vasoconstriction which results in shrinkage of swollen mucous membranes, reduction of tissue, hyeremia, edema and nasal congestion, and an increase in nasal airway patency. Phenylpropanolamine causes CNS stimulation and reportedly has an anorexigenic effect.
Pharmacokinetics: The active drugs, 12 mg of chlorpheniramine maleate and 75 mg of phenylpropanolamine hydrochloride, in each capsule of this special slow-release dosage form approximate the serum levels of two liquid doses containing 6 mg of chlorpheniramine maleate and 37.5 mg of phenylpropanolamine hydrochloride taken at six hour intervals. The absorption half-life of the drugs from a non-timed liquid is appreciably more rapid than from the slow-release formulation.
When studied under controlled conditions, the peak chlorpheniramine serum level occurs about 5.5 hours after administration and the peak phenylpropanolamine level occurs after about 3.5 hours. The average half-life of elimination is about 17.5 hours for chlorpheniramine and 5.0 hours for phenylpropanolamine.

INDICATIONS AND USAGE

For the treatment of the symptoms of seasonal and perennial allergic rhinitis and vasomotor rhinitis, including nasal obstruction (congestion).

CONTRAINDICATIONS

Hypersensitivity to either ingredient; severe hypertension; coronary artery disease; stenosing peptic ulcer; pyloroduodenal or bladder neck obstruction.
These capsules should NOT be used to treat lower respiratory tract conditions, including asthma.
As with any product containing a sympathomimetic, capsules should NOT be used in patients taking MAO inhibitors. Because of the higher risk of antihistamine side effects in infants generally, and for newborns and premature in particular, antihistamine therapy is contraindicated in nursing mothers. Capsules should NOT be used in newborns or premature infants.

WARNINGS

Caution patients about activities requiring alertness (e.g. operating vehicles or machinery). Patients should also be warned about the possible additive effects of alcohol and other CNS depressants (hypnotics, sedatives, tranquilizers, etc.).

PRECAUTIONS

General: Capsules should be used with considerable caution in patients with narrow angle glaucoma, stenosing peptic ulcer, pyloroduodenal obstruction, symptomatic prostatic hypertrophy, bladder neck obstruction, hypertension, thyroid disease, diabetes and heart disease. The risk of antihistamine induced dizziness, sedation and hypotension is greater in elderly patients (over 60 years).
Drug Interactions: These capsules should not be used in patients taking MAO inhibitors. Antihistamines have additive effects with alcohol and other CNS depressants (hypnotics, sedatives, tranquilizers, etc.).
Pregnancy: Pregnancy category C. Animal reproduction studies have not been conducted. It is also not known whether this product can cause fetal harm when administered to a pregnant woman or can affect reproduction capacity. Capsules should be given to pregnant women only if clearly needed.
Nursing Mothers: It is not known whether this drug is excreted in human milk. Because many drugs are excreted in human milk, caution should be exercised when this product is administered to a nursing mother.
Pediatric Use: Safety and effectiveness in children below the age of 12 have not been established.

ADVERSE REACTIONS

General: Urticaria, drug rash, anaphylactic shock, photosensitivity, excessive perspiration, chills, dryness of the mouth, nose and throat.
Cardiovascular System: Hypotension, hypertension, headache, palpitations, tachycardia, extrasystoles and angina pain.
Hematologic System: Hemolytic anemia, thrombocytopenia, agranulocytosis.
Nervous System: Sedation, dizziness, disturbed coordination, fatigue, confusion, restlessness, excitation, nervousness, tremor, irritability, insomnia, euphoria, paresthesias, blurred vision, diplopia, vertigo, tinnitus, acute labyrinthitis, hysteria, neuritis and convulsions.
Gastrointestinal System: Epigastric distress, anorexia, nausea, vomiting, diarrhea, constipation.
Genitourinary System: Urinary frequency, difficult urination, urinary retention, early menses.
Respiratory System: Thickening of bronchial secretions, tightness of chest and wheezing, nasal stuffiness.

Continued on next page

Boots—Cont.

OVERDOSAGE

Symptoms: Overdosage symptoms may vary from central nervous system depression to stimulation. Peripheral atropine-like signs and symptoms as well as gastrointestinal symptoms may occur. Marked cerebral irritation resulting in jerking of muscles and possible convulsions may be followed by deep stupor and respiratory failure. Acute hypertension or cardiovascular collapse with accompanying hypotension may occur.

Treatment: If spontaneous vomiting has not occurred, immediate evacuation of the stomach should be induced by emesis or gastric lavage. Saline cathartics, such as milk of magnesia, draw water into the bowel by osmosis, and therefore, are valuable for their action in rapid dilution of bowel content. Respiratory depression should be treated promptly with oxygen. Do not treat CNS depression with analeptics which might precipitate convulsion. If convulsions or marked CNS excitement occur, use only short-acting depressants.

DOSAGE AND ADMINISTRATION

Adults and children 12 years of age and older, one capsule every 12 hours. Should not be used in children under 12.

HOW SUPPLIED

RU-TUSS® II Capsules: No. 1 capsule, colorless body, transparent green cap, filled with white beads, printed "RU-TUSS II" over "31" and "BOOTS" over "31".
Bottles of 100   NDC 0048-0031-01
Store at controlled room temperature 15°–30°C (59°–86°F) and protect from moisture and light.

CAUTION

Federal (USA) law prohibits dispensing without prescription.

Manufactured for
Boots Pharmaceuticals, Inc.
Lincolnshire, Illinois 60069 USA
By
KV Pharmaceutical Company
St. Louis, Missouri 63144 USA
Rev. 4/16/90   0031-06
Shown in Product Identification Section, page 405

RU-TUSS®   Ⓒ Ⅲ
With Hydrocodone
[roo-tŭs]

DESCRIPTION

Each 5 mL (one teaspoonful) of RU-TUSS® with Hydrocodone contains:
Hydrocodone Bitartrate .... 1.7 mg
    (WARNING: MAY BE HABIT FORMING)
Phenylephrine Hydrochloride .... 5.0 mg
Phenylpropanolamine Hydrochloride .... 3.3 mg
Pheniramine Maleate .... 3.3 mg
Pyrilamine Maleate .... 3.3 mg
Alcohol 5%
Inactive Ingredients: citric acid, D&C Yellow No. 10, FD&C Blue No. 1, FD&C Yellow No. 6, flavors, glycerin, liquid glucose, menthol, methylparaben, propylene glycol, propylparaben, purified water, saccharin sodium, sorbitol solution.
RU-TUSS with Hydrocodone is an oral antitussive, antihistaminic and nasal decongestant preparation.

INDICATIONS AND USAGE

RU-TUSS with Hydrocodone is indicated for the temporary relief of symptoms associated with hay fever, allergies, nasal congestion and cough due to the common cold.

CONTRAINDICATIONS

Hypersensitivity to antihistamines. Concomitant use of antihypertensive or antidepressant drugs containing a monoamine oxidase inhibitor is contraindicated.
RU-TUSS with Hydrocodone is contraindicated in patients with glaucoma, bronchial asthma and in women who are pregnant.

WARNINGS

Patients should be warned of the potential that RU-TUSS with Hydrocodone may be habit forming.
RU-TUSS with Hydrocodone may cause drowsiness.
Patients should be warned of the possible additive effects caused by taking antihistamines with alcohol, hypnotics, sedatives and tranquilizers.

PRECAUTIONS

Patients taking RU-TUSS with Hydrocodone should avoid driving a motor vehicle or operating dangerous machinery (See **WARNINGS**).
Caution should be taken with patients having hypertension and cardiovascular disease.

ADVERSE REACTIONS

Gastrointestinal: nausea, vomiting, diarrhea, constipation, epigastric distress.
Genitourinary System: urinary frequency and dysuria.
Central Nervous System: drowsiness, giddiness, dizziness, headache, incoordination, faintness, hyperirritability, nervousness and insomnia, mydriasis.
Special Senses: tinnitus, visual disturbances, blurred vision.
Metabolic/Endocrine: anorexia, lassitude.
Cardiovascular: tightness of the chest, palpitations, tachycardia, hypotension/hypertension.
Miscellaneous: dryness of mucous membranes, xerostomia.
Respiratory: thickening of bronchial secretions.

OVERDOSAGE

Overdosing may cause restlessness, excitation, delirium, tremors, euphoria, stupor, tachycardia and even convulsions.

DOSAGE AND ADMINISTRATION

Adults and children 12 years and older: 2 teaspoonfuls every 4 to 6 hours.
Children 6 to under 12 years of age: 1 teaspoonful every 4 to 6 hours.
Children 2 to under 6 years of age: 1/2 to 1 teaspoonful every 4 to 6 hours, according to age.
NOTE: Doses for children should not be repeated more than 4 times in any 24 hour period.

HOW SUPPLIED

RU-TUSS® with Hydrocodone: clear, bright emerald green color, liquid.
16 oz bottles (473 mL)   NDC 0048-1007-16
Store at controlled room temperature 15°–30°C (59°–86°F).
Caution: Federal (USA) law prohibits dispensing without prescription.

Boots Pharmaceuticals, Inc.
Lincolnshire, Illinois 60069 USA
Rev. 4/16/90   7203-01

RU-TUSS® DE TABLETS   ℞
[roo-tŭs]

DESCRIPTION

Each prolonged action tablet contains:
Pseudoephedrine HCl.................................120 mg
Guaifenesin* ....600 mg
RU-TUSS DE is an oral decongestant-expectorant combination, formulated to provide prolonged therapeutic activity.
Inactive Ingredients: hydroxypropyl methylcellulose 2910, FD&C Blue No. 1 Lake, magnesium stearate, povidone, propylene glycol.

CLINICAL PHARMACOLOGY

Pseudoephedrine hydrochloride acts on alpha-adrenergic receptors in the mucosa of the respiratory tract producing vasoconstriction. Pseudoephedrine HCl shrinks swollen nasal mucous membranes, reduces tissue hyperemia, edema, nasal congestion and increases nasal airway patency. Drainage of sinus secretions is increased and obstructed Eustachian ostia may be opened. Pseudoephedrine produces little if any rebound congestion.
Guaifenesin enhances the flow of respiratory tract secretions. The enhanced flow of less viscid secretions lubricates irritated respiratory tract membranes, promotes ciliary action and facilitates the removal of inspissated mucus. As a result, sinus and bronchial drainage is improved and nonproductive coughs become more productive and less frequent.

INDICATIONS AND USAGE

RU-TUSS DE is indicated for the relief of nasal congestion due to the common cold, allergic rhinitis, hay fever or other upper respiratory allergies and nasal congestion associated with sinusitis. To promote nasal or sinus drainage; for the relief of Eustachian tube congestion; for adjunctive therapy in otitis media; for the symptomatic relief of respiratory conditions characterized by non-productive cough and in the presence of tenacious mucus and/or mucus plugs in the respiratory tract.

CONTRAINDICATIONS

RU-TUSS DE is contraindicated in patients with a known hypersensitivity to any of its ingredients or in patients with severe hypertension, coronary artery disease, prostatic hypertrophy or patients on MAO inhibitor therapy.

WARNINGS

Considerable caution should be exercised in patients with hypertension, diabetes mellitus, ischemic heart disease, hyperthyroidism, history of cardiac arrythmias, elevated intraocular pressure and prostatic hypertrophy.

*Guaifenesin is also known as glyceryl guaiacolate.

PRECAUTIONS

General: Hypertensive patients should use RU-TUSS DE only with medical advice, as they may experience a change in blood pressure due to added vasoconstriction. However, sustained action preparations may affect the cardiovascular system less.
Information for Patients: Excessive Use: May cause systemic effects (nervousness, dizziness, sleeplessness, lightheadedness, excitability, weakness, fear, anxiety, tremor, hallucinations, convulsions and respiratory difficulties) which are more likely in infants and in the elderly. Habituation and toxic psychosis have followed long-term usage. Excessive dosage may also cause nausea and vomiting.
Usage in Elderly: Patients 60 years and older are more likely to experience adverse reactions to sympathomimetics. Overdosage may cause hallucinations, convulsions, CNS depression, cardiovascular collapse and death. Demonstrate safe use of short-acting sympathomimetic before use of a sustained action formulation in elderly patients.
Persistent Cough: May indicate a serious condition. If cough persists for more than one week, tends to recur or is accompanied by a high fever, rash or persistent headache, consult a physician.
Drug Interactions: MAO inhibitors and beta adrenergic blockers increase effects of sympathomimetics. Sympathomimetics may reduce the antihypertensive effects of methyldopa, mecamylamine, reserpine and veratrum alkaloids.
Laboratory Test Interactions: Guaifenesin has been reported to interfere with clinical laboratory determinations or urinary 5-hydroxyindoleacetic acid (5-HIAA) and vanilmandelic acid (VMA).
Carcinogenesis, mutagenesis, impairment of fertility: Long-term studies in animals have not been performed to evaluate carcinogenic potential.
Pregnancy: Pregnancy category C. Animal reproduction studies have not been conducted with RU-TUSS DE. It is not known whether RU-TUSS DE can cause fetal harm when administered to a pregnant woman or can affect reproductive capacity. RU-TUSS DE should be given to a pregnant woman only if clearly needed.
Nursing Mothers: Because of the higher than usual risks to infants from sympathomimetic agents, RU-TUSS DE should not be given to nursing mothers.
Pediatric Use: Safety and effectiveness of RU-TUSS DE in children below the age of 6 has not been established (see **DOSAGE AND ADMINISTRATION**).

ADVERSE REACTIONS

Gastrointestinal: nausea and vomiting.
Central Nervous System: nervousness, dizziness, sleeplessness, lightheadedness, tremor, hallucinations, convulsions, CNS depression, fear, anxiety, headache, increased irritability or excitement.
Cardiovascular: palpitations, tachycardia, cardiovascular collapse and death.
General: weakness.
Respiratory: respiratory difficulties.

OVERDOSAGE

Symptoms: Overdosage may cause hallucinations, convulsions, CNS depression, cardiovascular collapse and death.
Treatment: Treatment of overdosage should provide both symptomatic and supportive care. If the amount ingested is considered dangerous or excessive, induce vomiting with ipecac syrup unless the patient is convulsing, comatose, or has lost the gag reflex, in which case, perform gastric lavage using a large bore tube. If indicated, follow with activated charcoal. Since the effects of RU-TUSS DE may last up to 12 hours, treatment should be continued for at least that length of time.

DOSAGE AND ADMINISTRATION

Adults and children 12 years of age and over, 1 tablet every 12 hours not to exceed 2,400 mg of guaifenesin in 24 hours.
Children 6 to under 12 years, ½ tablet every 12 hours not to exceed 1,200 mg of guaifenesin in 24 hours.
Not recommended for children under 6 years of age.

HOW SUPPLIED

RU-TUSS® DE Tablets: elongated, light blue, scored, film-coated tablet debossed with BOOTS logo and "90".
Bottles of 100   NDC 0048-0090-01
Store at controlled room temperature 15°–30° C (59°–86°F).

CAUTION

Federal (USA) law prohibits dispensing without prescription.

Boots Pharmaceuticals, Inc.
Lincolnshire, Illinois 60069 USA
Rev. 8/16/90   8463-02
Shown in Product Identification Section, page 405

SSD™ ℞
(1% Silver Sulfadiazine) Cream
SSD AF™*
(1% Silver Sulfadiazine) Cream

DESCRIPTION

SSD (1% Silver Sulfadiazine) Cream and SSD AF (1% Silver Sulfadiazine) Cream are topical antibacterial preparations which have as their active antimicrobial ingredient silver sulfadiazine. The active moiety is contained within an opaque, white, water-miscible cream base.

Each 1000 grams of SSD/SSD AF Cream contains 10 grams of silver sulfadiazine.

Inactive Ingredients: cetyl alcohol (SSD Cream only), isopropyl myristate, polyoxyl 40 stearate, propylene glycol, purified water, stearyl alcohol, sodium hydroxide, sorbitan monooleate, white petrolatum; with 0.3% methylparaben, as a preservative.

Silver sulfadiazine has an empirical formula of $C_{10}H_9AgN_4O_2S$, molecular weight of 357.14, and structural formula as shown:

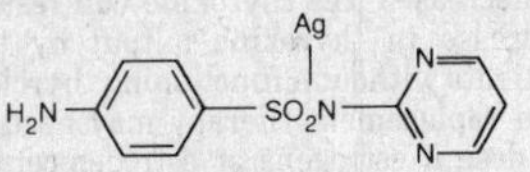

CLINICAL PHARMACOLOGY

Silver sulfadiazine has broad antimicrobial activity. It is bactericidal for many gram-negative and gram-positive bacteria as well as being effective against yeast. Results from *in vitro* testing are listed below.

Sufficient data have been obtained to demonstrate that silver sulfadiazine will inhibit bacteria that are resistant to other antimicrobial agents and that the compound is superior to sulfadiazine.

Studies utilizing radioactive micronized silver sulfadiazine, electron microscopy, and biochemical techniques have revealed that the mechanism of action of silver sulfadiazine on bacteria differs from silver nitrate and sodium sulfadiazine. Silver sulfadiazine acts only on the cell wall to produce its bactericidal effect.

Results of *In Vitro* Testing With Concentrations of Silver Sulfadiazine
Number of Sensitive Strains/Total Number of Strains Tested

Genus & Species	50 µg/mL	100 µg/mL
Pseudomonas aeruginosa	130/130	130/130
Pseudomonas maltophilia	7/7	7/7
Enterobacter species	48/50	50/50
Enterobacter cloacae	24/24	24/24
Klebsiella species	53/54	54/54
Escherichia coli	63/63	63/63
Serratia species	27/28	28/28
Providencia mirabilis	53/53	53/53
Morganella morganii	10/10	10/10
Proteus rettgeri	2/2	2/2
Proteus vulgaris	2/2	2/2
Providencia species	1/1	1/1
Citrobacter species	10/10	10/10
Acinetobacter calcoaceticus	10/11	11/11
Staphylococcus aureus	100/101	101/101
Staphylococcus epidermidis	51/51	51/51
β-Hemolytic Streptococcus	4/4	4/4
Enterococcus species	52/53	53/53
Corynebacterium diphtheriae	2/2	2/2
Clostridium perfringens	0/2	2/2
Candida albicans	43/50	50/50

Silver sulfadiazine is not a carbonic anhydrase inhibitor and may be useful in situations where such agents are contraindicated.

INDICATIONS AND USAGE

Silver Sulfadiazine Cream is a topical antimicrobial drug indicated as an adjunct for the prevention and treatment of wound sepsis in patients with second and third degree burns.

CONTRAINDICATIONS

Silver Sulfadiazine Cream is contraindicated in patients who are hypersensitive to silver sulfadiazine or any of the other ingredients in the preparation.

Because sulfonamide therapy is known to increase the possibility of kernicterus, Silver Sulfadiazine Cream should not be used on pregnant women approaching or at term, on premature infants, or on newborn infants during the first 2 months of life.

WARNINGS

There is potential cross-sensitivity between silver sulfadiazine and other sulfonamides. If allergic reactions attributable to treatment with silver sulfadiazine occur, continuation of therapy must be weighed against the potential hazards of the particular allergic reaction.

***Alternate Formula**

Fungal proliferation in and below the eschar may occur. However, the incidence of clinically reported fungal superinfection is low.

The use of Silver Sulfadiazine Cream in some cases of glucose-6-phosphate dehydrogenase-deficient individuals may be hazardous, as hemolysis may occur.

PRECAUTION

General: If hepatic and renal functions become impaired and elimination of drug decreases, accumulation may occur and discontinuation of Silver Sulfadiazine Cream should be weighed against the therapeutic benefit being achieved.

In considering the use of topical proteolytic enzymes in conjunction with Silver Sulfadiazine Cream, the possibility should be noted that silver may inactivate such enzymes.

Laboratory Tests: In the treatment of burn wounds involving extensive areas of the body, the serum sulfa concentrations may approach adult therapeutic levels (8 to 12 mg%). Therefore, in these patients it would be advisable to monitor serum sulfa concentrations. Renal function should be carefully monitored and the urine should be checked for sulfa crystals.

Absorption of the propylene glycol vehicle has been reported to affect serum osmolality, which may affect the interpretation of laboratory tests.

Carcinogenesis, Mutagenesis, Impairment of Fertility: Long-term dermal toxicity studies of 24 months duration in rats and 18 months in mice with concentrations of silver sulfadiazine three to ten times the concentration in Silver Sulfadiazine Cream revealed no evidence of carcinogenicity.

Pregnancy: Pregnancy category B. A reproductive study has been performed in rabbits at doses up to three to ten times the concentration of silver sulfadiazine in Silver Sulfadiazine Cream and has revealed no evidence of harm to the fetus due to silver sulfadiazine. There are, however, no adequate and well-controlled studies in pregnant women. Because animal reproduction studies are not always predictive of human response, this drug should be used during pregnancy only if clearly justified, especially in pregnant women approaching or at term (see **CONTRAINDICATIONS**).

Nursing Mothers: It is not known whether Silver Sulfadiazine Cream is excreted in human milk. However, sulfonamides are known to be excreted in human milk, and all sulfonamide derivatives are known to increase the possibility of kernicterus. Because of the possibility for serious adverse reactions in nursing infants from sulfonamides, a decision should be made whether to discontinue nursing or to discontinue the drug, taking into account the importance of the drug to the mother.

Pediatric Use: Safety and effectiveness in children have not been established (see **CONTRAINDICATIONS**).

ADVERSE REACTIONS

Several cases of transient leukopenia have been reported in patients receiving silver sulfadiazine therapy. Leukopenia associated with silver sulfadiazine administration is primarily characterized by decreased neutrophil count. Maximal white blood cell depression occurs within two to four days of initiation of therapy. Rebound to normal leukocyte levels follows onset within two to three days. Recovery is not influenced by continuation of silver sulfadiazine therapy. The incidence of leukopenia in various reports averages about 20%. A higher incidence has been seen in patients treated concurrently with cimetidine.

Other infrequently occurring events include skin necrosis, erythema multiforme, skin discoloration, burning sensation, rashes, and interstitial nephritis.

Reduction in bacterial growth after application of topical antibacterial agents has been reported to permit spontaneous healing of deep partial-thickness burns by preventing conversion of the partial thickness to full thickness by sepsis. However, reduction in bacterial colonization has caused delayed separation, in some cases necessitating escharotomy in order to prevent contracture.

Absorption of silver sulfadiazine varies depending upon the percent of body surface area and the extent of the tissue damage. Although few have been reported, it is possible that any adverse reaction associated with sulfonamides may occur. Some of the reactions which have been associated with sulfonamides are as follows: blood dyscrasias, including agranulocytosis, aplastic anemia, thrombocytopenia, leukopenia and hemolytic anemia; dermatologic and allergic reactions, including Stevens-Johnson syndrome and exfoliative dermatitis; gastrointestinal reactions; hepatitis and hepatocellular necrosis; CNS reactions; and toxic nephrosis.

DOSAGE AND ADMINISTRATION

FOR TOPICAL USE ONLY – NOT FOR OPHTHALMIC USE.

Prompt institution of appropriate regimens for care of the burned patient is of prime importance and includes the control of shock and pain. The burn wounds are then cleansed and debrided and Silver Sulfadiazine Cream is applied under sterile conditions. The burn areas should be covered with Silver Sulfadiazine Cream at all times. The cream should be applied once to twice daily to a thickness of approximately $\frac{1}{16}$ inch. Whenever necessary, the cream should be reapplied to any areas from which it has been removed by patient activity. Administration may be accomplished in minimal time because dressings are not required. However, if individual patient requirements make dressings necessary, they may be used.

Reapply immediately after hydrotherapy.

Treatment with Silver Sulfadiazine Cream should be continued until satisfactory healing has occurred or until the burn site is ready for grafting. The drug should not be withdrawn from the therapeutic regimen while there remains the possibility of infection except if a significant adverse reaction occurs.

HOW SUPPLIED

SSD™ (1% Silver Sulfadiazine) **Cream:** white to off-white cream.

50 gram jar 3P4000	NDC 0048-2100-71
400 gram jar 3P4007	NDC 0048-2100-70
1000 gram jar 3P4009	NDC 0048-2100-73
25 gram tube	NDC 0048-2100-77
50 gram tube	NDC 0048-2100-78
85 gram tube	NDC 0048-2100-79

SSD AF™* (1% Silver Sulfadiazine) **Cream:** white to off-white cream.

50 gram jar 3P4010	NDC 0048-2110-71
400 gram jar 3P4017	NDC 0048-2110-70
1000 gram jar 3P4019	NDC 0048-2110-73

Store at controlled room temperature 15°–30°C (59°–86°F).

CAUTION: Federal (USA) law prohibits dispensing without prescription.

Boots Pharmaceuticals, Inc.
Lincolnshire, Illinois 60069 USA

Rev. 9-13-91 7559-05

Shown in Product Identification Section, page 406

SYNTHROID® ℞
[*sin 'throid*]
(Levothyroxine Sodium, USP)
Synthroid Tablets—for oral administration
Synthroid Injection—for parenteral administration
7920-02

DESCRIPTION

SYNTHROID (Levothyroxine Sodium, USP) **Tablets** and **Injection** contain synthetic crystalline L-3,3',5,5'-tetraiodothyronine sodium salt [levothyroxine (T_4) sodium]. Synthetic T_4 is similar to that produced in the human thyroid gland. T_4 contains four iodine atoms and is formed by the coupling of two molecules of diiodotyrosine (DIT).

Levothyroxine (T_4) Sodium has an empirical formula of $C_{15}H_{10}I_4NNaO_4xH_2O$, molecular weight of 798.86 (anhydrous), and structural formula as shown:

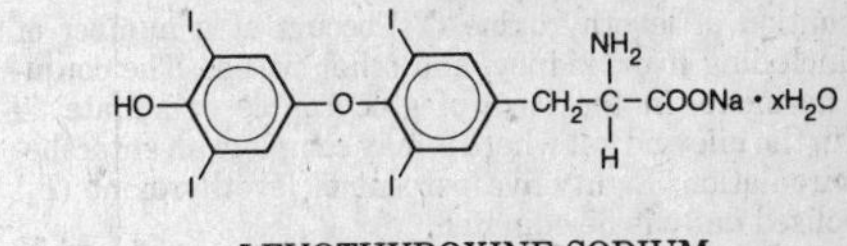

LEVOTHYROXINE SODIUM

Inactive Ingredients: acacia, lactose, magnesium stearate, povidone, confectioner's sugar, talc. The following are the color additives per tablet strength:

Strength (mcg)	Color Additive(s)
25	FD&C Yellow No. 6
50	None
75	FD&C Red No. 40, FD&C Blue No. 2
88	FD&C Blue No. 1, FD&C Yellow No. 6 D&C Yellow No. 10
100	D&C Yellow No. 10, FD&C Yellow No. 6
112	D&C Red No. 27 & 30
125	FD&C Yellow No. 6, FD&C Red No. 40, FD&C Blue No. 1
150	FD&C Blue No. 2
175	FD&C Blue No. 1, D&C Red No. 27 & 30
200	FD&C Red No. 40
300	D&C Yellow No. 10, FD&C Yellow No. 6, FD&C Blue No. 1

CLINICAL PHARMACOLOGY

The steps in the synthesis of thyroid hormones are controlled by thyrotropin (Thyroid Stimulating Hormone, TSH) secreted by the anterior pituitary. This hormone's secretion is in turn controlled by a feedback mechanism effected by the thyroid hormones themselves and by thyrotropin releasing hormone (TRH), a tripeptide of hypothalamic origin. Endogenous thyroid hormone secretion is suppressed when exogenous thyroid hormones are administered to euthyroid individuals in excess of the normal gland's secretion.

The mechanisms by which thyroid hormones exert their physiologic action are not well understood. These hormones

Continued on next page

Boots—Cont.

enhance oxygen consumption by most tissues of the body and increase the basal metabolic rate and the metabolism of carbohydrates, lipids, and proteins. Thus they exert a profound influence on every organ system in the body and are of particular importance in the development of the central nervous system.

The normal thyroid gland contains approximately 200 mcg of levothyroxine (T_4) per gram of gland, and 15 mcg of triiodothyronine (T_3) per gram. The ratio of these two hormones in the circulation does not represent the ratio in the thyroid gland, since about 80 percent of peripheral triiodothyronine comes from monodeiodination of levothyroxine at the 5 position (outer ring). Peripheral monodeiodination of levothyroxine at the 5 position (inner ring) results in the formation of reverse triiodothyronine (rT_3), which is calorigenically inactive. These facts would seem to advocate levothyroxine as the treatment of choice for the hypothyroid patient and to militate against the administration of hormone combinations which, while normalizing thyroxine levels may produce triiodothyronine levels in the thyrotoxic range.

Triiodothyronine (T_3) level is low in the fetus and newborn, in old age, in chronic caloric deprivation, hepatic cirrhosis, renal failure, surgical stress, and chronic illnesses representing what has been called the "low triiodothyronine syndrome."

PHARMACOKINETICS

Animal studies have shown that T_4 is only partially absorbed from the gastrointestinal tract. The degree of absorption is dependent on the vehicle used for its administration and by the character of the intestinal contents, the intestinal flora, including plasma protein, soluble dietary factors, all of which bind thyroid and thereby make it unavailable for diffusion.

Depending on other factors, absorption has varied from 48 to 79 percent of the administered dose. Fasting increases absorption. Malabsorption syndromes, as well as dietary factors, (children's soybean formula, concomitant use of anionic exchange resins such as cholestyramine) cause excessive fecal loss.

More than 99 percent of circulating hormones are bound to serum proteins, including thyroxine-binding globulin (TBG), thyroxine-binding prealbumin (TBPA), and albumin (TBa), whose capacities and affinities vary for the hormones. The higher affinity of levothyroxine (T_4) for both TBG and TBPA as compared to triiodothyronine (T_3) partially explains the higher serum levels and longer half-life of the former hormone. Both protein-bound hormones exist in equilibrium with minute amounts of free hormone, the latter accounting for the metabolic activity.

Deiodination of levothyroxine (T_4) occurs at a number of sites, including liver, kidney, and other tissues. The conjugated hormone, in the form of glucuronide or sulfate, is found in the bile and gut where it may complete an enterohepatic circulation. Eighty-five percent of levothyroxine (T_4) metabolized daily is deiodinated.

INDICATIONS AND USAGE

SYNTHROID is indicated:

1. As replacement or supplemental therapy in patients with hypothyroidism of any etiology, except transient hypothyroidism during the recovery phase of subacute thyroiditis. This category includes cretinism, myxedema, and ordinary hypothyroidism in patients of any age (children, adults, the elderly), or state (including pregnancy); primary hypothyroidism resulting from functional deficiency, primary atrophy, partial or total absence of thyroid gland, or the effects of surgery, radiation, or drugs, with or without the presence of goiter; and secondary (pituitary), or tertiary (hypothalamic) hypothyroidism (See **CONTRAINDICATIONS** and **PRECAUTIONS**). SYNTHROID **Injection** can be used intravenously whenever a rapid onset of effect is critical and either intravenously or intramuscularly in hypothyroid patients whenever the oral route is precluded for long periods of time.
2. As a pituitary TSH suppressant, in the treatment or prevention of various types of euthyroid goiters, including thyroid nodules, subacute or chronic lymphocytic thyroiditis (Hashimoto's), multinodular goiter, and in the management of thyroid cancer.
3. As a diagnostic agent in suppression tests to aid in the diagnosis of suspected mild hyperthyroidism or thyroid gland autonomy.

CONTRAINDICATIONS

Thyroid hormone preparations are generally contraindicated in patients with diagnosed but as yet uncorrected adrenal cortical insufficiency, untreated thyrotoxicosis, and apparent hypersensitivity to any of their active or extraneous constituents. There is no well documented evidence from the literature, however, of true allergic or idiosyncratic reactions to thyroid hormone.

WARNINGS

Drugs with thyroid hormone activity, alone or together with other therapeutic agents, have been used for the treatment of obesity. In euthyroid patients, doses within the range of daily hormonal requirements are ineffective for weight reduction. Larger doses may produce serious or even life threatening manifestations of toxicity, particularly when given in association with sympathomimetic amines such as those used for their anorectic effects.

The use of thyroid hormones in the therapy of obesity, alone or combined with other drugs, is unjustified and has been shown to be ineffective. Neither is their use justified for the treatment of male or female infertility unless this condition is accompanied by hypothyroidism.

PRECAUTIONS

General: Thyroid hormones should be used with great caution in a number of circumstances where the integrity of the cardiovascular system, particularly the coronary arteries, is suspected. These include patients with angina pectoris or the elderly, who have a greater likelihood of occult cardiac disease. In these patients, therapy should be initiated with low doses, i.e., 25–50 mcg levothyroxine (T_4). When, in such patients, a euthyroid state can only be reached at the expense of an aggravation of the cardiovascular disease, thyroid hormone dosage should be reduced.

Thyroid hormone therapy in patients with concomitant diabetes mellitus or insipidus or adrenal cortical insufficiency aggravates the intensity of their symptoms. Appropriate adjustments of the various therapeutic measures directed at these concomitant endocrine diseases are required. The therapy of myxedema coma may require simultaneous administration of glucocorticoids (See **DOSAGE AND ADMINISTRATION**).

Hypothyroidism decreases and hyperthyroidism increases the sensitivity to oral anticoagulants. Prothrombin time should be closely monitored in thyroid treated patients on oral anticoagulants and dosage of the latter agents adjusted on the basis of frequent prothrombin time determinations.

In infants, excessive doses of thyroid hormone preparations may produce craniosynostosis.

Information for the Patient: Patients on thyroid hormone preparations and parents of children on thyroid therapy should be informed that:

1. Replacement therapy is to be taken essentially for life, with the exception of cases of transient hypothyroidism, usually associated with thyroiditis, and in those patients receiving a therapeutic trial of the drug.
2. They should immediately report during the course of therapy any signs or symptoms of thyroid hormone toxicity, e.g., chest pain, increased pulse rate, palpitations, excessive sweating, heat intolerance, nervousness, or any other unusual event.
3. In case of concomitant diabetes mellitus, the daily dosage of antidiabetic medication may need readjustment as thyroid hormone replacement is achieved. If thyroid medication is stopped, a downward readjustment of the dosage of insulin or oral hypoglycemic agent may be necessary to avoid hypoglycemia. At all times, close monitoring of blood or urinary glucose levels is mandatory in such patients.
4. In case of concomitant oral anticoagulant therapy, the prothrombin time should be measured frequently to determine if the dosage of oral anticoagulants is to be readjusted.
5. Partial loss of hair may be experienced by children in the first few months of thyroid therapy, but this is usually a transient phenomenon and later recovery is usually the rule.

Laboratory Tests: Treatment of patients with thyroid hormones requires the periodic assessment of thyroid status by means of appropriate laboratory tests, by full clinical evaluation, or both. The TSH suppression test can be used to test the effectiveness of any thyroid preparation bearing in mind the relative insensitivity of the infant pituitary to the negative feedback effect of thyroid hormones. Serum T_4 levels can be used to test the effectiveness of levothyroxine sodium. When the total serum T_4 is low but TSH is normal, a test specific to assess unbound (free) T_4 levels is warranted. Specific measurements of T_4 and T_3 by competitive protein binding or radioimmunoassay are not influenced by blood levels of organic or inorganic iodine and have essentially replaced older tests of thyroid hormone measurements, i.e., PBI, BEI, and T_4 by column.

Drug Interactions: *Oral Anticoagulants*—Thyroid hormones appear to increase catabolism of vitamin K-dependent clotting factors. If oral anticoagulants are also being given, compensatory increases in clotting factor synthesis are impaired. Patients stabilized on oral anticoagulants who are found to require thyroid replacement therapy should be watched very closely when thyroid is started. If a patient is truly hypothyroid, it is likely that a reduction in anticoagulant dosage will be required. No special precautions appear to be necessary when oral anticoagulant therapy is begun in a patient already stabilized on maintenance thyroid replacement therapy.

Insulin or Oral Hypoglycemics—Initiating thyroid replacement therapy may cause increases in insulin or oral hypoglycemic requirements. The effects seen are poorly understood and depend upon a variety of factors such as dose and type of thyroid preparations and endocrine status of the patient. Patients receiving insulin or oral hypoglycemics should be closely watched during initiation of thyroid replacement therapy.

Cholestyramine—Cholestyramine binds both T_4 and T_3 in the intestine, thus impairing absorption of these thyroid hormones. *In vitro* studies indicate that the binding is not easily reversed. Therefore, four to five hours should elapse between administration of cholestyramine and thyroid hormones.

Estrogen, Oral Contraceptives—Estrogens tend to increase serum thyroxine-binding globulin (TBG). In a patient with a nonfunctioning thyroid gland who is receiving thyroid replacement therapy, free levothyroxine may be decreased when estrogens are started thus increasing thyroid requirements. However, if the patient's thyroid gland has sufficient function, the decreased free thyroxine will result in a compensatory increase in thyroxine output by the thyroid. Therefore, patients without a functioning thyroid gland who are on thyroid replacement therapy may need to increase their thyroid dose if estrogens or estrogen-containing oral contraceptives are given.

Drug/Laboratory Test Interactions: The following drugs or moieties are known to interfere with some laboratory tests performed in patients on thyroid hormone therapy: Androgens, corticosteroids, estrogens, oral contraceptives containing estrogens, iodine-containing preparations, and the numerous preparations containing salicylates.

1. Changes in TBG concentration should be taken into consideration in the interpretation of T_4 and T_3 values. Pregnancy, estrogens, and estrogen-containing oral contraceptives increase TBG concentrations. TBG may also be increased during infectious hepatitis. Decreases in TBG concentrations are observed in nephrosis, acromegaly, and after androgen or corticosteroid therapy. Familial hyper- or hypo-thyroxine-binding-globulinemias have been described. The incidence of TBG deficiency approximates 1 in 9000. The binding of thyroxine by TBPA is inhibited by salicylates. In such cases, the unbound (free) hormone should be measured. Alternatively, an indirect measure of free thyroxine, such as the Free Thyroxine Index (FTI) may be used.
2. Medicinal or dietary iodine interferes with all *in vivo* tests of radioiodine uptake, producing low uptakes which may not indicate a true decrease in hormone synthesis.
3. The persistence of clinical and laboratory evidence of hypothyroidism in spite of adequate dosage replacement indicates either poor patient compliance, poor absorption, or inactivity of the preparation. Intracellular resistance to thyroid hormone is quite rare, and is suggested by clinical signs and symptoms of hypothyroidism in the presence of high serum T_4 levels.

Carcinogenesis, Mutagenesis, and Impairment of Fertility: A reported association between prolonged thyroid therapy and breast cancer has not been confirmed and patients on thyroid therapy for established indications should not discontinue therapy. No confirmatory long-term studies in animals have been performed to evaluate carcinogenic potential, mutagenicity, or impairment of fertility in either males or females.

Pregnancy: Pregnancy category A. Thyroid hormones do not readily cross the placental barrier. The clinical experience to date does not indicate any adverse effect on fetuses when thyroid hormones are administered to pregnant women. On the basis of current knowledge, thyroid replacement therapy to hypothyroid women should not be discontinued during pregnancy.

Nursing Mothers: Minimal amounts of thyroid hormones are excreted in human milk. Thyroid is not associated with serious adverse reactions and does not have known tumorigenic potential. While caution should be exercised when thyroid is administered to a nursing woman, adequate replacement doses of levothyroxine are generally needed to maintain normal lactation.

Pediatric Use: Pregnant mothers provide little or no thyroid hormone to the fetus. The incidence of congenital hypothyroidism is relatively high (1 in 4,000) and the hypothyroid fetus would not derive any benefit from the small amounts of hormone crossing the placental barrier. Routine determinations of serum T_4 and/or TSH is strongly advised in neonates in view of the deleterious effects of thyroid deficiency on growth and development.

Treatment should be initiated immediately upon diagnosis, and maintained for life, unless transient hypothyroidism is suspected; in which case, therapy may be interrupted for 2 to 8 weeks after the age of 3 years to reassess the condition. Cessation of therapy is justified in patients who have maintained a normal TSH during those 2 to 8 weeks.

ADVERSE REACTIONS

Adverse reactions other than those indicative of hyperthyroidism because of therapeutic overdosage, either initially or during the maintenance periods, are rare (see **OVERDOSAGE**).

OVERDOSAGE

Signs and Symptoms: Excessive doses of thyroid result in hypermetabolic state resembling in every respect the condition of endogenous origin. The condition may be self-induced.

Treatment of Overdosage: Dosage should be reduced or therapy temporarily discontinued if signs and symptoms of overdosage appear. Treatment may be reinstated at a lower dosage. In normal individuals, normal hypothalamic-pituitary-thyroid axis function is restored in 6 to 8 weeks after thyroid suppression.

Treatment of acute massive thyroid hormone overdosage is aimed at reducing gastrointestinal absorption of the drugs and counteracting central and peripheral effects, mainly those of increased sympathetic activity. Vomiting may be induced initially if further gastrointestinal absorption can reasonably be prevented and barring contraindications such as coma, convulsions, or loss of the gagging reflex. Treatment is symptomatic and supportive. Oxygen may be administered and ventilation maintained. Cardiac glycosides may be indicated if congestive heart failure develops. Measures to control fever, hypoglycemia, or fluid loss should be instituted if needed. Antiadrenergic agents, particularly propranolol, have been used advantageously in the treatment of increased sympathetic activity. Propranolol may be administered intravenously at a dosage of 1 to 3 mg over a 10 minute period or orally, 80 to 160 mg/day, especially when no contraindications exist for its use. Other adjunctive measures may include administration of cholestyramine to interfere with thyroxine absorption, and glucocorticoids to inhibit conversion of T_4 to T_3.

DOSAGE AND ADMINISTRATION

The dosage and rate of administration of SYNTHROID® (Levothyroxine Sodium, USP) is determined by the indication and must in every case be individualized according to patient response and laboratory findings.

Hypothyroidism: SYNTHROID **Tablets** are usually instituted using low doses, with increments which depend on the cardiovascular status of the patient. The usual starting dose is 50 mcg, with increments of 25 mcg every 2 to 3 weeks. A lower starting dosage, 25 mcg/day or less, is recommended in patients with long standing hypothyroidism, particularly if cardiovascular impairment is suspected, in which case extreme caution is recommended. The appearance of angina is an indication for a reduction in dosage. Most patients require not more than 200 mcg/day. Failure to respond to doses of 300 mcg suggests lack of compliance or malabsorption. Adequate therapy usually results in normal TSH and T_4 levels after 2 to 3 weeks of the maintenance dose.

Readjustment of SYNTHROID **Tablet** dosage should be made within the first four weeks of therapy, after proper clinical and laboratory evaluations.

SYNTHROID **Injection** by intravenous or intramuscular routes can be substituted for the oral dosage form when ingestion of SYNTHROID **Tablets** is precluded for long periods of time. The initial parenteral dosage should be approximately one half of the previously established oral dosage of levothyroxine sodium tablets. Close observation of the patient, with individual adjustment of the dosage as needed, is recommended.

Myxedema Coma: Myxedema coma is usually precipitated in the hypothyroid patient by intercurrent illness or drugs such as sedatives and anesthetics and should be considered a medical emergency. Therapy should be directed at the correction of electrolyte disturbances and possible infection besides the administration of thyroid hormones. Corticosteroids should be administered routinely. T_4 may be administered via a nasogastric tube but the preferred route of administration is intravenous. Sodium levothyroxine (T_4) is given at a starting dose of 400 mcg (100 mcg/mL) given rapidly, and is usually well tolerated, even in the elderly. In the presence of concomitant heart disease, the sudden administration of such large doses of L-thyroxine intravenously is clearly not without its cardiovascular risks. Under such circumstances, intravenous therapy should not be undertaken without weighing the alternative risks of the myxedema coma and the cardiovascular disease. Clinical judgement in this situation may dictate smaller intravenous doses of SYNTHROID **Injection.** The initial dose is followed by daily supplements of 100 to 200 mcg given intravenously. Normal T_4 levels are achieved in 24 hours followed in 3 days by threefold evaluation of T_3. Continued daily administration of lesser amounts parenterally should be maintained until the patient is fully capable of accepting a daily oral dose. A daily maintenance dose of 50 to 100 mcg parenterally should suffice to maintain the euthyroid state, once established. Oral therapy would be resumed as soon as the clinical situation has been stabilized and the patient is able to take oral medication.

TSH Suppression in Thyroid Cancer, Nodules, and Euthyroid Goiters: Exogenous thyroid hormone may produce regression of metastases from follicular and papillary carcinoma of the thyroid and is used as ancillary therapy of these conditions following surgery or radioactive iodine. Medullary carcinoma of the thyroid is usually unresponsive to this therapy. TSH should be suppressed to low or undetectable levels. Therefore, larger amounts of thyroid hormone than those used for replacement therapy are frequently required. This therapy is also used in treating nontoxic solitary nodules and multinodular goiters, and to prevent thyroid enlargement in chronic (Hashimoto's) thyroiditis.

Thyroid Suppression Therapy: Administration of thyroid hormone in doses higher than those produced physiologically by the gland results in suppression of the production of endogenous hormone. This is the basis for the thyroid suppression test and is used as an aid in the diagnosis of patients with signs of mild hyperthyroidism in whom base line laboratory tests appear normal, or to demonstrate thyroid gland autonomy in patients with Graves' ophthalmopathy. ^{131}I uptake is determined before and after the administration of the exogenous hormone. A fifty percent or greater suppression of uptake indicates a normal thyroid-pituitary axis and thus rules out thyroid gland autonomy.

For adults, the average suppressive dose of levothyroxine (T_4) is 2.6 mcg/kg of body weight per day given for 7 to 10 days. These doses usually yield normal serum T_4 and T_3 levels and lack of response to TSH.

Levothyroxine sodium should be administered cautiously to patients in whom there is a strong suspicion of thyroid gland autonomy, in view of the fact that the exogenous hormone effects will be additive to the endogenous source.

Pediatric Dosage: Pediatric dosage should follow the recommendations summarized in Table I. In infants with congenital hypothyroidism, therapy with full doses should be instituted as soon as the diagnosis has been made. SYNTHROID **Tablets** may be given to infants and children who cannot swallow intact tablets by crushing the proper dose tablet and suspending the **freshly crushed** tablet in a small amount of water or formula. The suspension can be given by spoon or dropper. DO NOT STORE THE SUSPENSION FOR ANY PERIOD OF TIME. The crushed tablet may also be sprinkled over a small amount of food, such as cooked cereal or apple sauce.

Table I
Recommended Pediatric Dosage For Congenital Hypothyroidism*

	SYNTHROID (Levothyroxine Sodium Tablets, USP)	
Age	Dose per day	Daily dose per kg of body weight
0– 6 mos	25– 50 mcg	8–10 mcg
6–12 mos	50– 75 mcg	6– 8 mcg
1– 5 yrs	75–100 mcg	5– 6 mcg
6–12 yrs	100–150 mcg	4– 5 mcg

*To be adjusted on the basis of clinical response and laboratory tests (see **Laboratory Tests**).

HOW SUPPLIED

SYNTHROID® (Levothyroxine Sodium, USP), **Tablets:** round, color coded, scored tablet debossed with 'FLINT' and potency.

25 mcg, orange
Bottles of 100, Code 3P1023 NDC 0048-1020-03
Bottles of 1000, Code 3P1025 NDC 0048-1020-05
50 mcg, white
Bottles of 100, Code 3P1043 NDC 0048-1040-03
Bottles of 1000, Code 3P1045 NDC 0048-1040-05
Unit Dose Cartons of 100, Code 3P1033 NDC 0048-1040-13
75 mcg, violet
Bottles of 100, Code 3P1053 NDC 0048-1050-03
Bottles of 1000, Code 3P1055 NDC 0048-1050-05
Unit Dose Cartons of 100, Code 3P1003 NDC 0048-1050-13
88 mcg, olive
Bottles of 100, Code 3P0883 NDC 0048-1060-03
100 mcg, yellow
Bottles of 100, Code 3P1073 NDC 0048-1070-03
Bottles of 1000, Code 3P1075 NDC 0048-1070-05
Unit Dose Cartons of 100, Code 3P1063 NDC 0048-1070-13
112 mcg, rose
Bottles of 100, Code 3P1183 NDC 0048-1080-03
Bottles of 1000, Code 3P1185 NDC 0048-1080-05
Unit Dose Cartons of 100, Code 3P1193 NDC 0048-1080-13
125 mcg, brown
Bottles of 100, Code 3P1103 NDC 0048-1130-03
Bottles of 1000, Code 3P1105 NDC 0048-1130-05
Unit Dose Cartons of 100, Code 3P1113 NDC 0048-1130-13
150 mcg, blue
Bottles of 100, Code 3P1093 NDC 0048-1090-03
Bottles of 1000, Code 3P1095 NDC 0048-1090-05
Unit Dose Cartons of 100, Code 3P1083 NDC 0048-1090-13
175 mcg, lilac
Bottles of 100, Code 3P1153 NDC 0048-1100-03
200 mcg, pink
Bottles of 100, Code 3P1143 NDC 0048-1140-03
Bottles of 1000, Code 3P1145 NDC 0048-1140-05
Unit Dose Cartons of 100, Code 3P1133 NDC 0048-1140-13
300 mcg, green
Bottles of 100, Code 3P1173 NDC 0048-1170-03
Bottles of 1000, Code 3P1175 NDC 0048-1170-05
Unit Dose Cartons of 100, Code 3P1163 NDC 0048-1170-13

Store at controlled room temperature 15°–30°C (59°–86°F).

SYNTHROID® (Levothyroxine Sodium, USP) **Injection** is lyophilized with 10 mg Mannitol, USP and 0.7 mg tribasic sodium phosphate anhydrous in 10 mL vials. The pH may be adjusted with sodium hydroxide. It is supplied in color coded vials as follows:

200 mcg, gray
10 mL One Dose Vial, Code 3P1312 NDC 0048-1014-99
500 mcg, yellow
10 mL One Dose Vial, Code 3P1302 NDC 0048-1012-99

Store at controlled room temperature 15°–30° C (59°–86° F).

DIRECTIONS FOR RECONSTITUTION

Reconstitute the lyophilized levothyroxine sodium by aseptically adding 5 mL of 0.9% Sodium Chloride Injection, USP or Bacteriostatic Sodium Chloride Injection, USP with Benzyl Alcohol, only. Shake vial to insure complete mixing. **Use immediately** after reconstitution. Do not add to other intravenous fluids. Discard any unused portion.

Reference articles are available on request.

CAUTION: Federal (USA) law prohibits dispensing without a prescription.

Tablets
Manufactured by
Boots Pharmaceuticals PR, Inc.
Jayuya, Puerto Rico 00664-0795
Injection
Manufactured by
Baxter Healthcare Corporation
Cleveland, Mississippi 38732
For
Boots Pharmaceuticals, Inc.
Lincolnshire, Illinois 60069 USA
7920-03 Rev. 2/15/91

Shown in Product Identification Section, pages 405 & 406

TRAVASE® OINTMENT ℞

[*trāv'āz*]
(Sutilains Ointment, USP)

DESCRIPTION

TRAVASE® Ointment (Sutilains Ointment, USP) is a sterile topical preparation containing proteolytic enzymes, elaborated by *Bacillus subtilis*, in a hydrophobic ointment base consisting of 95% mineral oil and 5% polyethylene. One gram of ointment contains approximately 82,000 USP Casein Units* of proteolytic activity.

CLINICAL PHARMACOLOGY

TRAVASE Ointment selectively digests necrotic soft tissue by proteolytic action, thus facilitating the removal of necrotic tissue and purulent exudates that impair formation of granulation tissue and delay wound healing.

At body temperatures these proteolytic enzymes have optimal activity in the pH range from 6.0 to 6.8.

INDICATIONS AND USAGE

For wound debridement—TRAVASE Ointment is indicated as an adjunct to established methods of wound care for biochemical debridement of:

- Second and third degree burns,
- Decubitus ulcers,
- Incisional, traumatic, and pyogenic wounds,
- Ulcers secondary to peripheral vascular disease.

CONTRAINDICATIONS

Application of TRAVASE Ointment is contraindicated in:

- Wounds communicating with major body cavities,
- Wounds containing exposed major nerves or nervous tissue, and
- Fungating neoplastic ulcers.

WARNING

Do not permit TRAVASE Ointment to come into contact with the eyes. In the case of inadvertent contact, the eyes should be immediately rinsed with copious amounts of preferably sterile water.

*One USP Casein Unit of proteolytic activity is contained in the amount of sutilains which, when incubated with 35 mg of denatured casein at 37°C, produces in one minute a hydrolysate whose absorbance at 275 nm is equal to that of a tyrosine solution containing 1.5 micrograms of USP Tyrosine Reference Standard per mL.

Continued on next page

Boots—Cont.

PRECAUTIONS

A moist environment is essential for optimal activity of the enzyme. *In vitro*, several detergents and antiseptics (benzalkonium chloride, hexachlorophene, iodine, and nitrofurazone) may render the substrate indifferent to the action of the enzyme. Compounds such as thimerosal, containing metallic ions, interfere directly with enzyme activity to a slight degree, whereas neomycin, sulfamylon, streptomycin, and penicillin do not affect enzyme activity. If used concurrently with adjunctive topical therapy for 24–48 hours and no dissolution of slough occurs, then further therapy is not likely to be effective.

In cases of existent or threatening invasive infection, appropriate systemic antibiotic therapy should be instituted.

Although studies in humans have shown that there may be antibody response to absorbed enzyme material, there have been no reports of systemic allergic reaction to TRAVASE Ointment.

Pregnancy: Pregnancy category B: Studies in rabbits at doses up to two times the maximum human dose revealed no evidence of impaired fertility or fetal harm. There are, however, no adequate and well controlled studies in women. Because animal reproductive studies are not always predicative of human response, this drug should be used during pregnancy only if no adequate alternatives are available.

Pediatric Use: Safety and effectiveness in children have not been established.

ADVERSE REACTIONS

Adverse reactions consist of mild, transient pain, paresthesias, bleeding and transient dermatitis. Pain usually can be controlled by administration of mild analgesics. Side effects severe enough to warrant discontinuation of therapy have occurred occasionally.

If bleeding or dermatitis occurs as a result of the application of TRAVASE® Ointment (Sutilains Ointment, USP) therapy should be discontinued. No systemic toxicity has been observed as a result of the topical application of TRAVASE Ointment.

DOSAGE AND ADMINISTRATION

FOR TOPICAL USE ONLY—NOT FOR OPHTHALMIC USE.
ADHERENCE TO THE FOLLOWING IS SUGGESTED FOR OPTIMIZING THERAPEUTIC AFFECT:

1. Thoroughly cleanse and irrigate wound with sodium chloride solution or tap water. Wounds **MUST** be cleansed of antiseptics (e.g., hexachlorophene, benzalkonium chloride, nitrofurazone) or heavy-metal antibacterials (e.g., silver nitrate, thimerosal) which may alter substrate characteristics or denature the enzyme.
2. Thoroughly moisten wound area by tubbing, showering, or wet soaks (e.g., sodium chloride solution or tap water).
3. Apply approximately ⅛ inch (3mm) thick layer extending to ¼ to ½ inch (6mm to 12mm) beyond the area to be debrided, assuring intimate contact with necrotic tissue.
4. Apply a dressing that provides and maintains a moist environment.
5. Repeat entire procedure 3 to 4 times per day for best results.

HOW SUPPLIED

TRAVASE® Ointment (Sutilains Ointment, USP).
½ oz. (14.2 g) tube 3P3002 NDC 0048-1500-52
Refrigerate at 2° to 8°C (36°–46°F).
CAUTION: Federal (USA) law prohibits dispensing without prescription.

Boots Pharmaceuticals, Inc.
Lincolnshire, Illinois 60069 USA

8308-03 Rev. 10/16/91

Shown in Product Identification Section, page 406

EDUCATIONAL MATERIAL

Booklet-Pamphlet

"Thyroid Today" various authors, publication issued 4 times per year. Publication provides information written by physicians for physicians concerning thyroid disease diagnosis and treatment. Free to Physicians and Pharmacists.

Patient pamphlets on hypothyroidism. Free to Physicians and Pharmacists.

Educational Programs

Boots Pharmaceuticals, Inc. offers a modular series of educational programs on thyroid disease free to registered pharmacists, physicians.

Braintree Laboratories, Inc.
P.O. BOX 361
BRAINTREE, MA 02184

GoLYTELY® ℞
[*go-lit'lē*]
PEG-3350 and Electrolytes For Oral Solution

DESCRIPTION

A white powder for reconstitution containing 236 g polyethylene glycol 3350, 22.74 g sodium sulfate, 6.74 g sodium bicarbonate, 5.86 g sodium chloride, and 2.97 g potassium chloride. When dissolved in water to a volume of 4 liters, GoLYTELY is an isosmotic solution having a mildly salty taste. GoLYTELY is administered orally or via nasogastric tube.

CLINICAL PHARMACOLOGY

GoLYTELY induces a diarrhea which rapidly cleanses the bowel, usually within four hours. The osmotic activity of polyethylene glycol 3350 and the electrolyte concentration result in virtually no net absorption or excretion of ions or water. Accordingly, large volumes may be administered without significant changes in fluid or electrolyte balance.

INDICATIONS AND USAGE

GoLYTELY is indicated for bowel cleansing prior to colonoscopy and barium enema x-ray examination.

CONTRAINDICATIONS

GoLYTELY is contraindicated in patients with gastrointestinal obstruction, gastric retention, bowel perforation, toxic colitis, toxic megacolon or ileus.

WARNINGS

No additional ingredients, e.g. flavorings, should be added to the solution. GoLYTELY should be used with caution in patients with severe ulcerative colitis.

PRECAUTIONS

General: Patients with impaired gag reflex, unconscious or semiconscious patients, and patients prone to regurgitation or aspiration, should be observed during the administration of GoLYTELY, especially if it is administered via nasogastric tube. If a patient experiences severe bloating, distention or abdominal pain, administration should be slowed or temporarily discontinued until the symptoms abate. If gastrointestinal obstruction or perforation is suspected, appropriate studies should be performed to rule out these conditions before administration of GoLYTELY.

Information for patients: GoLYTELY produces a watery stool which cleanses the bowel before examination. Prepare the solution according to the instructions on the bottle. It is more palatable if chilled. For best results, no solid food should be consumed during the 3 to 4 hour period before drinking the solution, but in no case should solid foods be eaten within 2 hours of taking GoLYTELY.

Drink 240 ml (8 oz.) every 10 minutes. Rapid drinking of each portion is better than drinking small amounts continuously. The first bowel movement should occur approximately one hour after the start of GoLYTELY administration. You may experience some abdominal bloating and distention before the bowels start to move. If severe discomfort or distention occur, stop drinking temporarily or drink each portion at longer intervals until these symptoms disappear. Continue drinking until the watery stool is clear and free of solid matter. This usually requires at least 3 liters and it is best to drink all of the solution. Any unused portion should be discarded.

Drug Interactions: Oral medication administered within one hour of the start of administration of GoLYTELY may be flushed from the gastrointestinal tract and not absorbed.

Carcinogenesis, Mutagenesis, Impairment of Fertility: Carcinogenic and reproductive studies with animals have not been performed.

Pregnancy: Category C. Animal reproduction studies have not been conducted with GoLYTELY. It is also not known whether GoLYTELY can cause fetal harm when administered to a pregnant woman or can affect reproductive capacity. GoLYTELY should be given to a pregnant woman only if clearly needed.

Pediatric Use: Safety and effectiveness in children have not been established.

ADVERSE REACTIONS

Nausea, abdominal fullness and bloating are the most common adverse reactions (occurring in up to 50% of patients) to administration of GoLYTELY. Abdominal cramps, vomiting and anal irritation occur less frequently. These adverse reactions are transient and subside rapidly. Isolated cases of urticaria, rhinorrhea and dermatitis have been reported which may represent allergic reactions.

DOSAGE AND ADMINISTRATION

The recommended dose for adults is 4 liters of GoLYTELY solution prior to gastrointestinal examination, as ingestion of this dose produces a satisfactory preparation in over 95% of patients. Ideally the patient should fast for approximately three or four hours prior to GoLYTELY administration, but in no case should solid food be given for at least two hours before the solution is given.

GoLYTELY is usually administered orally, but may be given via nasogastric tube to patients who are unwilling or unable to drink the solution. **Oral administration** is at a rate of 240 ml (8 oz.) every 10 minutes, until 4 liters are consumed or the rectal effluent is clear. Rapid drinking of each portion is preferred to drinking small amounts continuously. **Nasogastric tube administration** is at the rate of 20–30 ml per minute (1.2–1.8 liters per hour). The first bowel movement should occur approximately one hour after the start of GoLYTELY administration.

Various regimens have been used. One method is to schedule patients for examination in midmorning or later, allowing the patients three hours for drinking and an additional one hour period for complete bowel evacuation. Another method is to administer GoLYTELY on the evening before the examination, particularly if the patient is to have a barium enema.

Preparation of the solution: GoLYTELY solution is prepared by filling the container to the 4 liter mark with water and shaking vigorously several times to insure that the ingredients are dissolved. Dissolution is facilitated by using lukewarm water. The solution is more palatable if chilled before administration. The reconstituted solution should be refrigerated and used within 48 hours. Discard any unused portion.

HOW SUPPLIED

In powdered form, for oral administration as a solution following reconstitution. Each disposable jug contains, in powdered form: polyethylene glycol 3350 236 g, sodium sulfate 22.74 g, sodium bicarbonate 6.74 g, sodium chloride 5.86 g, potassium chloride 2.97 g. When made up to 4 liters volume with water, the solution contains PEG 3350 17.6 mmol/L, sodium 125 mmol/L, sulfate 40 mmol/L, chloride 35 mmol/L, bicarbonate 20 mmol/L and potassium 10 mmol/L.

CAUTION

Federal law prohibits dispensing without prescription.

STORAGE

Store in sealed container at 59°–86°F. When reconstituted, keep solution refrigerated. Use within 48 hours. Discard unused portion.

NDC 52268-0100-01

Revised 7/1/87

Made by Lyne Laboratories, Stoughton, MA 02072 for BRAINTREE LABORATORIES, INC., Box 361, Braintree, MA 02184

Shown in Product Identification Section, page 406

NuLYTELY® ℞
PEG 3350, Sodium Chloride, Sodium Bicarbonate and Potassium Chloride for Oral Solution

DESCRIPTION

A white powder for reconstitution containing 420 g polyethylene glycol 3350, 5.72 g sodium bicarbonate, 11.2 g sodium chloride and 1.48 g potassium chloride. When dissolved in water to a volume of 4 liters, NuLYTELY is an isosmotic solution having a pleasant mineral water taste. NuLYTELY is administered orally or via nasogastric tube.

CLINICAL PHARMACOLOGY

NuLYTELY induces a diarrhea which rapidly cleanses the bowel, usually within four hours. The osmotic activity of polyethylene glycol 3350 and the electrolyte concentration result in virtually no net absorption of excretion of ions or water. Accordingly, large volumes may be administered without a significant changes in fluid or electrolyte balance.

INDICATIONS AND USAGE

NuLYTELY is indicated for bowel cleansing prior to colonoscopy.

CONTRAINDICATIONS

NuLYTELY is contraindicated in patients with gastrointestinal obstruction, gastric retention, bowel perforation, toxic colitis or toxic megacolon.

WARNINGS

No additional ingredients, e.g. flavorings, should be added to the solution. NuLYTELY should be used with caution in patients with severe ulcerative colitis.

PRECAUTIONS

General: Patients with impaired gag reflex, unconscious, or semiconscious patients, and patients prone to regurgitation or aspiration should be observed during the administration of NuLYTELY, especially if it is administered via nasogastric tubes. If a patient experiences severe bloating, distention or abdominal pain, administration should be slowed or temporarily discontinued until the symptoms abate. If gastrointestinal obstruction or perforation is suspected, appropriate

studies should be performed to rule out these conditions before administration of NuLYTELY.

Information for patients: NuLYTELY produces a watery stool which cleanses the bowel before examination. Prepare the solution according to the instructions on the bottle. It is more palatable if chilled. For best results, no solid foods should be consumed during the 3 to 4 hour period before drinking the solution, but in no case should solid foods be eaten within 2 hours of taking NuLYTELY.

Drink 240 ml (8 oz) every 10 minutes. Rapid drinking of each portion is better than drinking small amounts continuously. The first bowel movement should occur approximately one hour after the start of NuLYTELY administration. You may experience abdominal bloating and distention before the bowels start to move. If severe discomfort or distention occurs stop drinking temporarily or drink each portion at longer intervals until these symptoms disappear. Continue drinking until the water stool is clear and free of solid matter. This usually requires at least 3 liters. Any unused portion should be discarded.

Drug Interactions: Oral medication administered within one hour of the start of administration of NuLYTELY may be flushed from the gastrointestinal tract and not absorbed.

Carcinogenesis, Mutagenesis, Impairment of Fertility: Carcinogenic and reproductive studies with animals have not been performed. **Pregnancy:** Category C. Animal reproduction studies have not been conducted with NuLYTELY. It is also not known whether NuLYTELY can cause fetal harm when administered to a pregnant woman or can affect reproductive capacity. NuLYTELY should be given to a pregnant woman only if clearly needed.

Pediatric Use: Safety and effectiveness in children has not been established.

ADVERSE REACTIONS

Nausea, abdominal fullness and bloating are the most common adverse reactions (occurring in up to 50% of patients) to administration of NuLYTELY. Abdominal cramps, vomiting and anal irritation occur less frequently. These adverse reactions are transient and subside rapidly. Isolated cases of urticaria, rhinorrhea and dermatitis have been reported with a related drug (GoLYTELY®) which may represent allergic reactions.

DOSAGE AND ADMINISTRATION

NuLYTELY is usually administered orally, but may be given via nasogastric tube to patients who are unwilling or unable to drink the solution. Ideally, the patient should fast for approximately three or four hours prior to NuLYTELY administration, but in no case should solid food be given for at least two hours before the solution is given.

Oral administration is at a rate of 240 ml (8 oz.) every 10 minutes, until the rectal effluent is clear or 4 liters are consumed. Rapid drinking of each portion is preferred to drinking small amounts continuously. **Nasogastric tube administration** is at the rate of 20–30 ml per minute (1.2–1.8 liters per hour). The first bowel movement should occur approximately one hour after the start of NuLYTELY administration. Ingestion of 4 liters of NuLYTELY solution prior to gastrointestinal examination produces satisfactory preparation in over 95% of patients.

Various regimens have been used. One method is to schedule patients for examination in midmorning or later, allowing the patient three hours for drinking and an additional one hour period for complete bowel evacuation. Another method is to administer NuLYTELY on the evening before the examination.

Preparation of the solution: NuLYTELY solution is prepared by filling the container to the 4 liter mark with water and shaking vigorously several times to insure that the ingredients are dissolved. Dissolution is facilitated by using lukewarm water. The solution is more palatable if chilled before administration. The reconstituted solution should be refrigerated and used within 48 hours. Discard any unused portion.

HOW SUPPLIED

In powder form, for oral administration as a solution following reconstitution. Each disposable jug contains, in powdered form: polyethylene glycol 3350 420 g, sodium bicarbonate 5.72 g, sodium chloride 11.2 g, potassium chloride 1.48 g. When made up to 4 liters volumes with water, the solution contains PEG 3350 31.3 mmol/L, sodium 65 mmol/L, chloride 53 mmol/L, bicarbonate 17 mmol/L, and potassium 5 mmol/L.

CAUTION

Federal law prohibits dispensing without prescription.

STORAGE

Store in sealed container at 25°C. When reconstituted, keep solution refrigerated. Use within 48 hours. Discard unused portion.

NDC 52268-0300-01

Shown in Product Identification Section, page 406

PhosLo®   ℞
[phos "lō']
Calcium Acetate Tablets

DESCRIPTION

Each white round tablet (stamped "BRA 200") contains 667 mg of calcium acetate, USP (anhydrous; $Ca(CH_3COO)_2$; MW = 158.17 grams) equal to 169 mg (8.45 mEq) calcium, and 10 mg of the inert binder, polyethylene glycol 8000 NF.

CLINICAL PHARMACOLOGY

Patients with advanced renal insufficiency (creatinine clearance less than 30 ml/min) exhibit phosphate retention and some degree of hyperphosphatemia. The retention of phosphate plays a pivotal role in causing secondary hyperparathyroidism associated with osteodystrophy, and soft tissue calcification. The mechanism by which phosphate retention leads to hyperparathyroidism is not clearly delineated. Therapeutic efforts directed toward the control of hyperphosphatemia include reduction in the dietary intake of phosphate, inhibition of absorption of phosphate in the intestine with phosphate binders, and removal of phosphate from the body by more efficient methods of dialysis. The rate of removal of phosphate by dietary manipulation or by dialysis is insufficient. Dialysis patients absorb 40% to 80% of dietary phosphorous. Therefore, the fraction of dietary phosphate absorbed from the diet needs to be reduced by using phopsphate binders in most renal failure patients on maintenance dialysis. Calcium acetate (PhosLo) when taken with meals, combines with dietary phosphate to form insoluble phosphate which is excreted in the feces. Maintenance of serum phosphorus below 6.0 mg/dl is generally considered as a clinically acceptable outcome of treatment with phosphate binders. PhosLo is highly soluble at neutral pH, making the calcium readily available for binding to phosphate in the proximal small intestine.

Orally administered calcium acetate from pharmaceutical dosage forms has been demonstrated to be systemically absorbed up to approximately 40% under fasting conditions and up to approximately 30% under nonfasting conditions. This range represents data from both healthy subjects and renal dialysis patients under various conditions.

INDICATIONS AND USAGE

PhosLo is indicated for the control of hyperphosphatemia in end stage renal failure and does not promote aluminum absorption.

CONTRAINDICATIONS

Patients with hypercalcemia.

WARNINGS

Patients with end stage renal failure may develop hypercalcemia when given calcium with meals. No other calcium supplements should be given concurrently with PhosLo. Progressive hypercalcemia due to overdose of PhosLo may be severe as to require emergency measures. Chronic hypercalcemia may lead to vascular calcification, and other soft-tissue calcification. The serum calcium level should be monitored twice weekly during the early dose adjustment period. **The serum calcium times phosphate (CaXP) product should not be allowed to exceed 66.** Radiographic evaluation of suspect anatomical region may be helpful in early detection of soft-tissue calcification.

PRECAUTIONS

General: Excessive dosage of PhosLo induces hypercalcemia; therefore, early in the treatment during dosage adjustment serum calcium should be determined twice weekly. Should hypercalcemia develop, the dosage should be reduced or the treatment discontinued immediately depending on the severity of hypercalcemia. PhosLo should not be given to patients on digitalis, because hypercalcemia may precipitate cardiac arrhythmias. PhosLo therapy should always be started at low dose and should not be increased without careful monitoring of serum calcium. An estimate of daily calcium intake should be made initially and the intake adjusted as needed. Serum phosphorus should also be determined periodically.

Information for the patient: The patient should be informed about compliance with dosage instructions, adherence to instructions about diet and avoidance of the use of nonprescription anatacids. Patients should be informed about the symptoms of hypercalcemia (see ADVERSE REACTIONS section).

Drug interactions: PhosLo may decrease the bioavailability of tetracyclines.

Carcinogenesis, mutagenesis, impairment of fertility: Long term animal studies have not been performed to evaluate the carcinogenic potential or effect on fertility of PhosLo.

Pregnancy: teratogenic effects: Category C. Animal reproduction studies have not been conducted with PhosLo. It is also not known whether PhosLo can cause fetal harm when administered to a pregnant woman or can affect reproduction capacity. PhosLo should be given to a pregnant woman only if clearly needed.

Pediatric use: Safety and efficacy of PhosLo have not been established.

ADVERSE REACTIONS

In clinical studies, patients have occasionally experienced nausea during PhosLo therapy. Hypercalcemia may occur during treatment with PhosLo. Mild hypercalcemia (Ca > 10.5 mg/dl) may be asymptomatic or manifest itself as constipation, anorexia, nausea and vomiting. More severe hypercalcemia (Ca > 12 mg/dl) is associated with confusion, delerium, stupor and coma. Mild hypercalcemia is easily controlled by reducing the PhosLo dose or temporarily discontinuing therapy. Severe hypercalcemia can be treated by acute hemodialysis and discontinuing PhosLo therapy. Decreasing dialysate calcium concentration could reduce the incidence and severity of PhosLo-induced hypercalcemia. The long-term effect of PhosLo on the progression of vascular or soft-tissue calcification has not been determined. Isolated cases of pruritus have been reported which may represent allergic reactions.

OVERDOSAGE

Administration of PhosLo in excess of the appropriate daily dosage can cause severe hypercalcemia (See Adverse Reactions).

DOSAGE AND ADMINISTRATION

The recommended initial dose of PhosLo for the adult dialysis patient is 2 tablets with each meal. The dosage may be increased gradually to bring serum phosphate value below 6 mg/dl, as long as hypercalcemia does not develop. Most patients require 3–4 tablets with each meal.

Store at controlled room temperature, 15°–30°C.

HOW SUPPLIED

In tablet form for oral administration. Each white round tablet contains 667 mg calcium acetate (anhydrous; $Ca(CH_3COO)_2$; MW = 158.17 equal to 169 mg (8.45 mEq) calcium and 10 mg of the inert binder, polyethylene glycol 8000. NDC 52268-0200-01

Shown in Product Identification Section, page 406

EDUCATIONAL MATERIAL

GoLYTELY® and NuLYTELY®

Booklets
Complimentary patient booklets are available: "Bowel Preparation Before Your Colonoscopy."

Physician Support
GoLYTELY and NuLYTELY prescription pads and other materials are available.

PhosLo®

Brochures
Patient information booklets explaining importance of phosphate binding and PhosLo® therapy are available upon request.

Physician Support
PhosLo® prescription pads and other office/clinical material are also available.

Products are
listed alphabetically
in the
PINK SECTION.

Products are cross-indexed
by product classifications
in the
BLUE SECTION.

Products are cross-indexed by
generic and chemical names
in the
YELLOW SECTION.

Bristol Laboratories
A Bristol-Myers Squibb Company
P.O. BOX 4500
PRINCETON, NJ 08543-4500

CEFZIL™ ℞
(CEFPROZIL)
Tablets
250 mg and 500 mg
CEFZIL™
(CEFPROZIL)
for Oral Suspension
125 mg/5 mL and 250 mg/5mL

This is the full text of the latest Official Package Circular dated February 1992 (7718DIM-03).

DESCRIPTION
CEFZIL™ (cefprozil) is a semi-synthetic broad-spectrum cephalosporin antibiotic.
Cefprozil is a cis and trans isomeric mixture ($\geq 90\%$ cis). The chemical name for the monohydrate is (6R,7R)-7-[(R)-2-amino-2- (p-hydroxy-phenyl) acetamido]-8-oxo-3-propenyl-5-thia-1-azabicyclo [4.2.0]oct-2-ene-2- carboxylic acid monohydrate, and the structural formula is:

Cefprozil is a white to yellowish powder with a molecular formula for the monohydrate of $C_{18}H_{19}N_3O_5S \cdot H_2O$ and a molecular weight of 407.45.
CEFZIL tablets and CEFZIL for oral suspension are intended for oral administration.
CEFZIL tablets contain cefprozil equivalent to 250 mg or 500 mg of anhydrous cefprozil. In addition, each tablet contains the following inactive ingredients: cellulose, hydroxypropylmethylcellulose, magnesium stearate, methylcellulose, simethicone, sodium starch glycolate, polyethylene glycol, polysorbate 80, sorbic acid, and titanium dioxide. The 250 mg tablets also contain FD&C Yellow No. 6.
CEFZIL for oral suspension contains cefprozil equivalent to 125 mg or 250 mg anhydrous cefprozil per 5 mL constituted suspension. In addition, the oral suspension contains the following inactive ingredients: aspartame, cellulose, citric acid, colloidal silicone dioxide, FD&C Red No. 3, flavors (natural and artificial), glycine, polysorbate 80, simethicone, sodium benzoate, sodium carboxymethylcellulose, sodium chloride, and sucrose.

CLINICAL PHARMACOLOGY
Following oral administration of cefprozil to fasting subjects, approximately 95% of the dose was absorbed. Using the investigational capsule formulation, no food effect was observed. The food effect on the tablet and on the suspension formulations has not been studied.
The pharmacokinetic data were derived from the capsule dosing; however, bioequivalence has been demonstrated for the oral solution, capsule, tablet and suspension formulations under fasting conditions.
Average peak plasma concentrations after administration of 250 mg, 500 mg, or 1 g doses of cefprozil to fasting subjects were approximately 6.1, 10.5, and 18.3 mcg/mL respectively, and were obtained within 1.5 hours after dosing. Urinary recovery accounted for approximately 60% of the administered dose. (See Table.)
During the first 4-hour period after drug administration, the average urine concentrations following the 250 mg, 500 mg, and 1g doses were approximately 700 mcg/mL, 1000 mcg/mL, and 2900 mcg/mL.
Plasma protein binding is approximately 36% and is independent of concentration in the range of 2 mcg/mL to 20 mcg/mL.
The average plasma half-life in normal subjects is 1.3 hours. There was no evidence of accumulation of cefprozil in the plasma in individuals with normal renal function following multiple oral doses of up to 1000 mg every 8 hours for 10 days.

In patients with reduced renal function, the plasma half-life may be prolonged up to 5.2 hours depending on the degree of the renal dysfunction. In patients with complete absence of renal function the plasma half-life of cefprozil has been shown to be as long as 5.9 hours. The half-life is shortened during hemodialysis. Excretion pathways in patients with markedly impaired renal function have not been determined. (See PRECAUTIONS and DOSAGE AND ADMINISTRATION.)
The average AUC observed in elderly subjects (≥ 65 years of age) is approximately 35%–60% higher relative to young adults, and the average AUC in females is approximately 15%–20% higher than in males. The magnitude of these age and gender related changes in the pharmacokinetics of cefprozil are not sufficient to necessitate dosage adjustments.
In patients with impaired hepatic function, the half-life increases to approximately 2 hours. The magnitude of the changes does not warrant a dosage adjustment for patients with impaired hepatic function.
Adequate data on CSF levels of cefprozil are not available.

MICROBIOLOGY
Cefprozil has in vitro activity against a broad range of gram-positive and gram-negative bacteria. The bactericidal action of cefprozil results from inhibition of cell-wall synthesis. Cefprozil has been shown to be active against most strains of the following organisms both in vitro and in clinical infections. (See INDICATIONS AND USAGE.)
AEROBES, GRAM-POSITIVE:
Staphylococcus aureus
(including penicillinase-producing strains)
   NOTE: Cefprozil is inactive against methicillin-resistant staphylococci
Streptococcus pneumoniae
Streptococcus pyogenes
AEROBES, GRAM-NEGATIVE:
Moraxella (Branhamella) catarrhalis
Haemophilus influenzae
(including penicillinase-producing strains)
The following in vitro data are available; however, their clinical significance is unknown.
Cefprozil exhibits in vitro minimum inhibitory concentrations (MIC) of 8 mcg/mL or less against most strains of the following organisms. The safety and efficacy of cefprozil in treating infections due to these organisms have not been established in adequate and well-controlled trials.
AEROBES, GRAM-POSITIVE:
Enterococcus durans
Enterococcus faecalis
   NOTE: Cefprozil is inactive against *Enterococcus faecium*.
Listeria monocytogenes
Staphylococcus epidermidis
Staphylococcus saprophyticus
Staphylococcus warneri
Streptococci (Groups C, D, F, and G)
viridans group Streptococci
AEROBES, GRAM-NEGATIVE:
Citrobacter diversus
Escherichia coli
Klebsiella pneumoniae
Neisseria gonorrhoeae
(including penicillinase-producing strains)
Proteus mirabilis
Salmonella spp.
Shigella spp.
Vibrio spp.
   NOTE: Cefprozil is inactive against most strains of *Acinetobacter, Enterobacter, Morganella morganii, Proteus vulgaris, Providencia, Pseudomonas,* and *Serratia.*
ANAEROBES:
Bacteroides melaninogenicus
   NOTE: Most strains of the *Bacteroides fragilis* group are resistant to cefprozil.
Clostridium perfringens
Clostridium difficile
Fusobacterium spp.
Peptostreptococcus spp.
Propionibacterium acnes

SUSCEPTIBILITY TESTS
Diffusion Techniques
Quantitative methods that require measurement of zone diameters give the most precise estimate of the susceptibility of bacteria to antimicrobial agents. One such standardized

procedure recommended for use with the 30-mcg cefprozil disk is the National Committee for Clinical Laboratory Standards (NCCLS) approved procedure.[1] Interpretation involves correlation of the diameter obtained in the disk test with minimum inhibitory concentration (MIC) for cefprozil.
The class disk for cephalosporin susceptibility testing (the cephalothin disk) is not appropriate because of spectrum differences with cefprozil. The 30-mcg cefprozil disk should be used for all in vitro testing of isolates.
Reports from the laboratory giving results of the standard single-disk susceptibility test with a 30-mcg cefprozil disk should be interpreted according to the following criteria:

Zone diameter (mm)	Interpretation
≥ 18	(S) Susceptible
15–17	(MS) Moderately Susceptible
≤ 14	(R) Resistant

A report of "Susceptible" indicates that the pathogen is likely to be inhibited by generally achievable blood concentrations. A report of "Moderately Susceptible" indicates that the organism would be susceptible if high dosage is used or if the infection is confined to tissues and fluids (eg, urine) in which high antibiotic levels are attained. A report of "Resistant" indicates that the achievable concentration of the antibiotic is unlikely to be inhibitory and other therapy should be selected.
Standardized procedures require the use of laboratory control organisms. The 30-mcg cefprozil disk should give the following zone diameters:

Organism	Zone diameter (mm)
Escherichia coli ATCC 25922	21–27
Staphylococcus aureus ATCC 25923	27–33

Dilution Techniques
Use a standardized dilution method[2] (broth, agar, microdilution) or equivalent with cefprozil powder. The MIC values obtained should be interpreted according to the following criteria:

MIC (mcg/mL)	Interpretation
≤ 8	(S) Susceptible
16	(MS) Moderately Susceptible
≥ 32	(R) Resistant

As with standard diffusion techniques, dilution techniques require the use of laboratory control organisms. Standard cefprozil powder should give the following MIC values:

Organism	MIC (mcg/mL)
Enterococcus faecalis ATCC 29212	4–16
Escherichia coli ATCC 25922	1–4
Pseudomonas aeruginosa ATCC 27853	> 32
Staphylococcus aureus ATCC 29213	0.25–1

INDICATIONS AND USAGE
CEFZIL™ (cefprozil) is indicated for the treatment of patients with mild to moderate infections caused by susceptible strains of the designated microorganisms in the conditions listed below:
UPPER RESPIRATORY TRACT
Pharyngitis/Tonsillitis caused by *Streptococcus pyogenes.*
   NOTE: The usual drug of choice in the treatment and prevention of streptococcal infections, including the prophylaxis of rheumatic fever, is penicillin given by the intramuscular route. Cefprozil is generally effective in the eradication of *Streptococcus pyogenes* from the nasopharynx; however, substantial data establishing the efficacy of cefprozil in the subsequent prevention of rheumatic fever are not available at present.
Otitis Media caused by *Streptococcus pneumoniae, Haemophilus influenzae* and *Moraxella (Branhamella) catarrhalis.* (See CLINICAL STUDIES section.)
   NOTE: In the treatment of otitis media due to beta-lactamase producing organisms, cefprozil had bacteriologic eradication rates somewhat lower than those observed with a product containing a specific beta-lactamase inhibitor. In considering the use of cefprozil, lower overall eradication rates should be balanced against the susceptibility patterns of the common microbes in a given geographic area and the increased potential for toxicity with products containing beta-lactamase inhibitors.
LOWER RESPIRATORY TRACT
Secondary Bacterial Infection of Acute Bronchitis and Acute Bacterial Exacerbation of Chronic Bronchitis caused by *Streptococcus pneumoniae, Haemophilus influenzae,* (beta-lactamase positive and negative strains), and *Moraxella (Branhamella) catarrhalis.*
SKIN AND SKIN STRUCTURE
Uncomplicated Skin and Skin-Structure Infections caused by *Staphylococcus aureus* (including penicillinase-producing strains) and *Streptococcus pyrogenes.* Abscesses usually require surgical drainage.
Culture and susceptibility testing should be performed when appropriate to determine susceptibility of the causative organism to cefprozil.

CONTRAINDICATIONS
CEFZIL is contraindicated in patients with known allergy to the cephalosporin class of antibiotics.

Dosage (mg)	Mean Plasma Cefprozil* Concentrations (mcg/mL)			8-hour Urinary Excretion (%)
	Peak appx. 1.5 hr	4 hr	8 hr	
250 mg	6.1	1.7	0.2	60%
500 mg	10.5	3.2	0.4	62%
1000 mg	18.3	8.4	1.0	54%

* Data represent mean values of 12 healthy volunteers.

WARNINGS

BEFORE THERAPY WITH CEFZIL IS INSTITUTED, CAREFUL INQUIRY SHOULD BE MADE TO DETERMINE WHETHER THE PATIENT HAS HAD PREVIOUS HYPERSENSITIVITY REACTIONS TO CEFZIL, CEPHALOSPORINS, PENICILLINS, OR OTHER DRUGS. IF THIS PRODUCT IS TO BE GIVEN TO PENICILLIN-SENSITIVE PATIENTS, CAUTION SHOULD BE EXERCISED BECAUSE CROSS-SENSITIVITY AMONG BETA-LACTAM ANTIBIOTICS HAS BEEN CLEARLY DOCUMENTED AND MAY OCCUR IN UP TO 10% OF PATIENTS WITH A HISTORY OF PENICILLIN ALLERGY. IF AN ALLERGIC REACTION TO CEFZIL OCCURS, DISCONTINUE THE DRUG. SERIOUS ACTUE HYPERSENSITIVITY REACTIONS MAY REQUIRE TREATMENT WITH EPINEPHRINE AND OTHER EMERGENCY MEASURES, INCLUDING OXYGEN, INTRAVENOUS FLUIDS, INTRAVENOUS ANTIHISTAMINES, CORTICOSTEROIDS, PRESSOR AMINES, AND AIRWAY MANAGEMENT, AS CLINICALLY INDICATED.

Pseudomembranous colitis has been reported with nearly all antibacterial agents, and may range from mild to life-threatening. Therefore, it is important to consider this diagnosis in patients who present with diarrhea subsequent to the administration of antibacterial agents.

Treatment with antibacterial agents alters the normal flora of the colon and may permit overgrowth of clostridia. Studies indicate that a toxin produced by Clostridium difficile is a primary cause of "antibiotic-associated colitis".

After the diagnosis of pseudomembranous colitis has been established, therapeutic measures should be initiated. Mild cases of pseudomembranous colitis usually respond to discontinuation of the drug alone. In moderate to severe cases, consideration should be given to management with fluids and electrolytes, protein supplementation and treatment with an antibacterial drug effective against Clostridium difficile.

PRECAUTIONS

General

Evaluation of renal status before and during therapy is recommended, especially in seriously ill patients. In patients with known or suspected renal impairment (see DOSAGE AND ADMINISTRATION), careful clinical observation and appropriate laboratory studies should be done prior to and during therapy. The total daily dose of CEFZIL™ (cefprozil) should be reduced in these patients because high and/or prolonged plasma antibiotic concentrations can occur in such individuals from usual doses. Cephalosporins, including CEFZIL, should be given with caution to patients receiving concurrent treatment with potent diuretics since these agents are suspected of adversely affecting renal function. Prolonged use of CEFZIL may result in the overgrowth of nonsusceptible organisms. Careful observation of the patient is essential. If superinfection occurs during therapy, appropriate measures should be taken.

Cefprozil should be prescribed with caution in individuals with a history of gastrointestinal disease particularly colitis.

Positive direct Coombs' tests have been reported during treatment with cephalosporin antibiotics.

Information for Patients

Phenylketonurics: CEFZIL for oral suspension contains phenylalanine 28 mg per 5 mL (1 teaspoon) constituted suspension for both the 125 mg/5mL and 250 mg/5mL dosage forms.

Drug Interactions

Nephrotoxicity has been reported following concomitant administration of aminoglycoside antibiotics and cephalosporin antibiotics. Concomitant administration of probenecid doubled the AUC for cefprozil.

Drug/Laboratory Test Interactions

Cephalosporin antibiotics may produce a false positive reaction for glucose in the urine with copper reduction tests (Benedict's or Fehling's solution or with Clinitest®[3] tablets), but not with enzyme-based tests for glycosuria (eg, Tes-Tape®[4]). A false negative reaction may occur in the ferricyanide test for blood glucose. The presence of cefprozil in the blood does not interfere with the assay of plasma or urine creatinine by the alkaline picrate method.

Carcinogenesis, Mutagenesis, and Impairment of Fertility

No mutagenic potential of cefprozil was found in appropriate prokaryotic or eukaryotic cells in vitor or in vivo. No in vivo long-term studies have been performed to evaluate carcinogenic potential.

Reproductive studies revealed no impairment of fertility in animals.

Pregnancy: Teratogenic Effects. Pregnancy Category B

Reproduction studies have been performed in mice, rats, and rabbits at doses 14, 7, and 0.7 times the maximum daily human dose (1000 mg) based upon mg/m², and have revealed no evidence of harm to the fetus due to cefprozil. There are, however, no adequate and well-controlled studies in pregnant women. Because animal reproduction studies are not always predictive of human response, this drug should be used during pregnancy only if clearly needed.

Population/Infection	Dosage (mg)	Duration (days)
ADULTS (13 years and older)		
UPPER RESPIRATORY TRACT		
Pharyngitis/Tonsilitis	500 q 24h	10*
LOWER RESPIRATORY TRACT	500 q 12h	10
Secondary Bacterial Infection of Acute Bronchitis and Acute Bacterial Exacerbation of Chronic Bronchitis		
SKIN AND SKIN STRUCTURE		
Uncomplicated Skin and Skin Structure Infections	250 q 12h or 500 q 24h or 500 q 12h	10
INFANTS & CHILDREN (6 months–12 years)		
UPPER RESPIRATORY TRACT		
Otitis Media (See INDICATIONS AND USAGE and CLINICAL STUDIES sections)	15 mg/kg q 12h	10

*In the treatment of infections due to Streptococcus pyogenes, CEFZIL should be administered for at least 10 days.

Labor and Delivery

Cefprozil has not been studied for use during labor and delivery. Treatment should only be given if clearly needed.

Nursing Mothers

It is not known whether cefprozil is excreted in human milk. Because many drugs are excreted in human milk, caution should be exercised when CEFZIL™ (cefprozil) is administered to a nursing mother.

Pediatric Use

Safety and effectiveness in children below the age of 6 months have not been established. However, accumulation of other cephalosporin antibiotics in newborn infants (resulting from prolonged drug half-life in this age group) has been reported.

Geratric Use

Healthy geriatric volunteers (≥ 65 years old) who received a single 1 g dose of cefprozil had 35%–60% higher AUC and 40% lower renal clearance values when compared to healthy adult volunteers 20–40 years of age. In clinical studies, when geriatric patients received the usual recommended adult doses, clinical efficacy and safety were acceptable and comparable to results in nongeriatric adult patients.

ADVERSE REACTIONS

The adverse reactions to cefprozil are similar to those observed with other orally administered cephalosporins. Cefprozil was usually well tolerated in controlled clinical trials. Approximately 2% of patients discontinued cefprozil therapy due to adverse events.

The most common adverse effects observed in patients treated with cefprozil are:

Gastrointestinal—Diarrhea (2.9%), nausea (3.5%), vomiting (1%) and abdominal pain (1%).

Hepatobiliary—Elevation of AST (SGOT) (2%), ALT (SGPT) (2%), alkaline phosphatase (0.2%), and bilirubin values (<0.1%). As with some penicillins and some other cephalosporin antibiotics, cholestatic jaundice has been reported rarely.

Hypersensitivity—Rash (0.9%), urticaria (0.1%). Such reactions have been reported more frequently in children than in adults. Signs and symptoms usually occur a few days after initiation of therapy and subside within a few days after cessation of therapy.

CNS—Dizziness (1%), Hyperactivity, headache, nervousness, insomnia, confusion, and somnolence have been reported rarely (<1%). All were reversible.

Hematopoietic—Decreased leukocyte count (0.2%), eosinophilia (2.3%).

Renal—Elevated BUN (0.1%), serum creatinine (0.1%).

Other—Diaper rash and superinfection (1.5%), genital pruritus and vaginitis (1.6%).

Cephalosporin class paragraph

In addition to the adverse reactions listed above which have been observed in patients treated with cefprozil, the following adverse reactions and altered laboratory tests have been reported for cephalosporin-class antibiotics:

Anaphylaxis, Stevens-Johnson syndrome, erythema multiforme, toxic epidermal necrolysis, serum-sickness like reaction, fever, renal dysfunction, toxic nephropathy, aplastic anemia, hemolytic anemia, hemorrhage, prolonged prothrombin time, positive Coombs' test, elevated LDH, pancytopenia, neutropenia agranulocytosis, thrombocytopenia.

Several cephalosporins have been implicated in triggering seizures, particularly in patients with renal impairment, when the dosage was not reduced. (See DOSAGE AND ADMINISTRATION and OVERDOSAGE.) If seizures associated with drug therapy occur, the drug should be discontinued. Anticonvulsant therapy can be given if clinically indicated.

OVERDOSAGE

Cefprozil is eliminated primarily by the kidneys. In case of severe overdosage, especially in patients with comprised renal function, hemodialysis will aid in the removal of cefprozil from the body.

DOSAGE AND ADMINISTRATION

CEFZIL™ (cefprozil) is administered orally.
[See table above.]

Renal Impairment

Cefprozil may be administered to patients with impaired renal function. The following dosage schedule should be used

Creatinine Clearance (mL/min)	Dosage (mg)	Dosing Interval
30–120	standard	standard
0–30*	50% of standard	standard

*Cefprozil is in part removed by hemodialysis; therefore, cefprozil should be administered after the completion of hemodialysis.

Hepatic Impairment

No dosage adjustment is necessary for patients with impaired hepatic function.

HOW SUPPLIED

CEFZIL™ (cefprozil) Tablets

Each light orange film-coated tablet, imprinted with "BMS 7720 250", contains the equivalent of 250 mg anhydrous cefprozil.

Bottles of 100 Tablets	NDC 0087-7720-60
Cartons of 100 Tablets	NDC 0087-7720-66

(10 strips containing 10 tablets on each strip)

Each white film-coated tablet, imprinted with "BMS 7721 500", contains the equivalent of 500 mg anhydrous cefprozil.

Bottles of 100 Tablets	NDC 0087-7721-60
Cartons of 100 Tablets	NDC 0087-7721-66

(10 strips containing 10 tablets on each strip)

Store at controlled room temperature, 59° to 86°F (15° to 30°C).

CEFZIL™ (cefprozil) For Oral Suspension

Each 5 mL of constituted suspension contains the equivalent of 125 mg anhydrous cefprozil.

50 mL Bottle	NDC 0087-7718-40
100 mL Bottle	NDC 0087-7718-64

Each 5 mL of constituted suspension contains the equivalent of 250 mg anhydrous cefprozil.

50 mL Bottle	NDC 0087-7719-40
100 mL Bottle	NDC 0087-7719-64

All powder formulations for oral suspension contain cefprozil in a bubble-gum flavored mixture. Directions for mixing are included on the label. After mixing, store in a refrigerator, and discard unused portion after 14 days.

Store at controlled room temperature, 59° to 86°F (15° to 30°C) prior to constitution.

CLINICAL STUDIES

Study One:

In a controlled clinical study of acute otitis media performed in the United States, where significant rates of beta-lactamase producing organisms were found, cefprozil was compared to an oral antimicrobial agent that contained a specific beta-lactamase inhibitor. In this study, using very strict evaluability criteria and microbiologic and clinical response criteria at the 10–16 days post-therapy follow-up, the following presumptive bacterial eradication/clinical cure outcomes (ie, clinical success) and safety results were obtained:

Continued on next page

Bristol Laboratories—Cont.

U.S. Acute Otitis Media Study
Cefprozil vs. beta-lactamase inhibitor-containing control drug

Efficacy

Pathogen	% of Cases with Pathogen (n=155)	Outcome
S. pneumoniae	48.4%	cefprozil success rate 5% better than control
H. influenzae	35.5%	cefprozil success rate 17% less than control
M. catarrhalis	13.5%	cefprozil success rate 12% less than control
S. pyogenes	2.6%	cefprozil equivalent to control
Overall	100.0%	cefprozil success rate 5% less than control

Safety

The incidence of adverse events, primarily diarrhea and rash,* were clinically and statistically significantly higher in the control arm versus the cefprozil arm.

Age Group	Cefprozil	Control
6 months–2 years	21%	41%
3–12 years	10%	19%

Study Two:

In a controlled clinical study of acute otitis media performed in Europe, cefprozil was compared to an oral antimicrobial agent that contained a specific beta-lactamase inhibitor. As expected in a European population, this study had a lower incidence of beta-lactamase-producing organisms than usually seen in U.S. trials. In this study, using very strict evaluability criteria and microbiologic and clinical response criteria at the 10–16 days post-therapy follow-up, the following presumptive bacterial eradication/clinical cure outcomes (ie, clinical success) were obtained:

European Acute Otitis Media Study
Cefprozil vs. beta-lactamase inhibitor-containing control drug

Efficacy

Pathogen	% of Cases with Pathogen (n=47)	Outcome
S. pneumoniae	51.0%	cefprozil equivalent to control
H. influenzae	29.8%	cefprozil equivalent to control
M. catarrhalis	6.4%	cefprozil equivalent to control
S. pyogenes	12.8%	cefprozil equivalent to control
Overall	100.0%	cefprozil equivalent to control

Safety

The incidence of adverse events in the cefprozil arm was comparable to the incidence of adverse events in the control arm (agent that contained a specific beta-lactamase inhibitor).

REFERENCES

1. National Committee for Clinical Laboratory Standards, *Performance Standards for Antimicrobial Disk Susceptibility Tests—Fourth Edition.* Approved Standard NCCLS Document M2-A4, Vol. 10, No. 7, NCCLS, Villanova, PA, April, 1990.
2. National Committee for Clinical Laboratory Standards, *Methods for Dilution Antimicrobial Susceptibility Tests for Bacteria that Grow Aerobically—Second Edition.* Approved Standard NCCLS Document M7-A2, Vol. 10, No. 8, NCCLS, Villanova, PA, April, 1990.
3. Clinitest® is registered trademark of Miles Laboratories, Inc.
4. Tes-Tape® is a registered trademark of Eli Lilly and Company.

*The majority of these involved the diaper area in young children.

Shown in Product Identification Section, page 406

CORGARD® TABLETS ℞

[kor'gard]
Nadolol Tablets, USP

DESCRIPTION

CORGARD (nadolol) is a synthetic nonselective beta-adrenergic receptor blocking agent designated chemically as 1-(*tert*-butylamino)-3-[(5,6,7,8-tetrahydro-*cis*-6,7-dihydroxy-1-naphthyl)oxy]-2-propanol. Structural formula:
[See chemical structure at top of next column.]

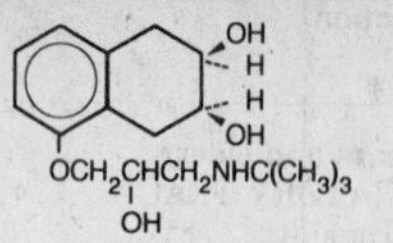

$C_{17}H_{27}NO_4$ MW 309.40 CAS-42200-33-9

Nadolol is a white crystalline powder. It is freely soluble in ethanol, soluble in hydrochloric acid, slightly soluble in water and in chloroform, and very slightly soluble in sodium hydroxide.

CORGARD (nadolol) is available for oral administration as 20 mg, 40 mg, 80 mg, 120 mg, and 160 mg tablets. Inactive ingredients: microcrystalline cellulose, colorant (FD&C Blue No. 2), corn starch, magnesium stearate, povidone (except 20 mg and 40 mg), and other ingredients.

CLINICAL PHARMACOLOGY

CORGARD (nadolol) is a nonselective beta-adrenergic receptor blocking agent. Clinical pharmacology studies have demonstrated beta-blocking activity by showing (1) reduction in heart rate and cardiac output at rest and on exercise, (2) reduction of systolic and diastolic blood pressure at rest and on exercise, (3) inhibition of isoproterenol-induced tachycardia, and (4) reduction of reflex orthostatic tachycardia.

CORGARD (nadolol) specifically competes with beta-adrenergic receptor agonists for available beta receptor sites; it inhibits both the $beta_1$ receptors located chiefly in cardiac muscle and the $beta_2$ receptors located chiefly in the bronchial and vascular musculature, inhibiting the chronotropic, inotropic, and vasodilator responses to beta-adrenergic stimulation proportionately. CORGARD has no intrinsic sympathomimetic activity and, unlike some other beta-adrenergic blocking agents, nadolol has little direct myocardial depressant activity and does not have an anesthetic-like membrane-stabilizing action. Animal and human studies show that CORGARD slows the sinus rate and depresses AV conduction. In dogs, only minimal amounts of nadolol were detected in the brain relative to amounts in blood and other organs and tissues. CORGARD has low lipophilicity as determined by octanol/water partition coefficient, a characteristic of certain beta-blocking agents that has been correlated with the limited extent to which these agents cross the blood-brain barrier, their low concentration in the brain, and low incidence of CNS-related side effects.

In controlled clinical studies, CORGARD (nadolol) at doses of 40 to 320 mg/day has been shown to decrease both standing and supine blood pressure, the effect persisting for approximately 24 hours after dosing.

The mechanism of the antihypertensive effects of beta-adrenergic receptor blocking agents has not been established; however, factors that may be involved include (1) competitive antagonism of catecholamines at peripheral (non-CNS) adrenergic neuron sites (especially cardiac) leading to decreased cardiac output, (2) a central effect leading to reduced tonic-sympathetic nerve outflow to the periphery, and (3) suppression of renin secretion by blockade of the beta-adrenergic receptors responsible for renin release from the kidneys.

While cardiac output and arterial pressure are reduced by nadolol therapy, renal hemodynamics are stable, with preservation of renal blood flow and glomerular filtration rate.

By blocking catecholamine-induced increases in heart rate, velocity and extent of myocardial contraction, and blood pressure, CORGARD (nadolol) generally reduces the oxygen requirements of the heart at any given level of effort, making it useful for many patients in the long-term management of angina pectoris. On the other hand, nadolol can increase oxygen requirements by increasing left ventricular fiber length and end diastolic pressure, particularly in patients with heart failure.

Although beta-adrenergic receptor blockade is useful in treatment of angina and hypertension, there are also situations in which sympathetic stimulation is vital. For example, in patients with severely damaged hearts, adequate ventricular function may depend on sympathetic drive. Beta-adrenergic blockade may worsen AV block by preventing the necessary facilitating effects of sympathetic activity on conduction. $Beta_2$-adrenergic blockade results in passive bronchial constriction by interfering with endogenous adrenergic bronchodilator activity in patients subject to bronchospasm and may also interfere with exogenous bronchodilators in such patients.

Absorption of nadolol after oral dosing is variable, averaging about 30%. Peak serum concentrations of nadolol usually occur in 3 to 4 hours after oral administration and the presence of food in the gastrointestinal tract does not affect the rate or extent of nadolol absorption. Approximately 30% of the nadolol present in serum is reversibly bound to plasma protein.

Unlike many other beta-adrenergic blocking agents, nadolol is not metabolized by the liver and is excreted unchanged, principally by the kidneys.

The half-life of therapeutic doses of nadolol is about 20 to 24 hours, permitting once-daily dosage. Because nadolol is excreted predominantly in the urine, its half-life increases in renal failure (see PRECAUTIONS and DOSAGE AND ADMINISTRATION). Steady-state serum concentrations of nadolol are attained in 6 to 9 days with once-daily dosage in persons with normal renal function. Because of variable absorption and different individual responsiveness, the proper dosage must be determined by titration.

Exacerbation of angina and, in some cases, myocardial infarction and ventricular dysrhythmias have been reported after abrupt discontinuation of therapy with beta-adrenergic blocking agents in patients with coronary artery disease. Abrupt withdrawal of these agents in patients without coronary artery disease has resulted in transient symptoms, including tremulousness, sweating, palpitation, headache, and malaise. Several mechanisms have been proposed to explain these phenomena, among them increased sensitivity to catecholamines because of increased numbers of beta receptors.

INDICATIONS AND USAGE

Angina Pectoris—CORGARD (nadolol) is indicated for the long-term management of patients with angina pectoris.

Hypertension—CORGARD (nadolol) is indicated in the management of hypertension; it may be used alone or in combination with other antihypertensive agents, especially thiazide-type diuretics.

CONTRAINDICATIONS

Nadolol is contraindicated in bronchial asthma, sinus bradycardia and greater than first degree conduction block, cardiogenic shock, and overt cardiac failure (see WARNINGS).

WARNINGS

Cardiac Failure—Sympathetic stimulation may be a vital component supporting circulatory function in patients with congestive heart failure, and its inhibition by beta-blockade may precipitate more severe failure. Although beta-blockers should be avoided in overt congestive heart failure, if necessary, they can be used with caution in patients with a history of failure who are well compensated, usually with digitalis and diuretics. Beta-adrenergic blocking agents do not abolish the inotropic action of digitalis on heart muscle.

IN PATIENTS WITHOUT A HISTORY OF HEART FAILURE, continued use of beta-blockers can, in some cases, lead to cardiac failure. Therefore, at the first sign or symptom of heart failure, the patient should be digitalized and/or treated with diuretics, and the response observed closely, or nadolol should be discontinued (gradually, if possible).

> **Exacerbation of Ischemic Heart Disease Following Abrupt Withdrawal**—Hypersensitivity to catecholamines has been observed in patients withdrawn from beta-blocker therapy; exacerbation of angina and, in some cases, myocardial infarction have occurred after *abrupt* discontinuation of such therapy. When discontinuing chronically administered nadolol, particularly in patients with ischemic heart disease, the dosage should be gradually reduced over a period of 1 to 2 weeks and the patient should be carefully monitored. If angina markedly worsens or acute coronary insufficiency develops, nadolol administration should be reinstituted promptly, at least temporarily, and other measures appropriate for the management of unstable angina should be taken. Patients should be warned against interruption or discontinuation of therapy without the physician's advice. Because coronary artery disease is common and may be unrecognized, it may be prudent not to discontinue nadolol therapy abruptly even in patients treated only for hypertension.

Nonallergic Bronchospasm (eg, chronic bronchitis, emphysema)—PATIENTS WITH BRONCHOSPASTIC DISEASES SHOULD IN GENERAL NOT RECEIVE BETA-BLOCKERS. Nadolol should be administered with caution since it may block bronchodilation produced by endogenous or exogenous catecholamine stimulation of $beta_2$ receptors.

Major Surgery—Because beta-blockade impairs the ability of the heart to respond to reflex stimuli and may increase the risks of general anesthesia and surgical procedures, resulting in protracted hypotension or low cardiac output, it has generally been suggested that such therapy should be withdrawn several days prior to surgery. Recognition of the increased sensitivity to catecholamines of patients recently withdrawn from beta-blocker therapy, however, has made this recommendation controversial. If possible, beta-blockers should be withdrawn well before surgery takes place. In the event of emergency surgery, the anesthesiologist should be informed that the patient is on beta-blocker therapy. The effects of nadolol can be reversed by administration of beta-receptor agonists such as isoproterenol, dopamine, dobutamine, or levarterenol. Difficulty in restarting and maintaining the heart beat has also been reported with beta-adrenergic receptor blocking agents.

Diabetes and Hypoglycemia—Beta-adrenergic blockade may prevent the appearance of premonitory signs and symptoms (eg, tachycardia and blood pressure changes) of acute hypoglycemia. This is especially important with labile diabetics.

Beta-blockade also reduces the release of insulin in response to hyperglycemia; therefore, it may be necessary to adjust the dose of antidiabetic drugs.

Thyrotoxicosis—Beta-adrenergic blockade may mask certain clinical signs (eg, tachycardia) of hyperthyroidism. Patients suspected of developing thyrotoxicosis should be managed carefully to avoid abrupt withdrawal of beta-adrenergic blockade which might precipitate a thyroid storm.

PRECAUTIONS

Impaired Renal Function—Nadolol should be used with caution in patients with impaired renal function (see DOSAGE AND ADMINISTRATION).

Information for Patients

Patients, especially those with evidence of coronary artery insufficiency, should be warned against interruption or discontinuation of nadolol therapy without the physician's advice. Although cardiac failure rarely occurs in properly selected patients, patients being treated with beta-adrenergic blocking agents should be advised to consult the physician at the first sign or symptom of impending failure. The patient should also be advised of a proper course in the event of an inadvertently missed dose.

Drug Interactions

When administered concurrently, the following drugs may interact with beta-adrenergic receptor blocking agents:

Anesthetics, general—exaggeration of the hypotension induced by general anesthetics (see WARNINGS, Major Surgery).

Antidiabetic drugs (oral agents and insulin)—hypoglycemia or hyperglycemia; adjust dosage of antidiabetic drug accordingly (see WARNINGS, Diabetes and Hypoglycemia).

Catecholamine-depleting drugs (eg, reserpine)—additive effect; monitor closely for evidence of hypotension and/or excessive bradycardia (eg, vertigo, syncope, postural hypotension).

Response to Treatment for Anaphylactic Reaction—

While taking beta-blockers, patients with a history of severe anaphylactic reaction to a variety of allergens may be more reactive to repeated challenge, either accidental, diagnostic, or therapeutic. Such patients may be unresponsive to the usual doses of epinephrine used to treat allergic reaction.

Carcinogenesis, Mutagenesis, Impairment of Fertility

In chronic oral toxicologic studies (1 to 2 years) in mice, rats, and dogs, nadolol did not produce any significant toxic effects. In 2-year oral carcinogenic studies in rats and mice, nadolol did not produce any neoplastic, preneoplastic, or nonneoplastic pathologic lesions. In fertility and general reproductive performance studies in rats, nadolol caused no adverse effects.

Pregnancy Category C

In animal reproduction studies with nadolol, evidence of embryo- and fetotoxicity was found in rabbits, but not in rats or hamsters, at doses 5 to 10 times greater (on a mg/kg basis) than the maximum indicated human dose. No teratogenic potential was observed in any of these species.

There are no adequate and well-controlled studies in pregnant women. Nadolol should be used during pregnancy only if the potential benefit justifies the potential risk to the fetus. Neonates whose mothers are receiving nadolol at parturition have exhibited bradycardia, hypoglycemia, and associated symptoms.

Nursing Mothers

Nadolol is excreted in human milk. Because of the potential for adverse effects in nursing infants, a decision should be made whether to discontinue nursing or to discontinue therapy taking into account the importance of CORGARD (nadolol) to the mother.

Pediatric Use

Safety and effectiveness in children have not been established.

ADVERSE REACTIONS

Most adverse effects have been mild and transient and have rarely required withdrawal of therapy.

Cardiovascular—Bradycardia with heart rates of less than 60 beats per minute occurs commonly, and heart rates below 40 beats per minute and/or symptomatic bradycardia were seen in about 2 of 100 patients. Symptoms of peripheral vascular insufficiency, usually of the Raynaud type, have occurred in approximately 2 of 100 patients. Cardiac failure, hypotension, and rhythm/conduction disturbances have each occurred in about 1 of 100 patients. Single instances of first degree and third degree heart block have been reported; intensification of AV block is a known effect of beta-blockers (see also CONTRAINDICATIONS, WARNINGS, and PRECAUTIONS).

Central Nervous System—Dizziness or fatigue has been reported in approximately 2 of 100 patients; paresthesias, sedation, and change in behavior have each been reported in approximately 6 of 1000 patients.

Respiratory—Bronchospasm has been reported in approximately 1 of 1000 patients (see CONTRAINDICATIONS and WARNINGS).

Gastrointestinal—Nausea, diarrhea, abdominal discomfort, constipation, vomiting, indigestion, anorexia, bloating, and flatulence have been reported in 1 to 5 of 1000 patients.

Miscellaneous—Each of the following has been reported in 1 to 5 of 1000 patients: rash; pruritus; headache; dry mouth, eyes, or skin; impotence or decreased libido; facial swelling; weight gain; slurred speech; cough; nasal stuffiness; sweating; tinnitus; blurred vision. Reversible alopecia has been reported infrequently.

The following adverse reactions have been reported in patients taking nadolol and/or other beta-adrenergic blocking agents, but no causal relationship to nadolol has been established.

Central Nervous System—Reversible mental depression progressing to catatonia; visual disturbances; hallucinations; an acute reversible syndrome characterized by disorientation for time and place, short-term memory loss, emotional lability with slightly clouded sensorium, and decreased performance on neuropsychometrics.

Gastrointestinal—Mesenteric arterial thrombosis; ischemic colitis; elevated liver enzymes.

Hematologic—Agranulocytosis; thrombocytopenic or nonthrombocytopenic purpura.

Allergic—Fever combined with aching and sore throat; laryngospasm; respiratory distress.

Miscellaneous—Pemphigoid rash; hypertensive reaction in patients with pheochromocytoma; sleep disturbances; Peyronie's disease.

The oculomucocutaneous syndrome associated with the beta-blocker practolol has not been reported with nadolol.

OVERDOSAGE

Nadolol can be removed from the general circulation by hemodialysis.

In addition to gastric lavage, the following measures should be employed, as appropriate. In determining the duration of corrective therapy, note must be taken of the long duration of the effect of nadolol.

Excessive Bradycardia—Administer atropine (0.25 to 1.0 mg). If there is no response to vagal blockade, administer isoproterenol cautiously.

Cardiac Failure—Administer a digitalis glycoside and diuretic. It has been reported that glucagon may also be useful in this situation.

Hypotension—Administer vasopressors, eg, epinephrine or levarterenol. (There is evidence that epinephrine may be the drug of choice.)

Bronchospasm—Administer a beta$_2$-stimulating agent and/or a theophylline derivative.

DOSAGE AND ADMINISTRATION

DOSAGE MUST BE INDIVIDUALIZED. CORGARD (NADOLOL) MAY BE ADMINISTERED WITHOUT REGARD TO MEALS.

Angina Pectoris—The usual initial dose is 40 mg CORGARD (nadolol) once daily. Dosage may be gradually increased in 40 to 80 mg increments at 3- to 7-day intervals until optimum clinical response is obtained or there is pronounced slowing of the heart rate. The usual maintenance dose is 40 or 80 mg administered once daily. Doses up to 160 or 240 mg administered once daily may be needed.

The usefulness and safety in angina pectoris of dosage exceeding 240 mg per day have not been established. If treatment is to be discontinued, reduce the dosage gradually over a period of 1 to 2 weeks (see WARNINGS).

Hypertension—The usual initial dose is 40 mg CORGARD (nadolol) once daily, whether it is used alone or in addition to diuretic therapy. Dosage may be gradually increased in 40 to 80 mg increments until optimum blood pressure reduction is achieved. The usual maintenance dose is 40 or 80 mg administered once daily. Doses up to 240 or 320 mg administered once daily may be needed.

Dosage Adjustment in Renal Failure—Absorbed nadolol is excreted principally by the kidneys and, although nonrenal elimination does occur, dosage adjustments are necessary in patients with renal impairment. The following dose intervals are recommended:

Creatinine Clearance ($mL/min/1.73m^2$)	Dosage Interval (hours)
>50	24
31–50	24–36
10–30	24–48
<10	40–60

HOW SUPPLIED

CORGARD TABLETS (Nadolol Tablets USP)

20 mg tablets in bottles of 100 (NDC 0003-0232-50), **40 mg tablets** in bottles of 100 (NDC 0003-0207-50) and 1000 (NDC 0003-0207-76), **80 mg tablets** in bottles of 100 (NDC 0003-0241-50) and 1000 (NDC 0003-0241-76), **120 mg tablets** in bottles of 100 (NDC 0003-0208-50) and 1000 (NDC 0003-0208-76), and **160 mg tablets** in bottles of 100 (NDC 0003-0246-49). Unimatic® unit-dose packs containing 100 tablets: **20 mg** (NDC 0003-0232-51); **40 mg** (NDC 0003-0207-53); **80 mg** (NDC 0003-0241-55).

All tablets are scored (bisect bar) and easy to break. Tablet identification numbers: 20 mg, **232**; 40 mg, **207**; 80 mg, **241**; 120 mg, **208**; and 160 mg, **246**.

Storage

Store at room temperature; avoid excessive heat. Protect from light. Keep bottle tightly closed.

Shown in Product Identification Section, page 406

CORZIDE® 40/5
CORZIDE® 80/5

℞

[kor'zīd]

Nadolol and Bendroflumethiazide Tablets

DESCRIPTION

CORZIDE (Nadolol and Bendroflumethiazide Tablets) for oral administration combines two antihypertensive agents: CORGARD® (nadolol), a nonselective beta-adrenergic blocking agent, and NATURETIN® (bendroflumethiazide), a thiazide diuretic-antihypertensive. Formulations: 40 mg and 80 mg nadolol per tablet combined with 5 mg bendroflumethiazide. Inactive ingredients: cellulose, colorant (FD&C Blue No. 2), lactose, magnesium stearate, povidone, sodium starch glycolate, and starch.

Nadolol

Nadolol is a white crystalline powder. It is freely soluble in ethanol, soluble in hydrochloric acid, slightly soluble in water and in chloroform, and very slightly soluble in sodium hydroxide.

Nadolol is designated chemically as 1-(*tert*-butylamino)-3-[(5,6,7,8-tetrahydro-*cis*-6,7-dihydroxy-1-naphthyl)oxy]-2-propanol. Structural formula:

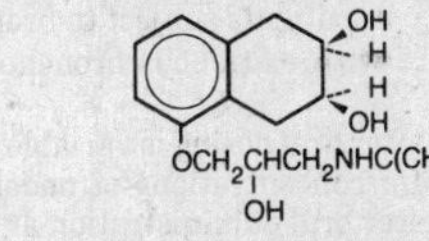

$C_{17}H_{27}NO_4$ MW 309.40 CAS-42200-33-9

Bendroflumethiazide

Bendroflumethiazide is a white crystalline powder. It is soluble in alcohol and in sodium hydroxide, and insoluble in hydrochloric acid, water, and chloroform.

Bendroflumethiazide is designated chemically as 3-benzyl-3,4-dihydro-6-(trifluoromethyl)-2*H*-1,2,4-benzothiadiazine-7-sulfonamide 1,1-dioxide. Structural formula:

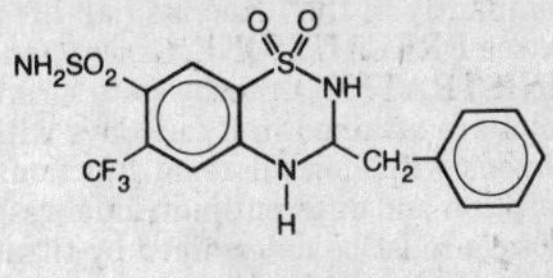

$C_{15}H_{14}F_3N_3O_4S_2$ MW 421.41 CAS-73-48-3

CLINICAL PHARMACOLOGY

Nadolol

Nadolol is a nonselective beta-adrenergic receptor blocking agent. Clinical pharmacology studies have demonstrated beta-blocking activity by showing (1) reduction in heart rate and cardiac output at rest and on exercise, (2) reduction of systolic and diastolic blood pressure at rest and on exercise, (3) inhibition of isoproterenol-induced tachycardia, and (4) reduction of reflex orthostatic tachycardia.

Nadolol specifically competes with beta-adrenergic receptor agonists for available beta receptor sites; it inhibits both the beta$_1$ receptors located chiefly in cardiac muscle and the beta$_2$ receptors located chiefly in the bronchial and vascular musculature, inhibiting the chronotropic, inotropic, and vasodilator responses to beta-adrenergic stimulation proportionately. Nadolol has no intrinsic sympathomimetic activity and, unlike some other beta-adrenergic blocking agents, nadolol has little direct myocardial depressant activity and does not have an anesthetic-like membrane-stabilizing action. Animal and human studies show that nadolol slows the sinus rate and depresses AV conduction. In dogs, only minimal amounts of nadolol were detected in the brain relative to amounts in blood and other organs and tissues. Nadolol has low lipophilicity as determined by octanol/water partition coefficient, a characteristic of certain beta-blocking agents that has been correlated with the limited extent to which these agents cross the blood-brain barrier, their low concentration in the brain, and low incidence of CNS-related side effects.

In controlled clinical studies, nadolol at doses of 40 to 320 mg/day has been shown to decrease both standing and supine blood pressure, the effect persisting for approximately 24 hours after dosing.

The mechanism of the antihypertensive effects of beta-adrenergic receptor blocking agents has not been established; however, factors that may be involved include (1) competitive antagonism of catecholamines at peripheral (non-CNS) adrenergic neuron sites (especially cardiac) leading to decreased cardiac output, (2) a central effect leading to reduced

Continued on next page

Bristol Laboratories—Cont.

tonic-sympathetic nerve outflow to the periphery, and (3) suppression of renin secretion by blockade of the beta-adrenergic receptors responsible for renin release from the kidneys.

While cardiac output and arterial pressure are reduced by nadolol therapy, renal hemodynamics are stable, with preservation of renal blood flow and glomerular filtration rate.

By blocking catecholamine-induced increases in heart rate, velocity and extent of myocardial contraction, and blood pressure, nadolol generally reduces the oxygen requirements of the heart at any given level of effort, making it useful for many patients in the long-term management of angina pectoris. On the other hand, nadolol can increase oxygen requirements by increasing left ventricular fiber length and end diastolic pressure, particularly in patients with heart failure.

Although beta-adrenergic receptor blockade is useful in treatment of angina and hypertension, there are also situations in which sympathetic stimulation is vital. For example, in patients with severely damaged hearts, adequate ventricular function may depend on sympathetic drive. Beta-adrenergic blockade may worsen AV block by preventing the necessary facilitating effects of sympathetic activity on conduction. $Beta_2$-adrenergic blockade results in passive bronchial constriction by interfering with endogenous adrenergic bronchodilator activity in patients subject to bronchospasm and may also interfere with exogenous bronchodilators in such patients.

Absorption of nadolol after oral dosing is variable, averaging about 30%. Peak serum concentrations of nadolol usually occur in 3 to 4 hours after oral administration and the presence of food in the gastrointestinal tract does not affect the rate or extent of nadolol absorption. Approximately 30% of the nadolol present in serum is reversibly bound to plasma protein.

Unlike many other beta-adrenergic blocking agents, nadolol is not metabolized by the liver and is excreted unchanged, principally by the kidneys.

The half-life of therapeutic doses of nadolol is about 20 to 24 hours, permitting once-daily dosage. Because nadolol is excreted predominantly in the urine, its half-life increases in renal failure (see **PRECAUTIONS,** *General,* and **DOSAGE AND ADMINISTRATION**). Steady state serum concentrations of nadolol are attained in 6 to 9 days with once-daily dosage in persons with normal renal function. Because of variable absorption and different individual responsiveness, the proper dosage must be determined by titration.

Exacerbation of angina and, in some cases, myocardial infarction and ventricular dysrhythmias have been reported after abrupt discontinuation of therapy with beta-adrenergic blocking agents in patients with coronary artery disease. Abrupt withdrawal of these agents in patients without coronary artery disease has resulted in transient symptoms, including tremulousness, sweating, palpitation, headache, and malaise. Several mechanisms have been proposed to explain these phenomena, among them increased sensitivity to catecholamines because of increased numbers of beta receptors.

Bendroflumethiazide

The mechanism of action of bendroflumethiazide results in an interference with the renal tubular mechanism of electrolyte reabsorption. At maximal therapeutic dosage all thiazides are approximately equal in their diuretic potency.

Thiazides increase excretion of sodium and chloride in approximately equivalent amounts. Natriuresis causes a secondary loss of potassium and bicarbonate.

The mechanism of the antihypertensive effect of thiazides is unknown. Thiazides do not affect normal blood pressure.

Onset of action of thiazides occurs in 2 hours and the peak effect at about 4 hours. Duration of action persists for approximately 6 to 12 hours. Thiazides are eliminated rapidly by the kidney.

INDICATIONS

CORZIDE (Nadolol and Bendroflumethiazide Tablets) is indicated in the management of hypertension.

This fixed combination drug is not indicated for initial therapy of hypertension. If the fixed combination represents the dose titrated to the individual patient's needs, it may be more convenient than the separate components.

CONTRAINDICATIONS

Nadolol

Nadolol is contraindicated in bronchial asthma, sinus bradycardia and greater than first degree conduction block, cardiogenic shock, and overt cardiac failure (see **WARNINGS**).

Bendroflumethiazide

Bendroflumethiazide is contraindicated in anuria. It is also contraindicated in patients who have previously demonstrated hypersensitivity to bendroflumethiazide or other sulfonamide-derived drugs.

WARNINGS

Nadolol

Cardiac Failure—Sympathetic stimulation may be a vital component supporting circulatory function in patients with congestive heart failure, and its inhibition by beta-blockade may precipitate more severe failure. Although beta-blockers should be avoided in overt congestive heart failure, if necessary, they can be used with caution in patients with a history of failure who are well compensated, usually with digitalis and diuretics. Beta-adrenergic blocking agents do not abolish the inotropic action of digitalis on heart muscle.

IN PATIENTS WITHOUT A HISTORY OF HEART FAILURE, continued use of beta-blockers can, in some cases, lead to cardiac failure. Therefore, at the first sign or symptom of heart failure, the patient should be digitalized and/or treated with diuretics, and the response observed closely, or nadolol should be discontinued (gradually, if possible).

Exacerbation of Ischemic Heart Disease Following Abrupt Withdrawal—Hypersensitivity to catecholamines has been observed in patients withdrawn from beta-blocker therapy; exacerbation of angina and, in some cases, myocardial infarction have occurred after *abrupt* discontinuation of such therapy. When discontinuing chronically administered nadolol, particularly in patients with ischemic heart disease, the dosage should be gradually reduced over a period of 1 to 2 weeks and the patient should be carefully monitored. If angina markedly worsens or acute coronary insufficiency develops, nadolol administration should be reinstituted promptly, at least temporarily, and other measures appropriate for the management of unstable angina should be taken. Patients should be warned against interruption or discontinuation of therapy without the physician's advice. Because coronary artery disease is common and may be unrecognized, it may be prudent not to discontinue nadolol therapy abruptly even in patients treated only for hypertension.

Nonallergic Bronchospasm (eg, chronic bronchitis, emphysema)—PATIENTS WITH BRONCHOSPASTIC DISEASES SHOULD IN GENERAL NOT RECEIVE BETA-BLOCKERS. Nadolol should be administered with caution since it may block bronchodilation produced by endogenous or exogenous catecholamine stimulation of $beta_2$ receptors.

Major Surgery—Because beta blockade impairs the ability of the heart to respond to reflex stimuli and may increase the risks of general anesthesia and surgical procedures, resulting in protracted hypotension or low cardiac output, it has generally been suggested that such therapy should be withdrawn several days prior to surgery. Recognition of the increased sensitivity to catecholamines of patients recently withdrawn from beta-blocker therapy, however, has made this recommendation controversial. If possible, beta-blockers should be withdrawn well before surgery takes place. In the event of emergency surgery, the anesthesiologist should be informed that the patient is on beta-blocker therapy. The effects of nadolol can be reversed by administration of beta-receptor agonists such as isoproterenol, dopamine, dobutamine, or levarterenol. Difficulty in restarting and maintaining the heart beat has also been reported with beta-adrenergic receptor blocking agents.

Diabetes and Hypoglycemia—Beta-adrenergic blockade may prevent the appearance of premonitory signs and symptoms (eg, tachycardia and blood pressure changes) of acute hypoglycemia. This is especially important with labile diabetics. Beta-blockade also reduces the release of insulin in response to hyperglycemia; therefore, it may be necessary to adjust the dose of antidiabetic drugs.

Thyrotoxicosis—Beta-adrenergic blockade may mask certain clinical signs (eg, tachycardia) of hyperthyroidism. Patients suspected of developing thyrotoxicosis should be managed carefully to avoid abrupt withdrawal of beta-adrenergic blockade which might precipitate a thyroid storm.

Bendroflumethiazide

Thiazides should be used with caution in severe renal disease. In patients with renal disease, thiazides may precipitate azotemia. Cumulative effects of the drug may develop in patients with impaired renal function.

Thiazides should be used with caution in patients with impaired hepatic function or progressive liver disease, since minor alterations of fluid and electrolyte balance may precipitate hepatic coma.

Sensitivity reactions may occur in patients with or without a history of allergy or bronchial asthma.

The possibility of exacerbation or activation of systemic lupus erythematosus has been reported.

Lithium generally should not be given with diuretics; diuretic agents reduce the renal clearance of lithium and add a high risk of lithium toxicity. Refer to the package insert for lithium preparations before use of such concomitant therapy.

PRECAUTIONS

General

Nadolol

Nadolol should be used with caution in patients with impaired renal function (see **DOSAGE AND ADMINISTRATION**).

Bendroflumethiazide

Periodic determination of serum electrolytes to detect possible electrolyte imbalance should be performed at appropriate intervals.

All patients receiving thiazide therapy should be observed for clinical signs of fluid or electrolyte imbalance, namely: hyponatremia, hypochloremic alkalosis, and hypokalemia. Serum and urine electrolyte determinations are particularly important when the patient is vomiting excessively or receiving parenteral fluids. Warning signs or symptoms of fluid and electrolyte imbalance may include: dryness of the mouth, thirst, weakness, lethargy, drowsiness, restlessness, muscle pains or cramps, muscular fatigue, hypotension, oliguria, tachycardia, and gastrointestinal disturbances, such as nausea and vomiting.

Hypokalemia may develop especially with brisk diuresis or when severe cirrhosis is present.

Interference with adequate oral electrolyte intake will also contribute to hypokalemia. Hypokalemia can sensitize or exaggerate the response of the heart to the toxic effects of digitalis (eg, increased ventricular irritability). Concurrent administration of a potassium-sparing diuretic or potassium supplements may be indicated in these patients.

Any chloride deficit is generally mild and usually does not require specific treatment except under extraordinary circumstances (as in liver disease or renal disease). Dilutional hyponatremia may occur in edematous patients in hot weather; appropriate therapy is water restriction, rather than administration of salt except in rare instances when the hyponatremia is life threatening. In actual salt depletion, appropriate replacement is the therapy of choice.

Hyperuricemia may occur or frank gout may be precipitated in certain patients receiving thiazide therapy.

Latent diabetes mellitus may become manifest during thiazide administration.

The antihypertensive effect of thiazide diuretics may be enhanced in the post-sympathectomy patient.

If progressive renal impairment becomes evident, as indicated by a rising nonprotein nitrogen or blood urea nitrogen (BUN), a careful reappraisal of therapy is necessary with consideration given to withholding or discontinuing diuretic therapy.

Thiazides may decrease serum PBI levels without signs of thyroid disturbance.

Calcium excretion is decreased by thiazides. Pathological changes in the parathyroid gland with hypercalcemia and hypophosphatemia have been observed in a few patients on prolonged thiazide therapy. The common complications of hyperparathyroidism such as renal lithiasis, bone resorption, and peptic ulceration have not been seen. Thiazides should be discontinued before carrying out tests for parathyroid function.

Thiazides have been shown to increase the urinary excretion of magnesium; this may result in hypomagnesemia.

Information for Patients

Patients, especially those with evidence of coronary artery insufficiency, should be warned against interruption or discontinuation of therapy without the physician's advice. Although cardiac failure rarely occurs in properly selected patients, patients being treated with beta-adrenergic blocking agents should be advised to consult the physician at the first sign or symptom of impending failure.

The patient should also be advised of a proper course in the event of an inadvertently missed dose.

The patient should be informed of symptoms that would suggest potential adverse effects and told to report them promptly.

Laboratory Tests

Serum electrolyte levels should be regularly monitored (see **WARNINGS,** *Bendroflumethiazide,* also **PRECAUTIONS,** *General, Bendroflumethiazide*).

Drug Interactions

Nadolol

When administered concurrently the following drugs may interact with beta-adrenergic receptor blocking agents:

Anesthetics, general—exaggeration of the hypotension induced by general anesthetics (see **WARNINGS,** *Nadolol, Major Surgery*).

Antidiabetic drugs (oral agents and insulin)—hypoglycemia or hyperglycemia; adjust dosage of antidiabetic drug accordingly (see **WARNINGS,** *Nadolol, Diabetes and Hypoglycemia*).

Catecholamine-depleting drugs (eg, reserpine)—additive effect; monitor closely for evidence of hypotension and/or excessive bradycardia (eg, vertigo, syncope, postural hypotension).

Response to Treatment for Anaphylactic Reaction—While taking beta-blockers, patients with a history of severe anaphylactic reaction to a variety of allergens may be more reac-

tive to repeated challenge, either accidental, diagnostic, or therapeutic. Such patients may be unresponsive to the usual doses of epinephrine used to treat allergic reaction.

Bendroflumethiazide

When administered concurrently, the following drugs may interact with bendroflumethiazide:

Alcohol, barbiturates, or narcotics —potentiation of orthostatic hypotension may occur.

Amphotericin B, corticosteroids, or corticotropin (ACTH) — may intensify electrolyte imbalance, particularly hypokalemia. Monitor potassium levels; use potassium replacements if necessary.

Anticoagulants (oral) —dosage adjustments of anticoagulant medication may be necessary since bendroflumethiazide may decrease their effects.

Antigout medications —dosage adjustments of antigout medication may be necessary since bendroflumethiazide may raise the level of blood uric acid.

Other antihypertensive medications (eg, ganglionic or peripheral adrenergic blocking agents) —dosage adjustments may be necessary since bendroflumethiazide may potentiate their effects.

Antidiabetic drugs (oral agents and insulin) —since thiazides may elevate blood glucose levels, dosage adjustments of antidiabetic agents may be necessary.

Calcium salts —increased serum calcium levels due to decreased excretion may occur. If calcium must be prescribed monitor serum calcium levels and adjust calcium dosage accordingly.

Cardiac glycosides —enchanced possibility of digitalis toxicity associated with hypokalemia. Monitor potassium levels; use potassium replacement if necessary.

Cholestyramine resin and colestipol HCL —may delay or decrease absorption of bendroflumethiazide. Sulfonamide diuretics should be taken at least 1 hour before or 4 to 6 hours after these medications.

Diazoxide —enhanced hyperglycemic, hyperuricemic, and antihypertensive effects. Be cognizant of possible interaction; monitor blood glucose and serum uric acid levels.

Lithium salts —may enhance lithium toxicity due to reduced renal clearance. Avoid concurrent use; if lithium must be prescribed monitor serum lithium levels and adjust lithium dosage accordingly. (see **WARNINGS**)

MAO inhibitors —dosage adjustments of one or both agents may be necessary since hypotensive effects are enhanced.

Nondepolarizing muscle relaxants, preanesthetics and anesthetics used in surgery (eg, tubocurarine chloride and gallamime triethiodide) —effects of these agents may be potentiated; dosage adjustments may be required. Monitor and correct any fluid and electrolye imbalances prior to surgery if feasible.

Nonsteroidal anti-inflammatory agents —in some patients the administration of a nonsteroidal anti-inflammatory agent can reduce the diuretic, natriuretic, and antihypertensive effect of loop, potassium-sparing or thiazide diuretics. Therefore, when bendroflumethiazide and nonsteroidal anti-inflammatory agents are used concomitantly, the patient should be observed closely to determine if the desired effect of the diuretic is obtained.

Methenamine —possible decrease effectiveness due to alkalinization of the urine.

Pressor amines (eg, norepinephrine) —decreased arterial responsiveness, but not sufficient to preclude effectiveness of the pressor agent for therapeutic use. Use caution in patients taking both medications who undergo surgery. Administer preanesthetic and anesthetic agents in reduced dosage and if possible, discontinue bendroflumethiazide 1 week prior to surgery.

Probenecid or sulfinpyrazone —increased dosage of these agents may be necessary since bendroflumethiazide may have hyperuricemic effects.

Drug/Laboratory Test Interactions

Bendroflumethiazide may produce false-negative results with the phentolamine and tyramine tests; may interfere with the phenosulfonphthalein test due to decreased excretion; and it may cause diagnostic interference of serum electrolyte levels, blood and urine glucose levels, and a decrease in serum PBI levels without signs of thyroid disturbance.

Carcinogenesis, Mutagenesis, Impairment of Fertility

Nadolol

In chronic oral toxicologic studies (1 to 2 years) in mice, rats, and dogs, nadolol did not produce any significant toxic effects. In 2-year oral carcinogenicity studies in rats and mice, nadolol did not produce any neoplastic, preneoplastic, or nonneoplastic pathologic lesions. In fertility and general reproductive performance studies in rats, nadolol caused no adverse effect.

Bendroflumethiazide

Studies have not been performed to evaluate carcinogenic potential, mutagenesis, or whether this drug adversely affects fertility in males or females.

Pregnancy—Teratogenic Effects

Nadolol

Category C. In animal reproduction studies with nadolol, evidence of embryo- and fetotoxicity was found in rabbits, but not in rats or hamsters, at doses 5 to 10 times greater (on

a mg/kg basis) than the maximum indicated human dose. No teratogenic potential was observed in any of these species. There are no adequate and well-controlled studies in pregnant women. Nadolol should be used during pregnancy only if the potential benefit justifies the potential risk to the fetus. Neonates whose mothers are receiving nadolol at parturition have exhibited bradycardia, hypoglycemia, and associated symptoms.

Bendroflumethiazide

Category C. Animal reproduction studies have not been conducted with bendroflumethiazide. It is also not known whether this drug can cause fetal harm when administered to a pregnant woman or can affect reproduction capacity. Bendroflumethiazide should be given to a pregnant woman only if clearly needed.

Pregnancy—Nonteratogenic Effects

Thiazides cross the placental barrier and appear in cord blood. The use of thiazides in pregnant women requires that the anticipated benefit be weighed against possible hazards to the fetus. These hazards include fetal or neonatal jaundice, thrombocytopenia, and possibly other adverse reactions which have occurred in the adult.

Nursing Mothers

Both nadolol and bendroflumethiazide are excreted in human milk. Because of the potential for serious adverse reactions in nursing infants from both drugs, a decision should be made whether to discontinue nursing or to discontinue therapy taking into account the importance of CORZIDE (Nadolol and Bendroflumethiazide Tablets) to the mother.

Pediatric Use

Safety and effectiveness in children have not been established.

ADVERSE REACTIONS

Nadolol

Most adverse effects have been mild and transient and have rarely required withdrawal of therapy.

Cardiovascular —Bradycardia with heart rates of less than 60 beats per minute occurs commonly, and heart rates below 40 beats per minute and/or symptomatic bradycardia were seen in about 2 of 100 patients. Symptoms of peripheral vascular insufficiency, usually of the Raynaud type, have occurred in approximately 2 of 100 patients. Cardiac failure, hypotension, and rhythm/conduction disturbances have each occurred in about 1 of 100 patients. Single instances of first degree and third degree heart block have been reported; intensification of AV block is a known effect of beta-blockers (see also **CONTRAINDICATIONS, WARNINGS,** and **PRECAUTIONS**).

Central Nervous System —Dizziness or fatigue has been reported in approximately 2 of 100 patients; paresthesias, sedation, and change in behavior have each been reported in approximately 6 of 1000 patients.

Respiratory —Bronchospasm has been reported in approximately 1 of 1000 patients (see **CONTRAINDICATIONS** and **WARNINGS**).

Gastrointestinal —Nausea, diarrhea, abdominal discomfort, constipation, vomiting, indigestion, anorexia, bloating, and flatulence have been reported in 1 to 5 of 1000 patients.

Miscellaneous —Each of the following has been reported in 1 to 5 of 1000 patients: rash; pruritus; headache; dry mouth, eyes, or skin; impotence or decreased libido; facial swelling; weight gain; slurred speech; cough; nasal stuffiness; sweating; tinnitus; blurred vision. Reversible alopecia has been reported infrequently.

The following adverse reactions have been reported in patients taking nadolol and/or other beta-adrenergic blocking agents, but no causal relationship to nadolol has been established.

Central Nervous System —Reversible mental depression progressing to catatonia; visual disturbances; hallucinations; an acute reversible syndrome characterized by disorientation for time and place, short-term memory loss, emotional lability with slightly clouded sensorium, and decreased performance on neuropsychometrics.

Gastrointestinal —Mesenteric arterial thrombosis; ischemic colitis; elevated liver enzymes.

Hematologic —Agranulocytosis; thrombocytopenic or nonthrombocytopenic purpura.

Allergic —Fever combined with aching and sore throat; laryngospasm; respiratory distress.

Miscellaneous —Pemphigoid rash; hypertensive reaction in patients with pheochromocytoma; sleep disturbances; Peyronie's disease.

The oculomucocutaneous syndrome associated with the betablocker practolol has not been reported with nadolol.

Bendroflumethiazide

Gastrointestinal System —nausea, vomiting, cramping and anorexia are not uncommon; diarrhea, constipation, gastric irritation, abdominal bloating, jaundice (intrahepatic cholestatic jaundice), hepatitis, and sialadenitis occasionally occur; and pancreatitis has been reported.

Central Nervous System —dizziness, vertigo, paresthesia, headache, and xanthopsia occasionally occur.

Hematologic —leukopenia, agranulocytosis, thrombocytopenia, hemolytic anemia, and aplastic anemia have been reported.

Dermatologic-Hypersensitivity —purpura, exfoliative dermatitis, pruritus, ecchymosis, urticaria, necrotizing, angiitis (vasculitis, cutaneous vasculitis), respiratory distress including pneumonitis, fever, and anaphylactic reactions occasionally occur; photosensitivity and rash have been reported.

Cardiovascular —Orthostatic hypotension may occur and may be potentiated by coadministration with certain other drugs (eg, alcohol, barbiturates, narcotics, other antihypertensive medications, etc.; (see **PRECAUTIONS**, Drug Interactions).

Other —muscle spasm, weakness, or restlessness is not uncommon; hyperglycemia, glycosuria, metabolic acidosis in diabetic patients, hyperuricemia, allergic glomerulonephritis, and transient blurred vision occasionally occur.

Whenever adverse reactions are moderate or severe, thiazide dosage should be reduced or therapy withdrawn.

OVERDOSAGE

In the event of overdosage, nadolol may cause excessive bradycardia, cardiac failure, hypotension, or bronchospasm. In addition to the expected diuresis, overdosage of bendroflumethiazide may produce varying degrees of lethargy which may progress to coma with minimal depression of respiration and cardiovascular function and without significant serum electrolyte changes or dehydration. The mechanism of thiazide-induced CNS depression is unknown. Gastrointestinal irritation may occur. Transitory increase in BUN has been reported, and serum electrolyte changes may occur, especially in patients with impaired renal function.

Treatment

Nadolol can be removed from the general circulation by hemodialysis. In determining the duration of corrective therapy, note must be taken of the long duration of the effect of nadolol. In addition to gastric lavage, the following measures should be employed, as appropriate.

Excessive Bradycardia—Administer atropine (0.25 to 1.0 mg). If there is no response to vagal blockade, administer isoproterenol cautiously.

Cardiac Failure—Administer a digitalis glycoside and diuretic. It has been reported that glucagon may also be useful in this situation.

Hypotension—Administer vasopressors, eg, epinephrine or levarterenol. (There is evidence that epinephrine may be the drug of choice.)

Bronchospasm—Administer a beta$_2$-stimulating agent and/or a theophylline derivative.

Stupor or Coma—Supportive therapy as warranted.

Gastrointestinal Effects—Symptomatic treatment as needed.

BUN and/or Serum Electrolyte Abnormalities—Institute supportive measures as required to maintain hydration, electrolyte balance, respiration, and cardiovascular and renal function.

DOSAGE AND ADMINISTRATION

DOSAGE MUST BE INDIVIDUALIZED (SEE INDICATIONS). CORZIDE MAY BE ADMINISTERED WITHOUT REGARD TO MEALS.

Bendroflumethiazide is usually given at a dose of 5 mg daily. The usual initial dose of nadolol is 40 mg once daily whether used alone or in combination with a diuretic. Bendroflumethiazide in CORZIDE is 30% more bioavailable than that of 5 mg NATURETIN tablets. Conversion from 5 mg NATURETIN to CORZIDE represents a 30% increase in dose of bendroflumethiazide.

The initial dose of CORZIDE (Nadolol and Bendroflumethiazide Tablets) may therefore be the 40 mg/5 mg tablet once daily. When the antihypertensive response is not satisfactory, the dose may be increased by administering the 80 mg/5 mg tablet once daily.

When necessary, another antihypertensive agent may be added gradually beginning with 50% of the usual recommended starting dose to avoid an excessive fall in blood pressure.

Dosage Adjustment in Renal Failure—Absorbed nadolol is excreted principally by the kidneys and, although nonrenal elimination does occur, dosage adjustments are necessary in patients with renal impairment. The following dose intervals are recommended:

Creatinine Clearance (ml/min/1.73m^2)	Dosage Interval (hours)
>50	24
31-50	24-36
10-30	24-48
<10	40-60

HOW SUPPLIED

CORZIDE (Nadolol and Bendroflumethiazide Tablets)

- **40 mg nadolol combined with 5 mg bendroflumethiazide** in bottles of 100 tablets (NDC 0003-0283-50).

- **80 mg nadolol combined with 5 mg bendroflumethiazide** in bottles of 100 tablets (NDC 0003-0284-50).

Continued on next page

Bristol Laboratories—Cont.

Round, biconvex tablets are white to bluish white with dark blue specks. Each tablet has a full bisect bar. Tablet identification numbers: 40 mg/5 mg combination, **283**; 80 mg/5 mg combination, **284**.

Storage

Keep bottle tightly closed. Store at room temperature; avoid excessive heat.

QUESTRAN® POWDER ℞

[*kwest'răn*]

(Cholestyramine for Oral Suspension, USP)

DESCRIPTION

QUESTRAN Powder, the chloride salt of a basic anion exchange resin, a cholesterol lowering agent, is intended for oral administration. Cholestyramine resin is quite hydrophilic, but insoluble in water. The cholestyramine resin in QUESTRAN is not absorbed from the digestive tract. Nine grams of QUESTRAN Powder contain 4 grams of anhydrous cholestyramine resin. It is represented by the following structural formula:

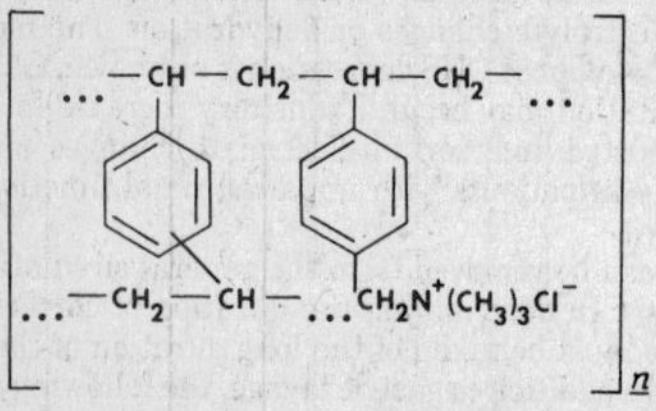

Representation of structure of main polymeric groups

This product contains the following inactive ingredients: acacia, citric acid, D&C Yellow No. 10, FD&C Yellow No. 6, flavor (natural and artificial), polysorbate 80, propylene glycol alginate, and sucrose.

CLINICAL PHARMACOLOGY

Cholesterol is probably the sole precursor of bile acids. During normal digestion, bile acids are secreted into the intestines. A major portion of the bile acids is absorbed from the intestinal tract and returned to the liver via the enterohepatic circulation. Only very small amounts of bile acids are found in normal serum.

QUESTRAN resin adsorbs and combines with the bile acids in the intestine to form an insoluble complex which is excreted in the feces. This results in a partial removal of bile acids from the enterohepatic circulation by preventing their absorption.

The increased fecal loss of bile acids due to QUESTRAN administration leads to an increased oxidation of cholesterol to bile acids, a decrease in beta lipoprotein or low density lipoprotein plasma levels and a decrease in serum cholesterol levels. Although in man, QUESTRAN produces an increase in hepatic synthesis of cholesterol, plasma cholesterol levels fall.

In patients with partial biliary obstruction, the reduction of serum bile acid levels by QUESTRAN reduces excess bile acids deposited in the dermal tissue with resultant decrease in pruritus.

INDICATIONS AND USAGE

1) QUESTRAN is indicated as adjunctive therapy to diet for the reduction of elevated serum cholesterol in patients with primary hypercholesterolemia (elevated low density lipoprotein [LDL] cholesterol) who do not respond adequately to diet. QUESTRAN may be useful to lower LDL cholesterol in patients who also have hypertriglyceridemia, but it is not indicated where hypertriglyceridemia is the abnormality of most concern.

In a large, placebo-controlled, multi-clinic study, the LRC-CPPT[a], hypercholesterolemic subjects treated with QUESTRAN had significant reductions in total and low-density lipoprotein cholesterol (LDL-C). Over the 7-year study period the QUESTRAN group experienced a 19% reduction in the combined rate of coronary heart disease death plus nonfatal myocardial infarction (cumulative incidences of 7% QUESTRAN and 8.6% placebo). The subjects included in the study were middle-aged men (age 35–59) with serum cholesterol levels above 265 mg/dL and no previous history of heart disease. It is not clear to what extent these findings can be extrapolated to other segments of the hypercholesterolemic population not studied.

Dietary therapy specific for the type of hyperlipoproteinemia is the initial treatment of choice. Excess body weight may be an important factor and caloric restriction for weight normalization should be addressed prior to drug therapy in the overweight. The use of drugs should be considered only when reasonable attempts have been made to obtain satisfactory results with nondrug methods. If the decision ultimately is to use drugs, the patient should be instructed that this does not reduce the importance of adhering to diet.

2) QUESTRAN is indicated for the relief of pruritus associated with partial biliary obstruction. QUESTRAN has been shown to have a variable effect on serum cholesterol in these patients. Patients with primary biliary cirrhosis may exhibit an elevated cholesterol as part of their disease.

CONTRAINDICATIONS

QUESTRAN is contraindicated in patients with complete biliary obstruction where bile is not secreted into the intestine and in those individuals who have shown hypersensitivity to any of its components.

PRECAUTIONS

General: Before instituting therapy with QUESTRAN, diseases contributing to increased blood cholesterol such as hypothyroidism, diabetes mellitus, nephrotic syndrome, dysproteinemias and obstructive liver disease should be looked for and specifically treated. A favorable trend in cholesterol reduction should occur during the first month of QUESTRAN therapy. The therapy should be continued to sustain cholesterol reduction. If adequate cholesterol reduction is not attained, QUESTRAN therapy should be discontinued.

Chronic use of QUESTRAN may be associated with increased bleeding tendency due to hypoprothrombinemia associated with Vitamin K deficiency. This will usually respond promptly to parenteral Vitamin K_1 and recurrences can be prevented by oral administration of Vitamin K_1. Reduction of serum or red cell folate has been reported over long term administration of QUESTRAN. Supplementation with folic acid should be considered in these cases.

There is a possibility that prolonged use of QUESTRAN, since it is a chloride form of anion exchange resin, may produce hyperchloremic acidosis. This would especially be true in younger and smaller patients where the relative dosage may be higher.

QUESTRAN may produce or worsen preexisting constipation. Dosage should be reduced or discontinued in such cases. Fecal impaction and aggravation of hemorrhoids may occur. Every effort should be made to avert severe constipation and its inherent problems in those patients with clinically symptomatic coronary artery disease.

Information for Patients: Inform your physician if you are pregnant or plan to become pregnant or are breastfeeding. Drink plenty of fluids and mix each 9-gram dose of QUESTRAN Powder in at least 2 to 6 ounces of fluid before taking.

Laboratory Tests: Serum cholesterol levels should be determined frequently during the first few months of therapy and periodically thereafter. Serum triglyceride levels should be measured periodically to detect whether significant changes have occurred.

The LRC-CPPT showed a dose-related increase in serum triglycerides of 10.7%–17.1% in the cholestyramine-treated group, compared with an increase of 7.9%–11.7% in the placebo group. Based on the mean values and adjusting for the placebo group, the cholestyramine-treated group showed an increase of 5% over pre-entry levels the first year of the study and an increase of 4.3% the seventh year.

Drug Interactions: QUESTRAN may delay or reduce the absorption of concomitant oral medication such as phenylbutazone, warfarin, chlorothiazide (acidic) or propranolol (basic), as well as tetracycline, penicillin G, phenobarbital, thyroid and thyroxine preparations, and digitalis. The discontinuance of QUESTRAN could pose a hazard to health if a potentially toxic drug such as digitalis has been titrated to a maintenance level while the patient was taking QUESTRAN.

Because cholestyramine binds bile acids, QUESTRAN may interfere with normal fat digestion and absorption and thus may prevent absorption of fat soluble vitamins such as A, D and K. When QUESTRAN is given for long periods of time, concomitant supplementation with water-miscible (or parenteral) form of vitamins A and D should be considered.

SINCE **QUESTRAN** MAY BIND OTHER DRUGS GIVEN CONCURRENTLY, PATIENTS SHOULD TAKE OTHER DRUGS AT LEAST 1 HOUR BEFORE OR 4 TO 6 HOURS AFTER **QUESTRAN** (OR AT AS GREAT AN INTERVAL AS POSSIBLE) TO AVOID IMPEDING THEIR ABSORPTION.

Carcinogenesis, Mutagenesis and Impairment of Fertility: In studies conducted in rats in which cholestyramine resin was used as a tool to investigate the role of various intestinal factors, such as fat, bile salts and microbial flora, in the development of intestinal tumors induced by potent carcinogens, the incidence of such tumors was observed to be greater in cholestyramine resin-treated rats than in control rats.

The relevance of this laboratory observation from studies in rats to the clinical use of QUESTRAN is not known. In the LRC-CPPT study referred to above, the total incidence of fatal and nonfatal neoplasms was similar in both treatment groups. When the many different categories of tumors are examined, various alimentary system cancers were somewhat more prevalent in the cholestyramine group. The small numbers and the multiple categories prevent conclusions from being drawn. However, in view of the fact that cholestyramine resin is confined to the GI tract and not absorbed, and in light of the animal experiments referred to above, further follow-up of the LRC-CPPT participants is planned for cause-specific mortality and cancer morbidity.

Pregnancy: Since QUESTRAN is not absorbed systemically, it is not expected to cause fetal harm when administered during pregnancy in recommended dosages. There are, however, no adequate and well-controlled studies in pregnant women, and the known interference with absorption of fat-soluble vitamins may be detrimental even in the presence of supplementation.

Nursing Mothers: Caution should be exercised when QUESTRAN is administered to a nursing mother. The possible lack of proper vitamin absorption described in the "Pregnancy" section may have an effect on nursing infants.

Pediatric Use: As experience in infants and children is limited, a practical dosage schedule has not been established. In calculating pediatric dosages, 44.4 mg of anhydrous cholestyramine resin are contained in 100 mg of QUESTRAN. The effects of long-term drug administration, as well as its effect in maintaining lowered cholesterol levels in pediatric patients, are unknown.

ADVERSE REACTIONS

The most common adverse reaction is constipation. When used as a cholesterol-lowering agent predisposing factors for most complaints of constipation are high dose and increased age (more than 60 years old). Most instances of constipation are mild, transient, and controlled with conventional therapy. Some patients require a temporary decrease in dosage or discontinuation of therapy.

Less Frequent Adverse Reactions: Abdominal discomfort and/or pain, flatulence, nausea, vomiting, diarrhea, eructation, anorexia, and steatorrhea, bleeding tendencies due to hypoprothrombinemia (Vitamin K deficiency) as well as Vitamin A (one case of night blindness reported) and D deficiencies, hyperchloremic acidosis in children, osteoporosis, rash and irritation of the skin, tongue and perianal area. One 10-month-old baby with biliary atresia had an impaction presumed to be due to QUESTRAN after 3 days administration of 9 grams daily. She developed acute intestinal sepsis and died.

Occasional calcified material has been observed in the biliary tree, including calcification of the gallbladder, in patients to whom cholestyramine resin has been given. However, this may be a manifestation of the liver disease and not drug related.

One patient experienced biliary colic on each of three occasions on which he took QUESTRAN. One patient diagnosed as acute abdominal symptom complex was found to have a "pasty mass" in the transverse colon on x-ray.

Other events (not necessarily drug related) reported in patients taking QUESTRAN include:

Gastrointestinal—GI-rectal bleeding, black stools, hemorrhoidal bleeding, bleeding from known duodenal ulcer, dysphagia, hiccups, ulcer attack, sour taste, pancreatitis, rectal pain, diverticulitis.

Laboratory test changes—Liver function abnormalities.

Hematologic—Prolonged prothrombin time, ecchymosis, anemia.

Hypersensitivity—Urticaria, asthma, wheezing, shortness of breath.

Musculoskeletal—Backache, muscle and joint pains, arthritis.

Neurologic—Headache, anxiety, vertigo, dizziness, fatigue, tinnitus, syncope, drowsiness, femoral nerve pain, paresthesia.

Eye—Uveitis.

Renal—Hematuria, dysuria, burnt odor to urine, diuresis.

Miscellaneous—Weight loss, weight gain, increased libido, swollen glands, edema, dental bleeding.

OVERDOSAGE

Overdosage of QUESTRAN has not been reported. Should overdosage occur, however, the chief potential harm would be obstruction of the gastrointestinal tract. The location of such potential obstruction, the degree of obstruction, and the presence or absence of normal gut motility would determine treatment.

DOSAGE AND ADMINISTRATION

The recommended starting adult dose for QUESTRAN is 1 packet or 1 level scoopful (9 grams of QUESTRAN contain 4 grams of anhydrous cholestyramine resin) once or twice a day. The recommended maintenance dose for QUESTRAN is 2 to 4 packets or scoopfuls daily (8–16 grams anhydrous cholestyramine resin) divided into two doses. It is recommended that increases in dose be gradual with periodic assessment of lipid/lipoprotein levels at intervals of not less than 4 weeks. The maximum recommended daily dose is 6 packets or scoopfuls of QUESTRAN (24 grams of anhydrous cholestyramine resin). The suggested time of administration is at mealtime but may be modified to avoid interference with absorption of other medications. Although the recommended dosing schedule is twice daily, QUESTRAN may be administered in 1 to 6 doses per day.

QUESTRAN Powder should not be taken in its dry form. Always mix QUESTRAN Powder with water or other fluids before ingesting. See Preparation Instructions.

Concomitant Therapy

Preliminary evidence suggests that the cholesterol-lowering effects of the HMG-CoA reductase inhibitor, lovastatin, and cholestyramine are additive. Additive effects on LDL and HDL cholesterol are seen with combined nicotinic acid-cholestyramine therapy.

PREPARATION

The color of QUESTRAN may vary somewhat from batch to batch, but this variation does not affect the performance of the product. Place the contents of one single-dose packet or one level scoopful of QUESTRAN in a glass or cup. Add at least 2 to 6 ounces of water or the beverage of your choice. Stir to a uniform consistency.

QUESTRAN may also be mixed with highly fluid soups or pulpy fruits with a high moisture content such as applesauce or crushed pineapple.

HOW SUPPLIED

QUESTRAN is available in cartons of sixty 9-gram packets and in cans containing 378 grams. Nine grams of QUESTRAN Powder contain 4 grams of anhydrous cholestyramine resin.

NDC 0087-0580-11 Cartons of 60 packets

NDC 0087-0580-05 Cans, 378 g

CLINICAL STUDIES

The NIH has concluded a 10-year randomized double-blind placebo-controlled study[a] in 12 lipid research clinics on the effect of lowering plasma cholesterol on coronary heart disease (CHD) risk (the risk of either coronary death or nonfatal myocardial infarction). Plasma cholesterol was lowered by a combination of a modest cholesterol-lowering diet and QUESTRAN. The dose response relationship between the amount of QUESTRAN ingested daily, the lowering of total plasma cholesterol, and the reduction in CHD risk is summarized below:

RELATION OF REDUCTION IN CHOLESTEROL TO REDUCTION IN CORONARY HEART DISEASE RISK

Packet Count	No.	Total Cholesterol Lowering	Reduction in CHD Risk
0–2	439	4.4%	10.9%
2–5	496	11.5%	26.1%
5–6	965	19.0%	39.3%

REFERENCE

[a]Anon: The Lipid Research Clinics Coronary Primary Prevention Trial Results: (I) Reduction in Incidence of Coronary Heart Disease; (II) The Relationship of Reduction in Incidence of Coronary Heart Disease to Cholesterol Lowering. *JAMA.* 1984; 251:351–374.

Shown in Product Identification Section, page 406

QUESTRAN® LIGHT ℞

[kwest'răn līt]

(Cholestyramine for Oral Suspension, USP)

This is the full text of the latest Official Package Circular dated September 1991 (58903DIM-03).

DESCRIPTION

QUESTRAN LIGHT (cholestyramine for oral suspension, USP), the chloride salt of a basic anion exchange resin, a cholesterol-lowering agent, is intended for oral administration. Cholestyramine resin is quite hydrophilic, but insoluble in water. The cholestyramine resin in QUESTRAN LIGHT is not absorbed from the digestive tract. Five grams of QUESTRAN LIGHT contain 4 grams of anhydrous cholestyramine resin. It is represented by the following structural formula:

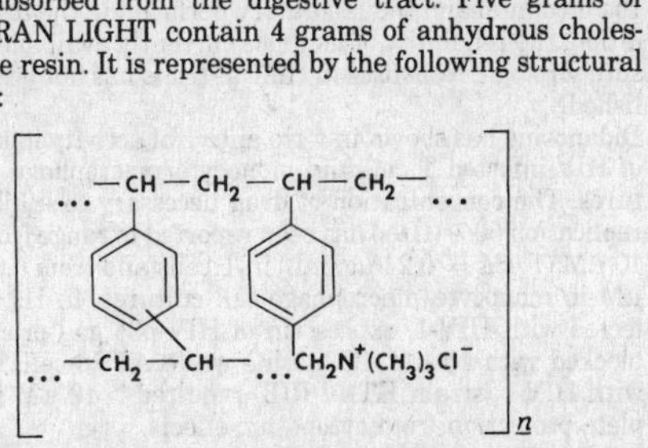

Representation of structure of main polymeric groups

This product contains the following inactive ingredients: aspartame, citric acid, D&C Yellow No. 10, FD&C Red No. 40, flavor (natural and artificial), propylene glycol alginate, colloidal silicon dioxide, sucrose, and xanthan gum.

CLINICAL PHARMACOLOGY

Cholesterol is probably the sole precursor of bile acids. During normal digestion, bile acids are secreted into the intestines. A major portion of the bile acids is absorbed from the intestinal tract and returned to the liver via the enterohepatic circulation. Only very small amounts of bile acids are found in normal serum.

Cholestyramine resin adsorbs and combines with the bile acids in the intestine to form an insoluble complex which is excreted in the feces. This results in a partial removal of bile acids from the enterohepatic circulation by preventing their absorption.

The increased fecal loss of bile acids due to cholestyramine resin administration leads to an increased oxidation of cholesterol to bile acids, a decrease in beta lipoprotein or low density lipoprotein plasma levels and a decrease in serum cholesterol levels. Although in man cholestyramine resin produces an increase in hepatic synthesis of cholesterol, plasma cholesterol levels fall.

In patients with partial biliary obstruction, the reduction of serum bile acid levels by cholestyramine resin reduces excess bile acids deposited in the dermal tissue with resultant decrease in pruritus.

INDICATIONS AND USAGE

1. QUESTRAN LIGHT is indicated as adjunctive therapy to diet for the reduction of elevated serum cholesterol in patients with primary hypercholesterolemia (elevated low density lipoprotein [LDL] cholesterol) who do not respond adequately to diet. Cholestyramine resin may be useful to lower LDL cholesterol in patients who also have hypertriglyceridemia, but it is not indicated where hypertriglyceridemia is the abnormality of most concern.

   In a large, placebo-controlled, multi-clinic study, the LRC-CPPT[a], hypercholesterolemic subjects treated with cholestyramine resin had significant reductions in total and low-density lipoprotein cholesterol (LDL-C). Over the 7-year study period the cholestyramine resin group experienced a 19% reduction in the combined rate of coronary heart disease death plus nonfatal myocardial infarction (cumulative incidences of 7% cholestyramine resin and 8.6% placebo). The subjects included in the study were middle-aged men (age 35-59) with serum cholesterol levels above 265 mg/dL and no previous history of heart disease. It is not clear to what extent these findings can be extrapolated to other segments of the hypercholesterolemic population not studied.

   Dietary therapy specific for the type of hyperlipoproteinemia is the initial treatment of choice. Excess body weight may be an important factor and caloric restriction for weight normalization should be addressed prior to drug therapy in the overweight. The use of drugs should be considered only when reasonable attempts have been made to obtain satisfactory results with nondrug methods. If the decision ultimately is to use drugs, the patient should be instructed that this does not reduce the importance of adhering to diet.

2. QUESTRAN LIGHT is indicated for the relief of pruritus associated with partial biliary obstruction. Cholestyramine resin has been shown to have a variable effect on serum cholesterol in these patients. Patients with primary biliary cirrhosis may exhibit an elevated cholesterol as part of their disease.

CONTRAINDICATIONS

Cholestyramine resin is contraindicated in patients with complete biliary obstruction where bile is not secreted into the intestine and in those individuals who have shown hypersensitivity to any of its components.

WARNING

PHENYLKETONURICS: QUESTRAN LIGHT CONTAINS 16.8 mg PHENYLALANINE PER 5-GRAM DOSE.

PRECAUTIONS

General

Before instituting therapy with cholestyramine resin, diseases contributing to increased blood cholesterol such as hypothyroidism, diabetes mellitus, nephrotic syndrome, dysproteinemias and obstructive liver disease should be looked for and specifically treated. A favorable trend in cholesterol reduction should occur during the first month of cholestyramine resin therapy. The therapy should be continued to sustain cholesterol reduction. If adequate cholesterol reduction is not attained, cholestyramine resin therapy should be discontinued.

Chronic use of cholestyramine resin may be associated with increased bleeding tendency due to hypoprothrombinemia associated with Vitamin K deficiency. This will usually respond promptly to parenteral Vitamin K_1 and recurrences can be prevented by oral administration of Vitamin K_1. Reduction of serum or red cell folate has been reported over long term administration of cholestyramine resin. Supplementation with folic acid should be considered in these cases.

There is a possibility that prolonged use of QUESTRAN LIGHT, since it is a chloride form of anion exchange resin, may produce hyperchloremic acidosis. This would especially be true in younger and smaller patients where the relative dosage may be higher.

Cholestyramine resin may produce or worsen preexisting constipation. Dosage should be reduced or discontinued in such cases. Fecal impaction and aggravation of hemorrhoids may occur. Every effort should be made to avert severe constipation and its inherent problems in those patients with clinically symptomatic coronary artery disease.

Information for Patients

Inform your physician if you are pregnant or plan to become pregnant or are breastfeeding. Drink plenty of fluids and mix each 5-gram dose of QUESTRAN LIGHT in at least 2 to 3 ounces of fluid before taking.

Laboratory Tests

Serum cholesterol levels should be determined frequently during the first few months of therapy and periodically thereafter. Serum triglyceride levels should be measured periodically to detect whether significant changes have occurred.

The LRC-CPPT showed a dose-related increase in serum triglycerides of 10.7% to 17.1% in the cholestyramine-treated group, compared with an increase of 7.9% to 11.7% in the placebo group. Based on the mean values and adjusting for the placebo group, the cholestyramine-treated group showed an increase of 5% over pre-entry levels the first year of the study and an increase of 4.3% the seventh year.

Drug Interactions

Cholestyramine resin may delay or reduce the absorption of concomitant oral medication such as phenylbutazone, warfarin, chlorothiazide (acidic), or propranolol (basic), as well as tetracycline, penicillin G, phenobarbital, thyroid and thyroxine preparations, and digitalis. The discontinuance of cholestyramine resin could pose a hazard to health if a potentially toxic drug such as digitalis has been titrated to a maintenance level while the patient was taking cholestyramine resin.

Because cholestyramine binds bile acids, cholestyramine resin may interfere with normal fat digestion and absorption and thus may prevent absorption of fat soluble vitamins such as A, D and K. When cholestyramine resin is given for long periods of time, concomitant supplementation with water-miscible (or parenteral) form of vitamins A and D should be considered.

SINCE CHOLESTYRAMINE RESIN MAY BIND OTHER DRUGS GIVEN CONCURRENTLY, PATIENTS SHOULD TAKE OTHER DRUGS AT LEAST 1 HOUR BEFORE OR 4 TO 6 HOURS AFTER CHOLESTYRAMINE RESIN (OR AT AS GREAT AN INTERVAL AS POSSIBLE) TO AVOID IMPEDING THEIR ABSORPTION.

Carcinogenesis, Mutagenesis and Impairment of Fertility

In studies conducted in rats in which cholestyramine resin was used as a tool to investigate the role of various intestinal factors, such as fat, bile salts and microbial flora, in the development of intestinal tumors induced by potent carcinogens, the incidence of such tumors was observed to be greater in cholestyramine resin-treated rats than in control rats.

The relevance of this laboratory observation from studies in rats to the clinical use of cholestyramine resin is not known. In the LRC-CPPT study referred to above, the total incidence of fatal and nonfatal neoplasms was similar in both treatment groups. When the many different categories of tumors are examined, various alimentary system cancers were somewhat more prevalent in the cholestyramine group. The small numbers and the multiple categories prevent conclusions from being drawn. However, in view of the fact that cholestyramine resin is confined to the GI tract and not absorbed, and in light of the animal experiments referred to above, further follow-up of the LRC-CPPT participants is planned for cause-specific mortality and cancer morbidity.

Pregnancy

Since cholestyramine resin is not absorbed systemically, it is not expected to cause fetal harm when administered during pregnancy in recommended dosages. There are, however, no adequate and well-controlled studies in pregnant women, and the known interference with absorption of fat soluble vitamins may be detrimental even in the presence of supplementation.

Nursing Mothers

Caution should be exercised when cholestyramine resin is administered to a nursing mother. The possible lack of proper vitamin absorption described in the "Pregnancy" section may have an effect on nursing infants.

Pediatric Use

As experience in infants and children is limited, a practical dosage schedule has not been established.

In calculating pediatric dosages, 80 mg of anhydrous cholestyramine resin are contained in 100 mg of QUESTRAN LIGHT.

The effects of long-term drug administration, as well as its effect in maintaining lowered cholesterol levels in pediatric patients, are unknown.

ADVERSE REACTIONS

The most common adverse reaction is constipation. When used as a cholesterol-lowering agent, predisposing factors for most complaints of constipation are high dose and increased age (more than 60 years old). Most instances of constipation are mild, transient, and controlled with conventional ther-

Continued on next page

Bristol Laboratories—Cont.

apy. Some patients require a temporary decrease in dosage or discontinuation of therapy.

Less Frequent Adverse Reactions: Abdominal discomfort and/or pain, flatulence, nausea, vomiting, diarrhea, dyspepsia, eructation, anorexia, indigestive feeling and steatorrhea, bleeding tendencies due to hypoprothrombinemia (Vitamin K deficiency) as well as Vitamin A (one case of night blindness reported) and D deficiencies, hyperchloremic acidosis in children, osteoporosis, rash and irritation of the skin, tongue and perianal area. One 10-month-old baby with biliary atresia had an impaction presumed to be due to cholestyramine resin after 3 days administration of 9 grams daily. She developed acute intestinal sepsis and died.

Occasional calcified material has been observed in the biliary tree, including calcification of the gallbladder, in patients to whom cholestyramine resin has been given. However, this may be a manifestation of the liver disease and not drug related.

One patient experienced biliary colic on each of three occasions on which he took cholestyramine resin. One patient diagnosed as acute abdominal symptom complex was found to have a "pasty mass" in the transverse colon on x-ray.

Other events (not necessarily drug related) reported in patients taking cholestyramine resin include:

Gastrointestinal—GI-rectal bleeding, black stools, hemorrhoidal bleeding, bleeding from known duodenal ulcer, dysphagia, hiccups, ulcer attack, sour taste, pancreatitis, rectal pain, diverticulitis.

Laboratory test changes—Liver function abnormalities.

Hematologic—Prolonged prothrombin time, ecchymosis, anemia.

Hypersensitivity—Urticaria, asthma, wheezing, shortness of breath.

Musculoskeletal—Backache, muscle and joint pains, arthritis.

Neurologic—Headache, anxiety, vertigo, dizziness, fatigue, tinnitus, syncope, drowsiness, femoral nerve pain, paresthesia.

Eye—Uveitis.

Renal—Hematuria, dysuria, burnt odor to urine, diuresis.

Miscellaneous—Weight loss, weight gain, increased libido, swollen glands, edema, dental bleeding.

OVERDOSAGE

Overdosage of cholestyramine resin has not been reported. Should overdosage occur, however, the chief potential harm would be obstruction of the gastrointestinal tract. The location of such potential obstruction, the degree of obstruction, and the presence or absence of normal gut motility would determine treatment.

DOSAGE AND ADMINISTRATION

The recommended starting adult dose for QUESTRAN LIGHT is one packet or one level scoopful (5 grams of QUESTRAN LIGHT contains 4 grams of anhydrous cholestyramine resin) once or twice a day. The recommended maintenance dose for QUESTRAN LIGHT is 2 to 4 packets or scoopfuls daily (8–16 grams anhydrous cholestyramine resin) divided into two doses. It is recommended that increases in dose be gradual with periodic assessment of lipid/lipoprotein levels at intervals of not less than 4 weeks. The maximum recommended daily dose is 6 packets or scoopfuls of QUESTRAN LIGHT (24 grams of anhydrous cholestyramine resin). The suggested time of administration is at mealtime but may be modified to avoid interference with absorption of other medications. Although the recommended dosing schedule is twice daily, QUESTRAN LIGHT may be administered in 1 to 6 doses per day.

QUESTRAN LIGHT should not be taken in its dry form. Always mix QUESTRAN LIGHT with water or other fluids before ingesting. See Preparation instructions.

Concomitant Therapy

Preliminary evidence suggests that the cholesterol-lowering effects of the HMG-CoA reductase inhibitor, lovastatin, and cholestyramine are additive. Additive effects on LDL and HDL cholesterol are seen with combined nicotinic acid-cholestyramine therapy.

PREPARATION

The color of QUESTRAN LIGHT may vary somewhat from batch to batch but this variation does not affect the performance of the product. Place the contents of one single-dose packet or one level scoopful of cholestyramine resin in a glass or cup. Add at least 2 to 3 ounces of water or the beverage of your choice. Stir to a uniform consistency.

QUESTRAN LIGHT may also be mixed with highly fluid soups or pulpy fruits with a high moisture content such as applesauce or crushed pineapple.

HOW SUPPLIED

QUESTRAN LIGHT is available in cartons of sixty 5-gram packets and in cans containing 210 grams. Five grams of QUESTRAN LIGHT contain 4 grams of anhydrous cholestyramine resin.

NDC 0087-0589-01 — 210 g cans, 42 doses
NDC 0087-0589-03 — Cartons of 60, 5 g packets

Store at room temperature.

CLINICAL STUDIES

The NIH has concluded a 10-year randomized double-blind placebo-controlled study[a] in 12 lipid research clinics on the effect of lowering plasma cholesterol on coronary heart disease (CHD) risk (the risk of either coronary death or nonfatal myocardial infarction). Plasma cholesterol was lowered by a combination of a modest cholesterol-lowering diet and cholestyramine resin. The dose response relationship between the amount of cholestyramine resin ingested daily, the lowering of total plasma cholesterol, and the reduction of CHD risk is summarized below:

RELATION OF REDUCTION IN CHOLESTEROL TO REDUCTION IN CORONARY HEART DISEASE RISK

No. of Doses* Per Day	No.	Total Cholesterol Lowering	Reduction in CHD Risk
0–2	439	4.4%	10.9%
2–5	496	11.5%	26.1%
5–6	965	19.0%	39.3%

*One dose contains 4 g cholestyramine resin.

REFERENCE

a. Anon: The Lipid Research Clinics Coronary Primary Prevention Trial Results: (I) Reduction in Incidence of Coronary Heart Disease; (II) The Relationship of Reduction in Incidence of Coronary Heart Disease to Cholesterol Lowering. *JAMA.* 1984; 251:351–374.

Shown in Product Identification Section, page 406

VIDEX® ℞
(didanosine)
VIDEX® (didanosine) Chewable/Dispersible Buffered Tablets
VIDEX® (didanosine) Buffered Powder for Oral Solution
VIDEX® (didanosine) Pediatric Powder for Oral Solution

WARNING

VIDEX IS INDICATED FOR THE TREATMENT OF ADULT AND PEDIATRIC PATIENTS (OVER 6 MONTHS OF AGE) WITH ADVANCED HIV INFECTION WHO ARE INTOLERANT OF ZIDOVUDINE THERAPY OR WHO HAVE DEMONSTRATED SIGNIFICANT CLINICAL OR IMMUNOLOGIC DETERIORATION DURING ZIDOVUDINE THERAPY. THIS INDICATION IS BASED PRIMARILY ON THE RESULTS OF NON-RANDOMIZED, PHASE 1 STUDIES IN WHICH AN INCREASE IN CD4 CELL COUNTS WAS OBSERVED FOR MANY PATIENTS DURING VIDEX THERAPY. THESE RESULTS WERE COMPARED WITH DATA FROM HISTORICAL CONTROLS AND WERE AUGMENTED BY AN INTERIM ANALYSIS OF CD4 DATA OBTAINED FROM A PORTION OF AN ONGOING CONTROLLED CLINICAL TRIAL. AT PRESENT THERE ARE NO RESULTS FROM CONTROLLED STUDIES REGARDING THE EFFECT OF VIDEX THERAPY ON THE CLINICAL PROGRESSION OF HIV INFECTION, SUCH AS INCIDENCE OF OPPORTUNISTIC INFECTIONS AND SURVIVAL. BECAUSE ZIDOVUDINE HAS BEEN SHOWN TO PROLONG SURVIVAL AND DECREASE THE INCIDENCE OF OPPORTUNISTIC INFECTIONS IN PATIENTS WITH ADVANCED HIV DISEASE, ZIDOVUDINE SHOULD BE CONSIDERED AS INITIAL THERAPY FOR THE TREATMENT OF ADVANCED HIV INFECTION, UNLESS CONTRAINDICATED.

THE MAJOR CLINICAL TOXICITIES OF VIDEX ARE PANCREATITIS AND PERIPHERAL NEUROPATHY. PANCREATITIS, WHICH CAN BE FATAL, OCCURRED IN 9% OF THE PHASE 1 PATIENTS TREATED WITH VIDEX AT OR BELOW THE RECOMMENDED DOSE. PANCREATITIS MUST BE CONSIDERED WHENEVER A PATIENT RECEIVING VIDEX DEVELOPS ABDOMINAL PAIN AND NAUSEA, VOMITING, OR ELEVATED BIOCHEMICAL MARKERS. UNDER THESE CIRCUMSTANCES, VIDEX USE SHOULD BE SUSPENDED UNTIL THE DIAGNOSIS OF PANCREATITIS IS EXCLUDED (SEE "WARNINGS").

PERIPHERAL NEUROPATHY OCCURRED IN 34% OF PHASE 1 PATIENTS TREATED WITH VIDEX AT OR BELOW THE RECOMMENDED DOSE (SEE "WARNINGS").

PATIENTS RECEIVING VIDEX OR ANY ANTIRETROVIRAL THERAPY MAY CONTINUE TO DEVELOP OPPORTUNISTIC INFECTIONS AND OTHER COMPLICATIONS OF HIV INFECTION, AND THEREFORE SHOULD REMAIN UNDER CLOSE CLINICAL OBSERVATION BY PHYSICIANS EXPERIENCED IN THE TREATMENT OF PATIENTS WITH HIV ASSOCIATED DISEASES.

DESCRIPTION

VIDEX® (didanosine) Chewable/Dispersible Buffered Tablets are available for oral administration in strengths of 25, 50, 100, or 150 mg of VIDEX. Each tablet is buffered with dihydroxyaluminum sodium carbonate, magnesium hydroxide, and sodium citrate. VIDEX tablets also contain: aspartame, confectioner's sugar, wintergreen flavor, polyplasdone, microcrystalline cellulose, silicon dioxide, and magnesium stearate.

VIDEX Buffered Powder for Oral Solution is supplied for oral administration in single-dose packets containing 100, 167, 250, or 375 mg of VIDEX. Packets of each product strength also contain a citrate-phosphate buffer (composed of dibasic sodium phosphate, sodium citrate, and citric acid) and sucrose.

VIDEX Pediatric Powder for Oral Solution is supplied for oral administration in 4- or 8-ounce glass bottles containing 2 or 4 g of VIDEX, respectively.

VIDEX is a synthetic purine nucleoside analogue active against the Human Immunodeficiency Virus (HIV). The chemical name for VIDEX is 2′,3′-dideoxyinosine; it is also called ddI. It has the following structural formula:

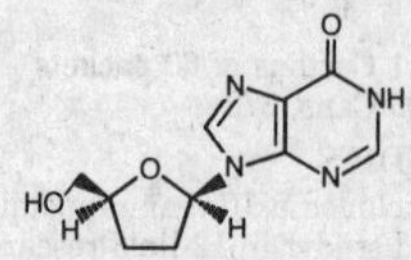

VIDEX is a white crystalline powder with the molecular formula $C_{10}H_{12}N_4O_3$ and a molecular weight of 236.2 daltons. The aqueous solubility of VIDEX at 25°C and pH of approximately 6 is 27.3 mg/mL. VIDEX is unstable in acidic solutions. For example, at pH <3 and 37°C, 10% of VIDEX decomposes to hypoxanthine in less than 2 minutes.

CLINICAL PHARMACOLOGY

Mechanism of Action

Didanosine, a nucleoside analogue of deoxyadenosine, is an inhibitor of the in vitro replication of HIV (also known as HTLV III or LAV) in human primary cell cultures and in established cell lines. After didanosine enters the cell, it is converted by cellular enzymes to the active antiviral metabolite, dideoxyadenosine triphosphate (ddATP). The intracellular half-life of ddATP, calculated from results obtained from the in vitro cell culture studies, varied from 8 to 24 hours.

A common feature of dideoxynucleosides (the class of compounds to which didanosine belongs) is the lack of a free 3′-hydroxyl group. In nucleic acid replication, the 3′-hydroxyl of a naturally occurring nucleoside is the acceptor for covalent attachment of subsequent nucleoside 5′-monophosphates; its presence is therefore requisite for continued DNA chain extension. Because ddATP lacks a 3′-hydroxyl group, incorporation of ddATP into viral DNA leads to chain termination and, thus, inhibition of viral replication. In addition, ddATP further contributes to inhibition of viral replication through interference with the HIV-RNA dependent DNA polymerase (reverse transcriptase) by competing with the natural nucleoside triphosphate, dATP, for binding to the active site of the enzyme.

Microbiology

The relationship between in vitro susceptibility of HIV to didanosine and the inhibition of HIV replication in man or clinical response to therapy has not been established. In vitro sensitivity results vary greatly depending upon the time between virus infection and didanosine treatment, the particular assay used, the cell type employed, the size of the virus inoculum and the laboratory performing the test. In addition, the reliability of methods currently available to measure virologic responses in clinical trials has not been established.

Didanosine has shown in vitro antiviral activity in a variety of HIV-infected T cell and monocyte/macrophage cell cultures. The concentration of drug necessary to inhibit viral replication 50% (ID_{50}) has been reported to range from 2.5 to 10 μM (1 μM = 0.24 μg/mL) in T cells and from 0.01 to 0.1 μM in monocyte/macrophage cell cultures. In H9 cells infected with HIV-1, expression of HIV-p24 gag protein was blocked with 10 μM didanosine while ATH8 cells infected with HIV-1 (strain HTLV-IIIB) required >10 μM for complete protection from cytopathic effects.

In a quantitative plaque (syncytium) reduction assay using HT4-6C cells, didanosine ID_{50} values of 2.1 μM for HIV-1 and 5.6 μM for HIV-2 have been reported. The ID_{50} values of zidovudine determined using this assay system were 0.05 and 0.08 μM for HIV-1 and HIV-2, respectively. However, in infected human MT-2 cells in culture, didanosine ID_{50} values reported for HIV-1 and HIV-2 were 1 and 10 μM, while ID_{50} values for zidovudine were 0.3 and >100 μM, respectively.

The development of clinically significant didanosine resistance in patients with HIV infection after receiving didanosine therapy has not been studied adequately and the fre-

quency of didanosine-resistant isolates in the general population remains unknown. Pre- and post-therapy clinical isolates of HIV obtained from 14 patients on long-term didanosine therapy have been evaluated in vitro for sensitivity to didanosine. Results obtained showed that 12 of 14 pretherapy isolates had ID_{50} values of $\leq 5\ \mu M$, whereas, 2 of the 14 pretherapy isolates had ID_{50} values of 30 and 50 μM, respectively. Comparisons of posttherapy to pretherapy ID_{50} values, determined in isolates taken from the same patient, revealed that in vitro sensitivity to didanosine decreased 15-fold in 1 patient, decreased 6-fold in 3 patients, and was not significantly altered in the remaining 10 patients evaluated. The clinical significance of these findings has not been established. In a quantitative plaque reduction assay using HT4-6C cells, didanosine has shown activity in vitro (ID_{50} 0.7 μM) against one zidovudine-resistant HIV-1 strain isolated from a patient who had received long-term therapy with zidovudine.

The results of cytotoxicity studies in various cell lines have shown little cytotoxic action with didanosine. In cultured human bone marrow progenitor cells the concentration of drug necessary to inhibit cell growth 50% (IC_{50}) was > 100 μM for didanosine. For zidovudine, IC_{50} values under similar assay conditions ranged from 0.13 to 5 μM.

Didanosine has shown antiviral activity in one mouse animal model. Mice with severe combined immundeficiency (SCID) of genetic origin have been shown to develop an immune system of human origin (SCID-hu) when transplanted with human fetal hematolymphoid organs. These SCID-hu mice, when inoculated with primary isolates of HIV become infected with HIV and subsequently develop viremia. It has been shown that antiretroviral agents can prevent development of HIV viremia in this animal model system. In an assay in which didanosine was administered to SCID-hu mice by intraperitoneal injection twice daily for 4 days commencing 24 hours prior to HIV infection and once daily for days 4 to 14 postinfection, the dose that protected 50% of the animals from developing viremia (PD_{50}) was reported to be 13.7 mg/kg/day. In a similar assay, the PD_{50} valued for zidovudine administered orally in drinking water was determined to be 40.4 mg/kg/day.

Didanosine has been shown to inhibit human hepatitis B virus (HBV) replication in vitro. In a cell culture assay using 2.2.15 (PR) cells which continuously produce HBV genome, the ID_{50} for didanosine was estimated to be 50 to 100 μM as demonstrated by reduction in extrachromosomal HBV DNA. The clinical significance of these findings is unknown.

Animal Toxicology

Evidence of a dose-limiting skeletal muscle toxicity has been observed in mice and rats (but not in dogs) following long-term (greater than 90 days) dosing with VIDEX® (didanosine) at doses that were approximately 1.2 to 12 times the estimated human exposure. The relationship of this finding to the potential of VIDEX to cause myopathy in humans is unclear. However, human myopathy has been associated with administration of other nucleoside analogues.

Pharmacokinetics

VIDEX is rapidly degraded at acidic pH. Therefore, all oral formulations contain buffering agents designed to increase the pH of the gastric environment. When VIDEX Chewable/Dispersible Buffered tablets are administered, each adult and pediatric dose must consist of 2 tablets in order to achieve adequate acid-neutralizing capacity for maximal absorption of VIDEX. The only exception is for pediatric patients who are less than 1 year of age; for these patients only 1 tablet is necessary to provide adequate acid neutralizing capacity.

Bioequivalence of Dosage Formulations: Results of a study in 18 asymptomatic, HIV seropositive patients comparing a 375-mg dose of VIDEX Powder for Oral Solution and VIDEX Chewable/Dispersible Buffered Tablets indicate that VIDEX is 20% to 25% more bioavailable from the tablet compared to the solution. A separate study in 24 asymptomatic, HIV seropositive patients demonstrated that a 375-mg dose of the VIDEX Buffered Powder for Oral Solution produced similar plasma concentrations to a 300-mg (2 × 150 mg tablets) dose of the VIDEX Chewable/Dispersible Buffered Tablets. Mean (±1 SD) peak plasma concentrations (C_{max}) were 1.6 (±0.6) μg/mL, range: 0.4 to 2.9 μg/mL, for the buffered solution and 1.6 (±0.5) μg/mL, range: 0.5 to 2.6 μg/mL, for the chewable tablet. Mean area under the plasma concentration versus time curve (AUC) values were 3.0 (±0.8) $\mu g \cdot hr$/mL, range: 1.6 to 5.1 $\mu g \cdot hr$/mL, for the buffered solution and 2.6 (±0.7) $\mu g \cdot hr$/mL, range: 1.1 to 3.9 $\mu g \cdot hr$/mL, for the chewable tablet.

Effect of Food on Oral Absorption: All VIDEX formulations should be administered on an empty stomach. A study in 8 asymptomatic HIV seropositive patients demonstrated that the administration of VIDEX® (didanosine) Chewable/Dispersible Buffered Tablets within 5 minutes of a meal resulted in a 50% decrease in mean C_{max} and AUC values. The mean C_{max} was 2.8 μg/mL (range: 1.1 to 4.2 μg/mL) in the fasting state, versus 1.3 μg/mL (range: 0.7 to 2.2 μg/mL) in the fed state. The AUC values averaged 3.9 $\mu g \cdot hr$/mL (range: 2.8 to 6.7 $\mu g \cdot hr$/mL) under fasting conditions, versus 2.1 $\mu g \cdot hr$/mL (range: 1.2 to 4.0 $\mu g \cdot hr$/mL) following a meal.

Study Design in Adults: The pharmacokinetics of VIDEX were evaluated in 69 adult patients with AIDS or severe AIDS-Related Complex after the administration of single and multiple intravenous (IV) and oral doses. These patients had creatinine clearance values of > 60 mL/min and no evidence of hepatic dysfunction. The oral doses were administered as a lyophilized formulation which was similar in composition to VIDEX Pediatric Powder for Oral Solution. Patients received a 60-minute IV infusion of VIDEX, administered once or twice a day for 2 weeks, at total daily doses ranging from 0.8 mg/kg to 33 mg/kg. Oral doses equivalent to twice the IV dose were administered for an additional 4 weeks. Plasma VIDEX concentrations were obtained on the first day of dosing and at steady state after intravenous and oral dosing.

Absorption and Dose Linearity in Adults: Although there was significant variability between patients, the C_{max} and AUC values increased in proportion to dose over the range of doses administered in clinical practice. At doses of 7 mg/kg or less, the average absolute bioavailability was 33 (±14)% after a single dose and 37 (±14)% after 4 weeks of VIDEX dosing. Pharmacokinetic parameters at steady state were not significantly different from values obtained after the initial IV or oral dose.

Distribution in Adults: The steady state volume of distribution after IV administration averaged 54 L (range: 22 to 103 L). In a study of 5 adults, the concentration of VIDEX in the cerebrospinal fluid 1 hour after infusion of VIDEX averaged 21% of simultaneous plasma concentration.[1]

Elimination in Adults: After oral administration of VIDEX, the average elimination half-life was 1.6 hours (range: 0.52 to 4.64 hours). Total body clearance averaged 800 mL/min (range: 412 to 1505 mL/min). Renal clearance represented approximately 50% of the total body clearance (average: 400, range: 95 to 860 mL/min), when VIDEX was administered either intravenously or orally. This indicates that active tubular secretion, in addition to glomerular filtration, is responsible for the renal elimination of VIDEX. Urinary recovery of VIDEX after a single dose was approximately 55% (range: 27 to 98%), and 20% (range: 3 to 31%) of the dose after IV and oral administration, respectively. There was no evidence of accumulation of VIDEX® (didanosine) after either IV or oral dosing.

Study Design in Children: The pharmacokinetics of VIDEX have been evaluated in two pediatric studies. In one study (ACTG/St. Jude), 16 children and 4 adolescents received a single IV dose ranging from 40 to 90 mg/m^2 and multiple, twice daily oral doses of 80 to 180 mg/m^2 of VIDEX. In another study (NCI), 48 pediatric patients received a single IV dose and then multiple, three times daily oral doses ranging from 20 to 180 mg/m^2.[2] In both studies, oral doses were administered as a lyophilized formula which was similar in composition to VIDEX Pediatric Powder for Oral Solution.

Absorption and Dose Linearity in Children: Although there was significant variability between patients, the C_{max} and AUC values increased in proportion to dose in both studies. These findings were similar to those in adult patients. The absolute bioavailability varied between patients in the ACTG/St. Jude study and averaged 32 (±12)%, range: 13 to 53%, and 42 (±18)%, range: 21 to 78%, after the first oral dose and at steady state, respectively. The NCI study also demonstrated significant variability in the oral absorption of VIDEX with an average absolute bioavailability of 19 (±17)%, range: 2 to 89%. In the ACTG/St. Jude study, the average steady state AUC was 1.4 (±0.4), 1.6 (±0.9) and 2.3 (±0.9) $\mu g \cdot hr$/mL after the administration of oral doses of 80, 120, and 180 mg/m^2, respectively. The average corresponding steady state C_{max} values were 0.8 (±0.4), 1.4 (±0.7), and 1.7 (±0.9) μg/mL, respectively.

Distribution in Children: In the ACTG/St. Jude study, the volume of distribution after IV administration averaged 35.6 L/m^2 (range: 18.4 to 60.7 L/m^2). In this study, the concentration of VIDEX ranged from 0.04 to 0.12 μg/mL in cerebrospinal fluid (CSF) samples collected from seven patients at times ranging from 1.5 to 3.5 hr after a single intravenous or oral dose. These CSF concentrations corresponded to 12 to 85% (mean: 46%) of the concentration in a simultaneous plasma sample.

Elimination in Children: In the ACTG/St. Jude study, the elimination half-life following oral administration average 0.8 hours (range: 0.51 to 1.2 hours). Total body clearance following IV administration averaged 532 mL/min/m^2 (range: 294 to 920 mL/min/m^2). Mean renal clearance ranged from 190 to 319 mL/min/m^2 after the first oral dose and from 231 to 265 mL/min/m^2 at steady state. Urinary recovery averaged 21% (range: 4 to 41%) at steady state. There was no evidence of accumulation of VIDEX after the administration of oral doses for an average of 26 days.

Metabolism: The metabolism of VIDEX has not been evaluated in man. When ^{14}C-radiolabeled VIDEX was administered to dogs as a single IV or oral dose, extensive metabolism occurred. The major metabolite identified in the urine, allantoin, represented approximately 61% of the administered radiolabel after oral administration. Three putative metabolites tentatively identified in the urine were hypoxanthine, xanthine, and uric acid. A similar metabolic profile was obtained using an isolated perfused rat liver preparation. The metabolic fate of the dideoxyribose moiety, released subsequent to enzymatic or chemical hydrolysis of the glycosidic bond, has not been determined. Based upon data from animal studies, it is presumed that the metabolism of VIDEX® (didanosine) in man will occur by the same pathways responsible for the elimination of endogenous purines.

The intracellular half-life of ddATP, the metabolite presumed to be responsible for the antiretroviral activity of VIDEX, is reported to be 8 to 24 hours in vitro. The half-life of intracellular ddATP in vivo has not been measured.

There are currently incomplete data concerning the effect of impaired renal or hepatic function on the pharmacokinetics of VIDEX. (See "**PRECAUTIONS.**")

In vitro human plasma protein binding is less than 5% with VIDEX, indicating that drug interactions involving binding site displacement are not anticipated.

INDICATIONS AND USAGE

VIDEX is indicated for the treatment of adult and pediatric patients (over 6 months of age) with advanced HIV infection who are intolerable of zidovudine therapy or who have demonstrated significant clinical or immunologic deterioration during zidovudine therapy. This indication is based primarily on the results of non-randomized, phase 1 studies in which an increase in CD4 cells counts was observed for many patients during VIDEX therapy. These results were compared with data from historical controls and were augmented by an interim analysis of CD4 data obtained from a portion of an ongoing controlled clinical trial (see "**Description of Studies**"). **At present there are no results from controlled studies regarding the effect of VIDEX therapy on the clinical progression of HIV infection, such as incidence of opportunistic infections and survival.** Because zidovudine has been shown to prolong survival and decrease the incidence of opportunistic infections in patients with advanced HIV disease, zidovudine should be considered as initial therapy for the treatment of advanced HIV infection, unless contraindicated.

Description of Studies

Adults: The activity of VIDEX was assessed using CD4 cell counts and p24 antigenemia as markers of biologic activity. Zidovudine therapy has been associated with increases in CD4 cells counts in controlled studies and clinical benefit (improved survival and decreased incidence of opportunistic infections). Absolute CD4 cells counts have been shown to have prognostic value. In adults, the primary evidence of VIDEX's efficacy is based on changes in CD4 cell counts. Other hematological parameters were, in general, stable during VIDEX therapy.

Decreases in p24 antigenemia were demonstrated in the VIDEX studies described below and provide evidence of antiviral activity. Decreases in p24 antigenemia have not been linked to clinical benefit.

Four phase 1 trials, three of which were dose escalation studies, were conducted at five institutions (see Table 1). One-hundred seventy patients were enrolled, 75% of whom had previously received zidovudine therapy. Patients were primarily male and caucasian, and most had a history of homosexual or bisexual contact as their HIV risk factor. Median CD4 count at entry was 62 cells/μL. Dosages in these studies ranged from 0.8 to 66 mg/kg/day, and were given using several schedules and by two routes of administration (IV and PO) for a median duration of 38 weeks (range: 0 to 99 weeks). The median average daily dose was 10.3 mg/kg/day.

[See Table 1 on next page.]

In the phase 1 studies, CD4 cell counts were obtained and analysed at varouis time intervals. For comparison, historical control groups consisted of patients from the placebo groups of three randomized, blinded trials that compared zidovudine therapy to placebo, and patients from one open trial of dextran sulfate (now known not to be orally absorbed and therefore considered a placebo).

Additional experience with VIDEX has been accumulated in the U.S. Expanded Access Program (7806 patients); part of the French Treatment IND program (103 patients); an open label study in Britain (105 patients).

Definitions of outcome were applied *post hoc* to data from patients receiving VIDEX in the phase 1 studies and to data from the historical control patients. These definitions of outcome had not been specified in the protocols and had not been previously correlated with clinical outcome. Analyses included the following:

a) Presence of a "response," where response was defined as i) the greater of a 50-cell or 50% increase over baseline CD4 cell count maintained for a minimum of any consecutive 4 weeks during therapy (50:50); ii) the greater of a 10-cell or 10% increase over baseline CD4 cell count maintained for a minimum of any consecutive 4 weeks during therapy (10:10);

b) % change from baseline in CD4 cell count at various time points on therapy;

c) Longitudinal changes during study weeks of 0 to 12: time weighted average of serial CD4 cell counts corrected for (nor-

Continued on next page

Bristol Laboratories—Cont.

malized by) baseline CD4 cell count (NAUC). [Normalized area under the curve (NAUC) = (Cumulative AUC of CD4 cell count up to time t)/(baseline CD4 count × t).] NAUCs that exceed a value of 1 indicate that the average CD4 level during therapy is increased over the baseline CD4 cell count; d) Dose response analyses.

Results

Comparisons of CD4 cell counts between patients receiving VIDEX® (didanosine) and historical controls must be considered with caution in light of the differences in their comparability, including entry CD4 cell counts, prior zidovudine therapy and standards of care for HIV patients over time (see Tables 1 and 2).

a) *Response:* i) 22% of patients receiving VIDEX had a 50:50 response in CD4 counts, in comparison to 2% to 12% of the historical control patients; ii) 50% of patients receiving VIDEX has a 10:10 response in CD4 counts, in comparison to 17% to 31% of the historical control patients.

b) *% change from baseline:* In patients receiving VIDEX the % increase from baseline CD4 cell counts was 29% at 4 weeks, 27% at 8 weeks, and 14% at 12 weeks. In comparison, historical control groups had progressive declines in CD4 cell counts, ranging from 6% to 24% below baseline at week 8 and 5% to 27% at week 12.

c) *Longitudinal changes during study weeks 0 to 12:* 70% of patients receiving VIDEX had NAUC values exceeding 1, compared to 34% to 46% of the historical control patients. The mean NAUC in patients receiving VIDEX was 1.38 versus 0.99 to 1.04 in the historical control groups.

d) *Dose Response:* Attempts to demonstrate a dose response among patients receiving VIDEX were inconclusive.

Results from an Ongoing Study: An interim analysis of summary CD4 data was obtained from an ongoing, randomized, double-blind study comparing continued zidovudine therapy (comparison group) to VIDEX therapy in patients previously treated with zidovudine. Data available from the first 12 weeks of study included information on 412 patients who had received a median of 13 months of zidovudine therapy and had a median CD4 cell count of 83 cells/μL at study entry. Preliminary results showed that the mean percent increase from baseline in CD4 cell counts after 12 weeks of VIDEX therapy was 11% compared to a decrease of 3.2% in the comparison group. Fifty-five percent of patients taking VIDEX® (didanosine) had NAUCs exceeding 1.0 compared to 39.7% of patients in the comparison group, while mean NAUCs were 1.14 and 0.97, respectively. The clinical significance of these differences is not known. No data on clinical outcome are currently available.

Children: Two pediatric phase 1 dose escalation clinical trials evaluated VIDEX in symptomatic patients with HIV disease (CDC P2 classification). The larger study was conducted at the National Cancer Institute (NCI), Pediatric Branch, and the smaller study conducted under the auspices of the AIDS Clinical Trials Group (ACTG) and St. Jude Children's Research Hospital. The pediatric data included a total of 98 patients, 89 of whom met the criteria for symptomatic HIV-disease (CDC Class P2). At the NCI, 69 of 78 patients had symptomatic HIV disease (9 treated later in the trial had documented infection but were asymptomatic, CDC class P1) and all of the 20 patients in the ACTG/St. Jude trial had CDC P2 disease (see Table 3).

Patients in these two studies received VIDEX at doses from 60 to 540 mg/m^2/day. Based on an increased incidence of pancreatitis observed at the higher doses administered, all patients treated at doses > 360 mg/m^2/day were dose reduced to this level or lower. Due to multiple dose adjustments, the majority of patients, 77%, received average daily doses $\leq$ 300 mg/m^2/day. Dosing information is provided in Table 4.

Activity of VIDEX® (didanosine) was based on the criteria previously described for the adult patients. CD4 cell count, p24 antigenemia, and weight were used to assess biologic activity of VIDEX; for the purpose of describing the results of these studies, changes in these measures were analyzed by classifying patients by retrospectively applied definitions of "response." These definitions have not been correlated with clinical outcome in controlled or uncontrolled studies, and do not reflect gross changes in response to drug. CD4 responses were defined as i) the greater of a 50 cell or 50% increase over baseline CD4 cell count maintained for a minimum of any consecutive 4 weeks during therapy (50:50) and ii) the greater of a 10 cell or 10% increase over baseline CD4 cell count maintained for a minimum of any consecutive 4 weeks during therapy (10:10). Percent change in CD4 cell count from baseline at various points in time was also analyzed. A response for p24 antigen was defined as a 50% reduction from baseline, or a decrease from between 32 to 64 pg/mL to < 32 pg/mL (assay sensitivity), occurring at any time during

therapy and maintained for at least 4 weeks. Weight gain in children was also analyzed as either a 10% increase in weight (for smaller children) to a 2.5 kg increase (for children > 25 kg), also occurring at any time during therapy and maintained for at least 4 weeks.

Separate analyses with patients pooled from both studies were performed for CD4, p24, and weight responses for the 89 patients with symptomatic HIV disease (CDC class P2) and for the subset of 40 children previously exposed to zidovudine (see Table 5). *Both of the studies from which these results were obtained were open-label studies without control patients. The effect of VIDEX on survival and the incidence of opportunistic infections in children could not be assessed in these studies. Data evaluating the impact of VIDEX therapy on clinical parameters of HIV infection in children are not currently available; therefore, zidovudine should be considered as initial therapy for the treatment of advanced HIV infection, unless contraindicated.*

In general, hematologic parameters were stable during treatment with VIDEX. In addition, improvement in platelet counts were seen in 3 of 6 patients with idiopathic thrombocytopenic purpura (ITP) who entered the pediatric studies with this diagnosis. Some children exhibited improvements in detailed neuropsychometric tests. Patients enrolled in the NCI trial underwent testing at entry and at 6 months on study. An increment in an individual's IQ score of 10% and a minimum of 8 points relative to baseline was considered a response. Improvement was seen in 12 of 43 evaluable patients with a baseline IQ < 115. In the absence of a control group the contribution of drug to this increase is uncertain.

[See Table 5 on next page.]

CONTRAINDICATION

VIDEX® (didanosine) is contraindicated in patients with previously demonstrated clinically significant hypersensitivity to any of the components of the formulations.

WARNINGS

THE MAJOR CLINICAL TOXICITIES OF VIDEX ARE PANCREATITIS AND PERIPHERAL NEUROPATHY.

1. Pancreatitis

PANCREATITIS OCCURRED IN 9% OF PATIENTS IN PHASE 1 STUDIES TREATED WITH VIDEX AT OR BELOW THE RECOMMENDED DOSE. THIS CONDITION CAN BE FATAL. PANCREATITIS MUST BE CONSIDERED WHENEVER A PATIENT RECEIVING VIDEX DEVELOPS ABDOMINAL PAIN AND NAUSEA, VOMITING, OR ELEVATED BIOCHEMICAL MARKERS. UNDER THESE CIRCUMSTANCES, VIDEX USE SHOULD BE SUSPENDED UNTIL THE DIAGNOSIS OF PANCREATITIS IS EXCLUDED. When treatment with other drugs known to cause pancreatic toxicity is required (for example,

Table 1
VIDEX® (didanosine) Adult Phase 1 Protocols

Study	Deaconess	ACTG 064	Boston City	NCI
N	30	44	39	57
Accrual Dates	6/89 to 10/89	10/88 to 9/89	10/88 to 10/89	7/88 to 3/90
Median CD4	22	77	69	44
Range	0–270	4–415	2–540	0–496
% Caucasian	97	89	67	88
% Homosexual	77	82	64	88
% IVDU	10	2	18	2
% Prior ZDV	100*	81	53	71
% AIDS	73	36	46	44
Dose range (mg/kg/day) and schedule	6 PO & 750/1500 mg/day PO BID	0.8 IV-66 PO BID	0.8 IV-30.4 PO QD	0.8 IV-51.2 PO BID or TID

* All patients had documented hematologic intolerance to ZDV.

Table 2
Pretreatment Patient Comparisons

Study	Historical Control Groups				
	All Phase 1	BW02	ACTG 001	ACTG 016	ACTG 060
Population	ARC & AIDS	ARC & AIDS	Kaposi's Sarcoma	Early ARC	HIV Infection
N: Placebo	170	137	89	344	60
Accrual Dates	7/88 to 3/90	2/86 to 7/86	1/87 to 11/87	8/87 to 5/89	8/88 to 3/89
Median CD4 cell/μL	62	68	277	397	204
Range	0–540	0–1069	14–1316	151–862	4–621
% Caucasian	85	NA*	87	83	74
% Prior ZDV	75	0	0	0	25
% AIDS	48	55	100	0	25

* NA = not available

Table 3
Baseline Characteristics of Pediatric Phase 1 Patients

	NCI	ACTG/St. Jude
Total patients	78	20
Male:female	48:30	12:8
Age (years)		
Median (Range)	6.9 (0.6–19)	6.3 (0.7–18)
Race		
Caucasian	52 (67)*	7 (35)
Black	17 (22)	11 (55)
Hispanic	4 (5)	2 (10)
Other	5 (6)	—
Prior ZDV	41 (52)	2 (10)
Mode of transmission		
Perinatal	39 (50)	10 (50)
Transfusion	21 (27)	4 (20)
Hemophiliac	18 (23)	6 (30)
Stage		
AIDS†	55 (70)	10 (50)
SHIV†	14 (18)	10 (50)
P1	9 (12)	—
Baseline CD4 cells/μL‡		
< 50	34 (45)	7 (35)
50–99	7 (9)	2 (10)
$\geq$ 100	35 (46)	11 (55)
Median	70	205

* Percentage of patients in this category for each study.
† CDC class P2.
‡ Two patients did not have baseline CD4 counts.

Table 4
Dosing and Duration of VIDEX Therapy in Children

	NCI N = 78	ACTG/St. Jude N = 20
Total Daily Dose		
Range (mg/m^2/day)	60–540	160–360
Regimen	TID	BID
Study Duration		
Median	35 weeks	37 weeks
Range	4–77 weeks	1–56 weeks
Cumulative Dose (mg/kg):		
Median (range)	2689 (3–7452)	2387 (29–3828)

Table 5
Responses
Pooled Pediatric Data (CDC P2)
N=89

	Prior zidovudine Pts (N=40)*	All Pts (N=89)
Baseline CD4 (cells/μL),	8	60
Median (range)	0–3140	0–3140
CD4 Response, 10:10 (%)	8/36 (22)	31/83 (37)
CD4 Response, 50:50 (%)	5/36 (14)	19/83 (23)
% CD4 Change at Week 8	+21	+27
p24 Response (%)†	10/18 (56)	36/49 (73)
CD4 (50:50) + weight (%)‡	1 (3)	4 (5)
p24 + weight (%)	4 (10)	9 (10)
CD4 (50:50) + p24 + weight (%)	1 (3)	9 (10)
Weight Response (%)	12/36 (33)	32/83 (39)
Neuropsychometric Response, NCI (%)§	7/21 (33)	12/43 (28)

* Patients for whom the drug is currently recommended.
† p24 response was assessable only in patients with detectable p24 antigen at entry; 5 of 34 patients with undetectable antigen at entry became antigenemic during study.
‡ Patients who had both a 50:50 CD4 response and a weight response; subsequent categories are defined similarly.
§ The denominator reflects those patients with a baseline IQ score <115; for the entire group, there was not a statistically significant change between entry and followup neuropsychometric scores.

Table 6
Incidence of Pancreatitis

	All Phase 1	Phase 1 ≤12.5 mg/kg/day*	Phase 1 >12.5 mg/kg/day
N	170	91	79
Pancreatitis	29 (17%)	8 (9%)	21 (27%)
Abdominal Pain	14 (8%)	9 (10%)	5 (6%)
Increased Amylase	26 (16%)	16 (18%)	12 (15%)
Abdominal Pain and Increased Amylase†	11 (6%)	6 (7%)	5 (6%)

* Patients entered at oral doses ≤12.5 mg/kg/day received an average daily dose similar to that expected from the recommended dosage.
† Some case reports recorded abdominal pain with elevated serum amylase, without reporting fully characterized pancreatitis.

Table 7
Incidence of Neuropathy

	All Phase 1	Phase 1 ≤12.5 mg/kg/day*	Phase 1 >12.5 mg/kg/day
N	170	91	79
Neuropathy	71 (42%)	31 (34%)	40 (51%)
Neuropathy requiring dose modification†	38 (22%)	11 (12%)	27 (34%)

* Patients entered at oral doses ≤12.5 mg/kg/day received average daily doses similar to that expected from the recommended dosage.
† Twenty-one of 38 subjects were rechallenged following dose modification and tolerated ddI for periods ranging from 3 days to 45 weeks.

IV pentamidine), suspension of VIDEX® (didanosine) should be considered.
The incidence of pancreatitis and potential manifestations of pancreatitis in the adult phase 1 studies are described in the table above.
[See Table 6.]
In the Expanded Access Program for VIDEX, where the median duration of exposure was shorter than in the phase 1 studies (5 months versus 8.5 months), lower incidences of pancreatitis (5%), and potential manifestations of pancreatitis (abdominal pain 5%, increased amylase 8%) were reported. Fatal pancreatitis occurred in 27 of 7806 treated patients (0.35%).
Eight of 27 (30%) subjects with a history of pancreatitis who were treated with VIDEX developed pancreatitis. VIDEX therapy should be used only with extreme caution in this population.
Patients with a history of pancreatitis should be followed closely, as should those with risk factors for pancreatitis such as a diagnosis of AIDS, CD4 cell counts below 100 cells/μl, and/or risk factors for pancreatitis in general, such as alcohol consumption and elevated triglycerides.
Positive relationships have been found between risk of pancreatitis and steady state plasma concentration of VIDEX, as well as with daily oral dose. Patients with renal impairment may be at greater risk for pancreatitis if treated without dose adjustment, although data are insufficient to recommended specific guidelines for dose adjustment at this time.
In pediatric studies, pancreatitis occurred in 2 of 60 (3%) patients treated at entry doses below 300 mg/m²/day and in 5 of 38 (13%) patients treated at higher doses. In pediatric patients with symptoms similar to those described above, VIDEX use should be suspended until the diagnosis of pancreatitis is excluded.

2. Peripheral Neuropathy
PERIPHERAL NEUROPATHY OCCURRED IN 34% OF PATIENTS IN PHASE 1 STUDIES TREATED WITH VIDEX DOSES AT OR BELOW THE CURRENTLY RECOMMENDED DOSE. PATIENTS SHOULD BE MONITORED FOR THE DEVELOPMENT OF A NEUROPATHY THAT IS USUALLY CHARACTERIZED BY DISTAL NUMBNESS, TINGLING, OR PAIN IN THE FEET OR HANDS.
Table 7 describes the incidence of neuropathy during VIDEX® (didanosine) therapy in the combined adult phase 1 studies.
Among the 91 adult phase 1 patients who received an average oral daily dose of VIDEX similar to the recomended dose, 12% had neuropathy requiring dose modification. In the Expanded Access Program, where the median duration of exposure to VIDEX was shorter than in the adult phase 1 studies, the incidence of neuropathy was 16%.
Neuropathy occurred more frequently in patients with a history of neuropathy or neurotoxic drug therapy. These patients may be at increased risk of neuropathy during VIDEX therapy.
Neuropathy has been reported rarely in children treated with VIDEX. However, because signs and symptoms of neuropathy are difficult to assess in children, physicians should be alerted to the possibility of this event.

3. Liver failure
Fatal liver failure of unknown etiology occurred during VIDEX therapy in 1/170 patients in the phase 1 studies and 14/7806 in the U.S. Expanded Access program.
4. Retinal depigmentation and vision
Four pediatric patients demonstrated retinal depigmentation at dosage of VIDEX above 300 mg/m²/day. Until further information is available from ongoing clinical trials with children treated at currently recommended lower doses of VIDEX, it has been proposed that children receiving VIDEX should undergo dilated retinal examination every 6 months or if a change in vision occurs. (See **"ADVERSE REACTIONS."**)

PRECAUTIONS
General
Patients receiving VIDEX or any other antiretroviral therapy may continue to develop opportunistic infections and other complications of HIV infection, and therefore should remain under close clinical observation by physicians experienced in the treatment of patients with associated HIV diseases.
Ingestion of VIDEX® (didanosine) with food reduces the absorption of VIDEX by as much as 50%. Therefore, VIDEX should be administered on an empty stomach.
Patients with Phenylketonuria: VIDEX Chewable/Dispersible Buffered Tablets contain the following quantities of phenylalanine:

Table 8

	150-mg Strength	All Other Strengths
Phenylalanine per 2-tablet dose	67.4 mg	45 mg
Phenylalanine per tablet	33.7 mg	22.5 mg

Patients on Sodium-Restricted Diets: VIDEX Chewable/Dispersible Buffered Tablets: Each VIDEX buffered tablet contains 264.5 mg sodium. A 2-tablet dose of VIDEX buffered tablets contains 529 mg sodium. VIDEX Buffered Powder for Oral Solution: Each single-dose packet of VIDEX Buffered Powder for Oral Solution contains 1380 mg sodium.
Patients With Renal Impairment: Patients with renal impairment (serum creatinine >1.5 mg/dL or creatinine clearance <60 mL/min) may be at greater risk of toxicity from VIDEX due to decreased drug clearance; a dose reduction should be considered. The magnesium hydroxide content of each VIDEX tablet is 15.7 mEq which may present an excessive load of magnesium to patients with significant renal impairment, particularly after prolonged dosing.
Patients With Hepatic Impairment: Patients with hepatic impairment may be at greater risk for toxicity related to VIDEX treatment due to altered metabolism; a dose reduction may be necessary.
Hyperuricemia: VIDEX has been associated with asymptomatic hyperuricemia; treatment suspension may be necessary if clinical measures aimed at reducing uric acids levels fail.
Diarrhea: VIDEX Buffered Powder for Oral Solution was associated with diarrhea in 34% of patients in the phase 1 adult studies (see **"ADVERSE REACTIONS"**). No data are available to demonstrate whether other formulations are associated with lower rates of diarrhea. However, if diarrhea develops in a patient receiving VIDEX Buffered Powder for Oral Solution, a trial of VIDEX Chewable/Dispersible Buffered Tablets should be considered.

Information for Patients
VIDEX is not a cure for HIV infection, and patients may continue to acquire illnesses associated with AIDS or ARC, including opportunistic infection. VIDEX has not been shown to reduce the incidence or frequency of such illnesses. Therefore, patients should remain under care of a physician when using VIDEX.
Patients should be informed that the major toxicities of VIDEX® (didanosine) are pancreatitis, which has been fatal in some patients, and peripheral neuropathy. Symptoms of pancreatitis include abdominal pain, and nausea and vomiting. Symptoms of peripheral neuropathy include tingling, burning, pain or numbness in the hands or feet. Patients should be advised that these symptoms should be reported to their physicians. They should be counseled that these toxicities occur with greatest frequency in patients with a history of these events, and that dose modification and/or discontinuation of VIDEX may be required if toxicity develops. They should be cautioned about the use of other medications that may exacerbate the VIDEX toxicity, including alcohol.
Patients should be told that the long-term effects of VIDEX are unknown at this time. Patients should be advised that

Continued on next page

Bristol Laboratories—Cont.

VIDEX therapy has not been shown to reduce the risk of transmission of HIV to other through sexual contact or blood contamination.

Drug Interactions

Drug interaction studies have demonstrated that there are no clinically significant interactions with VIDEX and ketoconazole or ranitidine. Drugs whose absorption can be affected by the level of acidity in the stomach (eg, ketoconazole, dapsone) should be administered at least 2 hours prior to dosing with VIDEX. Coadministration of VIDEX with drugs that are known to cause peripheral neuropathy or pancreatitis may increase the risk of these toxicities (see "**WARNINGS**"). Patients who receive these drugs should be observed closely. A study in 4 patients revealed that concomitant administration of ganciclovir does not significantly affect the pharmacokinetics of VIDEX. There is no evidence that VIDEX potentiates the myelosuppressive effects of ganciclovir.

As with other products containing magnesium and/or aluminum antacid components, VIDEX Chewable/Dispersible Buffered Tablets or VIDEX Pediatric Powder for Oral Solution should not be administered with a prescription antibiotic containing any form of tetracycline.

Plasma concentrations of some quinolone antibiotics are decreased when administered with antacids containing magnesium or aluminum. Therefore, doses of quinolone antibiotics should not be administered within 2 hours of taking VIDEX Chewable/Dispersible Buffered Tablets or Pediatric Powder for Oral Solution. Concomitant administration of antacids containing magnesium or aluminum with VIDEX Chewable/Dispersible Buffered Tablets or Pediatric Powder for Oral Solution may potentiate adverse effects associated with the antacid components.

Carcinogenesis and Mutagenesis

Long-term carcinogenicity studies of VIDEX in animals have not been completed. No evidence of mutagenicity (with or without metabolic activation) was observed in Ames *Salmonella* mutagenicity assays or in a mutagenicity assay conducted with *Escherichia coli* tester strain WP2 uvrA where only a slight increase in revertants was observed with VIDEX. In a mammalian cell gene mutation assay conducted in L5178Y/TK+/− mouse lymphoma cells, VIDEX was weakly positive both in the absence and presence of metabolic activation at concentrations of approximately 2000 μg/mL and above. In an in vitro cytogenic study performed in cultured human peripheral lymphocytes, high concentrations of VIDEX® (didanosine) ($\geq$ 500 μg/mL) elevated the frequency of cells bearing chromosome aberrations. Another in vitro mammalian cell chromosome aberration study using Chinese Hamster Lung cells revealed that VIDEX produces chromosome aberrations at $\geq$ 500 μg/mL after 48 hours of exposure. However, no significant elevations in the frequency of cells with chromosome aberrations were seen at VIDEX concentrations up to 250 μg/mL. Similar chromosomal aberration effects were induced by the natural nucleoside of didanosine (2'-deoxyinosine), suggesting that these effects of VIDEX were not due to a direct genotoxic interaction. In BALB/c 3T3 in vitro tranformation assay, VIDEX was considered positive only at concentrations of 3000 μg/

mL and above, whereas deoxyinosine induced a positive response in this assay at 1000 μg/mL and above. No evidence of genotoxicity was observed in rat and mouse micronucleus assays. The rats received oral VIDEX (up to 1000 mg/kg/day) for 7 days. The mice received oral VIDEX (up to 1000 mg/kg/day) for 4 weeks or intravenous VIDEX (up to 250 mg/kg/day) for 4 days.

The results from the genotoxicity studies suggest that VIDEX is not mutagenic at biologically and pharmacologically relevant doses. At significantly elevated doses in vitro, the genotoxic effects of VIDEX are similar in magnitude to those seen with natural DNA nucleosides.

Pregnancy, Reproduction and Fertility

Pregnancy Category B. Reproduction studies have been performed in rats and rabbits at doses up to 12 and 14.2 times the estimated human exposure (based upon plasma levels), respectively, and have revealed no evidence of impaired fertility or harm to the fetus due to VIDEX. At approximately 12 times the estimated human exposure, VIDEX was slightly toxic to female rats and their pups during mid and late lactation. These rats showed reduced food intake and body weight gains but the physical and functional development of the offspring was not impaired and there were no major changes in the F2 generation. There are no adequate and well-controlled studies in pregnant women. Because animal reproduction studies are not always predictive of human response, this drug should be used during pregnancy only if clearly needed.

Nursing Mothers

It is not known whether VIDEX is excreted in human milk. Because many drugs are excreted in human milk and because of the potential for serious adverse reactions from VIDEX in nursing infants, mothers should be instructed to discontinue nursing when taking VIDEX.

Pediatric Use

See "INDICATIONS," "WARNINGS," and "DOSAGE AND ADMINISTRATION" sections.

ADVERSE REACTIONS

THE MAJOR TOXICITIES OF VIDEX ARE PANCREATITIS AND PERIPHERAL NEUROPATHY (see "**WARNINGS**").

Adults: Data are reported here from patients in the U.S. phase 1 studies who received daily doses of an investigational formulation similar to VIDEX Pediatric Powder for Oral Solution below 12.5 mg/kg/day. Data are also provided for patients in the U.S. Expanded Access Program, all of whom received unit doses (VIDEX Buffered Powder for Oral Solution) adjusted for body weight to approximate 6 to 10 mg/kg/day.

Table 9 lists all adverse events reported from at least 5% of adult patients in the U.S. phase 1 studies. These adverse events should be considered as potential hazards of treatment with VIDEX® (didanosine) until controlled comparative data are available.

These adverse events were reported less frequently in the VIDEX Expanded Access program, where the median duration of exposure to VIDEX was shorter than in the combined U.S. adult phase 1 studies (5 versus 8.5 months). Differences in event rates may be due in part to differences in monitoring between phase 1 and Expanded Access studies. Pancreatitis occurred in 5% to 9% of patients across all studies (see

"**WARNINGS**"). Peripheral neuropathy requiring dose modification of VIDEX occurred in 5% to 12% of patients receiving recommended doses (see "**WARNINGS**"). Diarrhea was the most frequent clinical adverse event reported in the U.S. Expanded Access patients (18% of patients); 1.9% of episodes were reported as serious.

Clinical adverse events which occurred in greater than 1% and up to 5% of patients enrolled in the U.S. Expanded Access studies are listed below by body systems:

Adverse Event	%	Adverse Event	%
Body as a Whole		Nervous System	
Pneumonia	2	Seizure/Convulsions	3
Infection	2	Confusion	2
Anorexia	1	Anxiety	1
Weight Loss	1	Nervousness	1
Sepsis	1	Hypertonia	1
		Thinking Abnormal	1
Gastrointestinal			
Dyspepsia	1	Musculoskeleton	
GI Disorder	1	Myopathy	1
Liver Abnormalities	1		
Flatulence	1	Respiratory	
		Cough	1
Metabolic/Nutritional			
CPK Increase	1	Cardiovascular	
Edema	1	Hypertension	1
Hyperlipemia	1		

Events occurring in <1% of patients are listed below:

Body as a Whole	Respiratory
Ascites	Dyspnea
Face Edema	Pharyngitis
Enlarged Abdomen	Apnea
Flu Syndrome	Sinusitis
	Bronchitis
Nervous System	Pleural Effusion
Dementia	Rhinitis
Agitation	Pneumothorax
Ataxia	
Amnesia	Special Senses
Speech Disorder	Eye Disorder
Cerebrovascular	Amblyopia
Disorder	Deafness
Urogenital	Gastrointestinal
Kidney Failure	GI Hemorrhage
Polyuria	Dysphagia
	Oral Moniliasis
Cardiovascular	Colitis
Syncope	Esophagitis
Congestive Heart Failure	Sialadenitis
Pericardial Effusion	
Vasodilatation	Skin
Cardiomyopathy	Sweating
Palpitation	Herpes
	Acne

The proportion of 91 U.S. adult phase 1 patients experiencing serious laboratory abnormalities while receiving VIDEX® (didanosine) at a dose similar to the recommended dose is indicated below (see Table 10). Data are provided for those who began VIDEX therapy with normal or abnormal baseline values. The level of abnormality defined as serious is indicated for each parameter in parentheses.

Table 10
Adult Patient Laboratory Abnormalities

Lab Tests (Seriously Abnormal Level)	Normal Baseline	Abnormal Baseline
Leukopenia (<2000/μL)	5%	37%
Granulocytopenia (<1000/μL)	3%	56%
Thrombocytopenia (<50,000/μL)	1%	25%
Anemia (Hb <8.0 g/dL)	5%	0%
SGPT (>5×ULN)*	10%	12%
SGOT (>5×ULN)	10%	12%
Alkaline Phosphatase (>5×ULN)	4%	17%
Bilirubin (>5×ULN)	3%	0%
Uric Acid (>1.25×ULN)	6%	50%
Amylase (≥5×ULN)	3%	0%

*ULN=upper limits of normal.

Table 9
Adult Clinical Adverse Events

Adverse Events	Phase 1 ≤12.5 mg/kg/day N=91	Phase 1 All Patients N=170	U.S. Expanded Access N=7806
Headache	36%	32%	5%
Diarrhea (See "**PRECAUTIONS**")	34%	29%	18%
Peripheral Neuropathy (See "**WARNINGS**")	34%	42%	16%
Asthenia	25%	24%	3%
Insomnia	25%	22%	2%
Nausea/Vomiting (See "**WARNINGS**")	25%	25%	8%
Rash/Pruritus	24%	25%	4%
Abdominal Pain (See "**WARNINGS**")	21%	22%	5%
CNS Depression	19%	16%	<1%
Constipation	16%	13%	<1%
Stomatitis	14%	11%	<1%
Myalgia	13%	13%	1%
Arthritis	11%	11%	1%
Taste Loss/Perversion	10%	8%	<1%
Pain	10%	16%	4%
Dry Mouth	9%	8%	1%
Pancreatitis (See "**WARNINGS**")	9%	17%	5%
Alopecia	8%	7%	<1%
Dizziness	7%	8%	1%

Table 11
Pediatric Clinical Adverse Events

Adverse Events	Patients Receiving < 300 mg/m²/day (n=60)	All Patients (n=98)
Body as Whole		
Flu Syndrome	7%	7%
Malaise	38%	29%
Alopecia	7%	5%
Anorexia	52%	51%
Asthenia	42%	41%
Chills/Fever	82%	82%
Dehydration	7%	5%
Pain	27%	31%
Weight Loss	10%	8%
Increased Appetite	5%	2%
Change in Appetite	10%	6%
Failure to Thrive	13%	9%
GI System		
Liver Abnormalities	32%	38%
Melena	7%	7%
Oral Thrush	13%	9%
Abdominal Pain (see "**WARNINGS**")	32%	35%
Constipation	10%	12%
Diarrhea (see "**PRECAUTIONS**")	82%	81%
Dry Mouth	7%	4%
Nausea/Vomiting (see "**WARNINGS**")	57%	58%
Stomatitis/Mouth Sores	17%	16%
Pancreatitis (see "**WARNINGS**")	3%	7%
Lympho-Hematologic		
Ecchymosis	15%	15%
Hemorrhage	10%	10%
Petechiae	3%	7%
Musculoskeletal		
Muscle Atrophy	12%	8%
Myalgia	12%	9%
Arthritis	12%	11%
Decreased Strength	3%	6%
Cardiovascular		
Vasodilation	22%	22%
Arrhythmia	10%	6%
Nervous System		
Dizziness	5%	7%
Lethargy	7%	4%
Nervousness	33%	27%
Headache	58%	55%
Insomnia	10%	8%
Poor Coordination	8%	6%
Respiratory System		
Asthma	28%	21%
Cough	87%	85%
Dyspnea	27%	23%
Epistaxis	13%	14%
Hypoventilation	10%	8%
Pharyngitis	17%	14%
Rhinitis	48%	48%
Rhinorrhea	20%	21%
Rhonchi/Rales	8%	6%
Sinusitis	8%	7%
Congestion	5%	3%
Skin and Appendages		
Impetigo	5%	6%
Eczema	13%	12%
Excoriation	7%	4%
Skin Disorder	12%	13%
Sweating	8%	7%
Rash/Pruritus	72%	70%
Erythema	5%	4%
Special Senses		
Ear Pain/Otitis	13%	11%
Photophobia	8%	5%
Strabismus	8%	5%
Visual Impaired	5%	5%
Urogenital System		
Urinary Frequency	5%	4%

There was a higher incidence of serious laboratory toxicities in patients with abnormalities at baseline. This was confirmed in the Expanded Access Program. Until controlled, comparable data are available, these abnormalities should be considered as potential hazards of VIDEX® (didanosine) therapy.

Children: Adverse events reported in more than 5% of patients in the pediatric phase 1 trials (which includes all signs and symptoms on study) are listed in Table 11. There are no comparative controlled data to assess the incidence of adverse effects from VIDEX in children at this time; therefore, the adverse events reported in these pediatric studies should be considered as potential hazards of VIDEX treatment.

In pediatric studies, pancreatitis occurred in 2 of 60 (3%) patients treated at entry doses below 300 mg/m²/day and in 5 of 38 (13%) patients treated at higher doses.

Serious adverse events reported from less than 5% of patients in the pediatric phase 1 trials are listed in Table 12. Four pediatric patients developed depigmentation of the retina while being treated with VIDEX® (didanosine) at doses above 300 mg/m²/day. Two of the patients, treated at doses of 540 mg/m²/day, had progression of disease when treated with lower doses. One patient treated at lower doses has continued therapy without progression of disease. Until further information is available from ongoing clinical trials with children treated at currently recommended lower doses of VIDEX, it has been proposed that children receiving VIDEX should undergo dilated retinal examination every 6 months or if any change in vision occurs.

Table 12
Serious Pediatric Clinical Adverse Events
(< 5% of patients)

Event	%
Seizure	1
Neurologic	2
Pneumonia	1
Diabetes Melitus	1
Diabetes Insipidus	1

Serious laboratory abnormalities experienced by the pediatric patients are listed below (see Table 13). Laboratory abnormalities of grade 3 or 4 were observed more frequently among patients who began VIDEX therapy with abnormal values.

Table 13
Pediatric Patient Serious Laboratory Abnormalities
(Dose ≤ 300 mg/m²/day)
N=60

Laboratory Test (Seriously Abnormal Level)	Normal Baseline	Abnormal Baseline
Leukopenia (< 2000/μL)	3%	36%
Granulocytopenia (< 1000/μL)	24%	62%
Thrombocytopenia (< 50,000/μL)	2%	67%
Anemia (Hb < 8.0 g/dL)	4%	27%
SGPT (> 5 × ULN)	3%	25%
SGOT (> 5 × ULN)	0%	36%
Alkaline Phosphatase (> 5 × ULN)	0%	0%
Bilirubin (> 5 × ULN)	2%	0%
Uric Acid (> 1.25 × ULN)	0%	0%
Amylase (≥ 5 × ULN)	0%	0%

OVERDOSAGE

There is no known antidote for VIDEX® (didanosine) overdosage. Experience in the phase 1 studies in which VIDEX was initially administered at doses ten times the currently recommended dose indicates that the complications of chronic overdosage would include pancreatitis, peripheral neuropathy, diarrhea, hyperuricemia or, possibly, hepatic dysfunction. It is not known whether VIDEX is dialyzable by peritoneal or hemodialysis.

DOSAGE AND ADMINISTRATION

Dosage:
Adults: The dosing interval should be 12 hours. **All VIDEX formulations should be administered on an empty stomach. Adult patients should take 2 tablets at each dose so that adequate buffering is provided to prevent gastric acid degradation of VIDEX.** The recommended starting dose in adults is dependent on weight as outlined in the following table.

[See Table 14 top left next page.]

Continued on next page

Bristol Laboratories—Cont.

Table 14
Adult Dosing

Patient Weight	VIDEX Tablets	VIDEX Buffered Powder
≥ 75 kg	300 mg BID	375 mg BID
50–74 kg	200 mg BID	250 mg BID
35–49 kg	125 mg BID	167 mg BID

Children: The recommended dosing interval is 12 hours. **All VIDEX formulations should be administered on an empty stomach. To prevent gastric acid degradation, children older than 1 year of age should receive a 2-tablet dose; children under 1 year should receive a 1-tablet dose.** The recommended dose in children is dependent on body surface area as outlined in the table below (see Table 15). Doses equivalent to 100 mg/m²/day to 300 mg/m²/day of the VIDEX pediatric powder are currently being further evaluated in controlled clinical trials. **The optimal dose of VIDEX for children has not been established and some investigators recommend doses of up to 300 mg/m²/day divided into three daily doses.**

[See Table 15 below.]

Dose Adjustment:
Clinical signs suggestive of pancreatitis should prompt dose suspension and careful evaluation of the possibility of pancreatitis. Only after pancreatitis has been ruled out should dosing be resumed.
Many patients who have presented with symptoms of neuropathy will tolerate a reduced dose of VIDEX after resolution of these symptoms upon drug discontinuation.
There are insufficient data to recommend a specific dose adjustment of VIDEX in patients with impaired renal or hepatic function. A dose reduction should be considered in patients with renal insufficiency or hepatic impairment.

Method of Preparation:
VIDEX (didanosine) Chewable/Dispersible Buffered Tablets
Adult Dosing: Two tablets should be thoroughly chewed, manually crushed, or dispersed in at least 1 ounce of water prior to consumption. To disperse tablets, add 2 tablets to at least 1 ounce of drinking water. Stir until a uniform dispersion forms, and drink the entire dispersion immediately.
Pediatric Dosing: One or 2 tablets should be chewed, crushed, or dispersed in water prior to consumption, as described in the preceding **Adult-Dosing Method of Preparation.**
VIDEX (didanosine) Buffered Powder for Oral Solution
1. Open packet carefully and pour contents into a container with approximately 4 ounces of drinking water. Do not mix with fruit juice or other acid-containing liquid.
2. Stir until the powder completely dissolves (approximately 2 to 3 minutes).
3. Drink the entire solution immediately.
VIDEX (didanosine) Pediatric Powder for Oral Solution
Prior to dispensing, the pharmacist must constitute dry powder with Purified Water, USP, to an initial concentration of 20 mg/mL and immediately mix the resulting solution with antacid to a final concentration of 10 mg/mL as follows:
20 mg/mL Initial Solution: Constitute the product to 20 mg/mL by adding 100 mL or 200 mL of Purified Water, USP, to the 2 g or 4 g of VIDEX powder, respectively, in the product bottle.
10 mg/mL Final Admixture: 1. Immediately mix one part of the 20 mg/mL initial solution with one part of either Mylanta Double Strength (Mylanta is a registered trademark of Stuart Pharmaceuticals, Division of ICI Americas, Inc. Mylanta Double Strength, formerly Mylanta II, is distributed by Johnson & Johnson/Merck, Consumer Pharmaceuticals Company, Fort Washington, PA 19034 [USA]). Liquid or Maalox TC Suspension (Maalox is a registered trade-

mark of William H. Rorer Inc., Unit of Rhone-Poulenc.) for a final dispensing concentration of 10 mg VIDEX per mL. For patients home use, the admixture should be dispensed in appropriately sized, flint-glass bottles with child-resistant closures. This admixture is stable for 30 days under refrigeration, 36° to 46°F (2° to 8°C).
2. Instruct the patient to shake the admixture thoroughly prior to use and to store the tightly closed container in the refrigerator, 36° to 46°F (2° to 8°C), up to 30 days.

HOW SUPPLIED
VIDEX® (didanosine) Chewable/Dispersible Buffered Tablets are round, white, mint-flavored, embossed tablets with "VIDEX" above "BL" on one side and the product strength on the other. The tablets are available in the following strengths of VIDEX: 25, 50, 100, or 150 mg. Sixty tablets are packaged in bottles with child-resistant closures.
The tablets should be stored in tightly closed bottles at 59° to 86°F (15° to 30°C). If dispersed in water, the dose may be held for up to 1 hour at ambient temperature.
VIDEX (didanosine) Buffered Powder for Oral Solution is supplied in single-dose, child-resistant foil packets in the following strengths of VIDEX: 100, 167, 250, or 375 mg. Each product strength provides a sweetened, buffered solution of VIDEX.
The packets should be stored at 59° to 86°F (15° to 30°C). After dissolving in water, the solution may be stored at ambient room temperature for up to 4 hours.
VIDEX (didanosine) Pediatric Powder for Oral Solution is supplied in 4- and 8-ounce glass bottles containing 2 g or 4 g of VIDEX, respectively.
The bottles of powder should be stored at 59° to 86°F (15° to 30°C). The VIDEX admixture may be stored up to 30 days in a refrigerator, 36° to 46°F (2° to 8°C). Discard any unused portion after 30 days.
The NDC numbers for the previously described VIDEX products are:

[See Table 16 above.]

HANDLING AND DISPOSAL
Spill, Leak and Disposal Procedure
Avoid generating dust during clean-up of powdered products; use wet mop or damp sponge. Clean surface with soap and water as necessary. Containerize larger spills.
There is no single preferred method of disposal of containerized waste. Disposal options include incineration, landfill, or sewer as dictated by specific circumstances and relevant national, state, and local regulations.

REFERENCES
1. Hartman NR, et al. Pharmacokinetics of 2',3'-dideoxyadenosine and 2',3'-dideoxyinosine in patients with severe human immunodeficiency virus infection. *Clin Pharmacol Ther.* 1990;47;647–654.
2. Butler KM, et al. Dideoxyinosine in children with symptomatic human immunodeficiency virus infection. *New Eng J Med.* 1991;324;137–144.
Shown in Product Identification Section, page 406

Table 15
Pediatric Dosing
(Based on 200 mg/m²/day Average Recommended Dose)*

Body Surface Area (m²)	VIDEX® (didanosine) Tablets	VIDEX Pediatric Powder Dose	VIDEX Pediatric Powder Vol/10 mg/mL Admixture
1.1–1.4	100 mg BID	125 mg BID	12.5 mL BID
0.8–1.0	75 mg BID	94 mg BID	9.5 mL BID
0.5–0.7	50 mg BID	62 mg BID	6 mL BID
≤ 0.4	25 mg BID	31 mg BID	3 mL BID

* Based on VIDEX pediatric powder.

Table 16

NDC NO.	Packaging Information	Product Strength
VIDEX® Chewable/Dispersible Buffered Tablets		
0087-6628-43	60 tablets/bottle	25 mg/tablet
0087-6624-43	60 tablets/bottle	50 mg/tablet
0087-6627-43	60 tablets/bottle	100 mg/tablet
0087-6626-43	60 tablets/bottle	150 mg/tablet
VIDEX® Buffered Powder for Oral Solution		
0087-6614-43	One single-dose foil packet*	100 mg/packet
0087-6615-43	One single-dose foil packet*	167 mg/packet
0087-6616-43	One single-dose foil packet*	250 mg/packet
0087-6617-43	One single-dose foil packet*	375 mg/packet
VIDEX® Pediatric Powder for Oral Solution		
0087-6632-41	One bottle per carton	2 g/bottle
0087-6633-41	One bottle per carton	4 g/bottle

* Packaged as 30 packets per carton.

Bristol-Myers Oncology Division
A Bristol-Myers Squibb Company
P.O. BOX 4500
PRINCETON, NJ 08543-4500

BiCNU®   ℞
[bǐk 'nū]
(sterile carmustine [BCNU])

WARNINGS
BiCNU (sterile carmustine [BCNU]) should be administered under the supervision of a qualified physician experienced in the use of cancer chemotherapeutic agents.
Bone marrow suppression, notably thrombocytopenia and leukopenia, which may contribute to bleeding and overwhelming infections in an already compromised patient, is the most common and severe of the toxic effects of BiCNU (see "WARNINGS" and "ADVERSE REACTIONS").
Since the major toxicity is delayed bone marrow suppression, blood counts should be monitored weekly for at least 6 weeks after a dose (see "ADVERSE REACTIONS"). At the recommended dosage, courses of BiCNU should not be given more frequently than every 6 weeks.
The bone marrow toxicity of BiCNU is cumulative and therefore dosage adjustment must be considered on the basis of nadir blood counts from prior dose (see "Dosage Adjustment Table" under "DOSAGE AND ADMINISTRATION").
Pulmonary toxicity from BiCNU appears to be dose related. Patients receiving greater than 1400 mg/m² cumulative dose are at significantly higher risk than those receiving less.

DESCRIPTION
BiCNU (sterile carmustine [BCNU]) is one of the nitrosoureas used in the treatment of certain neoplastic diseases. It is 1,3-bis (2-chloroethyl)-1-nitrosourea. It is lyophilized pale yellow flakes or congealed mass with a molecular weight of 214.06. It is highly soluble in alcohol and lipids, and poorly soluble in water. BiCNU is administered by intravenous infusion after reconstitution as recommended.
The structural formula is:

$$Cl-CH_2-CH_2-\underset{\underset{NO}{|}}{N}-\overset{\overset{O}{\|}}{C}-NH-CH_2-CH_2-Cl$$

Sterile BiCNU is available in 100 mg single dose vials of lyophilized material.

CLINICAL PHARMACOLOGY
Although it is generally agreed that BiCNU alkylates DNA and RNA, it is not cross resistant with other alkylators. As with other nitrosoureas, it may also inhibit several key enzymatic processes by carbamoylation of amino acids in proteins.
Intravenously-administered BiCNU is rapidly degraded, with no intact drug detectable after 15 minutes. However, in studies with C−14 labeled drug, prolonged levels of the isotope were detected in the plasma and tissue, probably representing radioactive fragments of the parent compound.
It is thought that the antineoplastic and toxic activities of BiCNU may be due to metabolites. Approximately 60% to 70% of a total dose is excreted in the urine in 96 hours and about 10% as respiratory CO_2. The fate of the remainder is undetermined.
Because of the high lipid solubility and the relative lack of ionization at physiological pH, BiCNU crosses the blood-

brain barrier quite effectively. Levels of radioactivity in the CSF are ≥ 50% of those measured concurrently in plasma.

INDICATIONS AND USAGE

BiCNU is indicated as palliative therapy as a single agent or in established combination therapy with other approved chemotherapeutic agents in the following:

1. Brain tumors—glioblastoma, brainstem glioma, medulloblastoma, astrocytoma, ependymoma, and metastatic brain tumors.
2. Multiple myeloma—in combination with prednisone.
3. Hodgkin's Disease—as secondary therapy in combination with other approved drugs in patients who relapse while being treated with primary therapy, or who fail to respond to primary therapy.
4. Non-Hodgkin's lymphomas—as secondary therapy in combination with other approved drugs for patients who relapse while being treated with primary therapy, or who fail to respond to primary therapy.

CONTRAINDICATIONS

BiCNU should not be given to individuals who have demonstrated a previous hypersensitivity to it.

WARNINGS

Since the major toxicity is delayed bone marrow suppression, blood counts should be monitored weekly for at least 6 weeks after a dose (see "ADVERSE REACTIONS"). At the recommended dosage, courses of BiCNU should not be given more frequently than every 6 weeks.

The bone marrow toxicity of BiCNU is cumulative and therefore dosage adjustment must be considered on the basis of nadir blood counts from prior dose (see "Dosage Adjustment Table" under "DOSAGE AND ADMINISTRATION").

Pulmonary toxicity from BiCNU appears to be dose related. Patients receiving greater than 1400 mg/m^2 cumulative dose are at significantly higher risk than those receiving less. Additionally, delayed onset pulmonary fibrosis occurring up to 15 years after treatment has been reported in patients who received BiCNU in childhood and early adolescence (see "ADVERSE REACTIONS").

Long term use of nitrosoureas has been reported to be associated with the development of secondary malignancies.

Liver and renal function tests should be monitored periodically (see "ADVERSE REACTIONS").

BiCNU may cause fetal harm when administered to a pregnant woman. BiCNU has been shown to be embryotoxic in rats and rabbits and teratogenic in rats when given in doses equivalent to the human dose. There are no adequate and well-controlled studies in pregnant women. If this drug is used during pregnancy, or if the patient becomes pregnant while taking (receiving) this drug, the patient should be apprised of the potential hazard to the fetus. Women of childbearing potential should be advised to avoid becoming pregnant.

BiCNU has been administered through an intraarterial intracarotid route; this procedure is investigational and has been associated with ocular toxicity.

PRECAUTIONS

General: In all instances where the use of BiCNU is considered for chemotherapy, the physician must evaluate the need and usefulness of the drug against the risks of toxic effects or adverse reactions. Most such adverse reactions are reversible if detected early. When such effects or reactions do occur, the drug should be reduced in dosage or discontinued and appropriate corrective measures should be taken according to the clinical judgment of the physician. Reinstitution of BiCNU therapy should be carried out with caution, and with adequate consideration of the further need for the drug and alertness as to possible recurrence of toxicity.

Laboratory Tests: Due to delayed bone marrow suppression, blood counts should be monitored weekly for at least 6 weeks after a dose.

Baseline pulmonary function studies should be conducted along with frequent pulmonary function tests during treatment. Patients with a baseline below 70% of the predicted Forced Vital Capacity (FVC) or Carbon Monoxide Diffusing Capacity (DL$_{CO}$) are particularly at risk.

Since BiCNU may cause liver dysfunction, it is recommended that liver function tests be monitored.

Renal function tests should also be monitored periodically.

Carcinogenesis, Mutagenesis, Impairment of Fertility: BiCNU is carcinogenic in rats and mice, producing a marked increase in tumor incidence in doses approximating those employed clinically. Nitrosourea therapy does have carcinogenic potential in humans (see "ADVERSE REACTIONS"). BiCNU also affects fertility in male rats at doses somewhat higher than the human dose.

Pregnancy: Pregnancy "Category D," see "WARNINGS."

Nursing Mothers: It is not known whether this drug is excreted in human milk. Because many drugs are excreted in human milk and because of the potential for serious adverse reactions in nursing infants from BiCNU, a decision should be made whether to discontinue nursing or to discontinue the drug, taking into account the importance of the drug to the mother.

Pediatric Use: Safety and effectiveness in children have not been established.

ADVERSE REACTIONS

Hematologic Toxicity: The most frequent and most serious toxicity of BiCNU is delayed myelosuppression. It usually occurs 4 to 6 weeks after drug administration and is dose related. Thrombocytopenia occurs at about 4 weeks postadministration and persists for 1 to 2 weeks. Leukopenia occurs at 5 to 6 weeks after a dose of BiCNU and persists for 1 to 2 weeks. Thrombocytopenia is generally more severe than leukopenia. However, both may be dose-limiting toxicities. BiCNU may produce cumulative myelosuppression, manifested by more depressed indices or longer duration of suppression after repeated doses.

The occurrence of acute leukemia and bone marrow dysplasias have been reported in patients following long term nitrosourea therapy.

Anemia also occurs, but is less frequent and less severe than thrombocytopenia or leukopenia.

Pulmonary Toxicity: Pulmonary toxicity characterized by pulmonary infiltrates and/or fibrosis has been reported to occur from 9 days to 43 months after treatment with BiCNU and related nitrosoureas. Most of these patients were receiving prolonged therapy with total doses of BiCNU greater than 1400 mg/m^2. However, there have been reports of pulmonary fibrosis in patients receiving lower total doses. Other risk factors include past history of lung disease and duration of treatment. Cases of fatal pulmonary toxicity with BiCNU have been reported.

Additionally, delayed onset pulmonary fibrosis occurring up to 15 years after treatment has been reported in patient who received BiCNU in childhood and early adolescence in cumulative doses ranging from 770 to 1800 mg/m^2 combined with cranial radiotherapy for intracranial tumors. Chest x-rays have demonstrated pulmonary hypoplasia with upper zone contraction. Gallium scans have been normal in all cases. Thoracic CT scans have demonstrated an unusual pattern of upper zone fibrosis. There appears to be some late reduction of pulmonary function in a substantial percentage of these patients. This form of lung fibrosis may be slowly progressive and has resulted in death in some cases.

Gastrointestinal Toxicity: Nausea and vomiting after IV administration of BiCNU are noted frequently. This toxicity appears within 2 hours of dosing, usually lasting 4 to 6 hours, and is dose related. Prior administration of antiemetics is effective in diminishing and sometimes preventing this side effect.

Hepatotoxicity: A reversible type of hepatic toxicity, manifested by increased transaminase, alkaline phosphatase and bilirubin levels, has been reported in a small percentage of patients receiving BiCNU.

Nephrotoxicity: Renal abnormalities consisting of progressive azotemia, decrease in kidney size and renal failure have been reported in patients who received large cumulative doses after prolonged therapy with BiCNU and related nitrosoureas. Kidney damage has also been reported occasionally in patients receiving lower total doses.

Other Toxicities: Accidental contact of reconstituted BiCNU with skin has caused burning and hyperpigmentation of the affected areas.

Rapid IV infusion of BiCNU may produce intensive flushing of the skin and suffusion of the conjunctiva within 2 hours, lasting about 4 hours. It is also associated with burning at the site of injection although true thrombosis is rare. Neuroretinitis has been reported.

OVERDOSAGE

No proven antidotes have been established for BiCNU overdosage.

DOSAGE AND ADMINISTRATION

The recommended dose of BiCNU as a single agent in previously untreated patients is 150 to 200 mg/m^2 intravenously every 6 weeks. This may be given as a single dose or divided into daily injections such as 75 to 100 mg/m^2 on 2 successive days. When BiCNU is used in combination with other myelosuppressive drugs or in patients in whom bone marrow reserve is depleted, the doses should be adjusted accordingly. Doses subsequent to the initial dose should be adjusted according to the hematologic response of the patient to the preceding dose. The following schedule is suggested as a guide to dosage adjustment:

Nadir After Prior Dose		Percentage of Prior Dose to be Given
Leukocytes/mm^3	Platelets/mm^3	
> 4000	> 100,000	100%
3000–3999	75,000–99,999	100%
2000–2999	25,000–74,999	70%
< 2000	< 25,000	50%

A repeat course of BiCNU should not be given until circulating blood elements have returned to acceptable levels (platelets above 100,000/mm^3, leukocytes above 4,000/mm^3),

and this is usually in 6 weeks. Adequate number of neutrophils should be present on a peripheral blood smear. Blood counts should be monitored weekly and repeat courses should not be given before 6 weeks because the hematologic toxicity is delayed and cumulative.

Administration Precautions: As with other potentially toxic compounds, caution should be exercised in handling BiCNU and preparing the solution of BiCNU. Accidental contact of reconstituted BiCNU with the skin has caused transient hyperpigmentation of the affected areas. The use of gloves is recommended. If BiCNU lyophilized material or solution contacts the skin or mucosa, immediately wash the skin or mucosa thoroughly with soap and water.

The reconstituted solution should be used intravenously only and should be administered by IV drip. Injection of BiCNU over shorter periods of time than 1 to 2 hours may produce intense pain and burning at the site of injection.

Preparation of Intravenous Solutions: First, dissolve BiCNU with 3 mL of the supplied sterile diluent (Dehydrated Alcohol Injection, USP). Second, aseptically add 27 mL Sterile Water for Injection, USP. Each mL of resulting solution contains 3.3 mg of BiCNU in 10% ethanol, pH 5.6 to 6.0. Reconstitution as recommended results in a clear, colorless to yellowish solution which may be further diluted with 0.9% Sodium Chloride Injection, USP, or 5% Dextrose Injection, USP. Parenteral drug products should be inspected visually for particulate matter and discoloration prior to administration, whenever solution and container permit.

Important Note: The lyophilized dosage formulation contains no preservatives and is not intended as a multiple dose vial.

Stability: Unopened vials of the dry drug must be stored in a refrigerator (2°C to 8°C). The recommended storage of unopened vials provides a stable product for 2 years. After reconstitution as recommended, BiCNU is stable for 8 hours at room temperature (25°C) or 24 hours under refrigeration (4°C).

Vials reconstituted as directed and further diluted to a concentration of 0.2 mg/mL in 5% Dextrose Injection, USP, or 0.9% Sodium Chloride Injection, USP, should be utilized within 8 hours and protected from light. These solutions are also stable for 24 hours under refrigeration (4°C) and an additional 6 hours at room temperature (25°C) protected from light.

Glass containers were used for the stability data provided in this section. Only use glass containers for BiCNU administration.

Important Note: BiCNU has a low melting point (30.5° to 32.0°C or 86.9° to 89.6°F). Exposure of the drug to this temperature or above will cause the drug to liquefy and appear as an oil film on the vials. This is a sign of decomposition and vials should be discarded. If there is a question of adequate refrigeration upon receipt of this product, immediately inspect the larger vial in each individual carton. Hold the vial to a bright light for inspection. The BiCNU will appear as a very small amount of dry flakes or dry congealed mass. If this is evident, the BiCNU is suitable for use and should be refrigerated immediately.

Procedures for proper handling and disposal of anticancer drugs should be considered. Several guidelines on this subject have been published.[1-7] There is no general agreement that all of the procedures recommended in the guidelines are necessary or appropriate.

REFERENCES

1. Recommendations for the Safe Handling of Parenteral Antineoplastic Drugs, NIH Publication No. 83–2621. For sale by the Superintendent of Documents, US Government Printing Office, Washington, DC 20402.
2. AMA Council Report, Guidelines for Handling Parenteral Antineoplastics. *JAMA.* 1985; March 15.
3. National Study Commission on Cytotoxic Exposure—Recommendations for Handling Cytotoxic Agents. Available from Louis P. Jeffrey, ScD., Chairman, National Study Commission on Cytotoxic Exposure, Massachusetts College of Pharmacy and Allied Health Sciences, 179 Longwood Avenue, Boston, Massachusetts 02115.
4. Clinical Oncological Society of Australia. Guidelines and Recommendations for Safe Handling of Antineoplastic Agents. *Med J Australia.* 1983; 1:426–428.
5. Jones RB, et al: Safe handling of chemotherapeutic agents: a report from the Mount Sinai Medical Center, *CA—A Cancer J for Clinicians.* 1983; (Sept/Oct) 258–263.
6. American Society of Hospital Pharmacists Technical Assistance Bulletin on Handling Cytotoxic and Hazardous Drugs. *Am J Hosp Pharm.* 1990; 47:1033–1049.
7. OSHA Work-Practice Guidelines for Personnel Dealing with Cytotoxic (Antineoplastic) Drugs. *Am J Hosp Pharm.* 1986; 43:1193–1204.

SUPPLY

BiCNU (sterile carmustine [BCNU]). Each package contains a vial containing 100 mg carmustine and a vial containing 3 mL sterile diluent.

Continued on next page

Bristol-Myers Oncology—Cont.

NDC 0015-3012-18
Store dry powder in refrigerator (2° to 8°C).
For information on package sizes available refer to the current price schedule.
Manufactured by Ben Venue Laboratories, Inc., Bedford, Ohio 44146

BLENOXANE® ℞
[blĕ-nŏk 'săn]
(sterile bleomycin sulfate, USP)
vial, 15 units NSN 6505-01-060-4278(m)

> **WARNING**
> It is recommended that Blenoxane be administered under the supervision of a qualified physician experienced in the use of cancer chemotherapeutic agents.
> Appropriate management of therapy and complications is possible only when adequate diagnostic and treatment facilities are readily available.
> Pulmonary fibrosis is the most severe toxicity associated with Blenoxane. The most frequent presentation is pneumonitis occasionally progressing to pulmonary fibrosis. Its occurrence is higher in elderly patients and in those receiving greater than 400 units total dose, but pulmonary toxicity has been observed in young patients and those treated with low doses.
> A severe idiosyncratic reaction consisting of hypotension, mental confusion, fever, chills, and wheezing has been reported in approximately 1% of lymphoma patients treated with Blenoxane.

DESCRIPTION

Blenoxane (sterile bleomycin sulfate, USP) is a mixture of cytotoxic glycopeptide antibiotics isolated from a strain of *Streptomyces verticillus*. It is freely soluble in water.
Note: A unit of bleomycin is equal to the formerly used milligram activity. The term milligram activity is a misnomer and was changed to units to be more precise.

ACTION

Although the exact mechanism of action of Blenoxane is unknown, available evidence would seem to indicate that the main mode of action is the inhibition of DNA synthesis with some evidence of lesser inhibition of RNA and protein synthesis.
In mice, high concentrations of Blenoxane are found in the skin, lungs, kidneys, peritoneum, and lymphatics. Tumor cells of the skin and lungs have been found to have high concentrations of Blenoxane in contrast to the low concentrations found in hematopoietic tissue. The low concentrations of Blenoxane found in bone marrow may be related to high levels of Blenoxane degradative enzymes found in that tissue.
In patients with a creatinine clearance of >35 mL per minute, the serum or plasma terminal elimination half-life of bleomycin is approximately 115 minutes. In patients with a creatinine clearance of <35 mL per minute, the plasma or serum terminal elimination half-life increases exponentially as the creatinine clearance decreases. In humans, 60% to 70% of an administered dose is recovered in the urine as active bleomycin.

INDICATIONS

Blenoxane should be considered a palliative treatment. It has been shown to be useful in the management of the following neoplasms either as a single agent or in proven combinations with other approved chemotherapeutic agents:
Squamous Cell Carcinoma—Head and neck (including mouth, tongue, tonsil, nasopharynx, oropharynx, sinus, palate, lip, buccal mucosa, gingiva, epiglottis, larynx), skin, penis, cervix, and vulva. The response to Blenoxane is poorer in patients with head and neck cancer previously irradiated.
Lymphomas—Hodgkin's, reticulum cell sarcoma, lymphosarcoma.
Testicular Carcinoma—Embryonal cell, choriocarcinoma, and teratocarcinoma.

CONTRAINDICATIONS

Blenoxane is contraindicated in patients who have demonstrated a hypersensitive or an idiosyncratic reaction to it.

WARNINGS

Patients receiving Blenoxane must be observed carefully and frequently during and after therapy. It should be used with extreme caution in patients with significant impairment of renal function or compromised pulmonary function.
Pulmonary toxicities occur in 10% of treated patients. In approximately 1%, the nonspecific pneumonitis induced by Blenoxane progresses to pulmonary fibrosis, and death. Although this is age and dose related, the toxicity is unpredictable. Frequent roentgenograms are recommended.
Idiosyncratic reactions similar to anaphylaxis have been reported in 1% of lymphoma patients treated with Blenoxane. Since these usually occur after the first or second dose, careful monitoring is essential after these doses.
Renal or hepatic toxicity, beginning as a deterioration in renal or liver function tests, have been reported infrequently. These toxicities may occur, however, at any time after initiation of therapy.
Usage in Pregnancy: Safe use of Blenoxane in pregnant women has not been established.

ADVERSE REACTIONS

Pulmonary—This is potentially the most serious side effect, occurring in approximately 10% of treated patients. The most frequent presentation is pneumonitis occasionally progressing to pulmonary fibrosis. Approximately 1% of patients treated have died of pulmonary fibrosis. Pulmonary toxicity is both dose and age related, being more common in patients over 70 years of age and in those receiving over 400 units total dose. This toxicity, however, is unpredictable and has been seen occasionally in young patients receiving low doses.
Because of lack of specificity of the clinical syndrome, the identification of patients with pulmonary toxicity due to Blenoxane has been extremely difficult. The earliest symptom associated with Blenoxane pulmonary toxicity is dyspnea. The earliest sign is fine rales.
Radiographically, Blenoxane-induced pneumonitis produces nonspecific patchy opacities, usually of the lower lung fields. The most common changes in pulmonary function tests are a decrease in total lung volume and a decrease in vital capacity. However, these changes are not predictive of the development of pulmonary fibrosis.
The microscopic tissue changes due to Blenoxane toxicity include bronchiolar squamous metaplasia, reactive macrophages, atypical alveolar epithelial cells, fibrinous edema, and interstitial fibrosis. The acute stage may involve capillary changes and subsequent fibrinous exudation into alveoli producing a change similar to hyaline membrane formation and progressing to a diffuse interstitial fibrosis resembling the Hamman-Rich syndrome. These microscopic findings are nonspecific; eg, similar changes are seen in radiation pneumonitis and pneumocystic pneumonitis.
To monitor the onset of pulmonary toxicity, roentgenograms of the chest should be taken every 1 to 2 weeks. If pulmonary changes are noted, treatment should be discontinued until it can be determined if they are drug related. Recent studies have suggested that sequential measurement of the pulmonary diffusion capacity for carbon monoxide (DL_{co}) during treatment with Blenoxane may be an indicator of subclinical pulmonary toxicity. It is recommended that the DL_{co} be monitored monthly if it is to be employed to detect pulmonary toxicities, and thus the drug should be discontinued when the DL_{co} falls below 30% to 35% of the pretreatment value.
Because of bleomycin's sensitization of lung tissue, patients who have received bleomycin are at greater risk of developing pulmonary toxicity when oxygen is administered in surgery. While long exposure to very high oxygen concentrations is a known cause of lung damage, after bleomycin administration, lung damage can occur at lower concentrations that are usually considered safe. Suggestive preventive measures are:

(1) Maintain Fl O_2 at concentrations approximating that of room air (25%) during surgery and the postoperative period.
(2) Monitor carefully fluid replacement, focusing more on colloid administration rather than crystalloid.

Sudden onset of an acute chest pain syndrome suggestive of pleuropericarditis has been rarely reported during Blenoxane infusions. Although each patient must be individually evaluated, further courses of Blenoxane do not appear to be contraindicated.
Idiosyncratic Reactions—In approximately 1% of the lymphoma patients treated with Blenoxane an idiosyncratic reaction, similar to anaphylaxis clinically, has been reported. The reaction may be immediate or delayed for several hours, and usually occurs after the first or second dose. It consists of hypotension, mental confusion, fever, chills, and wheezing. Treatment is symptomatic including volume expansion, pressor agents, antihistamines, and corticosteroids.
Integument and Mucous Membranes—These are the most frequent side effects being reported in approximately 50% of treated patients. These consist of erythema, rash, striae, vesiculation, hyperpigmentation, and tenderness of the skin. Hyperkeratosis, nail changes, alopecia, pruritus, and stomatitis have also been reported. It was necessary to discontinue Blenoxane therapy in 2% of treated patients because of these toxicities.
Skin toxicity is a relatively late manifestation usually developing in the 2nd and 3rd week of treatment after 150 to 200 units of Blenoxane have been administered and appears to be related to the cumulative dose.
Other—Vascular toxicities coincident with the use of Blenoxane in combination with other antineoplastic agents have been reported rarely. The events are clinically heterogeneous and may include myocardial infarction, cerebrovascular accident, thrombotic microangiopathy (HUS) or cerebral arteritis. Various mechanisms have been proposed for these vascular complications. There are also reports of Raynaud's phenomenon occurring in patients treated with Blenoxane in combination with vinblastine with or without cisplatin or, in a few cases, with Blenoxane as a single agent. It is currently unknown if the cause of Raynaud's phenomenon in these cases is the disease, underlying vascular compromise. Blenoxane, vinblastine, hypomagnesemia, or a combination of any of these factors.
Fever, chills, and vomiting were frequently reported side effects. Anorexia and weight loss are common and may persist long after termination of this medication. Pain at tumor site, phlebitis, and other local reactions were reported infrequently.

DOSAGE

Because of the possibility of an anaphylactoid reaction, lymphoma patients should be treated with two units or less for the first two doses. If no acute reaction occurs, then the regular dosage schedule may be followed.
The following dose schedule is recommended: **Squamous cell carcinoma, lymphosarcoma, reticulum cell sarcoma, testicular carcinoma**—0.25 to 0.50 units/kg (10 to 20 units/m^2) given intravenously, intramuscularly, or subcutaneously weekly or twice weekly.
Hodgkin's Disease—0.25 to 0.50 units/kg (10 to 20 units/m^2) given intravenously, intramuscularly, or subcutaneously weekly or twice weekly. After a 50% response, a maintenance dose of one unit daily or five units weekly intravenously or intramuscularly should be given.
Pulmonary toxicity of Blenoxane appears to be dose related with a striking increase when the total dose is over 400 units. Total doses over 400 units should be given with great caution.
NOTE: When Blenoxane is used in combination with other antineoplastic agents, pulmonary toxicities may occur at lower doses.
Improvement of Hodgkin's Disease and testicular tumors is prompt and noted within 2 weeks. If no improvement is seen by this time, improvement is unlikely. Squamous cell cancers respond more slowly, sometimes requiring as long as 3 weeks before any improvement is noted.

ADMINISTRATION

Blenoxane may be given by the intramuscular, intravenous, or subcutaneous routes.
Intramuscular or Subcutaneous—Dissolve the contents of a Blenoxane vial in 1 to 5 mL of Sterile Water for Injection, USP, Sodium Chloride for Injection, USP, 5% Dextrose Injection, USP, or Bacteriostatic Water for Injection, USP.
Intravenous—Dissolve the contents of the vial in 5 mL or more of a solution suitable for injection, eg, physiologic saline or glucose, and administer slowly over a period of 10 minutes.

STABILITY

The sterile powder is stable under refrigeration (2°–8°C) and should not be used after the expiration date is reached.
Blenoxane is stable for 24 hours at room temperature in Sodium Chloride or 5% Dextrose Solution.
Blenoxane is stable for 24 hours in 5% Dextrose containing heparin 100 units per mL or 1000 units per mL.
Procedures for proper handling and disposal of anticancer drugs should be considered. Several guidelines on this subject have been published.[1–7] There is no general agreement that all of the procedures recommended in the guidelines are necessary or appropriate.

REFERENCES

1. Recommendations for the Safe Handling of Parenteral Antineoplastic Drugs. NIH Publication No. 83-2621. For sale by the Superintendent of Documents, US Government Printing Office, Washington, D.C. 20402.
2. AMA Council Report. Guidelines for Handling Parenteral Antineoplastics, *JAMA*. 1985 March 15.
3. National Study Commission on Cytotoxic Exposure—Recommendations for Handling Cytotoxic Agents. Available from Louis P. Jeffrey, Sc.D., Chairman, National Study Commission on Cytotoxic Exposure, Massachusetts College of Pharmacy and Allied Health Sciences, 179 Longwood Avenue, Boston, Massachusetts 02115.
4. Clinical Oncological Society of Australia. Guidelines and Recommendations for Safe Handling of Antineoplastic Agents. *Med J Australia*. 1983; 1:426-428.
5. Jones, RB, et. al. Safe handling of chemotherapeutic agents: A Report from the Mount Sinai Medical Center, *CA—A Cancer for Clinicians*. 1983; (Sept/Oct) 258-263.
6. American Society of Hospital Pharmacists Technical Assistance Bulletin on Handling Cytotoxic and Hazardous Drugs. *Am J Hosp Pharm*. 1990; 47:1033-1049.
7. OSHA Work-Practice Guidelines for Personnel Dealing with Cytotoxic (Antineoplasic) Drugs, *Am J Hosp Pharm*. 1986; 43:1193-1204.

SUPPLY

Each vial contains 15 units of Blenoxane as sterile bleomycin sulfate, USP.
NDC 0015-3010-20
Manufactured by Nippon Kayaku Co., Ltd.
Tokyo, Japan
For information on package sizes available, refer to the current price sheet.

CeeNU® ℞
[*cē'nū*]
(lomustine [CCNU]) capsules

> **WARNINGS**
> CeeNU (lomustine) should be administered under the supervision of a qualified physician experienced in the use of cancer chemotherapeutic agents.
> Bone marrow suppression, notably thrombocytopenia and leukopenia, which may contribute to bleeding and overwhelming infections in an already compromised patient, is the most common and severe of the toxic effects of CeeNU (see "WARNINGS" and "ADVERSE REACTIONS").
> Since the major toxicity is delayed bone marrow suppression, blood counts should be monitored weekly for at least 6 weeks after a dose (see "ADVERSE REACTIONS"). At the recommended dosage, courses of CeeNU should not be given more frequently than every 6 weeks.
> The bone marrow toxicity of CeeNU is cumulative and therefore dosage adjustment must be considered on the basis of nadir blood counts from prior dose (see Dosage Adjustment Table under "DOSAGE AND ADMINISTRATION").

DESCRIPTION

CeeNU (lomustine) (CCNU) is one of the nitrosoureas used in the treatment of certain neoplastic diseases. It is 1- (2-chloroethyl)- 3-cyclohexyl- 1 -nitrosourea. It is a yellow powder with the empirical formula of $C_9H_{16}ClN_3O_2$ and a molecular weight of 233.71. CeeNU is soluble in 10% ethanol (0.05 mg per mL) and in absolute alcohol (70 mg per mL). CeeNU is relatively insoluble in water (<0.05 mg per mL).
It is relatively unionized at a physiological pH.
Inactive ingredients in CeeNU capsules are: magnesium stearate and mannitol.
The structural formula is:

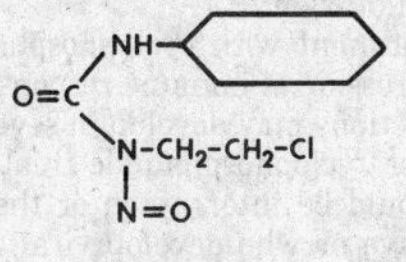

CeeNU is available in 10 mg, 40 mg and 100 mg capsules for oral administration.

CLINICAL PHARMACOLOY

Although it is generally agreed that CeeNU alkylates DNA and RNA, it is not cross resistant with other alkylators. As with other nitrosoureas, it may also inhibit several key enzymatic processes by carbamoylation of amino acids in proteins.
CeeNU may be given orally. Following oral administration of radioactive CeeNU at doses ranging from 30 mg/m^2 to 100 mg/m^2, about half of the radioactivity given was excreted in the form of degredation products within 24 hours.
The serum half-life of the metabolites ranges from 16 hours to 2 days. Tissue levels are comparable to plasma levels at 15 minutes after intravenous administration.
Because of the high lipid solubility and the relative lack of ionization at a physiological pH, CeeNU crosses the blood-brain barrier quite effectively. Levels of radioactivity in the CSF are 50% or greater than those measured concurrently in plasma.

INDICATIONS AND USAGE

CeeNU has been shown to be useful as a single agent in addition to other treatment modalities, or in established combination therapy with other approved chemotherapeutic agents in the following:
Brain tumors—both primary and metastatic, in patients who have already received appropriate surgical and/or radiotherapeutic procedures.
Hodgkin's Disease—secondary therapy in combination with other approved drugs in patients who relapse while being treated with primary therapy, or who fail to respond to primary therapy.

CONTRAINDICATIONS

CeeNU should not be given to individuals who have demonstrated a previous hypersensitivity to it.

WARNINGS

Since the major toxicity is delayed bone marrow suppression, blood counts should be monitored weekly for at least 6 weeks after a dose (see "ADVERSE REACTIONS"). At the recommended dosage, courses of CeeNU should not be given more frequently than every 6 weeks.
The bone marrow toxicity of CeeNU is cumulative and therefore dosage adjustment must be considered on the basis of nadir blood counts from prior dose (see Dosage Adjustment Table under "DOSAGE AND ADMINISTRATION").
Pulmonary toxicity from CeeNU appears to be dose related (see "ADVERSE REACTIONS").
Long term use in nitrosoureas has been reported to be possibly associated with the development of secondary malignancies.
Liver and renal function tests should be monitored periodically (see "ADVERSE REACTIONS").
Pregnancy Category D: CeeNU can cause fetal harm when administered to a pregnant woman. CeeNU is embryotoxic and teratogenic in rats and embryotoxic in rabbits at dose levels equivalent to the human dose. There are no adequate and well controlled studies in pregnant women. If this drug is used during pregnancy, or if the patient becomes pregnant while taking (receiving) this drug, the patient should be apprised of the potential hazard to the fetus. Women of childbearing potential should be advised to avoid becoming pregnant.

PRECAUTIONS

General: In all instances where the use of CeeNU is considered for chemotherapy, the physician must evaluate the need and usefulness of the drug against the risks of toxic effects or adverse reactions. Most such adverse reactions are reversible if detected early. When such effects or reactions do occur, the drug should be reduced in dosage or discontinued and appropriate corrective measures should be taken according to the clinical judgment of the physician. Reinstitution of CeeNU therapy should be carried out with caution and with adequate consideration of the further need for the drug and alertness as to possible recurrence of toxicity.
Laboratory Tests: Due to delayed bone marrow suppression, blood counts should be monitored weekly for at least 6 weeks after a dose.
Baseline pulmonary function studies should be conducted along with frequent pulmonary function tests during treatment. Patients with a baseline below 70% of the predicted Forced Vital Capacity (FVC) or Carbon Monoxide Diffusing Capacity (DL_{co}) are particularly at risk.
Since CeeNU may cause liver dysfunction, it is recommended that liver function tests be monitored periodically.
Renal function tests should also be monitored periodically.
Carcinogenesis, Mutagenesis, Impairment of Fertility: CeeNU is carcinogenic in rats and mice, producing a marked increase in tumor incidence in doses approximating those employed clinically. Nitrosourea therapy does have carcinogenic potential in humans (see "ADVERSE REACTIONS"). CeeNU also affects fertility in male rats at doses somewhat higher than the human dose.
Pregnancy: Pregnancy "Category D"—See "WARNINGS" section.
Nursing Mothers: It is not known whether this drug is excreted in human milk. Because many drugs are excreted in human milk and because of the potential for serious adverse reactions in nursing infants from CeeNU, a decision should be made whether to discontinue nursing or to discontinue the drug, taking into account the importance of the drug to the mother.
Information for the Patient: Patients receiving CeeNU should be given the following information and instructions by the physician:

1. Patients should be told that CeeNU is an anticancer drug and belongs to the group of medicines known as alkylating agents.
2. In order to provide the proper dose of CeeNU, patients should be aware that there may be two or more different types and colors of capsules in the container dispensed by the pharmacist.
3. Patients should be told that CeeNU is given as a single oral dose and will not be repeated for at least 6 weeks.
4. Patients should be told that nausea and vomiting usually last less than 24 hours, although loss of appetite may last for several days.
5. If any of the following reactions occur, notify the physician: fever, chills, sore throat, unusual bleeding or bruising, shortness of breath, dry cough, swelling of feet or lower legs, mental confusion or yellowing of eyes and skin.

ADVERSE REACTIONS

Hematologic Toxicity: The most frequent and most serious toxicity of CeeNU is delayed myelosuppression. It usually occurs 4 to 6 weeks after drug administration and is dose related. Thrombocytopenia occurs at about 4 weeks postadministration and persists for 1 to 2 weeks. Leukopenia occurs at 5 to 6 weeks after a dose of CeeNU and persists for 1 to 2 weeks. Approximately 65% of patients receiving 130 mg/m^2 develop white blood counts below 5000 wbc/mm^3. Thirty-six percent developed white blood counts below 3000 wbc/mm^3. Thrombocytopenia is generally more severe than leukopenia. However, both may be dose-limiting toxicities.
CeeNU may produce cumulative myelosuppression, manifested by more depressed indices or longer duration of suppression after repeated doses.
The occurrence of acute leukemia and bone marrow dysplasias have been reported in patients following long term nitrosourea therapy.
Anemia also occurs, but is less frequent and less severe than thrombocytopenia or leukopenia.
Pulmonary Toxicity: Pulmonary toxicity characterized by pulmonary infiltrates and/or fibrosis has been reported rarely with CeeNU. Onset of toxicity has occurred after an interval of 6 months or longer from the start of therapy with cumulative doses of CeeNU usually greater than 1100 mg/m^2. There is one report of pulmonary toxicity at a cumulative dose of only 600 mg.
Delayed onset pulmonary fibrosis occurring up to 15 years after treatment has been reported in patients who received related nitrosoureas in childhood and early adolescence combined with cranial radiotherapy for intracranial tumors.
Gastrointestinal Toxicity: Nausea and vomiting may occur 3 to 6 hours after an oral dose and usually lasts less than 24 hours. Prior administration of antiemetics is effective in diminishing and sometimes preventing this side effect. Nausea and vomiting can also be reduced if CeeNU is administered to fasting patients.
Hepatotoxicity: A reversible type of hepatic toxicity, manifested by increased transaminase, alkaline phosphatase and bilirubin levels, has been reported in a small percentage of patients receiving CeeNU.
Nephrotoxicity: Renal abnormalities consisting of progressive azotemia, decrease in kidney size and renal failure have been reported in patients who received large cumulative doses after prolonged therapy with CeeNU. Kidney damage has also been reported occasionally in patients receiving lower total doses.
Other Toxicities: Stomatitis and alopecia have been reported infrequently.
Neurological reactions such as disorientation, lethargy, ataxia, and dysarthria have been noted in some patients receiving CeeNU. However, the relationship to medication in these patients is unclear.

OVERDOSAGE

No proven antidotes have been established for CeeNU overdosage.

DOSAGE AND ADMINISTRATION

The recommended dose of CeeNU in adults and children as a single agent in previously untreated patients is 130 mg/m^2 as a single oral dose every 6 weeks. In individuals with compromised bone marrow function, the dose should be reduced to 100 mg/m^2 every 6 weeks. When CeeNU is used in combination with other myelosuppressive drugs, the doses should be adjusted accordingly.
Doses subsequent to the initial dose should be adjusted according to the hematologic response of the patient to the preceding dose. The following schedule is suggested as a guide to dosage adjustment:

Nadir After Prior Dose		Percentage of Prior Dose to be Given
Leukocytes	Platelets	
>4000	>100,000	100%
3000–3999	75,000–99,999	100%
2000–2999	25,000–74,999	70%
<2000	<25,000	50%

A repeat course of CeeNU should not be given until circulating blood elements have returned to acceptable levels (platelets above 100,000/mm^3; leukocytes above 4,000/mm^3) and this is usually in 6 weeks. Adequate number of neutrophils should be present on a peripheral blood smear. Blood counts should be monitored weekly and repeat courses should not be given before 6 weeks because the hematologic toxicity is delayed and cumulative.

HOW SUPPLIED

The dose pack of CeeNU (lomustine, CCNU) **NDC** 0015-3034-10 Capsules contains;
2—100 mg capsules (Green/Green)
2—40 mg capsules (White/Green)
2—10 mg capsules (White/White)
Stability: CeeNU Capsules are stable for the lot life indicated on package labeling when stored at room temperature in well closed containers. Avoid excessive heat (over 40°C).
Directions to the Pharmacist: The dose pack contains a total of 300 mg and will provide enough medication for titration of a single dose. The total dose prescribed by the physician can be obtained (to within 10 mg) by determining the appropriate combination of the enclosed capsule strengths.

Continued on next page

Bristol-Myers Oncology—Cont.

The appropriate number of capsules of each size should be placed in a single vial to which the patient information label (gummed label provided) explaining the differences in the appearance of the capsules is affixed. Each color-coded capsule is imprinted with the dose in milligrams.
A patient information sticker, to be placed on dispensing container, is enclosed.
Also available: Individual bottles of 20 capsules each.
NDC 0015-3032-20—100 mg capsules (Green/Green)
NDC 0015-3031-20—40 mg capsules (White/Green)
NDC 0015-3030-20—10 mg capsules (White/White)
Procedures for proper handling and disposal of anticancer drugs should be considered. Several guidelines on this subject have been published.[1–7] There is no general agreement that all of the procedures recommended in the guidelines are necessary or appropriate.

REFERENCES

1. Recommendations for the Safe Handling of Parenteral Antineoplastic Drugs. NIH Publication No. 83-2621. For sale by the Superintendent of Documents, U.S. Government Printing Office, Washington, D.C. 20402.
2. AMA Council Report. Guidelines for Handling Parenteral Antineoplastics. *JAMA.* 1985; March 15.
3. National Study Commission on Cytotoxic Exposure—Recommendations for Handling Cytotoxic Agents. Available from Louis P. Jeffrey, Sc.D., Chairman, National Study Commission on Cytotoxic Exposure, Massachusetts College of Pharmacy and Allied Health Sciences, 179 Longwood Avenue, Boston, Massachusetts 02115.
4. Clinical Oncological Society of Australia: Guidelines and Recommendations for Safe Handling of Antineoplastic Agents. *Med J Australia.* 1983; 1:426-428.
5. Jones, R. B., et. al. Safe Handling of Chemotherapeutic Agents: A report from the Mount Sinai Medical Center, *CA—A Cancer J for Clinicians.* 1983; Sept./Oct., 258-263.
6. American Society of Hospital Pharmacists Technical Assistance Bulletin on Handling Cytotoxic and Hazardous Drugs. *Am J Hosp Pharm.* 1990; 47:1033-1049.
7. OSHA Work-Practice Guidelines for Personnel Dealing with Cytotoxic (Antineoplastic) Drugs. *Am J Hosp Pharm.* 1986; 43:1193-1204.

CYTOXAN® for Injection ℞

[*sī-taks 'an*]
(cyclophosphamide for injection, USP)
Lyophilized CYTOXAN® for Injection
(cyclophosphamide for injection, USP)
CYTOXAN® Tablets (cyclophosphamide tablets, USP)

DESCRIPTION

CYTOXAN for Injection is a sterile white powder blend consisting of 45 mg sodium chloride per 100 mg cyclophosphamide (anhydrous). Lyophilized CYTOXAN for Injection is a sterile white lyophilized cake or partially broken cake containing 75 mg mannitol per 100 mg cyclophosphamide (anhydrous). CYTOXAN Tablets are for oral use and contain 25 mg or 50 mg cyclophosphamide (anhydrous). Inactive ingredients in CYTOXAN tablets are acacia, FD&C Blue No. 1, D&C Yellow No. 10 Aluminum Lake, lactose, magnesium stearate, starch, stearic acid, and talc. Cyclophosphamide is a synthetic antineoplastic drug chemically related to the nitrogen mustards. Cyclophosphamide is a white crystalline powder with the molecular formula of $C_7H_{15}Cl_2N_2O_2P \cdot H_2O$ and a molecular weight of 279.1. The chemical name for cyclophosphamide is 2-[bis(2-chloroethyl)amino]tetrahydro-2H-1,3,2-oxazaphosphorine 2-oxide monohydrate. Cyclophosphamide is soluble in water, saline, or ethanol and has the following structural formula:

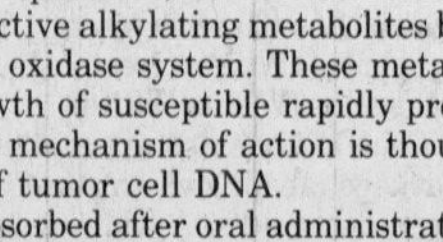

CLINICAL PHARMACOLOGY

CYTOXAN (cyclophosphamide) is biotransformed principally in the liver to active alkylating metabolites by a mixed function microsomal oxidase system. These metabolites interfere with the growth of susceptible rapidly proliferating malignant cells. The mechanism of action is thought to involve cross-linking of tumor cell DNA.
CYTOXAN is well absorbed after oral administration with a bioavailability greater than 75%. The unchanged drug has an elimination half-life of 3 to 12 hours. It is eliminated primarily in the form of metabolites, but from 5% to 25% of the dose is excreted in urine as unchanged drug. Several cytotoxic and noncytotoxic metabolites have been identified in urine and in plasma. Concentrations of metabolites reach a maximum in plasma 2 to 3 hours after an intravenous dose. Plasma protein binding of unchanged drug is low but some metabolites are bound to an extent greater than 60%. It has not been demonstrated that any single metabolite is responsible for either the therapeutic or toxic effects of cyclophosphamide. Although elevated levels of metabolites of cyclophosphamide have been observed in patients with renal failure, increased clinical toxicity in such patients has not been demonstrated.

INDICATION AND USAGE

Malignant Diseases—CYTOXAN, although effective alone in susceptible malignancies, is more frequently used concurrently or sequentially with other antineoplastic drugs.
The following malignancies are often susceptible to CYTOXAN treatment:
1. Malignant lymphomas (Stages III and IV of the Ann Arbor staging system), Hodgkin's disease, lymphocytic lymphoma (nodular or diffuse), mixed-cell type lymphoma, histiocytic lymphoma, Burkitt's lymphoma. **2.** Multiple myeloma. **3.** Leukemias: Chronic lymphocytic leukemia, chronic granulocytic leukemia (it is usually ineffective in acute blastic crisis), acute myelogenous and monocytic leukemia, acute lymphoblastic (stem-cell) leukemia in children (CYTOXAN given during remission is effective in prolonging its duration). **4.** Mycosis fungoides (advanced disease), **5.** Neuroblastoma (disseminated disease). **6.** Adenocarcinoma of the ovary. **7.** Retinoblastoma. **8.** Carcinoma of the breast.
Nonmalignant Disease: Biopsy Proven "Minimal Change" Nephrotic Syndrome in Children—CYTOXAN is useful in carefully selected cases of biopsy proven "minimal change" nephrotic syndrome in children but should not be used as primary therapy. In children whose disease fails to respond adequately to appropriate adrenocorticosteroid therapy or in whom the adrenocorticosteroid therapy produces or threatens to produce intolerable side effects. CYTOXAN may induce a remission. CYTOXAN is not indicated for the nephrotic syndrome in adults or for any other renal disease.

CONTRAINDICATIONS

Continued use of cyclophosphamide is contraindicated in patients with severely depressed bone marrow function. Cyclophosphamide is contraindicated in patients who have demonstrated a previous hypersensitivity to it. See WARNINGS and PRECAUTIONS sections.

WARNINGS

Carcinogenesis, Mutagenesis, Impairment of Fertility—Second malignancies have developed in some patients treated with cyclophosphamide used alone or in association with other antineoplastic drugs and/or modalities. Most frequently, they have been urinary bladder, myeloproliferative, or lymphoproliferative malignancies. Second malignancies most frequently were detected in patients treated for primary myeloproliferative or lymphoproliferative malignancies or nonmalignant disease in which immune processes are believed to be involved pathologically. In some cases, the second malignancy developed several years after cyclophosphamide treatment had been discontinued. Urinary bladder malignancies generally have occurred in patients who previously had hemorrhagic cystitis. One case of carcinoma of the renal pelvis was reported in a patient receiving long-term cyclophosphamide therapy for cerebral vasculitis. The possibility of cyclophosphamide-induced malignancy should be considered in any benefit-to-risk assessment for use of the drug.
Cyclophosphamide can cause fetal harm when administered to a pregnant woman and such abnormalities have been reported following cyclophosphamide therapy in pregnant women. Abnormalities were found in two infants and a 6-month-old fetus born to women treated with cyclophosphamide. Ectrodactylia was found in two of the three cases. Normal infants have also been born to women treated with cyclophosphamide during pregnancy, including the first trimester. If this drug is used during pregnancy, or if the patient becomes pregnant while taking (receiving) this drug, the patient should be apprised of the potential hazard to the fetus. Women of childbearing potential should be advised to avoid becoming pregnant.
Cyclophosphamide interferes with oogenesis and spermatogenesis. It may cause sterility in both sexes. Development of sterility appears to depend on the dose of cyclophosphamide, duration of therapy, and the state of gonadal function at the time of treatment. Cyclophosphamide-induced sterility may be irreversible in some patients.
Amenorrhea associated with decreased estrogen and increased gonadotropin secretion develops in a significant proportion of women treated with cyclophosphamide. Affected patients generally resume regular menses within a few months after cessation of therapy. Girls treated with cyclophosphamide during prepubescence generally develop secondary sexual characteristics normally and have regular menses. Ovarian fibrosis with apparently complete loss of germ cells after prolonged cyclophosphamide treatment in late prepubescence has been reported. Girls treated with cyclophosphamide during prepubescence subsequently have conceived.
Men treated with cyclophosphamide may develop oligospermia or azoospermia associated with increased gonadotropin but normal testosterone secretion. Sexual potency and libido are unimpaired in these patients. Boys treated with cyclophosphamide during prepubescence develop secondary sexual characteristics normally, but may have oligospermia or azoospermia and increased gonadotropin secretion. Some degree of testicular atrophy may occur. Cyclophosphamide-induced azoospermia is reversible in some patients, though the reversibility may not occur for several years after cessation of therapy. Men temporarily rendered sterile by cyclophosphamide have subsequently fathered normal children.
Urinary System—Hemorrhagic cystitis may develop in patients treated with cyclophosphamide. Rarely, this condition can be severe and even fatal. Fibrosis of the urinary bladder, sometimes extensive, also may develop with or without accompanying cystitis. Atypical urinary bladder epithelial cells may appear in the urine. These adverse effects appear to depend on the dose of cyclophosphamide and the duration of therapy. Such bladder injury is thought to be due to cyclophosphamide metabolites excreted in the urine. Forced fluid intake helps to assure an ample output of urine, necessitates frequent voiding, and reduces the time the drug remains in the bladder. This helps to prevent cystitis. Hematuria usually resolves in a few days after cyclophosphamide treatment is stopped, but it may persist. Medical and/or surgical supportive treatment may be required, rarely, to treat protracted cases of severe hemorrhagic cystitis. It is usually necessary to discontinue cyclophosphamide therapy in instances of severe hemorrhagic cystitis.
Cardiac Toxicity—Although a few instances of cardiac dysfunction have been reported following use of recommended doses of cyclophosphamide, no causal relationship has been established. Cardiotoxicity has been observed in some patients receiving high doses of cyclophosphamide ranging from 120 to 270 mg/kg administered over a period of a few days, usually as a portion of an intensive antineoplastic multidrug regimen or in conjunction with transplantation procedures. In a few instances with high doses of cyclophosphamide, severe, and sometimes fatal, congestive heart failure has occurred within a few days after the first cyclophosphamide dose. Histopathologic examination has primarily shown hemorrhagic myocarditis. Hemopericardium has occurred secondary to hemorrhagic myocarditis and myocardial necrosis. Pericarditis has been reported independent of any hemopericardium.
No residual cardiac abnormalities, as evidenced by electrocardiogram or echocardiogram appear to be present in patients surviving episodes of apparent cardiac toxicity associated with high doses of cyclophosphamide.
Cyclophosphamide has been reported to potentiate doxorubicin-induced cardiotoxicity.
Infections—Treatment with cyclophosphamide may cause significant suppression of immune responses. Serious, sometimes fatal, infections may develop in severely immunosuppressed patients. Cyclophosphamide treatment may not be indicated or should be interrupted or the dose reduced in patients who have or who develop viral, bacterial, fungal, protozoan, or helminthic infections.
Other—Rare instances of anaphylactic reaction including one death have been reported. One instance of possible cross-sensitivity with other alkylating agents has been reported.

PRECAUTIONS

General—Special attention to the possible development of toxicity should be exercised in patients being treated with cyclophosphamide if any of the following conditions are present.
1. Leukopenia. **2.** Thrombocytopenia. **3.** Tumor cell infiltration of bone marrow. **4.** Previous X-ray therapy. **5.** Previous therapy with other cytotoxic agents. **6.** Impaired hepatic function. **7.** Impaired renal function.
Laboratory Tests—During treatment, the patient's hematologic profile (particularly neutrophils and platelets) should be monitored regularly to determine the degree of hematopoietic suppression. Urine should also be examined regularly for red cells which may precede hemorrhagic cystitis.
Drug Interactions—The rate of metabolism and the leukopenic activity of cyclophosphamide reportedly are increased by chronic administration of high doses of phenobarbital.
The physician should be alert for possible combined drug actions, desirable or undesirable, involving cyclophosphamide even though cyclophosphamide has been used successfully concurrently with other drugs, including other cytotoxic drugs.
Cyclophosphamide treatment, which causes a marked and persistent inhibition of cholinesterase activity, potentiates the effect of succinylcholine chloride.
If a patient has been treated with cyclophosphamide within 10 days of general anesthesia, the anesthesiologist should be alerted.
Adrenalectomy—Since cyclophosphamide has been reported to be more toxic in adrenalectomized dogs, adjustment of the doses of both replacement steroids and cyclophosphamide may be necessary for the adrenalectomized patient.

Wound Healing—Cyclophosphamide may interfere with normal wound healing.

Carcinogenesis, Mutagenesis, Impairment of Fertility—See WARNINGS section for information on carcinogenesis, mutagenesis, and impairment of fertility.

Pregnancy—Pregnancy Category D. See WARNINGS section.

Nursing Mothers—Cyclophosphamide is excreted in breast milk. Because of the potential for serious adverse reactions and the potential for tumorigenicity shown for cyclophosphamide in humans, a decision should be made whether to discontinue nursing or to discontinue the drug, taking into account the importance of the drug to the mother.

ADVERSE REACTIONS

Information on adverse reactions associated with the use of CYTOXAN is arranged according to body system affected or type of reaction. The adverse reactions are listed in order of decreasing incidence. The most serious adverse reactions are described in the WARNINGS section.

Reproductive System—See WARNINGS section for information on impairment of fertility.

Digestive System—Nausea and vomiting commonly occur with cyclophosphamide therapy. Anorexia and, less frequently, abdominal discomfort or pain and diarrhea may occur. There are isolated reports of hemorrhagic colitis, oral mucosal ulceration and jaundice occurring during therapy. These adverse drug effects generally remit when cyclophosphamide treatment is stopped.

Skin and Its Structures—Alopecia occurs commonly in patients treated with cyclophosphamide. The hair can be expected to grow back after treatment with the drug or even during continued drug treatment, though it may be different in texture or color. Skin rash occurs occasionally in patients receiving the drug. Pigmentation of the skin and changes in nails can occur.

Hematopoietic System—Leukopenia occurs in patients treated with cyclophosphamide, is related to the dose of the drug, and can be used as a dosage guide. Leukopenia of less than 2000 cells/mm^3 develops commonly in patients treated with an initial loading dose of the drug, and less frequently in patients maintained on smaller doses. The degree of neutropenia is particularly important because it correlates with a reduction in resistance to infections.

Thrombocytopenia or anemia develop occasionally in patients treated with CYTOXAN. These hematologic effects usually can be reversed by reducing the drug dose or by interrupting treatment. Recovery from leukopenia usually begins in 7 to 10 days after cessation of therapy.

Urinary System—See WARNINGS section for information on cystitis and urinary bladder fibrosis.

Hemorrhagic ureteritis and renal tubular necrosis have been reported to occur in patients treated with cyclophosphamide. Such lesions usually resolve following cessation of therapy.

Infections—See WARNINGS section for information on reduced host resistance to infections.

Carcinogenesis—See WARNINGS section for information on carcinogenesis.

Respiratory System—Interstitial pulmonary fibrosis has been reported in patients receiving high doses of cyclophosphamide over a prolonged period.

Other—Rare instances of anaphylactic reaction including one death have been reported. One instance of possible cross-sensitivity with other alkylating agents has been reported.

OVERDOSAGE

No specific antidote for cyclophosphamide is known. Overdosage should be managed with supportive measures, including appropriate treatment for any concurrent infection, myelosuppression, or cardiac toxicity should it occur.

DOSAGE AND ADMINISTRATION

Treatment of Malignant Diseases: Adults and Children—When used as the only oncolytic drug therapy, the initial course of CYTOXAN for patients with no hematologic deficiency usually consists of 40 to 50 mg/kg given intravenously in divided doses over a period of 2 to 5 days. Other intravenous regimens include 10 to 15 mg/kg given every 7 to 10 days or 3 to 5 mg/kg twice weekly.

Oral CYTOXAN dosing is usually in the range of 1 to 5 mg/kg/day for both initial and maintenance dosing.

Many other regimens of intravenous and oral CYTOXAN have been reported. Dosages must be adjusted in accord with evidence of antitumor activity and/or leukopenia. The total leukocyte count is a good, objective guide for regulating dosage. Transient decreases in the total white blood cell count to 2000 cells/mm^3 (following short courses) or more persistent reduction to 3000 cells/mm^3 (with continuing therapy) are tolerated without serious risk of infection if there is no marked granulocytopenia.

When CYTOXAN is included in combined cytotoxic regimens, it may be necessary to reduce the dose of CYTOXAN as well as that of the other drugs.

CYTOXAN and its metabolites are dialyzable although there are probably quantitative differences depending upon the dialysis system being used. Patients with compromised renal function may show some measurable changes in pharmacokinetic parameters of CYTOXAN metabolism, but there is no consistent evidence indicating a need for CYTOXAN dosage modification in patients with renal function impairment.

Treatment of Nonmalignant Diseases: Biopsy Proven "Minimal Change" Nephrotic Syndrome in Children—An oral dose of 2.5 to 3 mg/kg daily for a period of 60 to 90 days is recommended. In males, the incidence of oligospermia and azoospermia increases if the duration of Cytoxan treatment exceeds 60 days. Treatment beyond 90 days increases the probability of sterility. Adrenocorticosteroid therapy may be tapered and discontinued during the course of CYTOXAN therapy. See PRECAUTIONS section concerning hematologic monitoring.

Preparation and Handling of Solutions—Parenteral drug products should be inspected visually for particulate matter and discoloration prior to administration, whenever solution and container permit.

CYTOXAN for Injection and Lyophilized CYTOXAN for Injection should be prepared for parenteral use by adding Sterile Water for Injection, USP, to the vial and shaking to dissolve. Use the quantity of diluent shown below to reconstitute the product.

	Cytoxan for Injection	**Lyophilized Cytoxan for Injection**
Dosage Strength	Quantity of Diluent	Quantity of Diluent
100 mg	5 mL	5 mL
200 mg	10 mL	10 mL
500 mg	25 mL	20–25 mL
1 g	50 mL	50 mL
2 g	100 mL	80–100 mL

Solutions of CYTOXAN for Injection and Lyophilized CYTOXAN for Injection may be injected intravenously, intramuscularly, intraperitoneally, or intrapleurally or they may be infused intravenously in the following:

Dextrose Injection, USP (5% dextrose)
Dextrose and Sodium Chloride Injection, USP (5% dextrose and 0.9% sodium chloride)
5% Dextrose and Ringer's Injection
Lactated Ringer's Injection, USP
Sodium Chloride Injection, USP (0.45% sodium chloride)
Sodium Lactate Injection, USP (1/6 molar sodium lactate)

Reconstituted CYTOXAN for Injection and Lyophilized CYTOXAN for Injection are chemically and physically stable for 24 hours at room temperature or for 6 days in the refrigerator; it does not contain any antimicrobial preservative and thus care must be taken to assure the sterility of prepared solutions.

The osmolarities of solutions of CYTOXAN for Injection, Lyophilized CYTOXAN for Injection, and normal saline are compared in the following table:

Lyophilized CYTOXAN for Injection	mOsm/L
4 mL diluent per 100 mg cyclophosphamide	219
5 mL diluent per 100 mg cyclophosphamide	172
CYTOXAN for Injection	352
Normal saline	287

Lyophilized CYTOXAN for Injection is slightly hypotonic with respect to normal saline.

Extemporaneous liquid preparations of CYTOXAN for oral administration may be prepared by dissolving CYTOXAN for Injection or Lyophilized CYTOXAN for Injection in Aromatic Elixir, N.F. Such preparations should be stored under refrigeration in glass containers and used within 14 days.

HOW SUPPLIED

CYTOXAN for Injection contains 45 mg of sodium chloride per 100 mg of cyclophosphamide (anhydrous) and is supplied in vials for single dose use.

CYTOXAN for Injection (cyclophosphamide for injection, USP).

NDC 0015-0500-41 100 mg vials, carton of 12, case of 1 carton
NDC 0015-0501-41 200 mg vials, carton of 12, case of 1 carton
NDC 0015-0502-41 500 mg vials, carton of 12, case of 1 carton
NDC 0015-0505-41 1.0 g vials, carton of 6
NDC 0015-0506-41 2.0 g vials, carton of 6

Lyophilized CYTOXAN for Injection contains 75 mg mannitol per 100 mg cyclophosphamide (anhydrous) and is supplied in vials for single-dose use.

Lyophilized CYTOXAN for Injection (cyclophosphamide for injection, USP)
U.S. Patent No. 4,537,883

NDC 0015-0539-41 100 mg vials, carton of 12, case of 1 carton
NDC 0015-0546-41 200 mg vials, carton of 12, case of 1 carton
NDC 0015-0547-41 500 mg vials, carton of 12, case of 1 carton
NDC 0015-0548-41 1.0 g vials, carton of 6
NDC 0015-0549-41 2.0 g vials, carton of 6

CYTOXAN Tablets, 25 mg, and CYTOXAN Tablets, 50 mg, are white tablets with blue flecks containing 25 mg and 50 mg cyclophosphamide (anhydrous), respectively.

CYTOXAN Tablets (cyclophosphamide tablets, USP)
NDC 0015-0503-01 50 mg, bottles of 100
NDC 0015-0503-02 50 mg, bottles of 1000
NDC 0015-0503-03 50 mg, Unit Dose, cartons of 100
NDC 0015-0503-48 50 mg, Compliance Pack, cartons of 28
NDC 0015-0504-01 25 mg, bottles of 100

Storage at or below 77°F (25°C) is recommended; this product will withstand brief exposure to temperatures up to 86°F (30°C) but should be protected from temperatures above 86°F (30°C).

Procedures for proper handling and disposal of anticancer drugs should be considered. Several guidelines on this subject have been published.[1–7] There is no general agreement that all of the procedures recommended in the guidelines are necessary or appropriate.

REFERENCES

1. Recommendations for the Safe Handling of Parenteral Antineoplastic Drugs. NIH Publication No. 83-2621. For sale by the Superintendent of Documents, US Government Printing Office, Washington, DC 20402.
2. AMA Council Report, Guidelines for Handling Parenteral Antineoplastics, *JAMA*. 1985 March 15.
3. National Study Commission on Cytotoxic Exposure—Recommendations for Handling Cytotoxic Agents. Available from Louis P. Jeffrey, Sc.D., Chairman, National Study Commission on Cytotoxic Exposure, Massachusetts College of Pharmacy and Allied Health Sciences, 179 Longwood Avenue, Boston, Massachusetts 02115.
4. Clinical Oncological Society of Australia. Guidelines and Recommendations for Safe Handling of Antineoplastic Agents. *Med J Australia*. 1983; 1:426–428.
5. Jones RB, et al: Safe handling of chemotherapeutic agents: A report from the Mount Sinai Medical Center. *CA—A Cancer J for Clinicians*. 1983; (Sept/Oct) 258–263.
6. American Society of Hospital Pharmacists Technical Assistance Bulletin on Handling Cytotoxic and Hazardous Drugs. *Am J Hosp Pharm*. 1990; 47:1033–1049.
7. OSHA Work-Practice Guidelines for Personnel Dealing with Cytotoxic (Antineoplastic) Drugs. *Am J Hosp Pharm*. 1986; 43:1193–1204.

Shown in Product Identification Section, page 406

IFEX® ℞
[*i-fĕx*]
(sterile ifosfamide)

> **WARNING**
>
> IFEX should be administered under the supervision of a qualified physician experienced in the use of cancer chemotherapeutic agents. Urotoxic side effects, especially hemorrhagic cystitis, as well as CNS toxicities such as confusion and coma have been assoicated with the use of IFEX. When they occur, they may require cessation of IFEX therapy. Severe myelosuppression has been reported. (See "Adverse Reactions" section.)

DESCRIPTION

IFEX (sterile ifosfamide) single-dose vials for constitution and administration by intravenous infusion each contain 1 gram or 3 grams of sterile ifosfamide. Ifosfamide is a chemotherapeutic agent chemically related to the nitrogen mustards and a synthetic analog of cyclophosphamide. Ifosfamide is 3-(2-chloroethyl)-2-[(2-chloroethyl)amino]-tetrahydro-2H-1,3,2-oxazaphosphorine 2-oxide. The molecular formula is $C_7H_{15}Cl_2N_2O_2P$ and its molecular weight is 261.1. Its structural formula is:

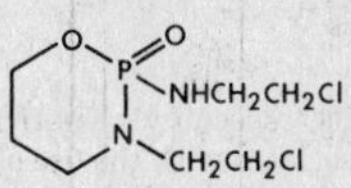

Ifosfamide is a white crystalline powder that is soluble in water.

CLINICAL PHARMACOLOGY

Ifosfamide has been shown to require metabolic activation by microsomal liver enzymes to produce biologically active metabolites. Activation occurs by hydroxylation at the ring carbon atom 4 to form the unstable intermediate 4-hydroxyifosfamide. This metabolite rapidly degrades to the stable urinary metabolite 4-ketoifosfamide. Opening of the ring results in formation of the stable urinary metabolite, 4-carboxyifosfamide. These urinary metabolites have not been

Continued on next page

Bristol-Myers Oncology—Cont.

found to be cytotoxic. N, N-*bis* (2-chloroethyl)-phosphoric acid diamide (ifosphoramide) and acrolein are also found. Enzymatic oxidation of the chloroethyl side chains and subsequent dealkylation produces the major urinary metabolites, dechloroethyl ifosfamide and dechloroethyl cyclophosphamide. The alkylated metabolites of ifosfamide have been shown to interact with DNA.
In vitro incubation of DNA with activated ifosfamide has produced phosphotriesters. The treatment of intact cell nuclei may also result in the formation of DNA-DNA cross-links. DNA repair most likely occurs in G-1 and G-2 stage cells.

Pharmacokinetics
Ifosfamide exhibits dose-dependent pharmacokinetics in humans. At single doses of 3.8–5.0 g/m^2, the plasma concentrations decay biphasically and the mean terminal elimination half-life is about 15 hours. At doses of 1.6–2.4 g/m^2/day, the plasma decay is monoexponential and the terminal elimination half-life is about 7 hours. Ifosfamide is extensively metabolized in humans and the metabolic pathways appear to be saturated at high doses.
After administration of doses of 5 g/m^2 of ^{14}C-labeled ifosfamide, from 70% to 86% of the dosed radioactivity was recovered in the urine, with about 61% of the dose excreted as parent compound. At doses of 1.6–2.4 g/m^2 only 12% to 18% of the dose was excreted in the urine as unchanged drug within 72 hours.
Two different dechloroethylated derivatives of ifosfamide, 4-carboxyifosfamide, thiodiacetic acid and cysteine conjugates of chloroacetic acid have been identified as the major urinary metabolites of ifosfamide in humans and only small amounts of 4-hydroxyifosfamide and acrolein are present. Small quantities (nmole/mL) of ifosfamide mustard and 4-hydroxyifosfamide are detectable in human plasma. Metabolism of ifosfamide is required for the generation of the biologically active species and while metabolism is extensive, it is also quite variable among patients.
In a study at Indiana University, 50 fully evaluable patients with germ cell testicular cancer were treated with IFEX in combination with cisplatin and either vinblastine or etoposide after failing (47 of 50 patients) at least two prior chemotherapy regimens consisting of cisplatin/vinblastine/bleomycin, (PVB), cisplatin/vinblastine/actinomycin D/bleomycin/cyclophosphamide, (VAB6), or the combination of cisplatin and etoposide. Patients were selected for remaining cisplatin sensitivity because they had previously responded to a cisplatin containing regimen and had not progressed while on the cisplatin containing regimen or within 3 weeks of stopping it. Patients served as their own control based on the premise that long term complete responses could not be achieved by retreatment with a regimen to which they had previously responded and subsequently relapsed.
Ten of 50 fully evaluable patients were still alive 2 to 5 years after treatment. Four of the 10 long term survivors were rendered free of cancer by surgical resection after treatment with the ifosfamide regimen; median survival for the entire group of 50 fully evaluable patients was 53 weeks.

INDICATION AND USAGE
IFEX, used in combination with certain other approved antineoplastic agents, is indicated for third line chemotherapy of germ cell testicular cancer. It should ordinarily be used in combination with a prophylactic agent for hemorrhagic cystitis, such as mesna.

CONTRAINDICATIONS
Continued use of IFEX is contraindicated in patients with severely depressed bone marrow function (See WARNINGS and PRECAUTIONS sections). IFEX is also contraindicated in patients who have demonstrated a previous hypersensitivity to it.

WARNINGS
Urinary System
Urotoxic side effects, especially hemorrhagic cystitis, have been frequently associated with the use of IFEX. It is recommended that a urinalysis should be obtained prior to each dose of IFEX. If microscopic hematuria (greater than 10 RBCs per high power field), is present, then subsequent administration should be withheld until complete resolution. Further administration of IFEX should be given with vigorous oral or parenteral hydration.

Hematopoietic System
When IFEX is given in combination with other chemotherapeutic agents, severe myelosuppression is frequently observed. Close hematologic monitoring is recommended. White blood cell (WBC) count, platelet count and hemoglobin should be obtained prior to each administration and at appropriate intervals. Unless clinically essential, IFEX should not be given to patients with a WBC count below 2000/μL and/or a platelet count below 50,000/μL.

Central Nervous System
Neurologic manifestations consisting of somnolence, confusion, hallucinations and in some instances, coma, have been reported following IFEX therapy. The occurrence of these symptoms requires discontinuing IFEX therapy. The symptoms have usually been reversible and supportive therapy should be maintained until their complete resolution.

Pregnancy
Animal studies indicate that the drug is capable of causing gene mutations and chromosomal damage *in vivo*. Embryotoxic and teratogenic effects have been observed in mice, rats and rabbits at doses 0.05–0.075 times the human dose. Ifosfamide can cause fetal damage when administered to a pregnant woman. If IFEX is used during pregnancy, or if the patient becomes pregnant while taking this drug, the patient should be apprised of the potential hazard to the fetus.

PRECAUTIONS
General
IFEX should be given cautiously to patients with impaired renal function as well as to those with compromised bone marrow reserve, as indicated by: leukopenia, granulocytopenia, extensive bone marrow metastases, prior radiation therapy, or prior therapy with other cytotoxic agents.

Laboratory Tests
During treatment, the patient's hematologic profile (particularly neutrophils and platelets) should be monitored regularly to determine the degree of hematopoietic suppression. Urine should also be examined regularly for red cells which may precede hemorrhagic cystitis.

Drug Interactions
The physician should be alert for possible combined drug actions, desirable or undesirable, involving ifosfamide even though ifosfamide has been used successfully concurrently with other drugs, including other cytotoxic drugs.

Wound Healing
Ifosfamide may interfere with normal wound healing.

Pregnancy
Pregnancy "Category D." See WARNINGS section.

Nursing Mothers
Ifosfamide is excreted in breast milk. Because of the potential for serious adverse events and the tumorigenicity shown for ifosfamide in animal studies, a decision should be made whether to discontinue nursing or to discontinue the drug, taking into account the importance of the drug to the mother.

Carcinogenesis, Mutagenesis, Impairment of Fertility
Ifosfamide has been shown to be carcinogenic in rats, with female rats showing a significant incidence of leiomyosarcomas and mammary fibroadenomas.
The mutagenic potential of ifosfamide has been documented in bacterial systems *in vitro* and mammalian cells *in vivo*. *In vivo,* ifosfamide has induced mutagenic effects in mice and *Drosophila melanogaster* germ cells, and has induced a significant increase in dominant lethal mutations in male mice as well as recessive sex-linked lethal mutations in Drosophila.
In pregnant mice, resorptions increased and anomalies were present at day 19 after 30 mg/m^2 dose of ifosfamide was administered on day 11 of gestation. Embryolethal effects were observed in rats following the administration of 54 mg/m^2 doses of ifosfamide from the 6th through the 15th day of gestation and embryotoxic effects were apparent after dams received 18 mg/m^2 doses over the same dosing period. Ifosfamide is embryotoxic to rabbits receiving 88 mg/m^2/day doses from the 6th through the 18th day after mating. The number of anomalies was also significantly increased over the control group.

Pediatric Use
Safety and effectiveness in children have not been established.

ADVERSE REACTIONS
In patients receiving IFEX as a single agent, the dose-limiting toxicities are myleosuppression and urotoxicity. Dose fractionation, vigorous hydration, and a protector such as mesna can significantly reduce the incidence of hematuria, especially gross hematuria, associated with hemorrhagic cystitis. At a dose of 1.2 g/m^2 daily for 5 consecutive days, leukopenia, when it occurs, is usually mild to moderate. Other significant side effects include alopecia, nausea, vomiting, and central nervous system toxicities.
[See table at top of next column.]

Adverse Reaction	*Incidence %
Alopecia	83
Nausea-Vomiting	58
Hematuria	46
Gross Hematuria	12
CNS Toxicity	12
Infection	8
Renal Impairment	6
Liver Dysfunction	3
Phlebitis	2
Fever	1
Allergic Reaction	<1
Anorexia	<1
Cardiotoxicity	<1
Coagulopathy	<1
Constipation	<1
Dermatitis	<1
Diarrhea	<1
Fatigue	<1
Hypertension	<1
Hypotension	<1
Malaise	<1
Polyneuropathy	<1
Pulmonary Symptoms	<1
Salivation	<1
Stomatitis	<1

*Based upon 2,070 patients from the published literature in 30 single agent studies.

Hematologic Toxicity
Myelosuppression was dose related and dose limiting. It consisted mainly of leukopenia and, to a lesser extent, thrombocytopenia. A WBC count <3000/μL is expected in 50% of the patients treated with IFEX single agent at doses of 1.2 g/m^2 per day for 5 consecutive days. At this dose level, thrombocytopenia (platelets < 100,000/μL) occurred in about 20% of the patients. At higher dosages, leukopenia was almost universal, and at total dosages of 10 to 12 g/m^2/cycle, one half of the patients had a WBC count below 1000/μL and 8% of patients had platelet counts less than 50,000/μL. Myelosuppression was usually reversible and treatment can be given every 3 to 4 weeks. When IFEX is used in combination with other myelosuppressive agents, adjustments in dosing may be necessary. Patients who experience severe myelosuppression are potentially at increased risk for infection.

Digestive System
Nausea and vomiting occurred in 58% of the patients who received IFEX. They were usually controlled by standard antiemetic therapy. Other gastrointestinal side effects include anorexia, diarrhea, and in some cases, constipation.

Urinary System
Urotoxicity consisted of hemorrhagic cystitis, dysuria, urinary frequency and other symptoms of bladder irritation. Hematuria occurred in 6% to 92% of patients treated with IFEX. The incidence and severity of hematuria can be significantly reduced by using vigorous hydration, a fractionated dose schedule and a protector such as mesna. At daily doses of 1.2 g/m^2 for 5 consecutive days without a protector, microscopic hematuria is expected in about one half of the patients and gross hematuria in about 8% of patients.
Renal toxicity occurred in 6% of the patients treated with ifosfamide as a single agent. Clinical signs, such as elevation in BUN or serum creatinine or decrease in creatinine clearance, were usually transient. They were most likely to be related to tubular damage. One episode of renal tubular acidosis which progressed into chronic renal failure was reported. Proteinuria and acidosis also occurred in rare instances. Metabolic acidosis was reported in 31% of patients in one study when IFEX was administered at doses of 2.0 to 2.5 g/m^2/day for 4 days. Renal tubular acidosis, Fanconi syndrome and renal rickets have been reported. Close clinical monitoring of serum and urine chemistries including phosphorus, potassium, alkaline phosphatase and other appropriate laboratory studies is recommended. Appropriate replacement therapy should be administered as indicated.

Central Nervous System
CNS side effects were observed in 12% of patients treated with IFEX. Those most commonly seen were somnolence, confusion, depressive psychosis, and hallucinations. Other less frequent symptoms include dizziness, disorientation, and cranial nerve dysfunction. Seizures and coma were occasionally reported. The incidence of CNS toxicity may be higher in patients with altered renal function.

Other
Alopecia occurred in approximately 83% of the patients treated with IFEX as a single agent. In combination, this incidence may be as high as 100%, depending on the other agents included in the chemotherapy regimen. Increases in liver enzymes and/or bilirubin were noted in 3% of the patients. Other less frequent side effects included phlebitis, pulmonary symptoms, fever of unknown origin, allergic reactions, stomatitis, cardiotoxicity, and polyneuropathy.

OVERDOSAGE
No specific antidote for IFEX is known. Management of overdosage would include general supportive measures to sustain the patient through any period of toxicity that might occur.

DOSAGE AND ADMINISTRATION
IFEX should be administered intravenously at a dose of 1.2 g/m^2 per day for 5 consecutive days. Treatment is repeated every 3 weeks or after recovery from hematologic toxicity (Platelets $\geq$ 100,000/μL, WBC $\geq$ 4,000/μL). In order to prevent bladder toxicity, IFEX should be given with extensive hydration consisting of at least two liters of oral or intravenous fluid per day. A protector, such as mesna, should also be used to prevent hemorrhagic cystitis. IFEX should be administered as a slow intravenous infusion lasting a minimum of

30 minutes. Although IFEX has been administered to a small number of patients with compromised hepatic and/or renal function, studies to establish optimal dose schedules of IFEX in such patients have not been conducted.

Preparation for Intravenous Administration/Stability

Injections are prepared for parenteral use by adding *Sterile Water for Injection USP, or Bacteriostatic Water for Injection USP* (benzyl alcohol or parabens preserved) to the vial and shaking to dissolve. Use the quantity of diluent shown below to reconstitute the product:

Dosage Strength	Quantity of Diluent	Final Concentration
1 gram	20 mL	50 mg/mL
3 grams	60 mL	50 mg/mL

Reconstituted solutions are chemically and physically stable for 1 week at 30°C or 3 weeks at 5°C.

Solutions of ifosfamide may be diluted further to achieve concentrations of 0.6 to 20 mg/mL in the following fluids:

5% Dextrose Injection, USP
0.9% Sodium Chloride Injection, USP
Lactated Ringer's Injection, USP
Sterile Water for Injection, USP

Such admixtures, when stored in large volume parenteral glass bottles, Viaflex bags, or PAB™ bags, are physically and chemically stable for at least 1 week at 30°C or 6 weeks at 5°C.

Because essentially identical stability results were obtained for Sterile Water admixtures as for the other admixtures (5% Dextrose Injection, 0.9% Sodium Chloride Injection, and Lactated Ringer's Injection), the use of large volume parenteral glass bottles, Viaflex bags or PAB™ bags that contain intermediate concentrations or mixtures of excipients (eg, 2.5% Dextrose Injection, 0.45% Sodium Chloride Injection, or 5% Dextrose and 0.9% Sodium Chloride Injection) is also acceptable.

The microbiological qualities of the constituted products or prepared admixtures should be considered, particularly where unpreserved vehicles are used.

Dilutions of IFEX not prepared by constitution with Bacteriostatic Water for Injection, USP (benzyl alcohol or parabens preserved), should be refrigerated and used within 6 hours.

Parenteral drug products should be inspected visually for particulate matter and discoloration prior to administration.

HOW SUPPLIED

IFEX (sterile ifosfamide) is only available in a combination package with the uroprotective agent Mesnex (mesna) injection.

IFEX (sterile ifosfamide)/Mesnex® (mesna) injection.

NDC 0015-3558-41 —5 × 1-gram Single Dose Vial of Ifex
—15 × 200-mg Single Dose Ampule of Mesnex

NDC 0015-3559-41 —2 × 3-gram Single Dose Vial of Ifex
—9 × 400-mg Single Dose Ampule of Mesnex

The dry powder may be stored at room temperature. Storage above 104°F (40°C) should be avoided.

Procedures for proper handling and disposal of anticancer drugs should be considered. Skin reactions associated with accidental exposure to IFEX may occur. The use of gloves is recommended. If IFEX solution contacts the skin or mucosa, immediately wash the skin thoroughly with soap and water or rinse the mucosa with copious amounts of water. Several guidelines on this subject have been published.[1–7] There is no general agreement that all of the procedures recommended in the guidelines are necessary or appropriate.

REFERENCES

1. Recommendations for the Safe Handling of Parenteral Antineoplastic Drugs. NIH Publication No. 83-2621. For sale by the Superintendent of Documents, U.S. Government Printing Office, Washington, DC 20402.
2. AMA Council Report, Guidelines for Handling Parenteral Antineoplastics, *JAMA.* 1985; March 15.
3. National Study Commission on Cytotoxic Exposure—Recommendations for Handling Cytotoxic Agents. Available from Louis P. Jeffrey, Sc.D., Chairman, National Study Commission on Cytotoxic Exposure, Massachusetts College of Pharmacy and Allied Health Sciences, 179 Longwood Avenue, Boston Massachusetts 02115.
4. Clinical Oncological Society of Australia: Guidelines and Recommendations for Safe Handling of Antineoplastic Agents. *Med J Australia.* 1983; 1:426–428.
5. Jones, RB, *et al:* Safe Handling of Chemotherapuetic Agents: A Report from the Mount Sinai Medical Center, *CA-A Cancer J for Clinicians.* 1983; Sept/Oct. 258–263.
6. American Society of Hospital Pharmacists Technical Assistance Bulletin on Handling Cytotoxic and Hazardous Drugs. *Am J Hosp Pharm.* 1990; 47:1033–1049.
7. OSHA Work-Practice Guidelines for Personnel Dealing with Cytotoxic (Antineoplastic) Drugs. *Am J Hosp Pharm.* 1986; 43:1193–1204.

U.S. Patent No. 3,732,340

Shown in Product Identification Section, page 406

LYSODREN® ℞

[*li 'sō-drĕn "*]
(mitotane tablets, USP)

> **WARNINGS**
>
> Lysodren (mitotane) should be administered under the supervision of a qualified physician experienced in the uses of cancer chemotherapeutic agents. Lysodren should be temporarily discontinued immediately following shock or severe trauma since adrenal suppression is its prime action. Exogenous steroids should be administered in such circumstances, since the depressed adrenal may not immediately start to secrete steroids.

DESCRIPTION

Lysodren (mitotane) is an oral chemotherapeutic agent. It is best known by its trivial name, o,p'-DDD, and is chemically, 1,1-dichloro-2-(o-chlorophenyl) -2- (p-chlorophenyl) ethane. The chemical structure is shown below.

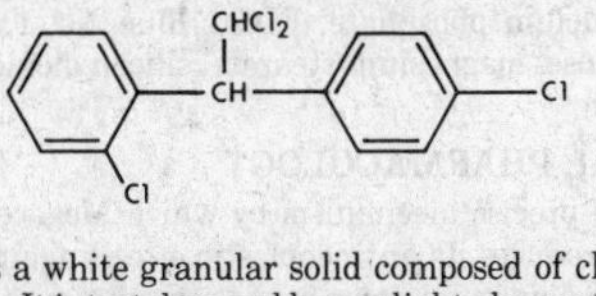

Lysodren is a white granular solid composed of clear colorless crystals. It is tasteless and has a slight pleasant aromatic odor. It is soluble in ethanol, isoctane and carbon tetrachloride. It has a molecular weight of 320.05.

Inactive ingredients in Lysodren tablets are: avicel, polyethylene glycol 3350, silicon dioxide, and starch.

Lysodren is available as 500 mg scored tablets for oral administration.

CLINICAL PHARMACOLOGY

Lysodren can best be described as an adrenal cytotoxic agent, although it can cause adrenal inhibition, apparently without cellular destruction. Its biochemical mechanism of action is unknown. Data are available to suggest that the drug modifies the peripheral metabolism of steroids as well as directly suppressing the adrenal cortex. The administration of Lysodren alters the extra-adrenal metabolism of cortisol in man, leading to a reduction in measurable 17-hydroxy corticosteroids, even though plasma levels of corticosteroids do not fall. The drug apparently causes increased formation of 6-β-hydroxyl cortisol.

Data in adrenal carcinoma patients indicate that about 40% of oral Lysodren is absorbed and approximately 10% of administered dose is recovered in the urine as a water-soluble metabolite. A variable amount of metabolite (1 to 17%) is excreted in the bile and the balance is apparently stored in the tissues.

Following discontinuation of Lysodren, the plasma terminal half life has ranged from 18 to 159 days. In most patients blood levels become undetectable after 6 to 9 weeks. Autopsy data have provided evidence that Lysodren is found in most tissues of the body; however, fat tissues are the primary site of storage. Lysodren is converted to a water-soluble metabolite.

No unchanged Lysodren has been found in urine or bile.

INDICATIONS AND USAGE

Lysodren is indicated in the treatment of inoperable adrenal cortical carcinoma of both functional and nonfunctional types.

CONTRAINDICATIONS

Lysodren should not be given to individuals who have demonstrated a previous hypersensitivity to it.

WARNINGS

Lysodren should be temporarily discontinued immediately following shock or severe trauma, since adrenal suppression is its prime action. Exogenous steroids should be administered in such circumstances, since the depressed adrenal may not immediately start to secrete steroids.

Lysodren should be administered with care to patients with liver disease other than metastatic lesions from the adrenal cortex, since the metabolism of Lysodren may be interfered with and the drug may accumulate.

All possible tumor tissues should be surgically removed from large metastatic masses before Lysodren administration is instituted. This is necessary to minimize the possibility of infarction and hemorrhage in the tumor due to a rapid cytotoxic effect of the drug.

Long-term continuous administration of high doses of Lysodren may lead to brain damage and impairment of function. Behavioral and neurological assessments should be made at regular intervals when continuous Lysodren treatment exceeds 2 years.

A substantial percentage of the patients treated show signs of adrenal insufficiency. It therefore appears necessary to watch for and institute steroid replacement in those patients. However, some investigators have recommended that steroid replacement therapy be administered concomitantly with Lysodren. It has been shown that the metabolism of exogenous steroids is modified and consequently somewhat higher doses than normal replacement therapy may be required.

PRECAUTIONS

General: Adrenal insufficiency may develop in patients treated with Lysodren, and adrenal steroid replacement should be considered for these patients.

Since sedation, lethargy, vertigo, and other CNS side effects can occur, ambulatory patients should be cautioned about driving, operating machinery, and other hazardous pursuits requiring mental and physical alertness.

Drug Interactions: Lysodren has been reported to accelerate the metabolism of warfarin by the mechanism of hepatic microsomal enzyme induction, leading to an increase in dosage requirements for warfarin. Therefore, physicians should closely monitor patients for a change in anticoagulant dosage requirements when administering Lysodren to patients on coumarin-type anticoagulants. In addition, Lysodren should be given with caution to patients receiving other drugs susceptible to the influence of hepatic enzyme induction.

Carcinogenesis, Mutagenesis, Impairment of Fertility: The carcinogenic and mutagenic potentials of Lysodren are unknown. However, the mechanism of action of this compound suggests that it probably has less carcinogenic potential than other cytotoxic chemotherapeutic drugs.

Pregnancy: Pregnancy "Category C." Animal reproduction studies have not been conducted with Lysodren. It is also not known whether Lysodren can cause fetal harm when administered to a pregnant woman or can affect reproduction capacity. Lysodren should be given to a pregnant woman only if clearly needed.

Nursing Mothers: It is not known whether this drug is excreted in human milk. Because many drugs are excreted in human milk and because of the potential for adverse reactions in nursing infants from mitotane, a decision should be made whether to discontinue nursing or to discontinue the drug, taking into account the importance of the drug to the mother.

ADVERSE REACTIONS

A very high percentage of patients treated with Lysodren has shown at least one type of side effect. The main types of adverse reactions consist of the following:

1. Gastrointestinal disturbances, which consist of anorexia, nausea or vomiting, and in some cases diarrhea, occur in about 80% of the patients.
2. Central nervous system side effects occur in 40% of the patients. These consist primarily of depression as manifested by lethargy and somnolence (25%), and dizziness or vertigo (15%).
3. Skin toxicity has been observed in about 15% of the cases. These skin changes consist primarily of transient skin rashes which do not seem to be dose related. In some instances, this side effect subsided while the patients were maintained on the drug without a change of dose.

Infrequently occurring side effects involve the eye (visual blurring, diplopia, lens opacity, toxic retinopathy); the genitourinary system (hematuria, hemorrhagic cystitis, and albuminuria); cardiovascular system (hypertension, orthostatic hypotension, and flushing); and some miscellaneous effects including generalized aching, hyperpyrexia, and lowered protein bound iodine (PBI).

OVERDOSAGE

No proven antidotes have been established for Lysodren overdosage.

DOSAGE AND ADMINISTRATION

The recommended treatment schedule is to start the patient at 2 to 6 g of Lysodren per day in divided doses, either three or four times a day. Doses are usually increased incrementally to 9 to 10 g per day. If severe side effects appear, the dose should be reduced until the maximum tolerated dose is achieved. If the patient can tolerate higher doses and improved clinical response appears possible, the dose should be increased until adverse reactions interfere. Experience has shown that the maximum tolerated dose (MTD) will vary from 2 to 16 g per day, but has usually been 9 to 10 g per day. The highest doses used in the studies to date were 18 to 19 g per day.

Treatment should be instituted in the hospital until a stable dosage regimen is achieved.

Treatment should be continued as long as clinical benefits are observed. Maintenance of clinical status or slowing of growth of metastatic lesions can be considered clinical benefits if they can clearly be shown to have occurred.

If no clinical benefits are observed after 3 months at the maximum tolerated dose, the case would generally be considered a clinical failure. However, 10% of the patients who showed a measurable response required more than 3 months at the

Continued on next page

Bristol-Myers Oncology—Cont.

MTD. Early diagnosis and prompt institution of treatment improve the probability of a positive clinical response. Clinical effectiveness can be shown by reduction in tumor mass; reduction in pain, weakness or anorexia; and reduction of symptoms and signs due to excessive steroid production.
A number of patients have been treated intermittently with treatment being restarted when severe symptoms have reappeared. Patients often do not respond after the third or fourth such course. Experience accumulated to date suggests that continuous treatment with the maximum possible dosage of Lysodren is the best approach.
Procedures for proper handling and disposal of anticancer drugs should be considered. Several guidelines on this subject have been published.[1–7] There is no general agreement that all of the procedures recommended in the guidelines are necessary or appropriate.

REFERENCES

1. Recommendations for the Safe Handling of Parenteral Antineoplastic Drugs. NIH Publication No. 83-2621. For sale by the Superintendent of Documents, U.S. Government Printing Office, Washington, D.C. 20402.
2. AMA Council Report. Guidelines for Handling Parenteral Antineoplastics. *JAMA.* 1985; March 15.
3. National Study Commission on Cytotoxic Exposure—Recommendations for Handling Cytotoxic Agents. Available from Louis P. Jeffrey, Sc.D., Chairman, National Study Commission on Cytotoxic Exposure, Massachusetts College of Pharmacy and Allied Health Sciences, 179 Longwood Avenue, Boston, Massachusetts 02115.
4. Clinical Oncological Society of Australia: Guidelines and Recommendations for Safe Handling of Antineoplastic Agents. *Med J Australia.* 1983; 1:426–428.
5. Jones, R. B., et. al. Safe Handling of Chemotherapeutic Agents: A Report from the Mount Sinai Medical Center, *CA—A Cancer J for Clinicians.* 1983; Sept./Oct., 258–263.
6. American Society of Hospital Pharmacists Technical Assistance Bulletin on Handling Cytotoxic Drugs in Hospitals. *Am J Hosp Pharm.* 1985; 42:131–137.
7. OSHA Work-Practice Guidelines for Personnel Dealing with Cytotoxic (Antineoplastic) Drugs. *Am J Hosp Pharm.* 1986; 43:1193–1204.

HOW SUPPLIED

Lysodren (mitotane) Tablets, USP
NDC 0015-3080-60—500 mg Tablets, bottle of 100
Tablets may be stored at room temperature.

MEGACE® ℞

[*měg'ace*]
(megestrol acetate tablets, USP)

> **WARNING**
> **The Use of MEGACE During the First 4 Months of Pregnancy is Not Recommended**
> Progestational agents have been used beginning with the first trimester of pregnancy in an attempt to prevent habitual abortion. There is no adequate evidence that such use is effective when such drugs are given during the first 4 months of pregnancy. Furthermore, in the vast majority of women, the cause of abortion is a defective ovum, which progestational agents could not be expected to influence. In addition, the use of progestational agents, with their uterine-relaxant properties, in patients with fertilized defective ova may cause a delay in spontaneous abortion. Therefore, the use of such drugs during the first 4 months of pregnancy is not recommended.
> Several reports suggest an association between intrauterine exposure to progestational drugs in the first trimester of pregnancy and genital abnormalities in male and female fetuses. The risk of hypospadias, 5 to 8 per 1,000 male births in the general population, may be approximately doubled with exposure to these drugs. There are insufficient data to quantify the risk to exposed female fetuses, but insofar as some of these drugs induce mild virilization of the external genitalia of the female fetus, and because of the increased association of hypospadias in the male fetus, it is prudent to avoid the use of these drugs during the first trimester of pregnancy.
> If the patient is exposed to Megace during the first 4 months of pregnancy or if she becomes pregnant while taking this drug, she should be apprised of the potential risks to the fetus.

DESCRIPTION

Megace, megestrol acetate, is a synthetic, antineoplastic and progestational drug. Megestrol acetate is a white, crystalline solid chemically designated as 17α-acetyloxy-6-methylpregna-4, 6-diene-3, 20-dione. Solubility at 37°C in water is 2 mcg per mL, solubility in plasma is 24 mcg per mL. Its molecular weight is 384.51. The empirical formula is $C_{24}H_{32}O_4$ and the structural formula is represented as follows:

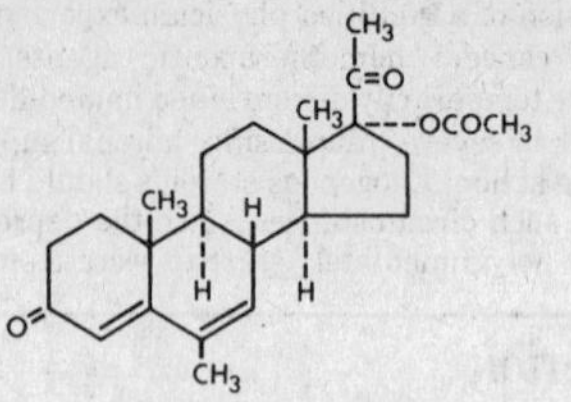

Megace is supplied for oral administration containing 20 mg and 40 mg megestrol acetate.
Megace Tablets contain the following inactive ingredients: acacia, calcium phosphate, FD&C Blue No. 1, Aluminum Lake, lactose, magnesium stearate, silicon dioxide colloidal, and starch.

CLINICAL PHARMACOLOGY

While the precise mechanism by which Megace (megestrol acetate) produces its antineoplastic effects against endometrial carcinoma is unknown at the present time, inhibition of pituitary gonadotropin production and resultant decrease in estrogen secretions may be factors. There is evidence to suggest a local effect as a result of the marked changes brought about by the direct instillation of progestational agents into the endometrial cavity. The antineoplastic action of megestrol acetate on carcinoma of the breast is effected by modifying the action of other steroid hormones and by exerting a direct cytotoxic effect on tumor cells.[1] In metastatic cancer, hormone receptors may be present in some tissues but not others. The receptor mechanism is a cyclic process whereby estrogen produced by the ovaries enters the target cell, forms a complex with cytoplasmic receptor and is transported into the cell nucleus. There it induces gene transcription and leads to the alteration of normal cell functions. Pharmacologic doses of megestrol acetate not only decrease the number of hormone-dependent human breast cancer cells but also is capable of modifying and abolishing the stimulatory effects of estrogen on these cells. It has been suggested[2] that progestins may inhibit in one of two ways: by interfering with either the stability, availability, or turnover of the estrogen receptor complex in its interaction with genes or in conjunction with the progestin receptor complex, by interacting directly with the genome to turn off specific estrogen-responsive genes.
There are several analytical methods used to estimate Megace plasma levels, including mass fragmentography, gas chromatography (GC), high pressure liquid chromatography (HPLC) and radioimmunoassay. The plasma levels by HPLC assay or radioimmunoassay methods are about one-sixth those obtained by the GC method. The plasma levels are dependent not only on the method used, but also on intestinal and hepatic inactivation of the drug, which may be affected by factors such as intestinal tract motility, intestinal bacteria, antibiotics administered, body weight, diet, and liver function.[3,4]
Metabolites account for only 5% to 8% of the administered dose and are considered negligible.[5] The major route of drug elimination in humans is the urine. When radiolabeled megestrol acetate was administered to humans in doses of 4 to 90 mg, the the urinary excretion within 10 days ranged from 56.5% to 78.4% (mean 66.4%) and fecal excretion ranged from 7.7% to 30.3% (mean 19.8%). The total recovered radioactivity varied between 83.1% and 94.7% (mean 86.2%). Respiratory excretion as labeled carbon dioxide and fat storage may have accounted for at least part of the radioactivity not found in the urine and feces.
In normal male volunteers (N-23) who received 160 mg of megestrol acetate given as a 40 mg qid regimen, the oral absorption of Megace appeared to be variable. Plasma levels were assayed by a high pressure liquid chromatographic (HPLC) procedure. Peak drug levels for the first 40 mg dose ranged from 10 to 56 ng/mL (mean 27.6 ng/mL) and the times to peak concentrations ranged from 1.0 to 3.0 hours (mean 2.2 hours). Plasma elimination half-life ranged from 13.0 to 104.9 hours (mean 34.2 hours). The steady state plasma concentrations for a 40 mg qid regimen have not been established.

INDICATIONS AND USAGE

Megace (megestrol acetate) is indicated for the palliative treatment of advanced carcinoma of the breast or endometrium (ie, recurrent, inoperable, or metastatic disease). It should not be used in lieu of currently accepted procedures such as surgery, radiation, or chemotherapy.

CONTRAINDICATIONS

As a diagnostic test for pregnancy.

WARNINGS

Megestrol acetate may cause fetal harm when administered to a pregnant woman. Fertility and reproduction studies with high doses of megestrol acetate have shown a reversible feminizing effect on some male rat fetuses.[6] There are not adequate and well-controlled studies in pregnant women. If this drug is used during pregnancy, or if the patient becomes pregnant while taking (receiving) this drug, the patient should be apprised of the potential hazard to the fetus. Women of childbearing potential should be advised to avoid becoming pregnant.
The use of Megace® (megestrol acetate) in other types of neoplastic disease is not recommended.
See also "Carcinogenesis, Mutagenesis, and Impairment of Fertility" section.

PRECAUTIONS

General:
Close surveillance is indicated for any patient treated for recurrent or metastatic cancer. Use with caution in patients with a history of thrombophlebitis.
Information for the Patients:
Patients using megestrol acetate should receive the following instructions.
1. This medication is to be used as directed by the physician.
2. Report any adverse reaction experiences while taking this medication.

Laboratory Tests:
Breast malignancies in which estrogen and/or progesterone receptors are positive are more likely to respond to Megace.[7,8,9]
Carcinogenesis, Mutagenesis, and Impairment of Fertility:
Administration for up to 7 years of megestrol acetate to female dogs is associated with an increased incidence of both benign and malignant tumors of the breast.[10] Comparable studies in rats and studies in monkeys are not associated with an increased incidence of tumors. The relationship of the dog tumors to humans is unknown but should be considered in assessing the benefit-to-risk ratio when prescribing Megace and in surveillance of patients on therapy.[10,11] Also see "WARNINGS" section.
Pregnancy:
Pregnancy Category D. See "WARNINGS" section.
Nursing Mothers:
Because of the potential for adverse effects on the newborn, nursing should be discontinued if Megace is required for treatment of cancer.
Pediatric Use:
Safety and effectiveness in children have not been established.

ADVERSE REACTIONS

Weight Gain:
Weight gain is a frequent side effect of Megace.[12,13] This gain has been associated with increased appetite and is not necessarily associated with fluid retention.
Thromboembolic Phenomena:
Thromboembolic phenomena including thrombophlebitis and pulmonary embolism have been rarely reported.
Other Adverse Reactions:
Nausea and vomiting, edema, breakthrough bleeding, dyspnea, tumor flare (with or without hypercalcemia), hyperglycemia, alopecia, hypertension, carpal tunnel syndrome, and rash.

OVERDOSAGE

No serious side effects have resulted from studies involving Megace (megestrol acetate) administered in dosages as high as 1600 mg/day. Oral administration of large, single doses of megestrol acetate (5 g/kg) did not produce toxic effects in mice.[6] Megestrol acetate has not been tested for dialyzability; however, due to its low solubility it is postulated that this would not be an effective means of treating overdose.

DOSAGE AND ADMINISTRATION

Breast cancer: 160 mg/day (40 mg qid)
Endometrial carcinoma: 40 to 320 mg/day in divided doses.
At least 2 months of continuous treatment is considered an adequate period for determining the efficacy of Megace (megestrol acetate).

HOW SUPPLIED

Megace® (megestrol acetate) is available as light blue, scored tablets containing 20 mg or 40 mg megestrol acetate.

NDC 0015-0595-01, 20 mg tablet	Bottles of 100
NDC 0015-0596-41, 40 mg tablet	Bottles of 100
NDC 0015-0596-45, 40 mg tablet	Bottles of 500
NDC 0015-0596-46 40 mg tablet	Bottles of 250

STORAGE

Store Megace at room temperature; protect from temperatures above 40°C (104°F).

SPECIAL HANDLING

Health Hazard Data

There is no threshold limit value established by OSHA, NIOSH, or ACGIH.

Exposure or "overdose" at levels approaching recommended dosing levels could result in side effects described above (WARNINGS, ADVERSE REACTIONS). Women at risk of pregnancy should avoid such exposure.

REFERENCES

1. Allegra JC, Kiefer SM. Mechanisms of Action of Progrestational Agents. *Semin Oncol.* 1985; 12(Suppl 1):3.
2. DeSombre ER, Kuivanen PC. Progestin Modulation of Estrogen-Dependent Marker Protein Synthesis in the Endometrium. *Semin Oncol.* 1985; 12(Suppl 1):6.
3. Alexieva-Figusch J, Blankenstein MA, Hop WCJ, et al. Treatment of Metastatic Breast Cancer Patients with Different Dosages of Megestrol Acetate: Dose Relations, Metabolic and Endocrine Effects. *Eur J Cancer Clin Oncol.* 1984; 20:33–40.
4. Gaver RC, Movahhed HS, Farmen RH, Pittman KA. Liquid Chromatographic Procedure for the Quantitative Analysis of Megestrol Acetate in Human Plasma. *J Pharm Sci.* 1985; 74:664.
5. Cooper JM, Kellie AE. The Metabolism of Megestrol Acetate (17-alpha-acetoxy-6-methylprega-4,6-diene-3,20-dione) in Women. *Steroids.* 1968;11:133.
6. David A, Edwards K, Fellowes KP, Plummer JM. Anti-Ovulatory and Other Biological Properties of Megestrol Acetate. *J Reprod Fertil.* 1963;5:331.
7. McGuire WL, Clark GM. The Prognostic Role of Progesterone Receptors in Human Breast Cancer. *Semin Oncol.* 1983;10(Suppl 4):2.
8. Horwitz KB. The Central Role of Progesterone Receptors and Progestational Agents in the Management and Treatment of Breast Cancer. *Semin Oncol.* 1988;15(Suppl 1):14.
9. Bonomi P, Johnson P, Anderson K, Wolter J, Bunting N, Strauss A, Roseman D, Shorey W, Econonou S. Primary Hormonal Therapy of Advanced Breast Cancer with Megestrol Acetate: Predictive Value of Estrogen Receptor and Progesterone Receptor Levels. *Semin Oncol.* 1985;12(1 Suppl 1):48–54.
10. Nelson LW, Weikel JH Jr., Reno FE. Mammary Nodules in Dogs during Four Years' Treatment with Megetrol Acetate or Chlormadionone Acetate. *J Natl Cancer Inst.* 1973;51:1303.
11. Owen LN, Briggs MH. Contraceptive Steroid Toxicology in the Beagle Dog and its Relevance to Human Carcinogenicity. *Curr Med Res Opin.* 1976;4:309.
12. Ansfield FJ, Kallas GJ, Singson JP. Clinical Results with Megestrol Acetate in Patients with Advanced Carcinoma of the Breast. *Surg Gynecol Obstet.* 1982;155:888.
13. Alexieva-Figusch J, van Gilse HA, Hop WCJ, et al. Progestin Therapy in Advanced Breast Cancer: Megestrol Acetate—An Evaluation of 160 Treated Cases. *Cancer.* 1980;46:2369.

Shown in Product Identification Section, page 406

MESNEX®   ℞
[mĕs-nĕx]
(Mesna) Injection

DESCRIPTION

Mesnex Injection is a detoxifying agent to inhibit the hemorrhagic cystitis induced by ifosfamide (Ifex®). The active ingredient mesna is a synthetic sulfhydryl compound designated as sodium 2-mercaptoethanesulfonate with a molecular formula of $C_2H_5NaO_3S_2$ and a molecular weight of 164.18. Its structural formula is as follows:

$$HS-CH_2-CH_2SO_3-Na^+$$

Mesnex Injection is a sterile preservative-free aqueous solution of clear and colorless appearance in clear glass ampules for intravenous administration. Mesnex Injection contains 100 mg/mL mesna, 0.25 mg/mL edetate disodium and sodium hydroxide for pH adjustment. The solution has a pH range of 6.5–8.5.

CLINICAL PHARMACOLOGY

Mesnex was developed as a prophylactic agent to prevent the hemorrhagic cystitis induced by ifosfamide.

Analogous to the physiological cysteine-cystine system, following intravenous administration, mesna is rapidly oxidized to its only metabolite, mesna disulfide (dimesna). Mesna disulfide remains in the intravascular compartment and is rapidly eliminated by the kidneys.

In the kidney, the mesna disulfide is reduced to the free thiol compound, mesna, which reacts chemically with the urotoxic ifosfamide metabolites (acrolein and 4-hydroxy-ifosfamide) resulting in their detoxification. The first step in the detoxification process is the binding of mesna to 4-hydroxy-ifosfamide forming a nonurotoxic 4-sulfoethylthioifosfamide.

Mesna also binds to the double bonds of acrolein and other urotoxic metabolites.

After administration of an 800 mg dose the half-lives of mesna and dimesna in the blood are 0.36 hours and 1.17 hours, respectively. Approximately 32% and 33% of the administered dose was eliminated in the urine in 24 hours as mesna and dimesna, respectively. The majority of the dose recovered was eliminated within 4 hours. Mesna has a volume of distribution of 0.652 L/kg and a plasma clearance of 1.23 L/kg/hour.

Ifosfamide has been shown to have dose-dependent pharmacokinetics in humans. At doses of 2–4 g, its terminal elimination half-life is about 7 hours. As a result, in order to maintain adequate levels of mesna in the urinary bladder during the course of elimination of the urotoxic ifosfamide metabolites, repeated doses of Mesnex are required.

Based on the pharmacokinetic profiles of mesna and ifosfamide as discussed above, Mesnex was given as bolus doses prior to ifosfamide and at 4 and 8 hours after ifosfamide administration. The hemorrhagic cystitis produced by ifosfamide is dose dependent. At a dose of 1.2 g/m² ifosfamide administered daily for 5 days, 16% to 26% of the patients who received conventional uroprophylaxis (high fluid intake, alkalinization of the urine and the administration of diuretics) developed hematuria (> 50 rbc/hpf or macrohematuria). In contrast none of the patients who received Mesnex together with this dose of ifosfamide developed hematuria. Higher doses of ifosfamide from 2 to 4 g/m² administered for 3 to 5 days, produced hematuria in 31% to 100% of the patients. When Mesnex was administered together with these doses of ifosfamide the incidence of hematuria was less than 7%.

INDICATIONS AND USAGE

Mesnex has been shown to be effective as a prophylactic agent in reducing the incidence of ifosfamide-induced hemorrhagic cystitis.

CONTRAINDICATIONS

Mesnex is contraindicated in patients known to be hypersensitive to mesna or other thiol compounds.

WARNINGS

Mesnex has been developed as an agent to prevent ifosfamide-induced hemorrhagic cystitis. It will not prevent or alleviate any of the other adverse reactions or toxicities associated with ifosfamide therapy.

Mesnex does not prevent hemorrhagic cystitis in all patients. Up to 6% of patients treated with mesna have developed hematuria (> 50 rbc/hpf or WHO grade 2 and above). As a result, a morning specimen of urine should be examined for the presence of hematuria (red blood cells) each day prior to ifosfamide therapy. If hematuria develops when Mesnex is given with ifosfamide according to the recommended dosage schedule, depending on the severity of the hematuria, dosage reductions or discontinuation of ifosfamide therapy may be initiated.

In order to obtain adequate protection, Mesnex must be administered with each dose of ifosfamide as outlined in the Dosage and Administration section. Mesnex is not effective in preventing hematuria due to other pathological conditions such as thrombocytopenia.

PRECAUTIONS

Laboratory Tests

A false positive test for urinary ketones may arise in patients treated with Mesnex. In this test, a red-violet color develops which, with the addition of glacial acetic acid, will return to violet.

Drug Interactions

In vitro and *in vivo* animal tumor models have shown that mesna does not have any effect on the antitumor efficacy of concomitantly administered cytotoxic agents.

Carcinogenesis, Mutagenesis and Impairment of Fertility

No long term animal studies have been performed to evaluate the carcinogenic potential of mesna. The Ames **Salmonella typhimurium** test, mouse micronucleus assay and frequency of sister chromatid exchange and chromosomal aberrations in PHA-stimulated lymphocytes *in vitro* assays revealed no mutagenic activity.

Pregnancy

Pregnancy Category B. Reproduction studies in rats and rabbits with oral doses up to 1000 mg/kg have revealed no harm to the fetus due to mesna. It is not known whether Mesnex can cause fetal harm when administered to a pregnant woman or can affect reproductive capacity. Mesnex should be given to a pregnant woman only if the benefits clearly outweigh any possible risks.

Teratology studies in rats and rabbits have shown no effects.

Nursing Mothers

It is not known whether mesna or dimesna is excreted in human milk. Because many drugs are excreted in human milk and because of the potential for adverse reactions in nursing infants, a decision should be made whether to discontinue nursing or discontinue the drug, taking into account the importance of the drug to the mother.

ADVERSE REACTIONS

Because Mesnex is used in combination with ifosfamide and other chemotherapeutic agents with documented toxicities, it is difficult to distinguish the adverse reactions which may be due to Mesnex from those caused by the concomitantly administered cytostatic agents. As a result, the adverse reaction profile of Mesnex was determined in three Phase I studies (16 subjects) utilizing intravenous and oral administration and two controlled studies in which ifosfamide and Mesnex were compared to ifosfamide and standard prophylaxis.

In Phase I studies in which IV bolus doses of 0.8 to 1.6 g/m² Mesnex were administered as single or three repeated doses to a total of 10 patients, a bad taste in the mouth (100%) and soft stools (70%) were reported. At intravenous and oral bolus doses of 2.4 g/m² which are approximately 10 times the recommended clinical doses (0.24 g/m²) headache (50%), fatigue (33%), nausea (33%), diarrhea (83%), limb pain (50%), hypotension (17%), and allergy (17%) have also been reported in the 6 patients who participated in this study.

In controlled clinical studies, adverse reactions which can be reasonably associated with Mesnex were vomiting, diarrhea and nausea.

OVERDOSAGE

There is no known antidote for Mesnex.

DOSAGE AND ADMINISTRATION

For the prophylaxis of ifosfamide-induced hemorrhagic cystitis, Mesnex may be given on a fractionated dosing schedule of bolus intravenous injections as outlined below.

Mesnex is given as intravenous bolus injections in a dosage equal to 20% of the ifosfamide dosage (w/w) at the time of ifosfamide administration and 4 and 8 hours after each dose of ifosfamide. The total daily dose of Mesnex is 60% of the ifosfamide dose.

The recommended dosing schedule is outlined below:

	0 Hours	4 Hours	8 Hours
Ifosfamide	1.2 g/m²	—	—
Mesnex	240 mg/m²	240 mg/m²	240 mg/m²

In order to maintain adequate protection, this dosing schedule should be repeated on each day that ifosfamide is administered. When the dosage of ifosfamide is adjusted (either increased or decreased), the dose of Mesnex should be modified accordingly. When exposed to oxygen, mesna is oxidized to the disulfide, dimesna. As a result, any unused drug remaining in the ampules after dosing should be discarded and new ampules used for each administration.

Preparation of Intravenous Solutions/Stability

For IV administration the drug can be diluted by adding the contents of a Mesnex ampule to any of the following fluids obtaining final concentrations of 20 mg mesna/mL fluid:

5% Dextrose Injection, USP
5% Dextrose and Sodium Chloride Injection, USP
0.9% Sodium Chloride Injection, USP
Lactated Ringer's Injection, USP

For example:

One ampule of Mesnex Injection 200 mg/2 mL may be added to 8 mL, or one ampule of Mesnex Injection 400 mg/4 mL may be added to 16 mL of any of the solutions listed above to create a final concentration of 20 mg mesna/mL fluid.

Diluted solutions are chemically and physically stable for 24 hours at 25°C (77°F).

It is recommended that solutions of Mesnex be refrigerated and used within 6 hours.

Mesna is not compatible with cisplatin.

Parenteral drug products should be inspected visually for particulate matter and discoloration prior to administration.

HOW SUPPLIED

Mesnex® (Mesna) Injection 100 mg/mL
NDC 0015-3560-41 200 mg Single Dose Ampule,
   Box of 15 Ampules of 2 mL (color-ring coding: turquoise/yellow)
NDC 0015-3561-41 400 mg Single Dose Ampule,
   Box of 15 Ampules of 4 mL (color-ring coding: blue/green)
NDC 0015-3562-41 1 g Single Dose Ampule,
   Box of 10 Ampules of 10 mL (color-ring coding: blue/green)
U.S. Patent No. 4,220,660
Store at room temperature.

Shown in Product Identification Section, page 406

MUTAMYCIN®   ℞
[mū"-tĕ-mī'-sĭn]
(mitomycin for injection) USP

WARNING

Mutamycin should be administered under the supervision of a qualified physician experienced in the use of cancer chemotherapeutic agents. Appropriate management of therapy and complications is possible only when

Continued on next page

Bristol-Myers Oncology—Cont.

adequate diagnostic and treatment facilities are readily available.

Bone marrow suppression, notably thrombocytopenia and leukopenia, which may contribute to overwhelming infections in an already compromised patient, is the most common and severe of the toxic effects of Mutamycin (see "Warnings" and "Adverse Reactions" sections).

Hemolytic Uremic Syndrome (HUS) a serious complication of chemotherapy, consisting primarily of microangiopathic hemolytic anemia, thrombocytopenia, and irreversible renal failure, has been reported in patients receiving systemic Mutamycin. The syndrome may occur at any time during systemic therapy with Mutamycin as a single agent or in combination with other cytotoxic drugs, however, most cases occur at doses ≥ 60 mg of Mutamycin. Blood product transfusion may exacerbate the symptoms associated with this syndrome.

The incidence of the syndrome has not been defined.

DESCRIPTION

Mutamycin (also known as mitomycin and/or mitomycin-C) is an antibiotic isolated from the broth of **Streptomyces caespitosus** which has been shown to have antitumor activity. The compound is heat stable, has a high melting point, and is freely soluble in organic solvents.

ACTION

Mutamycin selectively inhibits the synthesis of deoxyribonucleic acid (DNA). The guanine and cytosine content correlates with the degree of Mutamycin-induced cross-linking. At high concentrations of the drug, cellular RNA and protein synthesis are also suppressed.

In humans, Mutamycin is rapidly cleared from the serum after intravenous administration. Time required to reduce the serum concentration by 50% after a 30 mg. bolus injection is 17 minutes. After injection of 30 mg., 20 mg., or 10 mg. I.V., the maximal serum concentrations were 2.4 μg./mL, 1.7 μg./mL, and 0.52 μg./mL, respectively. Clearance is effected primarily by metabolism in the liver, but metabolism occurs in other tissues as well. The rate of clearance is inversely proportional to the maximal serum concentration because, it is thought, of saturation of the degradative pathways.

Approximately 10% of a dose of Mutamycin is excreted unchanged in the urine. Since metabolic pathways are saturated at relatively low doses, the percent of a dose excreted in urine increases with increasing dose. In children, excretion of intravenously administered Mutamycin is similar.

Animal Toxicology—Mutamycin has been found to be carcinogenic in rats and mice. At doses approximating the recommended clinical dose in man, it produces a greater than 100% increase in tumor incidence in male Sprague-Dawley rats, and a greater than 50% increase in tumor incidence in female Swiss mice.

INDICATIONS

Mutamycin is not recommended as single-agent, primary therapy. It has been shown to be useful in the therapy of disseminated adenocarcinoma of the stomach or pancreas in proven combinations with other approved chemotherapeutic agents and as palliative treatment when other modalities have failed. Mutamycin is not recommended to replace appropriate surgery and/or radiotherapy.

CONTRAINDICATIONS

Mutamycin is contraindicated in patients who have demonstrated a hypersensitive or idiosyncratic reaction to it in the past.

Mutamycin is contraindicated in patients with thrombocytopenia, coagulation disorder, or an increase in bleeding tendency due to other causes.

WARNINGS

Patients being treated with Mutamycin must be observed carefully and frequently during and after therapy.

The use of Mutamycin results in a high incidence of bone marrow suppression, particularly thrombocytopenia and leukopenia. Therefore, the following studies should be obtained repeatedly during therapy and for at least 8 weeks following therapy: platelet count, white blood cell count, differential, and hemoglobin. The occurrence of a platelet count below 100,000/mm^3 or a WBC below 4,000/mm^3 or a progressive decline in either is an indication to withhold further therapy until blood counts have recovered above these levels.

Patients should be advised of the potential toxicity of this drug, particularly bone marrow suppression. Deaths have been reported due to septicemia as a result of leukopenia due to the drug.

Patients receiving Mutamycin should be observed for evidence of renal toxicity. Mutamycin should not be given to patients with a serum creatinine greater than 1.7 mg %.

Usage in Pregnancy—Safe use of Mutamycin in pregnant women has not been established. Teratological changes have been noted in animal studies. The effect of Mutamycin on fertility is unknown.

PRECAUTIONS

Acute shortness of breath and severe bronchospasm have been reported following the administration of vinca alkaloids in patients who had previously or simultaneously received Mutamycin. The onset of this acute respiratory distress occurred within minutes to hours after the vinca alkaloid injection. The total number of doses for each drug has varied considerably. Bronchodilators, steroids and/or oxygen have produced symptomatic relief.

A few cases of adult respiratory distress syndrome have been reported in patients receiving Mutamycin in combination with other chemotherapy and maintained at FIO_2 concentrations greater than 50% perioperatively. Therefore, caution should be exercised using only enough oxygen to provide adequate arterial saturation since oxygen itself is toxic to the lungs. Careful attention should be paid to fluid balance and overhydration should be avoided.

ADVERSE REACTIONS

Bone Marrow Toxicity— This was the most common and most serious toxicity, occurring in 605 of 937 patients (64.4%). Thrombocytopenia and/or leukopenia may occur anytime within 8 weeks after onset of therapy with an average time of 4 weeks. Recovery after cessation of therapy was within 10 weeks. About 25% of the leukopenic or thrombocytopenic episodes did not recover. Mutamycin produces cumulative myelosuppression.

Integument and Mucous Membrane Toxicity— This has occurred in approximately 4% of patients treated with Mutamycin. Cellulitis at the injection site has been reported and is occasionally severe. Stomatitis and alopecia also occur frequently. Rashes are rarely reported. The most important dermatological problem with this drug, however, is the necrosis and consequent sloughing of tissue which results if the drug is extravasated during injection. Extravasation may occur with or without an accompanying stinging or burning sensation and even if there is adequate blood return when the injection needle is aspirated. There have been reports of delayed erythema and/or ulceration occurring either at or distant from the injection site, weeks to months after Mutamycin, even when no obvious evidence of extravasation was observed during administration. Skin grafting has been required in some cases.

Renal Toxicity—2% of 1,281 patients demonstrated a statistically significant rise in creatinine. There appeared to be no correlation between total dose administered or duration of therapy and the degree of renal impairment.

Pulmonary Toxicity—This has occurred infrequently but can be severe and may be life threatening. Dyspnea with a nonproductive cough and radiographic evidence of pulmonary infiltrates may be indicative of Mutamycin-induced pulmonary toxicity. If other etiologies are eliminated, Mutamycin therapy should be discontinued. Steroids have been employed as treatment of this toxicity, but the therapeutic value has not been determined. A few cases of adult respiratory distress syndrome have been reported in patients receiving Mutamycin in combination with other chemotherapy and maintained at FIO_2 concentrations greater than 50% perioperatively.

Hemolytic Uremic Syndrome (HUS)—This serious complication of chemotherapy, consisting primarily of microangiopathic hemolytic anemia (hematocrit ≤25%), thrombocytopenia (≤100,000/mm^3), and irreversible renal failure (serum creatinine ≥1.6 mg/dL) has been reported in patients receiving systemic Mutamycin. Microangiopathic hemolysis with fragmented red blood cells on peripheral blood smears has occurred in 98% of patients with the syndrome. Other less frequent complications of the syndrome may include pulmonary edema (65%), neurologic abnormalities (16%), and hypertension. Exacerbation of the symptoms associated with HUS has been reported in some patients receiving blood product transfusions. A high mortality rate (52%) has been associated with this syndrome.

The syndrome may occur at any time during systemic therapy with Mutamycin as a single agent or in combination with other cytotoxic drugs. Less frequently, HUS has also been reported in patients receiving combinations of cytotoxic drugs not including Mutamycin. Of 83 patients studied, 72 developed the syndrome at total doses exceeding 60 mg of Mutamycin. Consequently, patients receiving ≥60 mg of Mutamycin should be monitored closely for unexplained anemia with fragmented cells on peripheral blood smear, thrombocytopenia, and decreased renal function.

The incidence of the syndrome has not been defined.

Therapy for the syndrome is investigational.

Cardiac Toxicity—Congestive heart failure, often treated effectively with diuretics and cardiac glycosides, has rarely been reported. Almost all patients who experienced this side effect had received prior doxorubicin therapy.

Acute Side Effects Due to Mutamycin were fever, anorexia, nausea, and vomiting. They occurred in about 14% of 1,281 patients.

Other Undesirable Side Effects that have been reported during Mutamycin therapy have been headache, blurring of vision, confusion, drowsiness, syncope, fatigue, edema, thrombophlebitis, hematemesis, diarrhea, and pain. These did not appear to be dose related and were not unequivocally drug related. They may have been due to the primary or metastatic disease processes.

DOSAGE AND ADMINISTRATION

Mutamycin should be given intravenously only, using care to avoid extravasation of the compound. If extravasation occurs, cellulitis, ulceration, and slough may result.

Each vial contains either mitomycin 5 mg and mannitol 10 mg, mitomycin 20 mg and mannitol 40 mg, or mitomycin 40 mg and mannitol 80 mg. To administer, add Sterile Water for Injection, 10 mL, 40 mL or 80 mL, respectively. Shake to dissolve. If product does not dissolve immediately, allow to stand at room temperature until solution is obtained.

After full hematological recovery (see guide to dosage adjustment) from any previous chemotherapy, the following dosage schedule may be used at 6- to 8-week intervals:

20 mg/m^2 intravenously as a single dose via a functioning intravenous catheter.

Because of cumulative myelosuppression, patients should be fully reevaluated after each course of Mutamycin, and the dose reduced if the patient has experienced any toxicities. Doses greater than 20 mg/m^2 have not been shown to be more effective, and are more toxic than lower doses.

The following schedule is suggested as a guide to dosage adjustment:

Nadir After Prior Dose		
Leukocytes/ mm^3	**Platelets/ mm^3**	**Percentage of Prior Dose To be Given**
>4000	>100,000	100%
3000–3999	75,000–99,999	100%
2000–2999	25,000–74,999	70%
<2000	< 25,000	50%

No repeat dosage should be given until leukocyte count has returned to 4000/mm^3 and platelet count to 100,000/mm^3.

When Mutamycin is used in combination with other myelosuppressive agents, the doses should be adjusted accordingly. If the disease continues to progress after two courses of Mutamycin, the drug should be stopped since chances of response are minimal.

STABILITY

1. **Unreconstituted** Mutamycin stored at room temperature is stable for the lot life indicated on the package. Avoid excessive heat (over 40°C).
2. **Reconstituted** with Sterile Water for Injection to a concentration of 0.5 mg. per mL, Mutamycin is stable for 14 days refrigerated or 7 days at room temperature.
3. **Diluted** in various IV fluids at room temperature, to a concentration of 20 to 40 micrograms per mL:

IV Fluid	Stability
5% Dextrose Injection	3 hours
0.9% Sodium Chloride Injection	12 hours
Sodium Lactate Injection	24 hours

4. **The combination** of Mutamycin (5 mg. to 15 mg.) and heparin (1,000 units to 10,000 units) in 30 mL of 0.9% Sodium Chloride Injection is stable for 48 hours at room temperature.

Procedures for proper handling and disposal of anticancer drugs should be considered. Several guidelines on this subject have been published.[1–7] There is no general agreement that all of the procedures recommended in the guidelines are necessary or appropriate.

REFERENCES

1. Recommendations for the Safe Handling of Parenteral Antineoplastic Drugs. NIH Publication No. 83-2621. For sale by the Superintendent of Documents, U.S. Government Printing Office, Washington, D.C. 20402.
2. AMA Council Report. Guidelines for Handling Parenteral Antineoplastics, *JAMA.* 1985; March 15.
3. National Study Commission on Cytotoxic Exposure—Recommendations for Handling Cytotoxic Agents. Available from Louis P. Jeffrey, Sc.D., Chairman, National Study Commission on Cytotoxic Exposure, Massachusetts College of Pharmacy and Allied Health Sciences, 179 Longwood Avenue, Boston, Massachusetts 02115.

4. Clinical Oncological Society of Australia: Guidelines and Recommendations for Safe Handling of Antineoplastic Agents. *Med J Australia.* 1983; 1:426–428.
5. Jones, R. B., et. al. Safe Handling of Chemotherapeutic Agents: A Report from the Mount Sinai Medical Center, *CA—A Cancer J for Clinicians.* 1983; Sept./Oct., 258–263.
6. American Society of Hospital Pharmacists Technical Assistance Bulletin on Handling Cytotoxic and Hazardous Drugs. *Am J Hosp Pharm.* 1990; 47:1033–1049.
7. OSHA Work-Practice Guidelines for Personnel Dealing with Cytotoxic (antineoplastic) Drugs. *Am J Hosp Pharm.* 1986; 43:1193–1204.

SUPPLY
Mutamycin (mitomycin for Injection).
NDC 0015-3001-20—Each vial contains 5 mg. mitomycin.
NDC 0015-3002-20—Each vial contains 20 mg. mitomycin.
NDC 0015-3059-20—Each vial contains 40 mg mitomycin.
For information on package sizes available, refer to the current price schedule.
Shown in Product Identification Section, page 406

MYCOSTATIN® PASTILLES ℞
[mĭk 'ō-stat "in]
Nystatin

DESCRIPTION
Nystatin is a polyene antifungal antibiotic obtained from *Streptomyces noursei.* Structural formula:

$C_{47}H_{75}NO_{17}$ MW 926.13   CAS-1400-61-9

MYCOSTATIN (nystatin) Pastilles are round, light to dark gold-colored troches designed to dissolve slowly in the mouth. Each pastille provides 200,000 units nystatin. Inactive ingredients: anise oil, cinnamon oil, gelatin, sucrose, and other ingredients.

CLINICAL PHARMACOLOGY
Nystatin is both fungistatic and fungicidal *in vitro* against a wide variety of yeasts and yeast-like fungi. *Candida albicans* demonstrates no significant resistance to nystatin *in vitro* on repeated subculture in increasing levels of nystatin; other *Candida* species become quite resistant. Generally, resistance does not develop *in vivo*. Nystatin acts by binding to sterols in the cell membrane of susceptible fungi with a resultant change in membrane permeability allowing leakage of intracellular components. Nystatin exhibits no activity against bacteria, protozoa, trichomonads, or viruses.
Pharmacokinetics
Gastrointestinal absorption of nystatin is insignificant. Most orally administered nystatin is passed unchanged in the stool. Significant concentrations of nystatin may appear occasionally in the plasma of patients with renal insufficiency during oral therapy with conventional dosage forms. Mean nystatin concentrations in excess of those required *in vitro* to inhibit growth of clinically significant *Candida* persisted in saliva for approximately two hours after the start of oral dissolution of two nystatin pastilles (400,000 units nystatin) administered simultaneously to 12 healthy volunteers.

INDICATIONS AND USAGE
Mycostatin (nystatin) Pastilles are indicated for the treatment of candidiasis in the oral cavity.

CONTRAINDICATIONS
The pastille is contraindicated in those patients with a history of hypersensitivity to any of its components.

PRECAUTIONS
General
This medication is not to be used for the treatment of systemic mycoses.
In order to achieve maximum effect from the medication, pastilles must be allowed to dissolve slowly in the mouth; therefore, patients for whom the pastille is prescribed, including children and the elderly, must be competent to utilize the dosage form as intended.
If irritation or hypersensitivity develops with nystatin pastilles, treatment should be discontinued and appropriate therapy instituted.
Information for the Patient
Patients taking this medication should receive the following information and instructions:
1. Use as directed; the medication is not for any disorder other than that for which it was prescribed.
2. Allow pastille to dissolve slowly in the mouth; **do not chew or swallow the pastille.**

3. The patient should be advised regarding replacement of any missed doses.
4. There should be no interruption or discontinuation of medication until the prescribed course of treatment is completed even though symptomatic relief may occur within a few days.
5. If symptoms of local irritation develop, the physician should be notified promptly.
6. Good oral hygiene, including proper care of dentures, is particularly important for denture wearers.
Laboratory Tests
If there is a lack of therapeutic response, appropriate microbiological studies (eg, KOH smears and/or cultures) should be repeated to confirm the diagnosis of candidiasis and rule out other pathogens before instituting another course of therapy.
Carcinogenesis, Mutagenesis, Impairment of Fertility
Studies have not been performed to evaluate carcinogenic or mutagenic potential, or possible impairment of fertility in males or females.
Pregnancy: Teratogenic Effects
Category C. Animal reproduction studies have not been conducted with nystatin pastilles. It is also not known whether nystatin pastilles can cause fetal harm when administered to a pregnant woman or can affect reproduction capacity. Nystatin pastilles should be dispensed to a pregnant woman only if clearly needed.
Pediatric Use
See PRECAUTIONS, General.

ADVERSE REACTIONS
Nystatin is virtually nontoxic and nonsensitizing and is well-tolerated by all age groups, even during prolonged use. Rarely, oral irritation or sensitization may occur. Nausea has been reported occasionally during therapy.
Large oral doses of nystatin have occasionally produced diarrhea, gastrointestinal distress, nausea and vomiting.

OVERDOSAGE
Oral doses of nystatin in excess of five million units daily have caused nausea and gastrointestinal upset. There have been no reports of serious toxic effects or superinfections (see CLINICAL PHARMACOLOGY, Pharmacokinetics).

DOSAGE AND ADMINISTRATION
Children and Adults: The recommended dose is one or two pastilles (200,000 or 400,000 units nystatin) four or five times daily for as long as 14 days if necessary. The dosage regimen should be continued for at least 48 hours after disappearance of oral symptoms.
Dosage should be discontinued if symptoms persist after the initial 14 day period of treatment (see PRECAUTIONS, Laboratory Tests).
Administration: Pastilles must be allowed to dissolve slowly in the mouth, and should not be chewed or swallowed whole.

HOW SUPPLIED
Mycostatin (nystatin) Pastilles, 200,000 units nystatin each, in packages containing 30 pleasant-tasting pastilles (NDC 0003-0543-20).

ALSO AVAILABLE
Mycostatin (Nystatin, USP) is also available as a ready-to-use oral suspension, oral tablets, vaginal tablets, and topical powder, cream, and ointment (see package inserts accompanying those products for complete information).
Storage
Refrigerate between 2° and 8°C (36° and 46°F).

PARAPLATIN® ℞
[păr-a-plătin]
(carboplatin for injection)

> **WARNING**
> PARAPLATIN® (carboplatin for injection) should be administered under the supervision of a qualified physician experienced in the use of cancer chemotherapeutic agents. Appropriate management of therapy and complications is possible only when adequate treatment facilities are readily available.
> Bone marrow suppression is dose related and may be severe, resulting in infection and/or bleeding. Anemia may be cumulative and may require transfusion support. Vomiting is another frequent drug-related side effect.
> Anaphylactic-like reactions to PARAPLATIN have been reported and may occur within minutes of PARAPLATIN administration. Epinephrine, corticosteroids, and antihistamines have been employed to alleviate symptoms.

DESCRIPTION
PARAPLATIN® (carboplatin for injection) is supplied as a sterile lyophilized powder available in single-dose vials containing 50 mg, 150 mg, and 450 mg of carboplatin for administration by intravenous infusion. Each vial contains equal parts by weight of carboplatin and mannitol.
Carboplatin is a platinum coordination compound that is used as a cancer chemotherapeutic agent. The chemical name for carboplatin is platinum, diammine [1,1-cyclobutane-dicarboxylato(2-)-0,0']-, (SP-4-2), and has the following structural formula:

Carboplatin is a white to off-white crystalline powder with the molecular formula of $C_6H_{12}N_2O_4Pt$ and a molecular weight of 371.25. It is soluble in water at a rate of approximately 14 mg/mL, and the pH of a 1% solution is 5–7. It is virtually insoluble in ethanol, acetone, and dimethylacetamide.

CLINICAL PHARMACOLOGY
Carboplatin, like cisplatin, produces predominantly interstrand DNA cross-links rather than DNA-protein cross-links. This effect is apparently cell-cycle nonspecific. The aquation of carboplatin, which is thought to produce the active species, occurs at a slower rate than in the case of cisplatin. Despite this difference, it appears that both carboplatin and cisplatin induce equal numbers of drug-DNA cross-links, causing equivalent lesions and biological effects. The differences in potencies for carboplatin and cisplatin appear to be directly related to the difference in aquation rates.
In patients with creatinine clearances of about 60 mL/min or greater, plasma levels of intact carboplatin decay in a biphasic manner after a 30-minute intravenous infusion of 300 to 500 mg/m² of PARAPLATIN. The initial plasma half-life (alpha) was found to be 1.1 to 2.0 hours (N=6), and the postdistribution plasma half-life (beta) was found to be 2.6 to 5.9 hours (N=6). The total body clearance, apparent volume of distribution, and mean residence time for carboplatin are 4.4 L/hour, 16 L and 3.5 hours, respectively. The Cmax values and areas under the plasma concentration vs time curves from 0 to infinity (AUC inf) increase linearly with dose, although the increase was slightly more than dose proportional. Carboplatin, therefore, exhibits linear pharmacokinetics over the dosing range studied (300–500 mg/m²).
Carboplatin is not bound to plasma proteins. No significant quantities of protein-free, ultrafilterable platinum-containing species other than carboplatin are present in plasma. However, platinum from carboplatin becomes irreversibly bound to plasma proteins and is slowly eliminated with a minimum half-life of 5 days.
The major route of elimination of carboplatin is renal excretion. Patients with creatinine clearances of approximately 60 mL/min or greater excrete 65% of the dose in the urine within 12 hours and 71% of the dose within 24 hours. All of the platinum in the 24-hour urine is present as carboplatin. Only 3% to 5% of the administered platinum is excreted in the urine between 24 and 96 hours. There are insufficient data to determine whether biliary excretion occurs.
In patients with creatinine clearances below 60 mL/min the total body and renal clearances of carboplatin decrease as the creatinine clearance decreases. PARAPLATIN dosages should therefore be reduced in these patients (see "DOSAGE AND ADMINISTRATION").

CLINICAL STUDIES
Use with cyclophosphamide for initial treatment of ovarian cancer:
In two prospectively randomized, controlled studies conducted by the National Cancer Institute of Canada, Clinical Trials Group (NCIC) and the Southwest Oncology Group (SWOG), 789 chemotherapy naive patients with advanced ovarian cancer were treated with PARAPLATIN or cisplatin, both in combination with cyclophosphamide every 28 days for six courses before surgical re-evaluation. The following results were obtained from both studies:
COMPARATIVE EFFICACY
[See table on next page.]
COMPARATIVE TOXICITY
The pattern of toxicity exerted by the PARAPLATIN-containing regimen was significantly different from that of the cisplatin-containing combinations. Differences between the two studies may be explained by different cisplatin dosages and by different supportive care.
The PARAPLATIN-containing regimen induced significantly more thrombocytopenia and, in one study, significantly more leukopenia and more need for transfusional support. The cisplatin-containing regimen produced signifi-

Continued on next page

Bristol-Myers Oncology—Cont.

cantly more anemia in one study. However, no significant differences occurred in incidences of infections and hemorrhagic episodes.

Non-hematologic toxicities (emesis, neurotoxicity, ototoxicity, renal toxicity, hypomagnesemia, and alopecia) were significantly more frequent in the cisplatin-containing arms.

[See table on page 753 and table on page 754.]

Use as a single agent for secondary treatment of advanced ovarian cancer:

In two prospective, randomized controlled studies in patients with advanced ovarian cancer previously treated with chemotherapy, PARAPLATIN achieved six clinical complete responses in 47 patients. The duration of these responses ranged from 45 to 71+ weeks.

INDICATIONS

Initial treatment of advanced ovarian carcinoma:

PARAPLATIN is indicated for the initial treatment of advanced ovarian carcinoma in established combination with other approved chemotherapeutic agents. One established combination regimen consists of PARAPLATIN and cyclophosphamide (Cytoxan®). Two randomized controlled studies conducted by the NCIC and SWOG with PARAPLATIN vs cisplatin, both in combination with cyclophosphamide, have demonstrated equivalent overall survival between the two groups (see "CLINICAL STUDIES" section). There is limited statistical power to demonstrate equivalence in overall pathologic complete response rates and long-term survival (≥ 3 years) because of the small number of patients with these outcomes; the small number of patients with residual tumor < 2 cm after initial surgery also limits the statistical power to demonstrate equivalence in this subgroup.

Secondary treatment of advanced ovarian carcinoma:

PARAPLATIN is indicated for the palliative treatment of patients with ovarian carcinoma recurrent after prior chemotherapy, including patients who have been previously treated with cisplatin.

Within the group of patients previously treated with cisplatin, those who have developed progressive disease while receiving cisplatin therapy may have a decreased response rate.

CONTRAINDICATIONS

PARAPLATIN is contraindicated in patients with a history of severe allergic reactions to cisplatin or other platinum-containing compounds or mannitol.

PARAPLATIN should not be employed in patients with severe bone marrow depression or significant bleeding.

WARNINGS

Bone marrow suppression (leukopenia, neutropenia and thrombocytopenia) is dose dependent and is also the dose-limiting toxicity. Peripheral blood counts should be frequently monitored during PARAPLATIN treatment and, when appropriate, until recovery is achieved. Median nadir occurs at day 21 in patients receiving single-agent PARAPLATIN. In general, single intermittent courses of PARAPLATIN should not be repeated until leukocyte, neutrophil and platelet counts have recovered.

Since anemia is cumulative, transfusions may be needed during treatment with PARAPLATIN, particularly in patients receiving prolonged therapy.

Bone marrow suppression is increased in patients who have received prior therapy, especially regimens including cisplatin. Marrow suppression is also increased in patients with impaired kidney function. Initial PARAPLATIN dosages in these patients should be appropriately reduced (see "DOSAGE AND ADMINISTRATION") and blood counts should be carefully monitored between courses. The use of PARAPLATIN in combination with other bone marrow suppressing therapies must be carefully managed with respect to dosage and timing in order to minimize additive effects.

PARAPLATIN has limited nephrotoxic potential, but concomitant treatment with aminoglycosides has resulted in increased renal and/or audiologic toxicity, and caution must be exercised when a patient receives both drugs.

PARAPLATIN can induce emesis, which can be more severe in patients previously receiving emetogenic therapy. The incidence and intensity of emesis have been reduced by using premedication with antiemetics. Although no conclusive efficacy data exist with the following schedules of PARAPLATIN, lengthening the duration of single intravenous administration to 24 hours or dividing the total dose over five consecutive daily pulse doses has resulted in reduced emesis.

Although peripheral neurotoxicity is infrequent, its incidence is increased in patients older than 65 years and in patients previously treated with cisplatin. Pre-existing cisplatin-induced neurotoxicity does not worsen in about 70% of the patients receiving PARAPLATIN as secondary treatment.

As in the case of other platinum coordination compounds, allergic reactions to PARAPLATIN have been reported. These may occur within minutes of administration and should be managed with appropriate supportive therapy.

High dosages of PARAPLATIN (more than four times the recommended dose) have resulted in severe abnormalities of liver function tests.

PARAPLATIN may cause fetal harm when administered to a pregnant woman. PARAPLATIN has been shown to be embryotoxic and teratogenic in rats. There are no adequate and well-controlled studies in pregnant women. If this drug is used during pregnancy, or if the patient becomes pregnant while receiving this drug, the patient should be apprised of the potential hazard to the fetus. Women of childbearing potential should be advised to avoid becoming pregnant.

PRECAUTIONS

General: Needles or intravenous administration sets containing aluminum parts that may come in contact with PARAPLATIN should not be used for the preparation or administration of the drug. Aluminum can react with carboplatin causing precipitate formation and loss of potency.

Drug Interactions: The renal effects of nephrotoxic compounds may be potentiated by PARAPLATIN.

Carcinogenesis, mutagenesis, impairment of fertility: The carcinogenic potential of carboplatin has not been studied, but compounds with similar mechanisms of action and mutagenicity profiles have been reported to be carcinogenic. Carboplatin has been shown to be mutagenic both **in vitro** and **in vivo**. It has also been shown to be embryotoxic and teratogenic in rats receiving the drug during organogenesis.

Pregnancy: Pregnancy "category D": (see "**WARNINGS**").

Nursing mothers: It is not known whether carboplatin is excreted in human milk. Because there is a possibility of toxicity in nursing infants secondary to PARAPLATIN treatment of the mother, it is recommended that breastfeeding be discontinued if the mother is treated with PARAPLATIN.

ADVERSE REACTIONS

For a comparison of toxicities when carboplatin or cisplatin was given in combination with cyclophosphamide, see the COMPARATIVE TOXICITY subsection of the CLINICAL STUDIES section.

[See table on page 755.]

In the narrative section that follows, the incidences of adverse events are based on data from 1,893 patients with various types of tumors who received PARAPLATIN as single-agent therapy.

Hematologic toxicity: Bone marrow suppression is the dose-limiting toxicity of PARAPLATIN. Thrombocytopenia with platelet counts below 50,000/mm^3 occurs in 25% of the patients (35% of pretreated ovarian cancer patients); neutropenia with granulocyte counts below 1,000/mm^3 occurs in 16% of the patients (21% of pretreated ovarian cancer patients); leukopenia with WBC counts below 2,000/mm^3 occurs in 15% of the patients (26% of pretreated ovarian cancer patients). The nadir usually occurs about day 21 in patients receiving single-agent therapy. By day 28, 90% of patients have platelet counts above 100,000/mm^3; 74% have neutrophil counts above 2,000/mm^3; 67% have leukocyte counts above 4,000/mm^3.

Marrow suppression is usually more severe in patients with impaired kidney function. Patients with poor performance

Overview of Pivotal Trials

	NCIC	SWOG
Number of patients randomized	447	342
Median age (years)	60	62
Dose of cisplatin	75 mg/m^2	100 mg/m^2
Dose of carboplatin	300 mg/m^2	300 mg/m^2
Dose of cytoxan	600 mg/m^2	600 mg/m^2
Residual tumor <2 cm (number of patients)	39% (174/447)	14% (49/342)

Clinical Response in Measurable Disease Patients

	NCIC	SWOG
Carboplatin (number of patients)	60% (48/80)	58% (48/83)
Cisplatin (number of patients)	58% (49/85)	43% (33/76)
95% C.I. of difference (Carboplatin-Cisplatin)	(−13.9%, 18.6%)	(−2.3%, 31.1%)

Pathologic Complete Response*

	NCIC	SWOG
Carboplatin (number of patients)	11% (24/224)	10% (17/171)
Cisplatin (number of patients)	15% (33/223)	10% (17/171)
95% C.I. of difference (Carboplatin-Cisplatin)	(−10.7%, 2.5%)	(−6.9%, 6.9%)

*114 PARAPLATIN and 109 Cisplatin patients did not undergo second-look surgery in NCIC study
  90 PARAPLATIN and 106 Cisplatin patients did not undergo second-look surgery in SWOG study

Progression-Free Survival (PFS)

	NCIC	SWOG
Median		
Carboplatin	59 weeks	49 weeks
Cisplatin	61 weeks	47 weeks
2-year PFS*		
Carboplatin	31%	21%
Cisplatin	31%	21%
95% C.I. or difference (Carboplatin-Cisplatin)	(−9.3, 8.7)	(−9.0, 9.4)
3-year PFS*		
Carboplatin	19%	8%
Cisplatin	23%	14%
95% C.I. of difference (Carboplatin-Cisplatin)	(−11.5, 4.5)	(−14.1, 0.3)
Hazard Ratio**		
95% C.I.	1.10	1.02
(Carboplatin:Cisplatin)	(0.89, 1.35)	(0.81, 1.29)

 *Kaplan-Meier Estimates
  Unrelated deaths occurring in the absence of progression were counted as events (progression) in this analysis.
**Analysis adjusted for factors found to be of prognostic significance were consistent with unadjusted analysis.

Survival

	NCIC	SWOG
Median		
Carboplatin	110 weeks	86 weeks
Cisplatin	99 weeks	79 weeks
2-year Survival*		
Carboplatin	51.9%	40.2%
Cisplatin	48.4%	39.0%
95% C.I. of difference (Carboplatin-Cisplatin)	(−6.2, 13.2)	(−9.8, 12.2)
3-year Survival*		
Carboplatin	34.6%	18.3%
Cisplatin	33.1%	24.9%
95% C.I. of difference (Carboplatin-Cisplatin)	(−7.7, 10.7)	(−15.9, 2.7)
Hazard Ratio**		
95% C.I.	0.98	1.01
(Carboplatin:Cisplatin)	(0.78, 1.23)	(0.78, 1.30)

 * Kaplan-Meier Estimates
**Analysis adjusted for factors found to be of prognostic significance were consistent with unadjusted analysis.

status have also experienced a higher incidence of severe leukopenia and thrombocytopenia.

The hematologic effects, although usually reversible, have resulted in infectious or hemorrhagic complications in 5% of the patients treated with PARAPLATIN, with drug related death occurring in less than 1% of the patients.

Anemia with hemoglobin less than 11 g/dL has been observed in 71% of the patients who started therapy with a baseline above that value. The incidence of anemia increases with increasing exposure to PARAPLATIN. Transfusions have been administered to 26% of the patients treated with PARAPLATIN (44% of previously treated ovarian cancer patients).

Bone marrow depression may be more severe when PARAPLATIN is combined with other bone marrow suppressing drugs or with radiotherapy.

Gastrointestinal toxicity: Vomiting occurs in 65% of the patients (81% of previously treated ovarian cancer patients) and in about one-third of these patients it is severe. Carboplatin, as a single agent or in combination, is significantly less emetogenic than cisplatin; however, patients previously treated with emetogenic agents, especially cisplatin, appear to be more prone to vomiting. Nausea alone occurs in an additional 10%–15% of patients. Both nausea and vomiting usually cease within 24 hours of treatment and are often responsive to antiemetic measures. Although no conclusive efficacy data exist with the following schedules, prolonged administration of PARAPLATIN, either by continuous 24-hour infusion or by daily pulse doses given for 5 consecutive days, was associated with less severe vomiting than the single-dose intermittent schedule. Emesis was increased when PARAPLATIN was used in combination with other emetogenic compounds. Other gastrointestinal effects observed frequently were pain, in 17% of the patients; diarrhea, in 6%; and constipation, also in 6%.

Neurologic toxicity: Peripheral neuropathies have been observed in 4% of the patients receiving PARAPLATIN (6% of pretreated ovarian cancer patients) with mild paresthesias occurring most frequently. Carboplatin therapy produces significantly fewer and less severe neurologic side effects than does therapy with cisplatin. However, patients older than 65 years and/or previously treated with cisplatin appear to have an increased risk (10%) for peripheral neuropathies. In 70% of the patients with pre-existing cisplatin-induced peripheral neurotoxicity, there was no worsening of symptoms during therapy with PARAPLATIN. Clinical ototoxicity and other sensory abnormalities such as visual disturbances and change in taste have been reported in only 1% of the patients. Central nervous system symptoms have been reported in 5% of the patients and appear to be most often related to the use of antiemetics.

Although the overall incidence of peripheral neurologic side effects induced by PARAPLATIN is low, prolonged treatment, particularly in cisplatin pretreated patients, may result in cumulative neurotoxicity.

Nephrotoxicity: Development of abnormal renal function test results is uncommon, despite the fact that carboplatin, unlike cisplatin, has usually been administered without high-volume fluid hydration and/or forced diuresis. The incidences of abnormal renal function tests reported are 6% for serum creatinine and 14% for blood urea nitrogen (10% and 22%, respectively, in pretreated ovarian cancer patients). Most of these reported abnormalities have been mild and about one-half of them were reversible.

Creatinine clearance has proven to be the most sensitive measure of kidney function in patients receiving PARAPLATIN, and it appears to be the most useful test for correlating drug clearance and bone marrow suppression. Twenty-seven percent of the patients who had a baseline value of 60 mL/min or more demonstrated a reduction below this value during PARAPLATIN therapy.

Hepatic toxicity: The incidences of abnormal liver function tests in patients with normal baseline values were reported as follows: total bilirubin, 5%; SGOT, 15%; and alkaline phosphatase, 24%; (5%, 19%, and 37%, respectively, in pretreated ovarian cancer patients). These abnormalities have generally been mild and reversible in about one-half of the cases, although the role of metastatic tumor in the liver may complicate the assessment in many patients. In a limited series of patients receiving very high dosages of PARAPLATIN and autologous bone marrow transplantation, severe abnormalities of liver function tests were reported.

Electrolyte Changes: The incidences of abnormally decreased serum electrolyte values reported were as follows: sodium, 29%; potassium, 20%; calcium, 22%; and magnesium, 29%; (47%, 28%, 31%, and 43%, respectively, in pretreated ovarian cancer patients). Electrolyte supplementation was not routinely administered concomitantly with PARAPLATIN, and these electrolyte abnormalities were rarely associated with symptoms.

Allergic reactions: Hypersensitivity to PARAPLATIN has been reported in 2% of the patients. These allergic reactions have been similar in nature and severity to those reported with other platinum-containing compounds, i.e., rash, urticaria, erythema, pruritus, and rarely bronchospasm and

hypotension. These reactions have been successfully managed with standard epinephrine, corticosteroid and antihistamine therapy.

Other events: Pain and asthenia were the most frequently reported miscellaneous adverse effects; their relationship to the tumor and to anemia was likely. Alopecia was reported (3%). Cardiovascular, respiratory, genitourinary, and mucosal side effects have occurred in 6% or less of the patients. Cardiovascular events (cardiac failure, embolism, cerebrovascular accidents) were fatal in less than 1% of the patients and did not appear to be related to chemotherapy. Cancer-associated hemolytic uremic syndrome has been reported rarely.

OVERDOSAGE

There is no known antidote for PARAPLATIN overdosage. The anticipated complications of overdosage would be secondary to bone marrow suppression and/or hepatic toxicity.

DOSAGE AND ADMINISTRATION

NOTE: Aluminum reacts with carboplatin causing precipitate formation and loss of potency, therefore, needles or intravenous sets containing aluminum parts that may come in contact with the drug must not be used for the preparation or administration of PARAPLATIN.

Single agent therapy:
PARAPLATIN, as a single agent, has been shown to be effective in patients with recurrent ovarian carcinoma at a dosage of 360 mg/m² I.V. on day 1 every 4 weeks. In general, however, single intermittent courses of PARAPLATIN should not be repeated until the neutrophil count is at least 2,000 and the platelet count is at least 100,000.

Combination therapy with cyclophosphamide:
In the chemotherapy of advanced ovarian cancer, an effective combination for previously untreated patients consists of:
PARAPLATIN—300 mg/m² I.V. on day 1 every 4 weeks for six cycles.
Cyclophosphamide (Cytoxan®)—600 mg/m² I.V. on day 1 every 4 weeks for six cycles. For directions regarding the use and administration of cyclophosphamide (Cytoxan®) please refer to its package insert.

ADVERSE EXPERIENCES IN PATIENTS WITH OVARIAN CANCER NCIC STUDY

		Paraplatin Arm Percent[*]	Cisplatin Arm Percent[*]	P-Value[**]
Bone Marrow				
Thrombocytopenia,	< 100,000/mm³	70	29	< 0.001
	< 50,000/mm³	41	6	< 0.001
Neutropenia,	< 2,000 cells/mm³	97	96	n.s.
	< 1,000 cells/mm³	81	79	n.s.
Leukopenia,	< 4,000 cells/mm³	98	97	n.s.
	< 2,000 cells/mm³	68	52	0.001
Anemia,	< 11 g/dL	91	91	n.s.
	< 8 g/dL	18	12	n.s.
Infections		14	12	n.s.
Bleeding		10	4	n.s.
Transfusions		42	31	0.018
Gastrointestinal				
Nausea and vomiting		93	98	0.010
Vomiting		84	97	< 0.001
Other GI side effects		50	62	0.013
Neurologic				
Peripheral neuropathies		16	42	< 0.001
Ototoxicity		13	33	< 0.001
Other sensory side effects		6	10	n.s.
Central neurotoxicity		28	40	0.009
Renal				
Serum creatinine elevations		5	13	0.006
Blood urea elevations		17	31	< 0.001
Hepatic				
Bilirubin elevations		5	3	n.s.
SGOT elevations		17	13	n.s.
Alkaline phosphatase elevations		—	—	—
Electrolytes loss				
Sodium		10	20	0.005
Potassium		16	22	n.s.
Calcium		16	19	n.s.
Magnesium		63	88	< 0.001
Other side effects				
Pain		36	37	n.s.
Asthenia		40	33	n.s.
Cardiovascular		15	19	n.s.
Respiratory		8	9	n.s.
Allergic		12	9	n.s.
Genitourinary		10	10	n.s.
Alopecia[+]		50	62	0.017
Mucositis		10	9	n.s.

[*]Values are in percent of evaluable patients
[**]n.s. = not significant, p > 0.05
[+]May have been affected by cyclophosphamide dosage delivered

---

(See 'CLINICAL STUDIES' section).
Intermittent courses of PARAPLATIN in combination with cyclophosphamide should not be repeated until the neutrophil count is at least 2,000 and the platelet count is at least 100,000.

Dose Adjustment Recommendations:
The suggested dose adjustments for single agent or combination therapy shown in the table below are modified from controlled trials in previously treated and untreated patients with ovarian carcinoma. Blood counts were done weekly, and the recommendations are based on the lowest post-treatment platelet or neutrophil value.

Platelets	Neutrophils	Adjusted Dose[*] (From Prior Course)
> 100,000	> 2,000	125%
50–100,000	500–2,000	No Adjustment
< 50,000	< 500	75%

[*] Percentages apply to PARAPLATIN as a single agent or to both PARAPLATIN and cyclophosphamide in combination. In the controlled studies, dosages were also adjusted at a lower level (50 to 60%) for severe myelosuppression. Escalations above 125% were not recommended for these studies.

PARAPLATIN is usually administered by an infusion lasting 15 minutes or longer. No pre- or post-treatment hydration or forced diuresis is required.

Patients with impaired kidney function: Patients with creatinine clearance values below 60 mL/min are at increased risk of severe bone marrow suppression. In renally-impaired patients who received single-agent PARAPLATIN therapy, the incidence of severe leukopenia, neutropenia, or thrombocytopenia has been about 25% when the dosage modifications in the table below have been used.

Baseline Creatinine Clearance	Recommended Dose on Day 1
41–59 mL/min	250 mg/m²
16–40 mL/min	200 mg/m²

Continued on next page

Bristol-Myers Oncology—Cont.

The data available for patients with severely impaired kidney function (creatinine clearance below 15 mL/min) are too limited to permit a recommendation for treatment.[1,2]

These dosing recommendations apply to the initial course of treatment. Subsequent dosages should be adjusted according to the patient's tolerance based on the degree of bone marrow suppression.

PREPARATION OF INTRAVENOUS SOLUTIONS

Immediately before use, the content of each vial must be reconstituted with either Sterile Water for Injection, USP, 5% Dextrose in Water, or Sodium Chloride Injection, USP, according to the following schedule:

Vial Strength	Diluent Volume
50 mg	5 mL
150 mg	15 mL
450 mg	45 mL

These dilutions all produce a carboplatin concentration of 10 mg/mL.

PARAPLATIN can be further diluted to concentrations as low as 0.5 mg/mL with 5% Dextrose in Water (D_5W) or 0.9% Sodium Chloride Injection, USP.

STABILITY

Unopened vials of PARAPLATIN for Injection are stable for the life indicated on the package when stored at controlled room temperature 15°–30°C (59°–86°F), and protected from light.

When prepared as directed, PARAPLATIN solutions are stable for 8 hours at room temperature (25°C). Since no antibacterial preservative is contained in the formulation, it is recommended that PARAPLATIN solutions be discarded 8 hours after dilution.

Parenteral drug products should be inspected visually for particulate matter and discoloration prior to administration.

HOW SUPPLIED

NDC 0015-3213-30	50 mg vials, individually cartoned, shelf packs of 10 cartons, 10 shelf packs per case. (Yellow flip-off seals)
NDC 0015-3214-30	150 mg vials, individually cartoned, shelf packs of 10 cartons, 10 shelf packs per case. (Violet flip-off seals)
NDC 0015-3215-30	450 mg vials, individually cartoned, shelf packs of 6 cartons, 10 shelf packs per case. (Blue flip-off seals)

STORAGE

Store the unopened vials at controlled room temperature 15°–30°C (59°–86°F). Protect from light. Solutions for infusion should be discarded 8 hours after preparation.

HANDLING AND DISPOSAL

Procedures for proper handling and disposal of anticancer drugs should be considered. Several guidelines on this subject have been published.[3-9] There is no general agreement that all of the procedures recommended in the guidelines are necessary or appropriate.

REFERENCES

1. Egorin, M.J., et al: Pharmacokinetics and dosage reduction of cis-diammine (1,1-cyclobutanedicarboxylato) platinum in patients with impaired renal function. Cancer Res 1984; 44:5432–5438.
2. Carboplatin, Etoposide, and Bleomycin for Treatment of Stage IIC Seminoma Complicated by Acute Renal Failure. Cancer Treatment Reports, Vol. 71, No. 11, pp.1123–1124, November 1987.
3. Recommendations for the Safe Handling of Parenteral Antineoplastic Drugs. NIH Publication No. 83–2621. For sale by the Superintendent of Documents, U.S. Government Printing Office, Washington, DC 20402.
4. AMA Council Report. Guidelines for Handling Parenteral Antineoplastics. JAMA 1985 March 15.
5. National Study Commission Cytotoxic Exposure—Recommendations for Handling Cytotoxic Agents. Available from Louis P. Jeffrey, Chairman, National Study Commission on Cytotoxic Exposure, Massachusetts College of Pharmacy and Allied Health Sciences, 179 Longwood Avenue, Boston, Massachusetts, 02115.
6. Clinical Oncological Society of Australia: Guidelines and Recommendations for Safe Handling of Antineoplastic Agents. Med. J. Australia 1983; 1:426–428.
7. Jones, R.B., et al: Safe Handling of Chemotherapeutic agents: A Report from the Mount Sinai Medical Center. CA—A Cancer Journal for Clinicians, 1983; (Sept/Oct) 258–263.
8. American Society of Hospital Pharmacists Technical Assistance Bulletin on Handling Cytotoxic Drugs in Hospitals. Am. J. Hosp. Pharm. 1990; 47:1033–1049.
9. OSHA Work-Practice Guidelines for Personnel Dealing with Cytotoxic (Antineoplastic) Drugs. Am. J. Hosp. Pharm. 1986; 43:1193–1204.

U.S. Patent Nos. 4,140,707
4,657,927

Shown in Product Identification Section, page 406

PLATINOL®   ℞
[plă'tĭ-nŏl'']
(cisplatin for injection, USP)

This is the full text of the latest Official Package Circular dated January 1991 [3070DIM-32].

> ### WARNING
> PLATINOL should be administered under the supervision of a qualified physician experienced in the use of cancer chemotherapeutic agents. Appropriate management of therapy and complications is possible only when adequate diagnostic and treatment facilities are readily available.
> Cumulative renal toxicity associated with PLATINOL is severe. Other major dose-related toxicities are myelosuppression, nausea, and vomiting.
> Ototoxicity, which may be more pronounced in children, and is manifested by tinnitus, and/or loss of high frequency hearing and occasionally deafness, is significant.
> *Anaphylactic-like* reactions to PLATINOL have been reported. Facial edema, bronchoconstriction, tachycardia, and hypotension may occur within minutes of PLATINOL administration. Epinephrine, corticosteroids, and antihistamines have been effectively employed to alleviate symptoms (see "**WARNINGS**" and "**ADVERSE REACTIONS**" sections).

DESCRIPTION

PLATINOL (cis-diamminedichloroplatinum) is a heavy metal complex containing a central atom of platinum surrounded by two chloride atoms and two ammonia molecules in the cis position. It is a white lyophilized powder with the molecular formula Pt $Cl_2H_6N_2$, and a molecular weight of 300.1. It is soluble in water or saline at 1 mg/mL and in dimethylformamide at 24 mg/mL. It has a melting point of 207°C.

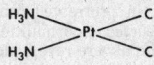

ACTION

PLATINOL has biochemical properties similar to that of bifunctional alkylating agents, producing interstrand and intrastrand cross-links in DNA. It is apparently cell-cycle nonspecific. Following a single IV dose, PLATINOL concentrates in liver, kidneys and large and small intestines in animals and humans. PLATINOL apparently has poor penetration into the CNS.

Plasma levels of radioactivity decay in a biphasic manner after an IV bolus dose of radioactive PLATINOL to patients. The initial plasma half-life is 25 to 49 minutes, and the postdistribution plasma half-life is 58 to 73 hours. During the postdistribution phase, greater than 90% of the radioactivity in the blood is protein bound. PLATINOL is excreted primarily in the urine. However, urinary excretion is incomplete with only 27% to 43% of the radioactivity being excreted within the first 5 days post dose in human beings. There are insufficient data to determine whether biliary or intestinal excretion occurs.

INDICATIONS

PLATINOL is indicated as palliative therapy to be employed as follows:

Metastatic Testicular Tumors—In established combination therapy with other approved chemotherapeutic agents in patients with metastatic testicular tumors who have already received appropriate surgical and/or radiotherapeutic procedures.

Metastatic Ovarian Tumors—In established combination therapy with other approved chemotherapeutic agents in patients with metastatic ovarian tumors who have already

---

ADVERSE EXPERIENCES IN PATIENTS WITH OVARIAN CANCER SWOG STUDY

		Paraplatin Arm Percent*	Cisplatin Arm Percent*	P-Values**
Bone Marrow				
Thrombocytopenia,	<100,000/mm³	59	35	<0.001
	<50,000/mm³	22	11	0.006
Neutropenia,	<2,000 cells/mm³	95	97	n.s.
	<1,000 cells/mm³	84	78	n.s.
Leukopenia,	<4,000 cells/mm³	97	97	n.s.
	<2,000 cells/mm³	76	67	n.s.
Anemia,	<11 g/dL	88	87	n.s.
	<8 g/dL	8	24	<0.001
Infections		18	21	n.s.
Bleeding		6	4	n.s.
Transfusions		25	33	n.s.
Gastrointestinal				
Nausea and vomiting		94	96	n.s.
Vomiting		82	91	0.007
Other GI side effects		40	48	n.s.
Neurologic				
Peripheral neuropathies		13	28	0.001
Ototoxicity		12	30	<0.001
Other sensory side effects		4	6	n.s.
Central neurotoxicity		23	29	n.s.
Renal				
Serum creatinine elevations		7	38	<0.001
Blood urea elevations		—	—	—
Hepatic				
Bilirubin elevations		5	3	n.s.
SGOT elevations		23	16	n.s.
Alkaline phosphatase elevations		29	20	n.s.
Electrolytes loss				
Sodium		—	—	—
Potassium		—	—	—
Calcium		—	—	—
Magnesium		58	77	<0.001
Other side effects				
Pain		54	52	n.s.
Asthenia		43	46	n.s.
Cardiovascular		23	30	n.s.
Respiratory		12	11	n.s.
Allergic		10	11	n.s.
Genitourinary		11	13	n.s.
Alopecia[+]		43	57	0.009
Mucositis		6	11	n.s.

*Values are in percent of evaluable patients
**n.s. = not significant, p > 0.05
[+]May have been affected by cyclophosphamide dosage delivered

PARAPLATIN®   **ADVERSE EXPERIENCES IN PATIENTS WITH OVARIAN CANCER**

		First Line Combination Therapy* Percent	Second Line Single Agent Therapy** Percent
Bone Marrow			
Thrombocytopenia,	$<100,000/mm^3$	66	62
	$<50,000/mm^3$	33	35
Neutropenia,	$<2,000$ cells/mm^3	96	67
	$<1,000$ cells/mm^3	82	21
Leukopenia,	$<4,000$ cells/mm^3	97	85
	$<2,000$ cells/mm^3	71	26
Anemia,	<11 g/dL	90	90
	<8 g/dL	14	21
Infections		16	5
Bleeding		8	5
Transfusions		35	44
Gastrointestinal			
Nausea and vomiting		93	92
Vomiting		83	81
Other GI side effects		46	21
Neurologic			
Peripheral neuropathies		15	6
Ototoxicity		12	1
Other sensory side effects		5	1
Central neurotoxicity		26	5
Renal			
Serum creatinine elevations		6	10
Blood urea elevations		17	22
Hepatic			
Bilirubin elevations		5	5
SGOT elevations		20	19
Alkaline phosphatase elevations		29	37
Electrolytes loss			
Sodium		10	47
Potassium		16	28
Calcium		16	31
Magnesium		61	43
Other side effects			
Pain		44	23
Asthenia		41	11
Cardiovascular		19	6
Respiratory		10	6
Allergic		11	2
Genitourinary		10	2
Alopecia		49	2
Mucositis		8	1

* **Use with cyclophosphamide for initial treatment of ovarian cancer:** Data are based on the experience of 393 patients with ovarian cancer (regardless of baseline status) who received initial combination therapy with PARAPLATIN and cyclophosphamide in two randomized controlled studies conducted by SWOG and NCIC (see "CLINICAL STUDIES" section). Combination with cyclophosphamide as well as duration of treatment may be responsible for the differences that can be noted in the adverse experience table.

** **Single agent use for the secondary treatment of ovarian cancer:** Data are based on the experience of 553 patients with previously treated ovarian carcinoma (regardless of baseline status) who received single-agent PARAPLATIN.

received appropriate surgical and/or radiotherapeutic procedures. An established combination consists of PLATINOL and doxorubicin hydrochloride. PLATINOL, as a single agent, is indicated as secondary therapy in patients with metastatic ovarian tumors refractory to standard chemotherapy who have not previously received PLATINOL therapy.

Advanced Bladder Cancer—PLATINOL is indicated as a single agent for patients with transitional cell bladder cancer which is no longer amenable to local treatments such as surgery and/or radiotherapy.

CONTRAINDICATIONS

PLATINOL is contraindicated in patients with preexisting renal impairment. PLATINOL should not be employed in myelosuppressed patients, or patients with hearing impairment.

PLATINOL is contraindicated in patients with a history of allergic reactions to PLATINOL or other platinum-containing compounds.

WARNINGS

PLATINOL produces cumulative nephrotoxicity which is potentiated by aminoglycoside antibiotics. The serum creatinine, BUN, creatinine clearance, and magnesium, sodium, potassium and calcium levels should be measured prior to initiating therapy, and prior to each subsequent course. At the recommended dosage, PLATINOL should not be given more frequently than once every 3 to 4 weeks (see "ADVERSE REACTIONS").

There are reports of severe neuropathies in patients in whom regimens are employed using higher doses of PLATINOL or greater dose frequencies than those recommended. These neuropathies may be irreversible and are seen as paresthesias in a stocking-glove distribution, areflexia, and loss of proprioception and vibratory sensation.

Loss of motor function has also been reported.

Anaphylactic-like reactions to PLATINOL have been reported. These reactions have occurred within minutes of administration to patients with prior exposure to PLATI-

NOL, and have been alleviated by administration of epinephrine, corticosteroids, and antihistamines.

Since ototoxicity of PLATINOL is cumulative, audiometric testing should be performed prior to initiating therapy and prior to each subsequent dose of drug (see "**ADVERSE REACTIONS**").

Safe use in human pregnancy has not been established. PLATINOL is mutagenic in bacteria and produces chromosome aberrations in animal cells in tissue culture. In mice PLATINOL is teratogenic and embryotoxic.

PLATINOL has not been studied for its carcinogenic potential but compounds with similar mechanisms of action and mutagenicity have been reported to be carcinogenic.

PRECAUTIONS

Peripheral blood counts should be monitored weekly. Liver function should be monitored periodically. Neurologic examination should also be performed regularly (see "**ADVERSE REACTIONS**").

Drug Interactions—Plasma levels of anticonvulsant agents may become subtherapeutic during cisplatin therapy.

ADVERSE REACTIONS

Nephrotoxicity—Dose-related and cumulative renal insufficiency is the major dose-limiting toxicity of PLATINOL® (cisplatin for injection, USP). Renal toxicity has been noted in 28% to 36% of patients treated with a single dose of 50 mg/m². It is first noted during the second week after a dose and is manifested by elevations in BUN and creatinine, serum uric acid and/or a decrease in creatinine clearance. **Renal toxicity becomes more prolonged and severe with repeated courses of the drug. Renal function must return to normal before another dose of PLATINOL can be given.** Impairment of renal function has been associated with renal tubular damage. The administration of PLATINOL using a 6- to 8-hour infusion with intravenous hydration, and mannitol has been used to reduce nephrotoxicity. However, renal toxicity still can occur after utilization of these procedures.

Ototoxicity—Ototoxicity has been observed in up to 31% of patients treated with a single dose of PLATINOL 50 mg/m², and is manifested by tinnitus and/or hearing loss in the high

frequency range (4,000 to 8,000 Hz). Decreased ability to hear normal conversational tones may occur occasionally. Deafness after the initial dose of PLATINOL has been reported rarely. Ototoxic effects may be more severe in children receiving PLATINOL. Hearing loss can be unilateral or bilateral and tends to become more frequent and severe with repeated doses. Ototoxicity may be enhanced with prior or simultaneous cranial irradiation. It is unclear whether PLATINOL-induced ototoxicity is reversible. Careful monitoring of audiometry should be performed prior to initiation of therapy and prior to subsequent doses of PLATINOL. Vestibular toxicity has also been reported.

Hematologic—Myelosuppression occurs in 25% to 30% of patients treated with PLATINOL. The nadirs in circulating platelets and leukocytes occur between days 18 to 23 (range 7.5 to 45) with most patients recovering by day 39 (range 13 to 62). Leukopenia and thrombocytopenia are more pronounced at higher doses (>50 mg/m²). Anemia (decrease of 2 g hemoglobin/100 mL) occurs at approximately the same frequency and with the same timing as leukopenia and thrombocytopenia.

In addition to anemia secondary to myelosuppression, a Coombs' positive hemolytic anemia has been reported. In the presence of cisplatin hemolytic anemia, a further course of treatment may be accompanied by increased hemolysis and this risk should be weighed by the treating physician.

Gastrointestinal—Marked nausea and vomiting occur in almost all patients treated with PLATINOL, and are occasionally so severe that the drug must be discontinued. Nausea and vomiting usually begin within 1 to 4 hours after treatment and last up to 24 hours. Various degrees of nausea and anorexia may persist for up to 1 week after treatment.

OTHER TOXICITIES

Vascular toxicities coincident with the use of PLATINOL in combination with other antineoplastic agents have been reported rarely. The events are clinically heterogeneous and may include myocardial infarction, cerebrovascular accident, thrombotic microangiopathy (HUS), or cerebral arteritis. Various mechanisms have been proposed for these vascular complications. There are also reports of Raynaud's phenomenon occurring in patients treated with the combination of bleomycin, vinblastine with or without PLATINOL. It has been suggested that hypomagnesemia developing coincident with the use of PLATINOL may be an added, although not essential, factor associated with this event. However, it is currently unknown if the cause of Raynaud's phenomenon in these cases is the disease, underlying vascular compromise, bleomycin, vinblastine, hypomagnesemia, or a combination of any of these factors.

Serum Electrolyte Disturbances—Hypomagnesemia, hypocalcemia, hyponatremia, hypokalemia and hypophosphatemia have been reported to occur in patients treated with PLATINOL and are probably related to renal tubular damage. Tetany has occasionally been reported in those patients with hypocalcemia and hypomagnesemia. Generally, normal serum electrolyte levels are restored by administering supplemental electrolytes and discontinuing PLATINOL. Inappropriate antidiuretic hormone syndrome has also been reported.

Hyperuricemia—Hyperuricemia has been reported to occur at approximately the same frequency as the increases in BUN and serum creatinine.

It is more pronounced after doses greater than 50 mg/m², and peak levels of uric acid generally occur between 3 to 5 days after the dose. Allopurinol therapy for hyperuricemia effectively reduces uric acid levels.

Neurotoxicity (see "**WARNINGS**" section)—Neurotoxicity, usually characterized by peripheral neuropathies, has been reported. The neuropathies usually occur after prolonged therapy (4 to 7 months); however, neurologic symptoms have been reported to occur after a single dose. PLATINOL therapy should be discontinued when the symptoms are first observed. Preliminary evidence suggests peripheral neuropathy may be irreversible in some patients.

Lhermitte's sign and autonomic neuropathy have also been reported.

Loss of taste and seizures have also been reported.

Ocular Toxicity—Optic neuritis, papilledema, and cerebral blindness have been reported infrequently in patients receiving standard recommended doses of PLATINOL. Improvement and/or total recovery usually occurs after discontinuing PLATINOL. Steroids with or without mannitol have been used; however, efficacy has not been established.

Blurred vision and altered color perception have been reported after the use of regimens with higher doses of PLATINOL or greater dose frequencies than those recommended in the package insert. The altered color perception manifests as a loss of color discrimination, particularly in the blue-yellow axis. The only finding on funduscopic exam is irregular retinal pigmentation of the macular area.

Anaphylactic-like Reactions—Anaphylactic-like reactions have been occasionally reported in patients previously ex-

Continued on next page

Bristol-Myers Oncology—Cont.

posed to PLATINOL. The reactions consist of facial edema, wheezing, tachycardia, and hypotension within a few minutes of drug administration. Reactions may be controlled by intravenous epinephrine, corticosteroids or antihistamines. Patients receiving PLATINOL should be observed carefully for possible anaphylactic-like reactions and supportive equipment and medication should be available to treat such a complication.

Other toxicities reported to occur infrequently are cardiac abnormalities, anorexia, elevated SGOT, and rash. Alopecia has also been reported.

DOSAGE AND ADMINISTRATION

Note: Needles or intravenous sets containing aluminum parts that may come in contact with PLATINOL® (cisplatin for injection, USP) should not be used for preparation or administration. Aluminum reacts with PLATINOL, causing precipitate formation and a loss of potency.

Metastatic Testicular Tumors—The usual PLATINOL dose for the treatment of testicular cancer in combination with other approved chemotherapeutic agents is 20 mg/m^2 IV daily for 5 days.

Metastatic Ovarian Tumors—An effective combination for the treatment of patients with metastatic ovarian tumors includes PLATINOL and doxorubicin hydrochloride in the following doses:

PLATINOL—50 mg/m^2 IV once every 3 weeks (day 1).

Doxorubicin hydrochloride—50 mg/m^2 IV once every 3 weeks (day 1).

For directions for the administration of doxorubicin hydrochloride, refer to the doxorubicin hydrochloride package insert.

In combination therapy, PLATINOL and doxorubicin hydrochloride are administered sequentially.

As a single agent, PLATINOL should be administered at a dose of 100 mg/m^2 IV once every 4 weeks.

Advanced Bladder Cancer—PLATINOL should be administered as a single agent at a dose of 50 to 70 mg/m^2 IV once every 3 to 4 weeks depending on the extent of prior exposure to radiation therapy and/or prior chemotherapy. For heavily pretreated patients an initial dose of 50 mg/m^2 repeated every 4 weeks is recommended.

Pretreatment hydration with 1 to 2 liters of fluid infused for 8 to 12 hours prior to a PLATINOL dose is recommended. The drug is then diluted in 2 liters of 5% Dextrose in ½ or ⅓ normal saline containing 37.5 g of mannitol, and infused over a 6- to 8-hour period. If diluted solution is not to be used within 6 hours, protect solution from light. Adequate hydration and urinary output must be maintained during the following 24 hours.

A repeat course of PLATINOL should not be given until the serum creatinine is below 1.5 mg/100 mL, and/or the BUN is below 25 mg/100 mL. A repeat course should not be given until circulating blood elements are at an acceptable level (platelets $\geq$100,000/mm^3, WBC $\geq$4,000/mm^3). Subsequent doses of PLATINOL should not be given until an audiometric analysis indicates that auditory acuity is within normal limits.

As with other potentially toxic compounds, caution should be exercised in handling the powder and preparing the solution of cisplatin. Skin reactions associated with accidental exposure to cisplatin may occur. The use of gloves is recommended. If cisplatin powder or solution contacts the skin or mucosae, immediately wash the skin or mucosae thoroughly with soap and water.

PREPARATION OF INTRAVENOUS SOLUTIONS

The 10 and 50 mg vials should be reconstituted with 10 mL or 50 mL of Sterile Water for Injection, USP, respectively. Each mL of the resulting solution will contain 1 mg of PLATINOL. Reconstitution as recommended results in a clear, colorless solution.

The reconstituted solution should be used intravenously only and should be administered by IV infusion over a 6- to 8-hour period. (See "**DOSAGE AND ADMINISTRATION.**")

STABILITY

Unopened vials of dry powder are stable for the lot life indicated on the package when stored at room temperature (27°C).

The reconstituted solution is stable for 20 hours at room temperature (27°C). Solution removed from the amber vial should be protected from light if it is not to be used within 6 hours.

Important note: Once reconstituted, the solution should be kept at room temperature (27°C). If the reconstituted solution is refrigerated, a precipitate will form.

Procedures for proper handling and disposal of anticancer drugs should be considered. Several guidelines on this subject have been published.[1–7] There is no general agreement that all of the procedures recommended in the guidelines are necessary or appropriate.

REFERENCES

1. Recommendations for the Safe Handling of Parenteral Antineoplastic Drugs. NIH Publication No. 83-2621. For sale by the Superintendent of Documents. US Government Printing Office, Washington, D.C. 20402.
2. AMA Council Report. Guidelines for Handling Parenteral Antineoplastics. *JAMA.* 1985; March 15.
3. National Study Commission on Cytotoxic Exposure—Recommendations for Handling Cytotoxic Agents. Available from Louis P. Jeffrey, ScD, Chairman, National Study Commission on Cytotoxic Exposure, Massachusetts College of Pharmacy and Allied Health Sciences, 179 Longwood Avenue, Boston, Massachusetts 02115.
4. Clinical Oncological Society of Australia. Guidelines and Recommendations for Safe Handling of Antineoplastic Agents. *Med J Australia.* 1983;1:426–428.
5. Jones RB, et al: Safe Handling of Chemotherapeutic Agents: A Report from the Mount Sinai Medical Center. *CA—A Cancer Journal for Clinicians.* 1983; (Sept/Oct);258–263.
6. American Society of Hospital Pharmacists Technical Assistance Bulletin on Handling Cytotoxic and Hazardous Drugs. *Am J Hosp Pharm.* 1990;47:1033–1049.
7. OSHA Work-Practice Guidelines for Personnel Dealing with Cytotoxic (Antineoplastic) Drugs. *Am J Hosp Pharm.* 1986;43:1193–1204.

HOW SUPPLIED

PLATINOL (cisplatin for injection, USP)

NDC 0015-3070-20—Each amber vial contains 10 mg of cisplatin.

NDC 0015-3072-20—Each amber vial contains 50 mg of cisplatin.

U.S. Patent No. 4,177,263
N-B312-A

PLATINOL®-AQ ℞

[pla-ti-nol -AQ]
(cisplatin injection, USP)

This is the full text of the latest Official Package Circular dated January 1991 [3072DIM-09].

WARNING

PLATINOL should be administered under the supervision of a qualified physician experienced in the use of cancer chemotherapeutic agents. Appropriate management of therapy and complications is possible only when adequate diagnostic and treatment facilities are readily available.

Cumulative renal toxicity associated with PLATINOL is severe. Other major dose-related toxicities are myelosuppression, nausea, and vomiting.

Ototoxicity, which may be more pronounced in children, and is manifested by tinnitus, and/or loss of high frequency hearing and occasionally deafness, is significant.

Anaphylactic-like reactions to PLATINOL have been reported. Facial edema, bronchoconstriction, tachycardia, and hypotension may occur within minutes of PLATINOL administration. Epinephrine, corticosteroids, and antihistamines have been effectively employed to alleviate symptoms (see "**WARNINGS**" and "**ADVERSE REACTIONS**" sections).

DESCRIPTION

Cisplatin (cis-diamminedichloroplatinum) is a heavy metal complex containing a central atom of platinum surrounded by two chloride atoms and two ammonia molecules in the cis position. It is a white powder with the molecular formula Pt $Cl_2H_6N_2$, and a molecular weight of 300.1. It is soluble in water or saline at 1 mg/mL and in dimethylformamide at 24 mg/mL. It has a melting point of 207°C. PLATINOL-AQ is a sterile aqueous solution, each mL containing 1 mg cisplatin and 9 mg sodium chloride. HCl and/or sodium hydroxide added to adjust pH.

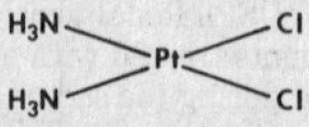

ACTION

PLATINOL has biochemical properties similar to that of bifunctional alkylating agents, producing interstrand and intrastrand cross-links in DNA. It is apparently cell-cycle nonspecific. Following a single IV dose, PLATINOL concentrates in liver, kidneys, and large and small intestines in animals and humans. PLATINOL apparently has poor penetration into the CNS.

Plasma levels of radioactivity decay in a biphasic manner after an IV bolus dose of radioactive PLATINOL to patients. The initial plasma half-life is 25 to 49 minutes, and the postdistribution plasma half-life is 58 to 73 hours. During the postdistribution phase, greater than 90% of the radioactivity in the blood is protein bound. PLATINOL is excreted primarily in the urine. However, urinary excretion is incomplete with only 27% to 43% of the radioactivity being excreted within the first 5 days post dose in human beings. There are insufficient data to determine whether biliary or intestinal excretion occurs.

INDICATIONS

PLATINOL is indicated as palliative therapy to be employed as follows:

Metastatic Testicular Tumors—In established combination therapy with other approved chemotherapeutic agents in patients with metastatic testicular tumors who have already received appropriate surgical and/or radiotherapeutic procedures.

Metastatic Ovarian Tumors—In established combination therapy with other approved chemotherapeutic agents in patients with metastatic ovarian tumors who have already received appropriate surgical and/or radiotherapeutic procedures. An established combination consists of PLATINOL-AQ and doxorubicin hydrochloride. PLATINOL, as a single agent, is indicated as secondary therapy in patients with metastatic ovarian tumors refractory to standard chemotherapy who have not previously received PLATINOL therapy.

Advanced Bladder Cancer—PLATINOL is indicated as a single agent for patients with transitional cell bladder cancer which is no longer amenable to local treatments such as surgery and/or radiotherapy.

CONTRAINDICATIONS

PLATINOL is contraindicated in patients with preexisting renal impairment. PLATINOL should not be employed in myelosuppressed patients, or patients with hearing impairment.

PLATINOL is contraindicated in patients with a history of allergic reactions to PLATINOL or other platinum-containing compounds.

WARNINGS

PLATINOL produces cumulative nephrotoxicity which is potentiated by aminoglycoside antibiotics. The serum creatinine, BUN, creatinine clearance, and magnesium, sodium, potassium, and calcium levels should be measured prior to initiating therapy, and prior to each subsequent course. At the recommended dosage, PLATINOL should not be given more frequently than once every 3 to 4 weeks (see "**ADVERSE REACTIONS**").

There are reports of severe neuropathies in patients in whom regimens are employed using higher doses of PLATINOL or greater dose frequencies than those recommended. These neuropathies may be irreversible and are seen as paresthesias in a stocking-glove distribution, areflexia, and loss of proprioception and vibratory sensation.

Loss of motor function has also been reported.

Anaphylactic-like reactions to PLATINOL have been reported. These reactions have occurred within minutes of administration to patients with prior exposure to PLATINOL, and have been alleviated by administration of epinephrine, corticosteroids, and antihistamines.

Since ototoxicity of PLATINOL is cumulative, audiometric testing should be performed prior to initiating therapy and prior to each subsequent dose of drug (see "**ADVERSE REACTIONS**").

Safe use in human pregnancy has not been established.

PLATINOL is mutagenic in bacteria and produces chromosome aberrations in animal cells in tissue culture. In mice PLATINOL® (cisplatin injection, USP) is teratogenic and embryotoxic.

PLATINOL has not been studied for its carcinogenic potential but compounds with similar mechanisms of action and mutagenicity have been reported to be carcinogenic.

PRECAUTIONS

Peripheral blood counts should be monitored weekly. Liver function should be monitored periodically. Neurologic examination should also be performed regularly (see "**ADVERSE REACTIONS**").

Drug Interactions—Plasma levels of anticonvulsant agents may become subtherapeutic during cisplatin therapy.

ADVERSE REACTIONS

Nephrotoxicity—Dose-related and cumulative renal insufficiency is the major dose-limiting toxicity of PLATINOL. Renal toxicity has been noted in 28% to 36% of patients treated with a single dose of 50 mg/m^2. It is first noted during the second week after a dose and is manifested by elevations in BUN and creatinine, serum uric acid, and/or a decrease in creatinine clearance. **Renal toxicity becomes more prolonged and severe with repeated courses of the drug. Renal function must return to normal before another dose of PLATINOL can be given.**

Impairment of renal function has been associated with renal tubular damage. The administration of PLATINOL using a 6- to 8-hour infusion with intravenous hydration, and manni-

tol has been used to reduce nephrotoxicity. However, renal toxicity still can occur after utilization of these procedures.

Ototoxicity—Ototoxicity has been observed in up to 31% of patients treated with a single dose of PLATINOL 50 mg/m^2, and is manifested by tinnitus and/or hearing loss in the high frequency range (4,000 to 8,000 Hz). Decreased ability to hear normal conversational tones may occur occasionally. Deafness after the initial dose of PLATINOL has been reported rarely. Ototoxic effects may be more severe in children receiving PLATINOL. Hearing loss can be unilateral or bilateral and tends to become more frequent and severe with repeated doses. Ototoxicity may be enhanced with prior or simultaneous cranial irradiation. It is unclear whether PLATINOL-induced ototoxicity is reversible. Careful monitoring of audiometry should be performed prior to initiation of therapy and prior to subsequent doses of PLATINOL.

Vestibular toxicity has also been reported.

Hematologic—Myelosuppression occurs in 25% to 30% of patients treated with PLATINOL. The nadirs in circulating platelets and leukocytes occur between days 18 to 23 (range 7.5 to 45) with most patients recovering by day 39 (range 13 to 62). Leukopenia and thrombocytopenia are more pronounced at higher doses (> 50 mg/m^2). Anemia (decrease of 2 g hemoglobin/100 mL) occurs at approximately the same frequency and with the same timing as leukopenia and thrombocytopenia.

In addition to anemia secondary to myelosuppression, a Coombs' positive hemolytic anemia has been reported. In the presence of cisplatin hemolytic anemia, a further course of treatment may be accompanied by increased hemolysis and this risk should be weighed by the treating physician.

Gastrointestinal—Marked nausea and vomiting occur in almost all patients treated with PLATINOL, and are occasionally so severe that the drug must be discontinued. Nausea and vomiting usually begin within 1 to 4 hours after treatment and last up to 24 hours. Various degrees of nausea and anorexia may persist for up to 1 week after treatment.

OTHER TOXICITIES

Vascular toxicities coincident with the use of PLATINOL in combination with other antineoplastic agents have been reported rarely. The events are clinically heterogeneous and may include myocardial infarction, cerebrovascular accident, thrombotic microangiopathy (HUS), or cerebral arteritis. Various mechanisms have been proposed for these vascular complications. There are also reports of Raynaud's phenomenon occurring in patients treated with the combination of bleomycin, vinblastine with or without PLATINOL. It has been suggested that hypomagnesemia developing coincident with the use of PLATINOL may be an added, although not essential, factor associated with this event. However, it is currently unknown if the cause of Raynaud's phenomenon in these cases is the disease, underlying vascular compromise, bleomycin, vinblastine, hypomagnesemia, or a combination of any of these factors.

Serum Electrolyte Disturbances—Hypomagnesemia, hypocalcemia, hyponatremia, hypokalemia and hypophosphatemia have been reported to occur in patients treated with PLATINOL®-AQ (cisplatin injection, USP) and are probably related to renal tubular damage. Tetany has occasionally been reported in those patients with hypocalcemia and hypomagnesemia. Generally, normal serum electrolyte levels are restored by administering supplemental electrolytes and discontinuing PLATINOL.

Inappropriate antidiuretic hormone syndrome has also been reported.

Hyperuricemia—Hyperuricemia has been reported to occur at approximately the same frequency as the increases in BUN and serum creatinine.

It is more pronounced after doses greater than 50 mg/m^2, and peak levels of uric acid generally occur between 3 to 5 days after the dose. Allopurinol therapy for hyperuricemia effectively reduces uric acid levels.

Neurotoxicity (see "**WARNINGS**" section)—Neurotoxicity, usually characterized by peripheral neuropathies, has been reported. The neuropathies usually occur after prolonged therapy (4 to 7 months); however, neurologic symptoms have been reported to occur after a single dose. PLATINOL therapy should be discontinued when the symptoms are first observed. Preliminary evidence suggests peripheral neuropathy may be irreversible in some patients.

Lhermitte's sign and autonomic neuropathy have also been reported.

Loss of taste and seizures have also been reported.

Ocular Toxicity—Optic neuritis, papilledema, and cerebral blindness have been reported infrequently in patients receiving standard recommended doses of PLATINOL. Improvement and/or total recovery usually occurs after discontinuing PLATINOL. Steroids with or without mannitol have been used; however, efficacy has not been established.

Blurred vision and altered color perception have been reported after the use of regimens with higher doses of PLATINOL or greater dose frequencies than those recommended in the package insert. The altered color perception manifests as a loss of color discrimination, particularly in the blue-yellow axis. The only finding on funduscopic exam is irregular retinal pigmentation of the macular area.

Anaphylactic-like Reactions—Anaphylactic-like reactions have been occasionally reported in patients previously exposed to PLATINOL® (cistplatin injection, USP). The reactions consist of facial edema, wheezing, tachycardia, and hypotension within a few minutes of drug administration. Reactions may be controlled by intravenous epinephrine, corticosteroids, or antihistamines. Patients receiving PLATINOL should be observed carefully for possible anaphylactic-like reactions and supportive equipment and medication should be available to treat such a complication.

Other toxicities reported to occur infrequently are cardiac abnormalities, anorexia, elevated SGOT, and rash. Alopecia has also been reported.

DOSAGE AND ADMINISTRATION

Note: Needles or intravenous sets containing aluminum parts that may come in contact with PLATINOL should not be used for preparation or administration. Aluminum reacts with PLATINOL, causing precipitate formation and a loss of potency.

Metastatic Testicular Tumors—The usual PLATINOL® (cisplatin injection, USP) dose for the treatment of testicular cancer in combination with other approved chemotherapeutic agents is 20 mg/m^2 IV daily for 5 days.

Metastatic Ovarian Tumors—An effective combination for the treatment of patients with metastatic ovarian tumors includes PLATINOL and doxorubicin hydrochloride in the following doses:

PLATINOL—50 mg/m^2 IV once every 3 weeks (day 1).

Doxorubicin hydrochloride—50 mg/m^2 IV once every 3 weeks (day 1).

For directions for the administration of doxorubicin hydrochloride, refer to the doxorubicin hydrochloride package insert.

In combination therapy, PLATINOL and doxorubicin hydrochloride are administered sequentially.

As a single agent, PLATINOL should be administered at a dose of 100 mg/m^2 IV once every 4 weeks.

Advanced Bladder Cancer—PLATINOL should be administered as a single agent at a dose of 50 to 70 mg/m^2 IV once every 3 to 4 weeks depending on the extent of prior exposure to radiation therapy and/or prior chemotherapy. For heavily pretreated patients an initial dose of 50 mg/m^2 repeated every 4 weeks is recommended.

Pretreatment hydration with 1 to 2 liters of fluid infused for 8 to 12 hours prior to a PLATINOL dose is recommended. The drug is then diluted in 2 liters of 5% Dextrose in $\frac{1}{2}$ or $\frac{1}{3}$ normal saline containing 37.5 g of mannitol, and infused over a 6- to 8-hour period. If diluted solution is not to be used within 6 hours, protect solution from light. Do not dilute PLATINOL®-AQ (cisplatin injection, USP) in just 5% Dextrose injection. Adequate hydration and urinary output must be maintained during the following 24 hours.

A repeat course of PLATINOL should not be given until the serum creatinine is below 1.5 mg/100 mL, and/or the BUN is below 25 mg/100 mL. A repeat course should not be given until circulating blood elements are at an acceptable level (platelets $\geq$ 100,000/mm^3, WBC $\geq$ 4,000/mm^3). Subsequent doses of PLATINOL should not be given until an audiometric analysis indicates that auditory acuity is within normal limits.

As with other potentially toxic compounds, caution should be exercised in handling the aqueous solution. Skin reactions associated with accidental exposure to cisplatin may occur. The use of gloves is recommended. If cisplatin solution contacts the skin or mucosae, immediately wash the skin or mucosae thoroughly with soap and water.

The aqueous solution should be used intravenously only and should be administered by IV infusion over a 6- to 8-hour period.

STABILITY

PLATINOL-AQ is a sterile, multidose vial without preservatives. Store at 15°C–25°C. Do not refrigerate. Protect unopened container from light.

The cisplatin remaining in the amber vial following initial entry is stable for 28 days protected from light or for seven days under fluorescent room light.

Procedures for proper handling and disposal of anticancer drugs should be considered. Several guidelines on this subject have been published.[1–7] There is no general agreement that all of the procedures recommended in the guidelines are necessary or appropriate.

REFERENCES

1. Recommendations for the Safe Handling of Parenteral Antineoplastic Drugs. NIH Publication No. 83-2621. For sale by the Superintendent of Documents, US Government Printing Office, Washington, DC 20402.
2. AMA Council Report. Guidelines for Handling Parenteral Antineoplastics. *JAMA*. 1985; March 15.
3. National Study Commission on Cytotoxic Exposure—Recommendations for Handling Cytotoxic Agents. Available from Louis P. Jeffrey, ScD, Chairman, National Study Commission on Cytotoxic Exposure, Massachusetts College of Pharmacy and Allied Health Sciences, 179 Longwood Avenue, Boston, Massachusetts 02115.
4. Clinical Oncological Society of Australia. Guidelines and Recommendations for Safe Handling of Antineoplastic Agents. *Med J Australia*. 1983;1:426–428.
5. Jones RB, et al: Safe Handling of Chemotherapeutic Agents: A Report from the Mount Sinai Medical Center. *CA—A Cancer Journal for Clinicians*. 1983; (Sept/Oct) 258–263.
6. American Society of Hospital Pharmacists Technical Assistance Bulletin on Handling Cytotoxic and Hazardous Drugs. *Am J Hosp Pharm*. 1990;47:1033–1049.
7. OSHA Work-Practice Guidelines for Personnel Dealing with Cytotoxic (Antineoplastic) Drugs. *Am J Hosp Pharm*. 1986; 43:1193–1204.

HOW SUPPLIED

PLATINOL-AQ (cisplatin injection).

NDC 0015-3220-22—Each multidose vial contains 50 mg of cisplatin.

NDC 0015-3221-22—Each multidose vial contains 100 mg of cisplatin.

U.S. Patent No. 4,177,263

N-B313-A

Shown in Product Identification Section, page 406

TESLAC® TABLETS ℞

[tez'lak]

Testolactone Tablets USP

DESCRIPTION

Teslac (Testolactone Tablets) is available for oral administration as tablets providing 50 mg testolactone per tablet. Testolactone is a synthetic antineoplastic agent that is structurally distinct from the androgen steroid nucleus in possessing a six-membered lactone ring in place of the usual five-membered carbocyclic D-ring. Testolactone is chemically designated as 13-hydroxy-3-oxo-13,17-secoandrosta-1,4-dien-17-oic acid δ-lactone. Graphic formula:

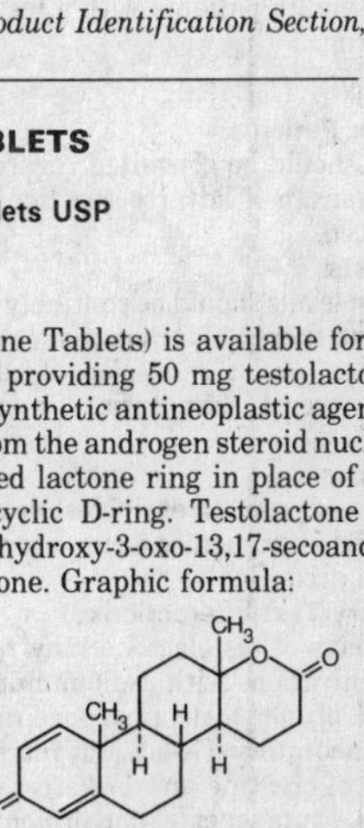

$C_{19}H_{24}O_3$ **MW 300.40** **CAS-968-93-4**

Inactive ingredients: calcium stearate, cornstarch, gelatin, and lactose.

Testolactone is a white, odorless, crystalline solid, soluble in ethanol and slightly soluble in water.

CLINICAL PHARMACOLOGY

Although the precise mechanism by which testolactone produces its clinical antineoplastic effects has not been established, its principal action is reported to be inhibition of steroid aromatase activity and consequent reduction in estrone synthesis from adrenal androstenedione, the major source of estrogen in postmenopausal women. Based on *in vitro* studies, the aromatase inhibition may be noncompetitive and irreversible. This phenomenon may account for the persistence of testolactone's effect on estrogen synthesis after drug withdrawal.

Despite some similarity to testosterone, testolactone has no *in vivo* androgenic effect. No other hormonal effects have been reported in clinical studies in patients receiving testolactone. In one study, testolactone administered orally (1000 mg/day) was reported to increase renal tubular reabsorption of calcium but to have no effect on serum calcium concentration. The mechanism of the hypocalciuric effect is unknown. No clinical effects in humans of testolactone on adrenal function have been reported; however, one study noted an increase in urinary excretion of 17-ketosteroids in most of the patients treated with 150 mg/day orally.

Testolactone is well absorbed from the gastrointestinal tract. It is metabolized to several derivatives in the liver, all of which preserve the lactone D-ring. These metabolites, as well as some unmetabolized drug, are excreted in the urine. Additional pharmacokinetic data in humans are unavailable.

For information concerning carcinogenesis, mutagenesis, pregnancy, and lactation, see the corresponding PRECAUTIONS sections.

In animals, parenteral but not oral testolactone reduced cortisone acetate induced hepatic glycogen deposits. In animal tests conducted to detect any hormonal activity for testolactone, some evidence of antiandrogenic and antiglucocorticoid activity was seen; increased growth rate in the newborn was suggested. However there was no clear manifestation of androgenic, estrogenic or antiestrogenic, progestational or antiprogestational, gonadotropin-like or antigonadotropic effects. Testolactone did not demonstrate anti-in-

Continued on next page

Bristol-Myers Oncology—Cont.

flammatory, mineralocorticoid-like, or glucocorticoid-like properties.

INDICATIONS AND USAGE

Teslac (Testolactone Tablets) is recommended as adjunctive therapy in the palliative treatment of advanced or disseminated breast cancer in postmenopausal women when hormonal therapy is indicated. It may also be used in women who were diagnosed as having had disseminated breast carcinoma when premenopausal, in whom ovarian function has been subsequently terminated.

Teslac (Testolactone Tablets) was found to be effective in approximately 15% of patients with advanced or disseminated mammary cancer evaluated according to the following criteria: 1) those with a measurable decrease in size of all demonstrable tumor masses; 2) those in whom more than 50% of non-osseous lesions decreased in size although all bone lesions remained static; and 3) those in whom more than 50% of total lesions improved while the remainder were static.

CONTRAINDICATIONS

Testolactone is contraindicated in the treatment of breast cancer in men and in patients with a history of hypersensitivity to the drug.

PRECAUTIONS

Information for Patients

The physician should be consulted regarding missed doses. Notify the physician if adverse reactions occur or become more pronounced.

Laboratory Tests

Plasma calcium levels should be routinely determined in any patient receiving therapy for mammary cancer, particularly during periods of active remission of bony metastases. If hypercalcemia occurs, appropriate measures should be instituted.

Drug Interactions

When administered concurrently, testolactone may increase the effects of oral anticoagulants; monitor and adjust anticoagulant dosage accordingly.

Drug/Laboratory Test Interactions

Physiologic effects of testolactone may result in decreased estradiol concentrations with radioimmunoassays for estradiol, increased plasma calcium concentrations (see PRECAUTIONS, Laboratory Tests), and increased 24-hour urinary excretion of creatine and 17-ketosteroids.

Carcinogenesis, Mutagenesis, Impairment of Fertility

No long-term animal studies have been performed to evaluate carcinogenic potential or mutagenesis. Testolactone did not affect fertility in male or female rats.

Pregnancy: Teratogenic Effects, Category C

In rats, testolactone has been shown to produce increased fetal mortality, increased abnormal fetal development, and increased mortality in growing pups when given at doses 5 to 15 times the recommended human dose. In rabbits, no teratologic effects were observed at doses 2.5 to 7.5 times the recommended human dose. There are no adequate and well controlled studies in pregnant women. Testolactone is intended for use only in postmenopausal women and should not be used during pregnancy.

Nursing Mothers

It is not known whether this drug is excreted in human milk. Because many drugs are excreted in human milk, a decision should be made whether or not to discontinue nursing.

Pediatric Use

Safety and effectiveness in children have not been established.

ADVERSE REACTIONS

Certain signs and symptoms have been reported in association with the use of this drug but, in these instances, it is often impossible to determine the relationship of the underlying disease and drug administration to the reported reaction. Such reactions include maculopapular erythema, increase in blood pressure, paresthesia, aches and edema of the extremities, glossitis, anorexia and nausea and vomiting. Alopecia alone and with associated nail growth disturbance have been reported rarely; these side effects subsided without interruption of treatment.

OVERDOSAGE

There have been no reports of acute overdosage with testolactone tablets.

DOSAGE AND ADMINISTRATION

The recommended oral dose is 250 mg qid.

In order to evaluate the response, therapy with testolactone should be continued for a minimum of three months unless there is active progression of the disease.

HOW SUPPLIED

TESLAC (Testolactone Tablets USP), **50 mg/tablet:** bottles of 100 (NDC 0003-0690-50). Each round, white, biconvex tablet is imprinted with the identification number **690.**

Storage

Store at room temperature; avoid excessive heat.

VEPESID® ℞
(ETOPOSIDE)
For Injection and Capsules

> **WARNINGS**
> VePesid (etoposide) should be administered under the supervision of a qualified physician experienced in the use of cancer chemotherapeutic agents. Severe myelosuppression with resulting infection or bleeding may occur.

DESCRIPTION

VePesid (etoposide) (also commonly known as VP-16) is a semisynthetic derivative of podophyllotoxin used in the treatment of certain neoplastic diseases. It is 4′-demethylepipodophyllotoxin 9-[4,6-0-(R)-ethylidene-β-D-glucopyranoside]. It is very soluble in methanol and chloroform, slightly soluble in ethanol, and sparingly soluble in water and ether. It is made more miscible with water by means of organic solvents. It has a molecular weight of 588.58 and a molecular formula of $C_{29}H_{32}O_{13}$.

VePesid may be administered either intravenously or orally. VePesid for Injection is available in 100 mg (5 mL) sterile, multiple dose vials. The pH of the clear yellow solution is 3 to 4. Each mL contains 20 mg etoposide, 2 mg citric acid, 30 mg benzyl alcohol, 80 mg polysorbate 80/tween 80, 650 mg polyethylene glycol 300, and 30.5 percent (v/v) alcohol. Vial headspace contains nitrogen.

VePesid is also available as 50 mg pink capsules. Each liquid filled, soft gelatin capsule contains 50 mg of etoposide in a vehicle consisting of citric acid, glycerin, purified water, and polyethylene glycol 400. The soft gelatin capsules contain gelatin, glycerin, sorbitol, purified water and parabens (ethyl and propyl) with the following dye system: iron oxide (red) and titanium dioxide; the capsules are printed with edible ink.

The structural formula is:

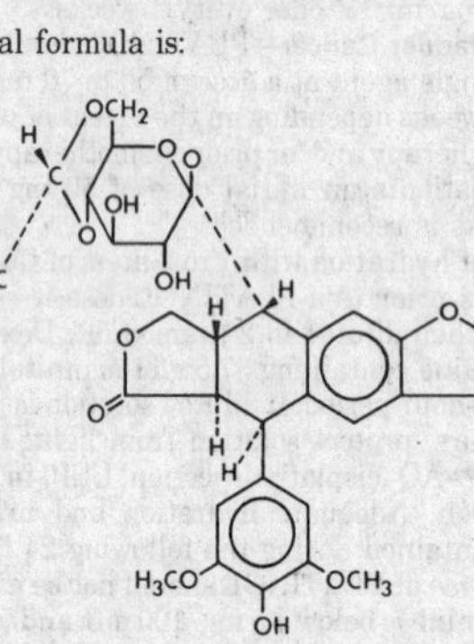

CLINICAL PHARMACOLOGY

VePesid has been shown to cause metaphase arrest in chick fibroblasts. Its main effect, however, appears to be at the G_2 portion of the cell cycle in mammalian cells. Two different dose-dependent responses are seen. At high concentrations (10 μg/mL or more), lysis of cells entering mitosis is observed. At low concentrations (0.3 to 10 μg/mL), cells are inhibited from entering prophase. It does not interfere with microtubular assembly. The predominant macromolecular effect of VePesid appears to be DNA synthesis inhibition.

Pharmacokinetics: On intravenous administration, the disposition of etoposide is best described as a biphasic process with a distribution half-life of about 1.5 hours and terminal elimination half-life ranging from 4 to 11 hours. Total body clearance values range from 33 to 48 mL/min or 16 to 36 mL/min/m^2 and, like the terminal elimination half-life, are independent of dose over a range 100–600 mg/m^2. Over the same dose range, the areas under the plasma concentration vs time curves (AUC) and the maximum plasma concentration (Cmax) values increase linearly with dose. Etoposide does not accumulate in the plasma following daily administration of 100 mg/m^2 for 4 to 5 days.

The mean volumes of distribution at steady state fall in the range of 18 to 29 liters or 7 to 17 L/m^2. Etoposide enters the CSF poorly. Although it is detectable in CSF and intracerebral tumors, the concentrations are lower than in extracerebral tumors and in plasma. Etoposide concentrations are higher in normal lung than in lung metastases and are similar in primary tumors and normal tissues of the myometrium. In vitro, etoposide is highly protein bound (97%) to human plasma proteins. An inverse relationship between plasma albumin levels and etoposide renal clearance is found in children. In a study determining the effect of other therapeutic agents on the *in vitro* binding of carbon-14 labeled etoposide to human serum proteins, only phenylbutazone, sodium salicylate and aspirin displaced protein-bound etoposide at concentrations achieved *in vivo.*[1]

Etoposide binding ratio correlates directly with serum albumin in patients with cancer and in normal volunteers. The unbound fraction of etoposide significantly correlated with bilirubin in a population of cancer patients.[2,3]

After intravenous administration of ^{3}H-etoposide (70–290 mg/m^2), mean recoveries of radioactivity in the urine range from 42 to 67%, and fecal recoveries range from 0 to 16% of the dose. Less than 50% of an intravenous dose is excreted in the urine as etoposide with mean recoveries of 8 to 35% within 24 hours.

In children, approximately 55% of the dose is excreted in the urine as etoposide in 24 hours. The mean renal clearance of etoposide is 7 to 10 mL/min/m^2 or about 35% of the total body clearance over a dose range of 80 to 600 mg/m^2. Etoposide, therefore, is cleared by both renal and nonrenal processes, ie, metabolism and biliary excretion. The effect of renal disease on plasma etoposide clearance is not known. Biliary excretion appears to be a minor route of etoposide elimination. Only 6% or less of an intravenous dose is recovered in the bile as etoposide. Metabolism accounts for most of the nonrenal clearance of etoposide. The major urinary metabolite of etoposide in adults and children is the hydroxy acid [4′-demethylepipodophyllic acid-9-(4, 6-0-(R)-ethylidene-β-D-glucopyranoside)], formed by opening of the lactone ring. It is also present in human plasma, presumably as the **trans** isomer. Glucuronide and/or sulfate conjugates of etoposide are excreted in human urine and represent 5 to 22% of the dose.

After either intravenous infusion or oral capsule administration, the Cmax and AUC values exhibit marked intra- and inter-subject variability. This results in variability in the estimates of the absolute oral bioavailability of etoposide oral capsules.

Cmax and AUC values for orally administered etoposide capsules consistently fall in the same range as the Cmax and AUC values for an intravenous dose of one-half the size of the oral dose. The overall mean value of oral capsule bioavailability is approximately 50% (range 25–75%). The bioavailability of etoposide capsules appears to be linear up to a dose of at least 250 mg/m^2.

There is no evidence of a first-pass effect for etoposide. For example, no correlation exists between the absolute oral bioavailability of etoposide capsules and nonrenal clearance. No evidence exists for any other differences in etoposide metabolism and excretion after administration of oral capsules as compared to intravenous infusion.

In adults, the total body clearance of etoposide is correlated with creatinine clearance, serum albumin concentration, and nonrenal clearance. In children, elevated serum SGPT levels are associated with reduced drug total body clearance. Prior use of cisplatin may also result in a decrease of etoposide total body clearance in children.

INDICATION AND USAGE

VePesid is indicated in the management of the following neoplasms:

Refractory Testicular Tumors—VePesid Injection in combination therapy with other approved chemotherapeutic agents in patients with refractory testicular tumors who have already received appropriate surgical, chemotherapeutic, and radiotherapeutic therapy.

Adequate data on the use of VePesid Capsules in the treatment of testicular cancer are not available.

Small Cell Lung Cancer—VePesid Injection and/or Capsules in combination with other approved chemotherapeutic agents as first line treatment in patients with small cell lung cancer.

CONTRAINDICATIONS

VePesid is contraindicated in patients who have demonstrated a previous hypersensitivity to etoposide or any component of the formulation.

WARNINGS

Patients being treated with VePesid must be frequently observed for myelosuppression both during and after therapy. Dose-limiting bone marrow suppression is the most significant toxicity associated with VePesid therapy. Therefore, the following studies should be obtained at the start of therapy and prior to each subsequent dose of VePesid: platelet count, hemoglobin, white blood cell count and differential. The occurrence of a platelet count below 50,000/mm^3 or an absolute neutrophil count below 500/mm^3 is an indication to withhold further therapy until the blood counts have sufficiently recovered.

Physicians should be aware of the possible occurrence of an anaphylactic reaction manifested by chills, fever, tachycardia, bronchospasm, dyspnea, and hypotension. (See "**ADVERSE REACTIONS**" section.) Treatment is symptomatic. The infusion should be terminated immediately, followed by the administration of pressor agents, corticosteroids, antihistamines, or volume expanders at the discretion of the physician.

For parenteral administration, VePesid should be given only by slow intravenous infusion (usually over a 30 to 60 minute

period) since hypotension has been reported as a possible side effect of rapid intravenous injection.

Pregnancy: Pregnancy "Category D." VePesid can cause fetal harm when administered to a pregnant woman. VePesid has been shown to be teratogenic in mice and rats. There are no adequate and well-controlled studies in pregnant women. If this drug is used during pregnancy, or if the patient becomes pregnant while receiving this drug, the patient should be apprised of the potential hazard to the fetus. Women of childbearing potential should be advised to avoid becoming pregnant.

VePesid is teratogenic and embryocidal in rats and mice at doses of 1 to 3% of the recommended clinical dose based on body surface area.

In a teratology study in SPF rats, VePesid was administered intravenously at doses of 0.13, 0.4, 1.2, and 3.6 mg/kg/day on days 6 to 15 of gestation. VePesid caused dose-related maternal toxicity, embryotoxicity, and teratogenicity at dose levels of 0.4 mg/kg/day and higher. Embryonic resorptions were 90 and 100% at the 2 highest dosages. At 0.4 and 1.2 mg/kg, fetal weights were decreased and fetal abnormalities including decreased weight, major skeletal abnormalities, exencephaly, encephalocele, and anophthalmia occurred. Even at the lowest dose tested, 0.13 mg/kg, a significant increase in retarded ossification was observed.

VePesid administered as a single intraperitoneal, injection in Swiss-Albino mice at dosages of 1, 1.5 and 2 mg/kg on days 6, 7, or 8 of gestation caused dose-related embryotoxicity, cranial abnormalities, and major skeletal malformations.

PRECAUTIONS

General: In all instances where the use of VePesid is considered for chemotherapy, the physician must evaluate the need and usefulness of the drug against the risk of adverse reactions. Most such adverse reactions are reversible if detected early. If severe reactions occur, the drug should be reduced in dosage or discontinued and appropriate corrective measures should be taken according to the clinical judgment of the physician. Reinstitution of VePesid therapy should be carried out with caution, and with adequate consideration of the further need for the drug and alertness as to possible recurrence of toxicity.

Laboratory Tests: Periodic complete blood counts should be done during the course of VePesid treatment. They should be performed prior to therapy and at appropriate intervals during and after therapy. At least one determination should be done prior to each dose of VePesid.

Carcinogenesis, Mutagenesis, Impairment of Fertility: Carcinogenicity tests with VePesid have not been conducted in laboratory animals. VePesid should be considered a potential carcinogen in humans. The occurrence of acute leukemia with or without a preleukemic phase has been reported rarely in patients treated with VePesid in association with other antineoplastic agents.

The mutagenic and genotoxic potential of VePesid has been established in mammalian cells. VePesid caused aberrations in chromosome number and structure in embryonic murine cells and human hematopoietic cells; gene mutations in Chinese hamster ovary cells; and DNA damage by strand breakage and DNA-protein cross-links in mouse leukemia cells. VePesid also caused a dose-related increase in sister chromatid exchanges in Chinese hamster ovary cells.

Treatment of Swiss-Albino mice with 1.5 mg/kg IP of VePesid on day 7 of gestation increased the incidence of intrauterine death and fetal malformations as well as significantly decreased the average fetal body weight. Maternal weight gain was not affected.

Treatment of pregnant SPF rats with 1.2 mg/kg/day IV of VePesid for 10 days led to a prenatal mortality of 92%, and 50% of the implanting fetuses were abnormal.

Pregnancy: Pregnancy "Category D." (See "**WARNINGS**" section.)

Nursing Mothers: It is not known whether this drug is excreted in human milk. Because many drugs are excreted in human milk and because of the potential for serious adverse reactions in nursing infants from VePesid, a decision should be made whether to discontinue nursing or to discontinue the drug, taking into account the importance of the drug to the mother.

Pediatric Use: Safety and effectiveness in children have not been established.

VePesid Injection contains polysorbate 80. In premature infants, a life-threatening syndrome consisting of liver and renal failure, pulmonary deterioration, thrombocytopenia, and ascites has been associated with an injectable vitamin E product containing polysorbate 80.

ADVERSE REACTIONS

The following data on adverse reactions are based on both oral and intravenous administration of VePesid as a single agent, using several different dose schedules for treatment of a wide variety of malignancies.

Hematologic Toxicity: Myelosuppression is dose related and dose limiting, with granulocyte nadirs occurring 7 to 14 days after drug administration and platelet nadirs occurring 9 to 16 days after drug administration. Bone marrow recovery is usually complete by day 20, and no cumulative toxicity has been reported.

The occurrence of acute leukemia with or without a preleukemic phase has been reported rarely in patients treated with VePesid in association with other antineoplastic agents.

Gastrointestinal Toxicity: Nausea and vomiting are the major gastrointestinal toxicities. The severity of such nausea and vomiting is generally mild to moderate with treatment discontinuation required in 1% of patients. Nausea and vomiting can usually be controlled with standard antiemetic therapy. Gastrointestinal toxicities are slightly more frequent after oral administration than after intravenous infusion.

Hypotension: Transient hypotension following rapid intravenous administration has been reported in 1% to 2% of patients. It has not been associated with cardiac toxicity or electrocardiographic changes. No delayed hypotension has been noted. To prevent this rare occurrence, it is recommended that VePesid be administered by slow intravenous infusion over a 30- to 60-minute period. If hypotension occurs, it usually responds to cessation of the infusion and administration of fluids or other supportive therapy as appropriate. When restarting the infusion, a slower administration rate should be used.

Allergic Reactions: Anaphylactic-like reactions characterized by chills, fever, tachycardia, bronchospasm, dyspnea and/or hypotension have been reported to occur in 0.7% to 2% of patients receiving intravenous VePesid and in less than 1% of the patients treated with the oral capsules. These reactions have usually responded promptly to the cessation of the infusion and administration of pressor agents, corticosteroids, antihistamines, or volume expanders as appropriate; however, the reactions can be fatal. Hypertension and/or flushing have also been reported. Blood pressure usually normalizes within a few hours after cessation of the infusion. Anaphylactic-like reactions have occurred during the initial infusion of VePesid.

Facial/tongue swelling, coughing, diaphoresis, cyanosis, tightness in throat, laryngospasm, back pain and/or loss of consciousness have sometimes occurred in association with the above reactions. In addition, an apparent hypersensitivity-associated apnea has been reported rarely.

Rash, urticaria, and/or pruritus have infrequently been reported at recommended doses. At investigational doses, a generalized pruritic erythematous maculopapular rash, consistent with perivasculitis, has been reported.

Alopecia: Reversible alopecia, sometimes progressing to total baldness, was observed in up to 66% of patients.

Other Toxicities: The following adverse reactions have been infrequently reported: aftertaste, fever, pigmentation, abdominal pain, constipation, dysphagia, transient cortical blindness, and optic neuritis, and a single report of radiation recall dermatitis.

Hepatic toxicity, generally in patients receiving higher doses of the drug than those recommended, has been reported with VePesid. Metabolic acidosis has also been reported in patients receiving higher doses.

The incidences of adverse reactions in the table that follows are derived from multiple data bases from studies in 2,081 patients when VePesid was used either orally or by injection as a single agent.

ADVERSE DRUG EFFECT	PERCENT RANGE OF REPORTED INCIDENCE
Hematologic toxicity	
Leukopenia (less than 1,000 WBC/mm^3)	3–17
Leukopenia (less than 4,000 WBC/mm^3)	60–91
Thrombocytopenia (less than 50,000 platelets/mm^3)	1–20
Thrombocytopenia (less than 100,000 platelets/mm^3)	22–41
Anemia	0–33
Gastrointestinal toxicity	
Nausea and vomiting	31–43
Abdominal pain	0–2
Anorexia	10–13
Diarrhea	1–13
Stomatitis	1–6
Hepatic	0–3
Alopecia	8–66
Peripheral neurotoxicity	1–2
Hypotension	1–2
Allergic reaction	1–2

OVERDOSAGE

No proven antidotes have been established for VePesid overdosage.

DOSAGE AND ADMINISTRATION

Note: Plastic devices made of acrylic or ABS (a polymer composed of acrylonitrile, butadiene, and styrene) have been reported to crack and leak when used with undiluted VePesid Injection.

VePesid for Injection: The usual dose of VePesid for Injection in testicular cancer in combination with other approved chemotherapeutic agents ranges from 50 to 100 mg/m^2/day on days 1 through 5 to 100 mg/m^2/day on days 1, 3, and 5. In small cell lung cancer, the VePesid for Injection dose in combination with other approved chemotherapeutic drugs ranges from 35 mg/m^2/day for 4 days to 50 mg/m^2/day for 5 days.

Chemotherapy courses are repeated at 3- to 4-week intervals after adequate recovery from any toxicity.

VePesid Capsules: In small cell lung cancer, the recommended dose of VePesid Capsules is two times the IV dose rounded to the nearest 50 mg.

The dosage, by either route, should be modified to take into account the myelosuppressive effects of other drugs in the combination or the effects of prior x-ray therapy or chemotherapy which may have compromised bone marrow reserve.

Administration Precautions: As with other potentially toxic compounds, caution should be exercised in handling and preparing the solution of VePesid. Skin reactions associated with accidental exposure to VePesid may occur. The use of gloves is recommended. If VePesid solution contacts the skin or mucosa, immediately wash the skin or mucosa thoroughly with soap and water.

Preparation for Intravenous Administration: VePesid for Injection must be diluted prior to use with either 5% Dextrose Injection, USP, or 0.9% Sodium Chloride Injection, USP, to give a final concentration of 0.2 or 0.4 mg/mL. If solutions are prepared at concentrations above 0.4 mg/mL, precipitation may occur. Hypotension following rapid intravenous administration has been reported, hence, it is recommended that the VePesid solution be administered over a 30- to 60-minute period. A longer duration of administration may be used if the volume of fluid to be infused is a concern.

VePesid should not be given by rapid intravenous injection.

Parenteral drug products should be inspected visually for particulate matter and discoloration (see "**DESCRIPTION**" section) prior to administration whenever solution and container permit.

Stability: Unopened vials of VePesid for Injection are stable for 24 months at room temperature (25°C). Vials diluted as recommended to a concentration of 0.2 or 0.4 mg/mL are stable for 96 and 24 hours, respectively, at room temperature (25°C) under normal room fluorescent light in both glass and plastic containers.

VePesid Capsules must be stored under refrigeration 2°–8°C (36°–46°F). The capsules are stable for 24 months under such refrigeration conditions.

Procedures for proper handling and disposal of anticancer drugs should be considered. Several guidelines on this subject have been published[4–10]. There is no general agreement that all of the procedures recommended in the guidelines are necessary or appropriate.

HOW SUPPLIED

VePesid (etoposide) For Injection

NDC 0015-3095-20—100 mg/5 mL Sterile Multiple Dose Vial, 10's

VePesid (etoposide) Capsules

NDC 0015-3091-45—50 mg pink capsules with "BRISTOL 3091" printed in black in blisterpacks of 20 individually labeled blisters, each containing one capsule.

Capsules are to be stored under refrigeration 2°–8°C (36°–46°F).

DO NOT FREEZE.

Dispense in child-resistant containers.

For information on package sizes available, refer to the current price schedule.

REFERENCES

1. Gaver RC; Deeb G; "The effect of other drugs on the *in vitro* binding of 14C-etoposide to human serum proteins." Proc Am Assoc Cancer Res; 30:A2132, 1989
2. Stewart CF; Pieper JA; Arbuck SG; Evans WE; "Altered protein binding of etoposide in patients with cancer." Clin Pharmacol Ther; 45:49–55 1989
3. Stewart CF; Arbuck SG; Fleming RA; Evans WE; "Prospective evaluation of a model for predicting etoposide plasma protein binding in cancer patients." Proc Am Assoc Cancer Res; 30:A958 1989
4. Recommendations for the Safe Handling of Parenteral Antineoplastic Drugs, NIH Publication No. 83-2621. For sale by the Superintendent of Documents, US Government Printing Office, Washington, D.C. 20402.
5. AMA Council Report. Guidelines for Handling Parenteral Antineoplastics. JAMA 1985 March 15.
6. National Study Commission on Cytotoxic Exposure—Recommendations for Handling Cytotoxic Agents. Available from Louis P. Jeffrey, Sc.D., Chairman, Na-

Continued on next page

Bristol-Myers Oncology—Cont.

tional Study Commission on Cytotoxic Exposure, Massachusetts College of Pharmacy and Allied Health Sciences, 179 Longwood Avenue, Boston, Massachusetts 02115.
7. Clinical Oncological Society of Australia. Guidelines and Recommendations for Safe Handling of Antineoplastic Agents. Med J Australia 1983; 1:426–428.
8. Jones RB, et al; Safe handling of chemotherapeutic agents: A report from the Mount Sinai Medical Center. CA—A Cancer Journal for Clinicians 1983; (Sept/Oct) 258–263.
9. American Society of Hospital Pharmacists Technical Assistance Bulletin on Handling Cytotoxic and Hazardous Drugs. Am J Hosp Pharm 1990; 47:1033–1049.
10. OSHA Work-Practice Guidelines for Personnel Dealing with Cytotoxic (Antineoplastic) Drugs. Am J Hosp Pharm 1986; 43:1193–1204.

Distributed by:
BRISTOL LABORATORIES
ONCOLOGY PRODUCTS
A Bristol-Myers Squibb Co.
Princeton, N.J. 08543
U.S.A.

Shown in Product Identification Section, page 406

Bristol-Myers Products
(A Bristol-Myers Squibb Company)
345 PARK AVENUE
NEW YORK, NY 10154

BUFFERIN® OTC
[*bŭf'fĕr-ĭn*]
Analgesic

COMPOSITION
Active Ingredient: Each coated tablet or caplet contains Aspirin 325 mg in a formulation buffered with Calcium Carbonate, Magnesium Oxide and Magnesium Carbonate.
Other Ingredients: Benzoic Acid, Citric Acid, Corn Starch, FD&C Blue No. 1, Hydroxypropyl Methylcellulose, Magnesium Stearate, Mineral Oil, Polysorbate 20, Povidone, Propylene Glycol, Simethicone Emulsion, Sodium Phosphate, Sorbitan Monolaurate, Titanium Dioxide. May also contain: Carnauba Wax, Zinc Stearate.

INDICATIONS
For temporary relief of headaches, pain and fever of colds, muscle aches, minor arthritis pain and inflammation, menstrual pain and toothaches.

WARNINGS
Children and teenagers should not use this medicine for chicken pox or flu symptoms before a doctor is consulted about Reye syndrome, a rare but serious illness reported to be associated with aspirin. KEEP THIS AND ALL OTHER MEDICATIONS OUT OF THE REACH OF CHILDREN. IN CASE OF ACCIDENTAL OVERDOSE, SEEK PROFESSIONAL ASSISTANCE OR CONTACT A POISON CONTROL CENTER IMMEDIATELY. As with any drug, if you are pregnant or nursing a baby, seek the advice of a health professional before using this product. IT IS ESPECIALLY IMPORTANT NOT TO USE ASPIRIN DURING THE LAST 3 MONTHS OF PREGNANCY UNLESS SPECIFICALLY DIRECTED TO DO SO BY A DOCTOR BECAUSE IT MAY CAUSE PROBLEMS IN THE UNBORN CHILD OR COMPLICATIONS DURING DELIVERY. Do not take this product for pain for more than 10 days (for adults) or 5 days (for children) or for fever for more than 3 days unless directed by a doctor. If pain or fever persists or gets worse, or new symptoms occur, or if redness or swelling is present, consult a doctor because these could be signs of a serious condition. Consult a dentist promptly for toothache. Do not give this product to children for the pain of arthritis unless directed by a doctor. Do not take this product if you are allergic to aspirin, have asthma, have stomach problems (such as heartburn, upset stomach or stomach pain) that persist or recur, or if you have ulcers or bleeding problems unless directed by a doctor. If ringing in the ears or loss of hearing occurs, consult a doctor before taking or giving any more of this product.

DRUG INTERACTION PRECAUTION
This product should not be taken by any adult or child who is taking a prescription drug for anticoagulation (thinning of blood) diabetes, gout or arthritis unless directed by a doctor.

DIRECTIONS
Adults: 2 tablets or caplets with water every 4 hours while symptoms persist, not to exceed 12 tablets or caplets in 24 hours, or as directed by a doctor. Children 6 to under 12 years of age: One tablet or caplet with water every 4 hours, not to exceed 5 tablets or caplets in 24 hours or as directed by a doctor. Children under 6: Consult a doctor.

HOW SUPPLIED
BUFFERIN is supplied as:
Coated circular white tablet with letter "B" debossed on one surface.
NDC 19810-0073-2 Bottle of 12's
NDC 19810-0093-3 Bottle of 30's
NDC 19810 0093-4 Bottle of 50's
NDC 19810-0073-5 Bottle of 100's
NDC 19810-0073-6 Bottle of 200's
NDC 19810-0093-2 Bottle of 275's
NDC 19810-0073-7 Bottle of 1000's for hospital and clinical use.
NDC 19810-0073-9 Boxed 150 × 2 tablet foil pack for hospital and clinical use.
Coated scored white caplet with letter "B" debossed on each side of scoring.
NDC 19810-0072-7 Bottle of 30's
NDC 19810-0072-8 Bottle of 50's
NDC 19810-0072-3 Bottle of 100's
All consumer sizes have child resistant closures except 100's for tablets and 50's for caplets which are sizes recommended for households without young children. Store at room temperature.
Professional samples available on request.
Also described in PDR For Nonprescription Drugs.

PROFESSIONAL LABELING

1. BUFFERIN® FOR RECURRENT TRANSIENT ISCHEMIC ATTACKS

INDICATION
For reducing the risk of recurrent transient ischemic attacks (TIA's) or stroke in men who have had transient ischemia of the brain due to fibrin platelet emboli. There is inadequate evidence that aspirin or buffered aspirin is effective in reducing TIA's in women at the recommended dosage. There is no evidence that aspirin or buffered aspirin is of benefit in the treatment of completed strokes in men or women.

CLINICAL TRIALS
The indication is supported by the results of a Canadian study (1) in which 585 patients with threatened stroke were followed in a randomized clinical trial for an average of 26 months to determine whether aspirin or sulfinpyrazone, singly or in combination, was superior to placebo in preventing transient ischemic attacks, stroke, or death. The study showed that, although sulfinpyrazone had no statistically significant effect, aspirin reduced the risk of continuing transient ischemic attacks, stroke, or death by 19 percent and reduced the risk of stroke or death by 31 percent. Another aspirin study carried out in the United States with 178 patients, showed a statistically significant number of "favorable outcomes," including reduced transient ischemic attacks, stroke, and death (2).

PRECAUTIONS
Patients presenting with signs and symptoms of TIA's should have a complete medical and neurologic evaluation. Consideration should be given to other disorders that resemble TIA's. Attention should be given to risk factors: it is important to evaluate and treat, if appropriate, other diseases associated with TIA's and stroke, such as hypertension and diabetes.
Concurrent administration of absorbable antacids at therapeutic doses may increase the clearance of salicylates in some individuals. The concurrent administration of nonabsorbable antacids may alter the rate of absorption of aspirin, thereby resulting in a decreased acetylsalicylic acid/salicylate ratio in plasma. The clinical significance of these decreases in available aspirin is unknown.
Aspirin at dosages of 1,000 milligrams per day has been associated with small increases in blood pressure, blood urea nitrogen, and serum uric acid levels. It is recommended that patients placed on long-term aspirin treatment be seen at regular intervals to assess changes in these measurements.

ADVERSE REACTIONS
At dosages of 1,000 milligrams or higher of aspirin per day, gastrointestinal side effects include stomach pain, heartburn, nausea and/or vomiting, as well as increased rates of gross gastrointestinal bleeding.

DOSAGE AND ADMINISTRATION
Adult oral dosage for men is 1,300 milligrams a day, in divided doses of 650 milligrams twice a day or 325 milligrams four times a day.

REFERENCES
(1) The Canadian Cooperative Study Group. "A Randomized Trial of Aspirin and Sulfinpyrazone in Threatened Stroke," *New England Journal of Medicine,* 299:53–59, 1978.
(2) Fields, W.S., et al., "Controlled Trial of Aspirin in Cerebral Ischemia," *Stroke* 8:301–316, 1977.

2. BUFFERIN® FOR MYOCARDIAL INFARCTION

INDICATION
Aspirin is indicated to reduce the risk of death and/or nonfatal myocardial infarction in patients with a previous infarction or unstable angina pectoris.

CLINICAL TRIALS
The indication is supported by the results of six, large, randomized multicenter, placebo-controlled studies[1–7] involving 10,816, predominantly male, post-myocardial infarction (MI) patients and one randomized placebo-controlled study of 1,266 men with unstable angina. Therapy with aspirin was begun at intervals after the onset of acute MI varying from less than 3 days to more than 5 years and continued for periods of from less than one year to four years. In the unstable angina study, treatment was started within 1 month after the onset of unstable angina and continued for 12 weeks and complicating conditions such as congestive heart failure were not included in the study.
Aspirin therapy in MI patients was associated with about a 20 percent reduction in the risk of subsequent death and/or nonfatal reinfarction, a median absolute decrease of 3 percent from the 12 to 22 percent event rates in the placebo groups. In the aspirin-treated unstable angina patients the reduction in risk was about 50 percent, a reduction in the event rate of 5% from the 10% rate in the placebo group over the 12 weeks of the study.
Daily dosage of aspirin in the post-myocardial infarction studies was 300 mg. in one study and 900 and 1500 mg. in five studies. A dose of 325 mg. was used in the study of unstable angina.

ADVERSE REACTIONS
Gastrointestinal Reactions: Doses of 1000 mg. per day of aspirin caused gastrointestinal symptoms and bleeding that in some cases were clinically significant. In the largest post-infarction study (The Aspirin Myocardial Infaraction Study (AMIS) with 4,500 people), the percentage incidences of gastrointestinal symptoms for the aspirin (1000 mg. of a standard, solid-tablet formulation) and placebo-treated subjects, respectively, were: stomach pain (14.5%; 4.4%); heartburn (11.9%; 4.8%); nausea and/or vomiting (7.6%; 2.1%); hospitalization for gastrointestinal disorder (4.8%; 3.5%). In the AMIS and other trials, aspirin treated patients had increased rates of gross gastrointestinal bleeding. Symptoms and signs of gastrointestinal irritation were not significantly increased in subjects treated for unstable angina with buffered aspirin in solution.
Cardiovascular and Biochemical:
In the AMIS trial, the dosage of 1000 mg. per day of aspirin was associated with small increases in systolic blood pressure (BP) (average 1.5 to 2.1 mm) and diastolic BP (0.5 to 0.6 mm), depending upon whether maximal or last available readings were used. Blood urea nitrogen and uric acid levels were also increased, but by less than 1.0 mg%.
Subjects with marked hypertension or renal insufficiency had been excluded from the trial so that the clinical importance of these observations for such subjects or for any subjects treated over more prolonged periods is not known. It is recommended that patients placed on long-term aspirin treatment, even at doses of 300 mg. per day, be seen at regular intervals to assess changes in these measurements.

REFERENCES
1. Elwood P.C., et al., "A Randomized Controlled Trial of Acetylsalicylic Acid in the Secondary Prevention of Mortality from Myocardial Infarction," British Medical Journal, 1:436–440, 1974. 2. The Coronary Drug Project Reserach Group, "Aspirin in Coronary Heart Disease," Journal of Chronic Disease, 29:625–642, 1976. 3. Breddin K, et al., "Secondary Prevention of Myocardial Infarction; Comparison of Acetylsalicylic Acid Phenprocoumon and Placebo," Thromb. Haemost., 41:225–236, 1979. 4. Aspirin Myocardial Infarction Study Research Group, "A Randomized, Controlled Trial of Aspirin in Persons Recovered from Myocardial Infarction," Journal American Medical Association, 243:661–669, 1980. 5. Elwood P.C., and Sweetnam, P.M., "Aspirin and Secondary Mortality after Myocardial Infarction," Lancet, pp. 1313–1315, December 22–29, 1979. 6. The Persantine-Aspirin Reinfarction Study Research Group. "Persantine and Aspirin in Coronary Heart Disease," Circulation 62;449–460, 1980. 7. Lewis H.D., et al., "Protective Effects of Aspirin Against Acute Myocardial Infarction and Death in Men with Unstable Angina, Results of a Veterans Administration Cooperative Study," New England Journal of Medicine, 309;396–403, 1983.

ADMINISTRATION AND DOSAGE
Although most of the studies used dosages exceeding 300 mg., two trials used only 300 mg. and pharmacologic data indicate that this dose inhibits platelet function fully. Therefore, 300 mg. or a conventional 325 mg. aspirin dose is a reasonable, routine dose that would minimize gastrointestinal adverse reactions.

Shown in Product Identification Section, page 406

BUFFERIN® AF Nite Time   OTC

COMPOSITION

Active Ingredients: Each caplet contains Acetaminophen 500 mg. and Diphenhydramine Citrate 38 mg.
Other Ingredients: Benzoic Acid, Carnauba Wax, Corn Starch, D&C Yellow No. 10, D&C Yellow No. 10 Aluminum Lake, FD&C Blue No. 1, FD&C Blue No. 1 Aluminum Lake, Hydroxypropyl Methylcellulose, Methylparaben, Magnesium Stearate, Propylene Glycol, Propylparaben, Simethicone Emulsion, Stearic Acid, Titanium Dioxide. Remove cotton and recap bottle.

INDICATIONS

For temporary relief of occasional minor aches and pains accompanied by sleeplessness.

WARNINGS

KEEP THIS AND ALL OTHER MEDICATIONS OUT OF THE REACH OF CHILDREN. IN CASE OF ACCIDENTAL OVERDOSE, SEEK PROFESSIONAL ASSISTANCE OR CONTACT A POISON CONTROL CENTER IMMEDIATELY. PROMPT MEDICAL ATTENTION IS CRITICAL FOR ADULTS AS WELL AS FOR CHILDREN EVEN IF YOU DO NOT NOTICE ANY SIGNS OR SYMPTOMS. As with any drug, if you are pregnant or nursing a baby, seek the advice of a health professional before using this product. Do not give this product to children under 12 years of age or use for more than 10 days unless directed by a doctor. Consult a doctor if symptoms persist or get worse or if new ones occur, or if sleeplessness persists continuously for more than 2 weeks because these may be symptoms of serious underlying medical illnesses. Do not take this product if you have asthma, glaucoma, emphysema, chronic pulmonary disease, shortness of breath, difficulty in breathing, or difficulty in urination due to enlargement of the prostate gland unless directed by a doctor. Avoid alcoholic beverages while taking this product. Do not take this product if you are taking sedatives or tranquilizers, without first consulting your doctor.

DIRECTIONS

Adults: 2 caplets at bedtime if needed or as directed by a doctor.

OVERDOSE

MUCOMYST (acetylcysteine) As An Antidote For Acetaminophen Overdose)

Acetaminophen is rapidly absorbed from the upper gastrointestinal tract with peak plasma levels occurring between 30 and 60 minutes after therapeutic doses and usually within 4 hours following an overdose. The parent compound, which is nontoxic, is extensively metabolized in the liver to form principally the sulfate and glucuronide conjugates which are also nontoxic and are rapidly excreted in the urine. A small fraction of an ingested dose is metabolized in the liver by the cytochrome P-450 mixed function oxidase enzyme system to form a reactive, potentially toxic, intermediate metabolite which preferentially conjugates with hepatic glutathione to form the nontoxic cysteine and mercapturic acid derivatives which are then excreted by the kidney. Therapeutic doses of acetaminophen do not saturate the glucuronide and sulfate conjugation pathways and do not result in the formation of sufficient reactive metabolite to deplete glutathione stores. However, following ingestion of a large overdose (150 mg/kg or greater) the glucuronide and sulfate conjugation pathways are saturated resulting in a larger fraction of the drug being metabolized via the P-450 pathway. The increased formation of reactive metabolite may deplete the hepatic stores of glutathione with subsequent binding of the metabolite to protein molecules within the hepatocyte resulting in cellular necrosis. Acetylcysteine has been shown to reduce the extent of liver injury following acetaminophen overdose. Early symptoms following a potentially hepatotoxic overdose may include: nausea, vomiting, diaphoresis and general malaise. Clinical and laboratory evidence of hepatic toxicity may not be apparent until 48 to 72 hours postingestion. In adults and adolescents, regardless of the quantity of acetaminophen reported to have been ingested, administer MUCOMYST® acetylcysteine immediately. MUCOMYST acetylcysteine therapy should be initiated and continued for a full course of therapy. Its effectiveness depends on early administration, with benefit seen principally in patients treated within 16 hours of the overdose.

If acetaminophen plasma assay capability is not available, and the estimated acetaminophen ingestion exceeds 150 mg/kg, MUCOMYST acetylcysteine therapy should be initiated and continued for a full course of therapy.

For full prescribing information, refer to the MUCOMYST package insert. Do not await the results of assays for acetaminophen level before initiating treatment with MUCOMYST acetylcysteine. The following additional procedures are recommended: The stomach should be emptied promptly by lavage or by induction of emesis with syrup of ipecac. A serum acetaminophen assay should be obtained as early as possible, but no sooner than four hours following ingestion. Liver function studies should be obtained initially and repeated at 24-hour intervals.

For additional emergency information call your regional poison center or toll-free (1-800-525-6115) to the Rocky Mountain Poison Center for assistance in diagnosis and for directions in the use of MUCOMYST acetylcysteine as an antidote.

HOW SUPPLIED

BUFFERIN® A/F Nite Time is supplied as: Light blue coated caplets with "BUFFERIN® Nite Time" imprinted in dark blue on one side.
NDC 19810-0084-1 Bottles of 24's
NDC 19810-0084-2 Bottles of 50's
The 50 caplet size does not have a child resistant closure and is recommended for households without young children.
Store at room temperature.
Shown in Product Identification Section, Page 406

Arthritis Strength BUFFERIN®   OTC

[*bŭf'fĕr-ĭn*]
Analgesic

COMPOSITION

Active Ingredients: Aspirin (500 mg) in a formulation buffered with Calcium Carbonate, Magnesium Oxide and Magnesium Carbonate.
Other Ingredients: Benzoic Acid, Citric Acid, Corn Starch, FD&C Blue No. 1, Hydroxypropyl Methylcellulose, Magnesium Stearate, Mineral Oil, Polysorbate 20, Povidone, Propylene Glycol, Simethicone Emulsion, Sodium Phosphate, Sorbitan Monolaurate, Titanium Dioxide. May also contain: Carnauba Wax, Zinc Stearate.

INDICATIONS

For temporary relief of the minor aches and pains, stiffness, swelling and inflammation of arthritis.

WARNINGS

Children and teenagers should not use this medicine for chicken pox or flu symptoms before a doctor is consulted about Reye syndrome, a rare but serious illness reported to be associated with aspirin. KEEP THIS AND ALL OTHER MEDICATIONS OUT OF THE REACH OF CHILDREN. IN CASE OF ACCIDENTAL OVERDOSE, SEEK PROFESSIONAL ASSISTANCE OR CONTACT A POISON CONTROL CENTER IMMEDIATELY. As with any drug, if you are pregnant or nursing a baby, seek the advice of a health professional before using this product.
IT IS ESPECIALLY IMPORTANT NOT TO USE ASPIRIN DURING THE LAST 3 MONTHS OF PREGNANCY UNLESS SPECIFICALLY DIRECTED TO DO SO BY A DOCTOR BECAUSE IT MAY CAUSE PROBLEMS IN THE UNBORN CHILD OR COMPLICATIONS DURING DELIVERY. Do not take this product for pain for more than 10 days or for fever for more than 3 days unless directed by a doctor. If pain or fever persists or gets worse, if new symptoms occur, or if redness or swelling is present, consult a doctor because these could be signs of a serious condition. Do not take this product if you are allergic to aspirin, have asthma, have stomach problems (such as heartburn, upset stomach or stomach pain) that persist or recur, or if you have ulcers or bleeding problems, unless directed by a doctor. If ringing in the ears or loss of hearing occurs, consult a doctor before taking any more of this product.

DRUG INTERACTION PRECAUTION

Do not take this product if you are taking a prescription drug for anticoagulation (thinning of blood), diabetes, gout or arthritis unless directed by a doctor.

DIRECTIONS

Adults: 2 caplets with water every 6 hours while symptoms persist, not to exceed 8 caplets in 24 hours, or as directed by a doctor. Children under 12 years of age: Consult a doctor.

HOW SUPPLIED

Arthritis Strength BUFFERIN® is supplied as:
White coated caplet "ASB" debossed on one side.
NDC 19810-0051-1 Bottle of 40's
NDC 19810-0051-2 Bottle of 100's
The 40 caplet size does not have a child resistant closure and is recommended for households without young children.
Store at room temperature.
Also described in PDR For Nonprescription Drugs.
Shown in Product Identification Section, page 406

Extra Strength BUFFERIN®   OTC

[*bŭf'fĕr-ĭn*]
Analgesic

COMPOSITION

Active Ingredients: Aspirin (500 mg) in a formulation buffered with Calcium Carbonate, Magnesium Oxide and Magnesium Carbonate.
Other Ingredients: Benzoic Acid, Citric Acid, Corn Starch, FD&C Blue No. 1, Hydroxypropyl Methylcellulose, Magnesium Stearate, Mineral Oil, Polysorbate 20, Povidone, Propylene Glycol, Simethicone Emulsion, Sodium Phosphate, Sorbitan Monolaurate, Titanium Dioxide. May also contain: Carnauba Wax, Zinc Stearate.

INDICATIONS

For temporary relief of headaches, pain and fever of colds, muscle aches, arthritis pain and inflammation, menstrual pain and toothaches.

WARNINGS

Children and teenagers should not use this medicine for chicken pox or flu symptoms before a doctor is consulted about Reye syndrome, a rare but serious illness reported to be associated with aspirin. KEEP THIS AND ALL OTHER MEDICATIONS OUT OF THE REACH OF CHILDREN. IN CASE OF ACCIDENTAL OVERDOSE, SEEK PROFESSIONAL ASSISTANCE OR CONTACT A POISON CONTROL CENTER IMMEDIATELY. As with any drug, if you are pregnant or nursing a baby, seek the advice of a health professional before using this product. IT IS ESPECIALLY IMPORTANT NOT TO USE ASPIRIN DURING THE LAST 3 MONTHS OF PREGNANCY UNLESS SPECIFICALLY DIRECTED TO DO SO BY A DOCTOR BECAUSE IT MAY CAUSE PROBLEMS IN THE UNBORN CHILD OR COMPLICATIONS DURING DELIVERY. Do not take this product for more than 10 days or for fever for more than 3 days unless directed by a doctor. If pain or fever persists or gets worse, if new symptoms occur, or if redness or swelling is present, consult a doctor because these could be signs of a serious condition. Consult a dentist promptly for toothache. Do not take this product if you are allergic to aspirin, have asthma, have stomach problems (such as heartburn, upset stomach or stomach pain) that persist or recur, or if you have ulcers or bleeding problems, unless directed by a doctor. If ringing in the ears or loss of hearing occurs, consult a doctor before taking any more of this product.

DRUG INTERACTION PRECAUTION

Do not take this product if you are taking a prescription drug for anticoagulation (thinning of blood), diabetes, gout or arthritis unless directed by a doctor.

DIRECTIONS

Adults: 2 tablets with water every 6 hours while symptoms persist, not to exceed 8 tablets in 24 hours, or as directed by a doctor. Children 12 years of age: Consult a doctor.

HOW SUPPLIED

Extra Strength BUFFERIN® is supplied as:
White elongated coated tablet with "ESB" debossed on one side.
NDC 19810-0074-1 Bottle of 30's
NDC 19810-0074-4 Bottle of 50's
NDC 19810-0074-3 Bottle of 100's
All sizes have child resistant closures except 60's which is recommended for households without young children.
Store at room temperature.
Also described in PDR For Nonprescription Drugs.
Shown in Product Identification Section, page 406

COMTREX®   OTC

[*cŏm'trĕx*]
Multi-Symptom Cold Reliever

COMPOSITION

Each tablet, caplet, liqui-gel and fluid ounce (30 ml.) contains:
[See table on next page.]

INDICATIONS

COMTREX® provides temporary relief of these major cold and flu symptoms: nasal and sinus congestion, runny nose, sneezing, coughing, minor sore throat pain, headache, fever, body aches and pain.

WARNINGS:

KEEP THIS AND ALL OTHER MEDICATIONS OUT OF THE REACH OF CHILDREN. IN CASE OF ACCIDENTAL OVERDOSE, SEEK PROFESSIONAL ASSISTANCE OR CONTACT A POISON CONTROL CENTER IMMEDIATELY. PROMPT MEDICAL ATTENTION IS CRITICAL FOR ADULTS AS WELL AS FOR CHILDREN EVEN IF YOU DO NOT NOTICE ANY SIGNS OR SYMPTOMS. As with any drug, if you are pregnant or nursing a baby, seek the advice of a health professional before using this product. Do not take this product for more than 7 days (for adults) or 5 days (for children), unless directed by a doctor. If symptoms do not improve or are accompanied by a fever that lasts for more than 3 days, or if new symptoms occur, consult a doctor. Do not exceed recommended dosage because at higher doses nervousness, dizziness or sleeplessness may occur. May cause excitability especially in children. A persistent cough may be a sign of a

Continued on next page

Bristol-Myers Products—Cont.

serious condition. If cough persists for more than 7 days, tends to recur, or is accompanied by rash, persistent headache, fever that lasts for more than 3 days, or if new symptoms occur, consult a doctor. Do not take this product for persistent or chronic cough such as occurs with smoking, asthma or emphysema, or if cough is accompanied by excessive phlegm (mucus/sputum) unless directed by a doctor. If sore throat is severe, persists for more than 2 days, is accompanied or followed by a fever, headache, rash, nausea or vomiting, consult a doctor promptly. This product should not be taken by persons who have asthma, glaucoma, emphysema, chronic pulmonary disease, high blood pressure, heart disease, thyroid disease, diabetes, shortness of breath, difficulty in breathing or difficulty in urination due to enlargement of the prostate gland unless directed by a doctor. May cause marked drowsiness; alcohol may increase the drowsiness effect. Avoid alcoholic beverages, and do not take this product if you are taking sedatives or tranquilizers without first consulting your doctor. Use caution when driving a motor vehicle or operating machinery.

DRUG INTERACTION PRECAUTION

This product should not be taken by any adult or child who is taking a prescription medication for high blood pressure or depression without first consulting a doctor.

DIRECTIONS

Tablets or Caplets: Adults: 2 tablets or caplets every 4 hours while symptoms persist, not to exceed 8 tablets or caplets in 24 hours, or as directed by a doctor. Children 6 to under 12 years of age: One tablet or caplet every 4 hours while symptoms persist, not to exceed 4 tablets or caplets in 24 hours, or as directed by a doctor. Children under 6: Consult a doctor.

Liqui-Gel: Adults: 2 liqui-gels every 4 hours while symptoms persist, not to exceed 12 liqui-gels in 24 hours, or as directed by a doctor. Children 6 to under 12 years of age: 1 liqui-gel every 4 hours while symptoms persist, not to exceed 5 liqui-gels in 24 hours, or as directed by a doctor. Children under 6: Consult a doctor.

Liquid: Adults: One fluid ounce (30 ml) in medicine cup provided or 2 tablespoons every 4 hours while symptoms persist, not to exceed 4 doses in 24 hours, or as directed by a doctor. Children 6 to under 12 years of age: ½ fluid ounce (15 ml) or one tablespoon every 4 hours while symptoms persist, not to exceed 4 doses in 24 hours, or as directed by a doctor. Children under 6: Consult a doctor.

OVERDOSE

MUCOMYST (acetylcysteine) As An Antidote For Acetaminophen Overdose)

Acetaminophen is rapidly absorbed from the upper gastrointestinal tract with peak plasma levels occurring between 30 and 60 minutes after therapeutic doses and usually within 4 hours following an overdose. The parent compound, which is nontoxic, is extensively metabolized in the liver to form principally the sulfate and glucuronide conjugates which are also nontoxic and are rapidly excreted in the urine. A small fraction of an ingested dose is metabolized in the liver by the cytochrome P-450 mixed function oxidase enzyme system to form a reactive, potentially toxic, intermediate metabolite which preferentially conjugates with hepatic glutathione to form the nontoxic cysteine and mercapturic acid derivatives which are then excreted by the kidney. Therapeutic doses of acetaminophen do not saturate the glucuronide and sulfate conjugation pathways and do not result in the formation of sufficient reactive metabolite to deplete glutathione stores. However, following ingestion of a large overdose (150 mg/kg or greater) the glucuronide and sulfate conjugation pathways are saturated resulting in a larger fraction of the drug being metabolized via the P-450 pathway. The increased formation of reactive metabolite may deplete the hepatic stores of glutathione with subsequent binding of the metabolite to protein molecules within the hepatocyte resulting in cellular necrosis. Acetylcysteine has been shown to reduce the extent of liver injury following acetaminophen overdose. Early symptoms following a potentially hepatotoxic overdose may include: nausea, vomiting, diaphoresis and general malaise. Clinical and laboratory evidence of hepatic toxicity may not be apparent until 48 to 72 hours postingestion. In adults and adolescents, regardless of the quantity of acetaminophen reported to have been ingested, administer MUCOMYST® acetylcysteine immediately. MUCOMYST acetylcysteine therapy should be initiated and continued for a full course of therapy. Its effectiveness depends on early administration, with benefit seen principally in patients treated within 16 hours of the overdose.

If acetaminophen plasma assay capability is not available, and the estimated acetaminophen ingestion exceeds 150 mg/kg, MUCOMYST acetylcysteine therapy should be initiated and continued for a full course of therapy.

For full prescribing information, refer to the MUCOMYST package insert. Do not await the results of assays for acetaminophen level before initiating treatment with MUCOMYST acetylcysteine. The following additional procedures are recommended: The stomach should be emptied promptly by lavage or by induction of emesis with syrup of ipecac. A serum acetaminophen assay should be obtained as early as possible, but no sooner than four hours following ingestion. Liver function studies should be obtained initially and repeated at 24-hour intervals.

For additional emergency information call your regional poison center or toll-free (1-800-525-6115) to the Rocky Mountain Poison Center for assistance in diagnosis and for directions in the use of MUCOMYST acetylcysteine as an antidote.

HOW SUPPLIED

COMTREX® is supplied as:

Yellow tablet with letter "C" debossed on one surface.
NDC 19810-0790-1 Blister packages of 24's
NDC 19810-0790-2 Bottles of 50's
NDC 19810-0790-3 Vials of 10's

Coated yellow caplet with "Comtrex" printed in red on one side.
NDC 19810-0792-3 Blister packages of 24's
NDC 19810-0792-4 Bottles of 50's

Yellow Liqui-gel with "Comtrex" printed in red on one side.
NDC 19810-0561-1 Blister packages of 24's
NDC 19810-0561-2 Blister packages of 50's

Clear Red Cherry Flavored liquid:
NDC 19810-0791-1 6 oz. plastic bottles

All sizes packaged in child resistant closures except for 24's for tablets, caplets and liqui-gels which are sizes recommended for households without young children. Store caplets, tablets and liquid at room temperature. Store liqui-gels below 86° F. (30° C.). Keep from freezing.

Also described in PDR For Nonprescription Drugs.

Shown in Product Identification Section, page 406

	COMTREX Per Tablet or Caplet	COMTREX Liquid-Gel per Liqui-Gel	COMTREX Liquid Per Fl. Ounce
Acetaminophen:	325 mg.	325 mg.	650 mg.
Pseudoephedrine HCl:	30 mg.	—	60 mg.
Phenylpropanolamine HCl:	—	12.5 mg.	—
Chlorpheniramine Maleate:	2 mg.	2 mg.	4 mg.
Dextromethorphan HBr:	10 mg.	10 mg.	20 mg.

Other Ingredients:

Tablet	**Caplet**	**Liqui-Gels**	**Liquid**
Corn Starch	Benzoic Acid	D&C Yellow No. 10	Alcohol (20% by volume)
D&C Yellow No. 10 Lake	Carnauba Wax	FD&C Red No. 40	Citric Acid
FD&C Red No. 40 Lake	Corn Starch	Gelatin	D&C Yellow No. 10
			FD&C Blue No. 1
Magnesium Stearate	D&C Yellow No. 10 Lake	Glycerin	FD&C Red No. 40
Methylparaben	FD&C Red No. 40 Lake	Polyethylene Glycol	Flavors
Propylparaben	Hydroxypropyl Methylcellulose	Povidone	Polyethylene Glycol
Stearic Acid	Magnesium Stearate	Propylene Glycol	Povidone
	Methylparaben	Silicon Dioxide	Sodium Citrate
May also contain:	Mineral Oil	Sorbitol	Sucrose
Povidone	Polysorbate 20	Titanium Dioxide	Water
	Povidone	Water	
	Propylene Glycol		
	Propylparaben		
	Simethicone Emulsion		
	Sorbitan Monolaurate		
	Stearic Acid		
	Titanium Dioxide		

ALLERGY-SINUS COMTREX **OTC**
[*cŏm ′trĕx*]
Multi-Symptom Allergy/Sinus Formula

COMPOSITION

ACTIVE INGREDIENTS

Each coated tablet or caplet contains 500 mg acetaminophen, 30 mg pseudoephedrine HCl, 2 mg chlorpheniramine maleate.

OTHER INGREDIENTS

Benzoic acid, carnauba wax, corn starch, D&C yellow No. 10 lake, FD&C blue No. 1 lake, FD&C Red No. 40 lake, hydroxypropyl methylcellulose, mineral oil, polysorbate 20, povidone, propylene glycol, simethicone emulsion, sodium citrate, sorbitan monolaurate, stearic acid, titanium dioxide. May also contain: crospovidone, D&C yellow No. 10, erythorbic acid, FD&C blue No. 1, magnesium stearate, methylparaben, microcrystalline cellulose, polysorbate 80, propylparaben, silicon dioxide, wood cellulose.

INDICATIONS

ALLERGY-SINUS COMTREX provides temporary relief of these upper respiratory allergy, hay fever, and sinusitis symptoms: sneezing, itchy, watery eyes, runny nose, headache, nasal and sinus pressure and congestion.

PRODUCT INFORMATION

Easy to swallow **ALLERGY-SINUS COMTREX** tablets and caplets contain three important ingredients for safe and effective relief. A maximum dose of **non-aspirin analgesic** —acetaminophen—to relieve sinus headache pain. A **decongestant**—pseudoephedrine HCl—to relieve nasal and sinus congestion. An **antihistamine**—chlorpheniramine maleate—to relieve sneezing, runny nose, and itchy eyes.

WARNINGS

KEEP THIS AND ALL OTHER MEDICATIONS OUT OF THE REACH OF CHILDREN. IN CASE OF ACCIDENTAL OVERDOSE, SEEK PROFESSIONAL ASSISTANCE OR CONTACT A POISON CONTROL CENTER IMMEDIATELY. PROMPT MEDICAL ATTENTION IS CRITICAL FOR ADULTS AS WELL AS FOR CHILDREN EVEN IF YOU DO NOT NOTICE ANY SIGNS OR SYMPTOMS. As with any drug, if you are pregnant or nursing a baby, seek the advice of a health professional before using this product. Do not take this product for more than 7 days unless directed by a doctor. If symptoms do not improve or are accompanied by a fever that lasts for more than 3 days, or if new symptoms occur, consult a doctor. Do not exceed recommended dosage because at higher doses nervousness, dizziness or sleeplessness may occur. May cause excitability especially in children. This product should not be taken by persons who have asthma, glaucoma, emphysema, chronic pulmonary disease, high blood pressure, heart disease, thyroid disease, diabetes, shortness of breath, difficulty in breathing or difficulty in urination due to enlargement of the prostate gland unless directed by a doctor. May cause drowsiness; alcohol may increase the drowsiness effect. Avoid alcoholic beverages, and do not take this product if you are taking sedatives or tranquilizers without first consulting your doctor. Use caution when driving a motor vehicle or operating machinery.

DRUG INTERACTION PRECAUTION

Do not take this product if you are presently taking a prescription drug for high blood pressure or depression, without first consulting your doctor.

OVERDOSE

MUCOMYST (acetylcysteine) As An Antidote For Acetaminophen Overdose)

Acetaminophen is rapidly absorbed from the upper gastrointestinal tract with peak plasma levels occurring between 30 and 60 minutes after therapeutic doses and usually within 4 hours following an overdose. The parent compound, which is nontoxic, is extensively metabolized in the liver to form principally the sulfate and glucuronide conjugates which are also nontoxic and are rapidly excreted in the urine. A small fraction of an ingested dose is metabolized in the liver by the cytochrome P-450 mixed function oxidase enzyme system to form a reactive, potentially toxic, intermediate metabolite which preferentially conjugates with hepatic glutathione to form the nontoxic cysteine and mercapturic acid derivatives which are then excreted by the kidney. Therapeutic doses of acetaminophen do not saturate the glucuronide and sulfate conjugation pathways and do not result in the formation of sufficient reactive metabolite to deplete glutathione stores. However, following ingestion of a large overdose (150 mg/kg or greater) the glucuronide and sulfate conjugation pathways are saturated resulting in a larger fraction of the drug being metabolized via the P-450 pathway. The increased formation of reactive metabolite may deplete the hepatic stores of glutathione with subsequent binding of the metabolite to protein molecules within the hepatocyte resulting in cellular necrosis. Acetylcysteine has been shown to reduce the extent of liver injury following acetaminophen overdose. Early symptoms following a potentially hepatotoxic overdose may include: nausea, vomiting, diaphoresis and general

malaise. Clinical and laboratory evidence of hepatic toxicity may not be apparent until 48 to 72 hours postingestion. In adults and adolescents, regardless of the quantity of acetaminophen reported to have been ingested, administer MUCOMYST® acetylcysteine immediately. MUCOMYST acetylcysteine therapy should be initiated and continued for a full course of therapy. Its effectiveness depends on early administration, with benefit seen principally in patients treated within 16 hours of the overdose.
If acetaminophen plasma assay capability is not available, and the estimated acetaminophen ingestion exceeds 150 mg/kg, MUCOMYST acetylcysteine therapy should be initiated and continued for a full course of therapy.
For full prescribing information, refer to the MUCOMYST package insert. Do not await the results of assays for acetaminophen level before initiating treatment with MUCOMYST acetylcysteine. The following additional procedures are recommended: The stomach should be emptied promptly by lavage or by induction of emesis with syrup of ipecac. A serum acetaminophen assay should be obtained as early as possible, but no sooner than four hours following ingestion. Liver function studies should be obtained initially and repeated at 24-hour intervals.
For additional emergency information call your regional poison center or toll-free (1-800-525-6115) to the Rocky Mountain Poison Center for assistance in diagnosis and for directions in the use of MUCOMYST acetylcysteine as an antidote.

DIRECTIONS

Adults: 2 tablets or caplets every 6 hours while symptoms persist, not to exceed 8 tablets or caplets in 24 hours, or as directed by a doctor. Children under 12 years of age: Consult a doctor.

HOW SUPPLIED

Allergy-Sinus COMTREX® is supplied as:
Coated green tablets with "Comtrex A/S" printed in black on one side.
NDC 19810-0774-1 Blister packages of 24's
NDC 19810-0774-2 Bottles of 50's
Coated green caplets with "A/S" debossed on one surface.
NDC 19810-0081-4 Blister packages of 24's
NDC 19810-0081-5 Bottles of 50's
All sizes packaged in child resistant closures except 24's for tablets and caplets which are sizes recommended for households without young children.
Store at room temperature.
Also described in PDR For Nonprescription Drugs.

Shown in Product Identification Section, page 406

Cough Formula COMTREX® OTC

[*cŏm 'trĕx*]
Multi-Symptom Cough Formula

COMPOSITION

ACTIVE INGREDIENTS
Each 4 teaspoonfuls (2/3 fl. oz.) contains:
—EXPECTORANT—200 mg Guaifenesin
—COUGH SUPPRESSANT—20 mg Dextromethorphan HBr
—ANALGESIC—500 mg Acetaminophen
—DECONGESTANT—60 mg Pseudoephedrine HCl

OTHER INGREDIENTS

Alcohol (20% by volume), Citric Acid, FD&C Red No. 40, Flavor, Menthol, Povidone, Saccharin Sodium, Sodium Citrate, Sucrose, Water.

INDICATIONS

For temporary relief of cough, nasal and upper chest congestion, minor sore throat pain and fever and pain due to a chest cold.

WARNINGS

KEEP THIS AND ALL OTHER MEDICATIONS OUT OF THE REACH OF CHILDREN. IN CASE OF ACCIDENTAL OVERDOSE, SEEK PROFESSIONAL ASSISTANCE OR CONTACT A POISON CONTROL CENTER IMMEDIATELY. PROMPT MEDICAL ATTENTION IS CRITICAL FOR ADULTS AS WELL AS FOR CHILDREN EVEN IF YOU DO NOT NOTICE ANY SYMPTOMS. As with any drug, if you are pregnant or nursing a baby, seek the advice of a health professional before using this product. Do not take this product for more than 7 days (for adults) or 5 days (for children) unless directed by a doctor. If symptoms do not improve or are accompanied by a fever that lasts for more than 3 days, or if new symptoms occur, consult a doctor. Do not exceed recommended dosage because at higher doses nervousness, dizziness or sleeplessness may occur. A persistent cough may be a sign of a serious condition. If cough persists for more than 7 days, tends to recur or is accompanied by rash, persistent headache, fever that lasts for more than 3 days, or if new symptoms occur, consult a doctor. Do not take this product for persistent or chronic cough such as occurs with smoking, asthma, chronic bronchitis or emphysema or if cough is accompanied by excessive phlegm (mucus/sputum) unless directed by a doctor. If sore throat is severe, persists for more than two days, is accompanied or followed by a fever, headache, rash, nausea or vomiting, consult a doctor promptly. This product should not be taken by persons who have heart disease, high blood pressure, thyroid disease, diabetes, difficulty in urination due to enlargement of the prostate gland unless directed by a doctor.

DRUG INTERACTION PRECAUTION

This product should not be taken by any adult or child who is taking a prescription medication for high blood pressure or depression without first consulting a doctor.

DIRECTIONS

ADULTS: 2/3 fluidounce (20 ml) in medicine cup provided or four teaspoons every 4 hours while symptoms persist, not to exceed 4 doses in 24 hours, or as directed by a doctor. Children 6 to under 12 years of age: 1/3 fluidounce (10 ml) in medicine cup provided or 2 teaspoons every 4 hours while symptoms persist, not exceed 4 doses in 24 hours, or as directed by a doctor. Children under 6: Consult a doctor.

OVERDOSE

MUCOMYST (acetylcysteine) As An Antidote For Acetaminophen Overdose)
Acetaminophen is rapidly absorbed from the upper gastrointestinal tract with peak plasma levels occurring between 30 and 60 minutes after therapeutic doses and usually within 4 hours following an overdose. The parent compound, which is nontoxic, is extensively metabolized in the liver to form principally the sulfate and glucuronide conjugates which are also nontoxic and are rapidly excreted in the urine. A small fraction of an ingested dose is metabolized in the liver by the cytochrome P-450 mixed function oxidase enzyme system to form a reactive, potentially toxic, intermediate metabolite which preferentially conjugates with hepatic glutathione to form the nontoxic cysteine and mercapturic acid derivatives which are then excreted by the kidney. Therapeutic doses of acetaminophen do not saturate the glucuronide and sulfate conjugation pathways and do not result in the formation of sufficient reactive metabolite to deplete glutathione stores. However, following ingestion of a large overdose (150 mg/kg or greater) the glucuronide and sulfate conjugation pathways are saturated resulting in a larger fraction of the drug being metabolized via the P-450 pathway. The increased formation of reactive metabolite may deplete the hepatic stores of glutathione with subsequent binding of the metabolite to protein molecules within the hepatocyte resulting in cellular necrosis. Acetylcysteine has been shown to reduce the extent of liver injury following acetaminophen overdose. Early symptoms following a potentially hepatotoxic overdose may include: nausea, vomiting, diaphoresis and general malaise. Clinical and laboratory evidence of hepatic toxicity may not be apparent until 48 to 72 hours postingestion. In adults and adolescents, regardless of the quantity of acetaminophen reported to have been ingested, administer MUCOMYST® acetylcysteine immediately. MUCOMYST acetylcysteine therapy should be initiated and continued for a full course of therapy. Its effectiveness depends on early administration, with benefit seen principally in patients treated within 16 hours of the overdose.
If acetaminophen plasma assay capability is not available, and the estimated acetaminophen ingestion exceeds 150 mg/kg, MUCOMYST acetylcysteine therapy should be initiated and continued for a full course of therapy.
For full prescribing information, refer to the MUCOMYST package insert. Do not await the results of assays for acetaminophen level before initiating treatment with MUCOMYST acetylcysteine. The following additional procedures are recommended: The stomach should be emptied promptly by lavage or by induction of emesis with syrup of ipecac. A serum acetaminophen assay should be obtained as early as possible, but no sooner than four hours following ingestion. Liver function studies should be obtained initially and repeated at 24-hour intervals.
For additional emergency information call your regional poison center or toll-free (1-800-525-6115) to the Rocky Mountain Poison Center for assistance in diagnosis and for directions in the use of MUCOMYST acetylcysteine as an antidote.

HOW SUPPLIED

Cough Formula COMTREX® is supplied as a clear red raspberry flavored liquid:
NDC 19810-0781-1 4 oz. plastic bottle
NDC 19810-0781-3 8 oz. plastic bottle
The 4 oz. size is not child resistant and is recommended for households without young children.
Store at room temperature.
Also described in PDR For Nonprescription Drugs.

DAY & NIGHT COMTREX® OTC

COMPOSITION

Active Ingredients: EACH DAYTIME CAPLET CONTAINS 325mg Acetaminophen, 30mg Pseudoephedrine HCl, 10mg Dextromethorphan HBr. EACH NIGHTTIME TABLET CONTAINS 325mg Acetaminophen, 30mg Pseudoephedrine HCl, 10mg Dextromethorphan HBr, 2mg Chlorpheniramine Maleate.
Other Ingredients: DAYTIME CAPLETS AND NIGHTTIME TABLETS BOTH CONTAIN: Corn Starch, D&C Yellow No. 10 Lake, FD&C Red No. 40 Lake, Magnesium Stearate, Methylparaben, Propylparaben, Stearic Acid. DAYTIME CAPLETS ALSO CONTAIN: Benzoic Acid, Carnauba Wax, Hydroxypropyl Methylcellulose, Mineral Oil, Polysorbate 20, Povidone, Propylene Glycol, Simethicone Emulsion, Sorbitan Monolaurate, Titanium Dioxide. NIGHTTIME TABLETS MAY ALSO CONTAIN: Povidone.

INDICATIONS

Day & Night COMTREX provides you with two different formulas. COMTREX Daytime Caplets (orange) and COMTREX Nighttime Tablets (yellow), for effective relief. COMTREX Daytime Caplets contain three ingredients for the temporary relief of these major cold and flu symptoms without causing drowsiness: a decongestant—to relieve stuffy nose and sinus congestion; a cough suppressant—to quiet cough; a non-aspirin analgesic—to relieve headache, fever, minor sore throat pain and body aches and pain. COMTREX Nighttime Tablets relieve all these symptoms plus they contain an antihistamine to temporarily relieve runny nose and sneezing.

WARNINGS for Daytime Caplets and Nighttime Tablets
KEEP THESE AND ALL OTHER MEDICATIONS OUT OF THE REACH OF CHILDREN. IN CASE OF ACCIDENTAL OVERDOSE, SEEK PROFESSIONAL ASSISTANCE OR CONTACT A POISON CONTROL CENTER IMMEDIATELY. PROMPT MEDICAL ATTENTION IS CRITICAL FOR ADULTS AS WELL AS FOR CHILDREN EVEN IF YOU DO NOT NOTICE ANY SIGNS OR SYMPTOMS. As with any drug, if you are pregnant or nursing a baby, seek the advice of a health professional before using these products. Do not take these products for more than 7 days or for fever for more than 3 days unless directed by a doctor. If symptoms do not improve or are accompanied by a fever that lasts for more than 3 days, or if new symptoms occur, consult a doctor. Do not exceed recommended dosage because at higher doses nervousness, dizziness or sleeplessness may occur. A persistent cough may be a sign of a serious condition. If cough persists for more than 7 days, tends to recur or is accompanied by rash, persistent headache, fever that lasts for more than 3 days, or if new symptoms occur, consult a doctor. Do not take these products for persistent or chronic cough such as occurs with smoking, asthma or emphysema, or if cough is accompanied by excessive phlegm (mucus/sputum) unless directed by a doctor. If sore throat is severe, persists for more than 2 days, is accompanied or followed by a fever, headache, rash, nausea or vomiting, consult a doctor promptly. These products should not be taken by persons who have asthma, glaucoma, emphysema, chronic pulmonary disease, high blood pressure, heart disease, thyroid disease, diabetes, shortness of breath, difficulty in breathing, or difficulty in urination due to an enlargement of the prostate gland unless directed by a doctor.
ADDITIONAL WARNINGS for Nighttime Tablets
May cause marked drowsiness; alcohol may increase the drowsiness effect. Avoid alcoholic beverages, and do not take this product if you are taking sedatives or tranquilizers without first consulting your doctor. Use caution when driving a motor vehicle or operating machinery. May cause excitability especially in children.
DRUG INTERACTION PRECAUTION: Do not take these products if you are presently taking a prescription medication for high blood pressure or depression without first consulting your doctor.

DIRECTIONS

Adults: 2 Daytime Caplets every 4 hours while symptoms persist, not to exceed 6 Daytime Caplets in 24 hours, or as directed by a doctor. 2 Nighttime Tablets at bedtime, if needed, to be taken no sooner than 4 hours after the last Daytime Caplets dose, or as directed by a doctor. **Children under 12:** Consult a doctor.

OVERDOSE

MUCOMYST (acetylcysteine) As An Antidote For Acetaminophen Overdose)
Acetaminophen is rapidly absorbed from the upper gastrointestinal tract with peak plasma levels occurring between 30 and 60 minutes after therapeutic doses and usually within 4 hours following an overdose. The parent compound, which is nontoxic, is extensively metabolized in the liver to form principally the sulfate and glucuronide conjugates which are

Continued on next page

Bristol-Myers Products—Cont.

also nontoxic and are rapidly excreted in the urine. A small fraction of an ingested dose is metabolized in the liver by the cytochrome P-450 mixed function oxidase enzyme system to form a reactive, potentially toxic, intermediate metabolite which preferentially conjugates with hepatic glutathione to form the nontoxic cysteine and mercapturic acid derivatives which are then excreted by the kidney. Therapeutic doses of acetaminophen do not saturate the glucuronide and sulfate conjugation pathways and do not result in the formation of sufficient reactive metabolite to deplete glutathione stores. However, following ingestion of a large overdose (150 mg/kg or greater) the glucuronide and sulfate conjugation pathways are saturated resulting in a larger fraction of the drug being metabolized via the P-450 pathway. The increased formation of reactive metabolite may deplete the hepatic stores of glutathione with subsequent binding of the metabolite to protein molecules within the hepatocyte resulting in cellular necrosis. Acetylcysteine has been shown to reduce the extent of liver injury following acetaminophen overdose. Early symptoms following a potentially hepatotoxic overdose may include: nausea, vomiting, diaphoresis and general malaise. Clinical and laboratory evidence of hepatic toxicity may not be apparent until 48 to 72 hours postingestion. In adults and adolescents, regardless of the quantity of acetaminophen reported to have been ingested, administer MUCOMYST® acetylcysteine immediately. MUCOMYST acetylcysteine therapy should be initiated and continued for a full course of therapy. Its effectiveness depends on early administration, with benefit seen principally in patients treated within 16 hours of the overdose.
If acetaminophen plasma assay capability is not available, and the estimated acetaminophen ingestion exceeds 150 mg/kg, MUCOMYST acetylcysteine therapy should be initiated and continued for a full course of therapy.
For full prescribing information, refer to the MUCOMYST package insert. Do not await the results of assays for acetaminophen level before initiating treatment with MUCOMYST acetylcysteine. The following additional procedures are recommended: The stomach should be emptied promptly by lavage or by induction of emesis with syrup of ipecac. A serum acetaminophen assay should be obtained as early as possible, but no sooner than four hours following ingestion. Liver function studies should be obtained initially and repeated at 24-hour intervals.
For additional emergency information call your regional poison center or toll-free (1-800-525-6115) to the Rocky Mountain Poison Center for assistance in diagnosis and for directions in the use of MUCOMYST acetylcysteine as an antidote.

HOW SUPPLIED

DAY & NIGHT COMTREX® is supplied as:
Day-Coated orange caplet with letter "C" debossed on one surface.
Night-Coated yellow tablet with letter "C" debossed on one surface.
NDC 19810-0078-1 Blister packages of 24's (18 caplets/6 tablets)
Store at room temperature.

Shown in Product Identification Section, page 406

Non-Drowsy COMTREX® OTC

COMPOSITION

Active Ingredients: Each caplet contains 325mg Acetaminophen, 30 mg Pseudoephedrine HCl, 10mg Dextromethorphan HBr. Other Ingredients: Benzoic Acid, Carnauba Wax, Corn Starch, D&C Yellow No. 10 Lake, FD&C Red No. 40 Lake, Hydroxypropyl Methylcellulose, Magnesium Stearate, Methylparaben, Mineral Oil, Polysorbate 20, Povidone, Propylene Glycol, Propylparaben, Simethicone Emulsion, Sorbitan Monolaurate, Stearic Acid, Titanium Dioxide.

INDICATIONS

For temporary relief of nasal and sinus congestion, coughing, minor sore throat pain, headache, fever, body aches and pain.

WARNINGS

KEEP THIS AND ALL OTHER MEDICATIONS OUT OF THE REACH OF CHILDREN. IN CASE OF ACCIDENTAL OVERDOSE, SEEK PROFESSIONAL ASSISTANCE OR CONTACT A POISON CONTROL CENTER IMMEDIATELY. PROMPT MEDICAL ATTENTION IS CRITICAL FOR ADULTS AS WELL AS FOR CHILDREN EVEN IF YOU DO NOT NOTICE ANY SIGNS OR SYMPTOMS. As with any drug, if you are pregnant or nursing a baby, seek the advice of a health professional before using this product. Do not take this product for more than 7 days (for adults) or 5 days (for children) or for fever for more than 3 days unless directed by a doctor. Do not exceed recommended dosage because at higher doses nervousness, dizziness or sleeplessness may occur. A persistent cough may be a sign of a serious condition. If cough persists for more than 7 days, tends to recur or is accompanied by rash, persistent headache, fever that lasts for more than 3 days, or if new symptoms occur, consult a doctor. Do not take this product for persistent or chronic cough such as occurs with smoking, asthma or emphysema, or if cough is accompanied by excessive phlegm (mucus/sputum) unless directed by a doctor. If sore throat is severe, persists for more than 2 days, is accompanied or followed by a fever, headache, rash, nausea or vomiting, consult a doctor promptly. This product should not be taken by persons who have high blood pressure, heart disease, thyroid disease, diabetes or difficulty in urination due to enlargement of the prostate gland unless directed by a doctor.
DRUG INTERACTION PRECAUTION: This product should not be taken by any adult or child who is taking a prescription medication for high blood pressure or depression without first consulting a doctor.

DIRECTIONS

Adults: 2 caplets every 4 hours while symptoms persist, not to exceed 8 caplets in 24 hours, or as directed by doctor. **Children 6 to under 12 years of age:** One caplet every 4 hours while symptoms persist, not to exceed 4 caplets in 24 hours, or as directed by a doctor. **Children under 6:** Consult a doctor.

OVERDOSE

MUCOMYST (acetylcysteine) As An Antidote For Acetaminophen Overdose)
Acetaminophen is rapidly absorbed from the upper gastrointestinal tract with peak plasma levels occurring between 30 and 60 minutes after therapeutic doses and usually within 4 hours following an overdose. The parent compound, which is nontoxic, is extensively metabolized in the liver to form principally the sulfate and glucuronide conjugates which are also nontoxic and are rapidly excreted in the urine. A small fraction of an ingested dose is metabolized in the liver by the cytochrome P-450 mixed function oxidase enzyme system to form a reactive, potentially toxic, intermediate metabolite which preferentially conjugates with hepatic glutathione to form the nontoxic cysteine and mercapturic acid derivatives which are then excreted by the kidney. Therapeutic doses of acetaminophen do not saturate the glucuronide and sulfate conjugation pathways and do not result in the formation of sufficient reactive metabolite to deplete glutathione stores. However, following ingestion of a large overdose (150 mg/kg or greater) the glucuronide and sulfate conjugation pathways are saturated resulting in a larger fraction of the drug being metabolized via the P-450 pathway. The increased formation of reactive metabolite may deplete the hepatic stores of glutathione with subsequent binding of the metabolite to protein molecules within the hepatocyte resulting in cellular necrosis. Acetylcysteine has been shown to reduce the extent of liver injury following acetaminophen overdose. Early symptoms following a potentially hepatotoxic overdose may include: nausea, vomiting, diaphoresis and general malaise. Clinical and laboratory evidence of hepatic toxicity may not be apparent until 48 to 72 hours postingestion. In adults and adolescents, regardless of the quantity of acetaminophen reported to have been ingested, administer MUCOMYST® acetylcysteine immediately. MUCOMYST acetylcysteine therapy should be initiated and continued for a full course of therapy. Its effectiveness depends on early administration, with benefit seen principally in patients treated within 16 hours of the overdose.
If acetaminophen plasma assay capability is not available, and the estimated acetaminophen ingestion exceeds 150 mg/kg, MUCOMYST acetylcysteine therapy should be initiated and continued for a full course of therapy.
For full prescribing information, refer to the MUCOMYST package insert. Do not await the results of assays for acetaminophen level before initiating treatment with MUCOMYST acetylcysteine. The following additional procedures are recommended: The stomach should be emptied promptly by lavage or by induction of emesis with syrup of ipecac. A serum acetaminophen assay should be obtained as early as possible, but no sooner than four hours following ingestion. Liver function studies should be obtained initially and repeated at 24-hour intervals.
For additional emergency information call your regional poison center or toll-free (1-800-525-6115) to the Rocky Mountain Poison Center for assistance in diagnosis and for directions in the use of MUCOMYST acetylcysteine as an antidote.

HOW SUPPLIED

Non-Drowsy Comtrex® is supplied as:
Coated yellow caplet with letter "C" debossed on one surface.
NDC 19810-0041-1 Blister packages of 24's
NDC 19810-0042-2 Botles of 50's
The 24 size does not have a child resistant closure and is recommended for households without young children.
Store at room temperature.

Shown in Product Identification Section, page 406

CONGESPIRIN® for Children Aspirin Free Chewable Cold Tablets OTC

[cŏn"gĕs'pir-in]

COMPOSITION

Each tablet contains acetaminophen 81 mg. (1¼ grains), phenylephrine hydrochloride 1¼ mg. Also Contains: Calcium Stearate, D&C Red No. 30 Aluminum Lake, D&C Yellow No. 10 Aluminum Lake, Ethyl Cellulose, Flavor, Mannitol, Microcrystalline Cellulose, Polyethylene, Saccharin Calcium, Sucrose.

INDICATIONS

A non-aspirin analgesic/nasal decongestant that temporarily reduces fever and relieves aches, pains and nasal congestion associated with colds and "flu."

WARNINGS

KEEP THIS AND ALL MEDICINES OUT OF CHILDREN'S REACH. IN CASE OF ACCIDENTAL OVERDOSE, CONTACT A PHYSICIAN IMMEDIATELY.

CAUTION

If child is under medical care, do not administer without consulting physician. Do not exceed recommended dosage. Consult your physician if symptoms persist or if high fever, high blood pressure, heart disease, diabetes or thyroid disease is present. Do not administer for more than 10 days unless directed by physician.

DIRECTIONS

Under 2, consult your physician.

2–3 years	2 tablets
4–5 years	3 tablets
6–8 years	4 tablets
9–10 years	5 tablets
11–12 years	6 tablets
over 12 years	8 tablets

Repeat dose in four hours if necessary. Do not give more than four doses per day unless prescribed by your physician.

OVERDOSE

MUCOMYST (acetylcysteine) As An Antidote For Acetaminophen Overdose)
Acetaminophen is rapidly absorbed from the upper gastrointestinal tract with peak plasma levels occurring between 30 and 60 minutes after therapeutic doses and usually within 4 hours following an overdose. The parent compound, which is nontoxic, is extensively metabolized in the liver to form principally the sulfate and glucuronide conjugates which are also nontoxic and are rapidly excreted in the urine. A small fraction of an ingested dose is metabolized in the liver by the cytochrome P-450 mixed function oxidase enzyme system to form a reactive, potentially toxic, intermediate metabolite which preferentially conjugates with hepatic glutathione to form the nontoxic cysteine and mercapturic acid derivatives which are then excreted by the kidney. Therapeutic doses of acetaminophen do not saturate the glucuronide and sulfate conjugation pathways and do not result in the formation of sufficient reactive metabolite to deplete glutathione stores. However, following ingestion of a large overdose (150 mg/kg or greater) the glucuronide and sulfate conjugation pathways are saturated resulting in a larger fraction of the drug being metabolized via the P-450 pathway. The increased formation of reactive metabolite may deplete the hepatic stores of glutathione with subsequent binding of the metabolite to protein molecules within the hepatocyte resulting in cellular necrosis. Acetylcysteine has been shown to reduce the extent of liver injury following acetaminophen overdose. Early symptoms following a potentially hepatotoxic overdose may include: nausea, vomiting, diaphoresis and general malaise. Clinical and laboratory evidence of hepatic toxicity may not be apparent until 48 to 72 hours postingestion. In adults and adolescents, regardless of the quantity of acetaminophen reported to have been ingested, administer MUCOMYST® acetylcysteine immediately. MUCOMYST acetylcysteine therapy should be initiated and continued for a full course of therapy. Its effectiveness depends on early administration, with benefit seen principally in patients treated within 16 hours of the overdose.
If acetaminophen plasma assay capability is not available, and the estimated acetaminophen ingestion exceeds 150 mg/kg, MUCOMYST acetylcysteine therapy should be initiated and continued for a full course of therapy.
For full prescribing information, refer to the MUCOMYST package insert. Do not await the results of assays for acetaminophen level before initiating treatment with MUCOMYST acetylcysteine. The following additional procedures are recommended: The stomach should be emptied promptly by lavage or by induction of emesis with syrup of ipecac. A serum acetaminophen assay should be obtained as early as possible, but no sooner than four hours following ingestion. Liver function studies should be obtained initially and repeated at 24-hour intervals.
For additional emergency information call your regional poison center or toll-free (1-800-525-6115) to the Rocky Mountain Poison Center for assistance in diagnosis and for

directions in the use of MUCOMYST acetylcysteine as an antidote.

HOW SUPPLIED

CONGESPIRIN Aspirin Free Chewable Cold Tablets are supplied as scored orange tablets with "C" on one side.
NDC 19810-0748-1 Bottles of 24's.
Bottles are child resistant.
Store at room temperature.
Also described in PDR For Nonprescription Drugs.

Aspirin Free EXCEDRIN®   OTC

COMPOSITION

Each caplet contains Acetaminophen 500 mg. and Caffeine 65 mg. Other Ingredients: Benzoic Acid, Carnauba Wax, Corn Starch, Croscarmellose Sodium, D&C Red No. 27 Lake, D&C Yellow No. 10 Lake, FD&C Blue No. 1 Lake, Hydroxypropyl Methylcellulose, Magnesium Stearate, Methylparaben, Microcrystalline Cellulose, Propylparaben, Saccharin Sodium, Simethicone Emulsion, Stearic Acid, Titanium Dioxide. May also contain: Erythorbic Acid, Mineral Oil, Polyethylene Glycol, Polysorbate 20, Polysorbate 80, Povidone, Propylene Glycol, Sorbitan Monolaurate.

INDICATIONS

For temporary relief of the pain of headache, sinusitis, colds, muscular aches, menstrual discomfort, toothaches and minor arthritis pain.

DIRECTIONS:

Adults: 2 caplets every 6 hours while symptoms persist, not to exceed 8 caplets in 24 hours, or as directed by a doctor. Children under 12 years of age: Consult a doctor.

WARNINGS

KEEP THIS AND ALL OTHER MEDICATIONS OUT OF THE REACH OF CHILDREN. IN CASE OF ACCIDENTAL OVERDOSE, SEEK PROFESSIONAL ASSISTANCE OR CONTACT A POISON CONTROL CENTER IMMEDIATELY. PROMPT MEDICAL ATTENTION IS CRITICAL FOR ADULTS AS WELL AS FOR CHILDREN EVEN IF YOU DO NOT NOTICE ANY SIGNS OR SYMPTOMS. As with any drug, if you are pregnant or nursing a baby, seek the advice of a health professional before using this product. Do not take this product for pain for more than 10 days or for fever for more than 3 days unless directed by a doctor. If pain or fever persists or gets worse, if new symptoms occur, of if redness or swelling is present, consult a doctor because these could be signs of a serious condition. Consult a dentist promptly for toothache.

OVERDOSE

MUCOMYST (acetylcysteine) As An Antidote For Acetaminophen Overdose)
Acetaminophen is rapidly absorbed from the upper gastrointestinal tract with peak plasma levels occurring between 30 and 60 minutes after therapeutic doses and usually within 4 hours following an overdose. The parent compound, which is nontoxic, is extensively metabolized in the liver to form principally the sulfate and glucuronide conjugates which are also nontoxic and are rapidly excreted in the urine. A small fraction of an ingested dose is metabolized in the liver by the cytochrome P-450 mixed function oxidase enzyme system to form a reactive, potentially toxic, intermediate metabolite which preferentially conjugates with hepatic glutathione to form the nontoxic cysteine and mercapturic acid derivatives which are then excreted by the kidney. Therapeutic doses of acetaminophen do not saturate the glucuronide and sulfate conjugation pathways and do not result in the formation of sufficient reactive metabolite to deplete glutathione stores. However, following ingestion of a large overdose (150 mg/kg or greater) the glucuronide and sulfate conjugation pathways are saturated resulting in a larger fraction of the drug being metabolized via the P-450 pathway. The increased formation of reactive metabolite may deplete the hepatic stores of glutathione with subsequent binding of the metabolite to protein molecules within the hepatocyte resulting in cellular necrosis. Acetylcysteine has been shown to reduce the extent of liver injury following acetaminophen overdose. Early symptoms following a potentially hepatotoxic overdose may include: nausea, vomiting, diaphoresis and general malaise. Clinical and laboratory evidence of hepatic toxicity may not be apparent until 48 to 72 hours postingestion. In adults and adolescents, regardless of the quantity of acetaminophen reported to have been ingested, administer MUCOMYST® acetylcysteine immediately. MUCOMYST acetylcysteine therapy should be initiated and continued for a full course of therapy. Its effectiveness depends on early administration, with benefit seen principally in patients treated within 16 hours of the overdose.
If acetaminophen plasma assay capability is not available, and the estimated acetaminophen ingestion exceeds 150 mg/kg, MUCOMYST acetylcysteine therapy should be initiated and continued for a full course of therapy.

For full prescribing information, refer to the MUCOMYST package insert. Do not await the results of assays for acetaminophen level before initiating treatment with MUCOMYST acetylcysteine. The following additional procedures are recommended: The stomach should be emptied promptly by lavage or by induction of emesis with syrup of ipecac. A serum acetaminophen assay should be obtained as early as possible, but no sooner than four hours following ingestion. Liver function studies should be obtained initially and repeated at 24-hour intervals.
For additional emergency information call your regional poison center or toll-free (1-800-525-6115) to the Rocky Mountain Poison Center for assistance in diagnosis and for directions in the use of MUCOMYST acetylcysteine as an antidote.

HOW SUPPLIED

Aspirin Free EXCEDRIN® is supplied as: Coated red caplets with "AF Excedrin" printed in white on one side.
NDC 19810-0089-1 Bottles of 24's
NDC 19810-0089-2 Bottles of 50's
NDC 19810-0089-3 Bottles of 100's
All sizes packaged in child resistant closures except 100's which is recommended for households without young children.
Store at room temperature.
Also described in PDR For Nonprescription Drugs.
Shown in Product Identification Section, page 406

EXCEDRIN® Extra-Strength   OTC
Analgesic
[ĕx″cĕd′rĭn]

COMPOSITION

Each tablet or caplet contains Acetaminophen 250 mg.; Aspirin 250 mg.; and Caffeine 65 mg.
Other ingredients: Benzoic Acid, FD&C Blue No. 1, Hydroxypropylcellulose, Hydroxypropyl Methylcellulose, Microcrystalline Cellulose, Mineral Oil, Polysorbate 20, Povidone, Propylene Glycol, Saccharin Sodium, Simethicone Emulsion, Sorbitan Monolaurate, Stearic Acid, Titanium Dioxide. May also contain: Carnauba wax.

INDICATIONS

For temporary relief of the pain of headache, sinusitis, colds, muscular aches, menstrual discomfort, toothaches and minor arthritis pain.

WARNINGS

Children and teenagers should not use this medicine for chicken pox or flu symptoms before a doctor is consulted about Reye syndrome, a rare but serious illness reported to be associated with aspirin. KEEP THIS AND ALL MEDICATIONS OUT OF THE REACH OF CHILDREN. IN CASE OF ACCIDENTAL OVERDOSE, SEEK PROFESSIONAL ASSISTANCE OR CONTACT A PHYSICIAN OR POISON CONTROL CENTER IMMEDIATELY. PROMPT MEDICAL ATTENTION IS CRITICAL FOR ADULTS AS WELL AS FOR CHILDREN EVEN IF YOU DO NOT NOTICE ANY SIGNS OR SYMPTOMS. As with any drug, if you are pregnant or nursing a baby, seek the advice of a health professional before using this product. IT IS ESPECIALLY IMPORTANT NOT TO USE ASPIRIN DURING THE LAST 3 MONTHS OF PREGNANCY UNLESS SPECIFICALLY DIRECTED TO DO SO BY A DOCTOR BECAUSE IT MAY CAUSE PROBLEMS IN THE UNBORN CHILD OR COMPLICATIONS DURING DELIVERY. Do not take this product for pain for more than 10 days or for fever for more than 3 days unless directed by a doctor. If pain or fever persists or gets worse, if new symptoms occur, or if redness or swelling is present, consult a doctor because these could be signs of a serious condition. Consult a dentist promptly for toothache. Do not take this product if you are allergic to aspirin, have asthma, have stomach problems (such as heartburn, upset stomach or stomach pain) that persist or recur, or if you have ulcers or bleeding problems, unless directed by a doctor. If ringing in the ears or loss of hearing occurs, consult a doctor before taking any more of this product.

DRUG INTERACTION PRECAUTION

Do not take this product if you are taking a prescription drug for anticoagulation (thinning of blood), diabetes, gout or arthritis unless directed by a doctor.

DIRECTIONS

Adults: 2 tablets or caplets with water every 6 hours while symptoms persist, not to exceed 8 tablets or caplets in 24 hours, or as directed by a doctor. Children under 12 years of age: Consult a doctor.

OVERDOSE

MUCOMYST (acetylcysteine) As An Antidote For Acetaminophen Overdose)
Acetaminophen is rapidly absorbed from the upper gastrointestinal tract with peak plasma levels occurring between 30 and 60 minutes after therapeutic doses and usually within 4

hours following an overdose. The parent compound, which is nontoxic, is extensively metabolized in the liver to form principally the sulfate and glucuronide conjugates which are also nontoxic and are rapidly excreted in the urine. A small fraction of an ingested dose is metabolized in the liver by the cytochrome P-450 mixed function oxidase enzyme system to form a reactive, potentially toxic, intermediate metabolite which preferentially conjugates with hepatic glutathione to form the nontoxic cysteine and mercapturic acid derivatives which are then excreted by the kidney. Therapeutic doses of acetaminophen do not saturate the glucuronide and sulfate conjugation pathways and do not result in the formation of sufficient reactive metabolite to deplete glutathione stores. However, following ingestion of a large overdose (150 mg/kg or greater) the glucuronide and sulfate conjugation pathways are saturated resulting in a larger fraction of the drug being metabolized via the P-450 pathway. The increased formation of reactive metabolite may deplete the hepatic stores of glutathione with subsequent binding of the metabolite to protein molecules within the hepatocyte resulting in cellular necrosis. Acetylcysteine has been shown to reduce the extent of liver injury following acetaminophen overdose. Early symptoms following a potentially hepatotoxic overdose may include: nausea, vomiting, diaphoresis and general malaise. Clinical and laboratory evidence of hepatic toxicity may not be apparent until 48 to 72 hours postingestion. In adults and adolescents, regardless of the quantity of acetaminophen reported to have been ingested, administer MUCOMYST® acetylcysteine immediately. MUCOMYST acetylcysteine therapy should be initiated and continued for a full course of therapy. Its effectiveness depends on early administration, with benefit seen principally in patients treated within 16 hours of the overdose.
If acetaminophen plasma assay capability is not available, and the estimated acetaminophen ingestion exceeds 150 mg/kg, MUCOMYST acetylcysteine therapy should be initiated and continued for a full course of therapy.
For full prescribing information, refer to the MUCOMYST package insert. Do not await the results of assays for acetaminophen level before initiating treatment with MUCOMYST acetylcysteine. The following additional procedures are recommended: The stomach should be emptied promptly by lavage or by induction of emesis with syrup of ipecac. A serum acetaminophen assay should be obtained as early as possible, but no sooner than four hours following ingestion. Liver function studies should be obtained initially and repeated at 24-hour intervals.
For additional emergency information call your regional poison center or toll-free (1-800-525-6115) to the Rocky Mountain Poison Center for assistance in diagnosis and for directions in the use of MUCOMYST acetylcysteine as an antidote.

HOW SUPPLIED

Extra Strength EXCEDRIN® is supplied as:
White circular tablet with letter "E" debossed on one side.
NDC 19810-0700-2 Bottles of 12's
NDC 19810-0772-9 Bottles of 30's
NDC 19810-0700-4 Bottles of 60's
NDC 19810-0700-5 Bottles of 100's
NDC 19810-0700-6 Bottles of 165's
NDC 19810-0700-7 Bottles of 225's
NDC 19810-0782-2 Bottles of 275's
NDC 19810-0700-1 A metal tin of 12's
NDC 19810-0772-1 Vials of 10's
Coated while caplets with "Excedrin" printed in red on one side.
NDC 19810-0002-1 Bottles of 24's
NDC 19810-0002-2 Bottles of 50's
NDC 19810-0002-8 Bottles of 100's
All sizes packaged in child resistant closures except 100's for tablets, 50's for caplets which are sizes recommended for households without young children.
Also described in PDR For Nonprescription Drugs.
Shown in Product Identification Section, page 406

EXCEDRIN P.M.®   OTC
[ĕx″cĕd′rĭn]
Analgesic Sleeping Aid

COMPOSITION

Each tablet, caplet and fluid ounce (30 ml.) contains:
[See table on next page.]

INDICATIONS

For temporary relief of occasional headaches and minor aches and pains with accompanying sleeplessness.

WARNINGS

KEEP THIS AND ALL OTHER MEDICATIONS OUT OF THE REACH OF CHILDREN. IN CASE OF ACCIDENTAL OVERDOSE, SEEK PROFESSIONAL ASSISTANCE OR CONTACT A POISON CONTROL CENTER IMMEDIATELY. PROMPT MEDICAL ATTENTION IS CRITICAL

Continued on next page

Bristol-Myers Products—Cont.

FOR ADULTS AS WELL AS FOR CHILDREN EVEN IF YOU DO NOT NOTICE ANY SIGNS OR SYMPTOMS. As with any drug, if you are pregnant or nursing a baby, seek the advice of a health professional before using this product. Do not give this product to children under 12 years of age or use for more than 10 days unless directed by a doctor. Consult a doctor if symptoms persist or get worse or if new ones occur, or if sleeplessness persists continuously for more than 2 weeks because these may be symptoms of serious underlying medical illnesses. Do not take this product if you have asthma, glaucoma, emphysema, chronic pulmonary disease, shortness of breath, difficulty in breathing, or difficulty in urination due to enlargement of the prostate gland unless directed by a doctor. Avoid alcoholic beverages while taking this product. Do not take this product if you are taking sedatives or tranquilizers, without first consulting your doctor.

DIRECTIONS

Tablets or Caplets:
Adults, 2 tablets or caplets at bedtime if needed or as directed by a doctor.
Liquid:
Adults, 1 fluid ounce (2 tablespoons) at bedtime if needed, or as directed by a doctor, using the dosage cup provided.

OVERDOSE

MUCOMYST (acetylcysteine) As An Antidote For Acetaminophen Overdose)
Acetaminophen is rapidly absorbed from the upper gastrointestinal tract with peak plasma levels occurring between 30 and 60 minutes after therapeutic doses and usually within 4 hours following an overdose. The parent compound, which is nontoxic, is extensively metabolized in the liver to form principally the sulfate and glucuronide conjugates which are also nontoxic and are rapidly excreted in the urine. A small fraction of an ingested dose is metabolized in the liver by the cytochrome P-450 mixed function oxidase enzyme system to form a reactive, potentially toxic, intermediate metabolite which preferentially conjugates with hepatic glutathione to form the nontoxic cysteine and mercapturic acid derivatives which are then excreted by the kidney. Therapeutic doses of acetaminophen do not saturate the glucuronide and sulfate conjugation pathways and do not result in the formation of sufficient reactive metabolite to deplete glutathione stores. However, following ingestion of a large overdose (150 mg/kg or greater) the glucuronide and sulfate conjugation pathways are saturated resulting in a larger fraction of the drug being metabolized via the P-450 pathway. The increased formation of reactive metabolite may deplete the hepatic stores of glutathione with subsequent binding of the metabolite to protein molecules within the hepatocyte resulting in cellular necrosis. Acetylcysteine has been shown to reduce the extent of liver injury following acetaminophen overdose. Early symptoms following a potentially hepatotoxic overdose may include: nausea, vomiting, diaphoresis and general malaise. Clinical and laboratory evidence of hepatic toxicity may not be apparent until 48 to 72 hours postingestion. In adults and adolescents, regardless of the quantity of acetaminophen reported to have been ingested, administer MUCOMYST® acetylcysteine immediately. MUCOMYST acetylcysteine therapy should be initiated and continued for a full course of therapy. Its effectiveness depends on early administration, with benefit seen principally in patients treated within 16 hours of the overdose.

If acetaminophen plasma assay capability is not available, and the estimated acetaminophen ingestion exceeds 150 mg/kg, MUCOMYST acetylcysteine therapy should be initiated and continued for a full course of therapy.
For full prescribing information, refer to the MUCOMYST package insert. Do not await the results of assays for acetaminophen level before initiating treatment with MUCOMYST acetylcysteine. The following additional procedures are recommended: The stomach should be emptied promptly by lavage or by induction of emesis with syrup of ipecac. A serum acetaminophen assay should be obtained as early as possible, but no sooner than four hours following ingestion. Liver function studies should be obtained initially and repeated at 24-hour intervals.
For additional emergency information call your regional poison center or toll-free (1-800-525-6115) to the Rocky Mountain Poison Center for assistance in diagnosis and for directions in the use of MUCOMYST acetylcysteine as an antidote.
For overdose treatment information, consult a regional poison control center.

HOW SUPPLIED

EXCEDRIN P.M.® is supplied as:
Light blue circular coated tablets with "PM" debossed on one side.
NDC 19810-0763-6 Bottles of 10's
NDC 19810-0764-3 Bottles of 24's
NDC 19810-0763-4 Bottles of 50's
NDC 19810-0764-4 Bottles of 100's
NDC 19810-0763-9 Vials of 10's
Light blue coated caplet with "Excedrin P.M." imprinted on one side.
NDC 19810-0032-5 Bottles of 24's
NDC 19810-0032-3 Bottles of 50's
NDC 19810-0032-6 Bottles of 100's
Light blue wild berry flavored liquid.
NDC 19810-0060-1 6 oz. (177 ml) Plastic Bottle
All sizes packaged in child resistant closures except 50's tablets and caplets which are recommended for households without young children.
Store at room temperature.
Also described in PDR For Nonprescription Drugs.

Sinus EXCEDRIN®   OTC
[ex "cĕd 'rĭn]
Analgesic, Decongestant

COMPOSITION
Each coated tablet or caplet contains 500 mg Acetaminophen and 30 mg Pseudoephedrine HCl.

OTHER INGREDIENTS
Corn Starch, D&C Yellow No. 10 Lake, FD&C Red No. 40 Lake, Hydroxypropyl Methylcellulose, Mineral Oil, Polysorbate 20, Povidone, Propylene Glycol, Simethicone Emulsion, Sorbitan Monolaurate, Stearic Acid, Titanium Dioxide. May also contain: Benzoic Acid, Carnauba Wax.

INDICATIONS
For temporary relief of headache, sinus pain and sinus pressure and congestion due to sinusitis or the common cold.

WARNINGS
KEEP THIS AND ALL OTHER MEDICATIONS OUT OF THE REACH OF CHILDREN. IN CASE OF ACCIDENTAL

OVERDOSE SEEK PROFESSIONAL ASSISTANCE OR CONTACT A POISON CONTROL CENTER IMMEDIATELY. PROMPT MEDICAL ATTENTION IS CRITICAL FOR ADULTS AS WELL AS FOR CHILDREN EVEN IF YOU DO NOT NOTICE ANY SIGNS OR SYMPTOMS. As with any drug, if you are pregnant or nursing a baby, seek the advice of a health professional before using this product. Do not take this product for more than 10 days unless directed by a doctor. If symptoms do not improve or are accompanied by a fever that lasts for more than 3 days, or if new symptoms occur, consult a doctor. Do not exceed recommended dosage because at higher doses nervousness, dizziness or sleeplessness may occur. Do not take this product if your have heart disease, high blood pressure, thyroid disease, diabetes, or difficulty in urination due to enlargement of the prostate gland unless directed by a doctor.

DRUG INTERACTION PRECAUTION
Do not take this product if you are taking a prescription medication for high blood pressure or depression without first consulting a doctor.

DIRECTIONS
Adults 2 tablets or caplets every 6 hours while symptoms persist, not to exceed 8 tablets or caplets in 24 hours, or as directed by a doctor. Children under 12 years of age: Consult a doctor.

OVERDOSE
MUCOMYST (acetylcysteine) As An Antidote For Acetaminophen Overdose)
Acetaminophen is rapidly absorbed from the upper gastrointestinal tract with peak plasma levels occurring between 30 and 60 minutes after therapeutic doses and usually within 4 hours following an overdose. The parent compound, which is nontoxic, is extensively metabolized in the liver to form principally the sulfate and glucuronide conjugates which are also nontoxic and are rapidly excreted in the urine. A small fraction of an ingested dose is metabolized in the liver by the cytochrome P-450 mixed function oxidase enzyme system to form a reactive, potentially toxic, intermediate metabolite which preferentially conjugates with hepatic glutathione to form the nontoxic cysteine and mercapturic acid derivatives which are then excreted by the kidney. Therapeutic doses of acetaminophen do not saturate the glucuronide and sulfate conjugation pathways and do not result in the formation of sufficient reactive metabolite to deplete glutathione stores. However, following ingestion of a large overdose (150 mg/kg or greater) the glucuronide and sulfate conjugation pathways are saturated resulting in a larger fraction of the drug being metabolized via the P-450 pathway. The increased formation of reactive metabolite may deplete the hepatic stores of glutathione with subsequent binding of the metabolite to protein molecules within the hepatocyte resulting in cellular necrosis. Acetylcysteine has been shown to reduce the extent of liver injury following acetaminophen overdose. Early symptoms following a potentially hepatotoxic overdose may include: nausea, vomiting, diaphoresis and general malaise. Clinical and laboratory evidence of hepatic toxicity may not be apparent until 48 to 72 hours postingestion. In adults and adolescents, regardless of the quantity of acetaminophen reported to have been ingested, administer MUCOMYST® acetylcysteine immediately. MUCOMYST acetylcysteine therapy should be initiated and continued for a full course of therapy. Its effectiveness depends on early administration, with benefit seen principally in patients treated within 16 hours of the overdose.
If acetaminophen plasma assay capability is not available, and the estimated acetaminophen ingestion exceeds 150 mg/kg, MUCOMYST acetylcysteine therapy should be initiated and continued for a full course of therapy.
For full prescribing information, refer to the MUCOMYST package insert. Do not await the results of assays for acetaminophen level before initiating treatment with MUCOMYST acetylcysteine. The following additional procedures are recommended: The stomach should be emptied promptly by lavage or by induction of emesis with syrup of ipecac. A serum acetaminophen assay should be obtained as early as possible, but no sooner than four hours following ingestion. Liver function studies should be obtained initially and repeated at 24-hour intervals.
For additional emergency information call your regional poison center or toll-free (1-800-525-6115) to the Rocky Mountain Poison Center for assistance in diagnosis and for directions in the use of MUCOMYST acetylcysteine as an antidote.

HOW SUPPLIED
Sinus EXCEDRIN® is supplied as:
Coated circular orange tablets with "Sinus Excedrin" imprinted in green on one side.
NDC 19810-0080-1 Blister packages of 24's
NDC 19810-0080-2 Bottles of 50's

	EXCEDRIN®PM Per Tablet or Caplet	EXCEDRIN®PM Per Fl. Ounce (30 ml.)
Tablet Ingredients		
Active Ingredients:		
Acetaminophen	500 mg.	1000 mg.
Diphenhydramine Citrate:	38 mg.	—
Diphenhydramine HCl:	—	50 mg
Other Ingredients:		
Per Tablet or Caplet		Liquid
Benzoic Acid		Alcohol (10% by volume)
Carnauba Wax		Benzoic Acid
Corn Starch		FD&C Blue No. 1
D&C Yellow No. 10 Aluminum Lake		
FD&C Blue No. 1 Aluminum Lake		Flavor
Hydroxypropyl Methylcellulose		Polyethylene Glycol
Magnesium Stearate		Povidone
Methylparaben		
Pregelatinized Starch		
Propylparaben		Sodium Citrate
Simethicone Emulsion		
Stearic Acid		Sucrose
Titanium Dioxide		Water
May Also Contain:		
D&C Yellow No. 10		
FD&C Blue No. 1		
Polyethylene Glycol		
Polysorbate 80		
Propylene Glycol		

Coated orange caplets with "Sinus Excedrin" imprinted in green on one side.
NDC 19810-0077-1 Blister packages of 24's
NDC 19810-0077-2 Bottles of 50's
All sizes have child resistant closures except 24's for tablets and caplets which are recommended for households without young children.
Store at room temperature.
Also described in PDR For Nonprescription Drugs.

4-WAY® Cold Tablets   OTC

COMPOSITION
Each tablet contains acetaminophen 325 mg., phenylpropanolamine HCl 12.5 mg., and chlorpheniramine maleate 2 mg. Other Ingredients: Corn Starch, Corn Starch Pregelatinized, Microcrystalline Cellulose, Sodium Starch Glycolate, Stearic Acid, Sucrose.

INDICATIONS
For temporary relief of nasal and sinus congestion, runny nose, sneezing, fever, minor sore throat pain, body aches and pain.

DIRECTIONS
Adults: 2 tablets every 4 hours while symptom persist, not to exceed 12 tablets in 24 hours, or as directed by a doctor. Children 6 to under 12 years of age: One tablet every 4 hours while symptoms persist, not to exceed 5 tablets in 24 hours, or as directed by a doctor. Children under 6: Consult a doctor.

WARNINGS
KEEP THIS AND ALL OTHER MEDICATIONS OUT OF THE REACH OF CHILDREN. IN CASE OF ACCIDENTAL OVERDOSE, SEEK PROFESSIONAL ASSISTANCE OR CONTACT A POISON CONTROL CENTER IMMEDIATELY. PROMPT MEDICAL ATTENTION IS CRITICAL FOR ADULTS AS WELL AS FOR CHILDREN EVEN IF YOU DO NOT NOTICE ANY SIGNS OR SYMPTOMS. As with any drug, if you are pregnant or nursing a baby, seek the advice of a health professional before using this product. Do not take this product for more than 10 days (for adults) or 5 days (for children) unless directed by a doctor. If symptoms do not improve or are accompanied by a fever that lasts for more than 3 days, or if new symptoms occur, consult a doctor. Do not exceed recommended dosage because at higher doses nervousness, dizziness or sleeplessness may occur. May cause excitablity especially in children. If sore throat is severe, persists for more than 2 days, is accompanied or followed by a fever, headache, rash, nausea or vomiting, consult a doctor promptly. This product should not be taken by persons who have asthma, glaucoma, emphysema, chronic pulmonary disease, high blood pressure, heart disease, thyroid disease, diabetes, shortness of breath, difficulty in breathing or difficulty in urination due to enlargment of the prostate gland unless directed by a doctor. May cause drowsiness; alcohol may increase the drowsiness effect. Avoid alcoholic beverages, and do not take this product if you are taking sedatives or tranquilizers without first consulting your doctor. Use caution when driving a motor vehicle or operating machinery.

DRUG INTERACTION PRECAUTION
This product should not be taken by any adult or child who is taking a prescription medication for high blood pressure or depression without first consulting your doctor.

OVERDOSE
MUCOMYST (acetylcysteine) As An Antidote For Acetaminophen Overdose)
Acetaminophen is rapidly absorbed from the upper gastrointestinal tract with peak plasma levels occurring between 30 and 60 minutes after therapeutic doses and usually within 4 hours following an overdose. The parent compound, which is nontoxic, is extensively metabolized in the liver to form principally the sulfate and glucuronide conjugates which are also nontoxic and are rapidly excreted in the urine. A small fraction of an ingested dose is metabolized in the liver by the cytochrome P-450 mixed function oxidase enzyme system to form a reactive, potentially toxic, intermediate metabolite which preferentially conjugates with hepatic glutathione to form the nontoxic cysteine and mercapturic acid derivatives which are then excreted by the kidney. Therapeutic doses of acetaminophen do not saturate the glucuronide and sulfate conjugation pathways and do not result in the formation of sufficient reactive metabolite to deplete glutathione stores. However, following ingestion of a large overdose (150 mg/kg or greater) the glucuronide and sulfate conjugation pathways are saturated resulting in a larger fraction of the drug being metabolized via the P-450 pathway. The increased formation of reactive metabolite may deplete the hepatic stores of glutathione with subsequent binding of the metabolite to protein molecules within the hepatocyte resulting in cellular necrosis. Acetylcysteine has been shown to reduce the extent of liver injury following acetaminophen overdose. Early symptoms following a potentially hepatotoxic overdose may include: nausea, vomiting, diaphoresis and general malaise. Clinical and laboratory evidence of hepatic toxicity may not be apparent until 48 to 72 hours postingestion. In adults and adolescents, regardless of the quantity of acetaminophen reported to have been ingested, administer MUCOMYST® acetylcysteine immediately. MUCOMYST acetylcysteine therapy should be initiated and continued for a full course of therapy. Its effectiveness depends on early administration, with benefit seen principally in patients treated within 16 hours of the overdose.
If acetaminophen plasma assay capability is not available, and the estimated acetaminophen ingestion exceeds 150 mg/kg, MUCOMYST acetylcysteine therapy should be initiated and continued for a full course of therapy.
For full prescribing information, refer to the MUCOMYST package insert. Do not await the results of assays for acetaminophen level before initiating treatment with MUCOMYST acetylcysteine. The following additional procedures are recommended: The stomach should be emptied promptly by lavage or by induction of emesis with syrup of ipecac. A serum acetaminophen assay should be obtained as early as possible, but no sooner than four hours following ingestion. Liver function studies should be obtained initially and repeated at 24-hour intervals.
For additional emergency information call your regional poison center or toll-free (1-800-525-6115) to the Rocky Mountain Poison Center for assistance in diagnosis and for directions in the use of MUCOMYST acetylcysteine as an antidote.

HOW SUPPLIED
4-WAY Cold Tablets are supplied as a white tablet with the number "4" debossed on one surface.
NDC 19810-0040-1 Bottle of 36's
All sizes packaged in child resistant bottle closures.
Store at room temperature.
Also described in PDR For Nonprescription Drugs.

4-WAY® Fast Acting Nasal Spray   OTC

COMPOSITION
New Formula: Phenylephrine hydrochloride 0.5%, naphazoline hydrochloride 0.05%, pyrilamine maleate 0.2%, in a buffered aqueous solution. Also Contains: Benzalkonium Chloride, Boric Acid, Sodium Borate, Water. Also available in a mentholated formula containing Phenylephrine hydrochloride 0.5%, naphazoline hydrochloride 0.05%, pyrilamine maleate 0.2%, in a buffered solution. Also Contains: Benzalkonium Chloride, Boric Acid, Camphor, Eucalyptol, Menthol, Poloxamer 188, Polysorbate 80, Sodium Borate, Water.

INDICATIONS
For prompt, temporary relief of nasal congestion due to the common cold, sinusitis, hay fever or other upper respiratory allergies.

DIRECTIONS AND USE INSTRUCTIONS:
Directions: Adults: Spray twice into each nostril not more often than every 6 hours. Do not give to children under 12 years of age unless directed by a doctor.
Use Instructions: For Metered Pump—
Remove protective cap. Hold bottle with thumb at base and nozzle between first and second fingers. With head upright, insert metered pump spray nozzle into nostril. Depress pump, twice all the way down, with a firm even stroke and sniff deeply. Repeat in other nostril. Do not tilt head backward while spraying. Wipe tip clean after each use. Note: This bottle is filled to correct level for proper pump action. Before using the first time, remove the protective cap from the tip and prime the metered pump by depressing pump firmly several times. Wipe nozzle clean after each use.
Use Instructions: For Atomizer—
With head in a normal, upright position, put atomizer tip into nostril. Squeeze bottle with firm, quick pressure while inhaling. Wipe nozzle clean after each use.

WARNINGS
KEEP THIS AND ALL OTHER MEDICATIONS OUT OF THE REACH OF CHILDREN. IN CASE OF ACCIDENTAL OVERDOSE OR INGESTION, SEEK PROFESSIONAL ASSISTANCE OR CONTACT A POISON CONTROL CENTER IMMEDIATELY. Do not exceed recommended dosage because burning, stinging, sneezing or increase of nasal discharge may occur. The use of this container by more than one person may spread infection. Do not use this product for more than 3 days. If symptoms persist, consult a doctor.
Do not use this product in children under 12 years of age because it may cause sedation if swallowed. Do not use this product if you have heart disease, high blood pressure, thyroid disease, diabetes or difficulty in urination due to enlargement of the prostate gland unless directed by a doctor.

HOW SUPPLIED
4-WAY® Fast Acting Nasal Spray is supplied as:
Original Regular formula:
NDC 19810-0001-1 Atomizer of ½ fluid ounce
NDC 19810-0001-2 Atomizer of 1 fluid ounce.
NDC 19810-0001-3 Metered pump of ½ fluid ounce.

Original Mentholated formula:
NDC 19810-0003-1 Atomizer of ½ fluid ounce.
NDC 19810-0003-2 Atomizer of 1 fluid ounce.
New Regular formula:
NDC 19810-0047-1. Atomizer of ½ fluid ounce.
NDC 19810-0047-2 Atomizer of 1 fluid ounce.
NDC 19810-0047-3 Metered pump of ½ fluid ounce.
New Mentholated formula:
NDC 19810-0049-1 Atomizer of ½ fluid ounce.
Store at room temperature.
Also described in the PDR For Nonprescription Drugs.

4-WAY® Long Lasting Nasal Spray   OTC

COMPOSITION
Oxymetazoline Hydrochloride 0.05% in a buffered isotonic aqueous solution. Phenylmercuric Acetate 0.002% added as a preservative. **Also Contains:** Benzalkonium Chloride, Glycine, Sorbitol, Water.

INDICATIONS
For prompt, temporary relief of nasal congestion due to the common cold, sinusitis, hay fever or other upper respiratory allergies.

DIRECTIONS AND USE INSTRUCTIONS
Directions: Adults and children 6 to under 12 years of age (with adult supervision): 2 or 3 sprays in each nostril not more often than every 10 to 12 hours. Do not exceed 2 applications in any 24-hour period. Children under 6 years of age: Consult a doctor.
Use Instruction: For Metered Pump—
Remove protective cap. Hold bottle with thumb at base and nozzle between first and second fingers. With head upright, insert metered pump spray nozzle into nostril. Depress pump all the way down, with a firm even stroke and sniff deeply. Repeat in other nostril. Do not tilt head backward while spraying. Wipe tip clean after each use. Note: This bottle is filled to correct level for proper pump action. Before using the first time, remove the protective cap from the tip and prime the metered pump by depressing pump firmly several times.
Use Instructions: For Atomizer—
With head in a normal, upright position, put atomizer tip into nostril. Squeeze bottle with firm, quick pressure while inhaling.

WARNINGS
KEEP THIS AND ALL OTHER MEDICATIONS OUT OF THE REACH OF CHILDREN. IN CASE OF ACCIDENTAL OVERDOSE OR INGESTION, SEEK PROFESSIONAL ASSISTANCE OR CONTACT A POISON CONTROL CENTER IMMEDIATELY. Do not exceed recommended dosage because burning, stinging, sneezing or increase of nasal discharge may occur. The use of this container by more than one person may spread infection. Do not use this product for more than 3 days. If symptoms persist, consult a doctor. Adults and children who have heart disease, high blood pressure, thyroid disease, diabetes, or difficulty in urination due to enlargement of the prostate gland should not use this product unless directed by a doctor.

HOW SUPPLIED
4-WAY Long Lasting Nasal Spray is supplied as:
Atomizers and a metered pump:
NDC 19810-0728-1 Atomizers of ½ fluid ounce.
NDC 19810-0728-3 Metered pump of ½ fluid ounce.
NDC 19810-0048-1 Atomizer of ½ fluid ounce.
Store at room temperature.
Also described in the PDR For Nonprescription Drugs.

NO DOZ® Tablets   OTC
[nō´dōz]

COMPOSITION
Each tablet contains 100 mg. Caffeine. Other Ingredients: Cornstarch, Flavors, Mannitol, Microcrystalline Cellulose, Stearic Acid, Sucrose.

INDICATIONS
Helps restore mental alertness or wakefulness when experiencing fatigue or drowsiness.

DIRECTIONS
Adults: One or two tablets not more often than every 3 to 4 hours.

WARNINGS
KEEP THIS AND ALL OTHER MEDICATIONS OUT OF THE REACH OF CHILDREN. IN CASE OF ACCIDENTAL OVERDOSE, SEEK PROFESSIONAL ASSISTANCE OR CONTACT A POISON CONTROL CENTER IMMEDI-

Continued on next page

Bristol-Myers Products—Cont.

ATELY. As with any drug, if you are pregnant or nursing a baby, seek the advice of a health professional before using this product. Do not give to children under 12 years of age. For occasional use only. Not intented for use as a substitute for sleep. If fatigue or drowsiness persists or continues to occur, consult a doctor. The recommended dose of this product contains about as much caffeine as a cup of coffee. Limit the use of caffeine-containing medications, foods, or beverages while taking this product because too much caffeine may cause nervousness, irritability, sleeplessness and, occasionally, rapid heart beat.

HOW SUPPLIED

NO DOZ® is supplied as:
A circular white tablet with "NoDoz" debossed on one side.
NDC 19810-0063-2 Blister pack of 16's
NDC 19810-0063-3 Blister pack of 36's
NDC 19810-0062-5 Bottle of 60's
NDC 19810-0063-1 Vials of 15's
Store at room temperature.
Also described in the PDR For Nonprescription Drugs.

NO DOZ® Maximum Strength Caplets   OTC

COMPOSITION

Each caplet contains 200 mg. Caffeine. Other ingredients: Benzoic Acid, Corn Starch, FD&C Blue No. 1, Flavors, Hydroxypropyl Methylcellulose, Microcrystalline Cellulose, Propylene Glycol, Simethicone Emulsion, Stearic Acid, Sucrose, Titanium Dioxide. May also contain: Carnauba Wax, Mineral Oil, Polysorbate 20, Povidone, Sorbitan Monolaurate.

INDICATIONS

Helps restore mental alertness or wakefulness when experiencing fatigue or drowsiness.

DIRECTIONS

Adults: one-half to one caplet not more often than every 3 to 4 hours.

WARNINGS

KEEP THIS AND ALL OTHER MEDICATIONS OUT OF THE REACH OF CHILDREN. IN CASE OF ACCIDENTAL OVERDOSE, SEEK PROFESSIONAL ASSISTANCE OR CONTACT A POISON CONTROL CENTER IMMEDIATELY. As with any drug, if you are pregnant or nursing a baby, seek the advice of a health professional before using this product. Do not give to children under 12 years of age. For occasional use only. Not intended for use as a substitute for sleep. If fatigue or drowsiness persists or continues to occur, consult a doctor. The recommended dose of this product contains about as much caffeine as a cup of coffee. Limit the use of caffeine-containing medications, foods, or beverages while taking this product because too much caffeine may cause nervousness, irritability, sleeplessness and, occasionally, rapid heart beat.

OVERDOSE

Typical of caffeine.

HOW SUPPLIED

NO DOZ® Maximum Strength is supplied as: White coated caplets with "NO DOZ" debossed on one side. The opposite side is scored.
NDC 19810-0064-1 Blister Packages of 12's
Store at room temperature.
Also described in PDR For Nonprescription Drugs.
NDC 19810-0064-3 Bottle of 30's .

NUPRIN®   OTC
(ibuprofen)
Analgesic

WARNING

ASPIRIN SENSITIVE PATIENTS. Do not take this product if you have had a severe allergic reaction to aspirin, e.g.—asthma, swelling, shock or hives, because even though this product contains no aspirin or salicylates, cross-reactions may occur in patients allergic to aspirin.

COMPOSITION

Each tablet or caplet contains ibuprofen USP, 200 mg. **Other Ingredients:** Carnauba wax, cornstarch, D&C Yellow No. 10, FD&C Yellow No. 6, hydroxypropyl methylcellulose, propylene glycol, silicon dioxide, stearic acid, titanium dioxide.

INDICATIONS

For the temporary relief of minor aches and pains associated with the common cold, headache, toothache, muscular aches, backache, for the minor pain of arthritis, for the pain of menstrual cramps and for reduction of fever.

WARNINGS

Do not take for pain for more than 10 days or for fever for more than 3 days unless directed by a doctor. If pain or fever persists or gets worse, if new symptoms occur, or if the painful area is red or swollen, consult a doctor. These could be signs of serious illness. If you are under a doctor's care for any serious condition, consult a doctor before taking this product. As with aspirin and acetaminophen, if you have any condition which requires you to take prescription drugs or if you have had any problems or serious side effects from taking any non-prescription pain reliever, do not take NUPRIN without first discussing it with your doctor. If you experience any symptoms which are unusual or seem unrelated to the condition for which you took ibuprofen, consult a doctor before taking any more of it. Although ibuprofen is indicated for the same conditions as aspirin and acetaminophen, it should not be taken with them except under a doctor's direction. Do not combine this product with any other ibuprofen-containing product. As with any drug, if you are pregnant or nursing a baby, seek the advice of a health professional before using this product. IT IS ESPECIALLY IMPORTANT NOT TO USE IBUPROFEN DURING THE LAST 3 MONTHS OF PREGNANCY UNLESS SPECIFICALLY DIRECTED TO DO SO BY A DOCTOR BECAUSE IT MAY CAUSE PROBLEMS IN THE UNBORN CHILD OR COMPLICATIONS DURING DELIVERY. Keep this and all drugs out of the reach of children. In case of accidental overdose, seek professional assistance or contact a poison control center immediately.

DIRECTIONS

Adults: Take 1 tablet or caplet every 4 to 6 hours while symptoms persist. If pain or fever does not respond to 1 tablet or caplet, 2 tablets or caplets may be used but do not exceed 6 tablets or caplets in 24 hours, unless directed by a doctor. The smallest effective dose should be used. Take with food or milk if occasional and mild heartburn, upset stomach, or stomach pain occurs with use. Consult a doctor if these symptoms are more than mild or if they persist. Children: Do not give this product to children under 12 except under the advice and supervision of a doctor.

OVERDOSE

For overdose treatment information, consult a regional poison control center.

HOW SUPPLIED

NUPRIN® is supplied as:
Golden yellow round tablets with "NUPRIN" printed in black on one side.
NDC 19810-0767-2 Bottles of 24's
NDC 19810-0767-3 Bottles of 50's
NDC 19810-0767-4 Bottles of 100's
NDC 19810-0767-7 Bottles of 150's
NDC 19810-0767-8 Bottles of 225's
NDC 19810-0767-9 Vials of 10's
Golden yellow caplets with "NUPRIN" printed in black on one side.
NDC 19810-0796-1 Bottles of 24's
NDC 19810-0796-2 Bottles of 50's
NDC 19810-0796-3 Bottles of 100's
All sizes packaged in child resistant closures except 24's for tablets and 24's for caplets, which are sizes recommended for households without young children.
Store at room temperature. Avoid excessive heat 40℃. (104°F.).
Also described in the PDR For Nonprescription Drugs.
Shown in Product Identification Section, page 406

PAZO® Hemorrhoid   OTC
Ointment/Suppositories

COMPOSITION

Ointment: Active Ingredients: Camphor, 2%; Ephedrine Sulphate, 0.2%; Zinc Oxide, 5%. Other Ingredients: Lanolin, Petrolatum.
Suppositories (per suppository): Active Ingredients: Ephedrine Sulfate, 3.86 mg; Zinc Oxide, 96.5 mg. Other Ingredients: Hydrogenated Vegetable Oil.

INDICATIONS

Ointment: For the temporary relief of local pain, itching, and discomfort associated with inflamed hemorrhoidal tissues. Temporarily shrinks hemorrhoidal tissue.
Suppositories: For the temporary relief of local itching and discomfort associated with inflamed hemorrhoidal tissues. Temporarily shrinks hemorrhoidal tissue.

DIRECTIONS

Ointment—Adults: When practical, cleanse the affected area with mild soap and warm water and rinse thoroughly. Gently dry by patting or blotting with toilet tissue or a soft cloth before application of this product. Apply externally to the affected area up to 4 times daily. Children under 12 years of age: consult a doctor.

Suppositories—Adults: When practical, cleanse the affected area with mild soap and warm water and rinse thoroughly. Gently dry by patting or blotting with toilet tissue or a soft cloth before application of this product. Remove foil wrapper and insert suppository into the rectum. Use rectally up to 4 times daily. Children under 12 years of age: consult a doctor.

WARNINGS

KEEP THIS AND ALL OTHER MEDICATIONS OUT OF THE REACH OF CHILDREN. IN CASE OF ACCIDENTAL INGESTION OR OVERDOSE, SEEK PROFESSIONAL ASSISTANCE OR CONTACT A POISON CONTROL CENTER IMMEDIATELY. As with any drug, if you are pregnant or nursing a baby, seek the advice of a health professional before using this product. If condition worsens or does not improve within 7 days, consult a doctor. Do not exceed the recommended daily dosage unless directed by a doctor. In case of bleeding consult a doctor promptly. Do not put this product into the rectum by using fingers or any mechanical device or applicator. Do not use this product if you have heart disease, high blood pressure, thyroid disease, diabetes, or difficulty in urination due to enlargement of the prostate gland unless directed by a doctor. Some users of this product may experience nervousness, tremor, sleeplessness, nausea, and loss of appetite. If these symptoms persist or become worse consult your doctor. DRUG INTERACTION PRECAUTION: Do not use this product if you are taking a prescription drug for high blood pressure or depression without first consulting your doctor.
Store at room temperature.

HOW SUPPLIED

PAZO® ointment is supplied with a plastic applicator as:
NDC 19810-0768-1 One ounce tubes
PAZO® suppositories are silver foil wrapped and supplied as:
NDC 19810-0703-1 Box of 12's
Also described in the PDR For Nonprescription Drugs.

THERAPEUTIC MINERAL ICE®   OTC
Pain Relieving Gel

COMPOSITION

Active Ingredient: Menthol 2%
Other Ingredients: Ammonium Hydroxide, Carbomer 934, Cupric Sulfate, FD&C Blue No. 1. Isopropyl Alcohol, Magnesium Sulfate, Sodium Hydroxide, Thymol, Water.

INDICATIONS

For the temporary relief of minor aches and pains of muscles and joints associated with arthritis, simple backache, strains, bruises, sprains and sports injuries. **USE ONLY AS DIRECTED. Read all warnings before use.**

WARNING

KEEP OUT OF THE REACH OF CHILDREN. For external use only. Not for internal use. Avoid contact with eyes and mucous membranes. Do not use with other ointments, creams, sprays, or liniments. **Do not use with Heating Pads or Heating Devices.** If condition worsens, or if symptoms persist for more than 7 days, or clear up and occur again within a few days, discontinue use of this product and consult your doctor. Do not apply to wounds or damaged skin. Do not bandage tightly. If you have sensitive skin, consult doctor **before** use. If skin irritation develops, discontinue use and consult your doctor. As with any drug, if you are pregnant or nursing a baby, seek the advice of a health professional **before** using this product. Keep cap tightly closed. Do not use, pour, spill or store near heat or open flame. **Note:** You can always use Mineral Ice as directed, but its use is never intended to replace your doctor's advice.

DIRECTIONS

Adults and children 2 years of age and older: Clean skin of all other ointments, creams, sprays, or liniments. Apply to affected areas not more than 3 to 4 times daily. May be used with wet or dry bandages or with ice packs. No protective cover needed. Children under 2 years of age: Consult a doctor.

HOW SUPPLIED

NDC 19810-0034-4 3.5 oz.
NDC 19810-0034-2 8 oz.
NDC 19810-0034-3 16 oz.
Store at room temperature.
Shown in Product Identification Section, page 406

Products are cross-indexed by
generic and chemical names in the
YELLOW SECTION.

The Brown Pharmaceutical Company, Inc.

See ICN PHARMACEUTICALS, INC.

Burroughs Wellcome Co.

3030 CORNWALLIS ROAD
RESEARCH TRIANGLE PARK, NC 27709

ACTIFED® Tablets and Syrup OTC
[ăk 'tĭ-fĕd]
Antihistamine/Nasal Decongestant

(See PDR For Nonprescription Drugs.)
Tablets Shown in Product Identification Section, page 406

ACTIFED® with CODEINE ℞ Ⓒ
[ăk 'tĭ-fed]
Cough Syrup

DESCRIPTION

Each 5 mL (1 teaspoonful) contains: codeine phosphate 10 mg (Warning—may be habit-forming), Actidil® (triprolidine hydrochloride) 1.25 mg, Sudafed® (pseudoephedrine hydrochloride) 30 mg and the inactive ingredients: alcohol 4.3%, methylparaben 0.1% and sodium benzoate 0.1% (added as preservatives), flavors, glycerin, and sorbitol. This medication is intended for oral administration.
Actifed with Codeine Cough Syrup has antitussive, antihistaminic and nasal decongestant effects. The components of Actifed with Codeine Cough Syrup have the following chemical names.
Codeine Phosphate, U.S.P.:
7,8-didehydro-4,5α-epoxy-3-methoxy-17-methyl-morphinan-6α-ol phosphate (1:1) (salt) hemihydrate
Triprolidine Hydrochloride Monohydrate:
(*E*)-2-[3-(1-pyrrolidinyl)-1-(*p-tolyl*) propenyl]pyridine monohydrochloride monohydrate
Pseudoephedrine Hydrochloride:
[*S*-(*R* *,*R* *)]-α-[1-(methylamino)ethyl]benzenemethanol hydrochloride

CLINICAL PHARMACOLOGY

Codeine: Codeine probably exerts its antitussive activity by depressing the medullary (brain) cough center, thereby raising its threshold for incoming cough impulses.
Codeine is readily absorbed from the gastrointestinal tract, with a therapeutic dose reaching peak antitussive effectiveness in about 2 hours and persisting for 4 to 6 hours. Codeine is rapidly distributed from blood to body tissues and taken up preferentially by parenchymatous organs such as liver, spleen and kidney. It passes the blood brain barrier and is found in fetal tissue and breast milk.
The drug is not bound by plasma proteins nor is it accumulated in body tissues. Codeine is metabolized in the liver to morphine and norcodeine, each representing about 10 percent of the administered codeine dose. About 90 percent of the dose is excreted within 24 hours, primarily through the kidneys. Urinary excretion products are free and glucuronide-conjugated codeine (about 70%), free and conjugated norcodeine (about 10%), free and conjugated morphine (about 10%), normorphine (under 4%) and hydrocodone (< 1%). The remainder of the dose appears in the feces.
Triprolidine: Antihistamines such as triprolidine hydrochloride act as antagonists of the H_1 histamine receptor. Consequently, they prevent histamine from eliciting typical immediate hypersensitivity responses in the nose, eyes, lungs and skin.
Animal distribution studies have shown localization of triprolidine in lung, spleen and kidney tissue. Liver microsome studies have revealed the presence of several metabolites with an oxidized product of the toluene methyl group predominating.
Pseudoephedrine: Pseudoephedrine acts as an indirect sympathomimetic agent by stimulating sympathetic (adrenergic) nerve endings to release norepinephrine. Norepinephrine in turn stimulates alpha and beta receptors throughout the body. The action of pseudoephedrine hydrochloride is apparently more specific for the blood vessels of the upper respiratory tract and less specific for the blood vessels of the systemic circulation. The vasoconstriction elicited at these sites results in the shrinkage of swollen tissues in the sinuses and nasal passages.
Pseudoephedrine is rapidly and almost completely absorbed from the gastrointestinal tract. Considerable variation in half-life has been observed (from about 4½ to 10 hours), which is attributed to individual differences in absorption and excretion. Excretion rates are also altered by urine pH, increasing with acidification and decreasing with alkalinization. As a result, mean half-life falls to about 4 hours at pH 5 and increases to 12 to 13 hours at pH 8.

Parameter	Codeine*	Triprolidine†	Pseudoephedrine‡
Elimination Half Life (hr)	2.7 ± 0.4§	4.0 ± 2.2	5.5 ± 0.9
Time to Maximum Concentration (hr)	1.2 ± 0.5	1.8 ± 0.7	2.6 ± 1.0
Maximum Plasma Concentration (ng/mL)	44.8 ± 11.7	4.9 ± 1.8	189 ± 44
Area Under Plasma Curve from t = 0 to t = ∞ (ng/mL·hr)	226 ± 41	42.5 ± 34.0	1938 ± 440

* 20 mg Codeine Phosphate hemihydrate (equivalent to 14.7 mg free base)
† 2.5 mg Triprolidine HCl monohydrate (equivalent to 2.1 mg free base)
‡ 60 mg Pseudoephedrine HCl (equivalent to 49.1 mg free base)
§ Means ± S.D.

After administration of a 60 mg tablet, 87 to 96% of the pseudoephedrine is cleared from the body within 24 hours. The drug is distributed to body tissues and fluids, including fetal tissue, breast milk and the central nervous system (CNS). About 55 to 75% of an administered dose is excreted unchanged in the urine; the remainder is apparently metabolized in the liver to inactive compounds by N-demethylation, parahydroxylation and oxidative deamination.
The pharmacokinetic properties of codeine, triprolidine and pseudoephedrine from 10 mL of Actifed with Codeine Cough Syrup were investigated compared to a reference preparation of equal component doses in 18 healthy adults. The results of this study showed that Actifed with Codeine Cough Syrup and the reference preparation were bioequivalent.
Pharmacokinetic parameters for Actifed with Codeine Cough Syrup are as follows:
[See table above.]

INDICATIONS AND USAGE

Actifed with Codeine Cough Syrup is indicated for temporary relief of coughs and upper respiratory symptoms, including nasal congestion, associated with allergy or the common cold.

CONTRAINDICATIONS

Actifed with Codeine Cough Syrup is contraindicated under the following conditions:
Use in Newborn or Premature Infants: This drug should *not* be used in newborn or premature infants.
Use in Lower Respiratory Disease: Antihistamines should *not* be used to treat lower respiratory tract symptoms, including asthma.
Hypersensitivity to: 1) codeine phosphate or other narcotics; 2) triprolidine hydrochloride or other antihistamines of similar chemical structure; or 3) sympathomimetic amines, including pseudoephedrine.
Sympathomimetic amines are contraindicated in patients with severe hypertension, severe coronary artery disease and in patients on monoamine oxidase (MAO) inhibitor therapy (see Drug Interaction Section).

WARNINGS

Actifed with Codeine Cough Syrup should be used with considerable caution in patients with increased intraocular pressure (narrow angle glaucoma), stenosing peptic ulcer, pyloroduodenal obstruction, symptomatic prostatic hypertrophy, bladder neck obstruction, hypertension, diabetes mellitus, ischemic heart disease, and hyperthyroidism.
In the presence of head injury or other intracranial lesions, the respiratory depressant effects of codeine and other narcotics may be markedly enhanced, as well as their capacity for elevating cerebrospinal fluid pressure.
Narcotics also produce other CNS depressant effects, such as drowsiness, that may further obscure the clinical course of patients with head injuries.
Codeine or other narcotics may obscure signs on which to judge the diagnosis or clinical course of patients with acute abdominal conditions.

PRECAUTIONS

General: Actifed with Codeine Cough Syrup should be prescribed with caution for certain special-risk patients, such as the elderly or debilitated, and for those with severe impairment of renal or hepatic function, gallbladder disease or gallstones, respiratory impairment, cardiac arrhythmias, history of bronchial asthma, prostatic hypertrophy or urethral stricture, and in patients known to be taking other antitussive, antihistamine or decongestant medications. Patients' self-medication habits should be investigated to determine their use of such medications. Actifed with Codeine Cough Syrup is intended for short-term use only.
Information for Patients:

1. Patients should be warned about engaging in activities requiring mental alertness such as driving a car, operating dangerous machinery or hazardous appliances.
2. Patients with a history of glaucoma, peptic ulcer, urinary retention or pregnancy should be cautioned before starting Actifed.
3. Patients should be told not to take alcohol, sleeping pills, sedatives or tranquilizers while taking Actifed.
4. Antihistamines as in Actifed, may cause dizziness, drowsiness, dry mouth, blurred vision, weakness, nausea, headache or nervousness in some patients.
5. Patients should be told to store this medicine in a tightly closed container in a dry, cool place away from heat or direct sunlight and out of the reach of children.
6. **Nursing Mothers** refer to following section titled "Nursing Mothers."

Actifed with Codeine Cough Syrup should not be used by persons intolerant to sympathomimetics used for the relief of nasal or sinus congestion. Such drugs include ephedrine, epinephrine, phenylpropanolamine, and phenylephrine. Symptoms of intolerance include drowsiness, dizziness, weakness, difficulty in breathing, tenseness, muscle tremors or palpitations.
Codeine may be habit-forming when used over long periods or in high doses. Patients should take the drug only for as long, in the amounts, and as frequently as prescribed.
Drug Interactions: Actifed with Codeine Cough Syrup may **enhance** the effects of:

1. monoamine oxidase (MAO) inhibitors;
2. other narcotic analgesics, alcohol, general anesthetics, tranquilizers, sedative-hypnotics, surgical skeletal muscle relaxants, or other CNS depressants, by causing increased CNS depression.

Actifed with Codeine Cough Syrup may **diminish:**
the antihypertensive effects of guanethidine, bethanidine, methyldopa, and reserpine.
Drug/Laboratory Test Interactions:
Codeine: Narcotic administration may increase serum amylase levels.
Carcinogenesis, Mutagenesis, Impairment of Fertility: No adequate studies have been conducted in animals to determine whether the components of Actifed with Codeine Cough Syrup have a potential for carcinogenesis, mutagenesis or impairment of fertility.
Pregnancy: *Teratogenic Effects:* Pregnancy Category C. Animal reproduction studies have not been conducted with Actifed with Codeine Cough Syrup. It is also not known whether Actifed with Codeine Cough Syrup can cause fetal harm when administered to a pregnant woman or can affect reproduction capacity. Actifed with Codeine Cough Syrup should be given to a pregnant woman only if clearly needed.
Teratology studies have been conducted with three ingredients of Actifed with Codeine Cough Syrup. Pseudoephedrine studies were conducted in rats at doses up to 150 times the human dose; triprolidine was studied in rats and rabbits at doses up to 125 times the human dose, and codeine studies were conducted in rats and rabbits at doses up to 150 times the human dose. No evidence of teratogenic harm to the fetus was revealed in any of these studies. However, overt signs of toxicity were observed in the dams which received pseudoephedrine. This was reflected in reduced average weight and length and rate of skeletal ossification in their fetuses.
Nursing Mothers: The components of Actifed with Codeine Cough Syrup are excreted in breast milk in small amounts, but the significance of their effects on nursing infants is not known. Because of the potential for serious adverse reactions in nursing infants from maternal ingestion of Actifed with Codeine Cough Syrup, a decision should be made whether to discontinue nursing or to discontinue the drug, taking into account the importance of the drug to the mother.
Pediatric Use: As in adults, the combination of an antihistamine, sympathomimetic amine and codeine can elicit either mild stimulation or mild sedation in children. In infants and children particularly, the ingredients in this drug product **in overdosage** may produce hallucinations, convulsions and death. Symptoms of toxicity in children may include fixed dilated pupils, flushed face, dry mouth, fever, excitation, hallucinations, ataxia, incoordination, athetosis, tonic clonic convulsions and postictal depression, (see CONTRAINDICATIONS and OVERDOSAGE sections).
Use in Elderly (approximately 60 years or older): The ingredients in Actifed with Codeine Cough Syrup are more likely to cause adverse reactions in elderly patients.

ADVERSE REACTIONS

(The most frequent adverse reactions are underlined.)
General: Dryness of mouth, dryness of nose, dryness of throat, urticaria, drug rash, anaphylactic shock, photosensitivity, excessive perspiration and chills.
Cardiovascular System: Hypotension, headache, palpitations, tachycardia, extrasystoles.

Continued on next page

Burroughs Wellcome—Cont.

Hematologic System: Hemolytic anemia, thrombocytopenia, agranulocytosis.
Nervous System: Sedation, sleepiness, dizziness, disturbed coordination, fatigue, confusion, restlessness, excitation, anxiety, nervousness, tremor, irritability, insomnia, euphoria, paresthesias, blurred vision, diplopia, vertigo, tinnitus, acute labyrinthitis, hysteria, neuritis, convulsions, CNS depression, hallucination.
G.I. System: Epigastric distress, anorexia, nausea, vomiting, diarrhea, constipation.
G.U. System: Urinary frequency, difficult urination, urinary retention, early menses.
Respiratory System: Thickening of bronchial secretions, tightness of chest and wheezing, nasal stuffiness, respiratory depression.

DRUG ABUSE AND DEPENDENCE

Like other medications containing a narcotic, Actifed with Codeine Cough Syrup is controlled by the Drug Enforcement Administration. It is classified under Schedule V.
Actifed with Codeine Cough Syrup can produce drug dependence of the morphine type, and therefore it has a potential for being abused. Psychic dependence, physical dependence and tolerance may develop on repeated administration.
The dependence liability of codeine has been found to be too small to permit a full definition of its characteristics. Studies indicate that addiction to codeine is extremely uncommon and requires very high parenteral doses.
When dependence on codeine occurs at therapeutic doses, it appears to require from one to two months to develop, and withdrawal symptoms are mild. Most patients on long-term oral codeine therapy show no signs of physical dependence upon abrupt withdrawal.

OVERDOSAGE

Since Actifed with Codeine Cough Syrup is comprised of three pharmacologically different compounds, it is difficult to predict the exact manifestation of symptoms in a given individual. Reaction to an overdosage of Actifed with Codeine Cough Syrup may vary from CNS depression to stimulation. A detailed description of symptoms which are likely to appear after ingestion of an excess of the individual components follows:
Overdosage with codeine can cause transient euphoria, drowsiness, dizziness, weariness, diminution of sensibility, loss of sensation, vomiting, transient excitement in children and occasionally in adult women, miosis progressing to nonreactive pinpoint pupils, itching sometimes with skin rashes and urticaria, and clammy skin with mottled cyanosis. In more severe cases, muscular relaxation with depressed or absent superficial and deep reflexes and a positive Babinski sign may appear. Marked slowing of the respiratory rate with inadequate pulmonary ventilation and consequent cyanosis may occur. Terminal signs include shock, pulmonary edema, hypostatic or aspiration pneumonia and respiratory arrest, with death occurring within 6–12 hours following ingestion.
Overdoses of antihistamines may cause hallucinations, convulsions, or possibly death, especially in infants and children. Antihistamines are more likely to cause dizziness, sedation, and hypotension in elderly patients.
Overdosage with triprolidine may produce reactions varying from depression to stimulation of the Central Nervous System (CNS); the latter is particularly likely in children. Atropine-like signs and symptoms (dry mouth, fixed dilated pupils, flushing, tachycardia, hallucinations, convulsions, urinary retention, cardiac arrthymias and coma) may occur.
Overdosage with pseudoephedrine can cause excessive CNS stimulation resulting in excitement, nervousness, anxiety, tremor, restlessness and insomnia. Other effects include tachycardia, hypertension, pallor, mydriasis, hyperglycemia and urinary retention. Severe overdosage may cause tachypnea or hyperpnea, hallucinations, convulsions, or delirium, but in some individuals there may be CNS depression with somnolence, stupor or respiratory depression. Arrhythmias (including ventricular fibrillation) may lead to hypotension and circulatory collapse. Severe hypokalemia can occur, probably due to compartmental shift rather than depletion of potassium. No organ damage or significant metabolic derangement is associated with pseudoephedrine overdosage.
The toxic plasma concentration of codeine is not known with certainty. Experimental production of mild to moderate CNS depression in healthy, nontolerant subjects occurs at plasma concentrations of 0.5–1.9 μg/mL when codeine is given by intravenous infusion. The single lethal dose of codeine in adults is estimated to be from 0.5 to 1.0 gram. It is also estimated that 5 mg/kg could be fatal in children.
The LD_{50} (single, oral dose) of triprolidine is 163 to 308 mg/kg in the mouse (depending upon strain) and 840 mg/kg in the rat.
Insufficient data are available to estimate the toxic and lethal doses of triprolidine in humans. No reports of acute poisoning with triprolidine have appeared.
The LD_{50} (single, oral dose) of pseudoephedrine is 726 mg/kg in the mouse, 2206 mg/kg in the rat and 1177 mg/kg in the rabbit. The toxic and lethal concentrations in human biologic fluids are not known. Excretion rates increase with urine acidification and decrease with alkalinization. Few reports of toxicity due to pseudoephedrine have been published and no case of fatal overdosage is known.
Therapy, if instituted within 4 hours of overdosage, is aimed at reducing further absorption of the drug. In the conscious patient, vomiting should be induced even though it may have occurred spontaneously. If vomiting cannot be induced, gastric lavage is indicated. Adequate precautions must be taken to protect against aspiration, especially in infants and children. Charcoal slurry or other suitable agents should be instilled into the stomach after vomiting or lavage. Saline cathartics or milk of magnesia may be of additional benefit.
In the unconscious patient, the airway should be secured with a cuffed endotracheal tube before attempting to evacuate the gastric contents. Intensive supportive and nursing care is indicated, as for any comatose patient.
If breathing is significantly impaired, maintenance of adequate airway and mechanical support of respiration is the most effective means of providing adequate oxygenation.
Hypotension is an early sign of impending cardiovascular collapse and should be treated vigorously.
Do not use CNS stimulants. Convulsions should be controlled by careful administration of diazepam or short-acting barbiturate, repeated as necessary. Physostigmine may be also considered for use in controlling centrally mediated convulsions.
Ice packs and cooling sponge baths, not alcohol, can aid in reducing the fever commonly seen in children.
For codeine, continuous stimulation that arouses, but does not exhaust, the patient is useful in preventing coma. Continuous or intermittent oxygen therapy is usually indicated, while Naloxone is useful as a codeine antidote. Close nursing care is essential.
Saline cathartics, such as milk of magnesia, help to dilute the concentration of the drugs in the bowel by drawing water into the gut, thereby hastening drug elimination.
Adrenergic receptor blocking agents are antidotes to pseudoephedrine. In practice, the most useful is the beta-blocker propranolol, which is indicated when there are signs of cardiac toxicity.
There are no specific antidotes to triprolidine. Histamine should not be given.
Pseudoephedrine and codeine are theoretically dialyzable, but the procedures have not been clinically established.
In severe cases of overdosage, it is essential to monitor both the heart (by electrocardiograph) and plasma electrolytes and to give intravenous potassium as indicated by these continuous controls. Vasopressors may be used to treat hypotension, and excessive CNS stimulation may be counteracted with parenteral diazepam. Stimulants should not be used.

DOSAGE AND ADMINISTRATION

DOSAGE SHOULD BE INDIVIDUALIZED ACCORDING TO THE NEEDS AND RESPONSE OF THE PATIENT.
Usual Dose:

	Teaspoonfuls (5 mL)	
Adults and children 12 years and older	2	every 4–6 hours not to exceed 4 doses in a 24-hour period
Children 6 to under 12 years	1	
Children 2 to under 6 years	½	

HOW SUPPLIED

Bottle of one pint (NDC 0081-0025-96).
Store at 15° to 25°C (59° to 77°F) and protect from light.
402624

ACTIFED® PLUS Tablets and Caplets OTC
[*ăk 'tĭ-fĕd*]
Analgesic/Antihistamine/Nasal Decongestant

(See PDR For Nonprescription Drugs.)
Tablets and Caplets Shown in Product Identification Section, page 406

ACTIFED® SINUS OTC
DAYTIME/NIGHTTIME
Caplets and Tablets
[*ăk '-tĭ-fĕd*]
Analgesic-Nasal Decongestant/
Analgesic-Nasal Decongestant-Antihistamine

(See PDR For Nonprescription Drugs.)
Caplets and Tablets Shown in Product Identification Section, pages 406 and 407

ALKERAN® ℞
[*al-kur 'an*]
(Melphalan)
2 mg Scored Tablets

> **WARNING:** Melphalan is leukemogenic in humans.
> Melphalan produces chromosomal aberrations *in vitro* and *in vivo* and therefore should be considered potentially mutagenic in humans.
> Melphalan produces amenorrhea.

DESCRIPTION

Alkeran (melphalan), also known as L-phenylalanine mustard, phenylalanine mustard, L-PAM, or L-sarcolysin, is a phenylalanine derivative of nitrogen mustard. Alkeran is a bifunctional alkylating agent which is active against selective human neoplastic diseases. It is known chemically as 4-[bis(2-chloroethyl)amino]-*L*-phenylalanine.
Melphalan is the active L-isomer of the compound and was first synthesized in 1953 by Bergel and Stock; the D-isomer, known as medphalan, is less active against certain animal tumors, and the dose needed to produce effects on chromosomes is larger than that required with the L-isomer. The racemic (DL-) form is known as merphalan or sarcolysin.
Melphalan is insoluble in water and has a pKa_1 of ~ 2.1.
Alkeran (melphalan) is available in tablet form for oral administration. Each scored tablet contains 2 mg melphalan and the inactive ingredients lactose, magnesium stearate, potato starch, povidone, and sucrose.

CLINICAL PHARMACOLOGY

Alberts *et al* [1] found that plasma melphalan levels are highly variable after oral dosing, both with respect to the time of the first appearance of melphalan in plasma (range 0 to 336 minutes) and to the peak plasma concentration (range 0.166 to 3.741 μg/mL) achieved.[2] These results may be due to incomplete intestinal absorption, a variable "first pass" hepatic metabolism, or to rapid hydrolysis. Five patients were studied after both oral and intravenous dosing with 0.6 mg/kg as a single bolus dose by each route. The areas under the plasma concentration-time curves after oral administration averaged 61 ± 26% (± standard deviation; range 25 to 89%) of those following intravenous administration. In 18 patients given a single oral dose of 0.6 mg/kg of melphalan, the terminal plasma half-disappearance time of parent drug was 89.5 ± 50 minutes. The 24-hour urinary excretion of parent drug in these patients was 10 ± 4.5%, suggesting that renal clearance is not a major route of elimination of parent drug.
Tattersall *et al*,[3] using universally labeled ^{14}C-melphalan, found substantially less radioactivity in the urine of patients given the drug by mouth (30% of administered dose in nine days) than in the urine of those given it intravenously (35 to 65% in seven days). Following either oral or intravenous administration, the pattern of label recovery was similar, with the majority being recovered in the first 24 hours. Following oral administration, peak radioactivity occurred in plasma at two hours and then disappeared with a half-life of approximately 160 hours. In one patient where parent drug (rather than just radiolabel) was determined, the melphalan half-disappearance time was 67 minutes.[3]

INDICATIONS AND USAGE

Alkeran (melphalan) is indicated for the palliative treatment of multiple myeloma and for the palliation of non-resectable epithelial carcinoma of the ovary.

CONTRAINDICATIONS

Melphalan should not be used in patients whose disease has demonstrated a prior resistance to this agent. Patients who have demonstrated hypersensitivity to melphalan should not be given the drug.

WARNINGS

As with other nitrogen mustard drugs, excessive dosage will produce marked bone marrow depression. Frequent blood counts are essential to determine optimal dosage and to avoid toxicity. The drug should be discontinued or the dosage reduced upon evidence of depression of the bone marrow.
There are many reports of patients with multiple myeloma who have developed acute, nonlymphocytic leukemia or myeloproliferative syndrome following therapy with alkylating agents (including melphalan). Evaluation of published reports strongly suggests that melphalan is leukemogenic (see PRECAUTIONS: Carcinogenesis). The potential benefits from the drug and potential risk of carcinogenesis must be evaluated on an individual basis.
Pregnancy: "Pregnancy Category D." Melphalan may cause fetal harm when administered to a pregnant woman. Animal reproduction studies have not been conducted with melphalan. There are no adequate and well-controlled studies in pregnant women. If this drug is used during pregnancy, or if the patient becomes pregnant while taking this drug, the patient should be apprised of the potential hazard to the fetus. Women of childbearing potential should be advised to avoid becoming pregnant.

PRECAUTIONS

General: Melphalan should be used with extreme caution in patients whose bone marrow reserve may have been compromised by prior irradiation or chemotherapy, or whose marrow function is recovering from previous cytotoxic therapy. If the leukocyte count falls below 3,000/µL, or the platelet count below 100,000 µL, the drug should be discontinued until the peripheral blood cell counts have recovered.

A recommendation as to whether or not dosage reduction should be made routinely in patients with impaired creatinine clearance cannot be made because:

(a) There is considerable inherent patient-to-patient variability in the systemic availability of melphalan in patients with normal renal function.

(b) There is only a small amount of the administered dose that appears as parent drug in the urine of patients with normal renal function.

Patients with azotemia should be closely observed, however, in order to make dosage reductions, if required, at the earliest possible time.

Information for Patients: Patients should be informed that the major toxicities of melphalan are related to myelosuppression, hypersensitivity, gastrointestinal toxicity, pulmonary toxicity, infertility, nonlymphocytic leukemia and myeloproliferative syndrome. Patients should never be allowed to take the drug without close medical supervision and should be advised to consult their physician if they experience skin rash, vasculitis, bleeding, fever, persistent cough, nausea, vomiting, amenorrhea, weight loss, or unusual lumps/masses. Women of childbearing potential should be advised to avoid becoming pregnant.

Laboratory Tests: Weekly examination of the blood should be made to determine hemoglobin levels, total and differential leukocyte counts, and platelet enumeration. Patients may develop symptoms of anemia if the hemoglobin falls below 9 to 10 gm/dL, and are at risk of severe infection if the absolute neutrophil count is below 1,000/mm^3, and may bleed if the platelet count falls below 50,000/mm^3.

Drug Interactions: There are no known drug/drug interactions with melphalan.

Carcinogenesis, Mutagenesis, Impairment of Fertility: In an animal study to evaluate carcinogenesis, rats were given melphalan i.p. 3 times weekly for six months in doses ten to twenty times greater than the recommended dose in man. Fifty percent (50%) of the animals developed peritoneal sarcomas. Males and females developed lung tumors in excess of controls.[4] In a 39-week test melphalan produced a dose-related increase in lung tumors in mice.[5]

Acute nonlymphocytic leukemia and myeloproliferative syndrome have been reported in patients with cancer treated with alkylating agents (including melphalan).[6,7,8] Some patients also received other chemotherapeutic agents or radiation therapy. Precise quantitation of the risk of acute leukemia, myeloproliferative syndrome or carcinoma is not possible. Published reports of leukemia in patients who have received melphalan (and other alkylating agents) suggest that the risk of leukemogenesis increases with chronicity of treatment and with cumulative dose. In one study,[7] the 10 year cumulative risk of developing acute leukemia or myeloproliferative syndrome after melphalan therapy was 19.5% for cumulative doses ranging from 730 mg to 9652 mg. In this same study, as well as in an additional study,[7,8] the 10 year cumulative risk of developing acute leukemia or myeloproliferative syndrome after melphalan therapy was less than 2% for cumulative doses under 600 mg. This does not mean that there is a cumulative dose below which there is no risk of the induction of secondary malignancy. The potential benefits from melphalan therapy must be weighed on an individual basis against the possible risk of the induction of a second malignancy.

Melphalan has been shown to cause chromatid or chromosome damage in man.[9] Melphalan causes suppression of ovarian function in pre-menopausal women, resulting in amenorrhea in a significant number of patients.[10,11]

Pregnancy: ***Teratogenic Effects:*** Pregnancy Category D: See WARNINGS section.

Nursing Mothers: It is not known whether this drug is excreted in human milk. Because many drugs are excreted in human milk and because of the potential for serious adverse reactions in nursing infants from melphalan, a decision should be made whether to discontinue nursing or to discontinue the drug, taking into account the importance of the drug to the mother.

Pediatric Use: The safety and effectiveness in children have not been established.

ADVERSE REACTIONS

Hematologic Effects: The most common side effect is bone marrow suppression.[12] Although bone marrow suppression frequently occurs, it is usually reversible if melphalan is withdrawn early enough. However, irreversible bone marrow failure has been reported.[13,14]

Gastrointestinal: Gastrointestinal disturbances such as nausea and vomiting, diarrhea and oral ulceration occur infrequently.

Miscellaneous: Other reported adverse reactions include: pulmonary fibrosis[15,16] and interstitial pneumonitis, skin hypersensitivity, vasculitis, alopecia, hemolytic anemia, and allergic reaction.

OVERDOSAGE

Immediate effects are likely to be vomiting, ulceration of the mouth, diarrhea and hemorrhage of the gastrointestinal tract. The main toxic effect is on the bone marrow, and there is no known antidote. The blood picture should be closely followed for three to six weeks. General supportive measures, together with appropriate blood transfusions and antibiotics, should be instituted if necessary. This drug is not removed from plasma to any significant degree by hemodialysis.[17]

The oral LD_{50} dose in mice is 21 mg/kg.

DOSAGE AND ADMINISTRATION

Multiple Myeloma: The usual oral dose is 6 mg (3 tablets) daily. The entire daily dose may be given at one time. It is adjusted, as required, on the basis of blood counts done at approximately weekly intervals. After two to three weeks of treatment, the drug should be discontinued for up to four weeks during which time the blood count should be followed carefully. When the white blood cell and platelet counts are rising, a maintenance dose of 2 mg daily may be instituted. Because of the patient-to-patient variation in melphalan plasma levels following oral administration of the drug, several investigators have recommended that melphalan dosage be cautiously escalated until some myelosuppression is observed, in order to assure that potentially therapeutic levels of the drug have been reached.[1,3]

Other dosage regimens have been used by various investigators. Osserman and Takatsuki have used an initial course of 10 mg/day for seven to ten days.[18,19] They report that maximal suppression of the leukocyte and platelet counts occurs within three to five weeks and recovery within four to eight weeks. Continuous maintenance therapy with 2 mg/day is instituted when the white blood cell count is greater than 4,000 and the platelet count is greater than 100,000. Dosage is adjusted to between 1 and 3 mg/day depending upon the hematological response. It is desirable to try to maintain a significant degree of bone marrow depression so as to keep the leukocyte count in the range of 3,000 to 3,500 cells/µL.

Hoogstraten *et al* have started treatment with 0.15 mg/kg/day for seven days.[20] This is followed by a rest period of at least 14 days, but it may be as long as five to six weeks. Maintenance therapy is started when the white blood cell and platelet counts are rising. The maintenance dose is 0.05 mg/kg per day or less and is adjusted according to the blood count.

Available evidence suggests that about one third to one half of the patients with multiple myeloma show a favorable response to oral administration of the drug.

One study by Alexanian *et al* has shown that the use of melphalan in combination with prednisone significantly improves the percentage of patients with multiple myeloma who achieve palliation.[21] One regimen has been to administer courses of melphalan at 0.25 mg/kg/day for four consecutive days (or, 0.20 mg/kg/day for five consecutive days) for a total dose of 1 mg/kg per course. These four- to five-day courses are then repeated every four to six weeks if the granulocyte count and the platelet count have returned to normal levels.

It is to be emphasized that response may be very gradual over many months; it is important that repeated courses or continuous therapy be given since improvement may continue slowly over many months, and the maximum benefit may be missed if treatment is abandoned too soon.

In patients with moderate to severe renal impairment, currently available pharmacokinetic data does not justify an absolute recommendation on dosage reduction to those patients, but it may be prudent to use a reduced dose initially.[22,23]

Epithelial Ovarian Cancer: One commonly employed regimen for the treatment of ovarian carcinoma has been to administer melphalan at a dose of 0.2 mg/kg daily for five days as a single course. Courses are repeated every four to five weeks depending upon hematologic tolerance.[24,25]

Procedures for proper handling and disposal of anti-cancer drugs should be considered. Several guidelines on this subject have been published.[26–32]

There is no general agreement that all of the procedures recommended in the guidelines are necessary or appropriate.

HOW SUPPLIED

White, scored tablets containing 2 mg melphalan, imprinted with "ALKERAN" and "A2A"; in bottle of 50 (NDC 0081-0045-35).

Store at 15° to 25°C (59° to 77°F) in a dry place, protect from light, and dispense in glass.

REFERENCES

1. Alberts DS, Chang SY, Chen H-SG, Evans TL, Moon TE. Oral melphalan kinetics. *Clin Pharmacol Ther.* 1979;86:737–745.
2. Unpublished data on file with Burroughs Wellcome Co.
3. Tattersall MHN, Jarman M, Newlands ES, Holyhead L, Milstead RA, Weinberg A. Pharmaco-kinetics of melphalan following oral or intravenous administration in patients with malignant disease. *Eur J Cancer.* 1978;14:507–513.
4. Weisburger JH, Griswold DP, Prejean JD, Casey AE, Wood HB, Weisburger EK. The carcinogenic properties of some of the principal drugs used in clinical cancer chemotherapy. *Recent Results Cancer Res.* 1975:52:1–17.
5. Shimkin MB, Weisburger JH, Weisburger EK, Gubareff N, Suntzeff V. Bioassay of 29 alkylating chemicals by the pulmonary-tumor response in strain A mice. *J Natl Cancer Inst.* 1966;36:915–935.
6. Einhorn N. Acute leukemia after chemotherapy (melphalan). *Cancer.* 1978;41:444–447.
7. Greene MH, Harris EL, Gershenson DM, et al. Melphalan may be a more potent leukemogen than cyclophosphamide. *Ann Intern Med* 1986;105:360–367.
8. Fisher B, Rockette H, Fisher ER, Wickerham DL, Redmond C, Brown A. Leukemia in breast cancer patients following adjuvant chemotherapy or postoperative radiation: the NSABP experience. *J Clin Oncol.* 1985;3:1640–1658.
9. Sharpe HB. Observations on the effect of therapy with nitrogen mustard or a derivative on chromosomes of human peripheral blood lymphocytes. *Cell Tissue Kinet.* 1971;4:501–504.
10. Rose DP, Davis TE. Ovarian function in patients receiving adjuvant chemotherapy for breast cancer. *Lancet.* 1977;1:1174–1176.
11. Ahmann DL, Payne WS, Scanlon PW. Repeated adjuvant chemotherapy with phenylalanine mustard or 5-fluorouracil, cyclophosphamide, and prednisone with or without radiation, after mastectomy for breast cancer. *Lancet.* 1978;1:893–896.
12. Speed DE, Galton DAG, Swan A. Melphalan in the treatment of myelomatosis. *Br Med J.* 1964;1:1664–1669.
13. Smith JP, Rutledge F. Chemotherapy in the treatment of cancer of the ovary. *Am J Obstet Gynecol.* 1970;107:691–703.
14. Bergsagel DE, Griffith KM, Haut A, Stuckey WJ Jr. The treatment of plasma cell myeloma. *Adv Cancer Res.* 1967;10:311–359.
15. Taetle R, Dickman PS, Feldman PS. Pulmonary histopathologic changes associated with melphalan therapy. *Cancer.* 1978;42:1239–1245.
16. Westerfield BT, Michalski JP, McCombs C, Light RW. Reversible melphalan-induced lung damage. *Am J Med.* 1980;68:767–771.
17. Pallante SL, Fenselau C, Mennel RG, et al. Quantitation by gas chromatography-chemical ionization-mass spectrometry of phenylalanine mustard in plasma of patients. *Cancer Res.* 1980;40:2268–2272.
18. Osserman EF. Therapy of plasma cell myeloma with melphalan (1-phenylalanine mustard). *Proc Am Assoc Cancer Res.* 1963;4:50. Abstract.
19. Osserman EF, Takatsuki K. Plasma cell myeloma: gamma globulin synthesis and structure. A review of biochemical and clinical data, with the description of a newly-recognized and related syndrome, "H-gamma-2-chain" (Franklin's) disease. *Medicine* (Balt). 1963;42:357–384.
20. Hoogstraten B, Sheehe PR, Cuttner J, et al. Melphalan in multiple myeloma. *Blood.* 1967;30:74–83.
21. Alexanian R, Haut A, Khan AU, et al. Treatment for multiple myeloma; combination chemotherapy with different melphalan dose regimens. *JAMA.* 1969;208:1680–1685.
22. Alberts DS, Chang SY, Chen H-SG, Larcom BJ, Evans TL. Comparative pharmacokinetics of chlorambucil and melphalan in man. *Recent Results Cancer Res.* 1980;74:124–131.
23. Alberts DS, Chen H-SG, Benz D, Mason NL. Effect of renal dysfunction in dogs on the disposition and marrow toxicity of melphalan. *Br J Cancer.* 1981;43:330–334.
24. Smith JP, Rutledge FN: Chemotherapy in advanced ovarian cancer. *Natl Cancer Inst Monogr.* 1975; 42:141–143.
25. Young RC, Chabner BA, Hubbard SP, et al. Advanced ovarian adenocarcinoma: a prospective clinical trial of melphalan (L-PAM) versus combination chemotherapy. *N Engl J Med* 1978;299:1261–1266.
26. Recommendations for the safe handling of parenteral antineoplastic drugs. Washington, DC: Division of Safety, National Institutes of Health; 1983. US Dept of Health and Human Services, Public Health Service publication NIH 83-2621.
27. AMA Council on Scientific Affairs. Guidelines for handling parenteral antineoplastics. *JAMA.* 1985; 253:1590–1591.

Continued on next page

Burroughs Wellcome—Cont.

28. National Study Commission on Cytotoxic Exposure. Recommendations for handling cytotoxic agents. 1984: Available from Louis P. Jeffrey, ScD, Director of Pharmacy Services, Rhode Island Hospital, 593 Eddy Street, Providence, Rhode Island 02902.
29. Clinical Oncological Society of Australia. Guidelines and recommendations for safe handling of antineoplastic agents. *Med J Australia.* 1983;1:426–428.
30. Jones RB, Frank R, Mass T. Safe handling of chemotherapeutic agents: a report from the Mount Sinai Medical Center. *CA-A Cancer J for Clin.* 1983;33 (Sept/Oct):258–263.
31. American Society of Hospital Pharmacists. Technical assistance bulletin on handling cytotoxic drugs in hospitals. *Am J Hosp Pharm.* 1985;42:131–137.
32. Yodaiken RE, Bennett D.: OSHA work-practice guidelines for personnel dealing with cytotoxic (antineoplastic) drugs. *Am J Hosp Pharm.* 1986;43:1193–1204.

403919

Shown in Product Identification Section, page 407

ANECTINE® ℞
[*ă-nĕk'tēn*]
(Succinylcholine Chloride)
Injection, USP

ANECTINE® ℞
(Succinylcholine Chloride)
Sterile Powder Flo-Pack®

This drug should be used only by individuals familiar with its actions, characteristics and hazards.

DESCRIPTION
Anectine (succinylcholine chloride) is an ultra short-acting depolarizing-type, skeletal muscle relaxant for intravenous administration.
Succinylcholine chloride is a white, odorless, slightly bitter powder and very soluble in water. The drug is unstable in alkaline solutions but relatively stable in acid solutions, depending upon the concentration of the solution and the storage temperature. Solutions of succinylcholine chloride should be stored under refrigeration to preserve potency.
Anectine Injection is a sterile non-pyrogenic solution for intravenous injection, containing 20 mg succinylcholine chloride in each ml and made isotonic with sodium chloride. The pH is adjusted to 3.5 with hydrochloric acid. Methylparaben (0.1%) is added as a preservative. Anectine Flo-Pack is a sterile powder, containing either 500 mg or 1000 mg of succinylcholine chloride in each vial.
The chemical name for succinylcholine chloride is 2,2′-[(1,4-dioxo-1,4-butanediyl)bis(oxy)]bis[*N,N,N*-trimethylethanaminium] dichloride.

CLINICAL PHARMACOLOGY
Succinylcholine is a depolarizing skeletal muscle relaxant. As does acetylcholine, it combines with the cholinergic receptors of the motor end plate to produce depolarization. This depolarization may be observed as fasciculations. Subsequent neuromuscular transmission is inhibited so long as adequate concentration of succinylcholine remains at the receptor site. Onset of flaccid paralysis is rapid (less than one minute after intravenous administration), and with single administration lasts approximately 4–6 minutes.
Succinylcholine is rapidly hydrolyzed by plasma pseudocholinesterase to succinylmonocholine (which possesses non-depolarizing muscle relaxant properties) and then more slowly to succinic acid and choline. About 10% of the drug is excreted unchanged in the urine. The paralysis following administration of succinylcholine is selective, initially involving consecutively the levator muscles of the face, muscles of the glottis and finally the intercostals and the diaphragm and all other skeletal muscles.
Succinylcholine has no direct action on the uterus or other smooth muscle structures. Because it is highly ionized and has low fat solubility, it does not readily cross the placenta.
Tachyphylaxis occurs with repeated administration.
When succinylcholine is given over a prolonged period of time, the characteristic depolarizing neuromuscular block (Phase I block) may change to a block with characteristics superficially resembling a non-depolarizing block (Phase II block). This may be associated with prolonged respiratory depression or apnea in patients who manifest the transition to Phase II block. When this diagnosis is confirmed by peripheral nerve stimulation, it may be reversed with anticholinesterase drugs such as neostigmine (See Precautions).
While succinylcholine has no direct effect on the myocardium, changes in rhythm may result from vagal stimulation, such as may result from surgical procedures (particularly in children) or from potassium-mediated alterations in electrical conductivity. These effects are enhanced by cyclopropane and halogenated anesthetics.
Succinylcholine causes a slight, transient increase in intraocular pressure immediately after its injection and during the fasciculation phase, and slight increases may persist after onset of complete paralysis. This suggests that the drug should not be used in the presence of open eye injuries.
As with other neuromuscular blockers, the potential for releasing histamine is present following succinylcholine administration. Serious histamine-mediated flushing, hypotension and bronchoconstriction are, however, uncommon in normal clinical usage.
Succinylcholine has no effect on consciousness, pain threshold or cerebration. It should be used only with adequate anesthesia.

INDICATIONS AND USAGE
Succinylcholine chloride is indicated as an adjunct to general anesthesia, to facilitate endotracheal intubation, and to provide skeletal muscle relaxation during surgery or mechanical ventilation.

CONTRAINDICATIONS
Succinylcholine is contraindicated for persons with genetically determined disorders of plasma pseudocholinesterase, personal or familial history of malignant hyperthermia, myopathies associated with elevated creatine phosphokinase (CPK) values, known hypersensitivity to the drug, acute narrow angle glaucoma, and penetrating eye injuries.

WARNINGS
Succinylcholine should be used only by those skilled in the management of artificial respiration and only when facilities are instantly available for endotracheal intubation and for providing adequate ventilation of the patient, including the administration of oxygen under positive pressure and the elimination of carbon dioxide. The clinician must be prepared to assist or control respiration.
Succinylcholine should not be mixed with short-acting barbiturates in the same syringe or administered simultaneously during intravenous infusion through the same needle. Solutions of succinylcholine have an acid pH, whereas those of barbiturates are alkaline. Depending upon the resultant pH of a mixture of solutions of these drugs, either free barbituric acid may be precipitated or succinylcholine hydrolyzed.
Succinylcholine administration has been associated with acute onset of fulminant hypermetabolism of skeletal muscle known as malignant hyperthermic crisis. This frequently presents as intractable spasm of the jaw muscles which may progress to generalized rigidity, increased oxygen demand, tachycardia, tachypnea and profound hyperpyrexia. Successful outcome depends on recognition of early signs, such as jaw muscle spasm, lack of laryngeal relaxation or generalized rigidity to initial administration of succinylcholine for endotracheal intubation, or failure of tachycardia to respond to deepening anesthesia. Skin mottling, rising temperature and coagulopathies occur late in the course of the hypermetabolic process. Recognition of the syndrome is a signal for discontinuance of anesthesia, attention to increased oxygen consumption, correction of metabolic acidosis, support of circulation, assurance of adequate urinary output and institution of measures to control rising temperature. Dantrolene sodium, intravenously, is recommended as an adjunct to supportive measures in the management of this problem. Consult literature references or the dantrolene prescribing information for additional information about the management of malignant hyperthermic crisis. Routine, continuous monitoring of temperature is recommended as an aid to early recognition of malignant hyperthermia.

PRECAUTIONS
General: Low levels or abnormal variants of pseudocholinesterase may be associated with prolonged respiratory depression or apnea following the use of succinylcholine. Low levels of pseudocholinesterase may occur in patients with the following conditions: burns, severe liver disease or cirrhosis, cancer, severe anemia, pregnancy, malnutrition, severe dehydration, collagen diseases, myxedema, and abnormal body temperature. Also, exposure to neurotoxic insecticides, antimalarial or anti-cancer drugs, monoamine oxidase inhibitors, contraceptive pills, pancuronium, chlorpromazine, ecothiopate iodide, or neostigmine may result in low levels of pseudocholinesterase. Succinylcholine should be administered with extreme care to such patients. If low pseudocholinesterase activity is suspected, a small test dose of from 5 to 10 mg of succinylcholine may be administered, or relaxation may be produced by the cautious administration of a 0.1% solution of the drug by intravenous drip. Apnea or prolonged muscle paralysis should be treated with controlled respiration.
Succinylcholine should be administered with great caution to patients recovering from severe trauma, those suffering from electrolyte imbalance, those receiving quinidine, and those who have been digitalized recently or who may have digitalis toxicity, because in these circumstances it may induce serious cardiac arrhythmias or cardiac arrest. Great caution should be observed also in patients with pre-existing hyperkalemia, those who are paraplegic, or have suffered extensive or severe burns, extensive denervation of skeletal muscle due to disease or injury of the central nervous system, or have degenerative or dystrophic neuromuscular disease, because such patients tend to become severely hyperkalemic when given succinylcholine.
When succinylcholine is given over a prolonged period of time, the characteristic depolarization block of the myoneural junction (Phase I block) may change to a block with characteristics superficially resembling a non-depolarizing block (Phase II block). Prolonged respiratory depression or apnea may be observed in patients manifesting this transition to Phase II block. The transition from Phase I to Phase II block has been reported in 7 of 7 patients studied under halothane anesthesia after an accumulated dose of 2 to 4 mg/kg succinylcholine (administered in repeated, divided doses). The onset of Phase II block coincided with the onset of tachyphylaxis and prolongation of spontaneous recovery. In another study, using balanced anesthesia (N_2O/O_2/narcotic-thiopental) and succinylcholine infusion, the transition was less abrupt, with great individual variability in the dose of succinylcholine required to produce Phase II block. Of 32 patients studied, 24 developed Phase II block. Tachyphylaxis was not associated with the transition to Phase II block, and 50% of the patients who developed Phase II block experienced prolonged recovery.
When Phase II block is suspected in cases of prolonged neuromuscular blockade, positive diagnosis should be made by peripheral nerve stimulation, prior to administration of any anticholinesterase drug. Reversal of Phase II block is a medical decision which must be made upon the basis of the individual clinical pharmacology and the experience and judgment of the physician. The presence of Phase II block is indicated by fade of responses to successive stimuli (preferably "train of four"). The use of anticholinesterase drugs to reverse Phase II block should be accompanied by appropriate doses of atropine to prevent disturbances of cardiac rhythm. After adequate reversal of Phase II block with an anticholinesterase agent, the patient should be continually observed for at least 1 hour for signs of return of muscle relaxation. Reversal should not be attempted unless: (1) a peripheral nerve stimulator is used to determine the presence of Phase II block (since anticholinesterase agents will potentiate succinylcholine-induced Phase I block), and (2) spontaneous recovery of muscle twitch has been observed for at least 20 minutes and has reached a plateau with further recovery proceeding slowly; this delay is to ensure complete hydrolysis of succinylcholine by pseudocholinesterase prior to administration of the anticholinesterase agent. Should the type of block be misdiagnosed, depolarization of the type initially induced by succinylcholine, that is depolarizing block, will be prolonged by an anticholinesterase agent.
Succinylcholine should be used with caution, if at all, during ocular surgery and in patients with glaucoma. The drug should be employed with caution in patients with fractures or muscle spasm because the initial muscle fasciculations may cause additional trauma.
Succinylcholine may increase intragastric pressure, which could result in regurgitation and possible aspiration of stomach contents.
Neuromuscular blockade may be prolonged in patients with hypokalemia or hypocalcemia.
Drug Interactions: Drugs which may enhance the neuromuscular blocking action of succinylcholine include: phenelzine, promazine, oxytocin, aprotinin, certain nonpenicillin antibiotics, quinidine, β-adrenergic blockers, procainamide, lidocaine, trimethaphan, lithium carbonate, magnesium salts, quinine, chloroquine, propanidid, diethylether, and isoflurane.
If other relaxants are to be used during the same procedure, the possibility of a synergistic or antagonistic effect should be considered.
Pregnancy: *Teratogenic Effects:* Pregnancy Category C. Animal reproduction studies have not been conducted with succinylcholine chloride. It is also not known whether succinylcholine can cause fetal harm when administered to a pregnant woman or can affect reproduction capacity. Succinylcholine should be given to a pregnant woman only if clearly needed.
Nonteratogenic Effects: Pseudocholinesterase levels are decreased by approximately 24% during pregnancy and for several days postpartum. Therefore, a higher proportion of patients may be expected to show sensitivity (prolonged apnea) to succinylcholine when pregnant than when nonpregnant.
Labor and Delivery: Succinylcholine is commonly used to provide muscle relaxation during delivery by caesarean section. While small amounts of succinylcholine are known to cross the placental barrier, under normal conditions the quantity of drug that enters fetal circulation after a single dose of 1 mg/kg to the mother will not endanger the fetus. However, since the amount of drug that crosses the placental barrier is dependent on the concentration gradient between the maternal and fetal circulations, residual neuromuscular blockade (apnea and flaccidity) may occur in the neonate

after repeated high doses to, or in the presence of atypical pseudocholinesterase in, the mother.

ADVERSE REACTIONS

Adverse reactions consist primarily of an extension of the drug's pharmacological actions. It causes profound muscle relaxation resulting in respiratory depression to the point of apnea; this effect may be prolonged. Hypersensitivity to the drug may exist in rare instances. The following additional adverse reactions have been reported: cardiac arrest, malignant hyperthermia, arrhythmias, bradycardia, tachycardia, hypertension, hypotension, hyperkalemia, prolonged respiratory depression or apnea, increased intraocular pressure, muscle fasciculation, postoperative muscle pain, rhabdomyolysis with possible myoglobinuric acute renal failure, excessive salivation, and rash.

DOSAGE AND ADMINISTRATION

The dosage of succinylcholine is essentially individualized and its administration should always be determined by the clinician after careful assessment of the patient. To avoid distress to the patient, succinylcholine should not be administered before unconsciousness has been induced. Succinylcholine should not be mixed with short-acting barbiturates in the same syringe or administered simultaneously during intravenous infusion through the same needle.

For Short Surgical Procedures: The average dose for relaxation of short duration is 0.6 mg/kg (~2.0 ml) Anectine (succinylcholine chloride) Injection given intravenously. The optimum dose will vary among individuals and may be from 0.3 to 1.1 mg/kg for adults (1.0 to 4.0 ml). Following administration of doses in this range, relaxation develops in about 1 minute; maximum muscular paralysis may persist for about 2 minutes, after which recovery takes place within 4 to 6 minutes. However, very large doses may result in more prolonged apnea. An initial test dose of 0.1 mg/kg (~0.5 ml) may be used to determine the sensitivity of the patient and the individual recovery time.

For Long Surgical Procedures: The dosage of succinylcholine administered by infusion depends upon the duration of the surgical procedure and the need for muscle relaxation. The average rate for an adult ranges between 2.5 and 4.3 mg per minute.

Solutions containing from 0.1% to 0.2% (1 to 2 mg per ml) succinylcholine have commonly been used for continuous intravenous drip. Solutions of 0.1% or 0.2% may conveniently be prepared by adding 1 g succinylcholine (the contents of one Anectine Sterile Powder Flo-Pack unit containing 1 g succinylcholine chloride) respectively to 1000 or 500 ml of sterile solution, such as sterile 5% dextrose solution or sterile isotonic saline solution. The more dilute solution (0.1% or 1 mg per ml) is probably preferable from the standpoint of ease of control of the rate of administration of the drug and, hence, of relaxation. This intravenous drip solution containing 1 mg per ml may be administered at a rate of 0.5 mg (0.5 ml) to 10 mg (10 ml) per minute to obtain the required amount of relaxation. The amount required per minute will depend upon the individual response as well as the degree of relaxation required. The 0.2% solution may be especially useful in those cases where it is desired to avoid overburdening the circulation with a large volume of fluid. It is recommended that neuromuscular function be carefully monitored with a peripheral nerve stimulator when using succinylcholine by infusion in order to avoid overdose, detect development of Phase II block, follow its rate of recovery, and assess the effects of reversing agents.

Solutions of succinylcholine must be used within 24 hours after preparation. Discard unused solutions.

Intermittent intravenous injections of succinylcholine may also be used to provide muscle relaxation for long procedures. An intravenous injection of 0.3 to 1.1 mg/kg may be given initially, followed, at appropriate intervals, by further injections of 0.04 to 0.07 mg/kg to maintain the degree of relaxation required.

Pediatric Use: For endotracheal intubation, the intravenous dose of succinylcholine is 2 mg/kg for infants and small children; for older children and adolescents the dose is 1 mg/kg.

Intravenous bolus administration of succinylcholine in infants or children may result in profound bradycardia or, rarely, asystole. As in adults, the incidence of bradycardia in children is higher following a second dose of succinylcholine. The occurrence of bradyarrhythmias may be reduced by pretreatment with atropine.

Intramuscular Use: If necessary, succinylcholine may be given intramuscularly to infants, older children or adults when a suitable vein is inaccessible. A dose of up to 3 to 4 mg/kg may be given, but not more than 150 mg total dose should be administered by this route. The onset of effect of succinylcholine given intramuscularly is usually observed in about 2 to 3 minutes.

Parenteral drug products should be inspected visually for particulate matter and discoloration prior to administration whenever solution and container permit.

HOW SUPPLIED

For immediate injection of single doses for short procedures: Anectine® Injection, 20 mg succinylcholine chloride in each ml.

Multiple-dose vials of 10 ml.

Box of 12 vials (NDC-0081-0071-95).

Store in refrigerator at 2° to 8°C (36° to 46°F). The multi-dose vials are stable for up to 14 days at room temperature without significant loss of potency.

For preparation of intravenous drip solutions only:

Anectine® Flo-Pack®, 500 mg sterile succinylcholine chloride powder.

Box of 12 vials (NDC-0081-0085-15).

Anectine® Flo-Pack®, 1000 mg sterile succinylcholine chloride powder.

Box of 12 vials (NDC-0081-0086-15).

Anectine Flo-Pack does not require refrigeration. Store at 15° to 30°C (59° to 86°F). Solutions of succinylcholine must be used within 24 hours after preparation. Discard unused solutions. 411001

CARDILATE® TABLETS ℞

[*kar'dĭ-lāt*]

(Erythrityl Tetranitrate)

DESCRIPTION

Cardilate (erythrityl tetranitrate) is an antianginal drug that belongs to the organic nitrate class of pharmaceutical agents. Erythrityl tetranitrate is soluble in alcohol, ether and glycerol, but insoluble in water. It has the empirical formula $C_4H_6N_4O_{12}$, molecular weight of 302.12 and melting point of 61°C.

Erythrityl tetranitrate is known chemically as (*R**S**)-1,2,3,4-butanetetrol tetranitrate.

In the pure state, erythrityl tetranitrate will explode upon percussion, but properly diluted with lactose, as in Cardilate tablets, it is nonexplosive. Since it is a low melting solid, erythrityl tetranitrate does not evaporate from the Cardilate tablets.

Cardilate Oral/Sublingual Tablets contain 10 mg erythrityl tetranitrate and the inactive ingredients lactose, magnesium stearate and potato starch, with disintegration characteristics that permit sublingual or oral (swallowed) administration.

CLINICAL PHARMACOLOGY

Cardilate exerts its effects by relaxation of vascular smooth muscle.[1] The action is maximal on the post-capillary vessels, including the large veins. Venodilatation results in peripheral blood pooling, which decreases venous return to the heart, central venous pressure and pulmonary capillary wedge pressure (preload reduction).[2] Pulmonary arteriolar dilatation causes a reduction in pulmonary vascular resistance.[2] A decrease in systemic arterial pressure (afterload reduction) can also occur, but is usually less pronounced. Augmentation of cardiac output generally occurs in those patients with increased filling pressures and high resting systemic vascular resistance.[2]

Mechanism of Action: The inadequate myocardial oxygenation that precipitates angina can be corrected by: (1) increasing the supply of oxygen to ischemic myocardium through direct dilatation of the large coronary conductance vessels or (2) decreasing the myocardial oxygen demand secondary to a reduction of cardiac work (preload and afterload reduction).[3] The beneficial effect of Cardilate probably involves both mechanisms.

Pharmacokinetics and Metabolism: Cardilate is readily absorbed from the sublingual, buccal and gastrointestinal mucosae. The peak effect from a swallowed dose is diminished but of longer duration when compared to the sublingual route.[4] The biotransformation of Cardilate is thought to occur by reductive hydrolysis catalyzed by the hepatic enzyme glutathione-organic nitrate reductase.[3] Differences in response among various nitrates may relate to both intrinsic potency at cardiovascular sites, as well as factors related to pharmacokinetics and biotransformation.[5]

Time to onset of effect is approximately 5 minutes for the sublingual route and 15 to 30 minutes for swallowed tablets, with peak effect in 15 minutes and 60 minutes, respectively. Duration of action will vary, but vasodilatory effects have been demonstrated for up to 3 hours after sublingual administration[4,6] and for 6 hours after the oral (swallowed) route.[4]

INDICATIONS AND USAGE

Cardilate (erythrityl tetranitrate) is intended for the prophylaxis and long-term treatment of patients with frequent or recurrent anginal pain and reduced exercise tolerance associated with angina pectoris, rather than for the treatment of the acute attack of angina pectoris, since its onset is somewhat slower than that of nitroglycerin.

CONTRAINDICATIONS

Cardilate should not be administered to individuals with a known hypersensitivity or idiosyncratic reaction to organic nitrates.

WARNINGS

The use of nitrates in acute myocardial infarction or congestive heart failure should be undertaken only under close clinical observation and/or in conjunction with hemodynamic monitoring.

PRECAUTIONS

General: Cardilate should be used with caution in patients with severe liver or renal disease. Development of tolerance and cross-tolerance to the effects of erythrityl tetranitrate and other organic nitrates may occur. However, recent studies in patients with chronic heart failure[1] indicate that nitrates produce sustained beneficial hemodynamic effects.

Carcinogenesis, Mutagenesis, Impairment of Fertility: No long-term studies in animals have been performed.

Pregnancy: ***Teratogenic Effects.*** Pregnancy Category C. Animal reproduction studies have not been conducted with Cardilate. It is also not known whether Cardilate can cause fetal harm when administered to a pregnant woman or can affect reproduction capacity. Cardilate should be given to a pregnant woman only if clearly needed.

Nursing Mothers: It is not known whether this drug is excreted in human milk. Because many drugs are excreted in human milk, caution should be exercised when Cardilate is administered to a nursing woman.

Pediatric Use: Safety and effectiveness in children have not been established.

ADVERSE REACTIONS

The most frequent adverse reaction in patients treated with Cardilate is headache. Lowering the dose and the use of analgesics will help control headaches, which usually diminish or disappear as therapy is continued. Other adverse reactions occurring are the following: cutaneous vasodilatation with flushing, and transient episodes of dizziness and weakness, plus other signs of cerebral ischemia associated with postural hypotension. Occasional individuals exhibit marked sensitivity to the hypotensive effects of organic nitrates, and severe responses (e.g., nausea, vomiting, weakness, restlessness, pallor, perspiration and collapse) can occur even with the usual therapeutic dose. Alcohol may enhance this effect. Drug rash and/or exfoliative dermatitis may occasionally occur.

OVERDOSAGE

Accidental overdosage of Cardilate may result in severe hypotension and reflex tachycardia, which can be treated by laying the patient down and elevating the legs. If further treatment is required, the administration of intravenous fluids or other means of treating hypotension should be considered.

DOSAGE AND ADMINISTRATION

The Cardilate Oral/ Sublingual Tablet can be placed under the tongue or swallowed. Sublingual therapy may be initiated with a dose of 5 to 10 mg prior to each anticipated physical or emotional stress, and at bedtime for patients subject to nocturnal attacks of angina. The dose may be increased as needed.

If the patient is to swallow the tablet, therapy may be initiated with 10 mg before each meal, as well as mid-morning and mid-afternoon if needed, and at bedtime for patients subject to nocturnal attacks. The dose may be increased or decreased as needed.

Dosage titration up to 100 mg daily has been well tolerated, but temporary headache is more apt to occur with increasing doses. When headache occurs, the dose should be reduced for a few days. If headache is troublesome during adjustment of dosage, it may be effectively relieved with an analgesic.

HOW SUPPLIED

Square, white, scored tablets containing 10 mg erythrityl tetranitrate, imprinted with "CARDILATE" and "X7A" on each tablet; bottle of 100 (NDC 0081-0168-55).

Store at 15°-25°C (59°- 77°F) in a dry place and dispense in glass.

REFERENCES

1. Chatterjee K, Parmley WW. Vasodilator therapy for chronic heart failure. *Ann Rev Pharmacol Toxicol.* 1980,20:475–512.
2. Goldberg S, Mann T, Grossman W. Nitrate therapy of heart failure in valvular heart disease. *Am J Med.* 1978;65:161–166.
3. Needleman P, Johnson EM. Vasodilators and the treatment of angina, in Gilman AG, Goodman LS, Gilman A (eds): *The Pharmacological Basis of Therapeutics*, ed 6. New York, Macmillan Publishing Co Inc, 1980, pp 819–833.

Continued on next page

Burroughs Wellcome—Cont.

4. Hanneman RE, Erb RJ, Stoltman WP, et al. Digital plethysmography for assessing erythrityl tetranitrate bioavailability. *Clin Pharmacol Ther.* 1981;29:35–39.
5. Wastila WB, Namm DH, Maxwell RA. Comparison of the vascular effects of several organic nitrates in anesthetized rats and dogs after intravenous and intraportal administration, in *Second International Symposium on Vascular Neuroeffector Mechanisms, Odense, 1975.* Basel, Karger, 1976, pp 216–225.
6. Haffty GB, Nakamura Y, Spodick DH, et al. Bioavailability of organic nitrates: A comparison of methods for evaluating plethysmographic responses. *J Clin Pharmacol.* 1982;22:117–124.   444611

Shown in Product Identification Section, page 407

CORTISPORIN® CREAM   ℞
[*kor'tĭ-spor"ĭn krēm*]
(Polymyxin B Sulfate-Neomycin
Sulfate-Hydrocortisone Acetate)

DESCRIPTION

Cortisporin® Cream (polymyxin B sulfate-neomycin sulfate-hydrocortisone acetate) is a topical antibacterial cream. Each gram contains: polymyxin B sulfate 10,000 units, neomycin sulfate equivalent to 3.5 mg neomycin base, and hydrocortisone acetate 5 mg (0.5%). The inactive ingredients are liquid petrolatum, white petrolatum, propylene glycol, polyoxyethylene polyoxypropylene compound, emulsifying wax, purified water, and 0.25% methylparaben added as a preservative. Sodium hydroxide or sulfuric acid may be added to adjust pH.

Polymyxin B sulfate is the sulfate salt of polymyxin B_1 and B_2, which are produced by the growth of *Bacillus polymyxa* (Prazmowski) Migula (Fam. Bacillaceae). It has a potency of not less than 6,000 polymyxin B units per mg, calculated on an anhydrous basis.

Neomycin sulfate is the sulfate salt of neomycin B and C, which are produced by the growth of *Streptomyces fradiae* Waksman (Fam. Streptomycetaceae). It has a potency equivalent of not less than 600 μg of neomycin standard per mg, calculated on an anhydrous basis.

Hydrocortisone acetate is the acetate ester of hydrocortisone, an anti-inflammatory hormone. Its chemical name is 21-(acetyloxy)-11β,17-dihydroxypregn-4-ene-3,20-dione.

The base is a smooth vanishing cream with a pH of approximately 5.0.

CLINICAL PHARMACOLOGY

Corticoids suppress the inflammatory response to a variety of agents and they may delay healing. Since corticoids may inhibit the body's defense mechanism against infection, a concomitant antimicrobial drug may be used when this inhibition is considered to be clinically significant in a particular case.

The anti-infective components in the combination are included to provide action against specific organisms susceptible to them. Polymyxin B sulfate and neomycin sulfate together are considered active against the following microorganisms: *Staphylococcus aureus, Escherichia coli, Haemophilus influenzae, Klebsiella-Enterobacter* species, *Neisseria* species and *Pseudomonas aeruginosa.* The product does not provide adequate coverage against *Serratia marcescens* and streptococci, including *Streptococcus pneumoniae.*

The relative potency of corticosteroids depends on the molecular structure, concentration and release from the vehicle. The acid pH helps restore normal cutaneous acidity. Owing to its excellent spreading and penetrating properties, the cream facilitates treatment of hairy and intertriginous areas. It may also be of value in selective cases where the lesions are moist.

INDICATIONS AND USAGE

For the treatment of corticosteroid-responsive dermatoses with secondary infection. It has not been demonstrated that this steroid-antibiotic combination provides greater benefit than the steroid component alone after 7 days of treatment (see WARNINGS section).

CONTRAINDICATIONS

Not for use in the eyes or in the external ear canal if the eardrum is perforated. This product is contraindicated in tuberculous, fungal or viral lesions of the skin (herpes simplex, vaccinia and varicella). This product is contraindicated in those individuals who have shown hypersensitivity to any of its components.

WARNINGS

Because of the concern of nephrotoxicity and ototoxicity associated with neomycin, this combination should not be used over a wide area or for extended periods of time.

PRECAUTIONS

General: As with any antibacterial preparation, prolonged use may result in overgrowth of nonsusceptible organisms, including fungi. Appropriate measures should be taken if this occurs. Use of steroids on infected areas should be supervised with care as anti-inflammatory steroids may encourage spread of infection. If this occurs, steroid therapy should be stopped and appropriate antibacterial drugs used. Generalized dermatological conditions may require systemic corticosteroid therapy.

Signs and symptoms of exogenous hyperadrenocorticism can occur with the use of topical corticosteroids, including adrenal suppression. Systemic absorption of topically applied steroids will be increased if extensive body surface areas are treated or if occlusive dressings are used. Under these circumstances, suitable precautions should be taken when long-term use is anticipated.

Information for Patients: If redness, irritation, swelling or pain persists or increases, discontinue use and notify physician. Do not use in the eyes.

Laboratory Tests: Systemic effects of excessive levels of hydrocortisone may include a reduction in the number of circulating eosinophils and a decrease in urinary excretion of 17-hydroxycorticosteroids.

Carcinogenesis, Mutagenesis, Impairment of Fertility: Long-term studies in animals (rats, rabbits, mice) showed no evidence of carcinogenicity attributable to oral administration of corticosteroids.

Pregnancy: *Teratogenic Effects:* Pregnancy Category C. Corticosteroids have been shown to be teratogenic in rabbits when applied topically at concentrations of 0.5% on days 6–18 of gestation and in mice when applied topically at a concentration of 15% on days 10–13 of gestation. There are no adequate and well controlled studies in pregnant women. Corticosteroids should be used during pregnancy only if the potential benefit justifies the potential risk to the fetus.

Nursing Mothers: Hydrocortisone acetate appears in human milk following oral administration of the drug. Since systemic absorption of hydrocortisone may occur when applied topically, caution should be exercised when Cortisporin Cream is used by a nursing woman.

Pediatric Use: Sufficient percutaneous absorption of hydrocortisone can occur in infants and children during prolonged use to cause cessation of growth, as well as other systemic signs and symptoms of hyperadrenocorticism.

ADVERSE REACTIONS

Neomycin occasionally causes skin sensitization. Ototoxicity and nephrotoxicity have also been reported (see WARNINGS section). Adverse reactions have occurred with topical use of antibiotic combinations including neomycin and polymyxin B. Exact incidence figures are not available since no denominator of treated patients is available. The reaction occurring most often is allergic sensitization. In one clinical study using a 20% neomycin patch, neomycin-induced allergic skin reactions occurred in two of 2,175 (0.09%) individuals in the general population.[1] In another study, the incidence was found to be approximately 1%.[2]

The following local adverse reactions have been reported with topical corticosteroids, especially under occlusive dressings: burning, itching, irritation, dryness, folliculitis, hypertrichosis, acneiform eruptions, hypopigmentation, perioral dermatitis, allergic contact dermatitis, maceration of the skin, secondary infection, skin atrophy, striae, and miliaria. When steroid preparations are used for long periods of time in intertriginous areas or over extensive body areas, with or without occlusive non-permeable dressings, striae may occur; also there exists the possibility of systemic side effects when steroid preparations are used over large areas or for a long period of time.

DOSAGE AND ADMINISTRATION

A small quantity of the cream should be applied 2 to 4 times daily, as required. The cream should, if conditions permit, be gently rubbed into the affected areas.

HOW SUPPLIED

Tube of 7.5 g (NDC 0081-0185-98).
Store at 15° to 25°C (59° to 77°F).

REFERENCES

1. Leyden JJ, Kligman AM: Contact dermatitis to neomycin sulfate. *JAMA* 1979;242:1276–1278.
2. Prystowsky SD, Allen AM, Smith RW, *et al:* Allergic contact hypersensitivity to nickel, neomycin, ethylenediamine, and benzocaine. *Arch Dermatol* 1979;115:959–962.   454425

CORTISPORIN® OINTMENT   ℞
[*kor'tĭ-spor"ĭn*]
(Polymyxin B Sulfate-Bacitracin Zinc-
Neomycin Sulfate-Hydrocortisone)

DESCRIPTION

Cortisporin® Ointment (polymyxin B sulfate-bacitracin zinc-neomycin sulfate-hydrocortisone) is a topical antibacterial ointment. Each gram contains: polymyxin B sulfate 5,000 units, bacitracin zinc 400 units, neomycin sulfate equivalent to 3.5 mg neomycin base, hydrocortisone 10 mg (1%), and special white petrolatum qs.

Polymyxin B sulfate is the sulfate salt of polymyxin B_1 and B_2, which are produced by the growth of *Bacillus polymyxa* (Prazmowski) Migula (Fam. Bacillaceae). It has a potency of not less than 6,000 polymyxin B units per mg, calculated on an anhydrous basis.

Bacitracin zinc is the zinc salt of bacitracin, a mixture of related cyclic polypeptides (mainly bacitracin A) produced by the growth of an organism of the *licheniformis* group of *Bacillis subtilis* (Fam. Bacillaceae). It has a potency of not less than 40 bacitracin units per mg.

Neomycin sulfate is the sulfate salt of neomycin B and C, which are produced by the growth of *Streptomyces fradiae* Waksman (Fam. Streptomycetaceae). It has a potency equivalent of not less than 600 μg of neomycin standard per mg, calculated on an anhydrous basis.

Hydrocortisone, 11β, 17, 21-trihydroxypregn-4-ene-3, 20-dione, is an anti-inflammatory hormone.

CLINICAL PHARMACOLOGY

Corticoids suppress the inflammatory response to a variety of agents and they may delay healing. Since corticoids may inhibit the body's defense mechanism against infection, a concomitant antimicrobial drug may be used when this inhibition is considered to be clinically significant in a particular case.

The anti-infective components in the combination are included to provide action against specific organisms susceptible to them. Polymyxin B sulfate, bacitracin zinc and neomycin sulfate together are considered active against the following microorganisms: *Staphylococcus aureus,* streptococci, including *Streptococcus pneumoniae, Escherichia coli, Haemophilus influenzae, Klebsiella-Enterobacter* species, *Neisseria* species and *Pseudomonas aeruginosa.*

The product does not provide adequate coverage against *Serratia marcescens.*

The relative potency of corticosteroids depends on the molecular structure, concentration and release from the vehicle.

INDICATIONS AND USAGE

For the treatment of corticosteroid-responsive dermatoses with secondary infection. It has not been demonstrated that this steroid-antibiotic combination provides greater benefit than the steroid component alone after 7 days of treatment (see WARNINGS section).

CONTRAINDICATIONS

Not for use in the eyes or in the external ear canal if the eardrum is perforated. This product is contraindicated in tuberculous, fungal or viral lesions of the skin (herpes simplex, vaccinia and varicella). This product is contraindicated in those individuals who have shown hypersensitivity to any of its components.

WARNINGS

Because of the concern of nephrotoxicity and ototoxicity associated with neomycin, this combination should not be used over a wide area or for extended periods of time.

PRECAUTIONS

General: As with any antibiotic preparation, prolonged use may result in the overgrowth of nonsusceptible organisms, including fungi. Appropriate measures should be taken if this occurs. Use of steroids on infected areas should be supervised with care as anti-inflammatory steroids may encourage spread of infection. If this occurs, steroid therapy should be stopped and appropriate antibacterial drugs used. Generalized dermatological conditions may require systemic corticosteroid therapy.

Signs and symptoms of exogenous hyperadrenocorticism can occur with the use of topical corticosteroids, including adrenal suppression. Systemic absorption of topically applied steroids will be increased if extensive body surface areas are treated or if occlusive dressings are used. Under these circumstances, suitable precautions should be taken when long-term use is anticipated.

Information for Patients: If redness, irritation, swelling or pain persists or increases, discontinue use and notify physician. Do not use in the eyes.

Laboratory Tests: Systemic effects of excessive levels of hydrocortisone may include a reduction in the number of circulating eosinophils and a decrease in urinary excretion of 17-hydroxycorticosteroids.

Carcinogenesis, Mutagenesis, Impairment of Fertility: Long-term studies in animals (rats, rabbits, mice) showed no evi-

dence of carcinogenicity attributable to oral administration of corticosteroids.

Pregnancy: ***Teratogenic Effects:*** Pregnancy Category C. Corticosteroids have been shown to be teratogenic in rabbits when applied topically at concentrations of 0.5% on days 6–18 of gestation and in mice when applied topically at a concentration of 15% on days 10–13 of gestation. There are no adequate and well-controlled studies in pregnant women. Corticosteroids should be used during pregnancy only if the potential benefit justifies the potential risk to the fetus.

Nursing Mothers: Hydrocortisone appears in human milk following oral administration of the drug. Since systemic absorption of hydrocortisone may occur when applied topically, caution should be exercised when Cortisporin Ointment is used by a nursing woman.

Pediatric Use: Sufficient percutaneous absorption of hydrocortisone can occur in infants and children during prolonged use to cause cessation of growth, as well as other systemic signs and symptoms of hyperadrenocorticism.

ADVERSE REACTIONS

Neomycin occasionally causes skin sensitization. Ototoxicity and nephrotoxicity have also been reported (see WARNINGS section). Adverse reactions have occurred with topical use of antibiotic combinations including neomycin, bacitracin and polymyxin B. Exact incidence figures are not available since no denominator of treated patients is available. The reaction occurring most often is allergic sensitization. In one clinical study, using a 20% neomycin patch, neomycin-induced allergic skin reactions occurred in two of 2,175 (0.09%) individuals in the general population.[1] In another study, the incidence was found to be approximately 1%.[2]

The following local adverse reactions have been reported with topical corticosteroids, especially under occlusive dressings: burning, itching, irritation, dryness, folliculitis, hypertrichosis, acneiform eruptions, hypopigmentation, perioral dermatitis, allergic contact dermatitis, maceration of the skin, secondary infection, skin atrophy, striae and miliaria.

When steroid preparations are used for long periods of time in intertriginous areas or over extensive body areas, with or without occlusive non-permeable dressings, striae may occur; also there exists the possibility of systemic side effects when steroid preparations are used over larger areas or for a long period of time.

DOSAGE AND ADMINISTRATION

A thin film is applied 2 to 4 times daily to the affected area.

HOW SUPPLIED

Tube of ½ oz with applicator tip (NDC 0081-0196-88). Store at 15° to 25°C (59° to 77°F).

REFERENCES

1. Leyden JJ, Kligman AM: Contact dermatitis to neomycin sulfate. *JAMA* 1979;242:1276–1278.
2. Prystowsky SD, Allen AM, Smith RW, et al: Allergic contact hypersensitivity to nickel, neomycin, ethylenediamine, and benzocaine. *Arch Dermatol* 1979;115: 959–962. 455056

CORTISPORIN® ℞

[*kor'tĭ-spor"ĭn*]

OPHTHALMIC OINTMENT Sterile

(Polymyxin B Sulfate-Bacitracin Zinc-Neomycin Sulfate-Hydrocortisone)

DESCRIPTION

Cortisporin® Ophthalmic Ointment (polymyxin B sulfate-bacitracin zinc-neomycin sulfate-hydrocortisone) is a sterile antimicrobial and anti-inflammatory ointment for ophthalmic use. Each gram contains: Aerosporin® (polymyxin B sulfate) 10,000 units, bacitracin zinc 400 units, neomycin sulfate equivalent to 3.5 mg neomycin base, hydrocortisone 10 mg (1%) and special white petrolatum, qs.

Polymyxin B sulfate is the sulfate salt of polymyxin B_1 and B_2, which are produced by the growth of *Bacillus polymyxa* (Prazmowski) Migula (Fam. Bacillaceae). It has a potency of not less than 6,000 polymyxin B units per mg, calculated on an anhydrous basis.

Bacitracin zinc is the zinc salt of bacitracin, a mixture of related cyclic polypeptides (mainly bacitracin A) produced by the growth of an organism of the *licheniformis* group of *Bacillus subtilis* (Fam. Bacillaceae). It has a potency of not less than 40 bacitracin units per mg.

Neomycin sulfate is the sulfate salt of neomycin B and C, which are produced by the growth of *Streptomyces fradiae* Waksman (Fam. Streptomycetaceae). It has a potency equivalent of not less than 600 µg of neomycin standard per mg, calculated on an anhydrous basis.

Hydrocortisone, 11β, 17, 21-trihydroxypregn-4-ene-3, 20-dione, is an anti-inflammatory hormone.

CLINICAL PHARMACOLOGY

Corticoids suppress the inflammatory response to a variety of agents and they may delay healing. Since corticoids may inhibit the body's defense mechanism against infection, a concomitant antimicrobial drug may be used when this inhibition is considered to be clinically significant in a particular case.

The anti-infective components in the combination are included to provide action against specific organisms susceptible to them.

Polymyxin B sulfate, bacitracin zinc and neomycin sulfate together are considered active against the following microorganisms: *Staphylococcus aureus*, streptococci, including *Streptococcus pneumoniae, Escherichia coli, Haemophilus influenzae, Klebsiella-Enterobacter* species, *Neisseria* species and *Pseudomonas aeruginosa.*

When used topically, polymyxin B, bacitracin and neomycin are rarely irritating, and absorption from the intact skin or mucous membrane is insignificant. The incidence of skin sensitization to this combination has been shown to be low on normal skin.[1,2] Since these antibiotics are seldom used systemically, the patient is spared sensitization to those antibiotics which might later be required systemically.

When a decision to administer both a corticoid and antimicrobials is made, the administration of such drugs in combination has the advantage of greater patient compliance and convenience, with the added assurance that the intended dosage of both drugs is administered, plus assured compatibility of ingredients when both types of drug are in the same formulation and particularly that the intended volume of each drug is delivered simultaneously, thereby avoiding dilution of either medication by successive applications.

The relative potency of corticosteroids depends on the molecular structure, concentration and release from the vehicle.

INDICATIONS AND USAGE

For steroid-responsive inflammatory ocular conditions for which a corticosteroid is indicated and where bacterial infection or a risk of bacterial ocular infection exists.

Ocular steroids are indicated in inflammatory conditions of the palpebral and bulbar conjunctiva, cornea and anterior segment of the globe where the inherent risk of steroid use in certain infective conjunctivitides is accepted to obtain a diminution in edema and inflammation. They are also indicated in chronic anterior uveitis and corneal injury from chemical, radiation, or thermal burns, or penetration of foreign bodies.

The use of a combination drug with an anti-infective component is indicated where the risk of infection is high or where there is an expectation that potentially dangerous numbers of bacteria will be present in the eye.

The particular anti-infective drugs in this product are active against the following common bacterial eye pathogens: *Staphylococcus aureus*, streptococci, including *Streptococcus pneumoniae, Escherichia coli, Haemophilus influenzae, Klebsiella-Enterobacter* species, *Neisseria* species, and *Pseudomonas aeruginosa.*

The product does not provide adequate coverage against *Serratia marcescens.*

CONTRAINDICATIONS

Epithelial herpes simplex keratitis (dendritic keratitis), vaccinia, varicella, and many other viral diseases of the cornea and conjunctiva. Mycobacterial infection of the eye. Fungal diseases of ocular structures. Hypersensitivity to a component of the medication. (Hypersensitivity to the antibiotic component occurs at a higher rate than for other components.)

The use of these combinations is always contraindicated after uncomplicated removal of a corneal foreign body.

WARNINGS

Prolonged use may result in glaucoma, with damage to the optic nerve, defects in visual acuity and fields of vision, and posterior subcapsular cataract formation. Prolonged use may suppress the host response and thus increase the hazard of secondary ocular infections. In those diseases causing thinning of the cornea or sclera, perforations have been known to occur with the use of topical steroids. In acute purulent conditions of the eye, steroids may mask infection or enhance existing infection. If these products are used for 10 days or longer, intraocular pressure should be routinely monitored even though it may be difficult in children and uncooperative patients.

Employment of steroid medication in the treatment of herpes simplex requires great caution.

Neomycin sulfate may cause cutaneous sensitization. A precise incidence of hypersensitivity reactions (primarily skin rash) due to topical neomycin is not known.

The manifestations of sensitization to neomycin are usually itching, reddening and edema of the conjunctiva and eyelid. It may be manifest simply as a failure to heal. During long-term use of neomycin-containing products, periodic examination for such signs is advisable, and the patient should be told to discontinue the product if they are observed. These symptoms subside quickly on withdrawing the medication. Neomycin-containing applications should be avoided for the patient thereafter.

PRECAUTIONS

General: The initial prescription and renewal of the medication order beyond 8 grams should be made by a physician only after examination of the patient with the aid of magnification, such as slit lamp biomicroscopy and, where appropriate, fluorescein staining.

The possibility of persistent fungal infections of the cornea should be considered after prolonged steroid dosing.

Allergic cross-reactions may occur which could prevent the use of any or all of the following antibiotics for the treatment of future infections: kanamycin, paromomycin, streptomycin, and possibly gentamicin.

Carcinogenesis, Mutagenesis, Impairment of Fertility: Long-term studies in animals (rats, rabbits, mice) showed no evidence of carcinogenicity attributable to oral administration of corticosteroids.

Pregnancy: ***Teratogenic Effects:*** Pregnancy Category C. Corticosteroids have been shown to be teratogenic in rabbits when applied topically at concentrations of 0.5% on days 6-18 of gestation and in mice when applied topically at a concentration of 15% on days 10-13 of gestation. There are no adequate and well-controlled studies in pregnant women. Corticosteroids should be used during pregnancy only if the potential benefit justifies the potential risk to the fetus.

Nursing Mothers: Hydrocortisone appears in human milk following oral administration of the drug. Since systemic absorption of hydrocortisone may occur when applied topically, caution should be exercised when Cortisporin Ophthalmic Ointment is used by a nursing woman.

ADVERSE REACTIONS

Adverse reactions have occurred with steroid/anti-infective combination drugs which can be attributed to the steroid component, the anti-infective component, or the combination. Reactions occurring most often from the presence of the anti-infective ingredient are localized hypersensitivity, including itching, swelling and conjunctival erythema. Local irritation on instillation has also been reported. Exact incidence figures are not available since no denominator of treated patients is available.

The reactions due to the steroid component in decreasing order of frequency are: elevation of intraocular pressure (IOP) with possible development of glaucoma, and infrequent optic nerve damage; posterior subcapsular cataract formation; and delayed wound healing.

Secondary Infection: The development of secondary infection has occurred after use of combinations containing steroids and antimicrobials. Fungal infections of the cornea are particularly prone to develop coincidentally with long-term applications of steroid. The possibility of fungal invasion must be considered in any persistent corneal ulceration where steroid treatment has been used.

Secondary bacterial ocular infection following suppression of host responses also occurs.

DOSAGE AND ADMINISTRATION

Apply the ointment in the affected eye every 3 or 4 hours, depending on the severity of the condition.

Not more than 8 grams should be prescribed initially and the prescription should not be refilled without further evaluation as outlined in PRECAUTIONS above.

HOW SUPPLIED

Tube of 1/8 oz with ophthalmic tip (NDC-0081-0197-86). Store at 15°-25°C (59°-77°F).

REFERENCES:

1. Leyden JJ and Kligman AM. Contact Dermatitis to Neomycin Sulfate. *JAMA 242 (12)*:1276-1278, 1979.
2. Prystowsky SD, Allen WA, Smith RW, Nonomura JH, Odom RB and Akers WA. Allergic Contact Hypersensitivity to Nickel, Neomycin, Ethylenediamine, and Benzocaine. *Arch Dermatol 115*:959-962, 1979. 454986

CORTISPORIN® ℞

[*kor'tĭ-spor"ĭn*]

OPHTHALMIC SUSPENSION Sterile

(Polymyxin B Sulfate-Neomycin Sulfate-Hydrocortisone)

DESCRIPTION

Cortisporin® Ophthalmic Suspension (polymyxin B sulfate-neomycin sulfate-hydrocortisone) is a sterile antimicrobial and anti-inflammatory suspension for ophthalmic use. Each ml contains: Aerosporin® (polymyxin B sulfate) 10,000 units, neomycin sulfate equivalent to 3.5 mg neomycin base and hydrocortisone 10 mg (1%). The vehicle contains thimerosal 0.001% (added as a preservative) and the inactive ingredients cetyl alcohol, glyceryl monostearate, mineral oil, polyoxyl 40 stearate, propylene gylcol and water for injection. Sulfuric acid may be added to adjust pH.

Polymyxin B sulfate is the sulfate salt of polymyxin B_1 and B_2, which are produced by the growth of *Bacillus polymyxa* (Prazmowski) Migula (Fam. Bacillaceae). It has a potency of not less than 6,000 polymyxin B units per mg, calculated on an anhydrous basis.

Continued on next page

Burroughs Wellcome—Cont.

Neomycin sulfate is the sulfate salt of neomycin B and C, which are produced by the growth of *Streptomyces fradiae* Waksman (Fam. Streptomycetaceae). It has a potency equivalent of not less than 600 μg of neomycin standard per mg, calculated on an anhydrous basis.
Hydrocortisone, 11β, 17, 21-trihydroxypregn-4-ene-3,20-dione, is an anti-inflammatory hormone.

CLINICAL PHARMACOLOGY

Corticoids suppress the inflammatory response to a variety of agents and they may delay healing. Since corticoids may inhibit the body's defense mechanism against infection, a concomitant antimicrobial drug may be used when this inhibition is considered to be clinically significant in a particular case.
The anti-infective components in the combination are included to provide action against specific organisms susceptible to them. Polymyxin B sulfate and neomycin sulfate together are considered active against the following microorganisms: *Staphylococcus aureus, Escherichia coli, Haemophilus influenzae, Klebsiella-Enterobacter* species, *Neisseria* species and *Pseudomonas aeruginosa.*
When used topically, polymyxin B and neomycin are rarely irritating, and absorption from the intact skin or mucous membrane is insignificant. The incidence of skin sensitization to this combination has been shown to be low on normal skin.[1,2] Since these antibiotics are seldom used systemically, the patient is spared sensitization to those antibiotics which might later be required systemically.
When a decision to administer both a corticoid and antimicrobials is made, the administration of such drugs in combination has the advantage of greater patient compliance and convenience, with the added assurance that the intended dosage of both drugs is administered, plus assured compatibility of ingredients when both types of drug are in the same formulation and, particularly that the intended volume of each drug is delivered simultaneously, thereby avoiding dilution of either medication by successive instillations.
The relative potency of corticosteroids depends on the molecular structure, concentration, and release from the vehicle.

INDICATIONS AND USAGE

For steroid-responsive inflammatory ocular conditions for which a corticosteroid is indicated and where bacterial infection or a risk of bacterial ocular infection exists.
Ocular steroids are indicated in inflammatory conditions of the palpebral and bulbar conjunctiva, cornea and anterior segment of the globe where the inherent risk of steroid use in certain infective conjunctivitides is accepted to obtain a diminution in edema and inflammation. They are also indicated in chronic anterior uveitis and corneal injury from chemical, radiation, or thermal burns, or penetration of foreign bodies.
The use of a combination drug with an anti-infective component is indicated where the risk of infection is high or where there is an expectation that potentially dangerous numbers of bacteria will be present in the eye.
The particular anti-infective drugs in this product are active against the following common bacterial eye pathogens: *Staphylococcus aureus, Escherichia coli, Haemophilus influenzae, Klebsiella-Enterobacter* species, *Neisseria* species, and *Pseudomonas aeruginosa.*
The product does not provide adequate coverage against *Serratia marcescens* and streptococci, including *Streptococcus pneumoniae.*

CONTRAINDICATIONS

Epithelial herpes simplex keratitis (dendritic keratitis), vaccinia, varicella, and many other viral diseases of the cornea and conjunctiva. Mycobacterial infection of the eye. Fungal diseases of ocular structures. Hypersensitivity to a component of the medication. (Hypersensitivity to the antibiotic component occurs at a higher rate than for other components.)
The use of these combinations is always contraindicated after uncomplicated removal of a corneal foreign body.

WARNINGS

Prolonged use may result in glaucoma, with damage to the optic nerve, defects in visual acuity and fields of vision, and posterior subcapsular cataract formation. Prolonged use may suppress the host response and thus increase the hazard of secondary ocular infections. In those diseases causing thinning of the cornea or sclera, perforations have been known to occur with the use of topical steroids. In acute purulent conditions of the eye, steroids may mask infection or enhance existing infection. If these products are used for 10 days or longer, intraocular pressure should be routinely monitored even though it may be difficult in children and uncooperative patients.
Employment of steroid medication in the treatment of herpes simplex requires great caution.
Neomycin sulfate may cause cutaneous sensitization. A precise incidence of hypersensitivity reactions (primarily skin rash) due to topical neomycin is not known.
The manifestations of sensitization to neomycin are usually itching, reddening and edema of the conjunctiva and eyelid. It may be manifest simply as a failure to heal. During long-term use of neomycin-containing products, periodic examination for such signs is advisable, and the patient should be told to discontinue the product if they are observed. These symptoms subside quickly on withdrawing the medication. Neomycin-containing applications should be avoided for the patient thereafter.

PRECAUTIONS

General: The initial prescription and renewal of the medication order beyond 20 milliliters should be made by a physician only after examination of the patient with the aid of magnification, such as slit lamp biomicroscopy and, where appropriate, fluorescein staining.
The possibility of persistent fungal infections of the cornea should be considered after prolonged steroid dosing.
Allergic cross-reactions may occur which could prevent the use of any or all of the following antibiotics for the treatment of future infections: kanamycin, paromomycin, streptomycin, and possibly gentamicin.
Carcinogenesis, Mutagenesis, Impairment of Fertility: Long-term studies in animals (rats, rabbits, mice) showed no evidence of carcinogenicity attributable to oral administration of corticosteroids.
Pregnancy: ***Teratogenic Effects:*** Pregnancy Category C. Corticosteroids have been shown to be teratogenic in rabbits when applied topically at concentrations of 0.5% on days 6–18 of gestation and in mice when applied topically at a concentration of 15% on days 10–13 of gestation. There are no adequate and well-controlled studies in pregnant women. Corticosteroids should be used during pregnancy only if the potential benefit justifies the potential risk to the fetus.
Nursing Mothers: Hydrocortisone appears in human milk following oral administration of the drug. Since systemic absorption of hydrocortisone may occur when applied topically, caution should be exercised when Cortisporin Ophthalmic Suspension is used by a nursing woman.

ADVERSE REACTIONS

Adverse reactions have occurred with steroid/anti-infective combination drugs which can be attributed to the steroid component, the anti-infective component, or the combination. Reactions occurring most often from the presence of the anti-infective ingredient are localized hypersensitivity, including itching, swelling and conjunctival erythema. Local irritation on instillation has also been reported. Exact incidence figures are not available since no denominator of treated patients is available.
The reactions due to the steroid component in decreasing order of frequency are: elevation of intraocular pressure (IOP) with possible development of glaucoma, and infrequent optic nerve damage; posterior subcapsular cataract formation; and delayed wound healing.
Secondary Infection: The development of secondary infection has occurred after use of combinations containing steroids and antimicrobials. Fungal infections of the cornea are particularly prone to develop coincidentally with long-term applications of steroid. The possibility of fungal invasion must be considered in any persistent corneal ulceration where steroid treatment has been used.
Secondary bacterial ocular infection following suppression of host responses also occurs.

DOSAGE AND ADMINISTRATION

One or two drops in the affected eye every 3 or 4 hours, depending on the severity of the condition. The suspension may be used more frequently if necessary.
Not more than 20 milliliters should be prescribed initially and the prescription should not be refilled without further evaluation as outlined in PRECAUTIONS above.
SHAKE WELL BEFORE USING.

HOW SUPPLIED

Plastic DROP DOSE® dispenser bottle of 7.5 ml (NDC-0081-0193-02).
Store at 15°–25°C (59°–77°F).

REFERENCES

1. Leyden JJ and Kligman AM. Contact Dermatitis to Neomycin Sulfate. *JAMA 242 (12)*: 1276–1278, 1979.
2. Prystowsky SD, Allen AM, Smith RW, Nonomura JH, Odom RB and Akers WA. Allergic Contact Hypersensitivity to Nickel, Neomycin, Ethylenediamine, and Benzocaine. *Arch Dermatol 115*:959–962, 1979. 455229

CORTISPORIN® OTIC SOLUTION Sterile ℞

[*kor'tĭ-spor"ĭn ō'tĭk*]
(Polymyxin B Sulfate-Neomycin Sulfate-Hydrocortisone)

DESCRIPTION

Cortisporin Otic Solution (polymyxin B sulfate-neomycin sulfate-hydrocortisone) is a sterile antibacterial and anti-inflammatory solution for otic use. Each ml contains: Aerosporin® (polymyxin B sulfate) 10,000 units, neomycin sulfate equivalent to 3.5 mg neomycin base, and hydrocortisone 10 mg (1%). The vehicle contains potassium metabisulfite 0.1% (added as a preservative) and the inactive ingredients cupric sulfate, glycerin, hydrochloric acid, propylene glycol, and Water for Injection.
Polymyxin B sulfate is the sulfate salt of polymyxin B_1 and B_2, which are produced by the growth of *Bacillus polymyxa* (Prazmowski) Migula (Fam. Bacillaceae). It has a potency of not less than 6,000 polymyxin B units per mg, calculated on an anhydrous basis.
Neomycin sulfate is the sulfate salt of neomycin B and C, which are produced by the growth of *Streptomyces fradiae* Waksman (Fam. Streptomycetaceae). It has a potency equivalent of not less than 600 μg of neomycin standard per mg, calculated on an anhydrous basis.
Hydrocortisone, 11β, 17, 21-trihydroxypregn-4-ene-3, 20-dione, is an anti-inflammatory hormone.

CLINICAL PHARMACOLOGY

Corticoids suppress the inflammatory response to a variety of agents and they may delay healing. Since corticoids may inhibit the body's defense mechanism against infection, a concomitant antimicrobial drug may be used when this inhibition is considered to be clinically significant in a particular case.
The anti-infective components in the combination are included to provide action against specific organisms susceptible to them. Polymyxin B sulfate and neomycin sulfate together are considered active against the following microorganisms: *Staphylococcus aureus, Escherichia coli, Haemophilus influenzae, Klebsiella-Enterobacter* species, *Neisseria* species, and *Pseudomonas aeruginosa.* This product does not provide adequate coverage against *Serratia marcescens* and streptococci, including *Streptococcus pneumonia.*
The relative potency of corticosteroids depends on the molecular structure, concentration, and release from the vehicle.

INDICATIONS AND USAGE

For the treatment of superficial bacterial infections of the external auditory canal caused by organisms susceptible to the action of the antibiotics.

CONTRAINDICATIONS

This product is contraindicated in those individuals who have shown hypersensitivity to any of its components, and in herpes simplex, vaccinia and varicella infections.

WARNINGS

This product should be used with care when the integrity of the tympanic membrane is in question because of the possibility of ototoxicity, and because stinging and burning may occur when this product gains access to the middle ear.
Neomycin sulfate may cause cutaneous sensitization. A precise incidence of hypersensitivity reactions (primarily skin rash) due to topical neomycin is not known.
When using neomycin-containing products to control secondary infection in the chronic dermatoses, such as chronic otitis externa or stasis dermatitis, it should be borne in mind that the skin in these conditions is more liable than is normal skin to become sensitized to many substances, including neomycin. The manifestation of sensitization to neomycin is usually a low-grade reddening with swelling, dry scaling and itching; it may be manifest simply as a failure to heal. Periodic examination for such signs is advisable, and the patient should be told to discontinue the product if they are observed. These symptoms regress quickly on withdrawing the medication. Neomycin-containing applications should be avoided for the patient thereafter.
Contains potassium metabisulfite, a sulfite that may cause allergic-type reactions including anaphylactic symptoms and life-threatening or less severe asthmatic episodes in certain susceptible people. The overall prevalence of sulfite sensitivity in the general population is unknown and probably low. Sulfite sensitivity is seen more frequently in asthmatic than in nonasthmatic people.

PRECAUTIONS

General: As with other antibiotic preparations, prolonged use may result in overgrowth of nonsusceptible organisms, including fungi.
If the infection is not improved after one week, cultures and susceptibility tests should be repeated to verify the identity of the organism and to determine whether therapy should be changed.
Treatment should not be continued for longer than ten days.
Allergic cross-reactions may occur which could prevent the use of any or all of the following antibiotics for the treatment of future infections: kanamycin, paromomycin, streptomycin, and possibly gentamicin.
Information for Patients: Avoid contaminating the dropper with material from the ear, fingers, or other source. This caution is necessary if the sterility of the drops is to be preserved.
If sensitization or irritation occurs, discontinue use immediately and contact your physician.
Do not use in the eyes.
Laboratory Tests: Systemic effects of excessive levels of hydrocortisone may include a reduction in the number of

circulating eosinophils and a decrease in urinary excretion of 17-hydroxycorticosteroids.

Carcinogenesis, Mutagenesis, Impairment of Fertility: Long-term studies in animals (rats, rabbits, mice) showed no evidence of carcinogenicity attributable to oral administration of corticosteroids.

Pregnancy: Teratogenic effects: Pregnancy Category C. Corticosteroids have been shown to be teratogenic in rabbits when applied topically at concentrations of 0.5% on days 6 to 18 of gestation and in mice when applied topically at a concentration of 15% on days 10 to 13 of gestation. There are no adequate and well-controlled studies in pregnant women. Corticosteroids should be used during pregnancy only if the potential benefit justifies the potential risk to the fetus.

Nursing Mothers: Hydrocortisone appears in human milk following oral administration of the drug. Since systemic absorption of hydrocortisone may occur when applied topically, caution should be exercised when Cortisporin Otic Solution is used by a nursing woman.

Pediatric Use: See **DOSAGE AND ADMINISTRATION**.

ADVERSE REACTIONS

Neomycin occasionally causes skin sensitization. Ototoxicity and nephrotoxicity have also been reported (See WARNINGS section). Adverse reactions have occurred with topical use of antibiotic combinations including neomycin and polymyxin B. Exact incidence figures are not available since no denominator of treated patients is available. The reaction occurring most often is allergic sensitization. In one clinical study, using a 20% neomycin patch, neomycin-induced allergic skin reactions occurred in two of 2,175 (0.09%) individuals in the general population.[1] In another study, the incidence was found to be approximately 1%.[2]

The following local adverse reactions have been reported with topical corticosteroids, especially under occlusive dressings: burning, itching, irritation, dryness, folliculitis, hypertrichosis, acneiform eruptions, hypopigmentation, perioral dermatitis, allergic contact dermatitis, maceration of the skin, secondary infection, skin atrophy, striae, and miliaria. Stinging and burning have been reported when this product has gained access to the middle ear.

DOSAGE AND ADMINISTRATION

The external auditory canal should be thoroughly cleansed and dried with a sterile cotton applicator.

For adults, 4 drops of the solution should be instilled into the affected ear 3 or 4 times daily. For infants and children, 3 drops are suggested because of the smaller capacity of the ear canal.

The patient should lie with the affected ear upward and then the drops should be instilled. This position should be maintained for 5 minutes to facilitate penetration of the drops into the ear canal.

Repeat, if necessary, for the opposite ear.

If preferred, a cotton wick may be inserted into the canal and then the cotton may be saturated with the solution. This wick should be kept moist by adding further solution every four hours. The wick should be replaced at least once every 24 hours.

HOW SUPPLIED

Bottle of 10 ml with sterilized dropper. (NDC 0081-0199-92). Store at 15° to 25°C (59° to 77°F).

Also Available: Cortisporin Otic Suspension bottle of 10 ml with sterilized dropper.

Pediotic™ Suspension bottle of 7.5 ml with sterilized dropper.

REFERENCES

1. Leyden JJ, Kligman AM. Contact dermatitis to neomycin sulfate, *JAMA* 1979;242(12):1276–1278.
2. Prystowsky SD, Allen AM, Smith RW, et al: Allergic contact hypersensitivity to nickel, neomycin, ethylenediamine, and benzocaine. *Arch Dermatol* 1979; 115: 959–962.　　　　455647

CORTISPORIN® OTIC SUSPENSION　　　℞
[kor'tĭ-spor "ĭn ō'tĭk]
Sterile
(Polymyxin B Sulfate-Neomycin Sulfate-Hydrocortisone)

DESCRIPTION

Cortisporin Otic Suspension (polymyxin B sulfate-neomycin sulfate-hydrocortisone) is a sterile antibacterial and anti-inflammatory suspension for otic use. Each ml contains: Aerosporin® (polymyxin B sulfate) 10,000 units, neomycin sulfate equivalent to 3.5 mg neomycin base, and hydrocortisone 10 mg (1%). The vehicle contains thimerosal 0.01% (added as a preservative) and the inactive ingredients cetyl alcohol, propylene glycol, polysorbate 80, and Water for Injection. Sulfuric acid may be added to adjust pH.

Polymyxin B sulfate is the sulfate salt of polymyxin B_1 and B_2, which are produced by the growth of *Bacillus polymyxa* (Prazmowski) Migula (Fam. Bacillaceae). It has a potency of

not less than 6,000 polymyxin B units per mg, calculated on an anhydrous basis.

Neomycin sulfate is the sulfate salt of neomycin B and C, which are produced by the growth of *Streptomyces fradiae* Waksman (Fam. Streptomycetaceae). It has a potency equivalent of not less than 600 μg of neomycin standard per mg, calculated on an anhydrous basis.

Hydrocortisone, 11β,17,21-trihydroxypregn-4-ene-3,20-dione, is an anti-inflammatory hormone.

CLINICAL PHARMACOLOGY

Corticoids suppress the inflammatory response to a variety of agents and they may delay healing. Since corticoids may inhibit the body's defense mechanism against infection, a concomitant antimicrobial drug may be used when this inhibition is considered to be clinically significant in a particular case.

The anti-infective components in the combination are included to provide action against specific organisms susceptible to them. Polymyxin B sulfate and neomycin sulfate together are considered active against the following microorganisms: *Staphylococcus aureus, Escherichia coli, Haemophilus influenzae, Klebsiella-Enterobacter* species, *Neisseria* species, and *Pseudomonas aeruginosa*. This product does not provide adequate coverage against *Serratia marcescens* and streptococci, including *Streptococcus pneumonia*.

The relative potency of corticosteroids depends on the molecular structure, concentration, and release from the vehicle.

INDICATIONS AND USAGE

For the treatment of superficial bacterial infections of the external auditory canal caused by organisms susceptible to the action of the antibiotics, and for the treatment of infections of mastoidectomy and fenestration cavities caused by organisms susceptible to the antibiotics.

CONTRAINDICATIONS

This product is contraindicated in those individuals who have shown hypersensitivity to any of its components, and in herpes simplex, vaccinia and varicella infections.

WARNINGS

This product should be used with care in cases of perforated eardrum and in long-standing cases of chronic otitis media because of the possibility of ototoxicity.

Neomycin sulfate may cause cutaneous sensitization. A precise incidence of hypersensitivity reactions (primarily skin rash) due to topical neomycin is not known.

When using neomycin-containing products to control secondary infection in the chronic dermatoses, such as chronic otitis externa or stasis dermatitis, it should be borne in mind that the skin in these conditions is more liable than is normal skin to become sensitized to many substances, including neomycin. The manifestation of sensitization to neomycin is usually a low-grade reddening with swelling, dry scaling and itching; it may be manifest simply as a failure to heal. Periodic examination for such signs is advisable, and the patient should be told to discontinue the product if they are observed. These symptoms regress quickly on withdrawing the medication. Neomycin-containing applications should be avoided for the patient thereafter.

PRECAUTIONS

General: As with other antibiotic preparations, prolonged use may result in overgrowth of nonsusceptible organisms, including fungi.

If the infection is not improved after one week, cultures and susceptibility tests should be repeated to verify the identity of the organism and to determine whether therapy should be changed.

Treatment should not be continued for longer than ten days. Allergic cross-reactions may occur which could prevent the use of any or all of the following antibiotics for the treatment of future infections: kanamycin, paromomycin, streptomycin, and possibly gentamicin.

Information for Patients: Avoid contaminating the dropper with material from the ear, fingers, or other source. This caution is necessary if the sterility of the drops is to be preserved.

If sensitization or irritation occurs, discontinue use immediately and contact your physician.

Do not use in the eyes.

SHAKE WELL BEFORE USING.

Laboratory Tests: Systemic effects of excessive levels of hydrocortisone may include a reduction in the number of circulating eosinophils and a decrease in urinary excretion of 17-hydroxycorticosteroids.

Carcinogenesis, Mutagenesis, Impairment of Fertility: Long-term studies in animals (rats, rabbits, mice) showed no evidence of carcinogenicity attributable to oral administration of corticosteroids.

Pregnancy: Teratogenic effects: Pregnancy Category C. Corticosteroids have been shown to be teratogenic in rabbits when applied topically at concentrations of 0.5% on days 6 to 18 of gestation and in mice when applied topically at a concentration of 15% on days 10 to 13 of gestation. There are no adequate and well-controlled studies in pregnant women.

Corticosteroids should be used during pregnancy only if the potential benefit justifies the potential risk to the fetus.

Nursing Mothers: Hydrocortisone appears in human milk following oral administration of the drug. Since systemic absorption of hydrocortisone may occur when applied topically, caution should be exercised when Cortisporin Otic Suspension is used by a nursing woman.

Pediatric Use: See DOSAGE AND ADMINISTRATION.

ADVERSE REACTIONS

Neomycin occasionally causes skin sensitization. Ototoxicity and nephrotoxicity have also been reported (See WARNINGS section). Adverse reactions have occurred with topical use of antibiotic combinations including neomycin and polymyxin B. Exact incidence figures are not available since no denominator of treated patients is available. The reaction occurring most often is allergic sensitization. In one clinical study, using a 20% neomycin patch, neomycin-induced allergic skin reactions occurred in two of 2,175 (0.09%) individuals in the general population.[1] In another study, the incidence was found to be approximately 1%.[2]

The following local adverse reactions have been reported with topical corticosteroids, especially under occlusive dressings: burning, itching, irritation, dryness, folliculitis, hypertrichosis, acneiform eruptions, hypopigmentation, perioral dermatitis, allergic contact dermatitis, maceration of the skin, secondary infection, skin atrophy, striae and miliaria. Stinging and burning have been reported rarely when this drug has gained access to the middle ear.

DOSAGE AND ADMINISTRATION

The external auditory canal should be thoroughly cleansed and dried with a sterile cotton applicator.

For adults, 4 drops of the suspension should be instilled into the affected ear 3 or 4 times daily.

For infants and children, 3 drops are suggested because of the smaller capacity of the ear canal.

The patient should lie with the affected ear upward and then the drops should be instilled. This position should be maintained for 5 minutes to facilitate penetration of the drops into the ear canal. Repeat, if necessary, for the opposite ear. If preferred, a cotton wick may be inserted into the canal and then the cotton may be saturated with the suspension. This wick should be kept moist by adding further suspension every four hours. The wick should be replaced at least once every 24 hours.

SHAKE WELL BEFORE USING.

HOW SUPPLIED

Bottle of 10 ml with sterilized dropper. (NDC 0081-0198-92). Store at 15° to 25°C (59° to 77°F).

Also Available: Cortisporin Otic Solution bottle of 10 ml with sterilized dropper.

Pediotic™ Suspension bottle of 7.5 ml with sterilized dropper.

REFERENCES

1. Leyden JJ, Kligman AM. Contact dermatitis to neomycin sulfate. *JAMA* 1979;242(12):1276–1278.
2. Prystowsky SD, Allen AM, Smith RW, et al: Allergic contact hypersensitivity to nickel, neomycin, ethylenediamine, and benzocaine. *Arch Dermatol* 1979;115:959–962.
　　　　455702

DARAPRIM®　　　℞
[dair'ah-prĭm ″]
(Pyrimethamine)
25 mg Scored Tablets

DESCRIPTION

Daraprim (pyrimethamine) is an antiparasitic available in tablet form for oral administration. Each scored tablet contains 25 mg pyrimethamine and the inactive ingredients corn and potato starch, lactose, and magnesium stearate. Pyrimethamine is known chemically as 2,4-diamino-5-(p-chlorophenyl)-6-ethylpyrimidine.

CLINICAL PHARMACOLOGY

Pyrimethamine is well absorbed, with peak levels occurring between 2 to 6 hours following administration. It is eliminated slowly and has a plasma half-life of approximately 96 hours. Pyrimethamine is 87% bound to human plasma proteins.

Microbiology: Pyrimethamine is a folic acid antagonist and the rationale for its therapeutic action is based on the differential requirement between host and parasite for nucleic acid precursors involved in growth. This activity is highly selective against plasmodia and *Toxoplasma gondii*.

Pyrimethamine possesses blood schizonticidal and some tissue schizonticidal activity against malaria parasites of man. However, its blood schizonticidal activity may be slower than that of 4-aminoquinoline compounds. It does not destroy gametocytes, but arrests sporogony in the mosquito.

Continued on next page

Burroughs Wellcome—Cont.

The action of Daraprim against *Toxoplasma gondii* is greatly enhanced when used in conjunction with sulfonamides. This was demonstrated by Eyles and Coleman[1] in the treatment of experimental toxoplasmosis in the mouse. Jacobs *et al*[2] demonstrated that combination of the two drugs effectively prevented the development of severe uveitis in most rabbits following the inoculation of the anterior chamber of the eye with toxoplasma.

INDICATIONS AND USAGE

Daraprim (Pyrimethamine) is indicated for the chemoprophylaxis of malaria due to susceptible strains of plasmodia. It should not be used alone to treat an acute attack of malaria. Fast-acting schizonticides such as chloroquine or quinine are indicated and preferable for the treatment of acute attacks. However, conjoint use of Daraprim will initiate *transmission control* and *suppressive cure* for susceptible strains of plasmodia.

Daraprim is also indicated for the treatment of toxoplasmosis. For this purpose the drug should be used conjointly with a sulfonamide since synergism exists with this combination.

CONTRAINDICATIONS

Use of Daraprim is contraindicated in patients with known hypersensitivity to pyrimethamine. Use of the drug is also contraindicated in patients with documented megaloblastic anemia due to folate deficiency.

WARNINGS

The dosage of pyrimethamine required for the treatment of toxoplasmosis is 10 to 20 times the recommended antimalaria dosage and approaches the toxic level. If signs of folate deficiency develop (see ADVERSE REACTIONS) reduce the dosage or discontinue the drug according to the response of the patient. Folinic acid (leucovorin) should be administered in a dosage of 5 to 15 mg daily (orally, I.V. or I.M.) until normal hematopoiesis is restored.

Daraprim should be kept out of the reach of children as children and infants are extremely susceptible to adverse effects from an overdose. Deaths in children have been reported after accidental ingestion.

PRECAUTIONS

General: The recommended dosage for chemoprophylaxis of malaria should not be exceeded. A small "starting" dose for toxoplasmosis is recommended in patients with convulsive disorders to avoid the potential nervous system toxicity of pyrimethamine. Daraprim should be used with caution in patients with impaired renal or hepatic function or in patients with possible folate deficiency, such as individuals with malabsorption syndrome, alcoholism or pregnancy, and those receiving therapy, such as phenytoin, affecting folate levels (see "Pregnancy" subsection).

Information for Patients: Patients should be warned that at the first appearance of a skin rash they should stop use of Daraprim and seek medical attention immediately. Patients should also be warned that the appearance of sore throat, pallor, purpura or glossitis may be early indications of serious disorders which require prophylactic treatment to be stopped, and medical treatment to be sought. Patients should be warned to keep Daraprim out of the reach of children. Patients should be warned that if anorexia and vomiting occur, they may be minimized by taking the drug with meals.

Laboratory Tests: In patients receiving high dosage, as for the treatment of toxoplasmosis, semiweekly blood counts, including platelet counts, should be done.

Drug Interactions: Pyrimethamine may be used with sulfonamides, quinine and other antimalarials, and with other antibiotics. However, the concomitant use of other antifolic drugs, such as sulfonamides or trimethoprim-sulfamethoxazole combinations, while the patient is receiving pyrimethamine for antimalarial prophylaxis, may increase the risk of bone marrow suppression. If signs of folate deficiency develop, pyrimethamine should be discontinued. Folinic acid (leucovorin) should be administered until normal hematopoiesis is restored (see WARNINGS). Mild hepatotoxicity has been reported in some patients when lorazepam and pyrimethamine were administered concomitantly.

Carcinogenesis, Mutagenesis, Impairment of Fertility:
Carcinogenesis: Pyrimethamine has been reported to produce a significant increase in the number of lung tumors per mouse when given intraperitoneally at high doses (0.025 g/kg).[3] There have been two reports of cancer associated with pyrimethamine administration: a 51-year-old female who developed chronic granulocytic leukemia after taking pyrimethamine for two years for toxoplasmosis,[4] and a 56-year-old patient who developed reticulum cell sarcoma after 14 months of pyrimethamine for toxoplasmosis.[5]
Mutagenesis: Pyrimethamine has been shown to be nonmutagenic in the following *in vitro* assays: the Ames point mutation assay, the Rec assay and the *E. coli* WP2 assay. It was positive in the L5178Y/TK +/− mouse lymphoma assay in the absence of exogenous metabolic activation.[6] Hu-

man blood lymphocytes cultured *in vitro* had structural chromosome aberrations induced by pyrimethamine.
In vivo, chromosomes analyzed from the bone marrow of rats dosed with pyrimethamine showed an increased number of structural and numerical aberrations.

Impairment of Fertility: The effects of pyrimethamine on rat pregnancy seem to indicate that the fertility index of rats treated with pyrimethamine is lowered only when the higher dosage is used, suggesting a possible toxic effect upon the whole organism and/or the conceptuses.[7]

Pregnancy: *Teratogenic Effects:* Pregnancy Category C. Pyrimethamine has been shown to be teratogenic in rats, hamsters and Goettingen miniature pigs. There are no adequate and well-controlled studies in pregnant women. Daraprim should be used during pregnancy only if the potential benefit justifies the potential risk to the fetus. Concurrent administration of folinic acid is strongly recommended when used for the treatment of toxoplasmosis during pregnancy.

Thiersch[8] reported that when rats were given an oral dose of pyrimethamine of 12.5 mg/kg from day 7 to 9 of the gestation period, there was 66.2% resorption and 32.8% of the live fetuses were stunted. When lower doses of 1 mg/kg and 0.5 mg/kg were given for 10 days, days 4 to 13 of gestation, there was 15% and 8.5% resorption, respectively, and 16.6% and 6.9% of the live fetuses were stunted. A daily oral dose as low as 0.3 mg/kg given for days 7 to 16 of gestation still resulted in 2.7% of the fetuses being stunted.

Sullivan and Takacs[9] found that less than 10% of hamster fetuses died or were malformed following single doses of 20 mg to the mother, which on a mg/kg basis was eight to nine times greater than that given to rats.

Hayama and Kokue[10] reported on the administration of pyrimethamine to pregnant female Goettingen miniature pigs. Sows given 0.9 mg/kg/day, during days 11 to 35 of pregnancy, i.e. the period of organogenesis in the pig, delivered normal offspring. Sows administered a high dose 3.6 mg/kg/day during the same gestational period delivered offspring with a high incidence of malformations including cleft palate, club foot, and micrognathia.

Nursing Mothers: Pyrimethamine is excreted in human milk. Milk samples obtained from lactating mothers after treatment with pyrimethamine were found to have measurable concentrations of the drug, with peak concentration at 6 hours postadministration. It is estimated that after a single 75 mg dose of oral pyrimethamine, approximately 3 to 4 mg of the drug would be passed on to the feeding child over a 48-hour period.

Because of the potential for serious adverse reactions in nursing infants from Daraprim, a decision should be made whether to discontinue nursing or to discontinue the drug, taking into account the importance of the drug to the mother. (See "Carcinogenesis, Mutagenesis, Impairment of Fertility" and "Pregnancy" subsections.)

Pediatric Use: See DOSAGE AND ADMINISTRATION.

ADVERSE REACTIONS

Hypersensitivity reactions, occasionally severe, can occur at any dose, particularly when pyrimethamine is administered concomitantly with a sulfonamide. With large doses of pyrimethamine, anorexia and vomiting may occur. Vomiting may be minimized by giving the medication with meals; it usually disappears promptly upon reduction of dosage. Doses used in toxoplasmosis may produce megaloblastic anemia, leukopenia, thrombocytopenia, pancytopenia, atrophic glossitis, hematuria and disorders of cardiac rhythm. Hematologic effects, however, may also occur at low doses in certain individuals (see PRECAUTIONS—General).

Insomnia, diarrhea, headache, light-headedness, dryness of the mouth or throat, fever, malaise, dermatitis, abnormal skin pigmentation, depression, seizures, pulmonary eosinophilia, and hyperphenylalaninemia have been reported rarely.

OVERDOSAGE

Acute intoxication may follow the ingestion of an excessive amount of pyrimethamine. Gastrointestinal and/or central nervous system signs may be present, including convulsions. The initial symptoms are usually gastrointestinal and may include abdominal pain, nausea, severe and repeated vomiting, possibly including hematemesis. Central nervous system toxicity may be manifest by initial excitability, generalized and prolonged convulsions which may be followed by respiratory depression, circulatory collapse and death within a few hours. Neurological symptoms appear rapidly (30 minutes to 2 hours after drug ingestion), suggesting that in gross overdosage pyrimethamine has a direct toxic effect on the central nervous system.

The fatal dose is variable, with the smallest reported fatal single dose being 250 mg to 300 mg. There are, however, reports of children who have recovered after taking 375 mg to 625 mg.

There is no specific antidote to acute pyrimethamine poisoning. Gastric lavage is recommended and is effective if carried out very soon after drug ingestion. A parenteral barbiturate may be indicated to control convulsions. Folinic acid may

also be given to counteract effects on the hematopoietic system (see WARNINGS).

DOSAGE AND ADMINISTRATION

For Chemoprophylaxis of Malaria:
Adults and children over 10 years—25 mg (1 tablet) once weekly
Children 4 through 10 years—12.5 mg (½ tablet) once weekly
Infants and children under 4 years—6.25 mg (¼ tablet) once weekly

Regimens planned to include *suppressive cure* should be extended through any characteristic periods of early recrudescence and late relapse for at least 10 weeks in each case.

For Treatment of Acute Attacks: Daraprim is recommended in areas where only susceptible plasmodia exist. This drug is not recommended alone in the treatment of acute attacks of malaria in nonimmune persons. Fast-acting schizonticides such as chloroquine or quinine are indicated for treatment of acute attacks. However, conjoint Daraprim dosage of 25 mg daily for 2 days will initiate *transmission control* and *suppressive cure.* Should circumstances arise wherein Daraprim must be used alone in semi-immune persons, the adult dosage for an acute attack is 50 mg for 2 days; children 4 through 10 years old may be given 25 mg daily for 2 days. In any event, clinical cure should be followed by the once-weekly regimen described above.

For Toxoplasmosis: The dosage of Daraprim for the treatment of toxoplasmosis must be carefully adjusted so as to provide maximum therapeutic effect and a minimum of side effects. At the high dosage required, there is a marked variation in the tolerance to the drug. Young patients may tolerate higher doses than older individuals.

The adult *starting* dose is 50 to 75 mg of the drug daily, together with 1 to 4 g daily of a sulfonamide of the sulfapyrimidine type, e.g., sulfadiazine. This dosage is ordinarily continued for 1 to 3 weeks, depending on the response of the patient and his tolerance of the therapy. The dosage may then be reduced to about one-half that previously given for each drug and continued for an additional 4 to 5 weeks.

The pediatric dosage of Daraprim is 1 mg/kg per day divided into 2 equal daily doses; after 2 to 4 days this dose may be reduced to one-half and continued for approximately one month. The usual pediatric sulfonamide dosage is used in conjunction with Daraprim.

HOW SUPPLIED

White, scored tablets containing 25 mg pyrimethamine, imprinted with "DARAPRIM" and "A3A" in bottles of 100 (NDC 0081-0201-55). Store at 15° to 25°C (59° to 77°F) in a dry place and protect from light.

REFERENCES

1. Eyles DE, Coleman N: Synergistic effect of sulfadiazine and Daraprim against experimental toxoplasmosis in the mouse. *Antibiot Chemother* 1953;3:483–490.
2. Jacobs L, Melton ML, Kaufman HE: Treatment of experimental ocular toxoplasmosis, *Arch Ophthalmol* 1964;71:111–118.
3. Bahna L: Pyrimethamine. *LARC Monogr Eval Carcinog Risk Chem* 1977; 13:233–242.
4. Jim RTS, Elizaga FV: Development of chronic granulocytic leukemia in a patient treated with pyrimethamine. *Hawaii Med J* 1977;36(6):173–176.
5. Sadoff L: Antimalarial drugs and Burkitt's lymphoma. *Lancet* 1973; 2(7840):1262–1263.
6. Clive D, Johnson KO, Spector JKS, et al.: Validation and characterization of the L5178Y/TK +/− mouse lymphoma mutagen assay system. *Mut Res* 1979;59:61–108.
7. Andrade ATL, Guerra MO, Silva NOG et al.: Antifertility effects of pyrimethamine. *Excerpta Med Int Cong Ser* 1976;370:317–321.
8. Thiersch JB: Effects of certain 2,4-diaminopyrimidine antagonists of folic acid on pregnancy and rat fetus. *Proc Soc Exp Biol Med* 1954;87:571–577.
9. Sullivan GE, Takacs E: Comparative teratogenicity of pyrimethamine in rats and hamsters. *Teratology* 1971;4:205–210.
10. Hayama T, Kokue E: Use of Goettingen miniature pigs for studying pyrimethamine teratogenesis, *CRC Crit Rev Toxicol* 1985;14(4):403–421.   462616
Shown in Product Identification Section, page 407

DIGIBIND®   ℞
[dĭ'gĭ-bĭnd]
Digoxin Immune Fab (Ovine)

DESCRIPTION

Digibind, Digoxin Immune Fab (Ovine), is a sterile lyophilized powder of antigen binding fragments (Fab) derived from specific antidigoxin antibodies raised in sheep. Production of antibodies specific for digoxin involves conjugation of digoxin as a hapten to human albumin. Sheep are immunized with this material to produce antibodies specific for the antigenic determinants of the digoxin molecule. The anti-

body is then papain digested and digoxin-specific Fab fragments of the antibody are isolated and purified by affinity chromatography. These antibody fragments have a molecular weight of approximately 50,000.

Each vial, which will bind approximately 0.6 mg of digoxin (or digitoxin), contains 40 mg of digoxin-specific Fab fragments derived from sheep plus 75 mg of sorbitol as a stabilizer and 28 mg of sodium chloride. The vial contains no preservatives.

Digibind is administered by intravenous injection after reconstitution with Sterile Water for Injection (4 ml per vial).

CLINICAL PHARMACOLOGY

After intravenous injection of Digoxin Immune Fab (Ovine) in the baboon, digoxin-specific Fab fragments are excreted in the urine with a biological half-life of about 9 to 13 hours.[1] In humans with normal renal function the half-life appears to be 15 to 20 hours.[2] Experimental studies in animals indicate that these antibody fragments have a large volume of distribution in the extracellular space, unlike whole antibody which distributes in a space only about twice the plasma volume.[1] Ordinarily, following administration of Digibind, improvement in signs and symptoms of digitalis intoxication begins within one-half hour or less.[2,3,4,5]

The affinity of Digibind for digoxin is in the range of 10^9 to 10^{10} M^{-1}, which is greater than the affinity of digoxin for (sodium, potassium) ATPase, the presumed receptor for its toxic effects. The affinity of Digibind for digitoxin is about 10^8 to 10^9 M^{-1}.[6]

Digibind binds molecules of digoxin, making them unavailable for binding at their site of action on cells in the body. The Fab fragment-digoxin complex accumulates in the blood, from which it is excreted by the kidney. The net effect is to shift the equilibrium away from binding of digoxin to its receptors in the body, thereby reversing its effects.

INDICATIONS AND USAGE

Digibind, Digoxin Immune Fab (Ovine), is indicated for treatment of potentially life-threatening digoxin intoxication.[3] Although designed specifically to treat life-threatening digoxin overdose, it has also been used successfully to treat life-threatening digitoxin overdose.[3] Since human experience is limited and the consequences of repeated exposures are unknown, Digibind is not indicated for milder cases of digitalis toxicity.

Manifestations of life-threatening toxicity include severe ventricular arrhythmias such as ventricular tachycardia or ventricular fibrillation, or progressive bradyarrhythmias such as severe sinus bradycardia or second or third degree heart block not responsive to atropine.

Ingestion of more than 10 mg of digoxin in previously healthy adults or 4 mg of digoxin in previously healthy children, or ingestion causing steady-state serum concentrations greater than 10 ng/ml, often results in cardiac arrest. Digitalis-induced progressive elevation of the serum potassium concentration also suggests imminent cardiac arrest. If the potassium concentration exceeds 5 mEq/L in the setting of severe digitalis intoxication, Digibind therapy is indicated.

CONTRAINDICATIONS

There are no known contraindications to the use of Digibind.

WARNINGS

Suicidal ingestion often involves more than one drug; thus toxicity from other drugs should not be overlooked.

One should consider the possibility of anaphylactic, hypersensitivity or febrile reactions. If an anaphylactoid reaction occurs, the drug infusion should be discontinued and appropriate therapy initiated using aminophylline, oxygen, volume expansion, diphenhydramine, corticosteroids and airway management as indicated. The need for epinephrine should be balanced against its potential risk in the setting of digitalis toxicity.

Since the Fab fragment of the antibody lacks the antigenic determinants of the Fc fragment, it should pose less of an immunogenic threat to patients than does an intact immunoglobulin molecule. Patients with known allergies would be particularly at risk, as would individuals who have previously received antibodies or Fab fragments raised in sheep. Papain is used to cleave the whole antibody into Fab and Fc fragments, and traces of papain or inactivated papain residues may be present in Digibind. Patients with allergies to papain, chymopapain, or other papaya extracts also may be particularly at risk.

Skin testing for allergy was performed during the clinical investigation of Digibind. Only one patient developed erythema at the site of skin testing, with no accompanying wheal reaction; this individual had no adverse reaction to systemic treatment with Digibind. Since allergy testing can delay urgently needed therapy, it is not routinely required before treatment of life-threatening digitalis toxicity with Digibind.

Skin testing may be appropriate for high risk individuals, especially patients with known allergies or those previously treated with Digoxin Immune Fab (Ovine). The intradermal skin test can be performed by: 1. Diluting 0.1 mL of reconstituted Digibind (10 mg/mL) in 9.9 mL sterile isotonic saline (1:100 dilution, 100 μg/mL). 2. Injecting 0.1 mL of the 1:100 dilution (10 μg) intradermally and observing for an urticarial wheal surrounded by a zone of erythema. The test should be read at 20 minutes.

The scratch test procedure is performed by placing one drop of a 1:100 dilution of Digibind on the skin and then making a ¼-inch scratch through the drop with a sterile needle. The scratch site is inspected at 20 minutes for an urticarial wheal surrounded by erythema.

If skin testing causes a systemic reaction, a tourniquet should be applied above the site of testing and measures to treat anaphylaxis should be instituted. Further administration of Digibind should be avoided unless its use is absolutely essential, in which case the patient should be pretreated with corticosteroids and diphenhydramine. The physician should be prepared to treat anaphylaxis.

PRECAUTIONS

General

Standard therapy for digitalis intoxication includes withdrawal of the drug and correction of factors that may contribute to toxicity, such as electrolyte disturbances, hypoxia, acid-base disturbances and agents such as catecholamines. Also, treatment of arrhythmias may include judicious potassium supplements, lidocaine, phenytoin, procainamide and/or propranolol; treatment of sinus bradycardia or atrioventricular block may involve atropine or pacemaker insertion. Massive digitalis intoxication can cause hyperkalemia; administration of potassium supplements in the setting of massive intoxication may be hazardous (see Laboratory Tests). After treatment with Digibind, the serum potassium concentration may drop rapidly[2] and must be monitored frequently, especially over the first several hours after Digibind is given (see Laboratory Tests).

The elimination half-life in the setting of renal failure has not been clearly defined. Patients with renal dysfunction have been successfully treated with Digibind.[4] There is no evidence to suggest the time-course of therapeutic effect is any different in these patients than in patients with normal renal function, but excretion of the Fab fragment-digoxin complex from the body is probably delayed. In patients who are functionally anephric, one would anticipate failure to clear the Fab fragment-digoxin complex from the blood by glomerular filtration and renal excretion. Whether failure to eliminate the Fab fragment-digoxin complex in severe renal failure can lead to reintoxication following release of newly unbound digoxin into the blood is uncertain. Such patients should be monitored for a prolonged period for possible recurrence of digitalis toxicity.

Patients with intrinsically poor cardiac function may deteriorate from withdrawal of the inotropic action of digoxin. Studies in animals have shown that the reversal of inotropic effect is relatively gradual, occurring over hours. When needed, additional support can be provided by use of intravenous inotropes, such as dopamine or dobutamine, or vasodilators. One must be careful in using catecholamines not to aggravate digitalis toxic rhythm disturbances. Clearly, other types of digitalis glycosides should not be used in this setting. Redigitalization should be postponed, if possible, until the Fab fragments have been eliminated from the body, which may require several days. Patients with impaired renal function may require a week or longer.

Laboratory Tests: Digibind will interfere with digitalis immunoassay measurements.[7] Thus, the standard serum digoxin concentration measurement can be clinically misleading until the Fab Fragment is eliminated from the body. Serum digoxin or digitoxin concentration should be obtained before Digibind administration if at all possible. These measurements may be difficult to interpret if drawn soon after the last digitalis dose, since at least 6 to 8 hours are required for equilibration of digoxin between serum and tissue. Patients should be closely monitored, including temperature, blood pressure, electrocardiogram and potassium concentration, during and after administration of Digibind. The total serum digoxin concentration may rise precipitously following administration of Digibind but this will be almost entirely bound to the Fab fragment and therefore not able to react with receptors in the body.

Potassium concentrations should be followed carefully. Severe digitalis intoxication can cause life-threatening elevation in serum potassium concentration by shifting potassium from inside to outside the cell. The elevation in serum potassium concentration can lead to increased renal excretion of potassium. Thus, these patients may have hyperkalemia with a total body deficit of potassium. When the effect of digitalis is reversed by Digibind, potassium shifts back inside the cell, with a resulting decline in serum potassium concentration.[4] Hypokalemia may thus develop rapidly. For these reasons, serum potassium concentration should be monitored repeatedly, especially over the first several hours after Digibind is given, and cautiously treated when necessary.

Carcinogenesis, Mutagenesis, Impairment of Fertility: There have been no long-term studies performed in animals to evaluate carcinogenic potential.

Pregnancy: Pregnancy Category C. Animal reproduction studies have not been conducted with Digibind. It is also not known whether Digibind can cause fetal harm when administered to a pregnant woman or can affect reproduction capacity. Digibind should be given to a pregnant woman only if clearly needed.

Nursing Mothers: It is not known whether this drug is excreted in human milk. Because many drugs are excreted in human milk, caution should be exercised when Digibind is administered to a nursing woman.

Pediatric Use: Digibind has been successfully used in infants with no apparent adverse sequelae. As in all other circumstances, use of this drug in infants should be based on careful consideration of the benefits of the drug balanced against the potential risk involved.

ADVERSE REACTIONS

Allergic reactions to Digibind have been reported rarely. Patients with a history of allergy, especially to antibiotics, appear to be at particular risk (see WARNINGS). In a few instances, low cardiac output states and congestive heart failure could have been exacerbated by withdrawal of the inotropic effects of digitalis. Hypokalemia may occur from re-activation of (sodium, potassium) ATPase (see Laboratory Tests). Patients with atrial fibrillation may develop a rapid ventricular response from withdrawal of the effects of digitalis on the atrioventricular node.[4]

DOSAGE AND ADMINISTRATION

GENERAL GUIDELINES:

The dosage of Digibind varies according to the amount of digoxin (or digitoxin) to be neutralized. The average dose used during clinical testing was 10 vials.

Dosage for Acute Ingestion of Unknown Amount: Twenty (20) vials (800 mg) of Digibind is adequate to treat most life-threatening ingestions in both **adults and children.** However, in children it is important to monitor for volume overload. In general, a large Digibind dose has a faster onset of effect but may enhance the possibility of a febrile reaction. The physician may consider administering 10 vials, observing the patient's response, and following with an additional 10 vials if clinically indicated.

Dosage for Toxicity During Chronic Therapy: For adults, 6 vials (240 mg) usually is adequate to reverse most cases of toxicity. This dose can be used in patients who are in acute distress or for whom a serum digoxin or digitoxin concentration is not available. In infants and small children (≤ 20 kg) a single vial usually should suffice.

Methods for calculating the dose of Digibind required to neutralize the known or estimated amount of digoxin or digitoxin in the body are given below (see DOSAGE CALCULATION section).

When determining the dose for Digibind, the following guidelines should be considered:

—Erroneous calculations may result from inaccurate estimates of the amount of digitalis ingested or absorbed or from nonsteady-state serum digitalis concentrations. Inaccurate serum digitalis concentration measurements are a possible source of error. Most serum digoxin assay kits are designed to measure values less than 5 ng/mL. Dilution of samples is required to obtain accurate measures above 5 ng/mL.

—Dosage calculations are based on a steady-state volume of distribution of approximately 6 L/kg for digoxin (0.6 L/kg for digitoxin) to convert serum digitalis concentration to the amount of digitalis in the body. The conversion is based on the principle that body load equals drug steady-state serum concentration multiplied by volume of distribution. These volumes are population averages and vary widely among individuals. Many patients may require higher doses for complete neutralization. Doses should ordinarily be rounded up to the next whole vial.

—If toxicity has not adequately reversed after several hours or appears to recur, readministration of Digibind at a dose guided by clinical judgment may be required.

—Failure to respond to Digibind raises the possibility that the clinical problem is not caused by digitalis intoxication. If there is no response to an adequate dose of Digibind, the diagnosis of digitalis toxicity should be questioned.

DOSAGE CALCULATION:

Acute Ingestion of Known Amount: Each vial of Digibind contains 40 mg of purified digoxin-specific Fab fragments which will bind approximately 0.6 mg of digoxin (or digitoxin). Thus one can calculate the total number of vials required by dividing the total digitalis body load in mg by 0.6 mg/vial (see Formula 1).

For toxicity from an acute ingestion, total body load in milligrams will be approximately equal to the amount ingested in milligrams for digoxin capsules and digitoxin, or the amount ingested in milligrams multiplied by 0.80 (to account for incomplete absorption) for digoxin tablets.

Table 1 gives dosage estimates in number of vials for **adults and children** who have ingested a single large dose of digoxin and for whom the approximate number of tablets or capsules is known. The Digibind dose (in number of vials) represented in Table 1 can be approximated using the following formula:

Continued on next page

Burroughs Wellcome—Cont.

Formula 1

$$\text{Dose (in \# of vials)} = \frac{\text{Total digitalis body load in mg}}{0.6 \text{ mg of digitalis bound/vial}}$$

TABLE 1: Approximate Digibind Dose for Reversal of a Single Large Digoxin Overdose

NUMBER OF DIGOXIN TABLETS OR CAPSULES INGESTED*	DIGIBIND DOSE # of Vials
25	9
50	17
75	25
100	34
150	50
200	67

*0.25 mg tablets with 80% bioavailability or 0.2 mg Lanoxicaps® Capsules with 100% bioavailability.

Calculations Based on Steady-State Serum Digoxin Concentrations: Table 2 gives dosage estimates in number of vials for **adult patients** for whom a steady-state serum digoxin concentration is known. The Digibind dose (in number of vials) represented in Table 2 can be approximated using the following formula:

Formula 2

$$\text{Dose (in \# of vials)} = \frac{(\text{Serum digoxin concentration in ng/mL}) \ (\text{weight in kg})}{100}$$

[See table below.]

Table 3 gives dosage estimates in milligrams **for infants and small children** based on the steady-state serum digoxin concentration. The Digibind dose represented in Table 3 can be estimated by multiplying the dose (in number of vials) calculated from Formula 2 by the amount of Digibind contained in a vial (40 mg/vial) (see Formula 3). Since infants and small children can have much smaller dosage requirements, it is recommended that the 40 mg vial be reconstituted as directed and administered with a tuberculin syringe. For very small doses, a reconstituted vial can be diluted with 36 mL of sterile isotonic saline to achieve a concentration of 1 mg/mL.

Formula 3

Dose (in mg) = (Dose [in # of vials]) (40 mg/vial)

[See table above.]

Calculation Based on Steady-State Digitoxin Concentration: The Digibind dose for digitoxin toxicity can be approximated using the following formula:

Formula 4

$$\text{Dose (in \# of vials)} = \frac{(\text{Serum digitoxin concentration in ng/mL}) \ (\text{weight in kg})}{1000}$$

If the dose based on ingested amount differs substantially from that calculated from the serum digoxin or digitoxin concentration, it may be preferable to use the higher dose.

ADMINISTRATION: The contents in each vial to be used should be dissolved with 4 mL of Sterile Water for Injection, by gentle mixing, to give a clear, colorless, approximately isosmotic solution with a protein concentration of 10 mg/mL. Reconstituted product should be used promptly. If it is not used immediately, it may be stored under refrigeration at 2 to 8°C (36 to 46°F) for up to 4 hours. The reconstituted product may be diluted with sterile isotonic saline to a convenient volume. Parenteral drug products should be inspected visually for particulate matter and discoloration prior to administration, whenever solution and container permit.

Digibind, Digoxin Immune Fab (Ovine), is administered by the intravenous route over 30 minutes. It is recommended that it be infused through a 0.22 micron membrane filter to ensure no undissolved particulate matter is administered. If cardiac arrest is imminent, it can be given as a bolus injection.

HOW SUPPLIED

Vials containing 40 mg of purified lyophilized digoxin-specific Fab fragments. Box of 1. (NDC 0081-0230-44).

TABLE 3: Infants and Small Children Dose Estimates of Digibind (in mg) from Steady-State Serum Digoxin Concentration

Patient Weight (kg)	SERUM DIGOXIN CONCENTRATION (ng/mL)						
	1	2	4	8	12	16	20
1	0.4* mg	1* mg	1.5* mg	3* mg	5 mg	7 mg	8 mg
3	1* mg	3* mg	5 mg	10 mg	15 mg	19 mg	24 mg
5	2* mg	4 mg	8 mg	16 mg	24 mg	32 mg	40 mg
10	4 mg	8 mg	16 mg	32 mg	48 mg	64 mg	80 mg
20	8 mg	16 mg	32 mg	64 mg	96 mg	128 mg	160 mg

*Dilution of reconstituted vial of 1 mg/mL may be desirable

STORAGE

Refrigerate at 2 to 8°C (36 to 46°F). Unreconstituted vials can be stored at up to 30°C (86°F) for a total of 30 days.

REFERENCES

1. Smith TW, Lloyd BL, Spicer N, Haber E. Immunogenicity and kinetics of distribution and elimination of sheep digoxin-specific IgG and Fab fragments in the rabbit and baboon. *Clin Exp Immunol* 1979; 36:384–396.
2. Smith TW, Haber E, Yeatman L, Butler VP Jr. Reversal of advanced digoxin intoxication with Fab fragments of digoxin-specific antibodies. *N Engl J Med* 1976; 294:797–800.
3. Smith TW, Butler VP Jr, Haber E, Fozzard H, Marcus Fl, Bremner WF, Schulman IC, Phillips A. Treatment of life-threatening digitalis intoxication with digoxin-specific Fab antibody fragments: Experience in 26 cases. *N Engl J Med* 1982; 307:1357–1362.
4. Wenger TL, Butler VP Jr, Haber E, Smith TW. Treatment of 63 severely digitalis-toxic patients with digoxin-specific antibody fragments. *J Am Coll Cardiol* 1985; 5:118A–123A.
5. Spiegel A, Marchlinski FE. Time course for reversal of digoxin toxicity with digoxin-specific antibody fragments. *Am Heart J* 1985; 109 :1397–1399.
6. Smith TW, Butler VP, Haber E. Characterization of antibodies of high affinity and specificity for the digitalis glycoside digoxin. *Biochemistry* 1970; 9:331–337.
7. Gibb I, Adams PC, Parnham AJ, Jennings K. Plasma digoxin: Assay anomalies in Fab-treated patients. *Br J Clin Pharmacol* 1983; 16:445–447.   465403

EMPIRIN® Tablets   **OTC**

[ĭm 'per-ĭn]

Analgesic

(See PDR For Nonprescription Drugs.)

Shown in Product Identification Section, page 407

EMPIRIN® with Codeine Tablets   R©

[ĭm'per-ĭn with kō 'dēn]

DESCRIPTION

Empirin with Codeine is supplied in tablet form for oral administration. Each tablet contains aspirin (acetylsalicylic acid) 325 mg, codeine phosphate in one of the following strengths: No. 3, 30 mg and No. 4, 60 mg (Warning—may be habit-forming), and the inactive ingredients colloidal silicon dioxide, microcrystalline cellulose, potato starch, and stearic acid.

Empirin with Codeine has analgesic, antipyretic and anti-inflammatory effects.

The components of Empirin with Codeine have the following chemical names:

a. Aspirin (acetylsalicylic acid): 2-(acetyloxy)benzoic acid
b. Codeine phosphate U.S.P.: 7,8-didehydro-4, 5α-epoxy-3-methoxy-17-methylmorphinan-6α-ol phosphate (1:1) (salt) hemihydrate

CLINICAL PHARMACOLOGY

Aspirin: The analgesic, anti-inflammatory and antipyretic effects of aspirin are believed to result from inhibition of the synthesis of certain prostaglandins. Aspirin interferes with clotting mechanisms primarily by diminishing platelet aggregation; at high doses prothrombin synthesis can be inhibited.

Aspirin in solution is rapidly absorbed from the stomach and from the upper small intestine. About 50 percent of an oral dose is absorbed in 30 minutes and peak plasma concentrations are reached in about 40 minutes. Higher than normal stomach pH or the presence of food slightly delays absorption.

Once absorbed, aspirin is mainly hydrolyzed to salicylic acid and distributed to all body tissues and fluids, including fetal tissue, breast milk and the central nervous system (CNS). Highest concentrations are found in plasma, liver, renal cortex, heart and lung.

From 50 to 80 percent of the salicylic acid and its metabolites in plasma are loosely bound to proteins. The plasma half-life of total salicylate is about 3.0 hours, with a 650 mg dose. Higher doses of aspirin cause increases in plasma salicylate half-life. Metabolism occurs primarily in the hepatocytes. The major metabolites are salicyluric acid (75%), the phenolic and acyl glucuronides of salicylate (15%), and gentisic and gentisuric acid (less than 1%).

Almost all of a therapeutic dose of aspirin is excreted through the kidneys, either as salicylic acid or the above-mentioned metabolic products. Renal clearance of salicylates is greatly augmented by an alkaline urine, as is produced by concurrent administration of sodium bicarbonate or potassium citrate.

Toxic salicylate blood levels are usually above 30 mg/100 mL. The single lethal dose of aspirin in normal adults is approximately 25 to 30 g, but patients have recovered from much larger doses with appropriate treatment.

Codeine: Codeine probably exerts its analgesic effect through actions on opiate receptors in the CNS.

Codeine is readily absorbed from the gastrointestinal tract, and a therapeutic dose reaches peak analgesic effectiveness in about 2 hours and persists for 4 to 6 hours. Oral codeine (60 mg) given to healthy males has been shown to achieve peak blood levels of 0.016 mg/100 mL at approximately one hour post-dose. The codeine plasma half-life for a 60 mg oral dose is about 2.9 hours. Blood levels causing CNS depression begin at 0.05 to 0.19 mg/100 mL. The single lethal dose of codeine in adults is estimated to be approximately 0.5 to 1.0 g.

Codeine is rapidly distributed from blood to body tissues and taken up preferentially by parenchymatous organs such as liver, spleen and kidney. It passes the blood-brain barrier and is found in fetal tissue and breast milk.

The drug is not bound by plasma proteins nor is it accumulated in body tissues. Codeine is metabolized in liver to morphine and norcodeine, each representing about 10 percent of the administered dose of codeine. About 90 percent of the dose is excreted within 24 hours, primarily through the kidneys. Urinary excretion products are free and glucuronide-conjugated codeine (about 70%), free and conjugated norcodeine (about 10%), free and conjugated morphine (about 10%), normorphine (under 4%) and hydrocodone (<1%). The remainder of the dose appears in the feces.

INDICATIONS AND USAGE

Empirin with Codeine is indicated for the relief of mild, moderate, and moderate to severe pain.

CONTRAINDICATIONS

Empirin with Codeine is contraindicated under the following conditions:

(1) hypersensitivity or intolerance to aspirin or codeine,
(2) severe bleeding, disorders of coagulation or primary hemostasis, including hemophilia, hypoprothrombinemia, von Willebrand's disease, the thrombocytopenias, thrombasthenia and other ill-defined hereditary platelet dysfunctions, as well as such associated conditions as severe vitamin K deficiency and severe liver damage,
(3) anticoagulant therapy, and
(4) peptic ulcer, or other serious gastrointestinal lesions.
(5) children or teenagers with the symptoms of chicken pox or influenza. Reye's Syndrome has been reported to be associated with aspirin use in this population.

WARNINGS

Therapeutic doses of aspirin can cause anaphylactic shock and other severe allergic reactions. A history of allergy is often lacking.

TABLE 2: Adult Dose Estimate of Digibind (in # of vials) from Steady-State Serum Digoxin Concentration

Patient Weight (kg)	SERUM DIGOXIN CONCENTRATION (ng/mL)						
	1	2	4	8	12	16	20
40	0.5 v	1 v	2 v	3 v	5 v	7 v	8 v
60	0.5 v	1 v	3 v	5 v	7 v	10 v	12 v
70	1 v	2 v	3 v	6 v	9 v	11 v	14 v
80	1 v	2 v	3 v	7 v	10 v	13 v	16 v
100	1 v	2 v	4 v	8 v	12 v	16 v	20 v

v = vials

Significant bleeding can result from aspirin therapy in patients with peptic ulcer or other gastrointestinal lesions, and in patients with bleeding disorders. Aspirin administered pre-operatively may prolong the bleeding time.

In the presence of head injury or other intracranial lesions, the respiratory depressant effects of codeine and other narcotics may be markedly enhanced, as well as their capacity for elevating cerebrospinal fluid pressure. Narcotics also produce other CNS depressant effects, such as drowsiness, that may further obscure the clinical course of patients with head injuries.

Codeine or other narcotics may obscure signs on which to judge the diagnosis or clinical course of patients with acute abdominal conditions.

PRECAUTIONS

General: Empirin with Codeine should be prescribed with caution for certain special-risk patients such as the elderly or debilitated, and those with severe impairment of renal or hepatic function, gallbladder disease or gallstones, respiratory impairment, cardiac arrhythmias, inflammatory disorders of the gastrointestinal tract, hypothyroidism, Addison's disease, prostatic hypertrophy or urethral stricture, coagulation disorders, head injuries, or acute abdominal conditions. Empirin with Codeine should not be prescribed for long-term therapy unless specifically indicated.

Precautions should be taken when administering salicylates to persons with known allergies. Hypersensitivity to aspirin is particularly likely in patients with nasal polyps, and relatively common in those with asthma.

Information for Patients: Empirin with Codeine may impair the mental and/or physical abilities required for the performance of potentially hazardous tasks such as driving a car or operating machinery. Such tasks should be avoided while taking Empirin with Codeine.

Alcohol and other CNS depressants may produce an additive CNS depression when taken with Empirin with Codeine, and should be avoided.

Codeine may be habit-forming when used over long periods or in high doses. Patients should take the drug only for as long as it is prescribed, in the amounts prescribed, and no more frequently than prescribed.

Laboratory Tests: Hypersensitivity to aspirin cannot be detected by skin testing or radioimmunoassay procedures. The primary screening tests for detecting a bleeding tendency are platelet count, bleeding time, activated partial thromboplastin time and prothrombin time.

In patients with severe hepatic or renal disease, effects of therapy should be monitored with serial liver and/or renal function tests.

Drug Interactions: Empirin with Codeine may *enhance* the effects of:

(1) monoamine oxidase (MAO) inhibitors,
(2) oral anticoagulants, causing bleeding by inhibiting prothrombin formation in the liver and displacing anticoagulants from plasma protein binding sites,
(3) oral antidiabetic agents and insulin, causing hypoglycemia by contributing an additive effect, and by displacing the oral antidiabetic agents from secondary binding sites,
(4) 6-mercaptopurine and methotrexate, causing bone marrow toxicity and blood dyscrasias by displacing these drugs from secondary binding sites,
(5) penicillins and sulfonamides, increasing their blood levels by displacing these drugs from protein binding sites,
(6) non-steroidal anti-inflammatory agents, increasing the risk of peptic ulceration and bleeding by contributing additive effects,
(7) other narcotic analgesics, alcohol, general anesthetics, tranquilizers such as chlordiazepoxide, sedative-hypnotics, or other CNS depressants, causing increased CNS depression,
(8) corticosteroids, potentiating steroid anti-inflammatory effects by displacing steroids from protein binding sites. Aspirin intoxication may occur with corticosteroid withdrawal because steroids promote renal clearance of salicylates.

Empirin with Codeine may *diminish* the effects of:

(1) uricosuric agents such as probenecid and sulfinpyrazone, reducing their effectiveness in the treatment of gout. Aspirin competes with these agents for protein binding sites.

Aspirin and its metabolites may be caused to accumulate in the body, perhaps to toxic levels, by para-aminosalicylic acid, furosemide, and vitamin C.

Drug/Laboratory Test Interactions:

Aspirin: Aspirin may interfere with the following laboratory determinations in blood: serum amylase, fasting blood glucose, carbon dioxide, cholesterol, protein, protein bound iodine, uric acid, prothrombin time, bleeding time, and spectrophotometric detection of barbiturates. Aspirin may interfere with the following laboratory determinations in urine: glucose, 5-hydroxyindoleacetic acid, Gerhardt ketone, vanillylmandelic acid (VMA), protein, uric acid, and diacetic acid.

Codeine: Codeine may increase serum amylase levels.

Carcinogenesis, Mutagenesis, Impairment of Fertility: No adequate long-term studies have been conducted in animals to determine whether codeine has a potential for carcinogenesis, mutagenesis, or impairment of fertility.

Adequate long-term studies have been conducted in mice and rats with aspirin, alone or in combination with other drugs, in which no evidence of carcinogenesis was seen. No adequate studies have been conducted in animals to determine whether aspirin has a potential for mutagenesis or impairment of fertility.

Pregnancy: *Teratogenic Effects:* Pregnancy Category C. Animal reproduction studies have not been conducted with Empirin with Codeine. It is also not known whether Empirin with Codeine can cause fetal harm when administered to a pregnant woman or can affect reproduction capacity. Empirin with Codeine should be given to a pregnant woman only if clearly needed.

Reproductive studies in rats and mice have shown aspirin to be teratogenic and embryocidal at four to six times the human therapeutic dose. Studies in pregnant women, however, have not shown that aspirin increases the risk of abnormalities when administered during the first trimester of pregnancy. In controlled studies involving 41,337 pregnant women and their offspring, there was no evidence that aspirin taken during pregnancy caused stillbirth, neonatal death or reduced birthweight. In controlled studies of 50,282 pregnant women and their offspring, aspirin administration in moderate and heavy doses during the first four lunar months of pregnancy showed no teratogenic effect.

Reproduction studies have been performed in rabbits and rats at doses up to 150 times the human dose and have revealed no evidence of impaired fertility or harm to the fetus due to codeine.

Nonteratogenic Effects: Therapeutic doses of aspirin in pregnant women close to term may cause bleeding in mother, fetus, or neonate. During the last 3 months of pregnancy regular use of aspirin may cause problems in the unborn child or complications during delivery.

Labor and Delivery: Ingestion of aspirin prior to delivery may prolong delivery or lead to bleeding in the mother or neonate. Use of codeine during labor may lead to respiratory depression in the neonate.

Nursing Mothers: Aspirin and codeine are excreted in breast milk in small amounts, but the significance of their effects on nursing infants is not known. Because of the potential for serious adverse reactions in nursing infants from Empirin with Codeine, a decision should be made whether to discontinue nursing or to discontinue the drug, taking into account the importance of the drug to the mother.

ADVERSE REACTIONS

Codeine: The most frequently observed adverse reactions to codeine include light-headedness, dizziness, drowsiness, nausea, vomiting, constipation and depression of respiration. Less common reactions to codeine include euphoria, dysphoria, pruritus and skin rashes.

Aspirin: Mild aspirin intoxication (salicylism) can occur in response to chronic use of large doses. Manifestations include nausea, vomiting, hearing impairment, tinnitus, diminished vision, headache, dizziness, drowsiness, mental confusion, hyperpnea, hyperventilation, tachycardia, sweating and thirst.

Therapeutic doses of aspirin can induce mild or severe allergic reactions manifested by skin rashes, urticaria, angioedema, rhinorrhea, asthma, abdominal pain, nausea, vomiting, or anaphylactic shock. A history of allergy is often lacking, and allergic reactions may occur even in patients who have previously taken aspirin without any ill effects. Allergic reactions to aspirin are most likely to occur in patients with a history of allergic disease, especially in patients with nasal polyps or asthma.

Some patients are unable to take aspirin or other salicylates without developing nausea or vomiting. Occasional patients respond to aspirin (usually in large doses) with dyspepsia or heartburn, which may be accompanied by occult bleeding. Excessive bruising or bleeding is sometimes seen in patients with mild disorders of primary hemostasis who regularly use low doses of aspirin.

Prolonged use of aspirin can cause painless erosion of gastric mucosa, occult bleeding and, infrequently, iron-deficiency anemia. High doses of aspirin can exacerbate symptoms of peptic ulcer and, occasionally, cause extensive bleeding. Excessive bleeding can follow injury or surgery in patients with or without known bleeding disorders who have taken therapeutic doses of aspirin within the preceding 10 days. Hepatotoxicity has been reported in association with prolonged use of large doses of aspirin in patients with lupus erythematosus, rheumatoid arthritis and rheumatic disease. Bone marrow depression, manifested by weakness, fatigue, or abnormal bruising or bleeding, has occasionally been reported.

In patients with glucose-6-phosphate dehydrogenase deficiency, aspirin can cause a mild degree of hemolytic anemia.

In hyperuricemic persons, low doses of aspirin may reduce the effectiveness of uricosuric therapy or precipitate an attack of gout.

DRUG ABUSE AND DEPENDENCE

Like other medications containing a narcotic analgesic, Empirin with Codeine is controlled by the Drug Enforcement Administration and is classified under Schedule III.

Empirin with Codeine can produce drug dependence of the morphine type, therefore, it has a potential for being abused. Psychic dependence, physical dependence and tolerance may develop on repeated administration.

The dependence liability of codeine has been found to be too small to permit a full definition of its characteristics. Studies indicate that addiction to codeine is extremely uncommon and requires very high parenteral doses.

When dependence on codeine occurs at therapeutic doses, it appears to require from one to two months to develop, and withdrawal symptoms are mild. Most patients on long-term oral codeine therapy show no signs of physical dependence upon abrupt withdrawal.

OVERDOSAGE

Severe intoxication, caused by overdose of Empirin with Codeine may produce: skin eruptions, dyspnea, vertigo, double vision, delusions, hallucinations, garbled speech, excitability, restlessness, delirium, constricted pupils, a positive Babinski sign, respiratory depression (slow and shallow breathing; Cheyne-Stokes respiration), cyanosis, clammy skin, muscle flaccidity, circulatory collapse, stupor and coma. In children, difficulty in hearing, tinnitus, dim vision, headache, dizziness, drowsiness, confusion, rapid breathing, sweating, thirst, nausea, vomiting, hyperpyrexia, dehydration and convulsions are prominent signs. The most severe manifestations from aspirin result from cardiovascular and respiratory insufficiency secondary to acid-base and electrolyte disturbances, complicated by hyperthermia and dehydration. The most severe manifestations from codeine are associated with respiratory depression.

Respiratory alkalosis is characteristic of the early phase of intoxication with aspirin while hyperventilation is occurring, but is quickly followed by metabolic acidosis in most people with severe intoxication. This occurs more readily in children. Hypoglycemia may occur in children who have taken large overdoses. Other laboratory findings associated with aspirin intoxication include ketonuria, hyponatremia, hypokalemia, and occasionally proteinuria. A slight rise in lactic dehydrogenase and hydroxybutyric dehydrogenase may occur.

Concentrations of aspirin in plasma above 30 mg/100 mL are associated with toxicity. (See Clinical Pharmacology section for information on factors influencing aspirin blood levels.) The single lethal dose of aspirin in adults is probably about 25 to 30 g, but is not known with certainty.

The toxic plasma concentration of codeine is not known with certainty. Experimental production of mild to moderate CNS depression in healthy, nontolerant subjects occurred at plasma concentrations of 0.05 to 0.19 mg/100 mL when codeine was given by intravenous infusion. The single lethal dose of codeine in adults is estimated to be from 0.5 to 1.0 g. It is also estimated that 5 mg/kg could be fatal in children. Hemodialysis and peritoneal dialysis can be performed to reduce the body aspirin content. Codeine is theoretically dialyzable but the procedure has not been clinically established.

Treatment of overdosage consists primarily of support of vital functions, management of codeine-induced respiratory depression, increasing salicylate elimination, and correcting the acid-base imbalance due primarily to salicylism.

In a comatose patient, primary attention should be given to establishment of adequate respiratory exchange through provisions of a patent airway and the institution of assisted or controlled ventilation. The narcotic antagonist naloxone is a specific antidote for respiratory depression which may result from overdose or unusual sensitivity to narcotics. Therefore, an appropriate dose of an antagonist should be administered, preferably by the intravenous route, simultaneously with efforts at respiratory resuscitation. Since the duration of action of Empirin with Codeine may exceed that of the antagonist, the patient should be kept under continued surveillance and repeated doses of the antagonist should be administered as needed to maintain adequate respiration. A narcotic antagonist should not be administered in the absence of clinically significant respiratory or cardiovascular depression.

Gastric emptying (Syrup of Ipecac) and/or lavage is recommended as soon as possible after ingestion, even if the patient has vomited spontaneously. (Apomorphine should not be used as an emetic for Empirin with Codeine, since it may potentiate hypotension and respiratory depression.) Administration of activated charcoal as a slurry is beneficial after lavage and/or emesis, if less than three hours have passed since ingestion. Charcoal adsorption should *not* be employed prior to emesis or lavage.

Continued on next page

Burroughs Wellcome—Cont.

Severity of aspirin intoxication is determined by measuring the blood salicylate level. Acid-base status should be closely followed with serial blood gas and serum pH measurements. Fluid and electrolyte balance should also be regularly monitored.

A serum salicylate level of 30 mg/100 mL or higher indicates a need for enhanced salicylate excretion that can be achieved through body-fluid supplementation and urine alkalinization if renal function is normal. In mild intoxication, urine flow can be increased by forcing oral fluids and giving potassium citrate capsules.

(DO NOT GIVE BICARBONATE BY MOUTH SINCE IT INCREASES THE RATE OF SALICYLATE ABSORPTION.) In severe cases, hyperthermia and hypovolemia, as well as respiratory depression are the major immediate threats to life. Children should be sponged with tepid water. Replacement fluid should be administered intravenously and augmented with sufficient bicarbonate to correct acidosis, with monitoring of plasma electrolytes and pH, to promote alkaline diuresis of salicylate if renal function is normal. Complete control may also require infusion of glucose to control hypoglycemia.

Potassium deficiency may also be corrected through the infusion, once adequate urinary output is assured. Plasma or plasma expanders may be needed if fluid replacement is insufficient to maintain normal blood pressure or adequate urinary output.

In patients with renal insufficiency or in cases of life-threatening intoxication, dialysis is usually required. Peritoneal dialysis or exchange transfusion is indicated in infants and young children, and hemodialysis in older patients.

Oxygen, intravenous fluids, vasopressors and other supportive measures should be employed as needed.

DOSAGE AND ADMINISTRATION

Dosage is adjusted according to the severity of pain and the response of the patient. It may occasionally be necessary to exceed the usual dosage recommended below when pain is severe or the patient has become tolerant to the analgesic effect of codeine. Empirin with Codeine is given orally. The usual adult dose for Empirin with Codeine No. 2 and No. 3 is one or two tablets every four hours as required. The usual adult dose for Empirin with Codeine No. 4 is one tablet every four hours as required.

Empirin with Codeine should be taken with food or a full glass of milk or water to lessen gastric irritation.

HOW SUPPLIED

Empirin with Codeine No. 3, 30 mg: (white tablet imprinted with "EMPIRIN" and "3")

Bottle of 100	NDC 0081-0220-55
Bottle of 500	NDC 0081-0220-70
Bottle of 1000	NDC 0081-0220-75
Dispenserpak®	
of 25	NDC 0081-0220-25

Empirin with Codeine No. 4, 60 mg: (white tablet imprinted with "EMPIRIN" and "4")

Bottle of 100	NDC 0081-0225-55
Bottle of 500	NDC 0081-0225-70

Store at 15° to 30°C (59° to 86°F) in a dry place and protect from light.   491269

Shown in Product Identification Section, page 407

EXOSURF® Neonatal™   ℞

[ĕx 'ō-sûrf nē-ō 'nātal]
(Colfosceril Palmitate, Cetyl Alcohol, Tyloxapol)
For intratracheal Suspension

DESCRIPTION

Exosurf Neonatal (colfosceril palmitate, cetyl alcohol, tyloxapol) for Intratracheal Suspension is a protein-free synthetic lung surfactant stored under vacuum as a sterile lyophilized powder. Exosurf Neonatal is reconstituted with preservative-free Sterile Water for Injection prior to administration by intratracheal instillation. Each 10 mL vial contains 108 mg colfosceril palmitate, commonly known as dipalmitoylphosphatidylcholine (DPPC). 12 mg cetyl alcohol, 8 mg tyloxapol, and 47 mg sodium chloride. Sodium hydroxide or hydrochloric acid may have been added to adjust pH. When reconstituted with 8 mL Sterile Water for Injection, the Exosurf Neonatal suspension contains 13.5 mg/mL colfosceril palmitate, 1.5 mg/mL cetyl alcohol, and 1 mg/mL tyloxapol in 0.1 N NaCl. The suspension appears milky white with a pH of 5 to 7 and an osmolality of 185 mOsm/L.

The chemical names of Exosurf Neonatal are **colfosceril palmitate** (1,2-dipalmitoyl-*sn*-3-phosphoglycerocholine), **cetyl alcohol** (1-hexadecanol), and **tyloxapol** (formaldehyde polymer with oxirane and 4-(1,1,3,3-tetramethylbutyl)-phenol).

CLINICAL PHARMACOLOGY

Surfactant deficiency is an important factor in the development of the neonatal respiratory distress syndrome (RDS). Thus, surfactant replacement therapy early in the course of RDS should ameliorate the disease and improve symptoms. Natural surfactant, a combination of lipids and apoproteins, exhibits not only surface tension reducing properties (conferred by the lipids), but also rapid spreading and adsorption (conferred by the apoproteins). The major fraction of the lipid component of natural surfactant is DPPC, which comprises up to 70% of natural surfactant by weight.

Although DPPC reduces surface tension, DPPC alone is ineffective in RDS because DPPC spreads and adsorbs poorly. In Exosurf Neonatal, which is protein free, cetyl alcohol acts as the spreading agent for the DPPC on the air-fluid interface. Tyloxapol, a polymeric long-chain repeating alcohol, is a nonionic surfactant which acts to disperse both DPPC and cetyl alcohol. Sodium chloride is added to adjust osmolality.

Pharmacokinetics: Exosurf Neonatal is administered directly into the trachea. Human pharmacokinetic studies of the absorption, biotransformation, and excretion of the components of Exosurf Neonatal have not been performed. Nonclinical studies, however, have shown that DPPC can be absorbed from the alveolus into lung tissue where it can be catabolized extensively and reutilized for further phospholipid synthesis and secretion. In the developing rabbit, 90% of alveolar phospholipids are recycled. In premature rabbits, the alveolar half-life of intratracheally administered H^3-labeled phosphatidylcholine is approximately 12 hours.

Animal Studies: In animal models of RDS, treatment with Exosurf Neonatal significantly improved lung volume, compliance and gas exchange in premature rabbits and lambs. The amount and distribution of lung water were not affected by Exosurf Neonatal treatment of premature rabbit pups. The extent of lung injury in premature rabbit pups undergoing mechanical ventilation was reduced significantly by Exosurf Neonatal treatment. In premature lambs, neither systemic blood flow nor flow through the ductus arteriosus were affected by Exosurf Neonatal treatment. Survival was

significantly better in both premature rabbits and premature lambs treated with Exosurf Neonatal.

Clinical Studies: Exosurf Neonatal has been studied in the U.S. and Canada in controlled clinical trials involving more than 4400 infants. Over 10,000 infants have received Exosurf Neonatal through an open, uncontrolled, North American study designed to provide the drug to premature infants who might benefit and to obtain additional safety information (Exosurf Neonatal Treatent IND).

Prophylactic Treatment; The efficacy of a single dose of Exosurf Neonatal in prophylactic treatment of infants at risk of developing respiratory distress syndrome (RDS) was examined in three double-blind, placebo-controlled studies, one involving 215 infants weighing 500 to 700 grams, one involving 385 infants weighing 700 to 1350 grams, and one involving 446 infants weighing 700 to 1100 grams. The infants were intubated and placed on mechanical ventilation, and received 5 mL/kg Exosurf Neonatal or placebo (air) within 30 minutes of birth.

The efficacy of one versus three doses of Exosurf Neonatal in prophylactic treatment of infants at risk of developing RDS was examined in a double-blind, placebo-controlled study of 823 infants weighing 700 to 1100 grams. The infants were intubated and placed on mechanical ventilation, and received a first 5 mL/kg dose of Exosurf Neonatal within 30 minutes. Repeat 5 mL/kg doses of Exosurf Neonatal or placebo (air) were given to all infants who remained on mechanical ventilation at approximately 12 and 24 hours of age. An initial analysis of 716 infants is available.

The major efficacy parameters from these studies are presented in Table 1.

[See table below.]

Rescue Treatment: The efficacy of Exosurf Neonatal in the rescue treatment of infants with RDS was examined in two double-blind, placebo-controlled studies. One study enrolled 419 infants weighing 700 to 1350 grams; the second enrolled 1237 infants weighing 1250 grams and above. In the rescue treatment studies, infants received an initial dose (5 mL/kg) of Exosurf Neonatal or placebo (air) between 2 and 24 hours of life followed by a second dose (5 mL/kg) approximately 12 hours later to infants who remained on mechanical ventilation. The major efficacy parameters from these studies are presented in Table 2.

[See table on next page.]

Clinical Results: In these six controlled clinical studies, infants in the Exosurf Neonatal group showed significant improvements in FiO_2 and ventilator settings which persisted for at least 7 days. Pulmonary air leaks were significantly reduced in each study. Five of these studies also showed a significant reduction in death from RDS. Further, overall mortality was reduced for all infants weighing > 700 grams. The one versus three-dose prophylactic treatment study in 700 to 1100 gram infants showed a further reduction in overall mortality with two additional doses.

Safety information is presented in Tables 3 and 4 (see ADVERSE REACTIONS). Beneficial effects in the Exosurf Neonatal group were observed for some safety assessments. Various forms of pulmonary air leak and use of pancuronium were reduced in infants receiving Exosurf Neonatal in all six studies.

Follow-up data at one year adjusted age are available on 1094 of 2470 surviving infants. Growth and development of infants who received Exosurf Neonatal in this sample were comparable to infants who received placebo.

Table 1
Efficacy Assessments—Prophylactic Treatment

	Single Dose 500 to 700 grams		Single Dose 700 to 1350 grams		Single Dose 700 to 1100 grams		One Versus Three Doses 700 to 1100 grams	
Number of Doses: Birth Weight Range:								
Treatment Group: Number of Infants:	Placebo (Air) N=106	EXOSURF N=109	Placebo (Air) N=185	EXOSURF N=176	Placebo (Air) N=222	EXOSURF N=224	One EXOSURF Dose N=356	Three EXOSURF Doses N=360
	% of Infants		% of Infants		% of Infants		% of Infants	
Death ≤ Day 28[a]	53	50	11	6	21	15	16	9*
Death through 1 Year[a]	59	60	14	11	30	20**	17	12*
Death from RDS[b]	25	13*	4	3	10	5§	3	2
Intact Cardiopulmonary Survival[a,c]	29	25	69	78*	65	68	74	78
Bronchopulmonary Dysplasia (BPD)[a,d]	43	44	23	18	19	21	8	12
RDS Incidence[b]	73	81	46	42	55	55	63	68

[a] "Intent-to-treat" analyses (as randomized) except for the 700 to 1350 gram, single dose study in which infants with congenital infections and anomalies were excluded
[b] "As-treated" analyses
[c] Defined by survival through 28 days of life without bronchopulmonary dysplasia
[d] Defined by a combination of clinical and radiographic criteria

*p < 0.05   **p < 0.01   §p = 0.051

Table 2
Efficacy Assessments—Rescue Treatment

Number of Doses: Birth Weight Range:	Two Doses 700 to 1350 grams		Two Doses 1250 grams and above	
Treatment Group Number of Infants:	Placebo (Air) N=213	EXOSURF N=206	Placebo (Air) N=623	EXOSURF N=614
	% of Infants		% of Infants	
Death ≤ Day 28[a]	23	11***	7	4*
Death through 1 Year[a]	27	15***	9	6§
Death from RDS[b]	10	3**	3	1*
Intact Cardiopulmonary Survival[a,c]	62	75**	88	93**
Bronchopulmonary Dysplasia (BPD)[a,d]	18	15	6	3*

[a] "Intent-to-treat" analyses (as randomized)
[b] "As-treated" analyses
[c] Defined by survival through 28 days of life without bronchopulmonary dysplasia
[d] Defined by a combination of clinical and radiographic criteria

* p<0.05　　** p<0.01　　*** p<0.001　　§p=0.067

INDICATIONS AND USAGE

Exosurf Neonatal is indicated for:

1. **Prophylactic** treatment of infants with birth weights of less than 1350 grams who are at risk of developing RDS (see PRECAUTIONS),
2. **Prophylactic** treatment of infants with birth weights greater than 1350 grams who have evidence of pulmonary immaturity, and
3. **Rescue** treatment of infants who have developed RDS.

For **prophylactic** treatment, the first dose of Exosurf Neonatal should be administered as soon as possible after birth (see DOSAGE AND ADMINISTRATION: General Guidelines for Administration).

Infants considered as candidates for **rescue** treatment with Exosurf Neonatal should be on mechanical ventilation and have a diagnosis of RDS by both of the following criteria:

1. Respiratory distress not attributable to causes other than RDS, based on clinical and laboratory assessments.
2. Chest radiographic findings consistent with the diagnosis of RDS.

During the clinical development of Exosurf Neonatal, all infants who received the drug were intubated and on mechanical ventilation. For three-dose prophylactic treatment with Exosurf Neonatal, the first dose of drug was administered as soon as possible after birth and repeat doses were given at approximately 12 and 24 hours after birth if infants remained on mechanical ventilaton at those times. For rescue treatment, two doses were given; one between 2 and 24 hours of life, and a second approximately 12 hours later if infants remained on mechanical ventilation. Infants who received rescue treatment with Exosurf Neonatal had a documented arterial to alveolar oxygen tension ratio (a/A) <0.22.

CONTRAINDICATIONS

There are no known contraindications to treatment with Exosurf Neonatal.

WARNINGS

Intratracheal Administration Only: Exosurf Neonatal should be administered only by instillation into the trachea (see DOSAGE AND ADMINISTRATION).

General:
The use of Exosurf Neonatal requires expert clinical care by experienced neonatologists and other clinicians who are accomplished at neonatal intubation and ventilatory management. Adequate personnel, facilities, equipment, and medications are required to optimize perinatal outcome in premature infants.

Instillation of Exosurf Neonatal should be performed **only** by trained medical personnel experienced in airway and clinical management of unstable premature infants. Vigilant clinical attention should be given to all infants prior to, during, and after administration of Exosurf Neonatal.

Acute Effects: Exosurf Neonatal can rapidly affect oxygenation and lung compliance.

Lung Compliance: If chest expansion improves substantially after dosing, peak ventilator inspiratory pressures should be reduced immediately, without waiting for confirmation of respiratory improvement by blood gas assessment. Failure to reduce inspiratory ventilator pressures rapidly in such instances can result in lung overdistention and fatal pulmonary air leak.

Hyperoxia: If the infant becomes pink and transcutaneous oxygen saturation is in excess of 95%, FiO_2 should be reduced in small but repeated steps (until saturation is 90 to 95%) without waiting for confirmation of elevated arterial pO_2 by blood gas assessment. Failure to reduce FiO_2 in such instances can result in hyperoxia.

Hypocarbia: If arterial or transcutaneous CO_2 measurements are <30 torr, the ventilator rate should be reduced at once. Failure to reduce ventilator rates in such instances can result in marked hypocarbia, which is known to reduce brain blood flow.

Table 3
Safety Assessments[3]—Prophylactic Treatment

Number of Doses: Birth Weight Range:	Single Dose 500 to 700 grams		Single Dose 700 to 1350 grams		Single Dose 700 to 1100 grams		One Versus Three Doses 700 to 1100 grams	
Treatment Group: Number of Infants:	Placebo (Air) N=108	EXOSURF N=107	Placebo (Air) N=193	EXOSURF N=192	Placebo (Air) N=222	EXOSURF N=224	One EXOSURF Dose N=356	Three EXOSURF Doses N=360
	% of Infants		% of Infants		% of Infants		% of Infants	
Intraventricular Hemorrhage (IVH)								
Overall	51	57	31	27	36	36	38	35
Severe IVH	26	25	10	8	13	14	9	9
Pulmonary Air Leak (PAL)								
Overall	52	48	16	11	32	25	29	27
Pneumothorax	23	10*	5	6	19	11*	14	12
Pneumopericardium	1	4	2	0	<1	1	1	1
Pneumomediastinum	2	1	2	3	7	1**	3	2
Pulmonary Interstitial Emphysema	43	44	13	7*	26	20	23	22
Death from PAL	4	6	<1	<1	2	1	2	1
Patent Ductus Arteriosus	49	53	66	70	50	55	59	57
Necrotizing Enterocolitis	2	4	11	13	3	4	6	2*
Pulmonary Hemorrhage	2	10**	2	4	1	4	4	6
Congenital Pneumonia	4	4	2	4	2	2	1	1
Nosocomial Pneumonia	10	10	2	4	4	7	14	15
Non-Pulmonary Infections	33	35	34	39	28	29	35	34
Sepsis	30	34	30	34	23	24	30	27
Death From Sepsis	4	4	3	3	1	2	3	2
Meningitis	4	6	3	1	2	3	1	2
Other Infections	7	4	5	3	6	10	10	11
Major Anomalies	3	1	2	4	7	4	4	4
Hypotension	70	77	52	47	59	62	54	50
Hyperbilirubinemia	22	21	63	61	27	31	20	21
Exchange Transfusion	4	3	1	2	2	2	3	1
Thrombocytopenia[b]	21	25	not available		9	8	12	10
Persistent Fetal Circulation	0	1	1	1	0	2*	1	<1
Seizures	11	8	2	2	11	9	6	5
Apnea	34	33	76	73	55	65*	62	68
Drug Therapy								
Antibiotics	96	99	98	96	98	99	>99	99
Diuretics	55	60	39	37	59	63	64	65
Anticonvulsants	14	18	23	24	20	20	9	8
Inotropes	46	40	20	20	26	20	28	27
Sedatives	62	71	65	64	63	57	52	52
Pancuronium	19	11	22	14*	19	13*	15	11
Methylxanthines	38	43	77	77	61	72*	75	82*

[a] All parameters were examined with "as-treated" analyses.
[b] Thrombocytopenia requiring platelet transfusion.

* p<0.05　　** p<0.01

Continued on next page

Burroughs Wellcome—Cont.

Pulmonary Hemorrhage: In the single study conducted in infants weighing <700 grams at birth, the incidence of pulmonary hemorrhage (10% vs 2% in the placebo group) was significantly increased in the Exosurf Neonatal group. None of the five studies involving infants with birth weights >700 grams showed a significant increase in pulmonary hemorrhage in the Exosurf Neonatal group. In a cross-study analysis of these five studies, pulmonary hemorrhage was reported for 1% (14/1420) of infants in the placebo group and 2% (27/1411) of infants in the Exosurf Neonatal group. Fatal pulmonary hemorrhage occurred in three infants; two in the Exosurf Neonatal group and one in the placebo group. Mortality from all causes among infants who developed pulmonary hemorrhage was 43% in the placebo group and 37% in the Exosurf Neonatal group.

Pulmonary hemorrhage in both Exosurf Neonatal and placebo infants was more frequent in infants who were younger, smaller, male, or who had a patent ductus arteriosus. Pulmonary hemorrhage typically occurred in the first 2 days of life in both treatment groups.

In more than 7700 infants in the open, uncontrolled study, pulmonary hemorrhage was reported in 4%, but fatal pulmonary hemorrhage was reported rarely (0.4%).

In the controlled clinical studies, Exosurf Neonatal treated infants who received steroids more than 24 hours prior to delivery or indomethacin postnatally had a lower rate of pulmonary hemorrhage than other Exosurf Neonatal treated infants. Attention should be paid to early and aggressive diagnosis and treatment (unless contraindicated) of patent ductus arteriosus during the first 2 days of life (while the ductus arteriosus is often clinically silent). Other potentially protective measures include attempting to decrease FiO_2 preferentially over ventilator pressures during the first 24 to 48 hours after dosing, and attempting to decrease PEEP minimally for at least 48 hours after dosing.

Mucous Plugs: Infants whose ventilation becomes markedly impaired during or shortly after dosing may have mucous plugging of the endotracheal tube, particularly if pulmonary secretions were prominent prior to drug administration. Suctioning of all infants prior to dosing may lessen the chance of mucous plugs obstructing the endotracheal tube. If endotracheal tube obstruction from such plugs is suspected, and suctioning is unsuccessful in removing the obstruction, the blocked endotracheal tube should be replaced immediately.

PRECAUTIONS

General: In the controlled clinical studies, infants known prenatally or postnatally to have major congenital anomalies, or who were suspected of having congenital infection, were excluded from entry. However, these disorders cannot be recognized early in life in all cases, and a few infants with these conditions were entered. The benefits of Exosurf Neonatal in the affected infants who received drug appeared to be similar to the benefits observed in infants without anomalies or occult infection.

Prophylactic Treatment—Infants <700 Grams: In infants weighing 500 to 700 grams, a single prophylactic dose of Exosurf Neonatal significantly: improved FiO_2 and ventilator settings, reduced pneumothorax, and reduced death from RDS, but increased pulmonary hemorrhage (see WARNINGS). Overall mortality did not differ significantly between the placebo and Exosurf Neonatal groups (see Table 1). Data on multiple doses in infants in this weight class are not yet available. Accordingly, clinicians should carefully evaluate the potential risks and benefits of Exosurf Neonatal administration in these infants.

Rescue Treatment—Number of Doses: A small number of infants with RDS have received more than two doses of Exosurf Neonatal as rescue treatment. Definitive data on the safety and efficacy of these additional doses are not available.

Carcinogenesis, Mutagenesis, Impairment of Fertility: Exosurf Neonatal at concentrations up to 10,000 μg/plate was not mutagenic in the Ames Salmonella assay.

Long-term studies have not been performed in animals to evaluate the carcinogenic potential of Exosurf Neonatal. The effects of Exosurf Neonatal on fertility have not been studied.

ADVERSE REACTIONS

General: Premature birth is associated with a high incidence of morbidity and mortality. Despite significant reductions in overall mortality associated with Exosurf Neonatal, some infants who received Exosurf Neonatal developed severe complications and either survived with permanent handicaps or died.

In controlled clinical studies evaluating the safety and efficacy of Exosurf Neonatal, numerous safety assessments were made. In infants receiving Exosurf Neonatal, pulmonary hemorrhage, apnea and use of methylxanthines were increased. A number of other adverse events were significantly reduced in the Exosurf Neonatal group, particularly

---

various forms of pulmonary air leak and use of pancuronium. (See CLINICAL PHARMACOLOGY: Clinical Results.) Tables 3 and 4 summarize the results of the major safety evaluations from the controlled clinical studies. [See Table 3 preceding page and Table 4 below.]

Pulmonary Hemorrhage: See WARNINGS.

Abnormal Laboratory Values: Abnormal laboratory values are common in critically ill, mechanically ventilated, premature infants. A higher incidence of abnormal laboratory values in the Exosurf Neonatal group was not reported.

Events During Dosing: Data on events during dosing are available from more than 8800 infants in the open, uncontrolled clinical study (Table 5). [See table on next page.]

Reflux: Reflux of Exosurf Neonatal into the endotracheal tube during dosing has been observed and may be associated with rapid drug administration. If reflux occurs, drug administration should be halted and, if necessary, peak inspiratory pressure on the ventilator should be increased by 4 to 5 cm H_2O until the endotracheal tube clears.

>20% Drop in Transcutaneous Oxygen Saturation: If transcutaneous oxygen saturation declines during dosing, drug administration should be halted and, if necessary, peak inspiratory pressure on the ventilator should be increased by 4 to 5 cm H_2O for 1 to 2 minutes. In addition, increases of FiO_2 may be required for 1 to 2 minutes.

Mucous Plugs: See WARNINGS.

OVERDOSAGE

There have been no reports of massive overdosage with Exosurf Neonatal.

DOSAGE AND ADMINISTRATION

Preparation of Suspension: Exosurf Neonatal is best reconstituted immediately before use because it does not contain antibacterial preservatives. However, the reconstituted suspension is chemically and physically stable and remains sterile (when reconstituted using aseptic techniques) when stored at 2° to 30°C (36° to 86°F) for up to 12 hours following reconstitution.

Solutions containing buffers or preservatives should not be used for reconstitution. **Do Not Use Bacteriostatic Water for Injection, USP.** Each vial of Exosurf Neonatal should be reconstituted only with **8 mL** of the accompanying diluent (preservative-free Sterile Water for Injection) as follows:

---

1. Fill a 10 mL or 12 mL syringe with 8 mL preservative-free Sterile Water for Injection using an 18 or 19 gauge needle;
2. Allow the vacuum in the vial to draw the sterile water into the vial;
3. Aspirate as much as possible of the 8 mL out of the vial into the syringe (while maintaining the vacuum), then SUDDENLY release the syringe plunger.

Step 3 should be repeated three or four times to assure adequate mixing of the vial contents. If vacuum is not present, the vial of Exosurf Neonatal should not be used.

The appropriate dosage volume for the entire dose (5 mL/kg) should then be drawn into the syringe from **below** the froth in the vial (again maintaining the vacuum). If the infant weighs less than 1600 grams, unused Exosurf Neonatal suspension will remain in the vial after the entire dose is drawn into the syringe. If the infant weighs more than 1600 grams, at least two vials will be required for each dose.

Reconstituted Exosurf Neonatal is a milky white suspension with a total volume of 8 mL per vial. Each mL of reconstituted Exosurf Neonatal contains 13.5 mg colfosceril palmitate, 1.5 mg cetyl alcohol, 1 mg tyloxapol, and sodium chloride to provide a 0.1 N concentration. If the suspension appears to separate, gently shake or swirl the vial to resuspend the preparation. The reconstituted product should be inspected visually for homogeneity immediately before administration; if persistent large flakes or particles are present, the vial should not be used.

Dosage: Accurate determination of weight at birth is the key to accurate dosing.

Prophylactic Treatment: The first dose of Exosurf Neonatal should be administered as a single 5 mL/kg dose as soon as possible after birth. Second and third doses should be administered approximately 12 and 24 hours later to all infants who remain on mechanical ventilation at those times.

Rescue Treatment: Exosurf Neonatal should be administered in two 5 mL/kg doses. The initial dose should be administered as soon as possible after the diagnosis of RDS is confirmed. The second dose should be administered approximately 12 hours following the first dose, provided the infant remains on mechanical ventilation. A small number of infants with RDS have received more than two doses of Exosurf Neonatal as rescue treatment. Definitive data on

---

Table 4
Safety Assessments[a]—Rescue Treatment

Number of Doses: Birth Weight Range:	Two Doses 700 to 1350 grams		Two Doses 1250 grams and above	
Treatment Group: Number of Infants:	Placebo (Air) N=213	EXOSURF N=206	Placebo (Air) N=622	EXOSURF N=615
	% of Infants		% of Infants	
Intraventricular Hemorrhage (IVH)				
Overall	48	52	23	18*
Severe IVH	13	9	5	4
Pulmonary Air Leak (PAL)				
Overall	54	34***	30	18***
Pneumothorax	29	20*	20	10***
Pneumopericardium	4	1	1	2
Pneumomediastinum	8	4	5	2**
Pulmonary Interstitial Emphysema	48	25***	24	13***
Death from PAL	7	3	<1	1
Patent Ductus Arteriosus	66	57	54	45*
Necrotizing Enterocolitis	3	3	1	2
Pulmonary Hemorrhage	3	1	<1	1
Congenital Pneumonia	2	3	2	2
Nosocomial Pneumonia	5	7	2	2
Non-Pulmonary Infections	19	22	13	13
Sepsis	15	17	8	8
Death From Sepsis	<1	<1	1	<1
Meningitis	1	<1	1	<1*
Other Infections	5	8	5	6
Major Anomalies	3	3	4	4
Hypotension	62	57	50	39**
Hyperbilirubinemia	17	19	12	10
Exchange Transfusion	3	4	1	2
Thrombocytopenia[b]	10	11	4	<1**
Persistent Fetal Circulation	1	1	6	2**
Seizures	10	10	6	3*
Apnea	48	65**	37	44*
Drug Therapy				
Antibiotics	100	99	98	98
Diuretics	60	65	45	34***
Anticonvulsants	17	17	10	5**
Inotropes	36	31	27	16***
Sedatives	72	68	76	64***
Pancuronium	34	17**	33	15***
Methylxanthines	62	74**	49	53

[a] All parameters were examined with "as-treated" analyses.
[b] Thrombocytopenia requiring platelet transfusion

* $p < 0.05$
** $p < 0.01$
*** $p < 0.001$

the safety and efficacy of these additional doses are not available (see PRECAUTIONS).

Use of Special Endotracheal Tube Adapter: With each vial of Exosurf Neonatal for Intratracheal Suspension, five different sized endotracheal tube adapters each with a special right angle Luer®-lock sideport are supplied. The adapters are clean but not sterile. The adapters should be used as follows:

1. Select an adapter size which correponds to the inside diameter of the endotracheal tube.
2. Insert the adapter into the endotracheal tube with a firm push-twist motion.
3. Connect the breathing circuit wye to the adapter.
4. Remove the cap from the sideport on the adapter. Attach the syringe containing drug to the sideport.
5. After completion of dosing, remove the syringe and RECAP THE SIDEPORT.

Administration: The infant should be suctioned prior to administration of Exosurf Neonatal.

Exosurf Neonatal suspension is administered via the sideport on the special endotracheal tube adapter **WITHOUT INTERRUPTING MECHANICAL VENTILATION.**

Each Exosurf Neonatal dose is administered in two 2.5 mL/kg half doses. Each half-dose is instilled slowly over 1 to 2 minutes (30 to 50 mechanical breaths) in small bursts timed with inspiration. After the first 2.5 mL/kg half-dose is administered in the midline position, the infant's head and torso are turned 45° to the **right** for 30 seconds while mechanical ventilation is continued. After the infant is returned to the midline position, the second 2.5 mL/kg half-dose is given in an identical fashion over another 1 to 2 minutes. The infant's head and torso are then turned 45° to the **left** for 30 seconds while mechanical ventilation is continued, and the infant is then turned back to the midline position. These maneuvers allow gravity to assist in the distribution of Exosurf Neonatal in the lungs.

During dosing, heart rate, color, chest expansion, facial expressions, the oximeter, and the endotracheal tube patency and position should be monitored. If heart rate slows, the infant becomes dusky or agitated, transcutaneous oxygen saturation falls more than 15%, or Exosurf Neonatal backs up in the endotracheal tube, dosing should be slowed or halted, and, if necessary, the peak inspiratory pressure, ventilator rate, and/or FiO_2 turned up. On the other hand, rapid improvements in lung function may require immediate reductions in peak inspiratory pressure, ventilator rate, and/or FiO_2. (See WARNINGS and see below for additional information concerning administration.)

Suctioning should not be performed for two hours after Exosurf Neonatal is administered, except when dictated by clinical necessity.

General Guidelines for Administration: Administration of Exosurf Neonatal should not take precedence over clinical assessment and stabilization of critically ill infants.

Intubation: Prior to dosing with Exosurf Neonatal, it is important to ensure that the endotracheal tube tip is in the trachea and not in the esophagus or right or left mainstem bronchus. Brisk and symmetrical chest movement with each mechanical inspiration should be confirmed prior to dosing, as should equal breath sounds in the two axillae. In prophylactic treatment, dosing with Exosurf Neonatal need not be delayed for radiographic confirmation of the endotracheal tube tip position. In rescue treatment, bedside confirmation of endotracheal tube tip position is usually sufficient, if at least one chest radiograph subsequent to the last intubation confirmed proper position of the endotracheal tube tip. Some lung areas will remain undosed if the endotracheal tube tip is too low.

Monitoring: Continuous ECG and transcutaneous oxygen saturation monitoring during dosing are essential. In most infants treated prophylactically, it should be possible to initiate such monitoring prior to administration of the first dose of Exosurf Neonatal. For subsequent prophylactic and all rescue doses, arterial blood pressure monitoring during dosing is also highly desirable. After both prophylactic and rescue dosing, frequent arterial blood gas sampling is required to prevent post-dosing hyperoxia and hypocarbia (see WARNINGS).

Ventilatory Support During Dosing: The 5 mL/kg dosage volume may cause transient impairment of gas exchange by physical blockage of the airway, particularly in infants on low ventilator settings. As a result, infants may exhibit a drop in oxygen saturation during dosing, especially if they are on low ventilator settings prior to dosing. These transient effects are easily overcome by increasing peak inspiratory pressure on the ventilator by 4 to 5 cm H_2O for 1 to 2 minutes during dosing. FiO_2 can also be increased if necessary. In infants who are particularly fragile or reactive to external stimuli, increasing peak inspiratory pressure by 4 to 5 cm H_2O and/or FiO_2 20% just prior to dosing may minimize any transient deterioration in oxygenation. However, in virtually all cases it should be possible to return the infant to pre-dose settings within a very short time of dose completion.

Table 5
Events During Dosing in the Open, Uncontrolled Study[a]

Treatment Type: Number of Infants:	Prophylactic Treatment N=1127	Rescue Treatment N=7711
	% of Infants	% of Infants
Reflux of Exosurf	20	31
Drop in O_2 saturation (≥20%)	6	22
Rise in O_2 saturation(≥10%)	5	6
Drop in transcutaneous pO_2 (≥20 mm Hg)	1	8
Rise in transcutaneous pO_2 (≥20 mm Hg)	2	5
Drop in transcutaneous pCO_2 (≥20 mm Hg)	<1	1
Rise in transcutaneous pCO_2 (≥20 mm Hg)	1	3
Bradycardia (<60 beats/min)	1	3
Tachycardia (>200 beats/min)	<1	<1
Gagging	1	5
Mucous Plugs	<1	<1

[a] Infants may have experienced more than one event.
Investigations were prohibited from adjusting FiO_2 and/or ventilator settings during dosing unless significant clinical deterioration occurred.

Post-Dosing: At the end of dosing, position of the endotracheal tube should be confirmed by listening for equal breath sounds in the two axillae. Attention should be paid to chest expansion, color, transcutaneous saturation, and arterial blood gases. Some infants who receive Exosurf Neonatal and other surfactants respond with rapid improvements in pulmonary compliance, minute ventilation, and gas exchange (see WARNINGS). Constant bedside attention of an experienced clinician for at least 30 minutes after dosing is essential. Frequent blood gas sampling also is absolutely essential. Rapid changes in lung function require immediate changes in peak inspiratory pressure, ventilator rate, and/or FiO_2.

HOW SUPPLIED

Exosurf Neonatal for Intratracheal Suspension is supplied in a carton containing one 10 mL vial of Exosurf Neonatal for Intratracheal Suspension, one 10 mL vial of Sterile Water for Injection, and five endotracheal tube adapters (2.5, 3.0, 3.5, 4.0, and 4.5 mm I.D.). (NDC 0081-0207-01)

Store Exosurf Neonatal for Intratracheal Suspension at 15° to 30°C (59° to 86°F) in a dry place.

EDUCATIONAL MATERIAL

A videotape on dosing is available from your Burroughs Wellcome Co. representative. This videotape demonstrates techniques for safe administration of Exosurf Neonatal and should be viewed by health care professionals who will administer the drug.

Licensed under U.S. Patent Nos. 4312860 and 4826821

500009

IMURAN® ℞

[ĭm'ū-ran"]

(Azathioprine)

50 mg Scored Tablets

100 mg (as the sodium salt) for I.V. injection, equivalent to 100 mg Azathioprine sterile lyophilized material.

> **WARNING**
>
> Chronic immunosuppression with this purine antimetabolite increases *risk of neoplasia* in humans. Physicians using this drug should be very familiar with this risk as well as with the mutagenic potential to both men and women and with possible hematologic toxicities. See WARNINGS.

DESCRIPTION

Imuran (Azathioprine), an immunosuppressive antimetabolite, is available in tablet form for oral administration and 100 mg vials for intravenous injection. Each scored tablet contains 50 mg azathioprine and the inactive ingredients lactose, magnesium stearate, potato starch, povidone, and stearic acid. Each 100 mg vial contains azathioprine, as the sodium salt, equivalent to 100 mg azathioprine sterile lyophilized material and sodium hydroxide to adjust pH.

Azathioprine is chemically 6-[(1-methyl-4-nitroimidazol-5-yl)thio] purine. It is an imidazolyl derivative of 6-mercaptopurine (Purinethol®) and many of its biological effects are similar to those of the parent compound.

Azathioprine is insoluble in water, but may be dissolved with addition of one molar equivalent of alkali. The sodium salt of azathioprine is sufficiently soluble to make a 10 mg/mL water solution which is stable for 24 hours at 59° to 77°F (15° to 25° C). Azathioprine is stable in solution at neutral or acid pH but hydrolysis to mercaptopurine occurs in excess sodium hydroxide (0.1N), especially on warming. Conversion to mercaptopurine also occurs in the presence of sulfhydryl compounds such as cysteine, glutathione and hydrogen sulfide.

CLINICAL PHARMACOLOGY AND ACTIONS

Metabolism[1]: Azathioprine is well absorbed following oral administration. Maximum serum radioactivity occurs at one to two hours after oral ^{35}S-azathioprine and decays with a half-life of five hours. This is not an estimate of the half-life of azathioprine itself but is the decay rate for all ^{35}S-containing metabolites of the drug. Because of extensive metabolism, only a fraction of the radioactivity is present as azathioprine. Usual doses produce blood levels of azathioprine, and of mercaptopurine derived from it, which are low (<1 μg/mL). Blood levels are of little predictive value for therapy since the magnitude and duration of clinical effects correlate with thiopurine nucleotide levels in tissues rather than with plasma drug levels. Azathioprine and mercaptopurine are moderately bound to serum proteins (30%) and are partially dialyzable.

Azathioprine is cleaved *in vivo* to mercaptopurine. Both compounds are rapidly eliminated from blood and are oxidized or methylated in erythrocytes and liver; no azathioprine or mercaptopurine is detectable in urine after eight hours. Conversion to inactive 6-thiouric acid by xanthine oxidase is an important degradative pathway, and the inhibition of this pathway in patients receiving allopurinol (Zyloprim®) is the basis for the azathioprine dosage reduction required in these patients (see Drug Interactions under PRECAUTIONS). Proportions of metabolites are different in individual patients, and this presumably accounts for variable magnitude and duration of drug effects. Renal clearance is probably not important in predicting biological effectiveness or toxicities, although dose reduction is practiced in patients with poor renal function.

Homograft Survival[1,2]: Summary information from transplant centers and registries indicates relatively universal use of Imuran with or without other immunosuppressive agents.[3,4,5] Although the use of azathioprine for inhibition of renal homograft rejection is well established, the mechanism(s) for this action are somewhat obscure. The drug suppresses hypersensitivities of the cell-mediated type and causes variable alterations in antibody production. Suppression of T-cell effects, including ablation of T-cell suppression, is dependent on the temporal relationship to antigenic stimulus or engraftment. This agent has little effect on established graft rejections or secondary responses.

Alterations in specific immune responses or immunologic functions in transplant recipients are difficult to relate specifically to immunosuppression by azathioprine. These patients have subnormal responses to vaccines, low numbers of T-cells, and abnormal phagocytosis by peripheral blood cells, but their mitogenic responses, serum immunoglobulins and secondary antibody responses are usually normal.

Immunoinflammatory Response: Azathioprine suppresses disease manifestations as well as underlying pathology in animal models of auto-immune disease. For example, the severity of adjuvant arthritis is reduced by azathioprine.

The mechanisms whereby azathioprine affects auto-immune diseases are not known. Azathioprine is immunosuppressive, delayed hypersensitivity and cellular cytotoxicity tests being suppressed to a greater degree than are antibody responses. In the rat model of adjuvant arthritis, azathioprine has been

Continued on next page

Burroughs Wellcome—Cont.

shown to inhibit the lymph node hyperplasia which precedes the onset of the signs of the disease. Both the immunosuppressive and therapeutic effects in animal models are dose-related. Azathioprine is considered a slow-acting drug and effects may persist after the drug has been discontinued.

INDICATIONS AND USAGE

Imuran is indicated as an adjunct for the prevention of rejection in renal homotransplantation. It is also indicated for the management of severe, active rheumatoid arthritis unresponsive to rest, aspirin or other nonsteroidal anti-inflammatory drugs, or to agents in the class of which gold is an example.

Renal Homotransplantation: Imuran is indicated as an adjunct for the prevention of rejection in renal homotransplantation. Experience with over 16,000 transplants shows a five-year patient survival of 35% to 55%, but this is dependent on donor, match for HLA antigens, anti-donor or anti B-cell alloantigen antibody and other variables. The effect of Imuran on these variables has not been tested in controlled trials.

Rheumatoid Arthritis[6,7]: Imuran is indicated only in adult patients meeting criteria for classic or definite rheumatoid arthritis as specified by the American Rheumatism Association.[8] Imuran should be restricted to patients with severe, active and erosive disease not responsive to conventional management including rest, aspirin or other non-steroidal drugs or to agents in the class of which gold is an example. Rest, physiotherapy and salicylates should be continued while Imuran is given, but it may be possible to reduce the dose of corticosteroids in patients on Imuran. The combined use of Imuran with gold, antimalarials or penicillamine has not been studied for either added benefit or unexpected adverse effects. The use of Imuran with these agents cannot be recommended.

CONTRAINDICATIONS

Imuran should not be given to patients who have shown hypersensitivity to the drug.

Imuran should not be used for treating rheumatoid arthritis in pregnant women.

Patients with rheumatoid arthritis previously treated with alkylating agents (cyclophosphamide, chlorambucil, melphalan or others) may have a prohibitive risk of neoplasia if treated with Imuran.[9]

WARNINGS

Severe *leukopenia and/or thrombocytopenia* may occur in patients on Imuran. Macrocytic anemia and severe bone marrow depression may also occur. Hematologic toxicities are dose related and may be more severe in renal transplant patients whose homograft is undergoing rejection. It is suggested that patients on Imuran have complete blood counts, including platelet counts, weekly during the first month, twice monthly for the second and third months of treatment, then monthly or more frequently if dosage alterations or other therapy changes are necessary. Delayed hematologic suppression may occur. Prompt reduction in dosage or temporary withdrawal of the drug may be necessary if there is a rapid fall in, or persistently low leukocyte count or other evidence of bone marrow depression. Leukopenia does not correlate with therapeutic effect; therefore the dose should not be increased intentionally to lower the white blood cell count.

Serious infections are a constant hazard for patients on chronic immunosuppression, especially for homograft recipients. Fungal, viral, bacterial and protozoal infections may be fatal and should be treated vigorously. Reduction of azathioprine dosage and/or use of other drugs should be considered.

Imuran is mutagenic in animals and humans, carcinogenic in animals, and may increase the patient's *risk of neoplasia.* Renal transplant patients are known to have an increased risk of malignancy, predominantly skin cancer and reticulum cell or lymphomatous tumors.[10] The risk of post-transplant lymphomas may be increased in patients who receive aggressive treatment with immonosuppressive drugs.[11] The degree of immunosuppression is determined not only by the immunosuppressive regimen but also by a number of other patient factors. The number of immunosuppressive agents may not necessarily increase the risk of post-transplant lymphomas. However, transplant patients who receive multiple immunosuppressive agents may be at risk for over-immunosuppression, therefore, immunosuppressive drug therapy should be maintained at lowest effective levels. Information is available on the spontaneous neoplasia risk in rheumatoid arthritis,[12,13] and on neoplasia following immunosuppressive therapy of other autoimmune diseases.[14,15] It has not been possible to define the precise risk of neoplasia due to Imuran.[16] The data suggest the risk may be elevated in patients with rheumatoid arthritis, though lower than for renal transplant patients.[11,13] However, acute myelogenous leukemia as well as solid tumors have been reported in patients with rheumatoid arthritis who have received azathioprine. Data on neoplasia in patients receiving Imuran can be found under ADVERSE REACTIONS.

Imuran has been reported to cause temporary depression in spermatogenesis and reduction in sperm viability and sperm count in mice at doses 10 times the human therapeutic dose[17]; a reduced percentage of fertile matings occurred when animals received 5 mg/kg.[18]

Pregnancy: "Pregnancy Category D": Imuran can cause fetal harm when administered to a pregnant woman. Imuran should not be given during pregnancy without careful weighing of risk versus benefit. Whenever possible, use of Imuran in pregnant patients should be avoided. This drug should not be used for treating rheumatoid arthritis in pregnant women.[19]

Imuran is teratogenic in rabbits and mice when given in doses equivalent to the human dose (5 mg/kg daily). Abnormalities included skeletal malformations and visceral anomalies.[18]

Limited immunologic and other abnormalities have occurred in a few infants born of renal allograft recipients on Imuran. In a detailed case report,[20] documented lymphopenia, diminished IgG and IgM levels, CMV infection, and a decreased thymic shadow were noted in an infant born to a mother receiving 150 mg azathioprine and 30 mg prednisone daily throughout pregnancy. At ten weeks most features were normalized. DeWitte et al[21] reported pancytopenia and severe immune deficiency in a pre-term infant whose mother received 125 mg azathioprine and 12.5 mg prednisone daily. There have been two published reports of abnormal physical findings. Williamson and Karp[22] described an infant born with preaxial polydactyly whose mother received azathioprine 200 mg daily and prednisone 20 mg every other day during pregnancy. Tallent et al[23] described an infant with a large myelomeningocele in the upper lumbar region, bilateral dislocated hips, and bilateral talipes equinovarus. The father was on long-term azathioprine therapy.

Benefit versus risk must be weighed carefully before use of Imuran in patients of reproductive potential. There are no adequate and well-controlled studies in pregnant women. If this drug is used during pregnancy or if the patient becomes pregnant while taking this drug, the patient should be apprised of the potential hazard to the fetus. Women of childbearing age should be advised to avoid becoming pregnant.

PRECAUTIONS

General: A gastrointestinal hypersensitivity reaction characterized by severe nausea and vomiting has been reported.[24,25,26] These symptoms may also be accompanied by diarrhea, rash, fever, malaise, myalgias, elevations in liver enzymes, and occasionally, hypotension. Symptoms of gastrointestinal toxicity most often develop within the first several weeks of Imuran therapy and are reversible upon discontinuation of the drug. The reaction can recur within hours after rechallenge with a single dose of Imuran.

Information for Patients:

Patients being started on Imuran should be informed of the necessity of periodic blood counts while they are receiving the drug and should be encouraged to report any unusual bleeding or bruising to their physician. They should be informed of the danger of infection while receiving Imuran and encouraged to report signs and symptoms of infection to their physician. Careful dosage instructions should be given to the patient, especially when Imuran is being administered in the presence of impaired renal function or concomitantly with allopurinol (see DOSAGE AND ADMINISTRATION and Drug Interactions under PRECAUTIONS). Patients should be advised of the potential risks of the use of Imuran during pregnancy and during the nursing period. The increased risk of neoplasia following Imuran therapy should be explained to the patient.

Laboratory Tests: See WARNINGS and ADVERSE REACTIONS.

Drug Interactions:

Use with Allopurinol: The principal pathway for detoxification of Imuran is inhibited by allopurinol. Patients receiving Imuran and allopurinol concomitantly should have a dose reduction of Imuran, to approximately $\frac{1}{3}$ to $\frac{1}{4}$ the usual dose.

Use with Other Agents Effecting Myelopoesis: Drugs which may affect leukocyte production, including co-trimoxazole, may lead to exaggerated leukopenia, especially in renal transplant recipients.[27]

Use with Angiotensin Converting Enzyme Inhibitors: The use of angiotensin converting enzyme inhibitors to control hypertension in patients on azathioprine has been reported to induce severe leukopenia.[28]

Carcinogenesis, Mutagenesis, Impairment of Fertility: See WARNINGS section.

Pregnancy: Teratogenic Effect. Pregnancy Category D. See WARNINGS section.

Nursing Mothers: The use of Imuran in nursing mothers is not recommended. Azathioprine or its metabolites are transferred at low levels, both transplacentally and in breast milk.[29,30,31] Because of the potential for tumorigenicity shown for azathioprine, a decision should be made whether to discontinue nursing or discontinue the drug, taking into account the importance of the drug to the mother.

Pediatric Use: Safety and efficacy of azathioprine in children have not been established.

ADVERSE REACTIONS

The principal and potentially serious toxic effects of Imuran are hematologic and gastrointestinal. The risks of secondary infection and neoplasia are also significant (see WARNINGS). The frequency and severity of adverse reactions depend on the dose and duration of Imuran as well as on the patient's underlying disease or concomitant therapies. The incidence of hematologic toxicities and neoplasia encountered in groups of renal homograft recipients is significantly higher than that in studies employing Imuran for rheumatoid arthritis. The relative incidences in clinical studies are summarized below:

Toxicity	*Renal Homograft*	*Rheumatoid Arthritis*
Leukopenia		
Any Degree	>50%	28%
$<2500/mm^3$	16%	5.3%
Infections	20%	<1%
Neoplasia		*
Lymphoma	0.5%	
Others	2.8%	

*Data on the rate and risk of neoplasia among persons with rheumatoid arthritis treated with azathioprine are limited. The incidence of lymphoproliferative disease in patients with RA appears to be significantly higher than that in the general population.[12] In one completed study, the rate of lymphoproliferative disease in RA patients receiving higher than recommended doses of azathioprine (5 mg/kg/day) was 1.8 cases per 1000 patient years of follow-up compared with 0.8 cases per 1000 patient years of follow-up, in those not receiving azathioprine.[13] However, the proportion of the increased risk attributable to the azathioprine dosage or to other therapies (ie, alkylating agents) received by azathioprine-treated patients cannot be determined.

Hematologic: Leukopenia and/or thrombocytopenia are dose dependent and may occur late in the course of Imuran therapy. Dose reduction or temporary withdrawal allows reversal of these toxicities. Infection may occur as a secondary manifestation of bone marrow suppression or leukopenia, but the incidence of infection in renal homotransplantation is 30 to 60 times that in rheumatoid arthritis. Macrocytic anemia and/or bleeding have been reported in two patients on Imuran.

Gastrointestinal: Nausea and vomiting may occur within the first few months of Imuran therapy, and occurred in approximately 12% of 676 rheumatoid arthritis patients. The frequency of gastric disturbance can be reduced by administration of the drug in divided doses and/or after meals. However, in some patients, nausea and vomiting may be severe and may be accompanied by symptoms such as diarrhea, fever, malaise, and myalgias (see PRECAUTIONS). Vomiting with abdominal pain may occur rarely with a hypersensitivity pancreatitis. Hepatotoxicity manifest by elevation of serum alkaline phosphatase, bilirubin and/or serum transaminases is known to occur following azathioprine use, primarily in allograft recipients. Hepatotoxicity has been uncommon (less than 1%) in rheumatoid arthritis patients. Hepatotoxicity following transplantation most often occurs within 6 months of transplantation and is generally reversible after interruption of Imuran. A rare, but life-threatening hepatic veno-occlusive disease associated with chronic administration of azathioprine has been described in transplant patients and in one patient receiving Imuran for panuveitis.[32,33,34] Periodic measurement of serum transaminases, alkaline phosphatase and bilirubin is indicated for early detection of hepatotoxicity. If hepatic veno-occlusive disease is clinically suspected, Imuran should be permanently withdrawn.

Others: Additional side effects of low frequency have been reported. These include skin rashes (approximately 2%), alopecia, fever, arthralgias, diarrhea, steatorrhea and negative nitrogen balance (all less than 1%).

OVERDOSAGE

The oral LD_{50}s for single doses of Imuran in mice and rats are 2500 mg/kg and 400 mg/kg, respectively. Very large doses of this antimetabolite may lead to marrow hypoplasia, bleeding, infection, and death. About 30% of Imuran is bound to serum proteins, but approximately 45% is removed during an 8 hour hemodialysis.[35] A single case has been reported of a renal transplant patient who ingested a single dose of 7500 mg Imuran. The immediate toxic reactions were nausea, vomiting, and diarrhea, followed by mild leukopenia and mild abnormalities in liver function. The white blood cell count, SGOT, and bilirubin returned to normal six days after the overdose.

DOSAGE AND ADMINISTRATION

Renal Homotransplantation: The dose of Imuran required to prevent rejection and minimize toxicity will vary with individual patients; this necessitates careful management. Initial dose is usually 3 to 5 mg/kg daily, beginning at the time of transplant. Imuran is usually given as a single daily dose on the day of, and in a minority of cases one to three days before, transplantation. Imuran is often initiated with the intravenous administration of the sodium salt, with subsequent use of tablets (at the same dose level) after the postoperative period. Intravenous administration of the sodium salt is indicated only in patients unable to tolerate oral medications. Dose reduction to maintenance levels of 1 to 3 mg/kg daily is usually possible. The dose of Imuran should not be increased to toxic levels because of threatened rejection. Discontinuation may be necessary for severe hematologic or other toxicity, even if rejection of the homograft may be a consequence of drug withdrawal.

Rheumatoid Arthritis: Imuran is usually given on a daily basis. The initial dose should be approximately 1.0 mg/kg (50 to 100 mg) given as a single dose or on a twice daily schedule. The dose may be increased, beginning at six to eight weeks and thereafter by steps at four-week intervals, if there are no serious toxicities and if initial response is unsatisfactory. Dose increments should be 0.5 mg/kg daily, up to a maximum dose of 2.5 mg/kg/day. Therapeutic response occurs after several weeks of treatment, usually six to eight; an adequate trial should be a minimum of 12 weeks. Patients not improved after twelve weeks can be considered refractory. Imuran may be continued long-term in patients with clinical response, but patients should be monitored carefully, and gradual dosage reduction should be attempted to reduce risk of toxicities.

Maintenance therapy should be at the lowest effective dose, and the dose given can be lowered decrementally with changes of 0.5 mg/kg or approximately 25 mg daily every four weeks while other therapy is kept constant. The optimum duration of maintenance Imuran has not been determined. Imuran can be discontinued abruptly, but delayed effects are possible.

Use in Renal Dysfunction: Relatively oliguric patients, especially those with tubular necrosis in the immediate postcadaveric transplant period, may have delayed clearance of Imuran or its metabolites, may be particularly sensitive to this drug and may require lower doses.

Parenteral Administration: Add 10 mL of Sterile Water for Injection, and swirl until a clear solution results. This solution, equivalent to 100 mg azathioprine, is for intravenous use only; it has a pH of approximately 9.6, and it should be used within twenty-four hours. Further dilution into sterile saline or dextrose is usually made for infusion; the final volume depends on time for the infusion, usually 30-60 minutes but as short as 5 minutes and as long as 8 hours for the daily dose.

Parenteral drug products should be inspected visually for particulate matter and discoloration prior to administration, whenever solution and container permit.

Procedures for proper handling and disposal of this immunosuppressive antimetabolite drug should be considered. Several guidelines on this subject have been published.[36–42] There is no general agreement that all of the procedures recommended in the guidelines are necessary or appropriate.

HOW SUPPLIED

50 mg overlapping circle-shaped, yellow to off-white, scored tablets imprinted with "IMURAN" and "50" on each tablet; bottle of 100 (NDC 0081-0597-55) and unit dose pack of 100 (NDC 0081-0597-56).

Store at 15° to 25°C (59° to 77°F) in a dry place and protect from light.

20 mL vial each containing the equivalent of 100 mg azathioprine (as the sodium salt) (NDC 0081-0598-71).

Store at 15° to 25°C (59° to 77°F) and protect from light. The sterile, lyophilized sodium salt is yellow, and should be dissolved in Sterile Water for Injection (see Parenteral Administration under DOSAGE AND ADMINISTRATION).

REFERENCES

1. Elion GB, Hitchings GH. Azathioprine. In: Sartorelli AC, Johns DG, eds. *Antineoplastic and Immunosuppressive Agents Pt II.* New York, NY: Springer Verlag; 1975: chap 48.
2. McIntosh J, Hansen P, Ziegler J, et al. Defective immune and phagocytic functions in uraemia and renal transplantation. *Int Arch Allergy Appl Immunol.* 1976;15:544–549.
3. Renal Transplant Registry Advisory Committee. The 12th report of the Human Renal Transplant Registry. *JAMA.* 1975;233:787–796.
4. McGeown M. Immunosuppression for kidney transplantation. *Lancet.* 1973;2:310–312.
5. Simmons RL, Thompson EJ, Yunis EJ, et al. 115 Patients with first cadaver kidney transplants followed two to seven and a half years: a multifactorial analysis. *Am J Med.* 1977;62:234–242.
6. Fye K, Talal N. Cytotoxic drugs in the treatment of rheumatoid arthritis. *Ration Drug Ther.* 1975;9(4):1–5.
7. Davis JD, Muss HB, Turner RA. Cytotoxic agents in the treatment of rheumatoid arthritis. *South Med J.* 1978;71:58–64.
8. McEwen C. The diagnosis and differential diagnosis of rheumatoid arthritis. In: Hollander JL, ed. *Arthritis and Allied Conditions: A Textbook of Rheumatology.* 8th ed. Philadelphia, PA: Lea and Febiger; 1972:403–418.
9. Hoover R, Fraumeni, JF. Drug-induced cancer. *Cancer.* 1981;47(5):1071–1080.
10. Hoover R, Fraumeni, JF Jr. Risk of cancer in renal transplant recipients. *Lancet.* 1973;2:55–57.
11. Wilkenson AH, Smith JL, Hunsicker LG, et al. Increased frequency of post-transplant lymphomas in patients treated with cyclosporine, azathioprine, and prednisone. *Transplantation.* 1989;47:293–296.
12. Prior P, Symmons DP, Hawkins CF, et al. Cancer morbidity in rheumatoid arthritis. *Ann Rheum Dis* 1984; 43:128–131.
13. Silman, AJ, Petrie J, Hazelman B, et al. Lymphoproliferative cancer and other malignancy in patients with rheumatoid arthritis treated with azathioprine: a 20 year follow up study. *Ann Rheum Dis.* 1988; 47:988–992.
14. Louie S, Schwartz RS. Immunodeficiency and pathogenesis of lymphoma and leukemia. *Semin Hematol.* 1978;15:117-138.
15. Wang KK, Czaja AJ, Beaver SJ, et al. Extra hepatic malignancy following long-term immunosuppressive therapy of severe hepatitis B surface antigen-negative chronic active hepatitis. *Hepatology.* 1989; 10:39–43.
16. Sieber SM, Adamson RH. Toxicity of antineoplastic agents in man: chromosomal aberrations, antifertility effects, congenital malformations, and carcinogenic potential. In: Klein G, Weinhouse S, eds. *Advances in Cancer Research,* v.22. New York, NY: Academic Press; 1975:57-155.
17. Clark JM. The mutagenicity of azathioprine in mice, *Drosophila Melanogaster* and *Neurospora Crassa. Mut Res.* 1975; 28(1):87–99.
18. Data on file, Burroughs Wellcome Co.
19. Tagatz GE, Simmons RL. Pregnancy after renal transplantion. *Ann Intern Med.* 1975:82:113-114, Editorial Notes.
20. Coté CJ, Meuwissen HJ, Pickering RJ. Effects on the neonate of prednisone and azathioprine administered to the mother during pregnancy. *J Pediatr.* 1974; 85(3):324–328.
21. DeWitte DB, Buick MK, Stephen EC, et al. Neonatal pancytopenia and severe combined immunodeficiency associated with antenatal administration of azathioprine and prednisone. *J Pediatr.* 1984;105(4):625–628.
22. Williamson RA, Karp LE. Azathioprine teratogenicity: review of the literature and case report. *Obstet Gynecol.* 1981;58:247–250.
23. Tallent MB, Simmons RL, Najarian JS. Birth defects in child of male recipient of kidney transplant. *JAMA.* 1970;211(11):1854–1855.
24. Assini JF, Hamilton R, Strosberg JM. Adverse reactions to azathioprine mimicking gastroenteritis. *J Rheumatol.* 1986;13:1117–1118.
25. Cochrane D, Adamson AR, Halsey JP. Adverse reactions to azathioprine mimicking gastroenteritis. *J Rheumatol.* 1987;14:1075.
26. Cox J, Daneshmend JK, Hawkey CJ, et al. Devastating diarrhea caused by azathioprine: management difficulty in inflammatory bowel disease. *Gut.* 1988;29(5):686–688.
27. Bradley PP, Warden GD, Maxwell JG, et al. Neutropenia and thrombocytopenia in renal allograft recipients treated with trimethoprim-sulfamethoxazole. *Ann Int Med.* 1980;93:560–562.
28. Kirchertz EJ, Grone HJ, Rieger J, et al. Successful low dose captopril rechallenge following drug-induced leucopenia. *Lancet.* 1981;8234:1362–1363.
29. Nelson D, Bugge C. Data on file, Burroughs Welcome Co.
30. Saarikoski S, Seppälä M. Immunosuppression during pregnancy: transmission of azathioprine and its metabolites from the mother to the fetus. *Am J Obstet Gynecol.* 1973;115:1100-1106.
31. Coulam CB, Moyer TP, Jiang NS, et al. Breast-feeding after renal transplantation. *Transplant Proc.* 1982;14:605–609.
32. Read AE, Wiesner RH, LaBrecque DR, et al. Hepatic veno-occlusive disease associated with renal transplantation and azathioprine therapy. *Ann Intern Med.* 1986;104:651-655.
33. Katzka DA, Saul SH, Jorkasky D, Sigal H. Reynolds JC, Soloway RD. Azathioprine and hepatic venocclusive disease in renal transplant patients. *Gastroenterology* 1986;90:446- 454.
34. Weitz H. Gokel JM, Loeschke K, et al. Veno-occlusive disease of the liver in patients receiving immunosuppressive therapy. *Virchows Arch A.* 1982:395:245-256.
35. Schusziarra V, Ziekursch V, Schlamp R, et al. Pharmacokinetics of azathioprine under haemodialysis. *Int J Clin Pharmacol Biopharm.* 1976;14(4):298–302.
36. Recommendations for the safe handling of parenteral antineoplastic drugs. Washington, DC: Division of Safety, National Institutes of Health; 1983. US Dept of Health and Human Services, Public Health Service publication NIH 83-2621.
37. AMA Council on Scientific Affairs. Guidelines for handling parenteral antineoplastics. *JAMA.* 1985;253:1590-1591.
38. National Study Commission on Cytotoxic Exposure. Recommendations for handling cytotoxic agents. 1984. Available from Louis P. Jeffrey, ScD, Director of Pharmacy Services, Rhode Island Hospital, 593 Eddy Street, Providence, Rhode Island 02902.
39. Clinical Oncological Society of Australia. Guidelines and recommendations for safe handling of antineoplastic agents. *Med J Australia.* 1983;1:426-428.
40. Jones RB, Frank R, Mass T. Safe handling of chemotherapeutic agents: a report from the Mount Sinai Medical Center. *CA-A Cancer J for Clin.* 1983;33(Sept/Oct):258-263.
41. American Society of Hospital Pharmacists. ASHP technical assistance bulletin on handling cytotoxic and hazardous drugs. *Am J Hosp Pharm.* 1990;47:1033–1049.
42. Yodaiken RE, Bennett D. OSHA work-practice guidelines for personnel dealing with cytotoxic (antineoplastic) drugs. *Am J Hosp Pharm.* 1986;43:1193–1204.

517079

Tablet Shown in Product Identification Section, page 407

KEMADRIN®   ℞

[kĕm'ah-drĭn]
(Procyclidine Hydrochloride)
5 mg Scored Tablets

DESCRIPTION

Kemadrin (Procyclidine Hydrochloride) is a synthetic antispasmodic compound of relatively low toxicity. It has been shown to be useful for the symptomatic treatment of parkinsonism (paralysis agitans) and extrapyramidal dysfunction caused by tranquilizer therapy. Procyclidine hydrochloride was developed at The Wellcome Research Laboratories as the most promising of a series of antiparkinsonism compounds produced by chemical modification of antihistamines. Procyclidine hydrochloride is a white crystalline substance which is soluble in water and almost tasteless. It is known chemically as α-cyclohexyl-α-phenyl-1-pyrrolidinepropanol hydrochloride.

Kemadrin® (Procyclidine Hydrochloride) is available in tablet form for oral administration. Each scored tablet contains 5 mg procyclidine hydrochloride and the inactive ingredients corn and potato starch, lactose, and magnesium stearate.

CLINICAL PHARMACOLOGY

Pharmacologic tests have shown that procyclidine hydrochloride has an atropine-like action and exerts an antispasmodic effect on smooth muscle. It is a potent mydriatic and inhibits salivation. It has no sympathetic ganglion blocking activity in doses as high as 4 mg/kg, as measured by the lack of inhibition of the response of the nictitating membrane to preganglionic electrical stimulation.

The intravenous LD_{50} in mice was about 60 mg/kg. Subcutaneously, doses of 300 mg/kg were not toxic. In dogs the intraperitoneal administration of procyclidine hydrochloride in doses of 5 mg/kg caused maximal dilation of the pupil and inhibition of salivation, but had no toxic action. When the dose was increased to 20 mg/kg the same symptoms occurred, and in addition there were tremors and ataxia lasting 4 to 5 hours. In one animal convulsions occurred which were controlled by pentobarbital. In all animals behavior returned to normal within 24 hours.

Chronic toxicity tests in rats showed that the compound caused only a very slight retardation in growth, and no change in the erythrocyte count or the histological appearance of the lungs, liver, spleen and kidney when as much as 10 mg/kg body weight was given subcutaneously daily for 9 weeks.

INDICATIONS

Kemadrin (Procyclidine Hydrochloride) is indicated in the treatment of parkinsonism including the postencephalitic, arteriosclerotic and idiopathic types. Partial control of the parkinsonism symptoms is the usual therapeutic accomplishment. Procyclidine hydrochloride is usually more efficacious in the relief of rigidity than tremor; but tremor, fatigue, weakness and sluggishness are frequently beneficially influenced. It can be substituted for all the previous medications in mild and moderate cases. For the control of more severe cases other drugs may be added to procyclidine therapy as indications warrant.

Clinical reports indicate that procyclidine often successfully relieves the symptoms of extrapyramidal dysfunction (dysto-

Continued on next page

Burroughs Wellcome—Cont.

nia, dyskinesia, akathisia and parkinsonism) which accompany the therapy of mental disorders with phenothiazine and rauwolfia compounds. In addition to minimizing the symptoms induced by tranquilizing drugs, the drug effectively controls sialorrhea resulting from neuroleptic medication. At the same time freedom from the side effects induced by tranquilizer drugs, as provided by the administration of procyclidine, permits a more sustained treatment of the patient's mental disorder.

Clinical results in the treatment of parkinsonism indicate that most patients experience subjective improvement characterized by a feeling of well-being and increased alertness, together with diminished salivation and a marked improvement in muscular coordination as demonstrated by objective tests of manual dexterity and by increased ability to carry out ordinary self-care activities. While the drug exerts a mild atropine-like action and therefore causes mydriasis, this may be kept minimal by careful adjustment of the daily dosage.

CONTRAINDICATIONS

Procyclidine hydrochloride should not be used in angle-closure glaucoma although simple type glaucomas do not appear to be adversely affected.

WARNINGS

Use in Children:

Safety and efficacy have not been established in the pediatric age group; therefore, the use of procyclidine hydrochloride in this age group requires that the potential benefits be weighed against the possible hazards to the child.

Pregnancy Warning: The safe use of this drug in pregnancy has not been established; therefore, the use of procyclidine hydrochloride in pregnancy, lactation or in women of childbearing age requires that the potential benefits be weighed against the possible hazards to the mother and child.

PRECAUTIONS

Conditions in which inhibition of the parasympathetic nervous system is undesirable such as tachycardia and urinary retention (such as may occur with marked prostatic hypertrophy) require special care in the administration of the drug. Hypotensive patients who receive the drug should be observed closely. Occasionally, particularly in older patients, mental confusion and disorientation may occur with the development of agitation, hallucinations and psychotic-like symptoms.

Patients with mental disorders occasionally experience a precipitation of a psychotic episode when the dosage of antiparkinsonism drugs is increased to treat the extrapyramidal side effects of phenothiazine and rauwolfia derivatives.

ADVERSE REACTIONS

Anticholinergic effects can be produced by therapeutic doses although these can frequently be minimized or eliminated by careful dosage. They include: dryness of the mouth, mydriasis, blurring of vision, giddiness, lightheadedness and gastrointestinal disturbances such as nausea, vomiting, epigastric distress and constipation. Occasionally an allergic reaction such as a skin rash may be encountered. Feelings of muscular weakness may occur. Acute suppurative parotitis as a complication of dry mouth has been reported.

DOSAGE AND ADMINISTRATION

For Parkinsonism: The dosage of the drug for the treatment of parkinsonism depends upon the age of the patient, the etiology of the disease, and individual responsiveness. Therefore, the dosage must remain flexible to permit adjustment to the individual tolerance and requirements of each patient. In general, younger and postencephalitic patients require and tolerate a somewhat higher dosage than older patients and those with arteriosclerosis.

For Patients Who Have Received No Other Therapy: The usual dose of procyclidine hydrochloride for initial treatment is 2.5 mg administered three times daily after meals. If well tolerated, this dose may be gradually increased to 5 mg three times a day and occasionally 5 mg given before retiring. In some cases smaller doses may be employed with good therapeutic results.

Occasionally a patient is encountered who cannot tolerate a bedtime dose of the drug. In such cases it may be desirable to adjust dosage so that the bedtime dose is omitted and the total daily requirement is administered in three equal daytime doses. It is best administered during or after meals to minimize the development of side reactions.

To Transfer Patients to Kemadrin (Procyclidine Hydrochloride) from Other Therapy: Patients who have been receiving other drugs may be transferred to procyclidine hydrochloride. This is accomplished gradually by substituting 2.5 mg three times a day for all or part of the original drug. The dose of procyclidine is then increased as required while that of the other drug is correspondingly omitted or decreased until complete replacement is achieved. The total daily dosage may then be adjusted to the level which produces maximum benefit.

For Drug-Induced Extrapyramidal Symptoms: For treatment of symptoms of extrapyramidal dysfunction induced by tranquilizer drugs during the therapy of mental disorders, the dosage of procyclidine hydrochloride will depend on the severity of side effects associated with tranquilizer administration. In general the larger the dosage of the tranquilizer the more severe will be the associated symptoms, including rigidity and tremors. Accordingly, the drug dosage should be adjusted to suit the needs of the individual patient and to provide maximum relief of the induced symptoms. A convenient method to establish the daily dosage of procyclidine is to begin with the administration of 2.5 mg three times daily. This may be increased by 2.5 mg daily increments until the patient obtains relief of symptoms. In most cases excellent results will be obtained with 10 to 20 mg daily.

HOW SUPPLIED

White, scored tablets containing 5 mg procyclidine hydrochloride imprinted with "KEMADRIN" and "S3A" in bottles of 100 (NDC 0081-0604-55).

Store at 15°–30°C (59°–86°F) in a dry place. 537992

Shown in Product Identification Section, page 407

LANOXICAPS® ℞

[*lă-nŏx 'ĭ-kăps"*]

(Digoxin Solution in Capsules)

50 μg (0.05 mg) I.D. Imprint A2C (red)
100 μg (0.1 mg) I.D. Imprint B2C (yellow)
200 μg (0.2 mg) I.D. Imprint C2C (green)

DESCRIPTION

Digoxin is one of the cardiac (or digitalis) glycosides, a closely related group of drugs having in common specific effects on the myocardium. These drugs are found in a number of plants. Digoxin is extracted from the leaves of *Digitalis lanata.* The term "digitalis" is used to designate the whole group. The glycosides are composed of two portions: a sugar and a cardenolide (hence "glycosides").

Digoxin has the molecular formula $C_{41}H_{64}O_{14}$, a molecular weight of 780.95 and melting and decomposition points above 235°C. The drug is practically insoluble in water and in ether; slightly soluble in diluted (50%) alcohol and in chloroform; and freely soluble in pyridine. Digoxin powder is composed of odorless white crystals.

Digoxin has the chemical name: 3β-[(*O*-2, 6-dideoxy-*β-D-ribo*-hexopyranosyl-(1→4)-*O*-2, 6-dideoxy-*β-D-ribo*-hexopyranosyl-(1→4)-2,6-dideoxy-*β-D-ribo*-hexopyranosyl) oxy]-12β, 14-dihydroxy-5β-card-20(22)-enolide.

Lanoxicaps is a stable solution of digoxin enclosed within a soft gelatin capsule for oral use. Each capsule contains the labeled amount of digoxin USP dissolved in a solvent comprised of polyethylene glycol 400 USP, 8 percent ethyl alcohol, propylene glycol USP and purified water USP. Inactive ingredients in the capsule shell include FD&C Red No. 40 (0.05 mg Capsule), D&C Yellow No. 10 (0.1 mg and 0.2 mg Capsules), FD&C Blue No. 1 (0.2 mg Capsule), gelatin, glycerin, methylparaben and propylparaben (added as preservatives), purified water, and sorbitol. Capsules printed with edible ink.

CLINICAL PHARMACOLOGY

Mechanism of Action: The influence of digitalis glycosides on the myocardium is dose-related, and involves both a direct action on cardiac muscle and the specialized conduction system, and indirect actions on the cardiovascular system mediated by the autonomic nervous system. The indirect actions mediated by the autonomic nervous system involve a vagomimetic action, which is responsible for the effects of digitalis on the sino-atrial (SA) and atrioventricular (AV) nodes; and also a baroreceptor sensitization which results in increased carotid sinus nerve activity and enhanced sympathetic withdrawal for any given increment in mean arterial pressure. The pharmacologic consequences of these direct and indirect effects are: 1) an increase in the force and velocity of myocardial systolic contraction (positive inotropic action); 2) a slowing of heart rate (negative chronotropic effect); and 3) decreased conduction velocity through the AV node. In higher doses, digitalis increases sympathetic outflow from the central nervous system (CNS) to both cardiac and peripheral sympathetic nerves. This increase in sympathetic activity may be an important factor in digitalis cardiac toxicity. Most of the extracardiac manifestations of digitalis toxicity are also mediated by the CNS.

Pharmacokinetics:

Absorption—Gastrointestinal absorption of digoxin is a passive process. Absorption of digoxin from Lanoxicaps capsules has been demonstrated to be 90 to 100% complete compared to an identical intravenous dose of digoxin. Conventional digoxin tablets are absorbed 60 to 80%. The enhanced absorption from Lanoxicaps compared to digoxin tablets and elixir is associated with reduced between-patient and within-patient variability in steady-state serum concentrations. The peak serum concentrations are higher than those observed after tablets. When digoxin tablets or capsules are taken after meals, the rate of absorption is slowed, but the total amount of digoxin absorbed is usually unchanged. When taken with meals high in bran fiber, however, the amount absorbed from an oral dose may be reduced. Comparisons of the systemic availability and equivalent doses for digoxin preparations are shown in the following table:

[See first table below.]

In some patients, orally administered digoxin is converted to cardioinactive reduction products (e.g., dihydrodigoxin) by colonic bacteria in the gut. Data suggest that one in ten patients treated with digoxin tablets will degrade 40% or more of the ingested dose. This phenomenon is minimized with Lanoxicaps because they are rapidly absorbed in the upper gastrointestinal tract.

Distribution—Following drug administration, a 6 to 8 hour distribution phase is observed. This is followed by a much more gradual serum concentration decline, which is dependent on digoxin elimination from the body. The peak height and slope of the early portion (absorption/distribution phases) of the serum concentration-time curve are dependent upon the route of administration and the absorption characteristics of the formulation. Clinical evidence indicates that the early high serum concentrations (particularly high for digoxin capsules) do not reflect the concentration of digoxin at its site of action, but that with chronic use, the steady-state post-distribution serum levels are in equilibrium with tissue levels and correlate with pharmacologic effects. In individual patients, these post-distribution serum concentrations are linearly related to maintenance dosage and may be useful in evaluating therapeutic and toxic effects (see Serum Digoxin Concentrations in DOSAGE AND ADMINISTRATION section).

Digoxin is concentrated in tissues and therefore has a large apparent volume of distribution. Digoxin crosses both the blood-brain barrier and the placenta. At delivery, serum digoxin concentration in the newborn is similar to the serum level in the mother. Approximately 20 to 25% of plasma digoxin is bound to protein. Serum digoxin concentrations are not significantly altered by large changes in fat tissue weight, so that its distribution space correlates best with lean (ideal) body weight, not total body weight.

Pharmacologic Response—The approximate times to onset of effect and to peak effect of all the Lanoxin and Lanoxicaps preparations are given in the following table:

[See bottom table.]

Excretion—Elimination of digoxin follows first-order kinetics (that is, the quantity of digoxin eliminated at any time is proportional to the total body content). Following intrave-

PRODUCT	BIOAVAILABILITY	EQUIVALENT DOSES (IN MG)*		
Lanoxin® Tablet	60–80%	0.125	0.25	0.5
Lanoxin Elixir	70–85%	0.125	0.25	0.5
Lanoxin Injection/IM	70–85%	0.125	0.25	0.5
Lanoxin Injection/IV	100%	0.1	0.2	0.4
Lanoxicaps Capsules	90–100%	0.1	0.2	0.4

*1 mg = 1000 μg

PRODUCT	TIME TO ONSET OF EFFECT*	TIME TO PEAK EFFECT*
Lanoxin® Tablet	0.5–2 hours	2–6 hours
Lanoxin Elixir	0.5–2 hours	2–6 hours
Lanoxin Injection/IM	0.5–2 hours	2–6 hours
Lanoxin Injection/IV	5–30 minutes†	1–4 hours
Lanoxicaps Capsules	0.5–2 hours	2–6 hours

*Documented for ventricular response rate in atrial fibrillation, inotropic effect and electrocardiographic changes.
†Depending upon rate of infusion.

nous administration to normal subjects, 50 to 70% of a digoxin dose is excreted unchanged in the urine. Renal excretion of digoxin is proportional to glomerular filtration rate and is largely independent of urine flow. In subjects with normal renal function, digoxin has a half-life of 1.5 to 2.0 days. The half-life in anuric patients is prolonged to 4 to 6 days. Digoxin is not effectively removed from the body by dialysis, exchange transfusion or during cardiopulmonary by-pass because most of the drug is in tissue rather than circulating in the blood.

INDICATIONS AND USAGE

Heart Failure: The increased cardiac output resulting from the inotropic action of digoxin ameliorates the disturbances characteristic of heart failure (venous congestion, edema, dyspnea, orthopnea and cardiac asthma).

Digoxin is more effective in "low output" (pump) failure than in "high output" heart failure secondary to arteriovenous fistula, anemia, infection or hyperthyroidism.

Digoxin is usually continued after failure is controlled, unless some known precipitating factor is corrected. Studies have shown, however, that even though hemodynamic effects can be demonstrated in almost all patients, corresponding improvement in the signs and symptoms of heart failure is not necessarily apparent. Therefore, in patients in whom digoxin may be difficult to regulate, or in whom the risk of toxicity may be great (e.g., patients with unstable renal function or whose potassium levels tend to fluctuate) a cautious withdrawal of digoxin may be considered. If digoxin is discontinued, the patient should be regularly monitored for clinical evidence of recurrent heart failure.

Atrial Fibrillation: Digoxin reduces ventricular rate and thereby improves hemodynamics. Palpitation, precordial distress or weakness are relieved and concomitant congestive failure ameliorated. Digoxin should be continued in doses necessary to maintain the desired ventricular rate.

Atrial Flutter: Digoxin slows the heart and regular sinus rhythm may appear. Frequently the flutter is converted to atrial fibrillation with a controlled ventricular response. Digoxin treatment should be maintained if atrial fibrillation persists. (Electrical cardioversion is often the treatment of choice for atrial flutter. See discussion of cardioversion in PRECAUTIONS section.)

Paroxysmal Atrial Tachycardia (PAT): Digoxin may convert PAT to sinus rhythm by slowing conduction through the AV node. If heart failure has ensued or paroxysms recur frequently, digoxin should be continued. In infants, digoxin is usually continued for 3 to 6 months after a single episode of PAT to prevent recurrence.

CONTRAINDICATIONS

Digitalis glycosides are contraindicated in ventricular fibrillation.

In a given patient, an untoward effect requiring permanent discontinuation of other digitalis preparations usually constitutes a contraindication to digoxin. Hypersensitivity to digoxin itself is a contraindication to its use. Allergy to digoxin, though rare, does occur. It may not extend to all such preparations, and another digitalis glycoside may be tried with caution.

WARNINGS

Digitalis alone or with other drugs has been used in the treatment of obesity. This use of digoxin or other digitalis glycosides is unwarranted. Moreover, since they may cause potentially fatal arrhythmias or other adverse effects, the use of these drugs solely for the treatment of obesity is dangerous.

It is recommended that digoxin in soft capsules be administered in divided daily doses to minimize any potential adverse reactions, since peak serum digoxin concentrations resulting from the capsules are approximately twice those after bioequivalent tablet doses (400 μg of Lanoxicaps are bioequivalent to 500 μg of tablets). Studies are underway to determine if there are any increased risks associated with the higher peaks that occur with single daily dosing of soft gelatin capsules.

Anorexia, nausea, vomiting and arrhythmias may accompany heart failure or may be indications of digitalis intoxication. Clinical evaluation of the cause of these symptoms should be attempted before further digitalis administration. In such circumstances determination of the serum digoxin concentration may be an aid in deciding whether or not digitalis toxicity is likely to be present. If the possibility of digitalis intoxication cannot be excluded, cardiac glycosides should be temporarily withheld, if permitted by the clinical situation.

Patients with renal insufficiency require smaller than usual maintenance doses of digoxin (see DOSAGE AND ADMINISTRATION section).

Heart failure accompanying acute glomerulonephritis requires extreme care in digitalization. Relatively low loading and maintenance doses and concomitant use of antihypertensive drugs may be necessary and careful monitoring is essential. Digoxin should be discontinued as soon as possible.

Patients with severe carditis, such as carditis associated with rheumatic fever or viral myocarditis, are especially sensitive to digoxin-induced disturbances of rhythm.

Newborn infants display considerable variability in their tolerance to digoxin. Premature and immature infants are particularly sensitive, and dosage must not only be reduced but must be individualized according to their degree of maturity.

Note: Digitalis glycosides are an important cause of accidental poisoning in children.

PRECAUTIONS

General: Digoxin toxicity develops more frequently and lasts longer in patients with renal impairment because of the decreased excretion of digoxin. Therefore, it should be anticipated that dosage requirements will be decreased in patients with moderate to severe renal disease (see DOSAGE AND ADMINISTRATION section). Because of the prolonged half-life, a longer period of time is required to achieve an initial or new steady-state concentration in patients with renal impairment than in patients with normal renal function.

In patients with hypokalemia, toxicity may occur despite serum digoxin concentrations within the "normal range", because potassium depletion sensitizes the myocardium to digoxin. Therefore, it is desirable to maintain normal serum potassium levels in patients being treated with digoxin. Hypokalemia may result from diuretic, amphotericin B or corticosteroid therapy, and from dialysis or mechanical suction of gastrointestinal secretions. It may also accompany malnutrition, diarrhea, prolonged vomiting, old age and long-standing heart failure. In general, rapid changes in serum potassium or other electrolytes should be avoided, and intravenous treatment with potassium should be reserved for special circumstances as described below (see TREATMENT OF ARRHYTHMIAS PRODUCED BY OVERDOSAGE section).

Calcium, particularly when administered rapidly by the intravenous route, may produce serious arrhythmias in digitalized patients. Hypercalcemia from any cause predisposes the patient to digitalis toxicity. On the other hand, hypocalcemia can nullify the effects of digoxin in man; thus, digoxin may be ineffective until serum calcium is restored to normal. These interactions are related to the fact that calcium affects contractility and excitability of the heart in a manner similar to digoxin.

Hypomagnesemia may predispose to digitalis toxicity. If low magnesium levels are detected in a patient on digoxin, replacement therapy should be instituted.

Quinidine, verapamil, amiodarone, and propafenone cause a rise in serum digoxin concentration, with the implication that digitalis intoxication may result. This rise appears to be proportional to the dose. The effect is mediated by a reduction in the digoxin clearance and, in the case of quinidine, decreased volume of distribution as well.

Certain antibiotics may increase digoxin absorption in patients who convert digoxin to inactive metabolites in the gut (see Pharmacokinetics portion of the CLINICAL PHARMACOLOGY section). Recent studies have shown that specific colonic bacteria in the lower gastrointestinal tract convert digoxin to cardioinactive reduction products, thereby reducing its bioavailability. Although inactivation of these bacteria by antibiotics is rapid, the serum digoxin concentration will rise at a rate consistent with the elimination half-life of digoxin. The magnitude of rise in serum digoxin concentration relates to the extent of bacterial inactivation, and may be as much as two-fold in some cases. This interaction is significantly reduced if digoxin is given as Lanoxicaps.

Patients with acute myocardial infarction or severe pulmonary disease may be unusually sensitive to digoxin-induced disturbances of rhythm.

Atrial arrhythmias associated with hypermetabolic states (e.g. hyperthyroidism) are particularly resistant to digoxin treatment. Large doses of digoxin are not recommended as the only treatment of these arrhythmias and care must be taken to avoid toxicity if large doses of digoxin are required. In hypothyroidism, the digoxin requirements are reduced. Digoxin responses in patients with compensated thyroid disease are normal.

Reduction of digoxin dosage may be desirable prior to electrical cardioversion to avoid induction of ventricular arrhythmias, but the physician must consider the consequences of rapid increase in ventricular response to atrial fibrillation if digoxin is withheld 1 to 2 days prior to cardioversion. If there is a suspicion that digitalis toxicity exists, elective cardioversion should be delayed. If it is not prudent to delay cardioversion, the energy level selected should be minimal at first and carefully increased in an attempt to avoid precipitating ventricular arrhythmias.

Incomplete AV block, especially in patients with Stokes-Adams attacks, may progress to advanced or complete heart block if digoxin is given.

In some patients with sinus node disease (i.e. Sick Sinus Syndrome), digoxin may worsen sinus bradycardia or sino-atrial block.

In patients with Wolff-Parkinson-White Syndrome and atrial fibrillation, digoxin can enhance transmission of impulses through the accessory pathway. This effect may result in extremely rapid ventricular rates and even ventricular fibrillation.

Digoxin may worsen the outflow obstruction in patients with idiopathic hypertrophic subaortic stenosis (IHSS). Unless cardiac failure is severe, it is doubtful whether digoxin should be employed.

Patients with chronic constrictive pericarditis may fail to respond to digoxin. In addition, slowing of the heart rate by digoxin in some patients may further decrease cardiac output.

Patients with heart failure from amyloid heart disease or constrictive cardiomyopathies respond poorly to treatment with digoxin.

Digoxin is not indicated for the treatment of sinus tachycardia unless it is associated with heart failure.

Digoxin may produce false positive ST-T changes in the electrocardiogram during exercise testing.

Intramuscular injection of digoxin is extremely painful and offers no advantages unless other routes of administration are contraindicated.

Laboratory Tests: Patients receiving digoxin should have their serum electrolytes and renal function (BUN and/or serum creatinine) assessed periodically; the frequency of assessments will depend on the clinical setting. For discussion of serum digoxin concentrations, see DOSAGE AND ADMINISTRATION section.

Drug Interactions: Potassium-depleting *corticosteroids* and *diuretics* may be major contributing factors to digitalis toxicity. *Calcium,* particularly if administered rapidly by the intravenous route, may produce serious arrhythmias in digitalized patients. *Quinidine, verapamil , amiodarone,* and *propafenone* cause a rise in serum digoxin concentration, with the implication that digitalis intoxication may result. Certain *antibiotics* increase digoxin absorption in patients who inactivate digoxin by bacterial metabolism in the lower intestine, so that digitalis intoxication may result. *Propantheline* and *diphenoxylate,* by decreasing gut motility, may increase digoxin absorption. *Antacids, kaolin-pectin, sulfasalazine, neomycin, cholestyramine* and certain *anticancer drugs* may interfere with intestinal digoxin absorption, resulting in unexpectedly low serum concentrations. There have been inconsistent reports regarding the effects of other drugs on the serum digoxin concentration. *Thyroid* administration to a digitalized, hypothyroid patient may increase the dose requirement of digoxin. Concomitant use of digoxin and *sympathomimetics* increases the risk of cardiac arrhythmias, because both enhance ectopic pacemaker activity. *Succinylcholine* may cause a sudden extrusion of potassium from muscle cells, and may thereby cause arrhythmias in digitalized patients. Although β adrenergic blockers or calcium channel blockers and digoxin may be useful in combination to control atrial fibrillation, their additive effects on AV node conduction can result in complete heart block.

Due to the considerable variability of these interactions, digoxin dosage should be carefully individualized when patients receive coadministered medications. Furthermore, caution should be exercised when combining digoxin with any drug that may cause a significant deterioration in renal function, since this may impair the excretion of digoxin.

Carcinogenesis, Mutagenesis, Impairment of Fertility: There have been no long-term studies performed in animals to evaluate carcinogenic potential.

Pregnancy: ***Teratogenic Effects:*** Pregnancy Category C. Animal reproduction studies have not been conducted with digoxin. It is also not known whether digoxin can cause fetal harm when administered to a pregnant woman or can affect reproduction capacity. Digoxin should be given to a pregnant woman only if clearly needed.

Nursing Mothers: Studies have shown that digoxin concentrations in the mother's serum and milk are similar. However, the estimated daily dose to a nursing infant will be far below the usual infant maintenance dose. Therefore, this amount should have no pharmacologic effect upon the infant. Nevertheless, caution should be exercised when digoxin is administered to a nursing woman.

ADVERSE REACTIONS

The frequency and severity of adverse reactions to digoxin depend on the dose and route of administration, as well as on the patient's underlying disease or concomitant therapies (see PRECAUTIONS section and Serum Digoxin Concentrations subsection of DOSAGE AND ADMINISTRATION). The overall incidence of adverse reactions has been reported as 5 to 20%, with 15 to 20% of them being considered serious (one to four percent of patients receiving digoxin). Evidence suggests that the incidence of toxicity has decreased since the introduction of the serum digoxin assay and improved standardization of digoxin tablets. Cardiac toxicity accounts for about one-half, gastrointestinal disturbances for about one-fourth, and CNS and other toxicity for about one-fourth of these adverse reactions.

Adults:

Cardiac—Unifocal or multiform ventricular premature contractions, especially in bigeminal or trigeminal patterns, are the most common arrhythmias associated with digoxin toxic-

Continued on next page

Burroughs Wellcome—Cont.

ity in adults with heart disease. Ventricular tachycardia may result from digitalis toxicity. Atrioventricular (AV) dissociation, accelerated junctional (nodal) rhythm and atrial tachycardia with block are also common arrhythmias caused by digoxin overdosage.

Excessive slowing of the pulse is a clinical sign of digoxin overdosage. AV block (Wenckebach) of increasing degree may proceed to complete heart block.

Note: The electrocardiogram is fundamental in determining the presence and nature of these cardiac disturbances. Digoxin may also induce other changes in the ECG (e.g. PR prolongation, ST depression), which represent digoxin effect and may or may not be associated with digitalis toxicity.

Gastrointestinal—Anorexia, nausea, vomiting and less commonly diarrhea are common early symptoms of overdosage. However, uncontrolled heart failure may also produce such symptoms. Digitalis toxicity very rarely may cause abdominal pain and hemorrhagic necrosis of the intestines.

CNS—Visual disturbances (blurred or yellow vision), headache, weakness, dizziness, apathy and psychosis can occur.

Other—Gynecomastia is occasionally observed. Maculopapular rash or other skin reactions are rarely observed.

Infants and Children: Toxicity differs from the adult in a number of respects. Anorexia, nausea, vomiting, diarrhea and CNS disturbances may be present but are rare as initial symptoms in infants. Cardiac arrhythmias are more reliable signs of toxicity. Digoxin in children may produce any arrhythmia. The most commonly encountered are conduction disturbances or supraventricular tachyarrhythmias, such as atrial tachycardia with or without block, and junctional (nodal) tachycardia. Ventricular arrhythmias are less common. Sinus bradycardia may also be a sign of impending digoxin intoxication, especially in infants, even in the absence of first degree heart block. Any arrhythmia or alteration in cardiac conduction that develops in a child taking digoxin should initially be assumed to be a consequence of digoxin intoxication.

OVERDOSAGE

Treatment of Arrhythmias Produced by Overdosage:

Adults: Digoxin should be discontinued until all signs of toxicity are gone. Discontinuation may be all that is necessary if toxic manifestations are not severe and appear only near the expected time for maximum effect of the drug.

Correction of factors that may contribute to toxicity such as electrolyte disturbances, hypoxia, acid-base disturbances and removal of aggravating agents such as catecholamines, should also be considered. Potassium salts may be indicated, particularly if hypokalemia in present. Potassium administration may be dangerous in the setting of massive digitalis overdosage (see Massive Digitalis Overdosage subsection below). Potassium chloride in divided oral doses totaling 3 to 6 grams of the salt (40 to 80 mEq K +) for adults may be given provided renal function is adequate (see below for potassium recommendations in Infants and Children).

When correction of the arrhythmia is urgent and the serum potassium concentration is low or normal, potassium should be administered intravenously in 5% dextrose injection. For adults, a total of 40 to 80 mEq (diluted to a concentration of 40 mEq per 500 mL) may be given at a rate not exceeding 20 mEq per hour, or slower if limited by pain due to local irritation. Additional amounts may be given if the arrhythmia is uncontrolled and potassium well-tolerated. ECG monitoring should be performed to watch for any evidence of potassium toxicity (e.g. peaking of T waves) and to observe the effect on the arrhythmia. The infusion may be stopped when the desired effect is achieved.

Note: Potassium should not be used and may be dangerous in heart block due to digoxin, unless primarily related to supraventricular tachycardia.

Other agents that have been used for the treatment of digoxin intoxication include lidocaine, procainamide, propranolol and phenytoin, although use of the latter must be considered experimental. In advanced heart block, atropine and/or temporary ventricular pacing may be beneficial. Digibind®, Digoxin Immune Fab (Ovine), can be used to reverse potentially life-threatening digoxin (or digitoxin) intoxication. Improvement in signs and symptoms of digitalis toxicity usually begins within ½ hour of Digibind administration. Each 40 mg vial of Digibind will neutralize 0.6 mg of digoxin (which is a usual body store of an adequately digitalized 70 kg patient).

Infants and Children: See Adult section for general recommendations for the treatment of arrhythmias produced by overdosage and for cautions regarding the use of potassium.

If a potassium preparation is used to treat toxicity, it may be given orally in divided doses totaling 1 to 1.5 mEq K+ per kilogram (kg) body weight (1 gram of potassium chloride contains 13.4 mEq K+).

When correction of the arrhythmia with potassium is urgent, approximately 0.5 mEq/kg of potassium per hour may be given intravenously, with careful ECG monitoring. The

$$\text{Maintenance Dose} = \text{Peak Body Stores (i.e. Loading Dose)} \times \frac{\text{\% Daily Loss}}{100}$$

$$\text{Where: \% Daily Loss} = 14 + \text{Ccr}/5$$

intravenous solution of potassium should be dilute enough to avoid local irritation; however, especially in infants, care must be taken to avoid intravenous fluid overload.

Massive Digitalis Overdosage: Manifestations of life-threatening toxicity include severe ventricular arrhythmias such as ventricular tachycardia or ventricular fibrillation, or progessive bradyarrhythmias such as severe sinus bradycardia or second or third degree heart block not responsive to atropine. An overdosage of more than 10 mg of digoxin in previously healthy adults or 4 mg in previously healthy children or overdosage resulting in steady-state serum concentrations greater than 10 ng/mL, often results in cardiac arrest.

Severe digitalis intoxication can cause life-threatening elevation in serum potassium concentration by shifting potassium from inside to outside the cell resulting in hyperkalemia. Administration of potassium supplements in the setting of massive intoxication may be hazardous.

Digibind®, Digoxin Immune Fab (Ovine), may be used at a dose equimolar to digoxin in the body to reverse the effects of ingestion of a massive overdose. The decision to administer Digibind before the onset of toxic manifestations will depend on the likelihood that life-threatening toxicity will occur (see above).

Patients with massive digitalis ingestion should receive large doses of activated charcoal to prevent absorption and bind digoxin in the gut during enteroenteric recirculation. Emesis or gastric lavage may be indicated especially if ingestion has occurred within 30 minutes of the patient's presentation at the hospital. Emesis should not be induced in patients who are obtunded. If a patient presents more than 2 hours after ingestion or already has toxic manifestations, it may be unsafe to induce vomiting or attempt passage of a gastric tube, because such maneuvers may induce an acute vagal episode that can worsen digitalis-toxic arrhythmias.

DOSAGE AND ADMINISTRATION

Recommended dosages are average values that may require considerable modification because of individual sensitivity or associated conditions. Diminished renal function is the most important factor requiring modification of recommended doses.

Due to the more complete absorption of digoxin from soft capsules, recommended oral doses are only 80 percent of those for Tablets, Elixir and I.M. Injection.

Because the significance of the higher peak serum concentrations associated with once daily capsules is not established, divided daily dosing is presently recommended for:

1. Infants and children under 10 years of age;
2. Patients requiring a daily dose of 300 µg (0.3 mg) or greater;
3. Patients with a previous history of digitalis toxicity;
4. Patients considered likely to become toxic;
5. Patients in whom compliance is not a problem.

Where compliance is considered a problem, single daily dosing may be appropriate.

In deciding the dose of digoxin, several factors must be considered:

1. The disease being treated. Atrial arrhythmias may require larger doses than heart failure.
2. The body weight of the patient. Doses should be calculated based upon lean or ideal body weight.
3. The patient's renal function, preferably evaluated on the basis of creatinine clearance.
4. Age is an important factor in infants and children.
5. Concomitant disease states, drugs or other factors likely to alter the expected clinical response to digoxin (see PRECAUTIONS and Drug Interactions sections).

Digitalization may be accomplished by either of two general approaches that vary in dosage and frequency of administration, but reach the same endpoint in terms of total amount of digoxin accumulated in the body.

1. Rapid digitalization may be achieved by administering a loading dose based upon projected peak body digoxin stores, then calculating the maintenance dose as a percentage of the loading dose.
2. More gradual digitalization may be obtained by beginning an appropriate maintenance dose, thus allowing digoxin body stores to accumulate slowly. Steady-state serum digoxin concentrations will be achieved in approximately 5 half-lives of the drug for the individual patient. Depending upon the patient's renal function, this will take between one and three weeks.

Adults:

Adults—Rapid Digitalization with a Loading Dose: Peak body digoxin stores of 8 to 12 µg/kg should provide therapeutic effect with minimum risk of toxicity in most patients with heart failure and normal sinus rhythm. Larger stores (10 to 15 µg/kg) are often required for adequate control of ventricular rate in patients with atrial flutter or fibrillation. Because of altered digoxin distribution and elimination, projected peak body stores for patients with renal insufficiency should be conservative (i.e. 6 to 10 µg/kg) [see PRECAUTIONS section].

The loading dose should be based on the projected peak body stores and administered in several portions, with roughly half the total given as the first dose. Additional fractions of this planned total dose may be given at 6 to 8 hour intervals, **with careful assessment of clinical response before each additional dose.**

If the patient's clinical response necessitates a change from the calculated dose of digoxin, then calculation of the maintenance dose should be based upon the amount actually given.

In previously undigitalized patients, a single initial Lanoxicaps dose of 400 to 600 µg (0.4 to 0.6 mg) usually produces a detectable effect in 0.5 to 2 hours that becomes maximal in 2 to 6 hours. Additional doses of 100 to 300 µg (0.1 to 0.3 mg) may be given cautiously at 6 to 8 hour intervals until clinical evidence of an adequate effect is noted.

The usual amount of Lanoxicaps that a 70 kg patient requires to achieve 8 to 15 µg/kg peak body stores is 600 to 1000 µg (0.6 to 1.0 mg).

Although peak body stores are mathematically related to loading doses and are utilized to calculate maintenance doses, they do not correlate with measured serum concentrations. This discrepancy is caused by digoxin distribution within the body during the first 6 to 8 hours following a dose. Serum concentrations drawn during this time are usually not interpretable.

The maintenance dose should be based upon the percentage of the peak body stores lost each day through elimination. The following formula has had wide clinical use:

[See above.]

Ccr is creatinine clearance, corrected to 70 kg body weight or 1.73 m^2 body surface area. **For adults,** if only serum creatinine concentrations (Scr) are available, a Ccr (corrected to 70 kg body weight) may be estimated in men as (140 − Age)/Scr. For women, this result should be multiplied by 0.85.

Note: This equation cannot be used for estimating creatinine clearance in infants or children.

A common practice involves the use of Lanoxin® Injection to achieve rapid digitalization, with conversion to Lanoxicaps or Lanoxin Tablets for maintenance therapy. If patients are switched from IV to oral digoxin formulations, allowances must be made for differences in bioavailability when calculating maintenance dosages (see table, CLINICAL PHARMACOLOGY section).

Adults—Gradual Digitalization with a Maintenance Dose: The following table provides average Lanoxicaps daily maintenance dose requirements for patients with heart failure based upon lean body weight and renal function:

[See table below.]

Example—based on the above table, a patient in heart failure with an estimated lean body weight of 70 kg and a Ccr of 60 mL/min, should be given 200 µg (0.2 mg) of Lanoxicaps per day, usually taken as a 100 µg (0.1 mg) capsule after the

Usual Lanoxicaps Daily Maintenance Dose Requirements (µg) for Estimated Peak Body Stores of 10 µg/kg

Corrected Ccr (mL/min per 70 kg)	Lean Body Weight (kg/lbs) 50/110	60/132	70/154	80/176	90/198	100/220	Number of Days Before Steady-State Achieved
0	50	100	100	100	150	150	22
10	100	100	100	150	150	150	19
20	100	100	150	150	150	200	16
30	100	150	150	150	200	200	14
40	100	150	150	200	200	250	13
50	150	150	200	200	250	250	12
60	150	150	200	200	250	300	11
70	150	200	200	250	250	300	10
80	150	200	200	250	300	300	9
90	150	200	250	250	300	350	8
100	200	200	250	300	300	350	7

morning and evening meals. Steady-state serum concentrations should not be anticipated before 11 days.

Infants and Children: Digitalization must be individualized. Divided daily dosing is recommended for infants and young children. In these patients, where dosage adjustment is frequent and outside the fixed dosages available, Lanoxicaps may not be the formulation of choice. Children over 10 years of age require adult dosages in proportion to their body weight.

In the newborn period, renal clearance of digoxin is diminished and suitable dosage adjustments must be observed. This is especially pronounced in the premature infant. Beyond the immediate newborn period, children generally require proportionally larger doses than adults on the basis of body weight or body surface area.

Lanoxin® Injection Pediatric can be used to achieve rapid digitalization, with conversion to an oral Lanoxin formulation for maintenance therapy. If patients are switched from IV to oral digoxin tablets or elixir, allowances must be made for differences in bioavailability when calculating maintenance dosages (see bioavailability table in CLINICAL PHARMACOLOGY section and dosing table below). Intramuscular injection of digoxin is extremely painful and offers no advantages unless other routes of administration are contraindicated.

Digitalizing and daily maintenance doses for each age group are given below and should provide therapeutic effect with minimum risk of toxicity in most patients with heart failure and normal sinus rhythm. Larger doses are often required for adequate control of ventricular rate in patients with atrial flutter or fibrillation.

The loading dose should be administered in several portions, with roughly half the total given as the first dose. Additional fractions of this planned total dose may be given at 6 to 8 hour intervals, **with careful assessment of clinical response before each additional dose.** If the patient's clinical response necessitates a change from the calculated maintenance dose of digoxin, then calculation of the maintenance dose should be based upon the amount actually given.

[See table below.]

More gradual digitalization can also be accomplished by beginning an appropriate maintenance dose. The range of percentages provided above can be used in calculating this dose for patients with normal renal function. In children with renal disease, digoxin dosing must be carefully titrated based upon desired clinical response.

Long-term use of digoxin is indicated in many children who have been digitalized for acute heart failure, unless the cause is transient. Children with severe congenital heart disease, even after surgery, may require digoxin for prolonged periods.

It cannot be overemphasized that both the adult and pediatric dosage guidelines provided are based upon average patient response and substantial individual variation can be expected. Accordingly, ultimate dosage selection must be based upon clinical assessment of the patient.

Serum Digoxin Concentrations: Measurement of serum digoxin concentrations can be helpful to the clinician in determining the state of digitalization and in assigning certain probabilities to the likelihood of digoxin intoxication. Studies in adults considered adequately digitalized (without evidence of toxicity) show that about two-thirds of such patients have serum digoxin levels ranging from 0.8 to 2.0 ng/mL. Patients with atrial fibrillation or atrial flutter require and appear to tolerate higher levels than do patients with other indications. On the other hand, in adult patients with clinical evidence of digoxin toxicity, about two-thirds will have serum digoxin levels greater than 2.0 ng/mL. Thus, whereas levels less than 0.8 ng/mL are infrequently associated with toxicity, levels greater than 2.0 ng/mL are often associated with toxicity. Values in between are not very helpful in deciding whether a certain sign or symptom is more likely caused by digoxin toxicity or by something else. There are rare patients who are unable to tolerate digoxin even at serum concentrations below 0.8 ng/mL. Some researchers suggest that infants and young children tolerate slightly higher serum concentrations than do adults.

To allow adequate time for equilibration of digoxin between serum and tissue, **sampling of serum concentrations for clinical use should be at least 6 or 8 hours after the last dose,** regardless of the route of administration or formulation

used. On a twice daily dosing schedule, there will be only minor differences in serum digoxin concentrations whether sampling is done at 8 or 12 hours after a dose. After a single daily dose, the concentration will be 10 to 25% lower when sampled at 24 versus 8 hours, depending upon the patient's renal function. Ideally, sampling for assessment of steady-state concentrations should be done just before the next dose.

If a discrepancy exists between the reported serum concentration and the observed clinical response, the clinician should consider the following possibilities:

1. Analytical problems in the assay procedure.
2. Inappropriate serum sampling time.
3. Administration of a digitalis glycoside other than digoxin.
4. Conditions (described in WARNINGS and PRECAUTIONS sections) causing an alteration in the sensitivity of the patient to digoxin.
5. The patient falls outside the norm in his response to or handling of digoxin. This decision should only be reached after exclusion of the other possibilities and generally should be confirmed by additional correlations of clinical observations with serum digoxin concentrations.

The serum concentration data should always be interpreted in the overall clinical context and an isolated serum concentration value should not be used alone as a basis for increasing or decreasing digoxin dosage.

Adjustment of Maintenance Dose in Previously Digitalized Patients: Lanoxicaps maintenance doses in individual patients on steady-state digoxin can be adjusted upward or downward in proportion to the ratio of the desired versus the measured serum concentration. For example, a patient at steady-state on 100 μg (0.1 mg) of Lanoxicaps per day with a measured serum concentration of 0.7 ng/mL, should have the dose increased to 200 μg (0.2 mg) per day to achieve a steady-state serum concentration of 1.4 ng/mL, **assuming the serum digoxin concentration measurement is correct, renal function remains stable during this time and the needed adjustment is not the result of a problem with compliance.**

Dosage Adjustment When Changing Preparations: The absolute bioavailability of the capsule formulation is greater than that of the standard tablets and very near that of the intravenous dosage form. As a result the doses recommended for Lanoxicaps capsules are the same as those for Lanoxin® Injection (see CLINICAL PHARMACOLOGY section).

Adjustments in dosage will seldom be necessary when converting a patient from intravenous to Lanoxicaps formulation. The differences in bioavailability between injectable Lanoxin or Lanoxicaps, and Lanoxin Elixir Pediatric or Lanoxin Tablets must be considered when changing patients from one dosage form to another.

Lanoxin Injection and Lanoxicaps doses of 100 μg (0.1 mg) and 200 μg (0.2 mg) are approximately equivalent to 125 μg (0.125 mg) and 250 μg (0.25 mg) doses of Lanoxin Tablets and Elixir Pediatric (see table in CLINICAL PHARMACOLOGY section). Intramuscular injection of digoxin is extremely painful and offers no advantages unless other routes of administration are contraindicated.

HOW SUPPLIED

LANOXICAPS® (DIGOXIN SOLUTION IN CAPSULES), 50 μg (0.05 mg): Bottle of 100 (NDC 0081-0270-55). Imprint A2C (red).

LANOXICAPS (DIGOXIN SOLUTION IN CAPSULES), 100 μg (0.1 mg)*: Bottles of 30 with child-resistant cap (NDC 0081-0272-30) and 100 (NDC 0081-0272-55).

LANOXICAPS (DIGOXIN SOLUTION IN CAPSULES), 200 μg (0.2 mg)*: Bottles of 30 with child-resistant cap (NDC 0081-0274-30) and 100 (NDC 0081-0274-55).

Store at 15° to 25°C (59° to 77°F) in a dry place and protect from light.

Also Available:

LANOXIN® (DIGOXIN) TABLETS, Scored 125 μg (0.125 mg): bottles of 30 (with child-resistant cap), 100 and 1000; unit dose pack of 100.

LANOXIN (DIGOXIN) TABLETS, Scored 250 μg (0.25 mg): bottles of 30 (with child-resistant cap), 100, 1000 and 5000; unit dose pack of 100.

LANOXIN (DIGOXIN) TABLETS, Scored 500 μg (0.5 mg): bottle of 100.

LANOXIN (DIGOXIN) ELIXIR PEDIATRIC, 50 μg (0.05 mg) per mL: bottle of 60 mL with calibrated dropper.

LANOXIN (DIGOXIN) INJECTION, 500 μg (0.5 mg) in 2 mL (250 μg [0.25 mg] per mL): boxes of 10 and 20 ampuls.

LANOXIN (DIGOXIN) INJECTION PEDIATRIC, 100 μg (0.1 mg) in 1 mL: box of 10 ampuls.

*U.S. Patent No. 4088750

Shown in Product Identification Section, page 407

LANOXIN® ELIXIR PEDIATRIC   ℞

[lă-nŏx 'ĭn ″]
(Digoxin)
50 μg (0.05 mg) per mL

DESCRIPTION

Digoxin is one of the cardiac (or digitalis) glycosides, a closely related group of drugs having in common specific effects on the myocardium. These drugs are found in a number of plants. Digoxin is extracted from the leaves of *Digitalis lanata.* The term "digitalis" is used to designate the whole group. The glycosides are composed of two portions: a sugar and a cardenolide (hence "glycosides").

Digoxin has the molecular formula $C_{41}H_{64}O_{14}$, a molecular weight of 780.95 and melting and decomposition points above 235°C. The drug is practically insoluble in water and in ether; slightly soluble in diluted (50%) alcohol and in chloroform; and freely soluble in pyridine. Digoxin powder is composed of odorless white crystals.

Digoxin has the chemical name: 3β-[(O -2,6-dideoxy-β -D-ribo -hexopyranosyl - (1 → 4) -O -2, -dideoxy   -β -D -ribo -hexopyranosyl-(1 → 4) -2,   6-dideoxy-β --D -ribo -hexopyranosyl) oxy]-12β,14-dihydroxy-5β -card-20(22)-enolide.

Lanoxin Elixir Pediatric is a stable solution of digoxin specially formulated for oral use in infants and children. Each mL contains 50 μg (0.05 mg) digoxin USP. The lime-flavored elixir contains the inactive ingredients alcohol 10%, methylparaben 0.1% (added as a preservative), citric acid, D&C Green No. 5 and Yellow No. 10, flavor, propylene glycol, sodium phosphate, and sucrose. Each package is supplied with a specially calibrated dropper to facilitate the administration of accurate dosage even in premature infants. Starting at 0.2 mL, this 1 mL dropper is marked in divisions of 0.1 mL, each corresponding to 5 μg (0.005 mg) digoxin.

CLINICAL PHARMACOLOGY

Mechanism of Action: The influence of digitalis glycosides on the myocardium is dose-related, and involves both a direct action on cardiac muscle and the specialized conduction system, and indirect actions on the cardiovascular system mediated by the autonomic nervous system. The indirect actions mediated by the autonomic nervous system involve a vagomimetic action, which is responsible for the effects of digitalis on the sino-atrial (SA) and atrioventricular (AV) nodes; and also a baroreceptor sensitization which results in increased carotid sinus nerve activity and enhanced sympathetic withdrawal for any given increment in mean arterial pressure. The pharmacologic consequences of these direct and indirect effects are: 1) an increase in the force and velocity of myocardial systolic contraction (positive inotropic action); 2) a slowing of heart rate (negative chronotropic effect); and 3) decreased conduction velocity through the AV node. In higher doses, digitalis increases sympathetic outflow from the central nervous system (CNS) to both cardiac and peripheral sympathetic nerves. This increase in sympathetic activity may be an important factor in digitalis cardiac toxicity. Most of the extracardiac manifestations of digitalis toxicity are also mediated by the CNS.

Pharmacokinetics: Note: The following data are from studies performed in adults, unless otherwise stated.

Absorption—Gastrointestinal absorption of digoxin is a passive process. Absorption of digoxin from the Lanoxin® Elixir Pediatric formulation has been demonstrated to be 70 to 85% complete compared to an identical intravenous dose of digoxin. When the Elixir is taken after meals, the rate of absorption is slowed, but the total amount of digoxin absorbed is usually unchanged. When taken with meals high in bran fiber, however, the amount absorbed from an oral dose may be reduced. Comparisons of the systemic availability and equivalent doses for digoxin preparations are shown in the following table:

[See table at bottom of next page.]

In some patients, orally administered digoxin is converted to cardioinactive reduction products (e.g., dihydrodigoxin) by

---

Usual Digitalizing and Maintenance Dosages for Lanoxicaps in Children with **Normal Renal Function Based on Lean Body Weight**

Age	Digitalizing* Dose (μg/kg)	Daily † Maintenance Dose (μg/kg)
2–5 Years	25–35	25–35% of the oral or IV loading dose ‡
5–10 Years	15–30	
Over 10 years	8–12	

*IV digitalizing doses are the same as Lanoxicaps digitalizing doses.
†Divided daily dosing is recommended for children under 10 years of age.
‡Projected or actual digitalizing dose providing desired clinical response.

Continued on next page

Burroughs Wellcome—Cont.

PRODUCT	TIME TO ONSET OF EFFECT*	TIME TO PEAK EFFECT*
Lanoxin® Tablet	0.5–2 hours	2–6 hours
Lanoxin Elixir	0.5–2 hours	2–6 hours
Lanoxin Injection/IM	0.5–2 hours	2–6 hours
Lanoxin Injection/IV	5–30 minutes†	1–4 hours
Lanoxicaps Capsules	0.5–2 hours	2–6 hours

*Documented for ventricular response rate in atrial fibrillation, inotropic effect and electrocardiographic changes.
†Depending upon rate of infusion.

colonic bacteria in the gut. Data suggest that one in ten patients treated with digoxin tablets will degrade 40% or more of the ingested dose.

Distribution—Following drug administration, a 6 to 8 hour distribution phase is observed. This is followed by a much more gradual serum concentration decline, which is dependent on digoxin elimination from the body. The peak height and slope of the early portion (absorption/distribution phases) of the serum concentration-time curve are dependent upon the route of administration and the absorption characteristics of the formulation. Clinical evidence indicates that the early high serum concentrations do not reflect the concentration of digoxin at its site of action, but that with chronic use, the steady-state post-distribution serum levels are in equilibrium with tissue levels and correlate with pharmacologic effects. In individual patients, these post-distribution serum concentrations are linearly related to maintenance dosage and may be useful in evaluating therapeutic and toxic effects (see Serum Digoxin Concentrations in DOSAGE AND ADMINISTRATION section).

Digoxin is concentrated in tissues and therefore has a large apparent volume of distribution. Digoxin crosses both the blood-brain barrier and the placenta. At delivery, serum digoxin concentration in the newborn is similar to the serum level in the mother. Approximately 20 to 25% of plasma digoxin is bound to protein. Serum digoxin concentrations are not significantly altered by large changes in fat tissue weight, so that its distribution space correlates best with lean (ideal) body weight, not total body weight.

Pharmacologic Response—The approximate times to onset of effect and to peak effect of all the Lanoxin® preparations are given in the following table:
[See table above.]

Excretion—Elimination of digoxin follows first-order kinetics (that is, the quantity of digoxin eliminated at any time is proportional to the total body content). Following intravenous administration to normal subjects, 50 to 70% of a digoxin dose is excreted unchanged in the urine. Renal excretion of digoxin is proportional to glomerular filtration rate and is largely independent of urine flow. In subjects with normal renal function, digoxin has a half-life of 1.5 to 2.0 days. The half-life in anuric patients is prolonged to 4 to 6 days. Digoxin is not effectively removed from the body by dialysis, exchange transfusion or during cardiopulmonary by-pass because most of the drug is in tissue rather than circulating in the blood.

INDICATIONS AND USAGE

Heart Failure: The increased cardiac output resulting from the inotropic action of digoxin ameliorates the disturbances characteristic of heart failure (venous congestion, edema, dyspnea, orthopnea and cardiac asthma).

Digoxin is more effective in "low output" (pump) failure than in "high output" heart failure secondary to arteriovenous fistula, anemia, infection or hyperthyroidism.

Digoxin is usually continued after failure is controlled, unless some known precipitating factor is corrected. Studies have shown, however, that even though hemodynamic effects can be demonstrated in almost all patients, corresponding improvement in the signs and symptoms of heart failure is not necessarily apparent. Therefore, in patients in whom digoxin may be difficult to regulate, or in whom the risk of toxicity may be great (e.g., patients with unstable renal function or whose potassium levels tend to fluctuate) a cautious withdrawal of digoxin may be considered. If digoxin is discontinued, the patient should be regularly monitored for clinical evidence of recurrent heart failure.

Atrial Fibrillation: Digoxin reduces ventricular rate and thereby improves hemodynamics. Palpitation, precordial distress or weakness are relieved and concomitant congestive failure ameliorated. Digoxin should be continued in doses necessary to maintain the desired ventricular rate.

Atrial Flutter: Digoxin slows the heart and regular sinus rhythm may appear. Frequently the flutter is converted to atrial fibrillation with a controlled ventricular response. Digoxin treatment should be maintained if atrial fibrillation persists. (Electrical cardioversion is often the treatment of choice for atrial flutter. See discussion of cardioversion in PRECAUTIONS section.)

Paroxysmal Atrial Tachycardia (PAT): Digoxin may convert PAT to sinus rhythm by slowing conduction through the AV node. If heart failure has ensued or paroxysms recur frequently, digoxin should be continued. In infants, digoxin is usually continued for 3 to 6 months after a single episode of PAT to prevent recurrence.

CONTRAINDICATIONS

Digitalis glycosides are contraindicated in ventricular fibrillation.

In a given patient, an untoward effect requiring permanent discontinuation of other digitalis preparations usually constitutes a contraindication to digoxin. Hypersensitivity to digoxin itself is a contraindication to its use. Allergy to digoxin, though rare, does occur. It may not extend to all such preparations, and another digitalis glycoside may be tried with caution.

WARNINGS

Anorexia, nausea, vomiting and arrhythmias may accompany heart failure or may be indications of digitalis intoxication. Clinical evaluation of the cause of these symptoms should be attempted before further digitalis administration. In such circumstances determination of the serum digoxin concentration may be an aid in deciding whether or not digitalis toxicity is likely to be present. If the possibility of digitalis intoxication cannot be excluded, cardiac glycosides should be temporarily withheld, if permitted by the clinical situation.

Patients with renal insufficiency require smaller than usual maintenance doses of digoxin (see DOSAGE AND ADMINISTRATION section).

Heart failure accompanying acute glomerulonephritis requires extreme care in digitalization. Relatively low loading and maintenance doses and concomitant use of antihypertensive drugs may be necessary and careful monitoring is essential. Digoxin should be discontinued as soon as possible.

Patients with severe carditis, such as carditis associated with rheumatic fever or viral myocarditis, are especially sensitive to digoxin-induced disturbances of rhythm.

Newborn infants display considerable variability in their tolerance to digoxin. Premature and immature infants are particularly sensitive, and dosage must not only be reduced but must be individualized according to their degree of maturity.

Note: Digitalis glycosides are an important cause of accidental poisoning in children.

PRECAUTIONS

General: Digoxin toxicity develops more frequently and lasts longer in patients with renal impairment because of the decreased excretion of digoxin. Therefore, it should be anticipated that dosage requirements will be decreased in patients with moderate to severe renal disease (see DOSAGE AND ADMINISTRATION section). Because of the prolonged half-life, a longer period of time is required to achieve an initial or new steady-state concentration in patients with renal impairment than in patients with normal renal function.

In patients with hypokalemia, toxicity may occur despite serum digoxin concentrations within the "normal range," because potassium depletion sensitizes the myocardium to digoxin. Therefore, it is desirable to maintain normal serum potassium levels in patients being treated with digoxin. Hypokalemia may result from diuretic, amphotericin B or corticosteroid therapy, and from dialysis or mechanical suction of gastrointestinal secretions. It may also accompany malnutrition, diarrhea, prolonged vomiting, old age and long-standing heart failure. In general, rapid changes in serum potassium or other electrolytes should be avoided, and intravenous treatment with potassium should be reserved for special circumstances as described below (see TREATMENT OF ARRHYTHMIAS PRODUCED BY OVERDOSAGE section).

Calcium, particularly when administered rapidly by the intravenous route, may produce serious arrhythmias in digitalized patients. Hypercalcemia from any cause predisposes the patient to digitalis toxicity. On the other hand, hypocalcemia can nullify the effects of digoxin in man; thus, digoxin may be ineffective until serum calcium is restored to normal. These interactions are related to the fact that calcium affects contractility and excitability of the heart in a manner similar to digoxin.

Hypomagnesemia may predispose to digitalis toxicity. If low magnesium levels are detected in a patient on digoxin, replacement therapy should be instituted.

Quinidine, verapamil, amiodarone, and propafenone cause a rise in serum digoxin concentration, with the implication that digitalis intoxication may result. This rise appears to be proportional to the dose. The effect is mediated by a reduction in the digoxin clearance and, in the case of quinidine, decreased volume of distribution as well.

Certain antibiotics may increase digoxin absorption in patients who convert digoxin to inactive metabolites in the gut (see Pharmacokinetics portion of the CLINICAL PHARMACOLOGY section). Recent studies have shown that specific colonic bacteria in the lower gastrointestinal tract convert digoxin to cardioinactive reduction products, thereby reducing its bioavailability. Although inactivation of these bacteria by antibiotics is rapid, the serum digoxin concentration will rise at a rate consistent with the elimination half-life of digoxin. The magnitude of rise in serum digoxin concentration relates to the extent of bacterial inactivation, and may be as much as two-fold in some cases.

Patients with acute myocardial infarction or severe pulmonary disease may be unusually sensitive to digoxin-induced disturbances of rhythm.

Atrial arrhythmias associated with hypermetabolic states (e.g. hyperthyroidism) are particularly resistant to digoxin treatment. Large doses of digoxin are not recommended as the only treatment of these arrhythmias and care must be taken to avoid toxicity if large doses of digoxin are required. In hypothyroidism, the digoxin requirements are reduced. Digoxin responses in patients with compensated thyroid disease are normal.

Reduction of digoxin dosage may be desirable prior to electrical cardioversion to avoid induction of ventricular arrhythmias, but the physician must consider the consequences of rapid increase in ventricular response to atrial fibrillation if digoxin is withheld 1 to 2 days prior to cardioversion. If there is a suspicion that digitalis toxicity exists, elective cardioversion should be delayed. If it is not prudent to delay cardioversion, the energy level selected should be minimal at first and carefully increased in an attempt to avoid precipitating ventricular arrhythmias.

Incomplete AV block, especially in patients with Stokes-Adams attacks, may progress to advanced or complete heart block if digoxin is given.

In some patients with sinus node disease (i.e. Sick Sinus Syndrome), digoxin may worsen sinus bradycardia or sino-atrial block.

In patients with Wolff-Parkinson-White Syndrome and atrial fibrillation, digoxin can enhance transmission of impulses through the accessory pathway. This effect may result in extremely rapid ventricular rates and even ventricular fibrillation.

Digoxin may worsen the outflow obstruction in patients with idiopathic hypertrophic subaortic stenosis (IHSS). Unless cardiac failure is severe, it is doubtful whether digoxin should be employed.

Patients with chronic constrictive pericarditis may fail to respond to digoxin. In addition, slowing of the heart rate by digoxin in some patients may further decrease cardiac output.

Patients with heart failure from amyloid heart disease or constrictive cardiomyopathies respond poorly to treatment with digoxin.

Digoxin is not indicated for the treatment of sinus tachycardia unless it is associated with heart failure.

Digoxin may produce false positive ST-T changes in the electrocardiogram during exercise testing.

Intramuscular injection of digoxin is extremely painful and offers no advantages unless other routes of administration are contraindicated.

Laboratory Tests: Patients receiving digoxin should have their serum electrolytes and renal function (BUN and/

PRODUCT	ABSOLUTE BIOAVAILABILITY	EQUIVALENT DOSES (IN MG)*		
Lanoxin® Tablet	60–80%	0.125	0.25	0.5
Lanoxin Elixir	70–85%	0.125	0.25	0.5
Lanoxin Injection/IM	70–85%	0.125	0.25	0.5
Lanoxin Injection/IV	100%	0.1	0.2	0.4
Lanoxicaps Capsules	90–100%	0.1	0.2	0.4

*1 mg = 1000 μg

or serum creatinine) assessed periodically; the frequency of assessments will depend on the clinical setting. For discussion of serum digoxin concentrations, see DOSAGE AND ADMINISTRATION section.

Drug Interactions: Potassium-depleting *corticosteroids* and *diuretics* may be major contributing factors to digitalis toxicity. *Calcium*, particularly if administered rapidly by the intravenous route, may produce serious arrhythmias in digitalized patients. *Quinidine, verapamil, amiodarone* and *propafenone* cause a rise in serum digoxin concentration, with the implication that digitalis intoxication may result. Certain *antibiotics* increase digoxin absorption in patients who inactivate digoxin by bacterial metabolism in the lower intestine, so that digitalis intoxication may result. *Propantheline* and *diphenoxylate*, by decreasing gut motility, may increase digoxin absorption. *Antacids, kaolin-pectin, sulfasalazine, neomycin, cholestyramine* and certain *anticancer drugs* may interfere with intestinal digoxin absorption, resulting in unexpectedly low serum concentrations. There have been inconsistent reports regarding the effects of other drugs on the serum digoxin concentration. *Thyroid* administration to a digitalized, hypothyroid patient may increase the dose requirement of digoxin. Concomitant use of digoxin and *sympathomimetics* increases the risk of cardiac arrhythmias, because both enhance ectopic pacemaker activity. *Succinylcholine* may cause a sudden extrusion of potassium from muscle cells, and may thereby cause arrhythmias in digitalized patients. Although β adrenergic blockers or calcium channel blockers and digoxin may be useful in combination to control atrial fibrillation, their additive effects on AV node conduction can result in complete heart block.

Due to the considerable variability of these interactions, digoxin dosage should be carefully individualized when patients receive coadministered medications. Furthermore, caution should be exercised when combining digoxin with any drug that may cause a significant deterioration in renal function, since this may impair the excretion of digoxin.

Carcinogenesis, Mutagenesis, Impairment of Fertility: There have been no long-term studies performed in animals to evaluate carcinogenic potential.

ADVERSE REACTIONS

The frequency and severity of adverse reactions to digoxin depend on the dose and route of administration, as well as on the patient's underlying disease or concomitant therapies (see PRECAUTIONS section and Serum Digoxin Concentrations subsection of DOSAGE AND ADMINISTRATION).

The overall incidence of adverse reactions has been reported as 5 to 20%, with 15 to 20% of them being considered serious (one to four percent of patients receiving digoxin). Evidence suggests that the incidence of toxicity has decreased since the introduction of the serum digoxin assay and improved standardization of digoxin tablets. Cardiac toxicity accounts for about one-half, gastrointestinal disturbances for about one-fourth, and CNS and other toxicity for about one-fourth of these adverse reactions.

Cardiac—Conduction disturbances or supraventricular tachyarrhythmias, such as atrioventricular (AV) block (Wenckebach), atrial tachycardia with or without block and junctional (nodal) tachycardia are the most common arrhythmias associated with digoxin toxicity in children. Ventricular arrhythmias, such as unifocal or multiform ventricular premature contractions, especially in bigeminal or trigeminal patterns, are less common. Ventricular tachycardia may result from digitalis toxicity. Sinus bradycardia may also be a sign of impending digoxin intoxication, especially in infants, even in the absence of first degree heart block. Any arrhythmias or alteration in cardiac conduction that develops in a child taking digoxin should initially be assumed to be a consequence of digoxin intoxication.

Note: The electrocardiogram is fundamental in determining the presence and nature of these cardiac disturbances. Digoxin may also induce other changes in the ECG (e.g. PR prolongation, ST depression), which represent digoxin effect and may or may not be associated with digitalis toxicity.

Gastrointestinal—Anorexia, nausea, vomiting and diarrhea may be early symptoms of overdosage. However, uncontrolled heart failure may also produce such symptoms. Digitalis toxicity very rarely may cause abdominal pain and hemorrhagic necrosis of the intestines.

CNS—Visual disturbances (blurred or yellow vision), headache, weakness, dizziness, apathy and psychosis can occur. These may be difficult to recognize in infants and children.

Other—Gynecomastia is occasionally observed. Maculopapular rash or other skin reactions are rarely observed.

OVERDOSAGE

Treatment of Arrhythmias Produced by Overdosage:

Digoxin should be discontinued until all signs of toxicity are gone. Discontinuation may be all that is necessary if toxic manifestations are not severe and appear only near the expected time for maximum effect of the drug.

Correction of factors that may contribute to toxicity such as electrolyte disturbances, hypoxia, acid-base disturbances and removal of aggravating agents such as catecholamines, should also be considered. Potassium salts may be indicated, particularly if hypokalemia is present. Potassium administration may be dangerous in the setting of massive digitalis overdosage (see Massive Digitalis Overdosage subsection below). Potassium chloride in divided oral doses totaling 1 to 1.5 mEq K+ per kilogram (kg) body weight may be given provided renal function is adequate (1 gram of potassium chloride contains 13.4 mEq K+).

When correction of the arrhythmia is urgent and the serum potassium concentration is low or normal, approximately 0.5 mEq/kg of potassium per hour may be given intravenously in 5% dextrose injection. The intravenous solution of potassium should be dilute enough to avoid local irritation; however, especially in infants, care must be taken to avoid intravenous fluid overload. ECG monitoring should be performed to watch for any evidence of potassium toxicity (e.g. peaking of T waves) and to observe the effect on the arrhythmia. The infusion may be stopped when the desired effect is achieved.

Note: Potassium should not be used and may be dangerous in heart block due to digoxin, unless primarily related to supraventricular tachycardia.

Other agents that have been used for the treatment of digoxin intoxication include lidocaine, procainamide, propranolol and phenytoin, although use of the latter must be considered experimental. In advanced heart block, atropine and/or temporary ventricular pacing may be beneficial.

Digibind®, Digoxin Immune Fab (Ovine), can be used to reverse potentially life-threatening digoxin (or digitoxin) intoxication. Improvement in signs and symptoms of digitalis toxicity usually begins within ½ hour of Digibind administration. Each 40 mg vial of Digibind will neutralize 0.6 mg of digoxin (which is a usual body store of an adequately digitalized 70 kg patient).

Massive Digitalis Overdosage: Manifestations of life-threatening toxicity include severe ventricular arrhythmias such as ventricular tachycardia or ventricular fibrillation, or progressive bradyarrhythmias such as severe sinus bradycardia or second or third degree heart block not responsive to atropine. An overdosage of more than 10 mg of digoxin in previously healthy adults or 4 mg in previously healthy children or overdosage resulting in steady-state serum concentrations greater than 10 ng/mL, often results in cardiac arrest.

Severe digitalis intoxication can cause life-threatening elevation in serum potassium concentration by shifting potassium from inside to outside the cell resulting in hyperkalemia. Administration of potassium supplements in the setting of massive intoxication may be hazardous.

Digibind®, Digoxin Immune Fab (Ovine), may be used at a dose equimolar to digoxin in the body to reverse the effects of ingestion of a massive overdose. The decision to administer Digibind before the onset of toxic manifestations will depend on the likelihood that life-threatening toxicity will occur (see above).

Patients with massive digitalis ingestion should receive large doses of activated charcoal to prevent absorption and bind digoxin in the gut during enteroenteric recirculation. Emesis or gastric lavage may be indicated especially if ingestion has occurred within 30 minutes of the patient's presentation at the hospital. Emesis should not be induced in patients who are obtunded. If a patient presents more than 2 hours after ingestion or already has toxic manifestations, it may be unsafe to induce vomiting or attempt passage of a gastric tube, because such maneuvers may induce an acute vagal episode that can worsen digitalis-toxic arrhythmias.

DOSAGE AND ADMINISTRATION

Recommended dosages are average values that may require considerable modification because of individual sensitivity or associated conditions. Diminished renal function is the most important factor requiring modification of recommended doses.

Adults: See the Lanoxin® Tablets package insert for specific recommendations.

Infants and Children: Digitalization must be individualized. Divided daily dosing is recommended for infants and young children. Children over 10 years of age require adult dosages in proportion to their body weight.

In the newborn period, renal clearance of digoxin is diminished and suitable dosage adjustments must be observed. This is especially pronounced in the premature infant. Beyond the immediate newborn period, children generally require proportionally larger doses than adults on the basis of body weight or body surface area.

In deciding the dose of digoxin, several factors must be considered:

1. The disease being treated. Atrial arrhythmias may require larger doses than heart failure.
2. The body weight of the patient. Doses should be calculated based upon lean or ideal body weight.
3. The patient's renal function, preferably evaluated on the basis of creatinine clearance.
4. Age is an important factor in infants and children.
5. Concomitant disease states, drugs or other factors likely to alter the expected clinical response to digoxin (see PRECAUTIONS and Drug Interactions sections).

Digitalization may be accomplished by either of two general approaches that vary in dosage and frequency of administration, but reach the same endpoint in terms of total amount of digoxin accumulated in the body.

1. Rapid digitalization may be achieved by administering a loading dose based upon projected peak body digoxin stores, then calculating the maintenance dose as a percentage of the loading dose.
2. More gradual digitalization may be obtained by beginning an appropriate maintenance dose, thus allowing digoxin body stores to accumulate slowly. Steady-state serum digoxin concentrations will be achieved in approximately 5 half-lives of the drug for the individual patient. Depending upon the patient's renal function, this will take between one and three weeks.

Infants and Children— Rapid Digitalization with a Loading Dose: Lanoxin Injection Pediatric can be used to achieve rapid digitalization, with conversion to an oral Lanoxin formulation for maintenance therapy. If patients are switched from IV to oral digoxin tablets or elixir, allowances must be made for differences in bioavailability when calculating maintenance dosages (see bioavailability table in CLINICAL PHARMACOLOGY section and dosing table below).

Intramuscular injection of digoxin is extremely painful and offers no advantages unless other routes of administration are contraindicated.

Digitalizing and daily maintenance doses for each age group are given below and should provide therapeutic effect with minimum risk of toxicity in most patients with heart failure and normal sinus rhythm. Larger doses are often required for adequate control of ventricular rate in patients with atrial flutter or fibrillation.

The loading dose should be administered in several portions, with roughly half the total given as the first dose. Additional fractions of this planned total dose may be given at 6 to 8 hour intervals, **with careful assessment of clinical response before each additional dose.** If the patient's clinical response necessitates a change from the calculated dose of digoxin, then calculation of the maintenance dose should be based upon the amount actually given.

[See table above.]

Usual Digitalizing and Maintenance Dosages for Lanoxin® Elixir Pediatric in Children with **Normal Renal Function Based on Lean Body Weight**

Age	Digitalizing* Dose (µg/kg)	Daily† Maintenance Dose (µg/kg)
Premature	20–30	20–30% of *oral* loading dose‡
Full Term	25–35	25–35% of *oral* loading dose‡
1–24 Months	35–60	
2–5 Years	30–40	
5–10 Years	20–35	
Over 10 Years	10–15	

*IV digitalizing doses are 80% of oral digitalizing doses.
†Divided daily dosing is recommended for children under 10 years of age.
‡Projected or actual digitalizing dose providing clinical response.

Infants and Children—Gradual Digitalization With A Maintenance Dose: More gradual digitalization can also be accomplished by beginning an appropriate maintenance dose. The range of percentages provided above can be used in calculating this dose for patients with normal renal function. In children with renal disease, digoxin dosing must be carefully titrated based upon desired clinical reponse.

Long-term use of digoxin is indicated in many children who have been digitalized for acute heart failure, unless the cause is transient. Children with severe congenital heart disease, even after surgery, may require digoxin for prolonged periods.

It cannot be overemphasized that these pediatric dosage guidelines are based upon average patient response and substantial individual variation can be expected. Accordingly,

Continued on next page

Burroughs Wellcome—Cont.

ultimate dosage selection must be based upon clinical assessment of the patient.

Serum Digoxin Concentrations: Measurement of serum digoxin concentrations can be helpful to the clinician in determining the state of digitalization and in assigning certain probabilities to the likelihood of digoxin intoxication. Studies in adults considered adequately digitalized (without evidence of toxicity) show that about two-thirds of such patients have serum digoxin levels ranging from 0.8 to 2.0 ng/mL. Patients with atrial fibrillation or atrial flutter require and appear to tolerate higher levels than do patients with other indications. On the other hand, in adult patients with clinical evidence of digoxin toxicity, about two-thirds will have serum digoxin levels greater than 2.0 ng/mL.

Thus, whereas levels less than 0.8 ng/mL are infrequently associated with toxicity, levels greater than 2.0 ng/mL are often associated with toxicity. Values in between are not very helpful in deciding whether a certain sign or symptom is more likely caused by digoxin toxicity or by something else. There are rare patients who are unable to tolerate digoxin even at serum concentrations below 0.8 ng/mL. Some researchers suggest that infants and young children tolerate slightly higher serum concentrations than do adults.

To allow adequate time for equilibration of digoxin between serum and tissue, **sampling of serum concentrations for clinical use should be at least 6 to 8 hours after the last dose,** regardless of the route of administration or formulation used. On a twice daily dosing schedule, there will be only minor differences in serum digoxin concentrations whether sampling is done at 8 or 12 hours after a dose. After a single daily dose, the concentration will be 10 to 25% lower when sampled at 24 versus 8 hours, depending upon the patient's renal function. Ideally, sampling for assessment of steady-state concentrations should be done just before the next dose.

If a discrepancy exists between the reported serum concentration and the observed clinical response, the clinician should consider the following possibilities:
1. Analytical problems in the assay procedure.
2. Inappropriate serum sampling time.
3. Administration of a digitalis glycoside other than digoxin.
4. Conditions (described in WARNINGS and PRECAUTIONS sections) causing an alteration in the sensitivity of the patient to digoxin.
5. The patient falls outside the norm in his response to or handling of digoxin. This decision should only be reached after exclusion of the other possibilities and generally should be confirmed by additional correlations of clinical observations with serum digoxin concentrations.

The serum concentration data should always be interpreted in the overall clinical context and an isolated serum concentration value should not be used alone as a basis for increasing or decreasing digoxin dosage.

Adjustment of Maintenance Dose in Previously Digitalized Patients: Lanoxin® Elixir Pediatric maintenance doses in individual patients on steady-state digoxin can be adjusted upward or downward in proportion to the ratio of the desired versus the measured serum concentration. For example, a patient at steady-state on 125 μg (0.125 mg) of Lanoxin Elixir per day with a measured serum concentration of 0.7 ng/mL, should have the dose increased to 250 μg (0.250 mg) per day to achieve a steady-state serum concentration of 1.4 ng/mL, **assuming the serum digoxin concentration measurement is correct, renal function remains stable during this time and the needed adjustment is not the result of a problem with compliance.**

Dosage Adjustment When Changing Preparations: The differences in bioavailability between injectable Lanoxin or Lanoxicaps and Lanoxin Elixir Pediatric or Lanoxin Tablets must be considered when changing patients from one dosage form to another.

Lanoxin Injection and Lanoxicaps doses of 100 μg (0.1 mg) and 200 μg (0.2 mg) are approximately equivalent to 125 μg (0.125 mg) and 250 μg (0.25 mg) doses of Lanoxin Elixir Pediatric and Lanoxin Tablets (see table in CLINICAL PHARMACOLOGY section). Intramuscular injection of digoxin is extremely painful and offers no advantages unless other routes of administration are contraindicated.

HOW SUPPLIED

LANOXIN® (DIGOXIN) ELIXIR PEDIATRIC, 50 μg (0.05 mg) per mL; Bottle of 60 mL with calibrated dropper. (NDC 0081-0264-27).
Store at 15° to 25°C (59° to 77°F) and protect from light.
Also Available:
LANOXIN® (DIGOXIN) TABLETS, Scored 125 μg (0.125 mg): bottles of 30 (with child-resistant cap), 100 and 1000; unit dose pack of 100.
LANOXIN (DIGOXIN) TABLETS, Scored 250 μg (0.25 mg): bottles of 30 (with child-resistant cap), 100, 1000 and 5000; unit dose pack of 100.

LANOXIN (DIGOXIN) TABLETS, Scored 500 μg (0.5 mg); bottle of 100.
LANOXIN (DIGOXIN) INJECTION, 500 μg (0.5 mg) in 2 mL (250 μg [0.25 mg] per mL): boxes of 10 and 50 ampuls.
LANOXIN (DIGOXIN) INJECTION PEDIATRIC, 100 μg (0.1 mg) in 1 mL: box of 10 ampuls.
LANOXICAPS® (DIGOXIN SOLUTION IN CAPSULES), 50 μg (0.05 mg) bottle of 100; 100 μg (0.1 mg) bottles of 30 (with child-resistant cap) and 100, 200 μg (0.2 mg) bottles of 30 (with child-resistant cap) and 100.

LANOXIN® INJECTION   ℞
[lă-nŏx 'in "]
(Digoxin)
500 μg (0.5 mg) in 2 mL (250 μg [0.25 mg] per mL)

DESCRIPTION

Digoxin is one of the cardiac (or digitalis) glycosides, a closely related group of drugs having in common specific effects on the myocardium. These drugs are found in a number of plants. Digoxin is extracted from the leaves of *Digitalis lanata*. The term "digitalis" is used to designate the whole group. The glycosides are composed of two portions: a sugar and a cardenolide (hence "glycosides"). Digoxin has the molecular formula $C_{41}H_{64}O_{14}$, a molecular weight of 780.95 and melting and decomposition points above 235°C. The drug is practically insoluble in water and in ether; slightly soluble in diluted (50%) alcohol and in chloroform; and freely soluble in pyridine. Digoxin powder is composed of odorless white crystals. Digoxin has the chemical name: 3β-[(O-2,6-dideoxy-β-D-ribo -hexopyranosyl-(1→4)-O-2,6-dideoxy-β-D-ribo-hexopyranosyl-(1→4)-2,6-dideoxy-β-D-ribo--hexopyranosyl)-oxy]-12β,14-dihydroxy-5β-card-20(22)-enolide.
Lanoxin (Digoxin) Injection is a sterile solution of digoxin for intravenous or intramuscular injection. The vehicle contains 40% propylene glycol and 10% alcohol. The injection is buffered to a pH of 6.8 to 7.2 with 0.3 percent sodium phosphate and 0.08 percent anhydrous citric acid. Each 2 mL ampul contains 500 μg (0.5 mg) digoxin (250 μg [0.25 mg] per mL). Dilution is not required.

CLINICAL PHARMACOLOGY

Mechanism of Action: The influence of digitalis glycosides on the myocardium is dose-related, and involves both a direct action on cardiac muscle and the specialized conduction system, and indirect actions on the cardiovascular system mediated by the autonomic nervous system. The indirect actions mediated by the autonomic nervous system involve a vagomimetic action, which is responsible for the effects of digitalis on the sino-atrial (SA) and atrioventricular (AV) nodes; and also a baroreceptor sensitization which results in increased carotid sinus nerve activity and enhanced sympathetic withdrawal for any given increment in mean arterial pressure. The pharmacologic consequences of these direct and indirect effects are: 1) an increase in the force and velocity of myocardial systolic contraction (positive inotropic action); 2) a slowing of heart rate (negative chronotropic effect); and 3) decreased conduction velocity through the AV node. In higher doses, digitalis increases sympathetic outflow from the central nervous system (CNS) to both cardiac and peripheral sympathetic nerves. This increase in sympathetic activity may be an important factor in digitalis cardiac toxicity. Most of the extracardiac manifestations of digitalis toxicity are also mediated by the CNS.

Pharmacokinetics:

Absorption—A comparison of the systemic availability and equivalent doses for digoxin preparations are shown in the following table:
[See first table below.]

Distribution—Following drug administration, a 6 to 8 hour distribution phase is observed. This is followed by a much more gradual serum concentration decline, which is dependent on digoxin elimination from the body. The peak height and slope of the early portion (absorption/distribution phases) of the serum concentration-time curve are dependent upon the route of administration and the absorption characteristics of the formulation. Clinical evidence indicates that the early high serum concentrations do not reflect the concentration of digoxin at its site of action, but that with chronic use, the steady-state post-distribution serum levels are in equilibrium with tissue levels and correlate with pharmacologic effects. In individual patients, these post-distribution serum concentrations are linearly related to maintenance dosage and may be useful in evaluating therapeutic and toxic effects (see Serum Digoxin Concentrations in DOSAGE AND ADMINISTRATION section).

Digoxin is concentrated in tissues and therefore has a large apparent volume of distribution. Digoxin crosses both the blood-brain barrier and the placenta. At delivery, serum digoxin concentration in the newborn is similar to the serum level in the mother. Approximately 20 to 25% of plasma digoxin is bound to protein. Serum digoxin concentrations are not significantly altered by large changes in fat tissue weight, so that its distribution space correlates best with lean (ideal) body weight, not total body weight.

Pharmacologic Response—The approximate times to onset of effect and to peak effect of all the Lanoxin® preparations are given in the following table:
[See bottom table.]

Excretion—Elimination of digoxin follows first-order kinetics (that is, the quantity of digoxin eliminated at any time is proportional to the total body content). Following intravenous administration to normal subjects, 50 to 70% of a digoxin dose is excreted unchanged in the urine. Renal excretion of digoxin is proportional to glomerular filtration rate and is largely independent of urine flow. In subjects with normal renal function, digoxin has a half-life of 1.5 to 2.0 days. The half-life in anuric patients is prolonged to 4 to 6 days. Digoxin is not effectively removed from the body by dialysis, exchange transfusion or during cardiopulmonary by-pass because most of the drug is in tissue rather than circulating in the blood.

INDICATIONS AND USAGE

Heart Failure: The increased cardiac output resulting from the inotropic action of digoxin ameliorates the disturbances characteristic of heart failure (venous congestion, edema, dyspnea, orthopnea and cardiac asthma). Digoxin is more effective in "low output" (pump) failure than in "high output" heart failure secondary to arteriovenous fistula, anemia, infection or hyperthyroidism. Digoxin is usually continued after failure is controlled, unless some known precipitating factor is corrected. Studies have shown, however, that even though hemodynamic effects can be demonstrated in almost all patients, corresponding improvement in the signs and symptoms of heart failure is not necessarily apparent. Therefore, in patients in whom digoxin may be difficult to regulate, or in whom the risk of toxicity may be great (e.g., patients with unstable renal function or whose potassium levels tend to fluctuate) a cautious withdrawal of digoxin may be considered. If digoxin is discontinued, the patient should be regularly monitored for clinical evidence of recurrent heart failure.

Atrial Fibrillation: Digoxin reduces ventricular rate and thereby improves hemodynamics. Palpitation, precordial distress or weakness are relieved and concomitant congestive failure ameliorated. Digoxin should be continued in doses necessary to maintain the desired ventricular rate.

Atrial Flutter: Digoxin slows the heart and regular sinus rhythm may appear. Frequently the flutter is converted to

PRODUCT	ABSOLUTE BIOAVAILABILITY	EQUIVALENT DOSES (IN MG)*		
Lanoxin Tablet	60–80%	0.125	0.25	0.5
Lanoxin Elixir	70–85%	0.125	0.25	0.5
Lanoxin Injection/IM	70–85%	0.125	0.25	0.5
Lanoxin Injection/IV	100%	0.1	0.2	0.4
Lanoxicaps Capsules	90–100%	0.1	0.2	0.4

*1 mg = 1000 μg

PRODUCT	TIME TO ONSET OF EFFECT*	TIME TO PEAK EFFECT*
Lanoxin Tablet	0.5–2 hours	2–6 hours
Lanoxin Elixir	0.5–2 hours	2–6 hours
Lanoxin Injection/IM	0.5–2 hours	2–6 hours
Lanoxin Injection/IV	5–30 minutes†	1–4 hours
Lanoxicaps Capsules	0.5–2 hours	2–6 hours

*Documented for ventricular response rate in atrial fibrillation, inotropic effect and electrocardiographic changes.
†Depending upon rate of infusion.

atrial fibrillation with a controlled ventricular response. Digoxin treatment should be maintained if atrial fibrillation persists. (Electrical cardioversion is often the treatment of choice for atrial flutter. See discussion of cardioversion in PRECAUTIONS section.)

Paroxysmal Atrial Tachycardia (PAT): Digoxin may convert PAT to sinus rhythm by slowing conduction through the AV node. If heart failure has ensued or paroxysms recur frequently, digoxin should be continued. In infants, digoxin is usually continued for 3 to 6 months after a single episode of PAT to prevent recurrence.

CONTRAINDICATIONS

Digitalis glycosides are contraindicated in ventricular fibrillation.

In a given patient, an untoward effect requiring permanent discontinuation of other digitalis preparations usually constitutes a contraindication to digoxin. Hypersensitivity to digoxin itself is a contraindication to its use. Allergy to digoxin, though rare, does occur. It may not extend to all such preparations, and another digitalis glycoside may be tried with caution.

WARNINGS

Digitalis alone or with other drugs has been used in the treatment of obesity. This use of digoxin or other digitalis glycosides is unwarranted. Moreover, since they may cause potentially fatal arrhythmias or other adverse effects, the use of these drugs solely for the treatment of obesity is dangerous.

It is recommended that digoxin in soft capsules be administered in divided daily doses to minimize any potential adverse reactions, since peak serum digoxin concentrations resulting from the capsules are approximately twice those after bioequivalent tablet doses (400 μg of Lanoxicaps are bioequivalent to 500 μg of tablets). Studies are underway to determine if there are any increased risks associated with the higher peaks that occur with single daily dosing of soft gelating capsules. Anorexia, nausea, vomiting and arrhythmias may accompany heart failure or may be indications of digitalis intoxication. Clinical evaluation of the cause of these symptoms should be attempted before further digitalis administration. In such circumstances determination of the serum digoxin concentration may be an aid in deciding whether or not digitalis toxicity is likely to be present. If the possibility of digitalis intoxication cannot be excluded, cardiac glycosides should be temporarily withheld, if permitted by the clinical situation.

Patients with renal insufficiency require smaller than usual maintenance doses of digoxin (see DOSAGE AND ADMINISTRATION section).

Heart failure accompanying acute glomerulonephritis requires extreme care in digitalization. Relatively low loading and maintenance doses and concomitant use of antihypertensive drugs may be necessary and careful monitoring is essential. Digoxin should be discontinued as soon as possible.

Patients with severe carditis, such as carditis associated with rheumatic fever or viral myocarditis, are especially sensitive to digoxin-induced disturbances of rhythm.

Newborn infants display considerable variability in their tolerance to digoxin. Premature and immature infants are particularly sensitive, and dosage must not only be reduced but must be individualized according to their degree of maturity.

Note: Digitalis glycosides are an important cause of accidental poisoning in children.

PRECAUTIONS

General: Digoxin toxicity develops more frequently and lasts longer in patients with renal impairment because of the decreased excretion of digoxin. Therefore, it should be anticipated that dosage requirements will be decreased in patients with moderate to severe renal disease (see DOSAGE AND ADMINISTRATION section). Because of the prolonged half-life, a longer period of time is required to achieve an initial or new steady-state concentration in patients with renal impairment than in patients with normal renal function.

In patients with hypokalemia, toxicity may occur despite serum digoxin concentrations within the "normal range," because potassium depletion sensitizes the myocardium to digoxin. Therefore, it is desirable to maintain normal serum potassium levels in patients being treated with digoxin. Hypokalemia may result from diuretic, amphotericin B or corticosteroid therapy, and from dialysis or mechanical suction of gastrointestinal secretions. It may also accompany malnutrition, diarrhea, prolonged vomiting, old age and long-standing heart failure. In general, rapid changes in serum potassium or other electrolytes should be avoided, and intravenous treatment with potassium should be reserved for special circumstances as described below (see TREATMENT OF ARRHYTHMIAS PRODUCED BY OVERDOSAGE section).

Calcium, particularly when administered rapidly by the intravenous route, may produce serious arrhythmias in digitalized patients. Hypercalcemia from any cause predisposes the patient to digitalis toxicity. On the other hand, hypocalcemia can nullify the effects of digoxin in man; thus, digoxin may be ineffective until serum calcium is restored to normal. These interactions are related to the fact that calcium affects contractility and excitability of the heart in a manner similar to digoxin.

Hypomagnesemia may predispose to digitalis toxicity. If low magnesium levels are detected in a patient on digoxin, replacement therapy should be instituted.

Quinidine, verapamil, and amoidarone cause a rise in serum digoxin concentration, with the implication that digitalis intoxication may result. This rise appears to be proportional to the dose. The effect is mediated by a reduction in the digoxin clearance and, in the case of quinidine, decreased volume of distribution as well.

Patients with acute myocardial infarction or severe pulmonary disease may be unusually sensitive to digoxin-induced disturbances of rhythm.

Atrial arrhythmias associated with hypermetabolic states (e.g. hyperthyroidism) are particularly resistant to digoxin treatment. Large doses of digoxin are not recommended as the only treatment of these arrhythmias and care must be taken to avoid toxicity if large doses of digoxin are required.

In hypothyroidism, the digoxin requirements are reduced. Digoxin responses in patients with compensated thyroid disease are normal.

Reduction of digoxin dosage may be desirable prior to electrical cardioversion to avoid induction of ventricular arrhythmias, but the physician must consider the consequences of rapid increase in ventricular response to atrial fibrillation if digoxin is withheld 1 to 2 days prior to cardioversion. If there is a suspicion that digitalis toxicity exists, elective cardioversion should be delayed. If it is not prudent to delay cardioversion, the energy level selected should be minimal at first and carefully increased in an attempt to avoid precipitating ventricular arrhythmias.

Incomplete AV block, especially in patients with Stokes-Adams attacks, may progress to advanced or complete heart block if digoxin is given.

In some patients with sinus node disease (i.e. Sick Sinus Syndrome), digoxin may worsen sinus bradycardia or sino-atrial block.

In patients with Wolff-Parkinson-White Syndrome and atrial fibrillation, digoxin can enhance transmission of impulses through the accessory pathway. This effect may result in extremely rapid ventricular rates and even ventricular fibrillation.

Digoxin may worsen the outflow obstruction in patients with idiopathic hypertrophic subaortic stenosis (IHSS). Unless cardiac failure is severe, it is doubtful whether digoxin should be employed.

Patients with chronic constrictive pericarditis may fail to respond to digoxin. In addition, slowing of the heart rate by digoxin in some patients may further decrease cardiac output.

Patients with heart failure from amyloid heart disease or constrictive cardiomyopathies respond poorly to treatment with digoxin.

Digoxin is not indicated for the treatment of sinus tachycardia unless it is associated with heart failure.

Digoxin may produce false positive ST-T changes in the electrocardiogram during exercise testing.

Intramuscular injection of digoxin is extremely painful and offers no advantages unless other routes of administration are contraindicated.

Laboratory Tests: Patients receiving digoxin should have their serum electrolytes and renal function (BUN and/or serum creatinine) assessed periodically; the frequency of assessments will depend on the clinical setting. For discussion of serum digoxin concentrations, see DOSAGE AND ADMINISTRATION section.

Drug Interactions: Potassium-depleting *corticosteroids* and *diuretics* may be major contributing factors to digitalis toxicity. *Calcium*, particularly if administered rapidly by the intravenous route, may produce serious arrhythmias in digitalized patients. *Quinidine, verapamil,* and *amiodarone* cause a rise in serum digoxin concentration, with the implication that digitalis intoxication may result. Certain *antibiotics* increase digoxin absorption in patients who inactivate digoxin by bacterial metabolism in the lower intestine, so that digitalis intoxication may result. *Propantheline* and *diphenoxylate*, by decreasing gut motility, may increase digoxin absorption. *Antacids, kaolin-pectin, sulfasalazine, neomycin, cholestyramine* and certain *anticancer drugs* may reduce intestinal digoxin absorption, resulting in unexpectedly low serum concentrations. There have been inconsistent reports regarding the effects of other drugs on the serum digoxin concentration. *Thyroid* administration to a digitalized, hypothyroid patient may increase the dose requirement of digoxin. Concomitant use of digoxin and *sympathomimetics* increases the risk of cardiac arrhythmias because both enhance ectopic pacemaker activity. *Succinylcholine* may cause a sudden extrusion of potassium from muscle cells, and may thereby cause arrhythmias in digitalized patients. Although β adrenergic blockers or calcium channel blockers and digoxin may be useful in combination to control atrial fibrillation, their additive effects on AV node conduction can result in complete heart block.

Due to the considerable variability of these interactions, digoxin dosage should be carefully individualized when patients receive coadministered medications. Furthermore, caution should be exercised when combining digoxin with any drug that may cause a significant deterioration in renal function, since this may impair the excretion of digoxin.

Carcinogenesis, Mutagenesis, Impairment of Fertility: There have been no long-term studies performed in animals to evaluate carcinogenic potential.

Pregnancy: ***Teratogenic Effects:*** Pregnancy Category C. Animal reproduction studies have not been conducted with digoxin. It is also not known whether digoxin can cause fetal harm when administered to a pregnant woman or can affect reproduction capacity. Digoxin should be given to a pregnant woman only if clearly needed.

Nursing Mothers: Studies have shown that digoxin concentrations in the mother's serum and milk are similar. However, the estimated daily dose to a nursing infant will be far below the usual infant maintenance dose. Therefore, this amount should have no pharmacologic effect upon the infant. Nevertheless, caution should be exercised when digoxin is administered to a nursing woman.

ADVERSE REACTIONS

The frequency and severity of adverse reactions to digoxin depend on the dose and route of administration, as well as on the patient's underlying disease or concomitant therapies (see PRECAUTIONS section and Serum Digoxin Concentrations subsection of DOSAGE AND ADMINISTRATION). The overall incidence of adverse reactions has been reported as 5 to 20%, with 15 to 20% of them being considered serious (one to four percent of patients receiving digoxin). Evidence suggests that the incidence of toxicity has decreased since the introduction of the serum digoxin assay and improved standardization of digoxin tablets. Cardiac toxicity accounts for about one-half, gastrointestinal disturbances for about one-fourth, and CNS and other toxicity for about one-fourth of these adverse reactions.

Adults:

Cardiac—Unifocal or multiform ventricular premature contractions, especially in bigeminal or trigeminal patterns, are the most common arrhythmias associated with digoxin toxicity in adults with heart disease. Ventricular tachycardia may result from digitalis toxicity. Atrioventricular (AV) dissociation, accelerated junctional (nodal) rhythm and atrial tachycardia with block are also common arrhythmias caused by digoxin overdosage.

Excessive slowing of the pulse is a clinical sign of digoxin overdosage. AV block (Wenckebach) of increasing degree may proceed to complete heart block.

Note: The electrocardiogram is fundamental in determining the presence and nature of these cardiac disturbances. Digoxin may also induce other changes in the ECG (e.g. PR prolongation, ST depression), which represent digoxin effect and may or may not be associated with digitalis toxicity.

Gastrointestinal—Anorexia, nausea, vomiting and less commonly diarrhea are common early symptoms of overdosage. However, uncontrolled heart failure may also produce such symptoms. Digitalis toxicity very rarely may cause abdominal pain and hemorrhagic necrosis of the intestines.

CNS—Visual disturbances (blurred or yellow vision), headache, weakness, dizziness, apathy and psychosis can occur.

Other—Gynecomastia is occasionally observed. Maculopapular rash or other skin reactions are rarely observed.

Infants and Children: Toxicity differs from the adult in a number of respects. Anorexia, nausea, vomiting, diarrhea and CNS disturbances may be present but are rare as initial symptoms in infants. Cardiac arrhythmias are more reliable signs of toxicity. Digoxin in children may produce any arrhythmia. The most commonly encountered are conduction disturbances or supraventricular tachyarrhythmias, such as atrial tachycardia with or without block, and junctional (nodal) tachycardia. Ventricular arrhythmias are less common. Sinus bradycardia may also be a sign of impending digoxin intoxication, expecially in infants, even in the absence of first degree heart block. Any arrhythmia or alteration in cardiac conduction that develops in a child taking digoxin should initially be assumed to be a consequence of digoxin intoxication.

OVERDOSAGE

Treatment of Arrhythmias Produced by Overdosage:

Adults: Digoxin should be discontinued until all signs of toxicity are gone. Discontinuation may be all that is necessary if toxic manifestations are not severe and appear only near the expected time for maximum effect of the drug.

Correction of factors that may contribute to toxicity such as electrolyte disturbances, hypoxia, acid-base disturbances and removal of aggravating agents such as catecholamines, should also be considered. Potassium salts may be indicated, particularly if hypokalemia is present. Potassium administration may be dangerous in the setting of massive digitalis overdosage (see Massive Digitalis Overdosage subsection below). Potassium chloride in divided oral doses totaling 3 to

Continued on next page

Burroughs Wellcome—Cont.

6 grams of the salt (40 to 80 mEq K+) for adults may be given provided renal function is adequate (see below for potassium recommendations in Infants and Children).

When correction of the arrhythmia is urgent and the serum potassium concentration is low or normal, potassium should be administered intravenously in 5% dextrose injection. For adults, a total of 40 to 80 mEq (diluted to a concentration of 40 mEq per 500 mL) may be given at a rate not exceeding 20 mEq per hour, or slower if limited by pain due to local irritation. Additional amounts may be given if the arrhythmia is uncontrolled and potassium well-tolerated. ECG monitoring should be performed to watch for any evidence of potassium toxicity (e.g. peaking of T waves) and to observe the effect on the arrhythmia. The infusion may be stopped when the desired effect is achieved.

Note: Potassium should not be used and may be dangerous in heart block due to digoxin, unless primarily related to supraventricular tachycardia.

Other agents that have been used for the treatment of digoxin intoxication include lidocaine, procainamide, propranolol and phenytoin, although use of the latter must be considered experimental. In advanced heart block, atropine and/or temporary ventricular pacing may be beneficial. Digibind®, Digoxin Immune Fab (Ovine), can be used to reverse potentially life-threatening digoxin (or digitoxin) intoxication. Improvement in signs and symptoms of digitalis toxicity usually begins within $\frac{1}{2}$ hour of Digibind administration. Each 40 mg vial of Digibind will neutralize 0.6 mg of digoxin (which is a usual body store of an adequately digitalized 70 kg patient).

Infants and Children: See Adult section for general recommendations for the treatment of arrhythmias produced by overdosage and for cautions regarding the use of potassium. If a potassium preparation is used to treat toxicity, it may be given orally in divided doses totaling 1 to 1.5 mEq K+ per kilogram (kg) body weight (1 gram of potassium chloride contains 13.4 mEq K+).

When correction of the arrhythmia with potassium is urgent, approximately 0.5 mEq/kg of potassium per hour may be given intravenously, with careful ECG monitoring. The intravenous solution of potassium should be dilute enough to avoid local irritation; however, especially in infants, care must be taken to avoid intravenous fluid overload.

Massive Digitalis Overdosage: Manifestations of life-threatening toxicity include severe ventricular arrhythmias such as ventricular tachycardia or ventricular fibrillation, or progressive bradyarrhythmias such as severe sinus bradycardia or second or third degree heart block not responsive to atropine. An overdosage of more than 10 mg of digoxin in previously healthy adults or 4 mg in previously healthy children or overdosage resulting in steady-state serum concentrations greater than 10 ng/mL, often results in cardiac arrest.

Severe digitalis intoxication can cause life-threatening elevation in serum potassium concentration by shifting potassium from inside to outside the cell resulting in hyperkalemia. Administration of potassium supplements in the setting of massive intoxication may be hazardous.

Digbind®, Digoxin Immune Fab (Ovine), may be used at a dose equimolar to digoxin in the body to reverse the effects of ingestion of a massive overdose. The decision to administer Digibind before the onset of toxic manifestations will depend on the likelihood that life-threatening toxicity will occur (see above).

Patients with massive digitalis ingestion should receive large doses of activated charcoal to prevent absorption and bind digoxin in the gut during enteroenteric recirculation. Emesis of gastric lavage may be indicated especially if ingestion has occurred within 30 minutes of the patient's presentation at the hospital. Emesis should not be induced in patients who are obtunded. If a patient presents more than 2 hours after ingestion or already has toxic manifestations, it may be unsafe to induce vomiting or attempt passage of a gastric tube, because such maneuvers may induce an acute vagal episode that can worsen digitalis-toxic arrhythmias.

DOSAGE AND ADMINISTRATION

Recommended dosages are average values that may require considerable modification because of individual sensitivity or associated conditions. Diminished renal function is the most important factor requiring modification of recommended doses.

Parenteral administration of digoxin should be used only when the need for rapid digitalization is urgent or when the drug cannot be taken orally. Intramuscular injection can lead to severe pain at the injection site, thus intravenous administration is preferred. If the drug must be administered by the intramuscular route, it should be injected deep into the muscle followed by massage. No more than 500 µg (2 mL) should be injected into a single site. Lanoxin® Injection can be administered undiluted or diluted with a 4-fold or greater volume of Sterile Water for Injection, 0.9% Sodium Chloride Injection or 5% Dextrose Injection. The use of less than a 4-fold volume of diluent could lead to precipitation of the digoxin. Immediate use of the diluted product is recommended.

If tuberculin syringes are used to measure very small doses, one must be aware of the problem of inadvertent overadministration of digoxin. The syringe should *not* be flushed with the parenteral solution after its contents are expelled into an indwelling vascular catheter.

Slow infusion of Lanoxin® Injection is preferable to bolus administration. Rapid infusion of digitalis glycosides has been shown to cause systemic and coronary arteriolar constriction, which may be clinically undesirable. Caution is thus advised and Lanoxin Injection should probably be administered over a period of 5 minutes or longer. Mixing of Lanoxin Injections with other drugs in the same container or simultaneous administration in the same intravenous line is not recommended.

In deciding the dose of digoxin, several factors must be considered:

1. The disease being treated. Atrial arrhythmias may require larger doses than heart failure.
2. The body weight of the patient. Doses should be calculated based upon lean or ideal body weight.
3. The patient's renal function, preferably evaluated on the basis of creatinine clearance.
4. Age is an important factor in infants and children.
5. Concomitant disease states, drugs or other factors likely to alter the expected clinical response to digoxin (see PRECAUTIONS and Drug Interactions sections).

Digitalization may be accomplished by either of two general approaches that vary in dosage and frequency of administration, but reach the same endpoint in terms of total amount of digoxin accumulated in the body.

1. Rapid digitalization may be achieved by administering a loading dose based upon projected peak body digoxin stores, then calculating the maintenance dose as a percentage of the loading dose.
2. More gradual digitalization may be obtained by beginning an appropriate maintenance dose, thus allowing digoxin body stores to accumulate slowly. Steady-state serum digoxin concentrations will be achieved in approximately 5 half-lives of the drug for the individual patient. Depending upon the patient's renal function, this will take between one and three weeks.

Adults:

Adults—Rapid Digitalization with a Loading Dose: Peak body digoxin stores of 8 to 12 µg/kg should provide therapeutic effect with minimum risk of toxicity in most patients with heart failure and normal sinus rhythm. Larger stores (10 to 15 µg/kg) are often required for adequate control of ventricular rate in patients with atrial flutter or fibrillation. Because of altered digoxin distribution and elimination, projected peak body stores for patients with renal insufficiency should be conservative (i.e. 6 to 10 µg/kg) [see PRECAUTIONS section].

The loading dose should be based on the projected peak body stores and administered in several portions, with roughly half the total given as the first dose. Additional fractions of this planned total dose may be given at 4 to 8 hour intervals, **with careful assessment of clinical response before each additional dose.**

If the patient's clinical response necessitates a change from the calculated dose of digoxin, then calculation of the maintenance dose should be based upon the amount actually given.

In previously undigitalized patients, a single initial intravenous Lanoxin® Injection dose of 400 to 600 µg (0.4 to 0.6 mg) usually produces a detectable effect in 5 to 30 minutes that becomes maximal in 1 to 4 hours. Additional doses of 100 to 300 µg (0.1 to 0.3 mg) may be given cautiously at 4 to 8 hour intervals until clinical evidence of an adequate effect is noted. The usual amount of Lanoxin Injection that a 70 kg patient requires to achieve 8 to 15 µg/kg peak body stores is 600 to 1000 µg (0.6 to 1.0 mg).

$$\text{Maintenance Dose} = \text{Peak Body Stores (i.e. Loading Dose)} \times \frac{\% \text{ Daily Loss}}{100}$$

$$\text{Where: } \% \text{ Daily Loss} = 14 + Ccr/5$$

Although peak body stores are mathematically related to loading doses and are utilized to calculate maintenance doses, they do not correlate with measured serum concentrations. This discrepancy is caused by digoxin distribution within the body during the first 6 to 8 hours following a dose. Serum concentrations drawn during this time are usually not interpretable.

The maintenance dose should be based upon the percentage of the peak body stores lost each day through elimination. The following formula has a wide clinical use:
[See above.]

Ccr is creatinine clearance, corrected to 70 kg body weight or 1.73 m² body surface area. *For adults*, if only serum creatinine concentrations (Scr) are available, a Ccr (corrected to 70 kg body weight) may be estimated in men as (140 –Age)/Scr. For women, this result should be multiplied by 0.85.

Note: This equation cannot be used for estimating creatinine clearance in infants or children.

A common practice involves the use of Lanoxin® Injection to achieve rapid digitalization, with conversion to Lanoxin Tablets or Lanoxicaps for maintenance therapy. If patients are switched from IV to oral digoxin formulations, allowances must be made for differences in bioavailability when calculating maintenance dosages (see table, CLINICAL PHARMACOLOGY section).

Infants and Children: Digitalization must be individualized. Divided daily dosing is recommended for infants and young children. Children over 10 years of age require adult dosages in proportion to their body weight.

In the newborn period, renal clearance of digoxin is diminished and suitable dosage adjustments must be observed. This is especially pronounced in the premature infant. Beyond the immediate newborn period, children generally require proportionally larger doses than adults on the basis of body weight or body surface area.

Infants and Children—Rapid Digitalization with a Loading Dose: Lanoxin Injection Pediatric can be used to achieve rapid digitalization, with conversion to an oral Lanoxin formulation for maintenance therapy. If patients are switched from IV to oral digoxin tablets or elixir, allowances must be made for differences in bioavailability when calculating maintenance dosages (see bioavailability table in CLINICAL PHARMACOLOGY section and dosing table next page). Intramuscular injection of digoxin is extremely painful and offers no advantages unless other routes of administration are contraindicated.

Digitalizing and daily maintenance doses for each age group are given below and should provide therapeutic effect with minimum risk of toxicity in most patients with heart failure and normal sinus rhythm. Larger doses are often required for adequate control of ventricular rate in patients with atrial flutter or fibrillation.

The loading dose should be administered in several portions, with roughly half the total given as the first dose. Additional fractions of this planned total dose may be given at 4 to 8 hour intervals, **with careful assessment of clinical response before each additional dose.** If the patient's clinical response necessitates a change from the calculated dose of digoxin, then calculation of the maintenance dose should be based upon the amount actually given.
[See table below.]

Infants and Children—Gradual Digitalization With A Maintenance Dose: More gradual digitalization can also be accomplished by beginning an appropriate maintenance dose. The range of percentages provided above can be used in calculating this dose for patients with normal renal function. In children with renal disease, digoxin dosing must be carefully titrated based upon clinical response.

Long-term use of digoxin is indicated in many children who have been digitalized for acute heart failure, unless the cause is transient. Children with severe congenital heart disease, even after surgery, may require digoxin for prolonged periods.

It cannot be overemphasized that both the adult and pediatric dosage guidelines provided are based upon average patient response and substantial individual variation can be

Usual Digitalizing and Maintenance Dosages for Lanoxin® Injection
in Children with **Normal Renal Function Based on Lean Body Weight**

Age	Digitalizing* Dose (µg/kg)	Daily† IV Maintenance Dose (µg/kg)
2 to 5 Years	25 to 35	
5 to 10 Years	15 to 30	25 to 35% of the IV loading dose‡
Over 10 years	8 to 12	

*   IV digitalizing doses are 80% of oral digitalizing doses.
†   Divided daily dosing is recommended for children under 10 years of age.
‡   Projected or actual digitalizing dose providing clinical response.

expected. Accordingly, ultimate dosage selection must be based upon clinical assessment of the patient.

Serum Digoxin Concentrations: Measurement of serum digoxin concentrations can be helpful to the clinician in determining the state of digitalization and in assigning certain probabilities to the likelihood of digoxin intoxication. Studies in adults considered adequately digitalized (without evidence of toxicity) show that about two-thirds of such patients have serum digoxin levels ranging from 0.8 to 2.0 ng/mL. Patients with atrial fibrillation or atrial flutter require and appear to tolerate higher levels than do patients with other indications. On the other hand, in adult patients with clinical evidence of digoxin toxicity, about two-thirds will have serum digoxin levels greater than 2.0 ng/mL. Thus, whereas levels less than 0.8 ng/mL are infrequently associated with toxicity, levels greater than 2.0 ng/mL are often associated with toxicity. Values in between are not very helpful in deciding whether a certain sign or symptom is more likely caused by digoxin toxicity or by something else. There are rare patients who are unable to tolerate digoxin even at serum concentrations below 0.8 ng/mL. Some researchers suggest that infants and young children tolerate slightly higher serum concentrations than do adults.

To allow adequate time for equilibration of digoxin between serum and tissue, **sampling of serum concentrations for clinical use should be at least 6 to 8 hours after the last dose,** regardless of the route of administration or formulation used. On a twice daily dosing schedule, there will be only minor differences in serum digoxin concentrations whether sampling is done at 8 or 12 hours after a dose. After a single daily dose, the concentration will be 10 to 25% lower when sampled at 24 versus 8 hours, depending upon the patient's renal function. Ideally, sampling for assessment of steady-state concentrations should be done just before the next dose.

If a discrepancy exists between the reported serum concentration and the observed clinical response, the clinician should consider the following possibilities:

1. Analytical problems in the assay procedure.
2. Inappropriate serum sampling time.
3. Administration of a digitalis glycoside other than digoxin.
4. Conditions (described in WARNINGS and PRECAUTIONS sections) causing an alteration in the sensitivity of the patient to digoxin.
5. The patient falls outside the norm in his response to or handling of digoxin. This decision should only be reached after exclusion of the other possibilities and generally should be confirmed by additional correlations of clinical observations with serum digoxin concentrations.

The serum concentration data should always be interpreted in the overall clinical context and an isolated serum concentration value should not be used alone as a basis for increasing or decreasing digoxin dosage.

Adjustment of Maintenance Dose in Previously Digitalized Patients: Lanoxin® Injection maintenance doses in individual patients on steady-state digoxin can be adjusted upward or downward in proportion to the ratio of the desired versus the measured serum concentration. For example, a patient at steady-state on 100 µg (0.1 mg) of Lanoxin Injection per day with a measured serum concentration of 0.7 ng/mL, should have the dose increased to 200 µg (0.2 mg) per day to achieve a steady-state serum concentration of 1.4 ng/mL, **assuming the serum digoxin concentration measurement is correct, renal function remains stable during this time and the needed adjustment is not the result of a problem with compliance.**

Dosage Adjustment When Changing Preparations: The difference in bioavailability between injectable Lanoxin or Lanoxicaps and Lanoxin Elixir Pediatric or Lanoxin Tablets must be considered when changing patients from one dosage form to another.

Lanoxin Injection and Lanoxicaps doses of 100 µg (0.1 mg) and 200 µg (0.2 mg) are approximately equivalent to 125 µg (0.125 mg) and 250 µg (0.25 mg) doses of Lanoxin Tablets and Elixir Pediatric (see table in CLINICAL PHARMACOLOGY section). Intramuscular injection of digoxin is extremely painful and offers no advantages unless other routes of administration are contraindicated.

HOW SUPPLIED

LANOXIN® (DIGOXIN) INJECTION, 500 µg (0.5 mg) in 2 mL (250 µg [0.25 mg] per mL); Boxes of 10 (NDC 0081-0260-10) and 50 ampuls (NDC 0081-0260-35).

Store at 15° to 25°C (59° to 77°F) and protect from light.

Also available:

LANOXIN (DIGOXIN) TABLETS, Scored 125 µg (0.125 mg): bottles of 30 (with child-resistant cap), 100 and 1000; unit dose pack of 100.

LANOXIN (DIGOXIN) TABLETS, Scored 250 µg (0.25 mg): bottles of 30 (with child-resistant cap), 100, 1000 and 5000; unit dose pack of 100.

LANOXIN (DIGOXIN) TABLETS, Scored 500 µg (0.5 mg): bottle of 100.

LANOXIN (DIGOXIN) ELIXIR PEDIATRIC, 50 µg (0.05 mg) per mL: bottle of 60 mL with calibrated dropper.

LANOXIN (DIGOXIN) INJECTION PEDIATRIC, 100 µg (0.1 mg) in 1 mL: box of 10 ampuls.

LANOXICAPS® (DIGOXIN SOLUTION IN CAPSULES), 50 µg (0.05 mg) bottle of 100; 100 µg (0.1 mg) bottles of 30 (with child-resistant cap) and 100, 200 µg (0.2 mg) bottles of 30 (with child-resistant cap) and 100.

LANOXIN® INJECTION PEDIATRIC ℞

[*lă-nŏx'ĭn"*]

(Digoxin)

100 µg (0.1 mg) in 1 mL

DESCRIPTION

Digoxin is one of the cardiac (or digitalis) glycosides, a closely related group of drugs having in common specific effects on the myocardium. These drugs are found in a number of plants. Digoxin is extracted from the leaves of *Digitalis lanata*. The term "digitalis" is used to designate the whole group. The glycosides are composed of two portions: a sugar and a cardenolide (hence "glycosides").

Digoxin has the molecular formula $C_{41}H_{64}O_{14}$, a molecular weight of 780.95 and melting and decomposition points above 235°C. The drug is practically insoluble in water and in ether; slightly soluble in diluted (50%) alcohol and in chloroform; and freely soluble in pyridine. Digoxin powder is composed of odorless white crystals.

Digoxin has the chemical name: 3β-[(*O*-2,6-dideoxy-β-*D-ribo*-hexopyranosyl-(1→4)-*O*-2,6-dideoxy-β-*D-ribo*-hexopyranosyl-(1→4)-2,6-dideoxy-β-*D-ribo*-hexopyranosyl)-oxy]-12β, 14-dihydroxy-5β-card-20(22)-enolide.

Lanoxin (Digoxin) Injection Pediatric is a sterile solution of digoxin for intravenous or intramuscular injection. The vehicle contains 40% propylene glycol and 10% alcohol. The injection is buffered to a pH of 6.8 to 7.2 with 0.17% sodium phosphate and 0.08% anhydrous citric acid. Each 1 mL ampul contains 100 µg (0.1 mg) digoxin. Dilution is not required.

CLINICAL PHARMACOLOGY

Mechanism of Action: The influence of digitalis glycosides on the myocardium is dose-related, and involves both a direct action on cardiac muscle and the specialized conduction system, and indirect actions on the cardiovascular system mediated by the autonomic nervous system. The indirect actions mediated by the autonomic nervous system involve a vagomimetic action, which is responsible for the effects of digitalis on the sino-atrial (SA) and atrioventricular (AV) nodes; and also a baroreceptor sensitization which results in increased carotid sinus nerve activity and enhanced sympathetic withdrawal for any given increment in mean arterial pressure. The pharmacologic consequences of these direct and indirect effects are: 1) an increase in the force and velocity of myocardial systolic contraction (positive inotropic action); 2) a slowing of heart rate (negative chronotropic effect); and 3) decreased conduction velocity through the AV node. In higher doses, digitalis increases sympathetic outflow from the central nervous system (CNS) to both cardiac and peripheral sympathetic nerves. This increase in sympathetic activity may be an important factor in digitalis cardiac toxicity. Most of the extracardiac manifestations of digitalis toxicity are also mediated by the CNS.

Pharmacokinetics: Note: The following data are from studies performed in adults, unless otherwise stated.

Absorption—A comparison of the systemic availability and equivalent doses for digoxin preparations are shown in the following table:

[See first table below.]

Distribution—Following drug administration, a 6 to 8 hour distribution phase is observed. This is followed by a much more gradual serum concentration decline, which is dependent on digoxin elimination from the body. The peak height and slope of the early portion (absorption/distribution phases) of the serum concentration-time curve are dependent upon the route of administration and the absorption characteristics of the formulation. Clinical evidence indicates that the early high serum concentrations do not reflect the concentration of digoxin at its site of action, but that with chronic use, the steady-state post-distribution serum levels are in equilibrium with tissue levels and correlate with pharmacologic effects. In individual patients, these post-distribution serum concentrations are linearly related to maintenance dosage and may be useful in evaluating therapeutic and toxic effects (see Serum Digoxin Concentrations in DOSAGE AND ADMINISTRATION section).

Digoxin is concentrated in tissues and therefore has a large apparent volume of distribution. Digoxin crosses both the blood-brain barrier and the placenta. At delivery, serum digoxin concentration in the newborn is similar to the serum level in the mother. Approximately 20 to 25% of plasma digoxin is bound to protein. Serum digoxin concentrations are not significantly altered by large changes in fat tissue weight, so that its distribution space correlates best with lean (ideal) body weight, not total body weight.

Pharmacologic Response—The approximate times to onset of effect and to peak effect of all the Lanoxin® preparations are given in the following table:

[See bottom table.]

Excretion—Elimination of digoxin follows first-order kinetics (that is, the quantity of digoxin eliminated at any time is proportional to the total body content). Following intravenous administration to normal subjects, 50 to 70% of a digoxin dose is excreted unchanged in the urine. Renal excretion of digoxin is proportional to glomerular filtration rate and is largely independent of urine flow. In subjects with normal renal function, digoxin has a half-life of 1.5 to 2.0 days. The half-life in anuric patients is prolonged to 4 to 6 days. Digoxin is not effectively removed from the body by dialysis, exchange transfusion or during cardiopulmonary by-pass because most of the drug is in tissue rather than circulating in the blood.

INDICATIONS AND USAGE

Heart Failure: The increased cardiac output resulting from the inotropic action of digoxin ameliorates the disturbances characteristic of heart failure (venous congestion, edema, dyspnea, orthopnea and cardiac asthma).

Digoxin is more effective in "low output" (pump) failure than in "high output" heart failure secondary to arteriovenous fistula, anemia, infection or hyperthyroidism.

Digoxin is usually continued after failure is controlled, unless some known precipitating factor is corrected. Studies have shown, however, that even though hemodynamic effects can be demonstrated in almost all patients, corresponding improvement in the signs and symptoms of heart failure is not necessarily apparent. Therefore, in patients in whom digoxin may be difficult to regulate, or in whom the risk of toxicity may be great (e.g., patients with unstable renal function or whose potassium levels tend to fluctuate) a cautious withdrawal of digoxin may be considered. If digoxin is discontinued, the patient should be regularly monitored for clinical evidence of recurrent heart failure.

Atrial Fibrillation: Digoxin reduces ventricular rate and thereby improves hemodynamics. Palpitation, precordial distress or weakness are relieved and concomitant conges-

PRODUCT	ABSOLUTE BIOAVAILABILITY	EQUIVALENT DOSES (IN MG*)		
Lanoxin Tablet	60–80%	0.125	0.25	0.5
Lanoxin Elixir	70–85%	0.125	0.25	0.5
Lanoxin Injection/IM	70–85%	0.125	0.25	0.5
Lanoxin Injection/IV	100%	0.1	0.2	0.4
Lanoxicaps Capsules	90–100%	0.1	0.2	0.4

*1 mg = 1000 µg

PRODUCT	TIME TO ONSET OF EFFECT*	TIME TO PEAK EFFECT*
Lanoxin Tablet	0.5–2 hours	2–6 hours
Lanoxin Elixir	0.5–2 hours	2–6 hours
Lanoxin Injection/IM	0.5–2 hours	2–6 hours
Lanoxin Injection/IV	5–30 minutes†	1–4 hours
Lanoxicaps Capsules	0.5–2 hours	2–6 hours

*Documented for ventricular response rate in atrial fibrillation, inotropic effect and electrocardiographic changes.

†Depending upon rate of infusion.

Continued on next page

Burroughs Wellcome—Cont.

tive failure ameliorated. Digoxin should be continued in doses necessary to maintain the desired ventricular rate.

Atrial Flutter: Digoxin slows the heart and regular sinus rhythm may appear. Frequently the flutter is converted to atrial fibrillation with a controlled ventricular response. Digoxin treatment should be maintained if atrial fibrillation persists. (Electrical cardioversion is often the treatment of choice for atrial flutter. See discussion of cardioversion in PRECAUTIONS section.)

Paroxysmal Atrial Tachycardia (PAT): Digoxin may convert PAT to sinus rhythm by slowing conduction through the AV node. If heart failure has ensued or paroxysms recur frequently, digoxin should be continued. In infants, digoxin is usually continued for 3 to 6 months after a single episode of PAT to prevent recurrence.

CONTRAINDICATIONS

Digitalis glycosides are contraindicated in ventricular fibrillation.

In a given patient, an untoward effect requiring permanent discontinuation of other digitalis preparations usually constitutes a contraindication to digoxin. Hypersensitivity to digoxin itself is a contraindication to its use. Allergy to digoxin, though rare, does occur. It may not extend to all such preparations, and another digitalis glycoside may be tried with caution.

WARNINGS

Anorexia, nausea, vomiting and arrhythmias may accompany heart failure or may be indications of digitalis intoxication. Clinical evaluation of the cause of these symptoms should be attempted before further digitalis administration. In such circumstances determination of the serum digoxin concentration may be an aid in deciding whether or not digitalis toxicity is likely to be present. If the possibility of digitalis intoxication cannot be excluded, cardiac glycosides should be temporarily withheld, if permitted by the clinical situation.

Patients with renal insufficiency require smaller than usual maintenance doses of digoxin (see DOSAGE AND ADMINISTRATION section).

Heart failure accompanying acute glomerulonephritis requires extreme care in digitalization. Relatively low loading and maintenance doses and concomitant use of antihypertensive drugs may be necessary and careful monitoring is essential. Digoxin should be discontinued as soon as possible.

Patients with severe carditis, such as carditis associated with rheumatic fever or viral myocarditis, are especially sensitive to digoxin-induced disturbances of rhythm.

Newborn infants display considerable variability in their tolerance to digoxin. Premature and immature infants are particularly sensitive, and dosage must not only be reduced but must be individualized according to their degree of maturity.

Note: Digitalis glycosides are an important cause of accidental poisoning in children.

PRECAUTIONS

General: Digoxin toxicity develops more frequently and lasts longer in patients with renal impairment because of the decreased excretion of digoxin. Therefore, it should be anticipated that dosage requirements will be decreased in patients with moderate to severe renal disease (see DOSAGE AND ADMINISTRATION section). Because of the prolonged half-life, a longer period of time is required to achieve an initial or new steady-state concentration in patients with renal impairment than in patients with normal renal function.

In patients with hypokalemia, toxicity may occur despite serum digoxin concentrations within the "normal range," because potassium depletion sensitizes the myocardium to digoxin. Therefore, it is desirable to maintain normal serum potassium levels in patients being treated with digoxin. Hypokalemia may result from diuretic, amphotericin B or corticosteroid therapy, and from dialysis or mechanical suction of gastrointestinal secretions. It may also accompany malnutrition, diarrhea, prolonged vomiting, old age and long-standing heart failure. In general, rapid changes in serum potassium or other electrolytes should be avoided, and intravenous treatment with potassium should be reserved for special circumstances as described below (see TREATMENT OF ARRHYTHMIAS PRODUCED BY OVERDOSAGE section).

Calcium, particularly when administered rapidly by the intravenous route, may produce serious arrythmias in digitalized patients. Hypercalcemia from any cause predisposes the patient to digitalis toxicity. On the other hand, hypocalcemia can nullify the effects of digoxin in man; thus, digoxin may be ineffective until serum calcium is restored to normal. These interactions are related to the fact that calcium affects contractility and excitability of the heart in a manner similar to digoxin.

Hypomagnesemia may predispose to digitalis toxicity. If low magnesium levels are detected in a patient on digoxin, replacement therapy should be instituted.

Quinidine, verapamil, amiodarone, and propafenone cause a rise in serum digoxin concentration, with the implication that digitalis intoxication may result. This rise appears to be proportional to the dose. The effect is mediated by a reduction in the digoxin clearance and, in the case of quinidine, decreased volume of distribution as well.

Patients with acute myocardial infarction or severe pulmonary disease may be unusually sensitive to digoxin-induced disturbances of rhythm.

Atrial arrhythmias associated with hypermetabolic states (e.g. hyperthyroidism) are particularly resistant to digoxin treatment. Large doses of digoxin are not recommended as the only treatment of these arrhythmias and care must be taken to avoid toxicity if large doses of digoxin are required.

In hypothyroidism, the digoxin requirements are reduced. Digoxin responses in patients with compensated thyroid disease are normal.

Reduction of digoxin dosage may be desirable prior to electrical cardioversion to avoid induction of ventricular arrhythmias, but the physician must consider the consequences of rapid increase in ventricular response to atrial fibrillation if digoxin is withheld 1 to 2 days prior to cardioversion. If there is a suspicion that digitalis toxicity exists, elective cardioversion should be delayed. If it is not prudent to delay cardioversion, the energy level selected should be minimal at first and carefully increased in an attempt to avoid precipitating ventricular arrhythmias.

Incomplete AV block, especially in patients with Stokes-Adams attacks, may progress to advanced or complete heart block if digoxin is given.

In some patients with sinus node disease (i.e. Sick Sinus Syndrome), digoxin may worsen sinus bradycardia or sinoatrial block.

In patients with Wolff-Parkinson-White Syndrome and atrial fibrillation, digoxin can enhance transmission of impulses through the accessory pathway. This effect may result in extremely rapid ventricular rates and even ventricular fibrillation.

Digoxin may worsen the outflow obstruction in patients with idiopathic hypertrophic subaortic stenosis (HSS). Unless cardiac failure is severe, it is doubtful whether digoxin should be employed.

Patients with chronic constrictive pericarditis may fail to respond to digoxin. In addition, slowing of the heart rate by digoxin in some patients may further decrease cardiac output.

Patients with heart failure from amyloid heart disease or constrictive cardiomyopathies respond poorly to treatment with digoxin.

Digoxin is not indicated for the treatment of sinus tachycardia unless it is associated with heart failure.

Digoxin may produce false positive ST-T changes in the electrocardiogram during exercise testing.

Intramuscular injection of digoxin is extremely painful and offers no advantages unless other routes of administration are contraindicated.

Laboratory Tests: Patients receiving digoxin should have their serum electrolytes and renal function (BUN and/or serum creatinine) assessed periodically; the frequency of assessments will depend on the clinical setting. For discussion of serum digoxin concentrations, see DOSAGE AND ADMINISTRATION section.

Drug Interactions: Potassium-depleting *corticosteroids* and *diuretics* may be major contributing factors to digitalis toxicity. *Calcium,* particularly if administered rapidly by the intravenous route, may produce serious arrhythmias in digitalized patients. *Quinidine, verapamil, amiodarone,* and *propafenone* cause a rise in serum digoxin concentration, with the implication that digitalis intoxication may result. Certain *antibiotics* increase digoxin absorption in patients who inactivate digoxin by bacterial metabolism in the lower intestine, so that digitalis intoxication may result. *Propantheline* and *diphenoxylate,* by decreasing gut motility, may increase digoxin absorption. *Antacids, kaolin-pectin, sulfasalazine, neomycin, cholestyramine* and certain *anticancer drugs* may interfere with intestinal digoxin absorption, resulting in unexpectedly low serum concentrations. There have been inconsistent reports regarding the effects of other drugs on the serum digoxin concentration. *Thyroid* administration to a digitalized, hypothyroid patient may increase the dose requirement of digoxin. Concomitant use of digoxin and *sympathomimetics* increases the risk of cardiac arrhythmias because both enhance ectopic pacemaker activity. *Succinylcholine* may cause a sudden extrusion of potassium from muscle cells, and may thereby cause arrhythmias in digitalized patients. Although β adrenergic blockers or calcium channel blockers and digoxin may be useful in combination to control atrial fibrillation, their additive effects on AV node conduction can result in complete heart block.

Due to the considerable variability of these interactions, digoxin dosage should be carefully individualized when patients receive coadministered medications. Furthermore, caution should be exercised when combining digoxin with any drug that may cause a significant deterioration in renal function, since this may impair the excretion of digoxin.

Carcinogenesis, Mutagenesis, Impairment of Fertility: There have been no long-term studies performed in animals to evaluate carcinogenic potential.

ADVERSE REACTIONS

The frequency and severity of adverse reactions to digoxin depend on the dose and route of administration, as well as on the patient's underlying disease or concomitant therapies (see PRECAUTIONS section and Serum Digoxin Concentrations subsection of DOSAGE AND ADMINISTRATION).

The overall incidence of adverse reactions in adults has been reported as 5 to 20%, with 15 to 20% of them being considered serious (one to four percent of patients receiving digoxin). Evidence suggests that the incidence of toxicity has decreased since the introduction of the serum digoxin assay and improved standardization of digoxin tablets. Cardiac toxicity accounts for about one-half, gastrointestinal disturbances for about one-fourth, and CNS and other toxicity for about one-fourth of these adverse reactions.

Cardiac—Conduction disturbances or supraventricular tachyarrhythmias, such as atrioventricular (AV) block (Wenckebach), atrial tachycardia with or without block and junctional (nodal) tachycardia are the most common arrhythmias associated with digoxin toxicity in children. Ventricular arrhythmias, such as unifocal or multiform ventricular premature contractions, especially in bigeminal or trigeminal patterns, are less common. Ventricular tachycardia may result from digitalis toxicity. Sinus bradycardia may also be a sign of impending digoxin intoxication, especially in infants, even in the absence of first degree heart block. Any arrhythmias or alteration in cardiac conduction that develops in a child taking digoxin should initially be assumed to be a consequence of digoxin intoxication.

Note: The electrocardiogram is fundamental in determining the presence and nature of these cardiac disturbances. Digoxin may also induce other changes in the ECG (e.g. PR prolongation, ST depression), which represent digoxin effect and may or may not be associated with digitalis toxicity.

Gastrointestinal—Anorexia, nausea, vomiting and diarrhea may be early symptoms of overdosage. However, uncontrolled heart failure may also produce such symptoms. Digitalis toxicity very rarely may cause abdominal pain and hemorrhagic necrosis of the intestines.

CNS—Visual disturbances (blurred or yellow vision), headache, weakness, dizziness, apathy and psychosis can occur. These may be difficult to recognize in infants and children.

Other—Gynecomastia is occasionally observed. Maculopapular rash or other skin reactions are rarely observed.

OVERDOSAGE

Treatment of Arrhythmias Produced by Overdosage:

Digoxin should be discontinued until all signs of toxicity are gone. Discontinuation may be all that is necessary if toxic manifestations are not severe and appear only near the expected time for maximum effect of the drug.

Correction of factors that may contribute to toxicity such as electrolyte disturbances, hypoxia, acid-base disturbances and removal of aggravating agents such as catecholamines, should also be considered. Potassium salts may be indicated, particularly if hypokalemia is present. Potassium administration may be dangerous in the setting of massive digitalis overdosage (see Massive Digitalis Overdosage subsection below). Potassium chloride in divided oral doses totaling 1 to 5 mEq K+ per kilogram (kg) body weight may be given provided renal function is adequate (1 gram of potassium chloride contains 13.4 mEq K+).

When correction of the arrhythmia with potassium is urgent and the serum potassium concentration is low or normal, approximately 0.5 mEq/kg of potassium per hour may be given intravenously in 5% dextrose injection. The intravenous solution of potassium should be dilute enough to avoid local irritation; however, especially in infants, care must be taken to avoid intravenous fluid overload. ECG monitoring should be performed to watch for any evidence of potassium toxicity (e.g. peaking of T waves) and to observe the effect on the arrhythmia. The infusion may be stopped when the desired effect is achieved.

Note: Potassium should not be used and may be dangerous in heart block due to digoxin, unless primarily related to supraventricular tachycardia.

Other agents that have been used for the treatment of digoxin intoxication include lidocaine, procainamide, propranolol and phenytoin, although use of the latter must be considered experimental. In advanced heart block, atropine and/or temporary ventricular pacing may be beneficial. Digibind®, Digoxin Immune Fab (Ovine), can be used to reverse potentially life-threatening digoxin (or digitoxin) intoxication. Improvement in signs and symptoms of digitalis toxicity usually begins within ½ hour of Digibind administration. Each 40 mg vial of Digibind will neutralize 0.6 mg of digoxin (which is a usual body store of an adequately digitalized 70 kg patient).

Massive Digitalis Overdosage: Manifestations of life-threatening toxicity include severe ventricular arrhythmias such as ventricular tachycardia or ventricular fibrillation, or progressive bradyarrhythmias such as severe sinus brady-

cardia or second or third degree heart block not responsive to atropine. An overdosage of more than 10 mg of digoxin in previously healthy adults or 4 mg in previously healthy children or overdosage resulting in steady-state serum concentrations greater than 10 ng/mL, often results in cardiac arrest.

Severe digitalis intoxication can cause life-threatening elevation in serum potassium concentration by shifting potassium from inside to outside the cell resulting in hyperkalemia. Administration of potassium supplements in the setting of massive intoxication may be hazardous.

Digibind®, Digoxin Immune Fab (Ovine), may be used at a dose equimolar to digoxin in the body to reverse the effects of ingestion of a massive overdose. The decision to administer Digibind before the onset of toxic manifestations will depend on the likelihood that life-threatening toxicity will occur (see above).

Patients with massive digitalis ingestion should receive large doses of activated charcoal to prevent absorption and bind digoxin in the gut during enteroenteric recirculation. Emesis or gastric lavage may be indicated especially if ingestion has occurred within 30 minutes of the patient's presentation at the hospital. Emesis should not be induced in patients who are obtunded. If a patient presents more than 2 hours after ingestion or already has toxic manifestations, it may be unsafe to induce vomiting or attempt passage of a gastric tube, because such maneuvers may induce an acute vagal episode that can worsen digitalis-toxic arrhythmias.

DOSAGE AND ADMINISTRATION

Recommended dosages are average values that may require considerable modification because of individual sensitivity or associated conditions. Diminished renal function is the most important factor requiring modification of recommended doses.

Parenteral administration of digoxin should be used only when the need for rapid digitalization is urgent or when the drug cannot be taken orally. Intramuscular injection can lead to severe pain at the injection site, thus intravenous administration is preferred. If the drug must be administered by the intramuscular route, it should be injected deep into the muscle followed by massage. No more than 200 μg (2 mL) should be injected into a single site.

Lanoxin® Injection Pediatric can be administered undiluted or diluted with a 4-fold or greater volume of Sterile Water for Injection, 0.9% Sodium Chloride Injection or 5% Dextrose Injection. The use of less than a 4-fold volume of diluent could lead to precipitation of the digoxin. Immediate use of the diluted product is recommended.

If tuberculin syringes are used to measure very small doses, one must be aware of the problem of inadvertent overadministration of digoxin. The syringe should *not* be flushed with the parenteral solution after its contents are expelled into an indwelling vascular catheter.

Slow infusion of Lanoxin Injection Pediatric is preferable to bolus administration. Rapid infusion of digitalis glycosides has been shown to cause systemic and coronary arteriolar constriction, which may be clinically undesirable. Caution is thus advised and Lanoxin Injection Pediatric should probably be administered over a period of 5 minutes or longer. Mixing of Lanoxin Injection Pediatric with other drugs in the same container or simultaneous administration in the same intravenous line is not recommended.

Adults: See the Lanoxin Injection package insert for specific recomendations.

Infants and Children: Digitalization must be individualized. Divided daily dosing is recommended for infants and young children. Children over 10 years of age require adult dosages in proportion to their body weight.

In the newborn period, renal clearance of digoxin is diminished and suitable dosage adjustments must be observed. This is especially pronounced in the premature infant. Beyond the immediate newborn period, children generally require proportionally larger doses than adults on the basis of body weight or body surface area.

In deciding the dose of digoxin, several factors must be considered:

1. The disease being treated. Atrial arrhythmias may require larger doses than heart failure.
2. The body weight of the patient. Doses should be calculated based upon lean or ideal body weight.
3. The patient's renal function, preferably evaluated on the basis of creatinine clearance.
4. Age is an important factor in infants and children.
5. Concomitant disease states, drugs or other factors likely to alter the expected clinical response to digoxin (see PRECAUTIONS and Drug Interactions sections).

Digitalization may be accomplished by either of two general approaches that vary in dosage and frequency of administration, but reach the same endpoint in terms of total amount of digoxin accumulated in the body.

1. Rapid digitalization may be achieved by administering a loading dose based upon projected peak body digoxin stores, then calculating the maintenance dose as a percentage of the loading dose.

Usual Digitalizing and Maintenance Dosages for Lanoxin® Injection Pediatric in Children with **Normal Renal Function Based on Lean Body Weight**

Age	Digitalizing* Dose (μg/kg)	Daily† IV Maintenance Dose (μg/kg)
Premature	15 to 25	20 to 30% of the IV loading dose‡
Full-Term	20 to 30	
1 to 24 Months	30 to 50	
2 to 5 Years	25 to 35	
5 to 10 Years	15 to 30	25 to 35% of the IV loading dose
Over 10 Years	8 to 12	

* IV digitalizing doses are 80% of oral digitalizing doses.
† Divided daily dosing is recommended for children under 10 years of age.
‡ Projected or actual digitalizing dose providing clinical response.

---

2. More gradual digitalization may be obtained by beginning an appropriate maintenance dose, thus allowing digoxin body stores to accumulate slowly. Steady-state serum digoxin concentrations will be achieved in approximately 5 half-lives of the drug for the individual patient. Depending upon the patient's renal function, this will take between one and three weeks.

Infants and Children—Rapid Digitalization with a Loading Dose: Lanoxin Injection Pediatric can be used to achieve rapid digitalization, with conversion to an oral Lanoxin formulation for maintenance therapy. If patients are switched from IV to oral digoxin tablets or elixir, allowances must be made for differences in bioavailability when calculating maintenance dosages (see bioavailability table in CLINICAL PHARMACOLOGY section and dosing table below).

Intramuscular injection of digoxin is extremely painful and offers no advantages unless other routes of administration are contraindicated.

Digitalizing and daily maintenance doses for each age group are given below and should provide therapeutic effect with minimum risk of toxicity in most patients with heart failure and normal sinus rhythm. Larger doses are often required for adequate control of ventricular rate in patients with atrial flutter or fibrillation.

The loading dose should be administered in several portions, with roughly half the total given as the first dose. Additional fractions of this planned total dose may be given at 4 to 8 hour intervals, **with careful assessment of clinical response before each additional dose.** If the patient's clinical response necessitates a change from the calculated dose of digoxin, then calculation of the maintenance dose should be based upon the amount actually given.

[See table above.]

Infants and Children—Gradual Digitalization With A Maintenance Dose: More gradual digitalization can also be accomplished by beginning an appropriate maintenance dose. The range of percentages provided above can be used in calculating this dose for patients with normal renal function. In children with renal disease, digoxin dosing must be carefully titrated based upon clinical response.

Long-term use of digoxin is indicated in many children who have been digitalized for acute heart failure, unless the cause is transient. Children with severe congenital heart disease, even after surgery, may require digoxin for prolonged periods.

It cannot be overemphasized that these pediatric dosage guidelines are based upon average patient response and substantial individual variation can be expected. Accordingly, ultimate dosage selection must be based upon clinical assessment of the patient.

Serum Digoxin Concentrations: Measurement of serum digoxin concentrations can be helpful to the clinician in determining the state of digitalization and in assigning certain probabilities to the likelihood of digoxin intoxication. Studies in adults considered adequately digitalized (without evidence of toxicity) show that about two-thirds of such patients have serum digoxin levels ranging from 0.8 to 2.0 ng/mL. Patients with atrial fibrillation or atrial flutter require and appear to tolerate higher levels than do patients with other indications. On the other hand, in adult patients with clinical evidence of digoxin toxicity, about two-thirds will have serum digoxin levels greater than 2.0 ng/mL. Thus, whereas levels less than 0.8 ng/mL are infrequently associated with toxicity, levels greater than 2.0 ng/mL are often associated with toxicity. Values in between are not very helpful in deciding whether a certain sign or symptom is more likely caused by digoxin toxicity or by something else. There are rare patients who are unable to tolerate digoxin even at serum concentrations below 0.8 ng/mL. Some researchers suggest that infants and young children tolerate slightly higher serum concentrations than do adults.

To allow adequate time for equilibration of digoxin between serum and tissue, **sampling of serum concentrations for clinical use should be at least 6 to 8 hours after the last dose,** regardless of the route of administration or formulation used. On a twice daily dosing schedule, there will be only minor differences in serum digoxin concentrations whether

---

sampling is done at 8 or 12 hours after a dose. After a single daily dose, the concentration will be 10 to 25% lower when sampled at 24 versus 8 hours, depending upon the patient's renal function. Ideally, sampling for assessment of steady-state concentrations should be done just before the next dose.

If a discrepancy exists between the reported serum concentration and the observed clinical response, the clinician should consider the following possibilities:

1. Analytical problems in the assay procedure.
2. Inappropriate serum sampling time.
3. Administration of a digitalis glycoside other than digoxin.
4. Conditions (described in WARNINGS and PRECAUTIONS sections) causing an alteration in the sensitivity of the patient to digoxin.
5. The patient falls outside the norm in his response to or handling of digoxin. This decision should only be reached after exclusion of the other possibilities and generally should be confirmed by additional correlations of clinical observations with serum digoxin concentrations.

The serum concentration data should always be interpreted in the overall clinical context and an isolated serum concentration value should not be used alone as a basis for increasing or decreasing digoxin dosage.

Adjustment of Maintenance Dose in Previously Digitalized Patients: Lanoxin® Injection Pediatric maintenance doses in individual patients on steady-state digoxin can be adjusted upward or downward in proportion to the ratio of the desired versus the measured serum concentrations. For example, a patient at steady-state on 100 μg (0.1 mg) of Lanoxin Injection Pediatric per day with a measured serum concentration of 0.7 ng/mL, should have the dose increased to 200 μg (0.2 mg) per day to achieve a steady-state serum concentration of 1.4 ng/mL, **assuming the serum digoxin concentration measurement is correct, renal function remains stable during this time and the needed adjustment is not the result of a problem with compliance.**

Dosage Adjustment When Changing Preparations: The differences in bioavailability between injectable Lanoxin or Lanoxicaps and Lanoxin Elixir Pediatric or Lanoxin Tablets must be considered when changing patients from one dosage form to another.

Lanoxin Injection and Lanoxicaps doses of 100 μg (0.1 mg) and 200 μg (0.2 mg) are approximately equivalent to 125 μg (0.125 mg) and 250 μg (0.25 mg) doses of Lanoxin Tablets and Lanoxin Elixir Pediatric (see table in CLINICAL PHARMACOLOGY section). Intramuscular injection of digoxin is extremely painful and offers no advantages unless other routes of administration are contraindicated.

HOW SUPPLIED

LANOXIN® (DIGOXIN) INJECTION PEDIATRIC, 100 μg (0.1 mg) in 1 mL; box of ampuls (NDC 0081-0262-10).
Store at 15° to 25°C (59° to 77°F) and protect from light.
Also available:

LANOXIN (DIGOXIN) TABLETS, Scored 125 μg (0.125 mg): bottles of 30 (with child-resistant cap), 100 and 1000; unit dose pack of 100.

LANOXIN (DIGOXIN) TABLETS, Scored 250 μg (0.25 mg): bottles of 30 (with child-resistant cap), 100, 1000 and 5000; unit dose pack of 100.

LANOXIN (DIGOXIN) TABLETS, Scored 500 μg (0.5 mg): bottle of 100.

LANOXIN (DIGOXIN) ELIXIR PEDIATRIC, 50 μg (0.05 mg) per mL; bottle of 60 mL with calibrated dropper.

LANOXIN (DIGOXIN) INJECTION, 500 μg (0.5 mg) in 2 mL (250 μg [0.25 mg] per mL): boxes of 10 and 50 ampuls.

LANOXICAPS® (DIGOXIN SOLUTION IN CAPSULES), 50 μg (0.05 mg) bottle of 100; 100 μg (0.1 mg) bottles of 30 (with child-resistant cap) and 100, 200 μg (0.2 mg) bottles of 30 (with child-resistant cap) and 100.

Continued on next page

Burroughs Wellcome—Cont.

PRODUCT	TIME TO ONSET OF EFFECT*	TIME TO PEAK EFFECT*
Lanoxin Tablet	0.5–2 hours	2–6 hours
Lanoxin Elixir	0.5–2 hours	2–6 hours
Lanoxin Injection/IM	0.5–2 hours	2–6 hours
Lanoxin Injection/IV	5–30 minutes†	1–4 hours
Lanoxicaps Capsules	0.5–2 hours	2–6 hours

*Documented for ventricular response rate in atrial fibrillation, inotropic effect and electrocardiographic changes.
†Depending upon rate of infusion.

LANOXIN® TABLETS ℞

[*lă-nŏx'ĭn"*]
(Digoxin)
125 μg (0.125 mg) Scored I.D. Imprint Y3B (yellow)
250 μg (0.25 mg) Scored I.D. Imprint X3A (white)
500 μg (0.5 mg) Scored I.D. Imprint T9A (green)

DESCRIPTION

Digoxin is one of the cardiac (or digitalis) glycosides, a closely related group of drugs having in common specific effects on the myocardium. These drugs are found in a number of plants. Digoxin is extracted from the leaves of *Digitalis lanata.* The term "digitalis" is used to designate the whole group. The glycosides are composed of two portions: a sugar and a cardenolide (hence "glycosides").

Digoxin has the molecular formula $C_{41}H_{64}O_{14}$, a molecular weight of 780.95 and melting and decomposition points above 235°C. The drug is practically insoluble in water and in ether; slightly soluble in diluted (50%) alcohol and in chloroform; and freely soluble in pyridine. Digoxin powder is composed of odorless white crystals.

Digoxin has the chemical name: 3β-[(*O*-2,6-dideoxy-β-*D-ribo*-hexopyranosyl-(1→4)-*O*-2, 6-dideoxy-β-*D-ribo*-hexopyranosyl-(1→4)-2,6-dideoxy-β-*D-ribo*-hexopyranosyl)oxy]-12β, 14-dihydroxy-5β-card-20(22)-enolide.

Lanoxin Tablets with 125 μg (0.125 mg), 250 μg (0.25 mg) or 500 μg (0.5 mg) digoxin USP are intended for oral use. Each tablet contains the labeled amount of digoxin USP and the inactive ingredients: 0.125 mg tablet–corn and potato starch, D&C Yellow No. 10, FD&C Yellow No. 6, lactose, and magnesium stearate; 0.25 mg tablet–corn and potato starch, lactose, magnesium stearate, and stearic acid; 0.5 mg tablet–corn and potato starch, D&C Green No. 5 and Yellow No. 10, FD&C Red No. 40, lactose, magnesium stearate, and stearic acid.

CLINICAL PHARMACOLOGY

Mechanism of Action: The influence of digitalis glycosides on the myocardium is dose-related, and involves both a direct action on cardiac muscle and the specialized conduction system, and indirect actions on the cardiovascular system mediated by the autonomic nervous system. The indirect actions mediated by the autonomic nervous system involve a vagomimetic action, which is responsible for the effects of digitalis on the sino-atrial (SA) and atrioventricular (AV) nodes; and also a baroreceptor sensitization which results in increased carotid sinus nerve activity and enhanced sympathetic withdrawal for any given increment in mean arterial pressure. The pharmacologic consequences of these direct and indirect effects are: 1) an increase in the force and velocity of myocardial systolic contraction (positive inotropic action); 2) a slowing of heart rate (negative chronotropic effect); and 3) decreased conduction velocity through the AV node. In higher doses, digitalis increases sympathetic outflow from the central nervous system (CNS) to both cardiac and peripheral sympathetic nerves. This increase in sympathetic activity may be an important factor in digitalis cardiac toxicity. Most of the extracardiac manifestations of digitalis toxicity are also mediated by the CNS.

Pharmacokinetics:

Absorption—Gastrointestinal absorption of digoxin is a passive process. Absorption of digoxin from the Lanoxin® tablet formulation has been demonstrated to be 60 to 80% complete compared to an identical intravenous dose of digoxin (absolute bioavailability). When digoxin tablets are taken after meals, the rate of absorption is slowed, but the total amount of digoxin absorbed is usually unchanged. When taken with meals high in bran fiber, however, the amount absorbed from an oral dose may be reduced. Comparison of the systemic availability and equivalent doses for digoxin preparations are shown in the following table:
[See table below.]

In some patients, orally administered digoxin is converted to cardioinactive reduction products (e.g., dihydrodigoxin) by colonic bacteria in the gut. Data suggest that one in ten patients treated with digoxin tablets will degrade 40% or more of the ingested dose.

Distribution—Following drug administration, a 6 to 8 hour distribution phase is observed. This is followed by a much more gradual serum concentration decline, which is dependent on digoxin elimination from the body. The peak height and slope of the early portion (absorption/distribution phases) of the serum concentration-time curve are dependent upon the route of administration and the absorption characteristics of the formulation. Clinical evidence indicates that the early high serum concentrations do not reflect the concentration of digoxin at its site of action, but that with chronic use, the steady-state post-distribution serum levels are in equilibrium with tissue levels and correlate with pharmacologic effects. In individual patients, these post-distribution serum concentrations are linearly related to maintenance dosage and may be useful in evaluating therapeutic and toxic effects (see Serum Digoxin Concentrations in DOSAGE AND ADMINISTRATION section).

Digoxin is concentrated in tissues and therefore has a large apparent volume of distribution. Digoxin crosses both the blood-brain barrier and the placenta. At delivery, serum digoxin concentration in the newborn is similar to the serum level in the mother. Approximately 20 to 25% of plasma digoxin is bound to protein. Serum digoxin concentrations are not significantly altered by large changes in fat tissue weight, so that its distribution space correlates best with lean (ideal) body weight, not total body weight.

Pharmacologic Response—The approximate times to onset of effect and to peak effect of all the Lanoxin® preparations are given in the following table:
[See table above.]

Excretion—Elimination of digoxin follows first-order kinetics (that is, the quantity of digoxin eliminated at any time is proportional to the total body content). Following intravenous administration to normal subjects, 50 to 70% of a digoxin dose is excreted unchanged in the urine. Renal excretion of digoxin is proportional to glomerular filtration rate and is largely independent of urine flow. In subjects with normal renal function, digoxin has a half-life of 1.5 to 2.0 days. The half-life in anuric patients is prolonged to 4 to 6 days. Digoxin is not effectively removed from the body by dialysis, exchange transfusion or during cardiopulmonary by-pass because most of the drug is in tissue rather than circulating in the blood.

INDICATIONS AND USAGE

Heart Failure: The increased cardiac output resulting from the inotropic action of digoxin ameliorates the disturbances characteristic of heart failure (venous congestion, edema, dyspnea, orthopnea and cardiac asthma).

Digoxin is more effective in "low output" (pump) failure than in "high output" heart failure secondary to arteriovenous fistula, anemia, infection or hyperthyroidism.

Digoxin is usually continued after failure is controlled, unless some known precipitating factor is corrected. Studies have shown, however, that even though hemodynamic effects can be demonstrated in almost all patients, corresponding improvement in the signs and symptoms of heart failure is not necessarily apparent. Therefore, in patients in whom digoxin may be difficult to regulate, or in whom the risk of toxicity may be great (e.g., patients with unstable renal function or whose potassium levels tend to fluctuate) a cautious withdrawal of digoxin may be considered. If digoxin is discontinued, the patient should be regularly monitored for clinical evidence of recurrent heart failure.

Atrial Fibrillation: Digoxin reduces ventricular rate and thereby improves hemodynamics. Palpitation, precordial distress or weakness are relieved and concomitant congestive failure ameliorated. Digoxin should be continued in doses necessary to maintain the desired ventricular rate.

Atrial Flutter: Digoxin slows the heart and regular sinus rhythm may appear. Frequently the flutter is converted to atrial fibrillation with a controlled ventricular response. Digoxin treatment should be maintained if atrial fibrillation persists. (Electrical cardioversion is often the treatment of choice for atrial flutter. See discussion of cardioversion in PRECAUTIONS section.)

PRODUCT	ABSOLUTE BIOAVAILABILITY	EQUIVALENT DOSES (IN MG*)		
Lanoxin Tablet	60–80%	0.125	0.25	0.5
Lanoxin Elixir	70–85%	0.125	0.25	0.5
Lanoxin Injection/IM	70–85%	0.125	0.25	0.5
Lanoxin Injection/IV	100%	0.1	0.2	0.4
Lanoxicaps Capsules	90–100%	0.1	0.2	0.4

*1 mg = 1000 μg

Paroxysmal Atrial Tachycardia (PAT): Digoxin may convert PAT to sinus rhythm by slowing conduction through the AV node. If heart failure has ensued or paroxysms recur frequently, digoxin should be continued. In infants, digoxin is usually continued for 3 to 6 months after a single episode of PAT to prevent recurrence.

CONTRAINDICATIONS

Digitalis glycosides are contraindicated in ventricular fibrillation.

In a given patient, an untoward effect requiring permanent discontinuation of other digitalis preparations usually constitutes a contraindication to digoxin. Hypersensitivity to digoxin itself is a contraindication to its use. Allergy to digoxin, though rare, does occur. It may not extend to all such preparations, and another digitalis glycoside may be tried with caution.

WARNINGS

Digitalis alone or with other drugs has been used in the treatment of obesity. This use of digoxin or other digitalis glycosides is unwarranted. Moreover, since they may cause potentially fatal arrhythmias or other adverse effects, the use of these drugs solely for the treatment of obesity is dangerous.

Anorexia, nausea, vomiting and arrhythmias may accompany heart failure or may be indications of digitalis intoxication. Clinical evaluation of the cause of these symptoms should be attempted before further digitalis administration. In such circumstances determination of the serum digoxin concentration may be an aid in deciding whether or not digitalis toxicity is likely to be present. If the possibility of digitalis intoxication cannot be excluded, cardiac glycosides should be temporarily withheld, if permitted by the clinical situation.

Patients with renal insufficiency require smaller than usual maintenance doses of digoxin (see DOSAGE AND ADMINISTRATION section).

Heart failure accompanying acute glomerulonephritis requires extreme care in digitalization. Relatively low loading and maintenance doses and concomitant use of antihypertensive drugs may be necessary and careful monitoring is essential. Digoxin should be discontinued as soon as possible.

Patients with severe carditis, such as carditis associated with rheumatic fever or viral myocarditis, are especially sensitive to digoxin-induced disturbances of rhythm.

Newborn infants display considerable variability in their tolerance to digoxin. Premature and immature infants are particularly sensitive, and dosage must not only be reduced but must be individualized according to their degree of maturity.

Note: Digitalis glycosides are an important cause of accidental poisoning in children.

PRECAUTIONS

General: Digoxin toxicity develops more frequently and lasts longer in patients with renal impairment because of the decreased excretion of digoxin. Therefore, it should be anticipated that dosage requirements will be decreased in patients with moderate to severe renal disease (see DOSAGE AND ADMINISTRATION section). Because of the prolonged half-life, a longer period of time is required to achieve an initial or new steady-state concentration in patients with renal impairment than in patients with normal renal function.

In patients with hypokalemia, toxicity may occur despite serum digoxin concentrations within the "normal range," because potassium depletion sensitizes the myocardium to digoxin. Therefore, it is desirable to maintain normal serum potassium levels in patients being treated with digoxin. Hypokalemia may result from diuretic, amphotericin B or corticosteroid therapy, and from dialysis or mechanical suction of gastrointestinal secretions. It may also accompany malnutrition, diarrhea, prolonged vomiting, old age and long-standing heart failure. In general, rapid changes in serum potassium or other electrolytes should be avoided, and intravenous treatment with potassium should be reserved for special circumstances as described below (see TREATMENT OF ARRHYTHMIAS PRODUCED BY OVERDOSAGE section).

Calcium, particularly when administered rapidly by the intravenous route, may produce serious arrhythmias in digitalized patients. Hypercalcemia from any cause predisposes the patient to digitalis toxicity. On the other hand, hypocal-

cemia can nullify the effects of digoxin in man; thus, digoxin may be ineffective until serum calcium is restored to normal. These interactions are related to the fact that calcium affects contractility and excitability of the heart in a manner similar to digoxin.
Hypomagnesemia may predispose to digitalis toxicity. If low magnesium levels are detected in a patient on digoxin, replacement therapy should be instituted.
Quinidine, verapamil, amiodarone, and propafenone cause a rise in serum digoxin concentration, with the implication that digitalis intoxication may result. This rise appears to be proportional to the dose. The effect is mediated by a reduction in the digoxin clearance and, in the case of quinidine, decreased volume of distribution as well.
Certain antibiotics may increase digoxin absorption in patients who convert digoxin to inactive metabolites in the gut (see Pharmacokinetics portion of the CLINICAL PHARMACOLOGY section). Recent studies have shown that specific colonic bacteria in the lower gastrointestinal tract convert digoxin to cardioinactive reduction products, thereby reducing its bioavailability. Although inactivation of these bacteria by antibiotics is rapid, the serum digoxin concentration will rise at a rate consistent with the elimination half-life of digoxin. The magnitude of rise in serum digoxin concentration relates to the extent of bacterial inactivation, and may be as much as two-fold in some cases. Patients with acute myocardial infarction or severe pulmonary disease may be unusually sensitive to digoxin-induced disturbances of rhythm.
Atrial arrhythmias associated with hypermetabolic states (e.g. hyperthyroidism) are particularly resistant to digoxin treatment. Large doses of digoxin are not recommended as the only treatment of these arrhythmias and care must be taken to avoid toxicity if large doses of digoxin are required. In hypothyroidism, the digoxin requirements are reduced. Digoxin responses in patients with compensated thyroid disease are normal.
Reduction of digoxin dosage may be desirable prior to electrical cardioversion to avoid induction of ventricular arrhythmias, but the physician must consider the consequences of rapid increase in ventricular response to atrial fibrillation if digoxin is withheld 1 to 2 days prior to cardioversion. If there is a suspicion that digitalis toxicity exists, elective cardioversion should be delayed. If it is not prudent to delay cardioversion, the energy level selected should be minimal at first and carefully increased in an attempt to avoid precipitating ventricular arrhythmias.
Incomplete AV block, especially in patients with Stokes-Adams attacks, may progress to advanced or complete heart block if digoxin is given.
In some patients with sinus node disease (i.e. Sick Sinus Syndrome), digoxin may worsen sinus bradycardia or sino-atrial block.
In patients with Wolff-Parkinson-White Syndrome and atrial fibrillation, digoxin can enhance transmission of impulses through the accessory pathway. This effect may result in extremely rapid ventricular rates and even ventricular fibrillation.
Digoxin may worsen the outflow obstruction in patients with idiopathic hypertrophic subaortic stenosis (IHSS). Unless cardiac failure is severe, it is doubtful whether digoxin should be employed.
Patients with chronic constrictive pericarditis may fail to respond to digoxin. In addition, slowing of the heart rate by digoxin in some patients may further decrease cardiac output.
Patients with heart failure from amyloid heart disease or constrictive cardiomyopathies respond poorly to treatment with digoxin.
Digoxin is not indicated for the treatment of sinus tachycardia unless it is associated with heart failure.
Digoxin may produce false positive ST-T changes in the electrocardiogram during exercise testing.
Intramuscular injection of digoxin is extremely painful and offers no advantages unless other routes of administration are contraindicated.

Laboratory Tests: Patients receiving digoxin should have their serum electrolytes and renal function (BUN and/or serum creatinine) assessed periodically; the frequency of assessments will depend on the clinical setting. For discussion of serum digoxin concentrations, see DOSAGE AND ADMINISTRATION section.

Drug Interactions: Potassium-depleting *corticosteroids* and *diuretics* may be major contributing factors to digitalis toxicity. *Calcium*, particularly if administered rapidly by the intravenous route, may produce serious arrhythmias in digitalized patients. *Quinidine, verapamil, amiodarone,* and *propafenone* cause a rise in serum digoxin concentration, with the implication that digitalis intoxication may result. Certain *antibiotics* increase digoxin absorption in patients who inactivate digoxin by bacterial metabolism in the lower intestine, so that digitalis intoxication may result. *Propantheline* and *diphenoxylate*, by decreasing gut motility, may increase digoxin absorption. *Antacids, kaolin-pectin, sulfasalazine, neomycin, cholestyramine* certain *anticancer drugs* and *metoclopramide* may reduce intestinal digoxin absorption, resulting in unexpectedly low serum concentrations. There have been inconsistent reports regarding the effects of other drugs on the serum digoxin concentration. *Thyroid* administration to a digitalized, hypothyroid patient may increase the dose requirement of digoxin. Concomitant use of digoxin and *sympathomimetics* increases the risk of cardiac arrhythmias because both enhance ectopic pacemaker activity. *Succinylcholine* may cause a sudden extrusion of potassium from muscle cells, and may thereby cause arrhythmias in digitalized patients. Although β adrenergic blockers or calcium channel blockers and digoxin may be useful in combination to control atrial fibrillation, their additive effects on AV node conduction can result in complete heart block.
Due to the considerable variability of these interactions, digoxin dosage should be carefully individualized when patients receive coadministered medications. Furthermore, caution should be exercised when combining digoxin with any drug that may cause a significant deterioration in renal function, since this may impair the excretion of digoxin.

Carcinogenesis, Mutagenesis, Impairment of Fertility: There have been no long-term studies performed in animals to evaluate carcinogenic potential.

Pregnancy: *Teratogenic Effects:* Pregnancy Category C. Animal reproduction studies have not been conducted with digoxin. It is also not known whether digoxin can cause fetal harm when administered to a pregnant woman or can affect reproduction capacity. Digoxin should be given to a pregnant woman only if clearly needed.

Nursing Mothers: Studies have shown that digoxin concentrations in the mother's serum and milk are similar. However, the estimated daily dose to a nursing infant will be far below the usual infant maintenance dose. Therefore, this amount should have no pharmacologic effect upon the infant. Nevertheless, caution should be exercised when digoxin is administered to a nursing woman.

ADVERSE REACTIONS

The frequency and severity of adverse reactions to digoxin depend on the dose and route of administration, as well as on the patient's underlying disease or concomitant therapies (see PRECAUTIONS section and Serum Digoxin Concentrations subsection of DOSAGE AND ADMINISTRATION). The overall incidence of adverse reactions has been reported as 5 to 20%, with 15 to 20% of them being considered serious (one to four percent of patients receiving digoxin). Evidence suggests that the incidence of toxicity has decreased since the introduction of the serum digoxin assay and improved standardization of digoxin tablets. Cardiac toxicity accounts for about one-half, gastrointestinal disturbances for about one-fourth, and CNS and other toxicity for about one-fourth of these adverse reactions.

Adults:

Cardiac—Unifocal or multiform ventricular premature contractions, especially in bigeminal or trigeminal patterns, are the most common arrhythmias associated with digoxin toxicity in adults with heart disease.
Ventricular tachycardia may result from digitalis toxicity. Atrioventricular (AV) dissociation, accelerated junctional (nodal) rhythm and atrial tachycardia with block are also common arrhythmias caused by digoxin overdosage.
Excessive slowing of the pulse is a clinical sign of digoxin overdosage. AV block (Wenckebach) of increasing degree may proceed to complete heart block.
Note: The electrocardiogram is fundamental in determining the presence and nature of these cardiac disturbances. Digoxin may also induce other changes in the ECG (e.g. PR prolongation, ST depression), which represent digoxin effect and may or may not be associated with digitalis toxicity.

Gastrointestinal—Anorexia, nausea, vomiting and less commonly diarrhea are common early symptoms of overdosage. However, uncontrolled heart failure may also produce such symptoms. Digitalis toxicity very rarely may cause abdominal pain and hemorrhagic necrosis of the intestines.

CNS—Visual disturbances (blurred or yellow vision), headache, weakness, dizziness, apathy and psychosis can occur.

Other—Gynecomastia is occasionally observed. Maculopapular rash or other skin reactions are rarely observed.

Infants and Children: Toxicity differs from the adult in a number of respects. Anorexia, nausea, vomiting, diarrhea and CNS disturbances may be present but are rare as initial symptoms in infants. Cardiac arrhythmias are more reliable signs of toxicity. Digoxin in children may produce any arrhythmia. The most commonly encountered are conduction disturbances or supraventricular tachyarrythmias, such as atrial tachycardia with or without block and junctional (nodal) tachycardia. Ventricular arrhythmias are less common. Sinus bradycardia may also be a sign of impending digoxin intoxication, especially in infants, even in the absence of first degree heart block. Any arrhythmia or alteration in cardiac conduction that develops in a child taking digoxin should initially be assumed to be a consequence of digoxin intoxication.

OVERDOSAGE

Treatment of Arrhythmias Produced by Overdosage:

Adults: Digoxin should be discontinued until all signs of toxicity are gone. Discontinuation may be all that is necessary if toxic manifestations are not severe and appear only near the expected time for maximum effect of the drug.
Correction of factors that may contribute to toxicity such as electrolyte disturbances, hypoxia, acid-base disturbances and removal of aggravating agents such as catecholamines, should also be considered. Potassium salts may be indicated, particularly if hypokalemia is present. Potassium administration may be dangerous in the setting of massive digitalis overdosage (see Massive Digitalis Overdosage subsection below). Potassium chloride in divided oral doses totaling 3 to 6 grams of the salt (40 to 80 mEq K+) for adults may be given provided renal function is adequate (see below for potassium recommendations in Infants and Children).
When correction of the arrhythmia is urgent and the serum potassium concentration is low or normal, potassium should be administered intravenously in 5% dextrose injection. For adults, a total of 40 to 80 mEq (diluted to a concentration of 40 mEq per 500 mL) may be given at a rate not exceeding 20 mEq per hour, or slower if limited by pain due to local irritation. Additional amounts may be given if the arrhythmia is uncontrolled and potassium well-tolerated. ECG monitoring should be performed to watch for any evidence of potassium toxicity (e.g. peaking of T waves) and to observe the effect on the arrhythmia. The infusion may be stopped when the desired effect is achieved.
Note: Potassium should not be used and may be dangerous in heart block due to digoxin, unless primarily related to supraventricular tachycardia.
Other agents that have been used for the treatment of digoxin intoxication include lidocaine, procainamide, propranolol and phenytoin, although use of the latter must be considered experimental. In advanced heart block, atropine and/or temporary ventricular pacing may be beneficial. Digibind®, Digoxin Immune Fab (Ovine), can be used to reverse potentially life-threatening digoxin (or digitoxin) intoxication. Improvement in signs and symptoms of digitalis toxicity usually begins within ½ hour of Digibind administration. Each 40 mg vial of Digibind will neutralize 0.6 mg of digoxin (which is a usual body store of an adequately digitalized 70 kg patient).

Infants and Children: See Adult section for general recommendations for the treatment of arrhythmias produced by overdosage and for cautions regarding the use of potassium.
If a potassium preparation is used to treat toxicity, it may be given orally in divided doses totaling 1 to 1.5 mEq K+ per kilogram (kg) body weight (1 gram of potassium chloride contains 13.4 mEq K+).
When correction of the arrhythmia with potassium is urgent, approximately 0.5 mEq/kg of potassium per hour may be given intravenously, with careful ECG monitoring. The intravenous solution of potassium should be dilute enough to avoid local irritation; however, especially in infants, care must be taken to avoid intravenous fluid overload.

Massive Digitalis Overdosage: Manifestations of life-threatening toxicity include severe ventricular arrhythmias such as ventricular tachycardia or ventricular fibrillation, or progressive bradyarrhythmias such as severe sinus bradycardia or second or third degree heart block not responsive to atropine. An overdosage of more than 10 mg of digoxin in previously healthy adults or 4 mg in previously healthy children or overdosage resulting in steady-state serum concentrations greater than 10 ng/mL, often results in cardiac arrest.
Severe digitalis intoxication can cause life-threatening elevation in serum potassium concentration by shifting potassium from inside to outside the cell resulting in hyperkalemia. Administration of potassium supplements in the setting of massive intoxication may be hazardous.
Digibind®, Digoxin Immune Fab (Ovine), may be used at a dose equimolar to digoxin in the body to reverse the effects of ingestion of a massive overdose. The decision to administer Digibind before the onset of toxic manifestations will depend on the likelihood that life-threatening toxicity will occur (see above).
Patients with massive digitalis ingestion should receive large doses of activated charcoal to prevent absorption and bind digoxin in the gut during enteroenteric recirculation. Emesis of gastric lavage may be indicated especially if ingestion has occurred within 30 minutes of the patient's presentation at the hospital. Emesis should not be induced in patients who are obtunded. If a patient presents more than 2 hours after ingestion or already has toxic manifestations, it may be unsafe to induce vomiting or attempt passage of a gastric tube, because such maneuvers may induce an acute vagal episode that can worsen digitalis-toxic arrhythmias.

DOSAGE AND ADMINISTRATION

Recommended dosages are average values that may require considerable modification because of individual sensitivity

Continued on next page

Burroughs Wellcome—Cont.

or associated conditions. Diminished renal function is the most important factor requiring modification of recommended doses.

In deciding the dose of digoxin, several factors must be considered:

1. The disease being treated. Atrial arrhythmias may require larger doses than heart failure.
2. The body weight of the patient. Doses should be calculated based upon lean or ideal body weight.
3. The patient's renal function, preferably evaluated on the basis of creatinine clearance.
4. Age is an important factor in infants and children.
5. Concomitant disease states, drugs or other factors likely to alter the expected clinical response to digoxin (see PRECAUTIONS and Drug Interactions sections).

Digitalization may be accomplished by either of two general approaches that vary in dosage and frequency of administration, but reach the same endpoint in terms of total amount of digoxin accumulated in the body.

1. Rapid digitalization may be achieved by administering a loading dose based upon projected peak body digoxin stores, then calculating the maintenance dose as a percentage of the loading dose.
2. More gradual digitalization may be obtained by beginning an appropriate maintenance dose, thus allowing digoxin body stores to accumulate slowly. Steady-state serum digoxin concentrations will be achieved in approximately 5 half-lives of the drug for the individual patient. Depending upon the patient's renal function, this will take between one and three weeks.

Adults:

Adults—Rapid Digitalization with a Loading Dose. Peak body digoxin stores of 8 to 12 μg/kg should provide therapeutic effect with minimum risk of toxicity in most patients with heart failure and normal sinus rhythm. Larger stores (10 to 15 μg/kg) are often required for adequate control of ventricular rate in patients with atrial flutter or fibrillation. Because of altered digoxin distribution and elimination, projected peak body stores for patients with renal insufficiency should be conservative (i.e. 6 to 10 μg/kg) [see PRECAUTIONS section].

The loading dose should be based on the projected peak body stores and administered in several portions, with roughly half the total given as the first dose. Additional fractions of this planned total dose may be given at 6 to 8 hour intervals, **with careful assessment of clinical response before each additional dose.**

If the patient's clinical response necessitates a change from the calculated dose of digoxin, then calculation of the maintenance dose should be based upon the amount actually given.

In previously undigitalized patients, a single initial Lanoxin® Tablet dose of 500 to 750 μg (0.5 to 0.75 mg) usually produces a detectable effect in 0.5 to 2 hours that becomes maximal in 2 to 6 hours. Additional doses of 125 to 375 μg (0.125 to 0.375 mg) may be given cautiously at 6 to 8 hour intervals until clinical evidence of an adequate effect is noted. The usual amount of Lanoxin Tablets that a 70 kg patient requires to achieve 8 to 15 μg/kg peak body stores is 750 to 1250 μg (0.75 to 1.25 mg).

Although peak body stores are mathematically related to loading doses and are utilized to calculate maintenance doses, they do not correlate with measured serum concentrations. This discrepancy is caused by digoxin distribution within the body during the first 6 to 8 hours following a dose. Serum concentrations drawn during this time are usually not interpretable.

The maintenance dose should be based upon the percentage of the peak body stores lost each day through elimination. The following formula has had wide clinical use:

[See formula at top of page.]

Ccr is creatinine clearance, corrected to 70 kg body weight or 1.73 m^2 body surface area. *For adults,* if only serum creatinine concentrations (Scr) are available, a Ccr (corrected to 70 kg body weight) may be estimated in men as (140 – Age)/Scr. For women, this result should be multiplied by 0.85.

Note: This equation cannot be used for estimating creatinine clearance in infants or children.

A common practice involves the use of Lanoxin® Injection to achieve rapid digitalization, with conversion to Lanoxin Tablets or Lanoxicaps for maintenance therapy. If patients are switched from IV to oral digoxin formulations, allowances must be made for differences in bioavailability when calculating maintenance dosages (see table, CLINICAL PHARMACOLOGY section).

Adults—Gradual Digitalization with a Maintenance Dose: The following table provides average Lanoxin Tablet daily maintenance dose requirements for patients with heart failure based upon lean body weight and renal function:

[See table above.]

Example—based on the above table, a patient in heart failure with an estimated lean body weight of 70 kg and a Ccr of

$$\text{Maintenance Dose} = \text{Peak Body Stores (i.e. Loading Dose)} \times \frac{\%\ \text{Daily Loss}}{100}$$

$$\text{Where: } \%\ \text{Daily Loss} = 14 + \text{Ccr}/5$$

Usual Lanoxin Daily Maintenance Dose Requirements (μg)
For Estimated Peak Body Stores of 10 μg/kg

Corrected Ccr (mL/min per 70 kg)	Lean Body Weight (kg/lbs) 50/110	60/132	70/154	80/176	90/198	100/220	Number of Days Before Steady-State Achieved
0	63*†	125	125	125	188††	188	22
10	125	125	125	188	188	188	19
20	125	125	188	188	188	250	16
30	125	188	188	188	250	250	14
40	125	188	188	250	250	250	13
50	188	188	250	250	250	250	12
60	188	188	250	250	250	375	11
70	188	250	250	250	250	375	10
80	188	250	250	250	375	375	9
90	188	250	250	250	375	500	8
100	250	250	250	375	375	500	7

* 63 μg = 0.063 mg
† ½ of 125 μg tablet or 125 μg every other day
‡ 1½ of 125 μg tablet.

60 mL/min, should be given a 250 μg (0.25 mg) Lanoxin® Tablet each day, usually taken after the morning meal. Steady-state serum concentrations should not be anticipated before 11 days.

Infants and Children: Digitalization must be individualized. Divided daily dosing is recommended for infants and young children. Children over 10 years of age require adult dosages in proportion to their body weight.

In the newborn period, renal clearance of digoxin is diminished and suitable dosage adjustments must be observed. This is especially pronounced in the premature infant. Beyond the immediate newborn period, children generally require proportionally larger doses than adults on the basis of body weight or body surface area.

Lanoxin Injection Pediatric can be used to achieve rapid digitalization, with conversion to an oral Lanoxin formulation for maintenance therapy. If patients are switched from IV to oral digoxin tablets or elixir, allowances must be made for differences in bioavailability when calculating maintenance dosages (see bioavailability table in CLINICAL PHARMACOLOGY section and dosing table below).

Intramuscular injection of digoxin is extremely painful and offers no advantages unless other routes of administration are contraindicated.

Digitalizing and daily maintenance doses for each age group are given below and should provide therapeutic effect with minimum risk of toxicity in most patients with heart failure and normal sinus rhythm. Larger doses are often required for adequate control of ventricular rate in patients with atrial flutter or fibrillation.

The loading dose should be administered in several portions, with roughly half the total given as the first dose. Additional fractions of this planned total dose may be given at 6 to 8 hour intervals, **with careful assessment of clinical response before each additional dose.** If the patient's clinical response necessitates a change from the calculated dose of digoxin, then calculation of the maintenance dose should be based upon the amount actually given.

[See table below.]

More gradual digitalization can also be accomplished by beginning an appropriate maintenance dose. The range of percentages provided above can be used in calculating this dose for patients with normal renal function. In children with renal disease, digoxin dosing must be carefully titrated based upon clinical response.

Long-term use of digoxin is indicated in many children who have been digitalized for acute heart failure, unless the cause is transient. Children with severe congenital heart disease, even after surgery, may require digoxin for prolonged periods.

It cannot be overemphasized that both the adult and pediatric dosage guidelines provided are based upon average patient response and substantial individual variation can be expected. Accordingly, ultimate dosage selection must be based upon clinical assessment of the patient.

Serum Digoxin Concentrations: Measurement of serum digoxin concentrations can be helpful to the clinician in determining the state of digitalization and in assigning certain probabilities to the likelihood of digoxin intoxication. Studies in adults considered adequately digitalized (without evidence of toxicity) show that about two-thirds of such patients have serum digoxin levels ranging from 0.8 to 2.0 ng/mL. Patients with atrial fibrillation or atrial flutter require and appear to tolerate higher levels than do patients with other indications. On the other hand, in adult patients with clinical evidence of digoxin toxicity, about two-thirds will have serum digoxin levels greater than 2.0 ng/mL. Thus, whereas levels less than 0.8 ng/mL are infrequently associated with toxicity, levels greater than 2.0 ng/mL are often associated with toxicity. Values in between are not very helpful in deciding whether a certain sign or symptom is more likely caused by digoxin toxicity or by something else. There are rare patients who are unable to tolerate digoxin even at serum concentrations below 0.8 ng/mL. Some researchers suggest that infants and young children tolerate slightly higher serum concentrations than do adults.

To allow adequate time for equilibration of digoxin between serum and tissue, **sampling of serum concentrations for clinical use should be at least 6 to 8 hours after the last dose,** regardless of the route of administration or formulation used. On a twice daily dosing schedule, there will be only minor differences in serum digoxin concentrations whether sampling is done at 8 or 12 hours after a dose. After a single daily dose, the concentration will be 10 to 25% lower when sampled at 24 versus 8 hours, depending upon the patient's renal function. Ideally, sampling for assessment of steady-state concentrations should be done just before the next dose.

If a discrepancy exists between the reported serum concentration and the observed clinical response, the clinician should consider the following possibilities:

1. Analytical problems in the assay procedure.
2. Inappropriate serum sampling time.
3. Administration of a digitalis glycoside other than digoxin.
4. Conditions (described in WARNINGS and PRECAUTIONS sections) causing an alteration in the sensitivity of the patient to digoxin.
5. The patient falls outside the norm in his response to or handling of digoxin. This decision should only be reached after exclusion of the other possibilities and generally should be confirmed by additional correlations of clinical observations with serum digoxin concentrations.

The serum concentration data should always be interpreted in the overall clinical context and an isolated serum concentration value should not be used alone as a basis for increasing or decreasing digoxin dosage.

Adjustment of Maintenance Dose in Previously Digitalized Patients:

Usual Digitalizing and Maintenance Dosages for Lanoxin Tablets
in Children **with Normal Renal Function Based on Lean Body Weight**

Age	Digitalizing* Dose (μg/kg)	Daily† Maintenance Dose (μg/kg)
2 to 5 Years	30 to 40	
5 to 10 Years	20 to 35	25 to 35% of *oral* loading dose‡
Over 10 years	10 to 15	

* IV digitalizing doses are 80% of oral digitalizing doses.
† Divided daily dosing is recommended for children under 10 years of age.
‡ Projected or actual digitalizing dose providing clinical response.

Lanoxin® Tablet maintenance doses in individual patients on steady-state digoxin can be adjusted upward or downward in proportion to the ratio of the desired versus the measured serum concentration. For example, a patient at steady-state on 125 μg (0.125 mg) of Lanoxin Tablets per day with a measured serum concentration of 0.7 ng/mL, should have the dose increased to 250 μg (0.25 mg) per day to achieve a steady-state serum concentration of 1.4 ng/mL, **assuming the serum digoxin concentration measurement is correct, renal function remains stable during this time and the needed adjustment is not the result of a problem with compliance.**

Dosage Adjustment When Changing Preparations: The difference in bioavailability between injectable Lanoxin or Lanoxicaps and Lanoxin Elixir Pediatric or Lanoxin Tablets must be considered when changing patients from one dosage form to another.

Lanoxin Injection and Lanoxicaps doses of 100 μg (0.1 mg) and 200 μg (0.2 mg) are approximately equivalent to 125 μg (0.125 mg) and 250 μg (0.25 mg) doses of Lanoxin Tablets and Elixir Pediatric (see table of CLINICAL PHARMACOLOGY section). Intramuscular injection of digoxin is extremely painful and offers no advantages unless other routes of administration are contraindicated.

HOW SUPPLIED

LANOXIN® (DIGOXIN) TABLETS, Scored 125 μg (0.125 mg): Bottles of 30 with child-resistant cap (NDC 0081-0242-30), 100 (NDC 0081-0242-55) and 1000 (NDC 0081-0242-75); unit dose pack of 100 (NDC 0081-0242-56). Imprinted with LANOXIN and Y3B (yellow). Store at 15° to 25°C (59° to 77°F) in a dry place and protect from light.

LANOXIN (DIGOXIN) TABLETS, Scored 250 μg (0.25 mg): Bottles of 30 with child-resistant cap (NDC 0081-0249-30), 100 (NDC 0081-0249-55), 1000 (NDC 0081-0249-75) and 5000 (NDC 0081-0249-80); unit dose pack of 100 (NDC 0081-0249-56). Imprinted with LANOXIN and X3A (white). Store at 15° to 25°C (59° to 77°F) in a dry place.

LANOXIN (DIGOXIN) TABLETS, Scored 500 μg (0.5 mg): Bottle of 100 (NDC 0081-0253-55). Imprinted with LANOXIN and T9A (green). Store at 15° to 25°C (59° to 77°F) in a dry place and protect from light.

Also Available:

LANOXIN (DIGOXIN) ELIXIR PEDIATRIC, 50 μg (0.05 mg) per mL; bottle of 60 mL with calibrated dropper.

LANOXIN (DIGOXIN) INJECTION, 500 μg (0.5 mg) in 2 mL (250 μg [0.25 mg] per mL); boxes of 10 and 50 ampuls.

LANOXIN (DIGOXIN) INJECTION PEDIATRIC, 100 μg (0.1 mg) in 1 mL; box of 10 ampuls.

LANOXICAPS® (DIGOXIN SOLUTION IN CAPSULES) 50 μg (0.05 mg) bottle of 100; 100 μg (0.1 mg) bottles of 30 (with child-resistant cap) and 100, 200 μg (0.2 mg) bottles of 30 (with child-resistant cap) and 100.

Shown in Product Identification Section, page 407

LEUCOVORIN CALCIUM FOR INJECTION ℞

WELLCOVORIN® brand STERILE POWDER
100 mg per vial

DESCRIPTION

Wellcovorin brand Leucovorin Calcium For Injection Sterile Powder is a sterile preparation containing leucovorin present as the calcium salt pentahydrate of *N*-[4-[[(2-amino-5-formyl-1, 4, 5, 6, 7, 8-hexahydro-4-oxo-6-pteridinyl)methyl] amino]benzoyl]-L-glutamic acid. Each 5 mg of leucovorin is equivalent to 5.40 mg of anhydrous leucovorin calcium.

Leucovorin is a water soluble vitamin in the folate group; it is useful as an antidote to drugs which act as folic acid antagonists.

Each 100 mg vial of Wellcovorin brand Leucovorin Calcium For Injection Sterile Powder, when reconstituted with 10 mL of sterile diluent, contains leucovorin (as the calcium salt) 10 mg/mL. The inactive ingredients are sodium chloride 80 mg per vial and sodium hydroxide and/or hydrochloric acid added to adjust the pH to approximately 8.1. The dry product contains no preservative. Dilute with Bacteriostatic Water for Injection, USP, which contains benzyl alcohol (see WARNINGS section), or with Sterile Water for Injection, USP.

Wellcovorin brand Leucovorin Calcium For Injection Sterile Powder, when reconstituted as directed, is suitable for IM or IV administration.

There is 0.004 mEq of calcium per mg leucovorin.

CLINICAL PHARMACOLOGY

Leucovorin is a mixture of the diastereoisomers of the 5-formyl derivative of tetrahydrofolic acid. The biologically active compound of the mixture is the (-)-L-isomer, known as Citrovorum factor or (-)-folinic acid. Leucovorin does not require reduction by the enzyme dihydrofolate reductase in order to participate in reactions utilizing folates as a source of "one-carbon" moieties. After intravenous administration of 25 mg calcium leucovorin, total reduced folate (as measured by *Lactobacillus casei* assay) reached a mean peak of 1259 ng/mL (range 897–1625).

The mean time to peak was 10 minutes. This initial rise in total reduced folate was primarily due to the parent compound 5- formyl THF (measured by S. *faecalis* assay) which rose to 1206 ng/mL at 10 minutes. A sharp drop in parent compound follows and coincides with the appearance of the metabolite (also active) 5-CH_3-THF which becomes the predominant circulating form of the drug. The mean peak of 5-CH_3-THF was 258 ng/mL occurring at 1.3 hours. The $t^{1/2}$ was 6.2 hours for total reduced folates. After intramuscular injection of 25 mg the mean peak total THF was 436 ng/mL (range 240–725) which occurred at a mean time of 52 minutes. Similar to IV administration, the initial sharp rise was due to the parent compound (5-CHO-THF) 360 ng/mL at 28 minutes and the level of the metabolite 5-CH_3-THF increased subsequently over time until at 1.5 hours it represented 50% of the circulating total folate. The mean peak of 5-CH_3-THF was 226 ng/mL at 2.8 hours. The $t^{1/2}$ of total reduced folate was 6.2 hours. There was no difference of statistical significance between IM and IV administration in the AUC for the total THF, 5-CHO-THF or 5-CH_3-THF.

INDICATIONS AND USAGE

Wellcovorin brand Leucovorin Calcium For Injection Sterile Powder is indicated (a) to diminish the toxicity and counteract the effect of inadvertently administered overdosages of folic acid antagonists and (b) in the treatment of the megaloblastic anemias due to sprue, nutritional deficiency, pregnancy, and infancy when oral therapy is not feasible.

CONTRAINDICATIONS

Leucovorin is improper therapy for pernicious anemia and other megaloblastic anemias secondary to the lack of vitamin B_{12}. A hematologic remission may occur while neurologic manifestations remain progressive.

WARNINGS

In the treatment of accidental overdosage of folic acid antagonists, leucovorin should be administered as promptly as possible. As the time interval between antifolate administration (e.g., methotrexate [MTX]) and leucovorin rescue increases, leucovorin's effectiveness in counteracting hematologic toxicity diminishes.

Monitoring of serum MTX concentration is essential in determining the optimal dose and duration of treatment with leucovorin which should be such that the resulting levels of tetrahydrofolate are equal to or greater than that of MTX.

In determining the dose and duration of leucovorin therapy, it should be remembered that there may be a delay of MTX excretion in the presence of a third space (i.e., ascites, pleural effusion) or if renal insufficiency or inadequate hydration exists. Under such circumstances, high doses of leucovorin are recommended. These doses are higher than those recommended for oral use and must be given intravenously.

If MTX is administered intrathecally as local therapy and leucovorin is administered concurrently, the presence of tetrahydrofolate which diffuses readily into the cerebrospinal fluid may negate the antineoplastic effect of MTX.

Leucovorin may enhance the toxicity of fluorouracil. Deaths from severe enterocolitis, diarrhea, and dehydration have been reported in elderly patients receiving leucovorin and fluorouracil. Concomitant granulocytopenia and fever were present in some but not all of patients.

Because of the preservative contained in Bacteriostatic Water for Injection, USP (benzyl alcohol preserved), doses greater than 10 mg/m^2 with this diluent are not recommended. If greater doses are required (see DOSAGE AND ADMINISTRATION) the desiccated powder should be reconstituted with Sterile Water for Injection, USP, and used immediately.

PRECAUTIONS

General: Following chemotherapy with folic acid antagonists, parenteral administration of leucovorin is preferable to oral dosing if there is a possibility that the patient may vomit and not absorb the leucovorin. In the presence of pernicious anemia, a hematologic remission may occur while neurologic manifestations remain progressive. Leucovorin has no effect on other established toxicities of MTX such as the nephrotoxicity resulting from drug precipitation in the kidney.

Drug Interactions: Folic acid in large amounts may counteract the antiepileptic effect of phenobarbital, phenytoin and primidone, and increase the frequency of seizures in susceptible children.

Leucovorin may enhance the toxicity of fluorouracil (see WARNINGS).

Pregnancy: ***Teratogenic Effects:*** Pregnancy Category C. Animal reproduction studies have not been conducted with leucovorin. It is also not known whether leucovorin can cause fetal harm when administered to a pregnant woman or can affect reproduction capacity. Leucovorin should be given to a pregnant woman only if clearly needed.

Nursing Mothers: It is not known whether this drug is excreted in human milk. Because many drugs are excreted in human milk, caution should be exercised when leucovorin is administered to a nursing mother.

Pediatric Use: See "Drug Interactions."

ADVERSE REACTIONS

Allergic sensitization has been reported following both oral and parenteral administration of folic acid.

OVERDOSAGE

Excessive amounts of leucovorin may nullify the chemotherapeutic effect of folic acid antagonists.

DOSAGE AND ADMINISTRATION

Inadvertent Overdosage of Antifol: As soon as possible after an inadvertent overdosage of the antifol, MTX, leucovorin should be given in a dosage regimen of 10 mg/m^2 every 6 hours IV or IM until the serum MTX levels are below 10^{-8} M. If there is adequate gastrointestinal function, doses subsequent to the initial dose may be given orally (see labeling of oral product). Concomitant hydration (3L/d) and urinary alkalinization with sodium bicarbonate should be employed. The bicarbonate dose should be adjusted to maintain a urinary pH at 7 or greater.

Serum samples should be assayed for creatinine levels and MTX levels at 24-hour intervals. If the 24-hour serum creatinine level has increased 50% over baseline or if the 24-hour MTX level is $> 5 \times 10^{-6}$ M or the 48-hour MTX level is $> 9 \times 10^{-7}$ M, the doses of leucovorin should be increased to 100 mg/m^2 q 3 hours IV until the MTX level is $< 10^{-8}$ M. When such doses are administered, a non-preserved diluent should be used (see WARNINGS). The rate of injection of leucovorin calcium should not exceed 17.5 mL (175 mg leucovorin) per minute.

Megaloblastic Anemia: No more than or up to 1 mg daily. There is no evidence that doses >1 mg daily have greater efficacy than those of 1 mg; additionally, loss of folate in urine becomes roughly logarithmic as the amount administered exceeds 1 mg.

Instructions for Reconstitution: Read WARNINGS for considerations in choice of diluent. The contents of each vial should be reconstituted with Bacteriostatic Water for Injection, USP (benzyl alcohol preserved) or with Sterile Water for Injection, USP. The 100 mg vial should be diluted with 10 mL, resulting in a solution containing 10 mg leucovorin per mL.

When reconstituted with Bacteriostatic Water for Injection, the resulting solution must be used within 7 days. If reconstituted with Sterile Water for Injection, use immediately and discard any unused portion.

Parenteral drug products should be inspected visually for particulate matter and discoloration prior to administration, whenever solution and container permit.

HOW SUPPLIED

100 mg/vial, Box of 1 (NDC 0081-0638-93).

Store dry powder and reconstituted solution at controlled room temperature 15° to 30°C (59° to 86°F). Protect from light.

LEUCOVORIN CALCIUM TABLETS ℞

WELLCOVORIN® brand

DESCRIPTION

Wellcovorin brand Leucovorin Calcium Tablets contain either 5 mg or 25 mg leucovorin as the calcium salt of *N*-[4-[[(2-amino-5-formyl-1, 4, 5, 6, 7, 8-hexahydro-4-oxo-6-pteridinyl)-methyl]amino]benzoyl]-*L*-glutamic acid and the inactive ingredients corn starch, FD&C Yellow No. 6 Lake (25 mg tablet only), lactose, povidone, and magnesium stearate. This is equivalent to 5.40 mg or 27.01 mg of anhydrous leucovorin calcium.

Leucovorin is a water soluble vitamin in the folate group; it is useful as an antidote to drugs which act as folic acid antagonists. These tablets are intended for oral administration only.

CLINICAL PHARMACOLOGY

Leucovorin is a mixture of the diastereoisomers of the 5-formyl derivative of tetrahydrofolic acid. The biologically active component of the mixture is the (-) -*L*-isomer, known as *Citrovorum factor,* or (-) -folinic acid. Leucovorin does *not* require reduction by the enzyme dihydrofolate reductase in order to participate in reactions utilizing folates as a source of "one-carbon" moieties. Following oral administration, leucovorin is rapidly absorbed and enters the general body pool of reduced folates.[1] The increase in plasma and serum folate activity (determined microbiologically with *Lactobacillus casei*) seen after oral administration of leucovorin is predominantly due to 5-methyltetrahydrofolate.[1,2,3,4,5]

Twenty normal men were given a single, oral 15 mg dose (7.5 mg/m^2) of leucovorin calcium and serum folate concentrations were assayed with *L casei.*[6] Mean values observed (± one standard error) were:[4]

Continued on next page

Burroughs Wellcome—Cont.

a) Time to peak serum folate concentration: 1.72 ± 0.08 hrs.,
b) Peak serum folate concentration achieved: 268 ± 18 ng/mL,
c) Serum folate half-disappearance time: 3.5 hours.

Oral tablets yielded areas under the serum folate concentration-time curves (AUC's) that were 12% greater than equal amounts of leucovorin given intramuscularly and equal to the same amounts given intravenously.

INDICATIONS AND USAGE

Wellcovorin brand Leucovorin Calcium Tablets are indicated for the prophylaxis and treatment of undesired hematopoietic effects of folic acid antagonists (see WARNINGS).

CONTRAINDICATIONS

Leucovorin is improper therapy for pernicious anemia and other megaloblastic anemias secondary to the lack of vitamin B_{12}. A hematologic remission may occur while neurologic manifestations remain progressive.

WARNINGS

In the treatment of accidental overdosage of folic acid antagonists, leucovorin should be administered as promptly as possible. As the time interval between antifolate administration (e.g. methotrexate [MTX]) and leucovorin rescue increases, leucovorin's effectiveness in counteracting hematologic toxicity diminishes.

Leucovorin may enhance the toxicity of fluorouracil. Deaths from severe enterocolitis, diarrhea, and dehydration have been reported in elderly patients receiving leucovorin and fluorouracil.[7] Concomitant granulocytopenia and fever were present in some but not all of the patients.

PRECAUTIONS

General: Following chemotherapy with folic acid antagonists, parenteral administration of leucovorin is preferable to oral dosing if there is a possibility that the patient may vomit and not absorb the leucovorin. In the presence of pernicious anemia a hematologic remission may occur while neurologic manifestations remain progressive. Leucovorin has no effect on other established toxicities of MTX, such as the nephrotoxicity resulting from drug precipitation in the kidney.

Drug Interactions: Folic acid in large amounts may counteract the antiepileptic effect of phenobarbital, phenytoin and primidone, and increase the frequency of seizures in susceptible children.

Leucovorin may enhance the toxicity of fluorouracil (see WARNINGS).

Pregnancy: ***Teratogenic Effects:*** Pregnancy Category C. Animal reproduction studies have not been conducted with leucovorin. It is also not known whether leucovorin can cause fetal harm when administered to a pregnant woman or can affect reproduction capacity. Leucovorin should be given to a pregnant woman only if clearly needed.

Nursing Mothers: It is not known whether this drug is excreted in human milk. Because many drugs are excreted in human milk, caution should be exercised when leucovorin is administered to a nursing mother.

Pediatric Use: See "Drug Interactions."

ADVERSE REACTIONS

Allergic sensitization has been reported following both oral and parenteral administration of folic acid.

OVERDOSAGE

Excessive amounts of leucovorin may nullify the chemotherapeutic effect of folic acid antagonists.

DOSAGE AND ADMINISTRATION

Leucovorin is a specific antidote for the hematopoietic toxicity of methotrexate and other strong inhibitors of the enzyme dihydrofolate reductase. Leucovorin rescue must begin within 24 hours of antifolate administration. A conventional leucovorin rescue dosage schedule is 10 mg/m^2 orally or parenterally followed by 10 mg/m^2 orally every six hours for seventy-two hours. If, however, at 24 hours following methotrexate administration the serum creatinine is increased by 50% or greater than the pre-methotrexate serum creatinine, the leucovorin dose should be immediately increased to 100 mg/m^2 every three hours until the serum methotrexate level is below 5×10^{-8} M.[8,9]

The recommended dose of leucovorin to counteract hematologic toxicity from folic acid antagonists with less affinity for mammalian dihydrofolate reductase than methotrexate (i.e. trimethoprim, pyrimethamine) is substantially less and 5 to 15 mg of leucovorin per day has been recommended by some investigators.[10,11,12]

HOW SUPPLIED

5 mg (off-white) scored tablets containing 5 mg leucovorin as the calcium salt imprinted with "WELLCOVORIN" and "5"; bottles of 20 (NDC 0081-0631-20) and 100 (NDC 0081-0631-55); unit dose pack of 50 (NDC 0081-0631-35).

25 mg (peach) scored tablets containing 25 mg leucovorin as the calcium salt imprinted with "WELLCOVORIN" and "25"; bottle of 25 (NDC 0081-0632-25); and Unit Dose Rescue Pak® of 10 (NDC 0081-0632-13).

Store at 15° to 25°C (59° to 77°F). Protect from light and moisture.

REFERENCES

1. Nixon PF, Bertino JR: Effective absorption and utilization of oral formyltetrahydrofolate in man. *N Engl J Med* 1972;*286*:175–179.
2. Ratanasthien K, Blair JA, Leeming RJ, Cooke WT, Melikian V: Folates in human serum. *J Clin Pathol* 1974;*27*:875–879.
3. Mehta BM, Gisolfi AL, Hutchison DJ, Nirenberg A, Kellick MG, Rosen G: Serum distribution of citrovorum factor and 5-methyltetrahydrofolate following oral and IM administration of calcium leucovorin in normal adults. *Cancer Treat Rep* 1978;*62*:345–350.
4. Data on file, Medical Division, Burroughs Wellcome Co., 3030 Cornwallis Rd., Research Triangle Park, NC 27709.
5. Whitehead VM, Pratt R, Viallet A, Cooper BA: Intestinal conversion of folinic acid to 5-methyltetrahydrofolate in man. *Br J Haematol* 1972;*22*:63–72.
6. Herbert V: Asceptic addition method for *Lactobacillus casei* assay of folate activity in human serum. *J Clin Pathol* 1966;*19*:12–16.
7. Grem JL, Shoemaker DD, Petrelli NJ, Douglass HO Jr: Severe and fatal toxic effects observed in treatment with high- and low-dose leucovorin plus 5-fluorouracil for colorectal carcinoma. *Cancer Treat Rep* 1987;*71*:1122.
8. Bleyer WA: The clinical pharmacology of methotrexate: new applications of an old drug. *Cancer* 1978;*41*:36–51.
9. Frei E, Blum RH, Pitman SW, et al: High dose methotrexate with leucovorin rescue: rationale and spectrum of antitumor activity. *Am J Med* 1980;*68*:370–376.
10. Golde DW, Bersch N, Quan SG: Trimethoprim and sulphamethoxazole inhibition of haematopoiesis *in vitro*. *Br J Haematol* 1978;*40*:363–367.
11. Steinberg SE, Campbell CL, Rabinovitch PS, Hillman RS: The effect of trimethoprim/sulfamethoxazole on Friend erythroleukemia cells. *Blood* 1980;*55*:501–504.
12. Mahmoud AAF, Warren KS: Algorithms in the diagnosis and management of exotic diseases, XX: toxoplasmosis. *J Infect Dis* 1977;*135*:493–496. 646324

Shown in Product Identification Section, page 407

LEUKERAN® ℞

[*lū'kŭh-răn*]
(Chlorambucil)
2 mg Sugar-coated Tablets

> **WARNING:** Leukeran (chlorambucil) can severely suppress bone marrow function. Chlorambucil is a carcinogen in humans. Chlorambucil is probably mutagenic and teratogenic in humans. Chlorambucil produces human infertility. See "WARNINGS" and "PRECAUTIONS" sections.

DESCRIPTION

Leukeran (chlorambucil) was first synthesized by Everett *et al.*[1] It is a bifunctional alkylating agent of the nitrogen mustard type that has been found active against selected human neoplastic diseases. Chlorambucil is known chemically as 4-[bis(2-chlorethyl)amino]benzenebutanoic acid.

Chlorambucil hydrolyzes in water and has a pKa of 5.8.

Leukeran (chlorambucil) is available in tablet form for oral administration. Each sugar-coated tablet contains 2 mg chlorambucil and the inactive ingredients corn and wheat starch, gum acacia, lactose, magnesium stearate, polysorbate 60, sucrose, and talc.

CLINICAL PHARMACOLOGY

Chlorambucil is rapidly and completely absorbed from the gastrointestinal tract. After single oral doses of 0.6–1.2 mg/kg, peak plasma chlorambucil levels are reached within one hour and the terminal half-life of the parent drug is estimated at 1.5 hours. Chlorambucil undergoes rapid metabolism to phenylacetic acid mustard, the major metabolite, and the combined chlorambucil and phenylacetic acid mustard urinary excretion is extremely low—less than 1% in 24 hours. The peak plasma levels of chlorambucil and phenylacetic acid mustard are similar, approximating 1 μg/mL; however, the metabolite's half-life is 1.6 times greater than the parent drug.[2,3]

Chlorambucil and its metabolites are extensively bound to plasma and tissue proteins. *In vitro*, chlorambucil is 99% bound to plasma proteins, specifically albumin.[4] Cerebrospinal fluid levels of chlorambucil have not been determined. Evidence of human teratogenicity suggests that the drug crosses the placenta.[5,6]

Chlorambucil is extensively metabolized in the liver primarily to phenylacetic acid mustard which has antineoplastic activity.[2,3] Chlorambucil and its major metabolite spontaneously degrade *in vivo* forming monohydroxy and dihydroxy derivatives.[2] After a single dose of radiolabeled chlorambucil (^{14}C) approximately 15% to 60% of the radioactivity appears in the urine after 24 hours. Again, less than 1% of the urinary radioactivity is in the form of chlorambucil or phenylacetic acid mustard.[2] In summary, the pharmacokinetic data suggest that oral chlorambucil undergoes rapid gastrointestinal absorption and plasma clearance and that it is almost completely metabolized, having extremely low urinary excretion.

INDICATIONS AND USAGE

Leukeran (chlorambucil) is indicated in the treatment of chronic lymphatic (lymphocytic) leukemia, malignant lymphomas including lymphosarcoma, giant follicular lymphoma and Hodgkin's disease. It is not curative in any of these disorders but may produce clinically useful palliation.

CONTRAINDICATIONS

Chlorambucil should not be used in patients whose disease has demonstrated a prior resistance to the agent. Patients who have demonstrated hypersensitivity to chlorambucil should not be given the drug.[7] There may be cross-hypersensitivity (skin rash) between chlorambucil and other alkylating agents.[8]

WARNINGS

Because of its carcinogenic properties, chlorambucil should not be given to patients with conditions other than chronic lymphatic leukemia or malignant lymphomas. Convulsions,[9] infertility,[10] leukemia[11,12] and secondary malignancies[13] have been observed when chlorambucil was employed in the therapy of malignant and non-malignant diseases.

There are many reports of acute leukemia arising in patients with both malignant[15] and non-malignant[16] diseases following chlorambucil treatment. In many instances, these patients also received other chemotherapeutic agents or some form of radiation therapy. The quantitation of the risk of chlorambucil-induction of leukemia or carcinoma in humans is not possible. Evaluation of published reports of leukemia developing in patients who have received chlorambucil (and other alkylating agents) suggests that the risk of leukemogenesis increases with both chronicity of treatment and large cumulative doses. However, it has proved impossible to define a cumulative dose below which there is no risk of the induction of secondary malignancy. The potential benefits from chlorambucil therapy must be weighed on an individual basis against the possible risk of the induction of a secondary malignancy.

Chlorambucil has been shown to cause chromatid or chromosome damage in man.[17,18] Both reversible and permanent sterility have been observed in both sexes receiving chlorambucil.

A high incidence of sterility has been documented when chlorambucil is administered to prepubertal and pubertal males.[19] Prolonged or permanent azoospermia has also been observed in adult males.[20] While most reports of gonadal dysfunction secondary to chlorambucil have related to males, the induction of amenorrhea in females with alkylating agents is well documented and chlorambucil is capable of producing amenorrhea. Autopsy studies of the ovaries from women with malignant lymphoma treated with combination chemotherapy including chlorambucil have shown varying degrees of fibrosis, vasculitis, and depletion of primordial follicles.[21,22]

Pregnancy: ***"Pregnancy Category D"***: Chlorambucil can cause fetal harm when administered to a pregnant woman. Unilateral renal agenesis has been observed in two offspring whose mothers received chlorambucil during the first trimester.[5,6] Urogenital malformations including absence of a kidney were found in fetuses of rats given chlorambucil.[14] There are no adequate and well-controlled studies in pregnant women. If this drug is used during pregnancy, or if the patient becomes pregnant while taking this drug, the patient should be apprised of the potential hazard to the fetus. Women of childbearing potential should be advised to avoid becoming pregnant.

PRECAUTIONS

General: Many patients develop a slowly progressive lymphopenia during treatment. The lymphocyte count usually rapidly returns to normal levels upon completion of drug therapy. Most patients have some neutropenia after the third week of treatment and this may continue for up to ten days after the last dose. Subsequently, the neutrophil count usually rapidly returns to normal. Severe neutropenia appears to be related to dosage and usually occurs only in patients who have received a total dosage of 6.5 mg/kg or more in one course of therapy with continuous dosing. About one-quarter of all patients receiving the continuous-dose schedule, and one-third of those receiving this dosage in eight weeks or less may be expected to develop severe neutropenia.[23]

While it is not necessary to discontinue chlorambucil at the first evidence of a fall in neutrophil count, it must be remembered that the fall may continue for ten days after the last

dose and that as the total dose approaches 6.5 mg/kg there is a risk of causing irreversible bone marrow damage. The dose of chlorambucil should be decreased if leukocyte or platelet counts fall below normal values and should be discontinued for more severe depression.

Chlorambucil should **not** be given at full dosages before four weeks after a full course of radiation therapy or chemotherapy because of the vulnerability of the bone marrow to damage under these conditions. If the pretherapy leukocyte or platelet counts are depressed from bone marrow disease process prior to institution of therapy, the treatment should be instituted at a reduced dosage.

Persistently low neutrophil and platelet counts or peripheral lymphocytosis suggest bone marrow infiltration. If confirmed by bone marrow examination, the daily dosage of chlorambucil should not exceed 0.1 mg/kg. Chlorambucil appears to be relatively free from gastrointestinal side effects or other evidence of toxicity apart from the bone marrow depressant action. In humans, single oral doses of 20 mg or more may produce nausea and vomiting.

Children with nephrotic syndrome[9] and patients receiving high pulse doses of chlorambucil[24] may have an increased risk of seizures. As with any potentially epileptogenic drug, caution should be exercised when administering chlorambucil to patients with a history of seizure disorder, head trauma or receiving other potentially epileptogenic drugs.

Information for Patients: Patients should be informed that the major toxicities of chlorambucil are related to hypersensitivity, drug fever, myelosuppression, hepatotoxicity, infertility, seizures, gastrointestinal toxicity, and secondary malignancies. Patients should never be allowed to take the drug without medical supervision and should consult their physician if they experience skin rash, bleeding, fever, jaundice, persistent cough, seizures, nausea, vomiting, amenorrhea, or unusual lumps/masses. Women of childbearing potential should be advised to avoid becoming pregnant.

Laboratory Tests: Patients must be followed carefully to avoid life-endangering damage to the bone marrow during treatment. Weekly examination of the blood should be made to determine hemoglobin levels, total and differential leukocyte counts, and quantitative platelet counts. Also, during the first 3 to 6 weeks of therapy, it is recommended that white blood cell counts be made 3 or 4 days after each of the weekly complete blood counts. Galton et al [23] have suggested that in following patients it is helpful to plot the blood counts on a chart at the same time that body weight, temperature, spleen size, etc., are recorded. It is considered dangerous to allow a patient to go more than two weeks without hematological and clinical examination during treatment.

Drug Interactions: There are no known drug/drug interactions with chlorambucil.

Carcinogenesis, Mutagenesis, Impairment of Fertility: See WARNINGS section for information on carcinogenesis, mutagenesis and impairment of fertility.

Pregnancy: *Teratogenic Effects:* Pregnancy Category D: See WARNINGS section.

Nursing Mothers: It is not known whether this drug is excreted in human milk. Because many drugs are excreted in human milk and because of the potential for serious adverse reactions in nursing infants from chlorambucil, a decision should be made whether to discontinue nursing or to discontinue the drug, taking into account the importance of the drug to the mother.

Pediatric Use: The safety and effectiveness in children have not been established.

ADVERSE REACTIONS
Hematologic: The most common side effect is bone marrow suppression.[25] Although bone marrow suppression frequently occurs, it is usually reversible if the chlorambucil is withdrawn early enough. However, irreversible bone marrow failure has been reported.[26,27]

Gastrointestinal: Gastrointestinal disturbances such as nausea and vomiting, diarrhea and oral ulceration occur infrequently.

CNS: Tremors, muscular twitching, confusion, agitation, ataxia, flaccid paresis and hallucinations have been reported as rare adverse experiences to chlorambucil which resolve upon discontinuation of drug. Rare, focal and/or generalized seizures have been reported to occur in both children[9,28,29] and adults[24,30–33] at both therapeutic daily doses, pulse dosing regimens and in acute overdose (see PRECAUTIONS-General).

Miscellaneous: Other reported adverse reactions include: pulmonary fibrosis, hepatotoxicity and jaundice, drug fever, skin hypersensitivity, peripheral neuropathy, interstitial pneumonia, sterile cystitis, infertility, leukemia and secondary malignancies (see WARNINGS).

OVERDOSAGE
Reversible pancytopenia was the main finding of inadvertent overdoses of chlorambucil.[34,35] Neurological toxicity ranging from agitated behavior and ataxia to multiple grand mal seizures has also occurred.[28,34] As there is no known antidote, the blood picture should be closely monitored and general supportive measures should be instituted, together with appropriate blood transfusions if necessary. Chlorambucil is not dialyzable.

Oral LD$_{50}$ single doses in mice are 123 mg/kg. In rats, a single intraperitoneal dose of 12.5 mg/kg of chlorambucil produces typical nitrogen-mustard effects; these include atrophy of the intestinal mucous membrane and lymphoid tissues, severe lymphopenia becoming maximal in four days, anemia and thrombocytopenia. After this dose, the animals begin to recover within three days and appear normal in about a week although the bone marrow may not become completely normal for about three weeks. An intraperitoneal dose of 18.5 mg/kg kills about 50% of the rats with development of convulsions. As much as 50 mg/kg has been given orally to rats as a single dose, with recovery. Such a dose causes bradycardia, excessive salivation, hematuria, convulsions, and respiratory dysfunction.

DOSAGE AND ADMINISTRATION
The usual oral dosage is 0.1 to 0.2 mg/kg body weight daily for three to six weeks as required. This usually amounts to 4 to 10 mg a day for the average patient. The entire daily dose may be given at one time. These dosages are for initiation of therapy or for short courses of treatment. The dosage must be carefully adjusted according to the response of the patient and must be reduced as soon as there is an abrupt fall in the white blood cell count. Patients with Hodgkin's disease usually require 0.2 mg/kg daily whereas patients with other lymphomas or chronic lymphocytic leukemia usually require only 0.1 mg/kg daily. When lymphocytic infiltration of the bone marrow is present, or when the bone marrow is hypoplastic, the daily dose should not exceed 0.1 mg/kg (about 6 mg for the average patient).

Alternate schedules for the treatment of chronic lymphocytic leukemia employing intermittent, bi-weekly or once monthly pulse doses of chlorambucil have been reported.[36,37] Intermittent schedules of chlorambucil begin with an initial single dose of 0.4 mg/kg. Doses are generally increased by 0.1 mg/kg until control of lymphocytosis or toxicity is observed. Subsequent doses are modified to produce mild hematologic toxicity. It is felt that the response rate of chronic lymphocytic leukemia to the bi-weekly or once monthly schedule of chlorambucil administration is similar or better to that previously reported with daily administration and that hematologic toxicity was less than or equal to that encountered in studies using daily chlorambucil.

Radiation and cytotoxic drugs render the bone marrow more vulnerable to damage and chlorambucil should be used with particular caution within four weeks of a full course of radiation therapy or chemotherapy. However, small doses of palliative radiation over isolated foci remote from the bone marrow will not usually depress the neutrophil and platelet count. In these cases chlorambucil may be given in the customary dosage.

It is presently felt that short courses of treatment are safer than continuous maintenance therapy although both methods have been effective. It must be recognized that continuous therapy may give the appearance of "maintenance" in patients who are actually in remission and have no immediate need for further drug. If maintenance dosage is used, it should not exceed 0.1 mg/kg daily and may well be as low as 0.03 mg/kg daily. A typical maintenance dose is 2 mg to 4 mg daily, or less, depending on the status of the blood counts. It may, therefore, be desirable to withdraw the drug after maximal control has been achieved since intermittent therapy reinstituted at time of relapse may be as effective as continuous treatment.

Procedures for proper handling and disposal of anti-cancer drugs should be considered. Several guidelines on this subject have been published.[38–44]

There is no general agreement that all of the procedures recommended in the guidelines are necessary or appropriate.

HOW SUPPLIED
White sugar-coated tablet containing 2 mg chlorambucil; bottle of 50 (NDC-0081-0635-35).
Store at 15°-25°C (59°-77°F) in a dry place.

REFERENCES
1. Everett JL, Roberts JJ, Ross WCJ: Aryl-2-halogenoalkylamines. Part XII. Some carboxylic derivatives of NN-Di-2-chloroethylaniline. *J Chem Soc* 1953, 3:2386–2392.
2. Alberts DS, Chang SY, Chen H-SG, et al: Pharmacokinetics and metabolism of chlorambucil in man: A preliminary report. *Cancer Treat Rev,* 1979;6 (suppl):9–17.
3. McLean A, Woods RL, Catovsky D, et al: Pharmacokinetics and metabolism of chlorambucil in patients with malignant disease. *Cancer Treat Rev,* 1979; 6(suppl):33–42.
4. Ehrsson H, Lönroth U, Wallin I, et al: Degradation of chlorambucil in aqueous solution: Influence of human albumin binding. *J Pharm Pharmacol,* 1981:33:313–315.
5. Shotton D, Monie IW: Possible teratogenic effect of chlorambucil on a human fetus. *JAMA* 1963;186:74–75.
6. Steege JF, Caldwell DS: Renal agenesis after first trimester exposure to chlorambucil. *South Med J* 1980;73:1414–1415.
7. Knisley RE, Settipane GA, Albala MM: Unusual reaction to chlorambucil in a patient with chronic lymphocytic leukemia. *Arch Dermatol* 1971;104:77–79.
8. Weiss RB, Bruno S: Hypersensitivity reactions to cancer chemotherapeutic agents. *Ann Intern Med* 1981; 94:66–72.
9. Williams SA, Makker SP, Grupe WE: Seizures: A significant side effect of chlorambucil therapy in children. *J Pediatr* 1978;93:516–518.
10. Freckman HA, Fry HL, Mendez FL, et al: Chlorambucil-prednisolone therapy for disseminated breast carcinoma. *JAMA* 1964;189:23–26.
11. Aymard JP, Frustin J, Witz F, et al: Acute leukemia after prolonged chlorambucil treatment for non-malignant disease: A report of a new case and literature survey. *Acta Haematol* 1980;63:283–285.
12. Berk PD, Goldberg JD, Silverstein MN, et al: Increased incidence of acute leukemia in polycythemia vera associated with chlorambucil therapy. *N Engl J Med.* 1981;304:441–447.
13. Lerner HJ: Acute myelogenous leukemia in patients receiving chlorambucil as long-term adjuvant chemotherapy for stage II breast cancer. *Cancer Treat Rep* 1978;62:1135–1138.
14. Monie IW: Chlorambucil-induced abnormalities of the urogenital system of rat fetuses. *Anat Rec* 1961;139:145–153.
15. Zarrabi MH, Grünwald HW, Rosner F: Chronic lymphocytic leukemia terminating in acute leukemia. *Arch Intern Med* 1977;137:1059–1064.
16. Cameron S: Chlorambucil and leukemia. *N Eng J Med* 1977; 296:1065.
17. Lawler SD, Lele KP: Chromosomal damage induced by chlorambucil in chronic lymphocytic leukemia. *Scand J Haematol* 1972;9:603–612.
18. Stevenson AC, Patel C: Effects of chlorambucil on human chromosomes. *Mutat Res* 1973;18:333–351.
19. Guesry P, Lenoir G, Broyer M: Gonadal effects of chlorambucil given to prepubertal and pubertal boys for nephrotic syndrome. *J Pediatr* 1978;92:299–303.
20. Richter P, Calamera JC, Morgenfeld MC, et al: Effect of chlorambucil on spermatogenesis in the human with malignant lymphoma. *Cancer* 1970;25:1026–1030.
21. Morgenfeld MC, Goldberg V, Parisier H, et al: Ovarian lesions due to cytostatic agents during the treatment of Hodgkin's disease. *Surg Gynecol Obstet* 1972; 134:826–828.
22. Sobrinho LG, Levine RA, DeConti RC: Amenorrhea in patients with Hodgkin's disease treated with antineoplastic agents. *Am J Obstet Gynecol* 1971;109:135–139.
23. Galton DAG, Israels LG, Nabarro JDN, et al: Clinical trials of p-(Di-2-chloroethylamino)-phenylbutyric acid (CB 1348) in malignant lymphoma. *Br Med. J* 1955;2:1172–1176.
24. Ciobanu N, Runowicz C, Gucalp R, et al: Reversible central nervous system toxicity associated with high-dose chlorambucil in autologous bone marrow transplantation for ovarian cancer. *Cancer Treat Rep* 1987;71:1324–1325.
25. Moore GE, Bross IDJ, Ausman R, et al: Effects of chlorambucil (NSC-3088) in 374 patients with advanced cancer. *Cancer Chemother Rep* 1968;52(pt 1):661–666.
26. Galton DAG, Wiltshaw E, Szur L, et al: The use of chlorambucil and steroids in the treatment of chronic lymphocytic leukemia. *Br J Haematol* 1961;7:73–98.
27. Rudd P, Fries JF, Epstein WV: Irreversible bone marrow failure with chlorambucil. *J Rheumatol* 1975;2:421–429.
28. Wolfson S, Olney MB: Accidental ingestion of a toxic dose of chlorambucil: Report of a case in a child. *JAMA* 1957;165:239–240.
29. Byrne TN, Moseley TAE, Finer MA: Myoclonic seizures following chlorambucil overdose. *Ann Neurol* 1981;9:191–194.
30. LaDelfa I, Myers BR, Hoffstein V: Chlorambucil induced myoclonic seizures in an adult. *J Clin Oncol* 1985;3:1691–1692.
31. Naysmith A, Robson RH: Focal fits during chlorambucil therapy. *Postgrad Med J* 1979;55:806–807.
32. Blank DW, Nanji AA, Schreiber DH, et al: Acute renal failure and seizures associated with chlorambucil overdose. *J Toxicol Clin Toxicol* 1983;20:361–365.
33. Ammenti A, Reitter B, Muller-Wiefel DE: Chlorambucil neurotoxicity: Report of two cases. *Helv Paediatr Acta* 1980;35:281–287.
34. Green AA, Naiman JL: Chlorambucil poisoning. *Am J Dis Child* 1968;116:190–191.
35. Enck RE, Bennett JM: Inadvertent chlorambucil overdose in adults. *NY State J Med* 1977;77:1480–1481.
36. Knospe WH, Loeb V Jr, Huguley CM: Bi-weekly chlorambucil treatment of chronic lymphocytic leukemia. *Cancer* 1974;33:555–562.

Continued on next page

Burroughs Wellcome—Cont.

37. Sawitsky A, Rai KR, Glidewell O, et al: Comparison of daily versus intermittent chlorambucil and prednisone therapy in the treatment of patients with chronic lymphocytic leukemia. *Blood* 1977;50:1049–1059.
38. Recommendations for the safe handling of parenteral antineoplastic drugs. US Dept of Health and Human Services publications No. (NIH) 83-2621. Government Printing Office, 1983.
39. Council on Scientific Affairs: Guidelines for handling parenteral antineoplastic drugs. AMA COUNCIL REPORT. *JAMA* 1985;253:1590–1592.
40. National Study Commission on Cytotoxic Exposure: Recommendations for Handling Cytotoxic Agents. (Available from L.P. Jeffrey, Director of Pharmacy Services, Rhode Island Hospital, 593 Eddy St, Providence, RI 02902.)
41. Clinical Oncological Society of Australia: Guidelines and recommendations for safe handling of antineoplastic agents. *Med J Australia* 1983;1:426–428.
42. Jones RB, Frank R, Mass T: Safe handling of chemotherapeutic agents: A report from the Mount Sinai Medical Center. *CA-A Cancer J for Clin* 1983;33:258–263.
43. American Society of Hospital Pharmacists technical assistance bulletin on handling cytotoxic drugs in hospitals. *Am J Hosp Pharm* 1985;42:131–137.
44. Yodaiken RE, Bennett D: OSHA work-practice guidelines for personnel dealing with cytotoxic (antineoplastic) drugs. *AM J Hosp Pharm* 1986;43:1193–1204.

542525

Shown in Product Identification Section, page 407

MANTADIL® CREAM ℞
[*măn'tah-dĭl"*]

DESCRIPTION
Mantadil® Cream contains the antihistamine chlorcyclizine hydrochloride 2% and the corticosteroid hydrocortisone acetate 0.5%, with methylparaben 0.25% (added as a preservative) in a vanishing cream base. The inactive ingredients are liquid and white petrolatum, emulsifying wax and purified water.

Mantadil Cream is an ANTIPRURITIC-ANTI-INFLAMMATORY-ANESTHETIC for topical administration.

Chlorcyclizine hydrochloride is known chemically as 1-[(4-chlorophenyl)phenylmethyl]- 4-methylpiperazine monohydrochloride.

Hydrocortisone acetate is the acetate ester of cortisol, known chemically as 21-(acetyloxy)-11β,17-dihydroxypregn-4-ene-3, 20-dione.

The pH of this product is approximately 4.5.

CLINICAL PHARMACOLOGY
Chlorcyclizine hydrochloride is an H_1 histamine-receptor antagonist that will occupy receptor sites in effector cells to the exclusion of histamine. It blocks most of the effects of histamine mediated by H_1 receptors, including contraction of smooth muscle and increased capillary permeability. Absorption of chlorcyclizine hydrochloride into the skin is rapid following topical application, whereas systemic absorption from the skin is minimal. Chlorcyclizine hydrochloride prevents local edema and provides local anesthetic and antipruritic action in the skin.

Hydrocortisone acetate administered topically suppresses most inflammatory and allergic responses in the skin. Following topical application, it is absorbed rapidly into the skin, where it reduces local heat, redness, swelling, and tenderness. A small part of the dose applied to broken skin is absorbed systemically and metabolized by the liver.

INDICATIONS AND USAGE
Mantadil Cream is indicated for the treatment of pruritic skin eruptions and other dermatoses including: eczema (allergic, nuchal and nummular); dermatitis (atopic, lichenoid and seborrheic); contact dermatitis including poison ivy, poison oak and poison sumac; localized neurodermatitis; insect bites; sunburn; intertrigo; and anogenital pruritus.

CONTRAINDICATIONS
This preparation is contraindicated in patients who are hypersensitive to any of its components; in tuberculosis of the skin, vaccinia, varicella, and herpes simplex. As with other topical products containing hydrocortisone, the cream should not be used in bacterial infections of the skin unless antibacterial therapy is concomitant.

Not for ophthalmic use.

WARNINGS
Oral chlorcyclizine is teratogenic in animals. Long-term reproduction studies of topical chlorcyclizine have not been conducted in humans.

PRECAUTIONS
General: If signs of irritation develop with use of this cream, treatment should be discontinued and appropriate therapy instituted.

Any of the side effects reported following systemic use of corticosteroids, including adrenal suppression, may also occur following their topical use, especially in infants and children. Systemic absorption of topically applied steroids will be increased if extensive body surface areas are treated or if the occlusive technique is used. Under these circumstances, suitable precautions should be taken when long-term use is anticipated, particularly in infants and children.

Carcinogenesis, Mutagenesis, Impairment of Fertility: Oral chlorcyclizine is teratogenic in animals. Long-term reproduction studies of topical chlorcyclizine have not been conducted. It is poorly absorbed percutaneously.

Pregnancy: ***Teratogenic Effects:*** Pregnancy Category C. Animal reproduction studies have not been conducted with Mantadil Cream. It is also not known whether Mantadil Cream can cause fetal harm when administered to a pregnant woman or can affect reproduction capacity. Mantadil Cream should be given to a pregnant woman only if clearly needed.

Nursing Mothers: Hydrocortisone acetate appears in human milk following oral administration of the drug.

Caution should be exercised when hydrocortisone acetate is administered to a nursing woman.

It is not known whether chlorcyclizine hydrochloride is excreted in human milk. Because many drugs are excreted in human milk, caution should be exercised when chlorcyclizine hydrochloride is administered to a nursing woman.

ADVERSE REACTIONS
Allergic contact dermatitis may occur with topical application of chlorcyclizine hydrochloride. Systemic side effects have been reported after topical application of antihistamines to large areas of skin.

The following local adverse reactions have been reported with topical corticosteroids, especially under occlusive dressings: irritation, folliculitis, hypertrichosis, acneiform eruptions, hypopigmentation, allergic contact dermatitis, secondary infection, skin atrophy, striae and miliaria.

OVERDOSAGE
With continued application of topical corticosteroid on large areas of damaged skin and under occlusion, there is a remote possibility that sufficient absorption could occur to produce Cushing's syndrome. This is more likely in children.

Systemic toxicity following topical application of chlorcyclizine has never been reported.

The oral LD_{50} of chlorcyclizine hydrochloride in the mouse is 300 mg/kg.

The intraperitoneal LD_{50} of hydrocortisone acetate in the mouse is 2300 mg/kg.

DOSAGE AND ADMINISTRATION
Apply to the skin two to five times daily. If the condition of the skin will permit, the cream should be well rubbed in.

HOW SUPPLIED
Mantadil Cream (Chlorcyclizine hydrochloride 2% and hydrocortisone acetate 0.5%) is available in 15 gram tubes (**NDC** 0081-0650-94).

Store at 15° to 25°C (59° to 77°F). 547129

MAREZINE® Tablets OTC
[*mâr'uh-zēn*]
Antiemetic
Motion Sickness Remedy

(See PDR For Nonprescription Drugs.)
Shown in Product Identification Section, page 407

MIVACRON® INJECTION ℞
MIVACRON PREMIXED INFUSION
[*mĭv'ah-krŏn*]
(Mivacurium Chloride)

This drug should be administered only by adequately trained individuals familiar with its actions, characteristics, and hazards.

DESCRIPTION
MIVACRON (mivacurium chloride) is a short-acting, nondepolarizing skeletal muscle relaxant for intravenous administration. Mivacurium chloride is [*R*-[*R**,*R**-(*E*)]]-2,2'-[(1,8-dioxo-4-octene-1,8-diyl)bis(oxy-3, 1-propanediyl)]bis[1,2, 3,4-tetrahydro-6,7-dimethoxy-2-methyl-1-[(3,4,5-trimethoxy-phenyl)methyl]isoquinolinium]dichloride. The molecular formula is $C_{58}H_{80}Cl_2N_2O_{14}$ and the molecular weight is 1100.18.

The partition coefficient of the compound is 0.015 in a 1-octanol/distilled water system at 25°C.

Mivacurium chloride is a mixture of three stereoisomers: (1*R*, 1'*R*, 2*S*, 2'*S*), the *trans-trans* diester; (1*R*, 1'*R*, 2*R*, 2'*S*), the *cis-trans* diester; and (1*R*, 1'*R*, 2*R*, 2'*R*), the *cis-cis* diester. The *trans-trans* and *cis-trans* stereoisomers comprise 92% to 96% of mivacurium chloride and their neuromuscular blocking potencies are not significantly different from each other or from mivacurium chloride. The *cis-cis* diester has been estimated from studies in cats to have one-tenth the neuromuscular blocking potency of the other two stereoisomers.

MIVACRON Injection is a sterile, non-pyrogenic solution (pH 3.5 to 5.0) containing mivacurium chloride equivalent to 2 mg/mL mivacurium in Water for Injection. Hydrochloric acid may have been added to adjust pH. MIVACRON Premixed Infusion is a sterile, non-pyrogenic solution (pH 3.5 to 5.0; 260 mOsmol/L-measured) containing mivacurium chloride equivalent to 0.5 mg/mL mivacurium in 5% Dextrose Injection USP. Hydrochloric acid may have been added to adjust pH.

CLINICAL PHARMACOLOGY
MIVACRON (a mixture of three stereoisomers) binds competitively to cholinergic receptors on the motor end-plate to antagonize the action of acetylcholine, resulting in a block of neuromuscular transmission. This action is antagonized by acetylcholinesterase inhibitors, such as neostigmine.

Pharmacodynamics: The time to maximum neuromuscular block is similar for recommended doses of MIVACRON and intermediate-acting agents (*e.g.*, atracurium), but longer than for the ultra-short-acting agent, succinylcholine. The clinically effective duration of action of the stereoisomers in MIVACRON (a mixture of three stereoisomers) is one-third to one-half that of intermediate-acting agents and 2 to 2.5 times that of succinylcholine.

The average ED_{95} (dose required to produce 95% suppression of the adductor pollicis muscle twitch response to ulnar nerve stimulation) of MIVACRON is 0.07 mg/kg (range: 0.06 to 0.09) in adults receiving opioid/nitrous oxide/oxygen anesthesia. The pharmacodynamics of doses of MIVACRON $\geq ED_{95}$ administered over 5 to 15 seconds during opioid/nitrous oxide/oxygen anesthesia are summarized in Table 1. The mean time for spontaneous recovery of the twitch response from 25% to 75% of control amplitude is about 6 minutes (range: 3 to 9, n=32) following an initial dose of 0.15 mg/kg MIVACRON and 7 to 8 minutes (range: 4 to 24, n=85) following initial doses of 0.20 or 0.25 mg/kg MIVACRON.

Volatile anesthetics may decrease the dosing requirement for MIVACRON and prolong the duration of action; the magnitude of these effects may be increased as the concentration of the volatile agent is increased. Isoflurane and enflurane (administered with nitrous oxide/oxygen to achieve 1.25 MAC [Minimum Alveolar Concentration]) may decrease the effective dose of MIVACRON by as much as 25%, and may prolong the clinically effective duration of action and decrease the average infusion requirement by as much as 35% to 40%. At equivalent MAC values, halothane has little or no effect on the ED_{50} of MIVACRON, but may prolong the duration of action and decrease the average infusion requirement by as much as 20% (**see Individualization of Dosages** subsection of CLINICAL PHARMACOLOGY and **Drug Interaction** subsections of PRECAUTIONS).

[See Table 1 on next page.]

Administration of MIVACRON over 60 seconds does not alter the time to maximum neuromuscular block or the duration of action. The duration of action of the stereoisomers in MIVACRON may be prolonged in patients with reduced plasma cholinesterase (pseudocholinesterase) activity (see **Reduced Plasma Cholinesterase Activity** subsection of PRECAUTIONS and **Individualization of Dosages** subsection of CLINICAL PHARMACOLOGY).

Interpatient variability in duration of action occurs with MIVACRON as with other neuromuscular blocking agents. However, analysis of data from 224 patients in clinical studies receiving various doses of MIVACRON during opioid/nitrous oxide/oxygen anesthesia with a variety of premedicants and varying lengths of surgery indicated that approximately 90% of the patients had clinically effective durations of block within 8 minutes of the median duration predicted from the dose-response data shown in Table 1. Variations in plasma cholinesterase activity, including values within the normal range and values as low as 20% below the lower limit of the normal range, were not associated with clinically significant effects on duration. The variability in duration, however, was greater in patients with plasma cholinesterase activity at or slightly below the lower limit of the normal range.

A dose of 0.15 mg/kg ($2 \times ED_{95}$) MIVACRON administered during the induction of thiopental/opioid/nitrous oxide/oxygen anesthesia produced generally good-to-excellent conditions for tracheal intubation in 2.5 minutes. Doses of 0.20 and 0.25 mg/kg (3 and $3.5 \times ED_{95}$) yielded similar conditions in 2.0 minutes.

Repeated administration of maintenance doses or continuous infusion of MIVACRON for up to 2.5 hours is not associated with development of tachyphylaxis or cumulative neu-

Table 1
Pharmacodynamic Dose Response During Opioid/Nitrous Oxide/Oxygen Anesthesia

Initial MIVACRON Dose (mg/kg)		Time to Maximum Block[1] (min)	Time to Spontaneous Recovery[1]			
			5% Recovery (min)	25% Recovery[2] (min)	95% Recovery[3] (min)	T_4/T_1 Ratio $\geq 75\%$[3] (min)
Adults						
0.07 to 0.10	[n=47]	4.9 (2.0–7.6)	11 (7–19)	13 (8–24)	21 (10–36)	21 (10–36)
0.15	[n=50]	3.3 (1.5–8.8)	13 (6–31)	16 (9–38)	26 (16–41)	26 (15–45)
0.20	[n=50]	2.5 (1.2–6.0)	16 (10–29)	20 (10–36)	31 (15–51)	34 (19–56)
0.25	[n=48]	2.3 (1.0–4.8)	19 (11–29)	23 (14–38)	34 (22–64)	43 (26–75)
Children 2 to 12 Years						
0.11 to 0.12	[n=17]	2.8 (1.2–4.6)	5 (3–9)	7 (4–10)	—	—
0.20	[n=18]	1.9 (1.3–3.3)	7 (3–12)	10 (6–15)	19 (14–26)	16 (12–23)
0.25	[n=9]	1.6 (1.0–2.2)	7 (4–9)	9 (5–12)	—	—

[1] Values shown are medians of means from individual studies (range of individual patient values).
[2] Clinically effective duration of neuromuscular block.
[3] Data available for as few as 40% of adults in specific dose groups and for 22% of children in the 0.20 mg/kg dose group due to administration of reversal agents or additional doses of MIVACRON prior to 95% recovery or T_4/T_1 ratio recovery to $\geq 75\%$.

romuscular blocking effects in ASA Physical Status I–II patients. Limited data are available from patients receiving infusions for longer than 2.5 hours. Spontaneous recovery of neuromuscular function after infusion is independent of the duration of infusion and comparable to recovery reported for single doses (Table 1).

The neuromuscular block produced by the stereoisomers in MIVACRON is readily antagonized by anticholinesterase agents. As seen with other nondepolarizing neuromuscular blocking agents, the more profound the neuromuscular block at the time of reversal, the longer the time and the greater the dose of anticholinesterase agent required for recovery of neuromuscular function.

In children (2 to 12 years), MIVACRON has a higher ED_{95} (0.10 mg/kg), faster onset, and shorter duration of action than in adults. The mean time for spontaneous recovery of the twitch response from 25% to 75% of control amplitude is about 5 minutes (n=4) following an initial dose of 0.20 mg/kg MIVACRON. Recovery following reversal is faster in children than in adults (Table 1).

Hemodynamics: Administration of MIVACRON in doses up to and including 0.15 mg/kg ($2 \times ED_{95}$) over 5 to 15 seconds to ASA Physical Status I–II patients during opioid/nitrous oxide/oxygen anesthesia is associated with minimal changes in mean arterial blood pressure (MAP) or heart rate (HR) (Table 2).

Table 2
Cardiovascular Dose Response During Opioid/Nitrous Oxide/Oxygen Anesthesia

Initial MIVACRON Dose (mg/kg)		% of Patients With $\geq 30\%$ Change			
		MAP		HR	
		Dec	Inc	Dec	Inc
Adults					
0.07 to 0.10	[n=49]	0%	2%	0%	0%
0.15	[n=53]	4%	4%	4%	2%
0.20	[n=53]	30%	0%	0%	8%
0.25	[n=44]	39%	2%	0%	14%
Children 2 to 12 years					
0.11 to 0.12	[n=17]	0%	6%	0%	0%
0.20	[n=17]	0%	0%	0%	0%
0.25	[n=8]	13%	0%	0%	0%

Higher doses of ≥ 0.20 mg/kg ($\geq 3 \times ED_{95}$) may be associated with transient decreases in MAP and increases in HR in some patients. These decreases in MAP are usually maximal within 1 to 3 minutes following the dose, typically resolve without treatment in an additional 1 to 3 minutes, and are usually associated with increases in plasma histamine concentration. Decreases in MAP can be minimized by administering MIVACRON over 30 or 60 seconds (see **Individualization of Dosages** subsection of CLINICAL PHARMACOLOGY and **General** subsection of PRECAUTIONS).

Analysis of 426 patients in clinical studies receiving initial doses of MIVACRON up to and including 0.30 mg/kg (i.e., 2 times the recommended intubating dose) during opioid/nitrous oxide/oxygen anethesia showed that high initial doses and a rapid rate of injection contributed to a greater proba-

bility of experiencing a decrease of $\geq 30\%$ in MAP after MIVACRON administration. Obese patients also had a greater probability of experiencing a decrease of $\geq 30\%$ in MAP when dosed on the basis of actual body weight, thereby receiving a larger dose than if dosed on the basis of ideal body weight (see **Individualization of Dosages** subsection of CLINICAL PHARMACOLOGY and the **General** subsection of PRECAUTIONS).

Children experience minimal changes in MAP or HR after administration of MIVACRON doses up to and including 0.20 mg/kg over 5 to 15 seconds, but higher doses (≥ 0.25 mg/kg) may be associated with transient decreases in MAP (Table 2).

Following a dose of 0.15 mg/kg MIVACRON administered over 60 seconds, adult patients with significant cardiovascular disease undergoing coronary artery bypass grafting or valve replacement procedures showed no clinically important changes in MAP or HR. Transient decreases in MAP were observed in some patients after doses of 0.20 to 0.25 mg/kg MIVACRON administered over 60 seconds. The number of patients in whom these decreases in MAP required treatment was small.

Pharmacokinetics: Table 3 describes the results from a study of 9 ASA Physical Status I–II adult patients (31 to 48 years) receiving an infusion of MIVACRON at 5 µg/kg/min for 60 minutes followed by 10 µg/kg/min for 60 minutes. MIVACRON is a mixture of isomers which do not interconvert in vivo. The mivacurium pharmacokinetic parameters presented in Table 3 were determined using a stereospecific assay. The two more potent isomers, cis-trans (36% of the mixture) and trans-trans (57% of the mixture), have very high clearances that exceed cardiac output reflecting the extensive metabolism by plasma cholinesterase. The volume of distribution is relatively small, reflecting limited tissue distribution secondary to the polarity and large molecular weight of mivacurium. The combination of high metabolic clearance and low distribution volume results in the short elimination half-life of approximately 2 minutes for the two active isomers. The short elimination half-lives and high metabolic clearances of the active isomers are consistent

Table 3
Stereoisomer Pharmacokinetic Parameters[1] of MIVACRON in ASA Physical Status I–II Adult Patients[2] [n=9] During Opioid/Nitrous Oxide/Oxygen Anesthesia

Parameter	trans-trans isomer	cis-trans isomer
Elimination Half-life ($t_{1/2}$, min)	2.3 (1.4–3.6)	2.1 (0.8–4.8)
Volume of Distribution (L/kg)	0.15 (0.06–0.24)	0.27 (0.08–0.56)
Plasma Clearance (mL/min/kg)	53 (32–105)	99 (52–230)

[1] Values shown are mean (range).
[2] Ages 31 to 48 years.

with the short duration of action of MIVACRON. The steady-state concentrations of the cis-trans and trans-trans isomers doubled after the infusion rate was increased from 5 to 10 µg/kg/min, indicating that their pharmacokinetics are dose-proportional.

The cis-cis isomer (6% of the mixture) has approximately one-tenth the neuromuscular blocking potency of the trans-trans and cis-trans isomers in cats. In the nine patients shown in Table 3, the volume of distribution of the cis-cis isomer averaged 0.31 L/kg (range: 0.18–0.46), the clearance averaged 4.2 mL/min/kg (range: 2.4–5.4), and the half-life averaged 55 minutes (range: 32–102). The neuromuscular blocking potency of the cis-cis isomer in humans has not been established; however, modeling of clinical pharmacokinetic-pharmacodynamic data suggests that the cis-cis isomer produces minimal (<5%) neuromuscular block during a two-hour infusion. In studies in which infusions of up to 2.5 hours were administered to ASA Physical Status I–II patients, the 25%–75% recovery times were independent of the duration of infusion, suggesting that the cis-cis isomer does not contribute significant neuromuscular block during use for up to 2.5 hours. Limited data are available from infusions of longer duration or from patients with compromised elimination capacities (hepatic or renal failure).

Metabolism and Excretion: *Enzymatic hydrolysis by plasma cholinesterase is the primary mechanism for inactivation of mivacurium and yields a quaternary alcohol and a quaternary monoester metabolite.* Renal and biliary excretion of unchanged mivacurium are minor elimination pathways; urine and bile are important elimination pathways for the two metabolites. Tests in which these two metabolites were administered to cats and dogs suggest that each metabolite is unlikely to produce clinically significant neuromuscular, autonomic, or cardiovascular effects following administration of MIVACRON.

Special Populations: The pharmacokinetics of mivacurium isomers has not been studied in the elderly or in patients with renal or hepatic disease using a stereospecific assay. The non-stereospecific, total mivacurium assay used in pharmacokinetic-pharmacodynamic studies in these populations provided preliminary evidence that reduced clearance of one or more isomers is responsible for the longer duration of action of MIVACRON seen in patients with end-stage kidney or liver disease. The data did not provide a pharmacokinetic explanation for the 15–20% longer duration of block seen in the elderly. Tables 4 and 5 summarize the pharmacodynamic results in these special populations as compared with young adults (ages 18 to 49 years). No data are available from patients with kidney or liver disease not requiring transplantation.

[See Table 4 on next page.]

Renal: The clinically effective duration of action of 0.15 mg/kg MIVACRON was about 1.5 times longer in patients with end-stage kidney disease than in healthy patients, presumably due to reduced clearance of one or more isomers.

Hepatic: The clinically effective duration of action of 0.15 mg/kg MIVACRON was three times longer in patients with end-stage liver disease than in healthy patients and is likely related to the markedly decreased plasma cholinesterase activity (30% of healthy patient values) which could decrease the clearance of one or more isomers (see **Reduced Plasma Cholinesterase Activity** subsection of PRECAUTIONS).

[See Table 5 on next page.]

Individualization of Dosages: DOSES OF MIVACRON SHOULD BE INDIVIDUALIZED AND A PERIPHERAL NERVE STIMULATOR SHOULD BE USED TO MEASURE NEUROMUSCULAR FUNCTION DURING MIVACRON ADMINISTRATION IN ORDER TO MONITOR DRUG EFFECT, DETERMINE THE NEED FOR ADDITIONAL DOSES, AND CONFIRM RECOVERY FROM NEUROMUSCULAR BLOCK.

Based on the known actions of MIVACRON (a mixture of three stereoisomers) and other neuromuscular blocking agents, the following factors should be considered when administering MIVACRON:

Renal or Hepatic Impairment: A dose of 0.15 mg/kg MIVACRON is recommended for facilitation of tracheal intubation in patients with renal or hepatic impairment. However, the clinically effective duration of block produced by this dose is about 1.5 times longer in patients with end-stage kidney disease and about 3 times longer in patients with end-stage liver disease than in patients with normal renal and hepatic function. Infusion rates should be decreased by as much as 50% in these patients depending on the degree of renal or hepatic impairment (see **Renal and Hepatic Disease** subsection of PRECAUTIONS).

Reduced Plasma Cholinesterase Activity: The possibility of prolonged neuromuscular block following administration of MIVACRON must be considered in patients with reduced plasma cholinesterase (pseudocholinesterase) activity.

Continued on next page

Burroughs Wellcome—Cont.

MIVACRON should be used with great caution, if at all, in patients known or suspected of being homozygous for the atypical plasma cholinesterase gene (see WARNINGS). Doses of 0.03 mg/kg produced complete neuromuscular block for 26 to 128 minutes in three such patients; thus initial doses greater than 0.03 mg/kg are not recommended in homozygous patients. Infusion of MIVACRON are not recommended in homozygous patients.

MIVACRON has been used safely in patients heterozygous for the atypical plasma cholinesterase gene and in genotypically normal patients with reduced plasma cholinesterase activity. After recommended intubating doses of MIVACRON, the clinically effective duration of block in heterozygous patients may be approximately 10 minutes longer than in patients with normal genotype and normal plasma cholinesterase activity. Lower MIVACRON infusion rates are recommended in these patients (see **Reduced Plasma Cholinesterase Activity** subsection of PRECAUTIONS).

Drugs or Conditions Causing Potentiation of or Resistance to Neuromuscular Block: As with other neuromuscular blocking agents, MIVACRON may have profound neuromuscular blocking effects in cachectic or debilitated patients, patients with neuromuscular diseases, and patients with carcinomatosis. In these or other patients in whom potentiation of neuromuscular block or difficulty with reversal may be anticipated, the recommended initial dose should be decreased. A test dose of not more than 0.015–0.020 mg/kg, which represents the lower end of the dose-response curve for MIVACRON, is recommended in such patients (see **General** subsection of PRECAUTIONS).

The neuromuscular blocking action of the stereoisomers in MIVACRON is potentiated by isoflurane or enflurane anesthesia. The recommended initial MIVACRON dose of 0.15 mg/kg may be used for intubation prior to the administration of these agents. If MIVACRON is first administered after establishment of stable-state isoflurane or enflurane anesthesia (administered with nitrous oxide/oxygen to achieve 1.25 MAC), the initial MIVACRON dose should be reduced by as much as 25%, and the infusion rate reduced by as much as 35% to 40%. A greater potentiation of the neuromuscular blocking action of the stereoisomers in MIVACRON may be expected with higher concentrations of enflurane or isoflurane. The use of halothane requires no adjustment of the initial dose of MIVACRON, but may prolong the duration of action and decrease the average infusion rate by as much as 20% (see **Drug Interactions** subsection of PRECAUTIONS).

When MIVACRON is administered to patients receiving certain antibiotics, magnesium salts, lithium, local anesthetics, procainamide and quinidine, longer durations of neuromuscular block may be expected and infusion requirements may be lower (see **Drug Interactions** subsection of PRECAUTIONS).

When MIVACRON is administered to patients chronically receiving phenytoin or carbamazepine, slightly shorter durations of neuromuscular block may be anticipated and infusion rate requirements may be higher (see **Drug Interactions** subsection of PRECAUTIONS).

Severe acid-base and/or electrolyte abnormalities may potentiate or cause resistance to the neuromuscular blocking action of the stereoisomers in MIVACRON. No data are available in such patients and no dosing recommendations can be made (see **General** subsection of PRECAUTIONS).

Burns: While patients with burns are known to develop resistance to nondepolarizing neuromuscular blocking agents, they may also have reduced plasma cholinesterase activity. Consequently, in these patients, a test dose of not more than 0.015–0.020 mg/kg MIVACRON is recommended, followed

by additional appropriate dosing guided by the use of a neuromuscular block monitor (see **General** subsection of PRECAUTIONS).

Cardiovascular Disease: In patients with clinically significant cardiovascular disease, the initial dose of MIVACRON should be 0.15 mg/kg or less, administered over 60 seconds (see **Hemodynamics** subsection of CLINICAL PHARMACOLOGY and **General** subsection of PRECAUTIONS).

Obesity: Obese patients (patients weighing $\geq$ 30% more than their ideal body weight) dosed on the basis of actual body weight, thereby receiving a larger dose than if dosed on the basis of ideal body weight, had a greater probability of experiencing a decrease of $\geq$ 30% in MAP (see **Hemodynamics** subsection of CLINICAL PHARMACOLOGY and **General** subsection of PRECAUTIONS). Therefore, in obese patients, the initial dose should be determined using the patient's ideal body weight (IBW), according to the following formulae:

Men: IBW in kg = [106 + (6 × inches in height above 5 feet)]/2.2

Women: IBW in kg = [100 + (5 × inches in height above 5 feet)]/2.2

Allergy and Sensitivity: In patients with any history suggestive of a greater sensitivity to the release of histamine or related mediators (*e.g.*, asthma), the initial dose of MIVACRON should be 0.15 mg/kg or less, administered over 60 seconds (see **General** subsection of PRECAUTIONS).

INDICATIONS AND USAGE

MIVACRON is a short-acting neuromuscular blocking agent indicated for inpatients and outpatients, as an adjunct to general anesthesia, to facilitate tracheal intubation and to provide skeletal muscle relaxation during surgery or mechanical ventilation.

CONTRAINDICATIONS

MIVACRON is contraindicated in patients known to have an allergic hypersensitivity to mivacurium chloride or other benzylisoquinolinium agents, as manifested by reactions such as urticaria or severe respiratory distress or hypotension. Use of MIVACRON from multi-dose vials is contraindicated in patients with a known allergy to benzyl alcohol.

WARNINGS

MIVACRON SHOULD BE ADMINISTERED IN CAREFULLY ADJUSTED DOSAGE BY OR UNDER THE SUPERVISION OF EXPERIENCED CLINICIANS WHO ARE FAMILIAR WITH THE DRUG'S ACTIONS AND THE POSSIBLE COMPLICATIONS OF ITS USE. THE DRUG SHOULD NOT BE ADMINISTERED UNLESS PERSONNEL AND FACILITIES FOR RESUSCITATION AND LIFE SUPPORT (TRACHEAL INTUBATION, ARTIFICIAL VENTILATION, OXYGEN THERAPY), AND AN ANTAGONIST OF MIVACRON ARE IMMEDIATELY AVAILABLE. IT IS RECOMMENDED THAT A PERIPHERAL NERVE STIMULATOR BE USED TO MEASURE NEUROMUSCULAR FUNCTION DURING THE ADMINISTRATION OF MIVACRON IN ORDER TO MONITOR DRUG EFFECT, DETERMINE THE NEED FOR ADDITIONAL DRUG, AND CONFIRM RECOVERY FROM NEUROMUSCULAR BLOCK.

MIVACRON HAS NO KNOWN EFFECT ON CONSCIOUSNESS, PAIN THRESHOLD, OR CEREBRATION. TO AVOID DISTRESS TO THE PATIENT, NEUROMUSCULAR BLOCK SHOULD NOT BE INDUCED BEFORE UNCONSCIOUSNESS.

MIVACRON IS METABOLIZED BY PLASMA CHOLINESTERASE AND SHOULD BE USED WITH GREAT CAUTION, IF AT ALL, IN PATIENTS KNOWN TO BE OR SUSPECTED OF BEING HOMOZYGOUS FOR THE ATYPICAL PLASMA CHOLINESTERASE GENE.

MIVACRON Injection and MIVACRON Premixed Infusion are acidic (pH 3.5 to 5.0) and may not be compatible with alkaline solutions having a pH greater than 8.5 (*e.g.*, barbiturate solutions).

PRECAUTIONS

General: Although MIVACRON (a mixture of three stereoisomers) is not a potent histamine releaser, the possibility of substantial histamine release must be considered. Release of histamine is related to the dose and speed of injection.

Caution should be exercised in administering MIVACRON to patients with clinically significant cardiovascular disease and patients with any history suggesting a greater sensitivity to the release of histamine or related mediators (*e.g.*, asthma). In such patients, the initial dose of MIVACRON should be 0.15 mg/kg or less, administered over 60 seconds; assurance of adequate hydration and careful monitoring of hemodynamic status are important (see **Hemodynamics** and **Individualization of Dosages** subsection of CLINICAL PHARMACOLOGY).

Obese patients may be more likely to experience clinically significant transient decreases in MAP than non-obese patients when the dose of MIVACRON is based on actual rather than ideal body weight. Therefore, in obese patients, the initial dose should be determined using the patient's ideal body weight (see **Hemodynamics** and **Individualization of Dosages** subsection of CLINICAL PHARMACOLOGY).

Recommended doses of MIVACRON have no clinically significant effects on heart rate; therefore, MIVACRON will not counteract the bradycardia produced by many anesthetic agents or by vagal stimulation.

Neuromuscular blocking agents may have a profound effect in patients with neuromuscular diseases (*e.g.*, myasthenia gravis and the myasthenic syndrome). In these and other conditions in which prolonged neuromuscular block is a possibility (*e.g.*, carcinomatosis), the use of a peripheral nerve stimulator and a dose of not more than 0.015–0.020 mg/kg MIVACRON is recommended to assess the level of neuromuscular block and to monitor dosage requirements (see **Individualization of Dosages** subsection of CLINICAL PHARMACOLOGY).

MIVACRON has not been studied in patients with burns. Resistance to nondepolarizing neuromuscular blocking agents may develop in patients with burns, depending upon the time elapsed since the injury and the size of the burn. Patients with burns may have reduced plasma cholinesterase activity which may offset this resistance (see **Individualization of Dosages** subsection of CLINICAL PHARMACOLOGY).

Acid-base and/or serum electrolyte abnormalities may potentiate or antagonize the action of neuromuscular blocking agents. The action of neuromuscular blocking agents may be

Table 5
Pharmacodynamic Parameters[1] of MIVACRON in ASA Physical Status I–II Patients and in Patients Undergoing Kidney or Liver Transplantation During Isoflurane/Nitrous Oxide/Oxygen Anesthesia

Parameter	Young Adult Patients	Kidney Transplant Patients	Liver Transplant Patients[3]
Initial Dose	0.15 mg/kg [n=8]	0.15 mg/kg [n=9]	0.15 mg/kg [n=8]
Maximum Block (%)	99.8 (98–100)	100 (100–100)	100 (100–100)
Time to Maximum Block (min)	1.9 (0.8–3.5)	2.6 (1.0–4.5)	2.1 (1.0 –4.0)
Clinically Effective Duration of Block[2] (min)	19 (12–30)	30 (19–58)	57 (29–80)

[1] Values shown are mean (range).
[2] Time from injection to 25% recovery of the control twitch height.
[3] Liver transplant patients received isoflurane without nitrous oxide.

Table 4
Pharmacodynamic Parameters[1] of MIVACRON in ASA Physical Status I–II Young Adult Patients and Elderly Patients During Isoflurane/Nitrous Oxide/Oxygen Anesthesia

Parameter	Young Adult Patients (18–49 years)		Elderly Patients (68–77 years)
Initial Dose	0.10 mg/kg [n=9]	0.25 mg/kg [n=9]	0.10 mg/kg [n=8]
Maximum Block (%)	98 (83–100)	100 (100–100)	99 (95–100)
Time to Maximum Block (min)	3.2 (2.0–6.0)	1.7 (1.3–2.5)	4.8 (3.0–7.0)
Clinically Effective Duration of Block[2] (min)	17 (9–29)	27 (18–34)	20 (14–28)

[1] Values shown are mean (range).
[2] Time from injection to 25% recovery of the control twitch height.

enhanced by magnesium salts administered for the management of toxemia of pregnancy (see **Individualization of Dosages** subsection of CLINICAL PHARMACOLOGY).

No data are available to support the use of MIVACRON by intramuscular injection.

Renal and Hepatic Disease: The possibility of prolonged neuromuscular block must be considered when MIVACRON is used in patients with renal or hepatic disease (see **Pharmacokinetics** subsection of CLINICAL PHARMACOLOGY). Most patients with chronic hepatic disease such as hepatitis, liver abscess, and cirrhosis of the liver exhibit a marked reduction in plasma cholinesterase activity. Patients with acute or chronic renal disease may also show a reduction in plasma cholinesterase activity (see **Individualization of Dosages** subsection of CLINICAL PHARMACOLOGY).

Reduced Plasma Cholinesterase Activity: The possibility of prolonged neuromuscular block following administration of MIVACRON must be considered in patients with reduced plasma cholinesterase (pseudocholinesterase) activity.

Plasma cholinesterase activity may be diminished in the presence of genetic abnormalities of plasma cholinesterase (e.g., patients heterozygous or homozygous for the atypical plasma cholinesterase gene), pregnancy, liver or kidney disease, malignant tumors, infections, burns, anemia, decompensated heart diseae, peptic ulcer, or myxedema. Plasma cholinesterase activity may also be diminished by chronic administration of oral contraceptives, glucocorticoids, or certain monoamine oxidase inhibitors and by irreversible inhibitors of plasma cholinesterase (e.g., organophosphate insecticides, echothiophate, and certain antineoplastic drugs).

MIVACRON has been used safely in patients heterozygous for the atypical plasma cholinesterase gene. At doses of 0.10 to 0.20 mg/kg MIVACRON, the clinically effective duration of action was 8 to 11 minutes longer in patients heterozygous for the atypical gene than in genotypically normal patients. As with succinylcholine, patients homozygous for the atypical plasma cholinesterase gene (1 in 2500 patients) are extremely sensitive to the neuromuscular blocking effect of MIVACRON. In three such adult patients, a small dose of 0.03 mg/kg (approximately the ED_{10-20} in genotypically normal patients) produced complete neuromuscular block for 26 to 128 minutes. Once spontaneous recovery had begun, neuromuscular block in these patients was antagonized with conventional doses of neostigmine. One adult patient, who was homozygous for the atypical plasma cholinesterase gene, received a dose of 0.18 mg/kg MIVACRON and exhibited complete neuromuscular block for about 4 hours. Response to post-tetanic stimulation was present after 4 hours, all four responses to train-of-four stimulation were present after 6 hours, and the patient was extubated after 8 hours. Reversal was not attempted in this patient.

Malignant Hyperthermia (MH): In a study of MH-susceptible pigs, MIVACRON did not trigger MH. MIVACRON has not been studied in MH-susceptible patients. Because MH can develop in the absence of established triggering agents, the clinician should be prepared to recognize and treat MH in any patient undergoing general anethesia.

Long-Term Use in the Intensive Care Unit (ICU): No data are available on the long-term use of MIVACRON in patients undergoing mechanical ventilation in the ICU.

Drug Interactions: Although MIVACRON (a mixture of three stereoisomers) has been administered safely following succinylcholine-facilitated tracheal intubation, the interaction between the stereoisomers in MIVACRON and succinylcholine has not been systematically studied. Prior administration of succinylcholine can potentiate the neuromuscular blocking effects of nondepolarizing agents. Evidence of spontaneous recovery from succinylcholine should be observed before the administration of MIVACRON.

The use of MIVACRON before succinylcholine to attenuate some of the side effects of succinylcholine has not been studied.

There are no clinical data on the use of MIVACRON with other nondepolarizing neuromuscular blocking agents.

Isoflurane and enflurane (administered with nitrous oxide/oxygen to achieve 1.25 MAC) decrease the ED_{50} of MIVACRON by as much as 25% (see **Pharmacodynamics** and **Individualization of Dosages** subsections of CLINICAL PHARMACOLOGY). These agents may also prolong the clinically effective duration of action and decrease the average infusion requirement of MIVACRON by as much as 35% to 40%. A greater potentiation of the neuromuscular blocking effects of the stereoisomers in MIVACRON may be expected with higher concentrations of enflurane or isoflurane. Halothane has little or no effect on the ED_{50}, but may prolong the duration of action and decrease the average infusion requirement by as much as 20%.

Other drugs which may enhance the neuromuscular blocking action of nondepolarizing agents such as the stereoisomers in MIVACRON include certain antibiotics (e.g., aminoglycosides, tetracyclines, bacitracin, polymyxins, lincomycin, clindamycin, colistin, and sodium colistimethate), magnesium salts, lithium, local anesthetics, procainamide, and quinidine. Drugs that may enhance the neuromuscular blocking effects of mivacurium by a reduction in plasma cho-

linesterase activity include chronic administration of oral contraceptives, glucocorticoids, or certain monamine oxidase inhibitors and by irreversible inhibitors of plasma cholinesterase (see **Reduced Plasma Cholinesterase Activity** subsection of PRECAUTIONS).

Resistance to the neuromuscular blocking action of nondepolarizing neuromuscular blocking agents has been demonstrated in patients chronically administered phenytoin or carbamazepine. While the effects of chronic phenytoin or carbamazepine therapy on the action of the stereoisomers in MIVACRON are unknown, slightly shorter durations of neuromuscular block may be anticipated and infusion rate requirements may be higher.

Carcinogenesis, Mutagenesis, Impairment of Fertility: Carcinogenesis and fertility studies have not been performed. MIVACRON was evaluated in a battery of four short-term mutagenicity tests. It was non-mutagenic in the Ames Salmonella assay, the mouse lymphoma assay, the human lymphocyte assay, and the in vivo rat bone marrow cytogenic assay.

Pregnancy: Teratogenic Effects: Pregnancy Category C. Teratology testing in nonventilated pregnant rats and mice treated subcutaneously with maximum subparalyzing doses of MIVACRON revealed no maternal or fetal toxicity or teratogenic effects. There are no adequate and well-controlled studies of MIVACRON in pregnant women. Because animal studies are not always predictive of human response, and the doses used were subparalyzing, MIVACRON should be used during pregnancy only if the potential benefit justifies the potential risk to the fetus.

Labor and Delivery: The use of MIVACRON during labor, vaginal delivery, or cesarean section has not been studied in humans and it is not known whether MIVACRON administered to the mother has effects on the fetus. Doses of 0.08 and 0.20 mg/kg MIVACRON given to female beagles undergoing cesarean section resulted in negligible levels of the stereoisomers in MIVACRON in umbilical vessel blood of neonates and no deleterious effects on the puppies.

Nursing Mothers: It is not known whether any of the stereoisomers of mivacurium are excreted in human milk. Because many drugs are excreted in human milk, caution should be exercised following administration of MIVACRON to a nursing woman.

Pediatric Use: MIVACRON has not been studied in children below the age of 2 years (see CLINICAL PHARMACOLOGY and DOSAGE AND ADMINISTRATION for clinical experience and recommendations for use in children 2 to 12 years of age).

Geriatric Use: MIVACRON was safely administered during clinical trials to 64 elderly (≥ 65 years) patients, including 31 patients with significant cardiovascular disease (see **General** subsection of PRECAUTIONS). The duration of neuromuscular block may be slightly longer in elderly patients than in young adult patients (see CLINICAL PHARMACOLOGY).

ADVERSE REACTIONS

Observed in Clinical Trials: MIVACRON (a mixture of three stereoisomers) was well tolerated during extensive clinical trials in inpatients and outpatients. Prolonged neuromuscular block, which is an important adverse experience associated with neuromuscular blocking agents as a class, was reported as an adverse experience in 3 of 2074 patients administered MIVACRON. The most commonly reported adverse experience following the administration of MIVACRON was transient, dose-dependent cutaneous flushing about the face, neck, and/or chest. Flushing was most frequently noted after the initial dose of MIVACRON and was reported in about 20% of adult patients who received the recommended dose of 0.15 mg/kg MIVACRON over 5 to 15 seconds. When present, flushing typically began within 1 to 2 minutes after the dose of MIVACRON and lasted for 3 to 5 minutes. Of 60 patients who experienced flushing after 0.15 mg/kg MIVACRON, one patient also experienced mild hypotension that was not treated, and one patient experienced moderate wheezing that was successfully treated.

Overall, hypotension was infrequently reported as an adverse experience in the clinical trials of MIVACRON. None of the 397 adults or 63 children who received recommended doses was treated for a decrease in blood pressure associated with the administration of MIVACRON. Above the recommended dosage range, 1% to 2% of healthy adults given ≥ 0.20 mg/kg over 5 to 15 seconds and 2% to 4% of cardiac surgery patients given ≥ 0.20 mg/kg over 60 seconds were treated for decreases in blood pressure associated with the administration of MIVACRON.

The following adverse experiences were reported in patients administered MIVACRON (all events judged by investigators during the clinical trials to have a possible causal relationship):

Incidence Greater Than 1%—
Cardiovascular: Flushing (15%)
Incidence Less Than 1%—
Cardiovascular: Hypotension, Tachycardia, Bradycardia, Cardiac Arrhythmia, Phlebitis

Respiratory: Bronchospasm, Wheezing, Hypoxemia
Dermatological: Rash, Urticaria, Erythema, Injection Site Reaction
Nonspecific: Prolonged Drug Effect
Neurologic: Dizziness
Musculoskeletal: Muscle Spasms

OVERDOSAGE

Overdosage with neuromuscular blocking agents may result in neuromuscular block beyond the time needed for surgery and anesthesia. The primary treatment is maintenance of a patent airway and controlled ventilation until recovery of normal neuromuscular function is assured. Once evidence of recovery from neuromuscular block is observed, further recovery may be facilitated by administration of an anticholinesterase agent (e.g., neostigmine, edrophonium) in conjunction with an appropriate anticholinergic agent. (see **Antagonism of Neuromuscular Block**). Overdosage may increase the risk of hemodynamic side effects, especially decreases in blood pressure. If needed, cardiovascular support may be provided by proper positioning of the patient, fluid administration, and/or vasopressor agent administration.

Antagonism of Neuromuscular Block:
ANTAGONISTS (SUCH AS NEOSTIGMINE) SHOULD NOT BE ADMINISTERED WHEN COMPLETE NEUROMUSCULAR BLOCK IS EVIDENT OR SUSPECTED. THE USE OF A PERIPHERAL NERVE STIMULATOR TO EVALUATE RECOVERY AND ANTAGONISM OF NEUROMUSCULAR BLOCK IS RECOMMENDED.

Administration of 0.030 to 0.064 mg/kg neostigmine or 0.5 mg/kg edrophonium at approximately 10% recovery from neuromuscular block (range: 1 to 15) produced 95% recovery of the muscle twitch response and a T_4/T_1 ratio ≥ 75% in about 10 minutes. The times from 25% recovery of the muscle twitch response to T_4/T_1 ratio ≥ 75% following these doses of antagonists averaged about 7 to 9 minutes. In comparison, average times for spontaneous recovery from 25% to T_4/T_1 ≥ 75% were 12 to 13 minutes.

Patients administered antagonists should be evaluated for adequate clinical evidence of antagonism, e.g., 5-second head lift and grip strength. Ventilation must be supported until no longer required.

Antagonism may be delayed in the presence of debilitation, carcinomatosis, and the concomitant use of certain broad spectrum antibiotics, or anesthetic agents and other drugs which enhance neuromuscular block or separately cause respiratory depression (see **Drug Interactions** subsection of PRECAUTIONS). Under such circumstances the management is the same as that of prolonged neuromuscular block (see OVERDOSAGE).

DOSAGE AND ADMINISTRATION

MIVACRON SHOULD ONLY BE ADMINISTERED INTRAVENOUSLY.
The dosage information provided below is intended as a guide only. Doses of MIVACRON should be individualized (see **Individualization of Dosages** subsection of CLINICAL PHARMACOLOGY). Factors that may warrant dosage adjustment include but may not be limited to: the presence of significant kidney, liver, or cardiovascular disease, obesity (patients weighing ≥ 30% more than ideal body weight for height), asthma, reduction in plasma cholinesterase activity, and the presence of inhalational anesthetic agents. The use of a peripheral nerve stimulator will permit the most advantageous use of MIVACRON, minimize the possibility of overdosage or underdosage, and assist in the evaluation of recovery.

Adults:
Initial Doses:
A dose of 0.15 mg/kg MIVACRON administered over 5 to 15 seconds is recommended for facilitation of tracheal intubation for most patients. When administered as a component of a thiopental/opioid/nitrous oxide/oxygen induction-intubation technique, 0.15 mg/kg ($2 \times ED_{95}$) MIVACRON produces generally good-to-excellent conditions for tracheal intubation in 2.5 minutes. Lower doses of MIVACRON may result in a longer time for development of satisfactory intubation conditions. Administration of MIVACRON doses above the recommended range (≥ 0.20 mg/kg) is associated with the development of transient decreases in blood pressure in some patients (see CLINICAL PHARMACOLOGY and ADVERSE REACTIONS).

In patients with clinically significant cardiovascular disease and in patients with any history suggesting a greater sensitivity to the release of histamine or other mediators (e.g., asthma), the dose of MIVACRON should be 0.15 mg/kg or less, administered over 60 seconds (see PRECAUTIONS). Clinically effective neuromuscular block may be expected to last for 15 to 20 minutes (range: 9 to 38) and spontaneous recovery may be expected to be 95% complete in 25 to 30 minutes (range: 16 to 41) following 0.15 mg/kg MIVACRON administered to patients receiving opioid/nitrous oxide/oxygen anesthesia. Maintenance dosing is generally required approximately 15 minutes following an initial dose of 0.15 mg/kg MIVACRON during opioid/nitrous oxide/oxy-

Continued on next page

Burroughs Wellcome—Cont.

gen anesthesia. Maintenance doses of 0.10 mg/kg each provide approximately 15 minutes of additional clinically effective block. For shorter or longer durations of action, smaller or larger maintenance doses may be administered.

The neuromuscular blocking action of MIVACRON is potentiated by isoflurane or enflurane anesthesia. The recommended initial MIVACRON dose of 0.15 mg/kg may be used to facilitate tracheal intubation prior to the administration of these agents; however, if MIVACRON is first administered after establishment of stable-state isoflurane or enflurane anesthesia (administered with nitrous oxide/oxygen to achieve 1.25 MAC), the initial MIVACRON dose may be reduced by as much as 25%. Greater reductions in the MIVACRON dose may be required with higher concentrations of enflurane or isoflurane. With halothane, which has only a minimal potentiating effect on MIVACRON, a smaller dosage reduction may be considered.

Continuous Infusion: Continuous infusion of MIVACRON may be used to maintain neuromuscular block. Upon early evidence of spontaneous recovery from an initial dose, an initial infusion rate of 9 to 10 μg/kg/min is recommended. If continuous infusion is initiated simultaneously with the administration of an initial dose, a lower initial infusion rate should be used (*e.g.,* 4 μg/kg/min). In either case, the initial infusion rate should be adjusted according to the response to peripheral nerve stimulation and to clinical criteria. On average, an infusion rate of 6 to 7 μg/kg/min (range: 1 to 15) may be expected to maintain neuromuscular block within the range of 89% to 99% for extended periods in adults receiving opioid/nitrous oxide/oxygen anesthesia. Reduction of the infusion rate by up to 35% to 40% should be considered when MIVACRON is administered during stable-state conditions of isoflurane or enflurane anesthesia (administered with nitrous oxide/oxygen to achieve 1.25 MAC). Greater reductions in the MIVACRON infusion rate may be required with greater concentrations of enflurane or isoflurane. With halothane, smaller reductions in infusion rate may be required.

Children:

Initial Doses: Dosage requirements for MIVACRON on a mg/kg basis are higher in children than adults. Onset and recovery of neuromuscular block occur more rapidly in children than adults (see CLINICAL PHARMACOLOGY).

The recommended dose of MIVACRON for facilitating tracheal intubation in children 2 to 12 years of age is 0.20 mg/kg administered over 5 to 15 seconds. When administered during stable opioid/nitrous oxide/oxygen anesthesia, 0.20 mg/kg of MIVACRON produces maximum neuromuscular block in an average of 1.9 minutes (range: 1.3 to 3.3) and clinically effective block for 10 minutes (range: 6 to 15). Maintenance doses are generally required more frequently in children than in adults. Administration of MIVACRON doses above the recommended range (>0.20 mg/kg) is associated with transient decreases in MAP in some children (see **Hemodynamics** subsection of CLINICAL PHARMACOLOGY). MIVACRON has not been studied in children below the age of 2 years.

Continuous Infusion: Children require higher MIVACRON infusion rates than adults. During opioid/nitrous oxide/oxygen anesthesia the infusion rate required to maintain 89% to 99% neuromuscular block averages 14 μg/kg/min (range: 5 to 31). The principles for infusion of MIVACRON in adults are also applicable to children (see above).

Infusion Rate Tables:

For adults and children the amount of infusion solution required per hour depends upon the clinical requirements of the patient, the concentration of MIVACRON in the infusion solution, and the patient's weight. The contribution of the infusion solution to the fluid requirements of the patient must be considered. Tables 6 and 7 provide guidelines for delivery in mL/hr (equivalent to microdrops/min when 60 microdrops = 1 mL) of MIVACRON Premixed Infusion (0.5 mg/mL) and of MIVACRON Injection (2 mg/mL).

[See Table 6 below.] [See Table 7 above.]

Table 7
Infusion Rates for Maintenance of Neuromuscular Block During Opioid/Nitrous Oxide/Oxygen Anesthesia Using MIVACRON Injection (2 mg/mL)

Patient Weight (kg)	Drug Delivery Rate (μg/kg/min) 4	5	6	7	8	10	14	16	18	20
	Infusion Delivery Rate (mL/hr)									
10	1.2	1.5	1.8	2.1	2.4	3.0	4.2	4.8	5.4	6.0
15	1.8	2.3	2.7	3.2	3.6	4.5	6.3	7.2	8.1	9.0
20	2.4	3.0	3.6	4.2	4.8	6.0	8.4	9.6	10.8	12.0
25	3.0	3.8	4.5	5.3	6.0	7.5	10.5	12.0	13.5	15.0
35	4.2	5.3	6.3	7.4	8.4	10.5	14.7	16.8	18.9	21.0
50	6.0	7.5	9.0	10.5	12.0	15.0	21.0	24.0	27.0	30.0
60	7.2	9.0	10.8	12.6	14.4	18.0	25.2	28.8	32.4	36.0
70	8.4	10.5	12.6	14.7	16.8	21.0	29.4	33.6	37.8	42.0
80	9.6	12.0	14.4	16.8	19.2	24.0	33.6	38.4	43.2	48.0
90	10.8	13.5	16.2	18.9	21.6	27.0	37.8	43.2	48.6	54.0
100	12.0	15.0	18.0	21.0	24.0	30.0	42.0	48.0	54.0	60.0

MIVACRON Premixed Infusion in Flexible Plastic Containers:

The flexible plastic container is fabricated from a specially formulated, nonplasticized, thermoplastic co-polyester (CR3). Water can permeate from inside the container into the overwrap but not in amounts sufficient to affect the solution significantly. Solutions inside the plastic container also can leach out certain of the chemical components in very small amounts before the expiration period is attained. However, the safety of the plastic has been confirmed by tests in animals according to USP biological standards for plastic containers.

Instructions for Use:

1. Tear outer wrap at notch and remove solution container. Check for minute leaks by squeezing container firmly. If leaks are found, discard solution as sterility may be impaired.
2. Close flow control clamp of administration set.
3. Remove cover from outlet port at bottom of container.
4. Insert piercing pin of administration set into port with a twisting motion until the pin is firmly seated. NOTE: See full directions on administration set carton.
5. Suspend container from hanger.
6. Squeeze and release drip chamber to establish proper fluid level in chamber during infusion.
7. Open flow control clamp to expel air from set. Close clamp.
8. Attach set to intravenous tubing.
9. Regulate rate of administration with flow control clamp.

Caution: Additives should not be introduced into this solution. Do not administer unless solution is clear and container is undamaged. MIVACRON Premixed Infusion is intended for single patient use only. The unused portion of the solution should be discarded.

Warning: Do not use flexible plastic container in series connections.

MIVACRON Injection Compatibility and Admixtures:

Y-site Administration: MIVACRON Injection may not be compatible with alkaline solutions having a pH greater than 8.5 (*e.g.,* barbiturate solutions).

Studies have shown that MIVACRON Injection is compatible with:

- 5% Dextrose Injection USP
- 0.9% Sodium Chloride Injection USP
- 5% Dextrose and 0.9% Sodium Chloride Injection USP
- Lactated Ringer's Injection USP
- 5% Dextrose in Lactated Ringer's Injection
- Sufenta® (sufentanil citrate) Injection, diluted as directed
- Alfenta® (alfentanil hydrochloride) Injection, diluted as directed
- Sublimaze® (fentanyl citrate) Injection, diluted as directed
- Versed® (midazolam hydrochloride) Injection, diluted as directed
- Inapsine® (droperidol) Injection, diluted as directed

Compatibility studies with other parenteral products have not been conducted.

Dilution Stability: MIVACRON Injection diluted to 0.5 mg mivacurium per mL in 5% Dextrose Injection USP, 5% Dextrose and 0.9% Sodium Chloride Injection USP, 0.9% Sodium Chloride Injection USP, Lactated Ringer's Injection USP, or 5% Dextrose in Lactated Ringer's Injection is physically and chemically stable when stored in PVC (polyvinyl chloride) bags at 5°C to 25°C (41°F to 77°F) for up to 24 hours. Aseptic techniques should be used to prepare the diluted product. Admixtures of MIVACRON should be prepared for single patient use only and used within 24 hours of preparation. The unused portion of diluted MIVACRON should be discarded after each case.

NOTE: Parenteral drug products should be inspected visually for particulate matter and discoloration prior to administration whenever solution and container permit. Solutions which are not clear and colorless should not be used.

Table 6
Infusion Rates for Maintenance of Neuromuscular Block During Opioid/Nitrous Oxide/Oxygen Anesthesia Using MIVACRON Premixed Infusion (0.5 mg/mL)

Patient Weight (kg)	Drug Delivery Rate (μg/kg/min) 4	5	6	7	8	10	14	16	18	20
	Infusion Delivery Rate (mL/hr)									
10	5	6	7	8	10	12	17	19	22	24
15	7	9	11	13	14	18	25	29	32	36
20	10	12	15	17	19	24	34	38	43	48
25	12	15	18	21	24	30	42	48	54	60
35	17	21	26	29	34	42	59	67	76	84
50	24	30	36	42	48	60	84	96	108	120
60	29	36	43	50	58	72	101	115	130	144
70	34	42	50	59	67	84	118	134	151	168
80	39	48	58	67	77	96	134	154	173	192
90	44	54	65	76	86	108	151	173	194	216
100	48	60	72	84	96	120	168	192	216	240

HOW SUPPLIED

MIVACRON Injection, 2 mg mivacurium in each mL.
5 mL Single Use Vials. Tray of 10 (NDC 0081-0705-44).
10 mL Single Use Vials. Tray of 10 (NDC 0081-0705-95).
MIVACRON Premixed Infusion in 5% Dextrose Injection USP, 0.5 mg mivacurium in each mL.
50 mL (in a 100 mL unit) Flexible Plastic Containers. (NDC 0081-0709-01).

STORAGE

Store MIVACRON Injection at room temperature of 15° to 25°C (59° to 77°F). Avoid exposure to direct ultraviolet light. DO NOT FREEZE.

Recommended storage for MIVACRON Premixed Infusion is room temperature (15° to 25°C/59° to 77°F). Avoid excessive heat. Avoid exposure to direct ultraviolet light. Protect from freezing.

U.S. Patent No. 4761418 554057

MYLERAN® ℞

[*mī'lah-răn"*]
(Busulfan)
2 mg Scored Tablets

> **WARNING**
>
> *Myleran ® (busulfan) is a potent drug. It should not be used unless a diagnosis of chronic myelogenous leukemia has been adequately established and the responsible physician is knowledgeable in assessing response to chemotherapy.*
>
> *Myleran (busulfan) can induce severe bone marrow hypoplasia. Reduce or discontinue the dosage immediately at the first sign of any unusual depression of bone marrow function as reflected by an abnormal decrease in any of the formed elements of the blood. A bone marrow examination should be performed if the bone marrow status is uncertain.*
>
> *SEE "WARNINGS" SECTION FOR INFORMATION REGARDING BUSULFAN-INDUCED LEUKEMOGENESIS IN HUMANS.*

DESCRIPTION

Myleran (busulfan) is a bifunctional alkylating agent. Busulfan is known chemically as 1,4-butanediol dimethanesulfonate.

Busulfan is *not* a structural analog of the nitrogen mustards. Myleran (busulfan) is available in tablet form for oral administration. Each scored tablet contains 2 mg busulfan and the inactive ingredients magnesium stearate and sodium chloride.

The activity of busulfan in chronic myelogenous leukemia was first reported by D.A.G. Galton in 1953.[1]

CLINICAL PHARMACOLOGY

No analytical method has been found which permits the quantitation of non-radiolabeled busulfan or its metabolites in biological tissues or plasma. All studies of the pharmacokinetics of busulfan in humans have employed radiolabeled drug using either sulfur-35 (labeling the "carrier" portion of the molecule) or carbon-14 or tritium in the alkane portion of

the 4-carbon chain (labels in the "alkylating" portion of the molecule).

Studies with ^{35}S-busulfan.[2] Following the intravenous administration of a single therapeutic dose of ^{35}S-busulfan, there was rapid disappearance of radioactivity from the blood; 90 to 95% of the ^{35}S-label disappeared within three to five minutes after injection. Thereafter, a constant, low level of radioactivity (1 to 3% of the injected dose) was maintained during the subsequent forty-eight hour period of observation. Following the oral administration of ^{35}S-busulfan, there was a lag period of one-half to two hours prior to the detection of radioactivity in the blood. However, at four hours the (low) level of circulating radioactivity was comparable to that obtained following intravenous administration.

After either oral or intravenous administration of ^{35}S-busulfan to humans, 45 to 60% of the radioactivity was recovered in the urine in the forty-eight hours after administration; the majority of the total urinary excretion occurred in the first twenty-four hours. In man, over 95% of the urinary sulfur-35 occurs as ^{35}S-methanesulfonic acid.

The fact that urinary recovery of sulfur-35 was equivalent, irrespective of whether the drug was given intravenously or orally, suggests virtually complete absorption by the oral route.

Studies with ^{14}C-busulfan.[2] Oral and intravenous administration of 1,4-^{14}C-busulfan showed the same rapid initial disappearance of plasma radioactivity with a subsequent low-level plateau as observed following the administration of ^{35}S-labeled drug. Cumulative radioactivity in the urine after forty-eight hours was 25 to 30% of the administered dose (contrasting with 45 to 60% for ^{35}S-busulfan) and suggests a slower excretion of the alkylating portion of the molecule and its metabolites than for the sulfonoxymethyl moieties. Regardless of the route of administration, 1,4-^{14}C-busulfan yielded a complex mixture of at least 12 radiolabeled metabolites in urine; the main metabolite being 3-hydroxy-tetrahydrothiophene-1, 1-dioxide.

Studies with ^{3}H-busulfan.[3] Human pharmacokinetic studies have been conducted employing busulfan labeled with tritium on the tetramethylene chain. These experiments confirmed a rapid initial clearance of the radioactivity from plasma, irrespective of whether the drug was given orally or intravenously, and showed a gradual accumulation of radioactivity in the plasma after repeated doses. Urinary excretion of less than 50% of the total dose given suggested a slow elimination of the metabolic products from the body.

There is no experience with the use of dialysis in an attempt to modify the clinical toxicity of busulfan. One technical difficulty would derive from the extremely poor water solubility of busulfan. Additionally, all studies of the metabolism of busulfan employing radiolabeled materials indicate rapid chemical reactivity of the parent compound with prolonged retention of some of the metabolites (particularly the metabolites arising from the "alkylating" portion of the molecule). The effectiveness of dialysis at removing significant quantities of unreacted drug would be expected to be minimal in such a situation.

No information is available regarding the penetration of busulfan into brain or cerebrospinal fluid.

Biochemical Pharmacology: In aqueous media, busulfan undergoes a wide range of nucleophilic substitution reactions. While this chemical reactivity is relatively non-specific, alkylation of the DNA is felt to be an important biological mechanism for its cytotoxic effect.[4] Coliphage T7 exposed to busulfan was found to have the DNA crosslinked by intrastrand crosslinkages, but no interstrand linkages were found.

The metabolic fate of busulfan has been studied in rats and humans using ^{14}C- and ^{35}S-labeled materials.[2,5,6] In man,[2] as in the rat,[6] almost all of the radioactivity in ^{35}S-labeled busulfan is excreted in the urine in the form of ^{35}S-methanesulfonic acid. No unchanged drug was found in human urine,[2] although a small amount has been reported in rat urine.[6] Roberts and Warwick demonstrated that the formation of methanesulfonic acid *in vivo* in the rat is not due to a simple hydrolysis of busulfan to 1,4-butanediol, since only about 4% of 2,3-^{14} C-busulfan was excreted as carbon dioxide whereas 2,3-^{14} C-1,4-butanediol was converted almost exclusively to carbon dioxide.[5] The predominant reaction of busulfan in the rat is the alkylation of sulfhydryl groups (particularly cysteine and cysteine-containing compounds) to produce a cyclic sulfonium compound which is the precursor of the major urinary metabolite of the 4-carbon portion of the molecule, 3-hydroxytetrahydrothiophene-1, 1-dioxide.[5] This has been termed a "sulfur-stripping" action of busulfan and it may modify the function of certain sulfur-containing amino acids, polypeptides, and proteins; whether this action makes an important contribution to the cytotoxicity of busulfan is unknown.

The biochemical basis for acquired resistance to busulfan is largely a matter of speculation. Although altered transport of busulfan into the cell is one possibility, increased intracellular inactivation of the drug before it reaches the DNA is also possible. Experiments with other alkylating agents have shown that resistance to this class of compounds may reflect an acquired ability of the resistant cell to repair alkylation damage more effectively.[4]

INDICATIONS AND USAGE

Myleran® (busulfan) is indicated for the palliative treatment of chronic myelogenous (myeloid, myelocytic, granulocytic) leukemia. Although not curative, busulfan reduces the total granulocyte mass, relieves symptoms of the disease, and improves the clinical state of the patient. Approximately 90% of adults with previously untreated chronic myelogenous leukemia will obtain hematologic remission with regression or stabilization of organomegaly following the use of busulfan. It has been shown to be superior to splenic irradiation with respect to survival times and maintenance of hemoglobin levels, and to be equivalent to irradiation at controlling splenomegaly.[7]

It is not clear whether busulfan unequivocally prolongs the survival of responding patients beyond the 31 months experienced by an untreated group of historical controls.[8] Median survival figures of 31–42 months have been reported for several groups of patients treated with busulfan, but concurrent control groups of comparable, untreated patients are not available.[7,9,10,11] The median survival figures reported from different studies will be influenced by the percentage of "poor risk" patients initially entered into the particular study. Patients who are alive two years following the diagnosis of chronic myelogenous leukemia, and who have been treated during that period with busulfan, are estimated to have a mean annual mortality rate during the second to fifth year which is approximately two-thirds that of patients who received either no treatment, conventional x-ray or ^{32}P-irradiation, or chemotherapy with minimally active drugs.[12]

Busulfan is clearly less effective in patients with chronic myelogenous leukemia who lack the Philadelphia (Ph^1) chromosome.[13] Also, the so-called "juvenile" type of chronic myelogenous leukemia, typically occurring in young children and associated with the absence of a Philadelphia chromosome, responds poorly to busulfan.[14] The drug is of no benefit in patients whose chronic myelogenous leukemia has entered a "blastic" phase.

CONTRAINDICATIONS

Myleran® (busulfan) should not be used unless a diagnosis of chronic myelogenous leukemia has been adequately established and the responsible physician is knowledgeable in assessing response to chemotherapy.

Myleran should not be used in patients whose chronic myelogenous leukemia has demonstrated prior resistance to this drug.

Myleran is of no value in chronic lymphocytic leukemia, acute leukemia, or in the "blastic crisis" of chronic myelogenous leukemia.

WARNINGS

The most frequent, serious side effect of treatment with busulfan is the induction of bone marrow failure (which may or may not be anatomically hypoplastic) resulting in severe pancytopenia. The pancytopenia caused by busulfan may be more prolonged than that induced with other alkylating agents. It is generally felt that the usual cause of busulfan-induced pancytopenia is the failure to stop administration of the drug soon enough; individual idiosyncrasy to the drug does not seem to be an important factor. *Myleran should be used with extreme caution and exceptional vigilance in patients whose bone marrow reserve may have been compromised by prior irradiation or chemotherapy, or whose marrow function is recovering from previous cytotoxic therapy.* Although recovery from busulfan-induced pancytopenia may take from one month to two years, this complication is potentially reversible and the patient should be vigorously supported through any period of severe pancytopenia.[15]

A rare, important complication of busulfan therapy is the development of bronchopulmonary dysplasia with pulmonary fibrosis.[16] Symptoms have been reported to occur within eight months to ten years after initiation of therapy—the average duration of therapy being four years. The histologic findings associated with "busulfan lung" mimic those seen following pulmonary irradiation. Clinically, patients have reported the insidious onset of cough, dyspnea, and low-grade fever. Pulmonary function studies have revealed diminished diffusion capacity and decreased pulmonary compliance. It is important to exclude more common conditions (such as opportunistic infections or leukemic infiltration of the lungs) with appropriate diagnostic techniques. If measures such as sputum cultures, virologic studies, and exfoliative cytology fail to establish an etiology for the pulmonary infiltrates, lung biopsy may be necessary to establish the diagnosis. Treatment of established busulfan-induced pulmonary fibrosis is unsatisfactory; in most cases the patients have died within six months after the diagnosis was established. There is no specific therapy for this complication other than the immediate discontinuation of busulfan. The administration of corticosteroids has been suggested, but the results have not been impressive or uniformly successful.

Busulfan may cause cellular dysplasia in many organs in addition to the lung. Cytologic abnormalities characterized by giant, hyperchromatic nuclei have been reported in lymph nodes, pancreas, thyroid, adrenal glands, liver, and bone marrow. This cytologic dysplasia may be severe enough to cause difficulty in interpretation of exfoliative cytologic examinations from the lung, bladder, breast, and the uterine cervix.

In addition to the widespread epithelial dysplasia that has been observed during busulfan therapy, chromosome aberrations have been reported in cells from patients receiving busulfan.

Busulfan is mutagenic in mice and, possibly, in man.

A number of malignant tumors have been reported in patients on busulfan therapy and this drug may be a human carcinogen. Four cases of acute leukemia occurred among 243 patients treated with busulfan as adjuvant chemotherapy following surgical resection of bronchogenic carcinoma. All four cases were from a subgroup of 19 of these 243 patients who developed pancytopenia while taking busulfan five to eight years before leukemia became clinically apparent. These findings suggest that busulfan is leukemogenic, although its mode of action is uncertain.[17]

Ovarian suppression and amenorrhea with menopausal symptoms commonly occur during busulfan therapy in premenopausal patients. Busulfan interferes with spermatogenesis in experimental animals, and there have been clinical reports of sterility, azoospermia and testicular atrophy in male patients.

A rare but life-threatening hepatic veno-occlusive disease has been reported following the investigational use of very high doses of busulfan in combination with cyclophosphamide or other chemotherapeutic agents prior to bone marrow transplantation.[18–24] A clear cause and effect relationship with busulfan has not been demonstrated. Periodic measurement of serum transaminases, alkaline phosphatase, and bilirubin is indicated for early detection of hepatotoxicity.

Pregnancy: "Pregnancy Category D." Busulfan may cause fetal harm when administered to a pregnant woman. Although there have been a number of cases reported where apparently normal children have been born after busulfan treatment during pregnancy,[25] one case has been cited where a malformed baby was delivered by a mother treated with busulfan. During the pregnancy that resulted in the malformed infant, the mother received x-ray therapy early in the first trimester, mercaptopurine until the third month, then busulfan until delivery.[26] In pregnant rats, busulfan produces sterility in both male and female offspring due to the absence of germinal cells in testes and ovaries.[27] Germinal cell aplasia or sterility in offspring of mothers receiving busulfan during pregnancy has not been reported in humans. There are no adequate and well-controlled studies in pregnant women. If this drug is used during pregnancy, or if the patient becomes pregnant while taking this drug, the patient should be apprised of the potential hazard to the fetus. Women of childbearing potential should be advised to avoid becoming pregnant.

PRECAUTIONS

General: The most consistent, dose-related toxicity is bone marrow suppression. This may be manifest by anemia, leukopenia, thrombocytopenia, or any combination of these. It is imperative that patients be instructed to report promptly the development of fever, sore throat, signs of local infection, bleeding from any site, or symptoms suggestive of anemia. Any one of these findings may indicate busulfan toxicity; however, they may also indicate transformation of the disease to an acute "blastic" form. Since busulfan may have a delayed effect, it is important to withdraw the medication temporarily at the first sign of an abnormally large or exceptionally rapid fall in any of the formed elements of the blood. *Patients should never be allowed to take the drug without close medical supervision.*

Seizures have been reported in patients receiving very high, investigational doses of busulfan.[18,28–32] As with any potentially epileptogenic drug, caution should be exercised when administering very high doses of busulfan to patients with a history of seizure disorder, head trauma, or receiving other potentially epileptogenic drugs. Some investigators have used prophylactic anticonvulsant therapy in this setting.

Information for Patients: Patients beginning therapy with busulfan should be informed of the importance of having periodic blood counts and to immediately report any unusual fever or bleeding. Aside from the major toxicity of myelosuppression, patients should be instructed to report any difficulty in breathing, persistent cough or congestion. They should be told that diffuse pulmonary fibrosis is an infrequent but serious and potentially life-threatening complication of long-term busulfan therapy. Patients should be alerted to report any signs of abrupt weakness, unusual fatigue, anorexia, weight loss, nausea and vomiting, and melanoderma that could be associated with a syndrome resembling adrenal insufficiency. Patients should never be allowed to take the drug without medical supervision and they should be informed that other encountered toxicities to bu-

Continued on next page

Burroughs Wellcome—Cont.

sulfan include infertility, amenorrhea, skin hyperpigmentation, drug hypersensitivity, dryness of the mucous membranes and rarely cataract formation. Women of childbearing potential should be advised to avoid becoming pregnant. The increased risk of a second malignancy should be explained to the patient.

Laboratory Tests: It is recommended that evaluation of the hemoglobin or hematocrit, total white blood cell count and differential count, and quantitative platelet count be obtained weekly while the patient is on busulfan therapy. In cases where the cause of fluctuation in the formed elements of the peripheral blood is obscure, bone marrow examination may be useful for evaluation of marrow status. A decision to increase, decrease, continue, or discontinue a given dose of busulfan must be based not only on the absolute hematologic values, but also on the rapidity with which changes are occurring. The dosage of busulfan may need to be reduced if this agent is combined with other drugs whose primary toxicity is myelosuppression. Occasional patients may be unusually sensitive to busulfan administered at standard dosage and suffer neutropenia or thrombocytopenia after a relatively short exposure to the drug. Busulfan should not be used where facilities for complete blood counts, including quantitative platelet counts, are not available at weekly (or more frequent) intervals.

Drug Interactions: Busulfan may cause additive myelosuppression when used with other myelosuppressive drugs.

In one study, 12 of approximately 330 patients receiving continuous busulfan and thioguanine therapy for treatment of chronic myelogenous leukemia were found to have esophageal varices associated with abnormal liver function tests.[33] Subsequent liver biopsies were performed in four of these patients, all of which showed evidence of nodular regenerative hyperplasia. Duration of combination therapy prior to the appearance of esophageal varices ranged from 6 to 45 months. With the present analysis of the data, no cases of hepatotoxicity have appeared in the busulfan alone arm of the study. Long-term continuous therapy with thioguanine and busulfan should be used with caution.

Carcinogenesis, Mutagenesis, Impairment of Fertility: See WARNINGS section.

Pregnancy: ***Teratogenic effects:*** Pregnancy Category D. See WARNINGS section.

Non-Teratogenic effects: There have been reports in the literature of small infants being born after the mothers received busulfan during pregnancy, in particular, during the third trimester.[34] One case was reported where an infant had mild anemia and neutropenia at birth after busulfan was administered to the mother from the eighth week of pregnancy to term.[25]

Nursing Mothers: It is not known whether this drug is excreted in human milk. Because of the potential for tumorigenicity shown for busulfan in animal and human studies, a decision should be made whether to discontinue nursing or to discontinue the drug, taking into account the importance of the drug to the mother.

ADVERSE REACTIONS

Hematological Effects: The most frequent, serious, toxic effect of busulfan is myelosuppression resulting in leukopenia, thrombocytopenia, and anemia. Myelosuppression is most frequently the result of a failure to discontinue dosage in the face of an undetected decrease in leukocyte or platelet counts.[15]

Pulmonary: Interstitial pulmonary fibrosis has been reported rarely, but it is a clinically significant adverse effect when observed and calls for immediate discontinuation of further administration of the drug. The role of corticosteroids in arresting or reversing the fibrosis has been reported to be beneficial in some cases and without effect in others.[16]

Cardiac: One case of endocardial fibrosis has been reported in a 79-year-old woman who received a total dose of 7,200 mg of busulfan over a period of nine years for the management of chronic myelogenous leukemia.[35] At autopsy, she was found to have endocardial fibrosis of the left ventricle in addition to interstitial pulmonary fibrosis.

Ocular: Busulfan is capable of inducing cataracts in rats and there have been several reports indicating that this is a rare complication in humans. In the few cases reported in humans, cataracts have occurred only after prolonged administration of busulfan.[36]

Dermatologic: Hyperpigmentation is the most common adverse skin reaction and occurs in 5–10% of patients, particularly those with a dark complexion.

Metabolic: In a few cases, a clinical syndrome closely resembling adrenal insufficiency and characterized by weakness, severe fatigue, anorexia, weight loss, nausea and vomiting, and melanoderma has developed after prolonged busulfan therapy. The symptoms have sometimes been reversible when busulfan was withdrawn. Adrenal responsiveness to exogenously administered ACTH has usually been normal. However, pituitary function testing with metyrapone revealed a blunted urinary 17-hydroxycorticosteroid excretion in two patients.[37] Following the discontinuation of busulfan (which was associated with clinical improvement), rechallenge with metyrapone revealed normal pituitary-adrenal function.

Hyperuricemia and/or hyperuricosuria are not uncommon in patients with chronic myelogenous leukemia. Additional rapid destruction of granulocytes may accompany the initiation of chemotherapy and increase the urate pool. Adverse effects can be minimized by increased hydration, urine alkalinization, and the prophylactic administration of a xanthine oxidase inhibitor such as Zyloprim® (allopurinol).

Hepatic Effects: Esophageal varices have been reported in patients receiving continuous busulfan and thioguanine therapy for treatment of chronic myelogenous leukemia (see PRECAUTIONS: Drug Interactions). Hepatic veno-occlusive disease has been observed in patients receiving higher than recommended doses of busulfan (see WARNINGS).

Miscellaneous: Other reported adverse reactions include: urticaria, erythema multiforme, erythema nodosum, alopecia, porphyria cutanea tarda, excessive dryness and fragility of the skin with anhidrosis, dryness of the oral mucous membranes and cheilosis, gynecomastia, cholestatic jaundice, and myasthenia gravis. Most of these are single case reports, and in many a clear cause and effect relationship with busulfan has not been demonstrated.

Seizures (see PRECAUTIONS-General) have been observed in patients receiving higher than recommended doses of busulfan.

OVERDOSAGE

There is no known antidote to busulfan. The principal toxic effect is on the bone marrow. Survival after a single 140 mg dose has been reported in an 18 kg, 4-year-old child,[38] but hematologic toxicity is likely to be more profound with chronic overdosage. The hematologic status should be closely monitored and vigorous supportive measures instituted if necessary. Induction of vomiting or gastric lavage followed by administration of charcoal would be indicated if ingestion were recent. It is not known whether busulfan is dialyzable (see CLINICAL PHARMACOLOGY).

Oral LD_{50} single doses in mice are 120 mg/kg. Two distinct types of toxic response are seen at median lethal doses given intraperitoneally. Within a matter of hours there are signs of stimulation of the central nervous system with convulsions and death on the first day. Mice are more sensitive to this effect than are rats. With doses at the LD_{50} there is also delayed death due to damage to the bone marrow. At three times the LD_{50}, atrophy of the mucosa of the large intestine is found after a week, whereas that of the small intestine is little affected.[39] After doses in the order of 10 times those used therapeutically were added to the diet of rats, irreversible cataracts were produced after several weeks. Small doses had no such effect.[40]

DOSAGE AND ADMINISTRATION

Busulfan is administered orally. The usual adult dose range for *remission induction* is four to eight mg, total dose, daily. Dosing on a weight basis is the same for both children and adults, approximately 60 μg per kg of body weight or 1.8 mg per square meter of body surface, daily. Since the rate of fall of the leukocyte count is dose related, daily doses exceeding four mg per day should be reserved for patients with the most compelling symptoms; the greater the total daily dose, the greater is the possibility of inducing bone marrow aplasia.

A decrease in the leukocyte count is not usually seen during the first ten to fifteen days of treatment; the leukocyte count may actually increase during this period and it should not be interpreted as resistance to the drug, nor should the dose be increased.[41] Since the leukocyte count may continue to fall for more than one month after discontinuing the drug, it is important that busulfan be discontinued *prior* to the total leukocyte count falling into the normal range. When the total leukocyte count has declined to approximately 15,000/μL the drug should be withheld.

With a constant dose of busulfan, the total leukocyte count declines exponentially; a weekly plot of the leukocyte count on semi-logarithmic graph paper aids in predicting the time when therapy should be discontinued.[42] With the recommended dose of busulfan, a normal leukocyte count is usually achieved in twelve to twenty weeks.

During remission, the patient is examined at monthly intervals and treatment resumed with the induction dosage when the total leukocyte count reaches approximately 50,000/μL. When remission is shorter than three months, maintenance therapy of 1 to 3 mg daily may be advisable in order to keep the hematological status under control and prevent rapid relapse.

Procedures for proper handling and disposal of anti-cancer drugs should be considered. Several guidelines on this subject have been published.[43–49]

There is no general agreement that all of the procedures recommended in the guidelines are necessary or appropriate.

HOW SUPPLIED

White, scored tablets containing 2 mg busulfan, imprinted with "MYLERAN" and "K2A" on each tablet; bottle of 25 (**NDC** 0081-0713-25). Store at 15° to 25°C (59° to 77°F) in a dry place.

REFERENCES

1. Galton DAG. Myleran in chronic myeloid leukemia: results of treatment. *Lancet.* 1953;1:208–213.
2. Nadkarni MV, Trams EG, Smith PK. Preliminary studies on the distribution and fate of TEM, TEPA, and Myleran in the human. *Cancer Res.* 1959;19:713–718.
3. Vodopick H, Hamilton HE, Jackson HL, Peng C-T, Sheets RF. Metabolic fate of tritiated busulfan in man. *J Lab Clin Med.* 1969;73:266–276.
4. Fox BW. Mechanism of action of methane sulfonates. In: Sartorelli AC, Johns DG, eds. *Antineoplastic and Immunosuppressive Agents,* Part II. Berlin: Springer Verlag; 1975:35–46.
5. Roberts JJ, Warwick GP. The mode of action of alkylating agents, III: the formation of 3-hydroxytetrahydrothiophene-1:1-dioxide from 1:4-dimethanesulphonyloxybutane (Myleran), S-β-L-alanyltetrahydrothiophenium mesylate, tetrahydrothiophene and tetrahydrothiophene-1:1-dioxide in the rat, rabbit and mouse. *Biochem Pharmacol.* 1961;6:217–227.
6. Peng C-T. Distribution and metabolic fate of S^{35}-labeled Myleran (busulfan) in normal and tumor-bearing rats. *J Pharmacol Exp Ther.* 1957;120:229–238.
7. Medical Research Council's Working Party for Therapeutic Trials in Leukemia. Chronic granulocytic leukaemia: comparison of radiotherapy and busulphan therapy. *Br Med J.* 1968;1:201–208.
8. Minot GR, Buckman TE, Isaacs R. Chronic myelogenous leukemia: age incidence, duration, and benefit derived from irradiation. *JAMA.* 1924;82:1489–1494.
9. Haut A, Abbott WS, Wintrobe MM, Cartwright GE. Busulfan in the treatment of chronic myelocytic leukemia: the effect of long term intermittent therapy. *Blood.* 1961;17:1–19.
10. Monfardini S, Gee T, Fried J, Clarkson B. Survival in chronic myelogenous leukemia: influence of treatment and extent of disease at diagnosis. *Cancer.* 1973;31:492–501.
11. Conrad FG. Survival in granulocytic leukemia. *Arch Intern Med.* 1973;131:684–685.
12. Sokal JE. Evaluation of survival data for chronic myelocytic leukemia. *Am J Hematol.* 1976;1:493–500.
13. Ezdinli EZ, Sokal JE, Crosswhite L, Sandberg AA. Philadelphia chromosome-positive and -negative chronic myelocytic leukemia. *Ann Intern Med.* 1970;72:175–182.
14. Smith KL, Johnson W. Classification of chronic myelocytic leukemia in children. *Cancer.* 1974; 34:670–679.
15. Stuart JJ, Crocker DL, Roberts HR. Treatment of busulfan-induced pancytopenia. *Arch Intern Med.* 1977; 136:1181–1183.
16. Sostman HD, Matthay RA, Putman CE. Cytotoxic drug-induced lung disease. *Am J Med.* 1977;62:608–615.
17. Stott H, Fox W, Girling DJ, Stephens RJ, Galton DAG. Acute leukaemia after busulphan. *Br Med J.* 1977;2:1513–1517.
18. Hartmann O, et al. High-dose busulfan and cyclophosphamide with autologous bone marrow transplantation support in advanced malignancies in children: A Phase II study. *J Clin Oncol* 1986;4:1804–10.
19. Copelan EA, et al. Marrow transplantation following busulfan and cyclophosphamide for chronic myelogenous leukemia in accelerated or blastic phase. *Br J Haematol* 1989; 71:487–91.
20. Kirchner H, et al. Allogeneic and autologous bone marrow transplantation (BMT) after high-dose busulfan and cyclophosphamide treatment. *Blut* 1988;57:198. (abstract)
21. Thompson J, et al. Allogeneic bone marrow transplantation (BMT) following transplant preparation with cyclophosphamide (CTX) and busulfan (BU). *Proc ASCO* 1989; 8:18. (abstract)
22. Geller RB, et al. Allogeneic bone marrow transplantation after high-dose busulfan and cyclophosphamide in patients with acute non-lymphocytic leukemia. *Blood* 1989; 73:2209–18.
23. Lu C, et al. Preliminary results of high-dose busulfan and cyclophosphamide with syngeneic or autologous bone marrow rescue. *Cancer Treat Rep* 1984; 68:711–7.
24. Groshow LB, et al. Pharmacokinetics of busulfan: correlation with veno-occlusive disease in patients undergoing bone marrow transplantation. *Cancer Chemother Pharmacol* 1989; 25:55–61.
25. Dugdale M, Fort AT. Busulfan treatment of leukemia during pregnancy: case report and review of the literature. *JAMA.* 1967; 199:131–133.
26. Diamond I, Anderson MM, McCreadie SR. Transplacental transmission of busulfan (Myleran) in a mother with leukemia: production of fetal malformation and cytomegaly. *Pediatrics.* 1960;25:85–90.

27. Bollag W. Cytostatica in der Schwangerschaft. *Schweiz Med Wochenschr.* 1954;84:393–395.
28. Marcus RE, et al. Convulsions due to high-dose busulfan. *Lancet* 1984;2:1463. (letter)
29. Martell RW, et al. High-dose busulfan and myoclonic epilepsy. *Ann Intern Med.* 1987; 106:173. (letter)
30. Sureda A, et al. High-dose busulfan and seizures. *Ann Intern Med* 1989; 111:543–4. (letter)
31. Grigg AP, et al. Busulfan and phenytoin. *Ann Intern Med* 1989; 111:1049–50. (letter)
32. Beelen DW, et al. Acute toxicity and first clinical results of intensive post-induction therapy using a modified busulfan and cyclophosphamide regimen with autologous bone marrow rescue in first remission of acute myeloid leukemia. *Blood* 1989; 74:1507–16.
33. Key NS, Kelly PMA, Emerson PM, Chapman RWG, Allan NC, McGee JO'D. Oesophageal varices associated with busulfan-thioguanine combination therapy for chronic myeloid leukaemia. *Lancet.* 1987;2:1050–1052.
34. Boros SJ, Reynolds JW. Intrauterine growth retardation following third-trimester exposure to busulfan. *Am J Obstet Gynecol.* 1977;129:111–112.
35. Weinberger A, Pinkhas J, Sandbank U, Shaklai M, deVries A. Endocardial fibrosis following busulfan treatment. *JAMA.* 1975;231:495.
36. Ravindranathan MP, Paul VJ, Kuriakose ET. Cataract after busulfan treatment. *Br Med J.* 1972;1:218–219.
37. Vivacqua RJ, Haurani Fl, Erslev AJ. "Selective"pituitary insufficiency secondary to busulfan. *Ann Intern Med.* 1967;67:380–387.
38. DeOliveira HP, Cruz E, Fonseca A de S, Medeiros M. Accidental ingestion of a toxic dose of Myleran by a child. *Acta Haematol* (Basel) 1963;29:249–255.
39. Sternberg SS, Phillips FS, Scholler J. Pharmacological and pathological effects of alkylating agents. *Ann NY Acad Sci.* 1958;68:811–825.
40. Solomon C, Light AE, deBeer EJ. Cataracts produced in rats by 1, 4-dimethanesulfonoxybutane (Myleran). *AMA Arch Ophthal.* 1955;54:850–852.
41. Stryckmans PA: Current concepts in chronic myelogenous leukemia. *Semin Hematol.* 1974;11:101–127.
42. Galton DAG. Chemotherapy of chronic myelocytic leukemia. *Semin Hematol.* 1969;6:323–343.
43. Recommendations for the safe handling of parenteral antineoplastic drugs. Washington, DC: Division of Safety, National Institutes of Health; 1983. US Dept of Health and Human Services, Public Health Service publication NIH 83-2621.
44. AMA Council on Scientific Affairs. Guidelines for handling parenteral antineoplastics. *JAMA.* 1985;253: 1590–1591.
45. National Study Commission on Cytotoxic Exposure. Recommendations for handling cytotoxic agents. 1984. Available from Louis P. Jeffrey, ScD, Director of Pharmacy Services, Rhode Island Hospital, 593 Eddy Street, Providence, Rhode Island 02902.
46. Clinical Oncological Society of Australia. Guidelines and recommendations for safe handling of antineoplastic agents. *Med J Australia.* 1983;1:426–428.
47. Jones RB, Frank R, Mass T. Safe handling of chemotherapeutic agents: a report from the Mount Sinai Medical Center. *CA-A Cancer J for Clin.* 1983;33(Sept/Oct): 258–263.
48. American Society of Hospital Pharmacists. ASHP technical assistance bulletin on handling cytotoxic and hazardous drugs. *AM J Hosp Pharm.* 1990;47:1033–1049.
49. Yodaiken RE, Bennett D. OSHA work-practice guidelines for personnel dealing with cytotoxic (antineoplastic) drugs. *Am J Hosp Pharm.* 1986;43:1193–1204.

558046

Shown in Product Identification Section, page 407

NEOSPORIN® G.U. IRRIGANT ℞

[*nē"ō-spor'in*]
Sterile
(Neomycin Sulfate-Polymyxin B Sulfate Solution for Irrigation)
NOT FOR INJECTION

DESCRIPTION

Neosporin G.U. Irrigant is a concentrated sterile antibiotic solution to be diluted for urinary bladder irrigation. Each ml contains neomycin sulfate equivalent to 40 mg neomycin base, 200,000 units polymyxin B sulfate and water for injection. The 20-ml multiple-dose vial contains, in addition to the above, 1 mg methylparaben (0.1%) added as a preservative.
Neomycin sulfate, an antibiotic of the aminoglycoside group, is the sulfate salt of neomycin B and C produced by *Streptomyces fradiae.* It has a potency equivalent to not less than 600 µg of neomycin per mg.
Polymyxin B sulfate, a polypeptide antibiotic, is the sulfate salt of polymyxin B_1 and B_2 produced by the growth of *Bacillus polymyxa.* It has a potency of not less than 6,000 polymyxin B units per mg.

CLINICAL PHARMACOLOGY

After prophylactic irrigation of the intact urinary bladder, neomycin and polymyxin B are absorbed in clinically insignificant quantities. A neomycin serum level of 0.1 µg/ml was observed in three of 33 patients receiving the rinse solution. This level is well below that which has been associated with neomycin-induced toxicity.
When used topically, polymyxin B sulfate and neomycin are rarely irritating.
Microbiology: The prepared Neosporin G.U. Irrigant Sterile solution is bactericidal. The aminoglycosides act by inhibiting normal protein synthesis in susceptible microorganisms. Polymyxins increase the permeability of bacterial cell wall membranes. The solution is active *in vitro* against
Escherichia coli
Staphylococcus aureus
Haemophilus influenzae
Klebsiella and *Enterobacter* species
Neisseria species, and
Pseudomonas aeruginosa
It is not active *in vitro* against *Serratia marcescens* and streptococci.
Bacterial resistance may develop following the use of the antibiotics in the catheter-rinse solution.

INDICATIONS AND USAGE

Neosporin G.U. Irrigant is indicated for short-term use (up to 10 days) as a continuous irrigant or rinse in the urinary bladder of abacteriuric patients to help prevent bacteriuria and gram-negative rod septicemia associated with the use of indwelling catheters.
Since organisms gain entrance to the bladder by way of, through, and around the catheter, significant bacteriuria is induced by bacterial multiplication in the bladder urine, in the mucoid film often present between catheter and urethra, and in other sites. Urinary tract infection may result from the repeated presence in the urine of large numbers of pathogenic bacteria. The use of closed systems with indwelling catheters has been shown to reduce the risk of infection. A three-way closed catheter system with constant neomycin-polymyxin B bladder rinse is indicated to prevent the development of infection while using indwelling catheters.
If uropathogens are isolated, they should be identified and tested for susceptibility so that appropriate antimicrobial therapy for systemic use can be initiated.

CONTRAINDICATIONS

Hypersensitivity to neomycin, the polymyxins, or any ingredient in the solution is a contraindication to its use. A history of hypersensitivity or serious toxic reaction to an aminoglycoside may also contraindicate the use of any other aminoglycoside because of the known cross-sensitivity of patients to drugs of this class.

WARNINGS

PROPHYLACTIC BLADDER CARE WITH NEOSPORIN G.U. IRRIGANT STERILE SHOULD NOT BE GIVEN WHERE THERE IS A POSSIBILITY OF SYSTEMIC AB-SORPTION. NEOSPORIN G.U. IRRIGANT STERILE SHOULD NOT BE USED FOR IRRIGATION OTHER THAN FOR THE URINARY BLADDER. Systemic absorption after topical application of neomycin to open wounds, burns, and granulating surfaces is significant and serum concentrations comparable to and often higher than those attained following oral and parenteral therapy have been reported. Absorption of neomycin from the denuded bladder surface has been reported.
However, the likelihood of toxicity following topical irrigation of the intact urinary bladder with Neosporin G.U. Irrigant Sterile is low since no appreciable amounts of these antibiotics enter the systemic circulation by this route if irrigation does not exceed ten days.
Neosporin G.U. Irrigant is intended for continuous prophylactic irrigation of the lumen of the intact urinary bladder of patients with indwelling catheters. Patients should be under constant supervision by a physician. Irrigation should be avoided in patients with defects in the bladder mucosa or bladder wall, such as vesical rupture, or in association with operative procedures on the bladder wall, because of the risk of toxicity due to systemic absorption following diffusion into absorptive tissues and spaces. When absorbed, neomycin and polymyxin B are nephrotoxic antibiotics, and the nephrotoxic potentials are additive. In addition, both antibiotics, when absorbed, are neurotoxins: neomycin can destroy fibers of the acoustic nerve causing permanent bilateral deafness; neomycin and polymyxin B are additive in their neuromuscular blocking effects, not only in terms of potency and duration but also in terms of characteristics of the blocks produced.
Aminoglycosides, when absorbed, can cause fetal harm when administered to a pregnant woman. Aminoglycoside antibiotics cross the placenta and there have been several reports of total, irreversible, bilateral, congenital deafness in children whose mothers received streptomycin during pregnancy. Although serious side effects have not been reported in the treatment of pregnant women with other aminoglycosides, the potential for harm exists. If Neosporin G.U. Irrigant Sterile is used during pregnancy, the patient should be apprised of the potential hazard to the fetus (See PRECAUTIONS).

PRECAUTIONS

General: Ototoxicity, nephrotoxicity, and neuromuscular blockade may occur if Neosporin G.U. Irrigant ingredients are systemically absorbed (See WARNINGS). Absorption of neomycin from the denuded bladder surface has been reported. Patients with impaired renal function, infants, dehydrated patients, elderly patients, and patients receiving high doses of prolonged treatment are especially at risk for the development of toxicity.
Irrigation of the bladder with Neosporin G.U. Irrigant may result in overgrowth of nonsusceptible organisms, including fungi. Appropriate measures should be taken if this occurs.
The safety and effectiveness of the preparation for use in the care of patients with recent lower urinary tract surgery have not been established.
Urine specimens should be collected during prophylactic bladder care for urinalysis, culture, and susceptibility testing. Positive cultures suggest the presence of organisms which are resistant to the bladder rinse antibiotics.
Pregnancy: ***Teratogenic Effects:*** Pregnancy Category D. (See WARNINGS section.)

ADVERSE REACTIONS

Neomycin occasionally causes skin sensitization when applied topically; however, topical application to mucus membranes rarely results in local or systemic hypersensitivity reactions.
Irritation of the urinary bladder mucosa has been reported.
Signs of ototoxicity and nephrotoxicity have been reported following parenteral use of these drugs and following the oral and topical use of neomycin (See WARNINGS).

DOSAGE AND ADMINISTRATION

This preparation is specifically designed for use with "three-way" catheters or with other catheter systems permitting **continuous** irrigation of the urinary bladder. The usual irrigation dose is one 1-ml ampul a day for up to ten days.
Using strict aseptic techniques, the contents of one 1-ml ampul of Neosporin G.U. Irrigant Sterile (Neomycin Sulfate-Polymyxin B Sulfate Solution for Irrigation) should be added to a 1,000-ml container of isotonic saline solution. This container should then be connected to the inflow lumen of the "three-way" catheter which has been inserted with full aseptic precautions; use of a sterile lubricant is recommended during insertion of the catheter. The outflow lumen should be connected, via a sterile disposable plastic tube, to a disposable plastic collection bag. Stringent procedures, such as taping the inflow and outflow junction at the catheter, should be observed when necessary to insure the junctional integrity of the system.
For most patients, the inflow rate of the 1,000-ml saline solution of neomycin and polymyxin B should be adjusted to a slow drip to deliver about 1,000 ml every twenty-four hours. If the patient's urine output exceeds 2 liters per day, it is recommended that the inflow rate be adjusted to deliver 2,000 ml of the solution in a twenty-four hour period.
It is important that the rinse of the bladder be **continuous;** the inflow or rinse solution should not be interrupted for more than a few minutes.
Preparation of the irrigation solution should be performed with strict aseptic techniques. The prepared solution should be stored at 4°C, and should be used within 48 hours following preparation to reduce the risk of contamination with resistant microorganisms.

HOW SUPPLIED

1-ml ampuls, boxes of 10 (NDC-0081-0748-10) and 50 ampuls (NDC-0081-0748-35); 20-ml multi-dose vial (NDC-0081-0748-93).
Store at 2° to 8°C (36° to 46°F). 561051

Professional Labeling

NEOSPORIN® OINTMENT OTC

[*nē"ō-spor'in*]
(Polymyxin B Sulfate-Bacitracin Zinc-Neomycin Sulfate)

DESCRIPTION

Neosporin Ointment (polymyxin B sulfate-bacitracin zinc-neomycin sulfate) is a topical first aid antibiotic ointment. Each gram of Neosporin Ointment contains: polymyxin B sulfate 5,000 units, bacitracin zinc 400 units and neomycin 3.5 mg in a special white petrolatum base.
Each gram of Maximum Strength Neosporin Ointment contains: polymyxin B sulfate 10,000 units, bacitracin zinc 500 units and neomycin 3.5 mg in a special white petrolatum base.

Continued on next page

Burroughs Wellcome—Cont.

INDICATIONS

First aid to help prevent infection in minor cuts, scrapes and burns.

CONTRAINDICATIONS

Not for use in the eyes or in the external ear canal if the eardrum is perforated. This product is contraindicated in those individuals who have shown hypersensitivity to any of its components.

WARNINGS

Because of the concern of nephrotoxicity and ototoxicity associated with neomycin, this combination should not be used over a wide area or for extended periods of time.

PRECAUTIONS

General: As with other antibacterial preparations, prolonged use may result in overgrowth of non-susceptible organisms, including fungi. Appropriate measures should be taken if this occurs.

Information for Patients: For external use only. Do not use in the eyes or apply over large areas of the body. In case of deep or puncture wounds, animal bites, or serious burns, consult a physician. Stop use and consult a physician if the condition persists or gets worse. Do not use longer than 1 week unless directed by a physician.

ADVERSE REACTIONS

Neomycin occasionally causes skin sensitization. Ototoxicity and nephrotoxicity have also been reported (see WARNINGS section). Adverse reactions have occurred with topical use of antibiotic combinations including neomycin and polymyxin B. Exact incidence figures are not available since no denominator of treated patients is available. The reaction occurring most often is allergic sensitization. In one clinical study, using a 20% neomycin patch, neomycin-induced allergic skin reactions occurred in two of 2,175 (0.09%) individuals in the general population.[1] In another study the incidence was found to be approximately 1%.[2]

DOSAGE AND ADMINISTRATION

Clean the affected area. Apply a small amount of this product (an amount equal to the surface area of the tip of a finger) on the area 1 to 3 times daily. May be covered with a sterile bandage.

HOW SUPPLIED

Neosporin Ointment:
Tubes of ½ oz and 1 oz; 1/32 oz (approx.) foil packets packed 144 per carton.

REFERENCES

1. Leyden JJ, Kligman AM: Contact dermatitis to neomycin sulfate. *JAMA* 1979; 242:1276–1278.
2. Prystowsky SD, Allen AM, Smith RW, et al: Allergic contact hypersensitivity to nickel, neomycin, ethylenediamine, and benzocaine. *Arch Dermatol* 1979; 115:959–962.
                                PL 5

NEOSPORIN®   ℞

[nē″ō-spor′in]
OPHTHALMIC OINTMENT Sterile
(Polymyxin B Sulfate-Bacitracin Zinc-Neomycin Sulfate)

DESCRIPTION

Neosporin Ophthalmic Ointment (polymyxin B sulfate-bacitracin zinc-neomycin sulfate) is a sterile antimicrobial ointment for ophthalmic use. Each gram contains: Aerosporin® (polymyxin B sulfate) 10,000 units, bacitracin zinc 400 units, neomycin sulfate equivalent to 3.5 mg neomycin base and special white petrolatum, qs.

Polymyxin B sulfate is the sulfate salt of polymyxin B_1 and B_2 which are produced by the growth of *Bacillus polymyxa* (Prazmowski) Migula (Fam. Bacillaceae). It has a potency of not less than 6,000 polymyxin B units per mg, calculated on an anhydrous basis.

Bacitracin zinc is the zinc salt of bacitracin, a mixture of related cyclic polypeptides (mainly bacitracin A) produced by the growth of an organism of the *licheniformis* group of *Bacillus subtilis* (Fam. Bacillaceae). It has a potency of not less than 40 bacitracin units per mg. The precise structural formula is not known.

Neomycin sulfate is the sulfate salt of neomycin B and C, which are produced by the growth of *Streptomyces fradiae* Waksman (Fam. Streptomycetaceae). It has a potency equivalent of not less than 600 μg of neomycin standard per mg, calculated on an anhydrous basis.

CLINICAL PHARMACOLOGY

A wide range of antibacterial action is provided by the overlapping spectra of polymyxin B sulfate, bacitracin and neomycin. The spectrum of action encompasses most bacterial pathogens capable of causing external infections of the eye and its adnexa.

Polymyxin B is bactericidal for a variety of gram-negative organisms. It increases the permeability of the bacterial cell membrane by interacting with the phospholipid components of the membrane.

Bacitracin is bactericidal for a variety of gram-positive and gram-negative organisms. It interferes with bacterial cell wall synthesis by inhibition of the regeneration of phospholipid receptors involved in peptidoglycan synthesis.

Neomycin is bactericidal for many gram-positive and gram-negative organisms. It is an aminoglycoside antibiotic which inhibits protein synthesis by binding with ribosomal RNA and causing misreading of the bacterial genetic code.

When used topically, polymyxin B, bacitracin and neomycin are rarely irritating, and absorption from the intact skin or mucous membrane is insignificant. The incidence of skin sensitization to this combination has been shown to be low on normal skin.[1,2] Since these antibiotics are seldom used systemically, the patient is spared sensitization to those antibiotics which might later be required systemically.

Microbiology: Polymyxin B sulfate, bacitracin zinc and neomycin sulfate together are considered active against the following microorganisms: *Staphylococcus aureus,* streptococci, including *Streptococcus pneumoniae, Escherichia coli, Haemophilus influenzae, Klebsiella-Enterobacter* species, *Neisseria* species and *Pseudomonas aeruginosa.* The product does not provide adequate coverage against *Serratia marcescens.*

INDICATIONS AND USAGE

Neosporin Ophthalmic Ointment is indicated in the short-term treatment of superficial external ocular infections caused by organisms susceptible to one or more of the antibiotics contained therein.

CONTRAINDICATIONS

This product is contraindicated in those individuals who have shown hypersensitivity to any of its components.

WARNINGS

The manifestations of sensitization to neomycin are usually itching, reddening and edema of the conjunctiva and eyelid. It may be manifest simply as a failure to heal. During long-term use of neomycin-containing products, periodic examination for such signs is advisable, and the patient should be told to discontinue the product if they are observed. These symptoms subside quickly on withdrawing the medication. Neomycin-containing applications should be avoided for the patient thereafter.

PRECAUTIONS

General: As with other antibiotic preparations, prolonged use may result in overgrowth of nonsusceptible organisms including fungi. Appropriate measures should be taken if this occurs.

Allergic cross-reactions may occur which could prevent the use of any or all of the following antibiotics for the treatment of future infections: kanamycin, paromomycin, streptomycin, and possibly gentamicin.

Information for Patients: If redness, irritation, swelling or pain persists or increases, discontinue use and contact your physician.

Avoid contaminating the applicator tip with material from the eye, fingers, or other source. This caution is necessary if the sterility of the ointment is to be preserved.

ADVERSE REACTIONS

Neomycin Sulfate may cause cutaneous and conjunctival sensitization. A precise incidence of hypersensivity reactions (primarily skin rash) due to topical neomycin is not known.

DOSAGE AND ADMINISTRATION

Apply the ointment every 3 or 4 hours for 7 to 10 days, depending on the severity of the infection.

HOW SUPPLIED

Tube of 1/8 oz with ophthalmic tip (NDC 0081-0732-86). Store at 15°–25°C (59°–77°F).

REFERENCES

1. Leyden JJ, and Kligman AM. Contact Dermatitis to Neomycin Sulfate, *JAMA* 242 (12): 1276–1278, 1979.
2. Prystowsky SD, Allen AM, Smith RW, Nonomura JH, Odom RB, and Akers WA. Allergic Contact Hypersensitivity to Nickel, Neomycin, Ethylenediamine, and Benzocaine. *Arch Dermatol* 115: 959–962, 1979.   561678

NEOSPORIN® OPHTHALMIC   ℞
SOLUTION Sterile

[nē′ō-spor′in]
(Polymyxin B Sulfate-Neomycin Sulfate-Gramicidin)

DESCRIPTION

Neosporin Ophthalmic Solution (polymyxin B sulfate-neomycin sulfate-gramicidin) is a sterile antimicrobial solution for ophthalmic use. Each ml contains: Aerosporin® (polymyxin B sulfate) 10,000 units, neomycin sulfate equivalent to 1.75 mg neomycin base and gramicidin 0.025 mg. The vehicle contains alcohol 0.5%, thimerosal 0.001% (added as a preservative) and the inactive ingredients propylene glycol, polyoxyethylene polyoxypropylene compound, sodium chloride and water for injection.

Polymyxin B sulfate is the sulfate salt of polymyxin B_1 and B_2 which are produced by the growth of *Bacillus polymyxa* (Prazmowski) Migula (Fam. Bacillaceae). It has a potency of not less than 6,000 polymyxin B units per mg, calculated on an anhydrous basis.

Neomycin sulfate is the sulfate salt of neomycin B and C, which are produced by the growth of *Streptomyces fradiae* Waksman (Fam. Streptomycetaceae). It has a potency equivalent of not less than 600 μg of neomycin standard per mg, calculated on an anhydrous basis.

Gramicidin (also called Gramicidin D) is a mixture of three pairs of antibacterial substances (Gramicidin A, B and C) produced by the growth of *Bacillus brevis* Dubos (Fam. Bacillaceae). It has a potency of not less than 900 μg of standard gramicidin per mg.

CLINICAL PHARMACOLOGY

A wide range of antibacterial action is provided by the overlapping spectra of polymyxin B sulfate, neomycin and gramicidin. The spectrum of action encompasses most bacterial pathogens capable of causing external infections of the eye and its adnexa.

Polymyxin B is bactericidal for a variety of gram-negative organisms. It increases the permeability of the bacterial cell membrane by interacting with the phospholipid components of the membrane.

Neomycin is bactericidal for many gram-positive and gram-negative organisms. It is an aminoglycoside antibiotic which inhibits protein synthesis by binding with ribosomal RNA and causing misreading of the bacterial genetic code.

Gramicidin is bactericidal for a variety of gram-positive organisms. It increases the permeability of the bacterial cell membrane to inorganic cations by forming a network of channels through the normal lipid bilayer of the membrane. When used topically, polymyxin B, neomycin and gramicidin are rarely irritating, and absorption from the intact skin or mucous membrane is insignificant. The incidence of skin sensitization to this combination has been shown to be low on normal skin.[1,2] Since these antibiotics are seldom used systemically, the patient is spared sensitization to those antibiotics which might later be required systemically.

Microbiology: Polymyxin B sulfate, neomycin sulfate and gramicidin together are considered active against the following microorganisms: *Staphylococcus aureus,* streptococci, including *Streptococcus pneumoniae, Escherichia coli, Haemophilus influenzae, Klebsiella-Enterobacter* species, *Neisseria* species and *Pseudomonas aeruginosa.* The product does not provide adequate coverage against *Serratia marcescens.*

INDICATIONS AND USAGE

Neosporin Ophthalmic Solution is indicated in the short-term treatment of superficial external ocular infections caused by organisms susceptible to one or more of the antibiotics contained therein.

CONTRAINDICATIONS

This product is contraindicated in those individuals who have shown hypersensitivity to any of its components.

WARNINGS

The manifestations of sensitization to neomycin are usually itching, reddening and edema of the conjunctiva and eyelid. It may be manifest simply as a failure to heal. During long-term use of neomycin-containing products, periodic examination for such signs is advisable, and the patient should be told to discontinue the product if they are observed. These symptoms subside quickly on withdrawing the medication. Neomycin-containing applications should be avoided for the patient thereafter.

PRECAUTIONS

General: As with other antibiotic preparations, prolonged use may result in overgrowth of nonsusceptible organisms including fungi. Appropriate measures should be taken if this occurs.

Allergic cross-reactions may occur which could prevent the use of any or all of the following antibiotics for the treatment of future infections: kanamycin, paromomycin, streptomycin, and possibly gentamicin.

Information for Patients: If redness, irritation, swelling or pain persists or increases, discontinue use and contact your physician.

Avoid contaminating the applicator tip with material from the eye, fingers, or other source. This caution is necessary if the sterility of the drops is to be preserved.

ADVERSE REACTIONS

Neomycin Sulfate may cause cutaneous and conjunctival sensitization. A precise incidence of hypersensitivity reactions (primarily skin rash) due to topical neomycin is not known.

DOSAGE AND ADMINISTRATION

The suggested dosage is one or two drops in the affected eye two to four times daily, or more frequently as required, for 7

to 10 days. In acute infections, initiate therapy with one or two drops every 15 to 30 minutes, reducing the frequency of instillation gradually as the infection is controlled.

HOW SUPPLIED
Drop Dose® of 10 ml (plastic dispenser bottle) (NDC-0081-0728-69).
Store at 15°–25°C (59°–77°F) and protect from light.

REFERENCES
1. Leyden JJ, and Kligman AM. Contact Dermatitis to Neomycin Sulfate. JAMA 242 (12): 1276–1278, 1979.
2. Prystowsky SD, Allen AM, Smith RW, Nonomura JH, Odom RB and Akers WA, Allergic Contact Hypersensitivity to Nickel, Neomycin, Ethylenediamine, and Benzocaine. Arch Dermatol 115: 959–962, 1979.   561834

NEOSPORIN® PLUS   OTC
MAXIMUM STRENGTH CREAM
[nē″ō-spor′in]
(Polymyxin B Sulfate-Neomycin Sulfate-Lidocaine)

First Aid Antibiotic/Topical Analgesic
(See PDR For Nonprescription Drugs.)

NEOSPORIN® PLUS MAXIMUM STRENGTH OINTMENT   OTC
[nē″ō-spor′in]
(Polymyxin B Sulfate-Bacitracin Zinc-Neomycin Sulfate-Lidocaine)

First Aid Antibiotic/Topical Analgesic
(See PDR For Nonprescription Drugs.)

NIX™ Creme Rinse   OTC
[nĭks]
Permethrin
Lice Treatment

(See PDR For Nonprescription Drugs.)

NUROMAX® INJECTION   ℞
[nōŏ′rō-măks]
(Doxacurium Chloride)

This drug should be administered only by adequately trained individuals familiar with its actions, characteristics, and hazards.

DESCRIPTION
Nuromax (doxacurium chloride) is a long-acting, nondepolarizing skeletal muscle relaxant for intravenous administration. Doxacurium chloride is *trans, trans*-2,2′-[succinylbis(oxytrimethylene)]bis[1,2,3,4-tetrahydro-6,7,8-trimethoxy-2-methyl-1-(3,4,5-trimethoxybenzyl)isoquinolinium] dichloride. The molecular formula is $C_{56}H_{78}Cl_2N_2O_{16}$ and the molecular weight is 1106.14. The compound does not partition into the 1-octanol phase of a distilled water/1-octanol system, *i.e.*, the n-octanol:water partition coefficient is 0. Doxacurium chloride is a mixture of the three *trans, trans* stereoisomers, a *dl* pair [(1R, 1′R, 2S, 2′S) and (1S, 1′S, 2R, 2′R)] and a meso form (1R, 1′S, 2S, 2′R).
Nuromax Injection is a sterile, non-pyrogenic aqueous solution (pH 3.9 to 5.0) containing doxacurium chloride equivalent to 1 mg/mL doxacurium in Water for Injection. Hydrochloric acid may have been added to adjust pH. Nuromax Injection contains 0.9% w/v benzyl alcohol.

CLINICAL PHARMACOLOGY
Nuromax binds competitively to cholinergic receptors on the motor end-plate to antagonize the action of acetylcholine, resulting in a block of neuromuscular transmission. This action is antagonized by acetylcholinesterase inhibitors, such as neostigmine.
Pharmacodynamics: Nuromax is approximately 2.5 to 3 times more potent than pancuronium and 10 to 12 times more potent than metocurine. Nuromax in doses of 1.5 to 2 x ED_{95} has a clinical duration of action (range and variability) similar to that of equipotent doses of pancuronium and metocurine (historic data and limited comparison). The average ED_{95} (dose required to produce 95% suppression of the adductor pollicis muscle twitch response to ulnar nerve stimulation) of Nuromax is 0.025 mg/kg (range: 0.020 to 0.033) in adults receiving balanced anesthesia.
The onset and clinically effective duration (time from injection to 25% recovery) of Nuromax administered alone or after succinylcholine during stable balanced anesthesia are shown in Table 1.

TABLE 1
Pharmacodynamic Dose Response*
Balanced Anesthesia

	Initial Nuromax Dose (mg/kg)		
	0.025† (n=34)	0.05 (n=27)	0.08 (n=9)
Time to Maximum Block (min)	9.3 (5.4–16)	5.2 (2.5–13)	3.5 (2.4–5)
Clinical Duration (min) (Time to 25% Recovery)	55 (9–145)	100 (39–232)	160 (110–338)

* Values shown are means (range).
† Nuromax administered after 10% to 100% recovery from an intubating dose of succinylcholine.

Initial doses of 0.05 mg/kg (2 x ED_{95}) and 0.08 mg/kg (3 x ED_{95}) Nuromax administered during the induction of thiopental-narcotic anesthesia produced good-to-excellent conditions for tracheal intubation in 5 minutes (13 of 15 cases studied) and 4 minutes (8 of 9 cases studied) (which are before maximum block), respectively.
As with other long-acting agents, the clinical duration of neuromuscular block associated with Nuromax shows considerable interpatient variability. An analysis of 390 cases in U.S. clinical trials utilizing a variety of premedications, varying lengths of surgery, and various anesthetic agents, indicates that approximately two-thirds of the patients had clinical durations within 30 minutes of the duration predicted by dose (based on mg/kg actual body weight). Patients ≥60 years old are approximately twice as likely to experience prolonged clinical duration (30 minutes longer than predicted) than patients <60 years old; thus, care should be used in older patients when prolonged recovery is undesirable (see **Geriatric Use** subsection of PRECAUTIONS and **Individualization of Dosages** subsection of CLINICAL PHARMACOLOGY). In addition, obese patients (patients weighing ≥30% more than ideal body weight for height) were almost twice as likely to experience prolonged clinical duration than non-obese patients; therefore, dosing should be based on ideal body weight (IBW) for obese patients (see **Individualization of Dosages** subsection of CLINICAL PHARMACOLOGY).
The mean time for spontaneous T_1 recovery from 25% to 50% of control following initial doses of Nuromax is approximately 26 minutes (range: 7 to 104, n=253) during balanced anesthesia. The mean time for spontaneous T_1 recovery from 25% to 75% is 54 minutes (range: 14 to 184, n=184).
Most patients receiving Nuromax in clinical trials required pharmacologic reversal prior to full spontaneous recovery from neuromuscular block (see **Antagonism of Neuromuscular Block** subsection of OVERDOSAGE); therefore, relatively few data are available on the time from injection to 95% spontaneous recovery of the twitch response. As with other long-acting neuromuscular blocking agents, Nuromax may be associated with prolonged times to full spontaneous recovery. Following an initial dose of 0.025 mg/kg Nuromax, some patients may require as long as 4 hours to exhibit full spontaneous recovery.
Cumulative neuromuscular blocking effects are not associated with repeated administration of maintenance doses of

Nuromax at 25% T_1 recovery. As with initial doses, however, the duration of action following maintenance doses of Nuromax may vary considerably among patients.
The Nuromax ED_{95} for children 2 to 12 years of age receiving halothane anesthesia is approximately 0.03 mg/kg. Children require higher Nuromax doses on a mg/kg basis than adults to achieve comparable levels of block. The onset time and duration of block are shorter in children than adults. During halothane anesthesia, doses of 0.03 mg/kg and 0.05 mg/kg Nuromax produce maximum block in approximately 7 and 4 minutes, respectively. The duration of clinically effective block is approximately 30 minutes after an initial dose of 0.03 mg/kg and approximately 45 minutes after 0.05 mg/kg. Nuromax has not been studied in children below the age of 2 years.
The neuromuscular block produced by Nuromax may be antagonized by anticholinesterase agents. As with other nondepolarizing neuromuscular blocking agents, the more profound the neuromuscular block at reversal, the longer the time and the greater the dose of anticholinesterase required for recovery of neuromuscular function.
Hemodynamics: Administration of Nuromax doses up to and including 0.08 mg/kg (~3 x ED_{95}) over 5 to 15 seconds to healthy adult patients during stable state balanced anesthesia and to patients with serious cardiovascular disease undergoing coronary artery bypass grafting, cardiac valvular repair, or vascular repair produced no dose-related effects on mean arterial blood pressure (MAP) or heart rate (HR).
No dose-related changes in MAP and HR were observed following administration of up to 0.05 mg/kg Nuromax over 5 to 15 seconds in 2- to 12-year-old children receiving halothane anesthesia.
Doses of 0.03 to 0.08 mg/kg (1.2 to 3 x ED_{95}) were not associated with dose-dependent changes in mean plasma histamine concentration. Clinical experience with more than 1,000 patients indicates that adverse experiences typically associated with histamine release (*e.g.*, bronchospasm, hypotension, tachycardia, cutaneous flushing, urticaria, *etc.*) are very rare following the administration of Nuromax (see ADVERSE REACTIONS).
Pharmacokinetics: Pharmacokinetic and pharmacodynamic results from a study of 24 healthy young adult patients and 8 healthy elderly patients are summarized in Table 2. The pharmacokinetics are linear over the dosage range tested (*i.e.*, plasma concentrations are approximately proportional to dose). The pharmacokinetics of Nuromax are similar in healthy young adult and elderly patients. Some healthy elderly patients tend to be more sensitive to the neuromuscular blocking effects of Nuromax than healthy young adult patients receiving the same dose. The time to maximum block is longer in elderly patients than in young adult patients (11.2 minutes versus 7.7 minutes at 0.025 mg/kg Nuromax). In addition, the clinically effective durations of block are more variable and tend to be longer in healthy elderly patients than in healthy young adult patients receiving the same dose.
[See table below.]
Table 3 summarizes the pharmacokinetic and pharmacodynamic results from a study of 9 healthy young adult patients, 8 patients with end-stage kidney disease undergoing kidney transplantation, and 7 patients with end-stage liver disease undergoing liver transplantation. The results suggest that a longer $t_{1/2}$ can be expected in patients with end-stage kidney disease; in addition, these patients may be more sensitive to

---

TABLE 2
Pharmacokinetic and Pharmacodynamic Parameters[1] of Nuromax in Young Adult and Elderly Patients
(Isoflurane Anesthesia)

Parameter	Healthy Young Adult Patients (22 to 49 yrs)			Healthy Elderly Patients (67 to 72 yrs)
	0.025 mg/kg (n=8)	0.05 mg/kg (n=8)	0.08 mg/kg (n=8)	0.025 mg/kg (n=8)
$t_{1/2}$ elimination (min)	86 (25–171)	123 (61–163)	98 (47–163)	96 (50–114)
Volume of Distribution at Steady State (L/kg)	0.15 (0.10–0.21)	0.24 (0.13–0.30)	0.22 (0.16–0.33)	0.22 (0.14–0.40)
Plasma Clearance (mL/min/kg)	2.22 (1.02–3.95)	2.62 (1.21–5.70)	2.53 (1.88–3.38)	2.47 (1.58–3.60)
Maximum Block (1%)	97 (88–100)	100 (100–100)	100 (100–100)	96 (90–100)
Clinically Effective Duration of Block[2] (min)	68 (35–90)	91 (47–132)	177 (74–268)	97 (36–179)

1 Values shown are means (range).
2 Time from injection to 25% recovery of the control twitch height.

Continued on next page

Burroughs Wellcome—Cont.

the neuromuscular blocking effects of Nuromax. The time to maximum block was slightly longer and the clinically effective duration of block was prolonged in patients with end-stage kidney disease.
[See table below.]
No data are available from patients with liver disease not requiring transplantation. There are no significant alterations in the pharmacokinetics of Nuromax in liver transplant patients. Sensitivity to the neuromuscular blocking effects of Nuromax was highly variable in patients undergoing liver transplantation. Three of 7 patients developed ≤50% block, indicating that a reduced sensitivity to Nuromax may occur in such patients. In those patients who developed >50% neuromuscular block, the time to maximum block and the clinically effective duration tended to be longer than in healthy young adult patients (see **Individualization of Dosages** subsection of CLINICAL PHARMACOLOGY).
Consecutively administered maintenance doses of 0.005 mg/kg Nuromax, each given at 25% T_1 recovery following the preceding dose, do not result in a progressive increase in the plasma concentration of doxacurium or a progressive increase in the depth or duration of block produced by each dose.
Nuromax is not metabolized *in vitro* in fresh human plasma. Plasma protein binding of Nuromax is approximately 30% in human plasma.
In vivo data from humans suggest that Nuromax is not metabolized and that the major elimination pathway is excretion of unchanged drug in urine and bile. In studies of healthy adult patients, 24% to 38% of an administered dose was recovered as parent drug in urine over 6 to 12 hours after dosing. High bile concentrations of Nuromax (relative to plasma) have been found 35 to 90 minutes after administration. The overall extent of biliary excretion is unknown. The data derived from analysis of human urine and bile are consistent with data from *in vivo* studies in the rat, cat, and dog, which indicate that all of an administered dose of Nuromax is recovered as parent drug in the urine and bile of these species.
Individualization of Dosages: In elderly patients or patients who have impaired renal function, the potential for a prolongation of block may be reduced by decreasing the initial Nuromax dose and by titrating the dose to achieve the desired depth of block. In obese patients (patients weighing ≥30% more than ideal body weight for height), the Nuromax dose should be determined using the patient's ideal body weight (IBW), according to the following formulae:
Men: IBW in kg=[106 +(6 x inches in height above 5 feet)]/2.2
Women: IBW in kg=[100 +(5 x inches in height above 5 feet)]/2.2
Dosage requirements for patients with severe liver disease are variable; some patients may require a higher than normal initial Nuromax dose to achieve clinically effective block. Once adequate block is established, the clinical duration of block may be prolonged in such patients relative to patients with normal liver function.
As with pancuronium, metocurine, and vecuronium, resistance to Nuromax, manifested by a reduced intensity and/or shortened duration of block, must be considered when Nuromax is selected for use in patients receiving phenytoin or carbamazepine (see **Drug Interactions** subsection of PRECAUTIONS).
As with other nondepolarizing neuromuscular blocking agents, a reduction in dosage of Nuromax must be considered in cachectic or debilitated patients, in patients with neuromuscular diseases, severe electrolyte abnormalities, or carcinomatosis, and in other patients in whom potentiation of neuromuscular block or difficulty with reversal is anticipated. Increased doses of Nuromax may be required in burn patients (see PRECAUTIONS).

INDICATIONS AND USAGE

Nuromax is a long-acting neuromuscular blocking agent, indicated as an adjunct to general anesthesia, to provide skeletal muscle relaxation during surgery. Nuromax can also be used to provide skeletal muscle relaxation for endotracheal intubation.

CONTRAINDICATIONS

Nuromax is contraindicated in patients known to have hypersensitivity to it.

WARNINGS

NUROMAX SHOULD BE ADMINISTERED IN CAREFULLY ADJUSTED DOSAGE BY OR UNDER THE SUPERVISION OF EXPERIENCED CLINICIANS WHO ARE FAMILIAR WITH THE DRUG'S ACTIONS AND THE POSSIBLE COMPLICATIONS OF ITS USE. THE DRUG SHOULD NOT BE ADMINISTERED UNLESS FACILITIES FOR INTUBATION, ARTIFICIAL RESPIRATION, OXYGEN THERAPY, AND AN ANTAGONIST ARE WITHIN IMMEDIATE REACH. IT IS RECOMMENDED THAT CLINICIANS ADMINISTERING LONG-ACTING NEUROMUSCULAR BLOCKING AGENTS SUCH AS NUROMAX EMPLOY A PERIPHERAL NERVE STIMULATOR TO MONITOR DRUG RESPONSE, NEED FOR ADDITIONAL RELAXANTS, AND ADEQUACY OF SPONTANEOUS RECOVERY OR ANTAGONISM.
NUROMAX HAS NO KNOWN EFFECT ON CONSCIOUSNESS, PAIN THRESHOLD, OR CEREBRATION. TO AVOID DISTRESS TO THE PATIENT, NEUROMUSCULAR BLOCK SHOULD NOT BE INDUCED BEFORE UNCONSCIOUSNESS.
Nuromax Injection is acidic (pH 3.9 to 5.0) and may not be compatible with alkaline solutions having a pH greater than 8.5 (*e.g.,* barbiturate solutions).
Nuromax Injection contains benzyl alcohol. In newborn infants, benzyl alcohol has been associated with an increased incidence of neurological and other complications which are sometimes fatal. See **Pediatric Use** subsection of PRECAUTIONS.

PRECAUTIONS

General: Nuromax has no clinically significant effects on heart rate; therefore, Nuromax will not counteract the bradycardia produced by many anesthetic agents or by vagal stimulation.
Neuromuscular blocking agents may have a profound effect in patients with neuromuscular diseases (*e.g.,* myasthenia gravis and the myasthenic syndrome). In these and other conditions in which prolonged neuromuscular block is a possibility (*e.g.,* carcinomatosis), the use of a peripheral nerve stimulator and a small test dose of Nuromax is recommended to assess the level of neuromuscular block and to monitor dosage requirements. Shorter acting muscle relaxants than Nuromax may be more suitable for these patients.
Resistance to nondepolarizing neuromuscular blocking agents may develop in patients with burns depending upon the time elapsed since the injury and the size of the burn. Nuromax has not been studied in patients with burns.
Acid-base and/or serum electrolyte abnormalities may potentiate or antagonize the action of neuromuscular blocking agents. The action of neuromuscular blocking agents may be enhanced by magnesium salts administered for the management of toxemia of pregnancy.
Nuromax has not been studied in patients with asthma.
No data are available to support the use of Nuromax by intramuscular injection.
Renal and Hepatic Disease: Nuromax has been studied in patients with end-stage kidney (n=8) or liver (n=7) disease undergoing transplantation procedures (see CLINICAL PHARMACOLOGY). The possibility of prolonged neuromuscular block in patients undergoing renal transplantation and the possibility of a variable onset and duration of neuromuscular block in patients undergoing liver transplantation must be considered when Nuromax is used in such patients.
Obesity: Administration of Nuromax on the basis of actual body weight is associated with a prolonged duration of action in obese patients (patients weighing ≥30% more than ideal body weight for height) (see CLINICAL PHARMACOLOGY). Therefore, the dose of Nuromax should be based upon ideal body weight in obese patients (see **Individualization of Dosages** subsection of CLINICAL PHARMACOLOGY).
Malignant Hyperthermia (MH): In a study of MH-susceptible pigs, Nuromax did not trigger MH. Nuromax has not been studied in MH-susceptible patients. Since MH can develop in the absence of established triggering agents, the clinician should be prepared to recognize and treat MH in any patient scheduled for general anesthesia.
Long-Term Use in the Intensive Care Unit (ICU): No data are available on the long-term use of Nuromax in patients undergoing mechanical ventilation in the ICU.
Drug Interactions: Prior administration of succinylcholine has no clinically important effect on the neuromuscular blocking action of Nuromax.
The use of Nuromax before succinylcholine to attenuate some of the side effects of succinylcholine has not been studied.
There are no clinical data on concomitant use of Nuromax and other nondepolarizing neuromuscular blocking agents.
Isoflurane, enflurane and halothane decrease the ED_{50} of Nuromax by 30% to 45%. These agents may also prolong the clinically effective duration of action by up to 25%.
Other drugs which may enhance the neuromuscular blocking action of nondepolarizing agents such as Nuromax include certain antibiotics (*e.g.,* aminoglycosides, tetracyclines, bacitracin, polymyxins, lincomycin, clindamycin, colistin, and sodium colistimethate), magnesium salts, lithium, local anesthetics, procainamide, and quinidine.
As with some other nondepolarizing neuromuscular blocking agents, the time of onset of neuromuscular block induced by Nuromax is lengthened and the duration of block is shortened in patients receiving phenytoin or carbamazepine.
Carcinogenesis, Mutagenesis, Impairment of Fertility: Carcinogenesis and fertility studies have not been performed. Nuromax was evaluated in a battery of four short-term mutagenicity tests. It was non-mutagenic in the Ames Salmonella assay, in the mouse lymphoma assay, and in the human lymphocyte assay. In the *in vivo* rat bone marrow cytogenic assay, statistically significant increases in the incidence of structural abnormalities, relative to vehicle controls, were observed in male rats dosed with 0.1 mg/kg (0.625 mg/m^2) Nuromax and sacrificed at 6 hours, but not at 24 or 48 hours, and in female rats dosed with 0.2 mg/kg (1.25 mg/m^2) Nuromax and sacrificed at 24 hours, but not at 6 or 48 hours. There was no increase in structural abnormalities in either male or female rats given 0.3 mg/kg (1.875 mg/m^2) Nuromax and sacrificed at 6, 24, or 48 hours. Thus, the incidence of abnormalities in the *in vivo* rat bone marrow cytogenetic assay was not dose-dependent and, therefore, the likelihood that the observed abnormalities were treatment-related or clinically significant is low.
Pregnancy: Teratogenic Effects: Pregnancy Category C. Teratology testing in nonventilated, pregnant rats and mice treated subcutaneously with maximum subparalyzing doses of Nuromax revealed no maternal or fetal toxicity or teratogenic effects. There are no adequate and well-controlled studies of Nuromax in pregnant women. Because animal studies are not always predictive of human response and the doses used were subparalyzing, Nuromax should be used during pregnancy only if the potential benefit justifies the potential risk to the fetus.
Labor and Delivery: The use of Nuromax during labor, vaginal delivery, or cesarean section has not been studied. It is not known whether Nuromax administered to the mother has immediate or delayed effects on the fetus. The duration of action of Nuromax exceeds the usual duration of operative obstetrics (cesarean section). Therefore, Nuromax is not recommended for use in patients undergoing C-section.
Nursing Mothers: It is not known whether Nuromax is excreted in human milk. Because many drugs are excreted in human milk, caution should be exercised following Nuromax administration to a nursing woman.

TABLE 3
Pharmacokinetic and Pharmacodynamic Parameters[1] of Nuromax in Healthy Patients and in Patients Undergoing Kidney or Liver Transplantation
(Isoflurane Anesthesia)

Parameter	Healthy Young Adult Patients 0.015 mg/kg (n=9)	Kidney Transplant Patients 0.015 mg/kg (n=8)	Liver Transplant Patients 0.015 mg/kg (n=7)
$t_{1/2}$ elimination (min)	99 (48–193)	221 (84–592)	115 (69–148)
Volume of Distribution at Steady State (L/kg)	0.22 (0.11–0.43)	0.27 (0.17–0.55)	0.29 (0.17–0.35)
Plasma Clearance (mL/min/kg)	2.66 (1.35–6.66)	1.23 (0.48–2.40)	2.30 (1.96–3.05)
Maximum Block (%)	86 (59–100)	98 (95–100)	70 (0-100)
Clinically Effective Duration of Block (min)	36 (19–80)	80 (29–133)	52 (20–91)

1 Values shown are means (range).

Pediatric Use: Nuromax has not been studied in children below the age of 2 years. See CLINICAL PHARMACOLOGY and DOSAGE AND ADMINISTRATION for clinical experience and recommendations for use in children 2 to 12 years of age.

Geriatric Use: Nuromax has been used in elderly patients, including patients with significant cardiovascular disease. In elderly patients the onset of maximum block is slower and the duration of neuromuscular block produced by Nuromax is more variable and, in some cases, longer than in young adult patients (see **Pharmacodynamics** and **Individualization of Dosages** subsections of CLINICAL PHARMACOLOGY).

ADVERSE REACTIONS

The most frequent adverse effect of nondepolarizing blocking agents as a class consists of an extension of the pharmacological action beyond the time needed for surgery and anesthesia. This effect may vary from skeletal muscle weakness to profound and prolonged skeletal muscle paralysis resulting in respiratory insufficiency and apnea which require manual or mechanical ventilation until recovery is judged to be clinically adequate (see OVERDOSAGE). Inadequate reversal of neuromuscular block from Nuromax is possible, as with all nondepolarizing agents. Prolonged neuromuscular block and inadequate reversal may lead to postoperative complications.

Observed in Clinical Trials: Adverse experiences were uncommon among the 1034 surgical patients and volunteers who received Nuromax and other drugs in U.S. clinical studies in the course of a wide variety of procedures conducted during balanced or inhalational anesthesia. The following adverse experiences were reported in patients administered Nuromax (all events judged by investigators during the clinical trials to have a possible causal relationship):

Incidence Greater than 1%—None

Incidence Less than 1%—

Cardiovascular*: hypotension,† flushing,† ventricular fibrillation, myocardial infarction

Respiratory: bronchospasm, wheezing

Dermatological: urticaria, injection site reaction

Special Senses: diplopia

Nonspecific: difficult neuromuscular block reversal, prolonged drug effect, fever

OVERDOSAGE

Overdosage with neuromuscular blocking agents may result in neuromuscular block beyond the time needed for surgery and anesthesia. The primary treatment is maintenance of a patent airway and controlled ventilation until recovery of normal neuromuscular function is assured. Once evidence of recovery from neuromuscular block is observed, further recovery may be facilitated by administration of an anticholinesterase agent (*e.g.,* neostigmine, edrophonium) in conjunction with an appropriate anticholinergic agent (see **Antagonism of Neuromuscular Block).**

Antagonism of Neuromuscular Block:

ANTAGONISTS (SUCH AS NEOSTIGMINE) SHOULD NOT BE ADMINISTERED PRIOR TO THE DEMONSTRATION OF SOME SPONTANEOUS RECOVERY FROM NEUROMUSCULAR BLOCK. THE USE OF A NERVE STIMULATOR TO DOCUMENT RECOVERY AND ANTAGONISM OF NEUROMUSCULAR BLOCK IS RECOMMENDED. T_4/T_1 SHOULD BE > ZERO BEFORE ANTAGONISM IS ATTEMPTED.

In an analysis of patients in whom antagonism of neuromuscular block was evaluated following administration of single doses of neostigmine averaging 0.06 mg/kg (range: 0.05 to 0.075) administered at approximately 25% T_1 spontaneous recovery during balanced anesthesia, 71% of patients exhibited $T_4/T_1 \geq 0.7$ before monitoring was discontinued. For these patients, the mean time to $T_4/T_1 \geq 0.7$ was 19 minutes (range: 7 to 55). As with other long-acting nondepolarizing neuromuscular blocking agents, the time for recovery of neuromuscular function following administration of neostigmine is dependent upon the level of residual neuromuscular block at the time of attempted reversal; longer recovery times than those cited above may be anticipated when neostigmine is administered at more profound levels of block (*i.e.,* at < 25% T_1 recovery).

Patients should be evaluated for adequate clinical evidence of antagonism, *e.g.,* 5-second head lift, and grip strength. Ventilation must be supported until no longer required. As with other neuromuscular blocking agents, physicians should be alert to the possibility that the action of the drugs used to antagonize neuromuscular block may wear off before the effects of Nuromax on the neuromuscular junction have declined sufficiently.

Antagonism may be delayed in the presence of debilitation, carcinomatosis, and the concomitant use of certain broad spectrum antibiotics, or anesthetic agents and other drugs which enhance neuromuscular block or separately cause respiratory depression (see **Drug Interactions** subsection of PRECAUTIONS). Under such circumstances the management is the same as that of prolonged neuromuscular block. In clinical trials, a dose of 1 mg/kg edrophonium was not as effective as a dose of 0.06 mg/kg neostigmine in antagonizing moderate to deep levels of neuromuscular block (i.e., < 60% T_1 recovery). Therefore, the use of 1 mg/kg edrophonium is not recommended for reversal from moderate to deep levels of block. The use of pyridostigmine has not been studied.

* Reports of ventricular fibrillation (n=1) and myocardial infarction (n=1) were limited to ASA Class 3–4 patients undergoing cardiac surgery (n=142).

† 0.3% incidence. All other reactions unmarked were ≤0.1%.

DOSAGE AND ADMINISTRATION

NUROMAX SHOULD ONLY BE ADMINISTERED INTRAVENOUSLY.

Nuromax, like other long-acting neuromuscular blocking agents, displays variability in the duration of its effect. The potential for a prolonged clinical duration of neuromuscular block must be considered when Nuromax is selected for administration. The dosage information provided below is intended as a guide only. Doses should be individualized (see **Individualization of Dosages** subsection of CLINICAL PHARMACOLOGY). Factors that may warrant dosage adjustment include: advancing age, the presence of kidney or liver disease, or obesity (patients weighing ≥30% more than ideal body weight for height). The use of a peripheral nerve stimulator will permit the most advantageous use of Nuromax, minimize the possibility of overdosage or underdosage, and assist in the evaluation of recovery.

Parenteral drug products should be inspected visually for particulate matter and discoloration prior to administration whenever solution and container permit.

Adults:

Initial Doses: When administered as a component of a thiopental/narcotic induction-intubation paradigm as well as for production of long-duration neuromuscular block during surgery, 0.05 mg/kg (2 x ED_{95}) Nuromax produces good-to-excellent conditions for tracheal intubation in 5 minutes in approximately 90% of patients. Lower doses of Nuromax may result in a longer time for development of satisfactory intubation conditions. Clinically effective neuromuscular block may be expected to last approximately 100 minutes on average (range: 39 to 232) following 0.05 mg/kg Nuromax administered to patients receiving balanced anesthesia.

An initial Nuromax dose of 0.08 mg/kg (3 x ED_{95}) should be reserved for instances in which a need for very prolonged neuromuscular block is anticipated. In approximately 90% of patients, good-to-excellent intubation conditions may be expected in 4 minutes after this dose; however, clinically effective block may be expected to persist for as long as 160 minutes or more (range: 110 to 338) (see CLINICAL PHARMACOLOGY).

If Nuromax is administered during steady-state isoflurane, enflurane, or halothane anesthesia, reduction of the Nuromax dose by one-third should be considered.

When succinylcholine is administered to facilitate tracheal intubation in patients receiving balanced anesthesia, an initial dose of 0.025 mg/kg (ED_{95}) Nuromax provides about 60 minutes (range: 9 to 145) of clinically effective neuromuscular block for surgery. For a longer duration of action, a larger initial dose may be administered.

Maintenance Doses: Maintenance dosing will generally be required about 60 minutes after an initial dose of 0.025 mg/kg Nuromax or 100 minutes after an initial dose of 0.05 mg/kg Nuromax during balanced anesthesia. Repeated maintenance doses administered at 25% T_1 recovery may be expected to be required at relatively regular intervals in each patient. The interval may vary considerably between patients. Maintenance doses of 0.005 and 0.01 mg/kg Nuromax each provide an average 30 minutes (range: 9 to 57) and 45 minutes (range: 14 to 108), respectively, of additional clinically effective neuromuscular block. For shorter or longer desired durations, smaller or larger maintenance doses may be administered.

Children:

When administered during halothane anesthesia, an initial dose of 0.03 mg/kg (ED_{95}) produces maximum neuromuscular block in about 7 minutes (range: 5 to 11) and clinically effective block for an average of 30 minutes (range: 12 to 54). Under halothane anesthesia, 0.05 mg/kg produces maximum block in about 4 minutes (range: 2 to 10) and clinically effective block for 45 minutes (range: 30 to 80). Maintenance doses are generally required more frequently in children than in adults. Because of the potentiating effect of halothane seen in adults, a higher dose of Nuromax may be required in children receiving balanced anesthesia than in children receiving halothane anesthesia to achieve a comparable onset and duration of neuromuscular block. Nuromax has not been studied in children below the age of 2 years.

Compatibility:

Y-site Administration: Nuromax Injection may not be compatible with alkaline solutions with a pH greater than 8.5 (*e.g.,* barbiturate solutions).

Nuromax is compatible with:

- 5% Dextrose Injection USP
- 0.9% Sodium Chloride Injection USP
- 5% Dextrose and 0.9% Sodium Chloride Injection USP
- Lactated Ringer's Injection USP
- 5% Dextrose and Lactated Ringer's Injection
- Sufenta® (sufentanil citrate) Injection, diluted as directed
- Alfenta® (alfentanil hydrochloride) Injection, diluted as directed
- Sublimaze® (fentanyl citrate) Injection, diluted as directed

Dilution Stability: Nuromax diluted up to 1:10 in 5% Dextrose Injection USP or 0.9% Sodium Chloride Injection USP has been shown to be physically and chemically stable when stored in polypropylene syringes at 5° to 25°C (41° to 77°F), for up to 24 hours. Since dilution diminishes the preservative effectiveness of benzyl alcohol, aseptic techniques should be used to prepare the diluted product. Immediate use of the diluted product is preferred, and any unused portion of diluted Nuromax should be discarded after 8 hours.

HOW SUPPLIED

Nuromax Injection, 1 mg doxacurium in each mL.

5 mL Multiple Dose vials containing 0.9% w/v benzyl alcohol as a preservative (see WARNINGS). Tray of 10 (NDC 0081-0763-44).

STORAGE

Store Nuromax Injection at room temperature of 15° to 25°C (59° to 77°F). DO NOT FREEZE.

U.S. Patent No. 4701460 562004

PEDIOTIC® SUSPENSION Sterile ℞

[pĕd-ē-ō 'tĭk]

(Polymyxin B Sulfate-Neomycin Sulfate-Hydrocortisone Otic Suspension)

DESCRIPTION

Pediotic (polymyxin B sulfate-neomycin sulfate-hydrocortisone otic suspension) is a sterile antibacterial and anti-inflammatory suspension for otic use. Each mL contains: polymyxin B sulfate 10,000 units, neomycin sulfate equivalent to 3.5 mg neomycin base, and hydrocortisone 10 mg (1%). The vehicle contains thimerosal 0.001% (added as a preservative) and the inactive ingredients cetyl alcohol, glyceryl monostearate, mineral oil, polyoxyl 40 stearate, propylene glycol, and Water for Injection. Sulfuric acid may be added to adjust pH. Pediotic Suspension has a minimum pH of 4.1, which is less acidic than the minimum pH of 3.0 for Cortisporin® Otic Suspension.

Polymyxin B sulfate is the sulfate salt of polymyxin B_1 and B_2, which are produced by the growth of *Bacillus polymyxa* (Prazmowski) Migula (Fam. Bacillaceae). It has a potency of not less than 6,000 polymyxin B units per mg, calculated on an anhydrous basis.

Neomycin sulfate is the sulfate salt of neomycin B and C, which are produced by the growth of *Streptomyces fradiae* Waksman (Fam. Streptomycetaceae). It has a potency equivalent of not less than 600 μg of neomycin standard per mg, calculated on an anhydrous basis.

Hydrocortisone, 11B, 17, 21-trihydroxypregn-4-ene-3, 20-dione, is an anti-inflammatory hormone.

CLINICAL PHARMACOLOGY

Corticoids suppress the inflammatory response to a variety of agents and they may delay healing. Since corticoids may inhibit the body's defense mechanism against infection, a concomitant antimicrobial drug may be used when this inhibition is considered to be clinically significant in a particular case.

The anti-infective components in the combination are included to provide action against specific organisms susceptible to them. Polymyxin B sulfate and neomycin sulfate together are considered active against the following microorganisms: *Staphylococcus aureus, Escherichia coli, Haemophilus influenzae, Klebsiella-Enterobacter* species, *Neisseria* species, and *Pseudomonas aeruginosa.* This product does not provide adequate coverage against *Serratia marcescens* and streptococci, including *Streptococcus pneumonia.*

The relative potency of corticosteroids depends on the molecular structure, concentration, and release from the vehicle.

INDICATIONS AND USAGE

For the treatment of superficial bacterial infections of the external auditory canal caused by organisms susceptible to the action of the antibiotics, and for the treatment of infections of mastoidectomy and fenestration cavities caused by organisms susceptible to the antibiotics.

CONTRAINDICATIONS

This product is contraindicated in those individuals who have shown hypersensitivity to any of its components, and in herpes simplex, vaccinia, and varicella infections.

WARNINGS

This product should be used with care in cases of perforated eardrum and in long-standing cases of chronic otitis media because of the possibility of ototoxicity.

Continued on next page

Burroughs Wellcome—Cont.

Neomycin sulfate may cause cutaneous sensitization. A precise incidence of hypersensitivity reactions (primarily skin rash) due to topical neomycin is not known.
When using neomycin-containing products to control secondary infection in the chronic dermatoses, such as chronic otitis externa or stasis dermatitis, it should be borne in mind that the skin in these conditions is more liable than is normal skin to become sensitized to many substances, including neomycin. The manifestation of sensitization to neomycin is usually a low-grade reddening with swelling, dry scaling and itching; it may be manifest simply as a failure to heal. Periodic examination for such signs is advisable, and the patient should be told to discontinue the product if they are observed. These symptoms regress quickly on withdrawing the medication. Neomycin-containing applications should be avoided for the patient thereafter.

PRECAUTIONS

General: As with other antibacterial preparations, prolonged use may result in overgrowth of non-susceptible organisms, including fungi.
If the infection is not improved after one week, cultures and susceptibility tests should be repeated to verify the identity of the organism and to determine whether therapy should be changed.
Treatment should not be continued for longer than ten days.
Allergic cross-reactions may occur which could prevent the use of any or all of the following antibiotics for the treatment of future infections: kanamycin, paromomycin, streptomycin, and possibly gentamicin.
Information for Patients: Avoid contaminating the dropper with material from the ear, fingers, or other source. This caution is necessary if the sterility of the drops is to be preserved. If sensitization or irritation occurs, discontinue use immediately and contact your physician. Do not use in the eyes.
SHAKE WELL BEFORE USING.
Laboratory Tests: Systemic effects of excessive levels of hydrocortisone may include a reduction in the number of circulating eosinophils and a decrease in urinary excretion of 17-hydroxycorticosteroids.
Carcinogenesis, Mutagenesis, Impairment of Fertility: Long-term studies in animals (rats, rabbits, mice) showed no evidence of carcinogenicity attributable to oral administration of corticosteroids.
Pregnancy: ***Teratogenic Effects:*** Pregnancy Category C. Corticosteroids have been shown to be teratogenic in rabbits when applied topically at concentrations of 0.5% on days 6–18 of gestation and in mice when applied topically at a concentration of 15% on days 10–13 of gestation. There are no adequate and well-controlled studies in pregnant women. Corticosteroids should be used during pregnancy only if the potential benefit justifies the potential risk to the fetus.
Nursing Mothers: Hydrocortisone appears in human milk following oral administration of the drug. Since systemic absorption of hydrocortisone may occur when applied topically, caution should be exercised when Pediotic is used by a nursing woman.
Pediatric Use: See DOSAGE AND ADMINISTRATION.

ADVERSE REACTIONS

Neomycin occasionally causes skin sensitization. Ototoxicity and nephrotoxicity have also been reported (see WARNINGS section). Adverse reactions have occurred with topical use of antibiotic combinations including neomycin and polymyxin B. Exact incidence figures are not available since no denominator of treated patients is available. The reaction occurring most often is allergic sensitization. In one clinical study, using a 20% neomycin patch, neomycin-induced allergic skin reactions occurred in two of 2,175 (0.09%) individuals in the general population.[1] In another study, the incidence was found to be approximately 1%.[2]
The following local adverse reactions have been reported with topical corticosteroids, especially under occlusive dressings: burning, itching, irritation, dryness, folliculitis, hypertrichosis, acneiform eruptions, hypopigmentation, perioral dermatitis, allergic contact dermatitis, maceration of the skin, secondary infection, skin atrophy, striae, and miliaria. Stinging and burning have been reported rarely when this drug has gained access to the middle ear.

DOSAGE AND ADMINISTRATION

The external auditory canal should be thoroughly cleansed and dried with a sterile cotton applicator.
For adults, 4 drops of the suspension should be instilled into the affected ear 3 or 4 times daily. For infants and children, 3 drops are suggested because of the smaller capacity of the ear canal.
The patient should lie with the affected ear upward and then the drops should be instilled. This position should be maintained for 5 minutes to facilitate penetration of the drops into the ear canal. Repeat, if necessary, for the opposite ear.
If preferred, a cotton wick may be inserted into the canal and then the cotton may be saturated with the suspension. This wick should be kept moist by adding further suspension every four hours. The wick should be replaced at least once every 24 hours.
SHAKE WELL BEFORE USING.

HOW SUPPLIED

Bottle of 7.5 ml with sterilized dropper. NDC 0081-0910-02.
Store at 15° to 25°C (59° to 77°F).

REFERENCES

1. Leyden JJ, Kligman AM: Contact dermatitis to neomycin sulfate. *JAMA* 1979;242:1276–1278.
2. Prystowsky SD, Allen AM, Smith RW, et al: Allergic contact hypersensitivity to nickel, neomycin, ethylenediamine, and benzocaine. *Arch Dermatol* 1979;115:959–962.
455741

POLYMYXIN B SULFATE ℞

AEROSPORIN® brand
Sterile Powder
Polymyxin B Sulfate for Parenteral and/or Ophthalmic Administration

> WARNING
> CAUTION: **WHEN THIS DRUG IS GIVEN INTRAMUSCULARLY AND/OR INTRATHECALLY, IT SHOULD BE GIVEN ONLY TO HOSPITALIZED PATIENTS, SO AS TO PROVIDE CONSTANT SUPERVISION BY A PHYSICIAN.**
> **RENAL FUNCTION SHOULD BE CAREFULLY DETERMINED AND PATIENTS WITH RENAL DAMAGE AND NITROGEN RETENTION SHOULD HAVE REDUCED DOSAGE. PATIENTS WITH NEPHROTOXICITY DUE TO POLYMYXIN B SULFATE USUALLY SHOW ALBUMINURIA, CELLULAR CASTS, AND AZOTEMIA. DIMINISHING URINE OUTPUT AND A RISING BUN ARE INDICATIONS FOR DISCONTINUING THERAPY WITH THIS DRUG.**
> **NEUROTOXIC REACTIONS MAY BE MANIFESTED BY IRRITABILITY, WEAKNESS, DROWSINESS, ATAXIA, PERIORAL PARESTHESIA, NUMBNESS OF THE EXTREMITIES, AND BLURRING OF VISION. THESE ARE USUALLY ASSOCIATED WITH HIGH SERUM LEVELS FOUND IN PATIENTS WITH IMPAIRED RENAL FUNCTION AND/OR NEPHROTOXICITY. THE CONCURRENT USE OF OTHER NEPHROTOXIC AND NEUROTOXIC DRUGS, PARTICULARLY KANAMYCIN, STREPTOMYCIN, CEPHALORIDINE, PAROMOMYCIN, TOBRAMYCIN, POLYMYXIN E (COLISTIN), NEOMYCIN, GENTAMICIN, AND VIOMYCIN, SHOULD BE AVOIDED.**
> **THE NEUROTOXICITY OF POLYMYXIN B SULFATE CAN RESULT IN RESPIRATORY PARALYSIS FROM NEUROMUSCULAR BLOCKADE, ESPECIALLY WHEN THE DRUG IS GIVEN SOON AFTER ANESTHESIA AND/OR MUSCLE RELAXANTS.**
> **USAGE IN PREGNANCY: THE SAFETY OF THIS DRUG IN HUMAN PREGNANCY HAS NOT BEEN ESTABLISHED.**

DESCRIPTION

Polymyxin B sulfate is one of a group of basic polypeptide antibiotics derived from *B polymyxa (B aerosporous).*
Aerosporin brand Polymyxin B Sulfate is in powder form suitable for preparation of sterile solutions for intramuscular, intravenous drip, intrathecal, or ophthalmic use.
In the medical literature, dosages have frequently been given in terms of equivalent weight of pure polymyxin B base. Each milligram of pure polymyxin B base is equivalent to 10,000 units of polymyxin B and each microgram of pure polymyxin B base is equivalent to 10 units of polymyxin B.
Aqueous solutions of Aerosporin brand Polymyxin B Sulfate may be stored up to 12 months without significant loss of potency if kept under refrigeration. In the interest of safety, solutions for parenteral use should be stored under refrigeration and any unused portion should be discarded after 72 hours. Polymyxin B sulfate should not be stored in alkaline solutions since they are less stable.

ACTIONS

Polymyxin B sulfate has a bactericidal action against almost all gram-negative bacilli except the Proteus group. Polymyxins increase the permeability of bacterial cell wall membranes. All gram-positive bacteria, fungi, and the gram-negative cocci, *N gonorrhoeae* and *N meningitidis,* are resistant.
Susceptibility plate testing: If the Kirby-Bauer method of disc susceptibility testing is used, a 300-unit polymyxin B disc should give a zone of over 11 mm when tested against a polymyxin B-susceptible bacterial strain.
Polymyxin B sulfate is not absorbed from the normal alimentary tract. Since the drug loses 50 percent of its activity in the presence of serum, active blood levels are low. Repeated injections may give a cumulative effect. Levels tend to be higher in infants and children. The drug is excreted slowly by the kidneys. Tissue diffusion is poor and the drug does not pass the blood brain barrier into the cerebrospinal fluid. In therapeutic dosage, polymyxin B sulfate causes some nephrotoxicity with tubule damage to a slight degree.

INDICATIONS

Acute Infections Caused by Susceptible Strains of *Pseudomonas aeruginosa.* Polymyxin B sulfate is a drug of choice in the treatment of infections of the urinary tract, meninges, and bloodstream caused by susceptible strains of *Ps aeruginosa.* It may also be used topically and subconjunctivally in the treatment of infections of the eye caused by susceptible strains of *Ps aeruginosa.*
It may be indicated in serious infections caused by susceptible strains of the following organisms, when less potentially toxic drugs are ineffective or contraindicated:
H influenzae, specifically meningeal infections.
Escherichia coli, specifically urinary tract infections.
Aerobacter aerogenes, specifically bacteremia.
Klebsiella pneumoniae, specifically bacteremia.
Note: In Meningeal Infections, Polymyxin B Sulfate Should Be Administered Only by the Intrathecal Route.

CONTRAINDICATIONS

This drug is contraindicated in persons with a prior history of hypersensitivity reactions to the polymyxins.

PRECAUTIONS

See "WARNING" box.
Baseline renal function should be done prior to therapy, with frequent monitoring of renal function and blood levels of the drug during parenteral therapy.
Avoid concurrent use of a curariform muscle relaxant and other neurotoxic drugs (ether, tubocurarine, succinylcholine, gallamine, decamethonium and sodium citrate) which may precipitate respiratory depression. If signs of respiratory paralysis appear, respiration should be assisted as required, and the drug discontinued.
As with other antibiotics, use of this drug may result in overgrowth of nonsusceptible organisms, including fungi. If superinfection occurs, appropriate therapy should be instituted.

ADVERSE REACTIONS

See "WARNING" box.
Nephrotoxic reactions: Albuminuria, cylinduria, azotemia, and rising blood levels without any increase in dosage.
Neurotoxic reactions: Facial flushing, dizziness progressing to ataxia, drowsiness, peripheral paresthesias (circumoral and stocking-glove), apnea due to concurrent use of curariform muscle relaxants and other neurotoxic drugs or inadvertent overdosage, and signs of meningeal irritation with intrathecal administration, e.g., fever, headache, stiff neck and increased cell count and protein cerebrospinal fluid.
Other reactions occasionally reported: Drug fever, urticarial rash, pain (severe) at intramuscular injection sites, and thrombophlebitis at intravenous injection sites.

DOSAGE AND ADMINISTRATION

PARENTERAL:
Intravenous. Dissolve 500,000 units polymyxin B sulfate in 300-500 cc of 5 percent dextrose in water for continuous intravenous drip.
Adults and children. 15,000-25,000 units/kg body weight/day in individuals with normal kidney function. This amount should be reduced from 15,000 units/kg downward for individuals with kidney impairment. Infusions may be given every 12 hours; however, the total daily dose must not exceed 25,000 units/kg/day.
Infants. Infants with normal kidney function may receive up to 40,000 units/kg/day without adverse effects.
Intramuscular. Not recommended routinely because of severe pain at injection sites, particularly in infants and children. Dissolve 500,000 units polymyxin B sulfate in 2 cc sterile distilled water. (Water for Injection, U.S.P.) or sterile physiologic saline (Sodium Chloride Injection, U.S.P.) or 1 percent procaine hydrochloride solution.
Adults and children. 25,000-30,000 units/kg/day. This should be reduced in the presence of renal impairment. The dosage may be divided and given at either 4- or 6-hour intervals.
Infants. Infants with normal kidney function may receive up to 40,000 units/kg/day without adverse effects.
Note: Doses as high as 45,000 units/kg/day have been used in limited clinical studies in treating prematures and newborn infants for sepsis caused by *Ps aeruginosa.*
Intrathecal. A treatment of choice for *Ps aeruginosa* meningitis. Dissolve 500,000 units polymyxin B sulfate in 10 cc of sterile physiologic saline (Sodium Chloride Injection, U.S.P.) for 50,000 units per ml dosage unit.
Adults and children over 2 years of age. Dosage is 50,000 units once daily intrathecally for 3-4 days, then 50,000 units once every other day for at least 2 weeks after cultures of the cerebrospinal fluid are negative and sugar content has returned to normal.
Children under 2 years of age. 20,000 units once daily, intrathecally for 3-4 days or 25,000 units once every other day.

Continue with a dose of 25,000 units once every other day for at least 2 weeks after cultures of the cerebrospinal fluid are negative and sugar content has returned to normal.

IN THE INTEREST OF SAFETY, SOLUTIONS FOR PARENTERAL USE SHOULD BE STORED UNDER REFRIGERATION, AND ANY UNUSED PORTIONS SHOULD BE DISCARDED AFTER 72 HOURS.

TOPICAL:

Ophthalmic. Dissolve 500,000 units polymyxin B sulfate in 20-50 cc sterile distilled water (Water for Injection, U.S.P.) or sterile physiologic saline (Sodium Chloride Injection, U.S.P.) for a 10,000-25,000 units per cc concentration.

For the treatment of *Ps aeruginosa* infections of the eye, a concentration of 0.1 percent to 0.25 percent (10,000 units to 25,000 units per cc) is administered 1-3 drops every hour, increasing the intervals as response indicates.

Subconjunctival injection of up to 10,000 units/day may be used for the treatment of *Ps aeruginosa* infections of the cornea and conjunctiva.

Note: Avoid total systemic and ophthalmic instillation over 25,000 units/kg/day.

HOW SUPPLIED

POLYMYXIN B SULFATE STERILE POWDER, AEROSPORIN brand, 500,000 units per vial

Rubber-stoppered glass vial with flip-off cap, tray of 10 (NDC 0081-0035-10).

Store at 15° to 25°C (59° to 77°F). 581111

POLYSPORIN® OINTMENT OTC

[*pah "lē-spor 'in*]

First Aid Antibiotic

(See PDR For Nonprescription Drugs.)

POLYSPORIN® OPHTHALMIC ℞

[*pah "lē-spor 'in*]

OINTMENT Sterile

(Polymyxin B-Bacitracin)

DESCRIPTION

Each gram contains Aerosporin® (Polymyxin B Sulfate) 10,000 units, bacitracin zinc 500 units, special white petrolatum qs.

ACTIONS

Polymyxin B attacks gram-negative bacilli, including virtually all strains of *Pseudomonas aeruginosa* and *H influenzae* species.

Bacitracin is active against most gram-positive bacilli and cocci, including hemolytic streptococci.

INDICATIONS

For the treatment of superficial ocular infections involving the conjunctiva and/or cornea caused by organisms susceptible to polymyxin B sulfate and bacitracin zinc.

CONTRAINDICATIONS

This product is contraindicated in those individuals who have shown hypersensitivity to any of its components.

WARNINGS

Ophthalmic ointments may retard corneal healing.

PRECAUTIONS

As with other antibiotic preparations, prolonged use may result in overgrowth of nonsusceptible organisms, including fungi. Appropriate measures should be taken if this occurs.

DOSAGE AND ADMINISTRATION

Apply the ointment every 3 or 4 hours, depending on the severity of the infection.

HOW SUPPLIED

Tube of 1/8 oz with ophthalmic tip. (NDC 0081-0797-86) 575940

POLYSPORIN® POWDER OTC

[*pah "lē-spor 'in*]

First Aid Antibiotic

(See PDR For Nonprescription Drugs.)

PROLOPRIM® ℞

[*prō 'lah-prim "*]

(Trimethoprim)

100 mg and 200 mg Scored Tablets

DESCRIPTION

Proloprim® (trimethoprim)* is a synthetic antibacterial available in tablet form for oral administration. Each scored white tablet contains 100 mg trimethoprim and the inactive ingredients corn starch, lactose, magnesium stearate, and sodium starch glycolate. Each scored yellow tablet contains 200 mg trimethoprim and the inactive ingredients corn starch, D&C Yellow No. 10, magnesium stearate, and sodium starch glycolate.

*Mfd. under U.S. Pat. No. 3,956,327.

Trimethoprim is 2, 4-diamino-5-(3,4,5,-trimethoxybenzyl)-pyrimidine. It is a white to light yellow, odorless, bitter compound with a molecular weight of 290.3 and the molecular formula $C_{14}H_{18}N_4O_3$.

CLINICAL PHARMACOLOGY

Trimethoprim is rapidly absorbed following oral administration. It exists in the blood as unbound, protein-bound and metabolized forms. Ten to twenty percent of trimethoprim is metabolized, primarily in the liver; the remainder is excreted unchanged in the urine. The principal metabolites of trimethoprim are the 1- and 3-oxides and the 3'- and 4'-hydroxy derivatives. The free form is considered to be the therapeutically active form. Approximately 44% of trimethoprim is bound to plasma proteins.

Mean peak plasma concentrations of approximately 1.0 μg/mL occur 1 to 4 hours after oral administration of a single 100 mg dose. A single 200 mg dose will result in serum levels approximately twice as high. The half-life of trimethoprim ranges from 8 to 10 hours. However, patients with severely impaired renal function exhibit an increase in the half-life of trimethoprim, which requires either dosage regimen adjustment or not using the drug in such patients (see DOSAGE AND ADMINISTRATION section). During a 13-week study of trimethoprim administered at a daily dosage of 200 mg (50 mg *q.i.d.*), the mean minimum steady-state concentration of the drug was 1.1 μg/mL. Steady-state concentrations were achieved within two to three days of chronic administration and were maintained throughout the experimental period.

Excretion of trimethoprim is primarily by the kidneys through glomerular filtration and tubular secretion. Urine concentrations of trimethoprim are considerably higher than are the concentrations in the blood. After a single oral dose of 100 mg, urine concentrations of trimethoprim ranged from 30 to 160 μg/mL during the 0 to 4 hour period and declined to approximately 18 to 91 μg/mL during the 8 to 24 hour period. A 200 mg single oral dose will result in trimethoprim urine levels approximately twice as high. After oral administration, 50% to 60% of trimethoprim is excreted in the urine within 24 hours, approximately 80% of this being unmetabolized trimethoprim.

Since normal vaginal and fecal flora are the source of most pathogens causing urinary tract infections, it is relevant to consider the distribution of trimethoprim into these sites. Concentrations of trimethoprim in vaginal secretions are consistently greater than those found simultaneously in the serum, being typically 1.6 times the concentrations of simultaneously obtained serum samples. Sufficient trimethoprim is excreted in the feces to markedly reduce or eliminate trimethoprim-susceptible organisms from the fecal flora.

Trimethoprim also passes the placental barrier and is excreted in human milk.

Microbiology: Proloprim blocks the production of tetrahydrofolic acid from dihydrofolic acid by binding to and reversibly inhibiting the required enzyme, dihydrofolate reductase. This binding is very much stronger for the bacterial enzyme than for the corresponding mammalian enzyme. Thus, Proloprim selectively interferes with bacterial biosynthesis of nucleic acids and proteins.

In vitro serial dilution tests have shown that the spectrum of antibacterial activity of Proloprim includes the common urinary tract pathogens with the exception of *Pseudomonas aeruginosa.*

The dominant non-*Enterobacteriaceae* fecal organisms, *Bacteroides* spp. and *Lactobacillus* spp., are not susceptible to trimethoprim concentrations obtained with the recommended dosage.

REPRESENTATIVE MINIMUM INHIBITORY CONCENTRATIONS FOR TRIMETHOPRIM-SUSCEPTIBLE ORGANISMS

Bacteria	Trimethoprim MIC—μg/mL (Range)
Escherichia coli	0.05–1.5
Proteus mirabilis	0.5 –1.5
Klebsiella pneumoniae	0.5 –5.0
Enterobacter species	0.5 –5.0
Staphylococcus species, coagulase-negative	0.15–5.0

Susceptibility Testing: The recommended quantitative disc susceptibility method[1,2] may be used for estimating the susceptibility of bacteria to Proloprim. With this procedure, reports from the laboratory giving results using the 5 μg trimethoprim disc should be interpreted according to the following criteria: Organisms producing zones of 16 mm or greater are classified as susceptible, whereas those producing zones of 11 to 15 mm are classified as having intermediate susceptibility. A report from the laboratory of "Susceptible to trimethoprim" or "Intermediate susceptibility to trimethoprim" indicates that the infection is likely to respond when, as in uncomplicated urinary tract infections, effective therapy is dependent upon the urine concentration of trimethoprim. Organisms producing zones of 10 mm or less are reported as resistant, indicating that other therapy should be selected.

Dilution methods for determining susceptibility are also used, and results are reported as the minimum drug concentration inhibiting microbial growth (MIC).[3] If the MIC is 8 μg/mL or less, the microorganism is considered "susceptible." If the MIC is 16 μg per mL or greater, the microorganism is considered "resistant."

INDICATIONS AND USAGE

For the treatment of initial episodes of uncomplicated urinary tract infections due to susceptible strains of the following organisms: *Escherichia coli, Proteus mirabilis, Klebsiella pneumoniae, Enterobacter* species and coagulase-negative *Staphylococcus* species, including *S. saprophyticus.*

Cultures and susceptibility tests should be performed to determine the susceptibility of the bacteria to trimethoprim. Therapy may be initiated prior to obtaining the results of these tests.

CONTRAINDICATIONS

Proloprim is contraindicated in individuals hypersensitive to trimethoprim and in those with documented megaloblastic anemia due to folate deficiency.

WARNINGS

Serious hypersensitivity reactions have been reported rarely in patients on trimethoprim therapy. Trimethoprim has been reported rarely to interfere with hematopoiesis, especially when administered in large doses and/or for prolonged periods.

The presence of clinical signs such as sore throat, fever, pallor or purpura may be early indications of serious blood disorders (see Chronic Overdosage).

Complete blood counts should be obtained if any of these signs are noted in a patient receiving trimethoprim and the drug discontinued if a significant reduction in the count of any formed blood element is found.

PRECAUTIONS

General: Trimethoprim should be given with caution to patients with possible folate deficiency. Folates may be administered concomitantly without interfering with the antibacterial action of trimethoprim. Trimethoprim should also be given with caution to patients with impaired renal or hepatic function (see CLINICAL PHARMACOLOGY and DOSAGE AND ADMINISTRATION).

Drug Interactions: Proloprim may inhibit the hepatic metabolism of phenytoin. Trimethoprim, given at a common clinical dosage, increased the phenytoin half-life by 51% and decreased the phenytoin metabolic clearance rate by 30%. When administering these drugs concurrently, one should be alert for possible excessive phenytoin effect.

Drug/Laboratory Test Interactions: Trimethoprim can interfere with a serum methotrexate assay as determined by the competitive binding protein technique (CBPA) when a bacterial dihydrofolate reductase is used as the binding protein. No interference occurs, however, if methotrexate is measured by a radioimmunoassay (RIA).

The presence of trimethoprim may also interfere with the Jaffé alkaline picrate reaction assay for creatinine resulting in overestimations of about 10% in the range of normal values.

Carcinogenesis, Mutagenesis, Impairment of Fertility:

Carcinogenesis: Long-term studies in animals to evaluate carcinogenic potential have not been conducted with trimethoprim.

Mutagenesis: Trimethoprim was demonstrated to be nonmutagenic in the Ames assay. In studies at two laboratories no chromosomal damage was detected in cultured Chinese hamster ovary cells at concentrations approximately 500 times human plasma levels; at concentrations approximately 1000 times human plasma levels in these same cells a low level of chromosomal damage was induced at one of the laboratories. No chromosomal abnormalities were observed in cultured human leukocytes at concentrations of trimethoprim up to 20 times human steady state plasma levels. No chromosomal effects were detected in peripheral lymphocytes of human subjects receiving 320 mg of trimethoprim in combination with up to 1600 mg of sulfamethoxazole per day for as long as 112 weeks.

Impairment of Fertility: No adverse effects on fertility or general reproductive performance were observed in rats given trimethoprim in oral dosages as high as 70 mg/kg/day for males and 14 mg/kg/day for females.

Pregnancy: ***Teratogenic Effects:*** Pregnancy Category C. Trimethoprim has been shown to be teratogenic in the rat when given in doses 40 times the human dose. In some rabbit studies, the overall increase in fetal loss (dead and resorbed

Continued on next page

Burroughs Wellcome—Cont.

and malformed conceptuses) was associated with doses 6 times the human therapeutic dose.
While there are no large well-controlled studies on the use of trimethoprim in pregnant women, Brumfitt and Pursell,[4] in a retrospective study, reported the outcome of 186 pregnancies during which the mother received either placebo or trimethoprim in combination with sulfamethoxazole. The incidence of congenital abnormalities was 4.5% (3 of 66) in those who received placebo and 3.3% (4 of 120) in those receiving trimethoprim and sulfamethoxazole. There were no abnormalities in the 10 children whose mothers received the drug during the first trimester. In a separate survey, Brumfitt and Pursell also found no congenital abnormalities in 35 children whose mothers had received trimethoprim and sulfamethoxazole at the time of conception or shortly thereafter.
Because trimethoprim may interfere with folic acid metabolism, Proloprim should be used during pregnancy only if the potential benefit justifies the potential risk to the fetus.
Nonteratogenic Effects: The oral administration of trimethoprim to rats at a dose of 70 mg/kg/day commencing with the last third of gestation and continuing through parturition and lactation caused no deleterious effects on gestation or pup growth and survival.
Nursing Mothers: Trimethoprim is excreted in human milk. Because trimethoprim may interfere with folic acid metabolism, caution should be exercised when Proloprim is administered to a nursing woman.
Pediatric Use: The safety of trimethoprim in infants under two months has not been demonstrated. The effectiveness of trimethoprim as a single agent has not been established in children under 12 years of age.

ADVERSE REACTIONS

The adverse effects encountered most often with trimethoprim were rash and pruritus.
Dermatologic: Rash, pruritus and phototoxic skin eruptions. At the recommended dosage regimens of 100 mg *b.i.d.*, or 200 mg *q.d.*, each for 10 days, the incidence of rash is 2.9% to 6.7%. In clinical studies which employed high doses of Proloprim, an elevated incidence of rash was noted. These rashes were maculopapular, morbilliform, pruritic and generally mild to moderate, appearing 7 to 14 days after the initiation of therapy.
Hypersensitivity: Rare reports of exfoliative dermatitis, erythema multiforme, Stevens-Johnson syndrome, toxic epidermal necrolysis (Lyell syndrome), and anaphylaxis have been received.
Gastrointestinal: Epigastric distress, nausea, vomiting, and glossitis. Elevation of serum transminase and bilirubin has been noted, but the significance of this finding is unknown. Cholestatic jaundice has been rarely reported.
Hematologic: Thrombocytopenia, leukopenia, neutropenia, megaloblastic anemia, and methemoglobinemia.
Neurologic: Aseptic meningitis has been rarely reported.
Miscellaneous: Fever, and increases in BUN and serum creatinine levels.

OVERDOSAGE

Acute: Signs of acute overdosage with trimethoprim may appear following ingestion of 1 gram or more of the drug and include nausea, vomiting, dizziness, headaches, mental depression, confusion and bone marrow depression (see Chronic Overdosage).
Treatment consists of gastric lavage and general supportive measures. Acidification of the urine will increase renal elimination of trimethoprim. Peritoneal dialysis is not effective and hemodialysis only moderately effective in eliminating the drug.
Chronic: Use of trimethoprim at high doses and/or for extended periods of time may cause bone marrow depression manifested as thrombocytopenia, leukopenia and/or megaloblastic anemia. If signs of bone marrow depression occur, trimethoprim should be discontinued and the patient should be given leucovorin; 5 to 15 mg leucovorin daily has been recommended by some investigators.

DOSAGE AND ADMINISTRATION

The usual oral adult dosage is 100 mg of Proloprim every 12 hours or 200 mg Proloprim every 24 hours, each for 10 days.
The use of trimethoprim in patients with a creatinine clearance of less than 15 mL/min is not recommended. For patients with a creatinine clearance of 15 to 30 mL/min, the dose should be 50 mg every 12 hours.
The effectiveness of trimethoprim has not been established in children under 12 years of age.

HOW SUPPLIED

100 mg Tablets (white, scored, round-shaped), containing 100 mg trimethoprim—bottle of 100 (NDC 0081-0820-55). Imprint on tablets "PROLOPRIM 09A." Store at 15° to 25°C (59° to 77°F) in a dry place.
200 mg Tablets (yellow, scored, round-shaped), containing 200 mg trimethoprim—bottle of 100 (NDC 0081-0825-55). Imprint on tablets "PROLOPRIM 200." Store at 15° to 25°C (59° to 77°F) in a dry place and protect from light.

REFERENCES

1. Bauer AW, Kirby WMM, Sherris JC, Turck M. Antibiotic susceptibility testing by a standardized single disk method. *Am J Clin Pathol.* 1966;45:493–496.
2. National Committee for Clinical Laboratory Standards. Performance standards for antimicrobial disk susceptibility tests, 2nd ed. Villanova, PA. 1979.
3. Ericsson HM, Sherris JC. Antibiotic sensitivity testing: report of an international collaborative study. *Acta Pathol Microbiol Scand* [B]. 1971;(suppl 217):1–90.
4. Brumfitt W, Pursell R. Trimethoprim-sulfamethoxazole in the treatment of bacteriuria in women. *J Infect Dis.* November 1973;128(suppl):S657–S663.

580389

Shown in Product Identification Section, page 407

PURINETHOL® ℞

[*pur'ĭn-eth-awl*]
(Mercaptopurine)
50 mg Scored Tablets

Caution: Purinethol (mercaptopurine) is a potent drug. It should not be used unless a diagnosis of acute lymphatic leukemia has been adequately established and the responsible physician is knowledgeable in assessing response to chemotherapy.

DESCRIPTION

Purinethol (mercaptopurine) was synthesized and developed by Hitchings, Elion, and associates at the Wellcome Research Laboratories.[1] It is one of a large series of purine analogues which interfere with nucleic acid biosynthesis and has been found active against human leukemias.
Mercaptopurine, known chemically as 1,7-dihydro-6*H*-purine-6-thione monohydrate, is an analogue of the purine bases adenine and hypoxanthine.
Purinethol (mercaptopurine) is available in tablet form for oral administration. Each scored tablet contains 50 mg mercaptopurine and the inactive ingredients corn and potato starch, lactose, magnesium stearate, and stearic acid.

CLINICAL PHARMACOLOGY

Clinical studies have shown that the absorption of an oral dose of mercaptopurine in man is incomplete and variable, averaging approximately 50% of the administered dose.[2] The factors influencing absorption are unknown. Intravenous administration of an investigational preparation of mercaptopurine revealed a plasma half-disappearance time of 21 minutes in children and 47 minutes in adults. The volume of distribution usually exceeded that of the total body water.[2]
Following the oral administration of ^{35}S-6-mercaptopurine in one subject, a total of 46% of the dose could be accounted for in the urine (as parent drug and metabolites) in the first 24 hours. Metabolites of mercaptopurine were found in urine within the first 2 hours after administration. Radioactivity (in the form of sulfate) could be found in the urine for weeks afterwards.[3]
There is negligible entry of mercaptopurine into cerebrospinal fluid.
Plasma protein binding averages 19% over the concentration range 10 to 50 micrograms per milliliter (a concentration only achieved by intravenous administration of mercaptopurine at doses exceeding 5 to 10 mg/kg).[2]
Monitoring of plasma levels of mercaptopurine during therapy is of questionable value.[3] There is technical difficulty in determining plasma concentrations which are seldom greater than 1 to 2 micrograms per ml after a therapeutic oral dose. More significantly, mercaptopurine enters rapidly into the anabolic and catabolic pathways for purines, and the active intracellular metabolites have appreciably longer half-lives than the parent drug. The biochemical effects of a single dose of mercaptopurine are evident long after the parent drug has disappeared from plasma. Because of this rapid metabolism of mercaptopurine to active intracellular derivatives, hemodialysis would not be expected to appreciably reduce toxicity of the drug. There is no known pharmacologic antagonist to the biochemical actions of mercaptopurine *in vivo*.
Mercaptopurine competes with hypoxanthine and guanine for the enzyme hypoxanthine-guanine phosphoribosyltransferase (HGPRTase) and is itself converted to thioinosinic acid (TIMP). This intracellular nucleotide inhibits several reactions involving inosinic acid (IMP), including the conversion of IMP to xanthylic acid (XMP) and the conversion of IMP to adenylic acid (AMP) via adenylosuccinate (SAMP). In addition, 6-methylthioinosinate (MTIMP) is formed by the methylation of TIMP. Both TIMP and MTIMP have been reported to inhibit glutamine-5-phosphoribosylpyrophosphate amidotransferase, the first enzyme unique to the *de novo* pathway for purine ribonucleotide synthesis.[3]
Experiments indicate that radiolabeled mercaptopurine may be recovered from the DNA in the form of deoxythioguanosine.[4] Some mercaptopurine is converted to nucleotide derivatives of 6-thioguanine (6-TG) by the sequential actions of inosinate (IMP) dehydrogenase and xanthylate (XMP) aminase, converting TIMP to thioguanylic acid (TGMP).
Animal tumors that are resistant to mercaptopurine often have lost the ability to convert mercaptopurine to TIMP. However, it is clear that resistance to mercaptopurine may be acquired by other means as well, particularly in human leukemias.
It is not known exactly which of any one or more of the biochemical effects of mercaptopurine and its metabolites are directly or predominantly responsible for cell death.[5]
The catabolism of mercaptopurine and its metabolites is complex. In man, after oral administration of ^{35}S-6-mercaptopurine, urine contains intact mercaptopurine, thiouric acid (formed by direct oxidation by xanthine oxidase, probably via 6-mercapto-8-hydroxypurine), and a number of 6-methylated thiopurines. The methylthiopurines yield appreciable amounts of inorganic sulfate.[3] The importance of the metabolism by xanthine oxidase relates to the fact that Zyloprim® (allopurinol) inhibits this enzyme and retards the catabolism of mercaptopurine and its active metabolites. A significant reduction in mercaptopurine dosage is mandatory if a potent xanthine oxidase inhibitor and Purinethol (mercaptopurine) are used simultaneously in a patient (see "PRECAUTIONS").

INDICATIONS AND USAGE

Purinethol (mercaptopurine) is indicated for remission induction and maintenance therapy of acute lymphatic leukemia. The response to this agent depends upon the particular subclassification of acute lymphatic leukemia and the age of the patient (child or adult).
Acute Lymphatic (Lymphocytic, Lymphoblastic) Leukemia: Given as a single agent for remission induction, mercaptopurine induces complete remission in approximately 25% of children and 10% of adults. However, reliance upon mercaptopurine alone is not justified for initial remission induction of acute lymphatic leukemia since combination chemotherapy with vincristine, prednisone, and L-asparaginase results in more frequent complete remission induction than with mercaptopurine alone or in combination. The duration of complete remission induced in acute lymphatic leukemia is so brief without the use of maintenance therapy that some form of drug therapy is considered essential. Mercaptopurine, as a single agent, is capable of significantly prolonging complete remission duration; however, combination therapy has produced remission duration longer than that achieved with mercaptopurine alone.
Acute Myelogenous (and Acute Myelomonocytic) Leukemia: As a single agent, mercaptopurine will induce complete remission in approximately 10% of children and adults with acute myelogenous leukemia or its subclassifications. These results are inferior to those achieved with combination chemotherapy employing optimum treatment schedules.
Central Nervous System Leukemia: Mercaptopurine is not effective for prophylaxis or treatment of central nervous system leukemia.
Other Neoplasms: Purinethol (mercaptopurine) is not effective in chronic lymphatic leukemia, the lymphomas (including Hodgkin's Disease), or solid tumors.

CONTRAINDICATIONS

Purinethol (mercaptopurine) should not be used unless a diagnosis of acute lymphatic leukemia has been adequately established and the responsible physician is knowledgeable in assessing response to chemotherapy.
Mercaptopurine should not be used in patients whose disease has demonstrated prior resistance to this drug. In animals and man, there is usually complete cross-resistance between Purinethol (mercaptopurine) and Tabloid® brand thioguanine.

WARNINGS

SINCE DRUGS USED IN CANCER CHEMOTHERAPY ARE POTENTIALLY HAZARDOUS, IT IS RECOMMENDED THAT ONLY PHYSICIANS EXPERIENCED WITH THE RISKS OF MERCAPTOPURINE AND KNOWLEDGEABLE IN THE NATURAL HISTORY OF ACUTE LEUKEMIAS ADMINISTER THIS DRUG.
Bone Marrow Toxicity: The most consistent, dose-related toxicity is bone marrow suppression. This may be manifest by anemia, leukopenia, thrombocytopenia, or any combination of these. Any of these findings may also reflect progression of the underlying disease. Since mercaptopurine may have a delayed effect, it is important to withdraw the medication temporarily at the first sign of an abnormally large fall in any of the formed elements of the blood.
Hepatotoxicity: Purinethol (mercaptopurine) is hepatotoxic in animals and man. A small number of deaths have been reported which may have been attributed to hepatic necrosis due to administration of mercaptopurine. Hepatic injury can occur with any dosage, but seems to occur with more frequency when doses of 2.5 mg/kg/day are exceeded.

The histologic pattern of mercaptopurine hepatotoxicity includes features of both intrahepatic cholestasis and parenchymal cell necrosis, either of which may predominate. It is not clear how much of the hepatic damage is due to direct toxicity from the drug and how much may be due to a hypersensitivity reaction. In some patients jaundice has cleared following withdrawal of mercaptopurine and reappeared with its reintroduction.[6]

Published reports have cited widely varying incidences of overt hepatotoxicity. In a large series of patients with various neoplastic diseases, mercaptopurine was administered orally in doses ranging from 2.5 mg/kg to 5.0 mg/kg without any evidence of hepatotoxicity. It was noted by the authors that no definite clinical evidence of liver damage could be ascribed to the drug, although an occasional case of serum hepatitis did occur in patients receiving 6-MP who previously had transfusions.[6] In reports of smaller cohorts of adult and pediatric leukemic patients, the incidence of hepatotoxicity ranged from 0 to 6%.[7,8,9] In an isolated report by Einhorn and Davidsohn, jaundice was observed more frequently (40%), especially when doses exceeded 2.5 mg/kg.[10] Usually, clinically detectable jaundice appears early in the course of treatment (one to two months). However, jaundice has been reported as early as one week and as late as eight years after the start of treatment with mercaptopurine.[11] Monitoring of serum transaminase levels, alkaline phosphatase, and bilirubin levels may allow early detection of hepatotoxicity. It is advisable to monitor these liver function tests at weekly intervals when first beginning therapy and at monthly intervals thereafter. Liver function tests may be advisable more frequently in patients who are receiving mercaptopurine with other hepatotoxic drugs or with known pre-existing liver disease.

The concomitant administration of mercaptopurine with other hepatotoxic agents requires especially careful clinical and biochemical monitoring of hepatic function. Combination therapy involving mercaptopurine with other drugs not felt to be hepatotoxic should nevertheless be approached with caution. The combination of mercaptopurine with doxorubicin (Adriamycin) was reported to be hepatotoxic in 19 of 20 patients undergoing remission-induction therapy for leukemia resistant to previous therapy.[12]

The hepatotoxicity has been associated in some cases with anorexia, diarrhea, jaundice, and ascites. Hepatic encephalopathy has occurred.

The onset of clinical jaundice, hepatomegaly, or anorexia with tenderness in the right hypochondrium are immediate indications for withholding mercaptopurine until the exact etiology can be identified. Likewise, any evidence of deterioration in liver function studies, toxic hepatitis, or biliary stasis should prompt discontinuation of the drug and a search for an etiology of the hepatotoxicity.

Immunosuppression: Mercaptopurine recipients may manifest decreased cellular hypersensitivities and impaired allograft rejection. Induction of immunity to infectious agents or vaccines will be subnormal in these patients; the degree of immunosuppression will depend on antigen dose and temporal relationship to drug. This immunosuppressive effect should be carefully considered with regard to intercurrent infections and risk of subsequent neoplasia.

Pregnancy: "Pregnancy Category D." Mercaptopurine can cause fetal harm when administered to a pregnant woman. Women receiving mercaptopurine in the first trimester of pregnancy have an increased incidence of abortion; the risk of malformation in offspring surviving first trimester exposure is not accurately known.[13] In a series of twenty-eight women receiving mercaptopurine after the first trimester of pregnancy, three mothers died undelivered, one delivered a stillborn child, and one aborted; there were no cases of macroscopically abnormal fetuses.[14] Since such experience cannot exclude the possibility of fetal damage, mercaptopurine should be used during pregnancy only if the benefit clearly justifies the possible risk to the fetus, and particular caution should be given to the use of mercaptopurine in the first trimester of pregnancy.

There are no adequate and well controlled studies in pregnant women. If this drug is used during pregnancy or if the patient becomes pregnant while taking the drug, the patient should be apprised of the potential hazard to the fetus. Women of childbearing potential should be advised to avoid becoming pregnant.

PRECAUTIONS

General: The safe and effective use of Purinethol demands a thorough knowledge of the natural history of the condition being treated. After selection of an initial dosage schedule, therapy will frequently need to be modified depending upon the patient's response and manifestations of toxicity.

The most frequent, serious, toxic effect of mercaptopurine is myelosuppression resulting in leukopenia, thrombocytopenia, and anemia. These toxic effects are often unavoidable during the induction phase of adult acute leukemia if remission induction is to be successful. Whether or not these manifestations demand modification or cessation of dosage depends both upon the response of the underlying disease and a careful consideration of supportive facilities (granulocyte

and platelet transfusions) which may be available. Life-threatening infections and bleeding have been observed as a consequence of mercaptopurine-induced granulocytopenia and thrombocytopenia. Severe hematologic toxicity may require supportive therapy with platelet transfusions for bleeding, and antibiotics and granulocyte transfusions if sepsis is documented.

If it is not the intent to deliberately induce bone marrow hypoplasia, it is important to discontinue the drug temporarily at the first evidence of an abnormally large fall in white blood cell count, platelet count, or hemoglobin concentration. In many patients with severe depression of the formed elements of the blood due to mercaptopurine, the bone marrow appears hypoplastic on aspiration or biopsy, whereas in other cases it may appear normocellular. The qualitative changes in the erythroid elements toward the megaloblastic series, characteristically seen with the folic acid antagonists and some other antimetabolites, are not seen with this drug. It is probably advisable to start with smaller dosages in patients with impaired renal function, since the latter might result in slower elimination of the drug and metabolites and a greater cumulative effect.

Information for Patients: Patients should be informed that the major toxicities of mercaptopurine are related to myelosuppression, hepatotoxicity and gastrointestinal toxicity. Patients should never be allowed to take the drug without medical supervision and should be advised to consult their physician if they experience fever, sore throat, jaundice, nausea, vomiting, signs of local infection, bleeding from any site, or symptoms suggestive of anemia. Women of childbearing potential should be advised to avoid becoming pregnant.

Laboratory Tests: It is recommended that evaluation of the hemoglobin or hematocrit, total white blood cell count and differential count, and quantitative platelet count be obtained weekly while the patient is on mercaptopurine therapy. In cases where the cause of fluctuations in the formed elements in the peripheral blood is obscure, bone marrow examination may be useful for the evaluation of marrow status. The decision to increase, decrease, continue, or discontinue a given dosage of mercaptopurine must be based not only on the absolute hematologic values, but also upon the rapidity with which changes are occurring. In many instances, particularly during the induction phase of acute leukemia, complete blood counts will need to be done more frequently than once weekly in order to evaluate the effect of the therapy.

Drug Interactions:

Interaction with allopurinol: When allopurinol and mercaptopurine are administered concomitantly, it is imperative that the dose of mercaptopurine be reduced to one-third to one-quarter of the usual dose. Failure to observe this dosage reduction will result in a delayed catabolism of mercaptopurine and the strong likelihood of inducing severe toxicity.

There is usually complete cross-resistance between Purinethol® (mercaptopurine) and Tabloid® brand thioguanine.

The dosage of mercaptopurine may need to be reduced when this agent is combined with other drugs whose primary or secondary toxicity is myelosuppression. Enhanced marrow suppression has been noted in some patients also receiving trimethoprim-sulfamethoxazole.[15,16]

Carcinogenesis, Mutagenesis, Impairment of Fertility: Purinethol (mercaptopurine) causes chromosomal aberrations in animals and man and induces dominant-lethal mutations in male mice. In mice, surviving female offspring of mothers who received chronic low doses of mercaptopurine during pregnancy were found sterile or if they became pregnant had smaller litters and more dead fetuses as compared to control animals.[17] Carcinogenic potential exists in man, but the extent of the risk is unknown.

The effect of mercaptopurine on human fertility is unknown for either males or females.

Pregnancy: *Teratogenic Effects:* Pregnancy Category D. See WARNINGS section.

Nursing Mothers: It is not known whether this drug is excreted in human milk. Because many drugs are excreted in human milk, and because of the potential for serious adverse reactions in nursing infants from mercaptopurine, a decision should be made whether to discontinue nursing or to discontinue the drug, taking into account the importance of the drug to the mother.

ADVERSE REACTIONS

The principal and potentially serious toxic effects of Purinethol are bone marrow toxicity and hepatotoxicity (see WARNINGS).

Hematologic Effects: The most frequent adverse reaction to mercaptopurine is myelosuppression. The induction of complete remission of acute lymphatic leukemia frequently is associated with marrow hypoplasia. Maintenance of remission generally involves multiple drug regimens whose component agents cause myelosuppression. Anemia, leukopenia, and thrombocytopenia are frequently observed. Dos-

ages and schedules are adjusted to prevent life-threatening cytopenias.

Renal: Hyperuricemia may occur in patients receiving mercaptopurine as a consequence of rapid cell lysis accompanying the antineoplastic effect. Adverse effects can be minimized by increased hydration, urine alkalinization, and the prophylactic administration of a xanthine oxidase inhibitor such as allopurinol. The dosage of mercaptopurine should be reduced to one-third to one-quarter of the usual dose if allopurinol is given concurrently.

Gastrointestinal: Intestinal ulceration has been reported.[18] Nausea, vomiting and anorexia are uncommon during initial administration. Mild diarrhea and sprue-like symptoms have been noted occasionally, but it is difficult at present to attribute these to the medication. Oral lesions are rarely seen, and when they occur they resemble thrush rather than antifolic ulcerations.

An increased risk of pancreatitis may be associated with the investigational use of Purinethol in inflammatory bowel disease.[19,20,21]

Miscellaneous: While dermatologic reactions can occur as a consequence of disease, the administration of Purinethol has been associated with skin rashes and hyperpigmentation.[22] Drug fever has been very rarely reported with mercaptopurine. Before attributing fever to mercaptopurine, every attempt should be made to exclude more common causes of pyrexia, such as sepsis, in patients with acute leukemia.

OVERDOSAGE

Signs and symptoms of overdosage may be immediate such as anorexia, nausea, vomiting and diarrhea; or delayed such as myelosuppression, liver dysfunction and gastroenteritis. Dialysis cannot be expected to clear mercaptopurine. Hemodialysis is thought to be of marginal use due to the rapid intracellular incorporation of mercaptopurine into active metabolites with long persistence. The oral LD_{50} of mercaptopurine was determined to be 480 mg/kg in the mouse and 425 mg/kg in the rat.[23]

There is no known pharmacologic antagonist of mercaptopurine. The drug should be discontinued immediately if unintended toxicity occurs during treatment. If a patient is seen immediately following an accidental overdosage of the drug, it may be useful to induce emesis.

DOSAGE AND ADMINISTRATION

Induction Therapy: Purinethol (mercaptopurine) is administered orally. The dosage which will be tolerated and be effective varies from patient to patient, and therefore careful titration is necessary to obtain the optimum therapeutic effect without incurring excessive, unintended toxicity. The usual initial dosage for children and adults is 2.5 mg/kg of body weight per day (100 to 200 mg in the average adult and 50 mg in an average 5-year-old child). Children with acute leukemia have tolerated this dose without difficulty in most cases; it may be continued daily for several weeks or more in some patients. If, after four weeks at this dosage, there is no clinical improvement and no definite evidence of leukocyte or platelet depression, the dosage may be increased up to 5 mg/kg daily. A dosage of 2.5 mg/kg per day may result in a rapid fall in leukocyte count within 1 to 2 weeks in some adults with acute lymphatic leukemia and high total leukocyte counts.

The total daily dosage may be given at one time. It is calculated to the nearest multiple of 25 mg. The dosage of mercaptopurine should be reduced to one-third to one-quarter of the usual dose if allopurinol is given concurrently. Because the drug may have a delayed action, it should be discontinued at the first sign of an abnormally large or rapid fall in the leukocyte or platelet count. If subsequently the leukocyte count or platelet count remains constant for two or three days, or rises, treatment may be resumed.

Maintenance Therapy: Once a complete hematologic remission is obtained, maintenance therapy is considered essential. Maintenance doses will vary from patient to patient. A usual daily maintenance dose of mercaptopurine is 1.5 to 2.5 mg/kg/day as a single dose. It is to be emphasized that in children with acute lymphatic leukemia in remission, superior results have been obtained when mercaptopurine has been combined with other agents (most frequently with methotrexate) for remission maintenance. Mercaptopurine should rarely be relied upon as a single agent for the maintenance of remissions induced in acute leukemia.

Procedures for proper handling and disposal of anti-cancer drugs should be considered. Several guidelines on this subject have been published.[18-23]

There is no general agreement that all of the procedures recommended in the guidelines are necessary or appropriate.

HOW SUPPLIED

Off-white, scored tablets containing 50 mg mercaptopurine, imprinted with "PURINETHOL" and "04A"; bottles of 25 (NDC 0081-0807-25) and 250 (NDC 0081-0807-65). Store at 15°–25°C (59°–77°F) in a dry place.

Continued on next page

Burroughs Wellcome—Cont.

REFERENCES

1. Hitchings GH, Elion GB: The chemistry and biochemistry of purine analogs. *Ann NY Acad Sci* 1954; 60:195–199.
2. Loo TL, Luce JK, Sullivan MP, et al: Clinical pharmacologic observations on 6-mercaptopurine and 6-methylthiopurine ribonucleoside. *Clin Pharmacol Ther* 1968; 9:180–194.
3. Elion GB: Biochemistry and pharmacology of purine analogs. *Fed Proc* 1967; 26:898–904.
4. Scannell JP, Hitchings GH: Thioguanine in deoxyribonucleic acid from tumors of 6-mercaptopurine-treated mice. *Proc Soc Exp Biol Med* 1966; 122:627–629.
5. Paterson ARP, Tidd DM: 6-thiopurines, in Sartorelli AC, Johns DG (eds): *Antineoplastic and Immunosuppressive Agents,* Part II. Berlin, Springer-Verlag, 1975, pp 384–403.
6. Burchenal JH, Ellison RR, Murphy ML, et al: Clinical studies on 6-mercaptopurine. *Ann NY Acad Sci* 1954; 60:359–368.
7. Farber S: Summary of experience with 6-mercaptopurine. *Ann NY Acad Sci* 1954; 60:412–414.
8. Fountain JR: Clinical observations of the treatment of leukemia and allied disorders with 6-mercaptopurine. *Ann NY Acad Sci* 1954; 60:439–446.
9. Hyman GA, Gellhorn A, Wolff JA: The therapeutic effect of mercaptopurine in a variety of human neoplastic diseases. *Ann NY Acad Sci* 1954; 60:430–435.
10. Einhorn M, Davidsohn I: Hepatotoxicity of mercaptopurine. *JAMA* 1964; 188:802–806.
11. Schein PS, Winokur SH: Immunosuppressive and cytotoxic chemotherapy: long-term complications. *Ann Intern Med* 1975; 82:84–95.
12. Stern MH, Minow RA, Casey JH, et al: Hepatotoxicity in patients treated with adriamycin and 6-mercaptopurine for refractory leukemia. *Am J Clin Pathol* 1975; 63:758–759.
13. Blatt J, Mulvihill JJ, Ziegler JL, et al: Pregnancy outcome following cancer chemotherapy. *Am J Med* 1980; 69:828–832.
14. Nicholson HO: Cytotoxic drugs in pregnancy. *J Obstet Gynaec Brit Cwlth* 1968; 75:307–312.
15. Woods WG, Daigle AE, Hutchinson RJ, et al: Myelosuppression associated with co-trimoxazole as a prophylactic antibiotic in the maintenance phase of childhood acute lymphocytic leukemia. *J Pediatr* 1984; 105:639–644.
16. Rees CA, Lennard L, Lilleyman JS, et al: Disturbance of 6-mercaptopurine metabolism by cotrimoxazole in childhood lymphoblastic leukaemia. *Cancer Chemother Pharmacol* 1984; 12:87–89.
17. Reimers TJ, Sluss PM: 6-mercaptopurine treatment of pregnant mice: effects on second and third generations. *Science* 1978; 201:65–67.
18. Clark PA, Hsia YE, Huntsman RG: Toxic complications of treatment with 6-mercaptopurine. *Br Med J* 1960; 1:393–395.
19. Present DH, Meltzer SJ, Wolke A, et al: Short and long term toxicity to 6-mercaptopurine in the management of inflammatory bowel disease. *Gastroenterology* 1985; 88:1545.
20. Bank L, Wright JP: 6-mercaptopurine-related pancreatitis in 2 patients with inflammatory bowel disease, abstract. *Dig Dis Sci* 1984; 29:357–359.
21. Singleton JW, Law DH, Kelley Jr ML, et al: National Cooperative Crohn's Disease Study: Adverse reactions to study drugs. *Gastroenterology* 1979; 77:870–882.
22. Dreizen S, Bodey GP, Rodriguez V, et al: Cutaneous complications of cancer chemotherapy. *Postgrad Med* 1975; 58:150–158.
23. Unpublished data on file with Burroughs Wellcome Co.
24. Recommendations for the Safe Handling of Parenteral Antineoplastic Drugs. NIH Publications No. 83-2321. For sale by the Superintendent of Documents, U.S. Government Printing Office, Washington, D.C. 20402.
25. AMA Council Report. Guidelines for Handling Parenteral Antineoplastics, *JAMA,* March 15, 1985.
26. National Study Commission on Cytotoxic Exposure—Recommendations for Handling Cytotoxic Agents. Available from Louis P. Jeffrey, Sc.D., Director of Pharmacy Services, Rhode Island Hospital, 593 Eddy Street, Providence, Rhode Island 02902.
27. Clinical Oncological Society of Australia: Guidelines and recommendations for safe handling of antineoplastic agents. *Med J Australia* 1983; 1:426–428.
28. Jones RB, et al: Safe handling of chemotherapeutic agents: A report from the Mount Sinai Medical Center. *Ca—A Cancer Journal for Clinicians* 1983; Sept/Oct:258–263.
29. American Society of Hospital Pharmacists technical assistance bulletin on handling cytotoxic drugs in hospitals. *Am J Hosp Pharm* 1985; 42:131–137. 579004

Shown in Product Identification Section, page 407

RETROVIR® Capsules ℞
[*ret-rō-vēr'*]
RETROVIR® Syrup ℞
(Zidovudine)

> **WARNING: THERAPY WITH RETROVIR (ZIDOVUDINE) MAY BE ASSOCIATED WITH HEMATOLOGIC TOXICITY INCLUDING GRANULOCYTOPENIA AND SEVERE ANEMIA REQUIRING TRANSFUSIONS (SEE WARNINGS).**
> IN ADDITION, PATIENTS TREATED WITH ZIDOVUDINE MAY CONTINUE TO DEVELOP OPPORTUNISTIC INFECTIONS (OI'S) AND OTHER COMPLICATIONS OF HIV INFECTION AND, THEREFORE SHOULD BE UNDER CLOSE CLINICAL OBSERVATION.

DESCRIPTION

Retrovir is the brand name for zidovudine [formerly called azidothymidine (AZT)], an antiretroviral drug active against human immunodeficiency virus (HIV).

Capsules: Retrovir Capsules are for oral administration. Each capsule contains 100 mg of zidovudine and the inactive ingredients corn starch, magnesium stearate, microcrystalline cellulose, and sodium starch glycolate. The 100 mg empty hard gelatin capsule, printed with edible black ink, consists of gelatin and titanium dioxide. The blue band around the capsule consists of gelatin and FD&C Blue No. 2.

Syrup: Retrovir Syrup is for oral administration. Each teaspoonful (5 mL) of Retrovir Syrup contains 50 mg of zidovudine and the inactive ingredients sodium benzoate 0.2% (added as a preservative), citric acid, flavors, glycerin, and liquid sucrose. Sodium hydroxide may be added to adjust pH.

The chemical name of zidovudine is 3′-azido-3′-deoxythymidine.

Zidovudine is a white to beige, odorless, crystalline solid with a molecular weight of 267.24 daltons and the molecular formula $C_{10}H_{13}N_5O_4$.

CLINICAL PHARMACOLOGY

Zidovudine is an inhibitor of the *in vitro* replication of some retroviruses including HIV (also known as HTLV III, LAV, or ARV). This drug is a thymidine analogue in which the 3′-hydroxy (-OH) group is replaced by an azido ($-N_3$) group. Cellular thymidine kinase converts zidovudine into zidovudine monophosphate. The monophosphate is further converted into the diphosphate by cellular thymidylate kinase and to the triphosphate derivative by other cellular enzymes. Zidovudine triphosphate interferes with the HIV viral RNA dependent DNA polymerase (reverse transcriptase) and thus, inhibits viral replication. Zidovudine triphosphate also inhibits cellular α-DNA polymerase, but at concentrations 100-fold higher than those required to inhibit reverse transcriptase. *In vitro,* zidovudine triphosphate has been shown to be incorporated into growing chains of DNA by viral reverse transcriptase. When incorporation by the viral enzyme occurs, the DNA chain is terminated. Studies in cell culture suggest that zidovudine incorporation by cellular α-DNA polymerase may occur, but only to a very small extent and not in all test systems. Chain termination has not been demonstrated with cellular α-DNA polymerase.

Microbiology: The relationship between *in vitro* susceptibility of HIV to zidovudine and the inhibition of HIV replication in man or clinical response to therapy has not been established. *In vitro* sensitivity results vary greatly depending upon the time between virus infection and zidovudine treatment of cell cultures, the particular assay used, the cell type employed, and the laboratory performing the test. In addition, the methods currently used to establish virologic responses in clinical trials may be relatively insensitive in detecting changes in the quantities of actively replicating HIV or reactivation of these viruses.

Zidovudine blocked 90% of detectable HIV replication *in vitro* at concentrations of $\leq$0.13 μg/mL (ID_{90}) when added shortly after laboratory infection of susceptible cells. This level of antiviral effect was observed in experiments measuring reverse transcriptase activity in H9 cells, PHA stimulated peripheral blood lymphocytes, and unstimulated peripheral blood lymphocytes. The concentration of drug required to produce a 50% decrease in supernatant reverse transcriptase was 0.013 μg/mL (ID_{50}) in both H9 cells and peripheral blood lymphocytes. Zidovudine at concentrations of 0.13 μg/mL also provided >90% protection from a strain of HIV (HTLV IIIB) induced cytopathic effects in two tetanus-specific T4 cell lines. p24 gag protein expression was also undetectable at the same concentration in these cells. Partial inhibition of viral activity in cells with chronic HIV infection (presumed to carry integrated HIV DNA) required concentrations of zidovudine (8.8 μg/mL in one laboratory to 13.3 μg/mL in another) which are approximately 100 times as high as those necessary to block HIV replication in acutely infected cells. HIV isolates from 18 untreated individuals with AIDS or ARC had ID_{50} sensitivity values between 0.003 to 0.013 μg/mL and ID_{95} sensitivity values between 0.03 to 0.3 μg/mL.

The development of resistance to zidovudine has not been adequately studied and the frequency of zidovudine-resistant isolates existing in the general population is unknown. Reduced *in vitro* sensitivity to zidovudine has been observed, however, in viral isolates from some individuals who have received prolonged courses of zidovudine treatment. For the small number of patients from whom isolates were studied, no correlations were evident between the development of reduced sensitivity in the laboratory and clinical response. Therefore, the quantitative relationship between *in vitro* susceptibility of HIV to zidovudine and clinical response to therapy has not been established. Studies of the development of resistance to zidovudine are incomplete and the frequency and degree of changes in *in vitro* sensitivity of virus isolates from HIV infected patients with differing severity of immune compromise are unknown.

The major metabolite of zidovudine, 3′-azido-3′-deoxy-5′-*O*-β-*D*-glucopyranuronosylthymidine (GAZT), does not inhibit HIV replication *in vitro.* GAZT does not antagonize the antiviral effect of zidovudine *in vitro* nor does GAZT compete with zidovudine triphosphate as an inhibitor of HIV reverse transcriptase.

The cytotoxicity of zidovudine for various cell lines was determined using a cell growth assay. ID_{50} values for several human cell lines showed little growth inhibition by zidovudine except at concentrations >50 μg/mL. However, one human T-lymphocyte cell line was sensitive to the cytotoxic effect of zidovudine with an ID_{50} of 5 μg/mL. Moreover, in a colony-forming unit assay designed to assess the toxicity of zidovudine for human bone marrow, an ID_{50} value of <1.25 μg/mL was estimated. Two of ten human lymphocyte cultures tested were found to be sensitive to zidovudine at 5 μg/mL or less.

Zidovudine has antiviral activity against some other mammalian retroviruses in addition to HIV. Human Immunodeficiency Virus-2 (HIV-2) replication *in vitro* is inhibited by zidovudine with an ID_{50} of 0.015 μg/mL, while HTLV-1 transmission to susceptible cells is inhibited by 1 to 3 μg/mL concentrations of drug. Several strains of simian immunodeficiency virus (SIV) are also inhibited by zidovudine with ID_{50} values ranging from 0.13 to 6.5 μg/mL, depending upon species of origin and assay method used. No significant inhibitory activity was exhibited against a variety of other human and animal viruses, except an ID_{50} of 1.4 to 2.7 μg/mL against the Epstein-Barr virus, the clinical significance of which is unknown.

The following microbiological activities of zidovudine have been observed *in vitro* but the clinical significance is unknown. Many *Enterobacteriaceae,* including strains of *Shigella, Salmonella, Klebsiella, Enterobacter, Citrobacter,* and *Escherichia coli* are inhibited *in vitro* by low concentrations of zidovudine (0.005 to 0.5 μg/mL). Synergy of zidovudine with trimethoprim has been observed against some of these bacteria *in vitro.* Limited data suggest that bacterial resistance to zidovudine develops rapidly. Zidovudine has no activity against gram positive organisms, anaerobes, mycobacteria, or fungal pathogens including *Candida albicans* and *Cryptococcus neoformans.* Although *Giardia lamblia* is inhibited by 1.9 μg/mL of zidovudine, no activity was observed against other protozoal pathogens.

Pharmacokinetics:

Adults: The pharmacokinetics of zidovudine has been evaluated in 22 adult HIV-infected patients in a Phase 1 dose-escalation study. Cohorts of 3 to 7 patients received 1 hour intravenous infusions of zidovudine ranging from 1 to 2.5 mg/kg every 8 hours to 2.5 to 7.5 mg/kg every 4 hours (3 to 45 mg/kg/day) for 14 to 28 days followed by oral dosing ranging from 2 to 5 mg/kg every 8 hours to 5 to 10 mg/kg every 4 hours (6 to 60 mg/kg/day) for an additional 32 days. After oral dosing, zidovudine was rapidly absorbed from the gastrointestinal tract with peak serum concentrations occurring within 0.5 to 1.5 hours. Dose-independent kinetics was observed over the range of 2 mg/kg every 8 hours to 10 mg/kg every 4 hours. The mean zidovudine half-life was approximately 1 hour and ranged from 0.78 to 1.93 hours following oral dosing.

Zidovudine is rapidly metabolized to 3′-azido-3′-deoxy-5′-*O*-β-*D*-glucopyranuronosylthymidine (GAZT) which has an apparent elimination half-life of 1 hour (range 0.61 to 1.73 hours). Following oral administration, urinary recoveries of zidovudine and GAZT accounted for 14 and 74% of the dose, respectively, and the total urinary recovery averaged 90% (range 63 to 95%), indicating a high degree of absorption. However, as a result of first-pass metabolism, the average oral capsule bioavailability of zidovudine is 65% (range 52 to 75%).

Additional pharmacokinetic data following intravenous dosing indicated dose-independent kinetics over the range of

1 to 5 mg/kg with a mean zidovudine half-life of 1.1 hours (range 0.48 to 2.86 hours). Total body clearance averaged 1900 mL/min/70 kg and the apparent volume of distribution was 1.6 L/kg. Renal clearance is estimated to be 400 mL/min/70 kg, indicating glomerular filtration and active tubular secretion by the kidneys. Zidovudine plasma protein binding is 34 to 38%, indicating that drug interactions involving binding site displacement are not anticipated.

The zidovudine cerebrospinal fluid (CSF)/plasma concentration ratio measured 1.8 hours following oral dosing at 2 mg/kg was 0.15 (n=1). The ratios measured at 2 to 4 hours following intravenous dosing of 2.5 mg/kg and 5.0 mg/kg were 0.20 (n=1) and 0.64 (n=3), respectively.

The pharmacokinetics of zidovudine have been evaluated in patients with impaired renal function following a single 200 mg oral dose. In five anuric patients, the half-life of zidovudine was 1.4 hours compared to 1.0 hour for control subjects with normal renal function; AUC values were approximately twice those of controls. However, in the anuric patients GAZT half-life was 8.0 hours (vs 0.9 hours for control) and AUC was 17 times higher than for control subjects. Hemodialysis appears to have a negligible effect on the removal of zidovudine, whereas GAZT elimination is enhanced.

Children: The pharmacokinetics and bioavailability of zidovudine have been evaluated in 21 HIV-infected children, aged 6 months through 12 years, following intravenous doses administered over the range of 80 to 160 mg/m² every 6 hours, and following oral doses of the intravenous solution administered over the range of 90 to 240 mg/m² every 6 hours. After discontinuation of the IV infusion, zidovudine plasma concentrations decayed biexponentially, consistent with two-compartment pharmacokinetics. Proportional increases in AUC and in zidovudine concentrations were observed with increasing dose, consistent with dose-independent kinetics over the dose range studied. The mean terminal half-life and total body clearance across all dose levels administered were 1.5 hours and 30.9 mL/min/kg, respectively. These values compare to mean half-life and total body clearance in adults of 1.1 hours and 27.1 mL/min/kg.

The mean oral bioavailability of 65% was independent of dose. This value is the same as the bioavailability in adults. Doses of 180 mg/m² four times daily in pediatric patients produced similar systemic exposure (24 hour AUC 10.7 hr μg/mL) as doses of 200 mg six times daily in adult patients (10.9 hr μg/mL).

Concentrations of zidovudine in cerebrospinal fluid were measured after both intermittent IV and oral drug administration in 21 children during Phase 1 and Phase 2 studies. The mean CSF/plasma zidovudine concentration ratio following intermittent IV and oral dosing ranged from 0.68 to 0.85 for the Phase 1 and Phase 2 participants, respectively. During continuous intravenous infusion the mean steady-state CSF/plasma ratio was 0.26.

As in adult patients, the major route of elimination in children was by metabolism to 5-glucuronylazidothymidine (GAZT). After IV dosing, about 29% of the dose was excreted in the urine unchanged and about 45% as GAZT. Overall, the pharmacokinetics of zidovudine in pediatric patients greater than 3 months of age is similar to that of zidovudine in adult patients.

Capsules: Steady-state serum concentrations of zidovudine following chronic oral administration of 250 mg every 4 hours (3.0 to 5.4 mg/kg) were determined in 21 adult patients (body weight ranged from 46.0 to 83.6 kg) in a controlled trial. Mean steady-state predose and 1.5 hours postdose zidovudine concentrations were 0.16 μg/mL (range 0 to 0.84 μg/mL) and 0.62 μg/mL (range 0.05 to 1.46 μg/mL), respectively.

Syrup: In a multiple dose bioavailability study conducted in 12 HIV-infected adults receiving doses of 100 or 200 mg every four hours, Retrovir Syrup was demonstrated to be bioequivalent to Retrovir Capsules with respect to area under the zidovudine plasma concentration-time curve (AUC). The rate of absorption of zidovudine syrup was greater than that of zidovudine capsules, as indicated by mean times to peak concentration of 0.5 and 0.8 hours, respectively. Mean values for steady-state peak concentration (dose-normalized to 200 mg) were 1.5 and 1.2 μg/mL for syrup and capsules, respectively.

INDICATIONS AND USAGE

Retrovir is indicated for the management of adult patients with HIV infection who have evidence of impaired immunity (CD4 cell count of 500/mm³ or less) before therapy is begun. Retrovir is also indicated for HIV-infected children over 3 months of age who have HIV-related symptoms or who are asymptomatic with abnormal laboratory values indicating significant HIV-related immunosuppression.

These indications are based on the results of three randomized, double-blind, placebo-controlled trials of oral zidovudine in HIV-infected adult patients with CD4 cell counts of 500/mm³ or less, and two open-label studies involving 124 children ages 3.5 months to 12 years with advanced HIV-associated disease. Specifically, separate studies evaluated zidovudine therapy in asymptomatic HIV-infected adults, in adults with early symptomatic disease, in adults with advanced symptomatic HIV disease (AIDS or advanced ARC), and in children with advanced symptomatic HIV disease (pediatric AIDS or advanced ARC).

Adults Asymptomatic HIV Infection: A randomized, double-blind, placebo-controlled trial of oral zidovudine was conducted in asymptomatic, HIV-infected adults at 32 medical centers.[1] Entry was dependent on the absence of signs and symptoms consistent with HIV disease, such as significant weight loss, fever, diarrhea, secondary infections and evidence of neurological dysfunction. In the study, 1338 asymptomatic individuals with absolute CD4(T4) lymphocyte counts of less than 500 cells/mm³ received a regimen of either 100 mg zidovudine, 300 mg zidovudine, or placebo, each administered five times a day. These study participants were monitored for the development of signs and symptoms of HIV disease and tolerance to the study regimens. The study was terminated early because of a statistically significant difference in progression to advanced symptomatic HIV disease (AIDS or advanced ARC) between the 500 mg/day zidovudine group and the placebo group. Of the 1338 patients enrolled in the study, 38 of the 428 patients receiving placebo, 17 of the 453 individuals receiving 500 mg zidovudine, and 19 of the 457 recipients of 1500 mg zidovudine progressed to advanced symptomatic HIV disease when followed for a mean of 55 weeks (range 19–107 weeks). Of the progressions noted above, AIDS occurred in 33 placebo recipients, 11 individuals receiving 500 mg and 14 patients receiving 1500 mg zidovudine. Changes in immunologic and virologic parameters (ie, CD4[T4] lymphocyte count and serum p24 antigen levels) paralleled the observed clinical benefits. Consistent with various epidemiologic studies of individuals with HIV infection, patients in this study with lower CD_4 cell counts or P24 antigenemia were more likely to progress to AIDS. Virtually all patients (for whom data are available) experienced a decline in CD_4 cell counts to less than 200 per mm³ before developing an AIDS-defining opportunistic infection. Although treatment of asymptomatic patients delays progression of disease in those patients at risk of progression over the initial 1–2 years of treatment, it is not known whether early treatment prolongs survival.

Zidovudine was well tolerated in a majority of patients. The following adverse clinical events were reported at a significantly greater incidence in individuals receiving 500 mg/day of zidovudine versus placebo: headache, malaise, anorexia, nausea and vomiting (see ADVERSE REACTIONS).

The two most common laboratory abnormalities reported were anemia and granulocytopenia, each of which occurred more often in patients receiving higher doses. These toxicities were easily managed in most cases by temporary dose interruption.

Early Symptomatic HIV Disease: This randomized, double-blind, placebo-controlled trial of oral zidovudine, conducted at 29 medical centers, studied 713 adults with early manifestations of HIV disease (ie, a baseline CD4[T4] cell count of 200 to 800/mm³ and symptoms such as oral thrush, oral hairy leukoplakia or intermittent diarrhea).[2] Patients received either placebo or 200 mg zidovudine every 4 hours (1200 mg/day). The trial was terminated early because of a statistically significant difference in the rates of development of advanced symptomatic HIV disease between the zidovudine and placebo groups. Of the 352 patients receiving placebo, 36 progressed to advanced symptomatic HIV disease, of whom 21 progressed to AIDS; whereas of the 361 zidovudine recipients, 13 progressed to advanced symptomatic HIV disease, of whom 5 progressed to AIDS.

Minimal toxicity was observed. Four percent of zidovudine recipients compared with none of the placebo recipients developed a hemoglobin concentration less than 8 g/dL and 4% of patients treated with zidovudine compared with 1% of placebo recipients developed a granulocyte count less than 750 cells/mm³. Asthenia, dyspepsia, nausea, and vomiting were the major adverse clinical events reported at significantly greater incidences in patients receiving zidovudine.

Advanced Symptomatic HIV Disease: This randomized, double-blind, placebo-controlled trial, conducted at 12 medical centers, was the original trial upon which the marketing of Retrovir was based. In this trial, 281 adults with advanced symptomatic HIV infection including AIDS were studied for a mean of four and a half months.[3,4]

The patient population of this controlled trial consisted of 160 patients with AIDS (85 Retrovir and 75 placebo) who had recovered from their first episode of PCP diagnosed within the previous four months[3,4] and 121 patients with ARC (59 Retrovir and 62 placebo) with multiple signs and symptoms of HIV infection, including mucocutaneous candidiasis and/or unexplained weight loss (≥15 lbs or >10% of prior body weight). All patients had evidence of impaired cellular immunity with an absence of delayed cutaneous hypersensitivity and CD4 (T4) lymphocytes less than 500 cells/mm³. All patients began therapy at a dose of 250 mg every 4 hours around the clock. This dosage was reduced or temporarily or permanently discontinued after serious marrow toxicity occurred. The trial was stopped early because of a statistically significant difference in mortality. There were 19 deaths in the placebo group and 1 in the Retrovir group. All deaths were apparently due to opportunistic infections (OI) or other complications of HIV infection. Treatment duration ranged from 12 weeks to 26 weeks, with a mean and median duration of 17 and 18 weeks, respectively.

Retrovir also significantly reduced the risk of acquiring an AIDS-defining OI in patients after 6 weeks of treatment. In addition, patients who received Retrovir generally did better than the placebo group in terms of several other measures of efficacy including performance level, neuropsychiatric function, maintenance of body weight and the number and severity of symptoms associated with HIV infection. A small, transient increase in mean CD4 (T4) counts was seen in the zidovudine group but the significance of this finding is unclear.

The most significant adverse reaction noted in the study was a depression of formed elements in the peripheral blood, which necessitated dose reduction or drug discontinuation in 34% of patients receiving Retrovir. Patients with lower CD4 counts were more likely to receive transfusions. 41% of Retrovir recipients and 16% of placebo recipients with <200 CD4 lymphocytes at entry were transfused (see ADVERSE REACTIONS). Only one of 30 Retrovir recipients and none of 30 placebo recipients with >200 CD4 lymphocytes required transfusion.

Although mean platelet counts in Retrovir recipients were statistically increased compared to mean baseline values, thrombocytopenia did occur in some patients. Twelve percent (12%) of Retrovir recipients compared to 5% of placebo recipients had >50% decreases from baseline platelet count.

At the conclusion of the placebo-controlled trial, approximately 80% of Retrovir and placebo recipients elected to enroll in an uncontrolled extension protocol in which all patients received Retrovir at a dose of 200 mg every four hours. This dose was chosen because of concern about hematologic toxicity and to allow for greater flexibility in dosing. These patients have been followed for variable periods of time. As the follow-up period lengthened, patient tracking became increasingly difficult. The intended treatment period of the original study was six months; however, some follow-up data are available for over 90% of patients originally enrolled in the trial. Data from patients in this and other studies show no new or unexpected clinical or laboratory adverse experiences for patients receiving Retrovir other than those listed (see ADVERSE REACTIONS), nor have previously reported adverse events increased significantly in frequency or severity with prolonged drug administration. At any time on study, approximately half of the patients received the recommended dose of zidovudine, while the remaining patients required reduction or interruption of their dosage regimen in response to myelosuppression and/or other clinical adverse events.

Benefits of therapy with Retrovir were observed during this extended period, although opportunistic infections continued to occur and additional patients died. Survival for all patients originally randomized to receive Retrovir was 96.5% at six months, 84.7% at one year, 68.3% at 18 months and 41.2% at two years. One year and two year survival for patients who entered the trial with AIDS was 79% and 31% when calculated since initiation of therapy (87% and 43%, respectively, since the first diagnosis of PCP). These survival rates were determined by the "intention to treat" method, which assumes all patients assigned to a drug actually took the drug throughout the study period.

While a direct comparison with survival data from other cohorts is not possible, untreated adult patients with AIDS diagnosed in San Francisco in 1985 who had survived 60 days after PCP had a one year survival of 34.7% and a two year survival of 4.2% from diagnosis of PCP. In a recent epidemiologic study of patients with AIDS diagnosed in San Francisco in 1986 and 1987, median survival was improved for patients receiving Retrovir compared to those not receiving therapy with Retrovir (21.6 vs. 14.9 months). Actual survival of untreated patients is likely to be lower than reported because of the difficulty in complete ascertainment of mortality. Caution is advised in making comparisons from such "natural history" experience since case definitions and follow-up practices vary.

Other, uncontrolled studies have shown that Retrovir may be of benefit in treating women, intravenous drug users, and racial minorities,[5] in addition to the patient population (primarily white males) included in the controlled trials.[3]

Dose Comparison Study: Results from a randomized, unblinded, dose comparison study of zidovudine, in adults with AIDS who had experienced an episode of PCP, indicate that an induction dose of zidovudine 200 mg administered orally every four hours (1200 mg/day) for one month, followed by chronic administration of 100 mg every 4 hours (600 mg/day), was associated with survival rates and frequency of opportunistic infections comparable to those observed in patients administered higher dosages as tolerated. The 600 mg per day regimen was also associated with a lower incidence of hematologic toxicity. The effectiveness of this lower dose in improving the neurologic dysfunction associated with

Continued on next page

Burroughs Wellcome—Cont.

HIV disease, however, is unknown (see DOSAGE AND ADMINISTRATION).

Pediatric Symptomatic HIV Disease: Two open-label studies have evaluated the pharmacokinetics, safety and efficacy of Retrovir in 124 children with advanced HIV disease (84 AIDS and 40 with other clinical and laboratory evidence of advanced HIV disease). The median age at entry was 3.3 years with 14% less than 12 months of age. In the majority of cases (73%), HIV was acquired by vertical transmission from an HIV-infected mother.

Thirty-six children were enrolled in the Phase 1 study, which evaluated three intravenous dosing regimens administered for 4 to 8 weeks. All children subsequently switched to an oral dose of 180 mg/m^2 every 6 hours and were followed for a mean of 465 days (range 121 to 855 days). Eighty-eight children participated in the Phase 2 study and these children were monitored for a mean of 186 days (range 3 to 352 days). In the Phase 2 study, oral zidovudine was initiated at a dose of 180 mg/m^2 every 6 hours.

Clinical, immunologic and virologic improvements were observed among some of the children receiving zidovudine in these open-label studies. Clinical improvements included reductions in hepatosplenomegaly and increases in weight percentiles in previously growth retarded children. The probability of remaining free of opportunistic infections through 12 months of follow-up was 0.76. Thirty-seven children developed one or more documented serious bacterial infections while participating in the studies. Seven of these children had more than one documented serious bacterial infection. The probability of survival at 12 months is 0.87 for the 124 patients enrolled in the Phase 1 and Phase 2 studies.

Improvements in the immunologic parameters CD4 cell counts and immunoglobulin concentration were observed among the study participants. For children with severely depressed CD4 cell counts (<500/mm^3) at entry, a mean increase of 148/mm^3 CD4$^+$ lymphocyte cell count was observed during the first two months of zidovudine therapy. Thereafter, CD4 cell counts declined but remained above baseline through 9 months of follow-up. A tendency towards normalization of elevated immunoglobulin concentrations (primarily IgG) was observed among study participants.

Substantial reductions in serum and CSF P_{24} antigen concentrations were observed in some patients, as well as a reduction in the number of patients with positive CSF HIV cultures, providing evidence of anti-retroviral effect.

The most frequently reported adverse events were anemia (Hgb <7.5 g/dL) and neutropenia (<750/mm^3), which occurred in forty-six percent of the children. Thirty-six percent of the patients had their dose modified due to the development of hematologic abnormalities and 30% received transfusions for anemia. Four patients had dosing permanently discontinued due to neutropenia (see ADVERSE REACTIONS).

CONTRAINDICATIONS

Retrovir Capsules and Syrup are contraindicated for patients who have potentially life-threatening allergic reactions to any of the components of the formulations.

WARNINGS

Zidovudine has been studied in controlled trials in significant numbers of asymptomatic and symptomatic HIV infected patients, but only for limited periods of time. Therefore, the full safety and efficacy profile of zidovudine has not been defined, particularly in regard to prolonged use and especially in HIV infected individuals who have less advanced disease (see following sections for more specific information: INDICATIONS AND USAGE, Microbiology, Carcinogenesis, Mutagenesis, Impairment of Fertility).

Insufficient clinical experience exists to recommend a dosing regimen in infants under 3 months of age. Preliminary evidence indicates that zidovudine clearance may be reduced in children less than one month of age.

A positive test for HIV-antibody in children under 15 months of age may represent passively acquired maternal antibodies, rather than an active antibody response to infection in the infant. Thus, the presence of HIV antibody in a child less than 15 months of age must be interpreted with caution, especially in the asymptomatic infant. Confirmatory tests such as serum P_{24} antigen or viral culture should be pursued in such children.

Zidovudine should be used with extreme caution in patients who have bone marrow compromise evidenced by granulocyte count <1000/mm^3 or hemoglobin <9.5 g/dL. In all of the placebo-controlled studies, but most frequently in patients with advanced symptomatic HIV disease, anemia and granulocytopenia were the most significant adverse events observed (see ADVERSE REACTIONS). There have been reports of pancytopenia associated with the use of zidovudine, which was reversible in most instances after discontinuance of the drug.

Significant anemia most commonly occurred after 4 to 6 weeks of therapy and in many cases required dose adjustment, discontinuation of zidovudine, and/or blood transfusions. Frequent blood counts are strongly recommended in patients with advanced HIV disease taking zidovudine. For asymptomatic HIV-infected individuals and patients with early HIV disease, most of whom have better marrow reserve, blood counts may be obtained less frequently, depending upon the patient's overall status. If anemia or granulocytopenia develops, dosage adjustments may be necessary (see DOSAGE AND ADMINISTRATION).

Sensitization reactions, including anaphylaxis in one patient, have been reported in individuals receiving zidovudine therapy. Patients experiencing a rash should undergo medical evaluation.

Coadministration of zidovudine with other drugs metabolized by glucuronidation should be avoided because the toxicity of either drug may be potentiated (see Drug Interactions under PRECAUTIONS). Zidovudine recipients who used acetaminophen during the controlled trial in advanced HIV disease, had an increased incidence of granulocytopenia which appeared to be correlated with the duration of acetaminophen use.

PRECAUTIONS

General: Zidovudine is eliminated from the body primarily by renal excretion following metabolism in the liver (glucuronidation). There are currently very little data available concerning the use of zidovudine in patients with impaired renal function (see Pharmacokinetics subsection of CLINICAL PHARMACOLOGY) and no data in patients with impaired hepatic function. These patients may be at greater risk of toxicity from zidovudine.

Information for Patients: Zidovudine is not a cure for HIV infections, and patients may continue to acquire illnesses associated with HIV infection, including opportunistic infections. Therefore, patients should be advised to seek medical care for any significant change in their health status.

Patients should be informed that the drug has been studied for limited periods of time, and that long term safety and efficacy are not known, particularly for patients with less advanced disease. Patients should be informed that the major toxicities of zidovudine are granulocytopenia and/or anemia. The frequency and severity of these toxicities are greater in patients with more advanced disease and those who initiate therapy later in the course of their infection. They should be told that if toxicity develops, they may require transfusions or dose modifications including possible discontinuation. They should be told of the extreme importance of having their blood counts followed closely while on therapy, especially for patients with advanced symptomatic HIV disease. They should be cautioned about the use of other medications, such as acetaminophen, that may exacerbate the toxicity of zidovudine (see WARNINGS).

Retrovir Capsules and Syrup are for oral ingestion only. Patients should be told of the importance of taking zidovudine exactly as prescribed. They should be told not to share medication and not to exceed the recommended dose. Patients should be told that the long-term effects of zidovudine are unknown at this time.

Patients should be advised that zidovudine therapy has not been shown to reduce the risk of transmission of HIV to others through sexual contact or blood contamination.

Drug Interactions: The interaction of other drugs with zidovudine has not been studied in a systematic manner. Coadministration of zidovudine with drugs that are nephrotoxic, cytotoxic, or which interfere with RBC/WBC number or function (eg, dapsone, pentamidine, amphotericin B, flucytosine, vincristine, vinblastine, adriamycin, or interferon) may increase the risk of toxicity. Limited data suggest that probenecid may inhibit glucuronidation and/or reduce renal excretion of zidovudine. In addition, other drugs (eg, acetaminophen, aspirin, or indomethacin) may competitively inhibit glucuronidation (see WARNINGS). Phenytoin levels have been reported to be low in some patients receiving zidovudine, while in one case a high level was documented. These observations suggest that phenytoin levels should be carefully monitored in patients receiving zidovudine since many patients with advanced HIV infections have CNS conditions which may predispose to seizure activity.

Some experimental nucleoside analogues which are being evaluated in HIV-infected patients may affect RBC/WBC number or function and may increase the potential for hematologic toxicity of zidovudine. Some experimental nucleoside analogues affecting DNA replication antagonize the *in vitro* antiviral activity of zidovudine against HIV and thus, concomitant use of such drugs should be avoided.

Some drugs such as trimethoprim-sulfamethoxazole, pyrimethamine, and acyclovir may be necessary for the management or prevention of opportunistic infections. In the controlled trial, in patients with advanced HIV disease, increased toxicity was not detected with limited exposure to these drugs. However, there is one published report of neurotoxicity (profound lethargy) associated with concomitant use of zidovudine and acyclovir.

Carcinogenesis, Mutagenesis, Impairment of Fertility: Zidovudine was administered orally at three dosage levels to separate groups of mice and rats (60 females and 60 males in each group). Initial single daily doses were 30, 60 and 120 mg/kg/day in mice and 80, 220 and 600 mg/kg/day in rats. The doses in mice were reduced to 20, 30 and 40 mg/kg/day after day 90 because of treatment-related anemia, whereas in rats only the high dose was reduced to 450 mg/kg/day on day 91 and then to 300 mg/kg/day on day 279.

In mice, seven late-appearing (after 19 months) vaginal neoplasms (5 non-metastasizing squamous cell carcinomas, one squamous cell papilloma and one squamous polyp) occurred in animals given the highest dose. One late-appearing squamous cell papilloma occurred in the vagina of a middle dose animal. No vaginal tumors were found at the lowest dose.

In rats, two late-appearing (after 20 months), non-metastasizing vaginal squamous cell carcinomas occurred in animals given the highest dose. No vaginal tumors occurred at the low or middle dose in rats.

No other drug-related tumors were observed in either sex of either species.

It is not known how predictive the results of rodent carcinogenicity studies may be for man. At doses that produced tumors in mice and rats, the estimated drug exposure (as measured by AUC) was approximately 3 times (mouse) and 24 times (rat) the estimated human exposure at the recommended therapeutic dose of 100 mg every 4 hours.

No evidence of mutagenicity (with or without metabolic activation) was observed in the Ames *Salmonella* mutagenicity assay. In a mutagenicity assay conducted in L5178Y/TK$^{+/-}$ mouse lymphoma cells, zidovudine was weakly mutagenic in the absence of metabolic activation only at the highest concentrations tested (4000 and 5000 μg/mL). In the presence of metabolic activation, the drug was weakly mutagenic at concentrations of 1000 μg/mL and higher. In an *in vitro* mammalian cell transformation assay, zidovudine was positive at concentrations of 0.5 μg/mL and higher. In an *in vitro* cytogenetic study performed in cultured human lymphocytes, zidovudine induced dose-related structural chromosomal abnormalities at concentrations of 3 μg/mL and higher. No such effects were noted at the two lowest concentrations tested, 0.3 and 1 μg/mL. In an *in vivo* cytogenetic study in rats given a single intravenous injection of zidovudine at doses of 37.5 to 300 mg/kg, there were no treatment-related structural or numerical chromosomal alterations in spite of plasma levels that were as high as 453 μg/mL five minutes after dosing.

In two *in vivo* micronucleus studies (designed to measure chromosome breakage or mitotic spindle apparatus damage) in male mice, oral doses of zidovudine of 100 to 1000 mg/kg/day administered once daily for approximately 4 weeks induced dose-related increases in micronucleated erythrocytes. Similar results were also seen after 4 or 7 days of dosing at 500 mg/kg/day in rats and mice.

No effect on male or female fertility (judged by conception rates) was seen in rats given zidovudine orally at doses up to 450 mg/kg/day.

Pregnancy: Pregnancy Category C. Oral teratology studies in the rat and in the rabbit at doses up to 500 mg/kg/day revealed no evidence of terogenicity with zidovudine. The incidence of fetal resorptions was increased in rats given 150 or 450 mg/kg/day and rabbits given 500 mg/kg/day. The doses used in the teratology studies resulted in peak plasma concentrations in rats of 68 to 234 times the peak human plasma concentrations and in rabbits 14 to 90 times the peak human plasma concentrations. It is not known whether zidovudine can cause fetal harm when administered to a pregnant woman or can affect reproductive capacity. Zidovudine should be given to a pregnant woman only if clearly needed.

Nursing Mothers: It is not known whether zidovudine is excreted in human milk. Because many drugs are excreted in human milk and because of the potential for serious adverse reactions from zidovudine in nursing infants, mothers should be instructed to discontinue nursing if they are receiving zidovudine.

Pediatric Use: See INDICATIONS, WARNINGS and DOSAGE AND ADMINISTRATION sections.

ADVERSE REACTIONS

Adults: The frequency and severity of adverse events associated with the use of zidovudine in adults are greater in patients with more advanced infection at the time of initiation of therapy. The following tables summarize the relative incidence of hematologic adverse events observed in the placebo-controlled clinical studies by severity of HIV disease present at the start of treatment.

[See first three tables on next page.]

The anemia reported in patients receiving zidovudine appeared to be the result of impaired erythrocyte maturation as evidenced by increased macrocytosis (MCV) while on drug.

The HIV-infected adults participating in these clinical trials often had baseline symptoms and signs of HIV disease and/or experienced adverse events at some time during study. It was often difficult to distinguish adverse events possibly associated with zidovudine administration from underlying

Asymptomatic HIV Infection Study (n = 1338)	Granulocytopenia (<750/mm³)			Anemia (Hgb < 8 g/dL)		
	Zidovudine		Placebo	Zidovudine		Placebo
	1500 mg*	500 mg		1500 mg*	500 mg	
CD4 ≤ 500	6.4% (n = 457)	1.8% (n = 453)	1.6% (n = 428)	6.4% (n = 457)	1.1% (n = 453)	0.2% (n = 428)

Early Symptomatic HIV Disease Study (n = 713)	Granulocytopenia (<750/mm³)		Anemia (Hgb < 8 g/dL)	
	Zidovudine 1200 mg	Placebo	Zidovudine 1200 mg	Placebo
CD4 > 200	4% (n = 361)	1% (n = 352)	4% (n = 361)	0% (n = 352)

Advanced Symptomatic HIV Disease Study (n = 281)	Granulocytopenia (<750/mm³)		Anemia (Hgb < 7.5 g/dL)	
	Zidovudine 1500 mg*	Placebo	Zidovudine 1500 mg*	Placebo
CD4 > 200	10% (n = 30)	3% (n = 30)	3% (n = 30)	0% (n = 30)
CD4 < 200	47% (n = 114)	10% (n = 107)	29% (n = 114)	5% (n = 107)

*Three times the currently recommended dose in asymptomatic patients.

Percentage (%) of Patients with Clinical Events in the Advanced HIV Disease Study

Adverse Event	Zidovudine (n = 144)%	Placebo (n = 137)%	Adverse Event	Zidovudine (n = 144)%	Placebo (n = 137)%
BODY AS A WHOLE			MUSCULOSKELETAL		
Asthenia	19	18	Myalgia	8	2
Diaphoresis	5	4	NERVOUS		
Fever	16	12	Dizziness	6	4
Headache	42	37	Insomnia	5	1
Malaise	8	7	Paresthesia	6	3
GASTROINTESTINAL			Somnolence	8	9
Anorexia	11	8	RESPIRATORY		
Diarrhea	12	18	Dyspnea	5	3
Dyspepsia	5	4	SKIN		
GI Pain	20	19	Rash	17	15
Nausea	46	18	SPECIAL SENSES		
Vomiting	6	3	Taste Perversion	5	8

Percentage (%) of Patients with Clinical Events in the Early Symptomatic HIV Disease Study

Adverse Event	Zidovudine (n = 361)%	Placebo (n = 352)%
BODY AS A WHOLE		
Asthenia	69	62
GASTROINTESTINAL		
Dyspepsia	6	1
Nausea	61	41
Vomiting	25	13

signs of HIV disease or intercurrent illnesses. The following table summarizes clinical adverse events or symptoms which occurred in at least 5% of all patients with advanced HIV disease treated with zidovudine in the original placebo-controlled study.[4] Of the items listed in the table, only severe headache, nausea, insomnia and myalgia were reported at a significantly greater rate in zidovudine recipients.
[See fourth table above.]
Clinical adverse events which occurred in less than 5% of all adult patients treated with zidovudine in the advanced HIV study are listed below. Since many of these adverse events were seen in placebo-treated patients as well as zidovudine recipients, their possible relationship to the drug is unknown.
Body as a whole: body odor, chills, edema of the lip, flu syndrome, hyperalgesia, back pain, chest pain, lymphadenopathy.
Cardiovascular: vasodilation.
Gastrointestinal: constipation, dysphagia, edema of the tongue, eructation, flatulence, bleeding gums, rectal hemorrhage, mouth ulcer.
Musculoskeletal: arthralgia, muscle spasm, tremor, twitch.
Nervous: anxiety, confusion, depression, emotional lability, nervousness, syncope, loss of mental acuity, vertigo.
Respiratory: cough, epistaxis, pharyngitis, rhinitis, sinusitis, hoarseness.
Skin: acne, pruritus, urticaria.
Special senses: amblyopia, hearing loss, photophobia.
Urogenital: dysuria, polyuria, urinary frequency, urinary hesitancy.
Subsequent to the initial trial, myopathy and sensitization reactions, including anaphylaxis in one patient, have been reported in adults receiving zidovudine therapy.
All unexpected events and expected events of a severe or life-threatening nature were monitored for adults in the placebo-

controlled studies in early HIV disease and asymptomatic HIV infection. Data concerning the occurrence of additional signs or symptoms were also collected. No distinction was made in reporting events between those possibly associated with the administration of the study medication and those due to the underlying disease. The following tables summarize all those events reported at a statistically significant greater incidence for zidovudine recipients in these studies:
[See small table first column and table at bottom left.]

The following events have been reported in adult patients treated with zidovudine: seizures, nail pigmentation, changes in liver function tests. They may also occur as part of the underlying disease process. As such, the relationship between these events and the use of zidovudine is uncertain.

Pediatrics: The incidences of anemia and granulocytopenia among children with advanced HIV disease receiving zidovudine were similar to the incidences which have been reported for adults with AIDS or advanced ARC (see above). Management of neutropenia and anemia included, in some cases, dose modification and/or blood product transfusions. In the open-label studies, seventeen percent had their dose modified (generally a reduction in dose by 30%) due to anemia and 25% had their dose modified (temporary discontinuation or dose reduction by 30%) for neutropenia. Four children had zidovudine permanently discontinued for neutropenia. The following table summarizes the occurrence of anemia (Hgb <7.5 g/dL) and granulocytopenia (<750/mm³) among 124 children receiving zidovudine for a mean of 267 days (range 3 to 855 days):

Advanced Pediatric	Granulocytopenia (<750/mm³)		Anemia (Hgb <7.5 g/dL)	
HIV disease	N	%	N	%
(N= 124)	48	39	28*	23

* Twenty-two children received one or more transfusions due to a decline in hemoglobin to <7.5 g/dL: an additional 15 children were transfused for hemoglobin levels >7.5 g/dL. Fifty-nine percent of the patients transfused had a pre-study history of anemia or transfusion requirement.
An increase in MCV (macrocytosis) was observed among the majority of children enrolled in the studies.
In the open-label studies involving 124 children, 16 clinical adverse events were reported by 24 children. No event was reported by more than 5.6% of the study populations. Due to the open-label design of the studies, it was difficult to determine possible zidovudine-related versus disease-related events. Therefore, all clinical events reported as associated with zidovudine therapy or of unknown relationship to zidovudine therapy are presented in the following table:

Percentage (%) of Pediatric Patients with Clinical Events in Open Label Studies

Adverse Event	N	%
BODY AS A WHOLE		
Fever	4	3.2
Phlebitis*/Bacteremia	2	1.6
Headache	2	1.6
GASTROINTESTINAL		
Nausea	1	0.8
Vomiting	6	4.8
Abdominal Pain	4	3.2
Diarrhea	1	0.8
Weight Loss	1	0.8
NERVOUS		
Insomnia	3	2.4
Nervousness/Irritability	2	1.6
Decreased Reflexes	7	5.6
Seizure	1	0.8
CARDIOVASCULAR		
Left Ventricular Dilation	1	0.8
Cardiomyopathy	1	0.8
S₃ Gallop	1	0.8
Congestive Heart Failure	1	0.8
Generalized Edema	1	0.8
ECG Abnormality	3	2.4
UROGENITAL		
Hematuria/Viral Cystitis	1	0.8

*Peripheral vein I.V. catheter site.
The clinical adverse events reported among adult zidovudine recipients may also occur in children.

Percentage (%) of Patients with Clinical Events* in an Asymptomatic HIV Infection Study

Adverse Event	1500 mg Zidovudine*** (n=457)%	500 mg Zidovudine (n=453)%	Placebo (n=428)%
BODY AS A WHOLE			
Asthenia	10.1	8.6**	5.8
Headache	58.0**	62.5	52.6
Malaise	55.6	53.2	44.9
GASTROINTESTINAL			
Anorexia	19.3	20.1	10.5
Constipation	8.1	6.4**	3.5
Nausea	57.3	51.4	29.9
Vomiting	16.4	17.2	9.8
NERVOUS			
Dizziness	20.8	17.9**	15.2

* Reported in ≥5% of study population.
** Not statistically significant versus placebo.
*** Three times the currently recommended dose in asymptomatic patients.

Continued on next page

Burroughs Wellcome—Cont.

OVERDOSAGE

Cases of acute overdoses in both children and adults have been reported with doses up to 50 grams. None were fatal. The only consistent finding in these cases of overdose was spontaneous or induced nausea and vomiting. Hematologic changes were transient and not severe. All patients recovered without permanent sequelae. Hemodialysis appears to have a negligible effect on the removal of zidovudine while elimination of its primary metabolite, GAZT, is enhanced.

DOSAGE AND ADMINISTRATION

Capsules and Syrup: Adults: For adults with symptomatic HIV infection, including AIDS, the recommended oral starting dose is 200 mg (two 100 mg capsules or four teaspoonfuls [20 mL] syrup) administered every four hours (1200 mg total daily dose). After one month, the dose may be reduced to 100 mg every four hours (600 mg total daily dose). The effectiveness of this lower dose in improving the neurologic dysfunction associated with HIV disease is unknown (see INDICATIONS AND USAGE).

For asymptomatic HIV infection, the recommended dose for adults is 100 mg administered orally every four hours while awake (500 mg/day).

Children: The recommended starting dose in children 3 months to 12 years of age is 180 mg/m^2 every six hours (720 mg/m^2 per day), not to exceed 200 mg every six hours.

Monitoring of Patients: Hematologic toxicities appear to be related to pretreatment bone marrow reserve and to dose and duration of therapy. In patients with poor bone marrow reserve, particularly in patients with advanced symptomatic HIV disease, frequent monitoring of hematologic indices is recommended to detect serious anemia or granulocytopenia (see WARNINGS). In patients who experience hematologic toxicity, reduction in hemoglobin may occur as early as 2 to 4 weeks, and granulocytopenia usually occurs after 6 to 8 weeks.

Dose Adjustment: Significant anemia (hemoglobin of <7.5 g/dL or reduction of >25% of baseline) and/or significant granulocytopenia (granulocyte count of <750/mm^3 or reduction of >50% from baseline) may require a dose interruption until evidence of marrow recovery is observed (see WARNINGS). For less severe anemia or granulocytopenia, a reduction in daily dose may be adequate. In patients who develop significant anemia, dose modification does not necessarily eliminate the need for transfusion. If marrow recovery occurs following dose modification, gradual increases in dose may be appropriate depending on hematologic indices and patient tolerance.

There are insufficient data to recommend dose adjustment of zidovudine in patients with impaired renal or hepatic function (see Pharmacokinetics).

HOW SUPPLIED

Retrovir Capsules 100 mg (white, opaque cap and body with a dark blue band) containing 100 mg zidovudine and printed with "Wellcome" and unicorn logo on cap and "Y9C" and "100" on body. Bottles of 100 (NDC 0081-0108-55) and Unit Dose Pack of 100 (NDC 0081-0108-56).

Retrovir Syrup (colorless to pale yellow, strawberry-flavored) containing 50 mg zidovudine in each teaspoonful (5 mL). Bottle of 240 mL (NDC 0081-0113-18) with child-resistant cap.

Capsules should be stored at 15° to 25°C (59° to 77°F) and protected from light and moisture.

Syrup should be stored at 15° to 25°C (59° to 77°F) and protected from light.

REFERENCES

1. Volberding PA, Lagakos SW, Koch MA, et al. Zidovudine in asymptomatic human immunodeficiency virus infection. A controlled trial in persons with fewer than 500 CD4-positive cells per cubic millimeter. *N Engl J Med* 1990:322(14):941–949.
2. Fischl MA, Richman DD, Hansen N, et al. The safety and efficacy of zidovudine in the treatment of patients with mildly symptomatic HIV infection. A double-blind, placebo-controlled trial. Submitted to *Annals Internal Med* 1990.
3. Fischl MA, Richman DD, Grieco MH, et al. The efficacy of azidothymidine (AZT) in the treatment of patients with AIDS and AIDS-related complex. A double-blind, placebo-controlled trial. *N Engl J Med* 1987;317:185–91.
4. Richman DD, Fischl MA, Grieco MH, et al. The toxicity of azidothymidine (AZT) in the treatment of patients with AIDS and AIDS-related complex. A double-blind, placebo-controlled trial. *N Engl J Med* 1987;317:192–7.
5. Creagh-Kirk T, Doi P, Andrews E, et al. Survival experience among patients with AIDS receiving zidovudine. Follow-up of patients in a compassionate plea program. *JAMA* 1988;260(20):3009–3015.

U.S. Patent No. 4724232 (Use Patent)

Other Pats. Pending 587013

Capsules Shown in Product Identification Section, page 407

RETROVIR® I.V. INFUSION ℞

[*rĕt-rō-vĕr'*]

(Zidovudine)

FOR INTRAVENOUS INFUSION ONLY

> **WARNING: THERAPY WITH RETROVIR (ZIDOVUDINE) IS OFTEN ASSOCIATED WITH HEMATOLOGIC TOXICITY INCLUDING GRANULOCYTOPENIA AND SEVERE ANEMIA REQUIRING TRANSFUSIONS (SEE WARNINGS).**
>
> IN ADDITION, PATIENTS TREATED WITH ZIDOVUDINE MAY CONTINUE TO DEVELOP OPPORTUNISTIC INFECTIONS (OI'S) AND OTHER COMPLICATIONS OF THE ACQUIRED IMMUNODEFICIENCY SYNDROME (AIDS) AND AIDS RELATED COMPLEX (ARC) CAUSED BY THE HUMAN IMMUNODEFICIENCY VIRUS (HIV). THEREFORE, PATIENTS ON ZIDOVUDINE SHOULD BE UNDER CLOSE CLINICAL OBSERVATION BY PHYSICIANS EXPERIENCED IN THE TREATMENT OF PATIENTS WITH DISEASES ASSOCIATED WITH HIV. THE SAFETY AND EFFICACY OF ZIDOVUDINE HAVE BEEN ESTABLISHED ONLY FOR CERTAIN ADULT AIDS AND ADVANCED ARC PATIENTS (SEE "INDICATIONS AND USAGE").

DESCRIPTION

Retrovir is the brand name for zidovudine [formerly called azidothymidine (AZT)], an antiretroviral drug active against human immunodeficiency virus (HIV). Retrovir I.V. Infusion is a sterile solution for intravenous infusion only. Each mL contains 10 mg zidovudine in Water for Injection. Hydrochloric acid and/or sodium hydroxide may have been added to adjust the pH to approximately 5.5. Retrovir I.V. Infusion contains no preservatives.

The chemical name of zidovudine is 3′-azido-3′-deoxythymidine.

Zidovudine is a white to beige, odorless, crystalline solid with a molecular weight of 267.24 daltons and the molecular formula $C_{10}H_{13}N_5O_4$.

CLINICAL PHARMACOLOGY

Zidovudine is an inhibitor of the *in vitro* replication of some retroviruses including HIV (also known as HTLV III, LAV, or ARV). This drug is a thymidine analogue in which the 3′-hydroxy (-OH) group is replaced by an azido (-N_3) group. Cellular thymidine kinase converts zidovudine into zidovudine monophosphate. The monophosphate is further converted into the diphosphate by cellular thymidylate kinase and to the triphosphate derivative by other cellular enzymes. Zidovudine triphosphate interferes with the HIV viral RNA dependent DNA polymerase (reverse transcriptase) and thus, inhibits viral replication. Zidovudine triphosphate also inhibits cellular α-DNA polymerase, but at concentrations 100-fold higher than those required to inhibit reverse transcriptase. *In vitro*, zidovudine triphosphate has been shown to be incorporated into growing chains of DNA by viral reverse transcriptase. When incorporation by the viral enzyme occurs, the DNA chain is terminated. Studies in cell culture suggest that zidovudine incorporation by cellular α-DNA polymerase may occur, but only to a very small extent and not in all test systems. Chain termination has not been demonstrated with cellular α-DNA polymerase.

Microbiology: The relationship between *in vitro* susceptibility of HIV to zidovudine and the inhibition of HIV replication in man or clinical response to therapy has not been established. *In vitro* sensitivity results vary greatly depending upon the time between virus infection and zidovudine treatment of cell cultures, the particular assay used, the cell type employed, and the laboratory performing the test. In addition, the methods currently used to establish virologic responses in clinical trials may be relatively insensitive in detecting changes in the quantities of actively replicating HIV or reactivation of these viruses.

Zidovudine blocked 90% of detectable HIV replication *in vitro* at concentrations of ≤0.13 μg/mL (ID_{90}) when added shortly after laboratory infection of susceptible cells. This level of antiviral effect was observed in experiments measuring reverse transcriptase activity in H9 cells, PHA stimulated peripheral blood lymphocytes, and unstimulated peripheral blood lymphocytes. The concentration of drug required to produce a 50% decrease in supernatant reverse transcriptase was 0.013 μg/mL (ID_{50}) in both H9 cells and peripheral blood lymphocytes. Zidovudine at concentrations of 0.13 μg/mL also provided >90% protection from a strain of HIV (HTLV IIIB) induced cytopathic effects in two tetanus-specific T4 cell lines. p24 gag protein expression was also undetectable at the same concentration in these cells. Partial inhibition of viral activity in cells with chronic HIV infection (presumed to carry integrated HIV DNA) required concentrations of zidovudine (8.8 μg/mL in one laboratory to 13.3 μg/mL in another) which are approximately 100 times as high as those necessary to block HIV replication in acutely infected cells. HIV isolates from 18 untreated individuals with AIDS or ARC had ID_{50} sensitivity values between 0.003 to 0.013 μg/mL and ID_{95} sensitivity values between 0.03 to 0.3 μg/mL.

The development of resistance to zidovudine has not been adequately studied and the frequency of zidovudine-resistant isolates existing in the general population is unknown. Reduced *in vitro* sensitivity to zidovudine has been observed, however, in viral isolates from some severely immunocompromised patients with AIDS or advanced ARC who have received prolonged courses of zidovudine treatment. In the small number of patients from whom isolates were studied, no correlations were evident between the development of reduced sensitivity in the laboratory and clinical response. Therefore, the quantitative relationship between *in vitro* susceptibility of HIV to zidovudine and clinical response to therapy has not been established. Studies of the development of resistance to zidovudine are incomplete and the frequency and degree of changes in *in vitro* sensitivity of virus isolates from HIV infected patients with differing severity of immune compromise are unknown.

The major metabolite of zidovudine, 3′-azido-3′-deoxy-5′-*O*-β-*D*-glucopyranuronosylthymidine (GAZT), does not inhibit HIV replication *in vitro*. GAZT does not antagonize the antiviral effect of zidovudine *in vitro* nor does GAZT compete with zidovudine triphosphate as an inhibitor of HIV reverse transcriptase.

The cytotoxicity of zidovudine for various cell lines was determined using a cell growth assay. ID_{50} values for several human cell lines showed little growth inhibition by zidovudine except at concentrations >50 μg/mL. However, one human T-lymphocyte cell line was sensitive to the cytotoxic effect of zidovudine with an ID_{50} of 5 μg/mL. Moreover, in a colony-forming unit assay designed to assess the toxicity of zidovudine for human bone marrow, an ID_{50} value of <1.25 μg/mL was estimated. Two of ten human lymphocyte cultures tested were found to be sensitive to zidovudine at 5 μg/mL or less.

Zidovudine has antiviral activity against some other mammalian retroviruses in addition to HIV. Human Immunodeficiency Virus-2 (HIV-2) replication *in vitro* is inhibited by zidovudine with an ID_{50} of 0.015 μg/mL, while HTLV-1 transmission to susceptible cells is inhibited by 1 to 3 μg/mL concentrations of drug. Several strains of simian immunodeficiency virus (SIV) are also inhibited by zidovudine with ID_{50} values ranging from 0.13 to 6.5 μg/mL, depending upon species of origin and assay method used. No significant inhibitory activity was exhibited against a variety of other human and animal viruses, except an ID_{50} of 1.4 to 2.7 μg/mL against the Epstein-Barr virus, the clinical significance of which is unknown.

The following microbiological activities of zidovudine have been observed *in vitro* but the clinical significance is unknown. Many *Enterobacteriaceae*, including strains of *Shigella, Salmonella, Klebsiella, Enterobacter, Citrobacter,* and *Escherichia coli* are inhibited *in vitro* by low concentrations of zidovudine (0.005 to 0.5 μg/mL). Synergy of zidovudine with trimethoprim has been observed against some of these bacteria *in vitro*. Limited data suggest that bacterial resistance to zidovudine develops rapidly. Zidovudine has no activity against gram positive organisms, anaerobes, mycobacteria, or fungal pathogens including *Candida albicans* and *Cryptococcus neoformans*. Although *Giardia lamblia* is inhibited by 1.9 μg/mL of zidovudine, no activity was observed against other protozoal pathogens.

Pharmacokinetics: General: The pharmacokinetics of zidovudine has been evaluated in 22 adult HIV-infected patients in a Phase I dose-escalation study. Cohorts of 3 to 7 patients received 1 hour intravenous infusions of zidovudine ranging from 1 to 2.5 mg/kg every 8 hours to 2.5 to 7.5 mg/kg every 4 hours (3 to 45 mg/kg/day) for 14 to 28 days. Following intravenous dosing, dose-independent kinetics was observed over the range of 1 to 5 mg/kg with a mean zidovudine half-life of 1.1 hours (range 0.48 to 2.86 hours). Total body clearance averaged 1900 mL/min/70 kg, and the apparent volume of distribution was 1.6 L/kg. At an experimental dose schedule of 7.5 mg/kg every 4 hours, total body clearance was calculated to be about 1200 mL/min/70 kg with no change in half-life. Renal clearance is estimated to be 400 mL/min/70 kg, indicating glomerular filtration and active tubular secretion by the kidneys. Zidovudine plasma protein binding is 34 to 38%, indicating that drug interactions involving binding site displacement are not anticipated. The mean steady-state peak and trough concentrations of zidovudine at 2.5 mg/kg every 4 hours were 1.06 and 0.12 g/mL, respectively. The simultaneous cerebrospinal fluid (CSF)/plasma concentration ratio of zidovudine measured at 2 to 4 hours following dosing of 2.5 mg/kg and 5.0 mg/kg were 0.20 (n = 1) and 0.64 (n = 3), respectively.

Zidovudine is rapidly metabolized to 3′-azido-3′-deoxy-5′-*O*-β-*D*-glucopyranuronosylthymidine (GAZT) which has an apparent elimination half-life of 1 hour (range 0.61 to 1.73 hours). Following intravenous administration, urinary recoveries of zidovudine and GAZT accounted for 18 and 60%

of the dose, respectively, and the total urinary recovery averaged 77% (range 64 to 98%). The pharmacokinetics of zidovudine have been evaluated in patients with impaired renal function following a single 200 mg oral dose. In five anuric patients, the half-life of zidovudine was 1.4 hours compared to 1.0 hour for control subjects with normal renal function; AUC values were approximately twice those of controls. However, in the anuric patients GAZT half-life was 8.0 hours (vs 0.9 hours for control) and AUC was 17 times higher than for control subjects. Hemodialysis appears to have a negligible effect on the removal of zidovudine, whereas GAZT elimination is enhanced.

INDICATIONS AND USAGE

Retrovir I.V. Infusion is indicated for the management of certain adult patients with symptomatic HIV infection (AIDS and advanced ARC) who have a history of cytologically confirmed *Pneumocystis carinii* pneumonia (PCP) or an absolute CD4 (T4 helper/inducer) lymphocyte count of less than 200/mm^3 in the peripheral blood before therapy is begun.

This indication is based primarily on the results of a randomized, double-blind, placebo-controlled trial of oral zidovudine conducted at 12 medical centers in the United States in which 281 patients with AIDS or advanced ARC were studied for an average of four and a half months. Additional data have been collected on patients who have received zidovudine in an open-label extension of this trial. Additional uncontrolled studies completed subsequently support the efficacy of Retrovir in prolonging survival in patients with AIDS and advanced ARC.

The patient population of the controlled trial consisted of 160 AIDS patients (85 Retrovir and 75 placebo) who had recovered from their first episode of PCP diagnosed within the previous four months and 121 ARC patients (59 Retrovir and 62 placebo) with multiple signs and symptoms of HIV infection, including mucocutaneous candidiasis and/or unexplained weight loss (≥ 15 lbs or > 10% of prior body weight). All patients had evidence of impaired cellular immunity with an absence of delayed cutaneous hypersensitivity and a decreased number of CD4 (T4) lymphocytes in the peripheral circulation. Two hundred twenty-one (79% of all patients) had fewer than 200 T4 cells/mm^3 at entry (95% of AIDS patients and 57% of ARC patients). All patients began therapy at a dose of 250 mg orally every 4 hours around the clock. This dosage was reduced or temporarily or permanently discontinued if serious marrow toxicity occurred. The trial was stopped because of a significant reduction in mortality before all patients had completed the planned 24 weeks of treatment. There were 19 deaths in the placebo group and 1 in the Retrovir group ($p < .001$). All deaths were apparently due to opportunistic infections (OI) or other complications of HIV infection. Treatment duration ranged from 12 weeks to 26 weeks, with a mean and median duration of 17 and 18 weeks, respectively.

Retrovir also significantly reduced the risk of acquiring an AIDS-defining OI in patients after 6 weeks of treatment ($p < .001$). In addition, patients who received Retrovir generally did better than the placebo group in terms of several other measures of efficacy including performance level, neuropsychiatric function, maintenance of body weight and the number and severity of symptoms associated with HIV infection. A modest increase in mean CD4 (T4) counts was seen in the zidovudine group but the significance of this finding is unclear as the CD4 (T4) counts declined again in some patients.

The most significant adverse reaction noted in the study was a depression of formed elements in the peripheral blood, which necessitated dose reduction or drug discontinuation in 49 of the 144 (34%) patients receiving Retrovir. Of those participants whose baseline CD4 (T4) lymphocyte counts were ≤ 200, 47% of those receiving Retrovir and 10% of those receiving placebo developed a granulocyte count of < 750/mm^3. Similarly, 45% of Retrovir recipients and only 14% of placebo recipients had a > 25% reduction in hemoglobin (see ADVERSE REACTIONS). Transfusions were administered to some patients with anemia. 47 of 114 (41%) Retrovir recipients and 17 of 107 (16%) placebo recipients with < 200 CD4 lymphocytes at entry were transfused. Only one of 30 Retrovir recipients and none of 30 placebo recipients with > 200 CD4 lymphocytes required transfusion.

Although mean platelet counts in Retrovir recipients were statistically increased compared to mean baseline values, thrombocytopenia did occur in some patients. Twelve percent (12%) of Retrovir recipients compared to 5% of placebo recipients had > 50% decreases from baseline platelet count.

At the conclusion of the placebo-controlled trial, 127 Retrovir recipients and 102 placebo recipients elected to enroll in an uncontrolled extension protocol in which all patients received Retrovir at an oral dose of 200 mg every four hours. This dose was chosen because of concern about cumulative hematologic toxicity and to allow for greater flexibility in dosing. These patients have been followed for variable periods of time. As the follow-up period lengthened, patient tracking became increasingly difficult. The intended treatment period of the original study was six months; however, some follow-up data are available for over 90% of patients originally enrolled in the trial. Data from patients in this and other studies show no new or unexpected clinical or laboratory adverse experiences for patients receiving Retrovir other than those listed (see ADVERSE REACTIONS), nor have previously reported adverse events increased significantly in frequency or severity with prolonged drug administration. At any time on study, approximately half of the patients received the recommended dose of zidovudine, while the remaining patients required reduction or interruption of their dosage regimen in response to myelosuppression and/or other clinical adverse events.

Benefits of therapy with Retrovir were observed during this extended period, although opportunistic infections continued to occur and additional patients died. Survival for all patients originally randomized to receive Retrovir was 96.5% at six months, 84.7% at one year, 68.3% at 18 months and 41.2% at two years. One year and two year survival for patients with AIDS was 79% and 31% when calculated since initiation of therapy (87% and 43%, respectively, since the first diagnosis of PCP). These survival rates were determined by the "intention to treat" method, which assumes all patients assigned to a drug actually took the drug throughout the study period.

While a direct comparison with survival data from other cohorts is not possible, untreated patients with AIDS diagnosed in San Francisco in 1985 who had survived 60 days after PCP had a one year survival of 34.7% and a two year survival of 4.2% from diagnosis of PCP. In a recent epidemiologic study of AIDS patients diagnosed in San Francisco in 1986 and 1987, median survival was improved for patients receiving Retrovir compared to those not receiving therapy with Retrovir (21.6 vs 14.9 months: $p < .001$). Actual survival of untreated patients is likely to be lower than reported because of the difficulty in complete ascertainment of mortality. Caution is advised in making comparisons from such "natural history" experience since case definitions and follow-up practices vary.

Other uncontrolled studies have shown that Retrovir is of benefit in treating women, intravenous drug users, and racial minorities, in addition to the specific patient population (primarily white males) included in the original controlled trial.

Data from a dose comparison study of zidovudine indicate that, in some patients with AIDS, an induction dose of zidovudine 200 mg administered orally every four hours (1200 mg/day) for one month, followed by chronic administration of 100 mg every 4 hours (600 mg/day), was associated with survival rates and frequency of opportunistic infections comparable to those observed in patients administered higher dosages as tolerated. The 600 mg per day regimen was also associated with a lower incidence of hematologic toxicity. The effectiveness of this lower dose in improving the neurologic dysfunction associated with HIV disease, however, is unknown (see DOSAGE AND ADMINISTRATION).

CONTRAINDICATIONS

Retrovir I.V. Infusion is contraindicated for patients who have potentially life-threatening allergic reactions to any of the components of the formulation.

WARNINGS

Zidovudine has been carefully studied in limited numbers of seriously ill HIV-infected patients treated for a limited period of time. Therefore, the full safety and efficacy profile of zidovudine has not been completely defined, particularly in regard to prolonged use, and especially in HIV-infected individuals who have less advanced disease.

Zidovudine should be used with extreme caution in patients who have bone marrow compromise evidenced by granulocyte count < 1000/mm^3 or hemoglobin < 9.5 g/dL. In the placebo-controlled study, anemia and granulocytopenia were the most significant adverse events observed (see ADVERSE REACTIONS). There have been reports of pancytopenia associated with the use of zidovudine, which was reversible in most instances after discontinuance of the drug. Significant anemia most commonly occurred after 4 to 6 weeks of therapy and in many cases required dose adjustment, discontinuation of zidovudine, and/or blood transfusions. Frequent (at least every 2 weeks) blood counts are strongly recommended in patients taking zidovudine. If anemia or granulocytopenia develops, dosage adjustments may be necessary (see DOSAGE AND ADMINISTRATION).

Sensitization reactions, including anaphylaxis in one patient, have been reported in individuals receiving zidovudine therapy. Patients experiencing a rash should undergo medical evaluation.

Coadministration of zidovudine with other drugs metabolized by glucuronidation should be avoided because the toxicity of either drug may be potentiated (see Drug Interactions under PRECAUTIONS). Zidovudine recipients who used acetaminophen during the controlled trial had an increased incidence of granulocytopenia which appeared to be correlated with the duration of acetaminophen use.

PRECAUTIONS

General: Zidovudine is eliminated from the body primarily by renal excretion following metabolism in the liver (glucuronidation). There are currently very little data available concerning the use of zidovudine in patients with impaired renal function (see Pharmacokinetics subsection of CLINICAL PHARMACOLOGY) and no data in patients with impaired hepatic function. These patients may be at greater risk of toxicity from zidovudine.

Information for Patients: Zidovudine is not a cure for HIV infections, and patients may continue to acquire illnesses associated with AIDS or ARC, including opportunistic infections. Therefore, patients should be advised to seek medical care for any significant change in their health status.

Patients should be informed that the major toxicities of zidovudine are granulocytopenia and/or anemia. They should be told that they may require transfusions or dose modifications including possible discontinuation if toxicity develops. They should be told of the extreme importance of having their blood counts followed closely while on therapy. They should be cautioned about the use of other medications such as acetaminophen that may exacerbate the toxicity of zidovudine. (See WARNINGS.)

Patients should be told that the long-term effects of zidovudine are unknown at this time. Patients should be advised that zidovudine therapy has not been shown to reduce the risk of transmission of HIV to others through sexual contact or blood contamination.

Drug Interactions: The interaction of other drugs with zidovudine has not been studied in a systematic manner. Coadministration of zidovudine with drugs that are nephrotoxic, cytotoxic, or which interfere with RBC/WBC number or function (e.g., dapsone, pentamidine, amphotericin B, flucytosine, vincristine, vinblastine, adriamycin, or interferon) may increase the risk of toxicity. Limited data suggest that probenecid may inhibit glucuronidation and/or reduce renal excretion of zidovudine. In addition, other drugs (e.g., acetaminophen, aspirin, or indomethacin) may competitively inhibit glucuronidation (see WARNINGS). Phenytoin levels have been reported to be low in some patients receiving zidovudine, while in one case a high level was documented. These observations suggest that phenytoin levels should be carefully monitored in patients receiving zidovudine since many patients with advanced HIV infections have CNS conditions which may predispose to seizure activity.

Some experimental nucleoside analogues which are being evaluated in AIDS and ARC patients may affect RBC/WBC number or function and may increase the potential for hematologic toxicity of zidovudine. Some experimental nucleoside analogues affecting DNA replication antagonize the *in vitro* antiviral activity of zidovudine against HIV and thus, concomitant use of such drugs should be avoided.

Some drugs such as trimethoprim-sulfamethoxazole, pyrimethamine, and acyclovir may be necessary for the management or prevention of opportunistic infections. In the controlled trial, increased toxicity was not detected with limited exposure to these drugs. However, there is one published report of neurotoxicity (profound lethargy) associated with concomitant use of zidovudine and acyclovir.

Carcinogenesis, Mutagenesis, Impairment of Fertility: Zidovudine was administered orally at three dosage levels to separate groups of mice and rats (60 females and 60 males in each group). Initial single daily doses were 30, 60 and 120 mg/kg/day in mice and 80, 220 and 600 mg/kg/day in rats. The doses in mice were reduced to 20, 30 and 40 mg/kg/day after day 90 because of treatment-related anemia, whereas in rats only the high dose was reduced to 450 mg/kg/day on day 91, and then 300 mg/kg/day on day 279.

In mice, seven late-appearing (after 19 months) vaginal neoplasms (5 non-metastasizing squamous cell carcinomas, one squamous cell papilloma and one squamous polyp) occurred at the highest dose. One late-appearing squamous cell papilloma occurred in the vagina of a middle dose animal. No vaginal tumors were found at the lowest dose.

In rats, two late-appearing (after 20 months), non-metastasizing vaginal squamous cell carcinomas occurred in animals given the highest dose. No vaginal tumors occurred at the low or middle dose in rats.

No other drug-related tumors were observed in either sex of either species.

It is not known how predictive the results of rodent carcinogenicity studies may be for man. At doses that produced tumors in mice and rats, the estimated drug exposure (as measured by AUC) was approximately 3 times (mouse) and 24 times (rat) the estimated human exposure at the recommended therapeutic dose of 100 mg every 4 hours.

No evidence of mutagenicity (with or without metabolic activation) was observed in the Ames *Salmonella* mutagenicity assay. In a mutagenicity assay conducted in L5178Y/TK$^{+/-}$ mouse lymphoma cells, zidovudine was weakly mutagenic in the absence of metabolic activation only at the highest concentrations tested (4000 and 5000 μg/mL). In the presence of metabolic activation, the drug was weakly mutagenic at concentrations of 1000 μg/mL and higher. In an *in vitro* mammalian cell transformation assay, zidovudine was positive at concentrations of 0.5 μg/mL and higher. In an *in vitro* cytogenetic study performed in cultured human lymphocytes,

Continued on next page

Burroughs Wellcome—Cont.

zidovudine induced dose-related structural chromosomal abnormalities at concentrations of 3 µg/mL and higher. No such effects were noted at the two lowest concentrations tested, 0.3 and 1 µg/mL. In an *in vivo* cytogenetic study in rats given a single intravenous injection of zidovudine at doses of 37.5 to 300 mg/kg, there were no treatment-related structural or numerical chromosomal alterations in spite of plasma levels that were as high as 453 µg/mL five minutes after dosing. In two *in vivo* micronucleus studies (designed to measure chromosome breakage or mitotic spindle apparatus damage) in male mice, oral doses of zidovudine of 100 to 1000 mg/kg/day administered once daily for approximately 4 weeks induced dose-related increases in micronucleated erythrocytes. Similar results were also seen after 4 or 7 days of dosing at 500 mg/kg/day in rats and mice.

No effect on male or female fertility (judged by conception rates) was seen in rats given zidovudine orally at doses up to 450 mg/kg/day.

Pregnancy: Pregnancy Category C. Oral teratology studies in the rat and in the rabbit at doses up to 500 mg/kg/day revealed no evidence of teratogenicity with zidovudine. The incidence of fetal resorptions was increased in rats given 150 or 450 mg/kg/day and rabbits given 500 mg/kg/day. The dose levels used in the teratology studies resulted in peak plasma concentrations in rats of 68 to 234 times the peak human plasma concentrations and in rabbits of 14 to 90 times the peak human plasma concentrations. It is not known whether zidovudine can cause fetal harm when administered to a pregnant woman or can affect reproductive capacity. Zidovudine should be given to a pregnant woman only if clearly needed.

Nursing Mothers: It is not known whether zidovudine is excreted in human milk. Because many drugs are excreted in human milk and because of the potential for serious adverse reactions from zidovudine in nursing infants, mothers should be instructed to discontinue nursing if they are receiving zidovudine.

Pediatric Use: The effectiveness of zidovudine in patients 12 years and younger has not been confirmed. Experience from Phase I studies shows that zidovudine administered orally at doses of 120 to 180 mg/m² every six hours (480 to 720 mg/m² per day) appears to give a side effect profile similar to adults. Overall, the pharmacokinetics of zidovudine in children, 6 months through 12 years of age, are similar to those observed in adult patients.

ADVERSE REACTIONS

The most frequent adverse events and abnormal laboratory values reported in the placebo-controlled clinical trial of oral zidovudine administration in 281 patients (144 patients zidovudine; 137 patients placebo) were granulocytopenia and anemia. The occurrence of these hematologic toxicities was inversely related to CD4 (T4) lymphocyte number, hemoglobin, and granulocyte count at study entry, and directly related to dose and duration of therapy. The frequency of granulocytopenia and anemia according to the patients' CD4 (T4) levels is shown in the following table:

[See first table above.]

Because many patients were anemic and/or granulocytopenic before starting therapy with zidovudine, examining the degree of change when compared to baseline, as shown in the table below, may be more informative.

[See second table.]

The anemia appeared to be the result of impaired erythrocyte maturation as evidenced by increasing macrocytosis (MCV) while on drug.

The 281 patients treated in this controlled trial of oral zidovudine had serious underlying disease with multiple baseline symptoms and clinical abnormalities. The following table summarizes those reported clinical adverse events which occurred in at least 5% of all patients treated with zidovudine. Severe headache, nausea, insomnia and myalgia were reported at a significantly greater rate in zidovudine recipients.

[See bottom table.]

Clinical adverse events which occurred in less than 5% of all patients treated with zidovudine are listed below. Since many of these adverse events were seen in placebo-treated patients as well as zidovudine recipients, their possible relationship to the drug is unknown.

Body as a whole: body odor, chills, edema of the lip, flu syndrome, hyperalgesia, back pain, chest pain, lymphadenopathy.

Cardiovascular: vasodilation.

Gastrointestinal: constipation, dysphagia, edema of the tongue, eructation, flatulence, bleeding gums, rectal hemorrhage, mouth ulcer.

Musculoskeletal: arthralgia, muscle spasm, tremor, twitch.

Nervous: anxiety, confusion, depression, emotional lability, nervousness, syncope, loss of mental acuity, vertigo.

Respiratory: cough, epistaxis, pharyngitis, rhinitis, sinusitis, hoarseness.

Skin: acne, pruritus, urticaria.

Special senses: amblyopia, hearing loss, photophobia.

Urogenital: dysuria, polyuria, urinary frequency, urinary hesitancy.

Subsequent to the initial trial, sensitization reactions, including anaphylaxis in one patient, have been reported in individuals receiving zidovudine therapy.

The following events have been reported in patients treated with zidovudine. They may also occur as part of the underlying disease process. As such, the relationship between these events and the use of zidovudine is uncertain: seizures, myopathy, nail pigmentation, changes in liver function tests.

The adverse events reported during intravenous administration of Retrovir IV Infusion are similar to those reported with oral administration; granulocytopenia and anemia were reported most frequently. Long-term intravenous administration beyond 2 to 4 weeks has not been studied in adults and may enhance hematologic adverse events. Local reaction, pain and slight irritation during intravenous administration occur infrequently.

OVERDOSAGE

Cases of acute overdoses in both children and adults have been reported with doses up to 50 grams. None were fatal. The only consistent finding in these cases of overdose was spontaneous or induced nausea and vomiting. Hematologic changes were transient and not severe. All patients recovered without permanent sequelae. Hemodialysis appears to have a negligible effect on the removal of zidovudine while elimination of its primary metabolite, GAZT, is enhanced.

DOSAGE AND ADMINISTRATION

Dosage: 1 to 2 mg/kg infused over 1 hour. This dose should be administered every 4 hours around the clock (6 times daily). Patients should receive Retrovir I.V. Infusion only until oral therapy can be administered (see recommended oral doses below).

The recommended oral starting dose in adults is 200 mg (two 100 mg capsules or four teaspoonfuls [20 mL] syrup) administered every four hours (1200 mg total daily dose). After one month, the dose may be reduced to 100 mg every four hours (600 mg total daily dose). The intravenous dosing regimen equivalent to the oral administration of 100 mg every four hours is approximately 1 mg/kg intravenously every four hours. The effectiveness of this lower dose in improving the neurologic dysfunction associated with HIV disease is unknown (see INDICATIONS AND USAGE).

Hematologic toxicities appear to be related to pretreatment bone marrow reserve and to dose and duration of therapy. Careful monitoring of hematologic indices every two weeks is recommended to detect serious anemia or granulocytopenia. In patients with hematologic toxicity, reduction in he-

Abnormality	Pretreatment CD4 (T4) Levels	
	≤ 200/mm³	
	Zidovudine (n=113)	Placebo (n=105)
Granulocytopenia (< 750/mm³)	47%	10%
Anemia (Hgb < 7.5 g/dL)	30%	6%
	> 200/mm³	
	(n=30)	(n=30)
Granulocytopenia (< 750/mm³)	10%	3%
Anemia (Hgb < 7.5 g/dL)	3%	0%

Abnormality	% Decrease from Baseline	Pretreatment CD4 (T4) Levels	
		≤ 200/mm³	
		Zidovudine (n=113)	Placebo (n=105)
Granulocytopenia	> 50%	55%	19%
Anemia	> 25%	45%	14%
		> 200/mm³	
		(n=30)	(n=30)
Granulocytopenia	> 50%	40%	13%
Anemia	> 25%	10%	10%

Percentage (%) of Patients with Clinical Events

Adverse Event	Zidovudine (n=144) %	Placebo (n=137) %
BODY AS A WHOLE		
Asthenia	19	18
Diaphoresis	5	4
Fever	16	12
Headache	42	37
Malaise	8	7
GASTROINTESTINAL		
Anorexia	11	8
Diarrhea	12	18
Dyspepsia	5	4
GI Pain	20	19
Nausea	46	18
Vomiting	6	3
MUSCULOSKELETAL		
Myalgia	8	2
NERVOUS		
Dizziness	6	4
Insomnia	5	1
Paresthesia	6	3
Somnolence	8	9
RESPIRATORY		
Dyspnea	5	3
SKIN		
Rash	17	15
SPECIAL SENSES		
Taste Perversion	5	8

moglobin may occur as early as 2 to 4 weeks, and granulocytopenia usually occurs after 6 to 8 weeks.

Dose Adjustment: Significant anemia (hemoglobin of <7.5 g/dL or reduction of $>25\%$ of baseline) and/or significant granulocytopenia (granulocyte count of $<750/mm^3$ or reduction of $>50\%$ from baseline) may require a dose interruption until some evidence of marrow recovery is observed. For less severe anemia or granulocytopenia, a reduction in daily dose may be adequate. In patients who develop significant anemia, dose modification does not necessarily eliminate the need for transfusion. If marrow recovery occurs following dose modification, gradual increases in dose may be appropriate depending on hematologic indices and patient tolerance.

There are insufficient data to recommend dose adjustment of zidovudine in patients with impaired renal or hepatic function (see Pharmacokinetics).

Method of Preparation: Retrovir I.V. Infusion must be diluted prior to administration. The calculated dose should be removed from the 20 mL vial and added to 5% Dextrose Injection solution to achieve a concentration no greater than 4 mg/mL. Admixture in biologic or colloidal fluids (e.g., blood products, protein solutions, etc.) is not recommended.

After dilution, the solution is physically and chemically stable for 24 hours at room temperature and 48 hours if refrigerated at 2° to 8°C (36° to 46°F). Care should be taken during admixture to prevent inadvertent contamination. As an additional precaution, the diluted solution should be administered within 8 hours if stored at 25°C (77°F) or 24 hours if refrigerated at 2° to 8°C to minimize potential administration of a microbially contaminated solution.

Parenteral drug products should be inspected visually for particulate matter and discoloration prior to administration whenever solution and container permit. Should either be observed, the solution should be discarded and fresh solution prepared.

Administration: Retrovir I.V. Infusion is administered intravenously at a constant rate over one hour. Rapid infusion or bolus injection should be avoided. Retrovir I.V. Infusion should not be given intramuscularly.

HOW SUPPLIED

Retrovir I.V. Infusion, 10 mg zidovudine in each mL. 20 mL Single-Use Vial, Tray of 10 (NDC 0081-0107-93).

Store vials at 15° to 25°C (59° to 77°F) and protect from light.

Also Available: Retrovir Capsules 100 mg, bottle of 100; Retrovir Syrup, bottle of 240 mL.

U.S. Patent No. 4724232 (Use Patent)

Other Pats. Pending   587054

SEPTRA® I.V. INFUSION   ℞
[sĕp'trah]
(Trimethoprim and Sulfamethoxazole)

DESCRIPTION

Septra I.V. Infusion (Trimethoprim and Sulfamethoxazole), a sterile solution for intravenous infusion only, is a synthetic antibacterial combination product. Each mL contains 16 mg trimethoprim* and 80 mg sulfamethoxazole compounded with 40% propylene glycol, 10% ethyl alcohol and 0.3% diethanolamine; 1% benzyl alcohol and 0.1% sodium metabisulfite added as preservatives, water for injection, and pH adjusted to approximately 10 with sodium hydroxide.

Trimethoprim is 2,4-diamino-5-(3,4,5-trimethoxybenzyl)-pyrimidine. It is a white to light yellow, odorless, bitter compound with a molecular weight of 290.3 and the molecular formula $C_{14}H_{18}N_4O_3$.

Sulfamethoxazole is N^1-(5-methyl-3-isoxazolyl)sulfanilamide. It is an almost white, odorless, tasteless compound with a molecular weight of 253.28 and the molecular formula $C_{10}H_{11}N_3O_3S$.

CLINICAL PHARMACOLOGY

Following a one-hour intravenous infusion of a single dose of 160 mg trimethoprim and 800 mg sulfamethoxazole to 11 patients whose weight ranged from 105 lbs. to 165 lbs. (mean, 143 lbs.), the mean peak plasma concentrations of trimethoprim and sulfamethoxazole were 3.4 ± 0.3 µg/mL and 46.3 ± 2.7 µg/mL, respectively. Following repeated intravenous administration of the same dose at eight-hour intervals, the mean plasma concentrations just prior to and immediately after each infusion at steady state were 5.6 ± 0.6 µg/mL and 8.8 ± 0.9 µg/mL for trimethoprim and 70.6 ± 7.3 µg/mL and 105.6 ± 10.9 µg/mL for sulfamethoxazole. The mean plasma half-life was 11.3 ± 0.7 hours for trimethoprim and 12.8 ± 1.8 hours for sulfamethoxazole. All of these 11 patients had normal renal function and their ages ranged from 17 to 78 years (median, 60 years)[1].

*Mfd. under U.S. Patent No. 3,956,327

REPRESENTATIVE MINIMUM INHIBITORY CONCENTRATION VALUES FOR SEPTRA SUSCEPTIBLE ORGANISMS (MIC-µg/mL)

Bacteria	TMP Alone	SMX Alone	TMP/SMX (1:19) TMP	TMP/SMX (1:19) SMX
Escherichia coli	0.05–1.5	1.0–245	0.05–0.5	0.95–9.5
Proteus species (indole positive)	0.5–5.0	7.35–300	0.05–1.5	0.95–28.5
Morganella morganii	0.5–5.0	7.35–300	0.05–1.5	0.95–28.5
Proteus mirabilis	0.5–1.5	7.35–30	0.05–0.15	0.95–2.85
Klebsiella species	0.15–5.0	2.45–245	0.05–1.5	0.95–28.5
Enterobacter species	0.15–5.0	2.45–245	0.05–1.5	0.95–28.5
Haemophilus influenzae	0.15–1.5	2.85–95	0.015–0.15	0.285–2.85
Streptococcus pneumoniae	0.15–1.5	7.35–24.5	0.05–0.15	0.95–2.85
Shigella flexneri †	<0.01–0.04	<0.16–>320	<0.002–0.03	0.04–0.625
Shigella sonnei †	0.02–0.08	0.625–>320	0.004–0.06	0.08–1.25

TMP = Trimethoprim   SMX = Sulfamethoxazole
†Rudoy RC, Nelson JD, Haltalin KC. *Antimicrobial Agents and Chemotherapy* 5:439-43, 1974.

Pharmacokinetic studies in children and adults suggest an age-dependent half-life of trimethoprim as indicated in the following table.[2]

Age (yrs.)	No. of Patients	Mean TMP Half-life (hours)
<1	2	7.67
1–10	9	5.49
10–20	5	8.19
20–63	6	12.82

Patients with severely impaired renal function exhibit an increase in the half-lives of both components, requiring dosage regimen adjustment (see DOSAGE AND ADMINISTRATION section).

Both trimethoprim and sulfamethoxazole exist in the blood as unbound, protein-bound and metabolized forms; sulfamethoxazole also exists as the conjugated form. The metabolism of sulfamethoxazole occurs predominately by N_4-acetylation, although the glucuronide conjugate has been identified. The principal metabolites of trimethoprim are the 1- and 3- oxides and the 3'- and 4'-hydroxy derivatives. The free forms of trimethoprim and sulfamethoxazole are considered to be the therapeutically active forms. Approximately 44% of trimethoprim and 70% of sulfamethoxazole are bound to plasma proteins. The presence of 10 mg percent sulfamethoxazole in plasma decreases the protein binding of trimethoprim by an insignificant degree; trimethoprim does not influence the protein binding of sulfamethoxazole.

Excretion of trimethoprim and sulfamethoxazole is primarily by the kidneys through both glomerular filtration and tubular secretion. Urine concentrations of both trimethoprim and sulfamethoxazole are considerably higher than are the concentrations in the blood. The percent of dose excreted in urine over a 12-hour period following the intravenous administration of the first dose of 240 mg of trimethoprim and 1200 mg of sulfamethoxazole on day 1 ranged from 17% to 42.4% as free trimethoprim; 7% to 12.7% as free sulfamethoxazole; and 36.7% to 56% as total (free plus the N_4-acetylated metabolite) sulfamethoxazole. When administered together as Septra, neither trimethoprim nor sulfamethoxazole affects the urinary excretion pattern of the other.

Both trimethoprim and sulfamethoxazole distribute to sputum and vaginal fluid; trimethoprim also distributes to bronchial secretions and both pass the placental barrier and are excreted in human milk.

Microbiology: Sulfamethoxazole inhibits bacterial synthesis of dihydrofolic acid by competing with *para*- aminobenzoic acid (PABA). Trimethoprim blocks the production of tetrahydrofolic acid from dihydrofolic acid by binding to and reversibly inhibiting the required enzyme, dihydrofolate reductase. Thus, Septra blocks two consecutive steps in the biosynthesis of nucleic acids and proteins essential to many bacteria.

In vitro studies have shown that bacterial resistance develops more slowly with Septra than with trimethoprim or sulfamethoxazole alone.

In vitro serial dilution tests have shown that the spectrum of antibacterial activity of Septra includes common bacterial pathogens with the exception of *Pseudomonas aeruginosa*. The following organisms are usually susceptible: *Escherichia coli*, *Klebsiella* species, *Enterobacter* species, *Morganella morganii*, *Proteus mirabilis*, indole-positive *Proteus* species, including *Proteus vulgaris*, *Haemophilus influenzae* (including ampicillin-resistant strains), *Streptococcus pneumoniae*, *Shigella flexneri* and *Shigella sonnei*. It should be noted, however, that there are little clinical data on the use of Septra I.V. Infusion in serious systemic infections due to *Haemophilus influenzae* and *Streptococcus pneumoniae*.
[See table above.]

Susceptibility Testing: The recommended quantitative disc susceptibility method may be used for estimating the suscep-

tibility of bacteria to Septra.[3,4] With this procedure, a report from the laboratory of "Susceptible to trimethoprim and sulfamethoxazole" indicates that the infection is likely to respond to therapy with Septra. If the infection is confined to the urine, a report of "Intermediate susceptibility to trimethoprim and sulfamethoxazole" also indicates that the infection is likely to respond. A report of "Resistant to trimethoprim and sulfamethoxazole" indicates that the infection is unlikely to respond to therapy with Septra.

INDICATIONS AND USAGE

PNEUMOCYSTIS CARINII PNEUMONIA: Septra I.V. Infusion is indicated in the treatment of *Pneumocystis carinii* pneumonia in children and adults.

SHIGELLOSIS: Septra I.V. Infusion is indicated in the treatment of enteritis caused by susceptible strains of *Shigella flexneri* and *Shigella sonnei* in children and adults.

URINARY TRACT INFECTIONS: Septra I.V. Infusion is indicated in the treatment of severe or complicated urinary tract infections due to susceptible strains of *Escherichia coli*, *Klebsiella* species, *Enterobacter* species, *Morganella morganii*, and *Proteus* species when oral administration of Septra is not feasible and when the organism is not susceptible to single agent antibacterials effective in the urinary tract.

Although appropriate culture and susceptibility studies should be performed, therapy may be started while awaiting the results of these studies.

CONTRAINDICATIONS

Hypersensitivity to trimethoprim or sulfonamides. Patients with documented megaloblastic anemia due to folate deficiency. Pregnancy at term and during the nursing period, because sulfonamides pass the placenta and are excreted in the milk and may cause kernicterus. Infants less than two months of age.

WARNINGS

FATALITIES ASSOCIATED WITH THE ADMINISTRATION OF SULFONAMIDES, ALTHOUGH RARE, HAVE OCCURRED DUE TO SEVERE REACTIONS, INCLUDING STEVENS-JOHNSON SYNDROME, TOXIC EPIDERMAL NECROLYSIS, FULMINANT HEPATIC NECROSIS, AGRANULOCYTOSIS, APLASTIC ANEMIA, OTHER BLOOD DYSCRASIAS AND HYPERSENSITIVITY OF THE RESPIRATORY TRACT.

SEPTRA SHOULD BE DISCONTINUED AT THE FIRST APPEARANCE OF SKIN RASH OR ANY SIGN OF ADVERSE REACTION. Clinical signs, such as rash, sore throat, fever, arthralgia, cough, shortness of breath, pallor, purpura or jaundice may be early indications of serious reactions. Cough, shortness of breath, and/or pulmonary infiltrates may be indicators of pulmonary hypersensitivity to sulfonamides. In rare instances, a skin rash may be followed by more severe reactions, such as Stevens-Johnson syndrome, toxic epidermal necrolysis, hepatic necrosis or serious blood disorder. Complete blood counts should be done frequently in patients receiving sulfonamides.

SEPTRA SHOULD NOT BE USED IN THE TREATMENT OF STREPTOCOCCAL PHARYNGITIS. Clinical studies have documented that patients with group A β-hemolytic streptococcal tonsillopharyngitis have a greater incidence of bacteriologic failure when treated with Septra than do those patients treated with penicillin, as evidenced by failure to eradicate this organism from the tonsillopharyngeal area. Contains sodium metabisulfite, a sulfite that may cause allergic-type reactions including anaphylactic symptoms and life-threatening or less severe asthmatic episodes in certain susceptible people. The overall prevalence of sulfite sensitiv-

Continued on next page

Burroughs Wellcome—Cont.

ity in the general population is unknown and probably low. Sulfite sensitivity is seen more frequently in asthmatic than in nonasthmatic people.

Contains benzyl alcohol. In newborn infants, benzyl alcohol has been associated with an increased incidence of neurological and other complications which are sometimes fatal.

PRECAUTIONS

General: Septra should be given with caution to patients with impaired renal or hepatic function, to those with possible folate deficiency (e.g., the elderly, chronic alcoholics, patients receiving anticonvulsant therapy, patients with malabsorption syndrome, and patients in malnutrition states) and to those with severe allergy or bronchial asthma. In glucose-6-phosphate dehydrogenase-deficient individuals, hemolysis may occur. This reaction is frequently dose-related. Adequate fluid intake must be maintained in order to prevent crystalluria and stone formation. (See CLINICAL PHARMACOLOGY and DOSAGE AND ADMINISTRATION.)

Local irritation and inflammation due to extravascular infiltration of the infusion has been observed with Septra I.V. Infusion. If these occur the infusion should be discontinued and restarted at another site.

Use in the Elderly: There may be an increased risk of severe adverse reactions in elderly patients, particularly when complicating conditions exist, e.g., impaired kidney and/or liver function, or concomitant use of other drugs. Severe skin reactions, or generalized bone marrow suppression (see WARNINGS and ADVERSE REACTIONS sections) or a specific decrease in platelets (with or without purpura) are the most frequently reported severe adverse reactions in elderly patients. In those concurrently receiving certain diuretics, primarily thiazides, an increased incidence of thrombocytopenia with purpura has been reported. Appropriate dosage adjustments should be made for patients with impaired kidney function (see DOSAGE AND ADMINISTRATION section).

Use in the Treatment of *Pneumocystis carinii* Pneumonia in Patients with Acquired Immunodeficiency Syndrome (AIDS): The incidence of side effects, particularly rash, fever, leukopenia, and elevated aminotransferase (transminase) values with Septra therapy in AIDS patients who are being treated for *Pneumocystis carinii* pneumonia has been reported to be greatly increased compared with the incidence normally associated with the use of Septra in non-AIDS patients.

Laboratory Tests: Appropriate culture and susceptibility studies should be performed before and throughout treatment. Complete blood counts should be done frequently in patients receiving Septra; if a significant reduction in the count of any formed blood element is noted, Septra should be discontinued. Urinalyses with careful microscopic examination and renal function tests should be performed during therapy, particularly for those patients with impaired renal function.

Drug Interactions: In elderly patients concurrently receiving certain diuretics, primarily thiazides, an increased incidence of thrombocytopenia with purpura has been reported. It has been reported that Septra may prolong the prothrombin time in patients who are receiving the anticoagulant warfarin. This interaction should be kept in mind when Septra is given to patients already on anticoagulant therapy, and the coagulation time should be reassessed.

Septra may inhibit the hepatic metabolism of phenytoin. Septra, given at a common clinical dosage, increased the phenytoin half-life by 39% and decreased the phenytoin metabolic clearance rate by 27%. When administering these drugs concurrently, one should be alert for possible excessive phenytoin effect.

Sulfonamides can also displace methotrexate from plasma protein binding sites, thus increasing free methotrexate concentrations.

Drug/Laboratory Test Interactions: Septra, specifically the trimethoprim component, can interfere with a serum methotrexate assay as determined by the competitive binding protein technique (CBPA) when a bacterial dihydrofolate reductase is used as the binding protein. No interference occurs, however, if methotrexate is measured by a radioimmunoassay (RIA).

The presence of trimethoprim and sulfamethoxazole may also interfere with the Jaffé alkaline picrate reaction assay for creatinine resulting in over-estimations of about 10% in the range of normal values.

Carcinogenesis, Mutagenesis, Impairment of Fertility:

Carcinogenesis: Long-term studies in animals to evaluate carcinogenic potential have not been conducted with Septra I.V. Infusion.

Mutagenesis: Bacterial mutagenic studies have not been performed with sulfamethoxazole and trimethoprim in combination. Trimethoprim was demonstrated to be non-mutagenic in the Ames assay. In studies at two laboratories no chromosomal damage was detected in cultured Chinese hamster ovary cells at concentrations approximately 500 times human plasma levels; at concentrations approximately 1000 times human plasma levels in these same cells a low level of chromosomal damage was induced at one of the laboratories. No chromosomal abnormalities were observed in cultured human leukocytes at concentrations of trimethoprim up to 20 times human steady state plasma levels. No chromosomal effects were detected in peripheral lymphocytes of human subjects receiving 320 mg of trimethoprim in combination with up to 1600 mg of sulfamethoxazole per day for as long as 112 weeks.

Impairment of Fertility: Septra I.V. Infusion has not been studied in animals for evidence of impairment of fertility. However, studies in rats at oral dosages as high as 70 mg/kg trimethoprim plus 350 mg/kg sulfamethoxazole daily showed no adverse effects on fertility or general reproductive performance.

Pregnancy: *Teratogenic Effects:* Pregnancy Category C. In rats, oral doses of 533 mg/kg sulfamethoxazole or 200 mg/kg trimethoprim produced teratological effects manifested mainly as cleft palates. The highest dose which did not cause cleft palates in rats was 512 mg/kg sulfamethoxazole or 192 mg/kg trimethoprim when administered separately. In two studies in rats, no teratology was observed when 512 mg/kg of sulfamethoxazole was used in combination with 128 mg/kg of trimethoprim. In one study, however, cleft palates were observed in one litter out of 9 when 355 mg/kg of sulfamethoxazole was used in combination with 88 mg/kg of trimethoprim.

In some rabbit studies, an overall increase in fetal loss (dead and resorbed and malformed conceptuses) was associated with doses of trimethoprim 6 times the human therapeutic dose.

While there are no large, well-controlled studies on the use of trimethoprim and sulfamethoxazole in pregnant women, Brumfitt and Pursell[5], in a retrospective study, reported the outcome of 186 pregnancies during which the mother received either placebo or oral trimethoprim and sulfamethoxazole. The incidence of congenital abnormalities was 4.5% (3 of 66) in those who received placebo and 3.3% (4 of 120) in those receiving trimethoprim and sulfamethoxazole. There were no abnormalities in the 10 children whose mothers received the drug during the first trimester. In a separate survey, Brumfitt and Pursell also found no congenital abnormalities in 35 children whose mothers had received oral trimethoprim and sulfamethoxazole at the time of conception or shortly thereafter.

Because trimethoprim and sulfamethoxazole may interfere with folic acid metabolism, Septra I.V. Infusion should be used during pregnancy only if the potential benefit justifies the potential risk to the fetus.

Nonteratogenic Effects: See CONTRAINDICATIONS section.

Nursing Mothers: See CONTRAINDICATIONS section.

Pediatric Use: Septra I.V. Infusion is not recommended for infants younger than two months of age (see CONTRAINDICATIONS section).

ADVERSE REACTIONS

The most common adverse effects are gastrointestinal disturbances (nausea, vomiting, anorexia) and allergic skin reactions (such as rash and urticaria). **FATALITIES ASSOCIATED WITH THE ADMINISTRATION OF SULFONAMIDES, ALTHOUGH RARE, HAVE OCCURRED DUE TO SEVERE REACTIONS, INCLUDING STEVENS-JOHNSON SYNDROME, TOXIC EPIDERMAL NECROLYSIS, FULMINANT HEPATIC NECROSIS, AGRANULOCYTOSIS, APLASTIC ANEMIA, OTHER BLOOD DYSCRASIAS AND HYPERSENSITIVITY OF THE RESPIRATORY TRACT (SEE WARNINGS SECTION).** Local reaction, pain and slight irritation on I.V. administration are infrequent. Thrombophlebitis has rarely been observed.

Hematologic: Agranulocytosis, aplastic anemia, thrombocytopenia, leukopenia, neutropenia, hemolytic anemia, megaloblastic anemia, hypoprothrombinemia, methemoglobinemia, eosinophilia.

Allergic: Stevens-Johnson syndrome, toxic epidermal necrolysis, anaphylaxis, allergic myocarditis, erythema multiforme, exfoliative dermatitis, angioedema, drug fever, chills, Henoch-Schoenlein purpura, serum sickness-like syndrome, generalized allergic reactions, generalized skin eruptions, conjunctival and scleral injection, photosensitivity, pruritus, urticaria and rash. In addition, periarteritis nodosa and systemic lupus erythematosus have been reported.

Gastrointestinal: Hepatitis including cholestatic jaundice and hepatic necrosis, elevation of serum transaminase and bilirubin, pseudomembranous enterocolitis, pancreatitis, stomatitis, glossitis, nausea, emesis, abdominal pain, diarrhea, anorexia.

Genitourinary: Renal failure, interstitial nephritis, BUN and serum creatinine elevation, toxic nephrosis with oliguria and anuria, and crystalluria.

Neurologic: Aseptic meningitis, convulsions, peripheral neuritis, ataxia, vertigo, tinnitus, headache.

Psychiatric: Hallucinations, depression, apathy, nervousness.

Endocrine: The sulfonamides bear certain chemical similarities to some goitrogens, diuretics (acetazolamide and the thiazides) and oral hypoglycemic agents. Cross-sensitivity may exist with these agents. Diuresis and hypoglycemia have occurred rarely in patients receiving sulfonamides.

Musculoskeletal: Arthralgia and myalgia.

Respiratory System: Pulmonary infiltrates, cough, shortness of breath.

Miscellaneous: Weakness, fatigue, insomnia.

OVERDOSAGE

Acute: Since there has been no extensive experience in humans with single doses of Septra I.V. Infusion in excess of 25 mL (400 mg trimethoprim and 2000 mg sulfamethoxazole), the maximum tolerated dose in humans is unknown. Signs and symptoms of overdosage reported with sulfonamides include anorexia, colic, nausea, vomiting, dizziness, headache, drowsiness and unconsciousness. Pyrexia, hematuria and crystalluria may be noted. Blood dyscrasias and jaundice are potential late manifestations of overdosage. Signs of acute overdosage with trimethoprim include nausea, vomiting, dizziness, headache, mental depression, confusion and bone marrow depression.

General principles of treatment include the administration of intravenous fluids if urine output is low and renal function is normal. Acidification of the urine will increase renal elimination of trimethoprim. The patient should be monitored with blood counts and appropriate blood chemistries, including electrolytes. If a significant blood dyscrasia or jaundice occurs, specific therapy should be instituted for these complications. Peritoneal dialysis is not effective and hemodialysis is only moderately effective in eliminating trimethoprim and sulfamethoxazole.

Chronic: Use of Septra I.V. Infusion at high doses and/or for extended periods of time may cause bone marrow depression manifested as thrombocytopenia, leukopenia, and/or megaloblastic anemia. If signs of bone marrow depression occur, the patient should be given leucovorin; 5 to 15 mg leucovorin daily has been recommended by some investigators.

Animal Toxicity: The LD_{50} of Septra I.V. Infusion in mice is 700 mg/kg or 7.3 mL/kg; in rats and rabbits the LD_{50} is > 500 mg/kg or > 5.2 mL/kg. The vehicle produced the same LD_{50} in each of these species as the active drug.

The signs and symptoms noted in mice, rats and rabbits with Septra I.V. Infusion or its vehicle at the high I.V. doses used in acute toxicity studies included ataxia, decreased motor activity, loss of righting reflex, tremors or convulsions, and/or respiratory depression.

DOSAGE AND ADMINISTRATION

CONTRAINDICATED IN INFANTS LESS THAN TWO MONTHS OF AGE. CAUTION—SEPTRA I.V. INFUSION MUST BE DILUTED IN 5% DEXTROSE IN WATER SOLUTION PRIOR TO ADMINISTRATION. DO NOT MIX SEPTRA I.V. INFUSION WITH OTHER DRUGS OR SOLUTIONS. RAPID INFUSION OR BOLUS INJECTION MUST BE AVOIDED.

DOSAGE

Children and Adults:

PNEUMOCYSTIS CARINII PNEUMONIA: Total daily dose is 15 to 20 mg/kg (based on the trimethoprim component) given in three to four equally divided doses every 6 or 8 hours for up to 14 days. One investigator noted that a total daily dose of 10 to 15 mg/kg was sufficient in 10 adult patients with normal renal function.[6]

SEVERE URINARY TRACT INFECTIONS AND SHIGELLOSIS: Total daily dose is 8 to 10 mg/kg (based on the trimethoprim component) given in two to four equally divided doses every 6, 8 or 12 hours for up to 14 days for severe urinary tract infections and 5 days for shigellosis. The maximum recommended daily dose is 60 mL per day.

For Patients with Impaired Renal Function: When renal function is impaired, a reduced dosage should be employed using the following table:

Creatinine Clearance (mL/min)	Recommended Dosage Regimen
Above 30	Use Standard Regimen
15–30	½ the Usual Regimen
Below 15	Use Not Recommended

Method of Preparation: Septra I.V. Infusion must be diluted. EACH 5 mL SHOULD BE ADDED TO 125 mL OF 5% DEXTROSE IN WATER. After diluting with 5% dextrose in water the solution should not be refrigerated and should be used within 6 hours. If a dilution of 5 mL per 100 mL of 5% dextrose in water is desired, it should be used within 4 hours. If upon visual inspection there is cloudiness or evidence of crystallization after mixing, the solution should be discarded and a fresh solution prepared.

Multiple Dose Vial: After initial entry into the vial, the remaining contents must be used within 48 hours.

The following infusion systems have been tested and found satisfactory: unit-dose glass containers; unit-dose polyvinyl chloride and polyolefin containers. No other systems have been tested and therefore no others can be recommended.

Dilution: EACH 5 mL OF SEPTRA I.V. INFUSION SHOULD BE ADDED TO 125 mL OF 5% DEXTROSE IN WATER.

NOTE: **In those instances where fluid restriction is desirable,** each 5 mL may be added to 75 mL of 5% dextrose in water. Under these circumstances the solution should be mixed just prior to use and should be administered within two (2) hours. If upon visual inspection there is cloudiness or evidence of crystallization after mixing, the solution should be discarded and a fresh solution prepared.

DO NOT MIX SEPTRA I.V. INFUSION-5% DEXTROSE IN WATER WITH DRUGS OR SOLUTIONS IN THE SAME CONTAINER.

ADMINISTRATION

The solution should be given by intravenous infusion over a period of 60 to 90 minutes. Rapid infusion or bolus injections must be avoided. Septra I.V. Infusion should not be given intramuscularly.

HOW SUPPLIED

5 mL vials, containing 80 mg trimethoprim (16 mg/mL) and 400 mg sulfamethoxazole (80 mg/mL) for infusion with 5% dextrose in water. Contains benzyl alcohol (see WARNINGS). Tray of 10 (NDC 0081-0856-44).

10 mL multiple dose vials, containing 160 mg trimethoprim (16 mg/mL) and 800 mg sulfamethoxazole (80 mg/mL) for infusion with 5% dextrose in water. Contains benzyl alcohol (see WARNINGS). Tray of 10 (NDC 0081-0856-95).

20 mL multiple dose vials, containing 320 mg trimethoprim (16 mg/mL) and 1600 mg sulfamethoxazole (80 mg/mL) for infusion with 5% dextrose in water. Contains benzyl alcohol (see WARNINGS). Tray of 10 (NDC 0081-0856-93).

STORE AT 15° to 25°C (59° to 77°F). DO NOT REFRIGERATE.

Also available in tablets containing 80 mg trimethoprim and 400 mg sulfamethoxazole (bottles of 100); DS (double strength) tablets containing 160 mg trimethoprim and 800 mg sulfamethoxazole (bottles of 100 and 250; unit dose pack of 100); and oral suspension containing 40 mg trimethoprim and 200 mg sulfamethoxazole in each 5 mL (pink, cherry-flavored: bottle of 1 pint [473 mL]; bottles of 20 mL—tray of 12, 100 mL—package of 6, 150 mL—package of 6 and 200 mL—tray of 6 with child-resistant caps; and purple, grape-flavored: bottle of 1 pint [473 mL]).

REFERENCES

1. Grose WE, Bodey GP, Loo TL. Clinical pharmacology of intravenously administered trimethoprim-sulfamethoxazole. *Antimicrob Agents Chemother.* 1979; 15:447–451.
2. Siber GR, Gorham C, Durbin W, Lesko L, Levin MJ. Pharmacology of intravenous trimethoprim-sulfamethoxazole in children and adults. In: Nelson JD, Grassi C, eds. *Current Chemotherapy of Infectious Disease.* Washington, DC: American Society for Microbiology, 1980; 1:691–692.
3. Bauer AW, Kirby WMM, Sherris JC, Turck M. Antibiotic susceptibility testing by standardized single disk method. *Am J Clin Pathol.* 1966; 45:493–496.
4. National Committee for Clinical Laboratory Standards. Performance standards for antimicrobial disk susceptibility tests, 2nd ed. Villanova, PA. 1979.
5. Brumfitt W, Pursell R. Trimethoprim-sulfamethoxazole in the treatment of bacteriuria in women. *J Infect Dis.* November 1973; 128(suppl):S657–S663.
6. Winston DJ, Lau WK, Gale RP, Young LS. Trimethoprim-sulfamethoxazole for the treatment of *Pneumocystis carinii* pneumonia. *Ann Int Med.* 1980; 92:762–769.

SEPTRA® I.V. INFUSION ℞

[*sĕp'trah*]

ADD-Vantage® Vials

(Trimethoprim and Sulfamethoxazole)

DESCRIPTION

Septra I.V. Infusion (Trimethoprim and Sulfamethoxazole), a sterile solution for intravenous infusion only, is a synthetic antibacterial combination product. Each mL contains 16 mg trimethoprim* and 80 mg sulfamethoxazole compounded with 40% propylene glycol, 10% ethyl alcohol and 0.3% diethanolamine; 1% benzyl alcohol and 0.1% sodium metabisulfite added as preservatives, water for injection, and pH adjusted to approximately 10 with sodium hydroxide.

Trimethoprim is 2,4-diamino-5-(3,4,5-trimethoxybenzyl) pyrimidine. It is a white to light yellow, odorless, bitter compound with a molecular weight of 290.3 and the molecular formula $C_{14}H_{18}N_4O_3$.

Sulfamethoxazole is N^1-(5-methyl-3-isoxazolyl) sulfanilamide. It is an almost white, odorless, tasteless compound with a molecular weight of 253.28 and the molecular formula $C_{10}H_{11}N_3O_3S$.

*Mfd. under U.S. Patent No. 3,956,327.

REPRESENTATIVE MINIMUM INHIBITORY CONCENTRATION VALUES FOR SEPTRA SUSCEPTIBLE ORGANISMS (MIC-μg/mL)

Bacteria	Trimethoprim Alone	Sulfamethoxazole Alone	Trimethoprim/Sulfamethoxazole (1:19)	
			Trimethoprim	Sulfamethoxazole
Escherichia coli	0.05–1.5	1.0–245	0.05–0.5	0.95–9.5
Proteus species (indole positive)	0.5–5.0	7.35–300	0.05–1.5	0.95–28.5
Morganella morganii	0.5–5.0	7.35–300	0.05–1.5	0.95–28.5
Proteus mirabilis	0.5–1.5	7.35–30	0.05–0.15	0.95–2.85
Klebsiella species	0.15–5.0	2.45–245	0.05–1.5	0.95–28.5
Enterobacter species	0.15–5.0	2.45–245	0.05–1.5	0.95–28.5
Haemophilus influenzae	0.15–1.5	2.85–95	0.015–0.15	0.285–2.85
Streptococcus pneumoniae	0.15–1.5	7.35–24.5	0.05–0.15	0.95–2.85
Shigella flexneri †	<0.01–0.04	<0.16–>320	<0.002–0.03	0.04–0.625
Shigella sonnei †	0.02–0.08	0.625–>320	0.004–0.06	0.08–1.25

† Rudoy RC, Nelson JD, Haltalin KC. *Antimicrobial Agents and Chemotherapy* 5:439–43, 1974.

CLINICAL PHARMACOLOGY

Following a one-hour intravenous infusion of a single dose of 160 mg trimethoprim and 800 mg sulfamethoxazole to 11 patients whose weight ranged from 105 lbs. to 165 lbs. (mean, 143 lbs.), the mean peak plasma concentrations of trimethoprim and sulfamethoxazole were 3.4 ± 0.3 μg/mL and 46.3 ± 2.7 μg/mL, respectively. Following repeated intravenous administration of the same dose at eight-hour intervals, the mean plasma concentrations just prior to and immediately after each infusion at steady state were 5.6 ± 0.6 μg/mL and 8.8 ± 0.9 μg/mL for trimethoprim and 70.6 ± 7.3 μg/mL and 105.6 ± 10.9 μg/mL for sulfamethoxazole. The mean plasma half-life was 11.3 ± 0.7 hours for trimethoprim and 12.8 ± 1.8 hours for sulfamethoxazole. All of these 11 patients had normal renal function and their ages ranged from 17 to 78 years (median, 60 years)[1].

Pharmacokinetic studies in children and adults suggest an age-dependent half-life of trimethoprim as indicated in the following table.[2]

Age (yrs.)	No. of Patients	Mean Trimethoprim Half-life (hours)
<1	2	7.67
1–10	9	5.49
10–20	5	8.19
20–63	6	12.82

Patients with severely impaired renal function exhibit an increase in the half-lives of both components, requiring dosage regimen adjustment (see DOSAGE AND ADMINISTRATION section).

Both trimethoprim and sulfamethoxazole exist in the blood as unbound, protein-bound and metabolized forms; sulfamethoxazole also exists as the conjugated form. The metabolism of sulfamethoxazole occurs predominately by N_4-acetylation, although the glucuronide conjugate has been identified. The principal metabolites of trimethoprim are the 1- and 3- oxides and the 3'- and 4'-hydroxy derivatives. The free forms of trimethoprim and sulfamethoxazole are considered to be the therapeutically active forms. Approximately 44% of trimethoprim and 70% of sulfamethoxazole are bound to plasma proteins. The presence of 10 mg percent sulfamethoxazole in plasma decreases the protein binding of trimethoprim by an insignificant degree; trimethoprim does not influence the protein binding of sulfamethoxazole.

Excretion of trimethoprim and sulfamethoxazole is primarily by the kidneys through both glomerular filtration and tubular secretion. Urine concentrations of both trimethoprim and sulfamethoxazole are considerably higher than are the concentrations in the blood. The percent of dose excreted in urine over a 12-hour period following the intravenous administration of the first dose of 240 mg of trimethoprim and 1200 mg of sulfamethoxazole on day 1 ranged from 17% to 42.4% as free trimethoprim; 7% to 12.7% as free sulfamethoxazole; and 36.7% to 56% as total (free plus the N_4-acetylated metabolite) sulfamethoxazole. When administered together as Septra, neither trimethoprim nor sulfamethoxazole affects the urinary excretion pattern of the other.

Both trimethoprim and sulfamethoxazole distribute to sputum and vaginal fluid; trimethoprim also distributes to bronchial secretions and both pass the placental barrier and are excreted in breast milk.

Microbiology: Sulfamethoxazole inhibits bacterial synthesis of dihydrofolic acid by competing with *para*-aminobenzoic acid (PABA). Trimethoprim blocks the production of tetrahydrofolic acid from dihydrofolic acid by binding to and reversibly inhibiting the required enzyme, dihydrofolate reductase. Thus, Septra blocks two consecutive steps in the biosynthesis of nucleic acids and proteins essential to many bacteria.

In vitro studies have shown that bacterial resistance develops more slowly with Septra than with trimethoprim or sulfamethoxazole alone.

In vitro serial dilution tests have shown that the spectrum of antibacterial activity of Septra includes common bacterial pathogens with the exception of *Pseudomonas aeruginosa*. The following organisms are usually susceptible: *Escherichia coli, Klebsiella* species, *Enterobacter* species, *Morganella morganii, Proteus mirabilis,* indole-positive *Proteus* species, including *Proteus vulgaris, Haemophilus influenzae* (including ampicillin-resistant strains), *Streptococcus pneumoniae, Shigella flexneri* and *Shigella sonnei*. It should be noted, however, that there are little clinical data on the use of Septra I.V. Infusion in serious systemic infections due to *Haemophilus influenzae* and *Streptococcus pneumoniae*.

[See table above.]

Susceptibility Testing: The recommended quantitative disc susceptibility method may be used for estimating the susceptibility of bacteria to Septra.[3,4] With this procedure, a report from the laboratory of "Susceptible to trimethoprim and sulfamethoxazole" indicates that the infection is likely to respond to therapy with Septra. If the infection is confined to the urine, a report of "Intermediate susceptibility to trimethoprim and sulfamethoxazole" also indicates that the infection is likely to respond. A report of "Resistant to trimethoprim and sulfamethoxazole" indicates that the infection is unlikely to respond to therapy with Septra.

INDICATIONS AND USAGE

PNEUMOCYSTIS CARINII PNEUMONIA: Septra I.V. Infusion is indicated in the treatment of *Pneumocystis carinii* pneumonia in children and adults.

SHIGELLOSIS: Septra I.V. Infusion is indicated in the treatment of enteritis caused by susceptible strains of *Shigella flexneri* and *Shigella sonnei* in children and adults.

URINARY TRACT INFECTIONS: Septra I.V. Infusion is indicated in the treatment of severe or complicated urinary tract infections due to susceptible strains of *Escherichia coli, Klebsiella* species, *Enterobacter* species, *Morganella morganii,* and *Proteus* species when oral administration of Septra is not feasible and when the organism is not susceptible to single agent antibacterials effective in the urinary tract.

Although appropriate culture and susceptibility studies should be performed, therapy may be started while awaiting the results of these studies.

CONTRAINDICATIONS

Hypersensitivity to trimethoprim or sulfonamides. Patients with documented megaloblastic anemia due to folate deficiency. Pregnancy at term and during the nursing period, because sulfonamides pass the placenta and are excreted in the milk and may cause kernicterus. Infants less than two months of age.

WARNINGS

FATALITIES ASSOCIATED WITH THE ADMINISTRATION OF SULFONAMIDES, ALTHOUGH RARE, HAVE OCCURRED DUE TO SEVERE REACTIONS, INCLUDING STEVENS-JOHNSON SYNDROME, TOXIC EPIDERMAL NECROLYSIS, FULMINANT HEPATIC NECROSIS, AGRANULOCYTOSIS, APLASTIC ANEMIA, OTHER BLOOD DYSCRASIAS AND HYPERSENSITIVITY OF THE RESPIRATORY TRACT.

SEPTRA SHOULD BE DISCONTINUED AT THE FIRST APPEARANCE OF SKIN RASH OR ANY SIGN OF ADVERSE REACTION. Clinical signs, such as rash, sore throat, fever, arthralgia, cough, shortness of breath, pallor, purpura or jaundice may be early indications of serious reactions. Cough, shortness of breath, and/or pulmonary infiltrates may be indicators of pulmonary hypersensitivity to sulfonamides. In rare instances, a skin rash may be followed by more severe reactions, such as Stevens-Johnson syndrome, toxic epidermal necrolysis, hepatic necrosis or serious blood disorder. Complete blood counts should be done frequently in patients receiving sulfonamides.

SEPTRA SHOULD NOT BE USED IN THE TREATMENT OF STREPTOCOCCAL PHARYNGITIS. Clinical studies have documented that patients with group A β-hemolytic

Continued on next page

Burroughs Wellcome—Cont.

streptococcal tonsillopharyngitis have a greater incidence of bacteriologic failure when treated with Septra than do those patients treated with penicillin, as evidenced by failure to eradicate this organism from the tonsillopharyngeal area. Contains sodium metabisulfite, a sulfite that may cause allergic-type reactions including anaphylactic symptoms and life-threatening or less severe asthmatic episodes in certain susceptible people. The overall prevalence of sulfite sensitivity in the general population is unknown and probably low. Sulfite sensitivity is seen more frequently in asthmatic than in nonasthmatic people.

Contains benzyl alcohol. In newborn infants, benzyl alcohol has been associated with an increased incidence of neurological and other complications which are sometimes fatal.

PRECAUTIONS

General: Septra should be given with caution to patients with impaired renal or hepatic function, to those with possible folate deficiency (e.g., the elderly, chronic alcoholics, patients receiving anticonvulsant therapy, patients with malabsorption syndrome, and patients in malnutrition states) and to those with severe allergy or bronchial asthma. In glucose-6-phosphate dehydrogenase-deficient individuals, hemolysis may occur. This reaction is frequently dose-related. Adequate fluid intake must be maintained in order to prevent crystalluria and stone formation. (See CLINICAL PHARMACOLOGY and DOSAGE AND ADMINISTRATION.)

Local irritation and inflammation due to extravascular infiltration of the infusion has been observed with Septra I.V. Infusion. If these occur the infusion should be discontinued and restarted at another site.

Use in the Elderly: There may be an increased risk of severe adverse reactions in elderly patients, particularly when complicating conditions exist, e.g., impaired kidney and/or liver function, or concomitant use of other drugs. Severe skin reactions, or generalized bone marrow suppression (see WARNINGS and ADVERSE REACTIONS sections) or a specific decrease in platelets (with or without purpura) are the most frequently reported severe adverse reactions in elderly patients. In those concurrently receiving certain diuretics, primarily thiazides, an increased incidence of thrombocytopenia with purpura has been reported. Appropriate dosage adjustments should be made for patients with impaired kidney function (see DOSAGE AND ADMINISTRATION section).

Use in the Treatment of *Pneumocystis carinii* Pneumonia in Patients with Acquired Immunodeficiency Syndrome (AIDS): The incidence of side effects, particularly rash, fever, leukopenia, and elevated aminotransferase (transaminase) values with Septra therapy in AIDS patients who are being treated for *Pneumocystis carinii* pneumonia has been reported to be greatly increased compared with the incidence normally associated with the use of Septra in non-AIDS patients.

Laboratory Tests: Appropriate culture and susceptibility studies should be performed before and throughout treatment. Complete blood counts should be done frequently in patients receiving Septra; if a significant reduction in the count of any formed blood element is noted, Septra should be discontinued. Urinalyses with careful microscopic examination and renal function tests should be performed during therapy, particularly for those patients with impaired renal function.

Drug Interactions: In elderly patients concurrently receiving certain diuretics, primarily thiazides, an increased incidence of thrombocytopenia with purpura has been reported. It has been reported that Septra may prolong the prothrombin time in patients who are receiving the anticoagulant warfarin. This interaction should be kept in mind when Septra is given to patients already on anticoagulant therapy, and the coagulation time should be reassessed.

Septra may inhibit the hepatic metabolism of phenytoin. Septra, given at a common clinical dosage, increased the phenytoin half-life by 39% and decreased the phenytoin metabolic clearance rate by 27%. When administering these drugs concurrently, one should be alert for possible excessive phenytoin effect.

Sulfonamides can also displace methotrexate from plasma protein binding sites, thus increasing free methotrexate concentrations.

Drug/Laboratory Test Interactions: Septra, specifically the trimethoprim component, can interfere with a serum methotrexate assay as determined by the competitive binding protein technique (CBPA) when a bacterial dihydrofolate reductase is used as the binding protein. No interference occurs, however, if methotrexate is measured by a radioimmunoassay (RIA).

The presence of trimethoprim and sulfamethoxazole may also interfere with the Jaffé alkaline picrate reaction assay for creatinine resulting in over-estimations of about 10% in the range of normal values.

Carcinogenesis, Mutagenesis, Impairment of Fertility:

Carcinogenesis: Long-term studies in animals to evaluate carcinogenic potential have not been conducted with Septra I.V. Infusion.

Mutagenesis: Bacterial mutagenic studies have not been performed with sulfamethoxazole and trimethoprim in combination. Trimethoprim was demonstrated to be non-mutagenic in the Ames assay. In studies at two laboratories no chromosomal damage was detected in cultured Chinese hamster ovary cells at concentrations approximately 500 times human plasma levels; at concentrations approximately 1000 times human plasma levels in these same cells a low level of chromosomal damage was induced at one of the laboratories. No chromosomal abnormalities were observed in cultured human leukocytes at concentrations of trimethoprim up to 20 times human steady state plasma levels. No chromosomal effects were detected in peripheral lymphocytes of human subjects receiving 320 mg of trimethoprim in combination with up to 1600 mg of sulfamethoxazole per day for as long as 112 weeks.

Impairment of Fertility: Septra I.V. Infusion has not been studied in animals for evidence of impairment of fertility. However, studies in rats at oral dosages as high as 70 mg/kg trimethoprim plus 350 mg/kg sulfamethoxazole daily showed no adverse effects on fertility or general reproductive performance.

Pregnancy: *Teratogenic Effects:* Pregnancy Category C. In rats, oral doses of 533 mg/kg sulfamethoxazole or 200 mg/kg trimethoprim produced teratological effects manifested mainly as cleft palates. The highest dose which did not cause cleft palates in rats was 512 mg/kg sulfamethoxazole or 192 mg/kg trimethoprim when administered separately. In two studies in rats, no teratology was observed when 512 mg/kg of sulfamethoxazole was used in combination with 128 mg/kg of trimethoprim. In one study, however, cleft palates were observed in one litter out of 9 when 355 mg/kg of sulfamethoxazole was used in combination with 88 mg/kg of trimethoprim.

In some rabbit studies, an overall increase in fetal loss (dead and resorbed and malformed conceptuses) was associated with doses of trimethoprim 6 times the human therapeutic dose.

While there are no large, well-controlled studies on the use of trimethoprim and sulfamethoxazole in pregnant women, Brumfitt and Pursell[5], in a retrospective study, reported the outcome of 186 pregnancies during which the mother received either placebo or oral trimethoprim and sulfamethoxazole. The incidence of congenital abnormalities was 4.5% (3 of 66) in those who received placebo and 3.3% (4 of 120) in those receiving trimethoprim and sulfamethoxazole. There were no abnormalities in the 10 children whose mothers received the drug during the first trimester. In a separate survey, Brumfitt and Pursell also found no congenital abnormalities in 35 children whose mothers had received oral trimethoprim and sulfamethoxazole at the time of conception or shortly thereafter.

Because trimethoprim and sulfamethoxazole may interfere with folic acid metabolism, Septra I.V. Infusion should be used during pregnancy only if the potential benefit justifies the potential risk to the fetus.

Nonteratogenic Effects: See CONTRAINDICATIONS section.

Nursing Mothers: See CONTRAINDICATIONS section.

Pediatric Use: Septra I.V. Infusion is not recommended for infants younger than two months of age (see CONTRAINDICATIONS section).

ADVERSE REACTIONS

The most common adverse effects are gastrointestinal disturbances (nausea, vomiting, anorexia) and allergic skin reactions (such as rash and urticaria). **FATALITIES ASSOCIATED WITH THE ADMINISTRATION OF SULFONAMIDES, ALTHOUGH RARE, HAVE OCCURRED DUE TO SEVERE REACTIONS, INCLUDING STEVENS-JOHNSON SYNDROME, TOXIC EPIDERMAL NECROLYSIS, FULMINANT HEPATIC NECROSIS, AGRANULOCYTOSIS, APLASTIC ANEMIA, OTHER BLOOD DYSCRASIAS AND HYPERSENSITIVITY OF THE RESPIRATORY TRACT (SEE WARNINGS SECTION).** Local reaction, pain and slight irritation on I.V. administration are infrequent. Thrombophlebitis has rarely been observed.

Hematologic: Agranulocytosis, aplastic anemia, thrombocytopenia, leukopenia, neutropenia, hemolytic anemia, megaloblastic anemia, hypoprothrombinemia, methemoglobinemia, eosinophilia.

Allergic: Stevens-Johnson syndrome, toxic epidermal necrolysis, anaphylaxis, allergic myocarditis, erythema multiforme, exfoliative dermatitis, angioedema, drug fever, chills, Henoch-Schoenlein purpura, serum sickness-like syndrome, generalized allergic reactions, generalized skin eruptions, conjunctival and scleral injection, photosensitivity, pruritus, urticaria and rash. In addition, periarteritis nodosa and systemic lupus erythematosus have been reported.

Gastrointestinal: Hepatitis including cholestatic jaundice and hepatic necrosis, elevation of serum transaminase and bilirubin, pseudomembranous enterocolitis, pancreatitis, stomatitis, glossitis, nausea, emesis, abdominal pain, diarrhea, anorexia.

Genitourinary: Renal failure, interstitial nephritis, BUN and serum creatinine elevation, toxic nephrosis with oliguria and anuria, and crystalluria.

Neurologic: Aseptic meningitis, convulsions, peripheral neuritis, ataxia, vertigo, tinnitus, headache.

Psychiatric: Hallucinations, depression, apathy, nervousness.

Endocrine: The sulfonamides bear certain chemical similarities to some goitrogens, diuretics (acetazolamide and the thiazides) and oral hypoglycemic agents. Cross-sensitivity may exist with these agents. Diuresis and hypoglycemia have occurred rarely in patients receiving sulfonamides.

Musculoskeletal: Arthralgia and myalgia.

Respiratory System: Pulmonary infiltrates, cough, shortness of breath.

Miscellaneous: Weakness, fatigue, insomnia.

OVERDOSAGE

Acute: Since there has been no extensive experience in humans with single doses of Septra I.V. Infusion in excess of 25 mL (400 mg trimethoprim and 2000 mg sulfamethoxazole), the maximum tolerated dose in humans is unknown. Signs and symptoms of overdosage reported with sulfonamides include anorexia, colic, nausea, vomiting, dizziness, headache, drowsiness and unconsciousness. Pyrexia, hematuria and crystalluria may be noted. Blood dyscrasias and jaundice are potential late manifestations of overdosage. Signs of acute overdosage with trimethoprim include nausea, vomiting, dizziness, headache, mental depression, confusion and bone marrow depression.

General principles of treatment include the administration of intravenous fluids if urine output is low and renal function is normal. Acidification of the urine will increase renal elimination of trimethoprim. The patient should be monitored with blood counts and appropriate blood chemistries, including electrolytes. If a significant blood dyscrasia or jaundice occurs, specific therapy should be instituted for these complications. Peritoneal dialysis is not effective and hemodialysis is only moderately effective in eliminating trimethoprim and sulfamethoxazole.

Chronic: Use of Septra I.V. Infusion at high doses and/or for extended periods of time may cause bone marrow depression manifested as thrombocytopenia, leukopenia, and/or megaloblastic anemia. If signs of bone marrow depression occur, the patient should be given leucovorin; 5 to 15 mg leucovorin daily has been recommended by some investigators.

Animal Toxicity: The LD_{50} of Septra I.V. Infusion in mice is 700 mg/kg or 7.3 mL/kg; in rats and rabbits the LD_{50} is > 500 mg/kg or > 5.2 mL/kg. The vehicle produced the same LD_{50} in each of these species as the active drug.

The signs and symptoms noted in mice, rats and rabbits with Septra I.V. Infusion or its vehicle at the high I.V. doses used in acute toxicity studies included ataxia, decreased motor activity, loss of righting reflex, tremors or convulsions, and/or respiratory depression.

DOSAGE AND ADMINISTRATION

CONTRAINDICATED IN INFANTS LESS THAN TWO MONTHS OF AGE. CAUTION—SEPTRA I.V. INFUSION MUST BE DILUTED IN 5% DEXTROSE IN WATER SOLUTION PRIOR TO ADMINISTRATION. DO NOT MIX SEPTRA I.V. INFUSION WITH OTHER DRUGS OR SOLUTIONS. RAPID INFUSION OR BOLUS INJECTION MUST BE AVOIDED.

DOSAGE

Children and Adults:

PNEUMOCYSTIS CARINII PNEUMONIA: Total daily dose is 15 to 20 mg/kg (based on the trimethoprim component) given in three to four equally divided doses every 6 to 8 hours for up to 14 days. One investigator noted that a total daily dose of 10 to 15 mg/kg was sufficient in 10 adult patients with normal renal function.[6]

SEVERE URINARY TRACT INFECTIONS AND SHIGELLOSIS: Total daily dose is 8 to 10 mg/kg (based on the trimethoprim component) given in two to four equally divided doses every 6, 8 or 12 hours for up to 14 days for severe urinary tract infections and 5 days for shigellosis. The maximum recommended daily dose is 60 mL per day.

For Patients with Impaired Renal Function: When renal function is impaired, a reduced dosage should be employed using the following table:

Creatinine Clearance (mL/min)	Recommended Dosage Regimen
Above 30	Use Standard Regimen
15–30	½ the Usual Regimen
Below 15	Use Not Recommended

Method of Preparation: Septra I.V. Infusion must be diluted. EACH 10 ML ADD-Vantage VIAL SHOULD BE

ADDED TO 250 ML OF 5% DEXTROSE IN WATER AND USED WITHIN SIX (6) HOURS. EACH 5 ML ADD-Vantage VIAL SHOULD BE ADDED TO 100 ML OF 5% DEXTROSE IN WATER AND USED WITHIN SIX (6) HOURS. If upon visual inspection there is cloudiness or evidence of crystallization after mixing, the solution should be discarded and a fresh solution prepared.

DO NOT MIX SEPTRA I.V. INFUSION-5% DEXTROSE IN WATER WITH DRUGS OR SOLUTIONS IN THE SAME CONTAINER.

After diluting with 5% dextrose in water, the solution should not be refrigerated and should be administered within the specified time.

ADMINISTRATION

The solution should be given by intravenous infusion over a period of 60 to 90 minutes. Rapid infusion or bolus injections must be avoided. Septra I.V. Infusion should not be given intramuscularly.

INSTRUCTIONS FOR USE

To Open Diluent Container:
Peel overwrap from the corner and remove container. Some opacity of the plastic due to moisture absorption during the sterilization process may be observed. This is normal and does not affect the solution quality or safety. The opacity will diminish gradually.

To Assemble ADD-Vantage® Vial and Flexible Diluent Container:

(Use Aseptic Technique)

1. Remove the protective covers from the top of the vial and the vial port on the diluent container as follows:
   a. To remove the breakaway vial cap, swing the pull ring over the top of the vial and pull down far enough to start the opening (SEE FIGURE 1), then pull straight up to remove the cap. (SEE FIGURE 2). **NOTE:** Once the breakaway cap has been removed, do not access vial with syringe.

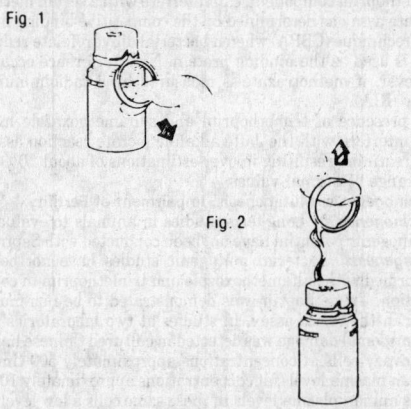

Fig. 1

Fig. 2

   b. To remove the vial port cover, grasp the tab on the pull ring, pull up to break the three tie strings, then pull back to remove the cover. (SEE FIGURE 3.)
2. Screw the vial into the vial port until it will go no further. THE VIAL MUST BE SCREWED IN TIGHTLY TO ASSURE A SEAL. This occurs approximately ½ turn (180°) after the first audible click. (SEE FIGURE 4.) The clicking sound does not assure a seal; the vial must be turned as far as it will go. **NOTE:** Once vial is seated, do not attempt to remove. (SEE FIGURE 4.)
3. Recheck the vial to assure that it is tight by trying to turn it further in the direction of assembly.
4. Label appropriately.

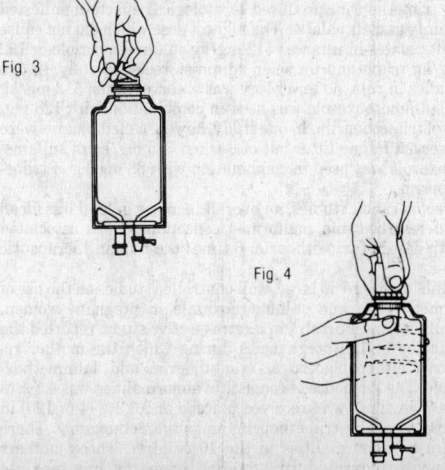

Fig. 3

Fig. 4

To Prepare Admixture:

1. Squeeze the bottom of the diluent container gently to inflate the portion of the container surrounding the end of the drug vial.
2. With the other hand, push the drug vial down into the container telescoping the walls of the container. Grasp the inner cap of the vial through the walls of the container. (SEE FIGURE 5.)
3. Pull the inner cap from the drug vial. (SEE FIGURE 6.) Verify that the rubber stopper has been pulled out, allowing the drug and diluent to mix.
4. Mix container contents thoroughly and use within the specified time.

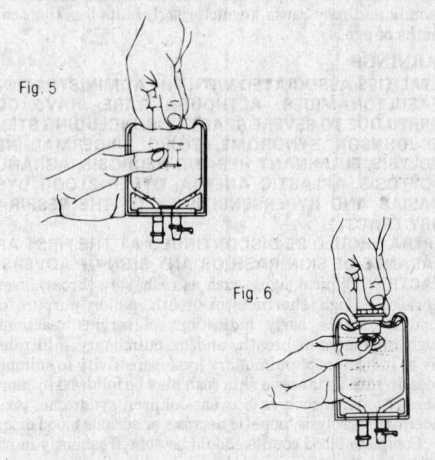

Fig. 5

Fig. 6

Preparation for Administration:

(Use Aseptic Technique)

1. Confirm the activation and admixture of vial contents.
2. Check for leaks by squeezing container firmly. If leaks are found, discard unit as sterility may be impaired.
3. Close flow control clamp of administration set.
4. Remove cover from outlet port at bottom of container.
5. Insert piercing pin of administration set into port with a twisting motion until the pin is firmly seated. **NOTE:** See full directions on administration set carton.
6. Lift the free end of the hanger loop on the bottom of the vial, breaking the two tie strings. Bend the loop outward to lock it in the upright position, then suspend container from hanger.
7. Squeeze and release drip chamber to establish proper fluid level in chamber.
8. Open flow control clamp and clear air from set. Close clamp.
9. Attach set to venipuncture device. If device is not indwelling, prime and make venipuncture.
10. Regulate rate of administration with flow control clamp.

WARNING

Do not use flexible container in series connections.

HOW SUPPLIED

10 mL ADD-Vantage® Vial containing 160 mg trimethoprim (16 mg/mL) and 800 mg sulfamethoxazole (80 mg/mL) for infusion with 5% dextrose in water. Contains benzyl alcohol (see WARNINGS). Box of 10 (NDC 0081-0856-47).
STORE AT 15° to 25°C (59° to 77°F).
DO NOT REFRIGERATE.

Also Available:
Septra I.V. infusion: 5 mL vials, containing 80 mg trimethoprim (16 mg/mL) and 400 mg sulfamethoxazole (80 mg/mL), tray of 10: 10 mL multiple dose vials containing 160 mg trimethoprim (16 mg/mL) and 800 mg sulfamethoxazole (80 mg/mL), tray of 10: 20 mL multiple dose vials containing 320 mg trimethoprim (16 mg/mL) and 1600 mg sulfamethoxazole (80 mg/mL), tray of 10.

REFERENCES

1. Grose WE, Bodey GP, Loo TL. Clinical pharmacology of intravenously administered trimethoprim-sulfamethoxazole. *Antimicrob Agents Chemother.* 1979:15:447–451.
2. Siber GR, Gorham C, Durbin W, Lesko L, Levin MJ. Pharmacology of intravenous trimethoprim-sulfamethoxazole in children and adults. In: Nelson JD, Grassi C, eds. *Current Chemotherapy of Infectious Disease.* Washington, DC: American Society for Microbiology; 1980:1:691–692.
3. Bauer AW, Kirby WMM, Sherris JC, Turck M. Antibiotic susceptibility testing by a standardized single disk method. *Am J Clin Pathol.* 1966:45:493–496.
4. National Committee for Clinical Laboratory Standards, Performance standards for antimicrobial disk susceptibility tests. 2nd ed. Villanova, PA. 1979.
5. Brumfitt W, Pursell R. Trimethoprim/sulfamethoxazole in the treatment of bacteriuria in women. *J Infect Dis.* November 1973:128(suppl):S657–S663.
6. Winston DJ, Lau WK, Gale RP, Young LS. Trimethoprim-sulfamethoxazole for the treatment of *Pneumocystis carinii* pneumonia. *Ann Int Med.* 1980:92:762–769.

SEPTRA® TABLETS   ℞
[sĕp´trah]
SEPTRA® DS (Double Strength) TABLETS   ℞
SEPTRA® SUSPENSION   ℞
SEPTRA® GRAPE SUSPENSION   ℞
(Trimethoprim and Sulfamethoxazole)

DESCRIPTION

Septra (Trimethoprim and Sulfamethoxazole) is a synthetic antibacterial combination product. Each Septra Tablet contains 80 mg trimethoprim* and 400 mg sulfamethoxazole and the inactive ingredients docusate sodium, FD&C Red No. 40, magnesium stearate, povidone, and sodium starch glycolate.

Each Septra DS (double strength) Tablet contains 160 mg trimethoprim* and 800 mg sulfamethoxazole and the inactive ingredients docusate sodium, FD&C Red No. 40, magnesium stearate, povidone, and sodium starch glycolate.

Each teaspoonful (5 mL) of Septra Suspension contains 40 mg trimethoprim* and 200 mg sulfamethoxazole and the inactive ingredients alcohol 0.26%, methylparaben 0.1% and sodium benzoate 0.1% (added as preservatives), carboxymethylcellulose sodium, citric acid, FD&C Red No. 40 and Yellow No. 6, flavor, glycerin, microcrystalline cellulose, polysorbate 80, saccharin sodium, and sorbitol. Each teaspoonful (5 mL) of Septra Grape Suspension contains 40 mg trimethoprim* and 200 mg sulfamethoxazole and the inactive ingredients alcohol 0.26%, methylparaben 0.1% and sodium benzoate 0.1% (added as preservatives), carboxymethylcellulose sodium, citric acid, FD&C Red No. 40 and Blue No. 1, flavor, glycerin, microcrystalline cellulose, polysorbate 80, saccharin sodium, and sorbitol. Both tablet and suspension forms are for oral administration.

Trimethoprim is 2,4-diamino-5-(3,4,5-trimethoxybenzyl)pyrimidine. It is a white to light yellow, odorless, bitter compound with a molecular weight of 290.3, and the molecular formula $C_{14}H_{18}N_4O_3$.

Sulfamethoxazole is N^1-(5-methyl-3-isoxazolyl) sulfanilamide. It is an almost white, odorless, tasteless compound with a molecular weight of 253.28, and the molecular formula $C_{10}H_{11}N_3O_3S$.

CLINICAL PHARMACOLOGY

Septra is rapidly absorbed following oral administration. Both sulfamethoxazole and trimethoprim exist in the blood as unbound, protein-bound and metabolized forms: sulfamethoxazole also exists as the conjugated form. The metabolism of sulfamethoxazole occurs predominately by N_4-acetylation, although the glucuronide conjugate has been identified. The principal metabolites of trimethoprim are the 1- and 3-oxides and the 3′- and 4′- hydroxy derivatives. The free forms of sulfamethoxazole and trimethoprim are considered to be the therapeutically active forms. Approximately 44% of trimethoprim and 70% of sulfamethoxazole are bound to plasma proteins. The presence of 10 mg percent sulfamethoxazole in plasma decreases the protein binding of trimethoprim by an insignificant degree; trimethoprim does not influence the protein binding of sulfamethoxazole.

Peak blood levels for the individual components occur 1 to 4 hours after oral administration. The mean serum half-lives of sulfamethoxazole and trimethoprim are 10 and 8 to 10 hours, respectively. However, patients with severely impaired renal function exhibit an increase in the half-lives of both components, requiring dosage regimen adjustment (see DOSAGE AND ADMINISTRATION section). Detectable amounts of trimethoprim and sulfamethoxazole are present in the blood 24 hours after drug administration. During administration of 160 mg trimethoprim and 800 mg sulfamethoxazole *b.i.d.,* the mean steady state plasma concentration of trimethoprim was 1.72 µg/mL. The steady state minimal plasma levels of free and total sulfamethoxazole were 57.4 µg/mL and 68.0 µg/mL, respectively. These steady state levels were achieved after three days of drug administration.[1]

Excretion of sulfamethoxazole and trimethoprim is primarily by the kidneys through both glomerular filtration and tubular secretion. Urine concentrations of both sulfamethoxazole and trimethoprim are considerably higher than are the

*Mfd. under U.S. Patent No. 3,956,327

Continued on next page

Burroughs Wellcome—Cont.

concentrations in the blood. The average percentage of the dose recovered in urine from 0 to 72 hours after a single oral dose is 84.5% for total sulfonamide and 66.8% for free trimethoprim. Thirty percent of the total sulfonamide is excreted as free sulfamethoxazole, with the remaining as N_4-acetylated metabolite.[2] When administered together as Septra, neither sulfamethoxazole nor trimethoprim affects the urinary excretion pattern of the other.

Both trimethoprim and sulfamethoxazole distribute to sputum, vaginal fluid, and middle ear fluid; trimethoprim also distributes to bronchial secretion and both pass the placental barrier and are excreted in human milk.

Microbiology: Sulfamethoxazole inhibits bacterial synthesis of dihydrofolic acid by competing with *para*-aminobenzoic acid (PABA). Trimethoprim blocks the production of tetrahydrofolic acid from dihydrofolic acid by binding to and reversibly inhibiting the required enzyme, dihydrofolate reductase. Thus, Septra blocks two consecutive steps in the biosynthesis of nucleic acids and proteins essential to many bacteria.

In vitro studies have shown that bacterial resistance develops more slowly with Septra than with either trimethoprim or sulfamethoxazole alone.

In vitro serial dilution tests have shown that the spectrum of antibacterial activity of Septra includes the common urinary tract pathogens with the exception of *Pseudomonas aeruginosa.* The following organisms are usually susceptible: *Escherichia coli, Klebsiella* species, *Enterobacter* species, *Morganella morganii, Proteus mirabilis* and indole-positive *Proteus* species including *Proteus vulgaris.*

The usual spectrum of antimicrobial activity of Septra includes bacterial pathogens isolated from middle ear exudate and from bronchial secretions (*Haemophilus influenzae,* including ampicillin-resistant strains, and *Streptococcus pneumoniae*), and enterotoxigenic strains of *Escherichia coli* (ETEC) causing bacterial gastroenteritis. *Shigella flexneri* and *Shigella sonnei* are also usually susceptible.

[See table below.]

Susceptibility Testing: The recommended quantitative disc susceptibility method may be used for estimating the susceptibility of bacteria to Septra.[3,4] With this procedure, a report from the laboratory of "Susceptible to trimethoprim and sulfamethoxazole" indicates that the infection is likely to respond to therapy with Septra. If the infection is confined to the urine, a report of "Intermediate susceptibility to trimethoprim and sulfamethoxazole" also indicates that the infection is likely to respond. A report of "Resistant to trimethoprim and sulfamethoxazole" indicates that the infection is unlikely to respond to therapy with Septra.

INDICATIONS AND USAGE

URINARY TRACT INFECTIONS: For the treatment of urinary tract infections due to susceptible strains of the following organisms: *Escherichia coli, Klebsiella* species, *Enterbacter* species, *Morganella morganii, Proteus mirabilis,* and *Proteus vulgaris.* It is recommended that initial episodes of uncomplicated urinary tract infections be treated with a single effective antibacterial agent rather than the combination.

ACUTE OTITIS MEDIA: For the treatment of acute otitis media in children due to susceptible strains of *Streptococcus pneumoniae* or *Haemophilus influenzae* when in the judgment of the physician Septra offers some advantage over the use of other antimicrobial agents. To date, there are limited data on the safety of repeated use of Septra in children under two years of age. Septra is not indicated for prophylactic or prolonged administration in otitis media at any age.

ACUTE EXACERBATIONS OF CHRONIC BRONCHITIS IN ADULTS: For the treatment of acute exacerbations of chronic bronchitis due to susceptible strains of *Streptococcus pneumoniae* or *Haemophilus influenzae* when in the judgment of the physician, Septra offers some advantage over the use of a single antimicrobial agent.

TRAVELERS' DIARRHEA IN ADULTS: For the treatment of travelers' diarrrhea due to susceptible strains of enterotoxigenic *E. coli.*

SHIGELLOSIS: For the treatment of enteritis caused by susceptible strains of *Shigella flexneri* and *Shigella sonnei* when antibacterial therapy is indicated.

PNEUMOCYSTIS CARINII PNEUMONIA: For the treatment of documented *pneumocystis carinii* pneumonia.

CONTRAINDICATIONS

Hypersensitivity to trimethoprim or sulfonamides. Patients with documented megaloblastic anemia due to folate deficiency. Pregnancy at term and during the nursing period, because sulfonamides pass the placenta and are excreted in the milk and may cause kernicterus. Infants less than two months of age.

WARNINGS

FATALITIES ASSOCIATED WITH THE ADMINISTRATION OF SULFONAMIDES, ALTHOUGH RARE, HAVE OCCURRED DUE TO SEVERE REACTIONS, INCLUDING STEVENS-JOHNSON SYNDROME, TOXIC EPIDERMAL NECROLYSIS, FULMINANT HEPATIC NECROSIS, AGRANULOCYTOSIS, APLASTIC ANEMIA, OTHER BLOOD DYSCRASIAS AND HYPERSENSITIVITY OF THE RESPIRATORY TRACT.

SEPTRA SHOULD BE DISCONTINUED AT THE FIRST APPEARANCE OF SKIN RASH OR ANY SIGN OF ADVERSE REACTION. Clinical signs, such as rash, sore throat, fever, arthralgia, cough, shortness of breath, pallor, purpura or jaundice may be early indications of serious reactions. Cough, shortness of breath, and/or pulmonary infiltrates may be indicators of pulmonary hypersensitivity to sulfonamides. In rare instances a skin rash may be followed by more severe reactions, such as Stevens-Johnson syndrome, toxic epidermal necrolysis, hepatic necrosis or serious blood disorder. Complete blood counts should be done frequently in patients receiving sulfonamides.

SEPTRA SHOULD NOT BE USED IN THE TREATMENT OF STREPTOCOCCAL PHARYNGITIS. Clinical studies have documented that patients with group A β-hemolytic streptococcal tonsillopharyngitis have a greater incidence of bacteriologic failure when treated with Septra than do those patients treated with penicillin, as evidenced by failure to eradicate this organism from the tonsillopharyngeal area.

PRECAUTIONS

General: Septra should be given with caution to patients with impaired renal or hepatic function, to those with possible folate deficiency (e.g., the elderly, chronic alcoholics, patients receiving anticonvulsant therapy, patients with malabsorption syndrome, and patients in malnutrition states) and to those with severe allergy or bronchial asthma. In glucose-6-phosphate dehydrogenase-deficient individuals, hemolysis may occur. This reaction is frequently dose-related. (See CLINICAL PHARMACOLOGY and DOSAGE AND ADMINISTRATION.)

Use in the Elderly: There may be an increased risk of severe adverse reactions in elderly patients, particularly when complicating conditions exist, e.g., impaired kidney and/or liver function, or concomitant use of other drugs. Severe skin reactions, or generalized bone marrow suppression (see WARNINGS and ADVERSE REACTIONS sections) or a specific decrease in platelets (with or without purpura) are the most frequently reported severe adverse reactions in elderly patients. In those concurrently receiving certain diuretics, primarily thiazides, an increased incidence of thrombocytopenia with purpura has been reported. Appropriate dosage adjustments should be made for patients with impaired kidney function (see DOSAGE AND ADMINISTRATION section).

Use in the Treatment of *Pneumocystis carinii* Pneumonia in Patients with Acquired Immunodeficiency Syndrome (AIDS): The incidence of side effects, particularly rash, fever, leukopenia, and elevated aminotransferase (transaminase) values with Septra therapy in AIDS patients who are being treated for *Pneumocystis carinii* pneumonia has been reported to be greatly increased compared with the incidence normally associated with the use of Septra in non-AIDS patients.

Information for Patients: Patients should be instructed to maintain an adequate fluid intake in order to prevent crystalluria and stone formation.

Laboratory Tests: Complete blood counts should be done frequently in patients receiving Septra; if a significant reduction in the count of any formed blood element is noted, Septra should be discontinued. Urinalysis with careful microscopic examination and renal function tests should be performed during therapy, particularly for those patients with impaired renal function.

Drug Interactions: In elderly patients concurrently receiving certain diuretics, primarily thiazides, an increased incidence of thrombocytopenia with purpura has been reported. It has been reported that Septra may prolong the prothrombin time in patients who are receiving the anticoagulant warfarin. This interaction should be kept in mind when Septra is given to patients already on anticoagulant therapy, and the coagulation time should be reassessed.

Septra may inhibit the hepatic metabolism of phenytoin. Septra, given at a common clinical dosage, increased the phenytoin half-life by 39% and decreased the phenytoin metabolic clearance rate by 27%. When administering these drugs concurrently, one should be alert for possible excessive phenytoin effect.

Sulfonamides can also displace methotrexate from plasma protein binding sites, thus increasing free methotrexate concentrations.

Drug/Laboratory Test Interactions: Septra, specifically the trimethoprim component, can interfere with a serum methotrexate assay as determined by the competitive binding protein technique (CBPA) when a bacterial dihydrofolate reductase is used as the binding protein. No interference occurs, however, if methotrexate is measured by a radioimmunoassay (RIA).

The presence of trimethoprim and sulfamethoxazole may also interfere with the Jaffé alkaline picrate reaction assay for creatinine resulting in over-estimations of about 10% in the range of normal values.

Carcinogenesis, Mutagenesis, Impairment of Fertility:

Carcinogenesis: Long-term studies in animals to evaluate carcinogenic potential have not been conducted with Septra.

Mutagenesis Bacterial mutagenic studies have not been performed with sulfamethoxazole and trimethoprim in combination. Trimethoprim was demonstrated to be non-mutagenic in the Ames assay. In studies at two laboratories no chromosomal damage was detected in cultured Chinese hamster ovary cells at concentrations approximately 500 times human plasma levels; at concentrations approximately 1000 times human plasma levels in these same cells a low level of chromosomal damage was induced at one of the laboratories. No chromosomal abnormalities were observed in cultured human leukocytes at concentrations of trimethoprim up to 20 times human steady state plasma levels. No chromosomal effects were detected in peripheral lymphocytes of human subjects receiving 320 mg of trimethoprim in combination with up to 1600 mg of sulfamethoxazole per day for as long as 112 weeks.

Impairment of Fertility: No adverse effects on fertility or general reproductive performance were observed in rats given oral dosages as high as 70 mg/kg/day trimethoprim plus 350 mg/kg/day sulfamethoxazole.

Pregnancy: ***Teratogenic Effects:*** Pregnancy Category C. In rats, oral doses of 533 mg/kg sulfamethoxazole or 200 mg/kg trimethoprim produced teratological effects manifested mainly as cleft palates. The highest dose which did not cause cleft palates in rats was 512 mg/kg sulfamethoxazole or 192 mg/kg trimethoprim when administered separately. In two studies in rats, no teratology was observed when 512 mg/kg of sulfamethoxazole was used in combination with 128 mg/kg of trimethoprim. In one study, however, cleft palates were observed in one litter out of 9 when 355 mg/kg of sulfamethoxazole was used in combination with 88 mg/kg of trimethoprim.

In some rabbit studies, an overall increase in fetal loss (dead and resorbed and malformed conceptuses) was associated with doses of trimethoprim 6 times the human therapeutic dose.

While there are no large, well-controlled studies on the use of trimethoprim and sulfamethoxazole in pregnant women, Brumfitt and Pursell[5], in a retrospective study, reported the outcome of 186 pregnancies during which the mother received either placebo or trimethoprim and sulfamethoxazole. The incidence of congenital abnormalities was 4.5% (3 of 66) in those who received placebo and 3.3% (4 of 120) in those receiving trimethoprim and sulfamethoxazole. There were no abnormalities in the 10 children whose mothers received the drug during the first trimester. In a separate

REPRESENTATIVE MINIMUM INHIBITORY CONCENTRATION VALUES FOR SEPTRA SUSCEPTIBLE ORGANISMS (MIC-μg/mL)

Bacteria	TMP Alone	SMX Alone	TMP/SMX (1:19) TMP	TMP/SMX (1:19) SMX
Escherichia coli	0.05-1.5	1.0-245	0.05-0.5	0.95-9.5
Escherichia coli (enterotoxigenic strains)	0.015-0.15	0.285->950	0.005-0.15	0.095-2.85
Proteus species (indole positive)	0.5-5.0	7.35-300	0.05-1.5	0.95-28.5
Morganella morganii	0.5-5.0	7.35-300	0.05-1.5	0.95-28.5
Proteus mirabilis	0.5-1.5	7.35-30	0.05-0.15	0.95-2.85
Klebsiella species	0.15-5.0	2.45-245	0.05-1.5	0.95-28.5
Enterobacter species	0.15-5.0	2.45-245	0.05-1.5	0.95-28.5
Haemophilus influenzae	0.15-1.5	2.85-95	0.015-0.15	0.285-2.85
Streptococcus pneumoniae	0.15-1.5	7.35-24.5	0.05-0.15	0.95-2.85
Shigella flexneri †	<0.01-0.04	<0.16->320	<0.002-0.03	0.04-0.625
Shigella sonnei †	0.02-0.08	0.625->320	0.004-0.06	0.08-1.25

TMP = Trimethoprim SMX = Sulfamethoxazole

†Rudoy RC, Nelson JD, Haltalin KC, *Antimicrobial Agents and Chemotherapy 5:* 439–43, 1974.

survey, Brumfitt and Pursell also found no congenital abnormalities in 35 children whose mothers had received oral trimethoprim and sulfamethoxazole at the time of conception or shortly thereafter.

Because trimethoprim and sulfamethoxazole may interfere with folic acid metabolism, Septra should be used during pregnancy only if the potential benefit justifies the potential risk to the fetus.

Nonteratogenic Effects: See CONTRAINDICATIONS section.

Nursing Mothers: See CONTRAINDICATIONS section.

Pediatric use: Septra is not recommended for infants younger than two months of age (see INDICATIONS AND USAGE and CONTRAINDICATIONS sections).

ADVERSE REACTIONS

The most common adverse effects are gastrointestinal disturbances (nausea, vomiting, anorexia) and allergic skin reactions (such as rash and urticaria). **FATALITIES ASSOCIATED WITH THE ADMINISTRATION OF SULFONAMIDES, ALTHOUGH RARE, HAVE OCCURRED DUE TO SEVERE REACTIONS, INCLUDING STEVENS-JOHNSON SYNDROME, TOXIC EPIDERMAL NECROLYSIS, FULMINANT HEPATIC NECROSIS, AGRANULOCYTOSIS, APLASTIC ANEMIA, OTHER BLOOD DYSCRASIAS AND HYPERSENSITIVITY OF THE RESPIRATORY TRACT (SEE WARNINGS SECTION).**

Hematologic: Agranulocytosis, aplastic anemia, thrombocytopenia, leukopenia, neutropenia, hemolytic anemia, megaloblastic anemia, hypoprothrombinemia, methemoglobinemia, eosinophilia.

Allergic: Stevens-Johnson syndrome, toxic epidermal necrolysis, anaphylaxis, allergic myocarditis, erythema multiforme, exfoliative dermatitis, angioedema, drug fever, chills, Henoch-Schoenlein purpura, serum sickness-like syndrome, generalized allergic reactions, generalized skin eruptions, photosensitivity, conjunctival and scleral injection, pruritus, urticaria and rash. In addition, periarteritis nodosa and systemic lupus erythematosus have been reported.

Gastrointestinal: Hepatitis including cholestatic jaundice and hepatic necrosis, elevation of serum transaminase and bilirubin, pseudomembranous enterocolitis, pancreatitis, stomatitis, glossitis, nausea, emesis, abdominal pain, diarrhea, anorexia.

Genitourinary: Renal failure, interstitial nephritis, BUN and serum creatinine elevation, toxic nephrosis with oliguria and anuria, and crystalluria.

Neurologic: Aseptic meningitis, convulsions, peripheral neuritis, ataxia, vertigo, tinnitus, headache.

Psychiatric: Hallucinations, depression, apathy, nervousness.

Endocrine: The sulfonamides bear certain chemical similarities to some goitrogens, diuretics (acetazolamide and the thiazides) and oral hypoglycemic agents. Cross-sensitivity may exist with these agents. Diuresis and hypoglycemia have occurred rarely in patients receiving sulfonamides.

Musculoskeletal: Arthralgia and myalgia.

Respiratory System: Pulmonary infiltrates, cough, shortness of breath.

Miscellaneous: Weakness, fatigue, insomnia.

OVERDOSAGE

Acute: The amount of a single dose of Septra that is either associated with symptoms of overdosage or is likely to be life-threatening has not been reported. Signs and symptoms of overdosage reported with sulfonamides include anorexia, colic, nausea, vomiting, dizziness, headache, drowsiness and unconsciousness. Pyrexia, hematuria and crystalluria may be noted. Blood dyscrasias and jaundice are potential late manifestations of overdosage. Signs of acute overdosage with trimethoprim include nausea, vomiting, dizziness, headache, mental depression, confusion and bone marrow depression. General principles of treatment include the institution of gastric lavage or emesis; forcing oral fluids; and the administration of intravenous fluids if urine output is low and renal function is normal. Acidification of the urine will increase renal elimination of trimethoprim. The patient should be monitored with blood counts and appropriate blood chemistries, including electrolytes. If a significant blood dyscrasia or jaundice occurs, specific therapy should be instituted for these complications. Peritoneal dialysis is not effective and hemodialysis is only moderately effective in eliminating trimethoprim and sulfamethoxazole.

Chronic: Use of Septra at high doses and/or for extended periods of time may cause bone marrow depression manifested as thrombocytopenia, leukopenia and/or megaloblastic anemia. If signs of bone marrow depression occur, the patient should be given leucovorin; 5 to 15 mg leucovorin daily has been recommended by some investigators.

DOSAGE AND ADMINISTRATION

Not recommended for use in infants less than two months of age.

URINARY TRACT INFECTIONS AND SHIGELLOSIS IN ADULTS AND CHILDREN AND ACUTE OTITIS MEDIA IN CHILDREN:

Adults: The usual adult dosage in the treatment of urinary tract infections is one Septra DS (double strength) tablet, two Septra tablets or four teaspoonfuls (20 mL) Septra Suspension every 12 hours for 10 to 14 days. An identical daily dosage is used for 5 days in the treatment of shigellosis.

Children: The recommended dose for children with urinary tract infections or acute otitis media is 8 mg/kg trimethoprim and 40 mg/kg sulfamethoxazole per 24 hours, given in two divided doses every 12 hours for 10 days. An identical daily dosage is used for 5 days in the treatment of shigellosis. The following table is a guideline for the attainment of this dosage:

Children: Two months of age or older

Weight		Dose—every 12 hours	
lb	kg	Teaspoonfuls	Tablets
22	10	1 (5 mL)	
44	20	2 (10 mL)	
66	30	3 (15 mL)	1½
88	40	4 (20 mL)	2 (or 1 DS Tablet)

For patients with impaired renal function: When renal function is impaired, a reduced dosage should be employed using the following table:

Creatinine Clearance (mL/min)	Recommended Dosage Regimen
Above 30	Use Standard Regimen
15–30	½ the Usual Regimen
Below 15	Use Not Recommended

ACUTE EXACERBATIONS OF CHRONIC BRONCHITIS IN ADULTS:

The usual adult dosage in the treatment of acute exacerbations of chronic bronchitis is one Septra DS (double strength) tablet, two Septra tablets or four teaspoonfuls (20 mL) Septra Suspension every 12 hours for 14 days.

TRAVELERS' DIARRHEA IN ADULTS:

For the treatment of travelers' diarrhea, the usual adult dosage is one Septra DS (double strength) tablet, two Septra tablets or four teaspoonfuls (20 mL) of Septra Suspension every 12 hours for 5 days.

PNEUMOCYSTIS CARINII PNEUMONIA:

The recommended dosage for patients with documented *Pneumocystis carinii* pneumonia is 20 mg/kg trimethoprim and 100 mg/kg sulfamethoxazole per 24 hours given in equally divided doses every 6 hours for 14 days. The following table is a guideline for the attainment of this dosage in children:

Weight		Dose—every 6 hours	
lb	kg	Teaspoonfuls	Tablets
18	8	1 (5 mL)	
35	16	2 (10 mL)	1
53	24	3 (15 mL)	1½
70	32	4 (20 mL)	2 (or 1 DS Tablet)

HOW SUPPLIED

TABLETS (pink, scored, round-shaped) containing 80 mg trimethoprim and 400 mg sulfamethoxazole: Bottles of 100 (NDC 0081-0852-55). Imprint on tablets "SEPTRA" and "Y2B."

DS (DOUBLE STRENGTH) TABLETS (pink, scored, oval-shaped) containing 160 mg trimethoprim and 800 mg sulfamethoxazole: Bottles of 100 (NDC 0081-0853-55) and 250 (NDC 0081-0853-65); unit dose pack of 100 (NDC 0081-0853-56). Imprint on tablets "SEPTRA DS" and O2C."

ORAL SUSPENSIONS (pink, cherry-flavored) containing 40 mg trimethoprim and 200 mg sulfamethoxazole in each teaspoonful (5 mL); Bottle of 1 pint (473 mL) (NDC 0081-0855-96); bottles of 20 mL—tray of 12 (NDC 0081-0855-93), 100 mL—package of 6 (NDC 0081-0855-03), 150 mL—package of 6 (NDC 0081-0855-01) and 200 mL—tray of 6 (NDC 0081-0855-02) with child-resistant caps; and (purple, grape-flavored) containing 40 mg trimethoprim and 200 mg sulfamethoxazole in each teaspoonful (5 mL); Bottle of 1 pint (473 mL) (NDC 0081-0854-96).

Tablets should be stored at 15° to 25°C (59° to 77°F) in a dry place and protected from light.

Suspensions should be stored at 15° to 25°C (59° to 77°F) and protected from light.

Also available:

SEPTRA I.V. Infusion: 5 mL vials, containing 80 mg trimethoprim (16 mg/mL) and 400 mg sulfamethoxazole (80 mg/mL), tray of 10; 10 mL multiple dose vials containing 160 mg trimethoprim (16 mg/mL) and 800 mg sulfamethoxazole (80 mg/mL), tray of 10; 20 mL multiple dose vials containing 320 mg trimethoprim (16 mg/mL) and 1600 mg sulfamethoxazole (80 mg/mL), tray of 10.

REFERENCES

1. Kremers P, Duvivier J, Heusghem C. Pharmacokinetic studies of co-trimoxazole in man after single and repeated doses. *J Clin Pharmacol*. 1974; 14:112–117.
2. Kaplan SA, Weinfeld RE, Abruzzo CW, McFaden K, Jack ML, Weissman L. Pharmacokinetic profile of trimethoprim-sulfamethoxazole in man. *J Infect Dis*. November 1973; 128(suppl):S547–S555.
3. Antibiotic susceptibility discs: certification procedure. Fed Reg. 37:20527–20529, 1972.
4. Bauer AW, Kirby WMM, Sherris JC, Turck M. Antibiotic susceptibility testing by standardized single disk method. *Am J Clin Pathol*. 1966; 45:493–496.
5. Brumfitt W, Pursell R. Trimethoprim-sulfamethoxazole in the treatment of bacteriuria in women. *J Infect Dis*. November 1973; 128(suppl):S657–S663.

U.S. Patent No. 4,209,513 (Tablet)
Shown in Product Identification Section, page 407

Children's SUDAFED® Liquid   OTC
[sū'dah-fĕd'']
Nasal Decongestant

(See PDR For Nonprescription Drugs.)

SUDAFED® Cough Syrup   OTC
[sū'dah-fĕd']
Nasal Decongestant/Cough Suppressant/Expectorant

(See PDR For Nonprescription Drugs.)

SUDAFED® SINUS Tablets and Caplets   OTC
[sū'dah-fĕd'']
Analgesic/Nasal Decongestant

(See PDR For Nonprescription Drugs.)
Shown in Product Identification Section, page 407

SUDAFED® Tablets 30 mg and 60 mg   OTC
[sū'dah-fĕd'']
Nasal Decongestant

(See PDR For Nonprescription Drugs.)
Shown in Product Identification Section, page 407

SUDAFED PLUS® Liquid and Tablets   OTC
[sū'dah-fĕd'']
Nasal Decongestant/Antihistamine

(See PDR For Nonprescription Drugs.)
Tablets shown in Product Identification Section, page 407

SUDAFED® 12 HOUR Caplets   OTC
[sū'dah-fĕd'']
Nasal Decongestant

(See PDR For Nonprescription Drugs.)
Shown in Product Identification Section, page 407

SUDAFED® Severe Cold Formula   OTC
[sū'dah-fĕd']
Tablets and Caplets
Nasal Decongestant/Cough Suppressant/Pain Reliever/Fever Reducer

(See PDR For Nonprescription Drugs.)
Shown in Product Identification Section, page 407

TABLOID® brand THIOGUANINE   ℞
[tab'loid]
40 mg Scored Tablets

CAUTION: Tabloid brand thioguanine is a potent drug. It should not be used unless a diagnosis of acute nonlymphocytic leukemia has been adequately established and the responsible physician is knowledgeable in assessing response to chemotherapy.

Continued on next page

Burroughs Wellcome—Cont.

DESCRIPTION

Tabloid brand thioguanine was synthesized and developed by Hitchings, Elion and associates at the Wellcome Research Laboratories. It is one of a large series of purine analogues which interfere with nucleic acid biosynthesis, and has been found active against selected human neoplastic diseases.[1]

Thioguanine, known chemically as 2-amino-1,7-dihydro-6*H*-purine-6-thione, is an analogue of the nucleic acid constituent guanine, and is closely related structurally and functionally to Purinethol® (mercaptopurine).

Tabloid brand thioguanine is available in tablets for oral administration. Each scored tablet contains 40 mg thioguanine and the inactive ingredients gum acacia, lactose, magnesium stearate, potato starch, and stearic acid.

CLINICAL PHARMACOLOGY

Clinical studies have shown that the absorption of an oral dose of thioguanine in man is incomplete and variable, averaging approximately 30% of the administered dose (range: 14–46%).[2,3] Following oral administration of ^{35}S-6-thioguanine, total plasma radioactivity reached a maximum at eight hours and declined slowly thereafter. Parent drug represented only a very small fraction of the total plasma radioactivity at any time, being virtually undetectable throughout the period of measurements.

The oral administration of radiolabeled thioguanine revealed only trace quantities of parent drug in the urine. However, a methylated metabolite, 2-amino-6-methylthiopurine (MTG), appeared very early, rose to a maximum six to eight hours after drug administration, and was still being excreted after 12 to 22 hours. Radiolabeled sulfate appeared somewhat later than MTG but was the principal metabolite after eight hours. Thiouric acid and some unidentified products were found in the urine in small amounts.[3] Intravenous administration of ^{35}S-6-thioguanine disclosed a median plasma half-disappearance time of 80 minutes (range: 25–240 minutes) when the compound was given in single doses of 65 to 300 mg/m^2. Although initial plasma levels of thioguanine did correlate with the dose level, there was no correlation between the plasma half-disappearance time and the dose.[2]

Thioguanine is incorporated into the DNA and the RNA of human bone marrow cells. Studies with intravenous ^{35}S-6-thioguanine have shown that the amount of thioguanine incorporated into nucleic acids is more than 100 times higher after five daily doses than after a single dose. With the 5-dose schedule, from one-half to virtually all of the guanine in the residual DNA was replaced by thioguanine.[2] Tissue distribution studies of ^{35}S-6-thioguanine in mice showed only traces of radioactivity in brain after oral administration. No measurements have been made of thioguanine concentrations in human cerebrospinal fluid, but observations on tissue distribution in animals, together with the lack of CNS penetration by the closely related compound, mercaptopurine, suggest that thioguanine does not reach therapeutic concentrations in the CSF.

Monitoring of plasma levels of thioguanine during therapy is of questionable value.[3] There is technical difficulty in determining plasma concentrations, which are seldom greater than 1 to 2 µg/mL after a therapeutic oral dose. More significantly, thioguanine enters rapidly into the anabolic and catabolic pathways for purines, and the active intracellular metabolites have appreciably longer half-lives than the parent drug. The biochemical effects of a single dose of thioguanine are evident long after the parent drug has disappeared from plasma. Because of this rapid metabolism of thioguanine to active intracellular derivatives, hemodialysis would not be expected to appreciably reduce toxicity of the drug.

Thioguanine competes with hypoxanthine and guanine for the enzyme hypoxanthine-guanine phosphoribosyltransferase (HGPRTase) and is itself converted to 6-thioguanylic acid (TGMP). This nucleotide reaches high intracellular concentrations at therapeutic doses. TGMP interferes at several points with the synthesis of guanine nucleotides. It inhibits *de novo* purine biosynthesis by pseudo-feedback inhibition of glutamine-5-phosphoribosylpyrophosphate amidotransferase—the first enzyme unique to the *de novo* pathway for purine ribonucleotide synthesis. TGMP also inhibits the conversion of inosinic acid (IMP) to xanthylic acid (XMP) by competition for the enzyme IMP dehydrogenase. At one time TGMP was felt to be a significant inhibitor of ATP:GMP phosphotransferase (guanylate kinase),[4] but recent results have shown this not to be so.[5]

Thioguanylic acid is further converted to the di- and tri-phosphates, thioguanosine diphosphate (TGDP) and thioguanosine triphosphate (TGTP) (as well as their 2′-deoxyribosyl analogues) by the same enzymes which metabolize guanine nucleotides.[6] Thioguanine nucleotides are incorporated into both the RNA and the DNA by phosphodiester linkages[2] and it has been argued that incorporation of such fraudulent bases contributes to the cytotoxicity of thioguanine.

Thus, thioguanine has multiple metabolic effects and at present it is not possible to designate one major site of action. Its tumor inhibitory properties may be due to one or more of its effects on (a) feedback inhibition of *de novo* purine synthesis; (b) inhibition of purine nucleotide interconversions; or (c) incorporation into the DNA and the RNA. The net consequence of its actions is a sequential blockade of the synthesis and utilization of the purine nucleotides.[4,6,7]

The catabolism of thioguanine and its metabolites is complex and shows significant differences between man and the mouse.[2,3] In both humans and mice, after oral administration of ^{35}S-6-thioguanine, urine contains virtually no detectable intact thioguanine. While deamination and subsequent oxidation to thiouric acid occurs only to a small extent in man, it is the main pathway in mice. The product of deamination by guanase, 6-thioxanthine is inactive, having negligible antitumor activity. This pathway of thioguanine inactivation is not dependent on the action of xanthine oxidase and an inhibitor of that enzyme (such as allopurinol), will not block the detoxification of thioguanine even though the inactive 6-thioxanthine is normally further oxidized by xanthine oxidase to thiouric acid before it is eliminated. In man, methylation of thioguanine is much more extensive than in the mouse. The product of methylation, 2-amino-6-methylthiopurine, is also substantially less active and less toxic than thioguanine and its formation is likewise unaffected by the presence of allopurinol. Appreciable amounts of inorganic sulfate are also found in both murine and human urine, presumably arising from further metabolism of the methylated derivatives.

In some animal tumors, resistance to the effect of thioguanine correlates with the loss of HGPRTase activity and the resulting inability to convert thioguanine to thioguanylic acid. However, other resistance mechanisms, such as increased catabolism of TGMP by a nonspecific phosphatase, may be operative. Although not invariable, it is usual to find cross-resistance between thioguanine and its close analogue, Purinethol® (mercaptopurine).

INDICATIONS AND USAGE

a) Acute Nonlymphocytic Leukemias: Tabloid brand thioguanine is indicated for remission induction, remission consolidation, and maintenance therapy of acute nonlymphocytic leukemias.[8,9] The response to this agent depends upon the age of the patient (younger patients faring better than older), and whether thioguanine is used in previously treated or previously untreated patients. Reliance upon thioguanine alone is seldom justified for initial remission induction of acute nonlymphocytic leukemias because combination chemotherapy including thioguanine results in more frequent remission induction and longer duration of remission than thioguanine alone.

b) Other Neoplasms: Tabloid brand thioguanine is not effective in chronic lymphocytic leukemia, Hodgkin's lymphoma, multiple myeloma or solid tumors. Although thioguanine is one of several agents with activity in the treatment of the chronic phase of chronic myelogenous leukemia, more objective responses are observed with Myleran® (busulfan), and therefore busulfan is usually regarded as the preferred drug.

CONTRAINDICATIONS

Thioguanine should not be used in patients whose disease has demonstrated prior resistance to this drug. In animals and man, there is usually complete cross-resistance between Purinethol® (mercaptopurine) and Tabloid® brand thioguanine.

WARNINGS

SINCE DRUGS USED IN CANCER CHEMOTHERAPY ARE POTENTIALLY HAZARDOUS, IT IS RECOMMENDED THAT ONLY PHYSICIANS EXPERIENCED WITH THE RISKS OF THIOGUANINE AND KNOWLEDGEABLE IN THE NATURAL HISTORY OF ACUTE NONLYMPHOCYTIC LEUKEMIAS ADMINISTER THIS DRUG.

The most consistent, dose-related toxicity is bone marrow suppression. This may be manifest by anemia, leukopenia, thrombocytopenia, or any combination of these. Any one of these findings may also reflect progression of the underlying disease. Since thioguanine may have a delayed effect, it is important to withdraw the medication temporarily at the first sign of an abnormally large fall in any of the formed elements of the blood.

It is recommended that evaluation of the hemoglobin concentration or hematocrit; total white blood cell count and differential count; and quantitative platelet count be obtained frequently while the patient is on thioguanine therapy. In cases where the cause of fluctuations in the formed elements in the peripheral blood is obscure, bone marrow examination may be useful for the evaluation of marrow status. The decision to increase, decrease, continue, or discontinue a given dosage of thioguanine must be based not only on the absolute hematologic values, but also upon the rapidity with which changes are occurring. In many instances, particularly during the induction phase of acute leukemia, complete blood counts will need to be done more frequently in order to evaluate the effect of the therapy. The dosage of thioguanine may need to be reduced when this agent is combined with other drugs whose primary toxicity is myelosuppression.

Myelosuppression is often unavoidable during the induction phase of adult acute nonlymphocytic leukemias if remission induction is to be successful. Whether or not this demands modification or cessation of dosage depends both upon the response of the underlying disease and a careful consideration of supportive facilities (granulocyte and platelet transfusions) which may be available. Life-threatening infections and bleeding have been observed as consequences of thioguanine-induced granulocytopenia and thrombocytopenia.

The effect of thioguanine on the immunocompetence of patients is unknown.

Pregnancy: *"Pregnancy Category D":* Drugs such as thioguanine are potential mutagens and teratogens. Thioguanine may cause fetal harm when administered to a pregnant woman. Thioguanine has been shown to be teratogenic in rats when given in doses five (5) times the human dose. When given to the rat on the 4th and 5th days of gestation, 13% of surviving placentas did not contain fetuses, and 19% of offspring were malformed or stunted. The malformations noted included generalized edema, cranial defects and general skeletal hypoplasia, hydrocephalus, ventral hernia, situs inversus, and incomplete development of the limbs.[10] There are no adequate and well-controlled studies in pregnant women. If this drug is used during pregnancy, or if the patient becomes pregnant while taking the drug, the patient should be apprised of the potential hazard to the fetus. Women of childbearing potential should be advised to avoid becoming pregnant.

PRECAUTIONS

General: Although the primary toxicity of thioguanine is myelosuppression, other toxicities have occasionally been observed, particularly when thioguanine is used in combination with other cancer chemotherapeutic agents.

A few cases of jaundice have been reported in patients with leukemia receiving thioguanine. Among these were two adult male patients and four children with acute myelogenous leukemia and an adult male with acute lymphocytic leukemia who developed veno-occlusive hepatic disease while receiving chemotherapy for their leukemia.[11,12] Six patients had received cytarabine prior to treatment with thioguanine, and some were receiving other chemotherapy in addition to thioguanine when they became symptomatic. While veno-occlusive hepatic disease has not been reported in patients treated with thioguanine alone, it is recommended that thioguanine be withheld if there is evidence of toxic hepatitis or biliary stasis, and that appropriate clinical and laboratory investigations be initiated to establish the etiology of the hepatic dysfunction. Deterioration in liver function studies during thioguanine therapy should prompt discontinuation of treatment and a search for an explanation of the hepatotoxicity.

Information For Patients: Patients should be informed that the major toxicities of thioguanine are related to myelosuppression, hepatotoxicity and gastrointestinal toxicity. Patients should never be allowed to take the drug without medical supervision and should be advised to consult their physician if they experience fever, sore throat, jaundice, nausea, vomiting, signs of local infection, bleeding from any site, or symptoms suggestive of anemia. Women of childbearing potential should be advised to avoid becoming pregnant.

Laboratory Tests: It is advisable to monitor liver function tests (serum transaminases, alkaline phosphatase, bilirubin) at weekly intervals when first beginning therapy and at monthly intervals thereafter. It may be advisable to perform liver function tests more frequently in patients with known pre-existing liver disease or in patients who are receiving thioguanine and other hepatotoxic drugs. Patients should be instructed to discontinue thioguanine immediately if clinical jaundice is detected. (See WARNINGS section.)

Drug Interactions: There is usually complete cross-resistance between Purinethol® (mercaptopurine) and Tabloid® brand thioguanine.

In one study, 12 of approximately 330 patients receiving continuous busulfan and thioguanine therapy for treatment of chronic myelogenous leukemia were found to have esophageal varices associated with abnormal liver function tests.[13] Subsequent liver biopsies were performed in four of these patients, all of which showed evidence of nodular regenerative hyperplasia. Duration of combination therapy prior to the appearance of esophageal varices ranged from 6 to 45 months. With the present analysis of the data, no cases of hepatotoxicity have appeared in the busulfan alone arm of the study. Long-term continuous therapy with thioguanine and busulfan should be used with caution.

Carcinogenesis, Mutagenesis, Impairment of Fertility: In view of its action on cellular DNA, thioguanine is potentially mutagenic and carcinogenic, and consideration should be given to the theoretical risk of carcinogenesis when thioguanine is administered. (See WARNINGS section.)

Pregnancy: Teratogenic Effects: Pregnancy Category D. See WARNINGS section.

Nursing Mothers: It is not known whether this drug is excreted in human milk. Because of the potential for tumorigenicity shown for thioguanine, a decision should be made whether to discontinue nursing or to discontinue the drug, taking into account the importance of the drug to the mother.

ADVERSE REACTIONS

The most frequent adverse reaction to thioguanine is myelosuppression. The induction of complete remission of acute myelogenous leukemia usually requires combination chemotherapy in dosages which produce marrow hypoplasia.[14]

Since consolidation and maintenance of remission are also effected by multiple drug regimens whose component agents cause myelosuppression, pancytopenia is observed in nearly all patients. Dosages and schedules must be adjusted to prevent life-threatening cytopenias whenever these adverse reactions are observed.

Hyperuricemia frequently occurs in patients receiving thioguanine as a consequence of rapid cell lysis accompanying the antineoplastic effect. Adverse effects can be minimized by increased hydration, urine alkalinization, and the prophylactic administration of a xanthine oxidase inhibitor such as Zyloprim® (allopurinol). Unlike Purinethol® (mercaptopurine) and Imuran® (azathioprine), thioguanine may be continued in the usual dosage when allopurinol is used conjointly to inhibit uric acid formation.

Less frequent adverse reactions include nausea, vomiting, anorexia and stomatitis. Intestinal necrosis and perforation have been reported in patients who received multiple drug chemotherapy including thioguanine.

Hepatic Effects: Liver enzyme and other liver function studies are occasionally abnormal. If jaundice, hepatomegaly or anorexia with tenderness in the right hypochondrium occurs, thioguanine should be withheld until the exact etiology can be determined. There have been reports of veno-occlusive liver disease occurring in patients who received combination chemotherapy including thioguanine.[11,12] Esophageal varices have been reported in patients receiving continuous busulfan and thioguanine therapy for treatment of chronic myelogenous leukemia. (See PRECAUTIONS: Drug Interactions section.)

OVERDOSAGE

Signs and symptoms of overdosage may be immediate, such as nausea, vomiting, malaise, hypertension and diaphoresis; or delayed, such as myelosuppression and azotemia.[15] It is not known whether thioguanine is dialyzable. Hemodialysis is thought to be of marginal use due to the rapid intracellular incorporation of thioguanine into active metabolites with long persistence. The oral LD_{50} of thioguanine was determined to be 823 mg/kg $\pm$ 50.73 mg/kg and 740 mg/kg $\pm$ 45.24 mg/kg for male and female rats respectively.[16]

Symptoms of overdosage may occur after a single dose of as little as 2.0 to 3.0 mg/kg thioguanine. As much as 35 mg/kg has been given in a single oral dose with reversible myelosuppression observed. There is no known pharmacologic antagonist of thioguanine. The drug should be discontinued immediately if unintended toxicity occurs during treatment. Severe hematologic toxicity may require supportive therapy with platelet transfusions for bleeding, and granulocyte transfusions and antibiotics if sepsis is documented. If a patient is seen immediately following an accidental overdosage of the drug, it may be useful to induce emesis.

DOSAGE AND ADMINISTRATION

Tabloid brand thioguanine is administered orally. The dosage which will be tolerated and effective varies according to the stage and type of neoplastic process being treated. Because the usual therapies for adult and childhood acute nonlymphocytic leukemias involve the use of thioguanine with other agents in combination, physicians responsible for administering these therapies should be experienced in the use of cancer chemotherapy and in the chosen protocol.

Ninety-six (59%) of one hundred sixty-three children with previously untreated acute nonlymphocytic leukemia obtained complete remission with a multiple drug protocol including thioguanine, prednisone, cytarabine, cyclophosphamide, and vincristine. Remission was maintained with daily thioguanine, four-day pulses of cytarabine and cyclophosphamide, and a single dose of vincristine every 28 days. The median duration of remission was 11.5 months.[8]

Fifty-three percent of previously untreated adults with acute nonlymphocytic leukemias attained remission following use of the combination of thioguanine and cytarabine according to a protocol developed at The Memorial Sloan-Kettering Cancer Center. A median duration of remission of 8.8 months was achieved with the multiple drug maintenance regimen which included thioguanine.[9]

On those occasions when single agent chemotherapy with thioguanine may be appropriate, the usual initial dosage for children and adults is approximately 2 mg/kg of body weight per day. If, after four weeks on this dosage, there is no clinical improvement and no leukocyte or platelet depression, the dosage may be cautiously increased to 3 mg/kg per day. The total daily dose may be given at one time.

The dosage of thioguanine used does not depend on whether or not the patient is receiving Zyloprim® (allopurinol); **this is in contradistinction to the dosage reduction which is mandatory when Purinethol® (mercaptopurine) or IMURAN® (azathioprine) is given simultaneously with allopurinol.**

Procedures for proper handling and disposal of anti-cancer drugs should be considered. Several guidelines on this subject have been published.[17–23]

There is no general agreement that all of the procedures recommended in the guidelines are necessary or appropriate.

HOW SUPPLIED

Greenish-yellow, scored tablets containing 40 mg thioguanine, imprinted with "WELLCOME" and "U3B" on each tablet; in bottle of 25 (NDC-0081-0880-25). Store at 15° to 25°C (59° to 77°F) in a dry place.

REFERENCES

1. Hitchings GH, Elion GB. The chemistry and biochemistry of purine analogs. *Ann NY Acad Sci.* 1954;60:195–199.
2. LePage GA, Whitecar JP Jr. Pharmacology of 6-thioguanine in man. *Cancer Res.* 1971;31:1627–1631.
3. Elion GB. Biochemistry and pharmacology of purine analogues. *Fed Proc.* 1967;26:898–904.
4. Miech RP, Parks RE Jr, Anderson JH Jr, Sartorelli AC. An hypothesis on the mechanism of action of 6-thioguanine. *Biochem Pharmacol.* 1967;16:2222–2227.
5. Miller RL, Adamczyk DL, Spector T, Agarwal KC, Miech RP, Panks RE Jr. Reassessment of the interactions of guanylate kinase and 6-thioguanine 5′-phosphate. *Biochem Pharmacol.* 1977;26:1573–1576.
6. Paterson ARP, Tidd DN. 6-Thiopurines. In: Sartorelli AC, Johns DG, eds. *Antineoplastic and Immunosuppressive Agents,* Part II. Berlin: Springer Verlag; 1975:384–403.
7. Nelson JA, Carpenter JW, Rose LM, Adamson DJ. Mechanisms of action of 6-thioguanine, 6-mercaptopurine, and 8-azaguanine. *Cancer Res.* 1975;35:2872–2878.
8. Chard RL Jr, Finklestein JZ, Sonley MJ, et al. Increased survival in childhood acute nonlymphocytic leukemia after treatment with prednisone, cytosine arabinoside, 6-thioguanine, cyclophosphamide, and oncovin (PATCO) combination therapy. *Med Ped Oncol.* 1978;4:263–273.
9. Mertelsmann R, Drapkin RL, Gee TS, et al. Treatment of acute nonlymphocytic leukemia in adults: response to 2,2-anhydro-1-B-D-arabinofuranosyl-5-fluorocytosine and thioguanine on the L-12 protocol. *Cancer.* 1981;48:2136–2142.
10. Thiersch JB: Effect of 2-6 diaminopurine (2-6DP): 6 chlorpurine (CIP) and thioguanine (ThG) on rat litter *in utero. Proc Soc Exp Biol Med.* 1957;94:40–43.
11. Griner PF, Elbadawi A, Packman CH. Veno-occlusive disease of the liver after chemotherapy of acute leukemia: report of two cases. *Ann Intern Med.* 1976;85:578–582.
12. Gill RA, Onstad GR, Cardamone JM, Maneval DC, Sumner HW. Hepatic veno-occlusive disease caused by 6-thioguanine. *Ann Intern Med.* 1982;96:58–60.
13. Key NS, Kelly PMA, Emerson PM, Chapman RWG, Allan NC, McGee JO'D. Oesophageal varices associated with busulfan-thioguanine combination therapy for chronic myeloid leukaemia. *Lancet.* 1987;2:1050–1052.
14. Clarkson BD, Dowling MD, Gee TS, Cunningham IB, Burchenal JH. Treatment of acute leukemia in adults. *Cancer.* 1975;36:775–795.
15. Presant CA, Denes AE, Klein L, Garrett S, Metter GE. Phase I and preliminary phase II observations of high-dose intermittent 6-thioguanine. *Cancer Treat Rep.* 1980;64:1109–1113.
16. Unpublished data on file with Burroughs Wellcome Co.
17. Recommendations for the safe handling of parenteral antineoplastic drugs. Washington, DC: Division of Safety, National Institutes of Health; 1983. US Dept. of Health and Human Services, Public Health Service publication NIH 83-2621.
18. AMA Council on Scientific Affairs. Guidelines for handling parenteral antineoplastics. *JAMA.* 1985;253: 1590–1591.
19. National Study Commission on Cytotoxic Exposure. Recommendations for handling cytotoxic agents. 1984. Available from Louis P. Jeffrey, ScD, Director of Pharmacy Services, Rhode Island Hospital, 593 Eddy Street, Providence, Rhode Island 02902.
20. Clinical Oncological Society of Australia. Guidelines and recommendations for safe handling of antineoplastic agents. *Med J Australia.* 1983;1:426–428.
21. Jones RB, Frank R, Mass T. Safe handling of chemotherapeutic agents: A report from the Mount Sinai Medical Center. *CA—A Cancer J for Clin.* 1983;33(Sept/Oct): 258–263.
22. American Society of Hospital Pharmacists. Technical assistance bulletin on handling cytotoxic drugs in hospitals. *Am J Hosp Pharm.* 1985;42:131–137.
23. Yodaiken RE, Bennett D. OSHA work-practice guidelines for personnel dealing with cytotoxic (antineoplastic) drugs. *Am. J Hosp Pharm.* 1986;43:1193–1204.

626027

Shown in Product Identification Section, page 407

TRACRIUM® INJECTION ℞

[trā ′krē ″um]

(Atracurium Besylate)

This drug should be used only by adequately trained individuals familiar with its actions, characteristics, and hazards.

DESCRIPTION

Tracrium (atracurium besylate) is an intermediate-duration, nondepolarizing, skeletal muscle relaxant for intravenous administration. Atracurium besylate is designated as 2,2′-[pentamethylenebis(oxycarbonylethylene)]bis(1,2,3,4-tetrahydro-6,7-dimethoxy-2-methyl-1-veratrylisoquinolinium) dibenzenesulfonate. It has a molecular weight of 1243.49, and its molecular formula is $C_{65}H_{82}N_2O_{18}S_2$.

Atracurium besylate is a complex molecule containing four sites at which different stereochemical configurations can occur. The symmetry of the molecule, however, results in only ten, instead of sixteen, possible different isomers. The manufacture of atracurium besylate results in these isomers being produced in unequal amounts but with a consistent ratio. Those molecules in which the methyl group attached to the quaternary nitrogen projects on the opposite side to the adjacent substituted-benzyl moiety predominate by approximately 3:1.

Tracrium Injection is a sterile, non-pyrogenic aqueous solution. Each mL contains 10 mg atracurium besylate. The pH is adjusted to 3.25–3.65 with benzenesulfonic acid. The multiple dose vial contains 0.9% benzyl alcohol added as a preservative. Tracrium slowly loses potency with time at the rate of approximately 6% per *year* under refrigeration (5°C). Tracrium Injection should be refrigerated at 2° to 8°C (36° to 46°F) to preserve potency. Rate of loss in potency increases to approximately 5% per *month* at 25°C (77°F). Upon removal from refrigeration to room temperature storage conditions (25°C/77°F), use Tracrium Injection within 14 days even if rerefrigerated.

CLINICAL PHARMACOLOGY

Tracrium is a nondepolarizing skeletal muscle relaxant. Nondepolarizing agents antagonize the neurotransmitter action of acetylcholine by binding competitively with cholinergic receptor sites on the motor end-plate. This antagonism is inhibited, and neuromuscular block reversed, by acetylcholinesterase inhibitors such as neostigmine, edrophonium, and pyridostigmine.

Tracrium can be used most advantageously if muscle twitch response to peripheral nerve stimulation is monitored to assess degree of muscle relaxation.

The duration of neuromuscular blockade produced by Tracrium is approximately one-third to one-half the duration of blockade by d-tubocurarine, metocurine, and pancuronium at initially equipotent doses. As with other nondepolarizing neuromuscular blockers, the time to onset of paralysis decreases and the duration of maximum effect increases with increasing Tracrium doses.

The ED_{95} (dose required to produce 95% suppression of the muscle twitch response with balanced anesthesia) has averaged 0.23 mg/kg (0.11 to 0.26 mg/kg in various studies). An initial Tracrium dose of 0.4 to 0.5 mg/kg generally produces maximum neuromuscular blockade within 3 to 5 minutes of injection, with good or excellent intubation conditions within 2 to 2.5 minutes in most patients. Recovery from neuromuscular blockade (under balanced anesthesia) can be expected to begin approximately 20 to 35 minutes after injection. Under balanced anesthesia, recovery to 25% of control is achieved approximately 35 to 45 minutes after injection, and recovery is usually 95% complete approximately 60–70 minutes after injection. The neuromuscular blocking action of Tracrium is enhanced in the presence of potent inhalation anesthetics. Isoflurane and enflurane increase the potency of Tracrium and prolong neuromuscular blockade by approximately 35%; however, halothane's potentiating effect (approximately 20%) is marginal (see DOSAGE AND ADMINISTRATION).

Repeated administration of maintenance doses of Tracrium has no cumulative effect on the duration of neuromuscular blockade if recovery is allowed to begin prior to repeat dosing. Moreover, the time needed to recover from repeat doses does not change with additional doses. Repeat doses can therefore be administered at relatively regular intervals with predictable results. After an initial dose of 0.4 to 0.5 mg/kg under balanced anesthesia, the first maintenance dose (suggested maintenance dose is 0.08 to 0.10 mg/kg) is

Continued on next page

Burroughs Wellcome—Cont.

generally required within 20 to 45 minutes, and subsequent maintenance doses are usually required at approximately 15 to 25 minute intervals.

Once recovery from Tracrium's neuromuscular blocking effects begins, it proceeds more rapidly than recovery from d-tubocurarine, metocurine, and pancuronium. Regardless of Tracrium dose, the time from start of recovery (from complete block) to complete (95%) recovery is approximately 30 minutes under balanced anesthesia, and approximately 40 minutes under halothane, enflurane or isoflurane. Repeated doses have no cumulative effect on recovery rate.

Reversal of neuromuscular blockade produced by Tracrium can be achieved with an anticholinesterase agent such as neostigmine, edrophonium, or pyridostigmine, in conjunction with an anticholinergic agent such as atropine or glycopyrrolate. Under balanced anesthesia, reversal can usually be attempted approximately 20 to 35 minutes after an initial Tracrium dose of 0.4 to 0.5 mg/kg, or approximately 10 to 30 minutes after a 0.08 to 0.10 mg/kg maintenance dose, when recovery of muscle twitch has started. Complete reversal is usually attained within 8–10 minutes of the administration of reversing agents. Rare instances of breathing difficulties, possibly related to incomplete reversal, have been reported following attempted pharmacologic antagonism of Tracrium-induced neuromuscular blockade. As with other agents in this class, the tendency for residual neuromuscular block is increased if reversal is attempted at deep levels of blockade or if inadequate doses of reversal agents are employed.

The pharmacokinetics of Tracrium in man are essentially linear within the 0.3 to 0.6 mg/kg dose range. The elimination half-life is approximately 20 minutes. THE DURATION OF NEUROMUSCULAR BLOCKADE PRODUCED BY TRACRIUM DOES NOT CORRELATE WITH PLASMA PSEUDOCHOLINESTERASE LEVELS AND IS NOT ALTERED BY THE ABSENCE OF RENAL FUNCTION. This is consistent with the results of *in vitro* studies which have shown that Tracrium is inactivated in plasma via two nonoxidative pathways: ester hydrolysis, catalyzed by nonspecific esterases; and Hofmann elimination, a nonenzymatic chemical process which occurs at physiological pH. Some placental transfer occurs in humans.

Radiolabel studies demonstrated that Tracrium undergoes extensive degradation in cats, and that neither kidney nor liver plays a major role in its elimination. Biliary and urinary excretion were the major routes of excretion of radioactivity (totaling > 90% of the labeled dose within 7 hours of dosing), of which Tracrium represented only a minor fraction. The metabolites in bile and urine were similar, including products of Hofmann elimination and ester hydrolysis.

Tracrium is a less potent histamine releaser than d-tubocurarine or metocurine. Histamine release is minimal with initial Tracrium doses up to 0.5 mg/kg, and hemodynamic changes are minimal within the recommended dose range. A moderate histamine release and significant falls in blood pressure have been seen following 0.6 mg/kg of Tracrium. The histamine and hemodynamic responses were poorly correlated. The effects were generally short-lived and manageable, but the possibility of substantial histamine release in sensitive individuals or in patients in whom substantial histamine release would be especially hazardous (e.g., patients with significant cardiovascular disease) must be considered.

It is not known whether the prior use of other nondepolarizing neuromuscular blocking agents has any effect on the activity of Tracrium. The prior use of succinylcholine decreases by approximately 2 to 3 minutes the time to maximum blockade induced by Tracrium, and may increase the depth of blockade. Tracrium should be administered only after a patient recovers from succinylcholine-induced neuromuscular blockade.

INDICATIONS AND USAGE

Tracrium is indicated, as an adjunct to general anesthesia, to facilitate endotracheal intubation and to provide skeletal muscle relaxation during surgery or mechanical ventilation.

CONTRAINDICATIONS

Tracrium is contraindicated in patients known to have a hypersensitivity to it.

WARNINGS

TRACRIUM SHOULD BE USED ONLY BY THOSE SKILLED IN AIRWAY MANAGEMENT AND RESPIRATORY SUPPORT. EQUIPMENT AND PERSONNEL MUST BE IMMEDIATELY AVAILABLE FOR ENDOTRACHEAL INTUBATION AND SUPPORT OF VENTILATION, INCLUDING ADMINISTRATION OF POSITIVE PRESSURE OXYGEN. ADEQUACY OF RESPIRATION MUST BE ASSURED THROUGH ASSISTED OR CONTROLLED VENTILATION. ANTICHOLINESTERASE REVERSAL AGENTS SHOULD BE IMMEDIATELY AVAILABLE.

DO NOT GIVE TRACRIUM BY INTRAMUSCULAR ADMINISTRATION.

Tracrium has no known effect on consciousness, pain threshold, or cerebration. It should be used only with adequate anesthesia.

Tracrium Injection, which has an acid pH, should not be mixed with alkaline solutions (e.g., barbiturate solutions) in the same syringe or administered simultaneously during intravenous infusion through the same needle. Depending on the resultant pH of such mixtures, Tracrium may be inactivated and a free acid may be precipitated.

Tracrium Injection 10 mL multiple dose vials contain benzyl alcohol. Benzyl alcohol has been associated with an increased incidence of neurological and other complications in newborn infants which are sometimes fatal. Tracrium Injection 5 mL single use vials do not contain benzyl alcohol.

PRECAUTIONS

General: Although Tracrium is a less potent histamine releaser than d-tubocurarine or metocurine, the possibility of substantial histamine release in sensitive individuals must be considered. Special caution should be exercised in administering Tracrium to patients in whom substantial histamine release would be especially hazardous (e.g., patients with clinically significant cardiovascular disease) and in patients with any history (e.g., severe anaphylactoid reactions or asthma) suggesting a greater risk of histamine release. In these patients, the recommended initial Tracrium dose is lower (0.3 to 0.4 mg/kg) than for other patients and should be administered slowly or in divided doses over one minute.

Since Tracrium has no clinically significant effects on heart rate in the recommended dosage range, it will not counteract the bradycardia produced by many anesthetic agents or vagal stimulation. As a result, bradycardia during anesthesia may be more common with Tracrium than with other muscle relaxants.

Tracrium may have profound effects in patients with myasthenia gravis, Eaton-Lambert syndrome, or other neuromuscular diseases in which potentiation of nondepolarizing agents has been noted. The use of a peripheral nerve stimulator is especially important for assessing neuromuscular blockade in these patients. Similar precautions should be taken in patients with severe electrolyte disorders or carcinomatosis.

Multiple factors in anesthesia practice are suspected of triggering malignant hyperthermia (MH), a potentially fatal hypermetabolic state of skeletal muscle. Halogenated anesthetic agents and succinylcholine are recognized as the principal pharmacologic triggering agents in MH-susceptible patients; however, since MH can develop in the absence of established triggering agents, the clinician should be prepared to recognize and treat MH in any patient scheduled for general anesthesia. Reports of MH have been rare in cases in which Tracrium has been used. In studies of MH-susceptible animals (swine) and in a clinical study of MH-susceptible patients, Tracrium did not trigger this syndrome.

Resistance to nondepolarizing neuromuscular blocking agents may develop in burn patients. Increased doses of nondepolarizing muscle relaxants may be required in burn patients and are dependent on the time elapsed since the burn injury and the size of the burn.

The safety of Tracrium has not been established in patients with bronchial asthma.

Long-Term Use in Intensive Care Unit (ICU): Tracrium has been used to facilitate mechanical ventilation in ICU patients. When there is a need for long-term medical ventilation, the benefits to risk ratio of neuromuscular blockade must be considered.

There is only limited information on the efficacy and safety of Tracrium administered by long-term (days to weeks) intravenous infusion to facilitate mechanical ventilation in intensive care facilities. For Tracrium, as with other neuromuscular blocking agents used in intensive care facilities, available evidence suggests that there is wide interpatient variability in dosage requirements and that these requirements may change with time. Limited data suggest that Tracrium infusion requirements may increase with prolonged administration in the ICU.

As with other neuromuscular blocking agents, little information is available on the plasma levels or clinical consequences of atracurium metabolites following long-term (days to weeks) infusion of Tracrium in the intensive care unit setting. One metabolite of atracurium, laudanosine, when administered alone to laboratory animals, has been associated with cerebral excitatory effects. Physiological effects of laudanosine in humans have not been demonstrated. The effects of hemodialysis, hemoperfusion and hemofiltration on plasma levels of atracurium and its metabolites are unknown.

Drug Interactions: Drugs which may enhance the neuromuscular blocking action of Tracrium include: enflurane; isoflurane; halothane; certain antibiotics, especially the aminoglycosides and polymyxins; lithium; magnesium salts; procainamide; and quinidine.

If other muscle relaxants are used during the same procedure, the possibility of a synergistic or antagonist effect should be considered.

The prior administration of succinylcholine does not enhance the duration, but quickens the onset and may increase the depth, of neuromuscular blockade induced by Tracrium. Tracrium should not be administered until a patient has recovered from succinylcholine-induced neuromuscular blockade.

Carcinogenesis, Mutagenesis, Impairment of Fertility: Carcinogenesis and fertility studies have not been performed. Atracurium was evaluated in a battery of three short-term mutagenicity tests. It was non-mutagenic in both the Ames Salmonella assay at concentrations up to 1000 μg/plate, and in a rat bone marrow cytogenicity assay at up to paralyzing doses. A positive response was observed in the mouse lymphoma assay under conditions (80 and 100 μg/mL, in the absence of metabolic activation) which killed over 80% of the treated cells; there was no mutagenicity at 60 μg/mL and lower, concentrations which killed up to half of the treated cells. A far weaker response was observed in the presence of metabolic activation at concentrations (1200 μg/mL and higher) which also killed over 80% of the treated cells.

Mutagenicity testing is intended to simulate chronic (years to lifetime) exposure in an effort to determine potential carcinogenicity. Thus, a single positive mutagenicity response for a drug used infrequently and/or briefly is of questionable clinical relevance.

Pregnancy: ***Teratogenic Effects:*** Pregnancy Category C. Tracrium has been shown to be potentially teratogenic in rabbits when given in doses up to approximately one-half the human dose. There are no adequate and well-controlled studies in pregnant women. Tracrium should be used during pregnancy only if the potential benefit justifies the potential risk to the fetus.

Tracrium was administered subcutaneously on days 6 through 18 of gestation to non-ventilated Dutch rabbits. Treatment groups were given either 0.15 mg/kg once daily or 0.10 mg/kg twice daily. Lethal respiratory distress occurred in two 0.15 mg/kg animals and in one 0.10 mg/kg animal, with transient respiratory distress or other evidence of neuromuscular blockade occurring in 10 of 19 and in 4 of 20 of the 0.15 mg/kg and 0.10 mg/kg animals, respectively. There was an increased incidence of certain spontaneously occurring visceral and skeletal anomalies or variations in one or both treated groups when compared to non-treated controls. The percentage of male fetuses was lower (41% vs. 51%) and the post-implantation losses were increased (15% vs. 8%) in the group given 0.15 mg/kg once daily when compared to the controls; the mean numbers of implants (6.5 vs. 4.4) and normal live fetuses (5.4 vs. 3.8) were greater in this group when compared to the control group.

Labor and Delivery: It is not known whether muscle relaxants administered during vaginal delivery have immediate or delayed adverse effects on the fetus or increase the likelihood that resuscitation of the newborn will be necessary. The possibility that forceps delivery will be necessary may increase.

Tracrium (0.3 mg/kg) has been administered to 26 pregnant women during delivery by cesarean section. No harmful effects were attributable to Tracrium in any of the newborn infants, although small amounts of Tracrium were shown to cross the placental barrier. The possibility of respiratory depression in the newborn infant should always be considered following cesarean section during which a neuromuscular blocking agent has been administered. In patients receiving magnesium sulfate, the reversal of neuromuscular blockade may be unsatisfactory and Tracrium dose should be lowered as indicated.

Nursing Mothers: It is not known whether this drug is excreted in human milk. Because many drugs are excreted in human milk, caution should be exercised when Tracrium is administered to a nursing woman.

Pediatric Use: Safety and effectiveness in children below the age of 1 month have not been established.

ADVERSE REACTIONS

Observed in Controlled Clinical Studies: Tracrium was well tolerated and produced few adverse reactions during extensive clinical trials. Most adverse reactions were suggestive of histamine release. In studies including 875 patients, Tracrium was discontinued in only one patient (who required treatment for bronchial secretions), and six other patients required treatment for adverse reactions attributable to Tracrium (wheezing in one, hypotension in five). Of the five patients who required treatment for hypotension, three had a history of significant cardiovascular disease. The overall incidence rate for clinically important adverse reactions, therefore, was 7/875 or 0.8%. The table below includes all adverse reactions reported attributable to Tracrium during clinical trials with 875 patients.

[See table at top of next page.]

Most adverse reactions were of little clinical significance unless they were associated with significant hemodynamic changes. The table below summarizes the incidences of substantial vital sign changes noted during Tracrium clinical

PERCENT OF PATIENTS REPORTING ADVERSE REACTIONS

Adverse Reaction	Initial Tracrium Dose (mg/kg)			
	0.00-0.30 (n = 485)	0.31-0.50* (n = 366)	≥ 0.60 (n = 24)	Total (n = 875)
Skin Flush	1.0%	8.7%	29.2%	5.0%
Erythema	0.6%	0.5%	0%	0.6%
Itching	0.4%	0%	0%	0.2%
Wheezing/Bronchial Secretions	0.2%	0.3%	0%	0.2%
Hives	0.2%	0%	0%	0.1%

*Includes the recommended initial dosage range for most patients.

trials with 530 patients, without cardiovascular disease, in whom these parameters were assessed.
[See table below.]

Observed in Clinical Practice: Based on initial clinical practice experience in approximately 3 million patients who received Tracrium in the U.S. and in the United Kingdom, spontaneously reported adverse reactions were uncommon (approximately 0.01–0.02%). The following adverse reactions are among the most frequently reported, but there are insufficient data to support an estimate of their incidence:

General: Allergic reactions (anaphylatic or anaphylactoid responses) which, in rare instances, were severe (e.g., cardiac arrest)

Musculoskeletal: Inadequate block, prolonged block

Cardiovascular: Hypotension, vasodilatation (flushing), tachycardia, bradycardia

Respiratory: Dyspnea, bronchospasm, laryngospasm

Integumentary: Rash, urticaria, reaction at injection site

OVERDOSAGE

There has been limited experience with Tracrium overdosage. The possibility of iatrogenic overdosage can be minimized by carefully monitoring muscle twitch response to peripheral nerve stimulation. Excessive doses of Tracrium can be expected to produce enhanced pharmacological effects. Overdosage may increase the risk of histamine release and cardiovascular effects, especially hypotension. If cardiovascular support is necessary, this should include proper positioning, fluid administration, and the use of vasopressor agents if necessary. The patient's airway should be assured, with manual or mechanical ventilation maintained as necessary. A longer duration of neuromuscular blockade may result from overdosage and a peripheral nerve stimulator should be used to monitor recovery. Recovery may be facilitated by administration of an anticholinesterase reversing agent such as neostigmine, edrophonium, or pyridostigmine, in conjunction with an anticholinergic agent such as atropine or glycopyrrolate. The appropriate package inserts should be consulted for prescribing information.

Three pediatric patients (3 weeks, 4 and 5 months of age) unintentionally received doses of 0.8 mg/kg to 1.0 mg/kg of Tracrium. The time to 25% recovery (50 to 55 minutes) following these doses, which were 5 to 6 times the ED₉₅ dose, was moderately longer than the corresponding time observed following doses 2.0 to 2.5 times the Tracrium ED₉₅ dose in infants (22 to 36 minutes). Cardiovascular changes were minimal. Nonetheless the possibility of cardiovascular changes must be considered in the case of overdose.

An adult patient (17 years of age) unintentionally received an initial dose of 1.3 mg/kg of Tracrium. The time from injection to 25% recovery (83 minutes) was approximately twice that observed following maximum recommended doses in adults (35–45 minutes). The patient experienced moderate hemodynamic changes (13% increase in mean arterial pressure and 27% increase in heart rate) which persisted for 40 minutes and did not require treatment.

The intravenous LD₅₀'s determined in non-ventilated male and female albino mice and male Wistar rats were 1.9, 2.01 and 1.31 mg/kg, respectively. Deaths occurred within 2 minutes and were caused by respiratory paralysis. The subcutaneous LD₅₀ determined in non-ventilated male Wistar rats was 282.8 mg/kg. Tremors, ptosis, loss of reflexes and respiratory failure preceded death which occurred 45–120 minutes after injection.

DOSAGE AND ADMINISTRATION

To avoid distress to the patient, Tracrium should not be administered before unconsciousness has been induced. Tracrium should not be mixed in the same syringe, or administered simultaneously through the same needle, with alkaline solutions (e.g., barbiturate solutions).

Tracrium should be administered intravenously. DO NOT GIVE TRACRIUM BY INTRAMUSCULAR ADMINISTRATION. Intramuscular administration of Tracrium may result in tissue irritation and there are no clinical data to support this route of administration.

The use of a peripheral nerve stimulator to monitor muscle twitch suppression and recovery will permit the most advantageous use of Tracrium and minimize the possibility of overdosage.

Parenteral drug products should be inspected visually for particulate matter and discoloration prior to administration, whenever solution and container permit.

Bolus Doses for Intubation and Maintenance of Neuromuscular Blockade:

Adults: A Tracrium dose of 0.4 to 0.5 mg/kg (1.7 to 2.2 times the ED₉₅), given as an intravenous bolus injection, is the recommended initial dose for most patients. With this dose, good or excellent conditions for nonemergency intubation can be expected in 2 to 2.5 minutes in most patients, with maximum neuromuscular blockade achieved approximately 3 to 5 minutes after injection. Clinically required neuromuscular blockade generally lasts 20 to 35 minutes under balanced anesthesia. Under balanced anesthesia, recovery to 25% of control is achieved approximately 35 to 45 minutes after injection, and recovery is usually 95% complete approximately 60 minutes after injection.

Tracrium is potentiated by isoflurane or enflurane anesthesia. The same initial Tracrium dose of 0.4 to 0.5 mg/kg may be used for intubation prior to administration of these inhalation agents; however, if Tracrium is first administered under steady state of isoflurane or enflurane, the initial Tracrium dose should be reduced by approximately one-third, i.e., to 0.25 to 0.35 mg/kg, to adjust for the potentiating effects of these anesthetic agents. With halothane, which has only a marginal (approximately 20%) potentiating effect on Tracrium, smaller dosage reductions may be considered. Tracrium doses of 0.08 to 0.10 mg/kg are recommended for maintenance of neuromuscular blockade during prolonged surgical procedures. The first maintenance dose will generally be required 20 to 45 minutes after the initial Tracrium injection, but the need for maintenance doses should be determined by clinical criteria. Because Tracrium lacks cumulative effects, maintenance doses may be administered at relatively regular intervals for each patient, ranging approximately from 15 to 25 minutes under balanced anesthesia, slightly longer under isoflurane or enflurane. Higher Tracrium doses (up to 0.2 mg/kg) permit maintenance dosing at longer intervals.

Children and Infants: No Tracrium dosage adjustments are required for pediatric patients two years of age or older. A Tracrium dose of 0.3 to 0.4 mg/kg is recommended as the initial dose for infants (1 month to 2 years of age) under halothane anesthesia. Maintenance doses may be required with slightly greater frequency in infants and children than in adults.

Special Considerations: An initial Tracrium dose of 0.3 to 0.4 mg/kg, given slowly or in divided doses over one minute,

is recommended for adults, children, or infants with significant cardiovascular disease and for adults, children, or infants with any history (e.g., severe anaphylactoid reactions or asthma) suggesting a greater risk of histamine release. Dosage reductions must be considered also in patients with neuromuscular disease, severe electrolyte disorders, or carcinomatosis in which potentiation of neuromuscular blockade or difficulties with reversal have been demonstrated. There has been no clinical experience with Tracrium in these patients, and no specific dosage adjustments can be recommended. No Tracrium dosage adjustments are required for patients with renal disease.

An initial Tracrium dose of 0.3 to 0.4 mg/kg is recommended for adults following the use of succinylcholine for intubation under balanced anesthesia. Further reductions may be desirable with the use of potent inhalation anesthetics. The patient should be permitted to recover from the effects of succinylcholine prior to Tracrium administration. Insufficient data are available for recommendation of a specific initial Tracrium dose for administration following the use of succinylcholine in children and infants.

Use by Infusion: After administration of a recommended initial bolus dose of Tracrium (0.3 to 0.5 mg/kg), a diluted solution of Tracrium can be administered by continuous infusion to adults and children aged 2 or more years for maintenance of neuromuscular blockade during extended surgical procedures. Long-term intravenous infusion to support mechanical ventilation in the intensive care unit has not been studied sufficiently to support dosage recommendations (see PRECAUTIONS: Long-Term Use in Intensive Care Unit).

Infusion of Tracrium should be individualized for each patient. The rate of administration should be adjusted according to the patient's response as determined by peripheral nerve stimulation. Accurate dosing is best achieved using a precision infusion device.

Infusion of Tracrium should be initiated only after early evidence of spontaneous recovery from the bolus dose. An initial infusion rate of 9 to 10 μg/kg/min may be required to rapidly counteract the spontaneous recovery of neuromuscular function. Thereafter, a rate of 5 to 9 μg/kg/min should be adequate to maintain continuous neuromuscular blockade in the range of 89 to 99% in most pediatric and adult patients under balanced anesthesia. Occasional patients may require infusion rates as low as 2 μg/kg/min or as high as 15 μg/kg/min.

The neuromuscular blocking effect of Tracrium administered by infusion is potentiated by enflurane or isoflurane and, to a lesser extent, by halothane. Reduction in the infusion rate of Tracrium should, therefore, be considered for patients receiving inhalation anesthesia. The rate of Tracrium infusion should be reduced by approximately one-third in the presence of steady-state enflurane or isoflurane anesthesia; smaller reductions should be considered in the presence of halothane.

In patients undergoing cardiopulmonary bypass with induced hypothermia, the rate of infusion of Tracrium required to maintain adequate surgical relaxation during hypothermia (25° to 28°C) has been shown to be approximately half the rate required during normothermia.

Spontaneous recovery from neuromuscular blockade following discontinuation of Tracrium infusion may be expected to proceed at a rate comparable to that following administration of a single bolus dose.

Tracrium infusion solutions may be prepared by admixing Tracrium Injection with an appropriate diluent such as 5% Dextrose Injection USP, 0.9% Sodium Chloride Injection USP, or 5% Dextrose and 0.9% Sodium Chloride Injection USP. Infusion solutions should be used within 24 hours of preparation. Unused solutions should be discarded. Solutions containing 0.2 mg/mL or 0.5 mg/mL Tracrium in the above diluents may be stored either under refrigeration or at room temperature for 24 hours without significant loss of potency. Care should be taken during admixture to prevent inadvertent contamination. Visually inspect prior to administration.

Spontaneous degradation of Tracrium has been demonstrated to occur more rapidly in lactated Ringer's solution than in 0.9% sodium chloride solution. Therefore, it is recommended that Lactated Ringer's Injection USP not be used as a diluent in preparing solutions of Tracrium for infusion.

The amount of infusion solution required per minute will depend upon the concentration of Tracrium in the infusion solution, the desired dose of Tracrium, and the patient's weight. The following tables provide guidelines for delivery, in mL/hr (equivalent to microdrops/min when 60 microdrops = 1 mL), of Tracrium solutions in concentrations of 0.2 mg/mL (20 mg in 100 mL) or 0.5 mg/mL (50 mg in 100 mL) with an infusion pump or a gravity flow device.

PERCENT OF PATIENTS SHOWING ≥ 30% VITAL SIGN CHANGES FOLLOWING ADMINISTRATION OF TRACRIUM

Vital Sign Change	Initial Tracrium Dose (mg/kg)			
	0.00-0.30 (n = 365)	0.31-0.50* (n = 144)	≥ 0.60 (n = 21)	Total (n = 530)
Mean Arterial Pressure				
Increase	1.9%	2.8%	0%	2.1%
Decrease	1.1%	2.1%	14.3%	1.9%
Heart Rate				
Increase	1.6%	2.8%	4.8%	2.1%
Decrease	0.8%	0%	0%	0.6%

*Includes the recommended initial dosage range for most patients.

Continued on next page

Burroughs Wellcome—Cont.

Tracrium (atracurium besylate) Infusion Rates for a Concentration of 0.2 mg/mL

Patient Weight (Kg)	Drug Delivery Rate (µg/kg/min)					
	5	6	7	8	9	10
	Infusion Delivery Rate (mL/hr)					
30	45	54	63	72	81	90
35	53	63	74	84	95	105
40	60	72	84	96	108	120
45	68	81	95	108	122	135
50	75	90	105	120	135	150
55	83	99	116	132	149	165
60	90	108	126	144	162	180
65	98	117	137	156	176	195
70	105	126	147	168	189	210
75	113	135	158	180	203	225
80	120	144	168	192	216	240
90	135	162	189	216	243	270
100	150	180	210	240	270	300

Tracrium (atracurium besylate) Infusion Rates for a Concentration of 0.5 mg/mL

Patient Weight (Kg)	Drug Delivery Rate (µg/kg/min)					
	5	6	7	8	9	10
	Infusion Delivery Rate (mL/hr)					
30	18	22	25	29	32	36
35	21	25	29	34	38	42
40	24	29	34	38	43	48
45	27	32	38	43	49	54
50	30	36	42	48	54	60
55	33	40	46	53	59	66
60	36	43	50	58	65	72
65	39	47	55	62	70	78
70	42	50	59	67	76	84
75	45	54	63	72	81	90
80	48	58	67	77	86	96
90	54	65	76	86	97	108
100	60	72	84	96	108	120

HOW SUPPLIED

Tracrium Injection, 10 mg atracurium besylate in each mL.
5 mL Single Use Vial (50 mg atracurium besylate per vial). Tray of 10 (NDC 0081-0940-44).
10 mL Multiple Dose Vial (100 mg atracurium besylate per vial). Contains benzyl alcohol (see WARNINGS). Tray of 10 (NDC 0081-0940-95).

STORAGE: Tracrium Injection should be refrigerated at 2° to 8°C (36° to 46°F) to preserve potency. DO NOT FREEZE. Upon removal from refrigeration to room temperature storage conditions (25°C/77°F), use Tracrium Injection within 14 days even if rerefrigerated.

U.S. Patent No. 4179507 627248

VASOXYL® INJECTION ℞

[*văz″ox′ĭl*]
(Methoxamine Hydrochloride)
20 mg in 1 ml

DESCRIPTION

Vasoxyl (methoxamine hydrochloride) Injection is a sterile solution for intravenous or intramuscular injection, made isotonic with sodium chloride. Each 1 ml ampul contains 20 mg methoxamine hydrochloride. Citric acid anhydrous 0.3% and sodium citrate 0.3% are added as buffers and potassium metabisulfite 0.1% is added as an antioxidant.

Methoxamine hydrochloride is a sympathomimetic amine. It has the empirical formula $C_{11}H_{17}NO_3 \cdot HCl$ and a molecular weight of 247.72. The drug is very soluble in water, soluble in ethanol, but practically insoluble in ether, benzene or chloroform. It is known chemically as α-(1-aminoethyl)-2,5-dimethoxybenzenemethanol hydrochloride.

CLINICAL PHARMACOLOGY

Vasoxyl is an alpha-receptor stimulant which produces a prompt and prolonged rise in blood pressure following parenteral administration. It is especially useful for maintaining blood pressure during operations under spinal anesthesia[1,2,3] and may also be used safely during general anesthesia. Vasoxyl does not increase the irritability of the cyclopropane-sensitized heart, making it useful during cyclopropane anesthesia.[4,5] Tachyphylaxis has not been a clinical problem.[1]

The major pharmacological effect of Vasoxyl is a potent, prolonged pressor action following parenteral administration. Vasoxyl differs from most other sympathomimetic amines both in animals[4,6,7] and in man[1,8] by having a predominantly peripheral action and lacking inotropic and chronotropic effects. Vasoxyl has less arrhythmogenic potential than other sympathomimetic amines and rarely causes ventricular tachycardia, fibrillation, or increased sinoatrial rate.[4] On occasion, a decrease in rate occurs as blood pressure increases,[1,9,10] apparently caused by a carotid sinus reflex. This bradycardia can be abolished by atropine.[9] The pressor action appears to be due to peripheral vasoconstriction rather than a centrally mediated effect. Evidence for direct action on blood vessels is provided in part by the observation of intense constriction along the course of a vein into which Vasoxyl has been injected.[1] Vasoxyl also increases venous pressure.[8]

Following intravenous administration of Vasoxyl in dogs[11] and humans,[9,12] the peak pressor effect occurs within 0.5 to 2 minutes. In a group of human surgical patients,[13] the duration of the pressor effect following a single intravenous dose of 2 to 4 mg of Vasoxyl was 10 to 15 minutes. No clinical pharmacology studies are available concerning the onset and duration of action after administration of recommended intramuscular doses (10 to 15 mg). With administration of 10 to 40 mg Vasoxyl intramuscularly to patients, however, the peak effect occurs within 15 to 20 minutes, and the duration of action is approximately one and a half hours.[14]

Data from pharmacokinetic studies of Vasoxyl following either intravenous or intramuscular administration are not available.

INDICATIONS AND USAGE

Vasoxyl is intended for supporting, restoring or maintaining blood pressure during anesthesia (including cyclopropane anesthesia). It can be used to terminate some episodes of supraventricular tachycardia.

CONTRAINDICATIONS

Vasoxyl is contraindicated in patients with severe hypertension, or in patients who are hypersensitive to methoxamine.

WARNINGS

The use of Vasoxyl in patients receiving monoamine oxidase inhibitors, tricyclic antidepressants or oxytocic agents such as vasopressin or certain ergot alkaloids may result in potentiation of the pressor effect (see "Drug Interactions" under PRECAUTIONS).

Contains potassium metabisulfite, a sulfite that may cause allergic-type reactions including anaphylactic symptoms and life-threatening or less severe asthmatic episodes in certain susceptible people. The overall prevalence of sulfite sensitivity in the general population is unknown and probably low. Sulfite sensitivity is seen more frequently in asthmatic than in nonasthmatic people.

PRECAUTIONS

General: Vasoxyl, like other vasopressor agents, should be used with caution in patients with hyperthyroidism, bradycardia, partial heart block, myocardial disease, or severe arteriosclerosis. Caution should be exercised to avoid overdosage, preventing undesirable high blood pressure and/or bradycardia. Note: Bradycardia may be abolished with atropine (see OVERDOSAGE). Also, caution should be taken when Vasoxyl is used closely following the parenteral injection of ergot alkaloids to avoid an excessive rise in blood pressure.

Drug Interactions: The pressor effect of Vasoxyl may be markedly potentiated when Vasoxyl is used in conjunction with monoamine oxidase inhibitors, tricyclic antidepressants, vasopressin or ergot alkaloids such as ergotamine, ergonovine or methylergonovine. Therefore, when initiating pressor therapy in patients receiving these drugs the initial dose should be small and given with caution (see WARNINGS).

Drug/Laboratory Test Interactions: Vasoxyl may increase plasma cortisol and ACTH levels. Caution should be used when interpreting plasma cortisol and ACTH levels in a patient concurrently receiving Vasoxyl.[15,16]

Carcinogenesis, Mutagenesis, Impairment of Fertility: No long-term studies have been performed to evaluate the potential of Vasoxyl in these areas.

Pregnancy: ***Teratogenic Effects:*** Pregnancy Category C: Vasoxyl has been shown to decrease uterine blood flow, decrease fetal heart rate and adversely affect the fetal acid-base status in pregnant ewes and monkeys at doses comparable to those used in humans. There are no adequate and well-controlled studies in pregnant women. There has been one report of a fetal death; the mother received Vasoxyl concomitantly with several other drugs. A direct causal relationship to Vasoxyl was not established. Vasoxyl should be used during pregnancy only if the potential benefit justifies the potential risk to the fetus.

Vasoxyl (2.5 mg I.V., 1 to 3 times over a 45 min. period) given to 7 pregnant ewes showed a significant deterioration in fetal acid-base status as evidenced by hypoxia, hypercarbia and metabolic acidosis.[17] An inverse relationship between pressor response to Vasoxyl and uteroplacental blood flow has been shown in 16 pregnant ewes studied at doses ranging from 0.025 mg/kg to 0.2 mg/kg.[18] Uterine blood flow was decreased at all doses, but no significant change in fetal blood gas or acid-base status was demonstrated. Vasoxyl administration to 4 fetuses (50 mcg/kg/min for 60 min) and to 4 ewes (25 mcg/kg/min for 30 min) was associated with a decrease in fetal heart rate and uterine blood flow.[19] Nine monkeys studied at an average Vasoxyl dose of 1.3 mg/kg administered over 57 min showed a decrease in uterine blood flow and a possible association with fetal asphyxia.[20]

Labor and Delivery: If vasopressor drugs are used to correct hypotension or added to the local anesthetic solution during labor and delivery, some oxytocic drugs (vasopressin, ergotamine, ergonovine, methylergonovine) may cause severe persistent hypertension (see WARNINGS and "Drug Interactions" under PRECAUTIONS).

"Note": In pregnant animals, Vasoxyl has been shown to decrease uterine blood flow, possibly resulting in fetal asphyxia. Uterine hypertonus and fetal bradycardia may also be produced. (See ADVERSE REACTIONS and "Pregnancy" under PRECAUTIONS).

Nursing Mothers: It is not known whether this drug is excreted in human milk. Because many drugs are excreted in human milk, caution should be exercised when Vasoxyl is administered to a nursing woman.

Pediatric Use: Safety and effectiveness in children have not been established.

ADVERSE REACTIONS

The following adverse reactions have been observed, but there are insufficient data to support an estimate of their frequency:

Cardiovascular: Excessive blood pressure elevations particularly with high dosage, ventricular ectopic beats
Gastrointestinal: Nausea, vomiting (often projectile)
Central Nervous System: Headache (often severe), anxiety
Integumentary: Sweating, pilomotor response
Genitourinary: Uterine hypertonus, fetal bradycardia (see "Labor and Delivery" under PRECAUTIONS), urinary urgency

OVERDOSAGE

Overdosage of Vasoxyl may be manifested as an undesirable elevation in blood pressure and/or bradycardia. Should a clinically significant elevation of blood pressure occur that requires treatment, it may be immediately reversed with an alpha-adrenergic blocking agent (e.g., phentolamine). Bradycardia may be abolished by atropine.

DOSAGE AND ADMINISTRATION

Blood volume depletion should always be corrected before any vasopressor is administered. The usual intravenous dose of Vasoxyl for emergencies is 3 to 5 mg, injected slowly. Intravenous injection may be supplemented by intramuscular injections to provide a more prolonged effect. The usual intramuscular dose is 10 to 15 mg given shortly before or at the time of administering spinal anesthesia to prevent a fall in blood pressure. The tendency for the blood pressure to fall is greater with higher levels of spinal anesthesia, hence the dosage may be adjusted accordingly; 10 mg may be adequate at lower spinal levels while 15 to 20 mg may be required at high levels of spinal anesthesia. Repeated doses may be given if necessary, but time should be allowed for the previous dose to act (about 15 minutes, see CLINICAL PHARMACOLOGY). For cases of only moderate hypotension, 5 to 10 mg intramuscularly may be adequate.

For purposes of correcting a fall in blood pressure, an intramuscular injection of 10 to 15 mg of Vasoxyl may be given depending upon the degree of fall. In cases where the systolic pressure falls to 60 mmHg or less, or whenever an emergency exists, an intravenous injection of 3 to 5 mg Vasoxyl is indicated. This intravenous dose may be accompanied by 10 to 15 mg intramuscularly to provide more prolonged effect.

For termination of episodes of supraventricular tachycardia not responsive to other modes of therapy, the usual dose of Vasoxyl is 10 mg intravenously, administered by slow push (i.e., 3 to 5 min).

Parenteral drug products should be inspected visually for particulate matter and discoloration prior to administration whenever solution and container permit.

HOW SUPPLIED

1 ml ampuls, containing 20 mg methoxamine hydrochloride. Box of 10 (NDC 0081-0957-10). Store at 15° to 30°C (59° to 86°F) and protect from light.

REFERENCES

1. King BD, Dripps RD: The use of methoxamine for maintenance of the circulation during spinal anesthesia. *Surg Gynecol Obstet* 1950;90:659–665.
2. Kistler EM, Ruben JE: Methoxamine in 1 percent procaine as a prophylactic vasopressor in spinal anesthesia. *Arch Surg* 1951;62:64–69.
3. Poe MF: Use of methoxamine hydrochloride as a pressor agent during spinal analgesia. *Anesthesiology* 1952; 13:89–93.
4. Lahti RE, Brill IC, McCawley EL: The effect of methoxamine hydrochloride (Vasoxyl) on cardiac rhythm. *J Pharmacol Exp Ther* 1955;115:268–274.

5. Stutzman JW, Pettinga FL, Fruggiero EJ: Cardiac effects of methoxamine (β-[2,5-dimethoxy-phenyl]-β-hydroxyisopropylamine HCl) and desoxyephedrine during cyclopropane anesthesia. *J Pharmacol Exp Ther* 1949; 97:385–387.

6. West JW, Faulk AT, Guzman SV: Comparative study of effects of levarterenol and methoxamine in shock associated with acute myocardial ischemia in dogs. *Circ Res* 1962;10:712–721.

7. Goldberg LI, Cotten M, Darby TD, Howell EV: Comparative heart contractile force effects of equipressor doses of several sympathomimetic amines. *J Pharmacol Exp Ther* 1953;108:177–185.

8. Aviado DM, Wnuck AL: Mechanisms for cardiac slowing by methoxamine. *J Pharmacol Exp Ther* 1957; 119:99–106.

9. Nathanson MH, Miller H: Clinical observations on a new epinephrin-like compound, methoxamine. *Am J Med Sci* 1952;223:270–279.

10. Stanfield CA, Yu PN: Hemodynamic effects of methoxamine in mitral valve disease. *Circ Res* 1960;8:859–864.

11. Imai S, Shigei T, Hashimoto K: Cardiac actions of methoxamine with special reference to its antagonist action to epinephrine. *Circ Res* 1961;9:552–560.

12. *The Extra Pharmacopoeia, Martindale* 28th Ed., Reynolds, JEF, ed., Pharmaceutical Press (London), pp. 19.

13. Goldberg LI, Bloodwell RD, Braunwald E, *et al.* The direct effects of norepinephrine, epinephrine, and methoxamine on myocardial contractile force in man. *Circ* 1960;22:1125–1132.

14. Data on File, Burroughs Wellcome Co.

15. Laurian L, Oberman Z, Hoerer E, *et al.*: Low cortisol and growth hormone secretion in response to methoxamine administration in obese subjects. *Isr J Med Sci* 1977;13:477–481.

16. Nakai Y, Imura H, Yoshimi T, Matsukura S: Adrenergic control mechanism for ACTH secretion in man. *Acta Endocrinol* 1973;74:263–270.

17. Shnider SM, DeLorimier AA, Asling JH, Morishima HO: Vasopressors in obstetrics. II. Fetal hazards of methoxamine administration during obstetric spinal anesthesia. *Am J Obstet Gynecol* 1970;106:680–686.

18. Ralston DH, Shnider SM, DeLorimier AA: Effects of equipotent ephedrine, metaraminol, mephentermine and methoxamine on uterine blood flow in the pregnant ewe. *Anesthesiology* 1974;40:354–370.

19. Oakes GK, Ehrenkranz RA, Walker AM, *et al.*: Effect of α-adrenergic agonist and antagonist infusion on the umbilical and uterine circulations of pregnant sheep. *Biol Neonate* 1980;38:229–237.

20. Eng M, Berges PU, Ueland K, *et al.*: The effects of methoxamine and ephedrine in normotensive pregnant primates. *Anesthesiology* 1971;35:354–360.   642729

VIROPTIC® OPHTHALMIC   ℞
[vī-rŏp´tĭk˝]
SOLUTION, 1% Sterile
(Trifluridine)

DESCRIPTION

Viroptic is the brand name for trifluridine (also known as trifluorothymidine, F_3TdR, F_3T), an antiviral drug for topical treatment of epithelial keratitis caused by Herpes simplex virus. The chemical name of trifluridine is 2'-deoxy-5-(trifluoromethyl)uridine.

Viroptic sterile ophthalmic solution contains 1% trifluridine in an aqueous solution with acetic acid and sodium acetate (buffers), sodium chloride, and thimerosal 0.001% (added as a preservative).

CLINICAL PHARMACOLOGY

Trifluridine is a fluorinated pyrimidine nucleoside with *in vitro* and *in vivo* activity against Herpes simplex virus, types 1 and 2 and vacciniavirus. Some strains of Adenovirus are also inhibited *in vitro*.

Trifluridine interferes with DNA synthesis in cultured mammalian cells. However, its antiviral mechanism of action is not completely known.

In vitro perfusion studies on excised rabbit corneas have shown that trifluridine penetrates the intact cornea as evidenced by recovery of parental drug and its major metabolite, 5-carboxy-2'-deoxyuridine, on the endothelial side of the cornea. Absence of the corneal epithelium enhances the penetration of trifluridine approximately two-fold.

Intraocular penetration of trifluridine occurs after topical instillation of Viroptic into human eyes. Decreased corneal integrity or stromal or uveal inflammation may enhance the penetration of trifluridine into the aqueous humor. Unlike the results of ocular penetration of trifluridine *in vitro*, 5-carboxy-2'-deoxyuridine was not found in detectable concentrations within the aqueous humor of the human eye.

Systemic absorption of trifluridine following therapeutic dosing with Viroptic appears to be negligible. No detectable concentrations of trifluridine or 5-carboxy-2'-deoxyuridine

were found in the sera of adult healthy normal subjects who had Viroptic instilled into their eyes seven times daily for 14 consecutive days.

INDICATIONS AND USAGE

Viroptic (Trifluridine) Ophthalmic Solution, 1% is indicated for the treatment of primary keratoconjunctivitis and recurrent epithelial keratitis due to Herpes simplex virus, types 1 and 2. Viroptic is also effective in the treatment of epithelial keratitis that has not responded clinically to the topical administration of idoxuridine or when ocular toxicity or hypersensitivity to idoxuridine has occurred. In a smaller number of patients found to be resistant to topical vidarabine, Viroptic was also effective.

The clinical efficacy of Viroptic in the treatment of stromal keratitis and uveitis due to Herpes simplex virus or ophthalmic infections caused by vacciniavirus and Adenovirus has not been established by well-controlled clinical trials. Viroptic has not been shown to be effective in the prophylaxis of Herpes simplex virus keratoconjunctivitis and epithelial keratitis by well-controlled clinical trials. Viroptic is not effective against bacterial, fungal or chlamydial infections of the cornea or nonviral trophic lesions.

During controlled multicenter clinical trials, 92 of 97 (95%) patients (78 of 81 with dendritic and 14 of 16 with geographic ulcers) responded to Viroptic therapy as evidenced by complete corneal re-epithelialization within the 14-day therapy period. In these controlled studies, 56 of 75 (75%) patients (49 of 58 with dendritic and 7 of 17 with geographic ulcers) responded to idoxuridine therapy. The mean time to corneal re-epithelialization of dendritic ulcers (6 days) and geographic ulcers (7 days) was similar for both therapies. In other clinical studies, Viroptic was evaluated in the treatment of Herpes simplex virus keratitis in patients who were unresponsive or intolerant to the topical administration of idoxuridine or vidarabine. Viroptic was effective in 138 of 150 (92%) patients (109 of 114 with dendritic and 29 of 36 with geographic ulcers) as evidenced by corneal re-epithelialization. The mean time to corneal re-epithelialization was 6 days for patients with dendritic ulcers and 12 days for patients with geographic ulcers.

CONTRAINDICATIONS

Viroptic (Trifluridine) Ophthalmic Solution, 1%, is contraindicated for patients who develop hypersensitivity reactions or chemical intolerance to trifluridine.

WARNINGS

The recommended dosage and frequency of administration should not be exceeded (see DOSAGE AND ADMINISTRATION).

PRECAUTIONS

General: Viroptic (Trifluridine) Ophthalmic Solution, 1% should be prescribed only for patients who have a clinical diagnosis of herpetic keratitis.

Viroptic may cause mild local irritation of the conjunctiva and cornea when instilled but these effects are usually transient.

Although documented *in vitro* viral resistance to trifluridine has not been reported following multiple exposure to Viroptic, the possibility exists of viral resistance development.

Drug Interactions: The following drugs have been administered topically to the eye and concurrently with Viroptic in a limited number of patients without apparent evidence of adverse interaction: antibiotics—chloramphenicol, erythromycin, polymyxin B sulfate, bacitracin, gentamicin sulfate, tetracycline HCl, sodium sulfacetamide, neomycin sulfate; steroids—dexamethasone, dexamethasone sodium phosphate, prednisolone acetate, prednisolone sodium phosphate, hydrocortisone, fluorometholone; and other ophthalmic drugs—atropine sulfate, scopolamine hydrobromide, naphazoline hydrochloride, cyclopentolate hydrochloride, homatropine hydrobromide, pilocarpine, 1-epinephrine hydrochloride, sodium chloride.

Carcinogenesis, Mutagenesis, Impairment of Fertility: *Mutagenic Potential.* Trifluridine has been shown to exert mutagenic, DNA-damaging and cell-transforming activities in various standard *in vitro* test systems, and clastogenic activity in *Vicia faba* cells. It did not induce chromosome aberrations in bone marrow cells of male or female rats following a single subcutaneous dose of 100 mg/kg, but was weakly positive in female, but not in male, rats following daily subcutaneous administration at 700 mg/kg/day for 5 days.

Although the significance of these test results is not clear or fully understood, there exists the possibility that mutagenic agents may cause genetic damage in humans.

Oncogenic Potential. Lifetime carcinogenicity bioassays in rats and mice given daily subcutaneous doses of trifluridine have been performed. Rats tested at 1.5, 7.5 and 15 mg/kg/day had increased incidences of adenocarcinomas of the intestinal tract and mammary glands, hemangiosarcomas of the speen and liver, carcinosarcomas of the prostate gland and granulosa-thecal cell tumors of the ovary. Mice were tested at 1, 5 and 10 mg/kg/day; those given 10 mg/kg/day trifluridine had significantly increased incidences of adeno-

carcinomas of the intestinal tract and uterus. Those given 10 mg/kg/day also had a significantly increased incidence of testicular atrophy as compared to vehicle control mice.

Pregnancy: *Teratogenic Effects:* Pregnancy Category C. Trifluridine was not teratogenic at doses up to 5.0 mg/kg/day (23 times the estimated human exposure) when given subcutaneously to rats and rabbits. However, fetal toxicity consisting of delayed ossification of portions of the skeleton occurred at dose levels of 2.5 and 5.0 mg/kg/day in rats and at 2.5 mg/kg/day in rabbits. In addition, both 2.5 and 5.0 mg/kg/day produced fetal death and resorption in rabbits. In both rats and rabbits, 1.0 mg/kg/day (5 times the estimated human exposure) was a no-effect level. There were no teratogenic or fetotoxic effects after topical application of Viroptic Ophthalmic Solution 1% (approximately 5 times the estimated human exposure) to the eyes of rabbits on the 6th through the 18th days of pregnancy.[1] In a non-standard test, trifluridine solution has been shown to be teratogenic when injected directly into the yolk sac of chicken eggs.[2] There are no adequate and well-controlled studies in pregnant women. Viroptic Ophthalmic Solution 1% should be used during pregnancy only if the potential benefit justifies the potential risk to the fetus.

Nursing Mothers: It is unlikely that trifluridine is excreted in human milk after ophthalmic instillation of Viroptic because of the relatively small dosage (≤ 5.0 mg/day), its dilution in body fluids and its extremely short half-life (approximately 12 minutes). The drug should not be prescribed for nursing mothers unless the potential benefits outweigh the potential risks.

ADVERSE REACTIONS

The most frequent adverse reactions reported during controlled clinical trials were mild, transient burning or stinging upon instillation (4.6%) and palpebral edema (2.8%). Other adverse reactions in decreasing order of reported frequency were superficial punctate keratopathy, epithelial keratopathy, hypersensitivity reaction, stromal edema, irritation, keratitis sicca, hyperemia, and increased intraocular pressure.

OVERDOSAGE

Overdosage by ocular instillation is unlikely because any excess solution should be quickly expelled from the conjunctival sac.

Acute overdosage by accidental oral ingestion of Viroptic has not occurred. However, should such ingestion occur, the 75 mg dosage of trifluridine in a 7.5 mL bottle of Viroptic is not likely to produce adverse effects. Single intravenous doses of 15–30 mg/kg/day in children and adults with neoplastic disease produce reversible bone marrow depression as the only potentially serious toxic effect and only after 3–5 courses of therapy.[3] The acute oral LD_{50} in the mouse and rat was 4379 mg/kg or higher.

DOSAGE AND ADMINISTRATION

Instill one drop of Viroptic Ophthalmic Solution, 1% onto the cornea of the affected eye every two hours while awake for a maximum daily dosage of nine drops until the corneal ulcer has completely re-epithelialized. Following re-epithelialization, treatment for an additional seven days of one drop every four hours while awake for a minimum daily dosage of five drops is recommended.

If there are no signs of improvement after seven days of therapy or complete re-epithelialization has not occurred after 14 days of therapy, other forms of therapy should be considered. Continuous administration of Viroptic for periods exceeding 21 days should be avoided because of potential ocular toxicity.

HOW SUPPLIED

Viroptic Ophthalmic Solution, 1% is supplied as a sterile ophthalmic solution in a plastic Drop Dose® dispenser bottle of 7.5 mL. (NDC 0081-0968-02)

Store under refrigeration 2° to 8°C (36° to 46°F).

ANIMAL PHARMACOLOGY AND ANIMAL TOXICOLOGY

Corneal wound healing studies in rabbits showed that Viroptic did not significantly retard closure of epithelial wounds. However, mild toxic changes such as intracellular edema of the basal cell layer, mild thinning of the overlying epithelium and reduced strength of stromal wounds were observed.

Whereas instillation of Viroptic into rabbit eyes during a subchronic toxicity study produced some degree of corneal epithelial thinning, a 12-month chronic toxicity study in rabbits in which Viroptic was instilled into eyes in intermittent, multiple, full-therapy courses showed no drug-related changes in the cornea.

REFERENCES

1. Itoi M, Getter JW, Kaneko N, et al: Teratogenicities of ophthalmic drugs. I. Antiviral ophthalmic drugs. *Arch Ophthalmol* 1975;93:46–51.

Continued on next page

Burroughs Wellcome—Cont.

2. Kury G, Crosby RJ: The teratogenic effect of 5-trifluoromethyl-2′-deoxyuridine in chicken embryos. *Toxicol Appl Pharmacol* 1967;11:72–80.
3. Ansfield FJ, Ramirez G: Phase I and II studies of 2′-deoxy-5-(trifluoromethyl)-uridine (NSC-75520). *Cancer Chemother Rep* 1971; 55(pt 1):205–208. 643060

WELLBUTRIN® Tablets ℞
[*wel ′byü-trin*]
(Bupropion Hydrochloride)

DESCRIPTION

Wellbutrin (bupropion hydrochloride),* an antidepressant of the aminoketone class, is chemically unrelated to tricyclic, tetracyclic, or other known antidepressant agents. Its structure closely resembles that of diethylpropion; it is related to phenylethylamines. It is designated as *2-tert-* butylamino-3′-chloropropiophenone hydrochloride. The molecular weight is 276.2. The empirical formula is $C_{13}H_{18}ClNO \cdot HCl$. Bupropion powder is white, crystalline, and highly soluble in water. It has a bitter taste and produces the sensation of local anesthesia on the oral mucosa.

Wellbutrin is supplied for oral administration as 75 mg (yellow-gold) and 100 mg (red) film-coated tablets. Each tablet contains the labeled amount of bupropion hydrochloride and the inactive ingredients: 75 mg tablet—D&C Yellow No. 10 Lake, FD&C Yellow No. 6 Lake, hydroxypropyl cellulose, hydroxypropyl methylcellulose, light mineral oil, microcrystalline cellulose, talc and titanium dioxide; 100 mg tablet—FD&C Red No. 40 Lake, FD&C Yellow No. 6 Lake, hydroxypropyl cellulose, hydroxypropyl methylcellulose, light mineral oil, microcrystalline cellulose, talc and titanium dioxide.

CLINICAL PHARMACOLOGY

Pharmacodynamics and Pharmacological Actions: The neurochemical mechanism of the antidepressant effect of bupropion is not known. Bupropion does not inhibit monoamine oxidase. Compared to classical tricyclic antidepressants, it is a weak blocker of the neuronal uptake of serotonin and norepinephrine; it also inhibits the neuronal reuptake of dopamine to some extent. Bupropion produces dose-related CNS stimulant effects in animals, as evidenced by increased locomotor activity, increased rates of responding in various schedule-controlled operant behavior tasks, and, at high doses, induction of mild stereotyped behavior.

Bupropion causes convulsions in rodents and dogs at doses approximately tenfold the dose recommended as the human antidepressant dose.

Absorption, Distribution, Pharmacokinetics, Metabolism, and Elimination:

Oral bioavailability and single dose pharmacokinetics: In man, following oral administration of Wellbutrin, peak plasma bupropion concentrations are usually achieved within 2 hours, followed by a biphasic decline. The average half-life of the second (post-distributional) phase is approximately 14 hours, with a range of 8 to 24 hours. Six hours after a single dose, plasma bupropion concentrations are approximately 30% of peak concentrations. Plasma bupropion concentrations are dose-proportional following single doses of 100 to 250 mg; however, it is not known if the proportionality between dose and plasma level is maintained in chronic use.

The absolute bioavailability of Wellbutrin tablets in man has not been determined because an intravenous formulation for human use is not available.

However, it appears likely that only a small proportion of any orally administered dose reaches the systemic circulation intact. For example, the absolute bioavailability of bupropion in animals (rats and dogs) ranges from 5–20%.

Metabolism: Following oral administration of 200 mg of ^{14}C-bupropion, 87% and 10% of the radioactive dose were recovered in the urine and feces, respectively. However, the fraction of the oral dose of Wellbutrin excreted unchanged was only 0.5%, a finding documenting the extensive metabolism of bupropion.

Several of the known metabolites of bupropion are pharmacologically active, but their potency and toxicity relative to bupropion have not been fully characterized. However, because of their longer elimination half-lives, the plasma concentrations of at least two of the known metabolites can be expected, especially in chronic use, to be very much higher than the plasma concentration of bupropion. This is of potential clinical importance because factors or conditions altering metabolic capacity (e.g., liver disease, congestive heart failure, age, concomitant medications, etc.) or elimination may be expected to influence the degree and extent of accumulation of these active metabolites.

Furthermore, bupropion has been shown to induce its own metabolism in three animal species (mice, rats, and dogs) following subchronic administration. If induction also occurs in humans, the relative contribution of bupropion and its metabolites to the clinical effects of Wellbutrin may be changed in chronic use.

Plasma and urinary metabolites so far identified include biotransformation products formed via reduction of the carbonyl group and/or hydroxylation of the *tert-* butyl group of bupropion. Four basic metabolites have been identified. They are the *erythro-* and *threo-* amino alcohols of bupropion, the *erythro-* amino diol of bupropion, and a morpholinol metabolite (formed from hydroxylation of the *tert-* butyl group of bupropion).

The morpholinol metabolite appears in the systemic circulation almost as rapidly as the parent drug following a single oral dose. Its peak level is three times the peak level of the parent drug; it has a half-life on the order of 24 hours; and its AUC 0–60 hrs is about 15 times that of bupropion.

The *threo-* amino alcohol metabolite has a plasma concentration-time profile similar to that of the morpholinol metabolite. The *erythro*-amino alcohol and the *erythro-* amino diol metabolites generally cannot be detected in the systemic circulation following a single oral dose of the parent drug. The morpholinol and the *threo-* amino alcohol metabolites have been found to be half as potent as bupropion in animal screening tests for antidepressant drugs.

During a chronic dosing study in 14 depressed patients with left ventricular dysfunction, it was found that there was substantial interpatient variability (two- to fivefold) in the trough steady-state concentrations of bupropion and the morpholinol and *threo-* amino alcohol metabolites. In addition, the steady-state plasma concentrations of these metabolites were 10–100 times the steady-state concentrations of the parent drug.

The effect of other disease states and altered organ function on the metabolism and/or elimination of bupropion has not been studied in detail. However, the elimination of the major metabolites of bupropion may be affected by reduced renal or hepatic function because they are moderately polar compounds and are likely to undergo conjugation in the liver prior to urinary excretion. The preliminary results of a comparative single-dose pharmacokinetic study in normal versus cirrhotic patients indicated that half-lives of the metabolites were prolonged by cirrhosis and that the metabolites accumulated to levels two to three times those in normals.

The effect of age on plasma concentrations of bupropion and its metabolites has not been characterized.

In vitro tests show that bupropion is 80% or more bound to human albumin at plasma concentrations up to 800 micromolar (200 μg/mL).

INDICATIONS AND USAGE

Wellbutrin is indicated for the treatment of depression. A physician considering Wellbutrin for the management of a patient's first episode of depression should be aware that the drug may cause generalized seizures with an approximate incidence of 0.4% (4/1000). This incidence of seizures may exceed that of other marketed antidepressants by as much as fourfold. This relative risk is only an approximate estimate because no direct comparative studies have been conducted.

The efficacy of Wellbutrin has been established in three placebo-controlled trials, including two of approximately three weeks duration in depressed inpatients, and one of approximately six weeks duration in depressed outpatients. The depressive disorder of the patients studied corresponds most closely to the Major Depression category of the APA Diagnostic and Statistical Manual III.

Major Depression implies a prominent and relatively persistent depressed or dysphoric mood that usually interferes with daily functioning (nearly every day for at least two weeks); it should include at least four of the following eight symptoms: change in appetite, change in sleep, psychomotor agitation or retardation, loss of interest in usual activities or decrease in sexual drive, increased fatigability, feelings of guilt or worthlessness, slowed thinking or impaired concentration, and suicidal ideation or attempts.

Effectiveness of Wellbutrin in long-term use, that is, for more than 6 weeks, has not been systematically evaluated in controlled trials. Therefore, the physician who elects to use Wellbutrin for extended periods should periodically reevaluate the long-term usefulness of the drug for the individual patient.

CONTRAINDICATIONS

Wellbutrin is contraindicated in patients with a seizure disorder. Wellbutrin is also contraindicated in patients with a current or prior diagnosis of bulimia or anorexia nervosa because of a higher incidence of seizures noted in such patients treated with Wellbutrin. The concurrent administration of Wellbutrin and a monoamine oxidase (MAO) inhibitor is contraindicated. At least 14 days should elapse between discontinuation of an MAO inhibitor and initiation of treatment with Wellbutrin. Wellbutrin is contraindicated in patients who have shown an allergic response to it.

WARNINGS

SEIZURES: Wellbutrin is associated with seizures in approximately 0.4% (4/1000) of patients treated at doses up to 450 mg/day. This incidence of seizures may exceed that of other marketed antidepressants by as much as fourfold. This relative risk is only an approximate estimate because no direct comparative studies have been conducted. The estimated seizure incidence for Wellbutrin increases almost tenfold between 450 and 600 mg/day, which is twice the usually required daily dose (300 mg) and one and one-third the maximum recommended daily dose (450 mg). Given the wide variability among individuals and their capacity to metabolize and eliminate drugs, this disproportionate increase in seizure incidence with dose incrementation calls for caution in dosing.

During the initial development, 25 among approximately 2400 patients treated with Wellbutrin experienced seizures. At the time of seizure, 7 patients were receiving daily doses of 450 mg or below, for an incidence of 0.33% (3/1000) within the recommended dose range. Twelve (12) patients experienced seizures at 600 mg per day (2.3% incidence); 6 additional patients had seizures at daily doses between 600 and 900 mg (2.8% incidence).

A separate, prospective study was conducted to determine the incidence of seizure during an 8 week treatment exposure in approximately 3200 additional patients who received daily doses of up to 450 mg. Patients were permitted to continue treatment beyond 8 weeks if clinically indicated. Eight (8) seizures occurred during the initial 8 week treatment period and 5 seizures were reported in patients continuing treatment beyond 8 weeks, resulting in a total seizure incidence of 0.4%.

The risk of seizure appears to be strongly associated with dose and the presence of predisposing factors. A significant predisposing factor (e.g., history of head trauma or prior seizure, CNS tumor, concomitant medications that lower seizure threshold, etc.) was present in approximately one-half of the patients experiencing a seizure. Sudden and large increments in dose may contribute to increased risk. While many seizures occurred early in the course of treatment, some seizures did occur after several weeks at fixed dose.

Recommendations for reducing the risk of seizure: **Retrospective analysis of clinical experience gained during the development of Wellbutrin suggests that the risk of seizure may be minimized if (1) the total daily dose of Wellbutrin does *not* exceed 450 mg, (2) the daily dose is administered t.i.d., with each single dose *not* to exceed 150 mg to avoid high peak concentrations of bupropion and/or its metabolites, and (3) the rate of incrementation of dose is very gradual. Extreme caution should be used when Wellbutrin is (1) administered to patients with a history of seizure, cranial trauma, or other predisposition(s) toward seizure, or (2) prescribed with other agents (e.g., antipsychotics, other antidepressants, etc.) or treatment regimens (e.g., abrupt discontinuation of a benzodiazepine) that lower seizure threshold.**

Potential for Hepatotoxicity: In rats receiving large doses of bupropion chronically, there was an increase in incidence of hepatic hyperplastic nodules and hepatocellular hypertrophy. In dogs receiving large doses of bupropion chronically, various histologic changes were seen in the liver, and laboratory tests suggesting mild hepatocellular injury were noted. Although scattered abnormalities in liver function tests were detected in patients participating in clinical trials, there is no clinical evidence that bupropion acts as a hepatotoxin in humans.

PRECAUTIONS

General:

Agitation and Insomnia: A substantial proportion of patients treated with Wellbutrin experience some degree of increased restlessness, agitation, anxiety, and insomnia, especially shortly after initiation of treatment. In clinical studies, these symptoms were sometimes of sufficient magnitude to require treatment with sedative/hypnotic drugs. In approximately 2% of patients, symptoms were sufficiently severe to require discontinuation of Wellbutrin treatment.

Psychosis, Confusion, and Other Neuropsychiatric Phenomena: Patients treated with Wellbutrin have been reported to show a variety of neuropsychiatric signs and symptoms including delusions, hallucinations, psychotic episodes, confusion, and paranoia. Because of the uncontrolled nature of many studies, it is impossible to provide a precise estimate of the extent of risk imposed by treatment with Wellbutrin. In several cases, neuropsychiatric phenomena abated upon dose reduction and/or withdrawal of treatment.

Activation of Psychosis and/or Mania: Antidepressants can precipitate manic episodes in Bipolar Manic Depressive patients during the depressed phase of their illness and may activate latent psychosis in other susceptible patients. Wellbutrin is expected to pose similar risks.

Altered Appetite and Weight: A weight loss of greater than 5 pounds occurred in 28% of Wellbutrin patients. This incidence is approximately double that seen in comparable patients treated with tricyclics or placebo. Furthermore, while 34.5% of patients receiving tricyclic antidepressants gained weight, only 9.4% of patients treated with Wellbutrin did. Consequently, if weight loss is a major presenting sign of a

*U.S. Patent No. 3819706

patient's depressive illness, the anorectic and/or weight reducing potential of Wellbutrin should be considered.

Suicide: The possibility of a suicide attempt is inherent in depression and may persist until significant remission occurs. Accordingly, prescriptions for Wellbutrin should be written for the smallest number of tablets consistent with good patient management.

Use in Patients with Systemic Illness: There is no clinical experience establishing the safety of Wellbutrin in patients with a recent history of myocardial infarction or unstable heart disease. Therefore, care should be exercised if it is used in these groups. Wellbutrin was well tolerated in patients who had previously developed orthostatic hypotension while receiving tricyclic antidepressants.

Because bupropion HCl and its metabolites are almost completely excreted through the kidney and metabolites are likely to undergo conjugation in the liver prior to urinary excretion, treatment of patients with renal or hepatic impairment should be initiated at reduced dosage as bupropion and its metabolites may accumulate in such patients beyond concentrations expected in patients without renal or hepatic impairment. The patient should be closely monitored for possible toxic effects of elevated blood and tissue levels of drug and metabolites.

Information for Patients: Physicians are advised to discuss the following issues with patients:

Patients should be instructed to take Wellbutrin in equally divided doses three or four times a day to minimize the risk of seizure.

Patients should be told that any CNS-active drug like Wellbutrin may impair their ability to perform tasks requiring judgment or motor and cognitive skills. Consequently, until they are reasonably certain that Wellbutrin does not adversely affect their performance they should refrain from driving an automobile or operating complex, hazardous machinery.

Patients should be told that the use and cessation of use of alcohol may alter the seizure threshold, and, therefore, that the consumption of alcohol should be minimized, and, if possible, avoided completely.

Patients should be advised to inform their physician if they are taking or plan to take any prescription or over-the-counter drugs. Concern is warranted because Wellbutrin and other drugs may affect each other's metabolism.

Patients should be advised to notify their physician if they become pregnant or intend to become pregnant during therapy.

Drug Interactions: No systematic data have been collected on the consequences of the concomitant administration of Wellbutrin and other drugs.

However, animal data suggest that Wellbutrin may be an inducer of drug metabolizing enzymes. This may be of potential clinical importance because the blood levels of co-administered drugs may be altered.

Alternatively, because bupropion is extensively metabolized, the co-administration of other drugs may affect its clinical activity. In particular, care should be exercised when administering drugs known to affect hepatic drug metabolizing enzyme systems (e.g., carbamazepine, cimetidine, phenobarbital, phenytoin).

Studies in animals demonstrate that the acute toxicity of bupropion is enhanced by the MAO inhibitor phenelzine (see CONTRAINDICATIONS).

Limited clinical data suggest a higher incidence of adverse experiences in patients receiving concurrent administration of Wellbutrin and L-dopa. Administration of Wellbutrin to patients receiving L-dopa concurrently should be undertaken with caution, using small initial doses and small gradual dose increases.

Concurrent administration of Wellbutrin and agents which lower seizure threshold should be undertaken only with extreme caution (see WARNINGS). Low initial dosing and small gradual dose increases should be employed.

Carcinogenesis, Mutagenesis, Impairment of Fertility: Lifetime carcinogenicity studies were performed in rats and mice at doses up to 300 and 150 mg/kg/day, respectively. In the rat study there was an increase in nodular proliferative lesions of the liver at doses of 100 to 300 mg/kg/day; lower doses were not tested. The question of whether or not such lesions may be precursors of neoplasms of the liver is currently unresolved. Similar liver lesions were not seen in the mouse study, and no increase in malignant tumors of the liver and other organs was seen in either study.

Bupropion produced a borderline positive response (2–3 times control mutation rate) in some strains in the Ames bacterial mutagenicity test, and a high oral dose (300, but not 100 or 200 mg/kg) produced a low incidence of chromosomal aberrations in rats. The relevance of these results in estimating the risk of human exposure to therapeutic doses is unknown.

A fertility study was performed in rats; no evidence of impairment of fertility was encountered at oral doses up to 300 mg/kg/day.

Pregnancy: ***Teratogenic Effects:*** Pregnancy Category B: Reproduction studies have been performed in rabbits and rats at doses up to 15–45 times the human daily dose and have revealed no definitive evidence of impaired fertility or harm to the fetus due to bupropion. (In rabbits, a slightly increased incidence of fetal abnormalities was seen in two studies, but there was no increase in any specific abnormality). There are no adequate and well-controlled studies in pregnant women. Because animal reproduction studies are not always predictive of human response, this drug should be used during pregnancy only if clearly needed.

TREATMENT EMERGENT ADVERSE EXPERIENCE INCIDENCE IN PLACEBO-CONTROLLED CLINICAL TRIALS*
(Percent of Patients Reporting)

Adverse Experience	Wellbutrin Patients (n = 323)	Placebo Patients (n = 185)
CARDIOVASCULAR		
Cardiac Arrhythmias	5.3	4.3
Dizziness	22.3	16.2
Hypertension	4.3	1.6
Hypotension	2.5	2.2
Palpitations	3.7	2.2
Syncope	1.2	0.5
Tachycardia	10.8	8.6
DERMATOLOGIC		
Pruritus	2.2	0.0
Rash	8.0	6.5
GASTROINTESTINAL		
Anorexia	18.3	18.4
Appetite Increase	3.7	2.2
Constipation	26.0	17.3
Diarrhea	6.8	8.6
Dyspepsia	3.1	2.2
Nausea/Vomiting	22.9	18.9
Weight Gain	13.6	22.7
Weight Loss	23.2	23.2
GENITOURINARY		
Impotence	3.4	3.1
Menstrual Complaints	4.7	1.1
Urinary Frequency	2.5	2.2
Urinary Retention	1.9	2.2
MUSCULOSKELETAL		
Arthritis	3.1	2.7
NEUROLOGICAL		
Akathisia	1.5	1.1
Akinesia/Bradykinesia	8.0	8.6
Cutaneous Temperature Disturbance	1.9	1.6
Dry Mouth	27.6	18.4
Excessive Sweating	22.3	14.6
Headache/Migraine	25.7	22.2
Impaired Sleep Quality	4.0	1.6
Increased Salivary Flow	3.4	3.8
Insomnia	18.6	15.7
Muscle Spasms	1.9	3.2
Pseudoparkinsonism	1.5	1.6
Sedation	19.8	19.5
Sensory Disturbance	4.0	3.2
Tremor	21.1	7.6
NEUROPSYCHIATRIC		
Agitation	31.9	22.2
Anxiety	3.1	1.1
Confusion	8.4	4.9
Decreased Libido	3.1	1.6
Delusions	1.2	1.1
Disturbed Concentration	3.1	3.8
Euphoria	1.2	0.5
Hostility	5.6	3.8
NONSPECIFIC		
Fatigue	5.0	8.6
Fever/Chills	1.2	0.5
RESPIRATORY		
Upper Respiratory Complaints	5.0	11.4
SPECIAL SENSES		
Auditory Disturbance	5.3	3.2
Blurred Vision	14.6	10.3
Gustatory Disturbance	3.1	1.1

*Events reported by at least 1% of Wellbutrin patients are included.

Labor and Delivery: The effect of Wellbutrin on labor and delivery in humans is unknown.

Nursing Mothers: Because of the potential for serious adverse reactions in nursing infants from Wellbutrin, a decision should be made whether to discontinue nursing or to discontinue the drug, taking into account the importance of the drug to the mother.

Pediatric Use: The safety and effectiveness of Wellbutrin in individuals under 18 years old have not been established.

Use in the Elderly: Wellbutrin has not been systematically evaluated in older patients.

ADVERSE REACTIONS

(See also WARNINGS and PRECAUTIONS) Adverse events commonly encountered in patients treated with Wellbutrin are agitation, dry mouth, insomnia, headache/migraine, nausea/vomiting, constipation, and tremor.

Adverse events were sufficiently troublesome to cause discontinuation of Wellbutrin treatment in approximately ten percent of the 2400 patients and volunteers who participated in clinical trials during the product's initial development. The more common events causing discontinuation include neuropsychiatric disturbances (3.0%), primarily agitation and abnormalities in mental status; gastrointestinal disturbances (2.1%), primarily nausea and vomiting; neurological disturbances (1.7%), primarily seizures, headaches, and sleep disturbances; and dermatologic problems (1.4%), primarily rashes. It is important to note, however, that many of these events occurred at doses that exceed the recommended daily dose.

Accurate estimates of the incidence of adverse events associated with the use of any drug are difficult to obtain. Estimates are influenced by drug dose, detection technique, setting, physician judgments, etc. Consequently, the table below is presented solely to indicate the relative frequency of adverse events reported in representative controlled clinical studies conducted to evaluate the safety and efficacy of Wellbutrin under relatively similar conditions of daily dosage (300–600 mg), setting, and duration (3–4 weeks). The figures cited cannot be used to predict precisely the incidence of untoward events in the course of usual medical practice where patient characteristics and other factors must differ from those which prevailed in the clinical trials. These incidence figures also cannot be compared with those obtained from other clinical studies involving related drug products as each group of drug trials is conducted under a different set of conditions.

Finally, it is important to emphasize that the tabulation does not reflect the relative severity and/or clinical importance of the events. A better perspective on the serious adverse events associated with the use of Wellbutrin is provided in the WARNINGS and PRECAUTIONS sections.

[See table above.]

Other Events Observed During the Development of Wellbutrin: The conditions and duration of exposure to Wellbutrin varied greatly and a substantial proportion of the experience was gained in open and uncontrolled clinical settings. During this experience, numerous adverse events were reported; however, without appropriate controls, it is impossible to determine with certainty which events were or were not caused by Wellbutrin. The following enumeration is organized by organ system and describes events in terms of their relative frequency of reporting in the data base. Events of major clinical importance are also described in the WARNINGS and PRECAUTIONS sections of the labeling.

The following definitions of frequency are used: Frequent adverse events are defined as those occurring in at least 1/100 patients. Infrequent adverse events are those occurring in 1/100 to 1/1000 patients, while rare events are those occurring in less than 1/1000 patients.

Cardiovascular: Frequent was edema; infrequent were chest pain, EKG abnormalities (premature beats and nonspecific ST-T changes), and shortness of breath/dyspnea; rare were flushing, pallor, phlebitis and myocardial infarction.

Dermatologic: Frequent were nonspecific rashes; infrequent were alopecia and dry skin; rare were change in hair color, hirsutism and acne.

Endocrine: Infrequent was gynecomastia; rare were glycosuria and hormone level change.

Gastrointestinal: Infrequent were dysphagia, thirst disturbance, and liver damage/jaundice; rare were rectal complaints, colitis, G.I. bleeding, intestinal perforation and stomach ulcer.

Genitourinary: Frequent was nocturia; infrequent were vaginal irritation, testicular swelling, urinary tract infection, painful erection, and retarded ejaculation; rare were dysuria, enuresis, urinary incontinence, menopause, ovarian disorder, pelvic infection, cystitis, dyspareunia, and painful ejaculation.

Hematologic/Oncologic: Rare were lymphadenopathy, anemia and pancytopenia.

Musculosketetal: Rare was musculosketetal chest pain.

Neurological: (see WARNINGS) Frequent were ataxia/incoordination, seizure, myoclonus, dyskinesia, and dystonia; infrequent were mydriasis, vertigo, and dysarthria; rare were EEG abnormality, abnormal neurological exam, impaired attention, sciatica and aphasia.

Continued on next page

Burroughs Wellcome—Cont.

Neuropsychiatric: (see PRECAUTIONS) Frequent were mania/hypomania, increased libido, hallucinations, decrease in sexual function, and depression; infrequent were memory impairment, depersonalization, psychosis, dysphoria, mood instability, paranoia, formal thought disorder, and frigidity; rare was suicidal ideation.
Oral Complaints: Frequent was stomatitis; infrequent were toothache, bruxism, gum irritation, and oral edema; rare was glossitis.
Respiratory: Infrequent were bronchitis and shortness of breath/dyspnea; rare were epistaxis, rate or rhythm disorder, pneumonia and pulmonary embolism.
Special Senses: Infrequent was visual disturbance; rare was diplopia.
Nonspecific: Frequent were flu-like symptoms; infrequent was nonspecific pain; rare were body odor, surgically related pain, infection, medication reaction and overdose.
Postintroduction Reports: Voluntary reports of adverse events temporally associated with Wellbutrin that have been received since market introduction and which may have no causal relationship with the drug include the following:
Cardiovascular: orthostatic hypotension, third degree heart block
Gastrointestinal: esophagitis, hepatitis
Hemic and Lymphatic: ecchymosis, leukocytosis, leukopenia
Musculoskeletal: arthralgia, myalgia, muscle rigidity/fever/rhabdomyolysis
Nervous: coma, delirium, dream abnormalities, paresthesia, unmasking of tardive dyskinesia
Skin and Appendages: angioedema, exfoliative dermatitis, urticaria
Special Senses: tinnitus

DRUG ABUSE AND DEPENDENCE

Humans: Controlled clinical studies conducted in normal volunteers, in subjects with a history of multiple drug abuse, and in depressed patients showed some increase in motor activity and agitation/excitement.
In a population of individuals experienced with drugs of abuse, a single dose of 400 mg Wellbutrin produced mild amphetamine-like activity as compared to placebo on the morphine-benzedrine subscale of the Addiction Research Center Index (ARCI) and a score intermediate between placebo and amphetamine on the Liking Scale of the ARCI. These scales measure general feelings of euphoria and drug desirability.
Findings in clinical trials, however, are not known to predict the abuse potential of drugs reliably. Nonetheless, evidence from single dose studies does suggest that the recommended daily dosage of bupropion when administered in divided doses is not likely to be especially reinforcing to amphetamine or stimulant abusers. However, higher doses, which could not be tested because of the risk of seizure, might be modestly attractive to those who abuse stimulant drugs.
Animals: Studies in rodents have shown that bupropion exhibits some pharmacologic actions common to psychostimulants, including increases in locomotor activity and the production of a mild stereotyped behavior and increases in rates of responding in several schedule-controlled behavior paradigms. Drug discrimination studies in rats showed stimulus generalization between bupropion and amphetamine and other psychostimulants. Rhesus monkeys have been shown to self-administer bupropion intravenously.

OVERDOSAGE

Lethal Doses in Animals: In rats, the acute oral LD_{50} values were 607 mg/kg (males) and 482 mg/kg (females). Respective values for mice were 544 mg/kg and 636 mg/kg. Signs of acute toxicity included labored breathing, salivation, arched back, ptosis, ataxia, and convulsions.
Human Overdose Experience: There has been limited clinical experience with overdosage of Wellbutrin. Thirteen overdoses occurred during clinical trials. Twelve patients ingested 850 to 4200 mg and recovered without significant sequelae. Another patient who ingested 9000 mg of Wellbutrin and 300 mg of tranylcypromine experienced a grand mal seizure and recovered without further sequelae.
Since introduction, Wellbutrin overdoses up to 17,500 mg have been reported. Seizure was reported in approximately one-third of all cases. Other serious reactions reported with overdoses of Wellbutrin alone included hallucinations, loss of consciousness, and tachycardia. Fever, muscle rigidity, rhabdomyolysis, hypotension, stupor, coma, and respiratory failure have been reported when Wellbutrin was part of multiple drug overdoses.
Although most patients recovered without sequelae, deaths associated with overdoses of Wellbutrin alone have been reported rarely in patients ingesting massive doses of Wellbutrin. Multiple uncontrolled seizures, bradycardia, cardiac failure, and cardiac arrest prior to death were reported in these patients.
Management of Overdose: Following suspected overdose, hospitalization is advised. If the patient is conscious, vomiting should be induced by syrup of ipecac. Activated charcoal also may be administered every 6 hours during the first 12 hours after ingestion. Baseline laboratory values should be obtained. Electrocardiogram and EEG monitoring also are recommended for the next 48 hours. Adequate fluid intake should be provided.
If the patient is stuporous, comatose, or convulsing, airway intubation is recommended prior to undertaking gastric lavage. Although there is little clinical experience with lavage following an overdose of Wellbutrin, it is likely to be of benefit within the first 12 hours after ingestion since absorption of the drug may not yet be complete.
While diuresis, dialysis, or hemoperfusion are sometimes used to treat drug overdosage, there is no experience with their use in the management of Wellbutrin overdose. Because diffusion of Wellbutrin from tissue to plasma may be slow, dialysis may be of minimal benefit several hours after overdose.
Based on studies in animals, it is recommended that seizures be treated with an intravenous benzodiazepine preparation and other supportive measures, as appropriate.
Further information about the treatment of overdoses may be available from a poison control center.

DOSAGE AND ADMINISTRATION

General Dosing Considerations: It is particularly important to administer Wellbutrin in a manner most likely to minimize the risk of seizure (see WARNINGS). Increases in dose should not exceed 100 mg/day in a 3 day period. Gradual escalation in dosage is also important if agitation, motor restlessness, and insomnia, often seen during the initial days of treatment, are to be minimized. If necessary, these effects may be managed by temporary reduction of dose or the short-term administration of an intermediate to long-acting sedative hypnotic. A sedative hypnotic usually is not required beyond the first week of treatment. Insomnia may also be minimized by avoiding bedtime doses. If distressing, untoward effects supervene, dose escalation should be stopped.
No single dose of Wellbutrin should exceed 150 mg. Wellbutrin should be administered t.i.d., preferably with at least 6 hours between successive doses.
Usual Dosage for Adults: The usual adult dose is 300 mg/day, given t.i.d. Dosing should begin at 200 mg/day, given as 100 mg b.i.d. Based on clinical response, this dose may be increased to 300 mg/day, given as 100 mg t.i.d., no sooner than 3 days after beginning therapy (see table below).
Increasing the Dosage Above 300 mg/Day: As with other antidepressants, the full antidepressant effect of Wellbutrin may not be evident until 4 weeks of treatment or longer. An increase in dosage, up to a maximum of 450 mg/day, given in divided doses of not more than 150 mg each, may be considered for patients in whom no clinical improvement is noted after several weeks of treatment at 300 mg/day. Dosing above 300 mg/day may be accomplished using the 75 or 100 mg tablets. The 100 mg tablet must be administered q.i.d. with at least 4 hours between successive doses, in order not to exceed the limit of 150 mg in a single dose. Wellbutrin should be discontinued in patients who do not demonstrate an adequate response after an appropriate period of treatment at 450 mg/day.
Elderly Patients: In general, older patients are known to metabolize drugs more slowly and to be more sensitive to the anticholinergic, sedative, and cardiovascular side effects of antidepressant drugs. Clinical trials enrolled several hundred patients 60 years of age and older. The experience with these patients and younger ones was similar.
Maintenance: The lowest dose that maintains remission is recommended. Although it is not known how long the patient should remain on Wellbutrin, it is generally recognized that acute episodes of depression require several months or longer of antidepressant drug treatment.

Dosing Regimen

Treatment Day	Total Daily Dose	Tablet Strength	Number of Tablets: Morning	Midday	Evening
1	200 mg	100 mg	1	0	1
4	300 mg	100 mg	1	1	1

HOW SUPPLIED

Wellbutrin (bupropion hydrochloride) Tablets are supplied as 75 mg (yellow-gold) round, biconvex tablets printed "WELLBUTRIN" and "75," bottles of 100 (NDC 0081-0177-55); and 100 mg (red) round, biconvex tablets printed "WELLBUTRIN" and "100," bottles of 100 (NDC 0081-0178-55).
Store at 15° to 25°C (59° to 77°F).
U.S. Patent No. 3885046 (Use Patent) 646502
Shown in Product Identification Section, page 407

ZOVIRAX® Capsules ℞
ZOVIRAX® Tablets ℞
ZOVIRAX® Suspension ℞
[zō″vī′răx]
(Acyclovir)

DESCRIPTION

Zovirax is the brand name for acyclovir, an antiviral drug. Zovirax Capsules, Tablets, and Suspension are formulations for oral administration. Each capsule of Zovirax contains 200 mg of acyclovir and the inactive ingredients corn starch, lactose, magnesium stearate, and sodium lauryl sulfate. The capsule shell consists of gelatin, FD&C Blue No. 2, and titanium dioxide. May contain one or more parabens. Printed with edible black ink.
Each 800 mg tablet of Zovirax contains 800 mg of acyclovir and the inactive ingredients FD&C Blue No. 2, magnesium stearate, microcrystalline cellulose, povidone, and sodium starch glycolate.
Each teaspoonful (5 mL) of Zovirax Suspension contains 200 mg of acyclovir and the inactive ingredients methylparaben 0.1% and propylparaben 0.02% (added as preservatives), carboxymethylcellulose sodium, flavor, glycerin, microcrystalline cellulose and sorbitol.
The chemical name of acyclovir is 9-[(2-hydroxyethoxy)methyl]guanine.
Acyclovir is a white, crystalline powder with a molecular weight of 225 daltons, and a maximum solubility in water of 2.5 mg/mL at 37°C.

CLINICAL PHARMACOLOGY

Mechanism of Antiviral Effects: Acyclovir is a synthetic purine nucleoside analogue with *in vitro* and *in vivo* inhibitory activity against human herpes viruses including herpes simplex types 1 (HSV-1) and 2 (HSV-2), varicella-zoster virus (VZV), Epstein-Barr virus (EBV) and cytomegalovirus (CMV).[1] In cell culture, acyclovir has the highest antiviral activity against HSV-1, followed in decreasing order of potency against HSV-2, VZV, EBV and CMV.[1]
The inhibitory activity of acyclovir for HSV-1, HSV-2, VZV and EBV is highly selective. The enzyme thymidine kinase (TK) of normal uninfected cells does not effectively use acyclovir as a substrate. However, TK encoded by HSV, VZV, and EBV[2] converts acyclovir into acyclovir monophosphate, a nucleotide analogue. The monophosphate is further converted into diphosphate by cellular guanylate kinase and into triphosphate by a number of cellular enzymes.[3] Acyclovir triphosphate interferes with herpes simplex virus DNA polymerase and inhibits viral DNA replication. Acyclovir triphosphate also inhibits cellular α-DNA polymerase, but to a lesser degree. *In vitro,* acyclovir triphosphate can be incorporated into growing chains of DNA by viral DNA polymerase and to a much smaller extent by cellular α-DNA polymerase.[4] When incorporation occurs, the DNA chain is terminated.[5,6] Acyclovir is preferentially taken up and selectively converted to the active triphosphate form by herpesvirus-infected cells. Thus, acyclovir is much less toxic *in vitro* for normal uninfected cells because: 1) less is taken up; 2) less is converted to the active form; 3) cellular α-DNA polymerase is less sensitive to the effects of the active form. The mode of acyclovir phosphorylation in cytomegalovirus-infected cells is not clearly established, but may involve virally induced cell kinases or an unidentified viral enzyme. Acyclovir is not efficiently activated in cytomegalovirus infected cells, which may account for the reduced susceptibility of cytomegalovirus to acyclovir *in vitro.*
Microbiology: The quantitative relationship between the *in vitro* susceptibility of herpes simplex and varicella-zoster viruses to acyclovir and the clinical response to therapy has not been established in man, and virus sensitivity testing has not been standardized. Sensitivity testing results, expressed as the concentration of drug required to inhibit by 50% the growth of virus in cell culture (ID_{50}), vary greatly depending upon the particular assay used,[7] the cell type employed,[8] and the laboratory performing the test.[1] The ID_{50} of acyclovir against HSV-1 isolates may range from 0.02 μg/mL (plaque reduction in Vero cells) to 5.9–13.5 μg/mL (plaque reduction in green monkey kidney [GMK] cells).[1] The ID_{50} against HSV-2 ranges from 0.01 μg/mL to 9.9 μg/mL (plaque reduction in Vero and GMK cells, respectively
Using a dye-uptake method in Vero cells,[9] which gives ID_{50} values approximately 5- to 10-fold higher than plaque reduction assays, 1417 HSV isolates (553 HSV-1 and 864 HSV-2) from approximately 500 patients were examined over a 5-year period.[10] These assays found that 90% of HSV-1 isolates

were sensitive to ≤ 0.9 μg/mL acyclovir and 50% of all isolates were sensitive to ≤ 0.2 μg/mL acyclovir. For HSV-2 isolates, 90% were sensitive to ≤ 2.2 μg/mL and 50% of all isolates were sensitive to ≤ 0.7 μg/mL of acyclovir. Isolates with significantly diminished sensitivity were found in 44 patients. It must be emphasized that neither the patients nor the isolates were randomly selected and, therefore, do not represent the general population.

Most of the less sensitive HSV clinical isolates have been relatively deficient in the viral TK.[11–19] Strains with alterations in viral TK[20] or viral DNA polymerase[21] have also been reported. Prolonged exposure to low concentrations (0.1 μg/mL) of acyclovir in cell culture has resulted in the emergence of a variety of acyclovir-resistant strains.[22]

The ID_{50} against VZV ranges from 0.17–1.53 μg/mL (yield reduction, human foreskin fibroblasts) to 1.85–3.98 μg/mL (foci reduction, human embryo fibroblasts [HEF]). Reproduction of EBV genome is suppressed by 50% in superinfected Raji cells or P3HR-1 lymphoblastoid cells by 1.5 μg/mL acyclovir. CMV is relatively resistant to acyclovir with ID_{50} values ranging from 2.3–17.6 μg/mL (plaque reduction, HEF cells) to 1.82–56.8 μg/mL (DNA hybridization, HEF cells). The latent state of the genome of any of the human herpesviruses is not known to be sensitive to acyclovir.[1]

Pharmacokinetics: The pharmacokinetics of acyclovir after oral administration have been evaluated in 6 clinical studies involving 110 adult patients. In one uncontrolled study of 35 immunocompromised patients with herpes simplex or varicella-zoster infection, Zovirax Capsules were administered in doses of 200 to 1000 mg every 4 hours, 6 times daily for 5 days, and steady-state plasma levels were reached by the second day of dosing. Mean steady-state peak and trough concentrations following the final 200 mg dose were 0.49 μg/mL (0.47 to 0.54 μg/mL) and 0.31 μg/mL (0.18 to 0.41 μg/mL), respectively, and following the final 800 mg dose were 2.8 μg/mL (2.3 to 3.1 μg/mL) and 1.8 μg/mL (1.3 to 2.5 μg/mL), respectively. In another uncontrolled study of 20 younger immunocompetent patients with recurrent genital herpes simplex infections, Zovirax Capsules were administered in doses of 800 mg every 6 hours, 4 times daily for 5 days; the mean steady-state peak and trough concentrations were 1.4 μg/mL (0.66 to 1.8 μg/mL) and 0.55 μg/mL (0.14 to 1.1 μg/mL), respectively.

In general, the pharmacokinetics of acyclovir in children is similar to adults. Mean half-life after oral doses of 300 mg/M^2 and 600 mg/M^2, in children ages 7 months to 7 years, was 2.6 hours (range 1.59 to 3.74 hours).

A single oral dose bioavailability study in 23 normal volunteers showed that Zovirax Capsules 200 mg are bioequivalent to 200 mg acyclovir in aqueous solution; and in a separate study in 20 volunteers, it was shown that Zovirax Suspension is bioequivalent to Zovirax Capsules. In a different single-dose bioavailability/bioequivalence study in 24 volunteers, one Zovirax 800 mg Tablet was demonstrated to be bioequivalent to four Zovirax 200 mg Capsules.

In a multiple-dose crossover study where 23 volunteers received Zovirax as one 200 mg capsule, one 400 mg tablet and one 800 mg tablet 6 times daily, absorption decreased with increasing dose and the estimated bioavailabilities of acyclovir were 20, 15, and 10%, respectively. The decrease in bioavailability is believed to be a function of the dose and not the dosage form. It was demonstrated that acyclovir is not dose proportional over the dosing range 200 mg to 800 mg. In this study, steady-state peak and trough concentrations of acyclovir were 0.83 and 0.46 μg/mL, 1.21 and 0.63 μg/mL, and 1.61 and 0.83 μg/mL for the 200, 400 and 800 mg dosage regimens, respectively.

In another study in 6 volunteers, the influence of food on the absorption of acyclovir was not apparent.

Following oral administration, the mean plasma half-life of acyclovir in volunteers and patients with normal renal function ranged from 2.5 to 3.3 hours. The mean renal excretion of unchanged drug accounts for 14.4% (8.6 to 19.8%) of the orally administered dose. The only urinary metabolite (identified by high performance liquid chromatography) is 9-[(carboxymethoxy)methyl]guanine. The half-life and total body clearance of acyclovir are dependent on renal function. A dosage adjustment is recommended for patients with reduced renal function (see DOSAGE AND ADMINISTRATION).

Orally administered acyclovir in children less than 2 years of age has not yet been fully studied.

INDICATIONS AND USAGE

Zovirax Capsules and Suspension are indicated for the treatment of initial episodes and the management of recurrent episodes of genital herpes in certain patients.

Zovirax Capsules, Tablets, and Suspension are indicated for the acute treatment of herpes zoster (shingles) and chickenpox (varicella).

Genital Herpes Infections: The severity of disease is variable depending upon the immune status of the patient, the frequency and duration of episodes, and the degree of cutaneous or systemic involvement. These factors should determine patient management, which may include symptomatic support and counseling only, or the institution of specific therapy. The physical, emotional and psycho-social difficulties posed by herpes infections as well as the degree of debilitation, particularly in immunocompromised patients, are unique for each patient, and the physician should determine therapeutic alternatives based on his or her understanding of the individual patient's needs. Thus orally administered Zovirax is not appropriate in treating all genital herpes infections. The following guidelines may be useful in weighing the benefit/risk considerations in specific disease categories:

First Episodes (primary and nonprimary infections—commonly known as initial genital herpes):

Double-blind, placebo-controlled studies[23,24,25] have demonstrated that orally administered Zovirax significantly reduced the duration of acute infection (detection of virus in lesions by tissue culture) and lesion healing. The duration of pain and new lesion formation was decreased in some patient groups. The promptness of initiation of therapy and/or the patient's prior exposure to Herpes simplex virus may influence the degree of benefit from therapy. Patients with mild disease may derive less benefit than those with more severe episodes. In patients with extremely severe episodes, in which prostration, central nervous system involvement, urinary retention or inability to take oral medication require hospitalization and more aggressive management, therapy may be best initiated with intravenous Zovirax.

Recurrent Episodes:

Double-blind, placebo-controlled studies[16,26–32] in patients with frequent recurrences (6 or more episodes per year) have shown that orally administered Zovirax given daily for 4 months to 3 years prevented or reduced the frequency and/or severity of recurrences in greater than 95% of patients.

In a study of 283 patients who received 400 mg (two 200 mg capsules) twice daily for 3 years, 45%, 52% and 63% of patients remained free of recurrences in the first, second and third years, respectively. Serial analyses of the 3 month recurrence rates for the 283 patients showed that 71% to 87% were recurrence-free in each quarter, indicating that the effects are consistent over time.

The frequency and severity of episodes of untreated genital herpes may change over time. After 1 year of therapy, the frequency and severity of the patient's genital herpes infection should be re-evaluated to assess the need for continuation of acyclovir therapy. Re-evaluation will usually require a trial off acyclovir to assess the need for reinstitution of suppressive therapy. Some patients, such as those with very frequent or severe episodes before treatment, may warrant uninterrupted suppression for more than a year.

Chronic suppressive therapy is most appropriate when, in the judgement of the physician, the benefits of such a regimen outweigh known or potential adverse effects. In general, orally administered Zovirax should not be used for the suppression of recurrent disease in mildly affected patients. Unanswered questions concerning the relevance to humans of *in vitro* mutagenicity studies and reproductive toxicity studies in animals given high parenteral doses of acyclovir for short periods (see Carcinogenesis, Mutagenesis, Impairment of Fertility) should be borne in mind when designing long-term management for individual patients. Discussion of these issues with patients will provide them the opportunity to weigh the potential for toxicity against the severity of their disease. Thus, this regimen should be considered only for appropriate patients with annual re-evaluation.

Limited studies[31,32] have shown that there are certain patients for whom intermittent short-term treatment of recurrent episodes is effective. This approach may be more appropriate than a suppressive regimen in patients with infrequent recurrences.

Immunocompromised patients with recurrent herpes infections can be treated with either intermittent or chronic suppressive therapy. Clinically significant resistance, although rare, is more likely to be seen with prolonged or repeated therapy in severely immunocompromised patients with active lesions.

Herpes Zoster Infections: In a double-blind, placebo-controlled study of 187 normal patients with localized cutaneous zoster infection (93 randomized to Zovirax and 94 to placebo), Zovirax (800 mg 5 times daily for 10 days) shortened the times to lesion scabbing, healing and complete cessation of pain, and reduced the duration of viral shedding and the duration of new lesion formation.[33]

In a similar double-blind, placebo-controlled study in 83 normal patients with herpes zoster (40 randomized to Zovirax and 43 to placebo), Zovirax (800 mg 5 times daily for 7 days) shortened the times to complete lesion scabbing, healing, and cessation of pain, reduced the duration of new lesion formation, and reduced the prevalence of localized zoster-associated neurologic symptoms (paresthesia, dysesthesia or hyperesthesia).[34]

Chickenpox: In a double-blind, placebo-controlled efficacy study in 110 normal patients, ages 5 to 16 years, who presented **within 24 hours** of the onset of a typical chickenpox rash, Zovirax was administered orally 4 times daily for 5 to 7 days at doses of 10, 15, or 20 mg/kg depending on the age group. Zovirax treatment reduced the maximum number of lesions (336 vs. greater than 500; lesions beyond 500 were not counted). Zovirax treatment also shortened the mean time to 50% healing (7.1 days vs. 8.7 days), reduced the number of vesicular lesions by the second day of treatment (49 vs. 113), and decreased the proportion of patients with fever (temperature greater than 100°F) by the second day (19% vs. 57%). Zovirax treatment did not affect the antibody response to varicella-zoster virus measured one month and one year following the treatment.[35]

In two concurrent double-blind, placebo-controlled studies, a total of 883 normal patients, ages 2 to 18 years, were enrolled **within 24 hours** of the onset of a typical chickenpox rash, and Zovirax was administered at 20 mg/kg orally up to 800 mg 4 times daily for 5 days. In the larger study of 815 children ages 2 to 12 years, Zovirax treatment reduced the median maximum number of lesions (277 vs. 386), reduced the median number of vesicular lesions by the second day of treatment (26 vs. 40), and reduced the proportion of patients with moderate to severe itching by the third day of treatment (15% vs. 34%).[36] In addition, in both studies (883 patients ages 2 to 18 years), Zovirax treatment also decreased the proportion of patients with fever (temperature greater than 100°F), anorexia, and lethargy by the second day of treatment, and decreased the mean number of residual lesions on Day 28.[36,37] There were no substantial differences in VZV-specific humoral or cellular immune responses measured at one month following treatment in patients receiving Zovirax compared to patients receiving placebo.[38]

Diagnosis: Diagnosis is confirmed by virus isolation. Accelerated viral culture assays or immunocytology allow more rapid diagnosis than standard viral culture. For patients with initial episodes of genital herpes, appropriate examinations should be performed to rule out other sexually transmitted diseases. While cutaneous lesions associated with herpes simplex and varicella-zoster infections are often characteristic, the finding of multinucleated giant cells in smears prepared from lesion exudate or scrapings may provide additional support to the clinical diagnosis.[35]

Multi-nucleated giant cells in smears do not distinguish varicella-zoster from herpes simplex infections.

CONTRAINDICATIONS

Zovirax Capsules, Tablets, and Suspension are contraindicated for patients who develop hypersensitivity or intolerance to the components of the formulations.

WARNINGS

Zovirax Capsules, Tablets, and Suspension are intended for oral ingestion only.

PRECAUTIONS

General: Zovirax has caused decreased spermatogenesis at high parenteral doses in some animals and mutagenesis in some acute studies at high concentrations of drug (see PRECAUTIONS—Carcinogenesis, Mutagenesis, Impairment of Fertility). The recommended dosage should not be exceeded (see DOSAGE AND ADMINISTRATION).

Exposure of Herpes simplex and varicella-zoster isolates to acyclovir *in vitro* can lead to the emergence of less sensitive viruses. The possibility of the appearance of less sensitive viruses in man must be borne in mind when treating patients. The relationship between the *in vitro* sensitivity of herpes simplex or varicella-zoster virus to acyclovir and clinical response to therapy has yet to be established (see CLINICAL PHARMACOLOGY-Microbiology).

Because of the possibility that less sensitive virus may be selected in patients who are receiving acyclovir, all patients should be advised to take particular care to avoid potential transmission of virus if active lesions are present while they are on therapy. In severely immunocompromised patients, the physician should be aware that prolonged or repeated courses of acyclovir may result in selection of resistant viruses which may not fully respond to continued acyclovir therapy.

Caution should be exercised when administering Zovirax to patients receiving potentially nephrotoxic agents since this may increase the risk of renal dysfunction.

Information for Patients: Patients are instructed to consult with their physician if they experience severe or troublesome adverse reactions, they become pregnant or intend to become pregnant, they intend to breastfeed while taking orally administered Zovirax, or they have any other questions.

Genital Herpes Infections: Genital herpes is a sexually transmitted disease and patients should avoid intercourse when visible lesions are present because of the risk of infecting intimate partners. Zovirax Capsules, Tablets, and Suspension are for oral ingestion only. Medication should not be shared with others. The prescribed dosage should not be exceeded. Zovirax does not eliminate latent viruses. Patients are instructed to consult with their physician if they do not receive sufficient relief in the frequency and severity of their genital herpes recurrences.

There are still unanswered questions concerning reproductive/gonadal toxicity and mutagenesis; long-term studies are continuing. Decreased sperm production has been seen at high doses in some animals; a placebo-controlled clinical

Continued on next page

Burroughs Wellcome—Cont.

study using 400 mg or 1000 mg of Zovirax per day for six months in humans did not show similar findings.[40] Chromosomal breaks were seen *in vitro* after brief exposure to high concentrations. Some other currently marketed medications also cause chromosomal breaks, and the significance of this finding is unknown. A placebo-controlled clinical study using 800 mg of Zovirax per day for one year in humans did not show any abnormalities in structure or number of chromosomes.[28]

Herpes Zoster Infections: Adults age 50 or older tend to have more severe shingles, and Zovirax treatment showed more significant benefit for older patients. Treatment was begun within 72 hours of rash onset in these studies, and was more useful if started within the first 48 hours.

Chickenpox: Although chickenpox in otherwise healthy children is usually a self-limited disease of mild to moderate severity, adolescents and adults tend to have more severe disease. Treatment was initiated within 24 hours of the typical chickenpox rash in the controlled studies, and there is no information regarding the effects of treatment begun later in the disease course. It is unknown whether the treatment of chickenpox in childhood has any effect on long-term immunity. However, there is no evidence to indicate that Zovirax treatment of chickenpox would have any effect on either decreasing or increasing the incidence or severity of subsequent recurrences of herpes zoster (shingles) later in life. Intravenous Zovirax is indicated for the treatment of varicella-zoster infections in immunocompromised patients.

Drug Interactions: Co-administration of probenecid with intravenous acyclovir has been shown to increase the mean half-life and the area under the concentration-time curve. Urinary excretion and renal clearance were correspondingly reduced.[41] The clinical effects of this combination have not been studied.

Carcinogenesis, Mutagenesis, Impairment of Fertility: The data presented below include references to peak steady state plasma acyclovir concentrations observed in humans treated with 800 mg given orally 6 times a day (dosing appropriate for treatment of herpes zoster) or 200 mg given orally 6 times a day (dosing appropriate for treatment of genital herpes). Plasma drug concentrations in animal studies are expressed as multiples of human exposure to acyclovir at the higher and lower dosing schedules (see Pharmacokinetics).

Acyclovir was tested in lifetime bioassays in rats and mice at single daily doses of up to 450 mg/kg administered by gavage. There was no statistically significant difference in the incidence of tumors between treated and control animals, nor did acyclovir shorten the latency of tumors. At 450 mg/kg/day, plasma concentrations were 3 to 6 times human levels in the mouse bioassay and 1 to 2 times human levels in the rat bioassay.

Acyclovir was tested in two *in vitro* cell transformation assays. Positive results were observed at the highest concentration tested (31 to 63 times human levels) in one system and the resulting morphologically transformed cells formed tumors when inoculated into immunosuppressed, syngeneic, weanling mice. Acyclovir was negative (40 to 80 times human levels) in the other, possibly less sensitive, transformation assay.

In acute cytogenetic studies, there was an increase, though not statistically significant, in the incidence of chromosomal damage at maximum tolerated parenteral doses of acyclovir (100 mg/kg) in rats (62 to 125 times human levels) but not in Chinese hamsters; higher doses of 500 and 1000 mg/kg were clastogenic in Chinese hamsters (380 to 760 times human levels). In addition, no activity was found after 5 days dosing in a dominant lethal study in mice (36 to 73 times human levels). In all 4 microbial assays, no evidence of mutagenicity was observed. Positive results were obtained in 2 of 7 genetic toxicity assays using mammalian cells *in vitro*. In human lymphocytes, a positive response for chromosomal damage was seen at concentrations 150 to 300 times the acyclovir plasma levels achieved in man. At one locus in mouse lymphoma cells, mutagenicity was observed at concentrations 250 to 500 times human plasma levels. Results in the other five mammalian cell loci follow: at 3 loci in a Chinese hamster ovary cell line, the results were inconclusive at concentrations at least 1850 times human levels; at 2 other loci in mouse lymphoma cells, no evidence of mutagenicity was observed at concentrations at least 1500 times human levels.

Acyclovir has not been shown to impair fertility or reproduction in mice (450 mg/kg/day, p.o.) or in rats (25 mg/kg/day, s.c.). In the mouse study plasma levels were 9 to 18 times human levels, while in the rat study they were 8 to 15 times human levels. At a higher dose in the rat (50 mg/kg/day, s.c.), there was a statistically significant increase in post-implantation loss, but no concomitant decrease in litter size. In female rabbits treated subcutaneously with acyclovir subsequent to mating, there was a statistically significant decrease in implantation efficiency but no concomitant decrease in litter size at a dose of 50 mg/kg/day (16 to 31 times human levels). No effect upon implantation efficiency was observed when the same dose was administered intravenously (53 to 106 times humans levels). In a rat peri- and postnatal study at 50 mg/kg/day s.c. (11 to 22 times human levels), there was a statistically significant decrease in the group mean numbers of corpora lutea, total implantation sites and live fetuses in the F_1 generation. Although not statistically significant, there was also a dose-related decrease in group mean numbers of live fetuses and implantation sites at 12.5 mg/kg/day and 25 mg/kg/day, s.c. The intravenous administration of 100 mg/kg/day, a dose known to cause obstructive nephropathy in rabbits, caused a significant increase in fetal resorptions and a corresponding decrease in litter size (plasma levels were not measured). However, at a maximum tolerated intravenous dose of 50 mg/kg/day in rabbits (53 to 106 times human levels), no drug-related reproductive effects were observed.

Intraperitoneal doses of 80 or 320 mg/kg/day acyclovir given to rats for 6 and 1 months, respectively, caused testicular atrophy. Plasma levels were not measured in the one month study and were 24 to 48 times human levels in the six month study. Testicular atrophy was persistent through the 4-week postdose recovery phase after 320 mg/kg/day; some evidence of recovery of sperm production was evident 30 days post-dose. Intravenous doses of 100 and 200 mg/kg/day acyclovir given to dogs for 31 days caused aspermatogenesis. At 100 mg/kg/day plasma levels were 47 to 94 times human levels, while at 200 mg/kg/day they were 159 to 317 times human levels. No testicular abnormalities were seen in dogs given 50 mg/kg/day i.v. for one month (21 to 41 times human levels) and in dogs given 60 mg/kg/day orally for one year (6 to 12 times human levels).

Pregnancy: *Teratogenic Effects:* Pregnancy Category C. Acyclovir was not teratogenic in the mouse (450 mg/kg/day, p.o.), rabbit (50 mg/kg/day, s.c. and i.v.) or in standard tests in the rat (50 mg/kg/day, s.c.). These exposures resulted in plasma levels 9 and 18, 16 and 106, and 11 and 22 times, respectively, human levels. In a non-standard test in rats, there were fetal abnormalities, such as head and tail anomalies, and maternal toxicity.[42] In this test, rats were given 3 s.c. doses of 100 mg/kg acyclovir on gestation day 10, resulting in plasma levels 63 and 125 times human levels. There are no adequate and well-controlled studies in pregnant women. Acyclovir should not be used during pregnancy unless the potential benefit justifies the potential risk to the fetus. Although acyclovir was not teratogenic in standard animal studies, the drug's potential for causing chromosome breaks at high concentration should be taken into consideration in making this determination.

Nursing Mothers: Acyclovir concentrations have been documented in breast milk in two women following oral administration of Zovirax and ranged from 0.6 to 4.1 times corresponding plasma levels.[43,44] These concentrations would potentially expose the nursing infant to a dose of acyclovir up to 0.3 mg/kg/day. Caution should be exercised when Zovirax is administered to a nursing woman.

Pediatric Use: Safety and effectiveness in children less than 2 years of age have not been adequately studied.

ADVERSE REACTIONS

Herpes Simplex: *Short-Term Administration:* The most frequent adverse events reported during clinical trials of treatment of genital herpes with orally administered Zovirax were nausea and/or vomiting in 8 of 298 patient treatments (2.7%) and headache in 2 of 298 (0.6%). Nausea and/or vomiting occurred in 2 of 287 (0.7%) patients who received placebo.

Less frequent adverse events, each of which occurred in 1 of 298 patient treatments with orally administered Zovirax (0.3%), included diarrhea, dizziness, anorexia, fatigue, edema, skin rash, leg pain, inguinal adenopathy, medication taste and sore throat.

Long-Term Administration: The most frequent adverse events reported in a clinical trial for the prevention of recurrences with continuous administration of 400 mg (two 200 mg capsules) 2 times daily for 1 year in 586 patients treated with Zovirax were: nausea (4.8%), diarrhea (2.4%), headache (1.9%) and rash (1.7%). The 589 control patients receiving intermittent treatment of recurrences with Zovirax for 1 year reported diarrhea (2.7%), nausea (2.4%), headache (2.2%) and rash (1.5%).

The most frequent adverse events reported during the second year by 390 patients who elected to continue daily administration of 400 mg (two 200 mg capsules) 2 times daily for 2 years were headache (1.5%), rash (1.3%) and paresthesia (0.8%). Adverse events reported by 329 patients during the third year include asthenia (1.2%), paresthesia (1.2%) and headache (0.9%).

Herpes Zoster: The most frequent adverse events reported during three clinical trials of treatment of herpes zoster (shingles) with 800 mg of oral Zovirax 5 times daily for 7 to 10 days in 323 patients were: malaise (11.5%), nausea (8.0%), headache (5.9%), vomiting (2.5%), diarrhea (1.5%) and constipation (0.9%). The 323 placebo recipients reported malaise (11.1%), nausea (11.5%), headache (11.1%), vomiting (2.5%), diarrhea (0.3%) and constipation (2.4%).

Chickenpox: The most frequent adverse events reported during three clinical trials of treatment of chickenpox with oral Zovirax in 495 patients were: diarrhea (3.2%), abdominal pain (0.6%), rash (0.6%), vomiting (0.6%), and flatulence (0.4%). The 498 patients receiving placebo reported: diarrhea (2.2%), flatulence (0.8%), and insomnia (0.4%).

Observed During Clinical Practice: Based on clinical practice experience in patients treated with oral Zovirax in the U.S., spontaneously reported adverse events are uncommon. Data are insufficient to support an estimate of their incidence or to establish causation. These events may also occur as part of the underlying disease process. Voluntary reports of adverse events which have been received since market introduction include:

General: fever, headache, pain, peripheral edema

Nervous: confusion, dizziness, hallucinations, paresthesia, somnolence (These symptoms may be marked in older adults.)

Digestive: diarrhea, elevated liver function tests, gastrointestinal distress, nausea

Hemic and Lymphatic: leukopenia, lymphadenopathy

Musculoskeletal: myalgia

Skin: alopecia, pruritus, rash, urticaria

Special Senses: visual abnormalities

OVERDOSAGE

Patients have ingested intentional overdoses of up to 100 capsules (20 g) of Zovirax, with no unexpected adverse effects.

Precipitation of acyclovir in renal tubules may occur when the solubility (2.5 mg/mL) in the intratubular fluid is exceeded. Renal lesions considered to be related to obstruction of renal tubules by precipitated drug crystals occurred in the following species: rats treated with i.v. and i.p. doses of 20 mg/kg/day for 21 and 31 days, respectively, and at s.c. doses of 100 mg/kg/day for 10 days; rabbits at s.c. and i.v. doses of 50 mg/kg/day for 13 days; and dogs at i.v. doses of 100 mg/kg/day for 31 days. A 6 hr hemodialysis results in a 60% decrease in plasma acyclovir concentration. Data concerning peritoneal dialysis are incomplete but indicate that this method may be significantly less efficient in removing acyclovir from the blood. In the event of acute renal failure and anuria, the patient may benefit from hemodialysis until renal function is restored (see DOSAGE AND ADMINISTRATION).

DOSAGE AND ADMINISTRATION

Treatment of initial genital herpes: 200 mg (one 200 mg capsule or one teaspoonful [5 mL] suspension) every 4 hours, 5 times daily for 10 days.

Chronic suppressive therapy for recurrent disease: 400 mg (two 200 mg capsules or two teaspoonfuls [10 mL] suspension) 2 times daily for up to 12 months, followed by re-evaluation. See INDICATIONS AND USAGE and PRECAUTIONS for considerations on continuation of suppressive therapy beyond 12 months. Alternative regimens have included doses ranging from 200 mg 3 times daily to 200 mg 5 times daily.

Intermittent Therapy: 200 mg (one 200 mg capsule or one teaspoonful [5 mL] suspension) every 4 hours, 5 times daily for 5 days. Therapy should be initiated at the earliest sign or symptom (prodrome) of recurrence.

Acute Treatment of Herpes Zoster: 800 mg (four 200 mg capsules or four teaspoonfuls [20 mL] suspension) every 4 hours orally 5 times daily for 7 to 10 days.

Treatment of Chickenpox: 20 mg/kg (not to exceed 800 mg) orally, 4 times daily for 5 days. Therapy should be initiated at the earliest sign or symptom.

Patients With Acute or Chronic Renal Impairment: Comprehensive pharmacokinetic studies have been completed following intravenous acyclovir infusions in patients with renal impairment. Based on these studies, dosage adjustments are recommended in the following chart for genital herpes and herpes zoster indications:

[See table on next page.]

Hemodialysis: For patients who require hemodialysis, the mean plasma half-life of acyclovir during hemodialysis is approximately 5 hours. This results in a 60% decrease in plasma concentrations following a six-hour dialysis period. Therefore, the patient's dosing schedule should be adjusted so that an additional dose is administered after each dialysis.[45,46]

Peritoneal Dialysis: No supplemental dose appears to be necessary after adjustment of the dosing interval.[47,48]

HOW SUPPLIED

Zovirax Capsules (blue, opaque cap and body) containing 200 mg acyclovir and printed with "Wellcome ZOVIRAX 200"—Bottle of 100 (NDC 0081-0991-55), and unit dose pack of 100 (NDC 0081-0991-56).

Zovirax Tablets (light blue, oval) containing 800 mg acyclovir and engraved with "ZOVIRAX 800"—Bottle of 100 (NDC 0081-0945-55).

Zovirax Suspension (off-white, banana-flavored) containing 200 mg acyclovir in each teaspoonful (5 mL)—Bottle of 1 pint (473 mL) (NDC 0081-0953-96).

Normal Dosage Regimen	Creatinine Clearance (mL/min/1.73m^2)	Adjusted Dosage Regimen	
		Dose (mg)	Dosing Interval
200 mg every 4 hours	>10	200	every 4 hours, 5x daily
	0–10	200	every 12 hours
400 mg every 12 hours	>10	400	every 12 hours
	0–10	200	every 12 hours
800 mg every 4 hours	>25	800	every 4 hours, 5x daily
	10–25	800	every 8 hours
	0–10	800	every 12 hours

Capsules should be stored at 15° to 25°C (59° to 77°F) and protected from light and moisture.
Tablets should be stored at 15° to 25°C (59° to 77°F) and protected from light and moisture.
Suspension should be stored at 15° to 25°C (59° to 77°F).

REFERENCES

1. O'Brien JJ, Campoli-Richards DM. Acyclovir—an updated review of its antiviral activity, pharmacokinetic properties, and therapeutic efficacy. *Drugs.* 1989;37:233–309.
2. Littler E, Zeuthen J, McBride AA, et al. Identification of an Epstein-Barr virus-coded thymidine kinase. *EMBO J.* 1986;5(8):1959–1966.
3. Miller WH, Miller RL. Phosphorylation of acyclovir (acycloguanosine) monophosphate by GMP kinase. *J Biol Chem.* 1980;255:7204–7207.
4. Furman PA, St Clair MH, Fyfe JA, et al. Inhibition of herpes simplex virus-induced DNA polymerase activity and viral DNA replication by 9-(2-hydroxyethoxymethyl)guanine and its triphosphate. *J Virol.* 1979;32:72–77.
5. Derse D, Cheng YC, Furman PA, et al. Inhibition of purified human and herpes simplex virus-induced DNA polymerases by 9-(2-hydroxyethoxymethyl)guanine triphosphate: effects on primer-template function. *J Biol Chem.* 1981;256:11447–11451.
6. McGuirt PV, Shaw JE, Elion GB, et al. Identification of small DNA fragments synthesized in herpes simplex virus-infected cells in the presence of acyclovir. *Antimicrob Agents Chemother.* 1984;25:507–509.
7. Barry DW, Blum MR. Antiviral drugs: acyclovir. In Turner P, Shand DG (eds). *Recent Advances in Clinical Pharmacology,* ed 3. New York, Churchill Livingstone, 1983, chap 4.
8. DeClercq E. Comparative efficacy of antiherpes drugs in different cell lines. *Antimicrob Agents Chemother.* 1982; 21:661–663.
9. McLaren C, Ellis MN, Hunter GA. A colorimetric assay for the measurement of the sensitivity of herpes simplex viruses to antiviral agents. *Antiviral Res.* 1983;3:223–234.
10. Barry DW, Nusinoff-Lehrman S. Viral resistance in clinical practice: Summary of five years experience with acyclovir. In Kono R, Nakajima A (eds): *Herpes Viruses and Virus Chemotherapy (Ex Med Int Congr Ser 667).* New York, *Excerpta Medica,* 1985;269–270.
11. Dekker C. Ellis MN, McLaren C, et al. Virus resistance in clinical practice. *J Antimicrob Chemother.* 1983;12 (suppl B);137–152.
12. Sibrack CD, Gutman LT, Wilfert CM, et al. Pathogenicity of acyclovir-resistant herpes simplex virus type 1 from an immunodeficient child. *J Infect Dis.* 1982;146: 673–682.
13. Crumpacker CS, Schnipper LE, Marlowe SI, et al. Resistance to antiviral drugs of herpes simplex virus isolated from a patient treated with acyclovir. *N Engl J Med.* 1982;306:343–346.
14. Wade JC, Newton B, McLaren C, et al. Intravenous acyclovir to treat mucocutenous herpes simplex virus infection after marrow transplantation. A double-blind trial. *Ann Intern Med.* 1982;96:265–269.
15. Burns WH, Saral R, Santos GW, et al. Isolation and characterization of resistant herpes simplex virus after acyclovir therapy. *Lancet.* 1982;1:421–423.
16. Straus SE, Takiff HE, Seidlin M, et al. Suppression of frequently recurring genital herpes: a placebo-controlled double-blind trial of oral acyclovir. *N Engl J Med.* 1984;310:1545–1550.
17. Collins, P. Viral sensitivity following the introduction of acyclovir. *Am J Med.* 1988;85(2A):129–134.
18. Erlich KS, Mills J, Chatis P, et al. Acyclovir-resistant herpes simplex virus infections in patients with the acquired immunodeficiency syndrome. *N Engl J Med.* 1989;320(5):293–296.
19. Hill EL, Ellis MN, Barry DW. In: *28th Intersci Conf on Antimicrob Agents Chemother.* Los Angeles 1988, Abst. No. 0840:260.
20. Ellis MN, Keller PM, Fyfe JA, et al. Clinical isolates of herpes simplex virus type 2 that induces thymidine kinase with alterated substrate specificity. *Antimicrob Agents Chemother.* 1987;31(7):1117–1125.
21. Collins P, Larder BA, Oliver NM, et al. Characterization of a DNA polymerase mutant of herpes simplex virus from a severely immunocompromised patient receiving acyclovir. *J gen Virol.* 1989;(70):375–382.
22. Field HJ, Darby G, Wildy P. Isolation and characterization of acyclovir-resistant mutants of herpes simplex virus. *J gen Virol.* 1980;49:115–124.
23. Bryson YJ, Dillon M, Lovett M, et al. Treatment of first episodes of genital herpes simplex virus infection with oral acyclovir: a randomized double-blind controlled trial in normal subjects. *N Engl J Med.* 1983:308:916–921.
24. Mertz GJ, Critchlow CW, Benedetti J, et al. Double-blind placebo-controlled trial of oral acyclovir in first-episode genital herpes simplex virus infection. *JAMA.* 1984; 252:1147–1151.
25. Nilsen AE, Aasen T, Halsos AM, et al. Efficacy of oral acyclovir in the treatment of initial and recurrent genital herpes. *Lancet.* 1982;2:571–573.
26. Douglas JM, Critchlow C, Benedetti J, et al. A double-blind study of oral acyclovir for suppression of recurrences of genital herpes simplex virus infection. *N Engl J Med.* 1984;310:1551–1556.
27. Mindel A, Weller IV, Faherty A, et al. Prophylactic oral acyclovir in recurrent genital herpes. *Lancet.* 1984;2: 57–59.
28. Mattison HR, Reichman RC, Benedetti J, et al. Double-blind, placebo-controlled trial comparing long-term suppressive with short-term oral acyclovir therapy for management of recurrent genital herpes. *Am J Med.* 1988;85(suppl 2A):20–25.
29. Straus SE, Croen KD, Sawyer MH, et al. Acyclovir suppression of frequently recurring genital herpes. *JAMA.* 1988;260:2227–2230.
30. Mertz GJ, Eron L, Kaufman R, et al. The Acyclovir Study Group. Prolonged continuous versus intermittent oral acyclovir treatment in normal adults with frequently recurring genital herpes simplex virus infection. *Amer J Med.* 1988;85(suppl 2A):14–19.
31. Data on file, Burroughs Wellcome Co.
32. Reichman RC, Badger GJ, Mertz GJ, et al. Treatment of recurrent genital herpes simplex infections with oral acyclovir: a controlled trial. *JAMA.* 1984;251:2103–2107.
33. Huff JC, Bean B, Balfour HH, Jr. et al. Therapy of herpes zoster with oral acyclovir. *Am J Med.* 1988;85(2A):85–89.
34. Morton P, Thompson AN. Oral acyclovir in the treatment of herpes zoster in general practice. *NZ Med J.* 1989;102:93–95.
35. Balfour HH Jr, Kelly JM, Suarez, CS, et al. Acyclovir treatment of varicella in otherwise healthy children. *J Pediatr.* 1990;116:633–639.
36. Dunkle LM, Arvin AM, Whitley RJ, et al. A controlled trial of acyclovir for chickenpox in normal children. *N Engl J Med.* 1991;325:1539–1544.
37. Balfour HH Jr, Rotbart HA, Feldman S, et al. Acyclovir treatment of varicella in otherwise healthy adolescents. *J Pediatr.* 1992. In press.
38. Data on file, Burroughs Wellcome Co.
39. Naib ZM, Nahmias AJ, Josey WE, et al. Relation of cytohistopathology of genital herpesvirus infection to cervical anaplasia. *Cancer Res* 1973;33:1452–1463.
40. Douglas JM, David LG, Remington ML, et al. A double-blind, placebo-controlled trial of the effect of chronically administered oral acyclovir on sperm production in man with frequently recurrent genital herpes. *J Infect Dis.* 1988;157:588–593.
41. Laskin OL, deMiranda P, King DH, et al. Effects of probenecid on the pharmacokinetics and elimination of acyclovir in humans. *Antimicrob Agents Chemother.* 1982;21:804–807.
42. Stahlmann R, Klug S, Lewandowski C, et al. Teratogenicity of acyclovir in rats. *Infection.* 1987;15:261–262.
43. Lau RJ, Emery MG, Galinsky RE, et al. Unexpected accumulation of acyclovir in breast milk with estimate of infant exposure. *Obstet Gynecol.* 1987;69(3):468–471.
44. Meyer LJ, deMiranda P, Sheth N, et al. Acyclovir in human breast milk. *Am J Obstet Gynecol.* 1988;158(3): 586–588.
45. Laskin OL, Longstreth JA, Whelton A, et al. Effect of renal failure on the pharmacokinetics of acyclovir. *Am J Med.* 1982;73:197–201.
46. Krasny HC, Liao SH, deMiranda P, et al. Influence of hemodialysis on acyclovir pharmacokinetics in patients with chronic renal failure. *Am J Med.* 1982;73:202–204.
47. Boelart J, Schurgers M, Daneels R, et al. Multiple dose pharmacokinetics of intravenous acyclovir in patients on continuous ambulatory peritoneal dialysis. *J Antimicrob Chemother.* 1987; 20:69–76.
48. Shah GM, Winer RL, Krasny HC. Acyclovir pharmacokinetics in a patient on continuous ambulatory peritoneal dialysis. *Am J Kidney Dis.* 1986;7:507–510.

U.S. Patent No. 4199574 647506

Shown in Product Identification Section, page 407

ZOVIRAX® Ointment 5% ℞
[*zō″vī′răx*]
(Acyclovir)

DESCRIPTION

Zovirax is the brand name for acyclovir, an antiviral drug active against herpes viruses. Zovirax Ointment 5% is a formulation for topical administration. Each gram of Zovirax Ointment 5% contains 50 mg of acyclovir in a polyethylene glycol (PEG) base.
The chemical name of acyclovir is 9-[(2-hydroxyethoxy)methyl]guanine.
Acyclovir is a white, crystalline powder with a molecular weight of 225 Daltons, and a maximum solubility in water of 1.3 mg/mL.

CLINICAL PHARMACOLOGY

Acyclovir is a synthetic acyclic purine nucleoside analogue with *in vitro* inhibitory activity against Herpes simplex types 1 and 2 (HSV-1 and HSV-2), varicella-zoster, Epstein-Barr and cytomegalovirus. In cell cultures, the inhibitory activity of acyclovir for Herpes simplex virus is highly selective. Cellular thymidine kinase does not effectively utilize acyclovir as a substrate. Herpes simplex virus-coded thymidine kinase, however, converts acyclovir into acyclovir monophosphate, a nucleotide. The monophosphate is further converted into diphosphate by cellular guanylate kinase and into triphosphate by a number of cellular enzymes.[1] Acyclovir triphosphate interferes with Herpes simplex virus DNA polymerase and inhibits viral DNA replication. Acyclovir triphosphate also inhibits cellular α-DNA polymerase but to a lesser degree. *In vitro,* acyclovir triphosphate can be incorporated into growing chains of DNA by viral DNA polymerase and to a much smaller extent by cellular α-DNA polymerase.[2] When incorporation occurs, the DNA chain is terminated.[3] Acyclovir is preferentially taken up and selectively converted to the active triphosphate form by herpesvirus-infected cells. Thus, acyclovir is much less toxic *in vitro* for normal uninfected cells because: 1) less is taken up; 2) less is converted to the active form; 3) cellular α-DNA polymerase is less sensitive to the effects of the active form.
The relationship between *in vitro* susceptibility of Herpes simplex virus to antiviral drugs and clinical response has not been established. The techniques and cell culture types used for determining *in vitro* susceptibility may influence the results obtained. Using a quantitative assay to determine the acyclovir concentration producing 50% inhibition of viral cytopathic effect (ID_{50}), 28 HSV-1 clinical isolates had a mean ID_{50} of 0.17 μg/mL and 32 HSV-2 clinical isolates had a mean ID_{50} of 0.46 μg/mL.* Results from other studies using different assays have yielded mean ID_{50} values for clinical HSV-1 isolates of 0.018, 0.03 and 0.043 μg/mL and for clinical HSV-2 isolates of 0.027, 0.36 and 0.03 μg/mL, respectively.[4,5,6]
Two clinical pharmacology studies were performed with Zovirax Ointment 5% in adult immunocompromised patients, at risk of developing mucocutaneous Herpes simplex virus infections or with localized varicella-zoster infections. These studies were designed to evaluate the dermal tolerance, systemic toxicity and percutaneous absorption of acyclovir.
In one of these studies, which included 16 inpatients, the complete ointment or its vehicle were randomly administered in a dose of 1 cm strips (25 mg acyclovir) four times a day for seven days to an intact skin surface area of 4.5 square inches. No local intolerance, systemic toxicity or contact dermatitis were observed. In addition, no drug was detected in blood and urine by radioimmunoassay (sensitivity, 0.01 μg/mL).
The other study included eleven patients with localized varicella-zoster. In this uncontrolled study, acyclovir was detected in the blood of 9 patients and in the urine of all patients tested. Acyclovir levels in plasma ranged from <0.01 to 0.28 μg/mL in eight patients with normal renal function, and from <0.01 to 0.78 μg/mL in one patient with impaired renal function. Acyclovir excreted in the urine ranged from

*Data on file at Burroughs Wellcome Co.

Continued on next page

Burroughs Wellcome—Cont.

<0.02 to 9.4 percent of the daily dose. Therefore, systemic absorption of acyclovir after topical application is minimal.

INDICATIONS AND USAGE

Zovirax (Acyclovir) Ointment 5% is indicated in the management of initial herpes genitalis and in limited nonlife-threatening mucocutaneous Herpes simplex virus infections in immunocompromised patients. In clinical trials of initial herpes genitalis, Zovirax Ointment 5% has shown a decrease in healing time and in some cases a decrease in duration of viral shedding and duration of pain. In studies in immunocompromised patients with mainly herpes labialis, there was a decrease in duration of viral shedding and a slight decrease in duration of pain.

By contrast, in studies of recurrent herpes genitalis and of herpes labialis in nonimmunocompromised patients, there was no evidence of clinical benefit; there was some decrease in duration of viral shedding.

Diagnosis: Whereas cutaneous lesions associated with Herpes simplex infections are often characteristic, the finding of multinucleated giant cells in smears prepared from lesion exudate or scrapings may assist in the diagnosis.[7] Positive cultures for Herpes simplex virus offer a reliable means for confirmation of the diagnosis. In genital herpes, appropriate examinations should be performed to rule out other sexually transmitted diseases.

CONTRAINDICATIONS

Zovirax Ointment 5% is contraindicated for patients who develop hypersensitivity or chemical intolerance to the components of the formulation.

WARNINGS

Zovirax Ointment 5% is intended for cutaneous use only and should not be used in the eye.

PRECAUTIONS

General: The recommended dosage, frequency of applications, and length of treatment should not be exceeded (see DOSAGE AND ADMINISTRATION). There exist no data which demonstrate that the use of Zovirax Ointment 5% will either prevent transmission of infection to other persons or prevent recurrent infections when applied in the absence of signs and symptoms. Zovirax Ointment 5% should not be used for the prevention of recurrent HSV infections. Although clinically significant viral resistance associated with the use of Zovirax Ointment 5% has not been observed, this possibility exists.

Drug Interactions: Clinical experience has identified no interactions resulting from topical or systemic administration of other drugs concomitantly with Zovirax Ointment 5%.

Carcinogenesis, Mutagenesis, Impairment of Fertility: Acyclovir was tested in lifetime bioassays in rats and mice at single daily doses of 50, 150 and 450 mg/kg/day given by gavage. These studies showed no statistically significant difference in the incidence of benign and malignant tumors produced in drug-treated as compared to control animals, nor did acyclovir induce the occurrence of tumors earlier in drug-treated animals as compared to controls. In 2 *in vitro* cell transformation assays, used to provide preliminary assessment of potential oncogenicity in advance of these more definitive lifetime bioassays in rodents, conflicting results were obtained. Acyclovir was positive at the highest dose used in one system and the resulting morphologically transformed cells formed tumors when inoculated into immunosuppressed, syngeneic, weanling mice. Acyclovir was negative in another transformation system.

No chromosome damage was observed at maximum tolerated parenteral doses of 100 mg/kg acyclovir in rats or Chinese hamsters; higher doses of 500 and 1000 mg/kg were clastogenic in Chinese hamsters. In addition, no activity was found in a dominant lethal study in mice. In 9 of 11 microbial and mammalian cell assays, no evidence of mutagenicity was observed. In 2 mammalian cell assays (human lymphocytes and L5178Y mouse lymphoma cells *in vitro*), positive response for mutagenicity and chromosomal damage occurred, but only at concentrations at least 1000 times the plasma levels achieved in man following topical application.

Acyclovir does not impair fertility or reproduction in mice at oral doses up to 450 mg/kg/day or in rats at subcutaneous doses up to 25 mg/kg/day. In rabbits given a high dose of acyclovir (50 mg/kg/day, s.c.), there was a statistically significant decrease in implantation efficiency.

Pregnancy: *Teratogenic Effects.* Pregnancy Category C. Acyclovir was not teratogenic in the mouse (450 mg/kg/day, p.o.), rabbit (50 mg/kg/day, s.c. and i.v.) or in standard tests in the rat (50 mg/kg/day, s.c.). In a non-standard test in rats, fetal abnormalities, such as head and tail anomalies, were observed following subcutaneous administration of acyclovir at very high doses associated with toxicity to the maternal rat. The clinical relevance of these findings is uncertain.[8] There are no adequate and well-controlled studies in pregnant women. Acyclovir should not be used during pregnancy unless the potential benefit justifies the potential risk to the fetus.

Nursing Mothers: It is not known whether topically applied acyclovir is excreted in breast milk. After oral administration of Zovirax, acyclovir concentrations have been documented in breast milk in two women and ranged from 0.6 to 4.1 times the corresponding plasma levels.[9,10] Caution should be exercised when Zovirax Ointment is administered to a nursing woman.

ADVERSE REACTIONS

Because ulcerated genital lesions are characteristically tender and sensitive to any contact or manipulation, patients may experience discomfort upon application of ointment. In the controlled clinical trials, mild pain (including transient burning and stinging) was reported by 103 (28.3%) of 364 patients treated with acyclovir and by 115 (31.1%) of 370 patients treated with placebo; treatment was discontinued in 2 of these patients. Other local reactions among acyclovir-treated patients included pruritis in 15 (4.1%), rash in 1 (0.3%) and vulvitis in 1 (0.3%). Among the placebo-treated patients, pruritus was reported by 17 (4.6%) and rash by 1 (0.3%).

In all studies, there was no significant difference between the drug and placebo group in the rate or type of reported adverse reactions nor were there any differences in abnormal clinical laboratory findings.

Observed During Clinical Practice: Based on clinical practice experience in patients treated with Zovirax Ointment in the U.S., spontaneously reported adverse events are uncommon. Data are insufficient to support an estimate of their incidence or to establish causation. These events may also occur as part of the underlying disease process. Voluntary reports of adverse events which have been received since market introduction include:

General: edema and/or pain at the application site

Skin: pruritus, rash

OVERDOSAGE

Overdosage by topical application of Zovirax Ointment 5% is unlikely because of limited transcutaneous absorption (see Clinical Pharmacology).

DOSAGE AND ADMINISTRATION

Apply sufficient quantity to adequately cover all lesions every 3 hours 6 times per day for 7 days. The dose size per application will vary depending upon the total lesion area but should approximate a one-half inch ribbon of ointment per 4 square inches of surface area. A finger cot or rubber glove should be used when applying Zovirax to prevent autoinoculation of other body sites and transmission of infection to other persons. **Therapy should be initiated as early as possible following onset of signs and symptoms.**

HOW SUPPLIED

Zovirax Ointment 5% is supplied in 15 g tubes (NDC 0081-0993-94) and 3 g tubes (NDC 0081-0993-41). Each gram contains 50 mg acyclovir in a polyethylene glycol base. Store at 15° to 25°C (59° to 77°F) in a dry place.

ANIMAL PHARMACOLOGY AND ANIMAL TOXICOLOGY

Topical treatment of guinea pigs with 10% acyclovir in polyethylene glycol ointment for three weeks did not result in cutaneous irritation or systemic toxicity. Also, a wide variety of animal tests by parenteral routes demonstrated that acyclovir has a low order of toxicity.

Acyclovir did not cause dermal sensitization in guinea pigs.

REFERENCES

1. Miller WH, Miller RL: Phosphorylation of acyclovir (acycloguanosine) monophosphate by GMP kinase. *J Biol Chem* 1980;255:7204–7207.
2. Furman PA, St. Clair MH, Fyfe JA, et al: Inhibition of herpes simplex virus-induced DNA polymerase activity and viral DNA replication by 9-(2-hydroxyethoxymethyl)guanine and its triphosphate. *J Virol* 1979; 32:72–77.
3. Derse D, Cheng YC, Furman PA, et al: Inhibition of purified human and herpes simplex virus-induced DNA polymerases by 9-(2-hydroxyethoxymethyl)guanine triphosphate: effects on primer-template function. *J Biol Chem* 1981;256:11447–11451.
4. Collins P, Bauer DJ: The activity *in vitro* against herpes virus of 9-(2-hydroxyethoxymethyl)guanine (acycloguanosine), a new antiviral agent. *J Antimicrob Chemother* 1979;5:431–436.
5. Crumpacker CS, Schnipper LE, Zaia JA, et al: Growth inhibition of acycloguanosine of herpesviruses isolated from human infections. *Antimicrob Agents Chemother* 1979;15:642–645.
6. DeClercq E, Descamps J, Verhelst G, et al: Comparative efficacy of antiherpes drugs against different strains of herpes simplex virus. *J Infect Dis* 1980; 141:563–574.
7. Naib ZM, Nahmias AJ, Josey WE, et al: Relation of cytohistopathology of genital herpesvirus infection to cervical anaplasia. *Cancer Res* 1973;33:1452–1463.
8. Stahlmann R, Klug S, Lewandowski C, et al: Teratogenicity of acyclovir in rats. *Infection* 1987;15:261–262.
9. Lau RJ, Emery MG, Galinsky RE, et al: Unexpected accumulation of acyclovir in breast milk with estimate of infant exposure. *Obstet Gynecol* 1987;69(3):468–471.
10. Meyer LJ, deMiranda P, Sheth N, et al: Acyclovir in human breast milk. *Am J Obstet Gynecol* 1988;158(3): 586–588.

U.S. Patent No. 4199574 647230

ZOVIRAX® Sterile Powder ℞
[zō″vī′răx]
(Acyclovir Sodium)
FOR INTRAVENOUS INFUSION ONLY

DESCRIPTION

Zovirax is the brand name for acyclovir, an antiviral drug active against herpesviruses. Zovirax Sterile Powder is a formulation for intravenous administration. Each 5.49 mg of sterile lyophilized acyclovir sodium is equivalent to 5 mg acyclovir.

The chemical name of acyclovir sodium is 9-[(2-hydroxyethoxy)methyl]guanine sodium.

Acyclovir sodium is a white, crystalline powder with a molecular weight of 247 daltons, and a solubility in water exceeding 100 mg/mL. Each 500 mg or 1000 mg vial of Zovirax Sterile Powder when reconstituted with 10 mL or 20 mL, respectively, sterile diluent yields 50 mg/mL acyclovir (pH approximately 11). Further dilution in any appropriate intravenous solution must be performed before infusion (see Method of Preparation). At physiologic pH, acyclovir exists as the unionized form with a molecular weight of 225 daltons and a maximum solubility of 2.5 mg/mL at 37°C.

CLINICAL PHARMACOLOGY

Mechanism of Antiviral Effects: Acyclovir is a synthetic purine nucleoside analogue with *in vitro* and *in vivo* inhibitory activity against human herpes viruses including herpes simplex types 1 (HSV-1) and 2 (HSV-2), varicella-zoster virus (VZV), Epstein-Barr virus (EBV) and cytomegalovirus (CMV). In cell culture, acyclovir has the highest antiviral activity against HSV-1, followed in decreasing order of potency against HSV-2, VZV, EBV and CMV.[1]

The inhibitory activity of acyclovir for HSV-1, HSV-2, VZV and EBV is highly selective. The enzyme thymidine kinase (TK) of normal uninfected cells does not effectively use acyclovir as a substrate. However, TK encoded by HSV, VZV and EBV[2] converts acyclovir into acyclovir monophosphate, a nucleotide analogue. The monophosphate is further converted into diphosphate by cellular guanylate kinase and into triphosphate by a number of cellular enzymes.[3] Acyclovir triphosphate interferes with Herpes simplex virus DNA polymerase and inhibits viral DNA replication. Acyclovir triphosphate also inhibits cellular α-DNA polymerase but to a lesser degree. *In vitro*, acyclovir triphosphate can be incorporated into growing chains of DNA by viral DNA polymerase and to a much smaller extent by cellular α-DNA polymerase.[4] When incorporation occurs, the DNA chain is terminated.[5,6] Acyclovir is preferentially taken up and selectively converted to the active triphosphate form by herpesvirus-infected cells. Thus, acyclovir is much less toxic *in vitro* for normal uninfected cells because: 1) less is taken up; 2) less is converted to the active form; 3) cellular α-DNA polymerase is less sensitive to the effects of the active form. The mode of acyclovir phosphorylation in cytomegalovirus-infected cells is not clearly established, but may involve virally induced cell kinases or an unidentified viral enzyme. Acyclovir is not efficiently activated in cytomegalovirus infected cells, which may account for the reduced susceptibility of cytomegalovirus to acyclovir *in vitro*.

Microbiology: The quantitative relationship between the *in vitro* susceptibility of herpes simplex virus to acyclovir and the clinical response to therapy has not been established in man, and virus sensitivity testing has not been standardized. Sensitivity testing results, expressed as the concentration of drug required to inhibit by 50% the growth of virus in cell culture (ID_{50}), vary greatly depending upon the particular assay used,[7] the cell type employed,[8] and the laboratory performing the test.[1] The ID_{50} of acyclovir against HSV-1 isolates may range from 0.02 μg/mL (plaque reduction in Vero cells) to 5.9–13.5μg/mL (plaque reduction in green monkey kidney [GMK] cells).[1] The ID_{50} against HSV-2 ranges from 0.01 μg/mL to 9.9 μg/mL (plaque reduction in Vero and GMK cells, respectively).[1]

Using a dye-uptake method in Vero cells,[9] which gives ID_{50} values approximately 5- to 10-fold higher than plaque reduction assays, 1417 isolates (553 HSV-1 and 864 HSV-2) from approximately 500 patients were examined over a 5-year period.[10] These assays found that 90% of HSV-1 isolates were sensitive to ≤ 0.9 μg/mL acyclovir and 50% of all isolates were sensitive to ≤ 0.2 μg/mL acyclovir. For HSV-2 isolates, 90% were sensitive to ≤ 2.2 μg/mL and 50% of all isolates were sensitive to ≤ 0.7 μg/mL of acyclovir. Isolates with significantly diminished sensitivity were found in 44 patients. It must be emphasized that neither the patients nor

the isolates were randomly selected and, therefore, do not represent the general population.
Most of the less sensitive clinical isolates have been relatively deficient in the viral TK.[11-19] Strains with alterations in viral TK[20] or viral DNA polymerase[21] have also been reported. Prolonged exposure to low concentrations (0.1 μg/mL) of acyclovir in cell culture has resulted in the emergence of a variety of acyclovir-resistant strains.[22]
The ID_{50} against VZV ranges from 0.17–1.53 μg/mL (yield reduction, human foreskin fibroblasts) to 1.85–3.98 μg/mL (foci reduction, human embryo fibroblasts [HEF]). Reproduction of EBV genome is suppressed by 50% in superinfected Raji cells or P3HR-1 lymphoblastoid cells by 1.5 μg/mL acyclovir. CMV is relatively resistant to acyclovir with ID_{50} values ranging from 2.3–17.6 μg/mL (plaque reduction, HEF cells) to 1.82–56.8 μg/mL (DNA hybridization, HEF cells). The latent state of the genome of any of the human herpesviruses is not known to be sensitive to acyclovir.[1]

Pharmacokinetics: The pharmacokinetics of acyclovir has been evaluated in 95 patients (9 studies). Results were obtained in adult patients with normal renal function during Phase I/II studies after single doses ranging from 0.5 to 15 mg/kg and after multiple doses ranging from 2.5 to 15 mg/kg every 8 hours. Pharmacokinetics was also determined in pediatric patients with normal renal function ranging in age from 1 to 17 years at doses of 250 mg/m^2 or 500 mg/m^2 every 8 hours. In these studies, dose-independent pharmacokinetics is observed in the range of 0.5 to 15 mg/kg. Proportionality between dose and plasma levels is seen after single doses or at steady state after multiple dosing.[23] When Zovirax was administered to adults at 5 mg/kg (approximately 250 mg/m^2) by 1-hr infusions every 8 hours, mean steady-state peak and trough concentrations of 9.8 μg/mL (5.5 to 13.8 μg/mL) and 0.7 μg/mL (0.2 to 1.0 μg/mL), respectively, were achieved. Similar concentrations are achieved in children over 1 year of age when doses of 250 mg/m^2 are given by 1-hr infusions every 8 hours. At a dose to 10 mg/kg given by 1-hr infusion every 8 hours, mean steady-state peak and trough concentrations were 22.9 μg/mL (14.1 to 44.1 μg/mL) and 1.9 μg/mL (0.5 to 2.9 μg/mL). Similar concentrations were achieved in children dosed at 500 mg/m^2 given by 1-hr infusion every 8 hours. Concentrations achieved in the cerebrospinal fluid are approximately 50% of plasma values. Plasma protein binding is relatively low (9% to 33%) and drug interactions involving binding site displacement are not anticipated.[23]
Renal excretion of unchanged drug by glomerular filtration and tubular secretion is the major route of acyclovir elimination accounting for 62 to 91% of the dose as determined by ^{14}C-labelled drug. The only major urinary metabolite detected is 9-carboxymethoxymethylguanine. This may account for up to 14.1% of the dose in patients with normal renal function. An insignificant amount of drug is recovered in feces and expired CO_2 and there is no evidence to suggest tissue retention.[23] However, postmortem examinations have shown that acyclovir is widely distributed in tissues and body fluids including brain, kidney, lung, liver, muscle, spleen, uterus, vaginal mucosa, vaginal secretions, cerebrospinal fluid and herpetic vesicular fluid.
The half-life and total body clearance of acyclovir is dependent on renal function as shown below.[23]

Creatinine Clearance (mL/min/1.73m^2)	Half-Life (hr)	Total Body Clearance (mL/min/1.73m^2)
>80	2.5	327
50–80	3.0	248
15–50	3.5	190
0 (Anuric)	19.5	29

Zovirax was administered at a dose of 2.5 mg/kg to 6 adult patients with severe renal failure. The peak and trough plasma levels during the 47 hours preceding hemodialysis were 8.5 μg/mL and 0.7 μg/mL, respectively.[24,25]
Consult DOSAGE AND ADMINISTRATION section for recommended adjustments in dosing based upon creatinine clearance.
The half-life and total body clearance of acyclovir in pediatric patients over 1 year of age is similar to those in adults with normal renal function (see DOSAGE AND ADMINISTRATION).

INDICATIONS AND USAGE

Zovirax Sterile Powder is indicated for the treatment of initial and recurrent mucosal and cutaneous Herpes simplex (HSV-1 and HSV-2) and varicella-zoster (shingles) infections in immunocompromised patients. It is also indicated for herpes simplex encephalitis in patients over 6 months of age and for severe initial clinical episodes of herpes genitalis in patients who are not immunocompromised.

Herpes Simplex Infections in Immunocompromised Patients
A multicenter trial of Zovirax Sterile Powder at a dose of 250 mg/m^2 every 8 hours (750 mg/m^2/day) for 7 days was conducted in 98 immunocompromised patients (73 adults and 25 children) with oro-facial, esophageal, genital and other localized infections (52 treated with Zovirax and 46 with placebo). Zovirax significantly decreased virus excretion, reduced pain, and promoted scabbing and rapid healing of lesions.[14,26,27,28]

Initial Episodes of Herpes Genitalis
In placebo-controlled trials, 58 patients with initial genital herpes were treated with intravenous Zovirax 5 mg/kg or placebo (27 patients treated with Zovirax and 31 treated with placebo) every eight hours for 5 days. Zovirax decreased the duration of viral excretion, new lesion formation, and duration of vesicles and promoted healing of lesions.[28,29,30]

Herpes Simplex Encephalitis
Sixty-two patients ages 6 months to 79 years with brain biopsy-proven herpes simplex encephalitis were randomized to receive either Zovirax (30 mg/kg/day) or adenine arabinoside (Vira-A) (15 mg/kg/day) for 10 days (28 were treated with Zovirax and 34 with Vira-A).[31] Overall mortality for Zovirax recipients at 6 months was 18% compared to 59% for Vira-A treated patients ($p = 0.003$). The proportion of Zovirax recipients functioning normally or with only mild sequelae (eg, decreased attention span) was 39% compared to 9% of Vira-A treated patients ($p = 0.01$). The remaining patients in both groups had moderate (eg, hemiparesis, speech impediment or seizure) or severe (continuous supportive care required) neurologic sequelae.
After 12 months of follow-up, two additional Zovirax recipients had died, resulting in an overall mortality of 25% compared to 59% for Vira-A treated patients ($p = 0.02$). Morbidity assessments at that time indicated that 32% of Zovirax recipients were functioning normally, or with only mild sequelae compared to 12% Vira-A patients ($p = 0.06$). Moderate to severe impairment was noted in all remaining patients in both groups who were available for evaluation. Patients less than 30 years of age and those who had the least severe neurologic involvement at time of entry into study had the best outcome with Zovirax treatment. An additional controlled study performed in Europe[32] demonstrated similar findings. The superiority of Zovirax over Vira-A for neonatal herpes encephalitis has not been demonstrated.

Varicella-Zoster Infections in Immunocompromised Patients
A multicenter trial of Zovirax Sterile Powder at a dose of 500 mg/m^2 every 8 hours for 7 days was conducted in immunocompromised patients with zoster infections (shingles). Ninety-four (94) patients were evaluated (52 patients were treated with Zovirax and 42 with placebo). Zovirax halted progression of infection as determined by significant reductions in cutaneous dissemination, visceral dissemination, or the proportion of patients deemed treatment failures.[28,33]
A comparative trial of Zovirax and vidarabine was conducted in 22 severely immunocompromised patients with zoster infections. Zovirax was shown to be superior to vidarabine as demonstated by significant differences in the time of new lesion formation, the time to pain reduction, the time to lesion crusting, the time to complete healing, the incidence of fever and the duration of positive viral cultures. In addition, cutaneous dissemination occurred in none of the 10 Zovirax recipients compared to 5 of the 10 vidarabine recipients who presented with localized dermatomal disease.[34]

Diagnosis
Diagnosis is confirmed by virus isolation. Accelerated viral culture assays or immunocytology allow more rapid diagnosis than standard viral culture. In initial episodes of genital herpes, appropriate examinations should be performed to rule out other sexually transmitted diseases. Whereas cutaneous lesions associated with Herpes simplex and varicella-zoster infections are often characteristic, the finding of multinucleated giant cells in smears prepared from lesion exudate or scrapings may assist in the diagnosis.[35]
The Tzanck smear does not distinguish varicella-zoster from herpes simplex infections. Culture of varicella-zoster is not widely available.
Herpes encephalitis should be confirmed by brain biopsy to obtain tissue for histologic examination and viral culture and to exclude other causes of neurologic disease. A presumptive diagnosis of herpes encephalitis may be made on the basis of focal changes in the temporal lobe visualized with various diagnostic methods including magnetic resonance imaging, computerized tomography, radionuclide scans or electroencephalography. Culture of the cerebrospinal fluid for herpes simplex virus is unreliable.

CONTRAINDICATIONS

Zovirax Sterile Powder is contraindicated for patients who develop hypersensitivity to the drug.

WARNINGS

Zovirax Sterile Powder is intended for intravenous infusion only, and should not be administered topically, intramuscularly, orally, subcutaneously, or in the eye. Intravenous infusions must be given over a period of at least 1 (one) hour to reduce the risk of renal tubular damage (see PRECAUTIONS and DOSAGE AND ADMINISTRATION).

PRECAUTIONS

General: The recommended dosage, frequency and length of treatment should not be exceeded (see DOSAGE AND ADMINISTRATION).
Although the aqueous solubility of acyclovir sodium (for infusion) is > 100 mg/mL, precipitation of acyclovir crystals in renal tubules can occur if the maximum solubility of free acyclovir (2.5 mg/mL at 37°C in water) is exceeded or if the drug is administered by bolus injection. This complication causes a rise in serum creatinine and blood urea nitrogen (BUN), and a decrease in renal creatinine clearance. Ensuing renal tubular damage can produce acute renal failure.
Abnormal renal function (decreased creatinine clearance) can occur as a result of acyclovir administration and depends on the state of the patient's hydration, other treatments, and the rate of drug administration. Bolus administration of the drug leads to a 10% incidence of renal dysfunction, while in controlled studies, infusion of 5 mg/kg (250 mg/m^2) and 10 mg/kg (500 mg/m^2) over an hour was associated with a lower frequency—3.8%. Concomitant use of other nephrotoxic drugs, pre-existing renal disease, and dehydration make further renal impairment with acyclovir more likely. In most instances, alterations of renal function were transient and resolved spontaneously or with improvement of water and electrolyte balance, drug dosage adjustment or discontinuation of drug administration. However, in some instances, these changes may progress to acute renal failure.
Administration of Zovirax by intravenous infusion must be accompanied by adequate hydration. Since maximum urine concentration occurs within the first 2 hours following infusion, particular attention should be given to establishing sufficient urine flow during that period in order to prevent precipitation in renal tubules. Recommended urine output is ≥ 500 mL per gram of drug infused. In patients with encephalitis, the recommended hydration should be balanced by the risk of cerebral edema.
When dosage adjustments are required they should be based on estimated creatinine clearance (see DOSAGE AND ADMINISTRATION).
Approximately 1% of patients receiving intravenous acyclovir have manifested encephalopathic changes characterized by either lethargy, obtundation, tremors, confusion, hallucinations, agitation, seizures or coma. Zovirax should be used with caution in those patients who have underlying neurologic abnormalities and those with serious renal, hepatic, or electrolyte abnormalities or significant hypoxia. It should also be used with caution in patients who have manifested prior neurologic reactions to cytotoxic drugs or those receiving concomitant intrathecal methotrexate or interferon.
Exposure of HSV isolates to acyclovir *in vitro* can lead to the emergence of less sensitive viruses. These viruses usually are deficient in thymidine kinase (required for acyclovir activation) and are less pathogenic in animals. Similar isolates have been observed in severely immunocompromised patients during the course of controlled and uncontrolled studies of intravenously administered Zovirax. These occurred in patients with severe combined immunodeficiencies or following bone marrow transplantation. The presence of these viruses was not associated with a worsening of clinical illness and, in some instances, the virus disappeared spontaneously. The possibility of the appearance of less sensitive viruses must be recognized when treating such patients.[11-19] The relationship between the *in vitro* sensitivity of herpes simplex or varicella-zoster virus to acyclovir and clinical response to therapy has not been established.

Drug Interactions: Co-administration of probenecid with acyclovir has been shown to increase the mean half-life and the area under the concentration-time curve. Urinary excretion and renal clearance were correspondingly reduced.[36] The clinical effects of this combination have not been studied.

Carcinogenesis, Mutagenesis, Impairment of Fertility: The data presented below include references to peak steady state plasma acyclovir concentrations observed in humans treated with 30 mg/kg/day (10 mg/kg/every 8 hr, dosing appropriate for treatment of herpes zoster or herpes encephalitis), or 15 mg/kg/day (5 mg/kg/every 8 hr, dosing appropriate for treatment of primary genital herpes or herpes simplex infections in immunocompromised patients). Plasma drug concentrations in animal studies are expressed as multiples of human exposure to acyclovir at the higher and lower dosing schedules (see Pharmacokinetics).
Acyclovir was tested in lifetime bioassays in rats and mice at single daily doses of up to 450 mg/kg given by gavage. There was no statistically significant difference in the incidence of tumors between treated and control animals, nor did acyclovir shorten the latency of tumors. At 450 mg/kg/day, plasma concentrations in both the mouse and rat bioassay were lower than concentrations in humans.
Acyclovir was tested in two *in vitro* cell transformation assays. Positive results were observed at the highest concentration tested (3 to 5 times human levels) in one system and the

Continued on next page

Burroughs Wellcome—Cont.

resulting morphologically transformed cells formed tumors when inoculated into immunosuppressed, syngeneic, weanling mice. Acyclovir was negative (3 to 6 times human levels) in the other, possibly less sensitive, transformation assay. In acute cytogenetic studies, there was an increase, not statistically significant, in the incidence of chromosomal damage at maximum tolerated parenteral doses of acyclovir (100 mg/kg) in rats (5 to 10 times human levels) but not in Chinese hamsters; higher doses of 500 and 1000 mg/kg were clastogenic in Chinese hamsters (31 and 61 times human levels). In addition, no activity was found after 5 days dosing in a dominant lethal study in mice (3 and 6 times human levels). In all 4 microbial assays, no evidence of mutagenicity was observed. Positive results were obtained in 2 of 7 genetic toxicity assays using mammalian cells *in vitro*. In human lymphocytes a positive response for chromosomal damage was seen at concentrations 13 to 25 times the acyclovir plasma levels achieved in man. At one locus in mouse lymphoma cells, mutagenicity was observed at concentrations 20 to 40 times human plasma levels. Results in the other five mammalian cell loci follow: at 3 loci in a Chinese hamster ovary cell line, the results were inconclusive at concentrations at least 150 times human levels. At 2 other loci in mouse lymphoma cells no evidence of mutagenicity was observed at concentrations at least 120 times human levels. Acyclovir has not been shown to impair fertility or reproduction in mice (450 mg/kg/day, p.o.) or in rats (25 mg/kg/day, s.c.). In the mouse study plasma levels were the same as human levels. At 50 mg/kg/day s.c. in the rat (1 to 2 times human levels), there was a statistically significant increase in post-implantation loss, but no concomitant decrease in litter size. In female rabbits treated subcutaneously with acyclovir subsequent to mating, there was a statistically significant decrease in implantation efficiency but no concomitant decrease in litter size at a dose of 50 mg/kg/day (1 to 3 times human levels). No effect upon implantation efficiency was observed when the same dose was administered intravenously (4 to 9 times human levels). In a rat peri- and postnatal study at 50 mg/kg/day s.c. (1 to 2 times human levels), there was a statistically significant decrease in the group mean numbers of corpora lutea, total implantation sites and live fetuses in the F$_1$ generation. Although not statistically significant, there was also a dose-related decrease in group mean numbers of live fetuses and implantation sites at 12.5 mg/kg/day and 25 mg/kg/day, s.c. The intravenous administration of 100 mg/kg/day, a dose known to cause obstructive nephropathy in rabbits, caused a significant increase in fetal resorptions and a corresponding decrease in litter size (plasma levels were not measured). However, at a maximum tolerated intravenous dose of 50 mg/kg/day in rabbits (4 to 9 times human levels), no drug-related reproductive effects were observed.

Intraperitoneal doses of 80 or 320 mg/kg/day acyclovir given to rats for 6 and 1 months, respectively, caused testicular atrophy. Plasma levels were not measured in the one month study and were 2 to 4 times human levels in the six-month study. Testicular atrophy was persistent through the 4-week postdose recovery phase after 320 mg/kg/day; some evidence of recovery of sperm production was evident 30 days postdose. Intravenous doses of 100 and 200 mg/kg/day acyclovir given to dogs for 31 days caused aspermatogenesis. At 100 mg/kg/day plasma levels were 4 to 8 times human levels, while at 200 mg/kg/day they were 13 to 25 times human levels. No testicular abnormalities were seen in dogs given 50 mg/kg/day i.v. for one month (2 to 3 times human levels) and in dogs given 60 mg/kg/day orally for one year (the same as human levels).

Pregnancy: *Teratogenic Effects:* Pregnancy Category C. Acyclovir was not teratogenic in the mouse (450 mg/kg/day, p.o.), rabbit (50 mg/kg/day, s.c. and i.v.) or in standard tests in the rat (50 mg/kg/day, s.c.). These exposures resulted in plasma levels the same as, 4 and 9, and 1 and 2 times, respectively, human levels. In a non-standard test in rats there were fetal abnormalities, such as head and tail anomalies, and maternal toxicity.[37] In this test, rats were given 3 s.c. doses of 100 mg/kg/acyclovir on gestation day 10, resulting in plasma levels 5 and 10 times human levels. There are no adequate and well-controlled studies in pregnant women. Acyclovir should not be used during pregnancy unless the potential benefit justifies the potential risk to the fetus. Although acyclovir was not teratogenic in standard animal studies, the drug's potential for causing chromosome breaks at high concentration should be taken into consideration in making this determination.

Nursing Mothers: Acyclovir concentrations have been documented in breast milk in two women following oral administration of Zovirax and ranged from 0.6 to 4.1 times corresponding plasma levels.[38,39] These concentrations would potentially expose the nursing infant to a dose of acyclovir up to 0.3 mg/kg/day. Caution should be exercised when Zovirax is administered to a nursing woman.

ADVERSE REACTIONS

The adverse reactions listed below have been observed in controlled and uncontrolled clinical trials in approximately 700 patients who received Zovirax at ~ 5 mg/kg (250 mg/m^2) three times daily, and approximately 300 patients who received ~ 10 mg/kg (500 mg/m^2) three times daily.

The most frequent adverse reactions reported during Zovirax administration were inflammation or phlebitis at the injection site in approximately 9% of the patients, and transient elevations of serum creatinine or BUN in 5% to 10% (the higher incidence occurred usually following rapid [less than 10 minutes] intravenous infusion). Nausea and/or vomiting occurred in approximately 7% of the patients (the majority occurring in nonhospitalized patients who received 10 mg/kg). Itching, rash or hives occurred in approximately 2% of patients. Elevation of transaminases occurred in 1–2% of patients.

Approximately 1% of patients receiving intravenous acyclovir have manifested encephalopathic changes characterized by either lethargy, obtundation, tremors, confusion, hallucinations, agitation, seizures or coma (see PRECAUTIONS).

Adverse reactions which occurred at a frequency of less than 1% and which were probably or possibly related to intravenous Zovirax administration were: anemia, anuria, hematuria, hypotension, edema, anorexia, lightheadedness, thirst, headache, diaphoresis, fever, neutropenia, thrombocytopenia, abnormal urinalysis (characterized by an increase in formed elements in urine sediment) and pain on urination. Other reactions have been reported with a frequency of less than 1% in patients receiving Zovirax, but a causal relationship between Zovirax and the reaction could not be determined. These include pulmonary edema with cardiac tamponade, abdominal pain, chest pain, thrombocytosis, leukocytosis, neutrophilia, ischemia of digits, hypokalemia, purpura fulminans, pressure on urination, hemoglobinemia and rigors.

Observed During Clinical Practice: Based on clinical practice experience in patients treated with Zovirax Sterile Powder in the U.S., spontaneously reported adverse events are uncommon. Data are insufficient to support an estimate of their incidence or to establish causation. These events may also occur as part of the underlying disease process. Voluntary reports of adverse events which have been received since market introduction include:

General: fever, pain
Digestive: elevated liver function tests, nausea
Hemic and Lymphatic: leukopenia
Nervous: agitation, coma, confusion, convulsions, hallucinations, obtundation, psychosis
Skin: rash
Urogenital: elevated blood urea nitrogen, elevated creatinine, renal failure

OVERDOSAGE

Overdosage has been reported following administration of bolus injections, or inappropriately high doses, and in patients whose fluid and electrolyte balance was not properly monitored. This has resulted in elevations in BUN, serum creatinine and subsequent renal failure. Lethargy, convulsions and coma have been reported rarely.

Precipitation of acyclovir in renal tubules may occur when the solubility (2.5 mg/mL) in the intratubular fluid is exceeded (see PRECAUTIONS). Renal lesions related to obstruction of renal tubules by precipitated drug crystals occurred in the following species: rats treated with i.v. and i.p. doses of 20 mg/kg/day for 21 and 31 days, respectively, and at s.c. doses of 100 mg/kg/day for 10 days; rabbits at s.c. and i.v. doses of 50 mg/kg/day for 13 days; and dogs at i.v. doses of 100 mg/kg/day for 31 days. In the event of overdosage, sufficient urine flow must be maintained to prevent precipitation of drug in renal tubules. Recommended urine output is ≥ 500 mL per gram of drug infused. A six-hour hemodialysis results in a 60% decrease in plasma acyclovir concentration. Data concerning peritoneal dialysis are incomplete but indicate that this method may be significantly less efficient in removing acyclovir from the blood. In the event of acute renal failure and anuria, the patient may benefit from hemodialysis until renal function is restored (see DOSAGE AND ADMINISTRATION).

DOSAGE AND ADMINISTRATION

CAUTION— RAPID OR BOLUS INTRAVENOUS AND INTRAMUSCULAR OR SUBCUTANEOUS INJECTION MUST BE AVOIDED. Therapy should be initiated as early as possible following onset of signs and symptoms. For diagnosis—see INDICATIONS.

Dosage:
HERPES SIMPLEX INFECTIONS
MUCOSAL AND CUTANEOUS HERPES SIMPLEX (HSV-1 and HSV-2) INFECTIONS IN IMMUNOCOMPROMISED PATIENTS — 5 mg/kg infused at a constant rate over 1 hour, every 8 hours (15 mg/kg/day) for 7 days in adult patients with normal renal function. In children under 12 years of age, more accurate dosing can be attained by infus-

ing 250 mg/m^2 at a constant rate over 1 hour, every 8 hours (750 mg/m^2/day) for 7 days.
SEVERE INITIAL CLINICAL EPISODES OF HERPES GENITALIS —The same dose given above—administered for 5 days.
HERPES SIMPLEX ENCEPHALITIS —10 mg/kg infused at a constant rate over at least 1 hour, every 8 hours for 10 days. In children between 6 months and 12 years of age, more accurate dosing is achieved by infusing 500 mg/m^2, at a constant rate over at least one hour, every 8 hours for 10 days.
VARICELLA ZOSTER INFECTIONS
ZOSTER IN IMMUNOCOMPROMISED PATIENTS —10 mg/kg infused at a constant rate over 1 hour, every 8 hours for 7 days in adult patients with normal renal function. In children under 12 years of age, equivalent plasma concentrations are attained by infusing 500 mg/m^2 at a constant rate over at least 1 hour, every 8 hours for 7 days. Obese patients should be dosed at 10 mg/kg (Ideal Body Weight). A maximum dose equivalent to 500 mg/m^2 every 8 hours should not be exceeded for any patient.
PATIENTS WITH ACUTE OR CHRONIC RENAL IMPAIRMENT: Refer to DOSAGE AND ADMINISTRATION section for recommended doses, and adjust the dosing interval as indicated in the table below.

Creatinine Clearance (mL/min/1.73m^2)	Percent of Recommended Dose	Dosing Interval (hours)
>50	100%	8
25–50	100%	12
10–25	100%	24
0–10	50%	24

Hemodialysis: For patients who require dialysis, the mean plasma half-life of acyclovir during hemodialysis is approximately 5 hours. This results in a 60% decrease in plasma concentrations following a six-hour dialysis period. Therefore, the patient's dosing schedule should be adjusted so that an additional dose is administered after each dialysis.[24,25]
Peritoneal Dialysis: No supplmental dose appears to be necessary after adjustment of the dosing interval.[40, 41]
Method of Preparation: Each 10 mL vial contains acyclovir sodium equivalent to 500 mg of acyclovir. Each 20 mL vial contains acyclovir sodium equivalent to 1000 mg of acyclovir. The contents of the vial should be dissolved in Sterile Water for Injection as follows:

Contents of Vial	Amount of Diluent
500 mg	10 mL
1000 mg	20 mL

The resulting solution in each case contains 50 mg acyclovir per mL (pH approximately 11). Shake the vial well to assure complete dissolution before measuring and transferring each individual dose. DO NOT USE BACTERIOSTATIC WATER FOR INJECTION CONTAINING BENZYL ALCOHOL OR PARABENS.
Administration: The calculated dose should then be removed and added to any appropriate intravenous solution at a volume selected for administration during each 1 hour infusion. Infusion concentrations of approximately 7 mg/mL or lower are recommended. In clinical studies, the average 70 kg adult received between 60 and 150 mL of fluid per dose. Higher concentrations (eg, 10 mg/mL) may produce phlebitis or inflammation at the injection site upon inadvertent extravasation. Standard, commercially available electrolyte and glucose solutions are suitable for intravenous administration; biologic or colloidal fluids (eg, blood products, protein solutions, etc.) are not recommended.
Once in solution in the vial at a concentration of 50 mg/mL, the drug should be used within 12 hours. Once diluted for administration, each dose should be used within 24 hours. Refrigeration of reconstituted solutions may result in formation of a precipitate which will redissolve at room temperature.

HOW SUPPLIED

10 mL sterile vials, each containing acyclovir sodium equivalent to 500 mg of acyclovir, tray of 10 (NDC 0081-0995-01).
20 mL sterile vials, each containing acyclovir sodium equivalent to 1000 mg of acyclovir, tray of 10 (NDC 0081-0952-01).
Store at 15° to 25°C (59° to 77°F).
Also available: ZOVIRAX Ointment, 5% in 3 g and 15 g tubes (each gram contains 50 mg acyclovir in a polyethylene glycol base), ZOVIRAX Capsules in bottles of 100 and unit dose pack of 100 (each capsule contains 200 mg acyclovir), ZOVIRAX Tablets in bottles of 100 (each tablet contains 800 mg acyclovir), and ZOVIRAX Suspension in 1 pint bottles (each 5 mL contains 200 mg acyclovir).

REFERENCES

1. O'Brien JJ, Campoli-Richards DM. Acyclovir—an updated review of its antiviral activity, pharmacokinetic properties and therapeutic efficacy. *Drugs* 1989; 37:233–309.
2. Littler E, Zeuthen J, McBride AA, et al. Identification of an Epstein-Barr virus-coded thymidine kinase. *The EMBO Journal* 1986;5(8):1959–1966.
3. Miller WH, Miller RL. Phosphorylation of acyclovir (acycloguanosine) monophosphate by GMP kinase. *J Biol Chem.* 1980;255:7204–7207.
4. Furman PA, St Clair MH, Fyfe JA, et al. Inhibition of herpes simplex virus-induced DNA polymerase activity and viral DNA replication by 9-(2-hydroxyethoxymethyl)guanine and its triphosphate. *J Virol.* 1979;32:72–77.
5. Derse D, Cheng YC, Furman PA, et al. Inhibition of purified human and herpes simplex virus-induced DNA polymerases by 9-(2-hydroxyethoxymethyl)guanine triphosphate: Effects on primer-template function. *J Biol Chem.* 1981;256:11447–11451.
6. McGuirt PV, Shaw JE, Elion GB, et al. Identification of small DNA fragments synthesized in herpes simplex virus-infected cells in the presence of acyclovir. *Antimicrob Agents Chemother.* 1984;25:507–509.
7. Barry DW, Blum MR. Antiviral drugs: acyclovir. In: Turner P, Shand DG eds. *Recent Advances in Clinical Pharmacology.* ed 3. New York: Churchill Livingstone, 1983: chap 4.
8. DeClercq E. Comparative efficacy of antiherpes drugs in different cell lines. *Antimicrob Agents Chemother.* 1982;21:661–663.
9. McLaren C, Ellis MN, Hunter GA. A colorimetric assay for the measurement of the sensitivity of herpes simplex viruses to antiviral agents. *Antiviral Res.* 1983; 3:223–234.
10. Barry DW, Nusinoff-Lehrman S. Viral resistance in clinical practice: summary of five years experience with acyclovir. In Kono R, Nakajima A eds. *Herpes Viruses and Virus Chemotherapy (Ex Med Int Congr Ser 667).* New York: *Excerpta Medica.* 1985:269–270.
11. Dekker C, Ellis MN, McLaren C, et al. Virus resistance in clinical practice. *J Antimicrob Chemother.* 1983;12 (suppl B):137–152.
12. Sibrack CD, Gutman LT, Wilfert CM, et al. Pathogenicity of acyclovir-resistant herpes simplex virus type 1 from an immunodeficient child. *J Infect Dis.* 1982; 146:673–682.
13. Crumpacker CS, Schnipper LE, Marlowe Sl, et al. Resistance to antiviral drugs of herpes simplex virus isolated from a patient treated with acyclovir. *N Engl J Med.* 1982;306:343–346.
14. Wade JC, Newton B, McLaren C, et al. Intravenous acyclovir to treat mucocutaneous herpes simplex virus infection after marrow transplantation. A double-blind trial. *Ann Intern Med.* 1982;96:265–269.
15. Burns WH, Saral R, Santos GW, et al. Isolation and characterization of resistant herpes simplex virus after acyclovir therapy. *Lancet.* 1982;1:421–423.
16. Straus SE, Takiff HE, Seidlin M, et al. Suppression of frequently recurring genital herpes: A placebo-controlled double-blind trial of oral acyclovir. *N Engl J Med.* 1984;310:1545–1550.
17. Collins P. Viral sensitivity following the introduction of acyclovir. *Am J Med.* 1988;85(2A):129–134.
18. Erlich KS, Mills J, Chatis P, et al. Acyclovir-resistant herpes simplex virus infections in patients with the acquired immunodeficiency syndrome. *N Engl J Med.* 1989;320(5):293–296.
19. Hill EL, Ellis MN, Barry DW. In: 28th Intersci Conf on Antimicrob Agents Chemother. Los Angeles, 1988, Abst. No. 0840:260.
20. Ellis MN, Keller PM, Fyfe JA, et al. Clinical isolates of herpes simplex virus type 2 that induces a thymidine kinase with altered substrate specificity. *Antimicrob Agents Chemother.* 1987;31(7):1117–1125.
21. Collins P, Larder BA, Oliver NM, et al. Characterization of a DNA polymerase mutant of herpes simplex virus from a severely immunocompromised patient receiving acyclovir. *J gen Virol.* 1989;(70):375–382.
22. Field HJ, Darby G, Wildy P. Isolation and characterization of acyclovir-resistant mutants of herpes simplex virus. *J gen Virol.* 1980;49:115–124.
23. Blum MR, Liao SH, deMiranda P. Overview of acyclovir pharmacokinetic disposition in adults and children. *Am J Med.* 1982;73:186–192.
24. Laskin OL, Longstreth JA, Whelton A, et al. Effect of renal failure on the pharmacokinetics of acyclovir. *Am J Med.* 1982;73:197–201.
25. Krasny HC, Liao SH, deMiranda P, et al. Influence of hemodialysis on acyclovir pharmacokinetics in patients with chronic renal failure. *Am J Med.* 1982;73:202–204.
26. Mitchell CD, Bean B, Gentry SR, et al. Acyclovir therapy for mucocutaneous herpes simplex infections in immunocompromised patients. *Lancet.* 1981;1:1389–1392.
27. Meyers JD, Wade JC, Mitchell CD, et al. Multicenter collaborative trial of intravenous acyclovir for treatment of mucocutaneous herpes simplex virus infection in the immunocompromised host. *Am J Med.* 1982:73: 229–235.
28. Data on file, Burroughs Wellcome Co.
29. Corey L, Fife KH, Benedetti JK, et al. Intravenous acyclovir for the treatment of primary genital herpes. *Ann Intern Med.* 1983;98(6):914–921.
30. Mindel A, Adler MW, Sutherland S, et al. Intravenous acyclovir treatment for primary genital herpes. *Lancet.* 1982;1:697–700.
31. Whitley RJ, Alford CA, Hirsch MS, et al. Vidarabine versus acyclovir therapy in herpes simplex encephalitis. *N Engl J Med.* 1986;314(3):144–149.
32. Sköldenberg B, Forsgren M, Alestig K, et al. Acyclovir versus vidarabine in herpes simplex encephalitis: randomized multicenter study in consecutive Swedish patients. *Lancet.* 1984;2(8405):707–711.
33. Balfour HH Jr, Bean B, Laskin OL, et al. Acyclovir halts progression of herpes zoster in immunocompromised patients. *N Engl J Med.* 1983;308(24):1448–1453.
34. Shepp DH, Danliker PS, Meyers JD. Treatment of varicella-zoster virus infection in severely immunocompromised patients. *N Engl J Med.* 1986;314:208–212.
35. Naib ZM, Nahmias AJ, Josey WE, et al. Relation of cytohistopathology of genital herpesvirus infection to cervical anaplasia. *Cancer Res.* 1973;33:1452–1463.
36. Laskin OL, deMiranda P, King DH, et al. Effects of probenecid on the pharmacokinetics and elimination of acyclovir in humans. *Antimicrob Agents Chemother.* 1982;21:804–807.
37. Stahlmann R, Klug S, Lewandowski C, et al. Teratogenicity of acyclovir in rats. *Infection.* 1987;15:261–262.
38. Lau RJ, Emery MG, Galinsky RE, et al. Unexpected accumulation of acyclovir in breast milk with estimate of infant exposure. *Obstet Gynecol.* 1987;69(3):468–471.
39. Meyer LJ, deMiranda P, Sheth N, et al. Acyclovir in human breast milk. *Am J Obstet Gynecol.* 1988; 158(3):586–588.
40. Boelart J, Schurgers M, Daneels R, et al. Multiple dose pharmacokinetics of intravenous acyclovir in patients on continuous ambulatory peritoneal dialysis. *J Antimicrob Chemother.* 1987;20:69–76.
41. Shah GM, Winer RL, Krasny HC. Acyclovir pharmacokinetics in a patient on continuous ambulatory peritoneal dialysis. *Am J Kidney Dis.* 1986;7:507–510.

U.S. Patent No. 4199574. 647338

ZYLOPRIM ® ℞
[*zī'lō-prĭm*]
(Allopurinol)
100 mg Scored Tablets and
300 mg Scored Tablets

DESCRIPTION

Zyloprim (Allopurinol) is known chemically as 1,5-dihydro-4*H*-pyrazolo[3,4-*d*]pyrimidin-4-one. It is a xanthine oxidase inhibitor which is administered orally. Each scored white tablet contains 100 mg allopurinol and the inactive ingredients lactose, magnesium stearate, potato starch, and povidone. Each scored peach tablet contains 300 mg allopurinol and the inactive ingredients corn starch, FD&C Yellow No. 6 Lake, lactose, magnesium stearate, and povidone. Its solubility in water at 37°C is 80.0 mg/dl and is greater in an alkaline solution.

CLINICAL PHARMACOLOGY

Zyloprim (allopurinol) acts on purine catabolism, without disrupting the biosynthesis of purines. It reduces the production of uric acid by inhibiting the biochemical reactions immediately preceding its formation.

Zyloprim is a structural analogue of the natural purine base, hypoxanthine. It is an inhibitor of xanthine oxidase, the enzyme responsible for the conversion of hypoxanthine to xanthine and of xanthine to uric acid, the end product of purine metabolism in man. Zyloprim is metabolized to the corresponding xanthine analogue, oxipurinol (alloxanthine), which also is an inhibitor of xanthine oxidase.

It has been shown that reutilization of both hypoxanthine and xanthine for nucleotide and nucleic acid synthesis is markedly enhanced when their oxidations are inhibited by Zyloprim and oxipurinol. This reutilization does not disrupt normal nucleic acid anabolism, however, because feedback inhibition is an integral part of purine biosynthesis. As a result of xanthine oxidase inhibition, the serum concentration of hypoxanthine plus xanthine in patients receiving Zyloprim for treatment of hyperuricemia is usually in the range of 0.3 to 0.4 mg/dl compared to a normal level of approximately 0.15 mg/dl. A maximum of 0.9 mg/dl of these oxypurines has been reported when the serum urate was lowered to less than 2 mg/dl by high doses of Zyloprim. These values are far below the saturation levels at which point their precipitation would be expected to occur (above 7 mg/dl).

The renal clearance of hypoxanthine and xanthine is at least 10 times greater than that of uric acid. The increased xanthine and hypoxanthine in the urine have not been accompanied by problems of nephrolithiasis. Xanthine crystalluria has been reported in only three patients. Two of the patients had Lesch-Nyhan syndrome, which is characterized by excessive uric acid production combined with a deficiency of the enzyme, hypoxanthine-guanine phosphoribosyltransferase (HGPRTase). This enzyme is required for the conversion of hypoxanthine, xanthine, and guanine to their respective nucleotides. The third patient had lymphosarcoma and produced an extremely large amount of uric acid because of rapid cell lysis during chemotherapy.

Zyloprim is approximately 90% absorbed from the gastrointestinal tract. Peak plasma levels generally occur at 1.5 hours and 4.5 hours for Zyloprim and oxipurinol respectively, and after a single oral dose of 300 mg Zyloprim, maximum plasma levels of about 3 μg/ml of Zyloprim and 6.5 μg/ml of oxipurinol are produced.

Approximately 20% of the ingested Zyloprim is excreted in the feces. Because of its rapid oxidation to oxipurinol and a renal clearance rate approximately that of glomerular filtration rate, Zyloprim has a plasma half-life of about 1–2 hours. Oxipurinol, however, has a longer plasma half-life (approximately 15.0 hours) and therefore effective xanthine oxidase inhibition is maintained over a 24-hour period with single daily doses of Zyloprim. Whereas Zyloprim is cleared essentially by glomerular filtration, oxipurinol is reabsorbed in the kidney tubules in a manner similar to the reabsorption of uric acid.

The clearance of oxipurinol is increased by uricosuric drugs, and as a consequence, the addition of a uricosuric agent reduces to some degree the inhibition of xanthine oxidase by oxipurinol and increases to some degree the urinary excretion of uric acid. In practice, the net effect of such combined therapy may be useful in some patients in achieving minimum serum uric acid levels provided the total urinary uric acid load does not exceed the competence of the patient's renal function.

Hyperuricemia may be primary, as in gout, or secondary to diseases such as acute and chronic leukemia, polycythemia vera, multiple myeloma, and psoriasis. It may occur with the use of diuretic agents, during renal dialysis, in the presence of renal damage, during starvation or reducing diets and in the treatment of neoplastic disease where rapid resolution of tissue masses may occur. Asymptomatic hyperuricemia is not an indication for Zyloprim treatment (see INDICATIONS AND USAGE).

Gout is a metabolic disorder which is characterized by hyperuricemia and resultant deposition of monosodium urate in the tissues, particularly the joints and kidneys. The etiology of this hyperuricemia is the overproduction of uric acid in relation to the patient's ability to excrete it. If progressive deposition of urates is to be arrested or reversed, it is necessary to reduce the serum uric acid level below the saturation point to suppress urate precipitation.

Administration of Zyloprim generally results in a fall in both serum and urinary uric acid within two to three days. The degree of this decrease can be manipulated almost at will since it is dose-dependent. A week or more of treatment with Zyloprim may be required before its full effects are manifested; likewise, uric acid may return to pretreatment levels slowly (usually after a period of seven to ten days following cessation of therapy). This reflects primarily the accumulation and slow clearance of oxipurinol. In some patients a dramatic fall in urinary uric acid excretion may not occur, particularly in those with severe tophaceous gout. It has been postulated that this may be due to the mobilization of urate from tissue deposits as the serum uric acid level begins to fall.

Zyloprim's action differs from that of uricosuric agents, which lower the serum uric acid level by increasing urinary excretion of uric acid. Zyloprim reduces both the serum and urinary uric acid levels by inhibiting the formation of uric acid. The use of Zyloprim to block the formation of urates avoids the hazard of increased renal excretion of uric acid posed by uricosuric drugs.

Zyloprim can substantially reduce serum and urinary uric acid levels in previously refractory patients even in the presence of renal damage serious enough to render uricosuric drugs virtually ineffective. Salicylates may be given conjointly for their antirheumatic effect without compromising the action of Zyloprim. This is in contrast to the nullifying effect of salicylates on uricosuric drugs.

Zyloprim also inhibits the enzymatic oxidation of mercaptopurine, the sulfur-containing analogue of hypoxanthine, to 6-thiouric acid. This oxidation, which is catalyzed by xanthine oxidase, inactivates mercaptopurine. Hence, the inhibition of such oxidation by Zyloprim may result in as much as a 75% reduction in the therapeutic dose requirement of

Continued on next page

Burroughs Wellcome—Cont.

mercaptopurine when the two compounds are given together.

INDICATIONS AND USAGE

THIS IS NOT AN INNOCUOUS DRUG. IT IS NOT RECOMMENDED FOR THE TREATMENT OF ASYMPTOMATIC HYPERURICEMIA.

Zyloprim (allopurinol) reduces serum and urinary uric acid concentrations. Its use should be individualized for each patient and requires an understanding of its mode of action and pharmacokinetics (see CLINICAL PHARMACOLOGY, CONTRAINDICATIONS, WARNINGS and PRECAUTIONS).

Zyloprim is indicated in:

(1) the management of patients with signs and symptoms of primary or secondary gout (acute attacks, tophi, joint destruction, uric acid lithiasis and/or nephropathy).

(2) the management of patients with leukemia, lymphoma and malignancies who are receiving cancer therapy which causes elevations of serum and urinary uric acid levels. Zyloprim treatment should be discontinued when the potential for overproduction of uric acid is no longer present.

(3) the management of patients with recurrent calcium oxalate calculi whose daily uric acid excretion exceeds 800 mg/day in male patients and 750 mg/day in female patients. Therapy in such patients should be carefully assessed initially and reassessed periodically to determine in each case that treatment is beneficial and that the benefits outweigh the risks.

CONTRAINDICATIONS

Patients who have developed a severe reaction to Zyloprim (allopurinol) should not be restarted on the drug.

WARNINGS

ZYLOPRIM (ALLOPURINOL) SHOULD BE DISCONTINUED AT THE FIRST APPEARANCE OF SKIN RASH OR OTHER SIGNS WHICH MAY INDICATE AN ALLERGIC REACTION. In some instances a skin rash may be followed by more severe hypersensitivity reactions such as exfoliative, urticarial and purpuric lesions as well as Stevens-Johnson syndrome (erythema multiforme exudativum), and/or generalized vasculitis, irreversible hepatotoxicity and on rare occasions death.

In patients receiving Purinethol® (mercaptopurine) or Imuran® (azathioprine), the concomitant administration of 300–600 mg of Zyloprim per day will require a reduction in dose to approximately one-third to one-fourth of the usual dose of mercaptopurine or azathioprine. Subsequent adjustment of doses of mercaptopurine or azathioprine should be made on the basis of therapeutic response and the appearance of toxic effects (see CLINICAL PHARMACOLOGY).

A few cases of reversible clinical hepatotoxicity have been noted in patients taking Zyloprim, and in some patients asymptomatic rises in serum alkaline phosphatase or serum transaminase have been observed. If anorexia, weight loss or pruritus develop in patients on Zyloprim, evaluation of liver function should be part of their diagnostic workup. In patients with pre-existing liver disease, periodic liver function tests are recommended during the early stages of therapy.

Due to the occasional occurrence of drowsiness, patients should be alerted to the need for due precaution when engaging in activities where alertness is mandatory.

The occurrence of hypersensitivity reactions to Zyloprim may be increased in patients with decreased renal function receiving thiazides and Zyloprim concurrently. For this reason, in this clinical setting, such combinations should be administered with caution and patients should be observed closely.

PRECAUTIONS

General: An increase in acute attacks of gout has been reported during the early stages of Zyloprim (allopurinol) administration, even when normal or subnormal serum uric acid levels have been attained. Accordingly, maintenance doses of colchicine generally should be given prophylactically when Zyloprim is begun. In addition, it is recommended that the patient start with a low dose of Zyloprim (100 mg daily) and increase at weekly intervals by 100 mg until a serum uric acid level of 6 mg/dl or less is attained but without exceeding the maximum recommended dose (800 mg per day). The use of colchicine or anti-inflammatory agents may be required to suppress gouty attacks in some cases. The attacks usually become shorter and less severe after several months of therapy. The mobilization of urates from tissue deposits which cause fluctuations in the serum uric acid levels may be a possible explanation for these episodes. Even with adequate Zyloprim therapy, it may require several months to deplete the uric acid pool sufficiently to achieve control of the acute attacks.

A fluid intake sufficient to yield a daily urinary output of at least two liters and the maintenance of a neutral or, preferably, slightly alkaline urine are desirable to (1) avoid the theoretical possibility of formation of xanthine calculi under the influence of Zyloprim therapy and (2) help prevent renal precipitation of urates in patients receiving concomitant uricosuric agents.

Some patients with pre-existing renal disease or poor urate clearance have shown a rise in BUN during Zyloprim administration. Although the mechanism responsible for this has not been established, patients with impaired renal function should be carefully observed during the early stages of Zyloprim administration and dosage decreased or the drug withdrawn if increased abnormalities in renal function appear and persist.

Renal failure in association with Zyloprim administration has been observed among patients with hyperuricemia secondary to neoplastic diseases. Concurrent conditions such as multiple myeloma and congestive myocardial disease were present among those patients whose renal dysfunction increased after Zyloprim was begun. Renal failure is also frequently associated with gouty nephropathy and rarely with Zyloprim-associated hypersensitivity reactions. Albuminuria has been observed among patients who developed clinical gout following chronic glomerulonephritis and chronic pyelonephritis.

Patients with decreased renal function require lower doses of Zyloprim than those with normal renal function. Lower than recommended doses should be used to initiate therapy in any patients with decreased renal function and they should be observed closely during the early stages of Zyloprim administration. In patients with severely impaired renal function or decreased urate clearance, the half-life of oxipurinol in the plasma is greatly prolonged. Therefore, a dose of 100 mg per day or 300 mg twice a week, or perhaps less, may be sufficient to maintain adequate xanthine oxidase inhibition to reduce serum urate levels.

Bone marrow depression has been reported in patients receiving Zyloprim, most of whom received concomitant drugs with the potential for causing this reaction. This has occurred as early as six weeks to as long as six years after the initiation of Zyloprim therapy. Rarely a patient may develop varying degrees of bone marrow depression, affecting one or more cell lines, while receiving Zyloprim alone.

Information for Patients: Patients should be informed of the following:

(1) They should be cautioned to discontinue Zyloprim (allopurinol) and to consult their physician immediately at the first sign of a skin rash, painful urination, blood in the urine, irritation of the eyes, or swelling of the lips or mouth. (2) They should be reminded to continue drug therapy prescribed for gouty attacks since optimal benefit of Zyloprim may be delayed for two to six weeks. (3) They should be encouraged to increase fluid intake during therapy to prevent renal stones. (4) If a single dose of Zyloprim is occasionally forgotten, there is no need to double the dose at the next scheduled time. (5) There may be certain risks associated with the concomitant use of Zyloprim and dicumarol, sulfinpyrazone, mercaptopurine, azathioprine, ampicillin, amoxicillin and thiazide diuretics, and they should follow the instructions of their physician. (6) Due to the occasional occurrence of drowsiness, patients should take precautions when engaging in activities where alertness is mandatory. (7) Patients may wish to take Zyloprim after meals to minimize gastric irritation.

Laboratory Tests: The correct dosage and schedule for maintaining the serum uric acid within the normal range is best determined by using the serum uric acid as an index.

In patients with pre-existing liver disease, periodic liver function tests are recommended during the early stages of therapy (see WARNINGS).

Zyloprim (allopurinol) and its primary active metabolite oxipurinol are eliminated by the kidneys; therefore, changes in renal function have a profound effect on dosage. In patients with decreased renal function or who have concurrent illnesses which can affect renal function such as hypertension and diabetes mellitus, periodic laboratory parameters of renal function, particularly BUN and serum creatinine or creatinine clearance, should be performed and the patient's Zyloprim dosage reassessed.

The prothrombin time should be reassessed periodically in the patients receiving dicumarol who are given Zyloprim.

Drug Interactions: In patients receiving Purinethol® (mercaptopurine) or Imuran® (azathioprine), the concomitant administration of 300-600 mg of Zyloprim (allopurinol) per day will require a reduction in dose to approximately one-third to one-fourth of the usual dose of mercaptopurine or azathioprine. Subsequent adjustment of doses of mercaptopurine or azathioprine should be made on the basis of therapeutic response and the appearance of toxic effects (see CLINICAL PHARMACOLOGY).

It has been reported that Zyloprim prolongs the half-life of the anticoagulant, dicumarol. The clinical basis of this drug interaction has not been established but should be noted when Zyloprim is given to patients already on dicumarol therapy.

Since the excretion of oxipurinol is similar to that of urate, uricosuric agents, which increase the excretion of urate, are also likely to increase the excretion of oxipurinol and thus lower the degree of inhibition of xanthine oxidase. The concomitant administration of uricosuric agents and Zyloprim has been associated with a decrease in the excretion of oxypurines (hypoxanthine and xanthine) and an increase in urinary uric acid excretion compared with that observed with Zyloprim alone. Although clinical evidence to date has not demonstrated renal precipitation of oxypurines in patients either on Zyloprim alone or in combination with uricosuric agents, the possibility should be kept in mind.

The reports that the concomitant use of Zyloprim and thiazide diuretics may contribute to the enhancement of allopurinol toxicity in some patients have been reviewed in an attempt to establish a cause-and-effect relationship and a mechanism of causation. Review of these case reports indicates that the patients were mainly receiving thiazide diuretics for hypertension and that tests to rule out decreased renal function secondary to hypertensive nephropathy were not often performed. In those patients in whom renal insufficiency was documented, however, the recommendation to lower the dose of Zyloprim was not followed. Although a causal mechanism and a cause-and-effect relationship have not been established, current evidence suggests that renal function should be monitored in patients on thiazide diuretics and Zyloprim even in the absence of renal failure, and dosage levels should be even more conservatively adjusted in those patients on such combined therapy if diminished renal function is detected.

An increase in the frequency of skin rash has been reported among patients receiving ampicillin or amoxicillin concurrently with Zyloprim compared to patients who are not receiving both drugs. The cause of the reported association has not been established.

Enhanced bone marrow suppression by cyclophosphamide and other cytotoxic agents has been reported among patients with neoplastic disease, except leukemia, in the presence of Zyloprim.

However, in a well-controlled study of patients with lymphoma on combination therapy, Zyloprim did not increase the marrow toxicity of patients treated with cyclophosphamide, doxorubicin, bleomycin, procarbazine and/or mechlorethamine.

Tolbutamide's conversion to inactive metabolites has been shown to be catalyzed by xanthine oxidase from rat liver. The clinical significance, if any, of these observations is unknown.

Chlorpropamide's plasma half-life may be prolonged by Zyloprim, since Zyloprim and chlorpropamide may compete for excretion in the renal tubule. The risk of hypoglycemia secondary to this mechanism may be increased if Zyloprim and chlorpropamide are given concomitantly in the presence of renal insufficiency.

Drug/Laboratory Test Interactions: Zyloprim (allopurinol) is not known to alter the accuracy of laboratory tests.

Pregnancy: ***Teratogenic Effects:*** Pregnancy Category C. Reproductive studies have been performed in rats and rabbits at doses up to twenty times the usual human dose (5 mg/kg/day), and it was concluded that there was no impaired fertility or harm to the fetus due to Zyloprim (allopurinol). There is a published report of a study in pregnant mice given 50 or 100 mg/kg allopurinol intraperitoneally on gestation days 10 or 13. There were increased numbers of dead fetuses in dams given 100 mg/kg allopurinol but not in those given 50 mg/kg. There were increased numbers of external malformations in fetuses at both doses of allopurinol on gestation day 10 and increased numbers of skeletal malformations in fetuses at both doses on gestation day 13. It cannot be determined whether this represented a fetal effect or an effect secondary to maternal toxicity. There are, however, no adequate or well-controlled studies in pregnant women. Because animal reproduction studies are not always predictive of human response, this drug should be used during pregnancy only if clearly needed.

Experience with Zyloprim during human pregnancy has been limited partly because women of reproductive age rarely require treatment with Zyloprim. There are two unpublished reports and one published paper of women giving birth to normal offspring after receiving Zyloprim during pregnancy.

Nursing Mothers: Zyloprim (allopurinol) and oxipurinol have been found in the milk of a mother who was receiving Zyloprim. Since the effect of Zyloprim on the nursing infant is unknown, caution should be exercised when Zyloprim is administered to a nursing woman.

Pediatric Use: Zyloprim (allopurinol) is rarely indicated for use in children with the exception of those with hyperuricemia secondary to malignancy or to certain rare inborn errors of purine metabolism (see INDICATIONS and DOSAGE AND ADMINISTRATION).

ADVERSE REACTIONS

Data upon which the following estimates of incidence of adverse reactions are made are derived from experiences reported in the literature, unpublished clinical trials and voluntary reports since marketing of Zyloprim (allopurinol) began. Past experience suggested that the most frequent event following the initiation of allopurinol treatment was

an increase in acute attacks of gout (average 6% in early studies). An analysis of current usage suggests that the incidence of acute gouty attacks has diminished to less than 1%. The explanation for this decrease has not been determined but may be due in part to initiating therapy more gradually (see PRECAUTIONS and DOSAGE AND ADMINISTRATION).

The most frequent adverse reaction to Zyloprim is skin rash. Skin reactions can be severe and sometimes fatal. Therefore, treatment with Zyloprim should be discontinued immediately if a rash develops (see WARNINGS). Some patients with the most severe reaction also had fever, chills, arthralgias, cholestatic jaundice, eosinophilia and mild leukocytosis or leukopenia. Among 55 patients with gout treated with Zyloprim for 3 to 34 months (average greater than 1 year) and followed prospectively, Rundles observed that 3% of patients developed a type of drug reaction which was predominantly a pruritic maculopapular skin eruption, sometimes scaly or exfoliative. However, with current usage, skin reactions have been observed less frequently than 1%. The explanation for this decrease is not obvious. The incidence of skin rash may be increased in the presence of renal insufficiency. The frequency of skin rash among patients receiving ampicillin or amoxicillin concurrently with Zyloprim has been reported to be increased (see PRECAUTIONS).

Most Common Reactions*
Probably Causally Related

Gastrointestinal: diarrhea, nausea, alkaline phosphatase increase, SGOT/SGPT increase
Metabolic and Nutritional: acute attacks of gout
Skin and Appendages: rash, maculopapular rash

Incidence Less Than 1%
Probably Causally Related

Body as a whole: ecchymosis, fever, headache
Cardiovascular: necrotizing angiitis, vasculitis
Gastrointestinal: hepatic necrosis, granulomatous hepatitis, hepatomegaly, hyperbilirubinemia, cholestatic jaundice, vomiting, intermittent abdominal pain, gastritis, dyspepsia
Hemic and Lymphatic: thrombocytopenia, eosinophilia, leukocytosis, leukopenia
Musculoskeletal: myopathy, arthralgias
Nervous: peripheral neuropathy, neuritis, paresthesia, somnolence
Repiratory: epistaxis
Skin and Appendages: erythema multiforme exudativum (Stevens-Johnson syndrome), toxic epidermal necrolysis (Lyell's syndrome), hypersensitivity vasculitis, purpura, vesicular bullous dermatitis, exfoliative dermatitis, eczematoid dermatitis, pruritus, urticaria, alopecia, onycholysis, lichen planus
Special Senses: taste loss/perversion
Urogenital: renal failure, uremia (see PRECAUTIONS)

Incidence Less Than 1%
Causal Relationship Unknown

Body as a whole: malaise
Cardiovascular: pericarditis, peripheral vascular disease, thrombophlebitis, bradycardia, vasodilation
Endocrine: infertility (male), hypercalcemia, gynecomastia (male)
Gastrointestinal: hemorrhagic pancreatitis, gastrointestinal bleeding, stomatitis, salivary gland swelling, hyperlipidemia, tongue edema, anorexia
Hemic and Lymphatic: aplastic anemia, agranulocytosis, eosinophilic fibrohistiocytic lesion of bone marrow, pancytopenia, prothrombin decrease, anemia, hemolytic anemia, reticulocytosis, lymphadenopathy, lymphocytosis
Musculoskeletal: myalgia
Nervous: optic neuritis, confusion, dizziness, vertigo, foot drop, decrease in libido, depression, amnesia, tinnitus, asthenia, insomnia
Respiratory: bronchospasm, asthma, pharyngitis, rhinitis
Skin and Appendages: furunculosis, facial edema, sweating, skin edema
Special Senses: cataracts, macular retinitis, iritis, conjunctivitis, amblyopia
Urogenital: nephritis, impotence, primary hematuria, albuminuria

OVERDOSAGE

Massive overdosing or acute poisoning by Zyloprim (allopurinol) has not been reported.

In mice the 50% lethal dose (LD_{50}) is 160 mg/kg given intraperitoneally (i.p.) with deaths delayed up to five days and 700 mg/kg orally (p.o.) (approximately 140 times the usual human dose) with deaths delayed up to three days. In rats the acute LD_{50} is 750 mg/kg i.p. and 6000 mg/kg p.o. (approximately 1200 times the human dose).

In the management of overdosage there is no specific antidote for Zyloprim. There has been no clinical experience in the management of a patient who has taken massive amounts of Zyloprim.

Both Zyloprim and oxipurinol are dialyzable; however, the usefulness of hemodialysis or peritoneal dialysis in the management of a Zyloprim overdose is unknown.

*Early clinical studies and incidence rates from early clinical experience with Zyloprim suggested that these adverse reactions were found to occur at a rate of greater than 1%. The most frequent event observed was acute attacks of gout following the initiation of therapy. Analyses of current usage suggest that the incidence of these adverse reactions is now less than 1%. The explanation for this decrease has not been determined, but it may be due to following recommended usage (see ADVERSE REACTIONS introduction, INDICATIONS, PRECAUTIONS and DOSAGE AND ADMINISTRATION).

DOSAGE AND ADMINISTRATION

The dosage of Zyloprim (allopurinol) to accomplish full control of gout and to lower serum uric acid to normal or near-normal levels varies with the severity of the disease. The average is 200 to 300 mg per day for patients with mild gout and 400 to 600 mg per day for those with moderately severe tophaceous gout. The appropriate dosage may be administered in divided doses or as a single equivalent dose with the 300 mg tablet. Dosage requirements in excess of 300 mg should be administered in divided doses. The minimal effective dosage is 100 to 200 mg daily and the maximal recommended dosage is 800 mg daily. To reduce the possibility of flare-up of acute gouty attacks, it is recommended that the patient start with a low dose of Zyloprim (100 mg daily) and increase at weekly intervals by 100 mg until a serum uric acid level of 6 mg/dl or less is attained but without exceeding the maximal recommended dosage.

Normal serum urate levels are usually achieved in one to three weeks. The upper limit of normal is about 7 mg/dl for men and postmenopausal women and 6 mg/dl for premenopausal women. Too much reliance should not be placed on a single serum uric acid determination since, for technical reasons, estimation of uric acid may be difficult. By selecting the appropriate dosage and, in certain patients, using uricosuric agents concurrently, it is possible to reduce serum uric acid to normal or, if desired, to as low as 2 to 3 mg/dl and keep it there indefinitely.

While adjusting the dosage of Zyloprim in patients who are being treated with colchicine and/or anti-inflammatory agents, it is wise to continue the latter therapy until serum uric acid has been normalized and there has been freedom from acute gouty attacks for several months.

In transferring a patient from a uricosuric agent to Zyloprim, the dose of the uricosuric agent should be gradually reduced over a period of several weeks and the dose of Zyloprim gradually increased to the required dose needed to maintain a normal serum uric acid level.

It should also be noted that Zyloprim is generally better tolerated if taken following meals. A fluid intake sufficient to yield a daily urinary output of at least two liters and the maintenance of a neutral or, preferably, slightly alkaline urine are desirable.

Since Zyloprim and its metabolites are primarily eliminated only by the kidney, accumulation of the drug can occur in renal failure, and the dose of Zyloprim should consequently be reduced. With a creatinine clearance of 10 to 20 ml/min, a daily dosage of 200 mg of Zyloprim is suitable. When the creatinine clearance is less than 10 ml/min the daily dosage should not exceed 100 mg. With extreme renal impairment (creatinine clearance less than 3 ml/min) the interval between doses may also need to be lengthened.

The correct size and frequency of dosage for maintaining the serum uric acid just within the normal range is best determined by using the serum uric acid level as an index.

For the prevention of uric acid nephropathy during the vigorous therapy of neoplastic disease, treatment with 600 to 800 mg daily for two or three days is advisable together with a high fluid intake. Otherwise similar considerations to the above recommendations for treating patients with gout govern the regulation of dosage for maintenance purposes in secondary hyperuricemia.

The dose of Zyloprim recommended for management of recurrent calcium oxalate stones in hyperuricosuric patients is 200 to 300 mg/day in divided doses or as the single equivalent. This dose may be adjusted up or down depending upon the resultant control of the hyperuricosuria based upon subsequent 24 hour urinary urate determinations. Clinical experience suggests that patients with recurrent calcium oxalate stones may also benefit from dietary changes such as the reduction of animal protein, sodium, refined sugars, oxalate-rich foods, and excessive calcium intake as well as an increase in oral fluids and dietary fiber.

Children, 6 to 10 years of age, with secondary hyperuricemia associated with malignancies may be given 300 mg Zyloprim daily while those under 6 years are generally given 150 mg daily. The response is evaluated after approximately 48 hours of therapy and a dosage adjustment is made if necessary.

HOW SUPPLIED

100 mg (white) scored, flat cylindrical tablets imprinted with "ZYLOPRIM 100" on a raised hexagon.
Bottles of 90 (NDC 0081-0996-19). 100 (NDC 0081-0996-55) and 1000 (NDC 0081-0996-75).
Store at 15° to 25°C (59° to 77°F) in a dry place.
300 mg (peach) scored, flat, cylindrical tablets imprinted with "ZYLOPRIM 300" on a raised hexagon.
Bottles of 90 (NDC 0081-0998-19), 100 (NDC 0081-0998-55) and 500 (NDC 0081-0998-70) and Unit Dose Pack of 100 (NDC 0081-0998-56).
Store at 15° to 25°C (59° to 77°F) in a dry place and protect from light.

Shown in Product Identification Section, page 407

Calgon Vestal Laboratories
Division of Calgon Corporation
Subsidiary of MERCK & CO., INC.
ST. LOUIS, MISSOURI 63133

EPI-LOCK®
WOUND DRESSING

Recommended Technique for Wounds With Light Exudate

1.
Dressing changes and cleansing of the wound should always be carried out as quickly as possible. . . . Cleanse the wound, if necessary, with Shur-Clens® (20% poloxamer 188) preferably warmed to 37°C or SĀF-Clens™ chronic wound cleanser. After cleansing, rinse surrounding skin with warm isotonic saline solution.

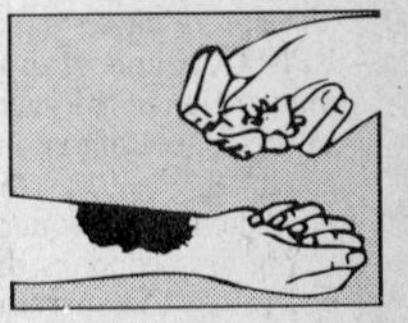

2.
Choose the proper size EPI-LOCK dressing, allowing at least 2 cm overlap at the wound edge. If necessary, cut EPI-LOCK to size. Several EPI-LOCK dressings may be overlapped if a large wound surface must be covered.

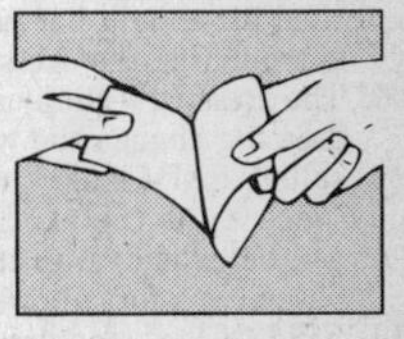

3.
Remove the paper from the back of the dressing and place the sterile surface in contact with the wound, overlapping the edges. A topical antimicrobial may be used under the EPI-LOCK dressing such as silver sulfadiazine cream.

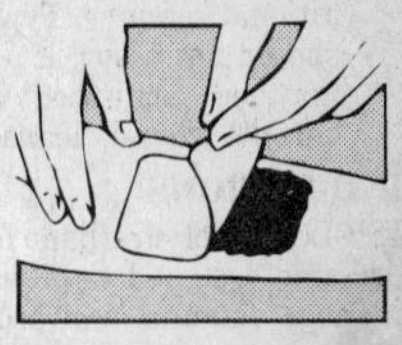

4.
Place the accompanying adhesive cover dressing over EPI-LOCK, allowing sufficient overlap to hold it securely in place. EPI-LOCK must conform closely to the wound surface; if necessary, utilize bulky bandaging to create gentle pressure.

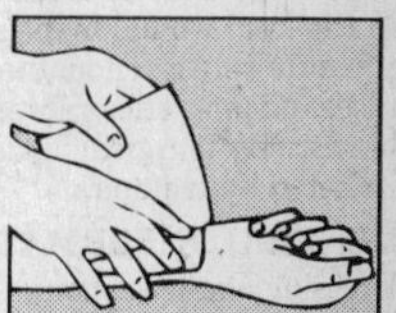

PLEASE NOTE: ABRASIONS, BURNS, AND LACERATIONS—At dressing change, the wound may have an unusual appearance. Instead of the usual dry eschar, a whitish or reddish exudate may cover the wound surface. This "liquid eschar" is normal, and is a collection of macrophages and new epithelial cells which should remain undisturbed while recovering the EPI-LOCK.

PRECAUTION: The reported incidence of infection when using "occlusive" dressings does not appear to be higher than with other conventional dressing techniques. If signs of infection should develop (strong odor, red streaking, strong pain, change in the color of the exudate, fever or tenderness in the area around the wound) use of EPI-LOCK should be discontinued and your physician contacted.

RECOMMENDED DRESSING TECHNIQUE FOR WOUNDS WITH MODERATE EXUDATE PRESSURE SORES & LEG ULCERS.

1. Lightly debride loose eschar and necrotic tissue as required, utilizing aseptic technique, prior to initial treatment with EPI-LOCK.
2. Choose the correct dressing size to allow at least 2 cm overlap at the wound edge in order to avoid leakage of exudate and loss of wound environment. The dressing should be trimmed to size before removal of the backing paper to insure the maintenance of sterility of the wound contact surface.
3. Cleanse the wound with warm isotonic (0.9%) saline solution, SĀF-Clens™ chronic wound cleanser, or with Shur-Clens® (20% poloxamer 188). Strong antiseptics such as surgical scrubs or solutions have been shown to cause tissue and blood cell damage, and should be avoided.

Continued on next page

Calgon Vestal Laboratories—Cont.

4. If inspection of the wound indicates that infection or colonization with pathogenic bacteria is present, proceed under standing orders of a physician. EPI-LOCK may be used in combination with a topical antibiotic for infected wounds.

5. Remove the paper from the back of the EPI-LOCK dressing and place the sterile dressing face in contact with the wound insuring at least 2 cm overlap at the wound edge. Avoid excessive overlap, as exudate may irritate healthy skin. Apply slight tension to eliminate air pockets and to provide intimate, wrinkle-free contact with the wound surface.

6. When wound exudate is expected to be minimal the EPI-LOCK dressing may be secured in place with the adhesive cover dressing supplied in each package (Adhesive Cover Dressing packaged with 4×4, 4×8, and 6×8 EPI-LOCK).

7. Where moderate amounts of exudate are anticipated, an absorptive gauze pad may be applied directly over the EPI-LOCK and wrapped with a stretch gauze bandage. If maceration of the surrounding skin becomes evident due to the degree of exudate, the following measures are advised:
   a. Make more frequent changes of the EPI-LOCK dressing or secondary dressing pad.
   b. Protect the surrounding skin with a barrier cream.
   c. Insure there is no more than 2 cm (¾ inch) overlap at the wound edge.

8. For optimum results, e.g., eliminating potential dehydration and minimizing or eliminating eschar formation, air should not penetrate the wound environment surrounding the dressing.

9. The dressing technique should be repeated as needed. At dressing change the wound may be washed with warm saline, SĀF-Clens™ chronic wound cleanser, or Shur-Clens.® As the exudate diminishes, dressing changes can be extended up to 7 days as wound condition and patient comfort allows.

10. EPI-LOCK wound dressings may be removed in the traditional manner. Typically, wound/dressing adherence should not occur. If adherence is encountered, removal may be facilitated with warm saline, SĀF-Clens™ chronic wound cleanser, or Shur-Clens.®

INDICATIONS

EPI-LOCK polyurethane foam dressing is an external wound dressing designed to provide a moist healing environment, manage exudate, and protect the wound from contamination.

EPI-LOCK is indicated as an external wound dressing for use in the local wound management of external wounds such as pressure sores, venous stasis ulcers, arterial ulcers, diabetic ulcers, donor sites, abrasions, lacerations and superficial burns, post surgical incisions and other external wounds inflicted by trauma.

GENERAL INFORMATION

Dressing changes should be carried out as quickly as possible.

Changing disturbs the wound environment and reduces the temperature at the wound site, resulting in a decrease in cell division and phagocytic activity which would lead to delayed healing.

During the course of treatment with EPI-LOCK the following may be observed and should be considered normal:

- At dressing change the wound may present an unpleasant odor and unusual appearance. A reddish-white or brown exudate may cover the wound surface.
- In the early state of treatment with EPI-LOCK, some ulcers may increase in size and serous exudate may increase due to active macrophage, increased enzymatic activity, and enzymatic liquefaction of necrotic or semi-necrotic tissues. This is part of the normal healing process encouraged by an environmental dressing and not a sign of wound deterioration.

All wounds can be expected to contain some microorganisms. However, if true clinical infection (fever, tenderness or redness in the area of the wound) should develop, appropriate steps as defined by the attending physician, should be taken to address that infection. Regular evaluation and cleansing of infected wounds should be practiced.

Some patients may experience discomfort, itching, erythema, or edema at the wound site for the first 24 hours of usage. This is due to the initiation of an inflammatory response.

As the healing progresses, the amount of exudate should diminish. EPI-LOCK can be left in place on the wound up to 7 days as wound condition and patient comfort allow.

Some wounds, such as leg ulcers and pressure sores, can be "non-healing" unless steps are taken to correct the underlying pathology. EPI-LOCK is designed for local wound management, and it can be part of the overall management program for these types of wounds.

EPI-LOCK is not indicated for wounds involving muscle, tendon or bone, nor for third degree burns.

INITIAL EXPECTATIONS OF EPI-LOCK IN WOUND HEALING*

CLINICAL OBSERVATION	EXPLANATION
—Increased wound exudate (wound may appear soupy, white/red, and foul odor)	—Active macrophage —Self debridement
—Discomfort, itching, erythema, edema (in some cases, usually decreases in 24 hours)	—Active macrophage —Increased/accelerated enzymatic activity
—Decreased exudate	—Healing matures

* Considered normal and customary when the proper moist wound healing environment is created.

CALGON VESTAL LABORATORIES
DIVISION OF CALGON CORPORATION
SUBSIDIARY OF MERCK & CO., Inc.
St. Louis, Missouri 63133
1-800-325-8005
EPI-LOCK® is a registered trademark of Derma-LOCK Medical Corporation

---

KALTOSTAT®
WOUND DRESSING
Calcium-Sodium Alginate Fiber

INSTRUCTIONS FOR USE

INTRODUCTION

The following notes are designed to help you and your patient take maximum advantage of the natural and beneficial wound healing properties of KALTOSTAT.

KALTOSTAT is a sterile, soft, white conformable material which is composed entirely of alginate fiber and is manufactured in the UK from a selected species of brown seaweed. It is totally different to traditional inert gauze products which tend to dry out and adhere to the wound surface causing damage on removal.

Research has shown that wounds respond best when maintained under moist conditions. This widely accepted fact led to the development of KALTOSTAT, a dressing which creates and maintains a moist wound environment.

KALTOSTAT is highly absorbent, and due to a process of ion exchange gradually forms a moist gel on contact with wound exudate.

In addition to its value in the treatment of exuding wounds it is also a natural haemostat and can be used in a wide variety of minor bleeding wounds.

HOW KALTOSTAT WORKS

The medicinal properties of raw seaweed have been known for centuries. KALTOSTAT has been developed using a sophisticated high technology process to enable the full healing potential of alginate to be realised.

Moist Wound Healing—Ion Exchange

When KALTOSTAT is placed directly onto a wound, e.g. a leg ulcer or pressure sore, the alginate fiber absorbs exudate. The calcium ions in the fiber react (through a process of ion exchange) with the sodium ions in the exudate, and the fibers gradually convert into a strong viscous gel which coats the wound surface. This creates a moist wound interface which provides the best possible environment for effective healing.

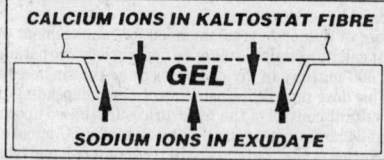

CALCIUM IONS IN KALTOSTAT FIBRE
↓ *GEL* ↓
↑ *SODIUM IONS IN EXUDATE* ↑

HAEMOSTASIS

The calcium ions released during ion exchange also aid the clotting process, and with the fiber matrix of the dressing brings about rapid staunching of bleeding.

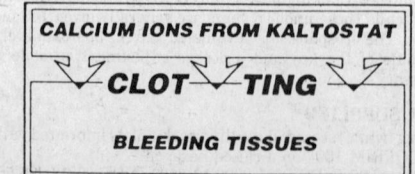

CALCIUM IONS FROM KALTOSTAT
CLOT TING
BLEEDING TISSUES

INDICATIONS

KALTOSTAT is approved for the management of exuding wounds with moderate to heavy exudate, e.g.

- Leg ulcers
- Pressure sores
- Fungating carcinomas

Being a natural haemostat KALTOSTAT is indicated in the management of minor bleeding wounds such as:

- Cuts
- Lacerations
- Grazes

It is not indicated for dry wounds or wounds with a greatly diminished output of exudate.

BENEFITS

● **High Absorbency—fewer dressing changes**
KALTOSTAT is extremely absorbent, 3.5 times more so than cotton gauze, and has the capacity to absorb on average 15 times its own weight of exudate. This results in less frequent dressing changes, allowing the wound to remain undisturbed for longer periods than under traditional products, thus increasing patient comfort and saving nursing time.

● **Tissue friendly**
KALTOSTAT is made entirely of natural calcium sodium alginate fiber. Any fibers remaining at the wound site at dressing changes need not be removed since they will simply disperse in the exudate.

● **Easy to apply and remove**
KALTOSTAT is simple to apply (see following instructions for use) and maintains its integrity on contact with exudate. It can easily be removed with forceps or gloved fingers.

APPLICATION/REMOVAL

KALTOSTAT may be applied to any moderate to heavily exuding wound.

1. Assess the wound. Remove any debris or slough. Cleanse the wound and surrounding skin by flushing with sterile normal saline, if appropriate. Dry the surrounding skin but leave the wound surface wet.

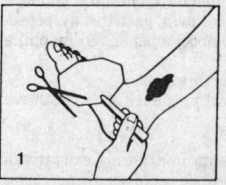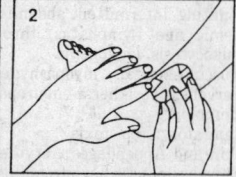

2. Cut or fold KALTOSTAT to the shape of the wound and apply. For wounds with a diminishing amount of exudate, moisten the dressing before application to help initiate gel formation. This is easily achieved by pouring sterile normal saline into the opened packet.

3. Apply a suitable secondary dressing to conserve moisture, and secure KALTOSTAT, e.g. layers of cotton gauze secured with a soft conforming bandage. For a very heavily exuding wound extra padding may be required. For wounds with diminishing exudate where the surrounding skin is healthy and intact, cover with a semi-permeable film dressing to prevent desiccation.

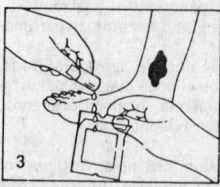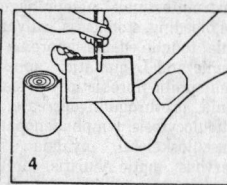

4. Initially, KALTOSTAT should be inspected daily without disturbing its relationship to the wound. Change KALTOSTAT only when maximum absorbency is reached (i.e. dressing is fully saturated with exudate) or when "strikethrough" of the secondary dressing is evident. Daily dressing changes may be necessary initially but reduce quickly to twice weekly as granulation tissue forms and exudate diminishes. Do not leave KALTOSTAT on longer than 7 days without changing.

If on inspection the dressing is moist but with a significant amount of unchanged fiber present, the interval between dressing changes may need to be increased. If the dressing appears to have formed a gel and then dried out, a more occlusive secondary dressing is required (e.g. semi-permeable adhesive film dressing). It may be necessary to re-moisten KALTOSTAT with sterile normal saline to ensure that the fiber directly in contact with the wound remains moist. **Advise the patient to avoid sitting too close to a direct heat source as this may cause KALTOSTAT to dry out.**

5. Simply remove KALTOSTAT with forceps or gloved fingers. Any stray fibers need not be removed as they will simply disperse in the exudate. A saline flush will aid removal if required. With continuous use of KALTOSTAT, a crust of alginate, dried exudate and skin scales may form around the edge of the wound. This should be removed using a saline soaked swab to aid softening.

6. When the wound is almost healed, with exudate diminished and epithelialisation occurring, it is time to discontinue KALTOSTAT and change to a dressing suitable for a low exuding wound.

NOTE: In the first few days of using KALTOSTAT it may appear that the wound has increased slightly in size. This is a normal occurrence and is caused by the removal of dead tissue around the edges of the wound.

DEEPER EXUDING CAVITIES, PRESSURE SORES

The KALTOSTAT 2g Cavity Dressing is specifically designed for the management of deeper exuding wounds. The full extent of the wound must be determined prior to application either visually or using a probe. Layer or coil fiber loosely in the wound up to the level of the surrounding skin. This will allow the alginate fiber to gel and expand to the size of the cavity. Apply a suitable secondary dressing (as before). For removal of KALTOSTAT from deeper cavities, a saline flush is recommended.

MINOR BLEEDING WOUNDS

For cuts and grazes, apply KALTOSTAT to the bleeding area to effect haemostasis. Remove once bleeding has ceased, and if appropriate, apply a fresh piece of KALTOSTAT covered by a suitable secondary dressing.

Infected Wounds

KALTOSTAT may be used to dress infected wounds but should be changed daily until infection is controlled. Concurrent systemic antimicrobial therapy may be given if indicated.

To apply, cleanse the wound as required, adding a final saline flush, then apply dressing as before.

NOTE: In general, creams, lotions, or powders should **not** be used with KALTOSTAT as they can act as a barrier between KALTOSTAT and wound exudate and may interfere with gel formation.

CALGON VESTAL LABORATORIES
DIVISION OF CALGON CORPORATION
SUBSIDIARY OF MERCK & CO., INC.
St. Louis, Missouri 63133
1-800-325-8005
Manufactured in the United Kingdom
by CV Laboratories Limited.

MITRAFLEX®
WOUND DRESSING

INSTRUCTIONS FOR USE

DESCRIPTION

MITRAFLEX® is a sterile, semi-occlusive, absorptive environmental dressing.

MITRAFLEX combines the moist wound environment properties of film dressings with the absorptive qualities of traditional therapies in a structure which is both adhesive and conformable.

MITRAFLEX dressings are constructed of three layers, each specifically engineered to give MITRAFLEX its unique blend of "easy to use" features while providing a microenvironment conducive to moist wound healing.

The wound contact surface of MITRAFLEX is a porous, nontoxic adhesive which facilitates ease of application to the wound site. A second layer consisting of a microporous polyurethane membrane absorbs and acts as a reservoir for wound exudate. The flexible outer layer is moisture vapor permeable which facilitates the reduction of exudate while maintaining a moist environment to promote optimal wound repair. The outer layer is impermeable to microorganisms and liquids.

INDICATIONS FOR USE

MITRAFLEX Wound Dressings are intended for use in the management of:
Venous stasis ulcers
Diabetic ulcers
Pressure sores
Donor sites
Partial-thickness wounds
Superficial burns
Abrasions and lacerations

CONTRAINDICATIONS

MITRAFLEX Wound Dressings should *not* be used on wounds involving exposed muscle, tendon or bone; lesions in patients with active vasculitis; patients with deep systemic infections; patients with arterial ischemic lesions.

Wounds treated with MITRAFLEX Wound Dressings should be examined at least every five to seven days (every two to three days for highly exudating wounds) for clinical signs of infection or unusual patient discomfort. The dressing should be changed if leakage of exudate occurs.

MITRAFLEX Wound Dressings absorb exudate which may cause the dressing to discolor in routine clinical use. The discoloration is not indicative of infection. Dressings displaying discoloration should be left in place unless accompanied by clinical signs of infection, unusual patient discomfort, or leakage.

Dressing Application:

1. Prior to application, thoroughly rinse or irrigate the wound with an appropriate cleansing solution. Gently dry the skin surrounding the wound to allow secure application of the dressing.
2. To ensure proper adherence to healthy skin, the dressing should extend at least one inch beyond the wound edge. The dressing may be overlapped or cut to accommodate the wound size. Size dressing to insure that the release paper split may still be utilized.
3. Fold dressing along split in release paper. Remove the release paper using minimal finger contact with the sterile dressing surface. Center the dressing over the wound and gently press it to the skin to smooth out any wrinkles.

Dressing Removal:

1. To remove the dressing, carefully lift an edge of the dressing while gently pressing against the skin. Continue pulling the dressing carefully from the skin.
2. Cleanse wound site prior to applying a new dressing.

Ordering Information:

Each MITRAFLEX Wound Dressing is supplied STERILE and individually packaged.

	Size	Contents	Reorder No.
MITRAFLEX			
Wound Dressing	2″ ×2″	10 per Box	1685-F5
MITRAFLEX			
Wound Dressing	4″ ×4″	5 per Box	1685-FA
MITRAFLEX			
Wound Dressing	4″ ×8″	5 per Box	1685-FD
MITRAFLEX			
Wound Dressing	8″ ×8″	5 per Box	1685-FB

DISTRIBUTED BY:
CALGON VESTAL LABORATORIES
DIVISION OF CALGON CORPORATION
SUBSIDIARY OF MERCK & CO., INC.
ST. LOUIS, MO 63133
1-800-325-8005
MITRAFLEX ® is a Registered trademark of PolyMedica Industries, Inc.

Campbell Laboratories Inc.
300 EAST 51st STREET
P.O. BOX 812, F.D.R. STATION
NEW YORK, NY 10150-0812

HERPECIN-L® Cold Sore Lip Balm Stick   OTC
[her "puh-sin-el"]

PRODUCT OVERVIEW

KEY FACTS

HERPECIN-L Lip Balm is a convenient, easy-to-use treatment for perioral *herpes simplex* infections with SPF 15.

MAJOR USES

HERPECIN-L not only treats cold sores, sun and fever blisters, but with prophylactic use, its sunscreens also protect to help prevent them. Users report early use at the *prodromal* stages of an attack will often abort the lesions and prevent scabbing. Prescribe: Apply "early and often".

SAFETY INFORMATION

For topical use only. A rare sensitivity may occur.

PRESCRIBING INFORMATION

HERPECIN-L® Cold Sore Lip Balm   OTC

COMPOSITION

A soothing, emollient, lip balm incorporating allantoin, the sunscreen, octyl-dimethyl-PABA (Padimate O), in a balanced, slightly acidic lipid base that includes petrolatum and titanium dioxide at a cosmetically acceptable level. (Has no caines, antibiotics, phenol or camphor.) (NDC 38083-777-31)

ACTIONS AND USES

HERPECIN-L relieves dryness and chapping by providing a lipid barrier to help restore normal moisture balance to the lips. Skin protectants help to soften the crusts and scabs of "cold sores". The sunscreen is effective in 2900-3200 AU range while titanium dioxide, though at low levels, helps to block, reflect the sun's rays and prevent sun-induced *herpes labialis*. Used as directed, SPF is over 15.

ADMINISTRATION

(1) Recurrent "*cold sores, sun and fever blisters*": Simply put, use **soon** and **often**. Frequent sufferers report that with *prophylactic* use (BID/PRN), attacks are fewer and less severe. Most recurrent *herpes labialis* patients are aware of the prodromal symptoms: tingling, itching, burning. At this stage, or if the lesion has already developed, HERPECIN-L should be applied liberally every hour, or as often as is convenient.

(2) *Outdoor protection:* Apply before and during sun exposure, after swimming and again at bedtime (h.s.). (3) *Dry, chapped lips:* Apply as needed.

ADVERSE REACTIONS

If sensitive to any of the ingredients, discontinue use.

CONTRAINDICATIONS

None.

HOW SUPPLIED

2.8 gm. swivel tubes.

SAMPLES AVAILABLE

Yes. (Please request on professional letterhead or Rx pad.)

J.R. Carlson Laboratories, Inc.
15 COLLEGE DR.
ARLINGTON HEIGHTS, IL 60004-1985

ACES®   OTC

DESCRIPTION

Each soft gel contains the antioxidants:

Beta-Carotene (pro-vitamin A)	5,000 IU
Vitamin C (calcium ascorbate)	500 mg
Vitamin E (d-alpha tocopherol)	200 IU
Selenium (L-selenomethionine)	50 mcg

ACES® provides the four major antioxidant nutrients in a convenient supplement form. The nutrient sources in ACES® are chosen with care. Beta-carotene is derived from algae. Calcium ascorbate is a form of vitamin C which is gentle to the stomach. Vitamin E is 100% natural-source from soy, the most biologically active form. Selenium is organically bound with an essential nutrient (methionine) to promote assimilation.

HOW SUPPLIED

In bottles of 50, 100, 200, and 360.
Also available as *ACES ® plus ZINC*.

BETA-CAROTENE SUPER D. SALINA   OTC

DESCRIPTION

Of the carotenoids found in plants, beta-carotene is the most biologically active. It is converted to vitamin A according to the body's need. As it does not accumulate in the liver, it is a safe, effective source of vitamin A.

Carlson *Super Beta-Carotene* is extracted from plant algae (*Dunaliella salina*), which produce 10,000 times more beta-carotene than carrot cells. Each soft gel contains 15 mg of beta-carotene, providing 25,000 IU vitamin A activity (500% US RDA).

HOW SUPPLIED

In bottles of 100 and 250.

E-GEMS®   OTC

DESCRIPTION

100% natural-source vitamin E (d-alpha tocopheryl acetate) soft gels. Available in 8 strengths: 30 IU, 100 IU, 200 IU, 400 IU, 600 IU, 800 IU, 1000 IU, 1200 IU.

HOW SUPPLIED

Supplied in a variety of bottle sizes.

KEY-E®   OTC

DESCRIPTION

Dry, 100% natural-source vitamin E (d-alpha tocopheryl succinate). Available in pleasant tasting, chewable tablets (100 IU, 200 IU, 400 IU) or gelatin capsules (200 IU, 400 IU).

HOW SUPPLIED

In bottles of 100, 250, and 500.

LIQUID CAL-600   OTC

DESCRIPTION

Each soft gelatin capsule provides 600 mg calcium from calcium carbonate.

HOW SUPPLIED

In bottles of 100 and 250.

Continued on next page

J.R. Carlson Laboratories—Cont.

NIACIN-TIME® OTC

DESCRIPTION

Niacin taken in a single 500 mg dose often causes flushing or itching. *Niacin-Time* ® is prepared by a patented process which minimizes these unpleasant side effects, often resulting in no flush. Each tablet provides a gradual release of 500 mg of Niacin over a period of 5–7 hours.

HOW SUPPLIED

In bottles of 100, 250, and 500.

SUPER OMEGA-3 FATTY ACIDS OTC

DESCRIPTION

Maximum potency Omega-3 fatty acids from deep, cold water fish. Each 1000 mg soft gel provides 330 mg EPA and 220 mg DHA.

HOW SUPPLIED

In bottles of 50, 100, and 200.

Carnrick Laboratories, Inc.
65 HORSE HILL ROAD
CEDAR KNOLLS, NJ 07927

AMEN® ℞
[*ā 'men '*]
(medroxyprogesterone acetate tablet USP 10 mg)

CAUTION

Federal Law Prohibits Dispensing Without Prescription

WARNING

THE USE OF AMEN® DURING THE FIRST 4 MONTHS OF PREGNANCY IS NOT RECOMMENDED.

Progestational agents have been used beginning with the first trimester of pregnancy in an attempt to prevent habitual abortion. There is no adequate evidence that such use is effective when such drugs are given during the first 4 months of pregnancy. Furthermore, in the vast majority of women, the cause of abortion is a defective ovum, which progestational agents could not be expected to influence. In addition, the use of progestational agents, with their uterine-relaxant properties, in patients with fertilized defective ova may cause a delay in spontaneous abortion. Therefore, the use of such drugs during the first 4 months of pregnancy is not recommended.

Several reports suggest an association between intrauterine exposure to progestational drugs in the first trimester of pregnancy and genital abnormalities in male and female fetuses. The risk of hypospadias, 5 to 8 per 1,000 male births in the general population, may be approximately doubled with exposure to these drugs. There are insufficient data to quantify the risk to exposed female fetuses, but insofar as some of these drugs induce mild virilization of the external genitalia of the female fetus, and because of the increased association of hypospadias in the male fetus, it is prudent to avoid the use of these drugs during the first trimester of pregnancy.

If the patient is exposed to Amen® during the first 4 months of pregnancy or if she becomes pregnant while taking this drug, she should be apprised of the potential risks to the fetus.

DESCRIPTION

Amen® tablets contain medroxyprogesterone acetate, a derivative of progesterone. It is a white to off-white, odorless crystalline powder, stable in air, melting between 200° and 210°C. It is freely soluble in chloroform, soluble in acetone and in dioxane, sparingly soluble in alcohol and in methanol, slightly soluble in ether, and insoluble in water.

The chemical name for medroxyprogesterone acetate is pregn-4-ene-3,20-dione, 17-(acetyloxy)-6-methyl-, (6α)-. The structural formula is:

[See chemical structure at top of next column.]

Amen tablets contain FD&C Yellow No. 6 as a color additive.

CLINICAL PHARMACOLOGY

Amen® (medroxyprogesterone acetate tablets), administered orally in the recommended dose to women with adequate endogenous estrogen, transforms proliferative endo-

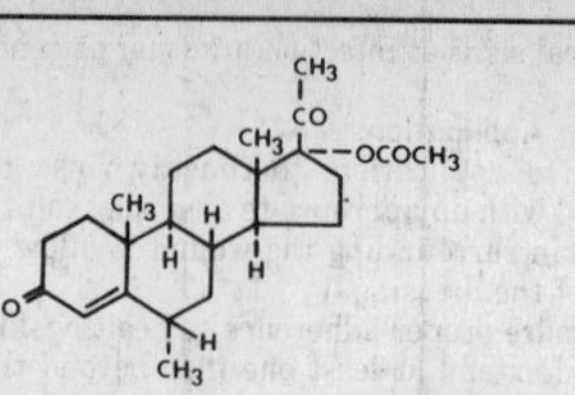

metrium into secretory endometrium. Androgenic and anabolic effects have been noted, but the drug is apparently devoid of significant estrogenic activity. While parenterally administered medroxyprogesterone acetate inhibits gonadotropin production, which in turn prevents follicular maturation and ovulation, available data indicate that this does not occur when the usually recommended oral dosage is given as single daily doses.

INDICATIONS AND USAGE

Amen® (medroxyprogesterone acetate tablets) is indicated in secondary amenorrhea and abnormal uterine bleeding due to hormonal imbalance in the absence of organic pathology, such as fibroids or uterine cancer.

CONTRAINDICATIONS

1. Thrombophlebitis, thromboembolic disorders, cerebral apoplexy or patients with a past history of these conditions. **2.** Liver dysfunction or disease. **3.** Known or suspected malignancy of breast or genital organs. **4.** Undiagnosed vaginal bleeding. **5.** Missed abortion. **6.** As a diagnostic test for pregnancy. **7.** Known sensitivity to Amen (medroxyprogesterone acetate tablets).

WARNINGS

1. The physician should be alert to the earliest manifestations of thrombotic disorders (thrombophlebitis, cerebrovascular disorders, pulmonary embolism, and retinal thrombosis). Should any of these occur or be suspected, the drug should be discontinued immediately.

2. Beagle dogs treated with medroxyprogesterone acetate developed mammary nodules, some of which were malignant. Although nodules occasionally appeared in control animals, they were intermittent in nature, whereas the nodules in the drug treated animals were larger, more numerous, persistent, and there were some breast malignancies with metastases. Their significance with respect to humans has not been established.

3. Discontinue medication pending examination if there is sudden partial or complete loss of vision, or if there is a sudden onset of proptosis, diplopia or migraine. If examination reveals papilledema, or retinal vascular lesions, medication should be withdrawn.

4. Detectable amounts of progestin have been identified in the milk of mothers receiving the drug. The effect of this on the nursing infant has not been determined.

5. Usage in pregnancy is not recommended (See WARNING Box).

6. Retrospective studies of morbidity and mortality in Great Britain and studies of morbidity in the United States have shown a statistically significant association between thrombophlebitis, pulmonary embolism, and cerebral thrombosis and embolism and the use of oral contraceptives.[6–9] The estimate of the relative risk of thromboembolism in the study by Vessey and Doll[8] was about sevenfold, while Sartwell and associates[9] in the United States found a relative risk of 4.4 meaning that the users are several times as likely to undergo thromboembolic disease without evident cause as nonusers. The American study also indicated that the risk did not persist after discontinuation of administration, and that it was not enhanced by long continued administration. The American study was not designed to evaluate a difference between products.

PRECAUTIONS

1. The pretreatment physical examination should include special reference to breasts and pelvic organs, as well as Papanicolaou smear.

2. Because progestogens may cause some degree of fluid retention, conditions which might be influenced by this factor, such as epilepsy, migraine, asthma, cardiac or renal dysfunction require careful observation.

3. In cases of breakthrough bleeding, as in all cases of irregular bleeding per vaginum, nonfunctional causes should be borne in mind. In cases of undiagnosed vaginal bleeding adequate diagnostic measures are indicated.

4. Patients who have a history of psychic depression should be carefully observed and the drug discontinued if the depression recurs to a serious degree.

5. Any possible influence of prolonged progestin therapy on pituitary, ovarian, adrenal, hepatic or uterine functions awaits further study.

6. A decrease in glucose tolerance has been observed in a small percentage of patients on estrogen-progestin combination drugs. The mechanism of this decrease is obscure. For this reason, diabetic patients should be carefully observed while receiving progestin therapy.

7. The age of the patient constitutes no absolute limiting factor although treatment with progestins may mask the onset of the climacteric.

8. The pathologist should be advised of progestin therapy when relevant specimens are submitted.

9. Because of the occasional occurence of thrombotic disorders, (thrombophlebitis, pulmonary embolism, retinal thrombosis, and cerebrovascular disorders) in patients taking estrogen-progestin combinations and since the mechanism is obscure, the physician should be alert to the earliest manifestation of these disorders.

10. Studies of the addition of a progestin product to an estrogen replacement regimen for seven or more days of a cycle of estrogen administration have reported a lowered incidence of endomentrial hyperplasia. Morphological and biochemical studies of endometrium suggest that 10–13 days of a progestin are needed to provide maximal maturation of the endometrium and to eliminate any hyperplastic changes. Whether this will provide protection from endometrial carcinoma has not been clearly established. There are possible additional risks which may be associated with the inclusion of progestin in estrogen replacement regimens. The potential risks include adverse effects on carbohydrate and lipid metabolism. The dosage used may be important in minimizing these adverse effects.

Information for the Patient

See Patient Information at end of insert.

ADVERSE REACTIONS

Pregnancy—(See WARNING Box for possible adverse effects on the fetus).

Breast—Breast tenderness or galactorrhea has been reported rarely.

Skin—Sensitivity reactions consisting of urticaria, pruritus, edema and generalized rash have occured in an occasional patient. Acne, alopecia and hirsutism have been reported in a few cases.

Thromboembolic Phenomena—Thromboembolic phenomena including thrombophlebitis and pulmonary embolism have been reported.

The following adverse reactions have been observed in women taking progestins including medroxyprogesterone acetate tablets: breakthrough bleeding; spotting; change in menstrual flow; amenorrhea; edema; change in weight (increase or decrease); changes in cervical erosion and cervical secretions; cholestatic jaundice; anaphylactoid reactions and anaphylaxis; rash (allergic) with and without pruritus; mental depression; pyrexia; insomnia; nausea; somnolence.

A statistically significant association has been demonstrated between use of estrogen-progestin combination drugs and the following serious adverse reactions: thrombophlebitis, pulmonary embolism and cerebral thrombosis and embolism. For this reason patients on progestin therapy should be carefully observed.

Although available evidence is suggestive of an association, such a relationship has been neither confirmed nor refuted for the following serious adverse reactions: neuro-ocular lesions, eg. retinal thrombosis and optic neuritis.

The following adverse reactions have been observed in patients receiving estrogen-progestin combination drugs: rise in blood pressure in susceptible individuals; premenstrual-like syndrome; changes in libido; changes in appetite; cystitis-like syndrome; headache; nervousness; dizziness; fatigue; backache; hirsutism; loss of scalp hair; erythema multiforme; erythema nodosum; hemorrhagic eruption; itching.

In view of these observations, patients on progestin therapy should be carefully observed.

The following laboratory results may be altered by the use of estrogen-progestin combination drugs:

Increased sulfobromophthalein retention and other hepatic function tests.

Coagulation tests: increase in prothrombin factors VII, VIII, IX and X.

Metyrapone test.

Pregnanediol determination.

Thyroid function: increase in PBI, and butanol extractable protein bound iodine and decrease in T^3 uptake values.

DOSAGE AND ADMINISTRATION

Secondary Amenorrhea—Amen® (medroxyprogesterone acetate tablets) may be given in dosages of 5 to 10 mg daily for from 5 to 10 days. A dose for inducing an optimum secretory transformation of an endometrium that has been adequately primed with either endogenous or exogenous estrogen is 10 mg of medroxyprogesterone acetate daily for 10 days. In cases of seconary amenorrhea, therapy may be started at any time. Progestin withdrawal bleeding usually occurs within three to seven days after discontinuing therapy with Amen.®

Abnormal Uterine Bleeding Due to Hormonal Imbalance in the Absence of Organic Pathology—Beginning on the calculated 16th or 21st day of the menstrual cycle, 5 to 10 mg of medroxyprogesterone acetate may be given daily for from 5 to 10 days. To produce an optimum secretory transformation of an endometrium that has been adequately primed with either endogenous or exogenous estrogen, 10 mg of Amen®

tablets daily for 10 days beginning on the 16th day of the cycle is suggested. Progestin withdrawal bleeding usually occurs within three to seven days after discontinuing therapy with Amen®. Patients with a past history of recurrent episodes of abnormal uterine bleeding may benefit from planned menstrual cycling with Amen®.

HOW SUPPLIED

Two-layered peach and white scored tablet with "C" on one side and "AMEN" on the other. Amen® tablets containing 10 mg of medroxyprogesterone acetate USP are available in bottles of 50 (NDC 0086-0049-05), 100 (NDC 0086-0049-10) and 1000 (NDC 0086-0049-90).

REFERENCES

1. Gal I, Kirman B, Stern J: Hormonal pregnancy tests and congenital malformation. Nature *216* :83, 1967.
2. Levy EP, Cohen A, Fraser FC: Hormone treatment during pregnancy and congenital heart defects. Lancet *1* :611, 1973.
3. Nora JJ, Nora AH: Birth defects and oral contraceptives. Lancet *1* :941–942, 1973.
4. Janerich DT, Piper JM, Glebatis DM: Oral contraceptives and congenital limb-reduction defects. N Engl J Med *291* :697-700, 1974.
5. Heinonen OP, Slone D, Monson RR, et al: Cardiovascular birth defects and antenatal exposure to female sex hormones. N Engl J Med *296* :67–70, 1977.
6. Royal College of General Practitioners: Oral contraception and thromboembolic disease. J Coll Gen Pract *13* :267–279, 1967.
7. Inman WHW, Vessey MP: Investigation of deaths from pulmonary, coronary, and cerebral thrombosis and embolism in women of child-bearing age. Br Med J *2* :193–199, 1968.
8. Vessey MP, Doll R: Investigation of relation between use of oral contraceptives and thromboembolic disease. A further report. Br Med J *2* :651–657, 1969.
9. Sartwell PE, Masi AT, Arthes FG, et al: Thromboembolism and oral contraceptives: An epidemiological case-control study. Am J Epidemiol *90* :365–380, 1969.

The text of the patient insert for progesterone and progesterone-like drugs is set forth below.

PATIENT INFORMATION: AMEN Tablets contain medroxyprogesterone acetate, a progesterone. The information below is that which the U.S. Food and Drug Administration requires be provided for all patients taking progesterones. The information below relates only to the risk to the unborn child associated with use of progesterone during pregnancy. For further information on the use, side effects and other risks associated with this product, ask your doctor.

WARNING FOR WOMEN

Progesterone or progesterone-like drugs have been used to prevent miscarriage in the first few months of pregnancy. No adequate evidence is available to show that they are effective for this purpose. Furthermore, most cases of early miscarriage are due to causes which could not be helped by these drugs.

There is an increased risk of minor birth defects in children whose mothers take this drug during the first 4 months of pregnancy. Several reports suggest an association between mothers who take these drugs in the first trimester of pregnancy and genital abnormalities in male and female babies. The risk to the male baby is the possibility of being born with a condition in which the opening of the penis is on the underside rather than the tip of the penis (hypospadias). Hypospadias occurs in about 5 to 8 per 1,000 male births and is about doubled with exposure to these drugs. There is not enough information to quantify the risk to exposed female fetuses, but enlargement of the clitoris and fusion of the labia may occur, although rarely.

Therefore, since drugs of this type may induce mild masculinization of the external genitalia of the female fetus, as well as hypospadias in the male fetus, it is wise to avoid using the drug during the first trimester of pregnancy.

These drugs have been used as a test for pregnancy but such use is no longer considered safe because of possible damage to a developing baby. Also, more rapid methods for testing for pregnancy are now available.

If you take Amen® (medroxyprogesterone acetate tablets) and later find you were pregnant when you took it, be sure to discuss this with your doctor as soon as possible.

Revised June 1990

Manufactured for Carnrick Laboratories, Inc.

Shown in Product Identification Section, page 407

BONTRIL® PDM Ⓒⅲ

[*bŏn 'tril*]

(phendimetrazine tartrate tablets, USP 35 mg)

HOW SUPPLIED

Three layered green, white and yellow tablet with 8648 on the scored side and the letter "C" on the other. Bontril® PDM tablets containing 35 mg of phendimetrazine tartrate are available in bottles of 100 (NDC 0086-0048-10) and 1,000 (NDC 0086-0048-90).

CAUTION

Federal law prohibits dispensing without prescription.

See product insert for complete information.

Manufactured for Carnrick Laboratories, Inc.

Shown in Product Identification Section, page 407

BONTRIL® SLOW-RELEASE Ⓒⅲ

[*bŏn 'tril*]

(brand of phendimetrazine tartrate slow-release capsules 105 mg

DESCRIPTION

Phendimetrazine tartrate, as the dextro isomer, has the chemical name of (+)-3,4-Dimethyl-2-phenylmorpholine Tartrate.

The structural formula is as follows:

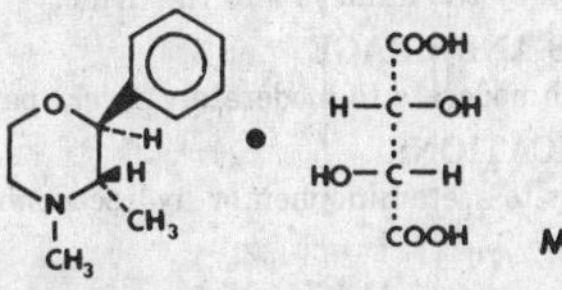

M.W. 341

Phendimetrazine tartrate is a white, odorless powder with a bitter taste. It is soluble in water, methanol and ethanol. Bontril Slow-Release capsules contain FD&C Yellow No. 6 as a color additive.

ACTIONS

Phendimetrazine tartrate is a sympathomimetic amine with pharmacological activity similar to the prototype drugs of this class used in obesity, the amphetamines. Actions include central nervous system stimulation and elevation of blood pressure. Tachyphylaxis and tolerance have been demonstrated with all drugs of this class in which these phenomena have been looked for.

Drugs of this class used in obesity are commonly known as "anorectics" or "anorexigenics". It has not been established, however, that the action of such drugs in treating obesity is primarily one of appetite suppression. Other central nervous system actions or metabolic effects may be involved.

Adult obese subjects instructed in dietary management and treated with anorectic drugs lose more weight on the average than those treated with placebo and diet, as determined in relatively short term clinical trials.

The magnitude of increased weight loss of drug-treated patients over placebo-treated patients is only a fraction of a pound a week. The rate of weight loss is greatest in the first weeks of therapy for both drug and placebo subjects and tends to decrease in succeeding weeks. The possible origin of the increased weight loss due to the various drug effects is not established. The amount of weight loss associated with the use of an anorectic drug varies from trial to trial, and the increased weight loss appears to be related in part to variables other than the drug prescribed, such as the physician investigator, the population treated, and the diet prescribed. Studies do not permit conclusions as to the relative importance of the drug and non-drug factors on weight loss.

The natural history of obesity is measured in years, whereas the studies cited are restricted to a few weeks duration; thus, the total impact of drug-induced weight loss over that of diet alone must be considered clinically limited.

The active drug 105 mg of phendimetrazine tartrate in each capsule of this special slow-release dosage form approximates the action of three 35 mg non-time release doses taken at 4 hours intervals.

The major route of elimination is via the kidneys where most of the drug and metabolites are excreted. Some of the drug is metabolized to phenmetrazine and also phendimetrazine-N-oxide.

The average half-life of elimination when studied under controlled conditions is about 1.9 hours for the non-time and 9.8 hours for the slow-release dosage form. The absorption half-life of the drug from conventional non-time 35 mg phendimetrazine tablets is approximately the same. These data indicate that the slow-release product has a similar onset of action to the conventional non-time-release product and, in addition, has a prolonged therapeutic effect.

INDICATIONS

Phendimetrazine tartrate is indicated in the management of exogenous obesity as a short term adjunct (a few weeks) in a regimen of weight reduction based on caloric restriction. The limited usefulness of agents of this class (see ACTIONS) should be measured against possible risk factors inherent in their use such as those described below.

CONTRAINDICATIONS

Advanced arteriosclerosis, symptomatic cardiovascular disease, moderate and severe hypertension, hyperthyroidism, known hypersensitivity, or idiosyncrasy to the sympathomimetic amines, glaucoma. Agitated states. Patients with a history of drug abuse. Use in patients taking other CNS stimulants including monoamine oxidase inhibitors.

WARNINGS

Tolerance to the anorectic effect usually develops within a few weeks. When this occurs, the recommended dose should not be exceeded in an attempt to increase the effect; rather, the drug should be discontinued.

Use of phendimetrazine within 14 days following the administration of monoamine oxidase inhibitors may result in a hypertensive crisis.

Abrupt cessation of administration following prolonged high dosage results in extreme fatigue and depression. Because of the effect on the central nervous system phendimetrazine tartrate may impair the ability of the patient to engage in potentially hazardous activities such as operating machinery or driving a motor vehicle; the patient should therefore be cautioned accordingly.

PRECAUTIONS

Caution is to be exercised in prescribing phendimetrazine for patients with even mild hypertension.

Insulin requirements in diabetes mellitus may be altered in association with the use of phendimetrazine and the concomitant dietary regimen.

Phendimetrazine may decrease the hypotensive effect of guanethidine.

The least amount feasible should be prescribed or dispensed at one time in order to minimize the possibility of overdosage.

Usage in Pregnancy: Safe use in pregnancy has not been established. Until more information is available, phendimetrazine tartrate should not be taken by women who are or may become pregnant unless, in the opinion of the physician, the potential benefits outweigh the possible hazards.

Usage in Children: Phendimetrazine tartrate is not recommended for use in children under 12 years of age.

ADVERSE REACTIONS

Cardiovascular: Palpitation, tachycardia, elevation of blood pressure.

Central Nervous System: Overstimulation, restlessness, dizziness, insomnia, tremor, headache; rarely psychotic episodes at recommended doses, agitation, flushing, sweating, blurring of vision.

Gastrointestinal: Dryness of the mouth, diarrhea, constipation, nausea, stomach pain.

Genitourinary: Changes in libido, urinary frequency, dysuria.

DRUG ABUSE AND DEPENDENCE

Controlled Substance: Phendimetrazine is a Schedule III controlled substance.

Dependence: Phendimetrazine Tartrate is related chemically and pharmacologically to the amphetamines. Amphetamines and related stimulant drugs have been extensively abused, and the possibility of abuse of phendimetrazine should be kept in mind when evaluating the desirability of including a drug as part of a weight reduction program. Abuse of amphetamines and related drugs may be associated with intense psychological dependence and severe social dysfunction. There are reports of patients who have increased the dosage to many times that recommended. Abrupt cessation following prolonged high dosage administration results in extreme fatigue and mental depression; changes are also noted on the sleep EEG. Manifestations of chronic intoxication with anorectic drugs include severe dermatoses, marked insomnia, irritability, hyperactivity and personality changes. The most severe manifestation of chronic intoxications is psychosis, often clinically indistinguishable from schizophrenia.

OVERDOSAGE

Manifestations of acute overdosage may include restlessness, tremor, hyperreflexia, rapid respiration, confusion, assaultiveness, hallucinations, panic states.

Fatigue and depression usually follow the central stimulation.

Cardiovascular effects include arrhythmias, hypertension, or hypotension and circulatory collapse. Gastrointestinal symptoms include nausea, vomiting, diarrhea, and abdominal cramps. Poisoning may result in convulsions, coma, and death.

Management of acute intoxication is largely symptomatic and includes lavage and sedation with a barbiturate. Experience with hemodialysis or peritoneal dialysis is inadequate to permit recommendation in this regard.

Acidification of the urine increases phendimetrazine tartrate excretion.

Intravenous phentolamine (Regitine) has been suggested for possible acute, severe hypertension, if this complicates overdosage.

Continued on next page

Carnrick Laboratories—Cont.

DOSAGE AND ADMINISTRATION
One Slow-Release Capsule (105 mg) in the morning, taken 30-60 minutes before the morning meal.
Phendimetrazine Tartrate is not recommended for use in children under twelve years of age.

HOW SUPPLIED
Phendimetrazine Slow-Release Capsules, 105 mg is supplied in bottles of 100 opaque green and clear yellow capsules, imprinted with the letter "C" and 8647. NDC # 0086-0047-10.
Store at controlled room temperature, 15°- 30°C(59°-86°F).
The most recent revision of this labeling is Nov. 1990.

CAUTION
Federal law prohibits dispensing without prescription.
Manufactured for Carnrick Laboratories, Inc.
Shown in Product Identification Section, page 407

CAPITAL® and CODEINE SUSPENSION Ⓒ
(acetaminophen and codeine phosphate oral suspension)

HOW SUPPLIED
CAPITAL® AND CODEINE SUSPENSION contains 120 mg of acetaminophen and 12 mg of codeine phosphate/5 mL and is given orally. CAPITAL® AND CODEINE SUSPENSION is a fruit punch-flavored pink suspension available in 16 fluid oz. (473 mL) bottles, NDC 0086-0046-16.
SHAKE WELL BEFORE USING
Store at controlled room temperature 15°-30°C (59°-86°F).
Dispense in tight, light-resistant glass container and label "Shake Well Before Using."

CAUTION
Federal law prohibits dispensing without prescription.
See product insert for complete information.
Manufactured for Carnrick Laboratories, Inc.
Shown in Product Identification Section, page 407

HYDROCET® CAPSULES Ⓒ III

CAUTION
Federal law prohibits dispensing without prescription.

DESCRIPTION
Each Hydrocet® capsule contains:
Hydrocodone Bitartrate, USP .... 5 mg
(WARNING: May be habit forming.)
Acetaminophen, USP .... 500 mg
Hydrocodone bitartrate is an opioid analgesic and antitussive and occurs as fine, white crystals or as a crystalline powder. It is affected by light. The chemical name is: 4,5α-epoxy-3-methoxy-17-methylmorphinan-6-one tartrate (1:1) hydrate (2:5). Its structure is as follows:

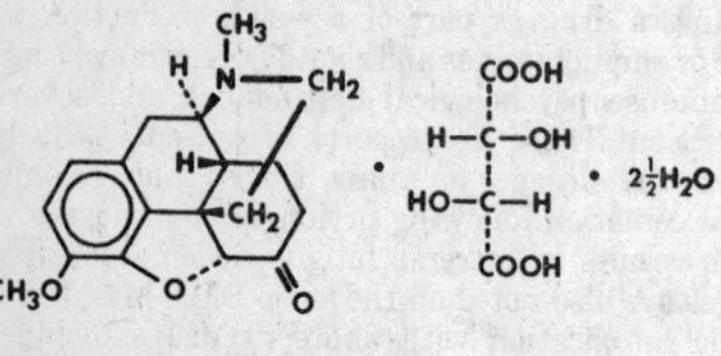

$C_{18}H_{21}NO_3 \cdot C_4H_6O_6 \cdot 2\frac{1}{2} H_2O$
M.W. 494.50

Acetaminophen, 4'-hydroxyacetanilide, is a nonopiate, nonsalicylate analgesic and antipyretic which occurs as a white, odorless crystalline powder possessing a slightly bitter taste. Its structure is as follows:

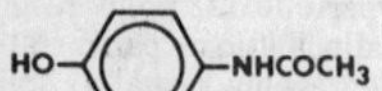

$C_8H_9NO_2$
M.W. 151.16

CLINICAL PHARMACOLOGY
Hydrocodone is a semisynthetic narcotic analgesic and antitussive with multiple actions qualitatively similar to those of codeine. Most of these involve the central nervous system and smooth muscle. The precise mechanism of action of hydrocodone and other opiates is not known, although it is believed to relate to the existence of opiate receptors in the central nervous system. In addition to analgesia, narcotics may produce drowsiness, changes in mood and mental clouding.
Radioimmunoassay techniques have recently been developed for the analysis of hydrocodone in human plasma. After a 10 mg oral dose of hydrocodone bitartrate, a mean peak serum drug level of 23.6 ng/ml and an elimination half-life of 3.8 hours were found.
The analgesic action of acetaminophen involves peripheral and central influences, but the specific mechanism is as yet undetermined. Antipyretic activity is mediated through hypothalamic heat regulating centers. Acetaminophen inhibits prostaglandin synthetase. Therapeutic doses of acetaminophen have negligible effects on the cardiovascular or respiratory systems; however, toxic doses may cause circulatory failure and rapid, shallow breathing. Acetaminophen is rapidly and almost completely absorbed from the gastrointestinal tract, producing maximum serum concentrations within 30 minutes to one hour. The plasma half-life in adults and children ranges from 0.90 hours to 3.25 hours with an average of approximately 2 hours. The drug distributes uniformly in most body fluids and is approximately 25% protein bound. Acetaminophen is conjugated in the liver, with less than 3% of the dose excreted unchanged in 24 hours. The primary metabolic pathway is conjugation to sulfate and glucuronide by-products. A minor oxidative pathway forms cysteine and mercapturic acid. These compounds are subsequently excreted by the kidneys into the urine.

INDICATIONS AND USAGE
For the relief of moderate to moderately severe pain.

CONTRAINDICATIONS
Hypersensitivity to acetaminophen or hydrocodone.

WARNINGS
Respiratory Depression: At high doses or in sensitive patients, hydrocodone may produce dose-related respiratory depression by acting directly on the brain stem respiratory center. Hydrocodone also affects the center that controls respiratory rhythm, and may produce irregular and periodic breathing.
Head Injury and Increased Intracranial Pressure: The respiratory depressant effects of narcotics and their capacity to elevate cerebrospinal fluid pressure may be markedly exaggerated in the presence of head injury, other intracranial lesions or a preexisting increase in intracranial pressure. Furthermore, narcotics produce adverse reactions which may obscure the clinical course of patients with head injuries.
Acute Abdominal Conditions: The administration of narcotics may obscure the diagnosis or clinical course of patients with acute abdominal conditions.

PRECAUTIONS
Special Risk Patients: As with any narcotic analgesic agent, HYDROCET® (Hydrocodone Bitartrate, USP 5 mg and Acetaminophen, USP 500 mg) capsules should be used with caution in elderly or debilitated patients and those with severe impairment of hepatic or renal function, hypothyroidism, Addison's disease, prostatic hypertrophy or urethral stricture. The usual precautions should be observed and the possibility of respiratory depression should be kept in mind.
Information for Patients: HYDROCET® (Hydrocodone Bitartrate, USP 5 mg and Acetaminophen, USP 500 mg) capsules like all narcotics, may impair the mental and/or physical abilities required for the performance of potentially hazardous tasks such as driving a car or operating machinery; patients should be cautioned accordingly.
Cough Reflex: Hydrocodone suppresses the cough reflex; as with all narcotics, caution should be exercised when HYDROCET® capsules are used postoperatively and in patients with pulmonary disease.
Drug Interactions: Patients receiving other narcotic analgesics, antipsychotics, antianxiety agents, or other CNS depressants (including alcohol) concomitantly with HYDROCET® capsules may exhibit an additive CNS depression. When combined therapy is contemplated, the dose of one or both agents should be reduced.
The use of MAO inhibitors or tricyclic antidepressants with hydrocodone preparations may increase the effect of either the antidepressant or hydrocodone.
The concurrent use of anticholinergics with hydrocodone may produce paralytic ileus.
Usage In Pregnancy:
Teratogenic Effects: Pregnancy Category C. Hydrocodone has been shown to be teratogenic in hamsters when given in doses 700 times the human dose. There are no adequate and well-controlled studies in pregnant women. HYDROCET® capsules should be used during pregnancy only if the potential benefit justifies the potential risk to the fetus.
Nonteratogenic Effects: Babies born to mothers who have been taking opioids regularly prior to delivery will be physically dependent. The withdrawal signs include irritability and excessive crying, tremors, hyperactive reflexes, increased respiratory rate, increased stools, sneezing, yawning, vomiting, and fever. The intensity of the syndrome does not always correlate with the duration of maternal opioid use or dose. There is no consensus on the best method of managing withdrawal. Chlorpromazine 0.7 to 1 mg/kg q6h, and paregoric 2 to 4 drops/kg q4h, have been used to treat withdrawal symptoms in infants. The duration of therapy is 4 to 28 days, with the dosage decreased as tolerated.
Labor and Delivery: As with all narcotics, administration of HYDROCET® capsules to the mother shortly before delivery may result in some degree of respiratory depression in the newborn, especially if higher doses are used.
Nursing Mothers: It is not known whether this drug is excreted in human milk. Because many drugs are excreted in human milk and because of the potential for serious adverse reactions in nursing infants from HYDROCET® (Hydrocodone Bitartrate, USP 5 mg and Acetaminophen, USP 500 mg) capsules, a decision should be made whether to discontinue nursing or to discontinue the drug, taking into account the importance of the drug to the mother.
Pediatric Use: Safety and effectiveness in children have not been established.

ADVERSE REACTIONS
The most frequently observed adverse reactions include lightheadedness, dizziness, sedation, nausea and vomiting. These effects seem to be more prominent in ambulatory than in nonambulatory patients and some of these adverse reactions may be alleviated if the patient lies down.
Other adverse reactions include:
Central Nervous System: Drowsiness, mental clouding, lethargy, impairment of mental and physical performance, anxiety, fear, dysphoria, psychic dependence, and mood changes.
Gastrointestinal System: The antiemetic phenothiazines are useful in suppressing the nausea and vomiting which may occur (see above); however, some phenothiazine derivatives seem to be antianalgesic and to increase the amount of narcotic required to produce pain relief, while other phenothiazines reduce the amount of narcotic required to produce a given level of analgesia. Prolonged administration of HYDROCET® capsules may produce constipation.
Genitourinary System: Ureteral spasm, spasm of vesical sphincters and urinary retention have been reported.
Respiratory Depression: Hydrocodone bitartrate may produce dose-related respiratory depression by acting directly on the brain stem respiratory center. Hydrocodone also affects the center that control respiratory rhythm, and may produce irregular and periodic breathing. If significant respiratory depression occurs, it may be antagonized by the use of naloxone hydrochloride. Apply other supportive measures when indicated.

DRUG ABUSE AND DEPENDENCE
HYDROCET® capsules are subject to the Federal Controlled Substances Act (Schedule III).
Psychic dependence, physical dependence, and tolerance may develop upon repeated administration of narcotics; therefore, HYDROCET® capsules should be prescribed and administered with caution. However, psychic dependence is unlikely to develop when HYDROCET® capsules are used for a short time for the treatment of pain.
Physical dependence, the condition in which continued administration of the drug is required to prevent the appearance of a withdrawal syndrome, assumes clinically significant proportions only after several weeks of continued narcotic use, although some mild degree of physical dependence may develop after a few days of narcotic therapy. Tolerance, in which increasingly large doses are required in order to produce the same degree of analgesia, is manifested initially by a shortened duration of analgesic effect, and subsequently by decreases in the intensity of analgesia. The rate of development of tolerance varies among patients.

OVERDOSAGE
Acetaminophen:
Signs and Symptoms: In acute acetaminophen overdosage, dose-dependent, potentially fatal hepatic necrosis is the most serious adverse effect. Renal tubular necrosis, hypoglycemic coma, and thrombocytopenia may also occur.
In adults, hepatic toxicity has rarely been reported with acute overdoses of less than 10 grams and fatalities with less than 15 grams. Importantly, young children seem to be more resistant than adults to the hepatotoxic effect of an acetaminophen overdose. Despite this, the measures outlined below should be initiated in any adult or child suspected of having ingested an acetaminophen overdose.
Early symptoms following a potentially hepatotoxic overdose may include: nausea, vomiting, diaphoresis and general malaise. Clinical and laboratory evidence of hepatic toxicity may not be apparent until 48 to 72 hours post-ingestion.
Treatment: The stomach should be emptied promptly by lavage or by induction of emesis with syrup of ipecac. Patients' estimates of the quantity of a drug ingested are notoriously unreliable. Therefore, if an acetaminophen overdose is suspected, a serum acetaminophen assay should be obtained as early as possible, but no sooner than four hours following ingestion. Liver function studies should be obtained initially and repeated at 24-hour intervals.
The antidote, N-acetylcysteine, should be administered as early as possible, preferably within 16 hours of the overdose ingestion for optimal results, but in any case, within 24 hours. Following recovery, there are no residual, structural or functional hepatic abnormalities.

Hydrocodone:

Signs and Symptoms: Serious overdose with hydrocodone is characterized by respiratory depression (a decrease in respiratory rate and/or tidal volume. Cheyne-Stokes respiration, cyanosis), extreme somnolence progressing to stupor or coma, skeletal muscle flaccidity, cold and clammy skin, and sometimes bradycardia and hypotension. In severe overdosage, apnea, circulatory collapse, cardiac arrest and death may occur.

Treatment: Primary attention should be given to the reestablishment of adequate respiratory exchange through provision of a patent airway and the institution of assisted or controlled ventilation. The narcotic antagonist naloxone is a specific antidote against respiratory depression which may result from overdosage or unusual sensitivity to narcotics, including hydrocodone. Therefore, an appropriate dose of naloxone hydrochloride (see package insert) should be administered, preferably by the intravenous route, and simultaneously with efforts at respiratory resuscitation. Since the duration of action of hydrocodone may exceed that of the antagonist, the patient should be kept under continued surveillance and repeated doses of the antagonist should be administered as needed to maintain adequate respiration.

An antagonist should not be administered in the absence of clinically significant respiratory or cardiovascular depression. Oxygen, intravenous fluids, vasopressors and other supportive measures should be employed as indicated.

Gastric emptying may be useful in removing unabsorbed drug.

DOSAGE AND ADMINISTRATION

Dosage should be adjusted according to the severity of the pain and the response of the patient. However, it should be kept in mind that tolerance to hydrocodone can develop with continued use and that the incidence of untoward effects is dose related.

The usual adult dosage is one or two capsules every four to six hours as needed for pain. The total 24 hour dose should not exceed 8 capsules.

HOW SUPPLIED

Blue and white, opaque capsules imprinted with the letter "C" and 8657.

Each capsule contains Hydrocodone Bitartrate, USP 5 mg (WARNING: MAY BE HABIT FORMING.) and Acetaminophen, USP 500 mg. Keep in tight, light resistant containers. Supplied in bottles of 100 capsules NDC 0086-0057-10. Store at controlled room temperature, 15°–30°C (59°–86°F). The most recent revision of this labeling is August 1990. Manufactured for Carnrick Laboratories, Inc.

Shown in Product Identification Section, page 407

MIDRIN®   ℞

[*mid′rin*]

CAUTION

Federal law prohibits dispensing without prescription.

DESCRIPTION

Each red capsule with pink band contains Isometheptene Mucate 65 mg., Dichloralphenazone 100 mg., and Acetaminophen 325 mg.

Isometheptene Mucate is a white crystalline powder having a characteristic aromatic odor and bitter taste. It is an unsaturated aliphatic amine with sympathomimetic properties.

Dichloralphenazone is a white, microcrystalline powder, with slight odor and tastes saline at first, becoming acrid. It is a mild sedative.

Acetaminophen, a non-salicylate, occurs as a white, odorless, crystalline powder possessing a slightly bitter taste.

Midrin capsules contain FD&C Yellow No. 6 as a color additive.

ACTIONS

Isometheptene Mucate, a sympathomimetic amine, acts by constricting dilated cranial and cerebral arterioles, thus reducing the stimuli that lead to vascular headaches. Dichloralphenazone, a mild sedative, reduces the patient's emotional reaction to the pain of both vascular and tension headaches. Acetaminophen raises the threshold to painful stimuli, thus exerting an analgesic effect against all types of headaches.

INDICATIONS

For relief of tension and vascular headaches.*

---

*Based on a review of this drug (isometheptene mucate) by the National Academy of Sciences-National Research Council and/or other information, FDA has classified the other indication as "possibly" effective in the treatment of migraine headache.

Final classification of the less-than-effective indication requires further investigation.

CONTRAINDICATIONS

Midrin is contraindicated in glaucoma and/or severe cases of renal disease, hypertension, organic heart disease, hepatic disease and in those patients who are on monoamine-oxidase (MAO) inhibitor therapy.

PRECAUTIONS

Caution should be observed in hypertension, peripheral vascular disease and after recent cardiovascular attacks.

ADVERSE REACTIONS

Transient dizziness and skin rash may appear in hypersensitive patients. This can usually be eliminated by reducing the dose.

DOSAGE AND ADMINISTRATION

FOR RELIEF OF MIGRAINE HEADACHE: The usual adult dosage is two capsules at once, followed by one capsule every hour until relieved, up to 5 capsules within a twelve hour period.

FOR RELIEF OF TENSION HEADACHE: The usual adult dosage is one or two capsules every four hours up to 8 capsules a day.

HOW SUPPLIED

Red capsules imprinted with pink band, the letter "C" and 86120. Bottles of 50 capsules, NDC 0086-0120-05. Bottles of 100 capsules, NDC 0086-0120-10. Store at controlled room temperature 15–30°C (59–86°F) in a dry place.

The most recent revision of this labeling is Nov. 1988. Manufactured for Carnrick Laboratories, Inc.

Shown in Product Identification Section, page 407

MOTOFEN®   ℞

Tablets
(difenoxin hydrochloride with atropine sulfate)
antidiarrheal

DESCRIPTION

Each five-sided dye free MOTOFEN tablet contains:

Difenoxin (as the hydrochloride) .... 1.0 mg

Warning—May be habit forming.

Atropine sulfate .... 0.025 mg

Difenoxin hydrochloride, 1-(3-cyano-3,3-diphenylpropyl)-4-phenyl-4-piperidinecarboxylic acid monohydrochloride, is an orally administered antidiarrheal agent which is chemically related to the narcotic meperidine.

The structural formula is:

Difenoxin Hydrochloride

Atropine sulfate is present to discourage deliberate overdosage.

Atropine sulfate, an anticholinergic, is endo ($\pm$)-α-(hydroxymethyl) benzeneacetic acid 8-methyl-8-azabicyclo[3.2.1] oct-3-yl ester sulfate (2:1) (salt) monohydrate and has the following structural formula:

Atropine Sulfate

Inactive ingredients: calcium stearate, cellulose, lactose, corn starch.

CLINICAL PHARMACOLOGY

Animal studies have shown that difenoxin hydrochloride manifests its antidiarrheal effect by slowing intestinal motility. The mechanism of action is by a local effect on the gastrointestinal wall.

Difenoxin is the principal active metabolite of diphenoxylate.

Following oral administration of MOTOFEN, difenoxin is rapidly and extensively absorbed. Mean peak plasma levels of approximately 160 ng/mL occurred within 40 to 60 minutes in most patients following an oral dose of 2mg. Plasma levels decline to less than 10% of their peak values within 24 hours and to less than 1% of their peak values within 72 hours. This decline parallels the appearance of difenoxin and its metabolites in the urine. Difenoxin is metabolized to an inactive hydroxylated metabolite. Both the drug and its me-

---

tabolites are excreted, mainly as conjugates, in urine and feces.

INDICATIONS AND USAGE

MOTOFEN (difenoxin hydrochloride with atropine sulfate) is indicated as adjunctive therapy in the management of acute nonspecific diarrhea and acute exacerbations of chronic functional diarrhea.

CONTRAINDICATIONS

MOTOFEN is contraindicated in patients with diarrhea associated with organisms that penetrate the intestinal mucosa (toxigenic *E. coli*, *Salmonella* species, *Shigella*) and pseudomembranous colitis associated with broad spectrum antibiotics. Antiperistaltic agents should not be used in these conditions because they may prolong and/or worsen diarrhea.

MOTOFEN is *contraindicated in children under 2 years of age* because of the decreased margin of safety of drugs in this class in younger age groups.

MOTOFEN is contraindicated in patients with a known hypersensitivity to difenoxin, atropine, or any of the inactive ingredients, and in patients who are jaundiced.

WARNINGS

MOTOFEN IS *NOT* AN INNOCUOUS DRUG AND DOSAGE RECOMMENDATIONS SHOULD BE STRICTLY ADHERED TO. MOTOFEN IS NOT RECOMMENDED FOR CHILDREN UNDER 2 YEARS OF AGE. OVERDOSAGE MAY RESULT IN SEVERE RESPIRATORY DEPRESSION AND COMA, POSSIBLY LEADING TO PERMANENT BRAIN DAMAGE OR DEATH (SEE *OVERDOSAGE*). THEREFORE, KEEP THIS MEDICATION OUT OF THE REACH OF CHILDREN.

FLUID AND ELECTROLYTE BALANCE—THE USE OF MOTOFEN DOES NOT PRECLUDE THE ADMINISTRATION OF APPROPRIATE FLUID AND ELECTROLYTE THERAPY. DEHYDRATION, PARTICULARLY IN CHILDREN, MAY FURTHER INFLUENCE THE VARIABILITY OF RESPONSE TO MOTOFEN AND MAY PREDISPOSE TO DELAYED DIFENOXIN INTOXICATION. DRUG-INDUCED INHIBITION OF PERISTALSIS MAY RESULT IN FLUID RETENTION IN THE COLON, AND THIS MAY FURTHER AGGRAVATE DEHYDRATION AND ELECTROLYTE IMBALANCE.

IF SEVERE DEHYDRATION OR ELECTROLYTE IMBALANCE IS MANIFESTED, MOTOFEN SHOULD BE WITHHELD UNTIL APPROPRIATE CORRECTIVE THERAPY HAS BEEN INITIATED.

Ulcerative Colitis—In some patients with acute ulcerative colitis, agents which inhibit intestinal motility or delay intestinal transit time have been reported to induce toxic megacolon. Consequently, patients with acute ulcerative colitis should be carefully observed and MOTOFEN therapy should be discontinued promptly if abdominal distention occurs or if other untoward symptoms develop.

Liver and Kidney Disease—MOTOFEN (difenoxin hydrochloride with atropine sulfate) should be used with extreme caution in patients with advanced hepatorenal disease and in all patients with abnormal liver function tests since hepatic coma may be precipitated.

Atropine—A subtherapeutic dose of atropine has been added to difenoxin hydrochloride to discourage deliberate overdosage. Usage of MOTOFEN in recommended doses is not likely to cause prominent anticholinergic side effects, but MOTOFEN should be avoided in patients in whom anticholinergic drugs are contraindicated. The warnings and precautions for use of anticholinergic agents should be observed. In children, signs of atropinism may occur even with recommended doses of MOTOFEN, particularly in patients with Down's Syndrome.

PRECAUTIONS

Information for Patients

CAUTION PATIENTS TO ADHERE STRICTLY TO RECOMMENDED DOSAGE SCHEDULES. THE MEDICATION SHOULD BE KEPT OUT OF REACH OF CHILDREN SINCE ACCIDENTAL OVERDOSAGE MAY RESULT IN SEVERE, EVEN FATAL, RESPIRATORY DEPRESSION. MOTOFEN may produce drowsiness or dizziness. The patient should be cautioned regarding activities requiring mental alertness, such as driving or operating dangerous machinery.

Drug Interactions

Since the chemical structure of difenoxin hydrochloride is similar to meperidine hydrochloride, the concurrent use of MOTOFEN with monoamine oxidase inhibitors may, in theory, precipitate a hypertensive crisis.

MOTOFEN may potentiate the action of barbiturates, tranquilizers, narcotics, and alcohol. When these medications are used concomitantly with MOTOFEN, the patient should be closely monitored.

Diphenoxylate hydrochloride, from which the principal active metabolite difenoxin is derived, was found to inhibit the hepatic microsomal enzyme system at a dose of 2 mg/kg/day

Continued on next page

Carnrick Laboratories—Cont.

in studies conducted with male rats. Therefore, difenoxin has the potential to prolong the biological half-lives of drugs for which the rate of elimination is dependent on the microsomal drug metabolizing enzyme system.

Carcinogenesis, Mutagenesis, Impairment of Fertility

No evidence of carcinogenesis was found in a long-term study of difenoxin hydrochloride/atropine in the rat. In this 104 week study, rats received dietary doses of 0, 1.25, 2.5, or 5 mg/kg/day difenoxin/atropine (20:1 ratio).

No experiments have been conducted to determine the mutagenic potential of MOTOFEN. MOTOFEN did not significantly impair fertility in rats.

Pregnancy/Teratogenic Effects

Pregnancy Category C. Reproduction studies in rats and rabbits with doses at 31 and 61 times the human therapeutic dose respectively, on a mg/kg basis, demonstrated no evidence of teratogenesis due to MOTOFEN (difenoxin hydrochloride with atropine sulfate).

Pregnant rats receiving oral doses of difenoxin hydrochloride/atropine 20 times the maximum human dose had an increase in delivery time as well as a significant increase in the percent of stillbirths.

Neonatal survival in rats was also reduced with most deaths occurring within four days of delivery.

There are no well controlled studies in pregnant women. MOTOFEN should be used during pregnancy only if the potential benefit justifies the potential risk to the fetus.

Nursing Mothers

Because of the potential for serious adverse reactions in nursing infants from MOTOFEN, a decision should be made whether to discontinue nursing or to discontinue the drug, taking into account the importance of the drug to the mother.

Pediatric Use

SAFETY AND EFFECTIVENESS IN CHILDREN BELOW THE AGE OF 12 HAVE NOT BEEN ESTABLISHED. MOTOFEN IS CONTRAINDICATED IN CHILDREN UNDER 2 YEARS OF AGE. See OVERDOSAGE section for information on hazards from accidental poisoning in children.

ADVERSE REACTIONS

In view of the small amount of atropine present (0.025 mg/tablet), effects such as dryness of the skin and mucous membranes, flushing, hyperthermia, tachycardia and urinary retention are very unlikely to occur, except perhaps in children.

Many of the adverse effects reported during clinical investigation of MOTOFEN are difficult to distinguish from symptoms associated with the diarrheal syndrome. However, the following events were reported at the stated frequencies:

Gastrointestinal: Nausea, 1 in 15 patients; vomiting, 1 in 30 patients; dry mouth, 1 in 30 patients; epigastric distress, 1 in 100 patients; and constipation, 1 in 300 patients.

Central Nervous System: Dizziness and light-headedness, 1 in 20 patients; drowsiness, 1 in 25 patients; and headache, 1 in 40 patients; tiredness, nervousness, insomnia and confusion ranged from 1 in 200 to 1 in 600 patients.

Other less frequent reactions: Burning eyes and blurred vision occurred in a few cases.

The following adverse reactions have been reported in patients receiving chemically-related drugs: numbness of extremities, euphoria, depression, sedation, anaphylaxis, angioneurotic edema, urticaria, swelling of the gums, pruritus, toxic megacolon, paralytic ileus, pancreatitis, and anorexia.

THIS MEDICATION SHOULD BE KEPT IN A CHILD-RESISTANT CONTAINER AND OUT OF THE REACH OF CHILDREN SINCE AN OVERDOSAGE MAY RESULT IN SEVERE RESPIRATORY DEPRESSION AND COMA, POSSIBLY LEADING TO PERMANENT BRAIN DAMAGE OR DEATH.

DRUG ABUSE AND DEPENDENCE

MOTOFEN (difenoxin hydrochloride with atropine sulfate) tablets are a Schedule IV controlled substance.

Addiction to (dependence on) difenoxin hydrochloride is theoretically possible at high dosage. Therefore, the recommended dosage should not be exceeded. Because of the structural and pharmacological similarities of difenoxin hydrochloride to drugs with a definite addiction potential, MOTOFEN should be administered with considerable caution to patients who are receiving addicting drugs, to individuals known to be addiction prone, or to those in whom histories suggest may increase the dosage on their own initiative.

OVERDOSAGE

Diagnosis and Treatment

In the event of overdosage (initial signs may include dryness of the skin and mucous membranes, flushing, hyperthermia and tachycardia followed by lethargy or coma, hypotonic reflexes, nystagmus, pinpoint pupils and respiratory depression) gastric lavage, establishment of a patent airway and possibly mechanically assisted respiration are advised.

The narcotic antagonist naloxone may be used in the treatment of respiratory depression caused by narcotic analgesics or pharmacologically related compounds such as MOTOFEN tablets. When naloxone is administered intravenously, the onset of action is generally apparent within two minutes. Naloxone may also be administered subcutaneously or intramuscularly providing a slightly less rapid onset of action but a more prolonged effect.

To counteract respiratory depression caused by MOTOFEN overdosage, the following dosage schedule for naloxone should be followed:

Adult Dosage: The usual initial adult dose of naloxone is 0.4 mg (one mL) administered intravenously. If respiratory function does not adequately improve after the initial dose, the same IV dose may be repeated at two-to-three minute intervals.

Children: The usual adult dose of naloxone for children is 0.01 mg/kg of body weight administered intravenously and repeated at two-to-three minute intervals if necessary.

Since the duration of action of difenoxin hydrochloride is longer than that of naloxone, improvement of respiration following administration may be followed by recurrent respiratory depression. Consequently, continuous observation is necessary until the effect of difenoxin hydrochloride on respiration (which effect may persist for many hours) has passed. Supplemental intramuscular doses of naloxone may be utilized to produce a longer lasting effect. TREAT ALL POSSIBLE MOTOFEN OVERDOSAGES AS SERIOUS AND MAINTAIN MEDICAL OBSERVATION FOR AT LEAST 48 HOURS, PREFERABLY UNDER CONTINUOUS HOSPITAL CARE.

Although signs of overdosage and respiratory depression may not be evident soon after ingestion of difenoxin hydrochloride, respiratory depression may occur from 12 to 30 hours later.

DOSAGE AND ADMINISTRATION

The recommended starting dose of MOTOFEN tablets in adults is 2 tablets (2 mg), then 1 tablet (1 mg) after each loose stool or 1 tablet (1 mg) every 3 to 4 hours as needed, but the total dosage during any 24-hour treatment period should not exceed 8 tablets (8 mg). In the treatment of diarrhea, if clinical improvement is not observed in 48 hours, continued administration of this type medication is not recommended. For acute diarrheas and acute exacerbations of functional diarrhea, treatment beyond 48 hours is usually not necessary.

Studies in children below the age of 12 have been inadequate to evaluate the safety and effectiveness of MOTOFEN in this age group. MOTOFEN is contraindicated in children under 2 years of age.

HOW SUPPLIED

MOTOFEN® is available as a white, dye-free, five-sided, scored tablet with "8674" on the scored side and "C" on the other. Each tablet contains 1.0 mg difenoxin (as the hydrochloride salt) and 0.025 mg atropine sulfate. Supplied in bottles of 100 tablets (NDC 0086-0074-10) and in bottles of 50 tablets (NDC 0086-0074-05).

Store at controlled room temperature, 15°–30°C (59°–86°F).

CAUTION: FEDERAL LAW PROHIBITS DISPENSING WITHOUT PRESCRIPTION

Manufactured for: Carnrick Laboratories, Inc.

12/91

Shown in Product Identification Section, page 407

NOLAHIST® OTC

[*nō 'lă-hist*]

(phenindamine tartrate)

ANTIHISTAMINE

Allergy/Cold Tablets

DESCRIPTION

Each dye-free NOLAHIST® tablet contains:

Phenindamine Tartrate .... 25 mg

INDICATIONS

Temporarily relieves runny nose, sneezing, itching of the nose or throat, and itchy, watery eyes due to hay fever or other upper respiratory allergies or allergic rhinitis. Temporarily relieves runny nose and sneezing associated with the common cold.

WARNINGS

May cause excitability especially in children. Do not take this product if you have asthma, glaucoma, emphysema, chronic pulmonary disease, shortness of breath, difficulty in breathing, or difficulty in urination due to enlargement of the prostate gland unless directed by a doctor. May cause drowsiness; alcohol may increase the drowsiness effect. Avoid alcoholic beverages while taking this product. Use caution when driving a motor vehicle or operating machinery. May cause nervousness and insomnia in some individuals. As with any drug, if you are pregnant or nursing a baby, seek the advice of a health professional before using this product. Keep this and all medication out of the reach of children. In case of accidental overdose, seek professional assistance or contact a Poison Control Center immediately.

DIRECTIONS

Adults: oral dosage is one tablet every 4 to 6 hours, not to exceed six tablets in 24 hours, or as directed by a doctor. Children 6 to under 12 years of age: oral dosage is one-half tablet every 4 to 6 hours, not to exceed 3 tablets in 24 hours, or as directed by a doctor. Children under 6 years of age: consult a doctor.

TAMPER-RESISTANT PACKAGE FEATURE

Bottle of 100—If printed outer wrap is broken or removed, do not purchase. Blisters—Tablets are individually sealed with Nolahist® identifying copy on the back. If seal is broken, do not use.

HOW SUPPLIED

White, capsule-shaped, scored tablet inscribed with 8652 on one side and C logo on the other side in bottles of 100 (NDC 0086-0052-10) and 7 boxes of 24 blisters (NDC 0086-0052-24). Each tablet contains phenindamine tartrate 25 mg. Store at 15°–30°C (59°–86°F) and keep tightly closed away from light.

Manufactured for Carnrick Laboratories, Inc. 9/92

Shown in Product Identification Section, page 407

NOLAMINE® ℞

[*nō 'lă-mēn '*]

DESCRIPTION

Each timed-release tablet contains:

Phenindamine tartrate .... 24 mg
Chlorpheniramine maleate .... 4 mg
Phenylpropanolamine hydrochloride .... 50 mg

Formulated to provide 8 to 12 hours of continuous relief.

CAUTION

Federal law prohibits dispensing without prescription.

INDICATIONS

As a nasal decongestant associated with the common cold, sinusitis, hay fever and other allergies.

CONTRAINDICATIONS

Hypersensitivity to any of the components. Contraindicated in concurrent MAO inhibitor therapy.

SIDE EFFECTS

Nervousness, insomnia, tremors, dizziness and drowsiness may occur occasionally.

PRECAUTIONS

Antihistamines may cause drowsiness and should be used with caution in patients who operate motor vehicles or dangerous machinery. Use with caution in patients with hypertension, cardiovascular disease, diabetes or hyperthyroidism. This product should be used with caution in patients with prostatic hypertrophy or glaucoma.

DOSAGE

Usual adult dose: Orally, one tablet every 8 hours. In mild cases, one tablet every 10 to 12 hours.

HOW SUPPLIED

Pink, timed release tablets coded C 86204 in bottles of 100 (NDC 0086-0204-10) and 250 (NDC 0086-0204-25). Store at controlled room temperature, 15°–30°C (59°–86°F) and keep away from light.

Manufactured for Carnrick Laboratories, Inc. 6/90

Shown in Product Identification Section, page 407

NOLEX® LA ℞

(phenylpropanolamine hydrochloride/guaifenesin)

DESCRIPTION

Each NOLEX LA white, blue-speckled, oval, scored, long-acting tablet for oral administration contains:

phenylpropanolamine hydrochloride .... 75 mg
guaifenesin .... 400 mg

in a special base to provide a prolonged therapeutic effect.

This product contains ingredients of the following therapeutic classes: decongestant and expectorant.

Phenylpropanolamine hydrochloride is a decongestant having the chemical name, benzenemethanol, α-(l-aminoethyl)-, hydrochloride (R*, S*), (±), with the following structure:

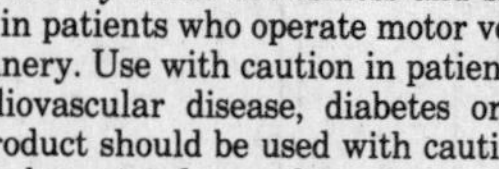

Guaifenesin is an expectorant having the chemical name, 1,2-propanediol, 3-(2-methoxyphenoxy)-, with the following structure:

[See chemical structure at top of next column.]

OCH₂CHCH₂OH / OH / OCH₃ (structural diagram)

CLINICAL PHARMACOLOGY

Phenylpropanolamine hydrochloride is an α-adrenergic receptor agonist (sympathomimetic) which produces vasoconstriction by stimulating α-receptors within the mucosa of the respiratory tract. Clinically, phenylpropanolamine shrinks swollen mucous membranes, reduces tissue hyperemia, edema, and nasal congestion, and increases nasal airway patency. Guaifenesin promotes lower respiratory tract drainage by thinning bronchial secretions, lubricates irritated respiratory tract membranes through increased mucus flow, and facilitates removal of viscous, inspissated mucus. As a result, sinus and bronchial drainage is improved, and dry, nonproductive coughs become more productive and less frequent.

INDICATIONS AND USAGE

NOLEX LA is indicated for the symptomatic relief of sinusitis, bronchitis, pharyngitis, and coryza when these conditions are associated with nasal congestion and viscous mucus in the lower respiratory tract.

CONTRAINDICATIONS

NOLEX LA is contraindicated in individuals with known hypersensitivity to sympathomimetics, severe hypertension, or in patients receiving monoamine oxidase inhibitors.

WARNINGS

Sympathomimetic amines should be used with caution in patients with hypertension, diabetes mellitus, heart disease, peripheral vascular disease, increased intraocular pressure, hyperthyroidism, or prostatic hypertrophy.

PRECAUTIONS

Information for Patients: Do not crush or chew NOLEX LA tablets prior to swallowing.
Drug Interactions: NOLEX LA should not be used in patients taking monoamine oxidase inhibitors or other sympathomimetics.
Drug/Laboratory Test Interactions: Guaifenesin has been reported to interfere with clinical laboratory determinations of urinary 5-hydroxyindoleacetic acid (5-HIAA) and urinary vanilmandelic acid (VMA).
Pregnancy: Pregnancy Category C. Animal reproduction studies have not been conducted with NOLEX LA. It is also not known whether NOLEX LA can cause fetal harm when administered to a pregnant woman or can affect reproduction capacity. NOLEX LA should be given to a pregnant woman only if clearly needed.
Nursing Mothers: It is not known whether the drugs in NOLEX LA are excreted in human milk. Because many drugs are excreted in human milk and because of the potential for serious adverse reactions in nursing infants, a decision should be made whether to discontinue nursing or to discontinue the product, taking into account the importance of the drug to the mother.
Pediatric Use: Safety and effectivness of NOLEX LA tablets in children below the age of 6 have not been established.

ADVERSE REACTIONS

Possible adverse reactions include nervousness, insomnia, restlessness, headache, nausea, or gastric irritation. These reactions seldom, if ever, require discontinuation of therapy. Urinary retention may occur in patients with prostatic hypertrophy.

OVERDOSAGE

The treatment of overdosage should provide symptomatic and supportive care. If the amount ingested is considered dangerous or excessive, induce vomiting with ipecac syrup unless the patient is convulsing, comatose, or has lost the gag reflex, in which case perform gastric lavage using a large-bore tube. If indicated, follow with activated charcoal and a saline cathartic. Since the effects of NOLEX LA may last up to 12 hours, treatment should be continued for at least that length of time.

DOSAGE AND ADMINISTRATION

Adults and children 12 years of age and older—one tablet twice daily (every 12 hours); children 6 to under 12 years —one-half (½) tablet twice daily (every 12 hours). NOLEX LA is not recommended for children under 6 years of age. Tablets may be broken in half for ease of administration without affecting release of medication but should not be crushed or chewed prior to swallowing.

HOW SUPPLIED

NOLEX LA is available as a white, blue-speckled, oval, scored, long-acting tablet for oral administration. It is inscribed with "8673" on the scored side and "C" on the other. Each long-acting tablet contains phenylpropanolamine hydrochloride 75 mg and guaifenesin 400 mg. Supplied in bottles of 100 tablets (NDC 0086-0073-10) and in bottles of 500 tablets (NDC 0086-0073-50).
Store at controlled room temperature, 15°–30°C (59°–86°F.)

CAUTION

Federal law prohibits dispensing without prescription.
Manufactured for Carnrick Laboratories, Inc.
2/91

Shown in Product Identification Section, page 407

PHRENILIN®　　℞
[fren´i-lin]
(Butalbital* 50 mg and Acetaminophen 325 mg Tablet) and
PHRENILIN® FORTE　　℞
(Butalbital* 50 mg and Acetaminophen 650 mg Capsule)
*(WARNING—May be habit forming)

DESCRIPTION

PHRENILIN®: Each PHRENILIN® tablet, an analgesic-sedative combination for oral administration, contains Butalbital*, USP 50 mg *(WARNING—May be habit forming), Acetaminophen, USP 325 mg.
PHRENILIN® FORTE: Each PHRENILIN® FORTE capsule, an analgesic-sedative combination for oral administration, contains Butalbital*, USP 50 mg *(WARNING—May be habit forming), Acetaminophen, USP 650 mg.

HO—⟨ ⟩—NHCOCH₃ (structural diagram)

Acetaminophen

$C_8H_9NO_2$
M.W. 151.16
Acetaminophen, 4'-hydroxy-acetanilide, is a non-opiate, non-salicylate analgesic and antipyretic which occurs as a white, odorless, crystalline powder possessing a slightly bitter taste.

(Butalbital structural diagram: CH₂=CHCH₂ / (CH₃)₂CHCH₂)

Butalbital

$C_{11}H_{16}N_2O_3$
M.W. 224.26
Butalbital, 5-Allyl-5-isobutyl-barbituric acid, a white odorless crystalline powder having a slightly bitter taste, is a short to intermediate-acting barbiturate.

CLINICAL PHARMACOLOGY

Pharmacologically, PHRENILIN® and PHRENILIN® FORTE (Butalbital and Acetaminophen) combine the analgesic properties of acetaminophen with the anxiolytic and muscle relaxant properties of butalbital.

INDICATIONS AND USAGE

PHRENILIN® and PHRENILIN® FORTE are indicated for the relief of the symptom complex of tension (or muscle contraction) headache.

CONTRAINDICATIONS

Hypersensitivity to acetaminophen or barbiturates. Patients with porphyria.

PRECAUTIONS

General
Barbiturates should be administered with caution, if at all, to patients who are mentally depressed, have suicidal tendencies, or a history of drug abuse.
Elderly or debilitated patients may react to barbiturates with marked excitement, depression, and confusion. In some persons, barbiturates repeatedly produce excitement rather than depression.
Information for Patients
Practitioners should give the following information and instructions to patients receiving barbiturates.
A. The use of barbiturates carries with it an associated risk of psychological and/or physical dependence. The patient should be warned against increasing the dose of the drug without consulting a physician.
B. Barbiturates may impair mental and/or physical abilities required for the performance of potentially hazardous tasks (e.g., driving, operating machinery, etc.)
C. Alcohol should not be consumed while taking barbiturates. Concurrent use of the barbiturates with other CNS depressants (e.g., alcohol, narcotics, tranquilizers, and antihistamines) may result in additional CNS depressant effects.
Drug Interactions:
Patients receiving narcotic analgesics, antipsychotics, anti-anxiety agents, or other CNS depressants (including alcohol) concomitantly with PHRENILIN® or PHRENILIN® FORTE (Butalbital and Acetaminophen) may exhibit additve CNS depressant effects.

DRUGS	EFFECT
Butalbital w/coumarin anticoagulants	Decreased effect of anticoagulant because of increased metabolism resulting from enzyme induction.
Butalbital w/tricyclic antidepressants	Decreased blood levels of the antidepressant

Usage in Pregnancy:
Adequate studies have not been performed in animals to determine whether this drug affects fertility in males or females, has teratogenic potential or has other adverse effects on the fetus. There are no well-controlled studies in pregnant women. Although there is no clearly defined risk, one cannot exclude the possibility of infrequent or subtle damage to the human fetus. PHRENILIN® or PHRENILIN® FORTE should be used in pregnant women only when clearly needed.
Nursing Mothers:
The effects of PHRENILIN® or PHRENILIN® FORTE on infants of nursing mothers are not known. Barbiturates are excreted in the breast milk of nursing mothers. The serum levels in infants are believed to be insignificant with therapeutic doses.
Pediatric Use:
Safety and effectiveness in children below the age of 12 have not been established.

ADVERSE REACTIONS

The most frequent adverse reactions are drowsiness and dizziness. Less frequent adverse reactions are lightheadedness and gastrointestinal disturbances including nausea, vomiting, and flatulence.
Mental confusion or depression can occur due to intolerance or overdosage of butalbital.
Several cases of dermatological reactions including toxic epidermal necrolysis and erythema multiforme have been reported.

DRUG ABUSE AND DEPENDENCE

Prolonged use of barbiturates can produce drug dependence, characterized by psychic dependence and tolerance. The abuse liability of PHRENILIN® or PHRENILIN® FORTE (Butalbital and Acetaminophen) is similar to that of other barbiturate-containing drug combinations. Caution should be exercised when prescribing medication for patients with a known propensity for taking excessive quantities of drugs, which is not uncommon in patients with chronic tension headache.

OVERDOSAGE

The toxic effects of acute overdosage of PHRENILIN® or PHRENILIN® FORTE are attributable mainly to its barbiturate component, and, to a lesser extent, acetaminophen.
Barbiturate
Symptoms: Drowsiness, confusion, coma; respiratory depression; hypotension; shock.
Treatment:
1. Maintenance of an adequate airway, with assisted respiration and oxygen administration as necessary.
2. Monitoring of vital signs and fluid balance.
3. If the patient is conscious and has not lost the gag reflex, emesis may be induced with ipecac. Care should be taken to prevent pulmonary aspiration of vomitus. After completion of vomiting, 30 grams of activated charcoal in a glass of water may be administered.
4. If emesis is contraindicated, gastric lavage may be performed with a cuffed endotracheal tube in place with the patient in the face down position. Activated charcoal may be left in the emptied stomach and a saline cathartic administered.
5. Fluid therapy and other standard treatment for shock, if needed.
6. If renal function is normal, forced diuresis may aid in the elimination of the barbiturate. Alkalinization of the urine increases renal excretion of some barbiturates, especially phenobarbital.
7. Although not recommended as a routine procedure, hemodialysis may be used in severe barbiturate intoxication or if the patient is anuric or in shock.
Acetaminophen
Signs and Symptoms: In acute acetaminophen overdosage, dose-dependent, potentially fatal hepatic necrosis is the most serious adverse effect. Renal tubular necrosis, hypoglycemic coma, and thrombocytopenia may also occur.
In adults, hepatic toxicity has rarely been reported with acute overdoses of less than 10 grams and fatalities with less than 15 grams. Importantly, young children seem to be more resistant than adults to the hepatoxic effect of an acetaminophen overdose.
Early symptoms following a potentially hepatotoxic overdose may include: nausea, vomiting, diaphoresis and general malaise. Clinical and laboratory evidence of hepatic toxicity may not be apparent until 48 to 72 hours post-ingestion.

Continued on next page

Carnrick Laboratories—Cont.

Treatment: The stomach should be emptied promptly by lavage or by induction of emesis with syrup of ipecac. Patients estimates of the quantity of a drug ingested are notoriously unreliable. Therefore, if an acetaminophen overdose is suspected, a serum acetaminophen assay should be obtained as early as possible, but no sooner than four hours following ingestion. Liver function studies should be obtained initially and repeated at 24-hour intervals.
The antidote, N-acetylcysteine, should be administered as early as possible, preferably within 16 hours of the overdose ingestion for optimal results, but in any case, within 24 hours. Following recovery, there are no residual, structural or functional hepatic abnormalities.

DOSAGE AND ADMINISTRATION

PHRENILIN®: Oral: One or two tablets every four hours as needed. Do not exceed six tablets per day.
PHRENILIN® FORTE : Oral: One capsule every four hours as needed. Do not exceed six capsules per day.

HOW SUPPLIED

PHRENILIN®: Pale violet scored tablets with the letter "C" on one side and 8650 on the other, in bottles of 100 (NDC 0086-0050-10). Each tablet contains butalbital, USP 50 mg (WARNING: May be habit forming) and acetaminophen, USP 325 mg.
PHRENILIN® FORTE: Amethyst, opaque capsules imprinted with the letter "C" and 8656, in bottles of 100 (NDC 0086-0056-10). Each capsule contains butalbital, USP 50 mg (WARNING: May be habit forming) and acetaminophen USP 650 mg.
Store PHRENILIN® and PHRENILIN® FORTE (Butalbital and Acetaminophen) at controlled room temperature, 15°-30°C (59°-86°F). Dispense in a tight container as defined in the USP.
Caution: Federal Law Prohibits Dispensing Without Prescription
The most recent revision of this labeling is February, 1992.
Manufactured for Carnrick Laboratories, Inc.
Shown in Product Identification Section, page 407

PROPAGEST® OTC
(Phenylpropanolamine HCl)
NASAL DECONGESTANT TABLETS

DESCRIPTION

Each tablet contains:
Phenylpropanolamine HCl .... 25 mg.

INDICATIONS

For the temporary relief of nasal congestion associated with the common cold, sinusitis, hay fever or other upper respiratory allergies.

DOSAGE

Adult oral dosage is one tablet every 4 hours not to exceed 6 tablets in 24 hours. Children 6 to under 12 years oral dosage is one-half tablet every 4 hours not to exceed 3 tablets in 24 hours. For children under 6 years, there is no recommended dosage except under the advice and supervision of a doctor.

WARNINGS

Do not exceed recommended dosage because at higher doses nervousness, dizziness, sleeplessness, rapid pulse or high blood pressure may occur.
Do not take this product for more than 7 days. If symptoms do not improve or are accompanied by fever, consult a doctor.
Do not take this product if you have heart disease, high blood pressure, thyroid disease, glaucoma, diabetes, or difficulty in urination due to enlargement of the prostate gland unless directed by a doctor.
As with any drug, if you are pregnant or nursing a baby, seek the advice of a health professional before using this product.
Keep this and all medication out of the reach of children.
In case of accidental overdose, seek professional assistance or contact a Poison Control Center immediately.
Drug Interaction Precaution: Do not take this product if you are presently taking a prescription drug for high blood pressure or depression, without first consulting your doctor. Do not take this product concurrently with other medication except on the advice of a doctor.
TAMPER-RESISTANT PACKAGE FEATURE:
Bottle of 100—If printed outer wrap is broken or removed, do not purchase.

HOW SUPPLIED

White, oval, scored tablets with "C" logo containing 25 mg. phenylpropanolamine HCl in bottles of 100. (NDC 0086-0051-10). Keep tightly closed, away from light and store at room temperature. 1/89

Manufactured for Carnrick Laboratories, Inc.
Shown in Product Identification Section, page 407

SALFLEX® ℞
(salsalate)
Tablets

DESCRIPTION

SALFLEX (salsalate) is a nonsteroidal anti-inflammatory agent for oral administration. Chemically, salsalate (salicylsalicylic acid or 2-hydroxy-benzoic acid, 2-carboxyphenyl ester) is a dimer of salicylic acid; its structural formula is shown below.
Chemical Structure:

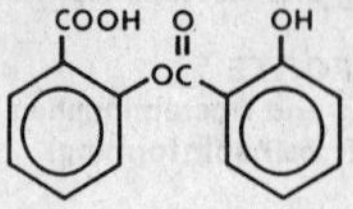

Each round, white, dye-free, film-coated SALFLEX tablet contains 500 mg salsalate.
Each oval, white, dye-free, film-coated SALFLEX tablet contains 750 mg salsalate. (See HOW SUPPLIED.)

CLINICAL PHARMACOLOGY

Salsalate is insoluble in acid gastric fluids (< 0.1 mg/ml at pH 1.0), but readily soluble in the small intestine where it is partially hydrolyzed to two molecules of salicylic acid. A significant portion of the parent compound is absorbed unchanged and undergoes rapid esterase hydrolysis in the body; its half-life is about one hour. About 13% is excreted through the kidneys as a glucuronide conjugate of the parent compound, the remainder as salicylic acid and its metabolites. Thus, the amount of salicylic acid available from SALFLEX (salsalate) is about 15% less than from aspirin, when the two drugs are administered on a salicylic acid molar equivalent basis (3.6 g salsalate/5 g aspirin). Salicylic acid biotransformation is saturated at anti-inflammatory doses of salsalate. Such capacity-limited biotransformation results in an increase in the half-life of salicylic acid from 3.5 to 16 or more hours. Thus, dosing with SALFLEX twice a day will satisfactorily maintain blood levels within the desired therapeutic range (10 to 30 mg/100 ml) throughout the 12-hour intervals. Therapeutic blood levels continue for up to 16 hours after the last dose. The parent compound does not show capacity-limited biotransformation, nor does it accumulate in the plasma on multiple dosing. Food slows the absorption of all salicylates including salsalate.
The mode of anti-inflammatory action of salsalate and other nonsteroidal anti-inflammatory drugs is not fully defined. Although salicylic acid (the primary metabolite of salsalate) is a weak inhibitor of prostaglandin synthesis **in vitro**, salsalate appears to selectively inhibit prostaglandin synthesis **in vivo**,[1] providing anti-inflammatory activity equivalent to aspirin[2] and indomethacin.[3] Unlike aspirin, salsalate does not inhibit platelet aggregation.[4]
The usefulness of salicylic acid, the active **in vivo** product of salsalate, in the treatment of arthritic disorders has been established.[5,6] In contrast to aspirin, salsalate causes no greater fecal gastrointestinal blood loss than placebo.[7]

INDICATIONS AND USAGE

SALFLEX (salsalate) is indicated for relief of the signs and symptoms of rheumatoid arthritis, osteoarthritis and related rheumatic disorders.

CONTRAINDICATIONS

SALFLEX is contraindicated in patients hypersensitive to salsalate.

WARNINGS

Reye Syndrome may develop in individuals who have chicken pox, influenza, or flu symptoms. Some studies suggest possible association between the development of Reye Syndrome and the use of medicines containing salicylate or aspirin. SALFLEX contains a salicylate and therefore is not recommended for use in patients with chicken pox, influenza or flu symptoms. See PRECAUTIONS.

PRECAUTIONS

General Precautions: Patients on treatment with SALFLEX should be warned not to take other salicylates so as to avoid potentially toxic concentrations. Great care should be exercised when SALFLEX is prescribed in the presence of chronic renal insufficiency or peptic ulcer disease. Protein binding of salicylic acid can be influenced by nutritional status, competitive binding of other drugs, and fluctuations in serum proteins caused by disease (rheumatoid arthritis, etc.). Although cross reactivity, including bronchospasm, has been reported occasionally with non-acetylated salicylates, including salsalate, in aspirin-sensitive patients,[8,9] salsalate is less likely than aspirin to induce asthma in such patients.[10]
Laboratory Tests: Plasma salicylic acid concentrations should be periodically monitored during long-term treatment with SALFLEX to aid maintenance of therapeutically effective levels: 10 to 30 mg/100 ml. Toxic manifestations are not usually seen until plasma concentrations exceed 30 mg/100 ml (see OVERDOSAGE). Urinary pH should also be regularly monitored: sudden acidification, as from pH 6.5 to 5.5, can double the plasma level, resulting in toxicity.
Drug Interactions: Salicylates antagonize the uricosuric action of drugs used to treat gout. ASPIRIN AND OTHER SALICYLATE DRUGS WILL BE ADDITIVE TO SALFLEX (salsalate) AND MAY INCREASE PLASMA CONCENTRATIONS OF SALICYLIC ACID TO TOXIC LEVELS. Drugs and foods that raise urine pH will increase renal clearance and urinary excretion of salicylic acid, thus lowering plasma levels; acidifying drugs or foods will decrease urinary excretion and increase plasma levels. Salicylates given concomitantly with anticoagulant drugs may predispose to systemic bleeding. Salicylates may enhance the hypoglycemic effect of oral antidiabetic drugs of the sulfonylurea class. Salicylate competes with a number of drugs for protein binding sites, notably penicillin, thiopental, thyroxine, triiodothyronine, phenytoin, sulfinpyrazone, naproxen, warfarin, methotrexate, and possibly corticosteroids.
Drug/Laboratory Test Interactions: Salicylate competes with thyroid hormone for binding to plasma proteins, which may be reflected in a depressed plasma T_4 value in some patients: thyroid function and basal metabolism are unaffected.
Carcinogenesis: No long-term animal studies have been performed with salsalate to evaluate its carcinogenic potential.
Use in Pregnancy: Pregnancy Category C: Salsalate and salicylic acid have been shown to be teratogenic and embryocidal in rats when given in doses 4 to 5 times the usual human dose. These effects were not observed at doses twice as great as the usual human dose. There are no adequate and well-controlled studies in pregnant women. SALFLEX should be used during pregnancy only if the potential benefit justifies the potential risk to the fetus.
Labor and Delivery: There exist no adequate and well-controlled studies in pregnant women. Although adverse effects on mother or infant have not been reported with salsalate use during labor, caution is advised when anti-inflammatory dosage is involved. However, other salicylates have been associated with prolonged gestation and labor, maternal and neonatal bleeding sequelae, potentiation of narcotic and barbiturate effects (respiratory or cardiac arrest in the mother), delivery problems and stillbirth.
Nursing Mothers: It is not known whether salsalate per se is excreted in human milk; salicylic acid, the primary metabolite of salsalate, has been shown to appear in human milk in concentrations approximating the maternal blood level. Thus the infant of a mother on SALFLEX therapy might ingest in mother's milk 30 to 80% as much salicylate per kg body weight as the mother is taking. Accordingly, caution should be exercised when SALFLEX (salsalate) is administered to a nursing woman.
Pediatric Use: Safety and effectiveness of SALFLEX use in children have not been established. (See WARNINGS section.)

ADVERSE REACTIONS

In two well-controlled clinical trials, the following reversible adverse experiences characteristic of salicylates were most commonly reported with salsalate (n = 280 pts; listed in descending order of frequency): tinnitus, nausea, hearing impairment, rash, and vertigo. These common symptoms of salicylates, i.e., tinnitus or reversible hearing impairment, are often used as a guide to therapy.
Although cause-and-effect relationships have not been established, spontaneous reports over a ten-year period have included the following additional medically significant adverse experiences: abdominal pain, abnormal hepatic function, anaphylactic shock, angioedema, bronchospasm, decreased creatinine clearance, diarrhea, G.I. bleeding, hepatatis, hypotension, nephritis and urticaria.

DRUG ABUSE AND DEPENDENCE

Drug abuse and dependence have not been reported with salsalate.

OVERDOSAGE

Death has followed ingestion of 10 to 30 g of salicylates in adults, but much larger amounts have been ingested without fatal outcome.
Symptoms: The usual symptoms of salicylism—tinnitus, vertigo, headache, confusion, drowsiness, sweating, hyperventilation, vomiting and diarrhea—will occur. More severe intoxication will lead to disruption of electrolyte balance and blood pH, and hyperthermia and dehydration.
Treatment: Further absorption of salsalate from the G.I. tract should be prevented by emesis (syrup of ipecac) and, if necessary, by gastric lavage.
Fluid and electrolyte imbalance should be corrected by the administration of appropriate I.V. therapy. Adequate renal

function should be maintained. Hemodialysis or peritoneal dialysis may be required in extreme cases.

DOSAGE AND ADMINISTRATION

Adults: The usual dosage is 3000 mg daily, given in divided doses as follows:
1) two doses of two 750 mg tablets;
2) two doses of three 500 mg tablets; or
3) three doses of two 500 mg tablets.

Some patients, e.g., the elderly, may require a lower dosage to achieve therapeutic blood concentrations and to avoid the more common side effects such as auditory.

Alleviation of symptoms is gradual, and full benefit may not be evident for 3 to 4 days, when plasma salicylate levels have achieved steady state. There is no evidence for development of tissue tolerance (tachyphylaxis), but salicylate therapy may induce increased activity of metabolizing liver enzymes, causing a greater rate of salicyluric acid production and excretion, with a resultant increase in dosage requirement for maintenance of therapeutic serum salicylate levels.

Children: Dosage recommendations and indications for SALFLEX use in children have not been established.

HOW SUPPLIED

SALFLEX 500 mg tablets:
Each round, white, dye-free, film-coated SALFLEX tablet is inscribed with 8671 on one side and "C" on the other. Each tablet contains 500 mg salsalate and is available in bottles of 100 tablets (NDC 0086-0071-10).

SALFLEX 750 mg tablets:
Each oval, white, dye-free, film-coated SALFLEX tablet is inscribed with 8672 on the scored side and "C" on the other. Each tablet contains 750 mg salsalate and is available in bottles of 100 tablets (NDC 0086-0072-10) and 500 tablets (NDC 0086-0072-50).

Store at controlled room temperature, 15°–30°C (59°–86°F).

CAUTION: Federal law prohibits dispensing without prescription.

REFERENCES

1. Morris HG, Sherman NA, McQuain C., et al: Effects of Salsalate (Non-Acetylated) Salicylate and Aspirin (ASA) on Serum and Urine Prostaglandins in Man. Clin. Pharm. Therap. **33**:(2) 197, 1983.
2. April PA, Curran NJ, Ekholm BP, et al: Multicenter Comparative Study of Salsalate (SSA) vs Aspirin (ASA) in Rheumatoid Arthritis (RA), Arthritis Rheumatism **50**(4 supplement):S93, 1987.
3. Deodhar SD, McLeod MM, Dick WC, et al: A Short-Term Comparative Trial of Salsalate and Indomethacin in Rheumatoid Arthritis. Curr. Med. Res. Opin. **5**:185–188, 1987.
4. Estes D, Kaplan K: Lack of Platelet Effect With the Aspirin Analog, Salsalate, Arthritis and Rheumatism, **23**:1303–1307, 1980.
5. Dick C, Dick PH, Nuki G, et al: Effect of Anti-inflammatory Drug Therapy on Clearance of ^{133}Xe from Knee Joints of Patients with Rheumatoid Arthritis. British Med. J. **3**:278–280, 1969.
6. Dick WC, Grayson MF, Woodburn A, et al: Indices of Inflammatory Activity. Ann. of the Rheum. Dis. **29**:643–648, 1970.
7. Cohen, A: Fecal Blood Loss and Plasma Salicylate Study of Salicylsalicylic Acid and Aspirin. J. Clin. Pharmacol. **19**:242–247, 1979.
8. Chudwin DS, Strub M, Golden HE, et al: Sensitivity to Non-Acetylated Salicylates in a Patient with Asthma, Nasal Polyps, and Rheumatoid Arthritis. Annals of Allergy **57**:133–134, 1986.
9. Spector SL, Wangaard CH, Farr RS: Aspirin and Concomitant Idiosyncrasies in Adult Asthmatic Patients. J. Allergy Clin. Immunol. **64**:500–506, 1979.
10. Stevenson DD, Schrank PJ, Hougham AJ, et al: Salsalate Cross Sensitivity in Aspirin-Sensitive Asthmatics. J. Allergy Clin. Immunol. **81**:181, 1988.

June 1989

Shown in Product Identification Section, page 407

SINULIN® OTC

Analgesic • Antihistamine • Decongestant

DESCRIPTION

SINULIN contains acetaminophen, an analgesic and antipyretic that relieves pain, sinus headache and reduces fever; phenylpropanolamine HCl, a decongestant that promotes nasal drainage and relieves sinus pressure; and chlorpheniramine maleate, an antihistamine that helps control allergic symptoms.

ACTIVE INGREDIENTS

Each tablet contains: acetaminophen 650 mg. (650 mg. is a nonstandard strength of acetaminophen per tablet compared to the established standard of 325 mg. acetaminophen per tablet), chlorpheniramine maleate 4 mg., phenylpropanolamine HCl 25 mg.

INDICATIONS

For the temporary relief of nasal and sinus congestion, runny nose, sneezing, itching of the nose or throat, itchy watery eyes, headache and fever associated with the common cold, sinusitis, hay fever or other upper respiratory allergies.

WARNINGS

Sinulin tablets contain FD&C Yellow No. 6 as a color additive.

Do not exceed recommended dosage because severe liver damage may occur and at higher doses, nervousness, dizziness, sleeplessness, rapid pulse or high blood pressure may occur.

Adults should not take this product for more than 7 days. Children 6 to under 12 years of age should not take this product for more than 5 days. If fever persists for more than 3 days, or recurs, consult a doctor. If symptoms persist, do not improve, or new ones occur, consult a doctor.

Do not take this product if you have high blood pressure, heart disease, diabetes, thyroid disease, glaucoma, asthma, emphysema, chronic pulmonary disease, shortness of breath, difficulty in breathing, or difficulty in urination due to enlargement of the prostate gland, or if you are presently taking a prescription drug for high blood pressure or depression, unless directed by a doctor.

This product may cause drowsiness; alcohol may increase the drowsiness effect. Avoid alcoholic beverages while taking this product. Use caution when driving a motor vehicle or operating machinery. May cause excitability especially in children.

If a rare sensitivity reaction occurs, discontinue use and consult a doctor.

As with any drug, if you are pregnant or nursing a baby, seek the advice of a health professional before using this product.

Keep this and all medication out of the reach of children.

In case of accidental overdose, seek professional assistance or contact a Poison Control Center immediately.

DRUG INTERACTION PRECAUTION

Do not take this product if you are presently taking a prescription drug for high blood pressure or depression without first consulting your doctor. Do not take this product concurrently with other medication except on the advice of a doctor.

DIRECTIONS

Adults: oral dosage is one tablet every 4 to 6 hours, or as directed by a doctor. Do not exceed 6 tablets in 24 hours.

Children 6 to under 12 years of age: oral dosage is one-half tablet every 4 to 6 hours, or as directed by a doctor. Do not exceed 3 tablets in 24 hours.

Children under 6 years of age: do not use unless directed by a doctor.

TAMPER-RESISTANT PACKAGE FEATURE

Bottles of 20's & 100's—If printed outer wrap is broken or removed, do not purchase. Blisters—Tablets are individually sealed with Sinulin® identifying copy on the back. If seal is broken, do not use.

HOW SUPPLIED

Peach color, scored tablets inscribed with 8666 on one side and C logo on the other. Bottles of 20 (NDC 0086-0066-02), 7 boxes of 24 blisters (NDC 0086-0066-24), and Bottles of 100 (NDC 0086-0066-10). Store at controlled room temperature (59°–86°F). 12/88

Manufactured for Carnrick Laboratories, Inc.

Shown in Product Identification Section, page 407

SKELAXIN® ℞

brand of metaxalone

CAUTION

Federal law prohibits dispensing without prescription.

DESCRIPTION

Each pale rose, scored tablet contains: metaxalone, 400 mg.

Skelaxin (metaxalone) has the following chemical structure and name:

5-[(3,4-dimethylphenoxy)methyl]-2 oxazolidinone

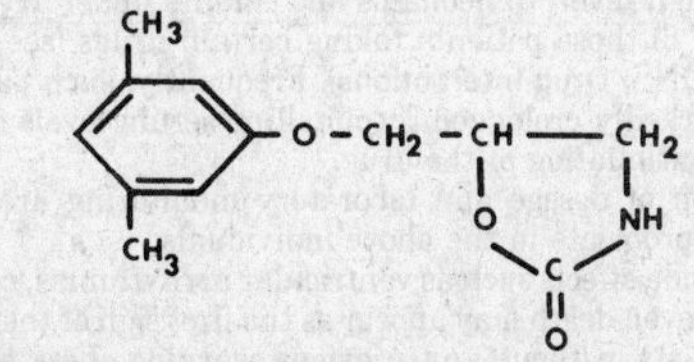

ACTIONS

The mechanism of action of metaxalone in humans has not been established, but may be due to general central nervous system depression. It has no direct action on the contractile mechanism of striated muscle, the motor end plate or the nerve fiber.

INDICATIONS

Skelaxin (metaxalone) is indicated as an adjunct to rest, physical therapy, and other measures for the relief of discomforts associated with acute, painful musculoskeletal conditions. The mode of action of this drug has not been clearly identified, but may be related to its sedative properties. Metaxalone does not directly relax tense skeletal muscles in man.

CONTRAINDICATIONS

Metaxalone is contraindicated in individuals who have shown hypersensitivity to the drug. Metaxalone should not be administered to patients with a known tendency to drug-induced, hemolytic, or other anemias. It is contraindicated in patients with significantly impaired renal or hepatic function.

PRECAUTIONS

Elevation in cephalin flocculation tests without concurrent changes in other liver function parameters have been noted. Hence, it is recommended that metaxalone be administered with great care to patients with pre-existing liver damage and that serial liver function studies be performed as required.

False-positive Benedict's tests, due to an unknown reducing substance, have been noted. A glucose-specific test will differentiate findings.

Pregnancy: Reproduction studies have been performed in rats and have revealed no evidence of impaired fertility or harm to the fetus due to metaxalone. Reactions reports from marketing experience have not revealed evidence of fetal injury, but such experience cannot exclude the possibility of infrequent or subtle damage to the human fetus. Safe use of metaxalone has not been established with regard to possible adverse effects upon fetal development. Therefore, metaxalone tablets should not be used in women who are or may become pregnant and particularly during early pregnancy unless in the judgment of the physician the potential benefits outweigh the possbile hazards.

Nursing Mothers: It is not known whether this drug is secreted in human milk. As a general rule, nursing should not be undertaken while a patient is on a drug since many drugs are excreted in human milk.

Pediatric Use: Safety and effectiveness in children 12 years of age and below have not been established.

ADVERSE REACTIONS

The most frequent reactions to metaxalone include nausea, vomiting, gastrointestinal upset, drowsiness, dizziness, headache, and nervousness or "irritability." Other adverse reactions are: hypersensitivity reaction, characterized by a light rash with or without pruritus; leukopenia; hemolytic anemia; jaundice.

DOSAGE

The recommended dose for adults and children over 12 years of age is two tablets (800 mg) three to four times a day.

MANAGEMENT OF OVERDOSAGE

Gastric lavage and supportive therapy as indicated. (When determining the LD_{50} in rats and mice, progressive sedation, hypnosis and finally respiratory failure were noted as the dosage increased. In dogs, no LD_{50} could be determined as the higher doses produced an emetic action in 15 to 30 minutes). No documented case of major toxicity has been reported.

HOW SUPPLIED

Skelaxin (metaxalone) is available as a 400 mg. pale rose tablet, inscribed with 8662 on the scored side and "C" on the other. Available in bottles of 100 (NDC 0086-0062-10) and in bottles of 500 (NDC 0086-0062-50).

Store at Controlled Room Temperature, between 15°C and 30°C (59°F and 86°F).

8/90

Manufactured for Carnrick Laboratories, Inc.

Shown in Product Identification Section, page 408

THEO-X™ ℞

EXTENDED-RELEASE TABLETS
THEOPHYLLINE ANHYDROUS

DESCRIPTION

Theophylline is a bronchodilator structurally classified as a xanthine derivative. It occurs as a white, odorless, crystalline powder having a bitter taste. Theophylline anhydrous has the chemical name 1*H*-Purine-2, 6-dione, 3,7-dihydro-1, 3-dimethyl-, and is represented by the following structural formula: [See chemical structure at top of next column.]

This product allows a 12-hour dosing interval for a majority of patients and a 24-hour dosing interval for selected patients (see DOSAGE AND ADMINISTRATION section for description of appropriate patient populations).

Continued on next page

Carnrick Laboratories—Cont.

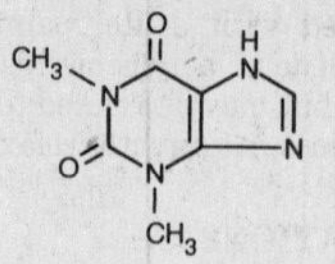

$C_7H_8N_4O_2$ 180.17

This product is available as extended-release tablets intended for oral administration, containing 100 mg, 200 mg, or 300 mg of theophylline anhydrous. Also contains Povidone, USP, Hydroxypropyl Methylcellulose, USP, Lactose Anhydrous, NF, and Magnesium Stearate, NF.

CLINICAL PHARMACOLOGY

Theophylline directly relaxes the smooth muscle of the bronchial airways and pulmonary blood vessels, thus acting mainly as a bronchodilator and smooth muscle relaxant. It has also been demonstrated that aminophylline has a potent effect on diaphragmatic contractility in normal persons and may then be capable of reducing fatigability and thereby improve contractility in patients with chronic obstructive airways disease. The exact mode of action remains unsettled. Although theophylline does cause inhibition of phosphodiesterase with a resultant increase in intracellular cyclic AMP, other agents similarly inhibit the enzyme, producing a rise of cyclic AMP, but are unassociated with any demonstrable bronchodilation. Other mechanisms proposed include an effect on translocation of intracellular calcium, prostaglandin antagonism, stimulation of catecholamines endogenously; inhibition of cyclic guanosine monophosphate metabolism, and adenosine receptor antagonism. None of these mechanisms has been proved, however.

In vitro, theophylline has been shown to act synergistically with beta agonists, and there are now available data which demonstrate an additive effect *in vivo* with combined use.

Pharmacokinetics: The half-life of theophylline is influenced by a number of known variables. It may be prolonged in chronic alcoholics, particularly those with liver disease (cirrhosis or alcoholic liver disease), in patients with congestive heart failure, and in those patients taking certain other drugs (see **PRECAUTIONS, Drug interactions**).

Newborns and neonates have extremely slow clearance rates compared to older infants and children, ie, those over 1 year. Older children have rapid clearance rates while most nonsmoking adults have clearance rates between these two extremes. In premature neonates the decreased clearance is related to oxidative pathways that have yet to be established.

Theophylline Elimination Characteristics
Theophylline

	Half-Life (in hours)	
	Range	Mean
Children	1–9	3.7
Adults	3–15	7.7

In cigarette smokers (1–2 packs/day) the mean half-life is 4–5 hours, much shorter than in nonsmokers. The increase in clearance associated with smoking is presumably due to stimulation of the hepatic metabolic pathway by components of cigarette smoke. The duration of this effect after cessation of smoking is unknown but may require 6 months to 2 years before the rate approaches that of the nonsmoker.

Single-Dose Study:

A single-dose crossover study was conducted in twelve healthy male volunteers to compare pharmacokinetic parameters when theophylline extended-release tablets were administered with and without food. Subjects were fasted overnight and received a single 300 mg tablet early the following morning.

When dosing was done under fed conditions, the subjects received a standard breakfast consisting of 2 fried eggs, 2 strips of bacon, 4 oz. hash brown potatoes, 1 slice of toast with a pat of butter, and 8 oz. whole milk 15 minutes pre-dosing. No food was allowed for five hours post-dosing then a standard lunch was served; at ten hours post-dosing a standard supper was served. Mean peak theophylline serum levels for the two treatments were 3.7 mcg/mL (fasting) and 4.4 mcg/mL (with food). The time of peak serum level varied from subject to subject, occurring from 4 to 14 hours after dosing. However, 92% of the subjects had serum levels at least 75% of the maximum value at 4 to 8 hours after dosing, during each phase.

Thus, blood samples taken 4 to 8 hours post-dosing should reference the peak serum level for most patients. The mean T_{max} was 6.2 hours (fasting) and 8.7 hours (with food). The respective AUC (0- inf.) for these treatments were 73.3 mcg × hr/mL and 82.2 mcg × hr/mL, respectively.

Multiple-Dose Study:

(300 mg)

A multiple-dose, steady-state study was conducted under fed conditions. Three high fat content meals were served at 6:30 a.m., 12 noon and 6:30 p.m. Nineteen normal subjects were dosed as 300 mg every 12 hours (7 p.m. and 7 a.m.) for eight doses. Dosing began one-half hour after the evening meal with the test dose occurring one-half hour after breakfast. At steady-state, the mean peak concentration was 8.8 mcg/mL and the mean trough concentration was 5.9 mcg/mL.

The time of peak concentration (T_{max}) was 6.2 hours. The average percent fraction of fluctuation [$(C_{max}$- $C_{min}/C_{min}) \times 100$] was 49% for this formulation and dosing regimen.

The subjects used for this study exhibited a mean half-life of 8.3 hours (range 5.2–12.2) and a mean clearance of 3.5 L/hour (range 2.3–5.6) as determined in a separate single-dose clearance study using 500 mg of immediate release theophylline, prior to this multiple-dose study.

(200 mg)

A multiple-dose steady-state study was conducted in sixteen normal subjects, with one 200 mg tablet given every 12 hours for eight doses. Three high fat content meals were served at 6:30 a.m., 12 noon and 6:30 p.m. Dosing began one-half hour after the evening meal with the test dose occurring one-half hour after breakfast. At steady-state following the eighth dose, the mean C_{max} was 5.1 mcg/mL and the mean C_{min} was 3.7 mcg/mL. The mean time to peak concentration was 6.2 hours. The average percent fraction of fluctuation was 39%.

The subjects used for this study exhibited a mean half-life of 8.7 hours (range 5.0–14.6) and a mean clearance of 3.6 L/hour (range 2.2–6.1).

(100 mg)

A multiple-dose steady-state study was conducted in sixteen normal subjects, with three 100 mg tablets given every 12 hours for eight doses. Three high fat content meals were served at 6:30 a.m., 12 noon and 6:30 p.m. Dosing began one-half hour after the evening meal with the test dose occurring one-half hour after breakfast. At steady-state following the eighth dose, the mean C_{max} was 8.1 mcg/mL and the mean C_{min} was 5.6 mcg/mL. The mean time to peak concentration was 6.2 hours. The average percent fraction of fluctuation was 45%.

The subjects used for this study were the same as those used in the previously cited 200 mg study.

Once-a-Day Dosing:

A multiple-dose, steady-state study was conducted under fed conditions with once-a-day dosing. Fed conditions were the same as those previously cited. Sixteen subjects were dosed as 2 × 300 mg tablets every morning at 8 a.m. for five doses. At steady-state, the mean C_{max} was 11.7 mcg/mL, and the mean C_{min} was 3.4 mcg/mL. The average percent fraction of fluctuation was 244%. The mean t_{max} was 8.7 hours.

The subjects used in the above study exhibited a mean half-life of 7.9 hours (range 5.3–13.4) and a mean clearance of 3.8 L/hour (range 2.3–5.7).

INDICATIONS AND USAGE

For relief and/or prevention of symptoms from asthma and reversible bronchospasm associated with chronic bronchitis and emphysema.

CONTRAINDICATIONS

This product is contraindicated in individuals who have shown hypersensitivity to its components. It is also contraindicated in patients with active peptic ulcer disease, and in individuals with underlying seizure disorders (unless receiving appropriate anticonvulsant medication).

WARNINGS

Serum levels above 20 mcg/mL are rarely found after appropriate administration of the recommended doses. However, in individuals in whom theophylline plasma clearance is reduced *for any reason*, even conventional doses may result in increased serum levels and potential toxicity. Reduced theophylline clearance has been documented in the following readily identifiable groups: 1) patients with impaired renal or liver function; 2) patients over 55 years of age, particularly males and those with chronic lung disease; 3) those with cardiac failure from any cause; 4) patients with sustained high fever; 5) neonates and infants under 1 year of age; and 6) those patients taking certain drugs (see **PRECAUTIONS, Drug Interactions**). Frequently, such patients have markedly prolonged theophylline serum levels following discontinuation of the drug.

Reduction of dosage and laboratory monitoring are especially appropriate in the above individuals.

Serious side effects such as ventricular arrhythmias, convulsions, or even death may appear as the first sign of theophylline toxicity without any previous warning. Less serious signs of theophylline toxicity (ie, nausea and restlessness) may occur frequently when initiating therapy, but are usually transient; when such signs are persistent during maintenance therapy, they are often associated with serum concentrations above 20 mcg/mL.

Stated differently, *serious toxicity is not reliably preceded by less severe side-effects.* A serum concentration measurement is the only reliable method of predicting potentially life-threatening toxicity.

Many patients who require theophylline may exhibit tachycardia due to their underlying disease process so that the cause/effect relationship to elevated serum theophylline concentrations may not be appreciated.

Theophylline products may cause or worsen arrhythmias and any significant change in rate and/or rhythm warrants monitoring and further investigation.

Studies in laboratory animals (minipigs, rodents, and dogs) recorded the occurrence of cardiac arrhythmias and sudden death (with histologic evidence of myocardial necrosis) when beta-agonists and methylxanthines were administered concurrently. The significance of these findings when applied to humans is currently unknown.

PRECAUTIONS

THEO-X TABLETS SHOULD NOT BE CHEWED OR CRUSHED.

General: On the average, theophylline half-life is shorter in cigarette and marijuana smokers than in non-smokers, but smokers can have half-lives as long as non-smokers. Theophylline should not be administered concurrently with other xanthines. Use with caution in patients with hypoxemia, hypertension, or those with history of peptic ulcer. Theophylline may occasionally act as a local irritant to the G.I. tract although gastrointestinal symptoms are more commonly centrally mediated and associated with serum drug concentrations over 20 mcg/mL.

Information for Patients: The importance of taking only the prescribed dose and time interval between doses should be reinforced. THEO-X Extended-Release Tablets should not be chewed or crushed. When dosing THEO-X on a once daily (q24h) basis, tablets should be taken whole and not split. The patient should alert the physician if symptoms occur repeatedly, especially near the end of a dosing interval.

Laboratory Tests: Serum levels should be monitored periodically to determine the theophylline level associated with observed clinical response and as the method of predicting toxicity. For such measurements, the serum sample should be obtained at the time of peak concentration, under steady-state conditions at approximately 6 hours after administration for this sustained-release product. It is important that the patient will not have missed or taken additional doses during the previous 48 hours and that dosing intervals will have been reasonably equally spaced. DOSAGE ADJUSTMENT BASED ON SERUM THEOPHYLLINE MEASUREMENTS WHEN THESE INSTRUCTIONS HAVE NOT BEEN FOLLOWED MAY RESULT IN RECOMMENDATIONS THAT PRESENT RISK OF TOXICITY TO THE PATIENT.

Drug Interactions:

Drug-Drug: Toxic synergism with ephedrine has been documented and may occur with some other sympathomimetic bronchodilators. In addition, the following drug interactions have been demonstrated:

Theophylline with:

Allopurinol (high-dose)	Increased serum theophylline levels
Cimetidine	Increased serum theophylline levels
Ciprofloxacin	Increased serum theophylline levels
Erythromycin, Troleandomycin	Increased serum theophylline levels
Lithium carbonate	Increased renal excretion of lithium
Oral contraceptives	Increased serum theophylline levels
Phenytoin	Decreased theophylline and pheyntoin serum levels
Propranolol	Increased serum theophylline levels
Rifampin	Decreased serum theophylline levels

Drug-Food: Taking THEO-X Extended-Release Tablets immediately after ingesting a high fat content meal (45 g fat, 55 g carbohydrates, 28 g protein, 789 calories) may result in a somewhat higher C_{max} and delayed T_{max}, and a somewhat greater extent of absorption when compared to taking in the fasting state. The influence of the type and amount of other foods, as well as the time interval between drug and food, has not been studied.

Drug-Laboratory Tests Interactions: Currently available analytical methods, including high pressure liquid chromatography and immunoassay techniques, for measuring serum theophylline levels are specific. Metabolites and other drugs generally do not affect the results. Other new analytic methods are also now in use. The physician should be aware of the laboratory method used and whether other drugs will interfere with the assay for theophylline.

Carcinogenesis, Mutagenesis, and Impairment of Fertility: Long-term carcinogenicity studies have not been performed with theophylline.

Chromosome-breaking activity was detected in human cell cultures at concentrations of theophylline up to 50 times the therapeutic serum concentrations in humans. Theophylline was not mutagenic in the dominant lethal assay in male mice given theophylline intraperitoneally in doses up to 30 times the maximum daily human oral dose.

Studies to determine the effect on fertility have not been performed with theophylline.

Pregnancy: Category C—Animal reproduction studies have not been conducted with theophylline. It is also not known whether theophylline can cause fetal harm when administered to a pregnant woman or can affect reproduction capacity. Xanthines should be given to a pregnant woman only if clearly needed.

Nursing Mothers: Theophylline is distributed into breast milk and may cause irritability or other signs of toxicity in nursing infants. Because of the potential for serious adverse reactions in nursing infants from theophylline, a decision should be made whether to discontinue nursing or to discontinue the drug, taking into account the importance of the drug to the mother.

Pediatric Use: Safety and effectiveness of THEO-X Extended-Release Tablets administered:

1. Every 24 hours in children under 12 years of age, have not been established.
2. Every 12 hours in children under 6 years of age, have not been established.

ADVERSE REACTIONS

The following adverse reactions have been observed, but there has not been enough systematic collection of data to support an estimate of their frequency. The most consistent adverse reactions are usually due to overdosage.

1. *Gastrointestinal:* nausea, vomiting, epigastric pain, hematemesis, diarrhea.
2. *Central nervous system:* headaches, irritability, restlessness, insomnia, reflex hyperexcitability, muscle twitching, clonic and tonic generalized convulsions.
3. *Cardiovascular:* palpitation, tachycardia, extrasystoles, flushing, hypotension, circulatory failure, ventricular arrhythmias.
4. *Respiratory:* tachypnea.
5. *Renal:* potentiation of diuresis.
6. *Others:* alopecia, hyperglycemia, inappropriate ADH syndrome, rash.

OVERDOSAGE

Management: It is suggested that the management principles (consistent with the clinical status of the patient when first seen) outlined below be instituted and that simultaneous contact with a Regional Poison Control Center be established. In this way both updated information and individualization regarding required therapy may be provided.

1. When potential oral overdose is established and seizure has not occurred:
   a. If patient is alert and seen within the early hours after ingestion, induction of emesis may be of value. Gastric lavage has been demonstrated to be of no value in influencing outcome in patients who present more than 1 hour after ingestion.
   b. Administer a cathartic. Sorbitol solution is reported to be of value.
   c. Administer repeated doses of activated charcoal and monitor theophylline serum levels.
   d. Prophylactic administration of phenobarbital has been shown to increase the seizure threshold in laboratory animals and administration of this drug can be considered.
2. If patient presents with a seizure:
   a. Establish an airway.
   b. Administer oxygen.
   c. Treat the seizure with intravenous diazepam, 0.1 to 0.3 mg/kg up to 10 mg. If seizures cannot be controlled, the use of general anesthesia should be considered.
   d. Monitor vital signs, maintain blood pressure, and provide adequate hydration.
3. If postseizure coma is present:
   a. Maintain airway and oxygenation.
   b. If a result of oral medication, follow above recommendations to prevent absorption of the drug, but intubation and lavage will have to be performed instead of inducing emesis, and the cathartic and charcoal will need to be introduced via a large bore gastric lavage tube.
   c. Continue to provide full supportive care and adequate hydration until the drug is metabolized. In general, drug metabolism is sufficiently rapid so as not to warrant dialysis. If repeated oral activated charcoal is ineffective (as noted by stable or rising serum levels) charcoal hemoperfusion may be indicated.

DOSAGE AND ADMINISTRATION

Taking THEO-X Extended-Release Tablets immediately after a high-fat content meal may result in a somewhat higher C_{max} and delayed T_{max}, and somewhat greater extent of absorption. However, the differences are usually not great and this product may normally be administered without regard to meals.

Effective use of theophylline (ie, the concentration of drug in the serum associated with optimal benefit and minimal risk of toxicity) is considered to occur when the theophylline concentration is maintained from 10 to 20 mcg/mL. The early studies from which these levels were derived were carried out in patients immediately or shortly after recovery from acute exacerbations of their disease (some hospitalized with status asthmaticus).

Although the 20 mcg/mL level remains appropriate as a critical value (above which toxicity is more likely to occur) for safety purposes, additional data are now available which indicate that the serum theophylline concentrations required to produce maximum physiologic benefit may, in fact, fluctuate with the degree of bronchospasm present and are variable. Therefore, the physician should individualize the range appropriate to the patient's requirements, based on both symptomatic response and improvement in pulmonary function. It should be stressed that serum theophylline concentrations maintained at the upper level of the 10 to 20 mcg/mL range may be associated with potential toxicity when factors known to reduce theophylline clearance are operative. (See **WARNINGS**).

If it is not possible to obtain serum level determinations, restriction of the daily dose (in otherwise healthy adults) to not greater than 13 mg/kg/day, to a maximum of 900 mg in divided doses will result in relatively few patients exceeding serum levels of 20 mcg/mL and the resultant greater risk of toxicity.

Caution should be exercised for younger children who cannot complain of minor side-effects. Older adults, those with cor pulmonale, congestive heart failure, and/or liver disease may have unusually low dosage requirements, and thus, may experience toxicity at the maximal dosage recommended below.

Theophylline does not distribute into fatty tissue. Dosage should be calculated on the basis of lean (ideal) body weight were mg/kg doses are presented.

THEO-X (Theophylline Extended-Release Tablets) are recommended for chronic or long-term management and prevention of symptoms, and not for use in treating acute symptoms of asthma and reversible bronchospasm.

Dosage Guidelines:

WARNING: DO NOT ATTEMPT TO MAINTAIN ANY DOSE THAT IS NOT TOLERATED.

Dosage guidelines are approximations only and the wide range of theophylline clearance between individuals (particularly those with concomitant disease) makes indiscriminate usage hazardous.

I. Acute Symptoms:

NOTE: Status asthmaticus should be considered a medical emergency and is defined as that degree of bronchospasm that is not rapidly responsive to usual doses of conventional bronchodilators. Optimal therapy for such patients frequently requires both **additional medication** parenterally administered, and **close monitoring**, preferably in an intensive care setting.

THEO-X (Theophylline Extended-Release Tablets) are not intended for patients experiencing an acute episode of bronchospasm (associated with asthma, chronic bronchitis, or emphysema). Such patients require rapid relief of symptoms and should be treated with an immediate-release or intravenous theophylline preparation (or other bronchodilators) and not with extended-release products.

II. Chronic Therapy:

A. Initiating Therapy with an Immediate-Release Product: It is recommended that the appropriate dosage be established using an immediate-release preparation. A dosage form which allows small incremental doses is desirable for initiating therapy. A liquid preparation should be considered for children to permit easier and more accurate dosage adjustment. Slow clinical titration is generally preferred to help aassure acceptance and safety of the medication and to allow the patient to develop tolerance to transient caffeine-like side-effects. Then, if the total 24-hour dose can be given by use of the available strengths of this product, the patient can usually be switched to THEO-X Extended-Release Tablets giving one-half of the daily dose at 12 hour intervals or one-third daily dose at 8-hour intervals. Patients who metabolize theophylline rapidly, such as the young, smokers, and some non-smoking adults, are the most likely candidates for dosing at 8-hour intervals. Such patients can generally be identified as having trough serum concentrations lower than desired or repeatedly exhibiting symptoms near the end of a dosing interval.

B. Initiating Therapy with THEO-X (Theophylline Extended-Release Tablets):

Alternatively, therapy can be initiated with THEO-X (Theophylline Extended-Release Tablets) since it is available in dosage forms/strengths which permit titration and adjustment of dosage as outlined in the following dosing guidelines. It is recommended that for children under 25 kg proper dosage be established with a liquid preparation to permit titration is small increments.

Initial Dose:

16 mg/kg/24 hours or 400 mg/24 hours (whichever is less) of theophylline in divided doses at 12 hours intervals.

Increasing Dose:

The above dosage may be increased in approximately 25 percent increments at 3 day intervals so long as the drug is tolerated. Following each adjustment, if the clinical response is satisfactory and serum levels can be measured, then such measurements should be obtained, then that dosage level should be maintained. Dosage increases may be made in this manner until the maximum dose indicated in section III below is reached.

It is important that no patient be maintained on any dosage that is not tolerated. When instructing patients to increase dosage according to the schedule above, they should be told not to take a subsequent dose if apparent side effects occur and to resume therapy at a lower dose once adverse effects have disappeared.

Titration and Adjustment and Chronic Maintenance:

If the desired response is not achieved with the above AVERAGE INITIAL DOSE recommendations, there are no adverse reactions and the serum theophylline level cannot be measured, dosage adjustment should proceed by increasing the dose in approximately 25% increments at three-day intervals. Following each adjustment, if the clinical response is satisfactory, then the dosage level should be maintained. DOSAGE increases may be made in this manner up to the following.

III. Maximum Dose of Theophylline Where the Serum Concentration is not Measured:

WARNING: DO NOT ATTEMPT TO MAINTAIN ANY DOSE THAT IS NOT TOLERATED.

Not to exceed the following: (or 900 mg, whichever is less)

Age 6 to under 9 years	24 mg/kg/day
Age 9 to under 12 years	20 mg/kg/day
Age 12 to under 16 Years	18 mg/kg/day
Age 16 years and older	13 mg/kg/day

IV. Measurement of Serum Theophylline Concentrations During Chronic Therapy:

If the above maximum doses are to be maintained or exceeded, serum theophylline measurement is essential (see **PRECAUTIONS, Laboratory Tests,** for guidance).

V. Final Adjustment of Dosage:

Dosage adjustment after serum theophylline measurement:

If serum theophylline is:		Directions:
Within desired range		Maintain dosage if tolerated.
Too high	20 to 25 mcg/mL	Decrease doses by about 10% and recheck serum level after 3 days.
	25 to 30 mcg/mL	Skip the next dose and decrease subsequent doses by about 25%. Recheck serum level after 3 days.
	Over 30 mcg/mL	Skip the next 2 doses and decrease subsequent doses by 50%. Recheck serum level after 3 days.
Too low		Increase dosage by 25% at 3-day intervals until either the desired serum concentration and/or clinical response is achieved. The total daily dose may need to be administered at more frequent intervals if symptoms occur repeatedly at the end of a dosing interval.

The serum concentration may be rechecked at appropriate intervals, but at least at the end of any adjustment period. When the patient's condition is otherwise clinically stable and none of the recognized factors which alter elimination are present, measurement of serum levels need be repeated only every 6 to 12 months.

DOSAGE ADJUSTMENT BASED ON SERUM THEOPHYLLINE CONCENTRATION MEASUREMENTS WHEN THESE INSTRUCTIONS HAVE NOT BEEN FOLLOWED MAY RESULT IN RECOMMENDATIONS THAT PRESENT RISK OF TOXICITY TO THE PATIENT.

Once-Daily Dosing: The slow absorption rate of this preparation may allow once-daily administration in adult non-smokers with appropriate total body clearance and other patients with low dosage requirements. Once-daily dosing should be considered only after the patient has been gradually and satisfactorily titrated to therapeutic levels with q12h dosing. Once-daily dosing should be based on twice the q12h dose and should be initiated at the end of the last q12h dosing interval. The trough concentration (C_{min}) obtained

Continued on next page

Carnrick Laboratories—Cont.

following conversion to once-daily dosing may be lower (especially in high clearance patients) and the peak concentration (C_{max}) may be higher (especially in low clearance patients) than that obtained with q12h dosing. If symptoms recur, or signs of toxicity appear during the once-daily dosing interval, dosing on the q12h basis should be reinstituted.

It is essential that serum theophylline concentrations be monitored before and after transfer to once-daily dosing. Food and posture, along with changes associated with circadian rhythm, may influence the rate of absorpiton and/or clearance rates of theophylline from extended-release dosage forms administered at night. The exact relationship of these and other factors to nightime serum concentrations and the clinical significance of such findings require additional study. Therefore, it is not recommended that THEO-X, when used as a once-a-day product, be administered at night.

HOW SUPPLIED

THEO-X (Theophylline Anhydrous Extended-Release Tablets) for oral administration is available as:

100 mg—White, dye-free, round, bisected, extended-release tablets inscribed with "C" on one side and "8631" on the scored side. Supplied in bottles of 100 (NDC 0086-0031-10) and 500 (NDC 0086-0031-50).

200 mg—White, dye-free, oval-shaped, bisected, extended-release tablets inscribed with "C" on one side and "8632" on the scored side. Supplied in bottles of 100 (NDC 0086-0032-10), 500 (NDC 0086-0032-50) and 1,000 (NDC 0086-0032-90).

300 mg—White, dye-free, capsule-shaped, bisected, extended-release tablets inscribed with "C" on one side and "8633" on the scored side. Supplied in bottles of 100 (NDC 0086-0033-10), 500 (NDC 0086-0033-50) and 1,000 (NDC 0086-0033-90).

Dispense in a well-closed container as defined in the USP. Store at controlled room temperature 15°–30°C (59°–86°F).

CAUTION: Federal law prohibits dispensing without prescription.

Issued 4/92

Shown in Product Identification Section, page 408

Center Laboratories
Division of EM Industries, Inc.
35 CHANNEL DRIVE
PORT WASHINGTON, NY 11050

EPIPEN®/EPIPEN® JR. Auto-Injectors   ℞
Epinephrine Auto-Injectors

Brief summary: Before prescribing, please consult package insert.

DESCRIPTION

The EpiPen Auto-Injectors contain 2 mL Epinephrine Injection for emergency intramuscular use. Each EpiPen Auto-Injector delivers a single dose of 0.3 mg epinephrine from Epinephrine Injection, USP, 1:1000 (0.3 mL) in a sterile solution. Each EpiPen Jr. Auto-Injector delivers a single dose of 0.15 mg epinephrine from Epinephrine Injection, USP, 1:2000 (0.3 mL) in a sterile solution. Each 0.3 mL also contains 1.8 mg sodium chloride, 0.5 mg sodium metabisulfite, hydrochloric acid to adjust pH, and water for injection. The pH range is 2.5–5.0.

CLINICAL PHARMACOLOGY

Epinephrine is a sympathomimetic drug, acting on both alpha and beta receptors. It is the drug of choice for the emergency treatment of severe allergic reactions (Type I) to insect stings or bites, foods, drugs, and other allergens. It can also be used in the treatment of idiopathic or exercise-induced anaphylaxis. Epinephrine when given subcutaneously or intramuscularly has a rapid onset and short duration of action.

INDICATIONS AND USAGE

Epinephrine is indicated in the emergency treatment of allergic reactions (anaphylaxis) to insect stings or bites, foods, drugs and other allergens as well as idiopathic or exercise-induced anaphylaxis. The EpiPen Auto-Injector is intended for immediate self-administration by a person with a history of an anaphylactic reaction. Such reactions may occur within minutes after exposure and consist of flushing, apprehension, syncope, tachycardia, thready or unobtainable pulse associated with a fall in blood pressure, convulsions, vomiting, diarrhea and abdominal cramps, involuntary voiding, wheezing, dyspnea due to laryngeal spasm, pruritis, rashes, urticaria or angioedema. The EpiPen is designed as emergency supportive therapy only and is not a replacement or substitute for immediate medical or hospital care.

CONTRAINDICATIONS

There are no absolute contraindications to the use of epinephrine in a life-threatening situation.

WARNINGS

Epinephrine is light sensitive and should be stored in the tube provided. Store at room temperature (15°–30°C/59°–86°F). Do not refrigerate. Before using, check to make sure solution in Auto-Injector is not discolored.

Replace the Auto-Injector if the solution is discolored or contains a precipitate. Avoid possible inadvertent intravascular administration. Select an appropriate injection site such as the thigh. DO NOT INJECT INTO BUTTOCK. Large doses or accidental intravenous injection of epinephrine may result in cerebral hemorrhage due to sharp rise in blood pressure. DO NOT INJECT INTRAVENOUSLY. Rapid acting vasodilators can counteract the marked pressor effects of epinephrine.

Epinephrine is the preferred treatment for serious allergic or other emergency situations even though this product contains sodium metabisulfite, a sulfite that may in other products cause allergic-type reactions including anaphylactic symptoms or life-threatening or less severe asthmatic episodes in certain susceptible persons. The alternatives to using epinephrine in a life-threatening situation may not be satisfactory. The presence of a sulfite in this product should not deter administration of the drug for treatment of serious allergic or other emergency situations.

PRECAUTIONS

Epinephrine is ordinarily administered with extreme caution to patients who have heart disease. Use of epinephrine with drugs that may sensitize the heart to arrhythmias, e.g., digitalis, mercurial diuretics, or quinidine, ordinarily is not recommended. Anginal pain may be induced by epinephrine in patients with coronary insufficiency. The effects of epinephrine may be potentiated by tricyclic antidepressants and monoamine oxidase inhibitors. Hyperthyroid individuals, individuals with cardiovascular disease, hypertension, or diabetes, elderly individuals, pregnant women, and children under 30 kg (66 lbs.) body weight may be theoretically at greater risk of developing adverse reactions after epinephrine administration. Despite these concerns, epinephrine is essential for the treatment of anaphylaxis. Therefore, patients with these conditions, and/or any other person who might be in a position to administer EpiPen or EpiPen Jr. to a patient experiencing anaphylaxis should be carefully instructed in regard to the circumstances under which this lifesaving medication should be used.

CARCINOGENESIS, MUTAGENESIS, IMPAIRMENT OF FERTILITY

Studies of epinephrine in animals to evaluate the carcinogenic and mutagenic potential or the effect on fertility have not been conducted.

USAGE IN PREGNANCY

Pregnancy Category C: Epinephrine has been shown to be teratogenic in rats when given in doses about 25 times the human dose. There are no adequate and well-controlled studies in pregnant women. Epinephrine should be used during pregnancy only if the potential benefit justifies the potential risk to the fetus.

PEDIATRIC USE

Epinephrine may be given safely to children at a dosage appropriate to body weight (see Dosage and Administration).

ADVERSE REACTIONS

Side effects of epinephrine may include palpitations, tachycardia, sweating, nausea and vomiting, respiratory difficulty, pallor, dizziness, weakness, tremor, headache, apprehension, nervousness and anxiety.

Cardiac arrhythmias may follow administration of epinephrine.

OVERDOSAGE

Overdosage or inadvertent intravascular injection of epinephrine may cause cerebral hemorrhage resulting from a sharp rise in blood pressure. Fatalities may also result from pulmonary edema because of peripheral vascular constriction together with cardiac stimulation.

DOSAGE AND ADMINISTRATION

Usual epinephrine adult dose for allergic emergencies is 0.3 mg. For pediatric use, the appropriate dosage may be 0.15 or 0.30 mg depending upon the body weight of the patient. However, the prescribing physician has the option of prescribing more or less than these amounts, based on careful assessment of each individual patient and recognizing the life-threatening nature of the reactions for which this drug is being prescribed. With severe persistant anaphylaxis, repeat injections with an additional EpiPen may be necessary.

HOW SUPPLIED

EpiPen and EpiPen Jr. Auto-Injectors are available singly or in packages of twelve.

CAUTION

Federal (U.S.A.) law prohibits dispensing without a prescription.

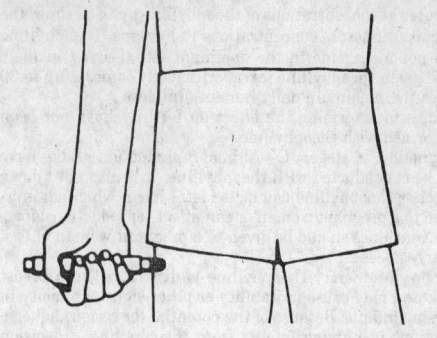

Issued: April 1988

HISTATROL®   ℞
Histamine Base 1 mg/mL
(Histamine Phosphate 2.75 mg/mL)
in Glycerin 50% (v/v)
For Percutaneous Testing

Histamine Base 0.1 mg/mL
(Histamine Phosphate 0.275 mg/mL)
For Intracutaneous (Intradermal) Testing

DESCRIPTION

The chemical formula for Histamine Phosphate is $C_5H_9N_3 \cdot 2H_3PO_4$; its molecular weight is 307.14. For prick, puncture or scratch testing, the product contains 1 mg/mL histamine base (2.75 mg/mL Histamine Phosphate) in Water for Injection; it also contains Glycerin 50% (v/v) as viscosity agent and Phenol 0.4% as preservative. For intracutaneous (intradermal) skin testing, the product contains 0.1 mg/mL histamine base (0.275 mg/mL Histamine Phosphate) in Water for Injection and Phenol 0.4% as preservative. The product should be stored refrigerated and protected from light.

CLINICAL PHARMACOLOGY

Histamine acts as a potent vasodilator when released from mast cells during an allergic reaction. It is largely responsible for the immediate skin test reaction of a sensitive patient when challenged with an offending allergen.

The effect of added Glycerin (50% v/v) to 1 mg/mL histamine base was studied by puncture testing using a bifurcated needle in twelve volunteer subjects. The mean sum of cross diameters of the wheals was 13.25mm for the non-glycerinated, and 12.54mm for the glycerinated formulation. Sum of cross-diameters of erythema was 52.88mm for the non-glycerinated, and 54.42mm for the glycerinated formulation. These differences are not statistically significant.

INDICATIONS AND USAGE

For use as a positive control in evaluation of allergenic (immediate hypersensitivity or "Type I") skin testing.

CONTRAINDICATIONS

Histamine should not be injected into individuals with hypotension, severe hypertension, severe cardiac, pulmonary, or renal disease. Not to be used for diagnosis of pheochromocytoma or to test the ability of the gastric mucosa to secrete hydrochloric acid.

WARNINGS

Care must be taken in intracutaneous testing to avoid injection into a venule or capillary. Pull back gently on the syringe plunger and note if blood is drawn. If blood is drawn, withdraw needle and inject into another skin site.

Small doses by any route of administration may precipitate asthma in patients with bronchial hyperactivity. This product is not intended for inhalation, intracutaneous or subcutaneous injection. The utmost caution is advised in using histamine in such patients and in those with a history of bronchial asthma.

PRECAUTIONS
General

A separate sterile needle or other percutaneous testing device should be used for each individual patient to prevent transmission of hepatitis and other infectious agents from one person to another.

Epinephrine Injection (1:1,000) and injectable antihistamines should be available for immediate use in the event the patient exhibits a severe response. A tourniquet can be applied above the test site to slow absorption if a severe response occurs.

Drug Interactions
Drugs can interfere with the performance of skin tests in general, and specifically with histamine[1].

Antihistamines: Response to histamine is suppressed by antihistamines. The length of suppression varies, and is dependent on individual patient, type of antihistamine and length of time the patient has been on antihistamines. The duration of this suppression may be as little as 24 hours (chlorpheniramine), and can be as long as 40 days (astemizole).

Tricyclic Antidepressants: These exert a potent and sustained decrease of skin reactivity to histamine, which may last for a few weeks.

$Beta_2$ Agonists: Oral terbutaline and parenteral ephedrine, in general, have been shown to decrease allergen induced wheal. Theoretically, this may also reduce whealing capacity to histamine.

Dopamine: Intravenous infusion of dopamine has been shown to inhibit skin test responses to histamine.

Beta Blocking Agents: Propranolol can significantly increase skin test reactivity, including histamine.

Other Drugs: Short acting steroids, inhaled $beta_2$ agonists, theophylline and cromolyn do not seem to affect skin test response.

Pregnancy Category C
There are no adequate and well-controlled studies in pregnant women. However, based on histamine's known ability to contract uterine muscle, exposure or repeated doses should be avoided. HISTATROL should be used during pregnancy only if the potential benefit justifies the potential risk to the fetus or mother.

Pediatric Use
Histamine solutions for percutaneous testing have been given safely in infants and young children.[2,3,4,5] Neonates and infants have lower skin test reactivity to histamines as well as common allergens.[3,4,5,6] About 20% of infants less than six months of age have been observed to have a negative reaction to histamine hydrochloride (1 mg/mL of salt).[4] Skin test reactivity gradually increases to age six and plateaus to age sixty.[2,3] Therefore small skin test reactions should be anticipated in children under age six.

ADVERSE REACTIONS
Following the injection of large doses of histamine, systemic reactions may include flushing, dizziness, headache, bronchial constriction, urticaria, asthma, marked hypertension or hypotension, abdominal cramps, vomiting, metallic taste, and local or generalized allergic manifestations.

OVERDOSAGE
A large subcutaneous dose of Histamine Phosphate may cause severe occipital headache, blurred vision, anginal pain, a rapid drop in blood pressure, and cyanosis of the face. Overdosage may cause severe symptoms including vasomotor collapse, shock, and even death.

Epinephrine Injection given subcutaneously or intramuscularly should be used in case of emergency due to severe reactions (see Precautions). An antihistamine preparation may be given intramuscularly to ameliorate systemic reaction to overdose.

DOSAGE AND ADMINISTRATION
For Prick, Puncture and Scratch Testing
Histamine base 1 mg/mL (Histamine Phosphate 2.75 mg/mL) should be used to give a reaction. (Refer to Interpretation Section.)

Prick, Puncture or Scratch Test Techniques
1. The skin in the test area should be cleansed with alcohol and air dried.
2. The histamine control skin test solution should be placed at the same site with the other skin test antigens, either on the patient's back or on the volar surface of the forearm. The patient should be placed in a comfortable position before the testing is begun.
3. For the prick test, a sharp needle is used to puncture the skin, but not to draw blood. If the scratch test is used, carefully break or scratch the skin with a sterile scarifier. Do not draw blood. Each scratch should be about 2 mm - 4 mm in length.
4. A small drop of the histamine base 1 mg/mL (Histamine Phosphate 2.75 mg/mL) is placed on the abraded skin site no closer than 4 or 5 cm from an adjacent test site. Some physicians prefer to place the solution on the test area and then prick through the drop with a sharp needle.
5. Use a separate sterile scarifier or needle for each patient.
6. The test should be read in 15–20 minutes; if a large wheal reaction occurs before that time the test site should be wiped free of histamine.

Interpretation
The patient's response is based on the size of: erythema (degree of redness) and/or size of wheal (smooth, slightly elevated area) which appear after 15–20 minutes.

For prick, puncture and scratch testing histamine base 1 mg/mL (Histamine Phosphate 2.75 mg/mL) should be used to give a positive reaction. In a large population, the NHANES II survey reports a mean diameter (average of length and width) wheal of 4.4 mm ± 1.65 mm (± standard deviation) and a mean erythema of 18.4 mm ± 8.55 mm (± standard deviation) when using 25 gauge B-D needle by prick puncture (Pepys) technique.[7] All positive reactions should be interpreted against an appropriate negative control.

For Intradermal Skin Testing
Histamine base 0.1 mg/mL (Histamine Phosphate 0.275 mg/mL) or 0.01 mg/mL should be used to give a reaction. (Refer to Interpretation Section.)

Intracutaneously (Intradermal) Test Techniques
1. The skin should be cleansed with alcohol and air dried.
2. A sterile one milliliter tuberculin syringe with 26 or 27 gauge needle should be used. A single sterile syringe should be used for each solution to assure sterility. Only the histamine base 0.1 mg/mL (Histamine Phosphate, 0.275 mg/mL) or greater dilution solution should be used.
3. The histamine base skin test solution should be injected at the same site with the other skin test allergens, either on the patient's back or on the arm. The patient should be placed in a comfortable position before the testing is begun.
4. The skin is held tense and the needle is inserted almost parallel to the skin, bevel side up, far enough to cover the beveled portion. Slowly inject 0.01 mL or 0.02 mL, making a small bleb approximately 3 mm - 5 mm in diameter.
5. The test should be read in 15–20 minutes.

Interpretation
The patient's response is based on the size of: erythema (degree of redness) and/or size of wheal (smooth, slightly elevated area) which appear after 15–20 minutes.

For intradermal skin testing histamine base 0.1 mg/mL (Histamine Phosphate 0.275 mg/mL) or 0.01 mg/mL should be used to give a positive reaction. The available 0.1 mg/mL concentration must be diluted ten-fold to achieve this dose. All positive reactions should be interpreted against an appropriate negative control. In two successive years of testing, the Committee on Standardization of the American College of Allergy reported positive reactions at histamine base doses of 0.01 mg/mL and higher.[7] Mean sum of wheal diameters was approximately 14 mm ± 4.8 mm and sum of erythema diameters was approximately 52 mm ± 21.6 mm following 0.01 mL intradermal doses of 0.01 mg/mL histamine base. When 0.01 mL of 0.1 mg/mL histamine base was injected, the sum of crossed diameters of wheal ranged from 15 - 20 mm and the sum of crossed diameters of erythema ranged from 60 - 80 mm.[8]

HOW SUPPLIED
Multidose vials containing 5 mL histamine base, 1 mg/mL (Histamine Phosphate 2.75 mg/mL) in Glycerin 50% (v/v) for prick, puncture, or scratch testing. Multidose vials containing 5 mL histamine base, 0.1 mg/mL (Histamine Phosphate 0.275 mg/mL) in aqueous solution for intradermal testing. Store at 2° -8°C.

REFERENCES

1. Bousquet, J.: In vivo methods for the study of allergy: skin test, techniques, and interpretation. In Allergy Principles and Practice, 3rd Edition, Middleton, et al eds., C.V. Mosby, St. Louis, MO, 1988.
2. Skassa-Brociek, W., et al.: Skin test reactivity to histamine from infancy to old age. J. Allergy Clin. Immunol. **80**:711, 1987.
3. Menardo, J.L. et al.: Skin test reactivity in infancy, J. Allergy Clin. Immunol. **75**:646, 1985.
4. Van Asperen, P.P., et al.: Skin test reactivity and clinical allergen sensitivity in infancy. J. Allergy Clin. Immunol. **73**: 381, 1984.
5. Matheson, A., et al.: Reactivity of the skin of the newborn infant. Pediatrics **10**:181, 1952.
6. Stevenson, D.D., et al.: Development of IgE in newborn human infants. J. Allergy **48**:61, 1971.
7. Committee on Standardization. Report of the Committee on Standardization: 1. A method of evaluating skin test response. Ann. Allergy **29**:30–34, 1971.
8. National Center for Health Statistics, P.J. Gergen and P.C. Turkeltaub: Percutaneous immediate hypersensitivity to eight allergens, United States, 1976–80. *Vital and Health Statistics.* Series 11, No. 235, DHHS Pub. No. (PHS) 86–1685. Public Health Service, Washington. U.S. Government Printing Office, July 1986.

Date of Issue: February, 1990.

Products are cross-indexed by generic and chemical names in the **YELLOW SECTION.**

Central Pharmaceuticals, Inc.
120 EAST THIRD STREET
SEYMOUR, IN 47274

AZDŌNE® TABLETS Ⓒ℞
[*ăz'dōn*]

DESCRIPTION
Each tablet contains:

Hydrocodone Bitartrate	5 mg
(WARNING—May be habit forming)	
Aspirin	500 mg

Hydrocodone bitartrate is an opioid analgesic and antitussive and occurs as fine, white crystals or as a crystalline powder. It is affected by light. The chemical name is: 4,5α-epoxy-3-methoxy-17-methylmorphinan-6-one tartrate (1:1) hydrate (2:5).

Aspirin, salicylic acid acetate, is a non-opiate salicylate analgesic, anti-inflammatory, and antipyretic which occurs as a white, crystalline tabular or needle-like powder and is odorless or has a faint odor.

Inactive Ingredients: D&C Red #7 Lake, Pregelatinized Starch and Stearic Acid.

HOW SUPPLIED
Flat, truncated oval, bisected mottled pink tablet containing 5 mg Hydrocodone Bitartrate (WARNING: May be habit formimg) and 500 mg of Aspirin. Each tablet is debossed with the Central logo on one side and the number 21 and the score on the other side.

Bottles of 100 tablets—NDC 0131-2821-37
Bottles of 1000 tablets—NDC 0131-2821-43

Shown in Product Identification Section, page 408

CODICLEAR® DH SYRUP Ⓒ℞
[*kō'dĭ-klēr"*]

DESCRIPTION
A clear, colorless, sweet-tasting syrup for oral administration, which is alcohol-free, sugar-free and dye-free.

Each teaspoonful (5 mL) contains:

Hydrocodone bitartrate	5 mg
(Warning—May be habit forming)	
Guaifenesin	100 mg

This product contains ingredients of the following therapeutic classes: antitussive and expectorant.

CAUTION
Federal law prohibits dispensing without prescription.

CLINICAL PHARMACOLOGY
Hydrocodone bitartrate is a potent antitussive which causes suppression of the cough reflex by a direct action on the cough center. Hydrocodone is approximately three times as potent as codeine on a weight basis, and has a higher addiction potential. Guaifenesin is used as an expectorant. It is thought to increase mucous flow in the lung by stimulation of gastric mucosal reflexes.

INDICATIONS
For the temporary relief of dry, non-productive cough associated with upper and lower respiratory tract congestion.

CONTRAINDICATIONS
Hypersensitivity to hydrocodone or guaifenesin. Hydrocodone is contraindicated in the presence of increased intracranial pressure and whenever ventilatory function is depressed.

WARNINGS
Hydrocodone can produce drug dependence and therefore has the potential for being abused. Codiclear DH should be prescribed and administered with the degree of caution appropriate for this type product.

PRECAUTIONS
General: The hydrocodone in this product may exhibit additive effects with other CNS depressants, including alcohol. Respiratory depression can be a real hazard so caution should be used, especially in patients with chronic obstructive pulmonary disease.

Information for Patients: The hydrocodone may cause drowsiness and ambulatory patients who operate machinery or motor vehicles should be cautioned accordingly.

Drug Interactions: Patients receiving other narcotic analgesics, general anesthetics, phenothiazines, other tranquilizers, sedative hypnotics or other CNS depressants (including alcohol) concomitantly with hydrocodone may exhibit an additive CNS depression. When such combined therapy is contemplated the dose of one or both agents should be reduced. (See WARNINGS.)

Laboratory Interactions: The metabolite of guaifenesin has been found to produce an apparent increase in urinary 5-

Continued on next page

Central—Cont.

hydroxyindoleacetic acid, and guaifenesin therefore may interfere with the interpretation of this test for the diagnosis of carcinoid syndrome. Guaifenesin administration should be discontinued 24 hours prior to the collection of urine specimens for the determination of 5-hydroxyindoleacetic acid.

Usage in Pregnancy: Pregnancy Category C. Hydrocodone has been shown to be teratogenic in hamsters when given in doses 700 times the human dose. There are no adequate and well-controlled studies in pregnant women. CODICLEAR DH Syrup should be used during pregnancy only if the potential benefit justifies the potential risk to the fetus.

ADVERSE REACTIONS

Adverse reactions include drowsiness, lassitude, nausea, giddiness, constipation, respiratory depression and addiction.

DRUG ABUSE AND DEPENDENCE

This product is a Schedule III Controlled Sustance. Because of the hydrocodone content, some abuse might be expected. Psychic dependence, physical dependence and tolerance may develop upon repeated administration. It should be prescribed and administered with the degree of caution appropriate for this type product.

OVERDOSAGE

Symptoms of overdosage include respiratory depression, extreme somnolence progressing to stupor or coma, skeletal muscle flaccidity, cold and clammy skin and other symptoms common with narcotic overdosage.

Primary treatment consists of insuring adequate respiration through provision of a patent airway and the institution of assisted or controlled ventilation. Naloxone hydrochloride should be administered in small intravenous doses (consult specific product labeling before use). In addition, oxygen, intravenous fluids, vasopressors and other supportive measures should be employed as indicated. Gastric emptying may be useful in removing unabsorbed drug. Activated charcoal may also be of benefit.

DOSAGE AND ADMINISTRATION

Usual Adult Dose—One teaspoonful (5 mL) after meals and at bedtime, not less than 4 hours apart (not to exceed 6 teaspoonful in a 24 hour period.) Treatment should be initiated with one teaspoonful and subsequent doses, up to a maximum single dose of 3 teaspoonsful, adjusted if required. Usual Children's Dose—Over 12 years: Initial dose 1 teaspoonful; maximum single dose, 2 teaspoonful. 2-12 years: Initial dose ½ teaspoonful: maximum single dose, 1 teaspoonful. Under 2 years: Narcotic antitussives are not recommended for use in children under 2 years of age. Children under 2 years may be more susceptible to the respiratory depressant effects of narcotics, including respiratory arrest, coma, and death. However, dosages based on hydrocodone, 0.3 mg/kg/24 hours divided into four equal doses have been suggested.

HOW SUPPLIED

Bottles of 4 fl. oz.—NDC 0131-5134-64
Bottles of one pint—NDC 0131-5134-70

CODIMAL® DH   ℃ ℞
[kō'di-mahl"]

DESCRIPTION

Each teaspoonful (5 mL) of CODIMAL DH contains: Hydrocodone Bitartrate 1.66 mg. (Warning—May be habit forming); Phenylephrine Hydrochloride 5.0 mg.; Pyrilamine Maleate 8.33 mg. Alcohol-Free.

HOW SUPPLIED

Codimal DH (Red Syrup)
4oz—NDC# 0131-5129-64
Pint—NDC# 0131-5129-70
Gallon—NDC# 0131-5129-72

CODIMAL® DM   OTC
[kō' di-mahl"]

DESCRIPTION

Each teaspoonful (5 mL) of CODIMAL® DM contains: Dextromethorphan hydrobromide 10 mg.; Phenylephrine hydrochloride 5 mg; Pyrilamine maleate 8.33 mg.; Sugar-Free, Dye-Free, Alcohol-Free

HOW SUPPLIED

Codimal® DM (Clear Syrup)
4 oz-NDC # 0131-5131-64
Pint-NDC# 0131-5131-70
Gallon-NDC# 0131-5131-72
For full information see product labeling.

CODIMAL®-L.A. CAPSULES   ℞
[kō'di-mahl"]

DESCRIPTION

Each Extended Release Capsule contains:
Chlorpheniramine maleate .... 8 mg
Pseudoephedrine
hydrochloride .... 120 mg
in a specially prepared base to provide prolonged action.

HOW SUPPLIED

No. 1 clear body, red cap printed with white Central logo and 40, filled with red, white, and blue beads.
Bottle of 100 Capsules-NDC 0131-4213-37
Bottle of 1000 Capsules-NDC 0131-4213-43
Shown in Product Identification Section, page 408

CODIMAL®–L.A. HALF CAPSULES   ℞

DESCRIPTION

Each Extended-Release Capsule contains:
Chlorpheniramine Maleate .... 4 mg
Pseudoephedrine Hydrochloride .... 60 mg
in a specially prepared base to provide prolonged action.

HOW SUPPLIED

Bottle of 100 Capsules
NDC 0131-4501-37
Shown in Product Identification Section, page 408

CODIMAL® PH   OTC
[kō' di-mahl"]

DESCRIPTION

Each teaspoonful (5 mL) of CODIMAL® PH contains: Codeine Phosphate 10 mg. (Warning-May be habit forming); Phenylephrine Hydrochloride 5 mg.; Pyrilamine Maleate 8.33 mg. Alcohol-Free

HOW SUPPLIED

Codimal® PH (Red Syrup)
4 oz-NDC# 0131-5038-64
Pint-NDC# 0131-5038-70
Gallon-NDC# 0131-5038-72

CO-GESIC®   ℃ ℞
TABLETS
(Hydrocodone Bitartrate and Acetaminophen Tablets)

DESCRIPTION

Each CO-GESIC® Tablet contains:
Hydrocodone Bitartrate* .... 5 mg
*WARNING: May be habit forming.
Acetaminophen.. 500 mg

DOSAGE AND ADMINISTRATION

Dosage should be adjusted according to the severity of the pain and the response of the patient. However, it should be kept in mind that tolerance to hydrocodone can develop with continued use and that the incidence of untoward effects is dose related.

The usual adult dosage is one or two tablets every four to six hours as needed for pain. The total 24 hour dose should not exceed 8 tablets.

HOW SUPPLIED

CO-GESIC® [Hydrocodone Bitartrate 5 mg (Warning: May be habit forming) and Acetaminophen 500 mg] Tablets are oval-shaped, white, scored compressed tablets debossed with 500 and 5 separated by bisect on one side and Central logo on the other.
Bottle of 100 tablets: NDC 0131-2104-37
Bottle of 500 tablets: NDC 0131-2104-41
Shown in Product Identification Section, page 408

GUAIMAX-D™   ℞
[guī'-max"]

DESCRIPTION

Each GUAIMAX-D™ white to off-white uncoated, scored, extended-release tablet for oral administration contains:
Pseudoephedrine
Hydrochloride .... 120 mg
Guaifenesin .... 600 mg
in a special base to provide a prolonged therapeutic effect. This product contains ingredients of the following therapeutic classes: nasal decongestant and expectorant.
Pseudoephedrine hydrochloride is a nasal decongestant having the chemical name, benzenemethanol, α[1-(me-

thylamino) ethyl]-, [S-(R^*,R^*)]-, hydrochloride, with the following structure:

$C_{10}H_{15}NO.HCl$ M.W. 201.70

Guaifenesin is an expectorant having the chemical name, 1, 2-propanediol, 3-(2-methoxyphenoxy)-, with the following structure:

$C_{10}H_{14}O_4$ M.W. 198.22

Inactive Ingredients: Each tablet contains Flavor, Magnesium Stearate, Microcrystalline Cellulose, Talc and other ingredients.

CLINICAL PHARMACOLOGY

Pseudoephedrine hydrochloride is an α-adrenergic receptor agonist (sympathomimetic) which produces vasoconstriction by stimulating α-receptors within the mucosa of the respiratory tract. Clinically, pseudoephedrine shrinks swollen mucous membranes, reduces tissue hyperemia, edema, and nasal congestion, and increases nasal airway patency. Guaifenesin promotes lower respiratory tract drainage by thinning bronchial secretions, lubricates irritated respiratory tract membranes through increased mucus flow, and facilitates removal of viscous, inspissated mucus. As a result of these drugs, sinus and bronchial drainage is improved, and dry, nonproductive coughs become more productive and less frequent.

INDICATIONS AND USAGE

GUAIMAX-D™ tablets are indicated for the relief of nasal congestion due to the common cold, hay fever or other upper respiratory allergies, and nasal congestion associated with sinusitis; to promote nasal or sinus drainage; for the symptomatic relief of respiratory conditions characterized by dry nonproductive cough and in the presence of tenacious mucus and/or mucous plugs in the respiratory tract.

CONTRAINDICATIONS

GUAIMAX-D™ tablets are contraindicated in patients with a known hypersensitivity to any of its ingredients, in nursing mothers, or in patients with severe hypertension, severe coronary artery disease, prostatic hypertrophy, or in patients on MAO inhibitor therapy.

WARNINGS

Sympathomimetic amines should be used with caution in patients with hypertension, diabetes mellitus, heart disease, peripheral vascular disease, increased intraocular pressure, hyperthyroidism, or prostatic hypertrophy.

PRECAUTIONS

General: Hypertensive patients should use GUAIMAX-D™ tablets only with medical advice, as they may experience a change in blood pressure due to added vasoconstriction.

Information for Patients: Persistent cough may indicate a serious condition. If cough persists for more than one week, tends to recur, or is accompanied by a high fever, rash, or persistent headache, consult a physician.

Drug Interactions: MAO inhibitors and beta adrenergic blockers increase effects of sympathomimetics. Sympathomimetics may reduce the antihypertensive effects of methyldopa, guanethidine, mecamylamine, reserpine and veratrum alkaloids.

Drug/Laboratory Test Interactions: Guaifenesin has been reported to interfere with clinical laboratory determinations of urinary 5-hydroxyindoleacetic acid (5-HIAA) and urinary vanillylmandelic acid (VMA).

Pregnancy: Pregnancy Category C. Animal reproduction studies have not been conducted with GUAIMAX-D™ tablets. It is also not known whether GUAIMAX-D™ tablets can cause fetal harm when administered to a pregnant woman or can affect reproduction capacity. GUAIMAX-D™ tablets should be given to a pregnant woman only if clearly needed.

Nursing Mothers: GUAIMAX-D™ tablets are contraindicated in the nursing mother because of the higher than usual risks to infants from sympathomimetic agents.

Usage in Elderly: Patients 60 years and older are more likely to experience adverse reactions to sympathomimetics. Overdose may cause hallucinations, convulsions, CNS depression and death. Demonstrate safe use of a short-acting sympathomimetic before use of a sustained action formulation in elderly patients.

Pediatric Use: Safety and effectiveness of GUAIMAX-D™ tablets in children below the age of 6 have not been established.

ADVERSE REACTIONS

Gastrointestinal: nausea and vomiting.
Central Nervous System: nervousness, dizziness, sleeplessness, lightheadedness, tremor, hallucinations, convulsions, CNS depression, fear, anxiety, headache, increased irritability or excitement.
Cardiovascular: palpitations, tachycardia, cardiovascular collapse and death.
General: weakness.
Respiratory: respiratory difficulties.

OVERDOSAGE

Symptoms: Overdosage may cause hallucinations, convulsions, CNS depression, cardiovascular collapse and death.
Treatment: Treatment of overdosage should provide symptomatic care. If the amount ingested is considered dangerous or excessive, induce vomiting with ipecac syrup unless the patient is convulsing, comatose, or has lost the gag reflex, in which case, perform gastric lavage using a large-bore tube. If indicated, follow with activated charcoal and a saline cathartic. Since the effects of GUAIMAX-D™ tablets may last up to 12 hours, treatment should be continued for at least that length of time.

DOSAGE AND ADMINISTRATION

Adults and children 12 years of age and older: one tablet twice daily (every 12 hours). Children 6 to under 12 years: one-half (½) tablet twice daily (every 12 hours). GUAIMAX-D™ tablets are not recommended for children under 6 years of age. Tablets may be broken in half for ease of administration without affecting release of medication but should not be crushed or chewed prior to swallowing.

HOW SUPPLIED

GUAIMAX-D™ tablets are uncoated white to off-white, debossed with the product name on one side and scored on the other with 131 on the left side and 2055 on the right side.
Bottles of 100 NDC 0131-2055-37

MONO-GESIC® TABLETS ℞

[mon″o-je′zik]
(salsalate)
(salicylsalicylic acid)

DESCRIPTION

Each oval, pink film-coated tablet contains:
Salsalate (salicylsalicylic acid) .... 750 mg
(see **HOW SUPPLIED**)
Mono-Gesic® (Salsalate) is a non-steroidal anti-inflammatory agent for oral administration. Chemically, salsalate (salicylsalicylic acid or 2-hydroxy-benzoic acid 2-carboxyphenyl ester) is a dimer of salicylic acid. It is represented by the following formula:

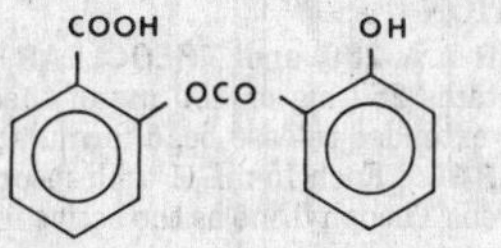

$C_{14}H_{10}O_5$ M.W. 258.2

The ingredient in this product is of the following classes: non-steroidal anti-inflammatory agent and analgesic.
Inactive Ingredients: Castor Oil, D&C Red #30 Lake, Hydroxypropyl Cellulose, Hydroxypropyl Methylcellulose, Microcrystalline Cellulose, Pharmaceutical Glaze, Polyethylene Glycol, Povidone, Propylene Glycol, Sodium Lauryl Sulfate, Sodium Starch Glycolate, Stearic Acid, Titanium Dioxide.

CLINICAL PHARMACOLOGY

Due to the poor solubility of salsalate in gastric fluid, most will pass through the stomach unhydrolyzed and unabsorbed. In the small intestine, it is partially hydrolyzed to two molecules of salicylic acid and rapidly and almost completely absorbed both as the parent compound and as salicylic acid. Salsalate is almost completely excreted in the urine with 7–13 percent of a single dose appearing as glucuronide conjugates of salsalate, less than 1 percent appearing as unchanged salsalate, and the remaining appearing as salicylic acid and its metabolites. The elimination half-life of salsalate is approximately one hour. However, salsalate produces more sustained serum salicylate levels than does acetylsalicylic acid. The reasons for this probably relate to the slower rate of hydrolysis of salsalate than acetylsalicylic acid.
The mode of action of salsalate and other non-steroidal anti-inflammatory drugs is unresolved. Although shown to have anti-inflammatory activity equal to that of aspirin and indomethacen, salsalate is a weak inhibitor of prostaglandin synthesis. Unlike aspirin, salsalate has not been associated with reactions causing asthmatic attacks in susceptible people. Also, it is not known to affect the platelet adhesiveness involved in the clotting mechanism and it causes little gastrointestinal blood loss as compared to other non-steroidal anti-inflammatory agents.

INDICATIONS AND USAGE

Mono-Gesic® is indicated for the temporary relief of symptoms of rheumatoid arthritis, osteoarthritis and related rheumatic disorders.

CONTRAINDICATIONS

Hypersensitivity to salsalate.

WARNINGS

Drugs of this class, salicylates, have been reported to be associated with the development of Reye Syndrome in children and teenagers with chicken pox, influenza, and influenza-like infections.

PRECAUTIONS

General: To avoid potentially toxic concentrations, the plasma salicylic acid levels should be monitored to maintain the therapeutically effective levels of 10 to 30 mg/100 mL. Changes in urinary pH can have significant effects on the plasma level of salicylic acid. Acidification can result in an increase in the plasma level resulting in toxicity while an increase in urinary pH will increase renal clearance and urinary excretion of salicylic acid, thus lowering plasma levels.
Information for Patients: Patients on long-term treatment should be warned not to take other salicylates. They should also be warned that if symptoms of overdosage, such as tinnitus, vertigo, headache, confusion, drowsiness, sweating, hyperventilation, vomiting or diarrhea appear, the drug should be stopped and physician notified.
Drug Interactions: Salicylates antagonize the uricosuric action of drugs used to treat gout. Salicylates will be additive to Mono-Gesic® and could increase plasma concentrations to toxic levels. Drugs and foods that raise urine pH will increase renal clearance and urinary excretion of salicylic acid, thus lowering plasma levels; acidifying drugs or foods will decrease urinary excretion and increase plasma levels. Salicylates may competitively displace anticoagulant drugs from plasma protein binding sites and thereby predispose to systemic bleeding. Salicylates may enhance the hypoglycemic effect of oral antidiabetic drugs of the sulfonylurea class. Salicylate competes with a number of drugs for protein binding sites, notably penicillin, thiopental, thyroxine, triiodothyronine, phenytoin, sulfinpyrazone, naproxen, warfarin, methotrexate, and possibly corticosteroids.
Drug/Laboratory Test Interactions: Salicylate competes with thyroid hormone for binding to plasma proteins, which may be reflected in a depressed plasma T_4 value in some patients; thyroid function and basal metabolism are unaffected.
Carcinogenesis: No long-term animal studies have been performed with Mono-Gesic® to evaluate its carcinogenic potential; however, several such studies using aspirin and other salicylates have failed to demonstrate any association of these agents with cancerous cell changes.
Use in Pregnancy: Pregnancy Category C: Salsalate and salicylic acid have been shown to be teratogenic and embryocidal in rats when given in doses four to five times the usual human dose. These effects were not observed at doses twice as great as the usual human dose. There are no adequate and well-controlled studies in pregnant women. Mono-Gesic® should be used during pregnancy only if the potential benefit justifies the potential risk to the fetus.
Labor and Delivery: There are no adequate and well-controlled studies in pregnant women. Although adverse effects on mother or infant have not been reported with Mono-Gesic® use during labor, caution is advised when anti-inflammatory dosage is involved. However, other salicylates have been associated with prolonged gestation and labor, maternal and neonatal bleeding sequelae, potentiation of narcotic and barbiturate effects (respiratory or cardiac arrest in the mother), delivery problems and stillbirth.
Nursing Mothers: It is not known whether salsalate per se is excreted in human milk; salicylic acid, the primary metabolite of Mono-Gesic®, has been shown to appear in human milk in concentrations approximating the maternal blood level. Thus the infant of a mother on Mono-Gesic® therapy might ingest in mother's milk 30 to 80 percent as much salicylate per kg body weight as the mother is taking. Accordingly, caution should be exercised when Mono-Gesic® is administered to a nursing woman.
Pediatric Use: Safety and effectiveness in children have not been established.

ADVERSE REACTIONS

Adverse reactions are usually the result of overdosage and may include tinnitus and temporary hearing loss, vertigo, headache, confusion, drowsiness, sweating, hyperventilation, vomiting and diarrhea.

DRUG ABUSE AND DEPENDENCE

Drug abuse and dependence have not been reported with Mono-Gesic®.

OVERDOSAGE

IN ALL CASES OF SUSPECTED OVERDOSE, IMMEDIATELY CALL YOUR REGIONAL POISON CENTER and/or SEEK PROFESSIONAL ASSISTANCE. No deaths after overdosage have been reported for Mono-Gesic®. Death has followed ingestion of 10 to 30 g of other salicylates in adults, but much larger amounts have been ingested without fatal outcome.
Signs and Symptoms: The usual symptoms of salicylism (tinnitus, vertigo, headache, confusion, drowsiness, sweating, hyperventilation, vomiting and diarrhea) will occur. More severe intoxication will lead to disruption of electrolyte balance and blood pH, hyperthermia and dehydration.
Treatment: Further absorption of Mono-Gesic® from the G.I. tract should be prevented by emesis (syrup of ipecac) and, if necessary, by gastric lavage.
Fluid and electrolyte imbalance should be corrected by the administration of appropriate I.V. therapy. Adequate renal function should be maintained. Hemodialysis or peritoneal dialysis may be required in extreme cases.

DOSAGE AND ADMINISTRATION

Dosage should be adjusted according to the severity of the disease and the response of the patient. Response will be gradual and full benefits may not be evident for three to four days when plasma salicylate levels have achieved steady state.
The usual dosage is 3,000 mg daily, given in divided doses, such as two 750 mg tablets twice daily or one tablet four times daily.

HOW SUPPLIED

MONO-GESIC® 750 mg tablets:
An oval, pink, film-coated tablet debossed with Central logo on one side and 750 bisect mg on the other side.
Bottles of 100 tablets—NDC 0131-2164-37
Bottles of 500 tablets—NDC 0131-2164-41
Shown in Product Identification Section, page 408

NIFEREX® DAILY TABLETS OTC

[ni′fer″ex]

DESCRIPTION

Each tablet contains:

Vitamin A (as acetate)	5000	IU
Vitamin E (as dl-alpha tocopheryl)	30	IU
Vitamin C (as ascorbic acid)	60	mg
Folic Acid	0.4	mg
B_1 (as thiamine mononitrate)	1.5	mg
B_2 (as riboflavin)	1.7	mg
Niacinamide	20	mg
Pantothenic Acid	10	mg
Biotin	0.3	mg
B_6 (as pyridoxine)	2	mg
B_{12} (as cyanocobalamin)	6	mcg
Vitamin D	400	IU
Calcium	259	mg
(as calcium carbonate and dicalcium phosphate)		
Iodine (as potassium iodide)	150	mcg
Iron (as polysaccharide-iron complex)	18	mg
Phosphorus (as dicalcium phosphate)	5.4	mg
Manganese (as manganese sulfate)	5	mg
Magnesium (as magnesium oxide)	100	mg
Zinc (as zinc sulfate)	15	mg
Copper (as copper sulfate)	2	mg

HOW SUPPLIED

Capsule shaped, lavendar film-coated tablet imprinted with 20 on one side and Central logo on other side.
Bottle of 100—NDC #0131-2210-37

NIFEREX® TABLETS/ELIXIR OTC

[ni′fer″ex]
NIFEREX® with VITAMIN C TABLETS
(polysaccharide-iron complex)

DESCRIPTION

NIFEREX is a highly water-soluble complex of iron and a low molecular weight polysaccharide. Each NIFEREX Film Coated Tablet and each NIFEREX with Vitamin C Chewable Tablet contains 50 mg elemental iron. In addition, each NIFEREX with Vitamin C tablet contains Ascorbic acid, U.S.P., 100 mg. and Sodium ascorbate, 168.75 mg. Each 5 mL (teaspoonful) NIFEREX Elixir contains 100 mg elemental iron, alcohol 10% (sugar free).

ACTION AND USES

NIFEREX is an easily assimilated source of iron for treatment of uncomplicated iron deficiency anemia. Because NIFEREX is a polysaccharide bound iron complex, it is relatively nontoxic and there are relatively few, if any, of the

Continued on next page

Central—Cont.

gastrointestinal side effects associated with iron therapy, thus permitting full therapeutic dosage (150 to 300 mg elemental iron daily) in a single dose if desirable. There is no staining of teeth and no metallic aftertaste.

INDICATIONS
For treatment of uncomplicated iron deficiency anemia.

CONTRAINDICATIONS
In patients with hemochromatosis and hemosiderosis, and in those with a known hypersensitivity to any of the ingredients.

DOSAGE AND ADMINISTRATION
ADULTS: One or two NIFEREX or NIFEREX with Vitamin C Tablets twice daily, or one to two teaspoonfuls NIFEREX Elixir daily or as directed by a physician. CHILDREN 6 to 12 years of age: One or two NIFEREX or one NIFEREX with Vitamin C Tablet daily, or one teaspoonful NIFEREX Elixir daily or as directed by a physician, Children 2 to 6 years of age: ½ teaspoonful NIFEREX Elixir daily or as directed by a physician.

HOW SUPPLIED
Niferex Elixir (dark brown liquid)
Bottles of 8 ounces—NDC 0131-5066-68
Niferex Tablets (round, brown film-coated)
Bottles of 100—NDC 0131-2200-37
Niferex with Vitamin C Tablets (round, brown, compressed, chewable tablet imprinted with Central logo)
Bottles of 50—NDC 0131-2202-34

NIFEREX®-150 CAPSULES   OTC
[ni' fer" ex]
(polysaccharide-iron complex)

DESCRIPTION
NIFEREX is a highly water-soluble complex of iron and a low molecular weight polysaccharide. Each NIFEREX-150 Capsule contains 150 mg elemental iron as polysaccharide-iron complex.

ACTIONS AND USES
NIFEREX is an easily assimilated source of iron for treatment of uncomplicated iron deficiency anemia. Because NIFEREX is a polysaccharide bound iron complex, it is relatively nontoxic and there are relatively few, if any, of the gastrointestinal side effects associated with iron therapy, thus permitting full therapeutic dosage (150 to 300 mg elemental iron daily) in a single dose if desirable. There is no staining of teeth and no metallic aftertaste.

INDICATIONS
For treatment of uncomplicated iron deficiency anemia.

CONTRAINDICATIONS
In patients with hemochromatosis and hemosiderosis, and in those with a known hypersensitivity to any of the ingredients.

DOSAGE AND ADMINISTRATION
ADULTS: One or two NIFEREX-150 Capsules daily.

HOW SUPPLIED
Niferex-150 Capsules (No. 1 opaque brown cap, opaque orange body printed with white Central logo and Central logo, filled with brown beads)
Bottles of 100-NDC 0131-4220-37
Bottles of 1000-NDC 0131-4220-43
Shown in Product Identification Section, page 408

NIFEREX®-150 FORTE CAPSULES   ℞
[ni'fer"ex for'ta]
NIFEREX® FORTE ELIXIR   ℞

DESCRIPTION
Each capsule Niferex®-150 Forte contains:
Iron (Elemental) .... 150 mg
  (as polysaccharide-iron complex)
Folic Acid .... 1 mg
Vitamin B₁₂ .... 25 mcg

Each teaspoon (5 ml) Niferex® Forte Elixir contains:
Iron (Elemental) .... 100 mg
  (as polysaccharide-iron complex)
Folic Acid .... 1 mg
Vitamin B₁₂ .... 25 mcg
Alcohol 10%
Sugar-Free

PRECAUTION
Folic acid, especially in doses above 0.1 mg–0.4 mg daily, may obscure pernicious anemia, in that hematologic remission

may occur while neurological manifestations remain progressive.

DOSAGE AND ADMINISTRATION
Adults—one capsule or one teaspoonful of elixir daily or as prescribed by a physician.

HOW SUPPLIED
Niferex-150 Forte Capsules (No. 1 opaque red cap, opaque brown body printed with white Central logo and 44, filled with brown beads)
Bottle of 100—NDC 0131-4330-37
Bottle of 1000—NDC 0131-4330-43
Niferex Forte Elixir (dark brown liquid)
Bottle of 4 fl. oz.—NDC 0131-5065-64
Capsules Shown in Product Identification Section, page 408

NIFEREX®—PN TABLETS   ℞
[ni'fer"ex]

DESCRIPTION
Each film-coated tablet contains:
Iron (Elemental) .... 60 mg
  (as polysaccharide-iron complex)
Folic acid .... 1 mg
Ascorbic acid .... 50 mg
  (as sodium ascorbate)
Cyanocobalamin (Vitamin B₁₂) .... 3 mcg
Vitamin A .... 4000 IU
Vitamin D .... 400 IU
Thiamine mononitrate .... 3 mg
Riboflavin .... 3 mg
Pyridoxine hydrochloride .... 2 mg
Niacinamide .... 10 mg
Calcium (as calcium carbonate) .... 125 mg
Zinc (as zinc sulfate monohydrate) .... 18 mg
This product contains ingredients of the following therapeutic classes: vitamins and minerals.

INACTIVE INGREDIENTS
Acetylated Monoglycerides, Castor Oil, Ethyl Cellulose, FD&C Blue #1 Lake, Hydrogenated Vegetable Oil, Hydroxypropyl Cellulose, Hydroxypropyl Methylcellulose, Magnesium Stearate, Microcrystalline Cellulose, Pharmaceutical Glaze, Polyethylene Glycol, Povidone, and Titanium Dioxide.

CLINICAL PHARMACOLOGY
This product is formulated to meet the needs of the pregnant or lactating patient with special consideration given to adequate amounts of hematopoietic factors, iron, folic acid and cyanocobalamin. Calcium (phosphorus-free) is also included in the formula to help supply the increased requirements of this mineral. The 60 mg of elemental iron is available in the form of Niferex® (polysaccharide-iron complex). This form of iron is especially useful in the pregnant patient because, although it is absorbed as well as ferrous sulfate, it does not produce the gastrointestinal irritation commonly associated with iron salts. In addition, folic acid and cyanocobalamin in therapeutic amounts are included to prevent or treat the significant number of pregnant patients who develop megaloblastic anemia of pregnancy.

INDICATIONS AND USAGE
For the prevention and/or treatment of dietary vitamin and mineral deficiencies associated with pregnancy and lactation.

CONTRAINDICATIONS
Hypersensitivity to any of the ingredients.

WARNINGS
Folic acid alone is improper therapy in the treatment of pernicious anemia and other megaloblastic anemias where vitamin B₁₂ is deficient.

PRECAUTIONS
Folic acid, especially in doses above 0.1 mg–0.4 mg daily may obscure pernicious anemia, in that hematologic remission may occur while neurological manifestations remain progressive.

ADVERSE REACTIONS
Allergic sensitization has been reported following both oral and parenteral administration of folic acid.

DOSAGE AND ADMINISTRATION
One tablet daily or as prescribed by a physician.

HOW SUPPLIED
(Oval, blue film coated tablet imprinted with 131/05)
Bottles of 100 tablets–NDC 0131-2209-37
Bottles of 1000 tablets–NDC 0131-2209-43
Shown in Product Identification Section, page 408

NIFEREX®-PN FORTE TABLETS   ℞

DESCRIPTION
Each tablet contains:
Iron (Elemental) .... 60 mg
  (as polysaccharide-iron complex)
Vitamin A acetate .... 5000 IU
Vitamin D .... 400 IU
Vitamin E .... 30 IU
  (as dl-alpha-tocopheryl acetate)
Vitamin C (ascorbic acid) .... 80 mg
Folic acid .... 1 mg
Thiamine (vitamin B₁) .... 3 mg
  (as thiamine mononitrate)
Riboflavin (vitamin B₂) .... 3.4 mg
Vitamin B₆ (as pyridoxine hydrochloride) .... 4 mg
Niacinamide .... 20 mg
Vitamin B₁₂ (Cyanocobalamin) .... 12 mcg
Calcium (as calcium carbonate) .... 250 mg
Iodine (as potassium iodide) .... 0.2 mg
Magnesium (as magnesium oxide) .... 10 mg
Copper (as cupric oxide) .... 2 mg
Zinc (as zinc sulfate) .... 25 mg

HOW SUPPLIED
Capsule shaped, white film coated tablet imprinted with Central logo on one side and 1 bisect O on the other.
Bottles of 100 Tablets—NDC 0131-2309-37
Shown in Product Identification Section, page 408

PREDNICEN®–M 21-Pak   ℞
[pred "nĭ-sĕn ']
(Prednisone Tablets, USP)

DESCRIPTION
Each white film-coated tablet imprinted with 131/07 contains:
Prednisone .... 5 mg

HOW SUPPLIED
Unit Pack 21 x 5 mg.—NDC # 0131-2228-81
Also Available in
Bottle of 100—NDC # 0131-2228-37
Bottle of 1000—NDC # 0131-2228-43

THEOCLEAR® L.A.–260 CAPSULES   ℞
[the 'ō-klēr "]
THEOCLEAR® L.A.–130 CAPSULES   ℞
THEOCLEAR®–80 Syrup   ℞
(theophylline syrup)

DESCRIPTION
THEOCLEAR L.A.-260 and **THEOCLEAR L.A.-130**: Each capsule contains 260 mg or 130 mg of theophylline anhydrous in an extended-release bead formulation.
THEOCLEAR-80: Each 15 mL (1 tablespoonful) contains 80 mg. Anhydrous Theophylline as the active ingredient. Other ingredients are saccharin sodium; tartaric acid; benzoic acid; citric acid; sorbitol; glycerin; propylene glycol; artificial flavor and purified water. This formulation provides an alcohol-free, dye-free, and sugar-free vehicle containing no corn by-products.

HOW SUPPLIED
Theoclear L.A.-260 Capsule (No. 0 clear cap, clear body printed with black Central logo and 260 mg, filled with white beads)
Bottle of 100—NDC 0131-4248-37
Bottle of 1000—NDC 0131-4248-43
Theoclear L.A.-130 Capsule (No. 1 clear cap, clear body printed with black Central logo and 130 mg, filled with white beads)
Bottle of 100—NDC 0131-4247-37
Theoclear-80 Syrup (Clear, colorless liquid with an anise odor)
One Pint—NDC 0131-5098-70
One Gallon—NDC 0131-5098-72
Capsules shown in Product Identification Section, page 408

Products are
listed alphabetically
in the
PINK SECTION.

Cerenex Pharmaceuticals
Division of Glaxo Inc.
FIVE MOORE DRIVE
RESEARCH TRIANGLE PARK, NC 27709

ZOFRAN® Injection   ℞
[zō'fran]
(ondansetron hydrochloride)
Dilute Before Using
For IV Injection Only

DESCRIPTION
The active ingredient in Zofran® Injection is ondansetron hydrochloride (HCl), the racemic form of ondansetron and a selective blocking agent of the serotonin 5-HT$_3$ receptor type. Chemically it is ($\pm$) 1,2,3,9-tetrahydro-9-methyl-3-[(2-methyl-1H-imidazol-1-yl)methyl] -4H-carbazol-4-one, monohydrochloride, dihydrate. It has the following structural formula:

The empirical formula is $C_{18}H_{19}N_3O \cdot HCl \cdot 2H_2O$, representing a molecular weight of 365.9.
Ondansetron HCl is a white to off-white powder that is soluble in water and normal saline.
Zofran Injection is a clear, colorless, nonpyrogenic, sterile solution for intravenous (IV) injection. Each 1 mL of aqueous solution contains 2 mg of ondansetron as the hydrochloride dihydrate; 8.3 mg of sodium chloride, USP; 0.5 mg of citric acid monohydrate, USP and 0.25 mg of sodium citrate dihydrate, USP as buffers; and 1.2 mg of methylparaben, NF and 0.15 mg of propylparaben, NF as preservatives in water for injection, USP. The pH of the injection solution is 3.3–4.0.

CLINICAL PHARMACOLOGY
Pharmacodynamics: Ondansetron is a selective 5-HT$_3$ receptor antagonist. While ondansetron's mechanism of action has not been fully characterized, it is not a dopamine-receptor antagonist. Serotonin receptors of the 5-HT$_3$ type are present both peripherally on vagal nerve terminals and centrally in the chemoreceptor trigger zone of the area postrema. It is not certain whether ondansetron's antiemetic action is mediated centrally, peripherally, or in both sites. However, cytotoxic chemotherapy appears to be associated with release of serotonin from the enterochromaffin cells of the small intestine. In humans, urinary 5-HIAA (5-hydroxyindoleacetic acid) excretion increases after cisplatin administration in parallel with the onset of emesis. The released serotonin may stimulate the vagal afferents through the 5-HT$_3$ receptors and initiate the vomiting reflex.
In animals, the emetic response to cisplatin can be prevented by pretreatment with an inhibitor of serotonin synthesis, bilateral abdominal vagotomy and greater splanchnic nerve section, or pretreatment with a serotonin 5-HT$_3$ receptor antagonist.
In normal volunteers, single IV doses of 0.15 mg/kg of ondansetron had no effect on esophageal motility, gastric motility, lower esophageal sphincter pressure, or small intestinal transit time. Multiday administration of ondansetron has been shown to slow colonic transit in normal volunteers. Ondansetron has no effect on plasma prolactin concentrations.
Pharmacokinetics: Ondansetron is extensively metabolized in humans, with approximately 5% of a radiolabeled dose recovered as the parent compound from the urine. The primary metabolic pathway is hydroxylation on the indole ring followed by glucuronide or sulfate conjugation.
In normal volunteers, the following mean pharmacokinetic data have been determined following a single 0.15-mg/kg IV dose.

Pharmacokinetics in Normal Volunteers

Age-group	n	Peak Plasma Concentration (ng/mL)	Mean Elimination Half-life (h)	Plasma Clearance (L/h/kg)
19-40	11	102	3.5	0.381
61-74	12	106	4.7	0.319
≥75	11	170	5.5	0.262

A reduction in clearance and increase in elimination half-life are seen in patients over 75 years old. In clinical trials, there was neither a difference in safety nor efficacy between patients over 65 years of age and those under 65 years of age; an insufficient number of patients were over 75 years of age to permit conclusions. No adjustment in dosage is recommended in the elderly.
In adult cancer patients, the mean elimination half-life was 4.0 hours, and there was no difference in the multidose phar-

macokinetics over a 4-day period. In a study of 21 pediatric cancer patients (aged 4–18 years) who received three IV doses of 0.15 mg/kg of ondansetron at 4-hour intervals, patients older than 15 years of age exhibited ondansetron pharmacokinetic parameters similar to those of adults. Patients aged 4–12 years generally showed higher clearance and somewhat larger volume of distribution than adults. Most pediatric patients younger than 15 years of age had a shorter (2.4 hours) ondansetron plasma half-life than patients older than 15 years of age. It is not known whether these differences in ondansetron plasma half-life may result in differences in efficacy between adults and some young children (see CLINICAL TRIALS: Pediatric Studies).
Plasma protein binding of ondansetron as measured in vitro was 70%-76%, with binding constant over the pharmacologic concentration range (10–500 ng/mL). Circulating drug also distributes into erythrocytes.

CLINICAL TRIALS
In a double-blind study of three different dosing regimens of Zofran® (ondansetron HCl) Injection, 0.015 mg/kg, 0.15 mg/kg, and 0.30 mg/kg, each given three times during the course of cancer chemotherapy, the 0.15-mg/kg dosing regimen was more effective than the 0.015-mg/kg dosing regimen. The 0.30-mg/kg dosing regimen was not shown to be more effective than the 0.15-mg/kg dosing regimen.
Cisplatin-Based Chemotherapy: In a double-blind study in 28 patients, Zofran Injection (three 0.15-mg/kg doses) was significantly more effective than placebo in preventing nau-

sea and vomiting induced by cisplatin-based chemotherapy. Treatment response was as follows:
[See table at top .]
Ondansetron was compared with metoclopramide in a single-blind trial in 307 patients receiving cisplatin ≥ 100 mg/m^2 with or without other chemotherapeutic agents. Patients received the first dose of ondansetron or metoclopramide 30 minutes before cisplatin. Two additional ondansetron doses were administered 4 and 8 hours later, or five additional metoclopramide doses were administered 2, 4, 7, 10, and 13 hours later. Cisplatin was administered over a period of 3 hours or less. Episodes of vomiting and retching were tabulated over the period of 24 hours after cisplatin. The results of this study are summarized below:
[See bottom table .]
Forty-one of the ondansetron patients were over 65 years of age. The complete response rate (zero emetic episodes) was 41% in this group compared with 40% in those 65 years old or younger.
Cyclophosphamide-Based Chemotherapy: In a double-blind, placebo-controlled study of Zofran Injection (three 0.15-mg/kg doses) in 20 patients receiving cyclophosphamide (500–600 mg/m^2) chemotherapy, Zofran Injection was significantly more effective than placebo in preventing nausea and vomiting. The results are summarized below:
[See first table on next page.]
Retreatment: In uncontrolled trials, 127 patients receiving cisplatin (median dose, 100 mg/m^2) and ondansetron who

---

Prevention of Chemotherapy-Induced Nausea and Emesis in Single-Day Cisplatin Therapy*

	Zofran Injection	Placebo	p Value†
Number of patients	14	14	
Treatment response			
0 Emetic episodes	2 (14%)	0 (0%)	
1–2 Emetic episodes	8 (57%)	0 (0%)	
3–5 Emetic episodes	2 (14%)	1 (7%)	
More than 5 emetic episodes/rescued	2 (14%)	13 (93%)	0.001
Median number of emetic episodes	1.5	Undefined‡	
Median time to first emetic episode (h)	11.6	2.8	0.001
Median nausea scores (0–100)§	3	59	0.034
Global satisfaction with control of nausea and vomiting (0–100)‖	96	10.5	0.009

* Chemotherapy was high dose (100 and 120 mg/m^2; Zofran Injection n=6, placebo n=5) or moderate dose (50 and 80 mg/m^2; Zofran Injection n=8, placebo n=9). Other chemotherapeutic agents included fluorouracil, doxorubicin and cyclophosphamide. There was no difference between treatments in the types of chemotherapy that would account for differences in response.
† Efficacy based on "all patients treated" analysis.
‡ Median undefined since at least 50% of the patients were rescued or had more than five emetic episodes.
§ Visual analog scale assessment of nausea: 0=no nausea, 100=nausea as bad as it can be.
‖ Visual analog scale assessment of satisfaction: 0=not at all satisfied, 100=totally satisfied.

Prevention of Emesis Induced by Cisplatin (≥ 100 mg/m²) Single-Day Therapy*

	Zofran Injection	Metoclopramide	p Value
Dose	0.15 mg/kg × 3	2 mg/kg × 6	
Number of patients in efficacy population	136	138	
Treatment response			
0 Emetic episodes	54 (40%)	41 (30%)	
1–2 Emetic episodes	34 (25%)	30 (22%)	
3–5 Emetic episodes	19 (14%)	18 (13%)	
More than 5 emetic episodes/rescued	29 (21%)	49 (36%)	
Comparison of treatments with respect to			
0 Emetic episodes	54/136	41/138	0.083
More than 5 emetic episodes/rescued	29/136	49/138	0.009
Median number of emetic episodes	1	2	0.005
Median time to first emetic episode (h)	20.5	4.3	<0.001
Global satisfaction with control of nausea and vomiting (0–100)†	85	63	0.001
Acute dystonic reactions	0	8	0.005
Akathisia	0	10	0.002

* In addition to cisplatin, 68% of patients received other chemotherapeutic agents, including cyclophosphamide, etoposide, and fluorouracil. There was no difference between treatments in the types of chemotherapy that would account for differences in response.
† Visual analog scale assessment: 0=not at all satisfied, 100=totally satisfied.

Continued on next page

Cerenex—Cont.

had two or fewer emetic episodes were retreated with ondansetron and chemotherapy, mainly cisplatin, for a total of 269 retreatment courses (median, 2; range, 1–10). No emetic episodes occurred in 160 (59%), and two or fewer emetic episodes occurred in 217 (81%) retreatment courses.

Pediatric Studies: Four open-label, noncomparative (one US, three foreign) trials have been performed with 209 pediatric cancer patients aged 4–18 years given a variety of cisplatin or noncisplatin regimens. In the three foreign trials, the initial Zofran Injection dose ranged from 0.04–0.87 mg/kg for a total dose of 2.16–12 mg. This was followed by the oral administration of ondansetron ranging from 4–24 mg daily for 3 days. In the US trial, Zofran was administered intravenously (only) in three doses of 0.15 mg/kg each for a total daily dose of 7.2–39 mg. In these studies, 58% of the 196 evaluable patients had a complete response (no emetic episodes) on day 1. Thus, prevention of emesis in these children was essentially the same as for patients older than 18 years of age. Overall, Zofran Injection was well tolerated in these pediatric patients.

INDICATIONS AND USAGE

Zofran® (ondansetron HCl) Injection is indicated for the prevention of nausea and vomiting associated with initial and repeat courses of emetogenic cancer chemotherapy, including high-dose cisplatin.

CONTRAINDICATIONS

Zofran® (ondansetron HCl) Injection is contraindicated for patients known to have hypersensitivity to the drug.

PRECAUTIONS

Drug Interactions: Ondansetron does not itself appear to induce or inhibit the cytochrome P-450 drug-metabolizing enzyme system of the liver. Because ondansetron is metabolized by hepatic cytochrome P-450 drug-metabolizing enzymes, inducers or inhibitors of these enzymes may change the clearance and, hence, the half-life of ondansetron. On the basis of available data, no dosage adjustment is recommended for patients on these drugs. Tumor response to chemotherapy in the P 388 mouse leukemia model is not affected by ondansetron. In humans, carmustine, etoposide, and cisplatin do not affect the pharmacokinetics of ondansetron.

Carcinogenesis, Mutagenesis, Impairment of Fertility: Carcinogenic effects were not seen in 2-year studies in rats and mice with oral ondansetron doses up to 10 and 30 mg/kg per day, respectively. Ondansetron was not mutagenic in standard tests for mutagenicity. Oral administration of ondansetron up to 15 mg/kg per day did not affect fertility or general reproductive performance of male and female rats.

Pregnancy: *Teratogenic Effects: Pregnancy Category B:* Reproduction studies were performed in pregnant rats and rabbits at daily doses up to 4 mg/kg per day and have revealed no evidence of impaired fertility or harm to the fetus due to ondansetron. There are, however, no adequate and well-controlled studies in pregnant women. Because animal reproduction studies are not always predictive of human response, this drug should be used during pregnancy only if clearly needed.

Nursing Mothers: Ondansetron is excreted in the breast milk of rats. It is not known whether ondansetron is excreted in human milk. Because many drugs are excreted in human milk, caution should be exercised when ondansetron is administered to a nursing woman.

Pediatric Use: Little information is available about dosage in children 3 years of age or younger (see DOSAGE AND ADMINISTRATION section for use in children 4–18 years of age).

Use in Elderly Patients: Dosage adjustment is not needed in patients over the age of 65 (see CLINICAL PHARMACOLOGY). Prevention of nausea and vomiting in elderly patients was no different than in younger age-groups.

ADVERSE REACTIONS

Clinical Trial Experience: The following adverse events have been reported in individuals receiving ondansetron at a dosage of three 0.15-mg/kg doses in clinical trials. These patients were receiving concomitant chemotherapy, primarily cisplatin, and IV fluids. Most were receiving a diuretic. [See second table above.]

Gastrointestinal: Constipation has been reported in 11% of chemotherapy patients receiving multiday ondansetron.

Integumentary: Rash has occurred in approximately 1% of patients receiving ondansetron.

Central Nervous System: There have been rare reports of grand mal seizure and a report consistent with, but not diagnostic of, an extrapyramidal reaction in a patient receiving ondansetron.

Hypersensitivity: Rare reports of of bronchospasm.

Altered Laboratory Findings: In comparative trials in cisplatin chemotherapy patients with normal baseline values of

Prevention of Chemotherapy-Induced Nausea and Emesis in Single-Day Cyclophosphamide Therapy*

	Zofran Injection	Placebo	p Value†
Number of patients	10	10	
Treatment response			
0 Emetic episodes	7 (70%)	0 (0%)	0.001
1–2 Emetic episodes	0 (0%)	2 (20%)	
3–5 Emetic episodes	2 (20%)	4 (40%)	
More than 5 emetic episodes/rescued	1 (10%)	4 (40%)	0.131
Median number of emetic episodes	0	4	0.008
Median time to first emetic episode (h)	Undefined‡	8.79	
Median nausea scores (0–100)§	0	60	0.001
Global satisfaction with control of nausea and vomiting (0–100)‖	100	52	0.008

*Chemotherapy consisted of cyclophosphamide in all patients, plus other agents, including fluorouracil, doxorubicin, methotrexate, and vincristine. There was no difference between treatments in the type of chemotherapy that would account for differences in response.
†Efficacy based on "all patients treated" analysis.
‡Median undefined since at least 50% of patients did not have any emetic episodes.
§Visual analog scale assessment of nausea: 0=no nausea, 100=nausea as bad as it can be.
‖Visual analog scale assessment of satisfaction: 0=not at all satisfied, 100=totally satisfied.

Principal Adverse Events in Comparative Trials

	Number of Patients with Event		
	Zofran® Injection n = 185 patients	Metoclopramide n = 156 patients	Placebo n = 34 patients
Diarrhea	41 (22%)	68 (44%)	6 (18%)
Headache	29 (16%)	11 (7%)	5 (15%)
Akathisia	0 (0%)	10 (6%)	0 (0%)
Acute dystonic reactions*	0 (0%)	8 (5%)	0 (0%)

*See Central Nervous System below.

aspartate transaminase (AST) and alanine transaminase (ALT), these enzymes have been reported to exceed twice the upper limit of normal in approximately 5% of patients. The increases were transient and did not appear to be related to dose or duration of therapy. On repeat exposure, similar transient elevations in transaminase values occurred in some courses, but symptomatic hepatic disease did not occur.

Postmarketing Experience: The following adverse events have been reported rarely in the routine management of patients.

Hepatic: From a foreign report, one 76-year-old male patient with lymphoma, who was a carrier of hepatitis B, developed liver failure 3 weeks after a second course of ondansetron (and cyclophosphamide) and subsequently died. The etiology of the liver failure is unclear.

Hypersensitivity: Hypersensitivity reactions (e.g., anaphylaxis, bronchospasm, shortness of breath, hypotension, angioedema, urticaria).

Cardiovascular: Tachycardia, angina (chest pain), and electrocardiographic alterations.

Central Nervous System: Reports consistent with, but not diagnostic of, extrapyramidal reactions.

Special Senses: Transient blurred vision.

Altered Laboratory Findings: Hypokalemia.

Drug Abuse and Dependence: Animal studies have shown that ondansetron is not discriminated as a benzodiazepine nor does it substitute for benzodiazepines in direct addiction studies.

OVERDOSAGE

There is no specific antidote for ondansetron overdose. Patients should be managed with appropriate supportive therapy. Individual doses as large as 145 mg and total daily dosages (three doses) as large as 252 mg have been administered intravenously without significant adverse events. These doses are more than 10 times the recommended daily dose.

DOSAGE AND ADMINISTRATION

The recommended IV dosage of Zofran® (ondansetron HCl) Injection is three 0.15-mg/kg doses. The first dose is infused over 15 minutes beginning 30 minutes before the start of emetogenic chemotherapy. Subsequent doses are administered 4 and 8 hours after the first dose of Zofran Injection. Zofran Injection should be diluted in 50 mL of 5% dextrose injection or 0.9% sodium chloride injection before administration. Zofran Injection should not be mixed with solutions for which physical and chemical compatibility have not been established. In particular, this applies to alkaline solutions as a precipitate may form.

Pediatric Use: On the basis of the limited available information (see CLINICAL TRIALS: Pediatric Studies and CLINICAL PHARMACOLOGY: Pharmacokinetics), the

dosage in children 4–18 years of age should be the same as for adults (see above). Little information is available about dosage in children 3 years of age or younger.

Use in the Elderly: The dosage is the same as for the general population.

Dosage Adjustment for Patients With Impaired Renal Function: No specific studies have been conducted in patients with renal insufficiency.

Dosage Adjustment for Patients With Impaired Hepatic Function: In patients with severe hepatic insufficiency, clearance is reduced and apparent volume of distribution is increased with a resultant increase in plasma half-life. In such patients, a total daily dose of 8 mg should not be exceeded.

Stability: Zofran Injection is stable at room temperature under normal lighting conditions for 48 hours after dilution with the following IV fluids: 0.9% sodium chloride injection, 5% dextrose injection, 5% dextrose and 0.9% sodium chloride injection, 5% dextrose and 0.45% sodium chloride injection, and 3% sodium chloride injection.

Note: Parenteral drug products should be inspected visually for particulate matter and discoloration before administration whenever solution and container permit.

HOW SUPPLIED

Zofran® (ondansetron HCl) Injection, 2 mg/mL, is supplied in 20-mL multidose vials (NDC 0173-0442-00).

Store between 2° and 30°C (36° and 86°F). Protect from light.
Shown in Product Identification Section, page 411

Cetus Oncology Corporation
4560 HORTON STREET
EMERYVILLE, CA 94608-2997

ACETYLCYSTEINE SOLUTION, USP ℞

HOW SUPPLIED

10% Acetylcysteine Solution, USP (100 mg acetylcysteine per mL).
Sterile, **NOT FOR INJECTION**
NDC 53905-211-03 10 mL vials; carton of 3 (with 1 plastic dropper)
NDC 53905-212-03 30 mL vials; carton of 3

20% Acetylcysteine Solution, USP (200 mg acetylcysteine per mL).
Sterile, **NOT FOR INJECTION**
NDC 53905-213-03 10 mL vials; carton of 3 (with 1 plastic dropper)
NDC 53905-214-03 30 mL vials; carton of 3
Store unopened vials at controlled room temperature 15° to 30°C (59° to 86°F). Store opened vial in refrigerator. Discard opened vial after 96 hours.
CAUTION—Federal law prohibits dispensing without prescription.
Revised August, 1992 KO-P-04

DOXORUBICIN Hydrochloride Injection, USP ℞

FOR INTRAVENOUS USE ONLY

WARNINGS

1. Severe local tissue necrosis will occur if there is extravasation during administration (See "**DOSAGE AND ADMINISTRATION**" Section). Doxorubicin must not be given by the intramuscular or subcutaneous route.
2. Serious irreversible myocardial toxicity with delayed congestive failure often unresponsive to any cardiac supportive therapy may be encountered as total dosage approaches 550 mg/m^2. This toxicity may occur at lower cumulative doses in patients with prior mediastinal irradiation or on concurrent cyclophosphamide therapy.
3. Dosage should be reduced in patients with impaired hepatic function.
4. Severe myelosuppression may occur.
5. Doxorubicin should be administered only under the supervision of a physician who is experienced in the use of cancer chemotherapeutic agents.

DESCRIPTION

Doxorubicin is a cytotoxic anthracycline antibiotic isolated from cultures of *Streptomyces peucetius* var. *caesius*. Doxorubicin consists of a naphthacenequinone nucleus linked through a glycosidic bond at ring atom 7 to an amino sugar, daunosamine.
Doxorubicin binds to nucleic acids, presumably by specific intercalation of the planar anthracycline nucleus with the DNA double helix. The anthracycline ring is lipophilic but the saturated end of the ring system contains abundant hydroxyl groups adjacent to the amino sugar, producing a hydrophilic center. The molecule is amphoteric, containing acidic functions in the ring phenolic groups and a basic function in the sugar amino group. It binds to cell membranes as well as plasma proteins.
Doxorubicin (Doxorubicin Hydrochloride Injection, USP) is a parenteral, isotonic solution containing no preservative, available in 5 mL (10 mg), 10 mL (20 mg), and 25 mL (50 mg) single dose vials.
Each mL contains doxorubicin hydrochloride and the following inactive ingredients: sodium chloride 0.9% and water for injection q.s. Hydrochloric acid is used to adjust pH to a target pH of 3.0.

CLINICAL PHARMACOLOGY

Though not completely elucidated, the mechanism of action of doxorubicin is related to its ability to bind to DNA and inhibit nucleic acid synthesis. Cell culture studies have demonstrated rapid cell penetration and perinucleolar chromatin binding, rapid inhibition of mitotic activity and nucleic acid synthesis, mutagenesis and chromosomal aberrations. Animal studies have shown activity in a spectrum of experimental tumors, immunosuppression, carcinogenic properties in rodents, induction of a variety of toxic effects, including delayed and progressive cardiac toxicity, myelosuppression in all species and atrophy to testes in rats and dogs.
Pharmacokinetic studies show the intravenous administration of normal or radiolabeled doxorubicin is followed by rapid plasma clearance and significant tissue binding. Urinary excretion, as determined by fluorimetric methods, accounts for approximately 4–5% of the administered dose in five days. Biliary excretion represents the major excretion route, 40–50% of the administered dose being recovered in the bile or the feces in seven days. Impairment of liver function results in slower excretion, and consequently, increased retention and accumulation in plasma and tissues. Doxorubicin does not cross the blood brain barrier.

INDICATIONS AND USAGE

Injectable doxorubicin hydrochloride has been used successfully to produce regression in disseminated neoplastic conditions such as acute lymphoblastic leukemia, acute myeloblastic leukemia, Wilms' tumor, neuroblastoma, soft tissue and bone sarcomas, breast carcinoma, ovarian carcinoma, transitional cell bladder carcinoma, thyroid carcinoma, lymphomas of both Hodgkin and non-Hodgkin types, bronchogenic carcinoma in which the small cell histologic type is the most responsive compared to other cell types and gastric carcinoma.
A number of other solid tumors have also shown some responsiveness but in numbers too limited to justify specific recommendation. Studies to date have shown malignant melanoma, kidney carcinoma, large bowel carcinoma, brain tumors and metastases to the central nervous system not to be significantly responsive to doxorubicin therapy.

CONTRAINDICATIONS

Doxorubicin therapy should not be started in patients who have marked myelosuppression induced by previous treatment with other antitumor agents or by radiotherapy. Conclusive data are not available on pre-existing heart disease as a co-factor of increased risk of doxorubicin induced cardiac toxicity. Preliminary data suggest that in such cases cardiac toxicity may occur at doses lower than the recommended cumulative limit. It is therefore not recommended to start doxorubicin in such cases. Doxorubicin treatment is contraindicated in patients who received previous treatment with complete cumulative doses of doxorubicin and/or daunorubicin.

WARNINGS

Special attention must be given to the cardiac toxicity exhibited by doxorubicin. Although uncommon, acute left ventricular failure has occurred, particularly in patients who have received total dosage of the drug exceeding the currently recommended limit of 550 mg/m^2. This limit appears to be lower (400 mg/m^2) in patients who received radiotherapy to the mediastinal area or concomitant therapy with other potentially cardiotoxic agents such as cyclophosphamide. The total dose of doxorubicin administered to the individual patient should also take into account a previous or concomitant therapy with related compounds such as daunorubicin. Congestive heart failure and/or cardiomyopathy may be encountered several weeks after discontinuation of doxorubicin therapy.
Cardiac failure is often not favorably affected by presently known medical or physical therapy for cardiac support.
Early clinical diagnosis of drug induced heart failure appears to be essential for successful treatment with digitalis, diuretics, low salt diet and bed rest. Severe cardiac toxicity may occur precipitously without antecedent EKG changes. A baseline EKG and EKGs performed prior to each dose or course after 300 mg/m^2 cumulative dose has been given is suggested. Transient EKG changes consisting of T-wave flattening, S-T depression and arrhythmias lasting for up to two weeks after a dose or course of doxorubicin are presently not considered indications for suspension of doxorubicin therapy. Doxorubicin cardiomyopathy has been reported to be associated with a persistent reduction in the voltage of the QRS wave, a prolongation of the systolic time interval and a reduction of the ejection fraction as determined by echocardiography or radionuclide angiography. None of these tests have yet been confirmed to consistently identify those individual patients that are approaching their maximally tolerated cumulative dose of doxorubicin. If test results indicate change in cardiac function associated with doxorubicin, the benefit of continued therapy must be carefully evaluated against the risk of producing irreversible cardiac damage.
Acute life-threatening arrhythmias have been reported to occur during or within a few hours after doxorubicin hydrochloride administration.
There is a high incidence of bone marrow depression, primarily of leukocytes, requiring careful hematologic monitoring. With the recommended dosage schedule, leukopenia is usually transient, reaching its nadir at 10–14 days after treatment with recovery usually occurring by the 21st day. White blood cell counts as low as 1000/mm^3 are to be expected during the treatment with appropriate doses of doxorubicin. Red blood cell and platelet levels should also be monitored since they may also be depressed. Hematologic toxicity may require dose reduction or suspension or delay of doxorubicin therapy. Persistent severe myelosuppression may result in superinfection and hemorrhage.
Doxorubicin may potentiate the toxicity of other anticancer therapies. Exacerbation of cyclophosphamide induced hemorrhagic cystitis and enhancement of the hepatotoxicity of 6-mercaptopurine have been reported. Radiation induced toxicity to the myocardium, mucosae, skin and liver have been reported to be increased by the administration of doxorubicin.
Toxicity to recommended doses of doxorubicin is enhanced by hepatic impairment, therefore, prior to the individual dosing, evaluation of hepatic function is recommended using conventional clinical laboratory tests such as SGOT, SGPT, alkaline phosphatase and bilirubin. (See "**DOSAGE AND ADMINISTRATION**" Section).
Necrotizing colitis manifested by typhlitis (cecal inflammation), bloody stools and severe and sometimes fatal infections have been associated with a combination of doxorubicin given by i.v. push daily for 3 days and cytarabine given by continuous infusion daily for 7 or more days.
On intravenous administration of doxorubicin, extravasation may occur with or without an accompanying stinging or burning sensation and even if blood returns well on aspiration of the infusion needle (See "**DOSAGE AND ADMINISTRATION**" Section). If any signs or symptoms of extravasation have occured the injection or infusion should be immediately terminated and restarted in another vein.
Doxorubicin and related compounds have also been shown to have mutagenic and carcinogenic properties when tested in experimental models.
Usage in Pregnancy—Safe use of doxorubicin in pregnancy has not been established. Doxorubicin is embryotoxic and teratogenic in rats and embryotoxic and abortifacient in rabbits. Therefore, the benefits to the pregnant patient should be carefully weighed against the potential toxicity to fetus and embryo. The possible adverse effects on fertility in males and females in humans or experimental animals have not been adequately evaulated.

PRECAUTIONS

Initial treatment with doxorubicin requires close observation of the patient and extensive laboratory monitoring. It is recommended, therefore, that patients be hospitalized at least during the first phase of the treatment.
Like other cytotoxic drugs, doxorubicin may induce hyperuricemia secondary to rapid lysis of neoplastic cells. The clinician should monitor the patient's blood uric acid level and be prepared to use such supportive and pharmacologic measures as might be necessary to control this problem.
Doxorubicin imparts a red coloration to the urine for 1–2 days after administration and patients should be advised to expect this during active therapy.
Doxorubicin is not an anti-microbial agent.

ADVERSE REACTIONS

Dose limiting toxicities of therapy are myelosuppression and cardiotoxicity (See "**WARNINGS** " Section). Other reactions reported are:
Cutaneous—Reversible complete alopecia occurs in most cases. Hyperpigmentation of nailbeds and dermal creases, primarily in children, and onycholysis have been reported in a few cases. Recall of skin reaction due to prior radiotherapy has occurred with doxorubicin administration.
Gastrointestinal—Acute nausea and vomiting occurs frequently and may be severe. This may be alleviated by antiemetic therapy. Mucositis (stomatitis and esophagitis) may occur 5–10 days after administration. The effect may be severe leading to ulceration and represents a site of origin for severe infections. The dosage regimen consisting of administration of doxorubicin on three consecutive days results in the greater incidence and severity of mucositis. Ulceration and necrosis of the colon, especially the cecum, may occur leading to bleeding or severe infections which can be fatal. This reaction has been reported in patients with acute nonlymphocytic leukemia treated with a 3-day course of doxorubicin combined with cytarabine. Anorexia and diarrhea have been occasionally reported.
Vascular—Phlebosclerosis has been reported especially when small veins are used or a single vein is used for repeated admininstration. Facial flushing may occur if the injection is given too rapidly.
Local—Severe cellulitis, vesication and tissue necrosis will occur if doxorubicin is extravasated during administration. Erythematous streaking along the vein proximal to the site of the injection has been reported (See "**DOSAGE AND ADMINISTRATION**" Section).
Hypersensitivity—Fever, chills, and urticaria have been reported occasionally. Anaphylaxis may occur. A case of apparent cross sensitivity to lincomycin has been reported.
Other—Conjunctivitis and lacrimation occur rarely.

OVERDOSAGE

Acute overdosage of doxorubicin enhances the toxic effects of mucositis, leukopenia and thrombopenia. Treatment of acute overdosage consists of treatment of the severely myelosuppressed patient with hospitalization, antibiotics, platelet and granulocyte transfusions and symptomatic treatment of mucositis.
Chronic overdosage with cumulative doses exceeding 500 mg/m^2 increases the risk of cardiomyopathy and resul-

Continued on next page

Cetus—Cont.

tant congestive heart failure. Treatment consists of vigorous management of congestive heart failure with digitalis preparations and diuretics. The use of peripheral vasodilators has been recommended.

DOSAGE AND ADMINISTRATION

Care in the administration of doxorubicin hydrochloride will reduce the chance of perivenous infiltration. It may also decrease the chance of local reactions such as urticaria and erythematous streaking. On intravenous administration of doxorubicin, extravasation may occur with or without any accompanying stinging or burning sensation and even if blood returns well on aspiration of the infusion needle. If any signs or symptoms of extravasation have occurred, the injection or infusion should be immediately terminated and restarted in another vein. If it is known or suspected that subcutaneous extravasation has occurred, local infiltration with an injectable corticosteroid and flooding the site with normal saline has been reported to lessen the local reaction. Because of the progressive nature of extravasation reactions, the area of injection should be frequently examined and plastic surgery consultation obtained. If ulceration begins, early wide excision of the involved areas should be considered.[1]

The most commonly used dosage schedule is 60–75 mg/m^2 as a single intravenous injection administered at 21-day intervals. The lower dose should be given to patients with inadequate marrow reserves due to old age, or prior therapy, or neoplastic marrow infiltration. An alternative dose schedule is weekly doses of 20 mg/m^2 which has been reported to produce a lower incidence of congestive heart failure. Thirty mg/m^2 on each of three successive days repeated every four weeks has also been used. Doxorubicin dosage must be reduced if the bilirubin is elevated as follows: Serum bilirubin 1.2 to 3.0 mg/dL—give ½ normal dose, > 3 mg/dL—give ¼ normal dose.

It is recommended that doxorubicin be slowly administered into a tubing of a freely running intravenous infusion of Sodium Chloride Injection, USP or 5% Dextrose Injection, USP. The tubing should be attached to a Butterfly® needle inserted preferably into a large vein. If possible, avoid veins over joints or in extremities with compromised venous or lymphatic drainage. The rate of administration is dependent on the size of the vein and the dosage. However, the dose should be administered in not less than 3 to 5 minutes. Local erythematous streaking along the vein as well as facial flushing may be indicative of too rapid an administration. A burning or stinging sensation may be indicative of perivenous infiltration and the infusion should be immediately terminated and restarted in another vein. Perivenous infiltration may occur painlessly.

Doxorubicin should not be mixed with heparin or 5-fluorouracil since it has been reported that these drugs are incompatible to the extent that a precipitate may form. Until specific compatibility data are available, it is not recommended that doxorubicin be mixed with other drugs.

Doxorubicin has been used concurrently with other approved chemotherapeutic agents. Evidence is available that in some types of neoplastic disease combination chemotherapy is superior to single agents. The benefits and risks of such therapy continue to be elucidated.

Handling and Disposal: Skin reactions associated with doxorubicin have been reported. Caution in the handling of solution must be exercised and the use of gloves is recommended. If doxorubicin contacts the skin or mucosae, immediately wash thoroughly with soap and water.

Procedures for proper handling and disposal of anti-cancer drugs should be considered. Several guidelines on this subject have been published.[2–7] There is no general agreement that all of the procedures recommended in the guidelines are necessary or appropriate.

HOW SUPPLIED

Doxorubicin Hydrochloride Injection. USP.
Sterile, single use only, contains no preservative.
NDC 53905-235-10 10 mg vial; 2 mg/mL, 5 mL, 10 vial packs.
NDC 53905-236-06 20 mg vial; 2 mg/mL, 10 mL, 6 vial packs.
NDC 53905-237-01 50 mg vial; 2 mg/mL, 25 mL, single vial packs.

Store under refrigeration, 2°–8°C (36°–46°F), protect from light and retain in carton until time of use. Discard unused portion.

CAUTION: Federal law prohibits dispensing without prescription.

REFERENCES

1. Rudolph R *et al:* Skin Ulcers Due to Adriamycin. *Cancer 38:*1087–1094, Sept. 1976.
2. Recommendations for the Safe Handling of Parenteral Antineoplastic Drugs. NIH Publication No. 83-2621. For sale by the Superintendent of Documents, U.S. Government Printing Office, Washington, D.C. 20402.
3. AMA Council Report. Guidelines for Handling Parenteral Antineoplastics. *JAMA,* March 15, 1985.
4. National Study Commission on Cytotoxic Exposure-Recommendations for Handling Cytotoxic Agents. Available from Louis P. Jeffrey, Sc.D., Director of Pharmacy Services, Rhode Island Hospital, 593 Eddy Street, Providence, Rhode Island 02902.
5. Clinical Oncological Society of Australia: Guidlines and recommendations for safe handling of antieoplastic agents. *Med J Australia 1:*426–428, 1983.
6. Jones RB, et al. Safe handling of chemotherapeutic agents: A report from the Mount Sinai Medical Center. *CA-A Cancer Journal for Clinicians* Sept/Oct, 258-263, 1983.
7. American Society of Hospital Pharmacists technical assistance bulletin on handling cytotoxic drugs in hospitals. *Am J Hosp Pharm 42:*131–137, 1985.

MANUFACTURED BY:
Farmitalia Carlo Erba
Milan, Italy
DISTRIBUTED BY:
Cetus Oncology Corporation
4650 Horton Street
Emeryville, CA 94608–2997
Revised February 1, 1991 057200291
NO-P-03

LEUCOVORIN Calcium for Injection ℞

HOW SUPPLIED

Leucovorin Calcium for Injection is supplied in packs of ten individually-boxed vials.
50 mg vial: NDC 53905-051-10. Each vial contains 50 mg leucovorin as the calcium salt and 45 mg sodium chloride.
100 mg vial: NDC 53905-052-10. Each vial contains 100 mg leucovorin as the calcium salt and 90 mg sodium chloride.
Caution: Federal law prohibits dispensing without prescription.
Revised April, 1991 DD-P-02

METOCLOPRAMIDE INJECTION, USP ℞

HOW SUPPLIED

Metoclopramide Injection, USP is supplied as a Pharmacy Bulk Package containing 5 mg metoclopramide (present as the hydrochloride) per mL in the following package strengths:
NDC 53905-195-01 250 mg in 50 mL
NDC 53905-196-01 500 mg in 100 mL
Store at controlled room temperature, 15° to 30°C (59° to 86°F). Do not permit to freeze. Contains no preservative.
PROTECT FROM LIGHT. Retain in carton until time of use. Discard unused portion no later than 4 hours after initial entry.
Dilutions may be stored unprotected from light under normal light conditions up to 24 hours after preparation.
Metoclopramide Injection, USP is also supplied as a 30 mL single-dose non-Pharmacy Bulk Package containing 5 mg metoclopramide (present as the hydrochloride) per mL in a carton of six flip-top vials.
NDC 53905-194-06 150 mg in 30 mL
Refer to the full prescribing information enclosed with this product for dosage and administration directions.

Container	Total Contents*	Concentration	Administration
30 mL (single-dose vial)	150 mg	5 mg/mL	For IV infusion Only—Dilute Before Using
50 mL Pharmacy Bulk Package	250 mg	5 mg/mL	For IV infusion Only—Dilute Before Using
100 mL Pharmacy Bulk Package	500 mg	5 mg/mL	For IV infusion Only—Dilute Before Using

*Metoclopramide (present as the hydrochloride)

CAUTION: Federal law prohibits dispensing without prescription.
Revised June, 1992 JB-P-04

PROLEUKIN® ℞

[*prō-lū′-kin*]
Aldesleukin
For Injection

WARNINGS

PROLEUKIN® (aldesleukin for injection) should be administered only in a hospital setting under the supervision of a qualified physician experienced in the use of anti-cancer agents. An intensive care facility and specialists skilled in cardiopulmonary or intensive care medicine must be available.

Proleukin administration has been associated with capillary leak syndrome (CLS). CLS results in hypotension and reduced organ perfusion which may be severe and can result in death.

Therapy with Proleukin should be restricted to patients with normal cardiac and pulmonary functions as defined by thallium stress testing and formal pulmonary function testing. Extreme caution should be used in patients with normal thallium stress tests and pulmonary function tests who have a history of prior cardiac or pulmonary disease.

Proleukin administration should be held in patients developing moderate to severe lethargy or somnolence; continued administration may result in coma.

DESCRIPTION

PROLEUKIN® (aldesleukin), a human recombinant interleukin-2 product, is a highly purified protein with a molecular weight of approximately 15,300 daltons. The chemical name is des-alanyl-1, serine-125 human interleukin-2. Proleukin, a lymphokine, is produced by recombinant DNA technology using a genetically engineered *E. coli* strain containing an analog of the human interleukin-2 gene. Genetic engineering techniques were used to modify the human IL-2 gene, and the resulting expression clone encodes a modified human interleukin-2. This recombinant form differs from native interleukin-2 in the following ways: a) Proleukin is not glycosylated because it is derived from *E. coli.*; b) The molecule has no N-terminal alanine; the codon for this amino acid was deleted during the genetic engineering procedure; c) The molecule has serine substituted for cysteine at amino acid position 125; this was accomplished by site specific manipulation during the genetic engineering procedure; and d) the aggregation state of Proleukin is likely to be different from that of native interleukin-2.

Biological activities tested *in vitro* for the native non-recombinant molecule have been reproduced with Proleukin.[1,2]

Proleukin for Injection is supplied as a sterile, white to off-white, lyophilized cake in single-use vials intended for intravenous (IV) administration. When reconstituted with 1.2 mL Sterile Water for Injection, USP, each mL contains 18 million IU (1.1 mg) Proleukin, 50 mg mannitol, and 0.18 mg sodium dodecyl sulfate, buffered with approximately 0.17 mg monobasic and 0.89 mg dibasic sodium phosphate to a pH of 7.5 (range 7.2 to 7.8). The manufacturing process for Proleukin involves fermentation in a defined medium containing tetracycline hydrochloride. The presence of the antibiotic is not detectable in the final product. Proleukin contains no preservatives in the final product.

Proleukin biological potency is determined by a lymphocyte proliferation bioassay and is expressed in International Units (IU) as established by the World Health Organization 1ST International Standard for interleukin 2 (human). The relationship between potency and protein mass is as follows:

18 million (18 × 10^6) IU Proleukin® = 1.1 mg protein

CLINICAL PHARMACOLOGY

Proleukin® has been shown to possess the biological activity of human native interleukin-2.[1,2] *In vitro* studies performed on human cell lines demonstrate the immunoregulatory properties of Proleukin, including: a) enhancement of lymphocyte mitogenesis and stimulation of long-term growth of human interleukin-2 dependent cell lines; b) enhancement of lymphocyte cytotoxicity; c) induction of killer cell [lymphokine-activated (LAK) and natural (NK)] activity; and d) induction of interferon-gamma production.

The *in vivo* administration of Proleukin in select murine tumor models and in the clinic produces multiple immunological effects in a dose dependent manner. These effects include activation of cellular immunity with profound lymphocytosis, eosinophilia, and thrombocytopenia, and the production of cytokines including tumor necrosis factor, IL-1 and gamma interferon.[3] *In vivo* experiments in murine tumor models have shown inhibition of tumor growth.[4] The exact mechanism by which Proleukin mediates its antitumor activity in animals and humans is unknown.

Pharmacokinetics: Proleukin exists as biologically active, non-covalently bound microaggregates with an average size of 27 recombinant interleukin-2 molecules. The solubilizing agent, sodium dodecyl sulfate, may have an effect on the kinetic properties of this product. The pharmacokinetic profile of Proleukin is characterized by high plasma concentrations following a short IV infusion, rapid distribution to extravascular, extracellular space and elimination from the body by metabolism in the kidneys with little or no bioactive protein excreted in the urine.

Studies of IV Proleukin in sheep and humans indicated that approximately 30% of the administered dose initially distributes to the plasma.

This is consistent with studies in rats that demonstrate a rapid (< 1 minute) and preferential uptake of approximately 70% of an administered dose into the liver, kidney and lung.

The serum half-life (T ½) curves of Proleukin remaining in the plasma are derived from studies done in 52 cancer patients following a 5 minute IV infusion.[5] These patients were shown to have a distribution and elimination T ½ of 13 and 85 minutes, respectively.

The relatively rapid clearance rate of Proleukin has led to dosage schedules characterized by frequent, short infusions. Observed serum levels are proportional to the dose of Proleukin.

Following the initial rapid organ distribution described above, the primary route of clearance of circulating Proleukin is the kidney. In humans and animals, Proleukin is cleared from the circulation by both glomerular filtration and peritubular extraction in the kidney.[6–9] This dual mechanism for delivery of Proleukin to the proximal tubule may account for the preservation of clearance in patients with rising serum creatinine values. Greater than 80% of the amount of Proleukin distributed to plasma, cleared from the circulation and presented to the kidney is metabolized to amino acids in the cells lining the proximal convoluted tubules. In humans, the mean clearance rate in cancer patients is 268 mL/min.[9]

Immunogenicity: Fifty-eight of 76 renal cancer patients (76%) treated with the every 8 hour Proleukin regimen developed low titers of non-neutralizing anti-interleukin-2 antibodies. Neutralizing antibodies were not detected in this group of patients, but have been detected in 1/106 (<1%) patients with IV Proleukin using a wide variety of schedules and doses. The clinical significance of anti-interleukin-2 antibodies is unknown.

Clinical Experience: Two hundred and fifty-five patients with metastatic renal cell cancer were treated with single agent Proleukin. Treatment was given by the every 8 hour regimen in 7 clinical studies conducted at 21 institutions. To be eligible for study, patients were required to have bidimensionally measurable disease; Eastern Cooperative Oncology Group (ECOG) Performance Status (PS) of 0 or 1 (see Table I); and normal organ function, including normal cardiac stress test and pulmonary function tests. Patients with brain metastases, active infections, organ allografts and diseases requiring steroid treatment were excluded. In addition, it was noted that 218 of the 225 (85%) patients had undergone nephrectomy prior to treatment with Proleukin.

Proleukin was given by 15 minute IV infusion every 8 hours for up to 5 days (maximum of 14 doses). No treatment was given on days 6 to 14 and then dosing was repeated for up to 5 days on days 15 to 19 (maximum of 14 doses). These 2 cycles constituted 1 course of therapy. All patients were treated with 28 doses or until dose-limiting toxicity occurred requiring ICU-level support. Patients received a median of 20 of 28 scheduled doses of Proleukin. Doses were held for specific toxicities (See "**DOSAGE AND ADMINISTRATION**" Section, "**Dose Modification**" Subsection). A variety of serious adverse events were encountered including: hypotension; oliguria/anuria; mental status changes including coma; pulmonary congestion and dyspnea; GI bleeding; respiratory failure leading to intubation; ventricular arrhythmias; myocardial ischemia and/or infarction; ileus or intestinal perforation, renal failure requiring dialysis; gangrene; seizures; sepsis and death (See "**ADVERSE REACTIONS**" Section).

Due to the toxicities encountered during the clinical trials, investigators used the following concomitant medications. Acetaminophen and indomethacin were started immediately prior to Proleukin to reduce fever. Renal function was particularly monitored because indomethacin may cause synergistic nephrotoxicity. Meperidine was added to control the rigors associated with fever. Ranitidine or cimetidine were given for prophylaxis of gastrointestinal irritation and bleeding. Antiemetics and antidiarrheals were used as needed to treat other gastrointestinal side effects. These medications were discontinued 12 hours after the last dose of Proleukin. Hydroxyzine or diphenhydramine used to control symptoms from pruritic rashes and continued until resolution of pruritus. **NOTE: Prior to the use of any product mentioned in this paragraph, the physician should refer to the package insert for the respective product.**

For the 255 patients in the Proleukin database, objective response was seen in 15% or 37 patients with nine (4%) complete and 28 (11%) partial responders. The 95% confidence interval for response was 11 to 20%. Onset of tumor regression has been observed as early as 4 weeks after completion of the first course of treatment and tumor regression may continue for up to 12 months after the start of treatment.

Durable responses were achieved with a median duration of objective (partial or complete) response by Kaplan-Meier projection at 23.2 months (1 to 50 months). The median duration of objective partial response was 18.8 months. The proportion of responding patients who will have response durations of 12 months or greater is projected to be 85% for all responders and 79% for patients with partial responses (Kaplan-Meier).

Complete Responders	Partial Responders	Response Rate	Onset of Response	Median Duration of Response
9 (4%)	28 (11%)	15%	1 to 12 mos.	23.2 months (range 1-50)

TABLE I
PERFORMANCE STATUS SCALE

Performance Status Equivalent: ECOG*	Karnofsky	Performance Status Definitions
0	100	Asymptomatic
1	80-90	Symptomatic: fully ambulatory
2	60-70	Symptomatic; in bed less than 50% of day
3	40-50	Symptomatic: in bed more than 50% of day
4	20-30	Bedridden

Zubrod, CG, et al. J Chron Dis 11:7-33, 1960

TABLE II
PROLEUKIN RESPONSE ANALYZED BY ECOG* PERFORMANCE STATUS (PS)

Pre-Treatment ECOG PS	No. of Patients Treated (n=255)	Response CR	Response PR	% of Patients Responding	On-Study Death Rate
0	166	9	21	18%	4%
1	80	0	7	9%	6%
≥2	9	0	0	0%	0%

* Eastern Cooperative Oncology Group

Response was observed in both lung and non-lung sites (e.g. liver, lymph node, renal bed recurrences, soft tissue). Patients with individual bulky lesions (> 5 × 5 cm) as well as large cumulative tumor burden (>25 cm² tumor area) achieved durable responses.

An analysis of prognostic factors showed that performance status as defined by the ECOG (see Table I) was a significant predictor of response. PS 0 patients had an 18% overall rate of objective response, which included all 9 complete response patients and 21 of 28 partial response patients. PS 1 patients had a lower rate of response (9%), all of which were partial responses. In this group it was notable that 6 of the 7 responders had resolution of tumor related symptoms and improved performance status to PS 0. All seven patients were fully functional and 4 of the 7 returned to work, suggesting that responses among the PS 1 patients were clinically meaningful as well (see Table II).

In addition, the frequency of toxicity was related to the performance status. As a group, PS 0 patients, when compared with PS 1 patients, had lower rates of adverse events with fewer on-study deaths (4% vs. 6%), less frequent intubations (8% vs. 25%), gangrene (0% vs. 6%), coma (1% vs. 6%), GI bleeding (4% vs. 8%), and sepsis (6% vs. 18%). These differences in toxicity are reflected in the shorter mean time to hospital discharge for PS 0 patients (2 vs. 3 days) as well as the smaller percentage of PS 0 patients experiencing a delayed (> 7 days) discharge from the hospital (8% vs. 19%). [See Table I and Table II above.]

INDICATIONS AND USAGE

Proleukin (aldesleukin) is indicated for the treatment of adults (≥ 18 years of age) with metastatic renal cell carcinoma.

Careful patient selection is mandatory prior to the administration of Proleukin. See "**CONTRAINDICATIONS**", "**WARNINGS**" and "**PRECAUTIONS**" Sections regarding patient screening, including recommended cardiac and pulmonary function tests and laboratory tests.

Evaluation of clinical studies to date reveals that patients with more favorable ECOG performance status (ECOG PS 0) at treatment initiation respond better to Proleukin, with a higher response rate and lower toxicity (See "**CLINICAL PHARMACOLOGY**" Section, "**Clinical Experience**" Subsection). Therefore, selection of patients for treatment should include assessment of performance status, as described in Table I.

Experience in patients with PS > 1 is extremely limited.

CONTRAINDICATIONS

Proleukin (aldesleukin) is contraindicated in patients with a known history of hypersensitivity to interleukin-2 or any component of the Proleukin formulation.

Patients with an abnormal thallium stress test or pulmonary function tests are excluded from treatment with Proleukin. Patients with organ allografts should be excluded as well. In addition, retreatment with Proleukin is contraindicated in patients who experienced the following toxicities while receiving an earlier course of therapy:

- Sustained ventricular tachycardia (≥ 5 beats)
- Cardiac rhythm disturbances not controlled or unresponsive to management
- Recurrent chest pain with ECG changes, consistent with angina or myocardial infarction
- Intubation required > 72 hours
- Pericardial tamponade
- Renal dysfunction requiring dialysis > 72 hours
- Coma or toxic psychosis lasting >48 hours
- Repetitive or difficult to control seizures
- Bowel ischemia/perforation
- GI bleeding requiring surgery

WARNINGS

See boxed "**WARNINGS**"

Proleukin (aldesleukin) administration has been associated with capillary leak syndrome (CLS) which results from extravasation of plasma proteins and fluid into the extravascular space and loss of vascular tone. CLS results in hypotension and reduced organ perfusion which may be severe and can result in death. The CLS may be associated with cardiac arrhythmias (supraventricular and ventricular), angina, myocardial infarction, respiratory insufficiency requiring intubation, gastrointestinal bleeding or infarction, renal insufficiency, and mental status changes.

Because of the severe adverse events which generally accompany Proleukin therapy at the recommended dosages, thorough clinical evaluation should be performed to exclude from treatment patients with significant cardiac, pulmonary, renal, hepatic or CNS impairment.

Should adverse events occur, which require dose modification, dosage should be withheld rather than reduced. (See "**DOSAGE AND ADMINISTRATION**" Section, "**Dose Modification**" Subsection).

Proleukin may exacerbate disease symptoms in patients with clinically unrecognized or untreated CNS metastases. All patients should have thorough evaluation and treatment of CNS metastases prior to receiving Proleukin therapy. They should be neurologically stable with a negative CT scan. In addition, extreme caution should be exercised in treating patients with a history of seizure disorder because Proleukin may cause seizures.

Intensive Proleukin treatment is associated with impaired neutrophil function (reduced chemotaxis) and with an increased risk of disseminated infection, including sepsis and bacterial endocarditis, in treated patients. Consequently, pre-existing bacterial infections should be adequately treated prior to initiation of Proleukin therapy. Additionally, all patients with indwelling central lines should receive antibiotic prophylaxis effective against *S. aureus*.[10–12] Antibiotic prophylaxis which has been associated with a reduced incidence of staphylococcal infections in Proleukin studies includes the use of: oxacillin, nafcillin, ciprofloxacin, or vancomycin. Disseminated infections acquired in the course of Proleukin treatment are a major contributor to treatment morbidity and use of antibiotic prophylaxis and aggressive treatment of suspected and documented infections may reduce the morbidity of Proleukin treatment. **NOTE: Prior to the use of any product mentioned in this paragraph, the physician should refer to the package insert for the respective product.**

PRECAUTIONS

General: Patients should have normal cardiac, pulmonary, hepatic and CNS function at the start of therapy. Patients who have had a nephrectomy are still eligible for treatment if they have serum creatinine levels ≤ 1.5 mg/dL.

Adverse events are frequent, often serious, and sometimes fatal.

Capillary leak syndrome (CLS) begins immediately after Proleukin treatment starts and is marked by increased capillary permeability to protein and fluids and reduced vascular tone. In most patients, this results in a concomitant drop in mean arterial blood pressure within 2 to 12 hours after the start of treatment. With continued therapy, clinically significant hypotension (defined as systolic blood pressure below 90 mm Hg or a 20 mm Hg drop from baseline systolic pressure) and hypoperfusion will occur. In addition, extravasation of protein and fluids into the extravascular space will lead to edema formation and creation of effusions.

Medical management of CLS begins with careful monitoring of the patient's fluid and organ perfusion status. This is

Continued on next page

Cetus—Cont.

achieved by frequent determination of blood pressure and pulse, and by monitoring organ function, which includes assessment of mental status and urine output. Hypovolemia is assessed by catheterization and central pressure monitoring.

Flexibility in fluid and pressor management is essential for maintaining organ perfusion and blood pressure. Consequently, extreme caution should be used in treating patients with fixed requirements for large volumes of fluid (e.g. patients with hypercalcemia).

Patients with hypovolemia are managed by administering IV fluids, either colloids or crystalloids. IV fluids are usually given when the central venous pressure (CVP) is below 3 to 4 mm H_2O. Correction of hypovolemia may require large volumes of IV fluids but caution is required because unrestrained fluid administration may exacerbate problems associated with edema formation or effusions.

With extravascular fluid accumulation, edema is common and some patients may develop ascites or pleural effusions. Management of these events depends on a careful balancing of the effects of fluid shifts so that neither the consequences of hypovolemia (e.g. impaired organ perfusion) nor the consequences of fluid accumulations (e.g. pulmonary edema) exceeds the patient's tolerance.

Clinical experience has shown that early administration of dopamine (1 to 5 μg/kg/min) to patients manifesting capillary leak syndrome, before the onset of hypotension, can help to maintain organ perfusion particularly to the kidney and thus preserve urine output. Weight and urine output should be carefully monitored. If organ perfusion and blood pressure are not sustained by dopamine therapy, clinical investigators have increased the dose of dopamine to 6 to 10 μg/kg/min or have added phenylephrine hydrochloride (1 to 5 μg/kg/min) to low dose dopamine. (See "**CLINICAL PHARMACOLOGY**" Section, "**Clinical Experience**" Subsection). Prolonged use of pressors, either in combination or as individual agents, at relatively high doses, may be associated with cardiac rhythm disturbances. **NOTE: Prior to the use of any product mentioned in this paragraph, the physician should refer to the package insert for the respective product.**

Failure to maintain organ perfusion, demonstrated by altered mental status, reduced urine output, a fall in the systolic blood pressure below 90 mm Hg or onset of cardiac arrhythmias, should lead to holding the subsequent doses until recovery of organ perfusion and a return of systolic blood pressure above 90 mm Hg are observed. (See "**DOSAGE AND ADMINISTRATION**" Section, "**Dose Modification**" Subsection).

Recovery from CLS begins soon after cessation of Proleukin therapy. Usually, within a few hours, the blood pressure rises, organ perfusion is restored and resorption of extravasated fluid and protein begins. If there has been excessive weight gain or edema formation, particularly if associated with shortness of breath from pulmonary congestion, use of diuretics, once blood pressure has normalized, has been shown to hasten recovery.

Oxygen is given to the patient if pulmonary function monitoring confirms that P_aO_2 is decreased.

Proleukin administration may cause anemia and/or thrombocytopenia. Packed red blood cell transfusions have been given both for relief of anemia and to insure maximal oxygen carrying capacity. Platelet transfusions have been given to resolve absolute thrombocytopenia and to reduce the risk of GI bleeding. In addition, leukopenia and neutropenia are observed.

Proleukin administration results in fever, chills, rigors, pruritus and gastrointestinal side effects in most patients treated at recommended doses. These side effects have been aggressively managed as described in the "**CLINICAL PHARMACOLOGY**" Section, "**Clinical Experience**" Subsection.

Renal and hepatic function are impaired during Proleukin treatment. Use of concomitant medications known to be nephrotoxic or hepatotoxic may further increase toxicity to the kidney or liver. In addition, reduced kidney and liver function secondary to Proleukin treatment may delay elimination of concomitant medications and increase the risk of adverse events from those drugs.

Patients may experience mental status changes including irritability, confusion, or depression while receiving Proleukin. These mental status changes may be indicators of bacteremia or early bacterial sepsis. Mental status changes due solely to Proleukin are generally reversible when drug administration is discontinued. However, alterations in mental status may progress for several days before recovery begins.

Impairment of thyroid function has been reported following Proleukin treatment. A small number of treated patients went on to require thyroid replacement therapy. This impairment of thyroid function may be a manifestation of auto-

TABLE III
Incidence of Adverse Events

Events by Body System	% of Patients	Events by Body System	% of Patients
Cardiovascular		**Gastrointestinal**	
Hypotension	85	Nausea and Vomiting	87
(requiring pressors)	71	Diarrhea	76
Sinus Tachycardia	70	Stomatitis	32
Arrhythmias	22	Anorexia	27
Atrial	8	GI Bleeding	13
Supraventricular	5	(requiring surgery)	2
Ventricular	3	Dyspepsia	7
Junctional	1	Constipation	5
Bradycardia	7	Intestinal Perforation/Ileus	2
Premature Ventricular Contractions	5	Pancreatitis	< 1
Premature Atrial Contractions	4	**Neurologic**	
Myocardial Ischemia	3	Mental Status Changes	73
Myocardial Infarction	2	Dizziness	17
Cardiac Arrest	2	Sensory Dysfunction	10
Congestive Heart Failure	1	Special Sensory Disorders	
Myocarditis	1	(vision, speech, taste)	7
Stroke	1	Syncope	3
Gangrene	1	Motor Dysfunction	2
Pericardial Effusion	1	Coma	1
Endocarditis	1	Seizure (grand mal)	1
Thrombosis	1		
Pulmonary		**Renal**	
Pulmonary Congestion	54	Oliguria/Anuria	76
Dyspnea	52	BUN Elevation	63
Pulmonary Edema	10	Serum Creatinine Elevation	61
Respiratory Failure		Proteinuria	12
(leading to intubation)	9	Hematuria	9
Tachypnea	8	Dysuria	3
Pleural Effusion	7	Renal Impairment Requiring Dialysis	2
Wheezing	6	Urinary Retention	1
Apnea	1	Urinary Frequency	1
Pneumothorax	1	**Dermatologic**	
Hemoptysis	1	Pruritus	48
Hepatic		Erythema	41
Elevated Bilirubin	64	Rash	26
Elevated Transaminase	56	Dry Skin	15
Elevated Alkaline Phosphatase	56	Exfoliative Dermatitis	14
Jaundice	11	Purpura/Petechiae	4
Ascites	4	Urticaria	2
Hepatomegaly	1	Alopecia	1
Hematologic		**Musculoskeletal**	
Anemia	77	Arthralgia	6
Thrombocytopenia	64	Myalgia	6
Leukopenia	34	Arthritis	1
Coagulation Disorders	10	Muscle Spasm	1
Leukocytosis	9	**Endocrine**	
Eosinophilia	6	Hypothyroidism	< 1
Abnormal Laboratory Findings		**General**	
Hypomagnesemia	16	Fever and/or Chills	89
Acidosis	16	Pain (all sites)	54
Hypocalcemia	15	Abdominal	15
Hypophosphatemia	11	Chest	12
Hypokalemia	9	Back	9
Hyperuricemia	9	Fatigue/Weakness/Malaise	53
Hypoalbuminemia	8	Edema	47
Hypoproteinemia	7	Infection	23
Hyponatremia	4	including urinary tract, injection site,	
Hyperkalemia	4	catheter tip, phlebitis, sepsis)	
Alkalosis	4	Weight Gain (≥ 10%)	23
Hypoglycemia	2	Headache	12
Hyperglycemia	2	Weight Loss (≥ 10%)	5
Hypocholesterolemia	1	Conjunctivitis	4
Hypercalcemia	1	Injection Site Reactions	3
Hypernatremia	1	Allergic Reactions (non-anaphylactic)	1
Hyperphosphatemia	1		

immunity, consequently, extra caution should be exercised when treating patients with known autoimmune disease.

Proleukin (aldesleukin) enhancement of cellular immune function may increase the risk of allograft rejection in transplant patients.

Laboratory Tests: The following clinical evaluations are recommended for all patients, prior to beginning treatment and then daily during drug administration.

- Standard hematologic tests—including CBC, differential and platelet counts
- Blood chemistries—including electrolytes, renal and hepatic function tests
- Chest x-rays

All patients should have baseline pulmonary function tests with arterial blood gases. Adequate pulmonary function should be documented (FEV_1 > 2 liters or ≥ 75% of predicted for height and age) prior to initiating therapy. All patients should be screened with a stress thallium study. Normal ejection fraction and unimpaired wall motion should be documented. If a thallium stress test suggests minor wall motion abnormalities of questionable significance, a stress echocardiogram to document normal wall motion may be useful to exclude significant coronary artery disease.

Daily monitoring during therapy with Proleukin should include vital signs (temperature, pulse, blood pressure and respiration rate) and weight. In a patient with a decreased blood pressure, especially less than 90 mm Hg, constant cardiac monitoring for rhythm should be conducted. If an abnormal complex or rhythm is seen, an ECG should be performed. Vital signs in these hypotensive patients should be taken hourly and central venous pressure (CVP) checked.

During treatment, pulmonary function should be monitored on a regular basis by clinical examination, assessment of vital signs and pulse oximetry. Patients with dyspnea or clinical signs of respiratory impairment (tachypnea or rales) should be further assessed with arterial blood gas determination. These tests are to be repeated as often as clinically indicated.

Cardiac function is assessed daily by clinical examination and assessment of vital signs. Patients with signs or symptoms of chest pain, murmurs, gallops, irregular rhythm or palpitations should be further assessed with an ECG examination and CPK evaluation. If there is evidence of cardiac ischemia or congestive heart failure, a repeat thallium study should be done.

Drug Interactions: Proleukin may affect central nervous function. Therefore, interactions could occur following concomitant administration of psychotropic drugs (e.g., narcotics, analgesics, antiemetics, sedatives, tranquilizers).

Organ System	Hold dose for	Subsequent doses may be given if
Cardiovascular	Atrial fibrillation, supraventricular tachycardia, or bradycardia that requires treatment or is recurrent or persistent	Patient is asymptomatic with full recovery to normal sinus rhythm.
	Systolic bp <90 mm Hg with increasing requirements for pressors	Systolic bp ≥90 mm Hg and stable or improving requirements for pressors
	Any ECG change consistent with MI or ischemia with or without chest pain; suspicion of cardiac ischemia	Patient is asymptomatic, MI has been ruled out, clinical suspicion of angina is low
Pulmonary	O_2 saturation <94% on room air or <90% with 2 liters O_2 by nasal prongs	O_2 saturation ≥94% on room air or ≥90% with 2 liters O_2 by nasal prongs
Central Nervous System	Mental status changes, including moderate confusion or agitation	Mental status changes completely resolved
Systemic	Sepsis syndrome, patient is clinically unstable	Sepsis syndrome has resolved, patient is clinically stable, infection is under treatment
Renal	Serum creatinine ≥4.5 mg/dL or a serum creatinine of 4 mg/dL in the presence of severe volume overload, acidosis, or hyperkalemia	Serum creatinine <4 mg/dL and fluid and electrolyte status is stable
	Persistent oliguria, urine output of ≤10 mL/hour for 16 to 24 hours with rising serum creatinine	Urine output >10 mL/hour with a decrease of serum creatinine ≥1.5 mg/dL or normalization of serum creatinine
Hepatic	Signs of hepatic failure including encephalopathy, increasing ascites, liver pain, hypoglycemia	All signs of hepatic failure have resolved*
Gastrointestinal	Stool guaiac repeatedly >3–4+	Stool guaiac negative
Skin	Bullous dermatitis or marked worsening of pre-existing skin condition (avoid topical steroid therapy)	Resolution of all signs of bullous dermatitis

*Discontinue all further treatment for that course. Consider starting a new course of treatment at least 7 weeks after cessation of adverse event and hospital discharge.

Concurrent administration of drugs possessing nephrotoxic (e.g. aminoglycosides, indomethacin), myelotoxic (e.g. cytotoxic chemotherapy), cardiotoxic (e.g. doxorubicin) or hepatotoxic (e.g. methotrexate, asparaginase) effects with Proleukin may increase toxicity in these organ systems. The safety and efficacy of Proleukin in combination with chemotherapies have not been established.

Although glucocorticoids have been shown to reduce Proleukin-induced side effects including fever, renal insufficiency, hyperbilirubinemia, confusion and dyspnea,[13] concomitant administration of these agents with Proleukin may reduce the antitumor effectiveness of Proleukin and thus should be avoided.

Beta-blockers and other antihypertensives may potentiate the hypotension seen with Proleukin (aldesleukin).

Carcinogenesis, Mutagenesis, Impairment of Fertility: There have been no studies conducted assessing the carcinogenic or mutagenic potential of Proleukin (aldesleukin).

There have been no studies conducted assessing the effect of Proleukin on fertility. It is recommended that this drug not be administered to fertile persons of either sex not practicing effective contraception.

Pregnancy: *Pregnancy Category C.* Animal reproduction studies have not been conducted with Proleukin. It is also not known whether Proleukin can cause fetal harm when administered to a pregnant woman or can affect reproduction capacity. In view of the known adverse effects of Proleukin, it should only be given to a pregnant woman with extreme caution, weighing the potential benefit with the risks associated with therapy.

Nursing Mothers: It is not known whether this drug is excreted in human milk. Because many drugs are excreted in human milk and because of the potential for serious adverse reactions in nursing infants from Proleukin, a decision should be made whether to discontinue nursing or to discontinue the drug, taking into account the importance of the drug to the mother.

Pediatric Use: Safety and effectiveness in children under 18 years of age have not been established.

ADVERSE REACTIONS

The rate of drug related deaths in the 255 metastatic renal cell carcinoma patients on study who received single-agent Proleukin was 4% (11/255).

Frequency and severity of adverse reactions to Proleukin have generally been shown to be dose-related and schedule-dependent. Most adverse reactions are self-limiting and are usually, but not invariably, reversible within 2 or 3 days of discontinuation of therapy.

Examples of adverse reactions with permanent sequelae include: myocardial infarction, bowel perforation/infarction, and gangrene.

The most frequently reported serious adverse reactions include hypotension, renal dysfunction with oliguria/anuria, dyspnea or pulmonary congestion, and mental status changes (i.e., lethargy, somnolence, confusion and agitation). Other serious toxicities have included: myocardial ischemia, myocarditis, gangrene, respiratory failure leading to intubation, GI bleeding requiring surgery, intestinal perforation/ ileus, coma, seizure, sepsis and renal impairment requiring dialysis. The incidence of these events has been higher in PS 1 patients than in PS 0 patients (See "CLINICAL PHARMACOLOGY" Section, "Clinical Experience" Subsection).

The following data on adverse reactions are based on 373 patients (255 with renal cell cancer and 118 with other tumors) treated with the recommended every 8 hour 15-minute infusion dosing regimen. These patients had metastatic or recurrent carcinoma and were enrolled in investigational trials in the United States.

Organ systems in which reactions occurred in a significant number of the patients treated are found in the following table: [See Table III preceding page.]

Other serious adverse events were derived from trials involving more than 1,800 patients treated with Proleukin-based regimens using a variety of doses and schedules. These events each occurred with a frequency of <1% and included: liver or renal failure resulting in death; duodenal ulceration; fatal intestinal perforation; bowel necrosis; fatal cardiac arrest, myocarditis, and supraventricular tachycardia; permanent or transient blindness secondary to optic neuritis; fatal malignant hyperthermia; pulmonary edema resulting in death; respiratory arrest; fatal respiratory failure; fatal stroke; transient ischemic attack; meningitis; cerebral edema; pericarditis; allergic interstitial nephritis; tracheoesophageal fistula; fatal pulmonary emboli; severe depression leading to suicide.

OVERDOSAGE

Side effects following the use of Proleukin are dose-related. Administration of more than the recommended dose has been associated with a more rapid onset of expected dose limiting toxicities. Adverse reactions generally will reverse when the drug is stopped, particularly because its serum half-life is short (See "CLINICAL PHARMACOLOGY" Section, "Pharmacokinetics" Subsection). Any continuing symptoms should be treated supportively. Life threatening toxicities have been ameliorated by the intravenous administration of dexamethasone,[13] which may result in loss of therapeutic effect from Proleukin. **NOTE: Prior to the use of dexamethasone, the physician should refer to the package insert for this product.**

DOSAGE AND ADMINISTRATION

Proleukin (aldesleukin for injection) should be administered by a 15-minute IV infusion every 8 hours. Before initiating treatment, carefully review the "INDICATIONS", "CONTRAINDICATIONS", "WARNINGS", "PRECAUTIONS", and "ADVERSE REACTIONS" Sections, particularly regarding patient selection, possible serious adverse events, patient monitoring and withholding dosage.

The following schedule has been used to treat adult patients with metastatic renal cell carcinoma. Each course of treatment consists of two 5-day treatment cycles separated by a rest period.

600,000 IU/kg (0.037 mg/kg) dose administered every 8 hours by a 15-minute IV infusion for a total of 14 doses. Following 9 days of rest, the schedule is repeated for another 14 doses, for a maximum of 28 doses per course. During clinical trials, doses were frequently held for toxicity (See "Dose Modification" Subsection). Patients treated with this schedule received a median of 20 of the 28 doses during the first course of therapy.

Retreatment: Patients should be evaluated for response approximately 4 weeks after completion of a course of therapy and again immediately prior to the scheduled start of the next treatment course. Additional courses of treatment may be given to patients only if there is some tumor shrinkage

following the last course and retreatment is not contraindicated (See "CONTRAINDICATIONS" Section). Each treatment course should be separated by a rest period of at least 7 weeks from the date of hospital discharge. Tumors have continued to regress up to 12 months following the initiation of Proleukin therapy.

Dose Modification: Dose modification for toxicity should be accomplished by holding or interrupting a dose rather than reducing the dose to be given. Decisions to stop, hold, or restart Proleukin therapy must be made after a global assessment of the patient. With this in mind, the following guidelines should be used:

Treatment with Proleukin (aldesleukin) should be permanently discontinued for:

Organ System	Permanently discontinue treatment for the following toxicities
Cardiovascular	Sustained ventricular tachycardia (≥5 beats)
	Cardiac rhythm disturbances not controlled or unresponsive to management
	Recurrent chest pain with ECG changes, documented angina or myocardial infarction
	Pericardial tamponade
Pulmonary	Intubation required >72 hours
Renal	Renal dysfunction requiring dialysis >72 hours
Central Nervous System	Coma or toxic psychosis lasting >48 hours.
	Repetitive or difficult to control seizures
Gastrointestinal	Bowel ischemia/perforation/GI bleeding requiring surgery

Doses should be held and restarted according to the following:

[See table above .]

Reconstitution and Dilution Directions:

Reconstitution and dilution procedures other than those recommended may alter the delivery and/or pharmacology of Proleukin and thus should be avoided.

1. Proleukin is a sterile, white to off-white, preservative-free, lyophilized powder suitable for IV infusion upon reconstitution and dilution. **EACH VIAL CONTAINS 22 MILLION IU (1.3 MG) OF PROLEUKIN AND SHOULD BE RECONSTITUTED ASEPTICALLY WITH 1.2 ML OF STERILE WATER FOR INJECTION, USP. WHEN RECONSTITUTED AS DIRECTED, EACH ML CONTAINS 18 MILLION IU (1.1 MG) OF PROLEUKIN.** The resulting solution should be a clear, colorless to slightly yellow liquid. The vial is for single-use only and any unused portion should be discarded.

2. During reconstitution, the Sterile Water for Injection, USP should be directed at the side of the vial and the contents gently swirled to avoid excess foaming. **DO NOT SHAKE.**

3. The dose of Proleukin, reconstituted in Sterile Water for Injection, USP (without preservative) should be diluted aseptically in 50 mL of 5% Dextrose Injection, USP and infused over a 15-minute period. Although glass bottles and plastic (polyvinyl chloride) bags have been used in clinical trials with comparable results, it is recommended that plastic bags be used as the dilution container since experimental studies suggest that use of plastic containers results in more consistent drug delivery. In-line filters should not be used when administering Proleukin.

4. Before and after reconstitution and dilution, store in a refrigerator at 2° to 8°C (36° to 46°F). Do not freeze. Administer Proleukin within 48 hours of reconstitution. The solution should be brought to room temperature prior to infusion in the patient.

5. Reconstitution or dilution with Bacteriostatic Water for Injection, USP, or 0.9% Sodium Chloride Injection, USP should be avoided because of increased aggregation. Animal studies have shown that dilution with albumin can alter the pharmacology of Proleukin. Proleukin for Injection should not be mixed with other drugs.

6. Parenteral drug products should be inspected visually for particulate matter and discoloration prior to administration, whenever solution and container permit.

HOW SUPPLIED

Proleukin (aldesleukin for injection) is supplied in packs of ten individually-boxed single-use vials. Each vial contains 22×10^6 IU of Proleukin. Discard unused portion.

NDC 53905-991-10

Store vials of lyophilized Proleukin for Injection in a refrigerator at 2° to 8°C (36° to 46°F).

Reconstituted or diluted Proleukin is stable for up to 48 hours at refrigerated and room temperatures, 2° to 25°C

Continued on next page

Cetus—Cont.

(36° to 77°F). However, since this product contains no preservative, the reconstituted and diluted solutions should be stored in the refrigerator.

Do not use beyond the expiration date printed on the vial.
Note: This product contains no preservative.
CAUTION: Federal law (USA) prohibits dispensing without a prescription.

REFERENCES

1. Doyle MV, Lee MT, Fong S. Comparison of the biological activities of human recombinant interleukin-2$_{125}$ and native interleukin-2. *J Biol Response Mod* 1985; **4**:96–109.
2. Ralph P, Nakoinz I, Doyle M, et al. Human B and T lymphocyte stimulating properties of interleukin-2 (IL-2) muteins. In: *Immune Regulation by Characterized Polypeptides.* Alan R. Liss, Inc. **1987**:453–62.
3. Winkelhake JL and Gauny SS. Human recombinant interleukin-2 as an experimental therapeutic. *Pharmacol Rev* 1990: **42**:1–28.
4. Rosenberg SA, Mule JJ, Spiess PJ, et al. Regression of established pulmonary metastases and subcutaneous tumor mediated by the systemic administration of high-dose recombinant interleukin-2. *J Exp Med* 1985; **161**:1169–88.
5. Konrad MW, Hemstreet G, Hersh EM, et al. Pharmacokinetics of recombinant interleukin-2 in humans. *Cancer Res* 1990; **50**:2009–17.
6. Donohue JH and Rosenberg SA. The fate of interleukin-2 after in vivo administration. *J Immunol* 1983; **130**:2203–8.
7. Koths K, Halenbeck R. Pharmacokinetic studies on ^{35}S-labeled recombinant interleukin-2 in mice. In: Sorg C and Schimpl A, eds. *Cellular and Molecular Biology of Lymphokines.* Academic Press: Orlando, Fl, **1985**:779.
8. Moyer BR, Young JD, Bauer RJ, et al. Renal mechanisms for the clearance of recombinant human IL-2 in the rat. *Pharmaceutical Res* 1990: **7**:S284 (abstract).
9. Cetus Corporation. Data on file. 1991.
10. Bock SN, Lee RE, Fisher B, et al. A prospective randomized trial evaluating prophylactic antibiotics to prevention triple-lumen catheter-related sepsis in patients treated with immunotherapy. *J Clin Oncol* 1990; **8**:161–69.
11. Hartman LC, Urba, WJ, Steis RG, et al. Use of prophylactic antibiotics for prevention of intravascular catheter-related infections in interleukin-2-treated patients. *J Natl Cancer Inst* 1989; **81**:1190–93.
12. Snydman DR, Sullivan B, Gill M, et al. Nosocomial sepsis associated with interleukin-2. *Ann Intern Med* 1990; **112**:102–07.
13. Mier JW, Vachino G, Klempner MS, et al. Inhibition of interleukin-2-induced tumor necrosis factor release by dexamethasone: Prevention of an acquired neutrophil chemotaxis defect and differential suppression of interleukin-2-associated side effects. *Blood* 1990; **76**:1933–40.

Manufactured by:
Chiron Corporation
Emeryville, CA 94608
Distributed by:
Cetus Oncology Corporation
Emeryville, CA 94608
Copyright 1992 Cetus Oncology Corporation
Issued May 1992
ZO-P-01 (PD 5486)
U.S. License No. 1106
U.S. Patent Nos. RE 33653; 4,530,787; 4,569,790; 4,604,377; 4,853,332; 4,748,234; 4,572,798; 4,959,314

Sterile VINBLASTINE Sulfate, USP ℞

HOW SUPPLIED

Sterile Vinblastine Sulfate, USP is supplied in packs of ten individually-boxed vials containing 10 mg lyophilized vinblastine sulfate. NDC 53905-091-10.

Store vials in a refrigerator, 2° to 8°C (36° to 46°F) to assure extended stability.

After reconstitution with 10 mL Bacteriostatic Sodium Chloride Injection, USP (preserved with benzyl alcohol), solution may be kept in a refrigerator, 2° to 8°C (36° to 46°F) for 30 days without significant loss of potency.

CAUTION—Federal law prohibits dispensing without a prescription.
Revised November, 1988　　　　　CO-P-02

Cetylite Industries, Inc.
9051 RIVER ROAD
P.O. BOX 90006
PENNSAUKEN, NJ 08110-0700

CETACAINE® ℞
[set 'a-cane ″]
TOPICAL ANESTHETIC

A BRAND OF
Benzocaine..14.0%
Butyl Aminobenzoate.. 2.0%
Tetracaine Hydrochloride...................................... 2.0%
Benzalkonium Chloride.. 0.5%
Cetyl Dimethyl Ethyl
　Ammonium Bromide..0.005%
In a bland water soluble base.

ACTION

Cetacaine produces anesthesia rapidly in approximately 30 seconds.

INDICATIONS

Cetacaine is a topical anesthetic indicated for the production of anesthesia of accessible mucous membrane.

Cetacaine Spray is indicated for use to control pain or gagging. Cetacaine in all forms is indicated for use to control pain.

DOSAGE AND ADMINISTRATION

Cetacaine Spray should be applied for approximately one second or less for normal anesthesia. Only limited quantity of Cetacaine is required for anesthesia and a spray in excess of 2 seconds is contraindicated. Average expulsion rate of residue from spray, at normal temperatures, is 200 mg. per second.

Tissue need not be dried prior to application of Cetacaine. Cetacaine should be applied directly to the site where pain control is required.

Cetacaine Liquid or Cetacaine Ointment may be applied with a cotton pledget or directly to tissue. Cotton pledget should not be held in position for extended periods of time, since local reactions to benzoate topical anesthetics are related to the length of time of application.

ADVERSE REACTIONS

Although systemic reactions to Cetacaine have not been reported, local reactions to benzoate topical anesthetics may be associated with the condition of the mucous membrane treated and the length of time of application. Dehydration of the epithelium or an escharotic effect may result from prolonged contact. Allergic reactions are known to occur in some patients with preparations containing benzocaine.

Usage in Pregnancy: Safe use of Cetacaine has not been established with respect to possible adverse effects upon fetal development. Therefore Cetacaine should not be used during early pregnancy, unless in the judgment of a physician the potential benefits outweigh the unknown hazards.

Routine precaution for the use of any topical anesthetic should be observed when Cetacaine is used.

CONTRAINDICATIONS

Cetacaine is not for injection.

Do not use on the eyes.

To avoid excessive systemic absorption, Cetacaine should not be applied to large areas of denuded or inflamed tissue.

Cetacaine should not be administered to patients who are hypersensitive to any of its ingredients.

Individual dosage of tetracaine hydrochloride in excess of 20 mg. is contraindicated. Cetacaine should not be used under dentures or cotton rolls, as retention of the active ingredients under a denture or cotton roll could possibly cause an escharotic effect.

Jetco-Spray® Cannula: The Jetco cannula for Cetacaine Spray is specially designed for accessibility and application of Cetacaine, at the required site of pain control.

The Jetco cannula is supplied in various sizes and shapes.

The Jetco cannula is inserted firmly onto the protruding plastic tubing on each bottle of Cetacaine Spray.

The Jetco cannula may be removed and re-inserted as many times as required for cleansing or sterilization.

PACKAGING AVAILABLE

Spray—Flavored, Aerosol 56 gm, including propellant with one J4 cannula...........................**NDC 10223-0201-1**
Medical Kit E—Flavored, Aerosol 56 gm, including propellant with two J4, one J6, one J8
cannula....................................**NDC 10223-0201-3**
Liquid—Flavored, 56 gm bottle.............**NDC 10223-0202-1**
Ointment—Flavored, 37 gm jar............**NDC 10223-0210-1**
Gel—29 gm in polyethylene tube.........**NDC 10223-0215-1**

CAUTION

Federal law prohibits dispensing Cetacaine without prescription.

Keep out of reach of children.

(REV. 5/88)

CETYLCIDE® SOLUTION
[see 'til-side ″]
**An instrument and hard surface disinfectant
for use in hospitals and dental/medical operatories.**

Active Ingredients:
Alkyl (85% C$_{16}$, 15% C$_{18}$) Dimethyl Ethyl
　Ammonium Bromide 6.5%
Alkyl (50% C$_{12}$, 30% C$_{14}$,
　17% C$_{16}$, 3% C$_{18}$) Dimethyl
　Benzyl Ammonium Chloride 6.5%
Isopropyl Alcohol 13.0%
Inert Ingredients 74.0%
Total Ingredients 100.0%
Formulation Contains Sodium Nitrite

Keep out of reach of children.

DIRECTIONS FOR USE

It is a violation of Federal Law to use this product in a manner inconsistent with its labeling.

Gently squeeze bottle until liquid fills upper chamber to appropriate black fill line [$\frac{1}{2}$ oz. (15 ml), 1 oz. (30 ml), or 2 oz. (60 ml)]. Pour directly into an appropriate amount of water to make a 1:32 or 1:64 dilution **Cetylcide** Use Solution.

Per Gallon: 1 oz. (30 ml) **Cetylcide** to one gallon (3.785 liters) tap water. In known hard water areas, use distilled water. Clean instruments thoroughly. . . rinse free of all soap before immersion, and allow them to remain in **Cetylcide** solution 15 minutes. Germicides containing a quaternary ammonium derivative should not be relied on to destroy spore forming bacteria, Mycobacterium tuberculosis or the etiologic agents of viral hepatitis. Thus, instruments suspected of such contamination should be sterilized by heat. Needles, hypodermic syringes, corroded instruments or those with deep narrow crevices, as well as hinged or defective plated instruments should be sterilized by heat. To maintain disinfection, they may then be immersed in **Cetylcide** solution. Discard the used solution daily.

Dilution directions for use against Pseudomonas aeruginosa.

Per Gallon: 2 oz. (60 ml) **Cetylcide** to one gallon (3.785 liters) tap water.

Per Quart: $\frac{1}{2}$ oz. (15 ml) **Cetylcide** to one quart (946 ml) tap water.

> **Storage and Disposal**
> Do not re-use empty container. Triple rinse (or equivalent) top section of the indented bottle, then puncture top section and discard in trash.

Cetylcide. . . when diluted as directed, is a potent bactericidal/bacteriostatic germicidal solution active against many kinds of pathogenic bacteria and human immunodeficiency virus (AIDS).

Cetylcide is stable in both concentrated and diluted form. When diluted for use as directed, **Cetylcide** makes a RUST-INHIBITING ● ODORLESS ● COLORLESS, efficient germicidal solution for the chemical disinfection of all METAL, RUBBER, and PLASTIC SURGICAL and DENTAL INSTRUMENTS and APPLIANCES.

Precautionary Statements
Hazards to Humans and Domestic Animals
Corrosive. Causes eye and skin damage. Do not get in eyes, on skin, or on clothing. Wear goggles or face shield and rubber gloves when handling. Harmful or fatal if swallowed. Avoid contamination of food.
Statement of Practical Treatment
Skin and Eyes: In case of contact, immediately flush eyes or skin with plenty of water for at least 15 minutes. For eyes, call a physician. Remove and wash contaminated clothing before reuse.
Ingestion: If swallowed, drink PROMPTLY a large quantity of milk, egg whites, gelatin solution or if these are not available, drink large quantities of water. Avoid alcohol. Call a physician immediately.
Note to Physician: Probable mucosal damage may contraindicate the use of gastric lavage.
EPA Reg. No. 3150-1, EPA Est. No. 3150-NJ-1
Made in U.S.A. Rev. 7/91-A

CETYLCIDE-G®
[see 'til-side ″]
**CONCENTRATE
FOR STERILIZATION AND DISINFECTION
For use in Hospitals, Medical, Dental, Veterinary and Other Health Care Facilities**

Bactericidal, Virucidal*, Tuberculocidal, Fungicidal, Sporicidal.

Cetylcide-G must be used with diluted (1:64) Cetylcide. Never use Cetylcide-G alone

Active Ingredient:

Glutaraldehyde	47.50%
Inert Ingredients:	52.50%
Total Ingredients:	100.00%

Keep out of reach of children
DANGER
Precautionary Statements
Wear goggles or safety glasses when handling.
Hazards to Humans and Domestic Animals
Causes severe eye and skin irritation; harmful if swallowed. Avoid contamination with eyes, skin and clothing. Avoid contamination of food.

Statement of Practical Treatment
In cases of eye contact, immediately flush with water and continue washing for at least 15 minutes. Obtain the advice of an ophthalmologist urgently. For skin contact, wash contaminated skin with soap and water. If contact has been widespread and prolonged, or if irritation persists, seek medical advice. Contaminated clothing should be washed before reuse. ***IF SWALLOWED:*** **DO NOT INDUCE VOMITING.** Do not give anything to drink. Obtain medical advice with urgency. ***NOTE TO PHYSICIAN:*** Probable mucosal damage may contraindicate the use of gastric lavage.

DIRECTIONS FOR USE
It is a violation of Federal Law to use this product in a manner inconsistent with its labeling.

Do not use this product on food or feed.
Cetylcide-G is an effective disinfectant/sterilant only when mixed with the correct dilution (1:64) of Cetylcide. Cetylcide is a registered quaternary disinfectant.
Prepare a dilution of Cetylcide using 1 part Cetylcide to 64 parts of tap water (The use-dilution of Cetylcide is 1:64 or 2 oz. of Cetylcide Concentrate to 128 oz. (1 gal.) of tap water.) In known hard water areas, use softened, deionized or distilled water.
To each quart of use-dilution Cetylcide, add one premeasured portion of Cetylcide-G (total 63 ml). To measure one portion of Cetylcide-G gently squeeze the lower portion of the bottle allowing solution to fill the top section to the fill line. Pour contents of this top section into a quart of diluted Cetylcide. The resulting disinfectant/sterilant mixture will be **green.** For one gallon of use dilution Cetylcide, add four pre-measured portions (total 252 ml) of Cetylcide-G.
Label the Cetylcide-G/Cetylcide mixture with the label(s) provided.
Clean instruments thoroughly. Rinse free of all soap before immersion. Clean and rinse the lumina of hollow instruments before filling with solution.

For use as a disinfectant; Immerse instruments in Cetylcide-G/Cetylcide solution for 20 minutes. This contact will kill bacteria in 3 minutes; fungi: *Trichophyton mentagrophytes, Candida parapsilosis, Candida albicans* and *Aspergillus fumigatus* in 10 minutes; viruses*: Herpes simplex type 1, Herpes simplex type 2, Poliovirus type I, Poliovirus type II, Poliovirus type III, Coxsackie virus B1, Coxsackie virus A9, Cytomegalovirus, Vaccinia virus, Adenovirus, Influenza A virus, Rhinovirus, Human Immunodeficiency virus (AIDS), Canine distemper virus and Canine parvovirus in 10 minutes, and *Mycobacterium tuberculosis* in 20 minutes at 20°C. Cetylcide-G/Cetylcide solution can be re-used as a disinfectant for up to 28 days.

For use as a sterilant; Immerse instruments in Cetylcide-G/Cetylcide solution for 3 hours. Remove instruments from the solution using aseptic technique to prevent recontamination. Rinse instruments thoroughly with sterile water. When sterile water is not available, use 70% isopropyl alcohol to rinse. This sterilization procedure kills bacterial spores. Cetylcide-G/Cetylcide solution can be re-used as a sterilant for up to 28 days.

Storage and Disposal
Do not contaminate water, food or feed by either storage or disposal. Pesticide wastes are toxic. Improper disposal or excess pesticide, spray, use mixture or rinsate is a violation of Federal Law. If these wastes cannot be disposed of by use according to label directions, contact your State Pesticide or your Environmental Control agency, or the Hazardous Waste representative at the nearest EPA Regional Office for guidance. Waste resulting from the use of this product may be disposed of on site.

Storage
This product should be stored at room temperature, preferably in a cool place.

Container Disposal
Do not re-use empty container. Triple rinse (or equivalent) top section of the indented bottle, then puncture top section and dispose of entire container in a sanitary landfill or by incineration if allowed by state and local authorities.

HOW SUPPLIED
32 ounce, 12 ounce dispenser bottle.
Manufactured By
CETYLITE
INDUSTRIES, INC.
9051 River Road
Pennsauken, NJ 08110-3293 1/91-A
EPA Reg. No. 3150-4 U.S. Pat. 4,923,899 Made in U.S.A.
EPA Establishment No. 3150-NJ-1 Foreign patents pend.

CIBA Consumer Pharmaceuticals
Division of CIBA-GEIGY Corporation
581 MAIN STREET
WOODBRIDGE, NJ 07095

DULCOLAX® **OTC**
[*dul 'co-lax*]
brand of bisacodyl USP

DESCRIPTION AND CLINICAL PHARMACOLOGY
Dulcolax is a contact stimulant laxative, administered either orally or rectally, which acts directly on the colonic mucosa to produce normal peristalsis throughout the large intestine. The active ingredient in Dulcolax, bisacodyl, is a colorless, tasteless compound that is practically insoluble in water or alkaline solution. Its chemical name is: bis(p-acetoxyphenyl)-2-pyridylmethane. Bisacodyl is very poorly absorbed, if at all, in the small intestine following oral administration, nor in the large intestine following rectal administration. On contact with the mucosa or submucosal plexi of the large intestine, bisacodyl stimulates sensory nerve endings to produce parasympathetic reflexes resulting in increased peristaltic contractions of the colon. It has also been shown to promote fluid and ion accumulation in the colon, which increases the laxative effect. A bowel movement is usually produced approximately 6 hours after oral administration (8–12 hours if taken at bedtime), and approximately 15 minutes to 1 hour after rectal administration, providing satisfactory cleansing of the bowel which may, under certain circumstances, obviate the need for colonic irrigation.
Dulcolax (brand of bisacodyl USP) is available as tablets of 5 mg each or as suppositories of 10 mg each. Each tablet also contains: acacia, acetylated monoglyceride, carnauba wax, cellulose acetate phthalate, corn starch, D&C Red No. 30 aluminum lake, D&C Yellow No. 10 aluminum lake, dibutyl phthalate, docusate sodium, gelatin, glycerin, iron oxides, kaolin, lactose, magnesium stearate, methylparaben, pharmaceutical glaze, polyethylene glycol, povidone, propylparaben, sodium benzoate, sorbitan monooleate, sucrose, talc, titanium dioxide, and white wax. Each suppository also contains hydrogenated vegetable oil. Tablets and suppositories contain less than 0.2 mg sodium per dosage unit and are thus dietetically sodium-free.

INDICATIONS AND USAGE
For the relief of occasional constipation and irregularity. For use as part of a bowel cleansing regimen in preparing the patient for surgery or for preparing the colon for x-ray endoscopic examination. Dulcolax will not replace the colonic irrigations usually given patients before intracolonic surgery, but is useful in the preliminary emptying of the colon prior to those procedures. Dulcolax may also be used in postoperative care (i.e., restoration of normal bowel hygiene), antepartum care, postpartum care, and in preparation for delivery.

CONTRAINDICATIONS
Stimulant laxatives, such as Dulcolax, are contraindicated for patients with acute surgical abdomen, appendicitis, rectal bleeding, gastroenteritis, or intestinal obstruction.

WARNINGS AND PRECAUTIONS
Use of Dulcolax is not recommended when abdominal pain, nausea, or vomiting are present. Long term administration of Dulcolax is not recommended in the treatment of chronic constipation. Rectal bleeding or failure to have a bowel movement after Dulcolax use may indicate a serious condition. If this occurs, the patient should discontinue use of the product.
Pregnancy Category B
Teratology
Reproduction studies of oral doses of Dulcolax (bisacodyl) have been performed in rats administered up to 70 times the human dose, and have revealed no evidence of impaired fertility or damage to the fetus. At the dose which equated to 70 times the human dose, there was some evidence of lower litter survival at weaning. There are, however, no adequate and well-controlled studies in pregnant women, hence Dulcolax should be used during pregnancy only at the discretion of the physician.
Extent of Drug Absorption
In a pharmacokinetic (crossover) study involving 12 patients (Roth, 1988), plasma levels of bisacodyl were measured following oral administration of a 10 mg reference solution and two 5 mg Dulcolax tablets, and following rectal administration of one 10 mg Dulcolax suppository. With the solution dose, the average Cmax was 237 ng/ml; with the tablet dose, the average Cmax was 26 ng/ml (11% of the solution Cmax); with the suppository dose, in six patients the plasma level was below the limit of detection, and in the remaining six patients, the average Cmax was 31 ng/ml (13% of the solution Cmax in those particular patients). These data demonstrate the low level of systemic absorption of bisacodyl resulting from Dulcolax use.
Clinical experience has shown that Dulcolax tablets or suppositories can be administered for constipation during pregnancy (Happert, 1963; Smith, 1964), apparently without the danger of stimulating the uterus (Smith, 1964), and postpartum (Sichel, 1961).
Due to the minimal extent of bisacodyl systemic absorption associated with Dulcolax usage, it is believed that the risk of harm to the fetus is very low. However, because animal reproduction studies are not always predictive of human response, Dulcolax should be used during pregnancy only at the discretion of the physician.

ADVERSE DRUG REACTIONS
The process of restoring normal bowel function by use of a laxative may result in some abdominal discomfort.

OVERDOSAGE
There are no specific antidotes that are required to be administered in the event of overdosage; however, supportive care may be required in order to prevent dehydration and/or electrolyte imbalance.

DOSAGE AND ADMINISTRATION
Tablets
Adults and children 12 years of age and over: Take 2 or 3 tablets (usually 2) in a single dose once daily.
Children 6 to under 12 years of age: Take 1 tablet once daily.
Expect results in 8–12 hours if taken at bedtime or within 6 hours if taken before breakfast. Do not chew or crush tablets. Do not administer tablets within 1 hour after taking an antacid or milk.
Children under 6 years of age: Oral administration is not recommended due to the requirement to swallow tablets whole.
Suppositories
Adults and children 12 years of age and over: Use 1 suppository once daily. Remove foil wrapper. Lie on your side and, with pointed end first, push suppository high into the rectum so it will not slip out. Retain it for 15 to 20 minutes. If you feel the suppository must come out immediately, it was not inserted high enough and should be pushed higher.
Children under 12 years of age: One half of one 10 mg suppository once daily.
If the suppository seems soft, hold in foil wrapper under cold water for one or two minutes. In the presence of anal fissures or hemorrhoids, suppository may be coated at the tip with petroleum jelly before insertion.
Preparation for x-ray endoscopy: For barium enemas, no food should be given following oral administration to prevent reaccumulation of material in the rectum, and a suppository should be administered one to two hours prior to examination.

HOW SUPPLIED
Dulcolax, brand of bisacodyl, is supplied as either orange tablets of 5 mg each in sample packages of 2 or boxes of 4, 10, 25, 50, 100 (OTC as well as hospital unit doses) and 1000, or as suppositories of 10 mg each in sample packages of 1 or boxes of 4, 8, 16, 50, and 500.
NDC 0083-6200 (tablets)
NDC 0083-6100 (suppositories)
Store Dulcolax tablets and suppositories at temperatures below 77°F (25°C). Avoid excessive humidity.
Dulcolax is also supplied in a Bowel Prep Kit. Each kit contains one Dulcolax suppository (10 mg), four Dulcolax tablets (5 mg each), and complete patient instructions.

BIBLIOGRAPHY
Happert, J.L.: "Clinical Trials of a New Contact Laxative, La 96a"; Gaz. Hop. 135, pp. 1145–1148 (1963).
Roth, V.W. et al: "Pharmacokinetics and Laxative Effect of Bisacodyl after Administration of Various Dosage Forms"; Arzneim.-Forsch. *38* (I), No. 4, pp. 570–4 (1988).

Continued on next page

CIBA Consumer—Cont.

Sichel, M.S.: "Postpartum and Postoperative Bowel Function"; Northwest Medicine 60, pp. 708-9 (1961).

Smith, J.J. et al: "Evaluation of a New Contact Laxative, Bisacodyl (Dulcolax), in Obstetrics and Gynecology"; West. J. Surgery, Obstet., and Gyn. 72, pp. 177–180 (1964).

Additional literature references available upon request.
July 1, 1992

NŌSTRIL® Nasal Decongestant Mild   OTC
NŌSTRIL® Nasal Decongestant 1/2% Regular
[nō'stril]
phenylephrine HCl, USP

DESCRIPTION
Nostril Nasal Decongestant contains phenylephrine HCl 0.25% (¼% Mild strengh) or phenylephrine HCl 0.5% (½% Regular strength).

ACTIONS
Nostril metered pump spray for nasal decongestion delivers measured, uniform doses. The medication constricts the smaller arterioles of the nasal passages, producing a gentle, predictable, decongestant effect. Nostril penetrates and shrinks swollen membranes, restoring freer breathing and unclogs sinus passages, bringing the effective medication in contact with inflamed, swollen tissues. It will not hurt tender membranes since it is formulated to match the pH of normal nasal secretions. The one-way pump helps prevent draw-back contamination of the medication.

INDICATIONS
For temporary relief of nasal congestion due to the common cold, hay fever, other upper respiratory allergies, or associated with sinusitis.

WARNINGS
Do not exceed recommended dosage because burning, stinging, sneezing, or increased nasal discharge may occur. Do not use for more than 3 days. If symptoms persist, consult a physician. Use of the dispenser by more than one person may spread infection. Do not use this product if you have heart disease, high blood pressure, thyroid disease, diabetes or difficulty in urination due to enlargement of the prostrate gland, unless directed by a physician. Keep this and all drugs out of reach of children.

SYMPTOMS AND TREATMENT OF ORAL OVERDOSAGE
In case of accidental ingestion, seek professional assistance or consult a poison control center immediately.

DOSAGE AND ADMINISTRATION
¼% Mild—Adults and children 6 to under 12 years of age (with adult supervision): 2 or 3 sprays in each nostril not more often than every 4 hours. Children under 6 years of age: consult a doctor.

½% Regular—Adults: 2 or 3 sprays in each nostril not more often than every 4 hours. Do not give to children under 12 years of age unless directed by a doctor.

Remove protective cap. Hold bottle with thumb at base and nozzle between first and second fingers. With head upright, insert nozzle into nostril. Depress pump 2 or 3 times, all the way down, and sniff deeply. Repeat in other nostril. Before using the first time, prime pump by depressing it firmly several times.

INACTIVE INGREDIENTS
Benzalkonium chloride 0.004% as a preservative, boric acid, sodium borate, water.

HOW SUPPLIED
Metered nasal pump spray in white plastic bottles of ½ fl. oz. (15 ml) packaged in tamper-resistant outer cartons.
0.25% (¼% Mild strength) for children 6 years and over and adults who prefer a milder decongestant (NDC 0083-7200-52).
0.5% (½% Regular strength) for adults and children 12 years or older (NDC 0083-7100-52).

NŌSTRILLA® Long Acting   OTC
[nō-stril 'a]
Nasal Decongestant
oxymetazoline HCl, USP

DESCRIPTION
Nōstrilla Long Acting Nasal Decongestant contains oxymetazoline HCl 0.05%.

ACTIONS
Nostrilla metered pump spray for nasal decongestion delivers measured, uniform doses. The medication constricts the smaller arterioles of the nasal passages, producing a pro-

---

longed (up to 12 hours), gentle, predictable, decongestant effect. Nōstrilla penetrates and shrinks swollen membrances, restoring freer breathing and unclogs sinus passages, bringing the effective medication in contact with inflamed, swollen tissues. It will not hurt tender membranes since it is formulated to match the pH of normal nasal secretions. Use at bedtime restores freer nasal breathing through the night. The one-way pump helps prevent draw-back contamination of the medication.

INDICATIONS
For temporary relief of nasal congestion due to the common cold, hay fever, other upper respiratory allergies, or associated with sinusitis.

WARNINGS
Do not exceed recommended dosage because burning, stinging, sneezing or increased nasal discharge may occur. Do not use for more than 3 days. If symptoms persist, consult a physician. Use of the dispenser by more than one person may spread infection. Do not use this product if you have heart disease, high blood pressure, thyroid disease, diabetes or difficulty in urination due to enlargement of the prostate gland unless directed by a doctor. Keep this and all drugs out of reach of children.

SYMPTOMS AND TREATMENT OF ORAL OVERDOSAGE
In case of accidental ingestion, seek professional assistance or contact a poison control center immediately.

DOSAGE AND ADMINISTRATION
Adults and children 6 to under 12 years of age (with adult supervision): 2 or 3 sprays in each nostril not more often than every 10 to 12 hours. Do not exceed 2 applications in any 24-hour period. Children under 6 years of age: consult a doctor. Remove protective cap. Hold bottle with thumb at base and nozzle between first and second fingers. With head upright, insert nozzle into nostril. Depress pump 2 or 3 times, all the way down, and sniff deeply. Repeat in other nostril. Before using the first time, prime pump by depressing it firmly several times.

INACTIVE INGREDIENTS
Benzalkonium chloride 0.02% as a preservative, glycine, sorbitol solution, water. (Mercury preservatives are not used in this product.)

HOW SUPPLIED
Metered nasal pump spray in white plastic bottles of ½ fl. oz. (15 ml) packaged in tamper-resistant outer cartons (NDC 0083-7300-52).

SLOW FE®   OTC
Slow Release Iron Tablets

DESCRIPTION
SLOW FE supplies ferrous sulfate, for the treatment of iron deficiency and iron deficiency anemia with a significant reduction in the incidence of the common side effects associated with taking oral iron preparations. The wax matrix delivery system of SLOW FE is designed to maximize the release of ferrous sulfate in the duodenum and the jejunum where it is best tolerated and absorbed. SLOW FE has been clinically shown to be associated with a lower incidence of constipation, diarrhea and abdominal discomfort when compared to an immediate release iron tablet[1] and a leading sustained release iron capsule.[2]

FORMULA
Each tablet contains 160 mg dried ferrous sulfate USP, equivalent to 50 mg elemental iron. Also contains cetostearyl alcohol, colloidal silicon dioxide, hydroxypropyl methylcellulose, shellac, lactose, magnesium stearate, polyethylene glycol.

DOSAGE
ADULTS—one or two tablets daily or as recommended by a physician. A maximum of four tablets daily may be taken. CHILDREN—one tablet daily. Tablets must be swallowed whole.

WARNING
The treatment of any anemic condition should be on the advice and under the supervision of a physician. As oral iron products interfere with absorption of oral tetracycline antibiotics, these products should not be taken within two hours of each other. As with any drug, if you are pregnant or nursing a baby, seek the advice of a health professional before using this product.

Keep this and all medicines out of reach of children. In case of accidental overdose, contact your physician or poison control center immediately.
Tamper Evident Packaging.

HOW SUPPLIED
Packages of 30, 60 and bottles of 100.
Packages of 30 supplied in non-child resistant packaging.
Packages of 60 and 100 supplied in Child-Resistant packaging.
Do not store above 86°F. Protect from moisture.

REFERENCES
1. Brock C et al. Adverse effects of iron supplementation: A comparative trial of a wax-matrix iron preparation and conventional ferrous sulfate tablets. *Clin Ther.* 1985; 7:I-VI.
2. Brock C, Curry H. Comparative incidence of side effects of a wax-matrix and a sustained-release iron preparation. *Clin Ther.* 1985;7:492–496.
Shown in Product Identification Section, page 408

TRANSDERM SCŌP®   ℞
[trans-derm scōpe]
scopolamine
(formerly Transderm-V)

Transdermal Therapeutic System

Programmed delivery *in vivo* of 0.5 mg of scopolamine over 3 days

This product is now marketed by CIBA Consumer Pharmaceuticals, Division of CIBA-GEIGY Corporation.

PRODUCT OVERVIEW

KEY FACTS
The active ingredient in the Transderm Scōp system is scopolamine, a belladonna alkaloid. The transdermal system contains 1.5 mg of scopolamine and is designed to deliver 0.5 mg of scopolamine at an approximately constant rate to the systemic circulation over the 3-day lifetime of the system.

MAJOR USES
Transderm Scōp system has proved to be clinically effective for the prevention of nausea and vomiting associated with motion sickness in adults when applied to the skin in the postauricular area.

SAFETY INFORMATION
Transderm Scōp system is contraindicated for patients with known hypersensitivity to scopolamine or any of the components of the adhesive matrix making up the therapeutic system, or in patients with glaucoma.
Before prescribing, please consult full prescribing information below.

PRESCRIBING INFORMATION

TRANSDERM SCŌP®   ℞
[trans-derm scōpe]
scopolamine
(formerly Transderm-V)

Transdermal Therapeutic System

DESCRIPTION
The Transderm Scōp system is a circular flat disc designed for continuous release of scopolamine following application to an area of intact skin on the head, behind the ear. Clinical evaluation has demonstrated that the system provides effective antiemetic and antinauseant actions when tested against motion-sickness stimuli in adults. The Transderm Scōp system is a film 0.2 mm thick and 2.5 cm², with four layers. Proceeding from the visible surface towards the surface attached to the skin, these layers are: (1) a backing layer of tan-colored, aluminized, polyester film; (2) a drug reservoir of scopolamine, mineral oil, and polyisobutylene; (3) a microporous polypropylene membrane that controls the rate of delivery of scopolamine from the system to the skin surface; and (4) an adhesive formulation of mineral oil, polyisobutylene, and scopolamine. A protective peel strip of siliconized polyester, which covers the adhesive layer, is removed before the system is used. The inactive components, mineral oil (12.4 mg) and polyisobutylene (11.4 mg), are not released from the system.

Cross section of the system:

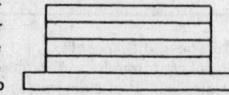

Backing Layer
Drug Reservoir
Rate-Controlling Membrane
Contact Adhesive
Protective Peel Strip

Release-Rate Concept: The Transderm Scōp system contains 1.5 mg of scopolamine. The system is programmed to deliver 0.5 mg of scopolamine at an approximately constant rate to the systemic circulation over the 3-day lifetime of the system. An initial priming dose of scopolamine, released from the adhesive layer of the system, saturates the skin binding sites and rapidly brings the plasma concentration of scopolamine to the required steady-state level. A continuous controlled release of scopolamine, which flows from the drug reservoir through the rate-controlling membrane, maintains the plasma level constant.

CLINICAL PHARMACOLOGY

The sole active agent of Transderm Scōp is scopolamine, a belladonna alkaloid with well-known pharmacological properties. The drug has a long history of oral and parenteral use for central anticholinergic activity, including prophylaxis of motion sickness. The mechanism of action of scopolamine in the central nervous system (CNS) is not definitely known but may include anticholinergic effects. The ability of scopolamine to prevent motion-induced nausea is believed to be associated with inhibition of vestibular input to the CNS, which results in inhibition of the vomiting reflex. In addition, scopolamine may have a direct action on the vomiting center within the reticular formation of the brain stem. Applied to the postauricular skin, Transderm Scōp provides for a gradual release of scopolamine from an adhesive matrix of mineral oil and polyisobutylene.

INDICATIONS AND USAGE

Transderm Scōp is indicated for prevention of nausea and vomiting associated with motion sickness in adults. The disc should be applied only to skin in the postauricular area.
Clinical Results: Transderm Scōp provides antiemetic protection within several hours following application of the disc behind the ear. In 195 adult subjects of different racial origins who participated in clinical efficacy studies at sea or in a controlled motion environment, there was a 75% reduction in the incidence of motion-induced nausea and vomiting. Transderm Scōp provided significantly greater protection than that obtained with oral dimenhydrinate.

CONTRAINDICATIONS

Transderm Scōp should not be used in patients with known hypersensitivity to scopolamine or any of the components of the adhesive matrix making up the therapeutic system, or in patients with glaucoma.

WARNINGS

Transderm Scōp should not be used in children and should be used with special caution in the elderly. See **PRECAUTIONS.**
Since drowsiness, disorientation, and confusion may occur with the use of scopolamine, patients should be warned of the possibility and cautioned against engaging in activities that require mental alertness, such as driving a motor vehicle or operating dangerous machinery.
Potentially alarming idiosyncratic reactions may occur with ordinary therapeutic doses of scopolamine.

PRECAUTIONS

General

Scopolamine should be used with caution in patients with pyloric obstruction, or urinary bladder neck obstruction. Caution should be exercised when administering an antiemetic or antimuscarinic drug to patients suspected of having intestinal obstruction.
Transderm Scōp should be used with special caution in the elderly or in individuals with impaired metabolic, liver, or kidney functions, because of the increased likelihood of CNS effects.

Information for Patients

Since scopolamine can cause temporary dilation of the pupils and blurred vision if it comes in contact with the eyes, patients should be strongly advised to wash their hands thoroughly with soap and water immediately after handling the disc.
Patients should be advised to remove the disc immediately and contact a physician in the unlikely event that they experience symptoms of acute narrow-angle glaucoma (pain in and reddening of the eyes accompanied by dilated pupils). Patients should be warned against driving a motor vehicle or operating dangerous machinery. A patient brochure is available.

Drug Interactions

Scopolamine should be used with care in patients taking drugs, including alcohol, capable of causing CNS effects. Special attention should be given to drugs having anticholinergic properties, e.g., belladonna alkaloids, antihistamines (including meclizine), and antidepressants.

Carcinogenesis, Mutagenesis, Impairment of Fertility

No long-term studies in animals have been performed to evaluate carcinogenic potential. Fertility studies were performed in female rats and revealed no evidence of impaired fertility or harm to the fetus due to scopolamine hydrobromide administered by daily subcutaneous injection. In the highest-dose group (plasma level approximately 500 times the level achieved in humans using a transdermal system), reduced maternal body weights were observed.

Pregnancy Category C

Teratogenic studies were performed in pregnant rats and rabbits with scopolamine hydrobromide administered by daily intravenous injection. No adverse effects were recorded in the rats. In the rabbits, the highest dose (plasma level approximately 100 times the level achieved in humans using a transdermal system) of drug administered had a

marginal embryotoxic effect. Transderm Scōp should be used during pregnancy only if the anticipated benefit justifies the potential risk to the fetus.

Nursing Mothers

It is not known whether scopolamine is excreted in human milk. Because many drugs are excreted in human milk, caution should be exercised when Transderm Scōp is administered to a nursing woman.

Pediatric Use

Children are particularly susceptible to the side effects of belladonna alkaloids. Transderm Scōp should not be used in children because it is not known whether this system will release an amount of scopolamine that could produce serious adverse effects in children.

ADVERSE REACTIONS

The most frequent adverse reaction to Transderm Scōp is dryness of the mouth. This occurs in about two thirds of the people. A less frequent adverse reaction is drowsiness, which occurs in less than one sixth of the people. Transient impairment of eye accommodation, including blurred vision and dilation of the pupils, is also observed.
The following adverse reactions have also been reported on infrequent occasions during the use of Transderm Scōp: disorientation; memory disturbances; dizziness; restlessness; hallucinations; confusion; difficulty urinating; rashes and erythema; acute narrow-angle glaucoma; and dry, itchy, or red eyes.
Drug Withdrawal: Symptoms including dizziness, nausea, vomiting, headache and disturbances of equilibrium have been reported in a few patients following discontinuation of the use of the Transderm Scōp system. These symptoms have occurred most often in patients who have used the systems for more than three days.

OVERDOSAGE

Overdosage with scopolamine may cause disorientation, memory disturbances, dizziness, restlessness, hallucinations, or confusion. Should these symptoms occur, the Transderm Scōp disc should be immediately removed. Appropriate parasympathomimetic therapy should be initiated if these symptoms are severe.

DOSAGE AND ADMINISTRATION

Initiation of Therapy: One Transderm Scōp disc (programmed to deliver 0.5 mg of scopolamine over 3 days) should be applied to the hairless area behind one ear at least 4 hours before the antiemetic effect is required. Only one disc should be worn at any time.
Handling: After the disc is applied on dry skin behind the ear, the hands should be washed thoroughly with soap and water and dried. Upon removal of the disc, it should be discarded, and the hands and application site washed thoroughly with soap and water and dried, to prevent any traces of scopolamine from coming into direct contact with the eyes. (A patient brochure is available.)
Continuation of Therapy: Should the disc become displaced, it should be discarded, and a fresh one placed on the hairless area behind the other ear. If therapy is required for longer than 3 days, the first disc should be discarded, and a fresh one placed on the hairless area behind the other ear.

HOW SUPPLIED

The Transderm Scōp system is a tan-colored disc, 2.5 cm², on a clear, oversized, hexagonal peel strip, which is removed prior to use.
Each Transderm Scōp system contains 1.5 mg of scopolamine and is programmed to deliver *in vivo* 0.5 mg of scopolamine over 3 days.
Transderm Scōp is available in packages of four discs. Each disc is foil wrapped. Patient instructions are included.
1 Package (4 discs) ....NDC 0083-4345-04
The system should be stored between 59° - 86°F (15° - 30°C).
C88-5 (Rev. 2/88)
Please read this instruction sheet carefully before opening the system package.

Information for the Patient About—

TRANSDERM SCŌP®
Generic Name: scopolamine,
pronounced skoe-POL-a-meen
(formerly Transderm-V)
Transdermal Therapeutic System

The Transderm Scōp system helps to prevent the nausea and vomiting of motion sickness for up to 3 days. It is an adhesive disc that you place behind your ear several hours before you travel. Wear only one disc at any time.
Be sure to wash your hands thoroughly with soap and water immediately after handling the disc, so that any drug that might get on your hands will not come into contact with your eyes.
Avoid drinking alcohol while using Transderm Scōp. Also, be careful about driving or operating any machinery while using the system because the drug might make you drowsy.

DO NOT USE TRANSDERM SCŌP IF YOU ARE ALLERGIC TO SCOPOLAMINE OR HAVE GLAUCOMA. TRANSDERM SCŌP SHOULD NOT BE USED IN CHILDREN AND SHOULD BE USED WITH SPECIAL CAUTION IN THE ELDERLY.

How the Transderm Scōp System Works

A group of nerve fibers deep inside the ear helps people keep their balance. For some people, the motion of ships, airplanes, trains, automobiles, and buses increases the activity of these nerve fibers. This increased activity causes the *dizziness, nausea, and vomiting* of motion sickness. People may have one, some, or all of these symptoms.
Transderm Scōp contains the drug scopolamine, which helps reduce the activity of the nerve fibers in the inner ear. When a Transderm Scōp disc is placed on the skin behind one of the ears, scopolamine passes through the skin and into the bloodstream. One disc may be kept in place for 3 days if needed.

Precautions

Before using Transderm Scōp be sure to tell your doctor if you—
● Are pregnant or nursing (or planning to become pregnant)
● Have (or have had) glaucoma (increased pressure in the eyeball)
● Have (or have had) any metabolic, liver, or kidney disease
● Have any obstructions of the stomach or intestine
● Have trouble urinating or any bladder obstruction
● Have any skin allergy or have had a skin reaction such as a rash or redness to any drug, especially scopolamine, or chemical or food substance.

Any of these conditions could make Transderm Scōp unsuitable for you. Also tell your doctor if you are taking any other medicines.
In the unlikely event that you experience pain in the eye and reddened whites of the eye, which may be accompanied by widening of the pupil and blurred vision, remove the disc immediately and consult your physician. As indicated below under Side Effects, widening of the pupils and blurred vision without pain or reddened whites of the eye is usually temporary and not serious.
Transderm Scōp should not be used in children. The safety of its use in children has not been determined. Children and the elderly may be particularly sensitive to the effects of scopolamine.

Side Effects

The most common side effect experienced by people using Transderm Scōp is dryness of the mouth. This occurs in about two thirds of the people. A less frequent side effect is drowsiness, which occurs in less than one sixth of the people. Temporary blurring of vision and dilation (widening) of the pupils may occur, especially if the drug is on your hands and comes in contact with the eyes. On infrequent occasions, disorientation, memory disturbances, dizziness, restlessness, hallucinations, confusion, difficulty urinating, skin rashes or redness, and dry, itchy, or red eyes and eye pain have been reported. If these effects do occur, remove the disc and call your doctor. Since drowsiness, disorientation, and confusion may occur with the use of scopolamine, be careful driving or operating any dangerous machinery, especially when you first start using the drug system.

Drug Withdrawal: Symptoms including dizziness, nausea, vomiting, headache and disturbances of equilibrium have been reported in a few people following discontinuation of the Transderm Scōp system. These symptoms have occurred most often in people who have used the Systems for more than three days. We recommend that you consult your doctor if these symptoms occur.

How to Use Transderm Scōp

Transderm Scōp should be stored between 59° - 86°F (15° - 30°C) until you are ready to use it.
1. Plan to apply one Transderm Scōp disc at least 4 hours before you need it. **Wear only one disc at any time.**
2. Select a hairless area of skin behind one ear, taking care to avoid any cuts or irritations. Wipe the area with a clean, dry tissue.
3. Peel the package open and remove the disc (Figure 1).

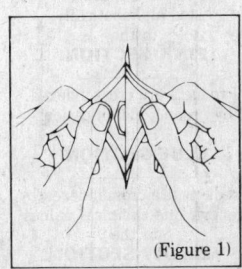

(Figure 1)

Continued on next page

CIBA Consumer—Cont.

4. Remove the clear plastic six-sided backing from the round system. Try not to touch the adhesive surface on the disc with your hands (Figure 2).

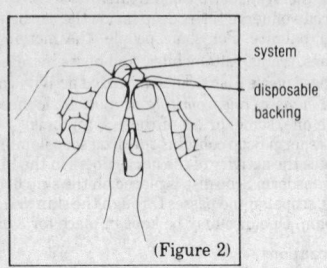

(Figure 2)

5. Firmly apply the adhesive surface (metallic side) to the dry area of skin behind the ear so that the tan-colored side is showing (Figure 3). Make good contact, especially around the edge. Once you have placed the disc behind your ear, do not move it for as long as you want to use it (up to 3 days).

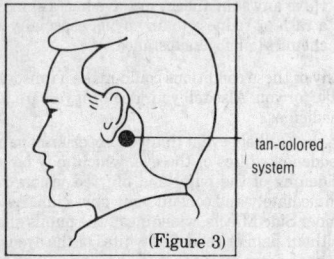

(Figure 3)

6. *Important:* **After the disc is in place, be sure to wash your hands thoroughly with soap and water to remove any scopolamine. If this drug were to contact your eyes, it could cause temporary blurring of vision and dilation (widening) of the pupils (the dark circles in the center of your eyes). This is not serious unless accompanied by eye pain and redness (see Precautions), and your pupils should return to normal.**

7. Remove the disc after 3 days and throw it away. (You may remove it sooner if you are no longer concerned about motion sickness.) After removing the disc, be sure to wash your hands and the area behind your ear thoroughly with soap and water.

8. If you wish to control nausea for longer than 3 days, *remove* the first disc after 3 days and place a new one *behind the other ear,* repeating instructions 2 to 7.

9. Keep the disc dry, if possible, to prevent it from falling off. Limited contact with water, however, as in bathing or swimming, will not affect the system. In the unlikely event that the disc falls off, throw it away and put a new one behind the other ear.

This leaflet presents a summary of information about Transderm Scōp. If you would like more information or if you have any questions, ask your doctor or pharmacist. A more technical leaflet is available, written for your doctor. If you would like to read the leaflet, ask your pharmacist to show you a copy. You may need the help of your doctor or pharmacist to understand some of the information.

Dist. by:
CIBA Consumer Pharmaceuticals
Division of CIBA-GEIGY Corp.
Summit, NJ 07901

C88-6 (Rev. 2/88)
Shown in Product Identification Section, page 408

Products are
listed alphabetically
in the
PINK SECTION.

Products are cross-indexed
by product classifications
in the
BLUE SECTION.

Products are cross-indexed by
generic and chemical names
in the
YELLOW SECTION.

CIBA Pharmaceutical Company
Division of CIBA-GEIGY Corporation
SUMMIT, NJ 07901

To provide a convenient and accurate means of identifying CIBA solid dosage form products, a code number has been imprinted on all tablets and capsules. To help you quickly identify a CIBA Tablet or Capsule by its code number, a numerical listing of codes (with corresponding product names) and an alphabetical listing of products (with corresponding codes and list numbers) have been compiled below.

CIBA Code #	ALPHABETICAL LISTING	List Number
	Anturane®	
	sulfinpyrazone USP	
41	TABLETS (white, single-scored) each containing 100 mg sulfinpyrazone USP	
	100s	1910
168	CAPSULES (green) each containing 200 mg sulfinpyrazone USP	
	100s	1920
	Apresazide®	
	hydralazine HCl and hydrochlorothiazide	
139	CAPSULES 25/25 (light blue and white opaque), each containing 25 mg hydralazine HCl and 25 mg hydrochlorothiazide	
	100s	3131
149	CAPSULES 50/50 (pink and white opaque), each containing 50 mg hydralazine HCl and 50 mg hydrochlorothiazide	
	100s	3132
159	CAPSULES 100/50 (pink flesh and white opaque), each containing 100 mg hydralazine HCl and 50 mg hydrochlorothiazide	
	100s	3133
	Apresoline® hydrochloride	
	hydralazine hydrochloride USP	
37	TABLETS, 10 mg (pale yellow, dry-coated)	
	100s	2629
	Consumer Pack	
	100s	2603
39	TABLETS, 25 mg (deep blue, dry-coated)	
	100s	2611
	1000s	2615
73	TABLETS, 50 mg (light blue, dry-coated)	
	100s	2619
	1000s	2623
101	TABLETS, 100 mg (peach, dry-coated)	
	100s	2638
	Cytadren®	
	aminoglutethimide USP	
24	TABLETS-250 mg (white, round, scored into quarters)	
	100s	2120
	Esidrix®	
	hydrochlorothiazide USP	
22	TABLETS, 25 mg (pink, scored)	
	100s	4310
	1000s	4313
	Accu-Pak®	
	100s	4312
	Consumer Pack	
	100s	4325
46	TABLETS, 50 mg (yellow, scored)	
	100s	4315
	1000s	4318
	Accu-Pak®	
	100s	4317
	Consumer Pack	
	30s	4328
	60s	4331
	100s	4330
192	TABLETS, 100 mg (blue, scored)	
	100s	4340
	Esimil®	
47	TABLETS (white, scored), each containing 10 mg guanethidine monosulfate USP and 25 mg hydrochlorothiazide USP	
	100s	4503
	Estraderm® 0.05 mg	
	estradiol transdermal system	
2310	Package of 6 Patient Calendar Packs (8 systems per Patient Calendar Pack)	0922
	Package of 1 Patient Calendar Pack (24 systems per Patient Calendar Pack)	0921
	Estraderm® 0.1 mg	
	estradiol transdermal system	
2320	Package of 6 Patient Calendar Packs (8 systems per Patient Calendar Pack)	0932
	Package of 1 Patient Calendar Pack (24 systems per Patient Calendar Pack)	0931

CIBA Code #		List Number
	Ismelin® sulfate	
	guanethidine monosulfate	
49	TABLETS, 10 mg (pale yellow, scored)	
103	TABLETS, 25 mg (white, scored)	5010
	100s	5020
	Lithobid®	
	lithium carbonate USP	
65	TABLETS, 300 mg (peach-colored)	
	100s	0210
	1000s	0220
	Accu-Pak® 100s	0230
	Lotensin®	
	benazepril hydrochloride	
59	TABLETS, 5 mg (round, light yellow, coated)	
	100s	4401
	Accu-Pak® 100s	4402
63	TABLETS, 10 mg (round, dark yellow, coated)	
	100s	4411
	Accu-Pak® 100s	4412
79	TABLETS, 20 mg (round, tan, coated)	
	100s	4421
	Accu-Pak® 100s	4422
94	TABLETS, 40 mg (round, dark rose, coated)	
	100s	4431
	Accu-Pak® 100s	4432
	Ludiomil®	
	maprotiline hydrochloride USP	
110	TABLETS, 25 mg (oval, dark orange, coated)	
	100s	1710
	Accu-Pak®	
	100s	1714
26	TABLETS, 50 mg (round, dark orange, coated)	
	100s	1720
	Accu-Pak®	
	100s	1721
135	TABLETS, 75 mg (oval, white, coated)	
	100s	1730
	Accu-Pak®	
	100s	1732
	Metopirone®	
	metyrapone USP	
130	TABLETS, 250 mg (white, scored)	
	18s	5403
	Rimactane®	
	rifampin USP	
154	CAPSULES, 300 mg (opaque scarlet and caramel)	
	30s	8903
	60s	8904
	100s	8901
	Rimactane®/INH Dual Pack	
	rifampin USP & isoniazid USP	
8912	Each Dual Pack contains two Rimactane 300-mg CAPSULES and one INH 300-mg TABLET	
		8912
	Ritalin® hydrochloride ℂ	
	methylphenidate hydrochloride USP	
07	TABLETS, 5 mg (yellow)	
	100s	7410
03	TABLETS, 10 mg (pale green, scored)	
	100s	7416
34	TABLETS, 20 mg (pale yellow, scored)	
	100s	7422
	Ritalin-SR® ℂ	
	methylphenidate hydrochloride sustained-release tablets	
16	TABLETS, 20 mg (round, white, scored)	
	100s	7442
	Ser-Ap-Es®	
71	TABLETS (light salmon pink, dry-coated), each containing 0.1 mg reserpine, 25 mg hydralazine hydrochloride and 15 mg hydrochlorothiazide	
	100s	6610
	1000s	6612
	Accu-Pak® 100s	6605
	Consumer Pack	
	100s	6617
	Transderm Scōp®	
	scopolamine	
4345	Package of 3 cartons (4 discs per carton)	5921

CIBA Code #		NUMERICAL LISTING
	Ritalin® hydrochloride ℂ	
	methylphenidate hydrochloride USP	
03	TABLETS, 10 mg (pale green, scored)	
07	TABLETS, 5 mg (yellow)	
	Ritalin-SR® ℂ	
	methylphenidate hydrochloride sustained-release tablets	
16	TABLETS, 20 mg (round, white, scored)	

Esidrix®
hydrochlorothiazide USP
22   TABLETS, 25 mg (pink, scored)
Cytadren®
aminoglutethamide
24   TABLETS, 250 mg (white, round, scored into quarters)
Ludiomil®
maprotiline hydrochloride
26   TABLETS, 50 mg (round, dark orange, coated)
Ritalin® hydrochloride Ⓒ
methylphenidate hydrochloride USP
34   TABLETS, 20 mg (pale yellow, scored)
Apresoline® hydrochloride
hydralazine hydrochloride USP
37   TABLETS, 10 mg (pale yellow, dry-coated)
39   TABLETS, 25 mg (deep blue, dry-coated)
Anturane®
sulfinpyrazone USP
41   TABLETS (white, single-scored) each containing 100 mg sulfinpyrazone USP
Esidrix®
hydrochlorothiazide USP
46   TABLETS, 50 mg (yellow, scored)
Esimil®
47   TABLETS (white, scored), each containing 10 mg guanethidine monosulfate and 25 mg hydrochlorothiazide
Ismelin® sulfate
guanethidine monosulfate
49   TABLETS, 10 mg (pale yellow, scored)
Lotensin®
benazepril hydrochloride
59   TABLETS, 5 mg (round, light yellow, coated)
63   TABLETS, 10 mg (round, dark yellow, coated)
Lithobid®
lithium carbonate
65   TABLETS, 300 mg (peach colored)
Ser-Ap-Es®
71   TABLETS (light salmon pink, dry-coated), each containing 0.1 mg reserpine, 25 mg hydralazine hydrochloride and 15 mg hydrochlorothiazide
Apresoline® hydrochloride
hydralazine hydrochloride USP
73   TABLETS, 50 mg (light blue, dry-coated)
Lotensin®
benazepril hydrochloride
79   TABLETS, 20 mg (round, tan, coated)
94   TABLETS, 40 mg (round, dark rose, coated)
Apresoline® hydrochloride
hydralazine hydrochloride USP
101   TABLETS, 100 mg (peach, dry-coated)
Ismelin® sulfate
guanethidine monosulfate
103   TABLETS, 25 mg (white, scored)
Ludiomil®
maprotiline hydrochloride USP
110   TABLETS, 25 mg (oval, dark orange coated)
Metopirone®
metyrapone USP
130   TABLETS, 250 mg (white, scored)
Ludiomil®
maprotiline hydrochloride USP
135   TABLETS, 75 mg (oval, white, coated)
Apresazide®
hydralazine HCl and hydrochlorothiazide
139   CAPSULES 25/25 (light blue and white opaque), each containing 25 mg hydralazine hydrochloride and 25 mg hydrochlorothiazide
149   CAPSULES 50/50 (pink and white opaque), each containing 50 mg hydralazine hydrochloride and 50 mg hydrochlorothiazide
Rimactane®
rifampin USP
154   CAPSULES, 300 mg (opaque scarlet and caramel)
Rimactane®/INH® Dual Pack
rifampin USP & isoniazid USP
8912   Each Dual Pack contains two Rimactane 300-mg CAPSULES and one INH 300-mg TABLET
Apresazide®
hydralazine HCl and hydrochlorothiazide
159   CAPSULES 100/50 (pink flesh and white opaque), each containing 100 mg hydralazine hydrochloride and 50 mg hydrochlorothiazide
Anturane®
sulfinpyrazone USP
168   CAPSULES (green) each containing 200 mg sulfinpyrazone USP
Esidrix®
hydrochlorothiazide USP
192   TABLETS, 100 mg (blue, scored)
Estraderm® 0.05 mg
estradiol transdermal system
2310   Package of 6 Patient Calendar Packs (8 systems per Patient Calendar Pack)

Estraderm® 0.1 mg
estradiol transdermal system
2320   Package of 6 Patient Calendar Packs (8 systems per Patient Calendar Pack)
Transderm Scōp®
scopolamine
4345   Package of 3 cartons (4 discs per carton)

ANTURANE® ℞
[ann 'too-rain]
sulfinpyrazone USP
Tablets, Capsules

DESCRIPTION
Anturane, sulfinpyrazone USP, is a uricosuric agent available as 100-mg tablets and 200-mg capsules for oral administration. Its chemical name is 1,2-diphenyl-4-[2-(phenylsulfinyl)ethyl]-3,5-pyrazolidinedione.
Sulfinpyrazone USP is a white to off-white powder practically insoluble in water and in solvent hexane, soluble in alcohol and in acetone, and sparingly soluble in dilute alkali. Its molecular weight is 404.48.
Inactive Ingredients. Anturane tablets: Colloidal silicon dioxide, gelatin, lactose, magnesium stearate, starch, stearic acid, and talc.
Anturane capsules: D&C Red No. 33, D&C Yellow No. 10, FD&C Blue No. 1, gelatin, lactose, magnesium stearate, methylparaben, propylparaben, silicon dioxide, sodium lauryl sulfate, starch, stearic acid, talc, and titanium dioxide.

CLINICAL PHARMACOLOGY
Its pharmacologic activity is the potentiation of the urinary excretion of uric acid. It is useful for reducing the blood urate levels in patients with chronic tophaceous gout and acute intermittent gout, and for promoting the resorption of tophi.

INDICATIONS
Anturane is indicated for the treatment of:
1. Chronic gouty arthritis
2. Intermittent gouty arthritis

CONTRAINDICATIONS
Patients with an active peptic ulcer or symptoms of gastrointestinal inflammation or ulceration should not receive the drug.
The drug is contraindicated in patients with a history or the presence of:
1. Hypersensitivity to phenylbutazone or other pyrazoles
2. Blood dyscrasias

WARNINGS
Studies on the teratogenicity of pyrazole compounds in animals have yielded inconclusive results. Up to the present time, however, there have been no reported cases of human congenital malformation proved to be due to the use of the drug.
It is suggested that Anturane be used with caution in pregnant women, weighing the potential risks against the possible benefits.

PRECAUTIONS
As with all pyrazole compounds, patients receiving Anturane should be kept under close medical supervision and periodic blood counts are recommended. It may be administered with care to patients with a history of healed peptic ulcer.
Recent reports have indicated that Anturane potentiates the action of certain sulfonamides, such as sulfadiazine and sulfisoxazole. In addition, other pyrazole compounds (phenylbutazone) have been observed to potentiate the hypoglycemic sulfonylurea agents, as well as insulin. In view of these observations, it is suggested that Anturane be used with caution in conjunction with sulfa drugs, the sulfonylurea hypoglycemic agents and insulin.
Because Anturane is a potent uricosuric agent, it may precipitate urolithiasis and renal colic, especially in the initial stages of therapy. For this reason, an adequate fluid intake and alkalinization of the urine are recommended. In cases with significant renal impairment, periodic assessment of renal function is indicated. Occasional cases of renal failure have been reported; but a cause-and-effect relationship has not always been clearly established.
Salicylates antagonize the uricosuric action of Anturane and for this reason their concomitant use is contraindicated in gouty arthritis.
Anturane may accentuate the action of coumarin-type anticoagulants and further depress prothrombin activity when these medications are employed simultaneously.

NOTE
Anturane has minimal anti-inflammatory effect and is not intended for the relief of an acute attack of gout.
In the initial stages of therapy, because of the marked ability of Anturane to mobilize urates, acute attacks of gouty arthritis may be precipitated.

ADVERSE REACTIONS
The most frequently reported adverse reactions with Anturane have been upper gastrointestinal disturbances. In these patients it is advisable to administer the drug with food, milk, or antacids. Despite this precaution, Anturane may aggravate or reactivate peptic ulcer.
Rash has been reported. In most instances, this reaction did not necessitate discontinuance of therapy. In general, Anturane has not been observed to affect electrolyte balance.
Blood dyscrasias (anemia, leukopenia, agranulocytosis, thrombocytopenia and aplastic anemia) have rarely been reported. There has also been a published report associating Anturane, administered concomitantly with other drugs including colchicine, with leukemia following long-term treatment of patients with gout. However, the circumstances involved in the two cases reported are such that a cause-and-effect relationship to Anturane has not been clearly established.

OVERDOSAGE
Symptoms: Nausea, vomiting, diarrhea, epigastric pain, ataxia, labored respiration, convulsions, coma. Possible symptoms, seen after overdosage with other pyrazolone derivatives: anemia, jaundice, ulceration.
Treatment: No specific antidote. Induce emesis; gastric lavage; supportive treatment (intravenous glucose infusions, analeptics).

DOSAGE AND ADMINISTRATION
Initial: 200–400 mg daily in two divided doses, with meals or milk, gradually increasing when necessary to full maintenance dosage in one week.
Maintenance: 400 mg daily, given in two divided doses, as above. This dosage may be increased to 800 mg daily, if necessary, and may sometimes be reduced to as low as 200 mg daily after the blood urate level has been controlled. Treatment should be continued without interruption even in the presence of acute exacerbations, which can be concomitantly treated with phenylbutazone or colchicine. Patients previously controlled with other uricosuric therapy may be transferred to Anturane at full maintenance dosage.

HOW SUPPLIED
Tablets 100 mg—round, white, scored (imprinted CIBA 41)
Bottles of 100 ....NDC 0083-0041-30
Capsules 200 mg—green (imprinted Anturane 200 CIBA 168)
Bottles of 100 ....NDC 0083-0168-30
Dispense in tight container (USP).

C87-5 (Rev. 2/87)

Shown in Product Identification Section, page 408

APRESAZIDE® ℞
[a-press 'a-zyde]
hydralazine hydrochloride and hydrochlorothiazide
Capsules

> **WARNING**
> This fixed-combination drug is not indicated for initial therapy of hypertension. Hypertension requires therapy titrated to the individual patient. If the fixed combination represents the dosage so determined, its use may be more convenient in patient management. The treatment of hypertension is not static but must be reevaluated as conditions in each patient warrant.

DESCRIPTION
Apresazide, hydralazine hydrochloride and hydrochlorothiazide, is an antihypertensive-diuretic combination available as capsules for oral administration. Apresazide capsules of 25/25 contain 25 mg of hydralazine hydrochloride USP and 25 mg of hydrochlorothiazide USP; capsules of 50/50 contain 50 mg of hydralazine hydrochloride USP and 50 mg of hydrochlorothiazide USP; and capsules of 100/50 contain 100 mg of hydralazine hydrochloride USP and 50 mg of hydrochlorothiazide USP.
Hydralazine hydrochloride is 1-hydrazinophthalazine monohydrochloride.
Hydralazine hydrochloride USP is a white to off-white, odorless crystalline powder. It is soluble in water, slightly soluble in alcohol, and very slightly soluble in ether. It melts at about 275°C, with decomposition, and has a molecular weight of 196.64.
Hydrochlorothiazide is 6-chloro-3,4-dihydro-2H -1,2,4-benzothiadiazine-7-sulfonamide 1,1-dioxide.

Continued on next page

The full prescribing information for each CIBA product is contained herein and is that in effect as of September 1, 1992 .

CIBA—Cont.

Hydrochlorothiazide USP is a white, or practically white, practically odorless crystalline powder. It is freely soluble in sodium hydroxide solution, in *n*-butylamine, and in dimethylformamide; sparingly soluble in methanol; slightly soluble in water; and insoluble in ether, in chloroform, and in dilute mineral acids. Its molecular weight is 297.73.

Inactive Ingredients: D&C Red No. 28 (25/25 and 50/50 capsules only); D&C Red No. 33 and D&C Yellow No. 10 (100/50 capsules only); FD&C Blue No. 1 (25/25 and 50/50 capsules only); FD&C Red No. 40 (50/50 capsules only); gelatin; magnesium stearate; methylparaben; propylparaben; silicon dioxide; sodium lauryl sulfate; starch; and titanium dioxide.

CLINICAL PHARMACOLOGY

Hydralazine

Although the precise mechanism of action of hydralazine is not fully understood, the major effects are on the cardiovascular system. Hydralazine apparently lowers blood pressure by exerting a peripheral vasodilating effect through a direct relaxation of vascular smooth muscle. Hydralazine, by altering cellular calcium metabolism, interferes with the calcium movements within the vascular smooth muscle that are responsible for initiating or maintaining the contractile state.

The peripheral vasodilating effect of hydralazine results in decreased arterial blood pressure (diastolic more than systolic); decreased peripheral vascular resistance; and an increased heart rate, stroke volume, and cardiac output. The preferential dilatation of arterioles, as compared to veins, minimizes postural hypotension and promotes the increase in cardiac output. Hydralazine usually increases renin activity in plasma, presumably as a result of increased secretion of renin by the renal juxtaglomerular cells in response to reflex sympathetic discharge. This increase in renin activity leads to the production of angiotensin II, which then causes stimulation of aldosterone and consequent sodium reabsorption. Hydralazine also maintains or increases renal and cerebral blood flow.

Hydrochlorothiazide

Thiazides affect the renal tubular mechanism of electrolyte reabsorption. At maximal therapeutic dosage, all thiazides are approximately equal in their diuretic potency. Thiazides increase excretion of sodium and chloride in approximately equivalent amounts. Natriuresis causes a secondary loss of potassium.

The mechanism of the antihypertensive effect of thiazides is unknown. Thiazides do not affect normal blood pressure.

Pharmacokinetics

Hydralazine. Hydralazine is rapidly absorbed after oral administration, and peak plasma levels are reached at 1–2 hours. Plasma levels decline with a half-life of 3–7 hours. Binding to human plasma protein is 87%. Plasma levels of hydralazine vary widely among individuals. Hydralazine is subject to polymorphic acetylation; slow acetylators generally have higher plasma levels of hydralazine and require lower doses to maintain control of blood pressure. Hydralazine undergoes extensive hepatic metabolism; it is excreted mainly in the form of metabolites in the urine.

Administration of hydralazine with food results in higher levels of the drug in plasma.

Hydrochlorothiazide. Onset of action of thiazides occurs in 2 hours and the peak effect at about 4 hours. The action persists for approximately 6–12 hours. Hydrochlorothiazide is rapidly absorbed, as indicated by peak concentrations 1–2.5 hours after oral administration. Plasma levels of the drug are proportional to dose; the concentration in whole blood is 1.6–1.8 times higher than in plasma. Thiazides are eliminated rapidly by the kidney. After oral administration of 25- to 100-mg doses, 72–97% of the dose is excreted in the urine, indicating dose-independent absorption. Hydrochlorothiazide is eliminated from plasma in a biphasic fashion with a terminal half-life of 10–17 hours. Plasma protein binding is 67.9%. Plasma clearance is 15.9–30.0 L/hr; volume of distribution is 3.6–7.8 L/kg.

Gastrointestinal absorption of hydrochlorothiazide is enhanced when administered with food. Absorption is decreased in patients with congestive heart failure, and the pharmacokinetics are considerably different in these patients.

INDICATIONS AND USAGE

Hypertension (see boxed **WARNING**).

CONTRAINDICATIONS

Hydralazine

Hypersensitivity to hydralazine; coronary artery disease; mitral valvular rheumatic heart disease.

Hydrochlorothiazide

Anuria; hypersensitivity to this or other sulfonamide-derived drugs.

WARNINGS

Hydralazine

In a few patients hydralazine may produce a clinical picture simulating systemic lupus erythematosus including glomerulonephritis. In such patients hydralazine should be discontinued unless the benefit-to-risk determination requires continued antihypertensive therapy with this drug. Signs and symptoms usually regress when the drug is discontinued, but residua have been detected many years later. Long-term treatment with steroids may be necessary. (See **PRECAUTIONS, Laboratory Tests.**)

Hydrochlorothiazide

Thiazides should be used with caution in patients with severe renal disease. In patients with renal disease, thiazides may precipitate azotemia. Cumulative effects of the drug may develop in patients with impaired renal function.

Thiazides should be used with caution in patients with impaired hepatic function or progressive liver disease, since minor alterations of fluid and electrolyte imbalance may precipitate hepatic coma.

Thiazides may add to or potentiate the action of other antihypertensive drugs. Potentiation occurs with ganglionic or peripheral adrenergic blocking drugs.

Sensitivity reactions are more likely to occur in patients with a history of allergy or bronchial asthma.

The possibility of exacerbation or activation of systemic lupus erythematosus has been reported.

PRECAUTIONS

General

Hydralazine. Myocardial stimulation produced by hydralazine can cause anginal attacks and ECG changes indicative of myocardial ischemia. The drug has been implicated in the production of myocardial infarction. It must, therefore, be used with caution in patients with suspected coronary artery disease.

The "hyperdynamic" circulation caused by hydralazine may accentuate specific cardiovascular inadequacies. For example, hydralazine may increase pulmonary artery pressure in patients with mitral valvular disease. The drug may reduce the pressor responses to epinephrine. Postural hypotension may result from hydralazine but is less common than with ganglionic blocking agents. It should be used with caution in patients with cerebral vascular accidents.

In hypertensive patients with normal kidneys who are treated with hydralazine, there is evidence of increased renal blood flow and a maintenance of glomerular filtration rate. In some instances where control values were below normal, improved renal function has been noted after administration of hydralazine. However, as with any antihypertensive agent, hydralazine should be used with caution in patients with advanced renal damage.

Peripheral neuritis, evidenced by paresthesia, numbness, and tingling, has been observed. Published evidence suggests that hydralazine has an antipyridoxine effect and that pyridoxine should be added to the regimen if symptoms develop.

Hydrochlorothiazide. All patients receiving thiazide therapy should be observed for clinical signs of fluid or electrolyte imbalance, namely hyponatremia, hypochloremic alkalosis, and hypokalemia (see **Laboratory Tests** and **Drug/Drug Interactions**). Warning signs are dryness of mouth, thirst, weakness, lethargy, drowsiness, restlessness, muscle pains or cramps, muscular fatigue, hypotension, oliguria, tachycardia, and gastrointestinal disturbance, such as nausea or vomiting.

Hypokalemia may develop, especially in cases of brisk diuresis or severe cirrhosis.

Interference with adequate oral intake of electrolytes will also contribute to hypokalemia. Hypokalemia may be avoided or treated by the use of potassium supplements or foods with a high potassium content.

Any chloride deficit is generally mild and usually does not require specific treatment, except under extraordinary circumstances (as in liver disease or renal disease). Dilutional hyponatremia may occur in edematous patients in hot weather; appropriate therapy is water restriction, rather than administration of salt, except in rare instances when the hyponatremia is life-threatening. In cases of actual salt depletion, appropriate replacement is the therapy of choice.

Hyperuricemia may occur or frank gout may be precipitated in certain patients receiving thiazide therapy.

Latent diabetes may become manifest during thiazide administration (see **Drug/Drug Interactions**).

The antihypertensive effects of the drug may be enhanced in the postsympathectomy patient.

If progressive renal impairment becomes evident, withholding or discontinuing diuretic therapy should be considered.

Calcium excretion is decreased by thiazides. Pathological changes in the parathyroid gland with hypercalcemia and hypophosphatemia have been observed in a few patients on prolonged thiazide therapy. The common complications of hyperparathyroidism, such as renal lithiasis, bone resorption, and peptic ulceration, have not been seen.

Information for Patients

Patients should be informed of possible side effects and advised to take the medication regularly and continuously as directed.

Laboratory Tests

Hydralazine. Complete blood counts and antinuclear antibody titer determinations are indicated before and periodically during prolonged therapy with hydralazine even though the patient is asymptomatic. These studies are also indicated if the patient develops arthralgia, fever, chest pain, continued malaise, or other unexplained signs or symptoms. A positive antinuclear antibody titer requires that the physician carefully weigh the implications of the test results against the benefits to be derived from antihypertensive therapy with a combination drug containing hydralazine.

Blood dyscrasias, consisting of reduction in hemoglobin and red cell count, leukopenia, agranulocytosis, and purpura, have been reported. If such abnormalities develop, therapy should be discontinued.

Hydrochlorothiazide. Initial and periodic determinations of serum electrolytes to detect possible electrolyte imbalance should be performed at appropriate intervals.

Serum and urine electrolyte determinations are particularly important when the patient is vomiting excessively or receiving parenteral fluids.

Drug/Drug Interactions

Hydralazine. MAO inhibitors should be used with caution in patients receiving hydralazine.

When other potent parenteral antihypertensive drugs, such as diazoxide, are used in combination with hydralazine, patients should be continously observed for several hours for any excessive fall in blood pressure. Profound hypotensive episodes may occur when diazoxide injections and hydralazine are used concomitantly.

Hydrochlorothiazide. Hypokalemia can sensitize or exaggerate the response of the heart to the toxic effects of digitalis (e.g., increased ventricular irritability).

Hypokalemia may develop during concomitant use of steroids or ACTH.

Insulin requirements in diabetic patients may be increased, decreased, or unchanged.

Thiazides may decrease arterial responsiveness to norepinephrine, but not enough to preclude effectiveness of the pressor agent for therapeutic use.

Thiazides may increase the responsiveness to tubocurarine.

Lithium renal clearance is reduced by thiazides, increasing the risk of lithium toxicity.

There have been rare reports in the literature of hemolytic anemia occurring with the concomitant use of hydrochlorothiazide and methyldopa.

Concurrent administration of some nonsteroidal anti-inflammatory agents may reduce the diuretic, natriuretic and antihypertensive effects of thiazide diuretics.

Drug/Laboratory Test Interactions

Thiazides may decrease serum levels of protein-bound iodine without signs of thyroid disturbance. Apresazide should be discontinued before tests for parathyroid function are made (See **General, *Hydrochlorothiazide,*** Calcium excretion).

Carcinogenesis, Mutagenesis, Impairment of Fertility

Hydralazine. In a lifetime study in Swiss albino mice, there was a statistically significant increase in the incidence of lung tumors (adenomas and adenocarcinomas) of both male and female mice given hydralazine continuously in their drinking water at a dosage of about 250 mg/kg per day (about 80 times the maximum recommended human dose). In a 2-year carcinogenicity study of rats given hydralazine by gavage at dosages of 15, 30, and 60 mg/kg per day (approximately 5 to 20 times the recommended human daily dose), microscopic examination of the liver revealed a small, but statistically significant, increase in benign neoplastic nodules in male and female rats from the high-dose group and in female rats from the intermediate-dose group. Benign interstitial cell tumors of the testes were also significantly increased in male rats from the high-dose group. The tumors observed are common in aged rats, and a significantly increased incidence was not observed until 18 months of treatment. Hydralazine was shown to be mutagenic in bacterial systems (Gene Mutation and DNA Repair) and in one of two rat and one rabbit hepatocyte in vitro DNA repair studies. Additional in vivo and in vitro studies using lymphoma cells, germinal cells, and fibroblasts from mice, bone marrow cells from chinese hamsters, and fibroblasts from human cell lines did not demonstrate any mutagenic potential for hydralazine.

The extent to which these findings indicate a risk to man is uncertain. While long-term clinical observation has not suggested that human cancer is associated with hydralazine use, epidemiologic studies have so far been insufficient to arrive at any conclusions.

Hydrochlorothiazide. Long-term carcinogenicity studies in animals have not been conducted with hydrochlorothiazide. Hydrochlorothiazide was not mutagenic in in vitro Ames Mutagenicity assay of *Salmonella typhimunium* strains TA 98, TA 100, TA 1535, TA 1537, and TA 1538 or in in vivo mutagenicity assays of mouse germinal cell chromosomes and Chinese Hamster bone marrow cell chromosomes. It was however, mutagenic in inducing nondisjunction (96% frequency) in diploid strains of *Aspergillus nidulans.*

Hydrochlorothiazide had no adverse effect on fertility of male or female mice or rats in studies in which these species were exposed to doses up to 4 and 100 mg/kg, respectively.

Pregnancy Category C

Animal reproduction studies have not been conducted with Apresazide.

Animal studies indicate that hydralazine is teratogenic in mice at 20–30 times the maximum daily human dose of 200–300 mg and possibly in rabbits at 10–15 times the maximum daily human dose, but that it is nonteratogenic in rats. Teratogenic effects observed were cleft palate and malformations of facial and cranial bones.

There are no adequate and well-controlled studies of Apresazide in pregnant women. However, thiazides cross the placental barrier and appear in cord blood, and there is a risk of fetal or neonatal jaundice, thrombocytopenia, and possibly other adverse reactions that have occurred in adults. Apresazide should be used during pregnancy only if the potential benefit justifies the potential risk to the fetus.

Nursing Mothers

It is not known whether hydralazine is excreted in human milk. Thiazides are excreted in human milk. Because of the potential for serious adverse reactions in nursing infants, a decision should be made whether to discontinue nursing or to discontinue the drug, taking into account the importance of the drug to the mother.

Pediatric Use

Safety and effectiveness of the combination drug in children have not been established.

ADVERSE REACTIONS

Adverse reactions are usually reversible upon reduction of dosage or discontinuation of Apresazide. Whenever adverse reactions are moderate or severe, it may be necessary to discontinue the drug.

The following adverse reactions have been observed, but there has not been enough systematic collection of data to support an estimate of their frequency.

Hydralazine

Common

Headache, anorexia, nausea, vomiting, diarrhea, palpitations, tachycardia, angina pectoris.

Less Frequent

Digestive: Constipation, paralytic ileus.

Cardiovascular: Hypotension, paradoxical pressor response, edema.

Respiratory: Dyspnea.

Neurologic: Peripheral neuritis, evidenced by paresthesia, numbness, and tingling; dizziness; tremors; muscle cramps; psychotic reactions characterized by depression, disorientation, or anxiety.

Genitourinary: Difficulty in urination.

Hematologic: Blood dyscrasias, consisting of reduction in hemoglobin and red cell count, leukopenia, agranulocytosis, purpura; lymphadenopathy; splenomegaly.

Hypersensitive Reactions: Rash, urticaria, pruritus, fever, chills, arthralgia, eosinophilia, and, rarely, hepatitis.

Other: Nasal congestion, flushing, lacrimation, conjunctivitis.

Hydrochlorothiazide

Digestive: Anorexia, gastric irritation, nausea, vomiting, cramping, diarrhea, constipation, jaundice (intrahepatic cholestatic), pancreatitis, sialadenitis.

Cardiovascular: Orthostatic hypotension (may be potentiated by alcohol, barbiturates, or narcotics).

Neurologic: Dizziness, vertigo, paresthesia, headache, xanthopsia.

Hematologic: Leukopenia, agranulocytosis, thrombocytopenia, aplastic anemia.

Hypersensitive Reactions: Purpura, photosensitivity, rash, urticaria, necrotizing angiitis, Stevens-Johnson syndrome.

Other: Hyperglycemia, glycosuria, hyperuricemia, muscle spasm, weakness, restlessness, transient blurred vision.

OVERDOSAGE

Acute Toxicity

Oral LD_{50}'s in rats (mg/kg): hydralazine, 173 and 187; hydrochlorothiazide, 2750.

Signs and Symptoms

Hydralazine. Signs and symptoms of overdosage include hypotension, tachycardia, headache, and generalized skin flushing.

Complications can include myocardial ischemia and subsequent myocardial infarction, cardiac arrhythmia, and profound shock.

Hydrochlorothiazide. The most prominent feature of poisoning is acute loss of fluid and electrolytes.

Cardiovascular: Tachycardia, hypotension, shock.

Neuromuscular: Weakness, confusion, dizziness, cramps of the calf muscles, paresthesia, fatigue, impairment of consciousness.

Digestive: Nausea, vomiting, thirst.

Renal: Polyuria, oliguria, or anuria (due to hemoconcentration).

Laboratory Findings: Hypokalemia, hyponatremia, hypochloremia, alkalosis; increased BUN (especially in patients with renal insufficiency).

Combined Poisoning: Signs and symptoms may be aggravated or modified by concomitant intake of antihypertensive medication, barbiturates, curare, digitalis (hypokalemia), corticosteroids, narcotics, or alcohol.

Treatment

There is no specific antidote.

The gastric contents should be evacuated, taking adequate precautions against aspiration and for protection of the airway. An activated charcoal slurry may be instilled if conditions permit. Dialysis may not be effective for elimination of Apresazide because of its plasma protein binding (see **CLINICAL PHARMACOLOGY**).

These manipulations may have to be omitted or carried out after cardiovascular status has been stabilized, since they might precipitate cardiac arrhythmias or increase the depth of shock.

Support of the cardiovascular system is of primary importance in suspected hydralazine overdosage. Shock should be treated with plasma expanders. The patient's legs should be kept raised and lost fluid and electrolytes (potassium, sodium) should be replaced. If possible, vasopressors should not be given, but if a vasopressor is required, care should be taken not to precipitate or aggravate cardiac arrhythmia. Tachycardia responds to beta blockers. Digitalization may be necessary, and renal function should be monitored and supported as required.

DOSAGE AND ADMINISTRATION

Dosage should be determined by individual titration (see boxed **WARNING**).

The usual dosage is one Apresazide capsule twice daily, the strength depending upon individual requirement following titration. For maintenance, the dosage should be adjusted to the lowest effective level.

When necessary, other antihypertensive agents such as sympathetic inhibitors may be added gradually in reduced dosages, and the effects should be watched carefully.

HOW SUPPLIED

Capsules 25/25—light blue and white opaque (imprinted APRESAZIDE® 25/25 CIBA 139)
25 mg of hydralazine hydrochloride and 25 mg of hydrochlorothiazide
Bottles of 100 .... NDC 0083-0139-30

Capsules 50/50—pink and white opaque (imprinted APRESAZIDE® 50/50 CIBA 149)
50 mg of hydralazine hydrochloride and 50 mg of hydrochlorothiazide
Bottles of 100 .... NDC 0083-0149-30

Capsules 100/50—flesh pink and white opaque (imprinted APRESAZIDE® 100/50 CIBA 159)
100 mg of hydralazine hydrochloride and 50 mg of hydrochlorothiazide
Bottles of 100 .... NDC 0083-0159-30

Samples, when available, are identified by the word *SAMPLE* appearing on each capsule.

Do not store above 86°F.

Dispense in tight, light-resistant container (USP).

C90-47 (Rev. 10/90)

Shown in Product Identification Section, page 408

APRESOLINE® hydrochloride ℞

[*a-press 'oh-leen*]

hydralazine hydrochloride USP

Tablets

DESCRIPTION

Apresoline, hydralazine hydrochloride USP, is an antihypertensive, available as 10-, 25-, 50-, and 100-mg tablets for oral administration. Its chemical name is 1-hydrazinophthalazine monohydrochloride.

Hydralazine hydrochloride USP is a white to off-white, odorless crystalline powder. It is soluble in water, slightly soluble in alcohol, and very slightly soluble in ether. It melts at about 275°C, with decomposition, and has a molecular weight of 196.64.

Inactive Ingredients: Acacia, D&C Yellow No. 10 (10-mg tablets), FD&C Blue No. 1 (25-mg and 50-mg tablets), FD&C Yellow No. 5 and FD&C Yellow No. 6 (100-mg tablets), lactose, magnesium stearate, mannitol, polyethylene glycol, sodium starch glycolate, starch and stearic acid.

CLINICAL PHARMACOLOGY

Although the precise mechanism of action of hydralazine is not fully understood, the major effects are on the cardiovascular system. Hydralazine apparently lowers blood pressure by exerting a peripheral vasodilating effect through a direct relaxation of vascular smooth muscle. Hydralazine, by altering cellular calcium metabolism, interferes with the calcium movements within the vascular smooth muscle that are responsible for initiating or maintaining the contractile state.

The peripheral vasodilating effect of hydralazine results in decreased arterial blood pressure (diastolic more than systolic); decreased peripheral vascular resistance; and an increased heart rate, stroke volume, and cardiac output. The preferential dilatation of arterioles, as compared to veins, minimizes postural hypotension and promotes the increase in cardiac output. Hydralazine usually increases renin activity in plasma, presumably as a result of increased secretion of renin by the renal juxtaglomerular cells in response to reflex sympathetic discharge. This increase in renin activity leads to the production of angiotensin II, which then causes stimulation of aldosterone and consequent sodium reabsorption. Hydralazine also maintains or increases renal and cerebral blood flow.

Hydralazine is rapidly absorbed after oral administration, and peak plasma levels are reached at 1–2 hours. Plasma levels of apparent hydralazine decline with a half-life of 3–7 hours. Binding to human plasma protein is 87%. Plasma levels of hydralazine vary widely among individuals. Hydralazine is subject to polymorphic acetylation; slow acetylators generally have higher plasma levels of hydralazine and require lower doses to maintain control of blood pressure. Hydralazine undergoes extensive hepatic metabolism; it is excreted mainly in the form of metabolites in the urine.

INDICATIONS AND USAGE

Essential hypertension, alone or as an adjunct.

CONTRAINDICATIONS

Hypersensitivity to hydralazine; coronary artery disease; mitral valvular rheumatic heart disease.

WARNINGS

In a few patients hydralazine may produce a clinical picture simulating systemic lupus erythematosus including glomerulonephritis. In such patients hydralazine should be discontinued unless the benefit-to-risk determination requires continued antihypertensive therapy with this drug. Symptoms and signs usually regress when the drug is discontinued but residua have been detected many years later. Long-term treatment with steroids may be necessary. (See **PRECAUTIONS, Laboratory Tests.**)

PRECAUTIONS

General: Myocardial stimulation produced by Apresoline can cause anginal attacks and ECG changes of myocardial ischemia. The drug has been implicated in the production of myocardial infarction. It must, therefore, be used with caution in patients with suspected coronary artery disease.

The "hyperdynamic" circulation caused by Apresoline may accentuate specific cardiovascular inadequacies. For example, Apresoline may increase pulmonary artery pressure in patients with mitral valvular disease. The drug may reduce the pressor responses to epinephrine. Postural hypotension may result from Apresoline but is less common than with ganglionic blocking agents. It should be used with caution in patients with cerebral vascular accidents.

In hypertensive patients wiith normal kidneys who are treated with Apresoline, there is evidence of increased renal blood flow and a maintenance of glomerular filtration rate. In some instances where control values were below normal, improved renal function has been noted after administration of Apresoline. However, as with any antihypertensive agent, Apresoline should be used with caution in patients with advanced renal damage.

Peripheral neuritis, evidenced by paresthesia, numbness, and tingling, has been observed. Published evidence suggests an antipyridoxine effect, and that pyridoxine should be added to the regimen if symptoms develop.

The Apresoline tablets (100 mg) contain FD&C Yellow No. 5 (tartrazine), which may cause allergic-type reactions (including bronchial asthma) in certain susceptible individuals. Although the overall incidence of FD&C Yellow No. 5 (tartrazine) sensitivity in the general population is low, it is frequently seen in patients who are also hypersensitive to aspirin.

Information for Patients: Patients should be informed of possible side effects and advised to take the medication regularly and continuously as directed.

Laboratory Tests: Complete blood counts and antinuclear antibody titer determinations are indicated before and periodically during prolonged therapy with hydralazine even though the patient is asymptomatic. These studies are also indicated if the patient develops arthralgia, fever, chest pain, continued malaise, or other unexplained signs or symptoms.

A positive antinuclear antibody titer requires that the physician carefully weigh the implications of the test results against the benefits to be derived from antihypertensive therapy with hydralazine.

Blood dyscrasias, consisting of reduction in hemoglobin and red cell count, leukopenia, agranulocytosis, and purpura, have been reported. If such abnormalities develop, therapy should be discontinued.

Drug/Drug Interactions: MAO inhibitors should be used with caution in patients receiving hydralazine.

Continued on next page

The full prescribing information for each CIBA product is contained herein and is that in effect as of September 1, 1992.

CIBA—Cont.

When other potent parenteral antihypertensive drugs, such as diazoxide, are used in combination with hydralazine, patients should be continuously observed for several hours for any excessive fall in blood pressure. Profound hypotensive episodes may occur when diazoxide injection and Apresoline are used concomitantly.

Drug/Food Interactions: Administration of hydralazine with food results in higher plasma levels.

Carcinogenesis, Mutagenesis, Impairment of Fertility: In a lifetime study in Swiss albino mice, there was a statistically significant increase in the incidence of lung tumors (adenomas and adenocarcinomas) of both male and female mice given hydralazine continuously in their drinking water at a dosage of about 250 mg/kg per day (about 80 times the maximum recommended human dose). In a 2-year carcinogenicity study of rats given hydralazine by gavage at dose levels of 15, 30, and 60 mg/kg/day (approximately 5 to 20 times the recommended human daily dosage), microscopic examination of the liver revealed a small, but statistically significant, increase in benign neoplastic nodules in male and female rats from the high-dose group and in female rats from the intermediate-dose group. Benign interstitial cell tumors of the testes were also significantly increased in male rats from the high-dose group. The tumors observed are common in aged rats and a significantly increased incidence was not observed until 18 months of treatment. Hydralazine was shown to be mutagenic in bacterial systems (Gene Mutation and DNA Repair) and in one of two rat and one rabbit hepatocyte *in vitro* DNA repair studies. Additional *in vivo* and *in vitro* studies using lymphoma cells, germinal cells, and fibroblasts from mice, bone marrow cells from chinese hamsters and fibroblasts from human cell lines did not demonstrate any mutagenic potential for hydralazine.

The extent to which these findings indicate a risk to man is uncertain. While long-term clinical observation has not suggested that human cancer is associated with hydralazine use, epidemiologic studies have so far been insufficient to arrive at any conclusions.

Pregnancy Category C: Animal studies indicate that hydralazine is teratogenic in mice at 20–30 times the maximum daily human dose of 200–300 mg and possibly in rabbits at 10–15 times the maximum daily human dose, but that it is nonteratogenic in rats. Teratogenic effects observed were cleft palate and malformations of facial and cranial bones. There are no adequate and well-controlled studies in pregnant women. Although clinical experience does not include any positive evidence of adverse effects on the human fetus, hydralazine should be used during pregnancy only if the expected benefit justifies the potential risk to the fetus.

Nursing Mothers: It is not known whether this drug is excreted in human milk. Because many drugs are excreted in human milk, caution should be exercised when Apresoline is administered to a nursing woman.

Pediatric Use: Safety and effectiveness in children have not been established in controlled clinical trials, although there is experience with the use of Apresoline in children. The usual recommended oral starting dosage is 0.75 mg/kg of body weight daily in four divided doses. Dosage may be increased gradually over the next 3–4 weeks to a maximum of 7.5 mg/kg or 200 mg daily.

ADVERSE REACTIONS

Adverse reactions with Apresoline are usually reversible when dosage is reduced. However, in some cases it may be necessary to discontinue the drug.

The following adverse reactions have been observed, but there has not been enough systematic collection of data to support an estimate of their frequency.

Common: Headache, anorexia, nausea, vomiting, diarrhea, palpitations, tachycardia, angina pectoris.
Less Frequent: *Digestive:* constipation, paralytic ileus.
Cardiovascular: hypotension, paradoxical pressor response, edema.
Respiratory: dyspnea.
Neurologic: peripheral neuritis, evidenced by paresthesia, numbness, and tingling; dizziness; tremors; muscle cramps; psychotic reactions characterized by depression, disorientation, or anxiety.
Genitourinary: difficulty in urination.
Hematologic: blood dyscrasias, consisting of reduction in hemoglobin and red cell count, leukopenia, agranulocytosis, purpura; lymphadenopathy; splenomegaly.
Hypersensitive Reactions: rash, urticaria, pruritus, fever, chills, arthralgia, eosinophilia, and, rarely, hepatitis.
Other: nasal congestion, flushing, lacrimation, conjunctivitis.

OVERDOSAGE

Acute Toxicity: No deaths due to acute poisoning have been reported.

Highest known dose survived: adults, 10 g orally.
Oral LD_{50} in rats: 173 and 187 mg/kg.
Signs and Symptoms: Signs and symptoms of overdosage include hypotension, tachycardia, headache, and generalized skin flushing.

Complications can include myocardial ischemia and subsequent myocardial infarction, cardiac arrhythmia, and profound shock.

Treatment: There is no specific antidote.
The gastric contents should be evacuated, taking adequate precautions against aspiration and for protection of the airway. An activated charcoal slurry may be instilled if conditions permit. These manipulations may have to be omitted or carried out after cardiovascular status has been stabilized, since they might precipitate cardiac arrhythmias or increase the depth of shock.

Support of the cardiovascular system is of primary importance. Shock should be treated with plasma expanders. If possible, vasopressors should not be given, but if a vasopressor is required, care should be taken not to precipitate or aggravate cardiac arrhythmia. Tachycardia responds to beta blockers. Digitalization may be necessary, and renal function should be monitored and supported as required.

No experience has been reported with extracorporeal or peritoneal dialysis.

DOSAGE AND ADMINISTRATION

Initiate therapy in gradually increasing dosages; adjust according to individual response. Start with 10 mg four times daily for the first 2–4 days, increase to 25 mg four times daily for the balance of the first week. For the second and subsequent weeks, increase dosage to 50 mg four times daily. For maintenance, adjust dosage to the lowest effective levels.

The incidence of toxic reactions, particularly the L.E. cell syndrome, is high in the group of patients receiving large doses of Apresoline.

In a few resistant patients, up to 300 mg of Apresoline daily may be required for a significant antihypertensive effect. In such cases, a lower dosage of Apresoline combined with a thiazide and/or reserpine or a beta blocker may be considered. However, when combining therapy, individual titration is essential to ensure the lowest possible therapeutic dose of each drug.

HOW SUPPLIED

Tablets 10 mg—round, pale yellow, dry-coated (imprinted CIBA 37)
    Bottles of 100—NDC 0083-0037-30
    Consumer Pack—One Unit
    12 bottles—100 tablets each—NDC 0083-0037-65
Tablets 25 mg—round, deep blue, dry-coated (imprinted CIBA 39)
    Bottles of 100—NDC 0083-0039-30
    Bottles of 1000—NDC 0083-0039-40
Tablets 50 mg—round, light blue, dry-coated (imprinted CIBA 73)
    Bottles of 100—NDC 0083-0073-30
    Bottles of 1000—NDC 0083-0073-40
Tablets 100 mg—round, peach, dry-coated (imprinted CIBA 101)
    Bottles of 100—NDC 0083-0101-30
Samples, when available, are identified by the word *SAMPLE* appearing on each tablet.
Do not store above 86°F (30°C).
Dispense in tight, light-resistant container (USP).
C92-19 (Rev. 4/92)
      Shown in Product Identification Section, page 408

APRESOLINE® hydrochloride   ℞
[a-press'oh-leen]
hydralazine hydrochloride USP
Parenteral

DESCRIPTION

Apresoline, hydralazine hydrochloride USP, is an antihypertensive available in 1-ml ampuls for intravenous and intramuscular administration. Each milliliter of the sterile, colorless solution contains hydralazine hydrochloride USP, 20 mg; methylparaben NF, 0.65 mg; propylparaben NF, 0.35 mg; propylene glycol USP, 103.6 mg. The pH of the solution is 3.4–4.0. Hydralazine hydrochloride is 1-hydrazinophthalazine monohydrochloride.

Hydralazine hydrochloride USP is a white to off-white, odorless crystalline powder. It is soluble in water, slightly soluble in alcohol, and very slightly soluble in ether. It melts at about 275°C, with decomposition, and has a molecular weight of 196.64.

CLINICAL PHARMACOLOGY

Although the precise mechanism of action of hydralazine is not fully understood, the major effects are on the cardiovascular system. Hydralazine apparently lowers blood pressure by exerting a peripheral vasodilating effect through a direct relaxation of vascular smooth muscle. Hydralazine, by altering cellular calcium metabolism, interferes with the calcium

movements within the vascular smooth muscle that are responsible for initiating or maintaining the contractile state. The peripheral vasodilating effect of hydralazine results in decreased arterial blood pressure (diastolic more than systolic); decreased peripheral vascular resistance; and an increased heart rate, stroke volume, and cardiac output. The preferential dilatation of arterioles, as compared to veins, minimizes postural hypotension and promotes the increase in cardiac output. Hydralazine usually increases renin activity in plasma, presumably as a result of increased secretion of renin by the renal juxtaglomerular cells in response to reflex sympathetic discharge. This increase in renin activity leads to the production of angiotensin II, which then causes stimulation of aldosterone and consequent sodium reabsorption. Hydralazine also maintains or increases renal and cerebral blood flow.

The average maximal decrease in blood pressure usually occurs 10–80 minutes after administration of parenteral Apresoline. No other pharamacokinetic data on parenteral Apresoline are available.

INDICATIONS AND USAGE

Severe essential hypertension when the drug cannot be given orally or when there is an urgent need to lower blood pressure.

CONTRAINDICATIONS

Hypersensitivity to hydralazine; coronary artery disease; mitral valvular rheumatic heart disease.

WARNINGS

In a few patients hydralazine may produce a clinical picture simulating systemic lupus erythematosus including glomerulonephritis. In such patients hydralazine should be discontinued unless the benefit-to-risk determination requires continued antihypertensive therapy with this drug. Symptoms and signs usually regress when the drug is discontinued but residua have been detected many years later. Long-term treatment with steroids may be necessary. (See PRECAUTIONS, Laboratory Tests.)

PRECAUTIONS

General: Myocardial stimulation produced by Apresoline can cause anginal attacks and ECG changes of myocardial ischemia. The drug has been implicated in the production of myocardial infarction. It must, therefore, be used with caution in patients with suspected coronary artery disease.

The "hyperdynamic" circulation caused by Apresoline may accentuate specific cardiovascular inadequacies. For example, Apresoline may increase pulmonary artery pressure in patients with mitral valvular disease. The drug may reduce the pressor responses to epinephrine. Postural hypotension may result from Apresoline but is less common than with ganglionic blocking agents. It should be used with caution in patients with cerebral vascular accidents.

In hypertensive patients with normal kidneys who are treated with Apresoline, there is evidence of increased renal blood flow and a maintenance of glomerular filtration rate. In some instances where control values were below normal, improved renal function has been noted after administration of Apresoline. However, as with any antihypertensive agent, Apresoline should be used with caution in patients with advanced renal damage.

Peripheral neuritis, evidenced by paresthesia, numbness, and tingling, has been observed. Published evidence suggests an antipyridoxine effect, and that pyridoxine should be added to the regimen if symptoms develop.

Laboratory Tests: Complete blood counts and antinuclear antibody titer determinations are indicated before and periodically during prolonged therapy with hydralazine even though the patient is asymptomatic. These studies are also indicated if the patient develops arthralgia, fever, chest pain, continued malaise, or other unexplained signs or symptoms. A positive antinuclear antibody titer requires that the physician carefully weigh the implications of the test results against the benefits to be derived from antihypertensive therapy with hydralazine.

Blood dyscrasias, consisting of reduction in hemoglobin and red cell count, leukopenia, agranulocytosis, and purpura, have been reported. If such abnormalities develop, therapy should be discontinued.

Drug/Drug Interactions: MAO inhibitors should be used with caution in patients receiving hydralazine.

When other potent parenteral antihypertensive drugs, such as diazoxide, are used in combination with hydralazine, patients should be continuously observed for several hours for any excessive fall in blood pressure. Profound hypotensive episodes may occur when diazoxide injection and Apresoline are used concomitantly.

Carcinogenesis, Mutagenesis, Impairment of Fertility: In a lifetime study in Swiss albino mice, there was a statistically significant increase in the incidence of lung tumors (adenomas and adenocarcinomas) of both male and female mice given hydralazine continuously in their drinking water at a dosage of about 250 mg/kg per day (about 80 times the maximum recommended human dose). In a 2-year carcinogenicity study of rats given hydralazine by gavage at dose levels of 15,

30, and 60 mg/kg/day (approximately 5 to 20 times the recommended human daily dosage), microscopic examination of the liver revealed a small, but statistically significant, increase in benign neoplastic nodules in male and female rats from the high-dose group and in female rats from the intermediate-dose group. Benign interstitial cell tumors of the testes were also significantly increased in male rats from the high-dose group. The tumors observed are common in aged rats and a significantly increased incidence was not observed until 18 months of treatment. Hydralazine was shown to be mutagenic in bacterial systems (Gene Mutation and DNA Repair) and in one of two rat and one rabbit hepatocyte *in vitro* DNA repair studies. Additional *in vivo* and *in vitro* studies using lymphoma cells, germinal cells, and fibroblasts from mice, bone marrow cells from chinese hamsters and fibroblasts from human cell lines did not demonstrate any mutagenic potential for hydralazine.

The extent to which these findings indicate a risk to man is uncertain. While long-term clinical observation has not suggested that human cancer is associated with hydralazine use, epidemiologic studies have so far been insufficient to arrive at any conclusions.

Pregnancy Category C: Animal studies indicate that hydralazine is teratogenic in mice at 20–30 times the maximum daily human dose of 200–300 mg and possibly in rabbits at 10–15 times the maximum daily human dose, but that it is nonteratogenic in rats. Teratogenic effects observed were cleft palate and malformations of facial and cranial bones. There are no adequate and well-controlled studies in pregnant women. Although clinical experience does not include any positive evidence of adverse effects on the human fetus, hydralazine should be used during pregnancy only if the expected benefit justifies the potential risk to the fetus.

Nursing Mothers: It is not known whether this drug is excreted in human milk. Because many drugs are excreted in human milk, caution should be exercised when Apresoline is administered to a nursing woman.

Pediatric Use: Safety and effectiveness in children have not been established in controlled clinical trials, although there is experience with the use of Apresoline in children. The usual recommended parenteral dosage, administered intramuscularly or intravenously, is 1.7–3.5 mg/kg of body weight daily, divided into four to six doses.

ADVERSE REACTIONS

Adverse reactions with Apresoline are usually reversible when dosage is reduced. However, in some cases it may be necessary to discontinue the drug.

The following adverse reactions have been observed, but there has not been enough systematic collection of data to support an estimate of their frequency.

Common: Headache, anorexia, nausea, vomiting, diarrhea, palpitations, tachycardia, angina pectoris.

Less Frequent: *Digestive:* constipation, paralytic ileus.
Cardiovascular: hypotension, paradoxical pressor response, edema.
Respiratory: dyspnea.
Neurologic: peripheral neuritis, evidenced by paresthesia, numbness, and tingling; dizziness; tremors; muscle cramps; psychotic reactions characterized by depression, disorientation, or anxiety.
Genitourinary: difficulty in urination.
Hematologic: blood dyscrasias, consisting of reduction in hemoglobin and red cell count, leukopenia, agranulocytosis, purpura; lymphadenopathy; splenomegaly.
Hypersensitive Reactions: rash, urticaria, pruritus, fever, chills, arthralgia, eosinophilia, and, rarely, hepatitis.
Other: nasal congestion, flushing, lacrimation, conjunctivitis.

OVERDOSAGE

Acute Toxicity: No deaths due to acute poisoning have been reported.

Highest known dose survived: adults, 10 g orally.

Oral LD$_{50}$ in rats: 173 and 187 mg/kg.

Signs and Symptoms: Signs and symptoms of overdosage include hypotension, tachycardia, headache, and generalized skin flushing.

Complications can include myocardial ischemia and subsequent myocardial infarction, cardiac arrhythmia, and profound shock.

Treatment: There is no specific antidote.

Support of the cardiovascular system is of primary importance. Shock should be treated with plasma expanders. If possible, vasopressors should not be given, but if a vasopressor is required, care should be taken not to precipitate or aggravate cardiac arrhythmia. Tachycardia responds to beta blockers. Digitalization may be necessary, and renal function should be monitored and supported as required.

No experience has been reported with extracorporeal or peritoneal dialysis.

DOSAGE AND ADMINISTRATION

When there is urgent need, therapy in the hospitalized patient may be initiated intramuscularly or as a rapid intravenous bolus injection directly into the vein. Parenteral Apresoline should be used only when the drug cannot be given orally. The usual dose is 20–40 mg, repeated as necessary. Certain patients (especially those with marked renal damage) may require a lower dose. Blood pressure should be checked frequently. It may begin to fall within a few minutes after injection, with the average maximal decrease occurring in 10–80 minutes. In cases where there has been increased intracranial pressure, lowering the blood pressure may increase cerebral ischemia. Most patients can be transferred to oral Apresoline within 24–48 hours.

The product should be used immediately after the ampul is opened. It should not be added to infusion solutions. Apresoline hydrochloride parenteral may discolor upon contact with metal; discolored solutions should be discarded. Parenteral drug products should be inspected visually for particulate matter and discoloration prior to administration, whenever solution and container permit.

HOW SUPPLIED

Ampuls 1 ml, containing 20 mg of hydralazine hydrochloride Cartons of 5 ampuls—NDC 0083-2626-05
See **Dosage and Administration.**
Store between 59° and 86°F (15°-30°C).

C86-15 (Rev. 4/86)

Dist. by:
CIBA Pharmaceutical Company
Division of CIBA-GEIGY Corporation
Summit, New Jersey 07901

AREDIA™ ℞
pamidronate disodium for injection
For Intravenous Infusion

Prescribing Information

DESCRIPTION

Aredia, pamidronate disodium, (APD), is a bone-resorption inhibitor available in vials for intravenous administration. Each vial contains 30 mg of sterile, lyophilized pamidronate disodium and 470 mg of mannitol, USP. The pH of a 1% solution of pamidronate disodium in distilled water is approximately 8.3. Aredia, a member of the group of chemical compounds known as bisphosphonates, is an analog of pyrophosphate. Pamidronate disodium is designated chemically as phosphonic acid (3-amino-1-hydroxypropylidene) bis-, disodium salt, pentahydrate, (APD).

Pamidronate disodium is a white-to-practically-white powder. It is soluble in water and in 2N sodium hydroxide, sparingly soluble in 0.1N hydrochloric acid and in 0.1N acetic acid, and practically insoluble in organic solvents. Its molecular formula is $C_3H_9NO_7P_2Na_2 \cdot 5H_2O$ and its molecular weight is 369.1.

Inactive Ingredients. Mannitol, USP, and phosphoric acid (for adjustment to pH 6.5 prior to lyophilization).

CLINICAL PHARMACOLOGY

The principal pharmacologic action of Aredia is inhibition of bone resorption. Although the mechanism of antiresorptive action is not completely understood, several factors are thought to contribute to this action. Aredia adsorbs to calcium phosphate (hydroxyapatite) crystals in bone and may directly block dissolution of this mineral component of bone. In vitro studies also suggest that inhibition of osteoclast activity contributes to inhibition of bone resorption. In animal studies, at doses recommended for the treatment of hypercalcemia, Aredia inhibits bone resorption apparently without inhibiting bone formation and mineralization. Of relevance to the treatment of hypercalcemia of malignancy is the finding that Aredia inhibits the accelerated bone resorption that results from osteoclast hyperactivity induced by various tumors in animal studies.

In cancer patients who had minimal or no bony involvement who were given an intravenous infusion of 60 mg of Aredia over 4 or 24 hours, a mean of 51% (32–80%) of the drug was excreted unchanged in the urine within 72 hours. Body retention during this period was calculated to be a mean of 49% (range 20–68%) of the dose, or 29.3 mg (12–41 mg). The urinary-excretion-rate profile after administration of 60 mg of Aredia over 4 hours exhibited biphasic disposition characteristics with an alpha half-life of 1.6 hours and a beta half-life of 27.2 hours. There are no human pharmacokinetic data for Aredia on the 90-mg dose or in patients who have either renal or hepatic insufficiency. The rate of elimination of Aredia from bone has not been determined.

After intravenous administration of radiolabeled Aredia in rats, approximately 50–60% of the compound was rapidly adsorbed by bone and slowly eliminated from the body by the kidneys. In rats given 10 mg/kg bolus injections of radiolabeled Aredia, approximately 30% of the compound was found in the liver shortly after administration and was then redistributed to bone or eliminated by the kidneys over 24–48 hours. Studies in rats injected with radiolabeled Aredia showed that the compound was rapidly cleared from the circulation and taken up mainly by bones, liver, spleen, teeth, and tracheal cartilage. Radioactivity was eliminated from most soft tissues within 1–4 days; was detectable in liver and spleen for 1 and 3 months, respectively; and remained high in bones, trachea, and teeth for 6 months after dosing. Bone uptake occurred preferentially in areas of high bone turnover. The terminal phase of elimination half-life in bone was estimated to be approximately 300 days.

Serum phosphate levels have been noted to decrease after administration of Aredia, presumably because of decreased release of phosphate from bone and increased renal excretion as parathyroid hormone levels, which are usually suppressed in hypercalcemia associated with malignancy, return towards normal. Phosphate therapy was administered in 30% of the patients in response to decrease in serum phosphate levels. Phosphate levels ususally returned towards normal within 7–10 days.

Urinary calcium/creatinine and urinary hydroxyproline/creatinine ratios decrease and usually return to within or below normal after treatment with Aredia. These changes occur within the first week after treatment, as do decreases in serum calcium levels, and are consistent with an antiresorptive pharmacologic action.

Hypercalcemia of Malignancy

Osteoclastic hyperactivity resulting in excessive bone resorption is the underlying pathophysiologic derangement in metastatic bone disease and hypercalcemia of malignancy. Excessive release of calcium into the blood as bone is resorbed results in polyuria and gastrointestinal disturbances, with progressive dehydration and decreasing glomerular filtration rate. This, in turn, results in increased renal resorption of calcium, setting up a cycle of worsening systemic hypercalcemia. Correction of excessive bone resorption and adequate fluid administration to correct volume deficits are therefore essential to the management of hypercalcemia.

Most cases of hypercalcemia associated with malignancy occur in patients who have breast cancer; squamous-cell tumors of the lung or head and neck; renal-cell carcinoma; and certain hematologic malignancies, such as multiple myeloma and some types of lymphomas. A few less-common malignancies, including vasoactive intestinal-peptide-producing tumors and cholangiocarcinoma, have a high incidence of hypercalcemia as a metabolic complication. Patients who have hypercalcemia of malignancy can generally be divided into two groups, according to the pathophysiologic mechanism involved.

In humoral hypercalcemia, osteoclasts are activated and bone resorption is stimulated by factors such as parathyroid-hormone-related protein, which are elaborated by the tumor and circulate systemically. Humoral hypercalcemia usually occurs in squamous-cell malignancies of the lung or head and neck or in genitourinary tumors such as renal-cell carcinoma or ovarian cancer. Skeletal metastases may be absent or minimal in these patients.

Extensive invasion of bone by tumor cells can also result in hypercalcemia due to local tumor products that stimulate bone resorption by osteoclasts. Tumors commonly associated with locally mediated hypercalcemia include breast cancer and multiple myeloma.

Total serum calcium levels in patients who have hypercalcemia of malignancy may not reflect the severity of hypercalcemia, since concomitant hypoalbuminemia is commonly present. Ideally, ionized calcium levels should be used to diagnose and follow hypercalcemic conditions; however, these are not commonly or rapidly available in many clinical situations. Therefore, adjustment of the total serum calcium value for differences in albumin levels if often used in place of measurement of ionized calcium; several nomograms are in use for this type of calculation (See DOSAGE AND ADMINISTRATION).

Clinical Trials

In one double-blind clinical trial, 52 patients who had hypercalcemia of malignancy were enrolled to receive 30 mg, 60 mg, or 90 mg of Aredia as a single 24-hour intravenous infusion if their corrected serum calcium levels were ≥ 12.0 mg/dL after 48 hours of saline hydration.

The mean baseline corrected serum calcium for the 30 mg, 60 mg and 90 mg groups were 13.8 mg/dL, 13.8 mg/dL and 13.3 mg/dL, respectively.

The majority of the patients (64%) had decreases in albumin-corrected serum calcium levels by 24 hours after initiation of treatment. Mean-corrected serum calcium levels at days 2–7 after initiation of treatment with Aredia were significantly reduced from baseline in all three dosage groups. As a result, by 7 days after initiation of treatment of Aredia, 40%, 61%, and 100% of the patients receiving 30 mg, 60 mg, and 90 mg of Aredia, respectively, had normal corrected serum calcium levels. Many patients (33–53%) in the 60-mg and 90-mg dosage groups continued to have normal-corrected serum calcium levels, or a partial response (≥ 15% decrease of corrected serum calcium from baseline), at day 14.

Continued on next page

The full prescribing information for each CIBA product is contained herein and is that in effect as of September 1, 1992.

CIBA—Cont.

In a second double-blind, controlled clinical trial, 65 cancer patients who had corrected serum calcium levels of ≥12.0 mg/dL after at least 24 hours of saline hydration were randomized to receive either 60 mg of Aredia as a single 24-hour intravenous infusion or 7.5 mg/kg of Didronel (etidronate disodium) as a 2-hour intravenous infusion daily for 3 days. Thirty patients were randomized to receive Aredia and 35 to receive Didronel.
The mean baseline corrected serum calcium for the Aredia 60 mg and Didronel groups were 14.6 mg/dL and 13.8 mg/dL, respectively.
By day 7, 70% of the patients in the Aredia group and 41% of the patients in the Didronel group had normal corrected serum calcium levels ($P < 0.05$). When partial responders (≥15% decrease of serum calcium from baseline) were also included, the response rates were 97% for the Aredia group and 65% for the Didronel group ($P < 0.01$). Mean corrected serum calcium for the Aredia and Didronel groups decreased from baseline values to 10.4 and 11.2 mg/dL, respectively, on day 7. At day 14, 43% of patients in the Aredia group and 18% of patients in the Didronel group still had normal corrected serum calcium levels, or maintenance of a partial response. For responders in the Aredia and Didronel groups, the median duration of response was similar (7 and 5 days, respectively). The time course of effect on corrected serum calcium is summarized in the following table.

Change in Corrected Serum Calcium by Time from Initiation of Treatment

Time (hr)	Mean Change from Baseline in Corrected Serum Calcium (mg/dL) Aredia	Didronel	p Value[1]
Baseline	14.6	13.8	
24	−0.3	−0.5	
48	− 1.5	− 1.1	
72	− 2.6	− 2.0	
96	− 3.5	− 2.0	<0.01
168	− 4.1	− 2.5	<0.01

[1] Comparison between treatment groups

In both trials, patients treated with Aredia had similar response rates in the presence or absence of bone metastases. Concomitant administration of furosemide did not affect response rates.
Twenty-five patients who had recurrent or refractory hypercalcemia of malignancy were given a second course of 60 mg of Aredia. Of these, 40% showed a complete response and 20% showed a partial response to the retreatment, and these responders had aboaut a 3 mg/dL fall in mean corrected serum calcium levels 7 days after treatment.

INDICTIONS AND USAGE

Aredia, in conjunction with adequate hydration, is indicated for the treatment of moderate or severe hypercalcemia associated with malignancy, with or without bone metastases. Patients who have either epidermoid or non-epidermoid tumors respond to treatment with Aredia. Vigorous saline hydration, an integral part of hypercalcemia therapy, should be initiated promptly and an attempt should be made to restore the urine output to about 2 L/day throughout treatment. Mild or asymptomatic hypercalcemia may be treated with conservative measures (i.e., saline hydration, with or without loop diuretics). Patients should be hydrated adequately throughout the treatment, but overhydration, especially in those patients who have cardiac failure, must be avoided. Diuretic therapy should not be employed prior to correction of hypovolemia. The safety and efficacy of Aredia in the treatment of hypercalcemia associated with hyperparathyroidism or with other non-tumor-related conditions has not been established.

CONTRAINDICATIONS

Aredia is contraindicated in patients with clinically significant hypersensitivity to Aredia or other bisphosphonates.

WARNINGS

In both rats and dogs, nephropathy has been associated with intravenous, bolus administration of Aredia. A 3-month study in rats found cortical tubular changes including epithelial degeneration with intravenous doses ≥5 g mg/kg, given once every two weeks. Following a recovery period (1 month), the degenerative changes were completely reversed. Focal fibrosis of renal tubules was partially reversed.
In two studies conducted in dogs, Aredia was given as a bolus intravenous injection either daily for 1 month or once a week for 3 months. In the 1-month study, tubulointerstitial nephritis, tubular degeneration and dilation occurred at 2 mg/kg. At recovery (1 month) the severity of these lesions was minimal or trace. Similar lesions (slight to marked severity) were noted in the 3-month study at 3 mg/kg and higher. However, no improvement of the lesions was observed following the 1-month recovery period.
Patients with hypercalcemia who receive an intravenous infusion of Aredia should have periodic evaluations of standard laboratory and clinical parameters of renal function. Studies conducted in young rats have reported the disruption of dental enamel formation with single-dose administration of bisphosphonates. The clinical significance of these findings is unknown.

PRECAUTIONS

General

Standard hypercalcemia-related metabolic parameters, such as serum levels of calcium, phosphate, magnesium, and potassium should be carefully monitored following initiation of therapy with Aredia. Cases of asymptomatic hypophosphatemia (16%), hypokalemia (9%), hypomagnesemia (12%), and hypocalcemia (6–12%), were reported in Aredia-treated patients. One case of hypocalcemia with symptomatic tetany has been reported during oral Aredia treatment. If hypocalcemia occurs, short-term calcium therapy may be necessary. Aredia has not been tested in patients who have class Dc renal impairment (creatinine >5.0 mg/dL). Clinical judgment should determine whether the potential benefit outweighs the potential risk in such patients.

Laboratory Tests

Serum calcium, electrolytes, phosphate, magnesium and creatinine, and CBC, differential, and hematocrit/hemoglobin must be closely monitored in patients treated with Aredia. Patients who have preexisting anemia, leukopenia, or thrombocytopenia should be monitored carefully in the first 2 weeks following treatment.

Drug Interactions

Concomitant administration of a loop diuretic had no effect on the calcium-lowering action of Aredia.

Carcinogenesis, Mutagenesis, Impairment of Fertility

In a 104-week carcinogenicity study (daily oral administration) in rats, there was a positive dose response relationship for benign adrenal pheochromocytoma in males ($p < 0.00001$). Although this condition was also observed in females, the incidence was not statistically significant. When the dose calculations were adjusted to account for the limited oral bioavailability of Aredia in rats, the lowest daily dose associated with adrenal pheochromocytoma was similar to the intended clinical dose. Aredia (daily oral administration) was not carcinogenic in an 80-week study in mice.
Aredia was nonmutagenic in four mutagenicity assays: Ames test, nucleus-anomaly test, sister-chromatid-exchange study, and point-mutation test.
In rats, decreased fertility occurred in first-generation offspring of parents who had received 150 mg/kg of Aredia orally; however, this occurred only when animals were mated with members of the same dose group. Aredia has not been administered intravenously in such a study.

Pregnancy Category C

Aredia has been shown to increase the length of gestation and parturition in rats resulting in an increasing pup mortality when given orally at daily doses of 60 and 150 mg/kg/day from before pregnancy until after parturition. When corrected for oral bioavailability, each daily dose is approximately 0.7 to 1.7 times the highest recommended human dose for a single intravenous infusion. Oral doses of 25 to 150 mg/kg/day during the period of gestation failed to demonstrate any teratogenic, fetotoxic, or embryotoxic effects in rats or rabbits. Animal reproduction studies have not been conducted with intravenously administered Aredia. It is not known if intravenous Aredia can cause fetal harm when administered to pregnant women or if it can affect reproduction capacity. There are no adequate and well-controlled studies in pregnant women. Aredia should be used during pregnancy only if the potential benefit justifies the potential risk to the fetus.

Nursing Mothers

It is not known whether Aredia is excreted in human milk. Because many drugs are excreted in human milk, caution should be exercised when Aredia is administered to a nursing woman.

Pediatric Use

Safety and effectiveness of Aredia in children have not been established.

ADVERSE REACTIONS

Transient mild elevation of temperature by at least 1°C was noted 24–48 hours after administration of Aredia in 27% of the patients in clinical trials.
Drug-related local soft-tissue symptoms (redness, swelling or induration and pain on palpation) at the site of catheter insertion were most common (18%) in patients treated with 90 mg of Aredia. When all on-therapy events are considered, that rate rises to 41%. Symptomatic treatment resulted in rapid resolution in all patients.
Uveitis was reported in 1 patient who had hypercalcemia of malignancy; another patient who had Paget's disease of bone developed mild iritis that was responsive to indomethacin and topical steroid. Both of these patients received Aredia in uncontrolled studies.
Four of 82 patients (4.9%) who received Aredia during the 2 U.S. controlled hypercalcemia clinical studies were reported to have had seizures; 2 of whom had preexisting seizure disorders. None of the seizures were considered to be drug-related by the investigators. However, a possible relationship between the drug and the occurrence of seizures cannot be ruled out.
At least 15% of patients treated with Aredia for hypercalcemia of malignancy also experienced the following adverse events during a clinical trial:
General: Fluid overload, generalized pain
Cardiovascular: Hypertension
Gastrointestinal: Abdominal pain, anorexia, constipation, nausea, vomiting
Genitourinary: Urinary tract infection
Musculoskeletal: Bone pain
Laboratory abnormality: Anemia, hypokalemia, hypomagnesemia, hypophosphatemia
Many of these adverse experiences may have been related to the underlying disease state.
The following table lists the adverse experiences considered to be related to treatment with bisphosphonates during comparative, controlled U.S. trials.

Bisphosphonate-Related Adverse Experiences In Two U.S. Controlled Clinical Trials

	Percent of Patients: Aredia (N=67) 60 mg	90 mg	Didronel (N=35) 7.5 mg/kg × 3 days
General			
Fatigue	0	12	0
Fever	20	18	9
Fluid overload	0	0	6
Infusion-site reaction	6	18	0
Moniliasis	0	6	0
Gastrointestinal			
Abdominal pain	2	0	0
Anorexia	2	12	0
Constipation	0	6	3
Gastrointestinal hemorrhage	0	6	0
Nausea	0	18	6
Ulcerative stomatitis	0	0	3
Respiratory System			
Dyspnea	0	0	3
Rales	0	6	0
Rhinitis	0	6	0
Upper respiratory infection	2	0	0
CNS			
Convulsions	0	0	3
Insomnia	2	0	0
Somnolence	2	6	0
Taste perversion	0	0	3
Abnormal vision	2	0	0
Cardiovascular			
Atrial fibrillation	0	6	0
Hypertension	0	6	0
Syncope	0	6	0
Tachycardia	0	6	0
Endocrine System			
Hypothyroidism	0	6	0
Hemic and Lymphatic System			
Anemia	0	6	0
Laboratory Abnormality			
Hypocalcemia	2	12	0
Hypokalemia	4	18	0
Hypomagnesemia	8	12	3
Hypophosphatemia	14	18	3
Abnormal hepatic function	0	0	3

OVERDOSAGE

One obese woman (95 kg) who was treated with 285 mg of Aredia/day for 3 days, experienced high fever (39.5°C), hypotension (from 170/190 mmHg to 90/60 mmHg), and transient taste perversion, noted about 6 hours after the first infusion. The fever and hypotension were rapidly corrected with steroids.
If overdosage occurs, symptomatic hypocalcemia could also result; such patients should be treated with short-term intravenous-calcium.

DOSAGE AND ADMINISTRATION

Consideration should be given to the severity of as well as the symptoms of hypercalcemia. The recommended dose of Aredia in moderate hypercalcemia (corrected serum calcium of approximately 12–13.5 mg/dL) is 60–90 mg, and in severe hypercalcemia (corrected serumn calcium, >13.5 mg/dL), is 90 mg, given as an initial, single-dose, intravenous infusion over 24 hours. Albumin-corrected serum calcium (CCa, mg/dL) = serum calcium, mg/dL + 0.8 (4.0 − serum albumin, g/dL).
Vigorous saline hydration alone may be sufficient for treating mild, asymptomatic hypercalcemia. Overhydration should be avoided in patients who have potential for cardiac

failure. In hypercalcemia associated with hematologic malignancies, the use of glucocorticoid therapy may be helpful.
A limited number of patients have received more than one treatment with Aredia for hypercalcemia. Retreatment with Aredia may be considered if hypercalcemia recurs. It is recommended that a minimum of 7 days elapse before retreatment, to allow for full response to the initial dose. The dose and manner of retreatment is identical to that of the initial therapy.

Preparation of Solution
Aredia is reconstituted by adding 10 mL of Sterile Water for Injection, USP, to each vial, resulting in a solution of 30 mg/10 mL. The pH of the reconstituted solution is 6.0–7.4. The drug should be completely dissolved before the solution is withdrawn. The daily dose must be administered as an intravenous infusion over 24 hours. The recommended dose should be diluted in 1000 mL of sterile 0.45% or 0.9% Sodium Chloride, USP, or 5% Dextrose Injection, USP. This infusion is stable for up to 24 hours at room temperature.
Aredia must not be mixed with calcium-containing Infusion solutions, such as Ringer's solution.
Note: **Parenteral drug products should be inspected visually for particulate matter and discoloration prior to administration, whenever solution and container permit.**
Aredia reconstituted with Sterile Water for Injection may be stored under refrigeration at 36–46°F (2–8°C) for up to 24 hours.

HOW SUPPLIED

Vials—each contains 30 mg of sterile, lyophilized, pamidronate disodium and 470 mg of mannitol, USP.
Carton of 4 vials ....NDC 0083-2601-04
Do not store above 86°F (30°C).
Caution: Federal law prohibits dispensing without prescription.

C91-47

CIBA
CIBA Pharmaceutical Company
Division of CIBA-GEIGY Corporation
Summit, New Jersey 07901

CIBACALCIN® ℞
calcitonin-human for injection
Syringes

DESCRIPTION

Cibacalcin, calcitonin-human for injection, is a synthetic polypeptide hormone consisting of 32 amino acids in the same linear sequence as found in naturally occurring human calcitonin.
All amino acids are in their optically active L configuration.
Cibacalcin is a white to off-white amorphous powder containing 3 moles of hydrochloric acid, bound to the basic peptide groups, and up to 8% (w/w) acetic acid and 10% (w/w) water. It is soluble in water, in physiological saline, in dilute acid, and in dilute base; sparingly soluble in methanol; and practically insoluble in chloroform. Its molecular formula is $C_{151}H_{226}N_{40}O_{45}S_3 \cdot 3HCl$ which corresponds to a molecular weight of 3527.2.
Cibacalcin is available in double-chambered, disposable, vial syringes for subcutaneous administration. The double-chambered syringes contain calcitonin-human for injection, 0.5 mg, and mannitol, 20 mg, in sterile, lyophilized form in one chamber, and a 1-ml solution of 30 mg of mannitol in Water for Injection in the other chamber.

CLINICAL PHARMACOLOGY

Calcitonins are polypeptide hormones secreted by the parafollicular or C-cells of the thyroid gland in mammals and by the ultimobranchial gland of birds and fish.
The precise physiologic functions of the calcitonins have not been completely defined; they appear to play a role in the regulation of calcium and bone metabolism. When Cibacalcin is given to normal subjects, serum calcium is lowered and urinary excretion of calcium, phosphorus, and sodium increases. Cibacalcin has also been shown to inhibit the pancreatic secretion of enzymes and gastric secretion during acute administration. The significance of these effects during chronic therapy, however, has not been investigated.
The metabolic clearance rate of exogenously administered immunoreactive Cibacalcin in normal subjects has been determined to be 8.4 ± 1.1 ml/kg per min. The half-life is 1.02 hours after single, subcutaneous doses of 0.5 mg. Evidence to date indicates that the kidney is the principal organ responsible for its degradation, with only small fractions of the parent substance (0.1%) appearing in the urine.
In Paget's disease (osteitis deformans), Cibacalcin causes a decrease in serum alkaline phosphatase and in urinary hydroxyproline excretion. Among 44 patients in clinical studies who had one or more determinations of serum alkaline phosphatase and 29 patients who had one or more determinations of urinary hydroxyproline during the first year of therapy, the following mean percent reductions from baseline were observed:

	Mean % Reduction (n*)	
Time Interval†	Serum Alkaline Phosphatase	Urinary Hydroxyproline
1–3 months	23.4(30)	21.4(20)
4–6 months	41.0(22)	47.4(12)
7–12 months	44.7(25)	56.1(14)

† Duration of treatment at time of observation
* Number of patients evaluated at each time interval

The mean reduction in serum alkaline phosphatase at the final visit compared to baseline for these patients was 36.1% (mean duration of treatment = 18.5 months) and for urinary hydroxyproline was 37.5% (mean duration of treatment = 21.2 months).
In a limited number of studies, patients treated with Cibacalcin have been reported to show radiological evidence of bone remodeling towards normal, including healing of lytic lesions. Serial biopsies of Pagetic bone indicate a decrease in the number of osteoclasts per square millimeter of bone during treatment.
The risk of diminishing effectiveness as a result of antibody formation or hypersensitivity reactions is less with Cibacalcin than with nonhuman forms of the hormone.
Long-term treatment (up to ten or more years in a few patients) with Cibacalcin has not been limited by antibody-mediated resistance.
Cibacalcin has been shown to be effective in patients who have developed resistance to nonhuman calcitonins.

INDICATIONS AND USAGE

Cibacalcin is indicated for the treatment of symptomatic Paget's disease of bone.
The effectiveness of Cibacalcin was demonstrated primarily in patients with moderate-to-severe disease characterized by multiple bone involvement and elevations of serum alkaline phosphatase and urinary hydroxyproline excretion.
Although reduction of serum alkaline phosphatase and urinary hydroxyproline excretion usually occurs within 3 months after initiation of treatment, maximum reductions may not occur until after 6–24 months of continuous treatment.
Cibacalcin has been reported to cause subjective relief of bone pain and tenderness and a reduction in elevated skin temperature over the affected skeletal areas in some patients.

CONTRAINDICATIONS

None known.

WARNINGS

Since Cibacalcin is a protein, the possibility of a systemic allergic reaction should not be disregarded. Therefore, appropriate materials for the emergency treatment of such a reaction should be available.
The incidence of osteogenic sarcoma is known to be increased in Paget's disease. Pagetic lesions, with or without therapy, may appear by X-ray to progress markedly, possibly with some loss of definition of periosteal margins. Such lesions must be evaluated carefully to differentiate them from osteogenic sarcoma.

PRECAUTIONS

General
The administration of Cibacalcin could lead to hypocalcemic tetany, under special circumstances. Calcium for parenteral administration should be available during the first few administrations of Cibacalcin.
Information for Patients
Patients and other persons who may administer Cibacalcin should receive careful instruction in sterile-injection techniques.
Carcinogenesis, Mutagenesis, Impairment of Fertility
No long-term carcinogenicity studies have been conducted with Cibacalcin.
Pregnancy Category C
Animal reproduction studies have not been conducted with Cibacalcin. However, salmon calcitonin has been shown to cause a decrease in fetal birth weight in rabbits when given in doses 14–56 times the dose recommended for human use. Calcitonin does not cross the placental barrier. This finding may be due to metabolic effects of the drug on the pregnant animal. It is also not known whether Cibacalcin can cause fetal harm when administered to a pregnant woman or can affect reproduction capacity. Cibacalcin should be given to a pregnant woman only if clearly needed.
Nursing Mothers
It is not known whether this drug is excreted in human milk. Because Cibacalcin is a peptide and subject to digestion in the gastrointestinal tract, it is unlikely that active drug will be absorbed by the nursing infant. However, studies of drug activity after ingestion have not been done in nursing infants and caution should be exercised when Cibacalcin is administered to a nursing woman. Calcitonin has been shown to inhibit lactation in animals.
Pediatric Use
The use of Cibacalcin has been reported in the rare disorders of bone in children referred to as juvenile Paget's disease. However, the safety and effectiveness of Cibacalcin in children have not been established.

ADVERSE REACTIONS

The adverse reaction rates listed below are based on studies that included a large proportion of patients with histories of unresponsiveness to nonhuman calcitonins, a number of whom also had displayed intolerance to those calcitonins.
Gastrointestinal: Nausea, with or without vomiting, was noted in about 14% to 21% of patients treated with the recommended dose of Cibacalcin. Anorexia, diarrhea, epigastric discomfort, or abdominal pain were reported in a few patients. Nausea improved in the majority of patients with continued therapy.
Dermatologic/Hypersensitivity: Flushing of face, ears, or hands occurred within minutes of injection in 16% to 21% of patients treated with the recommended dose. Flushing improved in the majority of patients with continued therapy. Skin rashes were reported rarely.
Genitourinary: Increased frequency of urination was noted in about 5% to 10% of patients.
Metabolic: Mild tetanic symptoms were reported rarely during Cibacalcin therapy. One patient developed asymptomatic mild hypercalcemia during a study.
Miscellaneous: Rare side effects included chills, chest pressure, weakness, headache, tenderness of palms and soles, dizziness, nasal congestion, shortness of breath, metallic taste, and paresthesia.

OVERDOSAGE

Dosages greater than 1 mg per day have not been administered chronically. In animals, single doses as high as 1,000 mg/kg produced no mortality or functional or structural organ changes.

DOSAGE AND ADMINISTRATION

The recommended starting dosage of Cibacalcin is 0.5 mg daily, given subcutaneously.
Some patients may obtain sufficient clinical and biochemical improvement with a dosage of 0.5 mg two or three times weekly or 0.25 mg daily.
As an aid in evaluating the efficacy of Cibacalcin, determination of serum alkaline phosphatase and urinary hydroxyproline excretion should be performed prior to initiation of therapy, during the first three months and at intervals (approximately 3–6 months) during chronic treatment.
Adjustments in dose should be guided by clinical and radiological evidence, as well as changes in serum alkaline phosphatase and urinary hydroxyproline excretion.
Side effects such as nausea and flushing may be minimized by administration at bedtime. Dose adjustment (e.g. from 0.5 mg to 0.25 mg) may also be helpful in this regard.
More severe cases (e.g., when there is evidence of mechanically weak bones with osteolytic lesions) may require dosages of up to 1 mg daily (0.5 mg twice daily).
Treatment should be continued for 6 months; if symptoms have been relieved, therapy may be discontinued until symptoms or radiologic signs recur. Biochemical parameters will relapse on cessation of therapy and should not be relied on as the basis for a decision to restart therapy with Cibacalcin.
The double-chambered syringe is intended primarily for subcutaneous administration by the patient. Reconstituted material should be used within 6 hours.
Note: **Parenteral drug products should be inspected visually for particulate matter and discoloration prior to administration, whenever solution and container permit.**
When the dosage is 0.25 mg (one-half of the solution), the remainder of the drug solution is to be discarded.

HOW SUPPLIED

Double-chambered syringes—each contains 0.5 mg of calcitonin-human for injection and 20 mg of mannitol, in sterile, lyophilized form, in one chamber and a 1-ml solution of 30 mg of mannitol in Water for Injection in the other chamber.
Unit Dose (blister pack)
Cartons of 5 syringes ....NDC 0083-6485-05
Do not store above 77°F (25°C). Protect from light.
Reconstituted material should be used within 6 hours.
No refrigeration required.

C87-50 (Rev. 2/88)

Information for the Patient
CIBACALCIN®
Calcitonin-human for injection
How to Prepare for Injection
1. Remove the foil covering from the double-chambered syringe.

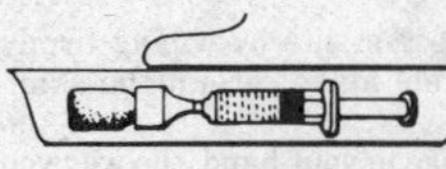

Continued on next page

The full prescribing information for each CIBA product is contained herein and is that in effect as of September 1, 1992.

CIBA—Cont.

2. Holding the barrel of the syringe, push it into the vial as far as it will go. Do not hold the plunger. If the red plastic collar positioned between the vial and the syringe is visible, then the syringe has **not** been pushed into the vial as far as it will go.

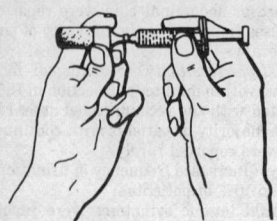

3. Hold the unit vertically as illustrated (vial up). Press firmly upward on the plunger as far as it will go, so the water in the syringe enters the vial containing the dry powder. Shake **gently** to mix. Whenever possible, inspect injectable products before use. If particles or discoloration are present, do not use.

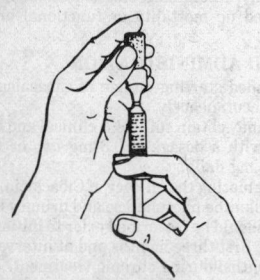

4. Pull the plunger **slowly** to the black line on the barrel of the syringe for a 0.25 mg dose. Withdraw the entire solution into the syringe for a 0.5 mg dose.
When the dosage of 0.25 mg (one-half of the solution) is used, the remainder of the drug solution in the vial is to be discarded.

5. Carefully pull the vial away from the syringe. Pointing syringe upward, tap barrel with fingertips to force any air bubbles to the surface. Push **gently** on plunger to expel air. Stop pushing when you see droplets of liquid at tip of needle.

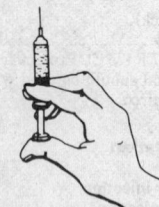

How to Inject

1. Clean the injection site by wiping firmly with a sterile alcohol swab. Make certain the skin is dry before injecting.
2. Hold the syringe in your hand, the way you would a pencil.
3. Using the thumb and index finger of your free hand, pinch up a two-inch fold of skin at the injection site.
4. Quickly plunge the needle all the way into the fold of skin, making sure the syringe is held at about a 60° angle. Let go of the skin fold with your free hand.

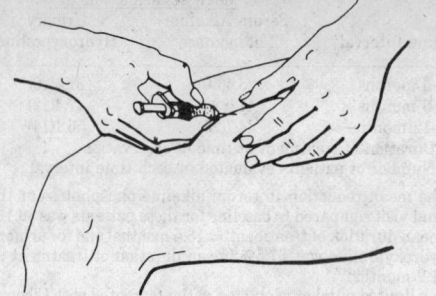

5. To check that the needle is not in a blood vessel, hold the syringe steady with your free hand and use the other hand to pull back slightly on the plunger.

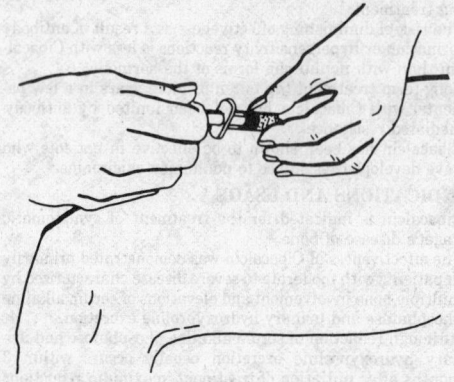

6. If blood appears in the syringe, remove the needle, discard the double-chambered syringe, and begin again with a new unit.
7. If no blood appears, inject the medication by **slowly** pushing down on the plunger.

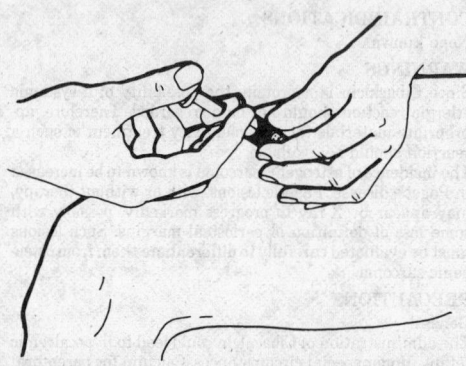

8. When you finish injecting the medication, take a fresh alcohol swab and press it against the skin with your free hand, as you quickly pull the needle out with your other hand. Remove the needle at the same 60° angle at which you inserted it.

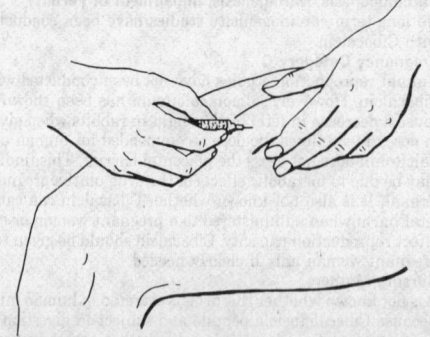

9. Gently rub the injection site with an alcohol swab to promote absorption of Cibacalcin.
10. Replace needle in used vial and bend both units back and forth until needle is broken. Discard entire unit.

Injection Sites

The figures above show the usual sites for your daily injection of Cibacalcin.

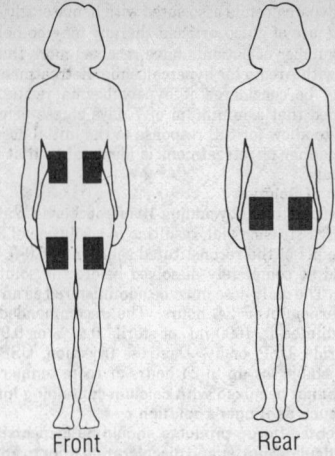

Front   Rear

- Carefully follow your doctor's instructions for injection
- Always remember to use a **different** injection site each day
- To help you remember which sites you have already used, you may find it helpful to keep a daily record
- If you have any questions, be sure to speak to your doctor Whenever possible, inspect injectable drug products for particles and discoloration before you use them.

Do not store above 77°F (25°C). Protect from light.
Once the solution has been made, it should be used within 6 hours.
No refrigeration required.

C87-51 (Rev. 2/88)

Dist. by:
CIBA Pharmaceutical Company
Division of CIBA-GEIGY Corporation
Summit, New Jersey 07901

CYTADREN® Tablets   ℞
[sight 'a-dren]
aminoglutethimide tablets USP

DESCRIPTION

Cytadren, aminoglutethimide tablets USP, is an inhibitor of adrenocortical steroid synthesis, available as 250-mg tablets for oral administration. Its chemical name is 3-(4-amino-phenyl)-3-ethyl-2, 6-piperidinedione.
Aminoglutethimide USP is a fine, white or creamy white, crystalline powder. It is very slightly soluble in water, and readily soluble in most organic solvents. It forms water-soluble salts with strong acids. Its molecular weight is 232.28.
Inactive Ingredients. Cellulose compounds, colloidal silicon dioxide, starch, stearic acid, and talc.

CLINICAL PHARMACOLOGY

Cytadren inhibits the enzymatic conversion of cholesterol to Δ^5-pregnenolone, resulting in a decrease in the production of adrenal glucocorticoids, mineralocorticoids, estrogens, and androgens.
Cytadren blocks several other steps in steroid synthesis, including the C-11, C-18, and C-21 hydroxylations and the hydroxylations required for the aromatization of androgens to estrogens, mediated through the binding of Cytadren to cytochrome P-450 complexes.
A decrease in adrenal secretion of cortisol is followed by an increased secretion of pituitary adrenocorticotropic hormone (ACTH), which will overcome the blockade of adrenocortical steroid synthesis by Cytadren. The compensatory increase in ACTH secretion can be suppressed by the simultaneous administration of hydrocortisone. Since Cytadren increases the rate of metabolism of dexamethasone but not that of hydrocortisone, the latter is preferred as the adrenal glucocorticoid replacement.
Although Cytadren inhibits the synthesis of thyroxine by the thyroid gland, the compensatory increase in thyroid-stimulating hormone (TSH) is frequently of sufficient magnitude to overcome the inhibition of thyroid synthesis due to Cytadren. In spite of an increase in TSH, Cytadren has not been associated with increased prolactin secretion.
Note: Cytadren was marketed previously as an anticonvulsant but was withdrawn from marketing for that indication in 1966 because of the effects on the adrenal gland.

Pharmacokinetics

Cytadren is rapidly and completely absorbed after oral administration. In 6 healthy male volunteers, maximum plasma levels of Cytadren averaged 5.9 µg/ml at a median of 1.5 hours after ingestion of two 250-mg tablets. The bioavailability of tablets is equivalent to equal doses given as a solution. After ingestion of a single oral dose, 34–54% is excreted in the urine as unchanged drug during the first 48 hours, and an additional fraction as the N-acetyl derivative.
The half-life of Cytadren in normal volunteers given single oral doses averaged 12.5 ± 1.6 hours.

Upon withdrawal of therapy with Cytadren, the ability of the adrenal glands to synthesize steroid returns, usually within 72 hours.

INDICATIONS AND USAGE

Cytadren is indicated for the suppression of adrenal function in selected patients with Cushing's syndrome. Morning levels of plasma cortisol in patients with adrenal carcinoma and ectopic ACTH-producing tumors were reduced on the average to about one half of the pretreatment levels, and in patients with adrenal hyperplasia to about two thirds of the pretreatment levels, during 1–3 months of therapy with Cytadren. Data available from the few patients with adrenal adenoma suggest similar reductions in plasma cortisol levels. Measurements of plasma cortisol showed reductions to at least 50% of baseline or to normal levels in one third or more of the patients studied, depending on diagnostic groups and time of measurement.

Because Cytadren does not affect the underlying disease process, it is used primarily as an interim measure until more definitive therapy such as surgery can be undertaken or in cases where such therapy is not appropriate. Only small numbers of patients have been treated for longer than 3 months. A decreased effect or "escape phenomenon" seems to occur more frequently in patients with pituitary-dependent Cushing's syndrome, probably because of increasing ACTH levels in response to decreasing glucocorticoid levels. Cytadren should be used only in those patients who are responsive to treatment.

CONTRAINDICATIONS

Cytadren is contraindicated in those patients with serious forms, and/or severe manifestations, of hypersensitivity to glutethimide or aminoglutethimide.

WARNINGS

Cytadren may cause adrenocortical hypofunction, especially under conditions of stress, such as surgery, trauma, or acute illness. Patients should be carefully monitored and given hydrocortisone and mineralocorticoid supplements as indicated. Dexamethasone should not be used. (See **PRECAUTIONS, Drug Interactions**.)

Cytadren also may suppress aldosterone production by the adrenal cortex and may cause orthostatic or persistent hypotension. The blood pressure should be monitored in all patients at appropriate intervals. Patients should be advised of the possible occurrence of weakness and dizziness as symptoms of hypotension, and of measures to be taken should they occur.

The effects of Cytadren may be potentiated if it is taken in combination with alcohol.

Cytadren can cause fetal harm when administered to a pregnant woman. In the earlier experience with the drug in about 5000 patients, two cases of pseudohermaphroditism were reported in female infants whose mothers were treated with Cytadren and concomitant anticonvulsants. Normal pregnancies have also occurred in patients treated with Cytadren.

When administered to rats at doses ½ and 1¼ times the maximum daily human dose, Cytadren caused a decrease in fetal implantation, an increase in fetal deaths, and a variety of teratogenic effects. The compound also caused pseudohermaphroditism in rats treated with approximately 3 times the maximum daily human dose. If this drug must be used during pregnancy, or if the patient becomes pregnant while taking the drug, the patient should be apprised of the potential hazard to the fetus.

PRECAUTIONS

General

This drug should be administered only by physicians familiar with its use and hazards. Therapy should be initiated in a hospital. (See **DOSAGE AND ADMINISTRATION**.)

Information for Patients

Patients should be warned that drowsiness may occur and that they should not drive, operate potentially dangerous machinery, or engage in other activities that may become hazardous because of decreased alertness.

Patients should also be warned of the possibility of hypotension and its symptoms (see **WARNINGS**).

Laboratory Tests

Hypothyroidism may occur in association with Cytadren; hence, appropriate clinical observations should be made and laboratory studies of thyroid function performed as indicated. Supplementary thyroid hormone may be required.

Hematologic abnormalities in patients receiving Cytadren have been reported (see **ADVERSE REACTIONS**). Therefore, baseline hematologic studies should be performed, followed by periodic hematologic evaluation.

Since elevations in SGOT, alkaline phosphatase, and bilirubin have been reported, appropriate clinical observations and regular laboratory studies should be performed before and during therapy.

Serum electrolyte levels should be determined periodically.

Drug Interactions

Cytadren accelerates the metabolism of dexamethasone; therefore, if glucocorticoid replacement is needed, hydrocortisone should be prescribed.

Aminoglutethimide diminishes the effect of coumarin and warfarin.

Carcinogenesis, Mutagenesis, Impairment of Fertility

Long-term carcinogenicity studies in animals and mutagenicity studies have not been performed with Cytadren. Cytadren affects fertility in female rats (see **WARNINGS**). The relevance of these findings to humans is not known.

Pregnancy Category D

See **WARNINGS**.

Nursing Mothers

It is not known whether this drug is excreted in human milk. Because many drugs are excreted in human milk and because of the potential for serious adverse reactions in nursing infants from Cytadren, a decision should be made whether to discontinue nursing or to discontinue the drug, taking into account the importance of the drug to the mother.

Pediatric Use

Safety and effectiveness in children have not been established (see **CLINICAL STUDIES IN CHILDREN**).

ADVERSE REACTIONS

Untoward effects have been reported in about 2 out of 3 patients with Cushing's syndrome who were treated for 4 or more weeks with Cytadren as the only adrenocortical suppressant.

The most frequent and reversible side effects were drowsiness (approximately 1 in 3 patients), morbilliform skin rash (1 in 6 patients), nausea and anorexia (each approximately 1 in 8 patients), and dizziness (about 1 in 20 patients). The dizziness was possibly caused by lowered vascular resistance or orthostasis. These reactions often disappear spontaneously with continued therapy.

Other Effects Observed

Hematologic: Single instances of neutropenia, leukopenia (patient received concomitant o,p'-DDD), pancytopenia (patient received concomitant 5-fluorouracil), and agranulocytosis occurred in 4 of 27 patients with Cushing's syndrome caused by adrenal carcinoma who were treated for at least 4 weeks. In 1 patient with adrenal hyperplasia, hemoglobin levels and hematocrit decreased during the course of treatment with Cytadren. From the earlier experience with the drug used as an anticonvulsant in 1,214 patients, transient leukopenia was the only hematologic effect and was reported once; Coombs'-negative hemolytic anemia also occurred once. In approximately 300 patients with nonadrenal malignancy, 1 in 25 showed some degree of anemia, and 1 in 150 developed pancytopenia during treatment with Cytadren.

Endocrine: Adrenal insufficiency occurred in about 1 in 30 patients with Cushing's syndrome who were treated with Cytadren for 4 or more weeks. This insufficiency tended to involve glucocorticoids as well as mineralocorticoids. Hypothyroidism is occasionally associated with thyroid enlargement and may be detected or confirmed by measuring plasma levels of the thyroid hormone. Masculinization and hirsutism have occasionally occurred in females, as has precocious sexual development in males.

Central Nervous System: Headache was reported in about 1 in 20 patients.

Cardiovascular: Hypotension, occasionally orthostatic, occurred in 1 in 30 patients receiving Cytadren. Tachycardia occurred in 1 in 40 patients.

Gastrointestinal and Liver: Vomiting occurred in 1 in 30 patients. Isolated instances of abnormal findings on liver function tests were reported. Suspected hepatotoxicity occurred in less than 1 in 1000 patients.

Skin: In addition to rash (1 in 6 patients, and often reversible with continued therapy), pruritus was reported in 1 in 20 patients. These may be allergic or hypersensitive reactions. Urticaria has occurred rarely.

Miscellaneous: Fever was reported in several patients who were treated with Cytadren for less than 4 weeks; some of these patients also received other drugs. Myalgia occurred in 1 in 30 patients.

OVERDOSAGE

Acute Toxicity

No deaths due to overdosage with Cytadren have been reported.

The highest known doses that have been survived are 7 g (33-year-old woman) and 7.5–10.0 g (16-year-old girl).

Oral LD$_{50}$'s (mg/kg): rats, 1800; dogs, >100. Intravenous LD$_{50}$'s (mg/kg): rats, 156; dogs > 100.

Signs and Symptoms

An acute overdose with Cytadren may reduce the production of steroids in the adrenal cortex to a degree that is clinically relevant. The following manifestations may be expected:

Respiratory Function: Respiratory depression, hyperventilation.

Cardiovascular System: Hypotension, hypovolemic shock due to dehydration.

Central Nervous System/Muscles: Somnolence, lethargy, coma, ataxia, dizziness, fatigue. (Extreme weakness has been reported with divided doses of 3 g daily.)

Gastrointestinal System: Nausea, vomiting.

Renal Function: Loss of sodium and water.

Laboratory Findings: Hyponatremia, hypochloremia, hyperkalemia, hypoglycemia.

The signs and symptoms of acute overdosage with Cytadren may be aggravated or modified if alcohol, hypnotics, tranquilizers, or tricyclic antidepressants have been taken at the same time.

Treatment

Symptomatic treatment of overdosage is recommended.

Since aminoglutethimide and glutethimide are chemically related, measures that have been used in successfully removing glutethimide from the body might be useful in removing aminoglutethimide.

Gastric lavage and unspecified supportive treatment have been employed. Full consciousness following deep coma was regained 40 hours or less after ingestion of 3 or 4 g without lavage. No evidence of hematologic, renal, or hepatic effects was subsequently found.

Close monitoring should be provided, and appropriate measures taken to support vital functions, if necessary.

If deficiency of circulating glucocorticoid develops, an intravenous infusion of a soluble hydrocortisone preparation (100 mg of hydrocortisone sodium succinate in 500 ml of isotonic sodium chloride solution) and 50 ml of 40% glucose solution should be given within 3 hours. After the initial infusion is completed, an intravenous administration of hydrocortisone, 10 mg per hour, should be continued until the patient is able to take oral cortisone.

If hypovolemia or hypotension occurs, an intravenous administration of norepinephrine, 10 mg, in 500 ml of isotonic sodium chloride should be administered according to the patient's needs and response. After rehydration, 500 ml of plasma or blood should be given for maintenance of sufficient circulatory volume.

Dialysis may be considered in severe intoxication.

DOSAGE AND ADMINISTRATION

Adults

Treatment should be instituted in a hospital until a stable dosage regimen is achieved. Therapy should be initiated with 250 mg orally four times daily, preferably at 6-hour intervals. Adrenocortical response should be followed by careful monitoring of plasma cortisol levels until the desired level of suppression is achieved. If the level of cortisol suppression is inadequate, the dosage may be increased in increments of 250 mg daily at intervals of 1–2 weeks to a total daily dose of 2 g. Dose reduction or temporary discontinuation of therapy may be required in the event of adverse effects, including extreme drowsiness, severe skin rash, or excessively low cortisol levels. If a skin rash persists for longer than 5–8 days or becomes severe, the drug should be discontinued. It may be possible to reinstate therapy at a lower dosage following the disappearance of a mild or moderate rash. Mineralocorticoid replacement (e.g., fludrocortisone) may be necessary. If glucocorticoid replacement therapy is needed, 20–30 mg of hydrocortisone orally in the morning will replace endogenous secretion.

HOW SUPPLIED

Tablets 250 mg — white, round, scored into quarters (imprinted CIBA 24)

Bottles of 100 ....NDC 0083-0024-30

Protect from light.

Dispense in tight, light-resistant container (USP).

CLINICAL STUDIES IN CHILDREN

Clinical investigations included 9 patients aged 2½ to 16 years; 4 of these were aged 10 or less. Seven of the patients received other therapies (drugs or irradiation) either with Cytadren or within a short period before initiation of therapy with Cytadren. Diagnoses included 5 patients with adrenal carcinoma, 3 with adrenal hyperplasia, and 1 with ectopic ACTH-producing tumor. Duration of treatment ranged from 3 days to 6½ months. Dosages ranged from 0.375 g to 1.5 g daily. In general, smaller doses were used for younger patients; for example, a 2½-year-old received 0.5–0.75 g daily, a 3½-year-old received 0.5 g daily, and all others over 10 years of age received 0.75–1.5 g daily. Results are difficult to evaluate because of the concomitant therapy, duration of therapy, or inadequate laboratory documentation. Most patients did show decreases in plasma or urinary steroids at some time during treatment, but these may have been due to other therapeutic modalities or their combinations.

C85-51 (Rev. 11/85)

Shown in Product Identification Section, page 408

Continued on next page

The full prescribing information for each CIBA product is contained herein and is that in effect as of September 1, 1992.

CIBA—Cont.

DESFERAL® ℞
[des'fer-all]
deferoxamine mesylate USP
Vials

DESCRIPTION

Desferal, deferoxamine mesylate USP, is an iron-chelating agent, available in vials for intramuscular, subcutaneous, and intravenous administration. Each vial contains 500 mg of deferoxamine mesylate USP in sterile, lyophilized form. Deferoxamine mesylate is N-[5-[3-[(5-aminopentyl)-hydroxycarbamoyl]propionamido]-pentyl]-3-[[5-(N-hydroxy-acetamido)-pentyl]carbamoyl] propionohydroxamic acid monomethanesulfonate (salt).

Deferoxamine mesylate USP is a white to off-white powder. It is freely soluble in water and slightly soluble in methanol. Its molecular weight is 656.79.

CLINICAL PHARMACOLOGY

Desferal chelates iron by forming a stable complex that prevents the iron from entering into further chemical reactions. It readily chelates iron from ferritin and hemosiderin but not readily from transferrin; it does not combine with the iron from cytochromes and hemoglobin. Desferal does not cause any demonstrable increase in the excretion of electrolytes or trace metals. Theoretically, 100 parts by weight of Desferal is capable of binding approximately 8.5 parts by weight of ferric iron.

Desferal is metabolized principally by plasma enzymes, but the pathways have not yet been defined. The chelate is readily soluble in water and passes easily through the kidney, giving the urine a characteristic reddish color. Some is also excreted in the feces via the bile.

INDICATIONS AND USAGE

Desferal is indicated for the treatment of acute iron intoxication and of chronic iron overload due to transfusion-dependent anemias.

Acute Iron Intoxication

Desferal is an adjunct to, and not a substitute for, standard measures used in treating acute iron intoxication, which may include the following: induction of emesis with syrup of ipecac; gastric lavage; suction and maintenance of a clear airway; control of shock with intravenous fluids, blood, oxygen, and vasopressors; and correction of acidosis.

Chronic Iron Overload

Desferal can promote iron excretion in patients with secondary iron overload from multiple transfusions (as may occur in the treatment of some chronic anemias, including thalassemia. Long-term therapy with Desferal slows accumulation of hepatic iron and retards or eliminates progression of hepatic fibrosis.

Iron mobilization with Desferal is relatively poor in patients under the age of 3 years with relatively little iron overload. The drug should ordinarily not be given to such patients unless significant iron mobilization (e.g., 1 mg or more of iron per day) can be demonstrated.

Desferal is not indicated for the treatment of primary hemochromatosis, since phlebotomy is the method of choice for removing excess iron in this disorder.

CONTRAINDICATIONS

Desferal is contraindicated in patients with severe renal disease or anuria, since the drug and the iron chelate are excreted primarily by the kidney.

WARNINGS

Ocular and auditory disturbances have been reported when Desferal was administered over prolonged periods of time, at high doses, or in patients with low ferritin levels. The ocular disturbances observed have been blurring of vision; cataracts after prolonged administration in chronic iron overload; decreased visual acuity including visual loss; impaired peripheral, color, and night vision; and retinal pigmentary abnormalities. The auditory abnormalities reported have been tinnitus and hearing loss including high frequency sensorineural hearing loss. In most cases, both ocular and auditory disturbances were reversible upon immediate cessation of treatment. Slit-lamp examinations performed in patients treated with Desferal for acute iron intoxication have not revealed cataracts.

Visual acuity tests, slit-lamp examinations, funduscopy and audiometry are recommended periodically in patients treated for prolonged periods of time. Toxicity is more likely to be reversed if symptoms or test abnormalities are detected early.

PRECAUTIONS

General

Flushing of the skin, urticaria, hypotension, and shock have occurred in a few patients when Desferal was administered by rapid intravenous injection. THEREFORE, DESFERAL SHOULD BE GIVEN INTRAMUSCULARLY OR BY SLOW SUBCUTANEOUS OR INTRAVENOUS INFUSION.

Iron overload increases susceptibility of patients to Yersinia enterocolitica infections. In some rare cases, treatment with Desferal has enhanced this susceptibility, resulting in generalized infections by providing this bacteria with a siderophore otherwise missing. In such cases, Desferal treatment should be discontinued until the infection is resolved.

In patients undergoing hemodialysis while receiving Desferal, there have been rare reports of fungal infections (i.e., mucormycosis) that have sometimes been fatal; however, a causal relationship to the drug has not been established.

Information for Patients

Patients should be informed that occasionally their urine may show a reddish discoloration.

Carcinogenesis, Mutagenesis, Impairment of Fertility

Long-term carcinogenicity studies in animals have not been performed with Desferal.

Cytotoxicity may occur, since Desferal has been shown to inhibit DNA synthesis in vitro.

Pregnancy Category C

Delayed ossification in mice and skeletal anomalies in rabbits were observed after Desferal was administered in daily doses up to 4.5 times the maximum daily human dose. No adverse effects were observed in similar studies in rats. There are no adequate and well-controlled studies in pregnant women. Desferal should be used during pregnancy only if the potential benefit justifies the potential risk to the fetus.

Nursing Mothers

It is not known whether this drug is excreted in human milk. Because many drugs are excreted in human milk, caution should be exercised when Desferal is administered to a nursing woman.

Pediatric Use

Safety and effectiveness in children under the age of 3 years have not been established (see INDICATIONS AND USAGE).

ADVERSE REACTIONS

The following adverse reactions have been observed, but there are not enough data to support an estimate of their frequency.

Skin: Localized irritation and pain, swelling and induration, pruritus, erythema, wheal formation.

Hypersensitive Reactions: Generalized erythema (rash), urticaria, anaphylactic reaction.

Cardiovascular: Tachycardia, hypotension, shock.

Digestive: Abdominal discomfort, diarrhea.

Special Senses: Ocular and auditory disturbances (see WARNINGS).

Other: Dysuria, leg cramps, fever.

OVERDOSAGE

Acute Toxicity

Intravenous LD$_{50}$'s (mg/kg): mice, 287; rats, 329.

Signs and Symptoms

Since Desferal is available only for parenteral administration, acute poisoning is unlikely to occur. However, tachycardia, hypotension, and gastrointestinal symptoms have occasionally developed in patients who received overdoses of Desferal.

Treatment

There is no specific antidote.

Signs and symptoms of overdosage may be eliminated by reducing the dosage.

Desferal is readily dialyzable.

DOSAGE AND ADMINISTRATION

Acute Iron Intoxication

Intramuscular Administration

This route is preferred and should be used for ALL PATIENTS NOT IN SHOCK.

Dosage. A dose of 1.0 g should be administered initially. This may be followed by 500 mg (one vial) every 4 hours for two doses. Depending upon the clinical response, subsequent doses of 500 mg may be administered every 4–12 hours. The total amount administered should not exceed 6.0 g in 24 hours.

Preparation of Solution. Desferal is dissolved by adding 2 ml of Sterile Water for Injection to each vial, resulting in a solution of 250 mg/ml. The drug should be completely dissolved before the solution is withdrawn. Desferal is then administered intramuscularly. See *NOTE* below.

Intravenous Administration

THIS ROUTE SHOULD BE USED ONLY FOR PATIENTS IN A STATE OF CARDIOVASCULAR COLLAPSE AND THEN ONLY BY SLOW INFUSION. THE RATE OF INFUSION SHOULD NOT EXCEED 15 MG/KG PER HOUR.

Dosage: An initial dose of 1.0 g should be administered at a rate NOT TO EXCEED 15 mg/kg per hour. This may be followed by 500 mg every 4 hours for two doses. Depending upon the clinical response, subsequent doses of 500 mg may be administered every 4–12 hours. The total amount administered should not exceed 6.0 g in 24 hours.

As soon as the clinical condition of the patient permits, intravenous administration should be discontinued and the drug should be administered intramuscularly.

Preparation of Solution. Desferal is dissolved by adding 2 ml of Sterile Water for Injection to each vial, resulting in a solution of 250 mg/ml. The drug should be completely dissolved before the solution is withdrawn. The solution is then added to physiologic saline, glucose in water, or Ringer's lactate solution and administered at a rate NOT TO EXCEED 15 mg/kg per hour. See *NOTE* below.

Chronic Iron Overload

The more effective of the following routes of administration must be chosen on an individual basis for each patient.

Intramuscular Administration

A daily dose of 0.5–1.0 g should be administered intramuscularly. In addition, 2.0 g should be administered intravenously with each unit of blood transfused; however, Desferal should be administered separately from the blood. The rate of intravenous infusion must not exceed 15 mg/kg per hour.

Subcutaneous Administration

A daily dose of 1.0–2.0 g (20–40 mg/kg per day) should be administered over 8–24 hours, utilizing a small portable pump capable of providing continuous mini-infusion. The duration of infusion must be individualized. In some patients, as much iron will be excreted after a short infusion of 8–12 hours as with the same dose given over 24 hours.

Preparation of Solution for Subcutaneous or Intramuscular Administration. Desferal is dissolved by adding 2.0 ml of Sterile Water for Injection to each vial, resulting in a solution of 250 mg/ml. The drug should be completely dissolved before the solution is withdrawn into the syringe to be used for administration. See *NOTE* below.

NOTE: Parenteral drug products should be inspected visually for particulate matter and discoloration prior to administration, whenever solution and container permit.

Desferal reconstituted with Sterile Water for Injection may be stored under sterile conditions and protected from light at room temperature for not longer than 1 week.

Reconstituting Desferal in solvents or under conditions other than indicated may result in precipitation. Turbid solutions should not be used.

HOW SUPPLIED

Vials —each containing 500 mg of sterile, lyophilized deferoxamine mesylate

Cartons of 4 vials ....NDC 0083-3801-04
C87-30 (Rev. 8/87)

Dist. by:
CIBA Pharmaceutical Company
Division of CIBA-GEIGY Corporation
Summit, New Jersey 07901

ESIDRIX® ℞
[ess'a-dricks]
hydrochlorothiazide USP

DESCRIPTION

Esidrix, hydrochlorothiazide USP, is a diuretic and antihypertensive available as 25-mg, 50-mg, and 100-mg tablets for oral administration. Its chemical name is 6-chloro-3,4-dihydro-2H-1,2,4-benzothiadiazine-7-sulfonamide 1,1-dioxide.

Hydrochlorothiazide USP is a white, or practically white, practically odorless, crystalline powder. It is slightly soluble in water, freely soluble in sodium hydroxide solution, in *n*-butylamine and in dimethylformamide, sparingly soluble in methanol, and insoluble in ether, in chloroform, and in dilute mineral acids. Its molecular weight is 297.73.

Inactive Ingredients: Colloidal silicon dioxide, D&C Yellow No. 10 (50-mg tablets), FD&C Blue No. 1 (100-mg tablets), FD&C Red No. 40 and FD&C Yellow No. 6 (25-mg tablets), lactose, starch, stearic acid, and sucrose.

CLINICAL PHARMACOLOGY

Thiazides affect the renal tubular mechanism of electrolyte reabsorption. At maximal therapeutic dosage all thiazides are approximately equal in their diuretic potency. Thiazides increase excretion of sodium and chloride in approximately equivalent amounts. Natriuresis causes a secondary loss of potassium.

The mechanism of the antihypertensive effect of thiazides is unknown. Thiazides do not affect normal blood pressure. Onset of action of thiazides occurs in 2 hours and the peak effect at about 4 hours. Its action persists for approximately 6 to 12 hours. Thiazides are eliminated rapidly by the kidney.

INDICATIONS AND USAGE

Hypertension

In the management of hypertension either as the sole therapeutic agent or to enhance the effect of other antihypertensive drugs in the more severe forms of hypertension.

Edema

As adjunctive therapy in edema associated with congestive heart failure, hepatic cirrhosis, and corticosteroid and estrogen therapy.

Esidrix has also been found useful in edema due to various forms of renal dysfunction, such as the nephrotic syndrome, acute glomerulonephritis, and chronic renal failure.

Usage in Pregnancy: The routine use of diuretics in an otherwise healthy woman is inappropriate and exposes mother and fetus to unnecessary hazard. Diuretics do not prevent development of toxemia of pregnancy, and there is no satisfactory evidence that they are useful in the treatment of developed toxemia.

Edema during pregnancy may arise from pathological causes or from the physiologic and mechanical consequences of pregnancy. Thiazides are indicated in pregnancy when edema is due to pathologic causes, just as they are in the absence of pregnancy (however, see **PRECAUTIONS, Pregnancy**). Dependent edema in pregnancy, resulting from restriction of venous return by the expanded uterus, is properly treated through elevation of the lower extremities and use of support hose; use of diuretics to lower intravascular volume in this case is illogical and unnecessary. There is hypervolemia during normal pregnancy which is not harmful to either the fetus or the mother (in the absence of cardiovascular disease) but which is associated with edema, including generalized edema, in the majority of pregnant women. If this edema produces discomfort, increased recumbency will often provide relief. In rare instances, this edema may cause extreme discomfort which is not relieved by rest. In these cases, a short course of diuretics may provide relief and may be appropriate.

CONTRAINDICATIONS

Anuria; hypersensitivity to this or other sulfonamide-derived drugs.

WARNINGS

Use with caution in severe renal disease. In patients with renal disease, thiazides may precipitate azotemia. Cumulative effects of the drug may develop in patients with impaired renal function.

Thiazides should be used with caution in patients with impaired hepatic function or progressive liver disease, since minor alterations of fluid and electrolyte imbalance may precipitate hepatic coma.

Thiazides may add to or potentiate the action of other antihypertensive drugs. Potentiation occurs with ganglionic or peripheral adrenergic blocking drugs.

Sensitivity reactions are more likely to occur in patients with a history of allergy or bronchial asthma.

The possibility of exacerbation or activation of systemic lupus erythematosus has been reported.

PRECAUTIONS

General

All patients receiving thiazide therapy should be observed for clinical signs of fluid or electrolyte imbalance: namely, hyponatremia, hypochloremic alkalosis, and hypokalemia (see **Laboratory Tests** and **Drug/Drug Interactions**). Warning signs are dryness of mouth, thirst, weakness, lethargy, drowsiness, restlessness, muscle pains or cramps, muscular fatigue, hypotension, oliguria, tachycardia, and gastrointestinal disturbance such as nausea or vomiting.

Hypokalemia may develop, especially with brisk diuresis or when severe cirrhosis is present.

Interference with adequate oral intake of electrolytes will also contribute to hypokalemia. Hypokalemia may be avoided or treated by use of potassium supplements or foods with a high potassium content.

Any chloride deficit is generally mild and usually does not require specific treatment except under extraordinary circumstances (as in liver disease or renal disease). Dilutional hyponatremia may occur in edematous patients in hot weather; appropriate therapy is water restriction rather than administration of salt, except in rare instances when the hyponatremia is life-threatening. In actual salt depletion, appropriate replacement is the therapy of choice.

Hyperuricemia may occur or frank gout may be precipitated in certain patients receiving thiazide therapy.

Latent diabetes may become manifest during thiazide administration (see **Drug/Drug Interactions**).

The antihypertensive effects of the drug may be enhanced in the postsympathectomy patient.

If progressive renal impairment becomes evident, withholding or discontinuing diuretic therapy should be considered.

Calcium excretion is decreased by thiazides. Pathological changes in the parathyroid gland with hypercalcemia and hypophosphatemia have been observed in a few patients on prolonged thiazide therapy. The common complications of hyperparathyroidism such as renal lithiasis, bone resorption, and peptic ulceration have not been seen.

Information for Patients

Patients should be informed of possible side effects and advised to take the medication regularly and continuously as directed.

Laboratory Tests

Initial and periodic determinations of serum electrolytes to detect possible electrolyte imbalance should be performed at appropriate intervals.

Serum and urine electrolyte determinations are particularly important when the patient is vomiting excessively or receiving parenteral fluids.

Drug/Drug Interactions

Hypokalemia can sensitize or exaggerate the response of the heart to the toxic effects of digitalis (e.g., increased ventricular irritability).

Hypokalemia may develop during concomitant use of steroids or ACTH.

Insulin requirements in diabetic patients may be increased, decreased, or unchanged.

Thiazides may decrease arterial responsiveness to norepinephrine. This diminution is not sufficient to preclude effectiveness of the pressor agent for therapeutic use.

Thiazide drugs may increase the responsiveness to tubocurarine.

Lithium renal clearance is reduced by thiazides, increasing the risk of lithium toxicity.

There have been rare reports in the literature of hemolytic anemia occurring with the concomitant use of hydrochlorothiazide and methyldopa.

Concurrent administration of some nonsteroidal anti-inflammatory agents may reduce the diuretic, natriuretic and antihypertensive effects of thiazide diuretics.

Drug/Laboratory Test Interactions

Thiazides may decrease serum PBI levels without signs of thyroid disturbance.

Thiazides should be discontinued before carrying out tests for parathyroid function (see **PRECAUTIONS, General,** calcium excretion).

Carcinogenesis, Mutagenesis, Impairment of Fertility

Long-term carcinogenicity studies in animals have not been conducted with Esidrix. Hydrochlorothiazide was not mutagenic in in vitro Ames mutagenicity assay of *Salmonella typhimurium* strains TA 98, TA 100, TA 1535, TA 1537, and TA 1538 or in in vivo mutagenicity assays of mouse germinal cell chromosomes and Chinese hamster bone marrow cell chromosomes. It was however, mutagenic in inducing nondisjunction (96% frequency) in diploid strains of *Aspergillus nidulans.*

Hydrochlorothiazide had no adverse effect on fertility of male or female mice or rats in studies in which these species were exposed to doses up to 4 and 100 mg/kg, respectively.

Pregnancy Category B

There are no adequate and well-controlled studies of Esidrix in pregnant women. Esidrix should be used during pregnancy only if clearly needed.

Nonteratogenic Effects. Thiazides cross the placental barrier and appear in cord blood, and there is a risk of fetal or neonatal jaundice, thrombocytopenia, and possibly other adverse reactions that have occurred in adults.

Nursing Mothers

Thiazides are excreted in breast milk. Because of the potential for serious adverse reactions in nursing infants, a decision should be made whether to discontinue nursing or to discontinue Esidrix, taking into account the importance of the drug to the mother.

Pediatric Use

Safety and effectiveness in children have not been established.

ADVERSE REACTIONS

Adverse reactions are usually reversible upon reduction of dosage or discontinuation of Esidrix. Whenever adverse reactions are moderate or severe, it may be necessary to discontinue the drug.

The following adverse reactions have been observed, but there has not been enough systematic collection of data to support an estimate of their frequency. Consequently the reactions are categorized by organ systems and are listed in decreasing order of severity and not frequency.

Digestive: Pancreatitis, jaundice (intrahepatic cholestatic), sialadenitis, vomiting, diarrhea, cramping, nausea, gastric irritation, constipation, anorexia.

Cardiovascular: Orthostatic hypotension (may be potentiated by alcohol, barbiturates, or narcotics).

Neurologic: Vertigo, dizziness, transient blurred vision, headache, paresthesia, xanthopsia, weakness, restlessness.

Musculoskeletal: Muscle spasm.

Hematologic: Aplastic anemia, agranulocytosis, leukopenia, thrombocytopenia.

Metabolic: Hyperglycemia, glycosuria, hyperuricemia.

Hypersensitive Reactions: Necrotizing angiitis, Stevens-Johnson syndrome, respiratory distress including pneumonitis and pulmonary edema, purpura, urticaria, rash, photosensitivity.

OVERDOSAGE

Acute Toxicity

No deaths due to acute poisoning with Esidrix have been reported.

Highest known doses ingested: children, 500 mg (14-year-old girl); young children, 125 mg (2½-year-old child).

Oral LD_{50} in rats: > 2750 mg/kg.

Signs and Symptoms

The most prominent feature of poisoning with Esidrix is acute loss of fluid and electrolytes.

Cardiovascular: Tachycardia, hypotension, shock.

Neuromuscular: Weakness, confusion, dizziness, cramps of the calf muscles, paresthesia, fatigue, impairment of consciousness.

Gastrointestinal: Nausea, vomiting, thirst.

Renal: Polyuria, oliguria or anuria (due to hemoconcentration).

Laboratory findings: Hypokalemia, hyponatremia, hypochloremia, alkalosis, increased BUN (especially in patients with renal insufficiency).

Combined poisoning: Signs and symptoms may be aggravated or modified by concomitant intake of antihypertensive medication, barbiturates, curare, digitalis (hypokalemia), corticosteroids, narcotics, or alcohol.

Treatment

There is no specific antidote.

Elimination of the drug: Induction of vomiting, gastric lavage.

Measures to reduce absorption: Activated charcoal.

Hypotension, shock: The patient's legs should be kept raised, and lost fluid and electrolytes (potassium, sodium) should be replaced.

Surveillance: Fluid and electrolyte balance (especially serum potassium) and renal function should be monitored until conditions become normal.

DOSAGE AND ADMINISTRATION

Therapy should be individualized according to patient response. Dosage should be titrated to gain maximal therapeutic response as well as the minimal dose possible to maintain that therapeutic response.

ADULTS

Hypertension

To Initiate Therapy: Usual dosage is 50–100 mg daily. May be given as a single dose every morning.

Maintenance: After a week dosage may be adjusted downward to as little as 25 mg a day, or upward. Rarely patients may require up to 200 mg daily in divided doses.

Combined Therapy: When necessary, other antihypertensive agents may be added cautiously. Since this drug potentiates the antihypertensive effect of other agents, such additions should be gradual. Dosages of ganglionic blockers in particular should be halved initially.

Edema

To Initiate Diuresis: 25 to 200 mg daily for several days, or until dry weight is attained.

Maintenance: 25 to 100 mg daily or intermittently depending on the patient's response. A few refractory patients may require up to 200 mg daily.

INFANTS AND CHILDREN

The usual pediatric dosage is administered twice daily.

The total daily dosage for infants up to 2 years of age: 12.5 to 37.5 mg; for children 2 to 12 years of age: 37.5 to 100 mg. Dosages should be based on body weight at the rate of 1 mg per pound, but infants below 6 months of age may require 1.5 mg per pound.

HOW SUPPLIED

Tablets 25 mg—round, pink, scored (imprinted CIBA 22)
    Bottles of 100 .... NDC 0083-0022-30
    Bottles of 1000 .... NDC 0083-0022-40
    Consumer Pack—One Unit
       12 bottles—100 tablets each .... NDC 0083-0022-65
    Accu-Pak® Unit Dose (blister pack)
       Box of 100 (strips of 10) .... NDC 0083-0022-32
Tablets 50 mg—round, yellow, scored (imprinted CIBA 46)
    Bottles of 100 .... NDC 0083-0046-30
    Bottles of 1000 .... NDC 0083-0046-40
    Consumer Pack—One Unit
       12 bottles—30 tablets each .... NDC 0083-0046-82
       12 bottles—60 tablets each .... NDC 0083-0046-73
       12 bottles—100 tablets each .... NDC 0083-0046-65
    Accu-Pak® Unit Dose (blister pack)
       Box of 100 (strips of 10) .... NDC 0083-0046-32
Tablets 100 mg—round, blue, scored (imprinted CIBA 192)
    Bottles of 100 .... NDC 0083-0192-30
Dispense in tight, light-resistant container (USP).
Do not store above 86°F (30°C)

C91-25 (Rev. 6/91)

Shown in Product Identification Section, page 408

Continued on next page

The full prescribing information for each CIBA product is contained herein and is that in effect as of September 1, 1992.

CIBA—Cont.

ESIMIL®   ℞
[ess'a-mill]
guanethidine monosulfate USP 10 mg
hydrochlorothiazide USP 25 mg
Combination Tablets

WARNING

This fixed-combination drug is not indicated for initial therapy of hypertension. Hypertension requires therapy titrated to the individual patient. If the fixed combination represents the dosage so determined, its use may be more convenient in patient management. The treatment of hypertension is not static but must be reevaluated as conditions in each patient warrant.

DESCRIPTION
Esimil is an antihypertensive-diuretic combination, available as tablets for oral administration. Each tablet contains Ismelin (guanethidine monosulfate USP), 10 mg, and Esidrix (hydrochlorothiazide USP), 25 mg.

Guanethidine monosulfate is [2-(hexahydro-1(2H)-azocinyl) ethyl]guanidine sulfate 1:1.

Guanethidine monosulfate USP is a white to off-white crystalline powder with a molecular weight of 296.38. It is very soluble in water, sparingly soluble in alcohol and practically insoluble in chloroform.

Hydrochlorothiazide is 6-chloro-3,4-dihydro-2H-1,2,4-benzo-thiadiazine-7-sulfonamide 1,1-dioxide.

Hydrochlorothiazide USP is a white, or practically white, practically odorless crystalline powder. It is slightly soluble in water; freely soluble in sodium hydroxide solution, in n-butylamine, and in dimethylformamide; sparingly soluble in methanol; and insoluble in ether, in chloroform, and in dilute mineral acids. Its molecular weight is 297.73.

Inactive Ingredients: Colloidal silicon dioxide, lactose, starch, stearic acid, and sucrose.

CLINICAL PHARMACOLOGY
Guanethidine
Guanethidine acts at the sympathetic neuroeffector junction by inhibiting or interfering with the release and/or distribution of the chemical mediator (presumably the catecholamine norepinephrine), rather than acting at the effector cell by inhibiting the association of the transmitter with its receptors. In contrast to ganglionic blocking agents, guanethidine suppresses equally the responses mediated by alpha- and beta-adrenergic receptors but does not produce parasympathetic blockade. Since sympathetic blockade results in modest decreases in peripheral resistance and cardiac output, guanethidine lowers blood pressure in the supine position. It further reduces blood pressure by decreasing the degree of vasoconstriction that normally results from reflex sympathetic nervous activity upon assumption of the upright posture, thus reducing venous return and cardiac output more. The inhibition of sympathetic venoconstrictive mechanisms results in venous pooling of blood. Therefore, the effect of guanethidine is especially pronounced when the patient is standing. Both the systolic and diastolic pressures are reduced.

Other actions at the sympathetic nerve terminal include depletion of norepinephrine. Once it gains access to the neuron, guanethidine accumulates within the intraneuronal storage vesicles and causes depletion of norepinephrine stores within the nerve terminal. Prolonged oral administration of guanethidine produces a denervation sensitivity of the neuroeffector junction, probably resulting from the chronic reduction in norepinephrine released by the sympathetic nerve endings. Systemic responses to catecholamines released from the adrenal medulla are not prevented and may even be augmented as a result of this denervation sensitivity. A paradoxical hypertensive crisis may occur if guanethidine is given to patients with pheochromocytoma or if norepinephrine is given to a patient receiving the drug.

Due to its poor lipid solubility, guanethidine does not readily cross the blood-brain barrier. In contrast to most neural blocking agents, guanethidine does not appear to suppress plasma renin activity in many patients.

Pharmacokinetics
The pharmacokinetics of guanethidine are complex. The amount of drug in plasma and in urine is linearly related to dose, although large differences occur between individuals because of variation in absorption and metabolism. Adrenergic blockade occurs with a minimum concentration in plasma of 8 ng/ml; this concentration is achieved in different individuals with doses of 10–50 mg per day at steady state. Guanethidine is eliminated slowly because of extensive tissue binding. After chronic oral administration, the initial phase of elimination with a half-life of 1.5 days is followed by a second phase of elimination with a half-life of 4–8 days. The renal clearance of guanethidine is 56 ml/min. Guanethidine

is converted by the liver to three metabolites, which are excreted in the urine. The metabolites are pharmacologically less active than guanethidine.

Hydrochlorothiazide
Thiazides affect the renal tubular mechanism of electrolyte reabsorption. At maximal therapeutic dosage, all thiazides are approximately equal in their diuretic potency. Thiazides increase excretion of sodium and chloride in approximately equivalent amounts. Natriuresis causes a secondary loss of potassium.

The mechanism of the antihypertensive effect of thiazides is unknown. Thiazides do not affect normal blood pressure.

Pharmacokinetics
The onset of action of thiazides occurs in 2 hours, and the peak effect at about 4 hours. The action persists for approximately 6–12 hours. Hydrochlorothiazide is rapidly absorbed, as indicated by peak plasma concentrations 1–2.5 hours after oral administration. Plasma levels of the drug are proportional to dose; the concentration in whole blood is 1.6–1.8 times higher than in plasma. Thiazides are eliminated rapidly by the kidney. After oral administration of 25- to 100-mg doses of hydrochlorothiazide, 72–97% of the dose is excreted in the urine, indicating dose-independent absorption. Hydrochlorothiazide is eliminated from plasma in a biphasic fashion with a terminal half-life of 10–17 hours. Plasma protein binding is 67.9%. Plasma clearance is 15.9–30.0 L/hr; volume of distribution is 3.6–7.8 L/kg.

Gastrointestinal absorption of hydrochlorothiazide is enhanced when administered with food. Absorption is decreased in patients with congestive heart failure, and the pharmacokinetics are considerably different in these patients.

INDICATIONS AND USAGE
Esimil is indicated for the treatment of hypertension (see boxed **WARNING**).

CONTRAINDICATIONS
Guanethidine
Known or suspected pheochromocytoma; hypersensitivity; frank congestive heart failure not due to hypertension; use of monoamine oxidase (MAO) inhibitors.

Hydrochlorothiazide
Anuria; hypersensitivity to this or other sulfonamide-derived drugs.

WARNINGS
Guanethidine and hydrochlorothiazide are potent drugs, and their use can lead to disturbing and serious clinical problems. Physicians should be familiar with both drugs and their combination before prescribing, and patients should be warned not to deviate from instructions.

Guanethidine

Orthostatic hypotension can occur frequently, and patients should be properly instructed about this potential hazard. Fainting spells may occur unless the patient is forewarned to sit or lie down with the onset of dizziness or weakness. Postural hypotension is most marked in the morning and is accentuated by hot weather, alcohol, or exercise. Dizziness or weakness may be particularly bothersome during the initial period of dosage adjustment and with postural changes, such as arising in the morning. The potential occurrence of these symptoms may require alteration of previous daily activity. The patient should be cautioned to avoid sudden or prolonged standing or exercise while taking the drug.

Inhibition of ejaculation has been reported in animals (see **PRECAUTIONS, Carcinogenesis, Mutagenesis, Impairment of Fertility**) as well as in men given guanethidine. This effect, which results from the sympathetic blockade caused by the drug's action, is reversible after guanethidine has been discontinued for several weeks. The drug does not cause parasympathetic blockade, and erectile potency is usually retained during administration of guanethidine. The possible occurrence of inhibition of ejaculation should be kept in mind when considering the use of guanethidine in men of reproductive age.

If possible, therapy should be withdrawn 2 weeks prior to surgery to reduce the possibility of vascular collapse and cardiac arrest during anesthesia. If emergency surgery is indicated, preanesthetic and anesthetic agents should be administered cautiously in reduced dosage. Oxygen, atropine, vasopressors, and adequate solutions for volume replacement should be ready for immediate use to counteract vascular collapse in the surgical patient. Vasopressors should be used only with extreme caution, since guanethidine augments responsiveness to exogenously administered norepinephrine and vasopressors; specifically, blood pressure may rise and cardiac arrhythmias may be produced.

Hydrochlorothiazide
Thiazides should be used with caution in patients with severe renal disease. In patients with renal disease, thiazides may precipitate azotemia. Cumulative effects of the drug may develop in patients with impaired renal function.

Thiazides should be used with caution in patients with impaired hepatic function or progressive liver disease, since minor alterations of fluid and electrolyte imbalance may precipitate hepatic coma.

Thiazides may add to or potentiate the action of other antihypertensive drugs. Potentiation occurs with ganglionic or peripheral adrenergic blocking drugs.

Sensitivity reactions are more likely to occur in patients with a history of allergy or bronchial asthma.

The possibility of exacerbation of activation of systemic lupus erythematosus has been reported.

PRECAUTIONS
General
Guanethidine. Dosage requirements may be reduced in the presence of fever.

Special care should be exercised when treating patients with a history of bronchial asthma; asthmatic patients are more apt to be hypersensitive to catecholamine depletion, and their condition may be aggravated.

The effects of guanethidine are cumulative over long periods; initial doses should be small and increased gradually in small increments.

Guanethidine should be used very cautiously in hypertensive patients with: renal disease and nitrogen retention or rising BUN levels, since decreased blood pressure may further compromise renal function; coronary insufficiency or recent myocardial infarction; and cerebrovascular disease, especially with encephalopathy.

Guanethidine should not be given to patients with severe cardiac failure except with extreme caution, since guanethidine may interfere with the compensatory role of the adrenergic system in producing circulatory adjustment in patients with congestive heart failure.

Patients with incipient cardiac decompensation should be watched for weight gain or edema.

Guanethidine should be used cautiously in patients with a history of peptic ulcer or other chronic disorders that may be aggravated by a relative increase in parasympathetic tone.

Hydrochlorothiazide. All patients receiving thiazide therapy should be observed for clinical signs of fluid or electrolyte imbalance, namely hyponatremia, hypochloremic alkalosis, and hypokalemia (see **Laboratory Tests** and **Drug/Drug Interactions**). Warning signs are dryness of mouth, thirst, weakness, lethargy, drowsiness, restlessness, muscle pains or cramps, muscular fatigue, hypotension, oliguria, tachycardia, and gastrointestinal disturbance, such as nausea or vomiting.

Hypokalemia may develop, especially in cases of brisk diuresis or severe cirrhosis.

Interference with adequate oral intake of electrolytes will also contribute to hypokalemia. Hypokalemia may be avoided or treated by use of potassium supplements or foods with a high potassium content.

Any chloride deficit is generally mild and usually does not require specific treatment, except under extraordinary circumstances (as in liver disease or renal disease). Dilutional hyponatremia may occur in edematous patients in hot weather; appropriate therapy is water restriction, rather than administration of salt, except in rare instances when the hyponatremia is life-threatening. In cases of actual salt depletion, appropriate replacement is the therapy of choice. Hyperuricemia may occur or frank gout may be precipitated in certain patients receiving thiazide therapy.

Latent diabetes may become manifest during thiazide administration (see **Drug/Drug Interactions**).

The antihypertensive effects of the drug may be enhanced in the postsympathectomy patient.

If progressive renal impairment becomes evident, withholding or discontinuing diuretic therapy should be considered.

Calcium excretion is decreased by thiazides. Pathological changes in the parathyroid gland with hypercalcemia and hypophosphatemia have been observed in a few patients on prolonged thiazide therapy. The common complications of hyperparathyroidism, such as renal lithiasis, bone resorption, and peptic ulceration, have not been seen.

Information for Patients
The patient should be advised to take this medication exactly as directed. If the patient misses a dose, he or she should be told to take only the next scheduled dose (without doubling it).

The patient should be advised to avoid sudden or prolonged standing or exercise and to arise slowly, especially in the morning, to reduce the orthostatic hypotensive effects of dizziness, lightheadedness, or fainting.

The patient should be cautioned about ingesting alcohol, since it aggravates the orthostatic hypotensive effects of guanethidine.

Male patients should be advised that guanethidine may interfere with ejaculation.

Laboratory Tests
Hydrochlorothiazide. Initial and periodic determinations of serum electrolytes to detect possible electrolyte imbalance should be performed at appropriate intervals.

Serum and urine electrolyte determinations are particularly important when the patient is vomiting excessively or receiving parenteral fluids.

Drug/Drug Interactions

Guanethidine. Concurrent use of guanethidine and rauwolfia derivatives may cause excessive postural hypotension, bradycardia, and mental depression.

Both digitalis and guanethidine slow the heart rate.

Amphetamine-like compounds, stimulants (e.g., ephedrine, methylphenidate), tricyclic antidepressants (e.g., amitriptyline, imipramine, desipramine) and other psychopharmacologic agents (e.g., phenothiazines and related compounds), as well as oral contraceptives, may reduce the hypotensive effect of guanethidine.

MAO inhibitors should be discontinued for at least 1 week before starting therapy with guanethidine.

Hydrochlorothiazide. Hypokalemia can sensitize or exaggerate the response of the heart to the toxic effects of digitalis (e.g., increased ventricular irritability).

Hypokalemia may develop during concomitant use of steroids or ACTH.

Insulin requirements in diabetic patients may be increased, decreased, or unchanged.

Thiazides may decrease arterial responsiveness to norepinephrine, but not enough to preclude effectiveness of the pressor agent for therapeutic use.

Thiazides may increase the responsiveness to tubocurarine.

Lithium renal clearance is reduced by thiazides, increasing the risk of lithium toxicity.

There have been rare reports in the literature of hemolytic anemia occurring with the concomitant use of hydrochlorothiazide and methyldopa.

Concurrent administration of some nonsteroidal anti-inflammatory agents may reduce the diuretic, natriuretic and antihypertensive effects of thiazide diuretics.

Drug/Laboratory Test Interactions

Thiazides may decrease serum levels of protein-bound iodine without signs of thyroid disturbance. Esimil should be discontinued before tests for parathyroid function are made (see **General, Hydrochlorothiazide,** Calcium excretion).

Carcinogenesis, Mutagenesis, Impairment of Fertility

Long-term carcinogenicity studies in animals have not been conducted with Esimil.

Guanethidine: While inhibition of sperm passage and accumulation of sperm debris have been reported in rats and rabbits after several weeks of administration of guanethidine, 5 or 10 mg/kg per day, subcutaneously or intraperitoneally, recovery of ejaculatory function and fertility has been demonstrated in rats given guanethidine intramuscularly, 25 mg/kg per day, for 8 weeks. Inhibition of ejaculation has also been reported in men (see **WARNINGS** and **ADVERSE REACTIONS**). This effect, which is attributable to the sympathetic blockade caused by the drug, is reversible several weeks after discontinuance of the drug.

Hydrochlorothiazide: Hydrochlorothiazide was not mutagenic in in vitro Ames Mutagenicity assay of Salmonella typhimurium strains TA 98, TA 100, TA 1535, TA 1537, and TA 1538 or in in vivo mutagenicity assays of mouse germinal cell chromosomes and Chinese hamster bone marrow cell chromosomes. It was however, mutagenic in inducing nondisjunction (96% frequency) in diploid strains of *Aspergillus nidulans.*

Hydrochlorothiazide had no adverse effect on fertility of male or female mice or rats in studies in which these species were exposed to doses up to 4 and 100 mg/kg, respectively.

Pregnancy Category B

A reproduction study performed in rats receiving doses at least 150 times the average daily human dose of Esimil has revealed no evidence of impaired fertility or harm to the fetus due to this drug.

There are no adequate and well-controlled studies of Esimil in pregnant women. Because animal reproduction studies are not always predictive of human response, this drug should be used during pregnancy only if clearly needed.

Nonteratogenic Effects. Thiazides cross the placental barrier and appear in cord blood, and there is a risk of fetal or neonatal jaundice, thrombocytopenia, and possibly other adverse reactions that have occurred in adults.

Nursing Mothers

Guanethidine is excreted in breast milk in very small quantity. Thiazides are also excreted in breast milk. Because of the potential for serious adverse reactions in nursing infants, a decision should be made whether to discontinue nursing or to discontinue Esimil, taking into account the importance of the drug to the mother.

Pediatric Use

Safety and effectiveness of the combination drug in children have not been established.

ADVERSE REACTIONS

Whenever adverse reactions are moderate or severe, it may be necessary to reduce the dosage of Esimil, discontinuing the drug, or administer the individual active components, reducing the dosage of either guanethidine or hydrochlorothiazide.

The following adverse reactions have been observed, but there are not enough data to support an estimate of their frequency. Consequently the reactions are categorized by organ system and are listed in decreasing order of severity and not frequency.

Guanethidine

Digestive: Diarrhea, which may be severe at times and necessitate discontinuance of medication; vomiting; nausea; increased bowel movements; dry mouth; parotid tenderness.

Cardiovascular: Chest pains (angina); bradycardia; a tendency toward fluid retention and edema with occasional development of congestive heart failure.

Respiratory: Dyspnea; asthma in susceptible individuals; nasal congestion.

Neurologic: Syncope resulting from either postural or exertional hypotension; dizziness; blurred vision; muscle tremor; ptosis of the lids; mental depression; chest paresthesias; weakness; lassitude; fatigue.

Muscular: Myalgia.

Genitourinary: Rise in BUN; urinary incontinence; inhibition of ejaculation; nocturia.

Metabolic: Weight gain.

Skin and Appendages: Dermatitis; scalp hair loss.

Although a causal relationship has not been established, a few instances of blood dyscrasias (anemia, thrombocytopenia, and leukopenia) and of priapism or impotence have been reported.

Hydrochlorothiazide

Digestive: Pancreatitis, jaundice (intrahepatic cholestatic), sialadenitis, vomiting, diarrhea, cramping, nausea, gastric irritation, constipation, anorexia.

Cardiovascular: Orthostatic hypotension (may be potentiated by alcohol, barbiturates, or narcotics).

Neurologic: Vertigo, dizziness, transient blurred vision, headache, paresthesia, xanthopsia, weakness, restlessness.

Musculoskeletal: Muscle spasm.

Hematologic: Aplastic anemia, agranulocytosis, leukopenia, thrombocytopenia.

Metabolic: Hyperglycemia, glycosuria, hyperuricemia.

Hypersensitive Reactions: Necrotizing angiitis, Stevens-Johnson syndrome, respiratory distress including pneumonitis and pulmonary edema, purpura, urticaria, rash, photosensitivity.

OVERDOSAGE

Acute Toxicity

No deaths due to acute poisoning with Esimil have been reported.

Oral LD_{50}'s in rats (mg/kg): guanethidine, 1262; hydrochlorothiazide, 2750.

Signs and Symptoms

Guanethidine. Postural hypotension (with dizziness, blurred vision, and possibly syncope when standing), shock, and bradycardia are most likely to occur; diarrhea (possibly severe), nausea, and vomiting may also occur. Unconsciousness is unlikely if adequate blood pressure and cerebral perfusion can be maintained by placing the patient in the supine position and by administering other treatment as required.

Hydrochlorothiazide. The most prominent feature of poisoning is acute loss of fluid and electrolytes.

Cardiovascular: Tachycardia, hypotension, shock.

Neuromuscular: Weakness, confusion, dizziness, cramps of the calf muscles, paresthesia, fatigue, impairment of consciousness.

Digestive: Nausea, vomiting, thirst.

Renal: Polyuria, oliguria, or anuria (due to hemoconcentration).

Laboratory Findings: Hypokalemia, hyponatremia, hypochloremia, alkalosis, increased BUN (especially in patients with renal insufficiency).

Combined Poisoning: Signs and symptoms may be aggravated or modified by concomitant intake of antihypertensive medication, barbiturates, digitalis (hypokalemia), corticosteroids, narcotics, or alcohol.

Treatment

There is no specific antidote.

The stomach contents should be evacuated. An activated charcoal slurry should be instilled and laxatives given, if conditions permit.

If hypotension or shock occurs, the patient's legs should be kept raised, and lost fluid and electrolytes (potassium, sodium) should be replaced. Renal function should be monitored until conditions become normal.

In sinus bradycardia, atropine should be administered.

In previously normotensive patients, treatment has consisted essentially of restoring blood pressure and heart rate to normal by keeping the patient in the supine position. Normal homeostatic control usually returns gradually over a 72-hour period in these patients.

In previously hypertensive patients, particularly those with impaired cardiac reserve or other cardiovascular-renal disease, intensive treatment may be required to support vital functions and to control cardiac irregularities that might be present. The supine position must be maintained; if vasopressors are required, they must be used with extreme caution, since guanethidine may increase responsiveness, causing a rise in blood pressure and development of cardiac arrhythmias.

Diarrhea, if severe or persistent, should be treated with anticholinergic agents to reduce intestinal hypermotility, and hydration and electrolyte balance should be maintained.

Since guanethidine is excreted slowly, cardiovascular and renal function should be monitored for a few days.

DOSAGE AND ADMINISTRATION

Dosage should be determined by individual titration (see boxed **WARNING**).

The usual dosage of Esimil is two tablets daily. Depending upon the degree of hypertension, the patient should be started on the lowest possible dose (usually one tablet daily) and the dose gradually increased at weekly intervals until the desired response is obtained. Blood pressure should be recorded with the patient in the supine position and again after 10 minutes of standing. Dosage should be increased only if standing blood pressure has not been reduced to desired levels. Dosage adjustment should be made at not less than weekly intervals; maximal dosage should not exceed four tablets daily. If additional effect is desirable, guanethidine tablets may be supplemented individually.

Before starting therapy with Esimil, at least 1 week should elapse after MAO inhibitors (see **CONTRAINDICATIONS**) or ganglionic blockers are discontinued.

When Esimil is to be substituted for other antihypertensive agents, the change should be made gradually. In general, dosage of the agent to be discontinued should be halved, and Esimil should be started at one tablet daily. This schedule should be followed for at least 1 week; then, dosage of the previous therapy may be halved again and the dosage of Esimil increased to two tablets daily. At the next weekly interval, the previously used drugs can generally be discontinued. The dosage of Esimil should be titrated at weekly intervals, as mentioned above.

Patients receiving more than 75 mg of guanethidine alone may do well on a smaller dose if also given hydrochlorothiazide. Because of the ratio of the combination, these patients are probably not candidates for Esimil.

HOW SUPPLIED

Tablets —round, white, scored (imprinted CIBA 47)
10 mg of guanethidine monosulfate
25 mg of hydrochlorothiazide
Bottles of 100 ....NDC 0083-0047-30

Do not store above 86°F (30°C).

Dispense in tight container (USP) C92-4 (Rev. 2/92)

Shown in Product Identification Section, page 408

ESTRADERM® ℞

[ess-tra-derm]

estradiol transdermal system

Continuous delivery for twice-weekly application

Prescribing Information

ESTROGENS HAVE BEEN REPORTED TO INCREASE THE RISK OF ENDOMETRIAL CARCINOMA.

Three independent case control studies have reported an increased risk of endometrial cancer in postmenopausal women exposed to exogenous estrogens for more than 1 year. This risk was independent of the other known risk factors for endometrial cancer. These studies are further supported by the finding that incidence rates of endometrial cancer have increased sharply since 1969 in eight different areas of the United States with population-based cancer-reporting systems, an increase which may be related to the rapidly expanding use of estrogens during the last decade.

The three case control studies reported that the risk of endometrial cancer in estrogen users was about 4.5–13.9 times greater than in nonusers. The risk appears to depend both on duration of treatment and on estrogen dose. In view of these findings, when estrogens are used for the treatment of menopausal symptoms, the lowest dose that will control symptoms should be utilized and medication should be discontinued as soon as possible. When prolonged treatment is medically indicated, the patient should be reassessed on at least a semiannual basis to determine the need for continued therapy. Although the evidence must be considered preliminary, one study suggests that cyclic administration of low doses of estrogen may carry less risk than continuous administration; it therefore appears prudent to utilize such a regimen.

Continued on next page

The full prescribing information for each CIBA product is contained herein and is that in effect as of September 1, 1992.

CIBA—Cont.

Close clinical surveillance of all women taking estrogens is important. In all cases of undiagnosed persistent or recurring abnormal vaginal bleeding, adequate diagnostic measures should be undertaken to rule out malignancy.

There is no evidence at present that "natural" estrogens are more or less hazardous than "synthetic" estrogens at equiestrogenic doses.

ESTROGENS SHOULD NOT BE USED DURING PREGNANCY.

The use of female sex hormones, both estrogens and progestogens, during early pregnancy may seriously damage the offspring. It has been shown that women who had been exposed *in utero* to diethylstilbestrol, a nonsteroidal estrogen, have an increased risk of developing in later life a form of vaginal or cervical cancer that is ordinarily extremely rare. This risk has been estimated as not greater than 4 per 1000 exposures. Furthermore, a high percentage of such exposed women (30–90%) have been found to have vaginal adenosis, epithelial changes of the vagina and cervix. Although these changes are histologically benign, it is not known whether they are precursors of malignancy. Although similar data on the use of other estrogens are not available, it cannot be presumed they would not induce similar changes.

Several reports suggest an association between intrauterine exposure to female sex hormones and congenital anomalies, including congenital heart defects and limb-reduction defects. One case control study estimated a 4.7-fold increased risk of limb-reduction defects in infants who had been exposed *in utero* to sex hormones (oral contraceptives, hormone withdrawal tests for pregnancy, or attempted treatment for threatened abortion). Some of these exposures were very short and involved only a few days of treatment. The data suggest that the risk of limb-reduction defects in exposed fetuses is somewhat less than 1 per 1000.

In the past, female sex hormones have been used during pregnancy in an attempt to treat threatened or habitual abortion. There is considerable evidence that estrogens are ineffective for these indications, and there is no evidence from well-controlled studies that progestogens are effective for these uses.

If Estraderm is used during pregnancy, or if the patient becomes pregnant while taking this drug, she should be apprised of the potential risks to the fetus and of the advisability of continuation of the pregnancy.

DESCRIPTION

Estraderm, estradiol transdermal system, is designed to release 17β-estradiol through a rate-limiting membrane continuously upon application to intact skin.

Two systems are available to provide nominal *in vivo* delivery of 0.05 or 0.1 mg of estradiol per day via skin of average permeability (interindividual variation in skin permeability is approximately 20%). Each corresponding system having a contact surface area of 10 or 20 cm² contains 4 or 8 mg of estradiol USP and 0.3 or 0.6 ml of alcohol USP, respectively. The composition of the systems per unit area is identical. Estradiol USP (17β-estradiol) is a white, crystalline powder, chemically described as estra-1,3,5(10)-triene-3, 17β-diol. The Estraderm system comprises four layers. Proceeding from the visible surface toward the surface attached to the skin, these layers are (1) a transparent polyester film, (2) a drug reservoir of estradiol USP and alcohol USP gelled with hydroxypropyl cellulose, and (3) an ethylene-vinyl acetate copolymer membrane, and (4) an adhesive formulation of light mineral oil and polyisobutylene. A protective liner (5) of siliconized polyethylene terephthalate film is attached to the adhesive surface and must be removed before the system can be used.

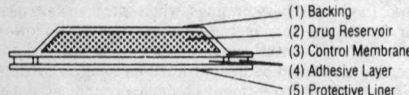

(1) Backing
(2) Drug Reservoir
(3) Control Membrane
(4) Adhesive Layer
(5) Protective Liner

The active component of the system is estradiol. The remaining components of the system are pharmacologically inactive. Alcohol is also released from the system during use.

CLINICAL PHARMACOLOGY

The Estraderm system releases estradiol, the major estrogenic hormone secreted by the human ovary. Estraderm provides systemic estrogen replacement therapy. Among numerous effects, estradiol is largely responsible for the development and maintenance of the female reproductive system and of secondary sexual characteristics. It promotes growth and development of the vagina, uterus, fallopian tubes, and breasts. Indirectly, estradiol contributes to the shaping of the skeleton, to the maintenance of tone and elasticity of urogenital structures, to changes in the epiphyses of the long bones that allow for the pubertal growth spurt and its termination, to the growth of axillary and pubic hair, and to the pigmentation of the nipples and genitals.

In the anovulatory cycle estrogen is the primary determinant in the onset of menstruation. Estradiol also affects the release of pituitary gonadotropins.

Loss of ovarian estradiol secretion after menopause can result in instability of thermoregulation, causing hot flushes associated with sleep disturbance and excessive sweating, and urogenital atrophy, causing dyspareunia and urinary incontinence. Estradiol replacement therapy alleviates many of these symptoms of estradiol deficiency in the menopausal woman.

Orally administered estradiol is rapidly metabolized by the liver to estrone and its conjugates, giving rise to higher circulating levels of estrone than estradiol. In contrast, the skin metabolizes estradiol only to a small extent. Therefore, transdermal administration produces therapeutic serum levels of estradiol with lower circulating levels of estrone and estrone conjugates, and requires smaller total doses than does oral therapy. Because estradiol has a short half-life (~1 hour), transdermal administration of estradiol allows a rapid decline in blood levels after an Estraderm system is removed, e.g., in a cycling regimen.

In a study using transdermally administered estradiol, 0.1 mg daily, plasma levels increased by 66 pg/ml resulting in an average plasma level of 73 pg/ml. There were no significant increases in the concentration of renin substrate or other hepatic proteins (sex-hormone-binding globulin, thyroxine-binding globulin and corticosteroid-binding globulin).

Pharmacokinetics

Administration of Estraderm produces mean serum concentrations of estradiol comparable to those produced by a daily oral administration of estradiol at about 20 times the daily transdermal dose. In single-application studies in 14 postmenopausal women using Estraderm systems that provided 0.05 and 0.1 mg of exogenous estradiol per day, these systems produced increased blood levels within 4 hours and maintained respective mean serum estradiol concentrations of 32 and 67 pg/ml above baseline over the application period. At the same time, increases in estrone serum concentration averaged only 9 and 27 pg/ml above baseline, respectively. Serum concentrations of estradiol and estrone returned to preapplication levels within 24 hours after removal of the system. The estimated daily urinary output of estradiol conjugates increased 5 to 10 times the baseline values and returned to near baseline within 2 days after removal of the system.

By comparison, estradiol (2 mg per day) administered orally to postmenopausal women resulted in increases in mean serum concentration of 59 pg/ml of estradiol and 302 pg/ml of estrone above baseline on the third consecutive day of dosing. Urinary output of estradiol conjugates after oral administration increased to about 100 times the baseline values and did not approach baseline until 7–8 days after the last dose.

In a 3-week multiple-application study of 14 postmenopausal women in which Estraderm 0.05 was applied twice weekly, the mean increments in steady-state serum concentration were 30 pg/ml for estradiol and 12 pg/ml for estrone. Urinary output of estradiol conjugates returned to baseline within 3 days after removal of the last (6th) system, indicating little or no estrogen accumulation in the body.

INDICATIONS AND USAGE

Estraderm is indicated for the treatment of the following: moderate-to-severe vasomotor symptoms associated with menopause; female hypogonadism; female castration; primary ovarian failure; and atrophic conditions caused by deficient endogenous estrogen production, such as atrophic vaginitis and kraurosis vulvae; and prevention of osteoporosis (loss of bone mass).

Estrogen replacement therapy is the most effective single modality for the prevention of postmenopausal osteoporosis in women. Case-controlled studies have shown a reduction of approximately 60% in the incidence of hip and wrist fractures in women who began estrogen replacement therapy within a few years of menopause. A recent, well-controlled, double-blind, prospective trial conducted at the Mayo Clinic has demonstrated that treatment with Estraderm prevents bone loss in postmenopausal women at dosage of 0.05 mg per day.

Treatment with Estraderm 0.05 mg showed full maintenance of bone density with a slight (0.8%), but not significant, increase. Placebo treatment resulted in a significant loss of more than 6% below baseline vertebral bone mass. Patients using either Estraderm 0.1 mg, or 0.05 mg, had significantly greater bone densities than those using placebo. Other studies suggest that estrogen replacement therapy reduces the rate of vertebral fractures.

Peak bone mass is reached at age 30 to 35 and can best be maximized by adequate calcium intake and exercise during the adolescent and early adult years. Early menopause is one of the best predictors for the development of osteoporosis. White women are at a higher risk for osteoporosis than white men, black women are at higher risk than black men, and thin women are at higher risk than obese women. Cigarette smoking may be an additional risk factor. Calcium deficiency has been implicated in the pathogenesis of this disease. Therefore, when not contraindicated, a calcium intake of 1000–1500 mg/day either by diet or supplements is recommended for postmenopausal women.

Immobilization and prolonged bedrest produce rapid bone loss, while weight-bearing exercise has been shown to both reduce bone loss and to increase bone mass. The optimal type and amount of physical activity that might lower the risk for osteoporosis have not been established.

CONTRAINDICATIONS

Estrogens should not be used in women or men with any of the following conditions:
1. known or suspected cancer of the breast;
2. known or suspected estrogen-dependent neoplasia;
3. known or suspected pregnancy (see Boxed Warning);
4. undiagnosed abnormal genital bleeding;
5. active thrombophlebitis or thromboembolic disorders;
6. history of thrombophlebitis, thrombosis, or thromboembolic disorders associated with previous estrogen use.

WARNINGS

1. *Induction of Malignant Neoplasms.* Long-term continuous administration of natural and synthetic estrogens in certain animal species increases the frequency of carcinomas of the breast, cervix, vagina, and liver. There are now reports that estrogens increase the risk of carcinoma of the endometrium in humans. (See Boxed Warning.)

At the present time, there is no satisfactory evidence that estrogens given to postmenopausal women increase the risk of breast cancer, although a recent long-term followup study has raised this possibility. Because of the animal data, there is a need for caution in prescribing estrogens for women with a strong family history of breast cancer or who have breast nodules, fibrocystic disease, or abnormal mammograms.

2. *Gallbladder Disease.* A recent study has reported a two- to threefold increase in the risk of surgically confirmed gallbladder disease in postmenopausal women receiving oral estrogens, similar to the twofold increase previously noted in users of oral contraceptives.

3. *Effects Similar to Those Caused by Estrogen-Progestogen Oral Contraceptives.* There are several serious adverse effects of oral contraceptives and other high-dose oral estrogen treatments, most of which have not, up to now, been documented as consequences of postmenopausal estrogen replacement therapy. This may reflect the comparatively low doses of estrogen used in postmenopausal women.

a. *Thromboembolic Disease.* It is now well established that users of oral contraceptives have an increased risk of various thromboembolic and thrombotic vascular diseases, such as thrombophlebitis, pulmonary embolism, stroke, and myocardial infarction. Cases of retinal thrombosis, mesenteric thrombosis, and optic neuritis have been reported in oral contraceptive users. There is evidence that the risk of several of these adverse reactions is related to the dose of the drug. An increased risk of postsurgery thromboembolic complications has also been reported in users of oral contraceptives. If feasible, estrogen should be discontinued at least 4 weeks before surgery of the type associated with an increased risk of thromboembolism, or during periods of prolonged immobilization.

While an increased rate of thromboembolic and thrombotic disease in postmenopausal users of estrogens has not been found, this does not rule out the possibility that such an increase may be present or that subgroups of women who have underlying risk factors or who are receiving relatively large doses of estrogens may have increased risk. Therefore, estrogens should not be used in persons with active thrombophlebitis or thromboembolic disorders, and they should not be used in persons with a history of such disorders in association with estrogen use. They should be used with caution in patients with cerebral vascular or coronary artery disease and only for those in whom estrogens are clearly needed.

Large doses of estrogen (5 mg conjugated estrogens per day), comparable to those used to treat cancer of the prostate and breast, have been shown in a large prospective clinical trial in men to increase the risk of nonfatal myocardial infarction, pulmonary embolism, and thrombophlebitis. When estrogen doses of this size are used, any of the thromboembolic and thrombotic adverse effects associated with oral contraceptive use should be considered a clear risk.

b. *Hepatic Adenoma.* Benign hepatic adenomas have been associated with the use of oral contraceptives. Although benign and rare, these tumors may rupture and cause death from intra-abdominal hemorrhage. Such lesions have not yet been reported in association with other estrogen or progestogen preparations, but they should be considered if abdominal pain and tenderness, abdominal

mass, or hypovolemic shock occurs in patients receiving estrogen. Hepatocellular carcinoma has also been reported in women taking estrogen-containing oral contraceptives. The causal relationship of this malignancy to these drugs is not known.

c. *Elevated Blood Pressure.* Women using oral contraceptives sometimes experience increased blood pressure which, in most cases, returns to normal upon discontinuing the drug. There is now a report that this may occur with use of oral estrogens in the menopause and blood pressure should be monitored with estrogen use, especially if high doses are used. Ethinyl estradiol and conjugated estrogens have been shown to increase renin substrate. In contrast to these oral estrogens, transdermally administered estradiol does not affect renin substrate.

d. *Glucose Tolerance.* A worsening of glucose tolerance has been observed in a significant percentage of patients on estrogen-containing oral contraceptives. For this reason, diabetic patients should be carefully observed while receiving estrogen.

4. *Hypercalcemia.* Administration of high doses of estrogens may lead to severe hypercalcemia in patients with breast cancer and bone metastases. If hypercalcemia occurs, use of the drug should be stopped and appropriate measures should be taken to reduce the serum calcium level.

PRECAUTIONS

General

1. A complete medical and family history should be taken before initiation of any estrogen therapy. The pretreatment and periodic physical examinations should include special reference to blood pressure, breasts, abdomen, and pelvic organs, as well as a cervical Papanicolaou test. As a general rule, estrogen should not be prescribed for longer than 1 year without another physical examination being performed.
2. Because estrogens may cause some degree of fluid retention, careful observation is required when conditions that might be influenced by this factor are present (e.g., asthma, epilepsy, migraine, and cardiac or renal dysfunction).
3. Certain patients may develop undesirable manifestations of excessive estrogenic stimulation, such as uterine bleeding, mastodynia, etc.
4. Prolonged administration of unopposed estrogen therapy has been reported to increase the risk of endometrial hyperplasia in some patients. Estrogens should be used with caution in patients who have or have had endometriosis.
5. Studies of the addition of a progestin for 7 or more days of a cycle of estrogen administration have reported a lowered incidence of endometrial hyperplasia. Morphological and biochemical studies of endometrium suggest that 12 to 13 days of progestin are needed to provide maximal maturation of the endometrium and to eliminate any hyperplastic changes. Whether this will provide protection from endometrial carcinoma has not been clearly established. There are possible additional risks that may be associated with the inclusion of progestin in estrogen replacement regimens. The potential risks include adverse effects on carbohydrate and lipid metabolism. The choice of progestin and dosage may be important in minimizing these adverse effects.
6. Oral contraceptives appear to be associated with an increased incidence of mental depression. Although it is not clear whether this is due to the estrogenic or progestogenic component of the contraceptive, patients with a history of depression should be carefully observed.
7. Preexisting uterine leiomyomata may increase in size during prolonged estrogen use. If this occurs, estrogen therapy should be discontinued while the cause is investigated.
8. In patients with a history of jaundice during pregnancy, there is an increased risk that jaundice will recur with the use of estrogen-containing oral contraceptives. If jaundice develops in any patient receiving estrogen, the medication should be discontinued while the cause is investigated.
9. Estrogens may be poorly metabolized in patients with impaired liver function and should be administered with caution in such patients.
10. Because the prolonged use of estrogens influences the metabolism of calcium and phosphorus, estrogens should be used with caution in patients with metabolic bone diseases associated with hypercalcemia and in patients with renal insufficiency.

Information for Patients

See Patient Package Insert printed below.

Drug/Laboratory Test Interactions

The results of certain endocrine and liver function tests may be affected by estrogen-containing oral contraceptives. The following changes have been observed with large doses of oral estrogen:

1. increased sulfobromophthalein retention;
2. increased prothrombin time; increased factors VII, VIII, IX, and X; decreased antithrombin 3; increased norepinephrine-induced platelet aggregability;
3. increased thyroxine-binding globulin (TBG), leading to increased circulating total thyroid hormone (T_4) as measured by column or radioimmunoassay; free T_3 resin uptake is decreased, reflecting the elevated TBG; free T_4 concentration is unaltered; TBG was not affected in clinical trials of Estraderm;
4. reduced response to the metyrapone test;
5. reduced serum folate concentration;
6. increased serum triglyceride and phospholipid concentration, and decreased pregnanediol excretion.

The pathologist should be informed that the patient is receiving estrogen therapy when relevant specimens are submitted.

Carcinogenesis, Mutagenesis, Impairment of Fertility

See WARNINGS and Boxed Warning.

Long-term continuous administration of natural and synthetic estrogens in certain animal species increases the frequency of carcinomas of the breast, cervix, vagina, and liver.

Pregnancy Category X

See CONTRAINDICATIONS and Boxed Warning.

Estrogens should not be used during pregnancy.

Nursing Mothers

As a general principle, the administration of any drug to nursing mothers should be done only when clearly necessary since many drugs are excreted in human milk.

ADVERSE REACTIONS

See WARNINGS and Boxed Warning regarding potential adverse effects on the fetus, induction of malignant neoplasms, increased incidence of gallbladder disease, and adverse effects similar to those of oral contraceptives, including thromboembolism.

The most commonly reported adverse reaction to Estraderm in clinical trials was redness and irritation at the application site. This occurred in about 17% of the women treated and caused approximately 2% to discontinue therapy. Reports of rash have been rare.

The following additional adverse reactions have been reported with estrogenic therapy, including oral contraceptives:

Genitourinary System: Breakthrough bleeding, spotting, change in menstrual flow; increase in size of uterine fibromyomata; change in cervical erosion and amount of cervical secretion.

Endocrine: Breast tenderness, breast enlargement.

Gastrointestinal: Nausea, vomiting; abdominal cramps, bloating; cholestatic jaundice have been observed with oral estrogen therapy.

Eyes: Steepening of corneal curvature; intolerance to contact lenses.

Central Nervous System: Headache, migraine, dizziness.

Miscellaneous: Change in weight, edema, change in libido.

OVERDOSAGE

Numerous reports of ingestion of large doses of estrogen-containing oral contraceptives by young children indicate that acute serious ill effects do not occur. Overdosage with estrogen may cause nausea, and withdrawal bleeding may occur in females.

DOSAGE AND ADMINISTRATION

The adhesive side of the Estraderm system should be placed on a clean, dry area of the skin on the trunk of the body (including the buttocks and abdomen.) *Estraderm should not be applied to the breasts.* The sites of application must be rotated, with an interval of at least 1 week allowed between applications to a particular site. The area selected should not be oily, damaged, or irritated. The waistline should be avoided, since tight clothing may rub the system off. The system should be applied immediately after opening the pouch and removing the protective liner. The system should be pressed firmly in place with the palm of the hand for about 10 seconds, making sure there is good contact, especially around the edges. In the unlikely event that a system should fall off, the same system may be reapplied. If necessary, a new system may be applied. In either case, the original treatment schedule should be continued.

Initiation of Therapy

Treatment of menopausal symptoms is usually initiated with Estraderm 0.05 mg applied to the skin twice weekly. The dosage should be adjusted as necessary to control symptoms. The lowest dosage necessary for the control of symptoms should be used, especially in women with an intact uterus. Attempts to taper or discontinue the medication should be made at 3-to 6-month intervals.

Prophylactic therapy with Estraderm to prevent postmenopausal bone loss should be initiated with the 0.05 mg/day dosage as soon as possible after menopause. The dosage may be adjusted if necessary to control concurrent menopausal symptoms. Discontinuation of estrogen replacement therapy may reestablish the natural rate of bone loss.

In women not currently taking oral estrogens, treatment with Estraderm can be initiated at once. In women who are currently taking oral estrogen, treatment with Estraderm can be initiated 1 week after withdrawal of oral hormone replacement therapy, or sooner if menopausal symptoms reappear in less than 1 week.

Therapeutic Regimen

Estraderm therapy may be given continuously in patients who do not have an intact uterus. In those patients with an intact uterus, Estraderm may be given on a cyclic schedule (e.g., 3 weeks on drug followed by 1 week off drug).

HOW SUPPLIED

Estraderm 0.05 (estradiol transdermal system)—each 10 cm^2 system contains 4 mg of estradiol USP for nominal* delivery of 0.05 mg of estradiol per day

Patient Calendar Pack
of 8 Systems ....NDC 0083-2310-08
Carton of 6 Patient Calendar Packs
of 8 Systems ....NDC 0083-2310-62
Carton of 1 Patient Calendar Pack
of 24 Systems ....NDC 0083-2310-24

Estraderm 0.1 (estradiol transdermal system—each 20 cm^2 system contains 8 mg of estradiol USP for nominal* delivery of 0.1 mg of estradiol per day

Patient Calendar Pack
of 8 Systems ....NDC 0083-2320-08
Carton of 6 Patient Calendar Packs
of 8 Systems ....NDC 0083-2320-62
Carton of 1 Patient Calendar Pack
of 24 Systems ....NDC 0083-2320-24

*See DESCRIPTION.

Do not store above 86°F (30°C).

Do not store unpouched. Apply immediately upon removal from the protective pouch.

C91-37/C91-38 (Rev. 9/91)

Information for the Patient

ESTRADERM®

Generic name: estradiol transdermal system
pronounced ess-tra-DYE-all

INTRODUCTION

Your doctor has prescribed Estraderm for the treatment of your menopausal symptoms, and/or to prevent osteoporosis, which is a thinning of your bones. During menopause, production of estrogen hormones by your body decreases well below the amounts normally produced during your fertile years. In many women this decrease in estrogen production causes uncomfortable symptoms, most noticeably hot flushes and sleep disturbance. Estrogens can be given to reduce or eliminate these symptoms.

The Estraderm system that your doctor has prescribed for you releases small amounts of estradiol through the skin in a continuous way. Estradiol is the same hormone that your ovaries produce abundantly before menopause. The dose of estradiol you require will depend upon your individual response. The dose is adjusted by the size of the Estraderm system used; the systems are available in two sizes.

This leaflet will provide you with general information about estrogens and with specific information about the Estraderm system. Please read it carefully. If you want to know more, you should ask your doctor for more information.

INFORMATION ABOUT ESTRADERM

How Estraderm Works

Estraderm contains estradiol. When applied to the skin as directed below, the Estraderm system releases estradiol, which flows through the skin into the bloodstream.

How and Where to Apply Estraderm

Each Estraderm system is individually sealed in a protective pouch. Tear open this pouch at the indentation (do not use scissors) and remove the system. Bubbles in the system are normal.

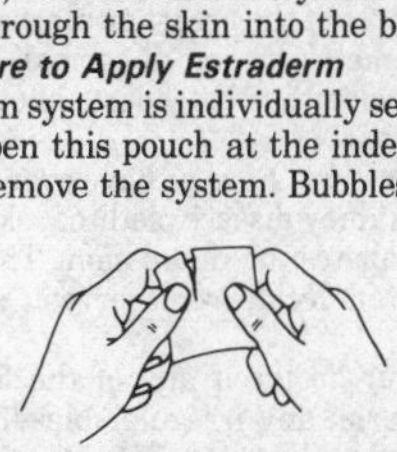

A stiff protective liner covers the adhesive side of the system—the side that will be placed against your skin. This liner must be removed before applying the system. Slide the protective liner sideways between your thumb and index finger. Then hold the system at one edge. Remove the protective liner and discard it. Try to avoid touching the adhesive.

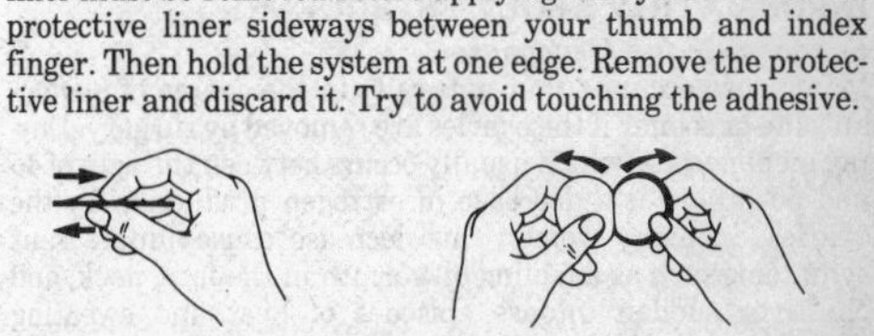

Continued on next page

The full prescribing information for each CIBA product is contained herein and is that in effect as of September 1, 1992.

CIBA—Cont.

Apply the adhesive side of the system to a clean, dry area of the skin on the trunk of your body, (including the buttocks and abdomen). Some women may find that is more comfortable to wear Estraderm on the buttocks. *Do not apply Estraderm to your breasts.* The sites of application must be rotated, with an interval of at least 1 week allowed between applications to a particular site. The area selected should not be oily, damaged, or irritated. Avoid the waistline, since tight clothing may rub the system off. Apply the system immediately after opening the pouch and removing the protective liner. Press the system firmly in place with the palm of your hand for about 10 seconds, making sure there is good contact, especially around the edges.

The Estraderm system should be worn continuously until it is time to replace it with a new system. You may wish to experiment with different locations when applying a new system, to find ones that are most comfortable for you and where clothing will not rub on the system.

When to Apply Estraderm

The Estraderm system should be changed twice weekly. Your Estraderm package contains a calendar check list on the back to help you remember a schedule. Mark the two-day schedule you plan to follow. Always change the system on the two days of the week you have marked.

When changing the system, remove the used Estraderm and discard it. Any adhesive that might remain on your skin can be easily rubbed off. Then place the new Estraderm on a different skin site. (The same skin site should not be used again for at least 1 week after removal of the system.)

Please note: Contact with water when you are bathing, swimming, or showering will not affect the system. In the unlikely event that a system should fall off, put this same system back on and continue to follow your original treatment schedule. If necessary, you may apply a new system but continue to follow your original schedule.

Benefits of Treatment With Estraderm

Regular use of Estraderm twice weekly offers relief of the symptoms of menopause and has been shown to help prevent osteoporosis, which is a thinning of the bones that makes them more fragile. In the years following the menopause, unless estrogen therapy is taken regularly, your bones can rapidly lose strength, possibly leading to osteoporosis and bone fractures. Estraderm may prevent this bone loss and the development of osteoporosis, and may help you to avoid fractures of your spine ("dowager's hump"), wrist, and hip later in life.

Small quantities of the naturally occurring hormone estradiol are absorbed through the skin from the Estraderm system, ensuring a continuous supply of circulating hormone in the body.

When estradiol is administered through your skin, the drug does not undergo the rapid chemical changes in the liver and stomach that would occur if you were taking it by mouth. There is no medical evidence that the use of any estrogen during menopause will keep you feeling young, keep your skin soft, or relieve nervousness.

PRECAUTIONS

The use of estrogens has benefits, but it has risks as well. Before using Estraderm, be sure to tell your doctor if you are pregnant. **ESTROGENS SHOULD NOT BE USED DURING PREGNANCY.** Also tell your doctor if you have ever had any of the following: cancer of the breast or uterus, unusual vaginal bleeding, endometriosis, or abnormal blood clotting. Your doctor may decide that Estraderm should not be used under these conditions.

Also tell your doctor if you have or have ever had high blood pressure, heart or kidney disease, asthma, skin allergy, epilepsy, migraine, diabetes, or depression. This information will help your doctor decide whether you should use Estraderm.

You should tell your doctor if any of the following occur while using Estraderm; any irregular bleeding; breast tenderness, enlargement, or lumps; pain or heaviness in the legs or chest; severe headache, dizziness, or changes in vision; or skin irritation, redness, or rash.

INFORMATION ABOUT ESTROGENS

Estrogens in the Menopause

Menopause occurs either naturally in the course of a woman's life or sooner if the ovaries are removed by surgery. During menopause—which usually occurs between the ages of 45 and 55—there is a decrease in estrogen production by the ovaries. In many women this decrease causes unpleasant symptoms such as a feeling of warmth in the face, neck, and chest, or sudden intense episodes of heat and sweating throughout the body (called "hot flashes" or "hot flushes"). Some women may also develop other changes: impaired bladder control and alterations in the vagina (such as dryness) that cause discomfort during and after intercourse.

Estrogens can be prescribed to treat menopausal symptoms. Some women have no symptoms or only mild ones and do not need estrogens; others may need estrogens for a few months;

and others will need treatment for longer periods. Usually treatment is cyclical and includes days when no estrogen is given. Other drugs called progestins, are sometimes given to offset the effects of estrogens on the lining of the uterus. You may wish to discuss the risks and benefits of such treatment with your doctor.

Estrogens in Osteoporosis

After age 40, and especially after menopause, some women develop osteoporosis. This is a thinning of the bones that makes them weaker and more likely to break, and often leads to fractures of spine, hip and wrist bones. Taking estrogens after the menopause slows down bone loss and may prevent bones from breaking. Eating foods that are high in calcium (such as milk products) or taking calcium supplements (1000–1500 milligrams per day), and certain types of exercise, may also help prevent osteoporosis.

Since estrogen use is associated with some risk, its use in the prevention of osteoporosis should be confined to women who appear to be susceptible to this condition. The following characteristics are often present in women who are likely to develop postmenopausal osteoporosis: underweight, sedentary, nicotine and alcohol abusers, Caucasian and Oriental women, surgical and spontaneous menopause at a young age. If you will be taking calcium supplements as part of the treatment to help prevent osteoporosis, check with your doctor about the amounts recommended.

Possible Risks and Discomforts From Treatment With Estrogens

The risk of endometrial cancer (cancer of the lining of the uterus) is greater in estrogen users than in nonusers. (If you have had your uterus removed by a total hysterectomy, this would not be a risk for you.) Recent studies have shown that this increased risk depends on estrogen dose, duration of treatment, and treatment regimen.

Despite numerous studies, there has been no definite link established between estrogen use and breast cancer. Nevertheless, women with a family history of breast cancer, or with breast nodules, fibrocystic breast disease (lumps), or abnormal mammograms should consult with their doctor before taking estrogens.

In certain animals treated with estrogen, cancer of the cervix, vagina, and liver occurred more frequently.

The following effects have also been reported in women taking estrogens: nausea (the most common side effect), retention of fluid, gallbladder disease, abnormal blood clotting, migraine, elevated serum calcium, growth of benign fibroid tumors in the uterus, jaundice, darkening of the skin, defects in the fetus, and liver tumors. Redness, irritation, or rash may occur at the site of Estraderm application.

Breast tenderness and excessive vaginal secretions may occur when the dose of estrogen administered is too high.

Based on a review of your medical needs, your doctor has prescribed Estraderm for you. Use it only as directed and do not give it to anyone else. Your doctor should reexamine you at least annually.

Do not store above 86°F (30°C).

Do not store unpouched. Apply immediately upon removal from the protective pouch.

C91-38 (Rev. 9/91)
C91-37/C91-38 (Rev. 9/91)

CIBA
CIBA Pharmaceutical Company
Division of CIBA-GEIGY Corporation
Summit, New Jersey 07901

Shown in Product Identification Section, page 408

INH™ isoniazid USP   ℞
Tablets

WARNING

Severe and sometimes fatal hepatitis associated with isoniazid therapy may occur and may develop even after many months of treatment. The risk of developing hepatitis is age related. Approximate case rates by age are: 0 per 1,000 for persons under 20 years of age, 3 per 1,000 for persons in the 20–34 year age group, 12 per 1,000 for persons in the 35–49 year age group, 23 per 1,000 for persons in the 50–64 year age group, and 8 per 1,000 for persons over 65 years of age. The risk of hepatitis is increased with daily consumption of alcohol. Precise data to provide a fatality rate for isoniazid-related hepatitis is not available; however, in a U.S. Public Health Service Surveillance Study of 13,838 persons taking isoniazid, there were 8 deaths among 174 cases of hepatitis. Therefore, patients given isoniazid should be carefully monitored and interviewed at monthly intervals. Serum transaminase concentration becomes elevated in about 10–20 percent of patients, usually during the first few months of therapy but it can occur at any time. Usually enzyme levels return to normal despite continuance of drug but in some cases progressive liver dysfunction occurs. Patients should be instructed to report immedi-

ately any of the prodromal symptoms of hepatitis, such as fatigue, weakness, malaise, anorexia, nausea, or vomiting. If these symptoms appear or if signs suggestive of hepatic damage are detected, isoniazid should be discontinued promptly, since continued use of the drug in these cases has been reported to cause a more severe form of liver damage.

Patients with tuberculosis should be given appropriate treatment with alternative drugs. If isoniazid must be reinstituted, it should be reinstituted only after symptoms and laboratory abnormalities have cleared. The drug should be restarted in very small and gradually increasing doses and should be withdrawn immediately if there is any indication of recurrent liver involvement. Preventive treatment should be deferred in persons with acute hepatic diseases.

DESCRIPTION

INH, isoniazid USP, is an antibiotic available as 300-mg tablets for oral administration. It is available in Dual Packs of Rimactane® rifampin USP/INH containing one 300-mg tablet of INH and two 300-mg capsules of Rimactane. Isoniazid is isonicotinic acid hydrazide.

Isoniazid USP is colorless or white crystals or white crystalline powder. It is odorless and slowly affected by exposure to air and light. It is freely soluble in water, sparingly soluble in alcohol, and slightly soluble in chloroform and in ether. Its molecular weight is 137.14.

Inactive Ingredients. Cellulose compounds, colloidal silicon dioxide, sodium starch glycolate, and stearic acid.

CLINICAL PHARMACOLOGY

Isoniazid acts against actively growing tubercle bacilli. Within 1 to 2 hours after oral administration isoniazid produces peak blood levels which decline to 50% or less within 6 hours. It diffuses readily into all body fluids (cerebrospinal, pleural, and ascitic fluids), tissues, organs, and excreta (saliva, sputum, and feces). The drug also passes through the placental barrier and into milk in concentrations comparable to those in the plasma. From 50 to 70% of a dose of isoniazid is excreted in the urine in 24 hours.

Isoniazid is metabolized primarily by acetylation and dehydrazination. The rate of acetylation is genetically determined. Approximately 50% of Blacks and Caucasians are "slow inactivators" and the rest are rapid inactivators; the majority of Eskimos and Orientals are "rapid inactivators." The rate of acetylation does not significantly alter the effectiveness of isoniazid. However, slow acetylation may lead to higher blood levels of the drug, and thus an increase in toxic reactions.

Pyridoxine (B_6) deficiency is sometimes observed in adults with high doses of isoniazid and is considered probably due to its competition with pyridoxal phosphate for the enzyme apotryptophanase.

INDICATIONS AND USAGE

For all forms of tuberculosis in which organisms are susceptible.

For preventive therapy for the following groups, in order of priority:

1. Household members and other close associates of persons with recently diagnosed tuberculous disease.
2. Positive tuberculin skin test reactors with findings on the chest roentgenogram consistent with nonprogressive tuberculous disease, in whom there are neither positive bacteriologic findings nor a history of adequate chemotherapy.
3. Newly infected persons.
4. Positive tuberculin skin test reactors in the following special clinical situations: prolonged therapy with adrenocorticosteroids; immunosuppressive therapy; some hematologic and reticuloendothelial diseases, such as leukemia or Hodgkin's disease; diabetes mellitus; silicosis; after gastrectomy.
5. Other positive tuberculin reactors under 35 years of age.

The risk of hepatitis must be weighed against the risk of tuberculosis in positive tuberculin reactors over the age of 35. However, the use of isoniazid is recommended for those with the additional risk factors listed above (1–4) and on an individual basis in situations where there is likelihood of serious consequences to contacts who may become infected.

CONTRAINDICATIONS

Isoniazid is contraindicated in patients who develop severe hypersensitivity reactions, including drug-induced hepatitis. Previous isoniazid-associated hepatic injury: severe adverse reactions to isoniazid, such as drug fever, chills, and arthritis; acute liver disease of any etiology.

WARNINGS

See the boxed warning.

PRECAUTIONS

All drugs should be stopped and an evaluation made at the first sign of a hypersensitivity reaction. If isoniazid therapy must be reinstituted, the drug should be given only after symptoms have cleared. The drug should be restarted in very

small and gradually increasing doses and should be withdrawn immediately if there is any indication of recurrent hypersensitivity reaction.

Use of isoniazid should be carefully monitored in the following:

1. Patients who are receiving phenytoin concurrently. Isoniazid may decrease the excretion of phenytoin or may enhance its effects. To avoid phenytoin intoxication, appropriate adjustment of the anticonvulsant should be made.
2. Daily users of alcohol. Daily ingestion of alcohol may be associated with a higher incidence of isoniazid hepatitis.
3. Patients with current chronic liver disease or severe renal dysfunction.

Ophthalmologic examinations (including ophthalmoscopy) should be done *before* INH is started and periodically thereafter, even without occurrence of visual symptoms.

Usage in Pregnancy and Lactation

It has been reported that in both rats and rabbits, isoniazid may exert an embryocidal effect when administered orally during pregnancy, although no isoniazid-related congenital anomalies have been found in reproduction studies in mammalian species (mice, rats, and rabbits). Isoniazid should be prescribed during pregnancy only when therapeutically necessary. The benefit of preventive therapy should be weighed against a possible risk to the fetus. Preventive treatment generally should be started after delivery because of the increased risk of tuberculosis for new mothers.

Since isoniazid is known to cross the placental barrier and to pass into maternal breast milk, neonates and breast-fed infants of isoniazid-treated mothers should be carefully observed for any evidence of adverse effects.

Carcinogenesis

Isoniazid has been reported to induce pulmonary tumors in a number of strains of mice.

ADVERSE REACTIONS

The most frequent reactions are those affecting the nervous system and the liver.

Nervous system reactions: Peripheral neuropathy is the most common toxic effect. It is dose-related, occurs most often in the malnourished and in those predisposed to neuritis (eg, alcoholics and diabetics), and is usually preceded by paresthesias of the feet and hands. The incidence is higher in "slow inactivators."

Other neurotoxic effects, which are uncommon with conventional doses, are convulsions, toxic encephalopathy, optic neuritis and atrophy, memory impairment, and toxic psychosis.

Gastrointestinal reactions: Nausea, vomiting, epigastric distress.

Hepatic reactions: Elevated serum transaminases (SGOT; SGPT), bilirubinemia, bilirubinuria, jaundice and occasionally severe and sometimes fatal hepatitis. The common prodromal symptoms are anorexia, nausea, vomiting, fatigue, malaise, and weakness. Mild and transient elevation of serum transaminase levels, occurs in 10 to 20 percent of persons taking isoniazid. The abnormality usually occurs in the first 4 to 6 months of treatment but can occur at any time during therapy. In most instances, enzyme levels return to normal with no necessity to discontinue medication. In occasional instances, progressive liver damage occurs, with accompanying symptoms. In these cases, the drug should be discontinued immediately. The frequency of progressive liver damage increases with age. It is rare in persons under 20, but occurs in up to 2.3 percent of those over 50 years of age.

Hematologic reactions: Agranulocytosis; hemolytic, sideroblastic, or aplastic anemia; thrombocytopenia; and eosinophilia.

Hypersensitivity reactions: Fever, skin eruptions (morbilliform, maculopapular, purpuric, or exfoliative), lymphadenopathy and vasculitis.

Metabolic and endocrine reactions: Pyridoxine deficiency, pellagra, hyperglycemia, metabolic acidosis, and gynecomastia.

Miscellaneous reactions: Rheumatic syndrome and systemic lupus erythematosus-like syndrome.

OVERDOSAGE

Signs and Symptoms

Isoniazid overdosage produces signs and symptoms within 30 minutes to 3 hours after ingestion. Nausea, vomiting, dizziness, slurring of speech, blurring of vision, and visual hallucinations (including bright colors and strange designs), are among the early manifestations. With marked overdosage, respiratory distress and CNS depression, progressing rapidly from stupor to profound coma, are to be expected, along with severe, intractable seizures. Severe metabolic acidosis, acetonuria, and hyperglycemia are typical laboratory findings.

Treatment

Untreated or inadequately treated cases of gross isoniazid overdosage can terminate fatally, but good response has been reported in most patients brought under adequate treatment within the first few hours after drug ingestion. Secure the airway and establish adequate respiratory exchange. Gastric lavage within the first 2 to 3 hours is ad-

vised, but should not be attempted until convulsions are under control. To control convulsions administer I.V. short-acting barbiturates and I.V. pyridoxine (usually 1 mg/1mg isoniazid ingested).

Obtain blood samples for immediate determination of gases, electrolytes, BUN, glucose, etc.; type and crossmatch blood in preparation for possible hemodialysis.

Rapid control of metabolic acidosis is fundamental to management. Give I.V. sodium bicarbonate at once and repeat as needed, adjusting subsequent dosage on the basis of laboratory findings (ie, serum sodium, pH, etc.).

Forced osmotic diuresis must be started early and should be continued for some hours after clinical improvement to hasten renal clearance of drug and help prevent relapse; monitor fluid intake and output.

Hemodialysis is advised for severe cases; if this is not available, peritoneal dialysis can be used along with forced diuresis.

Along with measures based on initial and repeated determination of blood gases and other laboratory tests as needed, utilize meticulous respiratory and other intensive care to protect against hypoxia, hypotension, aspiration pneumonitis, etc.

DOSAGE AND ADMINISTRATION [See also INDICATIONS]

NOTE—For preventive therapy of tuberculous infection it is recommended that physicians be familiar with the joint recommendations of the American Thoracic Society, American Lung Association, and the Center for Disease Control, as published in the American Review of Respiratory Diseases Vol. 110, No. 3, September 1974, or CDC's Morbidity and Mortality Weekly Report, Vol. 24, No. 8, February 22, 1975.

For treatment of active tuberculosis

Isoniazid is used in conjunction with other effective antituberculous agents.

If the bacilli become resistant, therapy must be changed to agents to which the bacilli are susceptible.

Usual oral dosage

Adults: 5 mg/kg up to 300 mg daily in a single dose.

Infants and children: 10–20 mg/kg depending on severity of infection, (up to 300–500 mg daily) in a single dose.

For preventive therapy

Adults: 300 mg/day in a single dose.

Infants and children: 10 mg/kg (up to 300 mg daily) in a single dose.

Continuous administration of isoniazid for a sufficient period is an essential part of the regimen because relapse rates are higher if chemotherapy is stopped prematurely. In the treatment of tuberculosis, resistant organisms may multiply and the emergence of resistant organisms during the treatment may necessitate a change in the regimen.

Concomitant administration of pyridoxine (B$_6$) is recommended in the malnourished and in those predisposed to neuropathy (eg, alcoholics and diabetics).

HOW SUPPLIED

Tablets, 300 mg (white, scored); available as Rimactane® rifampin USP/INH Dual Pack containing 30 INH Tablets and 60 Rimactane 300-mg Capsules.

NDC 0083-8912-23

Protect from heat, light and moisture (Rimactane/INH Dual Pack).

C87-32 (Rev. 8/87)

ISMELIN® sulfate   ℞

[iz'mel-lin]

guanethidine monosulfate USP

Tablets

DESCRIPTION

Ismelin, guanethidine monosulfate USP, is an antihypertensive, available as tablets of 10 mg and 25 mg for oral administration. Each 10-mg and 25-mg tablet contains guanethidine monosulfate USP equivalent to 10 mg and 25 mg of guanethidine sulfate, USP. Its chemical name is [2-(hexahydro-1(2H)-azocinyl)ethyl]guanidine sulfate 1:1.

Guanethidine monosulfate USP is a white to off-white crystalline powder with a molecular weight of 296.38. It is very soluble in water, sparingly soluble in alcohol, and practically insoluble in chloroform.

Inactive ingredients: Calcium stearate, colloidal silicon dioxide, D&C Yellow No. 10 (10-mg tablets), lactose, starch, stearic acid, and sucrose.

CLINICAL PHARMACOLOGY

Ismelin acts at the sympathetic neuroeffector junction by inhibiting or interfering with the release and/or distribution of the chemical mediator (presumably the catecholamine norepinephrine), rather than acting at the effector cell by inhibiting the association of the transmitter with its receptors. In contrast to ganglionic blocking agents, Ismelin suppresses equally the responses mediated by alpha- and beta-adrenergic receptors but does not produce parasympathetic blockade. Since sympathetic blockade results in modest de-

creases in peripheral resistance and cardiac output, Ismelin lowers blood pressure in the supine position. It further reduces blood pressure by decreasing the degree of vasoconstriction that normally results from reflex sympathetic nervous activity upon assumption of the upright posture, thus reducing venous return and cardiac output more. The inhibition of sympathetic venoconstrictive mechanisms results in venous pooling of blood. Therefore, the effect of Ismelin is especially pronounced when the patient is standing. Both the systolic and diastolic pressures are reduced.

Other actions at the sympathetic nerve terminal include depletion of norepinephrine. Once it gains access to the neuron, Ismelin accumulates within the intraneuronal storage vesicles and causes depletion of norepinephrine stores within the nerve terminal. Prolonged oral administration of Ismelin produces a denervation sensitivity of the neuroeffector junction, probably resulting from the chronic reduction in norepinephrine released by the sympathetic nerve endings. Systemic responses to catecholamines released from the adrenal medulla are not prevented and may even be augmented as a result of this denervation sensitivity. A paradoxical hypertensive crisis may occur if Ismelin is given to patients with pheochromocytoma or if norepinephrine is given to a patient receiving the drug.

Due to its poor lipid solubility, Ismelin does not readily cross the blood-brain barrier. In contrast to most neural blocking agents, Ismelin does not appear to suppress plasma renin activity in many patients.

Pharmacokinetics

The pharmacokinetics of Ismelin are complex. The amount of drug in plasma and in urine is linearly related to dose, although large differences occur between individuals because of variation in absorption and metabolism. Adrenergic blockade occurs with a minimum concentration in plasma of 8 ng/ml; this concentration is achieved in different individuals with dosages of 10–50 mg/day at steady state. Ismelin is eliminated slowly because of extensive tissue binding. After chronic oral administration, the initial phase of elimination with a half-life of 1.5 days is followed by a second phase of elimination with a half-life of 4–8 days. The renal clearance of Ismelin is 56 ml/min. Ismelin is converted by the liver to three metabolites, which are excreted in the urine. The metabolites are pharmacologically less active than Ismelin.

INDICATIONS AND USAGE

Ismelin is indicated for the treatment of moderate and severe hypertension, either alone or as an adjunct, and for the treatment of renal hypertension, including that secondary to pyelonephritis, renal amyloidosis, and renal artery stenosis.

CONTRAINDICATIONS

Known or suspected pheochromocytoma; hypersensitivity; frank congestive heart failure not due to hypertension; use of monoamine oxidase (MAO) inhibitors.

WARNINGS

Ismelin is a potent drug and its use can lead to disturbing and serious clinical problems. Before prescribing, physicians should familiarize themselves with the details of its use and warn patients not to deviate from instructions.

> Orthostatic hypotension can occur frequently, and patients should be properly instructed about this potential hazard. Fainting spells may occur unless the patient is forewarned to sit or lie down with the onset of dizziness or weakness. Postural hypotension is most marked in the morning and is accentuated by hot weather, alcohol, or exercise. Dizziness or weakness may be particularly bothersome during the initial period of dosage adjustment and with postural changes, such as arising in the morning. The potential occurrence of these symptoms may require alteration of previous daily activity. The patient should be cautioned to avoid sudden or prolonged standing or exercise while taking the drug.

Inhibition of ejaculation has been reported in animals (see **PRECAUTIONS, Carcinogenesis, Mutagenesis, Impairment of Fertility**) as well as in men given Ismelin. This effect, which results from the sympathetic blockade caused by the drug's action, is reversible after Ismelin has been discontinued for several weeks. The drug does not cause parasympathetic blockade, and erectile potency is usually retained during administration of Ismelin. The possible occurrence of inhibition of ejaculation should be kept in mind when considering the use of guanethidine in men of reproductive age. If possible, therapy should be withdrawn 2 weeks prior to surgery to reduce the possibility of vascular collapse and cardiac arrest during anesthesia. If emergency surgery is indicated, preanesthetic and anesthetic agents should be

Continued on next page

The full prescribing information for each CIBA product is contained herein and is that in effect as of September 1, 1992.

CIBA—Cont.

administered cautiously in reduced dosage. Oxygen, atropine, vasopressors, and adequate solutions for volume replacement should be ready for immediate use to counteract vascular collapse in the surgical patient. Vasopressors should be used only with extreme caution, since Ismelin augments responsiveness to exogenously administered norepinephrine and vasopressors; specifically, blood pressure may rise and cardiac arrhythmias may be produced.

PRECAUTIONS

General

Dosage requirements may be reduced in the presence of fever.

Special care should be exercised when treating patients with a history of bronchial asthma; asthmatic patients are more apt to be hypersensitive to catecholamine depletion, and their condition may be aggravated.

The effects of Ismelin are cumulative over long periods; initial doses should be small and increased gradually in small increments.

Ismelin should be used very cautiously in hypertensive patients with renal disease and nitrogen retention or rising BUN levels, since decreased blood pressure may further compromise renal function, coronary insufficiency or recent myocardial infarction, and cerebrovascular disease, especially with encephalopathy.

Ismelin should not be given to patients with severe cardiac failure except with extreme caution, since Ismelin may interfere with the compensatory role of the adrenergic system in producing circulatory adjustment in patients with congestive heart failure.

Patients with incipient cardiac decompensation should be watched for weight gain or edema, which may be averted by the concomitant administration of a thiazide.

Ismelin should be used cautiously in patients with a history of peptic ulcer or other chronic disorders that may be aggravated by a relative increase in parasympathetic tone.

Information for Patients

The patient should be advised to take Ismelin exactly as directed. If the patient misses a dose, he or she should be told to take only the next scheduled dose (without doubling it).

The patient should be advised to avoid sudden or prolonged standing or exercise and to arise slowly, especially in the morning, to reduce the orthostatic hypotensive effects of dizziness, lightheadedness, or fainting.

The patient should be cautioned about ingesting alcohol, since it aggravates the orthostatic hypotensive effects of Ismelin.

Male patients should be advised that guanethidine may interfere with ejaculation.

Drug Interactions

Concurrent use of Ismelin and rauwolfia derivatives may cause excessive postural hypotension, bradycardia, and mental depression.

Both digitalis and Ismelin slow the heart rate.

Thiazide diuretics enhance the antihypertensive action of Ismelin (see **DOSAGE AND ADMINISTRATION**).

Amphetamine-like compounds, stimulants (e.g., ephedrine, methylphenidate), tricyclic antidepressants (e.g., amitriptyline, imipramine, desipramine) and other psychopharmacologic agents (e.g., phenothiazines and related compounds), as well as oral contraceptives, may reduce the hypotensive effect of Ismelin.

MAO inhibitors should be discontinued for at least 1 week before starting therapy with Ismelin.

Carcinogenesis, Mutagenesis, Impairment of Fertility

Long-term carcinogenicity studies in animals have not been conducted with Ismelin.

While inhibition of sperm passage and accumulation of sperm debris have been reported in rats and rabbits after several weeks of administration of Ismelin, 5 or 10 mg/kg per day, subcutaneously or intraperitoneally, recovery of ejaculatory function and fertility has been demonstrated in rats given Ismelin intramuscularly, 25 mg/kg per day, for 8 weeks. Inhibition of ejaculation has also been reported in men (see **WARNINGS** and **ADVERSE REACTIONS**). This effect, which is attributable to the sympathetic blockade caused by the drug, is reversible several weeks after discontinuance of the drug.

Pregnancy Category C

Animal reproduction studies have not been conducted with Ismelin. It is also not known whether Ismelin can cause fetal harm when administered to a pregnant woman or can affect reproduction capacity. Ismelin should be given to a pregnant woman only if clearly needed.

Nursing Mothers

Ismelin is excreted in breast milk in very small quantity. Caution should be exercised when Ismelin is administered to a nursing woman.

Pediatric Use

Safety and effectiveness in children have not been established.

ADVERSE REACTIONS

The following adverse reactions have been observed, but there are not enough data to support an estimate of their frequency. Consequently the reactions are categorized by organ system and are listed in decreasing order of severity and not frequency.

Digestive: Diarrhea, which may be severe at times and necessitate discontinuance of medication; vomiting, nausea, increased bowel movements; dry mouth, parotid tenderness.

Cardiovascular: Chest pains (angina); bradycardia; a tendency toward fluid retention and edema with occasional development of congestive heart failure.

Respiratory: Dyspnea; asthma in susceptible individuals; nasal congestion.

Neurologic: Syncope resulting from either postural or exertional hypotension; dizziness; blurred vision; muscle tremor; ptosis of the lids; mental depression; chest paresthesias; weakness; lassitude; fatigue.

Muscular: Myalgia.

Genitourinary: Rise in BUN; urinary incontinence; inhibition of ejaculation; nocturia.

Metabolic: Weight gain.

Skin and Appendages: Dermatitis; scalp hair loss.

Although a causal relationship has not been established, a few instances of blood dyscrasia (anemia, thrombocytopenia, and leukopenia) and of priapism or impotence have been reported.

OVERDOSAGE

Acute Toxicity

No deaths due to acute poisoning have been reported.

Oral LD$_{50}$ in rats: 1262 mg/kg.

Signs and Symptoms

Postural hypotension (with dizziness, blurred vision, and possibly syncope when standing), shock, and bradycardia are most likely to occur, diarrhea (possibly severe), nausea and vomiting may also occur. Unconsciousness is unlikely if adequate blood pressure and cerebral perfusion can be maintained by placing the patient in the supine position and by administering other treatment as required.

Treatment

There is no specific antidote.

Treatment should consist of gastric lavage. An activated charcoal slurry should be instilled and laxatives given, if conditions permit.

In sinus bradycardia, atropine should be administered.

In previously normotensive patients, treatment has consisted essentially of restoring blood pressure and heart rate to normal by keeping the patient in the supine position. Normal homeostatic control usually returns gradually over a 72-hour period in these patients.

In previously hypertensive patients, particularly those with impaired cardiac reserve or other cardiovascular-renal disease, intensive treatment may be required to support vital functions and to control cardiac irregularities that might be present. The supine position must be maintained; if vasopressors are required, they must be used with extreme caution, since Ismelin may increase responsiveness, causing a rise in blood pressure and development of cardiac arrhythmias.

Diarrhea, if severe or persistent, should be treated with anticholinergic agents to reduce intestinal hypermotility; hydration and electrolyte balance should be maintained.

Since Ismelin is excreted slowly, cardiovascular and renal function should be monitored for a few days.

DOSAGE AND ADMINISTRATION

Better control may be obtained, especially in the initial phases of treatment, if the patient can have his blood pressure recorded regularly at home.

Ambulatory Patients

Initial doses should be small (10 mg) and increased gradually, depending upon the patient's response. Ismelin has a long duration of action; therefore, dosage increases should not be made more often than every 5–7 days, unless the patient is hospitalized.

Blood pressure should be measured in the supine position, after standing for 10 minutes, and immediately after exercise if feasible. Dosage may be increased only if there has been no decrease in the standing blood pressure from previous levels. The average daily dose is 25–50 mg; only one dose a day is usually required. [See chart above.]

The dosage should be reduced in any of the following situations: (1) normal supine pressure (2) excessive orthostatic fall in pressure (3) severe diarrhea.

Hospitalized Patients

Initial oral dose is 25–50 mg, increased by 25 mg or 50 mg daily or every other day, as indicated. This higher dosage is possible because hospitalized patients can be watched carefully. Unless absolutely impossible, the standing blood pressure should be measured regularly. Patients should not be discharged from the hospital until the effect of the drug on

Dosage Chart for Ambulatory Patients

Visits (Intervals of 5–7 Days)	*Daily Dose*
Visit 1 (Patient may be started on 10-mg tablets)	10 mg
Visit 2	20 mg
Visit 3 (Patient may be changed to 25-mg tablets whenever convenient)	30 mg
	(three 10-mg tablets) or 37.5 mg
	(one and one-half 25-mg tablets)
Visit 4	50 mg
Visit 5 and subsequent	Dosage may be increased by 12.5 mg or 25 mg if necessary.

the standing blood pressure is known. Patients should be told about the possibility of orthostatic hypotension and warned not to get out of bed without help during the period of dosage adjustment.

Combination Therapy

Ismelin may be added gradually to thiazides and/or hydralazine. Thiazide diuretics enhance the effectiveness of Ismelin and may reduce the incidence of edema. When thiazide diuretics are added to the regimen in patients taking Ismelin, it is usually necessary to reduce the dosage of Ismelin. After control is established, the dosage of all drugs should be reduced to the lowest effective level.

Note: When Ismelin is replacing MAO inhibitors, at least 1 week should elapse before commencing treatment with Ismelin (see **CONTRAINDICATIONS**). If ganglionic blockers have not been discontinued before Ismelin is started, they should be gradually withdrawn to prevent a spiking blood pressure response during the transfer period.

HOW SUPPLIED

Tablets 10 mg—round, pale yellow, scored (imprinted CIBA 49)

Bottles of 100 .... NDC 0083-0049-30

Tablets 25 mg—round, white, scored (imprinted CIBA 103)

Bottles of 100 .... NDC 0083-0103-30

Do not store above 86°F (30°C).

Dispense in tight container (USP).

C89-27 (Rev. 7/89)

Shown in Product Identification Section, page 408

LITHOBID® ℞

[*lith 'oh-bidd*]

lithium carbonate USP

slow-release tablets

CIBALITH-S® ℞

[*see 'ba-lith-ess*]

lithium citrate syrup USP

For Control of Manic Episodes in Manic-Depressive Psychosis

Caution: Federal law prohibits dispensing without prescription

---

> ### WARNING
> Lithium toxicity is closely related to serum lithium levels, and can occur at doses close to therapeutic levels. Facilities for prompt and accurate serum lithium determinations should be available before initiating therapy.

DESCRIPTION

Lithobid and Cibalith-S are two different forms of an antimanic medication for oral administration. Lithobid is a film-coated, slow-release, 300-mg lithium carbonate tablet. This slowly dissolving, film-coated tablet is designed to give lower serum lithium peaks than obtained with conventional oral lithium dosage forms.

Lithium carbonate USP is a white, granular, odorless powder, which is sparingly soluble in water and very slightly soluble in alcohol. It dissolves, with effervescence, in dilute mineral acids. Its molecular formula is Li$_2$CO$_3$, and its molecular weight is 73.89.

Cibalith-S is lithium citrate syrup containing 8 mEq of lithium per 5 ml, equivalent to the amount in 300 mg of lithium carbonate.

Lithium citrate is prepared in solution from lithium hydroxide and citric acid in a ratio approximating dilithium citrate.

Inactive Ingredients. Lithobid tablets 300 mg: Calcium stearate, carnauba wax, cellulose compounds, FD&C Blue No. 2 Aluminum Lake, FD&C Red No. 40 Aluminum Lake, FD&C Yellow No. 6 Aluminum Lake, povidone, propylene glycol, sodium chloride, sodium lauryl sulfate, sodium starch glycolate, sorbitol, and titanium dioxide.

Cibalith-S syrup. Citric acid, raspberry flavor, alcohol 0.3% v/v, purified water, sodium benzoate, sodium saccharin, and sorbitol.

INDICATIONS

Lithium is indicated in the treatment of manic episodes of manic-depressive illness. Maintenance therapy prevents or diminishes the intensity of subsequent episodes in those manic-depressive patients with a history of mania.

Typical symptoms of mania include pressure of speech, motor hyperactivity, reduced need for sleep, flight of ideas, grandiosity, elation, poor judgment, aggressiveness, and possibly hostility. When given to a patient experiencing a manic episode, lithium may produce a normalization of symptomatology within 1 to 3 weeks.

WARNINGS

Lithium should generally not be given to patients with significant renal or cardiovascular disease, severe debilitation or dehydration, or sodium depletion, and to patients receiving diuretics, since the risk of lithium toxicity is very high in such patients. If the psychiatric indication is life-threatening, and if such a patient fails to respond to other measures, lithium treatment may be undertaken with extreme caution, including daily serum lithium determinations and adjustment to the usually low doses ordinarily tolerated by these individuals. In such instances, hospitalization is a necessity.
Lithium toxicity is closely related to serum lithium levels, and can occur at doses close to the therapeutic levels (see DOSAGE AND ADMINISTRATION).
Lithium therapy has been reported in some cases to be associated with morphologic changes in the kidneys. The relationship between such changes and renal function has not been established.
Outpatients and their families should be warned that the patient must discontinue lithium therapy and contact his physician if such clinical signs of lithium toxicity as diarrhea, vomiting, tremor, mild ataxia, drowsiness, or muscular weakness occur.
Lithium may impair mental and/or physical abilities. Caution patients about activities requiring alertness (e.g., operating vehicles or machinery).
Lithium may prolong or potentiate the effects of neuromuscular blocking agents, such as decamethonium, pancuronium, and succinylcholine. Therefore, neuromuscular blocking agents should be given with caution to patients receiving lithium.
Combined use of haloperidol and lithium: An encephalopathic syndrome (characterized by weakness; lethargy; fever; tremulousness and confusion; extrapyramidal symptoms; leukocytosis; elevated serum enzymes, BUN, and fasting blood sugar), followed by irreversible brain damage, has occurred in a few patients treated with lithium plus haloperidol. A causal relationship between these events and the concomitant administration of lithium and haloperidol has not been established. However, patients receiving such combined therapy should be monitored closely for early evidence of neurological toxicity, and treatment discontinued promptly if such signs appear. The possibility of similar adverse interactions with other antipsychotic medications exists. In addition, concurrent use of lithium with chlorpromazine and possibly other phenothiazines decreases serum chlorpromazine levels as much as 40%.
Usage in Pregnancy: Adverse effects on nidation in rats, embryo viability in mice, and metabolism *in vitro* of rat testis and human spermatozoa have been attributed to lithium, as have teratogenicity in submammalian species and cleft palates in mice.
There are lithium birth registries in the United States and elsewhere; however there are at the present time insufficient data to determine the effects of lithium on human fetuses. Therefore, at this point, lithium should not be used in pregnancy, especially the first trimester, unless in the opinion of the physician, the potential benefits outweigh the possible hazards.
Usage in Nursing Mothers: Lithium is excreted in human milk. Nursing should not be undertaken during lithium therapy except in rare and unusual circumstances where, in the view of the physician, the potential benefits to the mother outweigh possible hazards to the child.
Usage in Children: Since information regarding the safety and effectivenss of lithium in children under 12 years of age is not available, its use in such patients is not recommended at this time (see OVERDOSAGE).

PRECAUTIONS

The ability to tolerate lithium is greater during the acute manic phase and decreases when manic symptoms subside (see DOSAGE AND ADMINISTRATION).
The distribution space of lithium approximates that of total body water. Lithium is primarily excreted in urine with insignificant excretion in feces. Renal excretion of lithium is proportional to its plasma concentration. The half-elimination time of lithium is approximately 24 hours. Lithium decreases sodium reabsorption by the renal tubules which could lead to sodium depletion. Therefore, it is essential for the patient to maintain a normal diet, including salt, and an adequate fluid intake (2500–3000 ml) at least during the initial stabilization period. Decreased tolerance to lithium has been reported to ensue from protracted sweating or diarrhea and, if such occur, supplemental fluid and salt should be administered.
In addition to sweating and diarrhea, concomitant infection with elevated temperatures may also necessitate a temporary reduction or cessation of medication.
Previously existing underlying disorders do not necessarily constitute a contraindication to lithium treatment; where hypothyroidism exists, careful monitoring of thyroid function during lithium stabilization and maintenance allows for correction of changing thyroid parameters, if any, where hypothyroidism occurs during lithium stabilization and maintenance, supplemental thyroid treatment may be used.
Drug Interactions: Concomitant administration of carbamazepine and lithium may increase the risk of neurotoxic side effects.
Aminophylline, caffeine, dyphylline, oxtriphylline, sodium bicarbonate, or theophylline used concurrently may decrease the therapeutic effect of lithium because of its increased urinary excretion.
Concurrent use of diuretics, especially thiazides, with lithium may provoke lithium toxicity due to reduced renal clearance.
Concurrent extended use of iodide preparations, especially potassium iodide, with lithium may produce hypothyroidism.
Indomethacin and piroxicam have been reported to increase significantly steady-state plasma lithium levels. In some cases, lithium toxicity has resulted from such interactions. There is also some evidence that other nonsteroidal, anti-inflammatory agents may have a similar effect. When such combinations are used, increased monitoring of plasma lithium levels is recommended (see WARNINGS).
There is evidence that angiotensin-converting enzyme inhibitors, such as enalapril and captopril, may substantially increase steady-state plasma lithium levels, sometimes resulting in lithium toxicity. When such combinations are used, lithium dosage may need to be decreased, and plasma lithium levels should be measured more often.

ADVERSE REACTIONS

Adverse reactions are seldom encountered at serum lithium levels below 1.5 mEq/l, except in the occasional patient sensitive to lithium. Mild-to-moderate toxic reactions may occur at levels from 1.5–2.5 mEq/l, and moderate-to-severe reactions may be seen at levels from 2.0–2.5 mEq/l, depending upon individual response to the drug.
Fine hand tremor, polyuria and mild thirst may occur during initial therapy for the acute manic phase, and may persist throughout treatment. Transient and mild nausea and general discomfort may also appear during the first few days of lithium administration.
These side effects are an inconvenience rather than a disabling condition, and usually subside with continued treatment or a temporary reduction or cessation of dosage. If persistent, a cessation of dosage is indicated.
Diarrhea, vomiting, drowsiness, muscular weakness and lack of coordination may be early signs of lithium intoxication, and can occur at lithium levels below 2.0 mEq/l. At higher levels, giddiness, ataxia, blurred vision, tinnitus and a large output of dilute urine may be seen. Serum lithium levels above 3.0 mEq/l may produce a complex clinical picture involving multiple organs and organ systems. Serum lithium levels should not be permitted to exceed 2.0 mEq/l during the acute treatment phase.
The following toxic reactions have been reported and appear to be related to serum lithium levels, including levels within the therapeutic range.
Neuromuscular: tremor, muscle hyperirritability (fasciculations, twitching, clonic movements of whole limbs), ataxia, choreoathetotic movements, hyperactive deep tendon reflexes.
Central Nervous System: blackout spells, epileptiform seizures, downbeat nystagmus, acute dystonia, slurred speech, dizziness, vertigo, incontinence of urine or feces, somnolence, psychomotor retardation, restlessness, confusion, stupor, coma. Cases of pseudotumor cerebri (increased intracranial pressure and papilledema) have been reported with lithium use. If undetected, this condition may result in enlargement of the blind spot, constriction of visual fields, and eventual blindness due to optic atrophy. If this syndrome occurs, lithium should be discontinued if clinically possible.
Cardiovascular: cardiac arrhythmia, hypotension, peripheral circulatory collapse.
Gastrointestinal: anorexia, nausea, vomiting, diarrhea.
Genitourinary: albuminuria, oliguria, polyuria, glycosuria.
Dermatologic: drying and thinning of hair, anesthesia of skin, chronic folliculitis, xerosis cutis, alopecia, exacerbation of psoriasis.
Autonomic Nervous System: blurred vision, dry mouth.
Miscellaneous: fatigue, lethargy, tendency to sleep, dehydration, weight loss, transient scotomata.
Thyroid Abnormalities: euthyroid goiter and/or hypothyroidism (including myxedema) accompanied by lower T_3 and T_4. I_{131} iodine uptake may be elevated (see PRECAUTIONS). Paradoxically, rare cases of hyperthyroidism have been reported.
EEG Changes: diffuse slowing, widening of frequency spectrum, potentiation and disorganization of background rhythm.
EKG Changes: reversible flattening, isoelectricity or inversion of T-waves.
Miscellaneous reactions unrelated to dosage are: transient electroencephalographic and electrocardiographic changes, leukocytosis, headache, diffuse nontoxic goiter with or without hypothyroidism, transient hyperglycemia, generalized pruritus with or without rash, cutaneous ulcers, albuminuria, worsening of organic brain syndromes, excessive weight gain, edematous swelling of ankles or wrists, metallic taste, and thirst or polyuria, sometimes resembling diabetes insipidus.
A single report has been received of the development of painful discoloration of fingers and toes and coldness of the extremities within one day of the starting of treatment of lithium. The mechanism through which these symptoms (resembling Raynaud's Syndrome) developed is not known. Recovery followed discontinuance.

DOSAGE AND ADMINISTRATION

Acute Mania: Optimal patient response can usually be established and maintained with the following dosages:

Lithobid ....900 mg b.i.d. or 600 mg t.i.d. (1800 mg per day)

Cibalith-S ....10 ml (2 teaspoons) (16 mEq of lithium) t.i.d.

Such doses will normally produce an effective serum lithium level ranging between 1.0 and 1.5 mEq/l. Dosage must be individualized according to serum levels and clinical response. Regular monitoring of the patient's clinical state and of serum lithium levels is necessary. Serum levels should be determined twice per week during the acute phase, and until the serum level and clinical condition of the patient have been stabilized.
Long-Term Control: The desirable serum lithium levels are 0.6 to 1.2 mEq/l. Dosage will vary from one individual to another, but usually the following dosages will maintain this level:

Lithobid..........................900 mg to 1200 mg per day given in two or three divided doses.

Cibalith-S......................5 ml (1 teaspoon) (8 mEq of lithium) t.i.d. or q.i.d.

Serum lithium levels in uncomplicated cases receiving maintenance therapy during remission should be monitored at least every two months. Patients abnormally sensitive to lithium may exhibit toxic signs at serum levels of 1.0 to 1.5 mEq/l. Elderly patients often respond to reduced dosage, and may exhibit signs of toxicity at serum levels ordinarily tolerated by other patients.
N.B.: Blood samples for serum lithium determinations should be drawn immediately prior to the next dose when lithium concentrations are relatively stable (i.e., 8–12 hours after previous dose). Total reliance must not be placed on serum levels alone. Accurate patient evaluation requires both clinical and laboratory analysis.
Lithobid slow-release tablets must be swallowed whole and never crushed or chewed.

OVERDOSAGE

The toxic levels for lithium are close to the therapeutic levels. It is therefore important that patients and their families be cautioned to watch for early toxic symptoms and to discontinue the drug and inform the physician should they occur. There has been a report of a transient syndrome of acute dystonia and hyperreflexia occurring in a 15 kg child who ingested 300 mg of lithium carbonate. Toxic symptoms are listed in detail under ADVERSE REACTIONS.
Treatment: No specific antidote for lithium poisoning is known. Early symptoms of lithium toxicity can usually be treated by reduction or cessation of dosage of the drug and resumption of the treatment at a lower dose after 24 to 48 hours. In severe cases of lithium poisoning, the first and foremost goal of treatment consists of elimination of this ion from the patient.
Treatment is essentially the same as that used in barbiturate poisoning: 1) gastric lavage 2) correction of fluid and electrolyte imbalance and 3) regulation of kidney functioning. Urea, mannitol, and aminophylline all produce significant increases in lithium excretion. Hemodialysis is an effective and rapid means of removing the ion from the severely toxic patient. Infection prophylaxis, regular chest x-rays, and preservation of adequate respiration are essential.

HOW SUPPLIED

Lithobid, lithium carbonate
Tablets—slow-release 300 mg—peach-colored (imprinted CIBA 65)
Bottles of 100 ....NDC 0083-0065-30
Bottles of 1000 ....NDC 0083-0065-40
Accu-Pak® Unit Dose (blister pack)
Box of 100 (strips of 10)..........................NDC 0083-0065-32

Continued on next page

The full prescribing information for each CIBA product is contained herein and is that in effect as of September 1, 1992.

CIBA—Cont.

Store between 59°–86°F (15°–30°C).
Protect from moisture.
Dispense in tight, child-resistant container (USP).
Shown in Product Identification Section, page 408

Cibalith-S, lithium citrate
Syrup—sugar-free, raspberry flavored, 8 mEq of lithium per 5 ml, equivalent to the amount in 300 mg of lithium carbonate.
Bottles of 480 ml ....NDC 0083-6565-76
Store between 59°–86°F (15°–30°C).
Dispense in tight, light-resistant, child-resistant container (USP).
C90-38 (Rev. 8/90)

Dist. by:
CIBA Pharmaceutical Co.
Division of CIBA-GEIGY Corporation
Summit, New Jersey 07901

LOTENSIN® ℞
benazepril hydrochloride
Tablets

Prescribing Information

> Use in Pregnancy
> When used in pregnancy during the second and third trimesters, ACE inhibitors can cause injury and even death to the developing fetus. When pregnancy is detected, Lotensin should be discontinued as soon as possible. See WARNINGS, Fetal/Neonatal Morbidity and Mortality.

DESCRIPTION
Benazepril hydrochloride is a white to off-white crystalline powder, soluble (> 100 mg/mL) in water, in ethanol, and in methanol. Benazepril's chemical name is 3-[[1-(ethoxy-carbonyl)-3-phenyl-(1S)-propyl]amino]-2,3,4,5-tetrahydro-2-oxo-1*H*-1-(3S)-benzazepine-1-acetic acid monohydrochloride. Its empirical formula is $C_{24}H_{28}N_2O_5 \cdot HCl$, and its molecular weight is 460.96.
Benazeprilat, the active metabolite of benazepril, is a non-sulfhydryl angiotensin-converting enzyme inhibitor. Benazepril is converted to benazeprilat by hepatic cleavage of the ester group.
Lotensin is supplied as tablets containing 5 mg, 10 mg, 20 mg, and 40 mg of benazepril for oral administration. The inactive ingredients are cellulose compounds, colloidal silicon dioxide, crospovidone, hydrogenated castor oil (5-mg, 10-mg, and 20-mg tablets), iron oxides, lactose, magnesium stearate (40-mg tablets), polysorbate 80, propylene glycol (5-mg and 40-mg tablets), starch, talc, and titanium dioxide.

CLINICAL PHARMACOLOGY
Mechanism of Action
Benazepril and benazeprilat inhibit angiotensin-converting enzyme (ACE) in human subjects and animals. ACE is a peptidyl dipeptidase that catalyzes the conversion of angiotensin I to the vasoconstrictor substance, angiotensin II. Angiotensin II also stimulates aldosterone secretion by the adrenal cortex.
Inhibition of ACE results in a decreased plasma angiotensin II, which leads to decreased vasopressor activity and to decreased aldosterone secretion. The latter decrease may result in a small increase in serum potassium. Hypertensive patients treated with Lotensin alone for up to 52 weeks had elevations of serum potassium of up to 0.2 mEq/L. Similar patients treated with Lotensin and hydrochlorothiazide for up to 24 weeks had no consistent changes in their serum potassium (see PRECAUTIONS).
Removal of angiotensin II negative feedback on renin secretion leads to increased plasma renin activity. In animal studies, benazepril had no inhibitory effect on the vasopressor response to angiotensin II and did not interfere with the hemodynamic effects of the autonomic neurotransmitters acetylcholine, epinephrine, and norepinephrine.
ACE is identical to kininase, an enzyme that degrades bradykinin. Whether increased levels of bradykinin, a potent vasodepressor peptide, play a role in the therapeutic effects of Lotensin remains to be elucidated.
While the mechanism through which benazepril lowers blood pressure is believed to be primarily suppression of the renin-angiotensin-aldosterone system, benazepril has an antihypertensive effect even in patients with low-renin hypertension. In particular, Lotensin was antihypertensive in all races studied, although it was somewhat less effective in blacks than in nonblacks.
Pharmacokinetics and Metabolism
Following oral administration of Lotensin, peak plasma concentrations of benazepril are reached within 0.5–1.0 hours. The extent of absorption is at least 37% as determined by urinary recovery and is not significantly influenced by the presence of food in the GI tract.
Cleavage of the ester group (primarily in the liver) converts benazepril to its active metabolite, benazeprilat. Peak plasma concentrations of benazeprilat are reached 1–2 hours after drug intake in the fasting state and 2–4 hours after drug intake in the nonfasting state. The serum protein binding of benazepril is about 96.7% and that of benazeprilat about 95.3%, as measured by equilbrium dialysis; on the basis of in vitro studies, the degree of protein binding should be unaffected by age, hepatic dysfunction, or concentration (over the concentration range of 0.24–23.6 μmol/L).
Benazepril is almost completely metabolized to benazeprilat, which has much greater ACE inhibitory activity than benazepril, and to the glucuronide conjugates of benazepril and benazeprilat. Only trace amounts of an administered dose of Lotensin can be recovered in the urine as unchanged benazepril, while about 20% of the dose is excreted as benazeprilat, 4% as benazepril glucuronide, and 8% as benazeprilat glucuronide.
The kinetics of benazepril are approximately dose-proportional within the dosage range of 10–80 mg.
The effective half-life of accumulation of benazeprilat following multiple dosing of benazepril hydrochloride is 10–11 hours. Thus, steady-state concentrations of benazeprilat should be reached after 2 or 3 doses of benazepril hydrochloride given once daily.
The kinetics did not change, and there was no significant accumulation during chronic administration (28 days) of once-daily doses between 5 mg and 20 mg. Accumulation ratios based on AUC and urinary recovery of benazeprilat were 1.19 and 1.27, respectively.
When dialysis was started two hours after ingestion of 10 mg of benazepril, approximately 6% of benazeprilat was removed in 4 hours of dialysis. The parent compound benazepril, was not detected in the dialysate.
The disposition of benazepril and benazeprilat in patients with mild-to-moderate renal insufficiency (creatinine clearance > 30 mL/min) is similar to that in patients with normal renal function. In patients with creatinine clearance ≤ 30 mL/min, peak benazeprilat levels and the initial (alpha phase) half-life increase, and time to steady-state may be delayed (see DOSAGE AND ADMINISTRATION).
Benazepril and benazeprilat are cleared predominantly by renal excretion in healthy subjects with normal renal function. Nonrenal (i.e., biliary) excretion accounts for approximately 11–12% of benazeprilat excretion in healthy subjects. In patients with renal failure, biliary clearance may compensate to an extent for deficient renal clearance.
In patients with hepatic dysfunction due to cirrhosis, levels of benazeprilat are essentially unaltered. The pharmacokinetics of benazepril and benazeprilat do not appear to be influenced by age.
In studies in rats given ^{14}C-benazepril, benazepril and its metabolites crossed the blood-brain barrier only to an extremely low extent. Multiple doses of benazepril did not result in accumulation in any tissue except the lung, where, as with other ACE inhibitors in similar studies, there was a slight increase in concentration due to slow elimination in that organ.
Some placental passage occurred when the drug was administered to pregnant rats.
Pharmacodynamics
Single and multiple doses of 10 mg or more of Lotensin cause inhibition of plasma ACE activity by at least 80–90% for at least 24 hours after dosing. Pressor responses to exogenous angiotensin I were inhibited by 60–90% (up to 4 hours post-dose) at the 10 mg dose.
Administration of Lotensin to patients with mild-to-moderate hypertension results in reduction of both supine and standing blood pressure to about the same extent with no compensatory tachycardia. Symptomatic postural hypotension is infrequent, although it can occur in patients who are salt- and/or volume-depleted (see WARNINGS).
In single-dose studies, Lotensin lowered blood pressure within 1 hour, with peak reductions achieved 2–4 hours after dosing. The antihypertensive effect of a single dose persisted for 24 hours. In multiple dose studies, once-daily doses of 20–80 mg decreased seated pressure (systolic/diastolic) 24 hours after dosing by about 6–12/4–7 mmHg. The trough values represent reductions of about 50% of that seen at peak.
Four dose-response studies using once-daily dosing were conducted in 470 mild-to-moderate hypertensive patients not using diuretics. The minimal effective once-daily dose of Lotensin was 10 mg; but further falls in blood pressure, especially at morning trough, were seen with higher doses in the studied dosing range (10–80 mg). In studies comparing the same daily dose of Lotensin given as a single morning dose or as a twice-daily dose, blood pressure reductions at the time of morning trough blood levels were greater with the divided regimen.
During chronic therapy, the maximum reduction in blood pressure with any dose is generally achieved after 1–2 weeks. The antihypertensive effects of Lotensin have continued during therapy for at least two years. Abrupt withdrawal of Lotensin has not been associated with a rapid increase in blood pressure.
In patients with mild-to-moderate hypertension, Lotensin 10–20 mg was similar in effectiveness to captopril, hydrochlorothiazide, nifedipine SR, and propranolol.
In antihypertensive effects of Lotensin were not appreciably different in patients receiving high- or low-sodium diets.
In hemodynamic studies in dogs, blood pressure reduction was accompanied by a reduction in peripheral arterial resistance, with an increase in cardiac output and renal blood flow and little or no change in heart rate. In normal human volunteers, single doses of benazepril caused an increase in renal blood flow but had no effect on glomerular filtration rate.
Use of Lotensin in combination with thiazide diuretics gives a blood-pressure-lowering effect greater than that seen with either agent alone. By blocking the renin-angiotensin-aldosterone axis, administration of Lotensin tends to reduce the potassium loss associated with the diuretic.

INDICATIONS AND USAGE
Lotensin is indicated for the treatment of hypertension. It may be used alone or in combination with thiazide diuretics.
In using Lotensin, consideration should be given to the fact that another angiotensin-converting enzyme inhibitor, captopril, has caused agranulocytosis, particularly in patients with renal impairment or collagen-vascular disease. Available data are insufficient to show that Lotensin does not have a similar risk (see WARNINGS).

CONTRAINDICATIONS
Lotensin is contraindicated in patients who are hypersensitive to this product or to any other ACE inhibitor.

WARNINGS
Angioedema
Angioedema of the face, extremities, lips, tongue, glottis, and larynx has been reported in patients treated with angiotensin-converting enzyme inhibitors. In U.S. clinical trials, symptoms consistent with angioedema were seen in none of the subjects who received placebo and in about 0.5% of the subjects who received Lotensin. Angioedema associated with laryngeal edema can be fatal. If laryngeal stridor or angioedema of the face, tongue, or glottis occurs, treatment with Lotensin should be discontinued and appropriate therapy instituted immediately. **Where there is involvement of the tongue, glottis, or larynx, likely to cause airway obstruction, appropriate therapy, e.g., subcutaneous epinephrine injection 1:1000 (0.3 mL to 0.5 mL) should be promptly administered (see ADVERSE REACTIONS).**
Hypotension
Lotensin can cause symptomatic hypotension. Like other ACE inhibitors, benazepril has been only rarely associated with hypotension in uncomplicated hypertensive patients. Symptomatic hypotension is most likely to occur in patients who have been volume- and/or salt-depleted as a result of prolonged diuretic therapy, dietary salt restriction, dialysis, diarrhea, or vomiting. Volume- and/or salt-depletion should be corrected before initiating therapy with Lotensin.
In patients with congestive heart failure, with or without associated renal insufficiency, ACE inhibitor therapy may cause excessive hypotension, which may be associated with oliguria or azotemia and, rarely, with acute renal failure and death. In such patients, Lotensin therapy should be started under close medical supervision; they should be followed closely for the first 2 weeks of treatment and whenever the dose of benazepril or diuretic is increased.
If hypotension occurs, the patient should be placed in a supine position, and, if necessary, treated with intravenous infusion of physiological saline. Lotensin treatment usually can be continued following restoration of blood pressure and volume.
Neutropenia/Agranulocytosis
Another angiotensin-converting enzyme inhibitor, captopril, has been shown to cause agranulocytosis and bone marrow depression, rarely in uncomplicated patients, but more frequently in patients with renal impairment, especially if they also have a collagen-vascular disease such as systemic lupus erythematosus or scleroderma. Available data from clinical trials of benazepril are insufficient to show that benazepril does not cause agranulocytosis at similar rates. Monitoring of white blood cell counts should be considered in patients with collagen-vascular disease, especially if the disease is associated with impaired renal function.
Fetal/Neonatal Morbidity and Mortality
ACE inhibitors can cause fetal and neonatal morbidity and death when administered to pregnant women.
Several dozen cases have been reported in the world literature. When pregnancy is detected, ACE inhibitors should be discontinued as soon as possible.
The use of ACE inhibitors during the second and third trimesters of pregnancy has been associated with fetal and neonatal injury, including hypotension, neonatal skull hypoplasia, anuria, reversible or irreversible renal failure, and death. Oligohydramnios has also been reported, presumably resulting from decreased fetal renal function; oligohydramnios in this setting has been associated with fetal limb con-

tractures, craniofacial deformation, and hypoplastic lung development. Prematurity, intrauterine growth retardation, and patent ductus arteriosus have also been reported, although it is not clear whether these occurrences were due to the ACE inhibitor exposure.

These adverse effects do not appear to have resulted from intrauterine ACE inhibitor exposure that has been limited to the first trimester. Mothers whose embryos and fetuses are exposed to ACE inhibitors only during the first trimester should be so informed. Nonetheless, when patients become pregnant, physicians should make every effort to discontinue the use of benazepril as soon as possible.

Rarely (probably less often than once in every thousand pregnancies), no alternative to ACE inhibitors will be found. In these rare cases, the mothers should be apprised of the potential hazards to their fetuses, and serial ultrasound examinations should be performed to assess the intraamniotic environment.

If oligohydramnios is observed, benazepril should be discontinued unless it is considered life-saving for the mother. Contraction stress testing (CST), a nonstress test (NST), or biophysical profiling (BPP) may be appropriate, depending upon the week of pregnancy. Patients and physicians should be aware, however, that oligohydramnios may not appear until after the fetus has sustained irreversible injury.

Infants with histories of *in utero* exposure to ACE inhibitors should be closely observed for hypotension, oliguria, and hyperkalemia. If oliguria occurs, attention should be directed toward support of blood pressure and renal perfusion. Exchange transfusion or dialysis may be required as means of reversing hypotension and/or substituting for disordered renal function. Benazepril, which crosses the placenta, can theoretically be removed from the neonatal circulation by these means; there are occasional reports of benefit from these maneuvers with another ACE inhibitor, but experience is limited.

No teratogenic effects of Lotensin were seen in studies of pregnant rats, mice, and rabbits. On a mg/m^2 basis, the doses used in these studies were 60 times (in rats), 9 times (in mice), and more than 0.8 times (in rabbits) the maximum recommended human dose (assuming a 50 kg woman). On a mg/kg basis these multiples are 300 times (in rats), 90 times (in mice) and more than 3 times (in rabbits) the maximum recommended human dose.

PRECAUTIONS

General

Impaired Renal Function: As a consequence of inhibiting the renin-angiotensin-aldosterone system, changes in renal function may be anticipated in susceptible individuals. In patients with severe congestive heart failure whose renal function may depend on the activity of the renin-angiotensin-aldosterone system, treatment with angiotensin-converting enzyme inhibitors, including Lotensin, may be associated with oliguria and/or progressive azotemia and (rarely) with acute renal failure and/or death. In a small study of hypertensive patients with renal artery stenosis in a solitary kidney or bilateral renal artery stenosis, treatment with Lotensin was associated with increases in blood urea nitrogen and serum creatinine; these increases were reversible upon discontinuation of Lotensin or diuretic therapy, or both. When such patients are treated with ACE inhibitors, renal function should be monitored during the first few weeks of therapy. Some hypertensive patients with no apparent preexisting renal vascular disease have developed increases in blood urea nitrogen and serum creatinine, usually minor and transient, especially when Lotensin has been given concomitantly with a diuretic. This is more likely to occur in patients with preexisting renal impairment. Dosage reduction of Lotensin and/or discontinuation of the diuretic may be required. **Evaluation of the hypertensive patient should always include assessment of renal function (see DOSAGE AND ADMINISTRATION).**

Hyperkalemia: In clinical trials, hyperkalemia (serum potassium at least 0.5 mEq/L greater than the upper limit of normal) occurred in approximately 1% of hypertensive patients receiving Lotensin. In most cases, these were isolated values which resolved despite continued therapy. Risk factors for the development of hyperkalemia include renal insufficiency, diabetes mellitus, and the concomitant use of potassium-sparing diuretics, potassium supplements, and/or potassium-containing salt substitutes, which should be used cautiously, if at all, with Lotensin (see Drug Interactions).

Cough: Cough has been reported with the use of ACE inhibitors. Characteristically, the cough is nonproductive, persistent, and resolves after discontinuation of therapy. ACE inhibitor-induced cough should be considered as part of the differential diagnosis of cough.

Impaired Liver Function: In patients with hepatic dysfunction due to cirrhosis, levels of benazeprilat are essentially unaltered.

Surgery/Anesthesia: In patients undergoing surgery or during anesthesia with agents that produce hypotension, benazepril will block the angiotensin II formation that could otherwise occur secondary to compensatory renin release. Hypotension that occurs as a result of this mechanism can be corrected by volume expansion.

Information for Patients

Pregnancy: Female patients of childbearing age should be told about the consequences of second- and third-trimester exposure to ACE inhibitors, and they should also be told that these consequences do not appear to have resulted from intrauterine ACE inhibitor exposure that has been limited to the first trimester. These patients should be asked to report pregnancies to their physicians as soon as possible.

Angioedema: Angioedema, including laryngeal edema, can occur with treatment with ACE inhibitors, especially following the first dose. Patients should be so advised and told to report immediately any signs or symptoms suggesting angioedema (swelling of face, eyes, lips, or tongue, or difficulty in breathing) and to take no more drug until they have consulted with the prescribing physician.

Symptomatic Hypotension: Patients should be cautioned that lightheadedness can occur, especially during the first days of therapy, and it should be reported to the prescribing physician. Patients should be told that if syncope occurs, Lotensin should be discontinued until the prescribing physician has been consulted.

All patients should be cautioned that inadequate fluid intake or excessive perspiration, diarrhea, or vomiting can lead to an excessive fall in blood pressure, with the same consequences of lightheadedness and possible syncope.

Hyperkalemia: Patients should be told not to use potassium supplements or salt substitutes containing potassium without consulting the prescribing physician.

Neutropenia: Patients should be told to promptly report any indication of infection (e.g., sore throat, fever), which could be a sign of neutropenia.

Drug Interactions

Diuretics: Patients on diuretics, especially those in whom diuretic therapy was recently instituted, may occasionally experience an excessive reduction of blood pressure after initiation of therapy with Lotensin. The possibility of hypotensive effects with Lotensin can be minimized by either discontinuing the diuretic or increasing the salt intake prior to initiation of treatment with Lotensin. If this is not possible, the starting dose should be reduced (see DOSAGE AND ADMINISTRATION).

Potassium Supplements and Potassium-Sparing Diuretics: Lotensin can attenuate potassium loss caused by thiazide diuretics. Potassium-sparing diuretics (spironolactone, amiloride, triamterene, and others) or potassium supplements can increase the risk of hyperkalemia. Therefore, if concomitant use of such agents is indicated, they should be given with caution, and the patient's serum potassium should be monitored frequently.

Oral Anticoagulants: Interaction studies with warfarin and acenocoumarol failed to identify any clinically important effects on the serum concentrations or clinical effects of these anticoagulants.

Lithium: Increased serum lithium levels and symptoms of lithium toxicity have been reported in patients receiving ACE inhibitors during therapy with lithium. These drugs should be coadministered with caution, and frequent monitoring of serum lithium levels is recommended. If a diuretic is also used, the risk of lithium toxicity may be increased.

Other: No clinically important pharmacokinetic interactions occurred when Lotensin was administered concomitantly with hydrochlorothiazide, chlorthalidone, furosemide, digoxin, propranolol, atenolol, naproxen, or cimetidine.

Lotensin has been used concomitantly with beta-adrenergic-blocking agents, calcium-channel-blocking agents, diuretics, digoxin, and hydralazine, without evidence of clinically important adverse interactions. Benazepril, like other ACE inhibitors, has had less than additive effects with beta-adrenergic blockers, presumably because both drugs lower blood pressure by inhibiting parts of the renin-angiotensin system.

Carcinogenesis, Mutagenesis, Impairment of Fertility

No evidence of carcinogenicity was found when benazepril was administered to rats and mice for up to two years at doses of up to 150 mg/kg/day. When compared on the basis of body weights, this dose is 110 times the maximum recommended human dose. When compared on the basis of body surface areas, this dose is 18 and 9 times (rats and mice, respectively) the maximum recommended human dose (calculations assume a patient weight of 60 kg). No mutagenic activity was detected in the Ames test in bacteria (with or without metabolic activation), in an in vitro test for forward mutations in cultured mammalian cells, or in a nucleus anomaly test. In doses of 50–500 mg/kg/day (6–60 times the maximum recommended human dose based on mg/m^2 comparison and 37–375 times the maximum recommended human dose based on a mg/kg comparison), Lotensin had no adverse effect on the reproductive performance of male and female rats.

Pregnancy Categories C (first trimester) and D (second and third trimesters)

See WARNINGS, Fetal/Neonatal Morbidity and Mortality.

Nursing Mothers

Minimal amounts of unchanged benazepril and of benazeprilat are excreted into the breast milk of lactating women treated with benazepril. A newborn child ingesting entirely breast milk would receive less than 0.1% of the mg/kg maternal dose of benazepril and benazeprilat.

Geriatric Use

Of the total number of patients who received benazepril in U.S. clinical studies of Lotensin, 18% were 65 or older while 2% were 75 or older. No overall differences in effectiveness or safety were observed between these patients and younger patients, and other reported clinical experience has not identified differences in responses between the elderly and younger patients, but greater sensitivity of some older individuals cannot be ruled out.

Pediatric Use

Safety and effectiveness in children have not been established.

ADVERSE REACTIONS

Lotensin has been evaluated for safety in over 6000 patients with hypertension; over 700 of these patients were treated for at least one year. The overall incidence of reported adverse events was comparable in Lotensin and placebo patients.

The reported side effects were generally mild and transient, and there was no relation between side effects and age, duration of therapy, or total dosage within the range of 2 to 80 mg. Discontinuation of therapy because of a side effect was required in approximately 5% of U.S. patients treated with Lotensin and in 3% of patients treated with placebo.

The most common reasons for discontinuation were headache (0.6%) and cough (0.5%). (See PRECAUTIONS, Cough).

The side effects considered possibly or probably related to study drug that occurred in U.S. placebo-controlled trials in more than 1% of patients treated with Lotensin are shown below.

PATIENTS IN U.S. PLACEBO-CONTROLLED STUDIES

	LOTENSIN (N=964)		PLACEBO (N=496)	
	N	%	N	%
Headache	60	6.2	21	4.2
Dizziness	35	3.6	12	2.4
Fatigue	23	2.4	11	2.2
Somnolence	15	1.6	2	0.4
Postural Dizziness	14	1.5	1	0.2
Nausea	13	1.3	5	1.0
Cough	12	1.2	5	1.0

Other adverse experiences reported in controlled clinical trials (in less than 1% of benazepril patients), and rarer events seen in postmarketing experience, include the following (in some, a causal relationship to drug use is uncertain):

Cardiovascular: Symptomatic hypotension was seen in 0.3% of patients, postural hypotension in 0.4%, and syncope in 0.1%; these reactions led to discontinuation of therapy in 4 patients who had received benazepril monotherapy and in 9 patients who had received benazepril with hydrochlorothiazide (see PRECAUTIONS and WARNINGS). Other reports include angina pectoris, palpitations, and peripheral edema.

Renal: Of hypertensive patients with no apparent preexisting renal disease, about 2% have sustained increases in serum creatinine to at least 150% of their baseline values while receiving Lotensin, but most of these increases have disappeared despite continuing treatment. A much smaller fraction of these patients (less than 0.1%) developed simultaneous (usually transient) increases in blood urea nitrogen and serum creatinine.

Fetal/Neonatal Morbidity and Mortality: See WARNINGS, Fetal/Neonatal Morbidity and Mortality.

Angioedema: Angioedema has been reported in patients receiving ACE inhibitors. During clinical trials in hypertensive patients with benazepril, 0.5% of patients experienced edema of the lips or face without other manifestations of angioedema. Angioedema associated with laryngeal edema and/or shock may be fatal. If angioedema of the face, extremities, lips, tongue, or glottis and/or larynx occurs, treatment with Lotensin should be discontinued and appropriate therapy instituted immediately (see WARNINGS).

Gastrointestinal: Constipation, gastritis, vomiting, and melena.

Dermatologic: Apparent hypersensitivity reactions (manifested by dermatitis, pruritis, or rash) and flushing.

Neurologic and Psychiatric: Anxiety, decreased libido, hypertonia, insomnia, nervousness, and paresthesia.

Continued on next page

The full prescribing information for each CIBA product is contained herein and is that in effect as of September 1, 1992.

CIBA—Cont.

Dose	Tablet Color	Bottle of 100	Accu-Pak® of 100
5 mg	light yellow	NDC 0083-0059-30	NDC 0083-0059-32
10 mg	dark yellow	NDC 0083-0063-30	NDC 0083-0063-32
20 mg	tan	NDC 0083-0079-30	NDC 0083-0079-32
40 mg	dark rose	NDC 0083-0094-30	NDC 0083-0094-32

Other: Arthralgia, arthritis, asthenia, asthma, bronchitis, dyspnea, impotence, infection, myalgia, sinusitis, sweating, and urinary tract infection.

Clinical Laboratory Test Findings

Creatinine and Blood Urea Nitrogen: Of hypertensive patients with no apparent preexisting renal disease, about 2% have sustained increases in serum creatinine to at least 150% of their baseline values while receiving Lotensin, but most of these increases have disappeared despite continuing treatment. A much smaller fraction of these patients (less than 0.1%) developed simultaneous (usually transient) increases in blood urea nitrogen and serum creatinine. None of these increases required discontinuation of treatment. Increases in these laboratory values are more likely to occur in patients with renal insufficiency or those pretreated with a diuretic and, based on experience with other ACE inhibitors, would be expected to be especially likely in patients with renal artery stenosis (see PRECAUTIONS, General).

Potassium: Since benazepril decreases aldosterone secretion, elevation of serum potassium can occur. Potassium supplements and potassium-sparing diuretics should be given with caution, and the patient's serum potassium should be monitored frequently (see PRECAUTIONS).

Hemoglobin: Decreases in hemoglobin (a low value and a decrease of 5 g/dL) were rare, occurring in only 1 of 2014 patients receiving Lotensin alone and in 1 of 1357 patients receiving Lotensin plus a diuretic. No U.S. patients discontinued treatment because of decreases in hemoglobin.

Other (causal relationships unknown): Clinically important changes in standard laboratory tests were rarely associated with Lotensin administration. Elevations of liver enzymes, serum bilirubin, uric acid, and blood glucose have been reported, as have scattered incidents of hyponatremia, electrocardiographic changes, leukopenia, eosinophilia, and proteinuria. In U.S. trials, less than 0.5% of patients discontinued treatment because of laboratory abnormalities.

OVERDOSAGE

Single oral doses of 3 g/kg benazepril were associated with significant lethality in mice. Rats however, tolerated single oral doses of up to 6 g/kg. Reduced activity was seen at 1 g/kg in mice and at 5 g/kg in rats. Human overdoses of benazepril have not been reported, but the most common manifestation of human benazepril overdosage is likely to be hypotension.

Laboratory determinations of serum levels of benazepril and its metabolites are not widely available, and such determinations have, in any event, no established role in the management of benazepril overdose.

No data are available to suggest physiological maneuvers (e.g., maneuvers to change the pH of the urine) that might accelerate elimination of benazepril and its metabolites. Benazeprilat can be removed from the body by dialysis, but this intervention should rarely, if ever, be required.

Angiotensin II could presumably serve as a specific antagonist-antidote in the setting of benazepril overdose, but angiotensin II is essentially unavailable outside of scattered research facilities. Because the hypotensive effect of benazepril is achieved through vasodilation and effective hypovolemia, it is reasonable to treat benazepril overdose by infusion of normal saline solution.

DOSAGE AND ADMINISTRATION

The recommended initial dose for patients not receiving a diuretic is 10 mg once-a-day. The usual maintenance dosage range is 20–40 mg per day administered as a single dose or in two equally divided doses. A dose of 80 mg gives an increased response, but experience with this dose is limited. The divided regimen was more effective in controlling trough (predosing) blood pressure than the same dose given as a once-daily regimen. Dosage adjustment should be based on measurement of peak (2–6 hours after dosing) and trough responses. If a once-daily regimen does not give adequate trough response an increase in dosage or divided administration should be considered. If blood pressure is not controlled with Lotensin alone, a diuretic can be added.

Total daily doses above 80 mg have not been evaluated.

Concomitant administration of Lotensin with potassium supplements, potassium salt substitutes, or potassium-sparing diuretics can lead to increases of serum potassium (see PRECAUTIONS).

In patients who are currently being treated with a diuretic, symptomatic hypotension occasionally can occur following the initial dose of Lotensin. To reduce the likelihood of hypotension, the diuretic should, if possible, be discontinued two to three days prior to beginning therapy with Lotensin (see WARNINGS). Then, if blood pressure is not controlled with Lotensin alone, diuretic therapy should be resumed.

If the diuretic cannot be discontinued, an initial dose of 5 mg Lotensin should be used to avoid excessive hypotension.

Dosage Adjustment in Renal Impairment

For patients with a creatinine clearance < 30 mL/min/1.73 m^2 (serum creatinine > 3 mg/dL), the recommended initial dose is 5 mg Lotensin once daily. Dosage may be titrated upward until blood pressure is controlled or to a maximum total daily dose of 40 mg.

HOW SUPPLIED

Lotensin is available in tablets of 5 mg, 10 mg, 20 mg, and 40 mg, packaged with a desiccant in bottles of 100 tablets. Lotensin is also supplied in blister packages (1 tablet/blister), in Accu-Pak® Unit Dose boxes containing 10 strips of 10 blisters each.

Each tablet is imprinted with LOTENSIN on one side and the tablet strength ("5", "10", "20", or "40") on the other. Samples, when available, are identified by the word *SAMPLE* on each tablet.

The National Drug Codes for the various packages are: [See table above.]

Storage: Do not store above 86°F (30°C). Protect from moisture.

Dispense in tight container (USP).

CIBA C92-18 (Rev. 3/92)

Dist. by:
CIBA Pharmaceutical Company
Division of CIBA-GEIGY Corporation
Summit, New Jersey 07901

Shown in Product Identification Section, page 408

LUDIOMIL® ℞

[loó-dee-oh-mill]

(maprotiline hydrochloride)
Tablets

DESCRIPTION

Ludiomil, maprotiline hydrochloride USP, is a tetracyclic antidepressant, available as 25-mg, 50-mg and 75-mg tablets for oral administration. Its chemical name is N-methyl-9,10-ethanoanthracene-9(10H)-propylamine hydrochloride.

Maprotiline hydrochloride USP is a fine, white to off-white, practically odorless crystalline powder. It is freely soluble in methanol and in chloroform, slightly soluble in water, and practically insoluble in isooctane. Its molecular weight is 313.87.

Inactive Ingredients. Calcium phosphate, cellulose compounds, colloidal silicon dioxide, FD&C Yellow No. 6 Aluminum Lake (25-mg and 50-mg tablets), lactose, magnesium stearate, povidone, shellac, starch, stearic acid, talc, and titanium dioxide.

CLINICAL PHARMACOLOGY

The mechanism of action of Ludiomil is not precisely known. It does not act primarily by stimulation of the central nervous system and is not a monoamine oxidase inhibitor. The postulated mechanism of Ludiomil is that it acts primarily by potentiation of central adrenergic synapses by blocking reuptake of norepinephrine at nerve endings. This pharmacologic action is thought to be responsible for the drug's antidepressant and anxiolytic effects.

The mean time to peak is 12 hours. The half-life of elimination averages 51 hours.

Steady-state levels measured prior to the morning dose on a one-dosage regimen are summarized as follows:

Regimen	Average Minimum Concentration ng/ml	95% Confidence Limits ng/ml
50 mg x 3 daily	238	181–295

INDICATIONS AND USAGE

Ludiomil is indicated for the treatment of depressive illness in patients with depressive neurosis (dysthymic disorder) and manic-depressive illness, depressed type (major depressive disorder). Ludiomil is also effective for the relief of anxiety associated with depression.

CONTRAINDICATIONS

Ludiomil is contraindicated in patients hypersensitive to Ludiomil and in patients with known or suspected seizure disorders. It should not be given concomitantly with monoamine oxidase (MAO) inhibitors. A minimum of 14 days should be allowed to elapse after discontinuation of MAO inhibitors before treatment with Ludiomil is initiated. Effects should be monitored with gradual increase in dosage until optimum response is achieved. The drug is not recommended for use during the acute phase of myocardial infarction.

WARNINGS

Seizures have been associated with the use of Ludiomil.

Most of the seizures have occurred in patients without a known history of seizures. However, in some of these cases, other confounding factors were present, including concomitant medications known to lower the seizure threshold, rapid escalation of the dosage of Ludiomil, and dosage that exceeded the recommended therapeutic range. The incidence of direct reports is less than $\frac{1}{10}$ of 1%. The risk of seizures may be increased when Ludiomil is taken concomitantly with phenothiazines, when the dosage of benzodiazepines is rapidly tapered in patients receiving Ludiomil or when the recommended dosage of Ludiomil is exceeded. While a cause-and-effect relationship has not been established, the risk of seizures in patients treated with Ludiomil may be reduced by (1) initiating therapy at a low dosage, (2) maintaining the initial dosage for 2 weeks before raising it gradually in small increments as necessitated by the long half-life of Ludiomil (average 51 hours), and (3) keeping the dosage at the minimally effective level during maintenance therapy. (See **DOSAGE AND ADMINISTRATION.)**

Extreme caution should be used when this drug is given to:
—patients with a history of myocardial infarction;
—patients with a history or presence of cardiovascular disease because of the possibility of conduction defects, arrhythmias, myocardial infarction, strokes and tachycardia.

PRECAUTIONS

General: The possibility of suicide in seriously depressed patients is inherent in their illness and may persist until significant remission occurs. Therefore, patients must be carefully supervised during all phases of treatment with Ludiomil, and prescriptions should be written for the smallest number of tablets consistent with good patient management.

Hypomanic or manic episodes have been known to occur in some patients taking tricyclic antidepressant drugs, particularly in patients with cyclic disorders. Such occurrences have also been noted, rarely, with Ludiomil.

Prior to elective surgery, Ludiomil should be discontinued for as long as clinically feasible, since little is known about the interaction between Ludiomil and general anesthetics.

Ludiomil should be administered with caution in patients with increased intraocular pressure, history of urinary retention, or history of narrow-angle glaucoma because of the drug's anticholinergic properties.

Information for Patients: Patients should be warned of the association between seizures and the use of Ludiomil. Moreover, they should be informed that this association is enhanced in patients with a known history of seizures and in those patients who are taking certain other drugs. (See **WARNINGS.)**

Warn patients to exercise caution about potentially hazardous tasks, or operating automobiles or machinery since the drug may impair mental and/or physical abilities.

Ludiomil may enhance the response to alcohol, barbiturates, and other CNS depressants, requiring appropriate caution of administration.

Laboratory Tests: Ludiomil should be discontinued if there is evidence of pathological neutrophil depression. Leukocyte and differential counts should be performed in patients who develop fever and sore throat during therapy.

Drug Interactions: Close supervision and careful adjustment of dosage are required when administering Ludiomil concomitantly with anticholinergic or sympathomimetic drugs because of the possibility of additive atropine-like effects.

Concurrent administration of Ludiomil with electroshock therapy should be avoided because of the lack of experience in this area.

Caution should be exercised when administering Ludiomil to hyperthyroid patients or those on thyroid medication because of the possibility of enhanced potential for cardiovascular toxicity of Ludiomil.

Ludiomil should be used with caution in patients receiving guanethidine or similar agents since it may block the pharmacologic effects of these drugs.

The risk of seizures may be increased when Ludiomil is taken concomitantly with phenothiazines or when the dosage of benzodiazepines is rapidly tapered in patients receiving Ludiomil.

Because of the pharmacologic similarity of Ludiomil to the tricyclic antidepressants, the plasma concentration of Ludiomil may be increased when the drug is given concomitantly with hepatic enzyme inhibitors (e.g., cemetidine, fluoxetine) and decreased by concomitant administration with hepatic enzyme enducers (e.g., barbiturates, phenytoin), as has occurred with tricyclic antidepressants. Adjustment of the dosage of Ludiomil may therefore be necessary in such cases. (See **Information for Patients.)**

Carcinogenesis, Mutagenesis, Impairment of Fertility: Carcinogenicity and chronic toxicity studies have been conducted in laboratory rats and dogs. No drug- or dose-related occurrence of carcinogenesis was evident in rats receiving

daily oral doses up to 60 mg/kg of Ludiomil for eighteen months or in dogs receiving daily oral doses up to 30 mg/kg of Ludiomil for one year. In addition, no evidence of mutagenic activity was found in offspring of female mice mated with males treated with up to 60 times the maximum daily human dose.

Pregnancy Category B: Reproduction studies have been performed in female laboratory rabbits, mice, and rats at doses up to 1.3, 7, and 9 times the maximum daily human dose respectively and have revealed no evidence of impaired fertility or harm to the fetus due to Ludiomil. There are, however, no adequate and well-controlled studies in pregnant women. Because animal reproduction studies are not always predictive of human response, this drug should be used during pregnancy only if clearly needed.

Labor and Delivery: Although the effect of Ludiomil on labor and delivery is unknown, caution should be exercised as with any drug with CNS depressant action.

Nursing Mothers: Ludiomil is excreted in breast milk. At steady state, the concentrations in milk correspond closely to the concentrations in whole blood. Caution should be exercised when Ludiomil is administered to a nursing woman.

Pediatric Use: Safety and effectiveness in children below the age of 18 have not been established.

ADVERSE REACTIONS

The following adverse reactions have been noted with Ludiomil and are generally similar to those observed with tricyclic antidepressants.

Cardiovascular: Rare occurrences of hypotension, hypertension, tachycardia, palpitation, arrhythmia, heart block, and syncope have been reported with Ludiomil.

Psychiatric: Nervousness (6%), anxiety (3%), insomnia (2%), and agitation (2%); rarely, confusional states (especially in the elderly), hallucinations, disorientation, delusions, restlessness, nightmares, hypomania, mania, exacerbation of psychosis, decrease in memory, and feelings of unreality.

Neurological: Drowsiness (16%), dizziness (8%), tremor (3%), and, rarely, numbness, tingling, motor hyperactivity, akathisia, seizures, EEG alterations, tinnitus, extrapyramidal symptoms, ataxia, and dysarthria.

Anticholinergic: Dry mouth (22%), constipation (6%), and blurred vision (4%); rarely, accommodation disturbances, mydriasis, urinary retention, and delayed micturition.

Allergic: Rare instances of skin rash, petechiae, itching, photosensitization, edema, and drug fever.

Gastrointestinal: Nausea (2%) and, rarely, vomiting, epigastric distress, diarrhea, bitter taste, abdominal cramps and dysphagia.

Endocrine: Rare instances of increased or decreased libido, impotence, and elevation or depression of blood sugar levels.

Other: Weakness and fatigue (4%) and headache (4%); rarely, altered liver function, jaundice, weight loss or gain, excessive perspiration, flushing, urinary frequency, increased salivation, nasal congestion and alopecia.

Note: Although there have been only isolated reports of the following adverse reactions with Ludiomil, its pharmacologic similarity to tricyclic antidepressants requires that each reaction be considered when administering Ludiomil.

—Bone marrow depression, including agranulocytosis, eosinophilia, purpura, and thrombocytopenia, myocardial infarction, stroke, peripheral neuropathy, sublingual adenitis, black tongue, stomatitis, paralytic ileus, gynecomastia in the male, breast enlargement and galactorrhea in the female, and testicular swelling.

Post-Introduction Reports: Several voluntary reports of interstitial pneumonitis, which were in some cases associated with eosinophilia and increased liver enzymes, have been received since market introduction. However, there is no clear causal relationship.

OVERDOSAGE

Animal Oral LD_{50}: The oral LD_{50} of Ludiomil is 600–750 mg/kg in mice, 760–900 mg/kg in rats, > 1000 mg/kg in rabbits, > 300 mg/kg in cats, and > 30 mg/kg in dogs.

Signs and Symptoms: Data dealing with overdosage in humans are limited with only a few cases on record. Symptoms are drowsiness, tachycardia, ataxia, vomiting, cyanosis, hypotension, shock, restlessness, agitation, hyperpyrexia, muscle rigidity, athetoid movements, mydriasis, cardiac arrhythmias, impaired cardiac condition. In severe cases, loss of consciousness and generalized convulsions may occur. Since congestive heart failure has been seen with overdosages of tricyclic antidepressants, it should be considered with Ludiomil overdosage.

Treatment: The recommended treatment for overdosage with heterocyclics may change periodically. Therefore, it is recommended that the physician contact a poison control center for current information on treatment. Because CNS involvement, respiratory depression, and cardiac arrhythmia can occur suddenly, hospitalization and close observation may be necessary, even when the amount ingested is thought to be small or the initial degree of intoxication appears slight or moderate. All patients with ECG abnormalities should have continuous cardiac monitoring and be closely observed until well after the cardiac status has returned to normal; relapses may occur after apparent recovery.

In the alert patient, the stomach should be emptied promptly by lavage. In the obtunded patient, the airway should be secured with a cuffed endotracheal tube before beginning lavage (do not induce emesis). Instillation of an activated charcoal slurry may help reduce the absorption of Ludiomil. The room should be darkened, allowing only minimal external stimulation to reduce the tendency to convulsions. If anticonvulsants are necessary, diazepam and phenytoin may be useful. Adequate respiratory exchange should be maintained, including intubation and artificial respiration, if necessary.

Since it has been reported that physostigmine increases the risk of seizures, its use is not recommended in cases of overdosage with Ludiomil.

Shock (circulatory collapse) should be treated with supportive measures such as appropriate position, intravenous fluids, and vasopressors if necessary.

Hyperpyrexia should be controlled by whatever means available, including ice packs if necessary.

Digitalis may increase conduction abnormalities and further irritate an already sensitized myocardium. If congestive heart failure necessitates rapid digitalization, particular care must be exercised.

Dialysis is of little value because of the low plasma concentration of this drug.

DOSAGE AND ADMINISTRATION

A single daily dose is an alternative to divided daily doses. Therapeutic effects are sometimes seen within 3 to 7 days, although as long as 2 to 3 weeks are usually necessary.

Initial Adult Dosage: An initial dosage of 75 mg daily is suggested for outpatients with mild-to-moderate depression. However, in some patients, particularly the elderly, an initial dosage of 25 mg daily may be used. Because of the long half-life of Ludiomil, the initial dosage should be maintained for two weeks. The dosage may then be increased gradually in 25-mg increments as required and tolerated. In most outpatients a maximum dose of 150 mg daily will result in therapeutic efficacy. It is recommended that this dose not be exceeded except in the most severely depressed patients. In such patients, dosage may be gradually increased to a maximum of 225 mg.

More severely depressed, hospitalized patients should be given an initial daily dose of 100 mg to 150 mg which may be gradually increased as required and tolerated. Most hospitalized patients with moderate-to-severe depression respond to a daily dosage of 150 mg although dosages as high as 225 mg may be required in some cases. Daily dosage of 225 mg should not be exceeded.

Elderly Patients: In general, lower dosages are recommended for patients over 60 years of age. Dosages of 50 mg to 75 mg daily are usually satisfactory as maintenance therapy for elderly patients who do not tolerate higher amounts.

Maintenance: Dosage during prolonged maintenance therapy should be kept at the lowest effective level. Dosage may be reduced to levels of 75 mg to 150 mg daily during such periods, with subsequent adjustment depending on therapeutic response.

HOW SUPPLIED

Tablets 25 mg—oval, dark orange, scored, coated (imprinted CIBA 110)

Bottle of 100 .... NDC 0083-0110-30
Accu-Pak® Unit Dose (blister pack)
Box of 100 (strips of 10) .... NDC 0083-0110-32

Tablets 50 mg—round, dark orange, scored, coated (imprinted CIBA 26)

Bottle of 100 .... NDC 0083-0026-30
Accu-Pak® Unit Dose (blister pack)
Box of 100 (strips of 10) .... NDC 0083-0026-32

Tablets 75 mg—oval, white, scored, coated (imprinted CIBA 135)

Bottle of 100 .... NDC 0083-0135-30

Do not store above 86°F (30°C).

Dispense in tight container (USP).

C91-41 (Rev. 1/92)

Shown in Product Identification Section, page 408

METOPIRONE® ℞

[met-oh-pie 'rone]
metyrapone USP
Tablets
Diagnostic Test of Pituitary Adrenocorticotropic Function

DESCRIPTION

Metopirone, metyrapone USP, is an inhibitor of endogenous adrenal corticosteroid synthesis, available as 250-mg tablets for oral administration. Its chemical name is 2-methyl-1,2-di-3-pyridyl-1-propanone.

Metyrapone USP is a white to light amber, fine, crystalline powder, having a characteristic odor. It is sparingly soluble in water, and soluble in methanol and in chloroform. It forms water-soluble salts with acids. Its molecular weight is 226.28.

Inactive Ingredients. Calcium phosphate, colloidal silicon dioxide, gelatin, and magnesium stearate.

CLINICAL PHARMACOLOGY

The pharmacological effect of Metopirone is to reduce cortisol and corticosterone production by inhibiting the 11-β-hydroxylation reaction in the adrenal cortex. Removal of the strong inhibitory feedback mechanism exerted by cortisol results in an increase in adrenocorticotropic hormone (ACTH) production by the pituitary. With continued blockade of the enzymatic steps leading to production of cortisol and corticosterone, there is a marked increase in adrenocortical secretion of their immediate precursors, 11-desoxycortisol and desoxycorticosterone, which are weak suppressors of ACTH release, and a corresponding elevation of these steroids in the plasma and of their metabolites in the urine. These metabolites are readily determined by measuring urinary 17-hydroxycorticosteroids (17-OHCS) or 17-ketogenic steroids (17-KGS). Because of these actions, Metopirone is used as a diagnostic test, with urinary 17-OHCS measured as an index of pituitary ACTH responsiveness. Metopirone may also suppress biosynthesis of aldosterone, resulting in a mild natriuresis.

The response to Metopirone does not occur immediately. Following oral administration, peak steroid excretion occurs during the subsequent 24-hour period. Metopirone is absorbed rapidly and well when administered orally as prescribed. Plasma concentrations during the period of treatment are 0.5–1 μg/ml. The major biotransformation is reduction of the ketone to an alcohol and conjugation of metyrapone and reduced metyrapone to the corresponding glucuronides. The apparent half-life of elimination averages 1–2.5 hours. Within 2 days after initiation of treatment, about 40% of the administered dose is excreted in the urine, mostly in the form of glucuronides.

INDICATIONS AND USAGE

A diagnostic drug for testing hypothalamic-pituitary ACTH function.

CONTRAINDICATIONS

Adrenal cortical insufficiency, hypersensitivity to Metopirone.

WARNINGS

Metopirone may induce acute adrenal insufficiency in patients with reduced adrenal secretory capacity.

PRECAUTIONS

General

Ability of adrenals to respond to exogenous ACTH should be demonstrated before Metopirone is employed as a test. In the presence of hypo- or hyperthyroidism, response to the Metopirone test may be subnormal.

Laboratory Tests

See **INTERPRETATION.**

Drug Interactions

All corticosteroid therapy must be discontinued prior to and during testing with Metopirone.

The metabolism of Metopirone is accelerated by phenytoin; therefore, results of the test may be inaccurate in patients taking phenytoin within two weeks before. A subnormal response may occur in patients on estrogen therapy.

Carcinogenesis, Mutagenesis, Impairment of Fertility

Long-term carcinogenicity and reproduction studies in animals have not been conducted.

Pregnancy Category C

A subnormal response to Metopirone may occur in pregnant women. Animal reproduction studies have not been conducted with Metopirone. The Metopirone test was administered to 20 pregnant women in their second and third trimester of pregnancy and evidence was found that the fetal pituitary responded to the enzymatic block. It is not known if Metopirone can affect reproduction capacity. Metopirone should be given to a pregnant woman only if clearly needed.

Nursing Mothers

It is not known whether this drug is excreted in human milk. Because many drugs are excreted in human milk, a decision should be made whether a woman undergoing the Metopirone test should discontinue nursing for the duration of the test.

Pediatric Use

See **DOSAGE AND ADMINISTRATION.**

Continued on next page

The full prescribing information for each CIBA product is contained herein and is that in effect as of September 1, 1992.

CIBA—Cont.

ADVERSE REACTIONS

Gastrointestinal System: Nausea, abdominal discomfort
Central Nervous System: Headache, dizziness, sedation
Dermatologic System: Allergic rash
Hematologic System: Rarely, decreased white blood cell count or bone marrow depression.

OVERDOSAGE

Acute Toxicity
One case has been recorded in which a 6-year-old girl died after two doses of Metopirone, 2 g.
Oral LD_{50} in animals (mg/kg): rats, 521; maximum tolerated intravenous dose in one dog, 300.

Signs and Symptoms
The clinical picture of poisoning with Metopirone is characterized by gastrointestinal symptoms and by signs of acute adrenocortical insufficiency.
Cardiovascular System: Cardiac arrhythmias, hypotension, dehydration.
Nervous System and Muscles: Anxiety, confusion, weakness, impairment of consciousness.
Gastrointestinal System: Nausea, vomiting, epigastric pain, diarrhea.
Laboratory Findings: Hyponatremia, hypochloremia, hyperkalemia.

Combined Poisoning
In patients under treatment with insulin or oral antidiabetics, the signs and symptoms of acute poisoning with Metopirone may be aggravated or modified.

Treatment
There is no specific antidote. Besides general measures to eliminate the drug and reduce its absorption, a large dose of hydrocortisone should be administered at once, together with saline and glucose infusions.
Surveillance: For a few days blood pressure and fluid and electrolyte balance should be monitored.

DOSAGE AND ADMINISTRATION

Day 1: Control period—Collect 24-hour urine for measurement of 17-OHCS or 17-KGS.
Day 2: ACTH test to determine the ability of adrenals to respond—Standard ACTH test such as infusion of 50 units ACTH over 8 hours and measurement of 24-hour urinary steroids. If results indicate adequate response, the Metopirone test may proceed.
Day 3–4: Rest period.
Day 5: Administration of Metopirone:
Recommended with milk or snack.
Adults: 750 mg orally, every 4 hours for 6 doses. A single dose is approximately equivalent to 15 mg/kg.
Children: 15 mg/kg orally every 4 hours for 6 doses. A minimal single dose of 250 mg is recommended.
Day 6: After administration of Metopirone— Determination of 24-hour urinary steroids for effect.

INTERPRETATION

ACTH Test
The normal 24-hour urinary excretion of 17-OHCS ranges from 3 to 12 mg. Following continuous intravenous infusion of 50 units ACTH over a period of 8 hours, 17-OHCS excretion increases to 15 to 45 mg per 24 hours.

Metopirone
Normal response: In patients with a normally functioning pituitary, administration of Metopirone is followed by a two- to four-fold increase of 17-OHCS excretion or doubling of 17-KGS excretion.
Subnormal response: Subnormal response in patients without adrenal insufficiency is indicative of some degree of impairment of pituitary function, either panhypopituitarism or partial hypopituitarism (limited pituitary reserve).

1. *Panhypopituitarism* is readily diagnosed by the classical clinical and chemical evidences of hypogonadism, hypothyroidism, and hypoadrenocorticism. These patients usually have subnormal basal urinary steroid levels. Depending upon the duration of the disease and degree of adrenal atrophy, they may fail to respond to exogenous ACTH in the normal manner. Administration of Metopirone is not essential in the diagnosis, but if given, it will not induce an appreciable increase in urinary steroids.
2. *Partial hypopituitarism* or limited pituitary reserve is the more difficult diagnosis as these patients do not present the classical signs and symptoms of hypopituitarism. Measurements of target organ functions often are normal under basal conditions. The response to exogenous ACTH is usually normal, producing the expected rise of urinary steroids (17-OHCS or 17-KGS). The response, however, to Metopirone is *subnormal;* that is, no significant increase in 17-OHCS or 17-KGS excretion occurs.

This failure to respond to metyrapone may be interpreted as evidence of impaired pituitary-adrenal reserve. In view of the normal response to exogenous ACTH, the failure to respond to metyrapone is inferred to be related to a defect in the CNS-pituitary mechanisms which normally regulate ACTH secretions. Presumably the ACTH secreting mechanisms of these individuals are already working at their maximal rates to meet everyday conditions and possess limited "reserve" capacities to secrete additional ACTH either in response to stress or to decreased cortisol levels occurring as a result of metyrapone administration.
Subnormal response in patients with Cushing's syndrome is suggestive of either autonomous adrenal tumors that suppress the ACTH-releasing capacity of the pituitary or nonendocrine ACTH-secreting tumors.
Excessive response: An excessive excretion of 17-OHCS or 17-KGS after administration of Metopirone is suggestive of Cushing's syndrome associated with adrenal hyperplasia. These patients have an elevated excretion of urinary corticosteroids under basal conditions and will often, but not invariably, show a "supernormal" response to ACTH and also to Metopirone, excreting more than 35 mg per 24 hours of either 17-OHCS or 17-KGS.

HOW SUPPLIED

Tablets 250 mg—round, white, scored (imprinted CIBA 130)
Bottles of 18 ....NDC 0083-0130-11
Dispense in tight, light-resistant container (USP).

C86-6 (Rev. 3/86)

Shown in Product Identification Section, page 408

NUPERCAINAL® OTC

[new-purr-cayne 'ull]
Hemorrhoidal and Anesthetic Ointment
Pain-Relief Cream

CAUTION
Nupercainal products are not for prolonged or extensive use and should never be applied in or near the eyes.
Consult labels before using.
Keep this and all medications out of reach of children.
NUPERCAINAL SHOULD NOT BE SWALLOWED. SWALLOWING OR USE OF A LARGE QUANTITY IS HAZARDOUS, PARTICULARLY TO CHILDREN. CONSULT A PHYSICIAN OR POISON CONTROL CENTER IMMEDIATELY. IF THE SYMPTOM BEING TREATED DOES NOT SUBSIDE, OR RASH, IRRITATION, SWELLING, PAIN, BLEEDING OR OTHER SYMPTOMS DEVELOP OR INCREASE, DISCONTINUE USE AND CONSULT A PHYSICIAN.

INDICATIONS

Nupercainal Ointment and Cream are fast-acting, long-lasting pain relievers that you can use for a number of painful skin conditions. **Nupercainal Hemorrhoidal and Anesthetic Ointment** is for hemorrhoids as well as for general use. **Nupercainal Pain-Relief Cream** is for general use only. The **Cream** is half as strong as the **Ointment.**
How to use Nupercainal Anesthetic Ointment (for general use). This soothing Ointment helps lubricate dry, inflamed skin and gives fast, temporary relief of pain, itching, and burning. It is recommended for sunburn, nonpoisonous insect bites, minor burns, cuts, and scratches. **DO NOT USE THIS PRODUCT IN OR NEAR YOUR EYES.**
Apply to affected areas gently. If necessary, cover with a light dressing for protection. Do not use more than 1 ounce of Ointment in a 24-hour period for an adult, do not use more than one-quarter of an ounce in a 24-hour period for a child. If irritation develops, discontinue use and consult your doctor.
How to use Nupercainal Hemorrhoidal and Anesthetic Ointment for fast, temporary relief of pain and itching due to hemorrhoids (also known as piles).
Remove cap from tube and set it aside. Attach the white plastic applicator to the tube. Squeeze the tube until you see the Ointment begin to come through the little holes in the applicator. Using your finger, lubricate the applicator with the Ointment. Now insert the entire applicator gently into the rectum. Give the tube a good squeeze to get enough Ointment into the rectum for comfort and lubrication. Remove applicator from rectum and wipe it clean. Apply additional Ointment to anal tissues to help relieve pain, burning, and itching. For best results use Ointment morning and night and after each bowel movement. After each use detach applicator, and wash it off with soap and water. Put cap back on tube before storing. In case of rectal bleeding, discontinue use and consult your doctor.
Pain-Relief Cream for general use. This Cream is particularly effective for fast, temporary relief of pain and itching associated with sunburn, cuts, scrapes, scratches, minor burns, and nonpoisonous insect bites. **DO NOT USE THIS PRODUCT IN OR NEAR YOUR EYES.** Apply liberally to affected area and rub in gently. This Cream is water-washable, so be sure to reapply after bathing, swimming, or sweating. If irritation develops, discontinue use and consult your doctor.
Nupercainal Hemorrhoidal and Anesthetic Ointment contains 1% dibucaine USP. Also contains acetone sodium bisulfite, lanolin, light mineral oil, purified water, and white petrolatum. Available in tubes of 1 and 2 ounces. Store between 59°–86°F.
Nupercainal Pain-Relief Cream contains 0.5% dibucaine USP. Also contains acetone sodium bisulfite, fragrance, glycerin, potassium hydroxide, purified water, stearic acid, and trolamine. Available in 1½ ounce tubes.
Dibucaine USP is officially classified as a "topical anesthetic" and is one of the strongest and longest lasting of all pain relievers. It is not a narcotic.

C86-62 (Rev. 12/86)

Distributed by:
CIBA CONSUMER PHARMACEUTICALS
EDISON, NEW JERSEY 08837

NUPERCAINAL® OTC

[new-purr-cayne 'ull]
Suppositories

CAUTION
Nupercainal Suppositories are not for prolonged or extensive use. Contact with the eyes should be avoided.
Consult labels before using.
Keep this and all medications out of reach of children.
NUPERCAINAL SUPPOSITORIES SHOULD NOT BE SWALLOWED. SWALLOWING CAN BE HAZARDOUS, PARTICULARLY TO CHILDREN. IN THE EVENT OF ACCIDENTAL SWALLOWING CONSULT A PHYSICIAN OR POISON CONTROL CENTER IMMEDIATELY.

INDICATIONS

Nupercainal Suppositories are for the temporary relief from itching, burning, and discomfort due to hemorrhoids or other anorectal disorders.
How to use Nupercainal Suppositories for hemorrhoids (also known as piles) or other anorectal disorders.
Tear off one suppository along the perforated line. Remove foil wrapper. Insert the suppository, rounded end first, well into the anus until you can feel it moving into your rectum. For best results, use one suppository after each bowel movement and as needed, but not to exceed 6 in a 24-hour period. Each suppository is sealed in its own foil packet to reduce danger of leakage when carried in pocket or purse. **To prevent melting, do not store above 86°F (30°C).**
Nupercainal Suppositories contain 2.4 gram cocoa butter and .25 gram zinc oxide. Also contains acetone sodium bisulfite and bismuth subgallate.

C86-42 (Rev. 9/86)

Distributed by:
CIBA CONSUMER PHARMACEUTICALS
EDISON, NEW JERSEY 08837

PRISCOLINE® hydrochloride ℞

[priss 'coe-leen]
tolazoline hydrochloride USP
Ampuls

DESCRIPTION

Priscoline, tolazoline hydrochloride USP, is a peripheral vasodilator available in ampuls for intravenous administration. Each milliliter of sterile, aqueous solution contains tolazoline hydrochloride USP, 25 mg; tartaric acid ACS, 6.5 mg; and hydrous sodium citrate USP, 6.5 mg. Tolazoline hydrochloride is 4,5-dihydro-2-(phenylmethyl)-1*H*-imidazole monohydrochloride.
Tolazoline hydrochloride USP is a white to off-white crystalline powder. Its solutions are slightly acid to litmus. It is freely soluble in water and in alcohol. Its molecular weight is 196.68.

CLINICAL PHARMACOLOGY

Priscoline is a direct peripheral vasodilator with moderate competitive alpha-adrenergic blocking activity. It decreases peripheral resistance and increases venous capacitance. It has the following additional actions: (1) sympathomimetic, including cardiac stimulation; (2) parasympathomimetic, including gastrointestinal tract stimulation that is blocked by atropine; and (3) histamine-like, including stimulation of gastric secretion and peripheral vasodilatation. Priscoline given intravenously produces vasodilatation, primarily due to a direct effect on vascular smooth muscle, and cardiac stimulation; the blood pressure response depends on the relative contributions of the two effects. Priscoline usually reduces pulmonary arterial pressure and vascular resistance.
In neonates the half-life of Priscoline ranges from 3 to 10 hours.

INDICATIONS AND USAGE

Priscoline is indicated for the treatment of persistent pulmonary hypertension of the newborn ("persistent fetal circulation") when systemic arterial oxygenation cannot be satis-

factorily maintained by usual supportive care (supplemental oxygen and/or mechanical ventilation).

Priscoline should be used in a highly supervised setting, where vital signs, oxygenation, acid-base status, fluid, and electrolytes can be monitored and maintained.

CONTRAINDICATIONS

Priscoline is contraindicated in patients with hypersensitivity to tolazoline.

WARNINGS

Priscoline stimulates gastric secretion and may activate stress ulcers. Through this mechanism, it can produce significant hypochloremic alkalosis. Pretreatment of infants with antacids may prevent gastrointestinal bleeding.

Patients should be observed closely for signs of systemic hypotension, and supportive therapy should be instituted if needed.

In patients with mitral stenosis, parenterally administered Priscoline may produce a rise or fall in pulmonary artery pressure and total pulmonary resistance; therefore, it must be used with caution in patients with known or suspected mitral stenosis.

PRECAUTIONS

General: The effects of Priscoline on pulmonary vessels may be pH dependent. Acidosis may decrease the effect of Priscoline.

Carcinogenesis, Mutagenesis, Impairment of Fertility: Long-term carcinogenicity studies in animals have not been performed with Priscoline.

Pregnancy Category C: Animal reproduction studies have not been conducted with Priscoline. It is also not known whether Priscoline can cause fetal harm when administered to a pregnant woman or can affect reproduction capacity. Priscoline should be given to a pregnant woman only if clearly needed.

Nursing Mothers: It is not known whether this drug is excreted in human milk. Because many drugs are excreted in human milk, caution should be exercised when Priscoline is administered to a nursing woman.

ADVERSE REACTIONS

The following adverse reactions have been observed, but there are insufficient data to support an estimate of their frequency:

Cardiovascular: Hypotension, tachycardia, cardiac arrhythmias, hypertension, pulmonary hemorrhage.

Digestive and Hepatic: Gastrointestinal hemorrhage, nausea, vomiting, diarrhea, hepatitis.

Skin: Flushing, increased pilomotor activity with tingling or chilliness, rash.

Hematologic: Thrombocytopenia, leukopenia.

Renal: Edema, oliguria, hematuria.

OVERDOSAGE

Acute Toxicity

Oral LD$_{50}$'s (mg/kg): mice, 400; rats, 1200.

Signs and Symptoms

Signs and symptoms of overdosage may include increased pilomotor activity, peripheral vasodilatation, skin flushing, and, in rare instances, hypotension and shock.

Treatment

In treating hypotension, it is most important to place the patient's head low and administer intravenous fluids. Epinephrine should not be used, since large doses of Priscoline may cause "epinephrine reversal" (further reduction in blood pressure, followed by an exaggerated rebound).

DOSAGE AND ADMINISTRATION

An initial dose of 1 to 2 mg/kg, via scalp vein, followed by an infusion of 1 to 2 mg/kg per hour have usually resulted in significant increases in arterial oxygen. There is very little experience with infusions lasting beyond 36 to 48 hours. Response, if it occurs, can be expected within 30 minutes after the initial dose.

Note: Parenteral drug products should be inspected visually for particulate matter and discoloration prior to administration, whenever solution and container permit.

HOW SUPPLIED

Ampuls—4 ml—each milliliter contains 25 mg of tolazoline hydrochloride.

Carton of 4 ampuls .... NDC 0083-6733-04
Store between 15° and 30°C (59°–86°F). Protect from light.
C89-33 (Rev. 8/89)

PRIVINE®   **OTC**
[pri-veen ']
0.05% Nasal Solution
0.05% Nasal Spray

CAUTION

Do not use Privine if you have glaucoma. Privine is an effective nasal decongestant **when you use it in the recommended dosage.** If you use too much, too long, or too often, Privine may be harmful to your nasal mucous membranes and cause

burning, stinging, sneezing or an increased runny nose. Do not use Privine by mouth.

Keep this and all medications out of the reach of children. Do not use Privine with children under 12 years of age, except with the advice and supervision of a doctor.

OVERDOSAGE IN YOUNG CHILDREN MAY CAUSE MARKED SEDATION AND IF SEVERE, EMERGENCY TREATMENT MAY BE NECESSARY.

IF NASAL STUFFINESS PERSISTS AFTER 3 DAYS OF TREATMENT, DISCONTINUE USE AND CONSULT A DOCTOR.

Privine is a nasal decongestant that comes in two forms: Nasal Solution (in a bottle with a dropper) and Nasal Spray (in a plastic squeeze bottle). Both are for prompt and prolonged relief of nasal congestion due to common colds, sinusitis, hay fever, etc.

How to use Nasal Solution. Squeeze rubber bulb to fill dropper with proper amount of medication. For best results, tilt head as far back as possible and put two drops of solution into your right nostril. Then lean head forward, inhaling and turning your head to the left. Refill dropper by squeezing bulb. Now tilt head as far back as possible and put two drops of solution into your left nostril. Then lean head forward, inhaling, and turning your head to the right.

Use only 2 drops in each nostril. Do not repeat this dosage more than every 3 hours.

The Privine dropper bottle is designed to make administration of the proper dosage easy and to prevent accidental overdosage. Privine will not cause sleeplessness, so you may use it before going to bed.

IMPORTANT

After use, be sure to rinse the dropper with very hot water. This helps prevent contamination of the bottle with bacteria from nasal secretions. Use of the dispenser by more than one person may spread infection.

NOTE

Privine Nasal Solution may be used on contact with glass, plastic, stainless steel and specially treated metals used in atomizers. Do not let the solution come in contact with reactive metals, especially aluminum. If solution becomes discolored, it should be discarded.

How to use Nasal Spray. For best results do **not** shake the plastic squeeze bottle.

Remove cap. With head held upright, spray twice into each nostril. Squeeze the bottle sharply and firmly while sniffing through the nose.

For best results use every 4 to 6 hours. Do not use more often than every 3 hours.

Avoid overdosage. Follow directions for use carefully.

Privine Nasal Solution contains 0.05% naphazoline hydrochloride, USP. It also contains benzalkonium chloride, disodium edetate dihydrate, hydrochloric acid, purified water, sodium chloride, and trolamine. It is available in bottles of .66 fl oz (20 ml) with dropper and bottles of 16 fl oz (473 ml). Privine Nasal Spray contains 0.05% naphazoline hydrochloride, USP. It also contains benzalkonium chloride, disodium edetate dihydrate, hydrochloric acid, purified water, sodium chloride, and trolamine. It is available in plastic squeeze bottles of $\frac{1}{2}$ fl oz (15 ml).

Store the nasal solution and nasal spray between 59°–86°F.
C86-43 (Rev. 9/86)

Distributed by:
CIBA CONSUMER PHARMACEUTICALS
Edison, New Jersey 08837

REGITINE®   ℞
[rej 'a-teen]
phentolamine mesylate USP
Vials

DESCRIPTION

Regitine, phentolamine mesylate USP, is an antihypertensive, available in vials for intravenous and intramuscular administration. Each vial contains phentolamine mesylate USP, 5 mg, and mannitol USP, 25 mg, in sterile, lyophilized form.

Phentolamine mesylate is 4,5-dihydro-2-[N- (m -hydroxyphenyl) -N- (p -methylphenyl) aminomethyl] -1H -imidazole 1:1 methanesulfonate.

Phentolamine mesylate USP is a white or off-white, odorless crystalline powder with a molecular weight of 377.46. Its solutions are acid to litmus. It is freely soluble in water and in alcohol, and slightly soluble in chloroform. It melts at about 178°C.

CLINICAL PHARMACOLOGY

Regitine produces an alpha-adrenergic block of relatively short duration. It also has direct, but less marked, positive inotropic and chronotropic effects on cardiac muscle and vasodilator effects on vascular smooth muscle.

Regitine has a half-life in the blood of 19 minutes following intravenous administration. Approximately 13% of a single intravenous dose appears in the urine as unchanged drug.

INDICATIONS AND USAGE

Regitine is indicated for the prevention or control of hypertensive episodes that may occur in a patient with pheochromocytoma as a result of stress or manipulation during preoperative preparation and surgical excision.

Regitine is indicated for the prevention or treatment of dermal necrosis and sloughing following intravenous administration or extravasation of norepinephrine.

Regitine is also indicated for the diagnosis of pheochromocytoma by the Regitine blocking test.

CONTRAINDICATIONS

Myocardial infarction, history of myocardial infarction, coronary insufficiency, angina, or other evidence suggestive of coronary artery disease; hypersensitivity to phentolamine or related compounds.

WARNINGS

Myocardial infarction, cerebrovascular spasm, and cerebrovascular occlusion have been reported to occur following the administration of Regitine, usually in association with marked hypotensive episodes.

For screening tests in patients with hypertension, the generally available urinary assay of catecholamines or other biochemical assays have largely replaced the Regitine and other pharmacological tests for reasons of accuracy and safety. None of the chemical or pharmacological tests is infallible in the diagnosis of pheochromocytoma. The Regitine blocking test is not the procedure of choice and should be reserved for cases in which additional confirmatory evidence is necessary and the relative risks involved in conducting the test have been considered.

PRECAUTIONS

General

Tachycardia and cardiac arrhythmias may occur with the use of Regitine or other alpha-adrenergic blocking agents. When possible, administration of cardiac glycosides should be deferred until cardiac rhythm returns to normal.

Drug Interactions

See **DOSAGE AND ADMINISTRATION, Diagnosis of pheochromocytoma,** *Preparation.*

Carcinogenesis, Mutagenesis, Impairment of Fertility

Long-term carcinogenicity studies, mutagenicity studies, and fertility studies have not been conducted with Regitine.

Pregnancy Category C

Administration of Regitine to pregnant rats and mice at oral doses 24–30 times the usual daily human dose (based on a 60-kg human) resulted in slightly decreased growth and slight skeletal immaturity of the fetuses. Immaturity was manifested by increased incidence of incomplete or unossified calcanei and phalangeal nuclei of the hind limb and of incompletely ossified sternebrae. At oral doses 60 times the usual daily human dose (based on a 60-kg human), a slightly lower rate of implantation was found in the rat. Regitine did not affect embryonic or fetal development in the rabbit at oral doses 20 times the usual daily human dose (based on a 60-kg human). No teratogenic or embryotoxic effects were observed in the rat, mouse, or rabbit studies.

There are no adequate and well-controlled studies in pregnant women. Regitine should be used during pregnancy only if the potential benefit justifies the potential risk to the fetus.

Nursing Mothers

It is not known whether this drug is excreted in human milk. Because many drugs are excreted in human milk and because of the potential for serious adverse reactions in nursing infants from Regitine, a decision should be made whether to discontinue nursing or to discontinue the drug, taking into account the importance of the drug to the mother.

Pediatric Use

See **DOSAGE AND ADMINISTRATION.**

ADVERSE REACTIONS

Acute and prolonged hypotensive episodes, tachycardia, and cardiac arrhythmias have been reported. In addition, weakness, dizziness, flushing, orthostatic hypotension, nasal stuffiness, nausea, vomiting, and diarrhea may occur.

OVERDOSAGE

Acute Toxicity

No deaths due to acute poisoning with Regitine have been reported.

Oral LD$_{50}$'s (mg/kg): mice, 1000; rats, 1250.

Signs and Symptoms

Overdosage with Regitine is characterized chiefly by cardiovascular disturbances, such as arrhythmias, tachycardia, hypotension, and possibly shock. In addition, the following might occur: excitation, headache, sweating, pupillary contraction, visual disturbances; nausea, vomiting, diarrhea; hypoglycemia.

Continued on next page

The full prescribing information for each CIBA product is contained herein and is that in effect as of September 1, 1992 .

CIBA—Cont.

Treatment

There is no specific antidote.

A decrease in blood pressure to dangerous levels or other evidence of shocklike conditions should be treated vigorously and promptly. The patient's legs should be kept raised and a plasma expander should be administered. If necessary, intravenous infusion of norepinephrine, titrated to maintain blood pressure at the normotensive level, and all available supportive measures should be included. Epinephrine should not be used, since it may cause a paradoxical reduction in blood pressure.

DOSAGE AND ADMINISTRATION

The reconstituted solution should be used upon preparation and should not be stored.

Note: Parenteral drug products should be inspected visually for particulate matter and discoloration prior to administration, whenever solution and container permit.

1. Prevention or control of hypertensive episodes in the patient with pheochromocytoma.

For preoperative reduction of elevated blood pressure, 5 mg of Regitine (1 mg for children) is injected intravenously or intramuscularly 1 or 2 hours before surgery, and repeated if necessary.

During surgery, Regitine (5 mg for adults, 1 mg for children) is administered intravenously as indicated, to help prevent or control paroxysms of hypertension, tachycardia, respiratory depression, convulsions, or other effects of epinephrine intoxication. (Postoperatively, norepinephrine may be given to control the hypotension that commonly follows complete removal of a pheochromocytoma.)

2. Prevention or treatment of dermal necrosis and sloughing following intravenous administration or extravasation of norepinephrine.

For Prevention: 10 mg of Regitine is added to each liter of solution containing norepinephrine. The pressor effect of norepinephrine is not affected.

For Treatment: 5–10 mg of Regitine in 10 ml of saline is injected into the area of extravasation within 12 hours.

3. Diagnosis of pheochromocytoma—Regitine blocking test.

The test is most reliable in detecting pheochromocytoma in patients with sustained hypertension and least reliable in those with paroxysmal hypertension. False-positive tests may occur in patients with hypertension without pheochromocytoma.

a. Intravenous

Preparation

The **CONTRAINDICATIONS, WARNINGS,** and **PRECAUTIONS** sections should be reviewed. Sedatives, analgesics, and all other medications except those that might be deemed essential (such as digitalis and insulin) are withheld for at least 24 hours, and preferably 48–72 hours, prior to the test. Antihypertensive drugs are withheld until blood pressure returns to the untreated, hypertensive level. This test is not performed on a patient who is normotensive.

Procedure

The patient is kept at rest in the supine position throughout the test, preferably in a quiet, darkened room. Injection of Regitine is delayed until blood pressure is stabilized, as evidenced by blood pressure readings taken every 10 minutes for at least 30 minutes.

Five milligrams of Regitine is dissolved in 1 ml of Sterile Water for Injection. The dose for adults is 5 mg; for children, 1 mg.

The syringe needle is inserted into the vein, and injection is delayed until pressor response to venipuncture has subsided. Regitine is injected rapidly. Blood pressure is recorded immediately after injection, at 30-second intervals for the first 3 minutes, and at 60-second intervals for the next 7 minutes.

Interpretation

A positive response, suggestive of pheochromocytoma, is indicated when the blood pressure is reduced more than 35 mm Hg systolic and 25 mm Hg diastolic. A typical positive response is a reduction in pressure of 60 mm Hg systolic and 25 mm Hg diastolic. Usually, maximal effect is evident within 2 minutes after injection. A return to preinjection pressure commonly occurs within 15–30 minutes but may occur more rapidly.

If blood pressure decreases to a dangerous level, the patient should be treated as outlined under **OVERDOSAGE.**

A positive response should always be confirmed by other diagnostic procedures, preferably by measurement of urinary catecholamines or their metabolites.

A negative response is indicated when the blood pressure is elevated, unchanged, or reduced less than 35 mm Hg systolic and 25 mm Hg diastolic after injection of Regitine. A negative reponse to this test does not exclude the diagnosis of pheochromocytoma, especially in patients with paroxysmal hypertension in whom the incidence of false-negative responses is high.

b. Intramuscular

If the intramuscular test for pheochromocytoma is preferred, preparation is the same as for the intravenous test. Five milligrams of Regitine is then dissolved in 1 ml of Sterile Water for Injection. The dose for adults is 5 mg intramuscularly; for children, 3 mg. Blood pressure is recorded every 5 minutes for 30–45 minutes following injection. A positive response is indicated when the blood pressure is reduced 35 mm Hg systolic and 25 mm Hg diastolic, or more, within 20 minutes following injection.

HOW SUPPLIED

Vials —each containing 5 mg of phentolamine mesylate USP and 25 mg of mannitol USP, in lyophilized form

Cartons of 2 .... NDC 0083-6830-02
Cartons of 6 .... NDC 0083-6830-06
The reconstituted solution should be used upon preparation and should not be stored.

Store between 59° and 86°F.

Dist. by:

CIBA Pharmaceutical Company
Division of CIBA-GEIGY Corporation
Summit, NJ 07901

C85-2 (Rev. 8/85)

RIMACTANE®   ℞

[re-mack 'tayne]
rifampin USP

DESCRIPTION

Rimactane, rifampin USP , is a semisynthetic antibiotic derivative of rifamycin B, available as 300-mg capsules for oral administration. It is also available in Dual Packs containing two 300-mg capsules of Rimactane and one 300-mg tablet of INH®, isoniazid USP. Rimactane is 3-[[(4-methyl-1-piperazinyl)imino] methyl] rifamycin.

Rifampin USP is a red-brown crystalline powder. It is very slightly soluble in water, freely soluble in chloroform, and soluble in ethyl acetate and in methanol. Its molecular weight is 822.95.

Inactive Ingredients: FD&C Blue No. 1, FD&C Red No. 40, FD&C Yellow No. 6, gelatin, lactose, magnesium stearate, methylparaben, propylparaben, silicon dioxide, sodium lauryl sulfate, starch, talc, and titanium dioxide.

ACTIONS

Rimactane inhibits DNA-dependent RNA polymerase activity in susceptible cells. Specifically, it interacts with bacterial RNA polymerase but does not inhibit the mammalian enzyme. This is the mechanism of action by which Rimactane exerts its therapeutic effect. Rimactane cross resistance has only been shown with other rifamycins.

Peak blood levels in normal adults vary widely from individual to individual. Peak levels occur between 2 and 4 hours following the oral administration of a 600-mg dose. The average peak value is 7 mcg/ml; however, the peak level may vary from 4 to 32 mcg/ml.

In normal subjects the $T\frac{1}{2}$ (biological half-life) of Rimactane in blood is approximately 3 hours. Elimination occurs mainly through the bile and, to a much lesser extent, the urine.

INDICATIONS

Pulmonary Tuberculosis

In the initial treatment and in the retreatment of pulmonary tuberculosis, Rimactane must be used in conjunction with at least one other antituberculous drug.

Frequently used regimens have been the following:

    isoniazid and Rimactane
    ethambutol and Rimactane
    isoniazid, ethambutol, and Rimactane

Neisseria Meningitidis Carriers

Rimactane is indicated for the treatment of asymptomatic carriers of *N. meningitidis* to eliminate meningococci from the nasopharynx.

Rimactane is not indicated for the treatment of meningococcal infection.

To avoid the indiscriminate use of Rimactane, diagnostic laboratory procedures, including serotyping and susceptibility testing, should be performed to establish the carrier state and the correct treatment. In order to preserve the usefulness of Rimactane in the treatment of asymptomatic meningococcal carriers, it is recommended that the drug be reserved for situations in which the risk of meningococcal meningitis is high.

Both in the treatment of tuberculosis and in the treatment of meningococcal carriers, small numbers of resistant cells, present within large populations of susceptible cells, can rapidly become the predominating type. Since rapid emergence of resistance can occur, culture and susceptibility tests should be performed in the event of persistent positive cultures.

CONTRAINDICATIONS

A history of previous hypersensitivity reaction to any of the rifamycins.

WARNINGS

Rifampin has been shown to produce liver dysfunction. There have been fatalities associated with jaundice in patients with liver disease or receiving rifampin concomitantly with other hepatotoxic agents. Since an increased risk may exist for individuals with liver disease, benefits must be weighed carefully against the risk of further liver damage. Periodic liver function monitoring is mandatory.

The possibility of rapid emergence of resistant meningococci restricts the use of Rimactane to short-term treatment of the asymptomatic carrier state. Rimactane is not to be used for the treatment of meningococcal disease.

Several studies of tumorigenicity potential have been done in rodents. In one strain of mice known to be particularly susceptible to the spontaneous development of hepatomas, rifampin given at a level 2–10 times the maximum dosage used clinically, resulted in a significant increase in the occurrence of hepatomas in female mice of this strain after one year of administration. There was no evidence of tumorigenicity in the males of this strain, in males or females of another mouse strain, or rats.

Usage in Pregnancy

Although rifampin has been reported to cross the placental barrier and appear in cord blood, the effect of Rimactane, alone or in combination with other antituberculous drugs, on the human fetus is not known. An increase in congenital malformations, primarily spina bifida and cleft palate, has been reported in the offspring of rodents given oral doses of 150-250 mg/kg/day of rifampin during pregnancy.

The possible teratogenic potential in women capable of bearing children should be carefully weighed against the benefits of therapy.

PRECAUTIONS

Rimactane is not recommended for intermittent therapy; the patient should be cautioned against intentional or accidental interruption of the daily dosage regimen since rare renal hypersensitivity reactions have been reported when therapy was resumed in such cases.

Rifampin has been observed to increase the requirements for anticoagulant drugs of the coumarin type. The cause of this phenomenon is unknown. In patients receiving anticoagulants and rifampin concurrently, it is recommended that the prothrombin time be performed daily or as frequently as necessary to establish and maintain the required dose of anticoagulant.

Urine, feces, saliva, sputum, sweat, and tears may be colored red-orange by rifampin and its metabolites. Soft contact lenses may be permanently stained. Individuals to be treated should be made aware of these possibilities.

It has been reported that the reliability of oral contraceptives may be affected in some patients being treated for tuberculosis with rifampin in combination with at least one other antituberculous drug. In such cases, alternative contraceptive measures may need to be considered.

Rifampin has been reported to diminish the effects of concurrently administered methadone, oral hypoglycemics, corticosteroids, dapsone, digitalis preparations and to reduce the bioavailability and efficacy of verapamil. Appropriate dosage adjustments may be necessary if indicated by the patient's clinical condition.

When rifampin is taken in combination with PAS, decreased rifampin serum levels may result. Therefore, the drugs should be given at least 4 hours apart.

Therapeutic levels of rifampin have been shown to inhibit standard assays for serum folate and vitamin B_{12}. Alternative methods must be considered when determining folate and vitamin B_{12} concentrations in the presence of rifampin.

Since rifampin has been reported to cross the placental barrier and appear in cord blood, neonates of rifampin-treated mothers should be carefully observed for any evidence of adverse effects. Rifampin is excreted in breast milk.

ADVERSE REACTIONS

Gastrointestinal disturbances such as heartburn, epigastric distress, anorexia, nausea, vomiting, gas, cramps, and diarrhea have been noted in some patients. Rarely, pseudomembranous enterocolitis has been reported. Headache, drowsiness, fatigue, ataxia, dizziness, inability to concentrate, mental confusion, visual disturbances, muscular weakness, fever, pains in extremities, generalized numbness, and menstrual disturbances have also been noted.

Hypersensitivity reactions have been reported. Encountered occasionally have been pruritus, urticaria, rash, pemphigoid reaction, eosinophilia, sore mouth, sore tongue, and exudative conjunctivitis. Rarely, hepatitis or a shock-like syndrome with hepatic involvement and abnormal liver function tests have been reported. Transient abnormalities in liver function tests (eg, elevations in serum bilirubin, BSP, alkaline phosphatase, serum transaminases) have also been observed. The BSP test should be performed prior to the morning dose of rifampin to avoid false-positive results.

Thrombocytopenia, transient leukopenia, hemolytic anemia, and decreased hemoglobin have been observed. Thrombocytopenia has occurred when rifampin and ethambutol were administered concomitantly according to an intermittent dose schedule twice weekly and in high doses.

Elevations in BUN and serum uric acid have occurred. Rarely, hemolysis, hemoglobinuria, hematuria, renal insufficiency or acute renal failure have been reported and are generally considered to be hypersensitivity reactions. These have usually occurred during intermittent therapy or when treatment was resumed following intentional or accidental interruption of a daily dosage regimen and were reversible when rifampin was discontinued and appropriate therapy instituted.

Although rifampin has been reported to have an immunosuppressive effect in some animal experiments, available human data indicate that this has no clinical significance.

DOSAGE AND ADMINISTRATION

It is recommended that Rimactane be administered once daily, either one hour before or two hours after a meal.

Data are not available for determination of dosage for children under 5.

Pulmonary Tuberculosis

Adults: 600 mg (two 300-mg Capsules) in a single daily administration.

Children: 10 to 20 mg/kg, not to exceed 600 mg/day.

In the treatment of pulmonary tuberculosis, Rimactane must be used in conjunction with at least one other antituberculous agent. In general, therapy should be continued until bacterial conversion and maximal improvement have occurred.

Meningococcal Carriers

It is recommended that Rimactane be administered once daily for four consecutive days in the following doses:

Adults: 600 mg (two 300-mg Capsules) in a single daily administration.

Children: 10 to 20 mg/kg, not to exceed 600 mg/day.

Susceptibility Testing

Pulmonary Tuberculosis: Rifampin susceptibility powders are available for both direct and indirect methods of determining the susceptibility of strains of mycobacteria. The MICs of susceptible clinical isolates when determined in 7H10 or other non-egg-containing media have ranged from 0.1 to 2 mcg/ml.

Meningococcal Carriers: Susceptibility discs containing 5 mcg rifampin are available for susceptibility testing of *N. meningitidis.*

Quantitative methods that require measurement of zone diameters give the most precise estimates of antibiotic susceptibility. One such procedure[1] has been recommended for use with discs for testing susceptibility to rifampin. Interpretations correlate zone diameters from the disc test with MIC (minimal inhibitory concentration) values for rifampin. A range of MIC's from 0.1 to 1 mcg/ml has been found *in vitro* for susceptible strains of *N. meningitidis.* With this procedure, a report from the laboratory of "resistant" indicates that the organism is not likely to be eradicated from the nasopharynx of asymptomatic carriers.

OVERDOSAGE

Signs and Symptoms

Nausea, vomiting, and increasing lethargy will probably occur within a short time after ingestion; actual unconsciousness may occur with severe hepatic involvement. Brownish-red or orange discoloration of the skin, urine, sweat, saliva, tears, and feces is proportional to amount ingested.

Liver enlargement, possibly with tenderness, can develop within a few hours after severe overdosage and jaundice may develop rapidly. Hepatic involvement may be more marked in patients with prior impairment of hepatic function. Other physical findings remain essentially normal.

Direct and total bilirubin levels may increase rapidly with severe overdosage; hepatic enzyme levels may be affected, especially with prior impairment of hepatic function. A direct effect upon hemopoietic system, electrolyte levels, or acid-base balance is unlikely.

Treatment

Since nausea and vomiting are likely to be present, gastric lavage is probably preferable to induction of emesis. Activated charcoal slurry instilled into the stomach following evacuation of gastric contents can help absorb any remaining drug in G.I. tract. Antiemetic medication may be required to control severe nausea/vomiting.

Active diuresis (with measured intake and output) will help promote excretion of the drug. Bile drainage may be indicated in presence of serious impairment of hepatic function lasting more than 24–48 hours; under these circumstances, extracorporeal hemodialysis may be required.

In patients with previously adequate hepatic function, reversal of liver enlargement and impaired hepatic excretory function probably will be noted within 72 hours, with rapid return toward normal thereafter.

HOW SUPPLIED

Capsules 300 mg—opaque, scarlet, caramel (imprinted CIBA 154)

Bottles of 30 .... NDC 0083-0154-26
Bottles of 60 .... NDC 0083-0154-29
Bottles of 100 .... NDC 0083-0154-30

Do not store above 86°F (30°C).

Keep tightly closed. Protect from heat and moisture.

Dispense in tight, light-resistant container (USP).

Also available—Rimactane®/INH® (isoniazid USP) Dual Pack. Each Dual Pack contains two Rimactane 300-mg capsules and one INH 300-mg tablet.

Cartons of 30 Dual Packs
(60 Rimactane capsules and
30 INH tablets) .... NDC 0083-8912-23

Store between 59°–86°F (15°–30°C). Protect from light and moisture.

REFERENCE

1. Bauer AW, Kirby WMM, Sherris JC, et al: Antibiotic susceptibility testing by a standardized single disk method. *Am J Clin Path* 1966;45:493–496.

C92-7 (Rev. 3/92)

Shown in Product Identification Section, page 408

RITALIN® hydrochloride Ⓒ II
[rit 'ah-lin]
methylphenidate hydrochloride
tablets USP

RITALIN-SR® Ⓒ II
methylphenidate hydrochloride USP
sustained-release tablets

DESCRIPTION

Ritalin hydrochloride, methylphenidate hydrochloride USP, is a mild central nervous system (CNS) stimulant, available as tablets of 5, 10, and 20 mg for oral administration; Ritalin-SR is available as sustained-release tablets of 20 mg for oral administration. Methylphenidate hydrochloride is methyl α-phenyl-2-piperidineacetate hydrochloride.

Methylphenidate hydrochloride USP is a white, odorless, fine crystalline powder. Its solutions are acid to litmus. It is freely soluble in water and in methanol, soluble in alcohol, and slightly soluble in chloroform and in acetone. Its molecular weight is 269.77.

Inactive Ingredients. Ritalin tablets: D&C Yellow No. 10 (5-mg and 20-mg tablets), FD&C Green No. 3 (10-mg tablets), lactose, magnesium stearate, polyethylene glycol, starch (5-mg and 10-mg tablets), sucrose, talc, and tragacanth (20-mg tablets).

Ritalin-SR tablets: Cellulose compounds, cetostearyl alcohol, lactose, magnesium stearate, mineral oil, povidone, titanium dioxide, and zein.

CLINICAL PHARMACOLOGY

Ritalin is a mild central nervous system stimulant.

The mode of action in man is not completely understood, but Ritalin presumably activates the brain stem arousal system and cortex to produce its stimulant effect.

There is neither specific evidence which clearly establishes the mechanism whereby Ritalin produces its mental and behavioral effects in children, nor conclusive evidence regarding how these effects relate to the condition of the central nervous system.

Ritalin in the SR tablets is more slowly but as extensively absorbed as in the regular tablets. Relative bioavailability of the SR tablet compared to the Ritalin tablet, measured by the urinary excretion of Ritalin major metabolite (α-phenyl-2-piperidine acetic acid) was 105% (49–168%) in children and 101% (85–152%) in adults. The time to peak rate in children was 4.7 hours (1.3–8.2 hours) for the SR tablets and 1.9 hours (0.3–4.4 hours) for the tablets. An average of 67% of SR tablet dose was excreted in children as compared to 86% in adults.

INDICATIONS

Attention Deficit Disorders, Narcolepsy

Attention Deficit Disorders (previously known as Minimal Brain Dysfunction in Children). Other terms being used to describe the behavioral syndrome below include: Hyperkinetic Child Syndrome, Minimal Brain Damage, Minimal Cerebral Dysfunction, Minor Cerebral Dysfunction.

Ritalin is indicated as an integral part of a total treatment program which typically includes other remedial measures (psychological, educational, social) for a stabilizing effect in children with a behavioral syndrome characterized by the following group of developmentally inappropriate symptoms: moderate-to-severe distractibility, short attention span, hyperactivity, emotional lability, and impulsivity. The diagnosis of this syndrome should not be made with finality when these symptoms are only of comparatively recent origin. Nonlocalizing (soft) neurological signs, learning disability, and abnormal EEG may or may not be present, and a diagnosis of central nervous system dysfunction may or may not be warranted.

Special Diagnostic Considerations

Specific etiology of this syndrome is unknown, and there is no single diagnostic test. Adequate diagnosis requires the use not only of medical but of special psychological, educational, and social resources.

Characteristics commonly reported include: chronic history of short attention span, distractibility, emotional lability, impulsivity, and moderate-to-severe hyperactivity; minor neurological signs and abnormal EEG. Learning may or may not be impaired. The diagnosis must be based upon a complete history and evaluation of the child and not solely on the presence of one or more of these characteristics.

Drug treatment is not indicated for all children with this syndrome. Stimulants are not intended for use in the child who exhibits symptoms secondary to environmental factors and/or primary psychiatric disorders, including psychosis. Appropriate educational placement is essential and psychosocial intervention is generally necessary. When remedial measures alone are insufficient, the decision to prescribe stimulant medication will depend upon the physician's assessment of the chronicity and severity of the child's symptoms.

CONTRAINDICATIONS

Marked anxiety, tension, and agitation are contraindications to Ritalin, since the drug may aggravate these symptoms. Ritalin is contraindicated also in patients known to be hypersensitive to the drug, in patients with glaucoma, and in patients with motor tics or with a family history or diagnosis of Tourette's syndrome.

WARNINGS

Ritalin should not be used in children under six years, since safety and efficacy in this age group have not been established.

Sufficient data on safety and efficacy of long-term use of Ritalin in children are not yet available. Although a causal relationship has not been established, suppression of growth (*ie,* weight gain, and/or height) has been reported with the long-term use of stimulants in children. Therefore, patients requiring long-term therapy should be carefully monitored.

Ritalin should not be used for severe depression of either exogenous or endogenous origin. Clinical experience suggests that in psychotic children, administration of Ritalin may exacerbate symptoms of behavior disturbance and thought disorder.

Ritalin should not be used for the prevention or treatment of normal fatigue states.

There is some clinical evidence that Ritalin may lower the convulsive threshold in patients with prior history of seizures, with prior EEG abnormalities in absence of seizures, and, very rarely, in absence of history of seizures and no prior EEG evidence of seizures. Safe concomitant use of anticonvulsants and Ritalin has not been established. In the presence of seizures, the drug should be discontinued.

Use cautiously in patients with hypertension. Blood pressure should be monitored at appropriate intervals in all patients taking Ritalin, especially those with hypertension.

Symptoms of visual disturbances have been encountered in rare cases. Difficulties with accommodation and blurring of vision have been reported.

Drug Interactions

Ritalin may decrease the hypotensive effect of guanethidine. Use cautiously with pressor agents and MAO inhibitors.

Human pharmacologic studies have shown that Ritalin may inhibit the metabolism of coumarin anticoagulants, anticonvulsants (phenobarbital, diphenylhydantoin, primidone), phenylbutazone, and tricyclic drugs (imipramine, clomipramine, desipramine). Downward dosage adjustments of these drugs may be required when given concomitantly with Ritalin.

Usage in Pregnancy

Adequate animal reproduction studies to establish safe use of Ritalin during pregnancy have not been conducted. Therefore, until more information is available, Ritalin should not be prescribed for women of childbearing age unless, in the opinion of the physician, the potential benefits outweigh the possible risks.

Drug Dependence

Ritalin should be given cautiously to emotionally unstable patients, such as those with a history of drug dependence or alcoholism, because such patients may increase dosage on their own initiative.

Chronically abusive use can lead to marked tolerance and psychic dependence with varying degrees of abnormal behavior. Frank psychotic episodes can occur, espe-

Continued on next page

The full prescribing information for each CIBA product is contained herein and is that in effect as of September 1, 1992.

CIBA—Cont.

cially with parenteral abuse. Careful supervision is required during drug withdrawal, since severe depression as well as the effects of chronic overactivity can be unmasked. Long-term follow-up may be required because of the patient's basic personality disturbances.

PRECAUTIONS

Patients with an element of agitation may react adversely; discontinue therapy if necessary.

Periodic CBC, differential, and platelet counts are advised during prolonged therapy.

Drug treatment is not indicated in all cases of this behavioral syndrome and should be considered only in light of the complete history and evaluation of the child. The decision to prescribe Ritalin should depend on the physician's assessment of the chronicity and severity of the child's symptoms and their appropriateness for his/her age. Prescription should not depend solely on the presence of one or more of the behavioral characteristics.

When these symptoms are associated with acute stress reactions, treatment with Ritalin is usually not indicated.

Long-term effects of Ritalin in children have not been well established.

ADVERSE REACTIONS

Nervousness and insomnia are the most common adverse reactions but are usually controlled by reducing dosage and omitting the drug in the afternoon or evening. Other reactions include hypersensitivity (including skin rash, urticaria, fever, arthralgia, exfoliative dermatitis, erythema multiforme with histopathological findings of necrotizing vasculitis, and thrombocytopenic purpura); anorexia; nausea; dizziness; palpitations; headache; dyskinesia; drowsiness; blood pressure and pulse changes, both up and down; tachycardia; angina; cardiac arrhythmia; abdominal pain; weight loss during prolonged therapy. There have been rare reports of Tourette's syndrome. Toxic psychosis has been reported. Although a definite causal relationship has not been established, the following have been reported in patients taking this drug: isolated cases of cerebral arteritis and/or occlusion; leukopenia and/or anemia; transient depressed mood, a few instances of scalp hair loss.

In children, loss of appetite, abdominal pain, weight loss during prolonged therapy, insomnia, and tachycardia may occur more frequently; however, any of the other adverse reactions listed above may also occur.

DOSAGE AND ADMINISTRATION

Dosage should be individualized according to the needs and responses of the patient.

Adults

Tablets: Administer in divided doses 2 or 3 times daily, preferably 30 to 45 minutes before meals. Average dosage is 20 to 30 mg daily. Some patients may require 40 to 60 mg daily. In others, 10 to 15 mg daily will be adequate. Patients who are unable to sleep if medication is taken late in the day should take the last dose before 6 p.m.

SR Tablets: Ritalin-SR tablets have a duration of action of approximately 8 hours. Therefore, Ritalin-SR tablets may be used in place of Ritalin tablets when the 8-hour dosage of Ritalin-SR corresponds to the titrated 8-hour dosage of Ritalin. Ritalin-SR tablets must be swallowed whole and never crushed or chewed.

Children (6 years and over)

Ritalin should be initiated in small doses, with gradual weekly increments. Daily dosage above 60 mg is not recommended.

If improvement is not observed after appropriate dosage adjustment over a one-month period, the drug should be discontinued.

Tablets: Start with 5 mg twice daily (before breakfast and lunch) with gradual increments of 5 to 10 mg weekly.

SR Tablets: Ritalin-SR tablets have a duration of action of approximately 8 hours. Therefore, Ritalin-SR tablets may be used in place of Ritalin tablets when the 8-hour dosage of Ritalin-SR corresponds to the titrated 8-hour dosage of Ritalin. Ritalin-SR tablets must be swallowed whole and never crushed or chewed.

If paradoxical aggravation of symptoms or other adverse effects occur, reduce dosage, or, if necessary, discontinue the drug.

Ritalin should be periodically discontinued to assess the child's condition. Improvement may be sustained when the drug is either temporarily or permanently discontinued.

Drug treatment should not and need not be indefinite and usually may be discontinued after puberty.

OVERDOSAGE

Signs and symptoms of acute overdosage, resulting principally from overstimulation of the central nervous system and from excessive sympathomimetic effects, may include the following: vomiting, agitation, tremors, hyperreflexia, muscle twitching, convulsions (may be followed by coma),

euphoria, confusion, hallucinations, delirium, sweating, flushing, headache, hyperpyrexia, tachycardia, palpitations, cardiac arrhythmias, hypertension, mydriasis, and dryness of mucous membranes.

Treatment consists of appropriate supportive measures. The patient must be protected against self-injury and against external stimuli that would aggravate overstimulation already present. If signs and symptoms are not too severe and the patient is conscious, gastric contents may be evacuated by induction of emesis or gastric lavage. In the presence of severe intoxication, use a carefully titrated dosage of a *short-acting* barbiturate *before* performing gastric lavage.

Intensive care must be provided to maintain adequate circulation and respiratory exchange; external cooling procedures may be required for hyperpyrexia.

Efficacy of peritoneal dialysis or extracorporeal hemodialysis for Ritalin overdosage has not been established.

HOW SUPPLIED

Tablets 5 mg—round, yellow (imprinted CIBA 7)

   Bottles of 100 .... NDC 0083-0007-30

Tablets 10 mg —round, pale green, scored (imprinted CIBA 3)

   Bottles of 100 .... NDC 0083-0003-30

Tablets 20 mg—round, pale yellow, scored (imprinted CIBA 34)

   Bottles of 100 .... NDC 0083-0034-30

Protect from light.

Do not store above 86°F (30°C)

Dispense in tight, light-resistant container (USP).

SR Tablets 20 mg—round, white, coated (imprinted CIBA 16)

   Bottles of 100 .... NDC 0083-0016-30

Note: SR Tablets are color-additive free.

Do not store above 86°F (30°C). Protect from moisture.

Dispense in tight, light-resistant container (USP).

C91-39 (Rev. 2/92)

Shown in Product Identification Section, page 408

SER-AP-ES®   ℞
[su-rapp'ess]
reserpine USP 0.1 mg
hydralazine hydrochloride USP 25 mg
hydrochlorothiazide USP 15 mg
Combination Tablets

> **WARNING**
>
> This fixed-combination drug is not indicated for initial therapy of hypertension. Hypertension requires therapy titrated to the individual patient. If the fixed combination represents the dosage so determined, its use may be more convenient in patient management. The treatment of hypertension is not static but must be reevaluated as conditions in each patient warrant.

DESCRIPTION

Ser-Ap-Es is an antihypertensive-diuretic combination, available as tablets for oral administration. Each tablet contains Serpasil (reserpine USP), 0.1 mg; Apresoline (hydralazine hydrochloride USP), 25 mg; and Esidrix (hydrochlorothiazide USP), 15 mg.

Reserpine is methyl 18β-hydroxy-11, 17α-dimethoxy-3β, 20α-yohimban-16β-carboxylate 3,4,5-trimethoxybenzoate (ester).

Reserpine USP, a pure crystalline alkaloid of rauwolfia, is a white or pale buff to slightly yellowish, odorless crystalline powder. It darkens slowly on exposure to light, but more rapidly when in solution. It is insoluble in water, freely soluble in acetic acid and in chloroform, slightly soluble in benzene, and very slightly soluble in alcohol and in ether. Its molecular weight is 608.69.

Hydralazine hydrochloride is 1-hydrazinophthalazine monohydrochloride.

Hydralazine hydrochloride USP is a white to off-white, odorless crystalline powder. It is soluble in water, slightly soluble in alcohol, and very slightly soluble in ether. It melts at about 275°C, with decomposition, and has a molecular weight of 196.64.

Hydrochlorothiazide is 6-chloro-3,4-dihydro-$2H$-1,2,4-benzothiadiazine-7-sulfonamide 1,1-dioxide.

Hydrochlorothiazide USP is a white, or practically white, practically odorless crystalline powder. It is slightly soluble in water; freely soluble in sodium hydroxide solution, in n-butylamine, and in dimethylformamide; sparingly soluble in methanol; and insoluble in ether, in chloroform, and in dilute mineral acids. Its molecular weight is 297.73.

Inactive Ingredients: Acacia, FD&C Blue No. 1, FD&C Green No. 3, FD&C Red No. 40, FD&C Yellow No. 6, lactose, polyethylene glycol, starch, stearic acid and sucrose.

CLINICAL PHARMACOLOGY

Reserpine: Reserpine depletes stores of catecholamines and 5-hydroxytryptamine in many organs, including the brain and adrenal medulla. Most of its pharmacological effects have been attributed to this action. Depletion is slower and less complete in the adrenal medulla than in other tissues. The depression of sympathetic nerve function results in a decreased heart rate and a lowering of arterial blood pressure. The sedative and tranquilizing properties of reserpine are thought to be related to depletion of catecholamines and 5-hydroxytryptamine from the brain.

Reserpine, like other rauwolfia compounds, is characterized by slow onset of action and sustained effects. Both cardiovascular and central nervous system effects may persist for a period of time following withdrawal of the drug.

Mean maximum plasma levels of 1.54 ng/ml were attained after a median of 3.5 hours in six normal subjects receiving a single oral dose of four 0.25-mg Serpasil tablets. Bioavailability was approximately 50% of that of a corresponding intravenous dose. Plasma levels of reserpine after intravenous administration declined with a mean half-life of 33 hours. Reserpine is extensively bound (96%) to plasma proteins. No definitive studies on the human metabolism of reserpine have been made.

Hydralazine: Although the precise mechanism of action of hydralazine is not fully understood, the major effects are on the cardiovascular system. Hydralazine apparently lowers blood pressure by exerting a peripheral vasodilating effect through a direct relaxation of vascular smooth muscle. Hydralazine, by altering cellular calcium metabolism, interferes with the calcium movements within the vascular smooth muscle that are responsible for initiating or maintaining the contractile state.

The peripheral vasodilating effect of hydralazine results in decreased arterial blood pressure (diastolic more than systolic); decreased peripheral vascular resistance; and an increased heart rate, stroke volume, and cardiac output. The preferential dilatation of arterioles, as compared to veins, minimizes postural hypotension and promotes the increase in cardiac output. Hydralazine usually increases renin activity in plasma, presumably as a result of increased secretion of renin by the renal juxtaglomerular cells in response to reflex sympathetic discharge. This increase in renin activity leads to the production of angiotensin II, which then causes stimulation of aldosterone and consequent sodium reabsorption. Hydralazine also maintains or increases renal and cerebral blood flow.

Hydralazine is rapidly absorbed after oral administration, and peak plasma levels are reached at 1–2 hours. Plasma levels decline with a half-life of 3–7 hours. Binding to human plasma protein is 87%. Plasma levels of hydralazine vary widely among individuals. Hydralazine is subject to polymorphic acetylation; slow acetylators generally have higher plasma levels of hydralazine and require lower doses to maintain control of blood pressure. Hydralazine undergoes extensive hepatic metabolism; it is excreted mainly in the form of metabolites in the urine.

Administration of hydralazine with food results in higher levels of the drug in plasma.

Hydrochlorothiazide: Thiazides affect the renal tubular mechanism of electrolyte reabsorption. At maximal therapeutic dosage, all thiazides are approximately equal in their diuretic potency. Thiazides increase excretion of sodium and chloride in approximately equivalent amounts. Natriuresis causes a secondary loss of potassium.

The mechanism of the antihypertensive effect of thiazides is unknown. Thiazides do not affect normal blood pressure.

The onset of action of thiazides occurs in 2 hours, and the peak effect at about 4 hours. The action persists for approximately 6–12 hours. Hydrochlorothiazide is rapidly absorbed, as indicated by peak plasma concentrations 1–2.5 hours after oral administration. Plasma levels of the drug are proportional to dose; the concentration in whole blood is 1.6–1.8 times higher than in plasma. Thiazides are eliminated rapidly by the kidney. After oral administration of 25- to 100-mg doses of hydrochlorothiazide, 72–97% of the dose is excreted in the urine, indicating dose-independent absorption. Hydrochlorothiazide is eliminated from plasma in a biphasic fashion with a terminal half-life of 10–17 hours. Plasma protein binding is 67.9%. Plasma clearance is 15.9–30.0 L/hr; volume of distribution is 3.6–7.8 L/kg.

Gastrointestinal absorption of hydrochlorothiazide is enhanced when administered with food. Absorption is decreased in patients with congestive heart failure, and the pharmacokinetics are considerably different in these patients.

INDICATIONS AND USAGE

Hypertension (see boxed **WARNING**).

CONTRAINDICATIONS

Reserpine: Hypersensitivity to reserpine; mental depression (especially with suicidal tendencies); active peptic ulcer; ulcerative colitis; patients receiving electroconvulsive therapy.

Hydralazine: Hypersensitivity to hydralazine; coronary artery disease; mitral valvular rheumatic heart disease.

Hydrochlorothiazide: Anuria; hypersensitivity to this or other sulfonamide-derived drugs.

WARNINGS

Reserpine: Extreme caution should be exercised in treating patients with a history of mental depression. The drug should be discontinued at the first sign of despondency, early morning insomnia, loss of appetite, impotence, or self-deprecation. Drug-induced depression may persist for several months after drug withdrawal and may be severe enough to result in suicide.

Hydralazine: In a few patients hydralazine may produce a clinical picture simulating systemic lupus erythematosus including glomerulonephritis. In such patients hydralazine should be discontinued unless the benefit-to-risk determination requires continued antihypertensive therapy with this drug. Signs and symptoms usually regress when the drug is discontinued, but residua have been detected many years later. Long-term treatment with steroids may be necessary. (See **PRECAUTIONS, Laboratory Tests.**)

Hydrochlorothiazide: Thiazides should be used with caution in patients with severe renal disease. In patients with renal disease, thiazides may precipitate azotemia. Cumulative effects of the drug may develop in patients with impaired renal function.

Thiazides should be used with caution in patients with impaired hepatic function or progressive liver disease, since minor alterations of fluid and electrolyte imbalance may precipitate hepatic coma.

Thiazides may add to or potentiate the action of other antihypertensive drugs. Potentiation occurs with ganglionic or peripheral adrenergic blocking drugs.

Sensitivity reactions are more likely to occur in patients with a history of allergy or bronchial asthma.

The possibility of exacerbation or activation of systemic lupus erythematosus has been reported.

PRECAUTIONS

General

Reserpine: Since reserpine increases gastrointestinal motility and secretion, it should be used cautiously in patients with a history of peptic ulcer, ulcerative colitis, or gallstones (biliary colic may be precipitated).

Caution should be exercised when treating hypertensive patients with renal insufficiency, since they adjust poorly to lowered blood pressure levels.

Preoperative withdrawal of reserpine does not assure that circulatory instability will not occur. It is important that the anesthesiologist be aware of the patient's drug intake and consider this in the overall management, since hypotension has occurred in patients receiving rauwolfia preparations. Anticholinergic and adrenergic drugs (e.g., metaraminol, norepinephrine) have been employed to treat adverse vago-circulatory effects.

Hydralazine: Myocardial stimulation produced by hydralazine can cause anginal attacks and ECG changes indicative of myocardial ischemia. The drug has been implicated in the production of myocardial infarction. It must, therefore, be used with caution in patients with suspected coronary artery disease.

The "hyperdynamic" circulation caused by hydralazine may accentuate specific cardiovascular inadequacies. For example, hydralazine may increase pulmonary artery pressure in patients with mitral valvular disease. The drug may reduce the pressor responses to epinephrine. Postural hypotension may result from hydralazine but is less common than with ganglionic blocking agents. It should be used with caution in patients with cerebral vascular accidents.

In hypertensive patients with normal kidneys who are treated with hydralazine, there is evidence of increased renal blood flow and a maintenance of glomerular filtration rate. In some instances where control values were below normal, improved renal function has been noted after administration of hydralazine. However, as with any antihypertensive agent, hydralazine should be used with caution in patients with advanced renal damage.

Peripheral neuritis, evidenced by paresthesia, numbness, and tingling, has been observed. Published evidence suggests that hydralazine has an antipyridoxine effect and that pyridoxine should be added to the regimen if symptoms develop.

Hydrochlorothiazide: All patients receiving thiazide therapy should be observed for clinical signs of fluid or electrolyte imbalance, namely hyponatremia, hypochloremic alkalosis, and hypokalemia (see **Laboratory Tests** and **Drug/Drug Interactions**). Warning signs are dryness of mouth, thirst, weakness, lethargy, drowsiness, restlessness, muscle pains or cramps, muscular fatigue, hypotension, oliguria, tachycardia, and gastrointestinal disturbance, such as nausea or vomiting.

Hypokalemia may develop, especially in cases of brisk diuresis or severe cirrhosis.

Interference with adequate oral intake of electrolytes will also contribute to hypokalemia. Hypokalemia may be avoided or treated by use of potassium supplements or foods with a high potassium content.

Any chloride deficit is generally mild and usually does not require specific treatment, except under extraordinary circumstances (as in liver disease or renal disease). Dilutional hyponatremia may occur in edematous patients in hot weather; appropriate therapy is water restriction, rather than administration of salt, except in rare instances when the hyponatremia is life-threatening. In cases of actual salt depletion, appropriate replacement is the therapy of choice. Hyperuricemia may occur or frank gout may be precipitated in certain patients receiving thiazide therapy.

Latent diabetes may become manifest during thiazide administration (see **Drug/Drug Interactions**).

The antihypertensive effects of the drug may be enhanced in the postsympathectomy patient.

If progressive renal impairment becomes evident, withholding or discontinuing diuretic therapy should be considered. Calcium excretion is decreased by thiazides. Pathological changes in the parathyroid gland with hypercalcemia and hypophosphatemia have been observed in a few patients on prolonged thiazide therapy. The common complications of hyperparathyroidism, such as renal lithiasis, bone resorption, and peptic ulceration, have not been seen.

Information for Patients: Patients should be informed of possible side effects and advised to take the medication regularly and continuously as directed.

Laboratory Tests

Hydralazine: Complete blood counts and antinuclear antibody titer determinations are indicated before and periodically during prolonged therapy with hydralazine even though the patient is asymptomatic. These studies are also indicated if the patient develops arthralgia, fever, chest pain, continued malaise, or other unexplained signs or symptoms. A positive antinuclear antibody titer requires that the physician carefully weigh the implications of the test results against the benefits to be derived from antihypertensive therapy with a combination drug containing hydralazine. Blood dyscrasias, consisting of reduction in hemoglobin and red cell count, leukopenia, agranulocytosis, and purpura, had been reported. If such abnormalities develop, therapy should be discontinued.

Hydrochlorothiazide: Initial and periodic determinations of serum electrolytes to detect possible electrolyte imbalance should be performed at appropriate intervals.

Serum and urine electrolyte determinations are particularly important when the patient is vomiting excessively or receiving parenteral fluids.

Drug/Drug Interactions

Reserpine: MAO inhibitors should be avoided or used with extreme caution.

Reserpine should be used cautiously with digitalis and quinidine, since cardiac arrhythmias have occurred with rauwolfia preparations.

Concurrent use of tricyclic antidepressants may decrease the antihypertensive effect of reserpine (see CONTRAINDICATIONS).

Concurrent use of reserpine and direct or indirect-acting sympathomimetics should be closely monitored. The action of direct-acting amines (epinephrine, isoproterenol, phenylephrine, metaraminol) may be prolonged when given to patients taking reserpine. The action of indirect-acting amines (ephedrine, tyramine, amphetamines) is inhibited.

Hydralazine: MAO inhibitors should be used with caution in patients receiving hydralazine.

When other potent parenteral antihypertensive drugs, such as diazoxide, are used in combination with hydralazine, patients should be continuously observed for several hours for any excessive fall in blood pressure. Profound hypotensive episodes may occur when diazoxide injections and hydralazine are used concomitantly.

Hydrochlorothiazide: Hypokalemia can sensitize or exaggerate the response of the heart to the toxic effects of digitalis (e.g., increased ventricular irritability).

Hypokalemia may develop during concomitant use of steroids or ACTH.

Insulin requirements in diabetic patients may be increased, decreased, or unchanged.

Thiazides may decrease arterial responsiveness to norepinephrine, but not enough to preclude effectiveness of the pressor agent for therapeutic use.

Thiazides may increase the responsiveness to tubocurarine.

Lithium renal clearance is reduced by thiazides, increasing the risk of lithium toxicity.

There have been rare reports in the literature of hemolytic anemia occurring with the concomitant use of hydrochlorothiazide and methyldopa.

Concurrent administration of some nonsteroidal anti-inflammatory agents may reduce the diuretic, natriuretic and antihypertensive effects of thiazide diuretics.

Drug/Laboratory Test Interactions: Thiazides may decrease serum levels of protein-bound iodine without signs of thyroid disturbance. Ser-Ap-Es should be discontinued before tests for parathyroid function are made (see **General, Hydrochlorothiazide,** Calcium excretion).

Carcinogenesis, Mutagenesis, Impairment of Fertility

Reserpine. *Animal Tumorigenicity:* Rodent studies have shown that reserpine is an animal tumorigen, causing an increased incidence of mammary fibroadenomas in female mice, malignant tumors of the seminal vesicles in male mice, and malignant adrenal medullary tumors in male rats. These findings arose in 2-year studies in which the drug was administered in the feed at concentrations of 5 and 10 ppm—about 100 to 300 times the usual human dose. The breast neoplasms are thought to be related to reserpine's prolactin-elevating effect. Several other prolactin-elevating drugs have also been associated with an increased incidence of mammary neoplasia in rodents.

The extent to which these findings indicate a risk to humans is uncertain. Tissue culture experiments show that about one third of human breast tumors are prolactin-dependent *in vitro*, a factor of considerable importance if the use of the drug is contemplated in a patient with previously detected breast cancer. The possibility of an increased risk of breast cancer in reserpine users has been studied extensively; however, no firm conclusion has emerged. Although a few epidemiologic studies have suggested a slightly increased risk (less than twofold in all studies except one) in women who have used reserpine, other studies of generally similar design have not confirmed this. Epidemiologic studies conducted using other drugs (neuroleptic agents) that, like reserpine, increase prolactin levels and therefore would be considered rodent mammary carcinogens have not shown an association between chronic administration of the drug and human mammary tumorigenesis. While long-term clinical observation has not suggested such an association, the available evidence is considered too limited to be conclusive at this time. An association of reserpine intake with pheochromocytoma or tumors of the seminal vesicles has not been explored.

Hydralazine: In a lifetime study in Swiss albino mice, there was a statistically significant increase in the incidence of lung tumors (adenomas and adenocarcinomas) of both male and female mice given hydralazine continuously in their drinking water at a dosage of about 250 mg/kg per day (about 80 times the maximum recommended human dose). In a 2-year carcinogenicity study of rats given hydralazine by gavage at dose levels of 15, 30, and 60 mg/kg/day (approximately 5 to 20 times the recommended human daily dosage), microscopic examination of the liver revealed a small, but statistically significant, increase in benign neoplastic nodules in male and female rats from the high-dose group and in female rats from the intermediate-dose group. Benign interstitial cell tumors of the testes were also significantly increased in male rats from the high-dose group. The tumors observed are common in aged rats and a significantly increased incidence was not observed until 18 months of treatment. Hydralazine was shown to be mutagenic in bacterial systems (Gene Mutation and DNA Repair) and in one of two rats and one rabbit hepatocyte *in vitro* DNA repair studies. Additional *in vivo* and *in vitro* studies using lymphoma cells, germinal cells, and fibroblasts from mice, bone marrow cells from Chinese hamsters and fibroblasts from human cell lines did not demonstrate any mutagenic potential for hydralazine.

The extent to which these findings indicate a risk to man is uncertain. While long-term clinical observation has not suggested that human cancer is associated with hydralazine use, epidemiologic studies have so far been insufficient to arrive at any conclusions.

Hydrochlorothiazide: Long-term carcinogenicity studies in animals have not been conducted with Esidrix. Hydrochlorothiazide was not mutagenic in in vitro Ames mutagenicity assay of Salmonella typhimurium strains TA 98, TA 100, TA 1535, TA 1537, and TA 1538 or in in vivo mutagenicity assays of mouse germinal cell chromosomes and chinese hamster bone marrow cell chromosomes. It was however, mutagenic in inducing nondisjunction (96% frequency) in diploid strains of Aspergillus nidulans.

Hydrochlorothiazide had no adverse effect on fertility of male or female mice or rats in studies in which these species were exposed to doses up to 4 and 100 mg/kg, respectively.

Pregnancy Category C: Animal reproduction studies have not been conducted with Ser-Ap-Es. Reserpine administered parenterally has been shown to be teratogenic in rats at doses up to 2 mg/kg and to have an embryocidal effect in guinea pigs given dosages of 0.5 mg daily. Animal studies indicate that hydralazine is teratogenic in mice at 20–30 times the maximum daily human dose of 200–300 mg and possibly in rabbits at 10–15 times the maximum daily human dose, but that it is nonteratogenic in rats. Teratogenic effects observed were cleft palate and malformations of facial and cranial bones.

Continued on next page

The full prescribing information for each CIBA product is contained herein and is that in effect as of September 1, 1992.

CIBA—Cont.

There are no adequate and well-controlled studies of Ser-Ap-Es in pregnant women. Ser-Ap-Es should be used during pregnancy only if the potential benefit justifies the potential risk to the fetus.
Nonteratogenic Effects: Reserpine crosses the placental barrier, and increased respiratory tract secretions, nasal congestion, cyanosis, and anorexia may occur in neonates of mothers treated with reserpine. Thiazides also cross the placental barrier and appear in cord blood, and there is a risk of fetal or neonatal jaundice, thrombocytopenia, and possibly other adverse reactions that have occurred in adults.
Nursing Mothers: Reserpine is excreted in maternal breast milk, and increased respiratory tract secretions, nasal congestion, cyanosis, and anorexia may occur in breast-fed infants. Thiazides are also excreted in breast milk. Because of the potential for serious adverse reactions in nursing infants and the potential for tumorigenicity shown for reserpine in animal studies, a decision should be made whether to discontinue nursing or to discontinue Ser-Ap-Es, taking into account the importance of the drug to the mother.
Pediatric Use: Safety and effectiveness of the combination drug in children have not been established.

ADVERSE REACTIONS

Adverse reactions are usually reversible upon reduction of dosage or discontinuation of Ser-Ap-Es. Whenever adverse reactions are moderate or severe, it may be necessary to discontinue the drug.
The following adverse reactions have been observed, but there has not been enough systematic collection of data to support an estimate of their frequency. Consequently the reactions are categorized by organ system and are listed in decreasing order of severity and not frequency.
Reserpine: The following have been observed with rauwolfia preparations:
Digestive: Vomiting, diarrhea, nausea, anorexia, dryness of mouth, hypersecretion.
Cardiovascular: Arrhythmias (particularly when used concurrently with digitalis or quinidine), syncope, angina-like symptoms, bradycardia, edema.
Respiratory: Dyspnea, epistaxis, nasal congestion.
Neurologic: Rare parkinsonian syndrome and other extrapyramidal tract symptoms; dizziness; headache; paradoxical anxiety; depression; nervousness; nightmares; dull sensorium; drowsiness.
Musculoskeletal: Muscular aches.
Genitourinary: Pseudolactation, impotence, dysuria, gynecomastia, decreased libido, breast engorgement.
Metabolic: Weight gain.
Special Senses: Deafness, optic atrophy, glaucoma, uveitis, conjunctival injection.
Hypersensitive Reactions: Purpura, rash, pruritus.
Hydralazine: *Digestive:* Hepatitis, paralytic ileus, vomiting, diarrhea, nausea, constipation, anorexia.
Cardiovascular: Angina pectoris, hypotension, paradoxical pressor response, tachycardia, palpitations, edema, flushing.
Respiratory: Dyspnea, nasal congestion.
Neurologic: Psychotic reactions characterized by depression, disorientation, or anxiety; peripheral neuritis, evidenced by paresthesia, numbness, and tingling; tremors; dizziness; headache.
Musculoskeletal: Muscle cramps, arthralgia.
Genitourinary: Difficulty in urination.
Hematologic: Blood dyscrasias, consisting of reduction in hemoglobin and red cell count, leukopenia, agranulocytosis; lymphadenopathy; splenomegaly; eosinophilia.
Special Senses: Conjunctivitis, lacrimation.
Hypersensitive Reactions: Purpura, fever, urticaria, rash, pruritus, chills.
Hydrochlorothiazide: *Digestive:* Pancreatitis, jaundice (intrahepatic cholestatic), sialadenitis, vomiting, diarrhea, cramping, nausea, gastric irritation, constipation, anorexia.
Cardiovascular: Orthostatic hypotension (may be potentiated by alcohol, barbiturates, or narcotics).
Neurologic: Vertigo, dizziness, transient blurred vision, headache, paresthesia, xanthopsia, weakness, restlessness.
Musculoskeletal: Muscle spasm.
Hematologic: Aplastic anemia, agranulocytosis, leukopenia, thrombocytopenia.
Metabolic: Hyperglycemia, glycosuria, hyperuricemia.
Hypersensitive Reactions: Necrotizing angiitis, Stevens-Johnson syndrome, respiratory distress including pneumonitis and pulmonary edema, purpura, urticaria, rash, photosensitivity.

OVERDOSAGE

Acute Toxicity: No deaths due to acute poisoning with Ser-Ap-Es have been reported.
Oral LD_{50}'s in animals (mg/kg): rats, 397; mice, 272.
Signs and Symptoms
Reserpine. The clinical picture of acute poisoning is characterized chiefly by signs and symptoms due to the reflex parasympathomimetic effect of reserpine.
Impairment of consciousness may occur and may range from drowsiness to coma, depending upon the severity of overdosage. Flushing of the skin, conjunctival injection, and pupillary constriction are to be expected. Hypotension, hypothermia, central respiratory depression, and bradycardia may develop in cases of severe overdosage. Increased salivary and gastric secretion and diarrhea may also occur.
Hydralazine. Signs and symptoms of overdosage include hypotension, tachycardia, headache, and generalized skin flushing.
Complications can include myocardial ischemia and subsequent myocardial infarction, cardiac arrhythmia, and profound shock.
Hydrochlorothiazide. The most prominent feature of poisoning is acute loss of fluid and electrolytes.
Cardiovascular: Tachycardia, hypotension, shock.
Neuromuscular: Weakness, confusion, dizziness, cramps of the calf muscles, paresthesia, fatigue, impairment of consciousness.
Digestive: Nausea, vomiting, thirst.
Renal: Polyuria, oliguria, or anuria (due to hemoconcentration).
Laboratory Findings: Hypokalemia, hyponatremia, hypochloremia, alkalosis; increased BUN (especially in patients with renal insufficiency).
Combined Poisoning: Signs and symptoms may be aggravated or modified by concomitant intake of antihypertensive medication, barbiturates, digitalis (hypokalemia), corticosteroids, narcotics, or alcohol.
Treatment: There is no specific antidote.
The gastric contents should be evacuated, taking adequate precautions against aspiration and for protection of the airway. An activated charcoal slurry may be instilled if conditions permit. Dialysis may not be effective for elimination of Ser-Ap-Es because of its plasma protein binding (see **CLINICAL PHARMACOLOGY**).
These manipulations may have to be omitted or carried out after cardiovascular status has been stabilized, since they might precipitate cardiac arrhythmias or increase the depth of shock.
If hypotension or shock occurs, the patient's legs should be kept raised and lost fluid and electrolytes (potassium, sodium) should be replaced.
Support of the cardiovascular system is of primary importance in suspected hydralazine overdosage. If possible, vasopressors should not be given, but if a vasopressor is required, care should be taken not to precipitate or aggravate cardiac arrhythmia. Tachycardia responds to beta blockers. Digitalization may be necessary.
If hypotension is severe enough to require treatment with a vasopressor, one having a direct action upon vascular smooth muscle (e.g., phenylephrine, levarterenol, metaraminol) should be used to treat the symptomatic effects of reserpine overdosage.
Fluid and electrolyte balance (especially serum potassium) and renal function should be monitored until conditions become normal. Since reserpine is long-acting, the patient should be observed carefully for at least 72 hours.

DOSAGE AND ADMINISTRATION

Dosage should be determined by individual titration (see boxed **WARNING**). Dosage regimens that exceed 0.25 mg of reserpine per day are not recommended.

HOW SUPPLIED

Tablets—round, salmon pink, dry-coated (imprinted CIBA 71) 0.1 mg of reserpine, 25 mg of hydralazine hydrochloride, 15 mg of hydrochlorothiazide
Bottles of 100—NDC 0083-0071-30
Bottles of 1000—NDC 0083-0071-40
Consumer Pack—One Unit
12 bottles—100 tablets each—NDC 0083-0071-99
Accu-Pak® Unit Dose (blister pack)
Box of 100 (strips of 10)—NDC 0083-0071-32
Do not store above 86°F (30°C).
Dispense in tight, light-resistant container (USP).
C91-48 (Rev. 11/91)
Shown in Product Identification Section, page 408

TRANSDERM SCŌP® ℞

[*trans-derm scōpe*]
scopolamine
(formerly Transderm-V)

Transdermal Therapeutic System

This product is now marketed by CIBA Consumer Pharmaceuticals, Division of CIBA-GEIGY Corporation. Please see the complete Prescribing Information on page 880.

VIOFORM® OTC

[*vye-oh-form*]
(clioquinol USP)
Antifungal/Antibacterial Ointment and Cream

Listed in USP, a Medicare designated compendium.

DESCRIPTION

Vioform is 5-chloro-7-iodo-8-quinolinol—an effective antifungal and antibacterial agent—available as 3% *Ointment* and 3% *Cream.*

INDICATIONS AND DIRECTIONS FOR USE

A soothing antifungal and antibacterial preparation for the treatment of inflamed conditions of the skin, such as eczema, athlete's foot and other fungal infections.
Apply to the affected area 2 or 3 times a day or use as directed by physician.

CONTRAINDICATIONS

Do not use in children under 2 years of age. Do not use for diaper rash.

PRECAUTIONS

May prove irritating to sensitized skin in rare cases. If this should occur, discontinue treatment and consult physician. May stain.
KEEP OUT OF REACH OF CHILDREN.

HOW SUPPLIED

Ointment, 3% clioquinol in a petrolatum base; tubes of 1 ounce.
Cream, 3% clioquinol in a water-washable base; tubes of 1 ounce.
Do not store above 86°F.
C90-17 (Rev. 3/90)

VIOFORM®-HYDROCORTISONE ℞

[*vye-oh-form*]
(clioquinol USP and hydrocortisone USP)

DESCRIPTION

Vioform-Hydrocortisone, a topical compound for dermatologic use, combines the antifungal and antibacterial actions of clioquinol USP and the anti-inflammatory and antipruritic effects of hydrocortisone USP to provide broad control of acute and chronic dermatoses. It is available as *Cream,* or *Ointment,* containing 3% clioquinol USP and 1% hydrocortisone USP and as *Mild Cream* containing 3% clioquinol USP and 0.5% hydrocortisone USP.
Vioform is 5-chloro-7-iodo-8-quinolinol.
Hydrocortisone is 11β,17,21-trihydroxypregn-4-ene-3,20-dione.

ACTIONS

In vitro studies have demonstrated that Vioform effectively inhibits the growth of various mycotic organisms such as Microsporons, Trichophytons, and Candida albicans and gram positive cocci such as staphylococci and enterococci. The role of steroids in alleviating the inflammation and pruritus associated with many dermatoses has been well established.

INDICATIONS

Based on a review of this drug by the National Academy of Sciences-National Research Council and/or other information, FDA has classified the indications as follows:
"Possibly" effective: Contact or atopic dermatitis; impetiginized eczema; nummular eczema; infantile eczema; endogenous chronic infectious dermatitis; stasis dermatitis; pyoderma; nuchal eczema and chronic eczematoid otitis externa; acne urticata; localized or disseminated neurodermatitis; lichen simplex chronicus; anogenital pruritus (vulvae, scroti, ani); folliculitis; bacterial dermatoses; mycotic dermatoses such as tinea (capitis, cruris, corporis, pedis); moniliasis; intertrigo.
Final classification of the less-than-effective indications requires further investigation.

CONTRAINDICATIONS

Hypersensitivity to Vioform-Hydrocortisone, or any of its ingredients or related compounds; lesions of the eye; tuberculosis of the skin; most viral skin lesions (including herpes simplex, vaccinia, and varicella).
Vioform should not be used in children under 2 years of age.
Vioform should not be used for diaper rash.

WARNINGS

This product is not for ophthalmic use.
In the presence of systemic infections, appropriate systemic antibiotics should be used.
Usage in Pregnancy: Although topical steroids have not been reported to have an adverse effect on pregnancy, the safety of their use in pregnant women has not been absolutely es-

tablished. In laboratory animals, increases in incidence of fetal abnormalities have been associated with exposure of gestating females to topical corticosteroids, in some cases at rather low dosage levels. Therefore, drugs of this class should not be used extensively on pregnant patients in large amounts or for prolonged periods of time.

PRECAUTIONS
May prove irritating to sensitized skin in rare cases. If irritation occurs, discontinue therapy. Staining of skin and fabrics may occur. Additionally, there are rare reports of discoloration of hair and nails.

Signs and symptoms of systemic toxicity, electrolyte imbalance, or adrenal suppression have not been reported with Vioform-Hydrocortisone. Nevertheless, the possibility of suppression of the pituitary-adrenal axis during therapy should be kept in mind, especially when the drug is used under occlusive dressings, for a prolonged period, or for treating extensive cutaneous areas since significant absorption of corticosteroid may occur under these conditions, particularly in children and infants.

Vioform may be absorbed through the skin and interfere with thyroid function tests. If such tests are contemplated, wait at least one month between discontinuation of therapy and performance of these tests. The ferric chloride test for phenylketonuria (PKU) can yield a false-positive result if Vioform is present in the diaper or urine.

Prolonged use may result in overgrowth of nonsusceptible organisms requiring appropriate therapy.

ADVERSE REACTIONS
There have been a few reports of rash and hypersensitivity. The following local adverse reactions have been reported with topical corticosteroids, especially under occlusive dressings: burning; itching; irritation; dryness; folliculitis; hypertrichosis; acneiform eruptions; hypopigmentation; perioral dermatitis; allergic contact dermatitis; maceration of the skin; secondary infection; skin atrophy; striae; miliaria. Discontinue therapy if any untoward reaction occurs.

DOSAGE AND ADMINISTRATION
Apply a thin layer to the affected parts 3 or 4 times daily. The *Cream*, because of its slight drying effect, is primarily useful for moist, weeping lesions; the *Ointment* is best used for dry lesions accompanied by thickening and scaling of the skin.

The *Mild Cream* should be used when treating lesions involving extensive body areas or less severe dermatoses.

HOW SUPPLIED
Cream, 3% clioquinol and 1% hydrocortisone in a water-washable base containing stearyl alcohol, cetyl alcohol, stearic acid, petrolatum, sodium lauryl sulfate, and glycerin in water; tubes of 5 and 20 Gm.

Ointment, 3% clioquinol and 1% hydrocortisone in a petrolatum base; tubes of 20 Gm.

Mild Cream, 3% clioquinol and 0.5% hydrocortisone in a water-washable base containing stearyl alcohol, cetyl alcohol, stearic acid, petrolatum, sodium lauryl sulfate, and glycerin in water; tubes of ½ and 1 ounce.

Do not store above 86°F.

C90-15 (Rev. 3/90)

Colgate-Hoyt/Gel-Kam
Division of Colgate-Palmolive Co.
1 COLGATE WAY
CANTON, MA 02021 U.S.A.

LURIDE® Drops   ℞
brand of Sodium Fluoride

DESCRIPTION
Each ml. (18 drops) contains 2.25 mg fluoride ion (F⁻) from 4.97 mg sodium fluoride (NaF), approximately 0.125 mg F per drop. For use as a dental caries preventive in children. Sugar-free. Saccharin-free.

CLINICAL PHARMACOLOGY
Sodium fluoride acts systemically (before tooth eruption) and topically (post-eruption) by increasing tooth resistance to acid dissolution, by promoting remineralization, and by inhibiting the cariogenic microbial process.

INDICATIONS AND USAGE
It has been established that ingestion of fluoridated drinking water (1 ppm F) during the period of tooth development results in a significant decrease in the incidence of dental caries.[1] LURIDE Drops was developed to provide systemic fluoride for use as a supplement in infants and children from birth to age 3 and older, living in areas where the drinking water fluoride level does not exceed 0.7 ppm.

CONTRAINDICATIONS
Do not use in areas where the drinking water exceeds 0.7 ppm F.

WARNINGS
See "Contraindications" above. As in the case of all medications, keep out of reach of children. Contains FD&C Yellow No. 6.

PRECAUTIONS
See "Overdosage" section below. Incompatibility of fluoride with dairy foods has been reported due to formation of calcium fluoride which is poorly absorbed.

ADVERSE REACTIONS
Allergic rash and other idiosyncrasies have been rarely reported.

OVERDOSAGE
Prolonged daily ingestion of excessive fluoride will result in varying degrees of dental fluorosis. (The total amount of sodium fluoride in a bottle of 30 ml LURIDE Drops (67.5 mg F) conforms with the recommendations of the American Dental Association for the maximum to be dispensed at one time for safety purposes.)

DOSAGE[2] AND ADMINISTRATION
Invert bottle vertically for proper drop delivery.

F-Content of Drinking Water	Daily Dosage Birth to Age 2	Age 2–3	Age 3–12
<0.3 ppm	2 drops	4 drops	8 drops
0.3–0.7 ppm	One-half above dosage.		
>0.7 ppm	Fluoride supplements contraindicated.		

LURIDE Drops may be administered orally undiluted or mixed with fluids.

HOW SUPPLIED
Squeeze-bottles of 30 ml. (peach flavor—NDC#0126-0003-31)

CAUTION
Federal (U.S.A.) law prohibits dispensing without prescription.

REFERENCES
1. *Accepted Dental Therapeutics*, Ed. 40, American Dental Association, Chicago, 1984, p. 399–402.
2. Ibid., p. 401; American Academy of Pediatrics, Pediatrics 63:150–152, 1979.

LURIDE® **Lozi–Tabs®** Tablets   ℞
brand of Sodium Fluoride
  Full–strength 1.0 mg F
  Luride–SF (no artificial flavor or color)
    1.0 mg F
  Half–strength 0.5 mg F
  Quarter–strength 0.25 mg F

DESCRIPTION
LURIDE® brand of sodium fluoride Lozi-Tabs® brand of lozenge/chewable tablets for use as a dental caries preventive in children. Sugar-free. Saccharin-free. Erythrosine (FDC Red dye #3)-free.

Each LURIDE 1.0 mg F tablet (full-strength) contains 1.0 mg fluoride (F) from 2.2 mg sodium fluoride (NaF).

Each LURIDE -SF 1.0 mg F tablet (SF for Special Formula: no artificial color or flavor) contains 1.0 mg F from 2.2 mg NaF.

Each LURIDE 0.5 mg F tablet (half-strength) contains 0.5 mg F from 1.1 mg NaF.

Each Luride 0.25 mg F tablet (quarter-strength) contains 0.25 mg F from 0.55 mg NaF.

CLINICAL PHARMACOLOGY
Sodium fluoride acts systemically (before tooth eruption) and topically (post-eruption) by increasing tooth resistance to acid dissolution, by promoting remineralization, and by inhibiting the cariogenic microbial process.

INDICATIONS AND USAGE
It is well established that ingestion of fluoridated drinking water (1 ppm F) during the period of tooth development results in a significant decrease in the incidence of dental caries.[1] LURIDE tablets were developed to provide fluoride for children living in areas where the water fluoride level is 0.7 ppm or less.

CONTRAINDICATIONS
LURIDE and LURIDE-SF 1.0 mg F tablets are contraindicated when the F-content of drinking water is 0.3 ppm or more and should not be administered to children under age 3. LURIDE 0.5 mg F and .25 mg F tablets are contraindicated when the F-content of drinking water exceeds 0.7 ppm.

WARNINGS
Do not use LURIDE or LURIDE-SF 1.0 mg F tablets for children under age 3, nor in areas where the F-content of the drinking water is 0.3 ppm or more. Do not use LURIDE 0.5 mg F or LURIDE 0.25 mg F in areas where the F-content of the drinking water is more than 0.7 ppm. As in the case of all medications, keep out of reach of children. LURIDE 1.0 mg F Orange Flavor and LURIDE 0.25 mg F contain FD&C Yellow No. 6.

PRECAUTIONS
See "Overdosage" section below. Incompatibility of fluoride with dairy foods has been reported due to formation of calcium fluoride which is poorly absorbed.

ADVERSE REACTIONS
Allergic rash and other idiosyncrasies have been rarely reported.

OVERDOSAGE
Prolonged daily ingestion of excessive fluoride will result in varying degrees of dental fluorosis. (The total amount of sodium fluoride in a bottle of 120 LURIDE tablets (all strengths) conforms with the recommendations of the American Dental Association for the maximum to be dispensed at one time for safety purposes.)

DOSAGE[2] AND ADMINISTRATION

F-Content of Drinking Water	Daily Dosage (F ion) Birth to Age 2	Age 2–3	Age 3–12
<0.3 ppm	0.25 mg	0.5 mg	1.0 mg.
0.3–0.7 ppm	One-half above dosages.		
>0.7 ppm	Fluoride supplements contraindicated.		

One tablet daily, to be dissolved in the mouth or chewed before swallowing, preferably at bedtime after brushing teeth.

HOW SUPPLIED
[See table below.]

CAUTION
Federal (U.S.A.) law prohibits dispensing without prescription.

LURIDE

Strength (F ion)	Tablets per Bottle	Flavor	NDC Number 0126-
1.0 mg F (full-strength)	120	cherry assorted[1] SF[2]	0006-21 0143-21 0007-21
	1000*	cherry assorted[1]	0006-10 0143-10
	5000*	cherry	0006-51
0.5 mg F (half-strength)	120	grape	0014-21
	1200*	grape	0014-81
0.25 mg F (quarter-strength)	120	vanilla	0186-21

(1) Cherry, orange, lemon, lime.
(2) Special Formula: no artificial flavor or coloring.
* FOR DISPENSING ONLY.

Continued on next page

Colgate-Hoyt/Gel-Kam—Cont.

REFERENCES

1. *Accepted Dental Therapeutics*, Ed. 40, American Dental Association, Chicago, 1984, p. 399–402.
2. Ibid., p. 401; American Academy of Pediatrics, Pediatrics 63:150–152, 1979

ORABASE® HCA ℞

Hydrocortisone Acetate 0.5%
Oral Paste

DESCRIPTION

ORABASE® HCA is an adrenocorticoid topical dental paste for application to the oral mucosa. Each gram contains hydrocortisone acetate 5mg (0.5%) in a paste vehicle containing pectin, gelatin, sodium carboxymethylcellulose dispersed in a plasticized hydrocarbon gel composed of 5% polyethylene in mineral oil, flavored with imitation vanilla.
Hydrocortisone acetate is also known as cortisol acetate. Structural formula: Pregn-4-ene-3,20-dione,21-(acetyloxy)-11,17 dihydroxy-, (11β)-.

CLINICAL PHARMACOLOGY

Hydrocortisone acetate is a natural corticosteroid and possesses properties of an anti-inflammatory, antipruritic, and vasoconstrictive nature. The paste acts as an adhesive vehicle for applying the active medication to oral tissues. The protective action of the adhesive vehicle may serve to reduce oral irritation.
The mechanism of anti-inflammatory activity of the topical corticosteroids is unclear. Various laboratory methods, including vasoconstrictor assays, are used to compare and predict potencies and/or clinical efficacies of the topical corticosteroids. There is some evidence to suggest that a recognizable correlation exists between vasoconstrictor potency and therapeutic efficacy in man.
Once absorbed, topical corticosteroids are handled through pharmacokinetic pathways similar to systemically administered corticosteroids. Corticosteroids are bound to plasma proteins in varying degrees. Corticosteroids are metabolized primarily in the liver and are then excreted by the kidneys. Some of the topical corticosteroids and their metabolites are also excreted into the bile.

INDICATIONS AND USAGE

Indicated for adjunctive treatment and for temporary relief of symptoms associated with oral inflammatory lesions and ulcerative lesions resulting from trauma.

CONTRAINDICATIONS

Topical corticosteroids are contraindicated in those patients with a history of hypersensitivity to any of the components of the preparation. Because it contains a corticosteroid the preparation is contraindicated in the presence of fungal, viral, or bacterial infections of the mouth or throat.

PRECAUTIONS

General: Systemic absorption of topical corticosteroids has produced reversible hypothalamic-pituitary-adrenal (HPA) axis suppression, manifestations of Cushing's syndrome, hyperglycemia, and glucosuria in some patients. Conditions which augment systemic absorption include the application of the more potent steroids, use over large surface areas, and prolonged use.
Therefore, patients receiving a large dose of a potent topical steroid applied to a large surface area should be evaluated periodically for evidence of HPA axis suppression by using the urinary free cortisol and ACTH stimulation tests. If HPA axis suppression is noted, an attempt should be made to withdraw the drug or to reduce the frequency of application. Recovery of HPA axis function is generally prompt and complete upon discontinuation of the drug. Infrequently, signs and symptoms of steroid withdrawal may occur, requiring supplemental systemic corticosteroids.
Children may absorb proportionally larger amounts of topical corticosteroids and thus be more susceptible to systemic toxicity (See PRECAUTIONS-Pediatric Use).
If irritation develops, topical corticosteroids should be discontinued and appropriate therapy instituted.
In the presence of infections, the use of an appropriate antifungal or antibacterial agent should be instituted. If a favorable response does not occur promptly, the corticosteroid should be discontinued until the infection has been adequately controlled.
Information for the Patient: Patients using topical corticosteroids should receive the following information and instructions:

1. This medication is to be used as directed by the dentist or physician. Avoid contact with the eyes.
2. Patients should be advised not to use this medication for any disorder other than for which it was prescribed.
3. The treated area should not be bandaged or otherwise covered or wrapped as to be occlusive unless directed by the dentist or physician.
4. Patients should report any signs of local adverse reactions especially under occlusive dressing.

Laboratory Tests: The following tests may be helpful in evaluating the HPA axis suppression:
Urinary free cortisol test
ACTH stimulation test
Carcinogenesis, Mutagenesis, and Impairment of Fertility: Long-term animal studies have not been performed to evaluate the carcinogenic potential or the affect on fertility of topical corticosteroids.
Studies to determine mutagenicity with hydrocortisone have revealed negative results.
Pregnancy Category C: Corticosteroids are generally teratogenic in laboratory animals when administered systemically at relatively low dosage levels. The more potent corticosteroids have been shown to be teratogenic after dermal application in laboratory animals. There are no adequate and well-controlled studies in pregnant women on teratogenic effects from topically applied corticosteroids. Therefore, topical corticosteroids should be used during pregnancy only if the potential benefit justifies the potential risk to the fetus. Drugs of this class should not be used extensively on pregnant patients, in large amounts, or for prolonged periods of time.
Nursing Mothers: It is not known whether topical administration of corticosteroids could result in sufficient systemic absorption to produce detectable quantities in breast milk. Systemically administered corticosteroids are secreted into breast milk in quantities not likely to have a deleterious effect on the infant. Nevertheless, caution should be exercised when topical corticosteroids are administered to a nursing woman.
Pediatric Use: Pediatric patients may demonstrate greater susceptibility to topical corticosteroid-induced HPA axis suppression and Cushing's syndrome than mature patients. Hypothalamic-pituitary-adrenal (HPA) axis suppression, Cushing's syndrome, and intracranial hypertension have been reported in children receiving topical corticosteroids. Manifestations of adrenal suppression in children include linear growth retardation, delayed weight gain, low plasma cortisol levels, and absence of response to ACTH stimulation. Manifestations of intracranial hypertension include bulging fontanelles, headaches, and bilateral papilledema.
Adminstration of topical corticosteroids to children should be limited to the least amount compatible with an effective therapeutic regimen. Chronic corticosteroid therapy may interfere with the growth and development of children.

ADVERSE REACTIONS

The following local adverse reactions are reported infrequently with topical corticosteroids. These reactions are listed in an approximate decreasing order of occurrence:
Burning
Itching
Irritation
Dryness
Hypopigmentation
Perioral dermatitis
Allergic contact dermatitis
Secondary infection
Striae
Miliaria

OVERDOSAGE

Topically applied corticosteroids can be absorbed in sufficient amounts to produce systemic effects (See PRECAUTIONS).

DOSAGE AND ADMINISTRATION

Dab, *do not rub*, on the lesion until the paste adheres. (Rubbing this preparation on lesions may result in a granular, gritty sensation.) After application, a smooth, slippery film develops.
Usual adult dose: Topical, to the oral mucous membrane, 2 or 3 times a day following meals and at bedtime.
Usual pediatric dose: Dosage has not been established.

HOW SUPPLIED

Net weight 5 g tubes (NDC#0126-0101-45) and 0.75 g patient starter packets in boxes of 100 (NDC#0126-0101-01).

CAUTION

Federal (U.S.A.) law prohibits dispensing without a prescription.

Keep Out of Reach of Children

Products are cross-indexed by generic and chemical names in the **YELLOW SECTION.**

Connaught Laboratories, Inc.

A Pasteur Mérieux Company
SWIFTWATER, PA 18370

CytoGam™ ℞

Cytomegalovirus Immune Globulin Intravaneous (Human)

DESCRIPTION

CytoGam™, Cytomegalovirus Immune Globulin Intravenous (Human) (CMV-IGIV), is a sterile lyophilized powder of immunoglobulin G (IgG), stabilized with 5% sucrose and 1% Albumin (Human). CytoGam™ contains no preservative. The purified immunoglobulin is derived from pooled adult human plasma selected for high titers of antibody for cytomegalovirus (CMV).[1] Source material for fractionation is obtained from another U.S. licensed manufacturer. Pooled plasma was fractionated by ethanol precipitation of the proteins according to Cohn Methods 6 and 9, modified to yield a product suitable for intravenous administration. Certain manufacturing operations have been performed by other firms. When reconstituted with Sterile Water for Injection, USP, each milliliter contains: 50 ± 10 mg of immunoglobulin, primarily IgG, and trace amounts of IgA and IgM; 50 mg of sucrose; 10 mg of Albumin (Human). The reconstituted solution should appear colorless and translucent.

CLINICAL PHARMACOLOGY

CytoGam™ contains IgG antibodies representative of the large number of normal persons who contributed to the plasma pools from which the product was derived. The globulin contains a relatively high concentration of antibodies directed against Cytomegalovirus (CMV). In the case of persons who may be exposed to CMV, CytoGam™ can raise the relevant antibodies to levels sufficient to attenuate or reduce the incidence of serious CMV disease.
In two separate clinical trials, CytoGam™ was shown to provide effective prophylaxis in renal-transplant recipients at risk for primary CMV disease. In the first randomized trial,[2] the incidence of virologically confirmed CMV-associated syndromes was reduced from 60% in controls ($n=35$) to 21% in recipients of CMV immune globulin ($n=24$) ($P<0.01$); marked leukopenia was reduced from 37% in controls to 4% in globulin recipients ($P<0.01$); and fungal or parasitic superinfections were not seen in globulin recipients but occurred in 20% of controls ($P = 0.05$). Serious CMV disease was reduced from 46% to 13%. There was a concomitant but not statistically significant reduction in the incidence of CMV pneumonia (17% of controls as compared with 4% of globulin recipients). There was no effect on rates of viral isolation or seroconversion although the rate of viremia was less in CytoGam™ recipients. In a subsequent non-randomized trial in renal transplant recipients ($n=36$),[3] the incidence of virologically confirmed CMV-associated syndrome was reduced to 36% in the globulin recipients. The rates of CMV-associated pneumonia, CMV-associated hepatitis, and concomitant fungal and parasitic superinfection were similar to those in the first trial.

INDICATIONS AND USAGE

Cytomegalovirus Immune Globulin Intravenous (Human) is indicated for the attenuation of primary (1°) Cytomegalovirus disease associated with kidney transplantation. Specifically, the product is indicated for kidney transplant recipients who are seronegative for CMV and who receive a kidney from a CMV seropositive donor. In a population of seronegative recipients of seropositive kidneys approximately 75% of the untreated recipients would be expected to develop CMV disease.[1,4] Clinical studies have shown a 50% reduction in 1° CMV disease in renal transplant patients given Cytomegalovirus Immune Globulin Intravenous (Human).[2,3]

CONTRAINDICATIONS

CytoGam™ should not be used in individuals with a history of a prior severe reaction associated with the administration of this or other human immunoglobulin preparations. Persons with selective immunoglobulin A deficiency have the potential for developing antibodies to immunoglobulin A and could have anaphylactic reactions to subsequent administration of blood products that contain immunoglobulin A.

WARNINGS

During administration, the patient's vital signs should be monitored continuously and careful observation made for any symptoms throughout the infusion. Epinephrine should be available for the treatment of an acute anaphylactic reaction (see PRECAUTIONS section).

PRECAUTIONS

Although systemic allergic reactions are rare (see ADVERSE REACTIONS section), epinephrine and diphenhydramine should be available for treatment of acute allergic symptoms. If hypotension or anaphylaxis occur, the administration of the immunoglobulin should be discontinued immediately and an antidote should be given as noted above.

CytoGam™ does not contain a preservative. After reconstitution of CytoGam™, the vial should be entered only once for administration purposes and the infusion should begin within 6 hours. The infusion schedule should be adhered to closely (see INFUSION section). Do not use if the solution is turbid.

Drug Interactions: Antibodies present in immune globulin preparations may interfere with the immune response to live virus vaccines such as measles, mumps, and rubella; therefore, vaccination with live virus vaccines should be deferred until approximately three months after administration of CytoGam™. If such vaccinations were given shortly after CytoGam™, a revaccination may be necessary. Admixtures of CytoGam™ with other drugs have not been evaluated. It is recommended that CytoGam™ be administered separately from other drugs or medications which the patient may be receiving (see ADMINISTRATION Section).

Pregnancy Category C. Animal reproduction studies have not been conducted with Cytomegalovirus Immune Globulin Intravenous (Human). It is also not known whether Cytomegalovirus Immune Globulin Intravenous (Human) can cause fetal harm when administered to a pregnant woman or can affect reproduction capacity. Cytomegalovirus Immune Globulin Intravenous (Human) should be given to a pregnant woman only if clearly needed.

ADVERSE REACTIONS

Minor reactions such as flushing, chills, muscle cramps, back pain, fever, nausea, vomiting, and wheezing were the most frequent adverse reactions observed during the clinical trials of CytoGam™. The incidence of these reactions during the clinical trials was less than 5.0% of all infusions and were most often related to infusion rates. A potential side reaction might be hypotension but this has not been observed in over 200 infusions. If a patient develops a minor side effect, *slow the rate* immediately or temporarily interrupt the infusion. Severe reactions such as angioneurotic edema and anaphylactic shock, although not observed during clinical trials, are a possibility. Clinical anaphylaxis may occur even when the patient is not known to be sensitized to immune globulin products. A reaction may be related to the rate of infusion; therefore, carefully adhere to the infusion rates as outlined under "DOSAGE AND ADMINISTRATION". If anaphylaxis or drop in blood pressure occurs, *discontinue infusion* and use antidote such as diphenhydramine and adrenalin.

OVERDOSAGE

Although little data are available, clinical experience with other immunoglobulin preparations suggests that the major manifestations would be those related to volume overload.

DOSAGE AND ADMINISTRATION

The maximum recommended total dosage per infusion is 150 mg/kg, administered according to the following schedule:

Within 72 hours of transplant:	150 mg/kg
2 weeks post transplant:	100 mg/kg
4 weeks post transplant:	100 mg/kg
6 weeks post transplant:	100 mg/kg
8 weeks post transplant:	100 mg/kg
12 weeks post transplant:	50 mg/kg
16 weeks post transplant:	50 mg/kg

Preparation for Administration. Remove the tab portion of the vial cap and clean the rubber stopper with 70% alcohol or equivalent. Reconstitute the lyophilized powder with 50 ml of Sterile Water for Injection, USP. DO NOT SHAKE VIAL; AVOID FOAMING. A double-ended transfer needle or large syringe are suitable for adding the water for reconstitution. When using a double-ended transfer needle, insert one end first into the vial of water. The lyophilized powder is supplied in an evacuated vial so the water should transfer by suction. After the water is transferred into the evacuated vial the residual vacuum should be released to hasten the dissolving process. Rotate the container gently to wet all the undissolved powder. A 30-minute interval should be allowed for dissolving the powder.

Parental drug products should be inspected visually for particulate matter and discoloration prior to administration whenever solution and container permit. Infuse the solution only if it is colorless, free of particulate matter and not turbid.

Infusion. Infusion should begin within 6 hours after reconstitution and should be completed within 12 hours of reconstitution. Vital signs should be taken preinfusion, mid-way and post-infusion as well as before any rate increase. CytoGam™ should be administered through an intravenous line using a constant infusion pump (i.e., IVAC pump or equivalent). Pre-dilution of CytoGam™ before infusion is not recommended. CytoGam™ should be administered through a separate intravenous line. If this is not possible, CytoGam™ may be "piggybacked" into a pre-existing line if that line contains either Sodium Chloride, Injection, USP, or one of the following dextrose solutions (with or without NaCl added): 2.5% dextrose in water, 5% dextrose in water, 10% dextrose in water, 20% dextrose in water. If a pre-existing line must be used, the CytoGam™ should not be diluted more than 1:2 with any of the above-named solutions. Admixtures of CytoGam™ with any other solutions have not

been evaluated. Filters are not necessary for the administration of CytoGam™.

Initial Dose. Administer intravenously at 15 mg per kg body weight per hour. If no adverse reactions occur after 30 minutes, the rate may be increased to 30 mg/kg/hr; if no adverse reactions occur after a subsequent 30 minutes then the infusion may be increased to 60 mg/kg/hr (volume not to exceed 75 ml/hour). DO NOT EXCEED THIS RATE OF ADMINISTRATION. The patient should be monitored closely during and after each rate change.

Subsequent Doses. Administer at 15 mg/kg/hr for 15 minutes. If no adverse reactions occur, increase to 30 mg/kg/hr for 15 minutes and then increase to a maximum rate of 60 mg/kg/hr (volume not to exceed 75 ml/hour). DO NOT EXCEED THIS RATE OF ADMINISTRATION. The patient should be monitored closely during each rate change.

Potential adverse reactions are: flushing, chills, muscle cramps, back pain, fever, nausea, vomiting, wheezing, drop in blood pressure. Minor adverse reactions have been infusion rate related—if the patient develops a minor side effect (i.e. nausea, back pain, flushing), slow the rate or temporarily interrupt the infusion. If anaphylaxis or drop in blood pressure occurs, discontinue infusion and use antidote such as diphenhydramine and adrenalin.

To prevent the transmission of hepatitis viruses or other infectious agents from one person to another, sterile disposable syringes and needles should be used. The syringes and needles should not be reused.

HOW SUPPLIED

CytoGam™ is supplied in a single dose vial containing 2500 mg ± 250 mg of lyophilized immunoglobulin for reconstitution with 50 ml of Sterile Water for Injection, USP—Product No. 14362-0119-1.

STORAGE

CytoGam™ should be stored between 2 and 8°C (35.6–46.4°F). Reconstituted CytoGam™ should be used within 6 hours. CytoGam™ should not be stored in the reconstituted state.

REFERENCES

1. Snydman, D.R., McIver, J., Leszczynski, J., Cho, S.I., Werner, B.G., Berardi, V.P., LoGerfo, F., Heinze-Lacey, B., Grady, G.F. A Pilot Trial of a Novel Cytomegalovirus Immune Globulin in Renal Transplant Recipients. Transplantation 38(5): 553–557, 1984.
2. Snydman, D.R., Werner, B.G. and Heinze-Lacey, B.H., et al. Use of Cytomegalovirus Immune Globulin to Prevent Cytomegalovirus Disease in Renal Transplant Recipients. NEJM 317: 1049–1054, 1987.
3. Snydman, D.R., Werner, B.G. and Tilney, N.L., et al. A Further Analysis of Primary Cytomegalovirus Disease Prevention in Renal Transplant Recipients with a Cytomegalovirus Immune Globulin: Interim Comparison of a Randomized and an Open-Label Trial. Transpl. Proced. Vol. XX, No. 6, Suppl. 8 (December), pp. 24–30, 1988.
4. Ho, M., Suwansirikul, S., Dowling, J.N., et al. The Transplanted Kidney as a Source of Cytomegalovirus Infection. NEJM 293 (2):1109–1112, 1975.

For additional information concerning the preparation and use of Cytomegalovirus Immune Globulin Intravenous (Human) contact:

Director of Medical Affairs
Connaught Laboratories, Inc.
Route 611
P.O. Box 187
Swiftwater, PA 18370
1-800-822-2463

Manufactured by:
MASSACHUSETTS PUBLIC HEALTH BIOLOGIC LABORATORIES
BOSTON, MASSACHUSETTS 02130
License No. 64
Distributed by;
CONNAUGHT LABORATORIES, INC.
Swiftwater, PA 18370, U.S.A.

Product Information
as of October, 1990
2075

DIPHTHERIA AND TETANUS TOXOIDS AND PERTUSSIS VACCINE ADSORBED USP (FOR PEDIATRIC USE)   ℞

Caution: Federal (U.S.A.) law prohibits dispensing without prescription.

DESCRIPTION

Diphtheria and Tetanus Toxoids and Pertussis Vaccine Adsorbed USP, for intramuscular use, combines diphtheria and tetanus toxoids, adsorbed with pertussis vaccine in a sterile isotonic sodium chloride solution containing sodium phosphate to control pH; each 0.5 ml injection contains not more than 0.25 mg of aluminum added in the form of aluminum potassium sulfate. Thimerosal (mercury derivative)

1:10,000 is added as a preservative. The vaccine, in suspension, is a turbid liquid, whitish in color. Each single dose of 0.5 ml is formulated to contain 6.7 Lf units of diphtheria toxoid and 5 Lf units of tetanus toxoid. The total human immunizing dose (the first three 0.5 ml doses given) contains an estimate of 12 units of pertussis vaccine.[1] Each component of the vaccine — diphtheria, tetanus and pertussis — meets the required potency standards.

CLINICAL PHARMACOLOGY

Simultaneous immunization against diphtheria, tetanus, and pertussis during infancy and childhood has been a routine practice in the United States since the late 1940s. This practice has played a major role in markedly reducing the incidence rates of cases and deaths from each of these diseases.[2]

DIPHTHERIA

Cornyebacterium diphtheriae may cause both a localized and a generalized disease. The systemic intoxication is caused by diphtheria exotoxin, an extracellular protein metabolite of toxigenic strains of *C. diphtheriae.*

At one time, diphtheria was common in the United States. More than 200,000 cases, primarily among children, were reported in 1921. Approximately 5%–10% of cases were fatal; the highest case-fatality ratios were in the very young and the elderly. Reported cases of diphtheria of all types declined from 306 in 1975 to 59 in 1979; most were cutaneous diphtheria reported from a single state. After 1979, cutaneous diphtheria was no longer reportable. From 1980 to 1983, only 15 cases of respiratory diphtheria were reported; 11 occurred among persons 20 years of age or older.[2]

The current rarity of diphtheria in the United States is due primarily to the high level of appropriate immunization among children (96% of children entering school have received three or more doses of Diphtheria and Tetanus Toxoids and Pertussis Vaccine [DTP]) and to an apparent reduction of the circulation of toxigenic strains of *C. diphtheriae.* Most cases occur among unimmunized or inadequately immunized persons. The age distribution of recent cases and the results of serosurveys indicate that many adults in the United States are not protected against diphtheria. Thus, it appears that in addition to continuing to immunize children more emphasis should be placed on adult immunization programs.[2]

Both toxigenic and non-toxigenic strains of *C. diphtheriae* can cause disease, but only strains that produce toxin cause myocarditis and neuritis. Furthermore, toxigenic strains are more often associated with severe or fatal illness in noncutaneous (respiratory or other mucosal surface) infections and are more commonly recovered from respiratory than from cutaneous infections.[2]

C. diphtheriae can contaminate the skin of certain individuals, usually at the site of a wound. Although a sharply demarcated lesion with a pseudomembraneous base often results, the appearance may not be distinctive and the infection can be confirmed only by culture. Usually other bacterial species can also be isolated. Cutaneous diphtheria has most commonly affected indigent adults and certain groups of Native Americans.[2]

Complete immunization significantly reduces the risk of developing diphtheria, and immunized persons who develop disease have milder illnesses. Protection is thought to last at least 10 years. Immunization does not, however, eliminate carriage of *C. diphtheriae* in the pharynx or nose or on the skin.[2]

TETANUS

Tetanus is an intoxication manifested primarily by neuromuscular dysfunction caused by a potent exotoxin elaborated by *Clostridium tetani.*

The occurrence of tetanus in the United States has decreased markedly because of the routine use of tetanus toxoid immunization. Nevertheless, the number of reported cases has remained relatively constant in the last decade at an annual average of 90 cases. In 1983, 91 tetanus cases were reported from 29 states. In recent years, approximately two-thirds of patients have been 50 years of age or older. The age distribution of recent cases and the results of serosurveys indicate that many United States adults are not protected against tetanus. The disease has occurred almost exclusively among persons who are unimmunized or inadequately immunized or whose immunization histories are unknown or uncertain.[2]

In 6% of tetanus cases reported during 1982 and 1983, no wound or other condition could be implicated. Non-acute skin lesions, such as ulcers, or medical conditions, such as abscesses, were reported in 17% of cases.[2]

Spores of *C. tetani* are ubiquitous. Serological tests indicate that naturally acquired immunity to tetanus toxin does not occur in the United States. Thus, universal primary immunization, with subsequent maintenance of adequate antitoxin levels by means of appropriately timed boosters, is necessary to protect all age groups. Tetanus toxoid is a highly effective antigen, and a completed primary series generally induces

Continued on next page

Connaught Laboratories—Cont.

protective levels of serum antitoxin that persist for 10 or more years.[2]

PERTUSSIS

Pertussis is a disease of the respiratory tract caused by *Bordetella pertussis.* This gram-negative coccobacillus produces a variety of biologically active components which have been associated with a number of effects such as lymphocytosis, leukocytosis, sensitivity to histamine, changes in glucose and/or insulin levels, neurological effects, and adjuvant activity.[3] The role of each of the different components in either the pathogenesis of or the immunity to pertussis is not well understood.

General use of standardized pertussis vaccine has resulted in a substantial reduction in cases and deaths from pertussis disease. However, the annual number of reported cases has changed relatively little during the last 10 years, when annual averages of 1,835 cases and 10 fatalities have occurred. In 1983, 2,463 cases were reported; in 1981, the latest year for which final national mortality statistics are available from the National Center for Health Statistics, six deaths were recorded. More precise data do not exist, since many cases go unrecognized or unreported, and diagnostic tests for *B. pertussis* — culture and direct-immunofluorescence assay (DFA) — may be unavailable, difficult to perform, or incorrectly interpreted.[2]

For 1982 and 1983, 53% of reported illnesses from *B. pertussis* occurred among children under 1 year of age and 78% in children less than 5 years of age; 13 of 15 deaths reported to the Centers for Disease Control (CDC) occurred in children less than 1 year old. Before widespread use of DTP, about 20% of cases and 50% of pertussis-related deaths occurred among children less than 1 year old.[2]

Pertussis is highly communicable (attack rates of over 90% have been reported for unimmunized household contacts) and can cause severe disease, particularly in very young children. Of patients under 1 year of age reported to CDC during 1982 and 1983, 75% were hospitalized; approximately 22% had pneumonia; 2% had one or more seizures; and 0.7% died.

Because of the substantial risks of complications of the disease, completion of a primary series of DTP early in life is recommended.[2]

In older children and adults, including in some instances those previously immunized, infection may result in nonspecific symptoms of bronchitis or an upper respiratory tract infection, and pertussis may not be diagnosed because classic signs, especially the inspiratory whoop, may be absent. Older preschool-aged children and school-aged siblings who are not fully immunized and develop pertussis can be important sources of infection for young infants, the group at highest risk of disease and disease severity. The importance of the infected adult in overall transmission remains to be defined.[2]

Controversy regarding use of pertussis vaccine led to a formal reevaluation of the benefits and risks of this vaccine. The analysis indicated that the benefits of the vaccine continue to outweigh its risks.[2,4]

Because the incidence and severity of pertussis decrease with age and because the vaccine may cause side effects and adverse reactions, pertussis immunization is not recommended for children after their seventh birthday.[2]

Evidence of the efficacy of pertussis vaccine can be provided by the recent British experience, where a reduction in the number of immunized individuals from 79% in 1973, to 31% in 1978 was associated with an epidemic of 102,500 pertussis cases and 36 deaths between late 1977 and 1980, and 1,440 cases per week reported during the winter of 1981–1982.[3] A similar situation occurred in Japan.[5,6]

The appropriate age for immunization of prematurely born infants is uncertain. Available data indicate that immunization with DTP is recommended to begin at a chronological age of 2 months.[7,8]

As with any vaccine, vaccination with DTP may not protect 100% of susceptible individuals.

INDICATIONS AND USAGE

For active immunization of infants and children to age 7 years against diphtheria, tetanus and pertussis (whooping cough) simultaneously. DTP is recommended for primary immunization of infants and children up to 7 years of age. However, in instances where the pertussis vaccine component is contraindicated, or where the physician decides that pertussis vaccine is not to be administered, Diphtheria and Tetanus Toxoids Adsorbed (For Pediatric Use) should be used. Immunization should be started at 6 weeks to 2 months of age and be completed before the seventh birthday.

CONTRAINDICATIONS

Persons 7 years of age and older must NOT be immunized with Pertussis Vaccine.

Absolute contraindications:[2]

1. Allergic hypersensitivity to any component of the vaccine.
2. Fever of 40.5°C (105°F) or greater within 48 hours.
3. Collapse or shock-like state (hypotonic-hyporesponsive episode) within 48 hours.
4. Persisting, inconsolable crying lasting 3 hours or more or an unusual, high-pitched cry occurring within 48 hours.
5. Convulsion(s) with or without fever occurring within 7 days.
6. Encephalopathy occurring within 7 days; this includes severe alterations in consciousness with generalized or local neurologic signs.

The presence of a neurologic condition characterized by changing developmental or neurologic findings, regardless of whether a definitive diagnosis has been made, is also considered an *absolute contraindication* to receipt of pertussis vaccine, because administration of DTP may coincide with or possibly even aggravate manifestations of the disease. Such disorders include uncontrolled epilepsy, infantile spasms, and progressive encephalopathy.[2]

Use of this product is also contraindicated if the child has a personal or family history of a seizure disorder. However, the ACIP does not accept family histories of convulsions or other central nervous system disorders as contraindications to pertussis vaccination.[2]

IT IS ALSO A CONTRAINDICATION TO ADMINISTER DTP TO INDIVIDUALS KNOWN TO BE SENSITIVE TO THIMEROSAL. IN ANY CASE, EPINEPHRINE INJECTION (1:1000) MUST BE IMMEDIATELY AVAILABLE, SHOULD AN ACUTE ANAPHYLACTIC REACTION OCCUR DUE TO ANY COMPONENT OF THE VACCINE.

Elective immunization procedures should be deferred during an outbreak of poliomyelitis.[9]

WARNINGS

This vaccine must NOT be used for immunizing persons 7 years of age and older.

IMMUNIZATION SHOULD BE DEFERRED DURING THE COURSE OF ANY ACUTE ILLNESS. THE OCCURRENCE OF ANY TYPE OF NEUROLOGICAL SYMPTOMS OR SIGNS, INCLUDING ONE OR MORE CONVULSIONS (SEIZURES) FOLLOWING ADMINISTRATION OF THIS PRODUCT IS *AN ABSOLUTE CONTRAINDICATION* TO FURTHER USE. THIS PRODUCT IS ALSO CONTRAINDICATED IF THE CHILD HAS A PERSONAL OR FAMILY HISTORY OF A SEIZURE DISORDER.

THE PRESENCE OF ANY EVOLVING OR CHANGING DISORDER AFFECTING THE CENTRAL NERVOUS SYSTEM IS A CONTRAINDICATION TO ADMINISTRATION OF DTP REGARDLESS OF WHETHER THE SUSPECTED NEUROLOGICAL DISORDER IS ASSOCIATED WITH OCCURRENCE OF SEIZURE ACTIVITY OF ANY TYPE.

The administration of DTP to children with proven or suspected underlying neurologic disorders, must be decided on an individual basis.

The ACIP recommends the following:

1. **Infants as yet unimmunized who are suspected of having underlying neurologic disease.** Possible latent central nervous system disorders that are suspected because of perinatal complications or other phenomena may become evident as they evolve over time. Because DTP administration may coincide with onset of overt manifestations of such disorders and result in confusion about causation, it is prudent to delay initiation of immunization with DTP or DT (but not OPV) until further observation and study have clarified the child's neurologic status. In addition, the effect of treatment, if any, can be assessed. The decision whether to commence immunization with DTP or DT should be made no later than the child's first birthday. In making this decision, it should be recognized that children with severe neurologic disorders may be at enhanced risk of exposure to pertussis from institutionalization or from attendance at clinics and special schools in which many of the children may be unimmunized. In addition, because of neurologic handicaps, these children may be in greater jeopardy from complications of the disease.[2]
2. **Infants and children with neurologic events temporally associated with DTP.** Infants and children who experience a seizure within 3 days of receipt of DTP or an encephalopathy within 7 days should not receive further pertussis vaccine, even though cause and effect may not be established (see CONTRAINDICATIONS).[2]
3. **Incompletely immunized children with neurologic events occurring between doses.** Infants and children who have received one or more doses of DTP and who experience a neurologic disorder, e.g., a seizure, temporally unassociated with the administration of vaccine but before the next scheduled dose, present a special problem. If the seizure or other disorder occurs before the first birthday and completion of the first three doses of the primary series of DTP, deferral of further doses of DTP or DT (but not OPV) is recommended until the infant's status has been clarified. The decision whether to use DTP or DT to complete the series should be made no later than the child's first birthday and should take into consideration the nature of the child's problem and the benefits and risks of the vaccine. If the seizure or other disorder occurs after the first birthday, the child's neurologic status should be evaluated to ensure the disorder is stable before a subsequent dose of DTP is given.[2]
4. **Infants and children with stable neurologic conditions.** Infants and children with stable neurologic conditions, including well-controlled seizures, may be vaccinated. The occurrence of single seizures (temporally unassociated with DTP) in infants and young children, while necessitating evaluation, need not contraindicate DTP immunization, particularly if the seizures can be satisfactorily explained.[2]
5. **Children with resolved or corrected neurologic disorders.** DTP administration is recommended for infants with certain neurologic problems that have clearly subsided without residua or have been corrected, such as neonatal hypocalcemic tetany or hydrocephalus (following placement of a shunt and without seizures).[2]

Immunosuppressive therapies, including irradiation, antimetabolites, alkylating agents, cytotoxic drugs, and corticosteroids (used in greater than physiologic doses), may reduce the immune response to vaccines. Short-term (less than 2 weeks) corticosteroid therapy or intra-articular, bursal, or tendon injections with corticosteroids should not be immunosuppressive. Although no specific studies with pertussis vaccine are available, if immunosuppressive therapy will be discontinued shortly, it would be reasonable to defer immunization until the patient has been off therapy for one month;[10] otherwise, the patient should be vaccinated while still on therapy.[2]

If Diphtheria and Tetanus Toxoids and Pertussis Vaccine Adsorbed USP (DTP) has been administered to persons receiving immunosuppressive therapy, a recent injection of immune globulin or having an immunodeficiency disorder, an adequate immunologic response may not be obtained.

DTP should not be given to infants or children with any coagulation disorder that would contraindicate intramuscular injection unless the potential benefit clearly outweighs the risk of administration.

The simultaneous administration of DTP, oral polio virus vaccine (OPV), and/or measles-mumps-rubella vaccine (MMR) has resulted in seroconversion rates and rates of side effects similar to those observed when the vaccines are administered separately.[2,10] Therefore, if there is any doubt that a vaccine recipient will return for further vaccine doses, the ACIP recommends the simultaneous administration of all vaccines appropriate to the age and previous vaccination status of the recipient. This would especially include the simultaneous administration of DTP, OPV, and MMR to such persons at 15 months of age or older.[2]

PRECAUTIONS

GENERAL

Epinephrine Injection (1:1000) must be immediately available should an acute anaphylactic reaction occur due to any component of the vaccine.

Prior to an injection of any vaccine, all known precautions should be taken to prevent side reactions. This includes a review of the patient's history with respect to possible sensitivity and any previous adverse reactions to the vaccine or similar vaccines (see CONTRAINDICATIONS), and a current knowledge of the literature concerning the use of the vaccine under consideration.

The vial of vaccine should be vigorously shaken to ensure a proper suspension of the antigen and adjuvant.

Special care should be taken to ensure that the injection does not enter a blood vessel.

A separate sterile syringe and needle or a sterile disposable unit should be used for each individual patient to prevent transmission of hepatitis or other infectious agents from one person to another.

PEDIATRIC USE

THIS VACCINE IS RECOMMENDED FOR IMMUNIZING CHILDREN 6 WEEKS THROUGH 6 YEARS (UP TO THE SEVENTH BIRTHDAY) OF AGE ONLY. Do NOT administer to persons 7 years of age and older.

INFORMATION FOR PATIENT

Parents should be fully informed of the benefits and risks of immunization with DTP.

Prior to administration of any dose of DTP, the parent or guardian should be asked about the recent health status of the infant or child to be injected.

The physician should inform the parents or guardian about the significant adverse reactions that need to be monitored.

As part of the infant's or child's immunization record, informed consent should be obtained and recorded. The lot number and manufacturer of the vaccine administered should be recorded in the event of the occurrence of any symptoms and/or signs of an adverse reaction. Vaccine information sheets are available from the CDC or the State Health Department which may serve as guidelines.

WHEN AN INFANT OR CHILD IS RETURNED FOR THE NEXT DOSE IN THE SERIES, THE PARENT SHOULD BE QUESTIONED CONCERNING OCCURRENCE OF ANY SYMPTOMS AND/OR SIGNS OF AN ADVERSE REACTION AFTER PREVIOUS DOSE (see CONTRAINDICATIONS; ADVERSE REACTIONS).

ADVERSE REACTIONS

Not all adverse events following administration of DTP are causally related to DTP vaccine.

Adverse reactions which may be local and include pain, erythema, heat, edema and induration with or without tenderness, are common after the administration of vaccines containing diphtheria, tetanus, or pertussis antigens. Some data suggest that febrile reactions are more likely to occur in those who have experienced such responses after prior doses.[11] However, these observations were not noted by Barkin, R.M., et al.[12] Occasionally, a nodule may be palpable at the injection site of adsorbed products for several weeks. Sterile abscesses at the site of injection have been reported (6–10 per million doses).

Mild systemic reactions, such as fever, drowsiness, fretfulness, and anorexia, occur quite frequently. These reactions are significantly more common following DTP than following DT, are usually self-limited, and need no therapy other than, perhaps, symptomatic treatment (e.g., antipyretics).[2]

Rash, allergic reactions, and respiratory difficulties, including apnea, have been observed.

Moderate to severe systemic events, such as fever of 40.5°C (105°F) or higher, persistent, inconsolable crying lasting 3 hours or more, unusual high-pitched crying, collapse, or convulsions, occur relatively infrequently. More severe neurologic complications, such as a prolonged convulsion or an encephalopathy, occasionally fatal, have been reported to be associated with DTP administration.[2]

Approximate rates for adverse events following receipt of DTP vaccine (regardless of dose number in the series) are indicated in Table 1.[2,13,14]

The frequency of local reactions and fever following DTP vaccination is significantly higher with increasing numbers of doses of DTP, while other mild to moderate systemic reactions (e.g., fretfulness, vomiting) are significantly less frequent.[13] If local redness of 2.5 cm or greater occurs, the likelihood of recurrence after another DTP dose increases significantly.[11]

In the National Childhood Encephalopathy Study (NCES), a large, case-control study in England,[14] children 2–35 months of age with serious, acute neurologic disorders, such as encephalopathy or complicated convulsion(s), were more likely to have received DTP in the 7 days preceding onset than their age-, sex-, and neighborhood-matched controls. Among children known to be neurologically normal before entering the study, the relative risk (estimated by odds ratio) of a neurologic illness occurring within the 7-day period following receipt of DTP dose, compared to children not receiving DTP vaccine in the 7-day period before onset of their illness, was 3.3 ($p < 0.001$). Within this 7-day period, the risk was significantly increased for immunized children only within 3 days of vaccination (relative risk 4.2, $p < 0.001$). The relative risk for illness occurring 4–7 days after vaccination was 2.1 ($0.05 < p < 0.1$). The attributable risk estimates for a serious acute neurologic disorder within 7 days after DTP vaccine (regardless of outcome) was one in 110,000 doses of DTP, and for a permanent neurologic deficit, one in 310,000 doses. No specific clinical syndrome was identified. Overall, DTP vaccine accounted for only a small proportion of cases of serious neurologic disorders reported in the population studied.[2]

Although there are uncertainties in the reported studies, recent data suggest that infants and young children who have had previous convulsions (whether febrile or nonfebrile) are more likely to have seizures following DTP than those without such histories.[2,15]

Rarely, an anaphylactic reaction (i.e., hives, swelling of the mouth, difficulty breathing, hypotension, or shock) has been reported after receiving preparations containing diphtheria, tetanus, and/or pertussis antigens.[2]

Arthus-type hypersensitivity reactions, characterized by severe local reactions (generally starting 2–8 hours after an injection), may follow receipt of tetanus toxoid, particularly in adults who have received frequent (e.g., annual) boosters of tetanus toxoid. A few cases of peripheral neuropathy have been reported following tetanus toxoid administration, although a causal relationship has not been established.[2]

Sudden infant death syndrome (SIDS) has occurred in infants following administration of DTP. A large case-control study of SIDS in the United States showed that receipt of DTP was not causally related to SIDS.[16] It should be recognized that the first three primary immunizing doses of DTP are usually administered to infants 2–6 months old and that approximately 85% of SIDS cases occur at ages 1–6 months, with the peak incidence occurring at 6 weeks–4 months of age. By chance alone, some SIDS victims can be expected to have recently received vaccine.[2]

Onset of infantile spasms has occurred in infants who have recently received DTP or DT. Analysis of data from the NCES on children with infantile spasms showed that receipt of DTP or DT was not causally related to infantile spasms.[17] The incidence of onset of infantile spasms increases at 3–9 months of age, the time period in which the second and third doses of DTP are generally given. Therefore, some cases of infantile spasms can be expected to be related by chance alone to recent receipt of DTP.[2]

TABLE 1.[2] Adverse events occurring within 48 hours of DTP Immunizations

Event	Frequency*
Local	
Redness	1/3 doses
Swelling	2/5 doses
Pain	1/2 doses
Mild/moderate systemic	
Fever > 38°C (100.4°F)	1/2 doses
Drowsiness	1/3 doses
Fretfulness	1/2 doses
Vomiting	1/15 doses
Anorexia	1/5 doses
More serious systemic	
Persistent, inconsolable crying (duration ≥ 3 hours)	1/100 doses
High-pitched, unusual cry	1/900 doses
Fever ≥ 40.5°C (≥ 105°F)	1/330 doses
Collapse (hypotonic-hyporesponsive episode)	1/1,750 doses
Convulsions (with or without fever)	1/1,750 doses
Acute encephalopathy†	1/110,000 doses
Permanent neurologic deficit†	1/310,000 doses

* Number of adverse events per total number of doses regardless of dose number in DTP series.
† Occurring within 7 days of DTP immunization.

Reporting of Adverse Events

Reporting by parents and patients of all adverse events occurring within 4 weeks of antigen administration should be encouraged. Adverse events that require a visit to a health-care provider should be reported by health-care providers to manufacturers and local or state health departments. The information will be forwarded to an appropriate federal agency (the Office of Biologics Research and Review, FDA, or CDC).[2]

The following illnesses have been reported as temporally associated with the vaccine; neurological complications[18] including cochlear lesion,[19] brachial plexus neuropathies,[19,20] paralysis of the radial nerve,[21] paralysis of the recurrent nerve,[19] accommodation paresis, and EEG disturbances with encephalopathy.[13] In the differential diagnosis of polyradiculoneuropathies following administration of a vaccine containing tetanus toxoid, tetanus toxoid should be considered as a possible etiology.[22]

DOSAGE AND ADMINISTRATION

Parenteral drug products should be inspected visually for extraneous particulate matter and/or discoloration prior to administration whenever solution and container permit. If these conditions exist, vaccine should not be administered.

Epinephrine Injection (1:1000) must be immediately available should an acute anaphylactic reaction occur due to any component of the vaccine.

SHAKE VIAL WELL *before withdrawing each dose. Vaccine contains a bacterial suspension. Vigorous agitation is required to resuspend the contents of the vial.*

Inject 0.5 ml intramuscularly. The vastus lateralis (mid-thigh laterally) is the preferred injection site for infants. The gluteus maximus should be avoided due to the potential for damage to the sciatic nerve. During the course of primary immunization, injections should not be made more than once at the same site.

Do NOT administer this product subcutaneously. Special care should be taken to ensure that the injection does not enter a blood vessel.

This vaccine is recommended for children 6 weeks through 6 years of age (up to seventh birthday) ideally beginning when the infant is 6 weeks to 2 months of age in accordance with the following schedules indicated in Table 2.[2]

Persons 7 years of age and older must NOT be immunized with Pertussis Vaccine.

HOW SUPPLIED

Vial, 7.5 ml — Product No. 49281-280-84

STORAGE

Store between 2° - 8°C (35° - 46°F). DO NOT FREEZE. Temperature extremes may adversely affect resuspendability of this vaccine.

REFERENCES

1. Code of Federal Regulations, 21CFR620.4(g), 1985
2. Recommendation of the Immunization Practices Advisory Committee. Diphtheria, Tetanus, and Pertussis: Guidelines for vaccine prophylaxis and other preventive measures. MMWR 34:405–426, 1985
3. Manclark, C.R., et al: Pertussis. In R. Germanier (ed), Bacterial Vaccines Academic Press Inc., NY 69–106, 1984
4. Hinman, A.R., et al: Pertussis and pertussis vaccine. Reanalysis of benefits, risks, and costs. JAMA 251:3109–3113, 1984
5. Aoyama, T., et al: Efficacy of an acellular pertussis vaccine in Japan. J Pediatr 107:180–183, 1985
6. Sato, Y., et al: Development of a pertussis component vaccine in Japan. Lancet 122–126, 1984
7. Report of the Committee on Infectious Diseases. Immunization of premature infants. American Academy of Pediatrics, 1982
8. Bernbaum, J.C., et al: Response of preterm infants to diphtheria-tetanus-pertussis immunizations. J Pediatr 107:184–188, 1985
9. Wilson, G.S.: The Hazards of Immunization. Provocation poliomyelitis. 270–274, 1967
10. Deforest, A., et al: Simultaneous administration of MMR, OPV and DTP vaccines. Presented at the 24th Interscience Conference on Antimicrobial Agents and Chemotherapy, Washington, DC (abstract #86). October, 1984
11. Baraff, L., et al: DTP—associated reactions: An analysis by injection site, manufacturer, prior reactions and dose. Pediatr 73:31, 1984
12. Barkin, R.M., et al: Diphtheria-pertussis-tetanus vaccine: Reactogenicity of commercial products. Pediatr 63:256, 1979
13. Cody, C.L., et al: Nature and rates of adverse reactions associated with DTP and DT immunizations in infants and children. Pediatr 68: 650–660, 1981
14. Miller, D.L., et al: Pertussis immunization and serious acute neurological illness in children. Br Med J [Clin Res] 282: 1595–1599, 1981
15. CDC. Adverse events following immunization surveillance. Surveillance Report No. 1, 1979–1982 (August 1984)
16. Hoffman, H.J.: SIDS and DTP. 17th Immunization Conference Proceedings, Atlanta, GA: Centers for Disease Control: 79–88, 1982
17. Bellman, M.H., et al: Infantile spasms and pertussis immunization. Lancet, i: 1031–1034, 1983
18. Fenichel, G.M., Neurological complications of immunization. Ann Neurol 12:119–128, 1982
19. Wilson, G.S.: The Hazards of Immunization. Allergic manifestations: Post-vaccinal neuritis. 153–156, 1967
20. Tsairis, P., et al: Natural history of brachial plexus neuropathy. Arch Neurol 27: 109–117, 1972
21. Blumstein, G.I., et al: Peripheral neuropathy following Tetanus toxoid administration. JAMA 198:1030–1031, 1966
22. Schlenska, G.K.: Unusual neurological complications following tetanus toxoid administration. J Neurol 215:299–302, 1977.

Product Information
as of July, 1986
0906

TABLE 2.[2] Routine diphtheria, tetanus, and pertussis immunization schedule summary for children under 7 years old — United States, 1985*

Dose	Age/Interval†	Product
Primary 1	6 weeks old or older	DTP†£
Primary 2	4–8 weeks after first dose§	DTP£
Primary 3	4–8 weeks after second dose§	DTP£
Primary 4	6–12 months after third dose§	DTP£
Booster	4–6 years old, before entering kindergarten or elementary school (not necessary if fourth primary immunizing dose administered on or after fourth birthday)	DTP£
Additional boosters	Every 10 years after last dose	Td

* Important details are in the text.
† Customarily begun at 8 weeks of age, with second and third doses given at 8-week intervals.
§ Prolonging the interval dose does not require restarting series.
£ DT, if pertussis vaccine is contraindicated. If the child is 1 year of age or older at the time the primary dose is given, a third dose 6–12 months after the second completes primary immunization with DT.

Continued on next page

Connaught Laboratories—Cont.

IMOGAM® RABIES ℞
[*ĭm 'o-găm*]
(Rabies Immune Globulin-Human)

NDC 50361-180-20 2ml (300IU) pediatric vial
NDC 50361-180-10 10ml (1500IU) adult vial
Supplied in tamper proof plastic box.

IMOVAX® RABIES ℞
[*ĭm 'o-vak*]
(Rabies Vaccine Human Diploid Cell)

NDC 50361-250-10 1ml IM pre-exposure/post-exposure single dose vial
Supplied in tamper proof unit dose plastic box containing disposable syringe with 1 ml of Sterile Water for Injection U.S.P. for reconstitution and sterile disposable needles for reconstitution and administration, and 1 ml vial of lyophilized vaccine.

IMOVAX® RABIES I.D. ℞
[*im 'o-vak I.D.*]
(Rabies Vaccine Human Diploid Cell)

NDC 50361-251-20 0.1ml I.D. pre-exposure immunization only intradermal syringe.
Supplied in a box containing tamperproof vacuum sealed glass tube holding syringe that contains 0.1ml of lyophilized Rabies Vaccine; a vial of Sterile Water for Injection U.S.P. for reconstitution of the vaccine.
The potency of IMOVAX® RABIES I.D. is equal to or greater than 2.5 I.U./ml of rabies antigen. A 0.1ml intradermal dose contains at least 0.25 I.U. Three 0.1ml I.D. are required for pre-exposure immunization.

IPOL™ ℞
POLIOVIRUS VACCINE INACTIVATED

DESCRIPTION
IPOL™, Poliovirus Vaccine Inactivated, produced by Pasteur Mérieux Sérums & Vaccins S.A., is a sterile suspension of three types of poliovirus: Type 1 (Mahoney), Type 2 (MEF-1), and Type 3 (Saukett). The viruses are grown in cultures of VERO cells, a continuous line of monkey kidney cells, by the microcarrier technique. The viruses are concentrated, purified, and made noninfectious by inactivation with formaldehyde. Each sterile immunizing dose (0.5 ml) of trivalent vaccine is formulated to contain 40 D antigen units of Type 1, 8 D antigen units of Type 2, and 32 D antigen units of Type 3 poliovirus, determined by comparison to a reference preparation. The poliovirus vaccine is dissolved in phosphate buffered saline. Also present are 0.5% of 2-phenoxyethanol and a maximum of 0.02% of formaldehyde per dose as preservatives. Neomycin, streptomycin and polymyxin B are used in vaccine production, and although purification procedures eliminate measurable amounts, less than 5 ng neomycin, 200 ng streptomycin and 25 ng polymyxin B per dose may still be present. The vaccine is clear and colorless and should be administered subcutaneously.

CLINICAL PHARMACOLOGY
IPOL is a highly purified, inactivated poliovirus vaccine produced by microcarrier culture.[1,2] This culture technique and improvements in purification, concentration and standardization of poliovirus antigen have resulted in a more potent and more consistently immunogenic vaccine than the Poliovirus Vaccine Inactivated which was available in the U.S. prior to 1988. These new methods allow for the production of vaccine that induces antibody responses in most children after administering fewer doses[3] than with vaccine available prior to 1988.
Studies in developed[3] and developing[4,5] countries with a similar inactivated poliovirus vaccine produced by the same technology have shown that a direct relationship exists between the antigenic content of the vaccine, the frequency of seroconversion, and resulting antibody titer.
A study in the U.S. was carried out, which involved 219 two-month old infants who had received three doses of a Poliovirus Vaccine Inactivated manufactured by the same process as IPOL except the cell substrate was primary monkey kidney cells. Seroconversion to all three Types of poliovirus was demonstrated in 99% of these infants after two doses of vaccine. Following a third dose of vaccine at 18 months of age, high titers of neutralizing antibody were present in 99.1% of children to Type 1 and 100% of children to Types 2 and 3 polioviruses.[6]
Additional studies were carried out in the U.S. with IPOL. Results were reported for 120 infants who received two doses of IPOL at 2 and 4 months of age. Of these 120 children, detectable serum neutralizing antibody was induced after two doses of vaccine in 98.3% (Type 1), 100% (Type 2) and 97.5% (Type 3) of the children. In 83 children receiving three doses at 2, 4, and 12 months of age detectable serum neutralizing antibodies were detected in 97.6% (Type 1) and 100% (Types 2 and 3) of the children.[7,8]
Poliovirus Vaccine Inactivated reduces pharyngeal excretion of poliovirus.[9–12] Field studies in Europe have demonstrated immunity in populations thoroughly immunized with another IPV.[13–17] A survey of Swedish children and young adults given a Swedish IPV demonstrated persistence of circulating antibodies for at least 10 years to all three types of poliovirus.[13]
Paralytic polio has not been reported in association with administration of Poliovirus Vaccine Inactivated.

INDICATIONS AND USAGE
Poliovirus Vaccine Inactivated is indicated for active immunization of infants, children and adults for the prevention of poliomyelitis. Recommendations on the use of live and inactivated poliovirus vaccines are described in the ACIP Recommendations[18,19] and the 1988 American Academy of Pediatrics Red Book.[20]

INFANTS, CHILDREN AND ADOLESCENTS

General Recommendations
It is recommended that all infants, unimmunized children and adolescents not previously immunized be vaccinated routinely against paralytic poliomyelitis.[18] Poliovirus Vaccine Inactivated should be offered to individuals who have refused Poliovirus Vaccine Live Oral Trivalent (OPV) or in whom OPV is contraindicated. Parents should be adequately informed of the risks and benefits of both inactivated and oral polio vaccines so that they can make an informed choice (Report of An Evaluation of Poliomyelitis Vaccine Policy Options, Institute of Medicine, National Academy of Sciences, Washington, D.C., 1988).
OPV should not be used in households with immunodeficient individuals because OPV is excreted in the stool by healthy vaccinees and can infect an immunocompromised household member, which may result in paralytic disease. In a household with an immunocompromised member, only Poliovirus Vaccine Inactivated should be used for all those requiring poliovirus immunization.[20]

Children Incompletely Immunized
Children of all ages should have their immunization status reviewed and be considered for supplemental immunization as follows for adults. Time intervals between doses longer than those recommended for routine primary immunization do not necessitate additional doses as long as a final total of four doses is reached (see DOSAGE AND ADMINISTRATION).
Previous clinical poliomyelitis (usually due to only a single poliovirus type) or incomplete immunization with OPV are not contraindications to completing the primary series of immunization with Poliovirus Vaccine Inactivated.

ADULTS

General Recommendations
Routine primary poliovirus vaccination of adults (generally those 18 years of age or older) residing in the U.S. is not recommended. Adults who have increased risk of exposure to either vaccine or wild poliovirus and have not been adequately immunized should receive polio vaccination in accordance with the schedule given in the DOSAGE AND ADMINISTRATION section.[18]
The following categories of adults run an increased risk of exposure to wild polioviruses:[19]

- Travelers to regions or countries where poliomyelitis is endemic or epidemic.
- Health care workers in close contact with patients who may be excreting polioviruses.
- Laboratory workers handling specimens that may contain polioviruses.
- Members of communities or specific population groups with disease caused by wild polioviruses.
- Incompletely vaccinated or unvaccinated adults in a household (or other close contacts) with children given OPV provided that the immunization of the child can be assured and not unduly delayed. The adult should be informed of the small OPV related risk to the contact.

IMMUNODEFICIENCY AND ALTERED IMMUNE STATUS

Patients with recognized immunodeficiency are at greater risk of developing paralysis when exposed to live poliovirus than persons with a normal immune system. Under no circumstances should oral live poliovirus vaccine be used in such patients or introduced into a household where such a patient resides.[18]
Poliovirus Vaccine Inactivated should be used in all patients with immunodeficiency diseases and members of such patients' households when vaccination of such persons is indicated. This includes patients with asymptomatic HIV infection, AIDS or AIDS Related Complex, severe combined immunodeficiency, hypogammaglobulinemia, or aggammaglobulinemia; altered immune states due to diseases such as leukemia, lymphoma, or generalized malignancy; or an immune system compromised by treatment with corticosteroids, alkylating drugs, antimetabolites or radiation. Patients with an altered immune state may or may not develop a protective response against paralytic poliomyelitis after administration of Poliovirus Vaccine Inactivated.[21]

CONTRAINDICATIONS
Poliovirus Vaccine Inactivated is contraindicated in persons with a history of hypersensitivity to any component of the vaccine, including neomycin, streptomycin and polymyxin B.
If anaphylaxis or anaphylactic shock occurs within 24 hours of administration of a dose of vaccine, no further doses should be given.
Vaccination of persons with any acute, febrile illness should be deferred until after recovery; however, minor illnesses such as mild upper respiratory infections, are not in themselves reasons for postponing vaccine administration.

WARNINGS
Neomycin, streptomycin, and polymyxin B are used in the producton of this vaccine. Although purification procedures eliminate measurable amounts of these substances, traces may be present (see DESCRIPTION) and allergic reactions may occur in persons sensitive to these substances.

PRECAUTIONS
General
Before injection of the vaccine, the physician should carefully review the recommendations for product use and the patient's medical history including possible hypersensitivities and side effects that may have occurred following previous doses of the vaccine.
Epinephrine hydrochloride (1:1000) and other appropriate agents should be available to control immediate allergic reactions.
Concerns have been raised that stimulation of the immune system of a patient with HIV infection by immunization with inactivated vaccines might cause deterioration in immunologic function. However, such effects have not been noted thus far among children with AIDS or among immunosuppressed individuals after immunizations with inactivated vaccines. The potential benefits of immunization of these children outweigh the undocumented risk of such adverse events.[18]

Drug Interactions
There are no known interactions of Poliovirus Vaccine Inactivated with drugs or foods. Simultaneous administration of other parenteral vaccines is not contraindicated.

Carcinogenesis, Mutagenesis, Impairment of Fertility
Long term studies in animals to evaluate carcinogenic potential or impairment of fertility have not been conducted.

PREGNANCY
REPRODUCTIVE STUDIES—PREGNANCY CATEGORY C

Animal reproduction studies have not been conducted with Poliovirus Vaccine Inactivated. It is also not known whether Poliovirus Vaccine Inactivated can cause fetal harm when administered to a pregnant woman or can affect reproduction capacity. Poliovirus Vaccine Inactivated should be given to a pregnant woman only if clearly needed.

PEDIATRIC USE
Safety and efficacy of IPOL have been shown in children 6 weeks of age and older[6,8] (see DOSAGE AND ADMINISTRATION).

ADVERSE REACTIONS
In earlier studies with the vaccine grown in primary monkey kidney cells, transient local reactions at the site of injection were observed during a clinical trial.[6] Erythema, induration and pain occurred in 3.2%, 1% and 13%, respectively, of vaccinees within 48 hours post-vaccination. Temperatures ≥ 39°C (≥ 102°F) were reported in up to 38% of vaccinees. Other symptoms noted included sleepiness, fussiness, crying, decreased appetite, and spitting up of feedings. Because Poliovirus Vaccine Inactivated was given in a different site but concurrently with Diphtheria and Tetanus Toxoids and Pertussis Vaccine Adsorbed (DTP), systemic reactions could not be attributed to a specific vaccine. However, these systemic reactions were comparable in frequency and severity to that reported for DTP given without IPV.
In another study using IPOL in the United States, there were no significant local or systemic reactions following injection of the vaccine. There were 7% (6/86), 12% (8/65) and 4% (2/45) of children with temperatures over 100.6°F, following the first, second and third doses respectively. Most of the children received DTP at the same time as IPV and therefore it was not possible to attribute reactions to a particular vaccine; however, such reactions were not significantly different than when DTP is given alone.
Although no causal relationship between Poliovirus Vaccine Inactivated and Guillain-Barré Syndrome (GBS) has been established,[22] GBS has been temporally related to administration of another Poliovirus Vaccine Inactivated.
NOTE: The National Childhood Vaccine Injury Act of 1986 requires the keeping of certain records and the reporting of certain events occurring after the administration of vaccine,

including the occurrence of any contraindicating reaction. Poliovirus Vaccines are listed vaccines covered by this Act and health care providers should ensure that they comply with the terms thereof.[23]

DOSAGE AND ADMINISTRATION

Parenteral drug products should be inspected visually for particulate matter and/or discoloration prior to administration. If these conditions exist, vaccine should not be administered.

After preparation of the injection site, immediately administer the vaccine subcutaneously. In infants and small children, the mid-lateral aspect of the thigh is the preferred site. In adults the vaccine should be administered in the deltoid area.

Care should be taken to avoid administering the injection into or near blood vessels and nerves. After aspiration, if blood or any suspicious discoloration appears in the syringe, do not inject but discard contents and repeat procedures using a new dose of vaccine administered at a different site. *DO NOT ADMINISTER VACCINE INTRAVENOUSLY.*

CHILDREN

Primary Immunization

A primary series of IPOL consists of three 0.5 ml doses administered subcutaneously. The interval between the first two doses should be at least four weeks, but preferably eight weeks. The first two doses are usually administered with DTP immunization and are given at two and four months of age. The third dose should follow at least six months but preferably 12 months after the second dose. It may be desirable to administer this dose with MMR and other vaccines, but at a different site, in children 15–18 months of age. All children who received a primary series of Poliovirus Vaccine Inactivated, or a combination of IPV and OPV, should be given a booster dose of OPV or IPV before entering school, unless the final (third dose) of the primary series was administered on or after the fourth birthday.[18]

The need to routinely administer additional doses is unknown at this time.[18]

A final total of four doses is necessary to complete a series of primary and booster doses. Children and adolescents with a previously incomplete series of IPV should receive sufficient additional doses to reach this number.

ADULTS

Unvaccinated Adults

For unvaccinated adults at increased risk of exposure to poliovirus, a primary series of Poliovirus Vaccine Inactivated is recommended. While the responses of adults to primary series have not been studied, the recommended schedule for adults is two doses given at a 1 to 2 month interval and a third dose given 6 to 12 months later. If less than 3 months but more than 2 months are available before protection is needed, 3 doses of Poliovirus Vaccine Inactivated should be given at least 1 month apart. Likewise, if only 1 or 2 months are available, two doses of Poliovirus Vaccine Inactivated should be given at least 1 month apart. If less than 1 month is available, a single dose of either OPV or IPV is recommended.

Incompletely Vaccinated Adults

Adults who are at an increased risk of exposure to poliovirus and who have had at least one dose of OPV, fewer than 3 doses of conventional IPV or a combination of conventional IPV or OPV totalling fewer than 3 doses should receive at least 1 dose of OPV or Poliovirus Vaccine Inactivated. Additional doses needed to complete a primary series should be given if time permits.

Completely Vaccinated Adults

Adults who are at an increased risk of exposure to poliovirus and who have previously completed a primary series with one or a combination of polio vaccines can be given a dose of either OPV or IPV.[19]

HOW SUPPLIED

Syringe, 0.5 ml with integrated needle (1 × 1 Dose package—Product No. 49281-8605-1 and 10 × 1 Dose package—Product No. 49281-8605-2)

STORAGE

The vaccine is stable if stored in the refrigerator between 2°C and 8°C (35°F and 46°F). *The vaccine must not be frozen.*

REFERENCES

1. van Wezel, A.L., et al: Inactivated poliovirus vaccine: Current production methods and new developments. Rev Infect Dis 6 (Suppl 2): S335–S340, 1984
2. Montagnon, B.J., et al: Industrial scale production of inactivated poliovirus vaccine prepared by culture of Vero cells on microcarrier. Rev Infect Dis 6 (Suppl 2): S341–S344, 1984
3. Salk, J., et al: Antigen content of inactivated poliovirus vaccine for use in a one- or two-dose regimen. Ann Clin Res 14: 204–212, 1982
4. Salk, J., et al: Killed poliovirus antigen titration in humans. Develop Biol Standard 41: 110–132, 1978
5. Salk, J., et al: Theoretical and practical considerations in the application of killed poliovirus vaccine for the control of paralytic poliomyelitis. Develop Biol Standard 47: 181–198, 1981
6. McBean, A.M., et al: Serologic response to oral polio vaccine and enhanced-potency inactivated polio vaccines. Am J Epidemiol 128: 615–628, 1988
7. Unpublished data available from Pasteur Mérieux Sérums & Vaccins S.A.
8. Faden, H., et al: Comparative evaluation of immunization with live attenuated and enhanced potency inactivated trivalent poliovirus vaccines in childhood: Systemic and local immune responses. J Infect Dis 162: 1291–1297, 1990
9. Marine, W.M., et al: Limitation of fecal and pharyngeal poliovirus excretion in Salk-vaccinated children. A family study during a Type 1 poliomyelitis epidemic. Amer J Hyg 76: 173–175, 1962
10. Bottiger, M., et al: Vaccination with attenuated Type 1 poliovirus, the Chat strain. II. Transmission of virus in relation to age. Acta Paed Scand 55: 416–421, 1966
11. Dick, G.W.A., et al: Vaccination against poliomyelitis with live virus vaccines. Effect of previous Salk vaccination on virus excretion. Brit Med J 2: 266–269, 1961
12. Wehrle, P.F., et al: Transmission of poliovirus; III. Prevalence of polioviruses in pharyngeal secretions of infected household contacts of patients with clinical disease. Pediatrics 27: 762–764, 1961
13. Bottiger, M.: Long-term immunity following vaccination with killed poliovirus vaccine in Sweden, a country with no circulating poliovirus. Rev Infect Dis 6 (Suppl 2): S545–551, 1984
14. Chin, T.D.Y.: Immunity induced by inactivated poliovirus vaccine and excretion of virus. Rev Infect Dis 6 (Suppl 2): S369–S370, 1984
15. Salk, D.: Herd effect and virus eradication with use of killed poliovirus vaccine. Develop Biol Standard 47: 247–255, 1981
16. Bijerk, H.: Surveillance and control of poliomyelitis in the Netherlands. Rev Infect Dis 6 (Suppl 2): S451–S456, 1984
17. Lapinleimu, K.: Elimination of poliomyelitis in Finland. Rev Infect Dis 6 (Suppl 2): S457–S460, 1984
18. Immunization Practices Advisory Committee (ACIP), Poliomyelitis Prevention: Enhanced-Potency Inactivated Poliomyelitis Vaccine Supplementary Statement. MMWR 36: 795–798, 1987
19. ACIP: Poliomyelitis Prevention, MMWR 31: 22–26 and 31–34, 1982
20. Report of the Committee on Infectious Diseases, American Academy of Pediatrics, 21st ed: 334–342, 1988
21. ACIP: Immunization of children infected with human T-lymphotropic virus type III/lymphadenopathy-associated virus. MMWR 35: 595–606, 1986
22. WHO: Weekly Epidemiology Record 54: 82–83, 1979
23. National Childhood Vaccine Injury Act: Requirements for permanent vaccination records and for reporting of selected events after vaccination. MMWR 37: 197–200, 1988

Product information as of December 1990

Manufactured by:
PASTEUR MÉRIEUX Sérums & Vaccins S.A.
Lyon, France
U.S. License No. 384
Distributed by:
Connaught Laboratories, Inc.
Swiftwater, Pennsylvania 18370, U.S.A.
800-VACCINE/800-822-2463

MONO-VACC® TEST (O.T.) ℞

[*mon'ō-vak*]

TUBERCULIN, MONO-VACC® TEST (O.T.)
(old tuberculin)
Multiple Puncture Device

NDC 50361-770-40 25 tests per box.

Supplied in plastic tamper proof box of 25 tests/box. Also available test reading cards in English, Spanish, Vietnamese and Chinese.

MULTITEST CMI® ℞

[*mul'tĭ-test*]

(Skin Test Antigens for Cellular Hypersensitivity)

NDC 50361-780-80

DESCRIPTION

Skin Test Antigens for Cellular Hypersensitivity, MULTITEST CMI® is a disposable, plastic applicator consisting of eight sterile test heads preloaded with the following seven delayed hypersensitivity skin test antigens and glycerin negative control for precutaneous administration: Tetanus Toxoid Antigen, Diphtheria Toxoid Antigen, Streptococcus Antigen, Old Tuberculin, Candida Antigen, Trichophyton Antigen, and Proteus Antigen.

MULTITEST CMI® provides a quick, convenient and uniform procedure for delayed cutaneous hypersensitivity testing.

Supplied in box of 10 individual cartons containing one preloaded MULTITEST CMI® per carton.

ProHIBiT® ℞
HAEMOPHILUS b CONJUGATE VACCINE

(Diphtheria Toxoid-Conjugate)

Caution: Federal (U.S.A.) law prohibits dispensing without prescription.

DESCRIPTION

ProHIBiT®, Haemophilus b Conjugate Vaccine (Diphtheria Toxoid-Conjugate), for intramuscular use, is a sterile solution, prepared from the purified capsular polysaccharide, a polymer of ribose, ribitol and phosphate (PRP) of the Eagen *Haemophilus influenzae* type b strain covalently bound to diphtheria toxoid (D) and dissolved in sodium phosphate buffered isotonic sodium chloride solution. The polysaccharide-protein conjugate molecule is referred to as PRP-D. Thimerosal (mercury derivative) 1:10,000 is added as a preservative. The vaccine is a clear, colorless solution. Each single dose of 0.5 ml is formulated to contain 25 mcg of purified capsular polysaccharide and 18 mcg of diphtheria toxoid protein.

CLINICAL PHARMACOLOGY

Haemophilus influenzae type b (Haemophilus b) is a leading cause of serious systemic bacterial disease in the United States. It is the most common cause of bacterial meningitis, accounting for an estimated 12,000 cases annually, primarily among children under 5 years of age. The mortality rate is 5%, and neurologic sequelae are observed in as many as 25%–35% of survivors.[1] Most cases of *Haemophilus influenzae* meningitis among children are caused by capsular strains of type b, although this capsular type represents only one of the six types known for this species. In addition to bacterial meningitis, Haemophilus b is responsible for other invasive diseases, including epiglottitis, sepsis, cellulitis, septic arthritis, osteomyelitis, pericarditis, and pneumonia.[1]

In the United States, approximately one of every 1,000 children under 5 years of age develops systemic Haemophilus b disease each year, and a child's cumulative risk of developing systemic Haemophilus b disease at some time during the first 5 years of life is approximately in 200. Attack rates peak between 6 months and 1 year of age and decline thereafter.[1] Approximately 30%–38% of Haemophilus b disease occurs among children 18 months of age or older, and 15%–25% occurs above 24 months of age.[2,3,4] Incidence rates of Haemophilus b disease are increased in certain high-risk groups, such as Native Americans (both American Indian and Eskimos), blacks, individuals of lower socioeconomic status, and patients with asplenia, sickle cell disease, Hodgkin's disease, and antibody deficiency syndromes.[1,4] Recent studies also have suggested that the risk of acquiring primary Haemophilus b disease for children under 5 years of age appears to be greater for those who attend day-care facilities than for those who do not.[5,6,7,8]

The potential for person-to-person transmission of the organism among susceptible individuals has been recognized. Studies of secondary spread of disease in household contacts of index patients have shown a substantially increased risk among exposed household contacts under 4 years of age.[9]

Adults can be colonized with *Haemophilus influenzae* type b from children infected with the organism.[10]

In 1974, a randomized controlled trial was conducted in Finland, which allowed the evaluation of clinical efficacy of a non-conjugated Haemophilus type b polysaccharide vaccine in children 3–71 months of age.[11] Approximately 98,000 children, half of whom received the Haemophilus b vaccine, were enrolled in the field trial and followed for a 4-year period for the occurrence of Haemophilus b disease. Among children 18–71 months of age, 90% protective efficacy (95% confidence limits, 55%–98%) in prevention of all forms of invasive Haemophilus b disease was demonstrated for the 4-year follow-up period.

Based on evidence from this 1974 Finnish efficacy trial, from passive protection in the infant rat model, and from experience with agammaglobulinemic children, an antibody concentration of ≥ 0.15 mcg/ml has been correlated with protection.[11,12,13,14] In three-week post-vaccination serum in the 1974 Finnish trial, antibody levels of ≥ 1 mcg/ml were correlated with long-term protection. In studies of children 18 months of age and older for functional activity, Anti-capsular antibodies induced by ProHIBiT® had bacterial activity, opsonic activity and were also active in passive protection assays.[15,16,17]

The development of stable humoral immunity requires the recognition of foreign material by at least two separate sets

Continued on next page

Connaught Laboratories—Cont.

of lymphocytes. These sets are the B-lymphocytes which are precursors of antibody forming cells, and the T-lymphocytes which modulate the function of B-cells. Some antigens such as polysaccharides are capable of stimulating B-cells directly to produce antibody (T-independent). The responses to many other antigens are augmented by helper T-lymphocytes (T-dependent).[18] The manufacturing process utilizes a new technology, covalent bonding of the capsular polysaccharide of *Haemophilus influenzae* type b to diphtheria toxoid, to produce an antigen which is postulated to convert the T-independent antigen into a T-dependent antigen.[19,20] The protein carries both its own antigenic determinants and those of the covalently bound polysaccharide. As a result of the conjugation to protein, the polysaccharide is postulated to be presented as a T-dependent antigen resulting in both an enhanced antibody response and an immunologic memory.

In studies conducted with ProHIBiT in several locations throughout the U.S., the antibody responses of 18–26 month old children were measured. (Table 1)[15] In other studies, the antibody responses to licensed Haemophilus b polysaccharide vaccines were measured in a comparable age group. (Table 1) [15] The data shown in Table 1 were obtained from sera tested in one laboratory using a single radioimmunoassay (RIA). Mean antibody levels induced by ProHIBiT in children 18–20 months of age are 30-fold higher than those induced by polysaccharide vaccines in the same age group.[15] The RIA procedure used by Connaught Laboratories, Inc. to estimate antibody responses to the Haemophilus b vaccines has been shown to correlate with the assay used by the Finland National Public Health Institute.[21] Antibody levels (≥1.0 mcg/ml) estimated by the Finnish assay were correlated with protection.[11]

[See table below.]

Following immunization of 16–24 month old children with a single dose of ProHIBiT, eighty-nine percent (109/123) had antibody levels ≥0.15 mcg/ml 12 months post immunization, compared to 93% 1 month post vaccination.[18]

No impairment of the immune response to ProHIBit® was observed in a group of 36 patients with sickle cell disease (SS, SC, S-tho-lassemia) aged 1.5 to 5.0 years (mean 3.3 years).[15,22,23] Satisfactory immune responses were obtained following administration of ProHIBit® in children 2 to 6 years of age with acute leukemia who had been on chemotherapy <1 year.[24] However, similar children with chemotherapy >1 year frequently failed to respond to the vaccine.

INDICATIONS AND USAGE

ProHIBiT is indicated for the routine immunization of children 18 months to 5 years of age against invasive diseases caused by *Haemophilus influenzae* type b.[25,26] Administration of ProHIBit® may be considered for children as young as 15 months of age when it is expected that the child will not return at 18 months for Haemophilus b immunization. It should be noted that the percentage of children 15 to 17 months of age producing anti-PRP levels ≥1.0 mcg/ml with administration of ProHIBit® is not as high as that seen in children 18 to 21 months of age, 53% compared to 75% (Table 1)[15]. The clinical significance of this difference is unknown. As with other vaccines, several days following administration of ProHIBiT are required for protective levels of antibody to be attained. Immunization with Haemophilus b conjugate is recommended by the Immunization Practices Advisory Committee (ACIP) for children who are immunosuppressed in association with AIDS or any other immunodeficiency disease.[27]

ProHIBiT will not protect against *Haemophilus influenzae* other than type b or other microorganisms that cause meningitis or septic disease.

No impairment of the immune response to the individual antigens was demonstrated when ProHIBiT and Diphtheria and Tetanus Toxoids and Pertussis Vaccine Adsorbed (DTP) were given in separate sites at the same time.[15,28]

Limited data are available on concomitant administration of ProHIBit® with MMR, OPV (IPV). Fourteen month old Finnish children boosted with PRP-D received MMR concomitantly. Pre and 4 weeks post sera from a small subset (11 patients) showed no significant difference in antibody response to measles, mumps, or Rubella antigens when compared to a group that received MMR alone. A group of 25 Finnish infants received concomitant DTP, PRP-D, and IPV was compared to a group of 25 receiving DTP and IPV only. No significant difference in response to Type 1, Type 2, or Type 3 polio antigens was noted. Response to oral polio vaccine was evaluated in 31 infants immunized with PRP-D who also received OPV concomitantly. No difference in response to Type 1, Type 2, or Type 3 antigens was observed when compared to 22 infants receiving placebo and OPV.[15,29]

ProHIBiT IS NOT RECOMMENDED FOR USE IN CHILDREN YOUNGER THAN 15 MONTHS OF AGE.

CONTRAINDICATIONS

HYPERSENSITIVITY TO ANY COMPONENT OF THE VACCINE, INCLUDING THIMEROSAL AND DIPHTHERIA TOXOID, IS A CONTRAINDICATION TO USE OF THIS VACCINE.

WARNINGS

If ProHIBiT is used in persons with malignancies or those receiving immunosuppressive therapy or who are otherwise immunocompromised, the expected immune response may not be obtained.

As with any vaccine, vaccination with ProHIBit® may not protect 100% of susceptible individuals.

PRECAUTIONS

GENERAL

As with the injection of any biological material, Epinephrine Injection (1:1000) should be available for immediate use should an anaphylactic or other allergic reaction occur.

Prior to an injection of any vaccine, all known precautions should be taken to prevent adverse reactions. This includes a review of the patient's history with respect to possible hypersensitivity to the vaccine or similar vaccines.

Any febrile illness or infection likely to be accompanied by fever is reason to delay the use of ProHIBit, since fever may result occasionally from administration of ProHIBit® alone.

As reported with Haemophilus b to polysaccharide vaccine,[30] cases of Haemophilus b disease may occur in the week after vaccination, prior to the onset of the protective effects of the vaccine.

Special care should be taken to ensure that the injection does not enter a blood vessel.[15]

A separate, sterile syringe and needle or a sterile disposable unit should be used for each individual patient to prevent transmission of hepatitis or other infectious agents from one person to another.

ALTHOUGH SOME IMMUNE RESPONSE TO THE DIPHTHERIA TOXOID COMPONENT MAY OCCUR, IMMUNIZATION WITH ProHIBiT DOES NOT SUBSTITUTE FOR ROUTINE DIPHTHERIA IMMUNIZATION.

CARCINOGENESIS, MUTAGENESIS, IMPAIRMENT OF FERTILITY

ProHIBiT has not been evaluated for its carcinogenic, mutagenic potential or impairment of fertility.

PREGNANCY

REPRODUCTIVE STUDIES — PREGNANCY CATEGORY C

Animal reproduction studies have not been conducted with ProHIBiT. It is also not known whether ProHIBiT can cause fetal harm when administered to a pregnant woman or can affect reproduction capacity. ProHIBiT is NOT recommended for use in a pregnant woman.

PEDIATRIC USE

ProHIBiT® IS NOT RECOMMENDED FOR USE IN CHILDREN YOUNGER THAN 15 MONTHS OF AGE

INFORMATION FOR PATIENT

Parent should be fully informed of the benefits and risk of immunization with Haemophilus b Conjugate Vaccine (Diphtheria Toxoid-Conjugate). Vaccine information booklets are available from Connaught Laboratories, Inc. Information sheets are available from the Centers for Disease Control (CDC) or the State Health Department which may serve as guidelines.

Prior to administration of Haemophilus b Conjugate Vaccine (Diphtheria Toxoid-Conjugate), the parent or guardian should be asked about the recent health status of the infant or child to be injected.

The physician should inform the parent or guardian about the significant adverse reactions that have been temporally associated with Haemophilus b Conjugate Vaccine (Diphtheria Toxoid-Conjugate) administration, informed consent should be obtained and recorded, and the parent should inform the physician if any of these events occur.

As part of the child's immunization record, the date, lot number and manufacturer of the vaccine administered should be recorded.[32,33]

ADVERSE REACTIONS

When ProHIBiT® alone was given to over 1,000 adults and children, no serious adverse reactions were observed.[15,20,25,34] Thrombocytopenia was seen in one adult but a causative relationship was not established.

When ProHIBiT® was given with DTP and Inactivated Poliovirus Vaccine to 55,000 Finnish children, the rate and extent of serious adverse reactions were not different from those seen when DTP or IPV were administered alone.[25,35]

Allergic reactions such as urticaria were infrequently observed.[15,35]

Selected adverse reactions following vaccination with ProHIBiT® (without DTP) in subjects 15–24 months of age are summarized in Table 2.[34]

TABLE 2[34]

Percentage of Subjects 15–24 Months Of Age Developing Local or Systemic Reactions to One Dose of Haemophilus b Conjugate Vaccine (Diphtheria Toxoid-Conjugate)

	No. of Subjects*	Reaction % 6 Hours	24 Hours	48 Hours
Fever >38.3°C	281	1.1	2.1	1.8
Erythema	285	—	2.5	0.4
Induration	285	—	1.0	0.4
Tenderness	285	—	4.6	0.7

*Not all subjects had measurements at all time periods.

Other adverse reactions temporally associated with administration of ProHIBiT® including diarrhea, vomiting, and crying were reported at a frequency of ≤1.2%. Fever of 39°C or more occured in <1%, while irritability, sleepiness, or anorexia were reported in 16.1%.[34]

Adverse reactions in clinical evaluations among 689 children, 7–14 months of age, 24 hours after receiving a single dose of ProHIBiT®, were observed and compared to 139 children who received a saline placebo. There were no significant differences in the reaction rates for fever, erythema, induration, and tenderness between the two groups.[15]

A post-marketing surveillance study was conducted between April 1988 and July 1989 in the United States in 50,007 children 16–60 months of age. At Southern California Kaiser Permanante, 29,309 of these children were followed closely to determine the number of systemic and local reactions occurring within 6, 24, and 48 hours post vaccination with ProHIBit® alone. These reactions are summarized in Table 3.[15]

TABLE 3[15]

Post-Marketing Surveillance Study in Subjects 16–60 Months of Age Experiencing Adverse Reactions (n = 29,309)

	Reaction % 6 Hours	24 Hours	48 Hours
Fever >38.9°C	2	2	2
Analgesic Given	23	12	8
Irritability	17	14	10
Drowsiness	13	8	5
Unusual Crying	2	2	2
Vomiting/Poor Eating	7	7	7
Redness	2	1	1
Swelling	2	2	1
Tenderness	25	12	5

Other adverse reactions reported with administration of ProHIBiT® included urticaria, seizure, and renal failure.[15,34] Guillain-Barré syndrome (GBS) rarely has been reported.[36] However, a cause and effect relationship for these adverse events has not been established.

TABLE 1

Immunogenicity Studies of ProHIBiT and Polysaccharide Vaccines*[18]

Vaccine	Age Group	No. of Subjects	Anti-Polysaccharide GMT (mcg/ml) Pre	Post	% Subjects Responding with ≥ 1.0 mcg/ml**
ProHIBiT	15–17 Mo.	43	0.017	1.12	53%
	18–21 Mo.	173	0.025	2.85	75%
POLYSACCHARIDE	22–26 Mo.	37	0.021	2.96	73%
	18–20 Mo.	51	0.021	0.100	24%
	24–27 Mo.	85	0.035	0.520	43%

* Only subjects whose sera had preimmunization levels ≤0.60 mcg/ml were included in this analysis.

** A subset of these data was obtained from a randomized comparison of the two vaccines, in which the percentage of children 18–20 months of age responding with ≥1.0 mcg/ml was 75% for ProHIBiT (n=12) and 27% for the polysaccharide (n=11).

Reporting of Adverse Events[32,33]
Reporting by parents and patients of all adverse events occurring within 4 weeks of vaccine administration should be encouraged. Adverse events that require a visit to a health-care provider should be reported by health-care providers to manufacturers and local or state health departments. The information will be forwarded to an appropriate federal agency (the Center for Biologics Evaluation and Research of the FDA or CDC).

Health Care Providers also should report these events to Director of Medical Affairs, Connaught Labortories, Inc., Route 611, P.O. Box 187, Swiftwater, PA 18370 or call 1-800-822-2463.

DOSAGE AND ADMINISTRATION

Parenteral drug products should be inspected visually for extraneous particulate matter and/or discoloration prior to administration whenever solution and container permit. If these conditions exist, vaccine should not be administered.
The immunizing dose is a single injection of 0.5 ml given intramuscularly in the outer aspect area of the vastus lateralis (mild-thigh) or deltoid.
Each 0.5 ml dose contains 25 mcg of purified capsular polysaccharide and 18 mcg of conjugated diphtheria toxoid protein.
Before injection, the skin over the site to be injected should be cleansed with a suitable germicide. After insertion of the needle, aspirate to ensure that the needle has not entered a blood vessel.
DO NOT INJECT INTRAVENOUSLY.

HOW SUPPLIED

Syringe, 1 Dose (6 per package)—Product No. 49281-541-61
Vial, 1 Dose (5 per package)—Product No. 49281-541-01
Vial, 5 Dose—Product No. 49281-541-05
Vial, 10 Dose—Product No. 49281-541-10

STORAGE

Store between 2°–8°C (35°–46°F). DO NOT FREEZE.

REFERENCES

1. Recommendation of the Immunization Practices Advisory Committee (ACIP). Polysaccharide vaccine for prevention of *Haemophilus influenzae* type b disease. MMWR 34: 201–205, 1985
2. Cochi, S.L., et al: Immunization of U.S. children with *Hemophilus influenzae* type b polysaccharide vaccine: A cost-effectiveness model of strategy assessment. JAMA 253: 521–529, 1985
3. Murphy, T.V., et al: Prospective surveillance of *Haemophilus influenzae* type b disease in Dallas County, Texas, and in Minnesota. Pediatr 79: 173–179, 1987
4. Broome, C.V.: Epidemiology of *Haemophilus influenzae* type b infections in the United States. Pediatr Infect Dis J 6: 779–782, 1987
5. Istre, G.R., et al: Risk factors for primary invasive *Haemophilus influenzae* disease: Increased risk from day care attendance and school-aged household members. J Pediatr 106: 190–195, 1985
6. Redmond, S.R., et al: *Hemophilus influenzae* type b disease. An epidemiologic study with special reference to day-care centers. JAMA 252: 2581–2584, 1984
7. Murphy, T.V., et al: County-wide surveillance of invasive *Haemophilus* infections: Risk of associated cases in child care programs (CCPs). Twenty-third Interscience Conference on Antimicrobial Agents and Chemotherapy (Abstract #788) 229, 1983
8. Fleming, D., et al: *Haemophilus influenzae* b (Hib) disease—secondary spread in day care. Twenty-fourth Interscience Conference on Antimicrobial Agents and Chemotherapy (Abstract #967) 261, 1984
9. CDC. Prevention of secondary cases of *Haemophilus influenzae* type b disease. MMWR 31: 672–680, 1982
10. Michaels, R.H., et al: Pharyngeal colonization with *Haemophilus influenzae* type b: A longitudinal study of families with a child with meningitis or epiglottitis due to *H. influenzae* type b. J Infec Dis 136: 222–227, 1977
11. Peltola, H., et al: Prevention of *Hemophilus influenzae* type b bacteremic infections with the capsular polysaccharide vaccine. N Engl J Med 310: 1561–1566, 1984
12. Smith, D.H., et al: Responses of children immunized with the capsular polysaccharide of *Hemophilus influenzae*, type b. Pediatr 52: 637–644, 1973
13. Robbins, J.B., et al: Quantitative measurement of "natural" and immunization-induced *Haemophilus influenzae* type b capsular polysaccharide antibodies. Pediatr Res 7: 103–110, 1973
14. Robbins, J.B., et al: A review of the efficacy trials with *Haemophilus influenzae* type b polysaccharide vaccines. In: Sell, S.H., Wright, P.E. eds. *Haemophilus influenzae.* New York: Elsevier Biomedical. 255–263, 1982
15. Unpublished data available from Connaught Laboratories, Inc.
16. Granoff, D.M., et al: Immunogenicity of *Haemophilus influenzae* type b polysaccharide-diphtheria toxoid conjugate vaccine in adults. J Pediatr 105: 22–27, 1984
17. Cates, K.L.: Serum opsonic activity for *Haemophilus influenzae* type b in infants immunized with polysaccharide-protein conjugate vaccines. J Infec Dis 152: 1076–1077, 1985
18. Benacerraf, B., et al: Textbook of Immunology. Cellular interactions. Williams and Wilkins, p. 22, 1979
19. Schneerson, R., et al: Preparation, characterization, and immunogenicity of *Haemophilus influenzae* type b polysaccharide-protein conjugates. J Exp Med 152: 361–376, 1980
20. Lepow, M.L., et al: Safety and immunogenicity of *Haemophilus influenzae* type b-polysaccharide diphtheria toxoid conjugate vaccine in infants 9 to 15 months of age. J Pediatr 106: 185–189, 1985
21. Greenberg, D.P., et al: Variability in quantitation of *Haemophilus influenzae* type b anticapsular antibody (anti-PRP) by radioimmunoassay (RIA). Twenty-sixth Interscience Conference on Antimicrobial Agents and Chemotherapy (Abstract #209) 133, 1986
22. Frank, A.L., et al: *Haemophilus influenzae* Type b immunization of children with sickle cell diseases. Pediatr 82: 571–575, 1988
23. Plotkin, S.A., et al: Vaccines, *Haemophilus influenzae* vaccines. W.B. Saunders Co. p 318, 1988
24. Gigliotti, F., et al: Response of children with acute lymphoblastic leukemia (ALL) to *H. influenzae* type b (Hib) conjugate vaccine. The Society for Pediatric Research (Serial #11595), 1988
25. ACIP—Update: Prevention of *Haemophilus influenzae* type b disease. MMWR 37: 13–16, 1988
26. Report of the Committee on Infectious Diseases, ed 21. Elk Grove Village, IL, American Academy of Pediatrics, p 209, 188
27. ACIP. Immunization of children infected with human immunodeficiency virus—Supplementary ACIP statement. MMWR 37: 181–183, 1988
28. Hendley, J.O., et al: Immunogenicity of *Haemophilus influenzae* type b capsular polysaccharide vaccines in 18-month-old infants. Pediatr 80: 351–354, 1987
29. Eskola, J., et al: Simultaneous administration of *Haemophilus influenzae* type b capsular polysaccharide-diphtheria toxoid conjugate vaccine with routine diphtheria-tetanus-pertussis and inactivated poliovirus vaccinations of childhood. Pediatr Infect Dis J 7: 480–484, 1988
30. FDA Workshop on Haemophilus b Polysaccharide Vaccine—A preliminary Report, MMWR 36: 529–531, 1987
31. Scheifele, D., et al: Antigenuria after receipt of Haemophilus b Diphtheria Toxoid Conjugate Vaccine. Pediatr Infect Dis J 8: 887–888, 1989
32. National Childhood Vaccine Injury Act of 1986 (Amended 1987)
33. National Childhood Vaccine Injury Act: Requirements for permanent vaccination records and for reporting of selected events after vaccination. MMWR 37: 197–200, 1988
34. Berkowitz, C.D., et al: Safety and immunogenicity of *Haemophilus influenzae* type b polysaccharide and polysaccharide diphtheria toxoid conjugate vaccines in children 15 to 24 months of age. J Pediatr 110: 509–514, 1987
35. Eskola, J., et al: Efficacy of *Haemophilus influenzae* type b polysaccharide-diphtheria toxoid conjugate vaccine in infancy. N Engl J Med 317: 717–722, 1987
36. D'Cruz, O.F., et al: Acute inflammatory demyelinating polyradiculoneuropathy (Guillain-Barré Syndrome) after immunization with *Haemophilus influenzae* type b conjugate vaccine. J Pediatr 115: 743–746, 1989

CONNAUGHT® is a trademark owned by Connaught Laboratories, Ltd.
Mfd. by: **CONNAUGHT** LABORATORIES, INC.
Swiftwater, Pennsylvania 18370, U.S.A.

Product Information
as of February, 1990
1746

BCG LIVE (INTRAVESICAL)
THERACYS® ℞

For Treatment of Carcinoma In-situ of the Urinary Bladder

DESCRIPTION

BCG Live (Intravesical), TheraCys®, as prepared by Connaught Laboratories Limited, is a freeze-dried suspension of an attenuated strain of *Mycobacterium bovis* (Bacillus Calmette and Giérin), which has been grown on Sauton medium (potato and glycerin based medium), used in the non-specific active therapy of carcinoma in-situ of the urinary bladder.
CAUTION: TheraCys® is NOT intended to be used as an immunizing agent for the prevention of tuberculosis. TheraCys® is NOT a vaccine for the prevention of cancer.
TheraCys® is formulated to contain 27 mg (dry weight)/vial Bacillus of Calmette and Guérin (BCG) and 5% w/v monosodium glutamate. This product contains no preservative. Each vial of TheraCys® is ready for use following reconstitution with the accompanying diluent (1.0 ml), which consists of approximately 0.85% sodium chloride, 0.025% Tween 80, 0.06% w/v sodium dihydrogen phosphate and 0.25% disodium hydrogen phosphate. The diluent contains no preservative. One dose consists of three pooled vials of reconstituted material further diluted in sterile, preservative-free saline. The reconstituted product contains $3.4 \pm 3.0 \times 10^8$ colony-forming units (CFU) per vial when resuspended in the diluent provided.
To ensure viability of the product through to its labeled expiration date, it is very important that TheraCys® and diluent be stored continuously between 2° and 8°C (35° and 46°F) until use (see STORAGE). It should be used immediately after reconstitution.

CLINICAL PHARMACOLOGY

TheraCys® promotes a local inflammatory reaction with histiocytic and leukocytic infiltration in the urinary bladder.[1,2,3] The local inflammatory effects are associated with an apparent elimination or reduction of superficial cancerous lesions of the urinary bladder. The exact mechanism by which this is accomplished is unknown.
In a randomized, actively controlled multicenter study TherCys® was compared to doxorubicin hydrochloride (Adriamycin) in the treatment of carcinoma in-situ of the urinary bladder. The response of 114 eligible patients for evaluation is given in Table 1 below. Among the 54 patients receiving TheraCys®, 74% had a complete response (negative by cystoscopic examination and by urine cytology). The estimated median time to treatment failure (recurrence, progression or death) was 48.2 months (Table 2).[4]

TABLE 1: RESPONSE OF PATIENTS WITH CARCINOMA IN-SITU TO TREATMENT WITH TheraCys® OR ADRIAMYCIN

	TheraCys® (n = 54)	Adriamycin (n = 60)
Complete Response†	74%*	42%*
No Response‡	11%	10%
Progressive Diseases§	13%	42%
No Evaluation	2%	7%
Total	100%	100%

* Difference is statistically significant (P < 0.01).
† Confirmed by cytology and cystoscopic examination.
‡ Less than a CR or stable disease.
§ Increase of stage or grade.

TABLE 2: TIME TO RECURRENCE, PROGRESSION OR DEATH: TIME TO TREATMENT FAILURE (TTF)

Treatment	Number Studied	Number Failures	Median TTF
TheraCys®	54	27	48.2 months*
Adriamycin	60	46	5.9 months*

* Difference is statistically significant (P < 0.01 by stratified logrank test).

The effect of chemotherapy (other than TheraCys® or Adriamycin) prior to entry into the controlled study was analysed. Patients in the TheraCys® treated arm who had received prior chemotherapy had a complete response rate of 81% (11/26) as compared to 68% (16/28) in the group who had not received prior chemotherapy (Table 3). This difference was not statistically significant.

TABLE 3: PRIOR VERSUS NO PRIOR TREATMENT

Prior Treatment*	Study Arm	Response Rate	Median TTF (# Events/N)
Yes	TheraCys®	81%	Not reached (11/26)
Yes	Adriamycin	53%	7.0 months (22/30)
No	TheraCys®	68%	32.8 months (16/28)
No	Adriamycin	30%	3.7 months (24/30)

* Other than TheraCys® and Adriamycin.

No survival advantage of TheraCys® therapy[4] over that for Adriamycin[4,5,6] was demonstrated after a 40–72 month follow-up. The median time to death for each group was 23 months and 21 months for TheraCys® and Adriamycin respectively.
The clinical trials carried out with TheraCys® included percutaneous administration of 0.5 ml of BCG Live (Intravesical) solution, which was reconstituted in the dilulent provided and further diluted in 50 ml sterile preservative-free

Continued on next page

Connaught Laboratories—Cont.

saline, with each intravesical dose.[4] Some studies have suggested that this may not be necessary[15] and if severe reactions, such as ulceration, occurred the percutaneous treatment was discontinued.

INDICATIONS AND USAGE

TheraCys® is indicated for intravesical use in the treatment of primary and relapsed carcimoma in-situ of the urinary bladder to eliminate residual tumor cells and to reduce the frequency of tumor recurrence. It is indicated for the treatment of carcinoma in-situ with or without associated papillary tumors. TheraCys® is not indicated for the treatment of papillary tumors occurring alone. TheraCys® is also indicated as a therapy for patients with carcinoma in-situ of the bladder following failure to respond to other treatment regimens. CAUTION: TheraCys® is NOT indicated as a immunizing agent for the prevention of tuberculosis. TheraCys® is NOT a vaccine for the prevention of cancer.

CONTRAINDICATIONS

Patients on immunosuppressive therapy or with compromised immune systems should not receive TheraCys® due to the risk of overwhelming systemic mycobacterial sepsis.

TheraCys® should not be administered to patients with fever unless the cause of the fever is determined and evaluated. If the fever is due to an infection, TheraCys® should be withheld until the patient is afebrile and off all therapy.

Patients with urinary tract infection should not receive TheraCys® treatment because administration may result in the risk of disseminated BCG infection or in an increased severity of bladder irritation.

TheraCys® should not be administered as an immunizing agent for the prevention of tuberculosis. TheraCys® is NOT a vaccine for the prevention of cancer.

WARNINGS

TheraCys® should NOT be administered as an immunizing agent for the prevention of tuberculosis. TheraCys® is NOT a vaccine for the prevention of cancer.

Since administration of intravesical TheraCys® causes an inflammatory response in the bladder and has been associated with hematuria, urinary frequency, dysuria and bacterial urinary tract infection, careful monitoring of urinary status is required. If there is an increase in the patient's existing symptoms, or if their symptoms persist or if any of these symptoms develop, the patient should be evaluated and managed for urinary tract infection or BCG toxicity.

Since death has occurred due to systemic BCG infection, patients should be closely monitored for symptoms of such an infection (see PRECAUTIONS). BCG therapy should be withheld upon any suspicion of systemic infection, e.g. granulomatous hepatitis.

Drug combinations containing bone marrow depressants and/or immunosuppressants and/or radiation may either impair the response to TheraCys® or increase the risk of osteomyelitis or disseminated BCG infection (see DRUG INTERACTIONS).

Patients undergoing antimicrobial therapy for other infections should be evaluated to assess whether the therapy will obviate the effects of TheraCys® actions.

For patients with small bladder capacity, increased risk of severity of local irritation should be considered in decisions to treat with TheraCys®.

Intravesical treatment of TheraCys® may induce a sensitivity to tuberculin which could complicate future interpretations of skin test reactions to tuberculin in the diagnosis of suspected mycobacterial infections. Determination of a patient's reactivity to tuberculin prior to administration of TheraCys® may be desirable in this regard.

PRECAUTIONS

General

Contains viable attentuated mycobacteria. Handle as infectious. Use aseptic technique.

The possibility of allergic reactions in individuals sensitive to the components of the product should be borne in mind.

After usage all equipment and materials (e.g. syringes, catheters and containers that may have come into contact with TheraCys®) used for instillation of the product into the bladder, should be placed immediately into plastic bags which are labelled "Infectious Waste" and disposed of accordingly as biohazardous waste.

Aseptic technique must be used during administration of intravesical TheraCys® so as not to introduce contanimants into the urinary tract or to traumatize unduly the urinary mucosa.

Urine voided for 6 hours after instillation should be disinfected with an equal volume of 5% hypochlorite solution (undiluted household bleach) and allowed to stand for 15 minutes before flushing.

It is recommended that intravesical TheraCys® not be administered any sooner than one week following transurethral resection because fatalities due to disseminated BCG infection have been reported with use of TheraCys® after traumatic catheterization.

If the physician believes that the bladder catheterization has been traumatic (e.g., associated with bleeding or possible false passage), then TheraCys® should not be administered and there must be a treatment delay of at least one week. Subsequent treatment should be resumed as if no interruption in the schedule had occurred. That is, all doses of TheraCys® should be administered even after a temporary halt in administration.

If systemic BCG infection is suspected (i.e., if patients have fever over 39°C (103°F) or persistent fever above 38°C (101°F) over two days or severe malaise), an infectious disease specialist should be consulted and fast acting antituberculosis therapy should be initiated. It should be noted that BCG systemic infections are rarely evidenced by positive cultures.

INFORMATION FOR PATIENTS

Patients should be advised to check with their doctor as soon as possible if there is an increase in their existing symptoms, or if their symptoms persist even after receiving a number of treatments, or if any of the following symptoms develop:

More Common	Rare
Blood in Urine	Cough
Fever and Chills	Skin Rash
Frequent Urge to Urinate	
Increased Frequency of Urination	
Joint Pain	
Nausea and vomiting	
Painful Urination	

A cough that develops after administration of TheraCys® could indicate a BCG systemic infection which is life-threatening. If systemic infection occurs it should be treated immediately with antituberculous antibiotics.

All patients should sit while voiding following instillation of solution.

Urine voided for 6 hours after instillation should be disinfected with an equal volume of 5% hypochlorite solution (undiluted household bleach) and allowed to stand for 15 minutes before flushing.

DRUG INTERACTIONS

Patients must also be advised that drug combinations containing bone marrow depressants and/or immunosuppressants and/or radiation may impair the response to TheraCys® or increase the risk of osteomyelitis or disseminated BCG infection.

PREGNANCY

Pregnancy Category C. TheraCys®. Animal reproduction studies have not been conducted with TheraCys®. It is also not known whether TheraCys® can cause fetal harm when administered to a pregnant woman or can affect reproduction capacity. TheraCys® should be given to a pregnant woman only if clearly needed. Women should be advised not be become pregnant while on therapy.

NURSING MOTHERS

It is not known whether TheraCys® is excreted in human milk. Because many drugs are excreted in human milk, caution should be exercised when TheraCys® is administered to a nursing mother.

PEDIATRIC USE

Safety and effectiveness for carcinoma in-situ of the urinary bladder in children have not been established.

ADVERSE REACTIONS

TheraCys® therapy can affect several organs (or parts) of the body in addition to the cancer cells.

In a controlled multi-center clinical trial comparing BCG therapy and doxorubicin hydrochloride (Adriamycin) for the intravesical treatment of superficial transitional cell carcinoma with and without carcinoma in-situ of the bladder, 112 patients received BCG.[4]

In another controlled study using TheraCys® for the treatment of superficial transitional cell carcinoma, with or without carcinoma in-situ, of the blader, similar adverse reactions were observed.[13] However, two deaths were noted in this study which may have been associated with traumatic catheterization.

The incidence of adverse reactions associated with intravesical TheraCys® therapy is given above. Most local adverse reactions occur following the third intravesical instillation. Symptoms usually begin two to four hours after instillation and persist for 24 to 72 hours. Systemic reactions usually last for 1–3 days after each intravesical instillation.[4,13,14]

[See Table 4 at top of next column.]

No fatalities associated with the use of TheraCys® were reported in this study. Two fatalities have been reported with the use of TheraCys® in another study after traumatic catheterization or in the presence of urinary infection.[13]

An increased risk of additional primary malignancies has been reported following radiotherapy and chemotherapy for many types of malignancies. No increase in second primary malignancies after treatment with TheraCys® was reported in these studies.[4]

TABLE 4: LOCAL REACTIONS (% OF 112 PATIENTS)

Reaction	Total	Severe*
Dysuria	51.8	3.6
Frequency	40.2	1.8
Hematuria	39.3	17.0
Cystitis	29.5	0.0
Urgency	17.9	0.0
Urinary Tract Infection	17.9	1.0
Urinary Incontinence	6.3	0.0
Cramps/Pain	6.3	0.0
Decreased Bladder Capacity	5.4	0.0
Tissue in Urine	0.9	0.0
Local Infection	0.9	0.0

*Severe is defined as grade 3 (severe) or grade 4 (life threatening).

TABLE 5: SYSTEMIC REACTIONS (% of 112 PATIENTS)

Reaction	Total	Severe*
Malaise	40.2	2.0
Fever (> 38°C)	38.4	2.6
Chills	33.9	2.6
Anemia	20.5	0.0
Nausea/Vomiting	16.1	0.0
Anorexia	10.7	0.0
Myalgia/Arthralgia/Arthritis	7.1	1.0
Diarrhea	6.3	0.0
Mild Liver Involvement	2.7	0.0
Mild Abdominal Pain	2.7	0.0
Systemic Infection**	2.7	2.0
Pulmonary Infection**	2.7	0.0
Cardiac	2.7	0.0
Headache	1.8	0.0
Hypersensitivity Skin Rash	1.8	0.0
Constipation	0.9	0.0
Dizziness	0.9	0.0
Fatigue	0.9	0.0
Leukopenia	5.4	0.0
Disseminated Intravascular Coagulation	2.7	0.0
Thrombocytopenia	0.9	0.0
Renal Toxicity	9.8	2.0
Genital Pain	9.8	0.0
Flank Pain	0.9	0.0

*Severe is defined as grade 3 (severe) or grade 4 (life threatening).

**Includes both BCG and other infections.

Irritative bladder symptoms associated with TheraCys® administration can be managed symptomatically with phenazopyridine hydrochloride (Pyridium), propantheline bromide (Pro-Banthine), and acetaminophen.[4]

Systemic side effects (such as malaise, fever and chills) may represent hypersensitivity reactions and can be treated with diphenhydramine hydrochloride.[4] Systemic infection as a result of the spread of BCG organisms has occasionally occurred with intravesical TheraCys® administration. The management of this condition is provided under PRECAUTIONS.

DOSAGE AND ADMINISTRATION

Intravesical treatment and prophylaxis for carcinoma in-situ of the urinary bladder should begin between 7 to 14 days after biopsy or transurethral resection if this procedure is done. A dose of **three** (3) vials of TheraCys® is given intravesically under aseptic conditions once weekly for 6 weeks (induction therapy). Each dose (3 reconstituted vials) is further diluted in an additional 50 ml sterile, preservative-free saline for a total of 53 ml (see below). A urethral catheter is inserted into the bladder under aseptic conditions, the bladder drained and then the 53 ml suspension of TheraCys® is instilled slowly by gravity following which the catheter is withdrawn. During the first hour following instillation, the patient should lie for 15 minutes each in the prone and supine positions and also on each side. The patient is then allowed to be up but retains the suspension for another 60 minutes for a total of two hours. All patients may not be able to retain the suspension for the 2 hours and should be instructed to void in less time if necessary. At the end of 2 hours all patients should void in a seated position for safety reasons. Patients should be instructed to maintain adequate hydration.

If the physician believes that the bladder catheterization has been traumatic (e.g., associated with bleeding or possible false passage), then TheraCys® should not be administered and there must be a treatment delay of at least one week. Subsequent treatment should be resumed as if no interruption in the schedule had occurred. That is, all doses of TheraCys® should be administered even after a temporary halt in administration.

The induction therapy should be followed by one treatment given 3, 6, 12, 18 and 24 months following the initial treatment.

After use, all equipment, materials and containers that may have come in contact with TheraCys® should be sterilized or disposed of properly as with any other biohazardous waste (see PRECAUTIONS).

Reconstitution of Freeze-Dried Product and Withdrawal from Rubber-Stoppered Vial.

TheraCys® SHOULD BE USED IMMEDIATELY AFTER RECONSTITUTION. KEEP REFRIGERATED UNTIL USE. DISCARD AFTER 2 HOURS.

DO NOT REMOVE THE RUBBER STOPPER FROM THE VIAL.

Reconstitute and dilute immediately prior to use.

Persons handling product should be masked and gloved.

TheraCys® should not be handled by persons with a known immunologic deficiency.

TheraCys® should be handled as infectious material.

Reconstitute and dilute using aseptic technique.

TheraCys® should be reconstituted only with the diluent provided to ensure proper dispersion of the organisms.

Apply a **sterile** pledget of cotton moistened with a suitable antiseptic to the surface of the rubber stoppers of the vials of diluent and TheraCys® product. Allow the antiseptic to act for at least 5 minutes. Draw into a **sterile** syringe a volume of air equal to the volume of the diluent in the vial. Pierce the centre of the rubber stopper in the vial containing diluent with the **sterile** needle of the syringe, invert the vial, slowly inject into it the air contained in the syringe and, keeping the point of the needle immersed, withdraw into the syringe 1.0 ml of diluent. Then holding the syringe-plunger steady, withdraw the needle from the vial. Inject this volume of diluent into the vial of freeze-dried material. Shake the vial gently until a fine, even suspension results. Withdraw the entire contents of the reconstituted material into the syringe.

The reconstituted material from three vials (1 dose) is further diluted in an additional 50 ml **sterile**, preservative-free saline to a final volume of 53 ml for intravesical instillation (and percutaneous injection if it is given, see CLINICAL PHARMACOLOGY).

HOW SUPPLIED

TheraCys® is supplied in packages containing three vials of the freeze-dried product containing 27 mg (dry weight)/vial ($3.4 \pm 3.0 \times 10^8$ CFU/vial) and three vials of diluent containing 1 ml/vial.

STORAGE

TheraCys® and the accompanying diluent should be kept in a refrigerator at a temperature between 2° and 8°C (35° and 46°F). It should not be used after the expiration date marked on the vial, otherwise it may be inactive. The product should be used **immediately** after reconstitution; however, it must not be used after 2 hours. Any reconstituted product which exhibits flocculation or clumping that cannot be dispersed with gentle shaking should not be used.

At no time should the freeze-dried or reconstituted TheraCys® be exposed to sunlight, direct or indirect. Exposure to artificial light should be kept to a minimum.[9]

REFERENCES

1. Old LJ, Clarke DA, Benacerraf B. Effect of bacillus Calmette-Guérin infection on transplanted tumors in the mouse. Nature 1959; 184:291.
2. Lamn DL, Harris SC, Gittes RF. Bacillus Calmette-Guérin and dinitrochlorobenzene immunotherapy of chemically induced bladder tumors. Investigative Urology 1977; 14: 369.
3. Morales A. Ottenhof P, Emerson L. Treatment of residual non-infiltrating bladder cancer with bacillus Calmette-Guérin. J Urol 1981; 125:649.
4. Unpublished clinical data available from Connaught Laboratories Limited.
5. Horn Y, Eidelman A, Walach N, Ilian M. Intravesical chemotherapy in a controlled trial with thiotepa versus doxorubicin hydrochloride. J Urol 1981; 125: 652–654.
6. Zincke H, Utz DC, Taylor WF, Myers RP, Leary FJ. Influence of thiotepa and doxorubicin instillation at time of transurethral surgical treatment of bladder cancer on tumor recurrence: a prospective, randomized, double-blind, controlled trial. J Urol 1983; 129: 505–509.
7. Unpublished clinical data available for Connaught Laboratories Limited.
8. Lamm DL, et al. Complications of Bacillus Calmette-Guérin immunotherapy: review of 2602 patients and comparison of chemotherapy complications. EORTIC GU Group Monograph 1989; 6: 335–355.
9. Landi S, Barbara C, Przykuta K, Held RH. Effect of light on freeze dried BCG Vaccines. J Biol Stand 1977; 5: 321–6.
10. Lamm DL, Blumenstein BA, Crawford ED, et al. South-West Oncology Group comparison of bacillus Calmette-Guérin and doxorubicin in the treatment and prophylaxis of superficial bladder cancer. J Urol 1987: 178A.
11. Mori K, Lamm DL, Crawford ED. A trial of Bacillus Calmette-Guérin versus Adriamycin in superficial bladder cancer: a South-West Oncology Group Study, Urol Int 1986; 41: 254–259.
12. Soloway M. Evaluation and management of patients with superficial bladder cancer. Urol Clin North Am 1987; 14: 771.
13. Lamm DL, BCG in carcinoma in-situ and superficial bladder tumors, EORTC GU Group Monograph 1988; 5: 497.
14. Lamm DL. Complications of Bacillus Calmette-Guérin immunotherapy in 1,278 patients with bladder cancer. J Urol 1986; 135: 272.
15. Lamm DL, Sarodosy MS, DeHaven JI. Percutaneous, oral, or intravesical BCG administration: what is the optimal route? EORTC Genitourinary Group Monograph 6: BCG in Superficial Bladder Cancer. 1989; 301–310.

Manufactured by
CONNAUGHT LABORATORIES LIMITED
Willowdale, Ontario, Canada
Distributed by:
CONNAUGHT LABORATORIES, INC.
Swiftwater, Pennsylvania 18370, U.S.A.
01-0590 CLI

ConvaTec
Division of E.R. Squibb & Sons, Inc.
PRINCETON, NJ 08543

DUODERM®   OTC
ADHESIVE COMPRESSION BANDAGE
Nonsterile
For the management of venous stasis leg ulcers where compression therapy is needed.
Apply over a primary wound dressing, such as DuoDERM® CGF® Control Gel Formula Dressing or DuoDERM® Hydroactive® Dressing

PRODUCT DESCRIPTRION
The DuoDERM Adhesive Compression Bandage is designed for use over a primary wound dressing, such as DuoDERM® CGF® Control Gel Formula Dressing or DuoDERM® Hydroactive® Dressing for patients with impaired venous return. It consists of a hydrocolloid adhesive skin contact layer and a woven cotton elastic support layer. This bandage is comfortable, allowing for more patient mobility and comfort, and does not slip, thereby maintaining compression more effectively.

INDICATIONS
● Venous stasis leg ulcer management where compression therapy is needed.

CONTRAINDICATIONS
● Do not use on an open wound.
● Arterial and mixed venous arterial ulcers.

PRECAUTIONS
See the instructions for use supplied with the primary wound dressing for the precautions of that product.
1. Initial use of this product should be under the direction of a health professional.
2. The DuoDERM Compression Bandage provides only local management of the wound site. In venous stasis ulcer care, lack of adequate rest in patients with vascular insufficiency can increase the amount of local edema and hinder potential healing.
3. If redness or irritation results, discontinue use and consult a health care professional.
4. Do not use on fragile or weeping eczematous skin.

INSTRUCTIONS FOR USE
IMPORTANT: Assure the leg is free of any oinments (including petrolatum-based ointments), sprays, creams, or powders.
PREPARING AND CLEANSING THE WOUND SITE
The ulcer should be cleansed and the surrounding skin dried carefully prior to the application of the primary wound dressing and the DuoDERM Compression Bandage.
APPLYING THE DRESSING
See instructions for use supplied with the primary wound dressing for application of that product. The dressing must be applied to the ulcer prior to the application of the compression bandage.
APPLYING THE ADHESIVE COMPRESSION BANDAGE
1. Start the bandage at the center of the ball of the foot, with the lower edge of the bandage at the base of the toes. Wrap the bandage using slight tension 1½ times around the foot.

[See Figure 1 above.]

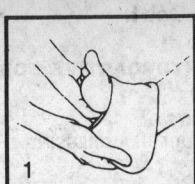

2. Anchor the attached bandage with the thumb and start the turn around the heel by pulling 6–7 inches of the bandage away from the roll. Relax the tension on the bandage and stretch the bandage about 50%. While the bandage is stretched, wrap around the heel area.

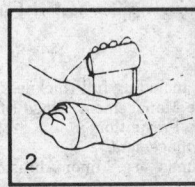

3. Anchor the attached bandage with the thumb, pull 6–7 inches of the bandage away from the roll, relax the tension on the bandage and stretch the bandage 50%. Wrap the bandage over the front of the ankle and under the arch to cover the gap.

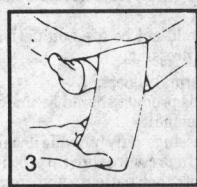

4. Anchor the attached bandage with your thumb, pull another 6–7 inches of bandage away from the roll, relax tension on the bandage and stretch the bandage 50% toward the ankle area. It is very important to maintain proper tension for two turns in the ankle area. This type of compression will aid venous return.
Overlap each turn by 50% as the bandage is wrapped up the leg, gradually decreasing the amount of stretch applied to the bandage.
Anchor the bandage with your thumb. Pull about 10 inches of the bandage away from the roll, relax the tension on the bandage and stretch only 25% of the bandage and wrap around the leg. Continue this technique, gradually decreasing the amount of stretch applied to the bandage, to just below the knee.

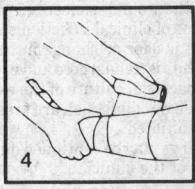

5. If necessary, cut any excess bandage and secure the end of the final turn of the bandage with pieces of tape.

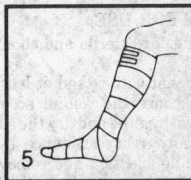

The DuoDERM Compression Bandage can be left undisturbed for up to 7 days, unless leakage of exudate is present, if signs of clinical infection are suspected, or if there is numbness or tingling in the toes.

REMOVING THE DRESSING AND THE BANDAGE
To remove the bandage, lift the free edge and carefully pull it off, while pressing on the adjacent skin with the other hand. Remove the primary wound dressing as described in that product's package insert.

HOW SUPPLIED
DuoDERM® Adhesive Compression Bandage
Individually packaged   **Order No.**
4 inches × 252 inches (7 yards) (stretched)   37340
ConvaTec
Division of E.R. Squibb & Sons, Inc.   ©1991
Princeton, NJ 08543   Made in U.S.A. J4399A

Continued on next page

ConvaTec—Cont.

DUODERM® HYDROACTIVE® DRESSING   OTC
Sterile

DuoDERM® CGF®
CONTROL GEL FORMULA DRESSING
Sterile

PRODUCT DESCRIPTION
DuoDERM Hydroactive Dressings and DuoDerm CGF Dressings interact with wound exudate producing a soft, moist gel at the wound interface. This gel enables removal of the dressing with little or no damage to newly formed tissue. They help isolate the wound against bacterial and other external contamination.

INDICATIONS
- Dermal Ulcers, including full thickness wounds
  - Pressure Sore Management, Stage I through IV
  - Pressure Sore Prevention
  - Leg Ulcer Management
- Superficial Wounds—e.g. Minor Abrasions
- Donor Sites
- Burns—Second Degree
- Occlusive Dressing Technique

PRECAUTIONS AND OBSERVATIONS
DuoDERM Dressings are not recommended for use on third degree burns.
The dressings should not be used on patients with a known sensitivity to the dressing.

When used on Dermal Ulcers:
1. Initial use of this product should be under the direction of a health professional.
2. DuoDERM Dressings only provide local management of the wound site. In pressure sore care, other aspects such as repositioning of the patient and nutritional support should not be neglected. In leg ulcer care, lack of adequate rest in patients with vascular (arterial or venous) insufficiency can increase the amount of local edema and hinder potential healing.
3. Increased Wound Size: Deeper tissue damage may have already occurred under an apparent superficial dermal ulcer. When using any occlusive dressing in the presence of necrotic material, the wound may increase in size and depth during the initial phase of management as the necrotic debris is cleaned away. Leg ulcers resulting from vasculitis may rapidly deteriorate during exacerbation of the underlying disorder.

Odor: Wounds, particularly those that are large or necrotic, are often accompanied by a disagreeable odor; however, this is not necessarily indicative of infection. The odor should disappear when the wound is cleansed (see infection).
Infection: If signs of clinical infection should develop, such as: uncharacteristic odor or change in the color of the exudate, fever or cellulitis (tenderness and erythema in the area of the wound), a bacterial culture of the wound site should be taken. If clinical signs of infection are present, medical treatment should be initiated.
DuoDERM dressings may be continued during the treatment at the discretion of the clinician.

Granulation: Excessive granulation tissue may develop in some wounds when using "occlusive" dressings.

INSTRUCTIONS FOR USE
DuoDERM dressings are sterile and should be handled appropriately.
Choose a dressing that will extend at least 1¼″ beyond the wound margin. Cleanse the wound according to hospital practice. Irrigate with saline and dry the surrounding skin to ensure it is free of any greasy substance. Use of the dressings help facilitate the liquefaction and removal of dead tissue; however, eschar that is particularly thick or fused to the wound margins should be removed prior to application of the dressing.

APPLYING THE DRESSING
1) Minimize finger contact with adhesive surface

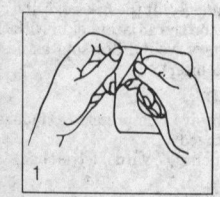

2) Apply in a rolling motion, avoid stretching

[See top of next column.]

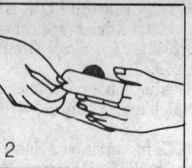

3) Smooth into place, especially around the edges

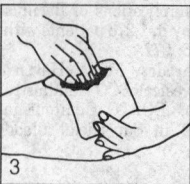

4) On a sacral ulcer, press into anal fold

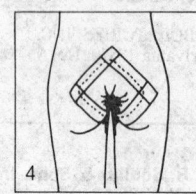

5) Use hypoallergenic tape around the edges to avoid peeling

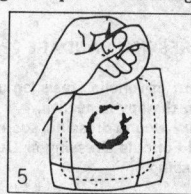

REMOVING THE DRESSING
1) Press down on the skin and carefully lift an edge of the dressing. Continue around until all edges are free.
Repeat cleansing procedure. It is unnecessary to remove all residual dressing material from the surrounding skin.

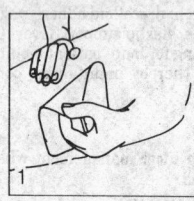

Leave the dressing in place (not more than 7 days) unless it is uncomfortable, leaking, or there are clinical signs of infection.
It is to be expected that large and necrotic wounds, or sacral ulcers, particularly in incontinent patients, will require more frequent dressing changes.
It is recommended to continue the use of DuoDERM dressings for one to two weeks after apparent healing.

HOW SUPPLIED
DuoDERM® Hydroactive® Dressing
Sterile

	ORDER #
4 × 4; Box of 5	187610
4 × 4; Box of 20 (Institutional Pack)	187611
8 × 8; Box of 3	187612

DuoDERM® CGF®
Control Gel Formula Dressing, Sterile
(Note: Use of this product will result in less gel deposition in the wound bed.

	ORDER #
4 × 4; Box of 5	187660
6 × 6; Box of 5	187661
6 × 8; Box of 5	187643
8 × 8; Box of 5	187662
8 × 12; Box of 5	187644
4 × 4; Box of 20	187658
6 × 6; Box of 20	187659

DuoDERM CGF Control Gel Formula Border Dressing Sterile, Individually blister packed

	ORDER #
2.5 × 2.5 (6cm × 6cm) Box of 5	187970
4 × 4 (10cm × 10cm) Box of 5	187971
6 × 6 (15cm × 15cm) Box of 5	187972
4 × 5 (10cm × 13cm) tri-angle shape: Box of 5	187973
6 × 7 (15cm × 18cm) tri-angle shape: Box of 5	187974

DuoDERM® Hydroactive® Granules
Sterile

5 gram tubes; Box of 5 tubes

DuoDERM® Hydroactive® Paste
Sterile
30 gram tube; Box of one tube
ConvaTec
Division of E.R. Squibb & Sons, Inc.
Princeton, NJ 08543   J3562E

DUODERM®   OTC
Hydroactive® Granules
Sterile

INDICATIONS
For use in the local management of exudating dermal ulcers in association with DuoDERM® Hydroactive® Dressing, DuoDERM® CGF® Control Gel Formula Dressing, or DuoDERM® CGF® Control Gel Formula Border Dressing (see package inserts accompanying those products for complete information).

CONTRAINDICATIONS
- Do not use on dermal ulcers involving muscle, tendon, or bone.

PRECAUTION
Do not use DuoDERM Granules on patients with a known sensitivity to the granules.

USING DuoDERM HYDROACTIVE GRANULES
In the presence of *excess* exudate the ability of DuoDERM dressings to remain in place with less frequent leakage may be improved by the application of DuoDERM granules directly into the wound site. Used in this way together with the dressings, DuoDERM Hydroactive Granules may reduce the frequency of dressing change.
DuoDERM granules are sterile and should be handled appropriately. Remove the tube from the blister pack and remove the cap from the tube.

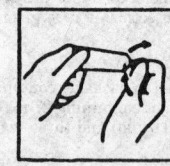

Dry the skin surrounding the wound to prevent the adhesion of excess granules. Fill the wound with granules.

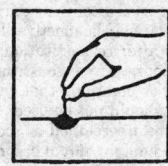

Do **not** overfill the wound—the level of granules should be slightly lower than the surrounding skin level.
Remove any excess granules from the surrounding skin and apply a DuoDERM dressing.

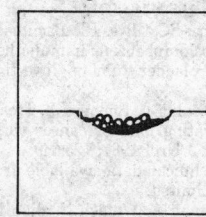

This package is for single use only. Any remaining granules should be discarded.
The location of the wound site or restricted mobility of the patient may render application of the granules by the above method difficult. In these cases, the following alternative method of application may be tried.
Place one side of a DuoDERM dressing in place as shown. Holding the dressing as level as possible, apply the granules to the dressing. Roll the dressing quickly into position over the wound.

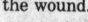

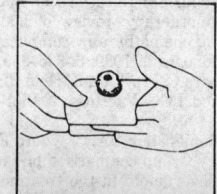

Removing The Granules

The granules are similar in composition to the hydroactive particles in the DuoDERM *Hydroactive* Dressing and will gradually form a gel in the presence of moisture. The granules soften continuously in the presence of moisture and can be easily removed with saline in the same way as the gelatinous dressing. Occasionally, some granules may adhere to the dry wound margins. These need not be completely removed if a new dressing is to be applied.

STORAGE AND AVAILABILITY
Store at room temperature; avoid exposure to high humidity.

HOW SUPPLIED
DuoDERM *Hydroactive* Granules
Sterile 5 grams/tube, box of 5 tubes
Order No: **187715**
ConvaTec
Division of E.R. Squibb & Sons, Inc.
Princeton, NJ 08543   ©1991 Squibb
PA125D

DUODERM®   OTC
Hydroactive® Paste
For dermal ulceration
Sterile

INSTRUCTIONS FOR USE
Note: Initial use of this product for dermal ulcers should be under the direction of a health professional.

PRODUCT DESCRIPTION
DuoDERM Paste is composed of natural hydrocolloids in a dermatologically approved vehicle and, like the DuoDERM Dressings, the paste is hypo-allergenic.

INDICATIONS
● The paste is designed to be used in association with DuoDERM® Dressings, DuoDERM® CGF® Control Gel Formula Dressings, or DuoDERM® CGF® Border Dressings for the local management of exudating dermal ulcers, including full thickness wounds. Used in this way, it may help extend the life of the dressing. (See package insert accompanying the dressing for complete information.)

PRECAUTIONS AND OBSERVATIONS
DuoDERM Paste is not recommended for use on third degree burns.
The paste should not be used on patients with a known sensitivity to the paste.
● Other aspects of pressure sore care, such as repositioning of the patient and nutritional support must not be neglected. Lack of adequate rest in patients with arterial or venous insufficiency can increase local edema and hinder healing.

INCREASED WOUND SIZE
● Use of any occlusive dressing in the presence of necrotic material may increase the wound size and depth during the initial phase of management as the necrotic debris is cleared away. This apparent deterioration is accompanied by gradual improvement. Deeper tissue damage may have already occurred under the apparent superficial pressure area. The initial deterioration that commonly occurs in these cases may be dramatic but is not in itself a contraindication for further use of DuoDERM Dressings or DuoDERM Paste.

INFECTION
If signs of clinical infection should develop, such as: uncharacteristic odor or change in the color of the exudate, fever or cellulitis (tenderness and erythema in the wound), a bacterial culture of the wound site should be taken. If clinical signs of infection are present, appropriate medical treatment should be initiated. DuoDERM Dressings may be continued during the treatment at the discretion of the clinician.

GRANULATION
● Excessive granulation tissue may develop when using occlusive dressings.

PREPARATION AND CLEANSING OF THE WOUND SITE
● Cleanse according to hospital practice.
● Irrigate with Saline.
● Dry surrounding skin carefully to remove any greasy substances since these will interfere with the DuoDERM Dressing's adhesion.

PASTE APPLICATION
● Swab the piercing spike (on cap) with alcohol.
● Remove the cap and puncture the tube's opening by inverting the cap and pressing on the metal membrane.
  NOTE: A small amount of clear liquid may be evident when the tube is opened. This is normal and is not an indication of product deterioration.

● Squeeze the paste into the wound. Smooth, if necessary, using a sterile spatula or a sterile gloved finger. The surface of the paste should not protrude above the level of the surrounding skin (excess paste should be removed).
  NOTE: Do not allow paste on the surrounding normal skin, otherwise the adherence of the dressing will be impaired.
● Select a DuoDERM dressing of appropriate size so that it extends at least 1¼ inches onto normal skin. Apply in a rolling motion and hold gently in place to ensure good adhesion.
  NOTE: Refer to the instructions accompanying DuoDERM Dressings for further information.

REMOVAL
● DuoDERM Paste is similar in composition to the DuoDERM Dressing and will gradually form a gel-like substance in the presence of moisture. This can be removed with saline when the dressing is changed. Material adhering to the wound margins need not be completely removed if a new dressing is to be applied.

HOW SUPPLIED
DuoDERM®
Hydroactive® Paste
Sterile 30 gram tube
ConvaTec
Division of E.R. Squibb & Sons, Inc.
Princeton, NJ 08543
©1991 Squibb   J8973 B

DuoDERM® CGF®   OTC
CONTROL GEL FORMULA <u>BORDER</u> DRESSING,
Sterile

PRODUCT DESCRIPTION
DuoDERM Control Gel Formula Border Dressings interact with wound exudate producing a soft mass that enables removal of the dressing with little or no damage to newly formed tissues. They help isolate the wound against bacterial and other external contamination. These dressings include an adhesive border so that additional taping (picture framing) is not required.

INDICATIONS
● Dermal Ulcers, including full thickness wounds
  ● Pressure Sore Management, Stage I through Stage IV
  ● Leg Ulcer Management
● Superficial Wounds—e.g. Minor Abrasions
● Burns—Second Degree
● Donor Sites

PRECAUTIONS AND OBSERVATIONS
DuoDERM CGF Border Dressings are not recommended for use on third degree burns.
The dressings should not be used on patients with a known sensitivity to the dressing.
When Used on Dermal Ulcers:
1. Initial use of this product should be under the direction of a health professional.
2. DuoDERM CGF Border Dressings only provide local management of the wound site. In pressure sore care, other aspects such as repositioning of the patient and nutritional support should not be neglected. In leg ulcer care, lack of adequate rest in patients with vascular (arterial or venous) insufficiency can increase the amount of local edema and hinder potential healing.
3. Increased Wound Size: Deeper tissue damage may have already occurred under an apparent superficial dermal ulcer. When using an occlusive dressing in the presence of necrotic material, the wound may increase in size and depth during the initial phase of management as the necrotic debris is cleared away. Leg ulcers resulting from vasculitis may rapidly deteriorate during exacerbation of the underlying disorder.
Odor: Wounds, particularly those that are large or necrotic, are often accompanied by a disagreeable odor; however, this is not necessarily indicative of infection. The odor should disappear when the wound is cleansed (see infection).
Infection: If signs of clinical infection should develop, such as: uncharacteristic odor or change in the color of the exudate, fever or cellulitis (tenderness and erythema in the area of the wound), a bacterial culture of the wound site should be taken. If clinical signs of infection are present, appropriate medical treatment should be initiated. DuoDERM dressings may be continued during the treatment at the discretion of the clinician.
Granulation: Excessive granulation tissue may develop in some wounds when using "occlusive" dressings.

INSTRUCTIONS FOR USE
Preparing and Cleansing the Wound Site
DuoDERM CGF Border dressings are sterile and should be handled appropriately.
Choose a dressing that allows the DuoDERM CGF mass to extend beyond the wound margin by at least 1¼", covering

---

all unhealthy tissue. Cleanse the wound according to hospital practice. Irrigate with saline and dry the surrounding skin to ensure it is free of any greasy substance. Use of the dressings help facilitate the liquefaction and removal of dead tissue; however, eschar that is particularly thick or fused to the wound margins should be removed prior to application of the dressing.
NOTE: DuoDERM® Paste or DuoDERM® Hydroactive® Granules may be used with this dressing. See the instructions for use with each product.

APPLYING THE DRESSING
1. Remove backing papers (1 and 2) from the center adhesive only.

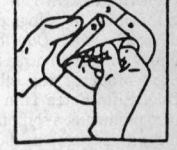

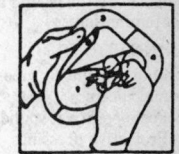

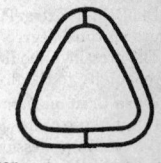

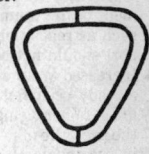

Note: The triangle shaped dressing can be applied in several directions depending on the location of the ulcer.

In sacral ulcers, the dressing may be folded in half lengthwise to make it easy to apply in the sacral folds.

2. Apply the dressing over the wound. Smooth into place, especially at edges.

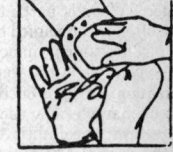

3. Fold back the border and remove the release paper from the border adhesive (3 and 4); press the borders into place.

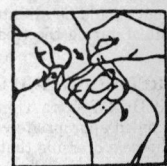

REMOVING THE DRESSING

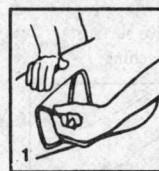

1) Press down on the skin and carefully lift an edge of the dressing. Continue around until all edges are free. Repeat cleansing procedure. It is unnecessary to remove all residual dressing material from the surrounding skin.

Leave the dressing in place (not more than 7 days) unless it is uncomfortable, leaking, or there are clinical signs of infection.

HOW SUPPLIED
DuoDERM® CGF®
Control Gel Formula Border Dressing, Sterile

Individually blister packed	Order No.
2.5 × 2.5 (6 cm × 6 cm); Box of 5	187970
4 × 4 (10 cm × 10 cm); Box of 5	187971
6 × 6 (15 cm × 15 cm); Box of 5	187972
4 × 5 (10 cm × 13 cm) tri-angle shape; Box of 5	187973
6 × 7 (15 cm × 18 cm) tri-angle shape; Box of 5	187974
4 × 4 Box of 20	187658
6 × 6 Box of 20	187659

ConvaTec
Division of   J4391B
E.R. Squibb & Sons, Inc.
Princeton, NJ 08543   © 1992 Squibb
Revised May 1992

Continued on next page

ConvaTec—Cont.

DUODERM®   OTC
EXTRA THIN CGF® DRESSING
Sterile

PRODUCT DESCRIPTION
DuoDERM Extra Thin dressings are highly flexible, control gel formula dressings designed for use on dry to lightly exudating wounds. DuoDERM Extra Thin dressings are particularly suitable in areas subject to friction and those requiring contouring, e.g., elbows, heels.

DuoDERM Extra Thin dressings interact with wound moisture producing a soft mass that enables removal of the dressing with little or no damage to newly formed tissues. They help isolate the wound against bacterial and other external contamination .

INDICATIONS
- Management of superficial, dry to lightly exudating dermal ulcers.
- Post-operative wounds.
- Protective dressings.

PRECAUTIONS AND OBSERVATIONS
DuoDERM Extra Thin dressings are not recommended for use on third degree burns.

The dressings should not be used on patients with a known sensitivity to the dressing.

When Used on Dermal Ulcers:
1. Initial use of this product should be under the direction of a health professional.
2. DuoDERM Extra Thin Dressing provides local management of the wound site. In chronic wounds, other aspects such as repositioning of the patient and nutritional support should not be neglected.
3. Increased Wound Size: Deeper tissue damage may have already occurred under an apparent superficial dermal ulcer. When using any occlusive dressing, particularly in the presence of necrotic material, the wound may increase in size and depth during the initial phase of management. Leg ulcers resulting from vasculitis may rapidly deteriorate during exacerbation of the underlying disorder.

Odor: Wounds, particularly those that are large or necrotic, are often accompanied by a disagreeable odor; however, this is not necessarily indicative of infection. The odor should disappear when the wound is cleansed (see infection).

Infection: If signs of clinical infection should develop, such as: uncharacteristic odor or change in the color of the exudate, fever or cellulitis (tenderness and erythema in the area of the wound), a bacterial culture of the wound site should be taken. If clinical signs of infection are present, medical treatment should be initiated. DuoDERM dressings may be continued during the treatment at the discretion of the clinician.

PREPARING AND CLEANSING THE WOUND SITE
DuoDERM Extra Thin dressings are sterile and should be handled appropriately.

Choose a dressing that will extend at least $1\frac{1}{4}''$ beyond the wound margin. Cleanse the wound according to hospital practice. Irrigate with saline and dry the surrounding skin to ensure it is free of any greasy substance.

APPLYING THE DRESSING
1) Minimize finger contact with adhesive surface
2) Apply in a rolling motion, avoid stretching

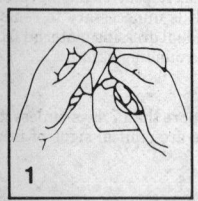
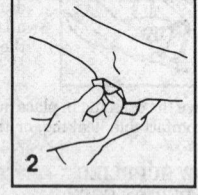

3) Smooth into place, especially around the edges
   When applying to a heel or elbow, it may be helpful to cut a slit approximately $\frac{1}{3}$ across each side of the dressing to facilitate application.
4) On a sacral ulcer, press into anal fold

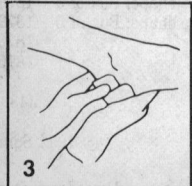
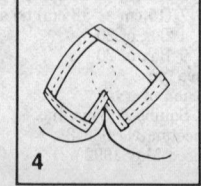

5) Use hypoallergenic tape around the edges to secure

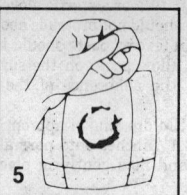

REMOVING THE DRESSING
1) Press down on the skin and carefully lift an edge of the dressing. Continue around until all edges are free. Repeat cleansing procedure It is unnecessary to remove all residual dressing material from the surrounding skin.

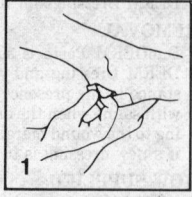

Leave the dressing in place (not more than 7 days) unless it is uncomfortable, leaking, or there are clinical signs of infection.

HOW SUPPLIED
DuoDERM® Extra Thin CGF® Dressing, Sterile

Individually Wrapped	Order #
4 × 4; Box of 10	187955
6 × 6; Box of 10	187957
2 × 4; Box of 20	187900
2 × 8; Box of 10	187961
3 × 3; Box of 20	187901
4 × 6; Box of 10	187902
6 × 7; Box of 10	187903

OTHER PRODUCTS
DuoDERM® CGF®
Control Gel Formula Dressing, Sterile

Individually blister packed	Order #
4 × 4, Box of 5	187660
6 × 6, Box of 5	187661
6 × 8, Box of 5	187643
8 × 8, Box of 5	187662
8 × 12, Box of 5	187644

DuoDERM CGF Control Gel Formula Border Dressing Sterile,

Individually blister packed	Order #
2.5 × 2.5 (6cm ×6cm) Box of 5	187970
4 × 4 (10cm ×10cm) Box of 5	187971
6 × 6 (15cm ×15cm) Box of 5	187972
4 × 5 (10cm ×13cm) tri-angle shape: Box of 5	187973
6 × 7 (15cm ×18cm) tri-angle shape: Box of 5	187974

DuoDERM® Hydroactive® Dressing

Sterile	Order #
4 × 4, Box of 5	187610
4 × 4, Box of 20 (Institutional Pack)	187611
8 × 8, Box of 3	187612

DuoDERM®Hydroactive® Paste
Sterile, 30 gram tube
DuoDERM® Hydroactive® Granules
Sterile, 5 grams per tube , Box of 5
ConvaTec

Division of E.R. Squibb & Sons, Inc.	J4362A
Princeton, NJ 08543 Made in USA ©1991	

Curatek Pharmaceuticals
1965 PRATT BOULEVARD
ELK GROVE VILLAGE, IL 60007

METROGEL®   ℞
(metronidazole)
0.75% Topical Gel
FOR TOPICAL USE ONLY
(NOT FOR OPHTHALMIC USE)

DESCRIPTION
METROGEL contains metronidazole, USP, at a concentration of 7.5 mg per gram (0.75%) in a gelled, purified water solution, containing methyl and propyl parabens, propylene glycol, carbomer 940, and edetate disodium. Metronidazole is classified therapeutically as an antiprotozoal and antibacterial agent. Chemically, metronidazole is named 2-methyl-5-nitro-1H-Imidazole-1-ethanol and has the following structure:

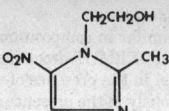

CLINICAL PHARMACOLOGY
Bioavailability studies on the topical administration of 1 gram of METROGEL to the face (7.5 mg of metronidazole) of 10 rosacea patients showed a maximum serum concentration of 66 nanograms per milliliter in one patient. This concentration is approximately 100 times less than concentrations afforded by a single 250 mg oral tablet. The serum metronidazole concentrations were below the detectable limits of the assay at the majority of time points in all patients. Three of the patients had no detectable serum concentrations of metronidazole at any time point. The mean dose of gel applied during clinical studies was 600 mg which represents 4.5 mg of metronidazole per application. Therefore, under normal usage levels, the formulation affords minimal serum concentrations of metronidazole.

The mechanisms by which METROGEL acts in reducing inflammatory lesions of rosacea are unknown, but may include an anti-bacterial and/or an anti-inflammatory effect.

INDICATIONS AND USAGE
METROGEL is indicated for topical application in the treatment of inflammatory papules, pustules, and erythema of rosacea.

CONTRAINDICATIONS
METROGEL is contraindicated in individuals with a history of hypersensitivity to metronidazole, parabens, or other ingredients of the formulations.

PRECAUTIONS
Because of the minimal absorption of metronidazole and consequently its insignificant plasma concentration after topical administration, the adverse experiences reported with the oral form of the drug have not been reported with METROGEL.

General
METROGEL has been reported to cause tearing of the eyes. Therefore, contact with the eyes should be avoided. If a reaction suggesting local irritation occurs, patients should be directed to use the medication less frequently, discontinue use temporarily, or discontinue use until further instructions. Metronidazole is a nitroimidazole and should be used with care in patients with evidence of, or history of, blood dyscrasia.

Information for the Patient
This medication is to be used as directed by the physician. It is for external use only. Avoid contact with the eyes.

Drug Interactions
Drug interactions are less likely with topical administration but should be kept in mind when METROGEL is prescribed for patients who are receiving anticoagulant treatment. Oral metronidazole has been reported to potentiate the anticoagulant effect of coumarin and warfarin resulting in a prolongation of prothrombin time.

Carcinogenesis: Tumorigenicity in Rodents
Metronidazole has shown evidence of carcinogenic activity in a number of studies involving chronic, oral administration in mice and rats but not in studies involving hamsters. These studies have not been conducted with 0.75% metronidazole gel, which would result in significantly lower systemic blood levels than oral formulations.

Mutagenicity Studies
Although metronidazole has shown mutagenic activity in a number of *in vitro* bacterial assay systems, studies in mammals *(in vivo)* have failed to demonstrate a potential for genetic damage.

Pregnancy: Pregnancy Category B
There has been no experience to date with the use of METROGEL in pregnant patients. Metronidazole crosses the placental barrier and enters the fetal circulation rapidly. No fetotoxicity was observed after oral metronidazole in rats or mice. However, because animal reproduction studies are not always predictive of human response and since oral metronidazole has been shown to be a carcinogen in some rodents, this drug should be used during pregnancy only if clearly needed.

Nursing Mothers
After oral administration, metronidazole is secreted in breast milk in concentrations similar to those found in the plasma. Even though METROGEL blood levels are significantly lower than those achieved after oral metronidazole, a decision should be made whether to discontinue nursing or to discontinue the drug, taking into account the importance of the drug to the mother.

Pediatric Use
Safety and effectiveness in children have not been established.

ADVERSE REACTIONS

Adverse conditions reported include watery (tearing) eyes if the gel is applied too closely to this area, transient redness, and mild dryness, burning, and skin irritation. None of the side effects exceeded an incidence of 2% of patients.

OVERDOSAGE

There is no human experience with overdosage of METROGEL. The acute oral toxicity of the METROGEL formulation was determined to be greater than 5 g/kg (the highest dose given) in albino rats.

DOSAGE AND ADMINISTRATION

Apply and rub in a thin film of METROGEL twice daily, morning and evening, to entire affected areas after washing. Significant therapeutic results should be noticed within three weeks. Clinical studies have demonstrated continuing improvement through nine weeks of therapy.

Areas to be treated should be cleansed before application of METROGEL. Patients may use cosmetics after application of METROGEL.

HOW SUPPLIED

METROGEL (0.75% metronidazole) is supplied in a 1 oz. (28.4 g) aluminum tube—NDC 55326-100-21.

Caution: Federal law prohibits dispensing without a prescription.

STORE AT CONTROLLED ROOM TEMPERATURES: 59° to 86° F; 15° to 30° C. Issued 10/88 ©1988

METROGEL-VAGINAL®

(metronidazole vaginal gel)
0.75% Vaginal Gel
FOR INTRAVAGINAL USE ONLY
NOT FOR OPHTHALMIC, DERMAL, OR ORAL USE

DESCRIPTION

METROGEL-VAGINAL is the intravaginal dosage form of the synthetic antibacterial agent, metronidazole, USP at a concentration of 0.75%. Metronidazole is a member of the imidazole class of antibacterial agents and is classified therapeutically as an anti-protozoal and anti-bacterial agent. Chemically, metronidazole is 2-methyl-5-nitroimidazole-1-ethanol. It has a chemical formula of $C_6H_9N_3O_3$, a molecular weight of 171.16.

METROGEL-VAGINAL is a gelled, purified water solution, containing metronidazole at a concentration of 7.5 mg/g (0.75%). The gel is formulated at pH 4.0. The gel also contains carbomer 934P, edetate disodium, methyl paraben, propyl paraben, propylene glycol, and sodium hydroxide. Each applicator full of 5 grams of vaginal gel contains approximately 37.5 mg of metronidazole.

CLINICAL PHARMACOLOGY

Normal Subjects:

Following a single, intravaginal 5-gram dose of metronidazole vaginal gel (equivalent to 37.5 mg of metronidazole) to 12 normal subjects, a mean maximum serum metronidazole concentration of 237 ng/mL was reported (range: 152 to 368 ng/mL). This is approximately 2% of the mean maximum serum metronidazole concentration reported in the same subjects administered a single, oral 500-mg dose of metronidazole (mean C_{max} = 12,785 ng/mL, range: 10,013 to 17,400 ng/mL). These peak concentrations were obtained in 6 to 12 hours after dosing with metronidazole vaginal gel and 1 to 3 hours after dosing with oral metronidazole.

The extent of exposure [area under the curve (A.U.C.)] of metronidazole, when administered as a single intravaginal 5-gram dose of metronidazole vaginal gel (equivalent to 37.5 mg of metronidazole), was approximately 4% of the A.U.C. of a single oral 500-mg metronidazole dose (4977 ng-hr/mL and approximately 125,000 ng-hr/mL, respectively). Dose adjusted comparisons of A.U.C.'s demonstrated that, on a mg to mg comparison basis, the absorption of metronidazole, when administered vaginally, was approximately half that of an equivalent oral dosage.

Patients with Bacterial Vaginosis:

Following single and multiple 5-gram doses of metronidazole vaginal gel to 4 patients with bacterial vaginosis, a mean maximum serum metronidazole concentration of 214 ng/mL on day 1 and 294 ng/mL (range: 228 to 349 ng/mL) on day five were reported. Steady state metronidazole serum concentrations following oral dosages of 400 to 500 mg B.I.D. have been reported to range from 6,000 to 20,000 ng/mL.

Microbiology:

The intracellular targets of action of metronidazole on anaerobes are largely unknown. The 5-nitro group of metronidazole is reduced by metabolically active anaerobes, and studies have demonstrated that the reduced form of the drug interacts with bacterial DNA. However, it is not clear whether interaction with DNA alone is an important component in the bactericidal action of metronidazole on anaerobic organisms.

Culture and sensitivity testing of bacteria are not routinely performed to establish the diagnosis of bacterial vaginosis. (See **INDICATIONS AND USAGE.**)

Standard methodology for the susceptibility testing of the potential bacterial vaginosis pathogens. *Gardnerella vaginalis, Mobiluncus* spp., and *Mycoplasma hominls,* has not been defined. Nonetheless, metronidazole is an antimicrobial agent active *in vitro* against most strains of the following organisms that have been reported to be associated with bacterial vaginosis:

Bacteroides spp. *Gardnerella vaginalis*
Mobiluncus spp. *Peptostreptococcus* spp.

INDICATIONS AND USAGE

METROGEL-VAGINAL is indicated in the treatment of bacterial vaginosis (formerly referred to as *Haemophilus* vaginitis, *Gardnerella* vaginitis, nonspecific vaginitis, *Corynebacterium* vaginitis, or anerobic vaginosis).

NOTE: For purposes of this indication, a clinical diagnosis of bacterial vaginosis is usually defined by the presence of a homogeneous vaginal discharge that (a) has a pH of greater than 4.5, (b) emits a "fishy" amine odor when mixed with a 10% KOH solution, and (c) contains clue cells on microscopic examination. Gram's stain results consistent with a diagnosis of bacterial vaginosis include (a) markedly reduced or absent *Lactobacillus* morphology, (b) predominace of *Gardnerella* morphotype, and (c) absent or few white blood cells. Other pathogens commonly associated with vulvovaginitis, e.g., *Trichomonas vaginalis, Chlamydia trachomatis, N. gonorrhoeae, Candida albicans,* and *Herpes simplex* virus should be ruled out.

CONTRAINDICATIONS

METROGEL-VAGINAL is contraindicated in patients with a prior history of hypersensitivity to metronidazole, parabens, other ingredients of the formulation, or other nitroimidazole derivatives.

WARNINGS

Convulsive Seizures and Peripheral Neuropathy:

Convulsive seizures and peripheral neuropathy, the latter characterized mainly by numbness or paresthesia of an extremity, have been reported in patients treated with oral metronidazole. The appearance of abnormal neurologic signs demands the prompt discontinuation of metronidazole vaginal gel therapy. Metronidazole vaginal gel should be administered with caution to patients with central nervous system diseases.

Psychotic Reactions:

Psychotic reactions have been reported in alcoholic patients who were using oral metronidazole and disulfiram concurrently. Metronidazole vaginal gel should not be administered to patients who have taken disulfiram within the last two weeks.

PRECAUTIONS

METROGEL-VAGINAL affords minimal peak serum levels and systemic exposure (A.U.C.'s) of metronidazole compared to 500 mg oral metronidazole dosing. Although these lower levels of exposure are less likely to produce the common reactions seen with oral metronidazole, the possibility of these and other reactions cannot be excluded presently. Data from well-controlled trials directly comparing metronidazole administered orally to metronidazole administered vaginally are not available.

General:

Patients with severe hepatic disease metabolize metronidazole slowly. This results in the accumulation of metronidazole and its metabolites in the plasma. Accordingly, for such patients, metronidazole vaginal gel should be administered cautiously.

Known or previously unrecognized vaginal candidiasis may present more prominent symptoms during therapy with metronidazole vaginal gel. Approximately 6% of patients treated with METROGEL-VAGINAL developed symptomatic *candida* vaginitis during or immediately after therapy.

Disulfiram-like reaction to alcohol has been reported with oral metronidazole, thus the possibility of such a reaction occurring while on metronidazole vaginal gel therapy cannot be excluded.

METROGEL-VAGINAL contains ingredients that may cause burning and irritation of the eye. In the event of accidental contact with the eye, rinse the eye with copious amounts of cool tap water.

Information for the Patient:

The patient should be informed not to drink alcohol while being treated with metronidazole vaginal gel. While blood levels are significantly lower with METROGEL-VAGINAL than with usual doses of oral metronidazole, a possible interaction with alcohol cannot be excluded.

The patient should also be instructed not to engage in vaginal intercourse during treatment with this product.

Drug Interactions:

Oral metronidazole has been reported to potentiate the anticoagulant effect of warfarin and other coumarin anticoagulants, resulting in a prolongation of prothrombin time. This possible drug interaction should be considered when metronidazole vaginal gel is prescribed for patients on this type of anticoagulant therapy.

Drug/Laboratory test interactions:

Metronidazole may interfere with certain types of determinations of serum chemistry values, such as aspartate aminotransferase (AST, SGOT), alanine aminotransferase (ALT, SGPT), lactate dehydrogenase (LDH), triglycerides, and glucose hexokinase. Values of zero may be observed. All of the assays in which interference has been reported involve enzymatic coupling of the assay to oxidation-reduction of nicotinamide-adenine dinucleotide (NAD+NADH). Interference is due to the similarity in absorbance peaks of NADH (340 nm) and metronidazole (322 nm) at pH 7.

Carcinogenesis, mutagenesis, impairment of fertility:

Metronidazole has shown evidence of carcinogenic activity in a number of studies involving chronic oral administration in mice and rats. Prominent among the effects in the mouse was the promotion of pulmonary tumorigenesis. This has been observed in all six reported studies in that species, including one study in which the animals were dosed on an intermittent schedule (administration during every fourth week only). At very high dose levels (approx. 500 mg/kg/day), there was a statistically significant increase in the incidence of malignant liver tumors in males. Also, the published results of one of the mouse studies indicate an increase in the incidence of malignant lymphomas as well as pulmonary neoplasms associated with lifetime feeding of the drug. All these effects are statistically significant. Several long-term oral dosing studies in the rat have been completed. There were statistically significant increases in the incidence of various neoplasms, particularly in mammary and hepatic tumors, among female rats administered metronidazole over those noted in the concurrent female control groups.

Two lifetime tumorigenicity studies in hamsters have been performed and reported to be negative. These studies have not been conducted with 0.75% metronidazole vaginal gel, which would result in significantly lower systemic blood levels than those obtained with oral formulations.

Although metronidazole has shown mutagenic activity in a number of *in vitro* assay systems, studies in mammals (*in vivo*) have failed to demonstrate a potential for genetic damage.

Fertility studies have been performed in mice up to six times the recommended human vaginal dose (based on mg/m^2) and have revealed no evidence of impaired fertility.

Pregnancy: Teratogenic Effects

Pregnancy Category B

There has been no experience to date with the use of METROGEL-VAGINAL in pregnant patients. Metronidazole crosses the placental barrier and enters the fetal circulation rapidly. No fetotoxicity or teratogenicity was observed when metronidazole was administered orally to pregnant mice at six times the recommended human vaginal dose (based on mg/m^2); however, in a single small study where the drug was administered intraperitoneally, some intrauterine deaths were observed. The relationship of these findings to the drug is unknown.

There are, however, no adequate and well-controlled studies in pregnant women. Because animal reproduction studies are not always predictive of human response, and because metronidazole is a carcinogen in rodents, this drug should be used during pregnancy only if clearly needed.

Nursing mothers:

Specific studies of metronidazole levels in human milk following intravaginally administered metronidazole have not been performed. However, metronidazole is secreted in human milk in concentrations similar to those found in plasma following oral administration of metronidazole.

Because of the potential for tumorigenicity shown for metronidazole in mouse and rat studies, a decision should be made whether to discontinue nursing or to discontinue the drug, taking into account the importance of the drug to the mother.

Pediatric use:

Safety and effectiveness in children have not been established.

ADVERSE REACTIONS

Clinical Trials:

There were no deaths or serious adverse events in clinical trials involving 295 patients; however, approximately 1% of non-pregnant patients treated with METROGEL-VAGINAL discontinued therapy early due to drug-related adverse events. One patient discontiued therapy due to abdominal pain after 2 days of therapy and one patient discontinued therapy due to a severe headache after 5 doses. Similar headaches of uncertain cause had been reported in the past by this patient.

Medical events judged to be related, probably related, or possibly related to administration of METROGEL-VAGINAL were reported for 50/295 (17%) non-pregnant patients. Unless percentages are otherwise stipulated, the incidence of individual adverse reactions listed below was less than 1%:

Genital tract:

Symptomatic *Candida* cervicitis/vaginitis (6.1%),
Vaginal, perineal, or vulvar itching (1.4%),
Urinary frequency, vaginal or vulvar burning or irritation, vaginal discharge (not *candida*), and vulvar swelling.

Gastrointestinal:

Cramps/pain (abdominal/uterine) (3.4%),

Continued on next page

Curatek—Cont.

Nausea (2.0%),
Metallic or bad taste (1.7%),
Constipation, decreased appetite, and diarrhea.
Central Nervous System:
Dizziness, headache, and lightheadedness.
Dermatologic:
Rash.
Laboratory:
Increased/decreased white blood cell counts (1.7%).

Other metronidazole formulations:
Other effects that have been reported in association with the use of **topical (dermal)** formulations of metronidazole include skin irritation, transient skin erythema, and mild skin dryness and burning. None of these adverse events exceeded an incidence of 2% of patients.
METROGEL-VAGINAL affords minimal peak serum levels and systemic exposure (A.U.C.'s) of metronidazole compared to 500 mg oral metronidazole dosing. Although these lower levels of exposure are less likely to produce the common reactions seen with oral metronidazole, the possibility of these and other reactions cannot be excluded presently. Data from well-controlled trials directly comparing metronidazole administered orally to metronidazole administered vaginally are not available.
The following adverse reactions and altered laboratory tests have been reported with the **oral or parenteral** use of metronidazole:
Cardiovascular: Flattening of the T-wave may be seen in electrocardiographic tracings.
Central Nervous System: (See **WARNINGS.**) Headache, dizziness, syncope, ataxia, confusion, convulsive seizures, peripheral neuropathy, vertigo, incoordination, irritability, depression, weakness, insomnia.
Gastrointestinal: Abdominal discomfort; nausea; vomiting; diarrhea; an unplesant metallic taste; anorexia; epigastric distress; abdominal cramping; constipation; "furry" tongue glossitis and stomatitis; pancreatitis; modification of taste of alcoholic beverages.
Genitourinary: Overgrowth of *Candida* in the vagina, dyspareunia, decreased libido, proctitis.
Hematopoietic: Reversible neutropenia, reversible thrombocytopenia.
Hypersensitivity Reactions: Urticaria; erythematous rash; flushing; nasal congestion; dryness of the mouth, vagina, or vulva; fever; pruritus; fleeting joint pains.
Renal: Dysuria, cystitis, polyuria, incontinence, a sense of pelvic pressure, darkened urine.

OVERDOSAGE

There is no human experience with overdosage of metronidazole vaginal gel. Vaginally applied metronidazole, 0.75% could be absorbed in sufficient amounts to produce systemic effect. (See **WARNINGS.**)

DOSAGE AND ADMINISTRATION

The recommended dose is one applicator full of METROGEL-VAGINAL (approximately 5 grams containing approximately 37.5 mg of metronidazole) intravaginally twice daily for 5 days. The medication should be applied once in the morning and once in the evening.

HOW SUPPLIED

METROGEL-VAGINAL (metronidazole vaginal gel) 0.75% Vaginal Gel is supplied in a 70 gram aluminum tube and packaged with a 5 gram vaginal applicator. NDC number is 55326-200-25.
Store at controlled room temperature 15° to 30°C (59° to 86°F). Protect from freezing.
Caution: Federal law prohibits dispensing without a prescription.
Issued 8/92.

Daniels Pharmaceuticals, Inc.
2517 25TH AVENUE NORTH
ST. PETERSBURG, FL 33713-3918

LEVOXINE® ℞
(LEVOTHYROXINE SODIUM TABLETS, USP)
FOR ORAL ADMINISTRATION

DESCRIPTION

Each LEVOXINE (Levothyroxine Sodium, USP) tablet contains synthetic crystalline levothyroxine sodium (L-thyroxine). L-thyroxine is the principle hormone secreted by the normal thyroid gland. Chemically, L-thyroxine is designated as L-tyrosine, O-(4-hydroxy-3,5-diiodophenyl)-3,5-diiodo-, monosodium salt, hydrate. The molecular formula is $C_{15}H_{10}I_4N\ NaO_4$ and the structural formula is:

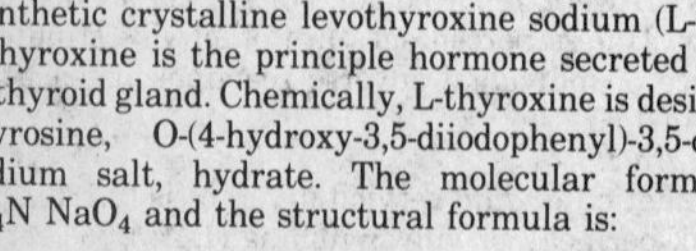

INACTIVE INGREDIENTS

Lactose, microcrystalline cellulose, pregelatinized starch, magnesium stearate. The following are the color additives per tablet strength:

Strength (mcg)	Color Additive(s)
25	FD&C Yellow No. 6
50	none
75	FD&C Blue No. 1
	D&C Red No. 30
88	FD&C Yellow No. 6
	FD&C Blue No. 1
	D&C Yellow No. 10
100	FD&C Yellow No. 6
	D&C Yellow No. 10
112	FD&C Yellow No. 6
	FD&C Red No. 40
	D&C Red No. 30
125	FD&C Red No. 40
	D&C Yellow No. 10
150	FD&C Blue No. 1
	D&C Red No. 30
175	FD&C Blue No. 1
	D&C Yellow No. 10
200	D&C Red No. 30
	D&C Yellow No. 10
300	FD&C Yelllow No. 6
	FD&C Blue No. 1
	D&C Yellow No. 10

CLINICAL PHARMACOLOGY

The principal effect of thyroid hormones is to increase the metabolic rate of body tissues.
The thyroid hormones are also concerned with growth and development of tissues in the young.
The major thyroid hormones are L-thyroxine (T_4) and L-triiodothyronine (T_3). The amounts of T_4 and T_3 released from the normally functioning thyroid gland are regulated by the amount of thyrotropin (TSH) secreted from the anterior pituitary gland. T_4 is the major component of normal thyroid gland secretions and is therefore the primary determinant of normal thyroid functions. T_4 acts as a substrate for physiologic deiodination to T_3 in the peripheral tissues. The physiologic effects of thyroid hormones are mediated at the cellular level primarily by T_3.
LEVOXINE (L-thyroxine) tablets taken orally provide T_4 which upon absorption cannot be distinguished from T_4 that is secreted endogenously.

INDICATIONS AND USAGE

LEVOXINE (L-thyroxine) tablets are indicated as replacement or supplemental therapy for diminished or absent thyroid function (e.g., cretinism, myxedema, nontoxic goiter or hypothyroidism generally, including the hypothyroid state in children, in pregnancy and in the elderly) resulting from functional deficiency, primary atrophy, from partial or complete absence of the gland or from the effects of surgery, radiation or antithyroid agents. Therapy must be maintained continuously to control the symptoms of hypothyroidism.

CONTRAINDICATIONS

L-thyroxine therapy is contraindicated in thyrotoxicosis, acute myocardial infarction and uncorrected adrenal insufficiency.

WARNINGS

Drugs with thyroid hormone activity, alone or together with other therapeutic agents, have been used for the treatment of obesity. In euthyroid patients, doses within the range of daily hormonal requirements are ineffective for weight reduction. Larger doses may produce serious or even life-threatening manifestations of toxicity, particularly when given in association with sympathomimetic amines such as those used for their anorectic effects.

PRECAUTIONS

General—Caution must be exercised in the administration of this drug to patients with cardiovascular disease. Development of chest pain or other aggravation of the cardiovascular disease requires a reduction of dosage.
Information For the Patient—Patients on thyroid preparations and parents of children on thyroid therapy should be informed that:

1. Replacement therapy is to be taken essentially for life, with the exception of cases of transient hypothyroidism, usually associated with thyroiditis, and in those patients receiving a therapeutic trial of the drug.
2. They should immediately report during the course of therapy any signs or symptoms of thyroid hormone toxicity, e.g., chest pain, increased pulse rate, palpitations, excessive sweating, heat intolerance, nervousness, or any other unusual event.
3. In case of concomitant diabetes mellitus, the daily dosage of antidiabetic medication may need readjustment as thyroid hormone replacement is achieved. If thyroid medication is stopped, a downward readjustment of the dosage of insulin or oral hypoglycemic agent may be necessary to avoid hypoglycemia. At all times, close monitoring of urinary or blood glucose levels is mandatory in such patients.
4. In case of concomitant oral anticoagulant therapy, the prothrombin time should be measured frequently to determine if the dosage of oral anticoagulants is to be readjusted.
5. Partial loss of hair may be experienced by children in the first few months of thyroid therapy, but this is usually a transient phenomenon and later recovery is usually the rule.

Laboratory Tests—The patient's response to thyroid replacement may be followed by laboratory tests such as serum thyroxine (T_4), serum triiodothyronine (T_3), free thyroxine index and thyroid stimulating hormone (TSH) blood levels.
Drug Interactions—In patients with diabetes mellitus, addition of thyroid hormone therapy may cause an increase in the required dosage of insulin or oral hypoglycemic agents. Therefore, patients with diabetes mellitus should be observed closely for possible changes in antidiabetic drug dosage requirements.
Patients stabilized on oral anticoagulants who are found to require thyroid replacement therapy should be watched very closely when therapy is started. If a patient is truly hypothyroid, it is likely that a reduction in anticoagulant dosage will be required. No special precautions appear to be necessary when oral anticoagulant therapy is begun in a patient already stabilized on maintenance thyroid replacement therapy.
Cholestyramine binds both T_4 and T_3 in the intestine, thus impairing absorption of these thyroid hormones. In vitro studies indicate that the binding is not easily removed. Therefore, four to five hours should elapse between administration of cholestyramine and thyroid hormones.
Estrogens tend to increase serum thyroxine-binding globulin (TBG). In a patient with a non-functioning thyroid gland who is receiving thyroid replacement therapy, free thyroxine may be decreased when estrogens are started thus increasing thyroid requirements. However, if the patient's thyroid gland has sufficient function the decreased free thyroxine will result in a compensatory increase in thyroxine output by the thyroid. Therefore, patients without a functioning thyroid gland who are on thyroid replacement therapy may need to increase their thyroid dose if estrogens or estrogen containing oral contraceptives are given.
Drug/Laboratory Test Interactions—The following drugs or moieties are known to interfere with laboratory tests performed on patients taking thyroid hormone: androgens, corticosteroids, estrogens, oral contraceptives containing estrogens, iodine-containing preparations, and the numerous preparations containing salicylates.

1. Changes in TBG concentration should be taken into consideration in the interpretation of T_4 and T_3 values. In such cases, the unbound (free) hormone should be measured. Pregnancy, estrogens, and estrogen-containing oral contraceptives increase TBG concentrations. TBG may also be increased during infectious hepatitis. Decreases in TBG concentrations are observed in nephrosis, acromegaly, and after androgen or corticosteroid therapy. Familial hyper- or hypo-thyroxine-binding-globulinemias have been described. The incidence of TBG deficiency approximates 1 in 9000. The binding of thyroxine by thyroid-binding pre-albumin (TBPA) is inhibited by salicylates.
2. Medical or dietary iodine interferes with all in vivo tests of radio-iodine uptake, producing low uptakes which may not be reflective of a true decrease in hormone synthesis.
3. The persistence of clinical and laboratory evidence of hypothyroidism in spite of adequate dosage replacement indicates either poor patient compliance, poor absorption, excessive fecal loss, or inactivity of the preparation. Intracellular resistance to thyroid hormone is quite rare.

Carcinogenesis, Mutagenesis, And Impairment Of Fertility—A reportedly apparent association between prolonged thyroid therapy and breast cancer has not been confirmed and patients on thyroid for established indications should not discontinue therapy. No confirmatory long-term studies in animals have been performed to evaluate carcinogenic potential, mutagenicity, or impairment of fertility in either males or females.
Pregnancy—Category A—Thyroid hormones do not readily cross the placental barrier. The clinical experience to date does not indicate any adverse effect on fetuses when thyroid hormones are administered to pregnant women. On the basis of current knowledge, thyroid replacement therapy to hypothyroid women should not be discontinued during pregnancy.
Nursing Mothers—Minimal amounts of thyroid hormones are excreted in human milk. Thyroid is not associated with serious adverse reactions and does not have a known tumorigenic potential. However, caution should be exercised when thyroid is administered to a nursing woman.
Pediatric Use—Pregnant mothers provide little or no thyroid hormone to the fetus. The incidence of congenital hypothyroidism is relatively high (1:4,000) and the hypothyroid fetus would not derive any benefit from the small amounts of

hormone crossing the placental barrier. Routine determinations of serum (T_4) and/or TSH is strongly advised in neonates in view of the deleterious effects of thyroid deficiency on growth and development.

Treatment should be initiated immediately upon diagnosis, and maintained for life, unless transient hypothyroidism is suspected; in which case, therapy may be interrupted for 2 to 8 weeks after the age of 3 years to reassess the condition. Cessation of therapy is justified in patients who have maintained a normal TSH during those 2 to 8 weeks.

ADVERSE REACTIONS

Adverse reactions are due to overdosage and are those of induced hyperthyroidism.

OVERDOSAGE—Excessive dosage of thyroid medication may result in symptoms of hyperthyroidism. Since, however, the effects do not appear at once, the symptoms may not appear for one to three weeks after the dosage regimen is begun. The most common signs and symptoms of overdosage are weight loss, palpitation, nervousness, diarrhea or abdominal cramps, sweating, tachycardia, cardiac arrhythmias, angina pectoris, tremors, headache, insomnia, intolerance to heat and fever. If symptoms of overdosage appear, discontinue medication for several days and reinstitute treatment at a lower dosage level.

Laboratory tests such as serum T_4, serum T_3 and the free thyroxine index will be elevated during the period of overdosage.

Complications as a result of the induced hypermetabolic state may include cardiac failure and death due to arrhythmia or failure.

TREATMENT OF OVERDOSAGE—Dosage should be reduced or therapy temporarily discontinued if signs and symptoms of overdosage appear. Treatment may be reinstituted at a lower dosage. In normal individuals, normal hypothalamic pituitary-thyroid axis function is restored in 6 to 8 weeks after thyroid suppression.

Treatment of acute massive thyroid hormone overdosage is aimed at reducing gastrointestinal absorption of the drugs and counteracting central and peripheral effects, mainly those of increased sympathetic activity. Vomiting may be induced initially if further gastrointestinal absorption can reasonably be prevented and barring contraindications such as coma, convulsions, or loss of the gagging reflex. Treatment is symptomatic and supportive. Oxygen may be administered and ventilation maintained. Cardiac glycosides may be indicated if congestive heart failure develops. Measures to control fever, hypoglycemia, or fluid loss should be instituted if needed.

Antiadrenergic agents, particularly propranolol, have been used advantageously in the treatment of increased sympathetic activity. Propranolol may be administered intravenously at a dosage of 1 to 3 mg over a 10 minute period or orally, 80 to 160 mg/day, especially when no contraindications exist for its use.

DOSAGE AND ADMINISTRATION

The goal of therapy should be the restoration of euthyroidism as judged by clinical response and confirmed by appropriate laboratory tests such as serum thyroxine (T_4), serum triiodothyronine (T_3), free thyroxine index and thyroid stimulating hormone (TSH) blood levels. The age and general condition of the patient and the severity and duration of hypothyroid symptoms determine the starting dosage and the rate of incremental dosage increase leading to a final maintenance dosage.

In otherwise healthy adults, the recommended initial dosage is 25 to 100 mcg (0.025 to 0.1 mg) daily, while the predicted full maintenance dose of 100 to 200 mcg (0.1 to 0.2 mg) daily may be achieved in two to three weeks.

In the elderly patient with long standing disease, evidence of myxedema, or evidence of cardiovascular dysfunction, the initial dose may be as little as 12.5 mcg (0.0125 mg) per day. Incremental increases of 25 mcg (0.025 mg) per day at 3 to 4 week intervals may be instituted depending on patient response. It is the physician's judgment of the severity of the disease and close observation of patient response which determine the rate and extent of dosage increase.

In infants and children there is a great urgency to achieve full thyroid replacement because of the critical importance of thyroid hormone in sustaining growth and maturation. Despite the smaller body size, the dosage needed to sustain a full rate of growth, development and general thriving is higher in the child than in the adult. The recommended daily replacement dosage of L-thyroxine in childhood is: 0–6 months: 5–6 mcg/kg; 6–12 months: 5–6 mcg/kg; 1–5 years: 3–5 mcg/kg; 6–10 years: 4–5 mcg/kg; over 10 years: 2–3 mcg/kg of body weight daily.

DOSAGE FORMS AVAILABLE

LEVOXINE (L-thyroxine) tablets are supplied as oval, color coded, potency marked tablets in 11 strengths: 25 mcg (0.025 mg)—orange, 50 mcg (0.05 mg)—white, 75 mcg (0.075 mg)—purple, 88 mcg (0.088 mg)—olive, 100 mcg (0.1 mg)—yellow, 112 mcg (0.112 mg)—rose, 125 mcg (0.125 mg)—brown, 150 mcg (0.15 mg)—blue, 175 mcg (0.175 mg)—turquoise, 200 mcg (0.2 mg)—pink and 300 mcg

(0.3 mg)—green, in bottles of 100 and 1000, and unit dose in cartons of 100 (10 strips of 10 tablets).

Revised April 1991
Shown in Product Identification Section, page 408

LEVOTHYROXINE SODIUM FOR INJECTION   ℞
Lyophilized
For Parenteral Administration
After Reconstitution

DESCRIPTION

Levothyroxine Sodium for Injection contains synthetic crystalline levothyroxine sodium (L-thyroxine), available as a sterile lyophilized powder. Each vial contains levothyroxine sodium—200 mcg (0.2 mg) or 500 mcg (0.5 mg).

HOW SUPPLIED

Levothyroxine Sodium for Injection—200 mcg NDC# 0689-0131-01 and 500 mcg NDC# 0689-0128-01 are available in 10 mL vials, individually boxed. This product is manufactured for Daniels Pharmaceuticals by Steris Laboratories, Phoenix, Arizona 85043.

TUSSIGON® Tablets   ℂ ℞
(Hydrocodone bitartrate and Homatropine methylbromide)

DESCRIPTION

Each blue, scored tablet contains Hydrocodone Bitartrate, USP, 5 mg, and Homatropine Methylbromide, USP 1.5 mg.

HOW SUPPLIED

Tussigon tablets are supplied in bottles of 100 count NDC# 0689-0082-01 and bottles of 500 count NDC# 0689-0082-05.

WARNING

Hydrocodone bitartrate may be habit forming.

Dartmouth Pharmaceuticals, Inc.
19 WHALER'S WAY
NORTH DARTMOUTH, MA 02747-1058

TOURO A&H CAPSULES   ℞
(Brompheniramine Maleate and Pseudoephedrine Hydrochloride)

DESCRIPTION

Each TOURO A&H green and clear capsule containing white beads for oral administration contains:

Brompheniramine Maleate	6 mg
Pseudoephedrine HCl	60 mg

in a special base to provide prolonged action.

HOW SUPPLIED

TOURO A&H is available as a green and clear capsule containing white beads.
NDC 58869-301-01   Bottle of 100

TOURO LA Caplets   ℞
(Pseudoephedrine Hydrochloride and Guaifenesin)

DESCRIPTION

Each TOURO LA white, scored time release caplet for oral administration contains:

Pseudoephedrine HCl	120 mg
Guaifenesin	400 mg

A special time-release base allows for caplets to be broken in half for ease of administration without affecting release medication but not crushed or chewed.

HOW SUPPLIED

TOURO LA is available as a white, scored caplet imprinted with "DP".
NDC 58869-436-01   Bottle of 100

ZARTAN   ℞
(Cephalexin capsules, USP)

DESCRIPTION

Each ZARTAN red and red capsule for oral administration contains:

Cephalexin	500 mg

HOW SUPPLIED

ZARTAN is available as a red and red capsule
NDC 58869-871-01   Bottle of 100

Dayton Laboratories, Inc.
3307 N.W. 74TH AVENUE
MIAMI, FL 33122

DAYTO HIMBIN TABLETS   ℞
DAYTO HIMBIN LIQUID   ℞
Yohimbine Hydrochloride 5.4 mg

DESCRIPTION

Each tablet contains 5.4 mg Yohimbine hydrochloride. Each 15 ml contains 5.4 mg Yohimbine hydrochloride, alcohol-free and sugar-free. Yohimbine is an indoalkylamine alkaloid with chemical similarity to reserpine.

ACTIONS

Yohimbine is primarily an alpha-2 adrenergic blocker, which blocks presynaptic alpha-2 adrenoreceptors.

CLINICAL PHARMACOLOGY

Its peripheral autonomic nervous system effect is to increase cholinergic and decrease adrenergic activity. Theoretically, increased penile blood inflow, decreased penile blood outflow or both, results since in the male sexual performance erection is linked to cholinergic activity, causing erectile stimulation without increasing libido. Yohimbine has a mild antidiuretic action, probably via stimulation of hypothalamic centers and release of posterior pituitary hormone. Yohimbine exerts a stimulating action on mood and may increase anxiety, although these actions have not been adequately studied and appear to require high doses. Its action on peripheral blood vessels resembles that of reserpine, though it is of short duration and weaker. Yohimbine, reportedly exerts no significant influence on cardiac stimulation and other effects mediated by beta-adrenergic receptors.

INDICATIONS

Mydriatic and sympatholytic agent. Male sexual dysfunction has been successfully treated with Yohimbine in patients with psychogenic, vascular or diabetic origins (18mg/day). Many physicians, specially Urologist, use Yohimbine experimentally in the treatment and, or, diagnostic classification of certain types of male erectile dysfunctions.

CONTRAINDICATIONS

Patients with renal disease; hypersensitivity to any of the components.

WARNINGS

The liquid form contains phenylalanine, phenylketonuric. Not for use in geriatric patients, psychiatric or cardio-renal patients. Generally not for use in women.

USAGE IN PREGNANCY

Do not use during pregnancy
USAGE IN CHILDREN
Do not use in children
DRUG INTERACTIONS
Do not use yohimbine with mood modifying drugs and antidepressants.

ADVERSE REACTIONS

CNS: Yohimbine readily penetrates the CNS and produces a complex pattern of responses in doses lower than those required to produce peripheral alpha-adrenergic blockade. These include, antidiuresis and central excitation including elevated blood pressure and heart rate, increased motor activity, irritability, tremor and nervousness. Headache, skin flushing and dizziness have been reported.

OVERDOSAGE

Daily doses of 20–30 mg daily may produce increased heart rate and blood pressure, rhinorrhea and piloerection. More severe symptoms may include incoordination, paresthesias, tremulousness and dissociative state.

DOSAGE AND ADMINISTRATION

USUAL ADULT DOSAGE: One tablet three times daily or one tablespoonful three times daily. If side effects occur the dosage may be reduced to ½ tablet or one teaspoonful three times daily. The therapy reported is not more than ten weeks.

HOW SUPPLIED

Tablets: Bottles of 60 pink scored and DL embossed tablets.
N.D.C. 52041-029-13
Liquid: Bottles of 12 oz (355 ml) red cherry flavored liquid.
N.D.C. 52041-035-37
Shown in Product Identification Section, page 408

Continued on next page

Dayton Laboratories—Cont.

FLATULEX   OTC
Simethicone plus Activated Charcoal

COMPOSITION:
Each DUAL-COATED tablet contains
OUTER LAYER (for gastric release)
Simethicone .... 80 mg.
INNER LAYER (for intestinal release)
Activated Charcoal .... 250 mg.

DESCRIPTION
Flatulex is a uniquely constructed tablet for the control and elimination of flatulence. It contains two active ingredients: Simethicone and Activated Charcoal. The tablets are constructed so that the 2 actives are independent of each other; Simethicone in a coated form for release in the stomach and Activated Charcoal in an enteric coated form for release in the intestine. This unique delivery system ensures that the Simethicone is released in the stomach while the Charcoal safely traverses the stomach to the intestine without being neutralized by acid.

ACTIONS
Simethicone (polydimethylsiloxane) is a surface active agent which acts as a dispersant of gas bubbles by reducing the surface tension of the bubbles, thus destroying mucosal pockets of gas which cause distress. It does not absorb gas per se, or reduce the quantity of gas present. This is done by movement of the gas into the intestine. Simethicone is not active in the intestine.
Activated Charcoal is a gas absorbent of high capacity. Its highly porous surface absorbs and adsorbs gases, poorly soluble substances, and toxins. It is widely used as a detoxicant. Activated Charcoal reduces the volume of intestinal gas, providing relief of symptoms and reducing or eliminating flatulence. It also absorbs microbial metabolites and toxins which may generate gas, thus reducing gas production, especially of hydrogen and methane. Charcoal is not effective in the stomach, due to absorption of HCl, which has a neutralizing effect. Flatulex is sodium-free, and safe, since ingredients are not absorbed into the bloodstream.

INDICATIONS
For relief of stomach gas, intestinal gas, and flatulence.

CONTRAINDICATIONS
No known contraindications other than hypersensitivity to Simethicone or Activated Charcoal.

PRECAUTIONS
Drug interaction: Activated Charcoal may absorb medication(s) while in the digestive tract. May cause temporary blackening of the stool. Do not exceed recommended dosage.

ADVERSE REACTIONS
No adverse reactions to this product have been reported.

DOSAGE
One tablet three times daily, preferably after meals. One tablet may be taken at bedtime to provide overnight relief.

HOW SUPPLIED
Supplied in bottles of 30
NDC 52041-028-09
Supplied in bottles of 100
NDC 52041-028-15
Shown in Product Identification Section, page 408

Delmont Laboratories, Inc.
P.O. BOX 269
SWARTHMORE, PA 19081

STAPHAGE LYSATE (SPL)®   ℞
[staf′faj lī′sāt]
BACTERIAL ANTIGEN MADE FROM STAPHYLOCOCCUS

DESCRIPTION
Bacterial Antigen Made from Staphylococcus, STAPHAGE LYSATE (SPL)®, is a bacteriologically sterile staphylococcal vaccine containing components of *S. aureus*, bacteriophage, and some culture medium ingredients (sodium chloride and ultrafiltered beef heart infusion broth).
SPL is prepared by lysing parent cultures of *S. aureus*, Serologic Types I & III,[1] with a polyvalent staphylococcus bacteriophage.[2] Bacteriologic sterility is achieved by ultrafiltration. Neither heat nor preservative is used in its preparation. SPL is standardized on the basis of bacterial cell content before phage lysis. Each milliliter contains: 120–180 million colony-forming units of *S. aureus* and 100–1000 million staphylococcus bacteriophage plaque-forming units.

SPL is administered by several routes, according to the directions of the physician. These include subcutaneous injection, intranasal aerosol inhalation or nasal drop instillation, oral administration, topical application or irrigation, and combinations of these routes.

CLINICAL PHARMACOLOGY
In experimental conditions, *S. aureus* or its cellular components may induce cell-mediated immunity.[3,4]
In uncontrolled studies in humans, favorable results have been reported using SPL for a variety of staphylococcal diseases,[5–9] as well as for Herpesvirus and aphthous ulcers (essentially treatment failures with other therapeutic modalities).[10]
In vitro, SPL has been shown to stimulate lymphoproliferative responses in both T- and B-cell subpopulations present in peripheral and cord blood of normal human subjects.[11–13] These findings appear to support the interpretation that SPL in staphylococcal-hypersensitive subjects acts as an immunopotentiator of nonspecific cell-mediated immunity. Pharmacokinetic data in humans are unavailable.

ANIMAL PHARMACOLOGY
An increased capability of macrophages to inactive staphylococci has been demonstrated in laboratory animals[4,14–16] following SPL treatment.
It further has been demonstrated that laboratory animals hypersensitized to staphylococcus and elicited specifically with SPL are protected nonspecifically against challenge with vaccinia virus,[17] influenza virus,[18] virulent field strains of *E. coli*,[19,20] and *K. pneumoniae*.[21]
In laboratory animals, SPL has been shown to act as an immunomodulator.[22]

INDICATIONS AND USAGE

> Based on a review by the Panel on Bacterial Vaccines and Bacterial Antigens with no U.S. Standard of Potency and other information, the Food and Drug Administration has directed that further investigation be conducted before this product is determined fully effective for the labeled indication(s).

SPL is indicated in the treatment of either staphylococcal infections or polymicrobial infections with a staphylococcal component.
Caution should be exercised when administering SPL intranasally to patients with known allergies (see "Intranasal Aerosol Inhalation" under *Dosage and Administration*).
Although SPL has been used in infants and children, its safety and effectiveness in these patient groups have not been established.
The use of SPL has not been shown to adversely affect other treatment modalities.

CONTRAINDICATIONS
During an acute asthmatic episode, SPL should not be used intranasally.

WARNINGS
In common with all antigens employed to stimulate the production of antibodies that are protective in the event of subsequent disease, SPL presents the remote potential of host sensitization to staphylococcal or bovine protein. Anaphylaxis has never been observed in the more than 10 million doses administered, but the physician must bear this possibility in mind and be prepared to deal with such an emergency by having at hand appropriate resuscitation equipment and medications.
Caution should be observed when administering SPL intranasally to patients with known allergies (see "Intranasal Aerosol Inhalation" under *Dosage and Administration*).

PRECAUTIONS

> SPL does not contain a preservative; therefore, it must be handled aseptically.
> SPL must not be used if it becomes cloudy or turbid. (This would indicate contamination.)
> SPL must be stored in the refrigerator (2–8°C). Do not freeze.

General—A separate, sterile tuberculin syringe and needle should be used for each patient to prevent transmission of homologous serum hepatitis and other disease entities from one patient to another.
SPL in the 1-ml ampule should be used for subcutaneous injection and intranasal aerosol inhalation. When a parenteral dose of SPL is withdrawn from the 1-ml ampule, the remainder must either be used immediately (by intranasal, oral, or topical administration depending on the condition being treated) or discarded.
SPL in the 10-ml vial should be used only for intranasal (aerosol or drop instillation), oral, or topical administration; it should not be used for subcutaneous injection.

When using the 10-ml vial, the rubber cap should be wiped carefully and completely with an appropriate antiseptic before introducing the needle to withdraw the solution.
Caution should be exercised when administering SPL intranasally to patients with known allergies (see "Intranasal Aerosol Inhalation" under *Dosage and Administration*).
In common with all antigens employed to stimulate the production of antibodies that are protective in the event of subsequent disease, SPL presents the remote potential of host sensitization to staphylococcal or bovine protein. Anaphylaxis has never been observed in the more than 10 million doses administered, but the physician must bear this possibility in mind and be prepared to deal with such an emergency by having at hand appropriate resuscitation equipment and medications.
Information for Patients—The physician may wish to inform the patient that SPL may cause vaccine-type or site-of-injection reactions (see under *Adverse Reactions*) and, if excessive, these reactions may be lessened by dose reduction at the discretion of the physician.
Pregnancy—Pregnancy Category B. Reproduction studies[23–26] have been performed in rats and rabbits at doses up to 250 times the human dose and have revealed no evidence of impaired fertility or harm to the fetus due to SPL. There are, however, no adequate and well-controlled studies in pregnant women. Because animal reproduction studies are not always predictive of human response, SPL should be used during pregnancy only if clearly indicated.
Nursing Mothers—It is not known whether SPL is excreted in human milk. Because many drugs are excreted in human milk, caution should be exercised when SPL is administered to a nursing woman.
Pediatric Use—Safety and effectiveness in children have not been established.

ADVERSE REACTIONS
SPL may cause general vaccine-type reactions (i.e., malaise, fever, or chills). If excessive, these reactions may be lessened by dose reduction at the discretion of the physician.
Reactions at the site of injection (i.e., redness, itching, and/or swelling) may occur in 2 to 3 hours and may last up to 3 days, steadily decreasing. These reactions indicate a normal response to SPL and, if excessive, may be lessened by dose reduction at the discretion of the physician.
Caution should be exercised when administering SPL intranasally to patients with known allergies (see "Intranasal Aerosol Inhalation" under *Dosage and Administration*).

DOSAGE AND ADMINISTRATION
SPL is administered by several routes, according to the directions of the physician. These include subcutaneous injection, intranasal aerosol inhalation or nasal drop instillation, oral administration, topical application or irrigation, and combinations of these routes. The severity of the infection and the response of the patient should be the guiding factors in determining the proper dosage regimen.
Parenteral drug products should be inspected visually for particulate matter and discoloration prior to administration, whenever solution and container permit.
It is highly recommended that all new patients first be skin-tested with 0.025 to 0.05 ml intracutaneously to assess their relative sensitivity to SPL. Based on relative sensitivity to the skin test, the initial dose of SPL is small, followed by incremental increases at prescribed intervals (according to urgency and tolerance), to a maximum dose. This dose is continued until improvement is certain, then the interval may be lengthened gradually to the longest interval that maintains adequte clinical control.
The limit of tolerance is the maximum quantity of SPL that can be given to a patient without producing signs of a general vaccine-type reaction (i.e., malaise, fever, or chills).
For chronic, recurrent, refractory, or deep-seated infections, it may be necessary to increase cautiously the frequency and/or the dose to achieve the desired therapeutic response. Children usually should receive about ½ the adult dose. Infants are best treated with nasal drop instillation, sprays, or topical application.
Subcutaneous Injection—SPL is administered in the deltoid region. Following the initial injection, subsequent injections are given in alternate arms, avoiding a previous site.
If an undue amount of local redness, itching, and/or swelling ensues, await a partial subsidence of the reactions, proceed with ½ the previous dose, and make incremental increases at longer intervals.
Following a subcutaneous injection, the unused contents of the 1-ml ampule may be given orally, topically, or intranasally to reinforce the subcutaneous dose.
Acute Infections: The initial dose varies from 0.05 to 0.2 ml, followed by incremental increases (according to urgency and tolerance) of 0.1 to 0.2 ml at 1- to 2-day intervals, to a maximum dose of up to 0.5 ml. This dose is continued until improvement is certain, then the interval may be lengthened gradually to the longest interval that maintains adequate clinical control.
Subacute and Chronic Infections: The initial dose varies from 0.05 to 0.1 ml, followed by incremental increases (ac-

cording to urgency and tolerance) of 0.1 to 0.2 ml at 2- to 4-day intervals, to a maximum dose of 0.2 to 0.5 ml. This dose is continued until improvement is certain, then the interval may be lengthened gradually to the longest interval that maintains adequate clinical control.

Intranasal Aerosol Inhalation—SPL is rapidly absorbed through the anterior nares, the main reservoir of pathogenic staphylococci. The nose often contains the identical strain isolated from infections in other parts of the body.

The importance of intranasal aerosol inhalation is stressed because of the high-absorptive characteristics of the nasal mucosa.

When using this route, some patients may experience transient general vaccine-type reactions (i.e., malaise, fever, or chills). If excessive, these reactions may be lessened by dose reduction at the discretion of the physician.

Intranasal aerosol inhalation allows direct access to the sinuses, throat and bronchi; when this route is combined with subcutaneous injection, better clinical results may be obtained.

A nebulizer with nasal tips is used, attached by rubber tubing having a hand-controlled air valve to an air supply (e.g., a DeVilbiss Air Compressor, 561 Series). The nebulizer should be cleaned after each use according to the manufacturer's directions.

A measured dose of SPL is placed in the nebulizer, adding sufficient sterile preservative-free water or isotonic saline to a total volume of 1.0 ml for efficient atomization. Nebulization is achieved by closing the air valve during inspiration, holding the breath a few seconds, and exhaling through the mouth, avoiding hyperventilation.

Patients without Allergies: The usual initial dose is 0.1 ml, followed by incremental increases (according to urgency and tolerance) of up to 0.2 ml at 1- to 3-day intervals, to a maximum dose of 0.5 to 1.0 ml. This dose is continued until improvement is certain, then the interval may be lengthened gradually to the longest interval that maintains adequate clinical control.

Patients with Known Allergies: Caution should be exercised when administering SPL by this route to patients with allergies such as bronchial asthma, pulmonary fibrosis, emphysema, bronchiectasis, hay fever, and multiple allergies.

It is highly recommended that these patients first be skin-tested with 0.025 to 0.05 ml intracutaneously to assess their relative sensitivity to SPL.

Based on relative sensitivity to the skin test, the initial dose varies from 0.05 to 0.1 ml, followed by incremental increases (according to urgency and tolerance) of 0.05 to 0.1 ml at weekly intervals, to a maximum dose of 0.25 to 0.5 ml. This dose is continued until improvement is certain, then the interval may be lengthened gradually to the longest interval that maintains adequate clinical control.

These doses can be increased cautiously at shorter intervals if the patient tolerates SPL well.

For faster immunologic response, SPL may be given concomitantly by subcutaneous injection or orally without aftereffects.

Nasal Drop Installation—If intranasal aerosol inhalation equipment is not available, the physician may administer SPL by nasal drop instillation, particularly to patients with upper respiratory symptoms. SPL may be given by this route either alone or concomitantly with other routes of administration.

Before using SPL by nasal drop instillation, review all information under "Intranasal Aerosol Inhalation."

When using this route, withdraw the appropriate dose (see under "Intranasal Aerosol Inhalation") with a sterile tuberculin syringe and needle, remove the needle, and use the syringe as a dropper. The dose should be divided equally between each nostril and should remain in contact with the nasal mucosa for a minimum of 2 minutes to achieve adequate absorption.

Oral Administration—The specific therapy of staphylococcal enterocolitis should include an oral dose of 1 to 2 ml, in water, 1 to 3 times a day as long as necessary to maintain adequate clinical control.

For systemic action, SPL by subcutaneous injection or intranasally will reinforce the oral dose.

Topical Application—Concomitantly with other routes of administration, SPL in the form of sprays, drops, packs, or irrigations may be used to treat accessible lesions of the skin and mucous membranes, including eye and ear infections, burns, sinus tracts, and ulcers. The usual dose varies from 0.25 to 2 ml, as often as indicated to maintain adequate clinical control.

HOW SUPPLIED

SPL is supplied in:

1-ml ampules, boxes of 10, for subcutaneous injection and intranasal aerosol inhalation.

10-ml multiple-dose vials for intranasal aerosol inhalation or nose drops, oral administration, and topical application.

SPL—Serologic Types I & III in equal parts—yellow label. Nebulizer outfits with rubber tubing, hand-controlled air valve, and nasal tips for use with air compressor.

Storage—SPL must be stored in the refrigerator (2–8°C). Do not freeze.

REFERENCES

Available on request.

P-108A   NOVEMBER 1982

Dermaide Research Corp.

P.O. BOX 562
PALOS HEIGHTS, IL 60463

DERMAIDE® ALOE CREAM   OTC
[*der'maid al"o cream*]

ACTIVE INGREDIENT

Aloe Vera Jel

INACTIVE INGREDIENTS

Mineral oil, stearic acid, petrolatum, triethanolamine, Beeswax, Cetyl esters, methylparaben, Propylparaben.

ACTIONS

Dermaide Aloe Cream is a soothing moisturizer for dry itchy skin, minor burns and sunburn, minor cuts, scrapes and mild skin irritations.

WARNINGS

If relief is not evident, consult your physician. Certain people may be allergic. If any skin reaction occurs, discontinue its use and wash off with soap and water.

PRECAUTION

Certain individuals may be allergic. If area become red and itchy, discontinue its use and wash off with soap and water.

DIRECTIONS

Wash and rinse the affected area thoroughly with luke warm water, apply Dermaide Aloe Cream generously over the affected area and continue to apply as often as necessary to keep the affected area covered.

HOW SUPPLIED

4 oz. jar.

Dermik Laboratories, Inc.

500 ARCOLA ROAD, P.O. BOX 1200
COLLEGEVILLE, PA 19426-0107

ANTHRA–DERM® Ointment   ℞
[*anthra-derm*]
(anthralin) 1%, ½%, ¼%, ¹⁄₁₀%
FOR TOPICAL USE ONLY

DESCRIPTION

Each gram of Anthra-Derm® (anthralin) Ointment ¹⁄₁₀%, ¼%, ½% and 1.0% contains 1 mg, 2.5 mg, 5 mg and 10 mg, respectively, of anthralin in a base consisting of mineral oil and white petrolatum. Anthralin is an anti-psoriatic agent with cytostatic, irritant and weak antimicrobial properties.

HOW SUPPLIED

Anthra-Derm® (anthralin) Ointment ¹⁄₁₀% (NDC 0066-0010-15), ¼% (NDC 0066-0025-15), ½% (NDC 0066-0050-15) and 1.0% (NDC-0066-0100-15) is available in 1.5 oz (42.5 g) tubes.

---

5 BENZAGEL®   ℞
[*ben-za-jel*]
(5% benzoyl peroxide) and
10 BENZAGEL®   ℞
(10% benzoyl peroxide)
MICROGEL™ FORMULA
Acne Gels

DESCRIPTION

Each gram of 5 Benzagel® and 10 Benzagel® contains 50 mg and 100 mg respectively, of benzoyl peroxide in a gel vehicle of purified water, carbomer 940, sodium hydroxide, docusate sodium, fragrance and alcohol 14%.

Benzoyl peroxide is an antibacterial and keratolytic agent.

HOW SUPPLIED

5 & 10 Benzagel® are available in 1.5 oz (42.5 g) and 3 oz (85 g) plastic tubes; 5 Benzagel® contains 50 mg benzoyl peroxide per gram and 10 Benzagel® contains 100 mg benzoyl peroxide per gram.

5-Benzagel 1.5 oz NDC 0066-0430-15
5-Benzagel 3.0 oz NDC 0066-0430-30
10-Benzagel 1.5 oz NDC 0066-0431-15
10 Benzagel 3.0 oz NDC 0066-0431-30

BENZAMYCIN® Topical Gel   ℞
[*ben'za-mi"sin*]
(erythromycin—benzoyl peroxide)

PRODUCT OVERVIEW

KEY FACTS

Benzamycin® is a topical gel containing 3% erythromycin and 5% benzoyl peroxide. Erythromycin is an antibiotic and benzoyl peroxide is an antibacterial and keratolytic agent.

MAJOR USES

Benzamycin® is indicated for the topical control of acne vulgaris.

SAFETY INFORMATION

Benzamycin® is contraindicated in patients with a history of hypersensitivity to erythromycin, benzoyl peroxide, or any of the other listed ingredients. Avoid contact with eyes and mucous membranes. Concomitant topical acne therapy should be used with caution. Adverse reactions may include dryness, erythema, and pruritus.

PRESCRIBING INFORMATION

BENZAMYCIN® Topical Gel   ℞
[*ben'za-mi"sin*]
(erythromycin—benzoyl peroxide)

Reconstitute Before Dispensing

DESCRIPTION

Each gram of Benzamycin® (erythromycin—benzoyl peroxide) topical gel contains, as dispensed, 30 mg (3%) of erythromycin and 50 mg (5%) of benzoyl peroxide in a gel vehicle of purified water, carbomer 940, alcohol 16%, sodium hydroxide, docusate sodium and fragrance.

Erythromycin ($C_{37}H_{67}NO_{13}$) is produced by a strain of *Streptomyces erythraeus* and belongs to the macrolide group of antibiotics.

Benzoyl peroxide ($C_{14}H_{10}O_4$), is an antibacterial and keratolytic agent.

CLINICAL PHARMACOLOGY

Erythromycin is a bacteriostatic macrolide antibiotic, but may be bactericidal in high concentrations. Although the mechanism by which erythromycin acts in reducing inflammatory lesions of acne vulgaris is unknown, it is presumably due to its antibiotic action. Antagonism has been demonstrated between clindamycin and erythromycin.

Benzoyl peroxide is an antibacterial agent which has been shown to be effective against *Propionibacterium acnes*, an anaerobe found in sebaceous follicles and comedones. The antibacterial action of benzoyl peroxide is believed to be due to the release of active oxygen. Benzoyl peroxide has a keratolytic and desquamative effect which may also contribute to its efficacy.

Benzoyl peroxide has been shown to be absorbed by the skin where it is converted to benzoic acid.

INDICATIONS AND USAGE

Benzamycin® Topical Gel is indicated for the topical control of acne vulgaris.

CONTRAINDICATIONS

Benzamycin® Topical Gel is contraindicated in those patients with a history of hypersensitivity to erythromycin, benzoyl peroxide or any of the other listed ingredients.

PRECAUTIONS

General—For external use only. Not for ophthalmic use. Avoid contact with eyes and mucous membranes. Concomitant topical acne therapy should be used with caution because a possible cumulative irritancy effect may occur, especially with peeling, desquamating or abrasive agents. If severe irritation develops, discontinue use and institute appropriate therapy.

The use of antibiotic agents may be associated with the overgrowth of antibiotic-resistant organisms. If this occurs, administration of this drug should be discontinued and appropriate measures taken.

Information for Patients—Patients using Benzamycin® Topical Gel should receive the following information and instructions:

1. Benzamycin® Topical Gel is for external use only. Avoid contact with the eyes and mucous membranes.
2. Patients should not use any other topical acne preparation unless otherwise directed by physician.
3. Benzamycin® Topical Gel may bleach hair or colored fabric.
4. If excessive irritation or dryness should occur, patient should discontinue medication and consult physician.
5. Discard product after 3 months and obtain fresh material.

Carcinogenesis, Mutagenesis and Impairment of Fertility: Long-term studies in animals have not been performed to evaluate carcinogenic potential or the effect on fertility.

Continued on next page

Dermik Laboratories—Cont.

Pregnancy Category C: Animal reproduction studies have not been conducted with Benzamycin® Topical Gel. It is also not known whether Benzamycin® Topical Gel can cause fetal harm when administered to a pregnant woman or can affect reproduction capacity. Benzamycin® Topical Gel should be given to a pregnant woman only if clearly needed.
Nursing Mothers: It is not known whether this drug is excreted in human milk. Because many drugs are excreted in human milk, caution should be exercised when Benzamycin® Topical Gel is administered to a nursing woman.
Pediatric Use: Safety and effectiveness in children under the age of 12 have not been established.

ADVERSE REACTIONS

Adverse reactions which may occur include dryness, erythema and pruritus. Of a total of 153 patients treated with Benzamycin® Topical Gel during clinical trials, 4 patients experienced adverse reactions, of whom three experienced dryness and one an urticarial reaction which responded well to symptomatic treatment.

DOSAGE AND ADMINISTRATION

Benzamycin® Topical Gel should be applied twice daily, morning and evening, or as directed by physician, to affected areas after the skin is thoroughly washed, rinsed with warm water and gently patted dry.
How Supplied and Dispensing Information: Benzamycin® Topical Gel is supplied in a package containing 20 g of benzoyl peroxide gel and a plastic vial containing 0.8 g of active erythromycin powder. Prior to dispensing, tap vial gently until powder flows freely, add 3 mL of ethyl alcohol 70% (to the mark) and shake well to dissolve erythromycin. Add this solution to gel and stir until homogeneous in appearance (1–1½ minutes). Benzamycin® Topical Gel should then be stored under refrigeration. Place a 3-month expiration date on the label.
Benzamycin® Topical Gel (NDC 0066-0510-23), as dispensed, is 23.3 g net weight.
Note: *Prior* to reconstitution, store at room temperature. *After* reconstitution, store in a cold place, preferably in a refrigerator. Do not freeze. Keep tightly closed. Keep out of the reach of children.
U.S. Patent Nos. 4,387,107 and 4,497,794. Other Patents Pending.

CAUTION

Federal law prohibits dispensing without prescription.

FLORONE® ℞
[flŏr-ōhn]
(brand of diflorasone diacetate cream and diflorasone diacetate ointment 0.05%)
FLORONE E® ℞
(brand of diflorasone diacetate emollient cream 0.05%)
Not For Ophthalmic Use

PRODUCT OVERVIEW

KEY FACTS

Florone is a topical corticosteroid containing 0.05% diflorasone diacetate in an emulsified, hydrophilic cream and in an ointment with an emollient, occlusive base. Florone Ointment contains no propylene glycol. Florone E Emollient Cream contains 0.5 mg diflorasone diacetate in a hydrophilic, vanishing cream base.

MAJOR USES

These products are indicated for the relief of the inflammatory and pruritic manifestations of corticosteroid-responsive dermatoses.

SAFETY INFORMATION

The Florone products are contraindicated in patients with a history of hypersensitivity to any of their components. Systemic absorption of topical corticosteroids has produced reversible HPA axis suppression. Therefore, patients receiving a large dose applied to a large area or under an occlusive dressing should be evaluated periodically. The most common adverse reactions are burning, itching, irritation, and dryness.

PRESCRIBING INFORMATION

FLORONE® ℞
[flŏr-ōhn]
(brand of diflorasone diacetate cream and diflorasone diacetate ointment 0.05%)
FLORONE E® ℞
(brand of diflorasone diacetate emollient cream 0.05%)
Not For Ophthalmic Use

DESCRIPTION

Each gram of FLORONE Cream and FLORONE Ointment contains 0.5 mg diflorasone diacetate in a cream or ointment base respectively. Each gram of Florone E Emollient Cream contains 0.5 mg diflorasone diacetate in an emollient cream base.
Chemically, diflorasone diacetate is: 6α, 9α-difluoro-11β, 17,21-trihydroxy-16β-methylpregna-1,4-diene-3,20-dione 17,21 diacetate.
FLORONE Cream contains diflorasone diacetate in an emulsified and hydrophilic cream base consisting of propylene glycol, stearic acid, polysorbate 60, sorbitan monostearate and monooleate, sorbic acid, citric acid and water. The corticosteroid is formulated as a solution in the vehicle using 15 percent propylene glycol to optimize drug delivery.
FLORONE Ointment contains diflorasone diacetate in an emollient, occlusive base consisting of polyoxypropylene 15-stearyl ether, stearic acid, lanolin alcohol and white petrolatum.
Florone E Emollient Cream contains diflorasone diacetate in a hydrophilic, vanishing cream base of propylene glycol, stearyl alcohol, cetyl alcohol, sorbitan monostearate, polysorbate 60, mineral oil and water.

CLINICAL PHARMACOLOGY

Topical corticosteroids share anti-inflammatory, antipruritic and vasoconstrictive actions.
The mechanism of anti-inflammatory activity of the topical corticosteroids is unclear. Various laboratory methods, including vasoconstrictor assays, are used to compare and predict potencies and/or clinical efficacies of the topical corticosteroids. There is some evidence to suggest that a recognizable correlation exists between vasoconstrictor potency and therapeutic efficacy in man.
Pharmacokinetics: The extent of percutaneous absorption of topical corticosteroids is determined by many factors including the vehicle, the integrity of the epidermal barrier and the use of occlusive dressings.
Topical corticosteroids can be absorbed from normal intact skin. Inflammation and/or other disease processes in the skin increase percutaneous absorption. Occlusive dressings substantially increase the percutaneous absorption of topical corticosteroids. Thus, occlusive dressings may be a valuable therapeutic adjunct for treatment of resistant dermatoses. (See DOSAGE AND ADMINISTRATION.)
Once absorbed through the skin, topical corticosteroids are handled through pharmacokinetic pathways similar to systemically administered corticosteroids. Corticosteroids are bound to plasma proteins in varying degrees. They are metabolized primarily in the liver and are then excreted by the kidneys. Some of the topical corticosteroids and their metabolites are also excreted into the bile.

INDICATIONS AND USAGE

Topical corticosteroids are indicated for relief of the inflammatory and pruritic manifestations of corticosteroid-responsive dermatoses.

CONTRAINDICATIONS

Topical steroids are contraindicated in those patients with a history of hypersensitivity to any of the components of the preparation.

PRECAUTIONS

General:
Systemic absorption of topical corticosteroids has produced reversible hypothalamic-pituitary-adrenal (HPA) axis suppression, manifestations of Cushing's syndrome, hyperglycemia, and glucosuria in some patients.
Conditions which augment systemic absorption include the application of the more potent steroids, use over large surface areas, prolonged use, and the addition of occlusive dressings.
Therefore, patients receiving a large dose of a potent topical steroid applied to a large surface area or under an occlusive dressing should be evaluated periodically for evidence of HPA axis suppression by using the urinary free-cortisol and ACTH stimulation tests. If HPA axis suppression is noted, an attempt should be made to withdraw the drug, to reduce the frequency of application, or to substitute a less potent steroid.
Recovery of HPA axis function is generally prompt and complete upon discontinuation of the drug. Infrequently, signs and symptoms of steroid withdrawal may occur, requiring supplemental systemic corticosteroids.
Children may absorb proportionally larger amounts of topical corticosteroids and thus be more susceptible to systemic toxicity. (See PRECAUTIONS—Pediatric Use.)
If irritation develops, topical corticosteroids should be discontinued and appropriate therapy instituted.
In the presence of dermatological infections, the use of an appropriate antifungal or antibacterial agent should be instituted. If a favorable response does not occur promptly, the corticosteroid should be discontinued until the infection has been adequately controlled.
Information for the Patient: Patients using topical corticosteroids should receive the following information and instructions:
1. This medication is to be used as directed by the physician. It is for external use only. Avoid contact with the eyes.
2. Patients should be advised not to use this medication for any disorder other than for which it was prescribed.
3. The treated skin area should not be bandaged or otherwise covered or wrapped as to be occlusive unless directed by the physician.
4. Patients should report any signs of local adverse reactions especially under occlusive dressing.
5. Parents of pediatric patients should be advised not to use tight-fitting diapers or plastic pants on a child being treated in the diaper area, as these garments may constitute occlusive dressings.

Laboratory Tests: The following tests may be helpful in evaluating the HPA axis suppression:
Urinary free cortisol test
ACTH stimulation test
Carcinogenesis, Mutagenesis, and Impairment of Fertility: Long-term animal studies have not been performed to evaluate the carcinogenic potential or the effect on fertility of topical corticosteroids.
Studies to determine mutagenicity with prednisolone and hydrocortisone have revealed negative results.
Pregnancy Category C: Corticosteroids are generally teratogenic in laboratory animals when administered systemically at relatively low dosage levels. The more potent corticosteroids have been shown to be teratogenic after dermal application in laboratory animals. There are no adequate and well-controlled studies in pregnant women on teratogenic effects from topically applied corticosteroids. Therefore, topical corticosteroids should be used during pregnancy only if the potential benefit justifies the potential risk to the fetus. Drugs of this class should not be used extensively on pregnant patients, in large amounts, or for prolonged periods of time.
Nursing Mothers: It is not known whether topical administration of corticosteroids could result in sufficient systemic absorption to produce detectable quantities in breast milk. Systemically administered corticosteroids are secreted into breast milk in quantities **not** likely to have a deleterious effect on the infant. Nevertheless, caution should be exercised when topical corticosteroids are administered to a nursing woman.
Pediatric Use: *Pediatric patients may demonstrate greater susceptibility to topical corticosteroid-induced HPA axis suppression and Cushing's syndrome than mature patients because of a larger skin surface area to body weight ratio.*
Hypothalamic-pituitary-adrenal (HPA) axis suppression, Cushing's syndrome, and intracranial hypertension have been reported in children receiving topical corticosteroids. Manifestations of adrenal suppression in children include linear growth retardation, delayed weight gain, low plasma cortisol levels, and absence of response to ACTH stimulation. Manifestations of intracranial hypertension include bulging fontanelles, headaches, and bilateral papilledema.
Administration of topical corticosteroids to children should be limited to the least amount compatible with an effective therapeutic regimen. Chronic corticosteroid therapy may interfere with the growth and development of children.

ADVERSE REACTIONS

The following local adverse reactions have been reported with topical corticosteroids, but may occur more frequently with the use of occlusive dressings. These reactions are listed in an approximate decreasing order of occurrence:
1. Burning
2. Itching
3. Irritation
4. Dryness
5. Folliculitis
6. Hypertrichosis
7. Acneiform eruptions
8. Hypopigmentation
9. Perioral dermatitis
10. Allergic contact dermatitis
11. Maceration of the skin
12. Secondary infection
13. Skin atrophy
14. Striae
15. Miliaria

OVERDOSAGE

Topically applied corticosteroids can be absorbed in sufficient amounts to produce systemic effects (See PRECAUTIONS).

DOSAGE AND ADMINISTRATION

Florone Cream and Florone Ointment are generally applied to the affected areas as a thin film from one to four times daily depending on the severity of the condition.
Florone E Emollient Cream should be applied to the affected areas as a thin film from one to three times daily depending on the severity or resistant nature of the condition.

Occlusive dressings may be used for the management of psoriasis or recalcitrant conditions.
If an infection develops, the use of occlusive dressings should be discontinued and appropriate antimicrobial therapy instituted.

HOW SUPPLIED

FLORONE Cream 0.05% is available as follows:
15 gram tube NDC 0066-0074-17
30 gram tube NDC 0066-0074-31
60 gram tube NDC 0066-0074-60
FLORONE Ointment 0.05% is available as follows:
15 gram tube NDC 0066-0075-17
30 gram tube NDC 0066-0075-31
60 gram tube NDC 0066-0075-60
Florone E Emollient Cream is available as follows:
15 gram tube NDC 0066-0072-17
30 gram tube NDC 0066-0072-31
60 gram tube NDC 0066-0072-60
Store at controlled room temperature 15°-30°C (59°-86°F).

CAUTION Federal law prohibits dispensing without prescription.

HYTONE® Cream, Lotion and Ointment ℞

[*hī-tōne*]
(hydrocortisone)

PRODUCT OVERVIEW

KEY FACTS

Hytone® contains 1% and 2½% Hydrocortisone and is available in a cream, a lotion, and an ointment.

MAJOR USES

Hytone® is indicated for the relief of the inflammatory and pruritic manifestations of corticosteroid-responsive dermatoses.

SAFETY INFORMATION

Hytone® is contraindicated in patients with a history of hypersensitivity to any of its components. Systemic absorption of topical corticosteroids has produced reversible HPA axis suppression. Therefore, patients receiving a large dose applied to a large area or under an occlusive dressing should be evaluated periodically. The most common adverse reactions are burning, itching, irritation, and dryness.

PRESCRIBING INFORMATION

HYTONE® Cream, Lotion and Ointment ℞

[*hī-tōne*]
(hydrocortisone)

DESCRIPTION

Cream—Each gram of 1% and 2½% Cream contains 10 mg or 25 mg, respectively, of hydrocortisone in a water-washable base of purified water, propylene glycol, glyceryl monostearate SE, cholesterol and related sterols, isopropyl myristate, polysorbate 60, cetyl alcohol, sorbitan monostearate, polyoxyl 40 stearate and sorbic acid.
Lotion—Each ml of 1% and 2½% Lotion contains 10 mg or 25 mg, respectively, of hydrocortisone in a vehicle consisting of carbomer 940, propylene glycol, polysorbate 40, propylene glycol stearate, cholesterol and related sterols, isopropyl myristate, sorbitan palmitate, cetyl alcohol, triethanolamine, sorbic acid, simethicone and purified water.
Ointment—Each gram of 1% and 2½% contains 10 mg or 25 mg, respectively, of hydrocortisone in a topical emollient base of mineral oil, white petrolatum and sorbitan sesquioleate.
Chemically, hydrocortisone is 11, 17, 21-trihydroxypregn-4-ene 3, 20-dione.
The topical corticosteroids including hydrocortisone, constitute a class of primarily synthetic steroids used as anti-inflammatory and antipruritic agents.

CLINICAL PHARMACOLOGY

Topical corticosteroids share anti-inflammatory, antipruritic and vasoconstrictive actions. The mechanism of anti-inflammatory activity of the topical corticosteroids is unclear. Various laboratory methods, including vasoconstrictor assays, are used to compare and predict potencies and/or clinical efficacies of the topical corticosteroids. There is some evidence to suggest that a recognizable correlation exists between vasoconstrictor potency and therapeutic efficacy in man.

Pharmacokinetics

The extent of percutaneous absorption of topical corticosteroids is determined by many factors including the vehicle, the integrity of the epidermal barrier, and the use of occlusive dressings.
Topical corticosteroids can be absorbed from normal intact skin. Inflammation and/or other disease processes in the skin increase percutaneous absorption. Occlusive dressings substantially increase the percutaneous absorption of topical Corticosteroids. Thus, occlusive dressings may be a valuable therapeutic adjunct for treatment of resistant dermatoses.
(See *DOSAGE AND ADMINISTRATION.*)
Once absorbed through the skin, topical corticosteroids are handled through pharmacokinetic pathways similar to systemically administered corticosteroids. Corticosteroids are bound to plasma proteins in varying degrees. Corticosteroids are metabolized primarily in the liver and are then excreted by the kidneys. Some of the topical corticosteroids and their metabolites are also excreted into the bile.

INDICATIONS AND USAGE

Topical corticosteroids are indicated for the relief of the inflammatory and pruritic manifestations of corticosteroid-responsive dermatoses.

CONTRAINDICATIONS

Topical corticosteroids are contraindicated in those patients with a history of hypersensitivity to any of the components of the preparation.

PRECAUTIONS

General—Systemic absorption of topical corticosteroids has produced reversible hypothalamic-pituitary-adrenal (HPA) axis suppression, manifestations of Cushing's syndrome, hyperglycemia, and glucosuria in some patients.
Conditions which augment systemic absorption include the application of the more potent steroids, use over large surface areas, prolonged use, and the addition of occlusive dressings.
Therefore, patients receiving a large dose of a potent topical steroid applied to a large surface area or under an occlusive dressing should be evaluated periodically for evidence of HPA axis suppression by using the urinary free cortisol and ACTH stimulation tests. If HPA axis suppression is noted, an attempt should be made to withdraw the drug, to reduce the frequency of application, or to substitute a less potent steroid.
Recovery of HPA axis function is generally prompt and complete upon discontinuation of the drug. Infrequently, signs and symptoms of steroid withdrawal may occur, requiring supplemental systemic corticosteroids.
Children may absorb proportionally larger amounts of topical corticosteroids and thus be more susceptible to systemic toxicity (See PRECAUTIONS—Pediatric Use).
If irritation develops, topical corticosteroids should be discontinued and appropriate therapy instituted.
In the presence of dermatological infections, the use of an appropriate antifungal or antibacterial agent should be instituted. If a favorable response does not occur promptly, the corticosteroid should be discontinued until the infection has been adequately controlled.
Information for the Patient—Patients using topical corticosteroids should receive the following information and instructions:

1. This medication is to be used as directed by the physician. It is for external use only. Avoid contact with the eyes.
2. Patients should be advised not to use this medication for any disorder other than for which it was prescribed.
3. The treated skin area should not be bandaged or otherwise covered or wrapped as to be occlusive unless directed by the physician.
4. Patients should report any signs of local adverse reactions, especially under occlusive dressing.
5. Parents of pediatric patients should be advised not to use tight-fitting diapers or plastic pants on a child being treated in the diaper area, as these garments may constitute occlusive dressings.

Laboratory Tests—The following tests may be helpful in evaluating the HPA axis suppression:
Urinary free cortisol test
ACTH stimulation test
Carcinogenesis, Mutagenesis, and Impairment of Fertility—Long-term animal studies have not been performed to evaluate the carcinogenic potential or the effect on fertility of topical corticosteroids.
Studies to determine mutagenicity with prednisolone and hydrocortisone have revealed negative results.
Pregnancy Category C—Corticosteroids are generally teratogenic in laboratory animals when administered systemically at relatively low dosage levels. The more potent corticosteroids have been shown to be teratogenic after dermal application in laboratory animals. There are no adequate and well-controlled studies in pregnant women on teratogenic effects from topically applied corticosteroids. Therefore, topical corticosteroids should be used during pregnancy only if the potential benefit justifies the potential risk to the fetus. Drugs of this class should not be used extensively on pregnant patients, in large amounts, or for prolonged periods of time.
Nursing Mothers—It is not known whether topical administration of corticosteroids could result in sufficient systemic absorption to produce detectable quantities in breast milk. Systemically administered corticosteroids are secreted into breast milk in quantities *not* likely to have a deleterious effect on the infant. Nevertheless, caution should be exercised when topical corticosteroids are administered to a nursing woman.
Pediatric Use—*Pediatric patients may demonstrate greater susceptibility to topical corticosteroid-induced HPA axis suppression and Cushing's syndrome than mature patients because of a larger skin surface area to body weight ratio.*
Hypothalamic-pituitary-adrenal (HPA) axis suppression, Cushing's syndrome, and intracranial hypertension have been reported in children receiving topical corticosteroids. Manifestations of adrenal suppression in children include linear growth retardation, delayed weight gain, low plasma cortisol levels, and absence of response to ACTH stimulation. Manifestations of intracranial hypertension include bulging fontanelles, headaches, and bilateral papilledema.
Administration of topical corticosteroids to children should be limited to the least amount compatible with an effective therapeutic regimen. Chronic corticosteroid therapy may interfere with the growth and development of children.

ADVERSE REACTIONS

The following local adverse reactions are reported infrequently with topical corticosteroids, but may occur more frequently with the use of occlusive dressings. These reactions are listed in an approximate decreasing order of occurrence:

Burning	Perioral dermatitis
Itching	Allergic contact dermatitis
Irritation	Maceration of the skin
Dryness	Secondary infection
Folliculitis	Skin atrophy
Hypertrichosis	Striae
Acneiform eruptions	Miliaria
Hypopigmentation	

OVERDOSAGE

Topically applied corticosteroids can be absorbed in sufficient amounts to produce systemic effects (See PRECAUTIONS).

DOSAGE AND ADMINISTRATION

Topical corticosteroids are generally applied to the affected area as a thin film from two to four times daily depending on the severity of the condition. Occlusive dressings may be used for the management of psoriasis or recalcitrant conditions.
If an infection develops, the use of occlusive dressings should be discontinued and appropriate antimicrobial therapy instituted.

HOW SUPPLIED

Cream—2½% - tube 1 oz NDC 0066-0095-01 and 2 oz NDC 0066-0095-02; 1% - tube 1 oz NDC 0066-0083-01 and jar 4 oz NDC 0066-0083-04.
Lotion—2½% - bottle 2 fl oz NDC 0066-0098-02; 1% - bottle 4 fl oz NDC 0066-0090-04.
Ointment—2 ½% - tube 1 oz NDC 0066-0085-01; 1% - tube 1 oz NDC 0066-0087-01.

CAUTION

Federal law prohibits dispensing without prescription.

PSORCON™ ℞

[*sŏr-kon*]
brand of diflorasone diacetate ointment
0.05%
Not For Ophthalmic Use

PRODUCT OVERVIEW

KEY FACTS

Psorcon® is a potent (Class I) topical corticosteroid containing 0.05% diflorasone diacetate in an optimized base.

MAJOR USES

Psorcon® is indicated for the relief of the inflammatory and pruritic manifestations of corticosteroid-responsive dermatoses.

SAFETY INFORMATION

Psorcon® is contraindicated in patients with a history of hypersensitivity to any of its components. Systemic absorption of topical corticosteroids has produced reversible HPA axis suppression. Therefore, patients receiving a large dose applied to a large area or under an occlusive dressing should be evaluated periodically. The most common adverse reactions are burning, itching, irritation, and dryness.

PRESCRIBING INFORMATION

PSORCON™ ℞

[*sŏr-kon*]
brand of diflorasone diacetate ointment
0.05%
Not For Ophthalmic Use

Continued on next page

Dermik Laboratories—Cont.

DESCRIPTION
Each gram of **psorcon** Ointment contains 0.5 mg diflorasone diacetate in an ointment base.
Chemically, diflorasone diacetate is 6α, 9α-difluoro-11β, 17, 21-trihydroxy-16β-methylpregna-1, 4-diene-3, 20-dione 17,21 diacetate.
Each gram of **psorcon** Ointment contains 0.5 mg diflorasone diacetate in an ointment base of propylene glycol, glyceryl monostearate and white petrolatum.

CLINICAL PHARMACOLOGY
Topical corticosteroids share anti-inflammatory, antipruritic and vasoconstrictive actions.
The mechanism of anti-inflammatory activity of the topical corticosteroids is unclear. Various laboratory methods, including vasoconstrictor assays, are used to compare and predict potencies and/or clinical efficacies of the topical corticosteroids. There is some evidence to suggest that a recognizable correlation exists between vasoconstrictor potency and therapeutic efficacy in man.

Pharmacokinetics
The extent of percutaneous absorption of topical corticosteroids is determined by many factors including the vehicle, the integrity of the epidermal barrier, and the use of occlusive dressings.
Topical corticosteroids can be absorbed from normal intact skin. Inflammation and/or other disease processes in the skin increase percutaneous absorption. Occlusive dressings substantially increase the percutaneous absorption of topical corticosteroids. Thus, occlusive dressings may be a valuable therapeutic adjunct for treatment of resistant dermatoses. (See DOSAGE AND ADMINISTRATION.)
Once absorbed through the skin, topical corticosteroids are handled through pharmacokinetic pathways similar to systemically administered corticosteroids. Corticosteroids are bound to plasma proteins in varying degrees. They are metabolized primarily in the liver and are then excreted by the kidneys. Some of the topical corticosteroids and their metabolites are also excreted into the bile.

INDICATIONS AND USAGE
Topical corticosteroids are indicated for relief of the inflammatory and pruritic manifestations of corticosteroid-responsive dermatoses.

CONTRAINDICATIONS
Topical steroids are contraindicated in those patients with a history of hypersensitivity to any of the components of the preparation.

PRECAUTIONS
General
Systemic absorption of topical corticosteroids has produced reversible hypothalamic-pituitary-adrenal (HPA) axis suppression, manifestations of Cushing's syndrome, hyperglycemia, and glucosuria in some patients.
Conditions which augment systemic absorption include the application of the more potent steroids, use over large surface areas, prolonged use, and the addition of occlusive dressings.
Therefore, patients receiving a large dose of a potent topical steroid applied to a large surface area or under an occlusive dressing should be evaluated periodically for evidence of HPA axis suppression by using the urinary free cortisol and ACTH stimulation tests. If HPA axis suppression is noted, an attempt should be made to withdraw the drug, to reduce the frequency of application, or to substitute a less potent steroid.
Recovery of HPA axis function is generally prompt and complete upon discontinuation of the drug. Infrequently, signs and symptoms of steroid withdrawal may occur, requiring supplemental systemic corticosteroids.
Children may absorb proportionally larger amounts of topical corticosteroids and thus be more susceptible to systemic toxicity. (See PRECAUTIONS—Pediatric Use.)
If irritation develops, topical corticosteroids should be discontinued and appropriate therapy instituted.
In the presence of dermatological infections, the use of an appropriate antifungal or antibacterial agent should be instituted. If a favorable response does not occur promptly, the corticosteroid should be discontinued until the infection has been adequately controlled.

Information for the Patient
Patients using topical corticosteroids should receive the following information and instructions:
1. This medication is to be used as directed by the physician. It is for external use only. Avoid contact with the eyes.
2. Patients should be advised not to use this medication for any disorder other than for which it was prescribed.
3. The treated skin area should not be bandaged or otherwise covered or wrapped as to be occlusive unless directed by the physician.
4. Patients should report any signs of local adverse reactions especially under occlusive dressing.
5. Parents of pediatric patients should be advised not to use tight-fitting diapers or plastic pants on a child being treated in the diaper area, as these garments may constitute occlusive dressings.

Laboratory Tests
The following tests may be helpful in evaluating the HPA axis suppression:
Urinary free cortisol test
ACTH stimulation test

Carcinogenesis, Mutagenesis, and Impairment of Fertility
Long-term animal studies have not been performed to evaluate the carcinogenic potential or the effect on fertility of topical corticosteroids.
Studies to determine mutagenicity with prednisolone and hydrocortisone have revealed negative results.

Pregnancy Category C
Corticosteroids are generally teratogenic in laboratory animals when administered systemically at relatively low dosage levels. The more potent corticosteroids have been shown to be teratogenic after dermal application in laboratory animals. There are no adequate and well-controlled studies in pregnant women on teratogenic effects from topically applied corticosteroids. Therefore, topical corticosteroids should be used during pregnancy only if the potential benefit justifies the potential risk to the fetus.

Nursing Mothers
It is not known whether topical administration of corticosteroids could result in sufficient systemic absorption to produce detectable quantities in breast milk. Systemically administered corticosteroids are secreted into breast milk in quantities **not** likely to have a deleterious effect on the infant. Nevertheless, caution should be exercised when topical corticosteroids are administered to a nursing woman.

Pediatric Use
Pediatric patients may demonstrate greater susceptibility to topical corticosteroid-induced HPA axis suppression and Cushing's syndrome than mature patients because of a large skin surface area to body weight ratio.
Hypothalamic-pituitary-adrenal (HPA) axis suppression, Cushing's syndrome, and intracranial hypertension have been reported in children receiving topical corticosteroids. Manifestations of adrenal suppression in children include linear growth retardation, delayed weight gain, low plasma cortisol levels, and absence of response to ACTH stimulation. Manifestations of intracranial hypertension include bulging fontanelles, headaches, and bilateral papilledema.
Administration of topical corticosteroids to children should be limited to the least amount compatible with an effective therapeutic regimen. Chronic corticosteroid therapy may interfere with the growth and development of children.

ADVERSE REACTIONS
The following local adverse reactions have been reported with topical corticosteroids, but may occur more frequently with the use of occlusive dressings. These reactions are listed in approximate decreasing order of occurrence.
1. Burning
2. Itching
3. Irritation
4. Dryness
5. Folliculitis
6. Hypertrichosis
7. Acneiform eruptions
8. Hypopigmentation
9. Perioral dermatitis
10. Allergic contact dermatitis
11. Maceration of the skin
12. Secondary infection
13. Skin atrophy
14. Striae
15. Miliaria

OVERDOSAGE
Topically applied corticosteroids can be absorbed in sufficient amounts to produce systemic effects. (See PRECAUTIONS.)

DOSAGE AND ADMINISTRATION
psorcon Ointment should be applied to the affected area as a thin film from one to three times daily depending on the severity or resistant nature of the condition.
Occlusive dressings may be used for the management of psoriasis or recalcitrant conditions.
If an infection develops, the use of occlusive dressings should be discontinued and appropriate antimicrobial therapy initiated.

HOW SUPPLIED
psorcon Ointment 0.05% is available in the following size tubes:

15 gram	NDC 0066-0071-17
30 gram	NDC 0066-0071-31
60 gram	NDC 0066-0071-60

Store at controlled room temperature 15°–30°C (59°–80°F).

CAUTION
Federal law prohibits dispensing without prescription.

SULFACET–R® Acne Lotion ℞
[sul-fa-set]
(sodium sulfacetamide 10% and sulfur 5%)

PRODUCT OVERVIEW

KEY FACTS
Sulfacet-R® contains sodium sulfacetamide 10% and sulfur 5% in a flesh-tinted lotion. Sodium sulfacetamide is an antibacterial, while sulfur acts as a keratolytic agent.

MAJOR USES
Sulfacet-R® is indicated in the topical control of acne vulgaris, acne rosacea, and seborrheic dermatitis.

SAFETY INFORMATION
Sulfacet-R® is contraindicated in patients with a known hypersensitivity to sulfonamides, sulfur, or any other of its ingredients. It should not be used in patients with kidney disease. Although rare, sensitivity to sodium sulfacetamide may occur. It contains sodium bisulfite which may cause allergic-type reactions. Sulfacet-R® may cause local irritation. If irritation develops, discontinue use of the product.

PRESCRIBING INFORMATION

SULFACET–R® Acne Lotion ℞
[sul-fa-set]
(sodium sulfacetamide 10% and sulfur 5%)

DESCRIPTION
Each mL of Sulfacet-R® Acne Lotion (sodium sulfacetamide 10% and sulfur 5%) as dispensed, contains 100 mg of sodium sulfacetamide and 50 mg of sulfur in a tinted lotion of purified water, alkylaryl sulfonic acid salts, hydroxyethylcellulose, propylene glycol, xanthan gum, lauric myristic diethanolamide, polyoxyethylene laurate, butylparaben, methylparaben, silicone emulsion, talc, zinc oxide, titanium dioxide, attapulgite, iron oxides, pH buffers and 2-bromo-2-nitropropane-1, 3-diol.
Sodium sulfacetamide is a sulfonamide with antibacterial activity while sulfur acts as a keratolytic agent. Chemically sodium sulfacetamide is N′-[(4-aminophenyl)sulfonyl]-acetamide, monosodium salt, monohydrate.

CLINICAL PHARMACOLOGY
The most widely accepted mechanism of action of sulfonamides is the Woods-Fildes theory which is based on the fact that sulfonamides act as competitive antagonists to para-aminobenzoic acid (PABA), an essential component for bacterial growth. While absorption through intact skin has not been determined, sodium sulfacetamide is readily absorbed from the gastrointestinal tract when taken orally and excreted in the urine, largely unchanged. The biological half-life has variously been reported as 7 to 12.8 hours.
The exact mode of action of sulfur in the treatment of acne is unknown, but it has been reported that it inhibits the growth of *p. acnes* and the formation of free fatty acids.

INDICATIONS
Sulfacet-R® is indicated in the topical control of acne vulgaris, acne rosacea and seborrheic dermatitis.

CONTRAINDICATIONS
Sulfacet-R® Acne Lotion is contraindicated for use by patients having known hypersensitivity to sulfonamides, sulfur, or any other component of this preparation. Sulfacet-R® Acne Lotion is not to be used by patients with kidney disease.

WARNINGS
Although rare, sensitivity to sodium sulfacetamide may occur. Therefore, caution and careful supervision should be observed when prescribing this drug for patients who may be prone to hypersensitivity to topical sulfonamides. Systemic toxic reactions such as agranulocytosis, acute hemolytic anemia, purpura hemorrhagica, drug fever, jaundice and contact dermatitis indicate hypersensitivity to sulfonamides. Particular caution should be employed if areas of denuded or abraded skin are involved. Contains sodium bisulfite, a sulfite that may cause allergic-type reactions including anaphylactic symptoms and life-threatening or less severe asthmatic episodes in certain susceptible people. The overall prevalence of sulfite sensitivity in the general population is unknown and probably low. Sulfite sensitivity is seen more frequently in asthmatic than in nonasthmatic people.

PRECAUTIONS
General—if irritation develops, use of the product should be discontinued and appropriate therapy instituted. For external use only. Keep away from eyes. Patients should be carefully observed for possible local irritation or sensitization during long-term therapy. The object of this therapy is to achieve desquamation without irritation, but sodium sulfacetamide and sulfur can cause reddening and scaling of epidermis. These side effects are not unusual in the treatment of acne vulgaris, but patients should be cautioned about the possibility. Keep out of the reach of children.

Carcinogenesis, Mutagenesis and Impairment of Fertility— Long-term studies in animals have not been performed to evaluate carcinogenic potential.

Pregnancy—Pregnancy Category C. Animal reproduction studies have not been conducted with Sulfacet-R® Acne Lotion. It is also not known whether Sulfacet-R® Acne Lotion can cause fetal harm when administered to a pregnant woman or can affect reproduction capacity. Sulfacet-R® Acne Lotion should be given to a pregnant woman only if clearly needed.

Nursing Mothers—It is not known whether sodium sulfacetamide is excreted in the human milk following topical use of Sulfacet-R® Acne Lotion. However, small amounts of orally administered sulfonamides have been reported to be eliminated in human milk. In view of this and because many drugs are excreted in human milk, caution should be exercised when Sulfacet-R® Acne Lotion is administered to a nursing woman.

Pediatric Use—Safety and effectiveness in children under the age of 12 have not been established.

ADVERSE REACTIONS

Although rare, sodium sulfacetamide may cause local irritation.

DOSAGE AND ADMINISTRATION

Shake well before using. Apply a thin film to affected areas with light massaging to blend in each application 1 to 3 times daily. Each package contains a Dermik Color Blender™ which enables the patient to alter the basic shade of the lotion so that it matches the skin color exactly.
(Important to the Pharmacist—At the time of dispensing, add contents of vial* to the bottle.
Shake well and/or stir with a glass rod to ensure uniform dispersion. Place expiration date of four (4) months on bottle label.)

HOW SUPPLIED

25g bottles
NDC 0066-0028-25

*Sulfa-Pak™ vial contains 2.1 grams of sodium sulfacetamide.

VANOXIDE–HC® Acne Lotion

[van-ox-īd]
(Clear) R

DESCRIPTION

Each gram of Vanoxide-HC® Lotion contains, as dispensed, 50 mg benzoyl peroxide, and 5 mg hydrocortisone, incorporated in a water-washable lotion of purified water, calcium phosphate, propylene glycol, caprylic/capric triglyceride, propylene glycol monostearate, laneth-10 acetate, decyl oleate, polysorbate 20, cetyl alcohol, mineral oil, lanolin alcohol, sodium phosphate, sodium biphosphate, stearyl heptanoate, hydroxyethylcellulose, tetrasodium EDTA, edetic acid, propylparaben, methylparaben, vegetable oil, monoglyceride citrate, silica, simethicone, BHT, sodium hydroxide, BHA, and propyl gallate.

HOW SUPPLIED

Bottles, 25 grams net weight as dispensed. Package contains a bottle of lotion base and a Benzie-Pak™ vial containing a mixture of benzoyl peroxide, 35%, and calcium phosphate, 64%, silica 1%. Net weight of vial is 3.8 grams.
To the Pharmacist—At the time of dispensing, add contents of Benzie-Pak™ to the lotion in the bottle. Shake well and/or stir with glass rod to ensure uniform dispersion. Place expiration date of three (3) months on bottle label.

VYTONE® CREAM R

[vī-tone]
(hydrocortisone-iodoquinol)

DESCRIPTION

Each gram of Vytone® Cream 1% contains 10 mg of hydrocortisone, and 10 mg of iodoquinol in a greaseless base of purified water, propylene glycol, glyceryl monostearate SE, cholesterol and related sterols, isopropyl myristate, polysorbate 60, cetyl alcohol, sorbitan monostearate, polyoxyl 40 stearate, sorbic acid, and polysorbate 20.
Chemically, hydrocortisone is 11, 17, 21-trihydroxypregn-4-ene-3, 20-dione and iodoquinol, 5,7-diiodo-8-quinolinol.
Hydrocortisone is an anti-inflammatory and antipruritic agent, while iodoquinol is an antifungal and antibacterial agent.

HOW SUPPLIED

1%-Tube 1 oz NDC 0066-0051-01

ZETAR® EMULSION (Coal Tar) R

[zē-tar]

DESCRIPTION

Zetar® Emulsion, coal tar, is a liquid for topical application, following dilution in aqueous media. Each ml contains 300 mg whole coal tar in polysorbates. It is a topical anti-eczematic. The complete chemical composition of coal tar has not been ascertained; components are grouped into six categories: aromatic hydrocarbons, acidic phenolic compounds, cyclic nitrogen compounds, organic sulfur compounds, nonacidic phenolics and nonbasic nitrogen compounds.

HOW SUPPLIED

Zetar® Emulsion (coal tar) is available in 6 fl oz (177 ml) plastic bottles. The strength of the preparation is 300 mg coal tar/mL.

Dey Laboratories, Inc.
2751 NAPA VALLEY CORPORATE DRIVE
NAPA, CA 94558

Brand Name or Generic Name	Concentration Or Size	NDC or Product #
Mucosil™-10(R)	Acetylcysteine Solution 10%	
	Twelve 4 mL Vials	49502-181-04
	Three 10 mL Vials	49502-181-10
	Three 30 mL Vials	49502-181-30
Mucosil™-20(R)	Acetylcysteine Solution 20%	
	Twelve 4 mL Vials	49502-182-04
	Three 10 mL Vials	49502-182-10
	Three 30 mL Vials	49502-182-30
	One 100 mL Vial	49502-182-00
Albuterol Sulfate Inhalation Solution R	Twenty-Five 3 mL Vials 0.083% (expressed as Albuterol)	49502-697-03
	Sixty 3 mL Vials 0.083% (expressed as Albuterol)	49502-697-60
Isoetharine Inhalation Solution S/F, USP (R)	Twenty-five 3 mL Vials 0.08%	49502-661-03
	Twenty-five 5 mL Vials 0.10%	49502-664-05
	Twenty-five 3 mL Vials 0.17%	49502-660-03
	Twenty-two 2 mL Vials 0.25%	49502-659-02
Metaproterenol Sulfate Inhalation Solution S/F, USP (R)	Twenty-five 2.5 mL Vials 0.4%	49502-678-03
	Twenty-five 2.5 mL Vials 0.6%	49502-676-03
	One 30 mL Vial 5%	49502-155-30
Racepinephrine Inhalation Solution S/F, USP (R)	One 15 mL Vial 2.25%	49502-154-15
Nebu-Sol™ Metered-Dose Dispenser™ OTC	Sodium Chloride Solution 0.9% Six 120 mL Aerosol Cans	49502-501-20
	Six 300 mL Aerosol Cans	49502-503-00
Dey-Wash™ Skin Wound Cleanser™ OTC	Sodium Chloride Solution 0.9% Twelve 220 mL Spray Cans	49502-282-20
Dey Vial® OTC	Sodium Chloride Solutions	
	Two Hundred Fifty 3 mL Vials 0.9%	49502-030-03
	Two Hundred Fifty 5 mL Vials 0.9%	49502-030-05
	One Hundred Twenty-five 10 mL Vials 0.9%	49502-030-10
	One Hundred 20 mL Vials 0.9%	49502-030-20
Dey-Pak® OTC	Sodium Chloride Solutions	
	One Hundred 3 mL Vials 0.45%	49502-620-03
	One Hundred 5 mL Vials 0.45%	49502-620-05
	Two Hundred Fifty 1 mL Vials 0.9%	49502-630-01
	One Hundred 3 mL Vials 0.9%	49502-630-03
	One Hundred 5 mL Vials 0.9%	49502-630-05
	Fifty 10 mL Vials 0.9%	49502-630-10
	Fifty 15 mL Vials 0.9%	49502-630-15
	Fifty 15 mL Vials 3%	49502-640-15
	Fifty 15 mL Vials 10%	49502-641-15
	Purified Water, USP	
	One Hundred 3 mL Vials	49502-610-03
	One Hundred 5 mL Vials	49502-610-05

Dista Products Company
Division of Eli Lilly and Company
LILLY CORPORATE CENTER
INDIANAPOLIS, IN 46285

LEGEND

Identi-Code®—Formula Identification Code, Dista
Identi-Dose®—Unit Dose Medication, Dista
Pulvules®—Filled Gelatin Capsules, Dista
RPak—Prescription Package, Dista

IDENTI-CODE® Index
(formula identification code, Dista)
Provides Positive Product Identification

A letter-number symbol, a 4-digit number, the name of the product, the strength of the product, or a combination of these appears on each Dista capsule and tablet and on each label of pediatric liquids and powders for oral suspension. The letter/number or 4-digit number identifies the product.

Identi-Code® Product Name

Coated Tablets

C19 Mi-Cebrin®
Composition (Each Coated Tablet): Thiamine (vitamin B_1), 10 mg; riboflavin (vitamin B_2), 5 mg; pyridoxine (vitamin B_6), 1.7 mg; pantothenic acid, 10 mg; niacinamide, 30 mg; vitamin B_{12} (activity equivalent), 3 μg; ascorbic acid (vitamin C) (as niacinamide ascorbate and sodium ascorbate), 100 mg; dl-alpha tocopheryl acetate (vitamin E), 5.5 IU (5.5 mg); vitamin A, 10,000 IU (3 mg); vitamin D, 400 IU (10 μg); contains also (approximately): iron (as ferrous fumarate), 15 mg; copper (as the sulfate), 1 mg; iodine (as calcium iodate), 0.15 mg; manganese (as the glycerophosphate), 1 mg; magnesium (as the hydroxide), 5 mg; zinc (as the sulfate), 1.5 mg

C20 Mi-Cebrin T®
Composition (Each Coated Tablet): Thiamine mononitrate (vitamin B_1), 15 mg; riboflavin (vitamin B_2), 10 mg; pyridoxine hydrochloride (vitamin B_6), 2 mg; pantothenic acid (as calcium pantothenate), 10 mg; niacinamide, 100 mg; vitamin B_{12} (activity equivalent), 7.5 μg; ascorbic acid (vitamin C) (as niacinamide ascorbate), 150 mg; dl-alpha tocopheryl acetate (vitamin E), 5.5 IU (5.5 mg); vitamin A, 10,000 IU (3 mg); vitamin D, 400 IU (10 μg); contains also (approximately): iron (as ferrous fumarate), 15 mg; copper (as the sulfate), 1 mg; iodine (as calcium iodate), 0.15 mg; manganese (as the glycerophosphate), 1 mg; magnesium (as the hydroxide), 5 mg; zinc (as the sulfate), 1.5 mg

C22 Becotin®-T
Composition (Each Coated Tablet): Thiamine mononitrate (vitamin B_1), 15 mg; riboflavin (vitamin B_2), 10 mg; pyridoxine hydrochloride (vitamin B_6), 5 mg; niacinamide, 100 mg; pantothenic acid (as calcium pantothenate), 20 mg; vitamin B_{12} (activity equivalent), 4 μg; ascorbic acid (vitamin C) (as niacinamide ascorbate), 300 mg

Continued on next page

This product information was prepared in June 1992. Current information on these and other products of Dista Products Company may be obtained by direct inquiry to Lilly Research Laboratories, Lilly Corporate Center, Indianapolis, Indiana 46285, (317) 276-3714.

Dista—Cont.

Pulvules®

3055 Cinobac®
Composition (Each Pulvule®): Cinoxacin, USP, 250 mg

3056 Cinobac®
Composition (Each Pulvule®): Cinoxacin, USP, 500 mg

3105 Prozac®
Composition (Each Pulvule®): fluoxetine hydrochloride, 20 mg (equiv. to fluoxetine)

3123 Co-Pyronil 2®
Composition (Each Pulvule®): chlorpheniramine maleate, 4 mg; pseudoephedrine hydrochloride, 60 mg

H09 Ilosone®
Composition (Each Pulvule®): Erythromycin Estolate, USP, 250 mg (equiv. to erythromycin)

H69 Keflex®
Composition (Each Pulvule®): Cephalexin, USP, 250 mg

H71 Keflex®
Composition (Each Pulvule®): Cephalexin, USP, 500 mg

H76 Nalfon® 200
Composition (Each Pulvule®): Fenoprofen Calcium, USP, 200 mg (equiv. to fenoprofen)

H77 Nalfon®
Composition (Each Pulvule®): Fenoprofen Calcium, USP, 300 mg (equiv. to fenoprofen)

Compressed Tablets

U26 Ilosone®
Composition (Each Compressed Tablet): Erythromycin Estolate, USP, 500 mg (equiv. to erythromycin)

U59 Nalfon®
Composition (Each Compressed Tablet): Fenoprofen Calcium, USP, 600 mg (equiv. to fenoprofen)

4142 Keftab®
Composition (Each Compressed Tablet): Cephalexin Hydrochloride, 250 mg (equiv. to cephalexin)

4143 Keftab®
Composition (Each Compressed Tablet): Cephalexin Hydrochloride, 500 mg (equiv. to cephalexin)

4202 Keflet®
Composition (Each Tablet): Cephalexin, 250 mg

4203 Keflet®
Composition (Each Tablet): Cephalexin, 500 mg

Miscellaneous

W14 Cordran® Tape
Composition: Flurandrenolide, USP, 4 µg/sq cm
W15 Ilosone® Liquid, Oral Suspension
Composition: Each 5 mL contain erythromycin estolate equivalent to 125 mg erythromycin (USP).
W17 Ilosone® Liquid, Oral Suspension
Composition: Each 5 mL contain erythromycin estolate equivalent to 250 mg erythromycin (USP).
W21 Keflex®, for Oral Suspension
Composition (When Mixed as Directed): Each 5 mL contain 125 mg cephalexin (USP).
W22 Keflex®, for Pediatric Drops
Composition (When Mixed as Directed): Each mL contains 100 mg cephalexin (USP).
W68 Keflex®, for Oral Suspension
Composition (When Mixed as Directed): Each 5 mL contain 250 mg cephalexin (USP).

UNIT-DOSE PACKAGING

Identi-Dose® (unit dose medication, Dista) Closed-circuit control of medication from pharmacy to nurse to patient and return. Simplifies counting and dispensing whether in single-unit or prescription-size quantities. Fits into any dispensing system for ready identification and legibility, better inventory control, protection from contamination, easier handling and recording under Medicare, prevention of drug loss through pilferage or spilling, better control of Federal Controlled Substances, and less chance of medication errors.

The following products are available through normal channels of supply:
Identi-Dose®
Pulvules®
No.
402 Keflex®, 250 mg
403 Keflex®, 500 mg
Ointments
No.
52 Ilotycin®, Ophthalmic
Miscellaneous
No.
M-202 Keflex®, for Oral Suspension, 250 mg/5 mL

ILOSONE® ℞
[ī'lō-sōn]
(erythromycin estolate)
USP

> ### WARNING
> Hepatic dysfunction with or without jaundice has occurred, chiefly in adults, in association with erythromycin estolate administration. It may be accompanied by malaise, nausea, vomiting, abdominal colic, and fever. In some instances, severe abdominal pain may simulate an abdominal surgical emergency.
> If the above findings occur, discontinue Ilosone® (Erythromycin Estolate, USP, Dista) promptly.
> Ilosone is contraindicated for patients with a known history of sensitivity to this drug and for those with preexisting liver disease.

DESCRIPTION
Erythromycin is produced by a strain of *Streptomyces erythraeus* and belongs to the macrolide group of antibiotics. It is basic and readily forms salts with acids. The base, the stearate salt, and the esters are poorly soluble in water and are suitable for oral administration.
Ilosone® (Erythromycin Estolate, USP, Dista) is the lauryl sulfate salt of the propionyl ester of erythromycin.
The Pulvules® contain 250 mg (0.237 mmol) erythromycin estolate. They also contain FD&C Red No. 3, FD&C Yellow No. 6, gelatin, iron oxides, magnesium stearate, mineral oil, silica gel, talc, titanium dioxide, and other inactive ingredients.
The tablets contain 500 mg (0.473 mmol) erythromycin estolate. They also contain cornstarch, magnesium stearate, povidone, titanium dioxide, and other inactive ingredients. The suspensions contain 125 mg (0.118 mmol) or 250 mg (0.237 mmol) of erythromycin estolate per 5 mL. The suspensions also contain butylparaben, carboxymethylcellulose, cellulose, citric acid, edetate calcium disodium, flavors, methylparaben, propylparaben, silicone, sodium chloride, sodium citrate, sodium lauryl sulfate, sucrose, and water. The 125-mg suspension also contains FD&C Yellow No. 6. The 250-mg suspension also contains FD&C Red No. 40.

ACTIONS
Erythromycin inhibits protein synthesis without affecting nucleic acid synthesis. Some strains of *Haemophilus influenzae* and staphylococci have demonstrated resistance to erythromycin. Some strains of *H. influenzae* that are resistant in vitro to erythromycin alone are susceptible to erythromycin and sulfonamides used concomitantly. Culture and susceptibility testing should be done. If the Bauer-Kirby method of disk susceptibility testing is used, a 15-µg erythromycin disk should give a zone diameter of at least 18 mm when tested against an erythromycin-susceptible organism.
Orally administered erythromycin estolate is readily and reliably absorbed. Because of acid stability, serum levels are comparable whether the estolate is taken in the fasting state or after food. After a single 250-mg dose, blood concentrations average 0.29, 1.2, and 1.2 µg/mL respectively at 2, 4, and 6 hours. Following a 500-mg dose, blood concentrations average 3, 1.9, and 0.7 µg/mL respectively at 2, 6, and 12 hours.
After oral administration, serum antibiotic levels consist of erythromycin base and propionyl erythromycin ester. The propionyl ester continuously hydrolyzes to the base form of erythromycin to maintain an equilibrium ratio of approximately 20% base and 80% ester in the serum.
After absorption, erythromycin diffuses readily into most body fluids. In the absence of meningeal inflammation, low concentrations are normally achieved in the spinal fluid, but passage of the drug across the blood-brain barrier increases in meningitis. In the presence of normal hepatic function, erythromycin is concentrated in the liver and excreted in the bile; the effect of hepatic dysfunction on excretion of erythromycin by the liver into the bile is not known. After oral ad-

ministration, less than 5% of the administered dose can be recovered as the active form in the urine.
Erythromycin crosses the placental barrier, but fetal plasma levels are low.

INDICATIONS
Streptococcus pyogenes (Group A β-hemolytic)—Upper and lower respiratory tract, skin, and soft-tissue infections of mild to moderate severity.
Injectable penicillin G benzathine is considered by the American Heart Association to be the drug of choice in the treatment and prevention of streptococcal pharyngitis and in long-term prophylaxis of rheumatic fever.
When oral medication is preferred for treating these conditions, penicillin G or V or erythromycin is the alternate drug of choice.
The importance of the patient's strict adherence to the prescribed dosage regimen must be stressed when oral medication is given. A therapeutic dose should be administered for at least 10 days.
α-Hemolytic Streptococci (viridans group) —Although no controlled clinical efficacy trials have been conducted, oral erythromycin has been suggested by the American Heart Association and American Dental Association for prophylactic use against bacterial endocarditis in patients hypersensitive to penicillin who have congenital heart disease or rheumatic or other acquired valvular heart disease when they undergo dental procedures and surgical procedures of the upper respiratory tract.[1] Erythromycin is not suitable for such prophylaxis prior to genitourinary or gastrointestinal tract surgery.
Note: When selecting antibiotics for the prevention of bacterial endocarditis, the physician or dentist should read the full joint statement of the American Heart Association and the American Dental Association.[1]
Staphylococcus aureus—Acute infections of skin and soft tissue that are mild to moderately severe. Resistance may develop during treatment.
Streptococcus pneumoniae —Infections of the upper respiratory tract (eg, otitis media, pharyngitis) and lower respiratory tract (eg, pneumonia) of mild to moderate severity.
Mycoplasma pneumoniae —In the treatment of respiratory tract infections due to this organism.
H. influenzae—May be used concomitantly with adequate doses of sulfonamides in treating upper respiratory tract infections of mild to moderate severity. Not all strains of this organism are susceptible at the erythromycin concentrations ordinarily achieved (see appropriate sulfonamide labeling for prescribing information).
Treponema pallidum—Erythromycin is an alternate choice of treatment for primary syphilis in penicillin-allergic patients. In primary syphilis, spinal-fluid examinations should be done before treatment and as part of follow-up after therapy.
Corynebacterium diphtheriae—As an adjunct to antitoxin, to prevent establishment of carriers, and to eradicate the organism in carriers.
Corynebacterium minutissimum—In the treatment of erythrasma.
Entamoeba histolytica —In the treatment of intestinal amebiasis only. Extraenteric amebiasis requires treatment with other agents.
Listeria monocytogenes —Infections due to this organism.
Bordetella pertussis —Erythromycin is effective in eliminating the organism from the nasopharynx of infected individuals, rendering them noninfectious. Some clinical studies suggest that erythromycin may be helpful in the prophylaxis of pertussis in exposed susceptible individuals.
Legionnaires' Disease —Although no controlled clinical efficacy studies have been conducted, in vitro and limited preliminary clinical data suggest that erythromycin may be effective in treating Legionnaires' disease.
Chlamydia trachomatis—Erythromycins are indicated for treatment of the following infections caused by *C. trachomatis*: conjunctivitis of the newborn, pneumonia of infancy, urogenital infections during pregnancy (*see* Precautions). When tetracyclines are contraindicated or not tolerated, erythromycin is indicated for the treatment of adults with uncomplicated urethral, endocervical, or rectal infections due to *C. trachomatis*.[2]

CONTRAINDICATION
Erythromycin is contraindicated in patients with known hypersensitivity to this antibiotic.

WARNINGS
(*See* boxed Warning.) The administration of erythromycin estolate has been associated with the infrequent occurrence of cholestatic hepatitis. Laboratory findings have been characterized by abnormal hepatic function test values, peripheral eosinophilia, and leukocytosis. Symptoms may include malaise, nausea, vomiting, abdominal cramps, and fever. Jaundice may or may not be present. In some instances, severe abdominal pain may simulate the pain of biliary colic, pancreatitis, perforated ulcer, or an acute abdominal surgical problem. In other instances, clinical symptoms and re-

sults of liver function tests have resembled findings in extrahepatic obstructive jaundice.
Initial symptoms have developed in some cases after a few days of treatment but generally have followed 1 or 2 weeks of continuous therapy. Symptoms reappear promptly, usually within 48 hours after the drug is readministered to sensitive patients. The syndrome seems to result from a form of sensitization, occurs chiefly in adults, and has been reversible when medication is discontinued.
Pseudomembranous colitis has been reported with virtually all broad-spectrum antibiotics (including macrolides, semisynthetic penicillins, and cephalosporins); therefore, it is important to consider its diagnosis in patients who develop diarrhea in association with the use of antibiotics. Such colitis may range in severity from mild to life threatening.
Treatment with broad-spectrum antibiotics alters the normal flora of the colon and may permit overgrowth of clostridia. Studies indicate that a toxin produced by *Clostridium difficile* is a primary cause of antibiotic-associated colitis.
Mild cases of pseudomembraneous colitis usually respond to drug discontinuance alone. In moderate to severe cases, management should include sigmoidoscopy, appropriate bacteriologic studies, and fluid, electrolyte, and protein supplementation. When the colitis does not improve after the drug has been discontinued, or when it is severe, oral vancomycin is the drug of choice for antibiotic-associated pseudomembranous colitis produced by *C. difficile.* Other causes of colitis should be ruled out.

PRECAUTIONS

General—Since erythromycin is excreted principally by the liver, caution should be exercised in administering the antibiotic to patients with impaired hepatic function.
Surgical procedures should be performed when indicated.
The antibacterial activity of erythromycin is markedly greater in alkaline than in neutral or acid media, and several investigators have recommended concomitant administration of urinary alkalinizing agents, such as sodium bicarbonate or acetazolamide (Diamox), when erythromycin is prescribed for treatment of urinary infections.
Laboratory Tests—There are reports that erythromycin interferes in some clinical laboratory tests and causes aberrant results. For example, evidence has been published indicating that high SGOT values recorded for some patients receiving erythromycin estolate may be artifacts and may not necessarily reflect changes in liver function.
Drug Interactions—Since probenecid inhibits tubular reabsorption of erythromycin in animals, it prolongs maintenance of plasma levels.
Erythromycin and lincomycin or clindamycin may under some conditions be antagonistic. Lincomycin or clindamycin therapy should be avoided in treatment of infections due to erythromycin-resistant organisms.
Erythromycin use in patients who are receiving high doses of theophylline may be associated with an increase in serum theophylline levels and potential theophylline toxicity. In case of theophylline toxicity and/or elevated serum theophylline levels, the dose of theophylline should be reduced while the patient is receiving concomitant erythromycin therapy.
Concomitant administration of erythromycin and digoxin has been reported to result in elevated digoxin serum levels.
There have been reports of increased anticoagulant effects when erythromycin and oral anticoagulants were used concomitantly. Increased anticoagulation effects due to this drug interaction may be more pronounced in the elderly.
Concurrent use of erythromycin and ergotamine or dihydroergotamine has been associated in some patients with acute ergot toxicity characterized by severe peripheral vasospasm and dysesthesia.
Erythromycin has been reported to decrease the clearance of triazolam and midazolam and thus may increase the pharmacologic effect of these benzodiazepines.
The use of erythromycin in patients concurrently taking drugs metabolized by the cytochrome P-450 system may be associated with elevations in serum concentrations of these other drugs. Elevated serum concentrations of the following drugs have been reported when administered concurrently with erythromycin: carbamazepine, cyclosporine, hexobarbital, phenytoin, alfentanil, disopyramide, lovastatin, and bromocriptine. Serum concentrations of these and other drugs metabolized by the cytochrome P-450 system should be monitored closely in patients concurrently receiving erythromycin.
Usage in Pregnancy—Pregnancy Category B—Reproduction studies have been performed in rats, mice, and rabbits using erythromycin and its various salts and esters at doses several times the usual human dose. No evidence of impaired fertility or harm to the fetus that appeared to be related to erythromycin was reported in these studies. There are, however, no adequate and well-controlled studies in pregnant women. Because animal reproductive studies are not always predictive of human response, this drug should be used during pregnancy only if clearly needed.
Nursing Mothers—Erythromycin is excreted in breast milk. Caution should be exercised when erythromycin is administered to a nursing woman.
Pediatric Use—See Indications *and* Dosage and Administration.

ADVERSE REACTIONS

The most frequent side effects of erythromycin preparations are gastrointestinal (eg, abdominal cramping and discomfort) and are dose related. Nausea, vomiting, and diarrhea occur infrequently with usual oral doses.
During prolonged or repeated therapy, there is a possibility of overgrowth of nonsusceptible bacteria or fungi. If such infections arise, the drug should be discontinued and appropriate therapy instituted.
Mild allergic reactions, such as urticaria and other skin rashes, have occurred. Serious allergic reactions, including anaphylaxis, have been reported.
There have been isolated reports of hearing loss and/or tinnitus in patients receiving erythromycin. The ototoxic effect of the drug is usually reversible with drug discontinuance; however, in rare instances involving intravenous administration, the ototoxic effect has been irreversible. Ototoxic effects occur chiefly in patients with renal or hepatic insufficiency and in patients receiving high doses of erythromycin.
Rarely, erythromycin has been associated with the production of ventricular arrhythmias, including ventricular tachycardia and torsade des pointes, in individuals with prolonged QT intervals.

OVERDOSAGE

Signs and Symptoms—Symptoms of oral overdose of erythromycin estolate may include nausea, vomiting, epigastric distress, and diarrhea. The severity of the epigastric distress and the diarrhea are dose related. Reversible mild acute pancreatitis has been reported. Hearing loss, with or without tinnitus and vertigo, may occur, especially in patients with renal or hepatic insufficiency.
Treatment—To obtain up-to-date information about the treatment of overdose, a good resource is your certified Regional Poison Control Center. Telephone numbers of certified poison control centers are listed in the *Physicians' Desk Reference (PDR).* In managing overdosage, consider the possibility of multiple drug overdoses, interaction among drugs, and unusual drug kinetics in your patient.
Unless 5 times the normal single dose of erythromycin estolate has been ingested, gastrointestinal decontamination should not be necessary. An accidental ingestion of erythromycin should not be predicted to have minimal toxicity unless there is a good approximation of how much was ingested and unless only a single medication was involved.
Protect the patient's airway and support ventilation and perfusion. Meticulously monitor and maintain, within acceptable limits, the patient's vital signs, blood gases, serum electrolytes, etc. Absorption of drugs from the gastrointestinal tract may be decreased by giving activated charcoal, which, in many cases, is more effective than emesis or lavage; consider charcoal instead of or in addition to gastric emptying. Repeated doses of charcoal over time may hasten elimination of some drugs that have been absorbed. Safeguard the patient's airway when employing gastric emptying or charcoal.
Forced diuresis, peritoneal dialysis, hemodialysis, or charcoal hemoperfusion have not been established as beneficial for an overdose of erythromycin estolate.

DOSAGE AND ADMINISTRATION

Adults —The usual dosage is 250 mg every 6 hours. This may be increased up to 4 g/day or more according to the severity of the infection.
Children —Age, weight, and severity of the infection are important factors in determining the proper dosage. The usual regimen is 30 to 50 mg/kg/day in divided doses. For more severe infections, this dosage may be doubled.
If administration is desired on a twice-a-day schedule in either adults or children, ½ of the total daily dose may be given every 12 hours.
Twice-a-day dosing is not recommended when doses larger than 1 g daily are administered.
Streptococcal Infections —For the treatment of streptococcal pharyngitis and tonsillitis, the usual dosage range is 20 to 50 mg/kg/day in divided doses.

Body Weight	Total Daily Dose
10 kg or less (less than 25 lb)	250 mg
11–18 kg (25–40 lb)	375 mg
18–25 kg (40–55 lb)	500 mg
25–36 kg (55–80 lb)	750 mg
36 kg or more (more than 80 lb)	1,000 mg (adult dose)

In the treatment of group A β-hemolytic streptococcal infections, a therapeutic dosage of erythromycin should be administered for at least 10 days. In continuous prophylaxis of streptococcal infections in persons with a history of rheumatic heart disease, the dosage is 250 mg twice a day.
For prophylaxis against bacterial endocarditis[1] in penicillin-allergic patients with congenital heart disease or rheumatic or other acquired valvular heart disease when undergoing dental procedures or surgical procedures of the upper respiratory tract, the dosage schedule for adults is 1 g (20 mg/kg for children) orally 1 hour before the procedure and then 500 mg (10 mg/kg for children) orally 6 hours later.
Primary Syphilis —A regimen of 20 g of erythromycin estolate in divided doses over a period of 10 days has been shown to be effective in the treatment of primary syphilis.
Dysenteric Amebiasis —Dosage for adults is 250 mg 4 times daily for 10 to 14 days; for children, 30 to 50 mg/kg/day in divided doses for 10 to 14 days.
Pertussis —Although optimum dosage and duration have not been established, the dosage of erythromycin utilized in reported clinical studies was 40 to 50 mg/kg/day, given in divided doses for 5 to 14 days.
Legionnaires' Disease —Although optimum doses have not been established, doses utilized in reported clinical data were those recommended above (1 to 4 g erythromycin estolate daily in divided doses).
Conjunctivitis of the Newborn Caused by C. trachomatis —Oral erythromycin suspension, 50 mg/kg/day in 4 divided doses for at least 2 weeks.[2]
Pneumonia of Infancy Caused by C. trachomatis —Although the optimum duration of therapy has not been established, the recommended therapy is oral erythromycin suspension, 50 mg/kg/day in 4 divided doses for at least 3 weeks.[2]
Urogenital Infections During Pregnancy Due to C. trachomatis—Although the optimum dose and duration of therapy have not been established, the suggested treatment is erythromycin, 500 mg orally 4 times a day for at least 7 days. For women who cannot tolerate this regimen, a decreased dose of 250 mg orally 4 times a day should be used for at least 14 days.[2]
For adults with uncomplicated urethral, endocervical, or rectal infections caused by *C. trachomatis* in whom tetracyclines are contraindicated or not tolerated: 500 mg orally 4 times a day for at least 7 days.[2]

REFERENCES

1. American Heart Association: Prevention of bacterial endocarditis. *Circulation,* 1984; 70:1123A.
2. Sexually Transmitted Diseases Treatment Guidelines 1982. Centers for Disease Control, Morbidity and Mortality Weekly Report, US Department of Health and Human Services, Atlanta, 1982; 31 (suppl): 355.

HOW SUPPLIED

℞ Pulvules, ivory and red
250 mg* (No. 375)—(100s) NDC 0777-0809-02
℞ Tablets, specially coated, white (capsule-shaped, scored)
500 mg* (No. 1863)—(50s) NDC 0777-2126-50
Store at controlled room temperature, 59° to 86°F (15° to 30°C).
℞ Liquid, Oral Suspension
125 mg*/5 mL, orange-flavored vehicle (M-148)†—(16 fl oz) NDC 0777-2315-05
250 mg*/5 mL, cherry-flavored vehicle (M-153)†—(100 mL) NDC 0777-2317-48; (16 fl oz) NDC 0777-2317-05

* Equivalent to erythromycin.
† Shake well before using. Refrigerate to maintain optimum taste.

[062591]

Shown in Product Identification Section, page 408

ILOTYCIN® ℞
[ī-lō-tī'-sĭn]
(erythromycin)
Ophthalmic Ointment, USP

DESCRIPTION

Ilotycin® (Erythromycin, USP, Dista) belongs to the macrolide group of antibiotics. It is basic and readily forms a salt when combined with an acid. The base, as crystals or powder, is slightly soluble in water, moderately soluble in ether, and readily soluble in alcohol or chloroform. The empirical formula for erythromycin is $C_{37}H_{67}NO_{13}$. Erythromycin (3R*, 4S*, 5S*, 6R*, 7R*, 9R*, 11R*, 12R*, 13S*, 14R*)-4-[(2,6-Dideoxy-3-*C* -methyl-3-*O* -methyl -α- L-*ribo* -hexopyranosyl]) oxy]-14-ethyl-7,12,13-trihydroxy-3,5,7,9,11,13-hexamethyl-6-[[3,4,6-trideoxy-3-(dimethylamino) -β-D-*xylo*-hexopyranosyl]

Continued on next page

This product information was prepared in June 1992. Current information on these and other products of Dista Products Company may be obtained by direct inquiry to Lilly Research Laboratories, Lilly Corporate Center, Indianapolis, Indiana 46285, (317) 276-3714.

Dista—Cont.

oxy]oxacyclotetradecane-2,10-dione is an antibiotic produced from a strain of *Streptomyces erythraeus.*
Each gram contains erythromycin, USP, 5 mg, in a sterile ophthalmic base of mineral oil and white petrolatum. The ⅛-oz tamper-resistant tubes also contain methylparaben and propylparaben. The special sterile ophthalmic ointment base flows freely over the conjunctiva.

CLINICAL PHARMACOLOGY

Microbiology—Erythromycin inhibits protein synthesis without affecting nucleic acid synthesis. Erythromycin is usually active against the following organisms in vitro and in clinical infections:

Streptococcus pyogenes (group A β-hemolytic)
Alpha-hemolytic streptococci (viridans group)
Staphylococcus aureus, including penicillinase-producing strains (methicillin-resistant staphylococci are uniformly resistant to erythromycin)
Streptococcus pneumoniae
Mycoplasma pneumoniae (Eaton Agent, PPLO)
Haemophilus influenzae (not all strains of this organism are susceptible at the erythromycin concentrations ordinarily achieved)
Treponema pallidum
Corynebacterium diphtheriae
Corynebacterium minutissimum
Listeria monocytogenes
Neisseria gonorrhoeae
Bordetella pertussis
Chlamydia trachomatis
Entamoeba histolytica

Disk Susceptibility Testing—Quantitative methods that require measurement for zone diameters give the most precise estimates of antibiotic susceptibility. One such procedure[1] has been recommended for use with disks to test susceptibility to erythromycin. Interpretation involves correlation of the diameters obtained in the disk test with minimum inhibitory concentration (MIC) values for erythromycin. Laboratory reports giving results of the standardized single-disk susceptibility test[1] using a 15-μg erythromycin disk should be interpreted according to the following criteria:
Susceptible organisms produce zones of 23 mm or greater, indicating that the test organism is likely to respond to therapy.
Organisms of intermediate susceptibility produce zones of 14 to 22 mm, indicating that the tested organism would be susceptible if high dosage is used or if the infection is confined to tissues and fluids in which high antibiotic levels are attained.
Resistant organisms produce zones of 13 mm or less, indicating other therapy should be selected.
A bacterial isolate may be considered susceptible if the MIC value for erythromycin is not more than 0.5 μg/mL. Organisms are considered resistant if the MIC is greater than 8 μg/mL.

INDICATIONS AND USAGE

For the treatment of superficial ocular infections involving the conjunctiva and/or cornea caused by organisms susceptible to Ilotycin® (Erythromycin, USP, Dista).
For prophylaxis of neonatal ophthalmia due to *N. gonorrhoeae* or *C. trachomatis.*
For prophylaxis of neonatal gonococcal ophthalmia, a 1% silver nitrate solution in single-dose ampoules or single-use tubes of an ophthalmic ointment containing 0.5% erythromycin or 1% tetracycline are each considered effective and acceptable by the American Academy of Pediatrics. The effectiveness of erythromycin or tetracycline in the prevention of ophthalmia caused by penicillinase-producing *N. gonorrhoeae* is not established.[2]
For prophylaxis of neonatal chlamydial ophthalmia, topical silver nitrate, erythromycin, and tetracycline are each considered equally acceptable for use.[2]

CONTRAINDICATION

This drug is contraindicated in patients with a history of hypersensitivity to erythromycin.

PRECAUTIONS

General—The use of antimicrobial agents may be associated with the overgrowth of antibiotic-resistant organisms; in such a case, antibiotic administration should be stopped and appropriate measures taken.
Usage in Pregnancy—Pregnancy Category B—Reproduction studies have been performed in rats, mice, and rabbits using erythromycin and its various salts and esters, at doses that were several multiples of the usual human dose. No evidence of impaired fertility or harm to the fetus that appeared related to erythromycin was reported in these studies. There are, however, no adequate and well-controlled studies in pregnant women. Because animal reproductive studies are not always predictive of human response, the erythromycins should be used during pregnancy only if clearly needed.
Pediatric Use—See Indications and Usage *and* Dosage and Administration.

ADVERSE REACTIONS

As with any other medicament intended for topical use, there is always the possibility that sensitivity reactions will occur in certain individuals. If such reactions develop, the medication should be discontinued. Eye irritation has been infrequently reported.

DOSAGE AND ADMINISTRATION

In the treatment of external ocular infections, Ophthalmic Ointment Ilotycin® (Erythromycin, USP, Dista) should be applied directly to the infected structure 1 or more times daily, depending on the severity of the infection.
For prophylaxis of neonatal gonococcal or chlamydial ophthalmia, a ribbon of ointment approximately 1 to 2 cm in length should be instilled into each lower conjunctival sac. The ointment should not be flushed from the eye following instillation. A new tube should be used for each infant. Infants born by cesarean section as well as those delivered by the vaginal route should receive prophylaxis.

HOW SUPPLIED

(℞) Ophthalmic Ointment, 5 mg/g (No. 52)—(⅛-oz tamper-resistant tubes), NDC 0777-1863-17; (ID24*—1-g plastic containers) NDC 0777-1863-52
Store at controlled room temperature, 59° to 86°F (15° to 30°C).

REFERENCES

1. National Committee for Clinical Laboratory Standards, M2-A4, Performance Standards for Antimicrobial Disk Susceptibility Tests—4th ed. 1991, NCCLS, Villanova, PA 19085.
2. Committee on Infectious Diseases. Report of the Committee on Infectious Diseases. Elk Grove Village, IL, American Academy of Pediatrics, 1988.

*Identi-Dose® (unit dose medication, Dista)

[050892]

ILOTYCIN® GLUCEPTATE ℞

[ī-lō-tī'sĭn gloo-sĕp'tāt]
(erythromycin gluceptate)
Sterile, USP
Intravenous

DESCRIPTION

Erythromycin is produced by a strain of *Streptomyces erythraeus* and belongs to the macrolide group of antibiotics. It is basic and readily forms a salt when combined with an acid.

ACTIONS

Erythromycin inhibits protein synthesis without affecting nucleic acid synthesis. Some strains of *Haemophilus influenzae* and staphylococci have demonstrated resistance to erythromycin. Culture and susceptibility testing should be done. If the Bauer-Kirby method of disk susceptibility testing is used, a 15-μg erythromycin disk should give a zone diameter of at least 18 mm when tested against an erythromycin-susceptible organism.
Intravenous injection of 200 mg of erythromycin produces peak serum levels of 3 to 4 μg/mL at 1 hour and 0.5 μg/mL at 6 hours.
Erythromycin diffuses readily into the body fluids. Only low concentrations are normally achieved in the spinal fluid, but passage of the drug across the blood-brain barrier increases in meningitis. In the presence of normal hepatic function, erythromycin is concentrated in the liver and excreted in the bile; the effect of hepatic dysfunction on excretion of erythromycin by the liver into the bile is not known. From 12% to 15% of intravenously administered erythromycin is excreted in active form in the urine.
Erythromycin crosses the placental barrier, but fetal plasma levels are low.

INDICATIONS

Streptococcus pyogenes (Group A β-hemolytic)—Upper and lower respiratory tract, skin, and soft-tissue infections of mild to moderate severity.
Injectable penicillin G benzathine is considered by the American Heart Association to be the drug of choice in the treatment and prevention of streptococcal pharyngitis and in long-term prophylaxis of rheumatic fever.
Staphylococcus aureus—Acute infections of skin and soft tissue that are mild to moderately severe. Resistance may develop during treatment.
Streptococcus pneumoniae—Infections of the upper respiratory tract (eg, otitis media and pharyngitis) and lower respiratory tract (eg, pneumonia) of mild to moderate severity.
Mycoplasma pneumoniae—In the treatment of respiratory tract infections due to this organism.
H. influenzae—May be used concomitantly with adequate doses of sulfonamides in treating upper respiratory tract infections of mild to moderate severity. Not all strains of this organism are susceptible at the erythromycin concentrations ordinarily achieved (see appropriate sulfonamide labeling for prescribing information).
Corynebacterium diphtheriae—As an adjunct to antitoxin.
Listeria monocytogenes—Infections due to this organism.
Neisseria gonorrhoeae—In female patients with a history of sensitivity to penicillin, a parenteral erythromycin (such as the gluceptate) may be administered in conjunction with an oral erythromycin as alternate therapy in acute pelvic inflammatory disease caused by *N. gonorrhoeae.* In the treatment of gonorrhea, patients suspected of having concomitant syphilis should have microscopic examinations (by immunofluorescence or dark-field) before receiving erythromycin and monthly serologic tests for a minimum of 4 months.
Legionnaires' Disease—Although no controlled clinical efficacy studies have been conducted, in vitro and limited preliminary clinical data suggest that erythromycin may be effective in treating Legionnaires' disease.

CONTRAINDICATION

Intravenous erythromycin is contraindicated in patients with known hypersensitivity to this antibiotic.

WARNINGS

Usage in Pregnancy—Safety of this drug for use during pregnancy has not been established.
Pseudomembranous colitis has been reported with virtually all broad-spectrum antibiotics (including macrolides, semisynthetic penicillins, and cephalosporins); therefore, it is important to consider its diagnosis in patients who develop diarrhea in association with the use of antibiotics. Such colitis may range in severity from mild to life threatening.
Treatment with broad-spectrum antibiotics alters the normal flora of the colon and may permit overgrowth of clostridia. Studies indicate that a toxin produced by *Clostridium difficile* is one primary cause of antibiotic-associated colitis.
Mild cases of pseudomembranous colitis usually respond to drug discontinuance alone. In moderate to severe cases, management should include sigmoidoscopy, appropriate bacteriologic studies, and fluid, electrolyte, and protein supplementation. When the colitis does not improve after the drug has been discontinued, or when it is severe, oral vancomycin is the drug of choice for antibiotic-associated pseudomembranous colitis produced by *C. difficile.* Other causes should be ruled out.

PRECAUTIONS

Surgical procedures should be performed when indicated.
Side effects following the use of intravenous erythromycin are rare. Occasional venous irritation has been encountered, but if the injection is given slowly, in dilute solution, preferably by continuous intravenous infusion over 20 to 60 minutes, pain and vessel trauma are minimized.
Since erythromycin is excreted principally by the liver, caution should be exercised in administering the antibiotic to patients with impaired hepatic function.
Drug Interactions—Erythromycin use in patients who are receiving high doses of theophylline may be associated with an increase in serum theophylline levels and potential theophylline toxicity. In case of theophylline toxicity and/or elevated serum theophylline levels, the dose of theophylline should be reduced while the patient is receiving concomitant erythromycin therapy.
Concomitant administration of erythromycin and digoxin has been reported to result in elevated digoxin serum levels.
There have been reports of increased anticoagulant effects when erythromycin and oral anticoagulants were used concomitantly. Increased anticoagulation effects due to this drug interaction may be more pronounced in the elderly.
Concurrent use of erythromycin and ergotamine or dihydroergotamine has been associated in some patients with acute ergot toxicity characterized by severe peripheral vasospasm and dysesthesia.
Erythromycin has been reported to decrease the clearance of triazolam and midazolam and thus may increase the pharmacologic effect of these benzodiazepines.
The use of erythromycin in patients concurrently taking drugs metabolized by the cytochrome P-450 system may be associated with elevations in serum concentrations of these other drugs. Elevated serum concentrations of the following drugs have been reported when administered concurrently with erythromycin: carbamazepine, cyclosporine, hexobarbital, phenytoin, alfentanil, disopyramide, lovastatin, and bromocriptine. Serum concentrations of these and other drugs metabolized by the cytochrome P-450 system should be monitored closely in patients concurrently receiving erythromycin.

ADVERSE REACTIONS

Allergic reactions, ranging from urticaria and mild skin eruptions to anaphylaxis, have occurred with intravenously administered erythromycin.
During prolonged or repeated therapy, there is a possibility of overgrowth of nonsusceptible bacteria or fungi. If such infections arise, the drug should be discontinued and appropriate therapy instituted.

Variations in liver function have been observed following daily doses at high levels or after prolonged therapy. Hepatic function tests should be performed when such therapy is given.
Reversible hearing loss associated with the intravenous infusion of 4 g/day or more of erythromycin has been reported rarely.
Rarely, erythromycin has been associated with the production of ventricular arrhythmias, including ventricular tachycardia and torsade des pointes, in individuals with prolonged QT intervals.

OVERDOSAGE

Signs and Symptoms—Experience with overdosage of Ilotycin® Gluceptate (Erythromycin Gluceptate, USP, Dista) is limited. Alterations in liver function tests and reversible hearing loss are possible, especially in patients with renal insufficiency.
Treatment—To obtain up-to-date information about the treatment of overdose, a good resource is your certified Regional Poison Control Center. Telephone numbers of certified poison control centers are listed in the *Physicians' Desk Reference (PDR)*. In managing overdosage, consider the possibility of multiple drug overdoses, interaction among drugs, and unusual drug kinetics in your patient.
Protect the patient's airway and support ventilation and perfusion. Meticulously monitor and maintain, within acceptable limits, the patient's vital signs, blood gases, serum electrolytes, etc.
Forced diuresis, peritoneal dialysis, hemodialysis, or charcoal hemoperfusion have not been established as beneficial for an overdose of erythromycin gluceptate.

DOSAGE AND ADMINISTRATION

Prepare the initial solution of Ilotycin® Gluceptate (Erythromycin Gluceptate, USP, Dista) by (1) adding at least 20 mL of Sterile Water for Injection to the 1-g vial of Ilotycin Gluceptate and (2) shaking the vial until all of the drug is dissolved.
It is important that the product be diluted only *with Sterile Water for Injection without preservatives.*
After reconstitution, the sterile solution should be stored in a refrigerator and used within 7 days.
When all of the drug is dissolved, the solution may then be added to 0.9% Sodium Chloride Injection or to 5% Dextrose in Water to give 1 g per liter for slow, continuous infusion. IV fluid admixtures with a pH below 5.5 tend to lose potency rapidly. Therefore, such solutions should be administered completely within 4 hours after dilution.
If the period of administration is prolonged, the pH of the infusion fluid should be buffered to neutrality with a sterile agent such as Neut® (Sodium Bicarbonate 4% Additive Solution, Abbott) or Buff™ (Phosphate-Carbonate Buffer, Travenol). For administration of the antibiotic in 500 or 1,000 mL of 5% Dextrose in Water, add 1 ampoule full-strength Buff or 5 mL of Neut; for administration of the antibiotic in the same volumes of 0.9% Sodium Chloride Injection, add 1 ampoule half-strength Buff or 5 mL of Neut. These solutions should be completely administered within 24 hours after dilution.
If the medication is to be given in 100 to 250 mL of fluid by a volume control set such as Metriset® (McGaw), Volu-Trole® "B" (Cutter), Soluset® (Abbott), or Buretrol® (Baxter-Travenol), the IV fluid should be buffered in its primary container before being added to the volumetric administration set.
If the medication is to be given by intermittent injection, one-fourth of the total daily dose can be given in 20 to 60 minutes by slow intravenous injection of 250 to 500 mg in 100 to 250 mL of 0.9% Sodium Chloride Injection or 5% Dextrose in Water. Injection should be sufficiently slow to avoid pain along the vein.
The recommended IV dosage for severe infections in adults and children is 15 to 20 mg/kg of body weight/day. Higher doses (up to 4 g/day) may be given in very severe infections. Continuous infusion is preferable, but administration in divided doses at intervals of no more than every 6 hours is also effective.
For treatment of acute pelvic inflammatory disease caused by *N. gonorrhoeae,* administer 500 mg Ilotycin® Gluceptate (Erythromycin Gluceptate, USP, Dista) intravenously every 6 hours for at least 3 days, followed by 250 mg oral erythromycin every 6 hours for 7 days.
Patients receiving intravenous erythromycin should be transferred to the oral dosage form as soon as possible.
For Treatment of Legionnaires' Disease—Although optimum doses have not been established, doses utilized in reported clinical data were those recommended above (1 to 4 g daily in divided doses).

HOW SUPPLIED

(℞) Vials:
1 g,* 30-mL size (No. 646)—(1s) NDC 0777-1441-01
Prior to reconstitution, store at controlled room temperature, 59° to 86°F (15° to 30°C).

* Equivalent to erythromycin.

[062591]

KEFLEX® ℞

[*kĕf'lĕks*]
(cephalexin)
USP

DESCRIPTION

Keflex® (Cephalexin, USP, Dista) is a semisynthetic cephalosporin antibiotic intended for oral administration. It is 7-(D-α-amino-α-phenylacetamido)-3-methyl-3-cephem-4-carboxylic acid monohydrate.
The nucleus of cephalexin is related to that of other cephalosporin antibiotics. The compound is a zwitterion; ie, the molecule contains both a basic and an acidic group. The isoelectric point of cephalexin in water is approximately 4.5 to 5.
The crystalline form of cephalexin which is available is a monohydrate. It is a white crystalline solid having a bitter taste. Solubility in water is low at room temperature; 1 or 2 mg/mL may be dissolved readily, but higher concentrations are obtained with increasing difficulty.
The cephalosporins differ from penicillins in the structure of the bicyclic ring system. Cephalexin has a *D*-phenylglycyl group as substituent at the 7-amino position and an unsubstituted methyl group at the 3-position.
Each Pulvule® contains cephalexin monohydrate equivalent to 250 mg (720 μmol) or 500 mg (1,439 μmol) of cephalexin. The Pulvules also contain cellulose, D & C Yellow No. 10, F D & C Blue No. 1, F D & C Yellow No. 6, gelatin, magnesium stearate, silicone, titanium dioxide, and other inactive ingredients.
After mixing, each 5 mL of Keflex, for Oral Suspension, will contain cephalexin monohydrate equivalent to 125 mg (360 μmol) or 250 mg (720 μmol) of cephalexin. The suspensions also contain flavors, methylcellulose, silicone, sodium lauryl sulfate, and sucrose. The 125-mg suspension contains F D & C Red No. 40, and the 250-mg suspension contains F D & C Yellow No. 6.
The pediatric drops contain cephalexin monohydrate equivalent to 100 mg (288 μmol) cephalexin/mL. The drops also contain D & C Yellow No. 10, flavors, and sucrose.

CLINICAL PHARMACOLOGY

Human Pharmacology—Keflex® (Cephalexin, USP, Dista) is acid stable and may be given without regard to meals. It is rapidly absorbed after oral administration. Following doses of 250 mg, 500 mg, and 1 g, average peak serum levels of approximately 9, 18, and 32 μg/mL respectively were obtained at 1 hour. Measurable levels were present 6 hours after administration. Cephalexin is excreted in the urine by glomerular filtration and tubular secretion. Studies showed that over 90% of the drug was excreted unchanged in the urine within 8 hours. During this period, peak urine concentrations following the 250-mg, 500-mg, and 1-g doses were approximately 1,000, 2,200, and 5,000 μg/mL respectively.
Microbiology—In vitro tests demonstrate that the cephalosporins are bactericidal because of their inhibition of cell-wall synthesis. Keflex is active against the following organisms in vitro:
β-hemolytic streptococci
Staphylococci, including coagulase-positive, coagulase-negative, and penicillinase-producing strains
Streptococcus pneumoniae
Escherichia coli
Proteus mirabilis
Klebsiella sp
Haemophilus influenzae
Moraxella (Branhamella) catarrhalis
Note—Most strains of enterococci (*Enterococcus faecalis* [formerly *Streptococcus faecalis*]) and a few strains of staphylococci are resistant to Keflex. It is not active against most strains of *Enterobacter* sp, *Morganella morganii* (formerly *Proteus morganii*), and *Proteus vulgaris*. It has no activity against *Pseudomonas* or *Acinetobacter calcoaceticus* (formerly *Mima* and *Herellea* sp). When tested by in vitro methods, staphylococci exhibit cross-resistance between Keflex and methicillin-type antibiotics.
Disk Susceptibility Tests—Quantitative methods that require measurement of zone diameters give the most precise estimates of antibiotic susceptibility. One such procedure* has been recommended for use with disks for testing susceptibility to cephalothin. Interpretations correlate zone diameters of the disk test with MIC values for Keflex. With this procedure, a report from the laboratory of "resistant" indicates that the infecting organism is not likely to respond to therapy. A report of "intermediate susceptibility" suggests that the organism would be susceptible if the infection is confined to the urine, in which high antibiotic levels can be obtained, or if high dosage is used in other types of infection.

*Bauer AW, Kirby WMM, Sherris JC, et al: Antibiotic susceptibility testing by a standardized single disk method. *Am J Clin Pathol* 1966;45:493; Standardized Disk Susceptibility Test. *Federal Register* 1974;39:19182–19184.

INDICATIONS AND USAGE

Keflex® (Cephalexin, USP, Dista) is indicated for the treatment of the following infections when caused by susceptible strains of the designated microorganisms:
Respiratory tract infections caused by *S. pneumoniae* and group A β-hemolytic streptococci (Penicillin is the usual drug of choice in the treatment and prevention of streptococcal infections, including the prophylaxis of rheumatic fever. Keflex is generally effective in the eradication of streptococci from the nasopharynx; however, substantial data establishing the efficacy of Keflex in the subsequent prevention of rheumatic fever are not available at present.)
Otitis media due to *S. pneumoniae, H. influenzae,* staphylococci, streptococci, and *M. catarrhalis*
Skin and skin structure infections caused by staphylococci and/or streptococci
Bone infections caused by staphylococci and/or *P. mirabilis*
Genitourinary tract infections, including acute prostatitis, caused by *E. coli, P. mirabilis,* and *Klebsiella* sp
Note—Culture and susceptibility tests should be initiated prior to and during therapy. Renal function studies should be performed when indicated.

CONTRAINDICATION

Keflex is contraindicated in patients with known allergy to the cephalosporin group of antibiotics.

WARNINGS

BEFORE CEPHALEXIN THERAPY IS INSTITUTED, CAREFUL INQUIRY SHOULD BE MADE CONCERNING PREVIOUS HYPERSENSITIVITY REACTIONS TO CEPHALOSPORINS AND PENICILLIN. CEPHALOSPORIN C DERIVATIVES SHOULD BE GIVEN CAUTIOUSLY TO PENICILLIN-SENSITIVE PATIENTS.
SERIOUS ACUTE HYPERSENSITIVITY REACTIONS MAY REQUIRE EPINEPHRINE AND OTHER EMERGENCY MEASURES.
There is some clinical and laboratory evidence of partial cross-allergenicity of the penicillins and the cephalosporins. Patients have been reported to have had severe reactions (including anaphylaxis) to both drugs.
Any patient who has demonstrated some form of allergy, particularly to drugs, should receive antibiotics cautiously. No exception should be made with regard to Keflex® (Cephalexin, USP, Dista).
Pseudomembranous colitis has been reported with virtually all broad-spectrum antibiotics (including macrolides, semisynthetic penicillins, and cephalosporins); therefore, it is important to consider its diagnosis in patients who develop diarrhea in association with the use of antibiotics. Such colitis may range in severity from mild to life-threatening.
Treatment with broad-spectrum antibiotics alters the normal flora of the colon and may permit overgrowth of clostridia. Studies indicate that a toxin produced by *Clostridium difficile* is a primary cause of antibiotic-associated colitis.
Mild cases of pseudomembranous colitis usually respond to drug discontinuance alone. In moderate to severe cases, management should include sigmoidoscopy, appropriate bacteriologic studies, and fluid, electrolyte, and protein supplementation. When the colitis does not improve after the drug has been discontinued, or when it is severe, oral vancomycin is the drug of choice for antibiotic-associated pseudomembranous colitis produced by *C. difficile*. Other causes of colitis should be ruled out.
Usage in Pregnancy—Safety of this product for use during pregnancy has not been established.

PRECAUTIONS

General—Patients should be followed carefully so that any side effects or unusual manifestations of drug idiosyncrasy may be detected. If an allergic reaction to Keflex® (Cephalexin, USP, Dista) occurs, the drug should be discontinued and the patient treated with the usual agents (eg, epinephrine or other pressor amines, antihistamines, or corticosteroids).
Prolonged use of Keflex may result in the overgrowth of nonsusceptible organisms. Careful observation of the patient is essential. If superinfection occurs during therapy, appropriate measures should be taken.
Positive direct Coombs' tests have been reported during treatment with the cephalosporin antibiotics. In hematologic studies or in transfusion cross-matching procedures

Continued on next page

This product information was prepared in June 1992. Current information on these and other products of Dista Products Company may be obtained by direct inquiry to Lilly Research Laboratories, Lilly Corporate Center, Indianapolis, Indiana 46285, (317) 276-3714.

Dista—Cont.

when antiglobulin tests are performed on the minor side or in Coombs' testing of newborns whose mothers have received cephalosporin antibiotics before parturition, it should be recognized that a positive Coombs' test may be due to the drug.

Keflex should be administered with caution in the presence of markedly impaired renal function. Under such conditions, careful clinical observation and laboratory studies should be made because safe dosage may be lower than that usually recommended.

Indicated surgical procedures should be performed in conjunction with antibiotic therapy.

As a result of administration of Keflex, a false-positive reaction for glucose in the urine may occur. This has been observed with Benedict's and Fehling's solutions and also with Clinitest® tablets but not with Tes-Tape® (Glucose Enzymatic Test Strip, USP, Lilly).

Broad-spectrum antibiotics should be prescribed with caution in individuals with a history of gastrointestinal disease, particularly colitis.

Usage in Pregnancy—*Pregnancy Category B*—The daily oral administration of cephalexin to rats in doses of 250 or 500 mg/kg prior to and during pregnancy, or to rats and mice during the period of organogenesis only, had no adverse effect on fertility, fetal viability, fetal weight, or litter size. Note that the safety of cephalexin during pregnancy in humans has not been established.

Cephalexin showed no enhanced toxicity in weanling and newborn rats as compared with adult animals. Nevertheless, because the studies in humans cannot rule out the possibility of harm, Keflex® (Cephalexin, USP, Dista) should be used during pregnancy only if clearly needed.

Nursing Mothers—The excretion of cephalexin in the milk increased up to 4 hours after a 500-mg dose; the drug reached a maximum level of 4 µg/mL, then decreased gradually, and had disappeared 8 hours after administration. Caution should be exercised when Keflex is administered to a nursing woman.

ADVERSE REACTIONS

Gastrointestinal—Symptoms of pseudomembranous colitis may appear either during or after antibiotic treatment. Nausea and vomiting have been reported rarely. The most frequent side effect has been diarrhea. It was very rarely severe enough to warrant cessation of therapy. Dyspepsia and abdominal pain have also occurred. As with some penicillins and some other cephalosporins, transient hepatitis and cholestatic jaundice have been reported rarely.

Hypersensitivity—Allergic reactions in the form of rash, urticaria, angioedema, and, rarely, erythema multiforme, Stevens-Johnson syndrome, or toxic epidermal necrolysis have been observed. These reactions usually subsided upon discontinuation of the drug. In some of these reactions, supportive therapy may be necessary. Anaphylaxis has also been reported.

Other reactions have included genital and anal pruritus, genital moniliasis, vaginitis and vaginal discharge, dizziness, fatigue, headache, agitation, confusion, hallucinations, arthralgia, arthritis, and joint disorder. Reversible interstitial nephritis has been reported rarely. Eosinophilia, neutropenia, thrombocytopenia, and slight elevations in SGOT and SGPT have been reported.

OVERDOSAGE

Signs and Symptoms—Symptoms of oral overdose may include nausea, vomiting, epigastric distress, diarrhea, and hematuria. If other symptoms are present, it is probably secondary to an underlying disease state, an allergic reaction, or toxicity due to ingestion of a second medication.

Treatment—To obtain up-to-date information about the treatment of overdose, a good resource is your certified Regional Poison Control Center. Telephone numbers of certified poison control centers are listed in the *Physicians' Desk Reference (PDR)*. In managing overdosage, consider the possibility of multiple drug overdoses, interaction among drugs, and unusual drug kinetics in your patient.

Unless 5 to 10 times the normal dose of cephalexin has been ingested, gastrointestinal decontamination should not be necessary.

Protect the patient's airway and support ventilation and perfusion. Meticulously monitor and maintain, within acceptable limits, the patient's vital signs, blood gases, serum electrolytes, etc. Absorption of drugs from the gastrointestinal tract may be decreased by giving activated charcoal, which, in many cases, is more effective than emesis or lavage; consider charcoal instead of or in addition to gastric emptying. Repeated doses of charcoal over time may hasten elimination of some drugs that have been absorbed. Safeguard the patient's airway when employing gastric emptying or charcoal.

Forced diuresis, peritoneal dialysis, hemodialysis, or charcoal hemoperfusion have not been established as beneficial for an overdose of cephalexin; however, it would be ex-

tremely unlikely that one of these procedures would be indicated.

The oral median lethal dose of cephalexin in rats is 5,000 mg/kg.

DOSAGE AND ADMINISTRATION

Keflex® (Cephalexin, USP, Dista) is administered orally.

Adults—The adult dosage ranges from 1 to 4 g daily in divided doses. The usual adult dose is 250 mg every 6 hours. For the following infections, a dosage of 500 mg may be administered every 12 hours: streptococcal pharyngitis, skin and skin-structure infections, and uncomplicated cystitis in patients over 15 years of age. Cystitis therapy should be continued for 7 to 14 days. For more severe infections or those caused by less susceptible organisms, larger doses may be needed. If daily doses of Keflex greater than 4 g are required, parenteral cephalosporins, in appropriate doses, should be considered.

Children—The usual recommended daily dosage for children is 25 to 50 mg/kg in divided doses. For streptococcal pharyngitis in patients over 1 year of age and for skin and skin-structure infections, the total daily dose may be divided and administered every 12 hours.

Keflex Suspension

Child's Weight	125 mg/5 mL	250 mg/5 mL
10 kg (22 lb)	1/2 to 1 tsp q.i.d.	1/4 to 1/2 tsp q.i.d.
20 kg (44 lb)	1 to 2 tsp q.i.d.	1/2 to 1 tsp q.i.d.
40 kg (88 lb)	2 to 4 tsp q.i.d.	1 to 2 tsp q.i.d.

or

Child's Weight	125 mg/5 mL	250 mg/5 mL
10 kg (22 lb)	1 to 2 tsp b.i.d.	1/2 to 1 tsp b.i.d.
20 kg (44 lb)	2 to 4 tsp b.i.d.	1 to 2 tsp b.i.d.
40 kg (88 lb)	4 to 8 tsp b.i.d.	2 to 4 tsp b.i.d.

In severe infections, the dosage may be doubled.

In the therapy of otitis media, clinical studies have shown that a dosage of 75 to 100 mg/kg/day in 4 divided doses is required.

In the treatment of β-hemolytic streptococcal infections, a therapeutic dosage of Keflex should be administered for at least 10 days.

HOW SUPPLIED

(℞) For Oral Suspension:
125 mg/5 mL (No. M-201)*—
  (100-mL size) NDC 0777-2321-48; (200-mL size) NDC 0777-2321-89
250 mg/5 mL (No. M-202)*—(100-mL size) NDC 0777-2368-48; (200-mL size) NDC 0777-2368-89; (5-mL size) (ID†100) NDC 0777-2368-33

(℞) For Pediatric Drops:
100 mg/mL (5 mg/drop) (No. M-204)*—(10-mL size, with dropper calibrated at 25 and 50 mg) NDC 0777-2322-37
(℞) Pulvules (white and dark green, size 2):
250 mg (No. 402)—(20s) NDC 0777-0869-20; (100s) NDC 0777-0869-02; (ID†100) NDC 0777-0869-33
(℞) Pulvules (light green and dark green, size 0):
500 mg (No. 403)—(20s) NDC 0777-0871-20; (100s) NDC 0777-0871-02; (ID†100) NDC 0777-0871-33

---

* After mixing, store in a refrigerator. May be kept for 14 days without significant loss of potency. Shake well before using. Keep tightly closed.

† Identi-Dose® (unit dose medication, Dista).

Keep Pulvules tightly closed. Store at controlled room temperature, 59° to 86°F (15° to 30°C).

[120591]

Shown in Product Identification Section, page 408

KEFTAB®   ℞
[kĕf′tăb]
(cephalexin hydrochloride)

DESCRIPTION

Keftab® (Cephalexin Hydrochloride, Dista) is a semisynthetic cephalosporin antibiotic intended for oral administration. Chemically, it is designated 7-(D-2-amino-2-phenylacetamido)-3-methyl-3-cephem-4-carboxylic acid hydrochloride monohydrate, and the chemical formula is $C_{16}H_{17}N_3O_4S \cdot HCl \cdot H_2O$. The molecular weight is 401.86.

The nucleus of cephalexin hydrochloride is related to that of other cephalosporin antibiotics. The compound is the hydrochloride salt of cephalexin. The isoelectric point of cephalexin in water is appropriately 4.5 to 5.

Cephalexin hydrochloride is in crystalline form and is a monohydrate. It is a white crystalline solid having a bitter taste. Solubility in water is high at room temperature; greater than 10 mg/mL may be dissolved readily.

The cephalosporins differ from penicillins in the structure of the bicyclic ring system. Cephalexin has a *D*-phenylglycyl group as substituent at the 7-amino position and an unsubstituted methyl group at the 3-position.

Each tablet contains cephalexin hydrochloride equivalent to 250 mg (720 µmol) or 500 mg (1,439 µmol) cephalexin. The tablets also contain D & C Yellow No. 10, F D & C Blue No. 1,

magnesium stearate, silicon dioxide, stearic acid, sucrose, and titanium dioxide. The 250-mg tablet also contains F D & C Blue No. 2, and the 500-mg tablet also contains F D & C Red No. 40.

CLINICAL PHARMACOLOGY

Human Pharmacology—Keftab® (Cephalexin Hydrochloride, Dista) is acid stable and may be given without regard to meals. It is rapidly absorbed after oral administration. Following doses of 250 mg and 500 mg, average peak serum levels of approximately 9 and 18 µg/mL respectively were obtained at 1 hour and declined to 1.6 and 3.4 µg/mL respectively at 3 hours. Measurable levels were present 6 hours after administration. Cephalexin is excreted in the urine by glomerular filtration and tubular secretion. Studies showed that approximately 70% of the drug was excreted unchanged in the urine within 12 hours. During the first 6 hours, average urine concentrations following the 250-mg and 500-mg doses were approximately 200 µg/mL (range, 54 to 663) and 500 µg/mL (range, 137 to 1,306) respectively. The average serum half-life is 1.1 hours.

Microbiology—In vitro tests demonstrate that the cephalosporins are bactericidal because of their inhibition of cell-wall synthesis. Keftab is active against the following organisms in vitro:

β-hemolytic streptococci
Staphylococcus aureus, including penicillinase-producing strains
Streptococcus pneumoniae
Escherichia coli
Proteus mirabilis
Klebsiella sp
Haemophilus influenzae
Moraxella (Branhamella) catarrhalis

Note—Most strains of enterococci (*Enterococcus faecalis* [formerly *Streptococcus faecalis*]) and a few strains of staphylococci are resistant to Keftab. When tested by in vitro methods, staphylococci exhibit cross-resistance between Keftab and methicillin-type antibiotics. Keftab is not active against most strains of *Enterobacter* sp, *Morganella morganii* (formerly *Proteus morganii*), *Serratia* sp, and *Proteus vulgaris*. It has no activity against *Pseudomonas* or *Acinetobacter* sp.

Disk Susceptibility Tests—Quantitative methods that require measurement of zone diameters give the most precise estimates of antibiotic susceptibility. One such procedure[1] has been recommended for use with cephalosporin class (cephalothin) disks for testing susceptibility to cephalexin. The currently accepted zone diameter interpretations for the cephalothin disks[1] are appropriate for determining susceptibility to cephalexin. Interpretations correlate zone diameters of the disk test with MIC values for cephalexin. With this procedure, a report from the laboratory of "resistant" indicates a zone diameter of 14 mm or less and that the infecting organism is not likely to respond to therapy. A report of "susceptibility" indicates a zone diameter of 18 mm or greater. A report of "intermediate susceptibility" indicates zone diameters between 15 and 17 mm and suggests that the organism would be susceptible if the infection is confined to the urine, in which high antibiotic levels can be obtained, or if high dosage is used in other types of infection.

Standardized procedures require use of control organisms.[1] The 30-µg cephalothin disk should give zone diameters between 18 and 23 mm and 25 and 37 mm for the reference strains *E. coli* ATCC 25922 and *S. aureus* ATCC 25923 respectively.

INDICATIONS AND USAGE

Keftab® (Cephalexin Hydrochloride, Dista) is indicated for the treatment of the following infections when caused by susceptible strains of the designated microorganisms:

Respiratory tract infections caused by *S. pneumoniae* and group A β-hemolytic streptococci (Penicillin is the usual drug of choice in the treatment and prevention of streptococcal infections, including the prophylaxis of rheumatic fever. Amoxicillin has been recommended by the American Heart Association as the standard regimen for the prophylaxis of bacterial endocarditis for dental, oral, and upper respiratory tract procedures, with penicillin V a rational and acceptable alternative in the prophylaxis against α-hemolytic streptococcal bacteremia in this setting. Keftab is generally effective in the eradication of streptococci from the nasopharynx; however, substantial data establishing the efficacy of Keftab in the subsequent prevention of either rheumatic fever or bacterial endocarditis are not available at present.)

Skin and skin structure infections caused by *S. aureus* and/or β-hemolytic streptococci.

Bone infections caused by *S. aureus* and/or *P. mirabilis*.

Genitourinary tract infections, including acute prostatitis, caused by *E. coli*, *P. mirabilis*, and *Klebsiella* sp.

Note—Culture and susceptibility tests should be initiated prior to and during therapy. Renal function studies should be performed when indicated.

---

1. 21 CFR 460.1, *Federal Register* 1987; 838–842.

CONTRAINDICATION

Keftab® (Cephalexin Hydrochloride, Dista) is contraindicated in patients with known allergy to the cephalosporin group of antibiotics.

WARNINGS

BEFORE CEPHALEXIN THERAPY IS INSTITUTED, CAREFUL INQUIRY SHOULD BE MADE CONCERNING PREVIOUS HYPERSENSITIVITY REACTIONS TO CEPHALOSPORINS AND PENICILLIN. CEPHALOSPORIN C DERIVATIVES SHOULD BE GIVEN CAUTIOUSLY TO PENICILLIN-SENSITIVE PATIENTS.
SERIOUS ACUTE HYPERSENSITIVITY REACTIONS MAY REQUIRE EPINEPHRINE AND OTHER EMERGENCY MEASURES.
There is some clinical and laboratory evidence of partial cross-allergenicity of the penicillins and the cephalosporins. Patients have been reported to have had severe reactions (including anaphylaxis) to both drugs.
Any patient who has demonstrated some form of allergy, particularly to drugs, should receive antibiotics cautiously. No exception should be made with regard to Keftab® (Cephalexin Hydrochloride, Dista).
Pseudomembranous colitis has been reported with virtually all broad-spectrum antibiotics (including macrolides, semisynthetic penicillins, and cephalosporins); therefore, it is important to consider its diagnosis in patients who develop diarrhea in association with the use of antibiotics. Such colitis may range in severity from mild to life threatening.
Treatment with broad-spectrum antibiotics alters the normal flora of the colon and may permit overgrowth of clostridia. Studies indicate that a toxin produced by *Clostridium difficile* is a primary cause of antibiotic-associated colitis. Mild cases of pseudomembranous colitis usually respond to drug discontinuance alone. In moderate to severe cases, management should include sigmoidoscopy, appropriate bacteriologic studies, and fluid, electrolyte, and protein supplementation. When the colitis does not improve after the drug has been discontinued or when it is severe, oral vancomycin is the drug of choice for antibiotic-associated pseudomembranous colitis produced by *C. difficile*. Other causes of colitis should be ruled out.

PRECAUTIONS

General —Patients should be followed carefully so that any side effects or unusual manifestations of drug idiosyncrasy may be detected. If an allergic reaction to Keftab® (Cephalexin Hydrochloride, Dista) occurs, the drug should be discontinued and the patient treated with the usual agents (eg, epinephrine or other pressor amines, antihistamines, or corticosteroids).
Prolonged use of Keftab may result in the overgrowth of nonsusceptible organisms. Careful observation of the patient is essential. If superinfection occurs during therapy, appropriate measures should be taken.
Positive direct Coombs' tests have been reported during treatment with the cephalosporin antibiotics. In hematologic studies or in transfusion cross-matching procedures when antiglobulin tests are performed on the minor side or in Coombs' testing of newborns whose mothers have received cephalosporin antibiotics before parturition, it should be recognized that a positive Coombs' test may be due to the drug.
Keftab should be administered with caution in the presence of markedly impaired renal function. Under such conditions, careful clinical observation and laboratory studies should be made because safe dosage may be lower than that usually recommended.
As a result of administration of Keftab, a false-positive reaction for glucose in the urine may occur. This has been observed with Benedict's and Fehling's solutions and also with Clinitest® tablets but not with Tes-Tape® (Glucose Enzymatic Test Strip, USP, Lilly).
Broad-spectrum antibiotics should be prescribed with caution in individuals with a history of gastrointestinal disease, particularly colitis.
Pregnancy —Pregnancy Category B —Reproduction studies have been performed on rats in doses of 250 or 500 mg/kg/day and have revealed no evidence of impaired fertility or harm to the fetus due to cephalexin. There are, however, no adequate and well-controlled studies in pregnant women. Because animal reproduction studies are not always predictive of human response, this drug should be used during pregnancy only if clearly needed.
Nursing Mothers —The excretion of cephalexin in the milk increased up to 4 hours after a 500-mg dose; the drug reached a maximum level of 4 µg/mL, then decreased gradually, and had disappeared 8 hours after administration. A decision should be considered to discontinue nursing temporarily during therapy with Keftab.
Pediatric Use —Safety and effectiveness in children have not been established.

ADVERSE REACTIONS

Gastrointestinal —Symptoms of pseudomembranous colitis may appear either during or after antibiotic treatment. Nau-

sea and vomiting have been reported rarely. The most frequent side effect has been diarrhea. It was very rarely severe enough to warrant cessation of therapy. Abdominal pain, gastritis, and dyspepsia have also occurred. As with some penicillins and some other cephalosporins, transient hepatitis and cholestatic jaundice have been reported rarely.
Hypersensitivity —Allergic reactions in the form of rash, urticaria, angioedema, and, rarely, erythema multiforme, Stevens-Johnson syndrome, or toxic epidermal necrolysis have been observed. These reactions usually subsided upon discontinuation of the drug. In some of these reactions, supportive therapy may be necessary. Anaphylaxis has also been reported.
Other reactions have included genital and anal pruritus, genital moniliasis, vaginitis and vaginal discharge, dizziness, fatigue, headache, agitation, confusion, hallucinations, arthralgia, arthritis, and joint disorder. Reversible interstitial nephritis has been reported rarely. Eosinophilia, neutropenia, thrombocytopenia, slight elevations in aspartate aminotransferase (AST, SGOT) and alanine aminotransferase (ALT, SGPT), and elevated creatinine and BUN have been reported.
In addition to the adverse reactions listed above that have been observed in patients treated with Keftab® (Cephalexin Hydrochloride, Dista), the following adverse reactions and altered laboratory tests have been reported for cephalosporin class antibiotics:
Adverse Reactions —Allergic reactions, including fever, colitis, renal dysfunction, toxic nephropathy, and hepatic dysfunction, including cholestasis.
Several cephalosporins have been implicated in triggering seizures, particularly in patients with renal impairment when the dosage was not reduced (*see* Indications and Usage *and* Precautions, General). If seizures associated with drug therapy should occur, the drug should be discontinued. Anticonvulsant therapy can be given if clinically indicated.
Altered Laboratory Tests —Increased prothrombin time, increased alkaline phosphatase, and leukopenia.

OVERDOSAGE

Signs and Symptoms —Symptoms of oral overdose may include nausea, vomiting, epigastric distress, diarrhea, and hematuria. If other symptoms are present, they are probably secondary to an underlying disease state, an allergic reaction, or toxicity due to ingestion of a second medication.
Treatment —To obtain up-to-date information about the treatment of overdose, a good resource is your certified Regional Poison Control Center. Telephone numbers of certified poison control centers are listed in the *Physicians' Desk Reference (PDR)*. In managing overdosage, consider the possibility of multiple drug overdoses, interaction among drugs, and unusual drug kinetics in your patient.
Unless 5 to 10 times the normal dose of cephalexin has been ingested, gastrointestinal decontamination should not be necessary.
Protect the patient's airway and support ventilation and perfusion. Meticulously monitor and maintain, within acceptable limits, the patient's vital signs, blood gases, serum electrolytes, etc. Absorption of drugs from the gastrointestinal tract may be decreased by giving activated charcoal, which, in many cases, is more effective than emesis or lavage; consider charcoal instead of or in addition to gastric emptying. Repeated doses of charcoal over time may hasten elimination of some drugs that have been absorbed. Safeguard the patient's airway when employing gastric emptying or charcoal.
Forced diuresis, peritoneal dialysis, hemodialysis, or charcoal hemoperfusion have not been established as beneficial for an overdose of cephalexin; however, it would be extremely unlikely that one of these procedures would be indicated.
The oral median lethal dose of cephalexin in rats is 5,000 mg/kg.

DOSAGE AND ADMINISTRATION

Keftab® (Cephalexin Hydrochloride, Dista) is administered orally.
The adult dosage ranges from 1 to 4 g daily in divided doses. For the following infections, a dosage of 500 mg may be administered every 12 hours: streptococcal pharyngitis, skin and skin structure infections, and uncomplicated cystitis. Cystitis therapy should be continued for 7 to 14 days. For other infections, the usual dose is 250 mg every 6 hours. For more severe infections or those caused by less susceptible organisms, larger doses may be needed. If daily doses of Keftab greater than 4 g are required, parenteral cephalosporins, in appropriate doses, should be considered.

HOW SUPPLIED

(℞) Tablets (elliptical-shaped):
250 mg* (light-green) (No. 4142)—(100s) NDC 0777-4142-02
500 mg* (dark-green) (No. 4143)—(100s) NDC 0777-4143-02

---

* Equivalent to cephalexin.

Store at controlled room temperature, 59° to 86°F (15° to 30°C).

[010992]

Shown in Product Identification Section, page 408

NALFON®   ℞
[năl′fŏn]
NALFON® 200
(fenoprofen calcium)
USP

DESCRIPTION

Nalfon® (Fenoprofen Calcium, USP, Dista) is a nonsteroidal, anti-inflammatory, antiarthritic drug. Pulvules® Nalfon contain fenoprofen calcium as the dihydrate in an amount equivalent to 200 mg (0.826 mmol) or 300 mg (1.24 mmol) of fenoprofen. The Pulvules also contain cellulose, gelatin, iron oxides, silicone, titanium dioxide, and other inactive ingredients. The 300-mg Pulvules also contain D & C Yellow No. 10 and F D & C Yellow No. 6.
Tablets Nalfon contain fenoprofen calcium as the dihydrate in an amount equivalent to 600 mg (2.48 mmol) of fenoprofen. The tablets also contain amberlite, benzyl alcohol, calcium phosphate, cornstarch, D & C Yellow No. 10, F D & C Yellow No. 6, hydroxypropyl methylcellulose, magnesium stearate, polyethylene glycol, stearic acid, titanium dioxide, and other inactive ingredients.
Chemically, Nalfon is an arylacetic acid derivative.
Nalfon is a white crystalline powder with a molecular weight of 558.64. At 25°C, it dissolves to a 15 mg/mL solution in alcohol (95%). It is slightly soluble in water and insoluble in benzene.
The *p* Ka of Nalfon is 4.5 at 25°C.

CLINICAL PHARMACOLOGY

Nalfon® (Fenoprofen Calcium, USP, Dista) is a nonsteroidal, anti-inflammatory, antiarthritic drug that also possesses analgesic and antipyretic activities. Its exact mode of action is unknown, but it is thought that prostaglandin synthetase inhibition is involved. Nalfon has been shown to inhibit prostaglandin synthetase isolated from bovine seminal vesicles. Reproduction studies in rats have shown Nalfon to be associated with prolonged labor and difficult parturition when given during late pregnancy. Evidence suggests that this may be due to decreased uterine contractility resulting from the inhibition of prostaglandin synthesis. Its action is not mediated through the adrenal gland.
Fenoprofen shows anti-inflammatory effects in rodents by inhibiting the development of redness and edema in acute inflammatory conditions and by reducing soft-tissue swelling and bone damage associated with chronic inflammation. It exhibits analgesic activity in rodents by inhibiting the writhing response caused by the introduction of an irritant into the peritoneal cavities of mice and by elevating pain thresholds that are related to pressure in edematous hindpaws of rats. In rats made febrile by the subcutaneous administration of brewer's yeast, fenoprofen produces antipyretic action. These effects are characteristic of nonsteroidal, anti-inflammatory, antipyretic, analgesic drugs.
The results in humans confirmed the anti-inflammatory and analgesic actions found in animals. The emergence and degree of erythemic response were measured in adult male volunteers exposed to ultraviolet irradiation. The effects of Nalfon, aspirin, and indomethacin were each compared with those of a placebo. All 3 drugs demonstrated antierythemic activity.
In patients with rheumatoid arthritis, the anti-inflammatory action of Nalfon has been evidenced by relief of pain, increase in grip strength, and reductions in joint swelling, duration of morning stiffness, and disease activity (as assessed by both the investigator and the patient). The anti-inflammatory action of Nalfon has also been evidenced by increased mobility (ie, a decrease in the number of joints having limited motion).
The use of Nalfon® (Fenoprofen Calcium, USP, Dista) in combination with gold salts or corticosteroids has been studied in patients with rheumatoid arthritis. The studies, however, were inadequate in demonstrating whether further improvement is obtained by adding Nalfon to maintenance therapy with gold salts or steroids. Whether or not Nalfon used in conjunction with partially effective doses of a corticosteroid has a "steroid-sparing" effect is unknown.
In patients with osteoarthritis, the anti-inflammatory and analgesic effects of Nalfon have been demonstrated by reduction in tenderness as a response to pressure and reductions

Continued on next page

This product information was prepared in June 1992. Current information on these and other products of Dista Products Company may be obtained by direct inquiry to Lilly Research Laboratories, Lilly Corporate Center, Indianapolis, Indiana 46285, (317) 276-3714.

Dista—Cont.

in night pain, stiffness, swelling, and overall disease activity (as assessed by both the patient and the investigator). These effects have also been demonstrated by relief of pain with motion and at rest and increased range of motion in involved joints.

In patients with rheumatoid arthritis and osteoarthritis, clinical studies have shown Nalfon to be comparable to aspirin in controlling the aforementioned measures of disease activity, but mild gastrointestinal reactions (nausea, dyspepsia) and tinnitus occurred less frequently in patients treated with Nalfon than in aspirin-treated patients. It is not known whether Nalfon causes less peptic ulceration than does aspirin.

In patients with pain, the analgesic action of Nalfon has produced a reduction in pain intensity, an increase in pain relief, improvement in total analgesia scores, and a sustained analgesic effect.

Under fasting conditions, Nalfon is rapidly absorbed, and peak plasma levels of 50 µg/mL are achieved within 2 hours after oral administration of 600-mg doses. Good dose proportionality was observed between 200-mg and 600-mg doses in fasting male volunteers. The plasma half-life is approximately 3 hours. About 90% of a single oral dose is eliminated within 24 hours as fenoprofen glucuronide and 4′-hydroxyfenoprofen glucuronide, the major urinary metabolites of fenoprofen. Fenoprofen is highly bound (99%) to albumin.

The concomitant administration of antacid (containing both aluminum and magnesium hydroxide) does not interfere with absorption of Nalfon.

There is less suppression of collagen-induced platelet aggregation with single doses of Nalfon than there is with aspirin.

INDICATIONS AND USAGE

Nalfon® (Fenoprofen Calcium, USP, Dista) is indicated for relief of the signs and symptoms of rheumatoid arthritis and osteoarthritis. It is recommended for the treatment of acute flare-ups and exacerbations and for the long-term management of these diseases.

Nalfon is also indicated for the relief of mild to moderate pain.

CONTRAINDICATIONS

Nalfon® (Fenoprofen Calcium, USP, Dista) is contraindicated in patients who have shown hypersensitivity to it.

The drug should not be administered to patients with a history of significantly impaired renal function.

Nalfon should not be given to patients in whom aspirin and other nonsteroidal anti-inflammatory drugs induce the symptoms of asthma, rhinitis, or urticaria, because cross-sensitivity to these drugs occurs in a high proportion of such patients.

WARNINGS

Risk of GI Ulceration, Bleeding, and Perforation with NSAID Therapy—Serious gastrointestinal toxicity, such as bleeding, ulceration, and perforation, can occur at any time, with or without warning symptoms, in patients treated chronically with NSAID therapy. Although minor upper gastrointestinal problems, such as dyspepsia, are common, usually developing early in therapy, physicians should remain alert for ulceration and bleeding in patients treated chronically with NSAIDs, even in the absence of previous GI tract symptoms. In patients observed in clinical trials of several months to 2 years duration, symptomatic upper GI ulcers, gross bleeding, or perforation appear to occur in approximately 1% of patients treated for 3 to 6 months, and in about 2% to 4% of patients treated for 1 year. Physicians should inform patients about the signs and/or symptoms of serious GI toxicity and what steps to take if they occur.

Studies to date have not identified any subset of patients not at risk of developing peptic ulceration and bleeding. Except for a prior history of serious GI events and other risk factors known to be associated with peptic ulcer disease, such as alcoholism, smoking, etc, no risk factors (eg, age, sex) have been associated with increased risk. Elderly or debilitated patients seem to tolerate ulceration or bleeding less well than other individuals and most spontaneous reports of fatal GI events are in this population. Studies to date are inconclusive concerning the relative risk of various NSAIDs in causing such reactions. High doses of any NSAID probably carry a greater risk of these reactions, although controlled clinical trials showing this do not exist in most cases. In considering the use of relatively large doses (within the recommended dosage range), sufficient benefit should be anticipated to offset the potential increased risk of GI toxicity.

Since Nalfon® (Fenoprofen Calcium, USP, Dista) has been marketed, there have been reports of genitourinary tract problems in patients taking it. The most frequently reported problems have been episodes of dysuria, cystitis, hematuria, interstitial nephritis, and nephrotic syndrome. This syndrome may be preceded by the appearance of fever, rash, arthralgia, oliguria, and azotemia and may progress to anuria. There may also be substantial proteinuria, and, on renal biopsy, electron microscopy has shown foot process fusion and T-lymphocyte infiltration in the renal interstitium. Early recognition of the syndrome and withdrawal of the drug have been followed by rapid recovery. Administration of steroids and the use of dialysis have also been included in the treatment. Because a syndrome with some of these characteristics has also been reported with other nonsteroidal anti-inflammatory drugs, it is recommended that patients who have had these reactions with other such drugs not be treated with Nalfon. In patients with possibly compromised renal function, periodic renal function examinations should be done.

PRECAUTIONS

General—Renal Effects—There have been reports of acute interstitial nephritis and nephrotic syndrome (*see* Contraindications *and* Warnings).

A second form of renal toxicity has been seen in patients with prerenal conditions leading to a reduction in renal blood flow or blood volume, in which renal prostaglandins play a supportive role in the maintenance of renal perfusion. In these patients, administration of an NSAID may cause a dose-dependent reduction in prostaglandin formation and may precipitate overt renal decompensation at any time. Patients at greatest risk for this reaction are those with impaired renal function, heart failure, liver dysfunction, those taking diuretics, and the elderly. Discontinuation of NSAID therapy is typically followed by recovery to the pretreatment state.

Since Nalfon® (Fenoprofen Calcium, USP, Dista) is primarily eliminated by the kidneys, patients with possibly compromised renal function (such as the elderly) should be monitored periodically, especially during long-term therapy. For such patients, it may be anticipated that a lower daily dosage will avoid excessive drug accumulation.

Miscellaneous—Peripheral edema has been observed in some patients taking Nalfon® (Fenoprofen Calcium, USP, Dista); therefore, Nalfon should be used with caution in patients with compromised cardiac function or hypertension. The possibility of renal involvement should be considered.

Studies to date have not shown changes in the eyes attributable to the administration of Nalfon. However, adverse ocular effects have been observed with other anti-inflammatory drugs. Eye examinations, therefore, should be performed if visual disturbances occur in patients taking Nalfon.

Caution should be exercised by patients whose activities require alertness if they experience CNS side effects while taking Nalfon.

Since the safety of Nalfon has not been established in patients with impaired hearing, these patients should have periodic tests of auditory function during prolonged therapy with Nalfon.

Information for Patients—Nalfon, like other drugs of its class, is not free of side effects. The side effects of these drugs can cause discomfort and, rarely, there are more serious side effects, such as gastrointestinal bleeding, which may result in hospitalization and even fatal outcomes.

NSAIDs (Nonsteroidal Anti-Inflammatory Drugs) are often essential agents in the management of arthritis and have a major role in the treatment of pain, but they also may be commonly employed for conditions which are less serious. Physicians may wish to discuss with their patients the potential risks (*see* Warnings, Precautions, *and* Adverse Reactions sections) and likely benefits of NSAID treatment, particularly when the drugs are used for less serious conditions where treatment without NSAIDs may represent an acceptable alternative to both the patient and physician.

Laboratory Tests—In chronic studies in rats, high doses of Nalfon caused elevation of serum transaminase and hepatocellular hypertrophy. In clinical trials, some patients developed elevation of serum transaminase, LDH, and alkaline phosphatase that persisted for some months and usually, but not always, declined despite continuation of the drug. The significance of this is unknown. It is recommended, therefore, that Nalfon be discontinued if any significant liver abnormality occurs.

As with other nonsteroidal anti-inflammatory drugs, borderline elevations in 1 or more liver tests may occur in up to 15% of patients. These abnormalities may progress, may remain essentially unchanged, or may be transient with continued therapy. The SGPT (ALT) test is probably the most sensitive indicator of liver dysfunction. Meaningful (ie, 3 times the upper limit of normal) elevations of SGPT or SGOT (AST) occurred in controlled clinical trials in less than 1% of patients. A patient with symptoms and/or signs suggesting liver dysfunction, or in whom an abnormal liver test has occurred, should be evaluated for evidence of the development of more severe hepatic reactions while using Nalfon. Severe hepatic reactions, including jaundice and cases of fatal hepatitis, have been reported with Nalfon, as with other nonsteroidal anti-inflammatory drugs. As a result, during long-term therapy, liver function tests should be monitored periodically. Although such reactions are rare, if liver tests continue to be abnormal or worsen, if clinical signs and symptoms consistent with liver disease develop, or if systemic manifestations occur (eg, eosinophilia and rash), Nalfon should be discontinued. If this drug is to be used in the presence of impaired liver function, it must be done under strict observation.

Patients with initial low hemoglobin values who are receiving long-term therapy with Nalfon should have a hemoglobin determination made at reasonable intervals.

Nalfon decreases platelet aggregation and may prolong bleeding time. Patients who may be adversely affected by prolongation of the bleeding time should be carefully observed when Nalfon is administered.

Because serious GI tract ulceration and bleeding can occur without warning symptoms, physicians should follow chronically treated patients for the signs and symptoms of ulceration and bleeding and should inform them of the importance of this follow-up (*see* Risk of GI Ulceration, Bleeding, and Perforation with NSAID Therapy *under* Warnings).

Laboratory Test Interactions—Amerlex-M kit assay values of total and free triiodothyronine in patients receiving Nalfon have been reported as falsely elevated on the basis of a chemical cross-reaction that directly interferes with the assay. Thyroid-stimulating hormone, total thyroxine, and thyrotropin-releasing hormone response are not affected.

Drug Interactions—The coadministration of aspirin decreases the biologic half-life of fenoprofen because of an increase in metabolic clearance that results in a greater amount of hydroxylated fenoprofen in the urine. Although the mechanism of interaction between fenoprofen and aspirin is not totally known, enzyme induction and displacement of fenoprofen from plasma albumin binding sites are possibilities. Because Nalfon® (Fenoprofen Calcium, USP, Dista) has not been shown to produce any additional effect beyond that obtained with aspirin alone and because aspirin increases the rate of excretion of Nalfon, the concomitant use of Nalfon and salicylates is not recommended.

Chronic administration of phenobarbital, a known enzyme inducer, may be associated with a decrease in the plasma half-life of fenoprofen. When phenobarbital is added to or withdrawn from treatment, dosage adjustment of Nalfon may be required.

In vitro studies have shown that fenoprofen, because of its affinity for albumin, may displace from their binding sites other drugs that are also albumin bound, and this may lead to drug interaction. Theoretically, fenoprofen could likewise be displaced. Patients receiving hydantoin, sulfonamides, or sulfonylureas should be observed for increased activity of these drugs and, therefore, signs of toxicity from these drugs. In patients receiving coumarin-type anticoagulants, the addition of Nalfon to therapy could prolong the prothrombin time. Patients receiving both drugs should be under careful observation. Patients treated with Nalfon may be resistant to the effects of loop diuretics.

In patients receiving Nalfon and a steroid concomitantly, any reduction in steroid dosage should be gradual in order to avoid the possible complications of sudden steroid withdrawal.

Usage in Pregnancy—Safe use of Nalfon during pregnancy and lactation has not been established; therefore, administration to pregnant patients and nursing mothers is not recommended. Reproduction studies have been performed in rats and rabbits. When fenoprofen was given to rats during pregnancy and continued until the time of labor, parturition was prolonged. Similar results have been found with other nonsteroidal anti-inflammatory drugs that inhibit prostaglandin synthetase.

Usage in Children—Fenoprofen calcium is not recommended for use in children because documented clinical experience has been insufficient to establish safety and a suitable dosage regimen in the pediatric age group.

ADVERSE REACTIONS

During clinical studies for rheumatoid arthritis, osteoarthritis, or mild to moderate pain and studies of pharmacokinetics, complaints were compiled from a checklist of potential adverse reactions, and the following data emerged. These encompass observations in 6,786 patients, including 188 observed for at least 52 weeks. For comparison, data are also presented from complaints received from the 266 patients who received placebo in these same trials. During short-term studies for analgesia, the incidence of adverse reactions was markedly lower than that seen in longer-term studies.

INCIDENCE GREATER THAN 1%

Probable Causal Relationship

Digestive System—During clinical trials with Nalfon® (Fenoprofen Calcium, USP, Dista), the most common adverse reactions were gastrointestinal in nature and occurred in 20.8% of patients receiving Nalfon as compared to 16.9% of patients receiving placebo. In descending order of frequency, these reactions included dyspepsia (10.3%, Nalfon, vs 2.3%, placebo), nausea (7.7% vs 7.1%), constipation (7% vs 1.5%), vomiting (2.6% vs 1.9%), abdominal pain (2% vs 1.1%), and diarrhea (1.8% vs 4.1%).

The drug was discontinued because of adverse gastrointestinal reactions in less than 2% of patients during premarketing studies.

Nervous System—The most frequent adverse neurologic reactions were headache (8.7% treated vs 7.5% placebo) and somnolence (8.5% vs 6.4%). Dizziness (6.5% vs 5.6%), tremor

(2.2% vs 0.4%), and confusion (1.4% vs none) were noted less frequently.

Nalfon was discontinued in less than 0.5% of patients because of these side effects during premarketing studies.

Skin and Appendages—Increased sweating (4.6% vs 0.4%), pruritus (4.2% vs 0.8%), and rash (3.7% vs 0.4%) were reported.

Nalfon was discontinued in about 1% of patients because of an adverse effect related to the skin during premarketing studies.

Special Senses—Tinnitus (4.5% vs 0.4%), blurred vision (2.2% vs none), and decreased hearing (1.6% vs none) were reported.

Nalfon was discontinued in less than 0.5% of patients because of adverse effects related to the special senses during premarketing studies.

Cardiovascular—Palpitations (2.5% vs 0.4%).

Nalfon was discontinued in about 0.5% of patients because of adverse cardiovascular reactions during premarketing studies.

Miscellaneous—Nervousness (5.7% vs 1.5%), asthenia (5.4% vs 0.4%), peripheral edema (5.0% vs 0.4%), dyspnea (2.8% vs none), fatigue (1.7% vs 1.5%), upper respiratory infection (1.5% vs 5.6%), and nasopharyngitis (1.2% vs none).

INCIDENCE LESS THAN 1%

Probable Causal Relationship

The following adverse reactions, occurring in less than 1% of patients, were reported in controlled clinical trials and voluntary reports made since Nalfon® (Fenoprofen Calcium, USP, Dista) was initially marketed. The probability of a causal relationship exists between Nalfon and these adverse reactions:

Digestive System—Gastritis, peptic ulcer with/without perforation, gastrointestinal hemorrhage, anorexia, flatulence, dry mouth, and blood in the stool. Increases in alkaline phosphatase, LDH, and SGOT, jaundice, and cholestatic hepatitis were observed (*see* Precautions).

Genitourinary Tract—Dysuria, cystitis, hematuria, oliguria, azotemia, anuria, interstitial nephritis, nephrosis, and papillary necrosis (*see* Warnings).

Hypersensitivity—Angioedema (angioneurotic edema).

Hematologic—Purpura, bruising, hemorrhage, thrombocytopenia, hemolytic anemia, aplastic anemia, agranulocytosis, and pancytopenia.

Miscellaneous—Anaphylaxis, urticaria, malaise, insomnia, and tachycardia.

INCIDENCE LESS THAN 1%

Causal Relationship Unknown

Other reactions reported either in clinical trials or spontaneously, occurred in circumstances in which a causal relationship could not be established. However, with these rarely reported reactions, the possibility of such a relationship cannot be excluded. Therefore, these observations are listed to alert the physician.

Skin and Appendages—Exfoliative dermatitis, toxic epidermal necrolysis, Stevens-Johnson syndrome, and alopecia.

Digestive System—Aphthous ulcerations of the buccal mucosa, metallic taste, and pancreatitis.

Cardiovascular—Atrial fibrillation, pulmonary edema, electrocardiographic changes, and supraventricular tachycardia.

Nervous System—Depression, disorientation, seizures, and trigeminal neuralgia.

Special Senses—Burning tongue, diplopia, and optic neuritis.

Miscellaneous—Personality change, lymphadenopathy, mastodynia, and fever.

OVERDOSAGE

Signs and Symptoms—Symptoms of overdose appear within several hours and generally involve the gastrointestinal and central nervous systems. They include dyspepsia, nausea, vomiting, abdominal pain, dizziness, headache, ataxia, tinnitus, tremor, drowsiness, and confusion. Hyperpyrexia, tachycardia, hypotension, and acute renal failure may occur rarely following overdose. Respiratory depression and metabolic acidosis have also been reported following overdose with certain NSAIDs.

Treatment—To obtain up-to-date information about the treatment of overdose, a good resource is your certified Regional Poison Control Center. Telephone numbers of certified poison control centers are listed in the *Physicians' Desk Reference (PDR)*. In managing overdosage, consider the possibility of multiple drug overdoses, interaction among drugs, and unusual drug kinetics in your patient.

Protect the patient's airway and support ventilation and perfusion. Meticulously monitor and maintain, within acceptable limits, the patient's vital signs, blood gases, serum electrolytes, etc. Absorption of drugs from the gastrointestinal tract may be decreased by giving activated charcoal, which, in many cases, is more effective than emesis or lavage; consider charcoal instead of or in addition to gastric emptying. Repeated doses of charcoal over time may hasten elimination of some drugs that have been absorbed. Safeguard the patient's airway when employing gastric emptying or charcoal.

Alkalinization of the urine, forced diuresis, peritoneal dialysis, hemodialysis, and charcoal hemoperfusion do not enhance systemic drug elimination.

DOSAGE AND ADMINISTRATION

Analgesia—For the treatment of mild to moderate pain, the recommended dosage is 200 mg every 4 to 6 hours, as needed.

Rheumatoid Arthritis and Osteoarthritis—The suggested dosage is 300 to 600 mg, 3 or 4 times a day. The dose should be tailored to the needs of the patient and may be increased or decreased depending on the severity of the symptoms. Dosage adjustments may be made after initiation of drug therapy or during exacerbations of the disease. Total daily dosage should not exceed 3,200 mg.

If gastrointestinal complaints occur, Nalfon® (Fenoprofen Calcium, USP, Dista) may be administered with meals or with milk. Although the total amount absorbed is not affected, peak blood levels are delayed and diminished.

Patients with rheumatoid arthritis generally seem to require larger doses of Nalfon than do those with osteoarthritis. The smallest dose that yields acceptable control should be employed.

Although improvement may be seen in a few days in many patients, an additional 2 to 3 weeks may be required to gauge the full benefits of therapy.

HOW SUPPLIED

℞ Pulvules:

200 mg* (white and ocher) (No. 415)—(Identi-Code† H76) (RxPak‡ of 100) NDC 0777-0876-02

300 mg* (yellow and ocher) (No. 416)—(Identi-Code† H77) (RxPak‡ of 100) NDC 0777-0877-02; (500s) NDC 0777-0877-03

℞ Tablets (DISTA imprinted on one side, NALFON on other side):

600 mg* (yellow, paracapsule-shaped, scored) (No. 1900)—(RxPak‡ of 100) NDC 0777-2159-02; (500s) NDC 0777-2159-03

Store at controlled room temperature, 59° to 86°F (15° to 30°C).

* Equivalent to fenoprofen.

† Identi-Code® (formula identification code, Dista).

‡ All RxPaks (prescription packages, Dista) have safey closures.

[121390]

Shown in Product Identification Section, pages 408 and 409

PROZAC® ℞

[*prō ʹzăk*]

(fluoxetine hydrochloride)

DESCRIPTION

Prozac® (Fluoxetine Hydrochloride, Dista) is an antidepressant for oral administration; it is chemically unrelated to tricyclic, tetracyclic, or other available antidepressant agents. It is designated (±)-N-methyl-3-phenyl-3-[(α,α,α-trifluoro-*p*-tolyl)oxy]propylamine hydrochloride and has the empirical formula of $C_{17}H_{18}F_3NO \cdot HCl$. Its molecular weight is 345.79. The structural formula is:

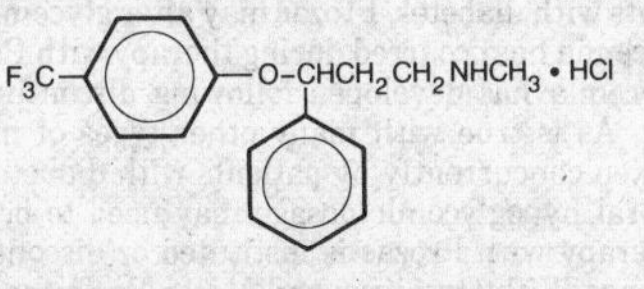
F3C
O-CHCH2CH2NHCH3 • HCl

Fluoxetine hydrochloride is a white to off-white crystalline solid with a solubility of 14 mg/mL in water.

Each Pulvule® contains fluoxetine hydrochloride equivalent to 20 mg (64.7 µmol) of fluoxetine. It also contains F D & C Blue No. 1, gelatin, iron oxide, silicone, starch, titanium dioxide, and other inactive ingredients.

The oral solution contains fluoxetine hydrochloride equivalent to 20 mg/5 mL (64.7 µmol) of fluoxetine. It also contains alcohol 0.23%, benzoic acid, flavoring agent, glycerin, purified water, and sucrose.

CLINICAL PHARMACOLOGY

Pharmacodynamics—The antidepressant action of fluoxetine is presumed to be linked to its inhibition of CNS neuronal uptake of serotonin. Studies at clinically relevant doses in man have demonstrated that fluoxetine blocks the uptake of serotonin into human platelets. Studies in animals also suggest that fluoxetine is a much more potent uptake inhibitor of serotonin than of norepinephrine.

Antagonism of muscarinic, histaminergic, and α_1-adrenergic receptors has been hypothesized to be associated with various anticholinergic, sedative, and cardiovascular effects of classical tricyclic antidepressant drugs. Fluoxetine binds to these and other membrane receptors from brain tissue much less potently in vitro than do the tricyclic drugs.

Absorption, Distribution, Metabolism, and Excretion:

Systemic Bioavailability—In man, following a single oral 40 mg dose, peak plasma concentrations of fluoxetine from 15 to 55 ng/mL are observed after 6 to 8 hours.

The Pulvule and oral solution dosage forms of fluoxetine are bioequivalent. Food does not appear to affect the systemic bioavailability of fluoxetine, although it may delay its absorption inconsequentially. Thus, fluoxetine may be administered with or without food.

Protein Binding—Over the concentration range from 200 to 1,000 ng/mL, approximately 94.5% of fluoxetine is bound in vitro to human serum proteins, including albumin and α_1-glycoprotein. The interaction between fluoxetine and other highly protein-bound drugs has not been fully evaluated, but may be important (*see* Precautions).

Metabolism—Fluoxetine is extensively metabolized in the liver to norfluoxetine and a number of other, unidentified metabolites. The only identified active metabolite, norfluoxetine, is formed by demethylation of fluoxetine. In animal models, norfluoxetine's potency and selectivity as a serotonin uptake blocker are essentially equivalent to fluoxetine's. The primary route of elimination appears to be hepatic metabolism to inactive metabolites excreted by the kidney.

Clinical Issues Related to Metabolism/Elimination—The complexity of the metabolism of fluoxetine has several consequences that may potentially affect fluoxetine's clinical use.

Accumulation and Slow Elimination—The relatively slow elimination of fluoxetine (elimination half-life of 2 to 3 days) and its active metabolite, norfluoxetine (elimination half-life of 7 to 9 days), assures significant accumulation of these active species in chronic use. After 30 days of dosing at 40 mg/day, plasma concentrations of fluoxetine in the range of 91 to 302 ng/mL and norfluoxetine in the range of 72 to 258 ng/mL have been observed. Plasma concentrations of fluoxetine were higher than those predicted by single-dose studies, presumably because fluoxetine's metabolism is not proportional to dose. Norfluoxetine, however, appears to have linear pharmacokinetics. Its mean terminal half-life after a single dose was 8.6 days and after multiple dosing was 9.3 days.

Thus, even if patients are given a fixed dose, steady state plasma concentrations are only achieved after continuous dosing for weeks. Nevertheless, plasma concentrations do **not** appear to increase without limit. Specifically, patients receiving fluoxetine at doses of 40 to 80 mg/day over periods as long as 3 years exhibited, on average, plasma concentrations similar to those seen among patients treated for 4 or 5 weeks.

The long elimination half-lives of fluoxetine and norfluoxetine assure that, even when dosing is stopped, active drug substance will persist in the body for weeks. This is of potential consequence when drug discontinuation is required or when drugs are prescribed that might interact with fluoxetine and norfluoxetine following the discontinuation of Prozac® (Fluoxetine Hydrochloride, Dista).

Liver Disease—As might be predicted from its primary site of metabolism, liver impairment can affect the elimination of fluoxetine. The elimination half-life of fluoxetine was prolonged in a study of cirrhotic patients, with a mean of 7.6 days compared to the range of 2 to 3 days seen in subjects without liver disease; norfluoxetine elimination was also delayed, with a mean duration of 12 days for cirrhotic patients compared to the range of 7 to 9 days in normal subjects. This suggests that the use of fluoxetine in patients with liver disease must be approached with caution. If fluoxetine is administered to patients with liver disease, a lower or less frequent dose should be used (*see* Precautions *and* Dosage and Administration).

Renal Disease—In single dose studies, the pharmacokinetics of fluoxetine and norfluoxetine were similar among subjects with all levels of impaired renal function including anephric patients on chronic hemodialysis. However, with chronic administration, additional accumulation of fluoxetine or its metabolites (possibly including some not yet identified) may occur in patients with severely impaired renal function and use of a lower or less frequent dose is advised (*see* Precautions).

Age—The effects of age upon the metabolism of fluoxetine have not been fully explored. The disposition of single doses of fluoxetine in healthy elderly subjects (greater than 65 years of age) did not differ significantly from that in younger normal subjects. However, given the long half-life and nonlinear disposition of the drug, a single-dose study is not adequate to rule out the possibility of altered pharmacokinetics

Continued on next page

This product information was prepared in June 1992. Current information on these and other products of Dista Products Company may be obtained by direct inquiry to Lilly Research Laboratories, Lilly Corporate Center, Indianapolis, Indiana 46285, (317) 276-3714.

Dista—Cont.

in the elderly, particularly if they have systemic illness or are receiving multiple drugs for concomitant diseases.

INDICATIONS AND USAGE

Prozac® (Fluoxetine Hydrochloride, Dista) is indicated for the treatment of depression. The efficacy of Prozac was established in 5- and 6-week trials with depressed outpatients whose diagnoses corresponded most closely to the DSM-III category of major depressive disorder.

A major depressive episode implies a prominent and relatively persistent depressed or dysphoric mood that usually interferes with daily functioning (nearly every day for at least 2 weeks); it should include at least 4 of the following 8 symptoms: change in appetite, change in sleep, psychomotor agitation or retardation, loss of interest in usual activities or decrease in sexual drive, increased fatigue, feelings of guilt or worthlessness, slowed thinking or impaired concentration, and a suicide attempt or suicidal ideation.

The antidepressant action of Prozac in hospitalized depressed patients has not been adequately studied.

The effectiveness of Prozac in long-term use, that is, for more than 5 to 6 weeks, has not been systematically evaluated in controlled trials. Therefore, the physician who elects to use Prozac for extended periods should periodically reevaluate the long-term usefulness of the drug for the individual patient.

CONTRAINDICATIONS

Prozac® (Fluoxetine Hydrochloride, Dista) is contraindicated in patients known to be hypersensitive to it.

Monoamine Oxidase Inhibitors—There have been reports of serious, sometimes fatal, reactions (including hyperthermia, rigidity, myoclonus, autonomic instability with possible rapid fluctuations of vital signs, and mental status changes that include extreme agitation progressing to delirium and coma) in patients receiving fluoxetine in combination with a monoamine oxidase inhibitor (MAOI), and in patients who have recently discontinued fluoxetine and are then started on an MAOI. Some cases presented with features resembling neuroleptic malignant syndrome. Therefore, Prozac should not be used in combination with an MAOI, or within 14 days of discontinuing therapy with an MAOI. Since fluoxetine and its major metabolite have very long elimination half-lives, at least 5 weeks should be allowed after stopping Prozac before starting an MAOI.

WARNINGS

Rash and Possibly Allergic Events—During premarketing testing of more than 5,600 US patients given fluoxetine, approximately 4% developed a rash and/or urticaria. Among these cases, almost a third were withdrawn from treatment because of the rash and/or systemic signs or symptoms associated with the rash. Clinical findings reported in association with rash include fever, leukocytosis, arthralgias, edema, carpal tunnel syndrome, respiratory distress, lymphadenopathy, proteinuria, and mild transaminase elevation. Most patients improved promptly with discontinuation of fluoxetine and/or adjunctive treatment with antihistamines or steroids, and all patients experiencing these events were reported to recover completely.

In premarketing clinical trials, 2 patients are known to have developed a serious cutaneous systemic illness. In neither patient was there an unequivocal diagnosis, but 1 was considered to have a leukocytoclastic vasculitis, and the other, a severe desquamating syndrome that was considered variously to be a vasculitis or erythema multiforme. Other patients have had systemic syndromes suggestive of serum sickness.

Since the introduction of Prozac, systemic events, possibly related to vasculitis, have developed in patients with rash. Although these events are rare, they may be serious, involving the lung, kidney, or liver. Death has been reported to occur in association with these systemic events.

Anaphylactoid events, including bronchospasm, angioedema, and urticaria alone and in combination, have been reported.

Pulmonary events, including inflammatory processes of varying histopathology and/or fibrosis, have been reported rarely. These events have occurred with dyspnea as the only preceding symptom.

Whether these systemic events and rash have a common underlying cause or are due to different etiologies or pathogenic processes is not known. Furthermore, a specific underlying immunologic basis for these events has not been identified. Upon the appearance of rash or of other possibly allergic phenomena for which an alternative etiology cannot be identified, Prozac should be discontinued.

PRECAUTIONS

General—Anxiety and Insomnia—Anxiety, nervousness, and insomnia were reported by 10% to 15% of patients treated with Prozac® (Fluoxetine Hydrochloride, Dista). These symptoms led to drug discontinuation in 5% of patients treated with Prozac.

Altered Appetite and Weight—Significant weight loss, especially in underweight depressed patients, may be an undesirable result of treatment with Prozac.

In controlled clinical trials, approximately 9% of patients treated with Prozac experienced anorexia. This incidence is approximately sixfold that seen in placebo controls. A weight loss of greater than 5% of body weight occurred in 13% of patients treated with Prozac compared to 4% of placebo and 3% of patients treated with tricyclics. However, only rarely have patients discontinued treatment with Prozac because of weight loss.

Activation of Mania/Hypomania—During premarketing testing, hypomania or mania occurred in approximately 1% of fluoxetine treated patients. Activation of mania/hypomania has also been reported in a small proportion of patients with Major Affective Disorder treated with other marketed antidepressants.

Seizures—Twelve patients among more than 6,000 evaluated worldwide in the course of premarketing development of fluoxetine experienced convulsions (or events described as possibly having been seizures), a rate of 0.2% that appears to be similar to that associated with other marketed antidepressants. Prozac should be introduced with care in patients with a history of seizures.

Suicide—The possibility of a suicide attempt is inherent in depression and may persist until significant remission occurs. Close supervision of high risk patients should accompany initial drug therapy. Prescriptions for Prozac should be written for the smallest quantity of capsules consistent with good patient management, in order to reduce the risk of overdose.

The Long Elimination Half-Lives of Fluoxetine and Its Metabolites—Because of the long elimination half-lives of the parent drug (2 to 3 days) and its major active metabolite (7 to 9 days), changes in dose will not be fully reflected in plasma for several weeks, affecting both strategies for titration to final dose and withdrawal from treatment (*see* Clinical Pharmacology *and* Dosage and Administration).

Use in Patients With Concomitant Illness—Clinical experience with Prozac® (Fluoxetine Hydrochloride, Dista) in patients with concomitant systemic illness is limited. Caution is advisable in using Prozac in patients with diseases or conditions that could affect metabolism or hemodynamic responses.

Fluoxetine has **not** been evaluated or used to any appreciable extent in patients with a recent history of myocardial infarction or unstable heart disease. Patients with these diagnoses were systematically excluded from clinical studies during the product's premarket testing. However, the electrocardiograms of 312 patients who received Prozac in double-blind trials were retrospectively evaluated; no conduction abnormalities that resulted in heart block were observed. The mean heart rate was reduced by approximately 3 beats/min.

In subjects with cirrhosis of the liver, the clearances of fluoxetine and its active metabolite, norfluoxetine, were decreased, thus increasing the elimination half-lives of these substances. A lower or less frequent dose should be used in patients with cirrhosis.

Since fluoxetine is extensively metabolized, excretion of unchanged drug in urine is a minor route of elimination. However, until adequate numbers of patients with severe renal impairment have been evaluated during chronic treatment with fluoxetine, it should be used with caution in such patients.

In patients with diabetes, Prozac may alter glycemic control. Hypoglycemia has occurred during therapy with Prozac, and hyperglycemia has developed following discontinuation of the drug. As is true with many other types of medication when taken concurrently by patients with diabetes, insulin and/or oral hypoglycemic dosage may need to be adjusted when therapy with Prozac is instituted or discontinued.

Interference With Cognitive and Motor Performance—Any psychoactive drug may impair judgment, thinking, or motor skills, and patients should be cautioned about operating hazardous machinery, including automobiles, until they are reasonably certain that the drug treatment does not affect them adversely.

Information for Patients—Physicians are advised to discuss the following issues with patients for whom they prescribe Prozac:

Because Prozac may impair judgment, thinking, or motor skills, patients should be advised to avoid driving a car or operating hazardous machinery until they are reasonably certain that their performance is not affected.

Patients should be advised to inform their physician if they are taking or plan to take any prescription or over-the-counter drugs, or alcohol.

Patients should be advised to notify their physician if they become pregnant or intend to become pregnant during therapy.

Patients should be advised to notify their physician if they are breast feeding an infant.

Patients should be advised to notify their physician if they develop a rash or hives.

Laboratory Tests—There are no specific laboratory tests recommended.

Drug Interactions—As with all drugs, the potential for interaction by a variety of mechanisms (eg, pharmacodynamic, pharmacokinetic drug inhibition or enhancement, etc) is a possibility (*see* Accumulation and Slow Elimination *under* Clinical Pharmacology).

Tryptophan—Five patients receiving Prozac® (Fluoxetine Hydrochloride, Dista) in combination with tryptophan experienced adverse reactions, including agitation, restlessness, and gastrointestinal distress.

Monoamine Oxidase Inhibitors—*See* Contraindications.

Other Antidepressants—There have been greater than 2-fold increases of previously stable plasma levels of other antidepressants when Prozac has been administered in combination with these agents (*see* Accumulation and Slow Elimination *under* Clinical Pharmacology).

Lithium—There have been reports of both increased and decreased lithium levels when lithium was used concomitantly with fluoxetine. Cases of lithium toxicity have been reported. Lithium levels should be monitored when these drugs are administered concomitantly.

Diazepam Clearance—The half-life of concurrently administered diazepam may be prolonged in some patients (*see* Accumulation and Slow Elimination *under* Clinical Pharmacology).

Potential Effects of Coadministration of Drugs Tightly Bound to Plasma Proteins—Because fluoxetine is tightly bound to plasma protein, the administration of fluoxetine to a patient taking another drug that is tightly bound to protein (eg, Coumadin, digitoxin) may cause a shift in plasma concentrations potentially resulting in an adverse effect. Conversely, adverse effects may result from displacement of protein bound fluoxetine by other tightly bound drugs (*see* Accumulation and Slow Elimination *under* Clinical Pharmacology).

CNS Active Drugs—The risk of using Prozac in combination with other CNS active drugs has not been systematically evaluated. Consequently, caution is advised if the concomitant administration of Prozac and such drugs is required (*see* Accumulation and Slow Elimination *under* Clinical Pharmacology).

Electroconvulsive Therapy—There are no clinical studies establishing the benefit of the combined use of ECT and fluoxetine. There have been rare reports of prolonged seizures in patients on fluoxetine receiving ECT treatment.

Carcinogenesis, Mutagenesis, Impairment of Fertility—There is no evidence of carcinogenicity, mutagenicity, or impairment of fertility with Prozac.

The dietary administration of fluoxetine to rats and mice for 2 years at levels equivalent to approximately 7.5 and 9.0 times the maximum human dose (80 mg) respectively produced no evidence of carcinogenicity.

Fluoxetine and norfluoxetine have been shown to have no genotoxic effects based on the following assays: bacterial mutation assay, DNA repair assay in cultured rat hepatocytes, mouse lymphoma assay, and in vivo sister chromatid exchange assay in Chinese hamster bone marrow cells.

Two fertility studies conducted in rats at doses of approximately 5 and 9 times the maximum human dose (80 mg) indicated that fluoxetine had no adverse effects on fertility. A slight decrease in neonatal survival was noted, but this was probably associated with depressed maternal food consumption and suppressed weight gain.

Pregnancy—Teratogenic Effects—Pregnancy Category B: Reproduction studies have been performed in rats and rabbits at doses 9 and 11 times the maximum daily human dose (80 mg) respectively and have revealed no evidence of harm to the fetus due to Prozac® (Fluoxetine Hydrochloride, Dista). There are, however, no adequate and well-controlled studies in pregnant women. Because animal reproduction studies are not always predictive of human response, this drug should be used during pregnancy only if clearly needed.

Labor and Delivery—The effect of Prozac on labor and delivery in humans is unknown.

Nursing Mothers—Because many drugs are excreted in human milk, caution should be exercised when Prozac is administered to a nursing woman. In 1 breast milk sample, the concentration of fluoxetine plus norfluoxetine was 70.4 ng/mL. The concentration in the mother's plasma was 295.0 ng/mL. No adverse effects on the infant were reported.

Usage in Children—Safety and effectiveness in children have not been established.

Usage in the Elderly—Prozac has not been systematically evaluated in older patients; however, several hundred elderly patients have participated in clinical studies with Prozac and no unusual adverse age-related phenomena have been identified. However, these data are insufficient to rule out possible age-related differences during chronic use, particularly in elderly patients who have concomitant systemic illnesses or who are receiving concomitant drugs.

Hyponatremia—Several cases of hyponatremia (some with serum sodium lower than 110 mmol/L) have been reported. The hyponatremia appeared to be reversible when Prozac was discontinued. Although these cases were complex with varying possible etiologies, some were possibly due to the syndrome of inappropriate antidiuretic hormone secretion (SIADH). The majority of these occurrences have been in

older patients and in patients taking diuretics or who were otherwise volume depleted.

Platelet Function —There have been rare reports of altered platelet function and/or abnormal results from laboratory studies in patients taking fluoxetine. While there have been reports of abnormal bleeding in several patients taking fluoxetine, it is unclear whether fluoxetine had a causative role.

ADVERSE REACTIONS

Commonly Observed —The most commonly observed adverse events associated with the use of Prozac® (Fluoxetine Hydrochloride, Dista) and not seen at an equivalent incidence among placebo-treated patients were: nervous system complaints, including anxiety, nervousness, and insomnia; drowsiness and fatigue or asthenia; tremor; sweating; gastrointestinal complaints, including anorexia, nausea, and diarrhea; and dizziness or lightheadedness.

Associated With Discontinuation of Treatment —Fifteen percent of approximately 4,000 patients who received Prozac in US premarketing clinical trials discontinued treatment due to an adverse event. The more common events causing discontinuation included: psychiatric (5.3%), primarily nervousness, anxiety, and insomnia; digestive (3.0%), primarily nausea; nervous system (1.6%), primarily dizziness; body as a whole (1.5%), primarily asthenia and headache; and skin (1.4%), primarily rash and pruritus.

Incidence in Controlled Clinical Trials —The table that follows enumerates adverse events that occurred at a frequency of 1% or more among patients treated with Prozac who participated in controlled trials comparing Prozac with placebo. The prescriber should be aware that these figures cannot be used to predict the incidence of side effects in the course of usual medical practice where patient characteristics and other factors differ from those that prevailed in the clinical trials. Similarly, the cited frequencies cannot be compared with figures obtained from other clinical investigations involving different treatments, uses, and investigators. The cited figures, however, do provide the prescribing physician with some basis for estimating the relative contribution of drug and nondrug factors to the side effect incidence rate in the population studied.
[See table at right.]

Other Events Observed During Premarketing Evaluation of Prozac® (Fluoxetine Hydrochloride, Dista) —During clinical testing in the US, multiple doses of Prozac were administered to approximately 5,600 subjects. Untoward events associated with this exposure were recorded by clinical investigators using descriptive terminology of their own choosing. Consequently, it is not possible to provide a meaningful estimate of the proportion of individuals experiencing adverse events without first grouping similar types of untoward events into a limited (ie, reduced) number of standardized event categories.

In the tabulations that follow, a standard COSTART Dictionary terminology has been used to classify reported adverse events. The frequencies presented, therefore, represent the proportion of the 5,600 individuals exposed to Prozac who experienced an event of the type cited on at least 1 occasion while receiving Prozac. All reported events are included except those already listed in tables, those COSTART terms so general as to be uninformative, and those events where a drug cause was remote. It is important to emphasize that, although the events reported did occur during treatment with Prozac, they were not necessarily caused by it.

Events are further classified within body system categories and enumerated in order of decreasing frequency using the following definitions: frequent adverse events are defined as those occurring on 1 or more occasions in at least 1/100 patients; infrequent adverse events are those occurring in 1/100 to 1/1,000 patients; rare events are those occurring in less than 1/1,000 patients.

Body as a Whole—*Frequent:* chills; *Infrequent:* chills and fever, cyst, face edema, hangover effect, jaw pain, malaise, neck pain, neck rigidity, and pelvic pain; *Rare:* abdomen enlarged, cellulitis, hydrocephalus, hypothermia, LE syndrome, moniliasis, and serum sickness.

Cardiovascular System—*Infrequent:* angina pectoris, arrhythmia, hemorrhage, hypertension, hypotension, migraine, postural hypotension, syncope, and tachycardia; *Rare:* AV block first degree, bradycardia, bundle branch block, cerebral ischemia, myocardial infarct, thrombophlebitis, vascular headache, and ventricular arrhythmia.

Digestive System—*Frequent:* increased appetite; *Infrequent:* aphthous stomatitis, dysphagia, eructation, esophagitis, gastritis, gingivitis, glossitis, liver function tests abnormal, melena, stomatitis, thirst; *Rare:* bloody diarrhea, cholecystitis, cholelithiasis, colitis, duodenal ulcer, enteritis, fecal incontinence, hematemesis, hepatitis, hepatomegaly, hyperchlorhydria, increased salivation, jaundice, liver tenderness, mouth ulceration, salivary gland enlargement, stomach ulcer, tongue discoloration, and tongue edema.

Endocrine System—*Infrequent:* hypothyroidism; *Rare:* goiter and hyperthyroidism.

Hemic and Lymphatic System—*Infrequent:* anemia and lymphadenopathy; *Rare:* bleeding time increased, blood dys-

TREATMENT-EMERGENT ADVERSE EXPERIENCE INCIDENCE IN PLACEBO-CONTROLLED CLINICAL TRIALS

Body System/ Adverse Event*	Percentage of Patients Reporting Event		Body System/ Adverse Event*	Percentage of Patients Reporting Event	
	Prozac† (N=1,730)	Placebo (N=799)		Prozac† (N=1,730)	Placebo (N=799)
Nervous			**Body as a Whole**		
Headache	20.3	15.5	Asthenia	4.4	1.9
Nervousness	14.9	8.5	Infection, viral	3.4	3.1
Insomnia	13.8	7.1	Pain, limb	1.6	1.1
Drowsiness	11.6	6.3	Fever	1.4	—
Anxiety	9.4	5.5	Pain, chest	1.3	1.1
Tremor	7.9	2.4	Allergy	1.2	1.1
Dizziness	5.7	3.3	Influenza	1.2	1.5
Fatigue	4.2	1.1	**Respiratory**		
Sedated	1.9	1.3	Upper respiratory infection	7.6	6.0
Sensation disturbance	1.7	2.0	Flu-like syndrome	2.8	1.9
Libido, decreased	1.6	—	Pharyngitis	2.7	1.3
Light-headedness	1.6	—	Nasal congestion	2.6	2.3
Concentration, decreased	1.5	—	Headache, sinus	2.3	1.8
Digestive			Sinusitis	2.1	2.0
Nausea	21.1	10.1	Cough	1.6	1.6
Diarrhea	12.3	7.0	Dyspnea	1.4	—
Mouth dryness	9.5	6.0	**Cardiovascular**		
Anorexia	8.7	1.5	Hot flushes	1.8	1.0
Dyspepsia	6.4	4.3	Palpitations	1.3	1.4
Constipation	4.5	3.3	**Musculoskeletal**		
Pain, abdominal	3.4	2.9	Pain, back	2.0	2.4
Vomiting	2.4	1.3	Pain, joint	1.2	1.1
Taste change	1.8	—	Pain, muscle	1.2	1.0
Flatulence	1.6	1.1	**Urogenital**		
Gastroenteritis	1.0	1.4	Menstruation, painful	1.9	1.4
Skin and Appendages			Sexual dysfunction	1.9	
Sweating, excessive	8.4	3.8	Frequent micturition	1.6	—
Rash	2.7	1.8	Urinary tract infection	1.2	—
Pruritus	2.4	1.4	**Special Senses**		
			Vision disturbance	2.8	1.8

* Events reported by at least 1% of patients treated with Prozac are included.
† Prozac® (Fluoxetine Hydrochloride Dista).
— Incidence less than 1%.

crasia, leukopenia, lymphocytosis, petechia, purpura, sedimentation rate increased, and thrombocythemia.

Metabolic and Nutritional—*Frequent:* weight loss; *Infrequent:* generalized edema, hypoglycemia, peripheral edema, and weight gain; *Rare:* dehydration, gout, hypercholesteremia, hyperglycemia, hyperlipemia, hypoglycemic reaction, hypokalemia, hyponatremia, and iron deficiency anemia.

Musculoskeletal System—*Infrequent:* arthritis, bone pain, bursitis, tenosynovitis, and twitching; *Rare:* bone necrosis, chondrodystrophy, muscle hemorrhage, myositis, osteoporosis, pathological fracture, and rheumatoid arthritis.

Nervous System—*Frequent:* abnormal dreams and agitation; *Infrequent:* abnormal gait, acute brain syndrome, akathisia, amnesia, apathy, ataxia, buccoglossal syndrome, CNS stimulation, convulsion, delusions, depersonalization, emotional lability, euphoria, hallucinations, hostility, hyperkinesia, hypesthesia, incoordination, libido increased, manic reaction, neuralgia, neuropathy, paranoid reaction, psychosis, and vertigo; *Rare:* abnormal electroencephalogram, antisocial reaction, chronic brain syndrome, circumoral paresthesia, CNS depression, coma, dysarthria, dystonia, extrapyramidal syndrome, hypertonia, hysteria, myoclonus, nystagmus, paralysis, reflexes decreased, stupor, and torticollis.

Respiratory System—*Frequent:* bronchitis, rhinitis, and yawn; *Infrequent:* asthma, epistaxis, hiccup, hyperventilation, and pneumonia; *Rare:* apnea, hemoptysis, hypoxia, larynx edema, lung edema, lung fibrosis/alveolitis, and pleural effusion.

Skin and Appendages—*Infrequent:* acne, alopecia, contact dermatitis, dry skin, herpes simplex, maculopapular rash, and urticaria; *Rare:* eczema, erythema multiforme, fungal dermatitis, herpes zoster, hirsutism, psoriasis, purpuric rash, pustular rash, seborrhea, skin discoloration, skin hypertrophy, subcutaneous nodule, and vesiculobullous rash.

Special Senses—*Infrequent:* amblyopia, conjunctivitis, ear pain, eye pain, mydriasis, photophobia, and tinnitus; *Rare:* blepharitis, cataract, corneal lesion, deafness, diplopia, eye hemorrhage, glaucoma, iritis, ptosis, strabismus, and taste loss.

Urogenital System—*Infrequent:* abnormal ejaculation, amenorrhea, breast pain, cystitis, dysuria, fibrocystic breast, impotence, leukorrhea, menopause, menorrhagia, ovarian

disorder, urinary incontinence, urinary retention, urinary urgency, urination impaired, and vaginitis; *Rare:* abortion, albuminuria, breast enlargement, dyspareunia, epididymitis, female lactation, hematuria, hypomenorrhea, kidney calculus, metrorrhagia, orchitis, polyuria, pyelonephritis, pyuria, salpingitis, urethral pain, urethritis, urinary tract disorder, urolithiasis, uterine hemorrhage, uterine spasm, and vaginal hemorrhage.

Postintroduction Reports —Voluntary reports of adverse events temporally associated with Prozac that have been received since market introduction and which may have no causal relationship with the drug include the following: aplastic anemia, cerebral vascular accident, confusion, dyskinesia (including, for example, a case of buccal-lingual-masticatory syndrome with involuntary tongue protrusion reported to develop in a 77-year-old female after 5 weeks of fluoxetine therapy and which completely resolved over the next few months following drug discontinuation), ecchymoses, eosinophilic pneumonia, gastrointestinal hemorrhage, hyperprolactinemia, immune-related hemolytic anemia, movement disorders developing in patients with risk factors including drugs associated with such events and worsening of preexisting movement disorders, neuroleptic malignant syndrome-like events, pancreatitis, pancytopenia, suicidal ideation, thrombocytopenia, thrombocytopenic purpura, vaginal bleeding after drug withdrawal, and violent behaviors.

DRUG ABUSE AND DEPENDENCE

Controlled Substance Class —Prozac® (Fluoxetine Hydrochloride, Dista) is not a controlled substance.
Physical and Psychologic Dependence —Prozac has not been systematically studied, in animals or humans, for its poten-

Continued on next page

This product information was prepared in June 1992. Current information on these and other products of Dista Products Company may be obtained by direct inquiry to Lilly Research Laboratories, Lilly Corporate Center, Indianapolis, Indiana 46285, (317) 276-3714.

Dista—Cont.

tial for abuse, tolerance, or physical dependence. While the premarketing clinical experience with Prozac did not reveal any tendency for a withdrawal syndrome or any drug seeking behavior, these observations were not systematic and it is not possible to predict on the basis of this limited experience the extent to which a CNS active drug will be misused, diverted, and/or abused once marketed. Consequently, physicians should carefully evaluate patients for history of drug abuse and follow such patients closely, observing them for signs of misuse or abuse of Prozac (eg, development of tolerance, incrementation of dose, drug-seeking behavior).

OVERDOSAGE
Human Experience—As of December 1987, there were 2 deaths among approximately 38 reports of acute overdose with fluoxetine, either alone or in combination with other drugs and/or alcohol. One death involved a combined overdose with approximately 1,800 mg of fluoxetine and an undetermined amount of maprotiline. Plasma concentrations of fluoxetine and maprotiline were 4.57 mg/L and 4.18 mg/L, respectively. A second death involved 3 drugs yielding plasma concentrations as follows: fluoxetine, 1.93 mg/L; norfluoxetine, 1.10 mg/L; codeine, 1.80 mg/L; temazepam, 3.80 mg/L.

One other patient who reportedly took 3,000 mg of fluoxetine experienced 2 grand mal seizures that remitted spontaneously without specific anticonvulsant treatment (*see Management of Overdose*). The actual amount of drug absorbed may have been less due to vomiting.

Nausea and vomiting were prominent in overdoses involving higher fluoxetine doses. Other prominent symptoms of overdose included agitation, restlessness, hypomania, and other signs of CNS excitation. Except for the 2 deaths noted above, all other overdose cases recovered without residua.

Since introduction, reports of death attributed to overdosage of fluoxetine alone have been extremely rare.

Animal Experience—Studies in animals do not provide precise or necessarily valid information about the treatment of human overdose. However, animal experiments can provide useful insights into possible treatment strategies.

The oral median lethal dose in rats and mice was found to be 452 and 248 mg/kg respectively. Acute high oral doses produced hyperirritability and convulsions in several animal species.

Among 6 dogs purposely overdosed with oral fluoxetine, 5 experienced grand mal seizures. Seizures stopped immediately upon the bolus intravenous administration of a standard veterinary dose of diazepam. In this short term study, the lowest plasma concentration at which a seizure occurred was only twice the maximum plasma concentration seen in humans taking 80 mg/day, chronically.

In a separate single-dose study, the ECG in dogs given high doses did not reveal prolongation of the PR, QRS, or QT intervals. Tachycardia and an increase in blood pressure were observed. Consequently, the value of the ECG in predicting cardiac toxicity is unknown. Nonetheless, the ECG should ordinarily be monitored in cases of human overdose (*see Management of Overdose*).

Management of Overdose—Establish and maintain an airway; ensure adequate oxygenation and ventilation. Activated charcoal, which may be used with sorbitol, may be as or more effective than emesis or lavage, and should be considered in treating overdose.

Cardiac and vital signs monitoring is recommended, along with general symptomatic and supportive measures. Based on experience in animals, which may not be relevant to humans, fluoxetine-induced seizures that fail to remit spontaneously may respond to diazepam.

There are no specific antidotes for Prozac® (Fluoxetine Hydrochloride, Dista).

Due to the large volume of distribution of Prozac, forced diuresis, dialysis, hemoperfusion, and exchange transfusion are unlikely to be of benefit.

In managing overdosage, consider the possibility of multiple drug involvement. The physician should consider contacting a poison control center on the treatment of any overdose. Telephone numbers of certified poison control centers are listed in the *Physicians' Desk Reference (PDR)*.

DOSAGE AND ADMINISTRATION
Initial Treatment—In controlled trials used to support the efficacy of fluoxetine, patients were administered morning doses ranging from 20 mg to 80 mg/day. Recent studies suggest that 20 mg/day may be sufficient to obtain a satisfactory antidepressant response. Consequently, a dose of 20 mg/day, administered in the morning, is recommended as the initial dose.

A dose increase may be considered after several weeks if no clinical improvement is observed. Doses above 20 mg/day should be administered on a b.i.d. schedule (ie, morning and noon) and should not exceed a maximum dose of 80 mg/day. As with other antidepressants, the full antidepressant effect may be delayed until 4 weeks of treatment or longer.

As with many other medications, a lower or less frequent dosage should be used in patients with renal and/or hepatic impairment. A lower or less frequent dosage should also be considered for patients, such as the elderly, with concurrent disease or on multiple medications.

Maintenance/Continuation/Extended Treatment—There is no body of evidence available to answer the question of how long the patient treated with fluoxetine should remain on it. It is generally agreed among expert psychopharmacologists (circa 1987) that acute episodes of depression require several months or longer of sustained pharmacologic therapy. Whether the dose of antidepressant needed to induce remission is identical to the dose needed to maintain and/or sustain euthymia is unknown.

HOW SUPPLIED
(℞) Pulvules: 20 mg* green and off-white (No. 3105)—(100s) NDC 0777-3105-02; (ID†100)NDC 0777-3105-33
(℞) Liquid, Oral Solution: 20 mg*/5 mL, mint flavor (M-5120‡)—(120 mL) NDC 0777-5120-58
Store at controlled room temperature, 59° to 86°F (15° to 30°C).

Animal Toxicology: Phospholipids are increased in some tissues of mice, rats, and dogs given fluoxetine chronically. This effect is reversible after cessation of fluoxetine treatment. Phospholipid accumulation in animals has been observed with many cationic amphiphilic drugs, including fenfluramine, imipramine, and ranitidine. The significance of this effect in humans is unknown.

* Fluoxetine base equivalent.
† Identi-Dose® (unit dose medication, Dista).
‡ Dispense in a tight, light-resistant container.

[032392]

Shown in Product Identification Section, page 409

Dorsey Pharmaceuticals

FOR DORSEY PRESCRIPTION PRODUCTS, PLEASE SEE SANDOZ PHARMACEUTICALS CORPORATION LISTING.

Du Pont Multi-Source Products
The Du Pont Merck Pharmaceutical Company
1000 STEWART AVENUE
GARDEN CITY, NY 11530

BRETYLOL®   ℞
[bre 'tĭ-lol "]
(bretylium tosylate)
INJECTION

For Intravenous or Intramuscular Use

DESCRIPTION
BRETYLOL (bretylium tosylate) Injection is an antifibrillatory and antiarrhythmic agent, intended for intravenous or intramuscular use.

BRETYLOL is a white, crystalline powder with an extremely bitter taste. It is freely soluble in water and alcohol. Each mL of sterile, non-pyrogenic solution contains 50 mg bretylium tosylate in Water for Injection, USP. The pH is adjusted when necessary, with dilute hydrochloric acid or sodium hydroxide. BRETYLOL contains no preservative.

CLINICAL PHARMACOLOGY
BRETYLOL is a bromobenzyl quaternary ammonium compound which selectively accumulates in sympathetic ganglia and their postganglionic adrenergic neurons where it inhibits norepinephrine release by depressing adrenergic nerve terminal excitability.

BRETYLOL also suppresses ventricular fibrillation and ventricular arrhythmias. The mechanisms of the antifibrillatory and antiarrhythmic actions of BRETYLOL are not established. In efforts to define these mechanisms, the following electrophysiologic actions of BRETYLOL have been demonstrated in animal experiments:
1. Increase in ventricular fibrillation threshold.
2. Increase in action potential duration and effective refractory period without changes in heart rate.
3. Little effect on the rate of rise or amplitude of the cardiac action potential (Phase 0) or in resting membrane potential (Phase 4) in normal myocardium. However, when cell injury slows the rate of rise, decreases amplitude, and lowers resting membrane potential, BRETYLOL transiently restores these parameters toward normal.
4. In canine hearts with infarcted areas BRETYLOL decreases the disparity in action potential duration between normal and infarcted regions.

5. Increase in impulse formation and spontaneous firing rate of pacemaker tissue as well as increased ventricular conduction velocity.

The restoration of injured myocardial cell electrophysiology toward normal, as well as the increase of the action potential duration and effective refractory period without changing their ratio to each other, may be important factors in suppressing re-entry of aberrant impulses and decreasing induced dispersion of local excitable states.

BRETYLOL induces a chemical sympathectomy-like state which resembles a surgical sympathectomy. Catecholamine stores are not depleted by BRETYLOL, but catecholamine effects on the myocardium and on peripheral vascular resistance are often seen shortly after administration because BRETYLOL causes an early release of norepinephrine from the adrenergic postganglionic nerve terminals. Subsequently, BRETYLOL blocks the release of norepinephrine in response to neuron stimulation. Peripheral adrenergic blockade regularly causes orthostatic hypotension but has less effect on supine blood pressure. The relationship of adrenergic blockade to the antifibrillatory and antiarrhythmic actions of BRETYLOL is not clear. In a study in patients with frequent ventricular premature beats, peak plasma concentration of BRETYLOL and peak hypotensive effects were seen within one hour of intramuscular administration, presumably reflecting adrenergic neuronal blockade. However, suppression of premature ventricular beats was not maximal until 6–9 hours after dosing, when mean plasma concentration had declined to less than one-half of peak level. This suggests a slower mechanism, other than neuronal blockade, was involved in suppression of the arrhythmia. On the other hand, antifibrillatory effects can be seen within minutes of an intravenous injection, suggesting that the effect on the myocardium may occur quite rapidly.

BRETYLOL has a positive inotropic effect on the myocardium, but it is not yet certain whether this effect is direct or is mediated by catecholamine release.

BRETYLOL is eliminated intact by the kidneys. No metabolites have been identified following administration of BRETYLOL in man and laboratory animals. In man, approximately 70 to 80% of a ^{14}C-labelled intramuscular dose is excreted in the urine during the first 24 hours, with an additional 10% excreted over the next three days.

The terminal half-life in four normal volunteers averaged 7.8 ± 0.6 hrs (range 6.9–8.1). In one patient with a creatinine clearance of 21.0 mL/min x 1.73 m², the half-life was 16 hours. In one patient with a creatinine clearance of 1.0 mL/min x 1.73 m² the half-life was 31.5 hours. During hemodialysis, this patient's arterial and venous BRETYLOL concentrations declined rapidly, resulting in a half-life of 13 hours. During dialysis there was a two-fold increase in total BRETYLOL clearance.

Effect on Heart Rate: There is sometimes an initial small increase in heart rate when BRETYLOL is administered, but this is an inconsistent and transient occurrence.

Hemodynamic Effects: Following intravenous administration of 5 mg/kg of BRETYLOL to patients with acute myocardial infarction, there was a mild increase in arterial pressure, followed by a modest decrease, remaining within normal limits throughout. Pulmonary artery pressures, pulmonary capillary wedge pressure, right atrial pressure, cardiac index, stroke volume index, and stroke work index were not significantly changed. These hemodynamic effects were not correlated with antiarrhythmic activity.

Onset of Action: Suppression of ventricular fibrillation is rapid, usually occurring within minutes following intravenous administration. Suppression of ventricular tachycardia and other ventricular arrhythmias develops more slowly, usually 20 minutes to 2 hours after parenteral administration.

INDICATIONS AND USAGE
BRETYLOL is indicated in the prophylaxis and therapy of ventricular fibrillation.

BRETYLOL is also indicated in the treatment of life-threatening ventricular arrhythmias, such as ventricular tachycardia, that have failed to respond to adequate doses of a first-line antiarrhythmic agent, such as lidocaine.

Use of BRETYLOL should be limited to intensive care units, coronary care units or other facilities where equipment and personnel for constant monitoring of cardiac arrhythmias and blood pressure are available.

Following injection of BRETYLOL there may be a delay of 20 minutes to 2 hours in the onset of antiarrhythmic action, although it appears to act within minutes in ventricular fibrillation. The delay in effect appears to be longer after intramuscular than after intravenous injection.

CONTRAINDICATIONS
There are no contraindications to use in treatment of ventricular fibrillation or life-threatening refractory ventricular arrhythmias.

WARNINGS
1. **Hypotension**
   Administration of BRETYLOL regularly results in postural hypotension, subjectively recognized by dizziness,

light-headedness, vertigo or faintness. Some degree of hypotension is present in about 50% of patients while they are supine. Hypotension may occur at doses lower than those needed to suppress arrhythmias.

Patients should be kept in the supine position until tolerance to the hypotensive effect of BRETYLOL develops. Tolerance occurs unpredictably but may be present after several days.

Hypotension with supine systolic pressure greater than 75 mm Hg need not be treated unless there are associated symptoms. If supine systolic pressure falls below 75 mm Hg, an infusion of dopamine or norepinephrine may be used to raise blood pressure. When catecholamines are administered, a dilute solution should be employed and blood pressure monitored closely because the pressor effects of the catecholamines are enhanced by BRETYLOL. Volume expansion with blood or plasma and correction of dehydration should be carried out where appropriate.

2. **Transient Hypertension and Increased Frequency of Arrhythmias**
Due to the initial release of norepinephrine from adrenergic postganglionic nerve terminals by BRETYLOL, transient hypertension or increased frequency of premature ventricular contractions and other arrhythmias may occur in some patients.
3. **Caution During Use with Digitalis Glycosides**
The initial release of norepinephrine caused by BRETYLOL may aggravate digitalis toxicity. When a life-threatening cardiac arrhythmia occurs in a digitalized patient, BRETYLOL should be used only if the etiology of the arrhythmia does not appear to be digitalis toxicity and other antiarrhythmic drugs are not effective. Simultaneous initiation of therapy with digitalis glycosides and BRETYLOL should be avoided.
4. **Patients with Fixed Cardiac Output**
In patients with fixed cardiac output (i.e., severe aortic stenosis or severe pulmonary hypertension), BRETYLOL should be avoided since severe hypotension may result from a fall in peripheral resistance without a compensatory increase in cardiac output. If survival is threatened by the arrhythmia, BRETYLOL may be used but vasoconstrictive catecholamines should be given promptly if severe hypotension occurs.

PRECAUTIONS

General

1. **Dilution for Intravenous Use**
BRETYLOL should be diluted (one part BRETYLOL with at least four parts of Dextrose Injection, USP or Sodium Chloride Injection, USP) prior to intravenous use. Rapid intravenous administration may cause severe nausea and vomiting. Therefore, the diluted solution should be infused over a period greater than 8 minutes. However, in treating existing ventricular fibrillation BRETYLOL should be given as rapidly as possible and may be given without dilution.
2. **Use Various Sites for Intramuscular Injection**
When injected intramuscularly, not more than 5 mL should be given in a site, and injection sites should be varied since repeated intramuscular injection into the same site may cause atrophy and necrosis of muscle tissue, fibrosis, vascular degeneration and inflammatory changes.
3. **Reduce Dosage in Impaired Renal Function**
Since BRETYLOL is excreted principally via the kidney, the dosage interval should be increased in patients with impaired renal function. See 'Clinical Pharmacology' section for information on the effect of reduced renal function on half-life.

Drug Interactions

1. Digitalis toxicity may be aggravated by the initial release of norepinephrine caused by BRETYLOL.
2. The pressor effects of catecholamines such as dopamine or norepinephrine are enhanced by BRETYLOL. When catecholamines are administered, dilute solutions should be used and blood pressure should be monitored closely. (See **WARNINGS.**)
3. Although there is little published information on concomitant administration of lidocaine and BRETYLOL, these drugs are often administered concurrently without any evidence of interactions resulting in adverse effects or diminished efficacy.

Carcinogenesis, Mutagenesis, Impairment of Fertility
No data are available on potential for carcinogenicity, mutagenicity or impairment of fertility in animals or humans.

Pregnancy Category C
Animal reproduction studies have not been conducted with bretylium tosylate. It is also not known whether bretylium tosylate can cause harm when administered to a pregnant woman or can affect reproduction capacity. Bretylium tosylate should be given to pregnant women only if clearly needed.

Suggested BRETYLOL Admixture Dilutions and Administration Rates for Continuous Infusion Maintenance Therapy Arranged in Descending Order of Concentration

PREPARATION				ADMINISTRATION		
Amount of BRETYLOL	Volume of IV Fluid*	Final Volume	Final Conc. (mg/mL)	Dose mg/min.	Microdrops per min.	mL/hr
FOR FLUID RESTRICTED PATIENTS:						
500 mg (10 mL)	50 mL	60 mL	8.3	1.0	7	7
				1.5	11	11
				2.0	14	14
2 g (40 mL)	500 mL	540 mL	3.7	1.0	16	16
1 g (20 mL)	250 mL	270 mL	3.7	1.5	24	24
				2.0	32	32
1 g (20 mL)	500 mL	520 mL	1.9	1.0	32	32
500 mg (10 mL)	250 mL	260 mL	1.9	1.5	47	47
				2.0	63	63

*IV fluid may be either Dextrose Injection, USP or Sodium Chloride Injection, USP.

Pediatric Use
The safety and efficacy of this drug in children has not been established. BRETYLOL has been administered to a limited number of pediatric patients, but such use has been inadequate to define fully proper dosage and limitations for use.

ADVERSE REACTIONS

Hypotension and postural hypotension have been the most frequently reported adverse reactions (see **WARNINGS** section). Nausea and vomiting occurred in about three percent of patients, primarily when BRETYLOL was administered rapidly by the intravenous route (see **PRECAUTIONS** section). Vertigo, dizziness, light-headedness and syncope, which sometimes accompanied postural hypotension, were reported in about 7 patients in 1000.

Bradycardia, increased frequency of premature ventricular contractions, transitory hypertension, initial increase in arrhythmias (see **WARNINGS** section), precipitation of anginal attacks, and sensation of substernal pressure have also been reported in a small number of patients, i.e., approximately 1–2 patients in 1000.

Renal dysfunction, diarrhea, abdominal pain, hiccups, erythematous macular rash, flushing, hyperthermia, confusion, paranoid psychosis, emotional lability, lethargy, generalized tenderness, anxiety, shortness of breath, diaphoresis, nasal stuffiness and mild conjunctivitis, have been reported in about 1 patient in 1000. The relationship of BRETYLOL administration to these reactions has not been clearly established.

OVERDOSAGE

In the presence of life threatening arrhythmias, underdosing with BRETYLOL probably presents a greater risk to the patient than potential overdosage. However, one case of accidental overdose has been reported in which a rapidly injected intravenous bolus of 30 mg/kg was given instead of an intended 10 mg/kg dose during an episode of ventricular tachycardia. Marked hypertension resulted, followed by protracted refractory hypotension. The patient expired 18 hours later in asystole, complicated by renal failure and aspiration pneumonitis. Bretylium serum levels were 8,000 ng/mL.

The exaggerated hemodynamic response was attributed to the rapid injection of a very large dose while some effective circulation was still present. Neither the total dose nor the serum levels observed in this patient are in themselves associated with toxicity. Total doses of 30 mg/kg are not unusual and do not cause toxicity when given incrementally during cardio-pulmonary resuscitation procedures. Similarly, patients maintained on chronic BRETYLOL therapy have had documented serum levels of 12,000 ng/mL. These levels were achieved after sequential dosage increases over time with no apparent ill effects.

If BRETYLOL is overdosed and symptoms of toxicity develop, administration of nitroprusside or another short acting intravenous antihypertensive agent should be considered for the treatment of the hypertensive response. Long acting drugs that might potentiate the subsequent hypotensive effects of BRETYLOL should not be used. Hypotension should be treated with appropriate fluid therapy and pressor agents such as dopamine or norepinephrine. Dialysis is probably not useful in the treatment of BRETYLOL overdose.

DOSAGE AND ADMINISTRATION

BRETYLOL is to be used clinically only for treatment of life-threatening ventricular arrhythmias under constant electrocardiographic monitoring. The clinical use of BRETYLOL is for short-term use only. Patients should either be kept supine during the course of BRETYLOL therapy or be closely observed for postural hypotension. The optimal dose schedule for parenteral administration of BRETYLOL has not been determined. There is comparatively little experience with dosages greater than 40 mg/kg/day, although such doses have been used without apparent adverse effects. The following schedule is suggested.

A. **For immediately Life-threatening Ventricular Arrhythmias such as Ventricular Fibrillation or Hemodynamically Unstable Ventricular Tachycardia:**
Administer undiluted BRETYLOL at a dosage of 5 mg/kg of body weight by rapid intravenous injection. Other usual cardiopulmonary resuscitative procedures, including electrical cardioversion, should be employed prior to and following the injection in accordance with good medical practice. If ventricular fibrillation persists, the dosage may be increased to 10 mg/kg and repeated as necessary.
For continuous suppression, dilute BRETYLOL with Dextrose Injection, USP or Sodium Chloride Injection, USP using the table below and administer the diluted solution as a constant infusion of 1 to 2 mg BRETYLOL per minute. When administering BRETYLOL (or any potent medication) by continuous intravenous infusion, it is advisable to use a precision volume control device. An alternative maintenance schedule is to infuse the diluted solution at a dosage of 5 to 10 mg BRETYLOL per kg body weight, over a period greater than 8 minutes, every 6 hours. More rapid infusion may cause nausea and vomiting.

B. **Other Ventricular Arrhythmias:**
1. Intravenous Use: **BRETYLOL must be diluted as described above before intravenous use.**
Administer the diluted solution at a dosage of 5 to 10 mg BRETYLOL per kg of body weight by intravenous infusion over a period greater than 8 minutes. More rapid infusion may cause nausea and vomiting. Subsequent doses may be given at 1 to 2 hour intervals if the arrhythmia persists.
For maintenance therapy, the same dosage may be administered every 6 hours, or a constant infusion of 1 to 2 mg BRETYLOL per minute may be given. (See table.)
2. For intramuscular Injection: **Do not dilute BRETYLOL prior to intramuscular injection.** Inject 5 to 10 mg BRETYLOL per kg of body weight. Subsequent doses may be given at 1 to 2 hour intervals if the arrhythmia persists. Thereafter maintain the same dosage every 6 to 8 hours.
Intramuscular injection should not be made directly into or near a major nerve, and the site of injection should be varied on repeated injection. No more than 5 mL should be injected intramuscularly in one site. (See **PRECAUTIONS.**)

As soon as possible, and when indicated, patients should be changed to an oral antiarrhythmic agent for maintenance therapy.

HOW SUPPLIED

NDC 0590-0012-10: 10 mL ampul containing 500 mg bretylium tosylate packaged in cartons of 20.

NDC 0590-0012-37: 10 mL prefilled syringe containing 500 mg bretylium tosylate packaged in cartons of 5.

NDC 0590-0012-71: 10 mL single use vial containing 500 mg bretylium tosylate packaged in cartons of 20.

NDC 0590-0012-79: 20 mL single use vial containing 1 g bretylium tosylate packaged in cartons of 20.

Store at controlled room temperature 15°–30°C (59°–86°F).

Caution: Federal (USA) law prohibits dispensing without prescription.

Du Pont Pharmaceuticals
Manati, Puerto Rico 00674
6229-1/Rev. Jan., 1991

Continued on next page

Du Pont Multi-Source—Cont.

CALCIPARINE® ℞

[*cal-cĭ'pŭ-rin*]
(heparin calcium)
INJECTION

For Subcutaneous and IV Use

DESCRIPTION

Heparin is a heterogenous group of straight-chain anionic mucopolysaccharides, called glycosaminoglycans having anticoagulant properties. Although others may be present, the main sugars occurring in heparin are: (1) α-L-iduronic acid 2-sulfate, (2) 2-deoxy-2-sulfamino-α-D-glucose 6-sulfate, (3) β-D-glucuronic acid, (4) 2-acetamido-2-deoxy-α-D-glucose, and (5) α-L-iduronic acid. These sugars are present in decreasing amounts, usually in the order (2) > (1) > (4) > (3) > (5), and are joined by glycosidic linkages, forming polymers of varying sizes. Heparin is strongly acidic because of its content of covalently linked sulfate and carboxylic acid groups. In heparin calcium, the acidic protons of the sulfate units are replaced by calcium ions.

Calciparine (heparin calcium injection) is a sterile solution of heparin calcium derived from porcine intestinal mucosa, standardized for anticoagulant activity. It is to be administered by intravenous or deep subcutaneous routes. The potency is determined by a biological assay using a USP reference standard based on units of heparin activity per milligram. Each mL of Calciparine contains 25,000 USP heparin units in Water for Injection. Calcium hydroxide and/or hydrochloric acid may have been added during manufacture to adjust pH to approximately 7.

CLINICAL PHARMACOLOGY

Heparin inhibits reactions that lead to the clotting of blood and the formation of fibrin clots both *in vitro* and *in vivo*. Heparin acts at multiple sites in the normal coagulation system. Small amounts of heparin in combination with antithrombin III (heparin cofactor) can inhibit thrombosis by inactivating activated Factor X and inhibiting the conversion of prothrombin to thrombin. Once active thrombosis has developed, larger amounts of heparin can inhibit further coagulation by inactivating thrombin and preventing the conversion of fibrinogen to fibrin. Heparin also prevents the formation of a stable fibrin clot by inhibiting the activation of the fibrin stabilizing factor.

Bleeding time is usually unaffected by heparin. Clotting time is prolonged by full therapeutic doses of heparin; in most cases, it is not measurably affected by low doses of heparin.

Peak plasma levels of heparin are achieved 2–4 hours following subcutaneous administration, although there are considerable individual variations. Loglinear plots of heparin plasma concentrations with time for a wide range of dose levels are linear which suggests the absence of zero order processes. Liver and the reticulo-endothelial system are the site of biotransformation. The biphasic elimination curve, a rapidly declining alpha phase ($t_{1/2} = 10$ minutes) and after the age of 40 a slower beta phase, indicates uptake in organs. The absence of a relationship between anticoagulant half-life and concentration half-life may reflect factors such as protein binding of heparin.

Heparin does not have fibrinolytic activity; therefore, it will not lyse existing clots.

INDICATIONS AND USAGE

Calciparine is indicated for:

Anticoagulant therapy in prophylaxis and treatment of venous thrombosis and its extension;

In a low-dose regimen for prevention of postoperative deep venous thrombosis and pulmonary embolism in patients undergoing major abdomino-thoracic surgery or who for other reasons are at risk of developing thromboembolic disease (see DOSAGE AND ADMINISTRATION);

Prophylaxis and treatment of pulmonary embolism;

Atrial fibrillation with embolization;

Diagnosis and treatment of acute and chronic consumption coagulopathies (disseminated intravascular coagulation);

Prevention of clotting in arterial and heart surgery;

Prophylaxis and treatment of peripheral arterial embolism;

As an anticoagulant in blood transfusions, extracorporeal circulation, and dialysis procedures and in blood samples for laboratory purposes.

CONTRAINDICATIONS

Heparin calcium should not be used in patients:

With severe thrombocytopenia;

In whom suitable blood coagulation tests—e.g., the whole-blood clotting time, partial thromboplastin time, etc.—cannot be performed at appropriate intervals (this contraindication refers to full-dose heparin; there is usually no need to monitor coagulation parameters in patients receiving low-dose heparin);

With an uncontrollable active bleeding state (see WARNINGS), except when this is due to disseminated intravascular coagulation.

WARNINGS

Heparin is not intended for intramuscular use.

Hypersensitivity: Patients with documented hypersensitivity to heparin should be given the drug only in clearly life-threatening situations.

Hemorrhage: Hemorrhage can occur at virtually any site in patients receiving heparin. An unexplained fall in hematocrit, fall in blood pressure, or any other unexplained symptom should lead to serious consideration of a hemorrhagic event.

Heparin calcium should be used with extreme caution in disease states in which there is increased danger of hemorrhage. Some of the conditions in which increased danger of hemorrhage exists are:

Cardiovascular—Subacute bacterial endocarditis. Severe hypertension.

Surgical—During and immediately following (a) spinal tap or spinal anesthesia or (b) major surgery, especially involving the brain, spinal cord, or eye.

Hematologic—Conditions associated with increased bleeding tendencies, such as hemophilia, thrombocytopenia, and some vascular purpuras.

Gastrointestinal—Ulcerative lesions and continuous tube drainage of the stomach or small intestine.

Other—Menstruation, liver disease with impaired hemostasis.

Coagulation Testing: When Calciparine is administered in therapeutic amounts, its dosage should be regulated by frequent blood coagulation tests. If the coagulation test is unduly prolonged or if hemorrhage occurs, Calciparine should be discontinued promptly (see OVERDOSAGE).

Thrombocytopenia: Thrombocytopenia has been reported to occur in patients receiving heparin with a reported incidence of 0 to 30%. Mild thrombocytopenia (count greater than 100,000/mm^3) may remain stable or reverse even if heparin is continued. However, thrombocytopenia of any degree should be monitored closely. If the count falls below 100,000/mm^3 or if recurrent thrombosis develops (see White Clot Syndrome, PRECAUTIONS), Calciparine should be discontinued. If continued heparin therapy is essential, administration of heparin from a different organ source can be reinstituted with caution.

PRECAUTIONS

1. *General:*

a. White Clot Syndrome:

Rare patients on heparin may develop new thrombus formation in association with thrombocytopenia resulting from irreversible aggregation of platelets induced by heparin, the so-called "white clot syndrome." The process may lead to severe thromboembolic complications like skin necrosis, gangrene of the extremities, myocardial infarction, pulmonary embolism, and stroke. Therefore, heparin administration should be promptly discontinued if a patient develops new thrombosis in association with thrombocytopenia.

b. Heparin Resistance:

Increased resistance to heparin is frequently encountered in fever, thrombosis, thrombophlebitis, infections with thrombosing tendencies, myocardial infarction, cancer and in postsurgical patients.

c. Increased Risk in Older Women:

A higher incidence of bleeding has been reported in women over 60 years of age.

2. *Laboratory Tests:*

Periodic platelet counts, hematocrits, and tests for occult blood in stool are recommended during the entire course of heparin therapy, regardless of the route of administration (see DOSAGE AND ADMINISTRATION).

3. *Drug Interactions:*

Oral anticoagulants: Calciparine may prolong the one-stage prothrombin time. Therefore, when Calciparine is given with dicumarol or warfarin sodium, a period of at least 5 hours after the last intravenous dose or 24 hours after the last subcutaneous dose should elapse before blood is drawn if a valid prothrombin time is to be obtained.

Platelet Inhibitors: Coadministration of drugs which interfere with platelet aggregation (the main hemostatic defense of heparinized patients) result in an additive or synergistic pharmacologic activity and can result in an increased risk of bleeding. They should be used with caution in patients receiving heparin calcium; these include:

Penicillins: High doses of parenteral penicillins should be avoided during coadministration of heparin.

Cephalosporins, especially those that possess methylthiotetrazole side chain (moxolactam, cefamandole, cefotetan and cefoperazone).

Salicylates, non-steroidal anti-inflammatory drugs, dextran and both ionic and non-ionic contract media agents.

Other interactions: Patients receiving intravenous nitroglycerin require higher doses of heparin for effective anticoagulation. On stopping nitroglycerin therapy, the partial thromboplastin time (PTT) can rise markedly, unless the heparin dosage is decreased. Close monitoring of the PTT is required to maintain adequate anticoagulant effect whenever these drugs are used in combination and to avoid excessive bleeding when therapy with nitroglycerin is terminated or the dosage decreased.

Antibiotics: Interactions between heparin and streptomycin, neomycin, polymyxin B and M, gentamicin, erythromycin and tetracyclines can result in the loss of antimicrobial activity of the antibiotic, loss of anticoagulant effect of heparin or both.

Phenothiazines, ascorbic acid, nicotine, antihistamines and digitaloids antagonize the antithrombotic activity of heparin.

4. *Drug/Laboratory Tests Interactions:*

Hyperaminotransferasemia:

Significant elevations of aminotransferase (SGOT [S-AST] and SGPT [S-ALT]) levels have occurred in a high percentage of patients (and healthy subjects) who have received heparin. Since aminotransferase determinations are important in the differential diagnosis of myocardial infarction, liver disease, and pulmonary emboli, rises that might be caused by drugs (like heparin) should be interpreted with caution.

5. *Carcinogenesis, Mutagenesis, Impairment of Fertility:*

No long-term studies in animals have been performed to evaluate carcinogenic potential of heparin. Also, no reproduction studies in animals have been performed concerning mutagenesis or impairment of fertility.

6. *Pregnancy:*

Teratogenic Effects: Pregnancy Category C. Animal reproduction studies have not been conducted with heparin calcium. It is also not known whether heparin calcium can cause fetal harm when administered to a pregnant woman or can affect reproduction capacity. Calciparine should be given to a pregnant woman only if clearly needed.

Nonteratogenic Effects: Heparin does not cross the placental barrier.

7. *Nursing Mothers:*

Heparin is not excreted in human milk.

8. *Pediatric Use:*

See DOSAGE AND ADMINISTRATION.

ADVERSE REACTIONS

1. Hemorrhage.

Hemorrhage from any tissue or organ is the chief complication that may result from heparin therapy (see WARNINGS). The signs and symptoms will vary according to the location and extent of bleeding and may present as paralysis, headache, chest, abdomen, joint or other pain, shortness of breath, difficult breathing or swallowing, unexplained swelling or unexplained shock. An overly prolonged clotting time or minor bleeding during therapy can usually be controlled by withdrawing the drug (see OVERDOSAGE). *It should be appreciated that gastrointestinal or urinary tract bleeding during anticoagulant therapy may indicate the presence of an underlying occult lesion.* Bleeding can occur at any site but certain specific hemorrhagic complications may be difficult to detect:

a. Adrenal hemorrhage, with resultant acute adrenal insufficiency, has occurred during anticoagulant therapy. Therefore, such treatment should be discontinued in patients who develop signs and symptoms of acute adrenal hemorrhage and insufficiency. Initiation of corrective therapy should not depend on laboratory confirmation of the diagnosis, since any delay in an acute situation may result in the patient's death.

b. Ovarian (corpus luteum) hemorrhage developed in a number of women of reproductive age receiving short- or long-term anticoagulant therapy. This complication if unrecognized may be fatal.

c. Retroperitoneal hemorrhage.

2. Local Irritation.

Local irritation, erythema, mild pain, hematoma or ulceration may follow deep subcutaneous (intrafat) injection of heparin calcium. These complications are much more common after intramuscular use, and such use is not recommended.

3. Hypersensitivity.

Generalized hypersensitivity reactions have been reported, with chills, fever, and urticaria as the most usual manifestations, and asthma, rhinitis, lacrimation, headache, nausea and vomiting, and anaphylactoid reactions, including shock, occurring more rarely. Itching and burning, especially on the plantar site of the feet, may occur.

Thrombocytopenia has been reported to occur in patients receiving heparin with a reported incidence of 0–30%. While often mild and of no obvious clinical significance, such thrombocytopenia can be accompanied by severe thromboembolic complications such as skin necrosis, gangrene of the extremities, myocardial infarction, pulmonary embolism, and stroke. (See WARNINGS, PRECAUTIONS.)

Certain episodes of painful, ischemic, and cyanosed limbs have in the past been attributed to allergic vasopastic reactions. Whether these are in fact identical to the thrombocytopenia associated complications remains to be determined.

METHOD OF ADMINISTRATION	FREQUENCY	RECOMMENDED DOSE*
Deep Subcuatneous (Intrafat) Injection A different site should be used for each injection to prevent the development of massive hematoma.	Initial Dose	5,000 units by I.V. injection, followed by 10,000–20,000 units of a concentrated solution, subcutaneously
	Every 8 hours or	8,000–10,000 units of a concentrated solution
	Every 12 hours	15,000–20,000 units of a concentrated solution
Intermittent Intravenous Injection	Initial dose	10,000 units, either undiluted or in 50–100 mL of 0.9% Sodium Chloride Injection, USP
	Every 4 to 6 Hours	5,000–10,000 units, either undiluted or in 50–100 mL of 0.9% Sodium Chloride Injection, USP
Continuous Intravenous Infusion	Initial Dose	5,000 units by I.V. Injection
	Continuous	20,000–40,000 units/24 hours in 1,000 mL of 0.9% Sodium Chloride Injection, USP (or in any compatible solution) for infusion

*Based on 150-lb. (68-kg) patient.

4. Miscellaneous
Osteoporosis following long-term administration of high-doses of heparin, cutaneous necrosis after systemic administration, suppression of aldosterone synthesis, delayed transient alopecia, priapism, and rebound hyperlipemia on discontinuation of heparin calcium have also been reported.
Significant elevations of aminotransferase (SGOT [S-AST] and SGPT [S-ALT]) levels have occurred in a high percentage of patients (and healthy subjects) who have received heparin.

OVERDOSAGE

Symptoms: Bleeding is the chief sign of heparin overdosage. Nosebleeds, blood in urine or tarry stools may be noted as the first sign of bleeding. Easy bruising or petechial formations may precede frank bleeding.
Treatment: Neutralization of heparin effect:
When clinical circumstances (bleeding) require reversal of heparinization, protamine sulfate (1% solution) by slow infusion will neutralize heparin calcium. *No more than 50 mg* should be administered, *very slowly,* in any 10 minute period. Each mg of protamine sulfate neutralizes approximately 100 USP heparin units. The amount of protamine required decreases over time as heparin is metabolized. Although the metabolism of heparin is complex, it may, for the purpose of choosing a protamine dose, be assumed to have a half-life of about ½ hour after intravenous injection.
Administration of protamine sulfate can cause severe hypotensive and anaphylactoid reactions. Because fatal reactions often resembling anaphylaxis have been reported, the drug should be given only when resuscitation techniques and treatment of anaphylactoid shock are readily available.
For additional information the labeling of Protamine Sulfate Injection, USP products should be consulted.

DOSAGE AND ADMINISTRATION

Parenteral drug products should be inspected visually for particulate matter and discoloration prior to administration, whenever solution and container permit. Slight discoloration does not alter potency.
When heparin is added to an infusion solution for continuous intravenous administration, the container should be inverted at least six times to insure adequate mixing and prevent pooling of the heparin in the solution.
Calciparine (heparin calcium) is not effective by oral administration and should be given by intermittent intravenous injection, intravenous infusion, or deep subcutaneous (intrafat, i.e., above the iliac crest or abdominal fat layer) injection. *The intramuscular route of administration should be avoided because of the frequent occurrence of hematoma at the injection site.*
The dosage of Calciparine should be adjusted according to the patient's coagulation test results. When heparin is given by continuous intravenous infusion, the coagulation time should be determined approximately every 4 hours in the early stages of treatment. When the drug is administered intermittently by intravenous injection, coagulation tests should be performed before each injection during the early stages of treatment and at appropriate intervals thereafter. Dosage is considered adequate when the activated partial thromboplastin time (APTT) is 1.5 to 2 times normal or when the whole blood clotting time is elevated approximately 2.5 to 3 times the control value. After deep subcutaneous (intrafat) injections, tests for adequacy of dosage are best performed on samples drawn 4–6 hours after the injections.
Periodic platelet counts, hematocrits, and tests for occult blood in stool are recommended during the entire course of heparin therapy, regardless of the route of administration.
Converting to Oral Anticoagulant When an oral anticoagulant of the coumarin or similar type is to be begun in patients already receiving Calciparine, baseline and subsequent tests of prothrombin activity must be determined at a time when heparin activity is too low to affect the prothrombin time. This is about 5 hours after the last I.V. bolus and 24 hours after the last subcutaneous dose. If continuous I.V. heparin infusion is used, prothrombin time can usually be measured at any time.
In converting from Calciparine to an oral anticoagulant, the dose of the oral anticoagulant should be the usual initial amount and thereafter prothrombin time should be determined at the usual intervals. To ensure continuous anticoagulation, it is advisable to continue full Calciparine therapy for several days after the prothrombin time has reached the therapeutic range. Calciparine therapy may then be discontinued without tapering.

Therapeutic Anticoagulant Effect with Full-Dose Calciparine

Although dosage must be adjusted for the individual patient according to the results of suitable laboratory tests, the following dosage schedules may be used as guidelines:
[See table above.]
Pediatric Use Follow recommendations of appropriate pediatric reference texts. In general, the following dosage schedule may be used as a guideline:
Initial Dose: 50 units/kg (I.V., drip)
Maintenance Dose: 100 units/kg (I.V., drip) every four hours, or 20,000 units/M^2/24 hours continuously
Surgery of the Heart and Blood Vessels Patients undergoing total body perfusion for open-heart surgery should receive an initial dose of not less than 150 units of heparin calcium per kilogram of body weight. Frequently, a dose of 300 units per kilogram is used for procedures estimated to last less than 60 minutes or 400 units per kilogram for those estimated to last longer than 60 minutes.
Low-Dose Prophylaxis of Postoperative Thromboembolism A number of well-controlled clinical trials have demonstrated that low-dose heparin prophylaxis, given just prior to and after surgery, will reduce the incidence of postoperative deep vein thrombosis in the legs (as measured by the I–125 fibrinogen technique and venography) and of clinical pulmonary embolism. The most widely used dosage has been 5,000 units 2 hours before surgery and 5,000 units every 8 to 12 hours thereafter for 7 days or until the patient is fully ambulatory, whichever is longer. The heparin is given by deep subcutaneous (intrafat, i.e., above the iliac crest or abdominal fat layer, arm or thigh) injection with a fine (25 to 26 gauge) needle to minimize tissue trauma. A concentrated solution of Calciparine (heparin calcium) is recommended. Such prophylaxis should be reserved for patients over the age of 40 who are undergoing major surgery. Patients with bleeding disorders and those having brain or spinal core surgery, spinal anesthesia, eye surgery, or potentially sanguineous operations should be excluded, as should patients receiving oral anticoagulants or platelet-active drugs (see WARNINGS). The value of such prophylaxis in hip surgery has not been established. The possibility of increased bleeding during surgery or postoperatively should be borne in mind. If such bleeding occurs, discontinuance of Calciparine and neutralization with protamine sulfate are advisable. If clinical evidence of thromboembolism develops despite low-dose prophylaxis, full therapeutic doses of anticoagulants should be given unless contraindicated. Prior to initiating heparinization, the physician should rule out bleeding disorders by appropriate history and laboratory tests, and appropriate coagulation tests should be repeated just prior to surgery. Coagulation tests values should be normal or only slightly elevated at these times.
Extracorporeal Dialysis Follow equipment manufacturers' operating directions carefully.
Blood Transfusion Addition of 400 to 600 USP units per 100 mL of whole blood is usually employed to prevent coagulation. Usually, 7,500 USP units of heparin calcium are added to 100 mL of 0.9% Sodium Chloride Injection, USP (or 75,000 USP units per 1,000 mL of 0.9% Sodium Chloride Injection, USP) and mixed; from this sterile solution, 6 to 8 mL are added per 100 mL of whole blood.
Laboratory Samples Addition of 70 to 150 units of heparin calcium per 10 to 20 mL sample of whole blood is usually employed to prevent coagulation of the sample. Leukocyte counts should be performed on heparinized blood within 2 hours after addition of the Calciparine. Heparinized blood should not be used for isoagglutinin, complement, or erythrocyte fragility tests or platelet counts.
Clearing Intermittent Infusion (Heparin Lock) Sets: To prevent clot formation in a heparin lock set following its proper insertion, dilute heparin solution (Heparin Lock Flush Solution, USP) is injected via the injection hub in a quantity sufficient to fill the entire set to the needle tip. This solution should be replaced each time the heparin lock is used. Aspirate before administering any solution via the lock in order to confirm patency and location of needle or catheter tip. If the drug to be administered is incompatible with heparin, the entire heparin lock set should be flushed with sterile water or normal saline before and after the medication is administered; following the second flush, the dilute heparin solution may be reinstilled into the set. The set manufacturer's instructions should be consulted for specifics concerning the heparin lock set in use at a given time.
NOTE: Since repeated injections of small doses of heparin can alter tests for activated partial thromboplastin time (APTT), a baseline value for APTT should be obtained prior to insertion of a heparin lock set.

HOW SUPPLIED

Calciparine (heparin calcium injection) is available as follows:
Calciparine 5,000 USP heparin units, 0.2 mL pre-filled disposable syringe, carton of 10, NDC 0056-0030-02.
Store at room temperature. Protect from freezing.
Caution: Federal law prohibits dispensing without prescription.
Distributed by
Du Pont Pharmaceuticals
Wilmington, Delaware 19880
Under license from Choay Laboratories Inc.
New York, NY
6267/Rev. Mar., 1991

INTROPIN® ℞
[in-trō'pin]
(dopamine HCl injection, USP)

DESCRIPTION

INTROPIN (dopamine HCl injection, USP) is a clear, practically colorless, aqueous, additive solution for intravenous infusion after dilution. Each mL contains either 40 mg, 80 mg, or 160 mg dopamine HCl, USP (equivalent to 32.3 mg, 64.6 mg and 129.2 mg dopamine base, respectively) in Water for Injection, USP containing 1% sodium metabisulfite, NF as an antioxidant. Hydrochloric acid or sodium hydroxide added to adjust pH when necessary. The solution is sterile and nonpyrogenic. The pH is 2.5-4.5. Dopamine HCl, a naturally occurring catecholamine, is an inotropic vasopressor agent. Its chemical name is 3,4-dihydroxyphenethylamine hydrochloride. The molecular weight is 189.65. Dopamine HCl is sensitive to alkalis, iron salts and oxidizing agents. **INTROPIN must be diluted in an appropriate, sterile parenteral solution** (see DOSAGE AND ADMINISTRATION section) **before intravenous administration.**

ACTIONS

INTROPIN exerts an inotropic effect on the myocardium resulting in an increased cardiac output. INTROPIN produces less increase in myocardial oxygen consumption than isoproterenol and its use is usually not associated with a tachyarrhythmia. Clinical studies indicate that INTROPIN usually increases systolic and pulse pressure with either no effect or a slight increase in diastolic pressure. Total peripheral resistance at low and intermediate therapeutic doses is usually unchanged. Blood flow to peripheral vascular beds may decrease while mesenteric flow increases. INTROPIN has also been reported to dilate the renal vasculature presumptively by activation of a "dopaminergic" receptor. This action is accompanied by increases in glomerular filtration rate, renal blood flow, and sodium excretion. An increase in urinary output produced by dopamine is usually not associated with a decrease in osmolality of the urine.

INDICATIONS

INTROPIN is indicated for the correction of hemodynamic imbalances present in the shock syndrome due to myocardial infarctions, trauma, endotoxic septicemia, open heart surgery, renal failure, and chronic cardiac decompensation as in congestive failure.

Continued on next page

Du Pont Multi-Source—Cont.

Where appropriate, restoration of blood volume with a suitable plasma expander or whole blood should be instituted or completed prior to administration of INTROPIN.
Patients most likely to respond adequately to INTROPIN are those in whom physiological parameters, such as urine flow, myocardial function, and blood pressure, have not undergone profound deterioration. Multiclinic trials indicate that the shorter the time interval between onset of signs and symptoms and initiation of therapy with volume correction and INTROPIN, the better the prognosis.
Poor Perfusion of Vital Organs—Urine flow appears to be one of the better diagnostic signs by which adequacy of vital organ perfusion can be monitored. Nevertheless, the physician should also observe the patient for signs of reversal of confusion or comatose condition. Loss of pallor, increase in toe temperature, and/or adequacy of nail bed capillary filling may also be used as indices of adequate dosage. Clinical studies have shown that when INTROPIN is administered before urine flow has diminished to levels approximating 0.3 mL/minute, prognosis is more favorable. Nevertheless, in a number of oliguric or anuric patients, administration of INTROPIN has resulted in an increase in urine flow which in some cases reached normal levels. INTROPIN may also increase urine flow in patients whose output is within normal limits and thus may be of value in reducing the degree of preexisting fluid accumulation. It should be noted that at doses above those optimal for the individual patient, urine flow may decrease, necessitating reduction of dosage. Concurrent administration of INTROPIN and diuretic agents may produce an additive or potentiating effect.
Low Cardiac Output—Increased cardiac output is related to the direct inotropic effect of INTROPIN on the myocardium. Increased cardiac output at low or moderate doses appears to be related to a favorable prognosis. Increase in cardiac output has been associated with either static or decreased systemic vascular resistance (SVR). Static or decreased SVR associated with low or moderate increments in cardiac output is believed to be a reflection of differential effects on specific vascular beds with increased resistance in peripheral beds (e.g. femoral) and concomitant decreases in mesenteric and renal vascular beds. Redistribution of blood flow parallels these changes so that an increase in cardiac output is accompanied by an increase in mesenteric and renal blood flow. In many instances the renal fraction of the total cardiac output has been found to increase. The increase in cardiac output produced by INTROPIN is not associated with substantial decreases in systemic vascular resistance as may occur with isoproterenol.
Hypotension—Hypotension due to inadequate cardiac output can be managed by administration of low to moderate doses of INTROPIN, which have little effect on SVR. At high therapeutic doses, the alpha adrenergic activity of INTROPIN becomes more prominent and thus may correct hypotension due to diminished SVR. As in the case of other circulatory decompensation states, prognosis is better in patients whose blood pressure and urine flow have not undergone profound deterioration. Therefore, it is suggested that the physician administer INTROPIN as soon as a definite trend toward decreased systolic and diastolic pressure becomes evident.

CONTRAINDICATIONS

INTROPIN should not be used in patients with pheochromocytoma.

WARNINGS

INTROPIN should not be administered in the presence of uncorrected tachyarrhythmias or ventricular fibrillation.
Do **NOT** add INTROPIN to any alkaline diluent solution, since the drug is inactivated in alkaline solution.
Patients who have been treated with monoamine oxidase (MAO) inhibitors prior to the administration of INTROPIN will require substantially reduced dosage. Dopamine is metabolized by MAO, and inhibition of this enzyme prolongs and potentiates the effect of INTROPIN. The starting dose in such patients should be reduced to at least one-tenth ($^1/_{10}$) of the usual dose.
Contains sodium metabisulfite, a sulfite that may cause allergic-type reactions including anaphylactic symptoms and life-threatening or less severe asthmatic episodes in certain susceptible people. The overall prevalence of sulfite sensitivity in the general population is unknown, and probably low. Sulfite sensitivity is seen more frequently in asthmatic than in nonasthmatic people.

PRECAUTIONS: General

Avoid Hypovolemia—Prior to treatment with INTROPIN, hypovolemia should be fully corrected, if possible, with either whole blood or plasma as indicated.
Decreased Pulse Pressure—If a disproportionate rise in the diastolic pressure (i.e., a marked decrease in the pulse pressure) is observed in patients receiving INTROPIN, the infusion rate should be decreased and the patient observed carefully for further evidence of predominant vasoconstrictor activity, unless such an effect is desired.
Extravasation—INTROPIN should be infused into a large vein whenever possible to prevent the possibility of extravasation into tissue adjacent to the infusion site. Extravasation may cause necrosis and sloughing of surrounding tissue. Large veins of the antecubital fossa are preferred to veins in the dorsum of the hand or ankle. Less suitable infusion sites should be used only if the patient's condition requires immediate attention. The physician should switch to more suitable sites as rapidly as possible. The infusion site should be continuously monitored for free flow.
Occlusive Vascular Disease—Patients with a history of occlusive vascular disease (for example, atherosclerosis, arterial embolism, Raynaud's disease, cold injury, diabetic endarteritis, and Buerger's disease) should be closely monitored for any changes in color or temperature of the skin in the extremities. If a change in skin color or temperature occurs and is thought to be the result of compromised circulation to the extremities, the benefits of continued INTROPIN infusion should be weighed against the risk of possible necrosis. This condition may be reversed by either decreasing or discontinuing the rate of infusion.

IMPORTANT—Antidote for Peripheral Ischemia: To prevent sloughing and necrosis in ischemic areas, the area should be infiltrated as soon as possible with 10 to 15 mL of saline solution containing from 5 to 10 mg of Regitine® (brand of phentolamine), an adrenergic blocking agent. A syringe with a fine hypodermic needle should be used, and the solution liberally infiltrated throughout the ischemic area. Sympathetic blockade with phentolamine causes immediate and conspicuous local hyperemic changes if the area is infiltrated within 12 hours. Therefore, phentolamine should be given as soon as possible after the extravasation is noted.

Avoid Cyclopropane or Halogenated Hydrocarbon Anesthetics—Cyclopropane or halogenated hydrocarbon anesthetics increase cardiac autonomic irritability and therefore may sensitize the myocardium to the action of certain intravenously administered catecholamines. This interaction appears to be related both to pressor activity and to beta adrenergic stimulating properties of these catecholamines. Therefore, as with certain other catecholamines, and because of the theoretical arrhythmogenic potential, INTROPIN should be used with EXTREME CAUTION in patients inhaling cyclopropane or halogenated hydrocarbon anesthetics.
Careful Monitoring Required—Close monitoring of the following indices—urine flow, cardiac output and blood pressure—during INTROPIN (dopamine HCl injection, USP) infusion is necessary as in the case of any adrenergic agent.
Pregnancy—Pregnancy Category C. Animal studies have revealed no evidence of teratogenic effects from INTROPIN. In one study, administration of INTROPIN to pregnant rats resulted in a decreased survival rate of the newborn and a potential for cataract formation in the survivors. There are no adequate and well-controlled studies in pregnant women. INTROPIN should be used during pregnancy only if the potential benefit justifies the potential risk to the fetus.
Pediatric Use—Safety and effectiveness in children have not been established.

ADVERSE REACTIONS

The most frequent adverse reactions observed in clinical evaluation of INTROPIN included ectopic beats, nausea, vomiting, tachycardia, anginal pain, palpitation, dyspnea, headache, hypotension, and vasoconstriction. Other adverse reactions which have been reported infrequently were aberrant conduction, bradycardia, piloerection, widened QRS complex, azotemia, and elevated blood pressure.

DOSAGE AND ADMINISTRATION

WARNING: This is a potent drug: It must be diluted before administration to patient.
Suggested Dilution—Transfer contents of one or more ampuls, vials or additive syringes by aseptic technique to either a 250 mL or 500 mL bottle of one of the following sterile intravenous solutions:
1) Sodium Chloride Injection, USP
2) Dextrose (5%) Injection, USP
3) Dextrose (5%) and Sodium Chloride (0.9%) Injection, USP
4) 5% Dextrose in 0.45% Sodium Chloride Solution
5) Dextrose (5%) in Lactated Ringer's Solution
6) Sodium Lactate ($^1/_6$ Molar) Injection, USP
7) Lactated Ringer's Injection, USP

INTROPIN has been found to be stable for a minimum of 24 hours after dilution in the sterile intravenous solutions listed above. However, as with all intravenous admixtures, dilution should be made just prior to administration.
Do **NOT** add INTROPIN Injection to Sodium Bicarbonate or other alkaline intravenous solutions, since the drug is inactivated in alkaline solution.
Rate of Administration—INTROPIN, after dilution, is administered intravenously through a suitable intravenous catheter or needle. An i.v. drip chamber or other suitable metering device is essential for controlling the rate of flow in drops/minute. Each patient must be individually titrated to the desired hemodynamic and/or renal response with INTROPIN. In titrating to the desired increase in systolic blood pressure, the optimum dosage rate for renal response may be exceeded, thus necessitating a reduction in rate after the hemodynamic condition is stablized.
Administration at rates greater than 50 mcg/kg/minute have safely been used in advanced circulatory decompensation states. If unnecessary fluid expansion is of concern, adjustment of drug concentration may be preferred over increasing the flow rate of a less concentrated dilution.
Suggested Regimen:
1. When appropriate, increase blood volume with whole blood or plasma until central venous pressure is 10 to 15 cm H_2O or pulmonary wedge pressure is 14–18 mm Hg.
2. Begin administration of diluted solution at doses of 2–5 mcg/kg/minute INTROPIN in patients who are likely to respond to modest increments of heart force and renal perfusion.
In more seriously ill patients, begin administration of diluted solution at doses of 5 mcg/kg/minute INTROPIN and increase gradually using 5 to 10 mcg/kg/minute increments up to 20 to 50 mcg/kg/minute as needed. If doses of INTROPIN in excess of 50 mcg/kg/minute are required, it is suggested that urine output be checked frequently. Should urine flow begin to decrease in the absence of hypotension, reduction of INTROPIN dosage should be considered. Multiclinic trials have shown that more than 50% of the patients were satisfactorily maintained on doses of INTROPIN less than 20 mcg/kg/minute. In patients who do not respond to these doses with adequate arterial pressures or urine flow, additional increments of INTROPIN may be employed in an effort to produce an appropriate arterial pressure and central perfusion.
3. Treatment of all patients requires constant evaluation of therapy in terms of the blood volume, augmentation of myocardial contractility, and distribution of peripheral perfusion. Dosage of INTROPIN should be adjusted according to the patient's response, with particular attention to diminution of established urine flow rate, increasing tachycardia or development of new dysrhythmias as indices for decreasing or temporarily suspending the dosage.
4. As with all potent intravenously administered drugs, care should be taken to control the rate of administration so as to avoid inadvertent administration of a bolus of drug.

OVERDOSAGE

In case of accidental overdosage, as evidenced by excessive blood pressure elevation, reduce rate of administration or temporarily discontinue INTROPIN until patient's condition stabilizes. Since the duration of action of INTROPIN is quite short, no additional remedial measures are usually necessary. If these measures fail to stabilize the patient's condition, use of the short-acting alpha adrenergic blocking agent, phentolamine, should be considered.

HOW SUPPLIED

—200 mg (5 mL containing 40 mg dopamine HCl, USP per mL)
NDC 0590-0040-05—Ampul
NDC 0590-0040-06—Single-dose vial (color coded white)
—400 mg (5 mL containing 80 mg dopamine HCl, USP per mL)
NDC 0590-0046-06—Single-dose vial (color coded green)
—800 mg (5 mL containing 160 mg dopamine HCl, USP per mL)
NDC 0590-0047-06—Single-dose vial (color coded yellow)
Store at controlled room temperature 15°–30°C (59°–86°F).
Caution: Federal law prohibits dispensing without prescription.
WARNING: NOT FOR DIRECT INTRAVENOUS INJECTION. MUST BE DILUTED BEFORE USE.

Du Pont Pharmaceuticals
Manati, Puerto Rico 00674
6227-1/Rev. Jan., 1991

MOBAN® ℞

[mō'ban]
(molindone hydrochloride)

DESCRIPTION

MOBAN (molindone hydrochloride) is a dihydroindolone compound which is not structurally related to the phenothiazines, the butyrophenones or the thioxanthenes.
MOBAN is 3-ethyl-6, 7-dihydro-2-methyl-5-(morpholinomethyl) indol-4 (5H)-one hydrochloride. It is a white to off-white crystalline powder, freely soluble in water and alcohol and has a molecular weight of 312.67.

MOBAN Tablets also contain:

All strengths: calcium sulfate, lactose, magnesium stearate, microcrystalline cellulose and povidone.

  5 mg:　alginic acid, colloidal silicon dioxide and FD&C Yellow 6.
 10 mg:　alginic acid, colloidal silicon dioxide, FD&C Blue 2 and FD&C Red 40.
 25 mg:　alginic acid, colloidal silicon dioxide, D&C Yellow 10, FD&C Blue 2, and FD&C Yellow 6.
 50 mg:　FD&C Blue 2 and sodium starch glycolate.
100 mg:　FD&C Blue 2, FD&C Yellow 6 and sodium starch glycolate.

MOBAN Concentrate contains: alcohol, artificial cherry flavor, artificial cover flavor, edetate disodium, glycerin, liquid sugar, methylparaben, propylparaben, sodium metabisulfite, sorbitol solution, and hydrochloric acid reagent grade for pH adjustment.

ACTIONS

MOBAN (molindone hydrochloride) has a pharmacological profile in laboratory animals which predominantly resembles that of major tranquilizers causing reduction of spontaneous locomotion and aggressiveness, suppression of a conditioned response and antagonism of the bizarre stereotyped behavior and hyperactivity induced by amphetamines. In addition, MOBAN antagonizes the depression caused by the tranquilizing agent tetrabenazine.

In human clinical studies tranquilization is achieved in the absence of muscle relaxing or incoordinating effects. Based on EEG studies, MOBAN exerts its effect on the ascending reticular activating system.

Human metabolic studies show MOBAN (molindone hydrochloride) to be rapidly absorbed and metabolized when given orally. Unmetabolized drug reached a peak blood level at 1.5 hours. Pharmacological effect from a single oral dose persists for 24-36 hours. There are 36 recognized metabolites with less than 2-3% unmetabolized MOBAN being excreted in urine and feces.

INDICATIONS

MOBAN is indicated for the management of the manifestations of psychotic disorders. The antipsychotic efficacy of MOBAN was established in clinical studies which enrolled newly hospitalized and chronically hospitalized, acutely ill, schizophrenic patients as subjects.

CONTRAINDICATIONS

MOBAN (molindone hydrochloride) is contraindicated in severe central nervous system depression (alcohol, barbiturates, narcotics, etc.) or comatose states, and in patients with known hypersensitivity to the drug.

WARNINGS

Tardive Dyskinesia: Tardive dyskinesia, a syndrome consisting of potentially irreversible, involuntary, dyskinetic movements may develop in patients treated with neuroleptic (antipsychotic) drugs. Although the prevalence of the syndrome appears to be highest among the elderly, especially elderly women, it is impossible to rely upon prevalence estimates to predict, at the inception of neuroleptic treatment, which patients are likely to develop the syndrome. Whether neuroleptic drug products differ in their potential to cause tardive dyskinesia is unknown.

Both the risk of developing the syndrome and the likelihood that it will become irreversible are believed to increase as the duration of treatment and the total cumulative dose of neuroleptic drugs administered to the patient increase. However, the syndrome can develop, although much less commonly, after relatively brief treatment periods at low doses.

There is no known treatment for established cases of tardive dyskinesia, although the syndrome may remit, partially or completely, if neuroleptic treatment is withdrawn. Neuroleptic treatment, itself, however, may suppress (or partially suppress) the signs and symptoms of the syndrome and thereby may possibly mask the underlying disease process. The effect that symptomatic suppression has upon the long-term course of the syndrome is unknown.

Given these considerations, neuroleptics should be prescribed in a manner that is most likely to minimize the occurrence of tardive dyskinesia. Chronic neuroleptic treatment should generally be reserved for patients who suffer from a chronic illness that, 1) is known to respond to neuroleptic drugs, and 2) for whom alternative, equally effective, but potentially less harmful treatments are not available or appropriate. In patients who do require chronic treatment, the smallest dose and the shortest duration of treatment producing a satisfactory clinical response should be sought. The need for continued treatment should be reassessed periodically.

If signs and symptoms of tardive dyskinesia appear in a patient on neuroleptics, drug discontinuation should be considered. However, some patients may require treatment despite the presence of the syndrome.

(For further information about the description of tardive dyskinesia and its clinical detection, please refer to the section on Adverse Reactions.)

Neuroleptic Malignant Syndrome (NMS)

A potentially fatal symptom complex sometimes referred to as Neuroleptic Malignant Syndrome (NMS) has been reported in association with antipsychotic drugs. Clinical manifestations of NMS are hyperpyrexia, muscle rigidity, altered mental status and evidence of autonomic instability (irregular pulse or blood pressure, tachycardia, diaphoresis, and cardiac dysrhythmias).

The diagnostic evaluation of patients with this syndrome is complicated. In arriving at a diagnosis, it is important to identify cases where the clinical presentation includes both serious medical illness (e.g., pneumonia, systemic infection, etc.) and untreated or inadequately treated extrapyramidal signs and symptoms (EPS). Other important considerations in the differential diagnosis include central anticholinergic toxicity, heat stroke, drug fever and primary central nervous system (CNS) pathology.

The management of NMS should include, 1) immediate discontinuation of antipsychotic drugs and other drugs not essential to concurrent therapy, 2) intensive symptomatic treatment and medical monitoring, and 3) treatment of any concomitant serious medical problems for which specific treatments are available. There is no general agreement about specific pharmacological treatment regimens for uncomplicated NMS.

If a patient requires antipsychotic drug treatment after recovery from NMS, the potential reintroduction of drug therapy should be carefully considered. The patient should be carefully monitored, since recurrences of NMS have been reported.

Usage in Pregnancy: Studies in pregnant patients have not been carried out. Reproduction studies have been performed in the following animals:

Pregnant Rats oral dose—	
no adverse effect	20 mg/kg/day—10 days
no adverse effect	40 mg/kg/day—10 days
Pregnant Mice oral dose—	
slight increase resorptions	20 mg/kg/day—10 days
slight increase resorptions	40 mg/kg/day—10 days
Pregnant Rabbits oral dose—	
no adverse effect	5 mg/kg/day—12 days
no adverse effect	10 mg/kg/day—12 days
no adverse effect	20 mg/kg/day—12 days

Animal reproductive studies have not demonstrated a teratogenic potential. The anticipated benefits must be weighed against the unknown risks to the fetus if used in pregnant patients.

Nursing Mothers: Data are not available on the content of MOBAN (molindone hydrochloride) in the milk of nursing mothers:

Usage in Children: Use of MOBAN (molindone hydrochloride) in children below the age of twelve years is not recommended because safe and effective conditions for its usage have not been established.

MOBAN has not been shown effective in the management of behavioral complications in patients with mental retardation.

Sulfites Sensitivity: MOBAN Concentrate contains sodium metabisulfite, a sulfite that may cause allergic-type reactions including anaphylactic symptoms and life-threatening or less severe asthmatic episodes in certain susceptible people. The overall prevalence of sulfite sensitivity in the general population is unknown and probably low. Sulfite sensitivity is seen more frequently in asthmatic than in nonasthmatic people.

PRECAUTIONS

Some patients receiving MOBAN (molindone hydrochloride) may note drowsiness initially and they should be advised against activities requiring mental alertness until their response to the drug has been established.

Increased activity has been noted in patients receiving MOBAN. Caution should be exercised where increased activity may be harmful.

MOBAN does not lower the seizure threshold in experimental animals to the degree noted with more sedating antipsychotic drugs. However, in humans convulsive seizures have been reported in a few instances.

The physician should be aware that this tablet preparation contains calcium sulfate as an excipient and that calcium ions may interfere with the absorption of preparations containing phenytoin sodium and tetracyclines.

MOBAN has an antiemetic effect in animals. A similar effect may occur in humans and may obscure signs of intestinal obstruction or brain tumor.

Neuroleptic drugs elevate prolactin levels; the elevation persists during chronic administration. Tissue culture experiments indicate that approximately one-third of human breast cancers are prolactin dependent in vitro, a factor of potential importance if the prescription of these drugs is contemplated in a patient with a previously detected breast cancer. Although disturbances such as galactorrhea, amenorrhea, gynecomastia, and impotence have been reported, the clinical significance of elevated serum prolactin levels is unknown for most patients. An increase in mammary neoplasms has been found in rodents after chronic administra-

tion of neuroleptic drugs. Neither clinical studies nor epidemiologic studies conducted to date, however, have shown an association between chronic administration of these drugs and mammary tumorigenesis; the available evidence is considered too limited to be conclusive at this time.

ADVERSE REACTIONS

CNS EFFECTS

The most frequently occurring effect is initial drowsiness that generally subsides with continued usage of the drug or lowering of the dose.

Noted less frequently were depression, hyperactivity and euphoria.

Neurological

Extrapyramidal Reactions

Extrapyramidal reactions noted below may occur in susceptible individuals and are usually reversible with appropriate management.

Akathisia

Motor restlessness may occur early.

Parkinson Syndrome

Akinesia, characterized by rigidity, immobility and reduction of voluntary movements and tremor, have been observed. Occurrence is less frequent than akathisia.

Dystonic Syndrome

Prolonged abnormal contractions of muscle groups occur infrequently. These symptoms may be managed by the addition of a synthetic antiparkinson agent (other than L-dopa), small doses of sedative drugs, and/or reduction in dosage.

Tardive Dyskinesia

Neuroleptic drugs are known to cause a syndrome of dyskinetic movements commonly referred to as tardive dyskinesia. The movements may appear during treatment or upon withdrawal of treatment and may be either reversible or irreversible (i.e., persistent) upon cessation of further neuroleptic administration.

The syndrome is known to have a variable latency for development and the duration of the latency cannot be determined reliably. It is thus wise to assume that any neuroleptic agent has the capacity to induce the syndrome and act accordingly until sufficient data has been collected to settle the issue definitively for a specific drug product. In the case of neuroleptics known to produce the irreversible syndrome, the following has been observed:

Tardive dyskinesia has appeared in some patients on long-term therapy and has also appeared after drug therapy has been discontinued. The risk appears to be greater in elderly patients on high-dose therapy, especially females. The symptoms are persistent and in some patients appear to be irreversible. The syndrome is characterized by rhythmical involuntary movements of the tongue, face, mouth or jaw (e.g., protrusion of tongue, puffing of cheeks, puckering of mouth, chewing movements). There may be involuntary movements of extremities.

There is no known effective treatment of tardive dyskinesia; antiparkinsonism agents usually do not alleviate the symptoms of this syndrome. It is suggested that all antipsychotic agents be discontinued if these symptoms appear. Should it be necessary to reinstitute treatment, or increase the dosage of the agent, or switch to a different antipsychotic agent, the syndrome may be masked. It has been reported that fine vermicular movements of the tongue may be an early sign of the syndrome and if the medication is stopped at that time the syndrome may not develop (see WARNINGS).

Autonomic Nervous System

Occasionally blurring of vision, tachycardia, nausea, dry mouth and salivation have been reported. Urinary retention and constipation may occur particularly if anticholinergic drugs are used to treat extrapyramidal symptoms. One patient being treated with MOBAN experienced priapism which required surgical intervention, apparently resulting in residual impairment of erectile function.

Laboratory Tests

There have been rare reports of leucopenia and leucocytosis. If such reactions occur, treatment with MOBAN may continue if clinical symptoms are absent. Alterations of blood glucose, B.U.N., and red blood cells have not been considered clinically significant.

Metabolic and Endrocrine Effects

Alteration of thyroid function has not been significant. Amenorrhea has been reported infrequently. Resumption of menses in previously amenorrheic women has been reported. Initially heavy menses may occur. Galactorrhea and gynecomastia have been reported infrequently. Increase in libido has been noted in some patients. Impotence has not been reported. Although both weight gain and weight loss have been in the direction of normal or ideal weight, excessive weight gain has not occurred with MOBAN.

Hepatic Effects

There have been rare reports of clinically significant alterations in liver function in association with MOBAN use.

Cardiovascular

Rare, transient, non-specific T wave changes have been reported on E.K.G. Association with a clinical syndrome has

Continued on next page

Du Pont Multi-Source—Cont.

not been established. Rarely has significant hypotension been reported.

Ophthalmological

Lens opacities and pigmentary retinopathy have not been reported where patients have received MOBAN (molindone hydrochloride). In some patients, phenothiazine induced lenticular opacities have resolved following discontinuation of the phenothiazine while continuing therapy with MOBAN.

Skin

Early, non-specific skin rash, probably of allergic origin, has occasionally been reported. Skin pigmentation has not been seen with MOBAN usage alone.

MOBAN (molindone hydrochloride) has certain pharmacological similarities to other antipsychotic agents. Because adverse reactions are often extensions of the pharmacological activity of a drug, all of the known pharmacological effects associated with other antipsychotic drugs should be kept in mind when MOBAN is used. Upon abrupt withdrawal after prolonged high dosage an abstinence syndrome has not been noted.

DOSAGE AND ADMINISTRATION

Initial and maintenance doses of MOBAN (molindone hydrochloride) should be individualized.

Initial Dosage Schedule

The usual starting dosage is 50-75 mg/day.

— Increase to 100 mg/day in 3 or 4 days.
— Based on severity of symptomatology, dosage may be titrated up or down depending on individual patient response.
— An increase to 225 mg/day may be required in patients with severe symptomatology.

Elderly and debilitated patients should be started on lower dosage.

Maintenance Dosage Schedule

1. Mild—5 mg-15 mg three or four times a day.
2. Moderate—10 mg-25 mg three or four times a day.
3. Severe—225 mg/day may be required.

DRUG INTERACTIONS

Potentiation of drugs administered concurrently with MOBAN (molindone hydrochloride) has not been reported. Additionally, animal studies have not shown increased toxicity when MOBAN is given concurrently with representative members of three classes of drugs (i.e., barbiturates, chloral hydrate and antiparkinson drugs).

MANAGEMENT OF OVERDOSAGE

Symptomatic, supportive therapy should be the rule.

Gastric lavage is indicated for the reduction of absorption of MOBAN (molindone hydrochloride) which is freely soluble in water.

Since the adsorption of MOBAN (molindone hydrochloride) by activated charcoal has not been determined, the use of this antidote must be considered of theoretical value.

Emesis in a comatose patient is contraindicated. Additionally, while the emetic effect of apomorphine is blocked by MOBAN in animals, this blocking effect has not been determined in humans.

A significant increase in the rate of removal of unmetabolized MOBAN from the body by forced diuresis, peritoneal or renal dialysis would not be expected. (Only 2% of a single ingested dose of MOBAN is excreted unmetabolized in the urine). However, poor response of the patient may justify use of these procedures.

While the use of laxatives or enemas might be based on general principles, the amount of unmetabolized MOBAN in feces is less than 1%. Extrapyramidal symptoms have responded to the use of diphenhydramine (Benadryl*), Amantadine HCl (Symmetrel®) and the synthetic anticholinergic antiparkinson agents, (i.e., Artane*, Cogentin*, Akineton*).

HOW SUPPLIED

As tablets in bottles of 100 with potencies and colors as follows:

5 mg orange	NDC 0056-0072-70
10 mg lavender	NDC 0056-0073-70
25 mg light green	NDC 0056-0074-70
50 mg blue	NDC 0056-0076-70
100 mg tan	NDC 0056-0077-70

As a concentrate containing 20 mg molindone hydrochloride per mL in 4 oz. (120 mL) bottles, NDC 0056-0460-04.

Store at controlled room temperature (59°–86°F, 15°–30°C). Protect from light.

Caution: Federal law prohibits dispensing without prescription.

* Benadryl-Trademark, Parke-Davis and Co.
* Artane-Trademark, Lederle Laboratories
* Cogentin-Trademark, Merck Sharp & Dohme
* Akineton-Trademark, Knoll Pharmaceutical Co.
* Symmetrel-Trademark of The Du Pont Merck Pharmaceutical Co.

MOBAN® is a Registered Trademark of The Du Pont Merck Pharmaceutical Co.

Du Pont Pharmaceuticals
Wilmington, Delaware 19880

6145-12/Rev. Nov., 1990

NARCAN® INJECTION   ℞

[nar'kan]

(naloxone hydrochloride)

Narcotic Antagonist

DESCRIPTION

NARCAN (naloxone hydrochloride injection, USP), a narcotic antagonist, is a synthetic congener of oxymorphone. In structure it differs from oxymorphone in that the methyl group on the nitrogen atom is replaced by an allyl group. Naloxone hydrochloride occurs as a white to slightly off-white powder, and is soluble in water, in dilute acids, and in strong alkali; slightly soluble in alcohol; practically insoluble in ether and in chloroform.

NARCAN injection is available as a sterile solution for intravenous, intramuscular and subcutaneous administration in three concentrations, 0.02 mg, 0.4 mg and 1.0 mg of naloxone hydrochloride per mL. One mL of the 0.02 mg and 0.4 mg strengths contains 8.6 mg of sodium chloride. One mL of the 1.0 mg strength contains 8.35 mg of sodium chloride. One mL of the 0.4 mg and 1.0 mg strengths also contains 2.0 mg of methylparaben and propylparaben as preservatives in a ratio of 9 to 1. pH is adjusted to 3.5 ± 0.5 with hydrochloric acid.

NARCAN injection is also available in a paraben-free formulation in three concentrations: 0.02 mg and 0.4 mg and 1.0 mg of naloxone hydrochloride per mL. One mL of each strength contains 9.0 mg of sodium chloride. pH is adjusted to 3.5 ± 0.5 with hydrochloric acid.

CLINICAL PHARMACOLOGY

NARCAN (naloxone hydrochloride injection, USP) prevents or reverses the effects of opioids including respiratory depression, sedation and hypotension. Also, it can reverse the psychotomimetic and dysphoric effects of agonist-antagonists such as pentazocine.

NARCAN (naloxone hydrochloride injection, USP) is an essentially pure narcotic antagonist, i.e., it does not possess the "agonistic" or morphine-like properties characteristic of other narcotic antagonists; NARCAN does not produce respiratory depression, psychotomimetic effects or pupillary constriction. In the absence of narcotics or agonistic effects of other narcotic antagonists it exhibits essentially no pharmacologic activity.

NARCAN has not been shown to produce tolerance nor to cause physical or psychological dependence.

In the presence of physical dependence on narcotics NARCAN will produce withdrawal symptoms.

Mechanisms of Action While the mechanism of action of NARCAN is not fully understood, the preponderance of evidence suggests that NARCAN antagonizes the opioid effects by competing for the same receptor sites.

When NARCAN is administered intravenously the onset of action is generally apparent within two minutes; the onset of action is only slightly less rapid when it is administered subcutaneously or intramuscularly. The duration of action is dependent upon the dose and route of administration of NARCAN. Intramuscular administration produces a more prolonged effect than intravenous administration. The requirement for repeat doses of NARCAN, however, will also be dependent upon the amount, type and route of administration of the narcotic being antagonized.

Following parenteral administration NARCAN is rapidly distributed in the body. It is metabolized in the liver, primarily by glucuronide conjugation and excreted in urine. In one study the serum half-life in adults ranged from 30 to 81 minutes (mean 64 ± 12 minutes). In a neonatal study the mean plasma half-life was observed to be 3.1 ± 0.5 hours.

INDICATIONS AND USAGE

NARCAN is indicated for the complete or partial reversal of narcotic depression, including respiratory depression, induced by opioids including natural and synthetic narcotics, propoxyphene, methadone and certain narcotic-antagonist analgesics: nalbuphine, pentazocine and butorphanol. NARCAN is also indicated for the diagnosis of suspected acute opioid overdosage.

CONTRAINDICATIONS

NARCAN is contraindicated in patients known to be hypersensitive to it.

WARNINGS

NARCAN should be administered cautiously to persons including newborns of mothers who are known or suspected to be physically dependent on opioids. In such cases an abrupt and complete reversal of narcotic effects may precipitate an acute abstinence syndrome.

The patient who has satisfactorily responded to NARCAN should be kept under continued surveillance and repeated doses of NARCAN should be administered, as necessary, since the duration of action of some narcotics may exceed that of NARCAN.

NARCAN is not effective against respiratory depression due to non-opioid drugs. Reversal of buprenorphine-induced respiratory depression may be incomplete. If an incomplete response occurs, respirations should be mechanically assisted.

PRECAUTIONS

In addition to NARCAN, other resuscitative measures such as maintenance of a free airway, artificial ventilation, cardiac massage, and vasopressor agents should be available and employed when necessary to counteract acute narcotic poisoning.

Several instances of hypotension, hypertension, ventricular tachycardia and fibrillation, and pulmonary edema have been reported. These have occurred in postoperative patients most of whom had pre-existing cardiovascular disorders or received other drugs which may have similar adverse cardiovascular effects. Although a direct cause and effect relationship has not been established, NARCAN should be used with caution in patients with pre-existing cardiac disease or patients who have received potentially cardiotoxic drugs.

Carcinogenesis, Mutagenesis, Impairment of Fertility Carcinogenicity and mutagenicity studies have not been performed with NARCAN. Reproductive studies in mice and rats demonstrated no impairment of fertility.

Use in Pregnancy Pregnancy Catagory B: Reproduction studies performed in mice and rats at doses up to 1,000 times the human dose, revealed no evidence of impaired fertility or harm to the fetus due to NARCAN. There are, however, no adequate and well controlled studies in pregnant women. Because animal reproduction studies are not always predictive of human response, NARCAN should be used during pregnancy only if clearly needed.

Nursing Mothers It is not known whether NARCAN is excreted in human milk. Because many drugs are excreted in human milk, caution should be exercised when NARCAN is administered to a nursing woman.

ADVERSE REACTIONS

Abrupt reversal of narcotic depression may result in nausea, vomiting, sweating, tachycardia, increased blood pressure, tremulousness, seizures and cardiac arrest. In postoperative patients, larger than necessary dosage of NARCAN may result in significant reversal of analgesia, and in excitement. Hypotension, hypertension, ventricular tachycardia and fibrillation, and pulmonary edema have been associated with the use of NARCAN postoperatively (see PRECAUTIONS & USAGE IN ADULTS-POSTOPERATIVE NARCOTIC DEPRESSION).

OVERDOSAGE

There is no clinical experience with NARCAN overdosage in humans.

In the mouse and rat the intravenous LD_{50} is 150 ± 5 mg/kg and 109 ± 4 mg/kg respectively. In acute subcutaneous toxicity studies in newborn rats the LD_{50} (95% CL) is 260 (228-296) mg/kg. Subcutaneous injection of 100 mg/kg/day in rats for 3 weeks produced only transient salivation and partial ptosis following injection; no toxic effects were seen at 10 mg/kg/day for 3 weeks.

DOSAGE AND ADMINISTRATION

NARCAN (naloxone hydrochloride injection, USP) may be administered intravenously, intramuscularly, or subcutaneously. The most rapid onset of action is achieved by intravenous administration and it is recommended in emergency situations.

Since the duration of action of some narcotics may exceed that of NARCAN the patient should be kept under continued surveillance and repeated doses of NARCAN should be administered, as necessary.

Intravenous Infusion NARCAN may be diluted for intravenous infusion in normal saline or 5% dextrose solutions. The addition of 2 mg of NARCAN in 500 mL of either solution provides a concentration of 0.004 mg/mL. Mixtures should be used within 24 hours. After 24 hours, the remaining unused solution must be discarded. The rate of administration should be titrated in accordance with the patient's response. Parenteral drug products should be inspected visually for particulate matter and discoloration prior to administration whenever solution and container permit. NARCAN should not be mixed with preparations containing bisulfite, metabisulfite, long-chain or high molecular weight anions, or any solution having an alkaline pH. No drug or chemical agent should be added to NARCAN unless its effect on the chemical and physical stability of the solution has first been established.

USAGE IN ADULTS

Narcotic Overdose—Known or Suspected An initial dose of 0.4 mg to 2 mg of NARCAN may be administered intravenously. If the desired degree of counteraction and improvement in respiratory functions is not obtained, it may be re-

peated at 2 to 3 minute intervals. If no response is observed after 10 mg of NARCAN have been administered, the diagnosis of narcotic induced or partial narcotic induced toxicity should be questioned. Intramuscular or subcutaneous administration may be necessary if the intravenous route is not available.

Postoperative Narcotic Depression For the partial reversal of narcotic depression following the use of narcotics during surgery, smaller doses of NARCAN are usually sufficient. The dose of NARCAN should be titrated according to the patient's response. For the initial reversal of respiratory depression, NARCAN should be injected in increments of 0.1 to 0.2 mg intravenously at two to three minute intervals to the desired degree of reversal i.e. adequate ventilation and alertness without significant pain or discomfort. Larger than necessary dosage of NARCAN may result in significant reversal of analgesia and increase in blood pressure. Similarly, too rapid reversal may induce nausea, vomiting, sweating or circulatory stress.

Repeat doses of NARCAN may be required within one to two hour intervals depending upon the amount, type (i.e., short or long acting) and time interval since last administration of narcotic. Supplemental intramuscular doses have been shown to produce a longer lasting effect.

USAGE IN CHILDREN

Narcotic Overdose—Known or Suspected The usual initial dose in children is 0.01 mg/kg body weight given I.V. If this dose does not result in the desired degree of clinical improvement, a subsequent dose of 0.1 mg/kg body weight may be administered. If an I.V. route of administration is not available, NARCAN may be administered I.M. or S.C. in divided doses. If necessary, NARCAN can be diluted with sterile water for injection.

Postoperative Narcotic Depression Follow the recommendations and cautions under **Adult Postoperative Depression.** For the initial reversal of respiratory depression NARCAN should be injected in increments of 0.005 mg to 0.01 mg intravenously at two to three minute intervals to the desired degree of reversal.

USAGE IN NEONATES

Narcotic-induced Depression The usual initial dose is 0.01 mg/kg body weight administered I.V., I.M., or S.C. This dose may be repeated in accordance with adult administration guidelines for postoperative narcotic depression.

HOW SUPPLIED

NARCAN (naloxone hydrochloride injection, USP) for intravenous, intramuscular and subcutaneous administration is available as:

0.4 mg/mL	1 mL disposable prefilled syringe—box of 10	NDC 0590-0365-15
	10 mL multiple dose vial—box of 1	NDC 0590-0365-05
0.4 mg/mL		
(paraben-free)	1 mL ampul—box of 10	NDC 0590-0358-10
1.0 mg/mL	10 mL multiple dose vial—box of 1	NDC 0590-0368-05
1.0 mg/mL	1 mL disposable prefilled syringe—box of 10	NDC 0590-0368-15
1.0 mg/mL	2 mL disposable prefilled syringe—box of 10	NDC 0590-0368-13
1.0 mg/mL		
(paraben-free)	2 mL ampul—box of 10	NDC 0590-0377-10
0.02 mg/mL		
(paraben-free)	2 mL ampul—box of 10	NDC 0590-0359-10

Store at controlled room temperature (59°–86°F, 15°–30°C).
Caution: Federal law prohibits dispensing without prescription.
Du Pont Pharmaceuticals
Manati, Puerto Rico 00674
NARCAN® is a Registered Trademark of The Du Pont Merck Pharmaceutical Co.   6108-11/Rev. Dec., 1990

NUBAIN®   ℞
[nū'bān]
(nalbuphine hydrochloride)

DESCRIPTION

NUBAIN (nalbuphine hydrochloride) is a synthetic narcotic agonist-antagonist analgesic of the phenanthrene series. It is chemically related to both the widely used narcotic antagonist, naloxone, and the potent narcotic analgesic, oxymorphone.

NALBUPHINE HYDROCHLORIDE

Nalbuphine hydrochloride is (-)-17-(cyclobutylmethyl)-4,5α-epoxymorphinan-3,6α,14-triol hydrochloride.
NUBAIN is available in two concentrations, 10 mg and 20 mg of nalbuphine hydrochloride per mL. Both strengths contain 0.94% sodium citrate hydrous, 1.26% citric acid anhydrous, 0.1% sodium metabisulfite, and 0.2% of a 9:1 mixture of methylparaben and propylparaben as preservatives; pH is

adjusted, if necessary, with hydrochloric acid. The 10 mg/mL strength contains 0.1% sodium chloride.
NUBAIN is also available in a sulfite and paraben-free formulation in two concentrations, 10 mg and 20 mg of nalbuphine hydrochloride per mL. One mL of each strength contains 0.94% sodium citrate hydrous, 1.26% citric acid anhydrous; pH is adjusted, if necessary, with hydrochloric acid. The 10 mg/mL strength contains 0.2% sodium chloride.

ACTIONS

NUBAIN is a potent analgesic. Its analgesic potency is essentially equivalent to that of morphine on a milligram basis. Its onset of action occurs within 2 to 3 minutes after intravenous administration, and in less than 15 minutes following subcutaneous or intramuscular injection. The plasma half-life of nalbuphine is 5 hours and in clinical studies the duration of analgesic activity has been reported to range from 3 to 6 hours.
The narcotic antagonist activity of NUBAIN is one-fourth as potent as nalorphine and 10 times that of pentazocine.

INDICATIONS

NUBAIN (nalbuphine hydrochloride) is indicated for the relief of moderate to severe pain. NUBAIN can also be used as a supplement to balanced anesthesia, for preoperative and postoperative analgesia, and for obstetrical analgesia during labor and delivery.

CONTRAINDICATIONS

NUBAIN should not be administered to patients who are hypersensitive to it.

WARNINGS

NUBAIN should be administered as a supplement to general anesthesia only by persons specifically trained in the use of intravenous anesthetics and management of the respiratory effects of potent opioids.

Naloxone, resuscitative and intubation equipment and oxygen should be readily available.

Drug Dependence NUBAIN has been shown to have a low abuse potential. When compared with drugs which are not mixed agonist-antagonists, it has been reported that nalbuphine's potential for abuse would be less than that of codeine and propoxyphene. Psychological and physical dependence and tolerance may follow the abuse or misuse of nalbuphine. Therefore, caution should be observed in prescribing it for emotionally unstable patients, or for individuals with a history of narcotic abuse. Such patients should be closely supervised when long-term therapy is contemplated.
Care should be taken to avoid increases in dosage or frequency of administration which in susceptible individuals might result in physical dependence.
Abrupt discontinuation of NUBAIN following prolonged use has been followed by symptoms of narcotic withdrawal, i.e., abdominal cramps, nausea and vomiting, rhinorrhea, lacrimation, restlessness, anxiety, elevated temperature and piloerection.
Use in Ambulatory Patients NUBAIN may impair the mental or physical abilities required for the performance of potentially dangerous tasks such as driving a car or operating machinery. Therefore, NUBAIN should be administered with caution to ambulatory patients who should be warned to avoid such hazards.
Use in Emergency Procedures Maintain patient under observation until recovered from NUBAIN effects that would affect driving or other potentially dangerous tasks.
Use in Children Clinical experience to support administration to patients under 18 years is not available at present.
Use in Pregnancy (other than labor) Safe use of NUBAIN in pregnancy has not been established. Although animal reproductive studies have not revealed teratogenic or embryotoxic effects, nalbuphine should only be administered to pregnant women when, in the judgement of the physician, the potential benefits outweigh the possible hazards.
Use During Labor and Delivery NUBAIN can produce respiratory depression in the neonate. It should be used with caution in women delivering premature infants.
Head Injury and Increased Intracranial Pressure The possible respiratory depressant effects and the potential of potent analgesics to elevate cerebrospinal fluid pressure (resulting from vasodilation following CO_2 retention) may be markedly exaggerated in the presence of head injury, intracranial lesions or a pre-existing increase in intracranial pressure. Furthermore, potent analgesics can produce effects which may obscure the clinical course of patients with head injuries. Therefore, NUBAIN should be used in these circumstances only when essential, and then should be administered with extreme caution.
Interaction With Other Central Nervous System Depressants Although NUBAIN possesses narcotic antagonist activity, there is evidence that in nondependent patients it will not antagonize a narcotic analgesic administered just before, concurrently, or just after an injection of NUBAIN. Therefore, patients receiving a narcotic analgesic, general anesthetics, phenothiazines, or other tranquilizers, sedatives, hypnotics, or other CNS depressants (including alcohol) concomitantly with NUBAIN may exhibit an additive effect.

When such combined therapy is contemplated, the dose of one or both agents should be reduced.
Sulfites Sensitivity NUBAIN contains sodium metabisulfite, a sulfite that may cause allergic-type reactions including anaphylactic symptoms and life-threatening or less severe asthmatic episodes in certain susceptible people. The overall prevalence of sulfite sensitivity in the general population is unknown and probably low. Sulfite sensitivity is seen more frequently in asthmatic than in nonasthmatic people.

PRECAUTIONS

Impaired Respiration At the usual adult dose of 10 mg/70 kg, NUBAIN causes some respiratory depression approximately equal to that produced by equal doses of morphine. However, in contrast to morphine, respiratory depression is not appreciably increased with higher doses of NUBAIN. Respiratory depression induced by NUBAIN can be reversed by NARCAN® (naloxone hydrochloride) when indicated. NUBAIN should be administered with caution at low doses to patients with impaired respiration (e.g., from other medication, uremia, bronchial asthma, severe infection, cyanosis or respiratory obstructions).
Impaired Renal or Hepatic Function Because NUBAIN is metabolized in the liver and excreted by the kidneys, patients with renal or liver dysfunction may over-react to customary doses. Therefore, in these individuals, NUBAIN should be used with caution and administered in reduced amounts.
Myocardial Infarction As with all potent analgesics, NUBAIN should be used with caution in patients with myocardial infarction who have nausea or vomiting.
Biliary Tract Surgery As with all narcotic analgesics, NUBAIN should be used with caution in patients about to undergo surgery of the biliary tract since it may cause spasm of the sphincter of Oddi.
Cardiovascular System During evaluation of NUBAIN in anesthesia, a higher incidence of bradycardia has been reported in patients who did not receive atropine pre-operatively or in the pre-operative period.

ADVERSE REACTIONS

The most frequent adverse reaction in 1066 patients treated with NUBAIN is sedation 381(36%).
Less frequent reactions are: sweaty/clammy 99(9%), nausea/vomiting 68(6%), dizziness/ vertigo 58(5%), dry mouth 44(4%), and headache 27(3%).
Other adverse reactions which may occur (reported incidence of 1% or less) are:
CNS Effects Nervousness, depression, restlessness, crying, euphoria, floating, hostility, unusual dreams, confusion, faintness, hallucinations, dysphoria, feeling of heaviness, numbness, tingling, unreality. The incidence of psychotomimetic effects, such as unreality, depersonalization, delusions, dysphoria and hallucinations has been shown to be less than that which occurs with pentazocine.
Cardiovascular Hypertension, hypotension, bradycardia, tachycardia, pulmonary edema.
Gastrointestinal Cramps, dyspepsia, bitter taste.
Respiration Depression, dyspnea, asthma.
Dermatological Itching, burning, urticaria.
Miscellaneous Speech difficulty, urinary urgency, blurred vision, flushing and warmth.

DOSAGE AND ADMINISTRATION

The usual recommended adult dose is 10 mg for a 70 kg individual, administered subcutaneously, intramuscularly or intravenously; this dose may be repeated every 3 to 6 hours as necessary. Dosage should be adjusted according to the severity of the pain, physical status of the patient, and other medications which the patient may be receiving. (See Interaction with Other Central Nervous System Depressants under WARNINGS). In non-tolerant individuals, the recommended single maximum dose is 20 mg, with a maximum total daily dose of 160 mg.
The use of NUBAIN as a supplement to balanced anesthesia requires larger doses than those recommended for analgesia. Induction doses of NUBAIN range from 0.3 mg/kg to 3.0 mg/kg intravenously to be administered over a 10 to 15 minute period with maintenance doses of 0.25 to 0.50 mg/kg in single intravenous administrations as required. The use of NUBAIN may be followed by respiratory depression which can be reversed with the narcotic antagonist NARCAN® (naloxone hydrochloride).
Patients Dependent on Narcotics Patients who have been taking narcotics chronically may experience withdrawal symptoms upon the administration of NUBAIN. If unduly troublesome, narcotic withdrawal symptoms can be controlled by the slow intravenous administration of small increments of morphine, until relief occurs. If the previous analgesic was morphine, meperidine, codeine, or other narcotic with similar duration of activity, one-fourth of the anticipated dose of NUBAIN can be administered initially and the patient observed for signs of withdrawal, i.e., abdominal cramps, nausea and vomiting, lacrimation, rhinorrhea, anxi-

Continued on next page

Du Pont Multi-Source—Cont.

ety, restlessness, elevation of temperature or piloerection. If untoward symptoms do not occur, progressively larger doses may be tried at appropriate intervals until the desired level of analgesia is obtained with NUBAIN.

Management of Overdosage The immediate intravenous administration of NARCAN® (naloxone hydrochloride) is a specific antidote. Oxygen, intravenous fluids, vasopressors and other supportive measures should be used as indicated. The administration of single doses of 72 mg of NUBAIN subcutaneously to eight normal subjects has been reported to have resulted primarily in symptoms of sleepiness and mild dysphoria.

HOW SUPPLIED

NUBAIN® (nalbuphine hydrochloride) injection for intramuscular, subcutaneous, or intravenous use is available in:
NDC 0590-0385-10 10 mg/mL, 1 mL ampuls (box of 10)
NDC 0590-0386-01 10 mg/mL, 10 mL multiple dose vials (box of 1)
NDC 0590-0395-10 (sulfite/paraben-free) 10 mg/mL, 1 mL ampuls (box of 10)
NDC 0590-0396-10 20 mg/mL, 1 mL ampuls (box of 10)
NDC 0590-0396-15 20 mg/mL, 1 mL disposable pre-filled syringes (box of 10)
NDC 0590-0399-01 20 mg/mL, 10 mL multiple dose vials (box of 1)
NDC 0590-0398-10 (sulfite/paraben-free) 20 mg/mL, 1 mL ampuls (box of 10)
Store at controlled room temperature (59°–86°F, 15°–30°C).
Caution: Federal law prohibits dispensing without prescription.
Du Pont Pharmaceuticals
Manati, Puerto Rico 00674
NUBAIN® is a Registered Trademark of The Du Pont Merck Pharmaceutical Co.
NARCAN® is a Registered Trademark of The Du Pont Merck Pharmaceutical Co.
6109-12/Rev. Dec., 1990

NUMORPHAN® Ⓒ

[nū-mor 'fan]
(oxymorphone hydrochloride)
injection

DESCRIPTION

NUMORPHAN (oxymorphone hydrochloride), a semi-synthetic narcotic substitute for morphine, is a potent analgesic. Oxymorphone hydrochloride is 4,5α-Epoxy-3,14- dihydroxy-17-methylmorphinan-6-one hydrochloride.
Oxymorphone hydrochloride occurs as a white or slightly off-white, odorless powder, sparingly soluble in alcohol and ether, but freely soluble in water.
NUMORPHAN injection is available in two concentrations, 1 mg and 1.5 mg of oxymorphone hydrochloride per mL. Both strengths contain sodium chloride 0.8%; with methylparaben 0.18%, propylparaben 0.02% and sodium dithionite 0.1%, as preservatives. pH is adjusted with sodium hydroxide.

ACTIONS

NUMORPHAN (oxymorphone hydrochloride) is a potent narcotic analgesic. Administered parenterally, 1 mg of NUMORPHAN is approximately equivalent in analgesic activity to 10 mg of morphine sulfate.
The onset of action is rapid; initial effects are usually perceived within 5 to 10 minutes. Its duration of action is approximately 3 to 6 hours.
NUMORPHAN produces mild sedation and causes little depression of the cough reflex. These properties make it particularly useful in postoperative patients.

INDICATIONS

NUMORPHAN (oxymorphone hydrochloride) is indicated for the relief of moderate to severe pain. This drug is also indicated parenterally for preoperative medication, for support of anesthesia, for obstetrical analgesia, and for relief of anxiety in patients with dyspnea associated with acute left ventricular failure and pulmonary edema.

CONTRAINDICATIONS

Safe use of NUMORPHAN (oxymorphone hydrochloride) in children under 12 years of age has not been established. This drug should not be used in patients known to be hypersensitive to morphine analogs.

WARNINGS

May be habit forming. As with other narcotic drugs, tolerance and addiction may develop. The addicting potential of the drug appears to be about the same as for morphine.
Like other narcotic-containing medications, NUMORPHAN is subject to the Federal Controlled Substances Act.
Interaction with other central nervous system depressants: Patients receiving other narcotic analgesics, general anesthetics, phenothiazines, other tranquilizers, sedatives, hypnotics or other CNS depressants (including alcohol) concomitantly with NUMORPHAN may exhibit an additive CNS depression. When such combined therapy is contemplated, the dose of one or both agents should be reduced.
Safe use in pregnancy has not been established (relative to possible adverse effects on fetal development). As with other analgesics, the use of NUMORPHAN (oxymorphone hydrochloride) in pregnancy, in nursing mothers, or in women of child-bearing potential requires that the possible benefits of the drug be weighed against the possible hazards to the mother and the child.
Sulfites Sensitivity: NUMORPHAN contains sodium dithionite, a sulfite that may cause allergic-type reactions including anaphylactic symptoms and life-threatening or less severe asthmatic episodes in certain susceptible people. The overall prevalence of sulfite sensitivity in the general population is unknown and probably low. Sulfite sensitivity is seen more frequently in asthmatic than in nonasthmatic people.

PRECAUTIONS

The same care and caution should be taken when administering NUMORPHAN (oxymorphone hydrochloride) as when other potent narcotic analgesics are used. It should be borne in mind that some respiratory depression may occur as with all potent narcotics especially when other analgesic and/or anesthetic drugs with depressant action have been given shortly before administration of NUMORPHAN.
The respiratory depressant effects of narcotics and their capacity to elevate cerebrospinal fluid pressure may be markedly exaggerated in the presence of head injury, other intracranial lesions or a pre-existing increase in intracranial pressure. Furthermore narcotics produce adverse reactions which may obscure the clinical course of patients with head injuries.
As with other analgesics, caution must also be exercised in elderly and debilitated patients and in patients who are known to be sensitive to central nervous system depressants, such as those with cardiovascular, pulmonary, or hepatic disease, in hypothyroidism (myxedema), acute alcoholism, delirium tremens, convulsive disorders, bronchial asthma and kyphoscoliosis. Debilitated and elderly patients and those with severe liver diseases should receive smaller doses of NUMORPHAN (oxymorphone hydrochloride).

ADVERSE REACTIONS

As with all potent narcotic analgesics, possible side effects include drowsiness, nausea, vomiting, miosis, itching, dysphoria, light-headedness, and headache. Respiratory depression may occur with oxymorphone as with other narcotics.

DOSAGE AND ADMINISTRATION

Usual Adult Dosage of NUMORPHAN (oxymorphone hydrochloride) Injection: Subcutaneous or intramuscular administration: initially 1 mg to 1.5 mg, repeated every 4 to 6 hours as needed. Intravenous: 0.5 mg initially. In nondebilitated patients the dose can be cautiously increased until satisfactory pain relief is obtained. For analgesia during labor 0.5 mg to 1 mg intramuscularly is recommended.

MANAGEMENT OF OVERDOSAGE

Signs and Symptoms: Serious overdosage with NUMORPHAN is characterized by respiratory depression, (a decrease in respiratory rate and/or tidal volume, Cheyne-Stokes respiration, cyanosis), extreme somnolence progressing to stupor or coma, skeletal muscle flaccidity, cold and clammy skin, and sometimes bradycardia and hypotension. In severe overdosage, apnea, circulatory collapse, cardiac arrest and death may occur.
Treatment: Primary attention should be given to the reestablishment of adequate respiratory exchange through provision of a patent airway and the institution of assisted or controlled ventilation. The narcotic antagonist naloxone hydrochloride (NARCAN®) is a specific antidote against respiratory depression which may result from overdosage or unusual sensitivity to narcotics including oxymorphone. Therefore, an appropriate dose of naloxone hydrochloride should be administered (usual initial adult dose 0.4 mg–2 mg) preferably by the intravenous route and simultaneously with efforts at respiratory resuscitation. Since the duration of action of oxymorphone may exceed that of the antagonist, the patient should be kept under continued surveillance and repeated doses of the antagonist should be administered as needed to maintain adequate respiration.
Oxygen, intravenous fluids, vasopressors and other supportive measures should be employed as indicated.

HOW SUPPLIED

For Injection: DEA Order Form Required
1 mg/mL 1 mL ampuls (box of 10)
NDC 0590-0370-10
1.5 mg/mL 1 mL ampuls (box of 10)
NDC 0590-0373-10
10 mL multiple dose vial (box of 1)
NDC 0590-0374-01
Store at controlled room temperature (59°–86°F, 15°–30°C).
Protect from light.
Caution: Federal law prohibits dispensing without prescription.
Du Pont Pharmaceuticals
Manati, Puerto Rico 00674
NUMORPHAN® is a Registered Trademark of The Du Pont Merck Pharmaceutical Co.
NARCAN® is a Registered Trademark of The Du Pont Merck Pharmaceutical Co.
6110-6/Rev. Dec., 1990

NUMORPHAN® Ⓒ ℞

(oxymorphone hydrochloride)
RECTAL SUPPOSITORIES
Narcotic
Analgesic

DESCRIPTION

NUMORPHAN (oxymorphone hydrochloride), a semi-synthetic narcotic substitute for morphine, is a potent analgesic. Oxymorphone hydrochloride occurs as a white or slightly off-white, odorless powder, sparingly soluble in alcohol and ether, but freely soluble in water.
The NUMORPHAN rectal suppository is available in a concentration of 5 mg of oxymorphone hydrochloride in a base consisting of polyethylene glycol 1000 and polyethylene glycol 3350.

ACTIONS

NUMORPHAN (oxymorphone hydrochloride) is a potent narcotic analgesic. Administered parenterally, 1 mg of NUMORPHAN is approximately equivalent in analgesic activity to 10 mg of morphine sulfate.
The onset of action of parenterally administered NUMORPHAN is rapid; initial effects are usually perceived within 5 to 10 minutes. Its duration of action is approximately 3 to 6 hours.
NUMORPHAN produces mild sedation and causes little depression of the cough reflex. These properties make it particularly useful in postoperative patients.

INDICATIONS

For the relief of moderate to severe pain.

CONTRAINDICATIONS

Safe use of NUMORPHAN (oxymorphone hydrochloride) in children under 12 years of age has not been established. This drug should not be used in patients known to be hypersensitive to morphine analogs.

WARNINGS

May be habit forming. As with other narcotic drugs, tolerance and addiction may develop. The addicting potential of the drug appears to be about the same as for morphine.
Like other narcotic-containing medications, NUMORPHAN is subject to the Federal Controlled Substances Act.
Interaction with other central nervous system depressants: Patients receiving other narcotic analgesics, general anesthetics, phenothiazines, other tranquilizers, sedatives, hypnotics or other CNS depressants (including alcohol) concomitantly with NUMORPHAN may exhibit an additive CNS depression. When such combined therapy is contemplated, the dose of one or both agents should be reduced.
Safe use in pregnancy has not been established (relative to possible adverse effects on fetal development). As with other potent analgesics, the use of NUMORPHAN (oxymorphone hydrochloride) in pregnancy, in nursing mothers, or in women of child-bearing potential requires that the possible benefits of the drug be weighed against the possible hazards to the mother and child.

PRECAUTIONS

The same care and caution should be taken when administering NUMORPHAN (oxymorphone hydrochloride) as when other potent narcotic analgesics are used. It should be borne in mind that some respiratory depression may occur as with all potent narcotics especially when other analgesic and/or anesthetic drugs with depressant action have been given shortly before administration of NUMORPHAN.
The respiratory depressant effects of narcotics and their capacity to elevate cerebrospinal fluid pressure may be markedly exaggerated in the presence of head injury, other intracranial lesions or a pre-existing increase in intracranial pressure. Furthermore, narcotics produce adverse reactions which may obscure the clinical course of patients with head injuries.
As with other analgesics, caution must also be exercised in elderly and debilitated patients and in patients who are known to be sensitive to central nervous system depressants, such as those with cardiovascular, pulmonary, or hepatic disease, in hypothyroidism (myxedema), acute alcoholism, delirium tremens, convulsive disorders, bronchial asthma and kyphoscoliosis. Debilitated and elderly patients and those with severe liver diseases should receive smaller doses of NUMORPHAN.

ADVERSE REACTIONS

As with all potent narcotic analgesics, possible side effects include drowsiness, nausea, vomiting, miosis, itching, dysphoria, light-headedness, and headache. Respiratory depression may occur with oxymorphone as with other narcotics.

DOSAGE AND ADMINISTRATION

Usual Adult Dosage of NUMORPHAN (oxymorphone hydrochloride) Rectal Suppositories: One suppository, 5 mg, every 4 to 6 hours. In nondebilitated patients the dose can be cautiously increased until satisfactory pain relief is obtained.

MANAGEMENT OF OVERDOSAGE

Signs and symptoms: Serious overdosage with NUMORPHAN is characterized by respiratory depression, (a decrease in respiratory rate and/or tidal volume, Cheyne-Stokes respiration, cyanosis), extreme somnolence progressing to stupor or coma, skeletal muscle flaccidity, cold and clammy skin, and sometimes bradycardia and hypotension. In severe overdosage, apnea, circulatory collapse, cardiac arrest and death may occur.

Treatment: Primary attention should be given to the reestablishment of adequate respiratory exchange through provision of a patent airway and the institution of assisted or controlled ventilation. The narcotic antagonist naloxone hydrochloride (NARCAN®) is a specific antidote against respiratory depression which may result from overdosage or unusual sensitivity to narcotics including oxymorphone. Therefore, an appropriate dose of naloxone hydrochloride should be administered (usual initial adult dose: 0.4 mg-2 mg) preferably by the intravenous route and simultaneously with efforts at respiratory resuscitation. Since the duration of action of oxymorphone may exceed that of the antagonist, the patient should be kept under continued surveillance and repeated doses of the antagonist should be administered as needed to maintain adequate respiration.

Oxygen, intravenous fluids, vasopressors and other supportive measures should be employed as indicated.

HOW SUPPLIED

Rectal Suppositories: DEA Order Form Required
5 mg, wrapped in gold foil, box of 6 NDC 0590-0761-06
Store under refrigeration (35°–46°F, 2°–8°C).
Caution: Federal law prohibits dispensing without prescription.

Du Pont Pharmaceuticals
Manati, Puerto Rico 00674
NUMORPHAN® is a Registered Trademark of The Du Pont Merck Pharmaceutical Co.
NARCAN® is a Registered Trademark of The Du Pont Merck Pharmaceutical Co.

6111-5/Rev. Dec., 1990

SYMMETREL®   ℞
[sim 'e-trel"]
(amantadine hydrochloride)

DESCRIPTION

SYMMETREL is designated generically as amantadine hydrochloride and chemically as 1-adamantanamine hydrochloride.

Amantadine hydrochloride is a stable white or nearly white crystalline powder, freely soluble in water and soluble in alcohol and in chloroform.

Amantadine hydrochloride has pharmacological actions as both an anti-Parkinson and an antiviral drug.

SYMMETREL is available in capsules and syrup.

SYMMETREL capsules contain: FD&C Red 40, gelatin, glycerin, hydrogenated vegetable oil, lecithin, methylparaben, propylparaben, soybean oil, titanium dioxide, vegetable shortening, white printing ink, and yellow wax.

SYMMETREL syrup contains: artificial raspberry flavor, citric acid, methylparaben, propylparaben, and sorbitol solution.

CLINICAL PHARMACOLOGY

SYMMETREL is readily absorbed, is not metabolized, and is excreted unchanged in the urine by glomerular filtration and tubular secretion.

After oral administration of a single dose of 100 mg, maximum blood levels are reached, based on the mean time of the peak urinary excretion rate, in approximately 4 hours; the peak excretion rate is approximately 5 mg/hr; the mean half-life of the excretion rate approximates 15 hours.

Compared with otherwise healthy adult individuals, the clearance of SYMMETREL is significantly reduced in adult patients with renal insufficiency. The elimination half-life increases two to three fold when creatinine clearance is less than 40 mL/min./1.73m², and averages eight days in patients on chronic maintenance hemodialysis.

The renal clearance of SYMMETREL is reduced and plasma levels are increased in otherwise healthy elderly patients age 65 years and older. The drug plasma levels in elderly patients receiving 100 mg daily have been reported to approximate those determined in younger adults taking 200

mg daily. Whether these changes are due to the normal decline in renal function or other age related factors is not known.

The mechanism of action of SYMMETREL in the treatment of Parkinson's disease and drug-induced extrapyramidal reactions is not known. It has been shown to cause an increase in dopamine release in the animal brain. The drug does not possess anticholinergic activity in animal tests at doses similar to those used clinically. The antiviral activity of SYMMETREL against influenza A virus is not completely understood. The mode of action of SYMMETREL appears to be the prevention of the release of infectious viral nucleic acid into the host cell. SYMMETREL does not appear to interfere with the immunogenicity of inactivated influenza A virus vaccine.

INDICATIONS AND USAGE

Parkinson's Disease/Syndrome: SYMMETREL is indicated in the treatment of idiopathic Parkinson's disease (Paralysis Agitans), postencephalitic parkinsonism, and symptomatic parkinsonism which may follow injury to the nervous system by carbon monoxide intoxication. It is indicated in those elderly patients believed to develop parkinsonism in association with cerebral arteriosclerosis. In the treatment of Parkinson's disease, SYMMETREL is less effective than levodopa, (−)-3-(3,4-dihydroxyphenyl)-L -alanine, and its efficacy in comparison with the anticholinergic antiparkinson drugs has not yet been established.

Drug-Induced Extrapyramidal Reactions: SYMMETREL is indicated in the treatment of drug-induced extrapyramidal reactions. Although anticholinergic-type side effects have been noted with SYMMETREL when used in patients with drug-induced extrapyramidal reactions, there is a lower incidence of these side effects than that observed with the anticholinergic antiparkinson drugs.

Influenza A Virus Respiratory Tract Illness:
Prophylaxis: SYMMETREL (amantadine hydrochloride) is indicated in the prevention or chemoprophylaxis of influenza A virus illness. SYMMETREL should be considered especially for high risk individuals, close household or hospital ward contacts of index cases, immunocompromised patients, health care and community services personnel. In the prophylaxis of influenza early vaccination as periodically recommended by the Centers for Disease Control's Immunization Practices Advisory Committee is the method of choice. When early vaccination is not feasible, or when the vaccine is contraindicated or not available, SYMMETREL can be used for chemoprophylaxis against influenza A virus illness. Because SYMMETREL does not appear to suppress antibody response, it can be used chemoprophylactically in conjunction with inactivated influenza A virus vaccine until protective antibody responses develop.

Treatment: SYMMETREL is also indicated in the treatment of uncomplicated respiratory tract illness caused by influenza A virus strains. There are as yet no well-controlled clinical studies demonstrating treatment with SYMMETREL will avoid the development of influenza A virus pneumonitis or other complications in high risk patients.

There is no clinical evidence indicating that SYMMETREL is effective in the prophylaxis or treatment of viral respiratory tract illnesses other than those caused by influenza A virus strains.

CONTRAINDICATIONS:

SYMMETREL is contraindicated in patients with known hypersensitivity to the drug.

WARNINGS:

Patients with a history of epilepsy or other "seizures" should be observed closely for possible increased seizure activity.
Patients with a history of congestive heart failure or peripheral edema should be followed closely as there are patients who developed congestive heart failure while receiving SYMMETREL.

Patients with Parkinson's disease improving on SYMMETREL should resume normal activities gradually and cautiously, consistent with other medical considerations, such as the presence of osteoporosis or phlebothrombosis.

Patients receiving SYMMETREL who note central nervous system effects or blurring of vision should be cautioned against driving or working in situations where alertness and adequate motor coordination are important.

PRECAUTIONS:

SYMMETREL (amantadine hydrochloride) should not be discontinued abruptly since a few patients with Parkinson's disease experienced a parkinsonian crisis, i.e., a sudden marked clinical deterioration when this medication was suddenly stopped. The dose of anticholinergic drugs or of SYMMETREL should be reduced if atropine-like effects appear when these drugs are used concurrently.

Neuroleptic Malignant Syndrome (NMS): Sporadic cases of possible Neuroleptic Malignant Syndrome (NMS) have been reported in association with dose reduction or withdrawal of SYMMETREL therapy.

NMS is an uncommon but life-threatening syndrome characterized by fever or hyperthermia; neurologic findings including muscle rigidity, involuntary movements, altered con-

sciousness; other disturbances such as autonomic dysfunction, tachycardia, tachypnea, hyper- or hypotension; laboratory findings such as creatine phosphokinase elevation, leukocytosis, and increased serum myoglobin.

The diagnostic evaluation of patients with this syndrome is complicated. In arriving at a diagnosis, it is important to identify cases where the clinical presentation includes both serious medical illness (e.g., pneumonia, systemic infection, etc.) and untreated or inadequately treated extrapyramidal signs and symptoms (EPS). Other important considerations in the differential diagnosis include central anticholinergic toxicity, heat stroke, drug fever and primary central nervous system (CNS) pathology.

The management of NMS should include: 1) intensive symptomatic treatment and medical monitoring, and 2) treatment of any concomitant serious medical problems for which specific treatments are available. There is no general agreement about specific pharmacological treatment regimens for uncomplicated NMS.

Because SYMMETREL is not metabolized and is mainly excreted in the urine, it accumulates in the plasma and in the body when renal function declines. Thus, the dose of SYMMETREL should be reduced in patients with renal impairment and in individuals who are 65 years of age or older. The dose of SYMMETREL may need careful adjustment in patients with congestive heart failure, peripheral edema, or orthostatic hypotension.

Care should be exercised when administering SYMMETREL to patients with liver disease, a history of recurrent eczematoid rash, or to patients with psychosis or severe psychoneurosis not controlled by chemotherapeutic agents. Rare instances of reversible elevation of liver enzymes have been reported in patients receiving SYMMETREL, though a specific relationship between the drug and such changes has not been established. Careful observation is required when SYMMETREL is administered concurrently with central nervous system stimulants.

No long-term studies in animals have been performed to evaluate the carcinogenic potential of SYMMETREL. The mutagenic potential of the drug has not yet been determined in experimental systems.

Pregnancy Category C: SYMMETREL (amantadine hydrochloride) has been shown to be embryotoxic and teratogenic in rats at 50 mg/kg/day, about 12 times the recommended human dose, but not at 37 mg/kg/day. Embryotoxic and teratogenic drug effects were not seen in rabbits which received up to 25 times the recommended human dose. There are no adequate and well-controlled studies in pregnant women. SYMMETREL should be used during pregnancy only if the potential benefit justifies the potential risk to the embryo or the fetus.

Nursing Mothers: SYMMETREL is excreted in human milk. Use is not recommended in nursing mothers.

Pediatric Use: The safety and efficacy of SYMMETREL in newborn infants, and infants below the age of 1 year have not been established.

ADVERSE REACTIONS:

The adverse reactions reported most frequently (5–10%) are: nausea, dizziness (lightheadedness), and insomnia.

Less frequently (1–5%) reported adverse reactions are: depression, anxiety, irritability, hallucinations, confusion, anorexia, dry mouth, constipation, ataxia, livedo reticularis, peripheral edema, orthostatic hypotension, headache, somnolence, nervousness, dream abnormality, agitation, dry nose, diarrhea and fatigue.

Infrequently (0.1–1%) occurring adverse reactions are: congestive heart failure, psychosis, urinary retention, dyspnea, fatigue, skin rash, vomiting, weakness, slurred speech, euphoria, confusion, thinking abnormality, amnesia, hyperkinesia, hypertension, decreased libido, and visual disturbance, including punctuate subepithelial or other corneal opacity, corneal edema, decreased visual acuity, sensitivity to light, and optic nerve palsy.

Rare (less than 0.1%) occurring adverse reactions are: instances of convulsion, leukopenia, neutropenia, eczematoid dermatitis and oculogyric episodes.

OVERDOSAGE:

There is no specific antidote. Deaths have been reported from overdose with SYMMETREL. The lowest reported acute lethal dose was 2 grams. However, slowly administered intravenous physostigmine in 1 and 2 mg doses in an adult[1] at 1 to 2 hour intervals and 0.5 mg doses in a child[2] at 5 to 10 minute intervals up to a maximum of 2 mg/hour have been reported to be effective in the control of central nervous system toxicity caused by amantadine hydrochloride. For acute overdosing, general supportive measures should be employed along with immediate gastric lavage or induction of emesis. Fluids should be forced, and if necessary, given intravenously. Hemodialysis does not remove significant amounts

---

[1] D.F. Casey, N. Engl. J. Med. 298:516, 1978.
[2] C.D. Berkowitz, J. Pediatr. 95:144, 1979.

Continued on next page

Du Pont Multi-Source—Cont.

of SYMMETREL; in patients with renal failure, a four hour hemodialysis removed 7 to 15 mg after a single 300 mg oral dose.[3] The pH of the urine has been reported to influence the excretion rate of SYMMETREL. Since the excretion rate of SYMMETREL increases rapidly when the urine is acidic, the administration of urine acidifying drugs may increase the elimination of the drug from the body. The blood pressure, pulse, respiration and temperature should be monitored. The patient should be observed for hyperactivity and convulsions; if required, sedation, and anticonvulsant therapy should be administered. The patient should be observed for the possible development of arrhythmias and hypotension; if required, appropriate antiarrhythmic and antihypotensive therapy should be given. The blood electrolytes, urine pH and urinary output should be monitored. If there is no record of recent voiding, catheterization should be done. The possibility of multiple drug ingestion by the patient should be considered.

DOSAGE AND ADMINISTRATION

Dosage for Parkinsonism:

Adult: The usual dose of SYMMETREL (amantadine hydrochloride) is 100 mg twice a day when used alone. SYMMETREL has an onset of action usually within 48 hours.

The initial dose of SYMMETREL is 100 mg daily for patients with serious associated medical illnesses or who are receiving high doses of other antiparkinson drugs. After one to several weeks at 100 mg once daily, the dose may be increased to 100 mg twice daily, if necessary.

Occasionally, patients whose responses are not optimal with SYMMETREL at 200 mg daily may benefit from an increase up to 400 mg daily in divided doses. However, such patients should be supervised closely by their physicians.

Patients initially deriving benefit from SYMMETREL not uncommonly experience a fall-off of effectiveness after a few months. Benefit may be regained by increasing the dose to 300 mg daily. Alternatively, temporary discontinuation of SYMMETREL for several weeks, followed by reinitiation of the drug, may result in regaining benefit in some patients. A decision to use other antiparkinson drugs may be necessary.

Dosage for Concomitant Therapy

Some patients who do not respond to anticholinergic antiparkinson drugs may respond to SYMMETREL. When SYMMETREL or anticholinergic antiparkinson drugs are each used with marginal benefit, concomitant use may produce additional benefit.

When SYMMETREL and levodopa are initiated concurrently, the patient can exhibit rapid therapeutic benefits. SYMMETREL should be held constant at 100 mg daily or twice daily while the daily dose of levodopa is gradually increased to optimal benefit.

When SYMMETREL is added to optimal well-tolerated doses of levodopa, additional benefit may result, including smoothing out the fluctuations in improvement which sometimes occur in patients on levodopa alone. Patients who require a reduction in their usual dose of levodopa because of development of side effects may possibly regain lost benefit with the addition of SYMMETREL.

Dosage for Drug-Induced Extrapyramidal Reactions:

Adult: The usual dose of SYMMETREL (amantadine hydrochloride) is 100 mg twice a day. Occasionally, patients whose responses are not optimal with SYMMETREL at 200 mg daily may benefit from an increase up to 300 mg daily in divided doses.

Dosage for Prophylaxis of Influenza A Virus Illness and Treatment of Uncomplicated Influenza A Virus Illness:

Normal Renal Function:

Adult: The adult daily dosage of SYMMETREL (amantadine hydrochloride) is 200 mg: two 100 mg capsules (or four teaspoonfuls of syrup) as a single daily dose, or the daily dosage may be split into one capsule of 100 mg (or two teaspoonfuls of syrup) twice a day. If central nervous system effects develop on once-a-day dosage, a split dosage schedule may reduce such complaints. In persons 65 years of age or older, the daily dosage of SYMMETREL is 100 mg.

Children: 1 yr.–9 yrs. of age: The total daily dose should be calculated on the basis of 2 to 4 mg/lb/day (4.4 to 8.8 mg/kg/day), but not to exceed 150 mg per day.

9 yrs.–12 yrs. of age: The total daily dose is 200 mg given as one capsule of 100 mg (or two teaspoonfuls of syrup) twice a day.

Impaired Renal Function: Depending upon creatinine clearance, the following dosage adjustments are recommended:

CREATININE CLEARANCE (ml/min./1.73m²)	SYMMETREL DOSAGE
30–50	200 mg 1st day and 100 mg each day thereafter
15–29	200 mg 1st day followed by 100 mg on alternate days
<15	200 mg every 7 days

The recommended dosage for patients on hemodialysis is 200 mg every 7 days.

Prophylactic dosing should be started in anticipation of an influenza A outbreak and before or after contact with individuals with influenza A virus respiratory tract illness.

SYMMETREL should be continued daily for at least 10 days following a known exposure. If SYMMETREL is used chemoprophylactically in conjunction with inactivated influenza A virus vaccine until protective antibody responses develop, then it should be administered for 2 to 3 weeks after the vaccine has been given. When inactivated influenza A virus vaccine is unavailable or contraindicated, SYMMETREL should be administered for up to 90 days in case of possible repeated and unknown exposures. Treatment of influenza A virus illness should be started as soon as possible, preferably within 24 to 48 hours, after onset of signs and symptoms, and should be continued for 24 to 48 hours after the disappearance of signs and symptoms.

HOW SUPPLIED

SYMMETREL (amantadine hydrochloride) is available as capsules (each red, soft gelatin capsule contains 100 mg amantadine hydrochloride) in:

Bottles of 100 NDC 0056-0105-70

Bottles of 500 NDC 0056-0105-85

Hospital Unit-Dose Blister Package of 100 NDC 0056-0105-75

As a syrup (each 5 mL (1 teaspoonful) contains 50 mg amantadine hydrochloride) in:

16 oz. (480 mL) bottles NDC 0056-0205-16.

Store at controlled room temperature (59°–86°F, 15°–30°C).

Caution: Federal law prohibits dispensing without prescription.

CAPSULES MANUFACTURED BY
R.P. Scherer—North America
St. Petersburg, Florida 33716
FOR
Du Pont Pharmaceuticals
Wilmington, Delaware 19880

SYMMETREL® is a Registered Trademark of The Du Pont Merck Pharmaceutical Co.

6043-23/Rev., 1991

TREXAN™ ℞

[*treks'an*]
(naltrexone hydrochloride)

DESCRIPTION

TREXAN (naltrexone hydrochloride), an opioid antagonist, is a synthetic congener of oxymorphone, and is technically, therefore, a thebaine derivative. However, it has no opioid agonist properties. Naltrexone differs in structure from oxymorphone in that the methyl group on the nitrogen atom is replaced by a cyclopropylmethyl group. TREXAN (naltrexone hydrochloride) is also related to the potent opioid antagonist, naloxone, or n-allylnoroxymorphone (NARCAN®).

TREXAN (naltrexone hydrochloride) is a white, crystalline compound. The hydrochloride salt is soluble in water to the extent of about 100 mg/cc. TREXAN is available in scored tablets containing 50 mg of naltrexone hydrochloride.

TREXAN Tablets also contain: alginic acid, FD&C Yellow 6, microcrystalline cellulose, stearic acid, and sugar.

CLINICAL PHARMACOLOGY

Pharmacodynamic actions: TREXAN (naltrexone hydrochloride) is a pure opioid antagonist. It markedly attenuates or completely blocks, reversibly, the subjective effects of intravenously administered opioids. [In this context, the term opioid is used to describe 1) classic morphine-like agonists and 2) analgesics possessing agonist and antagonist activity (e.g., butorphanol, nalbuphine and pentazocine).]

When co-administered with morphine, on a chronic basis, TREXAN blocks the physical dependence to morphine and presumably other opioids.

TREXAN has few, if any, intrinsic actions besides its opioid blocking properties. However, it does produce some pupillary constriction, by an unknown mechanism.

The administration of TREXAN is not associated with the development of tolerance or dependence.

In subjects physically dependent on opioids, TREXAN will precipitate withdrawal symptomatology.

Clinical studies indicate that 50 mg of TREXAN will block the pharmacologic effects of 25 mg of intravenously administered heroin for periods as long as 24 hours. Other data suggest that doubling the dose of TREXAN provides blockade for 48 hours, and tripling the dose of TREXAN provides blockade for about 72 hours.

While the mechanism of action is not fully understood, the preponderance of evidence suggests that TREXAN blocks the effects of opioids by competitive binding (i.e., analogous to competitive inhibition of enzymes) at opioid receptors. This makes the blockade produced potentially surmountable.

Bioavailability/Pharmacokinetics: Following oral administration, TREXAN (naltrexone hydrochloride) is subject to extensive "first pass" hepatic metabolism (its major route of elimination) with approximately 95% of the absorbed drug being converted to several metabolites. The major metabolite, 6-β-naltrexol, like TREXAN, is believed to be a pure antagonist and may contribute to the pharmacological blockade of opioid receptors. A minor metabolite is 2-hydroxy-3-methoxy-6-β-naltrexol. TREXAN and its metabolites are also conjugated to form additional metabolic products. TREXAN and its metabolites are excreted primarily by the kidney, with fecal excretion being a minor elimination pathway. The urinary excretion of unchanged TREXAN accounts for less than 1% of an oral dose; urinary excretion of unchanged and conjugated 6-β-naltrexol accounts for approximately 38% of an oral dose. The pharmacokinetic profile of TREXAN suggests that TREXAN and its metabolites undergo enterohepatic recycling.

Following the administration of 50 mg TREXAN tablets to 24 healthy adult male volunteers, the C_{max} for TREXAN and its major metabolite, 6-β-naltrexol were 8.6 ng/mL and 99.3 ng/mL, respectively. The maximum concentration (C_{max}), area under the curve (AUC), and amount excreted in the urine for both TREXAN and 6-β-naltrexol increased proportionally as the amount of TREXAN administered increased from 50 mg to 200 mg. The time to maximum concentration (T_{max}) is one hour for both TREXAN and 6-β-naltrexol. The mean elimination half-life (T-½) values for TREXAN and 6-β-naltrexol are 3.9 hours and 12.9 hours, respectively. The mean elimination half-life (T-½) and time to maximum concentration (T_{max}) for TREXAN and 6-β-naltrexol are independent of dose. TREXAN does not accumulate during chronic dosing. As predicted by its longer half-life, plasma levels of 6-β-naltrexol increase by 40% during chronic TREXAN dosing.

The total body clearance of TREXAN is 1.5 L/min, which approximates liver blood flow, and suggests TREXAN is a highly extracted compound. A renal clearance of 127 mL/min for TREXAN suggests it is solely cleared by glomerular filtration. A renal clearance of 283 mL/min for 6-β-naltrexol suggests an additional renal tubular secretory mechanism.

The volume of distribution for TREXAN following intravenous administration is estimated to be 1350 liters. *In vitro* tests with human plasma show TREXAN to be 21% bound to plasma protein over the therapeutic dose range.

In a relative bioavailability study in 24 healthy adult male volunteers, TREXAN tablets were found to be bioequivalent to TREXAN syrup; no differences were observed for C_{max}, AUC, and urinary excretion. As expected, the time to maximum concentration (T_{max}) occurred slightly earlier for the syrup (0.6 hours) than for the tablet (1.0 hr).

INDICATIONS AND USAGE

TREXAN (naltrexone hydrochloride) is indicated to provide blockade of the pharmacologic effects of exogenously administered opioids as an adjunct to the maintenance of the opioid free-state in detoxified formerly opioid-dependent individuals.

There are no data that demonstrate an unequivocally beneficial effect of TREXAN on rates of recidivism among detoxified, formerly opioid-dependent individuals.

CONTRAINDICATIONS

TREXAN is contraindicated in:

1) Patients receiving opioid analgesics.
2) Opioid dependent patients.
3) Patients in acute opioid withdrawal (see WARNINGS).
4) Any individual who has failed to pass the NARCAN challenge (see DOSAGE AND ADMINISTRATION section).
5) Any individual who has a positive urine screen for opioids.
6) Any individual with a history of sensitivity to TREXAN (naltrexone hydrochloride). It is not known if there is any cross-sensitivity with naloxone or other phenanthrene containing opioids.
7) Any individual with acute hepatitis or liver failure.

WARNINGS

Hepatotoxicity:

TREXAN has the capacity to cause dose related hepatocellular injury.

Prior to making a decision to initiate treatment with TREXAN, the physician should establish whether the patient has subclinical liver injury or disease. (See PRECAUTIONS; Laboratory Tests.) TREXAN is contraindicated in acute hepatitis or liver failure, but its use even in patients with evidence of less severe liver disease or a history of recent liver disease must be carefully considered in light of its hepatotoxic potential.

The evidence that identified TREXAN as a hepatotoxin was <u>not</u> obtained in studies involving its use at the doses recommended for opiate blockade, where the changes in serum levels of liver enzymes seen were similar to those present at baseline in the study population. However, the margin of separation between the apparently safe and the hepatotoxic doses appears to be only five-fold or less.

---

[3] V.W. Horadam, et al., Ann. Intern. Med. 94:454, 1981.

Evidence of TREXAN's hepatotoxic potential is derived primarily from a placebo controlled study in which TREXAN was administered to obese subjects at a dose approximately five-fold that recommended for the blockade of opiate receptors (300 mg per day). In the study, 5 of 26 TREXAN recipients developed elevations of serum transaminases (i.e., peak SGPT values ranging from a low of 121 to a high of 532; or 3 to 19 times their baseline values) after three to eight weeks of treatment. Although the patients involved were generally clinically asymptomatic and the transaminase levels of all patients on whom follow-up was obtained returned to (or toward) baseline values in a matter of weeks, the lack of any transaminase elevations of similar magnitude in any of the 24 placebo patients in the same study is persuasive evidence that TREXAN is a direct (i.e., not an idiosyncratic) hepatotoxin. This conclusion is also supported by evidence from other placebo controlled studies in which exposure to TREXAN at doses from one to two-fold the amount recommended for opiate blockade consistently produced more numerous and more significant elevations of serum transaminases than did placebo, and reports of transaminase elevations in 3 of 9 patients with Alzheimer's Disease who received TREXAN (up to 300 mg/day) for 5 to 8 weeks in an open clinical trial.

Unintended Precipitation of Abstinence: To prevent occurrence of an acute abstinence syndrome, or exacerbation of a pre-existing sub-clinical abstinence syndrome, patients should remain opioid-free for a minimum of 7–10 days before starting TREXAN. Since the absence of an opioid drug in the urine is often not sufficient proof that a patient is opioid-free, a NARCAN challenge should be employed to exclude the possibility of precipitating a withdrawal reaction following administration of TREXAN. The NARCAN challenge test is described in the DOSAGE AND ADMINISTRATION section.

While TREXAN is a potent antagonist with a prolonged pharmacologic effect (24 to 72 hours), the blockade produced by TREXAN is surmountable. This is useful in patients who may require analgesia, but poses a potential risk to individuals who attempt, on their own, to overcome the blockade by administering large amounts of exogenous opioids. Indeed, any attempt by a patient to overcome the antagonism by taking opioids is very dangerous and may lead to a fatal overdose. Injury may arise because the plasma concentration of exogenous opioids attained immediately following their acute administration may be sufficient to overcome the competitive receptor blockade. As a consequence, the patient may be in immediate danger of suffering life endangering opioid intoxication (e.g., respiratory arrest, circulatory collapse). Also, lesser amounts of exogenous opioids may prove dangerous if they are taken in a manner (i.e. relatively long after the last dose of naltrexone) and in an amount so that they persist in the body longer than effective concentrations of naltrexone and its metabolites. Patients should be told of the serious consequences of surmounting the opiate blockade. See Information for Patients section.

PRECAUTIONS

General:

Actions Suggested When Reversal of TREXAN Blockade is Required: In an emergency situation requiring analgesia which can only be achieved with opioids, the amount of opioid required may be greater than usual, and the resulting respiratory depression may be deeper and more prolonged. No methods to reverse overdose have been established by controlled clinical trials; therefore in such circumstances, a rapidly acting analgesic which minimizes respiratory depression is preferred. The amount of analgesic administered should be titrated to the needs of the patient.

Additionally, non-receptor mediated actions may occur (e.g., facial swelling, itching, generalized erythema presumably due to histamine release).

Irrespective of the drug chosen to reverse TREXAN (naltrexone hydrochloride) blockade, the patient should be monitored closely by appropriately trained personnel in a hospital setting.

Actions Suggested When Withdrawal is Accidentally Precipitated With TREXAN: Severe opioid withdrawal syndromes precipitated by the accidental ingestion of TREXAN have been reported in opioid-dependent individuals. Symptoms of withdrawal have usually appeared within five minutes of ingestion of TREXAN and have lasted for up to 48 hours. Mental status changes including confusion, somnolence and visual hallucinations have occurred. Significant fluid losses from vomiting and diarrhea have required intravenous fluid administration. In all cases patients were closely monitored and therapy tailored to meet individual requirements.

Interference With the Action of Narcotic Containing Drug Product: Patients taking TREXAN may not benefit from opioid containing medicines, such as cough and cold preparations, antidiarrheal preparations, and opioid analgesics. Where a non-opioid containing alternative is available, it should be used.

Information for Patients: It is suggested that the prescribing physician relate the following information to patients being treated with TREXAN:

You have been prescribed TREXAN (naltrexone hydrochloride) as part of the comprehensive treatment for your drug dependence. You should carry identification to alert medical personnel to the fact that you are taking TREXAN. A TREXAN medication card may be obtained from your physician and can be used for this purpose. Carrying the identification card should help to ensure that you can obtain adequate treatment in an emergency. If you require medical treatment, be sure to tell the treating physician that you are receiving TREXAN therapy.

You should take TREXAN as directed by your physician. If you attempt to self-administer heroin or any other opiate drug, in small doses, you will not perceive any effect. Most important, however, if you attempt to self-administer large doses of heroin or any other narcotic, you may die or sustain serious injury, including coma.

Laboratory tests: Tests designed to detect hepatic injury should be obtained prior to initiation of TREXAN therapy and periodically thereafter. (See WARNINGS section on Hepatotoxicity.)

Periodic testing of all patients after initiation of treatment is critical if the occurrence of TREXAN induced liver damage is to be detected at the earliest possible time. Evaluations, using appropriate batteries of tests to detect liver injury are recommended on a monthly basis during the first six months of use; thereafter, clinical judgment about the frequency of monitoring must be relied upon.

Laboratory tests which may be used for the separation and detection of morphine, methadone or quinine in the urine and with which TREXAN does not interfere include thin-layer, gas-liquid, and high pressure liquid chromatographic methods.

CARCINOGENESIS, MUTAGENESIS AND IMPAIRMENT OF FERTILITY:

Carcinogenesis: In a two-year carcinogenicity study in rats, there were small increases in the numbers of mesotheliomas in males, and tumors of vascular origin in both sexes. The number of tumors were within the range seen in historical control groups, except for the vascular tumors in females, where the 4% incidence exceeded the historical maximum of 2%.

Mutagenesis: A total of twenty-two distinct tests were performed using bacterial, mammalian, and tissue culture systems. All tests were negative except for weakly positive findings in the Drosophila recessive lethal assay and non-specific DNA repair tests with E. coli. The significance of these findings is undetermined.

Impairment of Fertility: TREXAN (100 mg/kg, approximately 140 times the human therapeutic dose) caused a significant increase in pseudopregnancy in the rat. A decrease in the pregnancy rate of mated female rats also occurred. The relevance of these observations to human fertility is not known.

Pregnancy: Category C. TREXAN has been shown to have an embryocidal effect in the rat and rabbit when given in doses approximately 140 times the human therapeutic dose. This effect was demonstrated in rats dosed with TREXAN (100 mg/kg) prior to and throughout gestation, and rabbits treated with 60 mg/kg of TREXAN during the period of organogenesis.

There are no adequate and well-controlled studies in pregnant women. TREXAN should be used in pregnancy only when the potential benefit justifies the potential risk to the fetus.

LABOR AND DELIVERY

Whether or not TREXAN affects the duration of labor and delivery is unknown.

NURSING MOTHERS

Whether or not TREXAN is excreted in human milk is unknown. Because many drugs are excreted in human milk, caution should be exercised when TREXAN is administered to a nursing mother.

PEDIATRIC USE

The safe use of TREXAN in subjects younger than 18 years old has not been established.

ADVERSE REACTIONS

While extensive clinical studies evaluating the use of TREXAN in detoxified, formerly opioid dependent individuals failed to identify any single, serious untoward risk of TREXAN use, placebo controlled studies employing up to five-fold higher doses of TREXAN (up to 300 mg per day) than that recommended for use in opiate receptor blockade have shown that TREXAN causes hepatocellular injury in a substantial proportion of patients exposed at this higher dose (See **WARNINGS** and **PRECAUTIONS**: Laboratory Tests).

Aside from this finding, however, available evidence does not incriminate TREXAN, used at any dose, as a cause of any other serious untoward event for the patient who is "opioid free." It is critical to recognize that TREXAN can precipitate or exacerbate abstinence signs and symptoms in any individual who is not completely free of exogenous opioids.

TREXAN used at the doses recommended to produce opiate receptor blockade does not appear to be the cause of any of the numerous adverse events and abnormal laboratory findings, including liver function abnormalities, that were observed in the course of the clinical trials that enrolled individuals with a history of both alcohol and substance abuse. In the one placebo controlled trial intended to assess the effects of opiate receptor blockade on drug abuse recidivism, observed untoward events and laboratory abnormalities occurred with nearly equal frequency among placebo and TREXAN recipients. In all open studies, the untoward events observed (e.g., lymphocytosis, transaminase elevations, GI disturbances) were findings that would be anticipated in any similar population not treated with naltrexone. Supporting this judgment, many of the abnormalities detected during the course of the clinical trials were present at baseline, and in some instances, baseline abnormalities, including transaminase elevations, improved or returned to normal during the course of treatment with naltrexone.

In summary, among opioid free individuals, TREXAN administration at the recommended dose has not been associated with a predictable profile of serious adverse or untoward events. However, as mentioned above, among individuals using opioids, TREXAN may cause serious reactions (see CONTRAINDICATIONS, WARNINGS, DOSAGE AND ADMINISTRATION).

Events other than hepatocellular injury reported during clinical testing:

The following adverse reactions have been reported both at baseline and during the TREXAN medication period at an incidence rate of more than 10%:

Difficulty sleeping, anxiety, nervousness, abdominal pain/cramps, nausea and/or vomiting, low energy, joint and muscle pain, and headache.

The incidence was less than 10% for:

Loss of appetite, diarrhea, constipation, increased thirst, increased energy, feeling down, irritability, dizziness, skin rash, delayed ejaculation, decreased potency, and chills.

The following events occurred in less than 1% of subjects:

Respiratory: nasal congestion, itching, rhinorrhea, sneezing, sore throat, excess mucus or phlegm, sinus trouble, heavy breathing, hoarseness, cough, shortness of breath.

Cardiovascular: nose bleeds, phlebitis, edema, increased blood pressure, non-specific ECG changes, palpitations, tachycardia.

Gastrointestinal: excessive gas, hemorrhoids, diarrhea, ulcer.

Musculoskeletal: painful shoulders, legs or knees; tremors, twitching.

Genitourinary: increased frequency of, or discomfort during urination; increased or decreased sexual interest.

Dermatologic: oily skin, pruritus, acne, athlete's foot, cold sores, alopecia.

Psychiatric: depression, paranoia, fatigue, restlessness, confusion, disorientation, hallucinations, nightmares, bad dreams.

Special senses: eyes-blurred, burning, light sensitive, swollen, aching, strained; ears "clogged", aching, tinnitus.

General: increased appetite, weight loss, weight gain, yawning, somnolence, fever, dry mouth, head "pounding", inguinal pain, swollen glands, "side" pains, cold feet, "hot spells."

Lethargy and somnolence have been reported following dosing of TREXAN (naltrexone hydrochloride) and thioridazine.

Laboratory tests: With the exception of liver test abnormalities in investigator studies (see WARNINGS, PRECAUTIONS, etc.), results of laboratory tests, like adverse reaction reports, have not shown consistent patterns of abnormalities that can be attributed to treatment with TREXAN.

In the trials evaluating TREXAN for the blockade of opiate receptors, abnormal liver function tests and lymphocytosis were the two most common categories of abnormalities reported. As noted earlier, these abnormalities are common among populations of parenteral opioid users and alcoholics. As is the case with the untoward events described above, a large proportion of patients had abnormal laboratory tests at baseline, further supporting the conclusion that the abnormalities observed are not attributable to TREXAN.

Idiopathic thrombocytopenic purpura was reported in one patient who may have been sensitized to TREXAN in a previous course of treatment with TREXAN. The condition cleared without sequelae after discontinuation of TREXAN and corticosteroid treatment.

DRUG ABUSE AND DEPENDENCE

TREXAN is a pure opioid antagonist. It does not lead to physical or psychological dependence. Tolerance to the opioid antagonist effect is not known to occur.

Continued on next page

Du Pont Multi-Source—Cont.

OVERDOSAGE

There is no clinical experience with TREXAN overdosage in humans. In one study, subjects who received 800 mg daily TREXAN for up to one week showed no evidence of toxicity.

In the mouse, rat and guinea pig, the oral LD_{50}s were 1,100 $\pm$ 96 mg/kg; 1,450 $\pm$ 265 mg/kg; and 1,490 $\pm$ 102 mg/kg, respectively.

In acute toxicity studies in the mouse, rat, and dog, cause of death was due to clonic-tonic convulsions and/or respiratory failure.

TREATMENT OF OVERDOSAGE

Consideration should be given to contacting a poison control center for the most up-to-date information.

In view of the lack of actual experience in the treatment of TREXAN overdose, patients should be treated symptomatically in a closely supervised environment.

DOSAGE AND ADMINISTRATION

Induction of TREXAN Therapy: DO NOT ATTEMPT TREATMENT UNTIL NARCAN CHALLENGE IS NEGATIVE (see below). Initiate treatment with TREXAN using the following guidelines:

1. Treatment should not be attempted until the patient has remained opioid-free for 7–10 days. Self-reporting of abstinence from opioids should be verified by analysis of the patient's urine for absence of opioids. The patient should not be manifesting withdrawal signs or reporting withdrawal symptoms.
2. A NARCAN challenge test (see below) should be administered to the patient. If signs of opioid withdrawal are still observed following NARCAN challenge, treatment with TREXAN should not be attempted. The NARCAN challenge can be repeated in 24 hours.
3. Treatment should be initiated carefully, slowly increasing the dose of TREXAN administered. This can be accomplished by administration of 25 mg of TREXAN initially. The patient should be observed for 1 hour. If no withdrawal signs occur, the patient may be given the rest of the daily dose.

NARCAN Challenge Test: The NARCAN challenge test should not be performed in a patient showing clinical signs or symptoms of opioid withdrawal, or in a patient whose urine contains opioids.

The NARCAN challenge test may be administered by either the intravenous or subcutaneous routes.

Intravenous challenge: Following appropriate screening of the patient, 0.8 mg of NARCAN should be drawn into a sterile syringe. If the intravenous route of administration is selected, 0.2 mg of NARCAN should be injected, and while the needle is still in the patient's vein, the patient should be observed for 30 seconds for evidence of withdrawal signs or symptoms. If there is no evidence of withdrawal, the remaining 0.6 mg of NARCAN should be injected, and the patient observed for an additional period of 20 minutes for signs and symptoms of withdrawal.

Subcutaneous challenge: If the subcutaneous route is selected, 0.8 mg should be administered subcutaneously, and the patient observed for signs and symptoms of withdrawal for 45 minutes.

Conditions and technique for observation of patient: During the appropriate period of observation, the patient's vital signs should be monitored and the patient should be monitored for signs of withdrawal. It is also important to question the patient carefully. The signs and symptoms of opioid withdrawal include, but are not limited to, the following:

WITHDRAWAL SIGNS: stuffiness or running nose, tearing, yawning, sweating, tremor, vomiting or piloerection.

WITHDRAWAL SYMPTOMS: feeling of temperature change, joint or bone and muscle pain, abdominal cramps, skin crawling, etc.

Interpretation of the Challenge: Warning: the elicitation of the enumerated signs or symptoms indicates a potential risk for the subject, and TREXAN should not be administered. If no signs or symptoms of withdrawal are observed, elicited, or reported, TREXAN MAY BE ADMINISTERED. If there is any doubt in the observer's mind that the patient is not in an opioid-free state, or is in continuing withdrawal, NARCAN should be readministered as follows:

Confirmatory rechallenge (if necessary): 1.6 mg of NARCAN should be injected intravenously and the patient again observed for signs and symptoms of withdrawal. If none are present, TREXAN may be administered. If signs and symptoms of withdrawal are present, administration of TREXAN should be delayed until repeated NARCAN challenge indicates the patient is no longer at risk.

Maintenance Treatment: Once the patient has been started on TREXAN, 50 mg every 24 hours will produce adequate clinical blockade of the actions of parenterally administered opioids (i.e., this dose will block the effects of a 25 mg intravenous heroin challenge). A flexible approach to a dosing regimen may be employed. Thus, patients may receive 50 mg of TREXAN every weekday with a 100 mg dose on Saturday or patients may receive 100 mg every other day, or 150 mg every third day. While the degree of opioid blockade may be somewhat reduced by using higher doses at longer dosing intervals, improved patient compliance may result from dosing every 48–72 hours.

Several of the clinical studies reported in the literature have employed the following dosing regimen: 100 mg on Monday, 100 mg on Wednesday, and 150 mg on Friday. This dosing schedule appeared to be acceptable to many TREXAN patients successfully maintaining their opioid free state.

HOW SUPPLIED

TREXAN (naltrexone hydrochloride) tablets are available in 50 mg round tablets, scored imprinted with DuPont on one side and TREXAN on the other. Bottles of 50 tablets (NDC 0056-0080-50).

Protect from excessive light.

Store at controlled room temperature (59°–86°F, 15°–30°C).

Dispense in a tight, light-resistant container as defined in the U.S.P.

Caution: Federal law prohibits dispensing without prescription.

NARCAN® is a Registered Trademark of The Du Pont Merck Pharmaceutical Co.

TREXAN® is a Registered Trademark of The Du Pont Merck Pharmaceutical Co.

Du Pont Pharmaceuticals
Wilmington, Delaware 19880

6162-4/Rev. Jan., 1991

TRIDIL® ℞

[tri 'dil]
(nitroglycerin)

FOR INTRAVENOUS USE ONLY. NOT FOR DIRECT INTRAVENOUS INJECTION. TRIDIL® MUST BE DILUTED IN DEXTROSE (5%) INJECTION, USP OR SODIUM CHLORIDE (0.9%) INJECTION, USP PRIOR TO ITS INFUSION (SEE DOSAGE AND ADMINISTRATION SECTION). THE ADMINISTRATION SET USED FOR INFUSION WILL AFFECT THE AMOUNT OF TRIDIL DELIVERED TO THE PATIENT. (SEE WARNINGS, AND DOSAGE AND ADMINISTRATION SECTIONS).

CAUTION

SEVERAL PREPARATIONS OF NITROGLYCERIN FOR INJECTION ARE AVAILABLE. THEY DIFFER IN CONCENTRATION AND/OR VOLUME PER VIAL. WHEN SWITCHING FROM ONE PRODUCT TO ANOTHER ATTENTION MUST BE PAID TO THE DILUTION AND DOSAGE AND ADMINISTRATION INSTRUCTIONS.

DESCRIPTION

Nitroglycerin in 1,2,3-propanetriol trinitrate, an organic nitrate whose empiric formula is $C_3H_5N_3O_9$, and whose molecular weight is 227.09. The organic nitrates are vasodilators, active on both arteries and veins.

TRIDIL (nitroglycerin) is a clear, practically colorless additive solution for intravenous infusion after dilution. Each mL of TRIDIL 5 mg contains 0.5 mg Nitroglycerin with 4.5 mg Lactose, USP; 10% Alcohol, USP; and 13.8 mg Monobasic Sodium Phosphate, USP as a buffer in Water for Injection, USP. Each mL of TRIDIL 25 mg, TRIDIL 50 mg, or TRIDIL 100 mg contains 5 mg Nitroglycerin in 30% Alcohol, USP; 30% Propylene Glycol, USP; and Water for Injection, USP. The solution is sterile, non-pyrogenic, and nonexplosive.

CLINICAL PHARMACOLOGY

The principal pharmacological action of TRIDIL (nitroglycerin) is relaxation of vascular smooth muscle and consequent dilatation of peripheral arteries and veins, especially the latter. Dilatation of the veins promotes peripheral pooling of blood and decreases venous return to the heart, thereby reducing left ventricular end-diastolic pressure and pulmonary capillary wedge pressure (preload). Arteriolar relaxation reduces systemic vascular resistance, systolic arterial pressure, and mean arterial pressure (afterload). Dilatation of the coronary arteries also occurs. The relative importance of preload reduction, afterload reduction, and coronary dilatation remains undefined.

Dosing regimens for most chronically used drugs are designed to provide plasma concentrations that are continuously greater than an minimally effective concentration. This strategy is inappropriate for organic nitrates. Several well-controlled clinical trials have used exercise testing to assess the anti-anginal efficacy of continuously-delivered nitrates. In the large majority of these trials, active agents were indistinguishable from placebo after 24 hours (or less) of continuous therapy. Attempts to overcome nitrate tolerance by dose escalation, even to doses far in excess of those used acutely, have consistently failed. Only after nitrates have been absent from the body for several hours has their anti-anginal efficacy been restored.

Pharmacokinetics: The volume of distribution of nitroglycerin is about 3 L/kg, and nitroglycerin is cleared from this volume at extremely rapid rates, with a resulting serum half-life of about 3 minutes. The observed clearance rates (close to 1 L/kg/min) greatly exceed hepatic blood flow; known sites of extrahepatic metabolism include red blood cells and vascular walls.

The first products in the metabolism of nitroglycerin are inorganic nitrate and the 1,2- and 1,3-dinitroglycerols. The dinitrates are less effective vasodilators than nitroglycerin, but they are longer-lived in the serum, and their net contribution to the overall effect of chronic nitroglycerin regimens is not known. The dinitrates are further metabolized to (non-vasoactive) mononitrates and, ultimately, to glycerol and carbon dioxide.

To avoid development of tolerance to nitroglycerin drug-free intervals of 10–12 hours are known to be sufficient; shorter intervals have not been well studied. In one well-controlled clinical trial, subjects receiving nitroglycerin appeared to exhibit a rebound or withdrawal effect, so that their exercise tolerance at the end of the daily drug-free interval was *less* than that exhibited by the parallel group receiving placebo.

Clinical Trials: Blinded, placebo-controlled trials of intravenous nitroglycerin have not been reported, but multiple investigators have reported open-label studies, and there are scattered reports of studies in which intravenous nitroglycerin was tested in blinded fashion against sodium nitroprusside.

In each of these studies, therapeutic doses of intravenous nitroglycerin were found to reduce systolic and diastolic arterial blood pressure. The heart rate was usually increased, presumably as a reflexive response to the fall in blood pressure. Coronary perfusion pressure was usually, but not always, maintained.

Intravenous nitroglycerin reduced central venous pressure (CVP), right atrial pressure (RAP), pulmonary arterial pressure (PAP), pulmonary-capillary wedge pressure (PCWP), pulmonary vascular resistance (PVR), and systemic vascular resistance (SVR). When these parameters were elevated, reducing them toward normal usually caused a rise in cardiac output. Conversely intravenous nitroglycerin usually *reduced* cardiac output when it was given to patients whose CVP, RAP, PAP, PCWP, PVR, and SVR were all normal.

Most clinical trials of intravenous nitroglycerin have been brief; they have typically followed hemodynamic parameters during a single surgical procedure. In one careful study, one of the few that lasted more than a few hours, continuous intravenous nitroglycerin had lost almost all of its hemodynamic effect after 48 hours. In the same study, patients who received nitroglycerin infusions for only 12 hours out of each 24 demonstrated no similar attenuation of effect. These results are consistent with those seen in multiple large, double-blind, placebo-controlled trials of other formulations of nitroglycerin and other nitrates.

INDICATIONS AND USAGE

TRIDIL (nitroglycerin) is indicated for treatment of perioperative hypertension; for control of congestive heart failure in the setting of acute myocardial infarction; for treatment of angina pectoris in patients who have not responded to sublingual nitroglycerin and B-blockers; and for induction of intraoperative hypotension.

CONTRAINDICATIONS

Allergic reactions to organic nitrates are extremely rare, but they do occur. TRIDIL is contraindicated in patients who are allergic to it.

WARNINGS

Nitroglycerin readily migrates into many plastics, including the polyvinyl chloride (PVC) plastics commonly used for intravenous administration sets. Nitroglycerin absorption by PVC tubing is increased when the tubing is long, the flow rates are low, and the nitroglycerin concentration of the solution is high. The delivered fraction of the solution's original nitroglycerin content has been 20–60% in published studies using PVC tubing; the fraction varies with time during a single infusion, and no simple correction factor can be used. PVC tubing has been used in most published studies of intravenous nitroglycerin, but the reported doses have been calculated by simply multiplying the flow rate of the solution by the solution's original concentration of nitroglycerin. *The actual doses delivered have been less, sometimes much less, than those reported.*

Some in-line intravenous filters also absorb nitroglycerin; these filters should be avoided.

Because of the absoprtion problem, the TRIDILSET® i.v. administration set and TRIDILSET V.I.P.® volumetric infusion pump connector set were developed to minimize the loss of TRIDIL. TRIDILSET or TRIDILSET V.I.P. are recommended for infusions of TRIDIL (see DOSAGE AND ADMINISTRATION).

DOSING INSTRUCTIONS MUST BE FOLLOWED WITH CARE. WHEN TRIDILSET/TRIDILSET V.I.P IS USED, THE CALCULATED DOSE WILL BE DELIVERED TO THE PATIENT, BECAUSE THE LOSS OF TRIDIL SEEN WITH STANDARD PVC TUBING WILL BE AVOIDED. THE DOSAGES REPORTED IN PUBLISHED STUDIES UTILIZED GENERAL-USE PVC ADMINISTRATION SETS, AND RECOMMENDED DOSES BASED ON THIS EXPERIENCE

WILL BE TOO HIGH WHEN TRIDILSET/TRIDILSET V.I.P. IS USED.

PRECAUTIONS

General Severe hypotension and shock may occur with even small doses of TRIDIL (nitroglycerin). This drug should therefore be used with caution in patients who may be volume depleted or who, for whatever reason, are already hypotensive. Hypotension induced by nitroglycerin may be accompanied by paradoxical bradycardia and increased angina pectoris.

Nitrate therapy may aggravate the angina caused by hypertrophic cardiomyopathy.

As tolerance to other forms of nitroglycerin develops, the effect of sublingual nitroglycerin on exercise tolerance, although still observable, is somewhat blunted.

In industrial workers who have had long-term exposure to unknown (presumably high) doses of organic nitrates, tolerance clearly occurs. Chest pain, acute myocardial infarction, and even sudden death have occurred during temporary withdrawal of nitrates from these workers, demonstrating the existence of true physical dependence.

Some clinical trials in angina patients have provided nitroglycerin for about 12 continuous hours of every 24-hour day. During the nitrate-free intervals in some of these trials, anginal attacks have been more easily provoked than before treatment, and patients have demonstrated hemodynamic rebound and *decreased* exercise tolerance. The importance of these observations to the routine, clinical use of intravenous nitroglycerin is not known.

Lower concentrations of nitroglycerin increase the potential precision of dosing, but these concentrations increase the total fluid volume that must be delivered to the patient. Total fluid load may be a dominant consideration in patients with compromised function of the heart, liver, and/or kidneys.

Nitroglycerin infusions should be administered only via a pump that can maintain a constant infusion rate.

Intracoronary injection of nitroglycerin infusions has not been studied.

Laboratory Tests: Because of the propylene glycol content of intravenous nitroglycerin, serum triglyceride assays that rely on glycerol oxidase may give falsely elevated results in patients receiving this medication.

Drug Interactions: The vasodilating effects of nitroglycerin may be additive with those of other vasodilators.

Administration of nitroglycerin infusions through the same infusion set as blood can result in pseudoagglutination and hemolysis. More generally, nitroglycerin in 5% dextrose or sodium chloride 0.9% should not be mixed with any other medication of any kind.

Intravenous nitroglycerin interferes, at least in some patients, with the anticoagulant effect of heparin. In patients receiving intravenous nitroglycerin, concomitant heparin therapy should be guided by frequent measurement of the activated partial thromboplastin time.

Carcinogenesis, Mutagenesis, and impairment of Fertility: No long-term studies in animals have been performed to evaluate the carcinogenic potential of TRIDIL. Studies to evaluate nitroglycerin's potential for mutagenicity or impairment of fertility have also not been performed.

Pregnancy Category C: Animal reproduction studies have not been conducted with TRIDIL. It is also not known whether TRIDIL can cause fetal harm when administered to a pregnant woman or whether it can affect reproductive capacity. TRIDIL should be given to a pregnant woman only if clearly needed.

Nursing Mothers: It is not known whether nitroglycerin is excreted in human milk. Because many drugs are excreted in human milk, caution should be exercised when TRIDIL is administered to a nursing woman.

Pediatric Use: Safety and effectiveness in children have not been established.

ADVERSE REACTIONS

Adverse reactions to TRIDIL (nitroglycerin) are generally dose-related and almost all of these reactions are the result of nitroglycerin's activity as a vasodilator. Headache, which may be severe, is the most commonly reported side effect. Headache may be recurrent with each daily dose, especially at higher doses. Transient episodes of lightheadedness, occasionally related to blood pressure changes, may also occur. Hypotension occurs infrequently, but in some patients it may be severe enough to warrant discontinuation of therapy. Syncope, crescendo angina, and rebound hypertension have been reported but are uncommon.

Extremely rarely, ordinary doses of organic nitrates have caused methemoglobinemia in normal-seeming patients. Methemoglobinemia is so infrequent at these doses that further discussion of its diagnosis and treatment is deferred (see OVERDOSAGE).

OVERDOSAGE

Hemodynamic Effects: The ill effects of TRIDIL (nitroglycerin) overdose are generally the results of nitroglycerin's capacity to induce vasodilatation, venous pooling, reduced cardiac output, and hypotension. These hemodynamic changes may have protean manifestations, including increased intracranial pressure, with any or all of persistent throbbing headache, confusion, and moderate fever; vertigo; palpitation; visual disturbances; nausea and vomiting (possibly with colic and even bloody diarrhea); syncope (especially in the upright posture); air hunger and dyspnea, later followed by reduced ventilatory effort; diaphoresis, with the skin either flushed or cold and clammy; heart block and bradycardia; paralysis; coma; seizures; and death.

Laboratory determinations of serum levels of TRIDIL and its metabolites are not widely available, and such determinations have, in any event, no established role in the management of TRIDIL overdose.

No data are available to suggest physiological maneuvers (e.g., maneuvers to change the pH of the urine) that might accelerate elimination of nitroglycerin and its active metabolites. Similarly, it is not known which—if any—of these substances can usefully be removed from the body by hemodialysis.

No specific antagonist to the vasodilator effects of TRIDIL is known, and no intervention has been subject to controlled study as a therapy of nitroglycerin overdose. Because the hypotension associated with nitroglycerin overdose is the result of venodilatation and arterial hypovolemia, prudent therapy in this situation should be directed toward increase in central fluid volume. Passive elevation of the patient's legs may be sufficient, but intravenous infusion of normal saline or similar fluid may also be necessary.

The use of epinephrine or other arterial vasoconstrictors in this setting is likely to do more harm than good.

In patients with renal disease or congestive heart failure, therapy resulting in central volume expansion is not without hazard. Treatment of TRIDIL overdose in these patients may be subtle and difficult, and invasive monitoring may be required.

Methemoglobinemia: Nitrate ions liberated during metabolism of nitroglycerin can oxidize hemoglobin into methemoglobin. Even in patients totally without cytochrome b_5 reductase activity, however, and even assuming that the nitrate moieties of nitroglycerin are quantitatively applied to oxidation of hemoglobin, about 1 mg/kg of nitroglycerin should be required before any of these patients manifests clinically significant ($\geq 10\%$) methemoglobinemia. In patients with normal reductase function, significant production of methemoglobin should require even larger doses of nitroglycerin. In one study in which 36 patients received 2–4 weeks of continuous nitroglycerin therapy at 3.1 to 4.4 mg/hr, the average methemoglobin level measured was 0.2%; this was comparable to that observed in parallel patients who received placebo.

Notwithstanding these observations, there are case reports of significant methemoglobinemia in association with moderate overdoses of organic nitrates. None of the affected patients had been thought to be unusually susceptible.

Methemoglobin levels are available from most clinical laboratories. The diagnosis should be suspected in patients who exhibit signs of impaired oxygen delivery despite adequate cardiac output and adequate arterial pO_2. Classically, methemoglobinemic blood is described as chocolate brown, without color change on exposure to air.

When methemoglobinemia is diagnosed, the treatment of choice is methylene blue, 1–2 mg/kg intravenously.

DOSAGE AND ADMINISTRATION

NOT FOR DIRECT INTRAVENOUS INJECTION

TRIDIL (NITROGLYCERIN) IS A CONCENTRATED, POTENT DRUG WHICH MUST BE DILUTED IN DEXTROSE (5%) INJECTION, USP OR SODIUM CHLORIDE (0.9%) INJECTION, USP PRIOR TO ITS INFUSION. TRIDIL SHOULD NOT BE MIXED WITH OTHER DRUGS.

1. Initial Dilution:

Aseptically transfer the contents of one TRIDIL ampul or vial (containing 25 or 50 mg of nitroglycerin) into a 500 mL *glass* bottle of either Dextrose (5%) Injection, USP or Sodium Chloride Injection (0.9%), USP. This yields a final concentration of 50 mcg/mL or 100 mcg/mL. Diluting 5 mg TRIDIL into 100 mL will also yield a final concentration of 50 mcg/mL.

2. Maintenance Dilution:

It is important to consider the fluid requirement of the patient as well as the expected duration of infusion in selecting the appropriate dilution of TRIDIL (nitroglycerin). After the initial dosage titration, the concentration of the solution may be increased, if necessary, to limit fluids given to the patient. The TRIDIL concentration should not exceed 400 mcg/mL. See chart.

Note: If the concentration is adjusted, it is imperative to flush TRIDILSET®/TRIDILSET V.I.P.® before a new concentration is utilized. The dead-space of the set is approximately 15 mL, and depending on the flow rate it could take from 10 minutes to 3 hours for the new concentration to reach the patient if the set were not flushed.

Invert the glass parenteral bottle several times to assure uniform dilution of TRIDIL. When stored in *glass* containers, the diluted solution is physically and chemically stable for up to 48 hours at room temperature, and up to seven days under refrigeration.

Dosage is affected by the type of container and administration set used. See WARNINGS.

Although the usual starting adult dose range reported in clinical studies was 25 mcg/min or more, these studies used PVC administration sets. THE USE OF NONABSORBING TUBING WILL RESULT IN THE NEED FOR REDUCED DOSES.

If a peristaltic action infusion pump is used, a TRIDILSET i.v. administration set should be selected. As the TRIDILSET drip chambers deliver approximately 60 microdrops/mL, the TRIDIL DILUTION AND ADMINISTRATION table below may be used to calculate TRIDIL dilution and flow rate in microdrops/minute to achieve the desired TRIDIL administration rate.

If a volumetric infusion pump is used, a TRIDILSET V.I.P. volumetric infusion pump connector set should be selected. The TRIDIL DILUTION AND ADMINISTRATION table below may still be used; however, flow rate will be determined directly by the infusion pump, independent of the drop size of the TRIDILSET V.I.P. drip chambers. Thus, the reference to "MICRODROPS/MIN" is not applicable, and the corresponding flow rate in mL/hr should be used to determine pump settings. NOTE: The TRIDILSET V.I.P. is not intended for use as an i.v. administration set independent of a volumetric infusion pump.

The dosage for TRIDILSET/TRIDILSET V.I.P. should initially be 5 mcg/min delivered through an infusion pump capable of exact and constant delivery of the drug. Subsequent titration must be adjusted to the clinical situation, with dose increments becoming more cautious as partial response is seen. Initial titration should be in 5 mcg/min increments, with increases every 3–5 minutes until some response is noted. If no response is seen at 20 mcg/min, increments of 10 and later 20 mcg/min can be used. Once a partial blood pressure response is observed, the dose increase should be reduced and the interval between increases should be lengthened.

Some patients with normal or low left ventricular filling pressures or pulmonary capillary wedge pressure (e.g., angina patients without other complications) may be hypersensitive to the effects of TRIDIL and may respond fully to doses

TRIDIL DILUTION AND ADMINISTRATION TABLE

	DILUTE			
	5 MG TRIDIL IN 100 ML OR 25 MG TRIDIL IN 500 ML	5 MG TRIDIL IN 50 ML OR 25 MG TRIDIL IN 250 ML OR 50 MG TRIDIL IN 500 ML	10 MG TRIDIL IN 50 ML OR 50 MG TRIDIL IN 250 ML OR 100 MG TRIDIL IN 500 ML	100 MG TRIDIL IN 250 ML 200 MG TRIDIL IN 500 ML
			TO YIELD	
	50 MCG/ML	100 MCG/ML	200 MCG/ML	400 MCG/ML
TRIDILSET ADMIXTURE FLOW RATE MICRO MIN = ML/HR	TRIDIL ADMINISTRATION RATE MCG I.V. NITROGLYCERIN/MIN			
3	—	5	10	20
6	5	10	20	40
12	10	20	40	80
24	20	40	80	160
48	40	80	160	320
72	60	120	240	480
96	80	160	320	640

Continued on next page

Du Pont Multi-Source—Cont.

as small as 5 mcg/min. These patients require especially careful titration and monitoring.
There is no fixed optimum dose of TRIDIL. Due to variations in the responsiveness of individual patients to the drug, each patient must be titrated to the desired level of hemodynamic function. Therefore, continuous monitoring of physiologic parameters (i.e., blood pressure and heart rate in all patients, other measurements such as pulmonary capillary wedge pressure, as appropriate) MUST be performed to achieve the correct dose. Adequate systemic blood pressure and coronary perfusion pressure must be maintained.

HOW SUPPLIED

NDC 0590-0092-10, 5 mg—10 mL ampul.
NDC 0590-0085-05, 25 mg—5 mL ampul.
NDC 0590-0085-86, 25 mg—5 mL single use vial.
NDC 0590-0090-10, 50 mg—10 mL ampul.
NDC 0590-0090-66, 50 mg—10 mL single use vial.
NDC 0590-0095-79, 100 mg—20 mL single use vial.
NDC 0590-0090-15, Tridilset® I.V. administration set with 50 mg—10 mL ampul.
NDC 0590-0090-71, Tridilset® I.V. administration set with 50 mg—10 mL single use vial.
NDC 0590-0090-20, Tridilset V.I.P.® volumetric infusion pump connector set with 50 mg—10 mL ampul.
NDC 0590-0090-76, Tridilset V.I.P.® volumetric infusion pump connector set with 50 mg—10 mL single use vial.
Protect from freezing.
Store at controlled room temperature 15°-30°C (59°-86°F).
Caution: Federal law prohibits dispensing without prescription.
Du Pont Pharmaceuticals
Manati, Puerto Rico 00674
6231-1/Rev., Mar., 1991

ZYDONE® Ⓒ III
[zī"dōn']
(Hydrocodone Bitartrate and Acetaminophen) Capsules

DESCRIPTION

Each ZYDONE capsule contains:

Hydrocodone Bitartrate	5 mg
WARNING: May be habit forming	
Acetaminophen	500 mg

Hydrocodone Bitartrate is an opioid analgesic and antitussive and occurs as fine, white crystals or as a crystalline powder. It is affected by light. The chemical name is: 4,5α-epoxy-3-methoxy-17-methylmorphinan-6-one tartrate (1:1) hydrate (2:5).
Acetaminophen, 4'-hydroxyacetanilide, is a non-opiate, non-salicylate analgesic and antipyretic which occurs as a white, odorless crystalline powder possessing a slightly bitter taste.
ZYDONE capsules also contain: FD&C Red 7, FD&C Yellow 6, gelatin, pharmaceutical glaze, silicon dioxide, sodium lauryl sulfate and titanium dioxide.

CLINICAL PHARMACOLOGY

Hydrocodone is a semisynthetic narcotic analgesic and antitussive with multiple actions qualitatively similar to those of codeine. Most of these involve the central nervous system and smooth muscle. The precise mechanism of action of hydrocodone and other opiates is not known, although it is believed to relate to the existence of opiate receptors in the central nervous system. In addition to analgesia, narcotics may produce drowsiness, changes in mood and mental clouding.
Radioimmunoassay techniques have recently been developed for the analysis of hydrocodone in human plasma. After a 10 mg oral dose of hydrocodone bitartrate, a mean peak serum drug level of 23.6 ng/mL and an elimination half-life of 3.8 hours were found.
The analgesic action of acetaminophen involves peripheral and central influences, but the specific mechanism is as yet undetermined. Antipyretic activity is mediated through hypothalamic heat regulating centers. Acetaminophen inhibits prostaglandin synthetase. Therapeutic doses of acetaminophen have negligible effects on the cardiovascular or respiratory systems; however, toxic doses may cause circulatory failure and rapid, shallow breathing. Acetaminophen is rapidly and almost completely absorbed from the gastrointestinal tract, producing maximum serum concentrations within 30 minutes to one hour. The plasma half-life in adults and children ranges from 0.90 hours to 3.25 hours with an average of approximately 2 hours. The drug distributes uniformly in most body fluids and is approximately 25% protein bound. Acetaminophen is conjugated in the liver, with less than 3% of the dose excreted unchanged in 24 hours. The primary metabolic pathway is conjugation to sulfate and glucuronide by-products. A minor oxidative pathway forms cysteine and mercapturic acid. These compounds are subsequently excreted by the kidneys into the urine.

INDICATIONS AND USAGE

For the relief of moderate to moderately severe pain.

CONTRAINDICATIONS

Hypersensitivity to acetaminophen or hydrocodone.

WARNINGS

Respiratory Depression: At high doses or in sensitive patients, hydrocodone may produce dose-related respiratory depression by acting directly on the brain stem respiratory center. Hydrocodone also affects the center that controls respiratory rhythm, and may produce irregular and periodic breathing.
Head Injury and Increased Intracranial Pressure: The respiratory depressant effects of narcotics and their capacity to elevate cerebrospinal fluid pressure may be markedly exaggerated in the presence of head injury, other intracranial lesions or a preexisting increase in intracranial pressure. Furthermore, narcotics produce adverse reactions which may obscure the clinical course of patients with head injuries.
Acute Abdominal Conditions: The administration of narcotics may obscure the diagnosis or clinical course of patients with acute abdominal conditions.

PRECAUTIONS

Special Risk Patients: As with any narcotic analgesic agent, Hydrocodone Bitartrate and Acetaminophen Capsules should be used with caution in elderly or debilitated patients and those with severe impairment of hepatic or renal function, hypothyroidism, Addison's disease, prostatic hypertrophy or urethral stricture. The usual precautions should be observed and the possibility of respiratory depression should be kept in mind.
Information for Patients: ZYDONE Capsules, like all narcotics, may impair the mental and/or physical abilities required for the performance of potentially hazardous tasks such as driving a car or operating machinery; patients should be cautioned accordingly.
Cough Reflex: Hydrocodone suppresses the cough reflex; as with all narcotics, caution should be exercised when ZYDONE Capsules are used postoperatively and in patients with pulmonary disease.
Drug Interactions: Patients receiving other narcotic analgesics, antipsychotics, antianxiety agents, or other CNS depressants (including alcohol) concomitantly with ZYDONE Capsules may exhibit an additive CNS depression. When combined therapy is contemplated, the dose of one or both agents should be reduced.
The use of MAO inhibitors or tricyclic antidepressants with hydrocodone preparations may increase the effect of either the antidepressant or hydrocodone.
The concurrent use of anticholinergics with hydrocodone may produce paralytic ileus.
Usage in Pregnancy: Teratogenic Effects: Pregnancy Category C. Hydrocodone has been shown to be teratogenic in hamsters when given in doses 700 times the human dose. There are no adequate and well-controlled studies in pregnant women. Hydrocodone Bitartrate and Acetaminophen Capsules should be used during pregnancy only if the potential benefit justifies the potential risk to the fetus.
Nonteratogenic Effects: Babies born to mothers who have been taking opioids regularly prior to delivery will be physically dependent. The withdrawal signs include irritability and excessive crying, tremors, hyperactive reflexes, increased respiratory rate, increased stools, sneezing, yawning, vomiting, and fever. The intensity of the syndrome does not always correlate with the duration of maternal opioid use or dose. There is no consensus on the best method of managing withdrawal. Chlorpromazine 0.7 to 1 mg/kg q6h, and paregoric 2 to 4 drops/kg q4h, have been used to treat withdrawal symptoms in infants. The duration of therapy is 4 to 28 days, with the dosage decreased as tolerated.
Labor and Delivery: As with all narcotics, administration of ZYDONE Capsules to the mother shortly before delivery may result in some degree of respiratory depression in the newborn, especially if higher doses are used.
Nursing Mothers: It is not known whether this drug is excreted in human milk. Because many drugs are excreted in human milk and because of the potential for serious adverse reactions in nursing infants from ZYDONE Capsules, a decision should be made whether to discontinue nursing or to discontinue the drug, taking into account the importance of the drug to the mother.
Pediatric Use: Safety and effectiveness in children have not been established.

ADVERSE REACTIONS

The most frequently observed adverse reactions include lightheadedness, dizziness, sedation, nausea and vomiting. These effects seem to be more prominent in ambulatory than in nonambulatory patients and some of these adverse reactions may be alleviated if the patient lies down.
Other adverse reactions include:
Central Nervous System: Drowsiness, mental clouding, lethargy, impairment of mental and physical performance, anxiety, fear, dysphoria, psychic dependence, mood changes.
Gastrointestinal System: The antiemetic phenothiazines are useful in suppressing the nausea and vomiting which may occur (see above); however, some phenothiazine derivatives seem to be antianalgesic and to increase the amount of narcotic required to produce pain relief, while other phenothiazines reduce the amount of narcotic required to produce a given level of analgesia. Prolonged administration of ZYDONE (Hydrocodone Bitartrate and Acetaminophen) Capsules may produce constipation.
Genitourinary System: Ureteral spasm, spasm of vesical sphincters and urinary retention have been reported.
Respiratory Depression: Hydrocodone Bitartrate may produce dose-related respiratory depression by acting directly on the brain stem respiratory center. Hydrocodone also affects the center that controls respiratory rhythm, and may produce irregular and periodic breathing. If significant respiratory depression occurs, it may be antagonized by the use of naloxone hydrochloride. Apply other supportive measures when indicated.

DRUG ABUSE AND DEPENDENCE

ZYDONE Capsules are subject to the Federal Controlled Substances Act (Schedule III).
Psychic dependence, physical dependence, and tolerance may develop upon repeated administration of narcotics; therefore, ZYDONE Capsules should be prescribed and administered with caution. However, psychic dependence is unlikely to develop when ZYDONE Capsules are used for a short time for the treatment of pain.
Physical dependence, the condition in which continued administration of the drug is required to prevent the appearance of a withdrawal syndrome, assumes clinically significant proportions only after several weeks of continued narcotic use, although some mild degree of physical dependence may develop after a few days of narcotic therapy. Tolerance, in which increasingly large doses are required in order to produce the same degree of analgesia, is manifested initially by a shortened duration of analgesic effect, and subsequently by decreases in the intensity of analgesia. The rate of development of tolerance varies among patients.

OVERDOSAGE

Hydrocodone: Signs and Symptoms: Serious overdose with hydrocodone is characterized by respiratory depression (a decrease in respiratory rate and/or tidal volume, Cheyne-Stokes respiration, cyanosis), extreme somnolence progressing to stupor or coma, skeletal muscle flaccidity, cold and clammy skin, and sometimes bradycardia and hypotension. In severe overdosage, apnea, circulatory collapse, cardiac arrest and death may occur.
Treatment: Primary attention should be given to the reestablishment of adequate respiratory exchange through provision of a patent airway and the institution of assisted or controlled ventilation. The narcotic antagonist naloxone is a specific antidote against respiratory depression which may result from overdosage or unusual sensitivity to narcotics, including hydrocodone. Therefore, an appropriate dose of naloxone hydrochloride (see package insert) should be administered, preferably by the intravenous route, and simultaneously with efforts at respiratory resuscitation. Since the duration of action of hydrocodone may exceed that of the antagonist, the patient should be kept under continued surveillance and repeated doses of the antagonist should be administered as needed to maintain adequate respiration.
An antagonist should not be administered in the absence of clinically significant respiratory or cardiovascular depression. Oxygen, intravenous fluids, vasopressors and other supportive measures should be employed as indicated.
Gastric emptying may be useful in removing unabsorbed drug.
Acetaminophen: Signs and Symptoms: In acute acetaminophen overdosage, dose-dependent, potentially fatal hepatic necrosis is the most serious adverse effect. Renal tubular necrosis, hypoglycemic coma and thrombocytopenia may also occur.
In adults, hepatic toxicity has rarely been reported with acute overdoses of less than 10 grams and fatalities with less than 15 grams. Importantly, young children seem to be more resistant than adults to the hepatotoxic effect of an acetaminophen overdose. Despite this, the measures outlined below should be initiated in any adult or child suspected of having ingested an acetaminophen overdose.
Early symptoms following a potentially hepatotoxic overdose may include: nausea, vomiting, diaphoresis and general malaise. Clinical and laboratory evidence of hepatic toxicity may not be apparent until 48 to 72 hours post-ingestion.
Treatment: The stomach should be emptied promptly by lavage or by induction of emesis with syrup of ipecac. Patients' estimates of the quantity of a drug ingested are notoriously unreliable. Therefore, if an acetaminophen overdose is suspected, a serum acetaminophen assay should be obtained as early as possible, but no sooner than four hours following

ingestion. Liver function studies should be obtained initially and repeated at 24-hour intervals.
The antidote, N-acetylcysteine, should be administered as early as possible, preferably within 16 hours of the overdose ingestion for optimal results, but in any case within 24 hours. Following recovery, there are no residual, structural or functional hepatic abnormalities.

DOSAGE AND ADMINISTRATION

Dosage should be adjusted according to the severity of the pain and the response of the patient. However, it should be kept in mind that tolerance to hydrocodone can develop with continued use and that the incidence of untoward effects is dose related.
The usual adult dosage is one or two capsules every four to six hours as needed for pain. The total 24 hour dose should not exceed eight capsules.

HOW SUPPLIED

ZYDONE (Hydrocodone Bitratrate 5 mg and Acetaminophen 500 mg) is a white, hard gelatin capsule with red band. Each capsule is imprinted in red, DU PONT ZYDONE.
Bottles of 100: NDC 0056-0091-70
Storage: Store at controlled room temperature 15°-30°C (59°-86°F).
CAUTION: Federal law prohibits dispensing without prescription.

Manufactured by
D.M. Graham Laboratories, Inc., Hobart, New York 13788
for
Du Pont Pharmaceuticals
Wilmington, Delaware 19880

ZYDONE® is a Registered Trademark of The Du Pont Merck Pharmaceutical Co.

6173-7/Rev. Dec., 1990

Du Pont Pharmaceuticals
WILMINGTON, DE 19880

BREVIBLOC® INJECTION ℞

[*brĕ'vĭ-blok*]
(esmolol hydrochloride)
10 mL Ampul—2.5 g
10 mL Single Dose Vial—100 mg

NOT FOR DIRECT INTRAVENOUS INJECTION. AMPUL MUST BE DILUTED PRIOR TO ITS INFUSION (SEE DOSAGE AND ADMINISTRATION SECTION).

DESCRIPTION

BREVIBLOC® (esmolol HCl) is a $beta_1$ selective (cardioselective) adrenergic receptor blocking agent with a very short duration of action (elimination half-life is approximately 9 minutes). Esmolol HCl is:
(±)-Methyl p-[2-hydroxy-3-(isopropylamino) propoxy] hydrocinnamate hydrochloride and has the following structure:

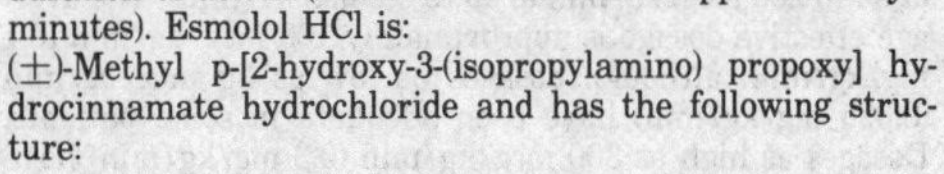
CH3O2CCH2CH2—
—OCH2CHOHCH2NHCH(CH3)2•HCl

Esmolol HCl has the empirical formula $C_{16}H_{26}NO_4Cl$ and a molecular weight of 331.8. It has one asymmetric center and exists as an enantiomeric pair.
Esmolol HCl is a white to off-white crystalline powder. It is a relatively hydrophilic compound which is very soluble in water and freely soluble in alcohol. Its partition coefficient (octanol/water) at pH 7.0 is 0.42 compared to 17.0 for propranolol.
BREVIBLOC® (esmolol HCl) INJECTION is a clear, colorless to light yellow, sterile, nonpyrogenic solution.
2.5 g, 10 mL Ampul - Each mL contains 250 mg esmolol HCl in 25% Propylene Glycol, USP, 25% Alcohol, USP and Water for Injection, USP; buffered with 17.0 mg Sodium Acetate, USP, and 0.00715 mL Glacial Acetic Acid, USP. Sodium hydroxide and/or hydrochloric acid added, as necessary, to adjust pH to 3.5-5.5.
100 mg, 10 mL Single Dose Vial - Each mL contains 10 mg esmolol HCl and Water for Injection, USP; buffered with 2.8 mg Sodium Acetate, USP, and 0.546 mg Glacial Acetic Acid, USP. Sodium hydroxide and/or hydrochloric acid added, as necessary, to adjust pH to 4.5-5.5.

CLINICAL PHARMACOLOGY

BREVIBLOC® (esmolol HCl) is a $beta_1$ selective (cardioselective) adrenergic receptor blocking agent with rapid onset, a very short duration of action, and no significant intrinsic sympathomimetic or membrane stabilizing activity at therapeutic dosages. Its elimination half-life after intravenous infusion is approximately 9 minutes. BREVIBLOC® inhibits the $beta_1$ receptors located chiefly in cardiac muscle, but this preferential effect is not absolute and at higher doses it begins to inhibit $beta_2$ receptors located chiefly in the bronchial and vascular musculature.

Pharmacokinetics and Metabolism
BREVIBLOC® (esmolol HCl) is rapidly metabolized by hydrolysis of the ester linkage, chiefly by the esterases in the cytosol of red blood cells and not by plasma cholinesterases or red cell membrane acetylcholinesterase. Total body clearance in man was found to be about 20 L/kg/hr, which is greater than cardiac output; thus the metabolism of BREVIBLOC® is not limited by the rate of blood flow to metabolizing tissues such as the liver or affected by hepatic or renal blood flow. BREVIBLOC® has a rapid distribution half-life of about 2 minutes and an elimination half-life of about 9 minutes.
Using an appropriate loading dose, steady-state blood levels of BREVIBLOC® for dosages from 50–300 mcg/kg/min (.05–0.3 mg/kg/min) are obtained within five minutes. (Steady-state is reached in about 30 minutes without the loading dose.) Steady-state blood levels of BREVIBLOC® increase linearly over this dosage range and elimination kinetics are dose-independent over this range. Steady-state blood levels are maintained during infusion but decrease rapidly after termination of the infusion. Because of its short half-life, blood levels of BREVIBLOC® can be rapidly altered by increasing or decreasing the infusion rate and rapidly eliminated by discontinuing the infusion.
Consistent with the high rate of blood-based metabolism of BREVIBLOC®, less than 2% of the drug is excreted unchanged in the urine. Within 24 hours of the end of infusion, approximately 73–88% of the dosage has been accounted for in the urine as the acid metabolite of BREVIBLOC®.
Metabolism of BREVIBLOC® results in the formation of the corresponding free acid and methanol. The acid metabolite has been shown in animals to have about 1/1500th the activity of esmolol and in normal volunteers its blood levels do not correspond to the level of beta blockade. The acid metabolite has an elimination half-life of about 3.7 hours and is excreted in the urine with a clearance approximately equivalent to the glomerular filtration rate. Excretion of the acid metabolite is significantly decreased in patients with renal disease, with the elimination half-life increased to about ten-fold that of normals, and plasma levels considerably elevated.
Methanol blood levels, monitored in subjects receiving BREVIBLOC® for up to 6 hours at 300 mcg/kg/min (0.3 mg/kg/min) and 24 hours at 150 mcg/kg/min (0.15 mg/kg/min), approximated endogenous levels and were less than 2% of levels usually associated with methanol toxicity.
BREVIBLOC® has been shown to be 55% bound to human plasma protein, while the acid metabolite is only 10% bound.

Pharmacodynamics
Clinical pharmacology studies in normal volunteers have confirmed the beta blocking activity of BREVIBLOC® (esmolol HCl), showing reduction in heart rate at rest and during exercise, and attenuation of isoproterenol-induced increases in heart rate. Blood levels of BREVIBLOC® have been shown to correlate with extent of beta blockade. After termination of infusion, substantial recovery from beta blockade is observed in 10–20 minutes.
In human electrophysiology studies, BREVIBLOC® produced effects typical of a beta blocker: a decrease in the heart rate, increase in sinus cycle length, prolongation of the sinus node recovery time, prolongation of the AH interval during normal sinus rhythm and during atrial pacing, and an increase in antegrade Wenckebach cycle length.
In patients undergoing radionuclide angiography, BREVIBLOC®, at dosages of 200 mcg/kg/min (0.2 mg/kg/min), produced reductions in heart rate, systolic blood pressure, rate pressure product, left and right ventricular ejection fraction and cardiac index at rest, which were similar in magnitude to those produced by intravenous propranolol (4 mg). During exercise, BREVIBLOC® produced reductions in heart rate, rate pressure product and cardiac index which were also similar to those produced by propranolol, but produced a significantly larger fall in systolic blood pressure. In patients undergoing cardiac catheterization, the maximum therapeutic dose of 300 mcg/kg/min (0.3 mg/kg/min) of BREVIBLOC® produced similar effects, and, in addition, there were small, clinically insignificant, increases in the left ventricular end diastolic pressure and pulmonary capillary wedge pressure. At thirty minutes after the discontinuation of BREVIBLOC® infusion, all of the hemodynamic parameters had returned to pretreatment levels.
The relative cardioselectivity of BREVIBLOC® was demonstrated in 10 mildly asthmatic patients. Infusions of BREVIBLOC® [100, 200 and 300 mcg/kg/min (0.1, 0.2 and 0.3 mg/kg/min)] produced no significant increases in specific airway resistance compared to placebo. At 300 mcg/kg/min (0.3 mg/kg/min), BREVIBLOC® produced slightly enhanced bronchomotor sensitivity to dry air stimulus. These effects were not clinically significant, and BREVIBLOC® was well tolerated by all patients. Six of the patients also received intravenous propranolol, and at a dosage of 1 mg, two experienced significant, symptomatic bronchospasm requiring bronchodilator treatment. One other propranolol-treated patient also experienced dry air-induced bronchospasm. No adverse pulmonary effects were observed in patients with COPD who received therapeutic dosages of BREVIBLOC® for treatment of supraventricular tachycardia (51 patients) or in perioperative settings (32 patients).

Supraventricular Tachycardia
In two multicenter, randomized, double-blind, controlled comparisons of BREVIBLOC® (esmolol HCl) with placebo and propranolol, maintenance doses of 50 to 300 mcg/kg/min (0.05 to 0.3 mg/kg/min) of BREVIBLOC® were found to be more effective than placebo and about as effective as propranolol, 3–6 mg given by bolus injections, in the treatment of supraventricular tachycardia, principally atrial fibrillation and atrial flutter. The majority of these patients developed their arrhythmias postoperatively. About 60–70% of the patients treated with BREVIBLOC® had a desired therapeutic effect (either a 20% reduction in heart rate, a decrease in heart rate to less than 100 bpm, or, rarely, conversion to NSR) and about 95% of those who responded did so at a dosage of 200 mcg/kg/min (0.2 mg/kg/min) or less. The average effective dosage of BREVIBLOC® was approximately 100–115 mcg/kg/min (0.1–0.115 mg/kg/min) in the two studies. Other multicenter baseline-controlled studies gave essentially similar results. In the comparison with propranolol, about 50% of patients in both the BREVIBLOC® and propanolol groups were on concomitant digoxin. Response rates were slightly higher with both beta blockers in the digoxin-treated patients.
In all studies significant decreases of blood pressure occurred in 20–50% of patients, identified either as adverse reaction reports by investigators, or by observation of systolic pressure less than 90 mmHg or diastolic pressure less than 50 mmHg. The hypotension was symptomatic (mainly diaphoresis or dizziness) in about 12% of patients, and therapy was discontinued in about 11% of patients, about half of whom were symptomatic. In comparison to propanolol, hypotension was about three times as frequent with BREVIBLOC®, 53% vs. 17%. The hypotension was rapidly reversible with decreased infusion rate or after discontinuation of therapy with BREVIBLOC®. For both BREVIBLOC® and propranolol, hypotension was reported less frequently in patients receiving concomitant digoxin.

INDICATIONS AND USAGE

Supraventricular Tachycardia
BREVIBLOC® (esmolol HCl) is indicated for the rapid control of ventricular rate in patients with atrial fibrillation or atrial flutter in perioperative, postoperative, or other emergent circumstances where short term control of ventricular rate with a short-acting agent is desirable. BREVIBLOC® is also indicated in noncompensatory sinus tachycardia where, in the physician's judgment, the rapid heart rate requires intervention. BREVIBLOC® is not intended for use in chronic settings where transfer to another agent is anticipated.

CONTRAINDICATIONS

BREVIBLOC® (esmolol HCl) is contraindicated in patients with sinus bradycardia, heart block greater than first degree, cardiogenic shock or overt heart failure (see WARNINGS).

WARNINGS

Hypotension: In clinical trials 20–50% of patients treated with BREVIBLOC® (esmolol HCl) have experienced hypotension, generally defined as systolic pressure less than 90 mmHg and/or diastolic pressure less than 50 mmHg. About 12% of the patients have been symptomatic (mainly diaphoresis or dizziness). Hypotension can occur at any dose but is dose-related so that doses beyond 200 mcg/kg/min (0.2 mg/kg/min) are not recommended. Patients should be closely monitored, especially if pretreatment blood pressure is low. Decrease of dose or termination of infusion reverses hypotension, usually within 30 minutes.
Cardiac Failure: Sympathetic stimulation is necessary in supporting circulatory function in congestive heart failure, and beta blockade carries the potential hazard of further depressing myocardial contractility and percipitating more severe failure. Continued depression of the myocardium with beta blocking agents over a period of time can, in some cases, lead to cardiac failure. At the first sign or symptom of impending cardiac failure, BREVIBLOC® should be withdrawn. Although withdrawal may be sufficient because of the short elimination half-life of BREVIBLOC®, specific treatment may also be considered. (see OVERDOSAGE.) The use of BREVIBLOC® for control of ventricular response in patients with supraventricular arrhythmias should be undertaken with caution when the patient is compromised hemodynamically or is taking other drugs that decrease any or all of the following: peripheral resistance, myocardial filling, myocardial contractility, or electrical impulse propagation in the myocardium. Despite the rapid onset and offset of BREVIBLOC®'s effects, several cases of death have been reported in complex clinical states where BREVIBLOC® was presumably being used to control ventricular rate.
Bronchospastic Diseases: PATIENTS WITH BRONCHOSPASTIC DISEASES SHOULD, IN GENERAL, NOT RECEIVE

Continued on next page

Du Pont—Cont.

BETA BLOCKERS. Because of its relative beta$_1$ selectivity and titrability, BREVIBLOC® may be used with caution in patients with bronchospastic diseases. However, since beta$_1$ selectivity is not absolute, BREVIBLOC® should be carefully titrated to obtain the lowest possible effective dose. In the event of bronchospasm, the infusion should be terminated immediately; a beta$_2$ stimulating agent may be administered if conditions warrant but should be used with particular caution as patients already have rapid ventricular rates.

Diabetes Mellitus and Hypoglycemia: BREVIBLOC® should be used with caution in diabetic patients requiring a beta blocking agent. Beta blockers may mask tachycardia occurring with hypoglycemia, but other manifestations such as dizziness and sweating may not be significantly affected.

PRECAUTIONS

General

Infusion concentrations of 20 mg/mL were associated with more serious venous irritation, including thrombophlebitis, than concentrations of 10 mg/mL. Extravasation of 20 mg/mL may lead to a serious local reaction and possible skin necrosis. Concentrations greater than 10 mg/mL or infusion into small veins or through a butterfly catheter should be avoided.

Because the acid metabolite of BREVIBLOC® is primarily excreted unchanged by the kidney, BREVIBLOC® (esmolol HCl) should be administered with caution to patients with impaired renal function. The elimination half-life of the acid metabolite was prolonged ten-fold and the plasma level was considerably elevated in patients with end-stage renal disease.

Care should be taken in the intravenous administration of BREVIBLOC® as sloughing of the skin and necrosis have been reported in association with infiltration and extravasation of intravenous infusions.

Drug Interactions

Catecholamine-depleting drugs, e.g., reserpine, may have an additive effect when given with beta blocking agents. Patients treated concurrently with BREVIBLOC® and a catecholamine depletor should therefore be closely observed for evidence of hypotension or marked bradycardia, which may result in vertigo, syncope, or postural hypotension.

A study of interaction between BREVIBLOC® and warfarin showed that concomitant administration of BREVIBLOC® and warfarin does not alter warfarin plasma levels. BREVIBLOC® concentrations were equivocally higher when given with warfarin, but this is not likely to be clinically important.

When digoxin and BREVIBLOC® (esmolol HCl) were concomitantly administered intravenously to normal volunteers, there was a 10–20% increase in digoxin blood levels at some time points. Digoxin did not affect BREVIBLOC® pharmacokinetics. When intravenous morphine and BREVIBLOC® were concomitantly administered in normal subjects, no effect on morphine blood levels was seen, but BREVIBLOC® steady-state blood levels were increased by 46% in the presence of morphine. No other pharmacokinetic parameters were changed.

The effect of BREVIBLOC® on the duration of succinylcholine-induced neuromuscular blockade was studied in patients undergoing surgery. The onset of neuromuscular blockade by succinylcholine was unaffected by BREVIBLOC®, but the duration of neuromuscular blockade was prolonged from 5 minutes to 8 minutes.

Although the interactions observed in these studies do not appear to be of major clinical importance, BREVIBLOC® should be titrated with caution in patients being treated concurrently with digoxin, morphine, succinylcholine or warfarin.

While taking beta-blockers, patients with a history of severe anaphylactic reaction to a variety of allergens may be more reactive to repeated challenge, either accidental, diagnostic, or therapeutic. Such patients may be unresponsive to the usual doses of epinephrine used to treat allergic reaction.

Caution should be exercised when considering the use of BREVIBLOC® and Verapamil in patients with depressed myocardial function. Fatal cardiac arrests have occurred in patients receiving both drugs. Additionally, BREVIBLOC® should not be used to control supraventricular tachycardia in the presence of agents which are vasoconstrictive and inotropic such as dopamine, epinephrine, and no repinephrine because of the danger of blocking cardiac contractility when systemic vascular resistance is high.

Carcinogenesis, Mutagenesis, Impairment of Fertility

Because of its short term usage no carcinogenicity, mutagenicity or reproductive performance studies have been conducted with BREVIBLOC®.

Pregnancy Category C

Teratogenicity studies in rats at intravenous dosages of BREVIBLOC® up to 3000 mcg/kg/min (3 mg/kg/min) (ten times the maximum human maintenance dosage) for 30 minutes daily produced no evidence of maternal toxicity, embryotoxicity or teratogenicity, while a dosage of 10,000 mcg/kg/min (10 mg/kg/min) produced maternal toxicity and lethality. In rabbits, intravenous dosages up to 1000 mcg/kg/min (1 mg/kg/min) for 30 minutes daily produced no evidence of maternal toxicity, embryotoxicity or teratogenicity, while 2500 mcg/kg/min (2.5 mg/kg/min) produced minimal maternal toxicity and increased fetal resorptions.

There are no adequate and well controlled studies in pregnant women. BREVIBLOC® should be used during pregnancy only if the potential benefit justifies the potential risk to the fetus.

Nursing Mothers

It is not known whether BREVIBLOC® is excreted in human milk, however, caution should be exercised when BREVIBLOC® is administered to a nursing woman.

Pediatric Use

The safety and effectiveness of BREVIBLOC® in children have not been established.

ADVERSE REACTIONS

Supraventricular Tachycardia

The following adverse reaction rates are based on use of BREVIBLOC® (esmolol HCl) in almost 400 clinical trial patients with supraventricular tachycardia. In addition, over 600 patients have been exposed in clinical studies of other conditions. The most important adverse effect has been hypotension (see WARNINGS). Most adverse effects have been mild and transient.

Cardiovascular—Symptomatic hypotension (diaphoresis, dizziness) occurred in 12% of patients, and therapy was discontinued in about 11%, about half of whom were symptomatic. Asymptomatic hypotension occurred in about 25% of patients. Hypotension resolved during BREVIBLOC® infusion in 63% of these patients and within 30 minutes after discontinuation of infusion in 80% of the remaining patients. Diaphoresis accompanied hypotension in 10% of patients. Peripheral ischemia occurred in approximately 1% of patients. Pallor, flushing, bradycardia (heart rate less than 50 beats per minute), chest pain, syncope, pulmonary edema and heart block have each been reported in less than 1% of patients. In two patients without supraventricular tachycardia but with serious coronary artery disease (post inferior myocardial infarction or unstable angina), severe bradycardia/sinus pause/asystole has developed, reversible in both cases with discontinuation of treatment.

Central Nervous System—Dizziness has occurred in 3% of patients; somnolence in 3%, confusion, headache, and agitation in about 2%, and fatigue in about 1% of patients. Paresthesia, asthenia, depression, abnormal thinking, anxiety, anorexia, and lightheadedness were reported in less than 1% of patients. Seizures were also reported in less than 1% of patients, with one death.

Respiratory—Bronchospasm, wheezing, dyspnea, nasal congestion, rhonchi, and rales have each been reported in less than 1% of patients.

Gastrointestinal—Nausea was reported in 7% of patients. Vomiting has occurred in about 1% of patients. Dyspepsia, constipation, dry mouth, and abdominal discomfort have each occurred in less than 1% of patients. Taste perversion has also been reported.

Skin (Infusion Site)—Infusion site reactions including inflammation and induration were reported in about 8% of patients. Edema, erythema, skin discoloration, burning at the infusion site, thrombophlebitis, and local skin necrosis from extravasation have each occurred in less than 1% of patients.

Miscellaneous—Each of the following has been reported in less than 1% of patients: Urinary retention, speech disorder, abnormal vision, midscapular pain, rigors, and fever.

OVERDOSAGE

Acute Toxicity

A few cases of massive accidental overdosage of BREVIBLOC® (esmolol HCl) have occurred due to errors in dilution. These intravenous bolus doses of BREVIBLOC® of 5000–6250 mcg/kg (5–6.25 mg/kg) over 1–2 minutes have produced hypotension, bradycardia, drowsiness and loss of consciousness. The effects have resolved within 10 minutes, in some cases with administration of a pressor agent.

Because of its approximately 9-minute elimination half-life, the first step in the management of toxicity should be to discontinue BREVIBLOC® infusion. Then, based on the observed clinical effects, the following general measures should also be considered:

Bradycardia: Intravenous administration of atropine or another anticholinergic drug.

Bronchospasm: Intravenous administration of a beta$_2$ stimulating agent and/or a theophylline derivative.

Cardiac Failure: Intravenous administration of a diuretic and/or digitalis glycoside. In shock resulting from inadequate cardiac contractility, intravenous administration of dopamine, dobutamine, isoproterenol, or amrinone may be considered.

Symptomatic Hypotension:

Intravenous administration of fluids and/or pressor agents.

DOSAGE AND ADMINISTRATION

2.5 g AMPUL

THE 2.5 g AMPUL IS NOT FOR DIRECT INTRAVENOUS INJECTION. THIS DOSAGE FORM IS A CONCENTRATED, POTENT DRUG WHICH MUST BE DILUTED PRIOR TO ITS INFUSION. BREVIBLOC® SHOULD NOT BE ADMIXED WITH SODIUM BICARBONATE. BREVIBLOC® SHOULD NOT BE MIXED WITH OTHER DRUGS PRIOR TO DILUTION IN A SUITABLE INTRAVENOUS FLUID. (See Compatibility Section below.)

Dilution: Aseptically prepare a 10 mg/mL infusion, by adding two 2.5 g ampuls to a 500 mL container, or one 2.5 g ampul to a 250 mL container, of a compatible intravenous solution listed below. (Remove overage prior to dilution as appropriate.) This yields a final concentration of 10 mg/mL. The diluted solution is stable for at least 24 hours at room temperature. Note: Concentrations of BREVIBLOC® greater than 10 mg/mL are likely to produce irritation on continued infusion (see PRECAUTIONS). BREVIBLOC® has, however, been well tolerated when administered via a central vein.

100 mg VIAL

This dosage form is prediluted to provide a ready-to-use 10 mg/mL concentration recommended for BREVIBLOC® intravenous administration. It may be used to administer the appropriate BREVIBLOC® loading dosage infusions by hand-held syringe while the maintenance infusion is being prepared.

When using the 100 mg vial, a loading dose of 0.5 mg/kg/min for a 70 kg patient would be 3.5 mL.

Supraventricular Tachycardia

In the treatment of supraventricular tachycardia, responses to BREVIBLOC® usually (over 95%) occur within the range of 50 to 200 mcg/kg/min (0.05 to 0.2 mg/kg/min). The average effective dosage is approximately 100 mcg/kg/min (0.1 mg/kg/min) although dosages as low as 25 mcg/kg/min (0.025 mg/kg/min) have been adequate in some patients. Dosages as high as 300 mcg/kg/min (0.3 mg/kg/min) have been used, but these provide little added effect and an increased rate of adverse effects, and are not recommended.

Dosage of BREVIBLOC® in supraventricular tachycardia must be individualized by titration in which each step consists of a loading dosage followed by a maintenance dosage.

To initiate treatment of a patient with supraventricular tachycardia, administer a loading infusion to 500 mcg/kg/min (0.5 mg/kg/min) over one minute followed by a four-minute maintenance infusion of 50 mcg/kg/min (0.05 mg/kg/min). If an adequate therapeutic effect is observed over the five minutes of drug administration, maintain the maintenance infusion dosage with periodic adjustments up or down as needed. If an adequate therapeutic effect is not observed, the same loading dosage is repeated over one minute followed by an increased maintenance rate infusion of 100 mcg/kg/min (0.1 mg/kg/min).

Time (minutes)	Loading Dose (over 1 minute) mcg/kg/min	Loading Dose (over 1 minute) mg/kg/min	Maintenance Dosage (over 4 minutes) mcg/kg/min	Maintenance Dosage (over 4 minutes) mg/kg/min
0–1	500	0.5		
1–5			50	0.05
5–6	500	0.5		
6–10			100	0.10
10–11	500	0.5		
11–15			150	0.15
15–16	*	*		
16–20			*200	*0.2
20–(24 hrs.)			Maintenance dose titrated to heart rate or other clinical endpoint.	

* As the desired heart rate or endpoint is approached, the loading infusion may be omitted and the maintenance infusion titrated to 300 mcg/kg/min (0.3 mg/kg/min) or downward as appropriate. Maintenance dosages above 200 mcg/kg/min (0.2 mg/kg/min) have not been shown to have significantly increased benefits. The interval between titration steps may be increased.

Continue titration procedure as above, repeating the original loading infusion of 500 mcg/kg/min (0.5 mg/kg/min) over 1 minute, but increasing the maintenance infusion rate over the subsequent four minutes by 50 mcg/kg/min (0.05 mg/kg/min) increments. As the desired heart rate or blood pressure is approached, omit subsequent loading doses and titrate the maintenance dosage up or down to endpoint. Also, if desired, increase the interval between steps from 5 to 10 minutes.

[See table on preceding page.]

This specific dosage regimen has not been studied intraoperatively and, because of the time required for titration, may not be optimal for intraoperative use.

The safety of dosages above 300 mcg/kg/min (0.3 mg/kg/min) has not been studied.

In the event of an adverse reaction, the dosage of BREVIBLOC® may be reduced or discontinued. If a local infusion site reaction develops, an alternative infusion site should be used and caution should be taken to prevent extravasation. The use of butterfly needles should be avoided.

Abrupt cessation of BREVIBLOC® in patients has not been reported to produce the withdrawal effects which may occur with abrupt withdrawal of beta blockers following chronic use in coronary artery disease (CAD) patients. However, caution should still be used in abruptly discontinuing infusions of BREVIBLOC® in CAD patients.

After achieving an adequate control of the heart rate and a stable clinical status in patients with supraventricular tachycardia, transition to alternative antiarrhythmic agents such as propranolol, digoxin, or verapamil, may be accomplished. A recommended guideline for such a transition is given below but the physician should carefully consider the labeling instructions for the alternative agent selected:

Alternative Agent	Dosage
Propranolol hydrochloride	10–20 mg q 4–6 h
Digoxin	0.125–0.5 mg q 6 h
	(p.o. or i.v.)
Verapamil	80 mg q 6 h

The dosage of BREVIBLOC® should be reduced as follows:
1. Thirty minutes following the first dose of the alternative agent, reduce the infusion rate of BREVIBLOC® by one-half (50%).
2. Following the second dose of the alternative agent, monitor the patient's response and if satisfactory control is maintained for the first hour, discontinue BREVIBLOC®.

The use of infusions of BREVIBLOC® up to 24 hours has been well documented; in addition, limited data from 24–48 hrs (N = 48) indicate that BREVIBLOC® is well tolerated up to 48 hours.

Compatibility with Commonly Use Intravenous Fluids
BREVIBLOC® (esmolol HCl) INJECTION was tested for compatibility with ten commonly used intravenous fluids at a final concentration of 10 mg esmolol HCl per mL. BREVIBLOC® INJECTION was found to be compatible with the following solutions and was stable for at least 24 hours at controlled room temperature or under refrigeration:

Dextrose (5%) Injection, USP
Dextrose (5%) in Lactated Ringer's Injection
Dextrose (5%) in Ringer's Injection
Dextrose (5%) and Sodium Chloride (0.45%) Injection, USP
Dextrose (5%) and Sodium Chloride (0.9%) Injection, USP
Lactated Ringer's Injection, USP
Potassium Chloride (40 mEq/liter) in Dextrose (5%) Injection, USP
Sodium Chloride (0.45%) Injection, USP
Sodium Chloride (0.9%) Injection, USP
BREVIBLOC® INJECTION was NOT compatible with Sodium Bicarbonate (5%) Injection, USP.

Note: Parenteral drug products should be inspected visually for particulate matter and discoloration prior to administration, whenever solution and container permit.

HOW SUPPLIED
NDC 0590-0015-71, 100 mg—10 mL vial, Box of 20
NDC 0590-0025-18, 2.5 g—10 mL ampul, Box of 10
STORE AT CONTROLLED ROOM TEMPERATURE (59°–86°F, 15°–30°C). Freezing does not adversely affect the product, but exposure to elevated temperatures should be avoided.

Du Pont Pharmaceuticals
Manati, Puerto Rico 00674

6224-2/Rev. Aug., 1991

COUMADIN®   ℞
[*ku'ma-din*]
(Crystalline Warfarin Sodium, U.S.P.)
TABLETS

DESCRIPTION
COUMADIN® (crystalline warfarin sodium), a vitamin K dependent factor anticoagulant, is chemically crystalline sodium warfarin isopropanol clathrate. The crystallization of warfarin sodium virtually eliminates trace impurities present in amorphous warfarin sodium, thus achieving a crystalline product of the highest purity. Warfarin is the coined generic name for 3-(α-acetonylbenzyl)-4-hydroxycoumarin. Its empirical formula is $C_{19}H_{15}NaO_4$ and its structural formula may be represented by the following:

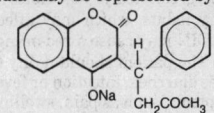

Warfarin sodium crystalline occurs as a white, odorless, crystalline powder, is discolored by light and is very soluble in water; freely soluble in alcohol; very slightly soluble in chloroform and in ether.

COUMADIN Tablets for oral use also contain:
All strengths:	Lactose, starch and other ingredients
1 mg:	D&C Red 6
2 mg:	FD&C Blue 2 and FD&C Red 40
2½ mg:	FD&C Blue 1 and D&C Yellow 10
5 mg:	FD&C Yellow 6
7½ mg:	D&C Yellow 10 and FD&C Yellow 6
10 mg:	Dye Free

CLINICAL PHARMACOLOGY
COUMADIN and other coumarin anticoagulants act by inhibiting the synthesis of vitamin K dependent coagulation factors. The resultant *in vivo* effect is a sequential depression of Factors VII, IX, X and II. The degree of depression is dependent upon the dosage administered. Anticoagulants have no direct effect on an established thrombus, nor do they reverse ischemic tissue damage. However, once a thrombosis has occurred, anticoagulant treatment aims to prevent further extension of the formed clot and prevents secondary thromboembolic complications which may result in serious and possible fatal sequelae.

After oral administration, absorption is essentially complete, and maximal plasma concentrations are reached in 1 to 9 hours. Approximately 97% is bound to albumin within the plasma. COUMADIN usually produces its anticoagulant effect in 36 to 72 hours, and its duration of action may persist for 4 to 5 days, thus producing a smooth, long lasting response curve. COUMADIN is metabolized by hepatic, microsomal enzymes to inactive metabolites that are excreted into the bile, reabsorbed and excreted into the urine.

INDICATIONS AND USAGE
COUMADIN is indicated for the prophylaxis and/or treatment of venous thrombosis and its extension, pulmonary embolism, atrial fibrillation with embolization, and as an adjunct in the prophylaxis of systemic embolism after myocardial infarction.

CONTRAINDICATIONS
Anticoagulation is contraindicated in any localized or general physical condition or personal circumstance in which the hazard of hemorrhage might be greater than the potential clinical benefits of anticoagulation, such as:
Pregnancy—COUMADIN is contraindicated in women who are or may become pregnant because the drug passes through the placental barrier and may cause fatal hemorrhage to the fetus in utero. Furthermore, there have been reports of birth malformations in children born to mothers who have been treated with warfarin during pregnancy. Women of childbearing potential who are candidates for anticoagulant therapy should be carefully evaluated and the indications critically reviewed with the patient. If the patient becomes pregnant while taking this drug, she should be apprised of the potential risks to the fetus, and the possibility of termination of the pregnancy should be discussed in light of those risks.
Hemorrhagic tendencies or blood dyscrasias.
Recent or contemplated surgery of: (1) central nervous system; (2) eye; (3) traumatic surgery resulting in large open surfaces.
Bleeding tendencies associated with active ulceration or overt bleeding of: (1) gastrointestinal, genitourinary or respiratory tracts; (2) cerebrovascular hemorrhage; (3) aneurysms—cerebral, dissecting aorta; (4) pericarditis and pericardial effusions; (5) bacterial endocarditis.
Threatened abortion, eclampsia and preeclampsia.
Inadequate laboratory facilities or unsupervised senility, alcoholism, psychosis; or lack of patient cooperation.
Spinal puncture and other diagnostic or therapeutic procedures with potential for uncontrollable bleeding.
Miscellaneous: major regional, lumbar block anesthesia and malignant hypertension.

WARNINGS
The most serious risks associated with anticoagulant therapy with sodium warfarin are hemorrhage in any tissue or organ and, less frequently, necrosis and/or gangrene of skin and other tissues. The risk of hemorrhage is related to the level of intensity and the duration of anticoagulant therapy. Hemorrhage and necrosis have in some cases been reported to result in death or permanent disability. Necrosis appears to be associated with local thrombosis and usually appears within a few days of the start of anticoagulant therapy. In severe cases of necrosis, treatment through debridement or amputation of the affected tissue, limb, breast or penis has been reported. Careful diagnosis is required to determine whether necrosis caused by an underlying disease. Warfarin therapy should be discontinued when warfarin is suspected to be the cause of developing necrosis and heparin therapy may be considered for anticoagulation. Although various treatments have been attempted, no treatment for necrosis has been considered uniformly effective. See below for information on predisposing conditions. These and other risks associated with anticoagulant therapy must be weighed against the risk of thrombosis or embolization in untreated cases.

COUMADIN is a potent drug with a half-life of 2½ days; therefore its effects may become more pronounced as daily maintenance doses overlap. It cannot be emphasized too strongly that treatment of each patient is a highly individualized matter. Dosage should be controlled by periodic determinations of prothrombin time or other suitable coagulation tests. Determinations of whole blood clotting and bleeding times are not effective measures for control of therapy. Heparin prolongs the one-stage prothrombin time. When heparin and COUMADIN are administered concomitantly, refer to CONVERSION FROM HEPARIN THERAPY for recommendations.

Caution should be observed when COUMADIN is administered in any situation or in the presence of any predisposing condition where added risk of hemorrhage or necrosis is present.

Anticoagulation therapy with COUMADIN may enhance the release of atheromatous plaque emboli, thereby increasing the risk of complications from systemic cholesterol microembolization, including the "purple toe syndrome." Discontinuation of COUMADIN therapy is recommended when such phenomena are observed. While the "purple toe syndrome" is reported to be reversible, other complications of microembolization may not be reversible.

Administration of anticoagulants in the following conditions will be based upon clinical judgment in which the risks of anticoagulant therapy are weighed against the risk of thrombosis or embolization in untreated cases. The following may be associated with these increased risks:
Lactation—COUMADIN appears in the milk of nursing mothers in an inactive form. Infants nursed by COUMADIN treated mothers had no change in prothrombin times. Effects in premature infants have not been evaluated.
Severe to moderate hepatic or renal insufficiency.
Infectious diseases or disturbances of intestinal flora—sprue, antibiotic therapy.
Trauma which may result in internal bleeding.
Surgery or trauma resulting in large exposed raw surfaces.
Indwelling catheters.
Severe to moderate hypertension.
Known or suspected deficiency in protein C—This hereditary or acquired condition, which should be suspected if there is a history of recurrent episodes of thromboembolic disorders in the patient or in the family, has been associated with an increased risk of developing necrosis following warfarin administration. Tissue necrosis may occur in the absence of protein C deficiency. It has been reported that concurrent anticoagulation therapy with heparin for 5 to 7 days during initiation of therapy with COUMADIN may minimize the incidence of this reaction. Warfarin therapy should be discontinued when warfarin is suspected to be the cause of developing necrosis and heparin therapy may be considered for anticoagulation.
Miscellaneous: polycythemia vera, vasculitis, severe diabetes, severe allergic and anaphylactic disorders.

Patients with congestive heart failure may become more sensitive to COUMADIN, thereby requiring more frequent laboratory monitoring, and reduced doses of COUMADIN. Concurrent use of anticoagulants with streptokinase or urokinase is not recommended and may be hazardous. (Please note recommendations accompanying these preparations.)

PRECAUTIONS
Periodic determination of prothrombin time or other suitable coagulation test is essential.
Numerous factors, alone or in combination, including travel, changes in diet, environment, physical state and medication may influence response of the patient to anticoagulants. It is generally good practice to monitor the patient's response with additional prothrombin time determinations in the period immediately after discharge from the hospital, and whenever other medications are initiated, discontinued or taken haphazardly. The following factors are listed for your reference; however, other factors may also affect the anticoagulant response.
The following factors, alone or in combination, may be responsible for INCREASED PT response.
[See table top left next page.]
Because a patient may be exposed to a combination of the above factors, the net effect of COUMADIN on PT response may be unpredictable. More frequent PT monitoring is therefore advisable. Medications of unknown interaction

Continued on next page

Du Pont—Cont.

ENDOGENOUS FACTORS:

cancer	hepatic disorders–
collagen disease	infectious hepatitis
congestive heart failure	jaundice
diarrhea	hyperthyroidism
elevated temperature	poor nutritional state
	steatorrhea
	vitamin K deficiency

EXOGENOUS FACTORS:

alcohol†	ibuprofen
allopurinol	indomethacin
aminosalicylic acid	influenza virus vaccine
amiodarone HCl	lovastatin
anabolic steroids	mefenamic acid
anesthetics, inhalation	methyldopa
antibiotics	methylphenidate
bromelains	metronidazole
chenodiol	miconazole
chloral hydrate†	monoamine oxidase inhibitors
chlorpropamide	nalidixic acid
chymotrypsin	naproxen
cimetidine	narcotics, prolonged
clofibrate	pentoxifylline
COUMADIN overdosage	phenylbutazone
dextran	phenytoin
dextrothyroxine	propafenone
diazoxide	pyrazolones
diflunisal	quinidine
diuretics†	quinine
disulfiram	ranitidine†
ethacrynic acid	salicylates
fenoprofen	sulfinpyrazone
fluoroquinolone antibiotics	sulfonamides, long acting
glucagon	sulindac
hepatotoxic drugs	tamoxifen
	thyroid drugs
	tolbutamide
	trimethoprim/sulfamethoxazole

also: other medications affecting blood elements which may modify hemostasis
- dietary deficiencies
- prolonged hot weather
- unreliable prothrombin time determinations

†Increased and decreased prothrombin time responses have been reported.

The following factors, alone or in combination, may be responsible for DECREASED PT response:

ENDOGENOUS FACTORS:
edema
hereditary coumarin resistance
hyperlipemia
hypothyroidism

EXOGENOUS FACTORS:

adrenocortical steroids	ethchlorvynol
alcohol†	glutethimide
aminoglutethimide	griseofluvin
antacids	haloperidol
antihistamines	meprobamate
barbiturates	nafcillin
carbamazepine	oral contraceptives
chloral hydrate†	paraldehyde
chlordiazepoxide	primidone
cholestyramine	ranitidine†
	rifampin
	sucralfate
COUMADIN underdosage	trazodone
diuretics†	vitamin C

also: diet high in vitamin K
unreliable PT determinations

†Increased and decreased prothrombin time responses have been reported.

with coumarins are best regarded with caution. When these medications are started or stopped, more frequent PT monitoring is advisable. Coumarins may also affect the action of other drugs. Hypoglycemic agents (chlorpropamide and tolbutamide) and anticonvulsants (phenytoin and phenobarbital) may accumulate in the body as a result of interference with either their metabolism or excretion.

Special Risk Patients: Caution should be observed when warfarin sodium is administered to certain patients such as the elderly or debilitated or when administered in any situation or physical condition where added risk of hemorrhage is present.

Information for Patients: The objective of anticoagulant therapy is to control the coagulation mechanism so that thrombosis is prevented, while avoiding spontaneous bleeding. Effective therapeutic levels with minimal complications are in part dependent upon cooperative and well-instructed patients who communicate effectively with their physician. Various COUMADIN patient educational guides are available to physicians on request. Patients should be advised: Strict adherence to prescribed dosage schedule is necessary. Do not take or discontinue any other medication, except on advice of physician. Avoid alcohol, salicylates (e.g. aspirin), large amounts of green leafy vegetables and/or drastic changes in dietary habits, which may affect COUMADIN therapy. COUMADIN may cause a red-orange discoloration of alkaline urine. The patient should notify the physician if any illness, such as diarrhea, infection or fever develops or if any unusual symptoms, such as pain, swelling or discomfort appear or if prolonged bleeding from cuts, increased menstrual flow or vaginal bleeding, nosebleeds or bleeding of gums from brushing, unusual bleeding or bruising, red or dark brown urine, red or tar black stools or diarrhea occurs.

Carcinogenesis, Mutagenesis, Impairment of Fertility: Carcinogenicity and mutagenicity studies have not been performed with COUMADIN. The reproductive effects of COUMADIN have not been evaluated.

Use in Pregnancy: Pregnancy Category X–"See CONTRAINDICATIONS."

Pediatric Use: Safety and effectiveness in children below the age of 18 have not been established.

ADVERSE REACTIONS

Potential adverse reactions to COUMADIN (crystalline warfain sodium) may include:

- Hemorrhage from any tissue or organ. This is a consequence of the anticoagulant effect. The signs and symptoms will vary according to the location and degree or extent of the bleeding. Hemorrhagic complications may present as paralysis; headache, chest, abdomen, joint or other pain; shortness of breath, difficult breathing or swallowing; unexplained swelling; or unexplained shock. Therefore, the possibility of hemorrhage should be considered in evaluating the condition of any anticoagulated patient with complaints which do not indicate an obvious diagnosis. Bleeding during anticoagulant therapy does not always correlate with prothrombin activity. (See OVERDOSAGE–Treatment.)
  Bleeding which occurs when the prothrombin time is within the therapeutic range warrants diagnostic investigation since it may unmask a previously unsuspected lesion, e.g. tumor, ulcer, etc.
- Necrosis of skin and other tissues. (See WARNINGS.)
- Other adverse reactions are infrequent and consist of alopecia, urticaria, dermatitis, fever, nausea, diarrhea, abdominal cramping, cramping, systemic cholesterol microembolization, a syndrome called "purple toes", cholestatic hepatic injury, and hypersensitivity reactions.
- Priapism has been associated with anticoagulant administration; however, a causal relationship has not been established.

OVERDOSAGE

Signs and Symptoms: Suspected or overt abnormal bleeding (i.e., appearance of blood in stools or urine, hematuria, excessive menstrual bleeding, melena, petechiae, excessive bruising or persistent oozing from superficial injuries) are early manifestations of anticoagulation beyond a safe and satisfactory level.

Treatment: Excessive anticoagulation, with or without bleeding, may be controlled by discontinuing COUMADIN therapy and if necessary, by administration of oral or parenteral vitamin K_1. (Please see recommendations accompanying vitamin K_1 preparations prior to use.)

Such use of vitamin K_1 reduces response to subsequent COUMADIN therapy. Patients may return to a pretreatment thrombotic status following the rapid reversal of a prolonged PT. Resumption of COUMADIN administration reverses the effect of vitamin K, and a therapeutic PT can again be obtained by careful dosage adjustment. If rapid anticoagulation is indicated, heparin may be preferable for initial therapy.

If minor bleeding progresses to major bleeding, give 5 to 25 mg (rarely up to 50 mg) parenteral vitamin K_1. In emergency situations of severe hemorrhage, clotting factors can be returned to normal by administering 200 to 500 ml of fresh whole blood or fresh frozen plasma, or by giving commercial Factor IX complex. Purified Factor IX preparations should not be used because they cannot increase the levels of prothrombin, Factor VII and Factor X which are also depressed along with the levels of Factor IX as a result of COUMADIN treatment. Packed red blood cells may also be given if significant blood loss has occurred. Infusions of blood or plasma should be monitored carefully to avoid precipitating pulmonary edema in elderly patients or patients with heart disease.

DOSAGE AND LABORATORY CONTROL

ADMINISTRATION The administration and dosage of COUMADIN must be individualized for each patient according to the particular patient's sensitivity to the drug. The dosage should be adjusted based upon the results of the one stage prothrombin time (PT). Different thromboplastin reagents vary substantially in their responsiveness to sodium warfarin-induced effects on prothrombin time. To define the appropriate therapeutic regimen it is important to be familiar with the sensitivity of the thromboplastin reagent used in the laboratory and its relationship to the International Reference Preparation (IRP)*, a sensitive thromboplastin reagent prepared from human brain.

Early clinical studies of oral anticoagulants, which formed the basis for recommended therapeutic ranges of 1.5 to 2.5 times control PT, used sensitive human brain thromboplastin. When using the less sensitive rabbit brain thromboplastins commonly employed in PT assays today, adjustments must be made to the targeted PT range that reflect this decrease in sensitivity. Available clinical evidence indicates that prolongation of the prothrombin time 1.2 to 1.5 times control, when measuring with the less sensitive thromboplastin reagents, is sufficient for prophylaxis and treatment of venous thromboembolism and minimizes the risk of hemorrhage associated with more prolonged PT values. In cases where the risk of thromboembolism is great, such as in patients with recurrent systemic embolism, a PT of 1.5 to 2.0 times control should be maintained. A ratio of greater than 2.0 appears to provide no additional therapeutic benefit in most patients and is associated with a higher risk of bleeding.

The proceedings and recommendations of the 1986 National Conference on Antithrombotic Therapy[1–3] review and evaluate issues related to oral anticoagulant therapy and the sensitivity of thromboplastin reagents and provide additional guidelines for defining the appropirate therapeutic regimen.

Initial Dosage COUMADIN therapy is commonly started above anticipated maintenance dosage levels. A commonly used regimen for COUMADIN is 10 mg/day for 2 to 4 days; with daily dosage adjustments based on the results of PT determinations. Use of a large loading dose (i.e., 30 mg) may increase the incidence of hemorrhagic and other complications, does not offer more rapid protection against thrombi formation, and is not recommended. Lower doses are recommended for elderly and/or debilitated patients and patients with increased sensitivity (see PRECAUTIONS section of this package insert).

Maintenance—Most patients are satisfactorily maintained at a dose of 2 to 10 mg daily. Flexibility of dosage is provided by breaking scored tablets in half. The individual dose and interval should be gauged by the patient's prothrombin response.

Duration of Therapy—The duration of therapy in each patient should be individualized. In general, anticoagulant therapy should be continued until the danger of thrombosis and embolism has passed.

LABORATORY CONTROL The prothrombin time (PT) reflects the depression of vitamin K dependent Factors VII, IX, X and II. There are several modifications of the one-stage PT and the physician should become familiar with the specific method used in his laboratory. The degree of anticoagulation indicated by any range of prothrombin times may be altered by the type of thromboplastin used; the appropriate therapeutic range must be based on the experience of each laboratory. The PT should be determined daily after the administration of the initial dose until PT results stabilize in the therapeutic range. Intervals between subsequent PT determinations should be based upon the physicians judgment of the patient's reliability and response to COUMADIN in order to maintain the individual within the therapeutic range. Acceptable intervals for PT determinations are normally within the range of one to four weeks. To ensure adequate control, it is recommended that additional prothrombin time tests are done when other warfarin products are interchanged with COUMADIN.

TREATMENT DURING DENTISTRY AND SURGERY The management of patients who undergo dental and surgical procedures requires close liaison between attending physicians, surgeons and dentists. In patients who must be anticoagulated prior to, during, or immediately following dental or surgical procedures, adjusting the dosage of COUMADIN to maintain the PT at the low end of the therapeutic range, may safely allow for continued anticoagulation. The operative site should be sufficiently limited and accessible to permit the effective use of local procedures for hemostasis. Under these conditions, dental and surgical procedures may be performed without undue risk of hemorrhage.

CONVERSION FROM HEPARIN THERAPY Since the onset of the COUMADIN effect is delayed, heparin is preferred initially for rapid anticoagulation. Conversion to COUMA-

**A system of standardizing the prothrombin time in oral anticoagulant control was introduced by the World Health Organization in 1983. It is based upon the determination of an International Normalized Ratio (INR) which provides a common basis for communication of PT results and interpretations of therapeutic ranges. The INR is derived from calibrations of commercial thromboplastin reagents against a sensitive human brain thromboplastin, the International Reference Preparation (IRP). For the three commercial rabbit brain thromboplastins, currently used in North America, a PT ratio of 1.3 to 2.0 is equivalent to an INR of 2.0 to 4.0. For other thromboplastins, the INR can be calculated as:*

$$INR = (observed\ PT\ ratio)^{ISI}$$

where the ISI (International Sensitivity Index) is the calibration factor and is available from the manufacturers of the thromboplastin reagent.[4]

DIN may begin concomitantly with heparin therapy or may be delayed 3 to 6 days. As heparin may affect the PT, patients receiving both heparin and COUMADIN should have blood for PT determination, drawn at least:

- 5 hours after the last IV bolus dose of heparin, or
- 4 hours after cessation of a continuous IV infusion of heparin, or
- 24 hours after the last subcutaneous heparin injection.

When COUMADIN has produced the desired therapeutic range or prothrombin activity, heparin may be discontinued. I.M. injections should be confined to the upper extremities which permits easy access for manual compression, inspections for bleeding and use of pressure bandages.

HOW SUPPLIED

Tablets: COUMADIN (crystalline warfarin sodium, USP). For oral use, single scored, imprinted numerically in bottles with potencies and colors as follows:

	100's	1000's
1 mg pink	NDC 0056-0169-70	NDC 0056-0169-90
2 mg lavender	NDC 0056-0170-70	NDC 0056-0170-90
2½ mg green	NDC 0056-0176-70	NDC 0056-0176-90
5 mg peach	NDC 0056-0172-70	NDC 0056-0172-90
7½ mg yellow	NDC 0056-0173-70	
10 mg white	NDC 0056-0174-70	

Also available in Hospital Unit-Dose blister package of 100:

1 mg	NDC 0056-0169-75
2 mg	NDC 0056-0170-75
2½ mg	NDC 0056-0176-75
5 mg	NDC 0056-0172-75
7½ mg	NDC 0056-0173-75
10 mg	NDC 0056-0174-75

COUMADIN oral tablet is available in 1, 2, 2½, 5, 7½ and 10 mg of crystalline warfarin sodium with one face inscribed with the word COUMADIN, single scored and imprinted numerically with the 1, 2, 2½, 5, 7½ and 10 superimposed, and on the other face inscribed with the Du Pont logo.

Protect from light. Store in carton until contents have been used.

REFERENCES

1. Sackett, D.L.: Rules of Evidence and Clinical Recommendations on the Use of Antithrombotic Agents. Chest, ACCP-NHLBI National Conference on Antithrombotic Therapy, Vol. 89, No. 2, pp. 2s–3s, 1986.
2. Hirsh, J., Deykin, D., Poller, L.: "Therapeutical Range" for Oral Anticoagulant Therapy. Chest, ACCP-NHLBI National Conference on Antithrombolic Therapy,. Vol. 89, No. 2, pp. 11s–15s, 1986.
3. Hirsh, J.: Is the Dose of Warfarin Prescribed by American Physicians Unnesessarily High? Arch Int Med, Vol. 147, pp. 769–771, 1987.
4. Poller, L.: Laboratory Control of Anticoagulant Therapy. Seminars in Thrombosis and Hemostasis, Vol. 12, No. 1, pp. 13–19, 1986.

COUMADIN® is a Registered Trademark of The Du Pont Merck Pharmaceutical Co.

6136-19/Rev. May, 1991

Shown in Product Identification Section, page 409

ETHMOZINE® ℞
(moricizine hydrochloride)
TABLETS

DESCRIPTION

ETHMOZINE (moricizine hydrochloride) is an orally active antiarrhythmic drug available for administration in tablets containing 200 mg, 250 mg and 300 mg of moricizine hydrochloride. The chemical name of moricizine hydrochloride is 10-(3-morpholinopropionyl) phenothiazine-2-carbamic acid ethyl ester hydrochloride and the structural formula is represented as follows:

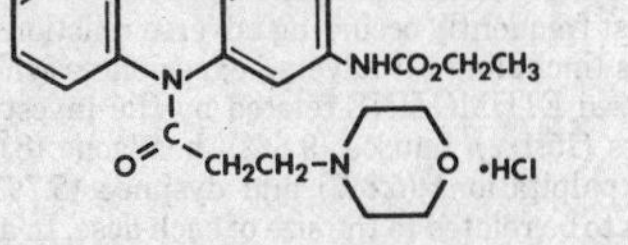

MW=464

Moricizine hydrochloride is a white to tan crystalline powder, freely soluble in water and has a pKa of 6.4 (weak base). ETHMOZINE tablets contain: lactose, microcrystalline cellulose, sodium starch glycolate, magnesium stearate and dyes (FD&C Blue 1, D&C Yellow 10 and FD&C Yellow 6 [200 mg tablet]; FD&C Yellow 6 and FD&C Red 40 [250 mg tablet]; FD&C Blue 1 [300 mg tablet]).

CLINICAL PHARMACOLOGY

Mechanism of Action

ETHMOZINE is a Class I antiarrhythmic agent with potent local anesthetic activity and myocardial membrane stabilizing effects. ETHMOZINE reduces the fast inward current carried by sodium ions.

In isolated dog Purkinje fibers, ETHMOZINE shortens Phase II and III repolarization, resulting in a decreased action potential duration and effective refractory period. A dose-related decrease in the maximum rate of Phase 0 depolarization (V_{max}) occurs without effect on maximum diastolic potential or action potential amplitude. The sinus node and atrial tissue of the dog are not affected.

Electrophysiology

Electrophysiology studies in patients with ventricular tachycardia have shown that ETHMOZINE, at daily doses of 750 mg and 900 mg, prolongs atrioventricular conduction. Both AV nodal conduction time (AH interval) and His-Purkinje conduction time (HV interval) are prolonged by 10–13% and 21–26%, respectively. The PR interval is prolonged by 16–20% and the QRS by 7–18%. Prolongations of 2–5% in the corrected QT interval result from widening of the QRS interval, but there is shortening of the JT interval, indicating an absence of significant effect on ventricular repolarization. Intra-atrial conduction or atrial effective refractory periods are not consistently affected. In patients without sinus node dysfunction, ETHMOZINE has minimal effects on sinus cycle length and sinus node recovery time. These effects may be significant in patients with sinus node dysfunction (see PRECAUTIONS: Electrocardiographic Changes/Conduction Abnormalities).

Hemodynamics

In patients with impaired left ventricular function, ETHMOZINE has minimal effects on measurements of cardiac performance such as cardiac index, stroke volume index, pulmonary capillary wedge pressure, systemic or pulmonary vascular resistance or ejection fraction, either at rest or during exercise. ETHMOZINE is associated with a small, but consistent increase in resting blood pressure and heart rate. Exercise tolerence in patients with ventricular arrhythmias is unaffected. In patients with a history of congestive heart failure or angina pectoris, exercise duration and rate-pressure product at maximal exercise are unchanged during ETHMOZINE administration. Nonetheless, in some cases worsened heart failure in patients with severe underlying heart disease has been attributed to ETHMOZINE.

Other Pharmacologic Effects

Although ETHMOZINE is chemically related to the neuroleptic phenothiazines, it has no demonstrated central or peripheral dopaminergic activity in animals. Moreover, in patients on chronic ETHMOZINE, serum prolactin levels did not increase.

Pharmacokinetics/Pharmacodynamics

The antiarrhythmic and electrophysiologic effects of ETHMOZINE are not related in time course or intensity to plasma moricizine concentrations or to the concentrations of any identified metabolite, all of which have short (2–3 hours) half-lives. Following single doses of ETHMOZINE, there is a prompt prolongation of the PR interval, which becomes normal within 2 hours, consistent with the rapid fall of plasma moricizine. JT interval shortening, however, peaks at about 6 hours and persists for at least 10 hours. Although an effect on VPD rates is seen within 2 hours after dosing, the full effect is seen after 10–14 hours and persists in full, when therapy is terminated, for more than 10 hours, after which the effect decays slowly, and is still substantial at 24 hours. This suggests either an unidentified, active, long half-life metabolite or a structural or functional "deep compartment" with slow entry from, and release to, the plasma. The following description of parent compound pharmacokinetics is therefore of uncertain relevance to clinical actions.

Following oral administration, ETHMOZINE undergoes significant first-past metabolism resulting in an absolute bioavailability of approximately 38%. Peak plasma concentrations of ETHMOZINE are usually reached within 0.5–2 hours. Administration 30 minutes after a meal delays the rate of absorption, resulting in lower peak plasma concentrations, but the extent of absorption is not altered. ETHMOZINE plasma levels are proportional to dose over the recommended therapeutic dose range.

The apparent volume of distribution after oral administration is very large ($\geq$ 300L) and is not significantly related to body weight. ETHMOZINE is approximately 95% bound to human plasma proteins. This binding interaction is independent of ETHMOZINE plasma concentration.

ETHMOZINE undergoes extensive biotransformation. Less than 1% of orally administered ETHMOZINE is excreted unchanged in the urine. There are at least 26 metabolites, but no single metabolite has been found to represent as much as 1% of the administered dose, and as stated above, antiarrhythmic response has relatively slow onset and offset. Two metabolites are pharmacologically active in at least one animal model: moricizine sulfoxide and phenothiazine-2-carbamic acid ethyl ester sulfoxide. Each of these metabolites represents a small percentage of the administered dose ($<$0.6%), is present in lower concentrations in the plasma than the parent drug, and has a plasma elimination half-life of approximately three hours.

ETHMOZINE has been shown to induce its own metabolism. Average ETHMOZINE plasma concentrations in patients decrease with multiple dosing. This decrease in plasma levels of parent drug does not appear to affect clinical outcome for patients receiving chronic ETHMOZINE therapy.

The plasma half-life of ETHMOZINE is 1.5–3.5 hours (most values about 2 hours) following single or multiple oral doses in patients with ventricular ectopy. Approximately 56% of the administered dose is execreted in the feces and 39% is excreted in the urine. Some ETHMOZINE is also recycled through enterohepatic circulation.

CLINICAL ACTIONS

ETHMOZINE at daily doses of 600–900 mg produces a dose-related reduction in the occurrence of frequent ventricular premature depolarizations (VPDs) and reduces the incidence of nonsustained and sustained ventricular tachycardia (VT). In controlled clinical trials, ETHMOZINE has been shown to have antiarrhythmic activity that is generally similar to that of disopyramide, propranolol and quinidine at the doses studied. In controlled and compassionate use programmed electrical stimulation studies (PES), ETHMOZINE prevented the induction of sustained ventricular tachycardia in approximately 25% of patients. In a post-marketing randomized comparative PES study, ETHMOZINE had a response rate of approximately 12% (7/59). Activity of ETHMOZINE is maintained during long-term use.

ETHMOZINE is effective in treating ventricular arrhythmias in patients with and without organic heart disease. ETHMOZINE may be effective in patients in whom other antiarrhythmic agents are ineffective, not tolerated and/or contraindicated.

Arrhythmia exacerbation or "rebound" is not noted following discontinuation of ETHMOZINE therapy.

INDICATIONS AND USAGE

ETHMOZINE is indicated for the treatment of documented ventricular arrhythmias, such as sustained ventricular tachycardia, that, in the judgement of the physician are life-threatening. Because of the proarrhythmic effects of ETHMOZINE, its use with lesser arrhythmias is generally not recommended. Treatment of patients with asymptomatic ventricular premature contractions should be avoided.

Initiation of ETHMOZINE treatment, as with other antiarrhythmic agents used to treat life-threatening arrhythmias, should be carried out in the hospital.

Antiarrhythmic drugs have not been shown to enhance survival in patients with ventricular arrhythmias.

CONTRAINDICATIONS

ETHMOZINE is contraindicated in patients with pre-existing second- or third-degree AV block and in patients with right bundle branch block when associated with left hemiblock (bifascicular block) unless a pacemaker is present. ETHMOZINE is also contraindicated in the presence of cardiogenic shock or known hypersensitivity to the drug.

WARNINGS

Mortality

ETHMOZINE was one of three antiarrhythmic drugs included in the National Heart Lung and Blood Institute's Cardiac Arrhythmia Suppression Trial (CAST I), a long-term multicenter, randomized, double-blind study in patients with asymptomatic non-life-threatening ventricular arrhythmias who had a myocardial infarction more than 6 days, but less than 2 years previously. An excessive mortality or nonfatal cardiac arrest rate was seen in patients treated with both of the Class IC agents included in the trial, which led to discontinuation of those 2 arms of the trial. The average duration of treatment with these agents was 10 months. The ETHMOZINE and placebo arms of the trial were continued in the NHLBI sponsored CAST II. In this randomized, double-blind trial, patients with asymptomatic non-life-threatening arrhythmias who had had a myocardial infarction within 4 to 90 days and left ventricular ejection fraction $\leq$0.40 prior to enrollment were evaluated. The average duration of treatment with ETHMOZINE in this study was 18 months. The study was discontinued because there was no possibility of demonstrating a benefit toward improved survival with ETHMOZINE and because of an evolving adverse trend after long-term treatment.

The applicability of the CAST results to other populations (e.g., those without recent myocardial infarction) is uncertain. Considering the known proarrhythmic properties of ETHMOZINE and the lack of evidence of improved survival for any antiarrhythmic drug in patients without life-threatening arrhythmias, the use of ETHMOZINE, as well as other antiarrhythmic agents, should be reserved for patients with life-threatening ventricular arrhythmias.

Proarrhythmia

Like other antiarrhythmic drugs, ETHMOZINE can provoke new rhythm disturbances or make existing arrhythmias worse. These proarrhythmic effects can range from an increase in the frequency of VPDs to the development of new or more severe ventricular tachycardia, e.g., tachycardia that is more sustained or more resistant to conversion to sinus rhythm, with potentially fatal consequences. It is often not possible to distinguish a proarrhythmic effect from the

Continued on next page

Du Pont—Cont.

patient's underlying rhythm disorder, so that the occurrence rates given below must be considered approximations. Note also that drug-induced arrhythmias can generally be identified only when they occur early after starting the drug and when the rhythm can be identified, usually because the patient is being monitored. It is clear from the NIH sponsored CAST (Cardiac Arrhythmia Suppression Trial) that some antiarrhythmic drugs can cause increased sudden death mortality, presumably due to new arrhythmias or asystole that do not appear early after treatment but that represent a sustained increased risk.

Domestic pre-marketing trials included 1072 patients given ETHMOZINE; 397 had baseline lethal arrhythmias (sustained VT or VF and non-sustained VT with hemodynamic symptoms) and 576 had potentially lethal arrhythmias (increased VPDs or NSVT in patients with known structural heart disease, active ischemia, congestive heart failure or an LVEF < 40% and/or CI < 2.0 $l/min/m^2$). In this population there were 40 (3.7%) identified proarrhythmic events, 26 (2.5%) of which were serious, either fatal (6), new hemodynamically significant sustained VT or VF (4), new sustained VT that was not hemodynamically significant (11) or sustained VT that became syncopal/presyncopal when it had not been before (5). Proarrhythmic effects described as incessant ventricular tachycardia were observed in the post-marketing PES study and in post-marketing adverse event reports.

In general, serious proarrhythmic effects in the domestic pre-marketing trials were equally common in patients with more and less severe arrhythmias, 2.5% in the patients with baseline lethal arrhythmias vs. 2.8% in patients with potentially lethal arrhythmias, although the patients with serious effects were more likely to have a history of sustained VT (38% vs. 23%). In the post-marketing comparative PES study, patients treated with ETHMOZINE (250–300 mg TID) had a proarrhythmia rate of 14% (8/59).

Five of the six fatal proarrhythmic events were in patients with baseline lethal arrhythmias; four had prior cardiac arrests. Rates and severity of proarrhythmic events were similar in patients given 600–900 mg of ETHMOZINE per day and those given higher doses. Patients with proarrhythmic events were more likely than the overall population to have coronary artery disease (85% vs. 67%), history of acute myocardial infarction (75% vs. 53%), congestive heart failure (60% vs. 43%), and cardiomegaly (55% vs. 33%). All of the six proarrhythmic deaths were in patients with coronary artery disease; 5/6 each had documented acute myocardial infarction, congestive heart failure, and cardiomegaly.

Electrolyte Disturbances

Hypokalemia, hyperkalemia or hypomagnesemia may alter the effects of Class I antiarrhythmic drugs. Electrolyte imbalances should be corrected before administration of ETHMOZINE.

Sick Sinus Syndrome

Ethmozine should be used only with extreme caution in patients with sick sinus syndrome, as it may cause sinus bradycardia, sinus pause or sinus arrest.

PRECAUTIONS

General:

Electrocardiographic Changes/Conduction Abnormalities

ETHMOZINE slows AV nodal and intraventricular conduction, producing dose-related increases in the PR and QRS intervals. In clinical trials, the average increase in the PR interval was 12% and the QRS interval was 14%. Although the QTC interval is increased, this is wholly because of QRS prolongation; the JT interval is shortened, indicating the absence of significant slowing of ventricular repolarization. The degree of lengthening of PR and QRS intervals does not predict efficacy.

In controlled clinical trials and in open studies, the overall incidence of delayed ventricular conduction, including new bundle branch block pattern, was approximately 9.4%. In patients without baseline conduction abnormalities, the frequency of second-degree AV block was 0.2% and third-degree AV block did not occur. In patients with baseline conduction abnormalities, the frequencies of second-degree AV block and third-degree AV block were 0.9% and 1.4%, respectively.

ETHMOZINE therapy was discontinued in 1.6% of patients due to electrocardiographic changes (0.6% due to sinus pause or asystole, 0.2% to AV block, 0.2% to junctional rhythm, 0.4% to intraventricular conduction delay, and 0.2% to wide QRS and/or PR interval).

In patients with pre-existing conduction abnormalities, ETHMOZINE therapy should be initiated cautiously. If second- or third-degree AV block occurs, ETHMOZINE therapy should be discontinued unless a ventricular pacemaker is in place. When changing the dose of ETHMOZINE or adding concomitant medications which may also affect cardiac conduction, patients should be monitored electrocardiographically.

Hepatic Impairment

Patients with significant liver dysfunction have reduced plasma clearance and an increased half-life of ETHMOZINE. Although the precise relationship of ETHMOZINE levels to effect is not clear, patients with hepatic disease should be treated with lower doses and closely monitored for excessive pharmacological effects, including effects on ECG intervals, before dosage adjustment. Patients with severe liver disease should be administered ETHMOZINE with particular care, if at all. (See DOSAGE AND ADMINISTRATION)

Renal Impairment

Plasma levels of intact ETHMOZINE are unchanged in hemodialysis patients, but a significant portion (39%) of ETHMOZINE is metabolized and excreted in the urine. Although no identified active metabolite is known to increase in people with renal failure, metabolites of unrecognized importance could be affected. For this reason, ETHMOZINE should be administered cautiously in patients with impaired renal function. Patients with significant renal dysfunction should be started on lower doses and monitored for excessive pharmacologic effects, including ECG intervals, before dosage adjustment. (See DOSAGE AND ADMINISTRATION)

Congestive Heart Failure

Most patients with congestive heart failure have tolerated the recommended ETHMOZINE daily doses without unusual toxicity or change in effect. Pharmacokinetic differences between ETHMOZINE patients with and without congestive heart failure were not apparent (See Hepatic Impairment above). In some cases, worsened heart failure has been attributed to ETHMOZINE. Patients with pre-existing heart failure should be monitored carefully when ETHMOZINE is initiated.

Effects on Pacemaker Threshold

The effect of ETHMOZINE on the sensing and pacing thresholds of artificial pacemakers has not been sufficiently studied. In such patients, pacing parameters must be monitored, if ETHMOZINE is used.

Drug Interactions

No significant changes in serum digoxin levels or pharmacokinetics have been observed in patients or healthy subjects receiving concomitant ETHMOZINE therapy. Concomitant use was associated with additive prolongation of the PR interval, but not with a significant increase in the rate of second- or third-degree AV block.

Concomitant administration of cimetidine resulted in a decrease in ETHMOZINE clearance of 49% and a 1.4 fold increase in plasma levels in healthy subjects. During clinical trials, no significant changes in the efficacy or tolerance of ETHMOZINE have been observed in patients receiving concomitant cimetidine therapy. Patients on cimetidine should have ETHMOZINE therapy initiated at relatively low doses, not more than 600 mg/day. Patients should be monitored when concomitant cimetidine therapy is instituted or discontinued or when the ETHMOZINE dose is changed.

Concomitant administration of beta blocker therapy did not reveal significant changes in overall electrocardiographic intervals in patients. In one controlled study, ETHMOZINE and propranolol administered concomitantly produced a small additive increase in the PR interval.

Theophylline clearance and plasma half-life were significantly affected by multiple dose ETHMOZINE administration when both conventional and sustained release theophylline were given to healthy subjects (clearance increased 44–66% and plasma half-life decreased 19–33%). Plasma theophylline levels should be monitored when concomitant ETHMOZINE is initiated or discontinued.

Because of possible additive pharmocologic effects, caution is indicated when ETHMOZINE is used with any drug that affects cardiac electrophysiology. Uncontrolled experience in patients indicates no serious adverse interaction during the concomitant use of ETHMOZINE and diuretics, vasodilators, antihypertensive drugs, calcium channel blockers, beta-blockers, angiotensin-converting enzyme inhibitors, or warfarin. Plasma warfarin levels, warfarin pharmacokinetics, and prothrombin times were unaffected during multiple dose ETHMOZINE administration to young, healthy, male subjects in a controlled study. However, there are isolated reports of the need to either increase or decrease warfarin doses after initiation of ETHMOZINE. Some patients who were taking warfarin with a stable prothrombin time experienced excessive prolongation of the prothrombin time following the initiation of ETHMOZINE. In some cases, liver enzymes also were elevated. Bleeding or bruising may occur. When ETHMOZINE is started or stopped in a patient stabilized on warfarin, more frequent prothrombin time monitoring is advisable.

Results from *in vitro* studies do not suggest alterations in ETHMOZINE plasma protein binding in the presence of other highly plasma protein bound drugs.

CARCINOGENESIS, MUTAGENESIS, IMPAIRMENT OF FERTILITY

In a 24-month mouse study in which ETHMOZINE was administered in the feed at concentrations calculated to provide doses ranging up to 320 mg/kg/day, ovarian tubular adenomas and granulosa cell tumors were limited in occurrence to ETHMOZINE treated animals. Although the findings were of borderline statistical significance, or not statistically significant, historical control data indicate that both of these tumors are uncommon in the strain of mouse studied.

In a 24-month study in which ETHMOZINE was administered by gavage to rats at doses of 25, 50 and 100 mg/kg/day, Zymbal's Gland Carcinoma was observed in one mid-dose and two high dose males. This tumor appears to be uncommon in the strain of rat studied. Rats of both sexes showed a dose-related increase in hepatocellular cholangioma (also described as bile ductile cystadenoma or cystic hyperplasia) along with fatty metamorphosis, possibly due to disruption of hepatic choline utilization for phospholipid biosynthesis. The rat is known to be uniquely sensitive to alteration in choline metabolism.

ETHMOZINE was not mutagenic when assayed for genotoxicity in *in vitro* bacterial (Ames test) and mammalian (Chinese hamster ovary/hypoxanthine-guanine phosphoribosyl transferase and sister chromatid exchange) cell systems or in *in vivo* mammalian systems (rat bone cytogenicity and mouse micronucleus).

A general reproduction and fertility study was conducted in rats at dose levels up to 6.7 times the maximum recommended human dose of 900 mg/day (based upon 50 kg human body weight) and revealed no evidence of impaired male or female fertility.

Pregnancy—Teratogenic Effects:

Pregnancy Category B

Teratology studies have been performed with ETHMOZINE in rats and in rabbits at doses up to 6.7 and 4.7 times the maximum recommended human daily dose, respectively, and have revealed no evidence of harm to the fetus. There are, however, no adequate and well-controlled studies in pregnant women. Because animal reproduction studies are not always predictive of human response, ETHMOZINE should be used during pregnancy only if clearly needed.

Pregnancy—Nonteratogenic Effects:

In a study in which rats were dosed with ETHMOZINE prior to mating, during mating and throughout gestation and lactation, dose levels 3.4 and 6.7 times the maximum recommended human daily dose produced a dose-related decrease in pup and maternal weight gain, possibly related to a larger litter size. In a study in which dosing was begun on Day 15 of gestation, ETHMOZINE, at a level 6.7 times the maximum recommended human daily dose, produced a retardation in maternal weight gain but no effect on pup growth.

Nursing Mothers

ETHMOZINE is secreted in the milk of laboratory animals and has been reported to be present in human milk. Because of the potential for serious adverse reactions in nursing infants from ETHMOZINE, a decision should be made whether to discontinue the drug, taking into account the importance of the drug to the mother.

Pediatric Use

The safety and effectiveness of ETHMOZINE in children less than 18 years of age have not been established.

ADVERSE REACTIONS

The most serious adverse reaction reported for ETHMOZINE is proarrhythmia (see WARNINGS). This occurred in 3.7% of 1072 patients with ventricular arrhythmias who received a wide range of doses under a variety of circumstances.

In addition to discontinuations because of proarrhythmias, in controlled clinical trials and in open studies, adverse reactions led to discontinuation of ETHMOZINE in 7% of 1105 patients with ventricular and supraventricular arrhythmias, including 3.2% due to nausea, 1.6% due to ECG abnormalities (principally conduction defects, sinus pause, junctional rhythm, or AV block), 1% due to congestive heart failure, and 0.3–0.4% due to dizziness, anxiety, drug fever, urinary retention, blurred vision, gastrointestinal upset, rash, and laboratory abnormalities.

The most frequently occurring adverse reactions in the 1072 patients (including all adverse experiences whether or not considered ETHMOZINE-related by the investigator) were dizziness (15.1%), nausea (9.6%), headache (8.0%), fatigue (5.9%), palpitations (5.8%) and dyspnea (5.7%). Dizziness appears to be related to the size of each dose. In a comparison of 900 mg/day given at 450 mg b.i.d. or 300 mg t.i.d., more than 20% of patients experienced dizziness on the b.i.d. regimen vs. 12% on the t.i.d. regimen.

Adverse reactions reported by less than 5%, but in 2% or greater of the patients were: sustained ventricular tachycardia, hypesthesias, abdominal pain, dyspepsia, vomiting, sweating, cardiac chest pain, asthenia, nervousness, paresthesias, congestive heart failure, musculoskeletal pain, diarrhea, dry mouth, cardiac death, sleep disorders, and blurred vision.

Adverse reactions infrequently reported (in less than 2% of the patients) were:

Cardiovascular hypotension, hypertension, syncope, supraventricular arrhythmias (including atrial fibrillation/flutter), cardiac arrest, bradycardia, pulmonary embolism,

INCIDENCE (%) OF THE MOST COMMON ADVERSE REACTIONS
(THERAPY DURATION = 1–14 DAYS)

Adverse Reactions	>2% Moricizine No.	%	>2% Placebo No.	%	>2% Quinidine No.	%	>5% Disopyramide No.	%	>5% Propranolol No.	%
Total No. of Patients	1072		618		110		31		24	
Dizziness	121	11.3	33	5.3	8	7.3	—		2	8.3
Nausea	74	6.9	18	2.9	7	6.4	3	9.7	—	
Headache	62	5.8	27	4.4	—		—		4	16.7
Pain	41	3.8	31	5.0	6	5.5	2	6.5	—	
Dyspnea	41	3.8	22	3.6	—		—		—	
Hypesthesia	40	3.7	—		3	2.7	—		—	
Fatigue	33	3.1	16	2.6	6	5.5	2	6.5	3	12.5
Vomiting	22	2.1	—		—		—		—	
Dry Mouth	—		—		—		11	35.5	—	
Nervousness	—		—		—		3	9.7	—	
Blurred vision	—		—		3	2.7	2	6.5	3	12.5
Diarrhea	—		—		25	22.7	—		—	
Constipation	—		—		—		2	6.5	—	
Somnolence	—		—		—		—		2	8.3
Urinary Retention	—		—		—		4	12.9	—	

myocardial infarction, vasodilation, cerebrovascular events, thrombophlebitis;

Nervous System tremor, anxiety, depression, euphoria, confusion, somnolence, agitation, seizure, coma, abnormal gait, hallucinations, nystagmus, diplopia, speech disorder, akathisia, loss of memory, ataxia, abnormal coordination, dyskinesia, vertigo, tinnitus;

Genitourinary urinary retention or frequency, dysuria, urinary incontinence, kidney pain, impotence, decreased libido;

Respiratory hyperventilation, apnea, asthma, pharyngitis, cough, sinusitus;

Gastrointestinal anorexia, bitter taste, dysphagia, flatulence, ileus;

Other drug fever, hypothermia, temperature intolerence, eye pain, rash, pruritus, dry skin, urticaria, swelling of the lips and tongue, periorbital edema.

During ETHMOZINE therapy, two patients developed thrombocytopenia that may have been drug-related. Clinically significant elevations in liver function tests (bilirubin, serum transaminases) and jaundice consistent with hepatitis were rarely reported. Although a cause and effect relationship has not been established, caution is advised in patients who develop unexplained signs of hepatic dysfunction, and consideration should be given to discontinuing therapy.

Three patients developed rechallenge-confirmed drug fever, with one patient experiencing an elevation above 103°F (to 105°F. with rigors). Fevers occurred at about 2 weeks in 2 cases, and after 21 weeks in the third. Fevers resolved within 48 hours of discontinuation of moricizine.

Adverse reactions were generally similar in patients over 65 (n=375) and under 65 (n=697), although discontinuation of therapy for reasons other than proarrhythmia was more common in older patients (13.9% vs. 7.7%). Overall mortality was greater in older patients (9.3% vs. 3.9%), but those were not deaths attributed to treatment and the older patients had more serious underlying heart disease.

The following table compares the most common (occurrence in more than 2% of the patients) non-cardiac adverse reactions (i.e., drug-related or of unknown relationship) in controlled clinical trials during the first one to two weeks of therapy with ETHMOZINE, quinidine, placebo, disopyramide, or propranolol in patients with ventricular arrhythmias.
[See table above.]

OVERDOSAGE
Deaths have occurred after accidental or intentional overdosages of 2,250 and 10,000 mg of ETHMOZINE, respectively.

Signs, Symptoms and Laboratory Findings Associated with an Overdosage of Drug
Overdosage with ETHMOZINE may produce emesis, lethargy, coma, syncope, hypotension, conduction disturbances, exacerbation of congestive heart failure, myocardial infarction, sinus arrest, arrhythmias (including junctional bradycardia, ventricular tachycardia, ventricular fibrillation, and asystole), and respiratory failure.

Lethal Dose in Animals
Oral doses of ETHMOZINE of about 200 mg/kg in dogs, 250 mg/kg in monkeys, 420 mg/kg in mice and 905 mg/kg in rats were lethal to about one-half of the animals exposed. Death was usually preceded by tremors, convulsions and respiratory depression.

Recommended General Treatment Procedures
A specific antidote for ETHMOZINE has not been identified. In the event of overdosage, treatment should be supportive.

Patients should be hospitalized and monitored for cardiac, respiratory and CNS changes. Advanced life support systems, including an intracardiac pacing catheter, should be provided where necessary. Acute overdosage should be treated with appropriate gastric evacuation, and with special care to avoid aspiration. Accidental introduction of ETHMOZINE into the lungs of monkeys resulted in rapid arrhythmic death.

DOSAGE AND ADMINISTRATION
The dosage of ETHMOZINE must be individualized on the basis of antiarrhythmic response and tolerance. Clinical, cardiac rhythm monitoring, electrocardiogram intervals, exercise testing, and/or programmed electrical stimulation testing may be used to guide antiarrhythmic response and dosage adjustment. In general, the patients will be at high risk and should be hospitalized for the initiation of therapy (see INDICATIONS AND USAGE).

The usual adult dosage is between 600 and 900 mg per day, given every 8 hours in three equally divided doses. Within this range, the dosage can be adjusted as tolerated, in increments of 150 mg/day at 3-day intervals, until the desired effect is obtained. Patients with life-threatening arrhythmias who exhibit a beneficial response as judged by objective criteria (Holter monitoring, programmed electrical stimulation, exercise testing, etc.) can be maintained on chronic ETHMOZINE therapy. As the antiarrhythmic effect of ETHMOZINE persists for more than 12 hours, some patients whose arrhythmias are well-controlled on a Q8H regimen may be given the same total daily dose in a Q12H regimen to increase convenience and help assure compliance. When higher doses are used, patients may experience more dizziness and nausea on the Q12 hour regimen.

Patients with Hepatic Impairment
Patients with hepatic disease should be started at 600 mg/day or lower and monitored closely, including measurement of ECG intervals, before dosage adjustment.

Patients with Renal Impairment
Patients with significant renal dysfunction should be started at 600mg/day or lower and monitored closely, including measurement of ECG intervals, before dosage adjustment.

Transfer to ETHMOZINE
Recommendations for transferring patients from another antiarrhythmic to ETHMOZINE can be given based on theoretical considerations. Previous antiarrhythmic therapy should be withdrawn for 1–2 plasma half-lives before starting ETHMOZINE at the recommended dosages. In patients in whom withdrawal of a previous antiarrhythmic is likely to produce life-threatening arrhythmias, hospitalization is recommended.

Transferred From	Start ETHMOZINE
Quinidine, Disopyramide	6–12 hours after last dose
Procainamide	3–6 hours after last dose
Encainide, Propafenone, Tocainide, or Mexiletine	8–12 hours after last dose
Flecainide	12–24 hours after last dose

HOW SUPPLIED
ETHMOZINE (moricizine hydrochloride) is available as oval, convex, film-coated tablets as follows:

200 mg (light green):	Bottles of 100 (NDC 0056-0061-70) Hospital Unit Dose Carton of 100 (NDC 0056-0061-75)
250 mg (light orange):	Bottles of 100 (NDC 0056-0062-70) Hospital Unit Dose Carton of 100 (NDC 0056-0062-75)
300 mg (light blue)	Bottles of 100 (NDC 0056-0064-70) Hospital Unit Dose Carton of 100 (NDC 0056-0064-75)

Store at controlled room temperature (59°–86°F, 15°–30°C) in a tightly-closed, light resistant container. Keep in carton until dispensed. Protect from light.

DuPont Pharmaceuticals
Wilmington, Delaware 19880
ETHMOZINE® is a Registered Trademark of The Du Pont Merck Pharmaceutical Co.
Printed in U.S.A.   6217-4/Rev. May, 1992
US Patent 3,864,487
Shown in Product Identification Section, page 409

HESPAN®   ℞
[hes′pan]
(6% hetastarch in 0.9% sodium chloride injection)

DESCRIPTION
HESPAN (6% hetastarch in 0.9% sodium chloride injection) is a sterile, nonpyrogenic solution. The composition of each 100 mL is as follows:

Hetastarch	6.0 g
Sodium Chloride, USP	0.9 g
Water for Injection, USP	qs

pH adjusted with Sodium Hydroxide NF
Concentration of Electrolytes (mEq/Liter): Sodium 154, Chloride 154
pH: 5.9 (3.5–7.0); Calc. Osmolarity: 310 mOsM/liter
Hetastarch is an artifical colloid derived from a waxy starch composed almost entirely of amylopectin. Hydroxyethyl ether groups are introduced into the glucose units of the starch and the resultant material is hydrolyzed to yield a product with a molecular weight suitable for use as a plasma volume expander and erythrocyte sedimenting agent. Hetastarch is characterized by its molar substitution, and also by its molecular weight. The molar substitution is 0.7 which means hetastarch has 7 hydroxyethyl groups for every 10 glucose units. The weight average molecular weight is approximately 480,000 with a range of 400,000 to 550,000 and with 80% of the polymers falling between the range of 30,000 and 2,400,000. Hydroxyethyl groups are attached by ether linkage primarily at C-2 of the glucose unit and to a lesser extent at C-3 and C-6. The polymer resembles glycogen, and the polymerized glucose units are joined primarily by 1–4 linkages with occasional 1–6 branching linkages. The degree of branching is approximately 1:20 which means that there is one 1–6 branch for every 20 glucose monomer units.
The chemical name for hetastarch is hydroxyethyl starch. The structural formula is as follows:

Amylopectin derivative in which R_2, R_3, and R_6 are H or CH_2CH_2OH, or R_6 is a branching point in the starch polymer connected through a 1–6 linkage to additional α-D-glucopyranosyl units.

HESPAN is a clear, pale yellow to amber solution. Exposure to prolonged adverse storage conditions may result in a change to a turbid deep brown or the formation of a crystalline precipitate. Do not use the solution if these conditions are evident.
The plastic container is made from a multi-layered film specifically developed for parenteral drugs. It contains no plasticizers and exhibits virtually no leachables. The solution contact layer is a rubberized copolymer of ethylene and propylene. The container is nontoxic and biologically inert. The container-solution unit is a closed system and is not dependent upon entry of external air during administration. The container is overwrapped to provide protection from the physical environment and to provide an additional moisture barrier when necessary.
The closure system has two ports; the one for the administration set has a tamper evident plastic protector.

CLINICAL PHARMACOLOGY
The plasma volume expansion produced by HESPAN approximate those of 5% human albumin. Intravenous infusion of HESPAN results in expansion of plasma volume that decreases over the succeeding 24 to 36 hours. The degree of plasma volume expansion and improvement in hemodynamic state depend upon the patient's intravascular status. Hetastarch molecules below 50,000 molecular weight are rapidly eliminated by renal excretion. A single dose of approximately 500 mL of HESPAN (approximately 30 g) results in elimination in the urine of approximately 33% of the dose within 24 hours. This is a variable process but generally results in an intravascular hetastarch concentration of less than 10% of the total dose injected by two weeks. The hy-

Continued on next page

Du Pont—Cont.

droxyethyl group is not cleaved by the body, but remains intact and attached to glucose units when excreted. Significant quantities of glucose are not produced as hydroxyethylation prevents complete metabolism of the smaller polymers.

The addition of HESPAN to whole blood increases the erythrocyte sedimentation rate. Therefore, HESPAN is used to improve the efficiency of granulocyte collection by centrifugal means.

INDICATIONS AND USAGE

HESPAN is indicated in the treatment of hypovolemia when plasma volume expansion is desired. It is not a substitute for blood or plasma.

The adjunctive use of HESPAN in leukapheresis has also been shown to be safe and efficacious in improving the harvesting and increasing the yield of granulocytes by centrifugal means.

CONTRAINDICATIONS

HESPAN is contraindicated in patients with known hypersensitivity to hydroxyethyl starch, or with bleeding disorders, or with congestive heart failure where volume overload is a potential problem. HESPAN should not be used in renal disease with oliguria or anuria not related to hypovolemia.

WARNINGS

Usage in Plasma Volume Expansion

Large volumes may alter the coagulation mechanism. Thus, administration of HESPAN may result in transient prolongation of prothrombin, partial thromboplastin and clotting times. With administration of large doses, the physician should also be alert to the possibility of transient prolongation of bleeding time.

Hematocrit may be decreased and plasma proteins diluted excessively by administration of large volumes of HESPAN. Administration of packed red cells, platelets, and fresh frozen plasma should be considered if excessive dilution occurs.

Use over extended periods: HESPAN has not been adequately evaluated to establish its safety in situations other than leukapheresis that require frequent use of colloidal solutions over extended periods. Certain conditions may affect the safe use of HESPAN on a chronic basis. For example, in patients with subarachnoid hemorrhage where HESPAN is used repeatedly over a period of days for the prevention of cerebral vasospasm, significant clinical bleeding may occur.

Usage in Leukapheresis

Slight declines in platelet counts and hemoglobin levels have been observed in donors undergoing repeated leukapheresis procedures using HESPAN due to the volume expanding effects of HESPAN and to the collection of platelets and erythrocytes. Hemoglobin levels usually return to normal within 24 hours. Hemodilution by HESPAN and saline may also result in 24 hour declines of total protein, albumin, calcium and fibrinogen values. None of these decreases are to a degree recognized to be clinically significant risks to healthy donors.

PRECAUTIONS

General

Regular and frequent clinical evaluation and complete blood counts (CBC) are necessary for proper monitoring of HESPAN use during leukapheresis. If the frequency of leukapheresis is to exceed the guidelines for whole blood donation, you may wish to consider the following additional studies: total leukocyte and platelet counts, leukocyte differential count, hemoglobin and hematocrit, prothrombin time (PT), and partial thromboplastin time (PTT) tests.

The possibility of circulatory overload should be kept in mind. Caution should be used when the risk of pulmonary edema and/or congestive heart failure is increased. Special care should be exercised in patients who have impaired renal clearance since this is the principal way in which hetastarch is eliminated.

Indirect bilirubin levels of 8.3 mg/L (normal 0.0–7.0 mg/L) have been reported in 2 out of 20 normal subjects who received multiple HESPAN infusions. Total bilirubin was within normal limits at all times; indirect bilirubin returned to normal by 96 hours following the final infusion. The significance, if any, of these elevations is not known; however, caution should be observed before administering HESPAN to patients with a history of liver disease.

HESPAN has been reported to produce hypersensitivity reactions such as wheezing and urticaria. However, hetastarch has not been observed to stimulate antibody formation. If hypersensitivity effects occur, they are readily controlled by discontinuation of the drug and, if necessary, administration of an antihistaminic agent.

Elevated serum amylase levels may be observed temporarily following administration of HESPAN, although no association with pancreatitis has been demonstrated.

Carcinogenesis, mutagenesis, impairment of fertility.

Long-term studies of animals have not been performed to evaluate the carcinogenic potential of hetastarch.

Teratogenic Effects

Pregnancy Category C. Animal reproduction studies have not been conducted with HESPAN. It is also not known whether HESPAN can cause fetal harm when administered to a pregnant woman or can affect reproduction capacity. HESPAN should be given to a pregnant woman only if clearly needed.

Nursing Mothers

It is not known whether hetastarch is excreted in human milk. Because many drugs are excreted in human milk, caution should be exercised when HESPAN is administered to a nursing woman.

Pediatric Use

The safety and effectiveness of HESPAN in children have not been established.

ADVERSE REACTIONS

The following have been reported: vomiting, fever, chills, pruritus, submaxillary and parotid glandular enlargement, mild influenza-like symptoms, headaches, muscle pains, peripheral edema of the lower extremities, anaphylactoid reactions (periorbital edema, urticaria, wheezing) bleeding due to hemodilution (see Warnings), and circulatory overload and pulmonary edema (see Precautions).

DOSAGE AND ADMINISTRATION

Dosage for Acute Use in Plasma Volume Expansion

HESPAN is administered by intravenous infusion only. Total dosage and rate of infusion depend upon the amount of blood or plasma lost and the resultant hemoconcentration. In adults, the amount usually administered is 500 to 1000 mL. Doses of more than 1500 mL per day for the typical 70 kg patient (approximately 20 mL per kg of body weight) are usually not required, although higher doses have been reported in postoperative and trauma patients where severe blood loss has occurred.

Dosage in Leukapheresis

250 to 700 mL of HESPAN to which citrate anticoagulant has been added is typically administered by aseptic addition to the input line of the centrifugation apparatus at a ratio of 1:8 to 1:13 to venous whole blood. The HESPAN and citrate should be thoroughly mixed to assure effective anticoagulation of blood as it flows through the leukapheresis machine. The safety and compatibility of other additives have not been established.

Parenteral drug products should be inspected for particulate matter and discoloration prior to administration whenever solution and container permit.

HOW SUPPLIED

HESPAN® (6% hetastarch in 0.9% sodium chloride injection) is supplied sterile and nonpyrogenic in 500 mL EXCEL® Containers packaged 12 per case (NDC 0056-0037-46). Exposure of pharmaceutical products to heat should be minimized. Avoid excessive heat. Protect from freezing. It is recommended that the product be stored at room temperature (25°C); however, brief exposure up to 40°C does not adversely affect the product.

CAUTION

Federal (USA) law prohibits dispensing without prescription.

To Open

Tear overwrap down at notch and remove solution container. Check for minute leaks by squeezing solution container firmly. If leaks are found, discard solution as sterility may be impaired.

Invert container and carefully inspect the solution in good light for cloudiness, haze, or particulate matter. Any container which is suspect should not be used.

Distributed by
Du Pont Pharmaceuticals
The Du Pont Merck Pharmaceutical Co.
Wilmington, Delaware 19880
Manufactured by
McGaw, Inc.
Irvine CA USA 92714-5895
Issued: October, 1991
Commodity Number
6253/October, 1991
U.S. Patent No. 4,803,102
EXCEL® is a registered trademark of McGaw, Inc.
HESPAN® is a registered trademark of The Du Pont Merck Pharmaceutical Co.

HYCODAN® Ⓒ III

[*hī-kō-dan*]
(hydrocodone bitartrate and homatropine methylbromide)
Tablets and Syrup
Antitussive

DESCRIPTION

HYCODAN contains hydrocodone (dihydrocodeinone) bitartrate, a semisynthetic centrally-acting narcotic antitussive. Homatropine methylbromide is included in a subtherapeutic amount to discourage deliberate overdosage.

Each HYCODAN tablet or teaspoonful (5 mL) contains:

Hydrocodone bitartrate, USP	5 mg
WARNING: May be habit forming.	
Homatropine methylbromide, USP	1.5 mg

HYCODAN tablets also contain: calcium phosphate dibasic, colloidal silicon dioxide, lactose, magnesium stearate, starch and stearic acid.

HYCODAN syrup: caramel coloring, FD&C Red 40, liquid sugar, methylparaben, propylparaben, sorbitol solution and wild cherry imitation flavor.

The hydrocodone component is 4,5α-epoxy-3-methoxy-17-methylmorphinan-6-one tartrate (1:1) hydrate (2:5), a fine white crystal or crystalline powder, which is derived from the opium alkaloid, thebaine, has a molecular weight of (494.50).

Homatropine methylbromide is 8-Azoniabicyclo-[3.2.1] octane, 3- [(hydroxyphenylacetyl) oxy] -8, 8-dimethyl-, bromide, endo-; a white crystal or fine white crystalline powder, with a molecular weight of (370.29).

CLINICAL PHARMACOLOGY

Hydrocodone is a semisynthetic narcotic antitussive and analgesic with multiple actions qualitatively similar to those of codeine. The precise mechanism of action of hydrocodone and other opiates is not known; however, hydrocodone is believed to act directly on the cough center. In excessive doses, hydrocodone, like other opium derivatives, will depress respiration. The effects of hydrocodone in therapeutic doses on the cardiovascular system are insignificant. Hydrocodone can produce miosis, euphoria, physical and physiological dependence.

Following a 10 mg oral dose of hydrocodone administered to five adult male subjects, the mean peak concentration was 23.6 ± 5.2 ng/mL. Maximum serum levels were achieved at 1.3 ± 0.3 hours and the half-life was determined to be 3.8 ± 0.3 hours. Hydrocodone exhibits a complex pattern of metabolism including O-demethylation, N-demethylation and 6-keto reduction to the corresponding 6-α- and 6-β- hydroxymetabolites.

INDICATIONS AND USAGE

HYCODAN is indicated for the symptomatic relief of cough.

CONTRAINDICATIONS

HYCODAN should not be administered to patients who are hypersensitive to hydrocodone or homatropine methylbromide.

WARNINGS

May be habit forming. Hydrocodone can produce drug dependence of the morphine type and, therefore, has the potential for being abused. Psychic dependence, physical dependence and tolerance may develop upon repeated administration of HYCODAN and it should be prescribed and administered with the same degree of caution appropriate to the use of other narcotic drugs (see DRUG ABUSE AND DEPENDENCE).

Respiratory Depression: HYCODAN produces dose-related respiratory depression by directly acting on brain stem respiratory centers. If respiratory depression occurs, it may be antagonized by the use of naloxone hydrochloride and other supportive measures when indicated.

Head Injury And Increased Intracranial Pressure: The respiratory depression properties of narcotics and their capacity to elevate cerebrospinal fluid pressure may be markedly exaggerated in the presence of head injury, other intracranial lesions or a pre-existing increase in intracranial pressure. Furthermore, narcotics produce adverse reactions which may obscure the clinical course of patients with head injuries.

Acute Abdominal Conditions: The administration of HYCODAN or other narcotics may obscure the diagnosis or clinical course of patients with acute abdominal conditions.

Pediatric Use: In young children, as well as adults, the respiratory center is sensitive to the depressant action of narcotic cough suppressants in a dose-dependent manner. Benefit to risk ratio should be carefully considered especially in children with respiratory embarrassment (e.g., croup).

PRECAUTIONS

General: Before prescribing medication to suppress or modify cough, it is important to ascertain that the underlying cause of cough is identified, that modification of cough does not increase the risk of clinical or physiological complications, and that appropriate therapy for the primary disease is provided.

Special Risk Patients: HYCODAN should be given with caution to certain patients such as the elderly or debilitated, and those with severe impairment of hepatic or renal functions, hypothyroidism, Addison's disease, prostatic hypertrophy or urethral stricture, asthma, and narrow-angle glaucoma.

Information For Patients: Hydrocodone may impair the mental and/or physical abilities required for the performance of potentially hazardous tasks such as driving a car or operating machinery. The patient using HYCODAN should be cautioned accordingly.

Drug Interactions: Patients receiving narcotics, antihistamines, antipsychotics, antianxiety agents or other CNS depressants (including alcohol) concomitantly with HYCODAN may exhibit an additive CNS depression. When combined therapy is contemplated, the dose of one or both agents should be reduced. The use of MAO inhibitors or tricyclic antidepressants with hydrocodone preparations may increase the effect of either the antidepressant or hydrocodone.

Carcinogenesis, Mutagenesis, Impairment Of Fertility: Studies of HYCODAN in animals to evaluate the carcinogenic and mutagenic potential and the effect on fertility have not been conducted.

Pregnancy:

Teratogenic Effects: Pregnancy Category C; Animal reproduction studies have not been conducted with HYCODAN (hydrocodone bitartrate and homatropine methylbromide). It is also not known whether HYCODAN can cause fetal harm when administered to a pregnant woman or can affect reproduction capacity. HYCODAN should be given to a pregnant woman only if clearly needed.

Nonteratogenic Effects: Babies born to mothers who have been taking opioids regularly prior to delivery will be physically dependent. The withdrawal signs include irritability and excessive crying, tremors, hyperactive reflexes, increased respiratory rate, increased stools, sneezing, yawning, vomiting and fever. The intensity of the syndrome does not always correlate with the duration of maternal opioid use or dose.

Labor and Delivery: As with all narcotics, administration of HYCODAN to the mother shortly before delivery may result in some degree of respiratory depression in the newborn, especially if higher doses are used.

Nursing Mothers: It is not known whether this drug is excreted in human milk. Because many drugs are excreted in human milk and because of the potential for serious adverse reactions in nursing infants from HYCODAN, a decision should be made whether to discontinue nursing or to discontinue the drug, taking into account the importance of the drug to the mother.

Pediatric Use: Safety and effectiveness of HYCODAN in children under six have not been established.

ADVERSE REACTIONS

Central Nervous System: Sedation, drowsiness, mental clouding, lethargy, impairment of mental and physical performance, anxiety, fear, dysphoria, dizziness, psychic dependence, mood changes.

Gastrointestinal System: Nausea and vomiting may occur; they are more frequent in ambulatory than in recumbent patients. Prolonged administration of HYCODAN may produce constipation.

Genitourinary System: Ureteral spasm, spasm of vesicle sphincters and urinary retention have been reported with opiates.

Respiratory Depression: HYCODAN may produce dose-related respiratory depression by acting directly on brain stem respiratory centers (see OVERDOSAGE).

Dermatological: Skin rash, pruritus.

DRUG ABUSE AND DEPENDENCE

HYCODAN is a Schedule III narcotic. Psychic dependence, physical dependence and tolerance may develop upon repeated administration of narcotics; therefore, HYCODAN should be prescribed and administered with caution. However, psychic dependence is unlikely to develop when HYCODAN is used for a short time for the treatment of cough. Physical dependence, the condition in which continued administration of the drug is required to prevent the appearance of a withdrawal syndrome, assumes clinically significant proportions only after several weeks of continued oral narcotic use, although some mild degree of physical dependence may develop after a few days of narcotic therapy.

OVERDOSAGE

Signs and Symptoms: Serious overdosage with hydrocodone is characterized by respiratory depression (a decrease in respiratory rate and/or tidal volume, Cheyne-Stokes respiration, cyanosis), extreme somnolence progressing to stupor or coma, skeletal muscle flaccidity, cold and clammy skin, and sometimes bradycardia and hypotension. In severe overdosage apnea, circulatory collapse, cardiac arrest and death may occur. The ingestion of very large amounts of HYCODAN may, in addition, result in acute homatropine intoxication.

Treatment: Primary attention should be given to the reestablishment of adequate respiratory exchange through provision of a patent airway and the institution of assisted or controlled ventilation. The narcotic antagonist naloxone hydrochloride is a specific antidote for respiratory depression which may result from overdosage or unusual sensitivity to narcotics including hydrocodone. Therefore, an appropriate dose of naloxone hydrochloride should be administered, preferably by the intravenous route, simultaneously with efforts at respiratory resuscitation. For further information, see full prescribing information for naloxone hydrochloride. An antagonist should not be administered in the absence of clinically significant respiratory depression. Oxygen, intravenous fluids, vasopressors and other supportive measures should be employed as indicated. Gastric emptying may be useful in removing unabsorbed drug.

DOSAGE AND ADMINISTRATION

Adults: One (1) tablet or one (1) teaspoonful (5 mL) of the syrup every 4 to 6 hours as needed; do not exceed six (6) tablets or six (6) teaspoonfuls in 24 hours.

Children 6 to 12 years of age: One-half (½) tablet or one-half (½) teaspoonful (2.5 mL) of the syrup every 4 to 6 hours as needed; do not exceed three (3) tablets or three (3) teaspoonfuls in 24 hours.

HOW SUPPLIED

As white tablets with one face scored and inscribed HYCODAN, and the other inscribed with Du Pont name is available in:

Bottles of 100	NDC 0056-0042-70
Bottles of 500	NDC 0056-0042-85

As a clear red colored, wild cherry flavored syrup in:

Bottles of one pint	NDC 0056-0234-16

Store at controlled room temperature (59°–86° F, 15°–30° C).

Caution: Federal law prohibits dispensing without prescription.

Oral prescription where permitted by state law.

Du Pont Pharmaceuticals
Wilmington, Delaware 19880

HYCODAN® is a Registered Trademark of The Du Pont Merck Pharmaceutical Co.

6014–17/Rev. Dec., 1990

HYCOMINE® Ⓒ III
(hydrocodone bitartrate and phenylpropanolamine hydrochloride)
Pediatric Syrup

HYCOMINE® Ⓒ III
(hydrocodone bitartrate and phenylpropanolamine hydrochloride)
Syrup

DESCRIPTION

HYCOMINE contains hydrocodone (dihydrocodeinone) bitartrate, a semi-synthetic centrally-acting narcotic antitussive and phenylpropanolamine hydrochloride, a sympathomimetic amine decongestant for oral administration. (See the approved package insert).

	HYCOMINE Pediatric Syrup	HYCOMINE Syrup
Each teaspoonful (5 mL) contains:		
Hydrocodone bitartrate, USP WARNING: May be habit forming	2.5 mg	5 mg
Phenylpropanolamine hydrochloride, USP	12.5 mg	25 mg

Also, HYCOMINE, both strengths, contain: artificial cherry flavor, glycerin, methylparaben, propylparaben, saccharin sodium, and sorbitol solution. HYCOMINE Pediatric Syrup contains: D&C Yellow 10 and FD&C Green 3. HYCOMINE Syrup: FD&C Red 40 and FD&C Yellow 6.

CLINICAL PHARMACOLOGY

Hydrocodone is a semisynthetic narcotic antitussive and analgesic with multiple actions qualitatively similar to those of codeine. The precise mechanism of action of hydrocodone and other opiates is not known; however, hydrocodone is believed to act directly on the cough center. In excessive doses, hydrocodone, like other opium derivatives, will depress respiration. The effects of hydrocodone in therapeutic doses on the cardiovascular system are insignificant. Hydrocodone can produce miosis, euphoria, physical and physiological dependence.

Following a 10 mg oral dose of hydrocodone administered to five adult male subjects, the mean peak concentration was 23.6 ± 5.2 ng/mL. Maximum serum levels were achieved at 1.3 ± 0.3 hours and the half-life was determined to be 3.8 ± 0.3 hours. Hydrocodone exhibits a complex pattern of metabolism including O-demethylation, N-demethylation and 6-keto reduction to the corresponding 6-α- and 6-β-hydroxymetabolites.

Phenylpropanolamine effects its vasoconstrictor activity by releasing noradrenaline from sympathetic nerve endings, and from direct stimulation of α-adrenoreceptors of blood vessels.

INDICATIONS AND USAGE

HYCOMINE is indicated for the symptomatic relief of cough and nasal congestion.

CONTRAINDICATIONS

HYCOMINE is contraindicated in patients hypersensitive to hydrocodone or phenylpropanolamine, and in patients on concurrent MAO inhibitor therapy. Patients known to be hypersensitive to other opioids or sympathomimetic amines may exhibit cross sensitivity to HYCOMINE. Phenylpropanolamine is contraindicated in patients with heart disease, hypertension, diabetes or hyperthyroidism. Hydrocodone is contraindicated in the presence of an intracranial lesion associated with increased intracranial pressure; and whenever ventilatory function is depressed.

WARNINGS

May be habit forming. Hydrocodone can produce drug dependence of the morphine type and, therefore, has the potential for being abused. Psychic dependence, physical dependence and tolerance may develop upon repeated administration of HYCOMINE and it should be prescribed and administered with the same degree of caution appropriate to the use of other narcotic drugs (see DRUG ABUSE AND DEPENDENCE).

Respiratory Depression: HYCOMINE produces dose-related respiratory depression by directly acting on brain stem respiratory centers. If respiratory depression occurs, it may be antagonized by the use of naloxone hydrochloride and other supportive measures when indicated.

Head Injury and Increased Intracranial Pressure: The respiratory depression properties of narcotics and their capacity to elevate cerebrospinal fluid pressure may be markedly exaggerated in the presence of head injury, other intracranial lesions or a preexisting increase in intracranial pressure. Furthermore, narcotics produce adverse reactions which may obscure the clinical course of patients with head injuries.

Acute Abdominal Conditions: The administration of HYCOMINE or other narcotics may obscure the diagnosis or clinical course of patients with acute abdominal conditions.

Pediatric Use: In young children, as well as adults, the respiratory center is sensitive to the depressant action of narcotic cough suppressants in a dose-dependent manner. Benefit to risk ratio should be carefully considered especially in children with respiratory embarrassment (e.g., croup).

Phenylpropanolamine: Hypertensive crises can occur with concurrent use of phenylpropanolamine and monoamine oxidase (MAO) inhibitors, indomethacin or with beta-blockers and methyldopa.

If a hypertensive crisis occurs, these drugs should be discontinued immediately and therapy to lower blood pressure should be instituted immediately. Fever should be managed by means of external cooling.

PRECAUTIONS

General: Before prescribing medication to suppress or modify cough, it is important to ascertain that the underlying cause of cough is identified, that modification of cough does not increase the risk of clinical or physiologic complications, and that appropriate therapy for the primary disease is provided.

Special Risk Patients: HYCOMINE should be given with caution to certain patients such as the elderly or debilitated, and those with severe impairment of hepatic or renal functions, hypothyroidism, Addison's disease, prostatic hypertrophy or urethral stricture, asthma, narrow-angle glaucoma, and uncontrolled hypertension.

Information for Patients: Hydrocodone may impair the mental and/or physical abilities required for the performance of potentially hazardous tasks such as driving a car or operating machinery; phenylpropanolamine may produce a rapid pulse, dizziness or palpitations. The patient using HYCOMINE should be cautioned accordingly.

Drug Interactions: Patients receiving other narcotic analgesics, general anesthetics, phenothiazines, other tranquilizers, sedative-hypnotics or other CNS depressants (including alcohol) concomitantly with hydrocodone may exhibit an additive CNS depression. When such combined therapy is contemplated, the dose of one or both agents should be reduced. The use of phenylpropanolamine with other sympathomimetic amines and MAO inhibitors may produce an additive elevation of blood pressure (see WARNINGS).

Carcinogenesis, Mutagenesis, Impairment of Fertility: Carcinogenicity, mutagenicity and reproduction studies have not been conducted with HYCOMINE.

Pregnancy: Teratogenic Effects: Pregnancy Category C: Animal reproduction studies have not been conducted with

Continued on next page

Du Pont—Cont.

HYCOMINE. It is also not known whether HYCOMINE can cause fetal harm when administered to a pregnant woman or can affect reproductive capacity. HYCOMINE should be given to a pregnant woman only if clearly needed.

Nonteratogenic Effects: Babies born to mothers who have been taking opioids regularly prior to delivery will be physically dependent. The withdrawal signs include irritability and excessive crying, tremors, hyperactive reflexes, increased respiratory rate, increased stools, sneezing, yawning, vomiting and fever. The intensity of the syndrome does not always correlate with the duration of maternal opioid use or dose.

Labor and Delivery: As with all narcotics, administration of HYCOMINE to the mother shortly before delivery may result in some degree of respiratory depression in the newborn, especially if higher doses are used.

Nursing Mothers: It is not known whether this drug is excreted in human milk. Because many drugs are excreted in human milk and because of the potential for serious adverse reactions in nursing infants from HYCOMINE, a decision should be made whether to discontinue nursing or discontinue the drug, taking into account the importance of the drug to the mother.

Pediatric Use: Safety and effectiveness of HYCOMINE in children under six have not been established.

ADVERSE REACTIONS

Respiratory System: Hydrocodone produces dose-related respiratory depression by acting directly on brain stem respiratory centers. (See **OVERDOSAGE**).

Cardiovascular System: Hypertension, postural hypotension, tachycardia and palpitations.

Genitourinary System: Ureteral spasm, spasm of vesical sphincters and urinary retention have been reported with opiates.

Central Nervous System: Sedation, drowsiness, mental clouding, lethargy, impairment of mental and physical performance, anxiety, fear, dysphoria, dizziness, psychic dependence, mood changes and blurred vision.

Gastrointestinal System: Nausea and vomiting occur more frequently in ambulatory than in recumbent patients. Prolonged administration of HYCOMINE may produce constipation.

Dermatological: Skin rash, pruritus.

DRUG ABUSE AND DEPENDENCE

Hycomine is a Schedule III narcotic. Psychic dependence, physical dependence, and tolerance may develop upon repeated administration of narcotics; therefore, Hycomine should be prescribed and administered with caution. However, psychic dependence is unlikely to develop when HYCOMINE is used for a short time for the treatment of cough. Physical dependence, the condition in which continued administration of the drug is required to prevent the appearance of a withdrawal syndrome, assumes clinically significant proportions only after several weeks of continued oral narcotic use, although some mild degree of physical dependence may develop after a few days of narcotic therapy.

OVERDOSAGE

Signs and Symptoms: Serious overdosage with HYCOMINE is characterized by respiratory depression (a decrease in respiratory rate and/or tidal volume, Cheyne-Stokes respiration, cyanosis), extreme somnolence progressing to stupor or coma, skeletal muscle flaccidity, cold and clammy skin, and sometimes bradycardia and hypotension. In severe overdosage apnea, circulatory collapse, cardiac arrest, and death may occur.

The signs and symptoms of overdosage of the individual components of HYCOMINE may be modified in varying degrees by the presence of other active ingredients. Overdosage with phenylpropanolamine alone may result in tremor, restlessness, increased motor activity, agitation and hallucinations.

Treatment: Primary attention should be given to the reestablishment of adequate respiratory exchange through provision of a patent airway and the institution of assisted or controlled ventilation. The narcotic antagonist naloxone hydrochloride is a specific antidote for respiratory depression which may result from overdosage or unusual sensitivity to narcotics including hydrocodone. Therefore, an appropriate dose of naloxone hydrochloride should be administered preferably by the intravenous route, simultaneously with efforts at respiratory resuscitation.

For further information, see full prescribing information for naloxone hydrochloride. An antagonist should not be administered in the absence of clinically significant respiratory depression. Oxygen, intravenous fluids, vasopressors, and other supportive measures should be employed as indicated. Gastric emptying may be useful in removing unabsorbed drug.

DOSAGE AND ADMINISTRATION

Adults: The usual dose for adults is one teaspoonful HYCOMINE Syrup (hydrocodone bitartrate 5 mg and phenylpropanolamine hydrochloride 25 mg/5 cc) every four hours as needed, not to exceed six teaspoonfuls in a 24 hour period.

Children 6 to 12 years of age: The usual dose for children 6 to 12 years of age is one teaspoonful HYCOMINE Pediatric Syrup (hydrocodone bitartrate 2.5 mg and phenylpropanolamine hydrochloride 12.5 mg/5 cc) every four hours as needed, not to exceed six teaspoonfuls in a 24 hour period.

HOW SUPPLIED

HYCOMINE Syrup (5 mg hydrocodone bitartrate, USP and 25 mg phenylpropanolamine hydrochloride, USP—per 5 mL teaspoonful) is available as an orange-colored, cherry-flavored syrup in bottles as follows:

One Pint (473.2 mL): NDC 0056-0246-16

HYCOMINE Pediatric Syrup (2.5 mg hydrocodone bitartrate, USP and 12.5 mg phenylpropanolamine hydrochloride, USP—per 5 mL teaspoonful) is available as a green-colored, cherry-flavored syrup in bottles as follows:

One Pint (473.2 mL): NDC 0056-0247-16

Store at controlled room temperature (59°–86°F, 15°–30°C).

Oral prescription where permitted by state law.

Du Pont Pharmaceuticals
Wilmington, Delaware 19880

HYCOMINE is a Registered Trademark of The Du Pont Merck Pharmaceutical Co.

6153-5/Rev. Dec., 1990

HYCOMINE® COMPOUND Ⓒ III

[*hī-ko-mēn kom 'pound*]

DESCRIPTION

HYCOMINE Compound tablets contain hydrocodone (dihydrocodeinone) bitartrate, a semi-synthetic centrally-acting narcotic antitussive; chlorpheniramine maleate, an antihistamine; phenylephrine hydrochloride, a sympathomimetic amine decongestant; acetaminophen, an analgesic/antipyretic; and caffeine, a centrally-acting stimulant; for oral administration.

Each HYCOMINE Compound tablet contains:

Hydrocodone bitartrate, USP	5 mg
WARNING: May be habit forming	
Chlorpheniramine maleate, USP	2 mg
Phenylephrine hydrochloride, USP	10 mg
Acetaminophen, USP	250 mg
Caffeine, anhydrous, USP	30 mg

HYCOMINE Compound tablets also contain: cherry flavor, colloidal silicon dioxide, FD&C Red 40, magnesium stearate, microcrystalline cellulose, povidone and starch.

CLINICAL PHARMACOLOGY

Clinical trials have proven hydrocodone bitartrate to be an effective antitussive agent which is pharmacologically 2 to 8 times as potent as codeine. At equi-effective doses, its sedative action is greater than codeine. The precise mechanism of action of hydrocodone and other opiates is not known, however, hydrocodone is believed to act by directly depressing the cough center. In excessive doses hydrocodone, like other opium derivatives, will depress respiration. The effects of hydrocodone in therapeutic doses on the cardiovascular system is insignificant. The constipation effects of hydrocodone are much weaker than that of morphine and no stronger than that of codeine. Hydrocodone can produce miosis, euphoria, physical and psychological dependence. At therapeutic antitussive doses, it does exert analgesic effects. Following a 10 mg oral dose of hydrocodone administered to five adult male human subjects, the mean peak concentration was 23.6 ± 5.2 ng/mL. Maximum serum levels were achieved at 1.3 ± 0.3 hours and the half-life was determined to be 3.8 ± 0.3 hours. Hydrocodone exhibits a complex pattern of metabolism including O-demethylation, N-demethylation and 6-keto reduction to the corresponding 6-α- and 6-β-hydroxymetabolites.

Chlorpheniramine maleate is a competitive H_1-receptor histamine blocking drug, thereby counteracting the effects of histamine release associated with allergic manifestations of upper respiratory tract inflammatory disorders. H_1-blocking drugs inhibit the actions of histamine on smooth muscle, capillary permeability, and can both stimulate and depress the central nervous system. Phenylephrine hydrochloride effects its vasoconstrictor activity by releasing noradrenaline from sympathetic nerve endings, and from direct stimulation of α-adrenoreceptors in blood vessels. Acetaminophen is an antipyretic and peripherally acting analgesic. Caffeine is a central nervous system stimulant.

INDICATIONS AND USAGE

HYCOMINE Compound is indicated for the symptomatic relief of cough, nasal congestion, and discomfort associated with upper respiratory tract infections.

CONTRAINDICATIONS

HYCOMINE Compound is contraindicated in patients hypersensitive to any component of the drug, and concurrent MAO inhibitor therapy. Patients known to be hypersensitive to other opioids, antihistamines, or sympathomimetic amines may exhibit cross sensitivity with HYCOMINE Compound. Phenylephrine is contraindicated in patients with heart disease, hypertension, diabetes or hyperthyroidism. Hydrocodone is contraindicated in the presence of an intracranial lesion associated with increased intracranial pressure, and whenever ventilatory function is depressed.

WARNINGS

May be habit forming. Hydrocodone can produce drug dependence of the morphine type and therefore has the potential for being abused. Psychic dependence, physical dependence and tolerance may develop upon repeated administration of HYCOMINE Compound and it should be prescribed and administered with the same degree of caution appropriate to the use of other narcotic drugs. (See DRUG ABUSE AND DEPENDENCE.)

Respiratory Depression: HYCOMINE Compound produces dose-related respiratory depression by directly acting on brain stem respiratory centers. If respiratory depression occurs, it may be antagonized by the use of NARCAN® (naloxone hydrochloride) and other supportive measures when indicated.

Head Injury and Increased Intracranial Pressure: The respiratory depressant properties of narcotics and their capacity to elevate cerebrospinal fluid pressure may be markedly exaggerated in the presence of head injury, other intracranial lesions or a pre-existing increase in intracranial pressure. Furthermore, narcotics produce adverse reactions which may obscure the clinical course of patients with head injuries.

Acute abdominal conditions: The administration of HYCOMINE Compound or other narcotics may obscure the diagnosis or clinical course of patients with acute abdominal conditions.

Phenylephrine: Hypertensive crises can occur with concurrent use of phenylephrine and monoamine oxidase (MAO) inhibitors, indomethacin or with beta-blockers and methyldopa.

If a hypertensive crisis occurs these drugs should be discontinued immediately and therapy to lower blood pressure should be instituted immediately. Fever should be managed by means of external cooling.

Chlorpheniramine: Antihistamines may produce drowsiness or excitation, particularly in children and elderly patients.

PRECAUTIONS

Before prescribing medication to suppress or modify cough, it is important to ascertain that the underlying cause of cough is identified, that modification of cough does not increase the risk of clinical or physiologic complications, and that appropriate therapy for the primary disease is provided.

Usage in Ambulatory Patients: Hydrocodone, like all narcotics, and antihistamines such as chlorpheniramine maleate, may impair the mental and/or physical abilities required for the performance of potentially hazardous tasks such as driving a car or operating machinery; phenylephrine may produce a rapid pulse, dizziness or palpitations; patients should be cautioned accordingly.

Drug Interactions: Patients receiving other narcotic analgesics, general anesthetics, phenothiazines, other tranquilizers, sedative-hypnotics or other CNS depressants (including alcohol) concomitantly with hydrocodone may exhibit an additive CNS depression. When such combined therapy is contemplated, the dose of one or both agents should be reduced. The use of phenylephrine with other sympathomimetic amines and MAO inhibitors may produce an additive elevation of blood pressure. MAO inhibitors may prolong the anticholinergic effects of antihistamines. (See WARNINGS.)

Carcinogenesis, mutagenesis, impairment of fertility: Carcinogenicity, mutagenicity, and reproduction studies have not been conducted with HYCOMINE Compound.

Usage in Pregnancy: Pregnancy Category C. Animal reproduction studies have not been conducted with HYCOMINE Compound. It is also not known whether HYCOMINE Compound can cause fetal harm when administered to a pregnant woman or can affect reproductive capacity. HYCOMINE Compound should be given to a pregnant woman only if clearly needed.

Nonteratogenic effects: Babies born to mothers who have been taking opioids regularly prior to delivery will be physically dependent. The withdrawal signs include irritability and excessive crying, tremors, hyperactive reflexes, increased respiratory rate, increased stools, sneezing, yawning, vomiting and fever. The intensity of the syndrome does not always correlate with the duration of maternal opioid use or dose. Chlorpromazine 0.7–1.0 mg/kg q 6 h, phenobarbital 2 mg/kg q 6 h, and paregoric 2–4 drops/kg q 4 h, have been used to treat withdrawal symptoms in infants. The duration of therapy is 4 to 28 days, with the dosages decreased as tolerated.

Nursing mothers: It is not known whether this drug is excreted in human milk. Because many drugs are excreted in human milk and because of the potential for serious adverse reactions in nursing infants from HYCOMINE Compound, a decision should be made whether to discontinue nursing or

discontinue the drug, taking into account the importance of the drug to the mother.

Pediatric use: Safety and effectiveness in children below the age of 2 years have not been established.

ADVERSE REACTIONS

Respiratory System: Hydrocodone produces dose-related respiratory depression by acting directly on brain stem respiratory centers.

Cardiovascular System: Hypertension, postural hypotension, tachycardia and palpitations.

Genitourinary System: Ureteral spasm, spasm of vesical sphincters and urinary retention have been reported with opiates.

Central Nervous System: Sedation, drowsiness, mental clouding, lethargy, impairment of mental and physical performance, anxiety, fear, dysphoria, dizziness, psychic dependence, mood changes, and blurred vision.

Gastrointestinal System: Nausea and vomiting occur more frequently in ambulatory than in recumbent patients.

DRUG ABUSE AND DEPENDENCE

Special care should be exercised in prescribing hydrocodone for emotionally unstable patients and for those with a history of drug misuse. Such patients should be closely supervised when long-term therapy is contemplated.

HYCOMINE Compound is a Schedule III narcotic. Psychic dependence, physical dependence, and tolerance may develop upon repeated administration of narcotics; therefore, HYCOMINE Compound should always be prescribed and administered with caution. Physical dependence is the condition in which continued administration of the drug is required to prevent the appearance of a withdrawal syndrome. Patients physically dependent on opioids will develop an abstinence syndrome upon abrupt discontinuation of the opioid or following the administration of a narcotic antagonist. The character and severity of the withdrawal symptoms are related to the degree of physical dependence. Manifestations of opioid withdrawal are similar to but milder than that of morphine and include lacrimation, rhinorrhea, yawning, sweating, restlessness, dilated pupils, anorexia, gooseflesh, irritability and tremor. In more severe forms, nausea, vomiting, intestinal spasm and diarrhea, increased heart rate and blood pressure, chills, and pains in bones and muscles of the back and extremities may occur. Peak effects will usually be apparent at 48 to 72 hours.

Treatment of withdrawal is usually managed by providing sufficient quantities of an opioid to suppress **severe** withdrawal symptoms and then gradually reducing the dose of opioid over a period of several days.

OVERDOSAGE

The signs and symptoms of overdosage of the individual components of HYCOMINE Compound may be modified in varying degrees by the presence of other active ingredients. Overdosage with phenylephrine alone may result in tremor, restlessness, increased motor activity, agitation and hallucinations.

Acetaminophen

Signs and Symptoms: In acute acetaminophen overdosage, dose-dependent, potentially fatal hepatic necrosis is the most serious adverse effect. Renal tubular necrosis, hypoglycemic coma and thrombocytopenia may also occur.

Acetaminophen in massive overdosage may cause hepatic toxicity in some patients. In cases of suspected overdose, you may wish to call your regional poison center for assistance in diagnosis and for directions in the use of N-acetylcysteine as an antidote.

In adults, hepatic toxicity has rarely been reported with acute overdoses of less than 10 grams and fatalities with less than 15 grams. Importantly, young children seem to be more resistant than adults to the hepatotoxic effect of an acetaminophen overdose. Despite this, the measures outlined below should be initiated in any adult or child suspected of having ingested an acetaminophen overdose.

Early symptoms following a potentially hepatotoxic overdose may include nausea, vomiting, diaphoresis and general malaise. Clinical and laboratory evidence of hepatic toxicity may not be apparent until 48 to 72 hours post-ingestion.

Treatment: The stomach should be emptied promptly by lavage or by induction of emesis with syrup of ipecac. Patient's estimates of the quantity of a drug ingested are notoriously unreliable. Therefore, if an acetaminophen overdose is suspected, a serum acetaminophen assay should be obtained as early as possible, but no sooner than four hours following ingestion. Liver function studies should be obtained initially and repeated at 24-hour intervals.

The antidote, N-acetylcysteine should be administered as early as possible, preferably within 16 hours of the overdose ingestions for optimal results, but in any case, within 24 hours. Following recovery, there are no residual structural or functional hepatic abnormalities.

Hydrocodone

Signs and Symptoms: Serious overdosage with hydrocodone is characterized by respiratory depression (a decrease in respiratory rate and/or tidal volume, Cheyne-Stokes respiration, cyanosis), extreme somnolence progressing to stupor or coma, skeletal muscle flaccidity, cold and clammy skin, and sometimes bradycardia and hypotension. In severe overdosage apnea, circulatory collapse, cardiac arrest and death may occur.

Treatment: Primary attention should be given to the reestablishment of adequate respiratory exchange through provision of a patent airway and the institution of assisted or controlled ventilation. The narcotic antagonist naloxone hydrochloride is a specific antidote for respiratory depression which may result from overdosage or unusual sensitivity to narcotics including hydrocodone. Therefore, an appropriate dose of naloxone hydrochloride should be administered, preferably by the intravenous route, simultaneously with efforts at respiratory resuscitation. For further information, see full prescribing information for naloxone hydrochloride. An antagonist should not be administered in the absence of clinically significant respiratory depression. Oxygen, intravenous fluids, vasopressors and other supportive measures should be employed as indicated. Gastric emptying may be useful in removing unabsorbed drug. Activated charcoal may be of benefit.

DOSAGE AND ADMINISTRATION

Usual dosage, not less than 4 hours apart:
Adults: 1 tablet 4 times a day.
Children: 6 to 12 years: 1/2 tablet 4 times a day.

HOW SUPPLIED

HYCOMINE® Compound is available as a coral pink, scored tablet in bottles as follows:

Bottles of 100	NDC 0056-0048-70
Bottles of 500	NDC 0056-0048-85

Store at controlled room temperature (59°–86° F, 15°–30° C)
Oral prescription where permitted by State Law.

Du Pont Pharmaceuticals
Wilmington, Delaware 19880
HYCOMINE® is a Registered Trademark of The Du Pont Merck Pharmaceutical Co.
NARCAN® is a Registered Trademark of The Du Pont Merck Pharmaceutical Co.
6015-12/Rev. Dec., 1990

HYCOTUSS® Ⓒ

[*hī-kō-tus*]
Expectorant

DESCRIPTION

HYCOTUSS Expectorant Syrup contains hydrocodone (dihydrocodeinone) bitartrate, a semi-synthetic centrally-acting narcotic antitussive and guaifenesin, an expectorant for oral administration.

Each teaspoonful (5 mL) contains:

Hydrocodone bitartrate, USP	5 mg
WARNING: May be habit forming	
Guaifenesin, USP	100 mg
Alcohol, USP	10% v/v

HYCOTUSS Expectorant Syrup also contains: artificial butterscotch flavor, FD&C Red 40, FD&C Yellow 6, glycerin, liquid sugar, methylparaben, propylparaben, saccharin sodium, and sorbitol solution.

CLINICAL PHARMACOLOGY

Clinical trials have proven hydrocodone bitartrate to be an effective antitussive agent which is pharmacologically 2 to 8 times as potent as codeine. At equi-effective doses, its sedative action is greater than codeine. The precise mechanism of action of hydrocodone and other opiates is not known, however, hydrocodone is believed to act by directly depressing the cough center. In excessive doses hydrocodone, like other opium derivatives, can depress respiration. The effects of hydrocodone in therapeutic doses on the cardiovascular system is insignificant. The constipation effects of hydrocodone are much weaker than that of morphine and no stronger than that of codeine. Hydrocodone can produce miosis, euphoria, physical and psychological dependence. At therapeutic antitussive doses, it does exert analgesic effects. Following a 10 mg oral dose of hydrocodone administered to five male human subjects, the mean peak concentration was 23.6 $\pm$ 5.2 ng/mL. Maximum serum levels were achieved at 1.3 $\pm$ 0.3 hours and half-life was determined to be 3.8 $\pm$ 0.3 hours. Hydrocodone exhibits a complex pattern of metabolism including O-demethylation, N-demethylation and 6-ketoreduction to the corresponding 6-α- and 6-β-hydroxymetabolites.

The exact mechanism of action is not established but guaifenesin is believed to act by stimulating receptors in the gastric mucosa that initiates a reflex secretion of respiratory tract fluid, thereby increasing the volume and decreasing the viscosity of bronchial secretions. Studies with guaifenesin indicate that it is rapidly absorbed from the gastrointestinal tract and has a half-life of one hour.

INDICATIONS AND USAGE

HYCOTUSS Expectorant is indicated for the symptomatic relief of irritating non-productive cough associated with upper and lower respiratory tract congestion.

CONTRAINDICATIONS

HYCOTUSS Expectorant is contraindicated in patients hypersensitive to hydrocodone or guaifenesin. Patients known to be hypersensitive to other opioids may exhibit cross sensitivity to HYCOTUSS Expectorant. Hydrocodone is contraindicated in the presence of an intracranial lesion associated with increased intracranial pressure; and whenever ventilatory function is depressed.

WARNINGS

May be habit forming. Hydrocodone can produce drug dependence of the morphine type and therefore has the potential for being abused. Psychic dependence, physical dependence and tolerance may develop upon repeated administration of HYCOTUSS Expectorant and it should be prescribed and administered with the same degree of caution appropriate to the use of other narcotic drugs (see DRUG ABUSE AND DEPENDENCE).

Respiratory Depression: HYCOTUSS Expectorant produces dose-related respiratory depression by directly acting on the brain stem respiratory centers. If respiratory depression occurs, it may be antagonized by the use of NARCAN® (naloxone hydrochloride) and other supportive measures when indicated.

Head Injury and Increased Intracranial Pressure: The respiratory depressant properties of narcotics and their capacity to elevate cerebrospinal fluid pressure may be markedly exaggerated in the presence of head injury, other intracranial lesions or a pre-existing increase in intracranial pressure. Furthermore, narcotics produce adverse reactions which may obscure the clinical course of patients with head injuries.

Acute Abdominal Conditions: The administration of HYCOTUSS Expectorant or other opioids may obscure the diagnosis or clinical course of patients with acute abdominal conditions.

PRECAUTIONS

Before prescribing medication to suppress or modify cough, it is important to ascertain that the underlying cause of cough is identified, that modification of cough does not increase the risk of clinical or physiologic complications, and that appropriate therapy for the primary disease is provided.

Usage in Ambulatory Patients: Hydrocodone, like all narcotics, may impair the mental and/or physical abilities required for the performance of potentially hazardous tasks such as driving a car or operating machinery, and patients should be warned accordingly.

Drug Interactions: Patients receiving other narcotics, analgesics, general anesthetics, phenothiazines, other tranquilizers, sedative hypnotics or other CNS depressants (including alcohol) concomitantly with hydrocodone may exhibit an additive CNS depression. When such combined therapy is contemplated, the dose of one or both agents should be reduced (see WARNINGS).

Laboratory Interactions: The metabolite of guaifenesin has been found to produce an apparent increase in urinary 5-hydroxyindoleacetic acid, and guaifenesin therefore may interfere with the interpretation of this test for the diagnosis of carcinoid syndrome. Guaifenesin administration should be discontinued 24 hours prior to the collection of urine specimens for the determination of 5-hydroxyindoleacetic acid.

Carcinogenesis, mutagenesis, impairment of fertility: Carcinogenicity, mutagenicity and reproduction studies have not been conducted with HYCOTUSS Expectorant.

Usage in Pregnancy: Pregnancy Category C. Animal reproduction studies have not been conducted with HYCOTUSS Expectorant. It is also not known whether HYCOTUSS Expectorant can cause fetal harm when administered to a pregnant woman or can affect reproductive capacity. HYCOTUSS Expectorant should be given to a pregnant woman only if clearly needed.

Nonteratogenic effects: Babies born to mothers who have been taking opioids regularly prior to delivery will be physically dependent. The withdrawal signs include irritability and excessive crying, tremors, hyperactive reflexes, increased respiratory rate, increased stools, sneezing, yawning, vomiting and fever. The intensity of the syndrome does not always correlate with the duration of maternal opioid use or dose. There is no consensus on the best method of managing withdrawal. Chlorpromazine 0.7–1.0 mg/kg q 6 h, phenobarbital 2 mg/kg q 6 h, and paregoric 2–4 drops/kg q 4 h, have been used to treat withdrawal symptoms in infants. The duration of therapy is 4 to 28 days, with the dosages decreased as tolerated.

Nursing mothers: It is not known whether this drug is excreted in human milk. Because many drugs are excreted in human milk and because of the potential for serious adverse reactions in nursing infants from HYCOTUSS Expectorant,

Continued on next page

Du Pont—Cont.

a decision should be made whether to discontinue nursing or discontinue the drug, taking into account the importance of the drug to the mother.

ADVERSE REACTIONS

Respiratory System: Hydrocodone produces dose-related respiratory depression by acting directly on brain stem respiratory centers.

Cardiovascular System: Hypertension, postural hypotension and palpitations.

Genitourinary System: Ureteral spasm, spasm of vesical sphincters and urinary retention have been reported with opiates.

Central Nervous System: Sedation, drowsiness, mental clouding, lethargy, impairment of mental and physical performance, anxiety, fear, dysphoria, dizziness, psychic dependence, mood changes and blurred vision.

Gastrointestinal System: Nausea and vomiting occur more frequently in ambulatory than in recumbent patients.

DRUG ABUSE AND DEPENDENCE

Special care should be exercised in prescribing hydrocodone for emotionally unstable patients and for those with a history of drug misuse. Such patients should be closely supervised when long-term therapy is contemplated.

HYCOTUSS Expectorant is a Schedule III narcotic. Psychic dependence, physical dependence and tolerance may develop upon repeated administration of narcotics; therefore, HYCOTUSS Expectorant should always be prescribed and administered with caution. Physical dependence is the condition in which continued administration of the drug is required to prevent the appearance of a withdrawal syndrome.

Patients physically dependent on opioids will develop an abstinence syndrome upon abrupt discontinuation of the opioid or following the administration of a narcotic antagonist. The character and severity of the withdrawal symptoms are related to the degree of physical dependence. Manifestations of opioid withdrawal are similar to but milder than that of morphine and include lacrimation, rhinorrhea, yawning, sweating, restlessness, dilated pupils, anorexia, gooseflesh, irritability and tremor. In more severe forms, nausea, vomiting, intestinal spasm and diarrhea, increased heart rate and blood pressure, chills, and pains in bones and muscles of the back and extremities may occur. Peak effects will usually be apparent at 48 to 72 hours.

Treatment of withdrawal is usually managed by providing sufficient quantities of an opioid to suppress **severe** withdrawal symptoms and then gradually reducing the dose of opioid over a period of several days.

OVERDOSAGE

Signs and Symptoms: Serious overdosage with HYCOTUSS Expectorant is characterized by respiratory depression (a decrease in respiratory rate and/or tidal volume, Cheyne-Stokes respiration, cyanosis), extreme somnolence progressing to stupor or coma, skeletal muscle flaccidity, cold and clammy skin, and sometimes bradycardia and hypotension. In severe overdosage apnea, circulatory collapse, cardiac arrest, and death may occur.

Treatment: Primary attention should be given to the reestablishment of adequate respiratory exchange through provision of a patent airway and the institution of assisted or controlled ventilation. The narcotic antagonist naloxone hydrochloride is a specific antidote for respiratory depression which may result from overdosage or unusual sensitivity to narcotics including hydrocodone. Therefore, an appropriate dose of naloxone hydrochloride should be administered, preferably by the intravenous route, simultaneously with efforts at respiratory resuscitation. For further information, see full prescribing information for naloxone hydrochloride. An antagonist should not be administered in the absence of clinically significant respiratory depression. Oxygen, intravenous fluids, vasopressors and other supportive measures should be employed as indicated. Gastric emptying may be useful in removing unabsorbed drug. Activated charcoal may be of benefit.

DOSAGE AND ADMINISTRATION

Usual Adult Dose: One teaspoonful (5 mL) after meals and at bedtime, not less than 4 hours apart (not to exceed 6 teaspoonful in a 24 hour period). Treatment should be initiated with one teaspoonful and subsequent doses, up to a maximum single dose of 3 teaspoonsful, adjusted if required.

Usual Children's Dose:

Over 12 years: Initial dose 1 teaspoonful; maximum single dose, 2 teaspoonsful.

6 to 12 years: Initial dose ½ teaspoonful; maximum single dose, 1 teaspoonful.

HOW SUPPLIED

HYCOTUSS Expectorant is available as an orange-colored, butterscotch flavored syrup in bottles as follows:

One pint: NDC 0056-0235-16

Store at controlled room temperature (59°–86° F, 15°–30° C).

Oral prescription where permitted by State Law.

Du Pont Pharmaceuticals
Wilmington, Delaware 19880

HYCOTUSS® is a Registered Trademark of The Du Pont Merck Pharmaceutical Co.

NARCAN® is a Registered Trademark of The Du Pont Merck Pharmaceutical Co.

6131-6/Rev. Dec., 1990

PENTASPAN® ℞

(10% pentastarch in 0.9% sodium chloride injection)

DESCRIPTION

PENTASPAN (10% pentastarch in 0.9% sodium chloride injection) is a sterile, nonpyrogenic solution. The composition of each 100 mL is as follows:

Pentastarch	10.0 g
Sodium Chloride USP	0.9 g
Water for Injection USP	qs

pH adjusted with Sodium Hydroxide NF

pH: 4.8 (3.5–7.0)

Calculated Osmolarity: 310 mOsM/liter

Concentration of Electrolytes (mEq/liter): Sodium 154; Chloride 154

Pentastarch is an artificial colloid derived from a waxy starch composed almost entirely of amylopectin. Hydroxyethyl ether groups are introduced into the glucose units of the starch and the resultant material is hydrolyzed to yield a product with a molecular weight suitable for use as an erythrocyte sedimenting agent. Pentastarch is characterized by its molar substitution, and also by its molecular weight. The degree of substitution is 0.45 which means pentastarch has 45 hydroxyethyl groups for every 100 glucose units. The weight average molecular weight of pentastarch is approximately 264,000 with a range of 150,000 to 350,000 and with 80% of the polymers falling between 10,000 and 2,000,000. Hydroxyethyl groups are attached by an ether linkage primarily at C-2 of the glucose unit and to a lesser extent at C-3 and C-6. The polymer resembles glycogen, and the polymerized glucose units are joined primarily by 1–4 linkages with occasional 1–6 branching linkages. The degree of branching is approximately 1:20 which means that there is one 1–6 branch for every 20 glucose monomer units.

The chemical name for pentastarch is hydroxyethyl starch. The structural formula is as follows:

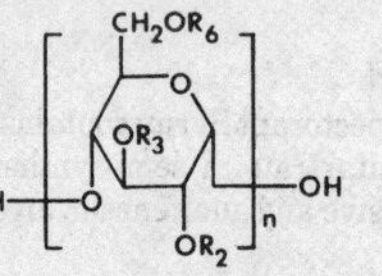

Amylopectin derivative in which R_2, R_3, and R_6 are H or CH_2CH_2OH, or R_6 is a branching point in the starch polymer connected through a 1–6 linkage to additional α-D-glucopyranosyl units.

PENTASPAN is a clear, pale yellow to amber solution. Exposure to prolonged adverse storage conditions may result in a change to a turbid deep brown or the formation of a crystalline precipitate. Do not use the solution if these conditions are evident.

The plastic container is made from a multilayered film specifically developed for parenteral drugs. It contains no plasticizers and exhibits virtually no leachables. The solution contact layer is a rubberized copolymer of ethylene and propylene. The container is nontoxic and biologically inert. The container-solution unit is a closed system and is not dependent upon entry of external air during administration. The container is overwrapped to provide protection from the physical environment and to provide an additional moisture barrier when necessary.

The closure system has two ports; the one for the administration set has a tamper evident plastic protector.

CLINICAL PHARMACOLOGY

The addition of PENTASPAN to whole blood increases the erythrocyte sedimentation rate. Therefore, 10% pentastarch in 0.9% sodium chloride injection is used to improve the efficiency of leukocyte collection by centrifugal means.

Pentastarch molecules below 50,000 molecular weight are rapidly eliminated by renal excretion. A single dose of approximately 500 mL of PENTASPAN (approximately 50 g) results in elimination in the urine of approximately 70% of the dose within 24 hours, and approximately 80% of the dose within one week. An additional 5–6% of the pentastarch dose is recovered in the leukapheresis collection bag. The remaining 12–15% (approximately 6.8 g) of an administered dose is presumed to undergo slower elimination. This is a variable process but generally results in an intravascular pentastarch concentration below the level of detection by one week. The hydroxyethyl group is not cleaved by the body, but remains intact and attached to glucose units when excreted.

The colloidal properties of the related product HESPAN® (6% hetastarch in 0.9% sodium chloride injection) approximate those of 5% human albumin. Intravenous infusion of HESPAN results in expansion of plasma volume that decreases over the succeeding 24 to 36 hours. Similar, although reduced duration, volume expansion may be expected to occur following use of PENTASPAN in leukapheresis procedures.

INDICATIONS AND USAGE

PENTASPAN is indicated as an adjunct in leukapheresis, to improve the harvesting and increase the yield of leukocytes by centrifugal means.

CONTRAINDICATIONS

PENTASPAN is contraindicated in donors with known hypersensitivity to hydroxyethyl starch, or with bleeding disorders, or with congestive heart failure where volume overload is a potential problem. PENTASPAN should not be used in renal disease with oliguria or anuria.

WARNINGS

Slight declines in platelet counts and hemoglobin levels have been observed in donors undergoing repeated leukapheresis procedures using HESPAN due to the volume expanding effects of HESPAN and to the collection of platelets and erythrocytes. Hemoglobin levels usually return to normal within 24 hours. Similar effects may be expected with PENTASPAN. Hemodilution by PENTASPAN and saline may also result in 24 hour declines of total protein, albumin, calcium and fibrinogen values. None of these decreases are to a degree recognized to be clinically significant risks to healthy donors.

Large volumes of PENTASPAN may slightly alter the coagulation mechanism; *i.e.,* transient prolongation of prothrombin, partial thromboplastin and clotting times. The physician should also be alert to the possibility of transient prolongation of bleeding time.

PRECAUTIONS

General

Regular and frequent clinical evaluation and complete blood counts (CBC) are necessary for proper monitoring of PENTASPAN use during leukapheresis. If the frequency of leukapheresis is to exceed the guidelines for whole blood donation, you may wish to consider the following additional studies: total leukocyte and platelet counts, leukocyte differential count, hemoglobin and hematocrit, prothrombin time (PT), and partial thromboplastin time (PTT) tests.

The possibility of circulatory overload should be kept in mind. Caution should be used when the risk of pulmonary edema and/or congestive heart failure is increased. Special care should be exercised in patients who have impaired renal clearance since this is the principal way in which pentastarch is eliminated.

The serum chemistries of sixteen normal volunteers who were given 500 to 2000 mL infusions of PENTASPAN were essentially unchanged pre- and post-infusion, except for dilutional effects. However, indirect bilirubin levels of 8.3 mg/L (normal 0–7 mg/L) have been reported in 2 out of 20 normal subjects who received multiple HESPAN infusions. Total bilirubin was within normal limits at all times; indirect bilirubin returned to normal by 96 hours following the final infusion. The significance, if any, of these elevations is not known; however, caution should be observed before administering PENTASPAN to patients with a history of liver disease.

PENTASPAN has been reported to produce hypersensitivity reactions such as wheezing and urticaria. However, pentastarch has not been observed to stimulate antibody formation. If hypersensitivity effects occur, they are readily controlled by discontinuation of the drug and, if necessary, administration of an antihistaminic agent.

Elevated serum amylase levels may be observed temporarily following administration of PENTASPAN, although no association with pancreatitis has been demonstrated.

Carcinogenesis, mutagenesis, impairment of fertility—

Long-term studies in animals have not been performed to evaluate the carcinogenic potential of pentastarch.

Teratogenic Effects—

Pregnancy Category C. PENTASPAN has been shown to be embryocidal in New Zealand rabbits and in Swiss Mice when given in doses 5 times the human dose. There are no adequate and well-controlled clinical studies using pentastarch in pregnant women. PENTASPAN should be used during pregnancy only if the potential benefits justify the potential risk to the fetus.

PENTASPAN was administered to mated New Zealand rabbits and Swiss Mice with intravenous doses of 10, 20, and 40 mL/kg/ day during the period of gestation. The results demonstrated that at 10 and 20 mL/kg/day pentastarch produced no higher incidence of teratogenicity or embryotoxicity in either species than normal saline did in control animals. At 40 mL/kg/day, however, pentastarch increased the number of resorptions and minor visceral anomalies (diffuse

edema of the trunk and extremities and diffuse whitish color of the heart, lungs, liver, and kidneys) in rabbits and reduced nidation in the mouse.

Nursing mothers—

It is not known whether pentastarch is excreted in human milk. Because many drugs are excreted in human milk, caution should be exercised when PENTASPAN is administered to a nursing woman.

Pediatric use—

The safety and effectiveness of PENTASPAN in children have not been established.

ADVERSE REACTIONS

The following have been reported in association with the use of PENTASPAN in leukapheresis: headache, diarrhea, nausea, weakness, temporary weight gain, insomnia, fatigue, fever, edema, paresthesia, acne, malaise, shakiness, dizziness, chest pain, chills, nasal congestion, anxiety, and increased heart rate. It is uncertain whether they are attributable to the drug, the procedure, additional adjunctive medication, or some combination of these factors.

DOSAGE AND ADMINISTRATION

250 to 700 mL of PENTASPAN to which citrate anticoagulant has been added is typically administered by aseptic addition to the input line of the centrifugation apparatus at a ratio of 1:8 to 1:13 to venous whole blood. PENTASPAN and citrate should be thoroughly mixed to assure effective anticoagulation of blood as it flows through the leukapheresis machine.

Do not use plastic container in series connection.

If administration is controlled by a pumping device, care must be taken to discontinue pumping action before the container runs dry or air embolism may result.

This solution is intended for intravenous administration using sterile equipment. It is recommended that intravenous administration apparatus be replaced at least once every 24 hours.

Use only if solution is clear and container and seals are intact.

The safety and compatibility of other additives have not been established.

Parenteral drug products should be inspected visually for particulate matter and discoloration prior to administration whenever solution and container permit.

HOW SUPPLIED

PENTASPAN (10% pentastarch in 0.9% sodium chloride injection) is supplied sterile and nonpyrogenic in 500 mL EXCEL® Containers packaged 12 per case (NDC 0056-0081-46).

Exposure of pharmaceutical products to heat should be minimized. Avoid excessive heat. Protect from freezing. It is recommended that the product be stored at room temperature (25°C); however, brief exposure up to 40°C does not adversely affect the product.

Caution: Federal (USA) law prohibits dispensing without prescription.

To Open

Tear overwrap down at notch and remove solution container. Check for minute leaks by squeezing solution container firmly. If leaks are found, discard solution as sterility may be impaired.

Invert container and carefully inspect the solution in good light for cloudiness, haze, or particulate matter. Any container which is suspect should not be used.

Distributed by
Du Pont Pharmaceuticals
Wilmington, Delaware 19880
Manufactured by
McGaw, Inc.
Irvine CA USA 92714-5895
Issued: October 1991
Commodity Number 6270-1/October, 1991
U.S. Patent No. 4,803,102
EXCEL® is a registered trademark of McGaw, Inc.
PENTASPAN® and HESPAN® are registered trademarks of The Du Pont Merck Pharmaceutical Co.

PERCOCET® CII

[perk 'o-set]
(oxycodone and acetaminophen tablets, USP)

DESCRIPTION

Each tablet of PERCOCET contains:

Oxycodone hydrochloride .... 5 mg†
WARNING: May be habit forming
Acetaminophen, USP .... 325 mg
† 5 mg oxycodone HCl is equivalent to 4.4815 mg of oxycodone.

PERCOCET Tablets also contain: microcrystalline cellulose, povidone, pregelatinized starch, stearic acid and other ingredients.

Acetaminophen occurs as a white, odorless, crystalline powder, possessing a slightly bitter taste.

The oxycodone component is 14-hydroxydihydrocodeinone, a white, odorless, crystalline powder having a saline, bitter taste. It is derived from the opium alkaloid thebaine.

CLINICAL PHARMACOLOGY

The principal ingredient, oxycodone, is a semisynthetic narcotic analgesic with multiple actions qualitatively similar to those of morphine; the most prominent of these involve the central nervous system and organs composed of smooth muscle. The principal actions of therapeutic value of the oxycodone in PERCOCET are analgesia and sedation.

Oxycodone is similar to codeine and methadone in that it retains at least one-half of its analgesic activity when administered orally.

Acetaminophen is a non-opiate, non-salicylate analgesic and antipyretic.

INDICATIONS AND USAGE

PERCOCET is indicated for the relief of moderate to moderately severe pain.

CONTRAINDICATIONS

PERCOCET should not be administered to patients who are hypersensitive to oxycodone or acetaminophen.

WARNINGS

Drug Dependence: Oxycodone can produce drug dependence of the morphine type and, therefore, has the potential for being abused. Psychic dependence, physical dependence and tolerance may develop upon repeated administration of PERCOCET, and it should be prescribed and administered with the same degree of caution appropriate to the use of other oral narcotic-containing medications. Like other narcotic-containing medications, PERCOCET is subject to the Federal Controlled Substances Act (Schedule II).

PRECAUTIONS

General

Head Injury and Increased Intracranial Pressure: The respiratory depressant effects of narcotics and their capacity to elevate cerebrospinal fluid pressure may be markedly exaggerated in the presence of head injury, other intracranial lesions or a pre-existing increase in intracranial pressure. Furthermore, narcotics produce adverse reactions which may obscure the clinical course of patients with head injuries.

Acute Abdominal Conditions: The administration of PERCOCET or other narcotics may obscure the diagnosis or clinical course in patients with acute abdominal conditions.

Special Risk Patients: PERCOCET should be given with caution to certain patients such as the elderly or debilitated, and those with severe impairment of hepatic or renal function, hypothyroidism, Addison's disease, and prostatic hypertrophy or urethral stricture.

Information for Patients Oxycodone may impair the mental and/or physical abilities required for the performance of potentially hazardous tasks such as driving a car or operating machinery. The patient using PERCOCET should be cautioned accordingly.

Drug Interaction Patients receiving other narcotic analgesics, general anesthetics, phenothiazines, other tranquilizers, sedative-hypnotics or other CNS depressants (including alcohol) concomitantly with PERCOCET may exhibit an additive CNS depression. When such combined therapy is contemplated, the dose of one or both agents should be reduced.

The use of MAO inhibitors or tricyclic antidepressants with oxycodone preparations may increase the effect of either the antidepressant or oxycodone.

The concurrent use of anticholinergics with narcotics may produce paralytic ileus.

Usage In Pregnancy Pregnancy Category C: Animal reproductive studies have not been conducted with PERCOCET. It is also not known whether PERCOCET can cause fetal harm when administered to a pregnant woman or can affect reproductive capacity. PERCOCET should not be given to a pregnant woman unless in the judgment of the physician, the potential benefits outweigh the possible hazards.

Nonteratogenic Effects: Use of narcotics during pregnancy may produce physical dependence in the neonate.

Labor and Delivery: As with all narcotics, administration of PERCOCET to the mother shortly before delivery may result in some degree of respiratory depression in the newborn and the mother, especially if higher doses are used.

Nursing Mothers It is not known whether PERCOCET is excreted in human milk. Because many drugs are excreted in human milk, caution should be exercised when PERCOCET is administered to a nursing woman.

Pediatric Use Safety and effectiveness in children have not been established.

ADVERSE REACTIONS

The most frequently observed adverse reactions include lightheadedness, dizziness, sedation, nausea and vomiting. These effects seem to be more prominent in ambulatory than in nonambulatory patients, and some of these adverse reactions may be alleviated if the patient lies down.

Other adverse reactions include euphoria, dysphoria, constipation, skin rash and pruritus. At higher doses, oxycodone has most of the disadvantages of morphine including respiratory depression.

DRUG ABUSE AND DEPENDENCE

PERCOCET Tablets are a Schedule II controlled substance. Oxycodone can produce drug dependence and has the potential for being abused. (See WARNINGS.)

OVERDOSAGE

Acetaminophen

Signs and Symptoms: In acute acetaminophen overdosage, dose-dependent, potentially fatal hepatic necrosis is the most serious adverse effect. Renal tubular necrosis, hypoglycemic coma and thrombocytopenia may also occur.

In adults, hepatic toxicity has rarely been reported with acute overdoses of less than 10 grams and fatalities with less than 15 grams. Importantly, young children seem to be more resistant than adults to the hepatotoxic effect of an acetaminophen overdose. Despite this, the measures outlined below should be initiated in any adult or child suspected of having ingested an acetaminophen overdose.

Early symptoms following a potentially hepatotoxic overdose may include: nausea, vomiting, diaphoresis and general malaise. Clinical and laboratory evidence of hepatic toxicity may not be apparent until 48 to 72 hours post-ingestion.

Treatment: The stomach should be emptied promptly by lavage or by induction of emesis with syrup of ipecac. Patient's estimates of the quantity of a drug ingested are notoriously unreliable. Therefore, if an acetaminophen overdose is suspected, a serum acetaminophen assay should be obtained as early as possible, but no sooner than four hours following ingestion. Liver function studies should be obtained initially and repeated at 24-hour intervals.

The antidote, N-acetylcysteine, should be administered as early as possible, preferably within 16 hours of the overdose ingestion for optimal results, but in any case, within 24 hours. Following recovery, there are no residual, structural, or functional hepatic abnormalities.

Oxycodone

Signs and Symptoms: Serious overdosage with oxycodone is characterized by respiratory depression (a decrease in respiratory rate and or tidal volume, Cheyne-Stokes respiration, cyanosis), extreme somnolence progressing to stupor or coma, skeletal muscle flaccidity, cold and clammy skin, and sometimes bradycardia and hypotension. In severe overdosage, apnea, circulatory collapse, cardiac arrest and death may occur.

Treatment: Primary attention should be given to the reestablishment of adequate respiratory exchange through provision of a patent airway and the institution of assisted or controlled ventilation. The narcotic antagonist naloxone hydrochloride (Narcan®) is a specific antidote against respiratory depression which may result from overdosage or unusual sensitivity to narcotics, including oxycodone. Therefore, an appropriate dose of naloxone hydrochloride (usual initial adult dose 0.4 mg to 2 mg) should be administered preferably by the intravenous route, and simultaneously with efforts at respiratory resuscitation (see package insert). Since the duration of action of oxycodone may exceed that of the antagonist, the patient should be kept under continued surveillance and repeated doses of the antagonist should be administered as needed to maintain adequate respiration.

An antagonist should not be administered in the absence of clinically significant respiratory or cardiovascular depression. Oxygen, intravenous fluids, vasopressors and other supportive measures should be employed as indicated.

Gastric emptying may be useful in removing unabsorbed drug.

DOSAGE AND ADMINISTRATION

Dosage should be adjusted according to the severity of the pain and the response of the patient. It may occasionally be necessary to exceed the usual dosage recommended below in cases of more severe pain or in those patients who have become tolerant to the analgesic effect of narcotics. PERCOCET (oxycodone and acetaminophen tablets) is given orally. The usual adult dosage is one tablet every 6 hours as needed for pain.

HOW SUPPLIED

PERCOCET (5 mg oxycodone hydrochloride and 325 mg acetaminophen tablets), supplied as a white tablet, with one face scored and inscribed PERCOCET, and the other inscribed with Du Pont name is available in:

Bottles of 100	NDC 0590-0127-70
Bottles of 500	NDC 0590-0127-85
Hospital Blister Pack of 25 (in units of 250 tablets)	NDC 0590-0127-65

Store at controlled room temperature (15°–30°C, 59°–86°F).

Caution: Federal law prohibits dispensing without prescription.

Continued on next page

Du Pont—Cont.

DEA Order Form Required
Du Pont Pharmaceuticals
Manati, Puerto Rico 00674
PERCOCET® is a Registered Trademark of The Du Pont Merck Pharmaceutical Co.
NARCAN® is a Registered Trademark of The Du Pont Merck Pharmaceutical Co.

6090-11/Rev. Dec., 1990
Shown in Product Identification Section, page 409

---

†PERCODAN®   ℂ

[perk 'o-dan]
(oxycodone and aspirin)
†PERCODAN®-DEMI
Tablets
(oxycodone and aspirin)

DESCRIPTION
Each tablet of PERCODAN® contains:
Oxycodone hydrochloride .... 4.50 mg*
   WARNING: May be habit forming
Oxycodone terephthalate .... 0.38 mg**
   WARNING: May be habit forming
Aspirin, U.S.P. .... 325 mg
*4.50 mg oxycodone HCl is equivalent to 4.0338 mg of oxycodone.
**0.38 mg oxycodone terephthalate is equivalent to 0.3008 mg of oxycodone.
PERCODAN Tablets also contain: D&C Yellow 10, FD&C Yellow 6, microcrystalline cellulose and starch.
Each tablet of PERCODAN®-Demi contains:
Oxycodone hydrochloride .... 2.25 mg*
   WARNING: May be habit forming
Oxycodone terephthalate .... 0.19 mg**
   WARNING: May be habit forming
Aspirin, U.S.P. .... 325 mg
*2.25 mg oxycodone HCl is equivalent to 2.0169 mg of oxycodone.
**0.19 mg oxycodone terephthalate is equivalent to 0.1504 mg of oxycodone.
PERCODAN-Demi Tablets also contain: microcrystalline cellulose and starch.
The oxycodone component is 14-hydroxydihydrocodeinone, a white odorless crystalline powder which is derived from the opium alkaloid, thebaine and may be represented by the following structural formula:

ACTIONS
The principal ingredient, oxycodone, is a semisynthetic narcotic analgesic with multiple actions qualitatively similar to those of morphine, the most prominent of these involve the central nervous system and organs composed of smooth muscle. The principal actions of therapeutic value of the oxycodone in PERCODAN® and PERCODAN®-Demi are analgesia and sedation.
Oxycodone is similar to codeine and methadone in that it retains at least one-half of its analgesic activity when administered orally.
PERCODAN® and PERCODAN®-Demi also contain the non-narcotic antipyretic-analgesic, aspirin.

INDICATIONS
For the relief of moderate to moderately severe pain.

CONTRAINDICATIONS
Hypersensitivity to oxycodone or aspirin.

WARNINGS
Drug Dependence: Oxycodone can produce drug dependence of the morphine type and, therefore, has the potential for being abused. Psychic dependence, physical dependence and tolerance may develop upon repeated administration of PERCODAN® and PERCODAN®-Demi, and it should be prescribed and administered with the same degree of caution appropriate to the use of other oral narcotic-containing medications. Like other narcotic-containing medications, PERCODAN® and PERCODAN®-Demi are subject to the Federal Controlled Substances Act.
Usage in ambulatory patients: Oxycodone may impair the mental and/or physical abilities required for the performance of potentially hazardous tasks such as driving a car or operating machinery. The patient using

†Products of DuPont Merck Pharma.

PERCODAN® and PERCODAN®-Demi should be cautioned accordingly.
Interaction with other central nervous system depressants: Patients receiving other narcotic analgesics, general anesthetics, phenothiazines, other tranquilizers, sedative-hypnotics or other CNS depressants (including alcohol) concomitantly with PERCODAN® and PERCODAN®-Demi may exhibit an additive CNS depression. When such combined therapy is contemplated, the dose of one or both agents should be reduced.
Usage in pregnancy: Safe use in pregnancy has not been established relative to possible adverse effects on fetal development. Therefore, PERCODAN® and PERCODAN®-Demi should not be used in pregnant women unless, in the judgment of the physician, the potential benefits outweigh the possible hazards.
Usage in children: PERCODAN® should not be administered to children. PERCODAN®-Demi, containing half the amount of oxycodone, can be considered. (See Dosage and Administration for PERCODAN®-Demi).
Reye Syndrome is a rare but serious disease which can follow flu or chicken pox in children and teenagers. While the cause of Reye Syndrome is unknown, some reports claim aspirin (or salicylates) may increase the risk of developing this disease.
Salicylates should be used with caution in the presence of peptic ulcer or coagulation abnormalities.

PRECAUTIONS
Head injury and increased intracranial pressure: The respiratory depressant effects of narcotics and their capacity to elevate cerebrospinal fluid pressure may be markedly exaggerated in the presence of head injury, other intracranial lesions or a pre-existing increase in intracranial pressure. Furthermore, narcotics produce adverse reactions which may obscure the clinical course of patients with head injuries.
Acute abdominal conditions: The administration of PERCODAN® and PERCODAN®-Demi or other narcotics may obscure the diagnosis or clinical course in patients with acute abdominal conditions.
Special risk patients: PERCODAN® and PERCODAN®-Demi should be given with caution to certain patients such as the elderly or debilitated, and those with severe impairment of hepatic or renal function, hypothyroidism, Addison's disease, and prostatic hypertrophy or urethral stricture.

ADVERSE REACTIONS
The most frequently observed adverse reactions include lightheadedness, dizziness, sedation, nausea and vomiting. These effects seem to be more prominent in ambulatory than in nonambulatory patients, and some of these adverse reactions may be alleviated if the patient lies down.
Other adverse reactions include euphoria, dysphoria, constipation and pruritus.

DRUG ABUSE AND DEPENDENCE
PERCODAN® and PERCODAN®-Demi tablets are a Schedule II controlled substance. Oxycodone can produce drug dependence and has the potential for being abused. (See WARNINGS.)

DOSAGE AND ADMINISTRATION
Dosage should be adjusted according to the severity of the pain and the response of the patient. It may occasionally be necessary to exceed the usual dose recommended below in cases of more severe pain or in those patients who have become tolerant to the analgesic effect of narcotics. PERCODAN® and PERCODAN®-Demi are given orally.
PERCODAN®: The usual adult dose is one tablet every 6 hours as needed for pain.
PERCODAN®-Demi: Adults—One or two tablets every six hours. Children 12 years and older—One-half tablet every six hours. Children 6 to 12 years—One-quarter tablet every six hours. PERCODAN®-Demi is not indicated for children under 6 years of age.

DRUG INTERACTIONS
The CNS depressant effects of PERCODAN® and PERCODAN®-Demi may be additive with that of other CNS depressants. (See WARNINGS.)
Aspirin may enhance the effect of anticoagulants and inhibit the uricosuric effects of uricosuric agents.

MANAGEMENT OF OVERDOSAGE
Signs and Symptoms: Serious overdose with PERCODAN® or PERCODAN®-Demi is characterized by respiratory depression (a decrease in respiratory rate and/or tidal volume, Cheyne-Stokes respiration, cyanosis), extreme somnolence progressing to stupor or coma, skeletal muscle flaccidity, cold and clammy skin, and sometimes bradycardia and hypotension. In severe overdosage, apnea, circulatory collapse, cardiac arrest and death may occur. The ingestion of very large amounts of PERCODAN® or PERCODAN®-Demi may, in addition, result in acute salicylate intoxication.
Treatment: Primary attention should be given to the reestablishment of adequate respiratory exchange through provision of a patent airway and the institution of assisted or

controlled ventilation. The narcotic antagonist naloxone hydrochloride (NARCAN®) is a specific antidote against respiratory depression which may result from overdosage or unusual sensitivity to narcotics, including oxycodone. Therefore, an appropriate dose of naloxone hydrochloride should be administered (usual initial adult dose: 0.4 mg–2 mg) preferably by the intravenous route, simultaneously with efforts at respiratory resuscitation. Since the duration of action of oxycodone may exceed that of the antagonist, the patient should be kept under continued surveillance and repeated doses of the antagonist should be administered as needed to maintain adequate respiration.
Oxygen, intravenous fluids, vasopressors and other supportive measures should be employed as indicated.
Gastric emptying may be useful in removing unabsorbed drug.

HOW SUPPLIED
Percodan®—As yellow, scored tablets, available in:

Bottles of 100	NDC 0590-0135-70
Bottles of 500	NDC 0590-0135-85
Bottles of 1000	NDC 0590-0135-90
Hospital blister pack of 25	NDC 0590-0135-65
(available in units of 250)	

Also available in Military Depot:
Btl's of 100 NSN 6505-01-030-9493
Blister Pack (250) NSN 6505-01-030-9492
Percodan®-Demi—White scored tablets available in:
Bottles of 100   NDC 0590-0166-70
Store At Controlled Room Temperature (59°–86°F, 15°–30°C).
Caution: Federal law prohibits dispensing without prescription.
DEA Order Form Required
Shown in Product Identification Section, page 409
PERCODAN is a Registered Trademark of The DuPont Merck Pharmaceutical Co.

NARCAN is a Registered Trademark of The DuPont Merck Pharmaceutical Co.
6190-1/Rev. Dec., 1990
6234-1/Rev. Oct., 1991

SINEMET®   ℞
(CARBIDOPA-LEVODOPA)
TABLETS

There has been a complete change of product marketing rights for SINEMET®. Effective January 1, 1990, Du Pont Pharmaceuticals assumed responsibility from Merck, Sharp & Dohme for marketing SINEMET® in the United States, Canada and Puerto Rico. The complete prescribing information follows:
® Registered trademark of MERCK & CO., Inc.

DESCRIPTION
When SINEMET* (Carbidopa-Levodopa) is to be given to patients who are being treated with levodopa, levodopa must be discontinued at least eight hours before therapy with SINEMET is started. In order to reduce adverse reactions, it is necessary to individualize therapy. See the WARNINGS and DOSAGE AND ADMINISTRATION sections before initiating therapy.
Carbidopa, an inhibitor of aromatic amino acid decarboxylation, is a white, crystalline compound, slightly soluble in water, with a molecular weight of 244.3. It is designated chemically as (—)-L-α-hydrazino-α-methyl-β-(3,4-dihydroxybenzene) propanoic acid monohydrate, and has the following structural formula:

Tablet content is expressed in terms of anhydrous carbidopa which has a molecular weight of 226.3.
Levodopa, an aromatic amino acid, is a white, crystalline compound, slightly soluble in water, with a molecular weight of 197.2. It is designated chemically as (—)-L-α-amino-β-(3,4-dihydroxybenzene) propanoic acid, and has the following structural formula:

SINEMET is supplied as tablets in three strengths:
SINEMET 25-100, containing 25 mg of carbidopa and 100 mg of levodopa.
SINEMET 10-100, containing 10 mg of carbidopa and 100 mg of levodopa.
SINEMET 25-250, containing 25 mg of carbidopa and 250 mg of levodopa.

Inactive ingredients are cellulose, magnesium stearate, and starch. Tablets SINEMET 10-100 and 25-250 also contain FD&C Blue 2. Tablets SINEMET 25-100 also contain D&C Yellow 10 and FD&C Yellow 6.

ACTIONS

Current evidence indicates that symptoms of Parkinson's disease are related to depletion of dopamine in the corpus striatum. Administration of dopamine is ineffective in the treatment of Parkinson's disease apparently because it does not cross the blood-brain barrier. However, levodopa, the metabolic precursor of dopamine, does cross the blood-brain barrier, and presumably is converted to dopamine in the basal ganglia. This is thought to be the mechanism whereby levodopa relieves symptoms of Parkinson's disease.

When levodopa is administered orally it is rapidly converted to dopamine in extracerebral tissues so that only a small portion of a given dose is transported unchanged to the central nervous system. For this reason, large doses of levodopa are required for adequate therapeutic effect and these may often be attended by nausea and other adverse reactions, some of which are attributable to dopamine formed in extracerebral tissues.

Since levodopa competes with certain amino acids, the absorption of levodopa may be impaired in some patients on a high protein diet.

Carbidopa inhibits decarboxylation of peripheral levodopa. It does not cross the blood-brain barrier and does not affect the metabolism of levodopa within the central nervous system.

Since its decarboxylase inhibiting activity is limited to extracerebral tissues, administration of carbidopa with levodopa makes more levodopa available for transport to the brain. In dogs, reduced formation of dopamine in extracerebral tissues, such as the heart, provides protection against the development of dopamine-induced cardiac arrhythmias. Clinical studies tend to support the hypothesis of a similar protective effect in humans although controlled data are too limited at the present time to draw firm conclusions.

Carbidopa reduces the amount of levodopa required by about 75 percent and, when administered with levodopa, increases both plasma levels and the plasma half-life of levodopa, and decreases plasma and urinary dopamine and homovanillic acid.

In clinical pharmacologic studies, simultaneous administration of carbidopa and levodopa produced greater urinary excretion of levodopa in proportion to the excretion of dopamine than administration of the two drugs at separate times.

Pyridoxine hydrochloride (vitamin B$_6$), in oral doses of 10 mg to 25 mg, may reverse the effects of levodopa by increasing the rate of aromatic amino acid decarboxylation. Carbidopa inhibits this action of pyridoxine.

INDICATIONS

SINEMET is indicated in the treatment of the symptoms of idiopathic Parkinson's disease (paralysis agitans), postencephalitic parkinsonism, and symptomatic parkinsonism which may follow injury to the nervous system by carbon monoxide intoxication and manganese intoxication. SINEMET is indicated in these conditions to permit the administration of lower doses of levodopa with reduced nausea and vomiting, with more rapid dosage titration, with a somewhat smoother response, and with supplemental pyridoxine (vitamin B$_6$).

The incidence of levodopa-induced nausea and vomiting is less with SINEMET than with levodopa. In many patients this reduction in nausea and vomiting will permit more rapid dosage titration.

In some patients a somewhat smoother antiparkinsonian effect results from therapy with SINEMET than with levodopa. However, patients with markedly irregular ("on-off") responses to levodopa have not been shown to benefit from SINEMET.

Since carbidopa prevents the reversal of levodopa effects caused by pyridoxine, SINEMET can be given to patients receiving supplemental pyridoxine (vitamin B$_6$).

Although the administration of carbidopa permits control of parkinsonism and Parkinson's disease with much lower doses of levodopa, there is no conclusive evidence at present that this is beneficial other than in reducing nausea and vomiting, permitting more rapid titration, and providing a somewhat smoother response to levodopa. *Carbidopa does not decrease adverse reactions due to central effects of levodopa. By permitting more levodopa to reach the brain, particularly when nausea and vomiting is not a dose-limiting factor, certain adverse CNS effects, e.g., dyskinesias, may occur at lower dosages and sooner during therapy with SINEMET than with levodopa.*

Certain patients who responded poorly to levodopa have improved when SINEMET was substituted. This is most likely due to decreased peripheral decarboxylation of levodopa which results from administration of carbidopa rather than to a primary effect of carbidopa on the nervous system. Carbidopa has not been shown to enhance the intrinsic efficacy of levodopa in parkinsonian syndromes.

In considering whether to give SINEMET to patients already on levodopa who have nausea and /or vomiting, the practitioner should be aware that, while many patients may be expected to improve, some do not. Since one cannot predict which patients are likely to improve, this can only be determined by a trial of therapy. It should be further noted that in controlled trials comparing SINEMET with levodopa, about half of the patients with nausea and/or vomiting on levodopa improved spontaneously despite being retained on the same dose of levodopa during the controlled portion of the trial.

CONTRAINDICATIONS

Monoamine oxidase inhibitors and SINEMET should not be given concomitantly. These inhibitors must be discontinued at least two weeks prior to initiating therapy with SINEMET.

SINEMET is contraindicated in patients with known hypersensitivity to this drug, and in narrow angle glaucoma.

Because levodopa may activate a malignant melanoma, it should not be used in patients with suspicious, undiagnosed skin lesions or a history of melanoma.

WARNINGS

When patients are receiving levodopa, it must be discontinued at least eight hours before SINEMET is started. SINEMET should be substituted at a dosage that will provide approximately 25 percent of the previous levodopa dosage (see DOSAGE AND ADMINISTRATION). Patients who are taking SINEMET should be instructed not to take additional levodopa unless it is prescribed by the physician.

As with levodopa, SINEMET may cause involuntary movements and mental disturbances. These reactions are thought to be due to increased brain dopamine following administration of levodopa. All patients should be observed carefully for the development of depression with concomitant suicidal tendencies. Patients with past or current psychoses should be treated with caution. *Because carbidopa permits more levodopa to reach the brain and, thus, more dopamine to be formed, dyskinesias may occur at lower dosages and sooner with SINEMET than with levodopa. The occurrence of dyskinesias may require dosage reduction.*

SINEMET should be administered cautiously to patients with severe cardiovascular or pulmonary disease, bronchial asthma, renal, hepatic or endocrine disease.

Care should be exercised in administering SINEMET, as with levodopa, to patients with a history of myocardial infarction who have residual atrial, nodal, or ventricular arrhythmias. In such patients, cardiac function should be monitored with particular care during the period of initial dosage adjustment, in a facility with provisions for intensive cardiac care.

As with levodopa there is a possibility of upper gastrointestinal hemorrhage in patients with a history of peptic ulcer.

A symptom complex resembling the neuroleptic malignant syndrome including muscular rigidity, elevated body temperature, mental changes, and increased serum creatine phosphokinase has been reported when antiparkinsonian agents were withdrawn abruptly. Therefore, patients should be observed carefully when the dosage of SINEMET is reduced abruptly or discontinued, especially if the patient is receiving neuroleptics.

Usage in Pregnancy and Lactation: Although the effects of SINEMET on human pregnancy and lactation are unknown, both levodopa and combinations of carbidopa and levodopa have caused visceral and skeletal malformations in rabbits. Use of SINEMET in women of childbearing potential requires that the anticipated benefits of the drug be weighed against possible hazards to mother and child. SINEMET should not be given to nursing mothers.

Usage in Children: The safety of SINEMET in patients under 18 years of age has not been established.

PRECAUTIONS

As with levodopa, periodic evaluations of hepatic, hematopoietic, cardiovascular, and renal function are recommended during extended therapy.

Patients with chronic wide angle glaucoma may be treated cautiously with SINEMET provided the intraocular pressure is well controlled and the patient is monitored carefully for changes in intraocular pressure during therapy.

Laboratory Tests

Abnormalities in laboratory tests may include elevations of liver function tests such as alkaline phosphatase, SGOT (AST), SGPT (ALT), lactic dehydrogenase, and bilirubin. Abnormalities in protein-bound iodine, blood urea nitrogen and positive Coombs test have also been reported. Commonly, levels of blood urea nitrogen, creatinine, and uric acid are lower during administration of SINEMET than with levodopa.

SINEMET may cause a false-positive reaction for urinary ketone bodies when a test tape is used for determination of ketonuria. This reaction will not be altered by boiling the urine specimen. False-negative tests may result with the use of glucose-oxidase methods of testing for glucosuria.

Drug Interactions

Caution should be exercised when the following drugs are administered concomitantly with SINEMET.

Symptomatic postural hypotension can occur when SINEMET is added to the treatment of a patient receiving antihypertensive drugs. Therefore, when therapy with SINEMET is started, dosage adjustment of the antihypertensive drug may be required. For patients receiving monoamine oxidase inhibitors, see CONTRAINDICATIONS.

There have been rare reports of adverse reactions, including hypertension and dyskinesia, resulting from the concomitant use of tricyclic antidepressants and SINEMET.

Phenothiazines and butyrophenones may reduce the therapeutic effects of levodopa. In addition, the beneficial effects of levodopa in Parkinson's disease have been reported to be reversed by phenytoin and papaverine. Patients taking these drugs with SINEMET should be carefully observed for loss of therapeutic response.

ADVERSE REACTIONS

The most common serious adverse reactions occurring with SINEMET are choreiform, dystonic, and other involuntary movements. Other serious adverse reactions are mental changes including paranoid ideation and psychotic episodes, depression with or without development of suicidal tendencies, and dementia. Convulsions also have occurred; however, a causal relationship with SINEMET has not been established.

A common but less serious effect is nausea.

Less frequent adverse reactions are cardiac irregularities and/or palpitation, orthostatic hypotensive episodes, bradykinetic episodes (the "on-off" phenomenon), anorexia, vomiting, and dizziness.

Rarely, gastrointestinal bleeding, development of duodenal ulcer, hypertension, phlebitis, hemolytic and nonhemolytic anemia, thrombocytopenia, leukopenia, and agranulocytosis have occurred.

Laboratory tests which have been reported to be abnormal are alkaline phosphatase, SGOT (AST), SGPT (ALT), lactic dehydrogenase, bilirubin, blood urea nitrogen, protein-bound iodine, and Coombs test.

Other adverse reactions that have been reported with levodopa are:

Nervous System: ataxia, numbness, increased hand tremor, muscle twitching, muscle cramps, blepharospasm (which may be taken as an early sign of excess dosage, consideration of dosage reduction may be made at this time), trismus, activation of latent Horner's syndrome.

Psychiatric: confusion, sleepiness, insomnia, nightmares, hallucinations, delusions, agitation, anxiety, euphoria.

Gastrointestinal: dry mouth, bitter taste, sialorrhea, dysphagia, bruxism, hiccups, abdominal pain and distress, constipation, diarrhea, flatulence, burning sensation of tongue.

Metabolic: weight gain or loss, edema.

Integumentary: malignant melanoma (see also CONTRAINDICATIONS), flushing, increased sweating, dark sweat, skin rash, loss of hair.

Genitourinary: urinary retention, urinary incontinence, dark urine, priapism.

Special Senses: diplopia, blurred vision, dilated pupils, oculogyric crises.

Miscellaneous: weakness, faintness, fatigue, headache, hoarseness, malaise, hot flashes, sense of stimulation, bizarre breathing patterns, neuroleptic malignant syndrome.

DOSAGE AND ADMINISTRATION

The optimum daily dosage of SINEMET must be determined by careful titration in each patient. SINEMET tablets are available in a 1:4 ratio of carbidopa to levodopa (SINEMET 25-100) as well as 1:10 ratio (SINEMET 25-250 and SINEMET 10-100). Tablets of the two ratios may be given separately or combined as needed to provide the optimum dosage. Studies show that peripheral dopa decarboxylase is saturated by carbidopa at approximately 70 to 100 mg a day. Patients receiving less than this amount of carbidopa are more likely to experience nausea and vomiting.

Usual Initial Dosage

Dosage is best initiated with one tablet of SINEMET 25-100 three times a day. This dosage schedule provides 75 mg of carbidopa per day. Dosage may be increased by one tablet every day or every other day, as necessary, until a dosage of eight tablets of SINEMET 25-100 a day is reached.

If SINEMET 10-100 is used, dosage may be initiated with one tablet three or four times a day. However, this will not provide an adequate amount of carbidopa for many patients. Dosage may be increased by one tablet every day or every other day until a total of eight tablets (2 tablets q.i.d.) is reached.

How to Transfer Patients from Levodopa

Levodopa must be discontinued at least eight hours before starting SINEMET (Carbidopa-Levodopa). A daily dosage of SINEMET should be chosen that will provide approximately 25 percent of the previous levodopa dosage. Patients who are taking less than 1500 mg of levodopa a day should be started on one tablet of SINEMET 25-100 three or four times a day. The suggested starting dosage for most patients taking more

Continued on next page

Du Pont—Cont.

than 1500 mg of levodopa is one tablet of SINEMET 25-250 three or four times a day.

Maintenance

Therapy should be individualized and adjusted according to the desired therapeutic response. At least 70 to 100 mg of carbidopa per day should be provided. When a greater proportion of carbidopa is required, one tablet of SINEMET 25-100 may be substituted for each tablet of SINEMET 10-100. When more levodopa is required, SINEMET 25-250 should be substituted for SINEMET 25-100 or SINEMET 10-100. If necessary, the dosage of SINEMET 25-250 may be increased by one-half or one tablet every day or every other day to a maximum of eight tablets a day. Experience with total daily dosages of carbidopa greater than 200 mg is limited.

Because both therapeutic and adverse responses occur more rapidly with SINEMET than with levodopa alone, patients should be monitored closely during the dose adjustment period. Specifically, involuntary movements will occur more rapidly with SINEMET than with levodopa. The occurrence of involuntary movements may require dosage reduction. Blepharospasm may be a useful early sign of excess dosage in some patients.

Current evidence indicates that other standard drugs for Parkinson's disease (except levodopa) may be continued while SINEMET is being administered, although their dosage may have to be adjusted.

If general anesthesia is required, SINEMET may be continued as long as the patient is permitted to take fluids and medication by mouth. If therapy is interrupted temporarily, the usual daily dosage may be administered as soon as the patient is able to take oral medication.

OVERDOSAGE

Management of acute overdosage with SINEMET is basically the same as management of acute overdosage with levodopa; however, pyridoxine is not effective in reversing the actions of SINEMET.

General supportive measures should be employed, along with immediate gastric lavage. Intravenous fluids should be administered judiciously and an adequate airway maintained. Electrocardiographic monitoring should be instituted and the patient carefully observed for the development of arrhythmias; if required, appropriate antiarrhythmic therapy should be given. The possibility that the patient may have taken other drugs as well as SINEMET should be taken into consideration. To date, no experience has been reported with dialysis; hence, its value in overdosage is not known.

HOW SUPPLIED

Tablets SINEMET 25-100 are yellow, oval, scored tablets, coded 650. They are supplied as follows:

NDC 0056-0650-68 bottles of 100

NDC 0056-0650-28 unit dose packages of 100.

Tablets SINEMET 10-100 are dark dapple-blue, oval, scored, uncoated tablets, coded 647. They are supplied as follows:

NDC 0056-0647-68 bottles of 100

NDC 0056-0647-28 unit dose packages of 100.

Tablets SINEMET 25-250 are light dapple-blue, oval, scored, uncoated tablets, coded 654. They are supplied as follows:

NDC 0056-0654-68 bottles of 100

NDC 0056-0654-28 unit dose packages of 100.

Storage

Tablets SINEMET 10-100 and Tablets SINEMET 25-250 must be protected from light.

Manufactured by:
MERCK SHARP & DOHME
DIV OF MERCK & CO., INC., WEST POINT, PA 19486, USA
For:
Du Pont Pharmaceuticals
The Du Pont Merck Pharmaceutical Co.
Wilmington, Delaware 19880
AHFS Category: 92:00
6219-1/April 1988

Shown in Product Identification Section, page 409

SINEMET® CR ℞
(Carbidopa-Levodopa)
Sustained-Release Tablets

DESCRIPTION

SINEMET* CR (Carbidopa-Levodopa) is a sustained-release combination of carbidopa and levodopa for the treatment of Parkinson's disease and syndrome.

Carbidopa, an inhibitor of aromatic amino acid decarboxylation, is a white, crystalline compound, slightly soluble in water, with a molecular weight of 244.3. It is designated chemically as (-)-L-α-hydrazino-α-methyl-β-(3,4-dihydroxybenzene) propanoic acid monohydrate. Its empirical formula is $C_{10}H_{14}N_2O_4 \cdot H_2O$ and its structural formula is:

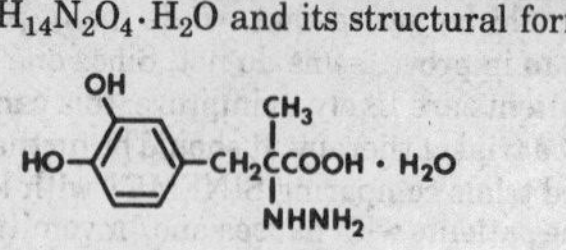

Tablet content is expressed in terms of anhydrous carbidopa, which has a molecular weight of 226.3.

Levodopa, an aromatic amino acid, is a white, crystalline compound, slightly soluble in water with a molecular weight of 197.2. It is designated chemically as (-)-L-α-amino-β-(3,4-dihydroxybenzene) propanoic acid. Its empirical formula is $C_9H_{11}NO_4$ and its structural formula is:

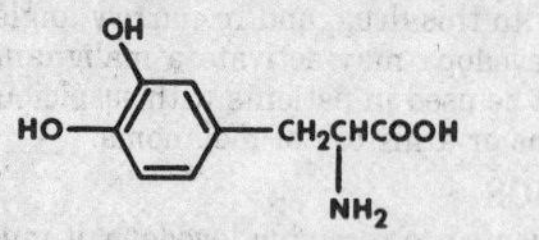

SINEMET CR is supplied as sustained-release tablets containing 50 mg of carbidopa and 200 mg of levodopa.

Inactive ingredients in SINEMET CR are: D&C Yellow 10, magnesium stearate, iron oxide, and other ingredients.

SINEMET CR is supplied as an oval, scored, biconvex, compressed tablet that is peach colored. The tablet is a polymeric-based drug delivery system which controls the release of carbidopa and levodopa as it slowly erodes.

CLINICAL PHARMACOLOGY

Pharmacodynamics

Current evidence indicates that symptoms of Parkinson's disease are related to depletion of dopamine in the corpus striatum. Administration of dopamine is ineffective in the treatment of Parkinson's disease apparently because it does not cross the blood-brain barrier. However, levodopa, the metabolic precursor of dopamine, does cross the blood-brain barrier, and presumably is converted to dopamine in the brain. This is thought to be the mechanism whereby levodopa relieves symptoms of Parkinson's disease.

When levodopa is administered orally it is rapidly decarboxylated to dopamine in extracerebral tissues so that only a small portion of a given dose is transported unchanged to the central nervous system. For this reason, large doses of levodopa are required for adequate therapeutic effect and these may often be attended by nausea and other adverse reactions, some of which are attributable to dopamine formed in extracerebral tissues.

Since levodopa competes with certain amino acids for transport across the gut wall, the absorption of levodopa may be impaired in some patients on a high protein diet.

Carbidopa inhibits decarboxylation of peripheral levodopa. It does not cross the blood-brain barrier and does not affect the metabolism of levodopa within the central nervous system.

Since its decarboxylase inhibiting activity is limited to extracerebral tissues, administration of carbidopa with levodopa makes more levodopa available for transport to the brain.

Patients treated with levodopa therapy for Parkinson's disease may develop motor fluctuations characterized by end-of-dose failure, peak dose dyskinesia, and akinesia. The advanced form of motor fluctuations ('on-off' phenomenon) is characterized by unpredictable swings from mobility to immobility. Although the causes of the motor fluctuations are not completely understood, *in some patients* they may be attenuated by treatment regimens that produce steady plasma levels of levodopa.

SINEMET CR contains 50 mg of carbidopa and 200 mg of levodopa in a sustained-release dosage form designed to release these ingredients over a 4 to 6 hour period. With SINEMET CR there is less variation in plasma levodopa levels than with SINEMET* (Carbidopa-Levodopa), the conventional formulation. *However, SINEMET CR (Carbidopa-Levodopa, Sustained-Release) is less systemically bioavailable than SINEMET (Carbidopa-Levodopa) and may require increased daily doses to achieve the same level of symptomatic relief as provided by SINEMET (Carbidopa-Levodopa).*

In clinical trials, patients with moderate to severe motor fluctuations who received SINEMET CR *did not experience quantitatively significant reductions* in 'off' time when compared to SINEMET (Carbidopa-Levodopa). However, global ratings of improvement as assessed by both patient and physician were better during therapy with SINEMET CR than with SINEMET (Carbidopa-Levodopa). In patients without motor fluctuations, SINEMET CR, under controlled conditions, provided the same therapeutic benefit with less frequent dosing when compared to SINEMET (Carbidopa-Levodopa).

Pyridoxine hydrochloride (vitamin B_6), in oral doses of 10 mg to 25 mg. may reverse the effects of levodopa by increasing the rate of aromatic amino acid decarboxylation. Carbidopa inhibits this action of pyridoxine.

Pharmacokinetics

Carbidopa reduces the amount of levodopa required to produce a given response by about 75 percent and, when administered with levodopa, increases both plasma levels and the plasma half-life of levodopa, and decreases plasma and urinary dopamine and homovanillic acid.

Elimination half-life of levodopa in the presence of carbidopa is about 1.5 hours. Following SINEMET CR, the apparent half-life of levodopa may be prolonged because of continuous absorption.

In healthy elderly subjects (56–67 years old) the mean time to peak concentration of levodopa after a single dose of SINEMET CR 50–200 was about 2 hours as compared to 0.5 hours after standard SINEMET (Carbidopa-Levodopa). The maximum concentration of levodopa after a single dose of SINEMET CR was about 35% of the standard SINEMET (Carbidopa-Levodopa) (1151 vs 3256 ng/mL). The extent of availability of levodopa from SINEMET CR was about 70–75% relative to intravenous levodopa or standard SINEMET (Carbidopa-Levodopa) in the elderly. The absolute bioavailability of levodopa from SINEMET CR (relative to I.V.) in young subjects was shown to be only about 44%. The extent of availability and the peak concentrations of levodopa were comparable in the elderly after a single dose and at steady state after t.i.d. administration of SINEMET CR 50–200. In elderly subjects, the average trough levels of levodopa at steady state after the CR tablet were about 2 fold higher than after the standard SINEMET (Carbidopa-Levodopa) (163 vs 74 ng/mL).

In these studies, using similar total daily doses of levodopa, plasma levodopa concentrations with SINEMET CR fluctuated in a narrower range than with SINEMET (Carbidopa-Levodopa). Because the bioavailability of levodopa from SINEMET CR relative to SINEMET (Carbidopa-Levodopa) is approximately 70–75%, the daily dosage of levodopa necessary to produce a given clinical response with the sustained-release formulation will usually be higher.

The extent of availability and peak concentrations of levodopa after a single dose of SINEMET CR 50–200 increased by about 50% and 25%, respectively, when administered with food.

INDICATIONS AND USAGE

SINEMET CR is indicated in the treatment of the symptoms of idiopathic Parkinson's disease (paralysis agitans), postencephalitic parkinsonism, and symptomatic parkinsonism which may follow injury to the nervous system by carbon monoxide intoxication and manganese intoxication.

CONTRAINDICATIONS

Nonselective MAO inhibitors are contraindicated for use with SINEMET CR. These inhibitors must be discontinued at least two weeks prior to initiating therapy with SINEMET CR. SINEMET CR may be administered concomitantly with the manufacturer's recommended dose of an MAO inhibitor with selectivity for MAO type B (e.g., selegiline HCl).

SINEMET CR is contraindicated in patients with known hypersensitivity to any component of this drug and in patients with narrow-angle glaucoma.

Because levodopa may activate a malignant melanoma, SINEMET CR should not be used in patients with suspicious, undiagnosed skin lesions or a history of melanoma.

WARNINGS

When patients are receiving levodopa without a decarboxylase inhibitor, levodopa must be discontinued at least eight hours before SINEMET CR is started. In order to reduce adverse reactions, it is necessary to individualize therapy. SINEMET CR should be substituted at a dosage that will provide approximately 25 percent of the previous levodopa dosage (see DOSAGE AND ADMINISTRATION).

Carbidopa does not decrease adverse reactions due to central effects of levodopa. By permitting more levodopa to reach the brain, particularly when nausea and vomiting is not a dose-limiting factor, certain adverse CNS effects, e.g., dyskinesias, will occur at lower dosages and sooner during therapy with SINEMET CR (Carbidopa-Levodopa. Sustained-Release) than with levodopa alone.

As with levodopa, SINEMET CR may cause involuntary movements and mental disturbances. These reactions are thought to be due to increased brain dopamine following administration of levodopa. All patients should be observed carefully for the development of depression with concomitant suicidal tendencies. Patients with past or current psychoses should be treated with caution. The occurrence of dyskinesias may require dosage reduction.

Patients receiving SINEMET CR may develop increased dyskinesia compared to SINEMET (Carbidopa-Levodopa).

SINEMET CR should be administered cautiously to patients with severe cardiovascular or pulmonary disease, bronchial asthma, renal, hepatic or endocrine disease.

As with levodopa, care should be exercised in administering SINEMET CR to patients with a history of myocardial infarction who have residual atrial, nodal, or ventricular arrhythmias. In such patients, cardiac function should be monitored with particular care during the period of initial dosage

*Registered trademark of MERCK & CO., INC.

adjustment, in a facility with provisions for intensive cardiac care.

As with levodopa, treatment with SINEMET CR may increase the possibility of upper gastrointestinal hemorrhage in patients with a history of peptic ulcer.

A symptom complex resembling the neuroleptic malignant syndrome including muscular rigidity, elevated body temperature, mental changes, and increased serum creatine phosphokinase has been reported when antiparkinsonian agents were withdrawn abruptly. Therefore, patients should be observed carefully when the dosage of SINEMET CR is reduced abruptly or discontinued, especially if the patient is receiving neuroleptics.

PRECAUTIONS

General

As with levodopa, periodic evaluations of hepatic, hematopoietic, cardiovascular, and renal function are recommended during extended therapy.

Patients with chronic wide-angle glaucoma may be treated cautiously with SINEMET CR provided the intraocular pressure is well controlled and the patient is monitored carefully for changes in intraocular pressure during therapy.

Information for Patients

The patient should be informed that SINEMET CR is a sustained-release formulation of carbidopa-levodopa which releases these ingredients over a 4 to 6 hour period. It is important that SINEMET CR be taken at regular intervals according to the schedule outlined by the physician. The patient should be cautioned not to change the prescribed dosage regimen and not to add any additional antiparkinson medications, including other carbidopa-levodopa preparations, without first consulting the physician.

If abnormal involuntary movements appear or get worse during treatment with SINEMET CR, the physician should be notified, as dosage adjustment may be necessary.

Patients should be advised that sometimes the onset of effect of the first morning dose of SINEMET CR may be delayed for up to 1 hour compared with the response usually obtained from the first morning dose of SINEMET (Carbidopa-Levodopa). The physician should be notified if such delayed responses pose a problem in treatment.

Patients must be advised that the whole or half tablet should be swallowed without chewing or crushing.

NOTE: The suggested advice to patients being treated with SINEMET CR is intended to aid in the safe and effective use of this medication. It is not a disclosure of all possible adverse or intended effects.

Laboratory Tests

Abnormalities in laboratory tests may include elevations of liver function tests such as alkaline phosphatase, SGOT (AST), SGPT (ALT), lactic dehydrogenase, and bilirubin. Abnormalities in blood urea nitrogen and positive Coombs test have also been reported. Commonly, levels of blood urea nitrogen, creatinine, and uric acid are lower during administration of carbidopa-levodopa preparations than with levodopa.

Carbidopa-levodopa preparations may cause a false-positive reaction for urinary ketone bodies when a test tape is used for determination of ketonuria. This reaction will not be altered by boiling the urine specimen. False-negative tests may result with the use of glucose-oxidase methods of testing for glucosuria.

Drug Interactions

Caution should be exercised when the following drugs are administered concomitantly with SINEMET CR (Carbidopa-Levodopa, Sustained-Release).

Symptomatic postural hypotension has occurred when carbidopa-levodopa preparations were added to the treatment of patients receiving some antihypertensive drugs. Therefore, when therapy with SINEMET CR is started, dosage adjustment of the antihypertensive drug may be required. For patients receiving monoamine oxidase inhibitors, see CONTRAINDICATIONS.

There have been rare reports of adverse reactions, including hypertension and dyskinesia, resulting from the concomitant use of tricyclic antidepressants and carbidopa-levodopa preparations.

Phenothiazines and butyrophenones may reduce the therapeutic effects of levodopa. In addition, the beneficial effects of levodopa in Parkinson's disease have been reported to be reversed by phenytoin and papaverine. Patients taking these drugs with SINEMET CR should be carefully observed for loss of therapeutic response.

Carcinogenesis, Mutagenesis, Impairment of Fertility

In a two-year bioassay of SINEMET (Carbidopa-Levodopa), no evidence of carcinogenicity was found in rats receiving doses of approximately two times the maximum daily human dose of carbidopa and four times the maximum daily human dose of levodopa (equivalent to 8 SINEMET CR tablets).

In reproduction studies with SINEMET (Carbidopa-Levodopa), no effects on fertility were found in rats receiving doses of approximately two times the maximum daily human dose of carbidopa and four times the maximum daily

human dose of levodopa (equivalent to 8 SINEMET CR tablets).

Pregnancy

Pregnancy Category C. No teratogenic effects were observed in a study in mice receiving up to 20 times the maximum recommended human dose of SINEMET (Carbidopa-Levodopa). There was a decrease in the number of live pups delivered by rats receiving approximately two times the maximum recommended human dose of carbidopa and approximately five times the maximum recommended human dose of levodopa during organogenesis. SINEMET (Carbidopa-Levodopa) caused both visceral and skeletal malformations in rabbits at all doses and ratios of carbidopa/levodopa tested, which ranged from 10 times/5 times the maximum recommended human dose of carbidopa/levodopa to 20 times/10 times the maximum recommended human dose of carbidopa/levodopa.

There are no adequate or well-controlled studies in pregnant women. Use of SINEMET CR in women of childbearing potential requires that the anticipated benefits of the drug be weighed against possible hazards to mother and child.

Nursing Mothers

It is not known whether this drug is excreted in human milk. Because many drugs are excreted in human milk, caution should be exercised when SINEMET CR is administered to a nursing mother.

Pediatric Use

Safety and effectiveness in infants and children have not been established, and use of the drug in patients below the age of 18 is not recommended.

ADVERSE REACTIONS

In controlled clinical trials, patients predominantly with moderate to severe motor fluctuations while on SINEMET (Carbidopa-Levodopa) were randomized to therapy with either SINEMET (Carbidopa-Levodopa) or SINEMET CR. The adverse experience frequency profile of SINEMET CR did not differ substantially from that of SINEMET (Carbidopa-Levodopa), as shown in Table I.

Table I.
Clinical Adverse Experiences Occurring
in 1% or Greater of Patients

Adverse Experience	SINEMET CR n=491 %	SINEMET (Carbidopa-Levodopa) n=524 %
Dyskinesia	16.5	12.2
Nausea	5.5	5.7
Hallucinations	3.9	3.2
Confusion	3.7	2.3
Dizziness	2.9	2.3
Depression	2.2	1.3
Urinary tract infection	2.2	2.3
Headache	2.0	1.9
Dream abnormalities	1.8	0.8
Dystonia	1.8	0.8
Vomiting	1.8	1.9
Upper respiratory infection	1.8	1.0
Dyspnea	1.6	0.4
'On-Off' phenomena	1.6	1.1
Back pain	1.6	0.6
Dry mouth	1.4	1.1
Anorexia	1.2	1.1
Diarrhea	1.2	0.6
Insomnia	1.2	1.0
Orthostatic hypotension	1.0	1.1
Shoulder pain	1.0	0.6
Chest pain	1.0	0.8
Muscle cramps	0.8	1.0
Paresthesia	0.8	1.1
Urinary frequency	0.8	1.1
Dyspepsia	0.6	1.1
Constipation	0.2	1.5

Abnormal laboratory findings occurring at a frequency of 1% or greater in approximately 443 patients who received SINEMET CR and 475 who received SINEMET (Carbidopa-Levodopa) during controlled clinical trials included: decreased hemoglobin and hematocrit; elevated serum glucose; white blood cells, bacteria and blood in the urine.

The adverse experiences observed in patients in uncontrolled studies were similar to those seen in controlled clinical studies.

Other adverse experiences reported overall in clinical trials in 748 patients treated with SINEMET CR, listed by body system in order of decreasing frequency, include:

Nervous System/Psychiatric: Chorea, somnolence, falling, anxiety disorder, disorientation, decreased mental acuity, gait abnormalities, extrapyramidal disorder, agitation, nervousness, sleep disorders, memory impairment.

Body as a Whole: Asthenia, fatigue, abdominal pain, orthostatic effects.

Digestive: Gastrointestinal pain, dysphagia, heartburn.

Cardiovascular: Palpitation, essential hypertension, hypotension, myocardial infarction.

Special Senses: Blurred vision.

Metabolic: Weight loss.

Skin: Rash.

Respiratory: Cough, pharyngeal pain, common cold.

Urogenital: Urinary incontinence.

Musculoskeletal: Leg pain.

Laboratory Tests: Decreased white blood cell count and serum potassium; increased BUN, serum creatinine and serum LDH; protein and glucose in the urine.

Other adverse experiences have been reported with various carbidopa-levodopa formulations and may occur with SINEMET CR:

Nervous System/Psychiatric: Mental changes including paranoid ideation, psychotic episodes, depression with suicidal tendencies and dementia; convulsions (however, a causal relationship has not been established); bradykinetic episodes.

Gastrointestinal: Gastrointestinal bleeding, development of duodenal ulcer.

Cardiovascular: Cardiac irregularities, phlebitis.

Hematologic: Hemolytic and nonhemolytic anemia, thrombocytopenia, leukopenia, agranulocytosis.

Laboratory Tests: Abnormalities in alkaline phosphatase, SGOT (AST), SGPT (ALT), lactic dehydrogenase, bilirubin, protein-bound iodine, Coombs test.

Other adverse reactions that have been reported with levodopa are:

Nervous System: Numbness, increased hand tremor, muscle twitching, blepharospasm (which may be taken as an early sign of excess dosage, consideration of dosage reduction may be made at this time), trismus, activation of latent Horner's syndrome.

Psychiatric: Delusions, euphoria.

Gastrointestinal: Bitter taste, sialorrhea, bruxism, hiccups, flatulence, burning sensation of tongue.

Metabolic: Weight gain, edema.

Integumentary: Malignant melanoma (see also CONTRAINDICATIONS), flushing, increased sweating, dark sweat, loss of hair.

Genitourinary: Urinary retention, urinary incontinence, dark urine, priapism.

Miscellaneous: Faintness, hoarseness, malaise, hot flashes, sense of stimulation, bizarre breathing patterns, neuroleptic malignant syndrome.

OVERDOSAGE

Management of acute overdosage with SINEMET CR is the same as with levodopa. Pyridoxine is not effective in reversing the actions of SINEMET CR.

General supportive measures should be employed, along with immediate gastric lavage. Intravenous fluids should be administered judiciously and an adequate airway maintained. Electrocardiographic monitoring should be instituted and the patient carefully observed for the development of arrhythmias; if required, appropriate antiarrhythmic therapy should be given. The possibility that the patient may have taken other drugs as well as SINEMET CR should be taken into consideration. To date, no experience has been reported with dialysis; hence, its value in overdosage is not known.

Based on studies in which high doses of levodopa and/or carbidopa were administered, a significant proportion of rats and mice given single oral doses of levodopa of approximately 1500–2000 mg/kg are expected to die. A significant proportion of infant rats of both sexes are expected to die at a dose of 800 mg/kg. A significant proportion of rats are expected to die after treatment with similar doses of carbidopa. The addition of carbidopa in a 1:10 ratio with levodopa increases the dose at which a significant proportion of mice are expected to die to 3360 mg/kg.

DOSAGE AND ADMINISTRATION

SINEMET CR tablets contain carbidopa (50 mg) and levodopa (200 mg) in a 1:4 ratio. The daily dosage of SINEMET CR must be determined by careful titration. Patients should be monitored closely during the dose adjustment period, particularly with regard to appearance or worsening of involuntary movements, dyskinesias or nausea. SINEMET CR may be administered as whole or as half-tablets which should not be chewed or crushed.

Standard drugs for Parkinson's disease, other than levodopa without a decarboxylase inhibitor, may be used concomitantly while SINEMET CR is being administered, although their dosage may have to be adjusted.

Since carbidopa prevents the reversal of levodopa effects caused by pyridoxine, SINEMET CR can be given to patients receiving supplemental pyridoxine (vitamin B_6).

Continued on next page

Du Pont—Cont.

Initial Dosage
Patients currently treated with conventional carbidopa-levodopa preparations: Dosage with SINEMET CR should be substituted at an amount that provides approximately 10% more levodopa per day, although this may need to be increased to a dosage that provides up to 30% more levodopa per day depending on clinical response (see DOSAGE AND ADMINISTRATION, *Titration*). The interval between doses of SINEMET CR should be 4–8 hours during the waking day. (See CLINICAL PHARMACOLOGY, *Pharmacodynamics.*)
A guideline for initiation of SINEMET CR is shown in Table II.

Table II.
Guidelines for Initial Conversion
from SINEMET (Carbidopa-Levodopa) to SINEMET CR

SINEMET (Carbidopa-Levodopa) Total Daily Dose* Levodopa (mg)	SINEMET CR Suggested Dosage Regimen
300–400	1 tab b.i.d.
500–600	1½ tab b.i.d. or 1 tab t.i.d.
700–800	A total of 4 tabs in 3 or more divided doses (e.g., 1½ tab a.m., 1½ tab early p.m., and 1 tab later p.m.)
900–1000	A total of 5 tabs in 3 or more divided doses (e.g., 2 tabs a.m., 2 tabs early p.m., and 1 tab later p.m.)

*For dosing ranges not shown in the table see DOSAGE AND ADMINISTRATION, *Initial Dosage—Patients currently treated with conventional carbidopa-levodopa preparations.*

Patients currently treated with levodopa without a decarboxylase inhibitor: Levodopa must be discontinued at least eight hours before therapy with SINEMET CR is started. SINEMET CR should be substituted at a dosage that will provide approximately 25% of the previous levodopa dosage. In patients with mild to moderate disease, the initial dose is usually 1 tablet of SINEMET CR b.i.d.
Patients not receiving levodopa: In patients with mild to moderate disease, the initial recommended dose is 1 tablet of SINEMET CR b.i.d. Initial dosage should not be given at intervals of less than 6 hours.
Titration
Following initiation of therapy, doses and dosing intervals may be increased or decreased depending upon therapeutic response. Most patients have been adequately treated with 2 to 8 tablets per day, administered as divided doses at intervals ranging from 4 to 8 hours during the waking day. Higher doses (12 or more tablets per day) and shorter intervals (less than 4 hours) have been used, but are not usually recommended.
When doses of SINEMET CR are given at intervals of less than 4 hours, and/or if the divided doses are not equal, it is recommended that the smaller doses be given at the end of the day.
An interval of at least 3 days between dosage adjustments is recommended.
Maintenance
Because Parkinson's disease is progressive, periodic clinical evaluations are recommended; adjustment of the dosage regimen of SINEMET CR may be required.
Addition of Other Antiparkinson Medications
Anticholinergic agents, dopamine agonists, and amantadine can be given with SINEMET CR. Dosage adjustment of SINEMET CR may be necessary when these agents are added.
A dose of SINEMET (Carbidopa-Levodopa) 25–100 or 10–100 (one half or a whole tablet) can be added to the dosage regimen of SINEMET CR in selected patients with advanced disease who need additional levodopa for a brief time during daytime hours.
Interruption of Therapy
Patients should be observed carefully if abrupt reduction or discontinuation of SINEMET CR is required, especially if the patient is receiving neuroleptics. (See WARNINGS.)
If general anesthesia is required, SINEMET CR may be continued as long as the patient is permitted to take oral medication. If therapy is interrupted temporarily, the usual dosage should be administered as soon as the patient is able to take oral medication.

HOW SUPPLIED
SINEMET CR 50–200 (Carbidopa-Levodopa) SUSTAINED-RELEASE TABLETS containing 50 mg of carbidopa and 200 mg of levodopa, are peach colored, oval, scored, biconvex, compressed tablets, coded 521. They are supplied as follows:
NDC 0056-0521-68 bottles of 100
NDC 0056-0521-28 unit dose package of 100.
Storage
Avoid temperatures above 30°C (86°F). Store in a tightly closed container.

Manufactured by:
MERCK SHARP & DOHME
DIV OF MERCK & CO., INC., WEST POINT, PA 19486, USA
For:
Du Pont Pharmaceuticals
The Du Pont Merck Pharmaceutical Co.
Wilmington, Delaware 19880

6251-3/Issued June 1991

AHFS Category: 92:00
Shown in Product Identification Section, page 409

EDUCATIONAL MATERIAL

BREVIBLOC®

Films/Slides/Videos
"Dosing and Administration of BREVIBLOC® (Esmolol) in the Critical Care Setting." This 11 minute video provides insight into the best approaches for dosing and administering a quick-acting, titratable beta-blocker. Available in ½" VHS tape—accompanied by an interactive D&A worksheet and a reusable, convenient dosing wall chart.

COUMADIN®

Books/Booklets/Brochures
"*COUMADIN® Patient Aid*". This booklet explains key points of anticoagulation therapy, how it affects the patient's lifestyle, warning signs, and Vitamin K information. It also includes a COUMADIN® ID card and a dosage calendar. Available in English and Spanish.
Slides/Video/Audio
"*Using COUMADIN® Safely and Effectively*". This 11 minute, ½-inch VHS video is designed to be shown by the physician or given to his/her patients on COUMADIN® in order to increase patient compliance and understanding of COUMADIN® therapy.
An audiocassette is also available as a patient give-away of the "Using COUMADIN® Safely and Effectively" video. Both items available in English and Spanish.
Pictures/Charts
"*COUMADIN® Patient Anticoagulant Record Charts*". This laminated 8-½" × 11" chart provide a convenient way to record patient prothrombin times and COUMADIN® doses.
"*COUMADIN® Patient Education Easel Flip Chart*". An easel that allows the physician or nurse to educate the patient about COUMADIN® therapy in a practical question-and-answer format. Available in English and Spanish.
All of the above is available at no charge to physicians, pharmacists, and other healthcare professionals involved with the management of patients on COUMADIN® therapy by writing to: Du Pont Company, Room G51962, P.O. Box 80010, Wilmington, DE 19880-0010.

SINEMET®

Booklets/Video
"Cornerstone" Patient & Medical Education Program: Medical education video, (H-24856), "Challenges of Early Diagnosis in Parkinson's Disease" featuring Dr. Matthew Stern, Asst. Prof. of Neurology, University of Pennsylvania and Co-Director of the Movement Disorder Center, Graduate Hospital, Philadelphia: Patient Education Booklets, (H-24857), "Parkinson's Disease and How It's Treated" and (H-24858), "Living with Parkinson's Disease". Available at no charge. Write Du Pont Pharmaceuticals and ask for materials by H # or call 1(800) 441-9861.

Dura Pharmaceuticals, Inc.
SAN DIEGO, CA 92121-1203

D.A. Chewable Tablets™   ℞

DESCRIPTION
Each D.A. Chewable Tablet for oral administration contains:
    Chlorpheniramine maleate .... 2 mg
    Phenylephrine HCl .... 10 mg
    Methscopolamine nitrate .... 1.25 mg
in an orange flavored and orange colored tablet.

HOW SUPPLIED
D.A. Chewable Tablets are available as orange flavored and orange colored scored tablets imprinted with "DURA" on one side and "DA JR" on the other.
NDC 51479-010-01   Bottle of 100
Dispense in tight containers as defined in USP/NF.
Store between 15°–30°C (59°–86°F).
Dispense in child-resistant containers.

DURA-GEST®   ℞

DESCRIPTION
Each Dura-Gest gray and white capsule for oral administration contains:
Phenylephrine hydrochloride .... 5 mg
Phenylpropanolamine hydrochloride .... 45 mg
Guaifenesin .... 200 mg

HOW SUPPLIED
DURA-GEST gray and white capsules are imprinted with DURA-GEST and 51479005.
NDC 51479-005-01 Bottle of 100
NDC 51479-005-05 Bottle of 500
Dispense in tight containers as defined in USP/NF.
Store between 15°–30°C (59°–86°F).
Dispense in child resistant containers.

DURA-TAP/PD® CAPSULES   ℞

DESCRIPTION
Each Dura-Tap/PD opaque blue and clear capsule containing white beads for oral administration contains:
Chlorpheniramine maleate .... 4 mg
Pseudoephedrine hydrochloride .... 60 mg
in a special base to provide prolonged action.

HOW SUPPLIED
Dura-Tap/PD is available as a opaque blue and clear capsule containing white beads imprinted with 51479007.
NDC 51479-007-01 Bottle of 100
Dispense in tight containers as defined in USP/NF.
Store between 15°–30°C (59°–86°F).
Dispense in child-resistant containers.

DURA-VENT® TABLETS   ℞

DESCRIPTION
Each Dura-Vent white, scored tablet for oral administration contains:
Phenylpropanolamine hydrochloride .... 75 mg
Guaifenesin .... 600 mg
in a special base to provide prolonged action.

HOW SUPPLIED
Dura-Vent is available as a white, scored tablet imprinted with DURA 7.5/7.5 .
NDC 51479-006-01 Bottle of 100
NDC 51479-006-06 Bottle of 600
Dispense in tight containers as defined in USP/NF.
Store between 15°–30°C (59°–86°F).
Dispense in child-resistant containers.

DURA-VENT/A® CAPSULES   ℞

DESCRIPTION
Each Dura-Vent/A clear capsule containing white beads for oral administration contains:
Phenylpropanolamine hydrochloride .... 75 mg
Chlorpheniramine maleate .... 10 mg
in a special base to provide prolonged action.

HOW SUPPLIED
Dura-Vent/A is available as a clear capsule containing white beads imprinted with Dura-Vent/A and 51479002.
NDC 51479-002-01 Bottle of 100
Dispense in tight containers as defined in USP/NF.
Store between 15°–30°C (59°–86°F).
Dispense in child-resistant containers.

DURA-VENT/DA® TABLETS   ℞

DESCRIPTION
Each Dura-Vent/DA light brown, scored tablet for oral administration contains:
Chlorpheniramine maleate .... 8 mg
Phenylephrine hydrochloride .... 20 mg
Methscopolamine nitrate .... 2.5 mg
in a special base to provide prolonged action.

HOW SUPPLIED
Dura-Vent/DA is available as a light brown, scored tablet imprinted with DURA DA.
NDC 51479-008-01 Bottle of 100
Dispense in tight containers as defined in USP/NF.
Store between 15°–30°C (59°–86°F).
Dispense in child-resistant containers.

FENESIN™ TABLETS ℞

DESCRIPTION

Each Fenesin light blue, scored tablet for oral administration contains:
Guaifenesin .... 600 mg
in a special base to provide prolonged action.

HOW SUPPLIED

Fenesin is available as a light blue, scored tablet imprinted with DURA 009.
NDC 51479-009-01 Bottle of 100
NDC 51479-009-06 Bottle of 600
Dispense in tight containers as defined in USP/NF.
Store between 15°–30°C (59°–86°F).
Dispense in child-resistant containers.

TORNALATE® ℞
(bitolterol mesylate)
Inhalation Solution, 0.2%

DESCRIPTION

Tornalate (bitolterol mesylate) is the di-p-toluate ester of the β-adrenergic agonist bronchodilator N-t-butylarterenol (colterol). It has a molecular weight of 557.7. Bitolterol mesylate is known chemically as 4-[2-[(1,1-dimethylethyl) aminol]-1-hydroxyethyl]-1,2-phenylene 4-methylbenzoate (ester) methanesulfonate (salt) and has the following structural formula:

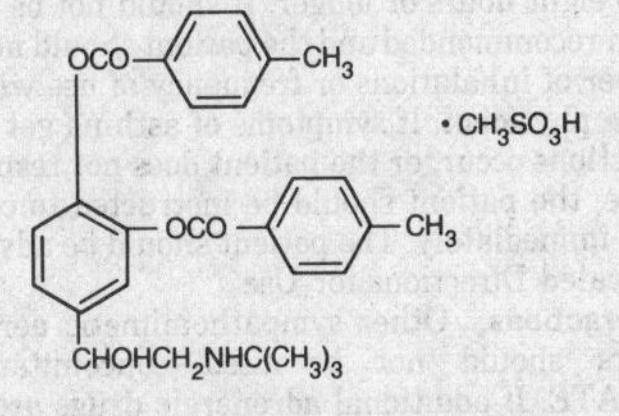

Tornalate Inhalation Solution contains 0.2% bitolterol mesylate in an aqueous vehicle containing alcohol 25% (v/v), citric acid, propylene glycol, and sodium hydroxide.
Each mL of Tornalate Inhalation Solution, 0.2% contains 2.0 mg of bitolterol mesylate.

CLINICAL PHARMACOLOGY

Tornalate is administered as a pro-drug which is hydrolyzed by esterases in tissue and blood to the active moiety colterol. Tornalate administered by nebulization has a rapid onset of activity (2 to 3 minutes) after administration in most patients based on interpolation between baseline and 5 minutes. The duration of action with Tornalate administered by nebulization is 6 hours or more in most patients and 8 hours in 40% of patients based on 15% or greater increase in forced expiratory volume in one second (FEV_1), as demonstrated in three-month isoproterenol controlled multicenter trials in nonsteroid dependent patients. Based on mid-maximal expiratory flow (MMEF) measurements, the duration of action is 7.5 to 8 hours in most patients. Median duration of effect in steroid-dependent asthmatic patients ranged from 4.3 to 7.1 hours based on 15% or greater increase in FEV_1. The mean maximum increase in FEV_1 over baseline in patients during the three-month studies was 49% to 55% and occurred by 30 to 60 minutes in most patients.

In vitro studies and in vivo pharmacologic studies have demonstrated that Tornalate has a preferential effect on beta-2 adrenergic receptors compared with isoproterenol. While it is recognized that beta-2 adrenergic receptors are the prominent receptors in bronchial smooth muscle, recent data indicate that there are between 10% to 50% beta-2 receptors in the human heart. The precise function of these, however, is not yet established. Tornalate has been shown in most controlled clinical trials to have more effect on the respiratory tract, in the form of bronchial smooth muscle relaxation than isoproterenol at comparable doses, while producing fewer cardiovascular effects. Controlled clinical studies and other clinical experience have shown the inhaled Tornalate, like other beta-adrenergic agonists, can produce a significant cardiovascular effect in some patients, as measured by pulse rate, blood pressure, symptoms and/or ECG changes.

The incidence of cardiovascular side effects such as tachycardia and palpitation was less in patients treated with bitolterol mesylate as compared with patients treated with isoproterenol hydrochloride. The incidence of tachycardia and palpitation was 3.7% and 3.1%, respectively, in patients treated with bitolterol mesylate as compared with an incidence of 12.3% and 12.6% for tachycardia and palpitation for patients treated with isoproterenol.

Blood levels of colterol formed by gradual release from the pro-drug (bitolterol) in the lungs are too low to be measured by currently available assay methods and the bioavailability, pharmacokinetics and metabolism of bitolterol following administration as a solution for inhalation are not known. Data on disposition are available from oral studies in man. Following oral administration of 5.9 mg tritiated bitolterol to man, radioactivity measurements indicated mean maximum colterol concentration in blood of approximately 2.1 $\mu g/mL$ one hour after medication. Urinary excretion data indicate that 83% of the radioactivity of this oral dose was excreted within the first 24 hours. By 72 hours, 85.6% of the tritium had been excreted in the urine and 8.1% in the feces. Most of the radioactivity was excreted as conjugated colterol; free colterol accounted for 2.1% to 3.7% of the total radioactivity excreted in the urine. No intact bitolterol was detected in urine.

The pharmacologic effects of β-adrenergic agonist drugs, including bitolterol mesylate, are at least in part attributable to stimulation through beta adrenergic receptors of intracellular adenyl cyclase, the enzyme which catalyzes the conversion of adenosine triphosphate (ATP) to cyclic-3′, 5′-adenosine monophosphate (c-AMP). Increased c-AMP levels are associated with relaxation of bronchial smooth muscle and inhibition of release of mediators of immediate hypersensitivity from cells, especially from mast cells.

In repetitive dosing studies, continued effectiveness was demonstrated throughout the three-month period of treatment in the majority of patients. In steroid-dependent asthmatics, the median duration of bronchodilator activity as measured by FEV_1 was greater on the first test day as compared with later test days, but patient response remained constant throughout the balance of the three-month period.

Recent studies in laboratory animals (minipigs, rodents, and dogs) recorded the occurrence of cardiac arrhythmias and sudden death (with histologic evidence of myocardial necrosis) when beta agonists and methylxanthines were administered concurrently. The significance of these findings when applied to humans is currently unknown.

INDICATIONS AND USAGE

Tornalate Inhalation Solution, 0.2% is indicated for both prophylaxis and treatment of asthma or other conditions characterized by reversible bronchospasm. It may be used with or without concurrent theophylline and/or steroid therapy.

CONTRAINDICATIONS

Tornalate Inhalation Solution, 0.2% is contraindicated in patients who are hypersensitive to bitolterol mesylate or any other ingredients of the formulation.

WARNINGS

As with other β-adrenergic agents, bitolterol mesylate should not be used in excess. Use of β-adrenergic drugs may have a deleterious cardiac effect. Paradoxical bronchoconstriction has been reported with administration of β-adrenergic agents. Immediate hypersensitivity reactions can occur after the administration of sympathomimetic agents. In such instances, the drug should be discontinued immediately and alternative therapy instituted.

In controlled clinical studies, clinically significant increases in pulse rate, increases and decreases in systolic and diastolic blood pressure have been demonstrated in individual patients after administration of Tornalate. Therefore, caution should be exercised when administering bitolterol mesylate to patients with underlying cardiovascular disease. Even though the changes may be significant in a small number of patients, these changes occur within a short period of time after administration and have not been shown to be persistent.

If an unusual smell or taste is noted with use of this product, the patient should discontinue use in consultation with his/her physician.

PRECAUTIONS

General As with all β-adrenergic stimulating agents, caution should be used when administering Tornalate to patients with cardiovascular disease such as ischemic heart disease or hypertension. Caution is also advised in patients with hyperthyroidism, diabetes mellitus, cardiac arrhythmias, convulsive disorders or unusual responsiveness to β-adrenergic agonists. Use of any β-adrenergic bronchodilator may produce significant changes in systolic and diastolic blood pressure in some patients.

Information for Patients The effects of Tornalate may last up to eight hours or longer. It should not be used more often than recommended and the patient should not increase the number of treatments or dose without first consulting with the physician. If symptoms of asthma increase, adverse reactions occur, or if the patient does not respond to the usual dose, the patient should immediately notify the physician. The patient should be advised as to the proper use of the equipment used for nebulization.

Drug Interactions Other sympathomimetic bronchodilators or epinephrine should not be used concomitantly with Tornalate because they may have additive effects.

Tornalate should be administered with caution to patients being treated with monoamine oxidase inhibitors or tricyclic antidepressants, since the action of bitolterol on the vascular system may be potentiated.

Carcinogenesis, Mutagenesis, and Impairment of Fertility No tumorigenicity (and specifically no increase in leiomyomas) was observed in a two year oral study in Sprague-Dawley CD rats at doses of Tornalate corresponding to 12 or 62 times the maximal total daily human inhalation dose (8.0 mg bitolterol mesylate per day). Tornalate was not tumorigenic in an 18 month oral study in Swiss-Webster mice at doses up to 312 times the maximal daily human inhalation dose. Ames Salmonella and mouse lymphoma mutation assays in vitro revealed no mutagenesis due to Tornalate. Reproductive studies in male and female rats revealed no significant effects on fertility at doses of Tornalate up to 241 times the maximal daily human inhalational dose.

Teratogenic Effects—Pregnancy Category C No teratogenic effects were seen in rats and rabbits after oral doses of Tornalate up to 361 times the maximal daily human inhalational dose and in mice after oral doses up to 188 times the maximal daily human inhalational dose.

When Tornalate (as base) was injected subcutaneously into mice in doses of 2 mg/kg, 10 mg/kg, and 20 mg/kg (corresponding to 15, 75, and 151 times the maximal daily human inhalational dose) the incidence of cleft palate was 5.7%, 3.8%, and 3.3%, respectively. Occurrence of cleft palate with isoproterenol (as base) at 10 mg/kg subcutaneously was 10.7%. Since well-controlled studies in pregnant women are not available, Tornalate should be used during pregnancy only if the potential benefit justifies the potential risk to the fetus.

Nursing Mothers It is not known whether Tornalate is excreted in human milk. Because many drugs are excreted in human milk, caution should be exercised when Tornalate is administered to a nursing woman.

Pediatric Use Safety and effectiveness of Tornalate in children 12 years of age or younger has not been established.

ADVERSE REACTIONS

The adverse reactions observed with Tornalate are consistent with those seen with other beta-adrenergic agonists. The frequency of most cardiovascular effects was less after bitolterol mesylate than after isoproterenol in 3-month repetitive dose studies.

Like the findings noted after the administration of other beta-adrenergic agonist drugs, infrequent laboratory abnormalities with undetermined clinical significance were noted after administration of Tornalate. These include decreases in hemoglobin and hematocrit, decreases in WBC, elevation of liver enzymes, increases in blood sugar, deceases in serum potassium and abnormal urinalysis. In addition, one patient in a Tornalate controlled clinical trial had increased liver function tests and documented hepatomegaly.

The results of all clinical trials with Tornalate (323 patients) showed the following side effects:

Central/Peripheral Nervous System: Tremors (26.6%), nervousness (11.1%), headache (8.4%), lightheadedness (6.8%), dizziness (4.0%), paresthesia (1.5%), somnolence (1.2%). In three-month studies, the incidence of tremors decreased from 22% during the first month to 9% during the third month.

Cardiovascular: Tachycardia (3.7%), palpitation (3.1%), irregular pulse (1.2%).

Respiratory: Coughing (2.5%), bronchospasm (1.5%), chest discomfort (1.5%), rhinitis (1.5%).

Oro-Pharyngeal: Throat irritation (2.5%), mouth irritation (1.9%).

Gastrointestinal: Nausea (1.9%).

Other: Fatigue (1.5%).

The incidence of the following adverse reactions was less than one percent.

CNS: Vertigo, insomnia, euphoria, incoordination, hyperkinesia, hypoesthesia, anxiety.

Cardiovascular: Transient ECG changes (ventricular premature contractions, atrial arrhythmia, inverted T waves, junctional rhythm), chest discomfort, increase in blood pressure, chills, heart rate decrease, flushing.

Respiratory: Dyspnea, sputum increase.

Gastrointestinal: Vomiting, hepatomegalia.

Others: Pruritus, urticaria, asthenia, arthralgia, eye irritation, facial discomfort, taste loss.

Clinical relevance or relationship to administration of Tornalate and rarely reported elevations of SGOT, SGPT, LDH are not known.

OVERDOSAGE

Overdosage with Tornalate may be expected to result in exaggeration of those drug effects listed in the ADVERSE REACTIONS section. In such cases therapy with Tornalate and all β-adrenergic stimulating drugs should be stopped, supportive therapy provided, and judicious use of a cardioselective β-adrenergic blocking agent should be considered bearing in mind the possibility that such agents can produce profound bronchospasm.

The oral LD_{50} of Tornalate in rats was 5,650 mg/kg and in mice it was 6,575 mg/kg.

Continued on next page

Dura—Cont.

DOSAGE AND ADMINISTRATION

Tornalate Inhalation Solution, 0.2% can be administered by nebulization to adults and children over 12 years of age. As with all medications, the physician should begin therapy with the lowest effective dose according to the individual patient's requirements following manufacturer's dosage recommendation. Tornalate should be administered during a ten to fifteen minute period. The treatment period can be adjusted by varying the amount of diluent placed in the nebulizer with the medication. The total volume (medication plus diluent) is usually adjusted to 2.0 mL to 4.0 mL. Safety of the treatment should be monitored by measuring blood pressure and pulse.

Clinical studies were conducted with two types of nebulizer systems.

Intermittent Aerosol Flow (Patient Activated Nebulizer) This nebulizer is operated by a patient activated valve to permit the release of aerosol mist only during inspiration.

Continuous Aerosol Flow Nebulizer This nebulizer generates a continuous flow of mist while the patient inhales and exhales through the nebulizer resulting in the loss of some medication through an exhaust port.

When using these types of nebulizer systems the following dosing regimens are recommended:

Tornalate Inhalation Solution, 0.2%

Doses	Intermittent Flow Nebulization		Continuous Flow Nebulization	
	Volume	Tornalate	Volume	Tornalate
Usual Dose	0.5 mL	1.0 mg	1.25 mL	2.5 mg
Decreased Dose	0.25 mL	0.5 mg	0.75 mL	1.5 mg
Increased dose	0.75 mL	1.5 mg	1.75 mL	3.5 mg

Up to 1.0 mL of Tornalate Inhalation Solution, 0.2% (2.0 mg Tornalate), can be administered with the intermittent flow system to severely obstructed patients.

The usual frequency of treatments is three times a day. Treatments may be increased up to four times daily, however the interval between treatments should not be less than four hours. For some patients two treatments a day may be adequate.

The maximum daily dose should not exceed 8.0 mg Tornalate with an intermittent flow nebulization system or 14.0 mg Tornalate with a continuous flow nebulization system.

Tornalate Inhalation Solution, 0.2% should be added to the nebulizer just prior to use and should not be left in the nebulizer.

Tornalate Inhalation Solution, 0.2% should not be mixed with other drugs such as cromolyn sodium or acetylcysteine at clinically recommended doses due to chemical and/or physical incompatibilities.

HOW SUPPLIED

Amber Glass Bottle of 10 mL (NDC 51479-011-01)
Amber Glass Bottle of 30 mL (NDC 51479-011-03)
Amber Glass Bottle of 60 mL (NDC 51479-011-06)

Included in each carton is a cellophane overwrapped graduated medicine dropper for use with Tornalate Inhalation Solution, 0.2%.

Do not use the solution if it is discolored or contains a precipitate.

Store at controlled room temperature between 15°C–30°C (59°F–86°F).

Caution: Federal law prohibits dispensing without a prescription.

DURA PHARMACEUTICALS

Distributed by DURA Pharmaceuticals, Inc., San Diego, CA 92121

Manufactured by Sterling Pharmaceuticals Inc., Barceloneata, Puerto Rico 00617

TS007A0292

TORNALATE® ℞
(bitolterol mesylate)
Metered Dose Inhaler
Bronchodilator for Oral Inhalation

DESCRIPTION

TORNALATE (bitolterol mesylate) is the di-*p*-toluate ester of the β-adrenergic bronchodilator *N-t*-butylarterenol (colterol). It has a molecular weight of 557.7. Bitolterol mesylate is known chemically as 4-[2-[(1,1-dimethylethyl) amino]-1-hydroxyethyl]-1,2-phenylene 4-methylbenzoate (ester) methanesulfonate (salt) and has the following structural formula:

[See chemical structure at top of next column.]

TORNALATE (bitolterol mesylate), Metered Dose Inhaler, is a complete aerosol unit for oral inhalation. It consists of a plastic-coated bottle of ready-to-use aerosol solution and a detachable plastic mouthpiece with built-in nebulizer. The bottle contains 16.4 g (15 mL) of 0.8% bitolterol mesylate in a

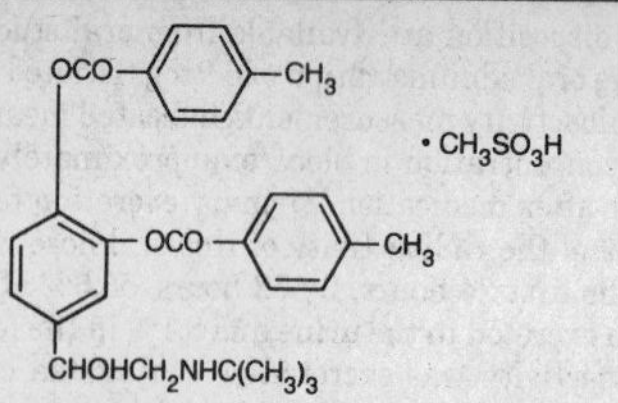

vehicle containing 38% alcohol (w/w), inert propellants (dichlorodifluoromethane and dichlorotetrafluoroethane), ascorbic acid, saccharin, and menthol.

Each bottle provides at least 300 actuations. Each actuation delivers a measured dose of 0.37 mg of bitolterol mesylate as a fine, even mist.

CLINICAL PHARMACOLOGY

TORNALATE (bitolterol mesylate) is administered as a pro-drug which is hydrolyzed by esterases in tissue and blood to the active moiety colterol. TORNALATE administered as an inhaled aerosol, has a rapid (3 to 4 minutes) onset of bronchodilator activity. The duration of action with TORNALATE is at least 5 hours in most patients and 8 or more hours in 25% to 35% of patients, based on 15% or greater increase in forced expiratory volume in one second (FEV_1), as demonstrated in 3 month isoproterenol controlled multicenter trials. Based on mean maximal expiratory flow (MMEF) measurements, the duration of action is 6 to 7 hours. The duration of bronchodilator action with TORNALATE in these trials is longer than that seen with isoproterenol, especially in steroid-dependent patients. Duration of effect was reduced over time in steroid-dependent asthmatic patients where the duration was 3.5 to 5 hours for FEV_1. The mean maximum increase in FEV_1 over baseline in the majority of patients was 39% to 42% and occurred by 30 to 60 minutes, similar to that seen in the isoproterenol group.

TORNALATE is a beta adrenergic agonist which has been shown by in vitro and in vivo pharmacological studies in animals to exert a preferential effect on $beta_2$ adrenergic receptors, such as those located in bronchial smooth muscle. However, controlled clinical trials in patients who were administered the drug have not revealed a preferential $beta_2$ adrenergic effect. At doses that produced long duration of bronchodilator activity (up to 8 hours in some patients) with a mean maximum bronchodilating effect of approximately 40% increase in FEV_1 (forced expiration volume in one second), a less than 10 beat per minute mean maximum increase in heart rate was seen. The effect on the heart rate was transient and similar to the increases seen in the isoproterenol treated patients in these studies.

Although blood levels of colterol formed by gradual release from the pro-drug (bitolterol) in the lungs are too low to be measured by currently available assay methods, data on disposition are available from oral studies in man. Following oral administration of 5.9 mg tritiated bitolterol mesylate to man, radioactivity measurements indicated mean maximum colterol concentration in blood of approximately 2.1 μg/mL one hour after medication. Urinary excretion data indicate that 83 percent of the radioactivity of this oral dose was excreted within the first 24 hours. By 72 hours, 85.6 percent of the tritium had been excreted in the urine and 8.1 percent in the feces. Most of the radioactivity was excreted as conjugated colterol; free colterol accounted for 2.1 to 3.7 percent of the total radioactivity excreted in the urine. No intact bitolterol was detected in urine.

The pharmacologic effects of β-adrenergic drugs including TORNALATE (bitolterol mesylate) are attributable to stimulation of adenyl cyclase, the enzyme which catalyzes the conversion of adenosine triphosphate (ATP) to cyclic-3′, 5′-adenosine monophosphate (c-AMP). Increased c-AMP levels are associated with relaxation of bronchial smooth muscle and with inhibition of release of mediators of immediate hypersensitivity.

In a six week clinical trial in which 24 asthmatic patients received TORNALATE and theophylline concurrently, improvement in pulmonary function was enhanced over that seen with either drug alone. No potentiation of side effects was observed, and 24-hour ECG recordings (Holter monitoring) indicated no greater degree of cardiac toxicity with TORNALATE alone or in combination with theophylline than that which occurred with theophylline alone.

TORNALATE did not adversely affect arterial oxygen tension in a blood-gas study in 24 asthmatic patients. However, a decrease in arterial oxygen tension has been reported with other adrenergic bronchodilators and could be anticipated to occur with TORNALATE as well.

In repetitive dosing studies, continued effectiveness was demonstrated throughout the 3 month period of treatment in the majority of patients. However, some overall decrease was observed in steroid dependent asthmatics.

INDICATIONS AND USAGE

TORNALATE (bitolterol mesylate) is indicated for both prophylactic and therapeutic use as a bronchodilator for bronchial asthma and for reversible bronchospasm. It may be used with or without concurrent theophylline and/or steroid therapy.

CONTRAINDICATIONS

TORNALATE (bitolterol mesylate) is contraindicated in patients who are hypersensitive to any of its ingredients.

WARNINGS

As with other β-adrenergic aerosols, TORNALATE (bitolterol mesylate) should not be used in excess. Use of aerosolized β-adrenergic drugs may have a deleterious cardiac effect. Paradoxical bronchoconstriction has been reported with administration of β-adrenergic agents. Immediate hypersensitivity (allergic) reactions can occur after the administration of TORNALATE. In such instances, the drug should be discontinued immediately and alternative therapy instituted.

PRECAUTIONS

General. As with all β-adrenergic stimulating agents, caution should be used when administering TORNALATE (bitolterol mesylate) to patients with cardiovascular disease such as ischemic heart disease or hypertension. Caution is also advised in patients with hyperthyroidism, diabetes mellitus, cardiac arrhythmias, convulsive disorders or unusual responsiveness to β-adrenergic agonists. Significant changes in systolic and diastolic blood pressure have been seen in individual patients and could be expected to occur in some patients after use of any β-adrenergic aerosol bronchodilator.

Information for Patients. The effects of TORNALATE may last up to eight hours or longer. It should not be used more often than recommended and the patient should not increase the number of inhalations or frequency of use without first asking the physician. If symptoms of asthma get worse, adverse reactions occur, or the patient does not respond to the usual dose, the patient should be instructed to contact the physician immediately. The patient should be advised to see the Illustrated Directions for Use.

Drug Interactions. Other sympathomimetic aerosol bronchodilators should not be used concomitantly with TORNALATE. If additional adrenergic drugs are to be administered by any route, they should be used with caution to avoid deleterious cardiovascular effects.

Carcinogenesis, Mutagenesis, and Impairment of Fertility. No tumorigenicity (and specifically no increase in leiomyomas) was observed in a two year oral study in Sprague-Dawley CD rats at doses of TORNALATE corresponding to 23 or 114 times the maximal daily human inhalational dose. TORNALATE was not tumorigenic in an 18 month oral study in Swiss-Webster mice at doses up to 568 times the maximal daily human inhalational dose.

Ames Salmonella and mouse lymphoma mutation assays in vitro revealed no mutagenesis due to TORNALATE. Reproductive studies in male and female rats revealed no significant effects on fertility at doses of TORNALATE up to 364 times the maximal daily human inhalational dose.

Teratogenic Effects—Pregnancy Category C. No teratogenic effects were seen in rats and rabbits after oral doses of TORNALATE up to 557 times the maximal daily human inhalational dose and in mice after oral doses up to 284 times the maximal daily human inhalational dose.

When TORNALATE was injected subcutaneously into mice at doses of 2 mg/kg, 10 mg/kg, and 20 mg/kg (corresponding to 23, 114, and 227 times the maximal daily human inhalational dose) cleft palate incidences of 5.7 percent, 3.8 percent, and 3.3 percent (compared with 0.9 percent in controls) were found. Cleft palate induction with isoproterenol at 10 mg/kg SC as the positive control was 10.7 percent. Since no well-controlled studies in pregnant women are available, TORNALATE should be used during pregnancy only if the potential benefit justifies the potential risk to the fetus.

Nursing Mothers. It is not known whether TORNALATE is excreted in human milk. Because many drugs are excreted in human milk, caution should be exercised when TORNALATE is administered to a nursing woman.

Pediatric Use. Safety and effectiveness of TORNALATE in children 12 years of age or younger has not been established.

ADVERSE REACTIONS

The results of all clinical trials with TORNALATE (bitolterol mesylate) in 492 patients showed the following side effects:

CNS: Tremors (14%), nervousness (5%), headache (4%), dizziness (3%), lightheadedness (3%), insomnia (<1%), hyperkinesia (<1%).

Gastrointestinal: Nausea (3%).

Oro-Pharyngeal: Throat irritation (5%).

Cardiovascular: The overall incidence of cardiovascular effects was approximately 5% of patients and these effects included palpitations (approximately 3%), and chest discomfort (approximately 1%). Tachycardia was seen in less than 1%. Premature ventricular contractions and flushing were rarely seen.

Respiratory: Coughing (4%), bronchospasm (<1%), dyspnea (<1%), chest tightness (<1%).

Clinical relevance or relationship to TORNALATE administration of rarely reported elevations of SGOT, decrease in platelets, decreases in WBC levels or proteinuria are not known.

In comparing the adverse reactions for bitolterol mesylate treated patients to those of isoproterenol treated patients, during three month clinical trials involving approximately 400 patients, the following moderate to severe reactions, as judged by the investigators, were reported for both steroid and non-steroid dependent patients. The table does not include mild reactions or those occurring only with the first dose.

PERCENT INCIDENCE OF MODERATE TO SEVERE ADVERSE REACTIONS

Reaction	Bitolterol N = 197	Isoproterenol N = 194
Central Nervous System		
Tremors	9.1%	1.5%
Nervousness	1.5%	1.0%
Headache	3.5%	6.1%
Dizziness	1.0%	1.5%
Insomnia	0.5%	0%
Cardiovascular		
Palpitations	1.5%	0%
PVC—Transient		
Increase	0.5%	0%
Chest Discomfort	0.5%	0%
Respiratory		
Cough	4.1%	1.0%
Bronchospasm	1.0%	0%
Dyspnea	1.0%	0%
Oro-Pharyngeal		
Throat Irritation	3.0%	3.1%
Gastrointestinal		
Nausea (Dyspepsia)	0.5%	0.5%

NOTE: In most patients, the total isoproterenol dosage was divided into three equally dosed inhalations, administered at three minute intervals. This procedure may have reduced the incidence of adverse reactions observed with isoproterenol.

OVERDOSAGE

Overdosage with TORNALATE (bitolterol mesylate) may be expected to result in exaggeration of those drug effects listed in the ADVERSE REACTIONS section. In such cases therapy with TORNALATE and all β-adrenergic stimulating drugs should be stopped, supportive therapy provided, and judicious use of a cardioselective β-adrenergic blocking agent should be considered bearing in mind the possibility that such agents can produce profound bronchospasm. As with all sympathomimetic aerosol medications, cardiac arrest and even death may be associated with abuse. The oral LD_{50} of TORNALATE in rats was greater than 5000 mg/kg and in mice greater than 6000 mg/kg.

DOSAGE AND ADMINISTRATION

The usual dose to relieve bronchospasm for adults and children over 12 years of age is two inhalations at an interval of at least one to three minutes followed by a third inhalation if needed. For prevention of bronchospasm, the usual dose is two inhalations every 8 hours. The dose of TORNALATE (bitolterol mesylate) should never exceed 3 inhalations every 6 hours or 2 inhalations every 4 hours. Medical consultation should be sought prior to an increase in the frequency of dosing because this may indicate a need for reevaluation of the patient's condition.

HOW SUPPLIED

TORNALATE (bitolterol mesylate), Metered Dose Inhaler, is supplied in 16.4 g (15 mL) self-contained aerosol units (NDC 51479-012-01).
Refill of 16.4 g (15 mL) NDC 51479-012-02.
Store at controlled room temperature between 15 °C and 30 °C (59 °F and 86 °F).

Distributed by DURA Pharmaceuticals, Inc.
San Diego, CA 92121
Manufactured by Sterling Pharmaceuticals Inc.
Barceloneta, Puerto Rico 00617

DURA 038A0792

Products are
listed alphabetically
in the
PINK SECTION.

Duramed Pharmaceuticals, Inc.
5040 LESTER ROAD
CINCINNATI, OH 45213

PRODUCT LIST

NDC # 51285-	Strength	Color	Description	Brand Equivalent	Pkg Size
Amantadine Capsules (R)					
803-02	100 mg.	Red	Capsule	Symmetrel	100
803-04					500
Aspirin 15gr Delayed Release (F.C.) (R)					
806-02	975 mg.	Yellow	Round	Easprin	100
Aspirin 800 mg. Tablets (C.T.) (R)					
824-02	800 mg.	White	Capsule-Shaped	Zorprin	100
Benztropine Mesylate Tablets (C.T.) (R)					
827-02	0.5 mg.	White	Round	Cogentin	100
828-02	1 mg.	White	Oval	Cogentin	100
828-05					1000
829-02	2 mg.	White	Round	Cogentin	100
829-05					1000
Duradrin Capsules (R)					
364-02	—	Scarlet & White	Capsule	Midrin	100
Duratex Capsules (R)					
293-02	—	Orange & Beige	Capsule	Entex	100
Iodur w/Codeine Liquid (R) (C-V)					
705-57		Red		Tussi-Organidin Liquid	Pint
705-59					Gal
Iodur DM Liquid (R)					
706-57		Yellow		Tussi-Organidin DM Liquid	Pint
706-59					Gal
Iodur Elixir Liquid (R)					
707-57		Amber		Organidin Elixir	Pint
Iodur Tablets (R)					
854-02	30 mg.	White	Round, Scored	Organidin	100
854-04					500
Isoniazid Tablets (R)					
274-02	100 mg.	White	Round, Scored	Isoniazid	100
274-05					1000
277-30	300 mg.	White	Round, Scored	Isoniazid	30
277-02					100
277-05					1000
Methylprednisolone Tablets (C.T.) (R)					
301-02	4 mg.	White	Oval, scored	Medrol	100
301-21					21 pk
Metoclopramide Tablets (C.T.) (R)					
834-02	5 mg.	White	Round	Reglan	100
834-04					500
Phenylpropanolamine HCl & Guaifenesin Long Acting Tablets (C.T.) (R)					
295-02	75/	Blue	Oval shaped, scored	Entex L.A.	100
295-04	400 mg.				500
Salsalate Tablets (F.C.) (R)					
296-02	500 mg.	Blue	Round	Disalcid	100
296-04					500
297-02	750 mg.	Blue	Capsule shaped, scored	Disalcid	100
297-04					500
Tricosal Tablets (C.T.) (R)					
832-02	500 mg.	White	Oval, scored	Trilisate	100
833-02	750 mg.	White	Oval, scored	Trilisate	100
Triotann Liquid (R)					
713-57	—	Med. Pink		Rynatan	pint
Triotann-S Pediatric Suspension (R)					
743-55	—	Med. Pink		Rynatan-S	4×4 oz.
Triotann (S.C.) (R)					
825-02	—	Buff	Capsule shaped	Rynatan	100

Products are cross-indexed by
generic and chemical names
in the
YELLOW SECTION.

Eastman Kodak Company
Dental Products
Health Sciences Division
343 STATE STREET
ROCHESTER, NEW YORK 14650

CARBOCAINE®   R
hydrochloride 3% Injection
(mepivacaine hydrochloride
injection, USP)
CARBOCAINE®   R
hydrochloride 2%
with **NEO–COBEFRIN®**
1:20,000 Injection
(mepivacaine hydrochloride
and levonordefrin injection, USP)

THESE SOLUTIONS ARE INTENDED FOR DENTAL USE ONLY.

DESCRIPTION

CARBOCAINE hydrochloride (mepivacaine hydrochloride), a tertiary amine used as a local anesthetic, is 1-methyl-2', 6'-pipecoloxylidide monohydrochloride with the following structural formula:

It is a white, crystalline, odorless powder soluble in water, but very resistant to both acid and alkaline hydrolysis.
Neo-Cobefrin (levonordefrin), a sympathomimetic amine used as a vasoconstrictor in local anesthetic solutions, is (−)-α-(1-Aminoethyl)-3, 4-dihydroxybenzyl alcohol with the following structural formula:

It is a white or buff-colored crystalline solid, freely soluble in aqueous solutions of mineral acids, but practically insoluble in water.
DENTAL CARTRIDGES MAY NOT BE AUTOCLAVED.
CARBOCAINE hydrochloride 3% Injection and CARBOCAINE hydrochloride 2% with Neo-Cobefrin 1:20,000 Injection are sterile solutions for injection.

COMPOSITION	CARTRIDGE	
Each mL contains:	2%	3%
mepivacaine hydrochloride	20 mg	30 mg
levonordefrin	0.05 mg	—
sodium chloride	4.0 mg	3.0 mg
acetone sodium bisulfite not more than	2.0 mg	—
water for injection, qs ad	1.0 mL	1.0 mL

The pH of the 2% cartridge solution is adjusted between 3.3 and 5.5 with NaOH or HCl.
The pH of the 3% cartridge solution is adjusted between 4.5 and 6.8 with NaOH or HCl.

CLINICAL PHARMACOLOGY

CARBOCAINE stabilizes the neuronal membrane and prevents the initiation and transmission of nerve impulses, thereby effecting local anesthesia.
CARBOCAINE is rapidly metabolized, with only a small percentage of the anesthetic (5 to 10 percent) being excreted unchanged in the urine. CARBOCAINE, because of its amide structure, is not detoxified by the circulating plasma esterases. The liver is the principal site of metabolism, with over 50 percent of the administered dose being excreted into the bile as metabolites. Most of the metabolized mepivacaine is probably resorbed in the intestine and then excreted into the urine since only a small percentage is found in the feces. The principal route of excretion is via the kidney. Most of the anesthetic and its metabolites are eliminated within 30 hours. It has been shown that hydroxylation and N-demethylation, which are detoxification reactions, play important roles in the metabolism of the anesthetic. Three metabolites of mepivacaine have been identified from adult humans: two phenols, which are excreted almost exclusively as their glucuronide conjugates, and the N-demethylated compound (2',6'-pipecoloxylidide).
The onset of action is rapid (30 to 120 seconds in the upper jaw; 1 to 4 minutes in the lower jaw) and CARBOCAINE hydrochloride 3% without vasoconstrictor will ordinarily provide operating anesthesia of 20 minutes in the upper jaw and 40 minutes in the lower jaw.

Continued on next page

Eastman Kodak—Cont.

CARBOCAINE hydrochloride 2% with Neo-Cobefrin 1:20,000 provides anesthesia of longer duration for more prolonged procedures, 1 hour to 2.5 hours in the upper jaw and 2.5 hours to 5.5 hours in the lower jaw.
CARBOCAINE does not ordinarily produce irritation or tissue damage.
Neo-Cobefrin is a sympathomimetic amine used as a vasoconstrictor in local anesthetic solutions. It has pharmacologic activity similar to that of epinephrine but it is more stable than epinephrine. In equal concentrations, Neo-Cobefrin is less potent than epinephrine in raising blood pressure, and as a vasoconstrictor.

INDICATIONS AND USAGE

CARBOCAINE is indicated for production of local anesthesia for dental procedures by infiltration or nerve block in adults and children.

CONTRAINDICATIONS

Mepivacaine is contraindicated in patients with a known hypersensitivity to amide-type local anesthetics.

WARNINGS

RESUSCITATIVE EQUIPMENT AND DRUGS SHOULD BE IMMEDIATELY AVAILABLE. (See Adverse Reactions.)
Reactions resulting in fatality have occurred on rare occasions with the use of local anesthetics, even in the absence of a history of hypersensitivity.
Fatalities may occur with use of local anesthetics in the head and neck region as the result of retrograde arterial flow to vital CNS areas even when maximum recommended doses are observed. The practitioner should be alert to early evidences of alteration in sensorium or vital signs.
The solution which contains a vasoconstrictor should be used with extreme caution for patients whose medical history and physical evaluation suggest the existence of hypertension, arteriosclerotic heart disease, cerebral vascular insufficiency, heart block, thyrotoxicosis and diabetes, etc.
CARBOCAINE hydrochloride 2% with Neo-Cobefrin 1:20,000 injection (mepivacaine hydrochloride and levonordefrin injection, USP) contains acetone sodium bisulfite, a sulfite that may cause allergic-type reactions including anaphylactic symptoms and life-threatening or less severe asthmatic episodes in certain susceptible people. The overall prevalence of sulfite sensitivity in the general population is unknown and probably low. Sulfite sensitivity is seen more frequently in asthmatic than in nonasthmatic people.
CARBOCAINE hydrochloride 3% injection (mepivacaine hydrochloride injection, USP) IS SULFITE FREE.

PRECAUTIONS

The safety and effectiveness of mepivacaine depend upon proper dosage, correct technique, adequate precautions, and readiness for emergencies.
The lowest dose that results in effective anesthesia should be used to avoid high plasma levels and possible adverse effects.
Injection of repeated doses of mepivacaine may cause significant increase in blood levels with each repeated dose due to slow accumulation of the drug or its metabolites, or due to slower metabolic degradation than normal.
Tolerance varies with the status of the patient. Debilitated, elderly patients, acutely ill patients, and children should be given reduced doses commensurate with their weight and physical status.
Mepivacaine should be used with caution in patients with a history of severe disturbances of cardiac rhythm or heart block.
INJECTIONS SHOULD ALWAYS BE MADE SLOWLY WITH ASPIRATION TO AVOID INTRAVASCULAR INJECTION AND THEREFORE SYSTEMIC REACTION TO BOTH LOCAL ANESTHETIC AND VASOCONSTRICTOR.
If sedatives are employed to reduce patient apprehension, use reduced doses, since local anesthetic agents, like sedatives, are central nervous system depressants which in combination may have an additive effect. Young children should be given minimal doses of each agent.
Changes in sensorium such as excitation, disorientation, drowsiness, may be early indications of a high blood level of the drug and may occur following inadvertent intravascular administration or rapid absorption of mepivacaine.
Local anesthetic procedures should be used with caution when there is inflammation and/or sepsis in the region of the proposed injection.
Information for Patients: The patient should be cautioned against loss of sensation and possibility of biting trauma should the patient attempt to eat or chew gum prior to return of sensation.
Clinically Significant Drug Interactions: The administration of local anesthetic solutions containing vasopressors, such as Neo-Cobefrin (levonordefrin), epinephrine or norepinephrine, to patients receiving tricyclic antidepressants or monoamine oxidase inhibitors *may* produce severe, prolonged hypertension. Concurrent use of these agents should generally be avoided. In situations when concurrent therapy is necessary, careful patient monitoring is essential.
Concurrent administration of vasopressor drugs and of ergot-type oxytocic drugs may cause severe, persistent hypertension or cerebrovascular accidents.
Phenothiazines and butyrophenones may reduce or reverse the pressor effect of epinephrine.
Solutions containing a vasoconstrictor should be used cautiously in the presence of diseases which may adversely affect the patient's cardiovascular system. Serious cardiac arrhythmias may occur if preparations containing a vasoconstrictor are employed in patients during or following the administration of potent inhalation anesthetics.
Mepivacaine SHOULD BE USED WITH CAUTION IN PATIENTS WITH KNOWN DRUG ALLERGIES AND SENSITIVITIES. A thorough history of the patient's prior experience with mepivacaine or other local anesthetics as well as concomitant or recent drug use should be taken (see Contraindications). Patients allergic to methylparaben or para-aminobenzoic acid derivatives (procaine, tetracaine, benzocaine, etc) have not shown cross-sensitivity to agents of the amide-type such as mepivacaine. Since mepivacaine is metabolized in the liver and excreted by the kidneys, it should be used cautiously in patients with liver and renal disease.
Carcinogenesis, Mutagenesis, Impairment of Fertility: Studies of CARBOCAINE hydrochloride, brand of mepivacaine hydrochloride injection, in animals to evaluate the carcinogenic and mutagenic potential or the effect on fertility have not been conducted.
Pregnancy Category C: Animal reproduction studies have not been conducted with this solution. It is also not known whether this solution can cause fetal harm when administered to a pregnant woman or can affect reproduction capacity. This solution should be given to a pregnant woman only if clearly needed.
Nursing Mothers: It is not known whether this drug is excreted in human milk. Because many drugs are excreted in human milk, caution should be exercised when this solution is administered to a nursing woman.
Pediatric Use: Great care must be exercised in adhering to safe concentrations and dosages for pedodontic administration (see Dosage and Administration).

ADVERSE REACTIONS

Systemic adverse reactions involving the central nervous system and the cardiovascular system usually result from high plasma levels due to excessive dosage, rapid absorption, or inadvertent intravascular injection.
A small number of reactions may result from hypersensitivity, idiosyncrasy, or diminished tolerance to normal dosage on the part of the patient.
Reactions involving the *central nervous system* are characterized by excitation and/or depression. Nervousness, dizziness, blurred vision, or tremors may occur followed by drowsiness, convulsions, unconsciousness, and possibly respiratory arrest. Since excitement may be transient or absent, the first manifestations may be drowsiness merging into unconsciousness and respiratory arrest.
Cardiovascular reactions are depressant. They may be the result of direct drug effect or more commonly in dental practice, the result of vasovagal reaction, particularly if the patient is in the sitting position. Failure to recognize premonitory signs such as sweating, feeling of faintness, changes in pulse or sensorium may result in progressive cerebral hypoxia and seizure or serious cardiovascular catastrophe. Management consists of placing the patient in the recumbent position and administration of oxygen. Vasoactive drugs such as ephedrine or methoxamine may be administered intravenously.
Allergic reactions are rare and may occur as a result of sensitivity to the local anesthetic and are characterized by cutaneous lesions of delayed onset or urticaria, edema, and other manifestations of allergy. The detection of sensitivity by skin testing is of limited value. As with other local anesthetics, anaphylactoid reactions to CARBOCAINE have occurred rarely. The reaction may be abrupt and severe and is not usually dose related. Localized puffiness and swelling may occur.

OVERDOSAGE

Treatment of a patient with toxic manifestations consists of assuring and maintaining a patent airway and supporting ventilation (respiration) as required. This usually will be sufficient in the management of most reactions. Should a convulsion persist despite ventilatory therapy, small increments of anticonvulsive agents may be given intravenously, such as benzodiazepine (eg, diazepam) or ultrashort-acting barbiturates (eg, thiopental or thiamylal) or short-acting barbiturates (eg, pentobarbital or secobarbital). Cardiovascular depression may require circulatory assistance with intravenous fluids and/or vasopressor (eg, ephedrine) as dictated by the clinical situation. Allergic reactions should be managed by conventional means.
IV and SC LD_{50}'s in mice for CARBOCAINE hydrochloride, brand of mepivacaine hydrochloride injection, 3% are 33 and 258 mg/kg respectively. The acute IV and SC LD_{50}'s in mice for CARBOCAINE hydrochloride 2% with Neo-Cobefrin 1:20,000 are 30 and 184 mg/kg respectively.

DOSAGE AND ADMINISTRATION

As with all local anesthetics, the dose varies and depends upon the area to be anesthetized, the vascularity of the tissues, individual tolerance and the technique of anesthesia. The lowest dose needed to provide effective anesthesia should be administered. For specific techniques and procedures, refer to standard dental manuals and textbooks.
For infiltration and block injections in the upper or lower jaw, the average dose of 1 cartridge will usually suffice.
Each cartridge contains 1.8 mL (36 mg of 2% or 54 mg of 3%). Five cartridges (180 mg of the 2% solution or 270 mg of the 3% solution) are usually adequate to affect anesthesia of the entire oral cavity. Whenever a larger dose seems to be necessary for an extensive procedure, the maximum dose should be calculated according to that patient's weight. A dose of up to 3 mg per pound of body weight may be administered. At any single dental sitting the total dose for all injected sites should not exceed 400 mg in adults.
The maximum pediatric dose should be *carefully calculated.*
Maximum Dose for Children =

$$\frac{\text{Child's Weight (lb)}}{150} \times \text{Maximum Recommended Dose for Adults (400 mg)}$$

The following table, approximating these calculations, may also be used as a guide. This table is based upon a recommended maximum for larger children of 5 cartridges (the maximum recommended adult dose) during any single dental sitting, regardless of the child's weight or (for 2% mepivacaine) calculated maximum amount of drug:
[See table at left.]
When using CARBOCAINE for infiltration or regional block anesthesia, injection should always be made slowly and with frequent aspiration.
Any unused portion of a cartridge should be discarded.
Parenteral drug products should be inspected visually for particulate matter and discoloration prior to administration, whenever solution and container permit.

DISINFECTION OF CARTRIDGES

As in the case of any cartridge, the diaphragm should be disinfected before needle puncture. The diaphragm should be thoroughly swabbed with either pure 91% isopropyl alcohol or 70% ethyl alcohol, USP, just prior to use. Many commercially available alcohol solutions contain ingredients which are injurious to container components, and therefore, should not be used. Cartridges should not be immersed in any solution.

Maximum Allowable Dosage

	3% Mepivacaine (Plain)		2% Mepivacaine 1:20,000 Levonordefrin	
	3 mg/lb (270 mg max.)		3 mg/lb (180 mg max.)	
Weight (lb)	Mg	Number of Cartridges	Mg	Number of Cartridges
20	60	1.1	60	1.6
30	90	1.7	90	2.5
40	120	2.2	120	3.3
50	150	2.8	150	4.2
60	180	3.3	180	5.0
80	240	4.4	180	5.0
100	270	5.0	180	5.0
120	270	5.0	180	5.0

Adapted from Malamed, Stanley F: Handbook of medical emergencies in the dental office, ed. 2, St. Louis, 1982. The C.V. Mosby Co.

HOW SUPPLIED

Both formulas are available in 1.8 mL cartridges, containers of 50, to fit the Carpule® Aspirator.

The 2% solution should be stored at controlled room temperature, between 15°C and 30°C (59°F and 86°F). **Protect from light.**

The 2% solution is not to be used if its color is pinkish or darker than slightly yellow or if it contains a precipitate.

CAT 144 9313	2% solution
Code 7101	NDC 58472-010-04
CAT 163 3130	3% solution
Code 7201	NDC 58472-020-04

Cook-Waite

Marketed by Eastman Kodak Company, Dental Products
Mfd. by Sterling Drug Inc., New York, NY 10016

Carbocaine, Carpule, Cook-Waite, and Neo-Cobefrin are the registered trademarks of Sterling Drug Inc.

Revised December 1991

For full prescribing information on the medical use of CARBOCAINE, see Sanofi Winthrop Pharmaceuticals product listing in this publication.

MARCAINE® hydrochloride 0.5% ℞
with epinephrine 1:200,000 (as bitartrate)
brand of bupivacaine and epinephrine injection, USP
THIS SOLUTION IS INTENDED FOR DENTAL USE.

DESCRIPTION

Bupivacaine hydrochloride is 1-butyl-2′, 6′-pipecoloxylidide hydrochloride, a white crystalline powder that is freely soluble in 95 per cent ethanol, soluble in water, and slightly soluble in chloroform or acetone. It has the following structural formula:

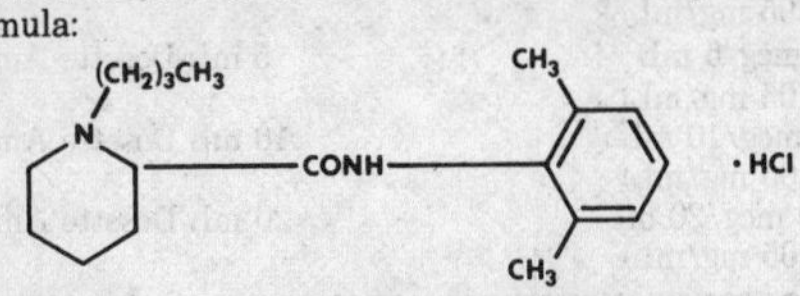

Epinephrine is (-)-3,4-Dihydroxy-α-[(methylamino)methyl] benzyl alcohol. It has the following structural formula:

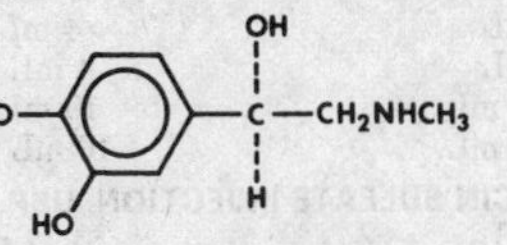

MARCAINE is available in a sterile isotonic solution with epinephrine (as bitartrate) 1:200,000. Solutions of MARCAINE containing epinephrine may not be autoclaved.

MARCAINE is related chemically and pharmacologically to the aminoacyl local anesthetics. It is a homologue of mepivacaine and is chemically related to lidocaine. All three of these anesthetics contain an amide linkage between the aromatic nucleus and the amino or piperidine group. They differ in this respect from the procaine-type local anesthetics, which have an ester linkage.

CLINICAL PHARMACOLOGY

MARCAINE stabilizes the neuronal membrane and prevents the initiation and transmission of nerve impulses, thereby effecting local anesthesia.

The onset of action following dental injections is usually 2 to 10 minutes and anesthesia may last two or three times longer than lidocaine and mepivacaine for dental use, in many patients up to 7 hours. The duration of anesthetic effect is prolonged by the addition of epinephrine 1:200,000. It has also been noted that there is a period of analgesia that persists after the return of sensation, during which time the need for strong analgesic is reduced.

After injection of MARCAINE for caudal, epidural, or peripheral nerve block in man, peak levels of MARCAINE in the blood are reached in 30 to 45 minutes, followed by a decline to insignificant levels during the next three to six hours. Because of its amide structure, MARCAINE is not detoxified by plasma esterases but is detoxified, via conjugation with glucuronic acid, in the liver. When administered in recommended doses and concentrations, MARCAINE does not ordinarily produce irritation or tissue damage, and does not cause methemoglobinemia.

Systemic absorption of local anesthetics produces effects on the cardiovascular and central nervous systems (CNS). At blood concentrations achieved with normal therapeutic doses, changes in cardiac conduction, excitability, refractoriness, contractility, and peripheral vascular resistance are minimal. However, toxic blood concentrations depress cardiac conduction and excitability, which may lead to atrioventricular block, ventricular arrhythmias, and cardiac arrest, sometimes resulting in fatalities. In addition, myocardial contractility is depressed and peripheral vasodilation occurs, leading to decreased cardiac output and arterial blood pressure. Recent clinical reports and animal research suggest that these cardiovascular changes are more likely to occur after unintended intravascular injection of bupivacaine. Therefore, incremental dosing is necessary.

Following systemic absorption, local anesthetics can produce central nervous system stimulation, depression, or both. Apparent central stimulation is manifested as restlessness, tremors and shivering progressing to convulsions, followed by depression and coma progressing ultimately to respiratory arrest. However, the local anesthetics have a primary depressant effect on the medulla and on higher centers. The depressed stage may occur without a prior excited state.

INDICATIONS AND USAGE

MARCAINE is indicated for the production of local anesthesia for dental procedures by infiltration injection or nerve block in adults.

MARCAINE is not recommended for children.

CONTRAINDICATION

MARCAINE is contraindicated in patients with a known hypersensitivity to it or to any local anesthetic agent of the amide-type or to other components of solutions of MARCAINE.

WARNINGS

LOCAL ANESTHETICS SHOULD BE EMPLOYED ONLY BY CLINICIANS WHO ARE WELL VERSED IN DIAGNOSIS AND MANAGEMENT OF DOSE-RELATED TOXICITY AND OTHER ACUTE EMERGENCIES WHICH MIGHT ARISE FROM THE BLOCK TO BE EMPLOYED, AND THEN ONLY AFTER INSURING THE *IMMEDIATE* AVAILABILITY OF OXYGEN, OTHER RESUSCITATIVE DRUGS, CARDIOPULMONARY RESUSCITATIVE EQUIPMENT, AND THE PERSONNEL RESOURCES NEEDED FOR PROPER MANAGEMENT OF TOXIC REACTIONS AND RELATED EMERGENCIES. (See also ADVERSE REACTIONS and PRECAUTIONS.) DELAY IN PROPER MANAGEMENT OF DOSE-RELATED TOXICITY, UNDERVENTILATION FROM ANY CAUSE, AND/OR ALTERED SENSITIVITY MAY LEAD TO THE DEVELOPMENT OF ACIDOSIS, CARDIAC ARREST AND, POSSIBLY, DEATH.

Small doses of local anesthetics injected into the head and neck area, as small as nine to eighteen milligrams, may produce adverse reactions similar to systemic toxicity seen with unintentional intravascular injections of larger doses. Confusion, convulsions, respiratory depression, and/or respiratory arrest, cardiovascular stimulation or depression and cardiac arrest have been reported. Reactions resulting in fatalities have occurred on rare occasions. In a few cases, resuscitation has been difficult or impossible despite apparently adequate preparation and appropriate management. These reactions may be due to intra-arterial injection of the local anesthetic with retrograde flow to the cerebral circulation. Patients receiving these blocks should have their circulation and respiration monitored and be constantly observed. Resuscitative equipment and personnel for treating adverse reactions should be immediately available. Dosage recommendations should not be exceeded (see DOSAGE AND ADMINISTRATION).

It is essential that aspiration for blood or cerebrospinal fluid (where applicable) be done prior to injecting any local anesthetic, both the original dose and all subsequent doses, to avoid intravascular injection. However, a negative aspiration does *not* ensure against an intravascular injection.

Reactions resulting in fatality have occurred on rare occasions with the use of local anesthetics, even in the absence of a history of hypersensitivity.

This solution which contains a vasoconstrictor should be used with extreme caution for patients whose medical history and physical evaluation suggest the existence of hypertension, arteriosclerotic heart disease, cerebral vascular insufficiency, heart block, thyrotoxicosis and diabetes, etc, as well as patients receiving drugs likely to produce alterations in blood pressure.

MARCAINE with epinephrine 1:200,000 or other vasopressors should not be used concomitantly with ergot-type oxytocic drugs, because a severe persistent hypertension may occur. Likewise, solutions of MARCAINE containing a vasoconstrictor, such as epinephrine, should be used with extreme caution in patients receiving monoamine oxidase inhibitors (MAOI) or antidepressants of the triptyline or imipramine types, because severe prolonged hypertension may result.

Until further experience is gained in children younger than 12 years, administration of MARCAINE in this age group is not recommended.

Contains sodium metabisulfite, a sulfite that may cause allergic-type reactions including anaphylactic symptoms and life-threatening or less severe asthmatic episodes in certain susceptible people. The overall prevalence of sulfite sensitivity in the general population is unknown and probably low. Sulfite sensitivity is seen more frequently in asthmatic than in nonasthmatic people.

PRECAUTIONS

The safety and effectiveness of local anesthetics depend upon proper dosage, correct technique, adequate precautions, and readiness for emergencies.

The lowest dosage that gives effective anesthesia should be used in order to avoid high plasma levels and serious systemic side effects. Injection of repeated doses of MARCAINE may cause significant increase in blood levels with each additional dose, due to accumulation of the drug or its metabolites or due to slow metabolic degradation. Tolerance varies with the status of the patient. Debilitated, elderly patients and acutely ill patients should be given reduced doses commensurate with age and physical condition.

Because of the long duration of anesthesia, when MARCAINE 0.5% with epinephrine, brand of bupivacaine and epinephrine injection, is used for dental injections, patients should be cautioned about the possibility of inadvertent trauma to tongue, lips, and buccal mucosa and advised not to chew solid foods or test the anesthetized area by biting or probing.

Changes in sensorium such as excitation, disorientation, drowsiness, may be early indications of a high blood level of the drug and may occur following inadvertent intravascular administration or rapid absorption of MARCAINE.

Solutions containing a vasoconstrictor should be used cautiously in areas with limited blood supply, in the presence of diseases that may adversely affect the patient's cardiovascular system, or in patients with peripheral vascular disease.

Caution is advised in administration of repeat doses of MARCAINE to patients with severe liver disease.

Local anesthetic procedures should be used with caution when there is inflammation and/or sepsis in the region of the proposed injection.

Drug Interactions: See WARNINGS concerning solutions containing a vasoconstrictor.

If sedatives are employed to reduce patient apprehension, use reduced doses, since local anesthetic agents, like sedatives, are central nervous system depressants which in combination may have an additive effect.

MARCAINE should be used cautiously in persons with known drug allergies or sensitivities, particularly to the amide-type local anesthetics.

Serious dose-related cardiac arrhythmias may occur if preparations containing a vasoconstrictor such as epinephrine are employed in patients during or following the administration of chloroform, halothane, cyclopropane, trichloroethylene, or other related agents. In deciding whether to use these products concurrently in the same patient, the combined action of both agents upon the myocardium, the concentration and volume of vasoconstrictor used, and the time since injection, when applicable, should be taken into account.

INFORMATION FOR PATIENTS: When appropriate, the dentist should discuss information including adverse reactions in the package insert for MARCAINE, brand of bupivacaine.

Clinically Significant Drug Interactions: The administration of local anesthetic solutions containing epinephrine or norepinephrine to patients receiving monoamine oxidase inhibitors or tricyclic antidepressants may produce severe, prolonged hypertension. Concurrent use of these agents should generally be avoided. In situations when concurrent therapy is necessary, careful patient monitoring is essential.

Concurrent administration of vasopressor drugs and of ergot-type oxytocic drugs may cause severe, persistent hypertension or cerebrovascular accidents.

Phenothiazines and butyrophenones may reduce or reverse the pressor effect of epinephrine.

Carcinogenesis, Mutagenesis, Impairment of Fertility: Long-term studies in animals of most local anesthetics including bupivacaine to evaluate the carcinogenic potential have not been conducted. Mutagenic potential or the effect on fertility has not been determined. There is no evidence from human data that MARCAINE may be carcinogenic or mutagenic or that it impairs fertility.

Pregnancy Category C: Decreased pup survival in rats and an embryocidal effect in rabbits have been observed when bupivacaine hydrochloride was administered to these species in doses comparable to nine and five times respectively the maximum recommended daily human dose (400 mg). There are no adequate and well-controlled studies in pregnant women of the effect of bupivacaine on the developing fetus. Bupivacaine hydrochloride should be used during pregnancy only if the potential benefit justifies the potential risk to the fetus. This does not exclude the use of MARCAINE at term for obstetrical anesthesia or analgesia.

Nursing Mothers: It is not known whether local anesthetic drugs are excreted in human milk. Because many drugs are excreted in human milk, caution should be exercised when local anesthetics are administered to a nursing woman.

Continued on next page

Eastman Kodak—Cont.

Pediatric Use: Until further experience is gained in children younger than 12 years, administration of MARCAINE in this age group is not recommended.

ADVERSE REACTIONS

Reactions to MARCAINE are characteristic of those associated with other amide-type local anesthetics. A major cause of adverse reactions to this group of drugs is excessive plasma levels, which may be due to overdosage, inadvertent intravascular injection, or slow metabolic degradation.

Excessive plasma levels of the amide-type local anesthetics cause systemic reactions involving the central nervous system and the cardiovascular system. The *central nervous system effects* are characterized by excitation or depression. The first manifestation may be nervousness, dizziness, blurred vision, or tremors, followed by drowsiness, convulsions, unconsciousness, and possibly respiratory arrest. Since excitement may be transient or absent, the first manifestation may be drowsiness, sometimes merging into unconsciousness and respiratory arrest. Other central nervous system effects may be nausea, vomiting, chills, constriction of the pupils, or tinnitus. The *cardiovascular manifestations* of excessive plasma levels may include depression of the myocardium, blood pressure changes (usually hypotension), and cardiac arrest. *Allergic reactions,* which may be due to hypersensitivity, idiosyncrasy, or diminished tolerance, are characterized by cutaneous lesions (eg, urticaria), edema, and other manifestations of allergy. Detection of sensitivity by skin testing is of doubtful value.

Transient facial swelling and puffiness may occur near the injection site.

Treatment of Reactions: Toxic effects of local anesthetics require symptomatic treatment; there is no specific cure. The dentist should be prepared to maintain an airway and to support ventilation with oxygen and assisted or controlled respiration as required. Supportive treatment of the cardiovascular system includes intravenous fluids and, when appropriate, vasopressors (preferably those that stimulate the myocardium). Convulsions may be controlled with oxygen and intravenous administration, in small increments, of a barbiturate, as follows: preferably, an ultrashort-acting barbiturate such as thiopental or thiamylal; if this is not available, a short-acting barbiturate (eg, secobarbital or pentobarbital) or diazepam. Intravenous barbiturates or anticonvulsant agents should only be administered by those familiar with their use.

DOSAGE AND ADMINISTRATION

As with all local anesthetics, the dosage varies and depends upon the area to be anesthetized, the vascularity of the tissues, the number of neuronal segments to be blocked, individual tolerance, and the technique of anesthesia. The lowest dosage needed to provide effective anesthesia should be administered. For specific techniques and procedures, refer to standard textbooks.

The 0.5% concentration with epinephrine is recommended for infiltration and block injection in the maxillary and mandibular area when a longer duration of local anesthetic action is desired, such as for oral surgical procedures generally associated with significant postoperative pain. The average dose of 1.8 mL (9 mg) per injection site will usually suffice; an occasional second dose of 1.8 mL (9 mg) may be used if necessary to produce adequate anesthesia after making allowance for 2 to 10 minutes onset time (see Clinical Pharmacology). The lowest effective dose should be employed and time should be allowed between injections; it is recommended that the total dose for all injection sites, *spread out* over a single dental sitting, should not ordinarily exceed 90 mg for a healthy adult patient (ten 1.8 mL injections of 0.5% MARCAINE with epinephrine, brand of bupivacaine and epinephrine injection). Injections should be made slowly and with frequent aspirations. Until further experience is gained, MARCAINE in dentistry is not recommended for children younger than 12 years.

Parenteral drug products should be inspected visually for particulate matter and discoloration prior to administration, whenever solution and container permit.

HOW SUPPLIED

Store at 25°C. May be stored for brief periods during shipment at temperatures not to exceed 30°C.

0.5% MARCAINE hydrochloride with epinephrine 1:200,000 (as bitartrate)—Sterile isotonic solutions containing sodium chloride. Each 1 mL contains 5 mg bupivacaine hydrochloride and 0.0091 mg epinephrine bitartrate, with 0.5 mg sodium metabisulfite, 0.001 mL monothioglycerol, and 2 mg ascorbic acid as antioxidants, 0.0017 mL 60% sodium lactate buffer, and 0.1 mg edetate calcium disodium as stabilizer. The pH of these solutions is adjusted with sodium hydroxide or hydrochloric acid. Solutions of MARCAINE that contain epinephrine should not be autoclaved and should be protected from light. Do not use the solution if its color is pinkish or darker than slightly yellow or if it contains a precipitate.

This solution is available in 1.8 mL cartridges, containers of 50, to fit the Carpule® Aspirator.

CAT 187 8297 Code 6301 **NDC 58472-230-50**

Cook-Waite

Marketed by Eastman Kodak Company, Dental Products
Mfd. by Sterling Drug Inc., New York, NY 10016

Carpule, Cook-Waite, and Marcaine are the registered trademarks of Sterling Drug Inc.

Revised November 1990

For full prescribing information on the medical use of MARCAINE, see Sanofi Winthrop Pharmaceuticals product listing in this publication.

Elder Pharmaceuticals Inc.

See ICN PHARMACEUTICALS, INC.

Elkins-Sinn, Inc.

2 ESTERBROOK LANE
CHERRY HILL, NJ 08003-4099

Elkins-Sinn's DOSETTE® line offers a broad spectrum of injectable products in a variety of unit-of-use containers—DOSETTE® vials, DOSETTE® ampuls, DOSETTE® syringes, and DOSETTE® cartridge-needle units. Easily adaptable to any hospital pharmacy set-up, the DOSETTE® system combines easily identifiable, clearly printed product labeling with space-conserving packaging. Each DOSETTE® container is characterized by product name and strength in large, bold-faced type, important usage and storage data, lot identification number, and expiration date.

Elkins-Sinn also produces a vast number of multiple dose vials. Listed below are the major ESI products. For prescribing information on products listed, write to Professional Service, Wyeth-Ayerst Laboratories, P.O. Box 8299, Philadelphia, PA 19101, or contact your local Wyeth-Ayerst representative.

AMIKACIN SULFATE INJECTION, USP

250 mg/mL	2 mL Dosette Vial
250 mg/mL	4 mL Vial

AMINOCAPROIC ACID INJECTION, USP

250 mg/mL	20 mL Multiple Dose Vial

AMINOPHYLLINE INJECTION, USP (Preservative-Free)

250 mg/10 mL	10 mL Single Use Vial
250 mg/10 mL	10 mL Dosette Ampul
500 mg/20 mL	20 mL Single Use Vial
500 mg/20 mL	20 mL Dosette Ampul

ATROPINE SULFATE INJECTION, USP

400 mcg/mL (0.4 mg, 1/150 gr)	1 mL Dosette Vial
400 mcg/mL (0.4 mg, 1/150 gr)	1 mL Dosette Ampul
400 mcg/mL (0.4 mg, 1/150 gr)	20 mL Multiple Dose Vial
1 mg/mL (1/60 gr)	1 mL Dosette Vial

BRETYLIUM TOSYLATE INJECTION (Preservative-Free)

500 mg/10 mL	10 mL Dosette Ampul
500 mg/10 mL	10 mL Single Use Vial

CHLORPROMAZINE HYDROCHLORIDE INJECTION, USP

25 mg/mL	1 mL Dosette Ampul
50 mg/2 mL	2 mL Dosette Ampul

CLINDAMYCIN PHOSPHATE INJECTION, USP

300 mg/2 mL	2 mL Dosette Vial
600 mg/4 mL	4 mL Single Use Vial
900 mg/6 mL	6 mL Single Use Vial
9 gram/60 mL (150 mg/mL)	Pharmacy Bulk Package

CODEINE PHOSPHATE INJECTION, USP ℂII

30 mg/mL	1 mL Dosette Vial
60 mg/mL	1 mL Dosette Vial

CYANOCOBALAMIN INJECTION, USP

1 mg/mL (1000 mcg)	1 mL Dosette Vial
1 mg/mL (1000 mcg)	10 mL Multiple Dose Vial
1 mg/mL (1000 mcg)	30 mL Multiple Dose Vial

CYCLOPHOSPHAMIDE FOR INJECTION, USP (Sterile Powder)

100 mg	Single Use Vial
200 mg	Single Use Vial
500 mg	Single Use Vial
1 gram	Single Use Vial

DEXAMETHASONE SODIUM PHOSPHATE INJECTION, USP

4 mg/mL	1 mL Dosette Vial
4 mg/mL	5 mL Multiple Dose Vial
10 mg/mL	1 mL Dosette Vial
10 mg/mL	10 mL Multiple Dose Vial

DEXTROSE INJECTION, USP

10% (100 mg/mL)	17 mL fill in 20 mL Single Dose Vial

DIAZEPAM INJECTION, USP ℂIV

5 mg/mL	1 mL Dosette Vial
5 mg/mL	10 mL Multiple Dose Vial
5 mg/mL	1 mL Dosette Syringe
10 mg/2 mL	2 mL Dosette Vial
10 mg/2 mL	2 mL Dosette Ampul
10 mg/2 mL	2 mL Dosette Syringe

DIAZEPAM INJECTION, USP ℂIV
DOSETTE CARTRIDGE NEEDLE UNITS

5 mg/mL	1 mL Dosette Cartridge
10 mg/2 mL	2 mL Dosette Cartridge

DIGOXIN INJECTION, USP

500 mcg/2 mL (0.5 mg)	2 mL Dosette Ampul

DIPHENHYDRAMINE HYDROCHLORIDE INJECTION, USP (High Potency)

50 mg/mL	1 mL Dosette Vial

DOPAMINE HYDROCHLORIDE INJECTION, USP

200 mg/5 mL	5 mL Dosette Ampul
200 mg/5 mL	5 mL Single Use Vial
400 mg/5 mL	5 mL Dosette Ampul
400 mg/5 mL	5 mL Single Use Vial

DOXYCYCLINE HYCLATE FOR INJECTION, USP

100 mg	Single Use Vial

DURAMORPH® (Morphine Sulfate Injection, USP) ℂII (Preservative-Free for Epidural & Intrathecal Administration)

5 mg/10 mL (0.5 mg/mL)	10 mL Dosette Ampul
10 mg/10 mL (1 mg/mL)	10 mL Dosette Ampul

EPINEPHRINE INJECTION, USP

1 mg/mL (1:1000)	1 mL Dosette Ampul

ERYTHROMYCIN LACTOBIONATE FOR INJECTION, USP

500 mg	Multiple Dose Vial
500 mg	100 mL Piggyback Vial
1 gram	Multiple Dose Vial

FENTANYL CITRATE INJECTION, USP (Preservative-Free)

100 mcg/2 mL (0.05 mg/mL)	2 mL Dosette Ampul
250 mcg/5 mL (0.05 mg/mL)	5 mL Dosette Ampul
500 mcg/10 mL (0.05 mg/mL)	10 mL Dosette Ampul
1000 mcg/20 mL (0.05 mg/mL)	20 mL Dosette Ampul

FUROSEMIDE INJECTION, USP (Preservative-Free)

20 mg/2 mL	2 mL Dosette Ampul
20 mg/2 mL	2 mL Single Use Vial
40 mg/4 mL	4 mL Dosette Ampul
40 mg/4 mL	4 mL Single Use Vial
100 mg/10 mL	10 mL Dosette Ampul
100 mg/10 mL	10 mL Single Use Vial

GENTAMICIN SULFATE INJECTION, USP

20 mg/2 mL (10 mg/mL—Pediatric)	2 mL Dosette Vial
80 mg/2 mL (40 mg/mL)	2 mL Dosette Vial
800 mg/20 mL (40 mg/mL)	20 mL Multiple Dose Vial

GENTAMICIN SULFATE INJECTION, USP
DOSETTE CARTRIDGE NEEDLE UNITS

60 mg/1.5 mL	1.5 mL Dosette Cartridge
80 mg/2 mL	2 mL Dosette Cartridge

HEPARIN SODIUM INJECTION, USP (Porcine Derived)

1,000 Units/mL	1 mL Dosette Vial
1,000 Units/mL	10 mL Multiple Dose Vial
1,000 Units/mL	30 mL Multiple Dose Vial
5,000 Units/mL	1 mL Dosette Vial
5,000 Units/mL	10 mL Multiple Dose Vial
10,000 Units/mL	1 mL Dosette Vial
10,000 Units/mL	4 mL Multiple Dose Vial

HEPARIN SODIUM INJECTION, USP (Porcine Derived)
DOSETTE CARTRIDGE NEEDLE UNITS

1,000 Units/1 mL	1 mL Dosette Cartridge
5,000 Units/0.5 mL	0.5 mL Dosette Cartridge
5,000 Units/1 mL	1 mL Dosette Cartridge
10,000 Units/1 mL	1 mL Dosette Cartridge

HEP-LOCK® (Heparin Lock Flush Solution, USP)

10 Units/mL	1 mL Dosette Vial
10 Units/mL	2 mL Dosette Vial
10 Units/mL	10 mL Multiple Dose Vial
10 Units/mL	30 mL Multiple Dose Vial
100 Units/mL	1 mL Dosette Vial
100 Units/mL	2 mL Dosette Vial
100 Units/mL	10 mL Multiple Dose Vial
100 Units/mL	30 mL Multiple Dose Vial

HEP-LOCK® (Heparin Lock Flush Solution, USP)
DOSETTE CARTRIDGE NEEDLE UNITS

10 Units/1 mL	1 mL Dosette Cartridge
25 Units/2.5 mL	2.5 mL Dosette Cartridge
100 Units/1 mL	1 mL Dosette Cartridge
250 Units/2.5 mL	2.5 mL Dosette Cartridge

HEP-LOCK®U/P (Preservative-Free Heparin Lock Flush Solution, USP)

10 Units/mL	1 mL Dosette Vial
100 Units/mL	1 mL Dosette Vial

HYDROMORPHONE HYDROCHLORIDE INJECTION, USP[℃]

2 mg/mL	1 mL Dosette Vial
2 mg/mL	20 mL Multiple Dose Vial

HYDROXYZINE HYDROCHLORIDE I.M. INJECTION, USP

25 mg/mL	1 mL Dosette Vial
50 mg/mL	1 mL Dosette Vial
100 mg/2 mL	2 mL Dosette Vial
50 mg/mL	10 mL Multiple Dose Vial

INFUMORPH™ 200
(Preservative-free Morphine Sulfate Sterile Solution)[℃]
For Use in Continuous Microinfusion Devices

200 mg/20 mL (10 mg/mL)	20 mL Dosette Ampul

INFUMORPH™ 500
(Preservative-free Morphine Sulfate Sterile Solution)[℃]
For Use in Continuous Microinfusion Devices

500 mg/20 mL (25 mg/mL)	20 mL Dosette Ampul

ISOPROTERENOL HYDROCHLORIDE INJECTION, USP
(Refrigeration not required)

0.2 mg/mL (1:5000)	5 mL Dosette Ampul

LEUCOVORIN CALCIUM FOR INJECTION (Lyophilized)

50 mg	Single Use Vial

LIDOCAINE HYDROCHLORIDE INJECTION, USP
(Preserved)

1% (10 mg/mL)	30 mL Multiple Dose Vial
1% (10 mg/mL)	50 mL Multiple Dose Vial
2% (20 mg/mL)	30 mL Multiple Dose Vial
2% (20 mg/mL)	50 mL Multiple Dose Vial

LIDOCAINE HYDROCHLORIDE INJECTION, USP
(Preservative-Free, Single Use)

1% (10 mg/mL)	5 mL Single Use Vial
2% (20 mg/mL)	5 mL Single Use Vial

LIDOCAINE HYDROCHLORIDE AND EPINEPHRINE INJECTION, USP   (1:100,000)
(Refrigeration not required)

1% (10 mg/mL)	30 mL Multiple Dose Vial
2% (20 mg/mL)	30 mL Multiple Dose Vial

MEPERIDINE HYDROCHLORIDE INJECTION, USP[℃]

25 mg/mL	1 mL Dosette Vial
25 mg/mL	1 mL Dosette Ampul
50 mg/mL	1 mL Dosette Vial
50 mg/mL	1 mL Dosette Ampul
75 mg/mL	1 mL Dosette Vial
75 mg/mL	1 mL Dosette Ampul
100 mg/mL	1 mL Dosette Vial
100 mg/mL	1 mL Dosette Ampul

METHYLDOPATE HYDROCHLORIDE INJECTION, USP

250 mg/5 mL	5 mL Single Use Vial
500 mg/10 mL	10 mL Single Use Vial

METRONIDAZOLE REDI-INFUSION™
(Preservative-Free, Single Use)

500 mg/100 mL	100 mL Single Use Vial
(5 mg/mL with disposable vented IV infusion set)	
500 mg/100 mL	100 mL Single Use Vial
500 mg/100 mL (5 mg/mL)	100 mL Plastic Bag

MORPHINE SULFATE INJECTION, USP[℃]

1 mg/mL	60 mL Single Use Vial
5 mg/mL (¹/₁₂ gr)	1 mL Dosette Vial
8 mg/mL (¹/₈ gr)	1 mL Dosette Vial
8 mg/mL (¹/₈ gr)	1 mL Dosette Ampul
10 mg/mL (¹/₆ gr)	1 mL Dosette Vial
10 mg/mL (¹/₆ gr)	1 mL Dosette Ampul
10 mg/mL (¹/₆ gr)	10 mL Multiple Dose Vial
15 mg/mL (¹/₄ gr)	1 mL Dosette Vial
15 mg/mL (¹/₄ gr)	1 mL Dosette Ampul
15 mg/mL (¹/₄ gr)	20 mL Multiple Dose Vial

NALOXONE HYDROCHLORIDE INJECTION, USP

400 mcg/mL	1 mL Dosette Vial
(0.4 mg/mL)	
400 mcg/mL	1 mL Dosette Ampul
(0.4 mg/mL)	
400 mcg/mL	10 mL Multiple Dose Vial
(0.4 mg/mL)	

NEOSTIGMINE METHYLSULFATE INJECTION, USP

1:1000 (1 mg/mL)	10 mL Multiple Dose Vial
1:2000 (0.5 mg/mL)	10 mL Multiple Dose Vial

PANCURONIUM BROMIDE INJECTION

1 mg/mL	10 mL Multiple Dose Vial
2 mg/mL	2 mL Dosette Vial
2 mg/mL	2 mL Dosette Ampul
2 mg/mL	5 mL Dosette Ampul
2 mg/mL	5 mL Single Use Vial

PHENOBARBITAL SODIUM INJECTION, USP[℃]

65 mg/mL (1 gr)	1 mL Dosette Vial
130 mg/mL (2 gr)	1 mL Dosette Vial

PHENYLEPHRINE HYDROCHLORIDE INJECTION, USP

10 mg/mL	1 mL Dosette Vial

PHENYTOIN SODIUM INJECTION, USP

100 mg/2 mL (50 mg/mL)	2 mL Dosette Vial
100 mg/2 mL (50 mg/mL)	2 mL Dosette Ampul
250 mg/5 mL (50 mg/mL)	5 mL Single Use Vial
250 mg/5 mL (50 mg/mL)	5 mL Dosette Ampul

PROCAINAMIDE HYDROCHLORIDE INJECTION, USP

100 mg/mL (1 gram/10 mL)	10 mL Multiple Dose Vial
500 mg/mL (1 gram/2 mL)	2 mL Multiple Dose Vial

PROCHLORPERAZINE EDISYLATE INJECTION, USP

10 mg/2 mL	2 mL Dosette Ampul
10 mg/2 mL	2 mL Dosette Vial

PROMETHAZINE HYDROCHLORIDE INJECTION, USP

25 mg/mL	1 mL Dosette Ampul
50 mg/mL	1 mL Dosette Ampul

PROTAMINE SULFATE INJECTION, USP
(Preservative-Free)
(Refrigeration not required)

50 mg/5 mL	5 mL Dosette Ampul
250 mg/25 mL	25 mL Single Use Vial

SODIUM CHLORIDE INJECTION, USP (Preservative-Free, Single Use)

0.9%	2 mL Dosette Vial
0.9%	5 mL Dosette Ampul
0.9%	10 mL Dosette Ampul

SODIUM CHLORIDE INJECTION, BACTERIOSTATIC, USP
(Preserved with 0.9% Benzyl Alcohol)

0.9%	30 mL Multiple Dose Vial
0.9%	2 mL Dosette Cartridge

SODIUM NITROPRUSSIDE, STERILE, USP

50 mg	Single Use Vial

SOTRADECOL® (Sodium Tetradecyl Sulfate Injection)

1%	2 mL Dosette Ampul
3%	2 mL Dosette Ampul

STERILE EMPTY VIAL

20 mL	20 mL Vial

SULFAMETHOXAZOLE & TRIMETHOPRIM CONCENTRATE FOR INJECTION, USP

80 mg/mL Sulfamethoxazole with 16 mg/mL Trimethoprim	5 mL Dosette Ampul
80 mg/mL Sulfamethoxazole with 16 mg/mL Trimethoprim	5 mL Single Use Vial
80 mg/mL Sulfamethoxazole with 16 mg/mL Trimethoprim	10 mL Single Use Vial
80 mg/mL Sulfamethoxazole with 16 mg/mL Trimethoprim	30 mL Multiple Dose Vial

THIAMINE HYDROCHLORIDE INJECTION, USP

100 mg/mL	1 mL Dosette Vial

TOBRAMYCIN SULFATE INJECTION, USP

10 mg/mL	2 mL Multiple Dose Vial
40 mg/mL	2 mL Multiple Dose Vial
40 mg/mL	30 mL Multiple Dose Vial
40 mg/mL	2 mL Dosette Syringe

VANCOMYCIN HYDROCHLORIDE, STERILE, USP

500 mg Vial	
1 gram Vial	

WATER FOR INJECTION, STERILE, USP (Preservative-Free)

	10 mL Dosette Ampul

WATER FOR INJECTION, BACTERIOSTATIC, USP
(Preserved with 0.9% Benzyl Alcohol)

	30 mL Multiple Dose Vial

AMIKACIN   ℞
[ă'mĭ-că-sĭn]
SULFATE INJECTION, USP

WARNINGS

Patients treated with parenteral aminoglycosides should be under close clinical observation because of the potential ototoxicity and nephrotoxicity associated with their use. Safety for treatment periods which are longer than 14 days has not been established.

Neurotoxicity, manifested as vestibular and permanent bilateral auditory ototoxicity, can occur in patients with preexisting renal damage and in patients with normal renal function treated at higher doses and/or for periods longer than those recommended. The risk of aminoglycoside-induced ototoxicity is greater in patients with renal damage. High frequency deafness usually occurs first and can be detected only by audiometric testing. Vertigo may occur and may be evidence of vestibular injury. Other manifestations of neurotoxicity may include numbness, skin tingling, muscle twitching and convulsions. The risk of hearing loss due to aminoglycosides increases with the degree of exposure to either high peak or high trough serum concentrations. Patients developing cochlear damage may not have symptoms during therapy to warn them of developing eighth-nerve toxicity, and total or partial irreversible bilateral deafness may occur after the drug has been discontinued. Aminoglycoside-induced ototoxicity is usually irreversible.

Aminoglycosides are potentially nephrotoxic. The risk of nephrotoxicity is greater in patients with impaired renal function and in those who receive high doses or prolonged therapy.

Neuromuscular blockade and respiratory paralysis have been reported following parenteral injection, topical instillation (as in orthopedic and abdominal irrigation or in local treatment of empyema) and following oral use of aminoglycosides. The possibility of these phenomena should be considered if aminoglycosides are administered by any route, especially in patients receiving anesthetics; neuromuscular blocking agents such as tubocurarine, succinylcholine, decamethonium; or in patients receiving massive transfusions of citrate-anticoagulated blood. If blockage occurs, calcium salts may reverse these phenomena, but mechanical respiratory assistance may be necessary.

Renal and eighth-nerve function should be closely monitored especially in patients with known or suspected renal impairment at the onset of therapy and also in those whose renal function is initially normal but who develop signs of renal dysfunction during therapy. Serum concentrations of amikacin should be monitored when feasible to assure adequate levels and to avoid potentially toxic levels and prolonged peak concentrations above 35 micrograms per mL. Urine should be examined for decreased specific gravity, increased excretion of proteins and the presence of cells or casts. Blood urea nitrogen, serum creatinine or creatinine clearance should be measured periodically. Serial audiograms should be obtained where feasible in patients old enough to be tested, particularly high risk patients. Evidence of ototoxicity (dizziness, vertigo, tinnitus, roaring in the ears and hearing loss) or nephrotoxicity requires discontinuation of the drug or dosage adjustment.

Concurrent and/or sequential systemic, oral or topical use of other neurotoxic or nephrotoxic products, particularly bacitracin, cisplatin, amphotericin B, cephaloridine, paromomycin, viomycin, polymyxin B, colistin, vancomycin or other aminoglycosides should be avoided. Other factors that may increase risk of toxicity are advanced age and dehydration.

The concurrent use of amikacin with potent diuretics (ethacrynic acid or furosemide) should be avoided since diuretics by themselves may cause ototoxicity. In addition, when administered intravenously, diuretics may enhance aminoglycoside toxicity by altering antibiotic concentrations in serum and tissue.

DESCRIPTION

Amikacin sulfate, a semi-synthetic aminoglycoside antibiotic derived from kanamycin, has the following structural formula:

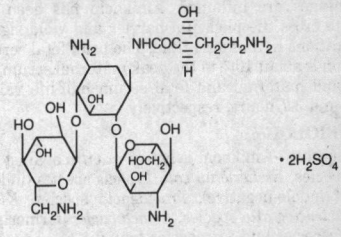

D-Streptamine,   O-3-amino-3-deoxy-α-D-glucopyranosyl-(1→6)-O-[6-amino-6-deoxy-α-D-glucopyranosyl-(1→4)]-N¹-(4-amino-2-hydroxy-1-oxobutyl)-2-deoxy-, (S)-, sulfate (1:2) (salt)

$C_{22}H_{43}N_5O_{13} \cdot 2H_2SO_4$ **Molecular weight 781.75**

The dosage form is supplied as a sterile, colorless to light straw-colored solution for IM or IV use.

Each mL contains 250 mg amikacin as the sulfate, sodium citrate (dihydrate) 28.5 mg and sodium metabisulfite 6.6 mg in Water for Injection. pH 3.5–5.5; sodium hydroxide and/or sulfuric acid added, if needed, for pH adjustment. Sealed under nitrogen.

CLINICAL PHARMACOLOGY
INTRAMUSCULAR ADMINISTRATION

Amikacin is rapidly absorbed after intramuscular administration. In normal adult volunteers, average peak serum concentrations of about 12, 16 and 21 mcg/mL are obtained 1 hour after intramuscular administration of 250 mg (3.7 mg/kg), 375 mg (5 mg/kg), 500 mg (7.5 mg/kg), single doses, respectively. At 10 hours, serum levels are about 0.3 mcg/mL, 1.2 mcg/mL and 2.1 mcg/mL, respectively.

Tolerance studies in normal volunteers reveal that amikacin is well tolerated locally following repeated intramuscular dosing, and when given at maximally recommended doses, no ototoxicity or nephrotoxicity has been reported. There is no evidence of drug accumulation with repeated dosing for 10 days when administered according to recommended doses.

Continued on next page

Elkins-Sinn—Cont.

With normal renal function, about 91.9% of an intramuscular dose is excreted unchanged in the urine in the first 8 hours and 98.2% within 24 hours. Mean urine concentrations for 6 hours are 563 mcg/mL following a 250 mg dose, 697 mcg/mL following a 375 mg dose and 832 mcg/mL following a 500 mg dose.

Preliminary intramuscular studies in newborns of different weights (less than 1.5 kg, 1.5 to 2 kg, over 2 kg) at a dose of 7.5 mg/kg revealed that, like other aminoglycosides, serum half-life values were correlated inversely with post-natal age and renal clearances of amikacin. The volume of distribution indicates that amikacin, like other aminoglycosides, remains primarily in the extracellular fluid space of neonates. Repeated dosing every 12 hours in all the above groups did not demonstrate accumulation after 5 days.

INTRAVENOUS ADMINISTRATION

Single doses of 500 mg (7.5 mg/kg) administered to normal adults as an infusion over a period of 30 minutes produced a mean peak serum concentration of 38 mcg/mL at the end of the infusion and levels of 24 mcg/mL, 18 mcg/mL and 0.75 mcg/mL at 30 minutes, 1 hour and 10 hours post-infusion, respectively. Eighty-four percent of the administered dose was excreted in the urine in 9 hours and about 94% within 24 hours.

Repeat infusions of 7.5 mg/kg every 12 hours in normal adults were well tolerated and caused no drug accumulation.

GENERAL

Pharmacokinetic studies in normal adult subjects reveal the mean serum half-life to be slightly over 2 hours with a mean total apparent volume of distribution of 24 liters (28% of the body weight). By the ultrafiltration technique, reports of serum protein binding range from 0 to 11%. The mean serum clearance rate is about 100 mL/min and the renal clearance rate is 94 mL/min in subjects with normal renal function.

Amikacin is excreted primarily by glomerular filtration. Patients with impaired renal function or diminished glomerular filtration pressure excrete the drug much more slowly (effectively prolonging the serum half-life). Therefore, renal function should be monitored carefully and dosage adjusted accordingly (see suggested dosage schedule under **DOSAGE AND ADMINISTRATION**).

Following administration at the recommended dose, therapeutic levels are found in bone, heart, gallbladder and lung tissue in addition to significant concentrations in urine; bile; sputum; bronchial secretions; interstitial, pleural and synovial fluids.

Spinal fluid levels in normal infants are approximately 10 to 20% of the serum concentrations and may reach 50% when the meninges are inflamed. Amikacin has been demonstrated to cross the placental barrier and yield significant concentrations in amniotic fluid. The peak fetal serum concentration is about 16% of the peak maternal serum concentration and maternal and fetal serum half-life values are about 2 and 3.7 hours, respectively.

MICROBIOLOGY

Gram-negative—Amikacin is active *in vitro* against *Pseudomonas* species, *Escherichia coli, Proteus* species (indole-positive and indole-negative), *Providencia* species, *Klebsiella-Enterobacter-Serratia* species, *Acinetobacter* (formerly *Mima-Herellea*) species and *Citrobacter freundii*.

When strains of the above organisms are found to be resistant to other aminoglycosides, including gentamicin, tobramycin and kanamycin, many are susceptible to amikacin *in vitro*.

Gram-positive—Amikacin is active *in vitro* against penicillinase and non-penicillinase-producing *Staphylococcus* species, including methicillin-resistant strains. However, aminoglycosides in general have a low order of activity against other gram-positive organisms, viz., *Streptococcus pyogenes*, enterococci and *Streptococcus pneumoniae* (formerly *Diplococcus pneumoniae*).

Amikacin resists degradation by most aminoglycoside inactivating enzymes known to affect gentamicin, tobramycin and kanamycin.

In vitro studies have shown that amikacin sulfate combined with a beta-lactam antibiotic acts synergistically against many clinically significant gram-negative organisms.

Disc Susceptibility Tests—Quantitative methods that require measurement of zone diameters give the most precise estimates of antibiotic susceptibility. One such procedure* has been recommended for use with discs to test susceptibility to amikacin. Interpretation involves correlation of the diameters obtained in the disc test with MIC values for amikacin. When the causative organism is tested by the Kirby-Bauer method of disc susceptibility, a 30 mcg amikacin disc should give a zone of 17 mm or greater to indicate susceptibility. Zone sizes of 14 mm or less indicate resistance. Zone sizes of 15 to 16 mm indicate intermediate susceptibility. With this procedure, a report from the laboratory of "susceptible" indicates that the infecting organism is likely to respond to therapy. A report of "resistant" indicates that the infecting organism is not likely to respond to therapy. A report of "intermediate susceptibility" suggests that the organism would be susceptible if the infection is confined to tissues and fluids (e.g., urine) in which high antibiotic levels are attained.

*Bauer, AW; Kirby, WMM; Sherris, JC and Turck, M: Antibiotic Testing by a Standardized Single Disc Method, AM J CLIN PATHOL, 45:493, 1966; Standardized Disc Susceptibility Test, *FEDERAL REGISTER*, 37:20527-29, 1972.

INDICATIONS AND USAGE

Amikacin Sulfate Injection is indicated in the short-term treatment of serious infections due to susceptible strains of gram-negative bacteria, including *Pseudomonas* species, *Escherichia coli*, species of indole-positive and indole-negative *Proteus, Providencia* species, *Klebsiella-Enterobacter-Serratia* species and *Acinetobacter (Mima-Herellea)* species.

Clinical studies have shown Amikacin Sulfate Injection to be effective in bacterial septicemia (including neonatal sepsis); in serious infections of the respiratory tract, bones and joints, central nervous system (including meningitis) and skin and soft tissue; intra-abdominal infections (including peritonitis); and in burns and post-operative infections (including post-vascular surgery). Clinical studies have shown amikacin also to be effective in serious complicated and recurrent urinary tract infections due to these organisms. Aminoglycosides, including amikacin, are not indicated in uncomplicated initial episodes of urinary tract infections unless the causative organisms are not susceptible to antibiotics having less potential toxicity.

Bacteriologic studies should be performed to identify causative organisms and their susceptibilities to amikacin. Amikacin may be considered as initial therapy in suspected gram-negative infections, and therapy may be instituted before obtaining the results of susceptibility testing. Clinical trials demonstrated that amikacin was effective in infections caused by gentamicin- and/or tobramycin-resistant strains of gram-negative organisms, particularly *Proteus rettgeri, Providencia stuartii, Serratia marcescens* and *Pseudomonas aeruginosa*. The decision to continue therapy with the drug should be based on results of the susceptibility tests, the severity of the infection and the response of the patient, as well as important additional considerations (see **WARNINGS** box).

Amikacin has also been shown to be effective in staphylococcal infections and may be considered as initial therapy under certain conditions in the treatment of known or suspected staphylococcal disease such as severe infections where the causative organism may be either a gram-negative bacterium or a staphylococcus, infections due to susceptible strains of staphylococci in patients allergic to other antibiotics and in mixed staphylococcal/gram-negative infections.

In certain severe infections such as neonatal sepsis, concomitant therapy with a penicillin-type drug may be indicated because of the possibility of infections due to gram-positive organisms such as streptococci or pneumococci.

CONTRAINDICATIONS

A history of hypersensitivity to amikacin is a contraindication for its use. A history of hypersensitivity or serious toxic reactions to aminoglycosides may contraindicate the use of any other aminoglycoside because of the known cross-sensitivities of patients to drugs in this class.

WARNINGS

See **WARNINGS** box above.

Aminoglycosides can cause fetal harm when administered to a pregnant woman. Aminoglycosides cross the placenta and there have been several reports of total irreversible, bilateral congenital deafness in children whose mothers received streptomycin during pregnancy. Although serious side effects to the fetus or newborns have not been reported in the treatment of pregnant women with other aminoglycosides, the potential for harm exists. Reproduction studies of amikacin have been performed in rats and mice and revealed no evidence of impaired fertility or harm to the fetus due to amikacin. There are no well-controlled studies in pregnant women, but investigational experience does not include any positive evidence of adverse effects to the fetus. If this drug is used during pregnancy, or if the patient becomes pregnant while taking this drug, the patient should be apprised of the potential hazard to the fetus.

Contains sodium metabisulfite, a sulfite that may cause allergic-type reactions including anaphylactic symptoms and life-threatening or less severe asthmatic episodes in certain susceptible people. The overall prevalence of sulfite sensitivity in the general population is unknown and probably low. Sulfite sensitivity is seen more frequently in asthmatic than nonasthmatic people.

PRECAUTIONS

Aminoglycosides are quickly and almost totally absorbed when they are applied topically, except to the urinary bladder, in association with surgical procedures. Irreversible deafness, renal failure and death due to neuromuscular blockade have been reported following irrigation of both small and large surgical fields with an aminoglycoside preparation.

Amikacin Sulfate Injection is potentially nephrotoxic, ototoxic and neurotoxic. The concurrent or serial use of other ototoxic or nephrotoxic agents should be avoided either systemically or topically because of the potential for additive effects. Increased nephrotoxicity has been reported following concomitant parenteral administration of aminoglycoside antibiotics and cephalosporins. Concomitant cephalosporins may spuriously elevate creatinine determinations.

Since amikacin is present in high concentrations in the renal excretory system, patients should be well-hydrated to minimize chemical irritation of the renal tubules. Kidney function should be assessed by the usual methods prior to starting therapy and daily during the course of treatment.

If signs of renal irritation appear (casts, white or red cells or albumin), hydration should be increased. A reduction in dosage (see **DOSAGE AND ADMINISTRATION**) may be desirable if other evidence of renal dysfunction occurs such as decreased creatinine clearance; decreased urine specific gravity; increased BUN, creatinine or oliguria. If azotemia increases or if a progressive decrease in urinary output occurs, treatment should be stopped.

Note: When patients are well hydrated and kidney function is normal, the risk of nephrotoxic reactions with amikacin is low if the dosage recommendations (see **DOSAGE AND ADMINISTRATION**) are not exceeded.

Elderly patients may have reduced renal function which may not be evident in routine screening tests such as BUN or serum creatinine. A creatinine clearance determination may be more useful. Monitoring of renal function during treatment with aminoglycosides is particularly important.

Aminoglycosides should be used with caution in patients with muscular disorders such as myasthenia gravis or parkinsonism since these drugs may aggravate muscle weakness because of their potential curare-like effect on the neuromuscular junction.

In vitro mixing of aminoglycosides with beta-lactam antibiotics (penicillin or cephalosporins) may result in a significant mutual inactivation. A reduction in serum half-life or serum level may occur when an aminoglycoside or penicillin-type drug is administered by separate routes. Inactivation of the aminoglycoside is clinically significant only in patients with severely impaired renal function. Inactivation may continue in specimens of body fluids collected for assay, resulting in inaccurate aminoglycoside readings. Such specimens should be properly handled (assayed promptly, frozen or treated with beta-lactamase).

Cross-allergenicity among aminoglycosides has been demonstrated.

As with other antibiotics, the use of amikacin may result in overgrowth of non-susceptible organisms. If this occurs, appropriate therapy should be instituted.

Aminoglycosides should not be given concurrently with potent diuretics (see **WARNINGS** box).

CARCINOGENESIS, MUTAGENESIS, IMPAIRMENT OF FERTILITY

Studies in humans have not been performed with the aminoglycosides to determine their effect on carcinogenesis, mutagenesis or impairment of fertility.

PREGNANCY

Pregnancy Category D (see **WARNINGS** section).

NURSING MOTHERS

It is not known whether this drug is excreted in human milk. As a general rule, nursing should not be undertaken while a patient is on a drug since many drugs are excreted in human milk.

PEDIATRIC USE

Aminoglycosides should be used with caution in premature and neonatal infants because of the renal immaturity of these patients and the resulting prolongation of serum half-life of these drugs.

ADVERSE REACTIONS

All aminoglycosides have the potential to induce auditory, vestibular and renal toxicity and neuromuscular blockade (see **WARNINGS** box). They occur more frequently in patients with present or past history of renal impairment, of treatment with other ototoxic or nephrotoxic drugs and in patients treated for longer periods and/or with higher doses than recommended.

Neurotoxicity-Ototoxicity—Toxic effects on the eighth cranial nerve can result in hearing loss, loss of balance or both. Amikacin primarily affects auditory function. Cochlear damage includes high frequency deafness and usually occurs before clinical hearing loss can be detected.

Neurotoxicity-Neuromuscular Blockage—Acute muscular paralysis and apnea can occur following treatment with aminoglycoside drugs.

Nephrotoxicity—Elevation of serum creatinine, albuminuria, presence of red and white cells, casts, azotemia and oliguria have been reported. Renal function changes are usually reversible when the drug is discontinued.

Other—In addition to those described above, other adverse reactions which have been reported on rare occasions are skin rash, drug fever, headache, paresthesia, tremor, nausea and vomiting, eosinophilia, arthralgia, anemia and hypotension.

OVERDOSAGE

In the event of overdosage or toxic reaction, peritoneal dialysis or hemodialysis will aid in the removal of amikacin from the blood. In the newborn infant, exchange transfusion may also be considered.

DOSAGE AND ADMINISTRATION

The patient's pretreatment body weight should be obtained for calculation of correct dosage. Amikacin Sulfate Injection may be given intramuscularly or intravenously.

The status of renal function should be estimated by measurement of the serum creatinine concentration or calculation of the endogenous creatinine clearance rate. The blood urea nitrogen (BUN) is much less reliable for this purpose. Reassessment of renal function should be made periodically during therapy.

Whenever possible, amikacin concentrations in serum should be measured to assure adequate but not excessive levels. It is desirable to measure both peak and trough serum concentrations intermittently during therapy. Peak concentrations (30–90 minutes after injection) above 35 micrograms per mL and trough concentrations (just prior to the next dose) above 10 micrograms per mL should be avoided. Dosage should be adjusted as indicated.

INTRAMUSCULAR ADMINISTRATION FOR PATIENTS WITH NORMAL RENAL FUNCTION

The recommended dosage for adults, children and older infants (see **WARNINGS** box) with normal renal function is 15 mg/kg/day divided into 2 or 3 equal doses administered at equally divided intervals, i.e., 7.5 mg/kg q12h or 5 mg/kg q8h. Treatment of patients in the heavier weight classes should not exceed 1.5 gram/day.

When amikacin is indicated in newborns (see **WARNINGS** box), it is recommended that a loading dose of 10 mg/kg be administered initially to be followed with 7.5 mg/kg every 12 hours.

The usual duration of treatment is 7 to 10 days. It is desirable to limit the duration of treatment to short-term whenever feasible. The total daily dose by all routes of administration should not exceed 15 mg/kg/day. In difficult and complicated infections where treatment beyond 10 days is considered, the use of amikacin should be reevaluated. If continued, amikacin serum levels and renal, auditory and vestibular functions should be monitored. At the recommended dosage level, uncomplicated infections due to amikacin-sensitive organisms should respond in 24 to 48 hours. If definite clinical response does not occur within 3 to 5 days, therapy should be stopped and the antibiotic susceptibility pattern of the invading organism should be rechecked. Failure of the infection to respond may be due to resistance of the organism or to the presence of septic foci requiring surgical drainage.

When amikacin is indicated in uncomplicated urinary tract infections, a dose of 250 mg twice daily may be used.

DOSAGE GUIDELINES
ADULTS AND CHILDREN WITH NORMAL RENAL FUNCTION

Patient Weight lbs	kg	Dosage 7.5 mg/kg q12h	OR	5 mg/kg q8h
99	45	337.5 mg		225 mg
110	50	375 mg		250 mg
121	55	412.5 mg		275 mg
132	60	450 mg		300 mg
143	65	487.5 mg		325 mg
154	70	525 mg		350 mg
165	75	562.6 mg		375 mg
176	80	600 mg		400 mg
187	85	637.5 mg		425 mg
198	90	675 mg		450 mg
209	95	712.5 mg		475 mg
220	100	750 mg		500 mg

INTRAMUSCULAR ADMINISTRATION FOR PATIENTS WITH IMPAIRED RENAL FUNCTION

Whenever possible, serum amikacin concentrations should be monitored by appropriate assay procedures. Doses may be adjusted in patients with impaired renal function either by administering normal doses at prolonged intervals or by administering reduced doses at a fixed interval.

Both methods are based on the patient's creatinine clearance or serum creatinine values since these have been found to correlate with aminoglycoside half-lives in patients with diminished renal function. These dosage schedules must be used in conjunction with careful clinical and laboratory observations of the patient and should be modified as necessary. Neither method should be used when dialysis is being performed.

Normal Dosage at Prolonged Intervals—If the creatinine clearance rate is not available and the patient's condition is stable, a dosage interval in hours for the normal dose can be calculated by multiplying the patient's serum creatinine by 9, e.g., if the serum creatinine concentration is 2 mg/100 mL, the recommended single dose (7.5 mg/kg) should be administered every 18 hours.

Reduced Dosage at Fixed Time Intervals—When renal function is impaired and it is desirable to administer amikacin at a fixed time interval, dosage must be reduced. In these patients, serum amikacin concentrations should be measured to assure accurate administration of amikacin and to avoid concentrations above 35 mcg/mL. If serum assay determinations are not available and the patient's condition is stable, serum creatinine and creatinine clearance values are the most readily available indicators of the degree of renal impairment to use as a guide for dosage.

First, initiate therapy by administering a normal dose, 7.5 mg/kg, as a loading dose. This loading dose is the same as the normally recommended dose which would be calculated for a patient with a normal renal function as described above.

To determine the size of maintenance doses administered every 12 hours, the loading dose should be reduced in proportion to the reduction in the patient's creatinine clearance rate:

$$\text{Maintenance Dose Every 12 hours} = \frac{\text{observed CC in mL/min}}{\text{normal CC in mL/min}} \times \text{calculated loading dose in mg}$$

(CC—creatinine clearance rate)

An alternate rough guide for determining reduced dosage at 12-hour intervals (for patients whose steady state serum creatinine values are known) is to divide the normally recommended dose by the patient's serum creatinine.

The above dosage schedules are not intended to be rigid recommendations but are provided as guides to dosage when the measurement of amikacin serum levels is not feasible.

INTRAVENOUS ADMINISTRATION

The individual dose, the total daily dose and the total cumulative dose of amikacin sulfate are identical to the dose recommended for intramuscular administration. The solution for intravenouis use is prepared by adding the contents of a 500 mg vial to 100–200 mL of sterile diluent such as Normal Saline or 5% Dextrose in Water or any other compatible solution.

The solution is administered to adults over a 30 to 60 minute period. The total daily dose should not exceed 15 mg/kg/day and may be divided into either 2 or 3 equally divided doses at equally divided intervals.

In pediatric patients, the amount of fluid used will depend on the amount ordered for the patient. It should be a sufficient amount to infuse the amikacin over a 30 to 60 minute period. Infants should receive a 1 to 2 hour infusion.

Amikacin should not be physically premixed with other drugs but should be administered separately according to the recommended dose and route.

Stability in IV Fluids—Amikacin sulfate is stable for 24 hours at room temperature at concentrations of 0.25 and 5 mg/mL in the following solutions:

- 5% Dextrose Injection, USP
- 5% Dextrose and 0.2% Sodium Chloride Injection, USP
- 5% Dextrose and 0.45% Sodium Chloride Injection, USP
- 0.9% Sodium Chloride Injection, USP
- Lactated Ringer's Injection, USP
- Normosol® M in 5% Dextrose Injection (or Plasma-Lyte 56 Injection in 5% Dextrose in Water)
- Normosol® R in 5% Dextrose Injection (or Plasma-Lyte 148 Injection in 5% Dextrose in Water)

Aminoglycosides administered by any of the above routes should not be physically premixed with other drugs but should be administered separately.

Because of the potential toxicity of aminoglycosides, "fixed dosage" recommendations which are not based upon body weight are not advised. Rather, it is essential to calculate the dosage to fit the needs of each patient.

Parenteral drug products should be inspected visually for particulate matter and discoloration prior to administration whenever the solution and container permit.

HOW SUPPLIED

Amikacin Sulfate Injection, USP is available in the following packages:

250 mg/mL

2 mL (500 mg) DOSETTE® vials packaged in 10s (*NDC* 0641-0123-23)

4 mL (1 gram) vials packaged in 10s (*NDC* 0641-2357-43)

STORAGE

Amikacin Sulfate Injection, USP is supplied as a colorless solution which requires no refrigeration. Store at controlled room temperature 15°–30°C (59°–86°F).

Store solutions for intravenous use as directed in **DOSAGE AND ADMINISTRATION.**

At times, the solution may become a very pale yellow; this does not indicate a decrease in potency.

DURAMORPH® Ⓒ

[dūr"a'mŏrf]

(morphine sulfate injection, USP)
Preservative-Free

DESCRIPTION

Morphine is the most important alkaloid of opium and is a phenanthrene derivative. It is available as the sulfate, having the following structural formula:

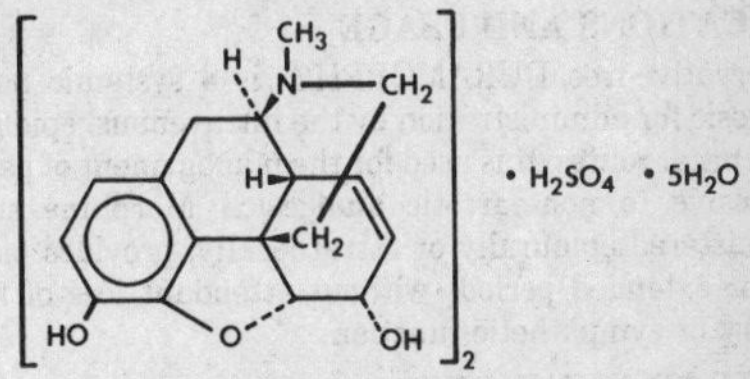

7,8 Didehydro-4,5-epoxy-17-methyl-(5α,6α)-morphinan-3,6-diol sulfate (2:1) (salt), pentahydrate

$(C_{17}H_{19}NO_3)_2 \cdot H_2SO_4 \cdot 5H_2O$ Molecular weight is 758.83.

Preservative-free DURAMORPH® (Morphine Sulfate Injection, USP) is a sterile, pyrogen-free, isobaric solution free of antioxidants, preservatives or other potentially neurotoxic additives, and is intended for intravenous, epidural or intrathecal administration as a narcotic analgesic. Each milliliter contains morphine sulfate 0.5 mg or 1 mg (Warning: May Be Habit Forming) and sodium chloride 9 mg in Water for Injection. pH range is 2.5–6.5. Ampuls are sealed under nitrogen. Each Dosette® ampul is intended for SINGLE USE ONLY. Discard any unused portion. DO NOT HEAT-STERILIZE.

CLINICAL PHARMACOLOGY

Morphine exerts its primary effects on the central nervous system and organs containing smooth muscle. Pharmacologic effects include analgesia, drowsiness, alteration in mood (euphoria), reduction in body temperature (at low doses), dose-related depression of respiration, interference with adrenocortical response to stress (at high doses), reduction in peripheral resistance with little or no effect on cardiac index and miosis.

Morphine, as other opioids, acts as an agonist interacting with stereospecific and saturable binding sites/receptors in the brain, spinal cord and other tissues. These sites have been classified as μ receptors and are widely distributed throughout the central nervous system being present in highest concentration in the limbic system (frontal and temporal cortex, amygdala and hippocampus), thalamus, striatum, hypothalamus, midbrain and laminae I, II, IV and V of the dorsal horn in the spinal cord. It has been postulated that exogenously administered morphine exerts its analgesic effect, in part, by altering the central release of neurotransmitter from afferent nerves sensitive to noxious stimuli. Peripheral threshold or responsiveness to noxious stimuli is unaffected leaving monosynaptic reflexes such as the patellar or the Achilles tendon reflex intact.

Autonomic reflexes are not affected by epidural or intrathecal morphine, however morphine exerts spasmogenic effects on the gastrointestinal tract that result in decreased peristaltic activity.

Central nervous system effects of intravenously administered morphine sulfate are influenced by ability to cross the blood-brain barrier.

The delay in the onset of analgesia following epidural or intrathecal injection may be attributed to its relatively poor lipid solubility (i.e., an oil/water partition coefficient of 1.42), and its slow access to the receptor sites. The hydrophilic character of morphine may also explain its retention in the CNS and its slow release into the systemic circulation, resulting in a prolonged effect.

Nausea and vomiting may be prominent and are thought to be the result of central stimulation of the chemoreceptor trigger zone. Histamine release is common; allergic manifestations of urticaria and, rarely, anaphylaxis may occur. Bronchoconstriction may occur either as an idiosyncratic reaction or from large dosages.

Approximately one-third of intravenous morphine is bound to plasma proteins. Free morphine is rapidly redistributed in parenchymatous tissues. The major metabolic pathway is through conjugation with glucuronic acid in the liver. Elimination half-life is approximately 1.5 to 2 hours in healthy volunteers. For intravenously administered morphine, 90% is excreted in the urine within 24 hours and traces are detectable in urine up to 48 hours. About 7–10% of administered morphine eventually appears in the feces as conjugated morphine.

Peak serum levels following epidural or intrathecal administration of DURAMORPH® are reached within 30 minutes in most subjects and decline to very low levels during the

Continued on next page

Elkins-Sinn—Cont.

next 2 to 4 hours. The onset of action occurs in 15 to 60 minutes following epidural administration or intrathecal administration; analgesia may last up to 24 hours. Due to this extended duration of action, sustained pain relief can be provided with lower daily doses (by these two routes) than are usually required with intravenous or intramuscular morphine administration.

INDICATIONS AND USAGE

Preservative-free DURAMORPH® is a systemic narcotic analgesic for administration by the intravenous, epidural or intrathecal routes. It is used for the management of pain not responsive to non-narcotic analgesics. Morphine sulfate, administered epidurally or intrathecally, provides pain relief for extended periods without attendant loss of motor, sensory or sympathetic function.

CONTRAINDICATIONS

DURAMORPH® is contraindicated in those medical conditions which would preclude the administration of opioids by the intravenous route—allergy to morphine or other opiates, acute bronchial asthma, upper airway obstruction.
Administration of morphine by the epidural or intrathecal route is contraindicated in the presence of infection at the injection site, anticoagulant therapy, bleeding diathesis, parenterally administered corticosteroids within a two week period or other concomitant drug therapy or medical condition which would contraindicate the technique of epidural or intrathecal analgesia.

WARNINGS

DURAMORPH® administration should be limited to use by those familiar with the management of respiratory depression, and in the case of epidural or intrathecal administration, familiar with the techniques and patient management problems associated with epidural or intrathecal drug administration. Because epidural administration has been associated with lessened potential for immediate or late adverse effects than intrathecal administration, the epidural route should be used whenever possible. Rapid intravenous administration may result in chest wall rigidity. FACILITIES WHERE DURAMORPH® IS ADMINISTERED MUST BE EQUIPPED WITH RESUSCITATIVE EQUIPMENT, OXYGEN, NALOXONE INJECTION, AND OTHER RESUSCITATIVE DRUGS. WHEN THE EPIDURAL OR INTRATHECAL ROUTE OF ADMINISTRATION IS EMPLOYED, PATIENTS MUST BE OBSERVED IN A FULLY EQUIPPED AND STAFFED ENVIRONMENT FOR AT LEAST 24 HOURS.
SEVERE RESPIRATORY DEPRESSION UP TO 24 HOURS FOLLOWING EPIDURAL OR INTRATHECAL ADMINISTRATION HAS BEEN REPORTED.
Morphine sulfate may be habit forming. (See DRUG ABUSE AND DEPENDENCE.)

PRECAUTIONS

GENERAL

Preservative-free DURAMORPH® (Morphine Sulfate Injection, USP) should be administered with extreme caution in aged or debilitated patients, in the presence of increased intracranial/intraocular pressure and in patients with head injury. Pupillary changes (miosis) may obscure the course of intracranial pathology. Care is urged in patients who have a decreased respiratory reserve (e.g., emphysema, severe obesity, kyphoscoliosis).
Seizures may result from high doses. Patients with known seizure disorders should be carefully observed for evidence of morphine-induced seizure activity.
It is recommended that administration of DURAMORPH® by the epidural or intrathecal routes be limited to the lumbar area. Intrathecal use has been associated with a higher incidence of respiratory depression than epidural use.
Smooth muscle hypertonicity may result in biliary colic, difficulty in urination and possible urinary retention requiring catheterization. Consideration should be given to risks inherent in urethral catheterization, e.g., sepsis, when epidural or intrathecal administration is considered, especially in the perioperative period.
Elimination half-life may be prolonged in patients with reduced metabolic rates and with hepatic or renal dysfunction. Hence, care should be exercised in administering morphine in these conditions, particularly with repeated dosing.
Patients with reduced circulating blood volume, impaired myocardial function or on sympatholytic drugs should be observed carefully for orthostatic hypotension, particularly in transport.
Patients with chronic obstructive pulmonary disease and patients with acute asthmatic attack may develop acute respiratory failure with administration of morphine. Use in these patients should be reserved for those whose conditions require endotracheal intubation and respiratory support or control of ventilation.

DRUG INTERACTIONS

Depressant effects of morphine are potentiated by either concomitant administration or in the presence of other CNS depressants such as alcohol, sedatives, antihistaminics or psychotropic drugs (e.g., MAO inhibitors, phenothiazines, butyrophenones and tricyclic antidepressants). Premedication or intra-anesthetic use of neuroleptics with morphine may increase the risk of respiratory depression.

CARCINOGENESIS, MUTAGENESIS, IMPAIRMENT OF FERTILITY

Studies of morphine sulfate in animals to evaluate the carcinogenic and mutagenic potential or the effect on fertility have not been conducted.

PREGNANCY

Teratogenic Effects—Pregnancy Category C. Animal reproduction studies have not been conducted with morphine. It is also not known whether morphine sulfate can cause fetal harm when administered to a pregnant woman or can affect reproduction capacity. Morphine sulfate should be given to a pregnant woman only if clearly needed.
Nonteratogenic Effects. Infants born from mothers who have been taking morphine chronically may exhibit withdrawal symptoms.

LABOR AND DELIVERY

Intravenous morphine readily passes into the fetal circulation and may result in respiratory depression in the neonate. Naloxone and resuscitative equipment should be available for reversal of narcotic-induced respiratory depression in the neonate. In addition, intravenous morphine may reduce the strength, duration and frequency of uterine contraction resulting in prolonged labor.
Epidurally and intrathecally administered morphine readily passes into the fetal circulation and may result in respiratory depression of the neonate. Controlled clinical studies have shown that *epidural* administration has little or no effect on the relief of labor pain.
However, studies have suggested that in most cases 0.2 to 1 mg of morphine *intrathecally* provides adequate pain relief with little effect on the duration of first stage labor. The second stage labor, though, may be prolonged if the parturient is not encouraged to bear down. A continuous intravenous infusion of naloxone, 0.6 mg/hr, for 24 hours after intrathecal injection may be employed to reduce the incidence of potential side effects.

NURSING MOTHERS

Morphine is excreted in maternal milk. Effect on the nursing infant is not known.

PEDIATRIC USE

Safety and effectiveness in children have not been established.

ADVERSE REACTIONS

The most serious side effect is respiratory depression. Because of delay in maximum CNS effect with intravenously administered drug (30 min), rapid administration may result in overdosing. Bolus administration by the epidural or intrathecal route may result in early respiratory depression due to direct venous redistribution of morphine to the respiratory centers in the brain. Late (up to 24 hours) onset of acute respiratory depression has been reported with administration by the epidural or intrathecal route and is believed to be the result of rostral spread. Reports of respiratory depression following intrathecal administration have been more frequent, but the dosage used in most of these cases has been considerably higher than that recommended. This depression may be severe and could require intervention. (See WARNINGS and OVERDOSAGE.) Even without clinical evidence of ventilatory inadequacy, a diminished CO_2 ventilation response may be noted for up to 22 hours following epidural or intrathecal administration.
While low doses of intravenously administered morphine have little effect on cardiovascular stability, high doses are excitatory, resulting from sympathetic hyperactivity and increase in circulating catecholamines. Excitation of the central nervous system resulting in convulsions may accompany high doses of morphine given intravenously. Dysphoric reactions may occur and toxic psychoses have been reported. Epidural or intrathecal administration is accompanied by a high incidence of pruritus which is dose related but not confined to site of administration. Nausea and vomiting are frequently seen in patients following morphine administration. Urinary retention which may persist for 10–20 hours following single epidural or intrathecal administration has been reported in approximately 90% of males. Incidence is somewhat lower in females. Patients may require catheterization. (See PRECAUTIONS.) Pruritus, nausea/vomiting and urinary retention frequently can be alleviated by the intravenous administration of low doses of naloxone (0.2 mg). Tolerance and dependence to chronically administered morphine, by whatever route, is known to occur. (See DRUG ABUSE AND DEPENDENCE.)
Miscellaneous side effects include constipation, headache, anxiety, depression of cough reflex, interference with thermal regulation and oliguria. Evidence of histamine release such as urticaria, wheals and/or local tissue irritation may occur. In general, side effects are amenable to reversal by

narcotic antagonists. NALOXONE INJECTION AND RESUSCITATIVE EQUIPMENT SHOULD BE IMMEDIATELY AVAILABLE FOR ADMINISTRATION IN CASE OF LIFE-THREATENING OR INTOLERABLE SIDE EFFECTS.

DRUG ABUSE AND DEPENDENCE

CONTROLLED SUBSTANCE

Morphine sulfate is a Schedule II substance under the Drug Enforcement Administration classification.

ABUSE

Morphine has recognized abuse and dependence potential.

DEPENDENCE

Cerebral and spinal receptors may develop tolerance/dependence independently, as a function of local dosage. Care must be taken to avert withdrawal in those patients who have been maintained on parenteral/oral narcotics when epidural or intrathecal administration is considered. Withdrawal may occur following chronic epidural or intrathecal administration, as well as the development of tolerance to morphine by these routes. (See Nonteratogenic Effects under PREGNANCY.)

OVERDOSAGE

Overdosage is characterized by respiratory depression with or without concomitant CNS depression. Since respiratory arrest may result either through direct depression of the respiratory center or as the result of hypoxia, primary attention should be given to the establishment of adequate respiratory exchange through provision of a patent airway and institution of assisted or controlled ventilation. The narcotic antagonist naloxone is a specific antidote. Naloxone (usually 0.4 mg) should be administered intravenously, simultaneously with respiratory resuscitation. *As the duration of effect of naloxone is considerably shorter than that of epidural or intrathecal morphine, repeated administration may be necessary.* Patients should be closely observed for evidence of renarcotization. *Note: Respiratory depression may be delayed in onset up to 24 hours* following epidural or intrathecal administration. In painful conditions, reversal of narcotic effect may result in acute onset of pain and release of catecholamines. Careful administration of naloxone may permit reversal of side effects without affecting analgesia. Parenteral administration of narcotics in patients receiving epidural or intrathecal morphine may result in overdosage.

DOSAGE AND ADMINISTRATION

Preservative-free DURAMORPH® (Morphine Sulfate Injection, USP) is intended for intravenous, epidural or intrathecal administration.

INTRAVENOUS ADMINISTRATION

Dosage: The initial dose of morphine should be 2 mg to 10 mg/70 kg of body weight. Patients under the age of 18; no information available.

EPIDURAL ADMINISTRATION

DURAMORPH® SHOULD BE ADMINISTERED EPIDURALLY ONLY BY PHYSICIANS EXPERIENCED IN THE TECHNIQUES OF EPIDURAL ADMINISTRATION AND WHO ARE THOROUGHLY FAMILIAR WITH THE LABELING. IT SHOULD BE ADMINISTERED ONLY IN SETTINGS WHERE ADEQUATE PATIENT MONITORING IS POSSIBLE. RESUSCITATIVE EQUIPMENT AND A SPECIFIC ANTAGONIST (NALOXONE INJECTION) SHOULD BE IMMEDIATELY AVAILABLE FOR THE MANAGEMENT OF RESPIRATORY DEPRESSION AS WELL AS COMPLICATIONS WHICH MIGHT RESULT FROM INADVERTENT INTRATHECAL OR INTRAVASCULAR INJECTION. [NOTE: INTRATHECAL DOSAGE IS USUALLY ¹/₁₀ THAT OF EPIDURAL DOSAGE.] PATIENT MONITORING SHOULD BE CONTINUED FOR AT LEAST 24 HOURS AFTER EACH DOSE, SINCE DELAYED RESPIRATORY DEPRESSION MAY OCCUR.
Proper placement of a needle or catheter in the epidural space should be verified before DURAMORPH® is injected. Acceptable techniques for verifying proper placement include: a) aspiration to check for absence of blood or cerebrospinal fluid, or b) administration of 5 mL (3 mL in obstetric patients) of 1.5% UNPRESERVED Lidocaine and Epinephrine (1:200,000) Injection and then observe the patient for lack of tachycardia (this indicates that vascular injection has *not* been made) and lack of sudden onset of segmental anesthesia (this indicates that intrathecal injection has *not* been made).

Epidural Adult Dosage: Initial injection of 5 mg in the lumbar region may provide satisfactory pain relief for up to 24 hours. If adequate pain relief is not achieved within one hour, careful administration of incremental doses of 1 to 2 mg at intervals sufficient to assess effectiveness may be given. No more than 10 mg/24 hr should be administered. Thoracic administration has been shown to dramatically increase the incidence of early and late respiratory depression even at doses of 1 to 2 mg.
For continuous infusion an initial dose of 2 to 4 mg/24 hours is recommended. Further doses of 1 to 2 mg may be given if pain relief is not achieved initially.

Aged or debilitated patients—Administer with extreme caution. (See PRECAUTIONS.) Doses of less than 5 mg may provide satisfactory pain relief for up to 24 hours.

Epidural Pediatric Use: No information on use in pediatric patients is available.

INTRATHECAL ADMINISTRATION

NOTE: INTRATHECAL DOSAGE IS USUALLY 1/10 THAT OF EPIDURAL DOSAGE.

DURAMORPH® SHOULD BE ADMINISTERED INTRATHECALLY ONLY BY PHYSICIANS EXPERIENCED IN THE TECHNIQUES OF INTRATHECAL ADMINISTRATION AND WHO ARE THOROUGHLY FAMILIAR WITH THE LABELING. IT SHOULD BE ADMINISTERED ONLY IN SETTINGS WHERE ADEQUATE PATIENT MONITORING IS POSSIBLE. RESUSCITATIVE EQUIPMENT AND A SPECIFIC ANTAGONIST (NALOXONE INJECTION) SHOULD BE IMMEDIATELY AVAILABLE FOR THE MANAGEMENT OF RESPIRATORY DEPRESSION AS WELL AS COMPLICATIONS WHICH MIGHT RESULT FROM INADVERTENT INTRAVASCULAR INJECTION. **PATIENT MONITORING SHOULD BE CONTINUED FOR AT LEAST 24 HOURS AFTER EACH DOSE, SINCE DELAYED RESPIRATORY DEPRESSION MAY OCCUR.** RESPIRATORY DEPRESSION (BOTH EARLY AND LATE ONSET) HAS OCCURRED MORE FREQUENTLY FOLLOWING INTRATHECAL ADMINISTRATION.

Intrathecal Adult Dosage: A single injection of 0.2 to 1 mg may provide satisfactory pain relief for up to 24 hours. (CAUTION: THIS IS ONLY 0.4 TO 2 ML OF THE 5 MG/10 ML AMPUL OR 0.2 TO 1 ML OF THE 10 MG/10 ML AMPUL OF DURAMORPH®). DO NOT INJECT INTRATHECALLY MORE THAN 2 ML OF THE 5 MG/10 ML AMPUL OR 1 ML OF THE 10 MG/10 ML AMPUL. USE IN THE LUMBAR AREA ONLY IS RECOMMENDED. Repeated intrathecal injections of DURAMORPH® are not recommended. A constant intravenous infusion of naloxone, 0.6 mg/hr, for 24 hours after intrathecal injection may be used to reduce the incidence of potential side effects.

Aged or debilitated patients—Administer with extreme caution. (See PRECAUTIONS.) A lower dosage is usually satisfactory.

Repeat Dosage: If pain recurs, alternative routes of administration should be considered, since experience with repeated doses of morphine by the intrathecal route is limited.

Intrathecal Pediatric Use: No information on use in pediatric patients is available.

Parenteral drug products should be inspected for particulate matter and discoloration prior to administration, whenever solution and container permit. Do not use if color is darker than pale yellow, if it is discolored in any other way or if it contains a precipitate.

HOW SUPPLIED

Preservative-free DURAMORPH® (Morphine Sulfate Injection, USP) is available in amber DOSETTE® ampuls for intravenous, epidural or intrathecal administration:

5 mg/10 mL (0.5 mg/mL) packaged in 10s (NDC 0641-1112-33)

10 mg/10 mL (1 mg/1 mL) packaged in 10s (NDC 0641-1114-33)

STORAGE

Protect from light. Store in carton at controlled room temperature, 15° to 30°C (59° to 86°F) until ready to use. DURAMORPH® contains no preservative. DISCARD ANY UNUSED PORTION. DO NOT HEAT-STERILIZE.

* * * *

Manufactured by
ELKINS-SINN, INC., Cherry Hill, NJ 08003-4099

INFUMORPH™ 200 Ⓒ
INFUMORPH™ 500 Ⓒ

(Preservative-free Morphine Sulfate Sterile Solution)
For Use in Continuous Microinfusion Devices

DESCRIPTION

Morphine is the most important alkaloid of opium and is a phenanthrene derivative. It is available as the sulfate salt, having the following structural formula:

[See structural formula at top of next column.]

INFUMORPH™ is a sterile, nonpyrogenic isobaric, **high potency solution of morphine sulfate,** free of antioxidants, preservatives or other potentially neurotoxic additives. **INFUMORPH™ is intended for use in continuous microinfusion devices for intraspinal administration in the management of pain.**

Each 20 mL ampul of INFUMORPH™ 200 contains morphine sulfate, USP 200 mg or 10 mg/mL (Warning: May be habit forming) and sodium chloride 8 mg/mL in Water for

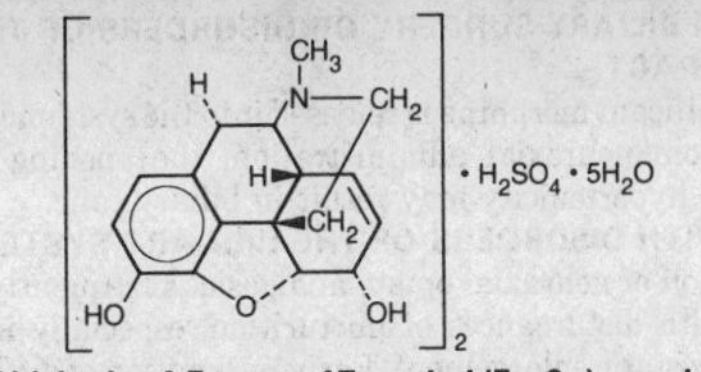

7,8-Didehydro-4,5-epoxy-17-methyl-(5α,6α)-morphinan-3,6-diol sulfate (2:1) (salt), pentahydrate $(C_{17}H_{19}NO_3)_2 \cdot H_2SO_4 \cdot 5H_2O$) Molecular Weight is 758.83.

Injection, USP. Each 20 mL ampul of INFUMORPH™ 500 contains morphine sulfate, USP 500 mg or 25 mg/mL (Warning: May be habit forming) and sodium chloride 6.25 mg/mL in Water for Injection, USP. If needed, sodium hydroxide and/or sulfuric acid are added for pH adjustment to 4.5. Ampuls are sealed under nitrogen. Each 20 mL DOSETTE® ampul of INFUMORPH™ is intended for **single use only.** *Discard any unused portion.* DO NO HEAT-STERILIZE.

CLINICAL PHARMACOLOGY

Morphine produces a wide spectrum of pharmacologic effects including analgesia, dysphoria, euphoria, somnolence, respiratory depression, diminished gastrointestinal motility and physical dependence. Opiate analgesia involves at least three anatomical areas of the central nervous system: the periaqueductal-periventricular gray matter, the ventromedial medulla and the spinal cord. A systemically administered opiate may produce analgesia by acting at any, all or some combination of these distinct regions. Morphine interacts predominantly with the μ-receptor. The μ-binding sites of opioids are very discretely distributed in the human brain, with high densities of sites found in the posterior amygdala, hypothalamus, thalamus, nucleus caudatus, putamen and certain cortical areas. They are also found on the terminal axons of primary afferents within laminae I and II (substantia gelatinosa) of the spinal cord and in the spinal nucleus of the trigeminal nerve.

Morphine has an apparent volume of distribution ranging from 1.0 to 4.7 L/kg after *intravenous* dosage. Protein binding is low, about 36%, and muscle tissue binding is reported as 54%. A blood-brain barrier exists, and when morphine is introduced outside of the CNS (e.g., *intravenously*), plasma concentrations of morphine remain higher than the corresponding CSF morphine levels. Conversely, when morphine is injected into the *intrathecal space,* it diffuses out into the systemic circulation slowly, accounting for the long duration of action of morphine administered by this route.

Morphine has a total plasma clearance which ranges from 0.9 to 1.2 L/kg/h (liters/kilogram/hour) in postoperative patients, but shows considerable interindividual variation. The major pathway of clearance is hepatic glucuronidation to morphine-3-glucuronide, which is pharmacologically inactive. The major excretion path of the conjugate is through the kidneys, with about 10% in the feces. Morphine is also eliminated by the kidneys, 2 to 12% being excreted unchanged in the urine. Terminal half-life is commonly reported to vary from 1.5 to 4.5 hours, although the longer half-lives were obtained when morphine levels were monitored over protracted periods with very sensitive radioimmunoassay methods. The accepted elimination half-life in normal subjects is 1.5 to 2 hours.

"Selective" blockade of pain sensation is possible by neuraxial application of morphine. In addition, duration of analgesia may be much longer by this route compared to systemic administration. However, CNS effects, associated with systemic administration, are still seen. These include respiratory depression, sedation, nausea and vomiting, pruritis and urinary retention. In particular, both early and late respiratory depression (up to 24 hours post dosing) have been reported following neuraxial administration. Circulation of the spinal fluid may also result in high concentrations of morphine reaching the brain stem directly.

The incidence of unwanted CNS effects, including delayed respiratory depression, associated with neuraxial application of morphine, is related to the circulatory dynamics of the epidural venous plexus and the spinal fluid. The lipid solubility and degree of ionization of morphine plays an important part in both the onset and duration of analgesia and the CNS effects. Morphine has a pH_a 7.9, with an octanol/water partition coefficient of 1.42 at pH 7.4. At this pH, the tertiary amino group in each of the opioids is mostly ionized, making the molecule water soluble. Morphine, with additional hydroxyl groups on the molecule, is significantly more water soluble than any other opioid in clinical use.

Morphine, injected into the *epidural space,* is rapidly absorbed into the general circulation. Absorption is so rapid that the plasma concentration-time profiles closely resembled those obtained after intravenous or intramuscular administration. Peak plasma concentrations averaging 33–40 ng/mL (range 5–62 ng/mL) are achieved within 10 to 15 minutes after administration of 3 mg of morphine. Plasma concentrations decline in a multiexponential fashion. The terminal half-life is reported to range from 39 to 249 minutes (mean of 90 ± 34.3 min) and, though somewhat shorter, is similar in magnitude as values reported after intravenous and intramuscular administration (1.5–4.5 h). CSF concentrations of morphine, after epidural doses of 2 to 6 mg in postoperative patients, have been reported to be 50 to 250 times higher than corresponding plasma concentrations. The CSF levels of morphine exceed those in plasma after only 15 minutes and are detectable for as long as 20 hours after the injection of 2 mg of epidural morphine. Approximately 4% of the dose injected epidurally reaches the CSF. This corresponds to the relative minimum effective epidural and intrathecal doses of 5 mg and 0.25 mg, respectively. The disposition of morphine in the CSF follows a biphasic pattern, with an early half-life of 1.5 h and a late phase half-life of about 6 h. Morphine crosses the dura slowly, with an absorption half-life across the dura averaging 22 minutes. Maximum CSF concentrations are seen 60–90 minutes after injection. Minimum effective CSF concentrations for postoperative analgesia average 150 ng/mL (range <1–380 ng/mL).

The *intrathecal route* of administration circumvents meningeal diffusion barriers and, therefore, lower doses of morphine produce comparable analgesia to that induced by the epidural route. After intrathecal bolus injection of morphine, there is a rapid initial distribution phase lasting 15–30 minutes and a half-life in the CSF of 42–136 min (mean 90 ± 16 min). Derived from limited data, it appears that the disposition of morphine in the CSF, from 15 minutes postintrathecal administration to the end of a six-hour observation period, represents a combination of the distribution and elimination phases. Morphine concentrations in the CSF averaged 332 ± 137 ng/mL at 6 hours, following a bolus dose of 0.3 mg of morphine. The apparent volume of distribution of morphine in the intrathecal space is about 22 ± 8 mL.

Time-to-peak plasma concentrations, however, is similar (5–10 min) after either epidural or intrathecal bolus administration of morphine. Maximum plasma morphine concentrations after 0.3 mg intrathecal morphine have been reported from <1 to 7.8 ng/mL. The minimum analgesic morphine plasma concentration during Patient-Controlled Analgesia (PCA) has been reported as 20–40 ng/mL, suggesting that any analgesic contribution from systemic redistribution would be minimal after the first 30–60 minutes with epidural administration and virtually absent with intrathecal administration of morphine.

INDICATION AND USAGE

INFUMORPH™ (Preservative-free Morphine Sulfate Sterile Solution) is indicated only for intrathecal or epidural infusion in the treatment of intractable chronic pain. It was developed for use in continuous microinfusion devices and may require dilution before use as dictated by the characteristics of the device and the dosage requirements of the individual patient.

INFUMORPH™ IS NOT RECOMMENDED FOR SINGLE-DOSE INTRAVENOUS, INTRAMUSCULAR OR SUBCUTANEOUS ADMINISTRATION DUE TO THE VERY LARGE AMOUNT OF MORPHINE IN THE AMPUL AND THE ASSOCIATED RISK OF OVERDOSAGE.

CONTRAINDICATIONS

The only absolute contraindication to the use of INFUMORPH™ is known allergy to morphine. Contraindications to the use of neuraxial analgesia include: the presence of infection at the injection microinfusion site, concomitant anticoagulant therapy, uncontrolled bleeding diathesis and the presence of any other concomitant therapy or medical condition which would render epidural or intrathecal administration of medication especially hazardous.

WARNINGS

THIS PRODUCT WAS DEVELOPED FOR USE (AFTER APPROPRIATE DILUTION, IF NECESSARY) IN CONTINUOUS MICROINFUSION DEVICES FOR INTRATHECAL OR EPIDURAL INFUSION OF NARCOTICS TO CONTROL SEVERE CANCER PAIN. CHRONIC NEURAXIAL OPIOID ANALGESIA IS APPROPRIATE ONLY WHEN LESS INVASIVE MEANS OF CONTROLLING PAIN HAVE FAILED AND SHOULD ONLY BE UNDERTAKEN BY THOSE WHO ARE EXPERIENCED IN APPLYING THE TREATMENT IN A SETTING WHERE ITS COMPLICATIONS CAN BE ADEQUATELY MANAGED.

BECAUSE OF THE RISK OF SEVERE ADVERSE EFFECTS, PATIENTS MUST BE OBSERVED IN A FULLY EQUIPPED AND STAFFED ENVIRONMENT FOR AT LEAST 24 HOURS AFTER THE INITIAL (SINGLE) TEST DOSE AND, AS APPROPRIATE, FOR THE FIRST SEVERAL DAYS AFTER CATHETER IMPLANTATION.

THE FACILITY MUST BE EQUIPPED TO RESUSCITATE PATIENTS WITH SEVERE OPIATE OVERDOSAGE, AND

Continued on next page

Elkins-Sinn—Cont.

THE PERSONNEL MUST BE FAMILIAR WITH THE USE AND LIMITATIONS OF SPECIFIC NARCOTIC ANTAGONISTS (NALOXONE, NALTREXONE) IN SUCH CASES.
RESERVOIR FILLING MUST BE PERFORMED BY FULLY TRAINED AND QUALIFIED PERSONNEL, FOLLOWING THE DIRECTIONS PROVIDED BY THE DEVICE MANUFACTURER. CARE SHOULD BE TAKEN IN SELECTING THE PROPER REFILL FREQUENCY TO PREVENT DEPLETION OF THE RESERVOIR, WHICH WOULD RESULT IN EXACERBATION OF SEVERE PAIN AND/OR REFLUX OF CSF INTO SOME DEVICES. STRICT ASEPTIC TECHNIQUE IN FILLING IS REQUIRED TO AVOID BACTERIAL CONTAMINATION AND SERIOUS INFECTION. **EXTREME CARE MUST BE TAKEN TO ENSURE THAT THE NEEDLE IS PROPERLY IN THE FILLING PORT OF THE DEVICE BEFORE ATTEMPTING TO REFILL THE RESERVOIR. INJECTING THE SOLUTION INTO THE TISSUE AROUND THE DEVICE OR (IN THE CASE OF DEVICES THAT HAVE MORE THAN ONE PORT) ATTEMPTING TO INJECT THE REFILL DOSE INTO THE DIRECT INJECTION PORT WILL RESULT IN A LARGE, CLINICALLY SIGNIFICANT, OVERDOSAGE TO THE PATIENT.**
A PERIOD OF OBSERVATION APPROPRIATE TO THE CLINICAL SITUATION SHOULD FOLLOW EACH REFILL OR MANIPULATION OF THE DRUG RESERVOIR. BEFORE DISCHARGE, THE PATIENT AND ATTENDANT(S) SHOULD RECEIVE INSTRUCTION IN THE PROPER HOME CARE OF THE DEVICE AND INSERTION SITE AND IN THE RECOGNITION AND PRACTICAL TREATMENT OF AN OVERDOSE OF NEURAXIAL MORPHINE.

TOLERANCE AND MYOCLONIC ACTIVITY
PATIENTS SOMETIMES MANIFEST UNUSUAL ACCELERATION OF NEURAXIAL MORPHINE REQUIREMENTS, WHICH MAY CAUSE CONCERN REGARDING SYSTEMIC ABSORPTION AND THE HAZARDS OF LARGE DOSES; THESE PATIENTS MAY BENEFIT FROM HOSPITALIZATION AND DETOXIFICATION. TWO CASES OF MYOCLONIC-LIKE SPASM OF THE LOWER EXTREMITIES HAVE BEEN REPORTED IN PATIENTS RECEIVING MORE THAN 20 MG/DAY OF INTRATHECAL MORPHINE. AFTER DETOXIFICATION, IT MIGHT BE POSSIBLE TO RESUME TREATMENT AT LOWER DOSES, AND SOME PATIENTS HAVE BEEN SUCCESSFULLY CHANGED FROM CONTINUOUS EPIDURAL MORPHINE TO CONTINUOUS INTRATHECAL MORPHINE. REPEAT DETOXIFICATION MAY BE INDICATED AT A LATER DATE. THE UPPER DAILY DOSAGE LIMIT FOR EACH PATIENT DURING CONTINUING TREATMENT MUST BE INDIVIDUALIZED.

PRECAUTIONS

Control of pain by neuraxial opiate delivery, using a continuous microinfusion device, is always accompanied by considerable risk to the patients and requires a high level of skill to be successfully accomplished. The task of treating these patients must be undertaken by experienced clinical teams, well-versed in patient selection, evolving technology and emerging standards of care. For reasons of safety, it is recommended that administration of INFUMORPH™ 200 and 500 (10 and 25 mg/mL, respectively) by the intrathecal route be limited to the lumber area

USE IN PATIENTS WITH INCREASED INTRACRANIAL PRESSURE OR HEAD INJURY
INFUMORPH™ (Preservative-free Morphine Sulfate Sterile Solution) should be used with extreme caution in patients with head injury or increased intracranial pressure. Pupillary changes (miosis) from morphine may obscure the existence, extent and course of intracranial pathology. High doses of neuraxial morphine may produce myoclonic events (see WARNINGS and ADVERSE REACTIONS). Clinicians should maintain a high index of suspicion for adverse drug reactions when evaluating altered mental status or movement abnormalities in patients receiving this modality of treatment.

USE IN CHRONIC PULMONARY DISEASE
Care is urged in using this drug in patients who have a decreased respiratory reserve (e.g., emphysema, severe obesity, kyphoscoliosis or paralysis of the phrenic nerve). INFUMORPH™ should not be given in cases of chronic asthma, upper airway obstruction or in any other chronic pulmonary disorder without due consideration of the known risk of acute respiratory failure following morphine administration in such patients.

USE IN HEPATIC OR RENAL DISEASE
The elimination half-life of morphine may be prolonged in patients with reduced metabolic rate and with hepatic and/or renal dysfunction. Hence, care should be exercised in administering INFUMORPH™ epidurally to patients with these conditions, since high blood morphine levels, due to reduced clearance, may take several days to develop.

USE IN BILIARY SURGERY OR DISORDERS OF THE BILIARY TRACT
As significant morphine is released into the systemic circulation from neuraxial administration, the ensuing smooth muscle hypertonicity may result in biliary colic.

USE WITH DISORDERS OF THE URINARY SYSTEM
Initiation of neuraxial opiate analgesia is frequently associated with disturbances of micturition, especially in males with prostatic enlargement. Early recognition of difficulty in urination and prompt intervention in cases of urinary retention is indicated.

USE IN AMBULATORY PATIENTS
Patients with reduced circulating blood volume, impaired myocardial function or on sympatholytic drugs should be monitored for the possible occurrence of orthostatic hypotension, a frequent complication in single-dose neuraxial morphine analgesia.

USE WITH OTHER CENTRAL NERVOUS SYSTEM DEPRESSANTS
The depressant effects of morphine are potentiated by the presence of other CNS depressants such as alcohol, sedatives, antihistaminics or psychotropic drugs. Use of neuroleptics in conjunction with neuraxial morphine may increase the risk of respiratory depression.

CARCINOGENESIS, MUTAGENESIS, IMPAIRMENT OF FERTILITY
Morphine is without known carcinogenic or mutagenic effects and is not known to impair fertility at non-narcotic doses in animals, but studies of the carcinogenic and mutagenic potential or the effect on fertility of INFUMORPH™ have not been conducted.

PREGNANCY CATEGORY C
Morphine sulfate is not teratogenic in rats at 35 mg/kg/day (thirty-five times the usual human dose) but does result in increased pup mortality and growth retardation at doses that narcotize the animal (> 10 mg/kg/day, ten times the usual human dose). INFUMORPH™ should only be given to pregnant women when no other method of controlling pain is available and means are at hand to manage the delivery and prenatal care of the opiate-dependent infant.

LABOR AND DELIVERY
INFUMORPH™ 200 and 500 (10 and 25 mg/mL, respectively) are too highly concentrated for routine use in obstetric neuraxial analgesia.

NURSING MOTHERS
Morphine is excreted in maternal milk. Effects on the nursing infant are not known.

PEDIATRIC USE
Adequate studies, to establish the safety and effectiveness of spinal morphine in children, have not been performed, and usage in this population is not recommended.

USE IN THE AGED
The pharmacodynamic effects of neuraxial morphine in the aged are more variable than in the younger population. Patients will vary widely in the effective initial dose, rate of development of tolerance and the frequency and magnitude of associated adverse effects as the dose is increased. Initial doses should be based on careful clinical observation following "test doses", after making due allowances for the effects of the patient's age and infirmity on their ability to clear the drug, particularly in patients receiving epidural morphine.

ADVERSE REACTIONS

IMPROPER OR ERRONEOUS SUBSTITUTION OF INFUMORPH™ 200 or 500 (10 or 25 mg/mL, respectively) FOR REGULAR DURAMORPH® (0.5 or 1 mg/mL) IS LIKELY TO RESULT IN SERIOUS OVERDOSAGE, LEADING TO SEIZURES, RESPIRATORY DEPRESSION AND, POSSIBLY, FATAL OUTCOME.

The most serious adverse experiences encountered during continuous intrathecal or epidural infusion of INFUMORPH™ are respiratory depression and myoclonus.

1. Single-dose neuraxial administration may result in acute or delayed respiratory depression for periods at least as long as 24 hours. **Severe respiratory depression, potentially life-threatening, can result from technical errors during refill, e.g., injection of INFUMORPH™ outside the filling port, unintentional injection into the direct bypass-dosing port featured on some devices or local infiltration.**
2. **Tolerance and myoclonus:** See WARNINGS for discussion of these and related hazards.

While low doses of intravenously administered morphine have little effect on cardiovascular stability, high doses are excitatory, resulting from **sympathetic hyperactivity** and increase in circulatory catecholamines. Excitation of the central nervous system, resulting in **convulsions**, may accompany high doses of morphine given intravenously.
Dysphoric reactions may occur after any size dose and **toxic psychoses** have been reported.
Pruritus: Single-dose epidural or intrathecal administration is accompanied by a high incidence of **pruritus** that is dose-related but not confined to the site of administration. Pruritus, following continuous infusion of epidural or intrathecal morphine, is occasionally reported in the literature; these reactions are poorly understood as to their cause.
Urinary retention: Urinary retention, which may persist 10 to 20 hours following single epidural or intrathecal administration, is a frequent side effect and must be anticipated primarily in male patients, with a somewhat lower incidence in females. Also frequently reported in the literature is the occurrence of urinary retention during the first several days of hospitalization for the initiation of continuous intrathecal or epidural morphine therapy. Patients who develop urinary retention have responded to cholinomimetic treatment and/or judicious use of catheters (see PRECAUTIONS).
Constipation: Constipation is frequently encountered during continuous infusion of morphine; this can usually be managed by conventional therapy.
Headache: Lumbar puncture-type headache is encountered in a significant minority of cases for several days following intrathecal catheter implantation; this, generally, responds to bed rest and/or other conventional therapy.
Peripheral edema: There are several reports of peripheral edema, including unexplained genital swelling in male patients, following infusion-device implant surgery.
Other: Other adverse experiences reported following morphine therapy include—**Dizziness, euphoria, anxiety, depression of cough reflex, interference with thermal regulation and oliguria.** Evidence of histamine release such as **urticaria, wheals** and/or **local tissue irritation** may occur.
Pruritus, nausea/vomiting and urinary retention, if associated with continuous infusion therapy, may respond to intravenous administration of a low dose of naloxone (0.2 mg). The risks of using narcotic antagonists in patients chronically receiving narcotic therapy should be considered.

NALOXONE INJECTION AND RESUSCITATIVE EQUIPMENT SHOULD BE IMMEDIATELY AVAILABLE FOR USE IN CASE OF LIFE-THREATENING OR INTOLERABLE SIDE EFFECTS AND WHENEVER INFUMORPH™ THERAPY IS BEING INITIATED, THE RESERVOIR IS BEING REFILLED OR ANY MANIPULATION OF THE RESERVOIR SYSTEM IS TAKING PLACE.

DRUG ABUSE AND DEPENDENCE

CONTROLLED SUBSTANCE
Morphine sulfate is a Schedule II narcotic under the United States Controlled Substance Act (21 U.S.C. 801–886).
Morphine is the most commonly cited prototype for narcotic substances that possess an addiction-forming or addiction-sustaining liability. A patient may be at risk for developing a dependence to morphine if used improperly or for overly long periods of time. As with all potent opioids which are μ-agonists, tolerance as well as psychological and physical dependence to morphine may develop irrespective of the route of administration (intravenous, intramuscular, intrathecal, epidural or oral). Individuals with a prior history of opioid or other substance abuse or dependence, being more apt to respond to the euphorogenic and reinforcing properties of morphine, would be considered to be a greater risk.
Care must be taken to avert withdrawal in patients who have been maintained on parenteral/oral narcotics when epidural or intrathecal administration is considered. Withdrawal symptoms may occur when morphine is discontinued abruptly or upon administration of a narcotic antagonist.

OVERDOSAGE

PARENTERAL ADMINISTRATION OF NARCOTICS IN PATIENTS RECEIVING EPIDURAL OR INTRATHECAL MORPHINE MAY RESULT IN OVERDOSAGE.
Overdosage of morphine is characterized by respiratory depression, with or without concomitant CNS depression. Since respiratory arrest may result either through direct depression of the respiratory center, or as the result of hypoxia, primary attention should be given to the establishment of adequate respiratory exchange through provision of a patent airway and institution of assisted, or controlled, ventilation. The narcotic antagonist, naloxone, is a specific antidote. An initial dose of 0.4 to 2 mg of naloxone should be administered intravenously, simultaneously with respiratory resuscitation. If the desired degree of counteraction and improvement in respiratory function is not obtained, naloxone may be repeated at 2- to 3-minute intervals. If no response is observed after 10 mg of naloxone has been administered, the diagnosis of narcotic-induced, or partial narcotic-induced, toxicity should be questioned. Intramuscular or subcutaneous administration may be used if the intravenous route is not available.
As the duration of effect of naloxone is considerably shorter than that of epidural or intrathecal morphine, repeated administration may be necessary. Patients should be closely observed for evidence of renarcotization.

DOSAGE AND ADMINISTRATION

INFUMORPH™ 200 AND 500 (10 AND 25 MG/ML, RESPECTIVELY) SHOULD NOT BE USED FOR SINGLE-DOSE NEURAXIAL INJECTION BECAUSE LOWER

DOSES CAN BE MORE RELIABLY ADMINISTERED WITH THE STANDARD PREPARATION OF DURAMORPH™ (0.5 AND 1 MG/ML).

CANDIDATES FOR NEURAXIAL ADMINISTRATION OF INFUMORPH™ IN A CONTINUOUS MICROINFUSION DEVICE SHOULD BE HOSPITALIZED TO PROVIDE FOR ADEQUATE PATIENT MONITORING DURING ASSESSMENT OF RESPONSE TO SINGLE DOSES OF INTRATHECAL OR EPIDURAL MORPHINE. HOSPITALIZATION SHOULD BE MAINTAINED FOR SEVERAL DAYS AFTER SURGERY INVOLVING THE INFUSION DEVICE FOR ADDITIONAL MONITORING AND ADJUSTMENT OF DAILY DOSAGE. THE FACILITY MUST BE EQUIPPED WITH RESUSCITATIVE EQUIPMENT, OXYGEN, NALOXONE INJECTION AND OTHER RESUSCITATIVE DRUGS. BECAUSE OF THE RISK OF DELAYED RESPIRATORY DEPRESSION, PATIENTS SHOULD BE OBSERVED IN A FULLY EQUIPPED AND STAFFED ENVIRONMENT FOR AT LEAST 24 HOURS AFTER EACH TEST DOSE AND, AS INDICATED, FOR THE FIRST SEVERAL DAYS AFTER SURGERY.

Familiarization with the continuous microinfusion device is essential. The desired amount of morphine should be withdrawn from the ampul through a microfilter. **To minimize risk from glass or other particles, the product must be filtered through a 5 μ (or smaller) microfilter before injecting into the microinfusion device.** If dilution is required, 0.9% Sodium Chloride Injection is recommended.

Intrathecal Dosage: The starting dose must be individualized, based upon in-hospital evaluation of the response to serial single-dose intrathecal bolus injections of regular DURAMORPH® 0.5 mg/mL or 1 mg/mL, with close observation of the analgesic efficacy and adverse effects *prior* to surgery involving the continuous microinfusion device. The recommended initial lumbar intrathecal dose range in patients with no tolerance to opioids is 0.2 to 1 mg/day. The published range of doses for individuals who have some degree of opioid tolerance varies from 1 to 10 mg/day. The upper daily dosage limit for each patient must be individualized.

Limited experience with continuous intrathecal infusion of morphine has shown that the daily doses have to be increased over time. Although the rate of increase, over time, in the dose required to sustain analgesia is highly variable, an estimate of the expected rate of increase is shown in the following Figure.

Figure: Dose Trend in Continuous Infusions of Intrathecal Morphine
(Mean and 95% Confidence Intervals)

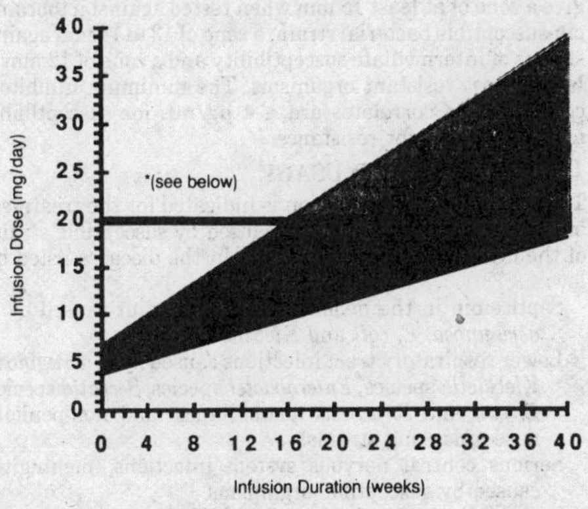
Infusion Dose (mg/day)
40
35
30
25
20
15
10
5
0
*(see below)
0 4 8 12 16 20 24 28 32 36 40
Infusion Duration (weeks)

*20 mg/day is the lowest dose for which regional myoclonus has been reported.
The rate of occurrence cannot be estimated.

Doses above 20 mg/day should be employed with caution since they may be associated with a higher likelihood of serious side effects (see WARNINGS concerning potential neurological hazards and ADVERSE REACTIONS).

Epidural Dosage: The starting dose must be individualized, based upon in-hospital evaluation of the response to serial single-dose epidural bolus injections of regular DURAMORPH® (Morphine Sulfate Injection, USP) 0.5 mg/mL or 1 mg/mL, with dose observation for analgesic efficacy and adverse effects *prior* to surgery involving the continuous microinfusion device.

The recommended initial epidural dose in patients who are not tolerant to opioids ranges from 3.5 to 7.5 mg/day. The usual starting dose for continuous epidural infusion, based upon limited data in patients who have some degree of opioid tolerance, is 4.5 to 10 mg/day. The dose requirements may increase significantly during treatment, frequently to 20–30 mg/day. The upper daily limit for each patient must be individualized.

SAFETY AND HANDLING INFORMATION

INFUMORPH™ is supplied in sealed ampuls. Accidental dermal exposure should be treated by the removal of any contaminated clothing and rinsing the affected area with water.

Each ampul of INFUMORPH™ contains a large amount of potent narcotic which has been associated with abuse and dependence among health care providers. **Due to the limited indications for this product, the risk of overdosage and the risk of its diversion and abuse, it is recommended that special measures be taken to control this product within the hospital or clinic. *INFUMORPH™ should be subject to rigid accounting, rigorous control of wastage and restrictive access.***

This parenteral drug product must be inspected for particulate matter before opening the amber ampul and again for color after removing contents from the ampul. Do not use if the solution in the unopened ampul contains a precipitate which does not disappear upon shaking. After removal, do not use unless the solution is colorless or pale yellow.

HOW SUPPLIED

Amber DOSETTE® ampuls for epidural or intrathecal via a continuous microinfusion device.

INFUMORPH™ 200 (Preservative-free Morphine Sulfate Sterile Solution) 200 mg/20 mL (10 mg/mL) packaged individually (*NDC* 0641-1131-31)

INFUMORPH™ 500 (Preservative-free Morphine Sulfate Sterile Solution) 500 mg/20 mL (25 mg/mL) packaged individually (*NDC* 0641-1132-31)

Also available from Elkins-Sinn, Inc. DURAMORPH® (Morphine Sulfate Injection, USP) 5 mg/10 mL (0.5 mg/mL) and 10 mg/10 mL (1 mg/mL). See insert J-1113.

STORAGE

Protect from light. Store in carton at controlled room temperature 15°–30°C (59°–86°F) until ready to use. DO NOT FREEZE. INFUMORPH™ contains no preservative or antioxidant. DISCARD ANY UNUSED PORTION. DO NOT HEAT-STERILIZE.

• • • • •

Additional package inserts may be obtained by contacting the Professional Service Department, Wyeth-Ayerst Laboratories, P.O. Box 8299, Philadelphia, PA 19101.

Manufactured by
ELKINS-SINN, INC. Cherry Hill, NJ 08003-4099

SOTRADECOL® ℞

[*sō 'trah "de 'kol "*]
(Sodium Tetradecyl Sulfate Injection)
For Intravenous Use Only

DESCRIPTION

Sodium tetradecyl sulfate is an anionic surfactant which occurs as a white, waxy solid. The structural formula is as follows:

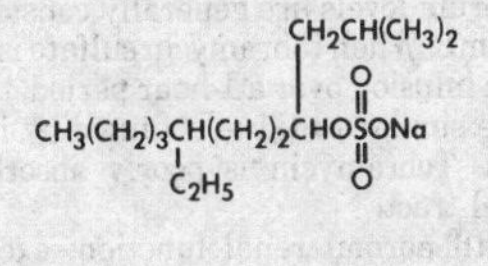
CH2CH(CH3)2
O
CH3(CH2)3CH(CH2)2CHOSONa
C2H5
O

$C_{14}H_{29}NaSO_4$
7-Ethyl-2-methyl-4-hendecanol sulfate sodium salt
M.W. 316.44

Sotradecol® (Sodium Tetradecyl Sulfate Injection) is a sterile nonpyrogenic solution for intravenous use as a sclerosing agent. Each mL contains sodium tetradecyl sulfate 10 mg or 30 mg, benzyl alcohol 0.02 mL and dibasic sodium phosphate, anhydrous 0.72 mg in Water for Injection. pH 7.9; monobasic sodium phosphate and/or sodium hydroxide added, if needed, for pH adjustment.

CLINICAL PHARMACOLOGY

Sotradecol® (Sodium Tetradecyl Sulfate Injection) is a mild sclerosing agent. Intravenous injection causes intima inflammation and thrombus formation. This usually occludes the injected vein. Subsequent formation of fibrous tissue results in partial or complete vein obliteration.

INDICATIONS AND USAGE

Indicated in the treatment of small uncomplicated varicose veins of the lower extremities that show simple dilation with competent valves. The benefit-to-risk ratio should be considered in selected patients who are great surgical risks due to conditions such as old age.

CONTRAINDICATIONS

Contraindicated in previous hypersensitivity reactions to the drug; in acute superficial thrombophlebitis; significant valvular or deep vein incompetence; huge superficial veins with wide open communications to deeper veins; phlebitis migrans; acute cellulitis; allergic conditions; acute infections; varicosities caused by abdominal and pelvic tumors unless the tumor has been removed; bedridden patients; such uncontrolled systemic diseases as diabetes, toxic hyperthyroidism, tuberculosis, asthma, neoplasm, sepsis, blood dyscrasias and acute respiratory or skin diseases.

WARNINGS

Since severe adverse local effects, including tissue necrosis, may occur following extravasation, Sotradecol® (Sodium Tetradecyl Sulfate Injection), should be administered only by a physician familiar with proper injection technique. Extreme care in needle placement and using the minimal effective volume at each injection site are, therefore, important. Allergic reactions have been reported. Therefore, as a precaution against anaphylactoid shock, it is recommended that 0.5 mL of Sotradecol® be injected into a varicosity, followed by observation of the patient for several hours before administration of a second or larger dose. The possibility of an anaphylactoid reaction should be kept in mind, and the physician should be prepared to treat it appropriately. In extreme emergencies, 0.25 mL of 1:1000 Epinephrine Injection (0.25 mg) intravenously should be used and side reactions controlled with antihistamines.

PRECAUTIONS

GENERAL

Venous sclerotherapy should not be undertaken if tests, such as the Trendelenberg and Perthes, and angiography show significant valvular or deep venous incompetence. The physician should bear in mind the fact that injection necrosis is likely to result from extravascular injection of sclerosing agents.

Extreme caution must be exercised in the presence of underlying arterial disease such as marked peripheral arteriosclerosis or thromboangiitis obliterans (Buerger's Disease).

The drug should only be administered by physicians who are familiar with an acceptable injection technique. Because of the danger of thrombosis extension into the deep venous system, thorough preinjection evaluation for valvular competency should be carried out and slow injections with a small amount (not over 2 mL) of the preparation should be injected into the varicosity. In particular, deep venous patency must be determined by angiography and/or the Perthes test before sclerotherapy is undertaken.

Embolism may occur as much as four weeks after injection of sodium tetradecyl sulfate.

The incidence of recurrence is low if the patient wears elastic stockings.

DRUG INTERACTIONS

No well-controlled studies have been performed on patients taking antiovulatory agents. The physician must use judgment and evaluate any patient taking antiovulatory drugs prior to initiating treatment with Sotradecol® (Sodium Tetradecyl Sulfate Injection). (See ADVERSE REACTIONS.)

Heparin should not be included in the same syringe as Sotradecol® since the two are incompatible.

CARCINOGENESIS, MUTAGENESIS, IMPAIRMENT OF FERTILITY

When tested in the L5178YTK$^{+}/^{-}$ mouse lymphoma assay, sodium tetradecyl sulfate did not induce a dose-related increase in the frequency of thymidine kinase-deficient mutants and, therefore, was judged to be nonmutagenic in this system. However, no long-term animal carcinogenicity studies with sodium tetradecyl sulfate have been performed.

PREGNANCY

Teratogenic Effects—Pregnancy Category C. Adequate reproduction studies have not been performed in animals to determine whether this drug affects fertility in males or females, has teratogenic potential, or has other adverse effects on the fetus. There are no well-controlled studies in pregnant women, but investigational and marketing experience does not include any positive evidence of adverse effects on the fetus. Although there is no clearly defined risk, such experience cannot exclude the possibility of infrequent or subtle damage to the human fetus.

NURSING MOTHERS

It is not known whether this drug is excreted in human milk. Because many drugs are excreted in human milk, caution should be exercised when Sodium Tetradecyl Sulfate Injection is administered to a nursing woman.

ADVERSE REACTIONS

Local reactions consisting of pain, urticaria or ulceration may occur at the site of injection. A permanent discoloration, usually small and hardly noticeable but which may be objectionable from a cosmetic viewpoint, may remain along the path of the sclerosed vein segment. Sloughing and necrosis of tissue may occur following extravasation of the drug. Systemic reactions, except for allergic ones, have been slight. These include headache, nausea and vomiting. Allergic reactions such as hives, asthma, hayfever and anaphylactoid shock have been reported. (See WARNINGS.)

Continued on next page

Elkins-Sinn—Cont.

One death has been reported in a patient who received Sotradecol® (Sodium Tetradecyl Sulfate Injection) and who had been receiving an antiovulatory agent.
Another death (fatal pulmonary embolism) has been reported in a 36-year-old female treated with sodium tetradecyl *acetate* and who was **not** taking oral contraceptives.

DOSAGE AND ADMINISTRATION

For intravenous use only. Do not use if precipitated or discolored. The strength of solution required depends on the size and degree of varicosity. In general, the 1% solution will be found most useful with the 3% solution preferred for larger varicosities. The dosage should be kept small, using 0.5 to 2 mL (preferably 1 mL maximum) for each injection, and the maximum single treatment should not exceed 10 mL.
Parenteral drug products should be inspected visually for particulate matter and discoloration prior to administration, whenever solution and container permit.

HOW SUPPLIED

Sotradecol® (Sodium Tetradecyl Sulfate Injection)
1%—2 mL DOSETTE® ampuls packaged in 5s (NDC 0641-1514-34)
3%—2 mL DOSETTE® ampuls packaged in 5s (NDC 0641-1516-34)
STORAGE
Store at controlled room temperature 15°-30°C (59°-86°F).

ANIMAL TOXICOLOGY

The intravenous LD_{50} of sodium tetradecyl sulfate in mice was reported to be 90 ± 5 mg/kg.
In the rat, the acute intravenous LD_{50} of sodium tetradecyl sulfate was estimated to be between 72 mg/kg and 108 mg/kg.
Purified sodium tetradecyl sulfate was found to have an LD_{50} of 2 g/kg when administered orally by stomach tube as a 25% aqueous solution to rats. In rats given 0.15 g/kg in drinking water for 30 days, no appreciable toxicity was seen although some growth inhibition was discernible.

* * * *

Manufactured by
ELKINS-SINN, INC., Cherry Hill, NJ 08003-4099

TOBRAMYCIN ℞
SULFATE INJECTION, USP

WARNINGS

Patients treated with tobramycin sulfate and other aminoglycosides should be under close clinical observation because these drugs have an inherent potential for causing ototoxicity and nephrotoxicity.
Neurotoxicity, manifested as both auditory and vestibular ototoxicity, can occur. The auditory changes are irreversible, are usually bilateral and may be partial or total. Eighth-nerve impairment and nephrotoxicity may develop, primarily in patients having preexisting renal damage and in those with normal renal function to whom aminoglycosides are administered for longer periods or in higher doses than those recommended.
Other manifestations of neurotoxicity may include numbness, skin tingling, muscle twitching and convulsions. The risk of aminoglycoside-induced hearing loss increases with the degree of exposure to either high peak or high trough serum concentrations. Patients who develop cochlear damage may not have symptoms during therapy to warn them of eighth-nerve toxicity, and partial or total irreversible bilateral deafness may continue to develop after the drug has been discontinued. Rarely, nephrotoxicity may not become manifest until the first few days after cessation of therapy. Aminoglycoside-induced nephrotoxicity usually is reversible.
Renal and eighth-nerve function should be closely monitored in patients with known or suspected renal impairment and also in those whose renal function is initially normal but who develop signs of renal dysfunction during therapy. Peak and trough serum concentrations of aminoglycosides should be monitored periodically during therapy to assure adequate levels and to avoid potentially toxic levels. Prolonged serum concentrations above 12 μg/mL should be avoided. Rising trough levels (above 2 μg/mL) may indicate tissue accumulation. Such accumulation, excessive peak concentrations, advanced age and cumulative dose may contribute to ototoxicity and nephrotoxicity (see PRECAUTIONS). Urine should be examined for decreased specific gravity and increased excretion of protein, cells and casts. Blood urea nitrogen, serum creatinine and creatinine clearance should be measured periodically. When feasible, it is recommended that serial audiograms be obtained in patients old enough to be tested, particularly high-risk patients. Evidence of impairment of renal, vestibular or auditory function requires discontinuation of the drug or dosage adjustment.
Tobramycin should be used with caution in premature and neonatal infants because of their renal immaturity and the resulting prolongation of serum half-life of the drug.
Concurrent and sequential use of other neurotoxic and/or nephrotoxic antibiotics, particularly other aminoglycosides (e.g., amikacin, streptomycin, neomycin, kanamycin, gentamicin and paromomycin), cephaloridine, viomycin, polymyxin B, colistin, cisplatin and vancomycin, should be avoided. Other factors that may increase patient risk are advanced age and dehydration.
Aminoglycosides should not be given concurrently with potent diuretics, such as ethacrynic acid and furosemide. Some diuretics themselves cause ototoxicity, and intravenously administered diuretics enhance aminoglycoside toxicity by altering antibiotic concentrations in serum and tissue.
Aminoglycosides can cause fetal harm when administered to a pregnant woman (see PRECAUTIONS).

DESCRIPTION

Tobramycin sulfate, a water-soluble antibiotic of the aminoglycoside group, is derived from the actinomycete *Streptomyces tenebrarius*. Tobramycin Sulfate Injection, USP is a clear and colorless sterile aqueous solution for intramuscular or intravenous (infusion) administration.
Each mL contains tobramycin sulfate equivalent to 10 mg (pediatric) or 40 mg tobramycin, methylparaben 1.8 mg, propylparaben 0.2 mg, sodium metabisulfite 1.2 mg and edetate disodium 0.1 mg in Water for Injection. pH 3.0–6.5; sulfuric acid and/or sodium hydroxide added, if needed, for pH adjustment. Sealed under nitrogen, Tobramycin is 4-0-[2,6-diamino-2, 3, 6-trideoxy -α- D-glucopyranosyl]- 6-0- [3-amino-3-deoxy-α-D-glucopyranosyl]-2-deoxy-streptamine. Its structural formula is as follows:

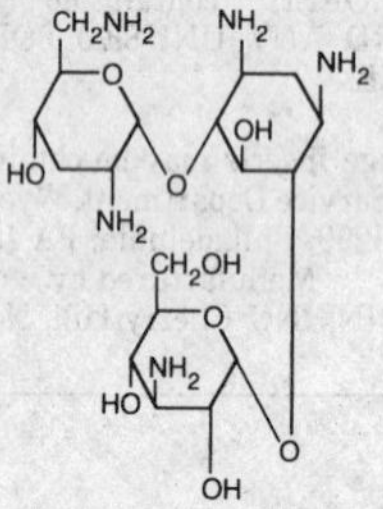

CLINICAL PHARMACOLOGY

Tobramycin is rapidly absorbed following intramuscular administration. Peak serum concentrations of tobramycin occur between 30 and 90 minutes after intramuscular administration. Following an intramuscular dose of 1 mg/kg of body weight, maximum serum concentrations reach about 4 μg/mL, and measurable levels persist for as long as 8 hours. Therapeutic serum levels are generally considered to range from 4 to 6 μg/mL. When tobramycin sulfate is administered by intravenous infusion over a 1-hour period, the serum concentrations are similar to those obtained by intramuscular administration. Tobramycin is poorly absorbed from the gastrointestinal tract.
In patients with normal renal function, except neonates, tobramycin administered every 8 hours does not accumulate in the serum. However, in those with reduced renal function and in neonates, the serum concentration of the antibiotic is usually higher and can be measured for longer periods of time than in normal adults. Dosage for such patients must, therefore, be adjusted accordingly (see DOSAGE AND ADMINISTRATION).
Following parenteral administration, little, if any, metabolic transformation occurs, and tobramycin is eliminated almost exclusively by glomerular filtration. Renal clearance is similar to that of endogenous creatinine. Ultrafiltration studies demonstrate that practically no serum protein binding occurs. In patients with normal renal function, up to 84% of the dose is recoverable from the urine in 8 hours and up to 93% in 24 hours.
Peak urine concentrations ranging from 75 to 100 μg/mL have been observed following the intramuscular injection of a single dose of 1 mg/kg. After several days of treatment, the amount of tobramycin excreted in the urine approaches the daily dose administered. When renal function is impaired, excretion of tobramycin is slowed, and accumulation of the drug may cause toxic blood levels.
The serum half-life in normal individuals is 2 hours. An inverse relationship exists between serum half-life and creatinine clearance, and the dosage schedule should be adjusted according to the degree of renal impairment (see DOSAGE AND ADMINISTRATION). In patients undergoing dialysis, 25% to 70% of the administered dose may be removed, depending on the duration and type of dialysis.
Tobramycin can be detected in tissues and body fluids after parenteral administration. Concentrations in bile and stools ordinarily have been low, which suggests minimum biliary excretion. Tobramycin has appeared in low concentration in the cerebrospinal fluid following parenteral administration, and concentrations are dependent on dose, rate of penetration and degree of meningeal inflammation. It has also been found in sputum, peritoneal fluid, synovial fluid and abscess fluids, and it crosses the placental membranes. Concentrations in the renal cortex are several times higher than the usual serum levels.
Probenecid does not affect the renal tubular transport of tobramycin.

Microbiology

In vitro tests demonstrate that tobramycin is bactericidal and that it acts by inhibiting the synthesis of protein in bacterial cells.
Tobramycin is usually active against most strains of the following organisms *in vitro* and in clinical infections:
Pseudomonas aeruginosa
Proteus species (indole-positive and indole-negative), including *Proteus mirabilis, P. morganii, P. rettgeri* and *P. vulgaris*
Escherichia coli
Klebsiella-Enterobacter-Serratia group
Citrobacter species
Providencia species
Staphylococci, including *Staphylococcus aureus* (coagulase-positive and coagulase-negative)
Aminoglycosides have a low order of activity against most gram-positive organisms, including *Streptococcus pyogenes, Streptococcus pneumoniae* and enterococci.
Although most strains of group D streptococci demonstrate *in vitro* resistance, some strains in this group are susceptible. *In vitro* studies have shown that an aminoglycoside combined with an antibiotic that interferes with cell-wall synthesis affects some group D streptococcal strains synergistically. The combination of penicillin G and tobramycin results in a synergistic bactericidal effect *in vitro* against certain strains of *Streptococcus faecalis*. However, this combination is not synergistic against other closely related organisms, e.g., *Streptococcus faecium*. Speciation of group D streptococci alone cannot be used to predict susceptibility. Susceptibility testing and tests for antibiotic synergism are emphasized.
Cross-resistance between aminoglycosides occurs and depends largely on inactivation by bacterial enzymes.

Susceptibility Tests

If the FDA Standardized Disc Test method (formerly the Bauer-Kirby-Sherris-Turck method) of disk susceptibility testing is used, a disk containing 10 μg tobramycin should give a zone of at least 15 mm when tested against a tobramycin-susceptible bacterial strain, a zone of 13 to 14 mm against strains of intermediate susceptibility and a zone of 12 mm or less against resistant organisms. The minimum inhibitory concentration correlates are ≤4 μg/mL for susceptibility and ≥8 μg/mL for resistance.

INDICATIONS AND USAGE

Tobramycin Sulfate Injection is indicated for the treatment of serious bacterial infections caused by susceptible strains of the designated microorganisms in the diseases listed below:
Septicemia in the neonate, child and adult caused by *P. aeruginosa, E. coli* and *Klebsiella* species
Lower respiratory tract infections caused by *P. aeruginosa, Klebsiella* species, *Enterobacter* species, *Serratia* species, *E. coli* and *S. aureus* (penicillinase and non-penicillinase-producing strains)
Serious central nervous system infections (meningitis) caused by susceptible organisms
Intra-abdominal infections, including peritonitis, caused by *E. coli, Klebsiella* species and *Enterobacter* species
Skin, bone and skin-structure infections caused by *P. aeruginosa, Proteus* species, *E. coli, Klebsiella* species, *Enterobacter* species and *S. aureus*
Complicated and recurrent urinary tract infections caused by *P. aeruginosa, Proteus* species (indole-positive and indole-negative), *E. coli, Klebsiella* species, *Enterobacter* species, *Serratia* species, *S. aureus, Providencia* species and *Citrobacter* species
Aminoglycosides, including tobramycin, are not indicated in uncomplicated initial episodes of urinary tract infections unless the causative organisms are not susceptibile to antibiotics having less potential toxicity. Tobramycin may be considered in serious staphylococcal infections when penicillin or other potentially less toxic drugs are contraindicated and when bacterial susceptibility testing and clinical judgment indicate its use.
Bacterial cultures should be obtained prior to and during treatment to isolate and identify etiologic organisms and to test their susceptibility to tobramycin. If susceptibility tests show that the causative organisms are resistant to tobramycin, other appropriate therapy should be instituted. In patients in whom a serious life-threatening gram-negative in-

TABLE 1
DOSAGE SCHEDULE GUIDE FOR ADULTS WITH NORMAL RENAL FUNCTION
(Dosage at 8-Hour Intervals)

For Patient Weighing		Usual Dose for Serious Infections 1 mg/kg q8h (Total, 3 mg/kg/day)		Maximum Dose for Life-Threatening Infections *(Reduce as soon as possible)* 1.66 mg/kg q8h (Total, 5 mg/kg/day)	
kg	lb	mg/dose	mL/dose*	mg/dose	mL/dose*
		q8h		q8h	
120	264	120 mg	3 mL	200 mg	5 mL
115	253	115 mg	2.9 mL	191 mg	4.75 mL
110	242	110 mg	2.75 mL	183 mg	4.5 mL
105	231	105 mg	2.6 mL	175 mg	4.4 mL
100	220	100 mg	2.5 mL	166 mg	4.2 mL
95	209	95 mg	2.4 mL	158 mg	4 mL
90	198	90 mg	2.25 mL	150 mg	3.75 mL
85	187	85 mg	2.1 mL	141 mg	3.5 mL
80	176	80 mg	2 mL	133 mg	3.3 mL
75	165	75 mg	1.9 mL	125 mg	3.1 mL
70	154	70 mg	1.75 mL	116 mg	2.9 mL
65	143	65 mg	1.6 mL	108 mg	2.7 mL
60	132	60 mg	1.5 mL	100 mg	2.5 mL
55	121	55 mg	1.4 mL	91 mg	2.25 mL
50	110	50 mg	1.25 mL	83 mg	2.1 mL
45	99	45 mg	1.1 mL	75 mg	1.9 mL
40	88	40 mg	1 mL	66 mg	1.6 mL

*Applicable to all product forms except Pediatric Tobramycin Sulfate Injection (see HOW SUPPLIED).

fection is suspected, including those in whom concurrent therapy with a penicillin or cephalosporin and an aminoglycoside may be indicated, treatment with tobramycin may be initiated before the results of susceptibility studies are obtained. The decision to continue therapy with tobramycin should be based on the results of susceptibility studies, the severity of the infection and the important additional concepts discussed in the WARNINGS box above.

CONTRAINDICATIONS
A hypersensitivity to any aminoglycoside is a contraindication to the use of tobramycin. A history of hypersensitivity or serious toxic reactions to aminoglycosides may also contraindicate the use of any other aminoglycoside because of the known cross-sensitivity of patients to drugs in this class.

WARNINGS
See WARNINGS box above.
Tobramycin Sulfate Injection contains sodium metabisulfite, a sulfite that may cause allergic-type reactions, including anaphylactic symptoms and life-threatening or less severe asthmatic episodes, in certain susceptible people. The overall prevalence of sulfite sensitivity in the general population is unknown and probably low. Sulfite sensitivity is seen more frequently in asthmatic than in nonasthmatic people.

PRECAUTIONS
Serum and urine specimens for examination should be collected during therapy, as recommended in the WARNINGS box. Serum calcium, magnesium and sodium should be monitored:
Peak and trough serum levels should be measured periodically during therapy. Prolonged concentrations above 12 μg/mL should be avoided. Rising trough levels (above 2 μg/mL) may indicate tissue accumulation. Such accumulation, advanced age and cumulative dosage may contribute to ototoxicity and nephrotoxicity. It is particularly important to monitor serum levels closely in patients with known renal impairment.
A useful guideline would be to perform serum level assays after 2 or 3 doses, so that the dosage could be adjusted if necessary, and also at 3- to 4-day intervals during therapy. In the event of changing renal function, more frequent serum levels should be obtained and the dosage or dosage interval adjusted according to the guidelines provided in the DOSAGE AND ADMINISTRATION section.
In order to measure the peak level, a serum sample should be drawn about 30 minutes following intravenous infusion or 1 hour after an intramuscular injection. Trough levels are measured by obtaining serum samples at 8 hours or just prior to the next dose of tobramycin. These suggested time intervals are intended only as guidelines and may vary according to institutional practices. It is important, however, that there be consistency within the individual patient program unless computerized pharmacokinetic dosing programs are available in the institution. These serum-level assays may be especially useful for monitoring the treatment of severely ill patients with changing renal function or of those infected with less sensitive organisms or those receiving maximum dosage.
Neuromuscular blockade and respiratory paralysis have been reported in cats receiving very high doses of tobramycin (40 mg/kg). The possibility that prolonged or secondary ap-

nea may occur should be considered if tobramycin is administered to anesthetized patients who are also receiving neuromuscular blocking agents, such as succinylcholine, tubocurarine or decamethonium, or to patients receiving massive transfusions of citrated blood. If neuromuscular blockade occurs, it may be reversed by the administration of calcium salts.
Cross-allergenicity among aminoglycosides has been demonstrated.
In patients with extensive burns, altered pharmacokinetics may result in reduced serum concentrations of aminoglycosides. In such patients treated with tobramycin, measurement of serum concentration is especially recommended as a basis for determination of appropriate dosage.
Elderly patients may have reduced renal function that may not be evident in the results of routine screening tests, such as BUN or serum creatinine. A creatinine clearance determination may be more useful. Monitoring of renal function during treatment with aminoglycosides is particularly important in such patients.
An increased incidence of nephrotoxicity has been reported following concomitant administration of aminoglycoside antibiotics and cephalosporins.
Aminoglycosides should be used with caution in patients with muscular disorders, such as myasthenia gravis or parkinsonism, since these drugs may aggravate muscle weakness because of their potential curare-like effect on neuromuscular function.
Aminoglycosides may be absorbed in significant quantities from body surfaces after local irrigation or application and may cause neurotoxicity and nephrotoxicity.
See WARNINGS box regarding concurrent use of potent diuretics and concurrent and sequential use of other neurotoxic or nephrotoxic drugs.
The inactivation of tobramycin and other aminoglycosides by β-lactam-type antibiotics (penicillins or cephalosporins) has been demonstrated *in vitro* and in patients with severe renal impairment. Such inactivation has not been found in patients with normal renal function who have been given the drugs by separate routes of administration.
Therapy with tobramycin may result in overgrowth of nonsusceptible organisms. If overgrowth of nonsusceptible organisms occurs, appropriate therapy should be initiated.

PREGNANCY
Pregnancy Category D. Aminoglycosides can cause fetal harm when administered to a pregnant woman. Aminoglycoside antibiotics cross the placenta, and there have been several reports of total irreversible bilateral congenital deafness in children whose mothers received streptomycin during pregnancy. Serious side effects to mother, fetus or newborn have not been reported in the treatment of pregnant women with other aminoglycosides. If tobramycin is used during pregnancy or if the patient becomes pregnant while taking tobramycin, she should be apprised of the potential hazard to the fetus.

USAGE IN CHILDREN
See INDICATIONS AND USAGE and DOSAGE AND ADMINISTRATION.

ADVERSE REACTIONS
Neurotoxicity—Adverse effects on both the vestibular and auditory branches of the eighth nerve have been noted, especially in patients receiving high doses or prolonged therapy,

in those given previous courses of therapy with an ototoxin and in cases of dehydration. Symptoms include dizziness, vertigo, tinnitus, roaring in the ears and hearing loss. Hearing loss is usually irreversible and is manifested initially by diminution of high-tone acuity. Tobramycin and gentamicin sulfates closely parallel each other in regard to ototoxic potential.
Nephrotoxicity—Renal function changes, as shown by rising BUN, NPN and serum creatinine and by oliguria, cylindruria and increased proteinuria, have been reported, especially in patients with a history of renal impairment who are treated for longer periods or with higher doses than those recommended. Adverse renal effects can occur in patients with initially normal renal function.
Clinical studies and studies in experimental animals have been conducted to compare the nephrotoxic potential of tobramycin and gentamicin. In some of the clinical studies and in the animal studies, tobramycin caused nephrotoxicity significantly less frequently than gentamicin. In some other clinical studies, no significant difference in the incidence of nephrotoxicity between tobramycin and gentamicin was found.
Other reported adverse reactions possibly related to tobramycin sulfate include anemia, granulocytopenia and thrombocytopenia; and fever, rash, itching, urticaria, nausea, vomiting, diarrhea, headache, lethargy, pain at the injection site, mental confusion and disorientation. Laboratory abnormalities possibly related to tobramycin include increased serum transaminases (SGOT, SGPT); increased serum LDH and bilirubin; decreased serum calcium, magnesium, sodium and potassium; and leukopenia, leukocytosis and eosinophilia.

OVERDOSAGE
In the event of overdosage or toxic reaction, hemodialysis or peritoneal dialysis will reduce serum levels. Hemodialysis is preferable because it is more efficient in reducing serum levels.

DOSAGE AND ADMINISTRATION
Tobramycin Sulfate Injection may be given intramuscularly or intravenously. Recommended dosages are the same for both routes. The patient's pretreatment body weight should be obtained for calculation of correct dosage. It is desirable to measure both peak and trough serum concentrations (see WARNINGS box and PRECAUTIONS).

**Administration for Patients with Normal Renal Function
—Adults with Serious Infections:** 3 mg/kg/day in 3 equal doses every 8 hours (see Table 1).
Adults with Life-Threatening Infections: Up to 5 mg/kg/day may be administered in 3 or 4 equal doses (see Table 1). The dosage should be reduced to 3 mg/kg/day as soon as clinically indicated. To prevent increased toxicity due to excessive blood levels, dosage should not exceed 5 mg/kg/day unless serum levels are monitored.

Children: 6 to 7.5 mg/kg/day in 3 or 4 equally divided doses (2 to 2.5 mg/kg every 8 hours or 1.5 to 1.89 mg/kg every 6 hours).

Premature or Full-Term Neonates 1 Week of Age or Less: Up to 4 mg/kg/day may be administered in 2 equal doses every 12 hours.

Continued on next page

Elkins-Sinn—Cont.

It is desirable to limit treatment to a short term. The usual duration of treatment is 7 to 10 days. A longer course of therapy may be necessary in difficult and complicated infections. In such cases, monitoring of renal, auditory and vestibular functions is advised, because neurotoxicity is more likely to occur when treatment is extended longer than 10 days.

Administration for Patients with Impaired Renal Function: Whenever possible, serum tobramycin concentrations should be monitored during therapy.

Following a loading dose of 1 mg/kg, subsequent dosage in these patients must be adjusted, either with reduced doses administered at 8-hour intervals or with normal doses given at prolonged intervals. Both of these methods are suggested as guides to be used when serum levels of tobramycin cannot be measured directly. They are based on either the creatinine clearance or the serum creatinine of the patient, because these values correlate with the half-life of tobramycin. The dosage schedules derived from either method should be used in conjunction with careful clinical and laboratory observations of the patient and should be modified as necessary. Neither method should be used when dialysis is being performed.

Reduced dosage at 8-hour intervals—When the creatinine clearance rate is 70 mL or less per minute or when the serum creatinine value is known, the amount of the reduced dose can be determined by multiplying the normal dose from Table 1 by the percent of normal dose from the accompanying nomogram.

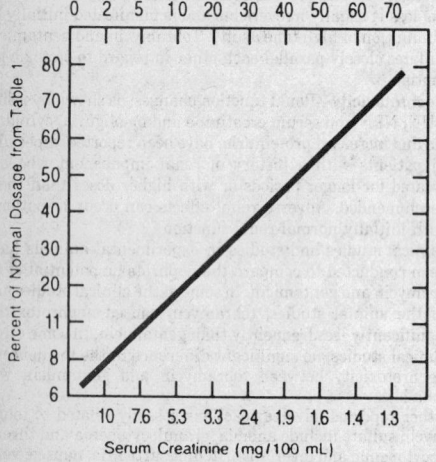

REDUCED DOSAGE NOMOGRAM*
Creatinine Clearance (mL/min/1.73 m²)

*Scales have been adjusted to facilitate dosage calculations.

An alternate rough guide for determining reduced dosage at 8-hour intervals (for patients whose steady-state serum creatinine values are known) is to divide the normally recommended dose by the patient's serum creatinine.

Normal dosage at prolonged intervals—If the creatinine clearance rate is not available and the patient's condition is stable, a dosage frequency *in hours* for the dosage given in Table 1 can be determined by multiplying the patient's serum creatinine by 6.

Dosage in Obese Patients: The appropriate dose may be calculated by using the patient's estimated lean body weight plus 40% of the excess as the basic weight on which to figure mg/kg.

Intramuscular Administration: Tobramycin sulfate may be administered by withdrawing the appropriate dose directly from a vial or by using a prefilled syringe.

Intravenous Administration: For intravenous administration, the usual volume of diluent (0.9% Sodium Chloride Injection or 5% Dextrose Injection) is 50 to 100 mL for adult doses. For children, the volume of diluent should be proportionately less than for adults. The diluted solution usually should be infused over a period of 20 to 60 minutes. Infusion periods of less than 20 minutes are not recommended because peak serum levels may exceed 12 µg/mL (see WARNINGS box).

Tobramycin should not be physically premixed with other drugs but should be administered separately according to the recommended dose and route.

Parenteral drug products should be inspected visually for particulate matter and discoloration prior to administration, whenever solution and container permit. Do not use if discolored.

HOW SUPPLIED

Tobramycin Sulfate Injection, USP is available in the following packages:

Pediatric—10 mg/mL (as tobramycin)
2 mL (20 mg) Multiple Dose vials packaged in 25s (*NDC* 0641-0585-25)
40 mg/mL (as tobramycin)
2 mL (80 mg) Multiple Dose vials packaged in 25s (*NDC* 0641-0587-25)
30 mL (1.2 g) Multiple Dose vial packaged individually (*NDC* 0641-2750-41)
2 mL (80 mg) DOSETTE® syringes (22 gauge, 1 1/4 inch) packaged in 25s (*NDC* 0641-6587-15)

STORAGE
Store at controlled room temperature 15°-30°C (59°-86°F). Avoid freezing. Do not use if discolored.

TUBEX®Closed Injection System
[*tū'beks*]

For TUBEX product information, directions, and a list of products available in the TUBEX Closed Injection System, please see Wyeth-Ayerst section on page 2647 of the 1993 PDR.

Enzon, Inc.
40 KINGSBRIDGE ROAD
PISCATAWAY, NJ 08854

ADAGEN™   ℞
[*ad-a-jen*]
(pegademase bovine)
Injection

PRODUCT OVERVIEW

KEY FACTS

Adagen (pegademase bovine injection) is a modified enzyme used to provide direct and specific replacement of adenosine deaminase, an enzyme that is deficient in patients with severe combined immunodeficiency disease (SCID). While regular administration of the compound can improve immune function and reduce the incidence of opportunistic infections in patients with SCID, it is of no value in patients with immunodeficiency due to other causes. Further, it is not an appropriate preparatory or support therapy for patients undergoing bone marrow transplantation.

MAJOR USES

Adagen is to be used as enzyme replacement therapy in patients who have SCID associated with a deficiency of ADA. Because the immune deficiency can be cured by bone marrow transplants, patients eligible for enzyme replacement must first have failed bone marrow transplant or be considered poor candidates for the procedure. It should be used in infants from birth or in children of any age at the time of diagnosis.

SAFETY INFORMATION

Adagen should be administered with caution to patients with thrombocytopenia and should not be given if thrombocytopenia is severe.

PRESCRIBING INFORMATION

ADAGEN™   ℞
[*ad-a-jen*]
(pegademase bovine) Injection

DESCRIPTION

ADAGEN™ (pegademase bovine) Injection is a modified enzyme used for enzyme replacement therapy for the treatment of severe combined immunodeficiency disease (SCID) associated with a deficiency of adenosine deaminase.

ADAGEN™ (pegademase bovine) Injection is supplied in an isotonic, pyrogen free, sterile solution, pH 7.2-7.4, for intramuscular injection only. The solution is clear and colorless. It is supplied in 1.5 mL single-dose vials.

The chemical name for **ADAGEN™** (pegademase bovine) Injection is (monomethoxypolyethylene glycol succinimidyl)$_{11-17}$-adenosine deaminase. It is a conjugate of numerous strands of monomethoxypolyethylene glycol (PEG), molecular weight 5,000, covalently attached to the enzyme adenosine deaminase (ADA). ADA (adenosine deaminase EC 3.5.4.4) used in the manufacture of **ADAGEN™** (pegademase bovine) Injection is derived from bovine intestine.

The structural formula of **ADAGEN™** (pegademase bovine) Injection is:

$$[CH_3-(OCH_2CH_2)_x-O-\overset{O}{\underset{\|}{C}}-CH_2CH_2-\overset{O}{\underset{\|}{C}}-NH]_y-\text{adenosine deaminase}$$

x = 114 oxyethylene groups per PEG strand.

y = 11–17 primary amino groups of lysine onto which succinyl PEG is attached.

Each milliliter of **ADAGEN™** (pegademase bovine) Injection contains:

Pegademase bovine ....250 units*
Monobasic sodium phosphate, USP ....1.20 mg
Dibasic sodium phosphate, USP ....5.58 mg
Sodium Chloride, USP ....8.50 mg
Water for Injection, USP ....q.s. to 1.0 mL

*One unit of activity is defined as the amount of ADA that converts 1 µM of adenosine to inosine per minute at 25°C and pH 7.3.

CLINICAL PHARMACOLOGY

Severe Combined Immunodeficiency Disease Associated with ADA Deficiency

Severe combined immunodeficiency disease (SCID) associated with a deficiency of ADA is a rare, inherited, and often fatal disease. In the absence of the ADA enzyme, the purine substrates adenosine and 2'-deoxyadenosine accumulate, causing metabolic abnormalities that are directly toxic to lymphocytes.

The immune deficiency can be cured by bone marrow transplantation. When a suitable bone marrow donor is unavailable or when bone marrow transplantation fails, non-selective replacement of the ADA enzyme has been provided by periodic irradiated red blood cell transfusions. However, transmission of viral infections and iron overload are serious risks associated with irradiated red blood cell transfusions, and relatively few ADA deficient patients have benefitted from chronic transfusion therapy.

ADAGEN™ (pegademase bovine) Injection provides specific and direct replacement of the deficient enzyme, but will not benefit patients with immunodeficiency due to other causes. In patients with ADA deficiency, rigorous adherence to a schedule of **ADAGEN™** (pegademase bovine) Injection administration can eliminate the toxic metabolites of ADA deficiency and result in improved immune function. It is imperative that treatment with **ADAGEN™** (pegademase bovine) Injection be carefully monitored by measurement of the level of ADA activity in plasma. Monitoring of the level of deoxyadenosine triphosphate (dATP) in erythrocytes is also helpful in determining that the dose of **ADAGEN™** (pegademase bovine) Injection is adequate.

Actions

ADAGEN™ (pegademase bovine) Injection provides specific replacement of the deficient enzyme.

In the absence of the enzyme ADA, the purine substrates adenosine, 2'-deoxyadenosine and their metabolites are toxic to lymphocytes. The direct action of **ADAGEN™** (pegademase bovine) Injection is the correction of these metabolic abnormalities. Improvement in immune function and diminished frequency of opportunistic infections compared with the natural history of combined immunodeficiency due to ADA deficiency only occurs after metabolic abnormalities are corrected. There is a lag between the correction of the metabolic abnormalities and improved immune function. This period of time is variable, and has been reported to be from a few weeks to as long as 6 months. In contrast to the natural history of combined immunodeficiency disease due to ADA deficiency, a trend toward diminished frequency of opportunistic infections and fewer complications of infections has occurred in patients receiving **ADAGEN™** (pegademase bovine) Injection.

Pharmacokinetics

The pharmacokinetics and biochemical effects of **ADAGEN™** (pegademase bovine) Injection have been studied in six children ranging in age from 6 weeks to 12 years with SCID associated with ADA deficiency.

After the intramuscular injection of **ADAGEN™** (pegademase bovine) Injection, peak plasma levels of ADA activity were reached 2 to 3 days following administration. The plasma elimination half-life of ADA following the administration of **ADAGEN™** (pegademase bovine) Injection was variable, even for the same child. The range was 3 to >6 days. Following weekly injections of **ADAGEN™** (pegademase bovine) Injection at 15 U/kg, the average trough level of ADA activity in plasma was between 20 and 25 µmol/hr/mL.

Biochemical Effects

The changes in red blood cell deoxyadenosine nucleotide (dATP) and S-adenosylhomocysteine hydrolase (SAHase) have been evaluated. In patients with ADA deficiency, inadequate elimination of 2'-deoxyadenosine caused a marked elevation in dATP and a decrease in SAHase level in red blood cells. Prior to treatment with **ADAGEN™** (pegademase bovine) Injection, the levels of dATP in the red blood cells ranged from 0.056 to 0.899 µmol/mL of erythrocytes. After 2 months of maintenance treatment with **ADAGEN™** (pegademase bovine) Injection, the levels decreased to 0.007 to 0.015 µmol/mL. The normal value of dATP is below 0.001 µmol/mL. In the same period of time, the levels of SAHase increased from the pretreatment range of 0.09 to 0.22 nmol/hr/mg protein to a range of 2.37 to 5.16 nmol/hr/mg protein. The normal value for SAHase is 4.18± 1.9 nmol/hr/mg protein.

The optimal dosage and schedule of administration of **ADAGEN™** (pegademase bovine) Injection should be established for each patient, based on monitoring of plasma ADA activity levels (trough levels before maintenance injection),

biochemical markers of ADA deficiency (primarily red cell dATP content), and parameters of immune function. Since improvement in immune function follows correction of metabolic abnormalities, maintenance dosage in individual patients should be aimed at achieving the following biochemical goals: 1) maintain plasma ADA activity (trough levels) in the range of 15–35 μmol/hr/mL (assayed at 37°C); and 2) decline in erythrocyte dATP to ≤ 0.005–0.015 μmol/mL packed erythrocytes, or ≤ 1% of the total erythrocyte adenine nucleotide (ATP + dATP) content, with a normal ATP level, as measured in a pre-injection sample.

In vitro immunologic data (lymphocyte response to mitogens and lymphocyte surface antigens) were obtained, but their clinical significance is unknown. Prior to treatment with **ADAGEN**™ (pegademase bovine) Injection, immune status was significantly below normal, as indicated by < 10% of normal mitogen responses and circulating mononuclear cells bearing T-cell surface antigens. These parameters improved, though not always to normal, within 2 to 6 months of therapy.

INDICATIONS AND USAGE

ADAGEN™ (pegademase bovine) Injection is indicated for enzyme replacement therapy for adenosine deaminase (ADA) deficiency in patients with severe combined immunodeficiency disease (SCID) who are not suitable candidates for—or who have failed—bone marrow transplantation. **ADAGEN**™ (pegademase bovine) Injection is recommended for use in infants from birth or in children of any age at the time of diagnosis. **ADAGEN**™ (pegademase bovine) Injection is not intended as a replacement for HLA indentical bone marrow transplant therapy. **ADAGEN**™ (pegademase bovine) Injection is also not intended to replace continued close medical supervision and the initiation of appropriate diagnostic tests and therapy (e.g., antibiotics, nutrition, oxygen, gammaglobulin) as indicated for intercurrent illnesses.

CONTRAINDICATIONS

There is no evidence to support the safety and efficacy of **ADAGEN**™ (pegademase bovine) Injection as preparatory or support therapy for bone marrow transplantation. Since **ADAGEN**™ (pegademase bovine) Injection is administered by intramuscular injection, it should be used with caution in patients with thrombocytopenia and should not be used if thrombocytopenia is severe.

PRECAUTIONS

Warnings

At present, testing prior to distribution may not assure the initial and continuing potency of each new lot of **ADAGEN**™ (pegademase bovine) Injection. Any laboratory or clinical indication of a decrease in potency of **ADAGEN**™ (pegademase bovine) Injection should be reported immediately by telephone to ENZON, Inc. Telephone 908-980-4500. Fax 908-980-5911.

General

There have been no reports of hypersensitivity reactions in patients who have been treated with **ADAGEN**™ (pegademase bovine) Injection.

One of 12 patients showed an enhanced rate of clearance of plasma ADA activity after 5 months of therapy at 15 U/kg/week. Enhanced clearance was correlated with the appearance of an antibody that directly inhibited both unmodified ADA and **ADAGEN**™ (pegademase bovine) Injection. Subsequently, the patient was treated with twice weekly intramuscular injections at an increased dose of 20 U/kg, or a total weekly dose of 40 U/kg. No adverse effects were observed at the higher dose and effective levels of plasma ADA were restored. After 4 months, the patient returned to a weekly dosage schedule of 20 U/kg and effective plasma levels have been maintained.

Appropriate care to protect immune deficient patients should be maintained until improvement in immune function has been documented. The degree of immune function improvement may vary from patient to patient and, therefore, each patient will require appropriate care consistent with immunologic status.

Laboratory Tests

The treatment of SCID associated with ADA deficiency with **ADAGEN**™ (pegademase bovine) Injection should be monitored by measuring plasma ADA activity and red blood cell dATP levels.

Plasma ADA activity and red cell dATP should be determined prior to treatment. Once treatment with **ADAGEN**™ (pegademase bovine) Injection has been initiated, a desirable range of plasma ADA activity (trough level before maintenance injection) should be 15–35 μmol/hr/mL. This minimum trough level will ensure that plasma ADA activity from injection to injection is maintained above the level of total erythrocyte ADA activity in the blood of normal individuals.

Plasma ADA activity (pre-injection) should be determined every 1–2 weeks during the first 8–12 weeks of treatment in order to establish an effective dose of **ADAGEN**™ (pegademase bovine) Injection. After two months of maintenance treatment with **ADAGEN**™ (pegademase bovine) Injection, red cell dATP levels should decrease to a range of ≤0.005 to 0.015 μmol/mL. The normal value of dATP is below 0.001 μmol/mL. Once the level of dATP has fallen adequately, it should be measured 2–4 times a year during the remainder of the first year and 2–3 times a year thereafter, assuming no interruption in therapy.

Between 3 and 9 months, plasma ADA should be determined twice a month, then monthly until after 18–24 months of treatment with **ADAGEN**™ (pegademase bovine) Injection.

Patients who have successfully been maintained on therapy for two years should continue to have plasma ADA measured every 2–4 months and red cell dATP measured twice yearly. More frequent monitoring would be necessary if therapy were interrupted or if an enhanced rate of clearance of plasma ADA activity develops.

Once effective ADA plasma levels have been established, should a patient's plasma ADA activity level fall below 10 μmol/hr/mL (which cannot be attributed to improper dosing, sample handling or antibody development) then all patients receiving this lot of **ADAGEN**™ (pegademase bovine) Injection will be required to have a blood sample for plasma ADA determination taken prior to their next injection of **ADAGEN**™ (pegademase bovine) Injection. The index patient will require re-testing for determination of plasma ADA activity prior to his/her next injection of **ADAGEN**™ (pegademase bovine) Injection. If this value, as well as the value from one of the other patients from a different site, is less than 10 μmol/hr/mL then the lot in use will be recalled and replaced with a new clinical lot by ENZON, Inc.

Immune function, including the ability to produce antibodies, generally improves after 2–6 months of therapy, and matures over a longer period. Compared with the natural history of combined immunodeficiency disease due to ADA deficiency, a trend toward diminished frequency of opportunistic infections and fewer complications of infections has occurred in patients receiving **ADAGEN**™ (pegademase bovine) Injection. However, the lag between the correction of the metabolic abnormalities and improved immune function with a trend toward diminished frequency of infections and complications of infection is variable, and has ranged from a few weeks to approximately 6 months. Improvement in the general clinical status of the patient may be gradual (as evidenced by improvement in various clinical parameters) but should be apparent by the end of the first year of therapy.

Antibody to **ADAGEN**™ (pegademase bovine) Injection may develop in patients and may result in more rapid clearance of **ADAGEN**™ (pegademase bovine) Injection. Antibody to **ADAGEN**™ (pegademase bovine) Injection should be suspected if a persistent fall in pre-injection levels of plasma ADA to ≤10 μmol/hr/mL occurs. If other causes for a decline in plasma ADA levels can be ruled out [such as improper storage of **ADAGEN**™ (pegademase bovine) Injection vials (freezing or prolonged storage at temperatures above 8°C), or improper handling of plasma samples (e.g., repeated freezing and thawing during transport to laboratory)], then a specific assay for antibody to ADA and **ADAGEN**™ (pegademase bovine) Injection (ELISA, enzyme inhibition) should be performed.

In patients undergoing treatment with **ADAGEN**™ (pegademase bovine) Injection, a decline in immune function, with increased risk of opportunistic infections and complications of infection, will result from failure to maintain adequate levels of plasma ADA activity [whether due to the development of antibody to **ADAGEN**™ (pegademase bovine) Injection, to improper calculation of **ADAGEN**™ (pegademase bovine) Injection dosage, to interruption of treatment or to improper storage of **ADAGEN**™ (pegademase bovine) Injection with subsequent loss of activity]. If a persistent decline in plasma ADA activity occurs, immune function and clinical status should be monitored closely and precautions should be taken to minimize the risk of infection. If antibody to ADA or **ADAGEN**™ (pegademase bovine) Injection is found to be the cause of a persistent fall in plasma ADA activity, then adjustment in the dosage of **ADAGEN**™ (pegademase bovine) Injection and other measures may be taken to induce tolerance and restore adequate ADA activity.

Drug Interactions

There are no known drug interactions with **ADAGEN**™ (pegademase bovine) Injection. However, Vidarbine is a substrate for ADA and 2′-deoxycoformycin is a potent inhibitor of ADA. Thus, the activities of these drugs and **ADAGEN**™ (pegademase bovine) Injection could be substantially altered if they are used in combination with one another.

Carcinogenesis, Mutagenesis, Impairment of Fertility

Long-term carcinogenic studies in animals have not been performed with **ADAGEN**™ (pegademase bovine) Injection nor have studies been performed on impairment of fertility. **ADAGEN**™ (pegademase bovine) Injection did not exhibit a mutagenic effect when tested against Salmonella typhimurium strains in the Ames assay.

Pregnancy

Pregnancy Category C. Animal reproduction studies have not been conducted with **ADAGEN**™ (pegademase bovine) Injection. It is also not known whether **ADAGEN**™ (pegademase bovine) Injection can cause fetal harm when administered to a pregnant woman or can affect reproduction capacity. **ADAGEN**™ (pegademase bovine) Injection should be given to a pregnant woman only if clearly needed.

Nursing Mothers

It is not known whether **ADAGEN**™ (pegademase bovine) Injection is excreted in human milk. Because many drugs are excreted in human milk, caution should be exercised when **ADAGEN**™ (pegademase bovine) Injection is administered to a nursing woman.

ADVERSE REACTIONS

Clinical experience with **ADAGEN**™ (pegademase bovine) Injection has been limited. The following adverse reactions have been reported: headache in one patient and pain at the injection site in two patients.

OVERDOSAGE

There is no documented experience with **ADAGEN**™ (pegademase bovine) Injection overdosage. An intraperitoneal dose of 50,000 U/kg of **ADAGEN**™ (pegademase bovine) Injection in mice resulted in weight loss up to 9%.

DOSAGE AND ADMINISTRATION

Before prescribing **ADAGEN**™ (pegademase bovine) Injection the physician should be thoroughly familiar with the details of this prescribing information. For further information concerning the essential monitoring of **ADAGEN**™ (pegademase bovine) Injection therapy, the prescribing physician should contact ENZON, Inc., 40 Kingsbridge Road, Piscataway, NJ 08854. Telephone 908-980-4500. Fax 908-980-5911.

ADAGEN™ (pegademase bovine) Injection is recommended for use in infants from birth or in children of any age at the time of diagnosis.

Parenteral drug products should be inspected visually for particulate matter and discoloration prior to administration, whenever solution and container permits.

ADAGEN™ (pegademase bovine) Injection should not be diluted nor mixed with any other drug prior to administration.

ADAGEN™ (pegademase bovine) Injection should be administered every 7 days as an intramuscular injection. The dosage of **ADAGEN**™ (pegademase bovine) Injection should be individualized. The recommended dosing schedule is 10 U/kg for the first dose, 15 U/kg for the second dose, and 20 U/kg for the third dose. The usual maintenance dose is 20 U/kg per week. Further increases of 5 U/kg/week may be necessary, but a maximum single dose of 30 U/kg should not be exceeded. Plasma levels of ADA more than twice the upper limit of 35 μmol/hr/mL have occurred on occasion in several patients, and have been maintained for several weeks in one patient who received twice weekly injections (20 U/kg per dose) of **ADAGEN**™ (pegademase bovine) Injection. No adverse effects have been observed at these higher levels; there is no evidence that maintaining pre-injection plasma ADA above 35 μmol/hr/mL produces any additional clinical benefits.

Dose proportionality has not been established and patients should be closely monitored when the dosage is increased. **ADAGEN**™ (pegademase bovine) Injection is not recommended for intravenous administration. The optimal dosage and schedule of administration should be established for each patient based on monitoring of plasma ADA activity levels (trough levels before maintenance injection) and biochemical markers of ADA deficiency (primarily red cell dATP content). Since improvement in immune function follows correction of metabolic abnormalities, maintenance dosage in individual patients should be aimed at achieving the following biochemical goasl: 1) maintain plasma ADA activity (trough levels before maintenance injection) in the range of 15–35 μmol/hr/mL (assayed at 37°C); and 2) decline in erythrocyte dATP to ≤0.005–0.015 μmol/mL packed erythrocytes, or ≤1% of the total erythrocyte adenine nucleotide (ATP + dATP) content, with a normal ATP level, as measured in a pre-injection sample. In addition, continued monitoring of immune function and clinical status is essential in any patient with a primary immunodeficiency disease and should be continued in patients undergoing treatment with **ADAGEN**™ (pegademase bovine) Injection.

HOW SUPPLIED

ADAGEN™ (pegademase bovine) Injection is a clear, colorless solution for intramuscular injection. Each vial contains 250 units/mL and is supplied as a 1.5 mL single-use vial, in boxes of 4 vials (NDC-57665-001-01).

Refrigerate. Store between +2°C and +8°C (36°F and 46°F). DO NOT FREEZE. **ADAGEN**™ (pegademase bovine) Injection should not be stored at room temperature. This product should not be used if there are any indications that it may have been frozen.

REFERENCES

1. Hershfield MS, Buckley RH, Greenberg ML, et al. Treatment of adenosine deaminase deficiency with polyethyl-

Continued on next page

Enzon—Cont.

ene glycol-modified adenosine deaminase. N Engl J Med 1987; 316:589–96.

2. Levy Y, Hershfield MS, Fernandez-Mejia C, Polmar ST, Scudiery D, Berger M, Sorensen RU. Adenosine deaminase deficiency with late onset of recurrent infections: response to treatment with polyethylene glycol-modified adenosine deaminase. J. Pediatr 1988; 113:312–17.

3. Kredich NM, Hershfield MS. Immunodeficiency diseases caused by adenosine deaminase deficiency and purine nucleoside phosphorylase deficiency. 6th ed. In: Scriver CR, Beaudet AL, Sly WS, Valle D, eds. The metabolic basis of inherited disease. New York: McGraw Hill, 1989; 1045–75.

4. Hirschhorn R. Inherited enzyme deficiencies and immunodeficiency: adenosine deaminase (ADA) and purine nucleoside phosphorylase (PNP) deficiencies. Clin Immunol Immunopathol 1986; 40:157–65.

5. Hirschhorn R, Roegner-Maniscalco V, Kuritsky L, Rosen FS. Bone marrow transplantation only partially restores purine metabolites to normal adenosine deaminase-deficient patients. J Clin Invest 1981; 68:1387–93.

6. Polmar AH, Stern RC, Schwartz AL, Wetzler EM, Chase PA, Hirschhorn R. Enzyme replacement therapy for adenosine deaminase deficiency and severe combined immunodeficiency. N Engl J Med 1976; 295:1337–43.

7. Rubinstein A, Hirschhorn R, Sicklick M, Murphy RA. In vivo and in vitro effects of thymosin and adenosine deaminase on adenosine-deaminase-deficient lymphocytes. N Engl J Med 1979; 300:387–92.

8. Hirschhorn R, Papageorgiou PS, Kesarwala HH, Taft LT. Amelioration of neurologic abnormalities after "enzyme replacement" in adenosine deaminase deficiency. N Engl J Med 1980; 303:377–80.

9. Hirshhorn R, Ratech H, Rubinstein A, et al. Increased excretion of modified adenine nucleosides by children with adenosine deaminase deficiency. Pediatr Res 1982; 16:362–9.

10. Polmar SH. Enzyme replacement and other biochemical approaches to the therapy of adenosine deaminase deficiency. In: Elliott K, Whelan J, eds. Enzyme defects and immune dysfunction. Amsterdam: Excerpta Medica, 1979; 213–30.

Everett Laboratories, Inc.
71 GLENWOOD PLACE
EAST ORANGE, NEW JERSEY 07017-3004

ĀCODA
Capsules   (III)

Each capsule contains:
Codeine Phosphate 30 mg
(WARNING: May be habit forming), Acetaminophen 150 mg, Aspirin 180 mg.
SUPPLIED
Bottles of 100 Black/Grey capsules imprinted EVERETT.

FLORVITE Drops 0.25 mg & 0.5 mg   ℞
FLORVITE Chewable Tablets 0.5 mg & 1 mg   ℞
Children's Vitamins + Fluoride

SUPPLIED
Bottles of 50 mL and tablets 100.

FLORVITE + IRON Drops 0.25 mg   ℞
FLORVITE + IRON Chewable Tablets
0.5 mg & 1 mg   ℞
Children's Vitamins + Iron + Fluoride

SUPPLIED
Bottles of 50 mL and tablets 100.

REPAN Tablets—REPAN Capsules   ℞

EACH TABLET AND EACH CAPSULE CONTAINS:
Butalbital 50 mg.
(Warning: May be habit forming), Caffeine (Anhydrous) 40 mg, Acetaminophen 325 mg.

SUPPLIED
Bottles of 100 tablets imprinted EVERETT and 162.
Bottles of 100 two-tone blue capsules imprinted EVERETT.

STROVITE TABLETS   ℞
Therapeutic Vitamins

SUPPLIED
Bottle of 100 tablets.

STROVITE PLUS CAPLETS   ℞
Therapeutic Multivitamin Mineral Supplement
Sugar Free

SUPPLIED
Bottles of 100 imprinted EV 201.

TUSSAFED DROPS & SYRUP   ℞
Antitussive-Decongestant-Antihistamine

Each dropperful (A) and each teaspoonful (B) contains:

	A	B
Dextromethorphan	4 mg	15 mg
Pseudoephedrine	25 mg	60 mg
Carbinoxamine	2 mg	4 mg

VITAFOL Caplets   ℞
Vitamins, Minerals, Iron, Folic Acid Supplement
Sugar Free

SUPPLIED
Bottles of 100 and 1000 tablets imprinted EV 0072.

VITAFOL Syrup   ℞
Vitamins, Minerals, Iron, Folic Acid Supplement
Sugar, Alcohol, and Yeast Free

SUPPLIED
Bottles of 16 oz.

ZE CAPS   OTC
Soft Gel Capsules
ANTIOXIDANT

EACH CAPSULE CONTAINS:
Zinc Gluconate 75 mg., Vitamin E 200 I.U.
SUPPLIED
Bottles of 60 sugar and salt free capsules.

Ferndale Laboratories, Inc.
780 W. EIGHT MILE ROAD
FERNDALE, MI 48220

ANALPRAM-HC® CREAM   ℞
Rectal Cream

DESCRIPTION
Contains Hydrocortisone acetate 1% or 2.5% and Pramoxine HCl 1% in a washable, nongreasy base containing stearic acid, cetyl alcohol, aquaphor, isopropyl palmitate, polyoxyl 40 stearate, propylene glycol, potassium sorbate 0.1%, sorbic acid 0.1%, triethanolamine lauryl sulfate and water.
Topical corticosteroids are anti-inflammatory and antipruritic agents. The structural formula, the chemical name, molecular formula and molecular weight for active ingredients are presented below.

Hydrocortisone acetate
(Pregn-4-ene-3,20-dione,21 - (acetyloxy)-11, 17-dihydroxy-,(11 β)-.)
$C_{23}H_{32}O_6$; mol wt: 404.50

Pramoxine hydrochloride
(4-(3-(p-butoxyphenoxy)propyl)morpholine hydrochloride)
$C_{17}H_{27}NO_3.HCl$; mol wt: 329.87

CLINICAL PHARMACOLOGY
Topical corticosteroids share anti-inflammatory, anti-pruritic and vasoconstrictive actions.
The mechanism of anti-inflammatory activity of the topical corticosteroids is unclear. Various laboratory methods, including vasoconstrictor assays, are used to compare and predict potencies and/or clinical efficacies of the topical corticosteroids. There is some evidence to suggest that a recognizable correlation exists between vasoconstrictor potency and therapeutic efficacy in man.
Pramoxine hydrochloride is a topical anesthetic agent which provides temporary relief from itching and pain. It acts by stabilizing the neuronal membrane of nerve endings with which it comes into contact.
Pharmacokinetics: The extent of percutaneous absorption of topical corticosteroids is determined by many factors including the vehicle, the integrity of the epidermal barrier, and the use of occlusive dressings.
Topical corticosteroids can be absorbed from normal intact skin. Inflammation and/or other disease processes in the skin increase percutaneous absorption. Occlusive dressings substantially increase the percutaneous absorption of topical corticosteroids. Thus, occlusive dressings may be a valuable therapeutic adjunct for treatment of resistant dermatoses (See DOSAGE AND ADMINISTRATION).
Once absorbed through the skin, topical corticosteroids are handled through pharmacokinetic pathways similar to systemically administered corticosteroids. Corticosteroids are bound to plasma proteins in varying degrees. Corticosteroids are metabolized primarily in the liver and are then excreted by the kidneys. Some of the topical corticosteroids and their metabolites are also excreted into the bile.

INDICATIONS AND USAGE
Topical corticosteroids are indicated for the relief of the inflammatory and pruritic manifestations of corticosteroid-responsive dermatoses of the anal region.

CONTRAINDICATIONS
Topical corticosteroids are contraindicated in those patients with a history of hypersensitivity to any of the components of the preparation.

PRECAUTIONS
General: Systemic absorption of topical corticosteroids has produced reversible hypothalamic-pituitary-adrenal (HPA) axis suppression, manifestations of Cushing's syndrome, hyperglycemia, and glucosuria in some patients.
Conditions which augment systemic absorption include the application of the more potent steroids, use over large surface areas, prolonged use, and the addition of occlusive dressings.
Therefore, patients receiving a large dose of a potent topical steroid applied to a large surface area and under an occlusive dressing should be evaluated periodically for evidence of HPA axis suppression by using the urinary free cortisol and ACTH stimulation tests. If HPA axis suppression is noted, an attempt should be made to withdraw the drug, to reduce the frequency of application, or to substitute a less potent steroid.
Recovery of HPA axis function is generally prompt and complete upon discontinuation of the drug. Infrequently, signs and symptoms of steroid withdrawal may occur, requiring supplemental systemic corticosteroids.
Children may absorb proportionally larger amounts of topical corticosteroids and thus be more susceptible to systemic toxicity. (See PRECAUTIONS—Pediatric Use).
If irritation develops, topical corticosteroids should be discontinued and appropriate therapy instituted.
In the presence of dermatological infections, the use of an appropriate antifungal or antibacterial agent should be instituted. If a favorable response does not occur promptly, the corticosteroid should be discontinued until the infection has been adequately controlled.
Information for the Patient: Patients using topical corticosteroids should receive the following information and instructions:
1. This medication is to be used as directed by the physician. It is for external use only. Avoid contact with the eyes.
2. Patients should be advised not to use this medication for any disorder other than for which it was prescribed.
3. The treated skin area should not be bandaged or otherwise covered or wrapped as to be occlusive unless directed by the physician.
4. Patients should report any signs of local adverse reactions especially under occlusive dressing.
5. Parents of pediatric patients should be advised not to use tightfitting diapers or plastic pants on a child being treated in the diaper area, as these sgarments may constitute occlusive dressings.
Laboratory Tests: The following tests may be helpful in evaluating the HPA axis suppression:
  Urinary free cortisol test
  ACTH stimulation test

Carcinogenesis, Mutagenesis, and Impairment of Fertility: Long-term animal studies have not been performed to evaluate the carcinogenic potential or the effect on fertility of topical corticosteroids.

Studies to determine mutagenicity with prednisolone and hydrocortisone have revealed negative results.

Pregnancy Category C: Corticosteroids are generally teratogenic in laboratory animals when administered systemically at relatively low dosage levels. The more potent corticosteroids have been shown to be teratogenic after dermal application in laboratory animals. There are no adequate and well-controlled studies in pregnant women on teratogenic effects from topically applied corticosteroids. Therefore, topical corticosteroids should be used during pregnancy only if the potential benefit justifies the potential risk to the fetus. Drugs of this class should not be used extensively on pregnant patients, in large amounts, or for prolonged periods of time.

Nursing Mothers: It is not known whether topical administration of corticosteroids could result in sufficient systemic absorption to produce detectable amounts in breast milk. Systemically administered corticosteroids are secreted into breast milk in quantities NOT likely to have a deleterious effect on the infant. Nevertheless, caution should be exercised when topical corticosteroids are administered to a nursing woman.

Pediatric Use: PEDIATRIC PATIENTS MAY DEMONSTRATE GREATER SUSCEPTIBILITY TO TOPICAL CORTICOSTEROID-INDUCED HPA AXIS SUPPRESSION AND CUSHING'S SYNDROME THAN MATURE PATIENTS BECAUSE OF A LARGER SKIN SURFACE AREA TO BODY WEIGHT RATIO.

Hypothalamic-pituitary-adrenal (HPA) axis suppression, Cushing's syndrome, and intracranial hypertension have been reported in children receiving topical corticosteroids. Manifestations of adrenal suppression in children include linear growth retardation, delayed weight gain, low plasma cortisol levels, and absence of response to ACTH stimulation. Manifestations of intracranial hypertension include bulging fontanelles, headaches, and bilateral papilledema.

Administration of topical corticosteroids to children should be limited to the least amount compatible with an effective therapeutic regimen. Chronic corticosteroid therapy may interfere with the growth and development of children.

ADVERSE REACTIONS

The following local adverse reactions are reported infrequently with topical corticosteroids, but may occur more frequently with the use of occlusive dressings. These reactions are listed in an approximate decreasing order of occurrence:

Burning	Hypopigmentation
Itching	Perioral dermatitis
Irritation	Allergic contact dermatitis
Dryness	Maceration of the skin
Folliculitis	Secondary infection
Hypertrichosis	Skin Atrophy
Acneiform eruptions	Striae
	Miliaria

OVERDOSAGE

Topically applied corticosteroids can be absorbed in sufficient amounts to produce systemic effects (See PRECAUTIONS).

DOSAGE AND ADMINISTRATION

Topical corticosteroids are generally applied to the affected area as a thin film three or four times daily depending on the severity of the condition.

Occlusive dressings may be used for the management of psoriasis or recalcitrant conditions. If an infection develops, the use of occlusive dressings should be discontinued and appropriate antimicrobial therapy instituted.

HOW SUPPLIED

ANALPRAM-HC® Cream 1% or 2.5% in a 1 oz. tube with six (6) rectal applicators.

Dispense in a tight container as defined in the USP.

Store at controlled room temperature 15°- 30°C (59°- 86°F).

KRONOFED-A® Kronocaps ℞
Dye-Free
Decongestant plus Antihistamine

Each sustained release, white and clear capsule contains:

Pseudoephedrine HCl	120 mg
Chlorpheniramine Maleate	8 mg

KRONOFED-A-JR® Kronocaps ℞
Dye-Free
Decongestant plus Antihistamine

Each sustained release, white and clear capsule contains:

Pseudoephedrine HCl	60 mg
Chlorpheniramine Maleate	4 mg

INDICATIONS

For temporary relief of upper respiratory and nasal congestion associated with the common cold, hay fever and allergies, sinusitis and vasomotor and allergic rhinitis.

CONTRAINDICATIONS

Severe hypertension or severe cardiac disease. Sensitivity to antihistamines or sympathomimetic agents.

PRECAUTIONS

Use with caution in patients with hyperthyroidism. Patients susceptible to the soporific effects of chlorpheniramine should be warned against driving or operating of machinery which requires complete mental alertness.

PREGNANCY

Pregnancy Category C: Animal reproduction studies have not been conducted with **KRONOFED-A®** medications. It is also not known whether **KRONOFED-A®** medications can cause fetal harm when administered to a pregnant woman or can affect reproduction capacity. **KRONOFED-A®** medications should be given to a pregnant woman only if clearly needed.

Nursing Mothers: Due to the possible passage of pseudoephedrine and chlorpheniramine into breast milk, and, because of the higher than usual risk for infants from sympathomimetic amines and antihistamines, the benefit to the mother vs. the potential risk should be considered and a decision should be made whether to discontinue nursing or to discontinue the drug.

CAUTION

Federal law prohibits dispensing without prescription.

DOSAGE

Kronofed-A® Capsules: Adults and children over 12 years of age—1 capsule every 12 hours. **Kronofed-A-JR®** Capsules: Children 6–12 years of age—1 capsule every 12 hours. Adults 1 or 2 capsules every 12 hours.

HOW SUPPLIED

Bottles of 100 and 500 Capsules.

LOCOID® ℞
(hydrocortisone butyrate)
Cream 0.1%
Ointment 0.1%
Topical Solution 0.1%

CAUTION: Federal law prohibits dispensing without prescription.

DESCRIPTION

LOCOID® cream, ointment and topical solution contain the topical corticosteroid, hydrocortisone butyrate, a non-fluorinated hydrocortisone ester. It has the chemical name: pregn-4-ene-3.20-dione, 11.21-dihydroxy-17-[(1-oxobutyl)oxy]-, 11β): the molecular formula: $C_{25}H_{36}O_6$; the molecular weight: 432.54; and the CAS registry number: 13609-67-1. Its structural formula is:

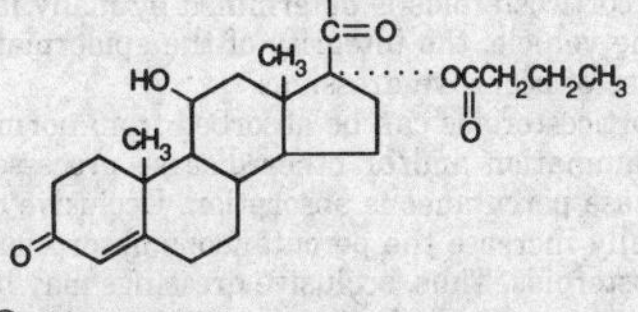

LOCOID® Cream 0.1%
Each gram of LOCOID® cream contains 1 mg of hydrocortisone butyrate in a hydrophilic base consisting of cetostearyl alcohol, ceteth-20, mineral oil, white petrolatum, citric acid, sodium citrate, methylparaben (preservative) and purified water.

LOCOID® Ointment 0.1%
Each gram of LOCOID® ointment contains 1 mg of hydrocortisone butyrate in a base consisting of mineral oil and polyethylene.

LOCOID® Solution 0.1%
Each mL of LOCOID® solution contains 1 mg of hydrocortisone butyrate in a vehicle consisting of isopropyl alcohol (50%), glycerin, povidone, citric acid, sodium citrate and purified water.

CLINICAL PHARMACOLOGY

Topical corticosteroids share anti-inflammatory, anti-pruritic and vasoconstrictive actions.

The mechanism of anti-inflammatory activity of the topical corticosteroids is unclear. Various laboratory methods, including vasoconstrictor assays, are used to compare and predict potencies and/or clinical efficacies of the topical corticosteroids. There is some evidence to suggest that a recognizable correlation exists between vasoconstrictor potency and therapeutic efficacy in man.

Pharmacokinetics
The extent of percutaneous absorption of topical corticosteroids is determined by many factors including the vehicle, the integrity of the epidermal barrier, and the use of occlusive dressings.

Topical corticosteroids can be absorbed from normal intact skin. Inflammation and/or other disease processes in the skin increase percutaneous absorption. Occlusive dressings substantially increase the percutaneous absorption of topical corticosteroids. Thus, occlusive dressings may be a valuable therapeutic adjunct for treatment of resistant dermatoses. (See DOSAGE AND ADMINISTRATION.)

Once absorbed through the skin, topical corticosteroids are handled through pharmacokinetic pathways similar to systemically administered corticosteroids. Corticosteroids are bound to plasma proteins in varying degrees. Corticosteroids are metabolized primarily in the liver and are then excreted by the kidneys. Some of the topical corticosteroids and their metabolites are also excreted into the bile.

INDICATIONS AND USAGE

LOCOID® cream 0.1% and ointment 0.1% (hydrocortisone butyrate) are indicated for the relief of the inflammatory and pruritic manifestations of corticosteroid-responsive dermatoses.

LOCOID® solution 0.1% (hydrocortisone butyrate) is indicated for the relief of the inflammatory and pruritic manifestations of seborrheic dermatitis.

CONTRAINDICATIONS

Topical corticosteroids are contraindicated in those patients with a history of hypersensitivity to any of the components of the preparation.

PRECAUTIONS

General: Systemic absorption of topical corticosteroids has produced reversible hypothalamic-pituitary-adrenal (HPA) axis suppression, manifestations of Cushing's syndrome, hyperglycemia, and glucosuria in some patients. Conditions which augment systemic absorption include the application of the more potent steroids, use over large surface areas, prolonged use, and the addition of occlusive dressings.

Therefore, patients receiving a large dose of a potent topical steroid applied to a large surface area or under an occlusive dressing should be evaluated periodically for evidence of HPA axis suppression by using the urinary free cortisol and ACTH stimulation tests. If HPA axis suppression is noted, an attempt should be made to withdraw the drug, to reduce the frequency of application, or to substitute a less potent steroid.

Recovery of HPA axis function is generally prompt and complete upon discontinuation of the drug. Infrequently, signs and symptoms of steroid withdrawal may occur, requiring supplemental systemic corticosteroids.

Children may absorb proportionally larger amounts of topical corticosteroids and thus be more susceptible to systemic toxicity (See PRECAUTIONS—PEDIATRIC USE.)

If irritation develops, topical corticosteroids should be discontinued and appropriate therapy instituted. In the presence of dermatological infections, the use of an appropriate antifungal or antibacterial agent should be instituted. If a favorable response does not occur promptly, the corticosteroid should be discontinued until the infection has been adequately controlled.

Information for the patient
Patients using topical corticosteroids should receive the following information and instructions:

1. This medication is to be used as directed by the physician. It is for external use only. Avoid contact with the eyes.
2. Patients should be advised not to use this medication for any disorder other than for which it was prescribed.
3. The treated skin area should not be bandaged or otherwise covered or wrapped as to be occlusive unless directed by the physician.
4. Patients should report any signs of local adverse reactions especially under occlusive dressing.
5. Parents of pediatric patients should be advised not to use tight-fitting diapers or plastic pants on a child being treated in the diaper area, as these garments may constitute occlusive dressings.

Laboratory tests
The following tests may be helpful in evaluating the HPA axis suppression:
Urinary free cortisol test
ACTH stimulation test

Carcinogenesis, Mutagenesis, and Impairment of Fertility
Long-term animal studies have not been performed to evaluate the carcinogenic potential or the effect on fertility of topical corticosteroids.

Studies to determine mutagenicity with prednisolone and hydrocortisone have revealed negative results.

Pregnancy Category C
Corticosteroids are generally teratogenic in laboratory animals when administered systemically at relatively low dosage levels. The more potent corticosteroids have been shown

Continued on next page

Ferndale Laboratories—Cont.

to be teratogenic after dermal application in laboratory animals. There are no adequate and well-controlled studies in pregnant women on teratogenic effects from topically applied corticosteroids. Therefore, topical corticosteroids should be used during pregnancy only if the potential benefit justifies the potential risk to the fetus. Drugs of this class should not be used extensively on pregnant patients, in large amounts, or for prolonged periods of time.

Nursing Mothers

It is not known whether topical administration of corticosteroids could result in sufficient systemic absorption to produce detectable quantities in breast milk. Systemically administered corticosteroids are secreted into breast milk, in quantities not likely to have a deleterious effect on the infant. Nevertheless, caution should be exercised when topical corticosteroids are administered to a nursing woman.

Pediatric Use

Pediatric patients may demonstrate greater susceptibility to topical corticosteroid-induced HPA axis suppression and Cushing's syndrome than mature patients because of a larger skin surface area to body weight ratio.

Hypothalamic-pituitary-adrenal (HPA) axis suppression, Cushing's syndrome, and intracranial hypertension have been reported in children receiving topical corticosteroids. Manifestations of adrenal suppression in children include linear growth retardation, delayed weight gain, low plasma cortisol levels, and absence of response to ACTH stimulation. Manifestations of intracranial hypertension include bulging fontanelles, headaches, and bilateral papilledema.

Administration of topical corticosteroids to children should be limited to the least amount compatible with an effective therapeutic regimen. Chronic corticosteroid therapy may interfere with the growth and development of children.

ADVERSE REACTIONS

The following local adverse reactions are reported infrequently with topical corticosteroids, but may occur more frequently with the use of occlusive dressings. These reactions are listed in an approximate decreasing order of occurrence: burning, itching, irritation, dryness, folliculitis, hypertrichosis, acneiform eruptions, hypopigmentation, perioral dermatitis, allergic contact dermatitis, maceration of the skin, secondary infection, skin atrophy, striae, miliaria.

OVERDOSAGE

Topically applied corticosteroids can be absorbed in sufficient amounts to produce systemic effects. (See PRECAUTIONS.)

DOSAGE AND ADMINISTRATION

LOCOID® cream 0.1% or LOCOID® ointment 0.1% (hydrocortisone butyrate) should be applied to the affected area as a thin film two to three times daily depending on the severity of the condition.

Occlusive dressings may be used for the management of psoriasis or recalcitrant conditions.

If an infection develops, the use of occlusive dressings should be discontinued and appropriate antimicrobial therapy instituted.

LOCOID® solution 0.1% (hydrocortisone butyrate) should be applied to the affected area as a thin film from two to three times daily depending on the severity of the condition.

HOW SUPPLIED

LOCOID® cream 0.1% (hydrocortisone butyrate) is supplied in tubes containing:

15 g NDC 0496-0802-15
45 g NDC 0496-0802-45

LOCOID® ointment 0.1% (hydrocortisone butyrate) is supplied in tubes containing:

15 g NDC 0496-0803-15
45 g NDC 0496-0803-45

LOCOID® solution 0.1% (hydrocortisone butyrate) is supplied in polyethylene bottles:

30 mL NDC 0496-0804-30
60 mL NDC 0496-0804-60

STORAGE

LOCOID® cream 0.1%: Store between 46° and 77°F (8° and 25°C).

LOCOID® ointment 0.1%: Store between 36°and 86°F (2°and 30°C).

LOCOID® solution 0.1%: Store between 41°and 77°F (5°and 25°C).

MARKETED BY:
FERNDALE LABORATORIES, INC.
FERNDALE, MICHIGAN 48220
MANUFACTURED BY:
Brocades Pharma by
Leiderdorp/Netherlands
Revised: June 1991

PRAMOSONE® CREAM, LOTION AND OINTMENT ℞

DESCRIPTION

Pramosone® Cream: Contains Hydrocortisone acetate 0.5%, 1% or 2.5% and Pramoxine HCl 1% in a hydrophilic base containing stearic acid, cetyl alcohol, aquaphor, isopropyl palmitate, polyoxyl 40 stearate, propylene glycol, potassium sorbate 0.1%, sorbic acid 0.1%, triethanolamine lauryl sulfate and water.

Pramosone® Lotion: Contains Hydrocortisone acetate 0.5%, 1% or 2.5% and Pramoxine HCl 1% in a base containing forlan-L, cetyl alcohol, stearic acid, di-isopropyl adipate, polyoxyl 40 stearate, silicon, triethanolamine, glycerine, polyvinylpyrolidone, potassium sorbate 0.1%, sorbic acid 0.1% and water.

Pramosone® Ointment: Contains Hydrocortisone acetate 1% or 2.5% and Pramoxine HCl 1% in an emollient ointment base containing Sorbitan sesquioleate, Water, Aquaphor and White petrolatum.

Topical corticosteroids are anti-inflammatory and antipruritic agents. The structural formula, the chemical name, molecular formula and molecular weight for active ingredients are presented below.

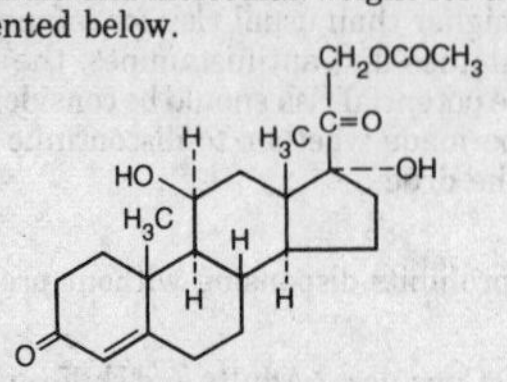

Hydrocortisone acetate
(Pregn-4-ene-3,20-dione,21 - (acetyloxy)-11, 17-dihydroxy-,(11 β)-.)
$C_{23}H_{32}O_6$; mol wt: 404.50

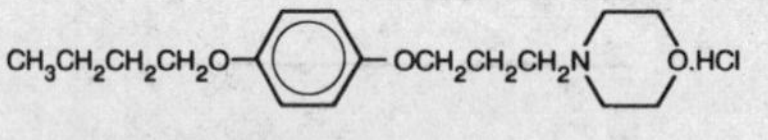

Pramoxine hydrochloride
(4-(3-(p-butoxyphenoxy)propyl)morpholine hydrochloride)
$C_{17}H_{27}NO_3.HCl$; mol wt: 329.87

CLINICAL PHARMACOLOGY

Topical corticosteroids share anti-inflammatory, anti-pruritic and vasoconstrictive actions.

The mechanism of anti-inflammatory activity of the topical corticosteroids is unclear. Various laboratory methods, including vasoconstrictor assays, are used to compare and predict potencies and/or clinical efficacies of the topical corticosteroids. There is some evidence to suggest that a recognizable correlation exists between vasoconstrictor potency and therapeutic efficacy in man.

Pramoxine hydrochloride is a topical anesthetic agent which provides temporary relief from itching and pain. It acts by stabilizing the neuronal membrane of nerve endings with which it comes into contact.

Pharmacokinetics: The extent of percutaneous absorption of topical corticosteroids is determined by many factors including the vehicle, the integrity of the epidermal barrier, and the use of occlusive dressings.

Topical corticosteroids can be absorbed from normal intact skin. Inflammation and/or other disease processes in the skin increase percutaneous absorption. Occlusive dressings substantially increase the percutaneous absorption of topical corticosteroids. Thus, occlusive dressings may be a valuable therapeutic adjunct for treatment of resistant dermatoses (See DOSAGE AND ADMINISTRATION).

Once absorbed through the skin, topical corticosteroids are handled through pharmacokinetic pathways similar to systemically administered corticosteroids. Corticosteroids are bound to plasma proteins in varying degrees. Corticosteroids are metabolized primarily in the liver and are then excreted by the kidneys. Some of the topical corticosteroids and their metabolites are also excreted into the bile.

INDICATIONS AND USAGE

Topical corticosteroids are indicated for the relief of the inflammatory and pruritic manifestations of corticosteroid-responsive dermatoses.

CONTRAINDICATIONS

Topical corticosteroids are contraindicated in those patients with a history of hypersensitivity to any of the components of the preparation.

PRECAUTIONS

General: Systemic absorption of topical corticosteroids has produced reversible hypothalamic-pituitary-adrenal (HPA) axis suppression, manifestations of Cushing's syndrome, hyperglycemia, and glucosuria in some patients.

Conditions which augment systemic absorption include the application of the more potent steroids, use over large surface areas, prolonged use, and the addition of occlusive dressings.

Therefore, patients receiving a large dose of a potent topical steroid applied to a large surface area and under an occlusive dressing should be evaluated periodically for evidence of HPA axis suppression by using the urinary free cortisol and ACTH stimulation tests. If HPA axis suppression is noted, an attempt should be made to withdraw the drug, to reduce the frequency of application, or to substitute a less potent steroid.

Recovery of HPA axis function is generally prompt and complete upon discontinuation of the drug. Infrequently, signs and symptoms of steroid withdrawal may occur, requiring supplemental systemic corticosteroids.

Children may absorb proportionally larger amounts of topical corticosteroids and thus be more susceptible to systemic toxicity. (See PRECAUTIONS—Pediatric Use).

If irritation develops, topical corticosteroids should be discontinued and appropriate therapy instituted.

In the presence of dermatological infections, the use of an appropriate antifungal or antibacterial agent should be instituted. If a favorable response does not occur promptly, the corticosteroid should be discontinued until the infection has been adequately controlled.

Information for the Patient: Patients using topical corticosteroids should receive the following information and instructions:

1. This medication is to be used as directed by the physician. It is for external use only. Avoid contact with the eyes.
2. Patients should be advised not to use this medication for any disorder other than for which it was prescribed.
3. The treated skin area should not be bandaged or otherwise covered or wrapped as to be occlusive unless directed by the physician.
4. Patients should report any signs of local adverse reactions especially under occlusive dressing.
5. Parents of pediatric patients should be advised not to use tightfitting diapers or plastic pants on a child being treated in the diaper area, as these garments may constitute occlusive dressings.

Laboratory Tests: The following tests may be helpful in evaluating the HPA axis suppression:

Urinary free cortisol test
ACTH stimulation test

Carcinogenesis, Mutagenesis, and Impairment of Fertility: Long-term animal studies have not been performed to evaluate the carcinogenic potential or the effect on fertility of topical corticosteroids.

Studies to determine mutagenicity with prednisolone and hydrocortisone have revealed negative results.

Pregnancy Category C: Corticosteroids are generally teratogenic in laboratory animals when administered systemically at relatively low dosage levels. The more potent corticosteroids have been shown to be teratogenic after dermal application in laboratory animals. There are no adequate and well-controlled studies in pregnant women on teratogenic effects from topically applied corticosteroids. Therefore, topical corticosteroids should be used during pregnancy only if the potential benefit justifies the potential risk to the fetus. Drugs of this class should not be used extensively on pregnant patients, in large amounts, or for prolonged periods of time.

Nursing Mothers: It is not known whether topical administration of corticosteroids could result in sufficient systemic absorption to produce detectable amounts in breast milk. Systemically administered corticosteroids are secreted into breast milk in quantities NOT likely to have a deleterious effect on the infant. Nevertheless, caution should be exercised when topical corticosteroids are administered to a nursing woman.

Pediatric Use: PEDIATRIC PATIENTS MAY DEMONSTRATE GREATER SUSCEPTIBILITY TO TOPICAL CORTICOSTEROID-INDUCED HPA AXIS SUPPRESSION AND CUSHING'S SYNDROME THAN MATURE PATIENTS BECAUSE OF A LARGER SKIN SURFACE AREA TO BODY WEIGHT RATIO.

Hypothalamic-pituitary-adrenal (HPA) axis suppression, Cushing's syndrome, and intracranial hypertension have been reported in children receiving topical corticosteroids. Manifestations of adrenal suppression in children include linear growth retardation, delayed weight gain, low plasma cortisol levels, and absence of response to ACTH stimulation. Manifestations of intracranial hypertension include bulging fontanelles, headaches, and bilateral papilledema.

Administration of topical corticosteroids to children should be limited to the least amount compatible with an effective therapeutic regimen. Chronic corticosteroid therapy may interfere with the growth and development of children.

ADVERSE REACTIONS

The following local adverse reactions are reported infrequently with topical corticosteroids, but may occur more frequently with the use of occlusive dressings. These reactions are listed in an approximate decreasing order of occurrence:

Burning	Hypopigmentation
Itching	Perioral dermatitis
Irritation	Allergic contact dermatitis
Dryness	Maceration of the skin
Folliculitis	Secondary infection
Hypertrichosis	Skin Atrophy
Acneiform eruptions	Striae
	Miliaria

OVERDOSAGE

Topically applied corticosteroids can be absorbed in sufficient amounts to produce systemic effects (See PRECAUTIONS).

DOSAGE AND ADMINISTRATION

Topical corticosteroids are generally applied to the affected area as a thin film three or four times daily depending on the severity of the condition.

Occlusive dressings may be used for the management of psoriasis or recalcitrant conditions. If an infection develops, the use of occlusive dressings should be discontinued and appropriate antimicrobial therapy instituted.

HOW SUPPLIED

CREAM: ½%, 1% or 2½% in 1 oz. tubes, 2 oz. tubes, 4 oz. jars and lb. jars.

LOTION: ½% or 1% in 2 fl. oz., 4 fl. oz. and 8 fl. oz. dispenser bottles. 2½% in 2 fl. oz. and 4 fl. oz. dispenser bottles.

OINTMENT: 1% or 2½% in 1 oz. tubes, 4 oz. jars and lb. jars.

Dispense in a tight container as defined in the official compendium.

Store at controlled room temperature 15°–30°C (59°–86°F).

PRAX® CREAM AND LOTION* OTC
(Pramoxine HCl 1% in an emollient hydrophilic base)

AVAILABLE

CREAM: 1 oz. tubes, 4 oz. jars and lb. jars. LOTION: 15 mL., 120 mL., and 240 mL. dispenser bottles.

*Additional information available upon request.

Ferring Laboratories, Inc.
400 RELLA BLVD, SUITE 201
SUFFERN, NY 10901

LUTREPULSE® for Injection ℞
(gonadorelin acetate)
Synthetic Gonadotropin-Releasing Hormone (GnRH)
For Pulsatile Intravenous Injection

DESCRIPTION

LUTREPULSE (gonadorelin acetate) for Injection is used for the induction of ovulation in women with primary hypothalamic amenorrhea. Gonadorelin acetate is a synthetic decapeptide that is identical in amino acid sequence to endogenous gonadotropin-releasing hormone (GnRH) synthesized in the human hypothalamus and in various neurons terminating in the hypothalamus. The molecular formula of gonadorelin acetate is:

$$C_{55}H_{75}N_{17}O_{13} \cdot xC_2H_4O_2 \cdot yH_2O$$

Its molecular weight is 1182.3 + x60 + y18, where x and y represent a non-stoichiometric ratio of acetate and water associated with the peptide, and x ranges from 1–2 and y ranges from 2–3. The amino acid sequence of GnRH is:

5-oxoPro-His-Trp-Ser-Tyr-Gly-Leu-Arg-Pro-Gly-NH_2

LUTREPULSE for Injection is a sterile, lyophilized powder intended for intravenous pulsatile injection after reconstitution. It is white and very soluble in water. Vials are available containing 0.8 mg or 3.2 mg gonadorelin acetate (expressed as the diacetate) and 10.0 mg mannitol as a carrier. After reconstituting with 8 mL of diluent (sterile 0.9% sodium chloride solution and hydrochloric acid to adjust the pH) for LUTREPULSE for Injection, the concentration of gonadorelin acetate is 5 μg per 50 μl in each vial containing 0.8 mg lyophilized hormone, and 20 μg per 50 μl in each vial containing 3.2 mg lyophilized hormone. LUTREPULSE (gonadorelin acetate) for Injection is intended for use with the LUTREPULSE for Injection KITS. The volumes and concentrations are specific for use with the LUTREPULSE PUMP for appropriate dosing.

CLINICAL PHARMACOLOGY

Under physiologic conditions, gonadotropin-releasing hormone (GnRH) is released by the hypothalamus in a pulsatile fashion. The primary effect of GnRH is the synthesis and release of luteinizing hormone (LH) in the anterior pituitary gland. GnRH also stimulates the synthesis and release of follicle stimulating hormone (FSH), but this effect is less pronounced. LH and FSH subsequently stimulate the gonads to produce steroids which are instrumental in regulating reproductive hormonal status. Unlike human menopausal gonadotropin (hMG) which supplies pituitary hormones, pulsatile administration of LUTREPULSE for Injection replaces defective hypothalamic secretion of GnRH. The pulsatile administration of LUTREPULSE for Injection approximates the natural hormonal secretory pattern, causing pulsatile release of pituitary gonadotropins. Accordingly, LUTREPULSE for Injection is useful in treating conditions of infertility caused by defective GnRH stimulation from the hypothalamus (See **INDICATIONS AND USAGE**). The following information summarizes clinical efficacy of gonadorelin acetate administered by pulsatile intravenous injection to patients with primary hypothalamic amenorrhea.

44 patients with primary hypothalamic amenorrhea (HA)
93% (41/44) patients ovulatory with gonadorelin acetate therapy
62% (24/39)* patients pregnant
100% (7/7) of those failing past attempts at ovulation induction by other methods were ovulatory on gonadorelin acetate.

Following intravenous injection of GnRH into normal subjects and/or hypogonadotropic patients, plasma GnRH concentrations rapidly decline with initial and terminal half-lives of 2–10 min. and 10–40 min., respectively. In these studies, high clearance values (500–1500 L/day) and low volumes of distribution (10–15 L) were calculated. The pharmacokinetics of GnRH in normal subjects and in hypogonadotropic patients were similar. GnRH was rapidly metabolized to various biologically inactive peptide fragments which are readily excreted in urine. Renal failure, but not hepatic disease, prolonged the half-life and reduced the clearance of GnRH.

INDICATIONS AND USAGE

LUTREPULSE (gonadorelin acetate) for Injection is indicated in the treatment of primary hypothalamic amenorrhea.

DIFFERENTIAL DIAGNOSIS: Proper diagnosis is critical for successful treatment with LUTREPULSE for Injection. It must be established that hypothalamic amenorrhea or hypogonadism is, in fact, due to a deficiency in quantity or pulsing of endogenous GnRH. The diagnosis of hypothalamic amenorrhea or hypogonadism is based on the exclusion of other causes of the dysfunction, since there is currently no practical technique to directly assess hypothalamic function. Prior to initiation of therapy with LUTREPULSE (gonadorelin acetate) for Injection, the physician should rule out disorders of general health, reproductive organs, anterior pituitary, and central nervous system, other than abnormalities of GnRH secretion.

CONTRAINDICATIONS

LUTREPULSE for Injection is contraindicated in women with any condition that could be exacerbated by pregnancy. For example, pituitary prolactinoma should be considered one such condition. Additionally, any history of sensitivity to gonadorelin acetate, gonadorelin hydrochloride or any component of LUTREPULSE for Injection is a contraindication. Patients who have ovarian cysts or causes of anovulation other than those of hypothalamic origin should not receive LUTREPULSE for Injection.

LUTREPULSE for Injection is intended to initiate events including the production of reproductive hormones (e.g. estrogens and progestins). Therefore, any condition that may be worsened by reproductive hormones, such as hormonally-dependent tumor, is a contraindication to the use of LUTREPULSE for Injection.

WARNINGS

Therapy with LUTREPULSE (gonadorelin acetate) for Injection should be conducted by physicians familiar with pulsatile GnRH delivery and the clinical ramifications of ovulation induction. While there have been few cases of hyperstimulation(<1%) this possibility must be considered. If hyperstimulation should occur, therapy should be discontinued and spontaneous resolution can be expected. The preservation of the endogenous feedback mechanisms makes severe hyperstimulation (with ascites and pleural effusion) rare. However, the physician shoud be aware of the possibility and be alert for any evidence of ascites, pleural effusion, hemoconcentration, rupture of a cyst, fluid or electrolyte imbalance, or sepsis.

Multiple pregnancy is a possibility that can be minimized by careful attention to the recommended doses and ultrasonographic monitoring of the ovarian response to therapy. Following a baseline pelvic ultrasound, follow-up studies should be conducted at a minimum on day 7 and day 14 of therapy.

Serious hypersensitivity reactions (anaphylaxis) have been reported following gonadotropin-releasing hormone administration, including gonadorelin acetate. Clinical manifestations may include: cardiovascular collapse, hypotension, tachycardia, loss of consciousness, angioedema, bronchospasm, dyspnea, urticaria, flushing and pruritus. If any allergic reaction occurs, therapy with gonadorelin should be dicontinued. Serious acute hypersensitivity reactions may require emergency medical treatment.

As with any intravenous medication, scrupulous attention to asepsis is important. The infusion area must be monitored as with all indwelling parenteral approaches. The cannula and IV site should be changed at 48-hour intervals.

*Five patients did not desire pregnancy.

PRECAUTIONS

GENERAL: Ovarian hyperstimulation has been reported. This may be related to pulse dosage or concomitant use of other ovulation stimulators. Hyperstimulation may be a greater risk in patients where spontaneous variations in endogenous GnRH secretion occur. Multiple follicle development, multiple pregnancy, and spontaneous termination of pregnancy have been reported. Multiple pregnancy can be minimized by appropriate monitoring of follicle formation; nonetheless, the patient and her partner should be advised of the frequency (12%) and potential risks of multiple pregnancy before starting treatment.

Ovarian hyperstimulation, a syndrome of sudden ovarian enlargement, ascites with or without pain, and/or pleural effusion, is rare with pulsatile GnRH therapy. Among 268 patients participating in clinical trials, one case of moderate hyperstimulation has been reported, but this cycle included the concomitant use of clomiphene citrate.

Antibody formation (IgE and IgG) has been reported following administration of gonadorelin. The safety and efficacy implication of antibody development are uncertain (see: **WARNINGS**).

LUTREPULSE (gonadorelin acetate) for Injection should be administered only with the LUTREPULSE PUMP. The patient should be provided with detailed oral and written instructions regarding infusion pump usage and potential sepsis in order to minimize the frequency of infusion pump malfunction and inflammation, infection, mild phlebitis, or hematoma at the catheter site.

INFORMATION FOR PATIENTS: The patient should be advised to discontinue the drug and seek medical attention at the first sign of skin rash, urticaria, rapid heart beat, difficulty in swallowing and breathing, or any swelling which may suggest angioedema (see: **WARNINGS** and **ADVERSE REACTIONS**).

LABORATORY TESTS: Following a diagnosis of primary hypothalamic amenorrhea, initiation of LUTREPULSE (gonadorelin acetate) for Injection therapy may be monitored by the following:

1) Ovarian ultrasound—baseline, therapy day 7, therapy day 14.
2) Mid-luteal phase serum progesterone.
3) Clinical observation of infusion site at each visit as needed.
4) Physical examination including pelvic at regularly scheduled visits.

DRUG INTERACTIONS: None are known. LUTREPULSE for Injection should not be used concomitantly with other ovulation stimulators.

DRUG/LABORATORY TEST INTERACTIONS: None are known.

CARCINOGENESIS, MUTAGENESIS, IMPAIRMENT OF FERTILITY: Since GnRH is a natural substance normally present in humans, long-term studies in animals have not been performed to evaluate carcinogenic potential. Mutagenicity testing was not done.

PREGNANCY: Pregnancy Category B

Reproduction studies (teratology and embryo-toxicity) performed in rats and rabbits have not revealed any evidence of harm to the fetus due to gonadorelin acetate. There was no evidence of teratogenicity when gonadorelin acetate was administered intravenously up to 120 μg/kg/day (>70 times the recommended human dose of 5 μg per pulse) in rats and rabbits.

Studies in pregnant women have shown that gonadorelin acetate does not increase the risk of abnormalities when administered during the first trimester of pregnancy. It appears that the possibility of fetal harm is remote, if the drug is used during pregnancy. In clinical studies, 47 pregnant patients have used gonadorelin acetate during the first trimester of pregnancy (51 pregnancies) and the drug had no apparent adverse effect on the course of pregnancy. Available follow-up reports on infants born to these women reveal no adverse effects or complications that were attributable to gonadorelin acetate. Nevertheless, because the studies in humans cannot rule out the possibility of harm, gonadorelin acetate should be used during pregnancy only for maintenance of the corpus luteum in ovulation induction cycles.

NURSING MOTHERS: It is not known whether this drug is excreted in human milk. There is no indication for use of LUTREPULSE (gonadorelin acetate) for Injection in a nursing woman.

PEDIATRIC USE: Safety and effectiveness in children under the age of 18 have not been established.

Continued on next page

Ferring Laboratories—Cont.

ADVERSE REACTIONS

Adverse reactions have been reported in approximately 10% of treatment regimens. Ten of 268 patients interrupted therapy because of an adverse reaction but subsequently resumed treatment. One other subject did not resume treatment.

In clinical studies involving 268 women, one case of moderate ovarian hyperstimulation has been reported. This cycle included concomitant use of clomiphene citrate. This low incidence of hyperstimulation appears to be due to the preservation of normal feedback mechanisms of the pituitary-ovarian axis.

Despite the preservation of feedback mechanisms, some incidents of multiple follicle development, multiple pregnancy, and spontaneous termination of pregnancy have been reported. Multiple pregnancy can be minimized by appropriate monitoring of follicle formation; nonetheless, the patient and her partner should be advised of the frequency and potential hazards of multiple pregnancy before starting treatment. In clinical studies involving 142 pregnancies, delivery information was available on 89 pregnancies. Eleven of these LUTREPULSE (gonadorelin acetate) for Injection-induced pregnancies (12%) were multiple (10 sets of twins, 1 set of triplets).

The following adverse reactions have occurred at the injection site: urticaria, pruritus, inflammation, infection, mild phlebitis, or hematoma at the catheter site. Additionally, infusion set malfunction and interruption of infusion may occur; this has no known adverse effect other than interruption of therapy. Acute generalized (anaphylaxis, angio edema, urticaria, etc.) hypersensitivity reactions have been reported (see: **WARNINGS** and **PRECAUTIONS**).

Anaphylaxis (bronchospasm, tachycardia, flushing, urticaria, induration at injection site) has been reported with the related polypeptide hormone gonadorelin hydrochloride (FACTREL®).

® Registered trademark of Wyeth-Ayerst Laboratories.

OVERDOSAGE

Continuous, non-pulsatile exposure to gonadorelin acetate could temporarily reduce pituitary responsiveness. If the pump should malfunction and deliver the entire contents of the 3.2 mg system, no harmful effects would be expected. Bolus doses as high as 3000 μg of gonadorelin hydrochloride have not been harmful. Pituitary hyperstimulation and multiple follicle development can be minimized by adhering to recommended doses, and appropriate monitoring of follicle formation (see **PRECAUTIONS**).

Administration of 640 μg/kg in monkeys as a single intravenous bolus resulted in no compound-related effects in clinical observations or gross morphologic evaluations.

DOSAGE AND ADMINISTRATION

DOSAGE: Dosages between 1 and 20 μg have been successfully used in clinical studies. The recommended dose in primary hypothalamic amenorrhea is 5 μg every 90 minutes. This is delivered by LUTREPULSE PUMP using the 0.8 mg solution at 50 μl per pulse (see physician pump manual). Sixty-eight percent of the 5 μg every 90 minute regimens induced ovulation in patients with primary hypothalamic amenorrhea.

The LUTREPULSE PUMP is capable of delivering 2.5, 5, 10, or 20 μg of gonadorelin acetate every 90 minutes. Some women may require a reduction in the recommended dose of 5 μg should laboratory testing and patient monitoring indicate an inappropriate response. While most primary hypothalamic amenorrhea patients will ovulate during the first cycle of 5 μg therapy, some may be refractory to this dose. The recommended treatment interval is 21 days. It may be necessary to raise the dose cautiously, and in stepwise fashion if there is no response after three treatment intervals. All dose changes should be carefully monitored for inappropriate response.

The following table can be used to calculate the dose per pulse when individualizing treatment:

Vial	Diluent	Volume/pulse	Dose/pulse
0.8 mg	8 mL	25 μL	2.5 μg
0.8 mg	8 mL	50 μL	5 μg
3.2 mg	8 mL	25 μL	10 μg
3.2 mg	8 mL	50 μL	20 μg

The response to LUTREPULSE (gonadorelin acetate) for Injection usually occurs within two to three weeks after therapy initiation. When ovulation occurs with the LUTREPULSE PUMP in place, therapy should be continued for another two weeks to maintain the corpus luteum. A comparison of LUTREPULSE for Injection to hCG or hCG + LUTREPULSE for Injection for corpus luteum maintenance revealed the following information:

hCG

Delivered = $\frac{43}{63}$ = 68%

Aborted = $\frac{20}{63}$ = 32%

LUTREPULSE for Injection

Delivered = $\frac{19}{26}$ = 73%

Aborted = $\frac{7}{26}$ = 27%

hCG + LUTREPULSE for Injection

Delivered = $\frac{19}{25}$ = 76%

Aborted = $\frac{6}{25}$ = 24%

LUTREPULSE (gonadorelin acetate) for Injection alone was able to maintain the corpus luteum during pregnancy.

ADMINISTRATION: LUTREPULSE for Injection is to be reconstituted aseptically with 8 mL of diluent for LUTREPULSE for Injection. *The drug product should be reconstituted immediately prior to use and transferred to the plastic reservoir.* First withdraw 8 mL of the saline diluent and then inject it onto the lyophile (drug product) cake. The product is shaken for a few seconds to produce a solution which should be clear, colorless, and free of particulate matter. Parenteral drug products should be inspected visually for particulate matter and discoloration prior to administration, whenever solution and container permit. If particulate matter or discoloration are present, the solution should not be used. A presterilized reservoir (bag) with the infusion catheter set supplied with the LUTREPULSE for Injection is filled with the reconstituted solution, and administered intravenously using the LUTREPULSE PUMP. The pump should be set to deliver 25 or 50 μL of solution, based upon the dose selected, over a pulse period of one minute and at a pulse frequency of 90 minutes. The 8 mL of solution will supply 90 minute pulsatile doses for approximately 7 consecutive days.

HOW SUPPLIED

LUTREPULSE (gonadorelin acetate) for Injection is supplied in a LUTREPULSE for Injection 0.8 mg (NDC 55566-7212-1) or 3.2 mg (NDC 55566-7211-1) KIT. Each kit contains one 10 mL vial of 0.8 mg or 3.2 mg LUTREPULSE for Injection as a lyophilized, sterile powder which should be stored at controlled room temperature (15–30°C, 59–86°F). The following components are included in each kit:

10 mL diluent for LUTREPULSE for Injection
Sterile catheter tubing
Sterile reservoir catheter with double-female luer adaptor
Sterile IV cannula units (four supplied)
Sterile 10 mL syringe
Sterile syringe needle
Alcohol swabs (four supplied)
Elastic belt
9-V battery
Physician package insert, physician pump manual, and patient instructions
The LUTREPULSE PUMP kit contains the following components:
LUTREPULSE Pump
9-V batteries (two supplied)
3-V lithium battery
Physician pump manual
Physician package insert
Warranty card
Manufactured for
FERRING LABORATORIES, INC.
Suffern, New York 10901
by FERRING ARZNEIMITTEL GmbH, Kiel, Germany
                 June, 1992—DC 110

Shown in Product Identification Section, page 409

RELEFACT® TRH   ℞
(protirelin)
Injection
FOR INTRAVENOUS ADMINISTRATION

HOW SUPPLIED

As 1 mL ampuls—boxes of 5 (NDC 55566-0081-5). Each mL contains Relefact TRH 0.50 mg (500 μg), sodium chloride 9.0 mg for isotonicity, hydrochloric acid and sodium hydroxide as needed to adjust pH.
Store at controlled room temperature (59–86°F).
Please see full prescribing information in the Diagnostic Product Information section.

Shown in Product Identification Section, page 409

SECRETIN–FERRING   ℞
[si-krē'tin]

HOW SUPPLIED

Secretin-Ferring is supplied as a lyophilized sterile powder in 10 ml vials (NDC 55566-1075-1) containing 75 CU. The unreconstituted product should be stored at −20°C (freezer). However, the biological activity of Secretin-Ferring will not be significantly decreased by storage at temperatures up to 25°C for up to 3 weeks. Expiration date is marked on the label.
Please see full prescribing information in the Diagnostic Product Information section.

Shown in Product Identification Section, page 409

The Fielding Company
94 WELDON PARKWAY
MARYLAND HEIGHTS, MO 63043

GERIMED® Tablets   OTC

DESCRIPTION

A multivitamin-multimineral supplement useful as adjunctive therapy in osteoporosis. Provides a balanced ratio of calcium and phosphorus (2.8 to 1) with adequate Vitamin D for proper absorption.

Each tablet contains:

		U.S. RDA
Dibasic Calcium Phosphate	600 mg.	*
Calcium Carbonate	500 mg.	*
Vitamin A	5000 I. U.	100%
Vitamin D	400 I. U.	100%
Vitamin E	30 I. U.	100%
Vitamin C	120 mg.	200%
Thiamine B$_2$	3 mg.	200%
Riboflavin B$_2$	3 mg.	176%
Niacinamide	25 mg.	100%
Pyridoxine B$_6$	2 mg.	100%
Vitamin B$_{12}$	6 mcg.	100%
Magnesium	50 mg.	11%
Zinc	15 mg.	100%

*Total Calcium	370 mg.	37%
*Total Phosphorus	130 mg.	13%
Calcium/Phosphorus ratio 2.8 - 1		

DOSAGE

One tablet daily, or as prescribed by the physician.

HOW SUPPLIED

Bottle of 60 tablets.
NDC 0421-0080-60

IROSPAN® Tablets/Capsules   OTC

Each tablet or capsule contains:
Ferrous Sulfate (exsic.)   200 mg.
Ascorbic Acid (Vit. C)   150 mg.

DESCRIPTION

Irospan is a unique presentation of sustained release ferrous sulfate and ascorbic acid. Irospan is of particular value during pregnancy and lactation providing excellent tolerance and absorption.

DOSAGE

One tablet or capsule daily or as prescribed by the physician.

HOW SUPPLIED

Irospan Tablets—bottles of 100. NDC 0421-0360-01
Irospan Capsules—bottles of 60. NDC 0421-0361-60

LURLINE® PMS Tablets   OTC

Each tablet contains:
Acetaminophen   500 mg.
Pamabrom   25 mg.
Pyridoxine   50 mg.

DESCRIPTION

Lurline PMS is a safe and effective approach for relief of the multi-symptom complex of premenstrual syndrome. The medication combines an analgesic, a mild diuretic and pyridoxine, representing a safe first line treatment.
Lurline PMS contains no hormones, no sedatives and is aspirin free.

DOSAGE

Start Lurline PMS at the first sign of pain or discomfort, usually 7 to 10 days before menses. Usual dosage is one tablet

3 or 4 times daily. Do not exceed the maximum dose of 8 tablets a day.

HOW SUPPLIED

Lurline PMS—bottles of 24. NDC 0421-8787-24
Lurline PMS—bottles of 50. NDC 0421-8787-50
Physician samples and literature available.

METRIC® 21   ℞
(metronidazole)

DESCRIPTION

An antiprotozoal and antibacterial agent for use in the treatment of trichomoniasis in both the female and male patient.

HOW SUPPLIED

Metric 21 (250 mg) in bottles of 100.
NDC 0421-8282-01

NESTABS® FA Tablets   ℞
Prenatal Tablets

DESCRIPTION

East tablet contains:

			U.S. RDA
Vitamin A	5000	Units	100%
Vitamin D	400	Units	100%
Vitamin E	30	Units	100%
Vitamin C	120	mg.	200%
Folic Acid	1	mg.	125%
Thiamine	3	mg.	176%
Riboflavin	3	mg.	125%
Niacinamide	20	mg.	100%
Pyridoxine	3	mg.	120%
Vitamin B12	8	mcg.	100%
Calcium Carbonate	500	mg.	15%
Iodine	150	mcg.	100%
Ferrous Fumarate	110	mg.	200%
Zinc	15	mg.	100%

A comprehensive vitamin-mineral supplement expressly formulated for use during pregnancy and lactation.

DOSAGE

One tablet daily, or as prescribed by the physician.

PRECAUTION

Folic acid may obscure pernicious anemia in that hematologic remission can occur while neurological manifestations remain progressive.

HOW SUPPLIED

Bottles of 100 tablets.
NDC 0421-1594-01

Fisons Consumer Health
Fisons Corporation
P.O. Box 1212
ROCHESTER, NY 14603

ALLEREST®   OTC
[al'e-rest]
Maximum Strength Tablets, Children's Chewable Tablets, Headache Strength Tablets, Sinus Pain Formula Tablets, No Drowsiness Tablets, Eye Drops, 12 Hour Caplets and 12 Hour Nasal Spray

(See PDR For Nonprescription Drugs.)

AMERICAINE®   OTC
[a-mer'i-kān]
Hemorrhoidal Ointment, Topical Spray, and First Aid Cream

(See PDR For Nonprescription Drugs.)

CALDECORT®   OTC
[kal'de-cort]
Hydrocortisone Multi-Purpose Anti-Itch Cream and Spray

(See PDR For Nonprescription Drugs.)

CALDECORT LIGHT®   OTC
[kal'de-cort līt]
Hydrocortisone in a Light Moisturizing Creme with Aloe

(See PDR For Nonprescription Drugs.)

CALDESENE®   OTC
[kal'de-sēn]
Medicated Powder and Ointment

(See PDR For Nonprescription Drugs.)

CRUEX®   OTC
[kru'ex]
Antifungal Powder, Spray Powder and Cream

(See PDR For Nonprescription Drugs.)

DESENEX®   OTC
[dess'i-nex]
Antifungal Powder, Spray Liquid, Spray Powder, Cream, Ointment, and Penetrating Foam, Foot & Sneaker Spray, Foot & Sneaker Powder Plus

(See PDR For Nonprescription Drugs.)

ISOCLOR®   OTC
[ī'so-klor]
Liquid, Tablets, and Timesule® Capsules

(See PDR For Nonprescription Drugs.)

SINAREST®   OTC
[sīn'a-rest]
Tablets, Extra Strength Tablets, No Drowsiness Tablets and 12 Hour Nasal Spray

(See PDR For Nonprescription Drugs.)

TING®   OTC
[tĭng]
Antifungal Cream, Powder, Spray Liquid and Spray Powder

Fisons Corporation
P.O. BOX 1710
ROCHESTER, NY 14603

AMERICAINE®   ℞
[uh-mer'ĭ-kān"]
(benzocaine)
Anesthetic Lubricant

DESCRIPTION

AMERICAINE Anesthetic Lubricant contains benzocaine 20% with benzethonium chloride 0.1% as a preservative in a water soluble base of polyethylene glycol 300 and 3350.
Benzocaine, a local anesthetic, is chemically ethyl p-aminobenzoate, $C_9H_{11}NO_2$, with a molecular weight of 165.19 and has the following structural formula:

$$NH_2-\bigcirc-COOC_2H_5$$

CLINICAL PHARMACOLOGY

Benzocaine reversibly stabilizes the neuronal membrane which decreases its permeability to sodium ions. Depolarization of the neuronal membrane is inhibited thereby blocking the initiation and conduction of nerve impulses.

INDICATIONS AND USAGE

AMERICAINE Anesthetic Lubricant is indicated for general use as a lubricant and topical anesthetic on intratracheal catheters and pharyngeal and nasal airways to obtund the pharyngeal and tracheal reflexes; on nasogastric and endoscopic tubes; urinary catheters; laryngoscopes; proctoscopes; sigmoidoscopes and vaginal specula.

CONTRAINDICATIONS

Known allergy or hypersensitivity to benzocaine.

PRECAUTIONS

General: Medication should be discontinued if sensitivity or irritation occurs.
Carcinogenesis, Mutagenesis, Impairment of Fertility: Long-term studies in animals or humans to evaluate the carcinogenic and mutagenic potential or the effect on fertility have not been conducted.

Pregnancy Category C: Animal reproduction studies have not been conducted with AMERICAINE Anesthetic Lubricant. It is also not known whether AMERICAINE Anesthetic Lubricant can cause fetal harm when administered to a pregnant woman or can affect reproduction capacity. AMERICAINE Anesthetic Lubricant should be given to a pregnant woman only if clearly needed.
Nursing Mothers: It is not known whether this drug is excreted in human milk. Because many drugs are excreted in human milk, caution should be exercised when AMERICAINE Anesthetic Lubricant is administered to a nursing woman.
Pediatric Use: Do not use in infants under 1 year of age.

ADVERSE REACTIONS

Contact dermatitis and/or hypersensitivity to benzocaine can cause burning, stinging, pruritus, tenderness, erythema, rash, urticaria and edema. Rarely, benzocaine may induce methemoglobinemia causing respiratory distress and cyanosis. Intravenous methylene blue is the specific therapy for this condition.

DOSAGE AND ADMINISTRATION

Apply evenly to exterior of tube or instrument prior to use. Store at 59°–86°F (15°–30°C).

HOW SUPPLIED

AMERICAINE (benzocaine) Anesthetic Lubricant is available in 1 oz. tubes (NDC 0585-0376-16) and 144 × 2.5 g unit-dose foil packs
(NDC 0585-0376-62).
Caution: Federal law prohibits dispensing without prescription.
FISONS Pharmaceuticals
Fisons Corporation
Rochester, NY 14623 USA
Americaine is a registered trademark of Fisons BV.
© 1991, Fisons Corporation.   11/88
RF238

AMERICAINE® OTIC   ℞
[uh-mer'ĭ-kān"]
(benzocaine)
Topical Anesthetic Ear Drops

DESCRIPTION

AMERICAINE Otic, topical anesthetic ear drops, contains benzocaine 20% (w/w) in a water soluble base of glycerin 1% (w/w) and polyethylene glycol 300 with benzethonium chloride 0.1% as a preservative.
Benzocaine, a local anesthetic, is chemically ethyl p-aminobenzoate, $C_9H_{11}NO_2$, with a molecular weight of 165.19 and has the following structural formula:

$$NH_2-\bigcirc-COOC_2H_5$$

CLINICAL PHARMACOLOGY

Benzocaine reversibly stabilizes the neuronal membrane which decreases its permeability to sodium ions. Depolarization of the neuronal membrane is inhibited thereby blocking the initiation and conduction of nerve impulses.

INDICATIONS AND USAGE

AMERICAINE Otic is indicated for relief of pain and pruritus in acute congestive and serous otitis media, acute swimmer's ear, and other forms of otitis externa.

CONTRAINDICATIONS

In the presence of a perforated tympanic membrane or ear discharge.
Known allergy or hypersensitivity to benzocaine.

WARNINGS

Indiscriminate use of anesthetic ear drops may mask symptoms of fulminating infection of the middle ear.

PRECAUTIONS

General: Medication should be discontinued if sensitivity or irritation occurs.
Carcinogenesis, Mutagenesis, Impairment of Fertility: Long-term studies in animals or humans to evaluate the carcinogenic and mutagenic potential or the effect on fertility have not been conducted.

Continued on next page

Information on Fisons' products appearing in these pages is current as of July 1992. For further information, please consult the package insert currently accompanying the product, or Fisons Corporation, P.O. Box 1710, Rochester, NY 14603, (716) 475-9000.

Fisons—Cont.

Pregnancy Category C: Animal reproduction studies have not been conducted with AMERICAINE Otic. It is also not known whether AMERICAINE Otic can cause fetal harm when administered to a pregnant woman or can affect reproduction capacity. AMERICAINE Otic should be given to a pregnant woman only if clearly needed.

Nursing Mothers: It is not known whether this drug is excreted in human milk. Because many drugs are excreted in human milk, caution should be exercised when AMERICAINE Otic is administered to a nursing woman.

Pediatric Use: Do not use in infants under 1 year of age.

ADVERSE REACTIONS

Contact dermatitis and/or hypersensitivity to benzocaine can cause burning, stinging, pruritus, tenderness, erythema, rash, urticaria and edema. Rarely, benzocaine may induce methemoglobinemia causing respiratory distress and cyanosis. Intravenous methylene blue is the specific therapy for this condition.

DOSAGE AND ADMINISTRATION

Instill 4–5 drops of AMERICAINE Otic in the external auditory canal, then insert a cotton pledget into the meatus. Application may be repeated every one to two hours if necessary.

Keep bottle tightly closed. Store at 59°–86°F (15°–30°C).

HOW SUPPLIED

AMERICAINE (benzocaine) Otic, topical anesthetic ear drops, is available in ½ fl. oz. dropper-top bottles (NDC 0585-0377-51).

Caution: Federal law prohibits dispensing without prescription.

Marketed by

FISONS Pharmaceuticals
Fisons Corporation
Rochester, NY 14623 USA
Manufactured by Taylor Pharmacal Co.,
Decatur, IL 62525
2/89   RF239
Americaine is a registered trademark of Fisons BV.
© 1991, FISONS CORPORATION.

BIPHETAMINE®   Ⓒ ℞

[bī-phet ' a-mēn "]
(amphetamine)

---

d- AND dl-AMPHETAMINE HAVE A HIGH POTENTIAL FOR ABUSE. THEY SHOULD THUS BE TRIED ONLY IN WEIGHT REDUCTION PROGRAMS FOR PATIENTS IN WHOM ALTERNATIVE THERAPY HAS BEEN INEFFECTIVE. ADMINISTRATION OF d- AND dl-AMPHETAMINE FOR PROLONGED PERIODS OF TIME IN OBESITY MAY LEAD TO DRUG DEPENDENCE AND MUST BE AVOIDED. PARTICULAR ATTENTION SHOULD BE PAID TO THE POSSIBILITY OF SUBJECTS OBTAINING d- AND dl -AMPHETAMINE FOR NON-THERAPEUTIC USE OR DISTRIBUTION TO OTHERS, AND THE DRUG SHOULD BE PRESCRIBED OR DISPENSED SPARINGLY.

DESCRIPTION

Biphetamine®
12½
Each capsule contains cationic exchange resin complexes equivalent to:

Amphetamine	6.25 mg
Dextroamphetamine	6.25 mg

Biphetamine®
20
Each capsule contains cationic exchange resin complexes equivalent to:

Amphetamine	10 mg
Dextroamphetamine	10 mg

Other ingredients in Biphetamine: dibasic calcium phosphate, FD&C Blue No. 1, FD&C Red No. 40, FD&C Yellow No. 6, gelatin, lactose, magnesium stearate, titanium dioxide and other ingredients in trace quantities.

ACTIONS

Amphetamine is a sympathomimetic amine with CNS stimulant activity. Peripheral actions include elevation of systolic and diastolic blood pressures and weak bronchodilator and respiratory stimulant action.

Behavioral effects in children —There is neither specific evidence which clearly establishes the mechanism whereby amphetamine produces its mental and behavioral effects in children, nor conclusive evidence regarding how these effects relate to the condition of the central nervous system.

Anorectic —Drugs of this class used in obesity are commonly known as "anorectics" or "anorexigenics". It has not been established, however, that the action of such drugs in treating obesity is primarily one of appetite suppression. For example, other central nervous system actions or metabolic effects may be involved.

Adult obese subjects instructed in dietary management and treated with "anorectic" drugs lose more weight, on the average, than those treated with placebo and diet, as determined in relatively short-term clinical trials.

The magnitude of increased weight loss of drug-treated patients over placebo-treated patients is, on the average, only a fraction of a pound a week. However, some patients lose more weight than this and some lose less. The rate of weight loss is greatest in the first weeks of therapy for both drug and placebo subjects and tends to decrease in succeeding weeks. The origins of the increased weight loss due to the various possible drug effects are not established. The amount of weight loss associated with the use of an "anorectic" drug varies from trial to trial, and may be related in part to variables other than the drug prescribed, such as the physician-investigator, the population treated, and the diet prescribed. Studies do not permit conclusions as to the relative importance of the drug and non-drug factors on weight loss.

The natural history of obesity is measured in years, whereas most studies cited are restricted to a few weeks duration; thus, the total impact of drug-induced weight loss over that of diet alone must be considered clinically limited.

Blood levels of amphetamine were determined in human subjects following the administration of Biphetamine Capsules and amphetamine phosphate capsules. Efficiency of absorption was the same for the resinate as for the soluble salt. The average absorption rate was slower and less variable for the resinate. Blood levels with the resinate reached a slightly lower, later, and flatter peak and a slightly higher blood level was maintained over a period of 16 hours. The clinical significance of these differences is not known. In efficacy studies a single dose of Biphetamine was given early in the day and the results obtained were comparable to those which have been reported for multiple daily doses of a soluble salt.

INDICATIONS

Behavioral syndrome in children —Biphetamine is indicated as an integral part of a total treatment program which typically includes other remedial measures (psychological, educational, social) for a stabilizing effect in children with a behavioral syndrome characterized by the following group of developmentally inappropriate symptoms: moderate to severe distractibility, short attention span, hyperactivity, emotional lability, and impulsivity. The diagnosis of this syndrome should not be made with finality when these symptoms are only of comparatively recent origin. Nonlocalizing (soft) neurological signs, learning disability, and abnormal EEG may not be present, and a diagnosis of central nervous system dysfunction may or may not be warranted.

Exogenous obesity —as a short-term (a few weeks) adjunct in a regimen of weight reduction based on caloric restriction for patients refractory to alternative therapy; e.g., repeated diets, group programs and other drugs. The limited usefulness of amphetamine (see ACTIONS) should be weighed against possible risks inherent in use of the drug, such as those described below.

CONTRAINDICATIONS

Advanced arteriosclerosis, symptomatic cardiovascular disease, moderate to severe hypertension, hyperthyroidism, known hypersensitivity or idiosyncrasy to the sympathomimetic amines, glaucoma.

Agitated states.

Patients with a history of drug abuse.

During or within 14 days following the administration of monoamine oxidase inhibitors (hypertensive crises may result).

WARNINGS

When tolerance to the "anorectic" effect develops, the recommended dose should not be exceeded in an attempt to increase the effect; rather the drug should be discontinued. Amphetamine may impair the ability of the patient to engage in potentially hazardous activities such as operating machinery or driving a motor vehicle; the patient should therefore be cautioned accordingly.

Drug Dependence: Amphetamine has been extensively abused. Tolerance, extreme psychological dependence, and severe social disability have occurred. There are reports of patients who have increased the dosage to many times that recommended. Abrupt cessation following prolonged high dosage administration results in extreme fatigue and mental depression; changes are also noted on the sleep EEG. Manifestations of chronic intoxication with amphetamine include severe dermatoses, marked insomnia, irritability, hyperactivity, and personality changes. The most severe manifestation of chronic intoxication is psychosis, often clinically indistinguishable from schizophrenia.

Usage in Pregnancy: Safe use in pregnancy has not been established. Reproduction studies in mammals at high multi-ples of the human dose have suggested both an embryotoxic and a teratogenic potential. Use of amphetamine by women who are or who may become pregnant, and especially by those in the first trimester of pregnancy, requires that the potential benefit be weighed against the possible hazard to mother and infant.

Usage in Children: Amphetamine is not recommended for use as an anorectic agent in children under 12 years of age or for behavior syndrome in children under 3 years of age. Clinical experience suggests that in psychotic children, administration of amphetamine may exacerbate symptoms of behavior disturbance and thought disorder.

Data are inadequate to determine whether chronic administration of amphetamine may be associated with growth inhibition; therefore, growth should be monitored during treatment.

PRECAUTIONS

Caution is to be exercised in prescribing amphetamine for patients with mild hypertension.

Insulin requirements in diabetes mellitus may be altered in association with the use of amphetamine and the concomitant dietary regimen.

Amphetamine may decrease the hypotensive effect of guanethidine.

The least amount feasible should be prescribed or dispensed at one time in order to minimize the possibility of overdosage.

Drug treatment is not indicated in all cases of this behavioral syndrome and should be considered only in light of the complete history and evaluation of the child. The decision to prescribe Biphetamine (amphetamine) should depend on the physician's assessment of the chronicity and severity of the child's symptoms and their appropriateness for his/her age. Prescription should not depend solely on the presence of one or more of the behavioral characteristics.

When these symptoms are associated with acute stress reactions, treatment with Biphetamine is usually not indicated.

Usage in Nursing Mothers: Amphetamines are excreted in human milk. Mothers taking amphetamines should be advised to refrain from nursing.

Long-term effects of Biphetamine in children have not been well-established.

ADVERSE REACTIONS

Cardiovascular: Palpitation, tachycardia, elevation of blood pressure. There have been isolated reports of cardiomyopathy associated with chronic amphetamine use.

Central nervous system: Overstimulation, restlessness, dizziness, insomnia, euphoria, dysphoria, tremor, headache; rarely psychotic episodes at recommended doses.

Gastrointestinal: Dryness of the mouth, unpleasant taste, diarrhea, constipation, other gastrointestinal disturbances.

Allergic: Urticaria.

Endocrine: Impotence, changes in libido.

DOSAGE AND ADMINISTRATION

Biphetamine should be administered at the lowest effective dosage and dosage should be individually adjusted. Late evening medication should be avoided because of possible insomnia.

Biphetamine capsules should be swallowed whole.

Behavioral Syndrome: Amphetamine is not recommended for children under 3 years of age.

Recommended regimen for establishment of optimal response with short acting dextroamphetamine product:

In children from 3 to 5 years of age, start with 2.5 mg daily; daily dosage may be raised in increments of 2.5 mg at weekly intervals until optimal response is obtained.

In children 6 years of age and older, start with 5 mg once or twice daily; daily dosage may be raised in increments of 5 mg at weekly intervals until optimal response is obtained. Only in rare cases will it be necessary to exceed a total of 40 milligrams per day.

Once the optimal response dosage level for amphetamine has been established, Biphetamine capsules may be used for once-a-day dosage wherever appropriate for reasons of convenience.

Biphetamine 12½ and 20 capsules are approximately equivalent to 10 mg and 15 mg, respectively, of dextroamphetamine administered as a single dose.

Where possible, drug administration should be interrupted occasionally to determine if there is a recurrence of behavioral symptoms sufficient to require continued therapy.

Obesity: One capsule daily, 10–14 hours before retiring; capsule strength may be adjusted to individual requirements.

OVERDOSAGE

Manifestations of acute overdosage with amphetamine include restlessness, tremor, hyperreflexia, rapid respiration, confusion, assaultiveness, hallucinations, panic states. Fatigue and depression usually follow the central stimulation. Cardiovascular effects include arrhythmias, hypertension or hypotension and circulatory collapse. Gastrointestinal symptoms include nausea, vomiting, diarrhea, and abdomi-

nal cramps. Fatal poisoning usually terminates in convulsions and coma.
While not reported to date with Biphetamine, hyperpyrexia and rhabdomyolysis can occur with amphetamine overdosage.
Management of acute amphetamine intoxication is largely symptomatic and includes lavage and sedation with a barbiturate. Experience with hemodialysis or peritoneal dialysis is inadequate to permit recommendation in this regard. Acidification of the urine increases amphetamine excretion. Intravenous phentolamine (Regitine) has been suggested on pharmacological grounds for possible acute, severe hypertension, if this complicates amphetamine overdosage.

HOW SUPPLIED

Two strengths: Biphetamine 12½ (black and white capsules, NDC 0585-0878-71); and Biphetamine 20 (black capsules, NDC 0585-0875-71). Stock bottles of 100.
Caution: Federal law prohibits dispensing without prescription.
***FISONS* Pharmaceuticals**
Fisons Corporation
Rochester, NY 14623 USA
RF192C
Rev. 2/89
Biphetamine is a registered trademark of Fisons BV.
© 1991, Fisons Corporation.

GASTROCROM® CAPSULES ℞

[*gas ' tro-krōm*]
(cromolyn sodium, USP)

DESCRIPTION

Each gelatin capsule of GASTROCROM (cromolyn sodium, USP) contains 100 mg cromolyn sodium. Cromolyn sodium is a hygroscopic, white powder having little odor. GASTROCROM may leave a slightly bitter aftertaste. It is soluble in water (1 part in 20) and the resulting solution is neutral. It is intended for oral use.
Chemically, cromolyn sodium is the disodium salt of 1,3-bis (2-carboxychromon-5-yloxy)-2-hydroxypropane. Its chemical structure is:

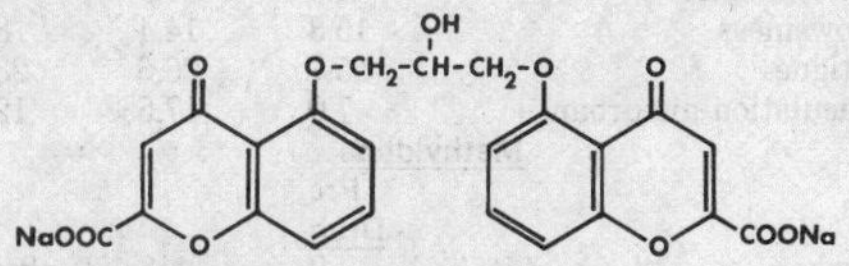

Pharmacologic Category: Mast cell stabilizer
Therapeutic Category: Antiallergic

CLINICAL PHARMACOLOGY

In vitro and *in vivo* animal studies have shown that cromolyn sodium inhibits the release of mediators from sensitized mast cells. Cromolyn sodium acts by inhibiting the release of histamine and leukotrienes (SRS-A) from the mast cell.
Cromolyn sodium has no intrinsic vasoconstrictor, antihistaminic or anti-inflammatory activity.
Cromolyn sodium is poorly absorbed from the gastrointestinal tract. No more than 1% of an administered dose is absorbed by humans after oral administration, the remainder being excreted in the feces. Very little absorption of cromolyn sodium was seen after oral administration of 500 mg by mouth to each of 12 volunteers. From 0.28 to 0.50% of the administered dose was recovered in the first 24 hours of urinary excretion in 3 subjects. The mean urinary excretion of an administered dose over 24 hours in the remaining 9 subjects was 0.45%.

INDICATIONS AND USAGE

GASTROCROM is indicated in the management of patients with mastocytosis. Use of this product has been associated with improvement in diarrhea, flushing, headaches, vomiting, urticaria, abdominal pain, nausea, and itching in some patients.

CONTRAINDICATIONS

GASTROCROM is contraindicated in those patients who have shown hypersensitivity to cromolyn sodium.

WARNINGS

The recommended dosage should be decreased in patients with decreased renal or hepatic function. Severe anaphylactic reactions may occur rarely in association with cromolyn sodium administration.

PRECAUTIONS

In view of the biliary and renal routes of excretion of GASTROCROM, consideration should be given to decreasing the dosage of the drug in patients with impaired renal or hepatic function.
Carcinogenesis, Mutagenesis, and Impairment of Fertility: Long term studies in mice (12 months intraperitoneal treatment followed by six months observation), hamsters (12 months intraperitoneal treatment followed by 12 months observation), and rats (18 months subcutaneous treatment) showed no neoplastic effect of cromolyn sodium.
No evidence of chromosomal damage or cytotoxicity was obtained in various mutagenesis studies.
No evidence of impaired fertility was shown in laboratory animal reproduction studies.
Pregnancy: Pregnancy Category B. Reproduction studies with cromolyn sodium administered parenterally to pregnant mice, rats and rabbits in doses up to 338 times the human clinical doses produced no evidence of fetal malformations. Adverse fetal effects (increased resorption and decreased fetal weight) were noted only at the very high parenteral doses that produced maternal toxicity. There are, however, no adequate and well controlled studies in pregnant women.
Because animal reproduction studies are not always predictive of human response, this drug should be used during pregnancy only if clearly needed.
Drug Interaction During Pregnancy: Cromolyn sodium and isoproterenol were studied following subcutaneous injections in pregnant mice. Cromolyn sodium alone in doses of 60 to 540 mg/kg (38 to 338 times the human dose) did not cause significant increases in resorptions or major malformations. Isoproterenol alone at a dose of 2.7 mg/kg (90 times the human dose) increased both resorptions and malformations. The addition of cromolyn sodium (338 times the human dose) to isoproterenol (90 times the human dose) appears to have increased the incidence of both resorptions and malformations.
Nursing Mothers: It is not known whether this drug is excreted in human milk. Because many drugs are excreted in human milk, caution should be exercised when GASTROCROM is administered to a nursing woman.
Pediatric Use: Animal studies suggest increased risk of toxicity in premature animals when given doses much higher than clinically recommended. In term infants up to six months of age, available clinical data suggest that the dose should not exceed 20 mg/kg/day. The use of this product in children less than two years should be reserved for patients with severe disease in which the potential benefits clearly outweigh the risks.

ADVERSE REACTIONS

Most of the adverse events reported in mastocytosis patients have been transient and could represent symptoms of the disease. The most frequently reported adverse events in mastocytosis patients who have received GASTROCROM during clinical studies were headache and diarrhea. Each occurred in 4 of the 87 patients. Pruritus, nausea and myalgia were each reported in 3 patients and abdominal pain, rash and irritability in 2 patients each. One report of malaise was also recorded.
A generally similar profile of adverse events has been reported during studies in other clinical conditions. Additional reports which have been received during the course of these studies and spontaneous reports during foreign marketing include: flushing, urticaria/angioedema, arthralgia, dizziness, fatigue, paresthesia, taste perversion, migraine, psychosis, anxiety, depression, insomnia, behavior change, esophagospasm, flatulence, dysphagia, hepatic function test abnormal, edema, dyspnea, polycythemia, neutropenia, dysuria, hallucinations, skin erythema and burning, burning mouth and throat, stiffness and weakness of the legs, and postprandial lightheadedness and lethargy. These events are infrequent, the majority representing only a single report, and in many cases the causal relationship to GASTROCROM is uncertain.

DOSAGE AND ADMINISTRATION

NOT FOR INHALATION. SEE DIRECTIONS FOR USE.
The usual starting dose is as follows:
Adults: Two capsules four times daily one-half hour before meals and at bedtime.
Premature to Term Infants: Not recommended.
Term to 2 years: 20 mg/kg/day in four divided doses. Use of this product in children less than 2 years is not recommended and should be attempted only in those patients with severe incapacitating diseases where the benefits clearly outweigh the risks.
Children: From 2–12 years: One capsule four times daily one-half hour before meals and bedtime.
If satisfactory control of symptoms is not achieved within two to three weeks the dosage may be increased but should not exceed 40 mg/kg/day (30 mg/kg/day for children six months to two years).
Patients should be advised that the effect of GASTROCROM therapy is dependent upon its administration at regular intervals, as directed.
Maintenance Dose: Once a therapeutic response has been achieved the dose may be reduced to the minimum required to maintain the patient with a lower degree of symptomatology. To prevent relapses, the dosage should be maintained.
Administration: GASTROCROM should be administered as a solution in water at least ½ hour before meals after preparation according to the following directions:

1. Open capsule(s) and pour powder contents of capsule(s) into ½ glass of hot water.
2. Stir until completely dissolved (clear solution).
3. Add equal quantity of cold water while stirring.
4. DO NOT MIX WITH FRUIT JUICE, MILK OR FOODS.
5. Drink all of the liquid.

HOW SUPPLIED

GASTROCROM Capsules, each containing 100 mg of cromolyn sodium, are supplied in aluminum cans containing 100 capsules.
Each capsule contains a precisely measured dose. The capsules are intentionally oversized to prevent the powder from spilling when the capsule is opened.
NDC 0585-0677-01
Keep tightly closed and out of the reach of children. Store between 15°C–30°C (59°F–86°F).
CAUTION: Federal law prohibits dispensing without prescription.
***FISONS* Pharmaceuticals**
Fisons Corporation
Rochester, NY 14623 USA
Made in England
GASTROCROM and FISONS are registered trademarks of FISONS plc.
© 1991, Fisons Corporation.
RF047B

HYLOREL® ℞

[*hi ' lō-rel "*]
brand of guanadrel sulfate tablets 814 438 101

DESCRIPTION

HYLOREL Tablets for oral administration contain guanadrel sulfate, an antihypertensive agent belonging to the class of adrenergic neuron blocking drugs. Guanadrel sulfate is (1,4-Dioxaspiro[4.5] dec-2-ylmethyl) guanidine sulfate with a molecular weight of 524.63. It is a white to off-white crystalline powder, which melts with decomposition at about 235°C. It is soluble in water to the extent of 76 mg/ml. The structural formula is represented as:

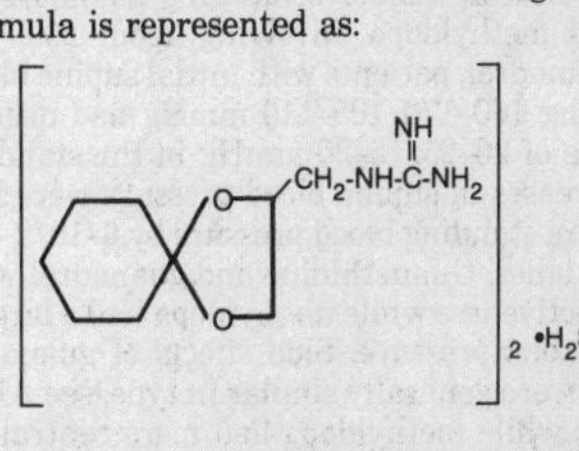

HYLOREL Tablets are available in two strengths: 10 mg and 25 mg. Inactive ingredients: colloidal silicon dioxide, corn starch, lactose, magnesium stearate, microcrystalline cellulose and talc. The 10 mg tablet also contains FD&C Yellow No. 6.

CLINICAL PHARMACOLOGY

Guanadrel sulfate is an orally effective antihypertensive agent that lowers both systolic and diastolic arterial blood pressures. Guanadrel sulfate inhibits sympathetic vasoconstriction by inhibiting norepinephrine release from neuronal storage sites in response to stimulation of the nerve and also causes depletion of norepinephrine from the nerve ending. This results in relaxation of vascular smooth muscle which decreases total peripheral resistance, and decreases venous return, both of which reduce the ability to maintain blood pressure in the upright position. The result is a hypotensive effect that is greater in the standing than in the supine position by about 10 mmHg systolic and 3.5 mmHg diastolic, on the average. Heart rate is also decreased usually by about 5 beats/minute. Fluid retention occurs during treatment with guanadrel, particularly when it is not accompanied by a diuretic. The drug does not inhibit parasympathetic nerve function nor does it enter the central nervous system.
Guanadrel sulfate is rapidly absorbed after oral administration. Plasma concentrations generally peak 1½ to 2 hours after ingestion. The half life is about 10 hours, but individual variability is great. Approximately 85% of the drug is eliminated in the urine. Urinary excretion is approximately 85% complete within 24 hours after administration; about 40% of the dose is excreted as unchanged drug. The disposition of guanadrel sulfate is significantly altered in patients with impaired renal function. A study in such patients has shown that as renal function (measured as creatinine clearance)

Continued on next page

Information on Fisons' products appearing in these pages is current as of July 1992. For further information, please consult the package insert currently accompanying the product, or Fisons Corporation, P.O. Box 1710, Rochester, NY 14603, (716) 475-9000.

Fisons—Cont.

declines, apparent total body clearance, renal and apparent nonrenal clearances decrease, and the terminal elimination half-life is prolonged. Dosage adjustments may be necessary, especially in patients with creatinine clearances of less than 60 mL/min (see DOSAGE AND ADMINISTRATION).

Guanadrel sulfate begins to decrease blood pressure within two hours and produces maximal decreases in four to six hours. No significant change in cardiac output accompanies the blood pressure decline in normal individuals.

Because drugs of the adrenergic neuron blocking class are transported into the neuron by the "norepinephrine pump", drugs that compete for the pump may block their effects. Tricyclic antidepressants have been shown to block the norepinephrine-depleting effect of guanadrel sulfate in rats and monkeys, and the blood pressure lowering effect of guanadrel sulfate in monkeys. Similar effects have been seen with guanethidine and inhibition of the antihypertensive effects of guanadrel sulfate by tricyclic antidepressants in humans should be presumed.

Therefore caution is recommended if guanadrel sulfate and a tricyclic antidepressant are used concomitantly. Should patients be on both a tricyclic antidepressant and guanadrel sulfate, caution is advised upon discontinuation of the tricyclic antidepressant, especially if discontinued abruptly, as an enhanced effect of guanadrel sulfate may occur.

Chlorpromazine seems to have a similar effect on guanethidine and may affect guanadrel as well. Indirectly acting adrenergic amines are transported into the neuron by the "norepinephrine pump" and may interfere with uptake or may displace blocking agents. Ephedrine rapidly reverses the effects of guanadrel but other agents have not been studied. Agents of the guanethidine class cause increased sensitivity to circulating norepinephrine, probably by preventing uptake of norepinephrine by adrenergic neurons, the usual mechanism for terminating norephinephrine effects. Agents of this class are thus dangerous in the presence of excess norephinephrine, e.g., in the presence of a pheochromocytoma.

In controlled clinical studies comparing guanadrel to guanethidine and methyldopa, involving about 2000 patients exposed to guanadrel, patients with initial supine blood pressures averaging 160–170/105–110 mmHg had decreases in blood pressure of 20–25/15–20 mmHg in the standing position. The decreases in supine blood pressure were less than the decreases in standing blood pressure by 6–10/2–7 mmHg in different studies. Guanethidine and guanadrel were very similar in effectiveness while methyldopa had a larger effect on supine systolic pressure. Side effects of guanadrel and guanethidine were generally similar in type (see ADVERSE REACTIONS) while methyldopa had more central nervous system effects (depression, drowsiness) but fewer orthostatic effects and less diarrhea.

INDICATIONS AND USAGE

HYLOREL Tablets are indicated for the treatment of hypertension in patients not responding adequately to a thiazide type diuretic. HYLOREL should be added to a diuretic regimen for optimum blood pressure control.

CONTRAINDICATIONS

HYLOREL Tablets are contraindicated in known or suspected pheochromocytoma.

HYLOREL should not be used concurrently with, or within one week of, monoamine oxidase inhibitors.

HYLOREL should not be used in patients hypersensitive to the drug.

HYLOREL should not be used in patients with frank congestive heart failure.

WARNINGS

a. *Orthostatic Hypotension*

Orthostatic hypotension and its consequences (dizziness and weakness) are frequent in people treated with HYLOREL Tablets. Rarely, fainting upon standing or exercise is seen. Careful instructions to the patient can minimize these symptoms, as can recognition by the physician that the supine blood pressure does not constitute an adequate assessment of the effects of this drug. Patients with known regional vascular disease (cerebral, coronary) are at particular risk from marked orthostatic hypotension and HYLOREL should be avoided in them unless drugs with lesser degrees of orthostatic hypotension are ineffective or unacceptable. In such patients hypotensive episodes should be avoided, even if this requires accepting a poorer degree of blood pressure control.

Instructions to patients: Patients should be advised about the risk of orthostatic hypotension and told to sit or lie down immediately at the onset of dizziness or weakness so that they can prevent loss of consciousness. They should be told that postural hypotension is worst in the morning and upon arising, and may be exaggerated by alcohol, fever, hot weather, prolonged standing, or exercise.

Surgery: To reduce the possibility of vascular collapse during anesthesia, guanadrel should be discontinued 48–72 hours before elective surgery. If emergency surgery is required, the anesthesiologist should be made aware that the patient has been taking HYLOREL and that preanesthetic and anesthetic agents should be administered cautiously in reduced dosage. If vasopressors are needed they must be used cautiously, as guanadrel can enhance the pressor response to such agents and increase their arrhythmogenicity.

b. *Drug Interactions*

As discussed above (CLINICAL PHARMACOLOGY), tricyclic antidepressants and indirect-acting sympathomimetics such as ephedrine or phenylpropanolamine, and possibly phenothiazines, can reverse the effects of neuronal blocking agents. IN VIEW OF THE PRESENCE OF SYMPATHOMIMETIC AMINES IN MANY NON-PRESCRIPTION DRUGS FOR THE TREATMENT OF COLDS, ALLERGY, OR ASTHMA, PATIENTS GIVEN GUANADREL SHOULD BE SPECIFICALLY WARNED NOT TO USE SUCH PREPARATIONS WITHOUT THEIR PHYSICIAN'S ADVICE.

Guanadrel enhances the activity of direct-acting sympathomimetics, like norepinephrine, by blocking neuronal uptake. Drugs that affect the adrenergic response by the same or other mechanisms would be expected to potentiate the effects of guanadrel, causing excessive postural hypotension and bradycardia. These include alpha- or beta-adrenergic blocking agents and reserpine. There is no clinical experience with the combination of HYLOREL with alpha-adrenergic blocking agents or reserpine.

When HYLOREL was added to the treatment regimen in hypertensive patients inadequately controlled with a diuretic and propranolol, no significant adverse effects, including bradycardia, were reported in the 26 patients treated concomitantly with the three drugs.

The use of HYLOREL with vasodilators has not been adequately studied and is not generally recommended because concomitant use may increase the potential for symptomatic orthostatic hypotension.

c. *Asthmatic patients*

Special care is needed in patients with bronchial asthma, as their condition may be aggravated by catecholamine depletion and sympathomimetic amines may interfere with the hypotensive effect of guanadrel.

PRECAUTIONS

General: Salt and water retention may occur with the use of HYLOREL Tablets. In clinical studies major problems did not arise because of concomitant diuretic use. Patients with heart failure have not been studied on HYLOREL, but guanadrel could interfere with the adrenergic mechanisms that maintain compensation.

In patients with a history of peptic ulcer, which could be aggravated by a relative increase in parasympathetic tone, HYLOREL should be used cautiously.

In patients with compromised renal function, decreases in renal and nonrenal clearances and in increase in the elimination half-life of guanadrel sulfate have been found. This could possibly lead to an increased incidence of side effects if standard doses are used in these patients. Titration of dose based on the blood pressure response is necessary because of marked interpatient variability (see DOSAGE AND ADMINISTRATION).

A transient increase in blood pressure has been observed in some patients.

Information for patients
See WARNINGS section.

Drug Interactions
See WARNINGS section.

Carcinogenesis, mutagenesis, impairment of fertility: No evidence of carcinogenic potential appeared in a 2-year mouse study of guanadrel sulfate. In a 2-year rat study, an increased number of benign testicular interstitial cell tumors was observed at dosages of 100 mg/kg/day and 400 mg/kg/day. These were common spontaneous tumors in aged rats and their significance to therapy with HYLOREL in man is unknown. Salmonella testing (Ames test) showed no evidence of mutagenic activity.

A reproduction study was performed in male and female rats at dosages of 0, 10, 30 and 100 mg/kg/day. Suppressed libido and reduced fertility were noted at 100 mg/kg/day (12 times the maximum human dose in a 50 kg subject) and libido was suppressed to a lesser extent at 30 mg/kg/day.

Pregnancy Category B

Teratology studies performed in rats and rabbits at doses up to 12 times the maximum recommended human dose (in a 50 kg subject) revealed no significant harm to the fetus due to guanadrel sulfate. There are, however, no adequate and well-controlled studies in pregnant women. Because animal reproduction studies are not always predictive, HYLOREL should be used in pregnant women only when the potential benefit outweighs the potential risk to mother and infant.

Nursing mothers: Whether guanadrel sulfate is excreted in human milk is not known, but because many drugs are excreted in human milk and because of the potential for serious adverse reactions in nursing infants from guanadrel, a decision should be made whether to discontinue nursing or discontinue the drug, taking into account the importance of the drug to the mother.

Pediatric Use: Safety and effectiveness in children have not been established.

ADVERSE REACTIONS

The adverse reaction data for guanadrel is derived principally from comparative long-term (6 months to 3 years) studies with methyldopa and guanethidine in which side effects were assessed through use of periodic questionnaires, a method that tends to give high adverse reaction rates. In the tables that follow, some of the adverse effects reported may not be drug-related, but in the absence of a placebo-treated group, these cannot be readily distinguished. Comparative results with two well-known drugs, methyldopa and guanethidine should aid in interpretation of these adverse reaction rates.

The following table displays the frequency of side effects which are believed to be related to sympathetic blocking agents: orthostatic faintness, increased bowel movements and ejaculation disturbances for peripherally acting drugs such as guanadrel and drowsiness for centrally acting drugs such as methyldopa. The frequencies observed were generally higher during the first 8 weeks of therapy. Week 0 frequencies, which were recorded just prior to administration of the antihypertensive drugs while the patients were receiving diuretics, serve as a reference point. Frequency while on therapy are shown for the first 8 weeks and for weeks 9 to 52.

FREQUENCY OF SIDE EFFECTS
Percent of Clinic Visits in
Which Side Effect was Reported

Guanadrel

Week	Pre Drug 0	1–8	9–52
Number of clinic visits analyzed	470	3003	4260
Side Effect			
Morning orthostatic faintness	6.6	9.4	6.8
Orthostatic faintness during the day	7.5	10.8	8.5
Other faintness	7.8	4.8	4.5
Increased bowel movements	4.9	7.9	6.1
Drowsiness	15.3	14.4	8.7
Fatigue	25.7	26.6	23.7
Ejaculation disturbance	7.0	17.5	12.0

Methyldopa

Week	Pre Drug 0	1–8	9–52
Number of clinic visits analyzed	266	1610	2216
Side Effect			
Morning orthostatic faintness	6.8	8.1	7.4
Orthostatic faintness during the day	7.5	8.0	7.8
Other faintness	6.2	3.7	3.8
Increased bowel movements	4.9	5.9	3.8
Drowsiness	13.2	21.2	18.6
Fatigue	32.9	22.6	27.6
Ejaculation disturbance	10.3	13.4	11.5

Guanethidine

Week	Pre Drug 0	1–8	9–52
Number of clinic visits analyzed	215	1421	2009
Side Effect			
Morning orthostatic faintness	4.6	10.7	7.9
Orthostatic faintness during the day	5.6	8.9	6.3
Other faintness	5.9	2.7	2.0
Increased bowel movements	3.7	7.9	9.4
Drowsiness	10.2	10.3	6.4
Fatigue	21.4	20.5	17.5
Ejaculation disturbance	6.9	16.6	18.2

The frequency of side effects over time may be reduced by the discontinuation of drugs in patients who experience intolerable side effects. Reasons for discontinuation of therapy with guanadrel are shown in the following table.

[See table top left next page.]

The following paragraph shows the incidence of reactions often associated with adrenergic neuron blockers as the percent of patients who reported the event at least once over the treatment periods of 6 months to 3 years. For such long-term studies these incidence rates of side effects, which are found often in untreated patients, tend to be high and accumulate with time. The incidence rates for two well-known comparison drugs, methyldopa and guanethidine should aid in interpreting the high rates. It can be seen that the serious conse-

PERCENT OF PATIENTS WHO DISCONTINUED

	Guana-drel	Methyl-dopa	Guanethi-dine
Orthostatic faintness	0.6	0.7	6.0*
Syncope	0.4	0.3	2.0
Other faintness	1.2	0.0	0.0
Increase bowel movements	0.8	0.7	1.4
Drowsiness	0.0	1.9*	0.0
Fatigue	0.2	2.6*	0.0
Ejaculation disturbances	0.4	0.0	0.0

*significantly greater than HYLOREL, p < 0.003

quences of the orthostatic effect of guanadrel, such as syncope, were very uncommon.

1544 guanadrel, 743 methyldopa and 330 guanethidine patients were evaluated in comparison studies. The observed incidence rates of major drug related side effects for guanadrel, methyldopa and guanethidine, respectively, are as follows: orthostatic faintness: 49%, 41%, 48%; other faintness: 47%, 46%, 45%; increased bowel movements: 31%, 28%, 36%; ejaculation disturbances: 18%, 21%, 22%; impotence: 5.1%, 12.2%, 7.2%: syncope: 0.4%, 0.3%, 2%; urine retention: 0.2%, 0%, 0%.

Apart from these adverse effects, many others were reported. Relationship to therapy is less clear, although some (such as peripheral edema with all three drugs, depression with methyldopa) are in part drug related. All adverse effects reported in at least 1% of guanadrel patients are listed in the following table:

Drug No. pts. treated Event	Guanadrel 1544 %	Methyl-dopa 743 %	Guanethi-dine 330 %
Cardiovascular-Respiratory			
Chest Pain	27.9	37.4	27.3
Coughing	26.9	36.2	21.5
Palpitations	29.5	35.0	24.5
Shortness of breath at rest	18.3	22.3	17.0
Shortness of breath on exertion	45.9	53.2	48.8
Central Nervous System-Special Senses			
Confusion	14.8	22.6	10.9
Depression	1.9	3.9	1.8
Drowsiness	44.6	64.1	28.5
Headache	58.1	69.0	49.7
Paresthesias	25.1	35.1	16.4
Psychological problems	3.8	4.8	3.9
Sleep disorders	2.1	2.3	2.7
Visual disturbances	29.2	35.3	26.1
Gastrointestinal			
Abdominal distress or pain	1.7	1.9	1.5
Anorexia	18.7	23.0	17.6
Constipation	21.0	29.1	20.3
Dry mouth, dry throat	1.7	4.0	0.6
Gas pain	32.0	39.7	29.4
Glossitis	8.4	10.8	4.8
Indigestion	23.7	30.8	18.5
Nausea and/or vomiting	3.9	4.8	3.6
Genitourinary			
Hematuria	2.3	4.2	2.1
Nocturia	48.4	52.4	41.5
Peripheral edema	28.6	37.4	22.7
Urinary urgency or frequency	33.6	39.8	27.6
Miscellaneous			
Excessive weight gain	44.3	53.7	42.4
Excessive weight loss	42.2	51.1	41.5
Fatigue	63.6	76.2	57.0
Musculoskeletal			
Aching limbs	42.9	51.7	33.9
Backache or neckache	1.5	1.1	1.8
Joint pain or inflammation	1.7	2.0	2.4
Leg cramps during the day	21.1	26.0	20.0
Leg cramps during the night	25.6	32.6	21.2

OVERDOSAGE

Overdosage usually produces marked dizziness and blurred vision related to postural hypotension and may progress to syncope on standing. The patient should lie down until these symptoms subside.

If excessive hypotension occurs and persists despite conservative treatment, intensive therapy may be needed to support vital functions. A vasoconstrictor such as phenylephrine will ameliorate the effect of HYLOREL Tablets, but great care must be used because patients may be hypersensitive to such agents.

DOSAGE AND ADMINISTRATION

As with other sympathetic suppressant drugs, the dose response to HYLOREL Tablets varies widely and must be adjusted for each patient until the therapeutic goal is achieved. With long-term therapy, some tolerance may occur and the dosage may have to be increased.

Because HYLOREL has a substantial orthostatic effect, monitoring both supine and standing pressures is essential, especially while dosage is being adjusted.

HYLOREL should be administered in divided doses. The usual starting dosage for treating hypertension is 10 mg per day, which can be given as 5 mg b.i.d. by breaking the 10 mg tablet. Because the half-life is approximately 10 hours, the dosage should be adjusted weekly or monthly until blood pressure is controlled. Most patients will require daily dosage in the range of 20 to 75 mg usually in twice daily doses. For larger doses 3 or 4 times daily dosing may be needed. A dosage of more than 400 mg/day is rarely required.

Dosage should be adjusted for patients with impaired renal function (see CLINICAL PHARMACOLOGY and PRECAUTIONS). As a general guideline, it is recommended that initial therapy with HYLOREL in patients with creatinine clearances of 30 to 60 mL/min be reduced to 5 mg every 24 hours. In patients with creatinine clearances less than 30 mL/min, the dosing interval should be increased to 48 hours. The time to achieve steady state will be increased. Dosage increases should be made cautiously at intervals not less than 7 days in patients with moderate renal insufficiency and not less than 14 days in patients with severe renal insufficiency. These recommendations are based upon human pharmacokinetic data and not clinical experience.

HOW SUPPLIED

HYLOREL Tablets are available as follows:
10 mg, scored elliptical tablets (light orange)
   Bottles of 100—NDC 0585-0787-71
25 mg, scored elliptical tablets (white)
   Bottles of 100—NDC 0585-0788-71
Store at controlled room temperature 15°–30° C (59°–86°F).
Caution: Federal law prohibits dispensing without prescription.
Mkt. by
***FISONS* Pharmaceuticals**
Fisons Corporation
Rochester, NY 14623 USA
Mfd. by The Upjohn Company   814 438 101
Kalamazoo, MI 49001, USA   691015
Revised August 1990
Hylorel is a registered trademark of Fisons Corporation.
© 1991, FISONS CORPORATION.

IMFERON®   ℞

[ĭm'fer-ŏn]
(iron dextran injection, USP)
Caution:
   Federal law prohibits dispensing without prescription.

WARNING

THE PARENTERAL USE OF COMPLEXES OF IRON AND CARBOHYDRATES HAS RESULTED IN ANAPHYLACTIC-TYPE REACTIONS. DEATHS ASSOCIATED WITH SUCH ADMINISTRATION HAVE BEEN REPORTED. THEREFORE, IMFERON SHOULD BE USED ONLY IN THOSE PATIENTS IN WHOM THE INDICATIONS HAVE BEEN CLEARLY ESTABLISHED AND LABORATORY INVESTIGATIONS CONFIRM AN IRON DEFICIENT STATE NOT AMENABLE TO ORAL IRON THERAPY.

DESCRIPTION

IMFERON (iron dextran injection, USP) is a dark brown, slightly viscous sterile liquid complex of ferric oxyhydroxide and low molecular weight dextran derivative in approximately 0.9% w/v sodium chloride for intravenous or intramuscular use. It contains the equivalent of 50 mg elemental iron (as an iron dextran complex) per mL. The pH of the solution is between 5.2 and 6.5. The multiple dose vial also contains 0.5% w/v phenol (for intramuscular use only).
Electron microscopy has shown the molecule to have an inner electron-dense FeOOH core with a diameter approximating 3 nm and an outer plastic (moldable) dextran shell with a diameter of approximately 13 nm. Almost all the iron (98–99%) is present as a stable ferric-dextran complex. The remaining iron represents a very weak ferrous complex.
Therapeutic Class: Hematinic

CLINICAL PHARMACOLOGY

General: After intramuscular injection, iron dextran is absorbed from the injection site into the capillaries and the lymphatic system. Circulating iron dextran is removed from the plasma by cells of the reticuloendothelial system, which split the complex into its components of iron and dextran. The iron is immediately bound to the available protein moieties to form hemosiderin or ferritin, the physiological forms of iron, or to a lesser extent to transferrin. This iron which is subject to physiological control replenishes hemoglobin and depleted iron stores.

Dextran, a polyglucose, is either metabolized or excreted. Negligible amounts of iron are lost via the urinary or alimentary pathways after administration of iron dextran. When iron dextran is administered during hemodialysis only negligible amounts may cross the dialysis membranes.

The major portion of intramuscular injections of iron dextran is absorbed within 72 hours; most of the remaining iron is absorbed over the ensuing 3 to 4 weeks. Staining from inadvertent deposition of iron dextran in subcutaneous and/or cutaneous tissues usually resolves or fades within several weeks or months; in some rare instances, however, such stains have been reported to persist for several years.

Various studies involving intravenously administered [59Fe] iron dextran to iron deficient subjects, some of whom had coexisting diseases, have yielded half-life values ranging from 5 hours to more than 20 hours. The 5-hour value was determined for [59Fe] iron dextran from a study that used laboratory methods to separate the circulating [59Fe] iron dextran from the transferrin-bound [59Fe]. The 20-hour value reflects a half-life determined by measuring total [59Fe], both circulating and bound. It should be understood that these half-life values do not represent clearance of iron from the body. Iron is not easily eliminated from the body and accumulation of iron can be toxic.

INDICATIONS

Intravenous or intramuscular injections of iron dextran are indicated for treatment of patients with documented iron deficiency in whom oral administration is unsatisfactory or impossible.

CONTRAINDICATIONS

Hypersensitivity to the product. All anemias not associated with iron deficiency.

WARNINGS

See Boxed WARNING.
A risk of carcinogenesis may attend the intramuscular injection of iron-carbohydrate complexes. Such complexes have been found under experimental conditions to produce sarcoma when large doses or small doses injected repeatedly at the same site were given to rats, mice, and rabbits, and possibly in hamsters.
The long latent period between the injection of a potential carcinogen and the appearance of a tumor makes it impossible to measure accurately the risk in man. There have, however, been several reports in the literature describing tumors at the injection site in humans who had previously received intramuscular injections of iron-carbohydrate complexes.
Large intravenous doses, such as used with total dose infusions (TDI), have been associated with an increased incidence of adverse effects. The adverse effects frequently are delayed (1–2 days) reactions typified by one or more of the following symptoms: arthralgia, backache, chills, dizziness, moderate to high fever, headache, malaise, myalgia, nausea, and vomiting. The onset is usually 24–48 hours after administration and symptoms generally subside within 3–4 days (such symptoms have been well recognized since iron dextran was first used). These symptoms have also been reported following intramuscular injection and usually subside within 3–7 days. The etiology of these reactions is not known. The potential for a delayed reaction must be considered when estimating the risk/benefit of treatment.
The maximum intravenous daily dose should not exceed 2 mL undiluted iron dextran.
This preparation should be used with extreme care in patients with serious impairment of liver function.
It should not be used during the acute phase of infectious kidney disease.
Patients with rheumatoid arthritis may have an acute exacerbation of joint pain and swelling following the intravenous administration of IMFERON.

PRECAUTIONS

General: Unwarranted therapy with parenteral iron will cause excess storage of iron with the consequent possibility

Continued on next page

Fisons—Cont.

of exogenous hemosiderosis. Such iron overload is particularly apt to occur in patients with hemoglobinopathies and other refractory anemias that might be erroneously diagnosed as iron deficiency anemias.

IMFERON should be used with caution in individuals with histories of significant allergies and/or asthma.

Epinephrine should be immediately available in the event of acute hypersensitivity reactions. (Usual adult dose: 0.5 mL of a 1:1000 solution, by subcutaneous or intramuscular injection.) Note: Patients using beta-blocking agents may not respond adequately to epinephrine. Isoproterenol or similar beta-agonist agents may be required in these patients.

Reports in the literature from countries outside the United States (in particular, New Zealand) have suggested that the use of intramuscular iron dextran in neonates has been associated with an increased incidence of gram-negative sepsis, primarily due to *E. coli.* This effect from the use of IMFERON in the United States has not been reported.

Information for Patients: Patients should be advised of the potential adverse reactions associated with the use of IMFERON.

Drug/Laboratory Test Interactions: Large doses of iron dextran (5 mL or more) have been reported to give a brown color to serum from a blood sample drawn 4 hours after administration.

The drug may cause falsely elevated values of serum bilirubin and falsely decreased values of serum calcium.

Serum iron determinations by colorimetric assays may not be meaningful for 3 weeks following the administration of iron dextran, particularly after large intravenous doses.

Serum ferritin peaks approximately 7 to 9 days after an intravenous dose of IMFERON and slowly returns to normal after about 3 weeks.

Examination of the bone marrow for iron stores may not be meaningful for prolonged periods following iron dextran therapy because residual iron dextran may remain in the reticuloendothelial cells.

Prolongation of the partial thromboplastin time has been reported to occur after intravenous administration of iron dextran when the blood sample for the test is mixed with anticoagulant citrate dextrose solution, USP. This interference apparently does not occur when anticoagulant sodium citrate solution, USP is used. Blood-typing and cross-matching are not affected by iron dextran.

Bone scans involving 99mTc-diphosphonate have been reported to show a dense, crescentic area of activity in the buttocks, following the contour of the iliac crest, 1 to 6 days after intramuscular injections of IMFERON.

Bone scans with 99mTc-labeled bone seeking agents, in the presence of high serum ferritin levels or following iron dextran infusions, have been reported to show reduction of bony uptake, marked renal activity, and excessive blood pool and soft tissue accumulation.

Caution should be used in interpreting results of serum iron measurements when blood samples are obtained within 1 or 2 weeks of administration of large doses of IMFERON.

Carcinogenesis, Mutagenesis, Impairment of Fertility: See WARNINGS.

Pregnancy: Pregnancy Category C. IMFERON has been shown to be teratogenic and embryocidal in mice, rats, rabbits, dogs, and monkeys when given in doses of about 3* times the maximum human dose. No consistent adverse fetal effects were observed in mice, rats, rabbits, dogs and monkeys at doses of 50 mg iron/kg or less. Fetal and maternal toxicity has been reported in monkeys at a total intravenous dose of 90 mg iron/kg over a 14 day period. Similar effects were observed in mice and rats on administration of a single dose of 125 mg iron/kg. Fetal abnormalities in rats and dogs were observed at doses of 250 mg iron/kg and higher. The animals used in these tests were not iron deficient. There are no adequate and well-controlled studies in pregnant women. IMFERON should be used during pregnancy only if the potential benefit justifies the potential risk to the fetus.

Placental Transfer: Various animal studies and studies in pregnant humans have demonstrated inconclusive results with respect to the placental transfer of iron dextran as iron dextran. It appears that some iron does reach the fetus, but the form in which it crosses the placenta is not clear.

Nursing Mothers: Caution should be exercised when IMFERON is administered to a nursing woman. Only traces of unmetabolized iron dextran are excreted in human milk.

Pediatric Usage: Not recommended for use in infants under 4 months of age (see DOSAGE AND ADMINISTRATION).

ADVERSE REACTIONS

Severe/fatal: Anaphylactic reactions have been reported with the use of IMFERON; on rare occasions these reactions

---

have been fatal. Such reactions, which occur most often within the first several minutes of administration, have been generally characterized by sudden onset of respiratory difficulty and/or cardiovascular collapse. The incidence of these acute hypersensitivity reactions has been estimated between 0.2% to 0.3%. (See boxed WARNING and PRECAUTIONS, *General,* pertaining to immediate availability of epinephrine.)

Mild/moderate: Delayed reactions (see WARNINGS). The incidence of delayed reactions reported in a longitudinal study of patients given multiple intravenous injections of IMFERON, usually 5 mL or greater, was approximately 8% (4% of the total number of injections given).

Other systemic/local: Isolated or multiple signs/symptoms with varying severity have been reported.

Cardiovascular: Chest pain, shock, hypotension, tachycardia, flushing.

(Flushing and hypotension may occur from too rapid injections by the I.V. route.)

Dermatologic: Urticaria, pruritus, purpura, rash.

Gastrointestinal: Abdominal pain, nausea, vomiting, diarrhea.

Hematologic/lymphatic: Leucocytosis, lymphadenopathy (generally inguinal and associated with I.M. injections).

Musculoskeletal/soft tissue: Arthralgia, arthritis (may represent reactivation in patients with quiescent rheumatoid arthritis—see PRECAUTIONS, *General*), myalgia, including backache; abscess formation (sterile); necrosis; atrophy/fibrosis (I.M. injection site); cellulitis, swelling; brown skin and/or underlying tissue discoloration (staining) (See CLINICAL PHARMACOLOGY), soreness or pain at or near intramuscular injection sites, which in some isolated instances was reported to persist for over a year; variable degree of inflammation; local phlebitis at or near I.V. injection site.

Neurologic: Convulsions (may accompany anaphylaxis), syncope, headache, weakness, paresthesia, febrile episodes, chills.

Respiratory: Bronchospasm, dyspnea.

Urologic: Hematuria.

Miscellaneous: Febrile episodes, sweating, chills.

OVERDOSAGE

Overdosage with IMFERON is unlikely to be associated with any acute manifestations. Excessive doses of IMFERON beyond the requirements for restoration of hemoglobin and replenishment of iron stores, may lead to hemosiderosis. Periodic monitoring of serum ferritin levels may be helpful in recognizing a deleterious progressive accumulation of iron resulting from impaired uptake of iron from the reticuloendothelial system in concurrent medical conditions such as chronic renal failure, Hodgkins disease, and rheumatoid arthritis. The LD_{50} of IMFERON is not less than 500 mg/kg in the mouse.

Dialysis: A study of [59Fe] iron dextran utilizing isotonic saline in a 4-hour in vitro dialysis run, indicated that less than 0.5% of the injected radiolabeled iron dextran traversed the dialysis membrane.

DOSAGE AND ADMINISTRATION

Oral iron should be discontinued prior to administration of IMFERON.

DOSAGE

I. *Iron Deficiency Anemia*

Periodic hematologic determination (hemoglobin and hematocrit) is a simple and accurate technique for monitoring hematological response, and should be used as a guide in therapy. It should be recognized that iron storage may lag behind the appearance of normal blood morphology. Serum iron, total iron binding capacity (TIBC) and percent saturation of transferrin are other important tests for detecting and monitoring the iron deficient state.

After administration of iron dextran complex, evidence of a therapeutic response can be seen in a few days as an increase in the reticulocyte count. If there has not been a 1 gram per 100 mL rise in hemoglobin within 2 weeks of starting iron dextran therapy, the diagnosis of iron deficiency anemia should be reviewed.

Although serum ferritin is usually a good guide to body iron stores, the correlation of body iron stores and serum ferritin may not be valid in patients on chronic renal dialysis who are also receiving iron dextran complex.

Although there are significant variations in body build and weight distribution among males and females, the accompanying table and formulae represent a convenient means for estimating the total iron required. This total iron requirement reflects the amount of iron needed to restore hemoglobin concentration to normal or near normal levels plus an additional allowance to provide adequate replenishment of iron stores in most individuals with moderately or severely reduced levels of hemoglobin. It should be remembered that iron deficiency anemia will not appear until essentially all iron stores have been depleted. Therapy, thus, should aim at not only replenishment of hemoglobin iron but iron stores as well.

Factors contributing to the formula are shown below.

$$\frac{\text{mg blood iron}}{\text{lb body weight}} = \frac{\text{mL blood}}{\text{lb body weight}} \times \frac{\text{g hemoglobin}}{\text{mL blood}} \times \frac{\text{mg iron}}{\text{g hemoglobin}}$$

a) Blood volume .... 7.0% body weight
b) Normal hemoglobin (males and females)
     over 15 kg (33 lbs.) .... 14.8 g/100 mL
     15 kg (33 lbs.) or less .... 12.0 g/100 mL
c) Iron content of hemoglobin 0.34%
d) Weight

Based on the above factors, individuals with normal hemoglobin levels will have approximately 35 mg of blood iron per kilogram of body weight (16 mg/lb).

Note: The table and accompanying formulae are applicable for dosage determinations only in patients with iron deficiency anemia; they are not to be used for dosage determinations in patients requiring iron replacement for blood loss.

TOTAL DOSE OF IMFERON IN ML
Observed Hemoglobin g/dL

Body Weight		3	4	5	6	7		9	10
kg	lb								
5	11	3	3	3	2	2	2	2	1
10	22	6	6	5	5	4	4	3	3
15	33	9	9	8	7	7	6	5	4
20	44	15	14	13	12	11	10	10	9
25	55	19	18	17	15	14	13	12	11
30	66	23	21	20	19	17	16	14	13
35	77	27	25	23	22	20	18	17	15
40	88	30	29	27	25	23	21	19	17
45	99	34	32	30	28	26	24	21	19
50	110	38	36	33	31	29	26	24	21
55	121	42	39	37	34	31	29	26	24
60	132	46	43	40	37	34	31	29	26
65	143	50	46	43	40	37	34	31	28
70	154	53	50	47	43	40	37	33	30
75	165	56	53	49	45	42	38	35	31
80	176	59	55	51	48	44	40	36	32
85	187	62	58	54	50	46	42	37	33
90	198	65	60	56	52	47	43	39	35
95	209	67	63	58	54	49	45	40	36
100	220	70	65	61	56	51	46	42	37
105	231	73	68	63	58	53	48	43	38
110	242	76	71	65	60	55	50	44	39
115	253	79	73	68	62	57	51	46	40
120	264	81	76	70	64	59	53	47	41

Dosage was calculated using the formula: Dose = 0.0476 × W × (Normal H − Observed H) + 1 mL per 5 kg to a maximum of 14 mL for iron stores.

Adults and Children over 15 kg (33 pounds):
See Dosage Table.

The total dose required may be calculated. If the patient's body weight in kilograms is W and the hemoglobin level is H g/dL:
Dose of IMFERON in mL required = 0.0476 × W × (14.8 − H) + iron stores.

Add 1 mL IMFERON for each 5 kg body weight to provide for the replenishment of iron stores to a maximum of 14 mL. For weight in pounds use the factor 0.0216.

Children 5–15 kg (11–33 pounds):
See Dosage Table.

Alternatively the total dose may be calculated.

IMFERON should not normally be given in the first four months of life. If the child's body weight in kilograms is W and hemoglobin level is H g/dL:
Dose of IMFERON required in mL = 0.0476 × W × (12 − H) + iron stores.

Add 1 mL IMFERON for each 5 kg body weight to provide for the replenishment of iron stores to a maximum of 14 mL. For weight in pounds use the factor 0.0216.

II. *Iron Replacement for Blood Loss*

Some individuals sustain blood losses on an intermittent or repetitive basis. Such blood losses may occur periodically in patients with hemorrhagic diatheses (familial telangiectasia; hemophilia; gastrointestinal bleeding) and on a repetitive basis from the procedures such as renal hemodialysis. Iron therapy in these patients should be directed toward replacement of the equivalent amount of iron represented in the lost blood. The table and formula presented under iron deficiency anemia are *not* applicable for simple iron replacement values.

Quantitative estimates of the individual's periodic blood loss and hematocrit during the bleeding episode provide a convenient method for the calculation of the required iron dose. The formula shown below is based on the approximation that 1 mL of normocytic, normochromic red cells contains 1 mg of elemental iron:

Replacement iron (in mg) = Blood loss (in mL) × hematocrit
     Example: Blood loss of 500 mL with 20% hematocrit
         Replacement iron = 500 × 0.20 = 100 mg
         IMFERON dose = $\dfrac{100 \text{ mg}}{50}$ = 2 mL

---

*The human dose presented here is the total iron required for treating an iron deficient state in a representative patient. The calculation represents a 50 kg patient with a hemoglobin value of 8 g/dL requiring 30 mL of IMFERON or 1500 mg iron—equivalent to 30 mg/kg.

Administration
The total amount of IMFERON required for the treatment of *iron deficiency anemia* or *iron replacement for blood loss* is determined from the table or appropriate formula. (See **Dosage.**)
I. *Intravenous Injection*
Prior to receiving their first intravenous IMFERON therapeutic dose, all patients should be given an intravenous *test dose* of 0.5 mL. Although anaphylactic reactions known to occur following IMFERON administration are usually evident within a few minutes, or sooner, it is recommended that a period of an hour or longer elapse before the remainder of the initial therapeutic dose is given.
Individual doses of 2 mL or less may be given on a daily basis until the calculated total amount required has been reached. IMFERON is given undiluted and *slowly* (1 mL or less per minute).
II. *Intramuscular Injection*
Prior to receiving their first intramuscular IMFERON therapeutic dose, all patients should be given an intramuscular *test dose* of 0.5 mL, administered in the same recommended test site and by the same technique as described below. Although anaphylactic reactions known to occur following IMFERON administration are usually evident within a few minutes or sooner, it is recommended that at least an hour or longer elapse before the remainder of the initial therapeutic dose is given.
If no adverse reactions are observed, IMFERON can be given according to the following schedule until the calculated total amount required has been reached. Each day's dose should ordinarily not exceed 0.5 mL (25 mg of iron) for infants under 5 kg (11 lbs.); 1.0 mL (50 mg of iron) for children under 10 kg (22 lbs.); and 2.0 mL (100 mg of iron) for other patients.
Daily doses larger than these have been associated with an increased number of reports of delayed reactions and should be utilized only in those situations where the potential benefits clearly outweigh the increased risk. A daily dose of 5 mL should not be exceeded.
IMFERON should be injected only into the muscle mass of the upper outer quadrant of the buttock—never into the arm or other exposed areas—and should be injected deeply, with a 2-inch or 3-inch 19 or 20 gauge needle. If the patient is standing, he/she should be bearing his/her weight on the leg opposite the injection site, or if in bed, he/she should be in the lateral position with injection site uppermost. To avoid injection or leakage into the subcutaneous tissue, a Z-track technique (displacement of the skin laterally prior to injection) is recommended.
NOTE: Do not mix IMFERON with other medications or add to parenteral nutrition solutions for intravenous infusion.

HOW SUPPLIED

For intramuscular or intravenous use:
2 mL ampules, boxes of 10:
NDC 0585-2226-10
For intramuscular use ONLY:
10 mL multiple dose vial containing
0.5% phenol as a preservative, boxes of 2:
NDC 0585-3226-20
CAUTION: Federal law prohibits dispensing without prescription.
Store at room temperature, preferably below 86°F. Do not freeze. Keep out of the reach of children.
***FISONS* Pharmaceuticals**
Fisons Corporation
Rochester, NY 14623 USA
IMFERON and FISONS are registered trademarks of FISONS plc. Revised 5/89
RF 042

Made in England

INTAL® Capsules ℞
[*in ' tal*]
(cromolyn sodium for inhalation, USP)

DESCRIPTION

Cromolyn sodium is the disodium salt of 1,3-bis (2-carboxychromon-5-yloxy)-2-hydroxypropane. The empirical formula is $C_{23}H_{14}Na_2O_{11}$; the molecular weight is 512.34. Each INTAL (cromolyn sodium for inhalation, USP) Capsule contains 20 mg cromolyn sodium and 20 mg lactose. The contents of the capsule are intended for inhalation use only with the SPINHALER® turbo-inhaler. Cromolyn sodium is a water-soluble, odorless, white, hydrated crystalline powder. It is tasteless at first, but leaves a slightly bitter aftertaste.
The molecular structure of cromolyn sodium is:
[See chemical structure at top of next column.]
Pharmacologic Category: Mast cell stabilizer/antiallergic.
Therapeutic Category: Antiasthmatic; reduces bronchial hyperreactivity.

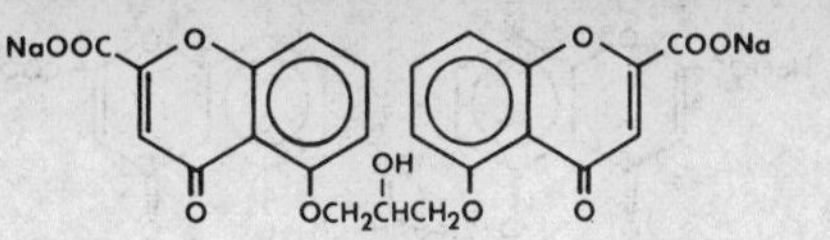

CLINICAL PHARMACOLOGY

In vitro and *in vivo* animal studies have shown that cromolyn sodium inhibits sensitized mast cell degranulation which occurs after exposure to specific antigens. Cromolyn sodium acts by inhibiting the release of mediators from mast cells. Studies show that cromolyn sodium indirectly blocks calcium ions from entering the mast cell, thereby preventing mediator release.
Cromolyn sodium inhibits both the immediate and non-immediate bronchoconstrictive reactions to inhaled antigen. Cromolyn sodium also attenuates bronchospasm caused by exercise, toluene diisocyanate, aspirin, cold air, sulfur dioxide and environmental pollutants.
Cromolyn sodium has no intrinsic bronchodilator, antihistaminic or anti-inflammatory activity.
After administration by inhalation, approximately 8% of the total cromolyn sodium dose administered is absorbed and rapidly excreted unchanged, approximately equally divided between urine and bile. The remainder of the dose is either exhaled or deposited in the oropharynx, swallowed, and excreted via the alimentary tract.

INDICATIONS AND USAGE

INTAL is a prophylactic agent indicated in the management of patients with bronchial asthma.
In patients whose symptoms are sufficiently frequent to require a continuous program of medication, INTAL is given by inhalation on a regular daily basis (see DOSAGE AND ADMINISTRATION). The effect of INTAL is usually evident after several weeks of treatment, although some patients show an almost immediate response.
In patients who develop acute bronchoconstriction in response to exposure to exercise, toluene diisocyanate, environmental pollutants, etc., INTAL should be given shortly before exposure to the precipitating factor (see DOSAGE AND ADMINISTRATION).

CONTRAINDICATIONS

INTAL is contraindicated in those patients who have shown hypersensitivity to cromolyn sodium or to lactose.

WARNINGS

INTAL has no role in the treatment of status asthmaticus.

PRECAUTIONS

General: Occasionally, patients may experience cough and/or bronchospasm following INTAL inhalation. At times, patients who develop bronchospasm may not be able to continue INTAL administration despite prior bronchodilator administration. Rarely, very severe bronchospasm has been encountered.
Symptoms of asthma may recur if INTAL is reduced below the recommended dosage or discontinued.
Information for Patients: INTAL is to be taken as directed by the physician. Because it is preventive medication, it may take up to four weeks before the patient experiences maximum benefit.
Patients may experience irritation of the throat or coughing after inhalation of the powder. In some cases, rinsing the mouth or taking a drink of water immediately before and/or after using the SPINHALER® will eliminate the throat irritation or cough.
If the patient experiences difficulty in emptying the capsule, which may require several deep inhalations, check to make certain the patient is following the directions carefully. A light dusting of powder remaining in the capsule is normal, and is not an indication that the SPINHALER or capsule is faulty or that the proper dose was not delivered. The SPINHALER should be washed in clean, warm water at least once a week, and dried thoroughly before use.
For additional information, see the accompanying leaflet entitled "Living a Full Life with Asthma."
Carcinogenesis, Mutagenesis, and Impairment of Fertility: Long term studies in mice (12 months intraperitoneal treatment followed by 6 months observation), hamsters (12 months intraperitoneal treatment followed by 12 months observation), and rats (18 months subcutaneous treatment) showed no neoplastic effect of cromolyn sodium.
No evidence of chromosomal damage or cytotoxicity was obtained in various mutagenesis studies.
No evidence of impaired fertility was shown in laboratory animal reproduction studies.
Pregnancy: Pregnancy Category B. Reproduction studies with cromolyn sodium administered parenterally to pregnant mice, rats, and rabbits in doses up to 338 times the human clinical dose produced no evidence of fetal malformations. Adverse fetal effects (increased resorptions and decreased fetal weight) were noted only at the very high parenteral doses that produced maternal toxicity. There are, however, no adequate and well-controlled studies in pregnant women. Because animal reproduction studies are not always predictive of human response, this drug should be used during pregnancy only if clearly needed.
Drug Interaction During Pregnancy: Cromolyn sodium and isoproterenol were studied following subcutaneous injections in pregnant mice. Cromolyn sodium alone in doses of 60 to 540 mg/kg (38 to 338 times the human dose) did not cause significant increases in resorptions or major malformations. Isoproterenol alone at a dose of 2.7 mg/kg (90 times the human dose) increased both resorptions and malformations. The addition of cromolyn sodium (338 times the human dose) to isoproterenol (90 times the human dose) appears to have increased the incidence of both resorptions and malformations.
Nursing Mothers: It is not known whether this drug is excreted in human milk. Because many drugs are excreted in human milk, caution should be exercised when INTAL is administered to a nursing woman.
Pediatric Use: Safety and effectiveness in children below the age of 2 years have not been established. For young children unable to utilize the SPINHALER, INTAL Nebulizer Solution is recommended.

ADVERSE REACTIONS

Clinical experience with the use of INTAL suggests that adverse reactions are rare events. The most common side effects are associated with inhalation of the powder and include transient cough (1 in 5 patients) and mild wheezing (1 in 25 patients). These effects rarely require treatment or discontinuation of the drug.
Information on the incidence of adverse reactions to INTAL has been derived from U.S. post-marketing surveillance experience. The following adverse reactions attributed to INTAL, based upon recurrence following readministration, have been reported in less than 1 in 10,000 patients: laryngeal edema, swollen parotid gland, angioedema, bronchospasm, joint swelling and pain, dizziness, dysuria and urinary frequency, nausea, cough, wheezing, headache, nasal congestion, rash, urticaria and lacrimation.
Other adverse reactions have been reported in less than 1 in 100,000 patients, and it is unclear whether these are attributable to the drug: anaphylaxis, nephrosis, periarteritic vasculitis, pericarditis, peripheral neuritis, pulmonary infiltrates with eosinophilia, polymyositis, exfoliative dermatitis, hemoptysis, anemia, myalgia, hoarsenesss, photodermatitis and vertigo.
The following adverse effects have been reported in less than 1 in 10,000 patients, and are a consequence of the SPINHALER® delivery system: inhalation of (capsule) gelatin particles and inhalation of mouthpiece or propeller.

OVERDOSAGE

There is no clinical syndrome associated with an overdosage of cromolyn sodium. Acute toxicity testing in a wide variety of species has demonstrated an extremely low order of toxicity for cromolyn sodium, regardless of whether administration was parenteral, oral or by inhalation. Parenteral administration in mice, rats, guinea pigs, hamsters and rabbits demonstrated an LD_{50} in the region of 4000 mg/kg. Intravenous administration in monkeys also indicated a similar order of toxicity. The highest dose administered by the oral route in rats and mice was 8000 mg/kg, and at this dose level no deaths occurred. By inhalation, even in long term studies, it proved impossible to achieve toxic dose levels of cromolyn sodium in a range of mammalian species.

DOSAGE AND ADMINISTRATION

For management of bronchial asthma in adults and children (two years of age and over) who are able to use the SPINHALER turbo-inhaler, the usual starting dosage is the contents of one INTAL Capsule inhaled four times daily at regular intervals.
Patients with chronic asthma should be advised that the effect of INTAL therapy is dependent upon its administration at regular intervals, as directed. INTAL should be introduced into the patient's therapeutic regimen when the acute episode has been controlled, the airway has been cleared and the patient is able to inhale adequately.
For the prevention of acute bronchospasm which follows exercise or exposure to cold dry air, environmental agents, (e.g., animal danders, toluene diisocyanate, pollutants), etc., the usual dose is the contents of one INTAL Capsule inhaled shortly before exposure to the precipitating factor.
It should be emphasized to the patient that the drug is poorly absorbed when swallowed and is not effective by this route of administration.
INTAL Therapy in Relation to Other Treatments for Asthma:
Non-steroidal agents: INTAL should be *added* to the pa-

Continued on next page

Information on Fisons' products appearing in these pages is current as of July 1992. For further information, please consult the package insert currently accompanying the product, or Fisons Corporation, P.O. Box 1710, Rochester, NY 14603, (716) 475-9000.

Fisons—Cont.

tient's existing treatment regimen (e.g., bronchodilators). When a clinical response to INTAL is evident, usually within two to four weeks, and if the asthma is under good control, an attempt may be made to decrease concomitant medication usage gradually.

If concomitant medications are eliminated or required on no more than a p.r.n. basis, the frequency of administration of INTAL may be titrated downward to the lowest level consistent with the desired effect. The usual decrease is from four capsules to three to two capsules per day. It is important that the dosage be reduced gradually to avoid exacerbation of asthma. It is emphasized that in patients whose dosage has been titrated to fewer than four capsules per day, an increase in the dosage of INTAL and the introduction of, or increase in, symptomatic medications may be needed if the patient's clinical condition deteriorates.

Corticosteroids: In patients chronically receiving corticosteroids for the management of bronchial asthma, the dosage should be maintained following the introduction of INTAL. If the patient improves, an attempt to decrease corticosteroids should be made. Even if the corticosteroid-dependent patient fails to show symptomatic improvement following INTAL administration, the potential to reduce corticosteroids may nonetheless be present. Thus, gradual tapering of corticosteroid dosage may be attempted. It is important that the dose be reduced slowly, maintaining close supervision of the patient to avoid an exacerbation of asthma.

It should be borne in mind that prolonged corticosteroid therapy frequently causes an impairment in the activity of the hypothalamic-pituitary-adrenal axis and a reduction in the size of the adrenal cortex. A potentially critical degree of impairment or insufficiency may persist asymptomatically for some time even after gradual discontinuation of adrenocortical steroids. Therefore, if a patient is subjected to significant stress, such as a severe asthmatic attack, surgery, trauma or severe illness while being treated or within one year (occasionally up to two years) after corticosteroid treatment has been terminated, consideration should be given to reinstituting corticosteroid therapy. When respiratory function is impaired, as may occur in severe exacerbation of asthma, a temporary increase in the amount of corticosteroids may be required to regain control of the patient's asthma.

It is particularly important that great care be exercised, if for any reason INTAL is withdrawn in cases where its use has permitted a reduction in the maintenance dose of corticosteroids. In such cases, continued close supervision of the patient is essential since there may be sudden reappearance of severe manifestations of asthma which will require immediate therapy and possible reintroduction of corticosteroids.

HOW SUPPLIED

INTAL Capsules, each containing 20 mg cromolyn sodium, are available in foil strip packs of 60 and 120 capsules. Each yellow and clear capsule is imprinted with the product identification code: FISONS 670. Store capsules between 15°C and 25°C (59°F and 77°F). Keep out of the reach of children. SPINHALER® turbo-inhalers are supplied separately in individual containers. The SPINHALER should be replaced after 6 months of use.

NDC 0585-0670-60   Pack of 60 INTAL Capsules
NDC 0585-0670-12   Pack of 120 INTAL Capsules
NDS 0585-1011-01   SPINHALER Turbo-Inhaler

CAUTION: Federal law prohibits dispensing without prescription.

FISONS Pharmaceuticals
Fisons Corporation
Rochester, NY 14623 USA
Made in England
INTAL, SPINHALER, and FISONS are registered trademarks of Fisons plc.
© 1992, Fisions Corporation

Revised 1/92
RF 025C

INTAL® Inhaler   ℞
[ĭn'tăl]
(cromolyn sodium inhalation aerosol)

DESCRIPTION

The active ingredient of INTAL Inhaler is cromolyn sodium. Cromolyn sodium is the disodium salt of 1,3 bis (2-carboxychromon-5-yloxy)-2-hydroxypropane. Cromolyn sodium has a molecular weight of 512.34. Cromolyn sodium is soluble in water.

The molecular structure of cromolyn sodium is:
[See chemical structure at top of next column.]
INTAL Inhaler is a metered dose aerosol unit for oral inhalation containing micronized cromolyn sodium, sorbitan trioleate with dichlorotetrafluoroethane and dichlorodifluoromethane as propellants. Each metered spray delivers to the

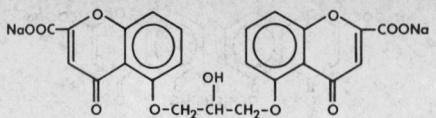

patient approximately 800 mcg of cromolyn sodium. Each 8.1 g canister delivers at least 112 metered sprays (56 doses); each 14.2 g canister delivers at least 200 metered sprays (100 doses).

Pharmacological Category: Mast cell stabilizer/anti-allergic.

Therapeutic Category: Prophylactic antiasthmatic; reduces bronchial hyperreactivity.

CLINICAL PHARMACOLOGY

In vitro and *in vivo* animal studies have shown that cromolyn sodium inhibits sensitized mast cell degranulation which occurs after exposure to specific antigens. Cromolyn sodium acts by inhibiting the release of mediators from mast cells. Studies show that cromolyn sodium indirectly blocks calcium ions from entering the mast cell, thereby preventing mediator release.

Cromolyn sodium inhibits both the immediate and non-immediate bronchoconstrictive reactions to inhaled antigen. Cromolyn sodium also attenuates bronchospasm caused by exercise, toluene diisocyanate, aspirin, cold air, sulfur dioxide and environmental pollutants, at least in some patients. Cromolyn sodium has no intrinsic bronchodilator, antihistaminic or anti-inflammatory activity.

After administration of cromolyn sodium capsules by inhalation, approximately 8% of the total dose administered is absorbed and rapidly excreted unchanged, approximately equally divided between urine and bile. The remainder of the dose is either exhaled or deposited in the oropharynx, swallowed, and excreted via the alimentary tract.

INDICATIONS AND USAGE

INTAL Inhaler is a prophylactic agent indicated in the management of patients with bronchial asthma.

In patients whose symptoms are sufficiently frequent to require a continuous program of medication, INTAL Inhaler is given by inhalation on a regular daily basis (see Dosage and Administration). The effect of INTAL Inhaler is usually evident after several weeks of treatment, although some patients show an almost immediate response.

If improvement occurs, it will ordinarily occur within the first 4 weeks of administration as manifested by a decrease in the severity of clinical symptoms of asthma, or in the need for concomitant therapy, or both.

In patients who develop acute bronchoconstriction in response to exposure to exercise, toluene diisocyanate, environmental pollutants, known antigens, etc., INTAL Inhaler should be used shortly before exposure to the precipitating factor, i.e., within 10–15 minutes but not more than 60 minutes (see Dosage and Administration). INTAL Inhaler may be effective in relieving bronchospasm in some, but not all, patients with exercise induced bronchospasm.

CONTRAINDICATIONS

INTAL Inhaler is contraindicated in those patients who have shown hypersensitivity to cromolyn sodium or other components.

WARNINGS

INTAL Inhaler has no role in the treatment of an acute attack of asthma, especially status asthmaticus. Severe anaphylactic reactions can occur after cromolyn sodium administration. The recommended dosage should be decreased in patients with decreased renal or hepatic function. INTAL Inhaler should be discontinued if the patient develops eosinophilic pneumonia (or pulmonary infiltrates with eosinophilia). Because of the propellants in this preparation, it should be used with caution in patients with coronary artery disease or a history of cardiac arrhythmias.

PRECAUTIONS

General: In view of the biliary and renal routes of excretion for cromolyn sodium, consideration should be given to decreasing the dosage or discontinuing the administration of the drug in patients with impaired renal or hepatic function. Occasionally, patients may experience cough and/or bronchospasm following cromolyn sodium inhalation. At times, patients who develop bronchospasm may not be able to continue administration despite prior bronchodilator administration. Rarely, very severe bronchospasm has been encountered.

Carcinogenesis, Mutagenesis, Impairment of Fertility: Long term studies in mice (12 months intraperitoneal treatment followed by 6 months observation), hamsters (12 months intraperitoneal treatment followed by 12 months observation), and rats (18 months subcutaneous treatment) showed no neoplastic effect of cromolyn sodium.

No evidence of chromosomal damage or cytotoxicity was obtained in various mutagenesis studies.

No evidence of impaired fertility was shown in laboratory animal reproduction studies.

Pregnancy: Pregnancy Category B. Reproduction studies with cromolyn sodium administered parenterally to pregnant mice, rats, and rabbits in doses up to 338 times the human clinical doses produced no evidence of fetal malformations. Adverse fetal effects (increased resorptions and decreased fetal weight) were noted only at the very high parenteral doses that produced maternal toxicity. There are, however, no adequate and well-controlled studies in pregnant women. Because animal reproduction studies are not always predictive of human response, this drug should be used during pregnancy only if clearly needed.

Drug Interaction During Pregnancy: Cromolyn sodium and isoproterenol were studied following subcutaneous injections in pregnant mice. Cromolyn sodium alone in doses of 60 to 540 mg/kg (38 to 338 times the human dose) did not cause significant increases in resorptions or major malformations. Isoproterenol alone at a dose of 2.7 mg/kg (90 times the human dose) increased both resorptions and malformations. The addition of cromolyn sodium (338 times the human dose) to isoproterenol (90 times the human dose) appears to have increased the incidence of both resorptions and malformations.

Nursing Mothers: It is not known whether this drug is excreted in human milk, therefore, caution should be exercised when INTAL Inhaler is administered to a nursing woman and the attending physician must make a benefit/risk assessment in regard to its use in this situation.

Pediatric Use: Safety and effectiveness in children below the age of 5 years have not been established. For young children unable to utilize the Inhaler, INTAL Nebulizer Solution (cromolyn sodium inhalation, USP) is recommended. Because of the possibility that adverse effects of this drug could become apparent only after many years, a benefit/risk consideration of the long-term use of INTAL Inhaler is particularly important in pediatric patients.

ADVERSE REACTIONS

In controlled clinical studies of INTAL Inhaler, the most frequently reported adverse reactions attributed to cromolyn sodium treatment were: Throat irritation or dryness, bad taste, cough, wheeze, nausea.

The most frequently reported adverse reactions attributed to other forms of cromolyn sodium (on the basis of reoccurrence following readministration) involve the respiratory tract and are: bronchospasm [sometimes severe, associated with a precipitous fall in pulmonary function (FEV_1)], cough, laryngeal edema (rare), nasal congestion (sometimes severe), pharyngeal irritation and wheezing.

Adverse reactions which occur infrequently and are associated with administration of the drug are: anaphylaxis, angioedema, dizziness, dysuria and urinary frequency, joint swelling and pain, lacrimation, nausea and headache, rash, swollen parotid gland, urticaria, pulmonary infiltrates with eosinophilia, substernal burning, and myopathy.

The following adverse reactions have been reported as rare events and it is unclear whether they are attributable to the drug: anemia, exfoliative dermatitis, hemoptysis, hoarseness, myalgia, nephrosis, periarteritic vasculitis, pericarditis, peripheral neuritis, photodermatitis, sneezing, drowsiness, nasal itching, nasal bleeding, nasal burning, serum sickness, stomach ache, polymyositis, vertigo, and liver disease.

OVERDOSAGE

No action other than medical observation should be necessary.

DOSAGE AND ADMINISTRATION

For management of bronchial asthma in adults and children (5 years of age and over) who are able to use the Inhaler, the usual starting dosage is two metered sprays inhaled four times daily at regular intervals. This dose should not be exceeded. Not all patients will respond to the recommended dose and there is evidence to suggest, at least in younger patients, that a lower dose may provide efficacy.

Patients with chronic asthma should be advised that the effect of INTAL Inhaler therapy is dependent upon its administration at regular intervals, as directed. INTAL Inhaler should be introduced into the patient's therapeutic regimen when the acute episode has been controlled, the airway has been cleared and the patient is able to inhale adequately.

For the prevention of acute bronchospasm which follows exercise, exposure to cold dry air or environmental agents, the usual dose is inhalation of two metered dose sprays shortly, i.e., 10–15 minutes but not more than 60 minutes, before exposure to the precipitating factor.

INTAL INHALER THERAPY IN RELATION TO OTHER TREATMENTS FOR ASTHMA: Non-steroidal agents: INTAL Inhaler should be **added** to the patient's existing treatment regimen (e.g., bronchodilators). When a clinical response to INTAL Inhaler is evident, usually within two to four weeks, and if the asthma is under good control, an attempt may be made to decrease concomitant medication usage gradually.

If concomitant medications are eliminated or required on no more than a p.r.n. basis, the frequency of administration of

INTAL Inhaler may be titrated downward to the lowest level consistent with the desired effect. The usual decrease is from four to three to two inhalations of two sprays per day. It is important that the dosage be reduced gradually to avoid exacerbation of asthma. It is emphasized that in patients whose dosage has been titrated to fewer than four inhalations per day, an increase in the dosage of INTAL Inhaler and the introduction of, or increase in, symptomatic medications may be needed if the patient's clinical condition deteriorates.

Corticosteroids: In patients chronically receiving corticosteroids for the management of bronchial asthma, the dosage should be maintained following the introduction of INTAL Inhaler. If the patient improves, an attempt to decrease corticosteroids should be made. Even if the corticosteroid-dependent patient fails to show symptomatic improvement following INTAL Inhaler administration, the potential to reduce corticosteroids may nonetheless be present. Thus, gradual tapering of corticosteroid dosage may be attempted. It is important that the dose be reduced slowly, maintaining close supervision of the patient to avoid an exacerbation of asthma.

It should be borne in mind that prolonged corticosteroid therapy frequently causes an impairment in the activity of the hypothalamic-pituitary-adrenal axis and a reduction in the size of the adrenal cortex. A potentially critical degree of impairment or insufficiency may persist asymptomatically for some time even after gradual discontinuation of adrenocortical steroids. Therefore, if a patient is subjected to significant stress, such as a severe asthmatic attack, surgery, trauma or severe illness while being treated or within one year (occasionally up to two years) after corticosteroid treatment has been terminated, consideration should be given to reinstituting corticosteroid therapy. When respiratory function is impaired, as may occur in severe exacerbation of asthma, a temporary increase in the amount of corticosteroids may be required to regain control of the patient's asthma.

It is particularly important that great care be exercised if for any reason cromolyn sodium is withdrawn in cases where its use has permitted a reduction in the maintenance dose of corticosteroids. In such cases, continued close supervision of the patient is essential since there may be sudden reappearance of severe manifestations of asthma which will require immediate therapy and possible reintroduction of corticosteroids.

HOW SUPPLIED

INTAL Inhaler, 8.1 g or 14.2 g canister, box of one. Supplied with inhalation adapter and patient instructions.

NDC 0585-0675-01	14.2 g canister
NDC 0585-0675-02	8.1 g canister

Store between 15°–30°C (59°–86°F). Contents under pressure. Do not puncture or incinerate. Keep out of the reach of children.

CAUTION: Federal law prohibits dispensing without prescription.

Manufactured for:
***FISONS* Pharmaceuticals**
Fisons Corporation
Rochester, NY 14623 USA
By: Health Care Specialties Division
3M Health Care Limited
Loughborough, England LE11 1EP

INTAL and FISONS are registered trademarks of FISONS plc.

Made in England

REV 6/90
RF043A

INTAL® Nebulizer Solution ℞
[*ĭn ′ tăl*]
(cromolyn sodium inhalation, USP)
For Inhalation Use Only—Not for Injection

DESCRIPTION

Cromolyn sodium is the disodium salt of 1,3-bis (2-carboxychromon-5-yloxy)-2-hydroxypropane. The empirical formula is $C_{23}H_{14}Na_2O_{11}$; the molecular weight is 512.34. Each 2 mL ampule of INTAL Nebulizer Solution (cromolyn sodium inhalation, USP) contains 20 mg cromolyn sodium in purified water. Cromolyn sodium is a water-soluble, odorless, white, hydrated crystalline powder. It is tasteless at first, but leaves a slightly bitter aftertaste. INTAL Nebulizer Solution is clear, colorless, sterile and has a pH of 4.0–7.0.

The molecular structure is:

[See chemical structure at top of next column.]

Pharmacologic Category: Mast cell stabilizer/antiallergic.

Therapeutic Category: Antiasthmatic; reduces bronchial hyperreactivity.

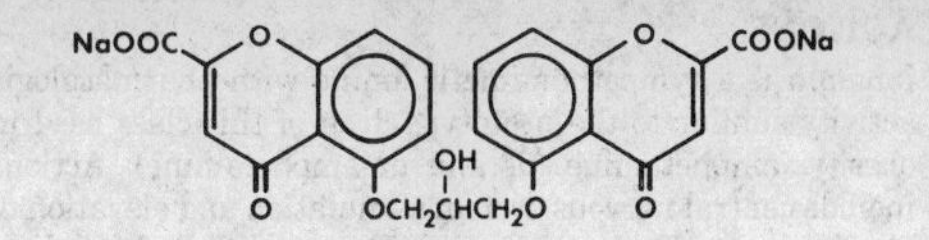

CLINICAL PHARMACOLOGY

In vitro and *in vivo* animal studies have shown that cromolyn sodium inhibits sensitized mast cell degranulation which occurs after exposure to specific antigens. Cromolyn sodium acts by inhibiting the release of mediators from mast cells. Studies show that cromolyn sodium indirectly blocks calcium ions from entering the mast cell, thereby preventing mediator release.

Cromolyn sodium inhibits both the immediate and non-immediate bronchoconstrictive reactions to inhaled antigen. Cromolyn sodium also attenuates bronchospasm caused by exercise, toluene diisocyanate, aspirin, cold air, sulphur dioxide and environmental pollutants.

Cromolyn sodium has no intrinsic bronchodilator, antihistaminic or anti-inflammatory activity.

After administration by inhalation, approximately 8% of the total cromolyn sodium dose administered is absorbed and rapidly excreted unchanged, approximately equally divided between urine and bile. The remainder of the dose is either exhaled or deposited in the oropharynx, swallowed and excreted via the alimentary tract.

INDICATIONS AND USAGE

INTAL is a prophylactic agent indicated in the management of patients with bronchial asthma.

In patients whose symptoms are sufficiently frequent to require a continuous program of medication, INTAL is given by inhalation on a regular daily basis (see **DOSAGE AND ADMINISTRATION**). The effect of INTAL is usually evident after several weeks of treatment, although some patients show an almost immediate response.

In patients who develop acute bronchoconstriction in response to exposure to exercise, toluene diisocyanate, environmental pollutants, etc., INTAL should be given shortly before exposure to the precipitating factor (see **DOSAGE AND ADMINISTRATION**).

CONTRAINDICATIONS

INTAL is contraindicated in those patients who have shown hypersensitivity to cromolyn sodium.

WARNINGS

INTAL has no role in the treatment of status asthmaticus.

PRECAUTIONS

General: Occasionally, patients may experience cough and/or bronchospasm following INTAL inhalation. At times, patients who develop bronchospasm may not be able to continue INTAL administration despite prior bronchodilator administration. Rarely, very severe bronchospasm has been encountered.

Symptoms of asthma may recur if INTAL is reduced below the recommended dosage or discontinued.

Information for Patients

INTAL is to be taken as directed by the physician. Because it is preventive medication, it may take up to four weeks before the patient experiences maximum benefit.

INTAL Nebulizer Solution should be used in a power-driven nebulizer with an adequate airflow rate equipped with a suitable face mask or mouthpiece.

The glass is an easy-break ampule. The glass is weakened at both ends so that they will break off easily by hand. As with all glass ampules, use caution when opening the ampule. Keep well away from nebulizer unit and face.

To open you should hold the ampule at an angle and break off the lower end (no solution will come out). Turn the ampule so the open end faces upward. Place your forefinger carefully over the open end of the ampule and now break off the other end.

To empty you should hold the ampule over the solution container and release your forefinger. The solution will flow out.

For additional information, see the accompanying leaflet entitled "Living a Full Life with Asthma."

Carcinogenesis, Mutagenesis, and Impairment of Fertility

Long term studies in mice (12 months intraperitoneal treatment followed by 6 months observation), hamsters (12 months intraperitoneal treatment followed by 12 months observation), and rats (18 months subcutaneous treatment) showed no neoplastic effect of cromolyn sodium.

No evidence of chromosomal damage or cytotoxicity was obtained in various mutagenesis studies.

No evidence of impaired fertility was shown in laboratory animal reproduction studies.

Pregnancy

Pregnancy Category B. Reproduction studies with cromolyn sodium administered parenterally to pregnant mice, rats, and rabbits in doses up to 338 times the human clinical dose produced no evidence of fetal malformations. Adverse fetal effects (increased resorptions and decreased fetal weight) were noted only at the very high parenteral doses that produced maternal toxicity. There are, however, no adequate and well-controlled studies in pregnant women. Because animal reproduction studies are not always predictive of human response, this drug should be used during pregnancy only if clearly needed.

Drug Interaction During Pregnancy

Cromolyn sodium and isoproterenol were studied following subcutaneous injections in pregnant mice. Cromolyn sodium alone in doses of 60 to 540 mg/kg (38 to 338 times the human dose) did not cause significant increases in resorptions or major malformations. Isoproterenol alone at a dose of 2.7 mg/kg (90 times the human dose) increased both resorptions and malformations. The addition of cromolyn sodium (338 times the human dose) to isoproterenol (90 times the human dose) appears to have increased the incidence of both resorptions and malformations.

Nursing Mothers

It is not known whether this drug is excreted in human milk. Because many drugs are excreted in human milk, caution should be exercised when INTAL is administered to a nursing woman.

Pediatric Use

Safety and effectiveness in children below the age of 2 years have not been established.

ADVERSE REACTIONS

Clinical experience with the use of INTAL suggests that adverse reactions are rare events. The following adverse reactions have been associated with INTAL Nebulizer Solution: cough, nasal congestion, nausea, sneezing and wheezing.

Other reactions have been reported in clinical trials; however, a causal relationship could not be established: drowsiness, nasal itching, nose bleed, nose burning, serum sickness, and stomachache.

In addition, adverse reactions have been reported with INTAL Capsules (cromolyn sodium for inhalation, USP). The most common side effects are associated with inhalation of the powder and include transient cough (1 in 5 patients) and mild wheezing (1 in 25 patients). These effects rarely require treatment or discontinuation of the drug.

Information on the incidence of adverse reactions to INTAL Capsules has been derived from U.S. postmarketing surveillance experience. The following adverse reactions attributed to INTAL, based upon recurrence following readministration, have been reported in less than 1 in 10,000 patients: laryngeal edema, swollen parotid gland, angioedema, bronchospasm, joint swelling and pain, dizziness, dysuria and urinary frequency, nausea, cough, wheezing, headache, nasal congestion, rash, urticaria and lacrimation.

Other adverse reactions have been reported in less than 1 in 100,000 patients, and it is unclear whether these are attributable to the drug: anaphylaxis, nephrosis, periarteritic vasculitis, pericarditis, peripheral neuritis, pulmonary infiltrates with eosinophilia, polymyositis, exfoliative dermatitis, hemoptysis, anemia, myalgia, hoarseness, photodermatitis and vertigo.

OVERDOSAGE

There is no clinical syndrome associated with an overdosage of cromolyn sodium. Acute toxicity testing in a wide variety of species has demonstrated an extremely low order of toxicity for cromolyn sodium, regardless of whether administration was parenteral, oral or by inhalation. Parenteral administration in mice, rats, guinea pigs, hamsters and rabbits demonstrated an LD_{50} in the region of 4000 mg/kg. Intravenous administration in monkeys also indicated a similar order of toxicity. The highest dose administered by the oral route in rats and mice was 8000 mg/kg, and at this dose level no deaths occurred. By inhalation, even in long term studies, it proved impossible to achieve toxic dose levels of cromolyn sodium in a range of mammalian species.

DOSAGE AND ADMINISTRATION

For management of bronchial asthma in adults and children (two years of age and over), the usual starting dosage is the contents of one ampule administered by nebulization four times a day at regular intervals.

Patients with chronic asthma should be advised that the effect of INTAL therapy is dependent upon its administration at regular intervals, as directed. INTAL should be introduced into the patient's therapeutic regimen when the acute episode has been controlled, the airway has been cleared and the patient is able to inhale adequately.

For the prevention of acute bronchospasm which follows exercise or exposure to cold dry air, environmental agents (e.g., animal danders, toluene diisocyanate, pollutants), etc., the usual dose is the contents of one ampule administered by

Continued on next page

Information on Fisons' products appearing in these pages is current as of July 1992. For further information, please consult the package insert currently accompanying the product, or Fisons Corporation, P.O. Box 1710, Rochester, NY 14603, (716) 475-9000.

Fisons—Cont.

nebulization shortly before exposure to the precipitating factor.

It should be emphasized to the patient that the drug is poorly absorbed when swallowed and is not effective by this route of administration.

INTAL Therapy in Relation to Other Treatments for Asthma: Non-steroidal agents

INTAL should be *added* to the patient's existing treatment regimen (e.g., bronchodilators). When a clinical response to INTAL is evident, usually within two to four weeks, and if the asthma is under good control, an attempt may be made to decrease concomitant medication usage gradually.

If concomitant medications are eliminated or required on no more than a prn basis, the frequency of administration of INTAL may be titrated downward to the lowest level consistent with the desired effect. The usual decrease is from four to three ampules per day. It is important that the dosage be reduced gradually to avoid exacerbation of asthma. It is emphasized that in patients whose dosage has been titrated to fewer than four ampules per day, an increase in the dose of INTAL and the introduction of, or increase in, symptomatic medications may be needed if the patient's clinical condition deteriorates.

Corticosteroids

In patients chronically receiving corticosteroids for the management of bronchial asthma, the dosage should be maintained following the introduction of INTAL. If the patient improves, an attempt to decrease corticosteroids should be made. Even if the corticosteroid-dependent patient fails to show symptomatic improvement following INTAL administration, the potential to reduce corticosteroids may nonetheless be present. Thus, gradual tapering of corticosteroid dosage may be attempted. It is important that the dose be reduced slowly, maintaining close supervision of the patient to avoid an exacerbation of asthma.

It should be borne in mind that prolonged corticosteroid therapy frequently causes an impairment in the activity of the hypothalamic-pituitary-adrenal axis and a reduction in the size of the adrenal cortex. A potentially critical degree of impairment or insufficiency may persist asymptomatically for some time even after gradual discontinuation of adrenocortical steroids. Therefore, if a patient is subjected to significant stress, such as a severe asthmatic attack, surgery, trauma or severe illness while being treated or within one year (occasionally up to two years) after corticosteroid treatment has been terminated, consideration should be given to reinstituting corticosteroid therapy. When respiratory function is impaired, as may occur in severe exacerbation of asthma, a temporary increase in the amount of corticosteroids may be required to regain control of the patient's asthma.

It is particularly important that great care be exercised if, for any reason, INTAL is withdrawn in cases where its use has permitted a reduction in the maintenance dose of corticosteroids. In such cases, continued close supervision of the patient is essential since there may be sudden reappearance of severe manifestations of asthma which will require immediate therapy and possible reintroduction of corticosteroids.

HOW SUPPLIED

INTAL Nebulizer Solution is supplied in a double-ended glass ampule. Each 2 mL ampule contains 20 mg cromolyn sodium in purified water.

NDC 0585-0673-02	60 ampules × 2 mL
NDC 0585-0673-03	120 ampules × 2 mL

INTAL Nebulizer Solution should be stored between 15°C and 25°C (59°F and 77°F) and protected from light. Do not use if it contains a precipitate.

CAUTION: Federal law prohibits dispensing without prescription.

FISONS Pharmaceuticals
Fisons Corporation
Rochester, NY 14623 USA
Made in France
INTAL and FISONS are Registered Trademarks Rev. 1/92
of Fisons plc   RF044A
© 1992, Fisons Corporation   332-1-80

IONAMIN®   Ⓒ ℞
[*i " on ' uh-min*]
(phentermine resin)

DESCRIPTION

Ionamin '15' and Ionamin '30' contain 15 mg and 30 mg respectively of phentermine as the cationic exchange resin complex. Phentermine is α, α-dimethyl phenethylamine (phenyl-tertiary-butylamine).

Other Ingredients in Ionamin: D&C Yellow No. 10, dibasic calcium phosphate, FD&C Yellow No. 6, gelatin, iron oxides (15 mg capsules only), lactose, magnesium stearate, titanium dioxide.

ACTIONS

Ionamin is a sympathomimetic amine with pharmacologic activity similar to the prototype drug of this class used in obesity, amphetamine (d- and dl-amphetamine). Actions include central nervous system stimulation and elevation of blood pressure. Tachyphylaxis and tolerance have been demonstrated with all drugs of this class in which these phenomena have been looked for.

Drugs of this class used in obesity are commonly known as "anorectics" or "anorexigenics." It has not been established, however, that the action of such drugs in treating obesity is primarily one of appetite suppression. Other central nervous system actions, or metabolic effects may be involved.

Adult obese subjects instructed in dietary management and treated with "anorectic" drugs, lose more weight on the average than those treated with placebo and diet, as determined in relatively short-term clinical trials.

The magnitude of increased weight loss of drug-treated patients over placebo-treated patients is only a fraction of a pound a week. The rate of weight loss is greatest in the first weeks of therapy for both drug and placebo subjects and tends to decrease in succeeding weeks. The possible origins of the increased weight loss due to the various drug effects are not established. The amount of weight loss associated with the use of an "anorectic" drug varies from trial to trial, and the increased weight loss appears to be related in part to variables other than the drugs prescribed, such as the physician-investigator, the population treated, and the diet prescribed. Studies do not permit conclusions as to the relative importance of the drug and non-drug factors on weight loss. The natural history of obesity is measured in years, whereas the studies cited are restricted to a few weeks' or months' duration; thus, the total impact of drug-induced weight loss over that of diet alone must be considered clinically limited. The bioavailability of Ionamin has been studied in humans in which blood levels of phentermine were measured by a gas chromatography method. Blood levels obtained with the 15 mg and 30 mg resin complex formulations indicated slower absorption with a reduced but prolonged peak concentration and without a significant difference in prolongation of blood levels when compared with the same doses of phentermine hydrochloride. The clinical significance of these differences is not known. In clinical trials establishing the efficacy of Ionamin, a single daily dose produced an effect comparable to that produced by other regimens of "anorectic" drug therapy.

INDICATION

Ionamin is indicated in the management of exogenous obesity as a short-term (a few weeks) adjunct in a regimen of weight reduction based on caloric restriction. The limited usefulness of agents of this class (see ACTIONS) should be measured against possible risk factors inherent in their use such as those described below.

CONTRAINDICATIONS

Advanced arteriosclerosis, symptomatic cardiovascular disease, moderate to severe hypertension, hyperthyroidism, known hypersensitivity, or idiosyncrasy to the sympathomimetic amines, glaucoma.

Agitated states.

Patients with a history of drug abuse.

During or within 14 days following the administration of monoamine oxidase inhibitors (hypertensive crises may result).

WARNINGS

If tolerance to the "anorectic" effect develops, the recommended dose should not be exceeded in an attempt to increase the effect; rather, the drug should be discontinued.

Ionamin may impair the ability of the patient to engage in potentially hazardous activities such as operating machinery or driving a motor vehicle; the patient should therefore be cautioned accordingly.

When using CNS active agents, consideration must always be given to the possibility of adverse interactions with alcohol.

Drug Dependence: Ionamin is related chemically and pharmacologically to amphetamine (d- and dl-amphetamine) and other stimulant drugs that have been extensively abused. The possibility of abuse of Ionamin should be kept in mind when evaluating the desirability of including a drug as part of a weight reduction program. Abuse of amphetamine (d- and dl-amphetamine) and related drugs may be associated with intense psychological dependence and severe social dysfunction. There are reports of patients who have increased the dosage of some of these drugs to many times that recommended. Abrupt cessation following prolonged high dosage administration results in extreme fatigue and mental depression; changes are also noted on the sleep EEG. Manifestations of chronic intoxication with anorectic drugs include severe dermatoses, marked insomnia, irritability, hyperactivity, and personality changes. The most severe manifestation of chronic intoxications is psychosis, often clinically indistinguishable from schizophrenia.

Usage in Pregnancy: Safe use in pregnancy has not been established. Use of Ionamin by women who are or may become pregnant requires that the potential benefit be weighed against the possible hazard to mother and infant.

Usage in Children: Ionamin is not recommended for use in children under 12 years of age.

PRECAUTIONS

Caution is to be exercised in prescribing Ionamin (phentermine resin) for patients with even mild hypertension. Insulin requirements in diabetes mellitus may be altered in association with the use of Ionamin and the concomitant dietary regimen.

Ionamin may decrease the hypotensive effect of adrenergic neuron blocking drugs.

The least amount feasible should be prescribed or dispensed at one time in order to minimize the possibility of overdosage.

ADVERSE REACTIONS

Cardiovascular: Palpitation, tachycardia, elevation of blood pressure.

Central Nervous System: Overstimulation, restlessness, dizziness, insomnia, euphoria, dysphoria, tremor, headache; rarely psychotic episodes at recommended doses with some drugs in this class.

Gastrointestinal: Dryness of the mouth, unpleasant taste, diarrhea, constipation, other gastrointestinal disturbances.

Allergic: Urticaria.

Endocrine: Impotence, changes in libido.

DOSAGE AND ADMINISTRATION

One capsule daily, before breakfast or 10–14 hours before retiring. For individuals exhibiting greater drug responsiveness, Ionamin '15' will usually suffice. Ionamin '30' is recommended for less responsive patients. Ionamin is not recommended for use in children under 12 years of age.

Ionamin capsules should be swallowed whole.

OVERDOSAGE

Manifestations of acute overdosage may include restlessness, tremor, hyperreflexia, rapid respiration, confusion, assaultiveness, hallucinations, panic states.

Fatigue and depression usually follow the central stimulation.

Cardiovascular effects include arrhythmias, hypertension, or hypotension and circulatory collapse. Gastrointestinal symptoms include nausea, vomiting, diarrhea, and abdominal cramps. Overdosage of pharmacologically similar compounds has resulted in fatal poisoning, usually terminating in convulsions and coma.

Management of acute Ionamin intoxication is largely symptomatic and includes lavage and sedation with a barbiturate. Experience with hemodialysis or peritoneal dialysis is inadequate to permit recommendation in this regard. Intravenous phentolamine (Regitine) has been suggested on pharmacologic grounds for possible acute, severe hypertension, if this complicates overdosage.

HOW SUPPLIED

Two strengths: Ionamin (phentermine resin) 15 mg (NDC 0585-0903) yellow and gray capsules; Ionamin (phentermine resin) 30 mg (NDC 0585-0904) yellow capsules. Stock bottles of 100 and 400.

Caution: Federal law prohibits dispensing without prescription.

FISONS Pharmaceuticals
Fisons Corporation
Rochester, NY 14623 USA
RF 195
Rev. 2/89
Ionamin is a registered trademark of Fisons BV.
© 1991, Fisons Corporation

ISOCLOR®   ℞ Ⓒ
[*īs ' ŏ-klŏr*]
Expectorant

DESCRIPTION

Each 5 mL (teaspoonful) contains:
Codeine phosphate, USP ....10 mg
(WARNING: May be habit forming)
Pseudoephedrine HCl, USP ....30 mg
Guaifenesin, USP ....100 mg
Other ingredients: Alcohol 5% v/v, artificial apricot flavor, benzoic acid, citric acid, FD&C Yellow No. 6, glycerin, menthol, purified water, sodium hydroxide, sucrose.

INDICATIONS

For temporary relief of troublesome, unproductive coughing associated with runny nose, nasal and sinus congestion, itching nose and throat.

CONTRAINDICATIONS

Severe hypertension or severe cardiac disease. Hypersensitivity to any of the components. Do not use in children under one year of age.

PRECAUTION

Use with caution in patients with hyperthyroidism.

DOSAGE

Adults .... 2 tsp
Children: 6–12 yrs .... ½ to 1 tsp
2–6 yrs .... ¼
1–2 yrs .... ⅛

Orally, 3 or 4 times a day.
Dispense in a tight container as defined in the USP.
CAUTION: Federal law prohibits dispensing without prescription.
Distributed by:
***FISONS* Pharmaceuticals**
Fisons Corporation
Rochester, NY 14623 USA
Manufactured by: Central Pharmaceuticals, Inc.
Seymour, IN 47247 U.S.A. LF087
Isoclor is a registered trademark of Fisons Corporation
© 1991, Fisons Corporation.

K–NORM® Capsules ℞
[*kā' nórm*]
(potassium chloride extended-release capsules, USP)

DESCRIPTION

K-Norm Capsules (potassium chloride extended-release capsules, USP) are a solid oral dosage form of potassium chloride containing 10 mEq (750 mg) of potassium chloride [equivalent to 10 mEq (390 mg) of potassium and 10 mEq (360 mg) of chloride] in a microencapsulated capsule. This formulation is intended to slow the release of potassium so that the likelihood of a high localized concentration of potassium chloride within the gastrointestinal tract is reduced.

K-Norm Capsules are an electrolyte replenisher. The chemical name is potassium chloride, and its structural formula is KCl. Potassium chloride, USP occurs as a white granular powder or as colorless crystals. It is odorless and has a saline taste. Its solutions are neutral to litmus. It is freely soluble in water and insoluble in alcohol.

Inactive ingredients: Calcium stearate, gelatin, pharmaceutical glaze, povidone, sugar spheres, talc.

CLINICAL PHARMACOLOGY

The potassium ion is the principal intracellular cation of most body tissues. Potassium ions participate in a number of essential physiological processes, including the maintenance of intracellular tonicity, the transmission of nerve impulses, the contraction of cardiac, skeletal and smooth muscle and the maintenance of normal renal function.

The intracellular concentration of potassium is approximately 150 to 160 mEq per liter. The normal adult plasma concentration is 3.5 to 5 mEq per liter. An active ion transport system maintains this gradient across the plasma membrane.

Potassium is a normal dietary constituent and under steady state conditions the amount of potassium absorbed from the gastrointestinal tract is equal to the amount excreted in the urine. The usual dietary intake of potassium is 50 to 100 mEq per day.

Potassium depletion may occur whenever the rate of potassium loss through renal excretion and/or loss from the gastrointestinal tract exceeds the rate of potassium intake. Such depletion usually develops as a consequence of therapy with diuretics, primary or secondary hyperaldosteronism, diabetic ketoacidosis, or inadequate replacement of potassium in patients on prolonged parenteral nutrition. Depletion can develop rapidly with severe diarrhea, especially if associated with vomiting. Potassium depletion due to these causes is usually accompanied by a concomitant loss of chloride and is manifested by hypokalemia and metabolic alkalosis. Potassium depletion may produce weakness, fatigue, disturbances of cardiac rhythm (primarily ectopic beats), prominent U-waves in the electrocardiogram, and, in advanced cases, flaccid paralysis and/or impaired ability to concentrate urine.

If potassium depletion associated with metabolic alkalosis cannot be managed by correcting the fundamental causes of the deficiency, e.g., where the patient requires long term diuretic therapy, supplementary potassium in the form of high potassium food or potassium chloride may be able to restore normal potassium levels.

In rare circumstances (e.g. patients with renal tubular acidosis) potassium depletion may be associated with metabolic acidosis and hyperchloremia. In such patients potassium replacement should be accomplished with potassium salts other than the chloride, such as potassium bicarbonate, potassium citrate, potassium acetate, or potassium gluconate.

INDICATIONS AND USAGE

BECAUSE OF REPORTS OF INTESTINAL AND GASTRIC ULCERATION AND BLEEDING WITH CONTROLLED RELEASE POTASSIUM CHLORIDE PREPARATIONS, THESE DRUGS SHOULD BE RESERVED FOR THOSE PATIENTS WHO CANNOT TOLERATE OR REFUSE TO TAKE LIQUIDS OR EFFERVESCENT POTASSIUM PREPARATIONS OR FOR PATIENTS IN WHOM THERE IS A PROBLEM OF COMPLIANCE WITH THESE PREPARATIONS.

1. For the treatment of patients with hypokalemia, with or without metabolic alkalosis; in digitalis intoxication; and in patients with hypokalemic familial periodic paralysis. If hypokalemia is the result of diuretic therapy, consideration should be given to the use of a lower dose of diuretic therapy, which may be sufficient without leading to hypokalemia.
2. For the prevention of hypokalemia in patients who would be at particular risk if hypokalemia were to develop, e.g., digitalized patients or patients with significant cardiac arrhythmias.

The use of potassium salts in patients receiving diuretics for uncomplicated essential hypertension is often unnecessary when such patients have a normal dietary pattern and when low doses of the diuretic are used. Serum potassium levels should be checked periodically, however, and if hypokalemia occurs, dietary supplementation with potassium-containing foods may be adequate to control milder cases. In more severe cases, and if dose adjustment of the diuretic is ineffective or unwarranted, supplementation with potassium salts may be indicated.

CONTRAINDICATIONS

Potassium supplements are contraindicated in patients with hyperkalemia, since a further increase in serum potassium concentration in such patients can produce cardiac arrest. Hyperkalemia may complicate any of the following conditions: chronic renal failure, systemic acidosis such as diabetic acidosis, acute dehydration, heat cramps, extensive tissue breakdown as in severe burns, adrenal insufficiency, or the administration of a potassium-sparing diuretic (e.g., spironolactone, triamterene, amiloride) (see OVERDOSAGE).

Controlled release formulations of potassium chloride have produced esophageal ulceration in certain cardiac patients with esophageal compression due to an enlarged left atrium. Potassium supplementation, when indicated in such patients, should be given as a liquid preparation.

All solid oral dosage forms of potassium chloride are contraindicated in any patient in whom there is structural, pathological (e.g., diabetic gastroparesis) or pharmacologic (use of anticholinergic agents or other agents with anticholinergic properties at sufficient doses to exert anticholinergic effects) cause for arrest or delay in capsule passage through the gastrointestinal tract; an oral liquid preparation should be used when indicated in these patients.

WARNINGS

Hyperkalemia: (see OVERDOSAGE) In patients with impaired mechanisms for excreting potassium, the administration of potassium salts can produce hyperkalemia and cardiac arrest. This occurs most commonly in patients given potassium by the intravenous route but may also occur in patients given potassium orally. Potentially fatal hyperkalemia can develop rapidly and be asymptomatic. The use of potassium salts in patients with chronic renal disease, or any other condition which impairs potassium excretion, requires particularly careful monitoring of the serum potassium concentration and appropriate dosage adjustment.

Interaction with Potassium-Sparing Diuretics: Hypokalemia should not be treated by the concomitant administration of potassium salts and a potassium-sparing diuretic (e.g., spironolactone, triamterene or amiloride) since the simultaneous administration of these agents can produce severe hyperkalemia.

Interaction with Angiotensin Converting Enzyme Inhibitors: Angiotensin converting enzyme (ACE) inhibitors (e.g., captopril, enalapril) will produce some potassium retention by inhibiting aldosterone production. Potassium supplements should be given to patients receiving ACE inhibitors only with close monitoring.

Gastrointestinal Lesions: Solid oral dosage forms of potassium chloride can produce ulcerative and/or stenotic lesions of the gastrointestinal tract and deaths. Based on spontaneous adverse reaction reports, enteric coated preparations of potassium chloride are associated with an increased frequency of small bowel lesions (40–50 per 100,000 patient years) compared to sustained release wax matrix formulations (less than one per 100,000 patient years). Because of the lack of extensive marketing experience with microencapsulated products, a comparison between such products and wax matrix or enteric coated products is not available. **K-Norm** Capsules are microencapsulated capsules formulated to provide a controlled rate of release of potassium chloride and thus to minimize the possibility of a high local concentration of potassium near the gastrointestinal wall.

Prospective trials have been conducted in normal human volunteers in which the upper gastrointestinal tract was evaluated by endoscopic inspection before and after one week of solid oral potassium chloride therapy. The ability of this model to predict events occurring in usual clinical practice is unknown. Trials which approximated usual clinical practice did not reveal any clear differences between the wax matrix and microencapsulated dosage forms. In contrast, there was a higher incidence of gastric and duodenal lesions in subjects receiving a high dose of a wax matrix controlled release formulation under conditions which did not resemble usual or recommended clinical practice (i.e., 96 mEq per day in divided doses of potassium chloride administered to fasted patients, in the presence of an anticholinergic drug to delay gastric emptying). The upper gastrointestinal lesions observed by endoscopy were asymptomatic and were not accompanied by evidence of bleeding (hemoccult testing). The relevance of these findings to the usual conditions (i.e., non-fasting, no anticholinergic agent, smaller doses) under which controlled release potassium chloride products are used is uncertain; epidemiologic studies have not identified an elevated risk, compared to microencapsulated products, for upper gastrointestinal lesions in patients receiving wax matrix formulations. **K-Norm** Capsules (potassium chloride extended-release capsules, USP) should be discontinued immediately and the possibility of ulceration, obstruction or perforation considered if severe vomiting, abdominal pain, distention, or gastrointestinal bleeding occurs.

Metabolic Acidosis: Hypokalemia in patients with metabolic acidosis should be treated with an alkalinizing potassium salt such as potassium bicarbonate, potassium citrate, potassium acetate or potassium gluconate.

PRECAUTIONS

General: The diagnosis of potassium depletion is ordinarily made by demonstrating hypokalemia in a patient with a clinical history suggesting some cause for potassium depletion. In interpreting the serum potassium level, the physician should bear in mind that acute alkalosis per se can produce hypokalemia in the absence of a deficit in total body potassium while acute acidosis per se can increase the serum potassium concentration into the normal range even in the presence of a reduced total body potassium. Regular serum potassium determinations are recommended. The treatment of potassium depletion, particularly in the presence of cardiac disease, renal disease, or acidosis requires careful attention to acid-base balance and appropriate monitoring of serum electrolytes, the electrocardiogram, and the clinical status of the patient. Potassium should generally not be given in the immediate postoperative period until urine flow is established.

Information for Patients: Physicians should consider reminding the patient of the following:

To take each dose with meals and with a full glass of water or other liquid.

To take this medicine following the frequency and amount prescribed by the physician. This is especially important if the patient is also taking diuretics and/or digitalis preparations.

To check with the physician if there is trouble swallowing capsules or if the capsules seem to stick in the throat.

To check with the physician at once if tarry stools or other evidence of gastrointestinal bleeding is noticed.

Laboratory Tests: When blood is drawn for analysis of plasma potassium it is important to recognize that artifactual elevations can occur after improper venipuncture technique or as a result of *in vitro* hemolysis of the sample. See PRECAUTIONS; General.

Drug Interactions: Potassium-sparing diuretics, angiotensin converting enzyme inhibitors: see WARNINGS.

Carcinogenesis, Mutagenesis, Impairment of Fertility: Carcinogenity, mutagenicity and fertility studies in animals have not been performed. Potassium is a normal dietary constituent.

Pregnancy: Teratogenic Effects—Pregnancy Category C: Animal reproduction studies have not been conducted with **K-Norm** Capsules. It is unlikely that potassium supplementation that does not lead to hyperkalemia would have an adverse effect on the fetus or would affect reproductive capacity.

Nursing Mothers: The normal potassium ion content of human milk is about 13 mEq per liter. Since oral potassium becomes part of the potassium pool, as long as body potassium is not excessive, the contribution of potassium chloride supplementation should have little or no effect on the level in human milk.

Continued on next page

Information on Fisons' products appearing in these pages is current as of July 1992. For further information, please consult the package insert currently accompanying the product, or Fisons Corporation, P.O. Box 1710, Rochester, NY 14603, (716) 475-9000.

Fisons—Cont.

Pediatric Use: Safety and effectiveness in children have not been established.

ADVERSE REACTIONS

One of the most severe adverse effects is hyperkalemia (see CONTRAINDICATIONS, WARNINGS, and OVERDOSAGE). There also have been reports of upper and lower gastrointestinal conditions including obstruction, bleeding, ulceration, and perforation (see CONTRAINDICATIONS and WARNINGS).

The most common adverse reactions to oral potassium salts are nausea, vomiting, flatulence, abdominal pain/discomfort, and diarrhea. These symptoms are due to irritation of the gastrointestinal tract and are best managed by diluting the preparation further, taking the dose with meals, or reducing the amount taken at one time.

Skin rash has been reported rarely.

OVERDOSAGE

The administration of oral potassium salts to persons with normal excretory mechanisms for potassium rarely causes serious hyperkalemia. However, if excretory mechanisms are impaired, or if potassium is administered too rapidly intravenously, potentially fatal hyperkalemia can result (see CONTRAINDICATIONS and WARNINGS). It is important to recognize that hyperkalemia is usually asymptomatic and may be manifested only by an increased serum potassium concentration (6.5–8.0 mEq/L) and characteristic electrocardiographic changes (peaking of T-waves, loss of P-wave, depression of S-T segment, prolongation of the QT interval), and widening and slurring of the QRS complex. Late manifestations include muscle paralysis and cardiovascular collapse from cardiac arrest. (9–12 mEq/L).

Treatment measures for hyperkalemia include the following:

1. Elimination of foods and medications containing potassium and of any agents with potassium-sparing properties;
2. Intravenous administration of 300 to 500 mL/hr of 10% dextrose solution containing 10–20 units of crystalline insulin per 1,000 mL;
3. Correction of acidosis, if present, with intravenous sodium bicarbonate;
4. Use of exchange resins, hemodialysis, or peritoneal dialysis.

In treating hyperkalemia, it should be recalled that in patients who have been stabilized on digitalis, too rapid a lowering of the serum potassium concentration can produce digitalis toxicity.

DOSAGE AND ADMINISTRATION

The usual dietary potassium intake by the average adult is 50 to 100 mEq per day. Potassium depletion sufficient to cause hypokalemia usually requires the loss of 200 or more mEq of potassium from the total body store.

Dosage must be adjusted to the individual needs of each patient. The dose for the prevention of hypokalemia is typically in the range of 20 mEq per day. Doses of 40–100 mEq per day or more are used for the treatment of potassium depletion. Dosage should be divided if more than 20 mEq per day is given such that no more than 20 mEq is given in a single dose.

K-Norm Capsules provide 10 mEq of potassium chloride.

K-Norm Capsules should be taken with meals and with a glass of water or other liquid. This product should not be taken on an empty stomach because of its potential for gastric irritation (see WARNINGS). Those patients having difficulty swallowing the capsules may be advised to sprinkle the contents onto a spoonful of soft food to facilitate ingestion.

HOW SUPPLIED

K-Norm Capsules are clear/clear hard gelatin capsules, imprinted with K-Norm 10, containing 10 mEq (750 mg) of potassium chloride [equivalent to 10 mEq (390 mg) of potassium and 10 mEq (360 mg) of chloride].

Store at controlled room temperature 15°- 30°C (59°- 86°F).

Packaged in bottles of 100's and 500's.

NDC 0585-0010-71—Bottle of 100's

NDC 0585-0010-85—Bottle of 500's

CAUTION: Federal law prohibits dispensing without prescription.

Marketed by
***FISONS* Pharmaceuticals**
Fisons Corporation
Rochester, NY 14623 U.S.A.
Mfd. by KV Pharmaceutical Company,
St. Louis, MO 63144
RF216B
Rev. 11/91

® Fisons BV
© 1991, Fisons Corporation

KOLYUM® LIQUID ℞

[ko ' lē-um "]
(potassium gluconate and potassium chloride)

DESCRIPTION

Potassium Supplement

Each tablespoonful (15 mL) of Kolyum Liquid provides 20 mEq potassium ion and 3.4 mEq chloride ion in a palatable sugar-free cherry-flavored vehicle. These mEq quantities are derived from the presence of potassium gluconate 3.9g and potassium chloride 0.25g. The blandness of the potassium gluconate and the presence of sorbitol in the formulation permit a high level of gastrointestinal tolerance.

Other Ingredients: Citric acid, D&C Red No. 33, FD&C Red No. 40, flavor, propylene glycol, saccharin sodium, sorbic acid, sorbitol solution, water.

CLINICAL PHARMACOLOGY

Potassium ion is the principal intracellular cation of most body tissues. Potassium ions participate in a number of essential physiological processes including the maintenance of intracellular tonicity, the transmission of nerve impulses, the contraction of cardiac, skeletal and smooth muscle, and the maintenance of normal renal function.

Potassium depletion may occur whenever the rate of potassium loss through renal excretion and/or loss from the gastrointestinal tract exceeds the rate of potassium intake. Such depletion usually develops slowly as a consequence of prolonged therapy with oral diuretics, primary or secondary hyperaldosteronism, diabetic ketoacidosis, severe diarrhea, or inadequate replacement of potassium in patients on prolonged parenteral nutrition. Potassium depletion due to these causes is usually accompanied by a concomitant deficiency of chloride and is manifested by hypokalemia and metabolic alkalosis. Potassium depletion may produce weakness, fatigue, disturbances of cardiac rhythm (primarily ectopic beats), prominent U-waves in the electrocardiogram and in advanced cases, flaccid paralysis and/or impaired ability to concentrate urine.

Potassium depletion associated with metabolic alkalosis is managed by correcting the fundamental causes of the deficiency whenever possible and administering supplemental potassium chloride, in the form of high potassium food, or a potassium salt supplement.

INDICATIONS AND USAGE

Kolyum is indicated for the prevention and treatment of hypokalemia which may occur secondary to diuretic or corticosteroid administration. Kolyum may be used in the treatment of cardiac arrhythmias due to digitalis intoxication. In hypokalemic states, especially in patients on salt-free diets, hypochloremic alkalosis may occur; treatment may then require chloride in addition to potassium supplementation. Kolyum provides 3.4 mEq of chloride per dose and therefore it may be used as an adjunct to the treatment of hypochloremic alkalosis.

CONTRAINDICATIONS

Hyperkalemia from any cause, severe renal impairment with oliguria or azotemia, untreated Addison's disease, adynamia episodica hereditaria (periodic paralysis, hyperkalemic type), acute dehydration, heat cramps, and patients receiving a potassium-sparing diuretic.

WARNINGS

Hyperkalemia

In patients with impaired mechanisms for excreting potassium, the administration of potassium salts can produce hyperkalemia and cardiac arrest. This occurs most commonly if one of these patients is given potassium by the intravenous route, but may also occur if potassium is given orally. Potentially fatal hyperkalemia can develop rapidly and be asymptomatic.

The use of potassium salts in patients with chronic renal disease, or any other condition which impairs potassium excretion, requires particularly careful monitoring of the serum potassium concentration and appropriate dosage adjustment.

Digitalis Intoxication

In the event that digitalis intoxication causes A-V block, potassium salts should not be given. In this situation potassium may potentiate the effect of digitalis on the conduction system, thus further depressing A-V conduction and ventricular responsiveness and inducing more dangerous arrhythmias.

Interaction with Potassium-Sparing Diuretics

Hypokalemia should not be treated by the concomitant administration of potassium salts and a potassium-sparing diuretic (e.g., spironolactone or triamterene), since the simultaneous administration of these agents can produce severe hyperkalemia.

Metabolic Acidosis

Hypokalemia in patients with metabolic acidosis should be treated with an alkalinizing potassium salt such as potassium bicarbonate, potassium citrate, or potassium acetate.

PRECAUTIONS

The treatment of potassium depletion, particularly in the presence of cardiac disease, renal disease, or acidosis, requires careful attention to acid-base balance and appropriate monitoring of serum electrolytes, the electrocardiogram, and the clinical status of the patient. In interpreting the serum potassium level, the physician should bear in mind that acute alkalosis per se can produce hypokalemia even in the absence of a deficit in total body potassium, while acute acidosis per se can increase the serum potassium into the normal range even in the presence of a reduced total body potassium. Potassium supplements must be administered with caution, since the amount of the deficiency and the daily intake are not accurately known. Extreme caution should be exercised in patients receiving aldosterone antagonists since potassium intoxication may occur.

ADVERSE REACTIONS

The most common adverse reactions to oral potassium salts are nausea, vomiting, abdominal discomfort, and diarrhea. These symptoms, due to irritation of the gastrointestinal tract, are best managed by additional dilution, administration with meals or reducing the dose. One of the most severe adverse effects is hyperkalemia (see Contraindications, Warnings and Overdosage).

OVERDOSAGE

Potassium intoxication may result from overdose of potassium or from ordinary therapeutic doses as in the conditions stated in "Contraindications". It is important to recognize that hyperkalemia is usually asymptomatic and may be manifested only by an increased serum potassium concentration and a clinical picture of A-V block (characteristic electrocardiograph changes may include peaking of T-waves, loss of P-wave, depression of S-T segment and prolongation of the QT interval). The symptoms and signs of potassium intoxication include paresthesias and weakness of the extremities, flaccid paralysis, listlessness, mental confusion, hypotension, cardiac arrhythmias and heart block. Hyperkalemia, when detected, must be treated immediately because lethal levels can be reached in a few hours.

Treatment of Hyperkalemia

1) Dextrose solution, 10% or 25%, containing 10 units of crystalline insulin per 20 g dextrose, given i.v. in a dose of 300–500 mL in one hour.
2) Absorption and exchange of potassium ions using cation exchange resins, orally and as retention enema. (Caution: Ammonium cycle exchange resins should not be used in patients with hepatic cirrhosis.)
3) Hemodialysis and peritoneal dialysis.
4) Ingestion of potassium-containing foods and medication should be stopped.
5) Transition from the hyperkalemic state to one of hypokalemia should be guarded against, especially in patients taking digitalis, as hypokalemia increases sensitivity to digitalis.

DOSAGE

The usual adult dose of Kolyum Liquid is one tablespoonful (15 mL) in 30 mL (one fluid ounce) or more of water twice daily.

This daily dose of Kolyum Liquid supplies 40 mEq of potassium ion, the approximate daily requirement, as well as 6.7 mEq of chloride ion. Deviations from this recommendation may be indicated; as no average total daily dose can be defined, the response of the patient to the dose of the drug must be assessed clinically. Larger doses may be required, but should be administered under close supervision because of the possibility of potassium intoxication.

HOW SUPPLIED

Kolyum Liquid

Stock bottles of 1 pint (NDC 0585-0858-67) and 1 gallon (NDC 0585-0858-93).

Dispense in a light-resistant container. **Store at room temperature.**

Caution: Federal law prohibits dispensing without prescription.

RF194
Rev. 3/89

Kolyum is a registered trademark of Fisons BV.
© 1991, Fisons Corporation.

***FISONS* Pharmaceuticals**
Fisons Corporation
Rochester, NY 14623 USA

MYKROX® TABLETS ℞

[mī'krahks]
(metolazone tablets, USP)

<u>DO NOT INTERCHANGE</u>

MYKROX® TABLETS ARE A RAPIDLY AVAILABLE FORMULATION OF METOLAZONE FOR ORAL ADMINISTRATION. MYKROX TABLETS AND OTHER FORMULATIONS OF METOLAZONE THAT SHARE ITS MORE RAPID AND

COMPLETE BIOAVAILABILITY ARE NOT THERAPEUTICALLY EQUIVALENT TO ZAROXOLYN® TABLETS AND OTHER FORMULATIONS OF METOLAZONE THAT SHARE ITS SLOW AND INCOMPLETE BIOAVAILABILITY. FORMULATIONS BIOEQUIVALENT TO MYKROX AND FORMULATIONS BIOEQUIVALENT TO ZAROXOLYN SHOULD NOT BE INTERCHANGED FOR ONE ANOTHER.

DESCRIPTION

MYKROX Tablets for oral administration contain ½ mg of metolazone, USP, a diuretic/saluretic/antihypertensive drug of the quinazoline class.

Metolazone has the molecular formula $C_{16}H_{16}ClN_3O_3S$, the chemical name 7-chloro-1,2,3,4-tetrahydro-2-methyl-3-(2-methylphenyl)-4-oxo-6-quinazoline-sulfonamide, and a molecular weight of 365.83. The structural formula is:

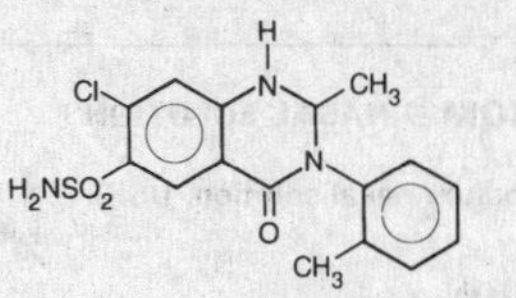

Metolazone is only sparingly soluble in water, but more soluble in plasma, blood, alkali and organic solvents.

Other ingredients in MYKROX Tablets: Dibasic calcium phosphate, magnesium stearate, microcrystalline cellulose, pregelatinized starch, sodium starch glycolate.

CLINICAL PHARMACOLOGY

MYKROX (metolazone) is a quinazoline diuretic, with properties generally similar to the thiazide diuretics. The actions of MYKROX result from interference with the renal tubular mechanism of electrolyte reabsorption. MYKROX acts primarily to inhibit sodium reabsorption at the cortical diluting site and to a lesser extent in the proximal convoluted tubule. Sodium and chloride ions are excreted in approximately equivalent amounts. The increased delivery of sodium to the distal-tubular exchange site results in increased potassium excretion. MYKROX does not inhibit carbonic anhydrase. A proximal action of metolazone has been shown in humans by increased excretion of phosphate and magnesium ions and by a markedly increased fractional excretion of sodium in patients with severely compromised glomerular filtration. This action has been demonstrated in animals by micropuncture studies.

The antihypertensive mechanism of action of metolazone is not fully understood but is presumed to be related to its saluretic and diuretic properties.

In two double-blind, controlled clinical trials of MYKROX Tablets, the maximum effect on mean blood pressure was achieved within 2 weeks of treatment and showed some evidence of an increased response at 1 mg compared to ½ mg. There was no indication of an increased response with 2 mg. After six weeks of treatment, the mean fall in serum potassium was 0.42 mEq/L at ½ mg, 0.66 mEq/L at 1 mg and 0.7 mEq/L at 2 mg. Serum uric acid increased by 1.1 to 1.4 mg/dL at increasing doses. There were small falls in serum sodium and chloride and a 1.3–2.1 mg/dL increase in BUN at increasing doses.

The rate and extent of absorption of metolazone from MYKROX Tablets were equivalent to those from an oral solution of metolazone. Peak blood levels are obtained within 2 to 4 hours of oral administration with an elimination half-life of approximately 14 hours. MYKROX Tablets have been shown to produce blood levels that are dose proportional between ½–2 mg. Steady state blood levels are usually reached in 4–5 days.

In contrast, other formulations of metolazone produce peak blood concentrations approximately 8 hours following oral administration; absorption continues for an additional 12 hours.

INDICATIONS AND USAGE

MYKROX Tablets are indicated for the treatment of hypertension, alone or in combination with other antihypertensive drugs of a different class.

MYKROX TABLETS HAVE NOT BEEN EVALUATED FOR THE TREATMENT OF CONGESTIVE HEART FAILURE OR FLUID RETENTION DUE TO RENAL OR HEPATIC DISEASE AND THE CORRECT DOSAGE FOR THESE CONDITIONS AND OTHER EDEMA STATES HAS NOT BEEN ESTABLISHED.

SINCE A SAFE AND EFFECTIVE DIURETIC DOSE HAS NOT BEEN ESTABLISHED, MYKROX TABLETS SHOULD NOT BE USED WHEN DIURESIS IS DESIRED.

Usage in Pregnancy

The routine use of diuretics in an otherwise healthy woman is inappropriate and exposes mother and fetus to unnecessary hazard. Diuretics do not prevent development of toxemia of pregnancy, and there is no evidence that they are useful in the treatment of developed toxemia (see PRECAUTIONS).

Edema during pregnancy may arise from pathologic causes or from the physiologic and mechanical consequences of pregnancy. MYKROX is not indicated for the treatment of edema in pregnancy. Dependent edema in pregnancy resulting from restriction of venous return by the expanded uterus is properly treated through elevation of the lower extremities and use of support hose; use of diuretics to lower intravascular volume in this case is illogical and unnecessary. There is hypervolemia during normal pregnancy which is harmful to neither the fetus nor the mother (in the absence of cardiovascular disease), but which is associated with edema, including generalized edema, in the majority of pregnant women. If this edema produces discomfort, increased recumbency will often provide relief. In rare instances, this edema may cause extreme discomfort which is not relieved by rest. In these cases, a short course of diuretics may be appropriate.

CONTRAINDICATIONS

Anuria, hepatic coma or pre-coma, known allergy or hypersensitivity to metolazone.

WARNINGS

Rapid Onset Hyponatremia

Rarely, the rapid onset of severe hyponatremia and/or hypokalemia has been reported following initial doses of thiazide and nonthiazide diuretics. When symptoms consistent with electrolyte imbalance appear rapidly, drug should be discontinued and supportive measures should be initiated immediately. Parenteral electrolytes may be required. Appropriateness of therapy with this class of drugs should be carefully re-evaluated.

Hypokalemia

Hypokalemia may occur, with consequent weakness, cramps, and cardiac dysrhythmias. Serum potassium should be determined at regular intervals, and dose reduction, potassium supplementation or addition of a potassium sparing diuretic instituted whenever indicated. Hypokalemia is a particular hazard in patients who are digitalized or who have or have had a ventricular arrhythmia; dangerous or fatal arrhythmias may be precipitated. Hypokalemia is dose related.

In controlled clinical trials, 1.5% of patients taking ½ mg and 3.1% of patients taking 1.0 mg of MYKROX daily developed clinical hypokalemia (defined as hypokalemia accompanied by signs or symptoms); 21% of the patients taking ½ mg and 30% of the patients taking 1.0 mg of MYKROX daily developed hypokalemia (defined as a serum potassium concentration below 3.5 mEq/L); in another controlled clinical trial in which the patients started therapy with a serum potassium level greater than 4.0 mEq/L, 8% of patients taking ½ mg of MYKROX daily developed hypokalemia (defined as a serum potassium concentration below 3.5 mEq/L).

Lithium

In general, diuretics should not be given concomitantly with lithium because they reduce its renal clearance and add a high risk of lithium toxicity. Read prescribing information for lithium preparations before use of such concomitant therapy.

Concomitant Therapy

Furosemide: Unusually large or prolonged losses of fluids and electrolytes may result when metolazone is administered concomitantly to patients receiving furosemide (see DRUG INTERACTIONS).

Other Antihypertensive Drugs: When MYKROX Tablets are used with other antihypertensive drugs, particular care must be taken to avoid excessive reduction of blood pressure, especially during initial therapy.

Cross-Allergy

Cross-allergy, while not reported to date, theoretically may occur when MYKROX Tablets are given to patients known to be allergic to sulfonamide-derived drugs, thiazides, or quinethazone.

PRECAUTIONS

DO NOT INTERCHANGE

MYKROX TABLETS ARE A RAPIDLY AVAILABLE FORMULATION OF METOLAZONE FOR ORAL ADMINISTRATION. MYKROX TABLETS AND OTHER FORMULATIONS OF METOLAZONE THAT SHARE ITS MORE RAPID AND COMPLETE BIOAVAILABILITY ARE NOT THERAPEUTICALLY EQUIVALENT TO ZAROXOLYN TABLETS AND OTHER FORMULATIONS OF METOLAZONE THAT SHARE ITS SLOW AND INCOMPLETE BIOAVAILABILITY. FORMULATIONS BIOEQUIVALENT TO MYKROX AND FORMULATIONS BIOEQUIVALENT TO ZAROXOLYN SHOULD NOT BE INTERCHANGED FOR ONE ANOTHER.

A. GENERAL:

Fluid and Electrolytes

All patients receiving therapy with MYKROX Tablets should have serum electrolyte measurements done at appropriate intervals and be observed for clinical signs of fluid and/or electrolyte imbalance: namely, hyponatremia, hypochloremic alkalosis, and hypokalemia. In patients with severe edema accompanying cardiac failure or renal disease, a low-salt syndrome may be produced, especially with hot weather and a low-salt diet. Serum and urine electrolyte determinations are particularly important when the patient has protracted vomiting, severe diarrhea, or is receiving parenteral fluids. Warning signs of imbalance are: dryness of mouth, thirst, weakness, lethargy, drowsiness, restlessness, muscle pains or cramps, muscle fatigue, hypotension, oliguria, tachycardia, and gastrointestinal disturbances such as nausea and vomiting. Hyponatremia may occur at any time during long term therapy and, on rare occasions, may be life threatening.

The risk of hypokalemia is increased when larger doses are used, when diuresis is rapid, when severe liver disease is present, when corticosteroids are given concomitantly, when oral intake is inadequate or when excess potassium is being lost extrarenally, such as with vomiting or diarrhea.

Glucose Tolerance

Metolazone may raise blood glucose concentrations possibly causing hyperglycemia and glycosuria in patients with diabetes or latent diabetes.

Hyperuricemia

MYKROX regularly causes an increase in serum uric acid and can occasionally precipitate gouty attacks even in patients without a prior history of them.

Azotemia

Azotemia, presumably pre-renal azotemia, may be precipitated during the administration of MYKROX Tablets. If azotemia and oliguria worsen during treatment of patients with severe renal disease, MYKROX Tablets should be discontinued.

Renal Impairment

Use caution when administering MYKROX Tablets to patients with severely impaired renal function. As most of the drug is excreted by the renal route, accumulation may occur.

Orthostatic Hypotension

Orthostatic hypotension may occur; this may be potentiated by alcohol, barbiturates, narcotics, or concurrent therapy with other antihypertensive drugs. In controlled clinical trials, 1.4% of patients treated with MYKROX Tablets (½ mg) had orthostatic hypotension; this effect was not reported in the placebo group.

Hypercalcemia

Use of other diuretics has been associated on rare occasions with pathological changes in the parathyroid glands. This possibility should be considered with clinical use of MYKROX Tablets. Hypercalcemia has been noted in a few patients treated with metolazone.

Systemic Lupus Erythematosus

Thiazide diuretics have exacerbated or activated systemic lupus erythematosus and this possibility should be considered with MYKROX Tablets.

B. INFORMATION FOR PATIENTS: Patients should be informed of possible adverse effects, advised to take the medication as directed and promptly report any possible adverse reactions to the treating physician.

C. DRUG INTERACTIONS:

Diuretics

Furosemide and probably other loop diuretics given concomitantly with metolazone can cause unusually large or prolonged losses of fluid and electrolytes (see WARNINGS).

Other Antihypertensives

When MYKROX Tablets are used with other antihypertensive drugs, care must be taken, especially during initial therapy. Dosage adjustments of other antihypertensives may be necessary.

Alcohol, Barbiturates, and Narcotics

The hypotensive effects of these drugs may be potentiated by the volume contraction that may be associated with metolazone therapy.

Digitalis Glycosides

Diuretic-induced hypokalemia can increase the sensitivity of the myocardium to digitalis. Serious arrhythmias can result.

Corticosteroids or ACTH

May increase the risk of hypokalemia and increase salt and water retention.

Lithium

Serum lithium levels may increase (see WARNINGS).

Curariform Drugs

Diuretic-induced hypokalemia may enhance neuromuscular blocking effects of curariform drugs (such as tubocurarine)—the most serious effect would be respiratory depression which could proceed to apnea. Accordingly, it may be advisable to discontinue MYKROX Tablets three days before elective surgery.

Continued on next page

Information on Fisons' products appearing in these pages is current as of July 1992. For further information, please consult the package insert currently accompanying the product, or Fisons Corporation, P.O. Box 1710, Rochester, NY 14603, (716) 475-9000.

Fisons—Cont.

Salicylates and Other Non-Steroidal Anti-Inflammatory Drugs
May decrease the antihypertensive effects of MYKROX Tablets.
Sympathomimetics
Metolazone may decrease arterial responsiveness to norepinephrine, but this diminution is not sufficient to preclude effectiveness of the pressor agent for therapeutic use.
Insulin and Oral Antidiabetic Agents
See Glucose Tolerance under GENERAL PRECAUTIONS.
Methenamine
Efficacy may be decreased due to urinary alkalizing effect of metolazone.
D. DRUG/LABORATORY TEST INTERACTIONS: None reported.
E. CARCINOGENESIS, MUTAGENESIS, IMPAIRMENT OF FERTILITY: Mice and rats given metolazone for 1½ to 2 years at daily doses of 2, 10 and 50 mg/kg (approximately 100, 500, and 2,500 times the recommended maximum daily dose of MYKROX 1 mg given to a 50 kg person) showed no evidence that metolazone caused an increased number of tumors. The small number of animals examined histologically and poor survival in the mice limit the conclusions that can be reached from these studies.
Reproductive performance has been evaluated in mice and rats. There is no evidence that metolazone possesses the potential for altering reproductive capacity in mice. In a rat study, in which males were treated orally with metolazone at doses of 2, 10 and 50 mg/kg for 127 days prior to mating with untreated females, an increased number of resorption sites was observed in dams mated with males from the 50 mg/kg group. In addition, the fetal weight of offspring was decreased and the pregnancy rate was reduced in dams mated with males from the 10 and 50 mg/kg groups.
F. PREGNANCY
Teratogenic Effects—Pregnancy Category B.
Reproduction studies performed in mice, rabbits and rats treated during the appropriate periods of gestation at doses up to 50 mg/kg/day (2,500 times the recommended maximum daily human dose of MYKROX) have revealed no evidence of harm to the fetus due to metolazone. There are, however, no adequate and well-controlled studies in pregnant women. Because animal reproduction studies are not always predictive of human response, MYKROX Tablets should be used during pregnancy only if clearly needed. Metolazone crosses the placental barrier and appears in cord blood.
Non-Teratogenic Effects
The use of MYKROX Tablets in pregnant women requires that the anticipated benefit be weighed against possible hazards to the fetus. These hazards include fetal or neonatal jaundice, thrombocytopenia, and possibly other adverse reactions which have occurred in the adult. It is not known what effect the use of the drug during pregnancy has on the later growth, development and functional maturation of the child. No such effects have been reported with metolazone.
G. LABOR AND DELIVERY: Based on clinical studies in which women received metolazone in late pregnancy until the time of delivery, there is no evidence that the drug has any adverse effects on the normal course of labor or delivery.
H. NURSING MOTHERS: Metolazone appears in breast milk. Because of the potential for serious adverse reactions in nursing infants from metolazone, a decision should be made whether to discontinue nursing or to discontinue the drug, taking into account the importance of the drug to the mother.
I. PEDIATRIC USE: Safety and effectiveness of MYKROX Tablets in children have not been established, and such use is not recommended.

ADVERSE REACTIONS

Adverse experience information is available from more than 14 years of accumulated marketing experience with other formulations of metolazone for which reliable quantitative information is lacking and from controlled clinical trials with MYKROX from which incidences can be calculated.
In controlled clinical trials with MYKROX, adverse experiences resulted in discontinuation of therapy in 6.7–6.8% of patients given ½ to 1 mg of MYKROX.
Adverse experiences occurring in controlled clinical trials with MYKROX with an incidence of > 2%, whether or not considered drug-related, are summarized in the following table.
[See table next column.]

Some of the adverse effects reported in association with MYKROX also occur frequently in untreated hypertensive patients, such as headache and dizziness, which occurred in 14.8 and 7.4% of patients in a smaller parallel placebo group. The following adverse effects were reported in less than 2% of the MYKROX treated patients.
Cardiovascular: Cold extremities, edema, orthostatic hypotension, palpitations.

Incidence of Adverse Experiences Volunteered or Elicited (by Patient in Percent)*

	MYKROX n=226†
Dizziness (lightheadedness)	10.2
Headaches	9.3
Muscle Cramps	5.8
Fatigue (malaise, lethargy, lassitude)	4.4
Joint Pain, swelling	3.1
Chest Pain (precordial discomfort)	2.7

* Percent of patients reporting an adverse experience one or more times.
† All doses combined (½, 1 and 2 mg).

Central and Peripheral Nervous System: Anxiety, depression, dry mouth, impotence, nervousness, neuropathy, weakness, "weird" feeling.
Dermatological: Pruritus, rash, skin dryness.
Eyes, Ears, Nose, Throat: Cough, epistaxis, eye itching, sinus congestion, sore throat, tinnitus.
Gastrointestinal: Abdominal discomfort (pain, bloating), bitter taste, constipation, diarrhea, nausea, vomiting.
Genitourinary: Nocturia.
Musculoskeletal: Back pain.
Other Adverse Experiences:
Adverse experiences reported with other marketed metolazone formulations and most thiazide diuretics, for which quantitative data are not available, are listed in decreasing order of severity within body systems. Several are single or rare occurrences.
Cardiovascular—excessive volume depletion, hemoconcentration, venous thrombosis.
Central and Peripheral Nervous System—syncope, paresthesias, drowsiness, restlessness (sometimes resulting in insomnia).
Dermatologic/Hypersensitivity—necrotizing angiitis (cutaneous vasculitis), purpura, dermatitis, photosensitivity, urticaria.
Gastrointestinal—hepatitis, intrahepatic cholestatic jaundice, pancreatitis, anorexia.
Hematologic—aplastic (hypoplastic) anemia, agranulocytosis, leukopenia.
Metabolic—hypokalemia (see WARNINGS, Hypokalemia), hyponatremia, hyperuricemia, hypochloremia, hypochloremic alkalosis, hyperglycemia, glycosuria, increase in serum urea nitrogen (BUN) or creatinine, hypophosphatemia.
Musculoskeletal—acute gouty attacks.
Other—transient blurred vision, chills.
In addition, rare adverse experiences reported in association with similar anti-hypertensive-diuretics but not reported to date for metolazone include: sialadenitis, xanthopsia, respiratory distress (including pneumonitis), thrombocytopenia and anaphylactic reactions. These experiences could occur with clinical use of metolazone.

OVERDOSAGE

Intentional overdosage has been reported rarely with metolazone and similar diuretic drugs.
Signs and Symptoms
Orthostatic hypotension, dizziness, drowsiness, syncope, electrolyte abnormalities, hemoconcentration and hemodynamic changes due to plasma volume depletion may occur. In some instances depressed respiration may be observed. At high doses, lethargy of varying degree may appear and may progress to coma within a few hours. The mechanism of CNS depression with thiazide overdosage is unknown. Also, GI irritation and hypermotility may occur. Temporary elevation of BUN has been reported, especially in patients with impairment of renal function. Serum electrolyte changes and cardiovascular and renal function should be closely monitored.
Treatment
There is no specific antidote available but immediate evacuation of the stomach contents is advised. Dialysis is not likely to be effective. Care should be taken when evacuating the gastric contents to prevent aspiration, especially in the stuporous or comatose patient. Supportive measures should be initiated as required to maintain hydration, electrolyte balance, respiration and cardiovascular and renal function.

DOSAGE AND ADMINISTRATION

Therapy should be individualized according to patient response.
For initial treatment of mild to moderate hypertension, the recommended dose is one MYKROX Tablet (½ mg) once daily, usually in the morning. If patients are inadequately controlled with one ½ mg tablet, the dose can be increased to two MYKROX Tablets (1 mg) once a day. An increase in hypokalemia may occur. Doses larger than one mg do not give increased effectiveness.
The same dose titration is necessary if MYKROX Tablets are to be substituted for other dosage forms of metolazone in the treatment of hypertension.
If blood pressure is not adequately controlled with two MYKROX Tablets alone, the dose should not be increased; rather, another antihypertensive agent with a different mechanism of action should be added to therapy with MYKROX Tablets.

HOW SUPPLIED

MYKROX Tablets (metolazone tablets, USP), ½ mg: White, flat-faced, round tablets embossed, MYKROX on one side and, ½, on reverse side.
Bottles of 100 NDC 0585-0847-71
Store at room temperature. Dispense in a tight, light-resistant container.
Caution: Federal law prohibits dispensing without prescription.
***FISONS* Pharmaceuticals**
Fisons Corporation
Rochester, NY 14623 U.S.A.
® FISONS BV
© 1991, Fisons Corporation
RF156B Rev. 12/91

NASALCROM® NASAL SOLUTION ℞
[*nāz 'ŭl-krōm* "]
(cromolyn sodium nasal solution, USP)

DESCRIPTION

Each milliliter of NASALCROM® Nasal Solution (cromolyn sodium nasal solution, USP) contains 40 mg cromolyn sodium in purified water with 0.01% benzalkonium chloride to preserve and 0.01% EDTA (edetate disodium) to stabilize the solution. NASALCROM possesses a natural pH of 4.5–6.5 and negligible titratable acidity. Chemically, cromolyn sodium is the disodium salt of 1,3-bis(2-carboxychromon-5-yloxy)-2-hydroxypropane. The empirical formula is $C_{23}H_{14}Na_2O_{11}$.
The molecular structure is:

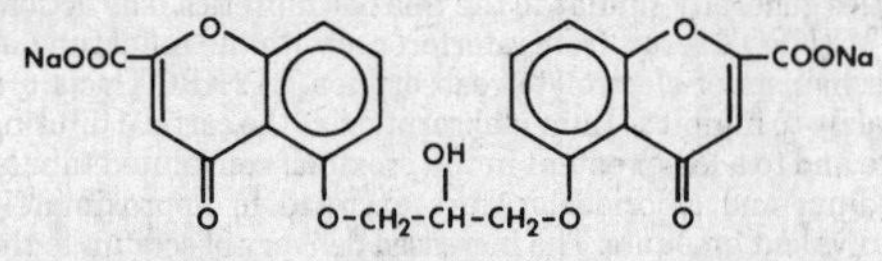

Pharmacologic Category: Mast cell stabilizer/ antiallergic.
Therapeutic Category: Antiallergic.
After priming the delivery system for NASALCROM, each actuation of the unit delivers a metered spray containing 5.2 mg of cromolyn sodium. The contents of one bottle delivers at least 100 sprays (13 mL bottle) or 200 sprays (26 mL bottle).

CLINICAL PHARMACOLOGY

In vitro and *in vivo* animal studies have shown that cromolyn sodium inhibits the degranulation of sensitized mast cells which occurs after exposure to specific antigens. Cromolyn sodium inhibits the release of histamine and SRS-A (the slow-reacting substance of anaphylaxis). Rhinitis induced by the inhalation of specific antigens can be inhibited to varying degrees by pretreatment with NASALCROM.
Another activity demonstrated *in vitro* is the capacity of cromolyn sodium to inhibit the degranulation of non-sensitized rat mast cells by phospholipase A and the subsequent release of chemical mediators. An additional *in vitro* study showed that cromolyn sodium did not inhibit the enzymatic activity of released phospholipase A on its specific substrate.
Cromolyn sodium has no intrinsic bronchodilator, antihistaminic or anti-inflammatory activity.
Cromolyn sodium is poorly absorbed from the gastrointestinal tract. After instillation of NASALCROM, less than 7% of the total dose administered is absorbed and is rapidly excreted unchanged in the bile and urine. The remainder of the dose is expelled from the nose, or swallowed and excreted via the alimentary tract.

INDICATIONS

NASALCROM is indicated for the prevention and treatment of the symptoms of allergic rhinitis.

CONTRAINDICATIONS

NASALCROM is contraindicated in those patients who have shown hypersensitivity to any of the ingredients.

PRECAUTIONS

General: Some patients may experience transient nasal stinging and/or sneezing immediately following instillation of NASALCROM. Except in rare occurrences, these experiences have not caused discontinuation of therapy.
In view of the biliary and renal routes of excretion for cromolyn sodium, consideration should be given to decreasing the dosage or discontinuing the administration of the drug in patients with impaired renal or hepatic function.
Carcinogenesis, Mutagenesis, and Impairment of Fertility: Long term studies in mice (12 months intraperitoneal treatment followed by 6 months observation), hamsters (12 months intraperitoneal treatment followed by 12 months observation), and rats (18 months subcutaneous treatment) showed no neoplastic effect of cromolyn sodium.
No evidence of chromosomal damage or cytotoxicity was obtained in various mutagenesis studies.

No evidence of impaired fertility was shown in laboratory animal reproduction studies.

Pregnancy: Pregnancy Category B. Reproduction studies with cromolyn sodium administered parenterally to pregnant mice, rats, and rabbits in doses up to 338 times the human clinical doses produced no evidence of fetal malformations. Adverse fetal effects (increased resorptions and decreased fetal weight) were noted only at the very high parenteral doses that produced maternal toxicity. There are, however, no adequate and well-controlled studies in pregnant women. Because animal reproduction studies are not always predictive of human response, this drug should be used during pregnancy only if clearly needed.

Drug Interaction During Pregnancy: Cromolyn sodium and isoproterenol were studied following subcutaneous injections in pregnant mice. Cromolyn sodium alone in doses of 60 to 540 mg/kg (38 to 338 times the human dose) did not cause significant increases in resorptions or major malformations. Isoproterenol alone at a dose of 2.7 mg/kg (90 times the human dose) increased both resorptions and malformations. The addition of cromolyn sodium (338 times the human dose) to isoproterenol (90 times the human dose) appears to have increased the incidence of both resorptions and malformations.

Nursing Mothers: It is not known whether this drug is excreted in human milk. Because many drugs are excreted in human milk, caution should be exercised when NASALCROM is administered to a nursing woman.

Pediatric Use: Safety and effectiveness in children below the age of 6 years have not been established.

ADVERSE REACTIONS

The most frequent adverse reactions occurring in the 430 patients included in the clinical trials with NASALCROM were sneezing (1 in 10 patients), nasal stinging (1 in 20), nasal burning (1 in 25), and nasal irritation (1 in 40). Headaches and bad taste were reported in about 1 in 50 patients. Epistaxis, postnasal drip, and rash were reported in less than one percent of the patients. One patient in the clinical trials developed anaphylaxis.

Adverse reactions which have occurred in the use of other cromolyn sodium formulations for inhalation include angioedema, joint pain and swelling, urticaria, cough, and wheezing. Other reactions reported rarely are serum sickness, periarteritic vasculitis, polymyositis, pericarditis, photodermatitis, exfoliative dermatitis, peripheral neuritis, and nephrosis.

DOSAGE AND ADMINISTRATION

The dose for adults and children 6 years and older is **one spray in each nostril** 3–4 times daily at regular intervals. If needed, this dose may be increased to one spray to each nostril 6 times daily. The patient should be instructed to clear the nasal passages before administering the spray and should inhale through the nose during administration.

In the management of seasonal (pollenotic) rhinitis, and for prevention of rhinitis caused by exposure to other types of specific inhalant allergens, treatment with NASALCROM will be more effective if started prior to expected contact with the offending allergen. Treatment should be continued throughout the period of exposure, i.e., until the pollen season is over or until exposure to the offending allergen is terminated.

In the management of perennial allergic rhinitis, the effects of treatment with NASALCROM may become apparent only after two to four weeks of treatment. The concomitant use of antihistamines and/or nasal decongestants may be necessary during the initial phase of treatment, but the need for this type of medication should diminish and may be eliminated when the full benefit of NASALCROM is achieved.

HOW SUPPLIED

NASALCROM is available in bottles of 13 mL and 26 mL. Each fully assembled unit consists of a pump unit and actuator with cover in position on the bottle of nasal solution. The amount of cromolyn sodium in each bottle is: 13 mL -520 mg (40 mg/mL); 26 mL -1040 mg (40 mg/mL).

NASALCROM should be stored between 15° and 25°C (59° and 77°F).Protect from light.

NDC 0585-0671-03 13 mL bottle (fully assembled unit)
NDC 0585-0671-04 26 mL bottle (fully assembled unit)

CAUTION

Federal law prohibits dispensing without prescription.

***FISONS* Pharmaceuticals**
Fisons Corporation
Rochester, NY 14623 USA
Made in England
NASALCROM, NASALMATIC and FISONS are Registered Trademarks of FISONS plc.
© 1992, Fisons Corporation.
All Rights Reserved
RF037C   Rev. 1/92

OPTICROM® 4%   ℞
[op 'ti-krŏm]
Ophthalmic Solution
(cromolyn sodium ophthalmic solution, USP)

DESCRIPTION

Each milliliter of OPTICROM 4% Ophthalmic Solution (cromolyn sodium ophthalmic solution, USP) contains 40 mg cromolyn sodium in purified water with 0.01% benzalkonium chloride to preserve and 0.1% EDTA (edetate disodium, USP) to stabilize the solution. OPTICROM is a clear, colorless, sterile solution with a pH of 4.0–7.0. It is intended for topical administration to the eye.

Chemically, cromolyn sodium is the disodium salt of 1,3-bis(2-carboxychromon-5-yloxy)-2-hydroxypropane. Its chemical structure is:

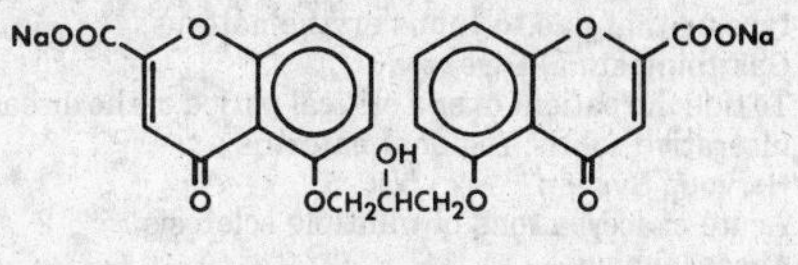

Pharmacologic Category: Mast cell stabilizer

CLINICAL PHARMACOLOGY

In vitro and *in vivo* animal studies have shown that cromolyn sodium inhibits the degranulation of sensitized mast cells which occurs after exposure to specific antigens. Cromolyn sodium acts by inhibiting the release of histamine and SRS-A (slow-reacting substance of anaphylaxis) from the mast cell. Another activity demonstrated *in vitro* is the capacity of cromolyn sodium to inhibit the degranulation of non-sensitized rat mast cells by phospholipase A and the subsequent release of chemical mediators. Another study showed that cromolyn sodium did not inhibit the enzymatic activity of released phospholipase A on its specific substrate.

Cromolyn sodium has no intrinsic vasoconstrictor, antihistaminic or anti-inflammatory activity.

Cromolyn sodium is poorly absorbed. When multiple doses of cromolyn sodium ophthalmic solution are instilled into normal rabbit eyes, less than 0.07% of the administered dose of cromolyn sodium is absorbed into the systemic circulation (presumably by way of the eye, nasal passages, buccal cavity and gastrointestinal tract). Trace amounts (less than 0.01%) of the cromolyn sodium dose penetrate into the aqueous humor and clearance from this chamber is virtually complete within 24 hours after treatment is stopped.

In normal volunteers, analysis of drug excretion indicates that approximately 0.03% of cromolyn sodium is absorbed following administration to the eye.

A study on corneal epithelial wound healing in albino rabbits failed to demonstrate any significant difference in the rate of corneal re-epithelialization between cromolyn sodium ophthalmic solution, sterile saline solution, no treatment and an ophthalmic corticosteroid.

INDICATIONS AND USAGE

OPTICROM is indicated in the treatment of vernal keratoconjunctivitis, vernal conjunctivitis, and vernal keratitis. Symptomatic response to therapy (decreased itching, tearing, redness and discharge) is usually evident within a few days, but longer treatment for up to six weeks is sometimes required. Once symptomatic improvement has been established, therapy should be continued for as long as needed to sustain improvement.

If required, corticosteroids may be used concomitantly with OPTICROM.

Users of soft (hydrophilic) contact lenses should refrain from wearing lenses while under treatment with OPTICROM (see **Contraindications**). Wear can be resumed within a few hours after discontinuation of the drug.

CONTRAINDICATIONS

OPTICROM is contraindicated in those patients who have shown hypersensitivity to cromolyn sodium or to any of the other ingredients.

As with all ophthalmic preparations containing benzalkonium chloride, patients are advised not to wear soft contact lenses during treatment with OPTICROM.

PRECAUTIONS

General: Patients may experience a transient stinging or burning sensation following application of OPTICROM.

The recommended frequency of administration should not be exceeded. The dose for adults and children is 1–2 drops in each eye 4–6 times a day at regular intervals.

Carcinogenesis, Mutagenesis, and Impairment of Fertility: Long term studies in mice (12 months intraperitoneal treatment followed by six months observation), hamsters (12 months intraperitoneal treatment followed by 12 months observation), and rats (18 months subcutaneous treatment) showed no neoplastic effect of cromolyn sodium.

No evidence of chromosomal damage or cytotoxicity was obtained in various mutagenesis studies.

No evidence of impaired fertility was shown in laboratory animal reproduction studies.

Pregnancy: Teratogenic effects: Pregnancy Category B. Reproduction studies with cromolyn sodium administered parenterally to pregnant mice, rats and rabbits in doses up to 338 times the human clinical doses produced no evidence of fetal malformations. Adverse fetal effects (increased resorption and decreased fetal weight) were noted only at the very high parenteral doses that produced maternal toxicity. There are, however, no adequate and well controlled studies in pregnant women. Because animal reproduction studies are not always predictive of human response, this drug should be used during pregnancy only if clearly needed.

Nursing Mothers: It is not known whether this drug is excreted in human milk. Because many drugs are excreted in human milk, caution should be exercised when OPTICROM is administered to a nursing woman.

Pediatric Use: Safety and effectiveness in children below the age of 4 years have not been established.

ADVERSE REACTIONS

The most frequently reported adverse reaction attributed to the use of OPTICROM, on the basis of reoccurrence following readministration, is transient ocular stinging or burning upon instillation.

The following adverse reactions have been reported as infrequent events. It is unclear whether they are attributable to the drug:
Conjunctival injection
Watery eyes
Itchy eyes
Dryness around the eye
Puffy eyes
Eye irritation
Styes

DOSAGE AND ADMINISTRATION

The dose for adults and children is 1–2 drops in each eye 4–6 times a day at regular intervals. One drop contains approximately 1.6 mg cromolyn sodium.

Patients should be advised that the effect of OPTICROM therapy is dependent upon its administration at regular intervals, as directed.

HOW SUPPLIED

OPTICROM is supplied as 10 mL of solution in an opaque polyethylene eye drop bottle.
    NDC 0585-0680-01   10 mL bottle
Keep tightly closed and out of the reach of children. Store below 30°C (86°F) and protect from light—store in original carton.

CAUTION: Federal law prohibits dispensing without prescription.

***FISONS* Pharmaceuticals**
Fisons Corporation
Rochester, NY 14623 USA
Made in England
         Rev. 11/91
OPTICROM and FISONS are Registered Trademarks of Fisons plc   RF046B
© 1991, Fisons Corporations.

PEDIAPRED®   ℞
[pĕd 'ē-uh-pred]
(prednisolone sodium phosphate, USP)
ORAL LIQUID

DESCRIPTION

PEDIAPRED Oral Liquid is a dye free, colorless to light straw colored, raspberry flavored solution. Each 5 mL (teaspoonful) of PEDIAPRED contains 6.70 mg prednisolone sodium phosphate (5.00 mg prednisolone base) in a palatable, aqueous vehicle.

Prednisolone sodium phosphate occurs as white or slightly yellow, friable granules or powder. It is freely soluble in water; soluble in methanol; slightly soluble in alcohol and in chloroform; and very slightly soluble in acetone and in dioxane. The chemical name of prednisolone sodium phosphate is pregna-1,4-diene-3,20-dione,11,17-dihydroxy-21- (phosphonooxy)-, disodium salt, (11β)-. Its chemical structure is:
[See chemical structure at top of next column.]
Pharmacological Category: Glucocorticoid

CLINICAL PHARMACOLOGY

Prednisolone is a synthetic adrenocortical steroid drug with predominantly glucocorticoid properties. Some of these properties reproduce the physiological actions of endogenous

Continued on next page

Information on Fisons' products appearing in these pages is current as of July 1992. For further information, please consult the package insert currently accompanying the product, or Fisons Corporation, P.O. Box 1710, Rochester, NY 14603, (716) 475-9000.

Fisons—Cont.

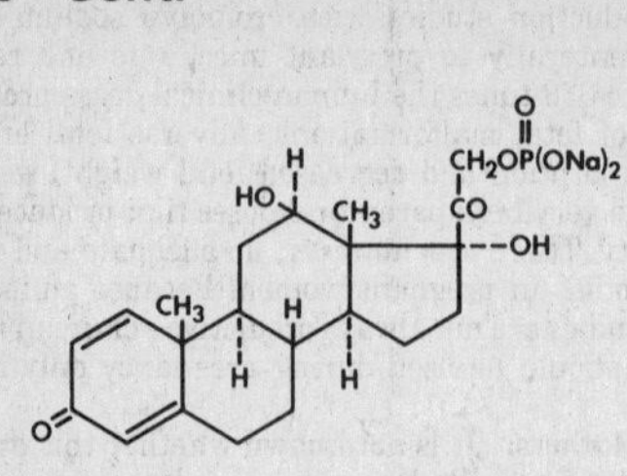

glucocorticosteroids, but others do not necessarily reflect any of the adrenal hormones' normal functions; they are seen only after administration of large therapeutic doses of the drug. The pharmacological effects of prednisolone which are due to its glucocorticoid properties include: promotion of gluconeogenesis; increased deposition of glycogen in the liver; inhibition of the utilization of glucose; anti-insulin activity; increased catabolism of protein; increased lipolysis; stimulation of fat synthesis and storage; increased glomerular filtration rate and resulting increase in urinary excretion of urate (creatinine excretion remains unchanged); and increased calcium excretion.

Depressed production of eosinophils and lymphocytes occurs, but erythropoiesis and production of polymorphonuclear leukocytes are stimulated. Anti-inflammatory processes (edema, fibrin deposition, capillary dilatation, migration of leukocytes and phagocytosis) and the later stages of wound healing (capillary proliferation, deposition of collagen, cicatrization) are inhibited. Prednisolone can stimulate secretion of various components of gastric juice. Stimulation of the production of corticotropin may lead to suppression of endogenous corticosteroids. Prednisolone has slight mineralocorticoid activity, whereby entry of sodium into cells and loss of intracellular potassium is stimulated. This is particularly evident in the kidney, where rapid ion exchange leads to sodium retention and hypertension.

Prednisolone is rapidly and well absorbed from the gastrointestinal tract following oral administration. PEDIAPRED Oral Liquid produces a 20% higher peak plasma level of prednisolone which occurs approximately 15 minutes earlier than the peak seen with tablet formulations. Prednisolone is 70–90% protein-bound in the plasma and it is eliminated from the plasma with a half-life of 2 to 4 hours. It is metabolized mainly in the liver and excreted in the urine as sulfate and glucuronide conjugates.

INDICATIONS AND USAGE

PEDIAPRED Oral Liquid is indicated in the following conditions:

1. **Endocrine Disorders**
Primary or secondary adrenocortical insufficiency (hydrocortisone or cortisone is the first choice; synthetic analogs may be used in conjunction with mineralocorticoids where applicable; in infancy mineralocorticoid supplementation is of particular importance); congenital adrenal hyperplasia; hypercalcemia associated with cancer; nonsuppurative thyroiditis
2. **Rheumatic Disorders**
As adjunctive therapy for short term administration (to tide the patient over an acute episode or exacerbation) in: psoriatic arthritis; rheumatoid arthritis, including juvenile rheumatoid arthritis (selected cases may require low dose maintenance therapy); ankylosing spondylitis; acute and subacute bursitis; acute nonspecific tenosynovitis; acute gouty arthritis; post-traumatic osteoarthritis; synovitis of osteoarthritis; epicondylitis
3. **Collagen Diseases**
During an exacerbation or as maintenance therapy in selected cases of: systemic lupus erythematosus; systemic dermatomyositis (polymyositis); acute rheumatic carditis
4. **Dermatologic Diseases**
Pemphigus; bullous dermatitis herpetiformis; severe erythema multiforme (Stevens-Johnson syndrome); exfoliative dermatitis; mycosis fungoides; severe psoriasis; severe seborrheic dermatitis
5. **Allergic States**
Control of severe or incapacitating allergic conditions intractable to adequate trials of conventional treatment in: seasonal or perennial allergic rhinitis; bronchial asthma; contact dermatitis; atopic dermatitis; serum sickness; drug hypersensitivity reactions
6. **Ophthalmic Diseases**
Severe acute and chronic allergic and inflammatory processes involving the eye and its adnexa such as: allergic conjunctivitis; keratitis; allergic corneal marginal ulcers; herpes zoster ophthalmicus; iritis and iridocyclitis; chorioretinitis; anterior segment inflammation; diffuse posterior uveitis and choroiditis; optic neuritis; sympathetic ophthalmia
7. **Respiratory Diseases**
Symptomatic sarcoidosis; Loeffler's syndrome not manageable by other means; berylliosis; fulminating or disseminated pulmonary tuberculosis when used concurrently with appropriate antituberculous chemotherapy; aspiration pneumonitis
8. **Hematologic Disorders**
Idiopathic thrombocytopenic purpura in adults; secondary thrombocytopenia in adults; acquired (autoimmune) hemolytic anemia; erythroblastopenia (RBC anemia); congenital (erythroid) hypoplastic anemia
9. **Neoplastic Diseases**
For palliative management of: leukemias and lymphomas in adults; acute leukemia of childhood
10. **Edematous States**
To induce a diuresis or remission of proteinuria in the nephrotic syndrome, without uremia, of the idiopathic type or that due to lupus erythematosus
11. **Gastrointestinal Diseases**
To tide the patient over a critical period of the disease in: ulcerative colitis; regional enteritis
12. **Nervous System**
Acute exacerbations of multiple sclerosis
13. **Miscellaneous**
Tuberculous meningitis with subarachnoid block or impending block when used concurrently with appropriate antituberculous chemotherapy; trichinosis with neurologic or myocardial involvement

CONTRAINDICATIONS

Systemic fungal infections.

WARNINGS

In patients on corticosteroid therapy subjected to unusual stress, increased dosage of rapidly acting corticosteroids before, during and after the stressful situation is indicated.

Corticosteroids may mask some signs of infection, and new infections may appear during their use. There may be decreased resistance and inability to localize infection when corticosteroids are used.

Prolonged use of corticosteroids may produce posterior subcapsular cataracts, glaucoma with possible damage to the optic nerves, and may enhance the establishment of secondary ocular infections due to fungi or viruses.

Average and large doses of hydrocortisone or cortisone can cause elevation of blood pressure, salt and water retention, and increased excretion of potassium. These effects are less likely to occur with the synthetic derivatives except when used in large doses. Dietary salt restriction and potassium supplementation may be necessary. All corticosteroids increase calcium excretion. **While on corticosteroid therapy patients should not be vaccinated against smallpox. Other immunization procedures should not be undertaken in patients who are on corticosteroids, especially on high doses, because of possible hazards of neurological complications and a lack of antibody response.**

The use of prednisolone in active tuberculosis should be restricted to those cases of fulminating or disseminated tuberculosis in which the corticosteroid is used for the management of the disease in conjunction with an appropriate antituberculous regimen.

If corticosteroids are indicated in patients with latent tuberculosis or tuberculin reactivity, close observation is necessary as reactivation of the disease may occur. During prolonged corticosteroid therapy these patients should receive chemoprophylaxis.

PRECAUTIONS

General: Drug-induced secondary adrenocortical insufficiency may be minimized by gradual reduction of dosage. This type of relative insufficiency may persist for months after discontinuation of therapy; therefore, in any situation of stress occurring during that period, hormone therapy should be reinstituted. Since mineralocorticoid secretion may be impaired, salt and/or a mineralocorticoid should be administered concurrently.

There is an enhanced effect of corticosteroids in patients with hypothyroidism and in those with cirrhosis.

Corticosteroids should be used cautiously in patients with ocular herpes simplex because of possible corneal perforation.

The lowest possible dose of corticosteroid should be used to control the condition under treatment, and when reduction in dosage is possible, the reduction should be gradual.

Psychic derangements may appear when corticosteroids are used, ranging from euphoria, insomnia, mood swings, personality changes, and severe depression, to frank psychotic manifestations. Also, existing emotional instability or psychotic tendencies may be aggravated by corticosteroids.

Aspirin should be used cautiously in conjunction with corticosteroids in hypoprothrombinemia.

Steroids should be used with caution in nonspecific ulcerative colitis, if there is a probability of impending perforation, abscess or other pyogenic infection; diverticulitis; fresh intestinal anastomoses; active or latent peptic ulcer; renal insufficiency; hypertension; osteoporosis; and myasthenia gravis.

Growth and development of infants and children on prolonged corticosteroid therapy should be carefully observed.

Although controlled clinical trials have shown corticosteroids to be effective in speeding the resolution of acute exacerbations of multiple sclerosis, they do not show that they affect the ultimate outcome or natural history of the disease. The studies do show that relatively high doses of corticosteroids are necessary to demonstrate a significant effect. (See DOSAGE AND ADMINISTRATION.)

Since complications of treatment with glucocorticoids are dependent on the size of the dose and the duration of treatment, a risk/benefit decision must be made in each individual case as to dose and duration of treatment and as to whether daily or intermittent therapy should be used.

Information for Patients: Patients should be warned not to discontinue the use of PEDIAPRED abruptly or without medical supervision, to advise any medical attendants that they are taking PEDIAPRED and to seek medical advice at once should they develop fever or other signs of infection.

Drug Interactions: Drugs such as barbiturates which induce hepatic microsomal drug metabolizing enzyme activity may enhance metabolism of prednisolone and require that the dosage of PEDIAPRED be increased.

Pregnancy: Pregnancy Category C—Prednisolone has been shown to be teratogenic in many species when given in doses equivalent to the human dose. There are no adequate and well controlled studies in pregnant women. PEDIAPRED should be used during pregnancy only if the potential benefit justifies the potential risk to the fetus. Animal studies in which prednisolone has been given to pregnant mice, rats and rabbits have yielded an increased incidence of cleft palate in the offspring.

Nursing Mothers: Prednisolone is excreted in breast milk, but only to a small (less than 1% of the administered dose) and probably clinically insignificant extent. Caution should be exercised when PEDIAPRED is administered to a nursing woman.

ADVERSE REACTIONS

Fluid and Electrolyte Disturbances
Sodium retention; fluid retention; congestive heart failure in susceptible patients; potassium loss; hypokalemic alkalosis; hypertension

Musculoskeletal
Muscle weakness; steroid myopathy; loss of muscle mass; osteoporosis; vertebral compression fractures; aseptic necrosis of femoral and humeral heads; pathologic fracture of long bones

Gastrointestinal
Peptic ulcer with possible perforation and hemorrhage; pancreatitis; abdominal distention; ulcerative esophagitis

Dermatologic
Impaired wound healing; thin fragile skin; petechiae and ecchymoses; facial erythema; increased sweating; may suppress reactions to skin tests

Metabolic
Negative nitrogen balance due to protein catabolism

Neurological
Convulsions; increased intracranial pressure with papilledema (pseudotumor cerebri) usually after treatment; vertigo; headache

Endocrine
Menstrual irregularities; development of cushingoid state; secondary adrenocortical and pituitary unresponsiveness, particularly in times of stress, as in trauma, surgery or illness; suppression of growth in children; decreased carbohydrate tolerance; manifestations of latent diabetes mellitus; increased requirements for insulin or oral hypoglycemic agents in diabetes

Ophthalmic
Posterior subcapsular cataracts; increased intraocular pressure; glaucoma; exophthalmos

OVERDOSAGE

The effects of accidental ingestion of large quantities of prednisolone over a very short period of time have not been reported, but prolonged use of the drug can produce mental symptoms, moon face, abnormal fat deposits, fluid retention, excessive appetite, weight gain, hypertrichosis, acne, striae, ecchymosis, increased sweating, pigmentation, dry scaly skin, thinning scalp hair, increased blood pressure, tachycardia, thrombophlebitis, decreased resistance to infection, negative nitrogen balance with delayed bone and wound healing, headache, weakness, menstrual disorders, accentuated menopausal symptoms, neuropathy, fractures, osteoporosis, peptic ulcer, decreased glucose tolerance, hypokalemia, and adrenal insufficiency. Hepatomegaly and abdominal distention have been observed in children.

Treatment of acute overdosage is by immediate gastric lavage or emesis. For chronic overdosage in the face of severe disease requiring continuous steroid therapy the dosage of prednisolone may be reduced only temporarily, or alternate day treatment may be introduced.

DOSAGE AND ADMINISTRATION

The initial dosage of PEDIAPRED may vary from 5 mL to 60 mL (5 to 60 mg prednisolone base) per day depending on

the specific disease entity being treated. In situations of less severity lower doses will generally suffice while in selected patients higher initial doses may be required. The initial dosage should be maintained or adjusted until a satisfactory response is noted. If after a reasonable period of time there is a lack of satisfactory clinical response, PEDIAPRED should be discontinued and the patient transferred to other appropriate therapy. **IT SHOULD BE EMPHASIZED THAT DOSAGE REQUIREMENTS ARE VARIABLE AND MUST BE INDIVIDUALIZED ON THE BASIS OF THE DISEASE UNDER TREATMENT AND THE RESPONSE OF THE PATIENT.** After a favorable response is noted, the proper maintenance dosage should be determined by decreasing the initial drug dosage in small decrements at appropriate time intervals until the lowest dosage which will maintain an adequate clinical response is reached. It should be kept in mind that constant monitoring is needed in regard to drug dosage. Included in the situations which may make dosage adjustments necessary are changes in clinical status secondary to remissions or exacerbations in the disease process, the patient's individual drug responsiveness, and the effect of patient exposure to stressful situations not directly related to the disease entity under treatment; in this latter situation it may be necessary to increase the dosage of PEDIAPRED for a period of time consistent with the patient's condition. If after long term therapy the drug is to be stopped, it is recommended that it be withdrawn gradually rather than abruptly.

In the treatment of acute exacerbations of multiple sclerosis daily doses of 200 mg of prednisolone for a week followed by 80 mg every other day or 4 to 8 mg dexamethasone every other day for one month have been shown to be effective.

For the purpose of comparison, the following is the equivalent milligram dosage of the various glucocorticoids: cortisone, 25; hydrocortisone, 20; prednisolone, 5; prednisone, 5; methylprednisolone, 4; triamcinolone, 4; paramethasone, 2; betamethasone, 0.75; dexamethasone, 0.75. These dose relationships apply only to oral or intravenous administration of these compounds. When these substances or their derivatives are injected intramuscularly or into joint spaces, their relative properties may be greatly altered.

HOW SUPPLIED

PEDIAPRED Oral Liquid is a colorless to light straw colored solution containing 6.70 mg prednisolone sodium phosphate (5.00 mg prednisolone base) per 5 mL (teaspoonful).

NDC 0585-2250-01 4 fl oz bottle

Store at room temperature. Do not refrigerate. Keep tightly closed and out of the reach of children.

CAUTION

Federal law prohibits dispensing without prescription.

***FISONS* Pharmaceuticals**
Fisons Corporation
Rochester, NY 14623 USA

Revised 3/89
RF 024

Pediapred is a registered trademark of Fisons Corporation.

TUSSIONEX® Ⓒ
Pennkinetic®
[*tus 'e-uh-nex*]
(hydrocodone polistirex
[Warning: may be habit forming]
and chlorpheniramine polistirex)
Extended-Release Suspension

DESCRIPTION

Each teaspoonful (5 mL) of TUSSIONEX® Pennkinetic® Extended-Release Suspension contains hydrocodone polistirex equivalent to 10 mg of hydrocodone bitartrate (Warning: May be habit-forming) and chlorpheniramine polistirex equivalent to 8 mg of chlorpheniramine maleate. TUSSIONEX Pennkinetic Extended-Release Suspension provides up to 12-hour relief per dose. Hydrocodone is a centrally-acting narcotic antitussive. Chlorpheniramine is an antihistamine. TUSSIONEX Pennkinetic Extended-Release Suspension is for oral use only.

Hydrocodone Polistirex: sulfonated styrene-divinylbenzene copolymer complex with 4,5α-epoxy-3-methoxy-17-methylmorphinan-6-one

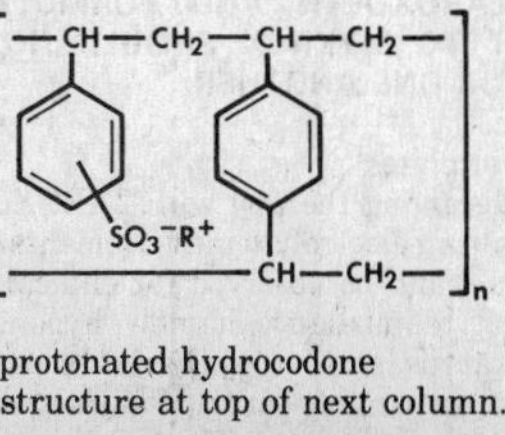

Where R^+ = protonated hydrocodone
[See chemical structure at top of next column.]

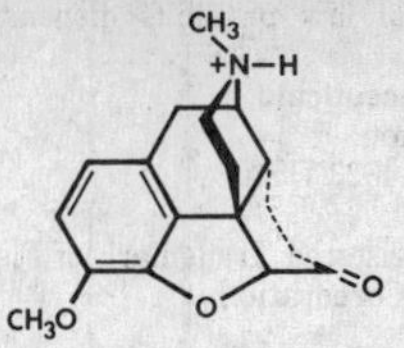

Chlorpheniramine Polistirex: sulfonated styrene-divinylbenzene copolymer complex with 2-[*p*-chloro-α-[2-(dimethylamino)ethyl]-benzyl]pyridine

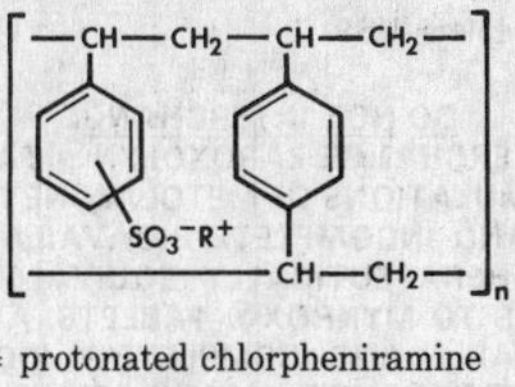

Where R^+ = protonated chlorpheniramine

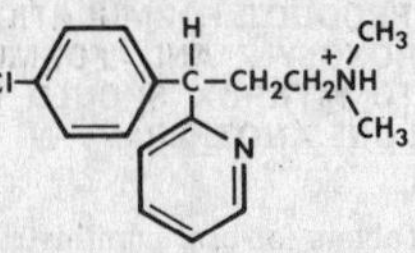

Other ingredients in TUSSIONEX Pennkinetic Extended-Release Suspension: Ascorbic acid, D&C Yellow No. 10, ethylcellulose, FD&C Yellow No. 6, flavor, high fructose corn syrup, methylparaben, polyethylene glycol 3350, polysorbate 80, pregelatinized starch, propylene glycol, propylparaben, purified water, sucrose, vegetable oil, xanthan gum.

CLINICAL PHARMACOLOGY

Hydrocodone is a semisynthetic narcotic antitussive and analgesic with multiple actions qualitatively similar to those of codeine. The precise mechanism of action of hydrocodone and other opiates is not known; however, hydrocodone is believed to act directly on the cough center. In excessive doses, hydrocodone, like other opium derivatives, will depress respiration. The effects of hydrocodone in therapeutic doses on the cardiovascular system are insignificant. Hydrocodone can produce miosis, euphoria, physical and psychological dependence.

Chlorpheniramine is an antihistamine drug (H_1 receptor antagonist) that also possesses anticholinergic and sedative activity. It prevents released histamine from dilating capillaries and causing edema of the respiratory mucosa.

Hydrocodone release from TUSSIONEX Pennkinetic Extended-Release Suspension is controlled by the Pennkinetic® System, an extended-release drug delivery system which combines an ion-exchange polymer matrix with a diffusion rate-limiting permeable coating. Chlorpheniramine release is prolonged by use of an ion-exchange polymer system.

Following multiple dosing with TUSSIONEX Pennkinetic Extended-Release Suspension, hydrocodone mean (S.D.) peak plasma concentrations of 22.8 (5.9) ng/mL occurred at 3.4 hours. Chlorpheniramine mean (S.D.) peak plasma concentrations of 58.4 (14.7) ng/mL occurred at 6.3 hours following multiple dosing. Peak plasma levels obtained with an immediate-release syrup occurred at approximately 1.5 hours for hydrocodone and 2.8 hours for chlorpheniramine. The plasma half-lives of hydrocodone and chlorpheniramine have been reported to be approximately 4 and 16 hours, respectively.

INDICATIONS AND USAGE

TUSSIONEX Pennkinetic Extended-Release Suspension is indicated for relief of cough and upper respiratory symptoms associated with allergy or a cold.

CONTRAINDICATIONS

Known allergy or sensitivity to hydrocodone or chlorpheniramine.

WARNINGS

Respiratory Depression: As with all narcotics, TUSSIONEX Pennkinetic Extended-Release Suspension produces dose-related respiratory depression by directly acting on brain stem respiratory centers. Hydrocodone affects the center that controls respiratory rhythm, and may produce irregular and periodic breathing. Caution should be exercised when TUSSIONEX Pennkinetic Extended-Release Suspension is used postoperatively and in patients with pulmonary disease or whenever ventilatory function is depressed. If respiratory depression occurs, it may be antagonized by the use of naloxone hydrochloride and other supportive measures when indicated (see OVERDOSAGE).

Head Injury and Increased Intracranial Pressure: The respiratory depressant effects of narcotics and their capacity to elevate cerebrospinal fluid pressure may be markedly exaggerated in the presence of head injury, other intracranial lesions or a pre-existing increase in intracranial pressure. Furthermore, narcotics produce adverse reactions which may obscure the clinical course of patients with head injuries.

Acute Abdominal Conditions: The administration of narcotics may obscure the diagnosis or clinical course of patients with acute abdominal conditions.

Obstructive Bowel Disease: Chronic use of narcotics may result in obstructive bowel disease especially in patients with underlying intestinal motility disorder.

Pediatric Use: In young children, as well as adults, the respiratory center is sensitive to the depressant action of narcotic cough suppressants in a dose-dependent manner. Benefit to risk ratio should be carefully considered especially in children with respiratory embarrassment (e.g., croup) (see PRECAUTIONS).

PRECAUTIONS

General: Caution is advised when prescribing this drug to patients with narrow-angle glaucoma, asthma or prostatic hypertrophy.

Special Risk Patients: As with any narcotic agent, TUSSIONEX Pennkinetic Extended-Release Suspension should be used with caution in elderly or debilitated patients and those with severe impairment of hepatic or renal function, hypothyroidism, Addison's disease, prostatic hypertrophy or urethral stricture. The usual precautions should be observed and the possibility of respiratory depression should be kept in mind.

Information for Patients: As with all narcotics, TUSSIONEX Pennkinetic Extended-Release Suspension may produce marked drowsiness and impair the mental and/or physical abilities required for the performance of potentially hazardous tasks such as driving a car or operating machinery; patients should be cautioned accordingly. TUSSIONEX Pennkinetic Extended-Release Suspension must not be diluted with fluids or mixed with other drugs as this may alter the resin-binding and change the absorption rate, possibly increasing the toxicity.

Keep out of the reach of children.

Cough Reflex: Hydrocodone suppresses the cough reflex; as with all narcotics, caution should be exercised when TUSSIONEX Pennkinetic Extended-Release Suspension is used postoperatively, and in patients with pulmonary disease.

Drug Interactions: Patients receiving narcotics, antihistaminics, antipsychotics, antianxiety agents or other CNS depressants (including alcohol) concomitantly with TUSSIONEX Pennkinetic Extended-Release Suspension may exhibit an additive CNS depression. When combined therapy is contemplated, the dose of one or both agents should be reduced.

The use of MAO inhibitors or tricyclic antidepressants with hydrocodone preparations may increase the effect of either the antidepressant or hydrocodone.

The concurrent use of other anticholinergics with hydrocodone may produce paralytic ileus.

Carcinogenesis, Mutagenesis, Impairment of Fertility: Carcinogenicity, mutagenicity and reproductive studies have not been conducted with TUSSIONEX Pennkinetic Extended-Release Suspension.

Pregnancy

Teratogenic Effects—Pregnancy Category C: Hydrocodone has been shown to be teratogenic in hamsters when given in doses 700 times the human dose. There are no adequate and well-controlled studies in pregnant women. TUSSIONEX Pennkinetic Extended-Release Suspension should be used during pregnancy only if the potential benefit justifies the potential risk to the fetus.

Nonteratogenic Effects: Babies born to mothers who have been taking opioids regularly prior to delivery will be physically dependent. The withdrawal signs include irritability and excessive crying, tremors, hyperactive reflexes, increased respiratory rate, increased stools, sneezing, yawning, vomiting and fever. The intensity of the syndrome does not always correlate with the duration of maternal opioid use or dose.

Labor and Delivery: As with all narcotics, administration of TUSSIONEX Pennkinetic Extended-Release Suspension to the mother shortly before delivery may result in some degree of respiratory depression in the newborn, especially if higher doses are used.

Nursing Mothers: It is not known whether this drug is excreted in human milk. Because many drugs are excreted in human milk and because of the potential for serious adverse reactions in nursing infants from TUSSIONEX Pennkinetic Extended-Release Suspension, a decision should be made whether to discontinue nursing or to discontinue the drug,

Continued on next page

Information on Fisons' products appearing in these pages is current as of July 1992. For further information, please consult the package insert currently accompanying the product, or Fisons Corporation, P.O. Box 1710, Rochester, NY 14603, (716) 475-9000.

Fisons—Cont.

taking into account the importance of the drug to the mother.

Pediatric Use: Safety and effectiveness of TUSSIONEX Pennkinetic Extended-Release Suspension in children under six have not been established.

ADVERSE REACTIONS

Central Nervous System: Sedation, drowsiness, mental clouding, lethargy, impairment of mental and physical performance, anxiety, fear, dysphoria, euphoria, dizziness, psychic dependence, mood changes.

Dermatologic System: Rash, pruritus.

Gastrointestinal System: Nausea and vomiting may occur; they are more frequent in ambulatory than in recumbent patients. Prolonged administration of TUSSIONEX Pennkinetic Extended-Release Suspension may produce constipation.

Genitourinary System: Ureteral spasm, spasm of vesicle sphincters and urinary retention have been reported with opiates.

Respiratory Depression: TUSSIONEX Pennkinetic Extended-Release Suspension may produce dose-related respiratory depression by acting directly on brain stem respiratory centers (see OVERDOSAGE).

Respiratory System: Dryness of the pharynx, occasional tightness of the chest.

DRUG ABUSE AND DEPENDENCE

TUSSIONEX Pennkinetic Extended-Release Suspension is a Schedule III narcotic. Psychic dependence, physical dependence and tolerance may develop upon repeated administration of narcotics; therefore, TUSSIONEX Pennkinetic Extended-Release Suspension should be prescribed and administered with caution. However, psychic dependence is unlikely to develop when TUSSIONEX Pennkinetic Extended-Release Suspension is used for a short time for the treatment of cough. Physical dependence, the condition in which continued administration of the drug is required to prevent the appearance of a withdrawal syndrome, assumes clinically significant proportions only after several weeks of continued oral narcotic use, although some mild degree of physical dependence may develop after a few days of narcotic therapy.

OVERDOSAGE

Signs and Symptoms: Serious overdosage with hydrocodone is characterized by respiratory depression (a decrease in respiratory rate and/or tidal volume, Cheyne-Stokes respiration, cyanosis), extreme somnolence progressing to stupor or coma, skeletal muscle flaccidity, cold and clammy skin, and sometimes bradycardia and hypotension. Although miosis is characteristic of narcotic overdose, mydriasis may occur in terminal narcosis or severe hypoxia. In severe overdosage apnea, circulatory collapse, cardiac arrest and death may occur. The manifestations of chlorpheniramine overdosage may vary from central nervous system depression to stimulation.

Treatment: Primary attention should be given to the reestablishment of adequate respiratory exchange through provision of a patent airway and the institution of assisted or controlled ventilation. The narcotic antagonist naloxone hydrochloride is a specific antidote for respiratory depression which may result from overdosage or unusual sensitivity to narcotics including hydrocodone. Therefore, an appropriate dose of naloxone hydrochloride should be administered, preferably by the intravenous route, simultaneously with efforts at respiratory resuscitation. Since the duration of action of hydrocodone in this formulation may exceed that of the antagonist, the patient should be kept under continued surveillance and repeated doses of the antagonist should be administered as needed to maintain adequate respiration. For further information, see full prescribing information for naloxone hydrochloride. An antagonist should not be administered in the absence of clinically significant respiratory depression. Oxygen, intravenous fluids, vasopressors and other supportive measures should be employed as indicated. Gastric emptying may be useful in removing unabsorbed drug.

DOSAGE AND ADMINISTRATION

Shake well before using.

Adults: 1 teaspoonful (5 mL) every 12 hours; do not exceed 2 teaspoonfuls in 24 hours.

Children 6–12: ½ teaspoonful every 12 hours; **do not exceed 1 teaspoonful in 24 hours.**

Not recommended for children under 6 years of age (see PRECAUTIONS).

HOW SUPPLIED

TUSSIONEX Pennkinetic (hydrocodone polistirex and chlorpheniramine polistirex) Extended-Release Suspension is a gold-colored suspension available in bottles of one pint (473 mL) (NDC 0585-0548-67) and 900 mL (NDC 0585-0548-91).

Shake well. Dispense in a well-closed container. Store at 59°–86°F (15°–30°C).

Caution: Federal law prohibits dispensing without prescription.

***FISONS* Pharmaceuticals**
Fisons Corporation
Rochester, NY 14623 USA
® Fisons BV
FISONS is a Registered Trademark of Fisons plc
© 1992, Fisons Corporation
RF240B Rev. 1/92

ZAROXOLYN® TABLETS ℞

[zar" ox ' uh-lin]
(metolazone tablets, USP)

DO NOT INTERCHANGE

DO NOT INTERCHANGE ZAROXOLYN® TABLETS AND OTHER FORMULATIONS OF METOLAZONE THAT SHARE ITS SLOW AND INCOMPLETE BIOAVAILABILITY AND ARE NOT THERAPEUTICALLY EQUIVALENT AT THE SAME DOSES TO MYKROX® TABLETS, A MORE RAPIDLY AVAILABLE AND COMPLETELY BIOAVAILABLE METOLAZONE PRODUCT. FORMULATIONS BIOEQUIVALENT TO ZAROXOLYN AND FORMULATIONS BIOEQUIVALENT TO MYKROX SHOULD NOT BE INTERCHANGED FOR ONE ANOTHER.

DESCRIPTION

ZAROXOLYN Tablets for oral administration contain 2½, 5 or 10 mg of metolazone, USP, a diuretic/saluretic/antihypertensive drug of the quinazoline class.

Metolazone has the molecular formula $C_{16}H_{16}ClN_3O_3S$, the chemical name 7-chloro-1,2,3,4-tetrahydro-2-methyl-3-(2-methylphenyl)-4-oxo-6- quinazolinesulfonamide and a molecular weight of 365.83. The structural formula is:

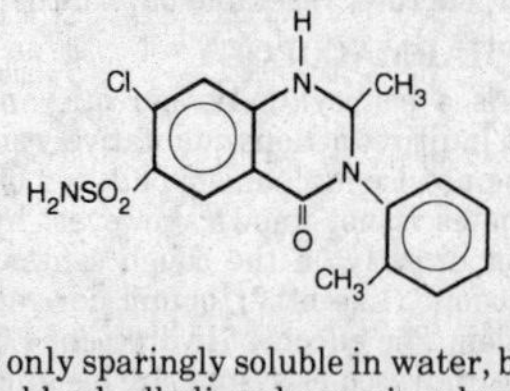

Metolazone is only sparingly soluble in water, but more soluble in plasma, blood, alkali and organic solvents.

ZAROXOLYN Tablets also contain magnesium stearate, microcrystalline cellulose and dye: 2½ mg-D&C Red No. 33; 5 mg-FD&C Blue No. 2; 10 mg-D&C Yellow No. 10 and FD&C Yellow No. 6.

CLINICAL PHARMACOLOGY

ZAROXOLYN (metolazone) is a quinazoline diuretic, with properties generally similar to the thiazide diuretics. The actions of ZAROXOLYN result from interference with the renal tubular mechanism of electrolyte reabsorption. ZAROXOLYN acts primarily to inhibit sodium reabsorption at the cortical diluting site and to a lesser extent in the proximal convoluted tubule. Sodium and chloride ions are excreted in approximately equivalent amounts. The increased delivery of sodium to the distal-tubular exchange site results in increased potassium excretion. ZAROXOLYN does not inhibit carbonic anhydrase. A proximal action of metolazone has been shown in humans by increased excretion of phosphate and magnesium ions and by a markedly increased fractional excretion of sodium in patients with severely compromised glomerular filtration. This action has been demonstrated in animals by micropuncture studies.

When ZAROXOLYN Tablets are given, diuresis and saluresis usually begin within one hour and may persist for 24 hours or more. For most patients, the duration of effect can be varied by adjusting the daily dose. High doses may prolong the effect. A single daily dose is recommended. When a desired therapeutic effect has been obtained, it may be possible to reduce dosage to a lower maintenance level.

The diuretic potency of ZAROXOLYN at maximum therapeutic dosage is approximately equal to thiazide diuretics. However, unlike thiazides, ZAROXOLYN may produce diuresis in patients with glomerular filtration rates below 20 mL/min.

ZAROXOLYN and furosemide administered concurrently have produced marked diuresis in some patients where edema or ascites was refractory to treatment with maximum recommended doses of these or other diuretics administered alone. The mechanism of this interaction is unknown (see DRUG INTERACTIONS and WARNINGS).

Maximum blood levels of metolazone are found approximately eight hours after dosing. A small fraction of metolazone is metabolized. Most of the drug is excreted in the unconverted form in the urine.

INDICATIONS AND USAGE

ZAROXOLYN is indicated for the treatment of salt and water retention including:

—edema accompanying congestive heart failure;

—edema accompanying renal diseases, including the nephrotic syndrome and states of diminished renal function.

ZAROXOLYN is also indicated for the treatment of hypertension, alone or in combination with other antihypertensive drugs of a different class. MYKROX Tablets, a more rapidly available form of metolazone, are intended for the treatment of new patients with mild to moderate hypertension. A dose titration is necessary if MYKROX Tablets are to be substituted for ZAROXOLYN in the treatment of hypertension. See package circular for MYKROX Tablets (Fisons).

Usage in Pregnancy

The routine use of diuretics in an otherwise healthy woman is inappropriate and exposes mother and fetus to unnecessary hazard. Diuretics do not prevent development of toxemia of pregnancy, and there is no evidence that they are useful in the treatment of developed toxemia.

Edema during pregnancy may arise from pathologic causes or from the physiologic and mechanical consequences of pregnancy. ZAROXOLYN is indicated in pregnancy when edema is due to pathologic causes, just as it is in the absence of pregnancy (see PRECAUTIONS). Dependent edema in pregnancy resulting from restriction of venous return by the expanded uterus is properly treated through elevation of the lower extremities and use of support hose; use of diuretics to lower intravascular volume in this case is illogical and unnecessary. There is hypervolemia during normal pregnancy which is harmful to neither the fetus nor the mother (in the absence of cardiovascular disease), but which is associated with edema, including generalized edema, in the majority of pregnant women. If this edema produces discomfort, increased recumbency will often provide relief. In rare instances, this edema may cause extreme discomfort which is not relieved by rest. In these cases, a short course of diuretics may be appropriate.

CONTRAINDICATIONS

Anuria, hepatic coma or pre-coma, known allergy or hypersensitivity to metolazone.

WARNINGS

Rapid Onset Hyponatremia

Rarely, the rapid onset of severe hyponatremia and/or hypokalemia has been reported following initial doses of thiazide and non-thiazide diuretics. When symptoms consistent with severe electrolyte imbalance appear rapidly, drug should be discontinued and supportive measures should be initiated immediately. Parenteral electrolytes may be required. Appropriateness of therapy with this class of drugs should be carefully re-evaluated.

Hypokalemia

Hypokalemia may occur with consequent weakness, cramps, and cardiac dysrhythmias. Serum potassium should be determined at regular intervals, and dose reduction, potassium supplementation or addition of a potassium-sparing diuretic instituted whenever indicated. Hypokalemia is a particular hazard in patients who are digitalized or who have or have had a ventricular arrhythmia; dangerous or fatal arrhythmias may be precipitated. Hypokalemia is dose related.

Lithium

In general, diuretics should not be given concomitantly with lithium because they reduce its renal clearance and add a high risk of lithium toxicity. Read prescribing information for lithium preparations before use of such concomitant therapy.

Concomitant Therapy

Furosemide: Unusually large or prolonged losses of fluids and electrolytes may result when ZAROXOLYN is administered concomitantly to patients receiving furosemide (see DRUG INTERACTIONS).

Other Antihypertensive Drugs: When ZAROXOLYN is used with other antihypertensive drugs, particular care must be taken to avoid excessive reduction of blood pressure, especially during initial therapy.

Cross-Allergy

Cross-allergy, while not reported to date, theoretically may occur when ZAROXOLYN is given to patients known to be allergic to sulfonamide-derived drugs, thiazides, or quinethazone.

PRECAUTIONS

DO NOT INTERCHANGE

DO NOT INTERCHANGE ZAROXOLYN TABLETS AND OTHER FORMULATIONS OF METOLAZONE THAT SHARE ITS SLOW AND INCOMPLETE BIOAVAILABILITY AND ARE NOT THERAPEUTICALLY EQUIVALENT AT THE SAME DOSES TO MYKROX TABLETS, A MORE RAPIDLY AVAILABLE AND COMPLETELY BIOAVAILABLE METOLAZONE PRODUCT. FORMULATIONS BIOEQUIVALENT TO ZAROXOLYN AND FORMULATIONS BIOEQUIVALENT TO MYKROX SHOULD NOT BE INTERCHANGED FOR ONE ANOTHER.

A. GENERAL:

Fluid and Electrolytes

All patients receiving therapy with ZAROXOLYN Tablets should have serum electrolyte measurements done at appropriate intervals and be observed for clinical signs of fluid and/or electrolyte imbalance: namely, hyponatremia, hypochloremic alkalosis, and hypokalemia. In patients with severe edema accompanying cardiac failure or renal disease, a

low-salt syndrome may be produced, especially with hot weather and a low-salt diet. Serum and urine electrolyte determinations are particularly important when the patient has protracted vomiting, severe diarrhea, or is receiving parenteral fluids. Warning signs of imbalance are: dryness of mouth, thirst, weakness, lethargy, drowsiness, restlessness, muscle pains or cramps, muscle fatigue, hypotension, oliguria, tachycardia, and gastrointestinal disturbances such as nausea and vomiting. Hyponatremia may occur at any time during long term therapy and, on rare occasions, may be life threatening.

The risk of hypokalemia is increased when larger doses are used, when diuresis is rapid, when severe liver disease is present, when corticosteroids are given concomitantly, when oral intake is inadequate or when excess potassium is being lost extrarenally, such as with vomiting or diarrhea.

Glucose Tolerance
Metolazone may raise blood glucose concentrations possibly causing hyperglycemia and glycosuria in patients with diabetes or latent diabetes.

Hyperuricemia
ZAROXOLYN regularly causes an increase in serum uric acid and can occasionally precipitate gouty attacks even in patients without a prior history of them.

Azotemia
Azotemia, presumably pre-renal azotemia, may be precipitated during the administration of ZAROXOLYN. If azotemia and oliguria worsen during treatment of patients with severe renal disease, ZAROXOLYN should be discontinued.

Renal Impairment
Use caution when administering ZAROXOLYN Tablets to patients with severely impaired renal function. As most of the drug is excreted by the renal route, accumulation may occur.

Orthostatic Hypotension
Orthostatic hypotension may occur; this may be potentiated by alcohol, barbiturates, narcotics, or concurrent therapy with other antihypertensive drugs.

Hypercalcemia
Use of other diuretics has been associated on rare occasions with pathological changes in the parathyroid glands. This possibility should be considered with clinical use of ZAROXOLYN Tablets. Hypercalcemia has been noted in a few patients treated with metolazone.

Systemic Lupus Erythematosus
Thiazide diuretics have exacerbated or activated systemic lupus erythematosus and this possibility should be considered with ZAROXOLYN Tablets.

B. INFORMATION FOR PATIENTS: Patients should be informed of possible adverse effects, advised to take the medication as directed and promptly report any possible adverse reactions to the treating physician.

C. DRUG INTERACTIONS:

Diuretics
Furosemide and probably other loop diuretics given concomitantly with metolazone can cause unusually large or prolonged losses of fluid and electrolytes (see WARNINGS).

Other Antihypertensives
When ZAROXOLYN Tablets are used with other antihypertensive drugs, care must be taken, especially during initial therapy. Dosage adjustments of other antihypertensives may be necessary.

Alcohol, Barbiturates, and Narcotics
The hypotensive effects of these drugs may be potentiated by the volume contraction that may be associated with metolazone therapy.

Digitalis Glycosides
Diuretic-induced hypokalemia can increase the sensitivity of the myocardium to digitalis. Serious arrhythmias can result.

Corticosteroids or ACTH
May increase the risk of hypokalemia and increase salt and water retention.

Lithium
Serum lithium levels may increase (see WARNINGS).

Curariform Drugs
Diuretic-induced hypokalemia may enhance neuromuscular blocking effects of curariform drugs (such as tubocurarine) — the most serious effect would be respiratory depression which could proceed to apnea. Accordingly, it may be advisable to discontinue ZAROXOLYN Tablets three days before elective surgery.

Salicylates and Other Non-Steroidal Anti-Inflammatory Drugs
May decrease the antihypertensive effects of ZAROXOLYN Tablets.

Sympathomimetics
Metolazone may decrease arterial responsiveness to norepinephrine, but this diminution is not sufficient to preclude effectiveness of the pressor agent for therapeutic use.

Insulin and Oral Antidiabetic Agents
See Glucose Tolerance under GENERAL PRECAUTIONS.

Methenamine
Efficacy may be decreased due to urinary alkalizing effect of metolazone.

D. DRUG/LABORATORY TEST INTERACTIONS: None reported.

E. CARCINOGENESIS, MUTAGENESIS, IMPAIRMENT OF FERTILITY: Mice and rats given metolazone for $1\frac{1}{2}$ to 2 years at daily doses of 2, 10 and 50 mg/kg (approximately 13, 67, and 333 times the average human dose of 0.15 mg/kg) showed no evidence that metolazone caused an increased number of tumors. The small number of animals examined histologically and poor survival in the mice limit the conclusions that can be reached from these studies.

Reproductive performance has been evaluated in mice and rats. There is no evidence that metolazone possesses the potential for altering reproductive capacity in mice. In a rat study, in which males were treated orally with metolazone at doses of 2, 10 and 50 mg/kg for 127 days prior to mating with untreated females, an increased number of resorption sites was observed in dams mated with males from the 50 mg/kg group. In addition, the fetal weight of offspring was decreased and the pregnancy rate was reduced in dams mated with males from the 10 and 50 mg/kg groups.

F. PREGNANCY:

Teratogenic Effects—Pregnancy Category B.
Reproduction studies performed in mice, rabbits and rats treated during the appropriate period of gestation at doses up to 50 mg/kg/day (333 times an average human dose of ZAROXOLYN) have revealed no evidence of harm to the fetus due to metolazone. There are, however, no adequate and well-controlled studies in pregnant women. Because animal reproduction studies are not always predictive of human response, ZAROXOLYN Tablets should be used during pregnancy only if clearly needed. Metolazone crosses the placental barrier and appears in cord blood.

Non-Teratogenic Effects
The use of ZAROXOLYN Tablets in pregnant women requires that the anticipated benefit be weighed against possible hazards to the fetus. These hazards include fetal or neonatal jaundice, thrombocytopenia, and possibly other adverse reactions which have occurred in the adult. It is not known what effect the use of the drug during pregnancy has on the later growth, development and functional maturation of the child. No such effects have been reported with metolazone.

G. LABOR AND DELIVERY: Based on clinical studies in which women received metolazone in late pregnancy until the time of delivery, there is no evidence that the drug has any adverse effects on the normal course of labor or delivery.

H. NURSING MOTHERS: Metolazone appears in breast milk. Because of the potential for serious adverse reactions in nursing infants from metolazone, a decision should be made whether to discontinue nursing or to discontinue the drug, taking into account the importance of the drug to the mother.

I. PEDIATRIC USE: Safety and effectiveness in children have not been established and such use is not recommended.

ADVERSE REACTIONS
ZAROXOLYN is usually well tolerated, and most reported adverse reactions have been mild and transient. Many ZAROXOLYN related adverse reactions represent extensions of its expected pharmacologic activity and can be attributed to either its antihypertensive action or its renal/metabolic actions. The following adverse reactions have been reported. Several are single or comparably rare occurrences. Adverse reactions are listed in decreasing order of severity within body systems.

Cardiovascular: Chest pain/discomfort, orthostatic hypotension, excessive volume depletion, hemoconcentration, venous thrombosis, palpitations.

Central and Peripheral Nervous System: Syncope, neuropathy, vertigo, paresthesias, psychotic depression, impotence, dizziness/light-headedness, drowsiness, fatigue, weakness, restlessness (sometimes resulting in insomnia), headache.

Dermatologic/Hypersensitivity: Necrotizing angiitis (cutaneous vasculitis), purpura, dermatitis (photosensitivity), urticaria and skin rashes.

Gastrointestinal: Hepatitis, intrahepatic cholestatic jaundice, pancreatitis, vomiting, nausea, epigastric distress, diarrhea, constipation, anorexia, abdominal bloating.

Hematologic: Aplastic/hypoplastic anemia, agranulocytosis, leukopenia.

Metabolic: Hypokalemia, hyponatremia, hyperuricemia, hypochloremia, hypochloremic alkalosis, hyperglycemia, glycosuria, increase in serum urea nitrogen (BUN) or creatinine, hypophosphatemia.

Musculoskeletal: Joint pain, acute gouty attacks, muscle cramps or spasm.

Other: Transient blurred vision, chills.

In addition, adverse reactions reported with similar antihypertensive-diuretics, but which have not been reported to date for ZAROXOLYN include: bitter taste, dry mouth, sialadenitis, xanthopsia, respiratory distress (including pneumonitis), thrombocytopenia and anaphylactic reactions. These reactions should be considered as possible occurrences with clinical usage of ZAROXOLYN.

Whenever adverse reactions are moderate or severe, ZAROXOLYN dosage should be reduced or therapy withdrawn.

OVERDOSAGE
Intentional overdosage has been reported rarely with metolazone and similar diuretic drugs.

Signs and Symptoms
Orthostatic hypotension, dizziness, drowsiness, syncope, electrolyte abnormalities, hemoconcentration and hemodynamic changes due to plasma volume depletion may occur. In some instances depressed respiration may be observed. At high doses, lethargy of varying degree may progress to coma within a few hours. The mechanism of CNS depression with thiazide overdosage is unknown. Also, GI irritation and hypermotility may occur. Temporary elevation of BUN has been reported, especially in patients with impairment of renal function. Serum electrolyte changes and cardiovascular and renal function should be closely monitored.

Treatment
There is no specific antidote available but immediate evacuation of the stomach contents is advised. Dialysis is not likely to be effective. Care should be taken when evacuating the gastric contents to prevent aspiration, especially in the stuporous or comatose patient. Supportive measures should be initiated as required to maintain hydration, electrolyte balance, respiration and cardiovascular and renal function.

DOSAGE AND ADMINISTRATION
Effective dosage of ZAROXOLYN should be individualized according to indication and patient response. A single daily dose is recommended. Therapy with ZAROXOLYN should be titrated to gain an initial therapeutic response and to determine the minimal dose possible to maintain the desired therapeutic response.

Usual Single Daily Dosage Schedules
Suitable initial dosages will usually fall in the ranges given.
Edema of cardiac failure:
ZAROXOLYN 5 to 20 mg once daily.
Edema of renal disease:
ZAROXOLYN 5 to 20 mg once daily.
Mild to moderate essential hypertension:
ZAROXOLYN $2\frac{1}{2}$ to 5 mg once daily.
New patients—MYKROX Tablets (metolazone tablets, USP) (see MYKROX package circular). If considered desirable to switch patients currently on ZAROXOLYN to MYKROX, the dose should be determined by titration starting at one tablet ($\frac{1}{2}$ mg) once daily and increasing to two tablets (1 mg) once daily if needed.

Treatment of Edematous States
The time interval required for the initial dosage to produce an effect may vary. Diuresis and saluresis usually begin within one hour and persist for 24 hours or longer. When a desired therapeutic effect has been obtained, it may be advisable to reduce the dose if possible. The daily dose depends on the severity of the patient's condition, sodium intake and responsiveness. A decision to change the daily dose should be based on the results of thorough clinical and laboratory evaluations. If antihypertensive drugs or diuretics are given concurrently with ZAROXOLYN, more careful dosage adjustment may be necessary. For patients who tend to experience paroxysmal nocturnal dyspnea, it may be advisable to employ a larger dose to ensure prolongation of diuresis and saluresis for a full 24-hour period.

Treatment of Hypertension
The time interval required for the initial dosage regimen to show effect may vary from three or four days to three to six weeks in the treatment of elevated blood pressure. Doses should be adjusted at appropriate intervals to achieve maximum therapeutic effect.

HOW SUPPLIED
ZAROXOLYN Tablets (metolazone tablets, USP) are provided as pink $2\frac{1}{2}$ mg tablets (NDC 0585-0975), blue 5 mg tablets (NDC 0585-0850), and yellow 10 mg tablets (NDC 0585-0835). The tablets are round and debossed on opposite sides with the tablet strength and ZAROXOLYN. All strengths available in bottles of 100, 500 and 1000, and unit dose packages of 100 (20 strips of 5).
Store at room temperature. Dispense in a tight, light-resistant container.
Caution: Federal law prohibits dispensing without prescription.

FISONS Pharmaceuticals
Fisons Corporation
Rochester, NY 14623 U.S.A.
RF241A   ® Fisons BV
Rev. 12/91   © 1991, Fisons Corporation

Continued on next page

Information on Fisons' products appearing in these pages is current as of July 1992. For further information, please consult the package insert currently accompanying the product, or Fisons Corporation, P.O. Box 1710, Rochester, NY 14603, (716) 475-9000.

Fisons—Cont.

┌─────────────────────────────────┐
│   **EDUCATIONAL MATERIAL**   │
└─────────────────────────────────┘

For educational information, please write to Fisons Corporation, PO Box 1710, Rochester, NY 14603.

C. B. Fleet Co., Inc.
4615 MURRAY PL.
LYNCHBURG, VA 24502-2235

FLEET® BABYLAX®, A LAXATIVE   **OTC**

ACTIVE INGREDIENT
Glycerin (USP)

INDICATIONS
For temporary relief of occasional constipation in young children. Children under 2 years old, consult physician.

ACTIONS
This product generally produces a bowel movement in 15 minutes to one hour. The exact mode of action of glycerin administered rectally as a laxative is not known. It has been suggested that glycerin causes dehydration of exposed tissues to produce an irritant effect which results in a laxative response.

WARNINGS
For rectal use only. Glycerin administered rectally may produce rectal discomfort or a burning sensation in some individuals. If use results in unusual pain or side effects, consult a physician.

GENERAL LAXATIVE WARNINGS
Do not use a laxative product when nausea, vomiting or abdominal pain are present unless directed by a physician. If you have noticed a sudden change in bowel habits that persists over two weeks, consult a physician before using a laxative. Laxative products should not be used longer than one week except under a physician's advice. Rectal bleeding or failure to have a bowel movement after use of a laxative may indicate a serious condition; discontinue use and consult a physician. Keep this and all drugs out of the reach of children. In case of accidental ingestion, seek professional assistance or contact a Poison Control Center immediately.

DOSAGE AND ADMINISTRATION
REMOVE PROTECTIVE SHIELD FROM TIP BEFORE ADMINISTERING.
Children under 2 years old: consult physician. Children 2–6 years of age: 1 rectal applicator containing 4 ml. of glycerin in a single daily dose or as directed by physician. Hold unit upright. Gently insert stem with tip pointing toward navel. Squeeze unit until nearly all liquid is expelled. Remove tip from rectum. Note: A small amount of liquid will remain in unit. Store and use at room temperature.

HOW SUPPLIED
Six 4 ml. rectal applicators per package.

IS THIS PRODUCT OTC?
Yes.

FLEET® BISACODYL ENEMA, A STIMULANT
LAXATIVE   **OTC**
(bisacodyl U.S.P.)

COMPOSITION
Each 30 ml (delivered dose) contains 10 mg. of bisacodyl, U.S.P. suspended in an aqueous medium. The FLEET® Bisacodyl Enema unit, with a 2-inch prelubricated Comfortip®, contains 1¼ fl. oz. of enema suspension in a ready-to-use plastic squeeze bottle. Designed for quick, convenient administration by nurse or patient according to instructions. Disposable after single use.

ACTION AND USES
FLEET® Bisacodyl Enema is a stimulant laxative acting directly on the colonic mucosa to produce peristalsis. FLEET® Bisacodyl Enema actually produces peristalsis and evacuation of the large intestine by stimulating sensory nerve endings in the colonic mucosa to produce parasympathetic reflexes. FLEET® Bisacodyl Enema is very effective usually producing an evacuation within 5 to 20 minutes. FLEET® Bisacodyl Enema may be used whenever a laxative or enema is indicated. It is useful as a laxative for occasional relief of constipation, in bowel cleansing in preparation for X-ray and endoscopic examination. May be used as a laxative in postoperative, antepartum, or postpartum care or in preparation for delivery.

WARNINGS
Do not use a laxative product when nausea, vomiting, or abdominal pain is present unless directed by a physician. If you have noticed a sudden change in bowel habits that persists over a period of 2 weeks, consult a physician before using a laxative. Rectal bleeding or failure to have a bowel movement after use of a laxative may indicate a serious condition. Discontinue use and consult a physician. Laxative products should not be used longer than 1 week unless directed by a physician. This product may cause abdominal discomfort, faintness, rectal burning, and mild cramps. Keep this and all drugs out of the reach of children. In case of accidental ingestion, seek professional assistance or contact a Poison Control Center immediately.

DOSAGE AND ADMINISTRATION
SHAKE BEFORE USING.
REMOVE PROTECTIVE SHIELD FROM TIP BEFORE ADMINISTERING.
Adults and children 12 years of age and older: 1 unit (30 ml) in a single daily dose.
Children 6 to under 12 years of age: one half unit (15 ml) in a single daily dose.
Children under 6 years of age: consult a physician.
Precaution: Do not administer to children under 2 years of age. **Administration:** Preferred position—Lying on left side with left knee slightly bent and the right leg drawn up, or knee-chest position. Rubber diaphragm at base of tube prevents accidental leakage and assures controlled flow of the enema solution. May be used at room temperature.

PROFESSIONAL ADMINISTRATION
See FLEET® Ready-to-Use Enema.

HOW SUPPLIED
FLEET® Bisacodyl Enema is supplied in 1¼ fl. oz. ready-to-use squeeze bottle.

IS THIS PRODUCT OTC?
Yes.

LITERATURE AVAILABLE
Professional literature mailed on request.

FLEET® ENEMA, A SALINE LAXATIVE   **OTC**

COMPOSITION
Each 118 ml. (delivered dose) contains 19 g. monobasic sodium phosphate and 7 g. dibasic sodium phosphate. The FLEET® Enema unit, with a 2-inch, pre-lubricated Comfortip®, contains 4½ fl. oz. of enema solution in a hand-size plastic squeeze bottle. Designed for quick, convenient administration by nurse or patient according to instructions. Disposable after single use.

ACTION AND USES
FLEET® Enema is useful as a laxative in the relief of occasional constipation, and as part of a bowel cleansing regimen in preparing the patient for surgery or for preparing the colon for x-ray and endoscopic examination. Used as directed, FLEET® Enema provides thorough yet safe cleansing action and induces complete emptying of the left colon usually within 2 to 5 minutes without pain or spasm. Also used for general postoperative care and to help relieve fecal or barium impaction.

GENERAL LAXATIVE WARNINGS
Do not use laxative products when nausea, vomiting, or abdominal pain is present. If you notice a sudden change in bowel habits that persists over a period of 2 weeks, consult a physician. Rectal bleeding or failure to have a bowel movement after use of a laxative may indicate a serious condition. Discontinue use and consult a physician. Laxative products should not be used longer than 1 week unless directed by a physician. As with any drug, if you are pregnant or nursing a baby, seek the advice of a health professional before using this product. Keep this and all drugs out of the reach of children. In case of accidental ingestion or overdose, seek professional assistance or contact a Poison Control Center immediately.

PROFESSIONAL USE WARNINGS
Do not use in patients with congenital megacolon, imperforate anus or congestive heart failure as hypernatremic dehydration may occur. Use with caution in patients with impaired renal function, heart disease, or pre-existing electrolyte disturbances (such as dehydration or those secondary to the use of diuretics) or in patients on calcium channel blockers, diuretics or other medications which may affect electrolyte levels — or where colostomy exists, as hypocalcemia, hyperphosphatemia, hypernatremia and acidosis may occur. Calcium and phosphorus levels should be carefully monitored. Since FLEET® Ready-to-Use Enema contains dibasic sodium phosphate and monobasic sodium phosphate, there is a risk of acute elevation of sodium concentration in the serum and consequent dehydration, particularly in children with megacolon or any other condition where there is retention of enema solution. Additional fluids by mouth are recommended where appropriate (Fonkalsrud, E. and Keen, J.: "Hypernatremic Dehydration Hypertonic Enemas in Congenital Megacolon," *JAMA* 199:584–586, 1967. Zumoff, B. and Hellman, L.: "Rectal Absorption of Sodium from Hypertonic Sodium Phosphate Solutions," data on file, C. B. Fleet Company, Inc. Gilman, A., Goodman, L., Gilman, A., eds., *The Pharmacological Basis of Therapeutics*, Sixth Edition, 1980, p. 1005.) In addition, elevated levels of serum phosphates and decreased levels of serum calcium have been reported in patients with renal disease (and with prolonged use). (McConnell, T. H., "Fatal Hypocalcemia from Phosphate Absorption from Laxative Preparation," *JAMA*, 216:147–148, 1971.). SINCE FLEET® BRAND ENEMAS ARE AVAILABLE IN ADULT AND CHILDREN'S SIZES, PRESCRIBE CAREFULLY.

PRECAUTIONS
DO NOT ADMINISTER 4½ oz. ADULT SIZE TO CHILDREN UNDER 12 YEARS OF AGE. DO NOT ADMINISTER 2¼ OZ CHILDREN'S SIZE TO CHILDREN UNDER 2 YEARS OF AGE. IF AFTER THE ENEMA SOLUTION IS ADMINISTERED THERE IS NO RETURN OF LIQUID, CONTACT A PHYSICIAN IMMEDIATELY AS DEHYDRATION COULD OCCUR.

OVERDOSAGE
Overdosage with Fleet® Enema may cause hypocalcemia, hyperphosphatemia, hypernatremia, hypernatremic dehydration and acidosis.

1. Hypocalcemia, hyperphosphatemia, hypernatremia and acidosis
   Calcium, Phosphate, Chloride and Sodium levels should be carefully monitored. Immediate corrective action should be taken to restore electrolyte balance with appropriate fluid replacements.

2. Hypernatremic Dehydration
   Calcium, Phosphate, Chloride and Sodium levels should be carefully monitored. Prompt parenteral administration of fluids with lower concentrations of Sodium and Chloride than extracellular fluid (40–50 mEq/liter) and moderate concentration of Potassium (20–30 mEq/liter) administered at a rate of 3,000 to 4,000 cc/sq. m of body surface during the first 12 to 24 hours dependent on the severity of dehydration and the clinical response (Fonkalsrud, E. and Keen, J.: Hypernatremic Dehydration from Hypertonic Enemas in Congenital Megacolon, *JAMA* 199:584-586, 1967). See article for more details.

ADMINISTRATION AND DOSAGE
REMOVE PROTECTIVE SHIELD FROM TIP BEFORE ADMINISTERING.
Preferred position: Lying on left side with left knee slightly bent and the right leg drawn up, or knee-chest position. Dosage: Adults, 4 fl. oz. in a single daily dose. Rubber diaphragm at base of tube prevents accidental leakage and assures controlled flow of the enema solution. May be used at room temperature. Each 118 ml. (delivered dose) contains 4.4 g. (191 mEq) sodium.

PROFESSIONAL DOSAGE AND ADMINISTRATION
Fleet® Ready-To-Use 4½ oz. Adult Size Enema should not be used in children under 12 years of age. In those cases where complications are reported, infants and young children are often involved. Fleet® Ready-To-Use Enema for Children should be used with caution in children of any age. Careful consideration of the use of enemas in general in children is recommended. The adult size enema should not be used in children under 12 years of age. For children 2 to 12 years of age, use Fleet® Ready-To-Use Enema for Children, which contains a dosage of one-half the adult size enema. For children less than 2 years of age, Fleet® Glycerin Suppositories for Children should be used.
Proper and safe use of Fleet® Ready-To-Use Enema also requires that the product be administered according to the Directions for Use. Health care professionals should remember, when administering the product, to *gently* insert the enema into the rectum with the tip pointing toward the navel. Insertion may be made easier by having the patient bear down as they would in having a bowel movement. Care during insertion is necessary due to lack of sensory innervation of the rectum and due to possibility of bowel perforation. Once inserted, squeeze the bottle until nearly all the liquid is expelled. If resistance is encountered on insertion of the nozzle or in administering the solution, the procedure should be discontinued. Forcing the enema can result in perforation and/or abrasion of the rectum.

HOW SUPPLIED
FLEET® Enema is supplied in a 4½ fl. oz. ready-to-use squeeze bottle. Children's size, 2¼ fl. oz. IMPORTANT: Fleet ® Enema, Adult and Child size, ARE NOT INTENDED FOR ORAL CONSUMPTION, in any dosage size.

IS THIS PRODUCT OTC?
Yes.

LITERATURE AVAILABLE
Professional literature mailed on request.

FLEET® MINERAL OIL ENEMA　　OTC
A LUBRICANT LAXATIVE

COMPOSITION
The FLEET® Mineral Oil Enema unit, with a 2-inch, pre-lubricated Comfortip®, delivers 118 ml of mineral oil USP in a hand-size plastic squeeze bottle.

ACTION AND INDICATIONS
Serves to soften and lubricate hard stools, easing their passage without irritating the mucosa. Results approximate a normal bowel movement in that only the rectum, sigmoid, and part or all of the descending colon are evacuated. Indicated for relief of fecal impaction; valuable in relief of occasional constipation when straining must be avoided (in hypertension, coronary occlusion, proctologic procedures, postoperative care); for removal of barium sulfate residues from the colon after barium administration for GI series or outlining the left atrium; to obtain the laxative benefits of mineral oil while avoiding possible untoward effects of oral administration such as (1) interference with intestinal absorption of fat-soluble vitamins A, D, E and K and other nutrients (2) danger of systemic absorption (3) possible risk of lipid pneumonia due to aspiration. Generally effective in 2 to 15 minutes.

WARNINGS
Do not use laxative products when nausea, vomiting, abdominal pain is present unless directed by a physician. If you have noticed a sudden change in bowel habits that persists over a period of 2 weeks, consult a physician. Rectal bleeding or failure to have a bowel movement after use of a laxative may indicate a serious condition. Discontinue use and consult a physician. Laxative products should not be used longer than 1 week unless directed by a physician. As with any drug, if you are pregnant or nursing a baby, seek the advice of a health professional before using this product. Keep this and all drugs out of the reach of children. In case of accidental ingestion, seek professional assistance or contact a Poison Control Center immediately.

PRECAUTIONS
DO NOT ADMINISTER TO CHILDREN UNDER 2 YEARS OF AGE.

ADMINISTRATION AND DOSAGE
REMOVE PROTECTIVE SHIELD FROM TIP BEFORE ADMINISTERING.
Preferred position: Lying on left side with left knee slightly bent and the right leg drawn up, or knee-chest position. Dosage: Adults and children 12 and over: one bottle (118 ml delivered dose) in a single daily dose. Children 2 to under 12: ½ bottle (59 ml delivered dose) in a single daily dose. Rubber diaphragm at base of tube prevents accidental leakage and assures controlled flow of the enema solution. May be used at room temperature. Follow with regular Fleet® Enema according to dosage instructions contained in PDR for more thorough cleansing.

PROFESSIONAL DOSAGE AND ADMINISTRATION
Fleet® Ready-To-Use Mineral Oil Enema should not be used in children under 2 years of age. Fleet® Ready-To-Use Mineral Oil Enema should be used with caution in children of any age. Careful consideration of the use of enemas in general in children is recommended.
Proper and safe use of Fleet® Ready-To-Use Mineral Oil Enema also requires that the product be administered according to the Directions for Use. Health care professionals should remember, when administering the product, to gently insert the enema into the rectum with the tip pointing toward the naval. Insertion may be made easier by having the patient bear down as they would in having a bowel movement. Care during insertion is necessary due to lack of sensory innervation of the rectum and due to possibility of bowel perforation. Once inserted, squeeze the bottle until nearly all the liquid is expelled. If resistance is encountered on insertion of the nozzle or in administering the solution, the procedure should be discontinued. Forcing the enema can result in perforation and/or abrasion of the rectum.

HOW SUPPLIED
FLEET® Mineral Oil Enema is supplied in 4½ fl.oz. ready-to-use squeeze bottle.

IS THIS PRODUCT OTC?
Yes.

FLEET® PHOSPHO®-SODA　　OTC
A BUFFERED ORAL SALINE LAXATIVE

COMPOSITION
Each 100 ml. of regular or flavored Phospho®-Soda contains 48 g. monobasic sodium phosphate and 18 g. dibasic sodium phosphate in a stable, buffered aqueous solution.

INDICATIONS
As a laxative, for the relief of occasional constipation. As a purgative, for use as part of a bowel cleansing regimen in preparing the patient for surgery or for preparing the colon for x-ray or endoscopic examination.

ACTION AND USES
Versatile in action as a gentle laxative or purgative, according to dosage. This product produces a bowel movement in ½ to 6 hours, depending on dosage. Especially useful as a preparation for colonoscopy. See DOSAGE AND ADMINISTRATION. Patient instruction pads available upon request.

CONTRAINDICATIONS
DO NOT USE THIS PRODUCT IF YOU HAVE KIDNEY DISEASE OR ARE ON A SODIUM RESTRICTED DIET UNLESS DIRECTED BY A PHYSICIAN.

PROFESSIONAL USE WARNINGS
Do not use in patients with congenital megacolon or congestive heart failure, as hypernatremic dehydration may occur. Use with caution in patients with impaired renal function as hypocalcemia, hyperphosphatemia, hypernatremia and acidosis may occur. Since Fleet® Phospho®-Soda contains dibasic sodium phosphate and monobasic sodium phosphate, there is a risk of acute elevation of sodium concentration in the serum and consequent dehydration, particularly in children with megacolon. Additional fluids by mouth are recommended where appropriate. (Fonkalsrud, E. and Keen, J.: "Hypernatremic Dehydration Hypertonic Enemas in Congenital Megacolon," *JAMA* 199:584–586, 1967. Zumoff, B. and Hellman, L.: "Rectal Absorption of Sodium from Hypertonic Sodium Phosphate Solutions," data on file, C. B. Fleet Company, Inc. Gilman, A., Goodman, L., Gilman, A., eds., *The Pharmacological Basis of Therapeutics*, Sixth Edition, 1980, p. 1005.) In addition, elevated levels of serum phosphates and decreased levels of serum calcium have been reported in patients with renal disease (and with prolonged use). (McConnell, T. H., "Fatal Hypocalcemia from Phosphate Absorption from Laxative Preparation," *JAMA*, 216:147–148, 1971.) SINCE FLEET® PHOSPHO®-SODA IS AVAILABLE IN THREE SIZES, PRESCRIBE BY VOLUMES. DO NOT PRESCRIBE "BY THE BOTTLE" AS SERIOUS SIDE EFFECTS FROM OVERDOSAGE MAY OCCUR.

GENERAL LAXATIVE WARNINGS
Do not use a laxative product when nausea, vomiting, or abdominal pain is present unless directed by a physician. If you have noticed a sudden change in bowel habits that persists over a period of 2 weeks, consult a physician before using a laxative. Rectal bleeding or failure to have a bowel movement may indicate a serious condition. Discontinue use and consult a physician. Laxative products should not be used longer than 1 week unless directed by a physician. Each teaspoonful (5 ml) contains 550 mg (24.1 milliequivalents) sodium. DO NOT USE THIS PRODUCT IF YOU ARE ON A SODIUM RESTRICTED DIET OR IF YOU HAVE KIDNEY DISEASE UNLESS DIRECTED BY A DOCTOR. SERIOUS SIDE EFFECTS FROM OVERDOSAGE MAY OCCUR. Keep this and all drugs out of the reach of children. In case of accidental overdose or ingestion, seek professional assistance or contact a Poison Control Center immediately. As with any drug, if you are pregnant or nursing a baby, seek the advice of a health professional before using this product.

OVERDOSAGE
Overdosage with Fleet® Phospho®-Soda may cause hypocalcemia, hyperphosphatemia, hypernatremia, hypernatremic dehydration and acidosis.
1. Hypocalcemia, hyperphosphatemia, hypernatremia and acidosis
   Calcium, Phosphate, Chloride and Sodium levels should be carefully monitored. Immediate corrective action should be taken to restore electrolyte balance with appropriate fluid replacements.
2. Hypernatremic Dehydration
   Calcium, Phosphate, Chloride and Sodium levels should be carefully monitored. Prompt parenteral administration of fluids with lower concentrations of Sodium and Chloride than extracellular fluid (40–50 mEq./liter) and moderate concentration of Potassium (20–30 mEq./liter) administered at a rate of 3,000 to 4,000 cc/sq. m of body surface during the first 12 to 24 hours dependent on the severity of dehydration and the clinical response (Fonkalsrud, E. and Keen, J.: "Hypernatremic Dehydration from Hypertonic Enemas in Congenital Megacolon." JAMA 199:584–586, 1967). See article for more details.

DOSAGE AND ADMINISTRATION
For purgative or laxative, best taken on an empty stomach. Most effective when taken upon rising, at least 30 minutes before a meal, or at bedtime for overnight action. Dilute recommended dosage with one-half glass (4 fl. oz.) cool water. Drink, then follow with one glass (8 fl. oz.) cool water.
DOSAGE: SINCE FLEET® PHOSPHO®-SODA IS AVAILABLE IN THREE SIZES, PRESCRIBE BY VOLUMES; DO NOT PRESCRIBE BY THE BOTTLE. DO NOT EXCEED RECOMMENDED DOSAGE AS SERIOUS SIDE EFFECTS MAY OCCUR.
SINGLE DAILY DOSAGE: DO NOT EXCEED.
LAXATIVE: Adults and children 12 years and over: 4 teaspoonfuls (20 ml).
Children 10 to under 12 years: 2 teaspoonfuls (10 ml).
Children 5 to under 10 years: 1 teaspoonful (5 ml).
PURGATIVE: Adults only: 3 tablespoonfuls (45 ml).
DO NOT GIVE TO CHILDREN UNDER 5 YEARS.
For colonoscopy, especially useful when taken as follows: 1½ fl. oz. (added to 4 fl. oz. water) 6 PM evening before exam (followed by three (3) 8 fl. oz. portions of clear liquids before retiring) and 1½ fl. oz. (added to 4 fl. oz. water) morning of exam. It is recommended that the prep be completed at least 3 hours in advance of appointment. Timing of dosage regimen can be adjusted by the physician.
Each teaspoonful (5 ml) contains: Active Ingredients: Monobasic Sodium Phosphate 2.4 g and Dibasic Sodium Phosphate 0.9 g. Each teaspoonful (5 ml) contains 550 mg (24.1 milliequivalents) sodium.

HOW SUPPLIED
Regular or Flavored, in bottles of 1½, 3, and 8 fl. oz. Fleet® Phospho®-Soda should not be confused with Fleet® Enema, a sodium phosphates disposable ready-to-use enema. Fleet® Enema, Adult and Child size, ARE NOT INTENDED FOR ORAL CONSUMPTION, in any dosage size.

IS THIS PRODUCT OTC?
Yes.

LITERATURE AVAILABLE
Professional literature mailed on request.

FLEET® PREP KITS　　OTC
Bowel Evacuant

DESCRIPTION
FLEET® Prep Kit No. 1 contains:
1. FLEET® Phospho®-Soda—1½ fl. oz. Ingredients: Each teaspoonful (5 ml) contains : Active Ingredients: Monobasic sodium phosphate 2.4 G and dibasic sodium phosphate 0.9 G.
2. FLEET® Bisacodyl—4 laxative tablets. Ingredients: Each enteric-coated tablet contains Bisacodyl, USP, 5 mg.
3. FLEET® Bisacodyl—1 laxative suppository. Ingredients: Bisacodyl, USP, 10 mg.
4. 1 Patient Instruction Sheet.
FLEET® Prep Kit No. 2 contains:
1. FLEET® Phospho®-Soda—1½ fl. oz.
2. FLEET® Bisacodyl—4 tablets.
3. FLEET® Bagenema—1. Ingredients: Liquid castile soap ⅔ fl. oz.
4. 1 Patient Instruction Sheet.
FLEET® Prep Kit No. 3 contains:
1. FLEET® Phospho®-Soda—1½ fl. oz.
2. FLEET® Bisacodyl—4 tablets.
3. FLEET® Bisacodyl Enema—1 laxative enema. Ingredients: 1–30 ml. dose containing 10 mg. of Bisacodyl.
4. 1 Patient Instruction Sheet.
FLEET® Prep Kit No. 4 contains:
1. FLEET® Flavored Castor Oil Emulsion-1½ fl. oz. Ingredients: Each tablespoonful (15 ml.) contains: Active Ingredients: Castor Oil U.S.P. 10 ml.
2. FLEET® Bisacodyl—4 tablets.
3. FLEET® Bisacodyl—1 suppository.
4. 1 Patient Instruction Sheet.
FLEET® Prep Kit No. 5 contains:
1. FLEET® Flavored Castor Oil Emulsion-1½ fl. oz.
2. FLEET® Bisacodyl—4 tablets.
3. FLEET® Bagenema—1.
4. 1 Patient Instruction Sheet.
FLEET® Prep Kit No. 6 contains:
1. FLEET® Flavored Castor Oil Emulsion-1½ fl. oz.
2. FLEET® Bisacodyl—4 tablets.
3. FLEET® Bisacodyl Enema—30 ml.
4. 1 Patient Instruction Sheet.

ACTIONS
Bowel Cleansing System

Continued on next page

Fleet—Cont.

INDICATIONS

For use as part of a bowel cleansing regimen in preparation of the colon for radiology (prior to barium enemas or I.V.P.'s), surgery, and many proctologic and colonoscopic procedures.

WARNINGS

Each recommended dose (1½ fl. oz.) (45 ml) of Phospho®-Soda contains 216.9 milli-equivalents (MEq) of sodium. Persons on a sodium restricted diet or with kidney disease should consult a health professional before use.

Castor oil affects the small intestine, and regular use may cause excessive loss of water and body salts which can have debilitating effects.

Bisacodyl products may cause abdominal discomfort, faintness, rectal burning, and mild cramps.

GENERAL LAXATIVE WARNINGS

Do not use a laxative product when nausea, vomiting, or abdominal pain is present unless directed by a physician. If you have noticed a sudden change in bowel habits that persists over a period of 2 weeks, consult a doctor before using a laxative. Rectal bleeding or failure to have a bowel movement may indicate a serious condition. Discontinue use and consult a physician. Laxative products should not be used longer than 1 week unless directed by a physician. Frequent or prolonged use of a laxative may result in dependence on laxatives. Keep this and all drugs out of the reach of children. In case of accidental overdose or ingestion, seek professional assistance or contact a Poison Control Center immediately.

PROFESSIONAL USE WARNINGS

Do not use in patients with congenital megacolon or congestive heart failure as hypernatremic dehydration may occur. Use with caution in patients with impaired renal function or where colostomy exists as hypocalcemia, hyperphosphatemia, hypernatremia and acidosis may occur. Since FLEET® Phospho®-Soda contains monobasic sodium phosphate and dibasic sodium phosphate, there is a risk of acute elevation of sodium concentration in the serum and consequent dehydration, particularly in children with megacolon. Additional fluids by mouth are recommended where appropriate. (Fonkalsrud, E. and Keen, J.: "Hypernatremic Dehydration Hypertonic Enemas in Congenital Megacolon," *JAMA* 199:584–586, 1967. Zumoff, B. and Hellman, L.: "Rectal Absorption of Sodium from Hypertonic Sodium Phosphate Solutions," data on file, C. B. Fleet Company, Inc. Gilman, A., Goodman, L., Gilman, A., eds., *The Pharmacological Basis of Therapeutics*, Sixth Edition, 1980, p. 1005.) In addition, elevated levels of serum phosphates and decreased levels of serum calcium have been reported in patients with renal disease (and with prolonged use). (McConnell, T. H., "Fatal Hypocalcemia from Phosphate Absorption from Laxative Preparation," *JAMA*, 216:147–148, 1971.) If any of these complications occur following administration of FLEET® Phospho®-Soda, immediate corrective action should be taken to restore electrolyte balance with appropriate fluid replacements. Calcium and phosphorous levels should be carefully monitored. **See individual listings (Fleet® Phospho®-Soda, Fleet® Bisacodyl Enema and Fleet® Flavored Castor Oil Emulsion) for additional warnings.**
THESE KITS SHOULD NOT BE USED BY PATIENTS UNDER 12 YEARS OF AGE.

DOSAGE AND ADMINISTRATION

SEE PATIENT INSTRUCTION SHEET FOR 12, 24, AND 48 HOUR PREPARATION SCHEDULE IN EACH KIT.

HOW SUPPLIED

See "Description" for contents of each kit.
Shipping Unit: 48 FLEET® Prep Kits per carton.
For full prescribing information on specific products, see individual listings (FLEET® Phospho®-Soda, FLEET® Bisacodyl Enema and FLEET® Flavored Castor Oil Emulsion).

IS THIS PRODUCT OTC?
Yes.

LITERATURE AVAILABLE
Yes.

FLEET® FLAVORED CASTOR OIL EMULSION, A STIMULANT LAXATIVE   OTC

INGREDIENTS

Each tablespoonful (15 ml.) contains:

ACTIVE INGREDIENTS

Castor Oil U.S.P. 10 ml.

INDICATIONS

As a laxative, for the relief of occasional constipation. As a purgative, for the preparation of the colon for x-ray or endoscopic examination. (See FLEET® Prep Kit listings.)

ACTIONS

Works directly on the small intestine to promote bowel movement. This product usually produces a bowel movement in 6 to 12 hours.

WARNINGS

Do not use laxative products when nausea, vomiting or abdominal pain is present unless directed by a physician. If you have noticed a sudden change in bowel habits that persists over a period of 2 weeks, consult a physician before using a laxative. Laxative products should not be used longer than 1 week unless directed by a physician. Rectal bleeding or failure to have a bowel movement may indicate a serious condition. Discontinue use and consult a physician. Castor oil affects the small intestine and regular use may cause excessive loss of water and body salts, which can have a debilitating effect. Keep this and all drugs out of the reach of children. In case of accidental overdose, seek professional assistance or contact a Poison Control Center immediately. As with any drug, if you are pregnant or nursing a baby, seek the advice of a health professional before using this product.

DOSAGE AND ADMINISTRATION

FLEET® Flavored Castor Oil Emulsion Stimulant Laxative is best taken on an empty stomach. May be chilled to enhance taste; avoid freezing. **Shake well before use.** Follow recommended dosage with one glass (8 fl. oz.) cool water.
SINGLE DAILY DOSAGE
LAXATIVE: Adults and children 12 years and over: 3 tablespoonfuls (45 ml).
Children 2 to under 12 years: 1 tablespoonful (15 ml).
Children under 2 years: consult a physician.
PURGATIVE: Adults and children 12 years and over: 6 tablespoonfuls (90 ml).

HOW SUPPLIED

Bottles of 1½ and 3 fl. oz.

IS THIS PRODUCT OTC?
Yes.

FLEET® RELIEF   OTC
Medicated Hemorrhoidal Ointment

ACTIVE INGREDIENT

Tube: Zinc Oxide, White Petrolatum, and Mineral Oil
Applicator: Zinc Oxide in a water-soluble ointment and White Petrolatum on the tip as a protectant and lubricant. An anorectal product.

INDICATIONS

FDA APPROVED USES. Applicator: An astringent in a lubricating base that gives temporary relief of itching and discomfort associated with inflamed hemorrhoidal tissues. **Tube:** A special combination of protectants and an astringent that gives temporary relief of itching and discomfort associated with inflamed hemorrhoidal tissues.

ACTIONS

Rapid action; temporarily coats and protects affected areas to ease pain, itching, and burning associated with hemorrhoids.

WARNING

Consult a doctor promptly if condition worsens or does not improve within seven days; if bleeding occurs; or if the introduction of the applicator into the rectum causes additional pain. As with any drug, if you are pregnant or nursing a baby, seek the advice of a health professional before using this product. In case of accidental ingestion, seek professional assistance or contact a Poison Control Center immediately. Keep this and all other drugs out of the reach of children. Do not exceed recommended dosage unless directed by a doctor.

DIRECTIONS FOR USE

When practical, cleanse the affected area with mild soap and warm water and rinse thoroughly. Gently dry by patting or blotting with toilet tissue or soft cloth before application of this product.
Applicator: Internal: Remove protective shield and gently insert prelubricated stem into the rectum. Squeeze the bulb gently, but firmly to expel the medication. While continuing to squeeze the bulb, remove the stem and discard the unit. **External:** Remove protective shield. Apply ointment to external areas. **Tube: Internal:** Attach enclosed applicator to tube. Lubricate with small amount of ointment, insert gently into rectum, and squeeze tube. **Caution: Applicator must be cleaned thoroughly after each use. External:** Apply ointment to external areas. Dosage: Tube and applicator Adults: Apply

---

to the affected area up to six times daily or after each bowel movement. Children under 12 years of age: Consult a doctor.

HOW SUPPLIED

Six 4 ml. rectal applicators or single one ounce tube with applicator.

IS THIS PRODUCT OTC?
Yes.

SUMMER'S EVE®   OTC
MEDICATED DOUCHE

ACTIVE INGREDIENT

Povidone-iodine provided as a .30 percent solution when packet and sanitized fluid are mixed.

INDICATIONS

For temporary relief of minor vaginal irritation and itching. Clinically effective in a program of treatment for vaginal moniliasis, T. vaginales vaginitis and non-specific vaginitis due to Candida albicans, Trichomonas vaginalis, and Gardnerella vaginalis.

ACTIONS

Povidone-iodine is an effective broad spectrum anti-microbial agent used in treatment of both gram negative and gram positive bacteria, fungi, yeast, and protozoa.

WARNINGS

DOUCHING DOES NOT PREVENT PREGNANCY.
Do not use during pregnancy or if nursing a baby except under the advice and supervision of a physician. If symptoms persist after seven days, discontinue use and consult a physician. If douching results in pain, soreness, swelling, redness, itching, excessive dryness or irritation, discontinue use. An association has been reported between frequent douching and pelvic inflammatory disease (PID), a serious infection of the reproductive system. It is not currently known whether frequent douching is causally related to PID, but women should be aware of this association. Douching should not be used for self-treatment if you have symptoms of PID or STD. PID symptoms include lower abdominal pain, fever, chills, nausea, vomiting, and/or a pus-like yellow cervical discharge. STD symptoms include vaginal discharge of an unusual amount, color or odor; painful and/or frequent urination; and genital sores or ulcers. If you have any of these symptoms or suspect you may have been exposed to a STD, do not use this product, or any douche, and consult a physician immediately. Women with iodine sensitivity should not use this product. The use of iodine as a douche may cause a transient rise of serum protein-bound iodine. Keep this and all drugs out of the reach of children. In case of accidental ingestion, seek professional assistance or contact a Poison Control Center immediately.

DOSAGE AND ADMINISTRATION

Dosage is contained in a single-unit concentrate packet to be added to 4.5 fluid ounces of sanitized solution supplied in a disposable unit. Use once daily for seven days even if symptoms disappear sooner. To use, remove sanitary overwrap. Unscrew nozzle cap. Carefully open the medicated packet and pour its contents into the bottle. (The contents may stain certain materials). Screw the nozzle cap back onto the bottle. Swirl bottle gently to assure complete mixing. Hold cap of bottle with one hand and grasp Comfortip™ nozzle with the other. IMPORTANT: Pull nozzle straight up until it clicks in place. This indicates the nozzle is locked and ready for use. (Unit is not ready to use until you hear this click). Gently insert nozzle into vagina, no more than 3 inches, and slowly squeeze the bottle. Do not close the vaginal opening; douching solution should flow freely out of vagina. Use while sitting on the toilet, in the tub, or while standing in the shower.

HOW SUPPLIED

4.5 fluid ounce single pack with one 0.14 fluid ounce medicated packet or twin pack containing two 4.5 fluid ounce units and two 0.14 fluid ounce packets.

IS THIS PRODUCT OTC?
Yes.

Products are cross-indexed
by product classifications
in the
BLUE SECTION.

Fleming & Company
1600 FENPARK DR.
FENTON, MO 63026

AEROLATE SR & JR & III Capsules   ℞
(theophylline, anhydrous T.D.)

AEROLATE LIQUID
(theophylline, anhydrous)

COMPOSITION
Contains theophylline 4 grs. (260 mg) as SR, 2 grs (130 mg) as JR, 1 gr. as III (65 mg) in red/clear capsules. Liquid has 150 mg theophylline/15cc in a non-sugar, non-alcoholic, non-saccharin tangerine flavored base.

ACTION AND USES
Timed action pellets by-pass stomach to prevent gastric upset. Bronchodilation is achieved through bowel absorption only. Liquid is for the acute attack primarily.

ADMINISTRATION AND DOSAGE
One capsule every 12 hours. Every 8 hours in severe attacks. Liquid—adults—40 ml (2.5 tablespoonfuls) for acute attack. Children—0.25 ml/lb. Maintainance therapy—adults—for the first 6 doses, 25 ml (1.5 tablespoonfuls) before breakfast, at 3 p.m., at bedtime. Then 15 ml doses at above times. Children—0.15 ml/lb at these times, then 0.1 ml/lb per dose.

SIDE EFFECTS
Nausea, vomiting, epigastric or substernal pain, palpitation, headache, dizziness may occur.

HOW SUPPLIED
Capsules in bottles of 100.
Liquid in pints and gallons.

CHLOR–3   OTC

DESCRIPTION
Medical condiment containing sodium chloride 50%; potassium chloride 30%; magnesium chloride 20%.

INDICATIONS AND USAGE
To reduce sodium intake for patients on diuretics; for potential hypertensives and cardiacs.
To encourage physicians to recommend a condiment to replace "table salt" for family use and gourmet cooking.

HOW SUPPLIED
Shaker 8 oz. plastic bottles.

CONGESS SR & JR Capsules   ℞
Expectorant/Decongestant T.D.

COMPOSITION
Contains guaifenesin 250 mgs/pseudoephedrine 120 mgs as SR; guaifenesin 125 mgs/pseudoephedrine 60 mgs as JR in blue/pink capsules.

ACTION AND USES
To loosen mucus plugs in upper respiratory tract and congestion in acute pulmonary disorders, and in coughing. Nasal decongestion and alleviation of bronchospasm is also achieved up to 12 hrs. that accompany most coughs, especially during the nocturnal period.

INDICATIONS
Nasal congestion, sinusitis, acute aerotitis media, bronchial asthma, serous otitis media, and symptoms of the common cold.

DOSAGE
Adults and children over 12 yrs. one SR capsule every 12 hrs. Under 12 yrs. one JR capsule as prescribed by physician.

PRECAUTION AND SIDE EFFECTS
Use with care in severe hypertension, heart disease, hyperthyroidism, diabetes. Low grade sensitivity to drugs may be experienced.

CONTRAINDICATIONS
Prostatic hypertrophy, patients receiving MAO inhibitors.

HOW SUPPLIED
Plastic bottles of 100 and 1000 capsules.

EXTENDRYL   ℞
T.D. Capsules SR & JR, Syrup and Tablets

Each timed action SR capsule contains phenylephrine HCl 20 mg; methscopolamine nitrate 2.5 mg; chlorpheniramine maleate 8 mg. The JR potency is exactly half-strength. Green/red color for both. Each 5 cc of root beer flavored syrup and tablet contains: phenylephrine HCl 10 mg; methscopolamine nitrate 1.25 mg; chlorpheniramine maleate 2 mg.

ACTION AND USES
Antihistaminic-decongestant for relief of respiratory congestion; allergic rhinitis; allergic skin reactions of urticaria and angioedema.

ADMINISTRATION AND DOSAGE
Capsules—one every 12 hrs of the SR for adults; one JR every 12 hrs for children 6–12 yrs. Syrup-two teaspoonfuls every 4 hrs for adults; children 1 teaspoonful every 4 hrs. Tablets—adults two and children one every 4 hrs. Do not exceed 4 doses in 24 hrs.
Children under 6 yrs. as recommended by a physician.

PRECAUTIONS
Withdraw therapy if drowsiness occurs. Patients are cautioned against driving or operating mechanical devices.

CONTRAINDICATIONS
Glaucoma, cardiac disease, hyperthyroidism and hypertension.

HOW SUPPLIED
Capsules and tablets in bottles of 100 and 1000. Syrup in pints and gallons.

IMPREGON Concentrate   OTC

ACTIVE INGREDIENT
Tetrachlorosalicylanilide 2%

INDICATIONS
Diaper Rash Relief, 'Staph' control, Mold inhibitor.

ACTIONS
This is a bacteriostatic/fungistatic agent for home usage and hospital usage.

WARNINGS
Impregon should not be exposed to direct sunlight for long periods after applications.

PRECAUTION
Addition of bleach prior to diaper treatment negates application effects.

DOSAGE AND ADMINISTRATION
One capful (5ml) per gallon of water to impregnate diapers in the diaper pail. Dilutions for many home areas accompany the full package.

NOTE
For disposable-type diapers, add one teaspoonful to 8 oz of water to a 'Windex-type' sprayer. Spray middle half area of diapers until damp, and allow to dry before using, to prevent rashes.

HOW SUPPLIED
Four ounce amber plastic bottles.

MAGONATE TABLETS   OTC
MAGONATE LIQUID
Magnesium Gluconate (Dihydrate)

ACTIVE INGREDIENTS
Each tablet contains magnesium gluconate (dihydrate) 500mg (27mg of Mg^{++}). Each 5cc of Magonate Liquid contains magnesium gluconate (dihydrate) 1000mg (54mg of Mg^{++}).

INDICATIONS
For all patients in negative magnesium balance.

PRECAUTION
Excessive dosage may cause loose stools.

DOSAGE AND ADMINISTRATION
Magonate is recommended during and for three weeks after a course in chemotherapy, then monitored regularly.
Adults and children over 12 yrs.—one or two tablets or ½ to 1 teaspoon of liquid t.i.d. Under 12 yrs.—one tablet or ½ teaspoon of liquid t.i.d. Dosage may be increased in severe cases.

HOW SUPPLIED
Magonate Tablets are supplied in bottles of 100 and 1000 tablets. Magonate Liquid is supplied in pints and gallons.

MARBLEN   OTC
(calcium and magnesium carbonates)
ANTACID SUSPENSIONS AND TABLET

(See PDR For Nonprescription Drugs.)

NEPHROCAPS   ℞
Dialysis Vitamin Supplement

DESCRIPTION
Each black oval gelatin 'liquid' capsule provides:
Thiamin 1.5 mg; Riboflavin 1.7 mg; Niacin 20 mg; Pantothenic acid 5 mg; Biotin 150 mcg; Cyanocobalamin 6 mcg; Pyridoxin 10 mg; Ascorbic acid 100 mg and Folic acid 1.0 mg.

INDICATIONS
The wasting syndrome in chronic renal failure; uremia; impaired metabolic functions of the kidney.

DOSAGE
One capsule daily. On dialysis days, one Nephrocap must be taken after treatment.

SUPPLIED
Plastic bottles of 100 only.

NEPHROX SUSPENSION   OTC
(aluminum hydroxide)
Antacid Suspension

(See PDR For Nonprescription Drugs.)

NICOTINEX Elixir   OTC
nicotinic acid

(See PDR For Nonprescription Drugs.)

OCEAN MIST   OTC
(buffered isotonic saline)

(See PDR For Nonprescription Drugs.)

PIMA Syrup   ℞
(potassium iodide)

COMPOSITION
Contains KI 5 grs./tsp., in a black raspberry flavored base.

ACTION AND USES
An expectorant in the symptomatic treatment of chronic pulmonary diseases where tenacious mucus complicates the problem, including bronchial asthma, bronchitis and pulmonary emphysema.

ADMINISTRATION AND DOSAGE
Children—one half to one tsp. and adults one or two tsp. every 4-6 hours.

SIDE EFFECTS
May include gastrointestinal upset, metallic taste, minor skin eruptions, nausea, vomiting and epigastric pain. Therapy should be withdrawn.

PRECAUTIONS
In patients sensitive to iodides, in hyperthyroidism, and in rare cases iodine-induced goiter may occur.

HOW SUPPLIED
Plastic pints and gallons.

PURGE   OTC
(flavored castor oil)

(See PDR For Nonprescription Drugs.)

RUM–K   ℞
(potassium chloride 15% conc.)

DESCRIPTION
Each 10 ml. contains 1.5 Gm. potassium chloride (20 mEq) in a butter/rum synthetic flavored base that is alcohol and sugar free.

INDICATIONS
Hypokalemic-hypochloremic alkalosis; digitalis toxicity; hypokalemia prevention secondary to corticosteroid or diuretic administration.

CONTRAINDICATIONS
Impaired renal function, untreated Addison's Disease, acute dehydration, heat cramps, hyperkalemia.

Continued on next page

Fleming—Cont.

PRECAUTIONS

Do not use in patients with low urinary output or renal decompensation. Potassium replacements vary and should be individualized. Patients should be checked frequently, ECG and plasma K^+ levels should be made. High serum concentrations of K^+ cause death thru cardiac depression, arrhythmias or arrest. Use with caution in cardiac disease.

ADVERSE REACTIONS

Vomiting, nausea, abdominal discomfort, diarrhea may occur. Symptoms and signs of potassium overdose include paresthesias of extremities, flaccid paralysis, listlessness, fall in blood pressure, weakness and heaviness of the legs, cardiac arrhythmias and heart block. Hyperkalemia may cause ECG changes as disappearance of the P wave, widening and slurring of QRS complex, changes of the S-T segment, tall peaked T waves.

DOSAGE AND ADMINISTRATION

Adults—two teaspoonsful (10ml) in 4–6 oz water 2 to 4 times daily after meals to supply 40–80 mEq of elemental potassium and chloride. Larger doses may be required and administered under close supervision due to possible potassium intoxication or saline laxative effect.

HOW SUPPLIED

2 oz; 4 oz; pints and gallons.

S-P-T   ℞
(Pork thyroid "liquid" capsules USP)

COMPOSITION

S-P-T is prepared by special process from cleaned, fresh pork thyroid glands, deprived of connective tissue, defatted and suspended in soy bean oil and encapsulated in gelatin for greater oral absorption. The active hormones (T4 and T3) are available in their natural state in a ratio of approximately 2.5:1, as in humans, to insure therapeutic availability. Capsules are standardized by USP method for iodine content and also biologically to insure 100% metabolic potency.

ACTION

To increase metabolic rate of body tissues. S-P-T is replacement therapy for diminished or absent thyroid function. Effect develops slowly and is fully reached in 10—14 days per grain increase in most instances.

INDICATIONS

As replacement therapy in hypothyroidism, cretinism, myxedema, and after surgery following complete thyroidectomy.

CONTRAINDICATIONS

In thyrotoxicosis, angina pectoris, myocardial infarction and hypertension unless complicated by hypothyroidism, and uncorrected adrenal insufficiency.

PRECAUTION AND SIDE EFFECTS

Overdosage may cause tachycardia, angina pectoris, diarrhea, nervousness, sweating, headache and increased pulse action. In most cases, reduction of dosage overcomes side effects.

DOSAGE AND ADMINISTRATION

Patients should be titrated starting at lower levels and increasing by 1 gr every 2 weeks until mild thyromimetic effects are noted. Then lower the dose to the level at which the patient felt best, as patients vary widely as to thyroid need.

> **WARNINGS**
>
> Drugs with thyroid hormone activity, alone or together with other therapeutic agents, have been used for the treatment of obesity. In euthyroid patients, doses within the range of daily hormonal requirements are ineffective for weight reduction. Larger doses may produce serious or even life-threatening manifestations of toxicity, particularly when given in association with sympathomimetic amines such as those used for their anorectic effects.

HOW SUPPLIED

As 1 gr (green); 2 gr (brown); 3 gr (red); 5 gr (black) gelatin sealed capsules in bottles of 100 and 1000.

Products are cross-indexed by
generic and chemical names in the
YELLOW SECTION.

Fluoritab Corporation
P.O. BOX 507
TEMPERANCE, MICHIGAN 48182-0507

FLUORITAB®   ℞
Sodium Fluoride supplements
Tablets, Full-strength 1.0 mg F
        Half-strength 0.5 mg F
Liquid, 0.25 mg F per drop

DESCRIPTION

FLUORITAB fluoride supplements are for use as a dental caries preventive in children. FLUORITAB TABLETS and FLUORITAB LIQUID provide the recommended fluoride to children in communities where water supplies are deficient in fluoride (less than 0.7 ppm F).

CLINICAL PHARMACOLOGY

Sodium Fluoride acts systemically and topically in the reduction of dental caries by promoting remineralization, by inhibiting the cariogenic microbial process, and by converting enamel hydroxapatite crystals to fluorapatite which is more resistant to acid dissolution.

ADMINISTRATION AND DOSAGE

	Fluoride in Drinking Water Supply		
Age of child	<0.3 ppm	0.3–0.7 ppm	>0.7 ppm
Birth to 2 yrs.	0.25*	0	0
2–3 yrs.	0.50	0.25	0
3–14 yrs.	1.00	0.50	0

* In mg. of fluoride ion per day

FLUORITAB TABLETS can be chewed or permitted to dissolve in the mouth. FLUORITAB LIQUID can be dropped directly into the mouth or added to most liquids.

CONTRAINDICATIONS

Dietary fluoride supplements should not be used where water with 0.7 ppm of fluoride is available.

OVERDOSAGE

Excess fluoride is to be avoided, as it may cause dental fluorosis.

HOW SUPPLIED

FLUORITAB TABLETS 1.0 mg F from 2.2 mg NaF in 100, 1000,* and 5000* tablet bottles. Available in pineapple and cherry flavors.
FLUORITAB TABLETS 0.5 mg F from 1.1 mg NaF in 1000* and 5000* tablet bottles available in pineapple flavor.
All Fluoritab tablets are dye-free and scored.
FLUORITAB LIQUID 0.25 mg F per drop, 22.8 ml—475 drop, squeeze drop bottle. No artificial flavor or color added.

REMARKS

FLUORITAB sodium fluoride supplements have been given American Dental Association "Acceptance" since 1958.

LITERATURE AVAILABLE

Prescription pads, ordering information, and educational folders will be sent free on request.

* For dispensing only

Forest Pharmaceuticals, Inc.
(Subsidiary of Forest Laboratories, Inc.)
2510 METRO BLVD.
ST. LOUIS, MO 63043

AEROBID®   ℞
AEROBID-M
(flunisolide)
Inhaler system
For oral inhalation only

PRODUCT OVERVIEW

KEY FACTS

The active component of the AEROBID/AEROBID-M Inhaler System is flunisolide which is an anti-inflammatory steroid. Each metered inhalation delivers about 250 mcg of flunisolide. Clinical studies indicate that recommended doses confer topical therapeutic activity on bronchial mucosa with minimal evidence of systemic action. Patients have been able to tolerate significant decreases in their systemic steroid dosages while using flunisolide.

MAJOR USES

AEROBID/AEROBID-M Inhaler System is to be used in patients who need chronic corticosteroid therapy in order to control their bronchial asthma symptoms.

SAFETY INFORMATION

Contraindicated in patients who are allergic to any of the ingredients used in the formulation of AEROBID/AEROBID-M. This product is not to be used in the primary treatment of status asthmaticus or other serious, acute episodes of asthma. Because AEROBID/AEROBID-M is not regarded as a bronchodilator, it should not be employed for rapid relief of bronchospasm.

PRESCRIBING INFORMATION

AEROBID®   ℞
AEROBID-M
(flunisolide)
Inhaler system
For oral inhalation only

DESCRIPTION

Flunisolide, the active component of AEROBID/AEROBID-M Inhaler System, is an anti-inflammatory steroid having the chemical name 6α-fluoro-11β, 16α, 17, 21-tetrahydroxypregna-1, 4-diene-3, 20-dione cyclic-16, 17-acetal with acetone. It has the following structure:

Flunisolide is a white to creamy white crystalline powder with a molecular weight of 434.49. It is soluble in acetone, sparingly soluble in chloroform, slightly soluble in methanol, and practically insoluble in water. It has a melting point of about 245℃.

AEROBID/AEROBID-M Inhaler is delivered in a metered-dose aerosol system containing a microcrystalline suspension of flunisolide as the hemihydrate in propellants (trichloromonofluoromethane, dichlorodifluoromethane and dichlorotetrafluoroethane) with sorbitan trioleate as a dispersing agent. AEROBID-M also contains menthol as a flavoring agent. Each activation delivers approximately 250 mcg of flunisolide to the patient. One AEROBID/AEROBID-M Inhaler System is designed to deliver at least 100 metered inhalations.

CLINICAL PHARMACOLOGY

Flunisolide has demonstrated marked anti-inflammatory and anti-allergic activity in classical test systems. It is a corticosteroid that is several hundred times more potent in animal anti-inflammatory assays than the cortisol standard. The molar dose of each activation of flunisolide in this preparation is approximately 2½ to 7 times that of comparable inhaled corticosteroid products marketed for the same indication. The dose of flunisolide delivered per activation in this preparation is 10 times that per activation of Nasalide® (flunisolide) nasal solution. Clinical studies have shown therapeutic activity on bronchial mucosa with minimal evidence of systemic activity at recommended doses.

After oral inhalation of 1 mg flunisolide, total systemic availability was 40%. The flunisolide that is swallowed is rapidly and extensively converted to the 6β-OH metabolite and to water-soluble conjugates during the first pass through the liver. This offers a metabolic explanation for the low systemic activity of oral flunisolide itself since the metabolite has low corticosteroid potency (on the order of the cortisol standard). The inhaled flunisolide absorbed through the bronchial tree is converted to the same metabolites. Repeated inhalation of 2.0 mg of flunisolide per day (the maximum recommended dose) for 14 days did not show accumulation of the drug in plasma. The plasma half-life of flunisolide is approximately 1.8 hours.

The following observations relevant to systemic absorption were made in clinical studies. In one uncontrolled study a statistically significant decrease in responsiveness to metyrapone was noted in 15 adult steroid-independent patients treated with 2.0 mg of flunisolide per day (the maximum recommended dose) for 3 months. A small but statistically significant drop in eosinophils from 11.5% to 7.4% of total circulating leucocytes was noted in another study in children who were not taking oral corticosteroids simultaneously. A 5% incidence of menstrual disturbances was reported during open studies, in which there were no control groups for comparison.

Aerosol administration of flunisolide 2.0 mg twice daily for one week to 6 healthy male subjects revealed neither suppression of adrenal function as measured by early morning cortisol levels nor impairment of HPA axis function as determined by insulin hypoglycemia tests.

Controlled clinical studies have included over 500 patients with asthma, among them 150 children age 6 and over. More than 120 patients have been treated in open trials for two

years or more. No significant adrenal suppression attributed to flunisolide was seen in these studies.

Significant decreases of systemic steroid dosages have been possible in flunisolide-treated patients. Asthma patients have had further symptomatic improvement with flunisolide treatment even while reducing concomitant medication.

INDICATIONS AND USAGE

AEROBID/AEROBID-M Inhaler is indicated only for patients who require chronic treatment with corticosteroids for control of the symptoms of bronchial asthma. Such patients would include those already receiving systemic corticosteroids, and selected patients who are inadequately controlled on a non-steroid regimen and in whom steroid therapy has been withheld because of concern over potential adverse effects.

As with any topically applied medication, flunisolide is absorbed through the mucous membrane and is systemically available. For these reasons, AEROBID/AEROBID-M Inhaler should be used with caution for initial therapy and the recommended dosage should not be exceeded. When the drug is used chronically at 2 mg/day, patients should be monitored periodically for effects on the hypothalamic-pituitary-adrenal axis.

AEROBID/AEROBID-M Inhaler is NOT indicated:
1. For relief of asthma that can be controlled by bronchodilators and other non-steroid medications.
2. In patients who require systemic corticosteroid treatment infrequently.
3. In the treatment of non-asthmatic bronchitis.

Insufficient information is available to warrant use in children under the age of 6.

CONTRAINDICATIONS

AEROBID/AEROBID-M Inhaler is contraindicated in the primary treatment of status asthmaticus or other acute episodes of asthma where intensive measures are required. Hypersensitivity to any of the ingredients of this preparation contraindicates its use.

WARNINGS

Particular care is needed in patients who are transferred from systemically active corticosteroids to AEROBID/AEROBID-M Inhaler because deaths due to adrenal insufficiency have occurred in asthmatic patients during and after transfer from systemic corticosteroids to aerosol corticosteroids. After withdrawal from systemic corticosteroids, a number of months are required for recovery of hypothalamic-pituitary-adrenal (HPA) function. During this period of HPA suppression, patients may exhibit signs and symptoms of adrenal insufficiency when exposed to trauma, surgery or infections, particularly gastroenteritis. Although AEROBID/AEROBID-M Inhaler may provide control of asthmatic symptoms during these episodes, it does NOT provide the systemic steroid that is necessary for coping with these emergencies.

During periods of stress or a severe asthmatic attack, patients who have been withdrawn from systemic corticosteroids should be instructed to resume systemic steroids (in large doses) immediately and to contact their physician for further instruction. These patients should also be instructed to carry a warning card indicating that they may need supplementary systemic steroids during periods of stress or a severe asthma attack. To assess the risk of adrenal insufficiency in emergency situations, routine tests of adrenal cortical function, including measurement of early morning resting cortisol levels, should be performed periodically in all patients. An early morning resting cortisol level may be accepted as normal if it falls at or near the normal mean level.

Localized infections with *Candida albicans* or *Aspergillus niger* have occurred in the mouth and pharynx and occasionally in the larynx. Positive cultures for oral *Candida* may be present in up to 34% of patients. Although the frequency of clinically apparent infection is considerably lower, these infections may require treatment with appropriate antifungal therapy or discontinuance of treatment with AEROBID/AEROBID-M inhaler.

AEROBID/AEROBID-M Inhaler is not to be regarded as a bronchodilator and is not indicated for rapid relief of bronchospasm.

Patients should be instructed to contact their physician immediately when episodes of asthma that are not responsive to bronchodilators occur during the course of treatment. During such episodes, patients may require therapy with systemic corticosteroids.

There is no evidence that control of asthma can be achieved by administration of the drug in amounts greater than the recommended doses, which appear to be the therapeutic equivalent of approximately 10 mg/day of oral prednisone. Theoretically, the use of inhaled corticosteroids with alternate day prednisone systemic treatment should be accompa-

---

nied by more HPA suppression than a therapeutically equivalent regimen of either alone.

Transfer of patients from systemic steroid therapy to AEROBID/AEROBID-M Inhaler may unmask allergic conditions previously suppressed by the systemic steroid therapy, e.g., rhinitis, conjunctivitis, and eczema.

Children who are on immunosuppressant drugs are more susceptible to infections than healthy children. Chicken pox and measles, for example, can have a more serious or even fatal course in children on immunosuppressant corticosteroids. In such children, or in adults who have not had these diseases, particular care should be taken to avoid exposure. If exposed, therapy with varicella zoster immune globulin (VZIG) or pooled intravenous immunoglobulin (IVIG), as appropriate, may be indicated. If chicken pox develops, treatment with antiviral agents may be considered.

PRECAUTIONS

General: Because of the relatively high molar dose of flunisolide per activation in this preparation, and because of the evidence suggesting higher levels of systemic absorption with flunisolide than with other comparable inhaled corticosteroids (see CLINICAL PHARMACOLOGY section), patients treated with AEROBID/AEROBID-M should be observed carefully for any evidence of systemic corticosteroid effect, including suppression of bone growth in children. Particular care should be taken in observing patients postoperatively or during periods of stress for evidence of a decrease in adrenal function. During withdrawal from oral steroids, some patients may experience symptoms of systemically active steroid withdrawal, e.g., joint and/or muscular pain, lassitude and depression, despite maintenance or even improvement of respiratory function (See DOSAGE AND ADMINISTRATION for details).

In responsive patients, flunisolide may permit control of asthmatic symptoms without suppression of HPA function. Since flunisolide is absorbed into the circulation and can be systemically active, the beneficial effects of AEROBID/AEROBID-M Inhaler in minimizing or preventing HPA dysfunction may be expected only when recommended dosages are not exceeded. The long-term effects of the drug in human subjects are still unknown. In particular, the local effects of the agent on developmental or immunologic processes in the mouth, pharynx, trachea, and lung are unknown. There is also no information about the possible long-term systemic effects of the agent.

The potential effects of the drug on acute, recurrent, or chronic pulmonary infections, including active or quiescent tuberculosis, are not known. Similarly, the potential effects of long-term administration of the drug on lung or other tissues are unknown.

Pulmonary infiltrates with eosinophilia may occur in patients on AEROBID/AEROBID-M Inhaler therapy. Although it is possible that in some patients this state may become manifest because of systemic steroid withdrawal when inhalational steroids are administered, a causative role for the drug and/or its vehicle cannot be ruled out.

Information for Patients

There is no evidence that better control of asthma can be achieved by the administration of AEROBID/AEROBID-M Inhaler in amounts greater than the recommended doses; higher doses may induce adrenal suppression.

Since the relief from AEROBID/AEROBID-M Inhaler depends on its regular use and on proper inhalation technique, patients must be instructed to take inhalations at regular intervals. They should also be instructed in the correct method of use (See Patient instruction Leaflet).

Patients receiving bronchodilators by inhalation should be advised to use the bronchodilator before AEROBID/AEROBID-M Inhaler in order to enhance penetration of flunisolide into the bronchial tree. After use of an aerosol bronchodilator, several minutes should elapse before using the AEROBID/AEROBID-M Inhaler.

Patients whose systemic corticosteroids have been reduced or withdrawn should be instructed to carry a warning card indicating that they may need supplemental systemic steroids during periods of stress or a severe asthmatic attack that is not responsive to bronchodilators.

Patients who are on immunosuppressant doses of corticosteroids should be warned to avoid exposure to chicken pox or measles and, if exposed, to obtain medical advice.

An illustrated leaflet of patient instructions for proper use accompanies each AEROBID/AEROBID-M Inhaler System.

CONTENTS UNDER PRESSURE

Do not puncture. Do not use or store near heat or open flame. Exposure to temperatures above 120°F (49°C) may cause container to explode. Never throw container into fire or incinerator. Keep out of reach of children.

Carcinogenesis: Long-term studies were conducted in mice and rats using oral administration to evaluate the carcinogenic potential of the drug. There was an increase in the incidence of pulmonary adenomas in mice, but not in rats. Female rats receiving the highest oral dose had an increased incidence of mammary adenocarcinoma compared to control rats. An increased incidence of this tumor type has been reported for other corticosteroids.

Impairment of Fertility: Female rats receiving high doses of flunisolide (200 mcg/kg/day) showed some evidence of impaired fertility. Reproductive performance in the low (8 mcg/kg/day) and mid-dose (40 mcg/kg/day) groups was comparable to controls.

Pregnancy: Pregnancy Category C. As with other corticosteroids, flunisolide has been shown to be teratogenic in rabbits and rats at doses of 40 and 200 mcg/kg/day respsectively. It was also fetotoxic in these animal reproductive studies. There are no adequate and well-controlled studies in pregnant women. Flunisolide should be used during pregnancy only if the potential benefit justifies the potential risk to the fetus.

Nursing Mothers: It is not known whether this drug is excreted in human milk. Because other corticosteroids are excreted in human milk, caution should be exercised when flunisolide is administered to nursing women.

ADVERSE REACTIONS

Adverse events reported in controlled clinical trials and long-term open studies in 514 patients treated with AEROBID/AEROBID-M are described below. Of those patients, 463 were treated for 3 months or longer, 407 for 6 months or longer, 287 for 1 year or longer, and 122 for 2 years or longer.

Musculoskeletal reactions were reported in 35% of steroid-dependent patients in whom the dose of oral steroid was being tapered. This is a well-known effect of steroid withdrawal.

Incidence 10% or greater:
Gastrointestinal: diarrhea (10%), nausea and/or vomiting (25%), upset stomach (10%)
General: flu (10%)
Mouth and Throat: sore throat (20%)
Nervous system: headache (25%)
Respiratory: cold symptoms (15%), nasal congestion (15%), upper respiratory infection (25%)
Special Senses: unpleasant taste (10%)
Incidence 3–9%
Cardiovascular: palpitations
Gastrointestinal: abdominal pain, heartburn
General: chest pain, decreased appetite, edema, fever
Mouth and Throat: *Candida* infection
Nervous System: dizziness, irritability, nervousness, shakiness
Reproductive: menstrual disturbances
Respiratory: chest congestion, cough*, hoarseness, rhinitis, runny nose, sinus congestion, sinus drainage, sinus infection, sinusitis, sneezing, sputum, wheezing*
Skin: eczema, itching (pruritus), rash
Special Senses: ear infection, loss of smell or taste
Incidence 1–3%
General: chills, increased appetite and weight gain, malaise, peripheral edema, sweating, weakness
Cardiovascular: hypertension, tachycardia
Gastrointestinal: constipation, dyspepsia, gas
Hemic/Lymph: capillary fragility, enlarged lymph nodes
Mouth and Throat: dry throat, glossitis, mouth irritation, pharyngitis, phlegm, throat irritation
Nervous System: anxiety, depression, faintness, fatigue, hyperactivity, hypoactivity, insomnia, moodiness, numbness, vertigo
Respiratory: bronchitis, chest tightness*, dyspnea, epistaxis, head stuffiness, laryngitis, nasal irritation, pleurisy, pneumonia, sinus discomfort
Skin: acne, hives, or urticaria
Special Senses: blurred vision, earache, eye discomfort, eye infection
Incidence less than 1%, judged by investigators as possibly or probably drug related: abdominal fullness, shortness of breath.

DOSAGE AND ADMINISTRATION

The AEROBID/AEROBID-M Inhaler System is for oral inhalation only.

Adults: The recommended starting dose is 2 inhalations twice daily morning and evening for a total daily dose of 1 mg. The maximum daily dose should not exceed 4 inhalations twice a day for a total daily dose of 2 mg. When the drug is used chronically at 2 mg/day, patients should be monitored periodically for effects on the hypothalamic-pituitary-adrenal axis.

Children: For children 6–15 years of age, two inhalations may be administered twice daily for a total daily dose of 1 mg. Higher doses have not been studied. Insufficient information is available to warrant use in children under age 6.

---

*The incidences as shown of cough, wheezing, and chest tightness were judged by investigators to be possibly or probably drug-related. In placebo-controlled trials, the *overall* incidences of these adverse events (regardless of investigators' judgment of drug relationship) were similar for drug and placebo-treated groups. They may be related to the vehicle or delivery system.

Continued on next page

Forest—Cont.

With chronic use, children should be monitored for growth as well as for effects on the HPA axis.

Rinsing the mouth after inhalation is advised. Patients receiving bronchodilators by inhalation should be advised to use the bronchodilator before **AEROBID/AEROBID-M** Inhaler in order to enhance penetration of flunisolide into the bronchial tree. After use of an aerosol bronchodilator, several minutes should elapse before use of the **AEROBID/AEROBID-M** inhaler to reduce the potential toxicity from the inhaled fluorocarbon propellants in the two aerosols.

Different considerations must be given to the following groups of patients in order to obtain the full therapeutic benefit of **AEROBID/AEROBID-M** Inhaler.

Patients not receiving systemic steroids: The use of **AEROBID/AEROBID-M** Inhaler is straightforward in patients who are inadequately controlled with non-steroid medications but in whom systemic steroid therapy has been withheld because of concern over potential adverse reactions. In patients who respond to the drug, an improvement in pulmonary function is usually apparent within one to four weeks after the start of treatment.

Patients receiving systemic steroids: In those patients dependent on systemic steroids, transfer to **AEROBID/AEROBID-M** and subsequent management may be more difficult because recovery from impaired adrenal function is usually slow. Such suppression has been known to last for up to 12 months. Clinical studies, however, have demonstrated that **AEROBID/AEROBID-M** may be effective in the management of these asthmatic patients and may permit replacement or significant reduction in the dosage of systemic corticosteroids.

Inhaled corticosteroids generally are not recommended for chronic use with alternate day prednisone regimens (see WARNINGS).

The patient's asthma should be reasonably stable before treatment with **AEROBID/AEROBID-M** Inhaler is started. Initially, the aerosol should be used concurrently with the patient's usual maintenance dose of systemic steroid. After approximately one week, gradual withdrawal of the systemic steroid is started by reducing the daily or alternate daily dose. The next reduction is made after an interval of one or two weeks, depending on the response of the patient. Generally, these decrements should not exceed 2.5 mg of prednisone or its equivalent. A slow rate of withdrawal cannot be overemphasized. During withdrawal, some patients may experience symptoms of systemically active steroid withdrawal, e.g., joint and/or muscular pain, lassitude and depression, despite maintenance or even improvement of respiratory function. Such patients should be encouraged to continue with the Inhaler but should be watched carefully for objective signs of adrenal insufficiency, such as hypotension and weight loss. If evidence of adrenal insufficiency occurs, the systemic steroid dose should be boosted temporarily and thereafter further withdrawal should continue more slowly. *During periods of stress or a severe asthma attack, transfer patients will require supplementary treatment with systemic steroids.* Exacerbations of asthma that occur during the course of treatment with **AEROBID/AEROBID-M** Inhaler should be treated with a short course of systemic steroid that is gradually tapered as these symptoms subside. There is no evidence that control of asthma can be achieved by administration of the drug in amounts greater than the recommended doses.

HOW SUPPLIED

AEROBID (flunisolide) Inhaler System is available in canisters of 100 metered inhalations.   NDC 0456-0672-99
AEROBID-M (flunisolide) Inhaler System is available in canisters of 100 metered inhalations.   NDC 0456-0670-99
Caution: FEDERAL LAW PROHIBITS DISPENSING WITHOUT PRESCRIPTION.
Revised 1/92

Shown in Product Identification Section, page 409

AEROCHAMBER®
with Inspiratory Flow Signal
Valved Aerosol Holding Chamber for use with Metered-Dose Inhalers.

Before using your AeroChamber, it is important to read these instructions very carefully, including the CAUTION sections that follow:

CAUTION
1. When cleaning, the only part of the AeroChamber to be removed is the rubber like ring that holds the Metered-Dose Inhaler.
2. Except as stated in 1 above, do not disassemble the AeroChamber, as the overall reliability and safety of the product may be affected.

3. Replace AeroChamber at once and do not use if the one-way valve becomes dislodged (partially or fully), or begins to harden or curl.
4. Running water through the AeroChamber at high pressures may harm the valve. Examine AeroChamber visually before and after cleaning to make sure the one-way valve and other parts are properly secured.
5. Disassembly may loosen or dislodge the one-way valve. Examine the AeroChamber visually before and after use to make sure the one-way valve and other parts are properly secured.
6. Do not allow children to play with the AeroChamber—allowing them to do so may alter its function and/or overall reliability. The one-way valve can be damaged as a result of pulling or poking.
7. As indicated, your AeroChamber should be inspected visually before and after daily use and may need to be replaced after 6 to 12 months of use.

INTRODUCTION
The AeroChamber is one of a family of valved aerosol holding chambers available from Forest Pharmaceuticals, Inc., designed to be used with virtually all Metered-Dose Inhalers [MDI's].
When you release a puff of aerosol into the AeroChamber, the puff will be held there for a few seconds.
The valved holding chamber selectively removes most large aerosol-drug particles that normally deposit in the mouth and throat, while allowing the smaller, therapeutic particles to pass through the patented one-way valve into the lungs. This provides effective treatment and helps to reduce unwanted side effects.
In addition, the AeroChamber is designed to make Metered-Dose Inhalers easier to use.

INSTRUCTIONS FOR USE
Please discuss the use of the AeroChamber with Mask with your physician, pharmacist, or other healthcare professional.

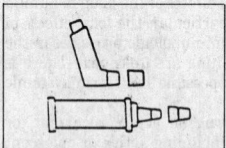 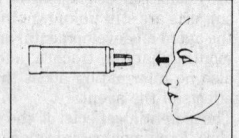

1. Remove the protective cap from the Metered-Dose Inhaler [MDI]. Remove the protective cap from the mouthpiece of AeroChamber.
2. Visually check the AeroChamber for foreign objects. Ensure that all parts are secure, including the one-way valve.

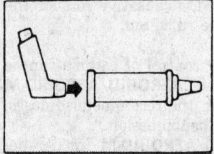 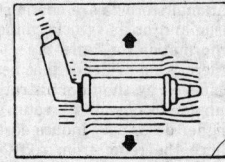

3. Insert inhaler mouthpiece into the round opening in the rubber like ring at the end of the AeroChamber.
4. Holding the AeroChamber and inhaler [MDI] firmly, shake vigorously 3 or 4 times.

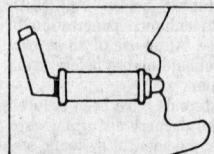 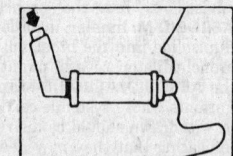

5. Place the AeroChamber mouthpiece in mouth and close lips.
6. Spray only one puff from the inhaler [MDI] into the AeroChamber per inhalation maneuver. Spraying more than one puff into the AeroChamber before or during an inhalation maneuver will result in delivery of improper dose of medication.

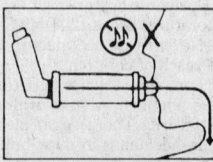

7. Breathe in slowly and deeply through mouth until you have taken a full breath. Do not breathe in so fast as to activate the flow signal whistle. A whistling sound from

the flow signal indicates that you are breathing in too quickly.
8. Hold breath for 5 to 10 seconds.
9. Repeat steps 4 to 8 as prescribed by your physician.
10. Remove inhaler and examine the AeroChamber to make certain that the one-way valve is properly secured.
11. Replace protective cap on AeroChamber and MDI.

HELPFUL HINTS
1. In order to obtain the maximum benefit from your Metered-Dose Inhaler, it is extremely important to fill your lungs during inhalation by taking a *slow*, deep breath. If the flow signal makes a whistling sound, it is an indication that you are breathing in too quickly.
2. The one-way valve allows you to inhale at your own rate so that coordination of inhalation with the actuation of the inhaler is not a problem.
3. If you have trouble inhaling through your mouth, with the AeroChamber mouthpiece between your lips, it may be necessary to gently pinch your nose while inhaling the medication.
4. For the elderly and small children who may have difficulty using the AeroChamber, there is also an Aerochamber available with Mask which allows another person to assist with coordination.
5. When using the AeroChamber with a corticosteroid Metered Dose Inhaler, it is recommended by the manufacturer of these drugs to rinse your mouth with water to remove any medication residue.

CLEANING INSTRUCTIONS
The AeroChamber is made of durable plastic materials and has only one moving part: the one-way valve. With repeated use, residue may accumulate inside the AeroChamber and around the valve. This eventually may interfere with effective use. We suggest cleaning the AeroChamber about once a week or more often, depending on your use of the product, per the following instructions.
To clean the AeroChamber:
1. Remove the rubber like ring from the end that holds the Metered-Dose Inhaler. Do not remove the mouthpiece from the AeroChamber body.
2. Remove the protective mouthpiece cap.
3. Soak AeroChamber and rubber like ring in basin filled with warm water, using mild detergent to dislodge or loosen any residue.
4. Rinse AeroChamber and rubber like ring in basin filled with clean warm water, using a gentle motion.
5. Lightly shake away excess water droplets and leave on clean surface to air-dry.
6. Be sure the AeroChamber is *completely dry* before use.
7. Replace the rubber like ring on the AeroChamber.
8. Replace the protective mouthpiece cap.

TECHNICAL INFORMATION
This apparently simple device is a product of considerable medical research and engineering. It was developed in a leading medical center.
The valve holding chamber selectively removes large aerosol particles that normally deposit in the mouth and throat, while allowing the smaller treatment particles to pass into the lungs. This provides effective treatment and helps reduce unwanted side effects.
This new device helps deliver aerosol medication to the lungs more reliably. Should you have any problem using the AeroChamber, please contact your doctor.

IMPORTANT INFORMATION
Package insert dosing instructions should be consulted for all metered-dose inhalers [MDIs] when used with AeroChamber®. Dosage and administration recommendations vary for different MDIs, and the limitations and conditions of use for each product should be considered before utilizing this device, particularly for younger and older patients.

BIBLIOGRAPHY
Corr D, Dolovich M, McCormack D, Ruffin R, Obeninski G, Newhouse M. Design and characteristics of a portable breath actuated, particle size selective medical aerosol inhaler. J Aerosol Sci. 1982; 13 No. (1):1–7.
Dolovich M, Eng P, Ruffin R, Corr D, Newhouse MT. Clinical evaluation of a simple demand inhalation MDI aerosol delivery device. Chest. 1983; 84 (1):36–41.
Berenberg MJ, Baigelman W, Cupples LA, Pearce L. Comparison of metered-dose inhaler attached to an AeroChamber with an updraft nebulizer for the administration of metaproterenol in hospitalized patients. Asthma. 1985; 22 (2):87–92.
Hodder RV, Calcutt LE, Leech JA, Metered dose inhaler with spacer is superior to wet nebulization for emergency room treatment of acute, severe asthma. Chest. 1988 94; 51S.
Newhouse MT. MDI plus AeroChamber: Aerosol dosing for controlling reversible airflow obstruction and managing acute exacerbations. Breathing Space. 1990:6-7, 12.

American Association for Respiratory Care, Aerosol Consensus Statement. Respiratory Care. 1991; 36: 1-6.
Assembled in USA of Canadian and USA Components/US Patent #s 4,470,412; 4,809,692; 4,832,015
Monaghan Medical Corporation, Plattsburgh, NY 12901
Distributed by:
FOREST PHARMACEUTICALS, INC.
Subsidiary of Forest Laboratories, Inc.
St. Louis, Missouri 63043-9979
UAD LABORATORIES
Division of Forest Pharmaceuticals, Inc.
Jackson, Mississippi 39209
REV 7/92

Shown in Product Identification Section, page 409

AEROCHAMBER®
with *Mask*
Valved Aerosol Holding Chamber with *Mask* for use with Metered-Dose Inhalers.

Before using your AeroChamber with *Mask*, it is important to read these instructions very carefully, including the CAUTION sections that follow:

CAUTION
1. When cleaning, the only part of the AeroChamber to be removed is the rubber like ring that holds the Metered-Dose Inhaler. Do not remove the white face mask from the AeroChamber body.
2. Except as stated in 1 above, do not disassemble the Aero-Chamber with Mask, as the overall reliability and safety of the product may be effected.
3. Replace AeroChamber with Mask at once and do not use if the one-way valve becomes dislodged (partially or fully), or begins to harden or curl.
4. Running water through the AeroChamber with Mask at high pressures may harm the valve. Examine AeroChamber with Mask visually before and after cleaning to make sure the one-way valve and other parts are properly secured.
5. Disassembly may loosen or dislodge the one-way valve. Examine the AeroChamber with Mask visually before and after use to make sure the one-way valve and other parts are properly secured.
6. Do not allow children to play with the AeroChamber with Mask—allowing them to do so may alter its function and/or overall reliability. The Mask membrane and the one-way valve can be damaged as a result of pulling or poking.
7. As indicated, your AeroChamber with Mask should be inspected visually before and after daily use and may need to be replaced after 6 to 12 months of use.

INTRODUCTION
The AeroChamber with Mask is one of a family of valved aerosol holding chambers available from Forest Pharmaceuticals, Inc., designed to be used with virtually all Metered-Dose Inhalers [MDI's].
When you release a puff of aerosol into the AeroChamber with Mask, the puff will be held there for a few seconds. The valved holding chamber selectively removes most large aerosol-drug particles that normally deposit in the mouth and throat, while allowing the smaller, therapeutic particles to pass through the patented one-way valve into the lungs. This provides effective treatment and helps to reduce unwanted side effects.
In addition, the AeroChamber with Mask is designed to make Metered-Dose Inhalers easier to use.

INSTRUCTIONS FOR USE
Please discuss the use of the AeroChamber with Mask with your physician, pharmacist, or other healthcare professional.

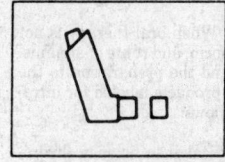 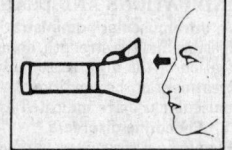

1. Remove protective cap from Metered-Dose Inhaler [MDI].
2. Visually check the AeroChamber with Mask for foreign objects. Ensure that all parts are secure, including the one-way valve.

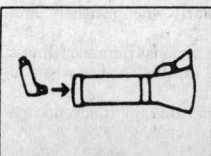 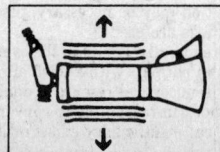

3. Insert inhaler mouthpiece into the round opening in the rubber like ring at the end of the AeroChamber with Mask.
4. Holding the AeroChamber with Mask and inhaler [MDI] firmly, shake vigorously 3 or 4 times.

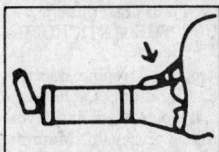 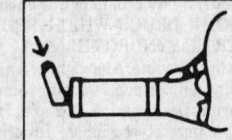

5. Place the soft mask gently to the face so that the mouth and nose are covered. Be certain to create a good seal. Leaks will inhibit the delivery of the medication. Seeing the diaphragm move is a helpful indication of a good seal.
6. Spray only one puff from the inhaler [MDI] into the Aero-Chamber with Mask per inhalation maneuver. The mask is to be held firmly to the face while inhaling at least [six] times. Spraying more than one puff into the AeroChamber with Mask before or during an inhalation maneuver will result in delivery of improper dose of medication.
7. Repeat steps 4 to 6 as prescribed by your Physician.
8. Remove inhaler and examine the AeroChamber with Mask to make certain that the one-way valve is properly secured.

HELPFUL HINTS
1. Some children may resist their treatment by grabbing at the mask. Place the child on your lap and wrap one arm around the child to simplify placing the mask on the child's face.
2. In the case of a smaller child, it may be more comfortable to lay the child on the bed while administering the medication.
3. If the child seems frightened by the AeroChamber with Mask, familiarize the child with the device by stroking his or her cheek with the soft mask. If the child cries during treatment with the AeroChamber with Mask, the medication will still be delivered as long as there is a good seal between the mask and the child's face. Remember, the child will breathe in after crying or screaming.
4. When using the AeroChamber with Mask with a corticosteroid Metered-Dose Inhaler, it is recommended that the patient's face be cleaned with soap and water to remove any medication residue.

CLEANING INSTRUCTIONS
The AeroChamber with Mask is made of durable plastic materials and has only one moving part: the one-way valve. With repeated use, residue may accumulate inside the Aero-Chamber with Mask and around the valve. This eventually may interfere with effective use. We suggest cleaning the AeroChamber with Mask about once a week or more often, depending on your use of the product, per the following instructions:
To clean the AeroChamber with Mask:
1. Remove the rubber like ring from the end that holds the Metered-Dose Inhaler. Do not remove the white face mask from the AeroChamber body.
2. Soak AeroChamber with Mask and rubber like ring in basin filled with warm water, using mild detergent to dislodge or loosen any residue.
3. Rinse AeroChamber with Mask and rubber like ring in basin filled with clean warm water, using a gentle motion.
4. Lightly shake away excess water droplets and leave on clean surface to air-dry.
5. Be sure the AeroChamber with Mask is *completely dry* before use.
6. Replace the rubber like ring on the AeroChamber with Mask.

TECHNICAL INFORMATION
This apparently simple device is a product of considerable medical research and engineering. It was developed in a leading medical center.
The valve holding chamber selectively removes large aerosol particles that normally deposit in the mouth and throat, while allowing the smaller treatment particles to pass into the lungs. This provides effective treatment and helps reduce unwanted side effects.
This new device helps deliver aerosol medication to the lungs more reliably. Should you have any problem using the AeroChamber, please contact your doctor.

IMPORTANT INFORMATION
Package insert dosing instructions should be consulted for all metered-dose inhalers [MDIs] when used with AeroChamber® with Mask. Dosage and administration recommendations vary for different MDIs, and the limitations and conditions of use for each product should be considered before utilizing this device, particularly for younger and older patients.

CAUTION: Federal law restricts this device to sale by, or on the order of, a physician.

BIBLIOGRAPHY
Conner WT, Dolovich MB, Frame R, Newhouse MT. Salbutamol administration to children under three by means of a mask and aerochamber. *J Clin Invest Med.* 1985; 8:A179.
Rachelefsky GS, Rohr AS, Wo J, et al. Use of a tube spacer to improve the efficacy of a metered-dose inhaler in asthmatic children. *Am J Dis Child.* 1986:140.
Salzman GA, Pyszczynski DR. Oropharyngeal candidiasis in patients treated with belcomethasone dipropionate delivered by metered-dose inhaler alone and with AeroChamber. *J Allergy Clin Immunol.* 1988; 81:424–428.
Sly RM, Barbera JM, Middleton HB, Eby DM. Delivery of albuterol aerosol by aerochamber to young children. *Ann Allergy.* 1988; 60:403–406.
Assembled in USA of Canadian and USA Components / US Patent #s 4,470,412; 4,809,692; 4,832,015 Monaghan Medical Corporation, Plattsburgh, NY 12901
Assembled in USA of Canadian and USA Components/US Patent #s 4,470,412; 4,809,692; 4,832,015
Monaghan Medical Corporation, Plattsburgh, NY 12901
Distributed by:
FOREST PHARMACEUTICALS, INC.
Subsidiary of Forest Laboratories, Inc.
St. Louis, Missouri 63043-9979
UAD LABORATORIES
Division of Forest Pharmaceuticals, Inc.
Jackson, Mississippi 39209
REV 7/92

Shown in Product Identification Section, page 409

AMBENYL® Cough Syrup   © ℞
[ăm'bĕn-ĭl]

DESCRIPTION
Each 5 ml of AMBENYL Cough Syrup contains:
Codeine phosphate
(Warning—May be habit-forming) .... 10 mg
Bromodiphenhydramine hydrochloride .... 12.5 mg
Alcohol, 5%
AMBENYL Cough Syrup also contains citric acid, D&C Red #33, ethyl alcohol, flavor, glucose liquid, glycerin, menthol, sodium citrate, sucrose, vanillin, water, and has a pH between 5.0 and 6.0.

HOW SUPPLIED
AMBENYL Cough Syrup is red and is supplied in 4 fl. oz. (NDC 0456-0681-04), 1 pint (NDC 0456-0681-16), and 1 gallon (NDC 0456-0681-28) bottles. Store at controlled room temperature 15°–30°C (59°–86°F).

Revised 3/90

ANTILIRIUM®   ℞
(physostigmine salicylate)

DESCRIPTION
ANTILIRIUM (Physostigmine Salicylate) is a derivative of the Calabar bean, and its active moiety, physostigmine, is also known as eserine.
It is soluble in water and a 0.5% aqueous solution has a pH of 5.8.
ANTILIRIUM Injection is available in 2 ml ampuls, each ml containing 1 mg of Physostigmine Salicylate in a vehicle composed of sodium bisulfite 0.1%, benzyl alcohol 2.0% as a preservative in water for injection.

CLINICAL PHARMACOLOGY
ANTILIRIUM is a reversible anticholinesterase which effectively increases the concentration of acetylcholine at the sites of cholinergic transmission. The action of acetylcholine is normally very transient because of its hydrolysis by the enzyme, acetylcholinesterase. ANTILIRIUM inhibits the destructive action of acetylcholinesterase and thereby prolongs and exaggerates the effect of the acetylcholine.
ANTILIRIUM contains a tertiary amine and easily penetrates the blood brain barrier, while an anticholinesterase, such as neostigmine, which has a quaternary ammonium ion is not capable of crossing the barrier. ANTILIRIUM can reverse both central and peripheral anticholinergia. The anticholinergic syndrome has both central and peripheral signs and symptoms. Central toxic effects include anxiety, delirium, disorientation, hallucinations, hyper-activity and seizures. Severe poisoning may produce coma, medullary paralysis and death. Peripheral toxicity is characterized by tachycardia, hyperpyrexia, mydriasis, vasodilatation, urinary

Continued on next page

Forest—Cont.

retention, diminution of gastrointestinal motility, decrease of secretion in salivary and sweat glands, and loss of secretions in the pharynx, bronchi, and nasal passages.

Dramatic reversal of the effects of anticholinergic symptoms can be expected in minutes after the intravenous administration of ANTILIRIUM, if the diagnosis is correct and the patient has not suffered anoxia or other insult. The duration of action of ANTILIRIUM is relatively short, approx. 45 to 60 minutes.

Numerous drugs and some plants produce the anticholinergic syndrome either directly or as a side effect; this undesirable or potentially dangerous phenomenon may be brought about by either therapeutic doses or overdoses of the drugs. Such drugs include among others, atropine, other derivatives of the belladonna alkaloids, tricyclic antidepressants, phenothiazines, and antihistamines.

INDICATIONS AND USAGES
To reverse the effect upon the central nervous system, caused by clinical or toxic dosages of drugs capable of producing the anticholinergic syndrome.

CONTRAINDICATIONS
ANTILIRIUM should not be used in the presence of asthma, gangrene, diabetes, cardiovascular disease, mechanical obstruction of the intestine or urogenital tract or any vagotonic state, and in patients receiving choline esters or depolarizing neuromuscular blocking agents (decamethonium succinylcholine).

For post-anesthesia, the concomitant use of atropine with the physostigmine salicylate is not recommended, since the atropine antagonizes the action of physostigmine.

WARNINGS
Contains sodium bisulfite, a sulfite that may cause allergic-type reactions including anaphylactic symptoms and life-threatening or less severe asthmatic episodes in certain susceptible people. The overall prevalence of sulfite sensitivity in the general population is unknown and probably low. Sulfite sensitivity is seen more frequently in asthmatic than in non-asthmatic people.

If excessive symptoms of salivation, emesis, urination and defecation occur, the use of ANTILIRIUM should be terminated. If excessive sweating or nausea occur, the dosage should be reduced.

Intravenous administration should be a slow, controlled rate, no more than 1 mg per minute (see dosage). Rapid administration can cause bradycardia, hypersalivation leading to respiratory difficulties and possible convulsions.

An overdosage of ANTILIRIUM can cause a cholinergic crisis.

PRECAUTIONS
Because of the possibility of hypersensitivity in an occasional patient, atropine sulfate injection should always be at hand since it is an antagonist and antidote for physostigmine.

USAGE IN PREGNANCY
Safe use in pregnancy and lactation has not been established; therefore, use in pregnant women, nursing mothers or women who may become pregnant requires that possible benefits be weighed against possible hazards to mother and child.

ADVERSE REACTIONS
Nausea, vomiting and salivation, can be offset by reducing dosage. Bradycardia and convulsions, if intravenous administration is too rapid. See DOSAGE AND ADMINISTRATION.

OVERDOSAGE
Can cause a cholinergic crisis. Appropriate antidote is atropine sulfate.

DOSAGE AND ADMINISTRATION
Post Anesthesia Care: 0.5 to 1.0 mg intramuscularly or intravenously. INTRAVENOUS ADMINISTRATION SHOULD BE AT A SLOW CONTROLLED RATE OF NO MORE THAN 1 MG PER MINUTE. Dosage may be repeated at intervals of 10 to 30 minutes if desired patient response is not obtained.

Overdosages of Drugs That Cause Anticholinergia: 2.0 mg intramuscularly or INTRAVENOUSLY AT SLOW CONTROLLED RATE (SEE ABOVE). Dosage may be repeated if life threatening signs, such as arrhythmia, convulsions or coma occurs.

Pediatric Dosage: Recommended dosage is 0.02 mg/kg, intramuscularly or by slow intravenous injection, no more than 0.5 mg per minute. If the toxic effects persist, and there is no sign of cholinergic effects, the dosage may be repeated at 5 to 10 minute intervals until a therapeutic effect is obtained or a maximum dose of 2 mg is attained.

IN ALL CASES OF POISONING, THE USUAL SUPPORTIVE MEASURES SHOULD BE UNDERTAKEN.

HOW SUPPLIED
Ampuls, 2 ml packed 12 per box, 1 mg per ml NDC-0456-1037-12.

CAUTION
Federal law prohibits dispensing without prescription.

SOME DRUGS WHICH PRODUCE THE ANTICHOLINERGIC SYNDROME

Amitriptyline, Amoxapine, Anisotropine, Atropine, Benztropine, Biperiden, Carbinoxamine, Clidinium, Cyclobenzaprine, Desipramine, Doxepin, Homatropine, Hyoscine, Hyoscyamine, Hyoscyamus, Imipramine, Lorazepam, Maprotiline, Mepenzolate, Nortriptyline, Propantheline, Protriptyline, Scopolamine, Trimipramine.

SOME PLANTS THAT PRODUCE THE ANTICHOLINERGIC SYNDROME

Black Henbane, Deadly Night Shade, Devil's Apple, Jimson Weed, Loco Seeds or Weeds, Matrimony Vine, Night Blooming Jessamine, Stinkweed.

ARMOUR® THYROID Tablets   ℞
[thī'roid]
(THYROID TABLETS, U.S.P.)

DESCRIPTION
Armour® Thyroid Tablets (Thyroid Tablets, USP) for oral use are natural preparations derived from porcine thyroid glands. (T_3 liothyronine is approximately four times as potent as T_4 levothyroxine on a microgram for microgram basis.) They provide 38 mcg levothyroxine (T_4) and 9 mcg liothyronine (T_3) per grain of thyroid. The inactive ingredients are calcium stearate, dextrose and mineral oil.

HOW SUPPLIED
Armour Thyroid tablets (thyroid tablets, USP) are supplied as follows: 15 mg (¼ gr) are available in bottles of 100 (NDC 0456-0457-01), 30 mg (½ gr) are available in bottles of 100 (NDC 0456-0458-01), 1000 (NDC 0456-0458-00), drums of 50,000 (NDC 0456-0458-69), and unit dose cartons of 100 (NDC 0456-0458-63). 60 mg (1 gr) are available in bottles of 100 (NDC 0456-0459-01), 1000 (NDC 0456-0459-00), 5000 (NDC 0456-0459-51), drums of 50,000 (NDC 0456-0459-69), and unit dose cartons of 100 (NDC 0456-0459-63). 90 mg (1½ gr) are available in bottles of 100 (NDC 0456-0460-01). 120 mg (2 gr) are available in bottles of 100 (NDC 0456-0461-01), 1000 (NDC 0456-0461-00), and drums of 50,000 (NDC 0456-0461-69). 180 mg (3 gr) are available in bottles of 100 (NDC 0456-0462-01), and 1000 (NDC 0456-0462-00). 240 mg (4 gr) are available in bottles of 100 (NDC 0456-0463-01). 300 mg (5 gr) are available in bottles of 100 (NDC 0456-0464-01). The bottles of 100 are special dispensing bottles with child-resistant closures.

Note: (T_3 liothyronine is approximately four times as potent as T_4 levothyroxine on a microgram for microgram basis.) Tablets should be stored at controlled room temperature, 59°–86°F (15°–30°C), in capped bottles or unbroken plastic strip packing.

Shown in Product Identification Section, Page 409

BANCAP HC® CAPSULES   Ⓒ ℞

DESCRIPTION
Each hard gelatin capsule contains:
Hydrocodone* Bitartrate .... 5 mg
  *(WARNING: May be habit forming)
Acetaminophen .... 500 mg
This product also contains FD&C Yellow No. 6
Hydrocodone bitartrate is an opioid analgesic and antitussive which occurs as fine, white crystals or as a crystalline powder. It is affected by light. The chemical name is: 4,5α-epoxy-3-methoxy-17-methylmorphinan-6-one tartrate (1:1) hydrate (2:5).

Acetaminophen, 4'-hydroxyacetanilide, is a non-opiate, non-salicylate analgesic and antipyretic which occurs as a white, odorless crystalline powder possessing a slightly bitter taste.

HOW SUPPLIED
Bancap HC (Hydrocodone Bitartrate 5 mg and Acetaminophen 500 mg) Capsules are black and red capsules imprinted FOREST 610. They are supplied as:
Bottles of 100—NDC 0456-0610-01
Bottles of 500—NDC 0456-0610-02
Store at controlled room temperature 15°–30°C (59°–86°F).
Dispense in a tight, light-resistant container as defined in the USP
CAUTION: Federal law prohibits dispensing without prescription.
Revised 4/90

DALALONE D.P.® INJECTION   ℞
(Dexamethasone acetate suspension)
Equivalent to Dexamethasone 16 mg/mL

PRODUCT OVERVIEW
KEY FACTS
Dalalone D.P. injection is a synthetic, long-acting, repository adrenocorticosteroid agent that provides a prompt onset of action. Each ml of suspension contains 16 mg of dexamethasone. It may be administered via intramuscular, intra-articular, or soft tissue injection, but must not be given intravenously or intralesionally.

MAJOR USES
Dexamethasone, a fluorinated derivative of prednisolone, is used primarily for its potent anti-inflammatory effects in disorders of many organ systems and other diseases responsive to glucocorticosteroids. At equipotent anti-inflammatory doses, dexamethasone almost lacks the sodium-retaining property of hydrocortisone.

SAFETY INFORMATION
Contraindicated in patients with systemic fungal infections. Corticosteroids can mask signs of existing or new infection. Repeated injections at the same site are to be avoided, as are subcutaneous injections, and injections into the deltoid muscle.

PRESCRIBING INFORMATION
DALALONE D.P.® INJECTION   ℞
(Dexamethasone acetate suspension)
Equivalent to Dexamethasone 16 mg/mL

NOT FOR INTRAVENOUS OR INTRALESIONAL USE
FOR INTRAMUSCULAR, INTRA-ARTICULAR AND
SOFT TISSUE USE

DESCRIPTION
Dexamethasone acetate, a synthetic adrenocortical steroid, is a white to practically white, odorless powder. It is a practically insoluble ester of dexamethasone.

It has a molecular weight of 434.5 and its empirical formula is $C_{24}H_{31}FO_6$.

Dexamethasone Acetate suspension is a sterile white suspension that settles on standing, but is easily resuspended by mild shaking.

Each ml. contains: Dexamethasone Acetate equivalent to Dexamethasone 16 mg.
6.67 mg. Sodium Chloride
5 mg. Creatinine
0.5 mg Edetate Disodium
5 mg Carboxymethylcellulose Sodium
0.75 mg Polysorbate 80
9 mg Benzyl Alcohol
1 mg Sodium Bisulfite
as preservatives in Water for Injection q.s., Sodium Hydroxide to adjust pH.

CLINICAL PHARMACOLOGY
Dexamethasone Acetate suspension is a long-acting, repository adrenocorticosteroid preparation with a prompt onset of action. It is suitable for intramuscular or local injection, but not when an immediate effect of short duration is desired. Naturally occurring glucocorticoids (hydrocortisone and cortisone), which also have salt-retaining properties, are used as replacement therapy in adrenocortical deficiency states. Their synthetic analogs, including dexamethasone, are primarily used for their potent anti-inflammatory effects in disorders of many organ systems.

Glucocorticoids cause profound and varied metabolic effects. In addition, they modify the body's immune responses to diverse stimuli.

At equipotent anti-inflammatory doses, dexamethasone almost completely lacks the sodium-retaining property of hydrocortisone.

INDICATIONS AND USAGE
A. Intramuscular administration. When oral therapy is not feasible and the strength, dosage form, and route of administration of the drug reasonably lend the preparation to the treatment of the condition, those products labeled for intramuscular use are indicated as follows:

1. Endocrine disorders
Primary or secondary adrenocortical insufficiency (hydrocortisone or cortisone is the drug of choice; synthetic analogs may be used in conjunction with mineralocorticoids where applicable; in infancy, mineralocorticoid supplementation is of particular importance).

Acute adrenocortical insufficiency (hydrocortisone or cortisone is the drug of choice; mineralocorticoid supplementation may be necessary, particularly when synthetic analogs are used).

Preoperatively and in the event of serious trauma or illness, in patients with known adrenal insufficiency or when adrenocortical reserve is doubtful.

Shock unresponsive to conventional therapy if adrenocortical insufficiency exists or is suspected.

Congenital adrenal hyperplasia.

Nonsuppurative thyroiditis.
Hypercalcemia associated with cancer.

2. Rheumatic disorders

As adjunctive therapy for short-term administration (to tide the patient over an acute episode or exacerbation) in:
Post-traumatic osteoarthritis
Synovitis of osteoarthritis
Rheumatoid arthritis, including juvenile rheumatoid arthritis (selected cases may require low-dose maintenance therapy).
Acute and subacute bursitis
Epicondylitis
Acute nonspecific tenosynovitis
Acute gouty arthritis
Psoriatic arthritis
Ankylosing spondylitis

3. Collagen diseases

During an exacerbation or as maintenance therapy in selected cases of:
Systemic lupus erythematosus
Acute rheumatic carditis

4. Dermatologic diseases

Pemphigus
Severe erythema multiforme (Stevens-Johnson syndrome)
Exfoliative dermatitis
Bullous dermatitis herpetiformis
Severe seborrheic dermatitis
Severe psoriasis
Mycosis fungoides.

5. Allergic states

Control of severe or incapacitating allergic conditions intractable to adequate trials of conventional treatment in:
Bronchial asthma
Contact dermatitis
Atopic dermatitis
Serum sickness
Seasonal or perennial allergic rhinitis
Drug hypersensitivity reactions
Urticarial transfusion reactions
Acute noninfectious laryngeal edema (epinephrine is the drug of first choice).

6. Ophthalmic diseases

Severe acute and chronic allergic and inflammatory processes involving the eye, such as:
Herpes zoster ophthalmicus
Iritis, Iridocyclitis
Chorioretinitis
Diffuse posterior uveitis and choroiditis
Optic neuritis
Sympathetic ophthalmia
Anterior segment inflammation
Allergic conjunctivitis
Allergic corneal marginal ulcers

7. Gastrointestinal diseases

To tide the patient over a critical period of disease in:
Ulcerative colitis—(Systemic therapy)
Regional enteritis—(Systemic therapy)

8. Respiratory diseases

Symptomatic sarcoidosis
Berylliosis
Fulminating or disseminated pulmonary tuberculosis when used concurrently with appropriate antituberculous chemotherapy.
Loeffler's syndrome not manageable by other means.
Aspiration pneumonitis.

9. Hematologic disorders

Acquired (autoimmune) hemolytic anemia
Idiopathic thrombocytopenic purpura in adults (I.V. only; I.M. administration is contraindicated)
Secondary thrombocytopenia in adults
Erythroblastopenia (RBC anemia)
Congenital (erythroid) hypoplastic anemia.

10. Neoplastic diseases

For palliative management of leukemias and lymphomas in adults
Acute leukemia of childhood.

11. Edematous state

To induce diuresis or remission of proteinuria in the nephrotic syndrome without uremia, of the idiopathic type, or that due to lupus erythematosus.

12. Miscellaneous

Tuberculous meningitis with subarachnoid block or impending block when used concurrently with appropriate antituberculous chemotherapy.
Trichinosis with neurologic or myocardial involvement
Diagnostic testing of adrenocortical hyperfunction.

B. By intra-articular or soft tissue injection as adjunctive therapy for short-term administration (to tide the patient over an acute episode of exacerbation) in:
Synovitis of osteoarthritis
Rheumatoid arthritis
Acute and subacute bursitis
Acute gouty arthritis
Epicondylitis
Acute nonspecific tenosynovitis
Post-traumatic osteoarthritis

CONTRAINDICATIONS

Systemic fungal infections.
Contraindicated in those persons who have shown hypersensitivity to any component of this preparation.

WARNINGS

Contains sodium metabisulfite, a sulfite that may cause allergic-type reactions including anaphylactic symptoms and life-threatening or less severe asthmatic episodes in certain susceptible people.
The overall prevalence of sulfite sensitivity in the general population is unknown and probably low. Sulfite sensitivity is seen more frequently in asthmatic than in non-asthmatic people.
DO NOT INJECT INTRAVENOUSLY. In patients on corticosteroid therapy subjected to any unusual stress, increased dosage of rapidly acting corticosteroids before, during, and after the stressful situation is indicated.
Corticosteroids may mask some signs of infection, and new infections may appear during their use. There may be decreased resistance and inability to localize infection when corticosteroids are used.
Prolonged use of corticosteroids may produce posterior subcapsular cataracts, glaucoma with possible damage to the optic nerves, and may enhance the establishment of secondary ocular infections due to fungi or viruses.
Usage in pregnancy. Since adequate human reproduction studies have not been done with corticosteroids, the use of these drugs in pregnancy, nursing mothers, or women of childbearing potential requires that the possible benefits of the drug be weighed against the potential hazards to the mother and embryo or fetus. Infants born of mothers who have received substantial doses of corticosteroids during pregnancy should be carefully observed for signs of hypoadrenalism.
Average and large doses of cortisone or hydrocortisone can cause elevation of blood pressure, salt and water retention, and increased excretion of potassium. These effects are less likely to occur with the synthetic derivatives except when used in large doses. Dietary salt restriction and potassium supplementation may be necessary. All corticosteroids increase calcium excretion.
While on corticosteroid therapy patients should not be vaccinated against smallpox. Other immunization procedures should not be undertaken in patients who are on corticosteroids, especially in high doses, because of possible hazards of neurologic complications and lack of antibody response.
If corticosteroids are indicated in patients with latent tuberculosis or tuberculin reactivity, close observation is necessary as reactivation of the disease may occur. During prolonged corticosteroid therapy, these patients should receive chemoprophylaxis.
Because rare instances of anaphylactoid reactions have occurred in patients receiving parenteral corticosteroid therapy, appropriate precautionary measures should be taken prior to administration, especially when the patient has a history of allergy to any drug.
Corticosteroids may suppress reaction to skin tests.
Repository adrenocorticosteroid preparations may cause atrophy at the site of injection. To minimize the likelihood and/or severity of atrophy, do not inject subcutaneously, avoid injection into the deltoid muscle, and avoid repeated intramuscular injections into the same site if possible.
Dosage in children under 12 has not been established.

PRECAUTIONS

Dexamethasone Acetate suspension is not recommended as initial therapy in acute, life-threatening situations.
This product, like many other steroid formulations, is sensitive to heat. Therefore, it should not be autoclaved when it is desirable to sterilize the exterior of the vial.
Drug-induced secondary adrenocortical insufficiency may be minimized by gradual reduction of dosage. This type of relative insufficiency may persist for months after discontinuation of therapy; therefore, in any situation of stress occurring during that period, hormone therapy should be reinstituted. If the patient is receiving steroids already, the dosage may have to be increased. Since mineralocorticoid secretion may be impaired, salt and/or a mineralocorticoid should be administered concurrently.
There is an enhanced effect of corticosteroids in patients with hypothyroidism and in those with cirrhosis.
Corticosteroids should be used cautiously in patients with ocular herpes simplex for fear of corneal ulceration and perforation.
Psychic derangements may appear when corticosteroids are used, ranging from euphoria, insomnia, mood swings, personality changes, and severe depression to frank psychotic manifestations. Also, existing emotional instability or psychotic tendencies may be aggravated by corticosteroids.
Aspirin should be used cautiously in conjunction with corticosteroids in hypoprothrombinemia.
Steroids should be used with caution in nonspecific ulcerative colitis, if there is a probability of impending perforation, abscess or other pyogenic infection, also in diverticuli-

tis, fresh intestinal anastomoses, active or latent peptic ulcer, renal insufficiency, hypertension, osteoporosis, and myasthenia gravis. Fat embolism has been reported as a possible complication of hypercortisonism.
An ulcer regimen including an antacid should be considered as a prophylactic measure during prolonged therapy.
Growth and development of infants and children on prolonged corticosteroid therapy should be carefully followed.
Steroids may increase or decrease motility and number of spermatozoa in some patients.
Since phenytoin, phenobarbital, ephedrine and rifampin may alter cortisol metabolism, glucocorticoid dosage adjustments may be required when any of these substances is started or stopped.
The prothrombin time should be checked frequently in patients who are receiving corticosteroids and coumarin anticoagulants at the same time because of reports that corticosteroids have altered the response to these anticoagulants. There are some reports of potentiation; others of inhibition.
Intra-articular injection of a corticosteroid may produce systemic as well as local effects.
Appropriate examination of any joint fluid present is necessary to exclude a septic process.
A marked increase in pain accompanied by local swelling, further restriction of joint motion, fever, and malaise are suggestive of septic arthritis. If this complication occurs and the diagnosis of sepsis is confirmed, appropriate antimicrobial therapy should be instituted.
Local injection of a steroid into an infected site is to be avoided.
Corticosteroids should not be injected into unstable joints.
Information for Patients:
Patients should be impressed strongly with the importance of not over-using joints in which symptomatic benefit has been obtained as long as the inflammatory process remains active.

ADVERSE REACTIONS

Fluid and electrolyte disturbances:
Sodium retention
Fluid retention
Congestive heart failure in susceptible patients
Potassium loss
Hypokalemic alkalosis
Hypertension
Hypotensive or shock-like reaction

Musculoskeletal:
Muscle weakness
Steroid myopathy
Loss of muscle mass
Osteoporosis
Vertebral compression fractures
Aseptic necrosis of femoral and humeral heads
Pathologic fracture of long bones

Gastrointestinal:
Peptic ulcer with possible subsequent perforation and hemorrhage
Pancreatitis
Abdominal distention
Ulcerative esophagitis

Dermatologic:
Impaired wound healing
Thin fragile skin
Petechiae and ecchymoses
Erythema
Increased sweating
Other cutaneous reactions

Neurologic:
Convulsions
Increased intracranial pressure with papilledema (pseudotumor cerebri) usually after treatment
Vertigo
Headache

Endocrine:
Menstrual irregularities
Development of cushingoid state
Suppression of growth in children
Secondary adrenocortical and pituitary unresponsiveness, particularly in times of stress, as in trauma, surgery or illness
Decreased carbohydrate tolerance
Manifestations of latent diabetes mellitus
Increased requirements for insulin or oral hypoglycemic agents in diabetics

Ophthalmic:
Posterior subcapsular cataracts
Increased intraocular pressure
Glaucoma
Exophthalmos

Metabolic:
Negative nitrogen balance due to protein catabolism

Continued on next page

Forest—Cont.

Other:
Hypersensitivity
Thromboembolism
Weight gain
Increased appetite
Nausea
Malaise
The following **additional** adverse reactions are related to parenteral corticosteroid therapy:
Rare instances of blindness associated with intralesional therapy around the face and head
Hyperpigmentation or hypopigmentation
Subcutaneous and cutaneous atrophy
Sterile abscess
Postinjection flare (following intra-articular use)
Charcot-like arthropathy
Scarring
Induration
Inflammation
Paresthesia
Ecchymosis
Delayed pain or soreness
Muscle twitching, ataxia, hiccups, and nystagmus have been reported in low incidence after injection of Dexamethasone Acetate suspension

DRUG ABUSE AND DEPENDENCE
(See WARNINGS section).

OVERDOSAGE
(See ADVERSE REACTION section).

DOSAGE AND ADMINISTRATION
Dosage Requirements Are Variable and Must Be Individualized on the Basis of the Disease Under Treatment and the Response of the Patient.
Dosage in children under 12 has not been established.
Intramuscular Injection
Dosage ranges from 0.5 to 1 mL, equivalent to 8 to 16 mg of Dexamethasone. If further treatment is needed, dosage may be repeated at intervals of 1 to 3 weeks.
Intra-articular and Soft Tissue Injection
The dose varies, depending on the location and the severity of inflammation. The usual dose is 0.25 to 1 mL, equivalent to 4 to 16 mg of Dexamethasone. If further treatment is needed, dosage may be repeated at intervals of 1 to 3 weeks.
Parenteral drug products should be inspected visually for particulate matter and discoloration prior to administration, whenever the solution and container permit.

HOW SUPPLIED
Single dose vials of 1 mL, containing Dexamethasone Acetate equivalent to Dexamethasone 16 mg. NDC 0456-1097-41.
Multiple dose vials of 5 mL, each mL containing Dexamethasone Acetate equivalent to Dexamethasone 16 mg. NDC 0456-1097-05.

PROTECT FROM LIGHT. Retain in carton until all contents are used.
STORE AT CONTROLLED ROOM TEMPERATURE 59°–86° F (15°–30° C). DO NOT PERMIT TO FREEZE. SENSITIVE TO HEAT—DO NOT AUTOCLAVE.
        SHAKE WELL.

CAUTION
Federal law prohibits dispensing without prescription.
Literature Revised: June 1992
Product No. 0669-01, 0669-05.
Mfd. by
Steris Laboratories, Inc.
Phoenix, AZ 85043 USA
Mfd. for
FOREST PHARMACEUTICALS, INC.
SUBSIDIARY OF FOREST LABORATORIES
ST. LOUIS, MISSOURI 63043
        6/92

ELIXOPHYLLIN®   **R**
[*ē"lix -off'fil-in*]
(theophylline anhydrous)
Capsules

ELIXOPHYLLIN® SR   **R**
(theophylline anhydrous)
Capsules

ELIXOPHYLLIN®   **R**
(theophylline anhydrous)
Elixir

DESCRIPTION
Elixophyllin® Capsules are available as Soft Gelatin Capsules intended for oral administration, containing 100 and 200 mg of Theophylline Anhydrous.

Each Elixophyllin® Capsule also contains the following inactive ingredients: gelatin, glycerin, methylparaben and sorbitol.
Elixophyllin® (theophylline anhydrous) SR Capsules
Elixophyllin® SR Capsules are designed to provide a prolonged therapeutic effect.
125 mg capsule—Each white, opaque, dye-free capsule contains 125 mg anhydrous theophylline.
250 mg capsule—Each clear, dye-free capsule contains 250 mg anhydrous theophylline.
Elixophyllin® SR Capsules also contain the following inactive ingredients: calcium stearate, gelatin, pharmaceutical glaze, povidone, starch, sucrose, talc, titanium dioxide (125 mg capsule only) and other ingredient(s).
Elixophyllin® (theophylline anhydrous) Elixir
ELIXOPHYLLIN Elixir is available as a liquid intended for oral administration, containing 80 mg of theophylline anhydrous and 20% alcohol in each 15 mL (tablespoonful).
ELIXOPHYLLIN Elixir also contains the following inactive ingredients: citric acid, FD&C Red #40, flavoring agent, glycerin, saccharin sodium and purified water. Elixophyllin Elixir has a pH of 3.0–4.0.
Theophylline is a bronchodilator structurally classified as a xanthine derivative. It occurs as a white, odorless, crystalline powder having a bitter taste. Theophylline anhydrous has the chemical name, 1H- Purine-2, 6-dione, 3,7-dihydro-1,3-dimethyl-, and is represented by the following structural formula:

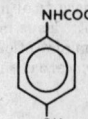

ANHYDROUS THEOPHYLLINE

HOW SUPPLIED
Elixophyllin® (brand of theophylline anhydrous) 100 mg Capsules are one piece, opaque, off-white to yellowish soft gelatin capsules imprinted with FOREST 642. They are supplied as:
  Bottles of 100 ....NDC 0456-0642-01
ELIXOPHYLLIN® (brand of theophylline anhydrous) 200 mg Capsules are one piece, opaque, off-white to yellowish soft gelatin capsules imprinted with FOREST 643. They are supplied as:
  Bottles of 100 ....NDC 0456-0643-01
  Bottles of 500 ....NDC 0456-0643-02
  Unit Dose boxes
  of 100 ....NDC 0456-0643-63
Elixophyllin® SR 125 mg Capsules—opaque, white, hard gelatin capsules, imprinted with FOREST 646.
125 mg Capsules
  Bottles of 100 ....NDC 0456-0646-01
  Bottles of 1000 ....NDC 0456-0646-00
  Unit Dose Boxes
  of 100 ....NDC 0456-0646-63
Elixophyllin® SR 250 mg Capsules—transparent, colorless, hard gelatin capsules, imprinted with FOREST 647.
250 mg Capsules
  Bottles of 100 ....NDC 0456-0647-01
  Bottles of 1000 ....NDC 0456-0647-00
  Unit Dose Boxes
  of 100 ....NDC 0456-0647-63
ELIXOPHYLLIN® Elixir is a clear red solution with a mixed fruit flavor. Each tablespoonful (15 mL) contains 80 mg anhydrous theophylline.
ELIXOPHYLLIN® Elixir is available in bottles of
  473 mL ....NDC 0456-0644-16
  946 mL ....NDC 0456-0644-32
  3785 mL ....NDC 0456-0644-28

ELIXOPHYLLIN®-GG   **R**
[*ē"lix-off'fil-in gēē-gēē*]
(theophylline-guaifenesin)
ORAL LIQUID

DESCRIPTION
Each 15 mL (tablespoonful) of ELIXOPHYLLIN®-GG (brand of theophylline-guaifenesin) Oral Liquid contains 100 mg anhydrous theophylline and 100 mg guaifenesin (glyceryl guaiacolate) in a cherry-berry flavored non-alcoholic liquid. ELIXOPHYLLIN®-GG Oral Liquid contains no sugar or dye.
Theophylline, a xanthine bronchodilator, is a white, odorless, crystalline powder having a bitter taste. Guaifenesin, a guaiacol compound is a white to slightly yellow crystalline powder with a bitter, aromatic taste.

HOW SUPPLIED
ELIXOPHYLLIN®-GG Oral Liquid is a clear, colorless, cherry-berry flavored non-alcoholic liquid. Each tablespoon-

ful (15 mL) contains 100 mg anhydrous theophylline and 100 mg guaifenesin.
ELIXOPHYLLIN®-GG Oral Liquid is available in bottles of:
237 mL .... NDC 0456-0648-08
473 mL .... NDC 0456-0648-16

RECOMMENDED STORAGE
Product should be stored at controlled room temperature 15–30°C (59–86°F).
Revised 7-87

ELIXOPHYLLIN-KI®   **R**
(brand of theophylline anhydrous
and potassium iodide)
Elixir

(PLEASE REFER TO ELIXOPHYLLIN® [THEOPHYLLINE ANHYDROUS] ELIXIR FOR COMPLETE INFORMATION ON THEOPHYLLINE.)

DESCRIPTION
Each 15 mL (tablespoonful) of ELIXOPHYLLIN-KI® (brand of theophylline anhydrous and potassium iodide) Elixir contains 80 mg anhydrous theophylline and 130 mg potassium iodide.

HOW SUPPLIED
ELIXOPHYLLIN-KI® Elixir is a clear yellowish amber solution with an anise aroma. Each tablespoonful (15 mL) contains 80 mg anhydrous theophylline and 130 mg potassium iodide.
ELIXOPHYLLIN-KI® Elixir is available in bottles of:
237 mL ....NDC 0456-0645-08

RECOMMENDED STORAGE
Product should be stored at controlled room temperature 15–30°C (59 –86°F).
Dispense in tight container.

ESGIC® Capsules   **R**
[*es'jik*]
(Butalbital, Acetaminophen and Caffeine Capsules)
50 mg/325 mg/40 mg
    Shown in Product Identification Section, page 409

ESGIC® Tablets   **R**
(Butalbital, Acetaminophen and Caffeine Tablets, USP)
50 mg/325 mg/40mg

ESGIC–PLUS™ TABLETS   **R**
[*es'jik*]
(Butalbital 50 mg, Acetaminophen 500 mg, and Caffeine 40 mg Tablets, USP)

DESCRIPTION
Each Esgic-Plus™ Tablet for oral administration contains:
Butalbital*   50 mg
  *WARNING: May be habit forming
  Acetaminophen   500 mg
  Caffeine   40 mg
Also contains colloidal silicon dioxide, croscarmellose sodium type A, microcrystalline cellulose and stearic acid.
Butalbital, 5-allyl-5-isobutylbarbituric acid, a white, odorless, crystalline powder having a lightly bitter taste, is a short to intermediate-acting barbiturate. Its structure is as follows:

$C_{11}H_{16}N_2O_3$ M.W. 224.26
Acetaminophen, 4'-hydroxyacetanilide, is a non-opiate, non-salicylate analgesic and antipyretic which occurs as a white, odorless, crystalline powder possessing a slightly bitter taste. Its structure is as follows:

$C_8H_9NO_2$ M.W. 151.16
Caffeine, 1, 3, 7-trimethylxanthine, is a central nervous system stimulant, which occurs as a white powder or white glis-

tening needles. It also has a bitter taste. Its structure is as follows:

$C_8H_{10}N_4O_2$ M.W. 194.19

CLINICAL PHARMACOLOGY

Pharmacologically, Esgic-Plus™ combines the analgesic properties of acetaminophen-caffeine with the anxiolytic and muscle relaxant properties of butalbital.

INDICATIONS AND USAGE

Esgic-Plus™ is indicated for the relief of the symptom complex of tension (or muscle contraction) headache.

CONTRAINDICATIONS

Hypersensitivity to acetaminophen, caffeine, or barbiturates. Patients with porphyria.

PRECAUTIONS

General

Barbiturates should be administered with caution, if at all, to patients who are mentally depressed, have suicidal tendencies, or a history of drug abuse.

Elderly or debilitated patients may react to barbiturates with marked excitement, depression, and confusion. In some persons, barbiturates repeatedly produce excitement rather than depression.

Information for Patients

Practitioners should give the following information and instructions to patients receiving barbiturates.

A. The use of barbiturates carries with it an associated risk of psychological and/or physical dependence. The patient should be warned against increasing the dose of the drug without consulting a physician.

B. Barbiturates may impair mental and/or physical abilities required for the performance of potentially hazardous tasks (e.g., driving, operating machinery, etc.).

C. Alcohol should not be consumed while taking barbiturates. Concurrent use of the barbiturates with other CNS depressants (e.g., alcohol, narcotics, tranquilizers, and antihistamines) may result in additional CNS depressant effects.

Drug Interactions

Patients receiving narcotic analgesics, antipsychotics, antianxiety agents, or other CNS depressants (including alcohol) concomitantly with Esgic-Plus™ (Butalbital, Acetaminophen, and Caffeine) may exhibit additive CNS depressant effects.

Drugs	Effect
Butalbital with coumarin anticoagulants	Decreased effect of anticoagulant because of increased metabolism resulting from enzyme induction.
Butalbital with tricyclic antidepressants	Decreased blood levels of the antidepressant.

Usage in Pregnancy

Adequate studies have not been performed in animals to determine whether this drug affects fertility in males or females, has teratogenic potential or has other adverse effects on the fetus. There are no well-controlled studies in pregnant women. Although there is no clearly defined risk, one cannot exclude the possibility of infrequent or subtle damage to the human fetus. Esgic-Plus™ should be used in pregnant women only when clearly needed.

Nursing Mothers

The effects of Esgic-Plus™ on infants of nursing mothers are not known.

Barbiturates are excreted in the breast milk of nursing mothers. The serum levels in infants are believed to be insignificant with therapeutic doses.

Pediatric Use

Safety and effectiveness in children below the age of 12 have not been established.

ADVERSE REACTIONS

The most frequent adverse reactions are drowsiness and dizziness. Less frequent adverse reactions are lightheadedness and gastrointestinal disturbances including nausea, vomiting and flatulence. Mental confusion or depression can occur due to intolerance or overdosage of butalbital.

Several cases of dermatological reactions including toxic epidermal necrolysis and erythema multiforme have been reported.

DRUG ABUSE & DEPENDENCE

Prolonged use of barbiturates can produce drug dependence, characterized by psychic dependence and tolerance. The abuse liability of Esgic-Plus™ is similiar to that of other barbiturate-containing drug combinations. Caution should be exercised when prescribing medication for patients with a known propensity for taking excessive quantities of drugs,

which is not uncommon in patients with chronic tension headache.

OVERDOSAGE

The toxic effects of acute overdosage of Esgic-Plus™ are attributable mainly to its barbiturate component, and, to a lesser extent, acetaminophen. Because toxic effects of caffeine occur in very high dosages only, the possibility of significant caffeine toxicity from Esgic-Plus™ overdosage is unlikely.

Barbiturate

Signs and Symptoms: Drowsiness, confusion, coma; respiratory depression; hypotension; shock.

Treatment:

1. Maintenance of an adequate airway, with assisted respiration and oxygen administration as necessary.
2. Monitoring of vital signs and fluid balance.
3. If the patient is conscious and has not lost the gag reflex, emesis may be induced with ipecac. Care should be taken to prevent pulmonary aspiration of vomitus. After completion of vomiting, 30 grams of activated charcoal in a glass of water may be administered.
4. If emesis is contraindicated, gastric lavage may be performed with a cuffed endotracheal tube in place with the patient in the facedown position. Activated charcoal may be left in the emptied stomach and a saline cathartic administered.
5. Fluid therapy and other standard treatment for shock, if needed.
6. If renal function is normal, forced diuresis may aid in the elimination of the barbiturate. Alkalinization of the urine increases renal excretion of some barbiturates, especially phenobarbital.
7. Although not recommended as a routine procedure, hemodialysis may be used in severe barbiturate intoxication or if the patient is anuric or in shock.

Acetaminophen

Signs and Symptoms: In acute acetaminophen overdosage, dose-dependent, potentially fatal hepatic necrosis is the most serious adverse effect. Renal tubular necrosis, hypoglycemic coma, and thrombocytopenia may also occur.

In adults, hepatic toxicity has rarely been reported with acute overdoses of less than 10 grams and fatalities with less than 15 grams. Importantly, young children seem to be more resistant than adults to the hepatotoxic effect of an acetaminophen overdose.

Early symptoms following a potentially hepatotoxic overdosage may include: nausea, vomiting, diaphoresis and general malaise. Clinical and laboratory evidence of hepatic toxicity may not be apparent until 48 to 72 hours post-ingestion.

Treatment: The stomach should be emptied promptly by lavage or by induction of emesis with syrup of ipecac. Patients' estimates of the quantity of a drug ingested are notoriously unreliable. Therefore, if an acetaminophen overdose is suspected, a serum acetaminophen assay should be obtained as early as possible, but no sooner than four hours following ingestion. Liver function studies should be obtained initially and repeated at 24-hour intervals.

The antidote, N-acetylcysteine, should be administered as early as possible, preferably within 16 hours of the overdose ingestion for optimal results, but in any case, within 24 hours. Following recovery, there are no residual, structural or functional hepatic abnormalities.

DOSAGE AND ADMINISTRATION

One tablet every four hours as needed. Do not exceed 6 tablets per day.

HOW SUPPLIED

Esgic-Plus™ (Butalbital 50 mg [WARNING - May be habit forming]. Acetaminophen 500mg and Caffeine 40mg) Tablets are white, capsule-shaped, single-scored, and are debossed "FOREST" on the upper side, "678" on one side of the score on the lower side. They are supplied as:

Bottles of 100—NDC 0456-0678-01

Storage:

Store at controlled room temperature 15°–30°C (59°–86°F).

Dispense in a tight, light-resistant container with a child-resistant closure.

CAUTION: Federal law prohibits dispensing without prescription.

Manufactured by:

MIKART, INC., Atlanta, GA 30318

Distributed by:

FOREST PHARMACEUTICALS, INC.

Subsidiary of Forest Laboratories, Inc.

St. Louis, MO 63043

Revised 10/91

Shown in Product Identification Section, page 409

KAY CIEL®   ℞
[kā'sēēl"]
(potassium chloride)
Oral Solution 10%

KAY CIEL®   ℞
(potassium chloride)
Powder

DESCRIPTION

ORAL SOLUTION—

Each 15 mL (tablespoonful) contains 1.5 g (20 mEq) potassium chloride in a palatable base.

KAY CIEL® Oral Solution also contains the following inactive ingredients; alcohol 4%, coloring agent, flavoring agent, methylparaben, propylparaben, saccharin sodium and water. Contains no sugar.

POWDER—

Each packet contains 1.5 g (20 mEq) potassium chloride. KAY CIEL® Powder also contains the following inactive ingredients; coloring agents, flavoring agent and saccharin sodium. Contains no sugar.

HOW SUPPLIED

Oral Solution in bottles of:

118 mL	NDC 0456-0661-04
473 mL	NDC 0456-0661-16
3785 mL	NDC 0456-0661-28

Powder in boxes of:

30 packets	NDC 0456-0662-70
100 packets	NDC 0456-0662-71

Revised 4-86

LEVOTHROID® TABLETS   ℞
[lēv'ō-throid"]
(levothyroxine sodium)

DESCRIPTION

LEVOTHROID® (levothyroxine sodium) provides crystalline sodium levothyroxine (T_4), a potent thyroid hormone, in nine different strengths to permit easy convenient dosage adjustment.

The structural formula for sodium levothyroxine is:

Sodium L-3, 3', 5, 5',-tetraiodothyronine

CLINICAL PHARMACOLOGY

The major thyroid hormones are L-thyroxine (T_4) and L-triiodothyronine (T_3). The amounts of T_4 and T_3 released into the circulation from the normally functioning thyroid gland are regulated by the amount of thyrotropin (TSH) secreted from the anterior pituitary gland. TSH secretion is in turn regulated by the levels of circulating T_4 and T_3 and by secretion of thyrotropin releasing factor (TRH) from the hypothalamus. Recognition of this complex feedback system is important in the diagnosis and treatment of thyroid dysfunction. The principal effect of exogenous thyroid hormones is to increase the metabolic rate of body tissues.

The thyroid hormones are also concerned with growth and differentiation of tissues. In deficiency states in the young there is retardation of growth and failure of maturation of the skeletal and other body systems, especially in failure of ossification in the epiphyses and in the growth and development of the brain.

The precise mechanism of action by which thyroid hormones affect thermogenesis and cellular growth and differentiation is not known. It is recognized that these physiologic effects are mediated at the cellular level primarily by T_3, a large part of which is derived from T_4 by deiodination in the peripheral tissues. Thyroxine (T_4) is the major component of normal secretions of the thyroid gland and is thus the primary determinant of normal thyroid function.

Depending on other factors, absorption has varied from 48 to 79 percent of the administered dose. Fasting increases absorption. Malabsorption syndromes, as well as dietary factors, (children's soybean formula, concomitant use of anionic exchange resins such as cholestyramine) cause excessive fecal loss.

More than 99 percent of circulating hormones are bound to serum proteins, including thyroid-binding globulin (TB$_g$), thyroid-binding prealbumin (TBPA), and albumin (TBa), whose capacities and affinities vary for the hormones.

L-thyroxine displays greater binding affinity than L-triiodothyronine, both in the circulation and at the cellular level, which explains its longer duration of action. The half-life of T_4 in normal plasma is 6–7 days while that of T_3 is about 1

Continued on next page

Forest—Cont.

day. The plasma half-lives of T_4 and T_3 are decreased in hyperthyroidism and increased in hypothyroidism.

INDICATIONS AND USAGE

Levothroid Tablets (levothyroxine sodium) are indicated as replacement or substitution therapy for diminished or absent thyroid function (e.g., cretinism, myxedema, non-toxic goiter or hypothyroidism generally, including the hypothyroid state in children, in pregnancy and in the elderly) resulting from functional deficiency, primary atrophy, from partial or complete absence of the gland or from the effects of surgery, radiation or antithyroid agents. Therapy must be maintained continuously to control the symptoms of hypothyroidism.

It may also be used to suppress the secretion of thyrotropin (TSH) action which may be beneficial in simple nonendemic goiter and in chronic lymphocytic thyroiditis. This may cause a reduction in the goiter size.

Thyroid hormone drugs are indicated as a diagnostic agent in suppression tests to differentiate suspected mild hyperthyroidism or thyroid gland autonomy.

Thyroid hormones may also be used with antithyroid drugs to treat thyrotoxicosis. This combination has been used to prevent goitrogenesis and hypothyroidism.

CONTRAINDICATIONS

Levothroid Tablets administration is contraindicated in untreated thyrotoxicosis and in acute myocardial infarction. Levothroid Tablets is contraindicated in the presence of uncorrected adrenal insufficiency because it increases the tissue demands for adrenocortical hormones and may cause an acute adrenal crisis in such patients. (See PRECAUTIONS.)

WARNINGS

Drugs with thyroid hormone activity, alone or together with other therapeutic agents, have been used for the treatment of obesity. In euthyroid patients, doses within the range of daily hormonal requirements are ineffective for weight reduction. Larger doses may produce serious or even life-threatening manifestations of toxicity, particularly when given in association with sympathomimetic amines such as those used for their anorectic effects.

The use of thyroid hormones in the therapy of obesity, alone or combined with other drugs, is unjustified and has been shown to be ineffective. Neither is their use justified for the treatment of male or female infertility unless this condition is accompanied by hypothyroidism.

PRECAUTIONS

General: Levothroid Tablets should be used with caution in patients with cardiovascular disease, including hypertension. The development of chest pain or other aggravation of cardiovascular disease will require a decrease in dosage.

Thyroid hormone therapy in patients with concomitant diabetes mellitus or diabetes insipidus or adrenal cortical insufficiency aggravates the intensity of their symptoms. Appropriate adjustments of the various therapeutic measures directed at these concomitant endocrine diseases are required.

The therapy of myxedema coma requires simultaneous administration of glucocorticoids. (See DOSAGE AND ADMINISTRATION.)

In infants, excessive doses of thyroid hormone preparations may produce craniosynostosis.

Information for the Patient: Patients on thyroid preparations and parents of children on thyroid therapy should be informed that:

1. Replacement therapy is to be taken essentially for life, with the exception of cases of transient hypothyroidism, usually associated with thyroiditis, and in those patients receiving a therapeutic trial of the drug.
2. They should immediately report during the course of therapy any signs or symptoms of thyroid hormone toxicity, e.g., chest pain, increased pulse rate, palpitations, excessive sweating, heat intolerance, nervousness, or any other unusual event.
3. In case of concomitant diabetes mellitus, the daily dosage of antidiabetic medication may need readjustment as thyroid hormone replacement is achieved. If thyroid medication is stopped, a downward readjustment of the dosage of insulin or oral hypoglycemic agent may be necessary to avoid hypoglycemia. At all times, close monitoring of urinary glucose levels is mandatory in such patients.
4. In case of concomitant oral anticoagulant therapy, the prothrombin time should be measured frequently to determine if the dosage of oral anticoagulants is to be readjusted.
5. Partial loss of hair may be experienced by children in the first few months of thyroid therapy, but this is usually a transient phenomenon and later recovery is usually the rule.

Laboratory Tests: The patient's response to thyroid replacement therapy may be followed by laboratory tests such as serum thyroxine (T_4), serum triiodothyronine (T_3), free thyroxine index and thyroid stimulating hormone (TSH) blood levels.

Drug Interactions: In patients with diabetes mellitus, addition of thyroid hormone therapy may cause an increase in the required dosage of insulin or oral hypoglycemic agents. Conversely, decreasing the dose of thyroid hormone may possibly cause hypoglycemic reactions if the dosage of insulin or oral hypoglycemic agents is not adjusted.

Thyroid replacement may potentiate anticoagulant effects with agents such as warfarin or bishydroxycoumarin and reduction of one-third in anticoagulant dosage should be undertaken upon initiation of Levothroid Tablets therapy. Subsequent anticoagulant dosage adjustment should be made on the basis of frequent prothrombin determinations.

Injection of epinephrine in patients with coronary artery disease may precipitate an episode of coronary insufficiency. This may be enhanced in patients receiving thyroid preparations. Careful observation is required if catecholamines are administered to patients in this category.

Cholestyramine or colestipol binds both T_4 and T_3 in the intestine, thus impairing absorption of these thyroid hormones. *In vitro* studies indicate that the binding is not easily removed. Therefore, four to five hours should elapse between administration of cholestyramine or colestipol and thyroid hormones.

Estrogens tend to increase serum thyroxine-binding globulin (TBg). In a patient with a non-functioning thyroid gland who is receiving thyroid replacement therapy, free levothyroxine may be decreased when estrogens are started thus increasing thyroid requirements. However, if the patient's thyroid gland has sufficient function the decreased free thyroxine will result in a compensatory increase in thyroxine output by the thyroid. Therefore, patients without a functioning thyroid gland who are on thyroid replacement therapy may need to increase their thyroid dose if estrogens or estrogen-containing oral contrceptives are given.

Drug/Laboratory Test Interactions: the following drugs or moieties are known to interfere with laboratory tests performed in patients on thyroid hormone therapy: androgens, corticosteroids, estrogens, oral contraceptives containing estrogens, iodine-containing preparations, and the numerous preparations containing salicylates.

1. Changes in TBg concentration should be taken into consideration in the interpretation of T_4 and T_3 values. In such cases, the unbound (free) hormone should be measured. Pregnancy, estrogens, and estrogen-containing oral contraceptives increase TBg concentrations. TBg may also be increased during infectious hepatitis. Decreases in TBg concentrations are observed in nephrosis, acromegaly, and after androgen or corticosteroid therapy. Familial hyper- or hypo-thyroxine-binding-globulinemias have been described. The incidence of TBg deficiency approximates 1 in 9000. The binding of thyroxine by thyroid-binding prealbumin (TBPA) is inhibited by salicylates.
2. Medical or dietary iodine interferes with all *in vivo* tests of radio-iodine uptake, producing low uptakes which may not be reflective of a true decrease in hormone synthesis.
3. The persistence of clinical and laboratory evidence of hypothyroidism in spite of adequate dosage replacement indicates either poor patient compliance, poor absorption, excessive fecal loss, or inactivity of the preparation. Intracellular resistance to thyroid hormone is quite rare.

Carcinogenesis, Mutagenesis, and Impairment of Fertility: A reportedly apparent association between prolonged thyroid therapy and breast cancer has not been confirmed and patients on thyroid for established indications should not discontinue therapy. No confirmatory long-term studies in animals have been performed to evaluate carcinogenic potential, mutagenicity, or impairment of fertility in either males or females.

Pregnancy—Category A: Thyroid hormones do not readily cross the placental barrier. The clinical experience to date does not indicate any adverse effect on fetuses when thyroid hormones are administered to pregnant women. On the basis of current knowledge, thyroid replacement therapy to hypothyroid women should not be discontinued during pregnancy.

Nursing Mothers: Minimal amounts of thyroid hormones are excreted in human milk. Thyroid is not associated with serious adverse reactions and does not have a known tumorigenic potential. However, caution should be exercised when thyroid is administered to a nursing woman.

Pediatric Use: The diagnosis and institution of therapy for cretinism should be done as soon after birth as feasible to prevent developmental deficiency. Screening tests for serum T_4 and TSH will identify this group of newborn patients.

ADVERSE REACTIONS

Patients who are sensitive to lactose may show intolerance to Levothroid Tablets since this substance is used in the manufacture of the product.

Adverse reactions other than those indicative of hyperthyroidism because of therapeutic overdosage, either initially or during the maintenance period, are rare. (See OVERDOSAGE.)

OVERDOSAGE

Excessive dosage of thyroid medication may result in symptoms of hyperthyroidism. Since, however, the effects do not appear at once, the symptoms may not appear for one to three weeks after the dosage regimen is begun. The most common signs and symptoms of overdosage are weight loss, palpitation, nervousness, diarrhea or abdominal cramps, sweating, tachycardia, cardiac arrhythmias, angina pectoris, tremors, headache, insomnia, intolerance to heat and fever. If symptoms of overdosage appear, discontinue medication for several days and reinstitute treatment at a lower dosage level.

Laboratory tests such as serum T_4, serum T_3 and the free thyroxine index will be elevated during the period of overdosage.

Complications as a result of the induced hypermetabolic state may include cardiac failure and death due to arrhythmia or failure.

Treatment of Overdosage: Dosage should be reduced or therapy temporarily discontinued if signs and symptoms of overdosage appear. Treatment may be reinstituted at a lower dosage. In normal individuals, normal hypothalamic-pituitary-thyroid axis function is restored in 6 to 8 weeks after thyroid suppression.

Treatment of acute massive thyroid hormone overdosage is aimed at reducing gastrointestinal absorption of the drugs and counteracting central and peripheral effects, mainly those of increased sympathetic activity. Vomiting may be induced initially if further gastrointestinal absorption can reasonably be prevented and barring contraindications such as coma, convulsions, or loss of the gagging reflex. Treatment is symptomatic and supportive. Oxygen may be administered and ventilation maintained. Cardiac glycosides may be indicated if congestive heart failure develops. Measures to control fever, hypoglycemia, or fluid loss should be instituted if needed. Antiadrenergic agents, particularly propranolol, have been used advantageously in the treatment of increased sympathetic activity. Propranolol may be administered intravenously at a dosage of 1 to 3 mg over a 10 minute period or orally, 80 to 160 mg/day, especially when no contraindications exist for its use. Other adjunctive measures may include administration of cholestyramine to interfere with thyroxine absorption, and glucocorticoids to inhibit conversion of T_4 to T_3.

DOSAGE AND ADMINISTRATION

The goal of therapy should be the restoration of euthyroidism as judged by clinical response and confirmed by appropriate laboratory values. In adults with no complicating endocrine or cardiovascular disease, the predicted full maintenance dose may be achieved immediately with adjustments made as indicated by clinical evaluation. The usual maintenance dose of Levothroid Tablets is 100 to 200 mcg.

In patients with known complications or in case of doubt, individual dose titration at 2- to 4-week intervals is recommended. The usual starting dose is 50 mcg with increases of 50 mcg at 2- to 4-week intervals until the patient is euthyroid or symptoms ensue which preclude further dose increase.

In adult myxedema or hypothyroid patients with angina, the starting dose should be 25 mcg with increases at 2- to 4-week intervals of 25 to 50 mcg as determined by clinical response.

Myxedema coma is usually precipitated in the hypothyroid patient of long-standing by intercurrent illness or drugs such as sedatives and anesthetics and should be considered a medical emergency. Therapy should be directed at the correction of electrolyte disturbances and possible infection besides the administration of thyroid hormones. Corticosteroids should be administered routinely. T_4 and T_3 may be administered via a nasogastric tube, but the preferred route of administration of both hormones is intravenous. Sodium levothyroxine (T_4) is given at a starting dose of 200–500 mcg (100 mcg/mL given rapidly), and is usually well tolerated, even in the elderly. This initial dose is followed by daily supplements of 100 to 200 mcg given IV. Normal T_4 levels are achieved in 24 hours followed in 3 days by threefold evaluation of T_3. Oral therapy with Levothroid Tablets should be resumed as soon as the clinical situation has been stablized and the patient is able to take oral medication.

Pediatric dosage should follow the recommendations summarized in Table I. In infants with congenital hypothyroidism, therapy with full doses should be instituted as soon as the diagnosis has been made. **Levothroid Tablets** may be given to infants and children who cannot swallow intact tablets by crushing the proper dose tablet and suspending the **freshly crushed** tablet in a small amount of water or formula. The suspension can be given by spoon or dropper. DO NOT STORE THE SUSPENSION FOR ANY PERIOD OF TIME. The crushed tablet may also be sprinkled over a small amount of food, such as cooked cereal or apple sauce.

TABLE I
Recommended Pediatric Dosage
For Congenital Hypothyroidism*
LEVOTHROID (Levothyroxine Sodium Tablets, USP)

Age	Dose per day	Daily dose per kg of body weight
0– 6 mos	25– 50 mcg	8–10 mcg
6–12 mos	50– 75 mcg	6– 8 mcg
1– 5 yrs	75–100 mcg	5– 6 mcg
6–12 yrs	100–150 mcg	4– 5 mcg

*To be adjusted on the basis of clinical response and laboratory tests (See **Laboratory Tests**).

HOW SUPPLIED

[See table at right.]

Tablets should be stored at controlled room temperature, 59°–86°F (15°–30°C) in capped bottles or unbroken plastic strip packing.

CAUTION: Federal law prohibits dispensing without prescription.

Mfd by: Rhône-Poulenc Rorer
Pharmaceuticals Inc.
Fort Washington, PA 19034
Mfd for: **Forest Pharmaceuticals, Inc.**
A Subsidiary of Forest Laboratories, Inc.
St. Louis, MO 63043
Rev. 3/91

Shown in Product Identification Section, page 409

Strength	Tablet	Markings	Package Size	NDC Number
25 mcg	Orange	LK	bottle of 100	0456-0320-01
50 mcg	White	LL	bottle of 100	0456-0321-01
50 mcg			unit dose cartons of 100	0456-0321-63
75 mcg	Grey	LT	bottle of 100	0456-0322-01
100 mcg	Yellow	LM	bottle of 100	0456-0323-01
100 mcg			unit dose cartons of 100	0456-0323-63
125 mcg	Purple	LH	bottle of 100	0456-0324-01
125 mcg			unit dose cartons of 100	0456-0324-63
150 mcg	Blue	LN	bottle of 100	0456-0325-01
150 mcg			unit dose cartons of 100	0456-0325-63
175 mcg	Turquoise	LP	bottle of 100	0456-0326-01
200 mcg	Pink	LR	bottle of 100	0456-0327-01
200 mcg			unit dose cartons of 100	0456-0327-63
300 mcg	Green	LS	bottle of 100	0456-0328-01
300 mcg			unit dose cartons of 100	0456-0328-63

LORCET®-10/650 Ⓒ III

HYDROCODONE BITARTRATE AND ACETAMINOPHEN TABLETS
10 mg/650 mg

DESCRIPTION

Each Lorcet® 10/650 tablet contains:

Hydrocodone* Bitartrate .... 10 mg
*(**WARNING:** May be habit forming)
Acetaminophen .... 650 mg

Also contains colloidal silicon dioxide, croscarmellose sodium, crospovidone, microcrystalline cellulose, povidone, pregelatinized starch, stearic acid and FD&C Blue #1 Lake.

Hydrocodone bitartrate is an opioid analgesic and antitussive which occurs as fine, white crystals or as a crystalline powder. It is affected by light. The chemical name is: 4,5α-epoxy-3-methoxy-17-methylmorphinan-6-one tartrate (1:1) hydrate (2:5). Its structure is as follows:

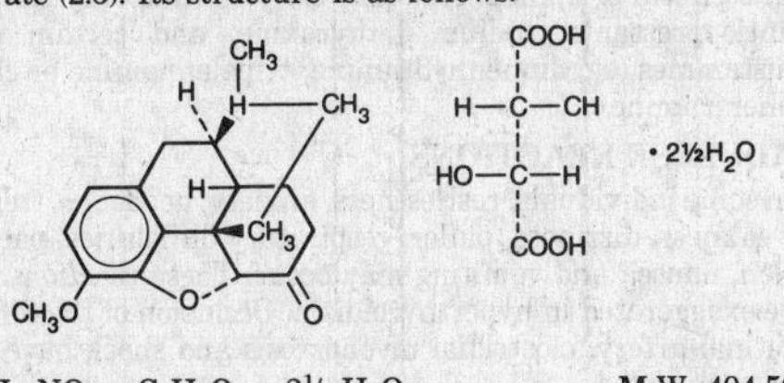

$C_{18}H_{21}NO_3 \cdot C_4H_6O_6 \cdot 2\frac{1}{2}\, H_2O$ M.W. 494.50

Acetaminophen, 4'-hydroxyacetanilide, is a non-opiate, non-salicylate analgesic and antipyretic which occurs as a white, odorless, crystalline powder possessing a slightly bitter taste. Its structure is as follows:

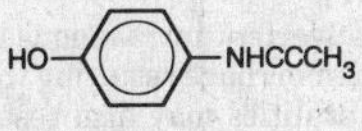

$C_8H_9NO_2$ M.W. 151.16

CLINICAL PHARMACOLOGY

Hydrocodone is a semisynthetic narcotic analgesic and antitussive with multiple actions qualitatively similar to those of codeine. Most of these involve the central nervous system and smooth muscle. The precise mechanism of action of hydrocodone and other opiates is not known, although it is believed to relate to the existence of opiate receptors in the central nervous system. In addition to analgesia, narcotics may produce drowsiness, changes in mood and mental clouding.

Radioimmunoassay techniques have recently been developed for the analysis of hydrocodone in human plasma. After a 10 mg oral dose of hydrocodone bitartrate, a mean peak serum drug level of 23.6 ng/mL and an elimination half-life of 3.8 hours were found.

The analgesic action of acetaminophen involves peripheral and central influences, but the specific mechanism is as yet undetermined. Antipyretic activity is mediated through hypothalamic heat regulating centers. Acetaminophen inhibits prostaglandin synthetase. Therapeutic doses of acetaminophen have negligible effects on the cardiovascular or respiratory systems; however, toxic doses may cause circulatory failure and rapid, shallow breathing. Acetaminophen is rapidly and almost completely absorbed from the gastrointestinal tract, producing maximum serum concentrations within 30 minutes to one hour. The plasma half-life in adults and children ranges from 0.90 hours to 3.25 hours with an average of approximately 2 hours. The drug distributes uniformly in most body fluids and is approximately 25% protein bound. Acetaminophen is conjugated in the liver, with less than 3% of the dose excreted unchanged in 24 hours. The primary metabolic pathway is conjugation to sulfate and glucuronide by-products. A minor oxidative pathway forms cysteine and mercapturic acid. These compounds are subsequently excreted by the kidneys into the urine.

INDICATIONS AND USAGE

For the relief of moderate to moderately severe pain.

CONTRAINDICATIONS

Hypersensitivity to acetaminophen or hydrocodone.

WARNINGS

Respiratory Depression: At high doses or in sensitive patients, hydrocodone may produce dose-related respiratory depression by acting directly on the brain stem respiratory center. Hydrocodone also affects the center that controls respiratory rhythm, and may produce irregular and periodic breathing.

Head Injury and Increased Intracranial Pressure: The respiratory depressant effects of narcotics and their capacity to elevate cerebrospinal fluid pressure may be markedly exaggerated in the presence of head injury, other intracranial lesions or a preexisting increase in intracranial pressure. Furthermore, narcotics produce adverse reactions which may obscure the clinical course of patients with head injuries.

Acute Abdominal Conditions: The administration of narcotics may obscure the diagnosis or clinical course of patients with acute abdominal conditions.

PRECAUTIONS

Special Risk Patients: As with any narcotic analgesic agent, Lorcet® 10/650 should be used with caution in elderly or debilitated patients and those with severe impairment of hepatic or renal function, hypothyroidism, Addison's disease, prostatic hypertrophy or urethral stricture. The usual precautions should be observed and the possibility of respiratory depression should be kept in mind.

Information for Patients: Lorcet® 10/650, like all narcotics, may impair the mental and/or physical abilities required for the performance of potentially hazardous tasks such as driving a car or operating machinery; patients should be cautioned accordingly.

Cough Reflex: Hydrocodone suppresses the cough reflex; as with all narcotics, caution should be exercised when Lorcet® 10/650 is used postoperatively and in patients with pulmonary disease.

Drug Interactions: Patients receiving other narcotic analgesics, antipsychotics, antianxiety agents, or other CNS depressants (including alcohol) concomitantly with Lorcet® 10/650 may exhibit an additive CNS depression. When combined therapy is contemplated, the dose of one or both agents should be reduced.

The use of MAO inhibitors or tricyclic antidepressants with hydrocodone preparations may increase the effect of either the antidepressant or hydrocodone.

The concurrent use of anticholinergics with hydrocodone may produce paralytic ileus.

Usage In Pregnancy:

Teratogenic Effects: Pregnancy Category C. Hydrocodone has been shown to be teratogenic in hamsters when given in doses 700 times the human dose. There are no adequate and well-controlled studies in pregnant women. Lorcet® 10/650 should be used during pregnancy only if the potential benefit justifies the potential risk to the fetus.

Nonteratogenic Effects: Babies born to mothers who have been taking opioids regularly prior to delivery will be physically dependent. The withdrawal signs include irritability and excessive crying, tremors, hyperactive reflexes, increased respiratory rate, increased stools, sneezing, yawning, vomiting, and fever. The intensity of the syndrome does not always correlate with the duration of maternal opioid use or dose. There is no consensus on the best method of managing withdrawal. Chlorpromazine 0.7 to 1 mg/kg q6h, and paregoric 2 to 4 drops/kg q4h, have been used to treat withdrawal symptoms in infants. The duration of therapy is 4 to 28 days, with the dosage decreased as tolerated.

Labor and Delivery: As with all narcotics, administration of Lorcet® 10/650 the mother shortly before delivery may result in some degree of respiratory depression in the newborn, especially if higher doses are used.

Nursing Mothers: It is not known whether this drug is excreted in human milk. Because many drugs are excreted in human milk and because of the potential for serious adverse reactions in nursing infants from Lorcet® 10/650, a decision should be made whether to discontinue nursing or to discontinue the drug, taking into account the importance of the drug to the mother.

Pediatric Use: Safety and effectiveness in children have not been established.

ADVERSE REACTIONS

The most frequently observed adverse reactions include lightheadedness, dizziness, sedation, nausea and vomiting. These effects seem to be more prominent in ambulatory than in nonambulatory patients and some of these adverse reactions may be alleviated if the patient lies down.

Other adverse reactions include:

Central Nervous System: Drowsiness, mental clouding, lethargy, impairment of mental and physical performance, anxiety, fear, dysphoria, psychic dependence, mood changes.

Gastrointestinal System: The antiemetic phenothiazines are useful in suppressing the nausea and vomiting which may occur (see above); however, some phenothiazine derivatives seem to be antianalgesic and to increase the amount of narcotic required to produce pain relief, while other phenothiazines reduce the amount of narcotic required to produce a given level of analgesia. Prolonged administration of Lorcet® 10/650 may produce constipation.

Genitourinary System: Ureteral spasm, spasm of vesical sphincters and urinary retention have been reported.

Respiratory Depression: Hydrocodone bitartrate may produce dose-related respiratory depression by acting directly on the brain stem respiratory center. Hydrocodone also affects the center that controls respiratory rhythm, and may produce irregular and periodic breathing. If significant respiratory depression occurs, it may be antagonized by the use of naloxone hydrochloride. Apply other supportive measures when indicated.

DRUG ABUSE AND DEPENDENCE

Lorcet® 10/650 is subject to the Federal Controlled Substances Act (Schedule III).

Psychic dependence, physical dependence, and tolerance may develop upon repeated administration of narcotics; therefore, Lorcet® 10/650 should be prescribed and administered with caution. However, psychic dependence is unlikely to develop when Lorcet® 10/650 is used for a short time for the treatment of pain.

Physical dependence, the condition in which continued administration of the drug is required to prevent the appearance of a withdrawal syndrome, assumes clinically significant proportions only after several weeks of continued narcotic use, although some mild degree of physical dependence may develop after a few days of narcotic therapy. Tolerance, in which increasingly large doses are required in order to produce the same degree of analgesia, is manifested initially by a shortened duration of analgesic effect, and subsequently by decreases in the intensity of analgesia. The rate of development of tolerance varies among patients.

OVERDOSAGE

Acetaminophen:

Signs and Symptoms: In acute acetaminophen overdosage, dose-dependent, potentially fatal hepatic necrosis is the most serious adverse effect. Renal tubular necrosis, hypoglycemic coma, and thrombocytopenia may also occur.

In adults, hepatic toxicity has rarely been reported with

Continued on next page

Forest—Cont.

acute overdoses of less than 10 grams and fatalities with less than 15 grams. Importantly, young children seem to be more resistant than adults to the hepatotoxic effect of an acetaminophen overdose. Despite this, the measures outlined below should be initiated in any adult or child suspected of having ingested an acetaminophen overdose.

Early symptoms following a potentially hepatotoxic overdose may include: nausea, vomiting, diaphoresis and general malaise. Clinical and laboratory evidence of hepatic toxicity may not be apparent until 48 to 72 hours post-ingestion.
Treatment: The stomach should be emptied promptly by lavage or by induction of emesis with syrup of ipecac. Patients' estimates of the quantity of a drug ingested are notoriously unreliable. Therefore, if an acetaminophen overdose is suspected, a serum acetaminophen assay should be obtained as early as possible, but no sooner than four hours following ingestion. Liver function studies should be obtained initially and repeated at 24-hour intervals.

The antidote, N-acetylcysteine, should be administered as early as possible, preferably within 16 hours of the overdose ingestion for optimal results, but in any case, within 24 hours. Following recovery, there are no residual, structural or functional hepatic abnormalities.

Hydrocodone:

Signs and Symptoms: Serious overdose with hydrocodone is characterized by respiratory depression (a decrease in respiratory rate and/or tidal volume, Cheyne-Stokes respiration, cyanosis), extreme somnolence progressing to stupor or coma, skeletal muscle flaccidity, cold and clammy skin, and sometimes bradycardia and hypotension. In severe overdosage, apnea, circulatory collapse, cardiac arrest and death may occur.

Treatment: Primary attention should be given to the reestablishment of adequate respiratory exchange through provision of a patent airway and the institution of assisted or controlled ventilation. The narcotic antagonist naloxone is a specific antidote against respiratory depression which may result from overdosage or unusual sensitivity to narcotics, including hydrocodone. Therefore, an appropriate dose of naloxone hydrochloride (see package insert) should be administered, preferably by the intravenous route, and simultaneously with efforts at respiratory resuscitation. Since the duration of action of hydrocodone may exceed that of the antagonist, the patient should be kept under continued surveillance and repeated doses of the antagonist should be administered as needed to maintain adequate respiration.

An antagonist should not be administered in the absence of clinically significant respiratory or cardiovascular depression. Oxygen, intravenous fluids, vasopressors and other supportive measures should be employed as indicated.

Gastric emptying may be useful in removing unabsorbed drug.

DOSAGE AND ADMINISTRATION

Dosage should be adjusted according to the severity of the pain and the response of the patient. However, it should be kept in mind that tolerance to hydrocodone can develop with continued use and that the incidence of untoward effects is dose related.

The usual adult dosage is one tablet every four to six hours as needed for pain. The total 24 hour dose should not exceed 6 tablets.

HOW SUPPLIED

Lorcet® 10/650, Hydrocodone* Bitartrate and Acetaminophen Tablets 10 mg/650 mg, each tablet of which contains hydrocodone* bitartrate 10 mg* (**WARNING:** May be habit forming) and acetaminophen 650 mg, are light-blue, capsule-shaped, scored tablets, debossed "UAD" on one side and "63 50" on the other side, and are supplied in containers of 20 tablets, NDC 0785-6350-30, in containers of 100 tablets. NDC 0785-6350-01, and containers of unit dose (4 × 25's), NDC 0785-6350-63.

Storage: Store at controlled room temperature 15–30°C (59–86°F).

Dispense in a tight, light-resistant container with a child-resistant closure.

CAUTION: Federal law prohibits dispensing without prescription.

A Schedule CIII Controlled Substance.
Manufactured by: MIKART, INC., ATLANTA, GA 30318.
Manufactured for:
UAD LABORATORIES, INC.
Division of Forest Pharmaceuticals Inc.
Jackson, MS 39209

Rev. 6/92
Code 558A00

Shown in Product Identification Section, page 433

NDC 0456-0686-01	Bottles of 100	1 mg off white round standard convex, imprint: 1
NDC 0456-0687-01	Bottles of 100	2 mg off white round standard convex, imprint: 2
NDC 0456-0683-01	Bottles of 100	3 mg off white round standard convex, imprint: 3

NITROGARD™   ℞
(Nitroglycerin
Extended-release)
Buccal Tables

DESCRIPTION

Nitroglycerin is 1,2,3-propanetriol trinitrate, an organic nitrate whose structural formula is:

$$H_2CONO_2$$
$$HCONO_2$$
$$H_2CONO_2$$

and whose molecular weight is 227.09. The organic nitrates are vasodilators, active on both arteries and veins.

NITROGARD (nitroglycerin) buccal tablets are an Extended-release preparation designed to deliver nitroglycerin through the oral mucosa over a sustained period of time. When a NITROGARD buccal tablet is placed under the lip or in the buccal pouch, it adheres to the mucosa. As the tablet gradually dissolves, it releases nitroglycerin to the systemic circulation.

Each extended-release tablet, for buccal administration contains 1 mg, 2 mg, or 3 mg of nitroglycerin.

HOW SUPPLIED

NITROGARD (Nitroglycerin Extended-release) Buccal tablets are supplied in three strengths as:
[See table above.]
CAUTION: Federal law prohibits dispensing without prescription.
Store at controlled room temperature 15°–30°C (59°–86°F).
Dispense in a tight container as defined in the USP.

FOREST PHARMACEUTICALS, INC.
Subsidiary of Forest Laboratories, Inc.
St. Louis, MO 63043

Rev. 3/91
MG #5832 (01)

SUS–PHRINE®   ℞
[*sŭs'frĭn''*]
(brand of epinephrine)
1:200
Aqueous Suspension for
Subcutaneous Injection

$$C_9H_{13}NO_3 \qquad M.W.\ 183.21$$

Epinephrine is a white to off-white, odorless, microcrystalline powder or granules. It is affected by light. The chemical name is:
1,2-Benzenediol, 4-[1-hydroxy-2-(methylamino)ethyl]-, (R)-,(-)-3,4-Dihydroxy-α [(methylamino)methyl] benzyl alcohol [51-43-4].

DESCRIPTION

Each mL of SUS-PHRINE® (brand of epinephrine) contains 5 mg epinephrine in a sterile aqueous vehicle containing ascorbic acid 10 mg and thioglycolic acid 6.6 mg (as sodium salts) phenol 5 mg and glycerin (USP) 325 mg. Sodium hydroxide is added to adjust the pH. Approximately 80% of the total epinephrine is in suspension.

CLINICAL PHARMACOLOGY

SUS-PHRINE® (epinephrine) acts at both the alpha and beta receptor sites. Beta stimulation provides bronchodilator action by relaxing bronchial muscle. Alpha stimulation increases vital capacity by relieving congestion of the bronchial mucosa and by constricting pulmonary vessels.

Recent studies in laboratory animals (minipigs, rodents, and dogs) recorded the occurrence of cardiac arrhythmias and sudden death (with histologic evidence of myocardial necrosis) when beta agonists and methylxanthines were administered concurrently. The significance of these findings when applied to humans is currently unknown.

SUS-PHRINE® (epinephrine) provides both rapid and sus-

tained epinephrine activity. The rapid action is due to the epinephrine in solution, while the sustained activity is due to the crystalline epinephrine free base in suspension.

INDICATIONS

For the symptomatic treatment of bronchial asthma, and reversible bronchospasm associated with chronic bronchitis and emphysema.

CONTRAINDICATIONS

Hypersensitivity to any of the components.

Narrow angle glaucoma, shock, cerebral arteriosclerosis and organic heart disease. Epinephrine is also contraindicated during general anesthesia with halogenated hydrocarbons or cyclopropane, and in local anesthesia of certain areas, e.g., fingers, toes, because of the danger of vasoconstriction producing sloughing of tissue, and in labor because the drug may delay the second stage.

WARNINGS

SUS-PHRINE (epinephrine) SHOULD NOT BE EMPLOYED TO CORRECT DRUG-INDUCED HYPOTENSION.

Administer with caution to elderly people; those with cardiovascular disease, diabetes, hypertension or hyperthyroidism; in psychoneurotic individuals and in pregnancy. Administer with extreme caution to patients with long-standing bronchial asthma and emphysema who have developed degenerative heart disease.

Cardiac arrhythmias may follow administration of epinephrine.

Anginal pain may be induced when coronary insufficiency is present.

PRECAUTIONS

DO NOT USE IF PRODUCT IS DISCOLORED. Discoloration indicates the oxidation of epinephrine and possible loss of potency.

Use of SUS-PHRINE® (epinephrine) with digitalis, mercurial diuretics or other drugs that sensitize the heart to arrhythmias is not recommended.

Patients should be instructed to contact a physician immediately if severe pain at the site of injection develops.

SUS-PHRINE® (epinephrine) should not be administered concomitantly with other sympathomimetic agents, since their combined effects on the cardiovascular system may be deleterious to the patient.

The effects of epinephrine may be potentiated by tricyclic antidepressants; sodium L-thyroxine, and certain antihistamines (eg, diphenhydramine, tripelennamine or chlorpheniramine).

ADVERSE REACTIONS

In some individuals, restlessness, anxiety, headache, tremor, weakness, dizziness, pallor, respiratory difficulties, palpitation, nausea and vomiting may occur. These reactions may be exaggerated in hyperthyroidism. Occlusion of the central retinal artery, clostridial myonecrosis and shock have also been reported.

Also, urticaria, wheal and hemorrhage at the site of injection may occur. Repeated injections at the same site may result in necrosis from vascular constriction.

Tolerance to epinephrine may occur with prolonged use.

OVERDOSAGE

Overdosage or inadvertent intravenous injection may cause cerebrovascular hemorrhage resulting from the sharp rise in blood pressure. Fatalities may also result from pulmonary edema because of peripheral constriction and cardiac stimulation produced. Rapidly acting vasodilators such as nitrites, or alpha blocking agents may counteract the marked pressor effects. Cardiac arrhythmias may be countered by administering rapidly acting antiarrhythmic or beta blocking agents.

DOSAGE AND ADMINISTRATION
NOTE: INJECT SUBCUTANEOUSLY.

As with all sterile products, failure to follow aseptic procedures may result in microbial contamination causing adverse consequences which could lead to life threatening illness.

It is suggested that SUS-PHRINE® (epinephrine) be administered with a tuberculin syringe and a 26 gauge, ½ inch needle.

A small initial test dose may be administered subcutaneously as a possible aid in determining patient sensitivity to epinephrine.

Site of injection should be varied to avoid necrosis at the site of injection.

Each time before withdrawing SUS-PHRINE® (epinephrine) into syringe, **SHAKE VIAL OR AMPUL THOROUGHLY** to disperse particles and obtain a uniform suspension. Inject

promptly subcutaneously to avoid settling of suspension in the syringe.

ADULTS:
Adult dosage range is 0.1 to 0.3 mL depending on patient response.
Subsequent doses should be administered only when necessary and not more frequently than every six hours.
Infants 1 month to 2 years and Children 2 to 12 years:
Pediatric dose is 0.005 mL/kg (2.2 lb) body weight injected subcutaneously.
FOR CHILDREN 30 kg OR LESS MAXIMUM SINGLE DOSE IS 0.15 mL
Subsequent doses should be administered only when necessary and not more frequently than every six hours.

CLINICAL STUDIES
Controlled studies comparing the effectiveness of SUS-PHRINE® (epinephrine) 1:200 and an aqueous solution of epinephrine 1:1000 were conducted in both pediatric and adult asthmatics. The studies demonstrated rapid bronchodilator activity following administration of either SUS-PHRINE® (epinephrine) or epinephrine 1:1000; however during the 6 hour study period, a greater improvement in FEV_1 and $FEF_{25-75\%}$ was observed 4 to 6 hours subsequent to SUS-PHRINE® (epinephrine) administration. Improvement in Wright Peak Expiratory Flow Rate was greater for SUSPHRINE® (epinephrine) than epinephrine 1:1000 3 to 8 hours following administration (10 hour study duration).

HOW SUPPLIED
In boxes of:
10 × 0.3 mL ampuls ....NDC 0456-0664-39
25 × 0.3 mL ampuls ....NDC 0456-0664-34
5.0 mL multiple dose vial...........................NDC 0456-0664-05
Store under refrigeration. Do not freeze. Do not expose to temperature above 30° C (86°F).
Revised 5/91
mfd by
Steris Laboratories, Inc.
Phoenix, AZ 85043
mfd for
Forest Pharmaceuticals, Inc.
Subsidiary of Forest Laboratories, Inc.
St. Louis, Missouri 83043

TESSALON®   ℞
(benzonatate USP)

PRODUCT OVERVIEW
KEY FACTS
Tessalon is a nonnarcotic, oral antitussive agent. It contains 100 mg of benzonatate per Perle. Chemically related to tetracaine and other topical anesthetics, Tessalon diminishes the cough reflex by anesthetizing the stretch receptors in the respiratory passages, lungs, and pleura.

MAJOR USES
Tessalon is used for the symptomatic relief of cough.

SAFETY INFORMATION
Contraindicated in patients who are allergic to benzonatate or related compounds. Tessalon should not be chewed or allowed to dissolve in the mouth.

PRESCRIBING INFORMATION
TESSALON®   ℞
(benzonatate USP)

DESCRIPTION
TESSALON®, a nonnarcotic oral antitussive agent, is 2, 5, 8, 11, 14, 17, 20, 23, 26-nonaoxaoctacosan-28-yl-p-(butylamino) benzoate; with a molecular weight of 603.7.

$$CH_3(CH_2)_2CH_2NH-\langle\rangle-COOCH_2CH_2(OCH_2CH_2)_nOCH_3$$
$$C_{30}H_{53}NO_{11}$$

Each TESSALON Perle contains:
Benzonatate, USP .... 100 mg
TESSALON Perles also contain: D&C Yellow 10, gelatin, glycerin, methylparaben and propylparaben.

CLINICAL PHARMACOLOGY
TESSALON acts peripherally by anesthetizing the stretch receptors located in the respiratory passages, lungs, and pleura by dampening their activity and thereby reducing the cough reflex at its source. It begins to act within 15 to 20 minutes and its effect lasts for 3 to 8 hours. TESSALON has no inhibitory effect on the respiratory center in recommended dosage.

INDICATIONS AND USAGE
TESSALON is indicated for the symptomatic relief of cough.

Name	Composition (T_3/T_4 per tablet)	Color	Armacode®
Thyrolar®—¼ (0456-0040-01)	3.1 mcg/12.5 mcg	Violet/White	YC
Thyrolar®—½ (0456-0045-01)	6.25 mcg/25 mcg	Peach/White	YD
Thyrolar®—1 (0456-0050-01)	12.5 mcg/50 mcg	Pink/White	YE
Thyrolar®—2 (0456-0055-01)	25 mcg/100 mcg	Green/White	YF
Thyrolar®—3 (0456-0060-01)	37.5 mcg/150 mcg	Yellow/White	YH

CONTRAINDICATIONS
Hypersensitivity to benzonatate or related compounds.

PRECAUTIONS
Information for patients: Release of TESSALON from the perle in the mouth can produce a temporary local anesthesia of the oral mucosa and choking could occur. Therefore, the perles should be swallowed without chewing.
Usage in Pregnancy: Pregnancy Category C. Animal reproduction studies have not been conducted with TESSALON. It is also not known whether TESSALON can cause fetal harm when administered to a pregnant woman or can affect reproduction capacity. TESSALON should be given to a pregnant woman only if clearly needed.
Nursing mothers: It is not known whether this drug is excreted in human milk. Because many drugs are excreted in human milk caution should be exercised when TESSALON is administered to a nursing woman.
Carcinogenesis, mutagenesis, impairment of fertility: Carcinogenicity, mutagenicity, and reproduction studies have not been conducted with TESSALON.

ADVERSE REACTIONS
Sedation, headache, mild dizziness, pruritus and skin eruptions, nasal congestion, constipation, nausea, gastrointestinal upset, sensation of burning in the eyes, a vague "chilly" sensation, numbness in the chest, and hypersensitivity have been reported.

OVERDOSAGE
No clinically significant cases have been reported, to our knowledge. The drug is chemically related to tetracaine and other topical anesthetics and shares various aspects of their pharmacology and toxicology. Drugs of this type are generally well absorbed after ingestion.
Signs and Symptoms
If perles are chewed or dissolved in the mouth, oropharyngeal anesthesia will develop rapidly. CNS stimulation may cause restlessness and tremors which may proceed to clonic convulsions followed by profound CNS depression.
Treatment
Evacuate gastric contents and administer copious amounts of activated charcoal slurry. Even in the conscious patient, cough and gag reflexes may be so depressed as to necessitate special attention to protection against aspiration of gastric contents and orally administered materials.
Convulsions should be treated with a short-acting barbiturate given intravenously and carefully titrated for the smallest effective dosage.
Intensive support of respiration and cardiovascular-renal function is an essential feature of the treatment of severe intoxication from overdosage.
Do not use CNS stimulants.

DOSAGE AND ADMINISTRATION
Adults and Children over 10: Usual dose is one 100 mg perle t.i.d. as required. If necessary, up to 6 perles daily may be given.

HOW SUPPLIED
Perles, 100 mg (yellow); bottles of 100 NDC 0456-0688-01.
Perles, 100 mg (yellow); bottles of 500 NDC 0456-0688-02
Store at controlled room temperature 15°–30°C (59°–86°F).
Revised August, 1988
Manufactured by
R.P. Scherer-North America
St. Petersburg, Florida 33702
for
Forest Pharmaceuticals, Inc.
Subsidiary of Forest Laboratories, Inc.
St. Louis, MO 63043-9979
Shown in Product Identification Section, page 409

THYROLAR® Tablets   ℞
[thī-rō-lär]
(Liotrix Tablets, USP)

DESCRIPTION
Thyrolar® Tablets (Liotrix Tablets, USP) contain triiodothyronine (T_3 liothyronine) sodium and tetraiodothyronine (T_4 levothyroxine) sodium in the amounts listed in the "How Supplied" section. (T_3 liothyronine sodium is approximately four times as potent at T_4 thyroxine on a microgram for microgram basis.)
The inactive ingredients are calcium phosphate, microcrystalline cellulose, cornstarch, lactose, and magnesium stearate. The tablets also contain the following dyes: Thyrolar® ¼-FD&C Blue #1 and FD&C Red #40; Thyrolar® ½-

---

FD&C Red #40 and D&C Yellow #10; Thyrolar® 1-FD&C Red #40; Thyrolar® 2-FD&C Blue #1, FD&C Red #40, and D&C Yellow #10; Thyrolar® 3-FD&C Red #40 and D&C Yellow #10.

STRUCTURAL FORMULAS

Liothyronine (T_3) Sodium

Levothyroxine (T_4) Sodium

HOW SUPPLIED
Thyrolar® Tablets (Liotrix Tablets, USP) are available in five potencies, coded as follows:
[See table above.]
Supplied in bottles of 100, two-layered compressed tablets. Tablets should be stored at controlled room temperature, 59°–86°F (15°–30°C) in tight, light-resistant containers.
Note: (T_3) liothyronine sodium is approximately four times as potent as T_4 thyroxine on a microgram for microgram basis.)
Shown in Product Identification Section, page 409

Fujisawa Pharmaceutical Company
Division of Fujisawa USA, Inc.
PARKWAY NORTH CENTER
3 PARKWAY NORTH
DEERFIELD, IL 60015-2548

ADENOCARD®   ℞
(adenosine)
For Rapid Bolus Intravenous Use

DESCRIPTION
Adenosine is an endogenous nucleoside occurring in all cells of the body. It is chemically 6-amino-9-β-D-ribofuranosyl-9-H-purine and has the following structural formula:

$C_{10}H_{13}N_5O_4$ 267.24

Adenosine is a white crystalline powder. It is soluble in water and practically insoluble in alcohol. Solubility increases by warming and lowering the pH. Adenosine is not chemically related to other antiarrhythmic drugs.
Adenocard® (adenosine) is a sterile solution for rapid bolus intravenous injection and is available in 6mg/2 mL vials. Each mL contains 3 mg adenosine and 9 mg sodium chloride in Water for Injection. The pH of the solution is between 5.5 and 7.5.

CLINICAL PHARMACOLOGY
Mechanism of Action
Adenocard (adenosine) slows conduction time through the A-V node, can interrupt the reentry pathways through the A-V node and can restore normal sinus rhythm in patients

Continued on next page

Fujisawa—Cont.

with paroxysmal supraventricular tachycardia (PSVT), including PSVT associated with Wolff-Parkinson-White Syndrome.

Adenocard is antagonized competitively by methylxanthines such as caffeine and theophylline and potentiated by blockers of nucleoside transport such as dipyridamole. Adenocard is not blocked by atropine.

Hemodynamics

The usual intravenous bolus dose of 6 or 12 mg Adenocard will have no systemic hemodynamic effects. When larger doses are given by infusion, adenosine decreases blood pressure by decreasing peripheral resistance.

Pharmacokinetics

Intravenously administered Adenocard (adenosine) is removed from the circulation very rapidly. Following an intravenous bolus, adenosine is taken up by erythrocytes and vascular endothelial cells. The half-life of intravenous adenosine is estimated to be less than 10 seconds. Adenosine enters the body pool and is primarily metabolized to inosine and adenosine monophosphate (AMP).

Hepatic and Renal Failure

Hepatic and renal failure should have no effect on the activity of a bolus Adenocard (adenosine) injection. Since Adenocard (adenosine) has a direct action, hepatic and renal function are not required for the activity or metabolism of a bolus adenosine injection.

Clinical Trial Results

In controlled studies in the United States, bolus doses of 3,6,9, and 12 mg were studied. A cumulative 60% of patients with paroxysmal supraventricular tachycardia had converted to normal sinus rhythm within one minute after an intravenous bolus dose of 6 mg Adenocard (some converted on 3 mg and failures were given 6 mg), and a cumulative 92% converted after a bolus dose of 12 mg. Seven to sixteen percent of patients converted after 1–4 placebo bolus injections. Similar responses were seen in a variety of patient subsets, including those using or not using digoxin, those with Wolff-Parkinson-White Syndrome, males, females, Caucasians, and Hispanics.

Adenosine is not effective in converting rhythms other than PSVT, such as atrial flutter, atrial fibrillation, or ventricular tachycardia to normal sinus rhythm. To date, such patients have not had adverse consequences following administration of adenosine.

INDICATIONS AND USAGE

Intravenous Adenocard (adenosine) is indicated for the following:

Conversion to sinus rhythm of paroxysmal supraventricular tachycardia (PSVT), including that associated with accessory bypass tracts (Wolff-Parkinson-White Syndrome). When clinically advisable, appropriate vagal maneuvers (e.g., Valsalva maneuver), should be attempted prior to Adenocard administration.

It is important to be sure that Adenocard solution actually reaches the systemic circulation (see **DOSAGE AND ADMINISTRATION**).

Adenocard does not convert atrial flutter, atrial fibrillation, or ventricular tachycardia to normal sinus rhythm. In the presence of atrial flutter or atrial fibrillation, a transient modest slowing of ventricular response may occur immediately following Adenocard administration.

CONTRAINDICATIONS

Intravenous Adenocard (adenosine) is contraindicated in:
1. Second- or third-degree A-V block (except in patients with a functioning artificial pacemaker).
2. Sick sinus syndrome (except in patients with a functioning artificial pacemaker).
3. Known hypersensitivity to adenosine.

WARNINGS

Heart Block

Adenocard (adenosine) exerts its effect by decreasing conduction through the A-V node and may produce a short-lasting first-, second- or third-degree heart block. In extreme cases, transient asystole may result (one case has been reported in a patient with atrial flutter who was receiving carbamazepine). Appropriate therapy should be instituted as needed. Patients who develop high-level block on one dose of Adenocard should not be given additional doses. Because of the very short half-life of adenosine, these effects are generally self-limiting.

Arrhythmias at Time of Conversion

At the time of conversion to normal sinus rhythm, a variety of new rhythms may appear on the electrocardiogram. They generally last only a few seconds without intervention, and may take the form of premature ventricular contractions, atrial premature contractions, sinus bradycardia, sinus tachycardia, skipped beats, and varying degrees of A-V nodal block. Such findings were seen in 55% of patients.

PRECAUTIONS

Drug Interactions

Intravenous Adenocard (adenosine) has been effectively administered in the presence of other cardioactive drugs, such as digitalis, quinidine, beta-adrenergic blocking agents, calcium-channel blocking agents, and angiotensin-converting enzyme inhibitors, without any change in the adverse reaction profile.

The effects of adenosine are antagonized by methylxanthines such as caffeine and theophylline. In the presence of methylxanthines, larger doses of adenosine may be required or adenosine may not be effective.

Adenosine effects are potentiated by dipyridamole. Thus, smaller doses of adenosine may be effective in the presence of dipyridamole. Carbamazepine has been reported to increase the degree of heart block produced by other agents. As the primary effect of adenosine is to decrease conduction through the A-V node, higher degrees of heart block may be produced in the presence of carbamazepine.

Asthma

Most patients with asthma who have received intravenous Adenocard (adenosine) have not experienced exacerbation of their asthma. Cases of bronchospasm have been reported rarely in both asthmatic and non-asthmatic patients. Inhaled adenosine has been reported to induce broncho-constriction in asthmatic patients but not in normal individuals.

Carcinogenesis, Mutagenesis

Studies in animals have not been performed to evaluate the carcinogenic potential of Adenocard (adenosine). Adenosine tested negative for mutagenic potential in the Salmonella/Mammalian Microsome Assay (Ames Test).

Adenosine, like other nucleosides at millimolar concentrations present for several doubling times of cells in culture, is known to produce a variety of chromosomal alterations. In rats and mice, adenosine administered intraperitoneally once a day for 5 days at 50, 100, and 150 mg/kg caused decreased spermatogenesis and increased numbers of abnormal sperm, a reflection of the ability of adenosine to produce chromosomal damage.

Pregnancy Category C

Animal reproduction studies have not been conducted with adenosine; nor have studies been performed in pregnant women. As adenosine is a naturally occurring material, widely dispersed throughout the body, no fetal effects would be anticipated. However, since it is not known whether Adenocard can cause fetal harm when administered to pregnant women, Adenocard should be used during pregnancy only if clearly needed.

Pediatrics

No controlled studies have been conducted in pediatric patients.

ADVERSE REACTIONS

The following reactions were reported with intravenous Adenocard (adenosine) used in controlled U.S. clinical trials. The placebo group had a *less than* 1% rate of all of these reactions.

Cardio-vascular	Facial flushing (18%), headache (2%), sweating, palpitations, chest pain, hypotension (less than 1%)
Respiratory	Shortness of breath/dyspnea (12%), chest pressure (7%), hyperventilation, head pressure (less than 1%)
Central Nervous System	Lightheadedness (2%), dizziness, tingling in arms, numbness (1%), apprehension, blurred vision, burning sensation, heaviness in arms, neck and back pain (less than 1%)
Gastro-intestinal	Nausea (3%), metallic taste, tightness in throat, pressure in groin (less than 1%)

In post-market clinical experience with Adenocard, cases of prolonged asystole, ventricular tachycardia, ventricular fibrillation, transient increase in blood pressure, and bronchospasm, in association with Adenocard use, have been reported.

OVERDOSAGE

The half-life of Adenocard (adenosine) is less than 10 seconds. Thus, adverse effects are generally rapidly self-limiting. Treatment of any prolonged adverse effects should be individualized and be directed toward the specific effect. Methylxanthines, such as caffeine and theophylline, are competitive antagonists of adenosine.

DOSAGE AND ADMINISTRATION

For rapid bolus intravenous use only.

Adenocard (adenosine) Injection should be given as a rapid bolus by the peripheral intravenous route. To be certain the solution reaches the systemic circulation, it should be administered either directly into a vein or, if given into an IV line, it should be given as close to the patient as possible and followed by a rapid saline flush.

The dose recommendation is based on clinical studies with peripheral venous bolus dosing. Central venous (CVP or other) administration of Adenocard has not been systematically studied.

The recommended intravenous doses for adults are as follows:

Initial dose 6 mg given as a rapid intravenous bolus (administered over a 1–2 second period).

Repeat administration If the first dose does not result in elimination of the supraventricular tachycardia within 1–2 minutes, 12 mg should be given as a rapid intravenous bolus. This 12 mg dose may be repeated a second time if required.

Doses greater than 12 mg are not recommended.

NOTE Parenteral drug products should be inspected visually for particulate matter and discoloration prior to administration.

HOW SUPPLIED

Adenocard (adenosine) Injection is supplied as a sterile solution in normal saline.

Product No.	NDC No.	
87102	57317-232-10	Adenocard® (adenosine) Injection 6mg/2 mL (3 mg/mL) in 2 mL flip-top vials, packaged in 10's.

Store at controlled room temperature 15°–30°C (59°–86°F).

DO NOT REFRIGERATE as crystallization may occur. If crystallization has occurred, dissolve crystals by warming to room temperature. The solution must be clear at the time of use.

Contains no preservatives. Discard unused portion.

CAUTION Federal (USA) law prohibits dispensing without prescription.

Manufactured for
Fujisawa Pharmaceutical Company
by Fujisawa USA, Inc.,
Deerfield, IL 60015

45514C
Revised: February 1992

ARISTOCORT® ℞
[*a-ris-tō-cort*]
triamcinolone
TABLETS

DESCRIPTION

ARISTOCORT triamcinolone is a synthetic adrenocorticosteroid. The tablets contain triamcinolone, 9-Fluoro-11β, 16α, 17,21-tetrahydroxypregna-1,4-diene-3,20-dione.
ARISTOCORT Triamcinolone Tablets contain 1, 2, 4, or 8 mg triamcinolone.

HOW SUPPLIED

ARISTOCORT® Triamcinolone Tablets are supplied as follows:

1 mg—oblong, flat, yellow tablet engraved with F on the unscored side and A1 on the scored side.
NDC 57317-602-50—Bottles of 50 Product Code 512150

2 mg—oblong, flat, pink tablet engraved with F on the unscored side and A2 on the scored side.
NDC 57317-601-10—Bottles of 100 Product Code 512271

4 mg—oblong, flat, white tablet engraved with F on the unscored side and A4 on the scored side.
NDC 57317-600-30—Bottles of 30 Product Code 512430
NDC 57317-600-10—Bottles of 100 Product Code 512471
NDC 57317-600-16—ARISTO-PAK®Product Code 512316 triamcinolone 16s (for 6 days therapy)

8 mg—oblong, flat, yellow tablet engraved with F on the unscored side and A8 on the scored side.
NDC 57317-603-50—Bottles of 50 Product Code 512550

Store at Controlled Room Temperature 15–30° C (59–86° F).
Manufactured for Fujisawa Pharmaceutical Company, Fujisawa USA, Inc., Deerfield, IL 60015, by Lederle Laboratories, Div. American Cyanamid Company, Pearl River, NY 10965   Rev. 11/91
10139-91

Suspensions
ARISTOCORT® ℞
[*a-ris-tō-cort*]
Sterile triamcinolone diacetate
Forte parenteral 40 mg/mL
Intralesional 25 mg/mL
NOT FOR INTRAVENOUS USE

DESCRIPTION

FORTE PARENTERAL

A sterile suspension of 40 mg/mL of triamcinolone diacetate (micronized) suspended in a vehicle consisting of:

Polysorbate 80 NF	0.20%
Polyethylene Glycol 3350 NF	3%
Sodium Chloride	0.85%
Benzyl Alcohol	0.90%
Water for Injection q.s.	100%

Hydrochloric acid and/or sodium hydroxide may be used during manufacture to adjust pH of suspension to approximately 6.

This preparation is a slightly soluble suspension suitable for parenteral administration through a 24-gauge needle (or larger), but NOT suitable for intravenous use. It may be administered by the intramuscular, intra-articular, or intrasynovial routes, depending upon the situation. The response to each glucocorticoid varies considerably with each type of disease indication and each corticosteroid prescribed. Irreversible clumping occurs when product is frozen. Chemically triamcinolone diacetate is 9-Fluoro-11β,16α,17,21-tetrahydroxypregna-1,4-diene-3,20-dione 16,21-diacetate.

ACTION

FORTE PARENTERAL

ARISTOCORT is primarily glucocorticoid in action and has potent anti-inflammatory, hormonal and metabolic effects common to cortisone-like drugs. It is essentially devoid of mineralocorticoid activity when administered in therapeutic doses, causing little or no sodium retention, with potassium excretion minimal or absent. The body's immune responses to diverse stimuli are also modified by its action.

INDICATIONS

FORTE PARENTERAL

Where oral therapy is not feasible or temporarily desirable in the judgment of the physician, sterile triamcinolone diacetate suspension, 40 mg/mL, is indicated for intramuscular use as follows:

1. Endocrine disorders
   Primary or secondary adrenocortical insufficiency (hydrocortisone or cortisone is the drug of choice; synthetic analogs may be used in conjunction with mineralocorticoids where applicable; in infancy, mineralocorticoid supplementation is of particular importance). Preoperatively and in the event of serious trauma or illness, in patients with known adrenal insufficiency or when adrenocortical reserve is doubtful
   Congenital adrenal hyperplasia
   Nonsuppurative thyroiditis
   Hypercalcemia associated with cancer
2. Rheumatic disorders. As adjunctive therapy for short-term administration (to tide the patient over an acute episode or exacerbation) in:
   Posttraumatic osteoarthritis
   Synovitis of osteoarthritis
   Rheumatoid arthritis, including juvenile rheumatoid arthritis (selected cases may require low-dose maintenance therapy)
   Acute and subacute bursitis
   Epicondylitis
   Acute nonspecific tenosynovitis
   Acute gouty arthritis
   Psoriatic arthritis
   Ankylosing spondylitis
3. Collagen diseases. During an exacerbation or as maintenance therapy in selected cases of:
   Systemic lupus erythematosus
   Acute rheumatic carditis
4. Dermatologic diseases. Pemphigus
   Severe erythema multiforme (Stevens-Johnson syndrome)
   Exfoliative dermatitis
   Bullous dermatitis herpetiformis
   Severe seborrheic dermatitis
   Severe psoriasis
   Mycosis fungoides
5. Allergic states. Control of severe or incapacitating allergic conditions intractable to adequate trials of conventional treatment in:
   Bronchial asthma
   Contact dermatitis
   Atopic dermatitis
   Serum sickness
   Seasonal or perennial allergic rhinitis
   Drug hypersensitivity reactions
   Urticarial transfusion reactions
   Acute noninfectious laryngeal edema (epinephrine is the drug of first choice).
6. Ophthalmic diseases. Severe acute and chronic allergic and inflammatory processes involving the eye, such as:
   Herpes zoster ophthalmicus
   Iritis, iridocyclitis
   Chorioretinitis
   Diffuse posterior uveitis and choroiditis
   Optic neuritis
   Sympathetic ophthalmia
   Allergic conjunctivitis
   Allergic corneal marginal ulcers
   Keratitis
7. Gastrointestinal disease. To tide the patient over a critical period of disease in:
   Ulcerative colitis - (Systemic therapy)
   Regional enteritis - (Systemic therapy)

8. Respiratory diseases
   Symptomatic sarcoidosis
   Berylliosis
   Fulminating or disseminated pulmonary tuberculosis when used concurrently with appropriate antituberculous chemotherapy
   Loeffler's syndrome not manageable by other means
   Aspiration pneumonitis
9. Hematologic disorders
   Acquired (autoimmune) hemolytic anemia
   Secondary thrombocytopenia in adults
   Erythroblastopenia (RBC anemia)
   Congenital (erythroid) hypoplastic anemia
10. Neoplastic diseases For palliative management of:
    Leukemias and lymphomas in adults
    Acute leukemia of childhood
11. Edematous state. To induce diuresis or remission of proteinuria in the nephrotic syndrome, without uremia, of the idiopathic type or that due to lupus erythematosus
12. Nervous System
    Acute exacerbations of multiple sclerosis
13. Miscellaneous. Tuberculous meningitis with subarachnoid block or impending block when used concurrently with appropriate antituberculous chemotherapy
    Trichinosis with neurologic or myocardial involvement

ARISTOCORT *triamcinolone diacetate* FORTE 40 mg/mL is indicated for intra-articular or soft tissue use as follows:
As adjunctive therapy for short-term administration (to tide the patient over an acute episode or exacerbation) in:
   Synovitis of osteoarthritis
   Rheumatoid arthritis
   Acute and subacute bursitis
   Acute gouty arthritis
   Epicondylitis
   Acute nonspecific tenosynovitis
   Posttraumatic osteoarthritis

ARISTOCORT FORTE is indicated for intralesional use as follows:
   Keloids
   Localized hypertrophic, infiltrated, inflammatory lesion of: Lichen planus, psoriatic plaques, granuloma annulare and lichen simplex chronicus (neurodermatitis)
   Discoid lupus erythematosus
   Necrobiosis lipoidica diabeticorum
   Alopecia areata
   It may also be useful in cystic tumors of an aponeurosis or tendon (ganglia).

DESCRIPTION

INTRALESIONAL

ARISTOCORT *triamcinolone diacetate* possesses glucocorticoid properties while being essentially devoid of mineralocorticoid activity thus causing little or no sodium retention. Supplied as a sterile suspension of 25 mg/mL micronized triamcinolone diacetate in the following vehicle:

Polysorbate 80 NF	0.20%
Polyethylene Glycol 3350 NF	3%
Sodium Chloride	0.85%
Benzyl Alcohol	0.90%
Water for Injection q.s.	100%

Hydrochloric acid and/or sodium hydroxide may be used during manufacture to adjust pH of suspension to approximately 6.

Chemically triamcinolone diacetate is Pregna - 1, 4 - diene - 3, 20 - dione, 16, 21 - bis(acetyloxy) - 9 - fluoro - 11, 17-dihydroxy-,(11β, 16α)- or 9-Fluoro-11β, 16α, 17, 21-tetrahydroxypregna-1, 4-diene-3,20-dione 16,21-diacetate. Molecular weight is 478.51.

ACTIONS

INTRALESIONAL

Naturally occurring glucocorticoids (hydrocortisone), which also have salt-retaining properties, are used as replacement therapy in adrenocortical deficiency states. Their synthetic analogs are primarily used for their potent anti-inflammatory effects in disorders of many organ systems.
Glucocorticoids cause profound and varied metabolic effects. In addition, they modify the body's immune responses to diverse stimuli.

INDICATIONS

INTRALESIONAL

ARISTOCORT *triamcinolone diacetate* Intralesional is indicated by the intralesional route for:
   Keloids
   Localized hypertrophic, infiltrated, inflammatory lesion of:
   lichen planus, psoriatic plaques, granuloma annulare and lichen simplex chronicus (neurodermatitis)

Discoid lupus erythematosus
Necrobiosis lipoidica diabeticorum
Alopecia areata
It may also be useful in cystic tumors of an aponeurosis or tendon (ganglia).
When used intra-articularly it is also indicated for:
Adjunctive therapy for short-term administration (to tide the patient over an acute episode or exacerbation) in:
   Synovitis of osteoarthritis
   Rheumatoid arthritis
   Acute and subacute bursitis
   Acute gouty arthritis
   Epicondylitis
   Acute nonspecific tenosynovitis
   Posttraumatic osteoarthritis

CONTRAINDICATIONS

FORTE PARENTERAL AND INTRALESIONAL

Systemic fungal infections.

WARNINGS

In patients on corticosteroid therapy subjected to any unusual stress, increased dosage of rapidly acting corticosteroids before, during, and after the stressful situation is indicated.

Corticosteroids may mask some signs of infection, and new infections may appear during their use. There may be decreased resistance and inability to localize infection when corticosteroids are used.

Prolonged use of corticosteroids may produce posterior subcapsular cataracts, glaucoma with possible damage to the optic nerves and may enhance the establishment of secondary ocular infections due to fungi or viruses.

Usage in Pregnancy

Since adequate human reproduction studies have not been done with corticosteroids, the use of these drugs in pregnancy, nursing mothers, or women of childbearing potential requires that the possible benefits of the drug be weighed against the potential hazards to the mother and embryo or fetus. Infants born of mothers who have received substantial doses of corticosteroids during pregnancy should be carefully observed for signs of hypoadrenalism.

Average and large doses of cortisone or hydrocortisone can cause elevation of blood pressure, salt and water retention, and increased excretion of potassium. These effects are less likely to occur with the synthetic derivatives except when used in large doses. Dietary salt restriction and potassium supplementation may be necessary. All corticosteroids increase calcium excretion.

While on Corticosteroid Therapy Patients Should Not Be Vaccinated Against Smallpox. Other Immunization Procedures Should Not Be Undertaken in Patients Who Are on Corticosteroids, Especially in High Doses, Because of Possible Hazards of Neurological Complications and Lack of Antibody Response.

The use of ARISTOCORT *triamcinolone diacetate* in active tuberculosis should be restricted to those cases of fulminating or disseminated tuberculosis in which the corticosteroid is used for the management of the disease in conjunction with appropriate antituberculous regimen.

If corticosteroids are indicated in patients with latent tuberculosis or tuberculin reactivity, close observation is necessary as reactivation of the disease may occur. During prolonged corticosteroid therapy, these patients should receive chemoprophylaxis.

Because rare instances of anaphylactoid reactions have occurred in patients receiving parenteral corticosteroid therapy, appropriate precautionary measures should be taken prior to administration, especially when the patient has a history of allergy to any drug.

Postinjection flare (following intra-articular use) and Charcot-like arthropathy have been associated with parenteral corticosteroid therapy.

Intralesional or sublesional injection of excessive dosage whether by single or multiple injection into any given area may cause cutaneous or subcutaneous atrophy.

PRECAUTIONS

FORTE PARENTERAL AND INTRALESIONAL

Drug-induced secondary adrenocortical insufficiency may be minimized by gradual reduction of dosage. This type of relative insufficiency may persist for months after discontinuation of therapy; therefore, in any situation of stress occurring during that period, hormone therapy should be reinstituted. Since mineralocorticoid secretion may be impaired, salt and/or a mineralocorticoid should be administered concurrently. There is an enhanced effect of corticosteroids in patients with hypothyroidism and in those with cirrhosis. Corticosteroids should be used cautiously in patients with ocular herpes simplex for fear of corneal perforation.

The lowest possible dose of corticosteroid should be used to control the condition under treatment, and when reduction in dosage is possible, the reduction must be gradual.

Continued on next page

Fujisawa—Cont.

Psychic derangements may appear when corticosteroids are used, ranging from euphoria, insomnia, mood swings, personality changes, and severe depression to frank psychotic manifestations. Also, existing emotional instability or psychotic tendencies may be aggravated by corticosteroids.

Aspirin should be used cautiously in conjunction with corticosteroids in hypoprothrombinemia.

Steroids should be used with caution in nonspecific ulcerative colitis, if there is a probability of impending perforation, abscess or other pyogenic infection, also in diverticulitis, fresh intestinal anastomoses, active or latent peptic ulcer, renal insufficiency, hypertension, osteoporosis, and myasthenia gravis.

Growth and development of infants and children on prolonged corticosteroid therapy should be carefully followed. The following additional precautions apply for parenteral corticosteroids.

Intra-articular injection of a corticosteroid may produce systemic as well as local effects.

Appropriate examination of any joint fluid present is necessary to exclude a septic process.

A marked increase in pain accompanied by local swelling, further restriction of joint motion, fever, and malaise are suggestive of septic arthritis. If this complication occurs and the diagnosis of sepsis is confirmed, appropriate antimicrobial therapy should be instituted.

Local injection of a steroid into a previously infected joint is to be avoided.

Corticosteroids should not be injected into unstable joints. The slower rate of absorption by intramuscular administration should be recognized.

Atrophy at the site of injection has been reported.

Routine laboratory studies, such as urinalysis, two-hour postprandial blood sugar, determination of blood pressure and body weight, and a chest X-ray should be made at regular intervals during prolonged therapy. Upper GI x-rays are desirable in patients with an ulcer history or significant dyspepsia.

FORTE PARENTERAL

Accidental injection into soft tissue during intra-articular administration decreases local effectiveness in the joint and, by increasing the rate of absorption, may produce systemic effects.

Although controlled clinical trials have shown corticosteroids to be effective in speeding the resolution of acute exacerbations of multiple sclerosis, they do not show that they affect the ultimate outcome or natural history of the disease. The studies do show that relatively high doses of corticosteroids are necessary to demonstrate a significant effect (See **DOSAGE AND ADMINISTRATION**).

Since complications of treatment with glucocorticoid are dependent on the size of the dose and the duration of treatment, a risk/benefit decision must be made in each individual case as to dose and duration of treatment and as to whether daily or intermittent therapy should be used.

ADVERSE REACTIONS

Fluid and electrolyte disturbances
  Sodium retention
  Fluid retention
  Congestive heart failure in susceptible patients
  Potassium loss
  Hypokalemic alkalosis
  Hypertension
Musculoskeletal
  Muscle weakness
  Steroid myopathy
  Loss of muscle mass
  Osteoporosis
  Vertebral compression fractures
  Aseptic necrosis of femoral and humeral heads
  Pathologic fracture of long bones
Gastrointestinal
  Peptic ulcer with possible subsequent perforation and hemorrhage
  Pancreatitis
  Abdominal distention
  Ulcerative esophagitis
Dermatologic
  Impaired wound healing
  Thin fragile skin
  Petechiae and ecchymoses
  Facial erythema
  Increased sweating
  May suppress reactions to skin tests
Neurological
  Convulsions
  Increased intracranial pressure with papilledema (pseudotumor cerebri) usually after treatment
  Vertigo
  Headache

Endocrine
  Menstrual irregularities
  Development of cushingoid state
  Suppression of growth in children
  Secondary adrenocortical and pituitary unresponsiveness, particularly in times of stress, as in trauma, surgery, or illness
  Decreased carbohydrate tolerance
  Manifestations of latent diabetes mellitus
  Increased requirements for insulin or oral hypoglycemic agents in diabetics
Ophthalmic
  Posterior subcapsular cataracts
  Increased intraocular pressure
  Glaucoma
  Exophthalmos
Metabolic
  Negative nitrogen balance due to protein catabolism
The following additional adverse reactions are related to parenteral and intralesional corticosteroid therapy:
  Rare instances of blindness associated with intralesional therapy around the face and head
  Hyperpigmentation or hypopigmentation
  Subcutaneous and cutaneous atrophy
  Sterile abscess
Anaphylactoid reactions have been reported rarely with products of this class.

DOSAGE AND ADMINISTRATION

General

The initial dosage of ARISTOCORT *triamcinolone diacetate* may vary from 3 to 48 mg per day, depending on the specific disease entity being treated. In situations of less severity, lower doses will generally suffice while in selected patients higher initial doses may be required. Usually the parenteral dosage ranges are one-third to one-half the oral dose given every 12 hours. However, in certain overwhelming, acute, life-threatening situations, administration in dosages exceeding the usual dosages may be justified and may be administered in multiples of the oral dosages.

The initial dosage should be maintained or adjusted until a satisfactory response is noted. If after a reasonable period of time there is a lack of satisfactory clinical response, ARISTOCORT should be discontinued and the patient transferred to other appropriate therapy. IT SHOULD BE EMPHASIZED THAT DOSAGE REQUIREMENTS ARE VARIABLE AND MUST BE INDIVIDUALIZED ON THE BASIS OF THE DISEASE UNDER TREATMENT AND THE RESPONSE OF THE PATIENT. After a favorable response is noted, the proper maintenance dosage should be determined by decreasing the initial drug dosage in small increments at appropriate time intervals until the lowest dosage that will maintain an adequate clinical response is reached. It should be kept in mind that constant monitoring is needed in regard to drug dosage. Included in the situations in which dosage adjustments may be necessary are changes in clinical status secondary to remissions or exacerbations in the disease process, the patient's individual drug responsiveness, and the effect of patient exposure to stressful situations not directly related to the disease entity under treatment. In this latter situation, it may be necessary to increase the dosage of ARISTOCORT for a period of time consistent with the patient's condition. If after long-term therapy the drug is to be stopped, it is recommended that it be withdrawn gradually rather than abruptly.

For intra-articular, intralesional and soft tissue use, a lesser initial dosage range of *triamcinolone diacetate* may produce the desired effect when the drug is administered to provide a localized concentration. The site of the injection and the volume of the injection should be carefully considered when *triamcinolone diacetate* is administered for this purpose.

Specific FORTE PARENTERAL—ARISTOCORT FORTE Parenteral is sterile *triamcinolone diacetate* (40 mg/mL) suspended in a suitable vehicle. The full-strength suspension may be employed. If preferred, the suspension may be diluted with normal saline or water. The diluent may also be prepared by mixing equal parts of normal saline and 1% procaine hydrochloride or other similar local anesthetics. The use of diluents containing preservatives such as methylparaben, propylparaben, phenol, etc. must be avoided as these preparations tend to cause flocculation of the steroid. These dilutions retain full potency for at least one week. Topical ethyl chloride spray may be used locally prior to injection.

Since this product has been designed for ease of administration, a small bore needle (not smaller than 24 gauge) may be used.

Intramuscular Although ARISTOCORT FORTE Parenteral may be administered intramuscularly for initial therapy, most physicians prefer to adjust the dose orally until adequate control is attained. Intramuscular administration provides a sustained or depot action that can be used to supplement or replace initial oral therapy. With intramuscular therapy, greater supervision of the amount of steroid used is made possible for the patient who is inconsistent in following an oral dosage schedule. In maintenance therapy, the pa-

tient-to-patient response is not uniform and, therefore, the dose must be individualized for optimal control.

Although *triamcinolone diacetate* may possess greater anti-inflammatory potency than many glucocorticoids, this is only dose-related since side effects, such as osteoporosis, peptic ulcer, etc., related to glucocorticoid activity, have not been diminished.

The average dose is 40 mg (1 mL) administered intramuscularly once a week for conditions in which anti-inflammatory action is desired.

In general, a single parenteral dose 4 to 7 times the oral daily dose may be expected to control the patient from 4 to 7 days up to 3 to 4 weeks. Dosage should be adjusted to the point where adequate but not necessarily complete relief of symptoms is obtained.

Intra-Articular and Intrasynovial The usual dose varies from 5 to 40 mg. The average for the knee, for example, is 25 mg. The duration of effect varies from one week to 2 months. However, acutely inflamed joints may require more frequent injections.

A lesser initial dosage range of sterile *triamcinolone diacetate* may produce the desired effect when the drug is administered to provide a localized concentration. The site of the injection and the volume of the injection should be carefully considered when *triamcinolone diacetate* is administered for this purpose.

A specific dose depends largely on the size of the joint. Strict surgical asepsis is mandatory. The physician should be familiar with anatomical relationships as described in standard text books. ARISTOCORT FORTE *triamcinolone diacetate* Parenteral may be used in any accessible joint except the intervertebrals. In general, intrasynovial therapy is suggested under the following circumstances:

1. When systemic steroid therapy is contraindicated because of side effects such as peptic ulcer.
2. When it is desirable to secure relief in one or two specific joints.
3. When good systemic maintenance fails to control flare-ups in a few joints and it is desirable to secure relief without increasing oral therapy.

Such treatment should not be considered to constitute a cure. Although this method will ameliorate the joint symptoms, it does not preclude the need for the conventional measures usually employed.

It is suggested that infiltration of the soft tissue by local anesthetic precede intra-articular injection. A 24-gauge or larger needle on a dry syringe may be inserted into the joint and excess fluid aspirated. For the first few hours following injection, there may be local discomfort in the joint, but this is usually followed rapidly by effective relief of pain and improvement in local function.

	Anti-inflammatory Relative Potency		Frequently Used Tablet Strength (mg)		Tablet × Potency Equivalent Value
Hydrocortisone	1	×	20	=	20
Prednisolone	4	×	5	=	20
ARISTOCORT *triamcinolone*	5	×	4	=	20
Dexamethasone	25	×	0.75	=	18.75

INTRALESIONAL

When ARISTOCORT Intralesional is administered by injection, strict aseptic technique is mandatory. Full strength suspensions may be employed, or if preferred, the suspension may be diluted, either to a 1:1 or 1:10 concentration, thus obtaining a working concentration of 12.5 mg/mL or approximately 2.5 mg/mL, respectively. Normal (isotonic) saline solution alone or equal parts of normal (isotonic) saline solution and 1% procaine or other local anesthetics may be used as diluents. These dilutions usually retain full potency for at least one week. Topical ethyl chloride spray may be used as a local anesthetic. The use of diluents containing preservatives such as methylparaben, propylparaben, phenol, etc. must be avoided as these preparations tend to cause flocculations of the steroid.

Since this product has been designed for ease of administration, a small bore needle (not smaller than 24 gauge) may be used.

Intralesional or Sublesional For small lesions, injection is usually well tolerated and a local anesthetic is not necessary. The location and type of lesion will determine the route of injection: intralesional, sublesional, intradermal, subdermal, intracutaneous, or subcutaneous. The size of the lesion will determine the total amount of drug needed, the concentration used, and the number and pattern of injection sites utilized (eg., from a total of 5 mg ARISTOCORT Intralesional in a 2 mL volume divided over several locations in small lesions, ranging up to 48 mg total ARISTOCORT Intralesional for large psoriatic plaques). Avoid injecting too superficially. In general, no more than 12.5 mg per injection site should be used. An average of 25 mg is the usual limit for any one lesion. Large areas require multiple injections with smaller doses per injection site.

For a majority of conditions, sublesional injection directly through the lesion into the deep dermal tissue is suggested.

In cases where it is difficult to inject intradermally, the suspension may be introduced subcutaneously, as superficially as possible.

Two or three injections at one to two week intervals may suffice as an average course of treatment for many conditions. Within 5-7 days after initial injection, involution of the lesion can usually be seen, with pronounced clearing towards normal tissue after 12-14 days. Multiple injections of small amounts of equal strength may be convenient in alopecia areata and in psoriasis where there are large or confluent lesions. This is best accomplished by a series of fan-like injections ½ to 1 inch apart.

Alopecia areata and totalis require an average dose of 25 to 30 mg in a concentration of 10 mg/mL subcutaneously, 1 to 2 times a week, to stimulate hair regrowth. Results may be expected in 3 to 6 weeks on this dosage, and hair growth may last 3-6 months after initial injection. No more than 0.5 mL should be given in any one site, because excessive deposition may produce local skin atrophy. Continued periodic local injections may be necessary to maintain response and continued hair growth. Use of more dilute solutions diminishes the incidence and degree of local atrophy in the injection site.

In keloids and similar dense scars, injections are usually made directly into the lesion.

Injections may be repeated as required, but probably a total of no more than 75 mg of ARISTOCORT *triamcinolone diacetate* a week should be given to any one patient. The need for repeated injections is best determined by clinical response. Remissions may be expected to last from a few weeks up to 11 months.

Intra-articular or Intrasynovial Strict surgical asepsis is mandatory. The physician should be familiar with anatomical relationships as described in standard text books. A recent paper details the anatomy and technical approach in arthrocentesis.

It is usually recommended that infiltration by local anesthetic of the soft tissue precede intra-articular injection. A 22-gauge or larger needle on a dry syringe should be inserted into the joint and excess fluid, if present, should be aspirated. The specific dose depends primarily on the size of the joint. The usual dose varies from 5 to 40 mg, with the average for the knee being 25 mg. Smaller joints as in the fingers require 2 to 5 mg. The duration of effect varies from one week to two months. However, acutely inflamed joints may require more frequent injections. Accidental injection into soft tissue is usually not harmful but decreases the local effectiveness. Injection into subcutaneous lipoid tissue may produce "pseudoatrophy" with a persistent depression of the overlying dermis, lasting several weeks or months.

Administration and dosage of ARISTOCORT Intralesional *triamcinolone diacetate* must be individualized according to the nature, severity, and chronicity of the disease or disorder treated, and should be undertaken with a view of the patient's entire clinical condition. Corticosteroid therapy is considered an adjunct to and not usually a replacement for conventional therapy. Therapy with ARISTOCORT Intralesional, as with all steroids, is of the suppressive type, related to its anti-inflammatory effect. The dose should be regulated during therapy according to the degree of therapeutic response, and should be reduced gradually to maintenance levels, whereby the patient obtains adequate or acceptable control of symptoms. When such control occurs, consideration should be given to a gradual decrease in dosage and eventual cessation of therapy. Remission of symptoms may be due to therapy or may be spontaneous, and a therapeutic test of gradual withdrawal of steroid treatment is usually indicated.

HOW SUPPLIED

Forte Parenteral (40 mg/mL): 1 mL Vial—NDC 57317-202-01, Product Code 511601, 5 mL Vial—NDC 57317-202-05, Product Code 511605

Intralesional (25 mg/mL) sterile suspension, Not For Intravenous Use: 5 ml Vial—NDC 57317-203-05, Product Code 511705

Store at Controlled Room Temperature 15°–30°C (59°–86°F). DO NOT FREEZE.

Manufactured for Fujisawa Pharmaceutical Company, Fujisawa USA, Inc., Deerfield, IL 60015, by Lederle Parenterals, Inc., Carolina, Puerto Rico 00630 Rev. 7/90

26455, 23274

ARISTOCORT A® ℞

[*a-ris-tō-cort*]

Triamcinolone Acetonide Topical Cream with AQUATAIN™ hydrophilic base

ARISTOCORT A® ℞

Triamcinolone Acetonide Topical Ointment with propylene glycol

DESCRIPTION

Each gram of 0.025% Topical Cream contains 0.25 mg of the highly active steroid, *triamcinolone acetonide* (a derivative of triamcinolone); each gram of 0.1% Topical Cream contains 1 mg *triamcinolone acetonide;* each gram of 0.5% Topical Cream contains 5 mg of *triamcinolone acetonide;* all in AQUATAIN™, a specially formulated cream base composed of emulsifying wax NF, isopropyl palmitate, glycerin USP, sorbitol solution USP, lactic acid, 2% benzyl alcohol, and purified water. AQUATAIN is non-staining, water-washable, paraben-free, spermaceti-free, and has a light texture and consistency.

Each gram of 0.1% Topical Ointment contains 1 mg *triamcinolone acetonide* (a derivative of triamcinolone) in a specially formulated ointment base composed of emulsifying wax NF, white petrolatum, and propylene glycol, Tenox II (butylated hydroxyanisole, propyl gallate, citric acid, propylene glycol) and lactic acid.

Chemically, *triamcinolone acetonide* is (11β,16α)-9-fluoro-11,21-dihydroxy-16,17- [(1-methylethylidene) bis (oxy)] pregna-1,4-diene-3,20-dione.

The topical corticosteroids constitute a class of primarily synthetic steroids used as anti-inflammatory and antipruritic agents.

CLINICAL PHARMACOLOGY

Topical corticosteroids share anti-inflammatory, antipruritic, and vasoconstrictive actions.

The mechanism of anti-inflammatory activity of the topical corticosteroids is unclear. Various laboratory methods, including vasoconstrictor assays, are used to compare and predict potencies and/or clinical efficacies of the topical corticosteroids. There is some evidence to suggest that a recognizable correlation exists between vasoconstrictor potency and therapeutic efficacy in man.

Pharmacokinetics

The extent of percutaneous absorption of topical corticosteroids is determined by many factors including the vehicle, the integrity of the epidermal barrier, and the use of occlusive dressings.

Topical corticosteroids can be absorbed from normal intact skin. Inflammation and/or other disease processes in the skin increase percutaneous absorption. Occlusive dressings substantially increase the percutaneous absorption of topical corticosteroids. Thus, occlusive dressings may be a valuable therapeutic adjunct for treatment of resistant dermatoses (See **DOSAGE AND ADMINISTRATION**).

Once absorbed through the skin, topical corticosteroids are handled through pharmacokinetic pathways similar to systemically administered corticosteroids. Corticosteroids are bound to plasma proteins in varying degrees. Corticosteroids are metabolized primarily in the liver and are then excreted by the kidneys. Some of the topical corticosteroids and their metabolites are also excreted into the bile.

INDICATIONS AND USAGE

Topical corticosteroids are indicated for the relief of the inflammatory and pruritic manifestations of corticosteroid-responsive dermatoses.

CONTRAINDICATIONS

Topical corticosteroids are contraindicated in those patients with a history of hypersensitivity to any of the components of the preparation.

PRECAUTIONS

General

Systemic absorption of topical corticosteroids has produced reversible hypothalamic-pituitary-adrenal (HPA) axis suppression, manifestations of Cushing's syndrome, hyperglycemia, and glucosuria in some patients.

Conditions that augment systemic absorption include the application of the more potent steroids, use over large surface areas, prolonged use, and the addition of occlusive dressings.

Therefore, patients receiving a large dose of a potent topical steroid applied to a large surface area or under an occlusive dressing should be evaluated periodically for evidence of HPA axis suppression by using the urinary free cortisol and ACTH stimulation tests. If HPA axis suppression is noted, an attempt should be made to withdraw the drug, to reduce the frequency of application, or to substitute a less potent steroid.

Recovery of HPA axis function is generally prompt and complete upon discontinuation of the drug. Infrequently, signs and symptoms of steroid withdrawal may occur, requiring supplemental systemic corticosteroids.

Children may absorb proportionally larger amounts of topical corticosteroids and thus be more susceptible to systemic toxicity (See **PRECAUTIONS—Pediatric Use**).

If irritation develops, topical corticosteroids should be discontinued and appropriate therapy instituted.

In the presence of dermatological infections, the use of an appropriate antifungal or antibacterial agent should be instituted. If a favorable response does not occur promptly, the corticosteroid should be discontinued until the infection has been adequately controlled.

Information for the Patient

Patients using topical corticosteroids should receive the following information and instructions.

1. This medication is to be used as directed by the physician. It is for external use only. Avoid contact with the eyes.
2. Patients should be advised not to use this medication for any disorder other than for which it was prescribed.
3. The treated skin area should not be bandaged or otherwise covered or wrapped as to be occlusive unless directed by the physician.
4. Patients should report any signs of local adverse reactions, especially under occlusive dressing.
5. Parents of pediatric patients should be advised not to use tight-fitting diapers or plastic pants on a child being treated in the diaper area, as these garments may constitute occlusive dressings.

Laboratory Tests

The following tests may be helpful in evaluating the HPA axis suppression:

Urinary free cortisol test
ACTH stimulation test

Carcinogenesis, Mutagenesis, and Impairment of Fertility

Long-term animal studies have not been performed to evaluate the carcinogenic potential or the effect on fertility of topical corticosteroids.

Studies to determine mutagenicity with prednisolone and hydrocortisone have revealed negative results.

Pregnancy Category C

Corticosteroids are generally teratogenic in laboratory animals when administered systemically at relatively low dosage levels. The more potent corticosteroids have been shown to be teratogenic after dermal application in laboratory animals. There are no adequate and well-controlled studies in pregnant women on teratogenic effects from topically applied corticosteroids. Therefore, topical corticosteroids should be used during pregnancy only if the potential benefit justifies the potential risk to the fetus. Drugs of this class should not be used extensively on pregnant patients, in large amounts, or for prolonged periods of time.

Nursing Mothers

It is not known whether topical administration of corticosteroids could result in sufficient systemic absorption to produce detectable quantities in breast milk. Systemically administered corticosteroids are secreted into breast milk in quantities *not* likely to have a deleterious effect on the infant. Nevertheless, caution should be exercised when topical corticosteroids are administered to a nursing woman.

Pediatric Use

Pediatric patients may demonstrate greater susceptibility to topical corticosteroid-induced HPA axis suppression and Cushing's syndrome than mature patients because of a larger skin surface area to body weight ratio.

Hypothalamic-pituitary-adrenal (HPA) axis suppression, Cushing's syndrome, and intracranial hypertension have been reported in children receiving topical corticosteroids. Manifestations of adrenal suppression in children include linear growth retardation, delayed weight gain, low plasma cortisol levels, and absence of response to ACTH stimulation. Manifestations of intracranial hypertension include bulging fontanelles, headaches, and bilateral papilledema.

Administration of topical corticosteroids to children should be limited to the least amount compatible with an effective therapeutic regimen. Chronic corticosteroid therapy may interfere with the growth and development of children.

ADVERSE REACTIONS

The following local adverse reactions are reported infrequently with topical corticosteroids, but may occur more frequently with the use of occlusive dressings. These reactions are listed in an approximate decreasing order of occurrence.

Burning
Itching
Irritation
Dryness
Folliculitis
Hypertrichosis
Acneiform eruptions
Hypopigmentation
Perioral dermatitis
Allergic contact dermatitis
Maceration of the skin
Secondary infection
Skin atrophy
Striae
Miliaria

OVERDOSAGE

Topically applied corticosteroids can be absorbed in sufficient amounts to produce systemic effects (See **PRECAUTIONS**).

DOSAGE AND ADMINISTRATION

Topical corticosteroids are generally applied to the affected area as a thin film from three to four times daily depending on the severity of the condition.

Occlusive dressings may be used for the management of psoriasis or recalcitrant conditions.

Continued on next page

Fujisawa—Cont.

If an infection develops, the use of occlusive dressings should be discontinued and appropriate antimicrobial therapy instituted.

HOW SUPPLIED

0.025% Cream
15 gram tubes—NDC 57317-042-15 Product code 510115
60 gram tubes—NDC 57317-042-60 Product code 510160

0.1% Cream
15 gram tubes—NDC 57317-052-15 Product code 510215
60 gram tubes—NDC 57317-052-60 Product code 510260
240 gram jars—NDC 57317-052-24 Product code 510324

0.5% Cream
15 gram tubes—NDC 57317-062-15 Product code 510415

0.1% Ointment
15 gram tubes—NDC 57317-072-15 Product code 510515
60 gram tubes—NDC 57317-072-60 Product code 510560

Store at Controlled Room Temperature 15–30°C (59–86°F), Do Not Freeze.

Military and VA depots: 0.1% cream, 60 gm tube, NSN 6505-01-107-1731

Manufactured for Fujisawa Pharmaceutical Company, Fujisawa USA, Inc., Deerfield, IL 60015 by Lederle Laboratories, Div. American Cyanamid Company, Pearl River, NY 10965   Rev. 7/90
26452, 23089, 23090, 23265

ARISTOSPAN®   ℞

[a-ris-tō-span]

Sterile Triamcinolone Hexacetonide Suspension, USP

5 mg/mL—Parenteral: for Intralesional Administration
20 mg/mL—Parenteral: for Intra-articular Administration
NOT FOR INTRAVENOUS USE

DESCRIPTION

Intralesional A sterile suspension containing 5 mg/mL of micronized *triamcinolone hexacetonide* in the following inactive ingredients:

Polysorbate 80 NF..0.20% w/v
Sorbitol Solution USP ....50.00% v/v
Water for Injection qs ad ....100.00%   V
Hydrochloric Acid and Sodium Hydroxide, if required, to adjust pH to 4.5–6.5.

Preservative
Benzyl Alcohol ....0.90% w/v

Intra-articular A sterile suspension containing 20 mg/mL of micronized *triamcinolone hexacetonide* in the following inactive ingredients:

Polysorbate 80 NF..0.40% w/v
Sorbitol Solution USP ....50.00% v/v
Water for Injection qs ad ....100.00%   V
Hydrochloric Acid and Sodium Hydroxide, if required, to adjust pH to 4.5–6.5.

Preservative
Benzyl Alcohol ....0.90% w/v

The hexacetonide ester of the potent glucocorticoid triamcinolone is relatively insoluble (0.0002% at 25° C in water). When injected intralesionally, sublesionally, or intra-articularly, it can be expected to be absorbed slowly from the injection site.

Chemically, *triamcinolone hexacetonide* USP is 9-Fluoro-11β, 16α, 17,21-tetrahydroxypregna-1,4-diene-3,20-dione cyclic 16,17-acetal with acetone 21-(3,3-dimethylbutyrate). Molecular weight 532.65.

ACTIONS

Naturally occurring glucocorticoids (hydrocortisone), which also have salt-retaining properties, are used as replacement therapy in adrenocortical deficiency states. Their synthetic analogs are primarily used for their potent anti-inflammatory effects in disorders of many organ systems. Glucocorticoids cause profound and varied metabolic effects. In addition, they modify the body's immune responses to diverse stimuli.

INDICATIONS

Intralesional

Intralesional or sublesional ARISTOSPAN *sterile triamcinolone hexacetonide suspension* is indicated for the following.

Keloids
Localized hypertrophic, infiltrated, inflammatory lesions of: lichen planus, psoriatic plaques, granuloma annulare, and lichen simplex chronicus (neurodermatitis)
Discoid lupus erythematosus
Necrobiosis lipoidica diabeticorum
Alopecia areata

Intralesional or sublesional ARISTOSPAN may also be useful in cystic tumors of an aponeurosis or tendon (ganglia).

Intra-articular

Intra-articular ARISTOSPAN *sterile triamcinolone hexacetonide suspension* is indicated as adjunctive therapy for short-term administration (to tide the patient over an acute episode or exacerbation) in:

Synovitis of osteoarthritis
Acute and subacute bursitis
Epicondylitis
Posttraumatic osteoarthritis
Rheumatoid arthritis
Acute gouty arthritis
Acute nonspecific tenosynovitis

CONTRAINDICATIONS

Systemic fungal infections

WARNINGS

In patients on corticosteroid therapy subjected to any unusual stress, increased dosage of rapidly acting corticosteroids before, during, and after the stressful situation is indicated.

Corticosteroids may mask some signs of infection, and new infections may appear during their use. There may be decreased resistance and inability to localize infection when corticosteroids are used.

Prolonged use of corticosteroids may produce posterior subcapsular cataracts, glaucoma with possible damage to the optic nerves, and may enhance the establishment of secondary ocular infections due to fungi or viruses.

Usage in Pregnancy

Since adequate human reproduction studies have not been done with corticosteroids, the use of these drugs in pregnancy, nursing mothers, or women of childbearing potential requires that the possible benefits of the drug be weighed against the potential hazards to the mother and embryo or fetus. Infants born of mothers who have received substantial doses of corticosteroids during pregnancy should be carefully observed for signs of hypoadrenalism.

Average and large doses of cortisone or hydrocortisone can cause elevation of blood pressure, salt and water retention, and increased excretion of potassium. These effects are less likely to occur with the synthetic derivatives, except when used in large doses. Dietary salt restriction and potassium supplementation may be necessary. All corticosteroids increase calcium excretion.

While on Corticosteroid Therapy Patients Should Not Be Vaccinated Against Smallpox. Other Immunization Procedures Should Not Be Undertaken in Patients Who Are on Corticosteroids, Especially in High Doses, Because of Possible Hazards of Neurological Complications and Lack of Antibody Response.

The use of ARISTOSPAN in active tuberculosis should be restricted to those cases of fulminating or disseminated tuberculosis in which the corticosteroid is used for the management of the disease in conjunction with an appropriate antituberculous regimen.

If corticosteroids are indicated in patients with latent tuberculosis or tuberculin reactivity, close observation is necessary as reactivation of the disease may occur. During prolonged corticosteroid therapy, these patients should receive chemoprophylaxis.

Because rare instances of anaphylactoid reactions have occurred in patients receiving parenteral corticosteroid therapy, appropriate precautionary measures should be taken prior to administration, especially when the patient has a history of allergy to any drug.

Intralesional or sublesional injection of excessive dosage, whether by single or multiple injection, into any given area, may cause cutaneous or subcutaneous atrophy.

Postinjection flare (following intra-articular use) and charcot-like arthropathy have been associated with parenteral corticosteroid therapy.

PRECAUTIONS

Drug-induced secondary adrenocortical insufficiency may be minimized by gradual reduction of dosage. This type of relative insufficiency may persist for months after discontinuation of therapy; therefore, in any situation of stress occurring during that period, hormone therapy should be reinstituted. Since mineralocorticoid secretion may be impaired, salt and/or a mineralocorticoid should be administered concurrently. There is an enhanced effect of corticosteroids in patients with hypothyroidism and in those with cirrhosis.

Corticosteroids should be used cautiously in patients with ocular herpes simplex for fear of corneal perforation.

The lowest possible dose of corticosteroids should be used to control the condition under treatment, and when reduction in dosage is possible, the reduction must be gradual.

Psychic derangements may appear when corticosteroids are used, ranging from euphoria, insomnia, mood swings, personality changes, and severe depression to frank psychotic manifestations. Also, existing emotional instability or psychotic tendencies may be aggravated by corticosteroids.

Aspirin should be used cautiously in conjunction with corticosteroids in hypoprothrombinemia.

Steroids should be used with caution in nonspecific ulcerative colitis, if there is a probability of impending perforation, abscess or other pyogenic infection, also in diverticulitis, fresh intestinal anastomoses, active or latent peptic ulcer, renal insufficiency, hypertension, osteoporosis, and myasthenia gravis.

Growth and development of infants and children on prolonged corticosteroid therapy should be carefully followed. The following additional precautions apply for parenteral corticosteroids.

Intra-articular injection of a corticosteroid may produce systemic as well as local effects.

Appropriate examination of any joint fluid present is necessary to exclude a septic process..

A marked increase in pain accompanied by local swelling, further restriction of joint motion, fever, and malaise are suggestive of septic arthritis. If this complication occurs and the diagnosis of sepsis is confirmed, appropriate antimicrobial therapy should be instituted.

Local injection of a steroid into a previously infected joint is to be avoided.

Corticosteroids should not be injected into unstable joints.

The slower rate of absorption by intramuscular administration should be recognized.

Atrophy at the site of injection has been reported.

Routine laboratory studies, such as urinalysis, two-hour postprandial blood sugar, determination of blood pressure and body weight, and a chest x-ray should be made at regular intervals during prolonged therapy. Upper GI x-rays are desirable in patients with an ulcer history or significant dyspepsia.

ADVERSE REACTIONS

Fluid and electrolyte disturbances
Sodium retention
Fluid retention
Congestive heart failure in susceptible patients
Potassium loss
Hypokalemic alkalosis
Hypertension

Musculoskeletal
Muscle weakness
Steroid myopathy
Loss of muscle mass
Osteoporosis
Vertebral compression fractures
Aseptic necrosis of femoral and humeral heads
Pathologic fracture of long bones

Gastrointestinal
Peptic ulcer with possible subsequent perforation and hemorrhage
Pancreatitis
Abdominal distention
Ulcerative esophagitis

Dermatologic
Impaired wound healing
Thin fragile skin
Petechiae and ecchymoses
Facial erythema
Increased sweating
May suppress reactions to skin tests

Neurological
Convulsions
Increased intracranial pressure with papilledema (pseudotumor cerebri) usually after treatment
Vertigo
Headache

Endocrine
Menstrual irregularities
Development of Cushingoid state
Suppression of growth in children
Secondary adrenocortical and pituitary unresponsiveness, particularly in times of stress, as in trauma, surgery, or illness
Decreased carbohydrate tolerance
Manifestations of latent diabetes mellitus
Increased requirements for insulin or oral hypoglycemic agents in diabetics

Ophthalmic
Posterior subcapsular cataracts
Increased intraocular pressure
Glaucoma
Exophthalmos

Metabolic
Negative nitrogen balance due to protein catabolism

The following additional adverse reactions are related to parenteral and intralesional corticosteroid therapy.

Rare instances of blindness associated with intralesional therapy around the orbit or intranasally

Hyperpigmentation or hypopigmentation
Subcutaneous and cutaneous atrophy
Sterile abscess

Anaphylactoid reactions have been reported rarely with products of this class.

DOSAGE AND ADMINISTRATION

General

The initial dosage of ARISTOSPAN *sterile triamcinolone hexacetonide suspension* may vary from 2 to 48 mg per day, depending on the specific disease entity being treated. In situations of less severity, lower doses will generally suffice, while in selected patients, higher initial doses may be required. Usually parenteral dosage ranges are one-third to one-half the oral dose given every 12 hours. However, in certain overwhelming, acute, life-threatening situations, administration in dosages exceeding the usual dosages may be justified and may be administered in multiples of the oral dosages.

The initial dosage should be maintained or adjusted until a satisfactory response is noted. If after a reasonable period of time there is a lack of satisfactory clinical response, ARISTOSPAN should be discontinued and the patient transferred to other appropriate therapy. It Should Be Emphasized That Dosage Requirements Are Variable and Must Be Individualized on the Basis of the Disease Under Treatment and the Response of the Patient. After a favorable response is noted, the proper maintenance dosage should be determined by decreasing the initial drug dosage in small increments at appropriate time intervals until the lowest dosage that will maintain an adequate clinical response is reached. It should be kept in mind that constant monitoring is needed in regard to drug dosage. Included in the situations in which dosage adjustments may be necessary are changes in clinical status secondary to remissions or exacerbations in the disease process, the patient's individual drug responsiveness, and the effect of patient exposure to stressful situations not directly related to the disease entity under treatment. In this latter situation, it may be necessary to increase the dosage of ARISTOSPAN for a period of time consistent with the patient's condition. If after long-term therapy the drug is to be stopped, it is recommended that it be withdrawn gradually rather than abruptly.

Directions for Use

Strict aseptic administration technique is mandatory. Topical ethyl chloride spray may be used locally before injection. The syringe should be gently agitated to achieve uniform suspension before use. Since this product has been designed for ease of administration, a small bore needle (not smaller than 24 gauge) may be used.

Dilution

Intralesional ARISTOSPAN suspension may be diluted, if desired, with Dextrose and Sodium Chloride Injection USP, (5% and 10% Dextrose), Sodium Chloride Injection USP, or Sterile Water for Injection USP.

The optimum dilution, ie, 1:1, 1:2, 1:4, should be determined by the nature of the lesion, its size, the depth of injection, the volume needed, and location of the lesion. In general, more superficial injections should be performed with greater dilution. Certain conditions, such as keloids, require a less dilute suspension such as 5 mg/mL, with variation in dose and dilution as dictated by the condition of the individual patient. Subsequent dosage, dilution, and frequency of injections are best judged by the clinical response.

The suspension may also be mixed with 1% or 2% Lidocaine Hydrochloride, using formulations that do not contain parabens. Similar local anesthetics may also be used. Diluents containing methylparaben, propylparaben, phenol, etc. should be avoided since these compounds may cause flocculation of the steroid. These dilutions will retain full potency for one week, but care should be exercised to avoid contamination of the vial's contents. The dilutions should be discarded after 7 days.

Intralesional or Sublesional Average Dose—Up to 0.5 mg per square inch of affected skin injected intralesionally or sublesionally. The frequency of subsequent injections is best determined by the clinical response. If desired, the vial may be diluted as indicated under **Directions for Use.**

A lesser initial dosage range of ARISTOSPAN *triamcinolone hexacetonide* may produce the desired effect when the drug is administered to provide a localized concentration. The site of the injection and the volume of the injection should be carefully considered when ARISTOSPAN is administered for this purpose.

Dilution

Intra-articular ARISTOSPAN suspension may be mixed with 1% or 2% Lidocaine Hydrochloride, using formulations that do not contain parabens. Similar local anesthetics may also be used. Diluents containing methylparaben, propylparaben, phenol, etc. should be avoided since these compounds may cause flocculation of the steroid. These dilutions will retain full potency for one week, but care should be exercised to avoid contamination.

Intra-articular Average Dose—2 to 20 mg (0.1 mL to 1.0 mL).

The dose depends on the size of the joint to be injected, the degree of inflammation, and the amount of fluid present. In general, large joints (such as knee, hip, shoulder) require 10 to 20 mg. For small joints (such as interphalangeal, metacarpophalangeal), 2 to 6 mg may be employed. When the amount of synovial fluid is increased, aspiration may be performed before administering ARISTOSPAN. Subsequent dosage and frequency of injections can best be judged by clinical response.

The usual frequency of injection into a single joint is every three or four weeks, and injection more frequently than that is generally not advisable. To avoid possible joint destruction from repeated use of intra-articular corticosteroids, injection should be as infrequent as possible, consistent with adequate patient care. Attention should be paid to avoiding deposition of drug along the needle path which might produce atrophy.

HOW SUPPLIED

Intralesional 5 mL, 12.5 mL vial—NDC 57317-206-05, Product Code 511805

Intra-articular 20 mg/mL, 1 mL vial—NDC 57317-205-01; Product Code 511901, 5 mL vial—NDC 57317-205-05, Product Code 511905

Color Code Violet Cap

Store at Controlled Room Temperature 15–30°C (59–86°F).

DO NOT FREEZE.

Military Depot: NSN-6505-00-148-6985, 5 mL vial Intra-articular

Manufactured for Fujisawa Pharmaceutical Company, Fujisawa USA, Inc., Deerfield, IL 60015, by Lederle Parenterals, Inc., Carolina, Puerto Rico 00630 Rev.7/90

27592

CEFIZOX® ℞

(sterile ceftizoxime sodium and ceftizoxime sodium injection)
For Intramuscular or Intravenous Use

DESCRIPTION

Cefizox® (sterile ceftizoxime sodium) is a sterile, semisynthetic, broad-spectrum, beta-lactamase resistant cephalosporin antibiotic for parenteral (I.V., I.M.) administration. It is the sodium salt of [6R-[6a, 7β(Z)]]-7-[[(2,3-dihydro-2-imino-4-thiazolyl) (methoxyimino) acetyl] amino]-8-oxo-5-thia-1-azabicyclo [4.2.0] oct-2-ene-2-carboxylic acid. Its sodium content is approximately 60 mg (2.6 mEq) per gram of ceftizoxime activity. It has the following structural formula:

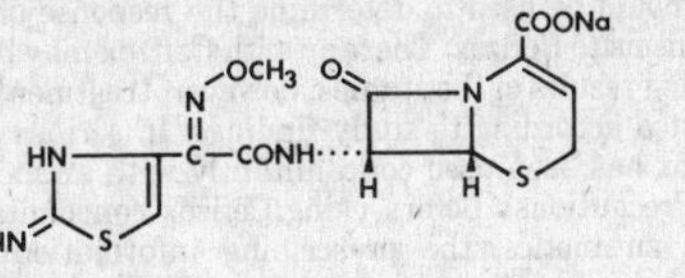

$C_{13}H_{12}N_5NaO_5S_2$ 405.38

Sterile ceftizoxime sodium is a white to pale yellow crystalline powder.

Cefizox is supplied in vials equivalent to 500 mg, 1 gram, 2 grams, or 10 grams of ceftizoxime, and in "Piggyback" Vials for intravenous admixture equivalent to 1 gram or 2 grams of ceftizoxime.

Cefizox, equivalent to 1 gram or 2 grams of ceftizoxime, is also supplied as a frozen, sterile, nonpyrogenic solution of ceftizoxime sodium in an iso-osmotic diluent in plastic containers. After thawing, the solution is intended for intravenous use.

The plastic container is fabricated from specially formulated polyvinyl chloride. Solutions in contact with the plastic container can leach out certain of its chemical components in very small amounts within the expiration period, e.g., di 2-ethylhexyl phthalate (DEHP), up to 5 parts per million. However, the suitability of the plastic has been confirmed in tests in animals according to the USP biological tests for plastic containers as well as by tissue culture toxicity studies.

CLINICAL PHARMACOLOGY

The table below demonstrates the serum levels and duration of Cefizox (sterile ceftizoxime sodium) following intramuscular administration of 500 mg and 1 gram doses, respectively, to normal volunteers.

Serum Concentrations After Intramuscular Administration
Serum Concentration (mcg/mL)

Dose	½ hr	1 hr	2 hr	4 hr	6 hr	8 hr
500 mg	13.3	13.7	9.2	4.8	1.9	0.7
1 gram	36.0	39.0	31.0	15.0	6.0	3.0

Following intravenous administration of 1, 2, and 3 gram doses of Cefizox to normal volunteers, the following serum levels were obtained.

Serum Concentrations After Intravenous Administration
Serum Concentration (mcg/mL)

Dose	5 min	10 min	30 min	1 hr	2 hr	4 hr	8 hr
1 gram	ND	ND	60.5	38.9	21.5	8.4	1.4
2 grams	131.8	110.9	77.5	53.6	33.1	12.1	2.0
3 grams	221.1	174.0	112.7	83.9	47.4	26.2	4.8

ND = Not Done

A serum half-life of approximately 1.7 hours was observed after intravenous or intramuscular administration.

Cefizox is 30% protein bound.

Cefizox is not metabolized, and is excreted virtually unchanged by the kidneys in 24 hours. This provides a high urinary concentration. Concentrations greater than 6000 mcg/mL have been achieved in the urine by 2 hours after a 1 gram dose of Cefizox intravenously. Probenecid slows tubular secretion and produces even higher serum levels, increasing the duration of measurable serum concentrations.

Cefizox achieves therapeutic levels in various body fluids, e.g., cerebrospinal fluid (in patients with inflamed meninges), bile, surgical wound fluid, pleural fluid, aqueous humor, ascitic fluid, peritoneal fluid, prostatic fluid and saliva, and in the following body tissues: heart, gallbladder, bone, biliary, peritoneal, prostatic, and uterine.

In clinical experience to date, no disulfiram-like reactions have been reported with Cefizox.

Microbiology

The bactericidal action of Cefizox results from inhibition of cell-wall synthesis. Cefizox is highly resistant to a broad spectrum of beta-lactamases (penicillinase and cephalosporinase), including Richmond types I, II, III, TEM, and IV, produced by both aerobic and anaerobic gram-positive and gram-negative organisms. Cefizox is active against a wide range of gram-positive and gram-negative organisms, and is usually active against the following organisms *in vitro* and in clinical situations. (see Indications and Usage)

Gram-Positive Aerobes
- *Staphylococcus aureus* (including penicillinase- and non-penicillinase-producing strains)
- NOTE: Methicillin-resistant staphylococci are resistant to cephalosporins, including ceftizoxime.
- *Staphylococcus epidermis* (including penicillinase- and nonpenicillinase-producing strains)
- *Streptococcus agalactiae*
- *Streptococcus pneumoniae*
- *Streptococcus pyogenes*
- NOTE: Ceftizoxime is usually inactive against most strains of *Enterococcus faecalis* (formerly *S. faecalis*).

Gram-Negative Aerobes
- *Acinetobacter* spp.
- *Enterobacter* spp.
- *Escherichia coli*
- *Haemophilus influenzae* (including ampicillin-resistant strains)
- *Klebsiella pneumoniae*
- *Morganella morganii* (formerly *Proteus morganii*)
- *Neisseria gonorrhoeae*
- *Proteus mirabilis*
- *Proteus vulgaris*
- *Providencia rettgeri* (formerly *Proteus rettgeri*)
- *Pseudomonas aeruginosa*
- *Serratia marcescens*

Anaerobes
- *Bacteroides* spp.
- *Peptococcus* spp.
- *Peptostreptococcus* spp.

Ceftizoxime is usually active against the following organisms *in vitro*, <u>but the clinical significance of these data is unknown.</u>

Gram-Positive Aerobes
- *Corynebacterium diphtheriae*

Gram-Negative Aerobes
- *Aeromonas hydrophila*
- *Citrobacter* spp.
- *Moraxella* spp.
- *Neisseria meningitidis*
- *Pasteurella multocida*
- *Providencia stuartii*
- *Salmonella* spp.
- *Shigella* spp.
- *Yersinia enterocolitica*

Anaerobes
- *Actinomyces* spp.
- *Bifidobacterium* spp.
- *Clostridium* spp.
- NOTE: Most strains of *Clostridium difficile* are resistant.
- *Eubacterium* spp.
- *Fusobacterium* spp.
- *Propionibacterium* spp.
- *Veillonella* spp.

Continued on next page

Fujisawa—Cont.

Susceptibility Testing: Diffusion Techniques

Quantitative methods that require measurement of zone diameters give the most precise estimate of susceptibility of bacteria to antimicrobial agents. One such standard procedure[1] has been recommended for use with disks to test susceptibility of organisms to ceftizoxime. Interpretation involves the correlation of the diameters obtained in the disk test with the minimum inhibitory concentration (MIC) for ceftizoxime.

Organisms should be tested with the ceftizoxime disk, since ceftizoxime has been shown by *in vitro* tests to be active against certain strains found resistant when other beta-lactam disks are used.

Reports from the laboratory giving results of the standard single-disk susceptibility test with a 30 mcg ceftizoxime disk should be interpreted according to the following criteria (with the exception of *Pseudomonas aeruginosa*).

Zone Diameter (mm)	Interpretation
≥ 20	(S) Susceptible
15–19	(MS) Moderately Susceptible
≤ 14	(R) Resistant

A report of "Susceptible" indicates that the pathogen is likely to be inhibited by generally achievable blood levels. A report of "Moderately Susceptible" suggests that the organism would be susceptible if high dosage is used or if the infection is confined to tissue and fluids (e.g., urine) in which high antibiotic levels are attained. A report of "Resistant" indicates that achievable concentrations of the antibiotic are unlikely to be inhibitory and other therapy should be selected.

Standardized procedures require the use of laboratory control organisms. The 30 mcg ceftizoxime disk should give the following zone diameters.

Organism	ATCC	Zone Diameter (mm)
Escherichia coli	25922	30–36
Pseudomonas aeruginosa	27853	12–17
Staphylococcus aureus	25923	27–35

Susceptibility Testing for Pseudomonas in Urinary Tract Infections

Most strains of *Pseudomonas aeruginosa* are moderately susceptible to ceftizoxime. Ceftizoxime achieves high levels in the urine (greater than 6000 mcg/mL at 2 hours with 1 gram IV) and, therefore, the following zone sizes should be used when testing ceftizoxime for treatment of urinary tract infections caused by *Pseudomonas aeruginosa*.

Susceptible organisms produce zones of 20 mm or greater, indicating that the test organism is likely to respond to therapy.

Organisms that produce zones of 11 to 19 mm are expected to be susceptible when the infection is confined to the urinary tract (in which high antibiotic levels are attained).

Resistant organisms produce zones of 10 mm or less, indicating that other therapy should be selected.

Susceptibility Testing: Dilution Techniques

When using the NCCLS agar dilution or broth dilution (including microdilution) method[2] or equivalent, the following MIC data should be used for interpretation.

MIC (mcg/mL)	Interpretation
≤ 8	(S) Susceptible
16–32	(MS) Moderately Susceptible
≥ 64	(R) Resistant

As with standard disk diffusion methods, dilution procedures require the use of laboratory control organisms. Standard Ceftizoxime powder should give MIC values in the following ranges.

Organism	ATCC	MIC (mcg/mL)
Escherichia coli	25922	0.03–0.12
Pseudomonas aeruginosa	27853	16–64
Staphylococcus aureus	29213	2–8

INDICATIONS AND USAGE

Cefizox (sterile ceftizoxime sodium) is indicated in the treatment of infections due to susceptible strains of the microorganisms listed below.

Lower Respiratory Tract Infections caused by *Klebsiella* spp.; *Proteus mirabilis; Escherichia coli; Haemophilus influenzae* including ampicillin-resistant strains; *Staphylococcus aureus* (penicillinase- and nonpenicillinase-producing); *Serratia* spp.; *Enterobacter* spp.; and *Bacteroides* spp.; and *Streptococcus* spp. including *S. pneumoniae*, but excluding enterococci.

Urinary Tract Infections caused by *Staphylococcus aureus* (penicillinase- and nonpenicillinase-producing); *Escherichia coli; Pseudomonas* spp. including *P. aeruginosa; Proteus mirabilis; P. vulgaris; Providencia rettgeri* (formerly *Proteus rettgeri*) and *Morganella morganii* (formerly *Proteus morganii*); *Klebsiella* spp.; *Serratia* spp. including *S. marcescens*; and *Enterobacter* spp.

Gonorrhea including uncomplicated cervical and urethral gonorrhea caused by *Neisseria gonorrhoeae*.

Pelvic Inflammatory Disease caused by *Neisseria gonorrhoeae, Escherichia coli* or *Streptococcus agalactiae*.

NOTE: Ceftizoxime, like other cephalosporins, has no activity against *Chlamydia trachomatis*. Therefore, when cephalosporins are used in the treatment of patients with pelvic inflammatory disease and *C. trachomatis* is one of the suspected pathogens, appropriate anti-chlamydial coverage should be added.

Intra-Abdominal Infections caused by *Escherichia coli; Staphylococcus epidermidis; Streptococcus* spp. (excluding enterococci); *Enterobacter* spp.; *Klebsiella* spp.; *Bacteroides* spp. including *B. fragilis;* and anaerobic cocci, including *Peptococcus* spp. and *Peptostreptococcus* spp.

Septicemia caused by *Streptococcus* spp. including *S. pneumoniae* (but excluding enterococci); *Staphylococcus aureus* (penicillinase- and nonpenicillinase-producing); *Escherichia coli; Bacteroides* spp. including *B. fragilis; Klebsiella* spp.; and *Serratia* spp.

Skin and Skin Structure Infections caused by *Staphylococcus aureus* (penicillinase- and nonpenicillinase-producing); *Staphylococcus epidermidis; Escherichia coli; Klebsiella* spp.; *Streptococcus* spp. including *Streptococcus pyogenes* (but excluding enterococci); *Proteus mirabilis; Serratia* spp.; *Enterobacter* spp.; *Bacteroides* spp. including *B. fragilis;* and anaerobic cocci, including *Peptococcus* spp. and *Peptostreptococcus* spp.

Bone and Joint Infections caused by *Staphylococcus aureus* (penicillinase- and nonpenicillinase-producing); *Streptococcus* spp. (excluding enterococci); *Proteus mirabilis; Bacteroides* spp.; and anaerobic cocci, including *Peptococcus* spp. and *Peptostreptococcus* spp.

Meningitis caused by *Haemophilus influenzae*. Cefizox has also been used successfully in the treatment of a limited number of pediatric and adult cases of meningitis caused by *Streptococcus pneumoniae*.

Cefizox has been effective in the treatment of seriously ill, compromised patients, including those who were debilitated, immunosuppressed or neutropenic.

Infections caused by aerobic gram-negative and by mixtures of organisms resistant to other cephalosporins, aminoglycosides, or penicillins have responded to treatment with Cefizox.

Because of the serious nature of some urinary tract infections due to *P. aeruginosa* and because many strains of *Pseudomonas* species are only moderately susceptible to Cefizox, higher dosage is recommended. Other therapy should be instituted if the response is not prompt.

Susceptibility studies on specimens obtained prior to therapy should be used to determine the response of causative organisms to Cefizox. Therapy with Cefizox may be initiated pending results of the studies; however, treatment should be adjusted according to study findings. In serious infections, Cefizox has been used concomitantly with aminoglycosides (see Precautions). Before using Cefizox concomitantly with other antibiotics, the prescribing information for those agents should be reviewed for contraindications, warnings, precautions, and adverse reactions. Renal function should be carefully monitored.

CONTRAINDICATIONS

Cefizox (sterile ceftizoxime sodium) is contraindicated in patients who have known allergy to the drug.

WARNINGS

BEFORE THERAPY WITH CEFIZOX (STERILE CEFTIZOXIME SODIUM) IS INSTITUTED, CAREFUL INQUIRY SHOULD BE MADE TO DETERMINE WHETHER THE PATIENT HAS HAD PREVIOUS HYPERSENSITIVITY REACTIONS TO CEPHALOSPORINS, PENICILLINS, OR OTHER DRUGS. THIS PRODUCT SHOULD BE GIVEN CAUTIOUSLY TO PENICILLIN-SENSITIVE PATIENTS. CAUTION SHOULD BE EXERCISED BECAUSE CROSS HYPERSENSITIVITY AMONG BETA-LACTAM ANTIBIOTICS HAVE BEEN CLEARLY DOCUMENTED AND MAY OCCUR IN UP TO 10% OF PATIENTS WITH A HISTORY OF PENICILLIN ALLERGY. IF AN ALLERGIC REACTION TO CEFIZOX OCCURS, DISCONTINUE THE DRUG. SERIOUS ACUTE HYPERSENSITIVITY REACTIONS MAY REQUIRE EPINEPHRINE AND OTHER EMERGENCY MEASURES, INCLUDING OXYGEN, INTRAVENOUS FLUIDS, INTRAVENOUS ANTIHISTAMINES, CORTICOSTEROIDS, PRESSOR AMINES, AND AIRWAY MANAGEMENT, AS CLINICALLY INDICATED.

Pseudomembranous colitis has been reported with the use of cephalosporins (and other broad-spectrum antibiotics); therefore, it is important to consider this diagnosis in patients who develop diarrhea in association with antibiotic use.

Treatment with broad-spectrum antibiotics alters normal flora of the colon and may permit overgrowth of *Clostridia*. Studies indicate a toxin produced by *Clostridium difficile* is one primary cause of antibiotic-associated colitis.

Mild cases of colitis may respond to drug discontinuance alone.

Moderate to severe cases should be managed with fluid, electrolyte, and protein supplementation as indicated.

When the colitis is not relieved by drug discontinuance or when it is severe, oral vancomycin is the treatment of choice for antibiotic-associated pseudomembranous colitis produced by *C. difficile*. Other causes of colitis should also be considered.

PRECAUTIONS

General

As with all broad-spectrum antibiotics, Cefizox (sterile ceftizoxime sodium) should be prescribed with caution in individuals with a history of gastrointestinal disease, particularly colitis.

Although Cefizox has not been shown to produce an alteration in renal function, renal status should be evaluated, especially in seriously ill patients receiving maximum dose therapy. As with any antibiotic, prolonged use may result in overgrowth of nonsusceptible organisms. Careful observation is essential; appropriate measures should be taken if superinfection occurs.

Drug Interactions

Although the occurrence has not been reported with Cefizox, nephrotoxicity has been reported following concomitant administration of other cephalosporins and aminoglycosides.

Carcinogenesis, Mutagenesis, Impairment of Fertility

Long term studies in animals to evaluate the carcinogenic potential of ceftizoxime have not been conducted.

In an *in vitro* bacterial cell assay (i.e., Ames test), there was no evidence of mutagenicity at ceftizoxime concentrations of 0.001–0.5 mcg/plate. Ceftizoxime did not produce increases in micronuclei in the *in vivo* mouse micronucleus test when given to animals at doses up to 7500 mg/kg, approximately six times greater than the maximum human daily dose on a mg/M^2 basis.

Ceftizoxime had no effect on fertility when administered subcutaneously to rats at daily doses of up to 1000 mg/kg/day, approximately two times the maximum human daily dose on a mg/M^2 basis. Ceftizoxime produced no histological changes in the sexual organs of male and female dogs when given intravenously for thirteen weeks at a dose of 1000 mg/kg/day, approximately five times greater than the maximum human daily dose on a mg/M^2 basis.

Pregnancy: Teratogenic Effects: Pregnancy Category B.

Reproduction studies performed in rats and rabbits have revealed no evidence of impaired fertility or harm to the fetus due to Cefizox. There are, however, no adequate and well-controlled studies in pregnant women. Because animal reproduction studies are not always predictive of human effects, this drug should be used during pregnancy only if clearly needed.

Labor and Delivery

Safety of Cefizox use during labor and delivery has not been established.

Nursing Mothers

Cefizox is excreted in human milk in low concentrations. Caution should be exercised when Cefizox is administered to a nursing woman.

Pediatric Use

Safety and efficacy in infants from birth to six months of age have not been established. In children six months of age and older, treatment with Cefizox has been associated with transient elevated levels of eosinophils, AST (SGOT), ALT (SGPT) and CPK (creatine phosphokinase). The CPK elevation may be related to I.M. administration.

The potential for the toxic effect in children from chemicals that may leach from the single-dose I.V. preparation has not been determined.

ADVERSE REACTIONS

Cefizox® (sterile ceftizoxime sodium) is generally well tolerated. The *most* frequent adverse reactions (*greater than 1% but less than 5%*) are:

Hypersensitivity—Rash, pruritus, fever.

Hepatic—Transient elevation in AST (SGOT), ALT (SGPT), and alkaline phosphatase.

Hematologic—Transient eosinophilia, thrombocytosis. Some individuals have developed a positive Coombs test.

Local—Injection site—Burning, cellulitis, phlebitis with I.V. administration, pain, induration, tenderness, paresthesia.

The *less* frequent adverse reactions (*less than 1%*) are:

Hypersensitivity—Numbness and anaphylaxis have rarely been reporte..

Hepatic—Elevation of bilirubin has been reported rarely.

Renal—Transient elevations of BUN and creatinine have been occasionally observed with Cefizox.

Hematologic—Anemia, leukopenia, neutropenia and thrombocytopenia have been reported rarely.

Urogenital—Vaginitis has occurred rarely.

Gastrointestinal—Diarrhea; nausea and vomiting have been reported occasionally.

Symptoms of pseudomembranous colitis can appear during or after antibiotic treatment (See Warnings).

In addition to the adverse reactions listed above which have been observed in patients treated with ceftizoxime, the fol-

lowing adverse reactions and altered laboratory tests have been reported for cephalosporinclass antibiotics:
Stevens-Johnson syndrome, erythema multiforme, toxic epidermal necrolysis, serum-sickness like reaction, toxic nephropathy, aplastic anemia, hemolytic anemia, hemorrhage, prolonged prothrombin time, elevated LDH, pancytopenia, and agranulocytosis.
Several cephalosporins have been implicated in triggering seizures, particularly in patients with renal impairment, when the dosage was not reduced. (See DOSAGE AND ADMINISTRATION.) If seizures associated with drug therapy occur, the drug should be discontinued. Anticonvulsant therpay can be given if clinically indicated.

DOSAGE AND ADMINISTRATION

The usual adult dosage is 1 or 2 grams of Cefizox (sterile ceftizoxime sodium) every 8 to 12 hours. Proper dosage and route of administration should be determined by the condition of the patient, severity of the infection, and susceptibility of the causative organisms.

General Guidelines for Dosage of Cefizox

Type of Infection	Daily Dose (Grams)	Frequency and Route
Uncomplicated		
Urinary Tract	1	500 mg q12h I.M. or I.V.
Other Sites	2–3	1 gram q8–12h I.M. or I.V.
Severe or Refractory	3–6	1 gram q8h I.M. or I.V.
		2 grams q8–12h I.M.[a] or I.V.
PID[b]	6	2 grams q8h I.V.
Life-Threatening[c]	9–12	3–4 grams q8h I.V.

a) When administering 2 gram I.M. doses, the dose should be divided and given in different large muscle masses.
b) If *C. trachomatis* is a suspected pathogen, appropriate antichlamydial coverage should be added, because ceftizoxime has no activity against this organism.
c) In life-threatening infections, dosages up to 2 grams every 4 hours have been given.

Because of the serious nature of urinary tract infections due to *P. aeruginosa* and because many strains of *Pseudomonas* species are only moderately susceptible to Cefizox, higher dosage is recommended. Other therapy should be instituted if the response is not prompt.
A single, 1 gram I.M. dose is the usual dose for treatment of uncomplicated gonorrhea.
The intravenous route may be preferable for patients with bacterial septicemia, localized parenchymal abscesses (such as intra-abdominal abscess), peritonitis, or other severe or life-threatening infections.
In those with normal renal function, the intravenous dosage for such infections is 2 to 12 grams of Cefizox daily. In conditions such as bacterial septicemia, 6 to 12 grams/day may be given initially by the intravenous route for several days, and the dosage may then be gradually reduced according to clinical response and laboratory findings.

Pediatric Dosage Schedule

	Unit Dose	Frequency
Children 6 months and older	50 mg/kg	q6-8h

Dosage may be increased to a total daily dose of 200 mg/kg (not to exceed the maximum adult dose for serious infection).

Impaired Renal Function

Modification of Cefizox dosage is necessary in patients with impaired renal function. Following an initial loading dose of 500 mg.–1 gram I.M. or I.V., the maintenance dosing schedule shown below should be followed. Further dosing should be determined by therapeutic monitoring, severity of the infection, and susceptibility of the causative organisms.
When only the serum creatinine level is available, creatinine clearance may be calculated from the following formula. The serum creatinine level should represent current renal function at the steady state.

Males

$$\text{Clcr} = \frac{\text{Weight (kg)} \times (140 - \text{age})}{72 \times \text{serum creatinine (mg/100 mL)}}$$

Females 0.85 of the calculated clearance values for males.

In patients undergoing hemodialysis, no additional supplemental dosing is required following hemodialysis; however, dosing should be timed so that the patient receives the dose (according to the table above) at the end of the dialysis.

[See first table next column.]

Preparation of Parenteral Solution

RECONSTITUTION
I.M. Administration: Reconstitute with Sterile Water for Injection. SHAKE WELL.

[See second table next column.]

Dosage in Adults with Reduced Renal Function

Creatinine Clearance mL/min	Renal Function	Less Severe Infections	Life-Threatening Infections
79–50	Mild impairment	500 mg q8h	0.75–1.5 grams q8H
49–5	Moderate to severe impairment	250–500 mg q12h	0.5–1 gram q12h
4–0	Dialysis patients	500 mg q48h or 250 mg q24h	0.5–1 gram q48h or 0.5 gram q24h

Vial Size	Diluent to Be Added	Approx. Avail. Vol.	Approx. Avg. Concentration
500 mg	1.5 mL	1.8 mL	280 mg/mL
1 gram	3.0 mL	3.7 mL	270 mg/mL
2 grams*	6.0 mL	7.4 mL	270 mg/mL

*When administering 2 gram I.M. doses, the dose should be divided and given in different large muscle masses.

I.V. Administration: Reconstitute with Sterile Water for Injection. SHAKE WELL.

Vial Size	Diluent to Be Added	Approx. Avail. Vol.	Approx. Avg. Concentration
500 mg	5 mL	5.3 mL	95 mg/mL
1 gram	10 mL	10.7 mL	95 mg/mL
2 grams	20 mL	21.4 mL	95 mg/mL

These solutions of Cefizox are stable 24 hours at room temperature or 96 hours if refrigerated (5°C).
Parenteral drug products should be inspected visually for particulate matter prior to administration. If particulate matter is evident in reconstituted fluids, then the drug solution should be discarded. Reconstituted solutions may range from yellow to amber without changes in potency.
Pharmacy Bulk Vials: For I.M. or I.V. direct injection, add Sterile Water for Injection to the 10 gram vial according to table below. SHAKE WELL. For I.V. intermittent or continuous infusion, add Sterile Water for Injection according to table below. SHAKE WELL. Add to parenteral fluids listed below under I.V. Administration.

Vial Size	Diluent to Be Added	Approx. Avail. Vol.	Approx. Avg. Concentration
10 grams	30 mL	37 mL	1 gram/3.5 mL
	45 mL	51 mL	1 gram/5 mL

These reconstituted solutions of Cefizox are stable 24 hours at room temperature or 96 hours if refrigerated (5°C).
"Piggyback" Vials: Reconstitute with 50 to 100 mL of Sodium Chloride Injection or any other I.V. solution listed below. SHAKE WELL.
Administer with primary I.V. fluids, as a single dose. These solutions of Cefizox are stable 24 hours at room temperature or 96 hours if refrigerated (5°C).
A solution of 1 gram Cefizox in 13 mL Sterile Water for Injection is isotonic.

I.M. Injection

Inject well within the body of a relatively large muscle. Aspiration is necessary to avoid inadvertent injection into a blood vessel. When administering 2 gram I.M. doses, the dose should be divided and given in different large muscle masses.

IV Administration

Direct (bolus) injection, slowly over 3 to 5 minutes, directly or through tubing for patients receiving parenteral fluids (see list below). Intermittent or continuous infusion, dilute reconstituted Cefizox in 50 to 100 mL of one of the following solutions:
- Sodium Chloride Injection
- 5% or 10% Dextrose Injection
- 5% Dextrose and 0.9%, 0.45%, or 0.2% Sodium Chloride Injection
- Ringer's Injection
- Lactated Ringer's Injection
- Invert Sugar 10% in Sterile Water for Injection
- 5% Sodium Bicarbonate in Sterile Water for Injection
- 5% Dextrose in Lactated Ringer's Injection (only when reconstituted with 4% Sodium Bicarbonate Injection)

In these fluids, Cefizox is stable 24 hours at room temperature or 96 hours if refrigerated (5°C).

Directions for Use of Cefizox in Viaflex® Plus Containers (PL 146® Plastic)

Viaflex and PL 146 are registered trademarks of Baxter International Inc.
Cefizox in Viaflex® Plus Containers (PL 146® Plastic) is to be administered either as a continuous or intermittent infusion using sterile equipment.

Storage

Store in freezer capable of maintaining a temperature of −20°C/−4°F.

Thawing of Plastic Container

Thaw frozen container at room temperature (25°C/77°F) or under refrigeration (5°C/41°F). DO NOT FORCE THAW BY IMMERSION IN WATER BATHS OR BY MICROWAVE IRRADIATION.
Containers may be thawed individually after separation from the frozen shingle. A shingle consists of stacked frozen containers. Remove frozen shingle from carton and allow to rest at room temperature until the containers can be easily separated (approximately 5 minutes). Then grasp the body of the container (not the ports, corner, or tail flap) to separate individual units.
Promptly return unneeded frozen containers to freezer.
Check for minute leaks by squeezing container firmly. If leaks are detected, discard solution as sterility may be impaired.
Do not add supplementary medication.
The container should be visually inspected. Components of the solution may precipitate in the frozen state and will dissolve upon reaching room temperature with little or no agitation. Potency is not affected. Agitate after solution has reached room temperature. If after visual inspection the solution remains cloudly or if an insoluble precipitate is noted or if any seal or outlet ports are not intact, the container should be discarded.
The thawed solution is stable for 10 days under refrigeration (5°C/41°F) or for 24 hours at room temperature (25°C/77°F).
Do not refreeze thawed antibiotics.
CAUTION Do not use plastic containers in series connections. Air embolism could result due to residual air being drawn from the primary container before administration of the fluid from the secondary container is complete.

Preparation for Intravenous Administration

1. Suspend container from eyelet support.
2. Remove plastic protector from outlet port at bottom of container.
3. Attach administration set. Refer to complete directions accompanying set.

HOW SUPPLIED

Cefizox® (sterile ceftizoxime sodium)
NDC 57317-250-01 Product No. 725001
Equivalent to 500 mg ceftizoxime in 10 mL, single-dose, flip-top vials, individually packaged
NDC 57317-251-01 Product No. 725101
Equivalent to 1 gram ceftizoxime in 20 mL single-dose, flip-top vials, individually packaged
NDC 57317-252-01 Product No. 725201
Equivalent to 1 gram ceftizoxime in 100 mL, single-dose Piggyback, flip-top vials, packaged in tens
NDC 57317-253-02 Product No. 725302
Equivalent to 2 grams ceftizoxime in 20 mL, single-dose, flip-top vials, individually packaged
NDC 57317-254-02 Product No. 725402
Equivalent to 2 grams ceftizoxime in 100 mL, single-dose, Piggyback, flip-top vials, packaged in tens
NDC 57317-255-10 Product No. 725510
Equivalent to 10 grams ceftizoxime in 100 mL, Pharmacy Bulk Package, packaged in tens
Unreconstituted Cefizox should be protected from excessive light, and stored at controlled room temperature (59°–86°F) in the original package until used.
Manufactured for Fujisawa Pharmaceutical Company, Division of Fujisawa USA, Inc., Deerfield, IL 60015, by SmithKline Beecham, Philadelphia, PA 19101, and by Baxter Healthcare Corporation, Deerfield, IL 60015.

REFERENCES

1. National Committee for Clinical Laboratory Standards, Approved Standard. *Performance Standards for Antimicrobial Disk Susceptibility Test*, 4th Edition, Vol 10 (7):M2-A4. Villanova, PA, April 1990.
2. National Committee for Clinical Laboratory Standards, Approved Standard. *Methods for Dilution Antimicrobial Susceptibility Tests for Bacteria that Grow Aerobically*, 2nd Edition, Vol 10 (8):M7-A2. Villanova, PA, April 1990.

45598C/Issued July 1992

CYCLOCORT® ℞
[amcinonide]

DESCRIPTION

The topical corticosteroids constitute a class of primarily synthetic steroids used as anti-inflammatory and antipruritic agents.
TOPICAL LOTION 0.1%
Each gram of Cyclocort (amcinonide) topical Lotion contains 1 mg of the active steroid amcinonide in Aquatain,™* a white, smooth, homogeneous, opaque emulsion composed of Benzyl Alcohol 1% (wt/wt) as preservative, Emulsifying Wax, Glycerin, Isopropyl Palmitate, Lactic Acid, Purified Water, and Sorbitol Solution. In addition, contains Polyethylene Glycol 400.

Continued on next page

Fujisawa—Cont.

Sodium hydroxide may be used to adjust pH to approximately 4.4 during manufacture.

TOPICAL CREAM 0.1%
Each gram of Cyclocort (amcinonide) topical Cream contains 1 mg of the active steroid amcinonide in Aquatain,* a white, smooth, homogeneous, opaque emulsion composed of Benzyl Alcohol 2% (wt/wt) as preservative, Emulsifying Wax, Glycerin, Isopropyl Palmitate, Lactic Acid, Purified Water, and Sorbitol Solution.

*Aquatain is non-staining, water-washable, paraben-free, spermaceti-free, and has a light texture and consistency.

TOPICAL OINTMENT 0.1%
Each gram of Cyclocort (amcinonide) topical Ointment contains 1 mg of the active steroid amcinonide in a specially formulated base composed of Benzyl Alcohol 2% (wt/wt) as preservative, White Petrolatum, Emulsifying Wax, and Tenox II (Butylated Hydroxyanisole, Propyl Gallate, Citric Acid, Propylene Glycol).
Chemically, amcinonide is:

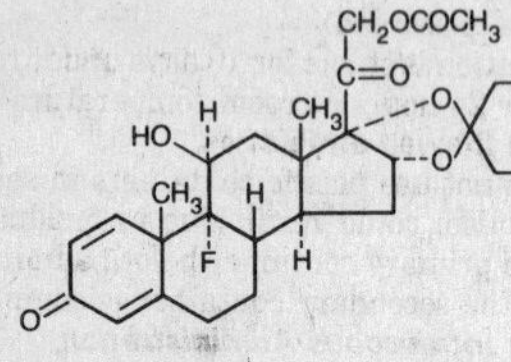

Molecular Weight 502.58 **$C_{28}H_{35}FO_7$**
Pregna-1,4-diene-3,20-dione, 21-(acetyloxy)-16,17-[cyclopentylidenebis(oxy)]-9-fluoro-11-hydroxy-, (11β, 16α).

CLINICAL PHARMACOLOGY
Topical corticosteroids have anti-inflammatory, antipruritic, and vasoconstrictive actions.
The mechanism of anti-inflammatory activity of the topical corticosteroids is unclear. Various laboratory methods, including vasoconstrictor assays, are used to compare and predict potencies and/or clinical efficacies of the topical corticosteroids. There is some evidence to suggest that a recognizable correlation exists between vasoconstrictor potency and therapeutic efficacy in man.

Pharmacokinetics
The extent of percutaneous absorption of topical corticosteroids is determined by many factors, including the vehicle, the integrity of the epidermal barrier, and the use of occlusive dressings.
Topical corticosteroids can be absorbed from normal intact skin. Inflammation and/or other disease processes in the skin increase percutaneous absorption. Occlusive dressings substantially increase the percutaneous absorption of topical corticosteroids (see DOSAGE AND ADMINISTRATION).
Once absorbed through the skin, topical corticosteroids are handled through pharmacokinetic pathways similar to systemically-administered corticosteroids. Corticosteroids are bound to plasma proteins in varying degrees.
Corticosteroids are metabolized primarily in the liver and are then excreted by the kidneys. Some of the topical corticosteroids and their metabolites are also excreted into the bile.

INDICATIONS AND USAGE
Topical corticosteroids are indicated for the relief of the inflammatory and pruritic manifestations of corticosteroid-responsive dermatoses.

CONTRAINDICATIONS
Topical corticosteroids are contraindicated in those patients with a history of hypersensitivity to any of the components of the preparation.

PRECAUTIONS
General
Systemic absorption of topical corticosteroids has produced reversible hypothalamic-pituitary-adrenal (HPA) axis suppression, manifestations of Cushing's syndrome, hyperglycemia, and glucosuria in some patients.
Conditions that augment systemic absorption include the application of the more potent steroids, use over large surface areas, prolonged use, and the addition of occlusive dressings. Therefore, patients receiving a large dose of a potent topical steroid applied to a large surface area or under an occlusive dressing should be evaluated periodically for evidence of HPA-axis suppression by using the urinary free-cortisol and ACTH stimulation tests. If HPA-axis suppression is noted, an attempt should be made to withdraw the drug, to reduce the frequency of application, or to substitute with a less potent steroid.
Recovery of HPA-axis function is generally prompt and complete upon discontinuation of the drug.
Infrequently, signs and symptoms of steroid withdrawal may occur, requiring supplemental systemic corticosteroids.
Children may absorb proportionally larger amounts of topical corticosteroids and thus be more susceptible to systemic toxicity (see PRECAUTIONS *Pediatric Use*).
If irritation develops, topical corticosteroids should be discontinued and appropriate therapy instituted.
In the presence of dermatological infections, the use of an appropriate antifungal or antibacterial agent should be instituted. If a favorable response does not occur promptly, the corticosteroid should be discontinued until the infection has been adequately controlled.
The products are not for ophthalmic use.

Information for the Patient
Patients using topical corticosteroids should receive the following information and instructions.
1. This medication is to be used as directed by the physician. It is for external use only. Avoid contact with the eyes.
2. Patients should be advised not to use this medication for any disorder other than for which it was prescribed.
3. The treated skin area should not be bandaged or otherwise covered or wrapped, as to be occlusive, unless directed by the physician.
4. Patients should report any signs of local adverse reactions, especially those that occur under occlusive dressings.
5. Parents of pediatric patients should be advised not to use tight-fitting diapers or plastic pants on a child being treated in the diaper area, as those garments may constitute occlusive dressings.

Laboratory Tests
The following tests may be helpful in evaluating the HPA-axis suppression.
Urinary free-cortisol test
ACTH stimulation test

Carcinogenesis, Mutagenesis, and Impairment of Fertility
Long-term animal studies have not been performed to evaluate the carcinogenic potential of topical corticosteroids or their effect on fertility.
Studies to determine mutagenicity with prednisolone and hydrocortisone have revealed negative results.

Pregnancy Category C
Corticosteroids are generally teratogenic in laboratory animals when administered systemically at relatively low dosage levels. The more potent corticosteroids have been shown to be teratogenic after dermal application in laboratory animals. There are no adequate and well-controlled studies in pregnant women on teratogenic effects from topically-applied corticosteroids. Therefore, topical corticosteroids should be used during pregnancy only if the potential benefit justifies the potential risk to the fetus. Drugs of this class should not be used extensively on pregnant patients, in large amounts, or for prolonged periods of time.

Nursing Mothers
It is not known whether topical administration of corticosteroids could result in sufficient systemic absorption to produce detectable quantities in breast milk. Systemically-administered corticosteroids are secreted into breast milk in quantities not likely to have a deleterious effect on the infant. Nevertheless, a decision should be made whether to discontinue nursing or to discontinue the drug, taking into account the importance of the drug to the mother.

Pediatric Use
Pediatric patients may demonstrate greater susceptibility to topical corticosteroid-induced HPA-axis suppression and Cushing's syndrome than mature patients because of a higher ratio of skin surface area to body weight.
Hypothalamic-pituitary-adrenal (HPA) axis suppression, Cushing's syndrome, and intracranial hypertension have been reported in children receiving topical corticosteroids. Manifestations of adrenal suppression in children include linear growth retardation, delayed weight gain, low plasma cortisol levels, and absence of response to ACTH stimulation. Manifestations of intracranial hypertension include bulging fontanelles, headaches, and bilateral papilledema.
Administration of topical corticosteroids to children should be limited to the least amount compatible with an effective therapeutic regimen. Chronic corticosteroid therapy may interfere with the growth and development of children.

ADVERSE REACTIONS
In the clinical trials with Cyclocort Lotion, the investigators reported a 4.7% incidence of side effects. In a weekly acceptability evaluation, approximately 20% of the patients treated with Cyclocort Lotion or placebo reported itching, stinging, soreness, or burning at one or more of the visits.
The following local adverse reactions are reported infrequently with topical corticosteroids, but may occur more frequently with the use of occlusive dressings. These reactions are listed in an approximate decreasing order of occurrence.

Burning	Perioral dermatitis
Itching	Allergic contact dermatitis
Irritation	Maceration of the skin
Dryness	Secondary infection
Folliculitis	Skin atrophy
Hypertrichosis	Striae
Acneiform eruptions	Miliaria
Hypopigmentation	

OVERDOSAGE
Topically-applied corticosteroids can be absorbed in sufficient amounts to produce systemic effects (see PRECAUTIONS).

DOSAGE AND ADMINISTRATION
Topical corticosteroids are generally applied to the affected area as a thin film from two to three times daily depending on the severity of the condition.
The lotion may be applied topically to the specified lesions, particularly to those in hairy areas, two times per day. The lotion should be rubbed into the affected area completely, and the area should be protected from washing, clothing, rubbing, etc. until the lotion has dried.
Occlusive dressings may be a valuable therapeutic adjunct for the management of psoriasis or recalcitrant conditions.
If an infection develops, the use of occlusive dressings should be discontinued and appropriate antimicrobial therapy instituted.

HOW SUPPLIED
Cyclocort® (amcinonide) Topical Lotion
0.1% (1 mg/g) qwith Aquatain™ hydrophilic base
NDC 57317-404-20 Product Code 740420
20 mL (19.6 g) Bottle
NDC 57317-404-60 Product Code 740460
60 mL (58.8 g) Bottle
Cyclocort® (amcinonide) Topical Cream
0.1% (1 mg/g) with Aquatain hydrophilic base
NDC 57317-054-15 Product Code 705415
15 gram Tube
NDC 57317-054-30 Product Code 705430
30 gram Tube
NDC 57317-054-60 Product Code 705460
60 gram Tube
Cyclocort® (amcinonide) Topical Ointment
0.1% (1 mg/g)
NDC 57317-115-15 Product Code 711515
15 gram Tube
NDC 57317-115-30 Product Code 711530
30 gram Tube
NDC 57317-115-60 Product Code 711560
60 gram Tube
Store at controlled room temperature 15°–30°C (59°–86°F).
DO NOT FREEZE.
Manufactured for Fujisawa Pharmaceutical Co., Division of Fujisawa USA, Inc., Deerfield, IL 60015 by Lederle Laboratories Division, American Cyanamid Company, Pearl River, NY 10965
20855-92/Issued April 1992
FP1

ELASE® ℞
[*ē'lāse"*]
(fibrinolysin and desoxyribonuclease, combined [bovine])

ELASE OINTMENT ℞
(fibrinolysin and desoxyribonuclease, combined [bovine], ointment)

ELASE-CHLOROMYCETIN® OINTMENT ℞
(fibrinolysin and desoxyribonuclease, combined [bovine], with chloramphenicol ointment)

DESCRIPTION
ELASE is a combination of two lytic enzymes, fibrinolysin and desoxyribonuclease, supplied as a lyophilized powder and in an ointment base of liquid petrolatum and polyethylene. The fibrinolysin component is derived from bovine plasma and the desoxyribonuclease is isolated in a purified form from bovine pancreas. The fibrinolysin used in the combination is activated by chloroform.

ELASE-CHLOROMYCETIN OINTMENT
Contains two lytic enzymes, fibrinolysin and desoxyribonuclease, combined with chloramphenicol in an ointment base. Chloramphenicol is a broad-spectrum antibiotic originally isolated from *Streptomyces venezuelae.* It is therapeutically active against a wide variety of susceptible organisms, both gram-positive and gram-negative. Chemically, chloramphenicol may be identified as D(-)- *threo*-1-*p*- nitrophenyl-2-dichloroacetamido-1, 3-propanediol.

ACTION
Combination of these two enzymes is based on the observation that purulent exudates consist largely of fibrinous material and nucleoprotein. Desoxyribonuclease attacks the desoxyribonucleic acid (DNA) and fibrinolysin attacks principally the fibrin of blood clots and fibrinous exudates.
The activity of desoxyribonuclease is limited principally to the production of large polynucleotides, which are less likely to be absorbed than the more diffusible protein fractions liberated by certain enzyme preparations obtained from

bacteria. The fibrinolytic action of ELASE and of the enzymes in ELASE OINTMENT and ELASE-CHLOROMYCETIN OINTMENT is directed mainly against denatured proteins, such as those found in devitalized tissue, while protein elements of living cells remain relatively unaffected.
ELASE, ELASE OINTMENT, and ELASE-CHLOROMYCETIN OINTMENT are combinations of active enzymes. This is an important consideration in treating patients suffering from lesions resulting from impaired circulation.
The enzymatic action of ELASE helps to produce clean surfaces and thus supports healing in a variety of exudative lesions.

ELASE-CHLOROMYCETIN OINTMENT
Chloramphenicol is a broad-spectrum antibiotic that is primarily bacteriostatic and acts by inhibition of protein synthesis by interfering with the transfer of activated amino acids from soluble RNA to ribosomes. Development of resistance to chloramphenicol can be regarded as minimal for staphylococci and many other species of bacteria.
The action of ELASE-CHLOROMYCETIN helps to produce clean surfaces and thus supports healing in a variety of exudative lesions.

INDICATIONS
ELASE and ELASE OINTMENT are indicated for topical use as debriding agents in a variety of inflammatory and infected lesions. These include: (1) general surgical wounds; (2) ulcerative lesions—trophic, decubitus, stasis, arteriosclerotic; (3) second- and third-degree burns; (4) circumcision and episiotomy. ELASE and ELASE OINTMENT are used intravaginally in: (1) cervicitis—benign, postpartum, and postconization; (2) vaginitis. ELASE is used as an irrigating agent in the following conditions: (1) infected wounds—abscesses, fistulae, and sinus tracts; (2) otorhinolaryngologic wounds; (3) superficial hematomas (except when the hematoma is adjacent to or within adipose tissue).

ELASE-CHLOROMYCETIN OINTMENT
Indicated for use in the treatment of infected lesions, such as burns, ulcers, and wounds where the actions of both a debriding agent and a topical antibiotic are desired. This dual-purpose approach is especially useful in the treatment of infections caused by organisms that utilize a process of fibrin deposition as protective device (ie, coagulase and staphylococcus). Appropriate measures should be taken to determine the susceptibility of the pathogen to chloramphenicol.

CONTRAINDICATIONS
These products (ELASE, ELASE OINTMENT, ELASE-CHLOROMYCETIN OINTMENT) are contraindicated in individuals with a history of hypersensitivity reactions to any of their components. ELASE is not recommended for parenteral use because the bovine fibrinolysin may be antigenic.

WARNINGS
ELASE-CHLOROMYCETIN OINTMENT
Bone marrow hypoplasia, including aplastic anemia and death, has been reported following the local application of chloramphenicol.

PRECAUTIONS
ELASE-CHLOROMYCETIN OINTMENT
The prolonged use of antibiotics may occasionally result in overgrowth of nonsusceptible organisms, including fungi. If new infections appear during medication, the drug should be discontinued and appropriate measures should be taken.
In all except very superficial infections, the topical use of chloramphenicol should be supplemented by appropriate systemic medication.
ELASE, ELASE OINTMENT, ELASE-CHLOROMYCETIN OINTMENT
The usual precautions against allergic reactions should be observed, particularly in persons with a history of sensitivity to materials of bovine origin.
ELASE
To be maximally effective, ELASE solutions must be freshly prepared before use. The loss in activity is reduced by refrigeration; however, even when stored in a refrigerator, the solution should not be used 24 hours or more after reconstitution.

ADVERSE REACTIONS
Side effects attributable to the enzymes have not been a problem at the dose and for the indications recommended herein. With higher concentrations, side effects have been minimal, consisting of local hyperemia.
Chills and fever attributable to antigenic action of profibrinolysin activators of bacterial origin are not a problem with ELASE, ELASE OINTMENT, or ELASE-CHLOROMYCETIN OINTMENT.
ELASE-CHLOROMYCETIN OINTMENT
Signs of local irritation, with subjective symptoms of itching or burning, angioneurotic edema, urticaria, vesicular and maculopapular dermatitis have been reported in patients sensitive to chloramphenicol and are causes for discontinuing the medication. Similar sensitivity reactions to other materials in topical preparations may also occur. Blood dys-

crasias have been associated with the use of chloramphenicol.
Preparation of ELASE Solution
The contents of each vial may be reconstituted with 10 mL of isotonic sodium chloride solution. Higher or lower concentrations can be prepared if desired by varying the amount of the diluent.

DOSAGE AND ADMINISTRATION
Since the conditions for which ELASE, ELASE OINTMENT, and ELASE-CHLOROMYCETIN OINTMENT are helpful vary considerably in severity, dosage must be adjusted to the individual case; however, the following general recommendations can be made.
Successful use of enzymatic debridement depends on several factors: (1) dense, dry eschar, if present, should be removed surgically before enzymatic debridement is attempted; (2) the enzyme must be in constant contact with the substrate; (3) accumulated necrotic debris must be periodically removed; (4) the enzyme must be replenished at least once daily; and (5) secondary closure or skin grafting must be employed as soon as possible after optimal debridement has been attained. It is further essential that wound-dressing techniques be performed carefully under aseptic conditions and that appropriate systemically acting antibiotics be administered concomitantly if, in the opinion of the physician, they are indicated.
General Topical Uses
ELASE OINTMENT
Local application should be repeated at intervals for as long as enzyme action is desired. After application, ELASE OINTMENT becomes rapidly and progressively less active and is probably exhausted for practical purposes at the end of 24 hours. A recommended procedure for application of ELASE OINTMENT follows.
1. Clean the wound with water, peroxide, or normal saline and dry area gently. If there is a dense, dry eschar present, it should be removed surgically before applying ELASE.
2. Apply a *thin* layer of ELASE OINTMENT.
3. Cover with petrolatum gauze or another type of nonadhering dressing.
4. Change the dressing at least ONCE a day, preferably two or three times daily. Frequency of application is more important than the amount of ELASE used. Flush away the necrotic debris and fibrinous exudates with saline, peroxide, or warm water so that newly applied ointment can be in direct contact with the substrate.
ELASE
Local application should be repeated at intervals for as long as enzyme action is desired. ELASE solution may be applied topically as a liquid, spray, or wet dressing. Application of a gentle spray of the solution can be accomplished by using a conventional atomizer. After application, ELASE, especially in solution, becomes rapidly and progressively less active and is probably exhausted for practical purposes at the end of 24 hours. The dry material for solution is stable at room temperature through the expiration date printed on the package. A recommended procedure for application of a solution of ELASE using a Wet-to-Dry method follows.
1. Mix one vial of ELASE powder with 10 to 50 mL of saline and saturate strips of fine-mesh gauze or an unfolded sterile gauze sponge with the ELASE solution.
2. Pack ulcerated area with the ELASE-saturated gauze, making sure the gauze remains in contact with the necrotic substrate (if the lesion is covered with a heavy eschar, it must be removed surgically before wet-to-dry debridement is begun).
3. ALLOW GAUZE TO DRY IN CONTACT WITH THE ULCERATED LESION (approximately six to eight hours). As the gauze dries, the necrotic tissues slough and become enmeshed in the gauze.
4. Remove dried gauze. This mechanically debrides the area. Repeat wet-to-dry procedure three or four times daily, since frequent dressing changes greatly enhance results. After two, three, or four days, the area becomes clean and starts to fill in with granulation tissue.
Intravaginal use
ELASE OINTMENT
In mild to moderate vaginitis and cervicitis, 5 mL of ELASE OINTMENT should be deposited deep in the vagina once nightly at bedtime for approximately five applications, or until the entire contents of one 30-g tube has been used. The patient should be checked by her physician to determine possible need for further therapy. In more severe cervicitis and vaginitis, some physicians prefer to initiate therapy with an application of ELASE (fibrinolysin and desoxyribonuclease, combined, [bovine]) in solution. See ELASE package insert.
ELASE
In severe cervicitis and vaginitis, the physician may instill 10 mL of the solution intravaginally, wait one or two minutes for the enzyme to disperse and then insert a cotton tampon in the vaginal canal. The tampon should be removed the next day. Continuing therapy should then be instituted with ELASE OINTMENT (fibrinolysin and desoxyribonuclease,

combined [bovine] ointment). See ELASE OINTMENT package insert.
Abscesses, empyema cavities, fistulae, sinus tracts, or subcutaneous hematomas
Despite the contraindication against parenteral use, ELASE has been used in irrigating these specific conditions. The ELASE solution should be drained and replaced at intervals of six to ten hours to reduce the amount of by-product accumulation and minimize loss of enzyme activity. Traces of blood in the discharge usually indicate active filling in of the cavity.

HOW SUPPLIED
ELASE (fibrinolysin and desoxyribonuclease, combined [bovine])
N 57317-030-10 ELASE—lyophilized powder for solution
ELASE is supplied in rubber diaphragm-capped vials of 30-mL capacity containing 25 units (Loomis) of fibrinolysin and 15,000 units (modified Christensen method) of desoxyribonuclease.
This product also contains sodium chloride and sucrose as incidental ingredients.

9030G020

ELASE OINTMENT (fibrinolysin and desoxyribonuclease, combined [bovine], ointment)
N 57317-011-12 ELASE OINTMENT, 10 g
The 10-g tube contains 10 units of fibrinolysin and 6,666 units of desoxyribonuclease in a special ointment base of liquid petrolatum and polyethylene.
N 57317-013-77 ELASE OINTMENT, 30 g
The 30-g tube contains 30 units of fibrinolysin and 20,000 units of desoxyribonuclease in a special ointment base of liquid petrolatum and polyethylene.
These products also contain sodium chloride and sucrose as incidental ingredients.

9011G020

ELASE-CHLOROMYCETIN OINTMENT (fibrinolysin and desoxyribonuclease, combined [bovine], with chloramphenicol ointment)
ELASE-CHLOROMYCETIN (fibrinolysin-desoxyribo-nuclease-chloramphenicol) is supplied in 30-g and 10-g ointment tubes. The 10-g tubes have an elongated nozzle to facilitate the application to surface lesions.
N 57317-023-77 ELASE-CHLOROMYCETIN OINTMENT, 30-g
The 30-g tubes contain 30 units (Loomis) of fibrinolysin (bovine) and 20,000 units** of desoxyribonuclease and 0.3 g† chloramphenicol in a special ointment base of liquid petrolatum and polyethylene.
N 57317-012-12 ELASE-CHLOROMYCETIN OINTMENT, 10-g
The 10-g tubes contain 10 units (Loomis) of fibrinolysin (bovine) and 6,666 units** of desoxyribonuclease and 0.1 g† chloramphenicol in a special ointment base of liquid petrolatum and polyethylene.
The ointment contains sodium chloride and sucrose used in its manufacture.

*Trademark
**Modified Christensen method.
†10 mg chloramphenicol per gram, or 1%

9021G010

Manufactured by
**Parke-Davis, Div of
Warner-Lambert Co.**
Morris Plains, NJ 07950
US License No. 1
Distributed by
**Fujisawa Pharmaceutical Company
Fujisawa USA, Inc.,**
Deerfield, IL 60015

GANITE™   ℞
(gallium nitrate injection)

> **WARNING**
> Concurrent use of gallium nitrate with other potentially nephrotoxic drugs (e.g., aminoglycosides, amphotericin B) may increase the risk for developing severe renal insufficiency in patients with cancer-related hypercalcemia. If use of a potentially nephrotoxic drug is indicated during gallium nitrate therapy, gallium nitrate administration should be discontinued and it is recommended that hydration be continued for several days after administration of the potentially nephrotoxic drug. Serum creatinine and urine output should be closely monitored during and subsequent to this period. GANITE™ therapy should be discontinued if the serum creatinine level exceeds 2.5 mg/dL.

Continued on next page

Fujisawa—Cont.

DESCRIPTION

Gallium nitrate injection is a clear, colorless, odorless, sterile solution of gallium nitrate, a hydrated nitrate salt of the group lIIa element, gallium. Gallium nitrate is formed by the reaction of elemental gallium with nitric acid, followed by crystallization of the drug from the solution. The stable, nonanhydrate, $[Ga(NO_3)_3 \cdot 9(H_2O)]$ is a white, slightly hygroscopic, crystalline powder of molecular weight 417.87, that is readily soluble in water.

Each mL of Ganite™ (gallium nitrate injection) contains gallium nitrate 25 mg (on an anhydrous basis) and sodium citrate dihydrate 28.75 mg. The solution may contain sodium hydroxide for pH adjustment to 6.0–7.0.

CLINICAL PHARMACOLOGY

Mechanism of Action

Ganite™ exerts a hypocalcemic effect by inhibiting calcium resorption from bone, possibly by reducing increased bone turnover. Although *in vitro* and animal studies have been performed to investigate the mechanism of action of gallium nitrate, the precise mechanism for inhibiting calcium resorption has not been determined. No cytotoxic effects were observed on bone cells in drug-treated animals.

Pharmacokinetics

Gallium nitrate was infused at a daily dose of 200 mg/m² for 5 (n=2) or 7 (n=10) consecutive days to 12 cancer patients. In most patients, apparent steady-state is achieved by 24 to 48 hours. The range of average steady-state plasma levels of gallium observed among 7 fully evaluable patients was between 1134 and 2399 ng/mL. The average plasma clearance of gallium (n=7) following daily infusion of gallium nitrate at a dose of 200 mg/m² for 5 or 7 days was 0.15 L/hr/kg (range: 0.12 to 0.20 L/hr/kg). In one patient who received daily infusion doses of 100, 150 and 200 mg/m², the apparent steady-state levels of gallium did not increase proportionally with an increase in dose. Gallium nitrate is not metabolized either by the liver or the kidney and appears to be significantly excreted via the kidney. Urinary excretion data for a dose of 200 mg/m² has not been determined.

Cancer-related Hypercalcemia

Hypercalcemia is a common problem in hospitalized patients with malignancy. It may affect 10–20% of patients with cancer. Different types of malignancy seem to vary in their propensity to cause hypercalcemia. A higher incidence of hypercalcemia has been observed in patients with non-small-cell lung cancer, breast cancer, multiple myeloma, kidney cancer, and cancer of head and neck. Hypercalcemia of malignancy seems to result from an imbalance between the net resorption of bone and urinary excretion of calcium. Patients with extensive osteolytic bone metastases frequently develop hypercalcemia; this type of hypercalcemia is common with primary breast cancer. Some of these patients have been reported to have increased renal tubular calcium resorption. Breast cancer cells have been reported to produce several potential bone-resorbing factors which stimulate the local osteoclast activity. Humoral hypercalcemia is common with the solid tumors of the lung, head and neck, kidney, and ovaries. Systemic factors (e.g., PTH-rP) produced either by the tumor or host cells have been implicated for the altered calcium fluxes between the extracellular fluid, the kidney, and the skeleton. About 30% of patients with myeloma develop hypercalcemia associated with extensive osteolytic lesions and impaired glomerular filtration. Myeloma cells have been reported to produce local factors that stimulate adjacent osteoclasts.

Hypercalcemia may produce a spectrum of signs and symptoms including: anorexia, lethargy, fatigue, nausea, vomiting, constipation, dehydration, renal insufficiency, impaired mental status, coma and cardiac arrest. A rapid rise in serum calcium may cause more severe symptoms for a given level of hypercalcemia. Since calcium is bound to serum proteins, which may fluctuate in concentration as a response to changes in blood volume, changes in total serum calcium (especially during rehydration) may not accurately reflect changes in the concentration of free-ionized calcium. In the absence of a direct measurement of free-ionized calcium, measurement of the serum albumin concentration and correction of the total serum calcium concentration may help in assessing the severity of hypercalcemia. The patient's acid-base status should also be taken into consideration while assessing the degree of hypercalcemia. Mild or asymptomatic hypercalcemia may be treated with conservative measures (i.e., saline hydration, with or without diuretics). The patient's cardiovascular status should be taken into consideration in the use of saline. In patients who have an underlying cancer type that may be sensitive to corticosteroids (e.g., hematologic cancers), the use or addition of corticosteroid therapy may be indicated.

Hypocalcemic Activity

A randomized double-blind clinical study comparing Ganite™ with calcitonin was conducted in patients with a serum calcium concentration (corrected for albumin) ≥12.0 mg/dL following 2 days of hydration. Ganite™ was given as a continuous intravenous infusion at a dose of 200 mg/m²/day for 5 days and calcitonin was given intramuscularly at a dose of 8 I.U./kg every 6 hours for 5 days. Elevated serum calcium (corrected for albumin) was normalized in 75% (18 of 24) of the patients receiving Ganite™ and in 27% (7 of 26) of the patients receiving calcitonin (p=0.0016). The time-course effect on serum calcium (corrected for albumin) is summarized in the following table.

Change in Corrected Serum Calcium by Time From Initiation of Treatment

Time Period[1] (hours)	Mean Change in Serum Calcium (mg/dL)[2] GANITE™	Calcitonin
24	−0.4	−1.6*
48	−0.9	−1.4
72	−1.5	−1.1
96	−2.9*	−1.1
120	−3.3*	−1.3

[1] Time after initiation of therapy in hours.
[2] Change from baseline in serum calcium (corrected for albumin).
*Comparison between treatment groups ($p < 0.01$).

The median duration of normocalcemia/hypocalcemia was 7.5 days for patients treated with Ganite™ and 1 day for patients treated with calcitonin. A total of 92% of patients treated with Ganite™ had a decrease in serum calcium (corrected for albumin) ≥2.0 mg/dL as compared to 54% of the patients treated with calcitonin (p=0.004).

An open-label, non-randomized study was conducted to examine a range of doses and dosing schedules of Ganite™ for control of cancer-related hypercalcemia. The principal dosing regimens were 100 and 200 mg/m²/day, administered as continuous intravenous infusions for 5 days. Ganite™ at a dose of 200 mg/m²/day for 5 days was found to normalize elevated serum calcium levels (corrected for albumin) in 83% of patients as compared to 50% of patients receiving a dose of 100 mg/m²/day for 5 days. A decrease in serum calcium (corrected for albumin) ≥2.0 mg/dL was observed in 83% and 94% of patients treated with Ganite™ at dosages of 100 and 200 mg/m²/day for 5 days, respectively. There were no significant differences in the proportion of patients responding to Ganite™ when considering either the presence or absence of bone metastasis, or whether the tumor histology was epidermoid or nonepidermoid.

INDICATIONS AND USAGE

Ganite™ is indicated for the treatment of clearly symptomatic cancer-related hypercalcemia that has not responded to adequate hydration. In general, patients with a serum calcium (corrected for albumin) <12 mg/dL would not be expected to be symptomatic. Mild or asymptomatic hypercalcemia may be treated with conservative measures (i.e., saline hydration, with or without diuretics). In the treatment of cancer-related hypercalcemia, it is important first to establish adequate hydration, preferably with intravenous saline, in order to increase the renal excretion of calcium and correct dehydration caused by hypercalcemia.

CONTRAINDICATIONS

Ganite™ should not be administered to patients with severe renal impairment (serum creatinine >2.5 mg/dL).

WARNINGS

(See boxed **WARNING**).

Severe hypophosphatemia secondary to Ganite has occasionally been encountered, and might require oral or intravenous phosphate treatment, as dictated by clinical circumstances.

The hypercalcemic state in cancer patients is commonly associated with impaired renal function. Abnormalities in renal function (elevated BUN and/or serum creatine) have been observed in clinical trials with Ganite™. **It is strongly recommended that serum creatinine be monitored during Ganite™ therapy.** Since patients with cancer-related hypercalcemia are frequently dehydrated, it is important that such patients be adequately hydrated with oral and/or intravenous fluids (preferably saline) and that a satisfactory urine output (2 L/day is recommended) be established before therapy with Ganite™ is started. Adequate hydration should be maintained throughout the treatment period, with careful attention to avoid overhydration in patients with compromised cardiovascular status. Diuretic therapy should not be employed prior to correction of hypovolemia. Ganite™ therapy should be discontinued if the serum creatinine level exceeds 2.5 mg/dL.

The use of Ganite™ in patients with marked renal insufficiency (serum creatinine >2.5 mg/dL) has not been systematically examined. If therapy is undertaken in patients with moderately impaired renal function (serum creatinine 2.0 to 2.5 mg/dL), frequent monitoring of the patient's renal status is recommended. Treatment should be discontinued if the serum creatinine level exceeds 2.5 mg/dL.

Combined use of Ganite™ with other potentially nephrotoxic drugs (e.g., aminoglycosides, amphotercin B) may increase the risk for developing renal insufficiency in patients with cancer-related hypercalcemia (see boxed **WARNING**).

PRECAUTIONS

General

Asymptomatic or mild to moderate hypocalcemia (6.5–8.0 mg/dL, corrected for serum albumin) occurred in approximately 38% of patients treated with Ganite™ in a controlled clinical trial. One patient exhibited a positive Chvostek's sign. If hypocalcemia occurs, Ganite™ therapy should be stopped and short-term calcium therapy may be necessary.

Laboratory Tests

Renal function (serum creatinine and BUN) and serum calcium must be closely monitored during Ganite™ therapy. In addition to baseline assessment, the suggested frequency of calcium and phosphorus determinations is daily and twice weekly, respectively. Ganite™ should be discontinued if the serum creatinine exceeds 2.5 mg/dL.

Drug Interactions

The concomitant use of highly nephrotoxic drugs in combination with Ganite™ may increase the risk for development of renal insufficiency (see **WARNINGS**). Available information does not indicate any adverse interaction with diuretics such as furosemide.

Carcinogenesis, Mutagenesis, Impairment of Fertility

Long-term studies in animals have not been performed to evaluate the carcinogenic potential of gallium nitrate. Gallium nitrate is not mutagenic in standard tests (i.e., Ames test and chromosomal aberration studies on human lymphocytes).

Use in Pregnancy

Pregnancy Category C

Animal reproduction studies have not been conducted with gallium nitrate. It is also not known whether gallium nitrate can cause fetal harm when administered to a pregnant woman or can affect reproductive capacity. Ganite™ should be administered to a pregnant woman only if clearly needed.

Nursing Mothers

It is not known whether gallium nitrate is excreted in human milk. Because of the potential for serious adverse reactions in nursing infants from gallium nitrate, a decision should be made whether to discontinue nursing or discontinue the drug, taking into account the importance of the drug to the mother.

Pediatric Use

The safety and effectiveness of Ganite™ in children have not been established.

ADVERSE REACTIONS

Kidney

Adverse renal effects, as demonstrated by rising BUN and creatinine, have been reported in about 12.5% of patients treated with Ganite™. In a controlled clinical trial of patients with cancer-related hypercalcemia, two patients receiving Ganite™ and one patient receiving calcitonin developed acute renal failure. Due to the serious nature of the patients' underlying conditions, the relationship of these events to the drug was unclear. Ganite™ should not be administered to patients with serum creatinine >2.5 mg/dL (see **CONTRAINDICATIONS** and **WARNINGS**).

Metabolic

Hypocalcemia may occur after Ganite™ treatment (see **PRECAUTIONS**).

Transient hypophosphatemia of mild-to-moderate degree may occur in up to 79% of hypercalcemic patients following treatment with Ganite™. In a controlled clinical trial, 33% of patients had at least 1 serum phosphorus measurement between 1.5–2.4 mg/dL, while 46% of patients had at least 1 serum phosphorus value <1.5 mg/dL. Severe hypophosphatemia was also reported in 7% of patients in controlled clincial trials (see **WARNINGS**). Patients who develop hypophosphatemia may require oral phosphorus therapy.

Decreased serum bicarbonate, possibly secondary to mild respiratory alkalosis, was reported in 40–50% of cancer patients treated with Ganite™. The cause for this effect is not clear. This effect has been asymptomatic and has not required specific treatment.

Hematologic

The use of very high doses of gallium nitrate (up to 1400 mg/m²) in treating patients for advanced cancer has been associated with anemia, and several patients have received red blood cell transfusions. Due to the serious nature of the underlying illness, it is uncertain whether the anemia was caused by gallium nitrate.

Blood Pressure

A decrease in mean systolic and diastolic blood pressure was observed several days after treatment with gallium nitrate in a controlled clinical trial. The decrease in blood pressure was asymptomatic and did not require specific treatment.

Visual and Auditory

In cancer chemotherapy trials, a small proportion (<1%) of patients treated with multiple high doses of gallium nitrate combined with other investigational anticancer drugs, have developed acute optic neuritis. While these patients were critically ill and had received multiple drugs, a reaction to high-dose gallium nitrate is possible. Most patients had full visual recovery; however, at least one case of persistent visual impairment has been reported. One patient with cancer-related hypercalcemia was reported to develop decreased hearing following gallium nitrate administration. Due to the patient's underlying condition and concurrent therapies, the relationship of this event to gallium nitrate administration is unclear. Tinnitus and partial loss of auditory acuity have been reported rarely (<1%) in patients who received high-dose gallium nitrate as anticancer treatment.

Miscellaneous

Other clinical events reported in association with gallium nitrate treatment for cancer as well as cancer-related hypercalcemia include: nausea and/or vomiting, tachycardia, lethargy, confusion, diarrhea, constipation, lower extremity edema, hypothermia, fever, dyspnea, rales and rhonchi, anemia, leukopenia, paresthesia, skin rash, pleural effusion, pulmonary infiltrates, and seizures. Due to the serious nature of the underlying condition of these patients, the relationship of these events to therapy with gallium nitrate is unknown.

OVERDOSAGE

Rapid intravenous infusion of gallium nitrate or use of doses higher than recommended (200 mg/m^2) may cause nausea and vomiting and a substantially increased risk of renal insufficiency. In the event of overdosage, further drug administration should be discontinued, serum calcium should be monitored, and the patient should receive vigorous intravenous hydration, with or without diuretics, for 2–3 days. During this time period, renal function and urinary output should be carefully monitored so that fluid intake and output are balanced.

DOSAGE AND ADMINISTRATION

The usual recommended dose of Ganite™ is 200 mg per square meter of body surface area (200 mg/m^2) daily for 5 consecutive days. In patients with mild hypercalcemia and few symptoms, a lower dosage of 100 mg/m^2/day for 5 days may be considered. If serum calcium levels are lowered into the normal range in less than 5 days, treatment may be discontinued early. The daily dose must be administered as an intravenous infusion over 24 hours. The daily dose should be diluted, preferably in 1,000 mL of 0.9% Sodium Chloride Injection, USP, or 5% Dextrose Injection, USP, for administration as an intravenous infusion over 24 hours. Adequate hydration must be maintained throughout the treatment period, with careful attention to avoid overhydration in patient with compromised cardiovascular status. Controlled studies have not been undertaken to evaluate the safety and effectiveness of retreatment with gallium nitrate.

When Ganite™ is added to either 0.9% Sodium Chloride Injection, USP, or 5% Dextrose Injection, USP, it is stable for at least 48 hours at room temperature (15°–30°C) and for seven (7) days if stored under refrigeration (2°–8°C). Parenteral drug products should be inspected visually for particulate matter and discoloration prior to administration whenever solution and container permit.

HOW SUPPLIED

Product No.	NDC No.	Ganite™ (gallium nitrate injection)
55120	57317-243-20	500 mg (25 mg/mL) in 20 mL single-dose, flip-top vials individually packaged.

Store at controlled room temperature 15°–30°C (59°–86°F). Contains no preservative. Discard unused portion.

CAUTION Federal law prohibits dispensing without prescription.

Manufactured for **Fujisawa Pharmaceutical Co.** by Fujisawa USA, Inc. Deerfield, IL 60015

Revised: July 1992

GRIVATE™   ℞

(griseofulvin microsize tablets) and
(griseofulvin microsize oral suspension)
Tablets/Suspension
Antifungal Agent for Ringworm Infections

DESCRIPTION

Griseofulvin is an antibiotic derived from a species of *Penicillium*. Each Grivate Tablet contains either 250 mg or 500 mg of griseofulvin microsize, and also contains calcium stearate, colloidal silicon dioxide, starch, and wheat gluten. Additionally, the 250 mg tablet also contains dibasic calcium phosphate. Each 5 mL of Grivate Suspension contains 125 mg of griseofulvin microsize and also contains alcohol 0.2%, docusate sodium, FD&C Red No. 40, FD&C Yellow No. 6, flavors, magnesium aluminum silicate, menthol, methylparaben, propylene glycol, propylparaben, saccharin sodium, simethicone emulsion, sodium alginate, sucrose, and purified water.

CLINICAL PHARMACOLOGY

Grivate (griseofulvin microsize) acts systematically to inhibit the growth of *Trichophyton, Microsporum,* and *Epidermophyton* genera of fungi. Fungistatic amounts are deposited in the keratin, which is gradually exfoliated and replaced by noninfected tissue.

Griseofulvin absorption from the gastrointestinal tract varies considerably among individuals, mainly because of insolubility of the drug in aqueous media of the upper G.I. tract. The peak serum level found in fasting adults given 0.5 gm occurs at about four hours and ranges between 0.5 and 2.0 mcg/mL.

It should be noted that some individuals are consistently "poor absorbers" and tend to attain lower blood levels at all times. This may explain unsatisfactory therapeutic results in some patients. Better blood levels can probably be attained in most patients if the tablets are administered after a meal with a high fat content.

INDICATIONS AND USAGE

Major indications for Grivate (griseofulvin microsize) are:
- Tinea capitis (ringworm of the scalp)
- Tinea corporis (ringworm of the body)
- Tinea pedis (athlete's foot)
- Tinea unguium (onychomycosis; ringworm of the nails)
- Tinea cruris (ringworm of the thigh)
- Tinea barbae (barber's itch)

Grivate (griseofulvin microsize) inhibits the growth of those genera of fungi that commonly cause ringworm infections of the hair, skin, and nails, such as:
- *Trichophyton rubrum*
- *Trichophyton tonsurans*
- *Trichophyton mentagrophytes*
- *Trichophyton interdigitalis*
- *Trichophyton verrucosum*
- *Trichophyton sulphureum*
- *Trichophyton schoenleini*
- *Microsporum audouini*
- *Microsporum canis*
- *Microsporum gypseum*
- *Epidermophyton floccosum*
- *Trichophyton megnini*
- *Trichophyton gallinae*
- *Trichophyton crateriform*

Prior to therapy, the type of fungi responsible for the infection should be identified. The use of the drug is not justified in minor or trivial infections which will respond to topical antifungal agents alone.

It is *not* effective in:
- Bacterial infections
- Candidiasis (Moniliasis)
- Histoplasmosis
- Actinomycosis
- Sporotrichosis
- Chromoblastomycosis
- Coccidioidomycosis
- North American Blastomycosis
- Cryptococcosis (Torulosis)
- Tinea versicolor
- Nocardiosis

CONTRAINDICATIONS

This drug is contraindicated in patients with porphyria, hepatocellular failure, and in individuals with a history of hypersensitivity to griseofulvin.

Two cases of conjoined twins have been reported in patients taking griseofulvin during the first trimester of pregnancy. Griseofulvin should not be prescribed to pregnant patients.

WARNINGS

Prophylactic Usage

Safety and efficacy of prophylactic use of this drug has not been established.

Chronic feeding of griseofulvin, at levels ranging from 0.5–2.5% of the diet, resulted in the development of liver tumors in several strains of mice, particularly in males. Smaller particle sizes result in an enhanced effect. Lower oral dosage levels have not been tested. Subcutaneous administration of relatively small doses of griseofulvin once a week during the first three weeks of life has also been reported to induce hepatomata in mice. Although studies in other animal species have not yielded evidence of tumorigenicity, these studies were not of adequate design to form a basis for conclusions in this regard.

In subacute toxicity studies, orally administered griseofulvin produced hepatocellular necrosis in mice, but this has not been seen in other species. Disturbances in porphyrin metabolism have been reported in griseofulvin-treated laboratory animals. Griseofulvin has been reported to have a colchicine-like effect on mitosis and cocarcinogenicity with methylcholanthrene in cutaneous tumor induction in laboratory animals.

Reports of animal studies in the Soviet literature state that a griseofulvin preparation was found to be embryotoxic and teratogenic on oral administration to pregnant Wistar rats. Rat reproduction studies done thus far in the United States and Great Britain have been inconclusive in this regard, and additional animal reproduction studies are underway. Pups with abnormalities have been reported in the litters of a few bitches treated with griseofulvin. Suppression of spermatogenesis has been reported to occur in rats but investigation in man failed to confirm this.

PRECAUTIONS

Patients on prolonged therapy with any potent medication should be under close observation. Periodic monitoring of organ system function, including renal, hepatic and hemopoietic, should be done.

Since griseofulvin is derived from species of penicillin, the possibility of cross sensitivity with penicillin exists; however, known penicillin-sensitive patients have been treated without difficulty.

Since a photosensitivity reaction is occasionally associated with griseofulvin therapy, patients should be warned to avoid exposure to intense natural or artifical sunlight. Should a photosensitivity reaction occur, lupus erythematosus may be aggravated.

Drug Interactions

Patients on warfarin-type anticoagulant therapy may require dosage adjustment of the anticoagulant during and after griseofulvin therapy. Concomitant use of barbiturates usually depresses griseofulvin activity and may necessitate raising the dosage.

The concomitant administration of griseofulvin has been reported to reduce the efficacy of oral contraceptives and to increase the incidence of breakthrough bleeding.

ADVERSE REACTIONS

When adverse reactions occur, they are most commonly of the hypersensitivity type such as skin rashes, urticaria and rarely, angioneurotic edema, and may necessitate withdrawal of therapy and appropriate countermeasures. Paresthesias of the hands and feet have been reported rarely after extended therapy. Other side effects reported occasionally are oral thrush, nausea, vomiting, epigastric distress, diarrhea, headache, fatigue, dizziness, insomnia, mental confusion and impairment of performance of routine activities. Proteinuria and leukopenia have been reported rarely. Administration of the drug should be discontinued if granulocytopenia occurs.

When rare, serious reactions occur with griseofulvin, they are usually associated with high dosages, long periods of therapy, or both.

DOSAGE AND ADMINISTRATION

Accurate diagnosis of the infecting organism is essential. Identification should be made either by direct microscopic examination of a mounting of infected tissue in a solution of potassium hydroxide or by culture on an appropriate medium.

Medication must be continued until the infecting organism is completely eradicated as indicated by appropriate clinical or laboratory examiniation. Representative treatment periods are: tinea capitis, 4 to 6 weeks; tinea corporis, 2 to 4 weeks; tinea pedis, 4 to 8 weeks; tinea unguium—depending on rate of growth—fingernails, at least 4 months; toenails, at least 6 months.

General measures in regard to hygiene should be observed to control sources of infection or reinfection. Concomitant use of appropriate topical agents is usually required, particularly in treatment of tinea pedis since in some forms of athlete's foot, yeasts and bacteria may be involved. Griseofulvin will not eradicate the bacterial or monilial infection.

Adults

A daily dose of 500 mg will give a satisfactory response in most patients with tinea corporis, tinea cruris, and tinea capitis.

For those fungus infections more difficult to eradicate such as tinea pedis and tinea unguium, a daily dose of 1.0 gram is recommended.

Children

Approximately 5 mg per pound of body weight per day is an effective dose for most children. On this basis the following dosage schedule for children is suggested:

Children weighing 30 to 50 pounds—125 mg to 250 mg daily.
Children weighing over 50 pounds—250 mg to 500 mg daily.

HOW SUPPLIED

(griseofulvin microsize)

NDC 57317-660-10 Product Code 766010 250 mg Tablets in bottles of 100

Tablets are white, scored, and imprinted Ortho 211.

NDC 57317-661-10 Product Code 766110 500 mg Tablets in bottles of 100

Tablets are white, scored, and imprinted Ortho 214.

Dispense Grivate tablets in a well-closed container as defined in the official compendia.

Continued on next page

Fujisawa—Cont.

NDC 57317-662-04 Product Code 766204 125 mg Suspension in 5 mL, 4 fl oz bottles
Dispense Grivate Suspension in a tight, light-resistant container as defined in the official compendia.
STORE AT ROOM TEMPERATURE
Manufactured for Fujisawa Pharmaceutical Co.,
Div. of Fujisawa USA, Inc., Deerfield, IL 60015
by Ortho Pharmaceutical Corp.,
Raritan, NJ 08869
Issued January 1992
U.S. Patents 2,900,304; 3,330,727

NebuPent™ ℞
(pentamidine isethionate)
For Inhalation Solution

DESCRIPTION

NebuPent™ (Pentamidine Isethionate), an anti-protozoal agent, is a sterile and nonpyrogenic lyophilized product. After reconstitution with Sterile Water for Injection, USP, NebuPent™ is administered by inhalation via the Respirgard® II nebulizer [Marquest, Englewood, CO] (see **DOSAGE AND ADMINISTRATION**).
Pentamidine isethionate, 4,4′-diamidinodiphenoxypentane di-(β-hydroxyethanesulfonate), is a white crystalline powder soluble in water and glycerin and insoluble in ether, acetone, and chloroform.

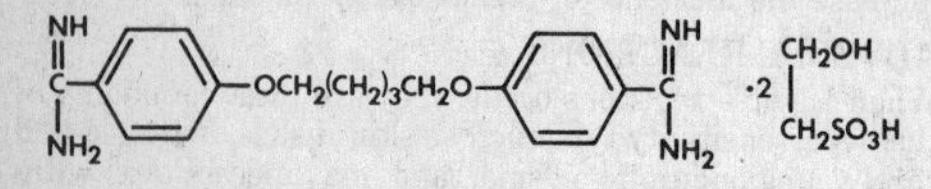

$C_{23}H_{36}N_4O_{10}S_2$ 592.68

Each vial contains 300 mg sterile pentamidine isethionate.

CLINICAL PHARMACOLOGY

Microbiology
Pentamidine isethionate, an aromatic diamidine, is known to have activity against *Pneumocystis carinii.* The mode of action is not fully understood. *In vitro* studies indicate that the drug interferes with protozoal nuclear metabolism by inhibition of DNA, RNA, phospholipid and protein synthesis.

Pharmacokinetics
In 5 AIDS patients with suspected *Pneumocystis carinii* pneumonia (PCP), the mean concentrations of pentamidine determined 18 to 24 hours after inhalation therapy were 23.2 ng/mL (range 5.1 to 43.0 ng/mL) in bronchoalveolar lavage fluid and 705 ng/mL (range 140 to 1336 ng/mL) in sediment after administration of a 300 mg single dose via the Respirgard® II nebulizer. In 3 AIDS patients with suspected PCP, the mean concentrations of pentamidine determined 18 to 24 hours after a 4 mg/kg intravenous dose were 2.6 ng/mL (range 1.5 to 4.0 ng/mL) in bronchoalveolar lavage fluid and 9.3 ng/mL (range 6.9 to 12.8 ng/mL) in sediment. In the patients who received aerosolized pentamidine, the peak plasma levels of pentamidine were at or below the lower limit of detection of the assay (2.3 ng/mL).
Following a single 2-hour intravenous infusion of 4 mg/kg of pentamidine isethionate to 6 AIDS patients, the mean plasma Cmax, T 1/2, and clearance were 612 ± 371 ng/mL, 6.4 ± 1.3 hr, and 248 ± 91 L/hr, respectively. In another study of aerosolized pentamidine in 13 AIDS patients with acute PCP who received 4 mg/kg/day administered via the Ultra Vent® jet nebulizer, peak plasma levels of pentamidine averaged 18.8 ± 11.9 ng/mL after the first dose. During the next 14 days of repeated dosing, the highest observed Cmax averaged 20.5 ± 21.2 ng/mL. In a third study, following daily administration of 600 mg of inhaled pentamidine isethionate with the Respirgard® II nebulizer for 21 days in 11 patients with acute PCP, mean plasma levels measured shortly after the 21st dose averaged 11.8 ± 10.0 ng/mL. Plasma concentrations after aerosol administration are substantially lower than those observed after a comparable intravenous dose. The extent of pentamidine accumulation and distribution following chronic inhalation therapy are not known.
In rats, intravenous administration of a 5 mg/kg dose resulted in concentrations of pentamidine in the liver and kidney that were 87.5- and 62.3-fold higher, respectively, than levels in those organs following 5 mg/kg administered as an aerosol.
No pharmacokinetic data are available following aerosol administration of pentamidine in humans with impaired hepatic or renal function.

INDICATIONS AND USAGE

NebuPent™ is indicated for the prevention of *Pneumocystis carinii* pneumonia (PCP) in high-risk, HIV-infected patients defined by one or both of the following criteria.

i. A history of one or more episodes of PCP
ii. A peripheral CD4+ (T4 helper/inducer) lymphocyte count less than or equal to 200/mm³.

These indications are based on the results of an 18-month randomized, dose-response trial in high-risk, HIV-infected patients and on existing epidemiological data from natural history studies.
The patient population of the controlled trial consisted of 408 patients, 237 of whom had a history of one or more episodes of PCP. The remaining patients without a history of PCP included 55 patients with Kaposi's sarcoma and 116 patients with other AIDS diagnoses, ARC or asymptomatic HIV infection. Patients were randomly assigned to receive NebuPent™ via the Respirgard® II nebulizer at one of the following three doses: 30 mg every two weeks (n=135), 150 mg every two weeks (n=134), or 300 mg every four weeks (n=139). The results of the trial demonstrated a significant protective effect ($p < 0.01$) against PCP with the 300 mg every four week dosage regimen compared to the 30 mg every two week dosage regimen. The 300 mg dose regimen reduced the risk of developing PCP by 50 to 70% compared to the 30 mg regimen. A total of 293 patients (72% of all patients) also received zidovudine at sometime during the trial. The analysis of the data demonstrated the efficacy of the 300 mg dose even after adjusting for the effect of zidovudine.
The results of the trial further demonstrate that the dose and frequency of dosing are important to the efficacy of NebuPent™ prophylaxis in that multiple analyses consistently demonstrated a trend toward greater efficacy with 300 mg every four weeks as compared to 150 mg every two weeks.
No dose-response was observed for reduction in overall mortality; however, mortality from PCP was low in all three dosage groups.

CONTRAINDICATIONS

NebuPent™ is contraindicated in patients with a history of an anaphylactic reaction to inhaled or parenteral pentamidine isethionate.

WARNINGS

The potential for development of acute PCP still exists in patients receiving NebuPent™ prophylaxis. Therefore, any patient with symptoms suggestive of the presence of a pulmonary infection, including but not limited to dyspnea, fever or cough, should receive a thorough medical evaluation and appropriate diagnostic tests for possible acute PCP as well as for other opportunistic and nonopportunistic pathogens. The use of NebuPent™ may alter the clinical and radiographic features of PCP and could result in an atypical presentation, including but not limited to mild disease or focal infection.
Prior to initiating NebuPent™ prophylaxis, symptomatic patients should be evaluated appropriately to exclude the presence of PCP. The recommended dose of NebuPent™ for the prevention of PCP is insufficient to treat acute PCP.

PRECAUTIONS

IMPORTANT: DO NOT MIX THE NEBUPENT™ SOLUTION WITH ANY OTHER DRUGS. DO NOT USE THE RESPIRGARD® II NEBULIZIER TO ADMINISTER A BRONCHODILATOR. (See DOSAGE AND ADMINISTRATION).

Pulmonary
Inhalation of NebuPent™ may induce bronchospasm or cough. This has been noted particularly in some patients who have a history of smoking or asthma. In clinical trials, cough and bronchospasm were the most frequently reported adverse experiences associated with NebuPent™ administration (38% and 15%, respectively, of patients receiving the 300 mg dose); however, less than 1% of the doses were interrupted or terminated due to these effects. For the majority of patients, cough and bronchospasm were controlled by administration of an aerosolized bronchodilator (only 1% of patients withdrew from the study due to treatment-associated cough or bronchospasm). In patients who experience bronchospasm or cough, administration of an inhaled bronchodilator prior to giving each NebuPent™ dose may minimize recurrence of the symptoms.

General
The extent and consequence of pentamidine accumulation following chronic inhalation therapy are not known. As a result, patients receiving NebuPent™ should be closely monitored for the development of serious adverse reactions that have occurred in patients receiving parenteral pentamidine, including hypotension, hypoglycemia, hyperglycemia, hypocalcemia, anemia, thrombocytopenia, leukopenia, hepatic or renal dysfunction, ventricular tachycardia, pancreatitis, and Stevens-Johnson syndrome.
Extrapulmonary infection with *P. carinii* has been reported infrequently. Most, but not all, of the cases have been reported in patients who have a history of PCP. The presence of extrapulmonary pneumocystosis should be considered when evaluating patients with unexplained signs and symptoms.
Cases of acute pancreatitis have been reported in patients receiving aerosolized pentamidine. NebuPent™ should be discontinued if signs or symptoms of acute pancreatitis develop.

Drug Interactions
While specific studies on drug interactions with NebuPent™ have not been conducted, the majority of patients in clinical trials received concomitant medications, including zidovudine, with no reported interactions.

Carcinogenesis, Mutagenesis and Impairment of Fertility
No studies have been conducted to evaluate the potential of pentamidine isethionate as a carcinogen or mutagen or to determine its effects on fertility.

Pregnancy. Pregnancy Category C
Animal reproduction studies have not been conducted with NebuPent™. It is also not known whether NebuPent™ can cause fetal harm when administered to a pregnant woman or can affect reproduction capacity. NebuPent™ should be given to a pregnant woman only if clearly needed. NebuPent™ should not be given to a pregnant woman unless the potential benefits are judged to outweigh the unknown risk.

Nursing Mothers
It is not known whether NebuPent™ is excreted in human milk. Because of the potential for serious adverse reactions in nursing infants from NebuPent™, a decision should be made whether to discontinue nursing or to discontinue the drug, taking into account the importance of the drug to the mother. Because many drugs are excreted in human milk, NebuPent™ should not be given to a nursing mother unless the potential benefits are judged to outweigh the unknown risk.

Pediatric Use
The safety and effectiveness of NebuPent™ in children have not been established.

ADVERSE REACTIONS

The most frequent adverse effects attributable to NebuPent™ administration are cough and bronchospasm (reported by 38% and 15%, respectively, of patients receiving 300 mg every four weeks).
The most frequently reported adverse experiences in the controlled clinical trials in which 607 patients were treated with NebuPent™ (139 patients at 300 mg every four weeks, 232 at 150 mg every two weeks, 101 at 100 mg every two weeks and 135 at 30 mg every two weeks) using the Respirgard® II nebulizer were as follows.

53–72% Fatigue, bad (metallic) taste, shortness of breath and decreased appetite
31–47% Dizziness and rash
10–23% Nausea, pharyngitis, chest pain or congestion, night sweats, chills and vomiting

In nearly all cases, neither the relationship to treatment or underlying disease nor the severity of adverse experiences was recorded.
Other less frequently occurring adverse experiences (reported by greater than 1% and up to 5% of patients in two clinical trials) were pneumothorax, diarrhea, headache, anemia (generally associated with zidovudine use), myalgia, abdominal pain and edema.
From a total experience with 1130 patients, adverse events reported with a frequency of 1% or less were as follows. No causal relationship to treatment has been established for these adverse events.

General Allergic reaction and extrapulmonary pneumocystosis
Cardiovascular Tachycardia, hypotension, hypertension, palpitations, syncope, cerebrovascular accident, vasodilatation, and vasculitis
Metabolic Hypoglycemia, hyperglycemia, and hypocalcemia
Gastrointestinal Gingivitis, dyspepsia, oral ulcer/abscess, gastritis, gastric ulcer, hypersalivation, dry mouth, splenomegaly, melena, hematochezia, esophagitis, colitis, and pancreatitis
Hematological Pancytopenia, neutropenia, eosinophilia and thrombocytopenia
Hepatorenal Hepatitis, hepatomegaly, hepatic dysfunction, renal failure, flank pain, and nephritis
Musculoskeletal Arthralgia
Neurological Tremors, confusion, anxiety, memory loss, seizure, neuropathy, paresthesia, insomnia, hypesthesia, drowsiness, emotional lability, vertigo, paranoia, neuralgia, hallucination, depression, and unsteady gait
Respiratory Rhinitis, laryngitis, laryngospasm, hyperventilation, hemoptysis, gagging, eosinophilic or interstitial pneumonitis, pleuritis, cyanosis, tachypnea, and rales
Skin Pruritis, erythema, dry skin, desquamation and urticaria
Special Senses Eye discomfort, conjunctivitis, blurred vision, blepharitis and loss of taste and smell
Urogenital Incontinence
Reproductive Miscarriage

OVERDOSAGE

Overdosage has not been reported with NebuPent™. The symptoms and signs of overdosage are not known.
A serious overdosage, to the point of producing systemic drug levels similar to those following parenteral administration, would have the potential of producing similar types of serious systemic toxicity (See **PRECAUTIONS**).

Available clinical pharmacology data (see **CLINICAL PHARMACOLOGY**) suggest that a dose up to 40 times the recommended NebuPent™ dosage would be required to produce systemic levels similar to a single 4 mg/kg intravenous dose.

DOSAGE AND ADMINISTRATION
IMPORTANT: NEBUPENT™ MUST BE DISSOLVED ONLY IN STERILE WATER FOR INJECTION, USP. DO NOT USE SALINE SOLUTION FOR RECONSTITUTION BECAUSE THE DRUG WILL PRECIPITATE. DO NOT MIX THE NEBUPENT™ SOLUTION WITH ANY OTHER DRUGS. DO NOT USE THE RESPIRGARD® II NEBULIZER TO ADMINISTER A BRONCHODILATOR.

Reconstitution
The contents of one vial (300 mg) must be dissolved in 6 mL Sterile Water for Injection, USP. Place the entire reconstituted contents of the vial into the Respirgard® II nebulizer reservoir for administration.

Dosage
The recommended adult dosage of NebuPent™ for the prevention of *Pneumocystis carinii* pneumonia is 300 mg once every four weeks administered via the Respirgard® II nebulizer.
The dose should be delivered until the nebulizer chamber is empty (approximately 30 to 45 minutes). The flow rate should be 5 to 7 liters per minute from a 40 to 50 pounds per square inch (PSI) air or oxygen source. Alternatively, a 40 to 50 PSI air compressor can be used with flow limited by setting the flowmeter at 5 to 7 liters per minute or by setting the pressure at 22 to 25 PSI. Low pressure (less than 20 PSI) compressors should not be used.

Stability
Freshly prepared solutions for aerosol use are recommended. After reconstitution with sterile water, the Nebupent™ solution is stable for 48 hours in the original vial at room temperature if protected from light.

HOW SUPPLIED

Product No.	NDC No.	
87715	57317-210-06	NebuPent™ (pentamidine isethionate) 300 mg lyophilized product in single-dose vials, individually packaged.

Store the dry product at controlled room temperature 15°-30°C (59°-86°F).
Protect the dry product and the reconstituted solution from light.
CAUTION Federal law prohibits dispensing without prescription.

Manufactured for **Fujisawa Pharmaceutical Co.,** by Fujisawa USA, Inc.
Deerfield, IL 60015
45474A
Revised: February 1991

PENTAM® 300   ℞
(sterile pentamidine isethionate)

DESCRIPTION
PENTAM® 300 (Sterile Pentamidine Isethionate), an antiprotozoal agent, is a nonpyrogenic, lyophilized product. After reconstitution, it should be administered by intramuscular or intravenous (IM or IV) routes (See **DOSAGE AND ADMINISTRATION**).
Pentamidine isethionate is a white crystalline powder soluble in water and glycerin and insoluble in ether, acetone, and chloroform. It is chemically designated as 4,4'-diamidino-diphenoxypentane di (β-hydroxyethanesulfonate) with the following structural formula:

$C_{23}H_{36}N_4O_{10}S_2$ 592.68

Each vial contains Pentamidine isethionate 300 mg.

CLINICAL PHARMACOLOGY
Pentamidine isethionate, an aromatic diamidine, is known to have activity against *Pneumocystis carinii*.
The mode of action of pentamidine is not fully understood. *In vitro* studies with mammalian tissues and the protozoan *Crithidia oncopelti* indicate that the drug interferes with nuclear metabolism, producing inhibition of the synthesis of DNA, RNA, phospholipids and proteins.
Little is known about the drug's pharmacokinetics. Preliminary studies have shown that in seven patients treated with daily IM doses of pentamidine at 4 mg/kg for 10 to 12 days, plasma concentrations were between 0.3 and 0.5 mcg/mL. The levels did not appreciably change with time after injec-

tion or from day to day. Higher plasma levels were encountered in patients with an elevated BUN. The patients continued to excrete decreasing amounts of pentamidine in urine up to six to eight weeks after cessation of the treatment. Tissue distribution has been studied in mice given a single intraperitoneal injection of pentamidine at 10 mg/kg. The concentration in the kidneys was the highest followed by that in the liver. In mice, pentamidine was excreted unchanged, primarily via the kidneys with some elimination in the feces. The ratio of amounts excreted in the urine and feces (4:1) was constant over the period of study.

INDICATIONS AND USAGE
PENTAM® 300 (Sterile Pentamidine Isethionate) is indicated for the treatment of pneumonia due to *Pneumocystis carinii*.

CONTRAINDICATIONS
Once the diagnosis of *Pneumocystis carinii* pneumonia has been firmly established, there are no absolute contraindications to the use of pentamidine isethionate.

WARNINGS
Fatalities due to severe hypotension, hypoglycemia, and cardiac arrhythmias have been reported in patients treated with pentamidine isethionate, both by the IM and IV routes. Severe hypotension may result after a single dose (see **PRECAUTIONS**). The administration of the drug should, therefore, be limited to the patients in whom *Pneumocystis carinii* has been demonstrated. Patients should be closely monitored for the development of serious adverse reactions (see **PRECAUTIONS and ADVERSE REACTIONS**).

PRECAUTIONS
General
Pentamidine isethionate should be used with caution in patients with hypertension, hypotension, hypoglycemia, hyperglycemia, hypocalcemia, leukopenia, thrombocytopenia, anemia, and hepatic or renal dysfunction.
Patients may develop sudden, severe hypotension after a single dose of pentamidine isethionate, whether given IV or IM. Therefore, patients receiving the drug should be lying down and the blood pressure should be monitored closely during administration of the drug and several times thereafter until the blood pressure is stable. Equipment for emergency resuscitation should be readily available. If pentamidine isethionate is administered IV, it should be infused over a period of 60 minutes.
Pentamidine isethionate-induced hypoglycemia has been associated with pancreatic islet cell necrosis and inappropriately high plasma insulin concentrations. Hyperglycemia and diabetes mellitus, with or without preceding hypoglycemia, have also occurred, sometimes several months after therapy with pentamidine isethionate. Therefore, blood glucose levels should be monitored daily during therapy with pentamidine isethionate, and several times thereafter.

Laboratory Tests
The following tests should be carried out before, during and after therapy.
a) Daily blood urea nitrogen and serum creatinine determinations
b) Daily blood glucose determinations
c) Complete blood count and platelet count
d) Liver function test, including bilirubin, alkaline phosphatase, AST (SGOT), and ALT (SGPT)
e) Serum calcium determinations
f) Electrocardiograms at regular intervals

Carcinogensis, Mutagensis, Impairment of Fertility
No studies have been conducted to evaluate the potential of pentamidine isethionate as a carcinogen, mutagen, or cause of impaired fertility.

Pregnancy Category C
Animal reproduction studies have not been conducted with pentamidine isethionate. It is also not known whether pentamidine isethionate can cause fetal harm when administered to a pregnant woman or can affect reproduction capacity. Pentamidine isethionate should be given to a pregnant woman only if clearly needed.

ADVERSE REACTIONS
CAUTION Fatalities due to severe hypotension, hypoglycemia, and cardiac arrhythmias have been reported in patients treated with pentamidine isethionate, both by the IM and IV routes. The administration of the drug should, therefore, be limited to the patients in whom *Pneumocystis carinii* has been demonstrated.
Of 424 patients treated with pentamidine isethionate, 244 (57.5%) developed some adverse reaction. Most of the patients had the acquired immunodeficiency syndrome (AIDS). In the following table, "Severe" refers to life-threatening reactions or reactions that required immediate corrective measures and led to discontinuation of pentamidine isethionate.

[See table at top of next column.]

Adverse Reactions	Number	%
Severe		
Leukopenia ($<1000/mm^3$)	12	2.8
Hypoglycemia (<25 mg/dL)	10	2.4
Thrombocytopenia ($<20,000/mm^3$)	7	1.7
Hypotension (<60 mm Hg systolic)	4	0.9
Acute renal failure (serum creatinine >6 mg/dL)	2	0.5
Hypocalcemia	1	0.2
Stevens-Johnson syndrome	1	0.2
Ventricular tachycardia	1	0.2
Total number of patients with severe effects*	37	8.7
Moderate		
Elevated serum creatinine (2.4 to 6.0 mg/dL)	98	23.1
Sterile abscess, pain, or induration at the site of IM injection	47	11.1
Elevated liver function tests	37	8.7
Leukopenia	32	7.5
Nausea, anorexia	25	5.9
Hypotension	17	4.0
Fever	15	3.5
Hypoglycemia	15	3.5
Rash	14	3.3
Bad taste in mouth	7	1.7
Confusion/hallucinations	7	1.7
Anemia	5	1.2
Neuralgia	4	0.9
Thrombocytopenia	4	0.9
Hyperkalemia	3	0.7
Phlebitis	3	0.7
Dizziness (without hypotension)	2	0.5
Other moderate adverse reactions**	5	1.2
Total number of patients with moderate adverse reactions*	207	48.8

*Patient total may not equal sum of reactions, since some patients had more than one reaction.

**Each of the following moderate adverse reactions was reported in one patient: hypocalcemia, abnormal ST segment of electrocardiogram, bronchospasm, diarrhea, and hyperglycemia.

DOSAGE AND ADMINISTRATION
Pentamidine isethionate should be administered IM or IV only. The recommended regimen for adults and children is 4 mg/kg once a day for 14 days. The benefits and risks of therapy with pentamidine isethionate for more than 14 days are not well defined.
Intramuscular Injection
The contents of one vial (300 mg) should be dissolved in 3 mL of Sterile Water for Injection, USP. The calculated daily dose should then be withdrawn and administered by deep IM injection.
Intravenous Injection
The contents of one vial should first be dissolved in 3 to 5 mL of Sterile Water for Injection, USP, or 5% Dextrose Injection, USP. The calculated dose of pentamidine isethionate should then be withdrawn and diluted further in 50 to 250 mL of 5% Dextrose Injection, USP. **The diluted IV solutions containing pentamidine isethionate should be infused over a period of 60 minutes.**
Aseptic technique should be employed in preparation of all solutions. Parenteral drug products should be inspected visually for particulate matter and discoloration prior to administration.
Stability—Intravenous infusion solutions of pentamidine isethionate at 1 mg and 2.5 mg/mL prepared in 5% Dextrose Injection, USP, are stable at room temperature for up to 24 hours.

HOW SUPPLIED

Product No.	NDC No.	
11310	57317-211-03	PENTAM® 300 (sterile pentamidine isethionate) 300 mg, lyophilized product in single-dose vials, packages of 10.

Store the dry product at controlled room temperature 15°-30°C (59°-86°F). Protect the dry product and reconstituted solution from light.
Discard unused portions.
CAUTION Federal law prohibits dispensing without prescription.
Manufactured for Fujisawa Pharmaceutical Co. by Fujisawa USA, Inc.
Deerfield, IL 60015
45485A
Revised: February 1991

Products are cross-indexed by generic and chemical names in the
YELLOW SECTION.

Galderma Laboratories, Inc.
3000 ALTAMESA BLVD.
SUITE 300
FT. WORTH, TX 76133

BENZAC® AC 2½, 5 & 10 Gel ℞
(benzoyl peroxide gel)
BENZAC®AC Wash 2½, 5 & 10 ℞
(benzoyl peroxide)

DESCRIPTION

Benzac®AC 2½, 5 and **10** (benzoyl peroxide gel), and **Benzac®AC Wash 2½, 5** and **10** (benzoyl peroxide) are topical, water-base, benzoyl peroxide containing preparations for use in the treatment of acne vulgaris. Benzoyl peroxide is an oxidizing agent which possesses antibacterial properties and is classified as a keratolytic. Benzoyl peroxide ($C_{14}H_{10}O_4$) is represented by the following chemical structure:

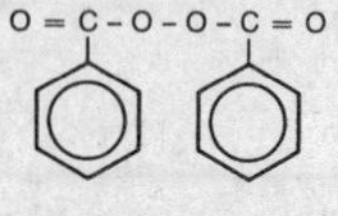

Benzac AC 2½, Benzac AC 5, and **Benzac AC 10** contain, respectively, benzoyl peroxide 2½%, 5% and 10% as the active ingredient in a gel base containing docusate sodium, edetate disodium, poloxamer 182, carbomer 940, propylene glycol, acrylates copolymer, glycerin, silicon dioxide, sodium hydroxide and purified water. May contain citric acid to adjust pH.

Benzac AC Wash 2½, Benzac AC Wash 5 and **Benzac AC Wash 10** contain, respectively, benzoyl peroxide 2½, 5% and 10% as the active ingredient in a vehicle consisting of purified water, sodium C14–16 olefin sulfonate, acrylates copolymer, glycerin, sodium hydroxide, and carbomer 940. May contain citric acid to adjust pH.

CLINICAL PHARMACOLOGY

The mechanism of action of benzoyl peroxide is not totally understood but its antibacterial activity against *Propionibacterium acnes* is thought to be a major mode of action. In addition, patients treated with benzoyl peroxide show a reduction in lipids and free fatty acids and mild desquamation (drying and peeling activity) with a simultaneous reduction in comedones and acne lesions.

Little is known about the percutaneous penetration, metabolism, and excretion of benzoyl peroxide, although it has been shown that benzoyl peroxide absorbed by the skin is metabolized to benzoic acid and then excreted as benzoate in the urine. There is no evidence of systemic toxicity caused by benzoyl peroxide in humans.

INDICATIONS AND USAGE

Benzac® AC 2½, 5 and **10** and **Benzac AC Wash 2½, 5** and **10** are indicated for the topical treatment of acne vulgaris.

CONTRAINDICATIONS

These preparations are contraindicated in patients with a history of hypersensitivity to any of their components.

PRECAUTIONS

General: For external use only. If severe irritation develops, discontinue use and institute appropriate therapy. After the reaction clears, treatment may often be resumed with less frequent application. These preparations should not be used in or near the eyes or on mucous membranes.

Information for patients: Avoid contact with eyes, eyelids, lips and mucous membranes. If accidental contact occurs, rinse with water. Contact with any colored material (including hair and fabric) may result in bleaching or discoloration. If excessive irritation develops, discontinue use and consult your physician.

Carcinogenesis, Mutagenesis, Impairment of Fertility: Data from several studies employing a strain of mice that are highly susceptible to developing cancer suggests that benzoyl peroxide acts as a tumor promoter. The clinical significance of these findings to humans is unknown. Benzoyl peroxide has not been found to be mutagenic (Ames Test) and there is no published data indicating it impairs fertility.

Pregnancy: Teratogenic Effects: *Pregnancy Category C:* Animal reproduction studies have not been conducted with benzoyl peroxide. It is not known whether benzoyl peroxide can cause fetal harm when administered to a pregnant woman or can affect reproduction capacity. Benzoyl peroxide should be used by a pregnant woman only if clearly needed. There are no available data on the effect of benzoyl peroxide on the later growth, development and functional maturation of the unborn child.

Nursing Mothers: It is not known whether this drug is excreted in human milk. Because many drugs are excreted in human milk, caution should be exercised when benzoyl peroxide is administered to a nursing woman.

Pediatric Use: Safety and effectiveness in children have not been established.

ADVERSE REACTIONS

Allergic contact dermatitis and dryness have been reported with topical benzoyl peroxide therapy.

OVERDOSAGE

If excessive scaling, erythema or edema occur, the use of this preparation should be discontinued. To hasten resolution of the adverse effects, cool compresses may be used. After symptoms and signs subside, a reduced dosage schedule may be cautiously tried if the reaction is judged to be due to excessive use and not allergenicity.

DOSAGE AND ADMINISTRATION

Benzac® AC 2½, 5 or **10** should be applied once or twice daily to cover affected areas after washing with a mild cleanser and water.

Benzac AC Wash 2½, 5 or **10.** Wash once or twice daily, avoiding contact with the eyes and mucous membranes. Wet the area of application. Apply **Benzac AC Wash 2½, 5** or **10** to the hands and wash the affected areas. Rinse with water and pat dry.

HOW SUPPLIED

Benzac AC 2½ Water Base Gel
60 g tubes—**NDC** 0299-3620-60
90 g tubes—**NDC** 0299-3620-90
Benzac AC 5 Water Base Gel
60 g tubes—**NDC** 0299-3625-60
90 g tubes—**NDC** 0299-3625-90
Benzac AC 10 Water Base Gel
60 g tubes—**NDC** 0299-3630-60
90 g tubes—**NDC** 0299-3630-90
Benzac AC Wash 2½
8 oz. plastic bottles—**NDC** 0299-3635-08
Benzac AC Wash 5
8 oz. plastic bottles—**NDC** 0299-3640-08
Benzac AC Wash 10
8 oz. plastic bottles—**NDC** 0299-3645-08

STORAGE

Store **Benzac AC** and **Benzac AC Wash** at controlled room temperature (59°–86°F).

CAUTION

Federal law prohibits dispensing without prescription.
Marketed by:
Owen/GALDERMA
LABORATORIES, INC. Fort Worth, Texas 76134
Mfd. by: Dermatological Products of Texas, Inc.
San Antonio, Texas 78296
OWEN and GALDERMA are registered trademarks.
126600-0491 Revised: April 1991

BENZAC® 5 & 10 Gel ℞
BENZAC W® 2½, 5 & 10 Water Base Gel ℞
BENZAC W® WASH 5 & 10 ℞
(benzoyl peroxide)

DESCRIPTION

Benzac® (benzoyl peroxide) 5 and 10 are topical alcohol-base preparations and Benzac W® 2½, 5 and 10 and Benzac W® Wash 5 and 10 are topical water-base preparations for use in the treatment of acne vulgaris. Benzoyl peroxide is an oxidizing agent which possesses antibacterial properties and is classified as keratolytic. Benzoyl peroxide ($C_{14}H_{10}O_4$) is represented by the following chemical structure:

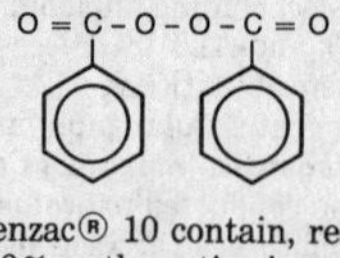

Benzac® 5 and Benzac® 10 contain, respectively, benzoyl peroxide 5% and 10% as the active ingredient in a gel base containing alcohol 12% (w/w), laureth 4, dimethicone, carbomer 940, sodium hydroxide, fragrance and purified water. May contain citric acid to adjust pH.

Benzac W® 2½, Benzac W® 5 and Benzac W® 10 contain, respectively, benzoyl peroxide 2½%, 5% and 10% as the active ingredient in a gel base containing docusate sodium, edetate disodium, poloxamer 182, carbomer 940, propylene glycol, silicon dioxide sodium hydroxide and purified water. May also contain citric acid to adjust pH.

Benzac W® Wash 5 and Benzac W® Wash 10 contain, respectively, benzoyl peroxide 5% and 10% as the active ingredient in a vehicle consisting of sodium C14–16 olefin sulfonate, carbomer 940, purified water, and citric acid.

CLINICAL PHARMACOLOGY

The mechanism of action of benzoyl peroxide is not totally understood, but its antibacterial activity against *Propionibacterium acnes* is thought to be a major mode of action. In addition, patients treated with benzoyl peroxide show a reduction in lipids and free fatty acids and mild desquamation (drying and peeling activity) with a simultaneous reduction in comedones and acne lesions. Little is known about the percutaneous penetration, metabolism, and excretion of benzoyl peroxide, although it has been shown that benzoyl peroxide absorbed by the skin is metabolized to benzoic acid and then excreted as benzoate in the urine. There is no evidence of systemic toxicity caused by benzoyl peroxide in humans.

INDICATIONS AND USAGE

Benzac® 5 and 10 and Benzac W® 2½, 5 and 10 are indicated for the topical treatment of acne vulgaris. Benzac W® Wash 5 and 10 are indicated for the topical treatment of mild to moderate acne vulgaris. In severe, complicated acne, Benzac W® Wash 5 and 10 may be used as an adjunct to other therapeutic regimens.

CONTRAINDICATIONS

These preparations are contraindicated in patients with a history of hypersensitivity to any of their components.

PRECAUTIONS

General: For external use only. If severe irritation develops, discontinue use and institute appropriate therapy. After the reaction clears, treatment may often be resumed with less frequent application. These preparations should not be used in or near the eyes or on mucous membranes.

Information for patients: Avoid contact with eyes, eyelids, lips and mucous membranes. If accidental contact occurs, rinse with water. Contact with any colored material (including hair and fabric) may result in bleaching or discoloration. If excessive irritation develops, discontinue use and consult your physician.

Carcinogensis, Mutagenesis, Impairment of Fertility: Data from several studies employing a strain of mice that are highly susceptible to developing cancer suggests that benzoyl peroxide acts as a tumor promoter. The clinical significance of these findings to humans is unknown. Benzoyl peroxide has been found not to be mutagenic (Ames test), and there is no published data indicating it impairs fertility.

Pregnancy: Teratogenic Effects: Pregnancy Category C: Animal reproduction studies have not been conducted with benzoyl peroxide. It is not known whether benzoyl peroxide can cause fetal harm when administered to a pregnant woman or can affect reproduction capacity. Benzoyl peroxide should be used by a pregnant woman only if clearly needed. There are no available data on the effect of benzoyl peroxide on the later growth, development and functional maturation of the unborn child.

Nursing Mothers: It is not known whether this drug is excreted in human milk. Because many drugs are excreted in human milk, caution should be exercised when benzoyl peroxide is administered to a nursing woman.

Pediatric Use: Safety and effectiveness in children have not been established.

ADVERSE REACTIONS

Allergic contact dermatitis and dryness have been reported with topical benzoyl peroxide therapy.

OVERDOSAGE

If excessive scaling, erythema or edema occur, the use of this preparation should be discontinued. To hasten resolution of the adverse effects, cool compresses may be used. After symptoms and signs subside, a reduced dosage schedule may be cautiously tried if the reaction is judged to be due to excessive use and not allergenicity.

DOSAGE AND ADMINISTRATION

Benzac® 5 or 10 or Benzac W® 2½, 5 or 10 should be applied once or twice daily to cover affected areas after washing with a mild cleanser and water. Wash with Benzac W® Wash 5 or 10 once or twice daily, avoiding contact with eyes and mucous membranes. Wet the area of application. Apply Benzac W® Wash 5 or 10 to the hands and wash the affected areas. Rinse with water and dry. The degree of drying and peeling can be adjusted by modification of the dosage schedule.

HOW SUPPLIED

Benzac® 5 Gel
60 g tubes—**NDC** 0299-3655-01
Benzac® 10 Gel
60 g tubes—**NDC** 0299-3665-01
Benzac W® 2½ Water Base Gel
60 g tubes—**NDC** 0299-3590-60
90 g tubes—**NDC** 0299-3590-90
Benzac W® 5 Water Base Gel
60 g tubes—**NDC** 0299-3600-01
90 g tubes—**NDC** 0299-3600-09
Benzac W® 10 Water Base Gel
60 g tubes—**NDC** 0299-3610-01
90 g tubes—**NDC** 0299-3610-09
Benzac W® Wash 5
4 oz. plastic bottles—**NDC** 0299-3670-04
8 oz. plastic bottles—**NDC** 0299-3670-08
Benzac W® Wash 10
8 oz. plastic bottles—**NDC** 0299-3672-08
Store Benzac W® and Benzac W® Wash at controlled room temperature (59°–86°F). Store Benzac® below 75°F.

CAUTION

Federal law prohibits dispensing without prescription.

CETAPHIL® OTC
Gentle Skin Cleanser—Soap Substitute

COMPOSITION

Contains water, cetyl alcohol, propylene glycol, sodium lauryl sulfate, stearyl alcohol, methylparaben, propylparaben and butylparaben.

ACTION AND USES

CETAPHIL® Cleanser was formulated for dermatologists as a gentle, non-irritating cleanser for sensitive skin. Unlike soap, **CETAPHIL** is completely non-alkaline, mild enough for all skin types. **CETAPHIL** soothes and softens as it cleanses, helping the skin retain needed moisture. **CETAPHIL** is also an excellent cleanser for the delicate skin of babies.

ADMINISTRATION AND DOSAGE

CETAPHIL can be used with or without water.
Without water: Apply a liberal amount to the skin and rub gently. The unique, low lathering formula allows gentle, yet thorough cleansing. Remove excess with a soft cloth, leaving a thin film of **CETAPHIL** on the skin. The emollient quality will leave the skin soft and moist.
With water: Apply to the skin and rub gently. Rinse.

HOW SUPPLIED

CETAPHIL® Cleanser 8 fl. oz. (UPC 0299-3921-08);
CETAPHIL® Cleanser 16 fl. oz. (UPC 0299-3921-16).

DESOWEN® ℞
(desonide)
Cream 0.05%/Ointment 0.05%/Lotion 0.05%

DESCRIPTION

DesOwen® Cream, Ointment and Lotion contain the topical corticosteroid, desonide, a nonfluorinated corticosteroid. It has the chemical name: Pregna-1,4-diene-3,20-dione,11, 21-dihydroxy-16,17-[(1-methylethylidene)bis(oxy)]-,(11β, 16α)-; the molecular formula: $C_{24}H_{32}O_6$; molecular weight: 416.51; *CAS-638-94-8*. The structural formula is:

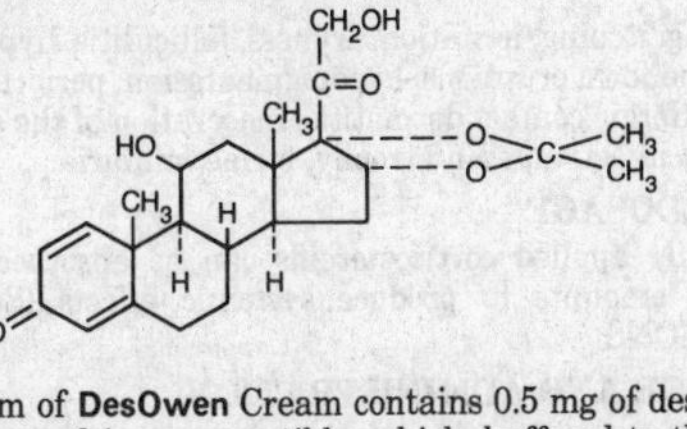

Each gram of **DesOwen** Cream contains 0.5 mg of desonide microdispersed in a compatible vehicle buffered to the pH range of normal skin. It contains purified water, emulsifying wax, propylene glycol, stearic acid, isopropyl palmitate, synthetic beeswax, polysorbate 60, citric acid, and sodium hydroxide. It is preserved with sorbic acid and potassium sorbate.
Each gram of **DesOwen** Ointment contains 0.5 mg of desonide in a base consisting of mineral oil and polyethylene.
Each gram of **DesOwen** Lotion contains 0.5 mg of desonide in a lotion vehicle consisting of sodium lauryl sulfate, light mineral oil, cetyl alcohol, stearyl alcohol, propylene glycol, methylparaben, propylparaben, sorbitan monostearate, glyceryl stearate SE, edetate sodium, and purified water. May contain citric acid and/or sodium hydroxide for pH adjustment.

CLINICAL PHARMACOLOGY

Topical corticosteroids share anti-inflammatory, anti-pruritic, and vasoconstrictive actions.
The mechanism of anti-inflammatory activity of the topical corticosteroids is unclear. Various laboratory methods, including vasoconstrictor assays, are used to compare and predict potencies and/or clinical efficacies of the topical corticosteroids. There is some evidence to suggest that a recognizable correlation exists between vasoconstrictor potency and therapeutic efficacy in man.
Pharmacokinetics: The extent of percutaneous absorption of topical corticosteroids is determined by many factors including the vehicle, the integrity of the epidermal barrier, and the use of occlusive dressings.
Topical corticosteroids can be absorbed from normal intact skin. Inflammation and/or other disease processes in the skin increase percutaneous absorption. Occlusive dressings substantially increase the percutaneous absorption of topical corticosteroids. Thus, occlusive dressings may be a valuable therapeutic adjunct for treatment of resistant dermatoses. (See DOSAGE AND ADMINISTRATION.)
Once absorbed through the skin, topical corticosteroids are handled through pharmacokinetic pathways similar to systemically administered corticosteroids. Corticosteroids are bound to plasma proteins in varying degrees. Corticosteroids are metabolized primarily in the liver and are then excreted by the kidneys. Some of the topical corticosteroids and their metabolites are also excreted into the bile.

INDICATIONS AND USAGE

DesOwen (desonide) Cream 0.05%, Ointment 0.05% and Lotion 0.05% are indicated for the relief of the inflammatory and pruritic manifestations of corticosteroid-responsive dermatoses.

CONTRAINDICATIONS

Topical corticosteroids are contraindicated in those patients with a history of hypersensitivity to any of the components of the preparation.

PRECAUTIONS

General: Systemic absorption of topical corticosteroids has produced reversible hypothalamic-pituitary-adrenal (HPA) axis suppression, manifestations of Cushing's syndrome, hyperglycemia, and glucosuria in some patients.
Conditions which augment systemic absorption include the application of the more potent steroids, use over large surface areas, prolonged use, and the addition of occlusive dressings.
Therefore, patients receiving a large dose of a potent topical steroid applied to a large surface area or under an occlusive dressing should be evaluated periodically for evidence of HPA axis suppression by using the urinary free cortisol and ACTH stimulation tests. If HPA axis suppression is noted, an attempt should be made to withdraw the drug, to reduce the frequency of application, or to substitute a less potent steroid.
Recovery of HPA axis function is generally prompt and complete upon discontinuation of the drug. Infrequently, signs and symptoms of steroid withdrawal may occur, requiring supplemental systemic corticosteroids.
Children may absorb proportionally larger amounts of topical corticosteroids and thus be more susceptible to systemic toxicity (See PRECAUTIONS—Pediatric Use).
If irritation develops, topical corticosteroids should be discontinued and appropriate therapy instituted.
In the presence of dermatological infections, the use of an appropriate antifungal or antibacterial agent should be instituted. If a favorable response does not occur promptly, the corticosteroids should be discontinued until the infection has been adequately controlled.
Information for the Patient: Patients using topical corticosteroids should receive the following information and instructions:

1. This medication is to be used as directed by the physician. It is for external use only. Avoid contact with the eyes.
2. Patients should be advised not to use this medication for any disorder other than for which it was prescribed.
3. The treated skin area should not be bandaged or otherwise covered or wrapped as to be occlusive unless directed by the physician.
4. Patients should report any signs of local adverse reactions especially under occlusive dressing.
5. Parents of pediatric patients should be advised not to use tight-fitting diapers or plastic pants on a child being treated in the diaper area, as these garments may constitute occlusive dressings.

Laboratory Tests: The following tests may be helpful in evaluating the HPA axis suppression:
Urinary free cortisol test
ACTH stimulation test
Carcinogenesis, Mutagenesis, and Impairment of Fertility: Long-term animal studies have not been performed to evaluate the carcinogenic potential or the effect on fertility of topical corticosteroids.
Studies to determine mutagenicity with prednisolone and hydrocortisone have revealed negative results.
Pregnancy Category C: Corticosteroids are generally teratogenic in laboratory animals when administered systemically at relatively low dosage levels. The more potent corticosteroids have been shown to be teratogenic after dermal application in laboratory animals. There are no adequate and well controlled studies in pregnant women on teratogenic effects from topically applied corticosteroids. Therefore, topical corticosteroids should be used during pregnancy only if the potential benefit justifies the potential risk to the fetus. Drugs of this class should not be used extensively on pregnant patients, in large amounts, or for prolonged periods of time.
Nursing Mothers: It is not known whether topical administration of corticosteroids could result in sufficient systemic absorption to produce detectable quantities in breast milk. Systemically administered corticosteroids are secreted into breast milk, in quantities *not* likely to have a deleterious effect on the infant. Nevertheless, caution should be exercised when topical corticosteroids are administered to a nursing woman.
Pediatric Use: *Pediatric patients may demonstrate greater susceptibility to topical corticosteroid-induced HPA axis suppression and Cushing's syndrome than mature patients because of a larger skin surface area to body weight ratio.*
Hypothalamic-pituitary-adrenal (HPA) axis suppression, Cushing's syndrome, and intracranial hypertension have been reported in children receiving topical corticosteroids. Manifestations of adrenal suppression in children include linear growth retardation, delayed weight gain, low plasma cortisol levels, and absence of response to ACTH stimulation. Manifestations of intracranial hypertension include bulging fontanelles, headaches, and bilateral papilledema.
Administration of topical corticosteroids to children should be limited to the least amount compatible with an effective therapeutic regimen. Chronic corticosteroid therapy may interfere with the growth and development of children.

ADVERSE REACTIONS

The following local adverse reactions are reported infrequently with topical corticosteroids, but may occur more frequently with the use of occlusive dressings. These reactions are listed in an approximate decreasing order of occurrence: burning, itching, irritation, dryness, folliculitis, hypertrichosis, acneiform eruptions, hypopigmentation, perioral dermatitis, allergic contact dermatitis, maceration of the skin, secondary infection, skin atrophy, striae and miliaria.

OVERDOSAGE

Topically applied corticosteroids can be absorbed in sufficient amounts to produce systemic effects (See PRECAUTIONS).

DOSAGE AND ADMINISTRATION

DesOwen®(desonide) Cream 0.05%, Ointment 0.05% or Lotion 0.05% should be applied to the affected area as a thin film two or three times daily depending on the severity of the condition. SHAKE LOTION WELL BEFORE USING.
Occlusive dressings may be used for the management of psoriasis or recalcitrant conditions.
If an infection develops, the use of occlusive dressings should be discontinued and appropriate antimicrobial therapy instituted.

HOW SUPPLIED

DesOwen (desonide) Cream 0.05% is supplied in tubes containing:
15 g **NDC** 0299-5770-15
60 g **NDC** 0299-5770-60
DesOwen (desonide) Ointment 0.05% is supplied in tubes containing:
15 g **NDC** 0299-5775-15
60 g **NDC** 0299-5775-60
DesOwen (desonide) Lotion 0.05% is supplied in bottles containing:
2 fl oz **NDC** 0299-5765-02
4 fl oz **NDC** 0299-5765-04
Storage Conditions: Store below 86° F (30° C). Avoid freezing.
CAUTION: Federal law prohibits dispensing without prescription.
Marketed by:
Owen/GALDERMA
LABORATORIES, INC.
Fort Worth,Texas 76134
Mfg. by: Dermatological
Products of Texas, Inc.
San Antonio, Texas 78296
OWEN and GALDERMA
are registered trademarks.
126500-0390 Revised: March, 1990

IONIL® PLUS Shampoo OTC
Therapeutic Salicylic Acid Shampoo

Controls dandruff, seborrheic dermatitis and psoriasis

CONTAINS

ACTIVE: salicylic acid 2% (W/W). **Inactive:** water, sodium laureth sulfate, lauramide DEA, quaternium-22, talloweth-60 myristyl glycol, laureth-23, TEA lauryl sulfate, glycol distearate, laureth-4, TEA-abietoyl hydrolyzed collagen, DMDM hydantoin, tetrasodium EDTA, sodium hydroxide, fragrance, FD&C Blue No. 1.

INDICATIONS

IONIL PLUS Shampoo relieves the itching, irritation and flaking associated with dandruff, seborrheic dermatitis, and psoriasis of the scalp.

DIRECTIONS

Wet hair, apply IONIL PLUS and massage into scalp. Let lather stand one minute, then rinse. Repeat application, if needed. For best results use at least twice a week or as directed by a physician.

WARNINGS

For external use only. Avoid contact with eyes. If contact occurs, rinse eyes thoroughly with water. If condition covers

Continued on next page

Galderma Laboratories—Cont.

a large area of the body, consult your physician before using this product. Use caution in exposing skin to sunlight after applying this product. If condition worsens or does not improve after regular use of this product as directed, consult a physician. Keep this and all drugs out of the reach of children. In case of accidental ingestion, seek professional assistance or contact a Poison Control Center immediately.

HOW SUPPLIED

8 fl. oz. (NDC 0299-3731-08) plastic bottles

IONIL T® PLUS Shampoo
Therapeutic Coal Tar Shampoo

Controls dandruff, seborrheic dermatitis and psoriasis

CONTAINS

Active: coal tar distillate 1% (equivalent to 1% w/v coal tar).

Inactive: water, sodium laureth sulfate, lauramide DEA, TEA-lauryl sulfate, laureth-23, talloweth-60 myristyl glycol, glycol distearate, laureth-4, quaternium-22 TEA-abietoyl hydrolyzed animal protein, DMDM hydantion, disodium EDTA, fragrance, FD&C blue No. 1, EXT. D&C yellow No. 7, may contain citric acid to adjust pH.

INDICATIONS

IONIL T PLUS Shampoo helps eliminate the symptoms of dandruff, seborrheic dermatitis and psoriasis. Will not discolor white or light colored hair. IONIL T PLUS leaves hair manageable.

DIRECTIONS

Wet hair, apply IONIL T PLUS, and massage into scalp. Let lather stand one minute and then rinse. Repeat application, if needed. For best results use at least twice a week or as directed by a physician.

WARNINGS

For external use only. Avoid contact with eyes. If contact occurs, rinse eyes thoroughly with water. If condition covers a large area of the body, consult your physician before using this product. Use caution in exposing skin to sunlight after applying this product. It may increase your tendency to sunburn for up to 24 hours after application. Do not use for prolonged periods without consulting a physician. Do not use this product with other forms of psoriasis therapy such as ultraviolet radiation or prescription drugs unless directed to do so by a physician. Keep this and all drugs out of the reach of children. In case of accidental ingestion, seek professional assistance or contact a Poison Control Center immediately.

HOW SUPPLIED

8 fl. oz. (NDC 0299-3752-08) plastic bottles

NUTRACORT® ℞
(hydrocortisone)
Cream 1%
Lotion 1% & 2.5%

DESCRIPTION

NUTRACORT® cream and lotion are topical hydrocortisone preparations. Hydrocortisone is therapeutically classed as an anti-inflammatory and anti-pruritic agent. Hydrocortisone is a white crystalline powder that is very slightly soluble in water and ether and sparingly soluble in acetone and alcohol.

Chemical Name:
Pregn-4-ene-3,20-dione, 11,17,21-trihydroxy-,(11β)-.
Empirical Formula: $C_{21}H_{30}O_5$
Molecular Weight: 362.47

NUTRACORT® Cream 1% contains: Hydrocortisone 1.0% (10 mg/g) in a cream base containing propylene glycol, polysorbate 60, emulsifying wax, synthetic beeswax, stearic acid, isopropyl palmitate, sorbic acid, potassium sorbate, propyl gallate, citric acid and/or sodium hydroxide (to adjust pH), purified water and certified color.

NUTRACORT® Lotion 1% contains: Hydrocortisone 1.0% (10 mg/mL) in a lotion base containing **Inactive:** purified water, light mineral oil, sorbitan monostearate, stearyl alcohol, cetyl alcohol, glyceryl stearate SE, sodium lauryl sulfate, edetate sodium, methylparaben, propylparaben, and certified color. May contain citric acid and/or sodium hydroxide for pH adjustment.

NUTRACORT® Lotion 2.5% contains: Hydrocortisone 2.5% (25 mg/mL) in a lotion base containing **Inactive:** purified water, light mineral oil, sorbitan monostearate, stearyl alcohol, glyceryl stearate SE, sodium lauryl sulfate, cetyl alcohol, edetate disodium, methylparaben, propylparaben, and certified colors. May contain citric acid and/or sodium hydroxide for pH adjustment.

CLINICAL PHARMACOLOGY

Topical corticosteroids share anti-inflammatory, anti-pruritic and vasoconstrictive actions.

The mechanism of anti-inflammatory activity of the topical corticosteroids is unclear. Various laboratory methods, including vasoconstrictor assays, are used to compare and predict potencies and/or clinical efficacies of the topical corticosteroids. There is some evidence to suggest that a recognizable correlation exists between vasoconstrictor potency and therapeutic efficacy in man.

Pharmacokinetics: The extent of percutaneous absorption of topical corticosteroids is determined by many factors including the vehicle, the integrity of the epidermal barrier, and the use of occlusive dressings.

Topical corticosteroids can be absorbed from normal intact skin. Inflammation and/or other disease processes in the skin increase percutaneous absorption. Occlusive dressings substantially increase the percutaneous absorption of topical corticosteroids. Thus, occlusive dressings may be a valuable therapeutic adjunct for treatment of resistant dermatoses. (See DOSAGE AND ADMINISTRATION.)

Once absorbed through the skin, topical corticosteroids are handled through pharmacokinetic pathways similar to systemically administered corticosteroids. Corticosteroids are bound to plasma proteins in varying degrees. Corticosteroids are metabolized primarily in the liver and are then excreted by the kidneys. Some of the topical corticosteroids and their metabolites are also excreted into the bile.

INDICATIONS AND USAGE

Topical corticosteroids are indicated for the relief of the inflammatory and pruritic manifestations of corticosteroid-responsive dermatoses.

CONTRAINDICATIONS

Topical corticosteroids are contraindicated in those patients with a history of hypersensitivity to any of the components of the preparation.

PRECAUTIONS

General: Systemic absorption of topical corticosteroids has produced reversible hypothalamic-pituitary-adrenal (HPA) axis suppression, manifestations of Cushing's syndrome, hyperglycemia, and glucosuria in some patients.

Conditions which augment systemic absorption include the application of the more potent steroids, use over large surface areas, prolonged use, and the addition of occlusive dressings.

Therefore, patients receiving a large dose of a potent topical steroid applied to a large surface area or under an occlusive dressing should be evaluated periodically for evidence of HPA axis suppression by using the urinary free cortisol and ACTH stimulation tests. If HPA axis suppression is noted, an attempt should be made to withdraw the drug, to reduce the frequency of application, or to substitute a less potent steroid. Recovery of HPA axis function is generally prompt and complete upon discontinuation of the drug. Infrequently, signs and symptoms of steroid withdrawal may occur, requiring supplemental systemic corticosteroids.

Children may absorb proportionally larger amounts of topical corticosteroids and thus be more susceptible to systemic toxicity. (See PRECAUTIONS—Pediatric Use.)

If irritation develops, topical corticosteroids should be discontinued and appropriate therapy instituted.

In the presence of dermatological infections, the use of an appropriate antifungal or antibacterial agent should be instituted. If a favorable response does not occur promptly, the corticosteroid should be discontinued until the infection has been adequately controlled.

Information for the Patient: Patients using topical corticosteroids should receive the following information and instructions:

1. This medication is to be used as directed by the physician. It is for external use only. Avoid contact with the eyes.
2. Patients should be advised not to use this medication for any disorder other than for which it was prescribed.
3. The treated skin area should not be bandaged or otherwise covered or wrapped as to be occlusive unless directed by the physician.
4. Patients should report any signs of local adverse reactions especially under occlusive dressing.
5. Parents of pediatric patients should be advised not to use tight-fitting diapers or plastic pants on a child being treated in the diaper area, as these garments may constitute occlusive dressings.

Laboratory Tests: The following tests may be helpful in evaluating the HPA axis suppression:
Urinary free cortisol test
ACTH stimulation test

Carcinogenesis, Mutagenesis, and Impairment of Fertility: Long-term animal studies have not been performed to evaluate the carcinogenic potential or the effect on fertility of topical corticosteroids.

Studies to determine mutagencity with prednisolone and hydrocortisone have revealed negative results.

Pregnancy Category C: Corticosteroids are generally teratogenic in laboratory animals when administered systemically at relatively low dosage levels. The more potent corticosteroids have been shown to be teratogenic after dermal application in laboratory animals. There are no adequate and well-controlled studies in pregnant women on teratogenic effects from topically applied corticosteroids. Therefore, topical corticosteroids should be used during pregnancy only if the potential benefit justifies the potential risk to the fetus. Drugs of this class should not be used extensively on pregnant patients, in large amounts, or for prolonged periods of time.

Nursing Mothers: It is not known whether topical administration of corticosteroids could result in sufficient systemic absorption to produce detectable quantities in breast milk. Systemically administered corticosteroids are secreted into breast milk in quantities *not* likely to have a deleterious effect on the infant. Nevertheless, caution should be exercised when topical corticosteroids are administered to a nursing woman.

Pediatric Use: *Pediatric patients may demonstrate greater susceptibility to topical corticosteroid-induced HPA axis suppression and Cushing's syndrome than mature patients because of a larger skin surface area to body weight ratio.*

Hypothalamic-pituitary-adrenal (HPA) axis suppression, Cushing's syndrome, and intracranial hypertension have been reported in children receiving topical corticosteroids. Manifestations of adrenal suppression in children include linear growth retardation, delayed weight gain, low plasma cortisol levels, and absence of response to ACTH stimulation. Manifestations of intracranial hypertension include bulging fontanelles, headaches, and bilateral papilledema.

Administration of topical corticosteroids to children should be limited to the least amount compatible with an effective therapeutic regimen. Chronic corticosteroid therapy may interfere with the growth and development of children.

ADVERSE REACTIONS

The following local adverse reactions are reported infrequently with topical corticosteroids, but may occur more frequently with the use of occlusive dressings. These reactions are listed in an approximate decreasing order of occurrence:

burning, itching, irritation, dryness, folliculitis, hypertrichosis, acneiform eruptions, hypopigmentation, perioral dermatitis, allergic contact dermatitis, maceration of the skin, secondary infection, skin atrophy, striae, miliaria.

OVERDOSAGE

Topically applied corticosteroids can be absorbed in sufficient amounts to produce systemic effects (See PRECAUTIONS).

DOSAGE AND ADMINISTRATION

Topical corticosteroids are generally applied to the affected area as a thin film from three to four times daily depending on the severity of the condition.

Occlusive dressings may be used for the management of psoriasis or recalcitrant conditions.

If an infection develops, the use of occlusive dressings should be discontinued and appropriate antimicrobial therapy instituted.

HOW SUPPLIED

NUTRACORT® Cream 1% is supplied in high density polyethylene (HDPE) tubes:
30g **NDC** 0299-5821-30
60g **NDC** 0299-5821-60
and in polypropylene jars:
4 oz. **NDC** 0299-5821-04

NUTRACORT® Lotion 1% is supplied in HDPE bottles:
2 fl. oz. **NDC** 0299-5830-01
4 fl. oz. **NDC** 0299-5830-02

NUTRACORT® Lotion 2.5% is supplied in HDPE bottles:
2 fl. oz. **NDC** 0299-5825-01
4 fl. oz. **NDC** 0299-5825-02

Store at room temperature.

NUTRADERM® Lotion
Therapeutic Dry Skin Lotion

NUTRADERM® Cream
Therapeutic Dry Skin Cream

COMPOSITION

Lotion contains purified water, mineral oil, sorbitan stearate, stearyl alcohol, sodium lauryl sulfate, cetyl alcohol, carbomer-940, methylparaben, triethanolamine, propylparaben and fragrance. Cream contains purified water, mineral oil, sorbitan stearate, stearyl alcohol, cetyl alcohol, sorbitol, isopropyl palmitate, cetyl esters wax, sodium lauryl sulfate, dimethicone, methylparaben, propylparaben, diazolidinyl urea, citric acid and fragrance.

ACTIONS AND USES

NUTRADERM® Lotion and Cream provides immediate moisture to dry skin while creating a barrier that seals in moisture.

NUTRADERM Lotion and Cream and lanolin free, and non-greasy.

ADMINISTRATION AND DOSAGE

Apply freely to dry skin as necessary, or as directed by your physician.

HOW SUPPLIED

NUTRADERM Lotion, 8 fl. oz. (UPC 0299-5880-04)
NUTRADERM Lotion, 16 fl. oz. (UPC 0299-5880-05) plastic bottles; also available as NUTRADERM Cream, 3 oz. (UPC 0299-5850-30) plastic tubes; NUTRADERM Cream, 1 lb. (UPC 0299-5850-05) plastic jar.

NUTRADERM® 30 Lotion
Therapeutic Dry Skin Lotion

COMPOSITION

Purified water, glycerin, petrolatum, cetearyl alcohol, ceteareth-20, dimethicone, C10–30 cholesterol/lanosterol esters, cyclomethicone, cetyl alcohol, sodium PCA, sodium lactate, malic acid, cetyl lactate, C12–C15 alcohols lactate, xanthan gum, sodium hydroxide, propylparaben, methylparaben, diazolidinyl urea, fragrance.

ACTIONS AND USES

NUTRADERM® 30 Lotion is specially formulated for the unique moisturizing needs of skin that is over 30 or prematurely dry. Emollients soothe, soften and form a protective barrier that resists washing off. Humectants help renew the skin's natural ability to retain moisture. Non-greasy. Absorbs quickly for immediate, long-lasting softness.

ADMINISTRATION AND USAGE

Apply to hands and body as needed.

HOW SUPPLIED

NUTRADERM 30 Lotion, 8 fl. oz. (UPC 0299-5870-08)
NUTRADERM 30 Lotion, 16 fl. oz. (UPC 0299-5870-16)

Gate Pharmaceuticals
Division of Lemmon Company
P.O. BOX 904
SELLERSVILLE, PA 18960

ADIPEX-P®   Ⓒ Ŗ
[ă 'dĭ-pĕx]
(phentermine hydrochloride 37.5 mg)

DESCRIPTION

Phentermine Hydrochloride has the chemical name of α, α-dimethylphenethylamine hydrochloride. The structural formula is as follows:

$C_{10}H_{15}N \cdot HCl$ M.W. 185.7

Phentermine hydrochloride is a white, odorless, hygroscopic, crystalline powder which is soluble in water and lower alcohols, slightly soluble in chloroform and insoluble in ether. ADIPEX-P, an anorectic agent for oral administration, is available as a capsule or tablet containing 37.5 mg of phentermine hydrochloride (equivalent to 30 mg of phentermine base).

ADIPEX-P capsules contain the inactive ingredients Corn Starch, Gelatin, Lactose, Magnesium Stearate, and Coloring. ADIPEX-P Tablets contain the inactive ingredients Acacia, Confectioner's Sugar, Corn Starch, Lactose, Magnesium Stearate, Stearic Acid, and Coloring.

CLINICAL PHARMACOLOGY

Phentermine hydrochloride is a sympathomimetic amine with pharmacologic activity similar to the prototype drugs of this class used in obesity, the amphetamines. Actions include central nervous system stimulation and elevation of blood pressure. Tachyphylaxis and tolerance have been demonstrated with all drugs of this class in which these phenomena have been looked for.

Drugs of this class used in obesity are commonly known as "anorectics" or "anorexigenics". It has not been established, however, that the action of such drugs in treating obesity is primarily one of appetite suppression. Other central nervous system actions, or metabolic effects may be involved, for example.

Adult obese subjects instructed in dietary management and treated with "anorectic" drugs, lose more weight on the aver-

age than those treated with placebo and diet, as determined in relatively short-term clinical trials.

The magnitude of increased weight loss of drug-treated patients over placebo-treated patients is only a fraction of a pound a week. The rate of weight loss is greatest in the first weeks of therapy for both drug and placebo subjects and tends to decrease in succeeding weeks. The possible origins of the increased weight loss due to the various drug effects are not established. The amount of weight loss associated with the use of "anorectic" drugs varies from trial to trial, and the increased weight loss appears to be related in part to variables other than the drug prescribed, such as the physician-investigator, the population treated, and the diet prescribed. Studies do not permit conclusions as to the relative importance of the drug and non-drug factors on weight loss.

The natural history of obesity is measured in years, whereas the studies cited are restricted to a few weeks duration; thus, the total impact of drug-induced weight loss over that of diet alone must be considered clinically limited.

INDICATIONS AND USAGE

Adipex-P® (phentermine hydrochloride) is indicated in the management of exogenous obesity as a short term adjunct (a few weeks) in a regimen of weight reduction based on caloric restriction.

The limited usefulness of agents of this class (see CLINICAL PHARMACOLOGY) should be measured against possible risk factors inherent in their use such as those described below.

CONTRAINDICATIONS

Advanced arteriosclerosis, symptomatic cardiovascular disease, moderate to severe hypertension, hyperthyroidism, known hypersensitivity or idiosyncrasy to the sympathomimetic amines, glaucoma.

Agitated states.

Patients with a history of drug abuse.

During or within 14 days following the administration of monoamine oxidase inhibitors (hypertensive crises may result).

WARNINGS

Tolerance to the anorectic effect usually develops within a few weeks. When this occurs, the recommended dose should not be exceeded in an attempt to increase the effect; rather, the drug should be discontinued.

Phentermine hydrochloride may impair the ability of the patient to engage in potentially hazardous activities such as operating machinery or driving a motor vehicle; the patient should therefore be cautioned accordingly.

Usage in Pregnancy: Safe use in pregnancy has not been established. Use of phentermine hydrochloride by women who are or who may become pregnant, and those in the first trimester of pregnancy, requires that the potential benefit be weighed against the possible hazard to mother and infant.

Usage in Children: Phentermine hydrochloride is not recommended for use in children under 12 years of age.

Usage with Alcohol: Concomitant use of alcohol with phentermine hydrochloride may result in an adverse drug interaction.

PRECAUTIONS

Caution is to be exercised in prescribing phentermine hydrochloride for patients with even mild hypertension.

Insulin requirements in diabetes mellitus may be altered in association with the use of phentermine hydrochloride and the concomitant dietary regimen.

Phentermine hydrochloride may decrease the hypotensive effect of guanethidine.

The least amount feasible should be prescribed or dispensed at one time in order to minimize the possibility of overdosage.

ADVERSE REACTIONS

Cardiovascular: Palpitation, tachycardia, elevation of blood pressure.

Central Nervous System: Overstimulation, restlessness, dizziness, insomnia, euphoria, dysphoria, tremor, headache; rarely psychotic episodes at recommended doses.

Gastrointestinal: Dryness of the mouth, unpleasant taste, diarrhea, constipation, other gastrointestinal disturbances.

Allergic: Urticaria.

Endocrine: Impotence, changes in libido.

DRUG ABUSE AND DEPENDENCE

Phentermine hydrochloride is a Schedule IV controlled substance. Phentermine hydrochloride is related chemically and pharmacologically to the amphetamines. Amphetamines and related stimulant drugs have been extensively abused, and the possibility of abuse of phentermine hydrochloride should be kept in mind when evaluating the desirability of including a drug as part of a weight reduction program. Abuse of amphetamines and related drugs may be associated with intense psychological dependence and severe social dysfunction. There are reports of patients who have increased the dosage to many times that recommended. Abrupt cessation following prolonged high dosage administration results in extreme fatigue and mental depression;

changes are also noted on the sleep EEG. Manifestations of chronic intoxication with anorectic drugs include severe dermatoses, marked insomnia, irritability, hyperactivity, and personality changes. The most severe manifestation of chronic intoxications is psychosis, often clinically indistinguishable from schizophrenia.

OVERDOSAGE

Manifestations of acute overdosage with phentermine hydrochloride include restlessness, tremor, hyperreflexia, rapid respiration, confusion, assaultiveness, hallucinations, panic states.

Fatigue and depression usually follow the central stimulation.

Cardiovascular effects include arrhythmias, hypertension or hypotension and circulatory collapse. Gastrointestinal symptoms include nausea, vomiting, diarrhea, and abdominal cramps. Fatal poisoning usually terminates in convulsions and coma.

Management of acute phentermine hydrochloride intoxication is largely symptomatic and includes lavage and sedation with a barbiturate. Experience with hemodialysis or peritoneal dialysis is inadequate to permit recommendation in this regard. Acidification of the urine increases phentermine excretion. Intravenous phentolamine has been suggested for possible acute, severe hypertension, if this complicates phentermine hydrochloride overdosage.

DOSAGE AND ADMINISTRATION

Dosage should be individualized to obtain an adequate response with the lowest effective dose.

The usual adult dose is one capsule or tablet (37.5 mg) daily, administered before breakfast or 1–2 hours after breakfast. For tablets, the dosage may be adjusted to the patient's need. For some patients $\frac{1}{2}$ tablet (18.75 mg) daily may be adequate, while in some cases it may be desirable to give $\frac{1}{2}$ tablet (18.75 mg) two times a day.

Late evening medication should be avoided because of the possibility of resulting insomnia.

Phentermine hydrochloride is NOT recommended for use in children under 12 years of age.

HOW SUPPLIED

Available in tablets and capsules containing 37.5 mg phentermine hydrochloride (equivalent to 30 mg phentermine base). Each blue and white, oblong, scored tablet is imprinted with "LEMMON"/"9"-"9". The #3 capsule has an opaque white body and an opaque light blue cap. Each capsule is imprinted with "Adipex-P"-"37.5" on the cap and two blue stripes on the body.

Tablets are packaged in bottles of 100 (NDC 57844-009-01); 400 (NDC 57844-009-26); and 1000 (NDC 57844-009-10). Capsules are packaged in bottles of 100 (NDC 57844-019-01). Store at controlled room temperature 15°-30°C (59°-86°F).

CAUTION: Federal law prohibits dispensing without prescription.

Manufactured for:
GATE PHARMACEUTICALS
Div. of Lemmon Company
Sellersville, PA 18960
Manufactured by:
Lemmon Company
Sellersville, Pa 18960

Printed in USA
Iss. 3/90

Shown in Product Identification Section, page 409

ORAP™   Ŗ
(Pimozide)
Tablets

DESCRIPTION

ORAP (pimozide) is an orally active antipsychotic agent of the diphenyl-butylpiperidine series. The structural formula of pimozide, 1-(1-(4,4- bis(4-fluorophenyl)butyl)-4-piperidinyl)-1,3-dihydro-2H-benzimidazol-2-one is:

The solubility of pimozide in water is less than 0.01 mg/ml; it is slightly soluble in most organic solvents.

Each white ORAP tablet contains 2 mg of pimozide and the following inactive ingredients: calcium stearate, cellulose, lactose and corn starch.

Continued on next page

Gate—Cont.

CLINICAL PHARMACOLOGY

Pharmacodynamic Actions

ORAP (pimozide) is an orally active antipsychotic drug product which shares with other antipsychotics the ability to blockade dopaminergic receptors on neurons in the central nervous system. Although its exact mode of action has not been established, the ability of pimozide to suppress motor and phonic tics in Tourette's Disorder is thought to be a function of its dopaminergic blocking activity. However, receptor blockade is often accompanied by a series of secondary alterations in central dopamine metabolism and function which may contribute to both pimozide's therapeutic and untoward effects. In addition, pimozide, in common with other antipsychotic drugs, has various effects on other central nervous system receptor systems which are not fully characterized.

Metabolism and Pharmacokinetics

More than 50% of a dose of pimozide is absorbed after oral administration. Based on the pharmacokinetic and metabolic profile, pimozide appears to undergo significant first pass metabolism. Peak serum levels occur generally six to eight hours (range 4–12 hours) after dosing. Pimozide is extensively metabolized, primarily by N-dealkylation in the liver. Two major metabolites have been identified, 1-(4-piperidyl)-2-benzimidazolinone and 4,4-bis(4-fluorophenyl) butyric acid. The antipsychotic activity of these metabolites is undetermined. The major route of elimination of pimozide and its metabolites is through the kidney.

The mean serum elimination half-life of pimozide in schizophrenic patients was approximately 55 hours. There was a 13-fold interindividual difference in the area under the serum pimozide level-time curve and an equivalent degree of variation in peak serum levels among patients studied. The significance of this is unclear since there are few correlations between plasma levels and clinical findings.

Effects of food, disease or concomitant medication upon the absorption, distribution, metabolism and elimination of pimozide are not known.

INDICATIONS AND USAGE

ORAP (pimozide) is indicated for the suppression of motor and phonic tics in patients with Tourette's Disorder who have failed to respond satisfactorily to standard treatment. ORAP is not intended as a treatment of first choice nor is it intended for the treatment for tics that are merely annoying or cosmetically troublesome. ORAP should be reserved for use in Tourette's Disorder patients whose development and/or daily life function is severely compromised by the presence of motor and phonic tics.

Evidence supporting approval of pimozide for use in Tourette's Disorder was obtained in two controlled clinical investigations which enrolled patients between the ages of 8 and 53 years. Most subjects in the two trials were 12 or older.

CONTRAINDICATIONS

1. ORAP (pimozide) is contraindicated in the treatment of simple tics or tics other than those associated with Tourette's Disorder.
2. ORAP should not be used in patients taking drugs that may, themselves, cause motor and phonic tics (e.g., pemoline, methylphenidate and amphetamines) until such patients have been withdrawn from these drugs to determine whether or not the drugs, rather than Tourette's Disorder, are responsible for the tics.
3. Because ORAP prolongs the QT interval of the electrocardiogram it is contraindicated in patients with congenital long QT syndrome, patients with a history of cardiac arrhythmias, or patients taking other drugs which prolong the QT interval of the electrocardiogram (see DRUG INTERACTIONS).
4. ORAP is contraindicated in patients with severe toxic central nervous system depression or comatose states from any cause.
5. ORAP is contraindicated in patients with hypersensitivity to it. As it is not known whether cross-sensitivity exists among the antipsychotics, pimozide should be used with appropriate caution in patients who have demonstrated hypersensitivity to other antipsychotic drugs.

WARNINGS

The use of ORAP (pimozide) in the treatment of Tourette's Disorder involves different risk/benefit considerations than when antipsychotic drugs are used to treat other conditions. Consequently, a decision to use ORAP should take into consideration the following (see also PRECAUTIONS—Information for Patients).

Tardive Dyskinesia

A syndrome consisting of potentially irreversible, involuntary, dyskinetic movements may develop in patients treated with antipsychotic drugs. Although the prevalence of the syndrome appears to be highest among the elderly, especially elderly women, it is impossible to rely upon prevalence estimates to predict, at the inception of antipsychotic treatment, which patients are likely to develop the syndrome.

Whether antipsychotic drug products differ in their potential to cause tardive dyskinesia is unknown.

Both the risk of developing tardive dyskinesia and the likelihood that it will become irreversible are believed to increase as the duration of treatment and the total cumulative dose of antipsychotic drugs administered to the patient increase. However, the syndrome can develop, although much less commonly, after relatively brief treatment periods at low doses.

There is no known treatment for established cases of tardive dyskinesia, although the syndrome may remit, partially or completely, if antipsychotic treatment is withdrawn. Antipsychotic treatment, itself, however, may suppress (or partially suppress) the signs and symptoms of the syndrome and thereby may possibly mask the underlying process. The effect that symptomatic suppression has upon the long-term course of the syndrome is unknown.

Given these considerations, antipsychotic drugs should be prescribed in a manner that is most likely to minimize the occurrence of tardive dyskinesia. Chronic antipsychotic treatment should generally be reserved for patients who suffer from a chronic illness that, 1) is known to respond to antipsychotic drugs, and 2) for whom alternative, equally effective, but potentially less harmful treatments are not available or appropriate. In patients who do require chronic treatment, the smallest dose and the shortest duration of treatment producing a satisfactory clinical response should be sought. The need for continued treatment should be reassessed periodically.

If signs and symptoms of tardive dyskinesia appear in a patient on antipsychotics, drug discontinuation should be considered. However, some patients may require treatment despite the presence of the syndrome.

(For further information about the description of tardive dyskinesia and its clinical detection, please refer to ADVERSE REACTIONS and PRECAUTIONS—Information for Patients.)

Neuroleptic Malignant Syndrome (NMS)

A potentially fatal symptom complex sometimes referred to as Neuroleptic Malignant Syndrome (NMS) has been reported in association with antipsychotic drugs. Clinical manifestations of NMS are hyperpyrexia, muscle rigidity, altered mental status (including catatonic signs) and evidence of autonomic instability (irregular pulse or blood pressure, tachycardia, diaphoresis, and cardiac dysrhythmias). Additional signs may include elevated creatine phosphokinase, myoglobinuria (rhabdomyolysis) and acute renal failure.

The diagnostic evaluation of patients with this syndrome is complicated. In arriving at a diagnosis, it is important to identify cases where the clinical presentation includes both serious medical illness (e.g., pneumonia, systemic infection, etc.) and untreated or inadequately treated extrapyramidal signs and symptoms (EPS). Other important considerations in the differential diagnosis include central anticholinergic toxicity, heat stroke, drug fever and primary central nervous system (CNS) pathology.

The management of NMS should include 1) immediate discontinuation of antipsychotic drugs and other drugs not essential to concurrent therapy, 2) intensive symptomatic treatment and medical monitoring, and 3) treatment of any concomitant serious medical problems for which specific treatments are available. There is no general agreement about specific pharmacological treatment regimens for uncomplicated NMS.

If a patient requires antipsychotic drug treatment after recovery from NMS, the potential reintroduction of drug therapy should be carefully considered. The patient should be carefully monitored, since recurrences of NMS have been reported.

Hyperpyrexia, not associated with the above symptom complex, has been reported with other antipsychotic drugs.

Other

Sudden, unexpected deaths have occurred in experimental studies of conditions other than Tourette's Disorder. These deaths occurred while patients were receiving dosages in the range of 1 mg per kg. One possible mechanism for such deaths is prolongation of the QT interval predisposing patients to ventricular arrhythmia. An electrocardiogram should be performed before ORAP treatment is initiated and periodically thereafter, especially during the period of dose adjustment.

ORAP may have a tumorigenic potential. Based on studies conducted in mice, it is known that pimozide can produce a dose related increase in pituitary tumors. The full significance of this finding is not known, but should be taken into consideration in the physician's and patient's decisions to use this drug product. This finding should be given special consideration when the patient is young and chronic use of pimozide is anticipated. (see PRECAUTIONS—Carcinogenesis, Mutagenesis, Impairment of Fertility)

PRECAUTIONS

General

ORAP (pimozide) may impair the mental and/or physical abilities required for the performance of potentially hazard-

ous tasks, such as driving a car or operating machinery, especially during the first few days of therapy.

ORAP produces anticholinergic side effects and should be used with caution in individuals whose conditions may be aggravated by anticholinergic activity.

ORAP should be administered cautiously to patients with impairment of liver or kidney function, because it is metabolized by the liver and excreted by the kidneys.

Antipsychotics should be administered with caution to patients receiving anticonvulsant medication, with a history of seizures, or with EEG abnormalities, because they may lower the convulsive threshold. If indicated, adequate anticonvulsant therapy should be maintained concomitantly.

Information for Patients

Treatment with ORAP exposes the patient to serious risks. A decision to use ORAP chronically in Tourette's Disorder is one that deserves full consideration by the patient (or patient's family) as well as by the treating physician. Because the goal of treatment is symptomatic improvement, the patient's view of the need for treatment and assessment of response are critical in evaluating the impact of therapy and weighing its benefits against the risks. Since the physician is the primary source of information about the use of a drug in any disease, it is recommended that the following information be discussed with patients and/or their families.

ORAP is intended only for use in patients with Tourette's Disorder whose symptoms are severe and who cannot tolerate, or who do not respond to HALDOL® (haloperidol).

Given the likelihood that a proportion of patients exposed chronically to antipsychotics will develop tardive dyskinesia, it is advised that all patients in whom chronic use is contemplated be given, if possible, full information about this risk. The decision to inform patients and/or their guardians must obviously take into account the clinical circumstances and the competency of the patient to understand the information provided.

There is *very* little information available on the use of ORAP in children under 12 years of age.

The information available on ORAP from foreign marketing experience and from U.S. clinical trials indicate that ORAP has a side effect profile similar to that of other antipsychotic drugs. Patients should be informed that all types of side effects associated with the use of antipsychotics may be associated with the use of ORAP.

In addition, sudden, unexpected deaths have occurred in patients taking high doses of ORAP for conditions other than Tourette's Disorder. These deaths may have been the result of an effect of ORAP upon the heart. Therefore, patients should be instructed not to exceed the prescribed dose of ORAP and they should realize the need for the initial ECG and for follow-up ECGs during treatment.

Also, pimozide, at a dose about 15 times that given humans, caused an increase in the number of benign tumors of the pituitary gland in female mice. It is not possible to say how important this is. Similar tumors were not seen in rats given pimozide, nor at lower doses in mice, which is reassuring. However, any such finding must be considered to suggest a possible risk of long term use of the drug.

Laboratory Tests

An ECG should be done at baseline and periodically thereafter throughout the period of dose adjustment. Any indication of prolongation of the QT$_c$ interval beyond an absolute limit of 0.47 seconds (children) or 0.52 seconds (adults), or more than 25% above the patient's original baseline should be considered a basis for stopping further dose increase (see CONTRAINDICATIONS) and considering a lower dose.

Since hypokalemia has been associated with ventricular arrhythmias, potassium insufficiency, secondary to diuretics, diarrhea, or other cause, should be corrected before ORAP therapy is initiated and normal potassium maintained during therapy.

Drug Interactions

Because ORAP prolongs the QT interval of the electrocardiogram, an additive effect on QT interval would be anticipated if administered with other drugs, such as phenothiazines, tricyclic antidepressants or antiarrhythmic agents, which prolong the QT interval. Such concomitant administration should not be undertaken (see CONTRAINDICATIONS).

ORAP may be capable of potentiating CNS depressants, including analgesics, sedatives, anxiolytics, and alcohol.

Carcinogenesis, Mutagenesis, Impairment of Fertility

Carcinogenicity studies were conducted in mice and rats. In mice, pimozide causes a dose-related increase in pituitary and mammary tumors.

When mice were treated for up to 18 months with pimozide, pituitary gland changes developed in females only. These changes were characterized as hyperplasia at doses approximating the human dose and adenoma at doses about fifteen times the maximum recommended human dose on a mg per kg basis. The mechanism for the induction of pituitary tumors in mice is not known.

Mammary gland tumors in female mice were also increased, but these tumors are expected in rodents treated with antipsychotic drugs which elevate prolactin levels. Chronic administration of an antipsychotic also causes elevated prolactin levels in humans. Tissue culture experiments indicate

that approximately one-third of human breast cancers are prolactin-dependent *in vitro*, a factor of potential importance if the prescription of these drugs is contemplated in a patient with a previously detected breast cancer. Although disturbances such as galactorrhea, amenorrhea, gynecomastia, and impotence have been reported with antipsychotic drugs, the clinical significance of elevated serum prolactin levels is unknown for most patients. Neither clinical studies nor epidemiologic studies conducted to date have shown an association between chronic administration of these drugs and mammary tumorigenesis. The available evidence, however, is considered too limited to be conclusive at this time.

In a 24 month carcinogenicity study in rats, animals received up to 50 times the maximum recommended human dose. No increased incidence of overall tumors or tumors at any site was observed in either sex. Because of the limited number of animals surviving this study, the meaning of these results is unclear.

Pimozide did not have mutagenic activity in the Ames test with four bacterial test strains, in the mouse dominant lethal test or in the micronucleus test in rats.

Reproduction studies in animals were not adequate to assess all aspects of fertility. Nevertheless, female rats administered pimozide had prolonged estrus cycles, an effect also produced by other antipsychotic drugs.

Pregnancy

Category C. Reproduction studies performed in rats and rabbits at oral doses up to 8 times the maximum human dose did not reveal evidence of teratogenicity. In the rat, however, this multiple of the human dose resulted in decreased pregnancies and in the retarded development of fetuses. These effects are thought to be due to an inhibition or delay in implantation which is also observed in rodents administered other antipsychotic drugs. In the rabbit, maternal toxicity, mortality, decreased weight gain, and embryotoxicity including increased resorptions were dose related. Because animal reproduction studies are not always predictive of human response, pimozide should be given to a pregnant woman only if the potential benefits of treatment clearly outweigh the potential risks.

Labor and Delivery

This drug has no recognized use in labor or delivery.

Nursing Mothers

It is not known whether pimozide is excreted in human milk. Because many drugs are excreted in human milk and because of the potential for tumorigenicity and unknown cardiovascular effects in the infant, a decision should be made whether to discontinue nursing or to discontinue the drug, taking into account the importance of the drug to the mother.

Pediatric Use

Although Tourette's Disorder most often has its onset between the ages of 2 and 15 years, information on the use and efficacy of ORAP in patients less than 12 years of age is limited.

Because its use and safety have not been evaluated in other childhood disorders, ORAP is not recommended for use in any condition other than Tourette's Disorder.

ADVERSE REACTIONS

General

Extrapyramidal reactions: Neuromuscular (extrapyramidal) reactions during the administration of ORAP (pimozide) have been reported frequently, often during the first few days of treatment. In most patients, these reactions involved Parkinson-like symptoms which, when first observed, were usually mild to moderately severe and usually reversible. Other types of neuromuscular reactions (motor restlessness, dystonia, akathisia, hyperreflexia, opisthotonos, oculogyric crises) have been reported far less frequently. Severe extrapyramidal reactions have been reported to occur at relatively low doses. Generally the occurrence and severity of most extrapyramidal symptoms are dose related since they occur at relatively high doses and have been shown to disappear or become less severe when the dose is reduced. Administration of antiparkinson drugs such as benztropine mesylate or trihexyphenidyl hydrochloride may be required for control of such reactions. It should be noted that persistent extrapyramidal reactions have been reported and that the drug may have to be discontinued in such cases.

Withdrawal Emergent Neurological Signs: Generally, patients receiving short term therapy experience no problems with abrupt discontinuation of antipsychotic drugs. However, some patients on maintenance treatment experience transient dyskinetic signs after abrupt withdrawal. In certain of these cases the dyskinetic movements are indistinguishable from the syndrome described below under "Tardive Dyskinesia" except for duration. It is not known whether gradual withdrawal of antipsychotic drugs will reduce the rate of occurrence of withdrawal emergent neurological signs but until further evidence becomes available, it seems reasonable to gradually withdraw use of ORAP.

Tardive Dyskinesia: ORAP may be associated with persistent dyskinesias. Tardive dyskinesia, a syndrome consisting of potentially irreversible, involuntary, dyskinetic movements, may appear in some patients on long-term therapy or

may occur after drug therapy has been discontinued. The risk appears to be greater in elderly patients on high-dose therapy, especially females. The symptoms are persistent and in some patients appear irreversible. The syndrome is characterized by rhythmical involuntary movements of tongue, face, mouth or jaw (e.g., protrusion of tongue, puffing of cheeks, puckering of mouth, chewing movements). Sometimes these may be accompanied by involuntary movements of extremities and the trunk.

There is no known effective treatment for tardive dyskinesia; antiparkinson agents usually do not alleviate the symptoms of this syndrome. It is suggested that all antipsychotic agents be discontinued if these symptoms appear. Should it be necessary to reinstitute treatment, or increase the dosage of the agent, or switch to a different antipsychotic agent, this syndrome may be masked.

It has been reported that fine vermicular movement of the tongue may be an early sign of tardive dyskinesia and if the medication is stopped at that time the syndrome may not develop.

Electrocardiographic Changes: Electrocardiographic changes have been observed in clinical trials of ORAP in Tourette's Disorder and schizophrenia. These have included prolongation of the QT interval, flattening, notching and inversion of the T wave and the appearance of U waves. Sudden, unexpected deaths and grand mal seizure have occurred at doses above 20 mg/day.

Neuroleptic Malignant Syndrome: Neuroleptic malignant syndrome (NMS) has been reported with ORAP. (See WARNINGS for further information concerning NMS.)

Hyperpyrexia: Hyperpyrexia has been reported with other antipsychotic drugs.

Clinical Trials

The following adverse reaction tabulation was derived from 20 patients in a 6 week long placebo controlled clinical trial of ORAP in Tourette's Disorder.

Body System/ Adverse Reaction	Pimozide (N = 20)	Placebo N = 20)
Body as a Whole		
Headache	1	2
Gastrointestinal		
Dry mouth	5	1
Diarrhea	1	0
Nausea	0	2
Vomiting	0	1
Constipation	4	2
Eructations	0	1
Thirsty	1	0
Appetite increase	1	0
Endocrine		
Menstrual disorder	0	1
Breast secretions	0	1
Musculoskeletal		
Muscle cramps	0	1
Muscle tightness	3	0
Stooped posture	2	0
CNS		
Drowsiness	7	3
Sedation	14	5
Insomnia	2	2
Dizziness	0	1
Akathisia	8	0
Rigidity	2	0
Speech disorder	2	0
Handwriting change	1	0
Akinesia	8	0
Psychiatric		
Depression	2	3
Excitement	0	1
Nervous	1	0
Adverse behavior effect	5	0
Special Senses		
Visual disturbance	4	0
Taste change	1	0
Sensitivity of eyes to light	1	0
Decreased accom- modation	4	1
Spots before eyes	0	1
Urogenital		
Impotence	3	0

Because clinical investigational experience with ORAP in Tourette's Disorder is limited, uncommon adverse reactions may not have been detected. The physician should consider that other adverse reactions associated with antipsychotics may occur.

Other Adverse Reactions

In addition to the adverse reactions listed above, those listed below have been reported in U.S. clinical trials of ORAP in conditions other than Tourette's Disorder.

Body as a Whole: Asthenia, chest pain, periorbital edema

Cardiovascular/Respiratory: Postural hypotension, hypotension, hypertension, tachycardia, palpitations

Gastrointestinal: Increased salivation, nausea, vomiting, anorexis, GI distress

Endocrine: Loss of libido

Metabolic/Nutritional: Weight gain, weight loss

Central Nervous System: Dizziness, tremor, parkinsonism, fainting, dyskinesia

Psychiatric: Excitement

Skin: Rash, sweating, skin irritation

Special Senses: Blurred vision, cataracts

Urogenital: Nocturia, urinary frequency

Postmarketing Reports

The following experiences were described in spontaneous postmarketing reports. These reports do not provide sufficient information to establish a clear causal relationship with the use of ORAP.

Hematologic: Hemolytic anemia.

Other: Seizure has been reported in one patient.

OVERDOSAGE

In general, the signs and symptoms of overdosage with ORAP (pimozide) would be an exaggeration of known pharmacologic effects and adverse reactions, the most prominent of which would be: 1) electrocardiographic abnormalities, 2) severe extrapyramidal reactions, 3) hypotension, 4) a comatose state with respiratory depression.

In the event of overdosage, gastric lavage, establishment of a patent airway and, if necessary, mechanically-assisted respiration are advised. Electrocardiographic monitoring should commence immediately and continue until the ECG parameters are within the normal range. Hypotension and circlatory collapse may be counteracted by use of intravenous fluids, plasma, or concentrated albumin, and vasopressor agents such as metaraminol, phenylephrine and norepinephrine. Epinephrine should not be used. In case of severe extrapyramidal reactions, antiparkinson medication should be administered. Because of the long half-life of pimozide, patients who take an overdose should be observed for at least 4 days. As with all drugs, the physician should consider contacting a poison control center for additional information on the treatment of overdose.

DOSAGE AND ADMINISTRATION

Reliable dose response data for the effects of ORAP (pimozide) on tic manifestations in Tourette's Disorder patients below the age of twelve are not available. Consequently, the suppression of tics by ORAP requires a slow and gradual introduction of the drug. The patient's dose should be carefully adjusted to a point where the suppression of tics and the relief afforded is balanced against the untoward side effects of the drug.

An ECG should be done at baseline and periodically thereafter especially during the period of dose adjustment (see WARNINGS and PRECAUTIONS-Laboratory Tests).

In general, treatment with ORAP should be initiated with a dose of 1 to 2 mg a day in divided doses. The dose may be increased thereafter every other day. Most patients are maintained at less than 0.2 mg/kg per day, or 10 mg/day, whichever is less. Doses greater than 0.2 mg/kg/day or 10 mg/day are not recommended.

Periodic attempts should be made to reduce the dosage of ORAP to see whether or not tics persist at the level and extent first identified. In attempts to reduce the dosage of ORAP, consideration should be given to the possibility that increases of tic intensity and frequency may represent a transient, withdrawal related phenomenon rather than a return of disease symptoms. Specifically, one to two weeks should be allowed to elapse before one concludes that an increase in tic manifestations is a function of the underlying disease syndrome rather than a response to drug withdrawal. A gradual withdrawal is recommended in any case.

ANIMAL PHARMACOLOGY

A chronic study in dogs indicated that pimozide caused gingival hyperplasia when administered for several months at about 5 times the maximum recommended human dose. This condition was reversible after withdrawal. This condition has not been observed following chronic administration of ORAP to man.

HOW SUPPLIED

ORAP™ (pimozide) 2 mg tablets, white, scored, imprinted "LEMMON" and "ORAP 2"—NDC 57844-187-01, bottles of 100.

Dispense in a tight, light-resistant container as defined in the official compendium.

Pharmacist: Dispense in a child-resistant container.

Shown in Product Identification Section, page 409

Gebauer Company
9410 ST. CATHERINE AVE.
CLEVELAND, OH 44104

ETHYL CHLORIDE, U.S.P. ℞
(Chloroethane)

INDICATIONS AND USAGE
Ethyl Chloride is a vapocoolant intended for topical application to control pain associated with minor surgical procedures (such as lancing boils, or incision and drainage of small abscesses), athletic injuries, injections, and for treatment of myofascial pain, restricted motion, and muscle spasm.

PRECAUTIONS
Inhalation of Ethyl Chloride should be avoided as it may produce narcotic and general anesthetic effects, and may produce deep anesthesia or fatal coma with respiratory or cardiac arrest. Ethyl Chloride is flammable and should never be used in the presence of an open flame, or electrical cautery equipment. When used to produce local freezing of tissues, adjacent skin areas should be protected by application of petrolatum. The thawing process may be painful, and freezing may lower local resistance to infection and delay healing.

ADVERSE REACTIONS
Cutaneous sensitization may occur, but appears to be extremely rare. Freezing can occasionally alter pigmentation.

CONTRAINDICATIONS
Ethyl Chloride is contraindicated in individuals with a history of hypersensitivity to it. This product should not be used on patients having vascular impairment of the extremities.

WARNINGS
For external use only.
Skin absorption of Ethyl Chloride can occur; no cases of chronic poisoning have been reported. Ethyl Chloride is known as a liver and kidney toxin; long term exposure may cause liver or kidney damage.
Contents under pressure. Store in a cool place. Do not store above 120°F. Do not store on or near high frequency ultrasound equipment.

DOSAGE AND ADMINISTRATION
To apply Ethyl Chloride from metal tube, invert nozzle 12 inches (30 cm.) above the treatment area. Open adjustable dispensing valve until the spray flows freely.
To apply Ethyl Chloride from amber bottle with dispenseal valve, invert over the treatment area approximately 12 inches (30 cm.) away from site of application. Open dispenseal spring valve completely allowing Ethyl Chloride to flow in a stream from the bottle.

1. TOPICAL ANESTHESIA IN MINOR SURGERY
The operative site should be cleansed with a suitable antiseptic. Apply petrolatum to protect the adjacent area. Spray Ethyl Chloride for a few seconds to the point of frost formation, when the tissue becomes white. Avoid prolonged spraying of skin beyond this state. The anesthetic action of Ethyl Chloride rarely lasts more than a few seconds to a minute. Quickly swab operative site with antiseptic and promptly make incision. Reapply as needed.

2. SPORTS INJURIES
The pain of bruises, contusions, abrasions, swelling, and minor sprains may be controlled with Ethyl Chloride.
Spray affected area for a few seconds until the tissue begins to frost and turn white. Avoid spraying of skin beyond this state. Use as you would ice. The amount of cooling depends on the dosage. The smallest dose needed to produce the desired effect should be used. Dosage varies with the nozzle size and duration of application.
Determine the extent of injury (fracture, sprain, etc.). The anesthetic effect of Ethyl Chloride rarely lasts more than a few seconds to a minute. This time interval is usually sufficient to help reduce or relieve the initial trauma of the injury.

3. FOR PRE-INJECTION ANESTHESIA
Prepare syringe and have it ready. Spray skin with Ethyl Chloride from a distance of about 12 inches (30 cm.) continuously for 3 to 5 seconds; do not frost skin. Swab skin with alcohol and quickly introduce needle with skin taut.

4. SPRAY and STRETCH TECHNIQUE for MYOFASCIAL PAIN
Ethyl Chloride may be used as a counterirritant in the management of myofascial pain, restricted motion, and muscle spasm. Clinical conditions that may respond to Ethyl Chloride include low back pain (due to muscle spasm), acute stiff neck, torticollis, acute bursitus of the shoulder, muscle spasm associated with osteoarthritis, tight hamstring, sprained ankle, masseter muscle spasm, certain types of headache, and referred pain due to irritated trigger point. Relief of pain facilitates early mobilization in restoration of muscle function. The Spray and Stretch technique is a therapeutic system which involves three stages: EVALUATION, SPRAYING, and STRETCHING.
The therapeutic value of Spray and Stretch becomes most effective when the practitioner has mastered all stages and applies them in the proper sequence.

I. EVALUATION
During the evaluation phase the cause of pain is determined as local spasm or an irritated trigger point. The method of applying the spray to a muscle spasm differs slightly from application to a trigger point. A trigger point is a deep hypersensitive localized spot in a muscle which causes a referred pain pattern. With trigger points the source of pain is seldom the site of the pain. A trigger point may be detected by a snapping palpation over the muscle, causing the muscle in which the irritated trigger point is situated to "jump".

II. SPRAYING
A. Patient should assume a comfortable position.
B. Take precautions to cover the patient's eyes, nose, mouth, if spraying near face.
C. Hold bottle in an upside down position 12 to 18 inches (30 to 45 cm.) away from the treatment surface allowing the jet stream of vapocoolant to meet the skin at an acute angle to lessen the shock of impact.
D. The spray is directed in parallel sweeps 1.5 to 2 cm. apart. The rate of spraying is approximately 10 cm/sec. and is continued until the entire muscle has been covered. The number of sweeps is determined by the size of the muscle. In the case of trigger point, the spray should be applied over the trigger point, through and over the reference zone. In the case of muscle spasm, the spray should be applied from origin to insertion.

III. STRETCHING
During application of the spray, the muscle is passively stretched. Force is gradually increased with successive sweeps, and the slack is smoothly taken up as the muscle relaxes, establishing a new stretch length.
Reaching the full normal length of the muscle is necessary to completely inactivate trigger points and relieve pain.
After rewarming, the procedure may be repeated as necessary. Moist heat should be applied for 10 to 15 minutes following treatment. For lasting benefit, any factors that perpetuate the trigger mechanism must be eliminated.

HOW SUPPLIED

100 gram metal tube	(NDC 0386-0001-05)
4 ounce amber glass bottle:	
Fine Spray	(NDC 0386-0001-04)
Medium Spray	(NDC 0386-0001-03)
Coarse Spray	(NDC 0386-0001-02)
"Spra Pak"	(NDC 0386-0001-01)

CAUTION
Federal law prohibits dispensing without a prescription.

FLUORI-METHANE® ℞
(Dichlorodifluoromethane 15%
Trichloromonofluoromethane 85%)

INDICATIONS AND USAGE
Fluori-Methane Spray is a vapocoolant intended for topical application in the management of myofascial pain, restricted motion, and muscle spasm, and for the control of pain associated with injections.
Clinical conditions that may respond to Spray and Stretch include low back pain (due to muscle spasm), acute stiff neck, torticollis, muscle spasm associated with osteoarthritis, ankle sprain, tight hamstring, masseter muscle spasm, certain types of headache, and referred pain due to trigger points. Relief of pain facilitates early mobilization in restoration of muscle function.

PRECAUTIONS
Care should be taken to minimize inhalation of vapors, especially with application around head or neck. Avoid contact with eyes. Fluori-Methane should not be applied to the point of frost formation.

ADVERSE REACTIONS
Cutaneous sensitization may occur, but appears to be extremely rare. Freezing can occasionally alter pigmentation.

CONTRAINDICATIONS
Fluori-Methane is contraindicated in individuals with a history of hypersensitivity to dichlorodifluoromethane, and/or trichloromonofluoromethane. This product should not be used on patients having vascular impairment of the extremities.

WARNINGS
For external use only.
Dichlorodifluoromethane and trichloromonofluoromethane are not classified as carcinogens. Based on animal studies and human experience, these fluorocarbons pose no hazard to man relative to systemic toxicity, carcinogenicity, mutagenicity, or teratogenicity when occupational exposures are below 1000 p.p.m. over an 8 hour time weighted average.
Contents under pressure. Store in a cool place. Do not store above 120°F. Do not store on or near high frequency ultrasound equipment.

DOSAGE AND ADMINISTRATION
To apply Fluori-Methane, invert the bottle over the treatment area approximately 12 inches (30 cm.) away from site of application. Open dispenseal spring valve completely, allowing the liquid to flow in a stream from the bottle.

1. SPRAY and STRETCH TECHNIQUE for MYOFASCIAL PAIN
Spray and Stretch technique is a therapeutic system which involves three stages: EVALUATION, SPRAYING, and STRETCHING.
The therapeutic value of Spray and Stretch becomes most effective when the practitioner has mastered all stages and applies them in proper sequence.

I. EVALUATION
During the evaluation phase the cause of pain is determined as local spasm or an irritated trigger point. The method of applying the spray to a muscle spasm differs slightly from application to a trigger point. A trigger point is a deep hypersensitive localized spot in a muscle which causes a referred pain pattern. With trigger points the source of pain is seldom the site of the pain. A trigger point may be detected by a snapping palpation over the muscle, causing the muscle in which the irritated trigger point is situated to "jump".

II. SPRAYING
A. Patient should assume a comfortable position.
B. Take precautions to cover the patient's eyes, nose, mouth, if spraying near face.
C. Hold bottle in an upside down position 12 to 18 inches (30 to 45 cm.) away from the treatment surface allowing the jet stream of vapocoolant to meet the skin at an acute angle to lessen the shock of impact.
D. The spray is directed in parallel sweeps 1.5 to 2 cm. apart. The rate of spraying is approximately 10 cm/sec. and is continued until the entire muscle has been covered. The number of sweeps is determined by the size of the muscle. In the case of a trigger point, the spray should be applied over the trigger point, through and over the reference zone. In the case of muscle spasm, the spray should be applied from origin to insertion.

III. STRETCHING
During application of the spray, the muscle is passively stretched. Force is gradually increased with successive sweeps, and the slack is smoothly taken up as the muscle relaxes, establishing a new stretch length.
Reaching the full normal length of the muscle is necessary to completely inactivate trigger points and relieve pain.
After rewarming, the procedure may be repeated as necessary. Moist heat should be applied for 10 to 15 minutes following treatment.
For lasting benefit, any factors that perpetuate the trigger mechanism must be eliminated.

2. PRE-INJECTION ANESTHESIA
Prepare syringe and have it ready. Spray skin with Fluori-Methane, from a distance of about 12 inches (30 cm.) continuously for 3 to 5 seconds; do not frost the skin. Swab skin with alcohol and quickly introduce needle with skin taut.

HOW SUPPLIED

4 ounce amber glass bottle.	
Calibrated Fine Spray	(NDC 0386-0003-04)
Calibrated Medium Spray	(NDC 0386-0003-05)

CAUTION
Federal law prohibits dispensing without a prescription.

FLURO-ETHYL® ℞
(Ethyl Chloride, U.S.P., 25%
Dichlorotetrafluoroethane, N.F., 75%)

INDICATIONS and USAGE
Fluro-Ethyl is a topical refrigerant anesthetic intended to control the pain associated with minor surgical procedures, dermabrasion, injections, contusions and minor strains.

PRECAUTIONS
Inhalation of Fluro-Ethyl should be avoided as it may produce narcotic and general anesthetic effects, and may produce deep anesthesia, or fatal coma with respiratory or cardiac arrest. When used to produce local freezing of tissues, adjacent skin areas should be protected by application of petrolatum. The thawing process may be painful, and freezing may lower local resistance to infection and delay healing.

ADVERSE REACTIONS
Cutaneous sensitization may occur, but appears to be extremely rare. Freezing can occasionally alter pigmentation. Frostbite may occur.

CONTRAINDICATIONS
Fluro-Ethyl is contraindicated in individuals with a history of hypersensitivity to Ethyl Chloride or Dichlorotetrafluoroethane. Fluro-Ethyl should not be used on patients having vascular impairment of the extremities.

WARNINGS

For external use only.

The components of Fluro-Ethyl are not listed as carcinogens by IARC, NTP or OSHA. Based on animal studies and human experiences this mixture poses no hazard to man relative to systemic toxicity, carcinogenicity, mutagenicity, or teratogenicity when occupational exposures are below its recommended exposure limits.

Skin absorption of Ethyl Chloride can occur; no cases of chronic poisoning have been reported. Ethyl Chloride is known as a liver and kidney toxin; long term exposure may cause liver or kidney damage.

Fluro-Ethyl can cause frostbite.

Contents under pressure. Store in a cool place, do not store above 120°F.

DOSAGE and ADMINISTRATION

To apply Fluro-Ethyl, invert the container over the treatment area approximately 2 to 4 inches (5-10cm) from the site of application. Press gently on side of the spray valve allowing the liquid to emerge as a fine mist spray.

1. TOPICAL ANESTHESIA IN MINOR SURGERY

The operative site should be cleansed with a suitable antiseptic. Apply petrolatum to protect the adjacent area. Spray Fluro-Ethyl for a few seconds to the point of frost formation, when the tissue becomes white. Avoid prolonged spraying of skin beyond this state. The anesthetic action of Fluro-Ethyl rarely lasts more than a few seconds to a minute. Quickly swab operative site with antiseptic and promptly make incision. Reapply as needed.

2. DERMABRASION

The operative site should be cleansed with a suitable antiseptic. Apply petrolatum to protect adjacent areas. Take precautions to cover the patient's eyes, nose, mouth, if spraying near the face. To firm the skin and numb the dermabrasion site, spray treatment area for 20 to 30 seconds prior to starting the dermabrasion procedure. Reapply as necessary during the procedure to maintain desired skin firmness.

3. FOR PRE-INJECTION ANESTHESIA

Prepare syringe and have it ready. Spray skin with Fluro-Ethyl from a distance of about 4 inches (10 cm) continuously for 2 to 3 seconds; do not frost skin. Swab skin with alcohol and quickly introduce needle with skin taut.

4. CONTUSIONS and MINOR STRAINS

The pain of bruises, contusions, and minor sprains may be controlled with Fluro-Ethyl.

Spray affected area from a distance of 6 to 12 inches (15 to 30 cm.) for a few seconds until the tissue begins to frost and turn white. Avoid spraying of skin beyond this state. Use as you would ice. The amount of cooling depends on the dosage. The smallest dose needed to produce the desired effect should be used.

Determine the extent of injury (fracture, sprain, etc.). The anesthetic effect of Fluro-Ethyl rarely lasts more than a few seconds to a minute. This time interval is usually sufficient to help reduce or relieve the initial trauma of the injury.

HOW SUPPLIED

Net weight 9 ounce aerosol spray can (NDC 0386-0002-09)

CAUTION

Federal law prohibits dispensing without a prescription.

For supporting educational materials contact Gebauer Company.

GEIGY Pharmaceuticals
Division of CIBA-GEIGY Corporation
ARDSLEY, NY 10502

GY-CODE® INDEX

Geigy Pharmaceuticals has established a Drug Identity Code System entitled GY-CODE. This system affords a convenient and accurate means of uniquely identifying each Geigy solid dosage form on which the GY-CODE number and the name "Geigy" appear. The GY-CODE number also appears as part of the National Drug Code number.

GY-CODE NUMBER	PROD. DESCRIPTION		NATIONAL DRUG CODE
20 Tofranil-PM® Capsules			
	imipramine pamoate	75 mg	
	Coral-colored capsules		
	30's		0028-0020-26
	100's		0028-0020-01
	100's Unit Dose Pkg.		0028-0020-61

22 Tofranil-PM® Capsules		
imipramine pamoate	150 mg	
Coral-colored capsules		
30's		0028-0022-26
100's		0028-0022-01
23 Lioresal® Tablets		
baclofen	10 mg	
White, oval, scored tablets		
100's		0028-0023-01
100's Unit Dose Pkg.		0028-0023-61
32 Tofranil® Tablets		
imipramine hydrochloride USP	10 mg	
Triangular, coral-colored, coated tablets		
100's		0028-0032-01
33 Lioresal® Tablets		
baclofen	20 mg	
White, capsule shaped, scored tablets		
100's		0028-0033-01
100's Unit Dose Pkg.		0028-0033-61
40 Tofranil-PM® Capsules		
imipramine pamoate	100 mg	
Dark yellow/coral-colored capsules		
30's		0028-0040-26
100's		0028-0040-01
42 Constant-T® Tablets		
theophylline (anhydrous)	200 mg	
Light pink, oval, scored tablets		
100's		0028-0042-01
100's Unit Dose Pkg.		0028-0042-61
Gy-Pak® 60's		
One Unit (12 × 60)		0028-0042-73
45 Tofranil-PM® Capsules		
imipramine pamoate	125 mg	
Light yellow/coral-colored capsules		
30's		0028-0045-26
100's		0028-0045-01
48 PBZ-SR® Tablets		
tripelennamine hydrochloride	100 mg	
Lavender-colored tablets		
100's		0028-0048-01
51 Lopressor® Tablets		
metoprolol tartrate	50 mg	
Light red, capsule-shaped, scored tablets		
100's		0028-0051-01
1000's		0028-0051-10
100's Unit Dose Pkg.		0028-0051-61
Gy-Pak® 60's		
One Unit (12 × 60)		0028-0051-73
Gy-Pak® 100's		
One Unit (12 × 100)		0028-0051-65
57 Constant-T® Tablets		
theophylline (anhydrous)	300 mg	
Light blue, oval, scored tablets		
100's		0028-0057-01
100's Unit Dose Pkg.		0028-0057-61
Gy-Pak® 60's		
One Unit (12 × 60)		0028-0057-73
Six Units (72 × 60)		0028-0057-73
58 Voltaren® Tablets		
diclofenac sodium	25 mg	
Yellow, biconvex with beveled edges, enteric-coated		
60's		0028-0058-60
100's		0028-0058-01
100's Unit Dose Pkg.		0028-0058-61
71 Lopressor® Tablets		
metoprolol tartrate	100 mg	
Light blue, capsule-shaped, scored tablets		
100's		0028-0071-01
1000's		0028-0071-10
100's Unit Dose Pkg.		0028-0071-61
Gy-Pak® 60's		
One Unit (12 × 60)		0028-0071-73
Six Units (72 × 60)		0028-0071-73
Gy-Pak® 100's		
One Unit (12 × 100)		0028-0071-65
Six Units (72 × 100)		0028-0071-65
72 Brethine® Tablets		
terbutaline sulfate USP	2.5 mg	
Oval, white, scored tablets		
100's		0028-0072-01
1000's		0028-0072-10
100's Unit Dose Pkg.		0028-0072-61
Gy-Pak® 100's		
One Unit (12 × 100)		0028-0072-65
Six Units (72 × 100)		0028-0072-65
105 Brethine® Tablets		
terbutaline sulfate USP	5 mg	
Round, scored, white tablets		
100's		0028-0105-01
1000's		0028-0105-10
100's Unit Dose Pkg.		0028-0105-61
Gy-Pak® 100's		
One unit (12 × 100)		0028-0105-65
Six units (72 × 100)		0028-0105-65

108 Lamprene® Capsules		
clofazimine	50 mg	
Brown, spherical capsules		
100's		0028-0108-01
109 Lamprene® Capsules		
clofazimine	100 mg	
Brown, oblong capsules		
100's		0028-0109-01
111 PBZ® Tablets		
tripelennamine hydrochloride USP	25 mg	
Round, white, scored tablets		
100's		0028-0111-01
117 PBZ® Tablets		
tripelennamine hydrochloride USP	50 mg	
Round, white, scored tablets		
100's		0028-0117-01
136 Tofranil® Tablets		
imipramine hydrochloride USP	50 mg	
Coral-colored (white Geigy imprint) coated tablets		
100's		0028-0136-01
1000's		0028-0136-10
Gy-Pak® 100's		
One unit (12 × 100)		0028-0136-65
140 Tofranil® Tablets		
imipramine hydrochloride USP	25 mg	
Coral-colored (black Geigy imprint) coated tablets		
100's		0028-0140-01
1000's		0028-0140-10
Gy-Pak® 100's		
One unit (12 × 100)		0028-0140-65
162 Voltaren® Tablets		
diclofenac sodium	50 mg	
Light brown, biconvex with beveled edges, enteric-coated		
60's		0028-0162-60
100's		0028-0162-01
1000's		0028-0162-10
100's Unit Dose Pkg.		0028-0162-61
164 Voltaren® Tablets		
diclofenac sodium	75 mg	
White, biconvex with beveled edges, enteric-coated		
60's		0028-0164-60
100's		0028-0164-01
1000's		0028-0164-10
100's Unit Dose Pkg.		0028-0164-61
6114 Otrivin® Nasal Drops (0.1%)		
xylometazoline hydrochloride USP		
20 ml		0028-6114-58
6116 Otrivin® Pediatric (0.05%)		
xylometazoline hydrochloride USP		
20 ml		0028-6116-58
6118 Otrivin® Spray (0.1%)		
xylometazoline hydrochloride USP		
15 ml		0028-6118-57
6946 PBZ® Antihistamine Cream		
tripelennamine hydrochloride		
Cream 2% (water-washable base)		
1 oz		0028-6946-76

BRETHAIRE®   ℞

[*breth-air'*]

terbutaline sulfate inhalation aerosol
Bronchodilator Aerosol
For Oral Inhalation Only

DESCRIPTION

Brethaire is a bronchodilator aerosol for oral inhalation. The active ingredient of Brethaire is terbutaline sulfate USP, (±)-α-[(*tert*-butylamino) methyl]-3,5-dihydroxybenzylalcohol sulfate (2:1) (salt), a beta-adrenergic agonist. The empirical formula is $(C_{12}H_{19}NO_3)_2 \cdot H_2SO_4$.

Terbutaline sulfate USP is a white to gray-white crystalline powder. It is odorless or has a faint odor of acetic acid. It is soluble in water and in 0.1N hydrochloric acid, slightly soluble in methanol, and insoluble in chloroform. Its molecular weight is 548.65.

Brethaire is a metered-dose dispenser containing micronized terbutaline sulfate in a suspension of the following composition:

	7.5-ml (10.5-g) Canister
terbutaline sulfate USP	0.075 g
sorbitan trioleate	0.105 g
trichloromonofluoromethane NF	2.58 g
dichlorotetrafluoroethane NF	2.58 g
dichlorodifluoromethane NF	5.16 g

Continued on next page

The full prescribing information for each GEIGY product is contained herein and is that in effect as of September 1, 1992.

GEIGY—Cont.

Each actuation delivers 0.20 mg of terbutaline sulfate from the mouthpiece (0.25 mg valve delivery). Each canister provides at least 300 inhalations.

CLINICAL PHARMACOLOGY

Brethaire is a beta-adrenergic-receptor agonist that has been shown by in vitro and in vivo studies in animals to exert a preferential effect on $beta_2$-adrenergic receptors. While it is recognized that $beta_2$-adrenergic receptors are the predominant receptors in bronchial smooth muscle, recent data indicate that there is a population of $beta_2$-receptors in the human heart existing in a concentration between 10–50%. The precise function of these, however, is not yet established (see PRECAUTIONS). Controlled clinical studies in patients who were administered Brethaire have not revealed a preferential $beta_2$-adrenergic effect.

The pharmacologic effects of beta-adrenergic agonists, including Brethaire, are at least in part attributable to stimulation through beta-adrenergic receptors of intracellular adenyl cyclase, the enzyme which catalyzes the conversion of adenosine triphosphate (ATP) to cyclic $3'5'$- adenosine monophosphate (cAMP). Increased cAMP levels are associated with relaxation of bronchial smooth muscle and inhibition of release of mediators of immediate hypersensitivity from cells, especially from mast cells.

Terbutaline sulfate by inhaler has been shown in controlled clinical studies to relieve bronchospasm associated with chronic obstructive pulmonary disease such as asthma, chronic bronchitis, and emphysema. This action was manifested by a clinically significant improvement in pulmonary function as demonstrated by an increase in FEV_1 of 15% or more in some patients. Terbutaline sulfate by inhaler also produced clinically significant increases in peak expiratory flow rate and instantaneous flow rates at 75, 50, and 25% of vital capacity. There were also clinically significant reductions in functional residual capacity, residual volume, and airway resistance in some patients. Clinically significant improvement in pulmonary function occurred within 5 to 30 minutes in most patients after administration of the drug. The response was well established by 5 minutes and the maximal effect usually occurred between 1 and 2 hours in most patients. Significant bronchodilator activity has been observed to persist for 3 to 4 hours after dosing in many patients in 3-month repetitive-dose studies. With continued administration of Brethaire, the duration of effectiveness decreases in most patients.

Recent studies in laboratory animals (minipigs, rodents, and dogs), recorded the occurrence of cardiac arrhythmias and sudden death (with histologic evidence of myocardial necrosis) when beta agonists and methylxanthines were administered concurrently. The significance of these findings when applied to humans is currently unknown.

INDICATIONS AND USAGE

Brethaire is indicated for the relief of bronchospasm in patients with reversible obstructive airway disease.

In controlled clinical trials the onset of improvement in pulmonary function was within 5 to 30 minutes. These studies also showed that maximum improvement in pulmonary function occurred at 120 minutes following two inhalations of Brethaire and that clinically significant improvement (i.e., 15% increase in FEV_1/predicted FEV_1) generally continued for 3 to 4 hours in most patients. In some studies there was a significant decrease in improvement of pulmonary function noted with continued administration of terbutaline sulfate aerosol. Continued effectiveness of Brethaire was demonstrated over a 14-week period in some patients in these clinical trials. Some patients with asthma, in single-dose studies only, have shown a therapeutic response that was still apparent at 6 hours.

CONTRAINDICATIONS

Brethaire is contraindicated in patients with a history of hypersensitivity to any of its components.

WARNINGS

As with other adrenergic aerosols, the potential for paradoxical bronchospasm (which can be life-threatening) should be kept in mind. If it occurs, the preparation should be discontinued immediately and alternative therapy instituted.

Fatalities have been reported in association with excessive use of inhaled sympathomimetic drugs. The exact cause of death is unknown. As with other beta-adrenergic aerosols, Brethaire should not be used in excess. Controlled clinical studies and other clinical experience have shown that Brethaire, like other inhaled beta-adrenergic agonists, can produce a significant cardiovascular effect in some patients, as measured by pulse rate, blood pressure, symptoms, and/or ECG changes.

There have been rare reports of seizures in patients receiving terbutaline; seizures did not recur in these patients after the drug was discontinued.

The contents of Brethaire are under pressure. Do not puncture the container. Do not use or store it near heat or open flame. Exposure to temperatures above 120°F may cause bursting. Never throw the container into a fire or incinerator. Keep it out of children's reach.

PRECAUTIONS

General

Terbutaline sulfate is a sympathomimetic amine and, as such, should be used with caution in patients with cardiovascular disorders, including coronary insufficiency and hypertension, in patients with hyperthyroidism or diabetes mellitus, and in patients who are unusually responsive to sympathomimetic amines.

Immediate hypersensitivity reactions and exacerbation of bronchospasm have been reported after terbutaline administration.

Large doses of intravenous terbutaline sulfate have been reported to aggravate preexisting diabetes and ketoacidosis. Terbutaline sulfate should not be used for tocolysis.

Although there have been no reports concerning the use of aerosol terbutaline sulfate during labor and delivery, it has been reported that high doses of terbutaline sulfate administered intravenously inhibit uterine contractions. Although this effect is extremely unlikely as a consequence of aerosol use, it should be kept in mind.

Information for Patients

The action of Brethaire may last up to 6 hours, and therefore, it should not be used more frequently than recommended. Patients should not increase the number or frequency of doses without consulting the physician. If symptoms get worse, patients should consult their physician promptly. While taking Brethaire, patients should not take other inhaled medicines that have not been prescribed by the physician.

See illustrated Instructions for Patients.

Drug Interactions

Other sympathomimetic aerosol bronchodilators or epinephrine should not be used concomitantly with terbutaline sulfate. Terbutaline sulfate should be administered with caution to patients being treated with monoamine oxidase inhibitors or tricyclic antidepressants, since the action of terbutaline sulfate on the vascular system may be potentiated. Beta-receptor-blocking agents and terbutaline sulfate inhibit the effect of each other.

Carcinogenesis, Mutagenesis, Impairment of Fertility

A 2-year oral carcinogenesis bioassay of terbutaline sulfate (50, 500, 1000, and 2000 mg/kg, corresponding to 1042, 10,417, 20,833, and 41,667 times the recommended daily adult dose) in Sprague-Dawley rats revealed drug-related changes in the female genital system. Female rats showed drug-related increases in leiomyomas of the mesovarium: 3 (5%) at 50 mg/kg, 17 (28%) at 500 mg/kg, 21 (35%) at 1000 mg/kg, and 23 (38%) at 2000 mg/kg, which were significant at the three highest levels. None occurred in female controls. The incidence of ovarian cysts was significantly elevated at all dose levels except 2000 mg/kg, and hyperplasia of the mesovarium was increased significantly at 500 and 2000 mg/kg.

A 21-month oral (feeding) study of terbutaline sulfate (5, 50, and 200 mg/kg, corresponding to 104, 1042, and 4167 times the recommended daily adult dose) in the mouse revealed no evidence of carcinogenicity.

Studies of terbutaline sulfate have not been conducted to determine mutagenic potential.

A Segment 1 oral reproduction study of terbutaline sulfate (up to 50 mg/kg corresponding to 1042 times the maximum clinical dose) in the rat revealed no adverse effects on fertility.

Pregnancy Category B

Reproduction studies have been performed in rats and rabbits at doses up to 1042 times the human dose and have revealed no evidence of impaired fertility or harm to the fetus due to terbutaline sulfate. There are, however, no adequate and well-controlled studies in pregnant women. Because animal reproduction studies are not always predictive of human response, this drug should be used during pregnancy only if clearly needed. For use in labor and delivery, see PRECAUTIONS, General.

Nursing Mothers

It is not known whether this drug is excreted in human milk. Because many drugs are excreted in human milk, caution should be exercised when terbutaline sulfate is administered to a nursing woman.

Pediatric Use

Safety and effectiveness in children below the age of 12 years have not been established.

ADVERSE REACTIONS

The adverse reactions of terbutaline sulfate are similar to those of other sympathomimetic agents. A 14-week double-blind study compared terbutaline sulfate and isoproterenol aerosols in 259 asthmatic patients. The results of this study showed that the incidence of cardiovascular effects was as follows: palpitations, none with terbutaline and fewer than 5 per 100 with isoproterenol; tachycardia, about 3 per 100 with terbutaline and about 2 per 100 with isoproterenol; and increased blood pressure, fewer than 1 per 100 with terbuta-line and about 2 per 100 with isoproterenol. In the same study, both drugs caused headache and nausea or digestive disorder in fewer than 10 patients per 100, tremor or nervousness in fewer than 5 patients per 100, and drowsiness in fewer than 5 patients per 100. About 4% of patients receiving terbutaline and about 1% of patients receiving isoproterenol had dysrhythmias. In addition, terbutaline sulfate, like other sympathomimetic agents, can cause adverse reactions such as angina, dyspnea and wheezing, vomiting, vertigo, central stimulation, insomnia, unusual taste, and drying or irritation of the oropharynx. Significantly more patients experienced dyspnea or wheezing, or both, after terbutaline than after isoproterenol administration. ECG changes such as sinus pause, atrial premature beats, AV block, ventricular premature beats, ST-T-wave depression, T-wave inversion, sinus bradycardia, and atrial escape beat with aberrant conduction were described after terbutaline administration. ECG changes were similar in frequency after isoproterenol administration.

OVERDOSAGE

Overdosage experience is limited. Excessive adrenergic-receptor stimulation may augment the signs and symptoms listed under ADVERSE REACTIONS and may be accompanied by other adrenergic effects. In the case of terbutaline overdosage, the patient should be treated symptomatically for the sympathomimetic overdosage with careful consideration given to the appropriateness of any chosen therapy and to the possible effect on the patient's underlying disease state.

DOSAGE AND ADMINISTRATION

The usual dosage for adults and children 12 years and older is two inhalations separated by a 60-second interval, repeated every 4 to 6 hours. Dosing should not be repeated more often than every 4 to 6 hours. The use of Brethaire can be continued as medically indicated to control recurring bouts of bronchospasm. During this time most patients gain optimal benefit from regular use of the inhaler. Safe usage for periods extending over several years has been documented.

If a previously effective dosage regimen fails to provide the usual relief, medical advice should be sought immediately, as this is often a sign of seriously worsening asthma, which would require reassessment of therapy.

HOW SUPPLIED

Brethaire contains 75 mg of terbutaline sulfate as a micronized powder in an inert propellant. This is sufficient medication for at least 300 actuations. Each actuation delivers approximately 0.20 mg of terbutaline sulfate from the mouthpiece (0.25 mg valve delivery).

Brethaire canister with mouthpiece, 7.5 ml (10.5 g)
....NDC 0028-5557-88
Brethaire canister refill, 7.5 ml (10.5 g)
....NDC 0028-5557-87
Store between 59°–86°F(15°–30°C).
Dispense with enclosed instructions for use.
Federal law prohibits dispensing without a prescription.

C88-19 (Rev. 7/88)

Dist. by:
GEIGY Pharmaceuticals
Division of CIBA-GEIGY Corporation
Ardsley, New York 10502

BRETHAIRE®   ℞
terbutaline sulfate inhalation aerosol

Instructions For Patients

Before using your BRETHAIRE inhaler, read complete instructions carefully.

1. **SHAKE THE INHALER WELL** immediately before each use. Then remove the cap from the mouthpiece. Test spray into the air before using for the first time and when the aerosol has not been used for a prolonged period. Inspect mouthpiece for possible foreign objects before each subsequent use.

2. **BREATHE OUT FULLY,** expelling as much air from your lungs as possible. Place the mouthpiece fully into the mouth holding the inhaler in its upright position (see Figure 1) and closing the lips around it.

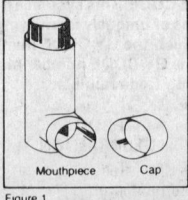
Figure 1

3. **WHILE BREATHING IN DEEPLY, FULLY DEPRESS THE TOP OF THE METAL CANISTER** with your index finger (see Figure 2 at top of next column).

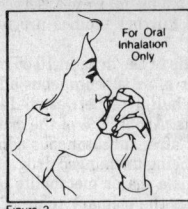

Figure 2

4. **HOLD YOUR BREATH AS LONG AS POSSIBLE.** Before breathing out, remove the inhaler from your mouth and release your finger from the canister.
5. Wait one minute and SHAKE the inhaler again. Repeat steps two through four for a second inhalation if prescribed by your doctor.
6. Replace cap after each use.
7. **CLEANSE THE INHALER THOROUGHLY AND FREQUENTLY.** Remove the metal canister and cleanse the plastic case and cap by rinsing thoroughly in warm running water at least once a day. After thoroughly drying the plastic case and cap, gently replace the canister into the case with a twisting motion and replace the cap.
DOSAGE: Use only as directed by your doctor.
WARNINGS: The action of BRETHAIRE inhaler may last up to six hours and therefore it should not be used more frequently than recommended. Do not increase the number or frequency of doses without consulting your physician. If symptoms do not improve, or get worse, consult your physician immediately. While taking BRETHAIRE inhaler, other inhaled medicines should be used only as prescribed by your physician.
Contents Under Pressure. Do not puncture.
Do not use or store near heat or open flame. Exposure to temperatures above 120°F may cause bursting.
Never throw container into fire or incinerator.
Keep out of reach of children.
Store between 59°–86°F (15°–30°C).

C90-50 (Rev. 11/90)

Dist. by:
GEIGY Pharmaceuticals
Div. of CIBA-GEIGY Corp.
Ardsley, NY 10502
Shown in Product Identification Section, page 409

BRETHANCER®   ℞

[*breth-anc'er*]
spacer-inhaler

The Brethancer spacer-inhaler is recommended for patients with difficulty coordinating conventional aerosol inhalers, so those patients may derive greater therapeutic benefit from their medication.
Although aerosol medications offer patients the benefits of rapidity of action, many patients have difficulty coordinating inhalation with aerosol activation. With Brethancer, the patient no longer requires this coordination but can inhale the aerosolized drug from the spacer tube after the canister is activated.
Unlike other devices designed to aid in the proper use of aerosol medications, Brethancer is compact and easy to carry in its closed form. The Brethancer has three interlocking and telescoping plastic components which, when extended, assist in improving the use of aerosol medications. Opening the device is accomplished in one motion, which simplifies use by the patient. As an additional feature, the breathing hole is closed when the Brethancer is telescoped, which prevents foreign matter from entering the unit.
The Brethancer unit will accommodate any of several currently available prescription aerosol bronchodilator medications.
The patient's inhalation technique should be checked regularly. See the patient package insert for operating instructions.
PATIENT PACKAGE INSERT—DIRECTIONS FOR USE PLEASE READ THESE INSTRUCTIONS BEFORE USING THE BRETHANCER®.
1. Remove the metal aerosol canister from the plastic mouthpiece, if so packaged.
2. Place the metal canister in the Brethancer so the narrow metal tip of the canister is inserted securely in the center hole of the Brethancer.
3. Shake well.
4. When opening Brethancer, do not push in the yellow plastic mouthpiece flap that appears behind the mouth hole of the gold outer section. Doing so can damage the unit and block the flow of medication when it is used.
Open the Brethancer by pulling firmly on the open end, so that all three sections are fully extended. Turn the light yellow section upwards until it locks in the upright position.
[See illustration at top of next column.]

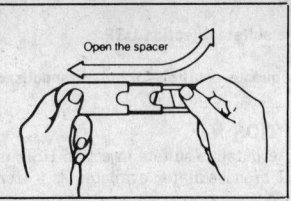

Open the spacer

DO NOT USE Brethancer if the mouthpiece flap is not fully opened *or* if you cannot see all the way through the inside of the fully extended and locked unit to the lightest colored inner section.
5. Place the open, dark yellow end of the Brethancer to your mouth and breathe out.

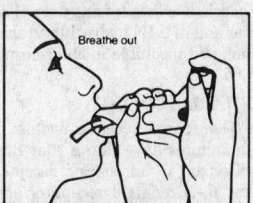

Breathe out

6. Press down on the canister one time.

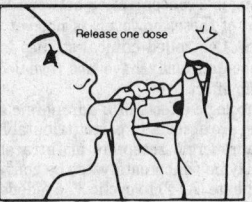

Release one dose

7. Then breathe in through the Brethancer, and try to hold your breath for a count of 10 before breathing out again. It is not necessary to press down on the canister and to breathe in at the same time.

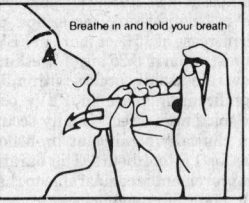

Breathe in and hold your breath

8. If another dose is needed, repeat steps 5 to 7.
To close the Brethancer completely, first press lightly on the sides of the middle yellow section and slide inside the dark yellow section. Then press lightly on the arrow on the bottom of the light yellow section and collapse all three sections together.

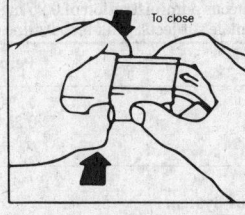

To close

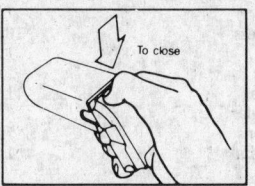

To close

PLEASE NOTE: Incorrectly closing Brethancer can damage it.
At least once a week, remove the canister and wash the extended Brethancer unit in hot water to keep the unit clean.
Be sure to use the Brethancer correctly so the inhaled drug reaches the lungs and produces its full effect. The Brethancer allows both time and distance for the aerosol to form a fine mist of small drug particles, which are carried into the lungs by the inhaled air. The Brethancer makes inhalation of the drug almost fail-safe.

Mfd by: Perlos, Finland
Dist. by: GEIGY Pharmaceuticals
Division of CIBA-GEIGY Corporation
Ardsley, New York 10502

C88-30 (Rev. 10/88)

BRETHINE®   ℞

[*breth-een'*]
terbutaline sulfate USP
Tablets of 5 mg
Tablets of 2.5 mg

DESCRIPTION
Brethine, terbutaline sulfate USP, is a bronchodilator available as tablets of 2.5 mg (2.05 mg of the free base) and 5 mg (4.1 mg of the free base) for oral administration. Terbutaline sulfate is α-[(*tert*-Butylamino) methyl]-3,5-dihydroxybenzyl alcohol sulfate (2:1) (salt).
Terbutaline sulfate USP is a white to gray-white crystalline powder. It is odorless or has a faint odor of acetic acid. It is soluble in water and in 0.1N hydrochloric acid, slightly soluble in methanol, and insoluble in chloroform. Its molecular weight is 548.65.
Inactive Ingredients. Cellulose compounds, lactose, magnesium stearate, povidone, and starch.

ACTIONS
Brethine is a β-adrenergic receptor agonist which has been shown by *in vitro* and *in vivo* pharmacological studies in animals to exert a preferential effect on β_2-adrenergic receptors such as those located in bronchial smooth muscle. Controlled clinical studies in patients who were administered the drug orally have revealed proportionally greater changes in pulmonary function parameters than in heart rate or blood pressure. While this *suggests* a relative preference for the β_2 receptor in man, the usual cardiovascular effects commonly associated with sympathomimetic agents were also observed with Brethine.
Brethine has been shown in controlled clinical studies to relieve bronchospasm in chronic obstructive pulmonary disease.
This action is manifested by a clinically significant increase in pulmonary function as demonstrated by an increase of 15% or more in FEV_1 and in $FEF_{25-75\%}$. Following administration of Brethine tablets, a measurable change in flow rate is usually observed in 30 minutes, and a clinically significant improvement in pulmonary function occurs at 60–120 minutes. The maximum effect usually occurs within 120-180 minutes. Brethine also produces a clinically significant decrease in airway and pulmonary resistance which persists for at least four hours or longer. Significant bronchodilator action, as measured by various pulmonary function determinations (airway resistance, $FEF_{25-75\%}$, or PEFR), has been demonstrated in some studies for periods up to eight hours. Clinical studies were conducted in which the effectiveness of Brethine was evaluated in comparison with ephedrine over periods up to three months. Both drugs continued to produce significant improvement in pulmonary function throughout this period of treatment.

INDICATIONS
Brethine is indicated as a bronchodilator for bronchial asthma and for reversible bronchospasm which may occur in association with bronchitis and emphysema.

CONTRAINDICATIONS
Brethine is contraindicated when there is known hypersensitivity to sympathomimetic amines.

WARNINGS
There have been rare reports of seizures in patients receiving terbutaline; seizures did not recur in these patients after the drug was discontinued.
Controlled clinical studies and other clinical experience have shown that Brethine, like other β-adrenergic agonists, can produce a significant cardiovascular effect in some patients, as measured by pulse rate, blood pressure, symptoms, and/or ECG changes.
Usage in Pregnancy: Animal reproductive studies have been negative with respect to adverse effects on fetal development. The safe use of Brethine has not, however, been established in human pregnancy. As with any medication, the use of the drug in pregnancy, lactation, or women of childbearing potential requires that the expected therapeutic benefit of the drug be weighed against its possible hazards to the mother or child.

Continued on next page

The full prescribing information for each GEIGY product is contained herein and is that in effect as of September 1, 1992.

GEIGY—Cont.

Usage in Pediatrics: Brethine tablets are not presently recommended for children below the age of 12 years due to insufficient clinical data in this pediatric group.

PRECAUTIONS

Brethine should be used with caution in patients with diabetes, hypertension, hyperthyroidism, and a history of seizures. Large doses of intravenous terbutaline sulfate have been reported to aggravate preexisting diabetes and ketoacidosis.

As with other sympathomimetic bronchodilator agents, Brethine should be administered cautiously to cardiac patients, especially those with associated arrhythmias.

The concomitant use of Brethine with other sympathomimetic agents is not recommended, since their combined effect on the cardiovascular system may be deleterious to the patient. However, this does not preclude the use of an aerosol bronchodilator of the adrenergic stimulant type for the relief of an acute bronchospasm in patients receiving chronic oral Brethine therapy.

Terbutaline sulfate should not be used for tocolysis. Serious adverse reactions may occur after administration of terbutaline sulfate to women in labor. In the mother, these include increased heart rate, transient hyperglycemia, hypokalemia, cardiac arrhythmias, pulmonary edema, and myocardial ischemia. Increased fetal heart rate and neonatal hypoglycemia may occur as a result of maternal administration.

Immediate hypersensitivity reactions and exacerbation of bronchospasm have been reported after terbutaline administration.

ADVERSE REACTIONS

Commonly observed side effects include nervousness and tremor. Other reported reactions include headache, increased heart rate, palpitations, drowsiness, nausea, vomiting, sweating, and muscle cramps. These reactions are generally transient in nature and usually do not require treatment. The frequency of these side effects appears to diminish with continued therapy. In general, all the side effects observed are characteristic of those commonly seen with sympathomimetic amines.

There have been rare reports of elevations in liver enzymes and of hypersensitivity vasculitis.

DOSAGE AND ADMINISTRATION

The usual oral dose of Brethine for adults is 5 mg administered at approximately six-hour intervals, three times daily, during the hours the patient is usually awake. If side effects are particularly disturbing, the dose may be reduced to 2.5 mg three times daily, and still provide a clinically significant improvement in pulmonary function. A dose of 2.5 mg, three times daily, also is recommended for children in the 12- to 15-year group. Brethine is not recommended at present for use in children below the age of 12 years. In adults, a total dose of 15 mg should not be exceeded in a 24-hour period. In children, a total dose of 7.5 mg should not be exceeded in a 24-hour period.

OVERDOSAGE

Overdosage experience is limited. Excessive beta-adrenergic receptor stimulation may augment the signs or symptoms listed under **ADVERSE REACTIONS** and they may be accompanied by other adrenergic effects. Treat the alert patient who has taken excessive oral medication by emptying the stomach by means of induced emesis, followed by gastric lavage. In the unconscious patient, secure the airway with a cuffed endotracheal tube before beginning lavage (do not induce emesis). Instillation of activated charcoal slurry may help reduce absorption of terbutaline sulfate. Maintain adequate respiratory exchange. Provide cardiac and respiratory support as needed. Continue observation until symptom-free.

HOW SUPPLIED

Tablets 2.5 mg—oval, white, scored (imprinted Geigy 72)
Bottles of 100 ....NDC 0028-0072-01
Bottles of 1000 ....NDC 0028-0072-10
Gy-Pak®—One Unit
12 bottles—100 tablets each ....NDC 0028-0072-65
Unit Dose (blister pack)
Box of 100 (strips of 10) ....NDC 0028-0072-61
Tablets 5 mg—round, white, scored (imprinted Geigy 105)
Bottles of 100 ....NDC 0028-0105-01
Bottles of 1000 ....NDC 0028-0105-10
Gy-Pak®—one Unit
12 bottles—100 tablets each ....NDC 0028-0105-65
Unit Dose (blister pack)
Box of 100 (strips of 10) ....NDC 0028-0105-61
Store at controlled room temperature 59°-86°F (15°-30°C).
Dispense in tight, light-resistant container (USP).

C91-4 (Rev. 2/91)

Shown in Product Identification Section, page 409

BRETHINE® ℞

[breth-een ']
terbutaline sulfate Injection USP
Ampuls
A sterile aqueous solution for subcutaneous injection.

DESCRIPTION

Brethine, terbutaline sulfate injection USP, is a β-adrenergic agonist bronchodilator available as a sterile, nonpyrogenic, aqueous solution in ampuls, for subcutaneous administration. Each milliliter of solution contains 1 mg of terbutaline sulfate USP (0.82 mg of the free base); sodium chloride ACS, for isotonicity; and hydrochloric acid ACS, for adjustment to a target pH of 4. Terbutaline sulfate is (±)-α-[(*tert*-butylamino)methyl]-3,5-dihydroxybenzyl alcohol sulfate (2:1) (salt). The empirical formula is $(C_{12}H_{19}NO_3)_2 \cdot H_2SO_4$. Terbutaline sulfate USP is a white to gray-white crystalline powder. It is odorless or has a faint odor of acetic acid. It is soluble in water and in 0.1N hydrochloric acid, slightly soluble in methanol, and insoluble in chloroform. Its molecular weight is 548.65.

CLINICAL PHARMACOLOGY

Brethine is a β-adrenergic receptor agonist. In vitro and in vivo studies in animals have shown that Brethine exerts a preferential effect on β_2-adrenergic receptors. While it is recognized that β_2-adrenergic receptors are the predominant receptors in bronchial smooth muscle, recent data indicate that there is a population of β_2-receptors in the human heart, existing in a concentration between 10–50%. The precise function of these, however, is not yet established (see WARNINGS). Controlled clinical studies in patients given Brethine subcutaneously have not revealed a preferential β_2-adrenergic effect.

The pharmacologic effects of β-adrenergic agonists, including Brethine, are at least in part attributable to stimulation through β-adrenergic receptors of intracellular adenylcyclase, the enzyme which catalyzes the conversion of adenosine triphosphate (ATP) to cyclic 3′, 5′-adenosine monophosphate (cAMP). Increased cAMP levels are associated with relaxation of bronchial smooth muscle and inhibition of release of mediators of immediate hypersensitivity from cells, especially from mast cells.

Controlled clinical studies have shown that Brethine relieves bronchospasm in acute and chronic obstructive pulmonary disease by significantly increasing pulmonary flow rates (e.g., an increase of 15% or more in FEV_1). After subcutaneous administration of 0.25 mg of Brethine, a measurable change in flow rate usually occurs within 5 minutes, and a clinically significant increase in FEV_1 occurs within 15 minutes. The maximum effect usually occurs within 30–60 minutes, and clinically significant bronchodilator activity may continue for 1.5 to 4 hours. The duration of clinically significant improvement is comparable to that observed with equimilligram doses of epinephrine.

Recent studies in laboratory animals (minipigs, rodents, and dogs) recorded the occurrence of cardiac arrhythmias and sudden death (with histological evidence of necrosis) when β-agonists and methylxanthines were administered concurrently. The significance of these findings when applied to humans is currently unknown.

Pharmacokinetics

After subcutaneous administration of 0.25 mg of terbutaline sulfate to two male subjects, peak terbutaline serum concentrations of 5.2 and 5.3 ng/ml were observed at about 20 minutes after dosing. Further studies are needed to confirm these results.

Elimination half-life of the drug in 10 of 14 patients was approximately 2.9 hr after subcutaneous administration, but longer elimination half-lives (between 6–14 hr) were found in the other 4 patients. About 90% of the drug was excreted in the urine at 96 hr after subcutaneous administration, with about 60% of this being unchanged drug. It appears that the sulfate conjugate is a major metabolite of terbutaline and urinary excretion is the primary route of elimination.

INDICATIONS AND USAGE

Brethine is indicated for the prevention and reversal of bronchospasm in patients with bronchial asthma and reversible bronchospasm associated with bronchitis and emphysema.

CONTRAINDICATIONS

Brethine is contraindicated in patients known to be hypersensitive to sympathomimetic amines or any component of this drug product.

WARNINGS

There have been rare reports of seizures in patients receiving terbutaline; seizures did not recur in these patients after the drug was discontinued.

Controlled clinical studies and other clinical experience have shown that Brethine, like other β-adrenergic agonists, can produce a significant cardiovascular effect in some patients, as measured by pulse rate, blood pressure, symptoms, and/or ECG changes.

PRECAUTIONS

General

Since Brethine is a sympathomimetic amine, it should be used with caution in patients with cardiovascular disorders, including ischemic heart disease, hypertension, and cardiac arrhythmias; in patients with hyperthyroidism or diabetes mellitus; and in patients who are unusually responsive to sympathomimetic amines or who have convulsive disorders.

Significant changes in systolic and diastolic blood pressure can be expected to occur in some patients after use of any β-adrenergic bronchodilator.

Immediate hypersensitivity reactions and exacerbations of bronchospasm have been reported after terbutaline administration.

Terbutaline sulfate should not be used for tocolysis.

Drug Interactions

The concomitant use of Brethine with other sympathomimetic agents is not recommended, since the combined effect on the cardiovascular system may be deleterious to the patient.

β-adrenergic agonists should be administered with caution to patients being treated with monoamine oxidase inhibitors or tricyclic antidepressants, since the action of β-adrenergic agonists on the vascular system may be potentiated.

Carcinogenesis, Mutagenesis, Impairment of Fertility

In a 2-year oral study in the rat, terbutaline sulfate caused a significant dose-related increase in the incidence of benign leiomyomas of the mesovarium at doses corresponding to 5,000, 50,000, 100,000, and 200,000 times the maximum recommended human subcutaneous dose (0.01 mg/kg). The relevance of these findings to humans is not known. An 18-month oral study in mice revealed no evidence of tumorigenicity at doses up to 200 mg/kg (20,000 times the maximum recommended human subcutaneous dose). Mutagenicity

Percent Incidence of Adverse Reactions

Reaction	Terbutaline 0.25 mg N=77	Terbutaline 0.5 mg N=205	Epinephrine 0.25 mg N=153	Epinephrine 0.5 mg N=61
Central Nervous System				
Tremors	7.8%	38.0%	16.3%	18.0%
Nervousness	16.9%	30.7%	8.5%	31.1%
Dizziness	1.3%	10.2%	7.8%	3.3%
Headache	7.8%	8.8%	3.3%	9.8%
Drowsiness	11.7%	9.8%	14.4%	8.2%
Cardiovascular				
Palpitations	7.8%	22.9%	7.8%	29.5%
Tachycardia	1.3%	1.5%	2.6%	0.0%
Respiratory				
Dyspnea	0.0%	2.0%	2.0%	0.0%
Chest Discomfort	1.3%	1.5%	2.6%	0.0%
Gastrointestinal				
Nausea/Vomiting	1.3%	3.9%	1.3%	11.5%
Systemic				
Weakness	1.3%	0.5%	2.6%	1.6%
Flushed Feeling	0.0%	2.4%	1.3%	0.0%
Sweating	0.0%	2.4%	0.0%	0.0%
Pain at Injection Site	2.6%	0.5%	2.6%	1.6%

Note: Some patients received more than one dosage strength of terbutaline sulfate and epinephrine. In addition, there were reports of anxiety, muscle cramps, and dry mouth (<0.5%).

studies have not been performed. A reproduction study in rats at oral doses up to 5000 times the maximum subcutaneous dose (0.01 mg/kg) revealed no evidence of impaired fertility.

Pregnancy Category B

Reproduction studies performed in mice, rats, or rabbits at doses up to 1500 times the subcutaneous maximum daily human dose of 0.01 mg/kg have revealed no evidence of impaired fertility or harm to the fetus due to Brethine. Increased levels of maternal and fetal blood glucose have been observed after intravenous administration of terbutaline to near-term pregnant baboons at doses up to 4 times the maximum recommended human subcutaneous dose.

There are, however, no adequate and well-controlled studies in pregnant women. Because animal reproduction studies are not always predictive of human response, this drug should be used during pregnancy only if clearly needed. Administration of the drug under these conditions requires careful benefit-to-risk determination.

Labor and Delivery

Terbutaline sulfate should not be used for tocolysis. Serious adverse reactions may occur after administration of terbutaline sulfate to women in labor. In the mother, these include increased heart rate, transient hyperglycemia, hypokalemia, cardiac arrhythmias, pulmonary edema, and myocardial ischemia. Increased fetal heart rate and neonatal hypoglycemia may occur as a result of maternal administration.

Nursing Mothers

It is not known whether this drug is excreted in human milk. Therefore, Brethine should be used during nursing only if the potential benefit justifies the possible risk to the newborn.

Pediatric Use

Brethine is not recommended for patients under the age of 12 years because of insufficient clinical data to establish safety and effectiveness.

ADVERSE REACTIONS

Adverse reactions observed with Brethine are similar to those commonly seen with other sympathomimetic agents. All these reactions are transient in nature and usually do not require treatment.

The following table compares adverse reactions seen in patients treated with terbutaline sulfate injection (0.25 mg and 0.5 mg) with those seen in patients treated with epinephrine injection (0.25 mg and 0.5 mg), during eight double-blind crossover studies involving a total of 214 patients.

[See table on preceding page.]

There have been rare reports of elevations of liver enzymes and of hypersensitivity vasculitis with terbutaline administration.

OVERDOSAGE

Acute Toxicity

Intravenous LD_{50}'s (mg/kg): rats, 61.5; mice, 48.4. Oral LD_{50} in rats is > 5000 mg/kg.

Signs and Symptoms

Excessive β-adrenergic receptor stimulation may augment the signs and symptoms listed under ADVERSE REACTIONS.

Treatment

There is no specific antidote. Treatment consists of discontinuation of Brethine along with the institution of appropriate symptomatic therapy.

DOSAGE AND ADMINISTRATION

Ampuls should be used only for subcutaneous administration and not intravenous infusion. Sterility and accurate dosing cannot be assured if the ampuls are not used in accordance with DOSAGE AND ADMINISTRATION.

The usual subcutaneous dose of Brethine is 0.25 mg injected into the lateral deltoid area. If significant clinical improvement does not occur within 15–30 minutes, a second dose of 0.25 mg may be administered. If the patient then fails to respond within another 15–30 minutes, other therapeutic measures should be considered. The total dose within 4 hours should not exceed 0.5 mg.

Note: Parenteral drug products should be inspected visually for particulate matter and discoloration prior to administration, whenever solution and container permit.

HOW SUPPLIED

Ampuls 1 mg/ml—The drug is supplied at a volume of 1 ml contained in a 2 ml clear glass ampul. Each ampul contains 1 mg of Brethine per 1 ml of solution; 0.25 ml of solution will provide the usual clinical dose of 0.25 mg. Ampuls are expiration-dated.

Box of 10 ampuls .... NDC 0028-7507-23
Box of 100 ampuls .... NDC 0028-7507-01

Keep at controlled room temperature 59°–86°F (15°–30°C).

Protect from light by storing ampuls in original carton until dispensed. Do not use if solution is discolored.

C91-3 (Rev. 2/91)

Shown in Product Identification Section, page 409

CONSTANT-T® ℞

[*kahn-stant 'tee'*]

theophylline (anhydrous) USP
Sustained-Action Tablets
Tablets
200 mg
300 mg

DESCRIPTION

Constant-T, theophylline (anhydrous) USP, is a xanthine bronchodilator available as sustained-action tablets of 200 mg and 300 mg for oral administration. Its chemical name is 3,7-Dihydro-1,3-dimethyl-,1*H*-purine-2,6-dione.

Theophylline (anhydrous) USP is a white, odorless crystalline powder having a bitter taste. It is stable in air. It is freely soluble in solutions of alkali hydroxides and in ammonia; sparingly soluble in alcohol, in chloroform, and in ether; and slightly soluble in water but more soluble in hot water. Its molecular weight is 180.17.

Inactive Ingredients. Cellulose compound, FD&C Blue No. 1 Aluminum Lake (300-mg tablets), FD&C Red No. 40 (200-mg tablets), lactose, magnesium stearate, povidone, and stearic acid.

ACTIONS

The pharmacologic actions of Constant-T are as a bronchodilator, pulmonary vasodilator and smooth muscle relaxant, since the drug directly relaxes the smooth muscle of the bronchial airways and pulmonary blood vessels. Theophylline also possesses other actions typical of the xanthine derivatives: coronary vasodilator, diuretic, cardiac stimulant, cerebral stimulant and skeletal muscle stimulant. The actions of theophylline may be mediated through inhibition of phosphodiesterase and a resultant increase in intracellular cyclic AMP which could mediate smooth muscle relaxation. No development of tolerance appears to occur with chronic use of theophylline.

The half-life is shortened with cigarette smoking and prolonged in alcoholism, reduced hepatic or renal function, congestive heart failure, and in patients receiving certain antibiotics (see Drug Interactions). High fever for prolonged periods may decrease theophylline elimination. Children over six months of age have rapid clearances with average half-lives of approximately 3–5 hours. Newborn infants have extremely slow clearances and half-lives exceeding 24 hours. Older adults with chronic obstructive pulmonary disease, any patients with cor pulmonale or other causes of heart failure, and patients with liver pathology may have much lower clearances with half-lives that exceed 24 hours. The half-life of theophylline in smokers (1–2 packs per day) averages 4–5 hours; the half-life in nonsmokers averages 7–9 hours.

In single-dose studies, adjusting the data to dosing equivalent to 8 mg/kg body weight, Constant-T produced mean peak theophylline blood levels of 9.1 ± 0.7 μg/mL at 5.0 ± 1.2 hours with the 200-mg dosage form, and 9.8 ± 0.9 μg/mL at 4.6 ± 0.9 hours with the 300-mg dosage form. In a multidose, steady-state, 5-day study, Constant-T achieved constant intrasubject theophylline levels with an average peak-trough difference of only 3.4 μg/mL. This is indicative of smooth and stable maintenance therapeutic theophylline levels throughout a 12-hour dosing interval.

INDICATIONS AND USAGE

Symptomatic relief and/or prevention of asthma and reversible bronchospasm associated with chronic bronchitis and emphysema.

CONTRAINDICATIONS

This product is contraindicated in individuals who have shown hypersensitivity to its components. It is also contraindicated in patients with active peptic ulcer disease, and in individuals with underlying seizure disorders (unless receiving appropriate anticonvulsant medication).

WARNINGS

Serum levels above 20 mcg/mL are rarely found after appropriate administration of the recommended doses. However, in individuals in whom theophylline plasma clearance is reduced **for any reason,** even conventional doses may result in increased serum levels and potential toxicity. Reduced theophylline clearance has been documented in the following readily identifiable groups: 1) patients with impaired liver function; 2) patients over 55 years of age, particularly males and those with chronic lung disease; 3) those with cardiac failure from any cause; 4) patients with sustained high fever; 5) neonates and infants under 1 year of age; and 6) those patients taking certain drugs (see PRECAUTIONS, Drug Interactions). Frequently, such patients have markedly prolonged theophylline serum levels following discontinuation of the drug. Decreased clearance of theophylline may be associated with either influenza immunization or active infection with influenza.

Reduction of dosage and laboratory monitoring is especially appropriate in the above individuals.

Serious side effects such as ventricular arrhythmias, convulsions or even death may appear as the first sign of toxicity without any previous warning. Less serious signs of theophylline toxicity (i.e., nausea and restlessness) may occur frequently when initiating therapy, but are usually transient; when such signs are persistent during maintenance therapy, they are often associated with serum concentrations above 20 mcg/mL.

Stated differently: **serious toxicity is not reliably preceded by less severe side effects.** A serum concentration measurement is the only reliable method of predicting potentially life-threatening toxicity.

Many patients who require theophylline exhibit tachycardia due to their underlying disease process so that the cause/effect relationship to elevated serum theophylline concentrations may not be appreciated.

Theophylline products may cause dysrhythmia and/or worsen preexisting arrhythmias and any significant change in rate and/or rhythm warrants monitoring and further investigation.

Studies in laboratory animals (minipigs, rodents, and dogs) recorded the occurrence of cardiac arrhythmias and sudden death (with histologic evidence of myocardial necrosis) when beta agonists and methylxanthines were administered concurrently. The significance of these findings when applied to humans is currently unknown.

PRECAUTIONS

General

On the average, theophylline half-life is shorter in cigarette and marijuana smokers than in nonsmokers, but smokers can have half-lives as long as nonsmokers. Theophylline should not be administered concurrently with other xanthines. Use with caution in patients with hypoxemia, hypertension, or those with history of peptic ulcer. Theophylline may occasionally act as a local irritant to G.I. tract although gastrointestinal symptoms are more commonly centrally mediated and associated with serum drug concentrations over 20 mcg/mL.

Information for Patients

PATIENTS SHOULD BE TOLD NOT TO CHEW OR CRUSH THEOPHYLLINE TABLETS IN THEIR MOUTHS.

The importance of taking only the prescribed dose and time interval between doses should be reinforced.

Contact your physician if symptoms occur repeatedly, especially at the end of a dosing interval.

Laboratory Tests

Serum levels should be monitored periodically to determine the theophylline level associated with observed clinical response and as the method of predicting toxicity. For such measurements, the serum sample should be obtained at the time of peak concentration, approximately 5 hours after administration of Constant-T. It is important that the patient will not have missed or taken additional doses during the previous 48 hours and that dosing intervals will have been reasonably equally spaced. DOSAGE ADJUSTMENT BASED ON SERUM THEOPHYLLINE MEASUREMENTS WHEN THESE INSTRUCTIONS HAVE NOT BEEN FOLLOWED MAY RESULT IN RECOMMENDATIONS THAT PRESENT RISK OF TOXICITY TO THE PATIENT.

Drug Interactions

Toxic synergism with ephedrine has been documented and may occur with other sympathomimetic bronchodilators. In addition, the following drug interactions have been demonstrated:

Theophylline with:	
Allopurinol (high-dose)	Increased serum theophylline levels
Cimetidine	Increased serum theophylline levels
Erythromycin, Troleandomycin	Increased serum theophylline levels
Lithium carbonate	Increased renal excretion of lithium
Oral Contraceptives	Increased serum theophylline levels
Phenytoin	Decreased theophylline and phenytoin serum levels
Rifampin	Decreased serum theophylline levels

Drug-Food Interactions

Taking Constant-T immediately after a high-fat content breakfast such as 2 scrambled eggs, 2 strips bacon, 2 blueberry muffins, 8 oz. grape juice, 8 oz. whole milk (about 775 calories including approximately 48.7 g of fat) may result in a different rate of absorption, but with no significant difference in the extent of absorption (see CLINICAL PHARMACOLOGY, Pharmacokinetics). The influence of the type and amount of other foods, as well as the time interval between drug and food has not been studied.

Continued on next page

The full prescribing information for each GEIGY product is contained herein and is that in effect as of September 1, 1992.

GEIGY—Cont.

Drug-Laboratory Test Interactions
Currently available analytical methods, including high pressure liquid chromatography and immunoassay techniques, for measuring serum theophylline levels are specific. Metabolites and other drugs generally do not affect the results. Other new analytic methods are also now in use. The physician should be aware of the laboratory method used and whether other drugs will interfere with the assay for theophylline.

Carcinogenesis, Mutagenesis, and Impairment of Fertility
Long-term carcinogenicity studies have not been performed with theophylline.
Chromosome-breaking activity was detected in human cell cultures at concentrations of theophylline up to 50 times the therapeutic serum concentration in humans. Theophylline was not mutagenic in the dominant lethal assay in male mice given theophylline intraperitoneally in doses up to 30 times the maximum daily human oral dose.
Studies to determine the effect on fertility have not been performed with theophylline.

Pregnancy Category C
Animal reproduction studies have not been conducted with theophylline. It is also not known whether theophylline can cause fetal harm when administered to a pregnant woman or can affect reproduction capacity. Xanthines should be given to a pregnant woman only if clearly needed.

Nursing Mothers
Theophylline is distributed into breast milk and may cause irritability or other signs of toxicity in nursing infants. Because of the potential for serious adverse reactions in nursing infants from theophylline, a decision should be made whether to discontinue nursing or to discontinue the drug, taking into account the importance of the drug to the mother.

Pediatric Use
The safey and effectiveness of theophylline in children below 6 years of age have not been established, and it is therefore not recommended for this age group.

ADVERSE REACTIONS
The following adverse reactions have been observed, but there has not been enough systematic collection of data to support an estimate of their frequency. The most consistent adverse reactions are usually due to overdosage.
Gastrointestinal: nausea, vomiting, epigastric pain, hematemesis, diarrhea.
Central nervous system: headaches, irritability, restlessness, insomnia, reflex hyperexcitability, muscle twitching, clonic and tonic generalized convulsions.
Cardiovascular: palpitation, tachycardia, extrasystoles, flushing, hypotension, circulatory failure, ventricular arrhythmias.
Respiratory: tachypnea.
Renal: albuminuria, increased excretion of renal tubular cells and red blood cells, potentiation of diuresis.
Others: alopecia, hyperglycemia, inappropriate ADH syndrome, rash.

OVERDOSAGE
Management
It is suggested that the management principles (consistent with the clinical status of the patient when first seen) outlined below be instituted and that simultaneous contact with a Regional Poison Control Center be established. In this way both updated information and individualization regarding required therapy may be provided.

1. When potential oral overdose is established and seizure has not occurred:
   a) If patient is alert and seen within the early hours after ingestion, induction of emesis may be of value. Gastric lavage has been demonstrated to be of no value in influencing outcome in patients who present more than 1 hour after ingestion.
   b) Administer a cathartic. Sorbitol solution is reported to be of value.
   c) Administer repeated doses of activated charcoal and monitor theophylline serum levels.
   d) Prophylactic administration of phenobarbital has been shown to increase the seizure threshold in laboratory animals, and administration of this drug can be considered.
2. If patient presents with a seizure:
   a) Establish an airway.
   b) Administer oxygen.
   c) Treat the seizure with intravenous diazepam, 0.1 to 0.3 mg/kg up to 10 mg. If seizures cannot be controlled, the use of general anesthesia should be considered.
   d) Monitor vital signs, maintain blood pressure and provide adequate hydration.
3. If post-seizure coma is present:
   a) Maintain airway and oxygenation.
   b) If a result of oral medication, follow above recommendations to prevent absorption of the drug, but intubation and lavage will have to be performed instead of inducing emesis, and the cathartic and charcoal will need to be introduced via a large bore gastric lavage tube.
   c) Continue to provide full supportive care and adequate hydration until the drug is metabolized. In general, drug metabolism is sufficiently rapid so as not to warrant dialysis. If repeated oral activated charcoal is ineffective (as noted by stable or rising serum levels) charcoal hemoperfusion may be indicated.

DOSAGE AND ADMINISTRATION
Taking Constant-T immediately after a high-fat content meal may alter its rate of absorption (see PRECAUTIONS, Drug-Food Interactions). The clinician should be aware of these potential differences. Most bioavailability studies with Constant-T were conducted in the fasting state and therefore, until more information is obtained, it is recommended that Constant-T be administered before meals.
Effective use of theophylline (i.e., the concentration of drug in the serum associated with optimal benefit and minimal risk of toxicity) is considered to occur when the theophylline concentration is maintained from 10 to 20 mcg/mL. The early studies from which these levels were derived were carried out in patients immediately or shortly after recovery from acute exacerbations of their disease (some hospitalized with status asthmaticus). Although the 20 mcg/mL level remains appropriate as a critical value (above which toxicity is more likely to occur) for safety purposes, additional data are now available which indicate that the serum theophylline concentrations required to produce maximum physiologic benefit may, in fact, fluctuate with the degree of bronchospasm present and are variable. Therefore, the physician should individualize the range appropriate to the patient's requirements, based on both symptomatic response and improvement in pulmonary function. It should be stressed that serum theophylline concentrations maintained at the upper level of the 10 to 20 mcg/mL range may be associated with potential toxicity when factors known to reduce theophylline clearance are operative. (See WARNINGS).
If it is not possible to obtain serum level determinations, restriction of the daily dose (in otherwise healthy adults) to not greater than 13 mg/kg/day, to a maximum of 900 mg, in divided doses will result in relatively few patients exceeding serum levels of 20 mcg/mL and the resultant greater risk of toxicity.
Caution should be exercised for younger children who cannot complain of minor side effects. Older adults, those with cor pulmonale, congestive heart failure, and/or liver disease may have unusually low dosage requirements and thus may experience toxicity at the maximal dosage recommended below.
Theophylline does not distribute into fatty tissue. Dosage should be calculated on the basis of lean (ideal) body weight where mg/kg doses are presented.

Frequency of Dosing
When immediate release products with rapid absorption are used, dosing to maintain serum levels generally requires administration every 6 hours. This is particularly true in children, but dosing intervals up to 8 hours may be satisfactory in adults since they eliminate the drug at a slower rate. Some children, and adults requiring higher than average doses (those having rapid rates of clearance, e.g., half-lives of under 6 hours) may benefit and be more effectively controlled during chronic therapy when given products with sustained-release characteristics since these provide longer dosing intervals and/or less fluctuation in serum concentration between dosing.
Dosage guidelines are approximations only and the wide range of theophylline clearance between individuals (particularly those with concomitant disease) makes indiscriminate usage hazardous.

Dosage Guidelines
Acute Symptoms of Asthma Requiring Rapid Theophyllinization: Contant-T is not intended for patients experiencing an acute episode of bronchospasm (associated with asthma, chronic bronchitis, or emphysema). Such patients require **rapid** relief of symptoms and should be treated with an immediate-release or intravenous theophylline preparation (or other bronchodilators) and not with sustained action products.

Chronic Therapy
Theophylline is a treatment for the management of reversible bronchospam (asthma, chronic bronchitis and emphysema) to prevent symptoms and maintain patent airways. A dosage form which allows small incremental doses is desirable for initiating therapy. A liquid preparation should be considered for children to permit both greater ease of and more accurate dosage adjustment. Slow clinical titration is generally preferred to assure acceptance and safety of the medication, and to allow the patient to develop tolerance to transient caffeine-like side effects. Then, if the total 24-hour dose can be given by use of the available strengths of Constant-T, the patient can usually be switched to one half of the daily dose of theophylline given at 12-hour intervals. However, certain patients, such as the young, smokers, and some nonsmoking adults, are likely to metabolize theophylline rapidly and require dosing at 8-hour intervals. Such patients can generally be identified as having trough serum concentrations lower than desired or repeatedly exhibiting symptoms near the end of a dosing interval.

Maximum Dose of Theophylline Where the Serum Concentration is Not Measured:
Warning: Do Not Attempt To Maintain Any Dose That Is Not Tolerated.
Not to exceed the following: (or 900 mg, whichever is less)

Age 6–9 years	24 mg/kg/day
Age 9–12 years	20 mg/kg/day
Age 12–16 years	18 mg/kg/day
Age 16 years and older	13 mg/kg/day

Measurement of Serum Theophylline Concentrations During Chronic Therapy: If the above maximum doses are to be maintained or exceeded, serum theophylline measurement is essential. (See PRECAUTIONS, Laboratory Tests, for guidance.)

Final Adjustment of Dosage: Dosage adjustment after serum theophylline measurement

If serum theophylline is:		Directions:
Within desired range		Maintain dosage if tolerated.
Too high	20 to 25 mcg/mL	Decrease doses by about 10% and recheck serum level after 3 days.
	25 to 30 mcg/mL	Skip the next dose and decrease subsequent doses by about 25%. Recheck serum level after 3 days.
	Over 30 mcg/mL	Skip next 2 doses and decrease subsequent doses by 50%. Recheck serum level after 3 days.
Too low		Increase dosage by 25% at 3 day intervals until either the desired serum concentration and/or clinical response is achieved. The total daily dose may need to be administered at more frequent intervals if symptoms occur repeatedly at the end of a dosing interval.

The serum concentration may be rechecked at appropriate intervals, but at least at the end of any adjustment period. When the patient's condition is otherwise clinically stable and none of the recognized factors which alter elimination are present, measurement of serum levels need be repeated only every 6 to 12 months.

HOW SUPPLIED
Sustained-Action Tablets 200 mg—light pink, oval, scored (imprinted Geigy 42)
Bottles of 100 ....NDC 0028-0042-01
Gy-Pak®—One Unit
12 bottles—60 tablets each ....NDC 0028-0042-73
Unit Dose (blister pack)
Box of 100 (strips of 10) ....NDC 0028-0042-61
Sustained-Action Tablets 300 mg—light blue, oval, scored (imprinted Geigy 57)
Bottles of 100 ....NDC 0028-0057-01
Gy-Pak®—One Unit
12 bottles—60 tablets each ....NDC 0028-0057-73
Unit Dose (blister pack)
Box of 100 (strips of 10) ....NDC 0028-0057-61
Store between 59°–86°F (15°–30°C). Protect from moisture.
Dispense in tight, light-resistant container (USP).
C91-9 (Rev. 7/91)
Shown in Product Identification Section, page 410

LAMPRENE® ℞
clofazimine
Capsules

DESCRIPTION
Lamprene, clofazimine, is an antileprosy agent available as capsules for oral administration. Each capsule contains 50 mg or 100 mg of micronized clofazimine suspended in an oil-wax base. Clofazimine is a substituted iminophenazine bright-red dye. Its chemical name is 3-(*p*-chloroanilino)-10-(*p*-chlorophenyl)-2, 10-dihydro-2-isopropyliminophenazine. Clofazimine is a reddish-brown powder. It is readily soluble in benzene; soluble in chloroform; poorly soluble in acetone and in ethyl acetate; sparingly soluble in methanol and in ethanol; and virtually insoluble in water. Its molecular weight is 473.4.
Inactive Ingredients. Beeswax, butylated hydroxytoluene, citric acid, ethyl vanillin, gelatin, glycerin, iron oxide, lecithin, p-methoxy acetophenone, parabens, plant oils, propylene glycol.

CLINICAL PHARMACOLOGY

Lamprene exerts a slow bactericidal effect on *Mycobacterium leprae* (Hansen's bacillus). Lamprene inhibits mycobacterial growth and binds preferentially to mycobacterial DNA. Lamprene also exerts anti-inflammatory properties in controlling erythema nodosum leprosum reactions. However, its precise mechanisms of action are unknown.

Pharmacokinetics

Lamprene has a variable absorption rate in leprosy patients, ranging from 45–62% after oral administration. The average serum concentrations in leprosy patients treated with 100 mg and 300 mg daily were 0.7 μg/ml and 1.0 μg/ml, respectively. After ingestion of a single dose of 300 mg, elimination of unchanged Lamprene and its metabolites in a 24-hour urine collection was negligible. Lamprene is retained in the human body for a long time. The half-life of Lamprene following repeated oral doses is estimated to be at least 70 days. Part of the ingested drug recovered from the feces may represent excretion via the bile. A small amount is also eliminated in the sputum, sebum, and sweat.

Lamprene is highly lipophilic and tends to be deposited predominantly in fatty tissue and in cells of the reticuloendothelial system. It is taken up by macrophages throughout the body. In autopsies performed on leprosy patients, clofazimine crystals were found predominantly in the mesenteric lymph nodes, adrenals, subcutaneous fat, liver, bile, gall bladder, spleen, small intestine, muscles, bones, and skin.

Microbiology

Measurement of the minimum inhibitory concentration (MIC) of Lamprene against leprosy bacilli *in vitro* is not yet feasible. In the mouse footpad system, the multiplication of *M. leprae* is inhibited by introducing 0.0001–0.001% Lamprene in the diet. Although bacterial killing may begin shortly after starting the drug, it cannot be measured in biopsy tissues taken from patients for mouse footpad studies until approximately 50 days after the start of therapy.

Lamprene does not show cross-resistance with dapsone or rifampin.

The following *in vitro* data are available, but their clinical significance is unknown. Lamprene has been shown *in vitro* to inhibit *M. avium* and *M. bovis* at concentrations of approximately 0.1–1.0 μg/ml. The MIC for *M. avium-intracellulare* isolated from patients with acquired immuno-deficiency syndrome (AIDS) ranged from 1.0 to 5.0 μg/ml. With a few exceptions, microorganisms other than mycobacteria are not inhibited by Lamprene.

INDICATIONS AND USAGE

Lamprene is indicated in the treatment of lepromatous leprosy, including dapsone-resistant lepromatous leprosy and lepromatous leprosy complicated by erythema nodosum leprosum. Lamprene has not been demonstrated to be effective in the treatment of other leprosy-associated inflammatory reactions.

Combination drug therapy has been recommended for initial treatment of multibacillary leprosy to prevent the development of drug resistance.

CONTRAINDICATIONS

There are no known contraindications.

WARNINGS

Severe abdominal symptoms (see below) have necessitated exploratory laparotomies in some patients receiving Lamprene. Rare reports have included splenic infarction, bowel obstruction, and gastrointestinal bleeding. There have also been reports of death following severe abdominal symptoms. Autopsies have revealed crystalline deposits of clofazimine in various tissues including the intestinal mucosa, liver, spleen, and mesenteric lymph nodes.

Lamprene should be used with caution in patients who have gastrointestinal problems such as abdominal pain and diarrhea. Dosages of Lamprene of more than 100 mg daily should be given for as short a period as possible and only under close medical supervision. If a patient complains of colicky or burning pain in the abdomen, nausea, vomiting, or diarrhea, the dose should be reduced, and if necessary, the interval between doses should be increased, or the drug should be discontinued.

PRECAUTIONS

General

Physicians should be aware that skin discoloration due to Lamprene may result in depression. Two suicides have been reported in patients receiving Lamprene. For skin dryness and ichthyosis, oil can be applied to the skin.

Information for Patients

Patients should be warned that Lamprene may cause a discoloration of the skin from red to brownish black, as well as discoloration of the conjunctivae, lacrimal fluid, sweat, sputum, urine, and feces. Patients should be advised that skin discoloration, although reversible, may take several months or years to disappear after the conclusion of therapy with Lamprene.

Patients should be told to take Lamprene with meals.

Drug Interactions

Preliminary data which suggest that dapsone may inhibit the anti-inflammatory activity of Lamprene have not been confirmed. If leprosy-associated inflammatory reactions develop in patients being treated with dapsone and clofazimine, it is still advisable to continue treatment with both drugs.

Carcinogenesis, Mutagenesis, Impairment of Fertility

Long-term carcinogenicity studies in animals have not been conducted with Lamprene. Results of mutagenicity studies (Ames test) were negative. There was some evidence of impaired fertility in one study in rats treated at a dose 25 times the usual human dose; the number of offspring was reduced and there was a lower proportion of implantations.

Pregnancy Category C

Lamprene was not teratogenic in laboratory animals at dose levels equivalent to 8 times (rabbit) and 25 times (rat) the usual human daily dose. However, there was evidence of fetotoxicity in the mouse at 12-25 times the human dose, i.e., retardation of fetal skull ossification, increased incidence of abortions and stillbirths, and impaired neonatal survival. The skin and fatty tissue of offspring became discolored approximately 3 days after birth, which was attributed to the presence of Lamprene in the maternal milk.

It has been found that Lamprene crosses the human placenta. The skin of infants born to women who had received the drug during pregnancy was found to be deeply pigmented at birth. No evidence of teratogenicity was found in these infants. There are no adequate and well-controlled studies in pregnant women. Lamprene should be used during pregnancy only if the potential benefit justifies the risk to the fetus.

Nursing Mothers

Lamprene is excreted in the milk of nursing mothers. Lamprene should not be administered to a nursing woman unless clearly indicated.

Pediatric Use

Safety and effectiveness in children have not been established. Several cases of children treated with Lamprene have been reported in the literature.

ADVERSE REACTIONS

In general, Lamprene is well tolerated when administered in dosages no greater than 100 mg daily. The most consistent adverse reactions are usually dose related and are usually reversible when Lamprene is discontinued.

Adverse Reactions Occuring in More Than 1% of Patients

Skin: Pigmentation from pink to brownish-black in 75–100% of the patients within a few weeks of treatment; ichthyosis and dryness (8–28%); rash and pruritus (1–5%).

Gastrointestinal: Abdominal and epigastric pain, diarrhea, nausea, vomiting, gastrointestinal intolerance (40–50%).

Ocular: Conjunctival and corneal pigmentation due to clofazimine crystal deposits; dryness; burning; itching; irritation.

Other: Discoloration of urine, feces, sputum, sweat; elevated blood sugar; elevated ESR.

Adverse Reactions Occurring in Less Than 1% of Patients

Skin: Phototoxicity, erythroderma, acneiform eruptions, monilial cheilosis.

Gastrointestinal: Bowel obstruction (see WARNINGS), gastrointestinal bleeding (see WARNINGS), anorexia, constipation, weight loss, hepatitis, jaundice, eosinophilic enteritis, enlarged liver.

Ocular: Diminished vision.

Nervous: Dizziness, drowsiness, fatigue, headache, giddiness, neuralgia, taste disorder.

Psychiatric: Depression secondary to skin discoloration; two suicides have been reported.

Laboratory: Elevated levels of albumin, serum bilirubin, and AST (SGOT); eosinophilia; hypokalemia.

Other: Splenic infarction (see WARNINGS), thromboembolism, anemia, cystitis, bone pain, edema, fever, lymphadenopathy, vascular pain.

OVERDOSAGE

No specific data are available on the treatment of overdosage with Lamprene. However, in case of overdose, the stomach should be emptied by inducing vomiting or by gastric lavage, and supportive symptomatic treatment should be employed.

DOSAGE AND ADMINISTRATION

Lamprene should be taken with meals.

Lamprene should be used preferably in combination with one or more other antileprosy agents to prevent the emergence of drug resistance.

For the treatment of proven dapsone-resistant leprosy, Lamprene should be given at a dosage of 100 mg daily in combination with one or more other antileprosy drugs for 3 years, followed by monotherapy with 100 mg of Lamprene daily. Clinical improvement usually can be detected between the first and third months of treatment and is usually clearly evident by the sixth month.

For dapsone-sensitive multibacillary leprosy, a combination therapy with two other antileprosy drugs is recommended. The triple-drug regimen should be given for at least 2 years and continued, if possible, until negative skin smears are obtained. At this time, monotherapy with an appropriate antileprosy drug can be instituted.

The treatment of erythema nodosum leprosum reactions depends on the severity of symptoms. In general, the basic antileprosy treatment should be continued, and if nerve injury or skin ulceration is threatened, corticosteriods should be given. Where prolonged corticosteroid therapy becomes necessary, Lamprene administered at dosages of 100 mg to 200 mg daily for up to 3 months may be useful in eliminating or reducing corticosteroid requirements. Dosages above 200 mg daily are not recommended, and the dosage should be tapered to 100 mg daily as quickly as possible after the reactive episode is controlled. The patient must remain under medical surveillance.

For advice about combination drug regimens, contact the USPHS Gillis W. Long Hansen's Disease Center, Carville, LA (504-642-7771).

HOW SUPPLIED

Capsules 50 mg—brown, spherical
Bottles of 100 ....NDC 0028-0108-01

Capsules 100 mg—brown, oblong (imprinted GEIGY GM)
Bottles of 100 ....NDC 0028-0109-01

Do not store above 86°F. Protect from moisture.

Dispense in tight container (USP).

C87-25 (Rev. 9/87)

Dist. by:
GEIGY Pharmaceuticals
Division of CIBA-GEIGY Corporation
Ardsley, New York 10502

Shown in Product Identification Section, page 410

LIORESAL® **Tablets** ℞
[lye-oar 'eh-sal]
baclofen USP **10 mg**
Muscle Relaxant, Antispastic **20 mg** ℞

DESCRIPTION

Lioresal, baclofen USP, is a muscle relaxant and antispastic, available as 10-mg and 20-mg tablets for oral administration. Its chemical name is 4-amino-3-(4-chlorophenyl)-butanoic acid.

Baclofen USP is a white to off-white, odorless or practically odorless crystalline powder, with a molecular weight of 213.66. It is slightly soluble in water, very slightly soluble in methanol, and insoluble in chloroform.

Inactive Ingredients. Cellulose compounds, magnesium stearate, povidone, and starch.

ACTIONS

The precise mechanism of action of Lioresal is not fully known. Lioresal is capable of inhibiting both monosynaptic and polysynaptic reflexes at the spinal level, possibly by hyperpolarization of afferent terminals, although actions at supraspinal sites may also occur and contribute to its clinical effect. Although Lioresal is an analog of the putative inhibitory neurotransmitter gamma-aminobutyric acid (GABA), there is no conclusive evidence that actions on GABA systems are involved in the production of its clinical effects. In studies with animals, Lioresal has been shown to have general CNS depressant properties as indicated by the production of sedation with tolerance, somnolence, ataxia, and respiratory and cardiovascular depression. Lioresal is rapidly and extensively absorbed and eliminated. Absorption may be dose-dependent, being reduced with increasing doses. Lioresal is excreted primarily by the kidney in unchanged form and there is relatively large intersubject variation in absorption and/or elimination.

INDICATIONS

Lioresal is useful for the alleviation of signs and symptoms of spasticity resulting from multiple sclerosis, particularly for the relief of flexor spasms and concomitant pain, clonus, and muscular rigidity.

Patients should have reversible spasticity so that Lioresal treatment will aid in restoring residual function.

Lioresal may also be of some value in patients with spinal cord injuries and other spinal cord diseases.

Lioresal is not indicated in the treatment of skeletal muscle spasm resulting from rheumatic disorders.

The efficacy of Lioresal in stroke, cerebral palsy, and Parkinson's disease has not been established and, therefore, it is not recommended for these conditions.

Continued on next page

The full prescribing information for each GEIGY product is contained herein and is that in effect as of September 1, 1992.

GEIGY—Cont.

CONTRAINDICATIONS
Hypersensitivity to baclofen.

WARNINGS
a. *Abrupt Drug Withdrawal:* Hallucinations and seizures have occurred on abrupt withdrawal of Lioresal. Therefore, except for serious adverse reactions, the dose should be reduced slowly when the drug is discontinued.

b. *Impaired Renal Function:* Because Lioresal is primarily excreted unchanged through the kidneys, it should be given with caution, and it may be necessary to reduce the dosage.

c. *Stroke:* Lioresal has not significantly benefited patients with stroke. These patients have also shown poor tolerability to the drug.

d. *Pregnancy:* Lioresal has been shown to increase the incidence of omphaloceles (ventral hernias) in fetuses of rats given approximately 13 times the maximum dose recommended for human use, at a dose which caused significant reductions in food intake and weight gain in dams. This abnormality was not seen in mice or rabbits. There was also an increased incidence of incomplete sternebral ossification in fetuses of rats given approximately 13 times the maximum recommended human dose, and an increased incidence of unossified phalangeal nuclei of forelimbs and hindlimbs in fetuses of rabbits given approximately 7 times the maximum recommended human dose. In mice, no teratogenic effects were observed, although reductions in mean fetal weight with consequent delays in skeletal ossification were present when dams were given 17 or 34 times the human daily dose. There are no studies in pregnant women. Lioresal should be used during pregnancy only if the benefit clearly justifies the potential risk to the fetus.

PRECAUTIONS
Safe use of Lioresal in children under age 12 has not been established, and it is, therefore, not recommended for use in children.

Because of the possibility of sedation, patients should be cautioned regarding the operation of automobiles or other dangerous machinery, and activities made hazardous by decreased alertness. Patients should also be cautioned that the central nervous system effects of Lioresal may be additive to those of alcohol and other CNS depressants.

Lioresal should be used with caution where spasticity is utilized to sustain upright posture and balance in locomotion or whenever spasticity is utilized to obtain increased function.

In patients with epilepsy, the clinical state and electroencephalogram should be monitored at regular intervals, since deterioration in seizure control and EEG have been reported occasionally in patients taking Lioresal.

It is not known whether this drug is excreted in human milk. As a general rule, nursing should not be undertaken while a patient is on a drug since many drugs are excreted in human milk.

A dose-related increase in incidence of ovarian cysts and a less marked increase in enlarged and/or hemorrhagic adrenal glands was observed in female rats treated chronically with Lioresal.

Ovarian cysts have been found by palpation in about 4% of the multiple sclerosis patients that were treated with Lioresal for up to one year. In most cases these cysts disappeared spontaneously while patients continued to receive the drug. Ovarian cysts are estimated to occur spontaneously in approximately 1% to 5% of the normal female population.

ADVERSE REACTIONS
The most common is transient drowsiness (10–63%). In one controlled study of 175 patients, transient drowsiness was observed in 63% of those receiving Lioresal compared to 36% of those in the placebo group. Other common adverse reactions are dizziness (5–15%), weakness (5–15%) and fatigue (2–4%). Others reported:

Neuropsychiatric: Confusion (1–11%), headache (4–8%), insomnia (2–7%); and, rarely, euphoria, excitement, depression, hallucinations, paresthesia, muscle pain, tinnitus, slurred speech, coordination disorder, tremor, rigidity, dystonia, ataxia, blurred vision, nystagmus, strabismus, miosis, mydriasis, diplopia, dysarthria, epileptic seizure.

Cardiovascular: Hypotension (0–9%). Rare instances of dyspnea, palpitation, chest pain, syncope.

Gastrointestinal: Nausea (4–12%), constipation (2–6%); and, rarely, dry mouth, anorexia, taste disorder, abdominal pain, vomiting, diarrhea, and positive test for occult blood in stool.

Genitourinary: Urinary frequency (2–6%); and, rarely, enuresis, urinary retention, dysuria, impotence, inability to ejaculate, nocturia, hematuria.

Other: Instances of rash, pruritus, ankle edema, excessive perspiration, weight gain, nasal congestion.

Some of the CNS and genitourinary symptoms may be related to the underlying disease rather than to drug therapy.

The following laboratory tests have been found to be abnormal in a few patients receiving Lioresal: increased SGOT, elevated alkaline phosphatase, and elevation of blood sugar.

OVERDOSAGE
Signs and Symptoms: Vomiting, muscular hypotonia, drowsiness, accommodation disorders, coma, respiratory depression, and seizures.

Treatment: In the alert patient, empty the stomach promptly by induced emesis followed by lavage. In the obtunded patient, secure the airway with a cuffed endotracheal tube before beginning lavage (do not induce emesis). Maintain adequate respiratory exchange, do not use respiratory stimulants.

DOSAGE AND ADMINISTRATION
The determination of optimal dosage requires individual titration. Start therapy at a low dosage and increase gradually until optimum effect is achieved (usually between 40–80 mg daily).

The following dosage titration schedule is suggested:
5 mg t.i.d. for 3 days
10 mg t.i.d. for 3 days
15 mg t.i.d. for 3 days
20 mg t.i.d. for 3 days

Thereafter additional increases may be necessary but the total daily dose should not exceed a maximum of 80 mg daily (20 mg q.i.d.).

The lowest dose compatible with an optimal response is recommended. If benefits are not evident after a reasonable trial period, patients should be slowly withdrawn from the drug (see **WARNINGS** *Abrupt Drug Withdrawal*).

HOW SUPPLIED
Tablets 10 mg —oval, white, scored (imprinted Lioresal on one side and 10 twice on the scored side)
  Bottles of 100 ....NDC 0028-0023-01
  Unit Dose (blister pack)
  Box of 100 (strips of 10) ....NDC 0028-0023-61
Tablets 20 mg —capsule-shaped, white, scored (imprinted Lioresal on one side and 20 twice on the scored side)
  Bottles of 100 ....NDC 0028-0033-01
  Unit Dose (blister pack)
  Box of 100 (strips of 10) ....NDC 0028-0033-61
Samples, when available, are identified by the word *Sample* appearing on each tablet.
Do not store above 86°F (30°C).
Dispense in tight container (USP).

C88-39 (Rev. 12/88)

Shown in Product Identification Section, page 410

LOPRESSOR®   ℞
metoprolol tartrate USP
Tablets
Ampuls

DESCRIPTION
Lopressor, metoprolol tartrate, is a selective beta$_1$-adrenoreceptor blocking agent, available as 50- and 100-mg tablets for oral administration and in 5-ml ampuls for intravenous administration. Each ampul contains a sterile solution of metoprolol tartrate USP, 5 mg, and sodium chloride USP, 45 mg. Metoprolol tartrate is 1-(isopropylamino)-3-[*p*-(2-methoxyethyl) phenoxy]-2-propanol (2:1) *dextro* -tartrate salt.

Metoprolol tartrate is a white, practically odorless, crystalline powder with a molecular weight of 684.82. It is very soluble in water; freely soluble in methylene chloride, in chloroform, and in alcohol; slightly soluble in acetone; and insoluble in ether.

Inactive Ingredients: Tablets contain cellulose compounds, colloidal silicon dioxide, D&C Red No. 30 aluminum lake (50-mg tablets), FD&C Blue No. 2 aluminum lake (100-mg tablets), lactose, magnesium stearate, polyethylene glycol, propylene glycol, povidone, sodium starch glycolate, talc, and titanium dioxide.

CLINICAL PHARMACOLOGY
Lopressor is a beta-adrenergic receptor blocking agent. *In vitro* and *in vivo* animal studies have shown that it has a preferential effect on beta$_1$ adrenoreceptors, chiefly located in cardiac muscle. This preferential effect is not absolute, however, and at higher doses, Lopressor also inhibits beta$_2$ adrenoreceptors, chiefly located in the bronchial and vascular musculature.

Clinical pharmacology studies have confirmed the beta-blocking activity of metoprolol in man, as shown by (1) reduction in heart rate and cardiac output at rest and upon exercise, (2) reduction of systolic blood pressure upon exercise, (3) inhibition of isoproterenol-induced tachycardia, and (4) reduction of reflex orthostatic tachycardia.

Relative beta$_1$ selectivity has been confirmed by the following: (1) In normal subjects, Lopressor is unable to reverse the beta$_2$-mediated vasodilating effects of epinephrine. This contrasts with the effect of nonselective (beta$_1$ plus beta$_2$) beta blockers, which completely reverse the vasodilating effects

of epinephrine. (2) In asthmatic patients, Lopressor reduces FEV$_1$ and FVC significantly less than a nonselective beta blocker, propranolol, at equivalent beta$_1$-receptor blocking doses.

Lopressor has no intrinsic sympathomimetic activity, and membrane-stabilizing activity is detectable only at doses much greater than required for beta blockade. Lopressor crosses the blood-brain barrier and has been reported in the CSF in a concentration 78% of the simultaneous plasma concentration. Animal and human experiments indicate that Lopressor slows the sinus rate and decreases AV nodal conduction.

In controlled clinical studies, Lopressor has been shown to be an effective antihypertensive agent when used alone or as concomitant therapy with thiazide-type diuretics, at dosages of 100–450 mg daily. In controlled, comparative, clinical studies, Lopressor has been shown to be as effective an antihypertensive agent as propranolol, methyldopa, and thiazide-type diuretics, and to be equally effective in supine and standing positions.

The mechanism of the antihypertensive effects of beta-blocking agents has not been elucidated. However, several possible mechanisms have been proposed: (1) competitive antagonism of catecholamines at peripheral (especially cardiac) adrenergic neuron sites, leading to decreased cardiac output; (2) a central effect leading to reduced sympathetic outflow to the periphery; and (3) suppression of renin activity.

By blocking catecholamine-induced increases in heart rate, in velocity and extent of myocardial contraction, and in blood pressure, Lopressor reduces the oxygen requirements of the heart at any given level of effort, thus making it useful in the long-term management of angina pectoris. However, in patients with heart failure, beta-adrenergic blockade may increase oxygen requirements by increasing left ventricular fiber length and end-diastolic pressure.

Although beta-adrenergic receptor blockade is useful in the treatment of angina and hypertension, there are situations in which sympathetic stimulation is vital. In patients with severely damaged hearts, adequate ventricular function may depend on sympathetic drive. In the presence of AV block, beta blockade may prevent the necessary facilitating effect of sympathetic activity on conduction. Beta$_2$-adrenergic blockade results in passive bronchial constriction by interfering with endogenous adrenergic bronchodilator activity in patients subject to bronchospasm and may also interfere with exogenous bronchodilators in such patients.

In controlled clinical trials, Lopressor, administered two or four times daily, has been shown to be an effective antianginal agent, reducing the number of angina attacks and increasing exercise tolerance. The dosage used in these studies ranged from 100 to 400 mg daily. A controlled, comparative, clinical trial showed that Lopressor was indistinguishable from propranolol in the treatment of angina pectoris.

In a large (1,395 patients randomized), double-blind, placebo-controlled clinical study, Lopressor was shown to reduce 3-month mortality by 36% in patients with suspected or definite myocardial infarction.

Patients were randomized and treated as soon as possible after their arrival in the hospital, once their clinical condition had stabilized and their hemodynamic status had been carefully evaluated. Subjects were ineligible if they had hypotension, bradycardia, peripheral signs of shock, and/or more than minimal basal rales as signs of congestive heart failure. Initial treatment consisted of intravenous followed by oral administration of Lopressor or placebo, given in a coronary care or comparable unit. Oral maintenance therapy with Lopressor or placebo was then continued for 3 months. After this double-blind period, all patients were given Lopressor and followed up to 1 year.

The median delay from the onset of symptoms to the initiation of therapy was 8 hours in both the Lopressor and placebo treatment groups. Among patients treated with Lopressor, there were comparable reductions in 3-month mortality for those treated early (≤ 8 hours) and those in whom treatment was started later. Significant reductions in the incidence of ventricular fibrillation and in chest pain following initial intravenous therapy were also observed with Lopressor and were independent of the interval between onset of symptoms and initiation of therapy.

The precise mechanism of action of Lopressor in patients with suspected or definite myocardial infarction is not known.

In this study, patients treated with metoprolol received the drug both very early (intravenously) and during a subsequent 3-month period, while placebo patients received no beta-blocker treatment for this period. The study thus was able to show a benefit from the overall metoprolol regimen but cannot separate the benefit of very early intravenous treatment from the benefit of later beta-blocker therapy. Nonetheless, because the overall regimen showed a clear beneficial effect on survival without evidence of an early adverse effect on survival, one acceptable dosage regimen is the precise regimen used in the trial. Because the specific benefit of very early treatment remains to be defined however, it is also reasonable to administer the drug orally to

patients at a later time as is recommended for certain other beta blockers.

Pharmacokinetics

In man, absorption of Lopressor is rapid and complete. Plasma levels following oral administration, however, approximate 50% of levels following intravenous administration, indicating about 50% first-pass metabolism.

Plasma levels achieved are highly variable after oral administration. Only a small fraction of the drug (about 12%) is bound to human serum albumin. Elimination is mainly by biotransformation in the liver, and the plasma half-life ranges from approximately 3 to 7 hours. Less than 5% of an oral dose of Lopressor is recovered unchanged in the urine; the rest is excreted by the kidneys as metabolites that appear to have no clinical significance. The systemic availability and half-life of Lopressor in patients with renal failure do not differ to a clinically significant degree from those in normal subjects. Consequently, no reduction in dosage is usually needed in patients with chronic renal failure.

Significant beta-blocking effect (as measured by reduction of exercise heart rate) occurs within 1 hour after oral administration, and its duration is dose-related. For example, a 50% reduction of the maximum registered effect after single oral doses of 20, 50, and 100 mg occurred at 3.3, 5.0, and 6.4 hours, respectively, in normal subjects. After repeated oral dosages of 100 mg twice daily, a significant reduction in exercise systolic blood pressure was evident at 12 hours.

Following intravenous administration of Lopressor, the urinary recovery of unchanged drug is approximately 10%. When the drug was infused over a 10-minute period, in normal volunteers, maximum beta blockade was achieved at approximately 20 minutes. Doses of 5 mg and 15 mg yielded a maximal reduction in exercise-induced heart rate of approximately 10% and 15%, respectively. The effect on exercise heart rate decreased linearly with time at the same rate for both doses, and disappeared at approximately 5 hours and 8 hours for the 5-mg and 15-mg doses, respectively.

Equivalent maximal beta-blocking effect is achieved with oral and intravenous doses in the ratio of approximately 2.5:1.

There is a linear relationship between the log of plasma levels and reduction of exercise heart rate. However, antihypertensive activity does not appear to be related to plasma levels. Because of variable plasma levels attained with a given dose and lack of a consistent relationship of antihypertensive activity to dose, selection of proper dosage requires individual titration.

In several studies of patients with acute myocardial infarction, intravenous followed by oral administration of Lopressor caused a reduction in heart rate, systolic blood pressure, and cardiac output. Stroke volume, diastolic blood pressure, and pulmonary artery end diastolic pressure remained unchanged.

In patients with angina pectoris, plasma concentration measured at 1 hour is linearly related to the oral dose within the range of 50 to 400 mg. Exercise heart rate and systolic blood pressure are reduced in relation to the logarithm of the oral dose of metoprolol. The increase in exercise capacity and the reduction in left ventricular ischemia are also significantly related to the logarithm of the oral dose.

INDICATIONS AND USAGE

Hypertension

Lopressor tablets are indicated for the treatment of hypertension. They may be used alone or in combination with other antihypertensive agents.

Angina Pectoris

Lopressor is indicated in the long-term treatment of angina pectoris.

Myocardial Infarction

Lopressor ampuls and tablets are indicated in the treatment of hemodynamically stable patients with definite or suspected acute myocardial infarction to reduce cardiovascular mortality. Treatment with intravenous Lopressor can be initiated as soon as the patient's clinical condition allows (see **DOSAGE AND ADMINISTRATION, CONTRAINDICATIONS,** and **WARNINGS**). Alternatively, treatment can begin within 3 to 10 days of the acute event (see **DOSAGE AND ADMINISTRATION**).

CONTRAINDICATIONS

Hypertension and Angina

Lopressor is contraindicated in sinus bradycardia, heart block greater than first degree, cardiogenic shock, and overt cardiac failure (see **WARNINGS**).

Myocardial Infarction

Lopressor is contraindicated in patients with a heart rate < 45 beats/min; second- and third-degree heart block; significant first-degree heart block (P-R interval ≥ 0.24 sec); systolic blood pressure < 100 mmHg; or moderate-to-severe cardiac failure (see **WARNINGS**).

WARNINGS

Hypertension and Angina

Cardiac Failure: Sympathetic stimulation is a vital component supporting circulatory function in congestive heart failure, and beta blockade carries the potential hazard of further depressing myocardial contractility and precipitating more severe failure. In hypertensive and angina patients who have congestive heart failure controlled by digitalis and diuretics, Lopressor should be administered cautiously. Both digitalis and Lopressor slow AV conduction.

In Patients Without a History of Cardiac Failure: Continued depression of the myocardium with beta-blocking agents over a period of time can, in some cases, lead to cardiac failure. At the first sign or symptom of impending cardiac failure, patients should be fully digitalized and/or given a diuretic. The response should be observed closely. If cardiac failure continues, despite adequate digitalization and diuretic therapy, Lopressor should be withdrawn.

Ischemic Heart Disease: Following abrupt cessation of therapy with certain beta-blocking agents, exacerbations of angina pectoris and, in some cases, myocardial infarction have occurred. When discontinuing chronically administered Lopressor, particularly in patients with ischemic heart disease, the dosage should be gradually reduced over a period of 1–2 weeks and the patient should be carefully monitored. If angina markedly worsens or acute coronary insufficiency develops, Lopressor administration should be reinstated promptly, at least temporarily, and other measures appropriate for the management of unstable angina should be taken. Patients should be warned against interruption or discontinuation of therapy without the physician's advice. Because coronary artery disease is common and may be unrecognized, it may be prudent not to discontinue Lopressor therapy abruptly even in patients treated only for hypertension.

Bronchospastic Diseases: PATIENTS WITH BRONCHO-SPASTIC DISEASES SHOULD, IN GENERAL, NOT RECEIVE BETA-BLOCKERS. Because of its relative beta$_1$ selectivity, however, Lopressor may be used with caution in patients with bronchospastic disease who do not respond to, or cannot tolerate, other antihypertensive treatment. Since beta$_1$ selectivity is not absolute, a beta$_2$-stimulating agent should be administered concomitantly, and the lowest possible dose of Lopressor should be used. In these circumstances it would be prudent initially to administer Lopressor in smaller doses three times daily, instead of larger doses two times daily, to avoid the higher plasma levels associated with the longer dosing interval. (See **DOSAGE AND ADMINISTRATION.**)

Major Surgery: The necessity or desirability of withdrawing beta-blocking therapy prior to major surgery is controversial; the impaired ability of the heart to respond to reflex adrenergic stimuli may augment the risks of general anesthesia and surgical procedures.

Lopressor, like other beta blockers, is a competitive inhibitor of beta-receptor agonists, and its effects can be reversed by administration of such agents, e.g., dobutamine or isoproterenol. However, such patients may be subject to protracted severe hypotension. Difficulty in restarting and maintaining the heart beat has also been reported with beta blockers.

Diabetes and Hypoglycemia: Lopressor should be used with caution in diabetic patients if a beta-blocking agent is required. Beta blockers may mask tachycardia occurring with hypoglycemia, but other manifestations such as dizziness and sweating may not be significantly affected.

Thyrotoxicosis: Beta-adrenergic blockade may mask certain clinical signs (e.g., tachycardia) of hyperthyroidism. Patients suspected of developing thyrotoxicosis should be managed carefully to avoid abrupt withdrawal of beta blockade, which might precipitate a thyroid storm.

Myocardial Infarction

Cardiac Failure: Sympathetic stimulation is a vital component supporting circulatory function, and beta blockade carries the potential hazard of depressing myocardial contractility and precipitating or exacerbating minimal cardiac failure.

During treatment with Lopressor, the hemodynamic status of the patient should be carefully monitored. If heart failure occurs or persists despite appropriate treatment, Lopressor should be discontinued.

Bradycardia: Lopressor produces a decrease in sinus heart rate in most patients; this decrease is greatest among patients with high initial heart rates and least among patients with low initial heart rates. Acute myocardial infarction (particularly inferior infarction) may in itself produce significant lowering of the sinus rate. If the sinus rate decreases to < 40 beats/min, particularly if associated with evidence of lowered cardiac output, atropine (0.25–0.5 mg) should be administered intravenously. If treatment with atropine is not successful, Lopressor should be discontinued, and cautious administration of isoproterenol or installation of a cardiac pacemaker should be considered.

AV Block: Lopressor slows AV conduction and may produce significant first- (P-R interval ≥ 0.26 sec), second-, or third-degree heart block. Acute myocardial infarction also produces heart block.

If heart block occurs, Lopressor should be discontinued and atropine (0.25–0.5 mg) should be administered intravenously. If treatment with atropine is not successful, cautious administration of isoproterenol or installation of a cardiac pacemaker should be considered.

Hypotension: If hypotension (systolic blood pressure ≤ 90 mmHg) occurs, Lopressor should be discontinued, and the hemodynamic status of the patient and the extent of myocardial damage carefully assessed. Invasive monitoring of central venous, pulmonary capillary wedge, and arterial pressures may be required. Appropriate therapy with fluids, positive inotropic agents, balloon counterpulsation, or other treatment modalities should be instituted. If hypotension is associated with sinus bradycardia or AV block, treatment should be directed at reversing these (see above).

Bronchospastic Diseases: PATIENTS WITH BRONCHO-SPASTIC DISEASES SHOULD, IN GENERAL, NOT RECEIVE BETA BLOCKERS. Because of its relative beta$_1$ selectivity, Lopressor may be used with extreme caution in patients with bronchospastic disease. Because it is unknown to what extent beta$_2$-stimulating agents may exacerbate myocardial ischemia and the extent of infarction, these agents should *not* be used prophylactically. If bronchospasm not related to congestive heart failure occurs, Lopressor should be discontinued. A theophylline derivative or a beta$_2$ agonist may be administered cautiously, depending on the clinical condition of the patient. Both theophylline derivatives and beta$_2$ agonists may produce serious cardiac arrhythmias.

PRECAUTIONS

General

Lopressor should be used with caution in patients with impaired hepatic function.

Information for Patients

Patients should be advised to take Lopressor regularly and continuously, as directed, with or immediately following meals. If a dose should be missed, the patient should take only the next scheduled dose (without doubling it). Patients should not discontinue Lopressor without consulting the physician.

Patients should be advised (1) to avoid operating automobiles and machinery or engaging in other tasks requiring alertness until the patient's response to therapy with Lopressor has been determined; (2) to contact the physician if any difficulty in breathing occurs; (3) to inform the physician or dentist before any type of surgery that he or she is taking Lopressor.

Laboratory Tests

Clinical laboratory findings may include elevated levels of serum transaminase, alkaline phosphatase, and lactate dehydrogenase.

Drug Interactions

Catecholamine-depleting drugs (e.g., reserpine) may have an additive effect when given with beta-blocking agents. Patients treated with Lopressor plus a catecholamine depletor should therefore be closely observed for evidence of hypotension or marked bradycardia, which may produce vertigo, syncope, or postural hypotension.

Risk of Anaphylactic Reaction. While taking beta-blockers, patients with a history of severe anaphylactic reaction to a variety of allergens may be more reactive to repeated challenge, either accidental, diagnostic, or therapeutic. Such patients may be unresponsive to the usual doses of epinephrine used to treat allergic reactions.

Carcinogenesis, Mutagenesis, Impairment of Fertility

Long-term studies in animals have been conducted to evaluate carcinogenic potential. In 2-year studies in rats at three oral dosage levels of up to 800 mg/kg per day, there was no increase in the development of spontaneously occurring benign or malignant neoplasms of any type. The only histologic changes that appeared to be drug related were an increased incidence of generally mild focal accumulation of foamy macrophages in pulmonary alveoli and a slight increase in biliary hyperplasia. In a 21-month study in Swiss albino mice at three oral dosage levels of up to 750 mg/kg per day, benign lung tumors (small adenomas) occurred more frequently in female mice receiving the highest dose than in untreated control animals. There was no increase in malignant or total (benign plus malignant) lung tumors, nor in the overall incidence of tumors or malignant tumors. This 21-month study was repeated in CD-1 mice, and no statistically or biologically significant differences were observed between treated and control mice of either sex for any type of tumor.

All mutagenicity tests performed (a dominant lethal study in mice, chromosome studies in somatic cells, a Salmonella/mammalian-microsome mutagenicity test, and a nucleus anomaly test in somatic interphase nuclei) were negative.

Continued on next page

The full prescribing information for each GEIGY product is contained herein and is that in effect as of September 1, 1992.

GEIGY—Cont.

No evidence of impaired fertility due to Lopressor was observed in a study performed in rats at doses up to 55.5 times the maximum daily human dose of 450 mg.

Pregnancy Category C

Lopressor has been shown to increase postimplantation loss and decrease neonatal survival in rats at doses up to 55.5 times the maximum daily human dose of 450 mg. Distribution studies in mice confirm exposure of the fetus when Lopressor is administered to the pregnant animal. These studies have revealed no evidence of impaired fertility or teratogenicity. There are no adequate and well-controlled studies in pregnant women. Because animal reproduction studies are not always predictive of human response, this drug should be used during pregnancy only if clearly needed.

Nursing Mothers

Lopressor is excreted in breast milk in very small quantity. An infant consuming 1 liter of breast milk daily would receive a dose of less than 1 mg of the drug. Caution should be exercised when Lopressor is administered to a nursing woman.

Pediatric Use

Safety and effectiveness in children have not been established.

ADVERSE REACTIONS

Hypertension and Angina

Most adverse effects have been mild and transient.

Central Nervous System: Tiredness and dizziness have occurred in about 10 of 100 patients. Depression has been reported in about 5 of 100 patients. Mental confusion and short-term memory loss have been reported. Headache, nightmares, and insomnia have also been reported.

Cardiovascular: Shortness of breath and bradycardia have occurred in approximately 3 of 100 patients. Cold extremities; arterial insufficiency, usually of the Raynaud type; palpitations; congestive heart failure; peripheral edema; and hypotension have been reported in about 1 of 100 patients. (See CONTRAINDICATIONS, WARNINGS, and PRECAUTIONS.)

Respiratory: Wheezing (bronchospasm) and dyspnea have been reported in about 1 of 100 patients (see WARNINGS).

Gastrointestinal: Diarrhea has occurred in about 5 of 100 patients. Nausea, dry mouth, gastric pain, constipation, flatulence, and heartburn have been reported in about 1 of 100 patients.

Hypersensitive Reactions: Pruritus or rash have occurred in about 5 of 100 patients. Worsening of psoriasis has also been reported.

Miscellaneous: Peyronie's disease has been reported in fewer than 1 of 100,000 patients. Musculoskeletal pain, blurred vision, and tinnitus have also been reported.

There have been rare reports of reversible alopecia, agranulocytosis, and dry eyes. Discontinuation of the drug should be considered if any such reaction is not otherwise explicable. The oculomucocutaneous syndrome associated with the beta blocker practolol has not been reported with Lopressor.

Myocardial Infarction

Central Nervous System: Tiredness has been reported in about 1 of 100 patients. Vertigo, sleep disturbances, hallucinations, headache, dizziness, visual disturbances, confusion, and reduced libido have also been reported, but a drug relationship is not clear.

Cardiovascular: In the randomized comparison of Lopressor and placebo described in the CLINICAL PHARMACOLOGY section, the following adverse reactions were reported:

	Lopressor	Placebo
Hypotension (systolic BP < 90 mmHg)	27.4%	23.2%
Bradycardia (heart rate < 40 beats/min)	15.9%	6.7%
Second- or third-degree heart block	4.7%	4.7%
First-degree heart block (P-R ≥ 0.26 sec)	5.3%	1.9%
Heart failure	27.5%	29.6%

Respiratory: Dyspnea of pulmonary origin has been reported in fewer than 1 of 100 patients.

Gastrointestinal: Nausea and abdominal pain have been reported in fewer than 1 of 100 patients.

Dermatologic: Rash and worsened psoriasis have been reported, but a drug relationship is not clear.

Miscellaneous: Unstable diabetes and claudication have been reported, but a drug relationship is not clear.

Potential Adverse Reactions

A variety of adverse reactions not listed above have been reported with other beta-adrenergic blocking agents and should be considered potential adverse reactions to Lopressor.

Central Nervous System: Reversible mental depression progressing to catatonia; an acute reversible syndrome characterized by disorientation for time and place, short-term

memory loss, emotional lability, slightly clouded sensorium, and decreased performance on neuropsychometrics.

Cardiovascular: Intensification of AV block (See CONTRAINDICATIONS).

Hematologic: Agranulocytosis, nonthrombocytopenic purpura, thrombocytopenic purpura.

Hypersensitive Reactions: Fever combined with aching and sore throat, laryngospasm, and respiratory distress.

OVERDOSAGE

Acute Toxicity

Several cases of overdosage have been reported, some leading to death.

Oral LD$_{50}$'s (mg/kg): mice, 1158–2460; rats, 3090–4670.

Signs and Symptoms

Potential signs and symptoms associated with overdosage with Lopressor are bradycardia, hypotension, bronchospasm, and cardiac failure.

Treatment

There is no specific antidote.

In general, patients with acute or recent myocardial infarction may be more hemodynamically unstable than other patients and should be treated accordingly (see WARNINGS, Myocardial Infarction).

On the basis of the pharmacologic actions of Lopressor, the following general measures should be employed:

Elimination of the Drug: Gastric lavage should be performed.

Bradycardia: Atropine should be administered. If there is no response to vagal blockade, isoproterenol should be administered cautiously.

Hypotension: A vasopressor should be administered, e.g., levarterenol or dopamine.

Bronchospasm: A beta$_2$-stimulating agent and/or a theophylline derivative should be administered.

Cardiac Failure: A digitalis glycoside and diuretic should be administered. In shock resulting from inadequate cardiac contractility, administration of dobutamine, isoproterenol, or glucagon may be considered.

DOSAGE AND ADMINISTRATION

Hypertension

The dosage of Lopressor should be individualized. Lopressor should be taken with or immediately following meals.

The usual initial dosage is 100 mg daily in single or divided doses, whether used alone or added to a diuretic. The dosage may be increased at weekly (or longer) intervals until optimum blood pressure reduction is achieved. In general, the maximum effect of any given dosage level will be apparent after 1 week of therapy. The effective dosage range is 100 to 450 mg per day. Dosages above 450 mg per day have not been studied. While once-daily dosing is effective and can maintain a reduction in blood pressure throughout the day, lower doses (especially 100 mg) may not maintain a full effect at the end of the 24-hour period, and larger or more frequent daily doses may be required. This can be evaluated by measuring blood pressure near the end of the dosing interval to determine whether satisfactory control is being maintained throughout the day. Beta$_1$ selectivity diminishes as the dose of Lopressor is increased.

Angina Pectoris

The dosage of Lopressor should be individualized. Lopressor should be taken with or immediately following meals.

The usual initial dosage is 100 mg daily, given in two divided doses. The dosage may be gradually increased at weekly intervals until optimum clinical response has been obtained or there is pronounced slowing of the heart rate. The effective dosage range is 100 to 400 mg per day. Dosages above 400 mg per day have not been studied. If treatment is to be discontinued, the dosage should be reduced gradually over a period of 1–2 weeks. (See WARNINGS.)

Myocardial Infarction

Early Treatment: During the early phase of definite or suspected acute myocardial infarction, treatment with Lopressor can be initiated as soon as possible after the patient's arrival in the hospital. Such treatment should be initiated in a coronary care or similar unit immediately after the patient's hemodynamic condition has stabilized.

Treatment in this early phase should begin with the intravenous administration of three bolus injections of 5 mg of Lopressor each; the injections should be given at approximately 2-minute intervals. During the intravenous administration of Lopressor, blood pressure, heart rate, and electrocardiogram should be carefully monitored.

In patients who tolerate the full intravenous dose (15 mg), Lopressor tablets, 50 mg every 6 hours, should be initiated 15 minutes after the last intravenous dose and continued for 48 hours. Thereafter, patients should receive a maintenance dosage of 100 mg twice daily (see *Late Treatment* below). Patients who appear not to tolerate the full intravenous dose should be started on Lopressor tablets either 25 mg or 50 mg every 6 hours (depending on the degree of intolerance) 15 minutes after the last intravenous dose or as soon as their clinical condition allows. In patients with severe intolerance, treatment with Lopressor should be discontinued (see WARNINGS).

Late Treatment: Patients with contraindications to treatment during the early phase of suspected or definite myocardial infarction, patients who appear not to tolerate the full early treatment, and patients in whom the physician wishes to delay therapy for any other reason should be started on Lopressor tablets, 100 mg twice daily, as soon as their clinical condition allows. Therapy should be continued for at least 3 months. Although the efficacy of Lopressor beyond 3 months has not been conclusively established, data from studies with other beta blockers suggest that treatment should be continued for 1–3 years.

Note: Parenteral drug products should be inspected visually for particulate matter and discoloration prior to administration, whenever solution and container permit.

HOW SUPPLIED

Tablets 50 mg—capsule-shaped, biconvex, pink, scored (imprinted GEIGY on one side and 51 twice on the scored side)

Bottles of 100 .... NDC 0028-0051-01
Bottles of 1000 .... NDC 0028-0051-10
Gy-Pak®—One Unit
  12 bottles—60 tablets each .... NDC 0028-0051-73
  12 bottles—100 tablets each .... NDC 0028-0051-65
Unit Dose (blister pack)
  Box of 100 (strips of 10) .... NDC 0028-0051-61

Tablets 100 mg—capsule-shaped, biconvex, light blue, scored (imprinted GEIGY on one side and 71 twice on the scored side)

Bottles of 100 .... NDC 0028-0071-01
Bottles of 1000 .... NDC 0028-0071-10
Gy-Pak®—One Unit
  12 bottles—60 tablets each .... NDC 0028-0071-73
  12 bottles—100 tablets each .... NDC 0028-0071-65
Unit Dose (blister pack)
  Box of 100 (strips of 10) .... NDC 0028-0071-61

Samples, when available, are identified by the word *SAMPLE* appearing on each tablet.

Store between 59°-86°F (15°-30°C). Protect from moisture.

Dispense in tight, light-resistant container (USP).

Ampuls 5 ml—each containing 5 mg of metoprolol tartrate
  Tray of 4 packs of 3 ampuls .... NDC 0028-4201-33
Do not store above 86°F (30°C). Protect from light.

C92-26 (Rev. 4/92)

Shown in Product Identification Section, page 410

LOPRESSOR HCT®   ℞
metoprolol tartrate USP and hydrochlorothiazide USP
50/25 Tablets
100/25 Tablets
100/50 Tablets
Beta Blocker/Diuretic Antihypertensive

DESCRIPTION

Lopressor HCT has the antihypertensive effect of Lopressor®, metoprolol tartrate, a selective beta$_1$-adrenoreceptor blocking agent, and the antihypertensive and diuretic actions of hydrochlorothiazide. It is available as tablets for oral administration. The 50/25 tablets contain 50 mg of metoprolol tartrate USP and 25 mg of hydrochlorothiazide USP; the 100/25 tablets contain 100 mg of metoprolol tartrate USP and 25 mg of hydrochlorothiazide USP; and the 100/50 tablets contain 100 mg of metoprolol tartrate USP and 50 mg of hydrochlorothiazide USP.

Metoprolol tartrate USP is (±)-1-Isopropylamino-3-[p-(2-methoxyethyl)phenoxy]-2-propanol 2:1 *dextro*-tartrate salt. Metoprolol tartrate USP is a white, crystalline powder with a molecular weight of 684.82. It is very soluble in water; freely soluble in methylene chloride, in chloroform, and in alcohol; slightly soluble in acetone; and insoluble in ether. Hydrochlorothiazide is 6-chloro-3,4-dihydro-2H-1,2,4-benzothiadiazine-7-sulfonamide, 1,1-dioxide.

Hydrochlorothiazide USP is a white, or practically white, practically odorless, crystalline powder. It is freely soluble in sodium hydroxide solution, in n-butylamine, and in dimethylformamide; sparingly soluble in methanol; slightly soluble in water; and insoluble in ether, in chloroform, and in dilute mineral acids. Its molecular weight is 297.73.

Inactive Ingredients: Cellulose compounds, colloidal silicon dioxide, D&C Yellow No. 10 (100/50-mg tablets), FD&C Blue No. 1 (50/25-mg tablets), FD&C Red No. 40 and FD&C Yellow No. 6 (100/25-mg tablets), lactose, magnesium stearate, povidone, sodium starch glycolate, starch, stearic acid, and sucrose.

CLINICAL PHARMACOLOGY

Lopressor

Lopressor is a beta-adrenergic receptor blocking agent. *In vitro* and *in vivo* animal studies have shown that it has a preferential effect on beta$_1$ adrenoreceptors, chiefly located in cardiac muscle. This preferential effect is not absolute, however, and at higher doses, Lopressor also inhibits beta$_2$ adrenoreceptors, chiefly located in the bronchial and vascular musculature.

Clinical pharmacology studies have confirmed the beta-blocking activity of metoprolol in man, as shown by (1) reduction in heart rate and cardiac output at rest and upon exercise, (2) reduction of systolic blood pressure upon exercise, (3) inhibition of isoproterenol-induced tachycardia, and (4) reduction of reflex orthostatic tachycardia.

Relative $beta_1$ selectivity has been confirmed by the following: (1) in normal subjects, Lopressor is unable to reverse the $beta_2$-mediated vasodilating effects of epinephrine. This contrasts with the effect of nonselective ($beta_1$ plus $beta_2$) beta blockers, which completely reverse the vasodilating effects of epinephrine. (2) In asthmatic patients, Lopressor reduces FEV_1 and FVC significantly less than a nonselective beta blocker, propranolol at equivalent $beta_1$-receptor blocking doses.

Lopressor has no intrinsic sympathomimetic activity and only weak membrane-stabilizing activity. Lopressor crosses the blood-brain barrier and has been reported in the CSF in a concentration 78% of the simultaneous plasma concentration. Animal and human experiments indicate that Lopressor slows the sinus rate and decreases AV nodal conduction.

In controlled clinical studies, Lopressor has been shown to be an effective antihypertensive agent when used alone or as concomitant therapy with thiazide-type diuretics, at dosages of 100–450 mg daily. In controlled, comparative, clinical studies, Lopressor has been shown to be as effective an antihypertensive agent as propranolol, methyldopa, and thiazide-type diuretics, and to be equally effective in supine and standing positions.

The mechanism of the antihypertensive effects of beta-blocking agents has not been elucidated. However, several possible mechanisms have been proposed: (1) competitive antagonism of catecholamines at peripheral (especially cardiac) adrenergic neuron sites, leading to decreased cardiac output; (2) a central effect leading to reduced sympathetic outflow to the periphery; and (3) suppression of renin activity.

In man, absorption of Lopressor is rapid and complete. Plasma levels following oral administration, however, approximate 50% of levels following intravenous administration, indicating about 50% first-pass metabolism. Plasma levels achieved are highly variable after oral administration. Only a small fraction of the drug (about 12%) is bound to human serum albumin. Elimination is mainly by biotransformation in the liver, and the plasma half-life ranges from approximately 3 to 7 hours. Less than 5% of an oral dose of Lopressor is recovered unchanged in the urine; the rest is excreted by the kidneys as metabolites that appear to have no clinical significance. The systemic availability and half-life of Lopressor in patients with renal failure do not differ to a clinically significant degree from those in normal subjects. Consequently, no reduction in dosage is usually needed in patients with chronic renal failure.

Significant beta-blocking effect (as measured by reduction of exercise heart rate) occurs within 1 hour after oral administration, and its duration is dose-related. For example, a 50% reduction of the maximum registered effect after single oral doses of 20, 50, and 100 mg occurred at 3.3, 5.0, and 6.4 hours, respectively, in normal subjects. After repeated oral dosages of 100 mg twice daily, a significant reduction in exercise systolic blood pressure was evident at 12 hours.

There is a linear relationship between the log of plasma levels and reduction of exercise heart rate. However, antihypertensive activity does not appear to be related to plasma levels. Because of variable plasma levels attained with a given dose and lack of a consistent relationship of antihypertensive activity to dose, selection of proper dosage requires individual titration.

Hydrochlorothiazide

Thiazides affect the renal tubular mechanism of electrolyte reabsorption. At maximal therapeutic dosage, all thiazides are approximately equal in their diuretic potency. Thiazides increase excretion of sodium and chloride in approximately equivalent amounts. Natriuresis causes a secondary loss of potassium.

The mechanism of the antihypertensive effect of thiazides is unknown. Thiazides do not affect normal blood pressure.

The onset of action of thiazides occurs in 2 hours and the peak effect at about 4 hours. The action persists for approximately 6–12 hours. Hydrochlorothiazide is rapidly absorbed, as indicated by peak plasma concentrations 1–2.5 hours after oral administration. Plasma levels of the drug are proportional to dose; the concentration in whole blood is 1.6–1.8 times higher than in plasma. Thiazides are eliminated rapidly by the kidney. After oral administration of 25- to 100-mg doses, 72–97% of the dose is excreted in the urine, indicating dose-independent absorption. Hydrochlorothiazide is eliminated from plasma in a biphasic fashion with a terminal half-life of 10–17 hours. Plasma protein binding is 67.9%. Plasma clearance is 15.9–30.0 L/hr; volume of distribution is 3.6–7.8 L/kg.

Gastrointestinal absorption of hydrochlorothiazide is enhanced when administered with food. Absorption is decreased in patients with congestive heart failure, and the pharmacokinetics are considerably different in these patients.

INDICATIONS AND USAGE

Lopressor HCT is indicated for the management of hypertension.

This fixed-combination drug is not indicated for initial therapy of hypertension. If the fixed combination represents the dose titrated to the individual patient's needs, therapy with the fixed combination may be more convenient than with the separate components.

CONTRAINDICATIONS

Lopressor

Lopressor is contraindicated in sinus bradycardia, heart block greater than first degree, cardiogenic shock, and overt cardiac failure (see **WARNINGS**).

Hydrochlorothiazide

Hydrochlorothiazide is contraindicated in patients with anuria or hypersensitivity to this or other sulfonamide-derived drugs (see **WARNINGS**).

WARNINGS

Lopressor

Cardiac Failure. Sympathetic stimulation is a vital component supporting circulatory function in congestive heart failure, and beta blockade carries the potential hazard of further depressing myocardial contractility and precipitating more severe failure. In hypertensive patients who have congestive heart failure controlled by digitalis and diuretics, Lopressor should be administered cautiously. Both digitalis and Lopressor slow AV conduction.

In Patients Without a History of Cardiac Failure. Continued depression of the myocardium with beta-blocking agents over a period of time can, in some cases, lead to cardiac failure. At the first sign or symptom of impending cardiac failure, patients should be fully digitalized and/or given a diuretic. The response should be observed closely. If cardiac failure continues, despite adequate digitalization and diuretic therapy, Lopressor should be withdrawn.

Ischemic Heart Disease. Following abrupt cessation of therapy with certain beta-blocking agents, exacerbations of angina pectoris and, in some cases, myocardial infarction have been reported. Even in the absence of overt angina pectoris, when discontinuing therapy, Lopressor should not be withdrawn abruptly, and patients should be cautioned against interruption of therapy without the physician's advice (see **PRECAUTIONS,** Information for Patients).

Bronchospastic Diseases. **PATIENTS WITH BRONCHOSPASTIC DISEASES SHOULD, IN GENERAL, NOT RECEIVE BETA BLOCKERS. Because of its relative $beta_1$ selectivity, however, Lopressor may be used with caution in patients with bronchospastic disease who do not respond to, or cannot tolerate, other antihypertensive treatment. Since $beta_1$ selectivity is not absolute, a $beta_2$-stimulating agent should be administered concomitantly, and the lowest possible dose of Lopressor should be used. In these circumstances it would be prudent initially to administer Lopressor in smaller doses three times daily, instead of larger doses two times daily, to avoid the higher plasma levels associated with the longer dosing interval. (See DOSAGE AND ADMINISTRATION.)**

Major Surgery. The necessity or desirability of withdrawing beta-blocking therapy prior to major surgery is controversial; the impaired ability of the heart to respond to reflex adrenergic stimuli may augment the risks of general anesthesia and surgical procedures.

Lopressor, like other beta blockers, is a competitive inhibitor of beta-receptor agonists, and its effects can be reversed by administration of such agents, e.g., dobutamine or isoproterenol. However, such patients may be subject to protracted severe hypotension. Difficulty in restarting and maintaining the heart beat has also been reported with beta blockers.

Diabetes and Hypoglycemia. Lopressor should be used with caution in diabetic patients if a beta-blocking agent is required. Beta blockers may mask tachycardia occurring with hypoglycemia, but other manifestations such as dizziness and sweating may not be significantly affected. Selective beta blockers do not potentiate insulin-induced hypoglycemia and, unlike nonselective beta blockers, do not delay recovery of blood glucose to normal levels.

Thyrotoxicosis. Beta-adrenergic blockade may mask certain clinical signs (e.g., tachycardia) or hyperthyroidism. Patients suspected of developing thyrotoxicosis should be managed carefully to avoid abrupt withdrawal of beta blockade, which might precipitate a thyroid storm.

Hydrochlorothiazide

Thiazides should be used with caution in patients with severe renal disease. In patients with renal disease, thiazides may precipitate azotemia. Cumulative effects of the drug may develop in patients with impaired renal function.

Thiazides should be used with caution in patients with impaired hepatic function or progressive liver disease, since minor alterations of fluid and electrolyte imbalance may precipitate hepatic coma.

Thiazides may add to or potentiate the action of other antihypertensive drugs. Potentiation occurs with ganglionic or peripheral adrenergic blocking drugs.

Sensitivity reactions are more likely to occur in patients with a history of allergy or bronchial asthma.

The possibility of exacerbation or activation of systemic lupus erythematosus has been reported.

PRECAUTIONS

General

Lopressor. Lopressor should be used with caution in patients with impaired hepatic function.

Hydrochlorothiazide. All patients receiving thiazide therapy should be observed for clinical signs of fluid or electrolyte imbalance, namely hyponatremia, hypochloremic alkalosis, and hypokalemia (see Laboratory Tests and Drug/Drug Interactions). Warning signs are dryness of mouth, thirst, weakness, lethargy, drowsiness, restlessness, muscle pains or cramps, muscular fatigue, hypotension, oliguria, tachycardia, and gastrointestinal disturbance, such as nausea or vomiting.

Hypokalemia may develop, especially in cases of brisk diuresis or severe cirrhosis.

Interference with adequate oral intake of electrolytes will also contribute to hypokalemia. Hypokalemia may be avoided or treated by the use of potassium supplements or foods with a high potassium content.

Any chloride deficit is generally mild and usually does not require specific treatment, except under extraordinary circumstances (as in liver disease or renal disease). Dilutional hyponatremia may occur in edematous patients in hot weather; appropriate therapy is water restriction, rather than administration of salt, except in rare instances when the hyponatremia is life-threatening. In cases of actual salt depletion, appropriate replacement is the therapy of choice.

Hyperuricemia may occur or frank gout may be precipitated in certain patients receiving thiazide therapy.

Latent diabetes may become manifest during thiazide administration (see Drug/Drug Interactions).

The antihypertensive effects of the drug may be enhanced in the postsympathectomy patient.

If progressive renal impairment becomes evident, withholding or discontinuing diuretic therapy should be considered.

Calcium excretion is decreased by thiazides. Pathological changes in the parathyroid gland with hypercalcemia and hypophosphatemia have been observed in a few patients on prolonged thiazide therapy. The common complications of hyperparathyroidism, such as renal lithiasis, bone resorption, and peptic ulceration, have not been seen.

Information for Patients

Patients should be advised to take Lopressor HCT regularly and continuously, as directed, with or immediately following meals. If a dose should be missed, the patient should take only the next scheduled dose (without doubling it). Patients should not discontinue Lopressor HCT without consulting the physician.

Patients should be advised (1) to avoid operating automobiles and machinery or engaging in other tasks requiring alertness until the patient's response to therapy with Lopressor has been determined; (2) to contact the physician if any difficulty in breathing occurs; (3) to inform the physician or dentist before any type of surgery that he or she is taking Lopressor HCT.

Laboratory Tests

Lopressor. Clinical laboratory findings may include elevated levels of serum transaminase, alkaline phosphatase, and lactate dehydrogenase.

Hydrochlorothiazide. Initial and periodic determinations of serum electrolytes to detect possible electrolyte imbalance should be performed at appropriate intervals.

Serum and urine electrolyte determinations are particularly important when the patient is vomiting excessively or receiving parenteral fluids.

Drug/Drug Interactions

Lopressor. Catecholamine-depleting drugs (e.g., reserpine) may have an additive effect when given with beta-blocking agents. Patients treated with Lopressor plus a catecholamine depletor should therefore be closely observed for evidence of hypotension or marked bradycardia, which may produce vertigo, syncope, or postural hypotension.

Risk of Anaphylactic Reaction. While taking beta-blockers, patients with a history of severe anaphylactic reaction to a variety of allergens may be more reactive to repeated challenge, either accidental, diagnostic, or therapeutic. Such patients may be unresponsive to the usual doses of epinephrine used to treat allergic reaction.

Hydrochlorothiazide. Hypokalemia can sensitize or exaggerate the response of the heart to the toxic effects of digitalis (e.g., increased ventricular irritability).

Hypokalemia may develop during concomitant use of steroids or ACTH.

Insulin requirements in diabetic patients may be increased, decreased, or unchanged.

Continued on next page

The full prescribing information for each GEIGY product is contained herein and is that in effect as of September 1, 1992.

GEIGY—Cont.

Thiazides may decrease arterial responsiveness to norepinephrine, but not enough to preclude effectiveness of the pressor agent for therapeutic use.
Thiazides may increase the responsiveness to tubocurarine.
Lithium renal clearance is reduced by thiazides, increasing the risk of lithium toxicity.
There have been rare reports in the literature of hemolytic anemia occurring with the concomitant use of hydrochlorothiazide and methyldopa.
Concurrent administration of some nonsteroidal anti-inflammatory agents may reduce the diuretic, natriuretic and antihypertensive effects of thiazide diuretics.

Drug/Laboratory Test Interactions

Hydrochlorothiazide. Thiazides may decrease serum levels of protein-bound iodine without signs of thyroid disturbance. Thiazides should be discontinued before tests for parathyroid function are made. (See General, *Hydrochlorothiazide,* Calcium excretion.)

Carcinogenesis, Mutagenesis, Impairment of Fertility

Lopressor. Long-term studies in animals have been conducted to evaluate carcinogenic potential. In a 2-year study in rats at three oral dosage levels of up to 800 mg/kg per day, there was no increase in the development of spontaneously occurring benign or malignant neoplasms of any type. The only histologic changes that appeared to be drug related were an increased incidence of generally mild focal accumulation of foamy macrophages in pulmonary alveoli and a slight increase in biliary hyperplasia. In a 21-month study in Swiss albino mice at three oral dosage levels of up to 750 mg/kg per day, benign lung tumors (small adenomas) occurred more frequently in female mice receiving the highest dose than in untreated control animals. There was no increase in malignant or total (benign plus malignant) lung tumors, nor in the overall incidence of tumors or malignant tumors. This 21-month study was repeated in CD-1 mice, and no statistically or biologically significant differences were observed between treated and control mice of either sex for any type of tumor.
All mutagenicity tests performed (a dominant lethal study in mice, chromosome studies in somatic cells, a *Salmonella*/mammalian-microsome mutagenicity test, and a nucleus anomaly test in somatic interphase nuclei) were negative.
No evidence of impaired fertility due to Lopressor was observed in a study performed in rats at doses up to 55.5 times the maximum daily human dose of 450 mg.

Hydrochlorothiazide. Long-term carcinogenicity studies in animals have not been conducted. Hydrochlorothiazide was not mutagenic in in vitro Ames mutagenicity assay of *Salmonella typhimurium* strains TA 98, TA 100, TA 1535, TA 1537, and TA 1538 or in in vivo mutagenicity assays of mouse germinal cell chromosomes and chinese hamster bone marrow cell chromosomes. It was however, mutagenic in inducing nondisjunction (96% frequency) in diploid strains of *Aspergillus nidulans.*
Hydrochlorothiazide had no adverse effect on fertility of male or female mice or rats in studies in which these species were exposed to doses up to 4 and 100 mg/kg, respectively.

Pregnancy Category C

Lopressor has been shown to increase postimplantation loss and decrease neonatal survival in rats at doses up to 55.5 times the maximum daily human dose of 450 mg. Distribution studies in mice confirm exposure of the fetus when Lopressor is administered to the pregnant animal. These studies have revealed no evidence of impaired fertility or teratogenicity.
There are no adequate and well-controlled studies in pregnant women with Lopressor HCT. Because animal reproduction studies are not always predictive of human response, this drug should be used during pregnancy only if clearly needed.
Nonteratogenic Effects. Thiazides cross the placental barrier and appear in cord blood, and there is a risk of fetal or neonatal jaundice, thrombocytopenia, and possibly other adverse reactions that have occurred in adults.

Nursing Mothers

Lopressor is excreted in breast milk in very small quantity. An infant consuming 1 liter of breast milk daily would receive a dose of metoprolol of less than 1 mg. Thiazides are also excreted in breast milk. If the use of Lopressor HCT is deemed essential, the patient should stop nursing.

Pediatric Use

Safety and effectiveness in children have not been established.

ADVERSE REACTIONS

Lopressor HCT

The following adverse reactions were reported in controlled clinical studies of the combination of Lopressor and hydrochlorothiazide.
Body as a Whole: Fatigue or lethargy and flu syndrome have each been reported in about 10 in 100 patients.
Nervous System: Dizziness or vertigo, drowsiness or somnolence, and headache have each occurred in about 10 in 100 patients. Nightmare has occurred in 1 in 100 patients.
Cardiovascular: Bradycardia has occurred in about 6 in 100 patients. Decreased exercise tolerance and dyspnea have each occurred in about 1 of 100 patients.
Digestive: Diarrhea, digestive disorder, dry mouth, nausea or vomiting, and constipation have each occurred in about 1 in 100 patients.
Metabolic and Nutritional: Hypokalemia has occurred in fewer than 10 in 100 patients. Edema, gout, and anorexia have each occurred in 1 in 100 patients.
Special Senses: Blurred vision, tinnitus, and earache have each been reported in 1 in 100 patients.
Skin: Sweating and purpura have each occurred in 1 in 100 patients.
Urogenital: Impotence has occurred in 1 in 100 patients.
Musculoskeletal: Muscle pain has occurred in 1 in 100 patients.

Lopressor

Most adverse effects have been mild and transient.
Central Nervous System: Tiredness and dizziness have occurred in about 10 of 100 patients. Depression has been reported in about 5 of 100 patients. Mental confusion and short-term memory loss have been reported. Headache, nightmares, and insomnia have also been reported, but a drug relationship is not clear.
Cardiovascular: Shortness of breath and bradycardia have occurred in approximately 3 of 100 patients. Cold extremities; arterial insufficiency, usually of the Raynaud type; palpitations; and congestive heart failure have been reported. (See **CONTRAINDICATIONS, WARNINGS,** and **PRECAUTIONS**).
Respiratory: Wheezing (bronchospasm) has been reported in fewer than 1 of 100 patients (see **WARNINGS**).
Gastrointestinal: Diarrhea has occurred in about 5 of 100 patients. Nausea, gastric pain, constipation, flatulence, and heartburn have been reported in 1 of 100, or fewer, patients.
Hypersensitive Reactions: Pruritus has occurred in fewer than 1 of 100 patients. Rash has been reported.
Miscellaneous: Peyronie's disease has been reported in fewer than 1 of 100,000 patients. Alopecia has been reported.
The oculomucocutaneous syndrome associated with the beta blocker practolol has not been reported with Lopressor.

Potential Adverse Reactions

A variety of adverse reactions not listed above have been reported with other beta-adrenergic blocking agents and should be considered potential adverse reactions to Lopressor.
Central Nervous System: Reversible mental depression progressing to catatonia; visual disturbances; hallucinations; an acute reversible syndrome characterized by disorientation for time and place, short-term memory loss, emotional lability, slightly clouded sensorium, and decreased performance on neuropsychometrics.
Cardiovascular: Intensification of AV block (see **CONTRAINDICATIONS**).
Hematologic: Agranulocytosis, nonthrombocytopenic purpura, thrombocytopenic purpura.
Hypersensitive Reactions: Fever combined with aching and sore throat, laryngospasm, and respiratory distress.

Hydrochlorothiazide

The following adverse reactions have been observed, but there has not been enough systematic collection of data to support an estimate of their frequency. Consequently the reactions are categorized by organ systems and are listed in decreasing order of severity and not frequency.
Digestive: Pancreatitis, jaundice (intrahepatic cholestatic), sialadenitis, vomiting, diarrhea, cramping, nausea, gastric irritation, constipation, anorexia.
Cardiovascular: Orthostatic hypotension (may be potentiated by alcohol, barbiturates, or narcotics).
Neurologic: Vertigo, dizziness, transient blurred vision, headache, paresthesia, xanthopsia, weakness, restlessness.
Musculoskeletal: Muscle spasm.
Hematologic: Aplastic anemia, agranulocytosis, leukopenia, thrombocytopenia.
Metabolic: Hyperglycemia, glycosuria, hyperuricemia.
Hypersensitive Reactions: Necrotizing angiitis, Stevens-Johnson syndrome, respiratory distress including pneumonitis and pulmonary edema, purpura, urticaria, rash, photosensitivity.

OVERDOSAGE

Acute Toxicity

Several cases of overdosage with Lopressor have been reported, some leading to death. No deaths have been reported with hydrochlorothiazide.
Oral LD_{50}'s (mg/kg): mice, 1158 (Lopressor); rats, 3090 (Lopressor), 2750 (hydrochlorothiazide).

Signs and Symptoms

Lopressor. Potential signs and symptoms associated with overdosage with Lopressor are bradycardia, hypotension, bronchospasm, and cardiac failure.
Hydrochlorothiazide. The most prominent feature of poisoning is acute loss of fluid and electrolytes.
Cardiovascular: Tachycardia, hypotension, shock.
Neuromuscular: Weakness, confusion, dizziness, cramps of the calf muscles, paresthesia, fatigue, impairment of consciousness.
Digestive: Nausea, vomiting, thirst.
Renal: Polyuria, oliguria, or anuria (due to hemoconcentration).
Laboratory Findings: Hypokalemia, hyponatremia, hypochloremia, alkalosis; increased BUN (especially in patients with renal insufficiency).
Combined Poisoning: Signs and symptoms may be aggravated or modified by concomitant intake of antihypertensive medication, barbiturates, curare, digitalis (hypokalemia), corticosteroids, narcotics, or alcohol.

Treatment

There is no specific antidote.
On the basis of the pharmacologic actions of Lopressor and hydrochlorothiazide, the following general measures should be employed:
Elimination of the Drug: Inducement of vomiting, gastric lavage, and activated charcoal.
Bradycardia: Atropine should be administered. If there is no response to vagal blockade, isoproterenol should be administered cautiously.
Hypotension: The patient's legs should be elevated, and lost fluid and electrolytes (potassium, sodium) should be replaced. A vasopressor should be administered, e.g., levarterenol or dopamine.
Bronchospasm: A $beta_2$-stimulating agent and/or a theophylline derivative should be administered.
Cardiac Failure: A digitalis glycoside and diuretic should be administered. In shock resulting from inadequate cardiac contractility, administration of dobutamine, isoproterenol, or glucagon may be considered.
Surveillance: Fluid and electrolyte balance (especially serum potassium) and renal function should be monitored until conditions become normal.

DOSAGE AND ADMINISTRATION

Dosage should be determined by individual titration (see **INDICATIONS AND USAGE**).
Hydrochlorothiazide is usually given at a dosage of 25 to 100 mg per day. The usual initial dosage of Lopressor is 100 mg daily in single or divided doses. Dosage may be increased gradually until optimum blood pressure control is achieved. The effective dosage range is 100 to 450 mg per day. While once-daily dosing is effective and can maintain a reduction in blood pressure throughout the day, lower doses (especially 100 mg) may not maintain a full effect at the end of the 24-hour period, and larger or more frequent daily doses may be required. This can be evaluated by measuring blood pressure near the end of the dosing interval to determine whether satisfactory control is being maintained thhroughout the day. $Beta_1$ selectivity diminishes as dosage of Lopressor is increased.
The following dosage schedule may be used to administer from 100 to 200 mg of Lopressor per day and from 25 to 50 mg of hydrochlorothiazide per day:

Lopressor HCT	*Dosage*
Tablets of 50/25	2 tablets per day in single or divided doses
Tablets of 100/25	1 to 2 tablets per day in single or divided doses
Tablets of 100/50	1 tablet per day in single or divided doses

Dosing regimens that exceed 50 mg of hydrochlorothiazide per day are not recommended. When necessary, another antihypertensive agent may be added gradually, beginning with 50% of the usual recommended starting dose to avoid an excessive fall in blood pressure.

HOW SUPPLIED

Tablets 50/25—capsule-shaped, white and blue, scored (imprinted Geigy on one side and 35 twice on the scored side) 50 mg of metoprolol tartrate and 25 mg of hydrochlorothiazide
Bottles of 100 .... NDC 0028-0035-01
Tablets 100/25—capsule-shaped, white and pink, scored (imprinted Geigy on one side and 53 twice on the scored side) 100 mg of metoprolol tartrate and 25 mg of hydrochlorothiazide
Bottles of 100 .... NDC 0028-0053-01
Tablets 100/50—capsule-shaped, white and yellow, scored (imprinted Geigy on one side and 73 twice on the scored side) 100 mg of metoprolol tartrate and 50 mg of hydrochlorothiazide
Bottles of 100 .... NDC 0028-0073-01
Samples, when available, are identified by the word *Sample* appearing on each tablet.
Store between 59°–86°F (15°–30°C). Protect from moisture.
Dispense in tight, light-resistant container (USP).
C91-32 (Rev. 9/91)
Shown in Product Identification Section, page 410

OTRIVIN®   OTC
xylometazoline hydrochloride USP
Nasal Spray and Nasal Drops 0.1%
Pediatric Nasal Drops 0.05%

One application provides rapid and long-lasting relief of nasal congestion for up to 10 hours.

Quickly clears stuffy noses due to common cold, sinusitis, hay fever.

Nasal congestion can make life miserable—you can't breathe, smell, taste, or sleep comfortably. That is why Otrivin is so helpful. It clears away that stuffy feeling, usually within 5 to 10 minutes, and your head feels clear for hours.

Otrivin has been prescribed by doctors for many years. Here is how you use it:

Nasal Spray 0.1%—Spray 2 or 3 times into each nostril every 8-10 hours. With head upright, squeeze sharply and firmly while inhaling (sniffing) through the nose.

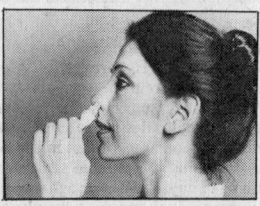

Nasal Drops 0.1%—for adults and children 12 years and older. Put 2 or 3 drops into each nostril every 8 to 10 hours. Tilt head as far back as possible. Immediately bend head forward toward knees, hold a few seconds, then return to upright position.

Do not give Nasal Spray 0.1% or Nasal Drops 0.1% to children under 12 years except under the advice and supervision of a physician.

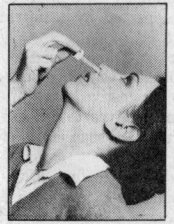
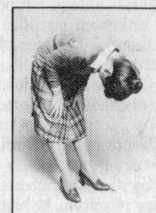
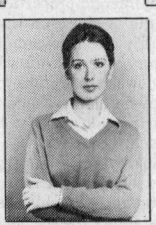

Pediatric Nasal Drops 0.05%—for children 2 to 12 years of age. Put 2 or 3 drops into each nostril every 8 to 10 hours. Tilt head as far back as possible. Immediately bend head forward toward knees, hold a few seconds, then return to upright position.

Do not give this product to children under 2 years except under the advice and supervision of a physician.

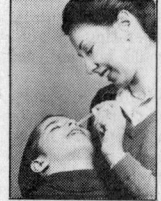
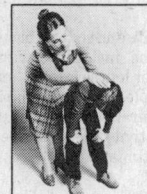
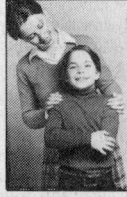

Otrivin Nasal Spray/Nasal Drops contain 0.1% xylometazoline hydrochloride, USP. Also contains benzalkonium chloride, potassium chloride, potassium phosphate monobasic, purified water, sodium chloride and sodium phosphate dibasic.

They are available in an unbreakable plastic spray package of ½ fl oz (15ml) and in a plastic dropper bottle of .66 fl oz (20ml).

Otrivin Pediatric Nasal Drops contain 0.05% xylometazoline hydrochloride, USP. Also contains benzalkonium chloride, potassium chloride, potassium phosphate monobasic, purified water, sodium chloride and sodium phosphate dibasic. It is available in a plastic dropper bottle of .66 fl oz (20ml).

WARNINGS
Do not exceed recommended dosage, because symptoms such as burning, stinging, sneezing, or increase of nasal discharge may occur. Do not use this product for more than 3 days. If symptoms persist, consult a physician. The use of this dispenser by more than one person may cause infection.

Keep this and all medicines out of the reach of children. In case of accidental ingestion, seek professional assistance or contact a Poison Control Center immediately.

C86–44 (Rev. 9/86)

Distributed by CIBA CONSUMER PHARMACEUTICALS EDISON, NEW JERSEY 08837

PBZ–SR®   ℞
tripelennamine hydrochloride USP
Extended-Release Tablets

DESCRIPTION
PBZ-SR, tripelennamine hydrochloride USP, is an antihistamine for oral administration available as 100-mg extended-release tablets that provide a gradual and prolonged release of drug from the wax matrix.

Tripelennamine hydrochloride is 2-[Benzyl[2-(dimethylamino)ethyl]amino] pyridine monohydrochloride.

Tripelennamine hydrochloride USP is a white, crystalline powder. Its solutions are practically neutral to litmus. It is freely soluble in water, in alcohol, and in chloroform; slightly soluble in acetone; and insoluble in benzene, in ether, and in ethyl acetate. Its molecular weight is 291.82.

Inactive Ingredients: Cellulose compounds, cetostearyl alcohol, D&C Red No. 30 lake, FD&C Blue No. 2 lake, magnesium stearate, mineral oil, titanium dioxide, and zein.

ACTIONS
Antihistamines are competitive antagonists of histamine, which also produce central nervous system effects (both stimulant and depressant) and peripheral anticholinergic, atropine-like effects (e.g., drying).

INDICATIONS
Perennial and seasonal allergic rhinitis; vasomotor rhinitis; allergic conjunctivitis due to inhalant allergens and foods; mild, uncomplicated allergic skin manifestations of urticaria and angioedema; amelioration of allergic reactions to blood or plasma; dermographism; anaphylactic reactions as adjunctive therapy to epinephrine and other standard measures after the acute manifestations have been controlled.

CONTRAINDICATIONS
PBZ-SR should not be used in premature infants, neonates, or nursing mothers; patients receiving MAO inhibitors; patients with narrow-angle glaucoma, stenosing peptic ulcer, symptomatic prostatic hypertrophy, bladder neck obstruction, pyloroduodenal obstruction, lower respiratory tract symptoms (including asthma), or hypersensitivity to tripelennamine or related compounds.

WARNINGS
Antihistamines often produce drowsiness and may reduce mental alertness in children and adults. Patients should be warned about engaging in activities requiring mental alertness (e.g., driving a car, operating machinery or hazardous appliances). In elderly patients, approximately 60 years or older, antihistamines are more likely to cause dizziness, sedation and hypotension. Patients should be warned that the central nervous system effects of PBZ-SR may be additive with those of alcohol and other CNS depressants (e.g., hypnotics, sedatives, tranquilizers, antianxiety agents).

Antihistamines may produce excitation, particularly in children.

Usage in Pregnancy: Although no tripelennamine-related teratogenic potential or other adverse effects on the fetus have been observed in limited animal reproduction studies, the safe use of this drug in pregnancy or during lactation has not been established. Therefore, the drug should not be used during pregnancy or lactation unless, in the judgment of the physician, the expected benefits outweigh the potential hazards.

Usage in Children: In infants and children particularly, antihistamines in overdosage may produce hallucinations, convulsions and/or death.

PRECAUTIONS
PBZ-SR, like other antihistamines, has atropine-like, anticholinergic activity and should be used with caution in patients with increased intraocular pressure, hyperthyroidism, cardiovascular disease, hypertension, or history of bronchial asthma.

ADVERSE REACTIONS
The most frequent adverse reactions to antihistamines are sedation or drowsiness; sleepiness; dryness of the mouth, nose, and throat; thickening of bronchial secretions; dizziness; disturbed coordination; epigastric distress.

Other adverse reactions which may occur are: fatigue; chills; confusion; restlessness; excitation; hysteria; nervousness; irritability; insomnia; euphoria; anorexia; nausea; vomiting; diarrhea; constipation; hypotension; tightness in the chest; wheezing; blurred vision; diplopia; vertigo; tinnitus; convulsions; headache; palpitations; tachycardia; extrasystoles; nasal stuffiness; urinary frequency; difficult urination; urinary retention; leukopenia; hemolytic anemia; thrombocytopenia; agranulocytosis; aplastic anemia; allergic or hypersensitivity reactions, including drug rash, urticaria, anaphylactic shock, and photosensitivity. Although the following may have been reported to occur in association with some antihistamines, they have not been known to result from the use of PBZ-SR: excessive perspiration, tremor, paresthesias, acute labyrinthitis, neuritis and early menses.

DOSAGE AND ADMINISTRATION
Dosage should be individualized according to the needs and response of the patient.

Adults: One 100-mg PBZ-SR tablet in the morning and one in the evening is generally adequate. In difficult cases, one 100-mg PBZ-SR tablet every 8 hours may be required.

Children: PBZ-SR tablets are not intended for use in children.

Note: PBZ-SR extended-release tablets must be swallowed whole and never crushed or chewed.

OVERDOSAGE
Signs and Symptoms: The greatest danger from acute overdosage with antihistamines is their central nervous system effects which produce depression and/or stimulation.

In children, stimulation predominates initially in a syndrome which may include excitement, hallucinations, ataxia, incoordination, athetosis, and convulsions followed by postictal depression. Dry mouth, fixed dilated pupils, flushing of the face, and fever are common and resemble the syndrome of atropine poisoning. In adults, CNS depression (i.e., drowsiness, coma) is more common. CNS stimulation is rare; fever and flushing are uncommon.

In both children and adults, there can be a terminal deepening of coma and cardiovascular collapse; death can occur, especially in infants and children.

Treatment: There is no specific therapy for acute overdosage with antihistamines. General symptomatic and supportive measures should be instituted promptly and maintained for as long as necessary.

In the conscious patient, vomiting should be induced even though it may have occurred spontaneously. If vomiting cannot be induced, gastric lavage is indicated. Adequate precautions must be taken to protect against aspiration, especially in infants and children. Charcoal slurry or other suitable agent should be instilled into the stomach after vomiting or lavage. Saline cathartics or milk of magnesia may be of additional benefit.

In the unconscious patient, the airway should be secured with a cuffed endotracheal tube before attempting to evacuate the gastric contents. Intensive supportive and nursing care is indicated, as for any comatose patient.

If breathing is significantly impaired, maintenance of an adequate airway and mechanical support of respiration is the safest and most effective means of providing for adequate oxygenation of tissues to prevent hypoxia (especially brain hypoxia during convulsions).

Hypotension is an early sign of impeding cardiovascular collapse and should be treated vigorously. Although general supportive measures are important, specific treatment with intravenous infusion of a vasopressor (e.g., levarterenol bitartrate) titrated to maintain adequate blood pressure may be necessary.

Do *not* use CNS stimulants.

Convulsions should be controlled by careful titration of a short-acting barbiturate, repeated as necessary.

Ice packs and cooling sponge baths can aid in reducing the fever commonly seen in children.

HOW SUPPLIED
Tablets (extended-release) 100 mg—round, lavender (imprinted Geigy 48)

Bottles of 100 ....NDC 0028-0048-01

Store at controlled room temperature (15°–30°C) (59°–86°F). Protect from moisture.

Dispense in tight container (USP).

C87-36 (Rev. 10/87)

Shown in Product Identification Section, page 410

Continued on next page

The full prescribing information for each GEIGY product is contained herein and is that in effect as of September 1, 1992.

GEIGY—Cont.

PBZ® ℞
tripelennamine hydrochloride
Tablets USP

Listed in USP, a Medicare designated compendium.

DESCRIPTION

PBZ, tripelennamine hydrochloride USP, is an antihistamine for oral administration. PBZ *tablets* contain 25 mg and 50 mg of the hydrochoride salt. Tripelennamine hydrochloride is 2-[Benzyl[2-(dimethylamino)ethyl]amino]pyridine monohydrochloride.
Tripelennamine hydrochloride USP is a white, crystalline powder. Its solutions are practically neutral to litmus. It is freely soluble in water, in alcohol, and in chloroform; slightly soluble in acetone; and insoluble in benzene, in ether, and in ethyl acetate. Its molecular weight is 291.82.
Inactive ingredients (PBZ Tablets 25 mg): Lactose, magnesium stearate, polyethylene glycol, starch, sucrose and talc. (PBZ Tablets 50 mg): Acacia, lactose, magnesium stearate, polyethylene glycol, talc and tragacanth.

ACTIONS

Antihistamines are competitive antagonists of histamine, which also produce central nervous system effects (both stimulant and depressant) and peripheral anticholinergic, atropine-like effects (e.g., drying).

INDICATIONS

Perennial and seasonal allergic rhinitis; vasomotor rhinitis; allergic conjunctivitis due to inhalant allergens and foods; mild, uncomplicated allergic skin manifestations of urticaria and angioedema; amelioration of allergic reactions to blood or plasma; dermographism; anaphylactic reactions as adjunctive therapy to epinephrine and other standard measures after the acute manifestations have been controlled.

CONTRAINDICATIONS

PBZ should not be used in premature infants, neonates, or nursing mothers; patients receiving MAO inhibitors; patients with narrow-angle glaucoma, stenosing peptic ulcer, symptomatic prostatic hypertrophy, bladder neck obstruction, pyloroduodenal obstruction, lower respiratory tract symptoms (including asthma), or hypersensitivity to tripelennamine or related compounds.

WARNINGS

Antihistamines often produce drowsiness and may reduce mental alertness in children and adults. Patients should be warned about engaging in activities requiring mental alertness (e.g., driving a car, operating machinery or hazardous appliances). In elderly patients, approximately 60 years or older, antihistamines are more likely to cause dizziness, sedation and hypotension.
Patients should be warned that the central nervous system effects of PBZ may be additive with those of alcohol and other CNS depressants (e.g., hypnotics, sedatives, tranquilizers, antianxiety agents).
Antihistamines may produce excitation, particularly in children.

Usage in Pregnancy
Although no tripelennamine-related teratogenic potential or other adverse effects on the fetus have been observed in limited animal reproduction studies, the safe use of this drug in pregnancy or during lactation has not been established. Therefore, the drug should not be used during pregnancy or lactation unless, in the judgment of the physician, the expected benefits outweigh the potential hazards.

Usage in Children
In infants and children particularly, antihistamines in overdosage may produce hallucinations, convulsions and/or death.

PRECAUTIONS

PBZ, like other antihistamines, has atropine-like, anticholinergic activity and should be used with caution in patients with increased intraocular pressure, hyperthyroidism, cardiovascular disease, hypertension, or history of bronchial asthma.

ADVERSE REACTIONS

The most frequent adverse reactions to antihistamines are sedation or drowsiness; sleepiness; dryness of the mouth, nose, and throat; thickening of bronchial secretions; dizziness; disturbed coordination; epigastric distress.
Other adverse reactions which may occur are: fatigue; chills; confusion; restlessness; excitation; hysteria; nervousness; irritability; insomnia; euphoria; anorexia; nausea; vomiting; diarrhea; constipation; hypotension; tightness in the chest; wheezing; blurred vision; diplopia; vertigo; tinnitus; convulsions; headache; palpitations; tachycardia; extrasystoles; nasal stuffiness; urinary frequency; difficult urination; urinary retention; leukopenia; hemolytic anemia; thrombocytopenia; agranulocytosis; aplastic anemia; allergic or hypersensitivity reactions, including drug rash, urticaria, anaphylactic shock, and photosensitivity. Although the following may have been reported to occur in association with some antihistamines, they have not been known to result from the use of PBZ: excessive perspiration, tremor, paresthesias, acute labyrinthitis, neuritis and early menses.

DOSAGE AND ADMINISTRATION

Dosage should be individualized.
Usual Adult Dose: 25 to 50 mg every four to six hours. As little as 25 mg may control symptoms, but as much as 600 mg daily may be given in divided doses, if necessary.
Children and Infants: 5 mg/kg/24 hours or 150 mg/m^2/24 hours divided into four to six doses. Do not exceed maximum total dose of 300 mg/24 hours.

OVERDOSAGE

Signs and Symptoms
The greatest danger from acute overdosage with antihistamines is their central nervous system effects which produce depression and/or stimulation.
In children, stimulation predominates initially in a syndrome which may include excitement, hallucinations, ataxia, incoordination, athetosis, and convulsions followed by postictal depression. Dry mouth, fixed dilated pupils, flushing of the face, and fever are common and resemble the syndrome of atropine poisoning.
In adults, CNS depression (i.e., drowsiness, coma) is more common. CNS stimulation is rare; fever and flushing are uncommon.
In both children and adults, there can be a terminal deepening of coma and cardiovascular collapse, death can occur, especially in infants and children.

Treatment
There is no specific therapy for acute overdosage with antihistamines. General symptomatic and supportive measures should be instituted promptly and maintained for as long as necessary.
In the conscious patient, vomiting should be induced even though it may have occurred spontaneously. If vomiting cannot be induced, gastric lavage is indicated. Adequate precautions must be taken to protect against aspiration, especially in infants and children. Charcoal slurry or other suitable agent should be instilled into the stomach after vomiting or lavage. Saline cathartics or milk of magnesia may be of additional benefit.
In the unconscious patient, the airway should be secured with a cuffed endotracheal tube before attempting to evacuate the gastric contents. Intensive supportive and nursing care is indicated, as for any comatose patient.
If breathing is significantly impaired, maintenance of an adequate airway and mechanical support of respiration is the safest and most effective means of providing for adequate oxygenation of tissues to prevent hypoxia (especially brain hypoxia during convulsions).
Hypotension is an early sign of impending cardiovascular collapse and should be treated vigorously. Although general supportive measures are important, specific treatment with intravenous infusion of a vasopressor (e.g., levarterenol bitartrate) titrated to maintain adequate blood pressure may be necessary.
Do *not* use CNS stimulants.
Convulsions should be controlled by careful titration of a short-acting barbiturate, repeated as necessary.
Ice packs and cooling sponge baths can aid in reducing the fever commonly seen in children.

HOW SUPPLIED

Tablets 25 mg—round, white to off-white, biconvex (scored on one side and imprinted Geigy 111 on the other side)
Bottles of 100 .... NDC 0028-0111-01
Tablets 50 mg—round, white to off-white, biconvex (scored on one side and imprinted Geigy 117 on the other side)
Bottles of 100 .... NDC 0028-0117-01
Do not store above 86°F (30°C). Protect from light.
Dispense in tight, light-resistant container.
C92-16 (Rev. 4/92)
Shown in Product Identification Section, page 410

TOFRANIL® ℞
[toe-fray'nill]
imipramine hydrochloride USP
Ampuls, 2 cc
For intramuscular administration

Each 2 cc ampul contains: imipramine hydrochloride USP, 25 mg; ascorbic acid, 2 mg; sodium bisulfite, 1 mg; sodium sulfite, anhydrous, 1 mg.

DESCRIPTION

Tofranil, imipramine hydrochloride USP, the original tricyclic antidepressant, is a member of the dibenzazepine group of compounds. It is designated 5-[3-(dimethylamino)propyl]-10, 11-dihydro-5H-dibenz[b,f] azepine monohydrochloride.
Imipramine hydrochloride USP is a white to off-white, odorless, or practically odorless crystalline powder. It is freely soluble in water and in alcohol, soluble in acetone, and insoluble in ether and in benzene. Its molecular weight is 316.87.

CLINICAL PHARMACOLOGY

The mechanism of action of Tofranil is not definitely known. However, it does not act primarily by stimulation of the central nervous system. The clinical effect is hypothesized as being due to potentiation of adrenergic synapses by blocking uptake of norepinephrine at nerve endings. The mode of action of the drug in controlling childhood enuresis is thought to be apart from its antidepressant effect.

INDICATIONS

Depression: For the relief of symptoms of depression. Endogenous depression is more likely to be alleviated than other depressive states. One to three weeks of treatment may be needed before optimal therapeutic effects are evident.

CONTRAINDICATIONS

The concomitant use of monoamine oxidase inhibiting compounds is contraindicated. Hyperpyretic crises or severe convulsive seizures may occur in patients receiving such combinations. The potentiation of adverse effects can be serious, or even fatal. When it is desired to substitute Tofranil in patients receiving a monoamine oxidase inhibitor, as long an interval should elapse as the clinical situation will allow, with a minimum of 14 days. Initial dosage should be low and increases should be gradual and cautiously prescribed.
The drug is contraindicated during the acute recovery period after a myocardial infarction. Patients with a known hypersensitivity to this compound should not be given the drug. The possibility of cross-sensitivity to other dibenzazepine compounds should be kept in mind.

WARNINGS

Children: A dose of 2.5 mg/kg/day of imipramine hydrochloride should not be exceeded in childhood. ECG changes of unknown significance have been reported in pediatric patients with doses twice this amount.
Extreme caution should be used when this drug is given to:
patients with cardiovascular disease because of the possibility of conduction defects, arrhythmias, congestive heart failure, myocardial infarction, strokes and tachycardia. These patients require cardiac surveillance at all dosage levels of the drug;
patients with increased intraocular pressure, history of urinary retention, or history of narrow-angle glaucoma because of the drug's anticholinergic properties;
hyperthyroid patients or those on thyroid medication because of the possibility of cardiovascular toxicity;
patients with a history of seizure disorder because this drug has been shown to lower the seizure threshold;
patients receiving guanethidine, clonidine, or similar agents, since imipramine hydrochloride may block the pharmacologic effects of these drugs;
patients receiving methylphenidate hydrochloride.
Since methylphenidate hydrochloride may inhibit the metabolism of imipramine hydrochloride, downward dosage adjustment of imipramine hydrochloride may be required when given concomitantly with methylphenidate hydrochloride.
Tofranil may enhance the CNS depressant effects of alcohol. Therefore, it should be borne in mind that the dangers inherent in a suicide attempt or accidental overdosage with the drug may be increased for the patient who uses excessive amounts of alcohol. (See **PRECAUTIONS.**)
Since imipramine hydrochloride may impair the mental and/or physical abilities required for the performance of potentially hazardous tasks, such as operating an automobile or machinery, the patient should be cautioned accordingly.
Contains sodium sulfite and sodium bisulfite, that may cause allergic-type reactions including anaphylactic symptoms and life-threatening or less severe asthmatic episodes in certain susceptible people. The overall prevalence of sulfite sensitivity in the general population is unknown and probably low. Sulfite sensitivity is seen more frequently in asthmatic than in nonasthmatic people.

PRECAUTIONS

An ECG recording should be taken prior to the initiation of larger-than-usual doses of imipramine hydrochloride and at appropriate intervals thereafter until steady state is achieved. (Patients with any evidence of cardiovascular disease require cardiac surveillance at all dosage levels of the drug. See **WARNINGS.**) Elderly patients and patients with cardiac disease or a prior history of cardiac disease are at special risk of developing the cardiac abnormalities associated with the use of imipramine hydrochloride.
It should be kept in mind that the possibility of suicide in seriously depressed patients is inherent in the illness and may persist until significant remission occurs. Such patients should be carefully supervised during the early phase of

treatment with imipramine hydrochloride, and may require hospitalization. Prescriptions should be written for the smallest amount feasible.
Hypomanic or manic episodes may occur, particularly in patients with cyclic disorders.
Such reactions may necessitate discontinuation of the drug. If needed, imipramine hydrochloride may be resumed in lower dosage when these episodes are relieved.
Administration of a tranquilizer may be useful in controlling such episodes.
An activation of the psychosis may occasionally be observed in schizophrenic patients and may require reduction of dosage and the addition of a phenothiazine.
Concurrent administration of imipramine hydrochloride with electroshock therapy may increase the hazards; such treatment should be limited to those patients for whom it is essential, since there is limited clinical experience.
Usage During Pregnancy and Lactation:
Animal reproduction studies have yielded inconclusive results. (See also **ANIMAL PHARMACOLOGY & TOXICOLOGY.**)
There have been no well-controlled studies conducted with pregnant women to determine the effect of imipramine hydrochloride on the fetus. However, there have been clinical reports of congenital malformations associated with the use of the drug. Although a causal relationship between these effects and the drug could not be established, the possibility of fetal risk from the maternal ingestion of imipramine hydrochloride cannot be excluded. Therefore, imipramine hydrochloride should be used in women who are or might become pregnant only if the clinical condition clearly justifies potential risk to the fetus.
Limited data suggest that imipramine hydrochloride is likely to be excreted in human breast milk. As a general rule, a woman taking a drug should not nurse since the possibility exists that the drug may be excreted in breast milk and be harmful to the child.
Usage in Children: The effectiveness of the drug in children for conditions other than nocturnal enuresis given orally has not been established.
Patients should be warned that imipramine hydrochloride may enhance the CNS depressant effects of alcohol. (See **WARNINGS.**)
Imipramine hydrochloride should be used with caution in patients with significantly impaired renal or hepatic function.
Patients who develop a fever and a sore throat during therapy with imipramine hydrochloride should have leukocyte and differential blood counts performed. Imipramine hydrochloride should be discontinued if there is evidence of pathological neutrophil depression.
Prior to elective surgery, imipramine hydrochloride should be discontinued for as long as the clinical situation will allow.
In occasional susceptible patients or in those receiving anticholinergic drugs (including antiparkinsonism agents) in addition, the atropine-like effects may become more pronounced (e.g., paralytic ileus).
Close supervision and careful adjustment of dosage is required when imipramine hydrochloride is administered concomitantly with anticholinergic drugs.
Avoid the use of preparations, such as decongestants and local anesthetics, which contain any sympathomimetic amine (e.g., epinephrine, norepinephrine), since it has been reported that tricyclic antidepressants can potentiate the effects of catecholamines.
Caution should be exercised when imipramine hydrochloride is used with agents that lower blood pressure.
Imipramine hydrochloride may potentiate the effects of CNS depressant drugs.
The plasma concentration of imipramine may increase when the drug is given concomitantly with hepatic enzyme inhibitors (e.g., cimetidine, fluoxetine) and decrease by concomitant administration with hepatic enzyme inducers (e.g., barbiturates, phenytoin), and adjustment of the dosage of imipramine may therefore be necessary.
Patients taking imipramine hydrochloride should avoid excessive exposure to sunlight since there have been reports of photosensitization.
Both elevation and lowering of blood sugar levels have been reported with imipramine hydrochloride use.

ADVERSE REACTIONS

Note: Although the listing which follows includes a few adverse reactions which have not been reported with this specific drug, the pharmacological similarities among the tricyclic antidepressant drugs require that each of the reactions be considered when imipramine is administered.
Cardiovascular: Orthostatic hypotension, hypertension, tachycardia, palpitation, myocardial infarction, arrhythmias, heart block, ECG changes, precipitation of congestive heart failure, stroke.
Psychiatric: Confusional states (especially in the elderly) with hallucinations, disorientation, delusions; anxiety, restlessness, agitation; insomnia and nightmares; hypomania; exacerbation of psychosis.
Neurological: Numbness, tingling, paresthesias of extremities; incoordination, ataxia, tremors; peripheral neuropathy; extrapyramidal symptoms; seizures, alterations in EEG patterns; tinnitus.
Anticholinergic: Dry mouth, and, rarely, associated sublingual adenitis; blurred vision, disturbances of accommodation, mydriasis; constipation, paralytic ileus; urinary retention, delayed micturition, dilation of the urinary tract.
Allergic: Skin rash, petechiae, urticaria, itching, photosensitization; edema (general or of face and tongue); drug fever; cross-sensitivity with desipramine.
Hematologic: Bone marrow depression including agranulocytosis; eosinophilia; purpura; thrombocytopenia.
Gastrointestinal: Nausea and vomiting, anorexia, epigastric distress, diarrhea; peculiar taste, stomatitis, abdominal cramps, black tongue.
Endocrine: Gynecomastia in the male; breast enlargement and galactorrhea in the female; increased or decreased libido, impotence; testicular swelling; elevation or depression of blood sugar levels; inappropriate antidiuretic hormone (ADH) secretion syndrome.
Other: Jaundice (simulating obstructive); altered liver function; weight gain or loss; perspiration; flushing; urinary frequency; drowsiness, dizziness, weakness and fatigue; headache; parotid swelling; alopecia; proneness to falling.
Withdrawal Symptoms: Though not indicative of addiction, abrupt cessation of treatment after prolonged therapy may produce nausea, headache and malaise.

DOSAGE AND ADMINISTRATION

Initially, up to 100 mg/day intramuscularly in divided doses. Parenteral administration should be used only for starting therapy in patients unable or unwilling to use oral medication. The oral form should supplant the injectable as soon as possible.
Lower dosages are recommended for elderly patients and adolescents. Lower dosages are also recommended for outpatients as compared to hospitalized patients who will be under close supervision. Dosage should be initiated at a low level and increased gradually, noting carefully the clinical response and any evidence of intolerance. Following remission, oral maintenance medication may be required for a longer period of time, at the lowest dose that will maintain remission.

OVERDOSAGE

Children have been reported to be more sensitive than adults to an acute overdosage of imipramine hydrochloride. An acute overdose of any amount in infants or young children, especially, must be considered serious and potentially fatal.
Signs and Symptoms: These may vary in severity depending upon factors such as the amount of drug absorbed, the age of the patient, and the interval between drug ingestion and the start of treatment. Blood and urine levels of imipramine may not reflect the severity of poisoning; they have chiefly a qualitative rather than quantitative value, and are unreliable indicators in the clinical management of the patient.
CNS abnormalities may include drowsiness, stupor, coma, ataxia, restlessness, agitation, hyperactive reflexes, muscle rigidity, athetoid and choreiform movements, and convulsions.
Cardiac abnormalities may include arrhythmia, tachycardia, ECG evidence of impaired conduction, and signs of congestive failure.
Respiratory depression, cyanosis, hypotension, shock, vomiting, hyperpyrexia, mydriasis, and diaphoresis may also be present.
Treatment: The recommended treatment for overdosage with tricyclic antidepressants may change periodically. Therefore, it is recommended that the physician contact a poison control center for current information on treatment. Because CNS involvement, respiratory depression and cardiac arrhythmia can occur suddenly, hospitalization and close observation may be necessary, even when the amount ingested is thought to be small or the initial degree of intoxication appears slight or moderate. All patients with ECG abnormalities should have continuous cardiac monitoring and be closely observed until well after cardiac status has returned to normal; relapses may occur after apparent recovery.
In the alert patient, empty the stomach promptly by lavage. In the obtunded patient, secure the airway with a cuffed endotracheal tube before beginning lavage (do not induce emesis). Instillation of activated charcoal slurry may help reduce absorption of imipramine.
Minimize external stimulation to reduce the tendency to convulsions. If anticonvulsants are necessary, diazepam and phenytoin may be useful.
Maintain adequate respiratory exchange. Do not use respiratory stimulants.
Shock should be treated with supportive measures, such as appropriate position, intravenous fluids, and, if necessary, a vasopressor agent. The use of corticosteroids in shock is controversial and may be contraindicated in cases of overdosage and tricyclic antidepressants. Digitalis may increase conduction abnormalities and further irritate an already sensitized myocardium. If congestive heart failure necessitates rapid digitalization, particular care must be exercised.
Hyperpyrexia should be controlled by whatever external means are available, including ice packs and cooling sponge baths, if necessary.
Hemodialysis, peritoneal dialysis, exchange transfusions and forced diuresis have been generally reported as ineffective because of the rapid fixation of imipramine in tissues. Blood and urine levels of imipramine may not correlate with the degree of intoxication, and are unreliable indicators in the clinical management of the patient.
The slow intravenous administration of physostigmine salicylate has been used as a last resort to reverse severe CNS anticholinergic manifestations of overdosage with tricyclic antidepressants; however, it should not be used routinely, since it may induce seizures and cholinergic crises.

HOW SUPPLIED

Ampuls 2 ml—*For intramuscular administration only*
25 mg imipramine hydrochloride, 2 mg ascorbic acid, 1 mg sodium bisulfite, 1 mg sodium sulfite
Boxes of 10 ....NDC 0028-0065-23
Store between 59°–86°F (15°–30°C).
Note: Upon storage, minute crystals may form in some ampuls. This has no influence on the therapeutic efficacy of the preparation, and the crystals redissolve when the affected ampuls are immersed in hot tap water for 1 minute.

ANIMAL PHARMACOLOGY & TOXICOLOGY

A. *Acute:* Oral LD_{50} ranges are as follows:

Rat	355 to 682 mg/kg
Dog	100 to 215 mg/kg

Depending on the dosage in both species, toxic signs proceeded progressively from depression, irregular respiration and ataxia to convulsions and death.
B. *Reproduction/Teratogenic:* The overall evaluation may be summed up in the following manner:
Oral: Independent studies in three species (rat, mouse and rabbit) revealed that when Tofranil is administered orally in doses up to approximately 2½ times the maximum human dose in the first 2 species and up to 25 times the maximum human dose in the third species, the drug is essentially free from teratogenic potential. In the three species studied, only one instance of fetal abnormality occurred (in the rabbit) and in that study there was likewise an abnormality in the control group. However, evidence does exist from the rat studies that some systemic and embryotoxic potential is demonstrable. This is manifested by reduced litter size, a slight increase in the stillborn rate and a reduction in the mean birth weight.
Parenteral: In contradistinction to the oral data, Tofranil does exhibit a slight but definite teratogenic potential when administered by the subcutaneous route. Drug effects on both the mother and fetus in the rabbit are manifested in higher resorption rates and decrease in mean fetal birth weights, while teratogenic findings occurred at a level of 5 times the maximum human dose. In the mouse, teratogenicity occurred at 1½ and 6½ times the maximum human dose, but no teratogenic effects were seen at levels 3 times the maximum human dose. Thus, in the mouse, the findings are equivocal.

C91-42 (Rev. 2/92)

Dist. by:
GEIGY Pharmaceuticals
Division of CIBA-GEIGY Corporation
Ardsley, New York 10502

TOFRANIL® ℞
[toe-fray'nill]
imipramine hydrochloride USP
Tablets of 10 mg
Tablets of 25 mg
Tablets of 50 mg
For oral administration

DESCRIPTION

Tofranil, imipramine hydrochloride USP, the original tricyclic antidepressant, is a member of the dibenzazepine group of compounds. It is designated 5-[3-(Dimethylamino)propyl]-10, 11-dihydro-5H-dibenz[b,f] azepine Monohydrochloride.
Imipramine hydrocloride USP is a white to off-white, odorless, or practically odorless crystalline powder. It is freely soluble in water and in alcohol, soluble in acetone, and insoluble in ether and in benzene. Its molecular weight is 316.87.
Inactive Ingredients. Calcium phosphate, cellulose compounds, docusate sodium, iron oxides, magnesium stearate,

Continued on next page

The full prescribing information for each GEIGY product is contained herein and is that in effect as of September 1, 1992.

GEIGY—Cont.

polyethylene glycol, povidone, sodium starch glycolate, sucrose, talc and titanium dioxide.

CLINICAL PHARMACOLOGY

The mechanism of action of Tofranil is not definitely known. However, it does not act primarily by stimulation of the central nervous system. The clinical effect is hypothesized as being due to potentiation of adrenergic synapses by blocking uptake of norepinephrine at nerve endings. The mode of action of the drug in controlling childhood enuresis is thought to be apart from its antidepressant effect.

INDICATIONS

Depression: For the relief of symptoms of depression. Endogenous depression is more likely to be alleviated than other depressive states. One to three weeks of treatment may be needed before optimal therapeutic effects are evident.

Childhood Enuresis: May be useful as temporary adjunctive therapy in reducing enuresis in children aged 6 years and older, after possible organic causes have been excluded by appropriate tests. In patients having daytime symptoms of frequency and urgency, examination should include voiding cystourethrography and cystoscopy, as necessary. The effectiveness of treatment may decrease with continued drug administration.

CONTRAINDICATIONS

The concomitant use of monoamine oxidase inhibiting compounds is contraindicated. Hyperpyretic crises or severe convulsive seizures may occur in patients receiving such combinations. The potentiation of adverse effects can be serious, or even fatal. When it is desired to substitute Tofranil in patients receiving a monoamine oxidase inhibitor, as long an interval should elapse as the clinical situation will allow, with a minimum of 14 days. Initial dosage should be low and increases should be gradual and cautiously prescribed.

The drug is contraindicated during the acute recovery period after a myocardial infarction. Patients with a known hypersensitivity to this compound should not be given the drug. The possibility of cross-sensitivity to other dibenzazepine compounds should be kept in mind.

WARNINGS

Children: A dose of 2.5 mg/kg/day of Tofranil should not be exceeded in childhood. ECG changes of unknown significance have been reported in pediatric patients with doses twice this amount.

Extreme caution should be used when this drug is given to:

patients with cardiovascular disease because of the possibility of conduction defects, arrhythmias, congestive heart failure, myocardial infarction, strokes and tachycardia. These patients require cardiac surveillance at all dosage levels of the drug;

patients with increased intraocular pressure, history of urinary retention, or history of narrow-angle glaucoma because of the drug's anticholinergic properties;

hyperthyroid patients or those on thyroid medication because of the possibility of cardiovascular toxicity;

patients with a history of seizure disorder because this drug has been shown to lower the seizure threshold;

patients receiving guanethidine, clonidine, or similar agents, since Tofranil may block the pharmacologic effects of these drugs;

patients receiving methylphenidate hydrochloride. Since methylphenidate hydrochloride may inhibit the metabolism of Tofranil, downward dosage adjustment of imipramine hydrochloride may be required when given concomitantly with methylphenidate hydrochloride.

Tofranil may enhance the CNS depressant effects of alcohol. Therefore, it should be borne in mind that the dangers inherent in a suicide attempt or accidental overdosage with the drug may be increased for the patient who uses excessive amounts of alcohol. (See **PRECAUTIONS.**)

Since Tofranil may impair the mental and/or physical abilities required for the performance of potentially hazardous tasks, such as operating an automobile or machinery, the patient should be cautioned accordingly.

PRECAUTIONS

An ECG recording should be taken prior to the initiation of larger-than-usual doses of Tofranil and at appropriate intervals thereafter until steady state is achieved. (Patients with any evidence of cardiovascular disease require cardiac surveillance at all dosage levels of the drug. See **WARNINGS.**)

Elderly patients and patients with cardiac disease or a prior history of cardiac disease are at special risk of developing the cardiac abnormalities associated with the use of Tofranil.

It should be kept in mind that the possibility of suicide in seriously depressed patients is inherent in the illness and may persist until significant remission occurs. Such patients should be carefully supervised during the early phase of treatment with Tofranil, and may require hospitalization. Prescriptions should be written for the smallest amount feasible.

Hypomanic or manic episodes may occur, particularly in patients with cyclic disorders. Such reactions may necessitate discontinuation of the drug. If needed, Tofranil may be resumed in lower dosage when these episodes are relieved. Administration of a tranquilizer may be useful in controlling such episodes.

An activation of the psychosis may occasionally be observed in schizophrenic patients and may require reduction of dosage and the addition of a phenothiazine.

Concurrent administration of Tofranil with electroshock therapy may increase the hazards; such treatment should be limited to those patients for whom it is essential, since there is limited clinical experience.

Usage During Pregnancy and Lactation:

Animal reproduction studies have yielded inconclusive results. (See also **ANIMAL PHARMACOLOGY & TOXICOLOGY.**)

There have been no well-controlled studies conducted with pregnant women to determine the effect of Tofranil on the fetus. However, there have been clinical reports of congenital malformations associated with the use of the drug. Although a causal relationship between these effects and the drug could not be established, the possibility of fetal risk from the maternal ingestion of Tofranil cannot be excluded. Therefore, Tofranil should be used in women who are or might become pregnant only if the clinical condition clearly justifies potential risk to the fetus.

Limited data suggest that Tofranil is likely to be excreted in human breast milk. As a general rule, a woman taking a drug should not nurse since the possibility exists that the drug may be excreted in breast milk and be harmful to the child.

Usage in Children: The effectiveness of the drug in children for conditions other than nocturnal enuresis has not been established.

The safety and effectiveness of the drug as temporary adjunctive therapy for nocturnal enuresis in children less than 6 years of age has not been established.

The safety of the drug for long-term, chronic use as adjunctive therapy for nocturnal enuresis in children 6 years of age or older has not been established; consideration should be given to instituting a drug-free period following an adequate therapeutic trial with a favorable response.

A dose of 2.5 mg/kg/day should not be exceeded in childhood. ECG changes of unknown significance have been reported in pediatric patients with doses twice this amount.

Patients should be warned that Tofranil may enhance the CNS depressant effects of alcohol. (See **WARNINGS.**)

Tofranil should be used with caution in patients with significantly impaired renal or hepatic function.

Patients who develop a fever and a sore throat during therapy with Tofranil should have leukocyte and differential blood counts performed. Tofranil should be discontinued if there is evidence of pathological neutrophil depression.

Prior to elective surgery, Tofranil should be discontinued for as long as the clinical situation will allow.

In occasional susceptible patients or in those receiving anticholinergic drugs (including antiparkinsonism agents) in addition, the atropine-like effects may become more pronounced (e.g., paralytic ileus).

Close supervision and careful adjustment of dosage is required when Tofranil is administered concomitantly with anticholinergic drugs.

Avoid the use of preparations, such as decongestants and local anesthetics, which contain any sympathomimetic amine (e.g., epinephrine, norepinephrine), since it has been reported that tricyclic antidepressants can potentiate the effects of catecholamines.

Caution should be exercised when Tofranil is used with agents that lower blood pressure.

Tofranil may potentiate the effects of CNS depressant drugs.

The plasma concentration of Tofranil may increase when the drug is given concomitantly with hepatic enzyme inhibitors (e.g., cimetidine, fluoxetine) and decrease by concomitant administration of hepatic enzyme inducers (e.g., barbiturates, phenytion), and adjustment of the dosage of Tofranil may therefore be necessary.

Patients taking Tofranil should avoid excessive exposure to sunlight since there have been reports of photosensitization.

Both elevation and lowering of blood sugar levels have been reported with Tofranil use.

ADVERSE REACTIONS

Note: Although the listing which follows includes a few adverse reactions which have not been reported with this specific drug, the pharmacological similarities among the tricyclic antidepressant drugs require that each of the reactions be considered when Tofranil is administered.

Cardiovascular: Orthostatic hypotension, hypertension, tachycardia, palpitation, myocardial infarction, arrhythmias, heart block, ECG changes, precipitation of congestive heart failure, stroke.

Psychiatric: Confusional states (especially in the elderly) with hallucinations, disorientation, delusions; anxiety, restlessness, agitation; insomnia and nightmares; hypomania; exacerbation of psychosis.

Neurological: Numbness, tingling, paresthesias of extremities; incoordination, ataxia, tremors; peripheral neuropathy; extrapyramidal symptoms; seizures, alterations in EEG patterns; tinnitus.

Anticholinergic: Dry mouth, and, rarely, associated sublingual adenitis; blurred vision, disturbances of accommodation, mydriasis; constipation, paralytic ileus; urinary retention, delayed micturition, dilation of the urinary tract.

Allergic: Skin rash, petechiae, urticaria, itching, photosensitization; edema (general or of face and tongue); drug fever; cross-sensitivity with desipramine.

Hematologic: Bone marrow depression including agranulocytosis; eosinophilia; purpura; thrombocytopenia.

Gastrointestinal: Nausea and vomiting, anorexia, epigastric distress, diarrhea; peculiar taste, stomatitis, abdominal cramps, black tongue.

Endocrine: Gynecomastia in the male; breast enlargement and galactorrhea in the female; increased or decreased libido, impotence; testicular swelling; elevation or depression of blood sugar levels; inappropriate antidiuretic hormone (ADH) secretion syndrome.

Other: Jaundice (simulating obstructive); altered liver function; weight gain or loss; perspiration; flushing; urinary frequency; drowsiness; dizziness, weakness and fatigue; headache; parotid swelling; alopecia; proneness to falling.

Withdrawal Symptoms: Though not indicative of addiction, abrupt cessation of treatment after prolonged therapy may produce nausea, headache and malaise.

Note: In enuretic children treated with Tofranil the most common adverse reactions have been nervousness, sleep disorders, tiredness, and mild gastrointestinal disturbances. These usually disappear during continued drug administration or when dosage is decreased. Other reactions which have been reported include constipation, convulsions, anxiety, emotional instability, syncope, and collapse. All of the adverse reactions reported with adult use should be considered.

DOSAGE AND ADMINISTRATION

Depression: Lower dosages are recommended for elderly patients and adolescents. Lower dosages are also recommended for outpatients as compared to hospitalized patients who will be under close supervision. Dosage should be initiated at a low level and increased gradually, noting carefully the clinical response and any evidence of intolerance. Following remission, maintenance medication may be required for a longer period of time, at the lowest dose that will maintain remission.

Usual Adult Dose:

Hospitalized patients— Initially, 100 mg/day in divided doses gradually increased to 200 mg/day as required. If no response after two weeks, increase to 250–300 mg/day.

Outpatients—Initially, 75 mg/day increased to 150 mg/day. Dosages over 200 mg/day are not recommended. Maintenance, 50–150 mg/day.

Adolescent and geriatric patients—Initially, 30–40 mg/day; it is generally not necessary to exceed 100 mg/day.

Childhood Enuresis: Initially, an oral dose of 25 mg/day should be tried in children aged 6 and older. Medication should be given one hour before bedtime. If a satisfactory response does not occur within one week, increase the dose to 50 mg nightly in children under 12 years; children over 12 may receive up to 75 mg nightly. A daily dose greater than 75 mg does not enhance efficacy and tends to increase side effects. Evidence suggests that in early night bedwetters, the drug is more effective given earlier and in divided amounts, i.e., 25 mg in midafternoon, repeated at bedtime. Consideration should be given to instituting a drug-free period following an adequate therapeutic trial with a favorable response. Dosage should be tapered off gradually rather than abruptly discontinued; this may reduce the tendency to relapse. Children who relapse when the drug is discontinued do not always respond to a subsequent course of treatment.

A dose of 2.5 mg/kg/day should not be exceeded. ECG changes of unknown significance have been reported in pediatric patients with doses twice this amount.

The safety and effectiveness of Tofranil as temporary adjunctive therapy for nocturnal enuresis in children less than 6 years of age has not been established.

OVERDOSAGE

Children have been reported to be more sensitive than adults to an acute overdosage of imipramine hydrochloride. An acute overdose of any amount in infants or young children, especially, must be considered serious and potentially fatal.

Signs and Symptoms: These may vary in severity depending upon factors such as the amount of drug absorbed, the age of the patient, and the interval between drug ingestion and the start of treatment. Blood and urine levels of Tofranil may not reflect the severity of poisoning; they have chiefly a qualitative rather than quantitative value, and are unreliable indicators in the clinical management of the patient.

CNS abnormalities may include drowsiness, stupor, coma, ataxia, restlessness, agitation, hyperactive reflexes, muscle rigidity, athetoid and choreiform movements, and convulsions.

Cardiac abnormalities may include arrhythmia, tachycardia, ECG evidence of impaired conduction, and signs of congestive failure.

Respiratory depression, cyanosis, hypotension, shock, vomiting, hyperpyrexia, mydriasis, and diaphoresis may also be present.

Treatment: The recommended treatment for overdosage with tricyclic antidepressants may change periodically. Therefore, it is recommended that the physician contact a poison control center for current information on treatment. Because CNS involvement, respiratory depression and cardiac arrhythmia can occur suddenly, hospitalization and close observation may be necessary, even when the amount ingested is thought to be small or the initial degree of intoxication appears slight or moderate. All patients with ECG abnormalities should have continuous cardiac monitoring and be closely observed until well after cardiac status has returned to normal; relapses may occur after apparent recovery.

In the alert patient, empty the stomach promptly by lavage. In the obtunded patient, secure the airway with a cuffed endotracheal tube before beginning lavage (do not induce emesis). Instillation of activated charcoal slurry may help reduce absorption of imipramine.

Minimize external stimulation to reduce the tendency to convulsions. If anticonvulsants are necessary, diazepam, and phenytoin may be useful.

Maintain adequate respiratory exchange. Do not use respiratory stimulants.

Shock should be treated with supportive measures, such as appropriate position, intravenous fluids, and, if necessary, a vasopressor agent. The use of corticosteroids in shock is controversial and may be contraindicated in cases of overdosage with tricyclic antidepressants. Digitalis may increase conduction abnormalities and further irritate an already sensitized myocardium. If congestive heart failure necessitates rapid digitalization, particular care must be exercised.

Hyperpyrexia should be controlled by whatever external means are available, including ice packs and cooling sponge baths, if necessary.

Hemodialysis, peritoneal dialysis, exchange transfusions and forced diuresis have been generally reported as ineffective because of the rapid fixation of Tofranil in tissues. Blood and urine levels of Tofranil may not correlate with the degree of intoxication, and are unreliable indicators in the clinical management of the patient.

The slow intravenous administration of physostigmine salicylate has been used as a last resort to reverse severe CNS anticholinergic manifestations of overdosage with tricyclic antidepressants; however, it should not be used routinely, since it may induce seizures and cholinergic crises.

HOW SUPPLIED

Tablets 10 mg — triangular, coral, sugar-coated (imprinted black Geigy 32)

Bottles of 100 ....NDC 0028-0032-01
Bottles of 1000 ....NDC 0028-0032-10

Tablets 25 mg — round, biconvex, coral, sugar-coated (imprinted black Geigy 140)

Bottles of 100 ....NDC 0028-0140-01
Bottles of 1000 ....NDC 0028-0140-10
Gy-Pak®—One Unit
12 bottles - 100 tablets each
....................NDC 0028-0140-65

Tablets 50 mg — round, biconvex, coral, sugar-coated (imprinted black Geigy 136)

Bottles of 100 ....NDC 0028-0136-01
Gy-Pak®—One Unit
12 bottles - 100 tablets each
....................NDC 0028-0136-65

Store between 59°–86°F (15°–30°C)
Dispense in tight container (USP).

ANIMAL PHARMACOLOGY & TOXICOLOGY

A. *Acute:* Oral LD_{50} ranges are as follows:

Rat	355 to 682 mg/kg
Dog	100 to 215 mg/kg

Depending on the dosage in both species, toxic signs proceeded progressively from depression, irregular respiration and ataxia to convulsions and death.

B. *Reproduction/Teratogenic:* The overall evaluation may be summed up in the following manner:

Oral: Independent studies in three species (rat, mouse and rabbit) revealed that when Tofranil is administered orally in doses up to approximately $2\frac{1}{2}$ times the maximum human dose in the first 2 species and up to 25 times the maximum human dose in the third species, the drug is essentially free from teratogenic potential. In the three species studied, only one instance of fetal abnormality occurred (in the rabbit) and in that study there was likewise an abnormality in the control group. However, evidence does exist from the rat studies that some systemic and embryotoxic potential is demonstrable. This is manifested by reduced litter size, a slight increase in the stillborn rate and a reduction in the mean birth weight.

C91-43 (Rev. 2/92)
Shown in Product Identification Section, page 410

For full prescribing information on Enuresis, please refer to Tofranil® imipramine hydrochloride USP, on page 1070.

TOFRANIL-PM® ℞

[toe-fray'nill]
imipramine pamoate
Capsules of 75 mg
Capsules of 100 mg
Capsules of 125 mg
Capsules of 150 mg
For oral administration

Each 75-mg capsule contains imipramine pamoate equivalent to 75 mg of imipramine hydrochloride.
Each 100-mg capsule contains imipramine pamoate equivalent to 100 mg of imipramine hydrochloride.
Each 125-mg capsule contains imipramine pamoate equivalent to 125 mg of imipramine hydrochloride.
Each 150-mg capsule contains imipramine pamoate equivalent to 150 mg of imipramine hydrochloride.

DESCRIPTION

Tofranil-PM, imipramine pamoate, is a tricyclic antidepressant, available as capsules for oral administration. The 75-, 100-, 125-, and 150-mg capsules contain imipramine pamoate equivalent to 75, 100, 125, and 150 mg of imipramine hydrochloride.

Imipramine pamoate is 5-(3-[dimethylamino)propyl]-10,11-dihydro-5H-dibenz[b,f]azepine 4,4′-methylenebis-(3-hydroxy-2-naphthoate) (2:1).

Imipramine pamoate is a fine, yellow, tasteless and odorless powder. It is soluble in ethanol, in acetone, in ether, in chloroform, and in carbon tetrachloride, and is insoluble in water. Its molecular weight is 949.21.

Inactive Ingredients. D&C Red No. 28, edetate calcium disodium, FD&C Blue No. 1, FD&C Yellow No. 6, gelatin, magnesium stearate, parabens, sodium lauryl sulfate, sodium propionate, starch, talc, and titanium dioxide.

CLINICAL PHARMACOLOGY

The mechanism of action of imipramine is not definitely known. However, it does not act primarily by stimulation of the central nervous system. The clinical effect is hypothesized as being due to potentiation of adrenergic synapses by blocking uptake of norepinephrine at nerve endings.

INDICATIONS

For the relief of symptoms of depression. Endogenous depression is more likely to be alleviated than other depressive states. One to three weeks of treatment may be needed before optimal therapeutic effects are evident.

CONTRAINDICATIONS

The concomitant use of monoamine oxidase inhibiting compounds is contraindicated. Hyperpyretic crises or severe convulsive seizures may occur in patients receiving such combinations. The potentiation of adverse effects can be serious, or even fatal. When it is desired to substitute Tofranil-PM in patients receiving a monoamine oxidase inhibitor, as long an interval should elapse as the clinical situation will allow, with a minimum of 14 days. Initial dosage should be low and increases should be gradual and cautiously prescribed.

The drug is contraindicated during the acute recovery period after a myocardial infarction. Patients with a known hypersensitivity to this compound should not be given the drug. The possibility of cross-sensitivity to other dibenzazepine compounds should be kept in mind.

WARNINGS

Extreme caution should be used when this drug is given to:

patients with cardiovascular disease because of the possibility of conduction defects, arrhythmias, congestive heart failure, myocardial infarction, strokes and tachycardia. These patients require cardiac surveillance at all dosage levels of the drug;

patients with increased intraocular pressure, history of urinary retention, or history of narrow-angle glaucoma because of the drug's anticholinergic properties;

hyperthyroid patients or those on thyroid medication because of the possibility of cardiovascular toxicity;

patients with a history of seizure disorder because this drug has been shown to lower the seizure threshold;

patients receiving guanethidine, clonidine, or similar agents, since imipramine pamoate may block the pharmacologic effects of these drugs;

patients receiving methylphenidate hydrochloride. Since methylphenidate hydrochloride may inhibit the metabolism of imipramine pamoate, downward dosage adjustment of imipramine pamoate may be required when given concomitantly with methylphenidate hydrochloride.

Since imipramine pamoate may impair the mental and/or physical abilities required for the performance of potentially hazardous tasks, such as operating an automobile or machinery, the patient should be cautioned accordingly.

Tofranil-PM may enhance the CNS depressant effects of alcohol. Therefore, it should be borne in mind that the dangers inherent in a suicide attempt or accidental overdosage with the drug may be increased for the patient who uses excessive amounts of alcohol. (See **PRECAUTIONS.**)

Usage in Children: Tofranil-PM should not be used in children of any age because of the increased potential for acute overdosage due to the high unit potency (75 mg, 100 mg, 125 mg and 150 mg). Each capsule contains imipramine pamoate equivalent to 75 mg, 100 mg, 125 mg or 150 mg imipramine hydrochloride.

PRECAUTIONS

An ECG recording should be taken prior to the initiation of larger-than-usual doses of imipramine pamoate and at appropriate intervals thereafter until steady state is achieved. (Patients with any evidence of cardiovascular disease require cardiac surveillance at all dosage levels of the drug. See **WARNINGS.**) Elderly patients and patients with cardiac disease or a prior history of cardiac disease are at special risk of developing the cardiac abnormalities associated with the use of imipramine pamoate. It should be kept in mind that the possibility of suicide in seriously depressed patients is inherent in the illness and may persist until significant remission occurs. Such patients should be carefully supervised during the early phase of treatment with imipramine pamoate and may require hospitalization. Prescriptions should be written for the smallest amount feasible.

Hypomanic or manic episodes may occur, particularly in patients with cyclic disorders. Such reactions may necessitate discontinuation of the drug. If needed, imipramine pamoate may be resumed in lower dosage when these episodes are relieved. Administration of a tranquilizer may be useful in controlling such episodes.

An activation of the psychosis may occasionally be observed in schizophrenic patients and may require reduction of dosage and the addition of a phenothiazine.

Concurrent administration of imipramine pamoate with electroshock therapy may increase the hazards; such treatment should be limited to those patients for whom it is essential, since there is limited clinical experience.

Usage During Pregnancy and Lactation:

Animal reproduction studies have yielded inconclusive results. (See also **ANIMAL PHARMACOLOGY & TOXICOLOGY.**)

There have been no well-controlled studies conducted with pregnant women to determine the effect of imipramine on the fetus. However, there have been clinical reports of congenital malformations associated with the use of the drug. Although a causal relationship between these effects and the drug could not be established, the possibility of fetal risk from the maternal ingestion of imipramine cannot be excluded. Therefore, imipramine should be used in women who are or might become pregnant only if the clinical condition clearly justifies potential risk to the fetus.

Limited data suggest that imipramine is likely to be excreted in human breast milk. As a general rule, a woman taking a drug should not nurse since the possibility exists that the drug may be excreted in breast milk and be harmful to the child.

Patients should be warned that imipramine pamoate may enhance the CNS depressant effects of alcohol. (See **WARNINGS.**)

Imipramine pamoate should be used with caution in patients with significantly impaired renal or hepatic function.

Patients who develop a fever and a sore throat during therapy with imipramine pamoate should have leukocyte and differential blood counts performed. Imipramine pamoate

Continued on next page

The full prescribing information for each GEIGY product is contained herein and is that in effect as of September 1, 1992.

GEIGY—Cont.

should be discontinued if there is evidence of pathological neutrophil depression.

Prior to elective surgery, imipramine pamoate should be discontinued for as long as the clinical situation will allow. In occasional susceptible patients or in those receiving anticholinergic drugs (including antiparkinsonism agents) in addition, the atropine-like effects may become more pronounced (e.g., paralytic ileus). Close supervision and careful adjustment of dosage is required when imipramine pamoate is administered concomitantly with anticholinergic drugs.

Avoid the use of preparations, such as decongestants and local anesthetics, which contain any sympathomimetic amine (e.g., epinephrine, norepinephrine), since it has been reported that tricyclic antidepressants can potentiate the effects of catecholamines.

Caution should be exercised when imipramine pamoate is used with agents that lower blood pressure.

Imipramine pamoate may potentiate the effects of CNS depressant drugs.

The plasma concentration of imipramine may increase when the drug is given concomitantly with hepatic enzyme inhibitors (e.g., cimetidine, fluoxetine) and decrease by concomitant administration with hepatic enzyme inducers (e.g., barbiturates, phenytoin), and adjustment of the dosage of imipramine may therefore be necessary.

Patients taking imipramine pamoate should avoid excessive exposure to sunlight since there have been reports of photosensitization.

Both elevation and lowering of blood sugar levels have been reported with imipramine pamoate use.

ADVERSE REACTIONS

Note: Although the listing which follows includes a few adverse reactions which have not been reported with this specific drug, the pharmacological similarities among the tricyclic antidepressant drugs require that each of the reactions be considered when imipramine is administered.

Cardiovascular: Orthostatic hypotension, hypertension, tachycardia, palpitation, myocardial infarction, arrhythmias, heart block, ECG changes, precipitation of congestive heart failure, stroke.

Psychiatric: Confusional states (especially in the elderly) with hallucinations, disorientation, delusions; anxiety, restlessness, agitation; insomnia and nightmares; hypomania; exacerbation of psychosis.

Neurological: Numbness, tingling, paresthesias of extremities; incoordination, ataxia, tremors; peripheral neuropathy; extrapyramidal symptoms; seizures, alterations in EEG patterns; tinnitus.

Anticholinergic: Dry mouth, and, rarely, associated sublingual adenitis; blurred vision, disturbances of accommodation, mydriasis; constipation, paralytic ileus; urinary retention, delayed micturition, dilation of the urinary tract.

Allergic: Skin rash, petechiae, urticaria, itching, photosensitization; edema (general or of face and tongue); drug fever; cross-sensitivity with desipramine.

Hematologic: Bone marrow depression including agranulocytosis; eosinophilia; purpura; thrombocytopenia.

Gastrointestinal: Nausea and vomiting, anorexia, epigastric distress, diarrhea; peculiar taste, stomatitis, abdominal cramps, black tongue.

Endocrine: Gynecomastia in the male; breast enlargement and galactorrhea in the female; increased or decreased libido, impotence; testicular swelling; elevation or depression of blood sugar levels; inappropriate antidiuretic hormone (ADH) secretion syndrome.

Other: Jaundice (simulating obstructive); altered liver function; weight gain or loss; perspiration; flushing; urinary frequency; drowsiness, dizziness, weakness and fatigue; headache; parotid swelling; alopecia; proneness to falling.

Withdrawal Symptoms: Though not indicative of addiction, abrupt cessation of treatment after prolonged therapy may produce nausea, headache and malaise.

DOSAGE AND ADMINISTRATION

The following recommended dosages for Tofranil-PM should be modified as necessary by the clinical response and any evidence of intolerance.

Initial Adult Dosage:

Outpatients—Therapy should be initiated at 75 mg/day. Dosage may be increased to 150 mg/day which is the dose level at which optimum response is usually obtained. If necessary, dosage may be increased to 200 mg/day.

Dosage higher than 75 mg/day may also be administered on a once-a-day basis after the optimum dosage and tolerance have been determined. The daily dosage may be given at bedtime. In some patients it may be necessary to employ a divided-dose schedule.

As with all tricyclics, the antidepressant effect of imipramine may not be evident for one to three weeks in some patients.

Hospitalized Patients—Therapy should be initiated at 100–150 mg/day and may be increased to 200 mg/day. If

there is no response after two weeks, dosage should be increased to 250–300 mg/day.

Dosage higher than 150 mg/day may also be administered on a once-a-day basis after the optimum dosage and tolerance have been determined. The daily dosage may be given at bedtime. In some patients it may be necessary to employ a divided-dose schedule.

As with all tricyclics, the antidepressant effect of imipramine may not be evident for one to three weeks in some patients.

Adult Maintenance Dosage: Following remission, maintenance medication may be required for a longer period of time at the lowest dose that will maintain remission after which the dosage should gradually be decreased.

The usual maintenance dosage is 75–150 mg/day. The total daily dosage can be administered on a once-a-day basis, preferably at bedtime. In some patients it may be necessary to employ a divided-dose schedule.

In cases of relapse due to premature withdrawal of the drug, the effective dosage of imipramine should be reinstituted.

Adolescent and Geriatric Patients: Therapy in these age groups should be initiated with Tofranil®, brand of imipramine hydrochloride, tablets at a total daily dosage of 25–50 mg, since Tofranil-PM capsules are not available in these strengths. Dosage may be increased according to response and tolerance, but it is generally unnecessary to exceed 100 mg/day in these patients. Tofranil-PM capsules may be used when total daily dosage is established at 75 mg or higher. The total daily dosage can be administered on a once-a-day basis, preferably at bedtime. In some patients it may be necessary to employ a divided-dose schedule.

As with all tricyclics, the antidepressant effect of imipramine may not be evident for one to three weeks in some patients.

Adolescent and geriatric patients can usually be maintained at lower dosage. Following remission, maintenance medication may be required for a longer period of time at the lowest dose that will maintain remission after which the dosage should gradually be decreased.

The total daily maintenance dosage can be administered on a once-a-day basis, preferably at bedtime. In some patients it may be necessary to employ a divided-dose schedule.

In cases of relapse due to premature withdrawal of the drug, the effective dosage of imipramine should be reinstituted.

OVERDOSAGE

Children have been reported to be more sensitive than adults to an acute overdosage of imipramine pamoate. An acute overdose of any amount in infants or young children, especially, must be considered serious and potentially fatal.

Signs and Symptoms: These may vary in severity depending upon factors such as the amount of drug absorbed, the age of the patient, and the interval between drug ingestion and the start of treatment. Blood and urine levels of imipramine may not reflect the severity of poisoning; they have chiefly a qualitative rather than a quantitative value, and are unreliable indicators in the clinical management of the patient.

CNS abnormalities may include drowsiness, stupor, coma, ataxia, restlessness, agitation, hyperactive reflexes, muscle rigidity, athetoid and choreiform movements, and convulsions.

Cardiac abnormalities may include arrhythmia, tachycardia, ECG evidence of impaired conduction, and signs of congestive failure.

Respiratory depression, cyanosis, hypotension, shock, vomiting, hyperpyrexia, mydriasis, and diaphoresis may also be present.

Treatment: The recommended treatment for overdosage with tricyclic antidepressants may change periodically. Therefore, it is recommended that the physician contact a poison control center for current information on treatment. Because CNS involvement, respiratory depression and cardiac arrhythmia can occur suddenly, hospitalization and close observation may be necessary, even when the amount ingested is thought to be small or the initial degree of intoxication appears slight or moderate. All patients with ECG abnormalities should have continuous cardiac monitoring and be closely observed until well after cardiac status has returned to normal; relapses may occur after apparent recovery.

In the alert patient, empty the stomach promptly by lavage. In the obtunded patient, secure the airway with a cuffed endotracheal tube before beginning lavage (do not induce emesis). Instillation of activated charcoal slurry may help reduce absorption of imipramine.

Minimize external stimulation to reduce the tendency to convulsions. If anticonvulsants are necessary, diazepam and phenytoin may be useful.

Maintain adequate respiratory exchange. Do not use respiratory stimulants.

Shock should be treated with supportive measures, such as appropriate position, intravenous fluids, and, if necessary, a vasopressor agent. Digitalis may increase conduction abnormalities and further irritate an already sensitized myocar-

dium. If congestive heart failure necessitates rapid digitalization, particular care must be exercised.

Hyperpyrexia should be controlled by whatever external means are available, including ice packs and cooling sponge baths, if necessary.

Hemodialysis, peritoneal dialysis, exchange transfusions and forced diuresis have been generally reported as ineffective because of the rapid fixation of imipramine in tissues. Blood and urine levels of imipramine may not correlate with the degree of intoxication, and are unreliable indicators in the clinical management of the patient.

The slow intravenous administration of physostigmine salicylate has been used as a last resort to reverse severe CNS anticholinergic manifestations of overdosage with tricyclic antidepressants; however, it should not be used routinely, since it may induce seizures and cholinergic crises.

HOW SUPPLIED

Capsules 75 mg — coral (imprinted Geigy 20) equivalent to 75 mg imipramine hydrochloride

    Bottles of 30 ....NDC 0028-0020-26
    Bottles of 100 ....NDC 0028-0020-01
    Unit Dose (blister pack)
      Box of 100 (strips of 10) ....NDC 0028-0020-61

Capsules 100 mg — dark yellow/coral (imprinted Geigy 40) equivalent to 100 mg imipramine hydrochloride

    Bottles of 30 ....NDC 0028-0040-26
    Bottles of 100 ....NDC 0028-0040-01

Capsules 125 mg — light yellow/coral (imprinted black Geigy 45) equivalent to 125 mg imipramine hydrochloride

    Bottles of 30 ....NDC 0028-0045-26
    Bottles of 100 ....NDC 0028-0045-01

Capsules 150 mg — coral (imprinted black Geigy 22) equivalent to 150 mg imipramine hydrochloride

    Bottles of 30 ....NDC 0028-0022-26
    Bottles of 100 ....NDC 0028-0022-01

Do not store above 86°F (30°C).

Dispense in tight container (USP).

ANIMAL PHARMACOLOGY & TOXICOLOGY

A. *Acute:* Oral LD_{50}:

Mouse	2185 mg/kg
Rat (F)	1142 mg/kg
(M)	1807 mg/kg
Rabbit	1016 mg/kg
Dog	693 mg/kg (Emesis ED_{50})

B. *Subacute:*

Two three-month studies in dogs gave evidence of an adverse drug effect on the testes, but only at the highest dose level employed, i.e., 90 mg/kg (10 times the maximum human dose). Depending on the histological section of the testes examined, the findings consisted of a range of degenerative changes up to and including complete atrophy of the seminiferous tubules, with spermatogenesis usually arrested.

Human studies show no definitive effect on sperm count, sperm motility, sperm morphology or volume of ejaculate.

Rat

One three-month study was done in rats at dosage levels comparable to those of the dog studies. No adverse drug effect on the testes was noted in this study, as confirmed by histological examination.

C. *Reproduction/Teratogenic:*

Oral: Imipramine pamoate was fed to male and female albino rats for 28 weeks through two breeding cycles at dose levels of 15 mg/kg/day and 40 mg/kg/day (equivalent to 2½ and 7 times the maximum human dose). No abnormalities which could be related to drug administration were noted in gross inspection. Autopsies performed on pups from the second breeding likewise revealed no pathological changes in organs or tissues; however, a decrease in mean litter size from both matings was noted in the drug-treated groups and significant growth suppression occurred in the nursing pups of both sexes in the high group as well as in the females of the low-level group. Finally, the lactation index (pups weaned divided by number left to nurse) was significantly lower in the second litter of the high-level group.

C91-44 (Rev. 2/92)

Shown in Product Identification Section, page 410

VOLTAREN®   ℞
diclofenac sodium
Enteric-Coated Tablets

DESCRIPTION

Voltaren, diclofenac sodium, is a nonsteroidal, anti-inflammatory benzeneacetic acid derivative, designated chemically as 2-[(2,6-dichlorophenyl)amino]benzeneacetic acid, monosodium salt.

Diclofenac sodium is a faintly yellow-white to light beige, virtually odorless, slightly hygroscopic crystalline powder. It is freely soluble in methanol, sparingly soluble in water, very slightly soluble in acetonitrile, and insoluble in chloroform and in 0.1N hydrochloric acid. Its molecular weight is 318.14.

In water, diclofenac sodium has a single dissociation constant (pKa) of 4.0.

Voltaren is available as enteric-coated tablets of 25 mg, 50 mg, and 75 mg for oral administration.

Inactive Ingredients. Cellulose acetate phthalate, colloidal silicon dioxide (25-mg and 50-mg enteric-coated tablets only), diethyl phthalate, hydroxypropyl methylcellulose, iron oxide (25-mg and 50-mg enteric-coated tablets only), lactose, magnesium stearate, microcrystalline cellulose, povidone, shellac, sodium starch glycolate (75-mg enteric-coated tablets only), starch (25-mg and 50-mg enteric-coated tablets only), talc (75-mg enteric-coated tablets only), titanium dioxide.

CLINICAL PHARMACOLOGY
Pharmacology
In pharmacologic studies, Voltaren has shown anti-inflammatory, analgesic, and antipyretic activity. As with other nonsteroidal anti-inflammatory agents, its mode of action is not known; however, its ability to inhibit prostaglandin synthesis may be involved in the anti-inflammatory effect.
Pharmacokinetics
Voltaren is completely absorbed from the gastrointestinal tract after fasting oral administration, with peak plasma levels occurring in 2–3 hours. However, due to first-pass metabolism, only about 50% of the absorbed dose is systemically available. The mean terminal half-life in plasma is approximately 2 hours, but early elimination is much more rapid. Area under the plasma concentration curve (AUC) is dose-proportional within the range of 25 mg to 150 mg. Peak plasma levels are less than dose-proportional and are approximately 1.0, 1.5, and 2 mcg/ml for 25-mg, 50-mg, and 75-mg doses, respectively. It should be noted that the administration of several individual tablets may not yield equivalent results in peak concentration as the administration of one tablet of a higher strength. This is due to the uncertainty of complete gastric emptying of all tablets at once to the duodenum. Clearance and volume of distribution were about 350 ml/min and 550 ml/kg, respectively. After repeated oral administration of 50 mg b.i.d., Voltaren did not accumulate in plasma. The degree of accumulation of diclofenac metabolites is unknown. Some of the metabolites may have activity. More than 99% of diclofenac is reversibly bound to human plasma albumin.

Voltaren is eliminated through metabolism and subsequent urinary and biliary excretion of the glucuronide and the sulfate conjugates of the metabolites. Approximately 65% of the dose is excreted in the urine, and approximately 35% in the bile.

Conjugates of the principal metabolite, 4'-hydroxy-diclofenac, account for 20–30% of the dose excreted in the urine and for 10–20% of the dose excreted in the bile. Conjugates of three other metabolites (5-hydroxy-,3'-hydroxy-, and 4',5-dihydroxy-diclofenac) together account for 10–20% of the dose excreted in the urine and for small amounts excreted in the bile. Conjugates of unchanged diclofenac account for 5–10% of the dose excreted in the urine and for less than 5% excreted in the bile. Little or no unchanged unconjugated drug is excreted. It is not known whether there is genetic polymorphism in the enzymes responsible for metabolism of diclofenac.

The extent of absorption of Voltaren is not significantly affected when the drug is taken with food; however, there is usually a delay in the onset of absorption of 1 to 4.5 hours, with delays as long as 10 hours in some patients. There is also a reduction in peak plasma levels.

A 4-week study comparing plasma level profiles of diclofenac (50 mg b.i.d.) in younger (26–46) versus older (66–81) adults did not show differences between age groups (10 patients per age group).

Single-dose studies of the effects of renal function impairment (50 mg intravenously) or hepatic impairment (100 mg oral solution) have been performed in small numbers of patients. To date no differences in the pharmacokinetics of diclofenac have been detected in patients with renal or hepatic impairment.

In patients with renal impairment (N=5, creatinine clearance 3 to 42 ml/min), AUC values and elimination rates were comparable to those in healthy subjects.

In patients with biopsy-confirmed cirrhosis or chronic active hepatitis (variably elevated transaminases and mildly elevated bilirubins, N=10), diclofenac concentrations and urinary elimination values were comparable to those in healthy subjects.

Voltaren diffuses into and out of the synovial fluid. Diffusion into the joint occurs during the first 4 hours following a dose, while plasma levels are higher than those in synovial fluid, after which the process reverses and synovial fluid levels are slightly higher than plasma levels. It is not known whether diffusion into the joint plays a role in the effectiveness of Voltaren.

In healthy subjects, the daily administration of 150 mg of Voltaren for 3 weeks resulted in a mean fecal blood loss less than that observed with 3.0 g of aspirin daily. In repeated-dose studies, mean fecal blood loss with 150 mg of Voltaren was also less than that observed with 750 mg of naproxen or

150 mg of indomethacin. Repeated-dose endoscopic studies in normal volunteers showed that daily doses of 75 mg or 100 mg of Voltaren for 1 week caused fewer gastric lesions, and those that did occur had lower scores than those which occurred following 500 mg daily doses of naproxen. The clinical significance of these findings is unknown since there is no evidence available to indicate that diclofenac is less likely than other drugs of its class to cause serious gastrointestinal lesions when used in chronic therapy.

In patients with rheumatoid arthritis, Voltaren has been administered safely in combination with gold or corticosteroids.

INDICATIONS AND USAGE
Voltaren is indicated for acute and chronic treatment of the signs and symptoms of rheumatoid arthritis, osteoarthritis, and ankylosing spondylitis.

CONTRAINDICATIONS
Voltaren is contraindicated in patients with hypersensitivity to it. Voltaren should not be given to patients in whom Voltaren, aspirin, or other nonsteroidal anti-inflammatory drugs induce asthma, urticaria, or other allergic-type reactions because severe, rarely fatal, anaphylactic-like reactions to Voltaren have been reported in such patients.

WARNINGS
Gastrointestinal Effects
Peptic ulceration and gastrointestinal bleeding have been reported in patients receiving Voltaren. Physicians and patients should therefore remain alert for ulceration and bleeding in patients treated chronically with diclofenac sodium, even in the absence of previous G.I. tract symptoms. It is recommended that patients be maintained on the lowest dose of diclofenac sodium possible consistent with achieving a satisfactory therapeutic response.

Risk of G.I. Ulcerations, Bleeding, and Perforation with NSAID Therapy: Serious gastrointestinal toxicity such as bleeding, ulceration, and perforation can occur at any time, with or without warning symptoms, in patients treated chronically with NSAID therapy. Although minor upper gastrointestinal problems, such as dyspepsia, are common, usually developing early in therapy, physicians should remain alert for ulceration and bleeding in patients treated chronically with NSAIDs even in the absence of previous G.I. tract symptoms. In patients observed in clinical trials of several months to 2 years duration, symptomatic upper G.I. ulcers, gross bleeding, or perforation appear to occur in approximately 1% of patients treated for 3–6 months, and in about 2–4% of patients treated for 1 year. Physicians should inform patients about the signs and/or symptoms of serious G.I. toxicity and what steps to take if they occur.

Studies to date have not identified any subset of patients not at risk of developing peptic ulceration and bleeding. Except for a prior history of serious G.I. events and other risk factors known to be associated with peptic ulcer disease, such as alcoholism, smoking, etc., no risk factors (e.g., age, sex) have been associated with increased risk. Elderly or debilitated patients seem to tolerate ulceration or bleeding less well than other individuals and most spontaneous reports of fatal G.I. events are in this population. Studies to date are inconclusive concerning the relative risk of various NSAIDs in causing such reactions. High doses of any NSAID probably carry a greater risk of these reactions, although controlled clinical trials showing this do not exist in most cases. In considering the use of relatively large doses (within the recommended dosage range), sufficient benefit should be anticipated to offset the potential increased risk of G.I. toxicity.

Hepatic Effects
As with other nonsteroidal anti-inflammatory drugs, elevations of one or more liver tests may occur during Voltaren therapy. These laboratory abnormalities may progress, may remain unchanged, or may be transient with continued therapy. Borderline elevations, (i.e., 1.2–3 times the upper limit of normal [ULN]), or greater elevations of transaminases occurred in about 15% of Voltaren-treated patients. The SGPT (ALT) test is probably the most sensitive indicator of liver injury. In clinical trials, meaningful elevations (i.e., more than 3 times the ULN) of SGOT (SGPT was not measured in all studies) occurred in about 2% of approximately 5700 patients at some time during Voltaren treatment. In a large, open, controlled trial, meaningful elevations of SGOT and/or SGPT occurred in about 4% of 3700 patients treated for 2–6 months, including marked elevations (i.e., more than 8 times the ULN) in about 1% of the 3700 patients. In that open-label study, a lower incidence of borderline (1.2–3 times the ULN), moderate (3–8 times the ULN), and marked (>8 times the ULN) elevations of SGOT or SGPT was observed in patients randomized to other NSAIDs. Transaminase elevations were seen more frequently in patients with osteoarthritis than in those with rheumatoid arthritis (see ADVERSE REACTIONS).

Transaminase elevations were reversible on cessation of therapy, and among 51 patients in all studies with marked elevations, signs and symptoms of liver disease occurred in only 3 cases, and only 1 patient developed jaundice. Most patients with borderline elevations did not have therapy

interrupted; transaminase elevations in most of these cases disappeared or did not progress. There were no identifying features to distinguish those patients who developed marked elevations from those who did not.

In addition to the enzyme elevations seen in clinical trials, rare cases of severe hepatic reactions, including jaundice and fatal fulminant hepatitis, have been reported.

Because severe hepatotoxicity may develop without a prodrome of distinguishing symptoms, physicians should measure transaminases periodically in patients receiving long-term therapy with Voltaren. The optimum times for making the first and subsequent transaminase measurements are not known. In the largest U.S. trial (open-label), which involved 3700 patients monitored first at 8 weeks and 1200 patients monitored again at 24 weeks, almost all meaningful elevations in transaminases were detected before patients became symptomatic. In 42 of the 51 patients in all trials who developed marked transaminase elevations, abnormal tests occurred during the first 2 months of therapy with Voltaren. Based on this experience the first transaminase measurement should be made no later than 8 weeks after the start of Voltaren treatment. As with other NSAIDs, if abnormal liver tests persist or worsen, if clinical signs and/or symptoms consistent with liver disease develop, or if systemic manifestations occur (e.g., eosinophilia, rash, etc.), Voltaren should be discontinued.

To minimize the possibility that hepatic injury will become severe between transaminase measurements, physicians should inform patients of the warning signs and symptoms of hepatotoxicity (e.g., nausea, fatigue, lethargy, pruritus, jaundice, right upper quadrant tenderness, and "flu-like" symptoms), and the appropriate action to take should these signs and symptoms appear.

PRECAUTIONS
General
Allergic Reactions: As with other nonsteroidal anti-inflammatory drugs, allergic reactions including anaphylaxis, have been reported with Voltaren. Specific allergic manifestations consisting of swelling of eyelids, lips, pharynx and larynx, urticaria, asthma, and bronchospasm, sometimes with a concomitant fall in blood pressure (severe at times) have been observed in clinical trials and/or the foreign marketing experience with Voltaren. Anaphylaxis has been reported rarely from foreign sources; in U.S. clinical trials with Voltaren in over 6000 patients, 1 case of anaphylaxis was reported. In controlled clinical trials, allergic reactions have been observed at an incidence of 0.5%. These reactions can occur without prior exposure to the drug.

Fluid Retention and Edema: Fluid retention and edema have been observed in some patients taking Voltaren. Therefore, as with other nonsteroidal anti-inflammatory drugs, Voltaren should be used with caution in patients with a history of cardiac decompensation, hypertension, or other conditions predisposing to fluid retention.

Renal Effects: As a class, nonsteroidal anti-inflammatory drugs have been associated with renal papillary necrosis and other abnormal renal pathology in long-term administration to animals. Papillary necrosis was observed only in 1 animal study with diclofenac, a 4-week study in baboons in which the drug was administered intramuscularly. In oral studies some evidence of renal toxicity was noted but papillary necrosis was not reported.

A second form of renal toxicity generally associated with nonsteroidal anti-inflammatory drugs is seen in patients with conditions leading to a reduction in renal blood flow or blood volume, where renal prostaglandins have a supportive role in the maintenance of renal perfusion. In these patients, administration of a nonsteroidal anti-inflammatory drug results in a dose-dependent decrease in prostaglandin synthesis and, secondarily, in a reduction of renal blood flow, which may precipitate overt renal failure. Patients at greatest risk of this reaction are those with impaired renal function, heart failure, liver dysfunction, those taking diuretics, and the elderly. Discontinuation of nonsteroidal anti-inflammatory drug therapy is typically followed by recovery to the pretreatment state.

Cases of significant renal failure in patients receiving Voltaren have been reported from postmarketing experience, but were not observed in over 4,000 patients in clinical trials during which serum creatinines and BUNs were followed serially. There were only 11 patients (0.28%) whose serum creatinines and concurrent serum BUNs were greater than 2.0 mg/dl and 40 mg/dl, respectively, while on diclofenac (mean rise in patients: creatinine 2.3 mg/dl and BUN 28.4 mg/dl).

Since Voltaren metabolites are eliminated primarily by the kidneys, patients with significantly impaired renal function

Continued on next page

The full prescribing information for each GEIGY product is contained herein and is that in effect as of September 1, 1992.

GEIGY—Cont.

should be more closely monitored than subjects with normal renal function.

Porphyria: The use of diclofenac in patients with hepatic porphyria should be avoided. To date, 1 patient has been described in whom diclofenac probably triggered a clinical attack of porphyria. The postulated mechanism for causing such attacks by diclofenac, as well as some other NSAIDs, is through stimulation of the porphyrin precursor delta-aminolevulinic acid (ALA, demonstrated in rats).

Information for Patients
Voltaren, like other drugs of its class, is not free of side effects. The side effects of these drugs can cause discomfort and, rarely, there are more serious side effects, such as gastrointestinal bleeding, which may result in hospitalization and even fatal outcomes.

NSAIDs are often essential agents in the management of arthritis, but they also may be commonly employed for conditions which are less serious.

Physicians may wish to discuss with their patients the potential risks (see WARNINGS, PRECAUTIONS, and ADVERSE REACTIONS) and likely benefits of NSAID treatment, particularly when the drugs are used for less serious conditions where treatment without NSAIDs may represent an acceptable alternative to both the patient and physician.

Laboratory Tests
Because serious G.I. tract ulceration and bleeding can occur without warning symptoms, physicians should follow chronically treated patients for the signs and symptoms of ulceration and bleeding and should inform them of the importance of this follow-up (see WARNINGS, *Risk of G.I. Ulcerations, Bleeding, and Perforation with NSAID Therapy*).

Drug Interactions
Aspirin: Concomitant administration of Voltaren and aspirin is not recommended because Voltaren is displaced from its binding sites during the concomitant administration of aspirin, resulting in lower plasma concentrations, peak plasma levels, and AUC values.

Anticoagulants: While studies have not shown Voltaren to interact with anticoagulants of the warfarin type, caution should be exercised, nonetheless, since interactions have been seen with other NSAIDs. Because prostaglandins play an important role in hemostasis, and NSAIDs affect platelet function as well, concurrent therapy with all NSAIDs, including Voltaren, and warfarin requires close monitoring of patients to be certain that no change in their anticoagulant dosage is required.

Digoxin, Methotrexate, Cyclosporine: Voltaren, like other NSAIDs, through effects on renal prostaglandins, may cause increased toxicity of certain drugs. Digoxin and methotrexate serum levels may be elevated as well as cyclosporine's nephrotoxicity. Patients receiving these drugs who are started on, or are given increased doses of, Voltaren or any other NSAID, and particularly those patients with altered renal function, should be observed for the development of the specific toxicities of these drugs. In the case of digoxin, serum levels should be monitored.

Lithium: Voltaren decreases lithium renal clearance and increases lithium plasma levels. In patients taking Voltaren and lithium concomitantly, lithium toxicity may develop.

Oral Hypoglycemics: Voltaren does not alter glucose metabolism in normal subjects nor are the effects of oral hypoglycemic agents altered by the concomitant administration of Voltaren. There are rare reports, however, from postmarketing experiences of changes in effects of insulin or oral hypoglycemic agents in the presence of diclofenac which necessitated changes in the doses of such agents. Both hypo- and hyperglycemic effects have been reported. A direct causal relationship has not been established, but physicians should consider the possibility that diclofenac may alter a diabetic patient's response to insulin or oral hypoglycemic agents.

Diuretics: Voltaren and other NSAIDs can inhibit the activity of diuretics. Concomitant treatment with potassium-sparing diuretics may be associated with increased serum potassium levels.

Other Drugs: In small groups of patients (7–10/interaction study), the concomitant administration of azathioprine, gold, chloroquine, D-penicillamine, prednisolone, doxycycline, or digitoxin did not significantly affect the peak levels and AUC values of Voltaren.

Protein Binding
In vitro, Voltaren interferes minimally or not at all with the protein binding of salicylic acid (20% decrease in binding), tolbutamide, prednisolone (10% decrease in binding), or warfarin. Benzylpenicillin, ampicillin, oxacillin, chlortetracycline, doxycycline, cephalothin, erythromycin, and sulfamethoxazole have no influence in vitro on the protein binding of Voltaren in human serum.

Drug/Laboratory Test Interactions
Effect on Blood Coagulation: Voltaren increases platelet aggregation time but does not affect bleeding time, plasma thrombin clotting time, plasma fibrinogen, or factors V and

VII to XII. Statistically significant changes in prothrombin and partial thromboplastin times have been reported in normal volunteers. The mean changes were observed to be less than 1 second in both instances, however, and are unlikely to be clinically important. Voltaren is a prostaglandin synthetase inhibitor, however, and all drugs that inhibit prostaglandin synthesis interfere with platelet function to some degree; therefore, patients who may be adversely affected by such an action should be carefully observed.

Carcinogenesis, Mutagenesis, Impairment of Fertility
Long-term carcinogenicity studies in rats given Voltaren up to 2 mg/kg/day (approximately the human dose) have revealed no significant increases in tumor incidence.

There was a slight increase in benign mammary fibroadenomas in mid-dose females (high-dose females had excessive mortality), but the increase was not significant for this common rat tumor. Voltaren did not show mutagenic potential in various mutagenicity studies including the Ames test. Voltaren administered to male and female rats at 4 mg/kg/day did not affect fertility. A 2-year mouse carcinogenicity study is underway.

Teratogenic Effects
Pregnancy Category B: Reproduction studies have been performed in mice given Voltaren (up to 20 mg/kg/day) and in rats and rabbits given Voltaren (up to 10 mg/kg/day), and have revealed no evidence of teratogenicity despite the induction of maternal toxicity and fetal toxicity. In rats, maternally toxic doses were associated with dystocia, prolonged gestation, reduced fetal weights and growth, and reduced fetal survival. Voltaren has been shown to cross the placental barrier in mice and rats.

There are no adequate and well-controlled studies in pregnant women. Voltaren should be used during pregnancy only if the benefits to the mother justify the potential risk to the fetus. Because of the known effects of prostaglandin-inhibiting drugs on the fetal cardiovascular system (closure of ductus arteriosus), use of Voltaren during late pregnancy should be avoided.

Labor and Delivery
The effects of Voltaren on labor and delivery in pregnant women are unknown. However, as with other nonsteroidal anti-inflammatory drugs, it is possible that Voltaren may inhibit uterine contraction.

Nursing Mothers
Voltaren has been found in the milk of nursing mothers. As with other drugs that are excreted in milk, Voltaren is not recommended for use in nursing women.

Pediatric Use
Dosage recommendations and indications for use in children have not been established.

ADVERSE REACTIONS

Adverse reaction information is derived from blinded-controlled and open-label clinical trials and worldwide marketing experience. In the description below, rates of the more common events represent clinical study results; rarer events are derived principally from marketing experience and publications, and accurate rate estimates are generally impossible.

The incidence of common adverse reactions (greater than 1%) is based upon controlled clinical trials in 1543 patients treated up to 13 weeks. By far the most common adverse effects were gastrointestinal symptoms, most of them minor, occurring in about 20%, and leading to discontinuation in about 3%, of patients. Peptic ulcer or G.I. bleeding occurred in clinical trials in less than 1% of approximately 1800 patients during their first 3 months of diclofenac treatment and in less than 2% of approximately 800 patients followed for 1 year. The only control group with sufficient patients for comparison received aspirin and only for the first 30 days of treatment. Comparative rates were 0.2% for peptic ulcer or G.I. bleeding in approximately 2000 diclofenac-treated patients and 0.6% in approximately 600 aspirin-treated patients.

In double-blind trials there were fewer minor gastrointestinal complaints in 1227 patients treated with Voltaren than in 721 patients treated with aspirin, 22% vs 33% (compared to 13% on placebo).

Gastrointestinal symptoms were followed in frequency by central nervous system side effects such as headache (7%) and dizziness (3%).

Meaningful (exceeding 3 times the upper limit of normal) elevations of SGPT (ALT) or SGOT (AST) occurred at an overall rate of about 2% during the first 2 months of Voltaren treatment. Unlike aspirin, where elevations occur more frequently in patients with rheumatoid arthritis, these elevations were more frequently observed in patients with osteoarthritis (2.6%) than in patients with rheumatoid arthritis (0.7%). Marked elevations (exceeding 8 times the upper limit of normal) were seen in about 1% of patients treated for 2–6 months (see WARNINGS).

The following adverse reactions were reported in patients treated with Voltaren:

Incidence Greater Than 1% (All derived from clinical trials.)
Body as a Whole: Abdominal pain or cramps*, headache*, fluid retention, abdominal distention.

Digestive: Diarrhea*, indigestion*, neausea*, constipation*, flatulence, liver test abnormalities, PUB, i.e., peptic ulcer, with or without bleeding and/or perforation, or bleeding without ulcer (see above and also WARNINGS).
Nervous System: Dizziness.
Skin and Appendages: Rash, pruritus.
Special Senses: Tinnitus.
Incidence Less Than 1%—Causal Relationship Probable (Adverse reactions reported only in worldwide postmarketing experience or in the literature, not seen in clinical trials, are considered rare and are italicized.)
Body as a Whole: Malaise, swelling of lips and tongue, photosensitivity, *anaphylaxis,* anaphylactoid reactions.
Cardiovascular: Hypertension, congestive heart failure.
Digestive: Vomiting, jaundice, melena, aphthous stomatitis, dry mouth and mucous membranes, bloody diarrhea, hepatitis, appetite change, pancreatitis with or without concomitant hepatitis. *colitis.*
Hemic and Lymphatic: Hemoglobin decrease, leukopenia, thrombocytopenia, hemolytic anemia *aplastic anemia, agranulocytosis,* purpura, *allergic purpura.*
Metabolic and Nutritional Disorders: Azotemia.
Nervous System: Insomnia, drowsiness, depression, diplopia, anxiety, irritability.
Respiratory: Epistaxis, asthma, laryngeal edema.
Skin and Appendages: Alopecia, urticaria, eczema, dermatitis, *bullous eruption, erythema multiforme major,* angioedema, *Stevens-Johnson syndrome.*
Special Senses: Blurred vision, taste disorder, reversible hearing loss, scotoma.
Urogenital: *Nephrotic syndrome,* proteinuria, *oliguria, interstital nephritis, papillary necrosis, acute renal failure.*
Incidence Less Than 1%—Causal Relationship Unknown (Adverse reactions reported only in worldwide postmarketing experience or in the literature, not seen in clinical trials, are considered rare and are italicized.)
Body as a Whole: Chest pain.
Cardiovascular: Palpitations, *flushing,* tachycardia, premature ventricular contractions, myocardial infarction.
Digestive: Esophageal lesions.
Hemic and Lymphatic: *Bruising.*
Metabolic and Nutritional Disorders: Hypoglycemia, *weight loss.*
Nervous System: Paresthesia, memory disturbance, nightmares, tremor, tic, *abnormal coordination,* convulsions, *disorientation, psychotic reaction.*
Respiratory: Dyspnea, hyperventilation, edema of pharynx.
Skin and Appendages: Excess perspiration, *exfoliative dermatitis.*
Special Senses: Vitreous floaters, night blindness, amblyopia.
Urogenital: Urinary frequency, nocturia, hematuria, impotence, vaginal bleeding.

OVERDOSAGE

Worldwide reports on overdosage with diclofenac cover 27 cases. In 10 of these 27 cases, diclofenac was the only drug taken; all of these patients recovered. The highest dose of diclofenac was 2.5 g in a 20-year-old male who suffered acute renal failure as a consequence, and who was treated with three dialysis sessions and recovered in 2 days. The next highest dose was 2.35 g in a 17-year-old girl who experienced vomiting and drowsiness. A dose of 2.0 g of diclofenac was taken by a woman of unspecified age who remained asymptomatic.

Animal LD$_{50}$'s show a wide range of susceptibilities to acute overdosage with primates being more resistant to acute toxicity than rodents (LD$_{50}$ in mg/kg—rats, 55; dogs, 500; monkeys, 3200).

In case of acute overdosage it is recommended that the stomach be emptied by vomiting or lavage. Forced diuresis may theoretically be beneficial because the drug is excreted in the urine. The effect of dialysis or hemoperfusion in the elimination of Voltaren (99% protein bound, see CLINICAL PHARMACOLOGY) remains unproven. In addition to supportive measures, the use of oral activated charcoal may help to reduce the absorption and reabsorption of Voltaren.

DOSAGE AND ADMINISTRATION

Voltaren may be administered as 25-mg, 50-mg, and 75-mg enteric-coated tablets. Patients should be generally maintained on the lowest dosage of Voltaren consistent with achieving a satisfactory therapeutic response.

In osteoarthritis, the recommended dosage is 100–150 mg/day in divided doses, 50 mg b.i.d. or t.i.d., or 75 mg b.i.d. Dosages above 150 mg/day have not been studied in patients with osteoarthritis.

In rheumatoid arthritis, the recommended dosage is 150–200 mg/day in divided doses, 50 mg t.i.d. or q.i.d., or 75 mg b.i.d. Dosages above 200 mg/day have not been studied in patients with rheumatoid arthritis.

In ankylosing spondylitis, the recommended dosage is 100–125 mg/day, administered as 25 mg q.i.d., with an extra

*Incidence, 3% to 9% (incidence of unmarked reactions is 1–3%)

25 mg dose at bedtime if necessary. Dosages above 125 mg/day have not been studied in patients with ankylosing spondylitis.

HOW SUPPLIED

Enteric-Coated Tablets 25 mg—yellow, round, biconvex with beveled edges (imprinted VOLTAREN 25)

    Bottles of 60...NDC 0028-0058-60

    Bottles of 100...NDC 0028-0058-01

    Unit Dose (blister pack)

        Box of 100 (strips of 10).....................NDC 0028-0058-61

Enteric-Coated Tablets 50 mg—light brown, round, biconvex with beveled edges (imprinted VOLTAREN 50)

    Bottles of 60...NDC 0028-0162-60

    Bottles of 100...NDC 0028-0162-01

    Bottles of 1000...NDC 0028-0162-10

    Unit Dose (blister pack)

        Box of 100 (strips of 10).....................NDC 0028-0162-61

Enteric-Coated Tablets 75 mg—white, round, biconvex with beveled edges (imprinted VOLTAREN 75)

    Bottles of 60...NDC 0028-0164-60

    Bottles of 100...NDC 0028-0164-01

    Bottles of 1000...NDC 0028-0164-10

    Unit Dose (blister pack)

        Box of 100 (strips of 10).....................NDC 0028-0164-61

Samples, when available, are identified by the word *SAMPLE* appearing on each enteric-coated tablet.

Do not store above 86°F (30°C). Protect from moisture.

Dispense in tight container (USP).

C92-29 (8/92)

Shown in Product Identification Section, page 410

GenDerm Corporation
**600 KNIGHTSBRIDGE PARKWAY
LINCOLNSHIRE, IL 60069**

OCCLUSAL®-HP   ℞

OCCLUSAL®   OTC

[ō-kloo′sal]

(Salicylic Acid USP)

Wart Remover

DESCRIPTION

Occlusal and Occlusal-HP are topical wart remover preparations containing 17% and 26% (w/w) Salicylic Acid USP, in a polyacrylic vehicle containing isopropyl alcohol, butyl acetate, polyvinyl butyral, dibutyl phthalate and acrylates copolymer. The pharmacologic activity of Occlusal and Occlusal-HP is generally attributed to the keratolytic action of Salicylic Acid. The structural formula of Salicylic Acid is:

CLINICAL PHARMACOLOGY

Although the exact mode of action of Salicylic Acid in the treatment of warts is not known, its activity appears to be associated with its keratolytic action which results in mechanical removal of epidermal cells infected with wart viruses.

INDICATIONS AND USAGE

Occlusal and Occlusal-HP are indicated for the treatment and removal of common warts and plantar warts. The common wart is easily recognized by the rough 'cauliflower-like' appearance of the surface. The plantar wart is recognized by its location only on the bottom of the foot, its tenderness, and the interruption of the footprint pattern.

WARNINGS

Occlusal and Occlusal-HP are for external use only. Occlusal and Occlusal-HP are flammable and should be kept away from fire or flame. Keep bottle tightly capped and store at room temperature away from heat when not in use.

Occlusal and Occlusal-HP should not be used on irritated skin, on any area that is infected or reddened, if you are a diabetic or if you have poor blood circulation. Occlusal and Occlusal-HP should not be used on moles, birthmarks, warts with hair growing from them, genital warts, or warts on the face or mucous membranes.

Do not permit Occlusal and Occlusal-HP to contact eyes or mucous membranes. If contact with eyes or mucous membranes occurs, immediately flush with water for 15 minutes. Occlusal and Occlusal-HP should not be allowed to contact normal skin surrounding wart. Treatment should be discontinued if excessive irritation occurs. If discomfort persists, see your doctor. Avoid inhaling vapors. Keep this and all drugs out of the reach of children.

ADVERSE REACTIONS

A localized irritant reaction may occur if Occlusal and Occlusal-HP are applied to the normal skin surrounding the wart. Any irritation may normally be controlled by temporarily discontinuing use of Occlusal and Occlusal-HP, and by applying the medication only to the wart site when treatment is resumed.

DIRECTIONS

Prior to application of Occlusal and Occlusal-HP, soak wart in warm water for five minutes. Remove any loosened tissue by rubbing with a brush, wash cloth, or emery board. Dry area thoroughly. Using the brush applicator supplied, apply twice to affected area, allowing the first application to dry before applying the second. Treatment should be once or twice (Occlusal-HP) a day and should continue as directed by physician. Be careful not to apply to surrounding skin.

OCCLUSAL: Clinically visible improvement will normally occur during the first 2 to 4 weeks. Maximum resolution may be expected after 6 to 12 weeks of drug use.

OCCLUSAL-HP: You should see improvement in 1 to 2 weeks. Maximum resolution may be expected after 4 to 6 weeks of daily Occlusal-HP use. If skin irritation develops or there is no improvement after several weeks, contact your physician.

HOW SUPPLIED

Occlusal in 15 mL bottles with brush applicator. (NDC 52761-121-15).

Occlusal-HP in 10 mL bottles with brush applicator (NDC 52761-135-10)

Store at controlled room temperature 15°–30°C (59°–86°F).

Occlusal-HP

Caution

Federal law prohibits dispensing without prescription.

PENTRAX®   OTC

[pen′trax]

Anti-dandruff Tar Shampoo

DESCRIPTION

Pentrax Tar Shampoo contains 7.71% Fractar® (equal to 4.3% coal tar), a standardized tar extract, a blend of highly concentrated detergents, and conditioning agents. Spectrophotometric standardization, based on hydrocarbon analysis, assures uniform therapeutic activity from batch to batch. Pentrax Tar Shampoo does not contain parabens or other preservatives. Pentrax Tar Shampoo contains the highest concentration of coal tar currently available. Fractar consists of the desirable crude coal tar fractions without undesirable residues. It has excellent lathering qualities and leaves hair clean and manageable.

ACTION AND INDICATIONS

Coal tar helps correct abnormalities of keratinization by decreasing epidermal proliferation and dermal infiltration. Pentrax Tar Shampoo is indicated for relief of itching, irritation, redness, flaking and/or scaling associated with dandruff, seborrheic dermatitis and psoriasis.

WARNINGS

FOR EXTERNAL USE ONLY. Avoid contact with the eyes —if this happens, rinse thoroughly with water. Do not use for prolonged periods without consulting a physician. If condition worsens or does not improve after regular use of this product as directed, consult a physician. Keep this and all drugs out of the reach of children.

DIRECTIONS

Massage into wet hair and scalp. Rinse. Reapply liberally allowing lather to remain on hair up to 10 minutes. Rinse thoroughly. For best results, use at least twice a week or as directed by a physician.

ACTIVE INGREDIENTS

Fractar®, a patented extract of coal tar, equivalent to coal tar 4.3%.

INACTIVE INGREDIENTS

Cocamide DEA, Diocty1 Sodium Sulfosuccinate, Lauramide Oxide, Laureth-23, PEG-8, Sodium Lauryl Sulfate.

HOW SUPPLIED

4 fl oz plastic bottle (NDC 52761-665-04)

8 fl oz plastic bottle (NDC 52761-665-08)

PRAMEGEL®   OTC

[pram′eh-gel]

Antipruritic

DESCRIPTION

PrameGel is an antipruritic containing pramoxine hydrochloride USP 1% and menthol USP 0.5% in a water soluble emollient base with a naturally derived humectant. PrameGel is propylene glycol, paraben and fragrance free.

INDICATIONS

PrameGel provides prompt temporary relief of itching associated with mild eczemas (including poison ivy and poison oak), insect bites, heat rash, sunburn, and other pruritic skin conditions, as well as for external anal itching.

WARNINGS

FOR EXTERNAL USE ONLY. Avoid contact with the eyes. If itching worsens or if symptoms persist for more than 7 days, discontinue use of this product and consult a physician. Stinging and burning may occur if applied to broken skin. Keep this and all drugs out of the reach of children.

DIRECTIONS

Adults and children 2 years of age and older: Apply PrameGel liberally to affected area no more than 3–4 times daily. Children under 2 years of age: Consult a physician.

ACTIVE INGREDIENTS

Pramoxine Hydrochloride 1% and Menthol 0.5%.

INACTIVE INCREGIENTS

Benzyl Alcohol, Carbomer 940, Methyl Gluceth-20, SD Alcohol 40, Sodium Hydroxide and Water.

HOW SUPPLIED

4 fl oz plastic bottle (NDC 52761-395-04).

SALAC®   OTC

[sal′ak]

Acne Medication Cleanser

DESCRIPTION

SalAc is an acne medication cleanser containing 2% salicylic acid USP in a surfactant blend especially formulated to remove excess sebum.

INDICATIONS

For the management of acne. Helps prevent new comedones (blackheads and whiteheads), papules, and pustules (acne pimples).

WARNINGS

For External Use Only. Using other topical acne medication at the same time or immediately following use of this product may increase dryness or irritation of skin. If this occurs, only one medication should be used unless directed by a physician.

Keep Cleanser Out of Eyes. Keep This and All Drugs Out of Reach of Children. If undue skin irritation develops or increases, adjust usage schedule or consult your physician.

DIRECTIONS

Wash affected area 2 to 3 times daily. Lather with warm water, massage into skin, rinse, and dry.

ACTIVE INGREDIENTS

Salicylic Acid USP 2%

INACTIVE INGREDIENTS

Benzyl Alcohol, Lauramide DEA, PEG-7 Glyceryl Cocoate, Polystyrene Dispersion, Purified Water, Sodium C_{14-16} Olefin Sulfonate and Sodium Chloride.

HOW SUPPLIED

6 fl oz plastic bottle (NDC 52761-077-06).

ZOSTRIX®   OTC

(Capsaicin 0.025%)

ZOSTRIX-®HP

High Potency

(Capsaicin 0.075%)

Formerly Axsain®

TOPICAL ANALGESIC CREAM

PRODUCT OVERVIEW

KEY FACTS

Zostrix/Zostrix-HP contain capsaicin which works via localized depletion of substance P, an endogenous neuropeptide involved in the transmission of pain impulses.

MAJOR USES

Zostrix/Zostrix-HP have proven to be clinically effective in controlling pain from rheumatoid arthritis, osteoarthritis, neuralgias such as the pain following shingles (herpes zoster) and painful diabetic neuropathy. Zostrix/Zostrix-HP are applied to the skin only after the zoster lesions have healed.

SAFETY INFORMATION

Patients may experience a warm, stinging, or burning sensation at the site of application, especially during the initial few days of use. This effect is related to the pharmacologic

Continued on next page

GenDerm—Cont.

action of capsaicin. Avoid contact with eyes or broken (open) or irritated skin.

PRESCRIBING INFORMATION

ZOSTRIX®
(Capsaicin 0.025%
ZOSTRIX®-HP
High Potency
(Capsaicin 0.075)
Formerly Axsain®
TOPICAL ANALGESIC CREAM

DESCRIPTION

Zostrix/Zostrix-HP contain capsaicin in an emollient base containing benzyl alcohol, cetyl alcohol, glyceryl monostearate, isopropyl myristate, PEG-100 stearate, purified water, sorbitol solution and white petrolatum. Capsaicin is a naturally occurring substance derived from plants of the Solanaceae family with the chemical name trans-8-methyl-N-vanillyl-6-nonenamide. Capsaicin is a white crystalline powder with a molecular weight of 305.4. It is practically insoluble in water but very soluble in alcohol, ether, and chloroform.

ACTION

Although the precise mechanism of action of capsaicin is not fully understood, current evidence suggests that capsaicin renders skin and joints insensitive to pain by depleting and preventing reaccumulation of substance P in peripheral sensory neurons. Substance P is thought to be the principal chemomediator of pain impulses from the periphery to the central nervous system. In addition, substance P has been shown to be released into joint tissues and activate inflammatory mediators involved with the pathogenesis of rheumatoid arthritis.

INDICATIONS

Zostrix/Zostrix-HP are indicated for the temporary relief of pain from rheumatoid arthritis, osteoarthritis and relief of neuralgias such as the pain following shingles (herpes zoster) or painful diabetic neuropathy.

WARNINGS

FOR EXTERNAL USE ONLY. Avoid contact with eyes and broken (open) or irritated skin. Do not bandage tightly. If condition worsens, or does not improve after 28 days, discontinue use of this product and consult your physician. **Keep this and all drugs out of the reach of children. In case of accidental ingestion, seek professional assistance or contact a Poison Control Center immediately.**

DIRECTIONS

Adults and children 2 years of age or older: Apply Zostrix/Zostrix-HP to affected area 3 to 4 times daily. Transient burning may occur upon application but generally disappears in several days. Application schedules of less than 3 to 4 times a day may not provide optimum pain relief and the burning sensation may persist. **Wash hands if possible after applying Zostrix/Zostrix-HP avoiding areas where drug was applied.**

HOW SUPPLIED

Zostrix
0.7 oz (20 g) tube (NDC 52761-552-20)
1.5 ox tube (NDC 52761-552-45)
3.0 oz tube (NDC 52761-552-85)
Zostrix-HP
1.0 oz tube (NDC 52761-501-30)
2.0 oz tube (NDC 52761-501-60)
Store at room temperature. 15°-30°C (59°-86°F).
U.S. Patents No. 4486450, 4536404

Genentech, Inc.

460 POINT SAN BRUNO BLVD.
SOUTH SAN FRANCISCO, CA 94080

ACTIMMUNE® ℞
(Interferon gamma-1b)
Injection

DESCRIPTION

ACTIMMUNE® (Interferon gamma-1b), a biologic response modifier, is a single-chain polypeptide containing 140 amino acids. Production of ACTIMMUNE is achieved by fermentation of a genetically engineered *Escherichia coli* bacterium containing the DNA which encodes for the human protein. Purification of the product is achieved by conventional column chromatography. ACTIMMUNE is a highly purified sterile solution consisting of non-covalent dimers of two identical 16,465 dalton monomers; with a specific activity of 30 million U/mg.

ACTIMMUNE (Interferon gamma-1b) is a sterile, clear, colorless solution filled in a single-dose vial for subcutaneous injection. Each 0.5 mL of ACTIMMUNE contains: **100 mcg (3 million U)** of Interferon gamma-1b formulated in 20 mg mannitol, 0.36 mg sodium succinate, 0.05 mg polysorbate 20 and Sterile Water for Injection.

CLINICAL PHARMACOLOGY

General

Interferons are a family of functionally related, species-specific proteins synthesized by eukaryotic cells in response to viruses and a variety of natural and synthetic stimuli. The most striking differences between interferon-gamma and other classes of interferon concern the immunomodulatory properties of this molecule. While gamma, alpha and beta interferons share certain properties, interferon-gamma has potent phagocyte-activating effects not seen with other interferon preparations. These effects include the generation of toxic oxygen metabolites within phagocytes, which are capable of mediating the killing of microorganisms such as *Staphylococcus aureus, Toxoplasma gondii, Leishmania donovani, Listeria monocytogenes,* and *Mycobacterium avium intracellulare.*

Clinical studies in patients using interferon-gamma have revealed a broad range of biological activities including the enhancement of the oxidative metabolism of tissue macrophages, enhancement of antibody-dependent cellular cytotoxicity (ADCC) and natural killer (NK) cell activity. Additionally, effects on Fc receptor expression on monocytes and major histocompatibility antigen expression have been noted.[1,2]

To the extent that interferon-gamma is produced by antigen-stimulated T lymphocytes and regulates the activity of immune cells, it is appropriate to characterize interferon-gamma as a lymphokine of the interleukin type. There is growing evidence that interferon-gamma interacts functionally with other interleukin molecules such as interleukin-2 and that all of the interleukins form part of a complex, lymphokine regulatory network.[3] For example, interferon-gamma and interleukin-4 appear to reciprocally interact to regulate murine lgE levels; interferon-gamma can suppress lgE levels in humans.[4,5] Interferon-gamma also inhibits the production of collagen at the transcription level in human systems.[6]

More specifically, with respect to Chronic Granulomatous Disease (an inherited disorder characterized by deficient phagocyte oxidative metabolism), pilot clinical trials of the systemic administration of ACTIMMUNE in patients with Chronic Granulomatous Disease were initiated which provided evidence for a treatment-related enhancement of phagocyte function including elevation of superoxide levels and improved killing of *Staphylococcus aureus.*[7,8] Based on this evidence, a randomized, double-blind, placebo-controlled clinical study was initiated to further delineate the effects of ACTIMMUNE in Chronic Granulomatous Disease.

Pharmacokinetics

The intravenous, intramuscular, and subcutaneous pharmacokinetics of ACTIMMUNE have been investigated in 24 healthy male subjects following single-dose administration of 100 mcg/m^2. ACTIMMUNE is rapidly cleared after intravenous administration (1.4 liters/minute) and slowly absorbed after intramuscular or subcutaneous injection. After intramuscular or subcutaneous injection, the apparent fraction of dose absorbed was greater than 89%. The mean elimination half-life after intravenous administration of 100 mcg/m^2 in healthy male subjects was 38 minutes. The mean elimination half-lives for intramuscular and subcutaneous dosing with 100 mcg/m^2 were 2.9 and 5.9 hours, respectively. Peak plasma concentrations, determined by ELISA, occurred approximately 4 hours (1.5 ng/mL) after intramuscular dosing and 7 hours (0.6 ng/mL) after subcutaneous dosing. Multiple dose subcutaneous pharmacokinetic studies were conducted in 38 healthy male subjects. There was no accumulation of ACTIMMUNE after 12 consecutive daily injections of 100 mcg/m^2. Pharmacokinetic studies in patients with Chronic Granulomatous Disease have not been performed.

Excretion studies of ACTIMMUNE have been performed. Trace amounts of interferon-gamma were detected in the urine of squirrel monkeys following intravenous administration of 500 mcg/kg. Interferon-gamma was not detected in the urine of healthy human volunteers following administration of 100 mcg/m^2 of ACTIMMUNE by the intravenous, intramuscular and subcutaneous routes. *In vitro* perfusion studies utilizing rabbit livers and kidneys demonstrate that these organs are capable of clearing interferon-gamma from perfusate. Studies of the administration of interferon-gamma to nephrectomized mice and squirrel monkeys demonstrate a reduction in clearance of interferon-gamma from blood; however, prior nephrectomy did not prevent elimination.

Effects of Chronic Granulomatous Disease

A randomized, double-blind, placebo-controlled study of ACTIMMUNE in patients with Chronic Granulomatous Disease, was performed to determine whether ACTIMMUNE administered subcutaneously on a three times weekly schedule could decrease the incidence of serious infectious episodes and improve existing infectious and inflammatory conditions in patients with Chronic Granulomatous Disease. One hundred twenty-eight eligible patients were enrolled on this study including patients with different patterns of inheritance. Most patients received prophylactic antibiotics. Patients ranged in age from 1 to 44 years with the mean age being 14.6 years. The study was terminated early following demonstration of a highly statistically significant benefit of ACTIMMUNE® (Interferon gamma-1b) therapy compared to placebo with respect to time to serious infection (p=0.0036), the primary endpoint of the investigation. Serious infection was defined as a clinical event requiring hospitalization and the use of parenteral antibiotics. The final analysis provided further support for the primary endpoint (p=0.0006). There was a 67 percent reduction in relative risk of serious infection in patients receiving ACTIMMUNE (n=63) compared to placebo (n=65). Additional supportive evidence of treatment benefit included a twofold reduction in the number of primary serious infections in the ACTIMMUNE group (30 on placebo versus 14 on ACTIMMUNE, p=0.002) and the total number and rate of serious infections including recurrent events (56 on placebo versus 20 on ACTIMMUNE, p= <0.0001). Moreover, the length of hospitalization for the treatment of all clinical events provided evidence highly supportive of an ACTIMMUNE treatment benefit. Placebo patients required three times as many inpatient hospitalization days for treatment of clinical events compared to patients receiving ACTIMMUNE (1493 versus 497 total days, p=0.02). An ACTIMMUNE treatment benefit with respect to time to serious infection was consistently demonstrated in all subgroup analyses according to stratification factors, including pattern of inheritance, use of prophylactic antibiotics, as well as age. There was a 67 percent reduction in relative risk of serious infection in patients receiving ACTIMMUNE compared to placebo across all groups. The beneficial effect of ACTIMMUNE therapy was observed throughout the entire study, in which the mean duration of ACTIMMUNE administration was 8.9 months/patient.

INDICATIONS AND USAGE

ACTIMMUNE is indicated for reducing the frequency and severity of serious infections associated with Chronic Granulomatous Disease. The safety and effectiveness in children under the age of 1 year has not been established.

CONTRAINDICATIONS

ACTIMMUNE is contraindicated in patients who develop or have known hypersensitivity to interferon-gamma, *E. coli* derived products, or any component of the product.

WARNINGS

ACTIMMUNE should be used with caution in patients with pre-existing cardiac disease, including symptoms of ischemia, congestive heart failure or arrhythmia. No direct cardiotoxic effect has been demonstrated but it is possible that acute and transient "flu-like" or constitutional symptoms such as fever and chills frequently associated with ACTIMMUNE administration at doses of 250 mcg/m^2/day or higher may exacerbate pre-existing cardiac conditions.

Caution should be exercised when treating patients with known seizure disorders and or compromised central nervous system function. Central nervous system adverse reactions including decreased mental status, gait disturbance and dizziness have been observed, particularly in patients receiving doses greater than 250 mcg/m^2/day. Most of these abnormalities were mild and reversible within a few days upon dose reduction or discontinuation of therapy.

Caution should be exercised when administering ACTIMMUNE to patients with myelosuppression. Reversible neutropenia and elevation of hepatic enzymes can be dose limiting above 250mcg/m^2/day. Thrombocytopenia and proteinuria have also been seen rarely.

PRECAUTIONS

General

Acute serious hypersensitivity reactions have not been observed in patients receiving ACTIMMUNE; however, if such an acute reaction develops the drug should be discontinued immediately and appropriate medical therapy instituted. Transient cutaneous rashes have occurred in some patients following injection but have rarely necessitated treatment interruption.

Information for Patients

Patients being treated with ACTIMMUNE and/or their parents should be informed regarding the potential benefits and risks associated with treatment. If home use is determined to be desirable by the physician, instructions on appropriate use should be given, including review of the contents of the Patient Information Insert. This information is intended to aid in the safe and effective use of the medication. It is not a disclosure of all possible adverse or intended effects.

If home use is prescribed, a puncture resistant container for the disposal of used syringes and needles should be supplied to the patient. Patients should be thoroughly instructed in the importance of proper disposal and cautioned against any reuse of needles and syringes. The full container should be

disposed of according to the directions provided by the physician (see Patient Information Insert).

The most common adverse experiences occurring with ACTIMMUNE therapy are "flu-like" or constitutional symptoms such as fever, headache, chills, myalgia or fatigue (see ADVERSE REACTIONS Section) which may decrease in severity as treatment continues. Some of the "flu-like" symptoms may be minimized by bedtime administration. Acetaminophen may be used to prevent or partially alleviate the fever and headache.

The long-term effects of ACTIMMUNE therapy on growth, development or other parameters, are not known.

Laboratory Tests

In addition to those tests normally required for monitoring patients with Chronic Granulomatous Disease, the following laboratory tests are recommended for all patients on ACTIMMUNE therapy prior to the beginning of and at three month intervals during treatment.

- Hematologic tests—including complete blood counts, differential and platelet counts.
- Blood chemistries—including renal and liver function tests.
- Urinalysis.

Drug Interactions

Interactions between ACTIMMUNE® (Interferon gamma-1b) and other drugs have not been fully evaluated. Caution should be exercised when administering ACTIMMUNE in combination with other potentially myelosuppressive agents (see WARNINGS).

Preclinical studies in rodents using species-specific interferon-gamma have demonstrated a decrease in hepatic microsomal cytochrome P-450 concentrations. This could potentially lead to a depression of the hepatic metabolism of certain drugs that utilize this degradative pathway.

Carcinogenesis, Mutagenesis, and Impairment of Fertility

Carcinogenesis: ACTIMMUNE has not been tested for its carcinogenic potential.

Mutagenesis: Ames tests using five different tester strains of bacteria with and without metabolic activation revealed no evidence of mutagenic potential. ACTIMMUNE was tested in a micronucleus assay for its ability to induce chromosomal damage in bone marrow cells of mice following two intravenous doses of 20 mg/kg. No evidence of chromosomal damage was noted.

Impairment of Fertility: Female cynomolgus monkeys treated with daily subcutaneous doses of 150 mcg/kg ACTIMMUNE (approximately 100 times the human dose) exhibited irregular menstrual cycles or absence of cyclicity during treatment. Similar findings were not observed in animals treated with 3 or 30 mcg/kg ACTIMMUNE. No studies have been performed assessing any potential effects of ACTIMMUNE on male fertility.

Pregnancy

Teratogenic Effects: Pregnancy Category C. ACTIMMUNE has shown an increased incidence of abortions in primates when given in doses approximately 100 × the human dose. A study in pregnant primates treated with intravenous doses 2-100 × the human dose failed to demonstrate teratogenic activity for ACTIMMUNE. There are no adequate and well-controlled studies in pregnant women. ACTIMMUNE should be used during pregnancy only if the potential benefit justifies the potential risk to the fetus. In addition, studies evaluating recombinant murine interferon-gamma in pregnant mice, revealed increased incidences of uterine bleeding and abortifacient activity and decreased neonatal viability at maternally toxic doses. The clinical significance of this latter observation with recombinant murine interferon-gamma tested in a homologus system is uncertain.

Nursing Mothers

It is not known whether ACTIMMUNE is excreted in human milk. Because many drugs are excreted in human milk and because of the potential for serious adverse reactions in nursing infants from ACTIMMUNE, a decision should be made whether to discontinue nursing or to discontinue the drug, dependent upon the importance of the drug to the mother.

Pediatric Use

Safety and effectiveness in children under the age of 1 year has not been established.

ADVERSE REACTIONS

The following data on adverse reactions are based on the subcutaneous administration of ACTIMMUNE at a dose of 50 mcg/m², three times weekly, in 63 patients with Chronic Granulomatous Disease during an investigational trial in the United States and Europe. Sixty-five additional patients with Chronic Granulomatous Disease received placebo on this study. The following table represents the percentage of patients experiencing common adverse reactions observed on this study. [See table at top of next column.]

Miscellaneous adverse events which occurred infrequently and may have been related to underlying disease included back pain (2 percent versus 0 percent), abdominal pain (8 percent versus 3 percent) and depression (3 percent versus 0 percent) for ACTIMMUNE and placebo treated patients, respectively.

Clinical Toxicity	Percent of Patients ACTIMMUNE	Placebo
Fever	52	28
Headache	33	9
Rash	17	6
Chills	14	0
Injection site erythema or tenderness	14	2
Fatigue	14	11
Diarrhea	14	12
Vomiting	13	5
Nausea	10	2
Weight loss	6	6
Myalgia	6	0
Anorexia	3	5
Arthralgia	2	0
Injection site pain	0	2

ACTIMMUNE has also been evaluated in additional disease states in studies in which patients have generally received higher doses (> 100 mcg/m²/day) administered by intramuscular injection or intravenous infusion. All of the previously described adverse reactions which occurred in patients with Chronic Granulomatous Disease have also been observed in patients receiving higher doses. Adverse reactions not observed in patients with Chronic Granulomatous Disease receiving doses less than 100 mcg/m²/day but seen rarely in patients receiving ACTIMMUNE in other studies include: *Cardiovascular* —hypotension, syncope, tachyarrhythmia, heart block, heart failure, and myocardial infarction. *Central Nervous System* —confusion, disorientation, gait disturbance, Parkinsonian symptoms, seizure, hallucinations, and transient ischemic attacks. *Gastrointestinal* —hepatic insufficiency, gastrointestinal bleeding, and pancreatitis. *Renal* —reversible renal insufficiency. *Hematologic* —deep venous thrombosis and pulmonary embolism. *Pulmonary* —tachypnea, bronchospasm, and interstitial pneumonitis. *Metabolic* —hyponatremia and hyperglycemia. *Other* —exacerbation of dermatomyositis.

Abnormal Laboratory Test Values: No statistically significant differences between the ACTIMMUNE® (Interferon gamma-1b) and placebo treatment groups were observed with regard to effect of treatment on hematologic, coagulation, hepatic and renal laboratory studies.

No neutralizing antibodies to ACTIMMUNE have been detected in any Chronic Granulomatous Disease patient receiving ACTIMMUNE.

DOSAGE AND ADMINISTRATION

The recommended dosage of ACTIMMUNE (Interferon gamma-1b) for the treatment of patients with Chronic Granulomatous Disease is 50 mcg/m² (1.5 million U/m²) for patients whose body surface area is greater than 0.5m² and 1.5 mcg/kg/dose for patients whose body surface area is equal to or less than 0.5 m². Injections should be administered subcutaneously three times weekly (for example, Monday, Wednesday, Friday). The optimum sites of injection are the right and left deltoid and anterior thigh. ACTIMMUNE can be administered by a physician, nurse, family member or patient when trained in the administration of subcutaneous injections. Parenteral drug products should be inspected visually for particulate matter and discoloration prior to administration, whenever solution and container permit.

The formulation does not contain a preservative. A vial of ACTIMMUNE is suitable for a single dose only. The unused portion of any vial should be discarded.

Higher doses are not recommended. Safety and efficacy has not been established for ACTIMMUNE given in doses greater or less than the recommended dose of 50 mcg/m². The minimum effective dose of ACTIMMUNE has not been established.

If severe reactions occur, the dosage should be modified (50 percent reduction) or therapy should be discontinued until the adverse reaction abates.

ACTIMMUNE (Interferon gamma-1b) may be administered using either sterilized glass or plastic disposable syringes.

HOW SUPPLIED

ACTIMMUNE® (Interferon gamma-1b) is a sterile, clear, colorless solution filled in a single-dose vial for subcutaneous injection. Each 0.5 mL of ACTIMMUNE contains: **100 mcg (3 million U)** of Interferon gamma-1b, formulated in 20 mg

mannitol, 0.36 mg sodium succinate, 0.05 mg polysorbate 20 and Sterile Water for Injection.

Single vial (NDC 50242-052-14)

Cartons of 12 (NDC 50242-052-23)

Stability and Storage

Vials of ACTIMMUNE (Interferon gamma-1b) must be placed in a 2–8°C (36–46°F) refrigerator immediately upon receipt to insure optimal retention of physical and biochemical integrity. DO NOT FREEZE. Avoid excessive or vigorous agitation. DO NOT SHAKE. An unentered vial of ACTIMMUNE should not be left at room temperature for a total time exceeding 12 hours prior to use. Vials exceeding this time period should not be returned to the refrigerator; such vials should be discarded.

Do not use beyond the expiration date stamped on the vial.

REFERENCES

1. Maluish AE, Urba WJ, Longo DL, *et al:* The determination of an immunologically active dose of interferon gamma in patients with melanoma. J Clin Onc *6:* 434–445, 1988.
2. Nathan CF, Kaplan G, Levis W, *et al:* Local and systemic effects of intradermal recombinant interferon gamma in patients with lepromatous leprosy. NEJM *315:* 6–11, 1986.
3. Fauci AS, Rosenberg SA, Sherwin SA, *et al:* Immunomodulators in clinical medicine. Ann Internal Med. *106:* 421–433, 1987.
4. Snapper CM, Paul WE: Interferon-gamma and B cell stimulatory factor-1 reciprocally regulate Ig isotype production. Science *236:* 944–947, 1987.
5. King CL, Gallin JI, Malech HL, *et al:* Regulation of immunoglobulin production in hyperimmunoglobulin E recurrent-infection syndrome by interferon gamma. PNAS USA *86:* 10085–10089, 1989.
6. Rosenbloom J, Feldman G, Freundlich B, Jimenez SA: Inhibition of excessive scleroderma fibroblast collagen production by recombinant gamma-interferon. Arth Rheum *29:* 851–856, 1986.
7. Ezekowitz RAB, Dinauer MC, Jaffe HS, *et al:* Partial correction of the phagocyte defect in patients with X-linked chronic granulomatous disease by subcutaneous interferon gamma. NEJM *319:* 146–151, 1988.
8. Sechler JMG, Malech HL, White CJ, Gallin JI: Recombinant human interferon-gamma reconstitutes defective phagocyte function in patients with chronic granulomatous disease of childhood. PNAS USA *85:* 4874–4878, 1988.

ACTIMMUNE®
(Interferon gamma-1b)
Injection
Manufactured by

GENENTECH, INC.   G48026-RO
460 Point San Bruno Blvd.   December, 1990
South San Francisco, CA 94080   ©1990 Genentech, Inc.
Shown in Product Identification Section, page 410

ACTIVASE®   ℞
Alteplase
recombinant

DESCRIPTION

Activase®, Alteplase, is a tissue plasminogen activator produced by recombinant DNA technology. It is a sterile, purified glycoprotein of 527 amino acids. It is synthesized using the complementary DNA (cDNA) for natural human tissue-type plasminogen activator obtained from a human melanoma cell line. The manufacturing process involves the secretion of the enzyme, alteplase, into the culture medium by an established mammalian cell line (Chinese Hamster Ovary cells) into which the cDNA for alteplase has been genetically inserted.

Phosphoric acid and/or sodium hydroxide may be used prior to lyophilization for pH adjustment.

Activase® is a sterile, white to off-white, lyophilized powder for intravenous administration after reconstitution with Sterile Water for Injection, USP.

[See table below.]

Biological potency is determined by an *in vitro* clot lysis assay and is expressed in International Units as tested against the WHO standard. The specific activity of Activase® is 580,000 IU/mg.

Quantitative Composition of the Lyophilized Product			
	100 mg Vial	50 mg Vial	20 mg Vial
Alteplase	100 mg (58 million IU)	50 mg (29 million IU)	20 mg (11.6 million IU)
L-Arginine	3.5 g	1.7 g	0.7 g
Phosphoric Acid	1 g	0.5 g	0.2 g
Polysorbate 80	less than 11 mg	less than 4 mg	less than 1.6 mg
Vacuum	No	Yes	Yes

Continued on next page

Genentech—Cont.

CLINICAL PHARMACOLOGY

Activase® is an enzyme (serine protease) which has the property of fibrin-enhanced conversion of plasminogen to plasmin. It produces limited conversion of plasminogen in the absence of fibrin. When introduced into the systemic circulation at pharmacologic concentration, Activase® binds to fibrin in a thrombus and converts the entrapped plasminogen to plasmin. This initiates local fibrinolysis with limited systemic proteolysis. Following administration of 100 mg Activase®, there is a decrease (16–36%) in circulating fibrinogen.[1,2] In a controlled trial, 8 of 73 patients (11%) receiving Activase® (1.25 mg/kg body weight over 3 hours) experienced a decrease in fibrinogen to below 100 mg/dL.[2]

Activase® is cleared rapidly from circulating plasma at a rate of 550–680 mL/min. Activase® is cleared primarily by the liver. More than 50% of Activase® present in plasma is cleared within 5 minutes after the infusion has been terminated, and approximately 80% is cleared within 10 minutes.

Coronary occlusion due to a thrombus is present in the infarct-related coronary artery in approximately 80% of patients experiencing a transmural myocardial infarction evaluated within four hours of onset of symptoms.[3,4]

In patients studied in a controlled trial with coronary angiography at 90 and 120 minutes following infusion of Activase®, infarct artery patency was observed in 71% and 85% of patients (n=85), respectively.[2] In a second study, where patients received coronary angiography prior to and following infusion of Activase® within six hours of the onset of symptoms, reperfusion of the obstructed vessel occurred within 90 minutes after the commencement of therapy in 71% of 83 patients.[1]

In a double-blind, randomized trial (138 patients) comparing Activase® to placebo, patients infused with Activase® within 4 hours of onset of symptoms experienced improved left ventricular function at day 10 compared to the placebo group, when ejection fraction was measured by gated blood pool scan (53.2% versus 46.4%, $p=0.018$). Relative to baseline (day 1) values, the net changes in ejection fraction were +3.6% and −4.7% for the treated and placebo group, respectively ($p=0.0001$). Also documented was a reduced incidence of clinical congestive heart failure in the treated group (14%) compared to the placebo group (33%) ($p=0.009$).[5]

In a second double-blind, randomized trial (145 patients) comparing Activase® to placebo, patients infused with Activase® within 2.5 hours of onset of symptoms experienced improved left ventricular function at a mean of 21 days compared to the placebo group, when ejection fraction was measured by gated blood pool scan (52% versus 48%, $p=0.08$) and by contrast ventriculogram (61% versus 54%, $p=0.006$). Although the contribution of Activase® alone is unclear, the incidence of nonischemic cardiac complications when taken as a group (i.e., congestive heart failure, pericarditis, atrial fibrillation, conduction disturbance) was reduced when compared to those patients treated with placebo ($p<0.01$).[6]

In a double-blind, randomized trial (5013 patients) comparing Activase® to placebo (ASSET study), patients infused with Activase® within five hours of the onset of symptoms of acute myocardial infarction experienced improved 30-day survival compared to those treated with placebo. At one month the overall mortality rates were 7.2% for the Activase® treated group and 9.8% for the placebo treated group ($p=0.001$).[7,8] This benefit was maintained at 6 months for Activase® treated patients (10.4%) compared to those treated with placebo (13.1%) ($p=0.008$).[8]

In a second double-blind, randomized trial (721 patients) comparing Activase® to placebo, patients infused with Activase® within five hours of the onset of symptoms experienced improved ventricular function 10–22 days after treatment compared to the placebo group, when global ejection fraction was measured by contrast ventriculography (50.7% versus 48.5%, $p=0.01$). Patients treated with Activase® had a 19% reduction in infarct size, as measured by cumulative release of HBDH (α-hydroxybutyrate dehydrogenase) activity compared to placebo treated patients ($p=0.001$). Patients treated with Activase® had significantly fewer episodes of cardiogenic shock ($p=0.02$), ventricular fibrillation ($p<0.04$) and pericarditis ($p=0.01$) compared to patients treated with placebo. Mortality at 21 days in Activase® treated patients was reduced to 3.7% compared to 6.3% in placebo treated patients (1p=0.05).[9] Although these data do not demonstrate unequivocally a significant reduction in mortality for this study, they do indicate a trend that is supported by the results of the ASSET study.

In a comparative randomized trial (n=45),[10] 59% of patients (n=22) treated with Activase® (100 mg over two hours) experienced moderate or marked lysis of pulmonary emboli when assessed by pulmonary angiography two hours after treatment initiation. Activase®-treated patients also experienced a significant reduction in pulmonary embolism-induced pulmonary hypertension within two hours of treatment ($p=0.003$). Pulmonary perfusion at 24 hours, as assessed by radionuclide scan, was significantly improved ($p=0.002$).

INDICATIONS AND USAGE

Acute Myocardial Infarction

Activase® is indicated for use in the management of acute myocardial infarction (AMI) in adults for the lysis of thrombi obstructing coronary arteries, the reduction of infarct size, the improvement of ventricular function following AMI, the reduction of the incidence of congestive heart failure and the reduction of mortality associated with AMI. Treatment should be initiated as soon as possible after the onset of AMI symptoms (see CLINICAL PHARMACOLOGY).

Pulmonary Embolism

Activase® is indicated in the management of acute massive pulmonary embolism (PE) in adults:

for the lysis of acute pulmonary emboli, defined as obstruction of blood flow to a lobe or multiple segments of the lungs, and

for the lysis of pulmonary emboli accompanied by unstable hemodynamics, e.g., failure to maintain blood pressure without supportive measures.

The diagnosis should be confirmed by objective means, such as pulmonary angiography or noninvasive procedures such as lung scanning.

CONTRAINDICATIONS

Because thrombolytic therapy increases the risk of bleeding, Activase® is contraindicated in the following situations:

- **Active internal bleeding**
- **History of cerebrovascular accident**
- **Recent (within two months) intracranial or intraspinal surgery or trauma (see WARNINGS)**
- **Intracranial neoplasm, arteriovenous malformation, or aneurysm**
- **Known bleeding diathesis**
- **Severe uncontrolled hypertension**

WARNINGS

Bleeding

The most common complication encountered during Activase® therapy is bleeding. The type of bleeding associated with thrombolytic therapy can be divided into two broad categories:

- Internal bleeding, involving the gastrointestinal tract, genitourinary tract, retroperitoneal or intracranial sites.
- Superficial or surface bleeding, observed mainly at invaded or disturbed sites (e.g., venous cutdowns, arterial punctures, sites of recent surgical intervention).

The concomitant use of heparin anticoagulation may contribute to bleeding. Some of the hemorrhagic episodes occurred one or more days after the effects of Activase® had dissipated, but while heparin therapy was continuing.

As fibrin is lysed during Activase® therapy, bleeding from recent puncture sites may occur. Therefore, thrombolytic therapy requires careful attention to all potential bleeding sites (including catheter insertion sites, arterial and venous puncture sites, cutdown sites and needle puncture sites).

Intramuscular injections and nonessential handling of the patient should be avoided during treatment with Activase®. Venipunctures should be performed carefully and only as required.

Should an arterial puncture be necessary during an infusion of Activase®, it is preferable to use an upper extremity vessel that is accessible to manual compression. Pressure should be applied for at least 30 minutes, a pressure dressing applied and the puncture site checked frequently for evidence of bleeding.

Should serious bleeding (not controllable by local pressure) occur, the infusion of Activase® and any concomitant heparin should be terminated immediately.

Each patient being considered for therapy with Activase® should be carefully evaluated and anticipated benefits weighed against potential risks associated with therapy.

In the following conditions, the risks of Activase® therapy may be increased and should be weighed against the anticipated benefits:

- Recent (within 10 days) major surgery, e.g., coronary artery bypass graft, obstetrical delivery, organ biopsy, previous puncture of noncompressible vessels
- Cerebrovascular disease
- Recent gastrointestinal or genitourinary bleeding (within 10 days)
- Recent trauma (within 10 days)
- Hypertension: systolic BP ≥ 180 mm Hg and/or diastolic BP ≥ 110 mm Hg
- High likelihood of left heart thrombus, e.g., mitral stenosis with atrial fibrillation
- Acute pericarditis
- Subacute bacterial endocarditis
- Hemostatic defects including those secondary to severe hepatic or renal disease
- Significant liver dysfunction
- Pregnancy
- Diabetic hemorrhagic retinopathy, or other hemorrhagic ophthalmic conditions
- Septic thrombophlebitis or occluded AV cannula at seriously infected site
- Advanced age, i.e., over 75 years old
- Patients currently receiving oral anticoagulants, e.g., warfarin sodium
- Any other condition in which bleeding constitutes a significant hazard or would be particularly difficult to manage because of its location

Arrhythmias

Coronary thrombolysis may result in arrhythmias associated with reperfusion. These arrhythmias (such as sinus bradycardia, accelerated idioventricular rhythm, ventricular premature depolarizations, ventricular tachycardia) are not different from those often seen in the ordinary course of acute myocardial infarction and may be managed with standard antiarrhythmic measures. It is recommended that antiarrhythmic therapy for bradycardia and/or ventricular irritability be available when infusions of Activase®, Alteplase, are administered.

Pulmonary Embolism

It should be recognized that the treatment of pulmonary embolism with Activase®, Alteplase, has not been shown to constitute adequate clinical treatment of underlying deep vein thrombosis. Furthermore, the possible risk of reembolization due to the lysis of underlying deep venous thrombi should be considered.

PRECAUTIONS

General

Standard management of myocardial infarction or pulmonary embolism should be implemented concomitantly with Activase® treatment. Noncompressible arterial puncture must be avoided (i.e., internal jugular and subclavian punctures should be avoided to minimize bleeding from noncompressible sites). Arterial and venous punctures should be minimized. In the event of serious bleeding, Activase® and heparin should be discontinued immediately. Heparin effects can be reversed by protamine.

Readministration

There is no experience with readministration of Activase®. If an anaphylactoid reaction occurs, the infusion should be discontinued immediately and appropriate therapy initiated.

Although sustained antibody formation in patients receiving one dose of Activase®, has not been documented, readministration should be undertaken with caution. Detectable levels of antibody (a single point measurement) were reported in one patient but subsequent antibody test results were negative.

Laboratory Tests

During Activase® therapy, if coagulation tests and/or measures of fibrinolytic activity are performed, the results may be unreliable unless specific precautions are taken to prevent *in vitro* artifacts. Activase® is an enzyme that when present in blood in pharmacologic concentrations remains active under *in vitro* conditions. This can lead to degradation of fibrinogen in blood samples removed for analysis. Collection of blood samples in the presence of aprotinin (150–200 units/mL) can to some extent mitigate this phenomenon.

Drug Interactions

The interaction of Activase® with other cardioactive drugs has not been studied. In addition to bleeding associated with heparin and vitamin K antagonists, drugs that alter platelet function (such as acetylsalicylic acid, dipyridamole) may increase the risk of bleeding if administered prior to, during or after Activase® therapy.

Use of Anticoagulants

Heparin has been administered concomitantly with and following infusions of Activase® to reduce the risk of rethrombosis. Because either heparin or Activase® alone may cause bleeding complications, careful monitoring for bleeding is advised, especially at arterial puncture sites.

Pregnancy (Category C)

Animal reproduction studies have not been conducted with Activase®. It is also not known whether Activase® can cause fetal harm when administered to a pregnant woman or can affect reproduction capacity. Activase® should be given to a pregnant woman only if clearly needed.

Pediatric Use

Safety and effectiveness of Activase® in children has not been established.

Carcinogenesis, Mutagenesis, Impairment of Fertility

Long-term studies in animals have not been performed to evaluate the carcinogenic potential or the effect on fertility. Short-term studies, which evaluated tumorigenicity of Activase® and effect on tumor metastases in rodents, were negative.

Studies to determine mutagenicity (Ames test) and chromosomal aberration assays in human lymphocytes were negative at all concentrations tested. Cytotoxicity, as reflected by a decrease in mitotic index, was evidenced only after pro-

longed exposure and only at the highest concentrations tested.

Nursing Mothers

It is not known whether Activase® is excreted in human milk. Because many drugs are excreted in human milk, caution should be exercised when Activase®, Alteplase, is administered to a nursing woman.

ADVERSE REACTIONS

Bleeding

The most frequent adverse reaction associated with Activase® is bleeding. The type of bleeding associated with thrombolytic therapy can be divided into two broad categories:
- Internal bleeding, involving the gastrointestinal tract, genitourinary tract, retroperitoneal or intracranial sites.
- Superficial or surface bleeding, observed mainly at invaded or disturbed sites (e.g., venous cutdowns, arterial punctures, sites of recent surgical intervention).

The following incidence of significant internal bleeding (estimated as > 250 cc blood loss) has been reported in studies in over 800 patients treated at all doses:

	Total Dose ≤ 100 mg	Total Dose > 100 mg
gastrointestinal	5%	5%
genitourinary	4%	4%
ecchymosis	1%	<1%
retroperitoneal	<1%	<1%
epistaxis	<1%	<1%
gingival	<1%	<1%

The incidence of intracranial bleeding (ICB) in patients treated with Activase® is as follows:

Dose	Number of Patients	%
100 mg	3272	0.4
150 mg	1779	1.3
1–1.4 mg/kg	237	0.4

These data indicate that a dose of 150 mg of Activase® should not be used because it has been associated with an increase in intracranial bleeding.

Recent data indicate that the incidence of stroke in 6 randomized double-blind placebo controlled trials[2,5-9,11] is not significantly different in the Activase® treated patients compared to those treated with placebo (37/3161, 1.2% versus 27/3092, 0.9%, respectively) (p=0.26).

Should serious bleeding in a critical location (intracranial, gastrointestinal, retroperitoneal, pericardial) occur, Activase® therapy should be discontinued immediately, along with any concomitant therapy with heparin.

Fibrin which is part of the hemostatic plug formed at needle puncture sites will be lysed during Activase® therapy. Therefore, Activase® therapy requires careful attention to potential bleeding sites, e.g., catheter insertion sites, arterial puncture sites.

Allergic Reactions

No serious or life-threatening allergic reactions have been reported. Other mild hypersensitivity reactions such as urticaria have been observed occasionally.

Other Adverse Reactions

Other adverse reactions have been reported, principally nausea and/or vomiting, hypotension, and fever. These reactions are frequent sequelae of myocardial infarction and may or may not be attributable to Activase® therapy.

DOSAGE AND ADMINISTRATION

Activase® is for intravenous administration only.

Acute Myocardial Infarction

Administer Activase® as soon as possible after the onset of symptoms.

The recommended dose is 100 mg administered as 60 mg (34.8 million IU) in the first hour (of which 6 to 10 mg is administered as a bolus over the first 1–2 minutes), 20 mg (11.6 million IU) over the second hour, and 20 mg (11.6 million IU) over the third hour. For smaller patients (less than 65 kg), a dose of 1.25 mg/kg administered over 3 hours, as described above, may be used.[12]

a. The bolus dose may be prepared in one of the following ways:
   1. By removing 6 to 10 mL from the vial of reconstituted (1 mg/mL) Activase® using a syringe and needle. If this method is used with the 20 mg or 50 mg vials, the syringe should not be primed with air and the needle should be inserted into the Activase® vial stopper. If the 100 mg vial is used, the needle should be inserted away from the puncture mark made by the transfer device.
   2. By removing 6 to 10 mL from a port (second injection site) on the infusion line after the infusion set is primed.
   3. By programming an infusion pump to deliver a 6 to 10 mL (1 mg/mL) bolus at the initiation of the infusion.

b. The remainder of the Activase® dose may be administered as follows:
   20 mg, 50 mg vials, administer using either a polyvinyl chloride bag or glass vial and infusion set
   100 mg vials, insert the spike end of an infusion set through the same puncture site created by the transfer device in the stopper of the vial of reconstituted

Activase®. Hang the Activase® vial from the plastic molded capping attached to the bottom of the vial.

Although the use of anticoagulants and antiplatelet drugs during and following administration of Activase® has not been shown to be of unequivocal benefit, heparin has been administered concomitantly for 24 hours or longer in more than 90% of patients. Aspirin and/or dipyridamole have been given either during and/or following heparin treatment.

Pulmonary Embolism

The recommended dose is 100 mg administered by intravenous infusion over two hours. Heparin therapy should be instituted or reinstituted near the end of or immediately following the Activase® infusion when the partial thromboplastin time or thrombin time returns to twice normal or less.

A DOSE OF 150 MG OF ACTIVASE®, ALTEPLASE, SHOULD NOT BE USED BECAUSE IT HAS BEEN ASSOCIATED WITH AN INCREASE IN INTRACRANIAL BLEEDING.

Reconstitution and Dilution

Activase® should be reconstituted by aseptically adding the appropriate volume of the accompanying Sterile Water for Injection, USP to the vial. It is important that Activase® be reconstituted only with Sterile Water for Injection, USP, without preservatives. Do not use Bacteriostatic Water for Injection, USP. The reconstituted preparation results in a colorless to pale yellow transparent solution containing Activase® 1 mg/mL at approximately pH 7.3. The osmolality of this solution is approximately 215 mOsm/kg.

Because Activase® contains no antibacterial preservatives, it should be reconstituted immediately before use. The solution may be used for intravenous administration within 8 hours following reconstitution when stored between 2–30°C (36–86°F). Before further dilution or administration, the product should be visually inspected for particulate matter and discoloration prior to administration whenever solution and container permit.

Activase® may be administered as reconstituted at 1 mg/mL. As an alternative, the reconstituted solution may be diluted further immediately before administration in an equal volume of 0.9% Sodium Chloride Injection, USP or 5% Dextrose Injection, USP to yield a concentration of 0.5 mg/mL. Either polyvinyl chloride bags or glass vials are acceptable. Activase® is stable for up to 8 hours in these solutions at room temperature. Exposure to light has no effect on the stability of these solutions. Excessive agitation during dilution should be avoided; mixing should be accomplished with gentle swirling and/or slow inversion. Do not use other infusion solutions, e.g., Sterile Water for Injection, USP or preservative-containing solutions for further dilution.

20 mg and 50 mg vials

Reconstitution should be carried out using a large bore needle (e.g., 18 gauge) and a syringe, directing the stream of Sterile Water for Injection, USP into the lyophilized cake. **DO NOT USE IF VACUUM IS NOT PRESENT.** Slight foaming upon reconstitution is not unusual; standing undisturbed for several minutes is usually sufficient to allow dissipation of any large bubbles.

No other medication should be added to infusion solutions containing Activase®, Alteplase. Any unused infusion solution should be discarded.

100 mg vials

Reconstitution should be carried out using the transfer device provided, adding the contents of the accompanying 100 mL vial of Sterile Water for Injection, USP to the contents of the 100 mg vial of Activase® powder. Slight foaming upon reconstitution is not unusual; standing undisturbed for several minutes is usually sufficient to allow dissipation of any large bubbles. Please refer to the accompanying Instructions for Reconstitution and Administration. **100 MG VIALS DO NOT CONTAIN VACUUM.**

100 MG VIAL RECONSTITUTION

1. Use aseptic technique throughout.
2. Remove the protective flip-caps from one vial of Activase® and one vial of Sterile Water for Injection, USP (SWFI).
3. Open the package containing the transfer device by peeling the paper label off the package.
4. Remove the protective cap from one end of the transfer device and keeping the vial of SWFI upright, insert the piercing pin vertically into the center of the stopper of the vial of SWFI.
5. Remove the protective cap from the other end of the transfer device. **DO NOT INVERT THE VIAL OF SWFI.**
6. Holding the vial of Activase® upside-down, position it so that the center of the stopper is directly over the exposed piercing pin of the transfer device.
7. Push the vial of Activase® down so that the piercing pin is inserted through the center of the Activase® vial stopper.
8. Invert the two vials so that the vial of Activase® is on the bottom (upright) and the vial of SWFI is upside-down, allowing the SWFI to flow down through the

transfer device. Allow the entire contents of the vial of SWFI to flow into the Activase® vial (approximately 0.5 cc of SWFI will remain in the diluent vial). Approximately two minutes are required for this procedure.
9. Remove the transfer device and the empty SWFI vial from the Activase® vial. Safely discard both the transfer device and the empty diluent vial according to institutional procedures.
10. Swirl gently to dissolve the Activase® powder. **DO NOT SHAKE.**

No other medication should be added to infusion solutions containing Activase®, Alteplase. Any unused infusion solution should be discarded.

HOW SUPPLIED

Activase® is supplied as a sterile, lyophilized powder in 20 mg and 50 mg vials containing vacuum and in 100 mg vials without vacuum.

Each 20 mg Activase® vial (11.6 million IU) is packaged with diluent for reconstitution. (20 mL Sterile Water for Injection, USP): NDC 50242-044-12.

Each 50 mg Activase® vial (29.0 million IU) is packaged with diluent for reconstitution. (50 mL Sterile Water for Injection, USP): NDC 50242-044-13.

Each 100 mg Activase® vial (58 million IU) is packaged with diluent for reconstitution (100 mL Sterile Water for Injection, USP), and one transfer device: NDC 50242-085-27.

Storage

Store lyophilized Activase® at controlled room temperature not to exceed 30°C (86°F), or under refrigeration (2–8°C/36–46°F). Protect the lyophilized material during extended storage from excessive exposure to light.

Do not use beyond the expiration date stamped on the vial.

REFERENCES

1. Mueller H, Rao AK, Forman SA, et al, Thrombolysis in Myocardial Infarction (TIMI): Comparative studies of coronary reperfusion and systemic fibrinogenolysis with two forms of recombinant tissue-type plasminogen activator. *J Am Coll Card* 1987; 10: 479–490.
2. Topol EJ, Morriss DC, Smalling RW, et al, A multicenter, randomized, placebo-controlled trial of a new form of intravenous recombinant tissue-type plasminogen activator (Activase®) in acute myocardial infarction. *J Am Coll Card* 1987; 9: 1205–1213.
3. De Wood MA, Spores J, Notske R, et al, Prevalence of total coronary occlusion during the early hours of transmural myocardial infarction. *New Engl J Med* 1980; 303: 897–902.
4. Chesebro JH, Knatterud G, Roberts R, et al, Thrombolysis in Myocardial Infarction (TIMI) Trial, Phase I: A comparison between intravenous tissue plasminogen activator and intravenous streptokinase. *Circulation* July, 1987; 76(1), 142–154.
5. Guerci AD, Gerstenblith G, Brinker JA, et al, A randomized trial of intravenous tissue plasminogen activator for acute myocardial infarction with subsequent randomization of elective coronary angioplasty. *New Engl J Med* 1987; 317: 1613–1618.
6. O'Rourke M, Baron D, Keogh A, et al, Limitation of myocardial infarction by early infusion of recombinant tissue-plasminogen activator. *Circulation* 1988; 77: 1311–1315.
7. Wilcox RG, von der Lippe G, Olsson CG, et al, Trial of tissue plasminogen activator for mortality reduction in acute myocardial infarction: ASSET. *Lancet* 1988; 2: 525–530.
8. Hampton JR, The University of Nottingham, Personal Communication.
9. Van de Werf F, Arnold AER, et al, Effect of intravenous tissue-plasminogen activator on infarct size, left ventricular function and survival in patients with acute myocardial infarction. *Br Med J* 1988; 297: 1374–1379.
10. Goldhaber SZ, Kessler CM, Heit J, et al, A randomized controlled trial of recombinant tissue plasminogen activator versus urokinase in the treatment of acute pulmonary embolism. *Lancet* 1988; 2: 293–298.
11. National Heart Foundation of Australia Coronary Thrombolysis Group: Coronary thrombolysis and myocardial infarction salvage by tissue plasminogen activator given up to 4 hours after onset of myocardial infarction. *Lancet* 1988; 1: 203–207.
12. Califf RM, Stump D, Thornton D, et al, Hemorrhagic complications after tissue plasminogen activator (t-PA) therapy for acute myocardial infarction. *Circulation* 1987; 76: IV-1.

Activase®, Alteplase, recombinant | G48005-R4
Manufactured by | Revised January, 1992
GENENTECH®, INC. | © 1992 Genentech, Inc.
460 Point San Bruno Boulevard
South San Francisco, CA 94080

Shown in Product Identification Section, page 410

Continued on next page

Genentech—Cont.

PROTROPIN® ℞
(somatrem for injection)

DESCRIPTION

Protropin is the Genentech trademark for somatrem, a polypeptide hormone which is of recombinant DNA origin. Protropin has 192 amino acid residues and a molecular weight of about 22,000 daltons. The product contains the identical sequence of 191 amino acids constituting pituitary-derived human growth hormone plus an additional amino acid, methionine, on the N-terminus of the molecule. Protropin growth hormone is synthesized in a special laboratory strain of *E. coli* bacteria which has been modified by the addition of the gene for human growth hormone production. Protropin growth hormone, a sterile, white, lyophilized powder, is intended for intramuscular or subcutaneous administration after reconstitution with Bacteriostatic Water for Injection, USP (benzyl alcohol preserved).

The quantitative composition of the lyophilized drug per vial is:

5 mg (approximately 13 IU) Vial
  Somatrem 5.0 mg (approximately 13 IU)
  Mannitol 40.0 mg
  Sodium Phosphates 1.7 mg
    (Monobasic Sodium Phosphate 0.1 mg and
    Dibasic Sodium Phosphate 1.6 mg)
10 mg (approximately 26 IU) Vial
  Somatrem 10.0 mg (approximately 26 IU)
  Mannitol 80.0 mg
  Sodium Phosphates 3.4 mg
    (Monobasic Sodium Phosphate 0.2 mg and
    Dibasic Sodium Phosphate 3.2 mg)

Phosphoric acid may be used for pH adjustment.

Protropin growth hormone is a highly purified preparation. Biological potency is determined by measuring the increase in body weight induced in hypophysectomized rats.

Bacteriostatic Water for Injection, USP (benzyl alcohol preserved) is a sterile water for injection packaged in a multiple dose vial. It contains an antimicrobial preservative. Each mL contains 0.9 percent benzyl alcohol. The pH is 4.5–7.0.

CLINICAL PHARMACOLOGY

Linear Growth—The primary and most intensively studied action of Protropin (somatrem for injection) is the stimulation of linear growth. This effect is demonstrated in patients lacking adequate endogenous growth hormone production. *In vitro*, preclinical, and clinical testing has demonstrated that Protropin growth hormone is therapeutically equivalent to somatropin (human growth hormone, pituitary origin). Short-term clinical studies in normal adults show equivalent pharmacokinetics. Treatment of growth hormone deficient children with Protropin growth hormone results in an increase in growth rate and somatomedin-C levels similar to that seen with somatropin therapy.

Other actions that have been demonstrated for Protropin (somatrem for injection) and/or somatropin include:

A. Tissue Growth—1) Skeletal Growth: Protropin (somatrem for injection) stimulates skeletal growth in patients with growth hormone deficiency. The measurable increase in body length after administration of somatropin results from its effect on the epiphyseal growth plates of long bones. Studies *in vitro* have shown that the incorporation of sulfate into proteoglycans is not due to a direct effect of somatropin, but rather is accomplished by a mediator called somatomedin-C. Somatomedin-C is low in the serum of growth hormone deficient children but increases during treatment with Protropin (somatrem for injection). 2) Cell Growth: It has been shown that the total number of skeletal muscle cells is markedly decreased in short-stature children lacking endogenous growth hormone compared with normal children. Treatment with somatropin results in an increase in both the number and the size of muscle cells. 3) Organ Growth: Somatropin influences the size of internal organs, and it also increases red cell mass.

B. Protein Metabolism—Linear growth is facilitated in part by increased cellular protein synthesis. This is reflected by nitrogen retention as demonstrated by a decline in urinary nitrogen excretion and blood urea nitrogen following the initiation of somatropin therapy. Treatment with Protropin (somatrem for injection) results in a similar decline in blood urea nitrogen.

C. Carbohydrate Metabolism—Both somatropin and Protropin (somatrem for injection) have been found to influence carbohydrate metabolism. It is recognized that children with hypopituitarism sometimes experience fasting hypoglycemia. In normal healthy subjects, large doses of Protropin growth hormone may impair glucose tolerance. Administration of either somatropin or Protropin to normal adults resulted in an increase in serum insulin levels. Although the precise mechanism by which somatropin and Protropin induce insulin resistance is pres-

ently not known, it is attributed to a decrease in insulin sensitivity. An increase in serum glucose levels is observed during treatment with somatropin.

D. Lipid Metabolism—In growth hormone deficient subjects, long-term administration of somatropin often results in a general reduction in body fat stores. Acute administration of somatropin to humans results in lipid mobilization. Nonesterified fatty acids increase in plasma within two hours of somatropin administration.

E. Mineral Metabolism—The retention of total body potassium and phosphorus, which is induced by somatropin administration, is thought to be due to cell growth. Sodium retention also occurs.

Serum levels of inorganic phosphate increase in patients with growth hormone deficiency after somatropin or Protropin (somatrem for injection) therapy due to metabolic activity associated with bone growth as well as increased tubular reabsorption of phosphate by the kidney. Serum calcium is not significantly altered in patients treated with either somatropin or Protropin.

Although calcium excretion in the urine is increased, there is a simultaneous increase in calcium absorption from the intestine.

F. Connective Tissue Metabolism—Somatropin stimulates the synthesis of chondroitin sulfate and collagen as well as the urinary excretion of hydroxyproline.

INDICATIONS AND USAGE

Protropin (somatrem for injection) is indicated only for the long-term treatment of children who have growth failure due to a lack of adequate endogenous growth hormone secretion. Other etiologies of short stature should be excluded.

CONTRAINDICATIONS

Protropin (somatrem for injection) should not be used in subjects with closed epiphyses.

Protropin growth hormone should not be used in patients with active neoplasia. Intracranial lesions must be inactive and antitumor therapy complete prior to instituting therapy. Protropin growth hormone should be discontinued if there is evidence of recurrent tumor growth.

Protropin growth hormone, when reconstituted with Bacteriostatic Water for Injection, USP (benzyl alcohol preserved) should not be used in patients with a known sensitivity to benzyl alcohol.

WARNINGS

Benzyl alcohol as a preservative in Bacteriostatic Water for Injection has been associated with toxicity in newborns. When administering Protropin to newborns, reconstitute with Sterile Water for Injection, USP. USE ONLY ONE DOSE PER VIAL AND DISCARD THE UNUSED PORTION.

PRECAUTIONS

General: Protropin (somatrem for injection) should be used only by physicians experienced in the diagnosis or management of patients with pituitary growth hormone deficiency. Patients with growth hormone deficiency secondary to an intracranial lesion should be examined frequently for progression or recurrence of the underlying disease process.

Because Protropin may induce a state of insulin resistance, patients should be observed for evidence of glucose intolerance.

Hypothyroidism may develop during Protropin treatment. Untreated hypothyroidism prevents optimal response to Protropin growth hormone. Therefore, patients should have periodic thyroid function tests and should be treated with thyroid hormone when indicated.

Leukemia has been reported in a small number of growth hormone deficient patients, treated with growth hormone. On the basis of current evidence, experts cannot conclude that growth hormone therapy is responsible for these occurrences. If there is any risk to an individual patient, it is minimal.

Slipped capital femoral epiphysis may occur more frequently in patients with endocrine disorders. Physicians and parents should be alert to the development of a limp or complaints of hip or knee pain in Protropin-treated patients.

As for any protein, a systemic allergic reaction may occur. See WARNINGS for use of Bacteriostatic Water for Injection, USP (benzyl alcohol preserved) in newborns.

Drug Interactions: Concomitant glucocorticoid therapy may inhibit the growth promoting effect of Protropin growth hormone. Patients with coexisting ACTH deficiency should have their glucocorticoid replacement dose carefully adjusted to avoid an inhibitory effect on growth.

Carcinogenesis, Mutagenesis, Impairment of Fertility: Carcinogenicity, mutagenicity and reproduction studies have not been conducted with Protropin growth hormone.

Pregnancy: Pregnancy (Category C). Animal reproduction studies have not been conducted with Protropin growth hormone. It is also not known whether Protropin growth hormone can cause fetal harm when administered to a pregnant woman or can affect reproduction capacity. Protropin growth hormone should be given to a pregnant woman only if clearly needed.

Nursing Mothers: It is not known whether this drug is excreted in human milk. Because many drugs are excreted in human milk, caution should be exercised when Protropin growth hormone is administered to a nursing woman.

ADVERSE REACTIONS

A. Protropin (somatrem for injection)

Approximately 30 percent of all Protropin-treated patients developed persistent antibodies to growth hormone.

In patients who had been previously treated with pituitary-derived growth hormone, one of twenty-two subjects developed persistent antibodies to growth hormone in response to Protropin therapy.

In children not previously treated with any exogenous growth hormone approximately 40 percent developed persistent antibodies to growth hormone.

In general, the growth hormone antibodies are not neutralizing and do not interfere with the growth response to Protropin growth hormone. One of eighty-four subjects treated with Protropin growth hormone for 6 to 36 months developed antibodies associated with high binding capacities and failed to respond to treatment with Protropin growth hormone.

In addition to an evaluation of compliance with treatment program and thyroid status, testing for antibodies to human growth hormone should be carried out in any patient who fails to respond to therapy.

Additional short-term immunologic and renal function studies were carried out in a group of patients after approximately two years of treatment to detect other potential adverse effects of antibodies to growth hormone. The antibody was determined to be of the IgG class; no antibodies to growth hormone of the IgE class were detected. Testing included immune complex determination, measurement of total hemolytic complement and specific complement components, and immunochemical analyses. No adverse effects of growth hormone antibody formation were observed.

These findings are supported by a toxicity study conducted in a primate model in which a similar antibody response to growth hormone was observed. Protropin (somatrem for injection), administered to monkeys by intramuscular injection at doses of 125 and 625 µg/kg TIW, was compared to pituitary-human growth hormone at the same doses and with placebo over a period of 90 days. Most monkeys treated with high-dose Protropin growth hormone developed persistent antibodies at week four. There were no biologically significant drug related changes in standard laboratory variables. Histopathologic examination of the kidney and other selected organs (pituitary, lungs, liver and pancreas) showed no treatment related toxicity. There was no evidence of immune complexes or immune complex toxicity when the kidney was also examined for the presence of immune complexes and possible toxic effects of immune complexes by immunohistochemistry and electron microscopy.

B. Bacteriostatic Water for Injection, USP (benzyl alcohol preserved)

Toxicity in newborns has been associated with benzyl alcohol as a preservative (see WARNINGS).

OVERDOSAGE

The recommended dosage of up to 0.1 mg (0.26 IU) per kg body weight three times per week should not be exceeded due to the potential risk of side effects.

DOSAGE AND ADMINISTRATION

The Protropin (somatrem for injection) dosage must be individualized for each patient. A dosage and schedule of up to 0.1 mg/kg (0.26 IU/kg) body weight administered three times per week (TIW) by intramuscular or subcutaneous injection is recommended.

After the dose has been determined, reconstitute as follows: each 5 mg vial with 1–5 mL of Bacteriostatic Water for Injection, USP (benzyl alcohol preserved); or each 10 mg vial with 1–10 mL of Bacteriostatic Water for Injection, USP (benzyl alcohol preserved) only. For use in newborns see WARNINGS. The pH of Protropin after reconstitution is approximately 7.8.

To prepare the Protropin solution, inject the Bacteriostatic Water for Injection, USP (benzyl alcohol preserved) into the vial of Protropin growth hormone, aiming the stream of liquid against the glass wall. Then swirl the product vial with a **GENTLE** rotary motion until the contents are completely dissolved. **DO NOT SHAKE.** Because Protropin growth hormone is a protein, shaking can result in a cloudy solution. Immediately after reconstitution, the Protropin solution should be clear. Occasionally, after refrigeration, you may notice that small colorless particles of protein are present in the Protropin solution. This is not unusual for proteins like Protropin growth hormone. If the solution is cloudy immediately after reconstitution or refrigeration, the contents **MUST NOT** be injected. Before and after injections the septum of the vial should be wiped with an antiseptic solution to prevent contamination of the contents after repeated needle insertions. It is recommended that Protropin growth hor-

mone be administered using sterile, disposable syringes and needles. The syringes should be of small enough volume that the prescribed dose can be drawn from the vial with reasonable accuracy.

STORAGE

Protropin (somatrem for injection), before and after reconstitution with Bacteriostatic Water for Injection, USP (benzyl alcohol preserved), must be stored at 2°–8°C/36°–46°F (refrigerator).

Reconstituted vials should be used within 14 days after reconstitution.

Avoid freezing the reconstituted vial of Protropin growth hormone and the Bacteriostatic Water for Injection, USP (benzyl alcohol preserved).

Expiration dates are stated on the labels.

HOW SUPPLIED

Protropin (somatrem for injection) is supplied as 5 mg (approximately 13 IU) or 10 mg (approximately 26 IU) of lyophilized, sterile somatrem per vial.

Each 5 mg carton contains two vials of Protropin (somatrem for injection) (5 mg per vial) and one 10 mL multiple dose vial of Bacteriostatic Water for Injection, USP (benzyl alcohol preserved). NDC 50242-015-02.

Each 10 mg carton contains two vials of Protropin (somatrem for injection) (10 mg per vial) and two 10 mL multiple dose vials of Bacteriostatic Water for Injection, USP (benzyl alcohol preserved). NDC 50242-016-20.

Protropin (somatrem for injection) Manufactured by:
Genentech, Inc.
460 Point San Bruno Boulevard
South San Francisco, CA 94080

Bacteriostatic Water for Injection, USP (benzyl alcohol preserved) Manufactured for:
Genentech, Inc.
G40053-R8
Revised March, 1991
PROTROPIN®
(somatrem for injection)
From Genentech®, Inc.
© 1991 Genentech, Inc.
Shown in Product Identification Section, page 410

Geneva Marsam
2555 W. MIDWAY BOULEVARD
P.O. BOX 446
BROOMFIELD, CO 80038-0446

ADDRESS INQUIRIES TO:
CUSTOMER SERVICE DEPARTMENT
1-800-525-8747

NDC # 0781-	Product	
3700	Sterile Ampicillin Sodium USP 125 mg	
3702	Sterile Ampicillin Sodium USP 250 mg	
3704	Sterile Ampicillin Sodium USP 500 mg	
3706	Sterile Ampicillin Sodium USP 500 mg	
3708	Sterile Ampicillin Sodium USP 1g	
3710	Sterile Ampicillin Sodium USP 1g	
3712	Sterile Ampicillin Sodium USP 2g	
3714	Sterile Ampicillin Sodium USP 2g	
3716	Sterile Ampicillin Sodium USP 10g	
3718	Sterile Cefazolin Sodium USP 500mg	
3722	Sterile Cefazolin Sodium USP 1g	
3724	Sterile Cefazolin Sodium USP 1g	
3726	Sterile Cefazolin Sodium USP 10g	
3740	Nafcillin Sodium For Injection USP 500mg	
3742	Nafcillin Sodium For Injection USP 1g	
3744	Nafcillin Sodium For Injection USP 1g	
3746	Nafcillin Sodium For Injection USP 2g	
3748	Nafcillin Sodium For Injection USP 2g	
3750	Nafcillin Sodium For Injection USP 10g	
3754	Neostigmine Methylsulfate Injection 0.5 mg/mL (1:2000)	
3756	Neostigmine Methylsulfate Injection 1mg/mL (1:1000)	
3758	Oxacillin Sodium For Injection USP 500mg	
3760	Oxacillin Sodium For Injection USP 1g	
3762	Oxacillin Sodium For Injection USP 1g	
3764	Oxacillin Sodium For Injection USP 2g	
3766	Oxacillin Sodium For Injection USP 2g	
3768	Oxacillin Sodium For Injection USP 10g	
3770	Tobramycin Sulfate Injection USP 10mg/mL	
3772	Tobramycin Sulfate Injection USP 40mg/mL	
3775	Tobramycin Sulfate Injection USP 30mg/mL	

Geneva Pharmaceuticals, Inc.
2555 WEST MIDWAY BLVD.
P.O. BOX 446
BROOMFIELD, CO 80038-0446

ADDRESS INQUIRIES TO:
CUSTOMER SERVICE DEPARTMENT
1-800-525-8747

NDC # 0781-	Product/Strength	Rx/OTC
1834	Acetaminophen Tablets USP E/S 500mg	OTC
1294	Acetaminophen Tablets USP 325mg	OTC
1752	Acetaminophen/Codeine Phosphate Tablets USP 300mg/30mg	Rx/CIII
1654	Acetaminophen/Codeine Phosphate Tablets USP 300mg/60mg	Rx/CIII
1870	Allergy Cold Tablets	OTC
1080	Allopurinol Tablets USP 100mg	Rx
1082	Allopurinol Tablets USP 300mg	Rx
1214	Aminophylline Tablets USP 100mg	Rx
1318	Aminophylline Tablets USP 200mg	Rx
1486	Amitriptyline HCl Tablets USP 10mg	Rx
1487	Amitriptyline HCl Tablets USP 25mg	Rx
1488	Amitriptyline HCl Tablets USP 50mg	Rx
1489	Amitriptyline HCl Tablets USP 75mg	Rx
1490	Amitriptyline HCl Tablets USP 100mg	Rx
1491	Amitriptyline HCl Tablets USP 150mg	Rx
1844	Amoxapine Tablets 25mg	Rx
1845	Amoxapine Tablets 50mg	Rx
1846	Amoxapine Tablets 100mg	Rx
1847	Amoxapine Tablets 150mg	Rx
1875	Aspirin and Codeine Phosphate Tablets USP 325mg/60mg	Rx/CIII
1078	Atenolol Tablets 25mg	Rx
1506	Atenolol Tablets 50mg	Rx
1507	Atenolol Tablets 100mg	Rx
1435	Butalbital Compound Tablets	Rx/CIII
1050	Carisoprodol Tablets USP 350mg	Rx
1148	Chlorpheniramine Maleate Tablets USP 4mg (OTC)	OTC
2698	Chlorpheniramine Maleate Extended-Release Capsules USP 12mg (OTC)	OTC
1140	Chlorpheniramine Maleate Tablets USP 4mg	Rx
2602	Chlorpheniramine Maleate Extended Release Capsules USP 8mg	Rx
4007	Chlorpromazine HCl Oral Concentrate 30mg/cc	Rx
4009	Chlorpromazine HCl Oral Concentrate 100mg/cc	Rx
4017	Chlorpromazine HCl Syrup 10mg/5cc	Rx
1715	Chlorpromazine HCl Tablets USP 10mg	Rx
1716	Chlorpromazine HCl Tablets USP 25mg	Rx
1717	Chlorpromazine HCl Tablets USP 50mg	Rx
1718	Chlorpromazine HCl Tablets USP 100mg	Rx
1719	Chlorpromazine HCl Tablets USP 200mg	Rx
1613	Chlorpropamide Tablets USP 100mg	Rx
1623	Chlorpropamide Tablets USP 250mg	Rx
1726	Chlorthalidone Tablets USP 25mg	Rx
1728	Chlorthalidone Tablets USP 50mg	Rx
1303	Chlorzoxazone Tablets USP 250mg	Rx
1304	Chlorzoxazone Tablets USP 500mg	Rx
2580	Clinoxide Capsules	Rx
1471	Clonidine HCl Tablets USP 0.1mg	Rx
1472	Clonidine HCl Tablets USP 0.2mg	Rx
1473	Clonidine HCl Tablets USP 0.3mg	Rx
1324	Cyclobenzaprine HCl Tablets 10mg	Rx
1576	Decongestant Sustained Release Tablets	Rx
1971	Desipramine HCl Tablets USP 10mg	Rx
1972	Desipramine HCl Tablets USP 25mg	Rx
1973	Desipramine HCl Tablets USP 50mg	Rx
1974	Desipramine HCl Tablets USP 75mg	Rx
1975	Desipramine HCl Tablets USP 100mg	Rx
1976	Desipramine HCl Tablets USP 150mg	Rx
1482	Diazepam Tablets USP 2mg	Rx/CIV
1483	Diazepam Tablets USP 5mg	Rx/CIV
1484	Diazepam Tablets USP 10mg	Rx/CIV
1527	Dimenhydrinate Tablets USP 50mg	OTC
2458	Diphenhydramine HCl Capsules USP 25mg	Rx
2498	Diphenhydramine HCl Capsules USP 50mg	Rx
1890	Dipyridamole Tablets USP 25mg	Rx

NDC # 0781-	Product/Strength	Rx/OTC
1678	Dipyridamole Tablets USP 50mg	Rx
1478	Dipyridamole Tablets USP 75mg	Rx
1600	Disobrom® Tablets	Rx
2110	Disopyramide Phosphate Capsules USP 100mg	Rx
2115	Disopyramide Phosphate Capsules USP 150mg	Rx
2800	Doxepin HCl Capsules USP 10mg	Rx
2801	Doxepin HCl Capsules USP 25mg	Rx
2802	Doxepin HCl Capsules USP 50mg	Rx
2803	Doxepin HCl Capsules USP 75mg	Rx
2804	Doxepin HCl Capsules USP 100mg	Rx
1995	Ercaf (Ergotamine Tartrate and Caffeine Tablets USP)	Rx
2861	Fenoprofen Calcium Capsules USP 200mg	Rx
2862	Fenoprofen Calcium Capsules USP 300mg	Rx
1863	Fenoprofen Calcium Tablets USP 600mg	Rx
1436	Fluphenazine HCl Tablets USP 1mg	Rx
1437	Fluphenazine HCl Tablets USP 2.5mg	Rx
1438	Fluphenazine HCl Tablets USP 5mg	Rx
1439	Fluphenazine HCl Tablets USP 10mg	Rx
1818	Furosemide Tablets USP 20mg	Rx
1966	Furosemide Tablets USP 40mg	Rx
1446	Furosemide Tablets USP 80mg	Rx
1391	Haloperidol Tablets USP 0.5mg	Rx
1392	Haloperidol Tablets USP 1mg	Rx
1393	Haloperidol Tablets USP 2mg	Rx
1396	Haloperidol Tablets USP 5mg	Rx
1397	Haloperidol Tablets USP 10mg	Rx
1398	Haloperidol Tablets USP 20mg	Rx
1480	Hydrochlorothiazide Tablets USP 25mg	Rx
1481	Hydrochlorothiazide Tablets USP 50mg	Rx
1332	Hydroxyzine HCl Tablets USP 10mg	Rx
1334	Hydroxyzine HCl Tablets USP 25mg	Rx
1336	Hydroxyzine HCl Tablets USP 50mg	Rx
2252	Hydroxyzine Pamoate Capsules 25mg	Rx
2254	Hydroxyzine Pamoate Capsules 50mg	Rx
2256	Hydroxyzine Pamoate Capsules 100mg	Rx
1762	Imipramine HCl Tablets USP 10mg	Rx
1764	Imipramine HCl Tablets USP 25mg	Rx
1766	Imipramine HCl Tablets USP 50mg	Rx
2325	Indomethacin Capsules USP 25mg	Rx
2350	Indomethacin Capsules USP 50mg	Rx
1515	Isosorbide Dinitrate Sublingual Tablets USP 2.5mg	Rx
1635	Isosorbide Dinitrate Tablets USP 5mg Oral	Rx
1565	Isosorbide Dinitrate Sublingual Tablets USP 5mg	Rx
1556	Isosorbide Dinitrate Tablets USP 10mg Oral	Rx
1695	Isosorbide Dinitrate Tablets USP 20mg Oral	Rx
1417	Isosorbide Dinitrate Extended-Release Tablets USP 40mg	Rx
1840	Isoxsuprine HCl Tablets USP 10mg	Rx
1842	Isoxsuprine HCl Tablets USP 20mg	Rx
1262	Lonox (Diphenoxylate HCl/Atropine Sulfate USP) Tablets	Rx/CV
1403	Lorazepam Tablets USP 0.5mg	Rx/CIV
1404	Lorazepam Tablets USP 1.0mg	Rx/CIV
1405	Lorazepam Tablets USP 2.0mg	Rx/CIV
1542	Meclizine HCl Tablets USP 12.5mg	Rx
1544	Meclizine HCl Tablets USP 25mg	Rx
1345	Meclizine HCl Tablets USP 12.5mg Layered (OTC)	OTC
1375	Meclizine HCl Tablets USP 25mg Layered (OTC)	OTC
2702	Meclofenamate Sodium Capsules USP 50mg	Rx
2703	Meclofenamate Sodium Capsules USP 100mg	Rx
1410	Meprobamate Tablets USP 400mg	Rx/CIV
1760	Methocarbamol Tablets USP 500mg	Rx
1750	Methocarbamol Tablets USP 750mg	Rx
1803	Methyclothiazide Tablets USP 2.5mg	Rx
1810	Methyclothiazide Tablets USP 5mg	Rx
1317	Methyldopa Tablets USP 125mg	Rx
1320	Methyldopa Tablets USP 250mg	Rx
1322	Methyldopa Tablets USP 500mg	Rx
1809	Methyldopa/Hydrochlorothiazide Tablets USP 250mg/15mg	Rx
1819	Methyldopa/Hydrochlorothiazide Tablets USP 250mg/25mg	Rx
1843	Methyldopa/Hydrochlorothiazide Tablets USP 500mg/30mg	Rx
1853	Methyldopa/Hydrochlorothiazide Tablets USP 500mg/50mg	Rx
1301	Metoclopramide HCl Tablets USP 10mg	Rx
1742	Metronidazole Tablets USP 250mg	Rx
1747	Metronidazole Tablets USP 500mg	Rx
2718	Nitroglycerin Sustained Release Capsules 2.5mg	Rx
2786	Nitroglycerin Sustained Release Capsules 6.5mg	Rx

Continued on next page

Geneva—Cont.

2798	Nitroglycerin Sustained Release Capsules 9mg	℞
2809	Oxazepam Capsules USP 10mg	℞/Ⓒ
2810	Oxazepam Capsules USP 15mg	℞/Ⓒ
2811	Oxazepam Capsules USP 30mg	℞/Ⓒ
2000	Papaverine HCl Sustained Release Capsules USP 150mg	℞
1265	Perphenazine and Amitriptyline HCl Tablets USP 2mg/10mg	℞
1273	Perphenazine and Amitriptyline HCl Tablets USP 2mg/25mg	℞
1266	Perphenazine and Amitriptyline HCl Tablets USP 4mg/10mg	℞
1267	Perphenazine and Amitriptyline HCl Tablets USP 4mg/25mg	℞
1268	Perphenazine and Amitriptyline HCl Tablets USP 4mg/50mg	℞
1046	Perphenazine Tablets USP 2mg	℞
1047	Perphenazine Tablets USP 4mg	℞
1048	Perphenazine Tablets USP 8mg	℞
1049	Perphenazine Tablets USP 16mg	℞
1540	Prednisolone Tablets USP 5mg	℞
1495	Prednisone Tablets USP 5mg	℞
1485	Prednisone Tablets USP 20mg	℞
1450	Prednisone Tablets USP 50mg	℞
1147	Procainamide HCl Extended-Release	℞
1157	Procainamide HCl Extended-Release Tablets 500mg	℞
1167	Procainamide HCl Extended-Release Tablets 750mg Tablets USP 250mg	℞
1720	Propoxyphene Napsylate/Acetaminophen Tablets USP 100mg/650mg	℞/Ⓒ
1378	Propoxyphene HCl/Acetaminophen Tablets USP 65mg/650mg	℞/Ⓒ
2367	Propoxyphene HCl/Aspirin and Caffeine Capsules USP 65mg/389mg/32.4mg	℞/Ⓒ
2140	Propoxyphene HCl Capsules 65mg	℞/Ⓒ
1344	Propranolol HCl Tablets USP 10mg	℞
1354	Propranolol HCl Tablets USP 20mg	℞
1364	Propranolol HCl Tablets USP 40mg	℞
1374	Propranolol HCl Tablets USP 60mg	℞
1384	Propranolol HCl Tablets USP 80mg	℞
1431	Propranolol HCl and Hydrochlorothiazide Tablets USP 40mg/25mg	℞
1432	Propranolol HCl and Hydrochlorothiazide Tablets USP 80mg/25mg	℞
1533	Pseudoephedrine HCl Tablets USP 30mg	OTC
1535	Pseudoephedrine HCl Tablets USP 60mg	OTC
1804	Quinidine Gluconate Extended Release Tablets 324mg	℞
1900	Quinidine Sulfate Tablets USP 200mg	℞
1902	Quinidine Sulfate Tablets USP 300mg	℞
2997	Quinine Sulfate Capsules USP 325mg	OTC
1926	Quiphile Tablets (Quinine Sulfate Tablets USP) 260mg	℞
2427	Resaid Sustained Release Capsules	℞
1108	Salsalate Tablets 500mg	℞
1109	Salsalate Tablets 750mg	℞
1149	Spironolactone/Hydrochlorothiazide Tablets USP 25mg/25mg	℞
1599	Spironolactone Tablets USP 25mg	℞
1015	Sulfisoxazole Tablets USP 500mg	℞
1811	Sulindac Tablets 150mg	℞
1812	Sulindac Tablets 200mg	℞
1988	T.E.H. Tablets	℞
1153	Tamine S.R. Tablets	℞
2201	Temazepam Capsules 15mg	℞/Ⓒ
2202	Temazepam Capsules 30mg	℞/Ⓒ
1604	Thioridazine HCl Tablets USP 10mg	℞
1614	Thioridazine HCl Tablets USP 15mg	℞
1624	Thioridazine HCl Tablets USP 25mg	℞
1634	Thioridazine HCl Tablets USP 50mg	℞
1644	Thioridazine HCl Tablets USP 100mg	℞
1664	Thioridazine HCl Tablets USP 150mg	℞
1674	Thioridazine HCl Tablets USP 200mg	℞
2226	Thiothixene Capsules USP 1mg	℞
2227	Thiothixene Capsules USP 2mg	℞
2228	Thiothixene Capsules USP 5mg	℞
2229	Thiothixene Capsules USP 10mg	℞
1126	Timolol Maleate Tablets USP 5mg	℞
1127	Timolol Maleate Tablets USP 10mg	℞
1128	Timolol Maleate Tablets USP 20mg	℞
1922	Tolazamide Tablets USP 100mg	℞
1932	Tolazamide Tablets USP 250mg	℞
1942	Tolazamide Tablets USP 500mg	℞
2182	Tolmetin Sodium 400mg	℞
1807	Trazodone HCl Tablets 50mg	℞
1808	Trazodone HCl Tablets 100mg	℞
1123	Triamterene/Hydrochlorothiazide Tablets 37.5mg/25mg	℞
2715	Triamterene/Hydrochlorothiazide Tablets 50mg/25mg	℞
1008	Triamterene/Hydrochlorothiazide Tablets USP 75mg/50mg	℞
4045	Trifluoperazine HCl Concentrate	℞
1030	Trifluoperazine HCl Tablets USP 1mg	℞
1032	Trifluoperazine HCl Tablets USP 2mg	℞
1034	Trifluoperazine HCl Tablets USP 5mg	℞
1036	Trifluoperazine HCl Tablets USP 10mg	℞
1016	Verapamil HCl Tablets USP 80mg	℞
1017	Verapamil HCl Tablets USP 120mg	℞

Genzyme Corporation
ONE KENDALL SQUARE
CAMBRIDGE, MA 02139

CEREDASE® ℞
[*sĕr 'ĕ-dāse*]
(alglucerase injection)

DESCRIPTION
Ceredase® (alglucerase injection) is a modified form of the enzyme, β-glucocerebrosidase (β-D-glucosyl-N-acylsphingosine glucohydrolase, EC 3.2.1.45). Alglucerase is a monomeric glycoprotein of 497 amino acids with carbohydrates making up approximately 6% of the molecule (M_r = 59,300 as determined by SDS-PAGE). The unmodified enzyme (β-glucocerebrosidase) also contains 497 amino acids and contains approximately 12% carbohydrate (M_r = 67,000). The carbohydrates on the unmodified enzyme consist of N-linked carbohydrate chains of the complex and high mannose type. Glucocerebrosidase and alglucerase catalyze the hydrolysis of the glycolipid, glucocerebroside, within the lysosomes of the reticuloendothelial system.

Alglucerase is prepared by modification of the oligosaccharide chains of human β-glucocerebrosidase. The modification alters the sugar residues at the non-reducing ends of the oligosaccharide chains of the glycoprotein so that they are predominantly terminated with mannose residues which are specifically recognized by carbohydrate receptors on macrophage cells. **Ceredase®** is supplied as a clear sterile non-pyrogenic solution of alglucerase in a citrate buffered solution (53 mM citrate, 143 mM sodium) containing 1% albumin human USP. The enzyme is supplied in two strengths, 400 international units/bottle (80 U/mL) and 50 international units/bottle (10 U/mL) with a fill volume of 5 mL per bottle. An international enzyme unit (U) is defined as the amount of enzyme required to hydrolyze in one minute one micromole of the synthetic substrate, 4 methylumbelliferyl-β-glucoside. **Ceredase®** is purified from a large pool of human placental tissue collected from selected donors. Steps have been introduced into the manufacturing process to reduce further the risk of viral contamination. However, no procedure has been shown to be totally effective in removing viral infectivity. (See PRECAUTIONS). Each lot of product has been tested and found negative for hepatits B surface antigen (HBsAg) and for antigens of the human immunodeficiency virus (HIV-1).

CLINICAL PHARMACOLOGY
Ceredase® (alglucerase injection) catalyzes the hydrolysis of the glycolipid, glucocerebroside, to glucose and ceramide as part of the normal degradation pathway for membrane lipids. Glucocerebroside is primarily derived from hematologic cell turnover. Gaucher disease is characterized by a functional deficiency in β-glucocerebrosidase enzymatic activity and the resultant accumulation of lipid glucocerebroside in tissue macrophages which become engorged and are termed Gaucher cells. Gaucher cells are typically found in liver, spleen and bone marrow and occasionally, as well, in lung, kidney and intestine. Secondary hematologic sequelae include severe anemia and thrombocytopenia in addition to the characteristic progressive hepatosplenomegaly. Skeletal complications, including osteonecrosis and osteopenia with secondary pathological fractures, are a common feature of Gaucher disease.

Pharmacokinetics

Following an intravenous infusion of different doses (between 0.6 and 234 U/kg) of **Ceredase®** (alglucerase injection) over a 4-hour period, steady-state enzymatic activity was achieved by 60 minutes. Individual steady-state enzymatic activity and area under the curve of the activity increased linearly with the infused dose (0.6 to 121 U/kg). Following infusion termination, plasma enzymatic activity declined rapidly with elimination half-life ranging between 3.6 and 10.4 minutes. Plasma clearance of **Ceredase®**, calculated from its plasma enzymatic activity, was variable and ranged between 6.34 and 25.39 mL/min/kg, whereas the volume of distribution ranged from 49.4 to 282.1 mL/kg. Within the dosage range of 0.6 and 121 U/kg, elimination half-life, plasma clearance, and volume of distribution values appear to be independent of the infused dose.

Pharmacologic Actions

Chronic administration of **Ceredase®** (alglucerase injection) in 13 patients with Type 1 Gaucher disease induced the following effects:

1. **Splenomegaly and hepatomegaly** were significantly reduced, presumably by disruption of the lysosomal storage sites and metabolism of glucocerebroside in Gaucher cells. This effect was demonstrated within 6 months of initiation of therapy.
2. **Hematologic deficiencies** in hemoglobin, hematocrit, erythrocyte and platelet counts were significantly improved. In most patients a change in hemoglobin was the first observable effect. In some patients hemoglobin levels were normalized after six months of therapy.
3. **Improved mineralization** occurred in four patients after prolonged treatment as a result of a reduction in the osteolytic actions of lipid-laden Gaucher cells in the marrow.
4. **Cachexia and wasting** in children were reduced.

INDICATIONS AND USAGE
Ceredase® (alglucerase injection) is indicated for use as long-term enzyme replacement therapy for patients with a confirmed diagnosis of Type 1 Gaucher disease who exhibit signs and symptoms that are severe enough to result in one or more of the following conditions:

a) moderate-to-severe anemia;
b) thrombocytopenia with bleeding tendency;
c) bone disease;
d) significant hepatomegaly or splenomegaly.

CONTRAINDICATIONS
There are no known contraindications to the use of **Ceredase®** (alglucerase injection). Treatment with **Ceredase®** should be discontinued if there is significant clinical evidence of hypersensitivity to the product.

PRECAUTIONS
General

Therapy with **Ceredase®** (alglucerase injection) should be directed by physicians knowledgeable in the management of patients with Gaucher disease.

Ceredase® is prepared from pooled human placental tissue that may contain the causative agents of some viral diseases. Manufacturing steps have been designed to reduce the risk of transmitting viral infectious agents. These steps have demonstrated *in vitro* inactivation of a panel of model viruses, including human immunodeficiency virus (HIV-1). The risk of contamination from slowly acting or latent viruses, including the Creutzfeldt-Jacob disease agent, is believed to be remote but has not been tested. Accordingly, the benefits and the risks of treatment with this product should be assessed prior to use.

Carcinogenesis, Mutagenesis, Impairment of Fertility

Studies have not been conducted to assess the potential effects of **Ceredase®** on carcinogenesis, mutagenesis, or impairment of fertility in animals or man.

Pregnancy Category C

Animal reproductive studies have not been conducted with **Ceredase®**. It is also not known whether **Ceredase®** can cause fetal harm when administered to a pregnant woman, or can affect reproductive capacity. **Ceredase®** should be given to a pregnant woman only if clearly needed.

Nursing Mothers

It is not known whether this drug is excreted in human milk. Because many drugs are excreted in human milk, caution should be exercised when **Ceredase®** is administered to a nursing woman.

ADVERSE REACTIONS
During clinical studies, involving 31 patients, 28 adverse experiences occurred that were possibly related to **Ceredase®** (alglucerase injection). Seven of these related to the route of administration and were claims of discomfort, burning and swelling at the site of venipuncture. The remaining 21 experiences (of which approximately 75% were reported by 2 patients) consisted of slight fever, chills, abdominal discomfort, nausea or vomiting. None of these events were judged to require medical intervention.

Most patients treated with **Ceredase®** on a chronic basis have not formed detectable antibodies. A 72 year old patient was found to demonstrate a positive response in testing procedures designed to detect antibodies to **Ceredase®**, 6 months after initiation of therapy. Close monitoring of this patient indicated no diminution of clinical response, and therapy has been continued. The clinical significance of this finding and its relationship to **Ceredase®** is unknown.

OVERDOSE
No obvious toxicity was detected after single doses up to 234 U/kg. There is no experience with higher doses.

DOSAGE AND ADMINISTRATION
Ceredase® (alglucerase injection) is administered by intravenous infusion over 1–2 hours. Dosage should be individualized for each patient. An initial dosage up to 60 U/kg of body weight per infusion may be used. The usual frequency of infusion is once every two weeks, but disease severity and patient convenience may dictate administration as often as once every other day or as infrequently as once every four

weeks. After patient response is well-established, dosage may be adjusted downward for maintenance therapy. Dosage can be progressively lowered at intervals of 3–6 months while closely monitoring response parameters. Ultrastructural evidence suggests that glucocerebroside lipid storage may respond to doses as low as 1 U/kg.

Ceredase® should not be shaken. Ceredase® should be stored at 2–8°C. Each bottle should be inspected visually for particulate matter and discoloration before use. Any bottles exhibiting particulate matter or discoloration should not be used. DO NOT USE Ceredase® after the expiration date on the bottle.

On the day of use, the appropriate amount of Ceredase® for each patient is diluted with normal saline to a final volume not to exceed 100 mL. Aseptic techniques should be used when diluting the dose. Ceredase® when diluted to 100 mL has been shown to be stable for up to 18 hours when stored at 2–8°C. The use of an in-line particulate filter is recommended for the infusion apparatus. Since Ceredase® does not contain any preservative, after opening, bottles should not be stored for subsequent use.

Relatively low toxicity, combined with the extended time course of response, allows small dosage adjustments to be made occasionally to avoid discarding partially used bottles. Thus, the dosage administered in individual infusions may be slightly increased or decreased to utilize fully each bottle as long as the monthly administered dosage remains substantially unaltered.

HOW SUPPLIED

Ceredase® (alglucerase injection) is supplied as a clear sterile citrate buffered solution (53 mM citrate, 143 mM sodium) containing 1% albumin human USP. The following packages are available:

—The 400 U bottle contains 5 mL in a 10 mL glass bottle. NDC 58468-1060-1.
—The 50 U bottle contains 5 mL in a 6 mL glass bottle. NDC 58468-1781-1. Store at 2–8°C.

CAUTION! FEDERAL (U.S.A.) LAW PROHIBITS DISPENSING WITHOUT A PRESCRIPTION.

Ceredase® (alglucerase injection) is manufactured by:

**Genzyme Corporation
One Kendall Square
Cambridge, MA 02139**

Certain manufacturing operations have been performed by other firms.

Revised February, 1992

Shown in Product Identification Section, page 410

Glaxo Dermatology
Division of Glaxo Inc.
**FIVE MOORE DRIVE
RESEARCH TRIANGLE PARK, NC 27709**

ACLOVATE®   ℞
[a'klō-vāt "]
(alclometasone dipropionate)
Cream, 0.05%
Ointment, 0.05%
For Dermatologic Use Only—
Not for Ophthalmic Use.

DESCRIPTION

Aclovate® Cream and Ointment contain alclometasone dipropionate for dermatologic use. Alclometasone dipropionate is a synthetic corticosteroid with anti-inflammatory activity.

Chemically, alclometasone dipropionate is 7α-chloro-11β, 17, 21-trihydroxy-16α-methylpregna-1, 4-diene-3, 20-dione 17, 21-dipropionate.

Alclometasone dipropionate has the empirical formula $C_{28}H_{37}ClO_7$ and a molecular weight of 521. It is a white powder, insoluble in water, slightly soluble in propylene glycol, and moderately soluble in hexylene glycol.

Aclovate Cream contains alclometasone dipropionate 0.5 mg/g in a hydrophilic, emollient cream base of propylene glycol, white petrolatum, cetearyl alcohol, glyceryl stearate, PEG 100 stearate, ceteth-20, monobasic sodium phosphate, chlorocresol, phosphoric acid, and purified water.

Aclovate Ointment contains alclometasone dipropionate 0.5 mg/g in an ointment base of hexylene glycol, white wax, propylene glycol stearate, and white petrolatum.

CLINICAL PHARMACOLOGY

The corticosteroids are a class of compounds comprising steroid hormones secreted by the adrenal cortex and their synthetic analogs. In pharmacologic doses, corticosteroids are used primarily for their anti-inflammatory and/or immunosuppressive effects. Topical corticosteroids such as alclometasone dipropionate are effective in the treatment of corticosteroid-responsive dermatoses primarily because of their anti-inflammatory, antipruritic, and vasoconstrictive actions. However, while the physiologic, pharmacologic, and

---

clinical effects of the corticosteroids are well known, the exact mechanisms of their actions in each disease are uncertain.

Alclometasone dipropionate, a corticosteroid, has been shown to have topical (dermatologic) and systemic pharmacologic and metabolic effects characteristic of this class of drugs.

Pharmacokinetics: The extent of percutaneous absorption of topical corticosteroids, including alclometasone dipropionate, is determined by many factors, including the vehicle, the integrity of the epidermal barrier, and the use of occlusive dressings (see DOSAGE AND ADMINISTRATION).

Topical corticosteroids can be absorbed from normal intact skin. A study utilizing a radio-labelled alclometasone dipropionate *ointment* formulation was performed to measure systemic absorption and excretion. Results indicated that approximately 3% of the steroid was absorbed during 8 hours of contact with intact skin of normal volunteers.

Inflammation and/or other disease processes in the skin may increase percutaneous absorption. Occlusive dressings substantially increase the percutaneous absorption of topical corticosteroids. Thus, occlusive dressings may be a valuable therapeutic adjunct for treatment of resistant dermatoses (see DOSAGE AND ADMINISTRATION).

The effects of Aclovate® (alclometasone dipropionate) Cream and Ointment on the hypothalamic-pituitary-adrenal (HPA) axis were studied under exaggerated conditions. In one study, Aclovate Ointment was applied to 30% of the body twice daily for 7 days, and occlusive dressings were used in selected patients either 12 hours or 24 hours daily. In another study, Aclovate Cream was applied to 80% of the body surface of normal subjects twice daily for 21 days with daily 12-hour periods of whole body occlusion. Average plasma and urinary free cortisol levels and urinary levels of 17-hydroxysteroids were slightly decreased (about 10%), suggesting slight suppression of the HPA axis under the exaggerated conditions of these studies.

Once absorbed through the skin, topical corticosteroids enter pharmacokinetic pathways similarly to systemically administered corticosteroids. Corticosteroids are bound to plasma proteins in varying degrees. Corticosteroids are metabolized primarily in the liver and are then excreted by the kidneys. Some of the topical corticosteroids, including alclometasone dipropionate and its metabolites, are also excreted into the bile.

INDICATIONS AND USAGE

Aclovate® (alclometasone dipropionate) Cream and Ointment are indicated for relief of the inflammatory and pruritic manifestations of corticosteroid-responsive dermatoses.

CONTRAINDICATIONS

Aclovate® (alclometasone dipropionate) Cream and Ointment are contraindicated in patients who are hypersensitive to alclometasone dipropionate, to other corticosteroids, or to any ingredient in these preparations.

PRECAUTIONS

General: Systemic absorption of topical corticosteroids has resulted in reversible HPA axis suppression, manifestations of Cushing's syndrome, hyperglycemia, and glucosuria in some patients.

Conditions that augment systemic absorption include the application of the more potent steroids, use over large surface areas, prolonged use, and the addition of occlusive dressings.

Children may absorb proportionally larger amounts of topical corticosteroids and thus be more susceptible to systemic toxicity (see PRECAUTIONS: Pediatric Use).

If irritation develops, topical corticosteroids should be discontinued and appropriate therapy instituted.

In the presence of dermatologic infections, the use of an appropriate antifungal or antibacterial agent should be instituted. If a favorable response does not occur promptly, the corticosteroid should be discontinued until the infection has been adequately controlled.

Information for Patients: Patients using Aclovate® (alclometasone dipropionate) Cream and Ointment should receive the following information and instructions:

1. This medication is to be used as directed by the physician. It is for external use only. Avoid contact with the eyes.
2. This medication should not be used for any disorder other than that for which it was prescribed.
3. The treated skin area should not be bandaged or otherwise covered or wrapped as to be occlusive unless directed by the physician.
4. Patients should report any signs of local adverse reactions, especially under occlusive dressings, to the physician.
5. Parents of pediatric patients should be advised not to use tight-fitting diapers or plastic pants on a child being treated in the diaper area, as these garments may constitute occlusive dressings.

Laboratory Tests: Although Aclovate Cream and Ointment were shown not to produce HPA axis suppression, the following tests may be helpful in evaluating if HPA axis suppression does occur: Urinary free cortisol test and ACTH stimulation test.

Carcinogenesis, Mutagenesis, Impairment of Fertility: Long-term animal studies have not been peformed to evaluate the carcinogenic potential or the effect on fertility of topical corticosteroids.

Studies to determine mutagenicity with prednisolone have revealed negative results.

Pregnancy: *Teratogenic Effects: Pregnancy Category C:* Corticosteroids are generally teratogenic in laboratory animals when administered systemically at relatively low dosage levels. The more potent corticosteroids have been shown to be teratogenic in animals after dermal application. There are no adequate and well-controlled studies of the teratogenic effects of topically applied corticosteroids in pregnant women. Therefore, topical corticosteroids should be used during pregnancy only if the potential benefit justifies the potential risk to the fetus. Drugs of this class should not be used extensively on pregnant patients, in large amounts, or for prolonged periods of time.

Nursing Mothers: It is not known whether topical administration of corticosteroids could result in sufficient systemic absorption to produce detectable quantities in breast milk. Systemically administered corticosteroids are secreted into breast milk in quantities not likely to have a deleterious effect on the infant. Nevertheless, caution should be exercised when topical corticosteroids are prescribed for a nursing woman.

Pediatric Use: Pediatric patients may demonstrate greater susceptibility to topical corticosteroid-induced HPA axis suppression and Cushing's syndrome than mature patients because of a larger skin surface area to body weight ratio. HPA axis suppression, Cushing's syndrome, and intracranial hypertension have been reported in children receiving topical corticosteroids. Manifestations of adrenal suppression in children include linear growth retardation, delayed weight gain, low plasma cortisol levels, and absence of response to ACTH stimulation. Manifestations of intracranial hypertension include bulging fontanelles, headaches, and bilateral papilledema.

Administration of topical corticosteroids to children should be limited to the least amount compatible with an effective therapeutic regimen. Chronic corticosteroid therapy may interfere with the growth and development of children.

ADVERSE REACTIONS

The following local adverse reactions have been reported with Aclovate® (alclometasone dipropionate) Cream: itching occurred in about 2 per 100 patients; burning, erythema, dryness, irritation, and papular rashes occurred in about 1 per 100 patients.

The following local adverse reactions have been reported with Aclovate® (alclometasone dipropionate) Ointment: itching or burning, 1 per 200 patients; erythema, 2 per 1,000 patients.

The following local adverse reactions are reported infrequently with the use of topical corticosteroids, but may occur more frequently with the use of occlusive dressings. These reactions are listed in an approximately decreasing order of occurrence: burning, itching, irritation, dryness, folliculitis, hypertrichosis, acneiform eruptions, hypopigmentation, perioral dermatitis, allergic contact dermatitis, maceration of the skin, secondary infection, skin atrophy, striae, and miliaria.

OVERDOSAGE

Topically applied Aclovate® (alclometasone dipropionate) Cream and Ointment can be absorbed in sufficient amounts to produce systemic effects (see PRECAUTIONS).

DOSAGE AND ADMINISTRATION

Apply a thin film of Aclovate® (alclometasone dipropionate) Cream or Ointment to the affected skin areas two or three times daily; massage gently until the medication disappears. Occlusive dressings may be used for the management of refractory lesions of psoriasis and other deep-seated dermatoses, such as localized neurodermatitis (lichen simplex chronicus).

Evaporation from the skin is reduced by use of the hydration technique with occlusive dressing as follows:

1. Cover the lesion with a thick layer of Aclovate Cream or Ointment and a light gauze dressing, then cover the area with a pliable plastic film.
2. Seal the edges to the normal skin by adhesive tape or other means.
3. Leave the dressing in place 1–4 days and repeat the procedure three or four times as needed.

With this method of treatment, marked improvement is often seen in a few days.

If an infection develops, the use of occlusive dressings should be discontinued and appropriate antimicrobial therapy instituted.

HOW SUPPLIED

Aclovate® (alclometasone dipropionate) Cream, 0.05% is supplied in 15-g (NDC 0173-0401-00), 45-g (NDC 0173-0401-01), and 60-g (NDC 0173-0401-06) tubes.

Continued on next page

Glaxo Dermatology—Cont.

Aclovate® (alclometasone dipropionate) Ointment, 0.05% is supplied in 15-g (NDC 0173-0402-00), 45-g (NDC 0173-0402-01), and 60-g (NDC 0173-0402-06) tubes.
Store between 2° and 30°C (36° and 86°F).
Shown in Product Identification Section, page 410

CUTIVATE® ℞
[*kyōōt'ə-vāt"*]
(fluticasone propionate)
Cream, 0.05%
For Dermatologic Use Only—
Not for Ophthalmic Use.

DESCRIPTION
Cutivate® Cream, 0.05% contains fluticasone propionate [(6α,11β,16α,17α)-6,9,-difluoro-11-hydroxy-16-methyl-3-oxo-17-(1-oxopropoxy) androsta-1,4-diene-17-carbothioic acid, S-fluoromethyl ester], a synthetic fluorinated corticosteroid, for topical dermatologic use. The topical corticosteroids constitute a class of primarily synthetic steroids used as anti-inflammatory and anti-pruritic agents.
Chemically, fluticasone propionate is $C_{25}H_{31}F_3O_5S$. It has the following structural formula:

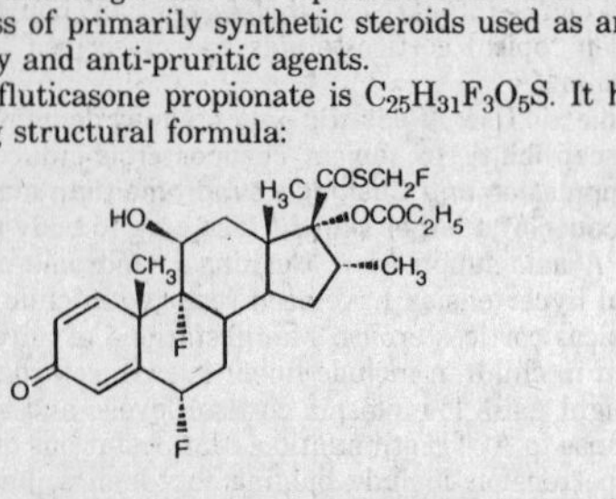

Fluticasone propionate has a molecular weight of 500.6. It is a white to off-white powder and is insoluble in water.
Each gram of Cutivate Cream, 0.05% contains fluticasone propionate 0.5 mg in a base of propylene glycol, mineral oil, cetostearyl alcohol, ceteth-20, isopropyl myristate, dibasic sodium phosphate, citric acid, purified water, and imidurea as preservative.

CLINICAL PHARMACOLOGY
Like other topical corticosteroids, fluticasone propionate has anti-inflammatory, antipruritic, and vasoconstrictive properties. The mechanism of the anti-inflammatory activity of the topical steroids, in general, is unclear. However, corticosteroids are thought to act by the induction of phospholipase A_2 inhibitory proteins, collectively called lipocortins. It is postulated that these proteins control the biosynthesis of potent mediators of inflammation such as prostaglandins and leukotrienes by inhibiting the release of their common precursor, arachidonic acid, which is released from membrane phospholipids by phospholipase A_2.
Pharmacokinetics: The extent of percutaneous absorption of topical corticosteroids is determined by many factors, including the vehicle and the integrity of the epidermal barrier. Occlusive dressing with hydrocortisone for up to 24 hours has not been demonstrated to increase penetration; however, occlusion of hydrocortisone for 96 hours markedly enhances penetration. Topical corticosteroids can be absorbed from normal intact skin, while inflammation and/or other disease processes in the skin increase percutaneous absorption.
Studies performed with Cutivate® (fluticasone propionate) Cream, 0.05% indicate that it is in the medium range of potency as compared with other topical corticosteroids.

INDICATIONS AND USAGE
Cutivate® (fluticasone propionate) Cream, 0.05% is a medium potency corticosteroid indicated for the relief of the inflammatory and pruritic manifestations of corticosteroid-responsive dermatoses.

CONTRAINDICATIONS
Fluticasone propionate cream, 0.05% is contraindicated in those patients with a history of hypersensitivity to any of the components of the preparation.

PRECAUTIONS
General: Systemic absorption of topical corticosteroids can produce reversible hypothalamic-pituitary-adrenal (HPA) axis suppression with the potential for glucocorticosteroid insufficiency after withdrawal from treatment. Manifestations of Cushing's syndrome, hyperglycemia, and glucosuria can also be produced in some patients by systemic absorption of topical corticosteroids while on therapy.
Patients receiving a large dose of a potent topical steroid applied to a large surface area or under an occlusive dressing should be evaluated periodically for evidence of HPA axis suppression. This may be done by using the ACTH stimulation, a.m. plasma cortisol, and urinary free cortisol tests.
Fluticasone propionate cream, 0.05% produced HPA axis suppression within 7 days when used at a dose of 30 g per day in diseased patients. In a study of the effects of fluticasone propionate cream, 0.05% on the HPA axis, a total of 30 g per day was used in two applications daily for 7 days to six patients with psoriasis or atopic dermatitis involving at least 30% of the body surface. One patient developed evidence of adrenal suppression after 6 days of treatment with a below normal plasma cortisol level that returned to low normal levels the following day. Another patient developed a 60% decrease (although never below normal) in the plasma cortisol level from pretreatment values after 2 days of treatment. This suppression persisted at this level for 48 hours before recovering by day 6 of treatment. The results of this study indicate that fluticasone propionate cream, 0.05% may be able to suppress the HPA axis within a few days with a dose of 30 g per day.
If HPA axis suppression is noted, an attempt should be made to withdraw the drug, to reduce the frequency of application, or to substitute a less potent steroid. Recovery of HPA axis function is generally prompt and complete upon discontinuation of topical corticosteroids. Infrequently, signs and symptoms of glucocorticosteroid insufficiency may occur that require supplemental systemic corticosteroids. For information on systemic supplementation, see prescribing information for those products.
Children may be more susceptible to systemic toxicity from equivalent doses due to their larger skin surface to body mass ratios (see PRECAUTIONS: Pediatric Use).
If irritation develops, fluticasone propionate cream, 0.05% should be discontinued and appropriate therapy instituted.
Allergic contact dermatitis with corticosteroids is usually diagnosed by observing *failure to heal* rather than noting a clinical exacerbation as with most topical products not containing corticosteroids. Such an observation should be corroborated with appropriate diagnostic patch testing.
If concomitant skin infections are present or develop, an appropriate antifungal or antibacterial agent should be used. If a favorable response does not occur promptly, use of fluticasone propionate cream, 0.05% should be discontinued until the infection has been adequately controlled.
Fluticasone propionate cream, 0.05% should not be used in the treatment of rosacea and perioral dermatitis.
Information for Patients: Patients using topical corticosteroids should receive the following information and instructions:
1. This medication is to be used as directed by the physician. It is for external use only. Avoid contact with the eyes.
2. This medication should not be used for any disorder other than that for which it was prescribed.
3. The treated skin area should not be bandaged or otherwise covered or wrapped so as to be occlusive unless directed by the physician.
4. Patients should report to their physician any signs of local adverse reactions.

Laboratory Tests: The following tests may be helpful in evaluating patients for HPA axis suppression:
ACTH stimulation test
A.M. plasma cortisol test
Urinary free cortisol test
Carcinogenesis, Mutagenesis, Impairment of Fertility: Long-term animal studies have not been performed to evaluate the carcinogenic potential of fluticasone propionate.
Fluticasone propionate was not mutagenic in the standard Ames test, *E. coli* fluctuation test, *S. cerevisiae* gene conversion test, or Chinese Hamster ovarian cell assay. It was not clastogenic in mouse micronucleus or cultured human lymphocyte tests.
In a fertility and general reproductive performance study in rats, fluticasone propionate administered subcutaneously to females at up to 50 μg/kg per day and to males at up to 100 μg/kg per day (later reduced to 50 μg/kg per day) had no effect upon mating performance or fertility. These doses are approximately 15 and 30 times, respectively, the human systemic exposure following use of the recommended human topical dose of fluticasone propionate cream, 0.05%, assuming human percutaneous absorption of approximately 3% and the use in a 70-kg person of 15 g per day.
Pregnancy: ***Teratogenic Effects: Pregnancy Category C:*** Corticosteroids have been shown to be teratogenic in laboratory animals when administered systemically at relatively low dosage levels. The more potent corticosteroids have been shown to be teratogenic after dermal application in laboratory animals. Teratology studies in the mouse demonstrated fluticasone propionate to be teratogenic (cleft palate) when administered subcutaneously in doses of 45 μg/kg per day and 150 μg/kg per day. This dose is approximately 14 and 45 times, respectively, the human topical dose of fluticasone propionate cream, 0.05%. There are no adequate and well-controlled studies in pregnant women. Fluticasone propionate cream, 0.05% should be used during pregnancy only if the potential benefit justifies the potential risk to the fetus.
Nursing Mothers: Systemically administered corticosteroids appear in human milk and could suppress growth, interfere with endogenous corticosteroid production, or cause other untoward effects. It is not known whether topical administration of corticosteroids could result in sufficient systemic absorption to produce detectable quantities in human milk. Because many drugs are excreted in human milk, caution should be exercised when fluticasone propionate cream, 0.05% is administered to a nursing woman.
Pediatric Use: Safety and effectiveness in children and infants have not been established. Because of a higher ratio of skin surface area to body mass, children are at a greater risk than adults of HPA axis suppression when they are treated with topical corticosteroids. They are therefore also at greater risk of glucocorticosteroid insufficiency after withdrawal of treatment and of Cushing's syndrome while on treatment. Adverse effects including striae have been reported with inappropriate use of topical corticosteroids in infants and children (see PRECAUTIONS).
HPA axis suppression, Cushing's syndrome, and intracranial hypertension have been reported in children receiving topical corticosteroids. Manifestations of adrenal suppression in children include linear growth retardation, delayed weight gain, low plasma cortisol levels, and absence of response to ACTH stimulation. Manifestations of intracranial hypertension include bulging fontanelles, headaches, and bilateral papilledema.

ADVERSE REACTIONS
In controlled clinical trials, the total incidence of adverse reactions associated with the use of fluticasone propionate cream, 0.05% was approximately 4%. These adverse reactions were mild, usually self-limiting, and consisted primarily of pruritus, dryness, numbness of fingers, and burning. These events occurred in 2.9%, 1.2%, 1.0%, and 0.6% of patients, respectively.
The following additional local adverse reactions have been reported infrequently with other topical corticosteroids, and they may occur more frequently with the use of occlusive dressings, especially with higher potency corticosteroids. These reactions are listed in an approximately decreasing order of occurrence: irritation, folliculitis, acneiform eruptions, hypopigmentation, perioral dermatitis, allergic contact dermatitis, secondary infection, skin atrophy, striae, and miliaria. Also, there are reports of the development of pustular psoriasis from chronic plaque psoriasis following reduction or discontinuation of potent topical corticosteroid products.

OVERDOSAGE
Topically applied fluticasone propionate cream, 0.05% can be absorbed in sufficient amounts to produce systemic effects (see PRECAUTIONS).

DOSAGE AND ADMINISTRATION
Apply a thin film of Cutivate® (fluticasone propionate) Cream, 0.05% to the affected skin areas twice daily. Rub in gently.

HOW SUPPLIED
Cutivate® (fluticasone propionate) Cream, 0.05% is supplied in 15-g (NDC 0173-0430-00), 30-g (NDC 0173-0430-01), and 60-g (NDC 0173-0430-02) tubes.
Store between 2° and 30°C (36° and 86°F).
Shown in Product Identification Section, page 410

CUTIVATE® ℞
[*kyōōt'ə-vāt"*]
(fluticasone propionate)
Ointment, 0.005%
For Dermatologic Use Only—
Not for Ophthalmic Use.

DESCRIPTION
Cutivate® Ointment, 0.005% contains fluticasone propionate [(6α,11β,16α,17α)-6,9,-difluoro-11-hydroxy-16-methyl-3-oxo-17-(1-oxopropoxy) androsta-1,4-diene-17-carbothioic acid, S-fluoromethyl ester], a synthetic fluorinated corticosteroid, for topical dermatologic use. The topical corticosteroids constitute a class of primarily synthetic steroids used as anti-inflammatory and anti-pruritic agents.
Chemically, fluticasone propionate is $C_{25}H_{31}F_3O_5S$. It has the following structural formula:

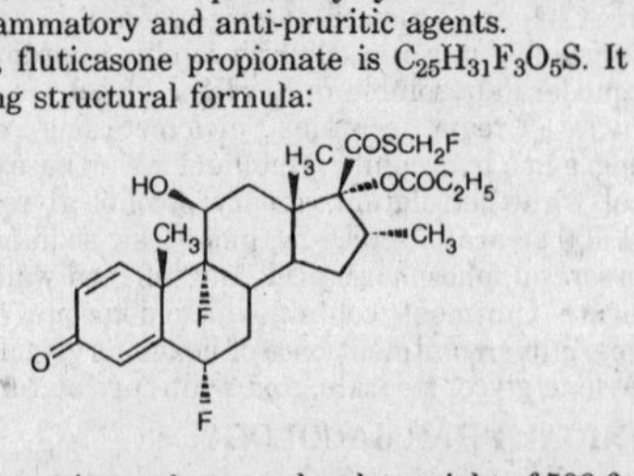

Fluticasone propionate has a molecular weight of 500.6. It is a white to off-white powder and is insoluble in water.
Each gram of Cutivate Ointment, 0.005% contains fluticasone propionate 0.05 mg in a base of propylene glycol, sorbitan sesquioleate, microcrystalline wax, and liquid paraffin.

CLINICAL PHARMACOLOGY
Like other topical corticosteroids, fluticasone propionate has anti-inflammatory, anti-pruritic, and vasoconstrictive prop-

erties. The mechanism of the anti-inflammatory activity of the topical steroids, in general, is unclear. However, corticosteroids are thought to act by the induction of phospholipase A_2 inhibitory proteins, collectively called lipocortins. It is postulated that these proteins control the biosynthesis of potent mediators of inflammation such as prostaglandins and leukotrienes by inhibiting the release of their common precursor, arachidonic acid, which is released from membrane phospholipids by phospholipase A_2.

Pharmacokinetics: The extent of percutaneous absorption of topical corticosteroids is determined by many factors, including the vehicle and the integrity of the epidermal barrier. Occlusive dressing with hydrocortisone for up to 24 hours has not been demonstrated to increase penetration; however, occlusion of hydrocortisone for 96 hours markedly enhances penetration. Topical corticosteroids can be absorbed from normal intact skin, while inflammation and/or other disease processes in the skin increase percutaneous absorption.

Studies performed with Cutivate® (fluticasone propionate) Ointment, 0.005% indicate that it is in the medium range of potency as compared with other topical corticosteroids.

INDICATIONS AND USAGE
Cutivate® (fluticasone propionate) Ointment, 0.005% is a medium potency corticosteroid indicated for the relief of the inflammatory and pruritic manifestations of corticosteroid-responsive dermatoses.

CONTRAINDICATIONS
Fluticasone propionate ointment, 0.005% is contraindicated in those patients with a history of hypersensitivity to any of the components of the preparation.

PRECAUTIONS
General: Systemic absorption of topical corticosteroids can produce reversible hypothalamic-pituitary-adrenal (HPA) axis suppression with the potential for glucocorticosteroid insufficiency after withdrawal from treatment. Manifestations of Cushing's syndrome, hyperglycemia, and glucosuria can also be produced in some patients by systemic absorption of topical corticosteroids while on therapy.

Patients receiving a large dose of a potent topical steroid applied to a large surface area or under an occlusive dressing should be evaluated periodically for evidence of HPA axis suppression. This may be done by using the ACTH stimulation, a.m. plasma cortisol, and urinary free cortisol tests. Fluticasone propionate ointment, 0.05% (a concentration 10 times that of fluticasone propionate ointment, 0.005%) did not suppress plasma cortisol in any of six patients but did moderately suppress 24-hour urinary free cortisol levels in two of six patients when used at a dose of 30 g per day for a week in patients with psoriasis or eczema. In a second study, fluticasone propionate ointment, 0.05% caused a minimal depression of a.m. plasma cortisol levels in 3 of 12 normal volunteers when applied at doses of 50 g per day for 21 days. Morning plasma levels returned to normal levels within the first week upon discontinuation of fluticasone propionate. In this study there was no corresponding decrease in 24-hour urinary free cortisol levels.

If HPA axis suppression is noted, an attempt should be made to withdraw the drug, to reduce the frequency of application, or to substitute a less potent steroid. Recovery of HPA axis function is generally prompt and complete upon discontinuation of topical corticosteroids. Infrequently, signs and symptoms of glucocorticosteroid insufficiency may occur that require supplemental systemic corticosteroids. For information on systemic supplementation, see prescribing information for those products.

Children may be more susceptible to systemic toxicity from equivalent doses due to their larger skin surface to body mass ratios (see PRECAUTIONS: Pediatric Use).

If irritation develops, fluticasone propionate ointment, 0.005% should be discontinued and appropriate therapy instituted. Allergic contact dermatitis with corticosteroids is usually diagnosed by observing *failure to heal* rather than noting a clinical exacerbation as with most topical products not containing corticosteroids. Such an observation should be corroborated with appropriate diagnostic patch testing.

If concomitant skin infections are present or develop, an appropriate antifungal or antibacterial agent should be used. If a favorable response does not occur promptly, use of fluticasone propionate ointment, 0.005% should be discontinued until the infection has been adequately controlled. Fluticasone propionate ointment, 0.005% should not be used in the treatment of rosacea and perioral dermatitis.

Information for Patients: Patients using topical corticosteroids should receive the following information and instructions:

1. This medication is to be used as directed by the physician. It is for external use only. Avoid contact with the eyes.
2. This medication should not be used for any disorder other than that for which it was prescribed.
3. The treated skin area should not be bandaged or otherwise covered or wrapped so as to be occlusive unless directed by the physician.

4. Patients should report to their physician any signs of local adverse reactions.

Laboratory Tests: The following tests may be helpful in evaluating patients for HPA axis suppression:
  ACTH stimulation test
  A.M. plasma cortisol test
  Urinary free cortisol test

Carcinogenesis, Mutagenesis, Impairment of Fertility: Long-term animal studies have not been performed to evaluate the carcinogenic potential of fluticasone propionate.

Fluticasone propionate was not mutagenic in the standard Ames test, *E. coli* fluctuation test, *S. cerevisiae* gene conversion test, or Chinese Hamster ovarian cell assay. It was not clastogenic in mouse micronucleus or cultured human lymphocyte tests.

In a fertility and general reproductive performance study in rats, fluticasone propionate administered subcutaneously to females at up to 50 µg/kg per day and to males at up to 100 µg/kg per day (later reduced to 50 µg/kg per day) had no effect upon mating performance or fertility. These doses are approximately 150 and 300 times, respectively, the human systemic exposure following use of the recommended human topical dose of fluticasone propionate ointment, 0.005%, assuming human percutaneous absorption of approximately 3% and the use in a 70-kg person of 15 g per day.

Pregnancy: *Teratogenic Effects: Pregnancy Category C:* Corticosteroids have been shown to be teratogenic in laboratory animals when administered systemically at relatively low dosage levels. The more potent corticosteroids have been shown to be teratogenic after dermal application in laboratory animals. Teratology studies in the mouse demonstrated fluticasone propionate to be teratogenic (cleft palate) when administered subcutaneously in doses of 45 µg/kg per day and 150 µg/kg per day. This dose is approximately 140 and 450 times, respectively, the human topical dose of fluticasone propionate ointment, 0.005%. There are no adequate and well-controlled studies in pregnant women. Fluticasone propionate ointment, 0.005% should be used during pregnancy only if the potential benefit justifies the potential risk to the fetus.

Nursing Mothers: Systemically administered corticosteroids appear in human milk and could suppress growth, interfere with endogenous corticosteroid production, or cause other untoward effects. It is not known whether topical administration of corticosteroids could result in sufficient systemic absorption to produce detectable quantities in human milk. Because many drugs are excreted in human milk, caution should be exercised when fluticasone propionate ointment, 0.005% is administered to a nursing woman.

Pediatric Use: Safety and effectiveness in children and infants have not been established. Because of a higher ratio of skin surface area to body mass, children are at a greater risk than adults of HPA axis suppression when they are treated with topical corticosteroids. They are therefore also at greater risk of glucocorticosteroid insufficiency after withdrawal of treatment and of Cushing's syndrome while on treatment. Adverse effects including striae have been reported with inappropriate use of topical corticosteroids in infants and children (see PRECAUTIONS).

HPA axis suppression, Cushing's syndrome, and intracranial hypertension have been reported in children receiving topical corticosteroids. Manifestations of adrenal suppression in children include linear growth retardation, delayed weight gain, low plasma cortisol levels, and absence of response to ACTH stimulation. Manifestations of intracranial hypertension include bulging fontanelles, headaches, and bilateral papilledema.

ADVERSE REACTIONS
In controlled clinical trials, the total incidence of adverse reactions associated with the use of fluticasone propionate ointment, 0.005% was approximately 4%. These adverse reactions were mild, usually self-limiting, and consisted primarily of pruritus, burning, hypertrichosis, increased erythema, hives, irritation, and lightheadedness. Each of these events occurred individually in less than 1% of patients.

The following additional local adverse reactions have been reported infrequently with other topical corticosteroids, and they may occur more frequently with the use of occlusive dressings, especially with higher potency corticosteroids. These reactions are listed in an approximately decreasing order of occurrence: dryness, folliculitis, acneiform eruptions, hypopigmentation, perioral dermatitis, allergic contact dermatitis, secondary infection, skin atrophy, striae, and miliaria. Also, there are reports of the development of pustular psoriasis from chronic plaque psoriasis following reduction or discontinuation of potent topical corticosteroid products.

OVERDOSAGE
Topically applied fluticasone propionate ointment, 0.005% can be absorbed in sufficient amounts to produce systemic effects (see PRECAUTIONS).

DOSAGE AND ADMINISTRATION
Apply a thin film of Cutivate® (fluticasone propionate) Ointment, 0.005% to the affected skin areas twice daily. Rub in gently.

HOW SUPPLIED
Cutivate® (fluticasone propionate) Ointment, 0.005% is supplied in 15-g (NDC 0173-0431-00), 30-g (NDC 0173-0431-01), and 60-g (NDC 0173-0431-02) tubes.
Store between 2° and 30°C (36° and 86°F).

Shown in Product Identification Section, page 410

EMGEL™ ℞
(erythromycin) 2%
Topical Gel
For Dermatologic Use Only—
Not for Ophthalmic Use.

DESCRIPTION
Emgel™ Topical Gel contains erythromycin. Erythromycin is a macrolide antibiotic obtained from cultures of *Streptomyces erythreus*. Erythromycin has the empirical formula $C_{37}H_{67}NO_{13}$ and a molecular weight of 733.94.
Emgel Topical Gel contains erythromycin, USP 2% (20 mg/g) with SD 40-2 alcohol 77%, propylene glycol, and hydroxypropyl cellulose.

CLINICAL PHARMACOLOGY
The exact mechanism by which erythromycin reduces lesions of acne vulgaris is not fully known; however, the effect appears to be due in part to the antibacterial activity of the drug.
Microbiology: Erythromycin appears to inhibit protein synthesis in susceptible organisms by reversibly binding to ribosomal subunits, thereby inhibiting translocation of aminoacyl transfer-RNA and inhibiting polypeptide synthesis. Antagonism has been demonstrated between erythromycin, lincomycin, chloramphenicol, and clindamycin.

INDICATIONS AND USAGE
Emgel™ (erythromycin) Topical Gel is indicated for the topical treatment of acne vulgaris.

CONTRAINDICATIONS
Emgel™ (erythromycin) Topical Gel is contraindicated in those individuals who have shown hypersensitivity to any of its components.

PRECAUTIONS
General: For topical use only; not for ophthalmic use. Concomitant topical acne therapy should be used with caution since a possible cumulative irritancy effect may occur, especially with the use of peeling, desquamating, or abrasive agents.
Avoid contact with eyes and all mucous membranes. The use of antibiotic agents may be associated with the overgrowth of antibiotic-resistant organisms. If this occurs, discontinue use and take appropriate measures.
Carcinogenesis, Mutagenesis, Impairment of Fertility: Animal studies to evaluate carcinogenic and mutagenic potential or effects on fertility have not been performed with erythromycin.
Pregnancy Category B: There was no evidence of teratogenicity or any other adverse effect on reproduction in female rats fed erythromycin base (up to 0.25% of diet) before and during mating, during gestation, and through weaning of two successive litters. There are, however, no adequate and well-controlled studies in pregnant women. Because animal reproduction studies are not always predictive of human response, this drug should be used in pregnancy only if clearly needed. Erythromycin has been reported to cross the placental barrier in humans, but fetal plasma levels are generally low.
Nursing Mothers: It is not known whether topically applied erythromycin is excreted in human milk. A decision should be made whether to discontinue nursing or to discontinue the drug, taking into account the importance of the drug to the mother.
Pediatric Use: Safety and effectiveness in children have not been established.

ADVERSE REACTIONS
The most common adverse reaction reported with Emgel™ (erythromycin) Topical Gel was burning. The following have been reported occasionally: peeling, dryness, itching, erythema, and oiliness. Irritation of the eyes and tenderness of the skin have also been reported with the topical use of erythromycin. A generalized urticarial reaction, possibly related to the use of erythromycin and which required systemic steroid therapy, has been reported.

DOSAGE AND ADMINISTRATION
Apply sparingly as a thin layer to affected area(s) twice a day, in the morning and the evening after the skin is thoroughly washed with soap and water and patted dry. The

Continued on next page

Glaxo Dermatology—Cont.

hands should be washed after application. If there has been no improvement after 6–8 weeks, or if the condition becomes worse, treatment should be discontinued, and the physician should be reconsulted. Spread the medication lightly rather than rubbing it in.

HOW SUPPLIED

Emgel™ (erythromycin) 2% Topical Gel is supplied in plastic bottles containing 27 g (NDC 0173-0440-01).

Note: FLAMMABLE: Keep away from heat and flame. Keep bottle tightly closed. Store at room temperature.

Shown in Product Identification Section, page 410

OXISTAT® ℞

[äx 'ē-stat "]
(oxiconazole nitrate)
Cream, 1%*
***Potency expressed as oxiconazole.**
For Dermatologic Use Only—
Not for Ophthalmic Use.

DESCRIPTION

Oxistat® Cream contains the active compound oxiconazole nitrate, a broad-spectrum antifungal, for topical dermatologic use.

Chemically, oxiconazole nitrate is 2′,4′-dichloro-2-imidazol-1-ylacetophenone (*Z*)-[*O*-(2,4-dichlorobenzyl)oxime], mononitrate, with the empirical formula $C_{18}H_{13}ON_3Cl_4 \cdot HNO_3$, a molecular weight of 492.16, and the following structural formula:

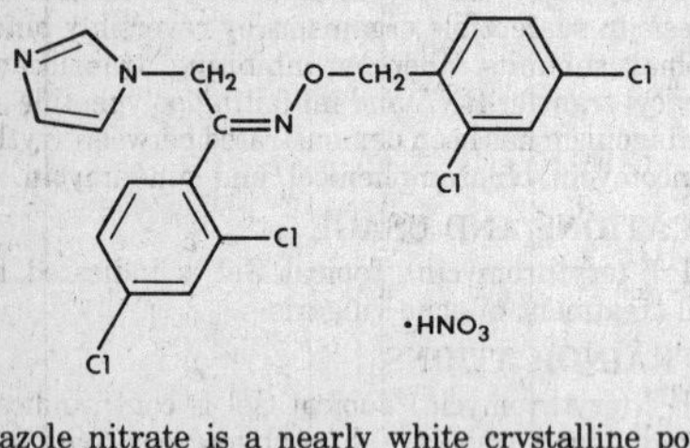

Oxiconazole nitrate is a nearly white crystalline powder, soluble in methanol; sparingly soluble in ethanol, chloroform, and acetone; and very slightly soluble in water.

Oxistat Cream contains 10 mg/g of oxiconazole as oxiconazole nitrate in a white to off-white, opaque cream base of purified water, white petrolatum, stearyl alcohol, propylene glycol, polysorbate 60, cetyl alcohol, and benzoic acid 0.2% as a preservative.

CLINICAL PHARMACOLOGY

Five hours after application of 2.5 mg/cm^2 of oxiconazole nitrate cream onto human skin, the concentration of oxiconazole nitrate was demonstrated to be 16.2 μmol in the epidermis, 3.64 μmol in the upper corium, and 1.29 μmol in the deeper corium. Systemic absorption of oxiconazole nitrate appears to be low. Less than 0.3% of the applied dose was recovered in the urine of volunteer subjects up to 5 days after application. Feces were not analyzed for the drug, and it is not known whether the absorption is higher than that estimated by recovery of drug in urine.

Microbiology: The fungicidal activity of oxiconazole results primarily from the inhibition of ergosterol synthesis, which is needed for cytoplasmic membrane integrity. It has *in vitro* activity against a wide range of organisms.

In vitro, oxiconazole is active against many strains of clinical isolates of the following dermatophytic organisms: *Trichophyton rubrum* and *Trichophyton mentagrophytes*.

Oxiconazole has been shown to be active against the following microorganisms *in vitro;* however, clinical efficacy has not been established: *Trichophyton tonsurans, Trichophyton violaceum, Microsporum canis, Microsporum audouini, Microsporum gypseum, Epidermophyton floccosum, Candida albicans,* and *Malassezia furfur.*

INDICATIONS AND USAGE

Oxistat® (oxiconazole nitrate) Cream is indicated for the topical treatment of the following dermal infections: tinea pedis, tinea cruris, and tinea corporis due to *Trichophyton rubrum* and *Trichophyton mentagrophytes.*

CONTRAINDICATIONS

Oxistat® (oxiconazole nitrate) Cream is contraindicated in individuals who have shown hypersensitivity to any of its components.

WARNINGS

Oxistat® (oxiconazole nitrate) Cream is not for ophthalmic use.

PRECAUTIONS

General: If a reaction suggesting sensitivity or chemical irritation should occur with the use of Oxistat® (oxiconazole nitrate) Cream, treatment should be discontinued and appropriate therapy instituted. Oxistat Cream is for external use only. Avoid introduction of Oxistat Cream into the eyes.

Carcinogenesis, Mutagenesis, Impairment of Fertility: Although no long-term studies in animals have been performed to evaluate carcinogenic potential, no evidence of mutagenic effect was found in two mutation assays (Ames test and Chinese hamster V79 *in vitro* cell mutation assay) or in two cytogenetic assays (human peripheral blood lymphocyte *in vitro* chromosome aberration assay and *in vivo* micronucleus assay in mice).

Reproductive studies revealed no impairment of fertility in rats at oral doses of 3 mg/kg per day in females and 15 mg/kg per day in males. However, at doses above this level, the following effects were observed: a reduction in the fertility parameters of males and females, a reduction in the number of sperm in vaginal smears, extended estrous cycle, and a decrease in mating frequency.

Pregnancy: *Teratogenic Effects: Pregnancy Category B:* Reproduction studies have been performed in rabbits, rats, and mice at oral doses up to 100, 150, and 200 mg/kg per day, respectively, and revealed no evidence of harm to the fetus due to oxiconazole nitrate. There are, however, no adequate and well-controlled studies in pregnant women. Because animal reproduction studies are not always predictive of human response, this drug should be used during pregnancy only if clearly needed.

Nursing Mothers: Since oxiconazole is excreted in human milk, caution should be exercised when the drug is administered to a nursing woman. Although human data relating concentrations of oxiconazole in milk were not obtained, after subcutaneous administration of 5 mg/kg to female rats, the milk:plasma ratio at 1.5–12 hours was in the range of 3.0–8.0.

ADVERSE REACTIONS

During clinical trials, 41 (4.3%) of 955 patients treated with oxiconazole nitrate 1% cream reported adverse reactions, including itching (1.6%), burning (1.4%), irritation and allergic contact dermatitis (0.4% each), folliculitis (0.3%), erythema (0.2%), and papules, fissuring, maceration, rash, stinging, and nodules (0.1% each).

OVERDOSAGE

Animal studies have shown oxiconazole nitrate to be a central nervous system depressant and tissue irritant when administered orally or by injection.

DOSAGE AND ADMINISTRATION

Oxistat® (oxiconazole nitrate) Cream should be applied to cover affected areas once daily (in the evening) in patients with tinea pedis, tinea corporis, and tinea cruris. Tinea corporis and tinea cruris should be treated for 2 weeks and tinea pedis for 1 month to reduce the possibility of recurrence. If a patient shows no clinical improvement after the treatment period, the diagnosis should be reviewed.

HOW SUPPLIED

Oxistat® (oxiconazole nitrate) Cream, 1% is supplied in 15-g (NDC 0173-0423-00), 30-g (NDC 0173-0423-01), and 60-g (NDC 0173-0423-04) tubes.

Store between 15° and 30°C (59° and 86°F).

Shown in Product Identification Section, page 410

TEMOVATE® ℞

[tim 'ō-vāt "]
(clobetasol propionate)
Cream, 0.05%*
Ointment, 0.05%*
Scalp Application, 0.05%*
***potency expressed as clobetasol propionate**
For Dermatologic Use Only—
Not for Ophthalmic Use.

DESCRIPTION

Temovate® Cream, Ointment, and Scalp Application contain the active compound clobetasol propionate, a synthetic corticosteroid, for topical dermatologic use. Clobetasol, an analog of prednisolone, has a high degree of glucocorticoid activity and a slight degree of mineralocorticoid activity.

Chemically, clobetasol propionate is (11β,16β)-21-chloro-9-fluoro-11-hydroxy-16-methyl-17-(1-oxopropoxy)pregna-1,4-diene-3,20-dione, and it has the following structural formula:

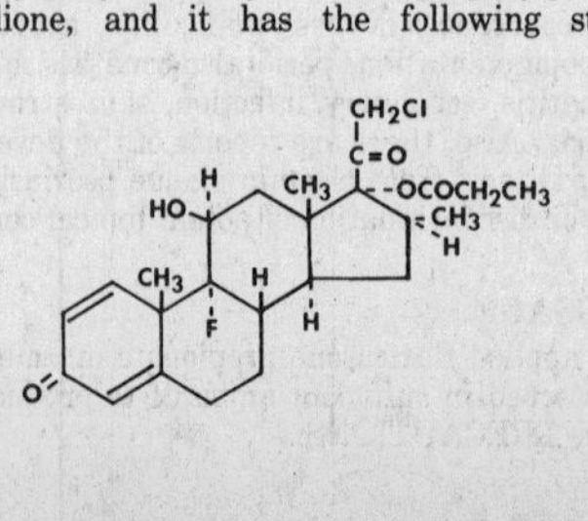

Clobetasol propionate has the empirical formula $C_{25}H_{32}ClFO_5$ and a molecular weight of 467. It is a white to cream-colored crystalline powder insoluble in water.

Temovate Cream contains clobetasol propionate 0.5 mg/g in a cream base of propylene glycol, glyceryl monostearate, cetostearyl alcohol, glyceryl stearate, PEG 100 stearate, white wax, chlorocresol, sodium citrate, citric acid monohydrate, and purified water.

Temovate Ointment contains clobetasol propionate 0.5 mg/g in a base of propylene glycol, sorbitan sesquioleate, and white petrolatum.

Temovate Scalp Application contains clobetasol propionate 0.5 mg/g in a base composed of purified water, isopropyl alcohol (39.3%), carbomer 934P, and sodium hydroxide.

CLINICAL PHARMACOLOGY:

The corticosteroids are a class of compounds comprising steroid hormones secreted by the adrenal cortex and their synthetic analogs. In pharmacologic doses, corticosteroids are used primarily for their anti-inflammatory and/or immunosuppressive effects. Topical corticosteroids such as clobetasol propionate are effective in the treatment of corticosteroid-responsive dermatoses primarily because of their anti-inflammatory, antipruritic, and vasoconstrictive actions. However, while the physiologic, pharmacologic, and clinical effects of the corticosteroids are well known, the exact mechanisms of their actions in each disease are uncertain.

Clobetasol propionate, a corticosteroid, has been shown to have topical (dermatologic) and systemic pharmacologic and metabolic effects characteristic of this class of drugs.

Pharmacokinetics: The extent of percutaneous absorption of topical corticosteroids, including clobetasol propionate, is determined by many factors, including the vehicle, the integrity of the epidermal barrier, and the use of occlusive dressings (see DOSAGE AND ADMINISTRATION).

As with all topical corticosteroids, clobetasol propionate can be absorbed from normal intact skin. Inflammation and/or other disease processes in the skin may increase percutaneous absorption. Occlusive dressings substantially increase the percutaneous absorption of topical corticosteroids (see DOSAGE AND ADMINISTRATION).

Once absorbed through the skin, topical corticosteroids enter pharmacokinetic pathways similarly to systemically administered corticosteroids. Corticosteroids are bound to plasma proteins in varying degrees. Corticosteroids are metabolized primarily in the liver and are then excreted by the kidneys. Some of the topical corticosteroids, including clobetasol propionate and its metabolites, are also excreted into the bile.

Temovate® (clobetasol propionate) Cream and Ointment have been shown to depress the plasma levels of adrenal cortical hormones following repeated nonocclusive application to diseased skin in patients with psoriasis and eczematous dermatitis. These effects have been shown to be transient and reversible upon completion of a 2-week course of treatment.

Following repeated nonocclusive application in the treatment of scalp psoriasis, there is some evidence that Temovate® (clobetasol propionate) Scalp Application has the potential to depress plasma cortisol levels in some patients. However, hypothalamic-pituitary-adrenal (HPA) axis effects produced by systemically absorbed clobetasol propionate have been shown to be transient and reversible upon completion of a 2-week course of treatment.

INDICATIONS AND USAGE

Temovate® (clobetasol propionate) Cream and Ointment are indicated for short-term treatment of inflammatory and pruritic manifestations of moderate to severe corticosteroid-responsive dermatoses. Temovate® (clobetasol propionate) Scalp Application is indicated for short-term topical treatment of inflammatory and pruritic manifestations of moderate to severe corticosteroid-responsive dermatoses of the scalp.

Treatment beyond 2 consecutive weeks is not recommended, and the total dosage should not exceed 50 g per week of cream and ointment and 50 mL per week of scalp application because of the potential for the drug to suppress the HPA axis.

These products are not recommended for use in children under 12 years of age.

CONTRAINDICATIONS

Temovate® (clobetasol propionate) Cream, Ointment, and Scalp Application are contraindicated in patients who are hypersensitive to clobetasol propionate, to other corticosteroids, or to any ingredient in these preparations. Temovate Scalp Application is also contraindicated in patients with primary infections of the scalp.

PRECAUTIONS

General: Clobetasol propionate is a highly potent topical corticosteroid that has been shown to suppress the HPA axis at doses as low as 2 g (of ointment) per day. Systemic absorption of topical corticosteroids has resulted in reversible HPA axis suppression, manifestations of Cushing's syndrome, hyperglycemia, and glucosuria in some patients.

Conditions that augment systemic absorption include the application of the more potent corticosteroids, use over large surface areas, prolonged use, and the addition of occlusive dressings. Therefore, patients receiving a large dose of a potent topical steroid applied to a large surface area should be evaluated periodically for evidence of HPA axis suppression by using the urinary free cortisol and ACTH stimulation tests. If HPA axis suppression is noted, an attempt should be made to withdraw the drug, to reduce the frequency of application, or to substitute a less potent steroid.
Recovery of HPA axis function is generally prompt and complete upon discontinuation of the drug. Infrequently, signs and symptoms of steroid withdrawal may occur, requiring supplemental systemic corticosteroids.
Children may absorb proportionally larger amounts of topical corticosteroids and thus be more susceptible to systemic toxicity (see PRECAUTIONS: Pediatric Use).
If irritation develops, topical corticosteroids should be discontinued and appropriate therapy instituted. Irritation is possible if Temovate® (clobetasol propionate) Scalp Application contacts the eye. If that should occur, immediate flushing of the eye with a large volume of water is recommended.
In the presence of dermatologic infections, the use of an appropriate antifungal or antibacterial agent should be instituted. If a favorable response does not occur promptly, the corticosteroid should be discontinued until the infection has been adequately controlled.
Although Temovate Scalp Application is intended for the treatment of inflammatory conditions of the scalp, it should be noted that certain areas of the body, such as the face, groin, and axillae, are more prone to atrophic changes than other areas of the body following treatment with corticosteroids. Frequent observation of the patient is important if these areas are to be treated.
As with other potent topical corticosteroids, Temovate® (clobetasol propionate) Cream, Ointment, and Scalp Application should not be used in the treatment of rosacea and perioral dermatitis. Topical corticosteroids in general should not be used in the treatment of acne or as sole therapy in widespread plaque psoriasis.

Information for Patients: Patients using Temovate Cream, Ointment, or Scalp Application should receive the following information and instructions:

1. This medication is to be used as directed by the physician and should not be used longer than the prescribed time period. It is for external use only. Avoid contact with the eyes.
2. This medication should not be used for any disorder other than that for which it was prescribed.
3. The treated skin area should not be bandaged or otherwise covered or wrapped so as to be occlusive.
4. Patients should report any signs of local adverse reactions to the physician.

Laboratory Tests: The following tests may be helpful in evaluating HPA axis suppression:
Urinary free cortisol test
ACTH stimulation test

Carcinogenesis, Mutagenesis, Impairment of Fertility: Long-term animal studies have not been performed to evaluate the carcinogenic potential or the effect on fertility of topical corticosteroids.
Studies to determine mutagenicity with prednisolone have revealed negative results.

Pregnancy: *Teratogenic Effects: Pregnancy Category C:* The more potent corticosteroids have been shown to be teratogenic in animals after dermal application. Clobetasol propionate has not been tested for teratogenicity by this route; however, it is absorbed percutaneously, and when administered subcutaneously it was a significant teratogen in both the rabbit and the mouse. Clobetasol propionate has greater teratogenic potential than steroids that are less potent.
There are no adequate and well-controlled studies of the teratogenic effects of topically applied corticosteroids, including clobetasol, in pregnant women. Therefore, clobetasol and other topical corticosteroids should be used during pregnancy only if the potential benefit justifies the potential risk to the fetus, and they should not be used extensively on pregnant patients, in large amounts, or for prolonged periods of time.

Nursing Mothers: It is not known whether topical administration of corticosteroids could result in sufficient systemic absorption to produce detectable quantities in breast milk. Systemically administered corticosteroids are secreted into breast milk in quantities not likely to have a deleterious effect on the infant. Nevertheless, caution should be exercised when topical corticosteroids are prescribed for a nursing woman.

Pediatric Use: Use of Temovate Cream, Ointment, and Scalp Application in children under 12 years of age is not recommended.
Pediatric patients may demonstrate greater susceptibility to topical corticosteroid-induced HPA axis suppression and Cushing's syndrome than mature patients because of a larger skin surface area to body weight ratio.
HPA axis suppression, Cushing's syndrome, and intracranial hypertension have been reported in children receiving topical corticosteroids. Manifestations of adrenal suppression in children include linear growth retardation, delayed weight gain, low plasma cortisol levels, and absence of response to ACTH stimulation. Manifestations of intracranial hypertension include bulging fontanelles, headaches, and bilateral papilledema.

ADVERSE REACTIONS

Temovate® (clobetasol propionate) Cream, Ointment, and Scalp Application are generally well tolerated when used for 2-week treatment periods.
The most frequent adverse reactions reported for Temovate Cream have been local and have included burning sensation in 4 of 421 patients and stinging sensation in 3 of 421 patients. Less frequent adverse reactions were itching, skin atrophy, and cracking and fissuring of the skin, which occurred in 1 of 421 patients.
The most frequent adverse events reported for Temovate Ointment have been local and have included burning sensation, irritation, and itching. These occurred in 2 of 366 patients. Less frequent adverse reactions were stinging, cracking, erythema, folliculitis, numbness of fingers, skin atrophy, and telangiectasia, which occurred in 1 of 366 patients.
The most frequent adverse events reported for Temovate Scalp Application have been local and have included burning and/or stinging sensation, which occurred in 29 of 294 patients; scalp pustules, which occurred in 3 of 294 patients; and tingling and folliculitis, each of which occurred in 2 of 294 patients. Less frequent adverse events were itching and tightness of the scalp, dermatitis, tenderness, headache, hair loss, and eye irritation, each of which occurred in 1 of 294 patients.
The following local adverse reactions are reported infrequently when topical corticosteroids are used as recommended. These reactions are listed in an approximately decreasing order of occurrence: burning, itching, irritation, dryness, folliculitis, hypertrichosis, acneiform eruptions, hypopigmentation, perioral dermatitis, allergic contact dermatitis, maceration of the skin, secondary infection, skin atrophy, striae, and miliaria. Systemic absorption of topical corticosteroids has produced reversible HPA axis suppression, manifestations of Cushing's syndrome, hyperglycemia, and glucosuria in some patients. In rare instances, treatment (or withdrawal of treatment) of psoriasis with corticosteroids is thought to have exacerbated the disease or provoked the pustular form of the disease, so careful patient supervision is recommended.

OVERDOSAGE

Topically applied Temovate® (clobetasol propionate) Cream, Ointment, and Scalp Application can be absorbed in sufficient amounts to produce systemic effects (see PRECAUTIONS).

DOSAGE AND ADMINISTRATION

A thin layer of Temovate® (clobetasol propionate) Cream or Ointment should be applied with gentle rubbing to the affected skin areas twice daily, once in the morning and once at night. Temovate Cream and Ointment are potent; therefore, **treatment must be limited to 2 consecutive weeks, and amounts greater than 50 g per week should not be used. Temovate Cream and Ointment are not to be used with occlusive dressings.**
Temovate® (clobetasol propionate) Scalp Application should be applied to the affected scalp areas twice daily, once in the morning and once at night. Temovate Scalp Application is potent; therefore, **treatment must be limited to 2 consecutive weeks, and amounts greater than 50 mL per week should not be used. Temovate Scalp Application is not to be used with occlusive dressings.**

HOW SUPPLIED

Temovate® (clobetasol propionate) Cream, 0.05% is supplied in 15-g (NDC 0173-0375-73), 30-g (NDC 0173-0375-72), and 45-g (NDC 0173-0375-01) tubes. Temovate® (clobetasol propionate) Ointment, 0.05% is supplied in 15-g (NDC 0173-0376-73), 30-g (NDC 0173-0376-72), and 45-g (NDC 0173-0376-01) tubes.
Store between 15° and 30°C (59° and 86°F). Temovate Cream should not be refrigerated.
Temovate® (clobetasol propionate) Scalp Application, 0.05% is supplied in plastic squeeze bottles, 25 mL (NDC 0173-0432-00) and 50 mL (NDC 0173-0432-01). **Store between 4° and 25°C (39° and 77°F). Do not use near an open flame.**
Shown in Product Identification Section, page 410

Products are cross-indexed by
generic and chemical names in the
YELLOW SECTION.

Glaxo Pharmaceuticals

Division of Glaxo Inc.
FIVE MOORE DRIVE
RESEARCH TRIANGLE PARK, NC 27709

CEPTAZ™ ℞

[sĕp' tăz]
(ceftazidime for injection, Glaxo)
L-arginine formulation
For Intravenous or Intramuscular Use

DESCRIPTION

Ceftazidime is a semisynthetic, broad-spectrum, beta-lactam antibiotic for parenteral administration. It is the pentahydrate of pyridinium, 1-[[7-[[(2-amino-4-thiazolyl)[(1-carboxy-1-methylethoxy) imino]acetyl] amino]-2-carboxy-8-oxo-5-thia -1- azabicyclo[4.2.0]oct-2-en-3-yl]methyl]-, hydroxide, inner salt, [6R-[6α,7β(Z)]]. It has the following structure:

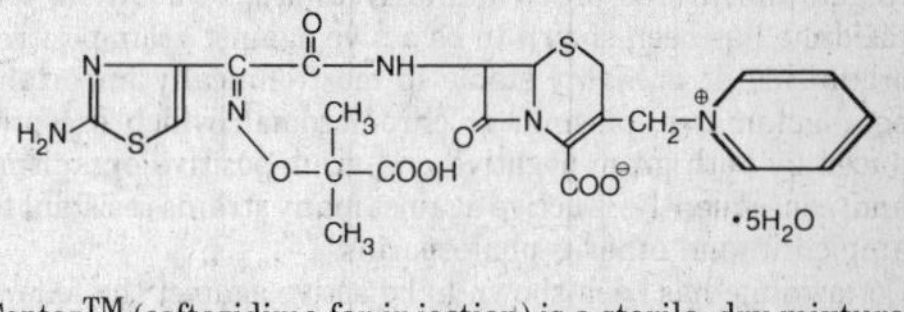

Ceptaz™ (ceftazidime for injection) is a sterile, dry mixture of ceftazidime pentahydrate and L-arginine. The L-arginine is at a concentration of 349 mg/g of ceftazidime activity. Ceptaz dissolves without the evolution of gas. The product contains no sodium ion. Solutions of Ceptaz range in color from light yellow to amber, depending on the diluent and volume used. The pH of freshly constituted solutions usually ranges from 5–7.5.

CLINICAL PHARMACOLOGY

After intravenous (IV) administration of 500-mg and 1-g doses of ceftazidime over 5 minutes to normal adult male volunteers, mean peak serum concentrations of 45 and 90 mcg/mL, respectively, were achieved. After IV infusion of 500-mg, 1-g, and 2-g doses of ceftazidime over 20–30 minutes to normal adult male volunteers, mean peak serum concentrations of 42, 69, and 170 mcg/mL, respectively, were achieved. The average serum concentrations following IV infusion of 500-mg, 1-g, and 2-g doses to these volunteers over an 8-hour interval are given in Table 1.

Table 1

Ceftazidime IV Dose	Serum Concentrations (mcg/mL) 0.5 h	1 h	2 h	4 h	8 h
500 mg	42	25	12	6	2
1 g	60	39	23	11	3
2 g	129	75	42	13	5

The absorption and elimination of ceftazidime were directly proportional to the size of the dose. The half-life following IV administration was approximately 1.9 hours. Less than 10% of ceftazidime was protein bound. The degree of protein binding was independent of concentration. There was no evidence of accumulation of ceftazidime in the serum in individuals with normal renal function following multiple IV doses of 1 and 2 g every 8 hours for 10 days.
Following intramuscular (IM) administration of 500-mg and 1-g doses of ceftazidime to normal adult volunteers, the mean peak serum concentrations were 17 and 39 mcg/mL, respectively, at approximately 1 hour. Serum concentrations remained above 4 mcg/mL for 6 and 8 hours after the IM administration of 500-mg and 1-g doses, respectively. The half-life of ceftazidime in these volunteers was approximately 2 hours.
The presence of hepatic dysfunction had no effect on the pharmacokinetics of ceftazidime in individuals administered 2 g intravenously every 8 hours for 5 days. Therefore, a dosage adjustment from the normal recommended dosage is not required for patients with hepatic dysfunction, provided renal function is not impaired.
Approximately 80%–90% of an IM or IV dose of ceftazidime is excreted unchanged by the kidneys over a 24-hour period. After the IV administration of single 500-mg or 1-g doses, approximately 50% of the dose appeared in the urine in the first 2 hours. An additional 20% was excreted between 2 and 4 hours after dosing, and approximately another 12% of the dose appeared in the urine between 4 and 8 hours later. The elimination of ceftazidime by the kidneys resulted in high therapeutic concentrations in the urine.
The mean renal clearance of ceftazidime was approximately 100 mL/min. The calculated plasma clearance of approximately 115 mL/min indicated nearly complete elimination of ceftazidime by the renal route. Administration of probene-

Continued on next page

Glaxo—Cont.

cid before dosing had no effect on the elimination kinetics of ceftazidime. This suggested that ceftazidime is eliminated by glomerular filtration and is not actively secreted by renal tubular mechanisms.

Since ceftazidime is eliminated almost solely by the kidneys, its serum half-life is significantly prolonged in patients with impaired renal function. Consequently, dosage adjustments in such patients as described in the DOSAGE AND ADMINISTRATION section are suggested.

Ceftazidime concentrations achieved in specific body tissues and fluids are depicted in Table 2.
[See table below.]

Microbiology: Ceftazidime is bactericidal in action, exerting its effect by inhibition of enzymes responsible for cell-wall synthesis. A wide range of gram-negative organisms is susceptible to ceftazidime *in vitro*, including strains resistant to gentamicin and other aminoglycosides. In addition, ceftazidime has been shown to be active against gram-positive organisms. It is highly stable to most clinically important beta-lactamases, plasmid or chromosomal, which are produced by both gram-negative and gram-positive organisms and, consequently, is active against many strains resistant to ampicillin and other cephalosporins.

Ceftazidime has been shown to be active against the following organisms both *in vitro* and in clinical infections (see INDICATIONS AND USAGE).

Aerobes, Gram-negative: *Citrobacter* spp., including *Citrobacter freundii* and *Citrobacter diversus; Enterobacter* spp., including *Enterobacter cloacae* and *Enterobacter aerogenes; Escherichia coli; Haemophilus influenzae,* including ampicillin-resistant strains; *Klebsiella* spp. (including *Klebsiella pneumoniae); Neisseria meningitidis; Proteus mirabilis; Proteus vulgaris; Pseudomonas* spp. (including *Pseudomonas aeruginosa*); and *Serratia* spp.

Aerobes, Gram-positive: *Staphylcoccus aureus,* including penicillinase- and non-penicillinase-producing strains; *Streptococcus agalactiae* (group B streptococci); *Streptococcus pneumoniae;* and *Streptococcus pyogenes* (group A beta-hemolytic streptococci).

Anaerobes: *Bacteroides* spp (NOTE: many strains of *Bacteroides fragilis* are resistant).

Ceftazidime has been shown to be active *in vitro* against most strains of the following organisms; however, the clinical significance of these data is unknown: *Acinetobacter* spp.; *Clostridium* spp. (not including *Clostridium difficile); Haemophilus parainfluenzae; Morganella morganii* (formerly *Proteus morganii); Neisseria gonorrhoeae; Peptococcus* spp., *Peptostreptococcus* spp., *Providencia* spp. (including *Providencia rettgeri,* formerly *Proteus rettgeri*); *Salmonella* spp.; *Shigella* spp.; *Staphylococcus epidermidis;* and *Yersinia enterocolitica.*

Ceftazidime and the aminoglycosides have been shown to be synergistic *in vitro* against *Pseudomonas aeruginosa* and the Enterobacteriaceae. Ceftazidime and carbenicillin have also been shown to be synergistic *in vitro* against *Pseudomonas aeruginosa.*

Ceftazidime is not active *in vitro* against methicillin-resistant staphylococci; *Streptococcus faecalis* and many other enterococci; *Listeria monocytogenes; Campylobacter* spp.; or *Clostridium difficile.*

Susceptibility Tests: *Diffusion Techniques:* Quantitative methods that require measurement of zone diameters give an estimate of antibiotic susceptibility. One such procedure[1-3] has been recommended for use with disks to test susceptibility to ceftazidime.

Reports from the laboratory giving results of the standard single-disk susceptibility test with a 30-mcg ceftazidime disk should be interpreted according to the following criteria:

Susceptible organisms produce zones of 18 mm or greater, indicating that the test organism is likely to respond to therapy.

Organisms that produce zones of 15–17 mm are expected to be susceptible if high dosage is used or if the infection is confined to tissues and fluids (e.g., urine) in which high antibiotic levels are attained.

Resistant organisms produce zones of 14 mm or less, indicating that other therapy should be selected.

Organisms should be tested with the ceftazidime disk since ceftazidime has been shown by *in vitro* tests to be active against certain strains found resistant when other beta-lactam disks are used.

Standardized procedures require the use of laboratory control organisms. The 30-mcg ceftazidime disk should give zone diameters between 25 and 32 mm for *Escherichia coli* ATCC 25922. For *Pseudomonas aeruginosa* ATCC 27853, the zone diameters should be between 22 and 29 mm. For *Staphylococcus aureus* ATCC 25923, the zone diameters should be between 16 and 20 mm.

Dilution Techniques: In other susceptibility testing procedures, e.g., ICS agar dilution or the equivalent, a bacterial isolate may be considered susceptible if the minimum inhibitory concentration (MIC) value for ceftazidime is not more than 16 mcg/mL. Organisms are considered resistant to ceftazidime if the MIC is equal to or greater than 64 mcg/mL. Organisms having an MIC value of less than 64 mcg/mL but greater than 16 mcg/mL are expected to be susceptible if high dosage is used or if the infection is confined to tissues and fluids (e.g., urine) in which high antibiotic levels are attained.

As with standard diffusion methods, dilution procedures require the use of laboratory control organisms. Standard ceftazidime powder should give MIC values in the range of 4–16 mcg/mL for *Staphylococcus aureus* ATCC 25923. For *Escherichia coli* ATCC 25922, the MIC range should be between 0.125 and 0.5 mcg/mL. For *Pseudomonas aeruginosa* ATCC 27853, the MIC range should be between 0.5 and 2 mcg/mL.

INDICATIONS AND USAGE

Ceptaz™ (ceftazidime for injection) is indicated for the treatment of patients with infections caused by susceptible strains of the designated organisms in the following diseases:

1. **Lower Respiratory Tract Infections,** including pneumonia, caused by *Pseudomonas aeruginosa* and other *Pseudomonas* spp; *Haemophilus influenzae,* including ampicillin-resistant strains; *Klebsiella* spp; *Enterobacter* spp; *Proteus mirabilis; Escherichia coli; Serratia* spp; *Citrobacter* spp; *Streptococcus pneumoniae;* and *Staphylococcus aureus* (methicillin-susceptible strains).

2. **Skin and Skin Structure Infections** caused by *Pseudomonas aeruginosa; Klebsiella* spp.; *Escherichia coli; Proteus* spp., including *Proteus mirabilis* and indole-positive *Proteus; Enterobacter* spp.; *Serratia* spp.; *Staphylococcus aureus* (methicillin-susceptible strains); and *Streptococcus pyogenes* (group A beta-hemolytic streptococci).

3. **Urinary Tract Infections,** both complicated and uncomplicated, caused by *Pseudomonas aeruginosa; Enterobacter* spp.; *Proteus* spp., including *Proteus mirabilis* and indole-positive *Proteus; Klebsiella* spp.; and *Escherichia coli.*

4. **Bacterial Septicemia** caused by *Pseudomonas aeruginosa; Klebsiella* spp.; *Haemophilus influenzae; Escherichia coli; Serratia* spp.; *Streptococcus pneumoniae;* and *Staphylococcus aureus* (methicillin-susceptible strains).

5. **Bone and Joint Infections** caused by *Pseudomonas aeruginosa; Klebsiella* spp.; *Enterobacter* spp.; and *Staphylococcus aureus* (methicillin-susceptible strains).

6. **Gynecologic Infections,** including endometritis, pelvic cellulitis, and other infections of the female genital tract caused by *Escherichia coli.*

7. **Intra-abdominal Infections,** including peritonitis caused by *Escherichia coli, Klebsiella* spp., and *Staphylococcus aureus* (methicillin-susceptible strains) and polymicrobial infections caused by aerobic and anaerobic organisms and *Bacteroides* spp. (many strains of *Bacteroides fragilis* are resistant).

8. **Central Nervous System Infections,** including meningitis, caused by *Haemophilus influenzae* and *Neisseria meningitidis.* Ceftazidime has also been used successfully in a limited number of cases of meningitis due to *Pseudomonas aeruginosa* and *Streptococcus pneumoniae.*

Specimens for bacterial cultures should be obtained before therapy in order to isolate and identify causative organisms and to determine their susceptibility to ceftazidime. Therapy may be instituted before results of susceptibility studies are known; however, once these results become available, the antibiotic treatment should be adjusted accordingly.

Ceptaz may be used alone in cases of confirmed or suspected sepsis. Ceftazidime has been used successfully in clinical trials as empiric therapy in cases where various concomitant therapies with other antibiotics have been used.

Ceptaz may also be used concomitantly with other antibiotics, such as aminoglycosides, vancomycin, and clindamycin; in severe and life-threatening infections; and in the immunocompromised patient (see COMPATIBILITY AND STABILITY). When such concomitant treatment is appropriate, prescribing information in the labeling for the other antibiotics should be followed. The dose depends on the severity of the infection and the patient's condition.

CONTRAINDICATIONS

Ceptaz™ (ceftazidime for injection) is contraindicated in patients who have shown hypersensitivity to ceftazidime or the cephalosporin group of antibiotics.

WARNINGS

BEFORE THERAPY WITH CEPTAZ™ (CEFTAZIDIME FOR INJECTION) IS INSTITUTED, CAREFUL INQUIRY SHOULD BE MADE TO DETERMINE WHETHER THE PATIENT HAS HAD PREVIOUS HYPERSENSITIVITY REACTIONS TO CEFTAZIDIME, CEPHALOSPORINS, PENICILLINS, OR OTHER DRUGS. IF THIS PRODUCT IS GIVEN TO PENICILLIN-SENSITIVE PATIENTS, CAUTION SHOULD BE EXERCISED BECAUSE CROSS-HYPERSENSITIVITY AMONG BETA-LACTAM ANTIBIOTICS HAS BEEN CLEARLY DOCUMENTED AND MAY OCCUR IN UP TO 10% OF PATIENTS WITH A HISTORY OF PENICILLIN ALLERGY. IF AN ALLERGIC REACTION TO CEPTAZ OCCURS, DISCONTINUE THE DRUG. SERIOUS ACUTE HYPERSENSITIVITY REACTIONS MAY REQUIRE TREATMENT WITH EPINEPHRINE AND OTHER EMERGENCY MEASURES, INCLUDING OXYGEN, IV FLUIDS, IV ANTIHISTAMINES, CORTICOSTEROIDS, PRESSOR AMINES, AND AIRWAY MANAGEMENT, AS CLINICALLY INDICATED.

Pseudomembranous colitis has been reported with nearly all antibacterial agents, including ceftazidime, and may range from mild to life-threatening. Therefore, it is important to consider this diagnosis in patients who present with diarrhea subsequent to the administration of antibacterial agents.

Treatment with antibacterial agents alters the normal flora of the colon and may permit overgrowth of clostridia. Studies indicate that a toxin produced by *Clostridium difficile* is a primary cause of "antibiotic-associated colitis."

After the diagnosis of pseudomembranous colitis has been established, therapeutic measures should be initiated. Mild cases of pseudomembranous colitis usually respond to discontinuation of the drug alone. In moderate to severe cases, consideration should be given to management with fluids and electrolytes, protein supplementation, and treatment with an oral antibacterial drug effective against *Clostridium difficile.*

Elevated levels of ceftazidime in patients with renal insufficiency can lead to seizures, encephalopathy, asterixis, and neuromuscular excitability (see PRECAUTIONS).

PRECAUTIONS

General: Ceftazidime has not been shown to be nephrotoxic; however, high and prolonged serum antibiotic concentrations can occur from usual doses in patients with transient or persistent reduction of urinary output because of renal insufficiency. The total daily dosage should be reduced when ceftazidime is administered to patients with renal insufficiency (see DOSAGE AND ADMINISTRATION). Elevated levels of ceftazidime in these patients can lead to seizures, encephalopathy, asterixis, and neuromuscular excitability. Continued dosage should be determined by degree of renal impairment, severity of infection, and susceptibility of the causative organisms.

Table 2: Ceftazidime Concentrations in Body Tissues and Fluids

Tissue or Fluid	Dose/ Route	No. of Patients	Time of Sample Post-dose	Average Tissue or Fluid Level (mcg/mL or mcg/g)
Urine	500 mg IM	6	0–2 h	2,100.0
	2 g IV	6	0–2 h	12,000.0
Bile	2 g IV	3	90 min	36.4
Synovial fluid	2 g IV	13	2 h	25.6
Peritoneal fluid	2 g IV	8	2 h	48.6
Sputum	1 g IV	8	1 h	9.0
Cerebrospinal fluid	2 g q8h IV	5	120 min	9.8
(inflamed meninges)	2 g q8h IV	6	180 min	9.4
Aqueous humor	2 g IV	13	1–3 h	11.0
Blister fluid	1 g IV	7	2–3 h	19.7
Lymphatic fluid	1 g IV	7	2–3 h	23.4
Bone	2 g IV	8	0.67 h	31.1
Heart muscle	2 g IV	35	30–280 min	12.7
Skin	2 g IV	22	30–180 min	6.6
Skeletal muscle	2 g IV	35	30–280 min	9.4
Myometrium	2 g IV	31	1–2 h	18.7

As with other antibiotics, prolonged use of Ceptaz™ (ceftazidime for injection) may result in overgrowth of nonsusceptible organisms. Repeated evaluation of the patient's condition is essential. If superinfection occurs during therapy, appropriate measures should be taken.

Cephalosporins may be associated with a fall in prothrombin activity. Those at risk include patients with renal and hepatic impairment, or poor nutritional state, as well as patients receiving a protracted course of antimicrobial therapy. Prothrombin time should be monitored in patients at risk and exogenous vitamin K administered as indicated.

Ceptaz should be prescribed with caution in individuals with a history of gastrointestinal disease, particularly colitis.

Arginine has been shown to alter glucose metabolism and elevate serum potassium transiently when administered at 50 times the recommended dose. The effect of lower dosing is not known.

Drug Interactions: Nephrotoxicity has been reported following concomitant administration of cephalosporins with aminoglycoside antibiotics or potent diuretics such as furosemide. Renal function should be carefully monitored, especially if higher dosages of the aminoglycosides are to be administered or if therapy is prolonged, because of the potential nephrotoxicity and ototoxicity of aminoglycosidic antibiotics. Nephrotoxicity and ototoxicity were not noted when ceftazidime was given alone in clinical trials.

Chloramphenicol in combination with cephalosporins, including ceftazidime, has been shown to be antagonistic *in vitro*. Due to the possibility of antagonism *in vivo*, this combination should be avoided.

Drug/Laboratory Test Interactions: The administration of ceftazidime may result in a false-positive reaction for glucose in the urine when using Clinitest® tablets. Benedict's solution, or Fehling's solution. It is recommended that glucose tests based on enzymatic glucose oxidase reactions (such as Clinistix® or Tes-Tape®) be used.

Carcinogenesis, Mutagenesis, Impairment of Fertility: Long-term studies in animals have not been performed to evaluate carcinogenic potential. However, a mouse Micronucleus test and an Ames test were both negative for mutagenic effects.

Pregnancy: ***Teratogenic Effects: Pregnancy Category B:*** Reproduction studies have been performed in mice and rats at doses up to 40 times the human dose and have revealed no evidence of impaired fertility or harm to the fetus due to ceftazidime. Ceptaz at 23 times the human dose was not teratogenic or embryotoxic in a rat reproduction study. There are, however, no adequate and well-controlled studies in pregnant women. Because animal reproduction studies are not always predictive of human response, this drug should be used during pregnancy only if clearly needed.

Nursing Mothers: Ceftazidime is excreted in human milk in low concentrations. It is not known whether the arginine component of this product is excreted in human milk. Because many drugs are excreted in human milk and because safety of the arginine component of Ceptaz in nursing infants has not been established, a decision should be made whether to discontinue nursing or to discontinue the drug, taking into account the importance of the drug to the mother.

Pediatric Use: Safety of the arginine component of Ceptaz in children has not been established. This product is for use in patients 12 years and older. If treatment with ceftazidime is indicated for pediatric patients, a sodium carbonate formulation should be used.

ADVERSE REACTIONS

The following adverse effects from clinical trials were considered to be either related to ceftazidime therapy or were of uncertain etiology. The most common were local reactions following IV injection and allergic and gastrointestinal reactions. No disulfiramlike reactions were reported.

Local Effects, reported in fewer than 2% of patients, were phlebitis and inflammation at the site of injection (1 in 69 patients).

Hypersensitivity Reactions, reported in 2% of patients, were pruritus, rash, and fever. Immediate reactions, generally manifested by rash and/or pruritus, occurred in 1 in 285 patients. Angioedema and anaphylaxis (bronchospasm and/or hypotension) have been reported very rarely.

Gastrointestinal Symptoms, reported in fewer than 2% of patients, were diarrhea (1 in 78), nausea (1 in 156), vomiting (1 in 500), and abdominal pain (1 in 416). The onset of pseudomembranous colitis symptoms may occur during or after treatment (see WARNINGS).

Central Nervous System Reactions (fewer than 1%) included headache, dizziness, and paresthesia. Seizures have been reported with several cephalosporins, including ceftazidime. In addition, encephalopathy, asterixis, and neuromuscular excitability have been reported in renally impaired patients treated with unadjusted dosage regimens of ceftazidime (see PRECAUTIONS: General).

Less Frequent Adverse Events (fewer than 1%) were candidiasis (including oral thrush) and vaginitis.

Hematologic: Exceedingly rare cases of hemolytic anemia have been reported.

Table 3: Recommended Dosage Schedule

	Dose	Frequency
Adults 12 years and older*		
Usual recommended dosage	**1 gram IV or IM**	**q8–12h**
Uncomplicated urinary tract infections	250 mg IV or IM	q12h
Bone and joint infections	2 grams IV	q12h
Complicated urinary tract infections	500 mg IV or IM	q8–12h
Uncomplicated pneumonia; mild skin and skin structure infections	500 mg–1 gram IV or IM	q8h
Serious gynecologic and intra-abdominal infections	2 grams IV	q8h
Meningitis	2 grams IV	q8h
Very severe life-threatening infections, especially in immunocompromised patients	2 grams IV	q8h
Lung infections caused by *Pseudomonas* spp. in patients with cystic fibrosis with normal renal function†	30–50 mg/kg IV to a maximum of 6 grams per day	q8h

*This product is for use in patients 12 years and older. If treatment with ceftazidime is indicated for pediatric patients, a sodium carbonate formulation should be used.

†Although clinical improvement has been shown, bacteriologic cures cannot be expected in patients with chronic respiratory disease and cystic fibrosis.

Laboratory Test Changes noted during ceftazidime clinical trials were transient and included: eosinophilia (1 in 13), positive Coombs' test without hemolysis (1 in 23), thrombocytosis (1 in 45), and slight elevations in one or more of the hepatic enzymes, aspartate aminotransferase (AST, SGOT) (1 in 16), alanine aminotransferase (ALT, SGPT) (1 in 15), LDH (1 in 18), GGT (1 in 19), and alkaline phosphatase (1 in 23). As with some other cephalosporins, transient elevations of blood urea, blood urea nitrogen, and/or serum creatinine were observed occasionally. Transient leukopenia, neutropenia, agranulocytosis, thrombocytopenia, and lymphocytosis were seen very rarely.

In addition to the adverse reactions listed above that have been observed in patients treated with ceftazidime, the following adverse reactions and altered laboratory tests have been reported for cephalosporin-class antibiotics:

Adverse Reactions: Urticaria, Stevens-Johnson syndrome, erythema multiforme, toxic epidermal necrolysis, colitis, renal dysfunction, toxic nephropathy, hepatic dysfunction including cholestasis, aplastic anemia, hemorrhage.

Altered Laboratory Tests: Prolonged prothrombin time, false-positive test for urinary glucose, elevated bilirubin, pancytopenia.

OVERDOSAGE

Ceftazidime overdosage has occurred in patients with renal failure. Reactions have included seizure activity, encephalopathy, asterixis, and neuromuscular excitability. Patients who receive an acute overdosage should be carefully observed and given supportive treatment. In the presence of renal insufficiency, hemodialysis or peritoneal dialysis may aid in the removal of ceftazidime from the body.

DOSAGE AND ADMINISTRATION

Dosage: The usual adult dosage is 1 gram administered intravenously or intramuscularly every 8–12 hours. The dosage and route should be determined by the susceptibility of the causative organisms, the severity of infection, and the condition and renal function of the patient.

The guidelines for dosage of Ceptaz™ (ceftazidime for injection) are listed in Table 3. The following dosage schedule is recommended.

Impaired Hepatic Function: No adjustment in dosage is required for patients with hepatic dysfunction.

Impaired Renal Function: Ceftazidime is excreted by the kidneys, almost exclusively by glomerular filtration. Therefore, in patients with impaired renal function (glomerular filtration rate [GFR] <50 mL per minute), it is recommended that the dosage of ceftazidime be reduced to compensate for its slower excretion. In patients with suspected renal insufficiency, an initial loading dose of 1 gram of Ceptaz may be given. An estimate of GFR should be made to determine the appropriate maintenance dosage. The recommended dosage is presented in Table 4.

When only serum creatinine is available, the following formula (Cockcroft's equation)[4] may be used to estimate creatinine clearance. The serum creatinine should represent a steady state of renal function:

Males:

$$\text{Creatinine clearance (mL/min)} = \frac{\text{Weight (kg)} \times (140-\text{age})}{72 \times \text{serum creatinine (mg/dL)}}$$

Females: 0.85 × male value

In patients with severe infections who would normally receive 6 grams of Ceptaz daily were it not for renal insufficiency, the unit dose given in the table above may be increased by 50% or the dosing frequency may be increased appropriately. Further dosing should be determined by therapeutic monitoring, severity of the infection, and susceptibility of the causative organism.

Table 4: Recommended Maintenance Dosages of Ceptaz in Renal Insufficiency

NOTE: IF THE DOSE RECOMMENDED IN TABLE 3 ABOVE IS LOWER THAN THAT RECOMMENDED FOR PATIENTS WITH RENAL INSUFFICIENCY AS OUTLINED IN TABLE 4, THE LOWER DOSE SHOULD BE USED.

Creatinine Clearance (mL/min)	Recommended Unit Dose of Ceptaz	Frequency of Dosing
50–31	1 gram	q12h
30–16	1 gram	q24h
15–6	500 mg	q24h
<5	500 mg	q48h

In patients undergoing hemodialysis, a loading dose of 1 gram is recommended, followed by 1 gram after each hemodialysis period.

Ceptaz can also be used in patients undergoing intraperitoneal dialysis and continuous ambulatory peritoneal dialysis. In such patients, a loading dose of 1 gram of Ceptaz may be given, followed by 500 mg every 24 hours. It is not known whether or not Ceptaz can be safely incorporated into dialysis fluid.

Note: Generally Ceptaz should be continued for 2 days after the signs and symptoms of infection have disappeared, but in complicated infections longer therapy may be required.

Administration: Ceptaz may be given intravenously or by deep IM injection into a large muscle mass such as the upper outer quadrant of the gluteus maximus or lateral part of the thigh.

Intramuscular Administration: For IM administration, Ceptaz should be constituted with one of the following diluents: sterile water for injection, bacteriostatic water for injection, or 0.5% or 1% lidocaine hydrochloride injection. Refer to Table 5 [on next page].

Intravenous Administration: The IV route is preferable for patients with bacterial septicemia, bacterial meningitis, peritonitis, or other severe or life-threatening infections, or for patients who may be poor risks because of lowered resistance resulting from such debilitating conditions as malnutrition, trauma, surgery, diabetes, heart failure, or malignancy, particularly if shock is present or pending.

For direct intermittent IV administration, constitute Ceptaz as directed in Table 5 with sterile water for injection, 5% dextrose injection, or 0.9% sodium chloride injection. Slowly inject directly into the vein over a period of 3 to 5 minutes or give through the tubing of an administration set while the patient is also receiving one of the compatible IV fluids (see COMPATIBILITY AND STABILITY).

For IV infusion, constitute the 1- or 2-gram infusion pack with 100 mL of sterile water for injection or one of the compatible IV fluids listed under the COMPATIBILITY AND STABILITY section. Alternatively, constitute the 1- or 2-gram vial and add an appropriate quantity of the resulting solution to an IV container with one of the compatible IV fluids.

Intermittent IV infusion with a Y-type administration set can be accomplished with compatible solutions. However, during

Continued on next page

Glaxo—Cont.

infusion of a solution containing ceftazidime, it is desirable to discontinue the other solution.
[See table below.]
Solutions of Ceptaz, like those of most beta-lactam antibiotics, should not be added to solutions of aminoglycoside antibiotics because of potential interaction.
However, if concurrent therapy with Ceptaz and an aminoglycoside is indicated, each of these antibiotics can be administered separately to the same patient.
Instructions for Constitution: Vials of Ceptaz as supplied are under a slightly reduced pressure. This may assist entry of the diluent. No gas-relief needle is required when adding the diluent, except for the infusion pack where it is required during the latter stages of addition (in order to preserve product sterility, a gas-relief needle should not be inserted until an overpressure is produced in the vial). No evolution of gas occurs on constitution. When the vial contents are dissolved, vials other than infusion packs may still be under a reduced pressure. This reduced pressure is particularly noticeable for the 10-g pharmacy bulk package.

COMPATIBILITY AND STABILITY

Intramuscular: Ceptaz™ (ceftazidime for injection), when constituted as directed with sterile water for injection, bacteriostatic water for injection, or 0.5% or 1% lidocaine hydrochloride injection, maintains satisfactory potency for 18 hours at room temperature or for 7 days under refrigeration. Solutions in sterile water for injection that are frozen immediately after constitution in the original container are stable for 6 months when stored at −20°C. Components of the solution may precipitate in the frozen state and will dissolve on reaching room temperature with little or no agitation. Potency is not affected. Frozen solutions should only be thawed at room temperature. Do not force thaw by immersion in water baths or by microwave irradiation. Once thawed, solutions should not be refrozen. Thawed solutions may be stored for up to 12 hours at room temperature or for 7 days in a refrigerator.
Intravenous: ***Ceftazidime concentration greater than 100 mg/mL (2-g vial or 10-g pharmacy bulk package):*** Ceptaz, when constituted as directed with sterile water for injection. 0.9% sodium chloride injection, or 5% dextrose injection, maintains satisfactory potency for 18 hours at room temperature or for 7 days under refrigeration. Solutions of a similar concentration in sterile water for injection that are frozen immediately after constitution in the original container are stable for 6 months when stored at −20°C. Components of the solution may precipitate in the frozen state and will dissolve on reaching room temperature with little or no agitation. Potency is not affected. Frozen solutions should only be thawed at room temperature. Do not force thaw by immersion in water baths or by microwave irradiation. Once thawed, solutions should not be refrozen. Thawed solutions may be stored for up to 12 hours at room temperature or for 7 days in a refrigerator.
Ceftazidime concentration of 100 mg/mL or less (1-g vial or infusion packs):
Ceptaz, when constituted as directed with sterile water for injection, 0.9% sodium chloride injection, or 5% dextrose injection maintains satisfactory potency for 24 hours at room temperature or for 7 days under refrigeration. Solutions, prepared by a pharmacist, of the approved arginine formulation of ceftazidime of a similar concentration in sterile water for injection, 0.9% sodium chloride injection, or 5% dextrose injection in the original container or in 0.9% sodium chloride injection in Viaflex® (PL 146® Plastic) small volume containers that are frozen immediately after constitution by the pharmacist are stable for 6 months when stored at −20°C. Solutions in the PL 146 Plastic small volume containers are in contact with the polyvinyl chloride layer of this container and can leach out certain chemical components of the plastic in very small amounts within the expiration period. The suitability of the plastic has been confirmed in tests in animals according to USP biological tests for plastic containers as well as by tissue culture toxicity studies. Stability of the frozen solution in other containers has not been confirmed. Frozen solutions should only be thawed at room temperature. Do not force thaw by immersion in water baths or by microwave irradiation. For the larger volumes of IV infusion solutions where it may be necessary to warm the frozen product, care should be taken to avoid heating after thawing is complete. Once thawed, solutions should not be refrozen. Thawed solutions may be stored for up to 18 hours at room temperature or for 7 days in a refrigerator.
Components of the solution may precipitate in the frozen state and will dissolve upon reaching room temperature with little or no agitation. Potency is not affected. Check for minute leaks in plastic containers by squeezing bag firmly. Discard bag if leaks are found as sterility may be impaired. Do not add supplementary medication to bags. Do not use unless solution is clear and seal is intact.
Use sterile equipment.
Caution: Do not use plastic containers in series connections. Such use could result in air embolism due to residual air being drawn from the primary container before administration of the fluid from the secondary container is complete.
Preparation for Administration:
1. Suspend container from eyelet support.
2. Remove protector from outlet port at bottom of container.
3. Attach administration set. Refer to complete directions accompanying set.

Ceptaz is compatible with the more commonly used IV infusion fluids. Solutions at concentrations between 1 and 40 mg/mL in 0.9% sodium chloride injection; 1/6 M sodium lactate injection; 5% dextrose injection; 5% dextrose and 0.225% sodium chloride injection; 5% dextrose and 0.45% sodium chloride injection; 5% dextrose and 0.9% sodium chloride injection; 10% dextrose injection; ringer's injection, USP; lactated ringer's injection, USP; 10% invert sugar in sterile water for injection; and Normosol®-M in 5% dextrose injection may be stored for up to 24 hours at room temperature or for 7 days if refrigerated.
Ceptaz is less stable in sodium bicarbonate injection than in other IV fluids. It is not recommended as a diluent. Solutions of Ceptaz in 5% dextrose injection and 0.9% sodium chloride injection are stable for at least 6 hours at room temperature in plastic tubing, drip chambers, and volume control devices of common IV infusion sets.
Ceftazidime at a concentration of 4 mg/mL has been found compatible for 24 hours at room temperature or for 7 days under refrigeration in 0.9% sodium chloride injection or 5% dextrose injection when admixed with: cefuroxime sodium (Zinacef®) 3 mg/mL; heparin sodium in concentrations up to 50 U/mL; or potassium chloride in concentrations up to 40 mEq/L. Ceftazidime may be constituted at a concentration of 20 mg/mL with metronidazole injection 5 mg/mL, and the resultant solution may be stored for 24 hours at room temperature or for 7 days under refrigeration. Ceftazidime at a concentration of 20 mg/mL has been found compatible for 24 hours at room temperature or for 7 days under refrigeration in 0.9% sodium chloride injection or 5% dextrose injection when admixed with 6 mg/mL clindamycin (as clindamycin phosphate).
Vancomycin solution exhibits a physical incompatibility when mixed with a number of drugs, including ceftazidime. The likelihood of precipitation with ceftazidime is dependent on the concentrations of vancomycin and ceftazidime present. It is therefore recommended, when both drugs are to be administered by intermittent IV infusion, that they be given separately, flushing the IV lines (with one of the compatible IV fluids) between the administration of these two agents.
Note: Parenteral drug products should be inspected visually for particulate matter before administration whenever solution and container permit.
As with other cephalosporins, Ceptaz powder as well as solutions tend to darken, depending on storage conditions; within the stated recommendations, however, product potency is not adversely affected.

Table 5: Preparation of Ceptaz Solutions

Size	Amount of Diluent to Be Added (mL)	Volume to Be Withdrawn (mL)	Approximate Ceftazidime Concentration (mg/mL)
Intramuscular			
1-gram vial	3.0	Total	250
Intravenous			
1-gram vial	10.0	Total	90
2-gram vial	10.0	Total	170
Infusion pack			
1-gram vial	100	—	10
2-gram vial	100	—	20
Pharmacy bulk package			
10-gram vial	40	Amount needed	200

Directions for Dispensing: ***Pharmacy Bulk Package—Not for Direct Infusion:*** The pharmacy bulk package is for use in a pharmacy admixture service only under a laminar flow hood. Entry into the vial must be made with a sterile transfer set or other sterile dispensing device, and the contents dispensed in aliquots using aseptic technique. The use of syringe and needle is not recommended as it may cause leakage (see DOSAGE AND ADMINISTRATION). GOOD PHARMACY PRACTICE DICTATES THAT THE CLOSURE BE PENETRATED ONLY ONE TIME AFTER CONSTITUTION. AFTER INITIAL PENETRATION OF THE CLOSURE, USE ENTIRE CONTENTS OF VIAL PROMPTLY. ANY UNUSED PORTION MUST BE DISCARDED WITHIN 18 HOURS OF CONSTITUTION.

HOW SUPPLIED

Ceptaz™ (ceftazidime for injection) in the dry state should be stored between 15° and 30°C (59° and 86°F) and protected from light. Ceptaz is a dry, white to off-white powder supplied in vials and infusion packs as follows:
NDC 0173-0414-00 1-g* Vial (Tray of 25)
NDC 0173-0415-00 2-g* Vial (Tray of 25)
NDC 0173-0416-00 1-g* Infusion Pack (Tray of 10)
NDC 0173-0417-00 2-g* Infusion Pack (Tray of 10)
NDC 0173-0418-00 10-g* Pharmacy Bulk Package (Tray of 6)

REFERENCES

1. Bauer AW, Kirby WMM, Sherris JC, Turck M. Antibiotic susceptibility testing by a standardized single disk method. *Am J Clin Pathol.* 1966;45:493–496.
2. National Committee for Clinical Laboratory Standards. *Approved Standard: Performance Standards for Antimicrobial Disc Susceptibility Tests.* (M2-A3). December 1984.
3. Certification procedure for antibiotic sensitivity discs (21 CFR 460.1). *Federal Register.* May 30, 1974;39: 19182–19184.
4. Cockcroft DW, Gault MH. Prediction of creatinine clearance from serum creatinine. *Nephron.* 1976;16:31–41.

Ceptaz is a trademark of Glaxo.
Clinitest and Clinistix are registered trademarks of Ames Division, Miles Laboratories, Inc.
Tes-Tape is a registered trademark of Eli Lilly and Company.
Viaflex and PL 146 Plastic are registered trademarks of Baxter International Inc.

* Equivalent to anhydrous ceftazidime.

Shown in Product Identification Section, pag 411

FORTAZ® ℞
[for' taz]
(ceftazidime for injection, Glaxo)
FORTAZ® ℞
(ceftazidime sodium injection)

For Intravenous or Intramuscular Use

DESCRIPTION

Ceftazidime is a semisynthetic, broad-spectrum, beta-lactam antibiotic for parenteral administration. It is the pentahydrate of pyridinium, 1-[[7-[[(2-amino-4-thiazolyl)[(1-carboxy-1-methylethoxy) imino]acetyl] amino]-2-carboxy-8-oxo-5-thia -1- azabicyclo[4.2.0]oct-2-en-3-yl]methyl]-, hydroxide, inner salt, [6R-[6α,7β(Z)]]. It has the following structure:

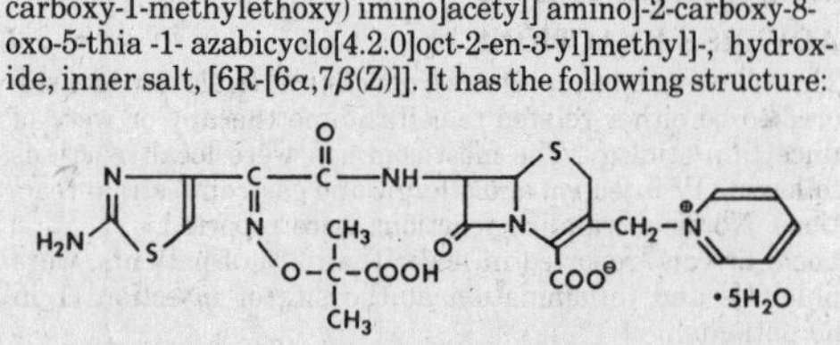

Fortaz® (ceftazidime for injection, Glaxo) is a sterile, dry, powdered mixture of ceftazidime pentahydrate and sodium carbonate. The sodium carbonate at a concentration of 118 mg/g of ceftazidime activity has been admixed to facilitate dissolution. The total sodium content of the mixture is approximately 54 mg (2.3 mEq)/g of ceftazidime activity.
Fortaz in sterile crystalline form is supplied in vials equivalent to 500 mg, 1 g, 2 g, or 6 g of anhydrous ceftazidime and in ADD-Vantage® vials equivalent to 1 or 2 g of anhydrous ceftazidime. Solutions of Fortaz range in color from light yellow to amber, depending on the diluent and volume used. The pH of freshly constituted solutions usually ranges from 5–8.
Fortaz® (ceftazidime sodium injection) is available as a frozen, iso-osmotic, sterile, nonpyrogenic solution with 1 or 2 g of ceftazidime as ceftazidime sodium premixed with approximately 2.2 or 1.6 g, respectively, of dextrose hydrous, USP. Dextrose has been added to adjust the osmolality. Sodium hydroxide is used to adjust pH and neutralize ceftazidime pentahydrate free acid to the sodium salt. The pH may have been adjusted with hydrochloric acid. Solutions of premixed

Fortaz range in color from light yellow to amber. The solution is intended for intravenous (IV) use after thawing to room temperature. The osmolality of the solution is approximately 300 mOsml/kg, and the pH of thawed solutions ranges from 5–7.5.
The plastic container for the frozen solution is fabricated from a specially designed multilayer plastic, PL 2040. Solutions are in contact with the polyethylene layer of this container and can leach out certain chemical components of the plastic in very small amounts within the expiration period. The suitability of the plastic has been confirmed in tests in animals according to USP biological tests for plastic containers as well as by tissue culture toxicity studies.

CLINICAL PHARMACOLOGY

After IV administration of 500-mg and 1-g doses of ceftazidime over 5 minutes to normal adult male volunteers, mean peak serum concentrations of 45 and 90 mcg/mL, respectively, were achieved. After IV infusion of 500-mg, 1-g, and 2-g doses of ceftazidime over 20–30 minutes to normal adult male volunteers, mean peak serum concentrations of 42, 69, and 170 mcg/mL, respectively, were achieved. The average serum concentrations following IV infusion of 500-mg, 1-g, and 2-g doses to these volunteers over an 8-hour interval are given in Table 1.

Table 1

Ceftazidime IV Dose	Serum Concentrations (mcg/mL)				
	0.5 h	1 h	2 h	4 h	8 h
500 mg	42	25	12	6	2
1 g	60	39	23	11	3
2 g	129	75	42	13	5

The absorption and elimination of ceftazidime were directly proportional to the size of the dose. The half-life following IV administration was approximately 1.9 hours. Less than 10% of ceftazidime was protein bound. The degree of protein binding was independent of concentration. There was no evidence of accumulation of ceftazidime in the serum in individuals with normal renal function following multiple IV doses of 1 and 2 g every 8 hours for 10 days.
Following intramuscular (IM) administration of 500-mg and 1-g doses of ceftazidime to normal adult volunteers, the mean peak serum concentrations were 17 and 39 mcg/mL, respectively, at approximately 1 hour. Serum concentrations remained above 4 mcg/mL for 6 and 8 hours after the IM administration of 500-mg and 1-g doses, respectively. The half-life of ceftazidime in these volunteers was approximately 2 hours.
The presence of hepatic dysfunction had no effect on the pharmacokinetics of ceftazidime in individuals administered 2 g intravenously every 8 hours for 5 days. Therefore, a dosage adjustment from the normal recommended dosage is not required for patients with hepatic dysfunction, provided renal function is not impaired.
Approximately 80%–90% of an IM or IV dose of ceftazidime is excreted unchanged by the kidneys over a 24-hour period. After the IV administration of single 500-mg or 1-g doses, approximately 50% of the dose appeared in the urine in the first 2 hours. An additional 20% was excreted between 2 and 4 hours after dosing, and approximately another 12% of the dose appeared in the urine between 4 and 8 hours later. The elimination of ceftazidime by the kidneys resulted in high therapeutic concentrations in the urine.
The mean renal clearance of ceftazidime was approximately 100 mL per minute. The calculated plasma clearance of approximately 115 mL per minute indicated nearly complete elimination of ceftazidime by the renal route. Administration of probenecid before dosing had no effect on the elimination kinetics of ceftazidime. This suggested that ceftazidime is eliminated by glomerular filtration and is not actively secreted by renal tubular mechanisms.
Since ceftazidime is eliminated almost solely by the kidneys, its serum half-life is significantly prolonged in patients with impaired renal function. Consequently, dosage adjustments in such patients as described in the DOSAGE AND ADMINISTRATION section are suggested.
Therapeutic concentrations of ceftazidime are achieved in the following body tissues and fluids.
[See table above.]

Table 2: Ceftazidime Concentrations in Body Tissues and Fluids

Tissue or Fluid	Dose/ Route	No. of Patients	Time of Sample Postdose	Average Tissue or Fluid Level (mcg/mL or mcg/g)
Urine	500 mg IM	6	0–2 h	2,100.0
	2 g IV	6	0–2 h	12,000.0
Bile	2 g IV	3	90 min	36.4
Synovial fluid	2 g IV	13	2 h	25.6
Peritoneal fluid	2 g IV	8	2 h	48.6
Sputum	1 g IV	8	1 h	9.0
Cerebrospinal fluid	2 g q8h IV	5	120 min	9.8
(inflamed meninges)	2 g q8h IV	6	180 min	9.4
Aqueous humor	2 g IV	13	1–3 h	11.0
Blister fluid	1 g IV	7	2–3 h	19.7
Lymphatic fluid	1 g IV	7	2–3 h	23.4
Bone	2 g IV	8	0.67 h	31.1
Heart muscle	2 g IV	35	30–280 min	12.7
Skin	2 g IV	22	30–180 min	6.6
Skeletal muscle	2 g IV	35	30–280 min	9.4
Myometrium	2 g IV	31	1–2 h	18.7

Microbiology: Ceftazidime is bactericidal in action, exerting its effect by inhibition of enzymes responsible for cell-wall synthesis. A wide range of gram-negative organisms is susceptible to ceftazidime *in vitro*, including strains resistant to gentamicin and other aminoglycosides. In addition, ceftazidime has been shown to be active against gram-positive organisms. It is highly stable to most clinically important beta-lactamases, plasmid or chromosomal, which are produced by both gram-negative and gram-positive organisms and, consequently, is active against many strains resistant to ampicillin and other cephalosporins.
Ceftazidime has been shown to be active against the following organisms both *in vitro* and in clinical infections (see INDICATIONS AND USAGE).
Aerobes, Gram-negative: *Citrobacter* spp., including *Citrobacter freundii* and *Citrobacter diversus; Enterobacter* spp., including *Enterobacter cloacae* and *Enterobacter aerogenes; Escherichia coli; Haemophilus influenzae,* including ampicillin-resistant strains; *Klebsiella* spp. (including *Klebsiella pneumoniae*); *Neisseria meningitidis; Proteus mirabilis; Proteus vulgaris; Pseudomonas* spp. (including *Pseudomonas aeruginosa*); and *Serratia* spp.
Aerobes, Gram-positive: *Staphylococcus aureus,* including penicillinase- and non–penicillinase-producing strains; *Streptococcus agalactiae* (group B streptococci); *Streptococcus pneumoniae;* and *Streptococcus pyogenes* (group A beta-hemolytic streptococci).
Anaerobes: *Bacteroides* spp (NOTE: many strains of *Bacteroides fragilis* are resistant).
Ceftazidime has been shown to be active *in vitro* against most strains of the following organisms; however, the clinical significance of these data is unknown: *Acinetobacter* spp.; *Clostridium* spp. (not including *Clostridium difficile*); *Haemophilus parainfluenzae; Morganella morganii* (formerly *Proteus morganii*); *Neisseria gonorrhoeae; Peptococcus* spp.; *Peptostreptococcus* spp.; *Providencia* spp. (including *Providencia rettgeri,* formerly *Proteus rettgeri*); *Salmonella* spp.; *Shigella* spp.; *Staphylococcus epidermidis;* and *Yersinia enterocolitica.*
Ceftazidime and the aminoglycosides have been shown to be synergistic *in vitro* against *Pseudomonas aeruginosa* and the enterobacteriaceae. Ceftazidime and carbenicillin have also been shown to be synergistic *in vitro* against *Pseudomonas aeruginosa.*
Ceftazidime is not active *in vitro* against methicillin-resistant staphylococci; *Streptococcus faecalis* and many other enterococci; *Listeria monocytogenes; Campylobacter* spp.; or *Clostridium difficile.*
Susceptibility Tests: ***Diffusion Techniques:*** Quantitative methods that require measurement of zone diameters give an estimate of antibiotic susceptibility. One such procedure[1–3] has been recommended for use with disks to test susceptibility to ceftazidime.
Reports from the laboratory giving results of the standard single-disk susceptibility test with a 30-mcg ceftazidime disk should be interpreted according to the following criteria:
Susceptible organisms produce zones of 18 mm or greater, indicating that the test organism is likely to respond to therapy.
Organisms that produce zones of 15–17 mm are expected to be susceptible if high dosage is used or if the infection is confined to tissues and fluids (e.g., urine) in which high antibiotic levels are attained.
Resistant organisms produce zones of 14 mm or less, indicating that other therapy should be selected.
Organisms should be tested with the ceftazidime disk since ceftazidime has been shown by *in vitro* tests to be active against certain strains found resistant when other beta-lactam disks are used.
Standardized procedures require the use of laboratory control organisms. The 30-mcg ceftazidime disk should give zone diameters between 25 and 32 mm for *Escherichia coli* ATCC 25922. For *Pseudomonas aeruginosa* ATCC 27853, the zone diameters should be between 22 and 29 mm. For *Staphylococcus aureus* ATCC 25923, the zone diameters should be between 16 and 20 mm.
Dilution Techniques: In other susceptibility testing procedures, e.g., ICS agar dilution or the equivalent, a bacterial isolate may be considered susceptible if the minimum inhibitory concentration (MIC) value for ceftazidime is not more than 16 mcg/mL. Organisms are considered resistant to ceftazidime if the MIC is equal to or greater than 64 mcg/mL. Organisms having an MIC value of less than 64 mcg/mL but greater than 16 mcg/mL are expected to be susceptible if high dosage is used or if the infection is confined to tissues and fluids (e.g., urine) in which high antibiotic levels are attained.
As with standard diffusion methods, dilution procedures require the use of laboratory control organisms. Standard ceftazidime powder should give MIC values in the range of 4–16 mcg/mL for *Staphylococcus aureus* ATCC 25923. For *Escherichia coli* ATCC 25922, the MIC range should be between 0.125 and 0.5 mcg/mL. For *Pseudomonas aeruginosa* ATCC 27853, the MIC range should be between 0.5 and 2 mcg/mL.

INDICATIONS AND USAGE

Fortaz® (ceftazidime for injection/ceftazidime sodium injection) is indicated for the treatment of patients with infections caused by susceptible strains of the designated organisms in the following diseases:

1. **Lower Respiratory Tract Infections,** including pneumonia, caused by *Pseudomonas aeruginosa* and other *Pseudomonas* spp.; *Haemophilus influenzae,* including ampicillin-resistant strains; *Klebsiella* spp.; *Enterobacter* spp.; *Proteus mirabilis; Escherichia coli; Serratia* spp.; *Citrobacter* spp.; *Streptococcus pneumoniae;* and *Staphylococcus aureus* (methicillin-susceptible strains).
2. **Skin and Skin Structure Infections** caused by *Pseudomonas aeruginosa; Klebsiella* spp.; *Escherichia coli; Proteus* spp., including *Proteus mirabilis* and indole-positive *Proteus; Enterobacter* spp.; *Serratia* spp.; *Staphylococcus aureus* (methicillin-susceptible strains); and *Streptococcus pyogenes* (group A beta-hemolytic streptococci).
3. **Urinary Tract Infections,** both complicated and uncomplicated, caused by *Pseudomonas aeruginosa; Enterobacter* spp.; *Proteus* spp., including *Proteus mirabilis* and indole-positive *Proteus; Klebsiella* spp.; and *Escherichia coli.*
4. **Bacterial Septicemia** caused by *Pseudomonas aeruginosa; Klebsiella* spp.; *Haemophilus influenzae; Escherichia coli; Serratia* spp.; *Streptococcus pneumoniae;* and *Staphylococcus aureus* (methicillin-susceptible strains).
5. **Bone and Joint Infections** caused by *Pseudomonas aeruginosa; Klebsiella* spp.; *Enterobacter* spp.; and *Staphylococcus aureus* (methicillin-susceptible strains).
6. **Gynecologic Infections,** including endometritis, pelvic cellulitis, and other infections of the female genital tract caused by *Escherichia coli.*
7. **Intra-abdominal Infections,** including peritonitis caused by *Escherichia coli, Klebsiella* spp., and *Staphylococcus aureus* (methicillin-susceptible strains) and polymicrobial infections caused by aerobic and anaerobic organisms and *Bacteroides* spp. (many strains of *Bacteroides fragilis* are resistant).
8. **Central Nervous System Infections,** including meningitis, caused by *Haemophilus influenzae* and *Neisseria meningitidis.* Fortaz has also been used successfully in a limited number of cases of meningitis due to *Pseudomonas aeruginosa* and *Streptococcus pneumoniae.*

Specimens for bacterial cultures should be obtained before therapy in order to isolate and identify causative organisms and to determine their susceptibility to ceftazidime. Therapy may be instituted before results of susceptibility studies are known; however, once these results become available, the antibiotic treatment should be adjusted accordingly.
Fortaz may be used alone in cases of confirmed or suspected sepsis. Fortaz has been used successfully in clinical trials as empiric therapy in cases where various concomitant therapies with other antibiotics have been used.

Continued on next page

Glaxo—Cont.

Fortaz may also be used concomitantly with other antibiotics, such as aminoglycosides, vancomycin, and clindamycin; in severe and life-threatening infections; and in the immunocompromised patient. When such concomitant treatment is appropriate, prescribing information in the labeling for the other antibiotics should be followed. The dose depends on the severity of the infection and the patient's condition.

CONTRAINDICATIONS

Fortaz® (ceftazidime for injection/ceftazidime sodium injection) is contraindicated in patients who have shown hypersensitivity to ceftazidime or the cephalosporin group of antibiotics.

WARNINGS

BEFORE THERAPY WITH FORTAZ® (CEFTAZIDIME FOR INJECTION, CEFTAZIDIME SODIUM INJECTION) IS INSTITUTED, CAREFUL INQUIRY SHOULD BE MADE TO DETERMINE WHETHER THE PATIENT HAS HAD PREVIOUS HYPERSENSITIVITY REACTIONS TO CEFTAZIDIME, CEPHALOSPORINS, PENICILLINS, OR OTHER DRUGS. IF THIS PRODUCT IS TO BE GIVEN TO PENICILLIN-SENSITIVE PATIENTS, CAUTION SHOULD BE EXERCISED BECAUSE CROSS-HYPERSENSITIVITY AMONG BETA-LACTAM ANTIBIOTICS HAS BEEN CLEARLY DOCUMENTED AND MAY OCCUR IN UP TO 10% OF PATIENTS WITH A HISTORY OF PENICILLIN ALLERGY. IF AN ALLERGIC REACTION TO FORTAZ OCCURS, DISCONTINUE THE DRUG. SERIOUS ACUTE HYPERSENSITIVITY REACTIONS MAY REQUIRE TREATMENT WITH EPINEPHRINE AND OTHER EMERGENCY MEASURES, INCLUDING OXYGEN, IV FLUIDS, IV ANTIHISTAMINES, CORTICOSTEROIDS, PRESSOR AMINES, AND AIRWAY MANAGEMENT, AS CLINICALLY INDICATED.

Pseudomembranous colitis has been reported with nearly all antibacterial agents, including ceftazidime, and may range from mild to life-threatening. Therefore, it is important to consider this diagnosis in patients who present with diarrhea subsequent to the administration of antibacterial agents.

Treatment with antibacterial agents alters the normal flora of the colon and may permit overgrowth of clostridia. Studies indicate that a toxin produced by *Clostridium difficile* is a primary cause of "antibiotic-associated colitis."

After the diagnosis of pseudomembranous colitis has been established, therapeutic measures should be initiated. Mild cases of pseudomembranous colitis usually respond to discontinuation of the drug alone. In moderate to severe cases, consideration should be given to management with fluids and electrolytes, protein supplementation and treatment with an antibacterial drug effective against *Clostridium difficile*.

Elevated levels of ceftazidime in patients with renal insufficiency can lead to seizures, encephalopathy, asterixis, and neuromuscular excitability (see PRECAUTIONS).

PRECAUTIONS

General: Ceftazidime has not been shown to be nephrotoxic; however, high and prolonged serum antibiotic concentrations can occur from usual doses in patients with transient or persistent reduction of urinary output because of renal insufficiency. The total daily dosage should be reduced when ceftazidime is administered to patients with renal insufficiency (see DOSAGE AND ADMINISTRATION). Elevated levels of ceftazidime in these patients can lead to seizures, encephalopathy, asterixis, and neuromuscular excitability. Continued dosage should be determined by degree of renal impairment, severity of infection, and susceptibility of the causative organisms.

As with other antibiotics, prolonged use of Fortaz® (ceftazidime for injection/ceftazidime sodium injection) may result in overgrowth of nonsusceptible organisms. Repeated evaluation of the patient's condition is essential. If superinfection occurs during therapy, appropriate measures should be taken.

Cephalosporins may be associated with a fall in prothrombin activity. Those at risk include patients with renal and hepatic impairment, or poor nutritional state, as well as patients receiving a protracted course of antimicrobial therapy. Prothrombin time should be monitored in patients at risk and exogenous vitamin K administered as indicated.

Fortaz should be prescribed with caution in individuals with a history of gastrointestinal disease, particularly colitis.

Drug Interactions: Nephrotoxicity has been reported following concomitant administration of cephalosporins with aminoglycoside antibiotics or potent diuretics such as furosemide. Renal function should be carefully monitored, especially if higher dosages of the aminoglycosides are to be administered or if therapy is prolonged, because of the potential nephrotoxicity and ototoxicity of aminoglycosidic antibiotics. Nephrotoxicity and ototoxicity were not noted when ceftazidime was given alone in clinical trials.

Chloramphenicol in combination with cephalosporins, including ceftazidime, has been shown to be antagonistic *in vitro*. Due to the possibility of an antagonism *in vivo*, this combination should be avoided.

Drug/Laboratory Test Interactions: The administration of ceftazidime may result in a false-positive reaction for glucose in the urine using Clinitest® tablets, Benedict's solution, or Fehling's solution. It is recommended that glucose tests based on enzymatic glucose oxidase reactions (such as Clinistix® or Tes-Tape®) be used.

Carcinogenesis, Mutagenesis, Impairment of Fertility: Long-term studies in animals have not been performed to evaluate carcinogenic potential. However, a mouse Micronucleus test and an Ames test were both negative for mutagenic effects.

Pregnancy: ***Teratogenic Effects: Pregnancy Category B:*** Reproduction studies have been performed in mice and rats at doses up to 40 times the human dose and have revealed no evidence of impaired fertility or harm to the fetus due to Fortaz. There are, however, no adequate and well-controlled studies in pregnant women. Because animal reproduction studies are not always predictive of human response, this drug should be used during pregnancy only if clearly needed.

Nursing Mothers: Ceftazidime is excreted in human milk in low concentrations. Caution should be exercised when Fortaz is administered to a nursing woman.

Pediatric Use: (see DOSAGE AND ADMINISTRATION).

ADVERSE REACTIONS

Ceftazidime is generally well tolerated. The incidence of adverse reactions associated with the administration of ceftazidime was low in clinical trials. The most common were local reactions following IV injection and allergic and gastrointestinal reactions. Other adverse reactions were encountered infrequently. No disulfiramlike reactions were reported.

The following adverse effects from clinical trials were considered to be either related to ceftazidime therapy or were of uncertain etiology:

Local Effects, reported in fewer than 2% of patients, were phlebitis and inflammation at the site of injection (1 in 69 patients).

Hypersensitivity Reactions, reported in 2% of patients, were pruritus, rash, and fever. Immediate reactions, generally manifested by rash and/or pruritus, occurred in 1 in 285 patients. Angioedema and anaphylaxis (bronchospasm and/or hypotension) have been reported very rarely.

Gastrointestinal Symptoms, reported in fewer than 2% of patients, were diarrhea (1 in 78), nausea (1 in 156), vomiting (1 in 500), and abdominal pain (1 in 416). The onset of pseudomembranous colitis symptoms may occur during or after treatment (see WARNINGS).

Central Nervous System Reactions (fewer than 1%) included headache, dizziness, and paresthesia. Seizures have been reported with several cephalosporins, including ceftazidime. In addition, encephalopathy, asterixis, and neuromuscular excitability have been reported in renally impaired patients treated with unadjusted dosage regimens of ceftazidime (see PRECAUTIONS: General).

Less Frequent Adverse Events (fewer than 1%) were candidiasis (including oral thrush) and vaginitis.

Hematologic: Exceedingly rare cases of hemolytic anemia have been reported.

Laboratory Test Changes noted during Fortaz clinical trials were transient and included: eosinophilia (1 in 13), positive Coombs' test without hemolysis (1 in 23), thrombocytosis (1 in 45), and slight elevations in one or more of the hepatic enzymes, aspartate aminotransferase (AST, SGOT) (1 in 16), alanine aminotransferase (ALT, SGPT) (1 in 15), LDH (1 in 18), GGT (1 in 19), and alkaline phosphatase (1 in 23). As with some other cephalosporins, transient elevations of blood urea, blood urea nitrogen, and/or serum creatinine were observed occasionally. Transient leukopenia, neutropenia, agranulocytosis, thrombocytopenia, and lymphocytosis were seen very rarely.

In addition to the adverse reactions listed above that have been observed in patients treated with ceftazidime, the following adverse reactions and altered laboratory tests have been reported for cephalosporin-class antibiotics:

Adverse Reactions: Urticaria, Stevens-Johnson syndrome, erythema multiforme, toxic epidermal necrolysis, colitis, renal dysfunction, toxic nephropathy, hepatic dysfunction including cholestasis, aplastic anemia, hemorrhage.

Altered Laboratory Tests: Prolonged prothrombin time, false-positive test for urinary glucose, elevated bilirubin, pancytopenia.

OVERDOSAGE

Ceftazidime overdosage has occurred in patients with renal failure. Reactions have included seizure activity, encephalopathy, asterixis, and neuromuscular excitability. Patients who receive an acute overdosage should be carefully observed and given supportive treatment. In the presence of renal insufficiency, hemodialysis or peritoneal dialysis may aid in the removal of ceftazidime from the body.

DOSAGE AND ADMINISTRATION

Dosage: The usual adult dosage is 1 gram administered intravenously or intramuscularly every 8–12 hours. The dosage and route should be determined by the susceptibility of the causative organisms, the severity of infection, and the condition and renal function of the patient.

The guidelines for dosage of Fortaz® (ceftazidime for injection/ceftazidime sodium injection) are listed in Table 3. The following dosage schedule is recommended. [See table.]

Impaired Hepatic Function: No adjustment in dosage is required for patients with hepatic dysfunction.

Impaired Renal Function: Ceftazidime is excreted by the kidneys, almost exclusively by glomerular filtration. Therefore, in patients with impaired renal function (glomerular filtration rate [GFR] <50 mL per minute), it is recommended that the dosage of ceftazidime be reduced to compensate for its slower excretion. In patients with suspected renal insufficiency, an initial loading dose of 1 gram of Fortaz may be given. An estimate of GFR should be made to determine the appropriate maintenance dose. The recommended dosage is presented in Table 4. [See next page.]

When only serum creatinine is available, the following formula (Cockcroft's equation)[4] may be used to estimate creatinine clearance. The serum creatinine should represent a steady state of renal function:

Males:

$$\text{Creatinine clearance (mL/min)} = \frac{\text{Weight (kg)} \times (140 - \text{age})}{72 \times \text{serum creatinine (mg/dL)}}$$

Females: 0.85 × male value

Table 3: Recommended Dosage Schedule

	Dose	Frequency
Adults		
Usual recommended dosage	**1 gram IV or IM**	**q8–12h**
Uncomplicated urinary tract infections	250 mg IV or IM	q12h
Bone and joint infections	2 grams IV	q12h
Complicated urinary tract infections	500 mg IV or IM	q8–12h
Uncomplicated pneumonia; mild skin and skin structure infections	500 mg–1 gram IV or IM	q8h
Serious gynecologic and intra-abdominal infections	2 grams IV	q8h
Meningitis	2 grams IV	q8h
Very severe life-threatening infections, especially in immunocompromised patients	2 grams IV	q8h
Lung infections caused by *Pseudomonas* spp. in patients with cystic fibrosis with normal renal function*	30–50 mg/kg IV to a maximum of 6 grams per day	q8h
Neonates (0–4 weeks)	30 mg/kg IV	q12h
Infants and children (1 month–12 years)	30–50 mg/kg IV to a maximum of 6 grams per day†	q8h

*Although clinical improvement has been shown, bacteriologic cures cannot be expected in patients with chronic respiratory disease and cystic fibrosis.

†The higher dose should be reserved for immunocompromised children or children with cystic fibrosis or meningitis.

Table 4: Recommended Maintenance Dosages of Fortaz in Renal Insufficiency
NOTE: IF THE DOSE RECOMMENDED IN TABLE 3 ABOVE IS LOWER THAN THAT RECOMMENDED FOR PATIENTS WITH RENAL INSUFFICIENCY AS OUTLINED IN TABLE 4, THE LOWER DOSE SHOULD BE USED.

Creatinine Clearance (mL/min)	Recommended Unit Dose of Fortaz	Frequency of Dosing
50–31	1 gram	q12h
30–16	1 gram	q24h
15–6	500 mg	q24h
<5	500 mg	q48h

In patients with severe infections who would normally receive 6 grams of Fortaz daily were it not for renal insufficiency, the unit dose given in the table above may be increased by 50% or the dosing frequency may be increased appropriately. Further dosing should be determined by therapeutic monitoring, severity of the infection, and susceptibility of the causative organism.
In children as for adults, the creatinine clearance should be adjusted for body surface area or lean body mass, and the dosing frequency should be reduced in cases of renal insufficiency.
In patients undergoing hemodialysis, a loading dose of 1 gram is recommended, followed by 1 gram after each hemodialysis period.
Fortaz can also be used in patients undergoing intraperitoneal dialysis and continuous ambulatory peritoneal dialysis. In such patients, a loading dose of 1 gram of Fortaz may be given, followed by 500 mg every 24 hours. In addition to IV use, Fortaz can be incorporated in the dialysis fluid at a concentration of 250 mg for 2 L of dialysis fluid.
Note: Generally Fortaz should be continued for 2 days after the signs and symptoms of infection have disappeared, but in complicated infections longer therapy may be required.
Administration: Fortaz may be given intravenously or by deep intramuscular injection into a large muscle mass such as the upper outer quadrant of the gluteus maximus or lateral part of the thigh.
Intramuscular Administration: For IM administration, Fortaz should be constituted with one of the following diluents: sterile water for injection, bacteriostatic water for injection, or 0.5% or 1% lidocaine hydrochloride injection. Refer to Table 5.
Intravenous Administration: The IV route is preferable for patients with bacterial septicemia, bacterial meningitis, peritonitis, or other severe or life-threatening infections, or for patients who may be poor risks because of lowered resistance resulting from such debilitating conditions as malnutrition, trauma, surgery, diabetes, heart failure, or malignancy, particularly if shock is present or pending.
For direct intermittent IV administration, constitute Fortaz as directed in Table 5 with sterile water for injection. Slowly inject directly into the vein over a period of 3–5 minutes or give through the tubing of an administration set while the patient is also receiving one of the compatible IV fluids (see COMPATIBILITY AND STABILITY).
For IV infusion, constitute the 1- or 2-gram infusion pack with 100 mL of sterile water for injection or one of the compatible IV fluids listed under the COMPATIBILITY AND STABILITY section. Alternatively, constitute the 500-mg, 1 gram, or 2-gram vial and add an appropriate quantity of the resulting solution to an IV container with one of the compatible IV fluids.
Intermittent IV infusion with a Y-type administration set can be accomplished with compatible solutions. However, during infusion of a solution containing ceftazidime, it is desirable to discontinue the other solution.
ADD-Vantage® vials are to be constituted only with 50 or 100 mL of 5% dextrose injection, 0.9% sodium chloride injection, or 0.45% sodium chloride injection in Abbott ADD-Vantage flexible diluent containers (see Instructions for Constitution). ADD-Vantage vials that have been joined to Abbott ADD-Vantage diluent containers and activated to dissolve the drug are stable for 24 hours at room temperature or for 7 days under refrigeration. Joined vials that have not been activated may be used within a 14-day period; this period corresponds to that for use of Abbott ADD-Vantage containers following removal of the outer packaging (overwrap).
Freezing solutions of Fortaz in the ADD-Vantage system is not recommended.
[See Table 5 above.]
All vials of Fortaz as supplied are under reduced pressure. When Fortaz is dissolved, carbon dioxide is released and a positive pressure develops. For ease of use please follow the recommended techniques of constitution described on the detachable Instructions for Constitution section of the product package insert.

Table 5: Preparation of Fortaz Solutions

Size	Amount of Diluent to Be Added (mL)	Approximate Available Volume (mL)	Approximate Ceftazidime Concentration (mg/mL)
Intramuscular			
500-mg vial	1.5	1.8	280
1-gram vial	3.0	3.6	280
Intravenous			
500-mg vial	5.0	5.3	100
1-gram vial	10.0	10.6	100
2-gram vial	10.0	11.5	170
Infusion pack			
1-gram vial	100*	100	10
2-gram vial	100*	100	20
Pharmacy bulk package			
6-gram vial	26	30	200

* **Note:** Addition should be in two stages (see Instructions for Constitution accompanying the product package insert).

Solutions of Fortaz, like those of most beta-lactam antibiotics, should not be added to solutions of aminoglycoside antibiotics because of potential interaction.
However, if concurrent therapy with Fortaz and an aminoglycoside is indicated, each of these antibiotics can be administered separately to the same patient.
Directions for Use of Fortaz® (ceftazidime sodium injection) Frozen in Galaxy® Plastic Containers: Fortaz supplied as a frozen, sterile, iso-osmotic, nonpyrogenic solution in plastic containers is to be administered after thawing either as a continuous or intermittent IV infusion. The thawed solution is stable for 24 hours at room temperature or for 7 days if stored under refrigeration. **Do not Refreeze.**
Thaw container at room temperature (25°C) or under refrigeration (5°C). Do not force thaw by immersion in water baths or by microwave irradiation. Components of the solution may precipitate in the frozen state and will dissolve upon reaching room temperature with little or no agitation. Potency is not affected. Mix after solution has reached room temperature. Check for minute leaks by squeezing bag firmly. Discard bag if leaks are found as sterility may be impaired. Do not add supplementary medication. Do not use unless solution is clear and seal is intact.
Use sterile equipment.
Caution: Do not use plastic containers in series connections. Such use could result in air embolism due to residual air being drawn from the primary container before administration of the fluid from the secondary container is complete.
Preparation for Administration:
1. Suspend container from eyelet support.
2. Remove protector from outlet port at bottom of container.
3. Attach administration set. Refer to complete directions accompanying set.

COMPATIBILITY AND STABILITY

Intramuscular: Fortaz® (ceftazidime for injection), when constituted as directed with sterile water for injection, bacteriostatic water for injection, or 0.5% or 1% lidocaine hydrochloride injection, maintains satisfactory potency for 24 hours at room temperature or for 7 days under refrigeration. Solutions in sterile water for injection that are frozen immediately after constitution in the original container are stable for 3 months when stored at −20°C. Once thawed, solutions should not be refrozen. Thawed solutions may be stored for up to 8 hours at room temperature or for 4 days in a refrigerator.
Intravenous: Fortaz, when constituted as directed with sterile water for injection, maintains satisfactory potency for 24 hours at room temperature or for 7 days under refrigeration. Solutions in sterile water for injection in the infusion vial or in 0.9% sodium chloride injection in Viaflex® small-volume containers that are frozen immediately after constitution are stable for 6 months when stored at −20°C. Do not force thaw by immersion in water baths or by microwave irradiation. Once thawed, solutions should not be refrozen. Thawed solutions may be stored for up to 24 hours at room temperature or for 7 days in a refrigerator. More concentrated solutions in sterile water for injection in the original container that are frozen immediately after constitution are stable for 3 months when stored at -20°C. Once thawed, solutions should not be refrozen. Thawed solutions may be stored for up to 8 hours at room temperature or for 4 days in a refrigerator.
Fortaz is compatible with the more commonly used IV infusion fluids. Solutions at concentrations between 1 and 40 mg/mL in 0.9% sodium chloride injection; 1/6 M sodium lactate injection; 5% dextrose injection; 5% dextrose and 0.225% sodium chloride injection; 5% dextrose and 0.45% sodium chloride injection; 5% dextrose and 0.9% sodium chloride injection; 10% dextrose injection; ringer's injection, USP; lactated ringer's injection, USP; 10% invert sugar in water for injection; and Normosol®-M in 5% dextrose injection may be stored for up to 24 hours at room temperature or for 7 days if refrigerated.
The 1- and 2-g Fortaz ADD-Vantage® vials, when diluted in 50 or 100 mL of 5% dextrose injection, 0.9% sodium chloride injection, or 0.45% sodium chloride injection, may be stored for up to 24 hours at room temperature or for 7 days under refrigeration.
Fortaz is less stable in sodium bicarbonate injection than in other IV fluids. It is not recommended as a diluent. Solutions of Fortaz in 5% dextrose injection and 0.9% sodium chloride injection are stable for at least 6 hours at room temperature in plastic tubing, drip chambers, and volume control devices of common IV infusion sets.
Ceftazidime at a concentration of 4 mg/mL has been found compatible for 24 hours at room temperature or for 7 days under refrigeration in 0.9% sodium chloride injection or 5% dextrose injection when admixed with: cefuroxime sodium (Zinacef®) 3 mg/mL; heparin 10 or 50 U/mL; or potassium chloride 10 or 40 mEq/L.
Vancomycin solution exhibits a physical incompatibility when mixed with a number of drugs, including ceftazidime. The likelihood of precipitation with ceftazidime is dependent on the concentrations of vancomycin and ceftazidime present. It is therefore recommended, when both drugs are to be administered by intermittent IV infusion, that they be given separately, flushing the IV lines (with one of the compatible IV fluids) between the administration of these two agents.
Note: Parenteral drug products should be inspected visually for particulate matter before administration whenever solution and container permit.
As with other cephalosporins, Fortaz powder as well as solutions tend to darken, depending on storage conditions; within the stated recommendations, however, product potency is not adversely affected.

HOW SUPPLIED

Fortaz® (ceftazidime for injection) in the dry state should be stored between 15° and 30°C (59° and 86°F) and protected from light. Fortaz is a dry, white to off-white powder supplied in vials and infusion packs as follows:
NDC 0173-0377-31 500-mg* Vial (Tray of 25)
NDC 0173-0378-35 1-g* Vial (Tray of 25)
NDC 0173-0379-34 2-g* Vial (Tray of 10)
NDC 0173-0380-32 1-g* Infusion Pack (Tray of 10)
NDC 0173-0381-32 2-g* Infusion Pack (Tray of 10)
NDC 0173-0382-37 6-g* Pharmacy Bulk Package (Tray of 6)
NDC 0173-0434-00 1-g ADD-Vantage® Vial (Tray of 25)
NDC 0173-0435-00 2-g ADD-Vantage® Vial (Tray of 10)
(The above ADD-Vantage vials are to be used only with Abbott ADD-Vantage diluent containers.)
Fortaz® (ceftazidime sodium injection) frozen as a premixed solution of ceftazidime sodium should not be stored above −20° C. Fortaz is supplied frozen in 50-mL, single-dose, plastic containers as follows:
NDC 0173-0412-00 1-g* Plastic Container
NDC 0713-0413-00 2-g* Plastic Container

REFERENCES: 1. Bauer AW, Kirby WMM, Sherris JC, Turck M. Antibiotic susceptibility testing by a standardized single disk method. *Am J Clin Pathol* 1966;45:493–496.
2. National Committee for Clinical Laboratory Standards. *Approved Standard: Performance Standards for Antimicrobial Disc Susceptibility Tests.* (M2-A3). December 1984.
3. Certification procedure for antibiotic sensitivity discs (21 CFR 460.1). *Federal Register.* May 30, 1974;39:19182-19184.
4. Cockcroft DW, Gault MH. Prediction of creatinine clearance from serum creatinine. *Nephron* 1976;16:31-41.

Fortaz is a registered trademark of Glaxo.
Galaxy is a trademark of Baxter International Inc.
ADD-Vantage is a registered trademark of Abbott Laboratories.
Clinitest and Clinistix are registered trademarks of Ames Division, Miles Laboratories, Inc.

*Equivalent to anhydrous ceftazidime.

Continued on next page

Glaxo—Cont.

Tes-Tape is a registered trademark of Eli Lilly and Company. Galaxy and Viaflex are registered trademarks of Baxter International Inc.

Shown in Product Identification Section, pages 410 and 411

ZANTAC® Injection ℞
[zan 'tak]
(ranitidine hydrochloride)

ZANTAC® Injection Premixed ℞
(ranitidine hydrochloride)

DESCRIPTION

The active ingredient in Zantac® Injection and Zantac® Injection Premixed is ranitidine hydrochloride (HCl), a histamine H_2-receptor antagonist. Chemically it is N[2-[[[5-[(dimethylamino)methyl]-2-furanyl]methyl]thio]ethyl]-N'-methyl-2-nitro-1,1-ethenediamine, hydrochloride. The empirical formula is $C_{13}H_{22}N_4O_3S \cdot HCl$, representing a molecular weight of 350.87.

Ranitidine HCl is a white to pale yellow, granular substance that is soluble in water.

Zantac Injection is a clear, colorless to yellow, nonpyrogenic liquid that tends to darken slightly without adversely affecting potency. The pH of the injection solution is 6.7–7.3.

Sterile Injection for Intramuscular or Intravenous Administration: Each 1 mL of aqueous solution contains ranitidine 25 mg (as the hydrochloride); phenol 5 mg as preservative; and 0.96 mg of monobasic potassium phosphate and 2.4 mg of dibasic sodium phosphate as buffers.

A pharmacy bulk package is a container of a sterile preparation for parenteral use that contains many single doses. The contents are intended for use in a pharmacy admixture program and are restricted to the preparation of admixtures for intravenous (IV) infusion.

Sterile, Premixed Solution for Intravenous Administration in Single-Dose, Flexible Plastic Containers: Each 50 mL contains ranitidine HCl equivalent to 50 mg of ranitidine, sodium chloride 225 mg, and citric acid 15 mg and dibasic sodium phosphate 90 mg as buffers in water for injection. It contains no preservatives. The osmolarity of this solution is 180 mOsm/L (approx.), and the pH is 6.7–7.3.

The flexible plastic container is fabricated from a specially formulated, nonplasticized, thermoplastic co-polyester (CR3). Water can permeate from inside the container into the overwrap but not in amounts sufficient to affect the solution significantly. Solutions inside the plastic container also can leach out certain of the chemical components in very small amounts before the expiration period is attained. However, the safety of the plastic has been confirmed by tests in animals according to USP biological standards for plastic containers.

CLINICAL PHARMACOLOGY

Zantac® (ranitidine HCl) is a competitive, reversible inhibitor of the action of histamine at the histamine H_2-receptors, including receptors on the gastric cells. Zantac does not lower serum Ca^{++} in hypercalcemic states. Zantac is not an anticholinergic agent.

Antisecretory Activity: 1. Effects on Acid Secretion: Zantac® (ranitidine HCl) Injection inhibits basal gastric acid secretion as well as gastric acid secretion stimulated by betazole and pentagastrin, as shown in the following table: [See table below.]

In a group of 10 known hypersecretors, ranitidine plasma levels of 71, 180, and 376 ng/mL inhibited basal acid secretion by 76%, 90%, and 99.5%, respectively.

It appears that basal- and betazole-stimulated secretions are most sensitive to inhibition by Zantac, while pentagastrin-stimulated secretion is more difficult to suppress.

2. Effects on Other Gastrointestinal Secretions:

Pepsin: Zantac does not affect pepsin secretion. Total pepsin output is reduced in proportion to the decrease in volume of gastric juice.

Intrinsic Factor: Zantac has no significant effect on pentagastrin-stimulated intrinsic factor secretion.

Serum Gastrin: Zantac has little or no effect on fasting or postprandial serum gastrin.

Other Pharmacologic Actions:

a. Gastric bacterial flora—increase in nitrate-reducing organisms, significance not known.

b. Prolactin levels—no effect in recommended oral or IV dosage, but small, transient, dose-related increases in serum prolactin have been reported after IV bolus injections of 100 mg or more.

c. Other pituitary hormones—no effect on serum gonadotropins, TSH, or GH. Possible impairment of vasopressin release.

d. No change in cortisol, aldosterone, androgen, or estrogen levels.

e. No antiandrogenic action.

f. No effect on count, motility, or morphology of sperm.

Pharmacokinetics: Serum concentrations necessary to inhibit 50% of stimulated gastric acid secretion are estimated to be 36–94 ng/mL. Following single IV or intramuscular (IM) 50-mg doses, serum concentrations of Zantac are in this range for 6–8 hours.

Following IV injection, approximately 70% of the dose is recovered in the urine as unchanged drug. Renal clearance averages 530 mL per minute, with a total clearance of 760 mL per minute. The volume of distribution is 1.4 L/kg, and the elimination half-life is 2–2.5 hours.

Four patients with clinically significant renal function impairment (creatinine clearance 25–35 mL per minute) administered 50 mg of ranitidine intravenously had an average plasma half-life of 4.8 hours, a ranitidine clearance of 29 mL per minute, and a volume of distribution of 1.76 L/kg. In general, these parameters appear to be altered in proportion to creatinine clearance (see DOSAGE AND ADMINISTRATION).

Zantac is absorbed very rapidly after IM injection. Mean peak levels of 576 ng/mL occur within 15 minutes or less following a 50-mg IM dose. Absorption from IM sites is virtually complete, with a bioavailability of 90%–100% compared with IV administration. Following oral administration, the relative bioavailability of Zantac® (ranitidine HCl) Tablets is 50%.

In man, the N-oxide is the principal metabolite in the urine; however, this amounts to less than 4% of the dose. Other metabolites are the S-oxide (1%) and the desmethyl ranitidine (1%). The remainder of the administered dose is found in the stool.

Studies in patients with hepatic dysfunction (compensated cirrhosis) indicate that there are minor, but clinically insignificant, alterations in ranitidine half-life, distribution, clearance, and bioavailability.

Serum protein binding averages 15%.

Clinical Trials: ***Active Duodenal Ulcer:*** In a multicenter, double-blind, controlled, US study of endoscopically diagnosed duodenal ulcers, earlier healing was seen in the patients treated with oral Zantac as shown in the following table:

[See table at top of page.]

	Oral Zantac*		Oral Placebo*	
	Number Entered	Healed/Evaluable	Number Entered	Healed/Evaluable
Outpatients				
Week 2	195	69/182 (38%)†	188	31/164 (19%)
Week 4		137/187 (73%)†		76/168 (45%)

*All patients were permitted p.r.n. antacids for relief of pain. †$p < 0.0001$.

In these studies, patients treated with oral Zantac reported a reduction in both daytime and nocturnal pain, and they also consumed less antacid than the placebo-treated patients.

[See second table above.]

Mean Daily Doses of Antacid

	Ulcer Healed	Ulcer Not Healed
Oral Zantac	0.06	0.71
Oral placebo	0.71	1.43

Pathological Hypersecretory Conditions (such as Zollinger-Ellison syndrome): Zantac inhibits gastric acid secretion and reduces occurrence of diarrhea, anorexia, and pain in patients with pathological hypersecretion associated with Zollinger-Ellison syndrome, systemic mastocytosis, and other pathological hypersecretory conditions (e.g., postoperative, "short-gut" syndrome, idiopathic). Use of oral Zantac was followed by healing of ulcers in 8 of 19 (42%) patients who were intractable to previous therapy.

In a retrospective review of 52 Zollinger-Ellison patients given Zantac as a continuous IV infusion for up to 15 days, no patients developed complications of acid-peptic disease such as bleeding or perforation. Acid output was controlled to less than or equal to 10 mEq per hour.

Effect of IV Zantac on Gastric Acid Secretion

	Time After Dose, h	% Inhibition of Gastric Acid Output by IV Dose, mg		
		20 mg	60 mg	100 mg
Betazole	Up to 2	93	99	99
Pentagastrin	Up to 3	47	66	77

INDICATIONS AND USAGE

Zantac® (ranitidine HCl) Injection and Zantac® (ranitidine HCl) Injection Premixed are indicated in some hospitalized patients with pathological hypersecretory conditions or intractable duodenal ulcers, or as an alternative to the oral dosage form for short-term use in patients who are unable to take oral medication.

CONTRAINDICATIONS

Zantac® (ranitidine HCl) Injection and Zantac® (ranitidine HCl) Injection Premixed are contraindicated for patients known to have hypersensitivity to the drug.

PRECAUTIONS

General: 1. Symptomatic response to Zantac® (ranitidine HCl) therapy does not preclude the presence of gastric malignancy.

2. Since Zantac is excreted primarily by the kidney, dosage should be adjusted in patients with impaired renal function (see DOSAGE AND ADMINISTRATION). Caution should be observed in patients with hepatic dysfunction since Zantac is metabolized in the liver.

3. In controlled studies in normal volunteers, elevations in SGPT have been observed when H_2-antagonists have been administered intravenously at greater than recommended dosages for 5 days or longer. Therefore, it seems prudent in patients receiving IV ranitidine at dosages greater than or equal to 100 mg q.i.d. for periods of 5 days or longer to monitor SGPT daily (from day 5) for the remainder of IV therapy.

4. Bradycardia in association with rapid administration of Zantac® (ranitidine HCl) Injection has been reported rarely, usually in patients with factors predisposing to cardiac rhythm disturbances. Recommended rates of administration should not be exceeded (see DOSAGE AND ADMINISTRATION).

Laboratory Tests: False-positive tests for urine protein with Multistix® may occur during Zantac therapy, and therefore testing with sulfosalicylic acid is recommended.

Drug Interactions: Although Zantac has been reported to bind weakly to cytochrome P-450 *in vitro*, recommended doses of the drug do not inhibit the action of the cytochrome P-450-linked oxygenase enzymes in the liver. However, there have been isolated reports of drug interactions that suggest that Zantac may affect the bioavailability of certain drugs by some mechanism as yet unidentified (e.g., a pH-dependent effect on absorption or a change in volume of distribution).

Increased or decreased prothrombin times have been reported during concurrent use of ranitidine and warfarin. However, in human pharmacokinetic studies with dosages of ranitidine up to 400 mg per day, no interaction occurred; ranitidine had no effect on warfarin clearance or prothrombin time. The possibility of an interaction with warfarin at dosages of ranitidine higher than 400 mg per day has not been investigated.

Carcinogenesis, Mutagenesis, Impairment of Fertility: There was no indication of tumorigenic or carcinogenic effects in lifespan studies in mice and rats at oral dosages up to 2,000 mg/kg per day.

Ranitidine was not mutagenic in standard bacterial tests *(Salmonella, Escherichia coli)* for mutagenicity at concentrations up to the maximum recommended for these assays.

In a dominant lethal assay, a single oral dose of 1,000 mg/kg to male rats was without effect on the outcome of two matings per week for the next 9 weeks.

Pregnancy: ***Teratogenic Effects: Pregnancy Category B:*** Reproduction studies have been performed in rats and rabbits at oral doses up to 160 times the human oral dose and have revealed no evidence of impaired fertility or harm to the fetus due to Zantac. There are, however, no adequate and well-controlled studies in pregnant women. Because animal reproduction studies are not always predictive of human response, this drug should be used during pregnancy only if clearly needed.

Nursing Mothers: Zantac is secreted in human milk. Caution should be exercised when Zantac is administered to a nursing mother.

Pediatric Use: Safety and effectiveness in children have not been established.

Use in Elderly Patients: Ulcer healing rates in elderly patients (65–82 years of age) treated with oral Zantac were no different from those in younger age-groups. The incidence rates for adverse events and laboratory abnormalities were also not different from those seen in other age-groups.

ADVERSE REACTIONS

Transient pain at the site of IM injection has been reported. Transient local burning or itching has been reported with IV administration of Zantac® (ranitidine HCl).

The following have been reported as events in clinical trials or in the routine management of patients treated with oral or parenteral Zantac. The relationship to Zantac therapy has been unclear in many cases. Headache, sometimes severe, seems to be related to Zantac administration.

Central Nervous System: Rarely, malaise, dizziness, somnolence, insomnia, and vertigo. Rare cases of reversible mental confusion, agitation, depression, and hallucinations have been reported, predominantly in severely ill elderly patients. Rare cases of reversible blurred vision suggestive of a change in accommodation have been reported. Rare reports of reversible involuntary motor disturbances have been received.

Cardiovascular: As with other H_2-blockers, rare reports of arrhythmias such as tachycardia, bradycardia, asystole, atrioventricular block, and premature ventricular beats.

Gastrointestinal: Constipation, diarrhea, nausea/vomiting, abdominal discomfort/pain, and rare reports of pancreatitis.

Hepatic: In normal volunteers, SGPT values were increased to at least twice the pretreatment levels in 6 of 12 subjects receiving 100 mg q.i.d. intravenously for 7 days, and in 4 of 24 subjects receiving 50 mg q.i.d. intravenously for 5 days. There have been occasional reports of hepatitis, hepatocellular or hepatocanalicular or mixed, with or without jaundice. In such circumstances, ranitidine should be immediately discontinued. These events are usually reversible, but in exceedingly rare circumstances death has occurred.

Musculoskeletal: Rare reports of arthralgias.

Hematologic: Blood count changes (leukopenia, granulocytopenia, and thrombocytopenia) have occurred in a few patients. These were usually reversible. Rare cases of agranulocytosis, pancytopenia, sometimes with marrow hypoplasia, and aplastic anemia and exceedingly rare cases of acquired immune hemolytic anemia have been reported.

Endocrine: Controlled studies in animals and man have shown no stimulation of any pituitary hormone by Zantac and no antiandrogenic activity, and cimetidine-induced gynecomastia and impotence in hypersecretory patients have resolved when Zantac has been substituted. However, occasional cases of gynecomastia, impotence, and loss of libido have been reported in male patients receiving Zantac, but the incidence did not differ from that in the general population.

Integumentary: Rash, including rare cases suggestive of mild erythema multiforme, and, rarely, alopecia.

Other: Rare cases of hypersensitivity reactions (e.g., bronchospasm, fever, rash, eosinophilia), anaphylaxis, angioneurotic edema, and small increases in serum creatinine.

OVERDOSAGE

There has been virtually no experience with overdosage with Zantac® (ranitidine HCl) Injection and limited experience with oral doses of ranitidine. Reported acute ingestions of up to 18 g orally have been associated with transient adverse effects similar to those encountered in normal clinical experience (see ADVERSE REACTIONS). In addition, abnormalities of gait and hypotension have been reported.

When overdosage occurs, clinical monitoring and supportive therapy should be employed.

Studies in dogs receiving dosages of Zantac® (ranitidine HCl) in excess of 225 mg/kg per day have shown muscular tremors, vomiting, and rapid respiration. Single oral doses of 1,000 mg/kg in mice and rats were not lethal. Intravenous LD_{50} values in mice and rats were 77 and 83 mg/kg, respectively.

DOSAGE AND ADMINISTRATION

Parenteral Administration: In some hospitalized patients with pathological hypersecretory conditions or intractable duodenal ulcers, or in patients who are unable to take oral medication, Zantac® (ranitidine HCl) may be administered parenterally according to the following recommendations:

Intramuscular Injection: 50 mg (2 mL) every 6–8 hours. (No dilution necessary.)

Intermittent Intravenous Injection:

a. Intermittent Bolus: 50 mg (2 mL) every 6–8 hours. Dilute Zantac® (ranitidine HCl) Injection, 50 mg, in 0.9% sodium chloride injection or other compatible IV solution (see Stability) to a concentration no greater than 2.5 mg/mL (20 mL). Inject at a rate no greater than 4 mL per minute (5 minutes).

b. Intermittent Infusion: 50 mg (2 mL) every 6–8 hours. Dilute Zantac Injection, 50 mg, in 5% dextrose injection or other compatible IV solution (see Stability) to a concentration no greater than 0.5 mg/mL (100 mL). Infuse at a rate no greater than 5–7 mL per minute (15–20 minutes).

Zantac® (ranitidine HCl) Injection Premixed solution, 50 mg, in 0.45% sodium chloride, 50 mL, requires no dilution and should be infused over 15–20 minutes.

In some patients it may be necessary to increase dosage. When this is necessary, the increases should be made by more frequent administration of the dose, but generally should not exceed 400 mg per day.

Continuous Intravenous Infusion: Add Zantac Injection to 5% dextrose injection or other compatible IV solution (see Stability). Deliver at a rate of 6.25 mg per hour (e.g., 150 mg [6 mL] Zantac Injection in 250 mL of 5% dextrose injection at 10.7 mL per hour).

For Zollinger-Ellison patients, dilute Zantac Injection in 5% dextrose injection or other compatible IV solution (see Stability) to a concentration no greater than 2.5 mg/mL. Start the infusion at a rate of 1.0 mg/kg per hour. If after 4 hours either a measured gastric acid output is greater than 10 mEq per hour or the patient becomes symptomatic, the dose should be adjusted upward in 0.5-mg/kg per hour increments, and the acid output should be remeasured. Dosages up to 2.5 mg/kg per hour and infusion rates as high as 220 mg per hour have been used.

Zantac Injection Premixed in Flexible Plastic Containers: Instructions for Use: ***To Open:*** Tear outer wrap at notch and remove solution container. Check for minute leaks by squeezing container firmly. If leaks are found, discard unit as sterility may be impaired.

Preparation for Administration: Use aseptic technique.

1. Close flow control clamp of administration set.
2. Remove cover from outlet port at bottom of container.
3. Insert piercing pin of administration set into port with a twisting motion until the pin is firmly seated. NOTE: See full directions on administration set carton.
4. Suspend container from hanger.
5. Squeeze and release drip chamber to establish proper fluid level in chamber during infusion of Zantac Injection Premixed.
6. Open flow control clamp to expel air from set. Close clamp.
7. Attach set to venipuncture device. If device is not indwelling, prime and make venipuncture.
8. Perform venipuncture.
9. Regulate rate of administration with flow control clamp.

Caution: Zantac Injection Premixed in flexible plastic containers is to be administered by slow IV drip infusion only. **Additives should not be introduced into this solution.** If used with a primary IV fluid system, the primary solution should be discontinued during Zantac Injection Premixed infusion. Do not administer unless solution is clear and container is undamaged.

Warning: Do not use flexible plastic container in series connections.

Dosage Adjustment for Patients with Impaired Renal Function: The administration of ranitidine as a continuous infusion has not been evaluated in patients with impaired renal function. On the basis of experience with a group of subjects with severely impaired renal function treated with Zantac, the recommended dosage in patients with a creatinine clearance less than 50 mL per minute is 50 mg every 18–24 hours. Should the patient's condition require, the frequency of dosing may be increased to every 12 hours or even further with caution. Hemodialysis reduces the level of circulating ranitidine. Ideally, the dosing schedule should be adjusted so that the timing of a scheduled dose coincides with the end of hemodialysis.

Stability: Zantac Injection is stable for 48 hours at room temperature when added to or diluted with most commonly used IV solutions, e.g., 0.9% sodium chloride injection, 5% dextrose injection, 10% dextrose injection, lactated ringer's injection, or 5% sodium bicarbonate injection.

Zantac Injection Premixed in flexible plastic containers is sterile through the expiration date on the label when stored under recommended conditions.

Note: Parenteral drug products should be inspected visually for particulate matter and discoloration before administration whenever solution and container permit.

Directions for Dispensing: ***Pharmacy Bulk Package—Not for Direct Infusion:*** The pharmacy bulk package is for use in a pharmacy admixture service only under a laminar flow hood. The closure should be penetrated only once with a sterile transfer set or other sterile dispensing device, and the contents dispensed in aliquots using aseptic technique. DISCARD ANY UNUSED PORTION WITHIN 24 HOURS OF FIRST ENTRY.

HOW SUPPLIED

Zantac® (ranitidine HCl) Injection, 25 mg/mL, containing phenol 0.5% as preservative, is available as follows:

NDC 0173-0362-38 2-mL single-dose vials (Tray of 10)
NDC 0173-0363-01 6-mL multidose vials (Singles)
NDC 0173-0363-00 40-mL pharmacy bulk packages (Singles)
NDC 0173-0362-00 2-mL single-dose, prefilled, disposable syringes (Singles)

Store between 4° and 30°C (39° and 86°F). Protect from light. Store the 40-mL pharmacy bulk vial in carton until time of use.

Note: To ensure patient safety, the needle with the prefilled syringes should be handled with care and should be destroyed and discarded if damaged in any manner. If the cannula is bent, no attempt should be made to straighten it. To prevent needle-stick injuries, needles should not be recapped, purposely bent, or broken by hand.

Zantac® (ranitidine HCl) Injection Premixed, 50 mg/50 mL, in 0.45% sodium chloride, is available as a sterile, premixed solution for IV administration in single-dose, flexible plastic containers (NDC 0173-0441-00). It contains no preservatives.

Store between 2° and 25°C (36° and 77°F). Protect from light. Exposure of pharmaceutical products to heat should be minimized. Avoid excessive heat; however, brief exposure up to 40°C does not adversely affect the product. Protect from freezing.

Shown in Product Identification Section, page 411

ZANTAC® 150 Tablets ℞
[zan 'tak]
(ranitidine hydrochloride)

ZANTAC® 300 Tabless ℞
(ranitidine hydrochloride)

ZANTAC® Syrup ℞
(ranitidine hydrochloride)

DESCRIPTION

The active ingredient in Zantac® 150 Tablets, Zantac® 300 Tablets, and Zantac® Syrup is ranitidine hydrochloride (HCl), a histamine H_2-receptor antagonist. Chemically it is N[2-[[[5-[(dimethylamino)methyl]-2-furanyl]methyl]thio]ethyl]-N′-methyl-2-nitro-1,1-ethenediamine, HCl.

The empirical formula is $C_{13}H_{22}N_4O_3S \cdot HCl$, representing a molecular weight of 350.87.

Ranitidine HCl is a white to pale yellow, granular substance that is soluble in water. It has a slightly bitter taste and sulfurlike odor.

Each Zantac 150 Tablet for oral administration contains 168 mg of ranitidine HCl equivalent to 150 mg of ranitidine. Each tablet also contains the inactive ingredients FD&C Yellow No. 6 Aluminum Lake, hydroxypropyl methylcellulose, magnesium stearate, microcrystalline cellulose, titanium dioxide, and yellow iron oxide.

Each Zantac 300 Tablet for oral administration contains 336 mg of ranitidine HCl equivalent to 300 mg of ranitidine. Each tablet also contains the inactive ingredients croscarmellose sodium, D&C Yellow No. 10 Aluminum Lake, hydroxypropyl methylcellulose, magnesium stearate, microcrystalline cellulose, titanium dioxide, and triacetin.

Each 1 mL of Zantac Syrup contains 16.8 mg of ranitidine HCl equivalent to 15 mg of ranitidine. Zantac Syrup also contains the inactive ingredients alcohol (7.5%), butylparaben, dibasic sodium phosphate, hydroxypropyl methylcellulose, peppermint flavor, monobasic potassium phosphate, propylparaben, purified water, saccharin sodium, sodium chloride, and sorbitol.

CLINICAL PHARMACOLOGY

Zantac® (ranitidine HCl) is a competitive, reversible inhibitor of the action of histamine at the histamine H_2-receptors, including receptors on the gastric cells. Zantac does not lower serum Ca^{++} in hypercalcemic states. Zantac is not an anticholinergic agent.

Antisecretory Activity: ***1. Effects on Acid Secretion:*** Zantac inhibits both daytime and nocturnal basal gastric acid secretions as well as gastric acid secretion stimulated by food, betazole, and pentagastrin, as shown in the following table: [See table below.]

Effect of Oral Zantac on Gastric Acid Secretion

	Time After Dose, h	% Inhibition of Gastric Acid Output by Dose, mg			
		75–80	100	150	200
Basal	Up to 4		99	95	
Nocturnal	Up to 13	95	96	92	
Betazole	Up to 3		97	99	
Pentagastrin	Up to 5	58	72	72	80
Meal	Up to 3		73	79	95

Continued on next page

Glaxo—Cont.

It appears that basal-, nocturnal-, and betazole-stimulated secretions are most sensitive to inhibition by Zantac, responding almost completely to doses of 100 mg or less, while pentagastrin- and food-stimulated secretions are more difficult to suppress.

2. Effects on Other Gastrointestinal Secretions:

Pepsin: Oral Zantac does not affect pepsin secretion. Total pepsin output is reduced in proportion to the decrease in volume of gastric juice.

Intrinsic Factor: Oral Zantac has no significant effect on pentagastrin-stimulated intrinsic factor secretion.

Serum Gastrin: Zantac has little or no effect on fasting or postprandial serum gastrin.

Other Pharmacologic Actions:

a. Gastric bacterial flora—increase in nitrate-reducing organisms, significance not known.

b. Prolactin levels—no effect in recommended oral or intravenous (IV) dosage, but small, transient, dose-related increases in serum prolactin have been reported after IV bolus injections of 100 mg or more.

c. Other pituitary hormones—no effect on serum gonadotropins, TSH, or GH. Possible impairment of vasopressin release.

d. No change in cortisol, aldosterone, androgen, or estrogen levels.

e. No antiandrogenic action.

f. No effect on count, motility, or morphology of sperm.

Pharmacokinetics: Zantac is 50% absorbed after oral administration, compared to an IV injection with mean peak levels of 440–545 ng/mL occurring at 2–3 hours after a 150-mg dose. The syrup and tablet formulations are bioequivalent. The elimination half-life is 2.5–3 hours.

Absorption is not significantly impaired by the administration of food or antacids. Propantheline slightly delays and increases peak blood levels of Zantac, probably by delaying gastric emptying and transit time. In one study, simultaneous administration of high-potency antacid (150 mmol) in fasting subjects has been reported to decrease the absorption of Zantac.

Serum concentrations necessary to inhibit 50% of stimulated gastric acid secretion are estimated to be 36–94 ng/mL. Following a single oral dose of 150 mg, serum concentrations of Zantac are in this range up to 12 hours. However, blood levels bear no consistent relationship to dose or degree of acid inhibition.

The principal route of excretion is the urine, with approximately 30% of the orally administered dose collected in the urine as unchanged drug in 24 hours. Renal clearance is about 410 mL per minute, indicating active tubular excretion. Four patients with clinically significant renal function impairment (creatinine clearance 25–35 mL per minute) administered 50 mg of ranitidine IV had an average plasma half-life of 4.8 hours, a ranitidine clearance of 29 mL per minute, and a volume of distribution of 1.76 L/kg. In general, these parameters appear to be altered in proportion to creatinine clearance (see DOSAGE AND ADMINISTRATION).

In man, the N-oxide is the principal metabolite in the urine; however, this amounts to less than 4% of the dose. Other metabolites are the S-oxide (1%) and the desmethyl ranitidine (1%). The remainder of the administered dose is found in the stool. Studies in patients with hepatic dysfunction (compensated cirrhosis) indicate that there are minor, but clinically insignificant, alterations in ranitidine half-life, distribution, clearance, and bioavailability.

The volume of distribution is about 1.4 L/kg. Serum protein binding averages 15%.

Clinical Trials: *Active Duodenal Ulcer:* In a multicenter, double-blind, controlled, US study of endoscopically diagnosed duodenal ulcers, earlier healing was seen in the patients treated with Zantac as shown in Table I:
[See table above.]

In these studies patients treated with Zantac reported a reduction in both daytime and nocturnal pain, and they also consumed less antacid than the placebo-treated patients.
[See Table II .]

Foreign studies have shown that patients heal equally well with 150 mg b.i.d. and 300 mg h.s. (85% versus 84%, respectively) during a usual 4-week course of therapy. If patients require extended therapy of 8 weeks, the healing rate may be higher for 150 mg b.i.d. as compared to 300 mg h.s. (92% versus 87%, respectively).

Studies have been limited to short-term treatment of acute duodenal ulcer. Patients whose ulcers healed during therapy had recurrences of ulcers at the usual rates. There have been no systematic studies to evaluate whether continued treatment with Zantac alters recurrence rates.

Maintenance Therapy in Duodenal Ulcer: Ranitidine has been found to be effective as maintenance therapy for patients following healing of acute duodenal ulcers. In two independent, double-blind, multicenter, controlled trials, the

Table I

	Zantac*		Placebo*	
	Number Entered	Healed/ Evaluable	Number Entered	Healed/ Evaluable
Outpatients				
Week 2	195	69/182 (38%)†	188	31/164 (19%)
Week 4		137/187 (73%)†		76/168 (45%)

*All patients were permitted p.r.n. antacids for relief of pain.   †$p < 0.0001$.

Table II

	Mean Daily Doses of Antacid	
	Ulcer Healed	Ulcer Not Healed
Zantac	0.06	0.71
Placebo	0.71	1.43

number of duodenal ulcers observed was significantly less in patients treated with Zantac (150 mg h.s.) than in patients treated with placebo over a 12-month period.

Duodenal Ulcer Prevalence

Double-blind, Multicenter, Placebo-Controlled Trials

Multicenter Trial	Drug	Duodenal Ulcer Prevalence			No. of Patients
		0–4 Months	0–8 Months	0–12 Months	
USA	RAN	20%*	24%*	35%*	138
	PLC	44%	54%	59%	139
Foreign	RAN	12%*	21%*	28%*	174
	PLC	56%	64%	68%	165

% = Life table estimate.
* = $p < 0.05$ (Zantac versus comparator).
RAN = ranitidine (Zantac).
PLC = placebo.

As with other H₂-antagonists, the factors responsible for the significant reduction in the prevalence of duodenal ulcers include prevention of recurrence of ulcers, more rapid healing of ulcers that may occur during maintenance therapy, or both.

Gastric Ulcer: In a multicenter, double-blind, controlled, US study of endoscopically diagnosed gastric ulcers, earlier healing was seen in the patients treated with Zantac as shown in the following table:

	Zantac*		Placebo*	
	Number Entered	Healed/ Evaluable	Number Entered	Healed/ Evaluable
Outpatients				
Week 2	92	16/83 (19%)	94	10/83 (12%)
Week 6		50/73 (68%)†		35/69 (51%)

*All patients were permitted p.r.n. antacids for relief of pain.
† $p = 0.009$.

In this multicenter trial, significantly more patients treated with Zantac became pain-free during therapy.

Pathological Hypersecretory Conditions (such as Zollinger-Ellison syndrome): Zantac inhibits gastric acid secretion and reduces occurrence of diarrhea, anorexia, and pain in patients with pathological hypersecretion associated with Zollinger-Ellison syndrome, systemic mastocytosis, and other pathological hypersecretory conditions (e.g., postoperative, "short-gut" syndrome, idiopathic). Use of Zantac was followed by healing of ulcers in 8 of 19 (42%) patients who were intractable to previous therapy.

Gastroesophageal Reflux Disease (GERD): In two multicenter, double-blind, placebo-controlled, 6-week trials performed in the United States and Europe, Zantac 150 mg b.i.d. was more effective than placebo for the relief of heartburn and other symptoms associated with GERD. Ranitidine-treated patients consumed significantly less antacid than did placebo-treated patients.

The US trial indicated that Zantac 150 mg b.i.d. significantly reduced the frequency of heartburn attacks and severity of heartburn pain within 1–2 weeks after starting therapy. The improvement was maintained throughout the 6-week trial period. Moreover, patient response rates demonstrated that the effect on heartburn extends through both the day and night time periods.

Erosive Esophagitis: In two multicenter, double-blind, randomized, placebo-controlled, 12-week trials performed in the

United States, Zantac® (ranitidine HCl) 150 mg q.i.d. was significantly more effective than placebo in healing endoscopically diagnosed erosive esophagitis and in relieving associated heartburn. The erosive esophagitis healing rates were as follows:

Erosive Esophagitis Patient Healing Rates

	Healed/Evaluable	
	Placebo* n=229	Zantac 150 mg q.i.d.* n=215
Week 4	43/198 (22%)	96/206 (47%)†
Week 8	63/176 (36%)	142/200 (71%)†
Week 12	92/159 (58%)	162/192 (84%)†

* All patients were permitted p.r.n. antacids for relief of pain.
†$p < 0.001$ versus placebo.

No additional benefit in healing of esophagitis or in relief of heartburn was seen with a ranitidine dose of 300 mg q.i.d.

INDICATIONS AND USAGE

Zantac® (ranitidine HCl) is indicated in:

1. Short-term treatment of active duodenal ulcer. Most patients heal within 4 weeks. Studies available to date have not assessed the safety of ranitidine in uncomplicated duodenal ulcer for periods of more than 8 weeks.

2. Maintenance therapy for duodenal ulcer patients at reduced dosage after healing of acute ulcers. No placebo-controlled comparative studies have been carried out for periods of longer than 1 year.

3. The treatment of pathological hypersecretory conditions (e.g., Zollinger-Ellison syndrome and systemic mastocytosis).

4. Short-term treatment of active, benign gastric ulcer. Most patients heal within 6 weeks and the usefulness of further treatment has not been demonstrated. Studies available to date have not assessed the safety of ranitidine in uncomplicated, benign gastric ulcer for periods of more than 6 weeks.

5. Treatment of GERD. Symptomatic relief commonly occurs within 1 or 2 weeks after starting therapy with Zantac 150 mg b.i.d.

6. Treatment of endoscopically diagnosed erosive esophagitis. Healing of endoscopically diagnosed erosive esophagitis occurs at 4 weeks (47%), 8 weeks (71%), and 12 weeks (84%) of therapy with Zantac 150 mg q.i.d. Symptomatic relief of heartburn commonly occurs within 24 hours of therapy initiation with Zantac.

Concomitant antacids should be given as needed for pain relief to patients with active duodenal ulcer; active, benign gastric ulcer; hypersecretory states; GERD; and erosive esophagitis.

CONTRAINDICATIONS

Zantac® (ranitidine HCl) is contraindicated for patients known to have hypersensitivity to the drug.

PRECAUTIONS

General: 1. Symptomatic response to Zantac® (ranitidine HCl) therapy does not preclude the presence of gastric malignancy.

2. Since Zantac is excreted primarily by the kidney, dosage should be adjusted in patients with impaired renal function (see DOSAGE AND ADMINISTRATION). Caution should be observed in patients with hepatic dysfunction since Zantac is metabolized in the liver.

Laboratory Tests: False-positive tests for urine protein with Multistix® may occur during Zantac therapy, and therefore testing with sulfosalicylic acid is recommended.

Drug Interactions: Although Zantac has been reported to bind weakly to cytochrome P-450 *in vitro*, recommended doses of the drug do not inhibit the action of the cytochrome P-450–linked oxygenase enzymes in the liver. However, there have been isolated reports of drug interactions that suggest that Zantac may affect the bioavailability of certain drugs by some mechanism as yet unidentified (e.g., a pH-dependent effect on absorption or a change in volume of distribution).

Increased or decreased prothrombin times have been reported during concurrent use of ranitidine and warfarin. However, in human pharmacokinetic studies with dosages of ranitidine up to 400 mg per day, no interaction occurred; ranitidine had no effect on warfarin clearance or prothrombin time. The possibility of an interaction with warfarin at dosages of ranitidine higher than 400 mg per day has not been investigated.

Carcinogenesis, Mutagenesis, Impairment of Fertility: There was no indication of tumorigenic or carcinogenic effects in life-span studies in mice and rats at dosages up to 2,000 mg/kg per day.

Ranitidine was not mutagenic in standard bacterial tests (*Salmonella, Escherichia coli*) for mutagenicity at concentrations up to the maximum recommended for these assays.

In a dominant lethal assay, a single oral dose of 1,000 mg/kg to male rats was without effect on the outcome of two matings per week for the next 9 weeks.

Pregnancy: *Teratogenic Effects: Pregnancy Category B:* Reproduction studies have been performed in rats and rabbits at doses up to 160 times the human dose and have revealed no evidence of impaired fertility or harm to the fetus due to Zantac. There are, however, no adequate and well-controlled studies in pregnant women. Because animal reproduction studies are not always predictive of human response, this drug should be used during pregnancy only if clearly needed.

Nursing Mothers: Zantac is secreted in human milk. Caution should be exercised when Zantac is administered to a nursing mother.

Pediatric Use: Safety and effectiveness in children have not been established.

Use in Elderly Patients: Ulcer healing rates in elderly patients (65–82 years of age) were no different from those in younger age-groups. The incidence rates for adverse events and laboratory abnormalities were also not different from those seen in other age-groups.

ADVERSE REACTIONS

The following have been reported as events in clinical trials or in the routine management of patients treated with Zantac® (ranitidine HCl). The relationship to Zantac therapy has been unclear in many cases. Headache, sometimes severe, seems to be related to Zantac administration.

Central Nervous System: Rarely, malaise, dizziness, somnolence, insomnia, and vertigo. Rare cases of reversible mental confusion, agitation, depression, and hallucinations have been reported, predominantly in severely ill elderly patients. Rare cases of reversible blurred vision suggestive of a change in accommodation have been reported. Rare reports of reversible involuntary motor disturbances have been received.

Cardiovascular: As with other H_2-blockers, rare reports of arrhythmias such as tachycardia, bradycardia, atrioventricular block, and premature ventricular beats.

Gastrointestinal: Constipation, diarrhea, nausea/vomiting, abdominal discomfort/pain, and rare reports of pancreatitis.

Hepatic: In normal volunteers, SGPT values were increased to at least twice the pretreatment levels in 6 of 12 subjects receiving 100 mg q.i.d. IV for 7 days, and in 4 of 24 subjects receiving 50 mg q.i.d. IV for 5 days. There have been occasional reports of hepatitis, hepatocellular or hepatocanalicular or mixed, with or without jaundice. In such circumstances, ranitidine should be immediately discontinued. These events are usually reversible, but in exceedingly rare circumstances death has occurred.

Musculoskeletal: Rare reports of arthralgias.

Hematologic: Blood count changes (leukopenia, granulocytopenia, and thrombocytopenia) have occurred in a few patients. These were usually reversible. Rare cases of agranulocytosis, pancytopenia, sometimes with marrow hypoplasia, and aplastic anemia and exceedingly rare cases of acquired immune hemolytic anemia have been reported.

Endocrine: Controlled studies in animals and man have shown no stimulation of any pituitary hormone by Zantac and no antiandrogenic activity, and cimetidine-induced gynecomastia and impotence in hypersecretory patients have resolved when Zantac has been substituted. However, occasional cases of gynecomastia, impotence, and loss of libido have been reported in male patients receiving Zantac, but the incidence did not differ from that in the general population.

Integumentary: Rash, including rare cases suggestive of mild erythema multiforme, and, rarely, alopecia.

Other: Rare cases of hypersensitivity reactions (e.g.. bronchospasm, fever, rash, eosinophilia), anaphylaxis, angioneurotic edema, and small increases in serum creatinine.

OVERDOSAGE

There has been limited experience with overdosage. Reported acute ingestions of up to 18 g orally have been associated with transient adverse effects similar to those encountered in normal clinical experience (see ADVERSE REAC-

TIONS). In addition, abnormalities of gait and hypotension have been reported.

When overdosage occurs, the usual measures to remove unabsorbed material from the gastrointestinal tract, clinical monitoring, and supportive therapy should be employed. Studies in dogs receiving dosages of Zantac® (ranitidine HCl) in excess of 225 mg/kg per day have shown muscular tremors, vomiting, and rapid respiration. Single oral doses of 1,000 mg/kg in mice and rats were not lethal. Intravenous LD_{50} values in mice and rats were 77 and 83 mg/kg, respectively.

DOSAGE AND ADMINISTRATION

Active Duodenal Ulcer: The current recommended adult oral dosage of Zantac® (ranitidine HCl) for duodenal ulcer is 150 mg or 10 mL (2 teaspoonfuls equivalent to 150 mg of ranitidine) twice daily. An alternative dosage of 300 mg or 20 mL (4 teaspoonfuls equivalent to 300 mg of ranitidine) once daily at bedtime can be used for patients in whom dosing convenience is important. The advantages of one treatment regimen compared to the other in a particular patient population have yet to be demonstrated (see Clinical Trials: *Active Duodenal Ulcer*). Smaller doses have been shown to be equally effective in inhibiting gastric acid secretion in US studies, and several foreign trials have shown that 100 mg b.i.d. is as effective as the 150-mg dose.

Antacid should be given as needed for relief of pain (see CLINICAL PHARMACOLOGY: Pharmacokinetics).

Maintenance Therapy: The current recommended adult oral dosage is 150 or 10 mL (2 teaspoonfuls equivalent to 150 mg of ranitidine) at bedtime.

Pathological Hypersecretory Conditions (such as Zollinger-Ellison syndrome): The current recommended adult oral dosage is 150 mg or 10 mL (2 teaspoonfuls equivalent to 150 mg of ranitidine) twice a day. In some patients it may be necessary to administer Zantac 150-mg doses more frequently. Dosages should be adjusted to individual patient needs, and should continue as long as clinically indicated. Dosages up to 6 g per day have been employed in patients with severe disease.

Benign Gastric Ulcer: The current recommended adult oral dosage is 150 mg or 10 mL (2 teaspoonfuls equivalent to 150 mg of ranitidine) twice a day.

GERD: The current recommended adult oral dosage is 150 mg or 10 mL (2 teaspoonfuls equivalent to 150 mg of ranitidine) twice a day.

Erosive Esophagitis: The current recommended adult oral dosage is 150 mg or 10 mL (2 teaspoonfuls equivalent to 150 mg of ranitidine) four times a day.

Dosage Adjustment for Patients With Impaired Renal Function: On the basis of experience with a group of subjects with severely impaired renal function treated with Zantac, the recommended dosage in patients with a creatinine clearance less than 50 mL per minute is 150 mg or 10 mL (2 teaspoonfuls equivalent to 150 mg of ranitidine) every 24 hours. Should the patient's condition require, the frequency of dosing may be increased to every 12 hours or even further with caution. Hemodialysis reduces the level of circulating ranitidine. Ideally, the dosing schedule should be adjusted so that the timing of a scheduled dose coincides with the end of hemodialysis.

HOW SUPPLIED

Zantac® 150 Tablets (ranitidine HCl equivalent to 150 mg of ranitidine) are peach, film-coated, five-sided tablets embossed with "ZANTAC 150" on one side and "Glaxo" on the other. They are available in bottles of 60 (NDC 0173-0344-42) and 100 (NDC 0173-0344-09) tablets and unit dose packs of 100 (NDC 0173-0344-47) tablets.

Zantac® 300 Tablets (ranitidine HCl equivalent to 300 mg of ranitidine) are yellow, film-coated, capsule-shaped tablets embossed with "ZANTAC 300" on one side and "Glaxo" on the other. They are available in bottles of 30 (NDC 0173-0393-40) tablets and unit dose packs of 100 (NDC 0173-0393-47) tablets.

Store between 15° and 30°C (59° and 86°F) in a dry place. Protect from light. Replace cap securely after each opening. Zantac® Syrup, a clear, peppermint-flavored liquid, contains 16.8 mg of ranitidine HCl equivalent to 15 mg of ranitidine per 1 mL in bottles of 16 fluid ounces (one pint) (NDC 0173-0383-54).

Store between 4° and 25°C (39° and 77°F). Dispense in tight, light-resistant containers as defined in the USP/NF.

Shown in Product Identification Section, page 411

ZINACEF® ℞
[*zin'ah-sef*]
(sterile cefuroxime sodium, Glaxo)

ZINACEF® ℞
(cefuroxime sodium injection)

DESCRIPTION

Cefuroxime is a semisynthetic, broad-spectrum cephalosporin antibiotic for parenteral administration. It is the sodium

salt of (6R, 7R)-3-carbamoyloxymethyl-7-[Z-2-methoxyimino-2-(fur-2-yl) acetamido]ceph-3-em-4-carboxylate.

Zinacef® (sterile cefuroxime sodium/cefuroxime sodium injection) contains approximately 54.2 mg (2.4 mEq) of sodium per gram of cefuroxime activity.

Zinacef® (sterile cefuroxime sodium) in sterile crystalline form is supplied in vials equivalent to 750 mg, 1.5 g, or 7.5 g of cefuroxime as cefuroxime sodium and in ADD-Vantage® vials equivalent to 750 mg or 1.5 g of cefuroxime as cefuroxime sodium. Solutions of Zinacef range in color from light yellow to amber, depending on the concentration and diluent used. The pH of freshly constituted solutions usually ranges from 6–8.5.

Zinacef® (cefuroxime sodium injection) is available as a frozen, iso-osmotic, sterile, nonpyrogenic solution with 750 mg or 1.5 g of cefuroxime as cefuroxime sodium. Approximately 1.4 g of dextrose hydrous, USP has been added to the 750-mg dose to adjust the osmolality. Sodium citrate hydrous, USP has been added as a buffer (300 mg and 600 mg to the 750-mg and 1.5-g doses, respectively). Zinacef contains approximately 111 mg (4.8 mEq) and 222 mg (9.7 mEq) of sodium in the 750-mg and 1.5-g doses, respectively. The pH has been adjusted with hydrochloric acid and may have been adjusted with sodium hydroxide. Solutions of premixed Zinacef range in color from light yellow to amber. The solution is intended for intravenous (IV) use after thawing to room temperature. The osmolality of the solution is approximately 300 mOsmol/kg, and the pH of thawed solutions ranges from 5–7.5.

The plastic container is fabricated from a specially designed multilayer plastic, PL 2040. Solutions are in contact with the polyethylene layer of this container and can leach out certain chemical components of the plastic in very small amounts within the expiration period. The suitability of the plastic has been confirmed in tests in animals according to USP biological tests for plastic containers as well as by tissue culture toxicity studies.

CLINICAL PHARMACOLOGY

After intramuscular (IM) injection of a 750-mg dose of cefuroxime to normal volunteers, the mean peak serum concentration was 27 mcg/mL. The peak occurred at approximately 45 minutes (range, 15–60 minutes). Following IV doses of 750 mg and 1.5 g, serum concentrations were approximately 50 and 100 mcg/mL, respectively, at 15 minutes. Therapeutic serum concentrations of approximately 2 mcg/mL or more were maintained for 5.3 hours and 8 hours or more, respectively. There was no evidence of accumulation of cefuroxime in the serum following IV administration of 1.5-g doses every 8 hours to normal volunteers. The serum half-life after either IM or IV injections is approximately 80 minutes.

Approximately 89% of a dose of cefuroxime is excreted by the kidneys over an 8-hour period, resulting in high urinary concentrations.

Following the IM administration of a 750-mg single dose, urinary concentrations averaged 1,300 mcg/mL during the first 8 hours. Intravenous doses of 750 mg and 1.5 g produced urinary levels averaging 1,150 and 2,500 mcg/mL, respectively, during the first 8-hour period. The concomitant oral administration of probenecid with cefuroxime slows tubular secretion, decreases renal clearance by approximately 40%, increases the peak serum level by approximately 30%, and increases the serum half-life by approximately 30%. Cefuroxime is detectable in therapeutic concentrations in pleural fluid, joint fluid, bile, sputum, bone, cerebrospinal fluid (in patients with meningitis), and aqueous humor.

Cefuroxime is approximately 50% bound to serum protein.

Microbiology: Cefuroxime has *in vitro* activity against a wide range of gram-positive and gram-negative organisms, and it is highly stable in the presence of beta-lactamases of certain gram-negative bacteria. The bactericidal action of cefuroxime results from inhibition of cell-wall synthesis. Cefuroxime is usually active against the following organisms *in vitro*.

Aerobes, Gram-positive: *Staphylococcus aureus; Staphylococcus epidermidis; Streptococcus pneumoniae;* and *Streptococcus pyogenes* (and other streptococci). NOTE: Most strains of enterococci, e.g., *Enterococcus faecalis* (formerly *Streptococcus faecalis*), are resistant to cefuroxime. Methicillin-resistant staphylococci and *Listeria monocytogenes* are resistant to cefuroxime.

Aerobes, Gram-negative: *Citrobacter* spp.; *Enterobacter* spp.; *Escherichia coli; Haemophilus influenzae* (including ampicillin-resistant strains); *Haemophilus parainfluenzae; Klebsiella* spp. (including *Klebsiella pneumoniae*); *Moraxella (Branhamella) catarrhalis* (including ampicillin- and cepha-

Continued on next page

Glaxo—Cont.

lothin-resistant strains); *Morganella morganii* (formerly *Proteus morganii*); *Neisseria gonorrhoeae* (including penicillinase- and non-penicillinase-producing strains); *Neisseria meningitidis; Proteus mirabilis; Providencia rettgeri* (formerly *Proteus rettgeri*); *Salmonella* spp.; and *Shigella* spp. NOTE: Some strains of *Morganella morganii, Enterobacter cloacae,* and *Citrobacter* spp. have been shown by *in vitro* tests to be resistant to cefuroxime and other cephalosporins. *Pseudomonas* and *Campylobacter* spp., *Acinetobacter calcoaceticus,* and most strains of *Serratia* spp. and *Proteus vulgaris* are resistant to most first- and second-generation cephalosporins.

Anaerobes: Gram-positive and gram-negative cocci (including *Peptococcus* and *Peptostreptococcus* spp.); gram-positive bacilli (including *Clostridium* spp.); and gram-negative bacilli (including *Bacteroides* and *Fusobacterium* spp.).

NOTE: *Clostridium difficile* and most strains of *Bacteroides fragilis* are resistant to cefuroxime.

Susceptibility Tests: *Diffusion Techniques:* Quantitative methods that require measurement of zone diameters give an estimate of antibiotic susceptibility. One such standard procedure[1] that has been recommended for use with disks to test susceptibility of organisms to cefuroxime uses the 30-mcg cefuroxime disk. Interpretation involves the correlation of the diameters obtained in the disk test with the minimum inhibitory concentration (MIC) for cefuroxime.

A report of "Susceptible" indicates that the pathogen is likely to be inhibited by generally achievable blood levels. A report of "Moderately Susceptible" suggests that the organism would be susceptible if high dosage is used or if the infection is confined to tissues and fluids in which high antibiotic levels are attained. A report of "Intermediate" suggests an equivocable or indeterminate result. A report of "Resistant" indicates that achievable concentrations of the antibiotic are unlikely to be inhibitory and other therapy should be selected.

Reports from the laboratory giving results of the standard single-disk susceptibility test for organisms other than *Haemophilus* spp. and *Neisseria gonorrhoeae* with a 30-mcg cefuroxime disk should be interpreted according to the following criteria:

Zone Diameter (mm)	Interpretation
≥ 18	(S) Susceptible
15–17	(MS) Moderately Susceptible
≤ 14	(R) Resistant

Results for *Haemophilus* spp. should be interpreted according to the following criteria:

Zone Diameter (mm)	Interpretation
≥ 24	(S) Susceptible
21–23	(I) Intermediate
≤ 20	(R) Resistant

Results for *Neisseria gonorrhoeae* should be interpreted according to the following criteria:

Zone Diameter (mm)	Interpretation
≥ 31	(S) Susceptible
26–30	(MS) Moderately Susceptible
≤ 25	(R) Resistant

Organisms should be tested with the cefuroxime disk since cefuroxime has been shown by *in vitro* tests to be active against certain strains found resistant when other beta-lactam disks are used. The cefuroxime disk should not be used for testing susceptibility to other cephalosporins.

Standardized procedures require the use of laboratory control organisms. The 30-mcg cefuroxime disk should give the following zone diameters.

1. Testing for organisms other than *Haemophilus* spp. and *Neisseria gonorrhoeae:*

Organism	Zone Diameter (mm)
Staphylococcus aureus ATCC 25923	27–35
Escherichia coli ATCC 25922	20–26

2. Testing for *Haemophilus* spp.:

Organism	Zone Diameter (mm)
Haemophilus influenzae ATCC 49766	28–36

3. Testing for *Neisseria gonorrhoeae:*

Organism	Zone Diameter (mm)
Neisseria gonorrhoeae ATCC 49226	33–41
Staphylococcus aureus ATCC 25923	29–33

Dilution Techniques: Use a standardized dilution method[1] (broth, agar, microdilution) or equivalent with cefuroxime powder. The MIC values obtained for bacterial isolates other than *Haemophilus* spp. and *Neisseria gonorrhoeae* should be interpreted according to the following criteria:

MIC (mcg/mL)	Interpretation
≤ 8	(S) Susceptible
16	(MS) Moderately Susceptible
≥ 32	(R) Resistant

MIC values obtained for *Haemophilus* spp. should be interpreted according to the following criteria:

MIC (mcg/mL)	Interpretation
≤ 4	(S) Susceptible
8	(I) Intermediate
≥ 16	(R) Resistant

MIC values obtained for *Neisseria gonorrhoeae* should be interpreted according to the following criteria:

MIC (mcg/mL)	Interpretation
≤ 1	(S) Susceptible
2	(MS) Moderately Susceptible
≥ 4	(R) Resistant

As with standard diffusion techniques, dilution methods require the use of laboratory control organisms. Standard cefuroxime powder should provide the following MIC values.

1. For organisms other than *Haemophilus* spp. and *Neisseria gonorrhoeae:*

Organism	MIC (mcg/mL)
Staphylococcus aureus ATCC 29213	0.5–2.0
Escherichia coli ATCC 25922	2.0–8.0

2. For *Haemophilus* spp.:

Organism	MIC (mcg/mL)
Haemophilus influenzae ATCC 49766	0.25–1.0

3. For *Neisseria gonorrhoeae:*

Organism	MIC (mcg/mL)
Neisseria gonorrhoeae ATCC 49226	0.25–1.0
Staphylococcus aureus ATCC 29213	0.25–1.0

INDICATIONS AND USAGE

Zinacef® (sterile cefuroxime sodium/cefuroxime sodium injection) is indicated for the treatment of patients with infections caused by susceptible strains of the designated organisms in the following diseases:

1. **Lower Respiratory Tract Infections,** including pneumonia, caused by *Streptococcus pneumoniae, Haemophilus influenzae* (including ampicillin-resistant strains), *Klebsiella* spp., *Staphylococcus aureus* (penicillinase- and non–penicillinase-producing strains), *Streptococcus pyogenes,* and *Escherichia coli.*

2. **Urinary Tract Infections** caused by *Escherichia coli* and *Klebsiella* spp.

3. **Skin and Skin Structure Infections** caused by *Staphylococcus aureus* (penicillinase- and non–penicillinase-producing strains), *Streptococcus pyogenes, Escherichia coli, Klebsiella* spp., and *Enterobacter* spp.

4. **Septicemia** caused by *Staphylococcus aureus* (penicillinase- and non–penicillinase-producing strains), *Streptococcus pneumoniae, Escherichia coli, Haemophilus influenzae* (including ampicillin-resistant strains), and *Klebsiella* spp.

5. **Meningitis** caused by *Streptococcus pneumoniae, Haemophilus influenzae* (including ampicillin-resistant strains), *Neisseria meningitidis,* and *Staphylococcus aureus* (penicillinase- and non–penicillinase-producing).

6. **Gonorrhea:** Uncomplicated and disseminated gonococcal infections due to *Neisseria gonorrhoeae* (penicillinase- and non–penicillinase-producing strains) in both males and females.

7. **Bone and Joint Infections** caused by *Staphylococcus aureus* (including penicillinase- and non–penicillinase-producing strains).

Clinical microbiological studies in skin and skin structure infections frequently reveal the growth of susceptible strains of both aerobic and anaerobic organisms. Zinacef has been used successfully in these mixed infections in which several organisms have been isolated. Appropriate cultures and susceptibility studies should be performed to determine the susceptibility of the causative organisms to Zinacef. Therapy may be started while awaiting the results of these studies; however, once these results become available, the antibiotic treatment should be adjusted accordingly. In certain cases of confirmed or suspected gram-positive or gram-negative sepsis or in patients with other serious infections in which the causative organism has not been identified, Zinacef may be used concomitantly with an aminoglycoside (see PRECAUTIONS). The recommended doses of both antibiotics may be given depending on the severity of the infection and the patient's condition.

Prevention: The preoperative prophylactic administration of Zinacef may prevent the growth of susceptible disease-causing bacteria and thereby may reduce the incidence of certain postoperative infections in patients undergoing surgical procedures (e.g., vaginal hysterectomy) that are classified as clean-contaminated or potentially contaminated procedures. Effective prophylactic use of antibiotics in surgery depends on the time of administration. Zinacef should usually be given one-half to 1 hour before the operation to allow sufficient time to achieve effective antibiotic concentrations in the wound tissues during the procedure. The dose should be repeated intraoperatively if the surgical procedure is lengthy.

Prophylactic administration is usually not required after the surgical procedure ends and should be stopped within 24 hours. In the majority of surgical procedures, continuing prophylactic administration of any antibiotic does not reduce the incidence of subsequent infections but will increase the possibility of adverse reactions and the development of bacterial resistance.

The perioperative use of Zinacef has also been effective during open heart surgery for surgical patients in whom infections at the operative site would present a serious risk. For these patients it is recommended that Zinacef therapy be continued for at least 48 hours after the surgical procedure ends. If an infection is present, specimens for culture should be obtained for the identification of the causative organism, and appropriate antimicrobial therapy should be instituted.

CONTRAINDICATIONS

Zinacef® (sterile cefuroxime sodium/cefuroxime sodium injection) is contraindicated in patients with known allergy to the cephalosporin group of antibiotics.

WARNINGS

BEFORE THERAPY WITH ZINACEF® (STERILE CEFUROXIME SODIUM/CEFUROXIME SODIUM INJECTION) IS INSTITUTED, CAREFUL INQUIRY SHOULD BE MADE TO DETERMINE WHETHER THE PATIENT HAS HAD PREVIOUS HYPERSENSITIVITY REACTIONS TO CEPHALOSPORINS, PENICILLINS, OR OTHER DRUGS. THIS PRODUCT SHOULD BE GIVEN CAUTIOUSLY TO PENICILLIN-SENSITIVE PATIENTS. ANTIBIOTICS SHOULD BE ADMINISTERED WITH CAUTION TO ANY PATIENT WHO HAS DEMONSTRATED SOME FORM OF ALLERGY, PARTICULARLY TO DRUGS. IF AN ALLERGIC REACTION TO ZINACEF OCCURS, DISCONTINUE THE DRUG. SERIOUS ACUTE HYPERSENSITIVITY REACTIONS MAY REQUIRE EPINEPHRINE AND OTHER EMERGENCY MEASURES.

Pseudomembranous colitis has been reported with the use of cephalosporins (and other broad-spectrum antibiotics); therefore, it is important to consider its diagnosis in patients who develop diarrhea in association with antibiotic use.
Treatment with broad-spectrum antibiotics alters the normal flora of the colon and may permit overgrowth of clostridia. Studies indicate that a toxin produced by *Clostridium difficile* is one primary cause of antibiotic-associated colitis. Cholestyramine and colestipol resins have been shown to bind the toxin *in vitro.*

Mild cases of colitis may respond to drug discontinuation alone. Moderate to severe cases should be managed with fluid, electrolyte, and protein supplementation as indicated. When the colitis is not relieved by drug discontinuation or when it is severe, oral vancomycin is the treatment of choice for antibiotic-associated pseudomembranous colitis produced by *Clostridium difficile.* Other causes of colitis should also be considered.

PRECAUTIONS

Although Zinacef® (sterile cefuroxime sodium/cefuroxime sodium injection) rarely produces alterations in kidney function, evaluation of renal status during therapy is recommended, especially in seriously ill patients receiving the maximum doses. Cephalosporins should be given with caution to patients receiving concurrent treatment with potent diuretics as these regimens are suspected of adversely affecting renal function.

The total daily dose of Zinacef should be reduced in patients with transient or persistent renal insufficiency (see DOSAGE AND ADMINISTRATION), because high and prolonged serum antibiotic concentrations can occur in such individuals from usual doses.

As with other antibiotics, prolonged use of Zinacef may result in overgrowth of nonsusceptible organisms. Careful observation of the patient is essential. If superinfection occurs during therapy, appropriate measures should be taken.

Broad-spectrum antibiotics should be prescribed with caution in individuals with a history of gastrointestinal disease, particularly colitis.

Nephrotoxicity has been reported following concomitant administration of aminoglycoside antibiotics and cephalosporins.

As with other therapeutic regimens used in the treatment of meningitis, mild-to-moderate hearing loss has been reported in a few pediatric patients treated with cefuroxime sodium. Persistence of positive CSF (cerebrospinal fluid) cultures at 18–36 hours has also been noted with cefuroxime sodium injection, as well as with other antibiotic therapies; however, the clinical relevance of this is unknown.

Drug/Laboratory Test Interactions: A false-positive reaction for glucose in the urine may occur with copper reduction tests (Benedict's or Fehling's solution or with Clinitest® tablets) but not with enzyme-based tests for glycosuria (e.g., Tes-Tape®). As a false-negative result may occur in the ferricyanide test, it is recommended that either the glucose oxidase or hexokinase method be used to determine blood plasma glucose levels in patients receiving Zinacef.

Cefuroxime does not interfere with the assay of serum and urine creatinine by the alkaline picrate method.

Carcinogenesis, Mutagenesis, Impairment of Fertility: Although no long-term studies in animals have been performed to evaluate carcinogenic potential, no mutagenic potential of cefuroxime was found in standard laboratory tests. Reproduction studies revealed no impairment of fertility in animals.

Pregnancy: ***Teratogenic Effects: Pregnancy Category B:*** Reproduction studies have been performed in mice and rabbits at doses up to 60 times the human dose and have revealed no evidence of impaired fertility or harm to the fetus due to cefuroxime. There are, however, no adequate and well-controlled studies in pregnant women. Because animal reproduction studies are not always predictive of human response, this drug should be used during pregnancy only if clearly needed.

Nursing Mothers: Since cefuroxime is excreted in human milk, caution should be exercised when Zinacef is administered to a nursing woman.

Pediatric Use: Safety and effectiveness in children below 3 months of age have not been established. Accumulation of other members of the cephalosporin class in newborn infants (with resulting prolongation of drug half-life) has been reported.

ADVERSE REACTIONS

Zinacef® (sterile cefuroxime sodium/cefuroxime sodium injection) is generally well tolerated. The most common adverse effects have been local reactions following IV administration. Other adverse reactions have been encountered only rarely.

Local Reactions: Thrombophlebitis has occurred with IV administration in 1 in 60 patients.

Gastrointestinal: Gastrointestinal symptoms occurred in 1 in 150 patients and included diarrhea (1 in 220 patients) and nausea (1 in 440 patients). Onset of pseudomembranous colitis symptoms may occur during or after antibiotic treatment (see WARNINGS).

Hypersensitivity Reactions: Hypersensitivity reactions have been reported in fewer than 1% of the patients treated with Zinacef and include rash (1 in 125). Pruritus, urticaria, and positive Coombs' test each occurred in fewer than 1 in 250 patients, and, as with other cephalosporins, rare cases of anaphylaxis, drug fever, erythema multiforme, toxic epidermal necrolysis, and Stevens-Johnson syndrome have occurred.

Blood: A decrease in hemoglobin and hematocrit has been observed in 1 in 10 patients and transient eosinophilia in 1 in 14 patients. Less common reactions seen were transient neutropenia (fewer than 1 in 100 patients) and leukopenia (1 in 750 patients). A similar pattern and incidence were seen with other cephalosporins used in controlled studies.

Hepatic: Transient rise in SGOT and SGPT (1 in 25 patients), alkaline phosphatase (1 in 50 patients), LDH (1 in 75 patients), and bilirubin (1 in 500 patients) levels has been noted.

Kidney: Elevations in serum creatinine and/or blood urea nitrogen and a decreased creatinine clearance have been observed, but their relationship to cefuroxime is unknown.

In addition to the adverse reactions listed above that have been observed in patients treated with cefuroxime, the following adverse reactions and altered laboratory tests have been reported for cephalosporin-class antibiotics:

Adverse Reactions: Vomiting, abdominal pain, colitis, vaginitis including vaginal candidiasis, toxic nephropathy, hepatic dysfunction including cholestasis, aplastic anemia, hemolytic anemia, hemorrhage.

Several cephalosporins have been implicated in triggering seizures, particularly in patients with renal impairment when the dosage was not reduced (see DOSAGE AND ADMINISTRATION). If seizures associated with drug therapy should occur, the drug should be discontinued. Anticonvulsant therapy can be given if clinically indicated.

Altered Laboratory Tests: Prolonged prothrombin time, pancytopenia, agranulocytosis, thrombocytopenia.

DOSAGE AND ADMINISTRATION

Dosage: ***Adults:*** The usual adult dosage range for Zinacef® (sterile cefuroxime sodium/cefuroxime sodium injection) is 750 mg to 1.5 grams every 8 hours, usually for 5–10 days. In uncomplicated urinary tract infections, skin and skin structure infections, disseminated gonococcal infections, and uncomplicated pneumonia, a 750-mg dose every 8 hours is recommended. In severe or complicated infections, a 1.5-gram dose every 8 hours is recommended.

In bone and joint infections, a 1.5-gram dose every 8 hours is recommended. In clinical trials, surgical intervention was performed when indicated as an adjunct to Zinacef therapy. A course of oral antibiotics was administered when appropriate following the completion of parenteral administration of Zinacef.

In life-threatening infections or infections due to less susceptible organisms, 1.5 grams every 6 hours may be required. In bacterial meningitis, the dosage should not exceed 3 grams every 8 hours. The recommended dosage for uncomplicated gonococcal infection is 1.5 grams given intramuscularly as a single dosage at two different sites together with 1 gram of oral probenecid. For preventive use for clean-contaminated or potentially contaminated surgical procedures, a 1.5-gram dose administered intravenously just before surgery (approximately one-half to 1 hour before the initial incision) is recommended. Thereafter, give 750 mg intravenously or intramuscularly every 8 hours when the procedure is prolonged.

For preventive use during open heart surgery, a 1.5-gram dose administered intravenously at the induction of anesthesia and every 12 hours thereafter for a total of 6 grams is recommended.

Impaired Renal Function: A reduced dosage must be employed when renal function is impaired. Dosage should be determined by the degree of renal impairment and the susceptibility of the causative organism (see Table 1).

Table 1: Dosage of Zinacef in Adults with Reduced Renal Function

Creatinine Clearance (mL/min)	Dose	Frequency
>20	750 mg–1.5 gram	q8h
10–20	750 mg	q12h
<10	750 mg	q24h*

* Since Zinacef is dialyzable, patients on hemodialysis should be given a further dose at the end of the dialysis.

When only serum creatinine is available, the following formula[2] (based on sex, weight, and age of the patient) may be used to convert this value into creatinine clearance. The serum creatinine should represent a steady state of renal function.

Males: $$\text{Creatinine Clearance (mL/min)} = \frac{\text{Weight (kg)} \times (140-\text{age})}{72 \times \text{serum creatinine (mg/dL)}}$$

Females: $0.85 \times$ male value

Note: As with antibiotic therapy in general, administration of Zinacef should be continued for a minimum of 48–72 hours after the patient becomes asymptomatic or after evidence of bacterial eradication has been obtained; a minimum of 10 days of treatment is recommended in infections caused by *Streptococcus pyogenes* in order to guard against the risk of rheumatic fever or glomerulonephritis; frequent bacteriologic and clinical appraisal is necessary during therapy of chronic urinary tract infection and may be required for several months after therapy has been completed; persistent infections may require treatment for several weeks; and doses smaller than those indicated above should not be used. In staphylococcal and other infections involving a collection of pus, surgical drainage should be carried out where indicated.

Infants and Children Above 3 Months of Age: Administration of 50–100 mg/kg per day in equally divided doses every 6–8 hours has been successful for most infections susceptible to cefuroxime. The higher dosage of 100 mg/kg per day (not to exceed the maximum adult dosage) should be used for the more severe or serious infections.

In bone and joint infections, 150 mg/kg per day (not to exceed the maximum adult dosage) is recommended in equally divided doses every 8 hours. In clinical trials, a course of oral antibiotics was administered to children following the completion of parenteral administration of Zinacef.

In cases of bacterial meningitis, a larger dosage of Zinacef is recommended, 200–240 mg/kg per day intravenously in divided doses every 6–8 hours.

In children with renal insufficiency, the frequency of dosage should be modified consistent with the recommendations for adults.

Preparation of Solution and Suspension: The directions for preparing Zinacef for both IV and IM use are summarized in Table 2.

Table 2: Preparation of Solution and Suspension

Strength	Amount of Diluent to Be Added (ml)	Volume to Be Withdrawn	Approximate Cefuroxime Concentration (mg/mL)
750-mg Vial	3.0 (IM)	Total*	220
750-mg Vial	8.0 (IV)	Total	90
1.5-gram Vial	16.0 (IV)	Total	90
750-mg Infusion pack	100 (IV)	—	7.5
1.5-gram Infusion pack	100 (IV)	—	15
7.5-gram Pharmacy bulk package	77 (IV)	Amount Needed†	95

***Note:** Zinacef is a suspension at IM concentrations.
†8 mL of solution contains 750 mg of cefuroxime; 16 mL of solution contains 1.5 grams of cefuroxime.

For Intramuscular Use: Each 750-mg vial of Zinacef should be constituted with 3 mL of sterile water for injection. Shake gently to disperse and withdraw completely the resulting suspension for injection.

For Intravenous Use: Each 750-mg vial should be constituted with 8.0 mL of sterile water for injection. Withdraw completely the resulting solution for injection.

Each 1.5-gram vial should be constituted with 16.0 mL of sterile water for injection, and the solution should be completely withdrawn for injection.

The 7.5-gram pharmacy bulk vial should be constituted with 77 mL of sterile water for injection; each 8 mL of the resulting solution contains 750 mg of cefuroxime.

Each 750-mg and 1.5-gram infusion pack should be constituted with 100 mL of sterile water for injection, 5% dextrose injection, 0.9% sodium chloride injection, or any of the solutions listed under the Intravenous portion of the COMPATIBILITY AND STABILITY section. [See table above.]

Administration: After constitution, Zinacef may be given intravenously or by deep IM injection into a large muscle mass (such as the gluteus or lateral part of the thigh). Before injecting intramuscularly, aspiration is necessary to avoid inadvertent injection into a blood vessel.

Intravenous Administration: The IV route may be preferable for patients with bacterial septicemia or other severe or life-threatening infections or for patients who may be poor risks because of lowered resistance, particularly if shock is present or impending.

For direct intermittent IV administration, slowly inject the solution into a vein over a period of 3–5 minutes or give it through the tubing system by which the patient is also receiving other IV solutions.

For intermittent IV infusion with a Y-type administration set, dosing can be accomplished through the tubing system by which the patient may be receiving other IV solutions. However, during infusion of the solution containing Zinacef, it is advisable to temporarily discontinue administration of any other solutions at the same site.

ADD-Vantage® vials are to be constituted only with 50 or 100 mL of 5% dextrose injection, 0.9% sodium chloride injection, or 0.45% sodium chloride injection in Abbott ADD-Vantage flexible diluent containers (see Instructions for Constitution section of the package insert). ADD-Vantage vials that have been joined to Abbott ADD-Vantage diluent containers and activated to dissolve the drug are stable for 24 hours at room temperature or for 7 days under refrigeration. Joined vials that have not been activated may be used within a 14-day period; this period corresponds to that for use of Abbott ADD-Vantage containers following removal of the outer packaging (overwrap).

Freezing solutions of Zinacef in the ADD-Vantage system is not recommended.

For continuous IV infusion, a solution of Zinacef may be added to an IV infusion pack containing one of the following fluids: 0.9% sodium chloride injection; 5% dextrose injection; 10% dextrose injection; 5% dextrose and 0.9% sodium chloride injection; 5% dextrose and 0.45% sodium chloride injection; or 1/6 M sodium lactate injection.

Solutions of Zinacef, like those of most beta-lactam antibiotics, should not be added to solutions of aminoglycoside antibiotics because of potential interaction.

However, if concurrent therapy with Zinacef and an aminoglycoside is indicated, each of these antibiotics can be administered separately to the same patient.

Directions for Use of Zinacef® (cefuroxime sodium injection) Frozen in Galaxy® Plastic Containers: Zinacef supplied as a frozen, sterile, iso-osmotic, nonpyrogenic solution in plastic containers is to be administered after thawing either as a continuous or intermittent IV infusion. The thawed solution of the premixed product is stable for 28 days if stored under refrigeration (5° C) or for 24 hours at room temperature (25° C). **Do not Refreeze.**

Thaw container at room temperature (25°C) or under refrigeration (5°C). Do not force thaw by immersion in water baths or by microwave irradiation. Components of the solution may precipitate in the frozen state and will dissolve upon reaching room temperature with little or no agitation. Potency is not affected. Mix after solution has reached room temperature. Check for minute leaks by squeezing bag firmly. Discard bag if leaks are found as sterility may be impaired. Do not add supplementary medication. Do not use unless solution is clear and seal is intact.

Use sterile equipment.

Caution: Do not use plastic containers in series connections. Such use could result in air embolism due to residual air being drawn from the primary container before administration of the fluid from the secondary container is complete.

Continued on next page

Glaxo—Cont.

Preparation for Administration:
1. Suspend container from eyelet support.
2. Remove protector from outlet port at bottom of container.
3. Attach administration set. Refer to complete directions accompanying set.

COMPATIBILITY AND STABILITY

Intramuscular: When constituted as directed with sterile water for injection, suspensions of Zinacef® (sterile cefuroxime sodium) for IM injection maintain satisfactory potency for 24 hours at room temperature and for 48 hours under refrigeration (5℃).
After the periods mentioned above any unused suspensions should be discarded.

Intravenous: When the 750-mg, 1.5-g, and 7.5-g pharmacy bulk vials are constituted as directed with sterile water for injection, the Zinacef solutions for IV administration maintain satisfactory potency for 24 hours at room temperature and for 48 hours (750-mg and 1.5-g vials) or for 7 days (7.5-g pharmacy bulk vial) under refrigeration (5℃). More dilute solutions, such as 750 mg or 1.5 g plus 100 mL of sterile water for injection, 5% dextrose injection, or 0.9% sodium chloride injection, also maintain satisfactory potency for 24 hours at room temperature and for 7 days under refrigeration.
These solutions may be further diluted to concentrations of between 1 and 30 mg/mL in the following solutions and will lose not more than 10% activity for 24 hours at room temperature or for at least 7 days under refrigeration: 0.9% sodium chloride injection; 1/6 M sodium lactate injection; ringer's injection, USP; lactated ringer's injection, USP; 5% dextrose and 0.9% sodium chloride injection; 5% dextrose injection; 5% dextrose and 0.45% sodium chloride injection; 5% dextrose and 0.225% sodium chloride injection; 10% dextrose injection; and 10% invert sugar in water for injection. Unused solutions should be discarded after the time periods mentioned above.
Zinacef has also been found compatible for 24 hours at room temperature when admixed in IV infusion with heparin (10 and 50 U/mL) in 0.9% sodium chloride injection and potassium chloride (10 and 40 mEq/L) in 0.9% sodium chloride injection. Sodium bicarbonate injection, USP is not recommended for the dilution of Zinacef.
The 750-mg and 1.5-g Zinacef ADD-Vantage® vials, when diluted in 50 or 100 mL of 5% dextrose injection, 0.9% sodium chloride injection, or 0.45% sodium chloride injection, may be stored for up to 24 hours at room temperature or for 7 days under refrigeration.
Frozen Stability: Constitute the 750-mg, 1.5-g, or 7.5-g vial as directed for IV administration in Table 2. Immediately withdraw the total contents of the 750-mg or 1.5-g vial or 8 or 16 mL from the 7.5-g bulk vial and add to a Baxter Viaflex® Mini-bag™ containing 50 or 100 mL of 0.9% sodium chloride injection or 5% dextrose injection and freeze. Frozen solutions are stable for 6 months when stored at −20℃. Frozen solutions should be thawed at room temperature and not refrozen. Do not force thaw by immersion in water baths or by microwave irradiation. Thawed solutions may be stored for up to 24 hours at room temperature or 7 days in a refrigerator.
Note: Parenteral drug products should be inspected visually for particulate matter and discoloration before administration whenever solution and container permit.
As with other cephalosporins, Zinacef powder as well as solutions and suspensions tend to darken, depending on storage conditions, without adversely affecting product potency.
Directions for Dispensing: *Pharmacy Bulk Package—Not for Direct Infusion:* The pharmacy bulk package is for use in a pharmacy admixture service only under a laminar flow hood. Entry into the vial must be made with a sterile transfer set or other sterile dispensing device, and the contents dispensed in aliquots using aseptic technique. The use of syringe and needle is not recommended as it may cause leakage (see DOSAGE AND ADMINISTRATION). AFTER INITIAL WITHDRAWAL USE ENTIRE CONTENTS OF VIAL PROMPTLY. ANY UNUSED PORTION MUST BE DISCARDED WITHIN 24 HOURS.

HOW SUPPLIED
Zinacef® (sterile cefuroxime sodium) in the dry state should be stored between 15° and 30℃ (59° and 86°F) and protected from light. Zinacef is a dry, white to off-white powder supplied in vials and infusion packs as follows:
NDC 0173-0352-31 750-mg* Vial (Tray of 25)
NDC 0173-0354-35 1.5-g* Vial (Tray of 25)
NDC 0173-0353-32 750-mg* Infusion Pack (Tray of 10)
NDC 0173-0356-32 1.5-g* Infusion Pack (Tray of 10)
NDC 0173-0400-00 7.5-g* Pharmacy Bulk Package (Tray of 6)
NDC 0173-0436-00 750-mg ADD-Vantage® Vial (Tray of 25)
NDC 0173-0437-00 1.5-g ADD-Vantage® Vial (Tray of 10)

---

*Equivalent to cefuroxime.

(The above ADD-Vantage vials are to be used only with Abbott ADD-Vantage diluent containers).
Zinacef frozen as a premixed solution of cefuroxime sodium should not be stored above −20° C. Zinacef is supplied frozen in 50-mL, single-dose, plastic containers as follows:
NDC 0173-0424-00 750-mg* Plastic Container (Carton of 24)
NDC 0173-0425-00 1.5-g* Plastic Container (Carton of 24)

REFERENCES
1. National Committee for Clinical Laboratory Standards. *Performance Standards for Antimicrobial Susceptibility Testing.* Third Informational Supplement. NCCLS Document M100-S3, Vol. 11, No. 17. Villanova, Pa: NCCLS; 1991.
2. Cockcroft DW, Gault MH: Prediction of creatinine clearance from serum creatinine. *Nephron.* 1976;16:31–41.
Zinacef is a registered trademark of Glaxo.
ADD-Vantage is a registered trademark of Abbott Laboratories.
Clinitest is a registered trademark of Ames Division, Miles Laboratories, Inc.
Tes-Tape is a registered trademark of Eli Lilly and Company.
Galaxy and Viaflex are registered trademarks of Baxter International Inc.

---

*Equivalent to cefuroxime.
Shown in Product Identification Section, page 411

Glenwood, Inc.
83 N. SUMMIT STREET
TENAFLY, NJ 07670

BICHLORACETIC ACID® KAHLENBERG   ℞
Dichloroacetic Acid—Topical

DESCRIPTION
BICHLORACETIC ACID (dichloroacetic acid) Kahlenberg $(CHCl_2COOH)$ is a clear, colorless liquid (sp. gr. 1.56) supplied full strength ready to use. It does not contain or require a solvent or diluent, is always uniform in potency. BICHLORACETIC ACID (dichloroacetic acid) remains colorless and retains its potency if kept in a tightly closed bottle and not contaminated with dissolved keratin or wooden applicators.

ACTIONS
BICHLORACETIC ACID (dichloroacetic acid) rapidly penetrates and cauterizes skin, keratin and other tissues. Its cauterizing effect is comparable to that obtained with such methods as electrocautery or freezing.

INDICATIONS
The lesions for which therapy with BICHLORACETIC ACID (dichloroacetic acid) is indicated are all types of verrucae: calluses; hard and soft corns; xanthoma palpebrarum; seborrheic keratoses; ingrown nails; cysts and benign erosion of the cervix including endocervicitis; epistaxis.

CONTRAINDICATION
Topically applied chemical cauterant-keratolytics should not be used for the treatment of malignant or premalignant lesions.

WARNING
BICHLORACETIC ACID (dichloroacetic acid) is an extremely powerful keratolytic and cauterant. It should be restricted to those areas where these effects are desired.

ADMINISTRATION AND DOSAGE
The amount of BICHLORACETIC ACID (dichloroacetic acid) which should be applied varies with the nature of the lesion. Dense horny lesions such as corns, warts, calluses, plantar warts, etc. require repeated intensive treatment. Lesions of light density such as pedunculated warts, xanthoma palpebrarum, soft corns, seborrheic keratoses, condyloma acuminata, etc. should receive lighter applications.
Similarly, the number of treatments necessary will vary depending on the particular lesion being treated.

COMPLETE TREATMENT KIT

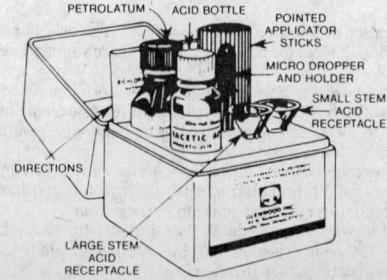

The treatment kit provides 10 ml. BICHLORACETIC ACID KAHLENBERG, 16 grams of petrolatum in a bottle, approximately 100 applicators, and a product insert with directions. Also included are a microdropper and holder and two sealed-stem acid receptacles of differing capacity.

HOW SUPPLIED
Bichloracetic Acid® Kahlenberg
Complete Treatment Kit, NDC 0516-1004-11
Restocking Unit, NDC 0516-1006-77, 75 ml. bottle
Replenishment Unit, NDC 0516-1007-11, 10 ml. bottle
Unit-Kit, NDC 0516-1010-05, 0.5 ml. single-use, disposable ampule

---

CALPHOSAN®   ℞
(calcium glycerophosphate/calcium lactate)
calcium/phosphorus solution in metabolic disorders involving low calcium

COMPOSITION
CALPHOSAN is a specially processed solution containing calcium glycerophosphate and calcium lactate. CALPHOSAN is isotonic, with a pH of about 7 or somewhat above. (Other calcium solutions are usually quite acid, with pH values of 4.5 to 5.5). Each 10 ml. CALPHOSAN contains calcium glycerophosphate 50 mg. and calcium lactate 50 mg. in a physiological solution of sodium chloride, with 0.25% phenol as a preservative.

ADVANTAGES
Intramuscular injections of CALPHOSAN raise blood serum calcium levels, do not raise the calcium levels above normal. Of conspicuous importance, intramuscular injections of CALPHOSAN are without pain, inflammatory reactions or sloughing.

INDICATIONS
Wherever calcium is indicated or in conditions associated with hypocalcemia.

ADMINISTRATION
10 ml. 1 to 4 times weekly or as determined by the physician.

USE IN PREGNANCY
Safety for use in pregnancy or during lactation has not been established.

CONTRAINDICATIONS
Hypercalcemia; and in view of the fact that hypercalcemia is associated with sarcoidosis and bone metastasis of neoplastic processes, it should not be used in those conditions. As there is a similarity in the actions of calcium and digitalis on the contractility and excitability of the heart muscle, CALPHOSAN is contraindicated in fully digitalized patients. **Do not use intramuscularly in infants and young children.**

AVAILABILITY
60 ml. multiple dose vials—NDC 0516-0060-60.

MYOTONACHOL™   ℞
Bethanechol Chloride—Oral USP

HOW SUPPLIED
Myotonachol.
    10 mg. tablets, flat, NDC 0516-0021-01 in bottles of 100s.
    25 mg. tablets, flat, NDC 0516-0022-01 in bottles of 100s.

POTABA®   ℞
Systemic ANTIFIBROSIS THERAPY

PRODUCT OVERVIEW
KEY FACTS
Potaba® (Aminobenzoate Potassium) is considered a member of the vitamin B complex. It has been suggested that the antifibrotic action of Potaba® is due to its mediation of increased oxygen uptake at the tissue level.

MAJOR USES
Potaba® offers a means of treatment of serious and often chronic entities, such as scleroderma and Peyronie's Disease.

SAFETY INFORMATION
Contraindicated in patients taking sulfonamides. Anorexia, nausea, fever and rash have occurred infrequently and subside with omission of the drug. Often, desensitization can be accomplished and treatment resumed.

PRODUCT ILLUSTRATION

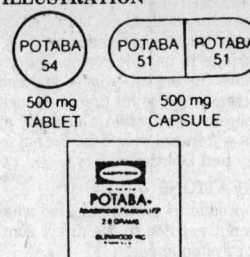

2.0 grams

PRESCRIBING INFORMATION

POTABA®   ℞
Systemic ANTIFIBROSIS THERAPY

FORMULA
POTABA is chemically Aminobenzoate Potassium, U.S.P.

INDICATIONS
Based on a review of this drug by the National Academy of Sciences-National Research Council and/or other information, FDA has classified the indications as follows:
"Possibly" effective: Potassium aminobenzoate is possibly effective in the treatment of scleroderma, dermatomyositis, morphea, linear scleroderma, pemphigus, and Peyronie's disease.
Final classification of the less-than-effective indications requires further investigation.

ADVANTAGES
POTABA offers a means of treatment of serious and often chronic entities involving fibrosis and nonsuppurative inflammation.

PHARMACOLOGY
P-Aminobenzoate is considered a member of the vitamin B complex. Small amounts are found in cereal, eggs, milk and meats. Detectable amounts are normally present in human blood, spinal fluid, urine, and sweat. PABA is a component of several biologically important systems, and it participates in a number of fundamental biological processes. It has been suggested that the antifibrosis action of POTABA is due to its mediation of increased oxygen uptake at the tissue level. Fibrosis is believed to occur from either too much serotonin or too little monoamine oxidase activity over a period of time. Monoamine oxidase requires an adequate supply of oxygen to function properly. By increasing oxygen supply at the tissue level POTABA may enhance MAO activity and prevent or bring about regression of fibrosis.

CLINICAL USES
PEYRONIE'S DISEASE: 21 patients with Peyronie's disease were placed on POTABA therapy for periods ranging from 3 months to 2 years. Pain disappeared from 16 of 16 cases in which it had been present. There was objective improvement in penile deformity in 10 of 17 patients, and decrease in plaque size in 16 of 21. The authors suggest that this medication offers no hazard of further local injury as may result from other therapy. There were no significant untoward effects encountered on long term POTABA therapy.
SCLERODERMA: Of 135 patients with diffuse systemic sclerosis treated with POTABA every patient but one has shown softening of the involved skin if treatment has been continued for 3 months or longer. The responses have been reported in a number of publications. The treatment program consists of systemic antifibrosis therapy with POTABA, physical therapy, including deep breathing exercises and dynamic traction splints where indicated, and bethanechol chloride (MYOTONACHOL, Glenwood) for relief of dysphagia as well as small doses of reserpine for amelioration of Raynaud's phenomena.
DERMATOMYOSITIS: Five patients with scleroderma and 2 with dermatomyositis were treated with POTABA. There was striking clinical improvement in each patient. Doses of 15-20 grams per day were well tolerated, and patients were easily able to take these doses.
MORPHEA and LINEAR SCLERODERMA: All 14 patients with localized forms of scleroderma placed on long-term POTABA treatment showed softening of the sclerotic component of their disorder. Treatment is particularly indicated in patients where persistent compressive sclerosis may contribute even greater disfigurement or functional embarrassment from secondary pressure atrophy.

DOSAGE AND ADMINISTRATION
The average adult daily dose of POTABA is 12 grams, usually given in four to six divided doses. Tablets and capsules 0.5 gram are given at the rate of 4 tablets or capsules 6 times daily, or 6 given four times daily, usually with meals, and at bed-time with a snack. Tablets must be dissolved in an adequate amount of liquid to prevent gastrointestinal upset. POTABA Envules contain 2 grams pure drug each, and 6 Envules are given for a total of 12 grams POTABA daily. POTABA Powder is used to prepare solutions, which are kept refrigerated, but for no longer than one week. 100 grams POTABA powder make 1 quart of 10% solution when dissolved in potable tap water. Children are given 1 gram POTABA daily in divided doses for each 10 lbs. of body weight.

SIDE EFFECTS
Anorexia, nausea, fever and rash have occurred infrequently and subside with omission of the drug. Often, desensitization can be accomplished and treatment resumed.

USAGE IN PREGNANCY
Safety for use in pregnancy or during lactation has not been established.

PRECAUTIONS
Should anorexia or nausea occur, therapy is interrupted until the patient is eating normally again. This permits prompt subsidence of symptoms and also avoids the possible development of hypoglycemia. Give cautiously to patients with renal disease. If a hypersensitivity reaction should occur, POTABA should be stopped.

CONTRAINDICATIONS
POTABA should not be administered to patients taking sulfonamides.

HOW SUPPLIED
POTABA Capsules—0.5 gm.
NDC 0516-0051-25 Bottle of 250
NDC 0516-0051-10 Bottle of 1000
POTABA Tablets—0.5 gm.
NDC 0516-0054-01 Bottle of 100
NDC 0516-0054-10 Bottle of 1000
POTABA Envules—2 gm.
NDC 0516-0052-50 Box of 50
POTABA Powder, pure
NDC 0516-0053-01 Bottle of 100 gms.
NDC 0516-0053-16 Bottle of 1 lb.
Shown in Product Identification Section, page 411

PRIMER® Unna Boot   OTC

COMPOSITION
Zinc Oxide, Acacia, Glycerin, Castor Oil and White Petrolatum. No preservatives.

ACTIONS AND USES
Treatment of venous insufficiency conditions such as stasis ulcers.

ADMINISTRATION AND DOSAGE
The combination of PRIMER and MEDIRIP elastic adhesive bandage produces a flexible cast boot. Apply the PRIMER over the entire lower leg, starting immediately behind the toes and continue up to the knee. Apply the elastic bandage over the PRIMER using firm evenly distributed pressure. Continue bandaging until the PRIMER is completely covered. The treatment is ambulatory and the patient should be encouraged to walk as much as possible.
Change bandage at least once a week for the first two or three weeks, then every two or three weeks until healing is complete.

PRECAUTIONS
If skin sensitivity or irritation develops discontinue use and consult a physician.

HOW SUPPLIED
3″ × 10 yards—Unna Boot-List No. 300-1
NDC 0516-1410-30
4″ × 10 yards—Unna Boot-List No. 400-1
NDC 0516-1410-40

YODOXIN®   ℞
210 mg. & 650 mg. Tablets
(IODOQUINOL TABLETS U.S.P.)

PRODUCT OVERVIEW

KEY FACTS
Yodoxin (Iodoquinol) is amebicidal against the cyst and trophozoite forms of Entaemoeba histolytica. Yodoxin® contains 64% organically bound iodine.

MAJOR USES
Yodoxin® is used in the treatment of intestinal amebiasis.

SAFETY INFORMATION
Contraindicated in patients with hepatic damage and in patients with known hypersensitivity to iodine and 8-hydroxyquinolines. Long term use of this drug should be avoided as optic neuritis, optic atrophy and peripheral neuropathy have been reported following prolonged high dosage with halogenated 8-hydroxyquinolines.

PRODUCT ILLUSTRATION

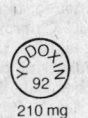 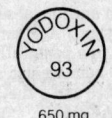

210 mg   650 mg

PRESCRIBING INFORMATION

YODOXIN®   ℞
210 mg. & 650 mg. Tablets
(IODOQUINOL TABLETS U.S.P.)

DESCRIPTION
Iodoquinol is of a light yellowish to tan color, nearly odorless and stable in air. The compound is practically insoluble in water, and sparingly soluble in most other solvents. It contains 64 per cent organically bound iodine.

ACTION
Iodoquinol is amebicidal against Entamoeba histolytica and is considered effective against the trophozoite and cyst forms.

INDICATIONS
Iodoquinol is used in the treatment of intestinal amebiasis.

CONTRAINDICATIONS
Known hypersensitivity to iodine and 8-hydroxyquinolines. Contraindicated in patients with hepatic damage.

WARNINGS
Optic neuritis, optic atrophy, and peripheral neuropathy have been reported following prolonged high dosage therapy with halogenated 8-hydroxyquinolines. Long term use of this drug should be avoided.

USE IN PREGNANCY
Safety for use in pregnancy or during lactation has not been established.

PRECAUTIONS
Iodoquinol should be used with caution in patients with thyroid disease.
Protein-bound serum iodine levels may be increased during treatment with iodoquinol and therefore interfere with certain thyroid function tests. These effects may persist for as long as six months after discontinuation of therapy. Discontinue the drug if hypersensitivity reactions occur.

ADVERSE REACTIONS
Skin: various forms of skin eruptions (acneiform papular and pustular; bullae; vegetating of tuberous iododerma), urticaria and pruritus. Gastrointestinal: nausea, vomiting, abdominal cramps, diarrhea, and pruritus ani.
Fever, chills, headache, vertigo and enlargement of thyroid have been reported. Optic neuritis, optic atrophy and peripheral neuropathy have been reported in association with prolonged high-dosage 8-hydroxyquinoline therapy.

DOSAGE AND ADMINISTRATION
Usual adult dose: (210 mg. each) 3 tablets three times daily, after meals for 20 days. Children 6 to 12 years: (210 mg. each) 2 tablets, t.i.d. Children under 6: (210 mg. each) one tablet per 15 pounds of body weight. Usual adult dose: (650 mg. each) one tablet three times a day for twenty days, to be taken after meals. Children (650 mg. each): For twenty days, 40 mg. per Kg. of body weight daily divided into 3 doses, not to exceed 1.95 grams in 24 hours, for 20 days.

HOW SUPPLIED
YODOXIN Tablets—210 mg.
NDC-0516-0092-01 Bottle of 100
NDC-0516-0092-10 Bottle of 1000
YODOXIN Tablets—650 mg.
NDC-0516-0093-01 Bottle of 100
NDC-0516-0093-10 Bottle of 1000

STORAGE
Store at Controlled Room Temperature 15–30°C. (59–86°F.)

CAUTION
Federal law prohibits dispensing without prescription.

Products are cross-indexed by
generic and chemical names
in the
YELLOW SECTION.

Gordon Laboratories, Inc.
STATE AND PARKVIEW ROADS
UPPER DARBY, PA 19082

GORDOCHOM™ Solution   ℞
[gŏrdō 'kŏm]

DESCRIPTION
Gordochom is an antifungal solution for topical use containing 25% Undecylenic Acid and 3% Chloroxylenol as its active ingredients in a penetrating oil base. Undecylenic Acid is chemically 10-hendecenoic acid having the empirical formula $C_{11}H_{20}O_2$ and the chemical bond structure $CH_2=CH(CH_2)_8CO_2H$.
Undecylenic Acid is a colorless to pale yellow liquid. It is soluble in water and soluble in alcohol, chloroform and ether.
Chloroxylenol is chemically 2-chloro-5-hydroxy-1,3-dimethylbenzene having the empirical formula C_8H_9ClO.

CLINICAL PHARMACOLOGY
Undecylenic Acid is a fungistatic agent employed in the treatment of tinea pedis, tinea capitis, ringworm and dermatophytosis.
Chloroxylenol is a topical antiseptic, germicide and antifungal agent effective against a wide variety of causitive fungi and yeast organisms. Among those affected by chloroxylenol are candida albicans, aspergillus niger, aspergillus flavus, trychophyton rubrum, tricophyton mentagrophytes, penicillum luteum and epidermophyton floccosum.
The penetrating oil base vehicle serves as a delivery system, enhancing the impregnation of Undecylenic Acid and Chloroxylenol as antimicrobial agents in the treatment of onychomycosis.

INDICATIONS
Gordochom is indicated in the treatment and prevention of onychomycosis, cutaneous fungus infections, as well as a softener for callous nail grooves.

CONTRAINDICATIONS
Gordochom is contraindicated in patients who are sensitive to Undecylenic Acid or Chloroxylenol.

WARNINGS
FOR EXTERNAL USE ONLY. Not for ophthalmic or optic use. Avoid inhaling and contact with eyes or other mucous membranes. Not to be applied over blistered, raw or oozing areas of skin or over deep puncture wounds.

PRECAUTIONS
If a reaction suggesting sensitivity or chemical irritation should occur with the use of Gordochom, treatment should be discontinued. Use of Gordochom in pregnancy has not been established.

ADVERSE REACTIONS
No significant adverse reactions have been reported. However, attention should be paid to localized hypersensitivity.

DOSAGE AND ADMINISTRATION
Cleanse the affected area thoroughly. Paint on affected area twice daily, morning and evening. As a precaution against relapse of the condition, continue therapy for several weeks after the condition has cleared.

HOW SUPPLIED
Gordochom is available in 1 oz. bottles with special brush applicator. (NDC# 10481-3010-2)
Store at controlled room temperatures (59°–86°F).
For external use only.
Keep out of reach of children.

CAUTION
Federal law prohibits dispensing without prescription.

IDENTIFICATION PROBLEM?
Consult PDR's
Product Identification Section
where you'll find over 1700
products pictured actual size
and in full color.

Gray Pharmaceutical Co.
affiliate, The Purdue Frederick Co.
100 CONNECTICUT AVENUE
NORWALK, CT 06850-3590

Senna
X-PREP® BOWEL EVACUANT LIQUID
[ĕx 'prep]
(standardized extract of senna fruit)

INDICATIONS
An easy-to-administer, palatable, highly effective bowel evacuant for cleansing the colon prior to x-ray, endoscopic examination or surgery. Permits excellent visualization without residual oil droplets. "Senna" X-PREP Liquid is fully prepared in a single dose container—all the patient has to do is drink the contents of one small bottle (2½ fl. oz.). Good patient cooperation is ensured because of highly pleasant taste. Predictable effectiveness helps reduce or eliminate the need for enemas prior to radiography.

DESCRIPTION
Each bottle contains 130 mg sennosides. Active Ingredient: Standaridized Senna Fruit Concentrate. Inactive Ingredients: Alcohol 7%, by volume, Methyl paraben, Potassium sorbate, Propyl paraben, Sodium lauryl sulfate, Sucrose, Water, Natural and Artificial Flavors and other ingredients.

CONTRAINDICATIONS
Acute surgical abdomen.

WARNINGS
Do not use this product unless directed by a physician. Do not use when abdominal pain, nausea or vomiting is present. As with any drug, if you are pregnant or nursing a baby, seek the advice of a health professional before using this product. In case of accidental overdose, seek professional assistance or contact a Poison Control Center immediately. Keep out of children's reach.

CAUTION
In diabetic patients, the physician should be aware of the sugar content of "Senna" X-PREP Liquid (50 grams per 2½ fl. oz. dose).

ADMINISTRATION AND DOSAGE
Recommended Dosage (or as directed by physician):
Adults and children 12 years of age and older: Take one bottle between 2 and 4 p.m. on day prior to x-ray or other diagnostic procedures. Drink entire contents. For children under 12 years of age, consult a doctor. A strong bowel action can be expected approximately 6 hours after drinking. After "Senna" X-PREP Liquid is taken, diet should be confined to clear fluids.

HOW SUPPLIED
2½ fl. oz. bottles (alcohol 7% by volume), each providing a single, complete adult dose.
Also Available—Two X-PREP® Bowel Evacuant Kits.
Kit #1 contains: Two SENOKOT-S® Tablets (standardized senna concentrate and docusate sodium), one bottle of X-PREP Liquid 2½ fl. oz., and one RECTOLAX® Suppository (bisacodyl 10 mg), plus easy-to-follow patient instructions for hydration, clear liquid diet, and the correct time-sequence for administering the above laxatives.
Kit #2 contains: One dose CITRALAX® Granules 1.06 oz. (effervescent citrate/sulfate of magnesia), one bottle of X-PREP Liquid 2½ fl. oz., and one RECTOLAX Suppository (bisacodyl 10 mg), plus easy-to-follow patient instructions.
Copyright © 1991, Gray Pharmaceutical Co., Norwalk, CT 06850-3590.

Guardian Laboratories
a division of United-Guardian, Inc.
P.O. Box 2500
SMITHTOWN, N.Y. 11787

CLORPACTIN® WCS-90   OTC
[klor-pak 'tin]
(brand of sodium oxychlorosene)

COMPOSITION
Stabilized organic derivative of hypochlorous acid. A white, water soluble powder with a characteristic smell of hypochlorous acid. Active chlorine derived from calcium hypochlorite: 3–4%.

ACTION AND USES
For use as a topical antiseptic for treating localized infections, particularly when resistant organisms are present. Complete spectrum (bacteria, fungi, viruses, mold, yeast and spores); effective in cases of antibiotic resistance; nontoxic and non-allergenic in use concentrations.

ADMINISTRATION AND DOSAGE
Applied by irrigation, instillations, spray, soaks or wet compresses, preferably thoroughly cleansing with gravity flow irrigation or syringe to provide copious quantities of fresh solution to remove the organic wastes and debris from the site of the involvement. Also for preoperative skin preparation and postoperative protection. Generally applied as the 0.4% solution in water, or isotonic saline, but as the 0.1% to 0.2% in Urology and Ophthalmology.

CONTRAINDICATIONS
The use of this product is contraindicated where the site of the infection is not exposed to the direct contact with the solution. Not for systemic use.

HOW SUPPLIED
In boxes containing 5 x 2 gram bottles.

LUBRASEPTIC® JELLY   OTC
[loo-bra "sep 'tik]

COMPOSITION
Active ingredients: Aryl phenols, as phenyl phenol 0.1%, Alkyl phenols, as amyl phenol 0.02%, in water miscible form as an acid complex. Phenyl mercuric nitrate 0.007%.

USES
For urethral instillation, prior to insertion of cystoscopes or sounds; for urethral dilations in the case of strictures. For proctologic use, in cases of hemorrhoids, or for post-hemorrhoidectomies, to provide increased comfort between and during the passage of stools. For endotracheal intubation. For use whenever a sterile water soluble lubricant is required: on cystoscopes and proctoscopes, in urological, rectal, and vaginal examinations or for use as a sterile dressing on burns, abrasions, and decubitus ulcers (bedsores).

PRECAUTIONS AND SIDE EFFECTS
No serious side effects or contraindications are known. Urethral instillation, in some individuals, may cause a temporary burning or stinging sensation but this usually disappears in several minutes. Excessive pressure should be avoided when instilling where strictures may exist.

HOW SUPPLIED
In boxes containing 24 packets each with a 10 gram sterile "bellows" shaped tube of jelly and a urethral Disposatip.

---

pHos-pHaid®   ℞
[fos 'fād]
(brand of urinary acidifier)

RENACIDIN® (Citric Acid,   ℞
Glucono-delta-lactone, and Magnesium Carbonate)
Irrigation

DESCRIPTION
Renacidin® (Citric Acid, Glucono-delta-lactone, and Magnesium Carbonate) Irrigation is a sterile, non-pyrogenic irrigation for use within the urinary tract in the prevention and dissolution of calculi.
Each 100 ml. of Renacidin Irrigation contains:
Active ingredients:

Citric Acid (anhydrous), U.S.P. $C_6H_8O_7$	6.602 grams
Glucono-delta-lactone $C_6H_{10}O_6$	0.198 grams
Magnesium Carbonate, U.S.P. $(MgCO_3)_4 \cdot Mg(OH)_2 \cdot 3H_2O$	3.177 grams

Citric Acid   **Glucono-delta-lactone**

Magnesium Carbonate
$(MgCO_3)_4 \cdot Mg(OH)_2 \cdot 3H_2O$
Inert ingredients:

Benzoic Acid, U.S.P.	0.023 grams

Solution pH: 3.85 (3.50–4.20)

HOW SUPPLIED
Renacidin Irrigation is available as a sterile, non-pyrogenic solution in 500 ml containers, packaged in cartons of six. Exposure of Renacidin Irrigation to heat or cold should be minimized. Renacidin Irrigation should be stored at controlled room temperature, 59° to 86°F (15° to 30°C). Avoid excessive heat or cold (keep from freezing). Brief exposure to

temperatures of up to 40°C or temperatures down to 5°C does not adversely affect the product.
NDC: 0327-0007-05
PRODUCT CODE: RN500

RENACIDIN® Powder   ℞
[ren "a-sē'din]

Gynex Pharmaceuticals, Inc.
1175 CORPORATE WOODS PARKWAY
VERNON HILLS, IL 60061

DELATESTRYL®   Ⓒ℞
Testosterone Enanthate Injection USP

DESCRIPTION
DELATESTRYL (Testosterone Enanthate Injection) provides testosterone enanthate, a derivative of the primary endogenous androgen testosterone, for intramuscualar administration. In their active form, androgens have a 17-beta-hydroxy group. Esterification of the 17-beta-hydroxy group increases the duration of action of testosterone; hydrolysis to free testosterone occurs *in vivo*. Each mL of sterile, colorless to pale yellow solution provides 200 mg testosterone enanthate in sesame oil with 5 mg chlorobutanol (chloral derivative) as a preservative.

HOW SUPPLIED
DELATESTRYL (Testosterone Enanthate Injection USP) is available in 5 mL (200 mg/mL) multiple-dose vials (NDC 54396-328-40) and in 1 mL (200 mg/mL) Unimatic® single dose syringes (NDC 54396-328-16). See package insert accompanying each Unimatic for complete information.
Storage
DELATESTRYL should be stored at room temperature. Warming and shaking the vial will redissolve any crystals that may have formed during storage at low temperatures.
Manufactured for
Gynex Pharmaceuticals, Inc.
Vernon Hills, IL 60061
by: Bristol-Myers Squibb
Princeton, NJ 08543

J4-468   Issued April 1992

GynoPharma Inc.
50 DIVISION STREET
SOMERVILLE, NJ 08876

PARAGARD® T380A   ℞
Intrauterine Copper Contraceptive

CAUTION: Federal law prohibits dispensing without prescription

NOTICE
You have received a Patient Information for an Informed Decision brochure that Federal Regulations (21 CFR 310.502) require you to furnish to each patient who is considering the use of the ParaGard®.
The Patient Information for an Informed Decision brochure contains information on the safety and efficacy of the Para-Gard®. It also contains the Patient Consent. You must not insert the ParaGard® until:
• You have read this physician prescription labeling and are familiar with all the information it contains.
• You and the patient have read the Patient Information for an Informed Decision brochure.
• You have counseled the patient and answered her questions about contraception, the ParaGard®, and the information in the brochure.
• You and the patient have reviewed and signed the Patient Consent.
The signed Patient Consent should be retained with the patient's records and a second copy of the signed brochure given to the patient for her records.

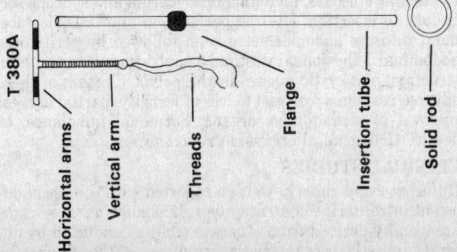

DESCRIPTION
The polyethylene body of the ParaGard® is wound with approximately 176 mg of copper wire and carries a copper collar of approximately 66.5 mg of copper on each of its transverse arms. The exposed surface areas of copper are 380 ± 23 mm². The dimensions of the ParaGard® are 36 mm in the vertical direction and 32 mm in the horizontal direction. The tip of the vertical arm of the ParaGard® is enlarged to form a bulb having a diameter of 3 mm. The ParaGard® is equipped with a monofilament polyethylene thread which is tied through the bulb, resulting in two threads at the tip to aid in removal of the IUD. The ParaGard® contains barium sulfate to render it radiopaque.
The ParaGard® is packaged together with an insertion tube and plunger in a Tyvek®-polyethylene pouch and then sterilized. The insertion tube is equipped with a movable flange to aid in gauging the depth to which the insertion tube is inserted through the cervical canal and into the uterine cavity.

CLINICAL PHARMACOLOGY
Available data indicate that the contraceptive effectiveness of the ParaGard® is enhanced by copper being released continuously from the copper coil and sleeves into the uterine cavity. The exact mechanism by which metallic copper enhances the contraceptive effect of an IUD has not been conclusively demonstrated. Various hypotheses have been advanced, including interference with sperm transport, fertilization, and implantation. Clinical studies with copper-bearing IUDs also suggest that fertilization is prevented either due to an altered number or lack of viability of spermatozoa.

INDICATIONS AND USAGE
The ParaGard® is indicated for intrauterine contraception. The ParaGard® is recommended for women who *have had at least one child* and are in a stable, mutually monogamous relationship, and have no history of pelvic inflammatory disease. The ParaGard® should not be kept in place longer than 8 years.

CONTRAINDICATIONS
The ParaGard® should not be inserted when one or more of the following conditions exist:
1. Pregnancy or suspicion of pregnancy.
2. Abnormalities of the uterus resulting in distortion of the uterine cavity.
3. Acute pelvic inflammatory disease or a history of pelvic inflammatory disease.
4. Postpartum endometritis or infected abortion in the past 3 months.
5. Known or suspected uterine or cervical malignancy, including unresolved, abnormal "Pap" smear.
6. Genital bleeding of unknown etiology.
7. Untreated acute cervicitis or vaginitis, including bacterial vaginosis, until infection is controlled.
8. Copper-containing IUDs should not be inserted in the presence of diagnosed Wilson's disease.
9. Known allergy to copper.
10. History of ectopic pregnancy.
11. Patient or her partner has multiple sexual partners.
12. Conditions associated with increased susceptibility to infections with microorganisms. Such conditions include, but are not limited to, leukemia, diabetes, acquired immune deficiency syndrome (AIDS), I.V. drug abuse, and those requiring chronic corticosteroid therapy.
13. Genital actinomycosis.
14. A previously inserted IUD that has not been removed.

WARNINGS
1. PREGNANCY
Effects on the offspring when pregnancy occurs with the ParaGard® in place are unknown.
a. Septic Abortion
Reports indicate an increased incidence of septic abortion with septicemia, septic shock, and death in patients becoming pregnant with an IUD in place. Most of these reports have been associated with, but not limited to, the mid-trimester of pregnancy. In some cases, the initial symptoms have been insidious and not easily recognized. If pregnancy should occur with a an IUD *in situ*, the IUD should be removed if the string is visible and removal is easily accomplished. Of course, manipulation may result in spontaneous abortion. If removal proves to be difficult, or if threads are not visible, interruption of the pregnancy should be considered and offered as an option.
b. Continuation of Pregnancy
If the patient elects to maintain the pregnancy and the IUD remains *in situ*, she should be warned that there is an increased risk of spontaneous abortion and sepsis. In addition, she is at increased risk of premature labor and delivery. As a consequence of premature birth, the fetus is at increased risk of damage. She should be followed

more closely than the usual obstetrical patient. The patient must be advised to report immediately all abnormal symptoms, such as flu-like syndrome, fever, abdominal cramping or pain, bleeding or vaginal discharge, because generalized symptoms of septicemia may be insidious.

2. ECTOPIC PREGNANCY
a. Although current data indicate that there is no increased risk of ectopic pregnancy in patients using the Para-Gard® and some data suggest there may be a lower risk than the general population using no method of contraception, a pregnancy which occurs with the ParaGard® in place is more likely to be ectopic than a pregnancy occurring without the ParaGard®[1-3]. Therefore, patients who become pregnant while using the ParaGard® should be carefully evaluated for the possibility of an ectopic pregnancy.
b. Special attention should be directed to patients with delayed menses, slight metrorrhagia and/or unilateral pelvic pain, and to those patients who wish to terminate a pregnancy because of IUD failure, to determine whether ectopic pregnancy has occurred.

3. PELVIC INFECTION (PELVIC INFLAMMATORY DISEASE, PID)
The ParaGard® is contraindicated in the presence of PID or in women with a history of PID. Use of all IUDs, including the ParaGard®, has been associated with an increased incidence of PID. Therefore a decision to use the ParaGard® must include consideration of the risks of PID. The highest rate of PID occurs shortly after insertion and up to four months thereafter. Administration of prophylactic antibiotics has been reported as useful (see INSERTION PRECAUTIONS). PID can necessitate hysterectomy and can also lead to tubo-ovarian abscesses, tubal occlusion and infertility and tubal damage that can predispose to ectopic pregnancy. PID can result in peritonitis and, infrequently, in death. The effect of PID on fertility is especially important for women who may wish to have children at a later date.
a. Women at special risk of PID
The risk of PID appears to be greater for women who have multiple sexual partners and also for those women whose sexual partners have multiple sexual partners. Women who have had PID are at high risk for a recurrence or re-infection.
b. PID warning to ParaGard® users
All women who choose the ParaGard® must be informed prior to insertion that IUD use has been associated with an increased incidence of PID and that PID can necessitate hysterectomy, can cause tubal damage leading to ectopic pregnancy or infertility or, in infrequent cases, can cause death. Patients must be taught to recognize and report to their physician promptly any symptoms of pelvic inflammatory disease. These symptoms include development of menstrual disorders (prolonged or heavy bleeding), unusual vaginal discharge, abdominal or pelvic pain or tenderness, dyspareunia, chills, and fever.
c. Asymptomatic PID
PID may be asymptomatic but still result in tubal damage and its sequelae.[4,5]
d. Treatment of PID
Following diagnosis of PID, or suspected PID, bacteriologic specimens should be obtained and antibiotic therapy should be initiated promptly. Removal of the ParaGard® after initiation of antibiotic therapy is usually appropriate. Time should be allowed for therapeutic blood levels to be reached prior to removal. Guidelines for PID treatment are available from the Center for Disease Control (CDC), Atlanta, Georgia. A copy of the printed guidelines has been provided to you by GynoPharma Inc. The guidelines were established after deliberation by a group of experts and staff of the CDC, but they should not be construed as rules suitable for use in all patients. Adequate PID treatment requires the application of current standards of therapy prevailing at the time of occurrence of the infection with reference to the prescription labeling of the antibiotic selected.
Genital actinomycosis has been associated primarily with long-term IUD use. If it occurs, promptly institute appropriate antibiotic therapy and remove the ParaGard®.

4. EMBEDMENT
Partial penetration or embedment of the ParaGard® in the endometrium or myometrium can result in difficult removal. In some cases this can result in breakage of the IUD, necessitating surgical removal.

5. PERFORATION
Partial or total perforation of the uterine wall or cervix may occur with the use of the ParaGard®. Insertions into patients after abortion or delivery should occur when the uterus is fully involuted. There is an increased risk of perforation in women who are lactating. The possibility of perforation must be kept in mind during insertion and at the time of any subsequent examination. If perforation occurs, the

Continued on next page

GynoPharma—Cont.

ParaGard® should be removed as soon as feasible. A surgical procedure may be required. Abdominal adhesions, intestinal penetration, intestinal obstruction, and local inflammatory reaction with abscess formation and erosion of adjacent viscera may result if the ParaGard® is left in the peritoneal cavity. There are reports that there has been migration after insertion, apparently in the absence of perforation at insertion.

6. MEDICAL DIATHERMY

The use of medical diathermy (short-wave and microwave) in a patient with a metal-containing IUD may cause heat injury to the surrounding tissue. Therefore, medical diathermy to the abdominal and sacral areas should not be used on patients with a ParaGard® in place.

7. EFFECTS OF COPPER

Additional amounts of copper available to the body from the ParaGard® may precipitate symptoms in women with Wilson's disease. The incidence of Wilson's disease is approximately 1 in 200,000. The long-term effects of intrauterine copper to a child conceived in the presence of an IUD are unknown.

8. RISKS OF MORTALITY

The available data from a variety of sources have been analyzed to estimate the risk of death associated with various methods of contraception. The estimates of risk of death include the combined risk of the contraceptive method plus the risk of pregnancy or abortion in the event of method failure. The findings of the analysis are shown in Table I.[6]

[See table below.]

PRECAUTIONS

1. Patient Counseling

Prior to insertion, the physician, nurse, or other trained health professional must provide the patient with the Patient Information for an Informed Decision brochure. The patient should be given the opportunity to read the leaflet and discuss fully any questions she may have concerning the ParaGard® as well as other methods of contraception.

2. Patient Evaluation and Clinical Considerations

a. A complete medical and social history, including that of the partner, should be obtained to determine conditions that might influence the selection of an IUD. A physical examination should include a pelvic examination, "Pap" smear, and appropriate tests for any other forms of genital disease, such as gonococcal and chlamydial laboratory evaluations if indicated. The physician should determine that the patient is not pregnant.

b. The uterus should be carefully sounded prior to the insertion to determine the degree of patency of the endocervical canal and the internal os, and the direction and depth of the uterine cavity. In occasional cases, severe cervical stenosis may be encountered. Do not use excessive force to overcome this resistance.

c. The uterus should sound to a depth of 6 to 8 centimeters (cm). Insertion of an IUD into a uterine cavity measuring less than 6.5 cm by sounding may increase the incidence of expulsion, bleeding, and pain.

d. Clinicians are cautioned that it is imperative for them to become thoroughly familiar with the instructions for use before attempting placement of the ParaGard®. To reduce the possibility of insertion in the presence of an existing undetermined pregnancy, the optimal time for insertion is the latter part of the menstrual period, or one or two days thereafter. The ParaGard® should not be inserted postpartum or postabortion until involution of the uterus is complete. The incidence of perforation and expulsion is greater if involution is not complete. Data also suggest that there may be an increased risk of perforation and expulsion if the woman is lactating.[7,8]

The ParaGard® should be placed at the fundus of the uterine cavity. Proper placement helps avoid partial or complete expulsion that could result in pregnancy. Contraceptive effectiveness is enhanced by proper placement.

e. Patients experiencing menorrhagia and/or metrorrhagia following IUD insertion may be at risk for the development of hypochromic microcytic anemia. Careful consideration of this risk must be given before insertion in patients with anemia or a history of menorrhagia or hypermenorrhea. Patients receiving anticoagulants or having a coagulopathy may have a greater risk of menorrhagia or hypermenorrhea.

f. Syncope, bradycardia, or other neurovascular episodes may occur during insertion or removal of IUDs, especially in patients with a previous disposition to these conditions or cervical stenosis.

g. Use of an IUD in patients with cervicitis should be postponed until treatment has eradicated the infection.

h. Patients with valvular or congenital heart disease are more prone to develop subacute bacterial endocarditis than patients who do not have valvular or congenital heart disease. Use of an IUD in these patients may represent a potential source of septic emboli. Patients with known congenital heart disease who may be at increased risk should be treated with appropriate antibiotics at the time of insertion.

i. Patients requiring short-term corticosteroid therapy should be carefully monitored for infection as a result of the insertion.

j. Since the ParaGard® may be partially or completely expelled, patients should be re-examined and evaluated shortly after the first postinsertion menses, but no later than 3 months afterwards. Thereafter, annual examination with appropriate evaluation, including a "Pap" smear, should be carried out. The ParaGard® should be kept in place no longer than 8 years.

k. The patient should be told that some bleeding or cramps may occur during the first few weeks after insertion. If these symptoms continue or are severe she should report them to her physician. She should be instructed on how to check to make certain that the threads still protrude from the cervix and cautioned that there is no contraceptive protection if the ParaGard® has been expelled. She should check frequently, at least after each menstrual period. She should be cautioned not to dislodge the ParaGard® by pulling on the thread. If a partial expulsion occurs, removal is indicated.

l. Rarely, a copper-induced urticarial allergic skin reaction may develop in women using a copper-containing IUD. If the symptoms of such an allergic response occur, the patient should be instructed to tell the consulting physician that a copper-containing device is being used.

m. The effect of magnetic resonance imaging of the pelvis was investigated in one study[9] in women with the CU-7® (Intrauterine Copper Contraceptive) and the Lippes Loop IUD. The CU-7® has a different configuration and contains less copper than the ParaGard® T380A. The results of the study indicate that neither the CU-7 nor the Lippes Loop were moved under the influence of the magnetic field nor did they heat during the spin-echo sequences usually employed for pelvic imaging.

3. Insertion Precautions

Because the presence of organisms capable of establishing PID cannot be determined by appearance, and because IUD insertion may be associated with introduction of vaginal bacteria into the uterus, clinicians may wish to consider the prophylactic administration of antibiotics. Regimens include doxycycline 200 mg orally one hour before insertion, or erythromycin 500 mg orally one hour before insertion and 500 mg orally six hours after insertion. The use of antibiotics in nursing mothers is not recommended. Before prescribing the above-mentioned antibiotics, refer to their prescription drug labeling and make certain that the patient is a suitable candidate for the drug.

TABLE I—Annual Number of Birth-related or Method-related Deaths Associated with Control of Fertility per 100,000 Nonsterile Women, by Fertility Control Method According to Age

Method of control and outcome	15–19	20–24	25–29	30–34	35–39	40–44
No fertility control methods*	7.0	7.4	9.1	14.8	25.7	28.2
Oral contraceptives non-smokers**	0.3	0.5	0.9	1.9	13.8	31.6
Oral contraceptives smokers**	2.2	3.4	6.6	13.5	51.1	117.2
IUD**	0.8	0.8	1.0	1.0	1.4	1.4
Condom*	1.1	1.6	0.7	0.2	0.3	0.4
Diaphragm/spermicide*	1.9	1.2	1.2	1.3	2.2	2.8
Periodic abstinence*	2.5	1.6	1.6	1.7	2.9	3.6

* Deaths are birth related

** Deaths are method related

4. Requirements for Continuation and Removal

a. The ParaGard® must be replaced before the end of the eighth year of use. There is no evidence of decreasing contraceptive efficacy with time before 8 years, but the contraceptive effectiveness at longer times has not been established; therefore, the patient should be informed of the known duration of contraceptive efficacy and be advised to return in 8 years for removal and possible insertion of a new ParaGard®.

b. The ParaGard® should be removed for the following medical reasons: menorrhagia- and/or metrorrhagia-producing anemia; pelvic infection; genital actinomycosis; intractable pelvic pain; dyspareunia; pregnancy; endometrial or cervical malignancy; uterine or cervical perforation; increase in length of the threads extending from the cervix, or any other indication of partial expulsion.

c. If the retrieval threads cannot be visualized, they may have retracted into the uterus or have been broken, or the ParaGard® may have been broken, or the ParaGard® may have been expelled. Localization may be made by feeling with a probe, X-ray, or sonography. When the physician elects to recover a ParaGard® with the threads not visible, the removal instructions should be reviewed.

d. Should the patient's relationship cease to be mutually monogamous, or should her partner become HIV positive, or acquire a sexually transmitted disease, she should be instructed to report this change to her clinician immediately. It may be advisable to recommend the use of a barrier method as a partial protection against acquiring sexually transmitted diseases until the ParaGard® T 380A can be removed.

5. Continuing Care of Patients Using ParaGard®

a. Any inquiries regarding pain, odorous discharge, bleeding, fever, genital lesions or sores, or a missed period should be promptly responded to and prompt examination is recommended.

b. If examination during visits subsequent to insertion reveals that the length of the threads has visibly or palpably changed from their length at time of insertion, the ParaGard® should be considered displaced and should be removed. A new ParaGard® may be inserted at that time or during the next menses or when it is certain that conception has not occurred. When the threads cannot be visualized by the physician, further investigation is necessary.

c. Since the ParaGard® may be partially or completely expelled, patients should be reexamined and evaluated shortly after the first postinsertion menses, but no later than 3 months afterwards. Thereafter, at least annual examination with appropriate evaluation, including a "Pap" smear, and if indicated, gonococcal and chlamydial laboratory evaluations, should be carried out. The ParaGard® should be kept in place no longer than 8 years.

d. In the event a pregnancy is confirmed during ParaGard® use, the following steps should be taken:

- Determine whether pregnancy is ectopic and take appropriate measures if it is.
- Inform patient of the risks of leaving an IUD *in situ* or removing it during pregnancy and of the lack of data on the long-term effects of the ParaGard® on the offspring of women who had it *in utero* during conception or gestation (see WARNINGS).
- If possible the ParaGard® should be removed after the patient has been warned of the risks of removal. If removal is difficult, the patient should be counseled about and offered pregnancy termination.
- If the ParaGard® is left in place, the patient's course should be followed closely.

ADVERSE REACTIONS

These adverse reactions are not listed in any order of frequency or severity.

Reported adverse reactions with intrauterine contraceptives include: endometritis; spontaneous abortion; septic abortion; septicemia; perforation of the uterus and cervix; embedment; fragmentation of the IUD; pelvic infection; tubo-ovarian abscess; tubal damage; vaginitis; leukorrhea; cervical erosion; pregnancy; ectopic pregnancy; fetal damage; difficult removal; complete or partial expulsion of the IUD, particularly in those patients with uteri measuring less than 6.5 cm by sounding; menstrual spotting; prolongation of menstrual flow; anemia; amenorrhea or delayed menses; pain and cramping; dysmenorrhea; backaches; dyspareunia; neurovascular episodes, including bradycardia and syncope secondary to insertion. Uterine perforation and IUD displacement into the abdomen have been followed by peritonitis, abdominal adhesions, intestinal penetration, intestinal obstruction, and cystic masses in the pelvis. (Certain of these adverse reactions can lead to loss of fertility, partial or total removal of reproductive organs, hormonal imbalance, or death). Urticarial allergic skin reaction may occur.

CLINICAL STUDIES

Different event rates have been reported with the use of different intrauterine contraceptives. Inasmuch as these rates are usually derived from separate studies conducted by different investigators in several populations, they cannot be

compared with precision. Considerably different rates are likely to be obtained because event rates per unit of time tend to decrease as studies are extended, since more susceptible subjects discontinue due to expulsions, adverse reactions, or pregnancy, leaving the study population richer in less susceptible subjects. In clinical trials conducted by The Population Council[10,11,12] and WHO, use-effectiveness of the ParaGard® as calculated by the life table method was determined through eight (8) years of use.

Data suggest a higher pregnancy rate in women under 20.[10,11]

[See Table II at right.]

The lowest expected and typical failure rates during the first year of continuous use of all contraceptive methods are listed in Table III. (adapted from reference 13).

TABLE III—Percentage of Women Experiencing an Accidental Pregnancy in the First Year of Continuous Use

Method	Lowest Expected*	Typical**
(No Contraception)	(85)	(85)
Oral Contraceptives		3.0
combined	0.1	N/A***
progestin only	0.5	N/A***
Diaphragm with spermicidal cream or jelly	6.0	18.0
Spermicides alone (foam, creams, jellies, and vaginal suppositories)	3.0	21.0
Vaginal Sponge		
nulliparous	6.0	18.0
multiparous	9.0	28.0
IUD		3.0
Copper T 380A (ParaGard® T380A)	0.8	N/A***
Medicated (Progestasert®)	2.0	N/A***
Condom	2.0	12.0
Periodic abstinence (all methods)	1.0–9.0	20.0
Female sterilization	0.2	0.4
Male sterilization	0.1	0.15

* The authors' best guess of the percentage of women expected to experience an accidental pregnancy among couples who initiate a method (not necessarily for the first time) and who use it consistently and correctly during the first year if they do not stop for any other reason.

** This term represents "typical" couples who initiate use of a method (not necessarily for the first time), who experience an accidental pregnancy during the first year if they do not stop use for any other reason.

*** N/A—Data not available.

HOW SUPPLIED

Available in cartons of one (NDC 54765-380-01) or five (NDC 54765-380-05) sterile units. Each ParaGard® is packaged in a Tyvek®-polyethylene pouch, together with an insertion tube and plunger rod.

INSTRUCTIONS FOR USE
PARAGARD® T380A
Intrauterine Copper Contraceptive

THERE IS DEBATE AS TO HOW MANY IUD INSERTIONS CONSTITUTE ADEQUATE TRAINING FOR A CLINICIAN. IT IS PROBABLY WISE TO HAVE DONE 15–25 INSERTIONS UNDER SUPERVISION PRIOR TO INSERTING AN IUD UNSUPERVISED. A PRACTITIONER WITH ONLY 4–6 INSERTIONS WOULD PROBABLY NOT HAVE HAD ADEQUATE EXPERIENCE WITH DIFFICULT INSERTIONS.

The ParaGard® (Intrauterine Copper Contraceptive) represents a different design in intrauterine contraceptives. Physicians are, therefore, cautioned that they should become thoroughly familiar with instructions for insertion before attempting placement of the ParaGard®. The insertion technique is different in several respects from that employed with other intrauterine contraceptives and the physician should pay particular attention to the drawings and commentary accompanying these instructions.

A single ParaGard® is placed at the fundus of the uterine cavity.

The ParaGard® may be inserted at any time during the cycle. However, it is essential that pregnancy be ruled out before insertion.

Present information indicates that the efficacy is retained for 8 years. Therefore, the ParaGard® must be removed and a new one inserted on or before 8 years from the date of insertion.

PRELIMINARY PREPARATION AND INSERTION

1. Before insertion, the patient must read each section of the Patient Information Brochure for an Informed Decision; the medical and social history and counseling of the patient must be completed; and the Patient Consent must be signed by the patient and by the physician.

TABLE II
ParaGard® T380A
(Intrauterine Copper Contraceptive)
GROSS CUMULATIVE RATES PER 100 CONTINUING USERS
BY YEAR AND PARITY

	1 Year		2 years		3 years		4 years		6 years		8 years	
	Parous	All	Parous	All	Parous	All	Parous	All	Parous	All	Parous	All
Pregnancy	0.5	0.6	0.8	0.9	1.1	1.5	1.2	1.6	1.7	2.1	1.9	2.3
Expulsion	5.3	5.7	7.0	8.0	8.1	9.4	9.3	10.5	9.5	10.8	11.2	12.5
Bleeding/Pain	9.7	11.9	17.0	20.6	22.1	26.1	24.3	28.6	28.9	33.0	32.2	36.0
Other Medical	1.6	2.5	3.2	4.5	4.2	5.9	5.6	7.4	6.1	7.9	7.3	9.0
Continuation	79.6	76.8	64.0	60.2	53.4	48.9	46.3	42.1	38.1	34.6	31.3	28.5
No. Completed	1837	3151	1294	2020	877	1123	721	874	570	570	297	297

Rates were calculated by combining the experience on a weighted basis from both The Population Council (PC, 3536 acceptors) and the World Health Organization's (WHO, 1396 acceptors) trials. 64%, 53%, 26%, and 18% of the women completed 1, 2, 3 and 4 years of use, respectively, were from the PC study. The rates in years 5 through 8 are derived solely from the WHO trials.

2. Refer to CONTRAINDICATIONS, WARNINGS, and PRECAUTIONS.

3. Pelvic examination is to be performed prior to insertion of the ParaGard®, including a cervical "Pap" smear, and gonococcal and chlamydial evaluations, if indicated, and any other necessary specific tests.

4. If appropriate, commence antibiotic prophylaxis one hour before insertion.

5. Use of aseptic technique during insertion is essential.

6. The endocervix should be cleansed with an antiseptic solution and a tenaculum applied to the cervix with downward traction for correction of the angulation as well as stabilization of the cervix.

7. With a speculum in place, gently insert a sterile sound to determine the depth and direction of the uterine canal. Be sure to determine the position of the uterus before insertion.

CAUTION

Any intrauterine procedure can result in severe pain, bradycardia, and syncope.

It is generally believed that perforations, if they occur, are encountered at the time of insertion, although the perforation may not be detected until some time later. The position of the uterus should be determined during the preinsertion examination. Great care must be exercised during the preinsertion sounding and subsequent insertion. No attempt should be made to force the insertion.

HOW TO INSERT ParaGard® T380A
STEP 1

To minimize chance of introducing contamination, do not remove the ParaGard® from the inserter tube prior to placement in the uterus. Do not bend the arms of the ParaGard® earlier than 5 minutes before it is to be introduced into the uterus.

In the absence of sterile gloves, this can be accomplished without destroying sterility by folding the arms in the partially opened package. Place the partially opened package on a flat surface and pull the solid rod partially from the package so it will not interfere with assembly. Place thumb and index finger on top of package on ends of the horizontal arms. Push insertion tube against arms of ParaGard® as indicated by arrow in Fig. 1 to start arms folding.

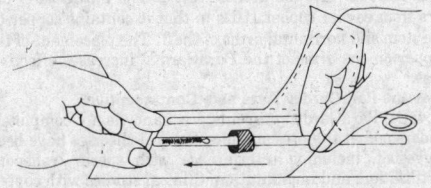

Fig. 1

Complete the bending by bringing thumb and index finger together while using the other hand to maneuver the insertion tube to pick up the arms of the ParaGard® (Fig. 2). Insert no further than necessary to insure retention of the arms. Introduce the solid rod into the insertion tube from the bottom alongside the threads until it touches the bottom of the ParaGard®.

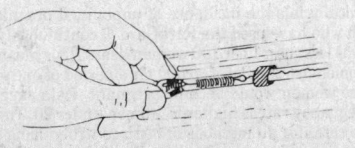

Fig. 2

STEP 2

Adjust the movable flange so that it indicates the depth to which the ParaGard® should be inserted and the direction in which the arms of the ParaGard® will open. At this point, make certain that the horizontal arms of the ParaGard® and the long axis of the flange lie in the same horizontal plane. Introduce the loaded inserter through the cervical canal and upwards until the ParaGard® lies in contact with the fundus. The movable flange should be at the cervix (Fig. 3).

DO NOT FORCE THE INSERTION.

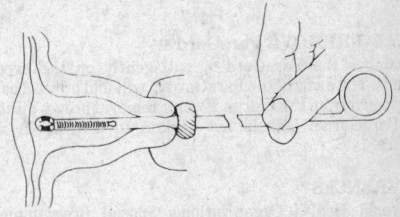

Fig. 3

STEP 3

To release the ParaGard®, withdraw the insertion tube not more than ½ inch while the solid rod is not permitted to move. This releases the arms of the ParaGard® (Fig. 4).

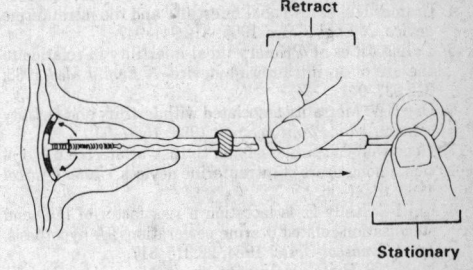

Retract

Stationary

Fig. 4

STEP 4

After the arms are released, the inserter tube should be moved upward gently until the resistance of the fundus is felt. This will assure placement of the T at the highest possible position within the endometrial cavity (Fig. 5).

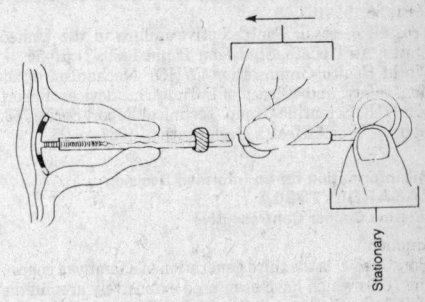

Stationary

Fig. 5

STEP 5

Withdraw the solid rod while holding the insertion tube stationary (Fig. 6).

[See top left next page.]

Continued on next page

GynoPharma—Cont.

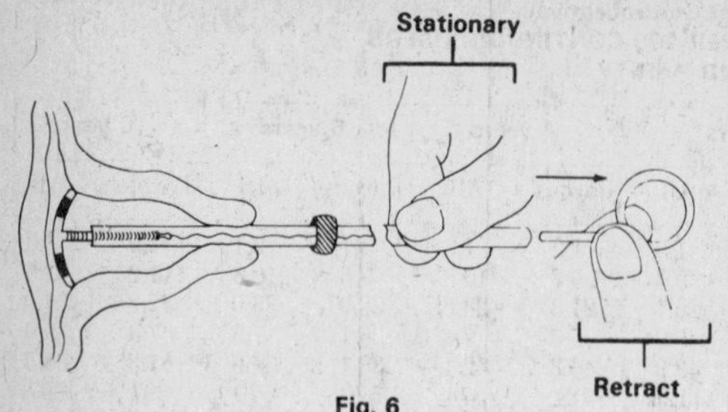

Fig. 6

STEP 6

Withdraw the insertion tube from the cervix. Be sure sufficient length of the threads are visible (1 in., or 2.5 cm) to facilitate checking for the presence of the ParaGard® (Fig. 7). Notation of length of the threads should be made in patient record.

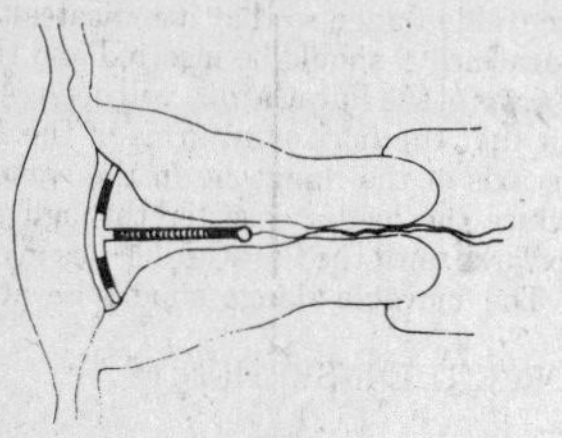

Fig. 7

HOW TO REMOVE ParaGard®

To remove the ParaGard®, pull gently on the exposed threads. The arms of the ParaGard® will fold upward as it is withdrawn from the uterus. Even if removal proves difficult, the ParaGard® should not remain in the uterus after 8 years.

REFERENCES

1. World Health Organization's Special Programme of Research, Development and Research Training in Human Reproduction: A multinational case-control study of ectopic pregnancy. *Clin Reprod Fertil* 1985; 3:131–143.
2. Ory HW, Women's Health Study: Ectopic pregnancy and intrauterine contraceptive devices: New perspectives. *Obstet Gynecol* 1981; 57:137–144.
3. Marchbanks PA et al: Risk factors for ectopic pregnancy: A population-based study. *JAMA* 1988; 259:1823–1827.
4. Cramer DW et al: Tubal infertility and the intrauterine device. *N Engl J Med* 1985; 312:941–947.
5. Daling JR et al: Primary tubal infertility in relation to the use of an intrauterine device. *N Engl J Med* 1985; 312:937–941.
6. Ory HW: Mortality associated with fertility and fertility control. *Fam Plann Perspect* 1983; 15:57–63.
7. Heartwell SF, Schlesselman S: Risk of uterine perforation among users of intrauterine devices. *Obstet Gynecol* 1983; 61:31–36.
8. Chi I-C, Kelly E: Is lactation a risk factor of IUD and sterilisation-related uterine perforations? A hypothesis. *Int J Gynaecol Obstet* 1984; 22:315–317.
9. Mark AS, Hricak H: Intrauterine contraceptove devices: MR imaging. *Radiology* 1987; 311–314.
10. Sivin, I, Stern J: Long-acting, more effective Copper T IUDs: A summary of US experience, 1970–1975, *Stud Fam Plann* 1979; 10:263–281.
11. Sivin I, Schmidt F: Effectiveness of IUDs: A review. *Contraception* 1987; 36:55–84.
12. Sivin I, Tatum HJ: Four years of experience with the TCu 380A intrauterine contraceptive device. *Fertil Steril* 1981; 36:159–163.
13. Trussell J, et al: Contraceptive failure in the United States: An Update. *Stud Fam Plann* 1990; 21:51–54.
14. World Health Organization (WHO): Mechanism of action, safety, and efficacy of intrauterine devices. Report of a WHO Scientific Group. Technical Report Series 753. Geneva; World Health Organization, 1987, p. 25.

Patient Information for an Informed Decision

PARAGARD® T380A

Intrauterine Copper Contraceptive

Introduction

The ParaGard® is the third generation of a family of copper-bearing IUDs which have been used extensively around the world. It is the first to contain copper on both the arms and the stem of the T. Tested in more than 3,500 women in the United States, the ParaGard® is the product of over a decade of research involving an international group of scientists and family-planning specialists. However, as with all methods of contraception, its use is associated with some risk. The purpose of this brochure is to explain those risks to you.

Important Notice

To understand the risks and benefits of the ParaGard® (Intrauterine Copper Contraceptive) you will need to read and understand this entire brochure and discuss it with your clinician. It contains information vital to your health. A more technical leaflet is available which is written for the medical professional. If you would like to read that leaflet, ask your clinician for a copy. You may need his/her help to understand some of the information.

If you have difficulty understanding any of the technical terms in this brochure, check the glossary on page 11 and ask your clinician for clarification.

Many clinicians consider IUDs to be the best contraceptive choice for certain women. The ParaGard® is most appropriately used in women who have had at least one child and are in a stable, mutually monogamous relationship, and those who require a reversible form of contraception, whether or not they feel they have completed their family.

In addition to reading this brochure, you should also learn about other reversible birth control methods. One of these methods may be more suitable or safer for you than the ParaGard®. In order to make the appropriate decision, you must discuss your questions about IUDs and other kinds of birth control with your clinician. Also, have the clinician explain to your satisfaction anything you do not understand in this brochure.

Under certain conditions you should not have the ParaGard® inserted; the risks to your health or your ability to bear children may be too great. Such conditions are described under *Special Risk Factors* and *What You Should Discuss With Your Clinician.* Even if none of these conditions applies to you, you may still experience serious problems while using the ParaGard® which will require immediate medical treatment. These medical problems could cause damage to your reproductive organs and the ability to bear children, or in some cases, could cause death. You may have to undergo major surgery, and you may become temporarily or permanently sterile (see *Special Risk Factors*). Prompt medical treatment, though absolutely necessary, may not be effective.

To become familiar with the danger signs of ParaGard® use, read *Side Effects, Adverse Reactions, and Warnings.* Always discuss these and other sections of the brochure with your clinician.

DESCRIPTION

The ParaGard® T380A (Intrauterine Copper Contraceptive) is a type of IUD that contains copper, and is inserted into the uterus (womb) to prevent pregnancy. Like all other contraceptives it is not 100% effective. (See *Effectiveness* for pregnancy rates.)

The ParaGard® is flexible and T-shaped with copper on both of the arms and stem of the T. The T itself is made of a flexible plastic material. The ParaGard® must be replaced every 8 years, to maintain its contraceptive effectiveness. Two white threads extend from the base of the ParaGard®. They will extend into your vagina to indicate the presence of the ParaGard®, and aid in its removal. The ParaGard® (Intrauterine Copper Contraceptive) is 36 mm in the vertical direction and 32 mm in the horizontal direction.

The Copper in the ParaGard®

Available data indicate that the contraceptive effectiveness of ParaGard® is enhanced by copper released continuously from the IUD into the uterine cavity. The ParaGard® differs from earlier copper IUDs in that it contains copper on the stem and horizontal arms of the T. The placement of the copper on the arms of the ParaGard® increases effectiveness.

How the ParaGard® Acts as a Contraceptive

How the ParaGard® prevents pregnancy is not completely understood at the present time. Several theories have been suggested, including interference with sperm transport, fertilization, and implantation. Clinical studies with copper-bearing IUDs suggest that fertilization is affected either due to an altered number or lack of viability of spermatozoa. IUDs do not prevent ovulation (production and release of an egg by the ovary).

The ParaGard® does not always prevent ectopic pregnancy (pregnancy outside the uterus, sometimes called tubal pregnancy). Ectopic pregnancy can require surgery, and can make you unable to bear children; in some cases it can cause death. (See *Special Risk Factors for Ectopic Pregnancy.*)

Effectiveness

In clinical trials the incidence of unplanned pregnancies in women who have used the ParaGard® continuously for one year was less than 1 per 100 woman-years. This means that if 100 women use the ParaGard® for a period of one year, one of these women would become pregnant. Data suggest that the pregnancy rate is higher in women under 20. The typical failure rates for all methods of birth control during the first year are listed below in Table 1. The failure rate tabulated below for IUDs includes *all* IUDs combined.

Table 1
Failure Rates for All Methods

Oral Contraceptives	less than 3%
IUD	up to 3%
Diaphragm with Spermicides	18%
Vaginal Sponge	18% to 28%
Condom alone	12%
Periodic abstinence	20%
No method	85%

Continuation Rates

In clinical trials 5 to 6 women out of 100 expelled the system during the first year. During the first year the number of women in the clinical trials who used the ParaGard® continuously for one year was 77 to 80 per 100 users. 12% of the women discontinued use because of bleeding and pain.

Lack of Contraceptive Effect After ParaGard® Removal

After discontinuation of ParaGard® use, its contraceptive effect on the uterus is reversed. Usually, but not always, a woman is able to become pregnant. In a study of 293 women, 78.4% of women seeking pregnancy became pregnant within a year following discontinuation.

Special Risk Factors

The conditions discussed below can significantly increase your chances of developing serious complications while using an IUD. Some of these conditions can necessitate surgery, can make you unable to have children, or can cause death. Read the information carefully and discuss it with your clinician.

Special Risk Factors for Pelvic Infection (Pelvic Inflammatory Disease)

Evidence indicates that ParaGard® users are more likely than other women to suffer a serious infection called pelvic inflammatory disease (PID), particularly in women with multiple sexual partners. PID is the medical term for infection in the upper pelvic area. This area includes the uterus (womb), fallopian tubes, ovaries, and surrounding tissues. (Vaginitis, a local infection of the vagina, is not PID, but may lead to it.) Studies indicate that the highest rate of PID occurs shortly after insertion and up to 4 months thereafter. PID can cause permanent blockage of the tubes; sterility; ectopic pregnancy; or, in infrequent cases, death. If you have now or have ever had PID, you must not use the ParaGard®. PID is an infection caused by gonorrhea, chlamydia, or other microscopic organisms. PID is frequently a sexually transmitted disease (STD or VD), and your chances of getting PID increase greatly if you have more than one sexual partner. Your risk of getting PID also increases if you have a sexual partner, who has sexual intercourse with others. If you are exposed to such situations, you have an increased risk of getting PID and must not use the ParaGard®. You should consider the use of a barrier method which may provide partial protection against sexually transmitted diseases. Treatment of PID may require surgical removal of your uterus (hysterectomy), tubes, and ovaries. Such surgery may have to be done on an emergency basis, and may result in death. Removing the ovaries may result in a lifelong need for hormonal treatments. Symptoms of PID include pelvic or lower abdominal pain, chills, fever, abnormal vaginal discharge, abnormal menstrual bleeding, or painful sexual intercourse. PID can occur even without these symptoms.

If you are using the ParaGard® and develop any of these symptoms, see your clinician as soon as possible. If you have PID, you should receive appropriate antibiotics promptly, and the IUD should be removed at the appropriate time. Failure to seek and receive prompt and adequate treatment will greatly increase the chances that you will become sterile, require surgery, or have life-threatening or fatal PID. Even prompt and adequate treatment cannot guarantee that these events will not occur.

Special Risk Factors for Ectopic Pregnancy

Ectopic pregnancy is an infrequent, but dangerous type of pregnancy that develops outside the uterus. Although current data indicate that the rate of ectopic pregnancy in patients using the ParaGard® is no higher, and some data suggest a lower rate than the general population, a pregnancy which occurs with the ParaGard® in place is more likely to be ectopic than a pregnancy occurring without the ParaGard®. If you have ever had an ectopic pregnancy, you have an increased risk of having another one. You also have an increased risk of an ectopic pregnancy if you have ever had certain types of infections. These infections include pelvic inflammatory disease (PID) or any venereal disease (VD) or sexually transmitted disease (STD) caused by, for example, gonorrhea or chlamydia. If you have ever had an ectopic pregnancy or these kinds of infections, you must not use the ParaGard®. Other contraceptive methods may be more suitable for you. Discuss this matter with your clinician.

	Yes	No	Not Sure
Heart disease	☐	☐	☐
Heart murmur	☐	☐	☐
Hepatitis or severe liver disease	☐	☐	☐
Wilson's disease	☐	☐	☐
Allergy to copper	☐	☐	☐
Diabetes	☐	☐	☐
Leukemia	☐	☐	☐
Fainting attacks	☐	☐	☐
Steroid therapy	☐	☐	☐
Anemia or blood clotting problems	☐	☐	☐
Current suspected or possible pregnancy	☐	☐	☐
Ectopic pregnancy (pregnancy outside of the uterus)			
Recent pregnancy	☐	☐	☐
Recent abortion or miscarriage	☐	☐	☐
Abnormalities of the uterus	☐	☐	☐
Bleeding between periods	☐	☐	☐
Cancer of the uterus (womb) or cervix	☐	☐	☐
Suspicious or abnormal Pap smear	☐	☐	☐
Prior IUD use	☐	☐	☐
IUD in place now	☐	☐	☐
Heavy menstrual flow	☐	☐	☐
Severe menstrual cramps	☐	☐	☐
Multiple sexual partners	☐	☐	☐
A sexual partner who has multiple sexual partners, or is at high risk for acquiring HIV	☐	☐	☐
Pelvic infection (including pus in fallopian tubes)	☐	☐	☐
Infection of the uterus (womb) or cervix	☐	☐	☐
Genital sores or lesions	☐	☐	☐
Sexually transmitted disease (venereal disease), such as herpes, gonorrhea, chlamydia, or acquired immune deficiency syndrome (AIDS)			
Unexplained genital bleeding	☐	☐	☐
Uterine or pelvic surgery	☐	☐	☐
Vaginal discharge or infection	☐	☐	☐
I.V. drug abuse	☐	☐	☐

Other Conditions That Increase Risk of Infection
Some conditions make you more susceptible to infection during ParaGard® use or following ParaGard® insertion. These conditions include leukemia and acquired immune deficiency syndrome (AIDS). In addition, certain defects or diseases of the heart valves, such as rheumatic heart disease, and diabetes and long-term steroid therapy, make you more likely than other ParaGard® users to develop an infection which may involve the heart. If you have any of these conditions you should probably not use the ParaGard®.

Side Effects
The following may occur while the ParaGard® is being inserted and while it is in place.
1. Pain, usually uterine cramps or low backache, occur at the time of insertion and may persist. (Pain and cramping may also occur at removal.) If pain is severe, becomes worse, or persists, contact your clinician.
2. Fainting may occur at the time of insertion or removal of the ParaGard®.
3. Some bleeding occurs following insertion in most women.
4. Partial or total perforation of the ParaGard® through the wall of the uterus may occur at the time of, or after, insertion. If you think the ParaGard® is displaced, check with your clinician (see *Warnings—tail or thread disappearance*). Perforation could result in abdominal adhesions, (scars) intestinal obstruction or penetration, inflammation, serious infection, and loss of contraceptive protection. Perforation and its complications may require surgery and, in infrequent cases, may result in serious illness or death.

5. Bleeding between menstrual periods may occur during the first 2 or 3 months after insertion. The first few menstrual periods after insertion may be heavier and longer than usual. If these conditions continue for longer than 2 or 3 months, consult your clinician.
6. Occasionally you may miss a menstrual period while using the ParaGard®. It is important to determine if you are pregnant; report this without delay to your clinician.
7. The ParaGard® may come out of your uterus through the cervical opening. This is called expulsion, and is most likely to occur during the first 2 or 3 menstrual cycles following insertion. Expulsion leaves you unprotected against pregnancy. Refer to the section called *Directions for Use* for information on how to check to see if your ParaGard® has been expelled. If you think the ParaGard® has come out or has been displaced, use another birth control method, such as contraceptive vaginal foam, cream, or jelly, or condoms (rubbers), until you can be checked by your clinician. (These alternative methods are usually not as effective in preventing uterine pregnancy as the ParaGard®.) Call your clinician for an examination.

What You Should Discuss With Your Clinician
Before you have the ParaGard® inserted, indicate below if you have ever had—or suspect you have ever had—any of the conditions listed below. Conditions listed are not necessarily contraindications. [See table above.]
Make certain you discuss any items you're not sure about.

Adverse Reactions
The following adverse reactions have been reported and may be caused by an IUD:

- Abdominal infection or adhesions (scar tissue)
- Anemia
- Backache
- Blood poisoning
- Bowel obstruction
- Cervical infection or erosion
- Cysts on ovaries and tubes
- Death
- Delayed menstruation
- Difficult removal
- Ectopic pregnancy
- Embedment (IUD surrounded by uterine tissue)
- Expulsion (IUD comes completely or partially out of the uterus)
- Fainting and pain at the time of insertion or removal
- Fragmentation (breakage) of the ParaGard®
- Infertility
- Spotting between periods
- Miscarriage
- Pain and cramps
- Painful intercourse
- Pelvic infection (PID), which may result in surgical removal of your reproductive organs, including hysterectomy
- Perforation of the uterus (womb) or cervix (IUD passes through uterine tissue)
- Pregnancy
- Prolonged or heavy menstrual flow
- Infected miscarriage followed, in some cases, by blood poisoning, which can lead to death
- Vaginal discharge

Warnings
If you have the ParaGard® inserted, call your clinician immediately for any of the following reasons:
1. A missed period. This may mean you are pregnant and the ParaGard® should be removed.
2. Unexplained or abnormal vaginal bleeding or discharge. This could indicate a serious complication, such as an infection or ectopic pregnancy.
3. A delayed period followed by scanty or irregular bleeding. This could indicate an ectopic pregnancy.
4. Pelvic or lower abdominal pain or cramps or unexplained fever. Such symptoms could mean an ectopic pregnancy or infection has developed requiring immediate treatment.
5. Exposure to venereal disease (VD), also called sexually transmitted disease (STD). The use of the ParaGard® does not prevent venereal disease. If exposure to venereal disease is suspected, report for examination and treatment promptly. Failure to do so could result in serious pelvic infection.
6. If your relationship ceases to be mutually monogamous or should your partner become HIV positive or acquire a sexually transmitted disease, you should report this change to your clinician immediately. It may be advisable to use a barrier method of contraception as a partial protection from acquiring STD until the ParaGard® T380A can be removed by your clinician.
7. Genital sores or lesions, or fever with vaginal discharge. These may indicate an infection.
8. Severe or prolonged menstrual bleeding. If the flow is heavier and lasts much longer than your usual menstrual flow, you may need to have the ParaGard® removed to prevent anemia.
9. Tail or thread disappearance or pain during sex. If you cannot feel the threads coming through the cervix, or have pain during sex, the ParaGard® may have been expelled or displaced, or may have perforated the uterus. If any of these has occurred, you are no longer protected from pregnancy. Use another birth control method, such as contraceptive vaginal foam, cream, or jelly, or condoms (rubbers) until you can be checked. (These alternative methods are not as effective against uterine pregnancy as the ParaGard®.) If perforation has occurred removal of the ParaGard® is necessary, usually by surgery.

[See Table 2 at left.]
Risk of death. Available data from a variety of sources have been analyzed to estimate the risk of death associated with various methods of contraception. The estimates of risk of death include the combined risk of the contraceptive method plus the risk of pregnancy or abortion in the event of method failure.

How the ParaGard® is Inserted and Removed
Before insertion, your clinician will perform a pelvic examination. Its purpose is to determine the size, shape, and position of the uterus. An instrument called a speculum will hold your vagina open so that the cervix (the entrance to the uterus) can be seen. (You will probably feel pressure from the speculum throughout the insertion procedure.)
The cervix is then cleaned with an antiseptic solution and an instrument called a tenaculum is attached to it. This instrument assists in holding the uterus steady during insertion. You may feel pain or a pinching sensation as the tenaculum is attached. Then the clinician will guide a narrow instru-

Table 2
Annual Number of Birth-Related or Method-Related Deaths Associated With Control of Fertility per 100,000 Nonsterile Women, by Fertility Control Method, According to Age

Method of control and outcome	15–19	20–24	25–29	30–34	35–39	40–44
No fertility control methods*	7.0	7.4	9.1	14.8	25.7	28.2
Oral contraceptives, nonsmokers**	0.3	0.5	0.9	1.9	13.8	31.6
Oral contraceptives, smokers**	2.2	3.4	6.6	13.5	51.1	117.2
IUD**	0.8	0.8	1.0	1.0	1.4	1.4
Condom*	1.1	1.6	0.7	0.2	0.3	0.4
Diaphragm/spermicide*	1.9	1.2	1.2	1.3	2.2	2.8
Periodic abstinence*	2.5	1.6	1.6	1.7	2.9	3.6

* Deaths are birth related
** Deaths are method related

Continued on next page

GynoPharma—Cont.

ment called a sound through the opening of the cervix into the uterus. The sound measures the depth and position of the uterus. You can expect to feel cramping similar to menstrual cramps as the sound is inserted and withdrawn.

Then your clinician will guide the ParaGard® (with the cross-arms of the T folded down) through the vagina and the cervix into the uterus.

As the ParaGard® is inserted, the arms of the T will unfold. During insertion you will have some pain or cramping. You may feel nauseated, weak, or faint. After the inserter is removed, the threads attached to the end of the ParaGard® will be clipped. The threads will extend into the vagina from the cervical opening. The tenaculum and speculum will then be removed. You may feel pain or pinching when the tenaculum is removed. You should remain lying down for a while and rise slowly to prevent fainting. During intercourse, neither you nor your partner should be aware of these threads. You should also not be aware of any other part of the ParaGard®. If you are, promptly follow the instructions under the heading, *Checking Your ParaGard®*, in the section *Directions for Use*.

When it is time to remove the ParaGard®, your clinician must remove it. Its removal may cause pain or cramping. The arms of the ParaGard® should fold upward as it is withdrawn from the uterus.

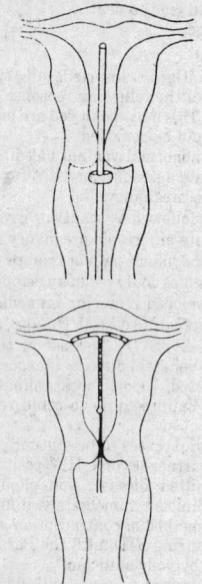

Directions for Use

Please read the following information and instructions carefully. Keep a copy of this brochure so that you may refer to it. If you have any questions, consult your clinician.

Checking Your ParaGard®

The ParaGard® can come out of the uterus (womb) without your knowing it. When this occurs, it is most often during or right after a menstrual period. Therefore at least after each menstrual period, check to make sure the threads can be felt at the cervix. You may check more often, and especially if you have some concern, or think you have an expulsion. Follow these steps to make sure that the ParaGard® has not been expelled without your knowing it:

1. Wash your hands.
2. Squat down or seat yourself on the toilet.
3. Insert the index or middle finger high into your vagina and locate your cervix. The cervix is the mouth of the uterus (womb). It feels firm, like the tip of your nose.

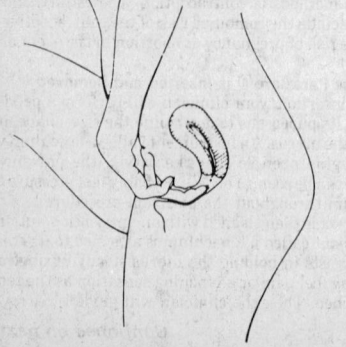

4. Feel for the threads of the ParaGard®. The threads should extend from the cervix and be high in your vagina. The threads may be difficult to feel.
5. If you can feel the threads, the ParaGard® is probably, but not always, in place. You should not pull on the threads. Doing so may displace the ParaGard®.
6. If you cannot feel threads, or if you can feel the ParaGard® itself, it has probably been displaced from the uterus. Also, if you or your partner can feel the ParaGard® during intercourse, it is displaced. If so, you are not being protected against pregnancy. Until you can be examined, use another birth control method, such as a contraceptive vaginal foam, cream, or jelly, or condoms (rubbers). (These alternative methods are not as effective against uterine pregnancy as the ParaGard®.) Call your clinician for an examination.

Follow-up Visits to the Clinician

1. You should return to see your clinician as soon as possible after your first menstrual period following insertion of your IUD, but no later than 3 months after insertion. This will allow the clinician to check on the location of the ParaGard®.
2. The ParaGard® requires replacement every 8 years. Check with your clinician concerning an appointment to have the ParaGard® replaced or removed.
3. The ParaGard® should not interfere with the proper use of tampons and douches. You may want to discuss this with your clinician.

Special Warning About Uterine Pregnancy With the ParaGard® in Place

Some women become pregnant while using the ParaGard®. If you miss your menstrual period, or if you suspect you are pregnant, see your clinician right away. When a pregnancy continues with the ParaGard® in place, serious complications may occur, including severe blood infection, spontaneous miscarriage, infected miscarriage, and death. These may occur at any time during the pregnancy.

When the ParaGard® remains in the uterus during conception or pregnancy, the long-term effects on the child (or fetus) are not known. Under such conditions some birth defects have occurred. Their relationship to the ParaGard® has not been established but has been suggested.

If your clinician confirms that you are pregnant, the ParaGard® should be removed. Removal of the ParaGard® may cause a miscarriage. However, successful ParaGard® removal in pregnancy decreases the likelihood of subsequent complications.

In some cases removal of the ParaGard® may prove to be difficult. If so, you and your clinician should discuss at that time the question of continuing the pregnancy in view of the serious complications [described above] that may occur. In reaching a decision about termination of pregnancy, you should be aware that the risks associated with abortion increase with the length of time you have been pregnant.

If you continue your pregnancy with the ParaGard® in place, your clinician will have to follow your course more closely than usual throughout your pregnancy. Be sure to report immediately to the clinician if you have any of the following symptoms or signs:

- Bleeding from the vagina
- Pelvic or lower abdominal pain or cramping
- Flu-like symptoms such as chills or fever
- Unusual vaginal discharge
- Ruptured membranes (your water breaks)
- Any other signs/symptoms which gives you concern

Any of these sympotoms could indicate that you are having a miscarriage or that you are beginning, or about to begin, premature labor. Premature labor may lead to delivery of a premature infant. Premature infants have a higher chance of dying, mental retardation, cerebral palsy, or other serious medical problems. Additionally, infection can cause infertility or death. Therefore, report any symptoms without delay to your clinician, so that you can obtain immediate treatment.

Patient Consent

I have read this brochure in its entirety and discussed its contents with my clinician. My clinician has answered all my questions and has advised me of the risks and benefits associated with the use of the ParaGard®, with other forms of contraception, and with no form of contraception at all. I have considered all factors and voluntarily choose to have the ParaGard® inserted by

_____
                                      Clinician

date _____

Patient Signature _____

The patient has signed this brochure in my presence after I counseled her and answered all her questions.

_____
    Clinician   Date

This ParaGard® is scheduled for removal on _____

Glossary

Cervix —Lower portion of the uterus visible in the vagina
Conception —Pregnancy
Contraceptive —Means of preventing conception
Ectopic Pregnancy —Pregnancy outside of the uterus
Expel —To force out
Fallopian Tubes —Tubes which carry the egg from the ovary to the uterus
Fertilization —The process of the sperm penetrating the egg of the female
Genital —Organs concerned with reproduction
HIV —Human Immunodeficiency Virus which causes AIDS
Implantation —Embedding of the fertilized egg into the lining of the uterus
Intrauterine —Within the uterus
Microscopic —Can be seen only by using a microscope
Monogamous —Practicing sexual relations with only one partner
Ovary —Almond-shaped organ. One ovary is located on each side of the uterus. Produces and releases human eggs.
Ovulation —Release of an egg by the ovary
STD —Sexually transmitted disease—also called venereal disease
Spermatozoa —Male reproductive cells
Uterus (womb) —Pear-shaped organ, located deep in the pelvis, that contains and nourishes a fetus during pregnancy
VD —Venereal disease—also called sexually transmitted disease
Viability —Ability to live

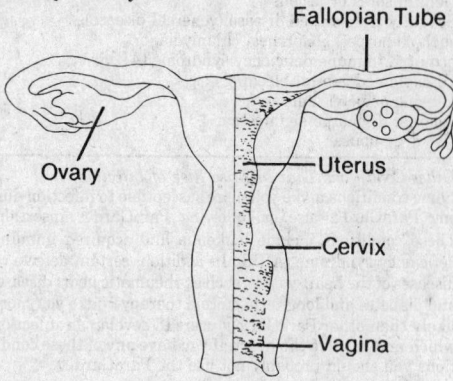

Shown in Product Identification Section, page 411

Health Maintenance Programs, Inc.
**7 WESTCHESTER PLAZA
ELMSFORD, NY 10523**

CALCIUM HEALTH PACKS™   OTC

Moderate-Dose Antioxidants and Vitamins plus High Dose Calcium, with Glutathione and Carotene

Each Packet Contains:

Antioxidants/Vitamins	Quantity	%RDA
1 Ascorbic-B/Yellow Cap		
Ascorbic Acid/C	800 mg	1333%
Calcium Pantothenate/B-5	120 mg	1200%
Thiamine HCl/B-1	40 mg	2666%
Pyridoxine HCl/B-6	20 mg	1000%
Niacinamide/B-3	20 mg	100%
Riboflavin/B-2	2 mg	118%
Cyanocobalamin/B-12	150 mcg	2500%
1 Combination/White Cap		
Calcium as the Carbonate	400 mg	40%
Ascorbic Acid/C	150 mg	250%
Glutathione	50 mg	
Cholecalciferol/D₃	125 IU	31%
1 Carotene-E/Red Cap		
Beta Carotene, crystalline	15 mg	
d,l-Alpha Tocopheryl Acetate/E	100 IU	333%

DIRECTIONS

Same as Performance Packs™
48 Packets/144 Capsules

CAROTENE–E Forté™   OTC

Each Capsule Contains:

Antioxidants/Vitamins	Quantity	%RDA
Beta Carotene, crystalline	30 MG	—
d,l-Alpha Tocopheryl Acetate/E	200 IU	667%

90 Capsules

CAROTENE–HEALTH PACKS™   OTC

Contains a Range of Antioxidant Vitamins, Carotene, Glutathione and Bone-promoting Calcium/Vitamin D₃ Nutritional Supplements.

Each Carotene Health Pack™ Blister Contains:

Antioxidants/Vitamins	Quantity	RDA
2 Ascorbic-B/Yellow Caps		
Ascorbic Acid/Vitamin C	1600 MG	2667%
Calcium Pantothenate/Vitamin B-5	240 MG	2400%
Thiamine HCl/Vitamin B-1	80 MG	5333%
Pyridoxine HCl/Vitamin B-6	40 MG	2000%
Niacinamide/Vitamin B-3	40 MG	200%
Riboflavin/Vitamin B-2	4 MG	236%
Cyanocobalamin/Vitamin B-12	300 MCG	5000%
1 White Capsule:		
Ascorbic Acid/Vitamin C	400 MG	667%
Calcium (as the carbonate)	250 MG	25%
Glutathione	100 MG	—
Cholecalciferol/Vitamin D₃	125 IU	31%
1 Carotene-E Forté/Red Cap		
Beta Carotene, crystalline	30 MG	—
d,l-Alpha Tocopheryl Acetate/Vitamin E	200 IU	667%

DIRECTIONS
One packet after meals or snacks, 1 to 3 times a day
48 Packets/192 Capsules

ENDURANCE PACKS™   OTC

High-Dose Antioxidants and Vitamins plus Calcium, *without Glutathione*

Each Packet Contains:

Antioxidants/Vitamins	Quantity	% RDA
2 Ascorbic-B/Yellow Caps		
Ascorbic Acid/C	1600 mg	2667%
Calcium Pantothenate/B-5	240 mg	2400%
Thiamine HCl/B-1	80 mg	5333%
Pyridoxine HCl/B-6	40 mg	2000%
Niacinamide/B-3	40 mg	200%
Riboflavin/B-2	4 mg	236%
Cyanocobalamin/B-12	300 mcg	5000%
1 Calcium-D/White Cap		
Calcium as the Carbonate	400 mg	40%
Cholecalciferol/D₃	125 IU	31%
1 Carotene-E/Red Cap		
Beta Carotene, crystalline	15 mg	—
d,l-Alpha Tocopheryl Acetate/E	100 IU	333%

DIRECTIONS
Same as Performance Packs
32 Packets/128 Capsules

FOR TWO™   OTC

Scientifically calculated, for pregnant/lactating women, to help provide the extra amounts of nutrients around the clock for mother and child

2 Capsules Contain:

Antioxidants/Vitamins	Quantity	RDA%
Retinyl Acetate/A	5000 IU	63%
Cholecalciferol/D₃	400 IU	100%
Ascorbic Acid/C	120 mg	200%
Niacinamide/B-3	40 mg	200%
d,l-Alpha Tocopheryl Acetate/E	30 IU	100%
Calcium Pantothenate/B-5	20 mg	200%
Pyridoxine HCl/B-6	6 mg	240%
Riboflavin/B-2	4 mg	200%
Thiamine HCl/B-1	3400 mcg	200%
Folic Acid	800 mcg	100%
Cyanocobalamin/B-12	8 mcg	100%
MINERALS:		
Calcium as the Carbonate	600 mg	60%
Magnesium as the Sulfate	200 mg	50%
Iron as Ferrous Fumarate	36 mg	200%
Iodine as Potassium Iodide	150 mcg	100%

DIRECTIONS
One with breakfast and one at bedtime.
120 Capsules

GLUTATHIONE–500™   OTC
Contains the Antioxidants Glutathione, Vitamin C, Minerals and Calcium/Vitamin D₃ Nutritional Supplements

Each Glutathione-500™ Capsule Contains:

Antioxidants/Vitamins	Quantity	RDA
Glutathione	500 MG	—
Ascorbic Acid/Vitamin C	125 MG	208%
Calcium (as the carbonate)	50 MG	5%
Zinc (as the oxide)	5 MG	33%
Manganese (as the sulfate)	1.33 MG	33%
Copper (as the oxide)	667 MCG	33%
Selenium (as sodium selenate)	18 MCG	33%
Cholecalciferol/Vitamin-D₃	85 IU	21%

ADULT FOOD SUPPLEMENT:
Take 1 capsule per day <u>after</u> meal <u>with</u> a <u>glass of water</u> or as directed by physician.
90 capsules

GLUTATHIONE–FORTÉ™   OTC
Pure glutathione antioxidant, and crystalline ascorbic acid

Each Capsule Contains:

Antioxidants/Vitamins	Quantity	%RDA
Ascorbic Acid/C	750 mg	1250%
Glutathione	250 mg	—

60 Capsules

GLUTATHIONE–HEALTH PACKS™   OTC
Contains a Range of Antioxidant Vitamins, Glutathione, Minerals and Calcium/Vitamin D₃ Nutritional Supplements

Each Glutathione Health Pack™ Blister Contains:

Antioxidants/Vitamins	Quantity	RDA
2 Ascorbic-B/Yellow Caps		
Ascorbic Acid/Vitamin C	1600 MG	2667%
Calcium Pantothenate/Vitamin B-5	240 MG	2400%
Thiamine HCl/Vitamin B-1	80 MG	5333%
Pyridoxine HCl/Vitamin B-6	40 MG	2000%
Niacinamide/Vitamin B-3	40 MG	200%
Riboflavin/Vitamin B-2	4 MG	236%
Cyanocobalamin/Vitamin B-12	300 MCG	5000%
1 White Capsule:		
Glutathione	500 MG	—
Ascorbic Acid/Vitamin C	125 MG	208%
Calcium (as the carbonate)	50 MG	5%
Zinc (as the oxide)	5 MG	33%
Manganese (as the sulfate)	1.33 MG	33%
Copper (as the oxide)	667 MCG	33%
Selenium (as sodium selenate)	18 MCG	33%
Cholecalciferol/Vitamin D₃	85 IU	21%
1 Carotene-E/Red Cap		
Beta Carotene, crystalline	15 MG	—
d,l-Alpha Tocopheryl Acetate/Vitamin E	100 IU	333%

DIRECTIONS
One packet per day <u>after a meal</u> or as directed by physician
48 Packets/192 Capsules

PERFORMANCE PACKS™   OTC
High-Dose Antioxidants and Vitamins plus Calcium, with Glutathione and Carotene

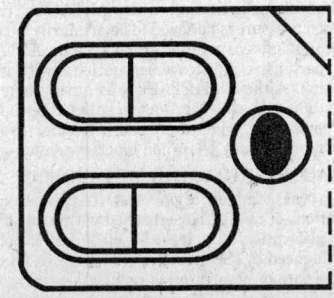

Unit dose blister pack has similar appearance to Glutathione Health Packs™, Carotene Health Packs™, Calcium Health Packs™, and Endurance Packs™

- Supplements During: Weight Loss Programs and Other Stresses
- For very Active Adults
- Strenuous Exercise
- Late Night Work
- Extensive Travel

Each Packet Contains:

Antioxidants/Vitamins	Quantity	%RDA
2 Ascorbic-B/Yellow Caps		
Ascorbic Acid/C	1600 mg	2667%
Calcium Pantothenate/B-5	240 mg	2400%
Thiamine HCl/B-1	80 mg	5333%
Pyridoxine HCl/B-6	40 mg	2000%
Niacinamide	40 mg	200%
Riboflavin/B-2	4 mg	236%
Cyanocobalamin/B-12	300 mcg	5000%
1 Combination/White Cap		
Ascorbic Acid/C	400 mg	667%
Calcium as the Carbonate	250 mg	25%
Glutathione	100 mg	—
Cholecalciferol/D₃	125 IU	31%
1 Carotene-E/Red Cap		
Beta Carotene, crystalline	15 mg	—
d,l-Alpha Tocopheryl Acetate/E	100 IU	333%

DIRECTIONS
One packet after meals or snacks, 1 to 3 times a day
48 Packets/192 Capsules

PURE–E™   OTC
Antioxidant Formulation of Pure Vitamin E, as capsules or as liquid

Each 0.3 cc = 300 IU:

Antioxidants/Vitamins	Quantity	%RDA
d,l-Alpha Tocopheryl Acetate/E	300 IU	1000%
d,l-Alpha Tocopheryl Acetate/E	600 IU	2000%

Two Ounces Liquid (60cc). Supplied with calibrated dropper

Each Capsule Contains:

Antioxidants/Vitamins	Quantity	%RDA
d,l-Alpha Tocopheryl Acetate/E	400 IU	1333%

90 Capsules

SUPERKIDS™   OTC
Scientifically developed, great tasting supplements. With extra water-soluble antioxidants and vitamins to help extend energy production.

	Children 2–4 yrs, 1 Tablet Contains:		Over 4 yrs 2 Tablets:
Antioxidants/Vitamins	Quantity	RDA%	RDA%
Retinyl Acetate/A	2500 IU	100%	100%
Cholecalciferol/D₃	200 IU	50%	100%
Ascorbic Acid/C	120 mg	300%	400%
Niacinamide/B-3	20 mg	222%	200%
d,l-Alpha Tocopheryl Acetate/E	15 IU	150%	100%
Calcium Pantothenate/B-5	10 mg	200%	200%
Pyridoxine HCl/B-6	4 mg	571%	400%
Thiamine NO₃/B-1	3 mg	428%	400%
Riboflavin/B-2	2 mg	250%	235%
Folic Acid	50 mcg	25%	25%
Cyanocobalamin/B-12	6 mcg	200%	200%
Minerals:			
Iron as Ferrous Fumarate			
Copper as Cupric Oxide			
Zinc as the Oxide		Provides less than	
Manganese as the Sulfate		25% of RDA	

DIRECTIONS
Over 4 years old, one in the morning and one in the afternoon. 2-4 years old ½ tablet twice a day.
60 Chewable tablets

Dow B. Hickam, Inc.
P.O. BOX 2006
SUGAR LAND, TX 77487-2006

GRANULEX ℞

COMPOSITION
Each 0.82 cc. of medication delivered to the wound site contains Trypsin crystallized 0.1 mg., Balsam Peru 72.5 mg., Castor Oil 650.0 mg., and an emulsifier.

ACTION
Trypsin is intended for debridement of eschar and other necrotic tissue. It appears that in many instances removal of wound debris strengthens humoral defense mechanisms sufficiently to retard proliferation of local pathogens. Balsam Peru is an effective capillary bed stimulant used to increase circulation in the wound site area. Also, Balsam Peru has a mildly bactericidal action. Castor Oil is used to improve epithelialization by reducing premature epithelial desiccation and cornification. Also, it can act as a protective covering and aids in the reduction of pain.

INDICATIONS
For the treatment of decubitus ulcers, varicose ulcers, debridement of eschar, dehiscent wounds and sunburn.

USES
Granulex is in aerosol form which can be important to healing. It must be remembered, healing starts with a thin sheath of epithelium no more than a cell or two thick. Any rough movement or trauma can quickly destroy the healing tissue. Aerosols have the advantage of eliminating all extraneous physical contact with the wound. Granulex is easy to apply and quickly reduces odor frequently accompanying a decubitus ulcer. The wound may be left open or a wet bandage may be applied. As a suggestion; keep in mind wounds heal poorly in the presence of hemoglobin or zinc deficiency.

WARNING
Do not spray on fresh arterial clots. Avoid spraying in eyes. Flammable, do not expose to fire or open flame. Contents under pressure. Do not puncture or incinerate. Do not store at temperature above 120°F. Keep out of reach of children. Use only as directed. Intentional misuse by deliberately concentrating and inhaling the contents can be harmful or fatal.

DOSAGE
Apply a minimum of twice daily or as often as necessary. Shake well, press the aerosol valve and coat the wound rapidly but not excessively.

HOW SUPPLIED
2 oz. Aerosol NDC 0514-0001-01
4 oz. Aerosol NDC 0514-0001-02

High Chemical Co.
1760 N. HOWARD ST.
PHILADELPHIA, PA 19122

SARAPIN ℞
[sar'a-pin]

COMPOSITION
An aqueous distillate of Sarracenia purpurea, pitcher plant, prepared for parenteral administration.

ACTION AND USES
Local injection therapy for the relief of pain of neuro-muscular or neuralgic origin.

ADMINISTRATION AND DOSAGE
Paravertebral nerve injection—2 to 10 cc. Local neuromuscular infiltration—5 to 10 cc.

SIDE EFFECTS
None.

PRECAUTIONS
Non-toxic.

CONTRAINDICATIONS
Local inflammation.

HOW SUPPLIED
50 cc. multi-dose vials NDC 10541-492-50.

LITERATURE AVAILABLE
Booklet "SARAPIN, Injection Technique in Pain Control."

Products are cross-indexed by generic and chemical names in the **YELLOW SECTION.**

Hoechst-Roussel Pharmaceuticals Inc.
SOMERVILLE, NJ 08876-1258

ALTACE™ ℞
(ramipril)*

USE IN PREGNANCY
When used in pregnancy during the second and third trimesters, ACE inhibitors can cause injury and even death to the developing fetus. When pregnancy is detected, ALTACE™ should be discontinued as soon as possible. **See WARNINGS. Fetal/neonatal morbidity and mortality.**

DESCRIPTION
Ramipril is a 2-aza-bicyclo [3.3.0]-octane-3-carboxylic acid derivative. It is a white, crystalline substance soluble in polar organic solvents and buffered aqueous solutions. Ramipril melts between 105°C and 112°C.
The CAS Registry Number is 87333-19-5. Ramipril's chemical name is (2*S*,3*aS*,6*aS*)-1[(*S*)-*N*-[(*S*)-1-Carboxy-3-phenylpropyl]alanyl]octahydrocyclopenta[*b*] pyrrole-2-carboxylic acid, 1-ethyl ester; its structural formula is:

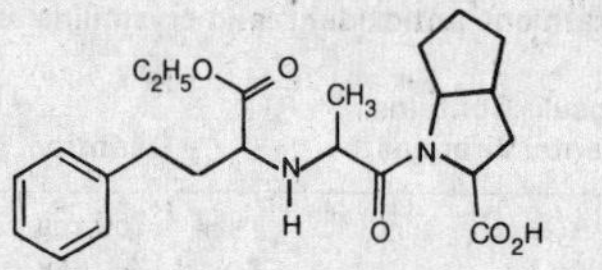

Its empiric formula is $C_{23}H_{32}N_2O_5$ and its molecular weight is 416.5.
Ramiprilat, the diacid metabolite of ramipril, is a non-sulfhydryl angiotensin converting enzyme inhibitor. Ramipril is converted to ramiprilat by hepatic cleavage of the ester group.
ALTACE™ (ramipril) is supplied as hard shell capsules containing 1.25 mg, 2.5 mg, 5 mg, and 10 mg of ramipril. The inactive ingredients present are pregelatinized starch NF, gelatin, and titanium dioxide. The 1.25 mg capsule shell contains yellow iron oxide, the 2.5 mg capsule shell contains D&C yellow #10 and FD&C red #40, the 5 mg capsule shell contains FD&C blue #1 and FD&C red #40, and the 10 mg capsule shell contains FD&C blue #1.

CLINICAL PHARMACOLOGY
Mechanism of Action
Ramipril and ramiprilat inhibit angiotensin-converting enzyme (ACE) in human subjects and animals. ACE is a peptidyl dipeptidase that catalyzes the conversion of angiotensin I to the vasoconstrictor substance, angiotensin II. Angiotensin II also stimulates aldosterone secretion by the adrenal cortex. Inhibition of ACE results in decreased plasma angiotensin II, which leads to decreased vasopressor activity and to decreased aldosterone secretion. The latter decrease may result in a small increase of serum potassium. In hypertensive patients with normal renal function treated with ALTACE alone for up to 56 weeks, approximately 4 percent of patients during the trial had an abnormally high serum potassium and an increase from baseline greater than 0.75 mEq/L, and none of the patients had an abnormally low potassium and a decrease from baseline greater than 0.75 mEq/L. In the same study, approximately 2% of patients treated with ALTACE and hydrochlorothiazide for up to 56 weeks had abnormally high potassium values and an increase from baseline of 0.75 mEq/L or greater, and approximately 2% had abnormally low values and decreases from baseline of 0.75 mEq/L or greater. (See PRECAUTIONS.)
Removal of angiotensin II negative feedback on renin secretion leads to increased plasma renin activity. ACE is identical to kininase, an enzyme that degrades bradykinin. Whether increased levels of bradykinin, a potent vasodepressor peptide, play a role in the therapeutic effects of ALTACE remains to be elucidated.
While the mechanism through which ALTACE™ (ramipril) lowers blood pressure is believed to be primarily suppression of the renin-angiotensin-aldosterone system, ALTACE has an antihypertensive effect even in patients with low-renin hypertension. Although ALTACE was antihypertensive in all races studied, black hypertensive patients (usually a low-renin hypertensive population) had a smaller average response to monotherapy than non-black patients.

PHARMACOKINETICS AND METABOLISM
Following oral administration of ALTACE, peak plasma concentrations of ramipril are reached within one hour. The extent of absorption is at least 50–60% and is not significantly influenced by the presence of food in the GI tract, although the rate of absorption is reduced.

*US Patent 4,587,258

Cleavage of the ester group (primarily in the liver) converts ramipril to its active diacid metabolite, ramiprilat. Peak plasma concentrations of ramiprilat are reached 2–4 hours after drug intake. The serum protein binding of ramipril is about 73% and that of ramiprilat about 56%; *in vitro*, these percentages are independent of concentration over the range of 0.01 to 10μg/ml.
Ramipril is almost completely metabolized to ramiprilat, which has about 6 times the ACE inhibitory activity of ramipril, and to the diketopiperazine ester, the diketopiperazine acid, and the glucuronides of ramipril and ramiprilat, all of which are inactive. After oral administration of ramipril, about 60% of the parent drug and its metabolites are eliminated in the urine, and about 40% is found in the feces. Less than 2% of the administered dose is recovered in urine as unchanged ramipril.
Blood concentrations of ramipril and ramiprilat increase with increased dose, but are not strictly dose-proportional. The 24-hour AUC for ramiprilat, however, is dose-proportional over the 2.5–20 mg dose range. The absolute bioavailabilities of ramipril and ramiprilat were 28% and 44%, respectively, when 5 mg of oral ramipril was compared with the same dose of ramipril given intravenously.
Plasma concentrations of ramiprilat decline in a triphasic manner (initial rapid decline, apparent elimination phase, terminal elimination phase). The initial rapid decline, which represents distribution of the drug into a large peripheral compartment and subsequent binding to both plasma and tissue ACE, has a half-life of 2–4 hours. Because of its potent binding to ACE and slow dissociation from the enzyme, ramiprilat shows two elimination phases. The apparent elimination phase corresponds to the clearance of free ramiprilat and has a half-life of 9–18 hours. The terminal elimination phase has a prolonged half-life (>50 hours) and probably represents the binding/dissociation kinetics of the ramiprilat/ACE complex. It does not contribute to the accumulation of the drug. After multiple daily doses of ramipril 5–10 mg, the half-life of ramiprilat concentrations within the therapeutic range was 13–17 hours.
After once-daily dosing, steady-state plasma concentrations of ramiprilat are reached by the fourth dose. Steady-state concentrations of ramiprilat are somewhat higher than those seen after the first dose of ALTACE™ (ramipril), especially at low doses (2.5 mg), but the difference is clinically insignificant.
The urinary excretion of ramipril, ramiprilat, and their metabolites is reduced in patients with impaired renal function. Compared to normal subjects, patients with creatinine clearance less than 40 ml/min/1.73m^2 had higher peak and trough ramiprilat levels and slightly longer times to peak concentrations. (See DOSAGE AND ADMINISTRATION.)
In patients with impaired liver function, the metabolism of ramipril to ramiprilat appears to be slowed, possibly because of diminished activity of hepatic esterases, and plasma ramipril levels in these patients are increased about 3-fold. Peak concentrations of ramiprilat in these patients, however, are not different from those seen in subjects with normal hepatic function, and the effect of a given dose on plasma ACE activity does not vary with hepatic function.

PHARMACODYNAMICS
Single doses of ramipril of 2.5–20 mg produce approximately 60–80% inhibition of ACE activity 4 hours after dosing with approximately 40–60% inhibition after 24 hours. Multiple oral doses of ramipril of 2.0 mg or more cause plasma ACE activity to fall by more than 90% 4 hours after dosing, with over 80% inhibition of ACE activity remaining 24 hours after dosing. The more prolonged effect of even small multiple doses presumably reflects saturation of ACE binding sites by ramiprilat and relatively slow release from those sites.
Administration of ALTACE to patients with mild to moderate hypertension results in a reduction of both supine and standing blood pressure to about the same extent with no compensatory tachycardia. Symptomatic postural hypotension is infrequent, although it can occur in patients who are salt- and/or volume-depleted. (See WARNINGS.) Use of ALTACE in combination with thiazide diuretics gives a blood pressure lowering effect greater than that seen with either agent alone.
In single-dose studies, doses of 5–20 mg of ALTACE lowered blood pressure within 1–2 hours, with peak reductions achieved 3–6 hours after dosing. The antihypertensive effect of a single dose persisted for 24 hours. In longer term (4–12 weeks) controlled studies, once-daily doses of 2.5–10 mg were similar in their effect, lowering supine or standing systolic and diastolic blood pressures 24 hours after dosing by about $^6/_4$ mm Hg more than placebo. In comparisons of peak vs trough effect, the trough effect represented about 50–60% of the peak response. In a titration study comparing divided (bid) vs qd treatment, the divided regimen was superior, indicating that for some patients the antihypertensive effect with once-daily dosing is not adequately maintained. (See DOSAGE AND ADMINISTRATION.)
In most trials, the antihypertensive effect of ALTACE increased during the first several weeks of repeated measurements. The antihypertensive effect of ALTACE has been

shown to continue during long-term therapy for at least 2 years. Abrupt withdrawal of ALTACE has not resulted in a rapid increase in blood pressure.

ALTACE has been compared with other ACE inhibitors, beta-blockers, and thiazide diuretics. It was approximately as effective as other ACE inhibitors and as atenolol. In both Caucasians and Blacks, hydrochlorothiazide (25 or 50 mg) was significantly more effective than ramipril.

Except for thiazides, no formal interaction studies of ramipril with other antihypertensive agents have been carried out. Limited experience in controlled and uncontrolled trials combining ramipril with a calcium channel blocker, a loop diuretic, or triple therapy (beta-blocker, vasodilator, and a diuretic) indicate no unusual drug-drug interactions. Other ACE inhibitors have had less than additive effects with beta adrenergic blockers, presumably because both drugs lower blood pressure by inhibiting parts of the renin-angiotensin system.

ALTACE™ (ramipril) was less effective in Blacks than in Caucasians. The effectiveness of ALTACE was not influenced by age, sex, or weight.

In a baseline controlled study of 10 patients with mild essential hypertension, blood pressure reduction was accompanied by a 15% increase in renal blood flow. In healthy volunteers, glomerular filtration rate was unchanged.

INDICATIONS AND USAGE

ALTACE is indicated for the treatment of hypertension. It may be used alone or in combination with thiazide diuretics.

In using ALTACE, consideration should be given to the fact that another angiotensin converting enzyme inhibitor, captopril, has caused agranulocytosis, particularly in patients with renal impairment or collagen-vascular disease. Available data are insufficient to show that ALTACE does not have a similar risk. (See WARNINGS.)

CONTRAINDICATIONS

ALTACE is contraindicated in patients who are hypersensitive to this product and in patients with history of angioneurotic edema.

WARNINGS

Angioedema

Angioedema of the face, extremities, lips, tongue, glottis, and larynx has been reported in patients treated with angiotensin converting enzyme inhibitors. Angioedema associated with laryngeal edema can be fatal. If laryngeal stridor or angioedema of the face, tongue, or glottis occurs, treatment with ALTACE should be discontinued and appropriate therapy instituted immediately. **Where there is involvement of the tongue, glottis, or larnyx, likely to cause airway obstruction, appropriate therapy, e.g., subcutaneous epinephrine solution 1:1,000 (0.3 ml to 0.5 ml) should be promptly administered.** (See ADVERSE REACTIONS.)

Hypotension

ALTACE can cause symptomatic hypotension, after either the initial dose or a later dose when the dosage has been increased. Like other ACE inhibitors, ramipril has been only rarely associated with hypotension in uncomplicated hypertensive patients. Symptomatic hypotension is most likely to occur in patients who have been volume- and/or salt-depleted as a result of prolonged diuretic therapy, dietary salt restriction, dialysis, diarrhea, or vomiting. Volume and/or salt depletion should be corrected before initiating therapy with ALTACE. In patients with congestive heart failure, with or without associated renal insufficiency, ACE inhibitor therapy may cause excessive hypotension, which may be associated with oliguria or azotemia and, rarely, with acute renal failure and death. In such patients, ALTACE therapy should be started under close medical supervision; they should be followed closely for the first 2 weeks of treatment and whenever the dose of ramipril or diuretic is increased.

If hypotension occurs, the patient should be placed in a supine position and, if necessary, treated with intravenous infusion of physiological saline. ALTACE™ (ramipril) treatment usually can be continued following restoration of blood pressure and volume.

Neutropenia/Agranulocytosis

Another angiotensin converting enzyme inhibitor, captopril, has been shown to cause agranulocytosis and bone marrow depression, rarely in uncomplicated patients, but more frequently in patients with renal impairment, especially if they also have a collagen-vascular disease such as systemic lupus erythematosus or scleroderma. Available data from clinical trials of ramipril are insufficient to show that ramipril does not cause agranulocytosis at similar rates. Monitoring of white blood cell counts should be considered in patients with collagen-vascular disease, especially if the disease is associated with impaired renal function.

Fetal/Neonatal Morbidity and Mortality

ACE inhibitors can cause fetal and neonatal morbidity and mortality when administered to pregnant women.

When ACE inhibitors have been used during the second and third trimesters of pregnancy, there have been reports of neonatal hypotension, renal failure, skull hypoplasia, and death. Oligohydramnios has also been reported, presumably resulting from decreased fetal renal function; oligohydramnios has been associated with fetal limb contractures, craniofacial malformations, hypoplastic lung development, and intrauterine growth retardation. Prematurity and patent ductus arteriosus have been reported, although it is not clear whether these occurrences were due to the ACE-inhibitor exposure or to the mother's underlying disease.

It is not known whether exposure limited to the first trimester can adversely affect fetal outcome.

A patient who becomes pregnant while taking ACE inhibitors, or who takes ACE inhibitors when already pregnant, should be apprised of the potential hazard to her fetus. If she continues to receive ACE inhibitors during the second or third trimester of pregnancy, frequent ultrasound examinations should be performed to look for oligohydramnios. When oligohydramnios is found, ACE inhibitors should generally be discontinued.

Infants with histories of *in utero* exposure to ACE inhibitors should be closely observed for hypotension, oliguria, and hypokalemia. If oliguria occurs, attention should be directed toward support of blood pressure and renal perfusion. Ramipril could theoretically be removed from the neonatal circulation by exchange transfusion, but no experience with this procedure has been reported.

Ramipril has been shown to increase the incidence of dilated renal pelvises in rat fetuses, to retard birth weights in mice, and to be toxic to pregnant rabbits and pregnant cynomolgus monkeys, but not, in any of these studies, to produce terata or to affect fertility, reproductive performance, or pregnancy. On a mg/kg basis, the doses used in these studies were 125–2500 times (in rats), 2500 times (in mice), more than 12 times (in monkeys), and more than twice (in rabbits) the maximum recommended human dose.

PRECAUTIONS

General

Impaired Renal Function: As a consequence of inhibiting the renin-angiotensin-aldosterone system, changes in renal function may be anticipated in susceptible individuals. In patients with severe congestive heart failure whose renal function may depend on the activity of the renin-angiotensin-aldosterone system, treatment with angiotensin converting enzyme inhibitors, including ALTACE™ (ramipril), may be associated with oliguria and/or progressive azotemia and (rarely) with acute renal failure and/or death.

In hypertensive patients with unilateral or bilateral renal artery stenosis, increases in blood urea nitrogen and serum creatinine may occur. Experience with another angiotensin converting enzyme inhibitor suggests that these increases are usually reversible upon discontinuation of ALTACE and/or diuretic therapy. In such patients renal function should be monitored during the first few weeks of therapy. Some hypertensive patients with no apparent pre-existing renal vascular disease have developed increases in blood urea nitrogen and serum creatinine, usually minor and transient, especially when ALTACE has been given concomitantly with a diuretic. This is more likely to occur in patients with pre-existing renal impairment. Dosage reduction of ALTACE and/or discontinuation of the diuretic may be required.

Evaluation of the hypertensive patient should always include assessment of renal function. (See DOSAGE AND ADMINISTRATION.)

Hyperkalemia: In clinical trials, hyperkalemia (serum potassium greater than 5.7 mEq/L) occurred in approximately 1% of hypertensive patients receiving ALTACE. In most cases, these were isolated values, which resolved despite continued therapy. None of these patients was discontinued from the trials because of hyperkalemia. Risk factors for the development of hyperkalemia include renal insufficiency, diabetes, mellitus, and the concomitant use of potassium-sparing diuretics, potassium supplements, and/or potassium-containing salt substitutes, which should be used cautiously, if at all, with ALTACE. (See DRUG INTERACTIONS.)

Impaired Liver Function: Since ramipril is primarily metabolized by hepatic esterases to its active moiety, ramiprilat, patients with impaired liver function could develop markedly elevated plasma levels of ramipril. No formal pharmacokinetic studies have been carried out in hypertensive patients with impaired liver function.

Surgery/Anesthesia: In patients undergoing surgery or during anesthesia with agents that produce hypotension, ramipril may block angiotensin II formation that would otherwise occur secondary to compensatory renin release. Hypotension that occurs as a result of this mechanism can be corrected by volume expansion.

Information for Patients

Angioedema: Angioedema, including laryngeal edema, can occur with treatment with ACE inhibitors, especially following the first dose. Patients should be so advised and told to report immediately any signs or symptoms suggesting angioedema (swelling of face, eyes, lips, or tongue, or difficulty in breathing) and to take no more drug until they have consulted with the prescribing physician.

Symptomatic Hypotension: Patients should be cautioned that light-headedness can occur, especially during the first days of therapy, and it should be reported. Patients should be told that if syncope occurs, ALTACE™ (ramipril) should be discontinued until the physician has been consulted.

All patients should be cautioned that inadequate fluid intake or excessive perspiration, diarrhea, or vomiting can lead to an excessive fall in blood pressure, with the same consequences of light-headedness and possible syncope.

Hyperkalemia: Patients should be told not to use salt substitutes containing potassium without consulting their physician.

Neutropenia: Patients should be told to promptly report any indication of infection (e.g., sore throat, fever), which could be a sign of neutropenia.

Drug Interactions

With diuretics: Patients on diuretics, especially those in whom diuretic therapy was recently instituted, may occasionally experience an excessive reduction of blood pressure after initiation of therapy with ALTACE. The possibility of hypotensive effects with ALTACE can be minimized by either discontinuing the diuretic or increasing the salt intake prior to initiation of treatment with ALTACE. If this is not possible, the starting dose should be reduced. (See DOSAGE AND ADMINISTRATION.)

With potassium supplements and potassium-sparing diuretics: ALTACE can attenuate potassium loss caused by thiazide diuretics. Potassium-sparing diuretics (spironolactone, amiloride, triamterene, and others) or potassium supplements can increase the risk of hyperkalemia. Therefore, if concomitant use of such agents is indicated, they should be given with caution, and the patient's serum potassium should be monitored frequently.

With lithium: Increased serum lithium levels and symptoms of lithium toxicity have been reported in patients receiving ACE inhibitors during therapy with lithium. These drugs should be coadministered with caution, and frequent monitoring of serum lithium levels is recommended. If a diuretic is also used, the risk of lithium toxicity may be increased.

Other: Neither ALTACE nor its metabolites have been found to interact with food, digoxin, or antacid.

Carcinogenesis, Mutagenesis, Impairment of Fertility

No evidence of a tumorigenic effect was found when ramipril was given by gavage to rats (up to 500 mg/kg/day for 24 months) or to mice (up to 1,000 mg/kg/day for 18 months). Dosages greatly in excess of those recommended for humans produced hypertrophy of the renal juxtaglomerular apparatus in mice, rats, dogs, and monkeys. No mutagenic activity was detected in the Ames test in bacteria, the micronucleus test in mice, unscheduled DNA synthesis in a human cell line, or a forward gene-mutation assay in a Chinese hamster ovary cell line. Several metabolites and degradation products of ramipril were also negative in the Ames test. A study in rats with dosages as great as 500 mg/kg/day did not produce adverse effects on fertility.

Pregnancy

Pregnancy Category D: See WARNINGS.

Nursing Mothers

Ingestion of a single 10 mg oral dose of ALTACE™ (ramipril) resulted in undetectable amounts of ramipril and its metabolites in breast milk. However, because multiple doses may produce low milk concentrations that are not predictable from single doses, ALTACE should not be administered to nursing mothers.

Geriatric Use

Of the total number of patients who received ramipril in US clinical studies of ALTACE 11.0% were 65 and over while 0.2% were 75 and over. No overall differences in effectiveness or safety were observed between these patients and younger patients, and other reported clinical experience has not identified differences in responses between the elderly and younger patients, but greater sensitivity of some older individuals cannot be ruled out.

One pharmacokinetic study conducted in hospitalized elderly patients indicated that peak ramiprilat levels and area under the plasma concentration time curve (AUC) for ramiprilat are higher in older patients.

Pediatric Use

Safety and effectiveness in children have not been established.

ADVERSE REACTIONS

ALTACE has been evaluated for safety in over 4,000 patients with hypertension; of these, 1,230 patients were studied in US controlled trials, and 1,107 were studied in foreign controlled trials. Almost 700 of these patients were treated for at least one year. The overall incidence of reported adverse events was similar in ALTACE and placebo patients. The most frequent clinical side effects (possibly or probably related to study drug) reported by patients receiving ALTACE in US placebo-controlled trials were: headache (5.4%), "dizziness" (2.2%) and fatigue or asthenia (2.0%), but only the last was more common in ALTACE patients than in patients

Continued on next page

Hoechst-Roussel—Cont.

given placebo. Generally, the side effects were mild and transient, and there was no relation to total dosage within the range of 1.25 to 20 mg. Discontinuation of therapy because of a side effect was required in approximately 3% of US patients treated with ALTACE. The most common reasons for discontinuation were: cough (1.0%), "dizziness" (0.5%), and impotence (0.4%).
The side effects considered possibly or probably related to study drug that occurred in US placebo-controlled trials in more than 1% of patients treated with ALTACE are shown below.

PATIENTS IN US PLACEBO CONTROLLED STUDIES

	Altace (N=651)		Placebo (N=286)	
	n	%	n	%
Headache	35	5.4	17	5.9
"Dizziness"	14	2.2	9	3.1
Asthenia (Fatigue)	13	2.0	2	0.7
Nausea/Vomiting	7	1.1	3	1.0

In placebo-controlled trials, there was also an excess of upper respiratory infection and flu syndrome in the ramipril group. As these studies were carried out before the relationship of cough to ACE inhibitors was recognized, some of these events may represent ramipril-induced cough. In a later 1-year study, increased cough was seen in almost 12% of ramipril patients, with about 4% of these patients, requiring discontinuation of treatment. Other adverse experiences reported in controlled clinical trials (in less than 1% of ramipril patients), or rarer events seen in postmarketing experience, include the following (in some, a causal relationship to drug use is uncertain.):
Cardiovascular: Symptomatic hypotension (reported in 0.5% of patients in US trials) (see PRECAUTIONS and WARNINGS), syncope (not reported in US trials), angina pectoris, arrhythmia, chest pain, palpitations, and myocardial infarction.
Renal: Some hypertensive patients with no apparent preexisting renal disease have developed minor, usually transient, increases in blood urea nitrogen and serum creatinine when taking ALTACE, particularly when ALTACE was given concomitantly with a diuretic. (See WARNINGS.)
Angioneurotic Edema: Angioneurotic edema has been reported in 0.3% of patients in US clinical trials. (See WARNINGS.)
Cough: A tickling, dry, persistent, nonproductive cough has been reported with the use of ACE inhibitors. Approximately 1% of patients treated with ALTACE have required discontinuation because of cough. The cough disappears shortly after discontinuation of treatment.
Gastrointestinal: Abdominal pain (sometimes with enzyme changes suggesting pancreatitis), anorexia, constipation, diarrhea, dry mouth, dyspepsia, dysphagia, gastroenteritis, nausea, increased salivation, taste disturbance, and vomiting.
Dermatologic: Apparent hypersensitivity reactions (manifested by dermatitis, pruritis, or rash, with or without fever), photosensitivity, and purpura.
Neurologic and Psychiatric: Anxiety, amnesia, convulsions, depression, hearing loss, insomnia, nervousness, neuralgia, neuropathy, paresthesia, somnolence, tinnitus, tremor, vertigo, and vision disturbances.
Other: arthralgia, arthritis, dyspnea, edema, epistaxis, impotence, increased sweating, malaise, myalgia, and weight gain.

Clinical Laboratory Test Findings:
Creatinine and Blood Urea Nitrogen: Increases in creatinine levels occurred in 1.2% of patients receiving ALTACE alone, and in 1.5% of patients receiving ALTACE and a diuretic. Increases in blood urea nitrogen levels occurred in 0.5% of patients receiving ALTACE alone and in 3% of patients receiving ALTACE with a diuretic. None of these increases required discontinuation of treatment. Increases in these laboratory values are more likely to occur in patients with renal insufficiency or those pretreated with a diuretic and, based on experience with other ACE inhibitors, would be expected to be especially likely in patients with renal artery stenosis. (See PRECAUTIONS and WARNINGS.)
Since ramipril decreases aldosterone secretion, elevation of serum potassium can occur. Potassium supplements and potassium-sparing diuretics should be given with caution, and the patient's serum potassium should be monitored frequently. (See PRECAUTIONS and WARNINGS.)
Hemoglobin and Hematocrit: Decreases in hemoglobin or hematocrit (a low value and a decrease of 5 g/dl or 5% respectively) were rare, occurring in 0.4% of patients receiving ALTACE alone and in 1.5% of patients receiving ALTACE plus a diuretic. No US patients discontinued treatment because of decreases in hemoglobin or hematocrit.
Other (causal relationships unknown): Clinically important changes in standard laboratory tests were rarely associated with ALTACE administration. Elevations of liver enzymes, serum bilirubin, uric acid, and blood glucose have been reported, as have scattered incidents of leukopenia, eosinophilia, and proteinuria. In US trials, less than 0.2% of patients discontinued treatment for laboratory abnormalities: all of these were cases of proteinuria or abnormal liver-function tests.

OVERDOSAGE

The oral LD_{50} of rats and mice is 10–11 g/kg. In dogs, oral doses as high as 1 g/kg induced only mild gastrointestinal distress. Human overdoses of ramipril have not been reported, but the most common manifestation of human ramipril overdosage is likely to be hypotension.
Laboratory determinations of serum levels of ramipril and its metabolites are not widely available, and such determinations have, in any event, no established role in the management of ramipril overdose.
No data are available to suggest physiological maneuvers (e.g., maneuvers to change the pH of the urine) that might accelerate elimination of ramipril and its metabolites. Similarly, it is not known which, if any, of these substances can be usefully removed from the body by hemodialysis.
Angiotensin II could presumably serve as a specific antagonist-antidote in the setting of ramipril overdose, but angiotensin II is essentially unavailable outside of scattered research facilities. Because the hypotensive effect of ramipril is achieved through vasodilation and effective hypovolemia, it is reasonble to treat ramipril overdose by infusion of normal saline solution.

DOSAGE AND ADMINISTRATION

The recommended initial dose for patients not receiving a diuretic is 2.5 mg once a day. Dosage should be adjusted according to the blood pressure response. The usual maintenance dosage range is 2.5 to 20 mg per day administered as a single dose or in two equally divided doses. In some patients treated once daily, the antihypertensive effect may diminish toward the end of the dosing interval. In such patients, an increase in dosage or twice daily administration should be considered. If blood pressure is not controlled with ALTACE alone, a diuretic can be added.
Concomitant administration of ALTACE with potassium supplements, potassium salt substitutes, or potassium-sparing diuretics can lead to increases of serum potassium. (See PRECAUTIONS.)
In patients who are currently being treated with a diuretic, symptomatic hypotension occasionally can occur following the initial dose of ALTACE. To reduce the likelihood of hypotension, the diuretic should, if possible, be discontinued two to three days prior to beginning therapy with ALTACE (see WARNINGS). Then, if blood pressure is not controlled with ALTACE alone, diuretic therapy should be resumed.
If the diuretic cannot be discontinued, an initial dose of 1.25 mg ALTACE should be used to avoid excess hypotension.
DOSAGE ADJUSTMENT IN RENAL IMPAIRMENT: For patients with a creatinine clearance <40 ml/min/1.73m^2 (serum creatinine >2.5 mg/dl), the recommended initial dose is 1.25 mg ALTACE once daily. Dosage may be titrated upward until blood pressure is controlled or to a maximum total daily dose of 5 mg.

HOW SUPPLIED

ALTACE is available in potencies of 1.25 mg, 2.5 mg, 5 mg, and 10 mg in hard gelatin capsules, packaged in bottles of 100 capsules. ALTACE is also supplied in blister packages (10 capsules/blister card).
ALTACE capsules are supplied as follows:
1.25 mg—yellow capsule
NDC 0039-0103-10—bottles of 100
NDC 0039-0103-11—Unit Dose Cartons of 100
2.5 mg—orange capsule
NDC 0039-0104-10—bottles of 100
NDC 0039-0104-11—Unit Dose Cartons of 100
5 mg—red capsule
NDC 0039-0105-10—bottles of 100
NDC 0039-0105-11—Unit Dose Cartons of 100
10 mg—Process Blue Capsules
NDC 0039-0106-10—bottles of 100
Dispense in well-closed container with safety closure.
Store at controlled room temperature (59° to 86°F).
Caution: Federal law prohibits dispensing without prescription.
Altace TM HOECHST AG
Made in USA
REG TM HOECHST AG 710300-2/91
Shown in Product Identification Section, page 411

A/T/S® ℞
(erythromycin)
2% Acne Topical Solution & Topical Gel

DESCRIPTION

A/T/S® contains erythromycin. Erythromycin is a macrolide antibiotic obtained from cultures of *Streptomyces erythreus.*

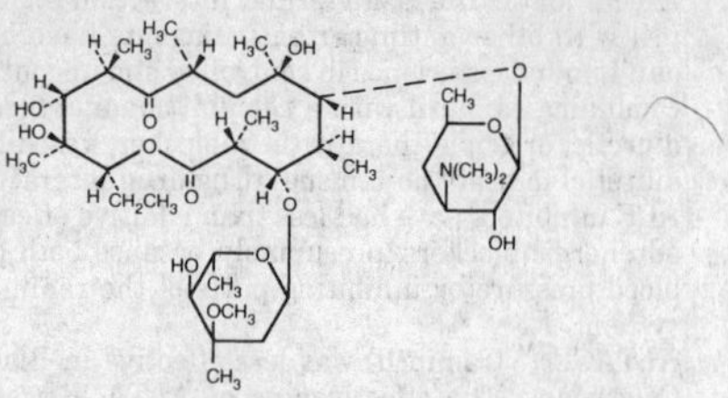

Empirical Formula: $C_{37}H_{67}NO_{13}$
Molecular Weight: 733.94
Each mL of A/T/S® (erythromycin) Topical Solution contains 20 mg of erythromycin base in a vehicle consisting of alcohol USP (66%), propylene glycol USP, and citric acid USP to adjust pH.
A/T/S® (erythromycin) Topical Gel contains erythromycin USP 2% (20 mg/g) with alcohol 92% and hydroxypropyl cellulose.

CLINICAL PHARMACOLOGY

The exact mechanism by which erythromycin reduces lesions of acne vulgaris is not fully known; however, the effect appears to be due in part to the antibacterial activity of the drug.

MICROBIOLOGY

Erythromycin appears to inhibit protein synthesis in susceptible organisms by reversibly binding to ribosomal subunits, thereby inhibiting translocation of aminoacyl transfer-RNA and inhibiting polypeptide synthesis.
Antagonism has been demonstrated between erythromycin, lincomycin, chloramphenicol, and clindamycin.

INDICATIONS AND USAGE

A/T/S® is indicated for the topical treatment of acne vulgaris.

CONTRAINDICATIONS

A/T/S® is contraindicated in those individuals who have shown hypersensitivity to any of its components.

PRECAUTIONS

General: For topical use only; not for ophthalmic use. Concomitant topical acne therapy should be used with caution since a possible cumulative irritancy effect may occur, especially with the use of peeling, desquamating or abrasive agents.
Avoid contact with eyes and all mucous membranes. The use of antibiotic agents may be associated with the overgrowth of antibiotic-resistant organisms. If this occurs, discontinue use and take appropriate measures.
Carcinogenesis, mutagenesis, impairment of fertility: Animal studies to evaluate carcinogenic and mutagenic potential, or effects on fertility have not been performed with erythromycin.
Pregnancy Category B:
There was no evidence of teratogenicity or any other adverse effect on reproduction in female rats fed erythromycin base (up to 0.25% of diet) prior to and during mating, during gestation and through weaning of two successive litters. There are, however, no adequate and well-controlled studies in pregnant women. Because animal reproduction studies are not always predictive of human response, this drug should be used in pregnancy only if clearly needed. Erythromycin has been reported to cross the placental barrier in humans, but fetal plasma levels are generally low.
Nursing Mothers:
It is not known whether topically applied erythromycin is excreted in human milk. A decision should be made whether to discontinue nursing or to discontinue the drug, taking into account the importance of the drug to the mother.
Pediatric Use:
Safety and effectiveness in children have not been established.

ADVERSE REACTIONS

Adverse conditions reported with the use of erythromycin topical solutions include dryness, tenderness, pruritus, desquamation, erythema, oiliness, and burning sensation. The most common adverse reaction reported with an erythromycin topical gel was burning. The following have been reported occasionally: peeling, dryness, itching, erythema, and oiliness. Irritation of the eyes and tenderness of the skin have also been reported with the topical use of erythromycin. A generalized urticarial reaction, possibly related to the use of erythromycin, which required systemic steroid therapy has been reported.

Of a total of 90 patients exposed to A/T/S® Topical Solution during clinical effectiveness studies, 17 experienced some type of adverse effect. These included dry skin, scaly skin, pruritus, irritation of the eye, and burning sensation.

DOSAGE AND ADMINISTRATION

A/T/S® (erythromycin) should be applied to the affected area(s) twice a day, in the morning and the evening after the skin is thoroughly washed with soap and water and patted dry. For A/T/S® Topical Solution, moisten the applicator or a pad with A/T/S®, then rub over the affected area. For A/T/S® Topical Gel, apply a thin film to affected area(s). Spread the medication lightly rather than rubbing it in. The hands should be washed after application. Acne lesions on the face, neck, shoulder, chest, and back may be treated in this manner. If there has been no improvement after 6 to 8 weeks, or if the condition becomes worse, treatment should be discontinued, and the physician should be reconsulted.

HOW SUPPLIED

A/T/S® 2% Topical Solution—60 mL bottles. A/T/S® 2% Topical Gel—30 gram tubes.

Note: FLAMMABLE. Keep away from heat and flame. Keep tube tightly closed. Store at room temperature (59°–86°F).

CAUTION

Federal law prohibits dispensing without prescription.

A/T/S REG TM Hoechst-Roussel Pharmaceuticals Inc.

711600-5/90

716000-4/86

Shown in Product Identification Section, page 411

CLAFORAN® ℞

[*klăf'or-an*]

(cefotaxime sodium)*

Sterile and Injection

DESCRIPTION

Sterile Claforan® (cefotaxime sodium) is a semisynthetic, broad spectrum cephalosporin antibiotic for parenteral administration. It is the sodium salt of 7-[2-(2-amino-4-thiazolyl) glyoxylamido]-3-(hydroxymethyl)-8-oxo-5-thia-1-azabicyclo [4.2.0] oct-2-ene-2-carboxylate 7^2-(Z)-(O-methyloxime), acetate (ester). Claforan contains approximately 50.5 mg (2.2 mEq) of sodium per gram of cefotaxime activity. Solutions of Claforan range from very pale yellow to light amber depending on the concentration and the diluent used. The pH of the injectable solutions usually ranges from 5.0 to 7.5.

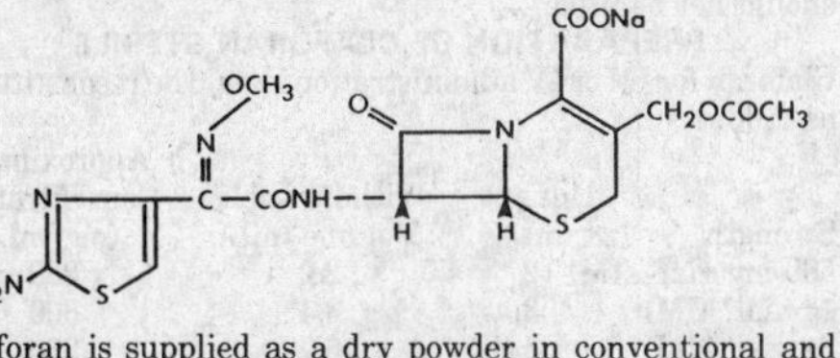

Claforan is supplied as a dry powder in conventional and ADD-Vantage® System compatible vials, infusion bottles, pharmacy bulk package bottles, and as a frozen, premixed injection in a buffered diluent solution in plastic containers. Claforan, equivalent to 1 gram and 2 grams cefotaxime, is supplied as frozen, premixed injections in plastic containers in 5% dextrose (containing dextrose hydrous, USP). The injections are buffered with sodium citrate hydrous, USP. The pH is adjusted with hydrochloric acid and may be adjusted with sodium hydroxide. The plastic container is fabricated from a specially formulated polyvinyl chloride. Solutions in contact with the plastic container can leach out certain of its chemical components in very small amounts within the expiration period, e.g., di-2-ethylhexyl phthalate (DEHP), up to 5 parts per million. However, the safety of the plastic has been confirmed in tests in animals according to USP biological tests for plastic containers as well as by tissue culture toxicity studies.

CLINICAL PHARMACOLOGY

Following IM administration of a single 500 mg or 1 g dose of Claforan to normal volunteers, mean peak serum concentrations of 11.7 and 20.5 μg/mL respectively were attained within 30 minutes and declined with an elimination half-life of approximately 1 hour. There was a dose-dependent increase in serum levels after the IV administration of 500 mg, 1 g and 2 g of Claforan (38.9, 101.7, and 214.4 μg/mL respectively) without alteration in the elimination half-life. There is no evidence of accumulation following repetitive IV infusion of 1 g doses every 6 hours for 14 days as there are no alterations of serum or renal clearance. About 60% of the administered dose was recovered from urine during the first 6 hours following the start of the infusion.

Approximately 20–36% of an intravenously administered dose of ^{14}C-cefotaxime is excreted by the kidney as unchanged cefotaxime and 15–25% as the desacetyl derivative, the major metabolite. The desacetyl metabolite has been shown to contribute to the bactericidal activity. Two other urinary metabolites (M_2 and M_3) account for about 20–25%. They lack bactericidal activity.

A single 50 mg/kg dose of Claforan was administered as an intravenous infusion over a 10- to 15-minute period to 29 newborn infants grouped according to birth weight and age. The mean half-life of cefotaxime in infants with lower birth weights (≤ 1500 grams), regardless of age, was longer (4.6 hours) than the mean half-life (3.4 hours) in infants whose birth weight was greater than 1500 grams. Mean serum clearance was also smaller in the lower birth weight infants. Although the differences in mean half-life values are statistically significant for weight, they are not clinically important. Therefore, dosage should be based solely on age. (See **Dosage and Administration** section.)

Additionally, no disulfiram-like reactions were reported in a study conducted in 22 healthy volunteers administered Claforan and ethanol.

Microbiology

The bactericidal activity of cefotaxime sodium results from inhibition of cell wall synthesis. Cefotaxime sodium has *in vitro* activity against a wide range of gram-positive and gram-negative organisms. Claforan has a high degree of stability in the presence of beta-lactamases, both penicillinases and cephalosporinases, of gram-negative and gram-positive bacteria. Cefotaxime sodium has been shown to be a potent inhibitor of β-lactamases produced by certain gram-negative bacteria. Cefotaxime sodium is usually active against the following microorganisms both *in vitro* and in clinical infections (see **Indications and Usage**).

Aerobes, Gram-positive: *Staphylococcus aureus,* including penicillinase and non-penicillinase producing strains, *Staphylococcus epidermidis, Enterococcus* species, *Streptococcus pyogenes* (Group A beta-hemolytic streptococci), *Streptococcus agalactiae* (Group B streptococci), *Streptococcus pneumoniae* (formerly *Diplococcus pneumoniae*).

Aerobes, Gram-negative: *Citrobacter* species, *Enterobacter* species, *Escherichia coli, Haemophilus influenzae* (including ampicillin-resistant *H. influenzae*), *Haemophilus parainfluenzae, Klebsiella* species (including *K. pneumoniae*), *Neisseria gonorrhoeae* (including penicillinase and non-penicillinase producing strains), *Neisseria meningitidis, Proteus mirabilis, Proteus vulgaris, Proteus inconstans,* Group B, *Morganella morganii, Providencia rettgeri, Serratia* species, and *Acinetobacter* species.

NOTE: Many strains of the above organisms that are multiply resistant to other antibiotics, e.g., penicillins, cephalosporins, and aminoglycosides, are susceptible to cefotaxime sodium.

Cefotaxime sodium is active against some strains of *Pseudomonas aeruginosa.*

Anaerobes: *Bacteroides* species, including some strains of *B. fragilis, Clostridium* species (NOTE: Most strains of *C. difficile* are resistant), *Peptococcus* species, *Peptostreptococcus* species, and *Fusobacterium* species (including *F. nucleatum*).

Cefotaxime sodium is highly stable *in vitro* to four of the five major classes of β-lactamases described by Richmond et al., including type IIIa (TEM) which is produced by many gram-negative bacteria. The drug is also stable to β-lactamase (penicillinase) produced by staphylococci. In addition, cefotaxime sodium shows high affinity for penicillin-binding proteins in the cell wall, including PBP, Ib and III.

Cefotaxime sodium also demonstrates *in vitro* activity against the following microorganisms although clinical significance is unknown: *Salmonella* species (including *S. typhi*), *Providencia* species, and *Shigella* species.

Cefotaxime sodium and aminoglycosides have been shown to be synergistic *in vitro* against some strains of *Pseudomonas aeruginosa.*

Susceptibility Tests

Quantitative methods that require measurement of zone diameters give the most precise estimate of antibiotic susceptibility. One such procedure[1] has been recommended for use with discs to test susceptibility to cefotaxime sodium. Interpretation involves correlation of the diameters obtained in the disc test with minimum inhibitory concentration (MIC) values for cefotaxime sodium.

Reports from the laboratory giving results of the standardized single-disc susceptibility test using a 30-μg cefotaxime sodium disc should be interpreted according to the following criteria:

Susceptible organisms produce zones of 20 mm or greater, indicating that the tested organism is likely to respond to therapy.

Organisms that produce zones of 15 to 19 mm are expected to be susceptible if high dosage is used or if the infection is confined to tissues and fluids (e.g., urine) in which high antibiotic levels are attained.

Resistant organisms produce zones of 14 mm or less, indicating that other therapy should be selected.

Organisms should be tested with the cefotaxime sodium disc, since cefotaxime sodium has been shown by *in vitro* tests to be active against certain strains found resistant when other beta lactam discs are used. The cefotaxime sodium disc should not be used for testing susceptibility to other cephalosporins. Organisms having zones of less than 18 mm around the cephalothin disc are not necessarily of intermediate susceptibility or resistant to cefotaxime sodium.

A bacterial isolate may be considered susceptible if the MIC value for cefotaxime sodium is not more than 16 μg/mL. Organisms are considered resistant to cefotaxime sodium if the MIC is equal to or greater than 64 μg/mL. Organisms having an MIC value of less than 64 μg/mL but greater than 16μg/mL are expected to be susceptible if high dosage is used or if the infection is confined to tissues and fluids (e.g., urine) in which high antibiotic levels are attained.

INDICATIONS AND USAGE

Treatment

Claforan is indicated for the treatment of patients with serious infections caused by susceptible strains of the designated microorganisms in the diseases listed below.

(1) **Lower respiratory tract infections,** including pneumonia, caused by *Streptococcus pneumoniae* (formerly *Diplococcus pneumoniae*), *Streptococcus pyogenes** (Group A streptococci) and other streptococci (excluding enterococci, e.g., *Streptococcus faecalis*), *Staphylococcus aureus* (penicillinase and non-penicillinase producing), *Escherichia coli, Klebsiella* species, *Haemophilus influenzae* (including ampicillin resistant strains), *Haemophilus parainfluenzae, Proteus mirabilis, Serratia marcescens*, Enterobacter* species, indole positive *Proteus* and *Pseudomonas* species (including *P. aeruginosa*).

(2) **Genitourinary infections.** Urinary tract infections caused by *Enterococcus* species, *Staphylococcus epidermidis, Staphylococcus aureus** (penicillinase and non-penicillinase producing), *Citrobacter* species, *Enterobacter* species, *Escherichia coli, Klebsiella* species, *Proteus mirabilis, Proteus vulgaris*, Proteus inconstans* Group B, *Morganella morganii*, Providencia rettgeri**, and *Serratia marcescens,* and *Pseudomonas* species (including *P. aeruginosa*). Also, uncomplicated gonorrhea of single or multiple sites caused by *Neisseria gonorrhoeae,* including penicillinase producing strains.

(3) **Gynecologic infections,** including pelvic inflammatory disease, endometritis and pelvic cellulitis caused by *Staphylococcus epidermidis, Streptococcus* species, *Enterococcus* species, *Enterobacter* species*, *Klebsiella* species*, *Escherichia coli, Proteus mirabilis, Bacteroides* species (including *Bacteroides fragilis**), *Clostridium* species, and anaerobic cocci (including *Peptostreptococcus* species and *Peptococcus* species) and *Fusobacterium* species (including *F. nucleatum**).

(4) **Bacteremia/Septicemia** caused by *Escherichia coli, Klebsiella* species, *Serratia marcescens, Staphylococcus aureus,* and *Streptococcus* species (including *S. pneumoniae*).

(5) **Skin and skin structure infections** caused by *Staphylococcus aureus* (penicillinase and non-penicillinase producing), *Staphylococcus epidermidis, Streptococcus pyogenes* (Group A streptococci) and other streptococci, *Enterococcus* species, *Acinetobacter* species*, *Escherichia coli, Citrobacter* species (including *C. freundii**). *Enterobacter* species, *Klebsiella* species, *Proteus mirabilis, Proteus vulgaris*, Morganella morganii, Providencia rettgeri*, Pseudomonas* species, *Serratia marcescens, Bacteroides* species, and anaerobic cocci (including *Peptostreptococcus** species and *Peptococcus* species).

(6) **Intra-abdominal infections** including peritonitis caused by *Streptococcus* species*, *Escherichia coli, Klebsiella* species, *Bacteroides* species, and anaerobic cocci (including *Peptostreptococcus** species and *Peptococcus** species), *Proteus mirabilis**, and *Clostridium* species* .

(7) **Bone and/or joint infections** caused by *Staphylococcus aureus* (penicillinase and non-penicillinase producing strains), *Streptococcus* species (including *S. pyogenes**), *Pseudomonas* species (including *P. aeruginosa**), and *Proteus mirabilis**.

(8) **Central nervous system infections,** e.g., meningitis and ventriculitis, caused by *Neisseria meningitidis, Haemophilus influenzae, Streptococcus pneumoniae, Klebsiella pneumoniae**, and *Escherichia coli**.

Although many strains of enterococci (e.g., *S. faecalis*) and *Pseudomonas* species are resistant to cefotaxime sodium *in vitro,* Claforan has been used successfully in treating patients with infections caused by susceptible organisms.

Specimens for bacteriologic culture should be obtained prior to therapy in order to isolate and identify causative organisms and to determine their susceptibilities to Claforan. Therapy may be instituted before results of susceptibility studies are known; however, once these results become available, the antibiotic treatment should be adjusted accordingly.

In certain cases of confirmed or suspected gram-positive or gram-negative sepsis or in patients with other serious infections in which the causative organism has not been identified, Claforan may be used concomitantly with an amino-

(*) Efficacy for this organism, in this organ system, has been studied in fewer than 10 infections.

*US Patent 4,152,432 Claforan REG TM ROUSSEL-UCLAF

Continued on next page

Hoechst-Roussel—Cont.

glycoside. The dosage recommended in the labeling of both antibiotics may be given and depends on the severity of the infection and the patient's condition. Renal function should be carefully monitored, especially if higher dosages of the aminoglycosides are to be administered or if therapy is prolonged, because of the potential nephrotoxicity and ototoxicity of aminoglycoside antibiotics. Some β-lactam antibiotics also have a certain degree of nephrotoxicity. Although, to date, this has not been noted when Claforan was given alone, it is possible that nephrotoxicity may be potentiated if Claforan is used concomitantly with an aminoglycoside.

Prevention

The administration of Claforan preoperatively reduces the incidence of certain infections in patients undergoing surgical procedures (e.g. abdominal or vaginal hysterectomy, gastrointestinal and genitourinary tract surgery) that may be classified as contaminated or potentially contaminated.

In patients undergoing cesarean section, intraoperative (after clamping the umbilical cord) and postoperative use of Claforan may also reduce the incidence of certain postoperative infections. See **Dosage and Administration** section.

Effective use for elective surgery depends on the time of administration. To achieve effective tissue levels, Claforan should be given ½ to 1½ hours before surgery. See **Dosage and Administration** section.

For patients undergoing gastrointestinal surgery, preoperative bowel preparation by mechanical cleansing as well as with a non-absorbable antibiotic (e.g., neomycin) is recommended.

If there are signs of infection, specimens for culture should be obtained for identification of the causative organism so that appropriate therapy may be instituted.

CONTRAINDICATIONS

Claforan is contraindicated in patients who have shown hypersensitivity to cefotaxime sodium or the cephalosporin group of antibiotics.

WARNINGS

BEFORE THERAPY WITH CLAFORAN IS INSTITUTED, CAREFUL INQUIRY SHOULD BE MADE TO DETERMINE WHETHER THE PATIENT HAS HAD PREVIOUS HYPERSENSITIVITY REACTIONS TO CEFOTAXIME SODIUM, CEPHALOSPORINS, PENICILLINS, OR OTHER DRUGS. THIS PRODUCT SHOULD BE GIVEN WITH CAUTION TO PATIENTS WITH TYPE 1 HYPERSENSITIVITY REACTIONS TO PENICILLIN. ANTIBIOTICS SHOULD BE ADMINISTERED WITH CAUTION TO ANY PATIENT WHO HAS DEMONSTRATED SOME FORM OF ALLERGY, PARTICULARLY TO DRUGS. IF AN ALLERGIC REACTION TO CLAFORAN OCCURS, DISCONTINUE TREATMENT WITH THE DRUG. SERIOUS HYPERSENSITIVITY REACTIONS MAY REQUIRE EPINEPHRINE AND OTHER EMERGENCY MEASURES.

Pseudomembranous colitis has been reported with the use of cephalosporins (and other broad spectrum antibiotics); therefore, it is important to consider its diagnosis in patients who develop diarrhea in association with antibiotic use.

Treatment with broad spectrum antibiotics alters normal flora of the colon and may permit overgrowth of Clostridia. Studies indicate a toxin produced by *Clostridium difficile* is one primary cause of antibiotic-associated colitis. Cholestyramine and colestipol resins have been shown to bind the toxin *in vitro*.

Mild cases of colitis may respond to drug discontinuance alone.

Moderate to severe cases should be managed with fluid, electrolyte, and protein supplementation as indicated.

When the colitis is not relieved by drug discontinuance or when it is severe, oral vancomycin is the treatment of choice for antibiotic-associated pseudomembranous colitis produced by *C. difficile*. Other causes of colitis should also be considered.

PRECAUTIONS

Claforan® (cefotaxime sodium) should be prescribed with caution in individuals with a history of gastrointestinal disease, particularly colitis.

Claforan has not been shown to be nephrotoxic; however, because high and prolonged serum antibiotic concentrations can occur from usual doses in patients with transient or persistent reduction of urinary output because of renal insufficiency, the total daily dosage should be reduced when Claforan is administered to such patients. Continued dosage should be determined by degree of renal impairment, severity of infection, and susceptibility of the causative organism.

Although there is no clinical evidence supporting the necessity of changing the dosage of cefotaxime sodium in patients with even profound renal dysfunction, it is suggested that, until further data are obtained, the dose of cefotaxime sodium be halved in patients with estimated creatinine clearances of less than 20 mL/min/1.73 m^2.

When only serum creatinine is available, the following formula[2] (based on sex, weight, and age of the patient) may be used to convert this value into creatinine clearance. The serum creatinine should represent a steady state of renal function.

Males $\dfrac{\text{Weight (kg)} \times (140 - \text{age})}{72 \times \text{serum creatinine}}$

Females $0.85 \times$ above value

As with other antibiotics, prolonged use of Claforan may result in overgrowth of nonsusceptible organisms. Repeated evaluation of the patient's condition is essential. If superinfection occurs during therapy, appropriate measures should be taken.

As with other beta-lactam antibiotics, granulocytopenia and, more rarely, agranulocytosis may develop during treatment with Claforan, particularly if given over long periods. For courses of treatment lasting longer than 10 days, blood counts should therefore be monitored.

Drug Interactions: Increased nephrotoxicity has been reported following concomitant administration of cephalosporins and aminoglycoside antibiotics.

Carcinogenesis, Mutagenesis: Long-term studies in animals have not been performed to evaluate carcinogenic potential. Mutagenic tests included a micronucleus and an Ames test. Both tests were negative for mutagenic effects.

Pregnancy (Category B): Reproduction studies have been performed in mice and rats at doses up to 30 times the usual human dose and have revealed no evidence of impaired fertility or harm to the fetus because of cefotaxime sodium. However, there are no well-controlled studies in pregnant women. Because animal reproductive studies are not always predictive of human response, this drug should be used during pregnancy only if clearly needed.

Nonteratogenic Effects: Use of the drug in women of childbearing potential requires that the anticipated benefit be weighed against the possible risks.

In perinatal and postnatal studies with rats, the pups in the group given 1200 mg/kg of Claforan were significantly lighter in weight at birth and remained smaller than pups in the control group during the 21 days of nursing.

Nursing Mothers: Claforan is excreted in human milk in low concentrations. Caution should be exercised when Claforan is administered to a nursing woman.

ADVERSE REACTIONS

Claforan is generally well tolerated. The most common adverse reactions have been local reactions following IM or IV injection. Other adverse reactions have been encountered infrequently.

The most frequent adverse reactions (greater than 1%) are:

Local (4.3%) - Injection site inflammation with IV administration. Pain, induration, and tenderness after IM injection.

Hypersensitivity (2.4%) - Rash, pruritus, fever, and eosinophilia.

Gastrointestinal (1.4%) - Colitis, diarrhea, nausea, and vomiting.

Symptoms of pseudomembranous colitis can appear during or after antibiotic treatment.

Nausea and vomiting have been reported rarely.

Less frequent adverse reactions (less than 1%) are:

Hematologic System - Neutropenia, transient leukopenia, eosinophilia, thrombocytopenia and agranulocytosis have been reported. Some individuals have developed positive direct Coombs Tests during treatment with Claforan and other cephalosporin antibiotics. Rare cases of hemolytic anemia have been reported.

Genitourinary System - Moniliasis, vaginitis.

Central Nervous System - Headache.

Liver - Transient elevations in SGOT, SGPT, serum LDH, and serum alkaline phosphatase levels have been reported.

Kidney - As with some other cephalosporins, transient elevations of BUN have been occasionally observed with Claforan.

DOSAGE AND ADMINISTRATION

Adults

Dosage and route of administration should be determined by susceptibility of the causative organisms, severity of the infection, and the condition of the patient (see table for dosage guideline). Claforan may be administered IM or IV after reconstitution. Premixed Claforan Injection is intended for IV administration after thawing. The maximum daily dosage should not exceed 12 grams.

[See table at bottom left.]

GUIDELINES FOR DOSAGE OF CLAFORAN

Type of Infection	Daily Dose (grams)	Frequency and Route
Gonorrhea	1	1 gram IM (single dose)
Uncomplicated infections	2	1 gram every 12 hours IM or IV
Moderate to severe infections	3–6	1–2 grams every 8 hours IM or IV
Infections commonly needing antibiotics in higher dosage (e.g., septicemia)	6–8	2 grams every 6–8 hours IV
Life-threatening infections	up to 12	2 grams every 4 hours IV

To prevent postoperative infection in contaminated or potentially contaminated surgery, the recommended dose is a single 1 gram IM or IV administered 30 to 90 minutes prior to start of surgery.

Cesarean Section Patients

The first dose of 1 gram is administered intravenously as soon as the umbilical cord is clamped. The second and third doses should be given as 1 gram intravenously or intramuscularly at 6 and 12 hours after the first dose.

Neonates, Infants and Children

The following dosage schedule is recommended:

Neonates (birth to 1 month):

0–1 week of age	50 mg/kg IV q 12 h
1–4 weeks of age	50 mg/kg IV q 8 h

It is not necessary to differentiate between premature and normal-gestational age infants.

Infants and Children (1 month to 12 years): For body weights less than 50 kg, the recommended daily dose is 50 to 180 mg/kg IM or IV of body weight divided into four to six equal doses. The higher dosages should be used for more severe or serious infections, including meningitis. For body weights 50 kg or more, the usual adult dosage should be used; the maximum daily dosage should not exceed 12 grams.

Impaired Renal Function - see **Precautions** section.

NOTE: As with antibiotic therapy in general, administration of Claforan should be continued for a minimum of 48 to 72 hours after the patient defervesces or after evidence of bacterial eradication has been obtained; a minimum of 10 days of treatment is recommended for infections caused by Group A beta-hemolytic streptococci in order to guard against the risk of rheumatic fever or glomerulonephritis; frequent bacteriologic and clinical appraisal is necessary during therapy of chronic urinary tract infection and may be required for several months after therapy has been completed; persistent infections may require treatment of several weeks and doses smaller than those indicated above should not be used.

PREPARATION OF CLAFORAN STERILE

Claforan for IM or IV administration should be reconstituted as follows:

Strength	Diluent (mL)	Withdrawable Volume (mL)	Approximate Concentration (mg/mL)
500 mg vial* (IM)	2	2.2	230
1g vial* (IM)	3	3.4	300
2g vial* (IM)	5	6.0	330
500 mg vial* (IV)	10	10.2	50
1g vial* (IV)	10	10.4	95
2g vial* (IV)	10	11.0	180
1g infusion	50–100	50–100	20–10
2g infusion	50–100	50–100	40–20
10g bottle	47	52.0	200
10g bottle	97	102.0	100

*in conventional vials

Shake to dissolve; inspect for particulate matter and discoloration prior to use. Solutions of Claforan range from light yellow to amber, depending on concentration, diluent used, and length and condition of storage.

For intramuscular use: Reconstitute VIALS with Sterile Water for Injection or Bacteriostatic Water for Injection as described above.

For intravenous use: Reconstitute VIALS with at least 10 mL of Sterile Water for Injection. Reconstitute INFUSION BOTTLES with 50 or 100 mL of 0.9% Sodium Chloride Injection or 5% Dextrose Injection. For other diluents, see **COMPATIBILITY and STABILITY** section.

Pharmacy Bulk Package: Reconstitute with 47 mL of diluent for an approximate concentration of 200 mg/mL or 97 mL of diluent for an approximate concentration of 100 mg/mL. Stock solutions may be further diluted for IV infusion with diluents as listed in **COMPATIBILITY and STABILITY** section.

NOTE: Solutions of Claforan must not be admixed with aminoglycoside solutions. If Claforan and aminoglycosides are to be administered to the same patient, they must be administered separately and not as mixed injection.

A SOLUTION OF 1 G CLAFORAN IN 14 ML OF STERILE WATER FOR INJECTION IS ISOTONIC.

IM Administration: As with all IM preparations, Claforan should be injected well within the body of a relatively large muscle such as the upper outer quadrant of the buttock (i.e.,

gluteus maximus); aspiration is necessary to avoid inadvertent injection into a blood vessel. Individual IM doses of 2 grams may be given if the dose is divided and is administered in different intramuscular sites.

IV Administration: The IV route is preferable for patients with bacteremia, bacterial septicemia, peritonitis, meningitis, or other severe or life-threatening infections, or for patients who may be poor risks because of lowered resistance resulting from such debilitating conditions as malnutrition, trauma, surgery, diabetes, heart failure, or malignancy, particularly if shock is present or impending.

For intermittent IV administration, a solution containing 1 gram or 2 grams in 10 mL of Sterile Water for Injection can be injected over a period of three to five minutes. With an infusion system, it may also be given over a longer period of time through the tubing system by which the patient may be receiving other IV solutions. However, during infusion of the solution containing Claforan, it is advisable to discontinue temporarily the administration of other solutions at the same site.

For the administration of higher doses by continuous IV infusion, a solution of Claforan may be added to IV bottles containing the solutions discussed below.

Preparation of Premixed Claforan Injection in Plastic Container

Premixed Claforan Injection may be used directly after thawing at room temperature. Solutions range from very pale yellow to light amber. After thawing, check for minute leaks by squeezing bag firmly and inspect for particulate matter, discoloration and solution clarity. Discard if leaks are found or seal is not intact. Additives should not be introduced into this solution.

Use sterile equipment.

WARNING: Do not use plastic containers in series connections. Such use could result in air embolism due to residual air being drawn from the primary container before administration of the fluid from the secondary container is complete.

Preparation for administration:

1. Suspend container from eyelet support.
2. Remove plastic protector from outlet port at bottom of container.
3. Attach administration set. Refer to complete directions accompanying set.

After thawing, premixed Claforan Injection, 1 gram and 2 grams in 50 mL plastic containers may be used for continuous or intermittent intravenous infusion.

PREPARATION OF CLAFORAN STERILE IN ADD-VANTAGE® SYSTEM

Claforan Sterile 1 g or 2 g may be reconstituted in 50 mL or 100 mL of 5% Dextrose or 0.9% Sodium Chloride in the ADD-Vantage® diluent container. Refer to enclosed, separate INSTRUCTIONS FOR ADD-VANTAGE® SYSTEM.

COMPATIBILITY AND STABILITY

Solutions of Claforan Sterile reconstituted as described above (**Preparation of Claforan Sterile**) maintain satisfactory potency for 24 hours at room temperature (at or below 22°C), 10 days under refrigeration (at or below 5°C), and for at least 13 weeks frozen. Solutions may be stored in disposable glass or plastic syringes for 24 hours at room temperature (at or below 22°C), 5 days under refrigeration (at or below 5°C), and 13 weeks frozen.

Reconstituted solutions may be further diluted up to 1000 mL with the following solutions and maintain satisfactory potency for 24 hours at room temperature (at or below 22°C), and at least 5 days under refrigeration (at or below 5°C); 0.9% Sodium Chloride Injection; 5 or 10% Dextrose Injection; 5% Dextrose and 0.9% Sodium Chloride Injection; 5% Dextrose and 0.45% Sodium Chloride Injection; 5% Dextrose and 0.2% Sodium Chloride Injection; Lactated Ringer's Solution; Sodium Lactate Injection (M/6); 10% Invert Sugar Injection, 8.5% TRAVASOL® (Amino Acid) Injection without Electrolytes.

Solutions of Claforan Sterile reconstituted in 0.9% Sodium Chloride Injection or 5% Dextrose Injection in Viaflex® plastic containers maintain satisfactory potency for 24 hours at room temperature (at or below 22°C), 5 days under refrigeration (at or below 5°C) and 13 weeks frozen. Solutions of Claforan Sterile reconstituted in 0.9% Sodium Chloride Injection or 5% Dextrose Injection in the ADD-Vantage® flexible containers maintain satisfactory potency for 24 hours at room temperature (at or below 22°C). DO NOT FREEZE.

NOTE: Claforan solutions exhibit maximum stability in the pH 5–7 range. Solutions of Claforan should not be prepared with diluents having a pH above 7.5, such as Sodium Bicarbonate Injection.

Claforan supplied as premixed, frozen injection is stable for the expiration dating period as indicated on the label. Thawed solutions of premixed Claforan Injection in plastic containers are stable for 24 hours at room temperature (at or below 22°C) or for 10 days under refrigeration (at or below 5°C).

Frozen samples should not be heated but should be thawed at room temperature before use. After the periods mentioned above, any unused solutions or frozen material should be discarded. DO NOT REFREEZE.

HOW SUPPLIED

Sterile Claforan is a dry off-white to pale yellow crystalline powder supplied in vials and bottles containing cefotaxime sodium as follows:

500 mg cefotaxime (free acid equivalent) in vials in packages of 10 (NDC 0039-0017-10).

1 g cefotaxime (free acid equivalent) in vials in packages of 10 (NDC 0039-0018-10), packages of 25 (NDC 0039-0018-25), packages of 50 (NDC 0039-0018-50); infusion bottles in packages of 10 (NDC 0039-0018-11)

2 g cefotaxime (free acid equivalent) in vials in packages of 10 (NDC 0039-0019-10), in packages of 25 (NDC 0039-0019-25), in packages of 50 (NDC 0039-0019-50); infusion bottles in packages of 10 (NDC 0039-0019-11)

10 g cefotaxime (free acid equivalent) in bottles (NDC 0039-0020-01)

1 g cefotaxime (free acid equivalent) in ADD-Vantage® System vials in packages of 25 (NDC 0039-0023-25) and 50 (NDC 0039-0023-50)

2 g cefotaxime (free acid equivalent) in ADD-Vantage® System vials in packages of 25 (NDC 0039-0024-25) and 50 (NDC 0039-0024-50).

ADD-Vantage® System diluents (5% Dextrose or 0.9% Sodium Chloride) are available from Abbott Laboratories.

NOTE: Claforan in the dry state should be stored below 30°C. The dry material as well as solutions tend to darken depending on storage conditions and should be protected from elevated temperatures and excessive light.

Premixed Claforan injection is supplied as a frozen, sterile, nonpyrogenic solution in 50 mL single dose plastic containers as follows:

1 g cefotaxime (free acid equivalent) in 5% dextrose solution in packages of 24 (NDC 0039-0043-50) 2B3518

2 g cefotaxime (free acid equivalent) in 5% dextrose solution in packages of 24 (NDC 0039-0044-50) 2B3519

NOTE: Premixed Claforan Injection in the frozen state should not be stored above −20°C.

Claforan injection supplied as a frozen, sterile, nonpyrogenic solution in plastic containers is manufactured for Hoechst-Roussel Pharmaceuticals Inc., by Baxter Healthcare Corporation.

References:

1) Bauer, A.W.; Kirby, W.M.M.; Sherris, J.C.; and Turck, M.: Antibiotic Susceptibility Testing by a Standardized Single Disk Method, Am. J. Clin. Pathol., 45:493, 1966; Standardized Disc Susceptibility Test, Federal Register, 39:19182-4, 1974. National Committee for Clinical Laboratory Standards, Approved Standard: ASM-2, Performance Standards for Antimicrobial Disc Susceptibility Tests, July, 1975.
2) Cockcroft, D.W. and Gault, M.H.: Prediction of Creatinine Clearance from Serum Creatinine. Nephron 16:31-41, 1976.

VIAFLEX REG TM BAXTER INTERNATIONAL INC.
ADD-Vantage REG TM ABBOTT LABORATORIES
Patent Pending
717890-10/90

DIAβETA® ℞
(glyburide)*
Tablets 1.25, 2.5 and 5.0 mg

DESCRIPTION

Diaβeta® (glyburide) is an oral blood-glucose-lowering drug of the sulfonylurea class. It is a white, crystalline compound, formulated as tablets of 1.25 mg, 2.5 mg, and 5 mg strengths for oral administration. Diaβeta® tablets contain the active ingredient glyburide and the following inactive ingredients: dibasic calcium phosphate USP, magnesium stearate NF, microcrystalline cellulose NF, sodium alginate NF, talc USP. Diaβeta® 2.5 mg tablets also contain FD&C Red #40. Diaβeta® 5 mg tablets also contain D&C Yellow #10 and FD&C Blue #1.

Chemically, Diaβeta® (glyburide) is identified as 1-[[p-[2-(5-chloro-O-anisamido)ethyl] phenyl] -sulfonyl] -3-cyclohexylurea. The structural formula is:

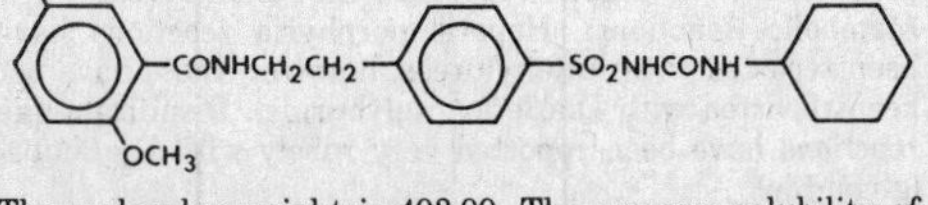

The molecular weight is 493.99. The aqueous solubility of Diaβeta® (glyburide) increases with pH as a result of salt formation.

CLINICAL PHARMACOLOGY

Diaβeta® (glyburide) appears to lower the blood glucose acutely by stimulating the release of insulin from the pancreas, an effect dependent upon functioning beta cells in the pancreatic islets. The mechanism by which Diaβeta® (glyburide) lowers blood glucose during long-term administration has not been clearly established.

With chronic administration in Type II diabetic patients, the blood glucose lowering effect persists despite a gradual decline in the insulin secretory response to the drug. Extrapancreatic effects may play a part in the mechanism of action of oral sulfonylurea hypoglycemic drugs.

In addition to its blood glucose lowering actions, Diaβeta® (glyburide) produces a mild diuresis by enhancement of renal free water clearance. Clinical experience to date indicates an extremely low incidence of disulfiram-like reactions in patients while taking Diaβeta® (glyburide).

Pharmacokinetics

Single-dose studies with Diaβeta® (glyburide) in normal subjects demonstrate significant absorption within one hour, peak drug levels at about four hours, and low but detectable levels at twenty-four hours. Mean serum levels of glyburide, as reflected by areas under the serum concentration-time curve, increase in proportion to corresponding increases in dose. Multiple-dose studies with Diaβeta® (glyburide) in diabetic patients demonstrate drug level concentration-time curves similar to single-dose studies, indicating no build-up of drug in tissue depots. The decrease of glyburide in the serum of normal healthy individuals is biphasic, the terminal half-life being about 10 hours. In single-dose studies in fasting normal subjects, the degree and duration of blood glucose lowering is proportional to the dose administered and to the area under the drug level concentration-time curve. The blood glucose lowering effect persists for 24 hours following single morning doses in non-fasting diabetic patients. Under conditions of repeated administration in diabetic patients, however, there is no reliable correlation between blood drug levels and fasting blood glucose levels. A one-year study of diabetic patients treated with Diaβeta® (glyburide) showed no reliable correlation between administered dose and serum drug level.

The major metabolite of Diaβeta® (glyburide) is the 4-trans-hydroxy derivative. A second metabolite, the 3-cis-hydroxy derivative, also occurs. These metabolites contribute no significant hypoglycemic action since they are only weakly active ($\frac{1}{400}$th and $\frac{1}{40}$th, respectively, as glyburide) in rabbits.

Diaβeta® (glyburide) is excreted as metabolites in the bile and urine, approximately 50% by each route. This dual excretory pathway is qualitatively different from that of other sulfonylureas, which are excreted primarily in the urine.

Sulfonylurea drugs are extensively bound to serum proteins. Displacement from protein binding sites by other drugs may lead to enhanced hypoglycemic action. *In vitro*, the protein binding exhibited by Diaβeta® (glyburide) is predominantly non-ionic, whereas that of other sulfonylureas (chlorpropamide, tolbutamide, tolazamide) is predominantly ionic. Acidic drugs such as phenylbutazone, warfarin, and salicylates displace the ionic-binding sulfonylureas from serum proteins to a far greater extent than the non-ionic binding Diaβeta® (glyburide). It has not been shown that this difference in protein binding will result in fewer drug-drug interactions with Diaβeta® (glyburide) in clinical use.

INDICATIONS AND USAGE

Diaβeta® (glyburide) is indicated as an adjunct to diet to lower the blood glucose in patients with non-insulin-dependent diabetes mellitus (Type II) whose hyperglycemia cannot be controlled by diet alone.

In initiating treatment for non-insulin-dependent diabetes, diet should be emphasized as the primary form of treatment. Caloric restriction and weight loss are essential in the obese diabetic patient. Proper dietary management alone may be effective in controlling the blood glucose and symptoms of hyperglycemia. The importance of regular physical activity should also be stressed, and cardiovascular risk factors should be identified and corrective measures taken where possible.

If this treatment program fails to reduce symptoms and/or blood glucose, the use of an oral sulfonylurea or insulin should be considered. Use of Diaβeta® (glyburide) must be viewed by both the physician and patient as a treatment in addition to diet, and not as a substitute for diet or as a convenient mechanism for avoiding dietary restraint. Furthermore, loss of blood glucose control on diet alone may be transient, thus requiring only short-term administration of Diaβeta® (glyburide).

During maintenance programs, Diaβeta® (glyburide) should be discontinued if satisfactory lowering of blood glucose is no longer achieved. Judgments should be based on regular clinical and laboratory evaluations.

In considering the use of Diaβeta® (glyburide) in asymptomatic patients, it should be recognized that controlling the blood glucose in non-insulin dependent diabetes has not been definitely established to be effective in preventing the long-term cardiovascular or neural complications of diabetes.

*U.S. Patents 3,454,635 and 3,507,954

Continued on next page

Hoechst-Roussel—Cont.

CONTRAINDICATIONS

Diaβeta® (glyburide) is contraindicated in patients with:
1. Known hypersensitivity to the drug.
2. Diabetic ketoacidosis, with or without coma. This condition should be treated with insulin.

WARNINGS:

SPECIAL WARNING ON INCREASED RISK OF CARDIOVASCULAR MORTALITY

The administration of oral hypoglycemic drugs has been reported to be associated with increased cardiovascular mortality as compared to treatment with diet alone or diet plus insulin. This warning is based on the study conducted by the University Group Diabetes Program (UGDP), a long-term prospective clinical trial designed to evaluate the effectiveness of glucose-lowering drugs in preventing or delaying vascular complications in patients with non-insulin-dependent diabetes. The study involved 823 patients who were randomly assigned to one of four treatment groups (Diabetes, 19 (supp. 2): 747-830, 1970).

UGDP reported that patients treated for 5 to 8 years with diet plus a fixed dose of tolbutamide (1.5 grams per day) had a rate of cardiovascular mortality approximately 2½ times that of patients treated with diet alone. A significant increase in total mortality was not observed, but the use of tolbutamide was discontinued based on the increase in cardiovascular mortality, thus limiting the opportunity for the study to show an increase in overall mortality. Despite controversy regarding the interpretation of these results, the findings of the UGDP study provide an adequate basis for this warning. The patient should be informed of the potential risks and advantages of Diaβeta® (glyburide) and of alternative modes of therapy.

Although only one drug in the sulfonylurea class (tolbutamide) was included in this study, it is prudent from a safety standpoint to consider that this warning may also apply to other oral hypoglycemic drugs in this class, in view of their close similarities in mode of action and chemical structure.

PRECAUTIONS

General

Hypoglycemia: All sulfonylurea drugs are capable of producing severe hypoglycemia. Proper patient selection, dosage, and instructions are important to avoid hypoglycemic episodes. Renal or hepatic insufficiency may cause elevated blood levels of Diaβeta® (glyburide) and the latter may also diminish gluconeogenic capacity, both of which increase the risk of serious hypoglycemic reactions. Elderly, debilitated or malnourished patients, and those with adrenal or pituitary insufficiency are particularly susceptible to the hypoglycemic action of glucose-lowering drugs. Hypoglycemia may be difficult to recognize in the elderly, and in people who are taking beta-adrenergic blocking drugs. Hypoglycemia is more likely to occur when caloric intake is deficient, after severe or prolonged exercise, when alcohol is ingested, or when more than one glucose-lowering drug is used.

Loss of control of blood glucose: When a patient stabilized on any diabetic regimen is exposed to stress such as fever, trauma, infection, or surgery, a loss of control may occur. At such times, it may be necessary to discontinue Diaβeta® (glyburide) and administer insulin.

The effectiveness of any oral hypoglycemic drug, including Diaβeta® (glyburide), in lowering blood glucose to a desired level decreases in many patients over a period of time, which may be due to progression of the severity of the diabetes or to diminished responsiveness to the drug. This phenomenon is known as secondary failure, to distinguish it from primary failure in which the drug is ineffective in an individual patient when first given.

Information for Patients

Patients should be informed of the potential risks and advantages of Diaβeta® (glyburide) and of alternative modes of therapy. They should also be informed about the importance of adherence to dietary instructions, of a regular exercise program, and of regular testing of urine and/or blood glucose.

The risks of hypoglycemia, its symptoms and treatment, and conditions that predispose to its development should be explained to patients and responsible family members. Primary and secondary failure should also be explained.

Laboratory Tests

Blood and urine glucose should be monitored periodically. Measurement of glycosylated hemoglobin may be useful.

Drug Interactions

The hypoglycemic action of sulfonylureas may be potentiated by certain drugs including nonsteroidal anti-inflammatory agents and other drugs that are highly protein bound, salicylates, sulfonamides, chloramphenicol, probenecid, coumarins, monoamine oxidase inhibitors, and beta adrenergic blocking agents. When such drugs are administered to a patient receiving Diaβeta® (glyburide), the patient should be observed closely for hypoglycemia. When such drugs are withdrawn from a patient receiving Diaβeta® (glyburide), the patient should be observed closely for loss of control.

Certain drugs tend to produce hyperglycemia and may lead to loss of control. These drugs include the thiazides and other diuretics, corticosteroids, phenothiazines, thyroid products, estrogens, oral contraceptives, phenytoin, nicotinic acid, sympathomimetics, calcium channel blocking drugs, and isoniazid. When such drugs are administered to a patient receiving Diaβeta® (glyburide), the patient should be closely observed for loss of control. When such drugs are withdrawn from a patient receiving Diaβeta® (glyburide), the patient should be observed closely for hypoglycemia.

A potential interaction between oral miconazole and oral hypoglycemic agents leading to severe hypoglycemia has been reported. Whether this interaction also occurs with the intravenous, topical or vaginal preparations of miconazole is not known.

Carcinogenesis, Mutagenesis, and Impairment of Fertility

Diaβeta® (glyburide) is non-mutagenic when studied in the Salmonella microsome test (Ames test) and in the DNA damage/alkaline elution assay. Studies in rats at doses up to 300 mg/kg/day for 18 months showed no carcinogenic effects.

Pregnancy

Teratogenic Effects: Pregnancy Category B

Reproduction studies have been performed in rats and rabbits at doses up to 500 times the human dose and have revealed no evidence of impaired fertility or harm to the fetus due to Diaβeta®(glyburide). There are, however, no adequate and well controlled studies in pregnant women. Because animal reproduction studies are not always predictive of human response, this drug should be used during pregnancy only if clearly needed.

Because recent information suggests that abnormal blood glucose levels during pregnancy are associated with a higher incidence of congenital abnormalities, many experts recommend that insulin be used during pregnancy to maintain blood glucose levels as close to normal as possible.

Nonteratogenic Effects

Prolonged severe hypoglycemia (4 to 10 days) has been reported in neonates born to mothers who were receiving a sulfonylurea drug at the time of delivery. This had been reported more frequently with the use of agents with prolonged half-lives. If Diaβeta® (glyburide) is used during pregnancy, it should be discontinued at least two weeks before the expected delivery date.

Nursing Mothers

Although it is not known whether Diaβeta® (glyburide) is excreted in human milk, some sulfonylureas are known to be excreted in human milk. Because the potential for hypoglycemia in nursing infants may exist, a decision should be made whether to discontinue nursing or to discontinue administering the drug, taking into account the importance of the drug to the mother. If Diaβeta® (glyburide) is discontinued and if diet alone is inadequate for controlling blood glucose, insulin therapy should be considered.

Pediatric Use: Safety and effectiveness in children have not been established.

ADVERSE REACTIONS

Hypoglycemia: See **Precautions** and **Overdosage** Sections.

Gastrointestinal Reactions: Cholestatic jaundice and hepatitis may occur rarely; Diaβeta® (glyburide) should be discontinued if this occurs. Liver function abnormalities, including isolated transaminase elevations, have been reported. Gastrointestinal disturbances, e.g., nausea, epigastric fullness, and heartburn, are the most common reactions and occur in 1.8% of treated patients. They tend to be dose-related and may disappear when dosage is reduced.

Dermatologic Reactions: Allergic skin reactions, e.g., pruritus, erythema, urticaria, and morbilliform or maculopapular eruptions, occur in 1.5% of treated patients. These may be transient and may disappear despite continued use of Diaβeta® (glyburide); if skin reactions persist, the drug should be discontinued.

Porphyria cutanea tarda and photosensitivity reactions have been reported with sulfonylureas.

Hematologic Reactions: Leukopenia, agranulocytosis, thrombocytopenia, hemolytic anemia, aplastic anemia, and pancytopenia have been reported with sulfonylureas.

Metabolic Reactions: Hepatic porphyria reactions have been reported with sulfonylureas; however, these have not been reported with Diaβeta® (glyburide). Disulfiram-like reactions have been reported very rarely with Diaβeta® (glyburide).

Cases of hyponatremia have been reported with glyburide and all other sulfonylureas, most often in patients who are on other medications or have medical conditions known to cause hyponatremia or increase release of antidiuretic hormone. The syndrome of inappropriate antidiuretic hormone (SIADH) secretion has been reported with certain other sulfonylureas, and it has been suggested that these sulfonylureas may augment the peripheral (antidiuretic) action of ADH and/or increase release of ADH.

OVERDOSAGE

Overdosage of sulfonylureas, including Diaβeta® (glyburide), can produce hypoglycemia. Mild hypoglycemic symptoms without loss of consciousness or neurologic findings should be treated aggressively with oral glucose and adjustments in drug dosage and/or meal patterns. Close monitoring should continue until the physician is assured that the patient is out of danger. Severe hypoglycemic reactions with coma, seizure, or other neurological impairment occur infrequently, but constitute medical emergencies requiring immediate hospitalization. If hypoglycemic coma is diagnosed or suspected, the patient should be given a rapid intravenous injection of concentrated (50%) glucose solution. This should be followed by a continuous infusion of a more dilute (10%) glucose solution at a rate that will maintain the blood glucose at a level above 100 mg/dL. Patients should be closely monitored for a minimum of 24 to 48 hours, since hypoglycemia may recur after apparent clinical recovery.

DOSAGE AND ADMINISTRATION

There is no fixed dosage regimen for the management of diabetes mellitus with Diaβeta® (glyburide) or any other hypoglycemic agent. In addition to the usual monitoring of urinary glucose, the patient's blood glucose must also be monitored periodically to determine the minimum effective dose for the patient; to detect primary failure, i.e., inadequate lowering of blood glucose at the maximum recommended dose of medication; and to detect secondary failure, i.e., loss of adequate blood glucose lowering response after an initial period of effectiveness. Glycosylated hemoglobin levels may also be of value in monitoring the patient's response to therapy.

Short-term administration of Diaβeta® (glyburide) may be sufficient during periods of transient loss of control in patients usually controlled well on diet.

1. **Usual Starting Dose**

   The usual starting dose of Diaβeta® (glyburide) as initial therapy is 2.5–5 mg daily, administered with breakfast or the first main meal. Those patients who may be more sensitive to hypoglycemic drugs should be started at 1.25 mg daily. (See **Precautions** Section for patients at increased risk). Failure to follow an appropriate dosage regimen may precipitate hypoglycemia. Patients who do not adhere to their prescribed dietary and drug regimen are more prone to exhibit unsatisfactory response to therapy.

   Transfer of patients from other oral antidiabetic regimens to Diaβeta® (glyburide) should be done conservatively and the initial daily dose should be 2.5 to 5 mg. When transferring patients from oral hypoglycemic agents other than chlorpropamide to Diaβeta® (glyburide), no transition period and no initial or priming dose is necessary. When transferring patients from chlorpropamide, particular care should be exercised during the first two weeks because the prolonged retention of chlorpropamide in the body and subsequent overlapping drug effects may provoke hypoglycemia.

   Some Type II diabetic patients being treated with insulin may respond satisfactorily to Diaβeta® (glyburide). If the insulin dose is less than 20 units daily, substitution of Diaβeta® (glyburide) 2.5 to 5 mg as a single daily dose may be tried. If the insulin dose is between 20 and 40 units daily, the patient may be placed directly on Diaβeta® (glyburide) 5 mg daily as a single dose. If the insulin dose is more than 40 units daily, a transition period is required for conversion to Diaβeta® (glyburide) In these patients, insulin dosage is decreased by 50% and Diaβeta® (glyburide) 5 mg daily is started. Please refer to Usual Maintenance Dose for further explanation.

2. **Usual Maintenance Dose**

   The usual maintenance dose is in the range of 1.25 to 20 mg daily, which may be given as a single dose or in divided doses (See Dosage Interval Section). Dosage increases should be made in increments of no more than 2.5 mg at weekly intervals based upon the patient's blood glucose response.

   No exact dosage relationship exists between Diaβeta® (glyburide) and the other oral hypoglycemic agents. Although patients may be transferred from the maximum dose of other sulfonylureas, the maximum starting dose of 5 mg of Diaβeta® (glyburide) should be observed. A maintenance dose of 5 mg Diaβeta® (glyburide) provides approximately the same degree of blood glucose control as 250 to 375 mg chlorpropamide, 250 to 375 mg tolazamide, 500 to 750 mg acetohexamide, or 1000 to 1500 mg tolbutamide.

   When transferring patients receiving more than 40 units of insulin daily, they may be started on a daily dose of Diaβeta® (glyburide) 5 mg concomitantly with a 50% reduction in insulin dose. Progressive withdrawal of insulin and increase of Diaβeta® (glyburide) in increments of 1.25 to 2.5 mg every 2 to 10 days is then carried out. During this conversion period when both insulin and Diaβeta® (glyburide) are being used, hypoglycemia may rarely occur. During insulin withdrawal, patients should test their urine for glucose and acetone at least three times daily

and report results to their physician. The appearance of persistent acetonuria with glycosuria indicates that the patient is a Type I diabetic who requires insulin therapy.

3. **Maximum Dose**
Daily doses of more than 20 mg are not recommended.

4. **Dosage Interval**
Once-a-day therapy is usually satisfactory, based upon usual meal patterns and a 10 hour half-life of Diaβeta® (glyburide). Some patients, particularly those receiving more than 10 mg daily, may have a more satisfactory response with twice-a-day dosage.

In elderly patients, debilitated or malnourished patients, and patients with impaired renal or hepatic function, the initial and maintenance dosing should be conservative to avoid hypoglycemic reactions. (See **Precautions** Section.)

HOW SUPPLIED

Diaβeta® (glyburide) tablets are supplied as white, oblong, monogrammed, scored tablets of 1.25 mg in bottles of 50 (NDC 0039-0050-05); pink, oblong, monogrammed, scored tablets of 2.5 mg in bottles of 30 (NDC 0039-0051-03); bottles of 60 (NDC 0039-0051-06); bottles of 100 (NDC 0039-0051-10, NSN 6505-01-187-6586); bottles of 500 (NDC 0039-0051-50; NSN 6505-01-313-3707); and in Unit Dose Cartons of 100 (NDC 0039-0051-11, NSN 6505-01-204-5416); and light green, oblong monogrammed, scored tablets of 5 mg in bottles of 30 (NDC 0039-0052-03, NSN 6505-01-259-1553); bottles of 60 (NDC 0039-0052-06, NSN 6505-01-258-7132); bottles of 100 (NDC 0039-0052-10, NSN 6505-01-187-6585); bottles of 500 (NDC 0039-0052-50, NSN 6505-01-190-4388), bottles of 1000 (NDC 0039-0052-70, NSN 6505-01-277-2804); and in Unit Dose Cartons of 100 (NDC 0039-0052-11, NSN 6505-01-203-6280).

Store at controlled room temperature (59°–86°F).
Dispense in well-closed containers with safety closures.
Caution: Federal law prohibits dispensing without a prescription.

Diaβeta REG TM HRPI

751010-2/90

Made in U.S.A.

Shown in Product Identification Section, page 411

LASIX® ℞

[*la' siks*]
(furosemide)
Oral Solution
Tablets/Injection
Diuretic

WARNING

Lasix (furosemide) is a potent diuretic which, if given in excessive amounts, can lead to a profound diuresis with water and electrolyte depletion. Therefore, careful medical supervision is required, and dose and dose schedule have to be adjusted to the individual patient's needs. (See under "DOSAGE AND ADMINISTRATION.")

DESCRIPTION

Lasix (furosemide) is a diuretic which is an anthranilic acid derivative. Chemically, it is 4-chloro-N-furfuryl-5-sulfamoylanthranilic acid.

Lasix® (furosemide) tablets for oral administration contain furosemide as the active ingredient and the following inactive ingredients: lactose USP, magnesium stearate NF, starch NF and talc USP.

Lasix® (furosemide) Injection is composed of 4-chloro-N-furfuryl-5-sulfamoylanthranilic acid, sodium chloride for isotonicity, sodium hydroxide to adjust pH, and in the single use vials and 10 mL syringe, 0.9% benzyl alcohol as preservative. Lasix® (furosemide) injection 10 mg/mL is a sterile, non-pyrogenic solution in ampules and disposable syringes for intravenous and intramuscular injection.

Lasix® (furosemide) Oral Solution contains furosemide as the active ingredient and the following inactive ingredients: alcohol USP 11.5%, D&C Yellow #10, FD&C Yellow #6 as color additives, flavors, glycerin USP, parabens NF, purified water USP, sorbitol NF; sodium hydroxide NF added to adjust pH. Lasix® (furosemide) Oral Solution 10 mg/mL is an orange flavored liquid for oral administration. Furosemide is a white to off-white odorless crystalline powder. It is practically insoluble in water, sparingly soluble in alcohol, freely soluble in dilute alkali solutions and insoluble in dilute acids.

The structural formula is as follows:

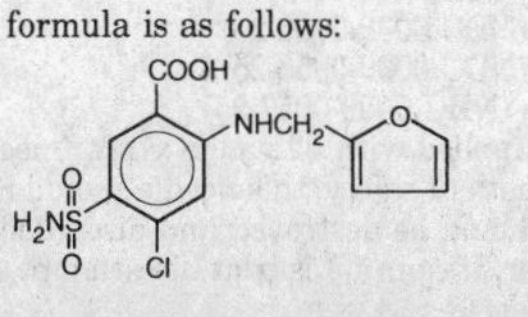

CLINICAL PHARMACOLOGY

Investigations into the mode of action of Lasix (furosemide) have utilized micropuncture studies in rats, stop flow experiments in dogs, and various clearance studies in both humans and experimental animals. It has been demonstrated that Lasix (furosemide) inhibits primarily the absorption of sodium and chloride not only in the proximal and distal tubules but also in the loop of Henle. The high degree of efficacy is largely due to this unique site of action. The action on the distal tubule is independent of any inhibitory effect on carbonic anhydrase and aldosterone.

Recent evidence suggests that furosemide glucuronide is the only or at least the major bio-transformation product of furosemide in man. Furosemide is extensively bound to plasma proteins, mainly to albumin. Plasma concentrations ranging from 1 to 400 ug/mL are 91 to 99% bound in healthy individuals. The unbound fraction averages 2.3 to 4.1% at therapeutic concentrations.

The onset of diuresis following oral administration is within 1 hour. The peak effect occurs within the first or second hour. The duration of diuretic effect is 6 to 8 hours.

The onset of diuresis following intravenous administration is within 5 minutes and somewhat later after intramuscular administration. The peak effect occurs within the first half hour. The duration of diuretic effect is approximately 2 hours.

In fasted normal men, the mean bioavailability of furosemide from Lasix® (furosemide) Tablets and Lasix® (furosemide) Oral Solution is 64% and 60%, respectively, of that from an intravenous injection of the drug. Although furosemide is more rapidly absorbed from the oral solution (50 minutes) than from the tablet (87 minutes), peak plasma levels and area under the plasma concentration-time curves do not differ significantly. Peak plasma concentrations increase with increasing dose but times-to-peak do not differ among doses. The terminal half-life of furosemide is approximately 2 hours.

Significantly more furosemide is excreted in urine following the IV injection than after the tablet or oral solution. There are no significant differences between the two oral formulations in the amount of unchanged drug excreted in urine.

INDICATIONS AND USAGE

Edema—Lasix (furosemide) is indicated in adults, infants, and children for the treatment of edema associated with congestive heart failure, cirrhosis of the liver, and renal disease, including the nephrotic syndrome. Lasix (furosemide) is particularly useful when an agent with greater diuretic potential is desired.

Parenteral therapy should be reserved for patients unable to take oral medication or for patients in emergency clinical situations.

Lasix (furosemide) Injection is also indicated as adjunctive therapy in acute pulmonary edema. The intravenous administration of Lasix (furosemide) is indicated when a rapid onset of diuresis is desired, eg, in acute pulmonary edema.

If gastrointestinal absorption is impaired or oral medication is not practical for any reason, Lasix (furosemide) is indicated by the intravenous or intramuscular route. Parenteral use should be replaced with oral Lasix (furosemide) as soon as practical.

Hypertension—Oral Lasix (furosemide) may be used in adults for the treatment of hypertension alone or in combination with other antihypertensive agents. Hypertensive patients who cannot be adequately controlled with thiazides will probably also not be adequately controlled with Lasix (furosemide) alone.

CONTRAINDICATIONS

Lasix® is contraindicated in patients with anuria and in patients with a history of hypersensitivity to furosemide.

WARNINGS

In patients with hepatic cirrhosis and ascites, Lasix® (furosemide) therapy is best initiated in the hospital. In hepatic coma and in states of electroyte depletion therapy should not be instituted until the basic condition is improved. Sudden alterations of fluid and electrolyte balance in patients with cirrhosis may precipitate hepatic coma; therefore, strict observation is necessary during the period of diuresis. Supplemental potassium chloride and, if required, an aldosterone antagonist are helpful in preventing hypokalemia and metabolic alkalosis.

If increasing azotemia and oliguria occur during treatment of severe progressive renal disease, Lasix® (furosemide) should be discontinued.

Cases of tinnitus and reversible or irreversible hearing impairment have been reported. Usually, reports indicate that Lasix® (furosemide) ototoxicity is associated with rapid injection, severe renal impairment, doses exceeding several times the usual recommended dose, or concomitant therapy with aminoglycoside antibiotics, ethacrynic acid, or other ototoxic drugs. If the physician elects to use high dose parenteral therapy, controlled intravenous infusion is advisable (for adults, an infusion rate not exceeding 4 mg Lasix® (furosemide) per minute has been used).

Pediatric Use

In premature neonates with respiratory distress syndrome, diuretic treatment with furosemide injection in the first few weeks of life may increase the risk of persistent patent ductus arteriosus (PDA), possibly through a prostaglandin E-mediated process.

PRECAUTIONS

General

Excessive diuresis may cause dehydration and blood volume reduction with circulatory collapse and possible vascular thrombosis and embolism, particularly in elderly patients. As with any effective diuretic, electrolyte depletion may occur during Lasix® (furosemide) therapy, especially in patients receiving higher doses and restricted salt intake. Hypokalemia may develop with Lasix® (furosemide), especially with brisk diuresis, inadequate oral electrolyte intake, when cirrhosis is present, or during concomitant use of corticosteroids or ACTH. Digitalis therapy may exaggerate metabolic effects of hypokalemia, especially myocardial effects.

All patients receiving Lasix® (furosemide) therapy should be observed for these signs or symptoms of fluid or electrolyte imbalance (hyponatremia, hypochloremic alkalosis, hypokalemia, hypomagnesemia or hypocalcemia); dryness of mouth, thirst, weakness, lethargy, drowsiness, restlessness, muscle pains or cramps, muscular fatigue, hypotension, oliguria, tachycardia, arrhythmia, or gastrointestinal disturbances such as nausea and vomiting.

Increases in blood glucose and alterations in glucose tolerance tests (with abnormalities of the fasting and 2-hour postprandial sugar) have been observed, and rarely, precipitation of diabetes mellitus has been reported.

Asymptomatic hyperuricemia can occur and gout may rarely be precipitated.

The sorbitol present in the vehicle may cause diarrhea (especially in children) when higher doses of Lasix® (furosemide) Oral Solution are given.

Patients allergic to sulfonamides may also be allergic to Lasix® (furosemide).

The possibility exists of exacerbation or activation of systemic lupus erythematosus.

As with many other drugs, patients should be observed regularly for the possible occurrence of blood dyscrasias, liver or kidney damage, or other idiosyncratic reactions.

Information for Patients

Patients receiving Lasix® (furosemide) should be advised that they may experience symptoms from excessive fluid and/or electrolyte losses. The postural hypotension that sometimes occurs can usually be managed by getting up slowly. Potassium supplements and/or dietary measures may be needed to control or avoid hypokalemia.

Patients with diabetes mellitus should be told that furosemide may increase blood glucose levels and thereby affect urine glucose tests. The skin of some patients may be more sensitive to the effects of sunlight while taking furosemide.

Hypertensive patients should avoid medications that may increase blood pressure, including over-the-counter products for appetite suppression and cold symptoms.

Laboratory Tests

Serum electrolytes (particularly potassium), CO_2, creatinine and BUN should be determined frequently during the first few months of Lasix® (furosemide) therapy and periodically thereafter.

Serum and urine electrolyte determinations are particularly important when the patient is vomiting profusely or receiving parenteral fluids. Abnormalities should be corrected or the drug temporarily withdrawn. Other medications may also influence serum electrolytes.

Reversible elevations of BUN may occur and are associated with dehydration, which should be avoided, particularly in patients with renal insufficiency.

Urine and blood glucose should be checked periodically in diabetics receiving Lasix® (furosemide), even in those suspected of latent diabetes.

Lasix® (furosemide) may lower serum levels of calcium (rarely cases of tetany have been reported) and magnesium. Accordingly, serum calcium levels should be determined periodically.

Drug Interactions

Lasix® (furosemide) may increase the ototoxic potential of aminoglycoside antibiotics, especially in the presence of impaired renal function. Except in life-threatening situations, avoid this combination.

Lasix® (furosemide) should not be used concomitantly with ethacrynic acid because of the possibility of ototoxicity.

Patients receiving high doses of salicylates concomitantly with Lasix® (furosemide), as in rheumatic disease, may experience salicylate toxicity at lower doses because of competative renal excretory sites.

Lasix® (furosemide) has a tendency to antagonize the skeletal muscle relaxing effect of tubocurarine and may potentiate the action of succinylcholine.

Continued on next page

Hoechst-Roussel—Cont.

Lithium generally should not be given with diuretics because they reduce lithium's renal clearance and add a high risk of lithium toxicity.
Lasix® (furosemide) may add to or potentiate the therapeutic effect of other antihypertensive drugs. Potentiation occurs with ganglionic or peripheral adrenergic blocking drugs.
Lasix® (furosemide) may decrease arterial responsiveness to norepinephrine. However, norepinephrine may still be used effectively.
One study in six subjects demonstrated that the combination of furosemide and acetylsalicylic acid temporarily reduced creatinine clearance in patients with chronic renal insufficiency. There are case reports of patients who developed increased BUN, serum creatinine and serum potassium levels, and weight gain when furosemide was used in conjunction with NSAIDs.
Literature reports indicate that coadministration of indomethacin may reduce the natriuretic and antihypertensive effects of Lasix® (furosemide) in some patients by inhibiting prostaglandin synthesis. Indomethacin may also affect plasma renin levels, aldosterone excretion, and renin profile evaluation. Patients receiving both indomethacin and Lasix® (furosemide) should be observed closely to determine if the desired diuretic and/or antihypertensive effect of Lasix® (furosemide) is achieved.

Carcinogenesis, Mutagenesis, Impairment of Fertility
No carcinogenic or mutagenic studies have been conducted with Lasix® (furosemide).
Lasix® (furosemide) produced no impairment of fertility in male or female rats, at 100 mg/kg/day (the maximum effective diuretic dose in the rat and 8 times the maximal human dose of 600 mg/day).

Pregnancy
Pregnancy Category C. Furosemide has been shown to cause unexplained maternal deaths and abortions in rabbits at 2, 4 and 8 times the human dose. There are no adequate and well-controlled studies in pregnant women. Lasix® (furosemide) should be used during pregnancy only if the potential benefit justifies the potential risk to the fetus.
The effects of furosemide on embryonic and fetal development and on pregnant dams were studied in mice, rats and rabbits.
Furosemide caused unexplained maternal deaths and abortions in the rabbit at the lowest dose of 25 mg/kg (2 times the maximal recommended human dose of 600 mg/day). In another study, a dose of 50 mg/kg (4 times the maximal recommended human dose of 600 mg/day) also caused maternal deaths and abortions when administered to rabbits between Days 12 and 17 of gestation. In a third study, none of the pregnant rabbits survived a dose of 100 mg/kg. Data from the above studies indicate fetal lethality that can precede maternal deaths.
The results of the mouse study and one of the three rabbit studies also showed an increased incidence of hydronephrosis (distention of the renal pelvis and, in some cases, of the ureters) in fetuses derived from treated dams as compared to the incidence in fetuses from the control group.

Nursing Mothers
Because it appears in breast milk, caution should be exercised when Lasix® (furosemide) is administered to a nursing mother.

Pediatric Use
Renal calcifications (from barely visible on x-ray to staghorn) have occurred in some severely premature infants treated with intravenous Lasix® (furosemide) for edema due to patent ductus arteriosus and hyaline membrane disease. The concurrent use of chlorothiazide has been reported to decrease hypercalciuria and dissolve some calculi.

ADVERSE REACTIONS

Adverse reactions are categorized below by organ system and listed by decreasing severity.

Gastrointestinal System Reactions

1. pancreatitis	5. cramping
2. jaundice (intrahepatic cholestatic jaundice)	6. diarrhea
	7. constipation
3. anorexia	8. nausea
4. oral and gastric irritation	9. vomiting

Systemic Hypersensitivity Reactions
Systemic Vasculitis, Interstitial Hephritis, Necrotizing Angiitis

Central Nervous System Reactions

1. tinnitus and hearing loss	4. dizziness
	5. headache
2. paresthesias	6. blurred vision
3. vertigo	7. xanthopsia

Hematologic Reactions

1. aplastic anemia (rare)	4. hemolytic anemia
2. thrombocytopenia	5. leukopenia
3. agranulocytosis (rare)	6. anemia

Dermatologic Reactions

1. exfoliative dermatis	5. urticaria
2. erythema multiforme	6. rash
3. purpura	7. pruritus
4. photosensitivity	

Cardiovascular Reaction
Orthostatic hypotension may occur and be aggravated by alcohol, barbiturates or narcotics.

Other Reactions

1. hyperglycemia	7. urinary bladder spasm
2. glycosuria	8. thrombophlebitis
3. hyperuricemia	9. transient injection site pain following intramuscular injection
4. muscle spasm	
5. weakness	
6. restlessness	10. fever

Whenever adverse reactions are moderate or severe, Lasix® (furosemide) dosage should be reduced or therapy withdrawn.

OVERDOSAGE

The principal signs and symptoms of overdose with Lasix® (furosemide) are dehydration, blood volume reduction, hypotension, electrolyte imbalance, hypokalemia and hypochloremic alkalosis, and are extensions of its diuretic action.
The acute toxicity of Lasix® (furosemide) has been determined in mice, rats and dogs. In all three, the oral LD_{50} exceeded 1000 mg/kg body weight, while the intravenous LD_{50} ranged from 300 to 680 mg/kg. The acute intragastric toxicity in neonatal rats is 7 to 10 times that of adult rats.
The concentration of Lasix® (furosemide) in biological fluids associated with toxicity or death is not known.
Treatment of overdosage is supportive and consists of replacement of excessive fluid and electrolyte losses.
Serum electrolytes, carbon dioxide level and blood pressure should be determined frequently. Adequate drainage must be assured in patients with urinary bladder outlet obstruction (such as prostatic hypertrophy). Hemodialysis does not accelerate furosemide elimination.

DOSAGE AND ADMINISTRATION

Oral Administration
Edema
Therapy should be individualized according to patient response to gain maximal therapeutic response and to determine the minimal dose needed to maintain that response.
Adults—The usual initial dose of Lasix® (furosemide) is 20 to 80 mg given as a single dose. Ordinarily a prompt diuresis ensues. If needed, the same dose can be administered 6 to 8 hours later or the dose may be increased. The dose may be raised by 20 or 40 mg and given not sooner than 6 to 8 hours after the previous dose until the desired diuretic effect has been obtained. This individually determined single dose should then be given once or twice daily (eg, at 8 am and 2 pm). The dose of Lasix® (furosemide) may be carefully titrated up to 600 mg/day in patients with clinically severe edematous states.
Edema may be most efficiently and safely mobilized by giving Lasix® (furosemide) on 2 to 4 consecutive days each week.
When doses exceeding 80 mg/day are given for prolonged periods, careful clinical observation and laboratory monitoring are particularly advisable. (See **PRECAUTIONS: Laboratory Tests.**)
Infants and Children—The usual initial dose of oral Lasix® (furosemide) in infants and children is 2 mg/kg body weight, given as a single dose. If the diuretic response is not satisfactory after the initial dose, dosage may be increased by 1 or 2 mg/kg no sooner than 6 to 8 hours after the previous dose. Doses greater than 6 mg/kg body weight are not recommended.
For maintenance therapy in infants and children, the dose should be adjusted to the minimum effective level.
Hypertension
Therapy should be individualized according to the patient's response to gain maximal therapeutic response and to determine the minimal dose needed to maintain that therapeutic response.
Adults—The usual initial daily dose of Lasix® (furosemide) for hypertension is 80 mg, usually divided into 40 mg twice a day. Dosage should then be adjusted according to response. If response is not satisfactory, add other antihypertensive agents.
Changes in blood pressure must be carefully monitored when Lasix® (furosemide) is used with other antihypertensive drugs, especially during initial therapy. To prevent excessive drop in blood pressure, the dosage of other agents should be reduced by at least 50 percent when Lasix® (furosemide) is added to the regimem. As the blood pressure falls under the potentiating effect of Lasix® (furosemide), a further reduction in dosage or even discontinuation of other antihypertensive drugs may be necessary.

Parenteral Administration
Adults—Parenteral therapy with Lasix® (furosemide) injection should be used only in patients unable to take oral medication or in emergency situations and should be replaced with oral therapy as soon as practical.
Edema
The usual initial dose of Lasix® (furosemide) is 20 to 40 mg given as a single dose, injected intramuscularly or intravenously. The intravenous dose should be given slowly (1 to 2 minutes). Ordinarily a prompt diuresis ensues. If needed, another dose may be administered in the same manner 2 hours later or the dose may be increased. The dose may be raised by 20 mg and given not sooner than 2 hours after the previous dose until the desired diuretic effect has been obtained. This individually determined single dose should then be given once or twice daily.
Therapy should be individualized according to patient response to gain maximal therapeutic response and to determine the minimal dose needed to maintain that response. Close medical supervision is necessary. If the physician elects to use high dose parenteral therapy, add the Lasix® (furosemide) to either Sodium Chloride Injection USP, Lactated Ringer's Injection USP, or Dextrose (5%) Injection USP after pH has been adjusted to above 5.5, and administer as a controlled intravenous infusion at a rate not greater than 4 mg/min. Lasix® (furosemide) Injection is a buffered alkaline solution.
Acute Pulmonary Edema
The usual initial dose of Lasix® (furosemide) is 40 mg injected slowly intravenously (over 1 to 2 minutes). If a satisfactory response does not occur within 1 hour, the dose may be increased to 80 mg injected slowly intravenously (over 1 to 2 minutes).
If necessary, additional therapy (eg, digitalis, oxygen) may be administered concomitantly.
Infants and Children—Parenteral therapy should be used only in patients unable to take oral medication or in emergency situations and should be replaced with oral therapy as soon as practical.
The usual initial dose of Lasix® (furosemide) Injection (intravenously or intramuscularly) in infants and children is 1 mg/kg body weight and should be given slowly under close medical supervision. If the diuretic response to the initial dose is not satisfactory, dosage may be increased by 1 mg/kg not sooner than 2 hours after the previous dose, until the desired diuretic effect has been obtained. Doses greater than 6 mg/kg body weight are not recommended.
Lasix® (furosemide) Injection should be inspected visually for particulate matter and discoloration before administration. Do not use if solution is discolored.

HOW SUPPLIED

Lasix® (furosemide) Tablets 20 mg are supplied as white, oval, monogrammed tablets in Bottles of 100 (NDC 0039-0067-10), 500 (NDC 0039-0067-50), 1000 (NDC 0039-0067-70), and in Unit Dose Packs of 100 (NDC 0039-0067-11). The 20 mg tablets are imprinted with "Lasix® " on one side and "HOECHST" on the other.
Lasix® (furosemide) Tablets 40 mg are supplied as white, round, monogrammed, scored tablets in Unit of Use Bottles of 100 (NDC 0039-0060-13), 500 (NDC 0039-0060-50), and 1000 (NDC 0039-0060-70), and in Unit Dose Packs of 100 (NDC 0039-0060-11). The 40 mg tablets are imprinted with "Lasix® 40" on one side and the Hoechst logo on the other.
Lasix® (furosemide) Tablets 80 mg are supplied as white, round, monogrammed, facetted edge tablets in Bottles of 50 (NDC 0039-0066-05), 500 (NDC 0039-0066-50), and in Unit Dose Packs of 100 (NDC 0039-0066-11). The 80 mg tablets are imprinted with "Lasix® 80" on one side and the Hoechst logo on the other.
Note: Dispense in well-closed, light-resistant containers. Exposure to light might cause a slight discoloration. Discolored tablets should not be dispensed.
Lasix® (furosemide) Oral Solution 10 mg/mL is supplied as orange-flavored liquid in Bottles of 60 mL (accompanied by graduated dropper) (NDC 0039-0063-06) and Bottles of 120 mL (accompanied by graduated dropper) (NDC 0039-0063-40).
Note: Store at controlled room temperature (59°–86°F).
Dispense in light-resistant containers. Discard opened bottle after 60 days.
Lasix® Injection, brand of furosemide, (10 mg/mL), is supplied as a sterile solution in 2 mL, 4 mL, and 10 mL amber ampules, single use vials, and in syringes.
Ampules:
2 mL 5's (NDC 0039-0061-15); 50's (NDC 0039-0061-05)
4 mL 5's (NDC 0039-0061-45); 25's (NDC 0039-0061-65)
10 mL 5's (NDC 0039-0061-08); 25's (NDC 0039-0061-25)
Syringes:
2 mL 5's (NDC 0039-0062-08)
4 mL 5's (NDC 0039-0064-08)
10 mL 5's (NDC 0039-0069-08)
Single Use Vials:
2 mL 25's (NDC 0039-0055-25)
4 mL 25's (NDC 0039-0056-25)
10 mL 25's (NDC 0039-0057-25)
Syringes supplied with 22 gauge x 1 1/4" needle.
To insure patient safety, this needle should be handled with care and should be destroyed and discarded if damaged in any manner. If cannula is bent, no attempt should be made to straighten.

To prevent needle-stick injuries, needles should not be recapped, purposely bent, or broken by hand.
Store at controlled room temperature (59°–86°F).
Do not use if solution is discolored.
Protect syringes from light. Do not remove syringes from individual package until time of use.
760010-1/91
763000-12/89
705060-1/91
Shown in Product Identification Section, pages 411 and 412

LOPROX® ℞
[lo' prahks]
(ciclopirox olamine) Cream 1%
Lotion 1%

DESCRIPTION
Loprox® (ciclopirox olamine) Cream 1% and Lotion 1% are for topical use. Each gram of Loprox® (ciclopirox olamine) Cream 1% contains 10 mg ciclopirox olamine in a water miscible vanishing cream base consisting of purified water USP, octyldodecanol NF, mineral oil USP, stearyl alcohol NF, cetyl alcohol NF, cocamide DEA, polysorbate 60 NF, myristyl alcohol NF, sorbitan monostearate NF, lactic acid USP, and benzyl alcohol NF (1%) as preservative.
Each gram of Loprox® (ciclopirox olamine) Lotion 1% contains 10 mg of ciclopirox olamine in a water miscible lotion base consisting of purified water USP, cocamide DEA, octyldodecanol NF, mineral oil USP, stearyl alcohol NF, cetyl alcohol NF, polysorbate 60 NF, myristyl alcohol NF, sorbitan monostearate NF, lactic acid USP, and benzyl alcohol NF (1%) as preservative. Loprox® (ciclopirox olamine) Cream and Lotion contain a synthetic, broad-spectrum, antifungal agent ciclopirox olamine. The chemical name is 6-cyclohexyl-1-hydroxy-4-methyl-2(*1H*)-pyridone, 2-aminoethanol salt.
The chemical structure is:

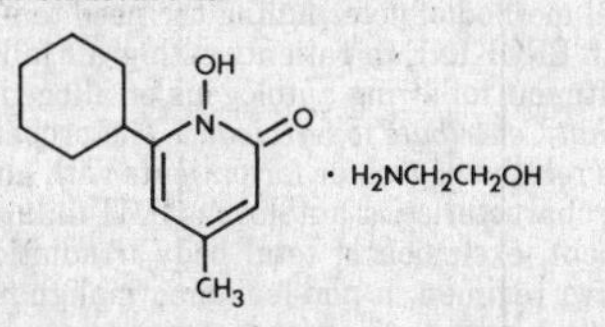

Loprox® (ciclopirox olamine) Cream 1% and Lotion 1% have a pH of 7.

CLINICAL PHARMACOLOGY
Ciclopirox olamine is a broad-spectrum, antifungal agent that inhibits the growth of pathogenic dermatophytes, yeasts, and *Malassezia furfur*. Ciclopirox olamine exhibits fungicidal activity *in vitro* against isolates of *Trichophyton rubrum, Trichophyton mentagrophytes, Epidermophyton floccosum, Microsporum canis,* and *Candida albicans*.
Pharmacokinetic studies in men with radiolabeled 1% ciclopirox olamine solution in polyethylene glycol 400 showed an average of 1.3% absorption of the dose when it was applied topically to 750 cm^2 on the back followed by occlusion for 6 hours. The biological half-life was 1.7 hours and excretion occurred via the kidney. Two days after application only 0.01% of the dose applied could be found in the urine. Fecal excretion was negligible.
Penetration studies in human cadaverous skin from the back, with Loprox® (ciclopirox olamine) Cream 1% with tagged ciclopirox olamine showed the presence of 0.8 to 1.6% of the dose in stratum corneum 1.5 to 6 hours after application. The levels in the dermis were still 10 to 15 times above the minimum inhibitory concentrations.
Autoradiographic studies with human cadaverous skin showed that ciclopirox olamine penetrates into the hair and through the epidermis and hair follicles into the sebaceous glands and dermis, while a portion of the drug remains in the stratum corneum.
Draize Human Sensitization Assay, 21-Day Cumulative Irritancy study, Phototoxicity study, and Photo-Draize study conducted in a total of 142 healthy male subjects showed no contact sensitization of the delayed hypersensitivity type, no irritation, no phototoxicity, and no photo-contact sensitization due to Loprox® (ciclopirox olamine) Cream 1%.
In vitro penetration studies in frozen or fresh excised human cadaver and pig skin indicated that the penetration of Loprox® (ciclopirox olamine) Lotion 1% is equivalent to that of Loprox® (ciclopirox olamine) Cream 1%. Therapeutic equivalence of cream and lotion formulations also was indicated by studies of experimentally induced guinea pig and human trichophytosis.

INDICATIONS AND USAGE
Loprox® (ciclopirox olamine) Cream 1% and Lotion 1% are indicated for the topical treatment of the following dermal infections: tinea pedis, tinea cruris and tinea corporis due to *Trichophyton rubrum, Trichophyton mentagrophytes, Epidermophyton floccosum,* and *Microsporum canis;* cutaneous candidiasis (moniliasis) due to *Candida albicans;* and tinea (pityriasis) versicolor due to *Malassezia furfur*.

CONTRAINDICATIONS
Loprox® (ciclopirox olamine) Cream 1% and Lotion 1% are contraindicated in individuals who have shown hypersensitivity to any of its components.

WARNINGS
General: Loprox® (ciclopirox olamine) Cream 1% and Lotion 1% are not for ophthalmic use.

PRECAUTIONS
If a reaction suggesting sensitivity or chemical irritation should occur with the use of Loprox® (ciclopirox olamine) Cream 1% or Lotion 1%, treatment should be discontinued and appropriate therapy instituted.
Information for patients—The patient should be told to:
1. Use the medication for the full treatment time even though symptoms may have improved and notify the physician if there is no improvement after four weeks.
2. Inform the physician if the area of application shows signs of increased irritation (redness, itching, burning, blistering, swelling, oozing) indicative of possible sensitization.
3. Avoid the use of occlusive wrappings or dressings.

Carcinogenesis, mutagenesis, impairment of fertility:
A carcinogenicity study in female mice dosed cutaneously twice per week for 50 weeks followed by a 6-month drug-free observation period prior to necropsy revealed no evidence of tumors at the application site. Several mutagenicity tests with ciclopirox olamine indicated no potential for mutagenesis. In a battery of *in vitro* genotoxicity tests with ciclopirox free acid, one assay was positive; however, the positive findings were not substantiated by *in vivo* testing.
Pregnancy Category B:
Reproduction studies have been performed in the mouse, rat, rabbit, and monkey, (via various routes of administration) at doses 10 times or more the topical human dose and have revealed no significant evidence of impaired fertility or harm to the fetus due to ciclopirox olamine. There are, however, no adequate or well-controlled studies in pregnant women. Because animal reproduction studies are not always predictive of human response this drug should be used during pregnancy only if clearly needed.
Nursing mothers:
It is not known whether this drug is excreted in human milk. Because many drugs are excreted in human milk, caution should be exercised when Loprox® (ciclopirox olamine) Cream 1% or Lotion 1% is administered to a nursing woman.
Pediatric use:
Safety and effectiveness in children below the age of 10 years have not been established.

ADVERSE REACTIONS
In all controlled clinical studies with 514 patients using Loprox® (ciclopirox olamine) Cream 1% and in 296 patients using the vehicle cream, the incidence of adverse reactions was low. This included pruritus at the site of application in one patient and worsening of the clinical signs and symptoms in another patient using ciclopirox olamine cream 1% and burning in one patient and worsening of the clinical signs and symptoms in another patient using the vehicle cream.
In the controlled clinical trial with 89 patients using Loprox® (ciclopirox olamine) Lotion 1% and 89 patients using the vehicle, the incidence of adverse reactions was low. Those considered possibly related to treatment or occurring in more than one patient were pruritus, which occurred in two patients using ciclopirox olamine lotion 1% and one patient using the lotion vehicle, and burning, which occurred in one patient using ciclopirox olamine lotion 1%.

DOSAGE AND ADMINISTRATION
Gently massage Loprox® (ciclopirox olamine) Cream 1% or Lotion 1% into the affected and surrounding skin areas twice daily, in the morning and evening. Clinical improvement with relief of pruritus and other symptoms usually occurs within the first week of treatment. If a patient shows no clinical improvement after four weeks of treatment with Loprox® (ciclopirox olamine) Cream 1% or Lotion 1%, the diagnosis should be redetermined. Patients with tinea versicolor usually exhibit clinical and mycological clearing after two weeks of treatment.

HOW SUPPLIED
Loprox® (ciclopirox olamine) Cream 1% is supplied in 15 gram, (NDC 0039-0009-15); 30 gram, (NDC 0039-0009-30); and 90 gram tubes, (NDC 0039-0009-90).
Loprox® (ciclopirox olamine) Lotion 1% is supplied in 30 mL bottles (NDC 0039-0008-30).
Shake lotion vigorously before each use.
Store at controlled room temperature (59°- 86°F).
Loprox® REG TM HOECHST AG 709000-8/90
U.S. Patent 3,883,545 708000-9/90
Shown in Product Identification Section, page 412

PROKINE™ ℞
(Sargramostim)

DESCRIPTION
PROKINE™ (Sargramostim) is a recombinant human granulocyte-macrophage colony stimulating factor (rhu GM-CSF) produced by recombinant DNA technology in a yeast (*S. cerevisiae*) expression system. GM-CSF is a hematopoietic growth factor which stimulates proliferation and differentiation of hematopoietic progenitor cells. PROKINE is a glycoprotein of 127 amino acids characterized by 3 primary molecular species having molecular masses of 19,500, 16,800, and 15,500 daltons. The amino acid sequence of PROKINE differs from the natural human GM-CSF by a substitution of leucine at position 23, and the carbohydrate moiety may be different from the native protein. Sargramostim has been selected as the proper name for yeast-derived rhu GM-CSF.
PROKINE is formulated as a sterile, white, preservative-free, lyophilized powder and is intended for IV infusion following reconstitution with 1 ml Sterile Water for Injection, USP. Each single use vial of PROKINE contains 500 mcg Sargramostim; 40 mg Mannitol, USP; 10 mg Sucrose, NF; and 1.2 mg Tromethamine, USP. The pH of the reconstituted, isotonic solution is 7.4 ± 0.3. The specific activity of PROKINE is approximately 5×10^7 colony forming units per mg in a normal human bone marrow colony formation assay.

CLINICAL PHARMACOLOGY
General
Granulocyte-macrophage colony stimulating factor belongs to a group of growth factors termed colony stimulating factors which support survival, clonal expansion, and differentiation of hematopoietic progenitor cells. GM-CSF induces partially committed progenitor cells to divide and differentiate in the granulocyte-macrophage pathways.
GM-CSF is also capable of activating mature granulocytes and macrophages. GM-CSF is a multilineage factor and, in addition to dose-dependent effects on the myelomonocytic lineage, can promote the proliferation of megakaryocytic and erythroid progenitors.[1] However, other factors are required to induce complete maturation in these two lineages. The various cellular responses (i.e., division, maturation, activation) are induced through GM-CSF binding to specific receptors expressed on the cell surface of target cells.[2]
***In vitro* Studies of PROKINE in Human Cells**
The biological activity of GM-CSF is species-specific. Consequently, *in vitro* studies have been performed on human cells to characterize the pharmacological activity of PROKINE. *In vitro* exposure of human bone marrow cells to PROKINE at concentrations ranging from 1–100 ng/ml results in the proliferation of hematopoietic progenitors and in the formation of pure granulocyte, pure macrophage, and mixed granulocyte-macrophage colonies.[3] Chemotactic, anti-fungal, and anti-parasitic[4] activities of granulocytes and monocytes are increased by exposure to PROKINE. PROKINE increases the cytotoxicity of monocytes toward certain neoplastic cell lines[3] and activates polymorphonuclear neutrophils to inhibit the growth of tumor cells.
***In vivo* Primate Studies of PROKINE**
Pharmacology/toxicology studies of PROKINE™ (Sargramostim) were performed in cynomolgus monkeys. An acute toxicity study revealed an absence of treatment-related toxicity following a single IV bolus injection at a dose of 300 mcg/kg. Two subacute studies were performed using IV injection (maximum dose 200 mcg/kg/day × 14 days) and subcutaneous injection (maximum dose 200 mcg/kg/day × 28 days). No major visceral organ toxicity was documented. Notable histopathology findings included increased cellularity in hematologic organs, heart, and lung tissues. A dose-dependent increase in leukocyte count occurred during the dosing period which consisted primarily of segmented neutrophils; increases in monocytes, basophils, eosinophils, and lymphocytes were also noted. Leukocyte counts decreased to pretreatment values over a 1–2 week recovery period.
Pharmacokinetics
Pharmacokinetic profiles have been analyzed in patients with various neoplastic diseases following intravenous administration of PROKINE. In 2 patients receiving 250 mcg/m^2 of PROKINE by 2 hour IV infusion, serum concentration ranged from 22,000 pg/ml to 23,000 pg/ml at the termination of the infusion. The pharmacokinetic profile, calculated on samples from 5 patients receiving 500–750 mcg/m^2 of PROKINE by 2 hour IV infusion, revealed a rapid initial decline in GM-CSF serum concentration ($t_{1/2\alpha}$~12 to 17 minutes) followed by a slower decrease ($t_{1/2\beta}$~2 hours). In four patients treated with PROKINE by subcutaneous injection (125 mcg/m^2 every 12 hours), PROKINE was detected in the serum within 5 minutes after administration (range 55–450 pg/ml). Peak levels were observed 2 hours after injection (range 350–3,900 pg/ml), and PROKINE remained at detectable levels 6 hours following injection (range 150–2,700 pg/ml).[5]

Continued on next page

Hoechst-Roussel—Cont.

Antibody Formation

Serum samples collected before and after PROKINE treatment from 137 patients with a variety of underlying diseases have been examined for the presence of antibodies. Neutralizing antibodies were detected in 5 of 137 patients (3.6%) after receiving PROKINE by continuous IV infusion (3 patients) or subcutaneous injection (2 patients) for 28 to 84 days in multiple courses. All 5 patients had impaired hematopoiesis before the administration of PROKINE and consequently the effect of the development of anti-GM-CSF antibodies on normal hematopoiesis could not be assessed. Drug-induced neutropenia, neutralization of endogenous GM-CSF activity, and diminution of the therapeutic effect of PROKINE secondary to formation of neutralizing antibody remain a theoretical possibility. A systematic screening program to evaluate antibody formation is ongoing for patients enrolled in clinical trials.

INDICATIONS AND USAGE

Use in Myeloid Reconstitution After Autologous Bone Marrow Transplantation

PROKINE is indicated for acceleration of myeloid recovery in patients with non-Hodgkin's lymphoma (NHL), acute lymphoblastic leukemia (ALL), and Hodgkin's disease undergoing autologous bone marrow transplantation (BMT). After autologous BMT in patients with NHL, ALL, or Hodgkin's disease, PROKINE has been found to be safe and effective in accelerating myeloid engraftment, decreasing median duration of antibiotic administration, reducing the median duration of infectious episodes and shortening the median duration of hospitalization. Hematologic response to PROKINE can be detected by complete blood count (CBC) with differential performed twice per week.

Insufficient data are presently available to support the efficacy of PROKINE in accelerating myeloid recovery following peripheral blood stem cell transplantation.

Use in Bone Marrow Transplantation Failure or Engraftment Delay

PROKINE™ is indicated in patients who have undergone allogeneic or autologous bone marrow transplantation (BMT) in whom engraftment is delayed or has failed. PROKINE™ has been found to be safe and effective in prolonging survival of patients who are experiencing graft failure or engraftment delay, in the presence or absence of infection, following autologous or allogeneic BMT. Survival benefit may be relatively greater in those patients who demonstrate one or more of the following characteristics: autologous BMT failure or engraftment delay, no previous total body irradiation, malignancy other than leukemia or a multiple organ failure (MOF) score ≥2 (See **CLINICAL EXPERIENCE**). Hematologic response to PROKINE™ can be detected by complete blood count (CBC) with differential performed twice per week.

CLINICAL EXPERIENCE

Effects of Myeloid Reconstitution After Autologous Bone Marrow Transplantation[6]

Following a dose-ranging Phase I/II trial in patients undergoing autologous BMT for lymphoid malignancies,[7,8] three single-center, randomized, placebo-controlled and double-blinded studies were conducted to evaluate the safety and efficacy of PROKINE for promoting hematopoietic reconstitution following autologous BMT. A total of 128 patients (65 PROKINE, 63 placebo) were enrolled in these 3 studies. The majority of the patients had lymphoid malignancy (87 NHL, 17 ALL), 23 patients had Hodgkin's disease, and 1 patient had acute myeloblastic leukemia (AML). In 72 patients with NHL or ALL, the bone marrow harvest was purged prior to storage with one of several monoclonal antibodies. No chemical agent was used for *in vitro* treatment of the bone marrow. Preparative regimens in the 3 studies included cyclophosphamide (total dose 120–150 mg/kg) and total body irradiation (total dose 1,200–1,575 rads). Other regimens used in patients with Hodgkin's disease and NHL without radiotherapy consisted of 3 or more of the following in combination (expressed as total dose): cytosine arabinoside (400 mg/m^2) and carmustine (300 mg/m^2), cyclophosphamide (140–150 mg/kg), hydroxyurea (4.5 gm/m^2) and etoposide (375–450 mg/m^2).

Median Survival by Multiple Organ Failure (MOF) Category
Median Survival (days)

	MOF ≤2 Organs	MOF >2 Organs	MOF (Composite of Both Groups)
Autologous BMT			
PROKINE	474 (n=58)	78.5 (n=10)	474 (n=68)
Historical	165 (n=14)	39 (n=3)	161 (n=17)
Allogeneic BMT			
PROKINE	174 (n=50)	27 (n=22)	97 (n=72)
Historical	52.5 (n=60)	15.5 (n=26)	35 (n=86)

Compared to placebo, administration of PROKINE in 2 studies (n=44 and 47) significantly improved the following hematologic and clinical endpoints: time to neutrophil engraftment, duration of hospitalization and infection experience or antibacterial usage. In the third study (n=37) there was a positive trend toward earlier myeloid engraftment in favor of PROKINE. This latter study differed from the other 2 in having enrolled a large number of patients with Hodgkin's disease who had also received extensive radiation and chemotherapy prior to harvest of autologous bone marrow. A subgroup analysis of the data from all 3 studies revealed that the median time to engraftment for patients with Hodgkin's disease, regardless of treatment, was 6 days longer when compared to patients with NHL and ALL, but that the overall beneficial PROKINE treatment effect was the same. In the following combined analysis of the 3 studies, these 2 subgroups (NHL and ALL vs. Hodgkin's disease) are presented separately.

Patients with Lymphoid Malignancy (Non-Hodgkin's Lymphoma and Acute Lymphoblastic Leukemia) Myeloid engraftment (absolute neutrophil count [ANC] ≥500 cells/mm^3) in 54 patients receiving PROKINE™ (Sargramostim) was observed 6 days earlier than in 50 patients treated with placebo (see table below). Accelerated myeloid engraftment was associated with significant clinical benefits. The median duration of hospitalization was 6 days shorter for the PROKINE group than for the placebo group. Median duration of infectious episodes (defined as fever and neutropenia; or 2 positive cultures of the same organism; or fever > 38°C and 1 positive blood culture; or clinical evidence of infection) was 3 days less in the group treated with PROKINE. The median duration of antibacterial administration in the post-transplantation period was 4 days shorter for the patients treated with PROKINE than for placebo-treated patients. The study was unable to detect a significant difference between the treatment groups in rate of disease relapse 24 months post-transplantation. As a group, leukemic subjects receiving PROKINE™ derived less benefit than NHL subjects. However, both the leukemic and NHL groups receiving PROKINE™ engrafted earlier than controls.

[See table below.]

Patients with Hodgkin's Disease If patients with Hodgkin's disease are analyzed separately, a trend toward earlier myeloid engraftment was noted. PROKINE-treated patients engrafted earlier (by 5 days) than the placebo-treated subjects (p=0.189, Wilcoxon) but the number of subjects was small (n=22); 1 patient (#23) from 1 site was non-controlled and was excluded from the analysis. Studies are in progress to confirm statistically the beneficial effect of PROKINE in patients with Hodgkin's disease.

Effects in Bone Marrow Transplantation Failure or Engraftment Delay

A historically-controlled study was conducted in patients experiencing graft failure following allogeneic or autologous BMT to determine whether PROKINE improved survival after BMT failure.

Three categories of patients were eligible for this study:

1) patients displaying a delay in engraftment (ANC ≤ 100 cells/mm^3 by day 28 post-transplantation);
2) patients displaying a delay in engraftment (ANC ≤ 100 cells/mm^3 by day 21 post-transplantation) and who had evidence of an active infection; and
3) patients who lost their marrow graft after a transient engraftment (manifested by an average of ANC ≥ 500 cells/mm^3 for at least one week followed by loss of engraftment with ANC ≤ 500 cells/mm^3 for at least one week beyond day 21 post-transplantation).

Autologous BMT: Combined Analysis from Placebo-Controlled Clinical Trials of Responses in Patients with NHL and ALL
Median Values (days)

	ANC ≥500/mm^3	ANC ≥1000/mm^3	Duration of Hospitalization	Duration of Infection	Duration of Antibacterial Therapy
PROKINE (n=54)	18*#	24*#	25*	1*	21*
Placebo (n=50)	24	32	31	4	25

* $p < 0.05$ Wilcoxon or CMH ridit chi squared
# $p < 0.05$ Log rank
Note: The single AML patient was not included

A total of 140 eligible patients from 35 institutions treated with PROKINE were evaluated in comparison to 103 historical control patients from a single institution. One hundred sixty-three patients had lymphoid or myeloid leukemia, 24 patients had non-Hodgkin's lymphoma, 19 patients had Hodgkin's disease and 37 patients had other diseases, such as aplastic anemia, myelodysplasia or non-hematologic malignancy. The majority of patients (223 out of 243) had received prior chemotherapy with or without radiotherapy and/or immunotherapy prior to preparation for transplantation.

One hundred day survival was improved in favor of the patients treated with PROKINE after graft failure following either autologous or allogeneic BMT. In addition, the median survival was improved by greater than 2-fold. The median survival of patients treated with PROKINE after autologous failure was 474 days versus 161 days for the historical patients. Similarly, after allogeneic failure, the median survival was 97 days with PROKINE treatment and 35 days for the historical controls. Improvement in survival was better in patients with fewer impaired organs.

[See table above.]

The MOF score is a simple clinical and laboratory assessment of 7 major organ systems: cardiovascular, respiratory, gastrointestinal, hematologic, renal, hepatic and neurologic.[9] Assessment of the MOF score is recommended as an additional method of determining the need to initiate treatment with PROKINE in patients with graft failure or delay in engraftment following autologous or allogeneic BMT.

Factors that Contribute to Survival: The probability of survival was relatively greater for patients with any one of the following characteristics: autologous BMT failure or delay in engraftment, exclusion of total body irradiation from the preparative regimen, a non-leukemic malignancy or MOF score ≤ 2 (0, 1 or 2 dysfunctional organ systems). Leukemic subjects derived less benefit than other subjects.

CONTRAINDICATIONS

PROKINE is contraindicated in patients with:

1) excessive leukemic myeloid blasts in the bone marrow or peripheral blood (≥ 10%).
2) known hypersensitivity to GM-CSF, yeast-derived products, or any component of the product.

WARNINGS

Fluid Retention

Peripheral edema, capillary leak syndrome, pleural and/or pericardial effusion have been reported in patients after PROKINE administration. In 156 patients enrolled in placebo-controlled studies using PROKINE at a dose of 250 mcg/m^2/day by 2 hour IV infusion, the reported incidences of fluid retention (PROKINE vs. placebo) were as follows: peripheral edema, 11% vs. 7%; pleural effusion, 1% vs. 0%; and pericardial effusion, 4% vs. 1%. Capillary leak syndrome was not observed in this limited number of studies; based on other uncontrolled studies and post-marketing reports, the incidence is estimated to be less than 1%. In patients with preexisting pleural and pericardial effusions, administration of PROKINE™ may aggravate fluid retention; however, fluid retention associated with or worsened by PROKINE has been reversible after interruption or dose reduction of PROKINE with or without diuretic therapy. PROKINE should be used with caution in patients with preexisting fluid retention, pulmonary infiltrates, or congestive heart failure.

Respiratory Symptoms

Sequestration of granulocytes in the pulmonary circulation has been documented following PROKINE infusion,[6] and dyspnea has been reported occasionally in patients treated with PROKINE. Special attention should be given to respiratory symptoms during or immediately following PROKINE infusion, especially in patients with preexisting lung disease. In patients displaying dyspnea during PROKINE administration, the rate of infusion should be reduced by half. If respiratory symptoms worsen despite infusion rate reduction, the infusion should be discontinued. Subsequent IV infusions may be administered following the standard dose schedule with careful monitoring. PROKINE should be administered with caution in patients with hypoxia.

Cardiovascular Symptoms

Occasional transient supraventricular arrhythmia has been reported in uncontrolled studies during PROKINE administration, particularly in patients with a previous history of cardiac arrhythmia. However, these arrhythmias have been

reversible after discontinuation of PROKINE. PROKINE should be used with caution in patients with preexisting cardiac disease.

Renal and Hepatic Dysfunction

In some patients with preexisting renal or hepatic dysfunction enrolled in uncontrolled clinical trials, administration of PROKINE has induced elevation of serum creatinine or bilirubin and hepatic enzymes. Dose reduction or interruption of PROKINE administration has resulted in a decrease to pretreatment values. However, in controlled clinical trials the incidences of renal and hepatic dysfunction were comparable between PROKINE (250 mcg/m²/day by 2 hour IV infusion) and placebo-treated patients. Monitoring of renal and hepatic function in patients displaying renal or hepatic dysfunction prior to initiation of treatment is recommended at least biweekly during PROKINE administration.

PRECAUTIONS

General

Parenteral administration of recombinant proteins should be attended by appropriate precautions in case an allergic or untoward reaction occurs. Transient rashes and local injection site reactions have occasionally been observed concomitantly with PROKINE treatment. Serious allergic or anaphylactic reactions have been reported rarely. If any serious allergic or anaphylactoid reaction occurs, PROKINE therapy should immediately be discontinued and appropriate therapy initiated (see WARNINGS).

Rarely, hypotension with flushing and syncope has been reported following the first administration of PROKINE. These signs have resolved with symptomatic treatment and have not recurred with subsequent doses in the same cycle of treatment.

Stimulation of marrow precursors with PROKINE may result in a rapid rise in white blood cell (WBC) count. If the ANC exceeds 20,000 cells/mm³ or if the platelet count exceeds 500,000/mm³, PROKINE administration should be interrupted or the dose reduced by half. The decision to reduce the dose or interrupt treatment should be based on the clinical condition of the patient. Excessive blood counts have returned to normal or baseline levels within 3 to 7 days following cessation of PROKINE™ therapy. Twice weekly monitoring of CBC with differential (including examination for the presence of blast cells) should be performed to preclude development of excessive counts.

Growth Factor Potential

PROKINE is a growth factor that primarily stimulates normal myeloid precursors. However, the possibility that PROKINE can act as a growth factor for any tumor type, particularly myeloid malignancies, cannot be excluded. Because of the possibility of tumor growth potentiation, precaution should be exercised when using this drug in any malignancy with myeloid characteristics.

PROKINE has been administered to patients with AML and myelodysplastic syndromes (MDS) in uncontrolled studies without evidence of increased relapse rates.[11,12,13] Controlled studies have not been performed in patients with AML or MDS. PROKINE™ may be administered to those patients with AML or MDS who experience graft failure or delay in engraftment after bone marrow ablation and transplantation.

Progression of the underlying neoplastic disease (NHL, ALL, or Hodgkin's disease) was not observed during PROKINE administration in clinical trials; however, should disease progression be detected during PROKINE treatment, PROKINE therapy should be discontinued. In controlled studies, the 24 month relapse rate was comparable in patients treated with PROKINE or placebo.

Use in Patients Receiving Purged Bone Marrow

PROKINE is effective in accelerating myeloid recovery in patients receiving bone marrow purged by anti-B lymphocyte monoclonal antibodies. Data obtained from uncontrolled studies suggest that if *in vitro* marrow purging with chemical agents causes a significant decrease in the number of responsive hematopoietic progenitors the patient may not respond to PROKINE. When the bone marrow purging process preserves a sufficient number of progenitors ($>1.2 \times 10^4$/kg), a beneficial effect of PROKINE on myeloid engraftment has been reported.[14]

Use in Patients Previously Exposed to Intensive Chemotherapy/Radiotherapy

In patients who before autologous BMT, have received extensive radiotherapy to hematopoietic sites for the treatment of primary disease in the abdomen or chest, or have been exposed to multiple myelotoxic agents (alkylating agents, anthracycline antibiotics, and antimetabolites), the effect of PROKINE on myeloid reconstitution may be limited.

Patient Monitoring

PROKINE can induce variable increases in WBC and/or platelet counts. In order to avoid potential complications of excessive leukocytosis (WBC >50,000 cells/mm³; ANC >20,000 cells/mm³), a CBC is recommended twice per week during PROKINE therapy. Monitoring of renal and hepatic function in patients displaying renal or hepatic dysfunction prior to initiation of treatment is recommended at least biweekly during PROKINE administration. Body weight and hydration status should be carefully monitored during PROKINE administration.

PERCENT OF PATIENTS REPORTING EVENT

Events by Body System	PROKINE (n=79)	Placebo (n=77)
Body, General		
Fever	95	96
Mucous membrane disorder	75	78
Asthenia	66	51
Malaise	57	51
Sepsis	11	14
Digestive System		
Nausea	90	96
Diarrhea	89	82
Vomiting	85	90
Anorexia	54	58
GI disorder	37	47
GI hemorrhage	27	33
Stomatitis	24	29
Liver damage	13	14
Skin and Appendages		
Alopecia	73	74
Rash	44	38
Metabolic/Nutritional Disorder		
Edema	34	35
Peripheral edema	11	7
Respiratory System		
Dyspnea	28	31
Lung disorder	20	23
Hemic and Lymphatic System		
Blood dyscrasia	25	27
Cardiovascular System		
Hemorrhage	23	30
Urogenital System		
Urinary tract disorder	14	13
Kidney function abnormal	8	10
Nervous System		
CNS disorder	11	16

Drug Interaction

Interactions between PROKINE and other drugs have not been fully evaluated. Drugs which may potentiate the myeloproliferative effects of PROKINE, such as lithium and corticosteroids, should be used with caution.

Concomitant Use with Chemotherapy and Radiotherapy

The safety and efficacy of PROKINE given simultaneously with cytotoxic chemotherapy or radiotherapy have not been established. Because of potential sensitivity of rapidly dividing hematopoietic progenitor cells to cytotoxic chemotherapeutic or radiologic therapies, PROKINE should not be administered within 24 hours preceding or following chemotherapy, or within 12 hours preceding or following radiotherapy.

Carcinogenesis, Mutagenesis, Impairment of Fertility

Animal studies have not been conducted with PROKINE to evaluate the carcinogenic potential or the effect on fertility.

Pregnancy (Category C)

Animal reproduction studies have not been conducted with PROKINE. It is not known whether PROKINE can cause fetal harm when administered to a pregnant woman or can affect reproductive capability. PROKINE should be given to a pregnant woman only if clearly needed.

Nursing Mothers

It is not known whether PROKINE is excreted in human milk. Because many drugs are excreted in human milk, PROKINE should be administered to a nursing woman only if clearly needed.

Pediatric Use

Safety and effectiveness in children have not been established; however, available safety data indicate that PROKINE does not exhibit any greater toxicity in children than adults. A total of 113 pediatric subjects between the ages of 4 months and 18 years have been treated with PROKINE in clinical trials at doses ranging from 60–1,000 mcg/m²/day intravenously and 4–1,500 mcg/m²/day subcutaneously. In 53 pediatric patients enrolled in controlled studies at a dose of 250 mcg/m²/day by 2 hour IV infusion, the type and frequency of adverse events were comparable to those reported for the adult population.

ADVERSE REACTIONS

PROKINE is generally well tolerated. In 3 placebo-controlled studies enrolling a total of 156 patients after autologous BMT or peripheral stem cell transplantation, events reported in at least 10% of patients in PROKINE or placebo groups were:

[See table above.]

The frequency and type of adverse events were similar between PROKINE™ and placebo control groups. Diarrhea, asthenia, rash, and malaise were the only events observed for 5% more subjects in the PROKINE group than in the placebo group.

No significant differences were observed between PROKINE and placebo-treated patients in the type or frequency of laboratory abnormalities, including renal and hepatic parameters. In some patients with preexisting renal or hepatic dysfunction enrolled in uncontrolled clinical trials, administration of PROKINE has induced elevation of serum creatinine or bilirubin and hepatic enzymes (see WARNINGS). In addition, there was no significant difference in relapse rate and 24 month survival between the PROKINE and placebo-treated patients.

Adverse events observed for the patients treated with PROKINE in the historically controlled BMT failure study were similar to those reported in the placebo-controlled studies. In addition, headache (26%), pericardial effusion (25%), arthralgia (21%) and myalgia (18%) were also reported in patients treated with PROKINE (Sargramostim) in the graft failure study.

In uncontrolled Phase I/II studies with PROKINE in 215 patients, the most frequent adverse events were fever, asthenia, headache, bone pain, chills, and myalgia. These systemic events were generally mild or moderate and were usually prevented or reversed by the administration of analgesics and antipyretics such as acetaminophen. In these uncontrolled trials, other infrequent events reported were dyspnea, peripheral edema, and rash.

In patients with preexisting peripheral edema, capillary leak syndrome, pleural and/or pericardial effusion, administration of PROKINE may aggravate fluid retention (see WARNINGS). Body weight and hydration status should be carefully monitored during PROKINE administration.

Adverse events observed in pediatric patients in controlled studies were comparable to those observed in adult patients.

OVERDOSAGE

The maximum amount of PROKINE that can be safely administered in single or multiple doses has not been determined. Doses up to 100 mcg/kg/day (4,000 mcg/m²/day or 16 times the recommended dose) were administered to 4 patients in a Phase I uncontrolled clinical study by continuous IV infusion for 7 to 18 days. Increases in WBC up to 200,000 cells/mm³ were observed. Adverse events reported were: dyspnea, malaise, nausea, fever, rash, sinus tachycardia, headache, and chills. All these events were reversible after discontinuation of PROKINE.

In case of overdosage, PROKINE therapy should be discontinued and the patient carefully monitored for WBC increase and respiratory symptoms.

DOSAGE AND ADMINISTRATION

Myeloid Reconstitution after Autologous Bone Marrow Transplantation

The recommended dose is 250 mcg/m²/day for 21 days as a 2 hour IV infusion beginning 2 to 4 hours after the autologous bone marrow infusion, and not less than 24 hours after the last dose of chemotherapy and 12 hours after the last dose of radiotherapy. If a severe adverse reaction occurs, the dose can be reduced or temporarily discontinued until the reaction abates. If blast cells appear or disease progression occurs, the treatment should be discontinued.

In order to avoid potential complications of excessive leukocytosis (WBC > 50,000 cells/mm³; ANC > 20,000 cells/mm³), a CBC with differential is recommended twice per week during PROKINE™ therapy. PROKINE treatment should be interrupted or the dose reduced by half if the ANC exceeds 20,000 cells/mm³.

Bone Marrow Transplantation Failure or Engraftment Delay

The recommended dose is 250 mcg/m²/day for 14 days as a 2 hour IV infusion. The dose can be repeated after 7 days off therapy if engraftment has not ccurred. If engraftment still has not occurred, a third course of 500 mcg/m²/day for 14 days may be tried after another 7 days off therapy. If there is still no improvement, it is unlikely that further dose escalation will be beneficial. If a severe adverse reaction occurs, the dose can be reduced or temporarily discontinued until the reaction abates. If blast cells appear or disease progression occurs, the treatment should be discontinued.

In order to avoid potential complications of excessive leukocytosis (WBC > 50,000 cells/mm³, ANC > 20,000 cells/mm³) a CBC with differential is recommended twice per week during PROKINE™ therapy. PROKINE treatment should be interrupted or the dose reduced by half if the ANC exceeds 20,000 cells/mm³.

Preparation of PROKINE

1. PROKINE is a sterile, white, preservative-free, lyophilized powder suitable for IV infusion upon reconstitution. PROKINE (250 mcg or 500 mcg vials) should be reconstituted aseptically with 1.0 ml Sterile Water for Injection, USP (without preservative). The reconstituted PROKINE

Continued on next page

Hoechst-Roussel—Cont.

solutions are clear, colorless, isotonic with a pH of 7.4±0.3, and contain 250 mcg or 500 mcg/ml of Sargramostim. The single-use vial should not be re-entered or reused. Do not save any unused portion for later administration.

2. During reconstitution the Sterile Water for Injection, USP should be directed at the side of the vial and the contents gently swirled to avoid foaming during dissolution. Avoid excessive or vigorous agitation; do not shake.
3. Dilution for IV infusion should be performed in 0.9% Sodium Chloride Injection, USP. If the final concentration of PROKINE is below 10 mcg/ml, Albumin (Human) at a final concentration of 0.1% should be added to the saline prior to addition of PROKINE to prevent adsorption to the components of the drug delivery system. To obtain a final concentration of 0.1% Albumin (Human), add 1 mg Albumin (Human) per 1 ml 0.9% Sodium Chloride Injection, USP (e.g. use 1 ml 5% Albumin (Human) in 50 ml 0.9% Sodium Chloride Injection, USP).
4. An in-line membrane filter should not be used for intravenous infusion of PROKINE.
5. PROKINE contains no antibacterial preservative and therefore should be administered as soon as possible, and within 6 hours following reconstitution and/or dilution for IV infusion. Store PROKINE solutions under refrigeration at 2–8°C (36–46°F); do not freeze. PROKINE vials are intended for single use only; discard any unused solution after 6 hours.
6. In the absence of compatibility and stability information, no other medication should be added to infusion solutions containing PROKINE. Use only 0.9% Sodium Chloride Injection, USP to prepare IV infusion solutions.
7. Aseptic technique should be employed in the preparation of all PROKINE™ solutions. To assure correct concentration following reconstitution, care should be exercised to eliminate any air bubbles from the needle hub of the syringe used to prepare the diluent. Parenteral drug products should be inspected visually for particulate matter and discoloration prior to administration whenever solution and container permit.

HOW SUPPLIED

PROKINE is available as a sterile, white, preservative-free, lyophilized powder in vials containing 250 mcg Sargramostim (1.25 × 10^7 units; NDC 0039-0113-01, NSN 6505-01-034-5511) or 500 mcg Sargramostim (2.50 × 10^7 units; NDC 0039-0114-01, NSN 6505-01-337-3121); 40 mg Mannitol, USP; 10 mg Sucrose, NF; and 1.2 mg Tromethamine, USP. Each dosage form is supplied packaged individually.

STORAGE

The sterile powder, the reconstituted solution and the diluted solution for injection should be refrigerated at 2–8°C (36–46°F). Do not freeze or shake. Do not use beyond the expiration date printed on the vial.

REFERENCES

1. Metcalf D. The molecular biology and functions of the granulocyte-macrophage colony-stimulating factors. Blood 1986; 67(2):257–267.
2. Park LS, Friend D, Gillis S, Urdal DL. Characterization of the cell surface receptor for human granulocyte/macrophage colony stimulating factor. J Exp Med 1986; 164:251–262.
3. Grabstein KH, Urdal DL, Tushinski RJ, *et al.* Induction of macrophage tumoricidal activity by granulocyte-macrophage colony-stimulating factors. Science 1986; 232:506–508.
4. Reed SG, Nathan CF, Pihl DL, *et al.* Recombinant granulocyte/macrophage colony-stimulating factor activates macrophages to inhibit *Trypanosoma cruzi* and release hydrogen peroxide. J Exp Med 1987; 166:1734–1746.
5. Shadduck RK, Waheed A, Evans C, *et al.* Serum and urinary levels of recombinant human granulocyte-macrophage colony stimulating factor: Assessment after intravenous infusion and subcutaneous injection. Exp Hem 1990; 18:601.
6. Nemunaitis J, Rabinowe SN, Singer JW, *et al.* Recombinant human granulocyte-macrophage colony-stimulating factor after autologous bone marrow transplantation for lymphoid malignancy: Pooled results of a randomized, double-blind, placebo controlled trial. NEJM 1991; 324(25):1773–1778.
7. Nemunaitis J, Singer JW, Buckner CD, *et al.* Use of recombinant human granulocyte-macrophage colony stimulating factor in autologous bone marrow transplantation for lymphoid malignancies. Blood 1988; 72(2):834–836.
8. Nemunaitis J, Singer JW, Buckner CD, *et al.* Long-term follow-up of patients who received recombinant human granulocyte-macrophage colony stimulating factor after autologous bone marrow transplantation for lymphoid malignancy. BMT 1991; 7:49–52.
9. Goris RJA, Boekhorst TPA, Nuytinck JKS, *et al.* Multiple organ failure: Generalized auto-destructive inflammation? Arch Sur 1985; 120:1109–1115.
10. Herrmann F, Schulz G, Lindemann A, *et al.* Yeast-expressed granulocyte-macrophage colony-stimulating factor in cancer patients: A phase Ib clinical study. In Behring Institute Research Communications, Colony Stimulating Factors-CSF. International Symposium, Garmisch-Partenkirchen, West Germany. 1988; 83:107–118.
11. Estey EH, Dixon D, Kantarjian H, *et al.* Treatment of poor-prognosis, newly diagnosed acute myeloid leukemia with Ara-C and recombinant human granulocyte-macrophage colony-stimulating factor. Blood 1990; 75(9):1766–1769.
12. Vadhan-Raj S, Keating M, LeMaistre A, *et al.* Effects of recombinant human granulocyte-macrophage colony-stimulating factor in patients with myelodysplastic syndromes. NEJM 1987; 317:1545–1552.
13. Buchner T, Hiddemann W, Koenigsmann M, *et al.* Recombinant human granulocyte-macrophage colony stimulating factor after chemotherapy in patients with acute myeloid leukemia at higher age or after relapse. Blood 1991; 78(5):1190–1197.
14. Blazar BR, Kersey JH, McGlave PB, *et al. In vivo* administration of recombinant human granulocyte/macrophage colony-stimulating factor in acute lymphoblastic leukemia patients receiving purged autografts. Blood 1989; 73(3):849–857.

Prokine is a trademark of Hoechst-Roussel Pharmaceuticals Inc., Somerville, NJ 08876-1258.

Manufactured by: IMMUNEX CORPORATION
Seattle, WA 98101
Distributed by: HOECHST-ROUSSEL
Pharmaceuticals Inc.
Somerville, NJ 08876-1258

US License No: 1132 711400-6/92

TOPICORT® ℞

[top' i-kort"]
(desoximetasone)
EMOLLIENT CREAM 0.25%

TOPICORT® LP

(desoximetasone)
EMOLLIENT CREAM 0.05%

TOPICORT® GEL

(desoximetasone) 0.05%

TOPICORT® OINTMENT

(desoximetasone) 0.25%

DESCRIPTION

Topicort® (desoximetasone) Emollient Cream 0.25%, Topicort® LP (desoximetasone) Emollient Cream 0.05%, Topicort® Gel (desoximetasone) 0.05%, and Topicort® Ointment (desoximetasone) 0.25% contain the active synthetic corticosteroid desoximetasone. The topical corticosteroids constitute a class of primarily synthetic steroids used as anti-inflammatory and anti-pruritic agents. Each gram of Topicort® (desoximetasone) Emollient Cream 0.25% contains 2.5 mg of desoximetasone in an emollient cream consisting of white petrolatum USP, purified water USP, isopropyl myristate NF, lanolin alcohols NF, mineral oil USP, cetostearyl alcohol NF, aluminum stearate and magnesium stearate.

Each gram of Topicort® LP (desoximetasone) Emollient Cream 0.05% contains 0.5 mg of desoximetasone in an emollient cream consisting of white petrolatum USP, purified water USP, isopropyl myristate NF, lanolin alcohols NF, mineral oil USP, cetostearyl alcohol NF, aluminum stearate, edetate disodium USP, lactic acid USP and magnesium stearate.

Each gram of Topicort® Gel (desoximetasone) 0.05% contains 0.5 mg desoximetasone in a gel consisting of purified water USP, SD alcohol 40 (20% w/w), isopropyl myristate NF, carbomer 940, trolamine NF, edetate disodium USP, and docusate sodium USP.

Each gram of Topicort® Ointment (desoximetasone) 0.25% contains 2.5 mg of desoximetasone in a base consisting of white petrolatum USP, propylene glycol USP, sorbitan sesquioleate, beeswax, fatty alcohol citrate, fatty acid pentaerythritol ester, aluminum stearate, citric acid, and butylated hydroxyanisole.

The chemical name of desoximetasone is Pregna-1, 4-diene-3, 20-dione, 9-fluoro-11, 21-dihydroxy-16-methyl-, (11β,16α)-.

Desoximetasone has the empirical formula $C_{22}H_{29}FO_4$ and a molecular weight of 376.47. The CAS Registry Number is 382-67-2.

The chemical structure is:

[See chemical structure at top of next column.]

CLINICAL PHARMACOLOGY

Topical corticosteroids share anti-inflammatory, anti-pruritic and vasoconstrictive actions.

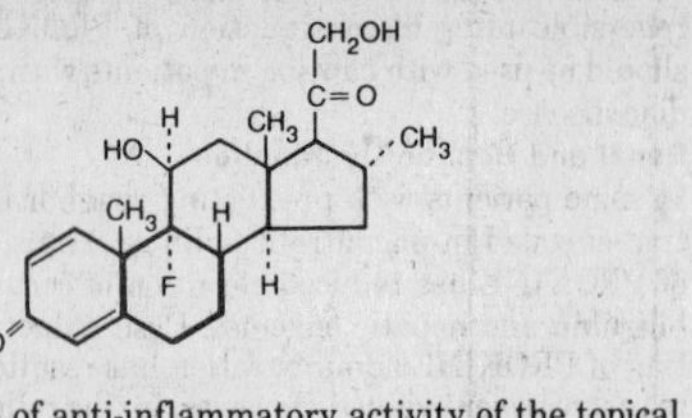

The mechanism of anti-inflammatory activity of the topical corticosteroids is unclear. Various laboratory methods, including vasoconstrictor assays, are used to compare and predict potencies and/or clinical efficacies of the topical corticosteroids. There is some evidence to suggest that a recognizable correlation exists between vasoconstrictor potency and therapeutic efficacy in man.

Pharmacokinetics

The extent of percutaneous absorption of topical corticosteroids is determined by many factors including the vehicle, the integrity of the epidermal barrier, and the use of occlusive dressings.

Topical corticosteroids can be absorbed from normal intact skin. Inflammation and/or other disease processes in the skin increase percutaneous absorption. Occlusive dressings substantially increase the percutaneous absorption of topical corticosteroids. Thus, occlusive dressings may be a valuable therapeutic adjunct for treatment of resistant dermatoses.

Once absorbed through the skin, topical corticosteroids are handled through pharmacokinetic pathways similar to systemically administered corticosteroids. Corticosteroids are bound to plasma proteins in varying degrees. Corticosteroids are metabolized primarily in the liver and are then excreted by the kidneys. Some of the topical corticosteroids and their metabolites are also excreted into the bile.

Pharmacokinetic studies in men with Topicort® (desoximetasone) Emollient Cream 0.25% with tagged desoximetasone showed a total of 5.2% ± 2.9% excretion in urine (4.1% ± 2.3%) and feces (1.1% ± 0.6%) and no detectable level (limit of sensitivity: 0.005 μg/mL) in the blood when it was applied topically on the back followed by occlusion for 24 hours. Seven days after application, no further radioactivity was detected in urine or feces. The half-life of the material was 15 ± 2 hours (for urine) and 17 ± 2 hours (for feces) between the third and fifth trial day.

Pharmacokinetic studies in men with Topicort® Ointment (desoximetasone) 0.25% with tagged desoximetasone showed no detectable level (limit of sensitivity: 0.003 μg/mL) in 1 subject and 0.004 and 0.006 μg/mL in the remaining 2 subjects in the blood when it was applied topically on the back followed by occlusion for 24 hours. The extent of absorption for the ointment was 7% based on radioactivity recovered from urine and feces. Seven days after application, no further radioactivity was detected in urine or feces.

Studies with other similarly structured steroids have shown that predominant metabolite reaction occurs through conjugation to form the glucuronide and sulfate ester.

INDICATIONS AND USAGE

Topicort® (desoximetasone) Emollient Cream 0.25%, Topicort® LP (desoximetasone) Emollient Cream 0.05%, Topicort® Gel (desoximetasone) 0.05% and Topicort® Ointment (desoximetasone) 0.25% are indicated for the relief of the inflammatory and pruritic manifestations of corticosteroid-responsive dermatoses.

CONTRAINDICATIONS

Topical corticosteroids are contraindicated in those patients with a history of hypersensitivity to any of the components of the preparation.

PRECAUTIONS

General

Systemic absorption of topical corticosteroids has produced reversible hypothalamic-pituitary-adrenal (HPA) axis suppression, manifestations of Cushing's syndrome, hyperglycemia, and glucosuria in some patients.

Conditions which augment systemic absorption include the application of the more potent steroids, use over large surface areas, prolonged use, and the addition of occlusive dressings.

Therefore, patients receiving a large dose of a potent topical steroid applied to a large surface area or under an occlusive dressing should be evaluated periodically for evidence of HPA axis suppression by using the urinary free cortisol and ACTH stimulation tests. If HPA axis suppression is noted, an attempt should be made to withdraw the drug, to reduce the frequency of application, or to substitute a less potent steroid.

Recovery of HPA axis function is generally prompt and complete upon discontinuation of the drug. Infrequently, signs and symptoms of steroid withdrawal may occur, requiring supplemental systemic corticosteroids.

Children may absorb proportionally larger amounts of topical corticosteroids and thus be more susceptible to systemic toxicity. (See **Precautions—Pediatric Use.**)

If irritation develops, topical corticosteroids should be discontinued and appropriate therapy instituted.

In the presence of dermatological infections, the use of an appropriate antifungal or antibacterial agent should be instituted. If a favorable response does not occur promptly, the corticosteroid should be discontinued until the infection has been adequately controlled.

Information for the Patient

Patients using topical corticosteroids should receive the following information and instructions:

1. This medication is to be used as directed by the physician. It is for external use only. Avoid contact with the eyes.
2. Patients should be advised not to use this medication for any disorder other than for which it was prescribed.
3. The treated skin area should not be bandaged or otherwise covered or wrapped as to be occlusive unless directed by the physician.
4. Patients should report any signs of local adverse reactions especially under occlusive dressing.
5. Parents of pediatric patients should be advised not to use tight-fitting diapers or plastic pants on a child being treated in the diaper area, as these garments may constitute occlusive dressings.

Laboratory Tests

The following tests may be helpful in evaluating the HPA axis suppression:

Urinary free cortisol test
ACTH stimulation test

Carcinogenesis, Mutagenesis, and Impairment of Fertility

Long-term animal studies have not been performed to evaluate the carcinogenic potential or the effect on fertility of topical corticosteroids.

Studies to determine mutagenicity with prednisolone and hydrocortisone have revealed negative results.

Pregnancy Category C

Corticosteroids are generally teratogenic in laboratory animals when administered systemically at relatively low dosage levels. The more potent corticosteroids have been shown to be teratogenic after dermal application in laboratory animals.

Desoximetasone has been shown to be teratogenic and embryotoxic in mice, rats, and rabbits when given by subcutaneous or dermal routes of administration in doses 3 to 30 times the human dose of Topicort® (desoximetasone) Emollient Cream 0.25% and Topicort® Ointment (desoximetasone) 0.25%, or 15 to 150 times the human dose of Topicort® LP (desoximetasone) Emollient Cream 0.05% and Topicort® Gel (desoximetasone) 0.05%.

There are no adequate and well-controlled studies in pregnant women on teratogenic effects from topically applied corticosteroids. Therefore, Topicort® (desoximetasone) Emollient Cream 0.25%, Topicort® LP (desoximetasone) Emollient Cream 0.05%, Topicort® Gel (desoximetasone) 0.05% and Topicort® Ointment (desoximetasone) 0.25% should be used during pregnancy only if the potential benefit justifies the potential risk to the fetus. Drugs of this class should not be used extensively on pregnant patients, in large amounts, or for prolonged periods of time.

Nursing Mothers

It is not known whether topical administration of corticosteroids could result in sufficient systemic absorption to produce detectable quantities in breast milk. Systemically administered corticosteroids are secreted into breast milk in quantities not likely to have a deleterious effect on the infant. Nevertheless, caution should be exercised when topical corticosteroids are administered to a nursing woman.

Pediatric Use

Pediatric patients may demonstrate greater susceptibility to topical corticosteroid-induced HPA axis suppression and Cushing's syndrome than mature patients because of a larger skin surface area to body weight ratio.

Hypothalamic-pituitary-adrenal (HPA) axis suppression, Cushing's syndrome, and intracranial hypertension have been reported in children receiving topical corticosteroids. Manifestations of adrenal suppression in children include linear growth retardation, delayed weight gain, low plasma cortisol levels, and absence of response to ACTH stimulation. Manifestations of intracranial hypertension include bulging fontanelles, headaches, and bilateral papilledema.

Administration of topical corticosteroids to children should be limited to the least amount compatible with an effective therapeutic regimen. Chronic corticosteroid therapy may interfere with the growth and development of children. The safety and effectiveness of Topicort® Ointment (desoximetasone) 0.25% in children below the age of 10 have not been established.

ADVERSE REACTIONS

The following local adverse reactions are reported infrequently with topical corticosteroids, but may occur more frequently with the use of occlusive dressings. These reactions are listed in an approximate decreasing order of occurrence:

Burning	Perioral dermatitis
Itching	Allergic contact dermatitis
Irritation	Maceration of the skin
Dryness	Secondary infection
Folliculitis	Skin Atrophy
Hypertrichosis	Striae
Acneiform eruptions	Miliaria
Hypopigmentation	

In controlled clinical studies the incidence of adverse reactions was low (0.8%) for Topicort® (desoximetasone) Emollient Cream 0.25% and included burning, folliculitis and folliculo-pustular lesions. The incidence of adverse reactions was also 0.8% for Topicort® LP (desoximetasone) Emollient Cream 0.05% and included pruritus, erythema, vesiculation and burning sensation. In controlled clinical studies the incidence of adverse reactions was low (0.3%) for Topicort® Ointment (desoximetasone) 0.25% and consisted of development of comedones at the site of application.

OVERDOSAGE

Topically applied corticosteroids can be absorbed in sufficient amounts to produce systemic effects. (See **Precautions**.)

DOSAGE AND ADMINISTRATION

Apply a thin film of Topicort® (desoximetasone) Emollient Cream 0.25%, Topicort® LP (desoximetasone) Emollient Cream 0.05%, Topicort® Gel (desoximetasone) 0.05% or Topicort® Ointment (desoximetasone) 0.25% to the affected skin areas twice daily. Rub in gently.

HOW SUPPLIED

Topicort® (desoximetasone) Emollient Cream 0.25% is supplied in 15 gram (NDC 0039-0011-23), 60 gram (NDC 0039-0011-60) and 4 ounce (NDC 0039-0011-04) tubes.

Topicort® LP (desoximetasone) Emollient Cream 0.05% is supplied in 15 gram (NDC 0039-0012-23) and 60 gram (NDC 0039-0012-60) tubes.

Topicort® Gel (desoximetasone) 0.05% is supplied in 15 gram (NDC 0039-0014-23) and 60 gram (NDC 0039-0014-60) tubes.

Topicort® Ointment (desoximetasone) 0.25% is supplied in 15 gram (NDC 0039-0025-15) and 60 gram (NDC 0039-0025-60) tubes.

Store at controlled room temperature (59°-86°F).

Topicort® REG TM Roussel Uclaf

711000-1/89
725000-2/89
714000-2/89

Shown in Product Identification Section, page 412

TRENTAL® ℞
(pentoxifylline)*
Tablets, 400 mg

DESCRIPTION

Trental® (pentoxifylline) tablets for oral administration contain 400 mg of the active drug and the following inactive ingredients: benzyl alcohol NF, D&C Red #27 Aluminum Lake or FD&C Red No. 30, hydroxypropyl methylcellulose USP, magnesium stearate NF, polyethylene glycol NF, povidone USP, talc USP, titanium dioxide USP, and other ingredients in a controlled-release formulation. Trental® (pentoxifylline) is a trisubstituted xanthine derivative designated chemically as 1-(5-oxohexyl)-3, 7-dimethylxanthine that, unlike theophylline, is a hemorheologic agent, i.e. an agent that affects blood viscosity. Pentoxifylline is soluble in water and ethanol, and sparingly soluble in toluene.

The chemical structure is:

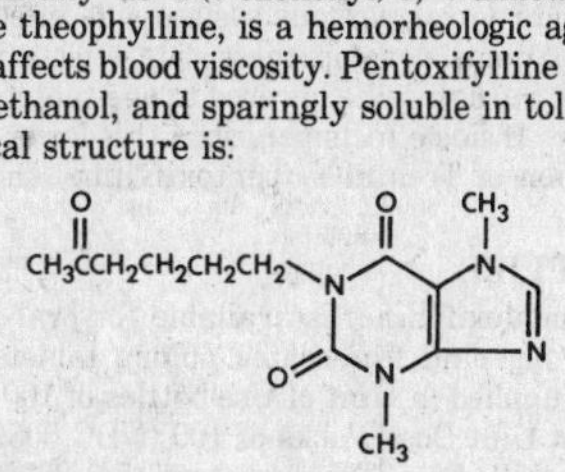

$CH_3\overset{O}{\overset{\|}{C}}CH_2CH_2CH_2CH_2$
O
CH_3
N
N
N
N
O
CH_3

CLINICAL PHARMACOLOGY

Mode of Action

Pentoxifylline and its metabolites improve the flow properties of blood by decreasing its viscosity. In patients with chronic peripheral arterial disease, this increases blood flow to the affected microcirculation and enhances tissue oxygenation. The precise mode of action of pentoxifylline and the sequence of events leading to clinical improvement are still to be defined. Pentoxifylline administration has been shown to produce dose related hemorheologic effects, lowering blood viscosity, and improving erythrocyte flexibility. Tissue oxygen levels have been shown to be significantly increased by therapeutic doses of pentoxifylline in patients with peripheral arterial disease.

Pharmacokinetics and Metabolism

After oral administration in aqueous solution pentoxifylline is almost completely absorbed. It undergoes a first-pass effect and the various metabolites appear in plasma very soon after dosing. Peak plasma levels of the parent compound and its metabolites are reached within 1 hour. The major metabolites are Metabolite I (1-[5-hydroxyhexyl]-3,7-dimethylxanthine) and Metabolite V (1-[3-carboxypropyl]-3,-7-dimethylxanthine), and plasma levels of these metabolites are 5 and 8 times greater, respectively, than pentoxifylline.

Following oral administration of aqueous solutions containing 100 to 400 mg of pentoxifylline, the pharmacokinetics of the parent compound and Metabolite I are dose-related and not proportional (non-linear), with half-life and area under the blood-level time curve (AUC) increasing with dose. The elimination kinetics of Metabolite V are not dose-dependent. The apparent plasma half-life of pentoxifylline varies from 0.4 to 0.8 hours and the apparent plasma half-lives of its metabolites vary from 1 to 1.6 hours. There is no evidence of accumulation or enzyme induction (Cytochrome P_{450}) following multiple oral doses.

Excretion is almost totally urinary; the main biotransformation product is Metabolite V. Essentially no parent drug is found in the urine. Despite large variations in plasma levels of parent compound and its metabolites, the urinary recovery of Metabolite V is consistent and shows dose proportionality. Less than 4% of the administered dose is recovered in feces. Food intake shortly before dosing delays absorption of an immediate release dosage form but does not affect total absorption. The pharmacokinetics and metabolism of Trental® (pentoxifylline) have not been studied in patients with renal and/or hepatic dysfunction, but AUC was increased and elimination rate decreased in an older population (60–68 years) compared to younger individuals (22–30 years).

After administration of the 400 mg controlled-release Trental® (pentoxifylline) tablet, plasma levels of the parent compound and its metabolites reach their maximum within 2 to 4 hours and remain constant over an extended period of time. The controlled release of pentoxifylline from the tablet eliminates peaks and troughs in plasma levels for improved gastrointestinal tolerance.

INDICATIONS AND USAGE

Trental® (pentoxifylline) is indicated for the treatment of patients with intermittent claudication on the basis of chronic occlusive arterial disease of the limbs. Trental® (pentoxifylline) can improve function and symptoms but is not intended to replace more definitive therapy, such as surgical bypass, or removal of arterial obstructions when treating peripheral vascular disease.

CONTRAINDICATIONS

Trental® (pentoxifylline) should not be used in patients who have previously exhibited intolerance to this product or methylxanthines such as caffeine, theophylline, and theobromine.

PRECAUTIONS

General: Patients with chronic occlusive arterial disease of the limbs frequently show other manifestations of arteriosclerotic disease. Trental® (pentoxifylline) has been used safely for treatment of peripheral arterial disease in patients with concurrent coronary artery and cerebrovascular diseases, but there have been occasional reports of angina, hypotension, and arrhythmia. Controlled trials do not show that Trental® (pentoxifylline) causes such adverse effects more often than placebo, but, as it is a methylxanthine derivative, it is possible some individuals will experience such responses.

Drug Interactions: Although a causal relationship has not been established, there have been reports of bleeding and/or prolonged prothrombin time in patients treated with Trental® (pentoxifylline) with and without anticoagulants or platelet aggregation inhibitors. Patients on warfarin should have more frequent monitoring of prothrombin times, while patients with other risk factors complicated by hemorrhage (e.g., recent surgery, peptic ulceration) should have periodic examinations for bleeding including hematocrit and/or hemoglobin. Trental® (pentoxifylline) has been used concurrently with antihypertensive drugs, beta blockers, digitalis, diuretics, antidiabetic agents, and antiarrhythmics, without observed problems. Small decreases in blood pressure have been observed in some patients treated with Trental® (pentoxifylline); periodic systemic blood pressure monitoring is recommended for patients receiving concomitant antihypertensive therapy. If indicated, dosage of the antihypertensive agents should be reduced.

Carcinogenesis, Mutagenesis and Impairment of Fertility: Long-term studies of the carcinogenic potential of pentoxifylline were conducted in mice and rats by dietary administration of the drug at doses up to approximately 24 times (570 mg/kg) the maximum recommended human daily dose (MRHD) of 24 mg/kg for 18 months in mice and 18 months in rats with an additional 6 months without drug exposure in the latter. No carcinogenic potential for pentoxifylline was noted in the mouse study. In the rat study, there was a

Continued on next page

*U.S. Patents 3,737,433 and 4,189,469

Hoechst-Roussel—Cont.

INCIDENCE (%) OF SIDE EFFECTS

	Controlled-Release Tablets Commercially Available		Immediate-Release Capsules Used only for Controlled Clinical Trials	
	Trental®	Placebo	Trental®	Placebo
(Numbers of Patients at Risk)	(321)	(128)	(177)	(138)
Discontinued for Side Effect	3.1	0	9.6	7.2
CARDIOVASCULAR SYSTEM				
Angina/Chest pain	0.3	—	1.1	2.2
Arrhythmia/Palpitation	—	—	1.7	0.7
Flushing	—	—	2.3	0.7
DIGESTIVE SYSTEM				
Abdominal Discomfort	—	—	4.0	1.4
Belching/Flatus/Bloating	0.6	—	9.0	3.6
Diarrhea	—	—	3.4	2.9
Dyspepsia	2.8	4.7	9.6	2.9
Nausea	2.2	0.8	28.8	8.7
Vomiting	1.2	—	4.5	0.7
NERVOUS SYSTEM				
Agitation/Nervousness	—	—	1.7	0.7
Dizziness	1.9	3.1	11.9	4.3
Drowsiness	—	—	1.1	5.8
Headache	1.2	1.6	6.2	5.8
Insomnia	—	—	2.3	2.2
Tremor	0.3	0.8	—	—
Blurred Vision	—	—	2.3	1.4

statistically significant increase in benign mammary fibroadenomas in females in the high dose group (24 × MRHD). The relevance of this finding to human use is uncertain since this was only a marginal statistically significant increase for a tumor that is common in aged rats. Pentoxifylline was devoid of mutagenic activity in various strains of *Salmonella* (Ames test) when tested in the presence and absence of metabolic activation.

Pregnancy: Category C. Teratogenic studies have been performed in rats and rabbits at oral doses up to about 25 and 10 times the maximum recommended human daily dose (MRHD) of 24 mg/kg, respectively. No evidence of fetal malformation was observed. Increased resorption was seen in rats at 25 times MRHD. There are, however, no adequate and well controlled studies in pregnant women. Because animal reproduction studies are not always predictive of human response, Trental® (pentoxifylline) should be used during pregnancy only if clearly needed.

Nursing Mothers: Pentoxifylline and its metabolites are excreted in human milk. Because of the potential for tumorigenicity shown for pentoxifylline in rats, a decision should be made whether to discontinue nursing or discontinue the drug, taking into account the importance of the drug to the mother.

Pediatric Use: Safety and effectiveness in children below the age of 18 years have not been established.

ADVERSE REACTIONS

Clinical trials were conducted using either controlled-release Trental® (pentoxifylline) tablets for up to 60 weeks or immediate-release Trental® (pentoxifylline) capsules for up to 24 weeks. Dosage ranges in the tablet studies were 400 mg bid to tid and in the capsule studies, 200–400 mg tid.

The table summarizes the incidence (in percent) of adverse reactions considered drug related, as well as the numbers of patients who received controlled-release Trental® (pentoxifylline) tablets, immediate-release Trental® (pentoxifylline) capsules, or the corresponding placebos. The incidence of adverse reactions was higher in the capsule studies (where dose related increases were seen in digestive and nervous system side effects) than in the tablet studies. Studies with the capsule include domestic experience, whereas studies with the controlled-release tablets were conducted outside the U.S. The table indicates that in the tablet studies few patients discontinued because of adverse effects.

[See table above.]

Trental® (pentoxifylline) has been marketed in Europe and elsewhere since 1972. In addition to the above symptoms, the following have been reported spontaneously since marketing or occurred in other clinical trials with an incidence of less than 1%; the causal relationship was uncertain:

Cardiovascular—dyspnea, edema, hypotension.

Digestive—anorexia, cholecystitis, constipation, dry mouth/thirst.

Nervous—anxiety, confusion.

Respiratory—epistaxis, flu-like symptoms, laryngitis, nasal congestion.

Skin and Appendages—brittle fingernails, pruritus, rash, urticaria, angioedema.

Special Senses—blurred vision, conjunctivitis, earache, scotoma.

Miscellaneous—bad taste, excessive salivation, leukopenia, malaise, sore throat/swollen neck glands, weight change.

A few rare events have been reported spontaneously worldwide since marketing in 1972. Although they occurred under circumstances in which a causal relationship with pentoxifylline could not be established, they are listed to serve as information for physicians: Cardiovascular—angina, arrhythmia, tachycardia; Digestive—hepatitis, jaundice, increased liver enzymes; and Hemic and Lymphatic—decreased serum fibrinogen, pancytopenia, aplastic anemia, purpura, thrombocytopenia.

OVERDOSAGE

Overdosage with Trental® (pentoxifylline) has been reported in children and adults. Symptoms appear to be dose related. A report from a poison control center on 44 patients taking overdoses of enteric-coated pentoxifylline tablets noted that symptoms usually occurred 4–5 hours after ingestion and lasted about 12 hours. The highest amount ingested was 80 mg/kg; flushing, hypotension, convulsions, somnolence, loss of consciousness, fever, and agitation occurred. All patients recovered.

In addition to symptomatic treatment and gastric lavage, special attention must be given to supporting respiration, maintaining systemic blood pressure, and controlling convulsions. Activated charcoal has been used to adsorb pentoxifylline in patients who have overdosed.

DOSAGE AND ADMINISTRATION

The usual dosage of Trental® (pentoxifylline) in controlled-release tablet form is one tablet (400 mg) three times a day with meals.

While the effect of Trental® (pentoxifylline) may be seen within 2 to 4 weeks, it is recommended that treatment be continued for at least 8 weeks. Efficacy has been demonstrated in double-blind clinical studies of 6 months duration. Digestive and central nervous system side effects are dose related. If patients develop these side effects it is recommended that the dosage be lowered to one tablet twice a day (800 mg/day). If side effects persist at this lower dosage, the administration of Trental® (pentoxifylline) should be discontinued.

HOW SUPPLIED

Trental® (pentoxifylline) is available for oral administration as 400 mg pink film-coated oblong tablets imprinted Trental®; supplied in Unit of Use bottles of 100 (NDC 0039-0078-10) and Unit Dose Packs of 100 (NDC 0039-0078-11). Store at controlled room temperature (59°–86°F). Dispense in well closed, light resistant containers. Protect blisters from light.

778010-2/91

The CAS Registry Number is 6493-05-6.

Trental® REG TM Hoechst AG

Shown in Product Identification Section, page 412

Products are
listed alphabetically
in the
PINK SECTION.

ICI Pharma
A Business Unit of ICI Americas Inc.
WILMINGTON, DE 19897 USA

NOLVADEX® 10 mg Tablets ℞
[*nol'va-dex"*]
(tamoxifen citrate)

DESCRIPTION

NOLVADEX® (tamoxifen citrate) tablets for oral administration contain 15.2 mg of tamoxifen citrate, which is equivalent to 10 mg of tamoxifen. It is a nonsteroidal antiestrogen. Chemically, NOLVADEX is the trans-isomer of a triphenylethylene derivative. The chemical name is (Z) 2-[4-(1,2-diphenyl-1-butenyl) phenoxy]-N, N-dimethylethanamine 2-hydroxy-1,2,3-propanetricarboxylate (1:1). The structural and empirical formulas are:

$$(CH_3)_2N(CH_2)_2O \cdots C{=}C \cdots \cdot C_6H_8O_7$$
$$C_2H_5$$

$$(C_{32}H_{37}NO_8)$$

Tamoxifen citrate has a molecular weight of 563.62, the pKa' is 8.85, the equilibrium solubility in water at 37°C is 0.5 mg/mL and in 0.02 N HCl at 37°C, it is 0.2 mg/mL. NOLVADEX is intended only for oral administration; the tablets should be protected from heat and light.

Inactive ingredients: carboxymethylcellulose calcium, magnesium stearate, mannitol, starch.

CLINICAL PHARMACOLOGY

NOLVADEX is a nonsteroidal agent which has demonstrated potent antiestrogenic properties in animal test systems. The antiestrogenic effects may be related to its ability to compete with estrogen for binding sites in target tissues such as breast. Tamoxifen inhibits the induction of rat mammary carcinoma induced by dimethylbenzanthracene (DMBA) and causes the regression of already established DMBA-induced tumors. In this rat model, tamoxifen appears to exert its antitumor effects by binding to estrogen receptors.

In cytosols derived from human breast adenocarcinomas, tamoxifen competes with estradiol for estrogen receptor protein. Preliminary pharmacokinetics in women using radiolabeled tamoxifen has shown that most of the radioactivity is slowly excreted in the feces, with only small amounts appearing in urine. The drug is excreted mainly as conjugates, with unchanged drug and hydroxylated metabolites accounting for 30% of the total.

Blood levels of total radioactivity following single oral doses of approximately 0.3 mg/kg reached peak values of 0.06–0.14 μg/mL at 4–7 hours after dosing, with only 20%–30% of the drug present as tamoxifen. There was an initial half-life of 7–14 hours with secondary peaks four or more days later. The prolongation of blood levels and fecal excretion is believed to be due to enterohepatic circulation.

Two studies (Hubay and NSABP B-09) demonstrated an improved disease-free survival following radical or modified radical mastectomy in postmenopausal women or women 50 years of age or older with surgically curable breast cancer with positive axillary nodes when NOLVADEX was added to adjuvant cytotoxic chemotherapy. In the Hubay study, NOLVADEX was added to "low-dose" CMF (cyclophosphamide, methotrexate and fluorouracil). In the NSABP B-09 study, NOLVADEX was added to melphalan [L-phenylalanine mustard (P)] and fluorouracil (F).

Tumor hormone receptors may help predict which patients will benefit from the adjuvant therapy, but not all breast cancer adjuvant NOLVADEX studies have shown a clear relationship between hormone receptor status and treatment effect. In the Hubay study, patients with a positive (more than 3 fmol) estrogen receptor were more likely to benefit. In the NSABP B-09 study in women age 50–59 years, only women with both estrogen and progesterone receptor levels 10 fmol or greater clearly benefited, while there was a nonstatistically significant trend toward adverse effect in women with both estrogen and progesterone receptor levels less than 10 fmol. In women age 60–70 years, there was a trend toward a beneficial effect of NOLVADEX without any clear relationship to estrogen or progesterone receptor status.

Three prospective studies (ECOG-1178, Toronto, NATO) using NOLVADEX adjuvantly as a single agent demonstrated an improved disease-free survival following total mastectomy and axillary dissection for postmenopausal women with positive axillary nodes compared to placebo/no treatment controls. The NATO study also demonstrated an overall survival benefit.

One prospective, double-blind, randomized study (NSABP-14) demonstrated a significant improvement in disease-free

survival for NOLVADEX compared to placebo when used adjuvantly following total mastectomy and axillary dissection or segmental resection, axillary dissection, and breast radiation in women with axillary node-negative breast cancer whose tumors were estrogen receptor positive (≥ 10 fmol/mg cytosol protein). The benefit was apparent in both women under age 50 and those aged 50 years or more. One additional randomized study (NATO) demonstrated improved disease-free survival for NOLVADEX compared to no adjuvant therapy following total mastectomy and axillary dissection in postmenopausal women with axillary node-negative breast cancer. In this study, the benefits of NOLVADEX appeared to be independent of estrogen receptor status.

Three prospective, randomized studies (Ingle, Pritchard, Buchanan) compared NOLVADEX to ovarian ablation (oophorectomy or ovarian irradiation) in premenopausal women with advanced breast cancer. Although the objective response rate, time to treatment failure, and survival were similar with both treatments, the limited patient accrual prevented a demonstration of equivalence. In an overview analysis of survival data from the three studies, the hazard ratio for death (NOLVADEX/ovarian ablation) was 1.00 with two-sided 95% confidence intervals of 0.73 to 1.37. Elevated serum and plasma estrogens have been observed in premenopausal women receiving NOLVADEX. However, the data from the randomized studies do not suggest an adverse effect. A limited number of premenopausal patients with disease progression during NOLVADEX therapy responded to subsequent ovarian ablation.

INDICATIONS AND USAGE

Adjuvant Therapy: NOLVADEX is effective in delaying recurrence following total mastectomy and axillary dissection or segmental mastectomy, axillary dissection, and breast irradiation in women with axillary node-negative breast cancer. Data are insufficient to predict which women are most likely to benefit and to determine if NOLVADEX provides any benefit in women with tumors less than 1 cm. NOLVADEX is effective in delaying recurrence following total mastectomy and axillary dissection in postmenopausal women with breast cancer (T_{1-3}, N_1, M_0). In some NOLVADEX adjuvant studies, most of the benefit to date has been in the subgroup with 4 or more positive axillary nodes.

The estrogen and progesterone receptor values may help to predict whether adjuvant NOLVADEX therapy is likely to be beneficial.

Therapy for Advanced Disease: NOLVADEX is effective in the treatment of metastatic breast cancer in women. In premenopausal women with metastatic breast cancer, NOLVADEX is an alternative to oophorectomy or ovarian irradiation. Available evidence indicates that patients whose tumors are estrogen receptor positive are more likely to benefit from NOLVADEX therapy.

CONTRAINDICATIONS

NOLVADEX is contraindicated in patients with known hypersensitivity to the drug.

WARNINGS

Visual disturbance including corneal changes, cataracts and retinopathy have been reported in patients receiving NOLVADEX.

As with other additive hormonal therapy (estrogens and androgens), hypercalcemia has been reported in some breast cancer patients with bone metastases within a few weeks of starting treatment with NOLVADEX. If hypercalcemia does occur, appropriate measures should be taken and, if severe, NOLVADEX should be discontinued.

A small number of cases of endometrial hyperplasia and endometrial polyps have been reported in association with NOLVADEX treatment. A definitive relationship to NOLVADEX therapy has not been established.

In a single large randomized trial in Sweden of adjuvant tamoxifen 40 mg/day for 2–5 years, an increased incidence of endometrial cancer was noted. Thirteen of 931 tamoxifen treated patients versus 2 of 915 controls developed cancer of the body of the uterus [RR = 6.4 (1.4 − 28), P < 0.01]. However, in a review of more than 12,000 patients entered into twelve other large ongoing adjuvant studies (including NSABP B-14) in which patients have received NOLVADEX 20–40 mg/day for periods of 1–5+ years versus control, no increased incidence of cancer of the uterus was seen.

In the same Swedish trial, the incidence of second primary breast tumors was reduced in the tamoxifen arm (P < 0.05). In the NSABP B-14 trial in which patients were randomized to NOLVADEX 20 mg/day for 5 years versus placebo, the incidence of second primary breast cancers is also reduced.

Pregnancy Category D: NOLVADEX may cause fetal harm when administered to a pregnant woman. Individuals should not become pregnant while taking NOLVADEX and should use barrier or nonhormonal contraceptive measures. Effects on reproductive functions are expected from the antiestrogenic properties of the drug. In reproductive studies in rats at dose levels equal to or below the human dose, nonteratogenic developmental skeletal changes were seen and were found to be reversible. In addition, in fertility studies in rats and in teratology studies in rabbits using doses at or below those used in humans, a lower incidence of embryo implantation and a higher incidence of fetal death or retarded in utero growth were observed, with slower learning behavior in some rat pups. The impairment of learning behavior did not achieve statistical significance in one study, and, in another study where significance was reported, this was by comparing dosed animals with controls of another study. Several pregnant marmosets were dosed during organogenesis or in the last half of pregnancy. No deformations were seen, and although the dose was high enough to terminate pregnancy in some animals, those that did maintain pregnancy showed no evidence of teratogenic malformations. There are no adequate and well-controlled studies in pregnant women. There have been reports of spontaneous abortions, birth defects, fetal deaths, and vaginal bleeding. If this drug is used during pregnancy or the patient becomes pregnant while taking this drug, the patient should be apprised of the potential hazard to the fetus.

PRECAUTIONS

General: NOLVADEX should be used cautiously in patients with existing leukopenia or thrombocytopenia. Observations of leukopenia and thrombocytopenia occasionally have been reported. Decreases in platelet counts, usually to 50,000–100,000/mm³, infrequently lower, have been occasionally reported in patients taking NOLVADEX for breast cancer. In patients with significant thrombocytopenia, rare hemorrhagic episodes have occurred, but it is uncertain if these episodes are due to NOLVADEX therapy.

Information for Patients: Women taking NOLVADEX should be instructed to report abnormal vaginal bleeding which should be promptly investigated.

Laboratory Tests: Periodic complete blood counts, including platelet counts, may be appropriate.

Drug Interactions: When NOLVADEX is used in combination with coumarin-type anticoagulants, a significant increase in anticoagulant effect may occur. Where such coadministration exists, careful monitoring of the patient's prothrombin time is recommended.

Drug/Laboratory Testing Interactions: During postmarketing surveillance, T_4 elevations were reported for a few postmenopausal patients which may be explained by increases in thyroid-binding globulin. These elevations were not accompanied by clinical hyperthyroidism.

Variations in the karyopyknotic index on vaginal smears and various degrees of estrogen effect on Pap smears have been infrequently seen in postmenopausal patients given NOLVADEX.

In the postmarketing experience with NOLVADEX, infrequent cases of hyperlipidemias have been reported. Periodic monitoring of plasma triglycerides and cholesterol may be indicated in patients with pre-existing hyperlipidemias.

Carcinogenesis: A conventional carcinogenesis study in rats, (doses of 5, 20, and 35 mg/kg/day for up to 2 years) revealed hepatocellular carcinoma at all doses, and the incidence of these tumors was significantly greater among rats given 20 or 35 mg/kg/day (69%) than those given 5 mg/kg/day (14%). The incidence of these tumors in rats given 5 mg/kg/day (29.5 mg/m²) was significantly greater than in controls.

In addition, preliminary data from 2 independent reports of 6-month studies in rats reveal liver tumors which in one study are classified as malignant.

Endocrine changes in immature and mature mice were investigated in a 13-month study. Granulosa cell ovarian tumors and interstitial cell testicular tumors were found in mice receiving NOLVADEX, but not in the controls.

Mutagenesis: No genotoxic potential has been found in a battery of in vivo and in vitro tests with pro- and eukaryotic test systems with drug metabolizing systems present.

Impairment of Fertility: Fertility in female rats was decreased following administration of 0.04 mg/kg for two weeks prior to mating through day 7 of pregnancy. There was a decreased number of implantations, and all fetuses were found dead.

Following administration to rats of 0.16 mg/kg from day 7–17 of pregnancy, there were increased numbers of fetal deaths. Administration of 0.125 mg/kg to rabbits during days 6–18 of pregnancy resulted in abortion or premature delivery. Fetal deaths occurred at higher doses. There were no teratogenic changes in either rat or rabbit segment II studies. Several pregnant marmosets were dosed with 10 mg/kg/day either during organogenesis or in the last half of pregnancy. No deformations were seen, and although the dose was high enough to terminate pregnancy in some animals, those that did maintain pregnancy showed no evidence of teratogenic malformations. Rats given 0.16 mg/kg from day 17 of pregnancy to 1 day before weaning demonstrated increased numbers of dead pups at parturition. It was reported that some rat pups showed slower learning behavior, but this did not achieve statistical significance in one study, and in another study where significance was reported, this was obtained by comparing dosed animals with controls of another study.

The recommended daily human dose of 20–40 mg corresponds to 0.4–0.8 mg/kg for an average 50 kg woman.

Pregnancy Category D: See WARNINGS.

Nursing Mothers: It is not known whether this drug is excreted in human milk. Because many drugs are excreted in human milk and because of the potential for serious adverse reactions in nursing infants from NOLVADEX, a decision should be made whether to discontinue nursing or to discontinue the drug, taking into account the importance of the drug to the mother.

ADVERSE REACTIONS

Adverse reactions to NOLVADEX are relatively mild and rarely severe enough to require discontinuation of treatment. If adverse reactions are severe, it is sometimes possible to control them by a simple reduction of dosage without loss of control of the disease.

In patients treated with NOLVADEX for metastatic breast cancer, the most frequent adverse reactions to NOLVADEX are hot flashes and nausea and/or vomiting. These may occur in up to one-fourth of patients.

Less frequently reported adverse reactions are vaginal bleeding, vaginal discharge, menstrual irregularities and skin rash. Usually these have not been of sufficient severity to require dosage reduction or discontinuation of treatment. Increased bone and tumor pain and, also, local disease flare have occurred, which are sometimes associated with a good tumor response. Patients with increased bone pain may require additional analgesics. Patients with soft tissue disease may have sudden increases in the size of preexisting lesions, sometimes associated with marked erythema within and surrounding the lesions and/or the development of new lesions. When they occur, the bone pain or disease flare are seen shortly after starting NOLVADEX and generally subside rapidly.

Other adverse reactions which are seen infrequently are hypercalcemia, peripheral edema, distaste for food, pruritus vulvae, depression, dizziness, light-headedness and headache.

There have been infrequent reports of thromboembolic events occurring during NOLVADEX therapy. Since for cancer patients in general an increased incidence of thromboembolic events is known to occur, a causal relationship to NOLVADEX remains conjectural. An increased incidence has been reported when cytotoxic agents are combined with NOLVADEX.

Ovarian cysts have been observed in a small number of premenopausal patients with advanced breast cancer who have been treated with NOLVADEX.

Continued clinical studies have resulted in further information which better indicates the incidence of adverse reactions with NOLVADEX as compared to placebo.

In the ongoing NSABP study B-14, patients with axillary node-negative breast cancer were randomized to 5 years of NOLVADEX or placebo following primary surgery. The reported adverse effects are tabulated below (mean follow-up of 29 months). The incidence of hot flashes (57% v 41%), vaginal discharge (24% v 12%), and irregular menses (19% v 15%) were higher with NOLVADEX compared with placebo. The incidence of all other adverse effects were similar in the two treatment groups with the exception of thromboembolic events (phlebitis), which although rare, were more common with NOLVADEX than with placebo.

[See table at top of next page.]

In the Eastern Cooperative Oncology Group (ECOG) adjuvant breast cancer trial, NOLVADEX or placebo was administered for 2 years to patients following mastectomy. When compared to placebo, NOLVADEX showed a significantly higher incidence of hot flashes (19% versus 8% for placebo). The incidence of all other adverse reactions was similar in the 2 treatment groups with the exception of thrombocytopenia where the incidence for NOLVADEX was 10% versus 3% for placebo, an observation of borderline statistical significance.

The other adverse reactions reported equally in the ECOG study for NOLVADEX and placebo include abnormal renal function tests, fatigue, dyspnea, anorexia, cough, and abdominal cramps. A relationship of these reactions to the administration of NOLVADEX has not been demonstrated since the frequency was not significantly different from that reported in placebo treated patients.

In other adjuvant studies, Toronto and NOLVADEX Adjuvant Trial Organization (NATO), patients received either NOLVADEX or no therapy. In the Toronto study, hot flashes and nausea and/or vomiting were observed in 29% and 19% of patients, respectively, for NOLVADEX versus 1% and 0% in the untreated group. In the NATO trial, hot flashes, nausea and/or vomiting and vaginal bleeding were reported in 2.8%, 2.1%, and 2.0% of patients, respectively, for NOLVADEX versus 0.2% for each in the untreated group. The following table summarizes the incidence of adverse reactions reported at a frequency of 2% or greater from clinical trials (Ingle, Pritchard, Buchanan) which compared

Continued on next page

ICI Pharma—Cont.

NSABP B-14 STUDY

Adverse Effect	No. of Patients (%)			
	NOLVADEX (n=1376)		Placebo (n=1396)	
Hot flashes	787	(57)	566	(41)
Fluid retention	339	(25)	326	(23)
Vaginal discharge	330	(24)	160	(12)
Irregular menses	264	(19)	203	(15)
Nausea	255	(19)	235	(17)
Skin rash	180	(13)	150	(11)
Diarrhea	106	(8)	129	(9)
Vomiting	25	(2)	16	(1)
Phlebitis	15	(1)	2	(<1)
Thrombocytopenia*	10	(1)	4	(<1)
Leukopenia**	7	(1)	10	(1)

*Defined as a platelet count of <100,000/mm³
**Defined as a white blood cell count of <3000/mm³

Adverse Reactions*	NOLVADEX All Effects Number of Patients (%) n=104		OVARIAN ABLATION All Effects Number of Patients (%) n=100	
Flush	34	(32.7)	46	(46)
Amenorrhea	17	(16.3)	69	(69)
Altered Menses	13	(12.5)	5	(5)
Oligomenorrhea	9	(8.7)	1	(1)
Bone Pain	6	(5.7)	6	(6)
Menstrual Disorder	6	(5.7)	4	(4)
Nausea	5	(4.8)	4	(4)
Cough/Coughing	4	(3.8)	1	(1)
Edema	4	(3.8)	1	(1)
Fatigue	4	(3.8)	1	(1)
Musculoskeletal Pain	3	(2.8)	0	(0)
Pain	3	(2.8)	4	(4)
Ovarian Cyst(s)	3	(2.8)	2	(2)
Depression	2	(1.9)	2	(2)
Abdominal Cramps	1	(1)	2	(2)
Anorexia	1	(1)	2	(2)

*Some patients had more than one adverse reaction.

NOLVADEX therapy to ovarian ablation in premenopausal patients with metastatic breast cancer.
[See second above.]

OVERDOSAGE

Acute overdosage in humans has not been reported. Signs observed at the highest doses following studies to determine LD₅₀ in animals were respiratory difficulties and convulsions. No specific treatment for overdosage is known; treatment must be symptomatic.

DOSAGE AND ADMINISTRATION

One or two 10 mg tablets twice a day (morning and evening). In three single agent adjuvant studies, one 10 mg NOLVADEX tablet was administered two (ECOG and NATO) or three (Toronto) times a day for two years (see Clincial Pharmacology). In the ongoing NSABP study B-14, one 10 mg NOLVADEX tablet is being given twice a day for five years. The optimal duration of adjuvant therapy is not known.

HOW SUPPLIED

Tablets containing tamoxifen as the citrate in an amount equivalent to 10 mg of tamoxifen (round, biconvex, uncoated, white tablet identified with NOLVADEX 600 debossed on one side and a cameo debossed on the other side) are supplied in bottles of 60 tablets and 250 tablets. Protect from heat and light. NDC 0310-0600.

Rev E 11/91

ICI Pharma
A business unit of ICI Americas Inc.
Wilmington, DE 19897 USA
Shown in Product Identification Section, page 412

SORBITRATE®
[*sorb′i-trate*]
(Isosorbide Dinitrate)

℞

DESCRIPTION

SORBITRATE® (isosorbide dinitrate), an organic nitrate, is a vasodilator with effects on both arteries and veins.
SORBITRATE is available as:
SORBITRATE® SUBLINGUAL
2.5 mg Sublingual Tablet. Each tablet contains 2.5 mg of isosorbide dinitrate.

Inactive ingredients: corn starch, lactose (hydrous), magnesium stearate, pregelatinized starch.
5 mg Sublingual Tablet. Each tablet contains 5 mg of isosorbide dinitrate.
Inactive ingredients: corn starch, lactose (hydrous), magnesium stearate, pregelatinized starch, Red 7.
10 mg Sublingual Tablet. Each tablet contains 10 mg of isosorbide dinitrate.
Inactive ingredients: corn starch, lactose (hydrous), magnesium stearate, Yellow 10.

SORBITRATE® CHEWABLE
5 mg Chewable Tablet. Each tablet contains 5 mg of isosorbide dinitrate.
Inactive ingredients: Blue 1, confectioner's sugar, corn starch, flavor, hydrogenated vegetable oil, magnesium stearate, mannitol, povidone, Yellow 10.
10 mg Chewable Tablet. Each tablet contains 10 mg of isosorbide dinitrate.
Inactive ingredients: confectioner's sugar, corn starch, flavor, hydrogenated vegetable oil, magnesium stearate, mannitol, povidone, Yellow 10.

SORBITRATE® ORAL
5 mg Oral Tablet. Each tablet contains 5 mg of isosorbide dinitrate.
Inactive ingredients: Blue 1, corn starch, lactose (hydrous), magnesium stearate, pregelatinized starch, Yellow 10.
10 mg Oral Tablet. Each tablet contains 10 mg of isosorbide dinitrate.
Inactive ingredients: corn starch, lactose (hydrous), magnesium stearate, pregelatinized starch, Yellow 10.
20 mg Oral Tablet. Each tablet contains 20 mg of isosorbide dinitrate.
Inactive ingredients: Blue 1, corn starch, lactose (hydrous), magnesium stearate, pregelatinized starch.
30 mg Oral Tablet. Each tablet contains 30 mg of isosorbide dinitrate.
Inactive ingredients: corn starch, lactose (hydrous), magnesium stearate, pregelatinized starch.
40 mg Oral Tablet. Each tablet contains 40 mg of isosorbide dinitrate.
Inactive ingredients: Blue 1, corn starch, lactose (hydrous), magnesium stearate, pregelatinized starch.

SORBITRATE® SA
Sustained Action Tablet. Each tablet contains 10 mg of isosorbide dinitrate in the outer coat and 30 mg in the inner core (sustained action base).
Inactive ingredients: carbomer 934P, ethylcellulose, lactose (hydrous), magnesium stearate, polyethylene glycol, Yellow 10.

The chemical name for isosorbide dinitrate is 1,4,3,6- dianhydrosorbitol-2.5-dinitrate and the compound has the following structural formula:

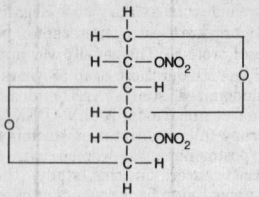

Molecular Weight: 236.14
Isosorbide dinitrate is a white, crystalline, odorless compound which is stable in air and in solution, has a melting point of 70°C and has an optical rotation of +134° (c = 1.0, alcohol, 20°C). Isosorbide dinitrate is freely soluble in organic solvents such as acetone, alcohol, and ether; but is only sparingly soluble in water.

CLINICAL PHARMACOLOGY

The principal pharmacological action of isosorbide dinitrate is relaxation of vascular smooth muscle, producing a vasodilatory effect on both peripheral arteries and veins, with predominant effects on the latter. Dilation of the postcapillary vessels, including large veins, promotes peripheral pooling of blood and decreases venous return to the heart, thereby reducing left-ventricular end-diastolic pressure (preload). Arteriolar relaxation reduces systemic vascular resistance and arterial pressure (after-load).

The mechanism by which isosorbide dinitrate relieves angina pectoris is not fully understood. Myocardial oxygen consumption or demand (as measured by the pressure-rate product, tension-time index, and stroke-work index) is decreased by both the arterial and venous effects of isosorbide dinitrate and, presumably, a more favorable supply-demand ratio is achieved. While the large epicardial coronary arteries are also dilated by isosorbide dinitrate, the extent to which this contributes to relief of exertional angina is unclear.

Therapeutic doses of isosorbide dinitrate may reduce systolic, diastolic, and mean arterial blood pressures, especially in the upright posture. Effective coronary perfusion is usually maintained. The decrease in systemic blood pressure may result in reflex tachycardia, an effect which results in an unfavorable influence on myocardial oxygen demand. Hemodynamic studies indicate that isosorbide dinitrate may reduce the abnormally elevated left ventricular end-diastolic and pulmonary capillary wedge pressures that occur during an acute episode of angina pectoris.

Isosorbide dinitrate is metabolized by enzymatic denitration to the intermediate products isosorbide-2-mononitrate and isosorbide-5-mononitrate. Both metabolites have biological activity, especially the 5-mononitrate which is also the principal metabolite. The liver is a principal site of metabolism and isosorbide dinitrate is subject to a large first-pass effect. The systemic clearance of the drug following intravenous infusion is about 3.4 liters/min. Since the clearance exceeds hepatic blood flow, considerable extrahepatic metabolism must also occur.

The average bioavailability of isosorbide dinitrate is 59 and 22 percent following sublingual and oral administration, respectively. The terminal half-life is about 20 minutes, 60 minutes, and 4 hours following i.v., sublingual, and oral administration, respectively. The dependence of half-life on the route of administration is not understood. Over limited ranges of i.v. dosing, the pharmacokinetics of isosorbide dinitrate appear linear. However, both the 2- and 5-mononitrate metabolites have been shown to decrease the rate of disappearance of the dinitrate from the blood and the half-lives of isosorbide-5-mononitrate and isosorbide-2-mononitrate range from 4.0–5.6 and 1.5–3.1 hours, respectively.

The pharmacokinetics and/or bioavailability of isosorbide dinitrate during multiple dosing have not been well studied. Because the metabolites influence the clearance of isosorbide dinitrate, prediction of blood levels of parent compound to metabolites from single-dose studies is uncertain.

INDICATIONS AND USAGE

SORBITRATE (isosorbide dinitrate) is indicated for the treatment and prevention of angina pectoris. Controlled clinical trials have demonstrated that the sublingual, chewable, immediate release, and controlled release oral dosage forms of isosorbide dinitrate are effective in improving exercise tolerance in patients with angina pectoris. When single sublingual or chewable doses (5 mg) of isosorbide dinitrate were administered prophylactically to patients with angina pectoris in various clinical studies, duration of exercise until chest pain or fatigue was significantly improved for at least 45 minutes (and as long as 2 hours in some studies) following dosing. Similar studies after single oral (15 to 120 mg) and oral controlled-release (40 to 80 mg) doses of isosorbide dinitrate have shown significant improvement in exercise tolerance for up to 8 hours following dosing. The exercise electro-

cardiographic evidence suggests that improved exercise tolerance with isosorbide dinitrate is not at the expense of greater myocardial ischemia. All dosage forms of isosorbide dinitrate may therefore be used prophylactically to decrease frequency and severity of anginal attacks and can be expected to decrease the need for sublingual nitroglycerin.
The sublingual and chewable forms of the drug are indicated for acute prophylaxis of angina pectoris when taken a few minutes before situations likely to provoke anginal attacks. Because of a slower onset of effect, the oral forms of isosorbide dinitrate are not indicated for acute prophylaxis.
In controlled clinical trials, chewable and sublingual isosorbide dinitrate were effective in relieving an acute attack of angina pectoris. Relief occurred with a mean time of 2.9 and 3.4 minutes (chewable and sublingual respectively) compared to relief of angina with a mean time of 1.9 minutes following sublingual nitroglycerin. Because of the more rapid relief of chest pain with sublingual nitroglycerin, the use of sublingual or chewable isosorbide dinitrate for aborting an acute anginal attack should be limited to patients intolerant or unresponsive to sublingual nitroglycerin.

CONTRAINDICATIONS

SORBITRATE is contraindicated in patients who have shown purported hypersensitivity or idiosyncrasy to it or other nitrates or nitrites.

WARNINGS

The benefits of SORBITRATE during the early days of an acute myocardial infarction have not been established. If one elects to use organic nitrates in early infarction, hemodynamic monitoring and frequent clinical assessment should be used because of the potential deleterious effects of hypotension.

PRECAUTIONS

General: Severe hypotensive response, particularly with upright posture, may occur with even small doses of SORBITRATE. The drug should therefore be used with caution in subjects who may have blood volume depletion from diuretic therapy or in subjects who have low systolic blood pressure (eg, below 90 mmHg). Paradoxical bradycardia and increased angina pectoris may accompany nitrate-induced hypotension.
Nitrate therapy may aggravate the angina caused by hypertrophic cardiomyopathy. Tolerance to this drug and cross-tolerance to other nitrates and nitrites may occur.
Marked symptomatic, orthostatic hypotension has been reported when calcium channel blockers and organic nitrates were used in combination. Dose adjustment of either class of agents may be necessary.
Tolerance to the vascular and antianginal effects of isosorbide dinitrate or nitroglycerin has been demonstrated in clinical trials, experience through occupational exposure, and in isolated tissue experiments in the laboratory. The importance of tolerance to the appropriate use of isosorbide dinitrate in the management of patients with angina pectoris has not been determined. However, one clinical trial using treadmill exercise tolerance (as an endpoint) found an 8-hour duration of action of oral isosorbide dinitrate following the first dose (after a 2-week placebo washout) and only a 2-hour duration of effect of the same dose after 1 week of repetitive dosing at conventional dosing intervals. On the other hand, several trials have been able to differentiate isosorbide dinitrate from placebo after 4 weeks of therapy, and in open trials, an effect seems detectable for as long as several months.
Tolerance clearly occurs in industrial workers continuously exposed to nitroglycerin. Moreover, physical dependence also occurs since chest pain, acute myocardial infarction, and even sudden death have occurred during temporary withdrawal of nitroglycerin from the workers. In clinical trials in angina patients, there are reports of anginal attacks being more easily provoked and of rebound in the hemodynamic effects soon after nitrate withdrawal. The relative importance of these observations to the routine, clinical use of isosorbide dinitrate is not known. However, it seems prudent to gradually withdraw patients from isosorbide dinitrate when the therapy is being terminated, rather than stopping the drug abruptly.
Information for Patients: Headache may occur during initial therapy with SORBITRATE. Headache is usually relieved by the use of standard headache remedies, or by lowering the dose, and tends to disappear after the first week or two of use.
Drug Interactions: Alcohol may enhance any marked sensitivity to the hypotensive effect of nitrates.
Isosorbide dinitrate acts directly on vascular smooth muscle; therefore, any other agent that depends on vascular smooth muscle as the final common path can be expected to have decreased or increased effect depending on the agent.
Carcinogenesis, Mutagenesis, Impairment of Fertility: No long-term studies in animals have been performed to evaluate the carcinogenic potential of this drug. A modified two-litter reproduction study in rats fed isosorbide dinitrate at 25 or 100 mg/kg/day did not reveal any effects on fertility or gestation or any remarkable gross pathology in any parent or offspring fed isosorbide dinitrate as compared with rats fed a basal-controlled diet.
Pregnancy Category C: Isosorbide dinitrate has been shown to cause a dose-related increase in embryotoxicity (increase in mummified pups) in rabbits at oral doses 35 and 150 times the maximum recommended human daily dose. There are no adequate and well-controlled studies in pregnant women. SORBITRATE should be used during pregnancy only if the potential benefit justifies the potential risk to the fetus.
Nursing Mothers: It is not known whether this drug is excreted in human milk. Because many drugs are excreted in human milk, caution should be exercised when SORBITRATE is administered to a nursing woman.
Pediatric Use: The safety and effectiveness of SORBITRATE in children has not been established.

ADVERSE REACTIONS

Adverse reactions, particularly headache and hypotension, are dose related. In clinical trials at various doses, the following have been observed.
Headache is the most common adverse reaction and may be severe and persistent; reported incidence varies widely, apparently being dose-related, with an average occurrence of about 25%. Cutaneous vasodilation with flushing may occur. Transient episodes of dizziness and weakness, as well as other signs of cerebral ischemia associated with postural hypotension, may occasionally develop (the incidence of reported symptomatic hypotension ranges from 2% to 36%). An occasional individual will exhibit marked sensitivity to the hypotensive effects of nitrates and severe responses (nausea, vomiting, weakness, restlessness, pallor, perspiration, and collapse) may occur even with the usual therapeutic dose. Drug rash and/or exfoliative dermatitis may occasionally occur. Nausea and vomiting appear to be uncommon.

OVERDOSAGE

Signs and Symptoms: These may include the following: a prompt fall in blood pressure, persistent and throbbing headache, vertigo, palpitation, visual disturbances, flushed and perspiring skin (later becoming cold and cyanotic), nausea and vomiting (possibly with colic and even bloody diarrhea), syncope (especially in the upright position), methemoglobinemia with cyanosis and anoxia, initial hyperpnea, dyspnea and slow breathing, slow pulse (dicrotic and intermittent), heart block, increased intracranial pressure with cerebral symptoms of confusion and moderate fever, paralysis and coma followed by clonic convulsions and possibly death due to circulatory collapse.
It is not known what dose of the drug is associated with symptoms of overdosing or what dose of the drug would be life-threatening. The acute oral LD_{50} of isosorbide dinitrate in rats was found to be approximately 1100 mg/kg of body weight. These animal experiments indicate that approximately 500 times the usual therapeutic dose would be required to produce such toxic symptoms in humans. It is not known whether the drug is dialyzable.
Treatment of Overdose: Prompt removal of the ingested material by gastric lavage is reasonable, but not documented to be useful. Keep the patient recumbent in a shock position and comfortably warm. Passive movements of the extremities may aid venous return. Administer oxygen and artificial respiration if necessary. If methemoglobinemia is present, administer methylene blue (1% solution), 1 to 2 mg/kg intravenously.
Methemoglobin: Case reports of clinically-significant methemoglobinemia are rare at conventional doses of organic nitrates. The formation of methemoglobin is dose related and in the case of genetic abnormalities of hemoglobin that favor methemoglobin formation, even conventional doses of organic nitrate could produce harmful concentrations of methemoglobin.

WARNING

Epinephrine is ineffective in reversing the severe hypotensive events associated with overdose. It and related compounds are contraindicated in this situation.

DOSAGE AND ADMINISTRATION

For the treatment of angina pectoris, the usual starting dose for sublingual isosorbide dinitrate is 2.5 to 5 mg; and for chewable tablets, 5 mg.
Isosorbide dinitrate should be titrated upward until angina is relieved or side effects limit the dose. In ambulatory patients, the magnitude of the incremental dose increase should be guided by measurements of standing blood pressure.
The initial dosage of sublingual or chewable isosorbide dinitrate for acute prophylactic therapy in angina pectoris patients is generally 5 or 10 mg every 2 to 3 hours. Adequate, controlled clinical studies demonstrating the effectiveness of chronic maintenance therapy with these dosage forms have not been reported.
For the treatment of chronic stable angina pectoris, the usual starting dose for immediate-release oral (swallowed) tablets is 5 to 20 mg; and for controlled-release forms, 40 mg. For maintenance, oral doses of 10 to 40 mg given every 6 hours; or oral controlled-release doses of 40 to 80 mg given every 8 to 12 hours is generally recommended. The extent to which development of tolerance should modify the dosage program has not been defined. **The oral controlled-release forms of isosorbide dinitrate should not be chewed.**

HOW SUPPLIED

SORBITRATE Sublingual
2.5 mg Sublingual Tablets. (NDC-0310-0853) White, round tablets (identified front "S", reverse "853") are supplied in bottles of 100.
5 mg Sublingual Tablets. (NDC-0310-0760) Pink, round tablets (identified front "S", reverse "760") are supplied in bottles of 100.
10 mg Sublingual Tablets. (NDC-0310-0761) Yellow, round tablets (identified front "S", reverse "761") are supplied in bottles of 100.
SORBITRATE Chewable
5 mg Chewable Tablets. (NDC-0310-0810) Green, round, scored tablets (identified front "S", reverse "810") are supplied in bottles of 100 and 500.
10 mg Chewable Tablets. (NDC-0310-0815) Yellow, round, scored tablets (identified front "S", reverse "815") are supplied in bottles of 100.
SORBITRATE Oral
5 mg Oral Tablets. (NDC-0310-0770) Green, oval-shaped, scored tablets (identified front "S", reverse "770") are supplied in bottles of 100, 500, and Unit Dose 100.
10 mg Oral Tablets. (NDC-0310-0780) Yellow, oval-shaped, scored tablets (identified front "S", reverse "780") are supplied in bottles of 100, 500, and Unit Dose 100.
20 mg Oral Tablets. (NDC-0310-0820) Blue, oval-shaped, scored tablets (identified front "S", reverse "820") are supplied in bottles of 100 and Unit Dose 100.
30 mg Oral Tablets. (NDC-0310-0773) White, oval-shaped, scored tablets (identified front "S", reverse "773") are supplied in bottles of 100 and Unit Dose 100.
40 mg Oral Tablets. (NDC-0310-0774) Light blue, oval-shaped, scored tablets (identified front "S", reverse "774") are supplied in bottles of 100 and Unit Dose 100.
SORBITRATE SA
40 mg Sustained Action Tablets. (NDC-0310-0880) Yellow, round, compression-coated tablets (identified front "S", reverse "880") are supplied in bottles of 100 and Unit Dose 100.

Avoid storage at temperatures above 25°C (77°F).
Rev F 01/92
ICI Pharma
A business unit of ICI Americas Inc.
Wilmington, DE 19897 USA
Shown in Product Identification Section, page 412

TENORETIC® (atenolol and chlorthalidone) ℞
[ten "o-ret 'ic]

DESCRIPTION

TENORETIC® (atenolol and chlorthalidone) is for the treatment of hypertension. It combines the antihypertensive activity of two agents: a $beta_1$-selective (cardioselective) hydrophilic blocking agent (atenolol, TENORMIN®) and a monosulfonamyl diuretic (chlorthalidone). Atenolol is Benzeneacetamide, 4-[2'-hydroxy-3'-[(1-methylethyl) amino] propoxy].-.
$C_{14}H_{22}N_2O_3$

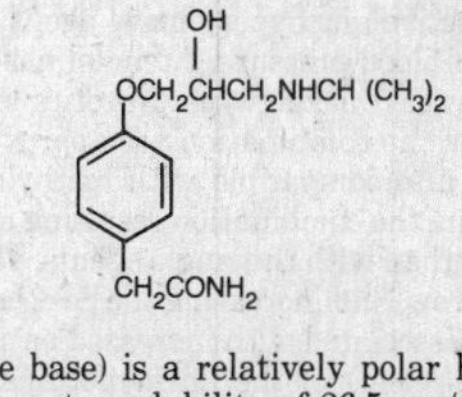

Atenolol (free base) is a relatively polar hydrophilic compound with a water solubility of 26.5 mg/mL at 37°C. It is freely soluble in 1N HCl (300 mg/mL at 25°C) and less soluble in chloroform (3 mg/mL at 25°C).
Chlorthalidone is 2-Chloro-5-(1-hydroxy-3-oxo-1 isoindolinyl) benzene sulfonamide:
$C_{14}H_{11}ClN_2O_4S$

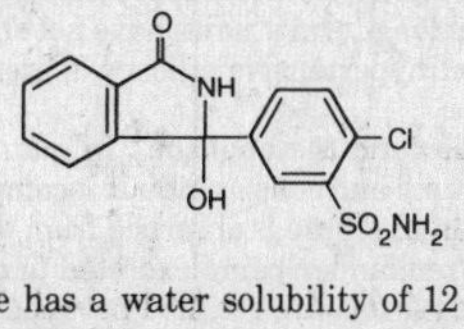

Chlorthalidone has a water solubility of 12 mg/100 mL at 20°C.
Each TENORETIC 100 Tablet contains:

Atenolol (TENORMIN®)	100 mg
Chlorthalidone	25 mg

Continued on next page

ICI Pharma—Cont.

Each TENORETIC 50 Tablet contains:

Atenolol (TENORMIN®)	50 mg
Chlorthalidone	25 mg

Inactive ingredients: magnesium stearate, microcrystalline cellulose, povidone, sodium starch glycolate.

CLINICAL PHARMACOLOGY

TENORETIC

Atenolol and chlorthalidone have been used singly and concomitantly for the treatment of hypertension. The antihypertensive effects of these agents are additive, and studies have shown that there is no interference with bioavailability when these agents are given together in the single combination tablet. Therefore, this combination provides a convenient formulation for the concomitant administration of these two entities. In patients with more severe hypertension, TENORETIC may be administered with other antihypertensives such as vasodilators.

Atenolol

Atenolol is a $beta_1$-selective (cardioselective) beta-adrenergic receptor blocking agent without membrane stabilizing or intrinsic sympathomimetic (partial agonist) activities. This preferential effect is not absolute, however, and at higher doses, atenolol inhibits $beta_2$-adrenoreceptors, chiefly located in the bronchial and vascular musculature.

Pharmacodynamics: In standard animal or human pharmacological tests, beta-adrenoreceptor blocking activity of atenolol has been demonstrated by: (1) reduction in resting and exercise heart rates and cardiac output, (2) reduction of systolic and diastolic blood pressure at rest and on exercise, (3) inhibition of isoproterenol induced tachycardia and (4) reduction in reflex orthostatic tachycardia.

A significant beta-blocking effect of atenolol, as measured by reduction of exercise tachycardia, is apparent within one hour following oral administration of a single dose. This effect is maximal at about 2 to 4 hours and persists for at least 24 hours. The effect at 24 hours is dose related and also bears a linear relationship to the logarithm of plasma atenolol concentration. However, as has been shown for all beta-blocking agents, the antihypertensive effect does not appear to be related to plasma level.

In normal subjects, the $beta_1$-selectivity of atenolol has been shown by its reduced ability to reverse the $beta_2$-mediated vasodilating effect of isoproterenol as compared to equivalent beta-blocking doses of propranolol. In asthmatic patients, a dose of atenolol producing a greater effect on resting heart rate than propranolol resulted in much less increase in airway resistance. In a placebo controlled comparison of approximately equipotent oral doses of several beta blockers, atenolol produced a significantly smaller decrease of FEV_1 than nonselective beta blockers, such as propranolol and unlike those agents did not inhibit bronchodilation in response to isoproterenol.

Consistent with its negative chronotropic effect due to beta blockade of the SA node, atenolol increases sinus cycle length and sinus node recovery time. Conduction in the AV node is also prolonged. Atenolol is devoid of membrane stabilizing activity, and increasing the dose well beyond that producing beta blockade does not further depress myocardial contractility. Several studies have demonstrated a moderate (approximately 10%) increase in stroke volume at rest and exercise.

In controlled clinical trials, atenolol given as a single daily dose, was an effective antihypertensive agent providing 24-hour reduction of blood pressure. Atenolol has been studied in combination with thiazide-type diuretics and the blood pressure effects of the combination are approximately additive. Atenolol is also compatible with methyldopa, hydralazine and prazosin, the combination resulting in a larger fall in blood pressure than with the single agents. The dose range of atenolol is narrow, and increasing the dose beyond 100 mg once daily is not associated with increased antihypertensive effect. The mechanisms of the antihypertensive effects of beta-blocking agents have not been established. Several mechanisms have been proposed and include: (1) competitive antagonism of catecholamines at peripheral (especially cardiac) adrenergic neuron sites, leading to decreased cardiac output, (2) a central effect leading to reduced sympathetic outflow to the periphery and (3) suppression of renin activity. The results from long-term studies have not shown any diminution of the antihypertensive efficacy of atenolol with prolonged use.

Pharmacokinetics and Metabolism: In man, absorption of an oral dose is rapid and consistent but incomplete. Approximately 50% of an oral dose is absorbed from the gastrointestinal tract, the remainder being excreted unchanged in the feces. Peak blood levels are reached between 2 and 4 hours after ingestion. Unlike propranolol or metoprolol, but like nadolol, hydrophilic atenolol undergoes little or no metabolism by the liver, and the absorbed portion is eliminated primarily by renal excretion. Atenolol also differs from propranolol in that only a small amount (6–16%) is bound to proteins in the plasma. This kinetic profile results in relatively consistent plasma drug levels with about a fourfold interpatient variation. There is no information as to the pharmacokinetic effect of atenolol on chlorthalidone.

The elimination half-life of atenolol is approximately 6 to 7 hours and there is no alteration of the kinetic profile of the drug by chronic administration. Following doses of 50 mg or 100 mg, both beta-blocking and antihypertensive effects persist for at least 24 hours. When renal function is impaired, elimination of atenolol is closely related to the glomerular filtration rate; but significant accumulation does not occur until the creatinine clearance falls below 35 mL/min/1.73m^2 (see circular for atenolol [TENORMIN®]).

Chlorthalidone

Chlorthalidone is a monosulfonamyl diuretic which differs chemically from thiazide diuretics in that a double ring system is incorporated in its structure. It is an oral diuretic with prolonged action and low toxicity. The diuretic effect of the drug occurs within 2 hours of an oral dose. It produces diuresis with greatly increased secretion of sodium and chloride. At maximal therapeutic dosage, chlorthalidone is approximately equal in its diuretic effect to comparable maximal therapeutic doses of benzothiadiazine diuretics. The site of action appears to be the cortical diluting segment of the ascending limb of Henle's loop of the nephron.

INDICATIONS AND USAGE

TENORETIC is indicated in the treatment of hypertension. This fixed dose combination drug is not indicated for initial therapy of hypertension. If the fixed dose combination represents the dose appropriate to the individual patient's needs, it may be more convenient than the separate components.

CONTRAINDICATIONS

TENORETIC is contraindicated in patients with: sinus bradycardia; heart block greater than first degree; cardiogenic shock; overt cardiac failure (see WARNINGS); anuria; hypersensitivity to this product or to sulfonamide-derived drugs.

WARNINGS

Cardiac Failure: Sympathetic stimulation is necessary in supporting circulatory function in congestive heart failure, and beta blockade carries the potential hazard of further depressing myocardial contractility and precipitating more severe failure. In patients who have congestive heart failure controlled by digitalis and/or diuretics, TENORETIC should be administered cautiously. Both digitalis and atenolol slow AV conduction.

IN PATIENTS WITHOUT A HISTORY OF CARDIAC FAILURE, continued depression of the myocardium with beta-blocking agents over a period of time can, in some cases, lead to cardiac failure. At the first sign or symptom of impending cardiac failure, patients receiving TENORETIC should be digitalized and/or be given additional diuretic therapy. Observe the patient closely. If cardiac failure continues despite adequate digitalization and diuretic therapy, TENORETIC therapy should be withdrawn.

Renal and Hepatic Disease and Electrolyte Disturbances: Since atenolol is excreted via the kidneys, TENORETIC should be used with caution in patients with impaired renal function.

In patients with renal disease, thiazides may precipitate azotemia. Since cumultive effects may develop in the presence of impaired renal function, if progressive renal impairment becomes evident, TENORETIC should be discontinued.

In patients with impaired hepatic function or progressive liver disease, minor alterations in fluid and electrolyte balance may precipitate hepatic coma. TENORETIC should be used with caution in these patients.

Ischemic Heart Disease: Following abrupt cessation of therapy with certain beta-blocking agents in patients with coronary artery disease, exacerbations of angina pectoris and, in some cases, myocardial infarction have been reported. Therefore, such patients should be cautioned against interruption of therapy without the physician's advice. Even in the absence of overt angina pectoris, when discontinuation of TENORETIC is planned, the patient should be carefully observed and should be advised to limit physical activity to a minimum. TENORETIC should be reinstated if withdrawal symptoms occur. Because coronary artery disease is common and may be unrecognized, it may be prudent not to discontinue TENORETIC therapy abruptly even in patients treated only for hypertension.

Bronchospastic Diseases: PATIENTS WITH BRONCHOSPASTIC DISEASE SHOULD, IN GENERAL, NOT RECEIVE BETA BLOCKERS. Because of its relative $beta_1$-selectivity, however, TENORETIC may be used with caution in patients with bronchospastic disease who do not respond to or cannot tolerate, other antihypertensive treatment. Since $beta_1$-selectivity is not absolute, the lowest possible dose of TENORETIC should be used and a $beta_2$-stimulating agent (bronchodilator) should be made available. If dosage must be increased, dividing the dose should be considered in order to achieve lower peak blood levels.

Anesthesia and Major Surgery: It is not advisable to withdraw beta-adrenoreceptor blocking drugs prior to surgery in the majority of patients. However, care should be taken when using anesthetic agents such as those which may depress the myocardium. Vagal dominance, if it occurs, may be corrected with atropine (1–2 mg IV).

Beta blockers are competitive inhibitors of beta-receptor agonists and their effects on the heart can be reversed by administration of such agents; eg, dobutamine or isoproterenol with caution (see section on Overdosage).

Metabolic and Endocrine Effects: TENORETIC may be used with caution in diabetic patients. Beta blockers may mask tachycardia occurring with hypoglycemia, but other manifestations such as dizziness and sweating may not be significantly affected. At recommended doses atenolol does not potentiate insulin-induced hypoglycemia and, unlike nonselective beta blockers, does not delay recovery of blood glucose to normal levels.

Insulin requirements in diabetic patients may be increased, decreased or unchanged; latent diabetes mellitus may become manifest during chlorthalidone administration.

Beta-adrenergic blockade may mask certain clinical signs (eg, tachycardia) of hyperthyroidism. Abrupt withdrawal of beta blockade might precipitate a thyroid storm; therefore, patients suspected of developing thyrotoxicosis from whom TENORETIC therapy is to be withdrawn should be monitored closely.

Because calcium excretion is decreased by thiazides, TENORETIC should be discontinued before carrying out tests for parathyroid function. Pathologic changes in the parathyroid glands, with hypercalcemia and hypophosphatemia, have been observed in a few patients on prolonged thiazide therapy; however, the common complications of hyperparathyroidism such as renal lithiasis, bone resorption, and peptic ulceration have not been seen.

Hyperuricemia may occur, or acute gout may be precipitated in certain patients receiving thiazide therapy.

PRECAUTIONS

General: TENORETIC may aggravate peripheral arterial circulatory disorders.

Electrolyte and Fluid Balance Status: Periodic determination of serum electrolytes to detect possible electrolyte imbalance should be performed at appropriate intervals.

Patients should be observed for clinical signs of fluid or electrolyte imbalance; ie, hyponatremia, hypochloremic alkalosis, and hypokalemia. Serum and urine electrolyte determinations are particularly important when the patient is vomiting excessively or receiving parenteral fluids. Warning signs or symptoms of fluid and electrolyte imbalance include dryness of the mouth, thirst, weakness, lethargy, drowsiness, restlessness, muscle pains or cramps, muscular fatigue, hypotension, oliguria, tachycardia, and gastrointestinal disturbances such as nausea and vomiting.

Measurement of potassium levels is appropriate especially in elderly patients, those receiving digitalis preparations for cardiac failure, patients whose dietary intake of potassium is abnormally low, or those suffering from gastrointestinal complaints.

Hypokalemia may develop especially with brisk diuresis, when severe cirrhosis is present, or during concomitant use of corticosteroids or ACTH.

Interference with adequate oral electrolyte intake will also contribute to hypokalemia. Hypokalemia can sensitize or exaggerate the response of the heart to the toxic effects of digitalis (eg, increased ventricular irritability). Hypokalemia may be avoided or treated by use of potassium supplements or foods with a high potassium content.

Any chloride deficit during thiazide therapy is generally mild and usually does not require specific treatment except under extraordinary circumstances (as in liver disease or renal disease). Dilutional hyponatremia may occur in edematous patients in hot weather; appropriate therapy is water restriction rather than administration of salt except in rare instances when the hyponatremia is life-threatening. In actual salt depletion, appropriate replacement is the therapy of choice.

Drug Interactions: TENORETIC may potentiate the action of other antihypertensive agents used concomitantly. Patients treated with TENORETIC plus a catecholamine depletor (eg, reserpine) should be closely observed for evidence of hypotension and/or marked bradycardia which may produce vertigo, syncope or postural hypotension.

Thiazides may decrease arterial responsiveness to norepinephrine. This diminution is not sufficient to preclude the therapeutic effectiveness of norepinephrine. Thiazides may increase the responsiveness to tubocurarine.

Lithium generally should not be given with diuretics because they reduce its renal clearance and add a high risk of lithium toxicity. Read circulars for lithium preparations before use of such preparations with TENORETIC.

Beta blockers may exacerbate the rebound hypertension which can follow the withdrawal of cloridine. If the two drugs are coadministered, the beta blocker should be withdrawn several days before the gradual withdrawal of clonidine. If replacing clonidine by beta-blocker therapy, the introduction of beta blockers should be delayed for several days after clonidine administration has stopped.

While taking beta blockers, patients with a history of anaphylactic reaction to a variety of allergens may have a more severe reaction on repeated challenge, either accidental, diagnostic or therapeutic. Such patients may be unresponsive to the usual doses of epinephrine used to treat the allergic reaction.

Other Precautions: In patients receiving thiazides, sensitivity reactions may occur with or without a history of allergy or bronchial asthma. The possible exacerbation or activation of systemic lupus erythematosus has been reported. The antihypertensive effects of thiazides may be enhanced in the postsympathectomy patient.

Carcinogenesis, Mutagenesis, Impairment of Fertility: Two long-term (maximum dosing duration of 18 or 24 months) rat studies and one long-term (maximum dosing duration of 18 months) mouse study, each employing dose levels as high as 300 mg/kg/day or 150 times the maximum recommended human antihypertensive dose,* did not indicate a carcinogenic potential of atenolol. A third (24 month) rat study, employing doses of 500 and 1,500 mg/kg/day (250 and 750 times the maximum recommended human antihypertensive dose*) resulted in increased incidences of benign adrenal medullary tumors in males and females, mammary fibroadenomas in females, and anterior pituitary adenomas and thyroid parafollicular cell carcinomas in males. No evidence of a mutagenic potential of atenolol was uncovered in the dominant lethal test (mouse), in vivo cytogenetics test (Chinese hamster) or Ames test (*S typhimurium*).

Fertility of male or female rats (evaluated at dose levels as high as 200 mg/kg/day or 100 times the maximum recommended human dose*) was unaffected by atenolol administration.

Animal Toxicology: Six month oral studies were conducted in rats and dogs using TENORETIC doses up to 12.5 mg/kg/day (atenolol/chlorthalidone 10/2.5 mg/kg/day—approximately five times the maximum recommended human antihypertensive dose*). There were no functional or morphological abnormalities resulting from dosing either compound alone or together other than minor changes in heart rate, blood pressure and urine chemistry which were attributed to the known pharmacologic properties of atenolol and/or chlorthalidone.

Chronic studies of atenolol performed in animals have revealed the occurrence of vacuolation of epithelial cells of Brunner's glands in the duodenum of both male and female dogs at all tested dose levels (starting at 15 mg/kg/day or 7.5 times the maximum recommended human antihypertensive dose*) and increased incidence of atrial degeneration of hearts of male rats at 300 but not 150 mg atenolol/kg/day (150 and 75 times the maximum recommended human antihypertensive dose*, respectively).

Use in Pregnancy: Pregnancy Category C. TENORETIC was studied for tetatogenic potential in the rat and rabbit. Doses of atenolol/chlorthalidone of 8/2, 80/20, and 240/60 mg/kg/day were administered orally to pregnant rats with no evidence of embryofetotoxicty observed. Two studies were conducted in rabbits. In the first study, pregnant rabbits were dosed with 8/2, 80/20, and 160/40 mg/kg/day of atenolol/chlorthalidone. No teratologenic effects were noted, but embryonic resorptions were observed at all dose levels (ranging from approximately 5 times to 100 times the maximum recommended human dose*). In the second rabbit study, doses of atenolol/chlorthalidone were 4/1, 8/2, and 20/5 mg/kg/day. No teratogenic or embryotoxic effects were demonstrated. TENORETIC should be used during pregnancy only if the potential benefit justifies the potential risk to the fetus.

Atenolol—Atenolol has been shown to produce a dose-related increase in embryo/fetal resorptions in rats at doses equal to or greater than 50 mg/kg or 25 or more times the maximum recommended human antihypertensive dose.* Although similar effects were not seen in rabbits, the compound was not evaluated in rabbits at doses above 25 mg/kg or 12.5 times the maximum recommended human antihypertensive dose.* There are no adequate and well-controlled studies in pregnant women.

Chlorthalidone—Thiazides cross the placental barrier and appear in cord blood. The use of chlorthalidone and related drugs in pregnant women requires that the anticipated benefits of the drug be weighed against possible hazards to the fetus. These hazards include fetal or neonatal jaundice, thrombocytopenia and possibly other adverse reactions which have occurred in the adult.

Nursing Mothers: Atenolol is excreted in human breast milk at a ratio of 1.5 to 6.8 when compared to the concentration in plasma. Caution should be exercised when atenolol is administered to a nursing woman. Clinically significant bradycardia has been reported in breast fed infants. Premature infants, or infants with impaired renal function, may be more likely to develop adverse effects.

Pediatric Use: Safety and effectiveness in children have not been established.

*Based on the maximum dose of 100 mg/day in a 50 kg patient.

	Volunteered (US Studies) Atenolol n=164 %	Placebo n=206 %	Total—Volunteered and Elicited (Foreign + US Studies) Atenolol n=399 %	Placebo n=407 %
CARDIOVASCULAR				
Bradycardia	3	0	3	0
Cold Extremities	0	0.5	12	5
Postural Hypotension	2	1	4	5
Leg Pain	0	0.5	3	1
CENTRAL NERVOUS SYSTEM/ NEUROMUSCULAR				
Dizziness	4	1	13	6
Vertigo	2	0.5	2	0.2
Light-Headedness	1	0	3	0.7
Tiredness	0.6	0.5	26	13
Fatigue	3	1	6	5
Lethargy	1	0	3	0.7
Drowsiness	0.6	0	2	0.5
Depression	0.6	0.5	12	9
Dreaming	0	0	3	1
GASTROINTESTINAL				
Diarrhea	2	0	3	2
Nausea	4	1	3	1
RESPIRATORY (see Warnings)				
Wheeziness	0	0	3	3
Dyspnea	0.6	1	6	4

ADVERSE REACTIONS

TENORETIC is usually well tolerated in properly selected patients. Most adverse effects have been mild and transient. The adverse effects observed for TENORETIC are essentially the same as those seen with the individual components.

Atenolol: The frequency estimates in the following table were derived from controlled studies in which adverse reactions were either volunteered by the patient (US studies) or elicited, eg, by checklist (foreign studies). The reported frequency of elicited adverse effects was higher for both atenolol and placebo-treated patients than when these reactions were volunteered. Where frequency of adverse effects for atenolol and placebo is similar, causal relationship to atenolol is uncertain.

[See table above.]

MISCELLANEOUS: There have been reports of skin rashes and/or dry eyes associated with the use of beta-adrenergic blocking drugs. The reported incidence is small, and, in most cases, the symptoms have cleared when treatment was withdrawn. Discontinuance of the drug should be considered if any such reaction is not otherwise explicable. Patients should be closely monitored following cessation of therapy.

During postmarketing experience, the following have been reported in temporal relationship to the use of the drug: elevated liver enzymes and/or bilirubin, headache, impotence, Peyronie's disease, psoriasiform rash or exacerbation of psoriasis, purpura, reversible alopecia, and thrombocytopenia. TENORETIC, like other beta blockers, has been associated with the development of antinuclear antibodies (ANA) and lupus syndrome.

Chlorthalidone: Cardiovascular: orthostatic hypotension; Gastrointestinal: anorexia, gastric irritation, vomiting, cramping, constipation, jaundice (intrahepatic cholestatic jaundice), pancreatitis; CNS: vertigo, paresthesias, xanthopsia; Hematologic: leukopenia, agranulocytosis, thrombocytopenia, aplastic anemia; Hypersensitivity: purpura, photosensitivity, rash, urticaria, necrotizing angiitis (vasculitis) (cutaneous vasculitis), Lyell's syndrome (toxic epidermal necrolysis); Miscellaneous: hyperglycemia, glycosuria, hyperuricemia, muscle spasm, weakness, restlessness. Clinical trials of TENORETIC conducted in the United States (89 patients treated with TENORETIC) revealed no new or unexpected adverse effects.

POTENTIAL ADVERSE EFFECTS: In addition, a variety of adverse effects not observed in clinical trials with atenolol but reported with other beta-adrenergic blocking agents should be considered potential adverse effects of atenolol. Nervous System: Reversible mental depression progressing to catatonia; hallucinations; an acute reversible syndrome characterized by disorientation for time and place, short-term memory loss, emotional lability, slightly clouded sensorium, and decreased performance on neuropsychometrics; Cardiovascular: Intensification of AV block (see CONTRAINDICATIONS); Gastrointestinal: Mesenteric arterial thrombosis, ischemic colitis; Hematologic: Agranulocytosis; Allergic: Erythematous rash, fever combined with aching and sore throat, laryngospasm and respiratory distress.

There have been reports of a syndrome comprising psoriasiform skin rash, conjunctivitis sicca, otitis, and sclerosing serositis attributed to the beta-adrenergic receptor blocking agent, practolol. This syndrome has not been reported with TENORETIC or TENORMIN® (atenolol).

Clinical Laboratory Test Findings: Clinically important changes in standard laboratory parameters were rarely associated with the administration of TENORETIC. The changes in laboratory parameters were not progressive and usually were not associated with clinical manifestations. The most common changes were increases in uric acid and decreases in serum potassium.

OVERDOSAGE

No specific information is available with regard to overdosage and TENORETIC in humans. Treatment should be symptomatic and supportive and directed to the removal of any unabsorbed drug by induced emesis, or administration or activated charcoal. Atenolol can be removed from the general circulation by hemodialysis. Further consideration should be given to dehydration, electrolyte imbalance and hypotension by established procedures.

Atenolol: Overdosage with atenolol has been reported with patients surviving acute doses as high as 5 g. One death was reported in a man who may have taken as much as 10 g acutely.

The predominant symptoms reported following atenolol overdose are lethargy, disorder of respiratory drive, wheezing, sinus pause, and bradycardia. Additionally, common effects associated with overdosage of any beta-adrenergic blocking agent are congestive heart failure, hypotension, bronchospasm, and/or hypoglycemia. Other treatment modalities should be employed at the physician's discretion and may include:

BRADYCARDIA: Atropine 1–2 mg intravenously. If there is no response to vagal blockade, give isoproterenol cautiously. In refractory cases, a transvenous cardiac pacemaker may be indicated. Glucagon in a 10 mg intravenous bolus has been reported to be useful. If required, this may be repeated or followed by an intravenous infusion of glucagon 1–10 mg/h depending on response.

HEART BLOCK (SECOND OR THIRD DEGREE): Isoproterenol or transvenous pacemaker.

CONGESTIVE HEART FAILURE: Digitalize the patient and administer a diuretic. Glucagon has been reported to be useful.

HYPOTENSION: Vasopressors such as dopamine or norepinephrine (levarterenol). Monitor blood pressure continuously.

BRONCHOSPASM: A $beta_2$-stimulant such as isoproterenol or terbutaline and/or aminophylline.

HYPOGLYCEMIA: Intravenous glucose.

ELECTROLYTE DISTURBANCE: Monitor electrolyte levels and renal function. Institute measures to maintain hydration and electrolytes.

Based on the severity of symptoms, management may require intensive support care and facilities for applying cardiac and respiratory support.

Chlorthalidone: Symptoms of chlorthalidone overdose include nausea, weakness, dizziness and disturbances of electrolyte balance.

DOSAGE AND ADMINISTRATION

DOSAGE MUST BE INDIVIDUALIZED (SEE INDICATIONS)

Chlorthalidone is usually given at a dose of 25 mg daily; the usual initial dose of atenolol is 50 mg daily. Therefore, the initial dose should be one TENORETIC 50 tablet given once a day. If an optimal response is not achieved, the dosage should be increased to one TENORETIC 100 tablet given once a day. When necessary, another antihypertensive agent may be

Continued on next page

ICI Pharma—Cont.

added gradually beginning with 50 percent of the usual recommended starting dose to avoid an excessive fall in blood pressure.
Since atenolol is excreted via the kidneys, dosage should be adjusted in cases of severe impairment of renal function. No significant accumulation of atenolol occurs until creatinine clearance falls below 35 mL/min/1.73m² (normal range is 100–150 mL/min/1.73m²); therefore, the following maximum dosages are recommended for patients with renal impairment.

Creatinine Clearance (mL/min/1.73m²)	Atenolol Elimination Half-life (hrs)	Maximum Dosage
15–35	16–27	50 mg daily
< 15	> 27	50 mg every other day

HOW SUPPLIED

TENORETIC 50 Tablets (atenolol 50 mg and chlorthalidone 25 mg), NDC 0310-0115, (white, round, biconvex, uncoated tablets with ICI on one side and 115 on the other side, bisected) are supplied in bottles of 100 tablets.
TENORETIC 100 Tablets (atenolol 100 mg and chlorthalidone 25 mg), NDC 0310-0117, (white, round, biconvex, uncoated tablets with ICI on one side and 117 on the other side) are supplied in bottles of 100 tablets.
Store at controlled room temperature, 15°–30°C (59°–86°F). Dispense in well-closed, light-resistant containers.
Manufactured by ICI Pharmaceuticals P.R. Inc.
Distributed by:
ICI Pharma
A business unit of ICI Americas Inc.
Wilmington, DE 19897 USA

Rev 0 02/92

Shown in Product Identification Section, page 412

TENORMIN® Tablets ℞
TENORMIN® I.V. Injection
[ten-or' min]
(atenolol)

DESCRIPTION

TENORMIN (atenolol), a synthetic, beta$_1$-selective (cardioselective) adrenoreceptor blocking agent, may be chemically described as benzeneacetamide, 4-[2'-hydroxy-3'-[(1-methylethyl)amino]propoxy]-. The molecular and structural formulas are:
$C_{14}H_{22}N_2O_3$

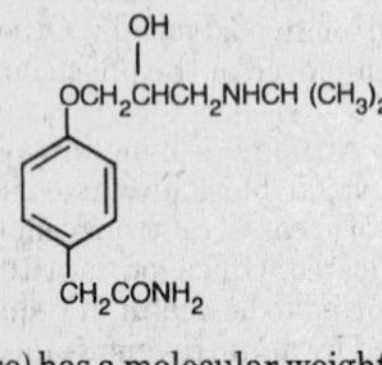
OH
OCH2CHCH2NHCH (CH3)2
CH2CONH2

Atenolol (free base) has a molecular weight of 266. It is a relatively polar hydrophilic compound with a water solubility of 26.5 mg/mL at 37°C and a log partition coefficient (octanol/water) of 0.23. It is freely soluble in 1N HCl (300 mg/mL at 25°C) and less soluble in chloroform (3 mg/mL at 25°C).
TENORMIN is available as 25, 50 and 100 mg tablets for oral administration. TENORMIN for parenteral administration is available as TENORMIN I.V. Injection containing 5 mg atenolol in 10 mL sterile, isotonic, citrate-buffered, aqueous solution. The pH of the solution is 5.5–6.5.
Inactive Ingredients: TENORMIN Tablets: Magnesium stearate, microcrystalline cellulose, povidone, sodium starch glycolate. TENORMIN I.V. Injection: Sodium chloride for isotonicity and citric acid and sodium hydroxide to adjust pH.

CLINICAL PHARMACOLOGY

TENORMIN is a beta$_1$-selective (cardioselective) beta-adrenergic receptor blocking agent without membrane stabilizing or intrinsic sympathomimetic (partial agonist) activities. This preferential effect is not absolute, however, and at higher doses, TENORMIN inhibits beta$_2$-adrenoreceptors, chiefly located in the bronchial and vascular musculature.
Pharmacokinetics and Metabolism: In man, absorption of an oral dose is rapid and consistent but incomplete. Approximately 50% of an oral dose is absorbed from the gastrointestinal tract, the remainder being excreted unchanged in the feces. Peak blood levels are reached between two (2) and four (4) hours after ingestion. Unlike propranolol or metoprolol, but like nadolol, TENORMIN undergoes little or no metabolism by the liver, and the absorbed portion is eliminated primarily by renal excretion. Over 85% of an intravenous dose is excreted in urine within 24 hours compared with approximately 50% for an oral dose. TENORMIN also differs from propranolol in that only a small amount (6%–16%) is bound to proteins in the plasma. This kinetic profile results in relatively consistent plasma drug levels with about a fourfold interpatient variation.
The elimination half-life of oral TENORMIN is approximately 6 to 7 hours, and there is no alteration of the kinetic profile of the drug by chronic administration. Following intravenous administration, peak plasma levels are reached within 5 minutes. Declines from peak levels are rapid (5- to 10-fold) during the first 7 hours; thereafter, plasma levels decay with a half-life similar to that of orally administered drug. Following oral doses of 50 mg or 100 mg, both beta-blocking and antihypertensive effects persist for at least 24 hours. When renal function is impaired, elimination of TENORMIN is closely related to the glomerular filtration rate; significant accumulation occurs when the creatinine clearance falls below 35 mL/min/1.73m². (See DOSAGE AND ADMINISTRATION).
Pharmacodynamics: In standard animal or human pharmacological tests, beta-adrenoreceptor blocking activity of TENORMIN has been demonstrated by: (1) reduction in resting and exercise heart rate and cardiac output, (2) reduction of systolic and diastolic blood pressure at rest and on exercise, (3) inhibition of isoproterenol induced tachycardia, and (4) reduction in reflex orthostatic tachycardia.
A significant beta-blocking effect of TENORMIN, as measured by reduction of exercise tachycardia, is apparent within one hour following oral administration of a single dose. This effect is maximal at about 2 to 4 hours, and persists for at least 24 hours. Maximum reduction in exercise tachycardia occurs within 5 minutes of an intravenous dose. For both orally and intravenously administered drug, the duration of action is dose related and also bears a linear relationship to the logarithm of plasma TENORMIN concentration. The effect on exercise tachycardia of a single 10 mg intravenous dose is largely dissipated by 12 hours, whereas beta-blocking activity of single oral doses of 50 mg and 100 mg is still evident beyond 24 hours following administration. However, as has been shown for all beta-blocking agents, the antihypertensive effect does not appear to be related to plasma level.
In normal subjects, the beta$_1$-selectivity of TENORMIN has been shown by its reduced ability to reverse the beta$_2$-mediated vasodilating effect of isoproterenol as compared to equivalent beta-blocking doses of propranolol. In asthmatic patients, a dose of TENORMIN producing a greater effect on resting heart rate than propranolol resulted in much less increase in airway resistance. In a placebo controlled comparison of approximately equipotent oral doses of several beta blockers, TENORMIN produced a significantly smaller decrease of FEV_1 than nonselective beta blockers such as propranolol and, unlike those agents, did not inhibit bronchodilation in response to isoproterenol.
Consistent with its negative chronotropic effect due to beta blockade of the SA node, TENORMIN increases sinus cycle length and sinus node recovery time. Conduction in the AV node is also prolonged. TENORMIN is devoid of membrane stabilizing activity, and increasing the dose well beyond that producing beta blockade does not further depress myocardial contractility. Several studies have demonstrated a moderate (approximately 10%) increase in stroke volume at rest and during exercise.
In controlled clinical trials, TENORMIN, given as a single daily oral dose, was an effective antihypertensive agent providing 24-hour reduction of blood pressure. TENORMIN has been studied in combination with thiazide-type diuretics, and the blood pressure effects of the combination are approximately additive. TENORMIN is also compatible with methyldopa, hydralazine, and prazosin, each combination resulting in a larger fall in blood pressure than with the single agents. The dose range of TENORMIN is narrow and increasing the dose beyond 100 mg once daily is not associated with increased antihypertensive effect. The mechanisms of the antihypertensive effects of beta-blocking agents have not been established. Several possible mechanisms have been proposed and include: (1) competitive antagonism of catecholamines at peripheral (especially cardiac) adrenergic neuron sites, leading to decreased cardiac output, (2) a central effect leading to reduced sympathetic outflow to the periphery, and (3) suppression of renin activity. The results from long-term studies have not shown any diminution of the antihypertensive efficacy of TENORMIN with prolonged use.
By blocking the positive chronotropic and inotropic effects of catecholamines and by decreasing blood pressure, atenolol generally reduces the oxygen requirements of the heart at any given level of effort, making it useful for many patients in the long-term management of angina pectoris. On the other hand, atenolol can increase oxygen requirements by increasing left ventricular fiber length and end diastolic pressure, particularly in patients with heart failure.
In a multicenter clinical trial (ISIS-1) conducted in 16,027 patients with suspected myocardial infarction, patients presenting within 12 hours (mean = 5 hours) after the onset of pain were randomized to either conventional therapy plus TENORMIN (n = 8,037), or conventional therapy alone (n = 7,990). Patients with a heart rate of < 50 bpm or systolic blood pressure < 100 mm Hg, or with other contraindications to beta blockade, were excluded. Thirty-eight percent of each group were treated within 4 hours of onset of pain. The mean time from onset of pain to entry was 5.0 ± 2.7 hours in both groups. Patients in the TENORMIN group were to receive TENORMIN I.V. Injection 5–10 mg given over 5 minutes plus TENORMIN Tablets 50 mg every 12 hours orally on the first study day (the first oral dose administered about 15 minutes after the IV dose) followed by either TENORMIN Tablets 100 mg once daily or TENORMIN Tablets 50 mg twice daily on days 2–7. The groups were similar in demographic and medical history characteristics and in electrocardiographic evidence of myocardial infarction, bundle branch block, and first degree atrioventricular block at entry.
During the treatment period (days 0–7), the vascular mortality rates were 3.89% in the TENORMIN group (313 deaths) and 4.57% in the control group (365 deaths). This absolute difference in rates, 0.68%, is statistically significant at the P < 0.05 level. The absolute difference translates into a proportional reduction of 15% (3.89-4.57/4.57 = −0.15). The 95% confidence limits are 1%–27%. Most of the difference was attributed to mortality in days 0-1 (TENORMIN—121 deaths; control—171 deaths).
Despite the large size of the ISIS-1 trial, it is not possible to identify clearly subgroups of patients most likely or least likely to benefit from early treatment with atenolol. Good clinical judgment suggests, however, that patients who are dependent on sympathetic stimulation for maintenance of adequate cardiac output and blood pressure are not good candidates for beta blockade. Indeed, the trial protocol reflected that judgment by excluding patients with blood pressure consistently below 100 mm Hg systolic. The overall results of the study are compatible with the possibility that patients with borderline blood pressure (less than 120 mm Hg systolic), especially if over 60 years of age, are less likely to benefit.
The mechanism through which atenolol improves survival in patients with definite or suspected acute myocardial infarction is unknown, as is the case for other beta blockers in the postinfarction setting. Atenolol, in addition to its effects on survival, has shown other clinical benefits including reduced frequency of ventricular premature beats, reduced chest pain, and reduced enzyme elevation.

INDICATIONS AND USAGE

Hypertension: TENORMIN is indicated in the management of hypertension. It may be used alone or concomitantly with other antihypertensive agents, particularly with a thiazide-type diuretic.
Angina Pectoris Due to Coronary Atherosclerosis: TENORMIN is indicated for the long-term management of patients with angina pectoris.
Acute Myocardial Infarction: TENORMIN is indicated in the management of hemodynamically stable patients with definite or suspected acute myocardial infarction to reduce cardiovascular mortality. Treatment can be initiated as soon as the patient's clinical condition allows. (See DOSAGE AND ADMINISTRATION, CONTRAINDICATIONS, AND WARNINGS.) In general, there is no basis for treating patients like those who were excluded from the ISIS-1 trial (blood pressure less than 100 mm Hg systolic, heart rate less than 50 bpm) or have other reasons to avoid beta blockade. As noted above, some subgroups (eg, elderly patients with systolic blood pressure below 120 mm Hg) seemed less likely to benefit.

CONTRAINDICATIONS

TENORMIN is contraindicated in sinus bradycardia, heart block greater than first degree, cardiogenic shock, and overt cardiac failure. (See WARNINGS.)

WARNINGS

Cardiac Failure: Sympathetic stimulation is necessary in supporting circulatory function in congestive heart failure, and beta blockade carries the potential hazard of further depressing myocardial contractility and precipitating more severe failure. In patients who have congestive heart failure controlled by digitalis and/or diuretics, TENORMIN should be administered cautiously. Both digitalis and atenolol slow AV conduction.
In patients with acute myocardial infarction, cardiac failure which is not promptly and effectively controlled by 80 mg of intravenous furosemide or equivalent therapy is a contraindication to beta-blocker treatment.
In Patients Without a History of Cardiac Failure: Continued depression of the myocardium with beta-blocking agents over a period of time can, in some cases, lead to cardiac failure. At the first sign or symptom of impending cardiac failure, patients should be fully digitalized and/or be given a diuretic and the response observed closely. If cardiac failure continues despite adequate digitalization and diuresis, TENORMIN should be withdrawn. (SEE DOSAGE AND ADMINISTRATION.)

Cessation of Therapy with TENORMIN: Patients with coronary artery disease, who are being treated with TENORMIN, should be advised against abrupt discontinuation of therapy. Severe exacerbation of angina and the occurrence of myocardial infarction and ventricular arrhythmias have been reported in angina patients following the abrupt discontinuation of therapy with beta blockers. The last two complications may occur with or without preceding exacerbation of the angina pectoris. As with other beta blockers, when discontinuation of TENORMIN is planned, the patients should be carefully observed and advised to limit physical activity to a minimum. If the angina worsens or acute coronary insufficiency develops, it is recommenced that TENORMIN be promptly reinstituted, at least temporarily. Because coronary artery disease is common and may be unrecognized, it may be prudent not to discontinue TENORMIN therapy abruptly even in patients treated only for hypertension. (See DOSAGE AND ADMINISTRATION.)

Bronchospastic Diseases: PATIENTS WITH BRONCHOSPASTIC DISEASE SHOULD, IN GENERAL, NOT RECEIVE BETA BLOCKERS. Because of its relative beta$_1$ selectivity, however, TENORMIN may be used with caution in patients with bronchospastic disease who do not respond to, or cannot tolerate, other antihypertensive treatment. Since beta$_1$ selectivity is not absolute, the lowest possible dose of TENORMIN should be used with therapy initiated at 50 mg and a beta$_2$-stimulating agent (bronchodilator) should be made available. If dosage must be increased, dividing the dose should be considered in order to achieve lower peak blood levels.

Anesthesia and Major Surgery: It is not advisable to withdraw beta-adrenoreceptor blocking drugs prior to surgery in the majority of patients. However, care should be taken when using anesthetic agents such as those which may depress the myocardium. Vagal dominance, if it occurs, may be corrected with atropine (1-2 mg IV).

Additionally, caution should be used when TENORMIN I.V. Injection is administered concomitantly with such agents.

TENORMIN, like other beta blockers, is a competitive inhibitor of beta-receptor agonists and its effects on the heart can be reversed by administration of such agents: eg, dobutamine or isoproterenol with caution (see section on OVERDOSAGE).

Diabetes and Hypoglycemia: TENORMIN should be used with caution in diabetic patients if a beta-blocking agent is required. Beta blockers may mask tachycardia occurring with hypoglycemia, but other manifestations such as dizziness and sweating may not be significantly affected. At recommended doses TENORMIN does not potentiate insulin-induced hypoglycemia and, unlike nonselective beta blockers, does not delay recovery of blood glucose to normal levels.

Thyrotoxicosis: Beta-adrenergic blockade may mask certain clinical signs (eg, tachycardia) of hyperthyroidism. Patients suspected of having thyroid disease should be monitored closely when adminstering TENORMIN I.V. Injection. Abrupt withdrawal of beta blockade might precipitate a thyroid storm; therefore, patients suspected of developing thyrotoxicosis from whom TENORMIN therapy is to be withdrawn should be monitored closely. (See DOSAGE AND ADMINISTRATION.)

PRECAUTIONS

General: Patients already on a beta blocker must be evaluated carefully before TENORMIN is administered. Initial and subsequent TENORMIN dosages can be adjusted downward depending on clinical observations including pulse and blood pressure. TENORMIN may aggravate peripheral arterial circulatory disorders.

Impaired Renal Function: The drug should be used with caution in patients with impaired renal function. (See DOSAGE AND ADMINISTRATION.)

Drug Interactions: Catecholamine-depleting drugs (eg, reserpine) may have an additive effect when given with beta-blocking agents. Patients treated with TENORMIN plus a catecholamine depletor should therefore be closely observed for evidence of hypotension and/or marked bradycardia which may produce vertigo, syncope or postural hypotension.

Should it be decided to discontinue therapy in patients receiving beta blockers and clonidine concurrently, the beta blocker should be discontinued several days before the gradual withdrawal of clonidine.

Caution should be exercised with TENORMIN I.V. Injection when given in close proximity with drugs that may also have a depressant effect on myocardial contractility. On rare occasions, concomitant use of intravenous beta blockers and intravenous verapamil has resulted in serious adverse reactions, especially in patients with severe cardiomyopathy, congestive heart failure, or recent myocardial infarction.

	Volunteered (US Studies)		Total—Volunteered and Elicited (Foreign + US Studies)	
	Atenolol (n = 164) %	Placebo (n = 206) %	Atenolol (n = 399) %	Placebo (n = 407) %
CARDIOVASCULAR				
Bradycardia	3	0	3	0
Cold Extremities	0	0.5	12	5
Postural Hypotension	2	1	4	5
Leg Pain	0	0.5	3	1
CENTRAL NERVOUS SYSTEM/NEUROMUSCULAR				
Dizziness	4	1	13	6
Vertigo	2	0.5	2	0.2
Light-headedness	1	0	3	0.7
Tiredness	0.6	0.5	26	13
Fatigue	3	1	6	5
Lethargy	1	0	3	0.7
Drowsiness	0.6	0	2	0.5
Depression	0.6	0.5	12	9
Dreaming	0	0	3	1
GASTROINTESTINAL				
Diarrhea	2	0	3	2
Nausea	4	1	3	1
RESPIRATORY (see WARNINGS)				
Wheeziness	0	0	3	3
Dyspnea	0.6	1	6	4

Information on concurrent usage of atenolol and aspirin is limited. Data from several studies, ie, TIMI-II, ISIS-2, currently do not suggest any clinical interaction between aspirin and beta blockers in the acute myocardial infarction setting.

While taking beta blockers, patients with a history of anaphylactic reaction to a variety of allergens may have a more severe reaction on repeated challenge, either accidental, diagnostic or therapeutic. Such patients may be unresponsive to the usual doses of epinephrine used to treat the allergic reaction.

Carcinogenesis, Mutagenesis, Impairment of Fertility: Two long-term (maximum dosing duration of 18 or 24 months) rat studies and one long-term (maximum dosing duration of 18 months) mouse study, each employing dose levels as high as 300 mg/kg/day or 150 times the maximum recommended human antihypertensive dose,* did not indicate a carcinogenic potential of atenolol. A third (24 month) rat study, employing doses of 500 and 1,500 mg/kg/day (250 and 750 times the maximum recommended human antihypertensive dose*) resulted in increased incidences of benign adrenal medullary tumors in males and females, mammary fibroadenomas in females, and anterior pituitary adenomas and thyroid parafollicular cell carcinomas in males. No evidence of a mutagenic potential of atenolol was uncovered in the dominant lethal test (mouse), in vivo cytogenetics test (Chinese hamster) or Ames test (*S typhimurium*).

Fertility of male or female rats (evaluated at dose levels as high as 200 mg/kg/day or 100 times the maximum recommended human dose*) was unaffected by atenolol administration.

Animal Toxicology: Chronic studies employing oral atenolol performed in animals have revealed the occurrence of vacuolation of epithelial cells of Brunner's glands in the duodenum of both male and female dogs at all tested dose levels of atenolol (starting at 15 mg/kg/day or 7.5 times the maximum recommended human antihypertensive dose*) and increased incidence of atrial degeneration of hearts of male rats at 300 but not 150 mg atenolol/kg/day (150 and 75 times the maximum recommended human antihypertensive dose,* respectively).

Usage in Pregnancy: Pregnancy Category C: Atenolol has been shown to produce a dose-related increase in embryo/fetal resorptions in rats at doses equal to or greater than 50 mg/kg/day or 25 or more times the maximum recommended human antihypertensive dose*. Although similar effects were not seen in rabbits, the compound was not evaluated in rabbits at doses above 25 mg/kg/day or 12.5 times the maximum recommended human antihypertensive dose*. There are no adequate and well-controlled studies in pregnant women. TENORMIN should be used during pregnancy only if the potential benefit justifies the potential risk to the fetus.

Nursing Mothers: Atenolol is excreted in human breast milk at a ratio of 1.5 to 6.8 when compared to the concentration in plasma. Caution should be exercised when TENORMIN is administered to a nursing woman. Clinically significant bradycardia has been reported in breast fed infants. Premature infants, or infants with impaired renal function, may be more likely to develop adverse effects.

Pediatric Use: Safety and effectiveness in children have not been established.

*Based on the maximum dose of 100 mg/day in a 50 kg patient.

ADVERSE REACTIONS

Most adverse effects have been mild and transient.

The frequency estimates in the following table were derived from controlled studies in hypertensive patients in which adverse reactions were either volunteered by the patient (US studies) or elicited, eg, by checklist (foreign studies). The reported frequency of elicited adverse effects was higher for both TENORMIN and placebo-treated patients than when these reactions were volunteered. Where frequency of adverse effects of TENORMIN and placebo is similar, causal relationship to TENORMIN is uncertain.

[See table above.]

Acute Myocardial Infarction: In a series of investigations in the treatment of acute myocardial infarction, bradycardia and hypotension occurred more commonly, as expected for any beta blocker, in atenolol-treated patients than in control patients. However, these usually responded to atropine and/or to withholding further dosage of atenolol. The incidence of heart failure was not increased by atenolol. Inotropic agents were infrequently used. The reported frequency of these and other events occurring during these investigations is given in the following table.

In a study of 477 patients, the following adverse events were reported during either intravenous and/or oral atenolol administration:

[See table on bottom left next page.]

In the subsequent International Study of Infarct Survival (ISIS-1) including over 16,000 patients of whom 8,037 were randomized to receive TENORMIN treatment, the dosage of intravenous and subsequent oral TENORMIN was either discontinued or reduced for the following reasons:

[See table on top right next page.]

During postmarketing experience with TENORMIN, the following have been reported in temporal relationship to the use of the drug: elevated liver enzymes and/or bilirubin, headache, impotence, Peyronie's disease, psoriasiform rash or exacerbation of psoriasis, purpura, reversible alopecia, and thrombocytopenia. TENORMIN, like other beta blockers, has been associated with the development of antinuclear antibodies (ANA) and lupus syndrome.

POTENTIAL ADVERSE EFFECTS

In addition, a variety of adverse effects have been reported with other beta-adrenergic blocking agents, and may be considered potential adverse effects of TENORMIN.

Hematologic: Agranulocytosis.

Allergic: Fever, combined with aching and sore throat, laryngospasm, and respiratory distress.

Central Nervous System: Reversible mental depression progressing to catatonia; visual disturbances; hallucinations; an acute reversible syndrome characterized by disorientation of time and place; short-term memory loss; emotional lability with slightly clouded sensorium; and, decreased performance on neuropsychometrics.

Gastrointestinal: Mesenteric arterial thrombosis, ischemic colitis.

Other: Erythematous rash, Raynaud's phenomenon.

Miscellaneous: There have been reports of skin rashes and/or dry eyes associated with the use of beta-adrenergic blocking drugs. The reported incidence is small, and in most cases, the symptoms have cleared when treatment was withdrawn. Discontinuance of the drug should be considered if any such reaction is not otherwise explicable. Patients should be

Continued on next page

ICI Pharma—Cont.

closely monitored following cessation of therapy. (See DOSAGE AND ADMINISTRATION.)

The oculomucocutaneous syndrome associated with the beta blocker practolol has not been reported with TENORMIN. Furthermore, a number of patients who had previously demonstrated established practolol reactions were transferred to TENORMIN therapy with subsequent resolution or quiescence of the reaction.

OVERDOSAGE

Overdosage with TENORMIN has been reported with patients surviving acute doses as high as 5 g. One death was reported in a man who may have taken as much as 10 g acutely.

The predominant symptoms reported following TENORMIN overdose are lethargy, disorder of respiratory drive, wheezing, sinus pause and bradycardia. Additionally, common effects associated with overdosage of any beta-adrenergic blocking agent and which might also be expected in TENORMIN overdose are congestive heart failure, hypotension, bronchospasm and/or hypoglycemia.

Treatment of overdose should be directed to the removal of any unabsorbed drug by induced emesis, gastric lavage, or administration of activated charcoal. TENORMIN can be removed from the general circulation by hemodialysis. Other treatment modalities should be employed at the physician's discretion and may include:

BRADYCARDIA: Atropine intravenously. If there is no response to vagal blockade, give isoproterenol cautiously. In refractory cases, a transvenous cardiac pacemaker may be indicated.

HEART BLOCK (SECOND OR THIRD DEGREE): Isoproterenol or transvenous cardiac pacemaker.

CARDIAC FAILURE: Digitalize the patient and administer a diuretic. Glucagon has been reported to be useful.

HYPOTENSION: Vasopressors such as dopamine or norepinephrine (levarterenol). Monitor blood pressure continuously.

BRONCHOSPASM: A $beta_2$ stimulant such as isoproterenol or terbutaline and/or aminophylline.

HYPOGLYCEMIA: Intravenous glucose.

Based on the severity of symptoms, management may require intensive support care and facilities for applying cardiac and respiratory support.

DOSAGE AND ADMINISTRATION

Hypertension: The initial dose of TENORMIN is 50 mg given as one tablet a day either alone or added to diuretic therapy. The full effect of this dose will usually be seen within one to two weeks. If an optimal response is not achieved, the dosage should be increased to TENORMIN 100 mg given as one tablet a day. Increasing the dosage beyond 100 mg a day is unlikely to produce any further benefit. TENORMIN may be used alone or concomitantly with other antihypertensive agents including thiazide-type diuretics, hydralazine, prazosin, and alpha-methyldopa.

Angina Pectoris: The initial dose of TENORMIN is 50 mg given as one tablet a day. If an optimal response is not achieved within one week, the dosage should be increased to TENORMIN 100 mg given as one tablet a day. Some patients may require a dosage of 200 mg once a day for optimal effect. Twenty-four hour control with once daily dosing is achieved by giving doses larger than necessary to achieve an immediate maximum effect. The maximum early effect on exercise tolerance occurs with doses of 50 to 100 mg, but at these doses the effect at 24 hours is attenuated, averaging about 50% to 75% of that observed with once a day oral doses of 200 mg.

	Reasons for Reduced Dosage			
	IV Atenolol Reduced Dose (<5 mg)*		Oral Partial Dose	
Hypotension/Bradycardia	105	(1.3%)	1168	(14.5%)
Cardiogenic Shock	4	(.04%)	35	(.44%)
Reinfarction	0	(0%)	5	(.06%)
Cardiac Arrest	5	(.06%)	28	(.34%)
Heart Block (> first degree)	5	(.06%)	143	(1.7%)
Cardiac Failure	1	(.01%)	233	(2.9%)
Arrhythmias	3	(.04%)	22	(.27%)
Bronchospasm	1	(.01%)	50	(.62%)

*Full dosage was 10 mg and some patients received less than 10 mg but more than 5 mg.

Acute Myocardial Infarction: In patients with definite or suspected acute myocardial infarction, treatment with TENORMIN I.V. Injection should be initiated as soon as possible after the patient's arrival in the hospital and after eligibility is established. Such treatment should be initiated in a coronary care or similar unit immediately after the patient's hemodynamic condition has stabilized. Treatment should begin with the intravenous administration of 5 mg TENORMIN over 5 minutes followed by another 5 mg intravenous injection 10 minutes later. TENORMIN I.V. Injection should be administered under carefully controlled conditions including monitoring of blood pressure, heart rate, and electrocardiogram. Dilutions of TENORMIN I.V. Injection in Dextrose Injection USP, Sodium Chloride Injection USP, or Sodium Chloride and Dextrose Injection may be used. These admixtures are stable for 48 hours if they are not used immediately.

In patients who tolerate the full intravenous dose (10 mg), TENORMIN Tablets 50 mg should be initiated 10 minutes after the last intravenous dose followed by another 50 mg oral dose 12 hours later. Thereafter, TENORMIN can be given orally either 100 mg once daily or 50 mg twice a day for a further 6–9 days or until discharge from the hospital. If bradycardia or hypotension requiring treatment or any other untoward effects occur, TENORMIN should be discontinued.

Data from other beta blocker trials suggest that if there is any question concerning the use of IV beta blocker or clinical estimate that there is a contraindication, the IV beta blocker may be eliminated and patients fulfilling the safety criteria may be given TENORMIN Tablets 50 mg twice daily or 100 mg once a day for at least seven days (if the IV dosing is excluded).

Although the demonstration of efficacy of TENORMIN is based entirely on data from the first seven postinfarction days, data from other beta blocker trials suggest that treatment with beta blockers that are effective in the postinfarction setting may be continued for one to three years if there are no contraindications.

TENORMIN is an additional treatment to standard coronary care unit therapy.

Elderly Patients or Patients with Renal Impairment: TENORMIN is excreted by the kidneys; consequently dosage should be adjusted in cases of severe impairment of renal function. Some reduction in dosage may also be appropriate for the elderly, since decreased kidney function is a physiologic consequence of aging. Atenolol excretion would be expected to decrease with advancing age.

No significant accumulation of TENORMIN occurs until creatinine clearance falls below 35 mL/min/1.73 m². Accumulation of atenolol and prolongation of its half-life were studied in subjects with creatinine clearance between 5

and 105 mL/min. Peak plasma levels were significantly increased in subjects with creatinine clearances below 30 mL/min.

The following maximum oral dosages are recommended for elderly, renally-impaired patients and for patients with renal impairment due to other causes:

Creatinine Clearance (mL/min/1.73m²)	Atenolol Elimination Half-Life (h)	Maximum Dosage
15–35	16–27	50 mg daily
<15	>27	25 mg daily

Some renally-impaired or elderly patients being treated for hypertension may require a lower starting dose of TENORMIN: 25 mg given as one tablet a day. If this 25 mg dose is used, assessment of efficacy must be made carefully. This should include measurement of blood pressure just prior to the next dose ("trough" blood pressure) to ensure that the treatment effect is present for a full 24 hours.

Although a similar dosage reduction may be considered for elderly and/or renally-impaired patients being treated for indications other than hypertension, data are not available for these patient populations.

Patients on hemodialysis should be given 25 mg or 50 mg after each dialysis; this should be done under hospital supervision as marked falls in blood pressure can occur.

Cessation of Therapy in Patients with Angina Pectoris: If withdrawal of TENORMIN therapy is planned, it should be achieved gradually and patients should be carefully observed and advised to limit physical activity to a minimum.

Parenteral drug products should be inspected visually for particulate matter and discoloration prior to administration, whenever solution and container permit.

HOW SUPPLIED

TENORMIN Tablets: Tablets of 25 mg atenolol, NDC 0310-0107 (round, flat, uncoated white tablets with "T" debossed on one side and 107 debossed on the other side) are supplied in bottles of 100 tablets.

Tablets of 50 mg atenolol, NDC 0310-0105 (round, flat, uncoated white tablets identified with ICI debossed on one side and 105 debossed on the other side, bisected) are supplied in bottles of 100 tablets and 1000 tablets, and unit dose packages of 100 tablets. These tablets are distributed by ICI Pharma.

Tablets of 100 mg atenolol, NDC 0310-0101 (round, flat, uncoated white tablets with ICI debossed on one side and 101 debossed on the other side) are supplied in bottles of 100 tablets and unit dose packages of 100 tablets. These tablets are distributed by ICI Pharma.

Store at controlled room temperature, 15°–30°C (59°–86°F). Dispense in well-closed, light resistant containers.

TENORMIN I.V. Injection:
TENORMIN I.V. Injection, NDC 0310-0108, is supplied as 5 mg atenolol in 10 mL ampules of isotonic citrate-buffered aqueous solution.

Protect from light. Keep ampules in outer packaging until time of use. Store at room temperature.

ICI Pharma
A business unit of ICI Americas Inc.
Wilmington, DE 19897 USA
Rev X 02/92

Shown in Product Identification Section, page 412

	Conventional Therapy Plus Atenolol (n=244)		Conventional Therapy Alone (n=233)	
Bradycardia	43	(18%)	24	(10%)
Hypotension	60	(25%)	34	(15%)
Bronchospasm	3	(1.2%)	2	(0.9%)
Heart Failure	46	(19%)	56	(24%)
Heart Block	11	(4.5%)	10	(4.3%)
BBB + Major Axis Deviation	16	(6.6%)	28	(12%)
Supraventricular Tachycardia	28	(11.5%)	45	(19%)
Atrial Fibrillation	12	(5%)	29	(11%)
Atrial Flutter	4	(1.6%)	7	(3%)
Ventricular Tachycardia	39	(16%)	52	(22%)
Cardiac Reinfarction	0	(0%)	6	(2.6%)
Total Cardiac Arrests	4	(1.6%)	16	(6.9%)
Nonfatal Cardiac Arrests	4	(1.6%)	12	(5.1%)
Deaths	7	(2.9%)	16	(6.9%)
Cardiogenic Shock	1	(0.4%)	4	(1.7%)
Development of Ventricular Septal Defect	0	(0%)	2	(0.9%)
Development of Mitral Regurgitation	0	(0%)	2	(0.9%)
Renal Failure	1	(0.4%)	0	(0%)
Pulmonary Emboli	3	(1.2%)	0	(0%)

ZOLADEX®   ℞
(goserelin acetate implant)
Equivalent to 3.6 mg goserelin

DESCRIPTION

ZOLADEX® (goserelin acetate implant) contains a potent synthetic decapeptide analogue of luteinizing hormone-releasing hormone (LHRH). Goserelin acetate is chemically described as an acetate salt of [D-Ser(Bu^t)^6,Azgly^{10}]LHRH. Its chemical structure is pyro-Glu-His-Trp-Ser-Tyr-D-Ser(Bu^t)-Leu-Arg-Pro-Azgly-NH$_2$ acetate [C$_{59}$H$_{84}$N$_{18}$O$_{14}$ ·(C$_2$H$_4$O$_2$)$_x$ where x = 1 to 2.4].

Goserelin acetate is an off-white powder with a molecular weight of 1269 (free base). It is freely soluble in glacial acetic acid. It is soluble in water, 0.1M hydrochloric acid, 0.1M sodium hydroxide, dimethylformamide and dimethyl sulfoxide. Goserelin acetate is practically insoluble in acetone, chloroform and ether.

ZOLADEX is supplied as a sterile, biodegradable product containing goserelin acetate equivalent to 3.6 mg of goserelin. ZOLADEX is designed for subcutaneous injection with continuous release over a 28-day period. Goserelin acetate is dispersed in a matrix of D,L-lactic and glycolic acids copolymer (13.3–14.3 mg/dose) containing less than 2.5% acetic acid and up to 15% goserelin-related substances and presented as a sterile, white to cream colored 1-mm diameter cylinder, preloaded in a special single use syringe with a 16 gauge needle and overwrapped in a sealed, light and moisture proof, aluminum foil laminate pouch containing a desiccant capsule. Studies of the D,L-lactic and glycolic acids copolymer have indicated that it is completely biodegradable and has no demonstrable antigenic potential.

CLINICAL PHARMACOLOGY

Mechanism of Action: ZOLADEX is a synthetic decapeptide analogue of LHRH. ZOLADEX acts as a potent inhibitor of pituitary gonadotropin secretion when administered in the biodegradable formulation. Following initial administration, ZOLADEX causes an initial increase in serum luteinizing hormone (LH) and follicle stimulating hormone (FSH) values with subsequent increases in serum levels of testosterone. Chronic administration of ZOLADEX leads to sustained suppression of pituitary gonadotropins, and serum levels of testosterone consequently fall into the range normally seen in surgically castrated men approximately 2–4 weeks after initiation of therapy. This leads to accessory sex organ regression. In animal and in in vitro studies, administration of ZOLADEX resulted in the regression or inhibition of growth of the hormonally sensitive dimethylbenzanthracene (DMBA)-induced rat mammary tumor and Dunning R3327 prostate tumor. In clinical trials with follow-up of more than 2 years, suppression of serum testosterone to castrate levels has been maintained for the duration of therapy.

Pharmacokinetics and Metabolism: In clinical trials with the 3.6 mg formulation of ZOLADEX, peak concentrations in serum were achieved 12 to 15 days after subcutaneous administration. The mean peak serum concentration was approximately 2.5 ng/mL. Pharmacokinetic data were obtained using a nonspecific RIA method.

Goserelin is absorbed at a much slower rate initially for the first 8 days, and then there is more rapid and continuous absorption for the remainder of the 28-day dosing period. Despite the change in the absorption rate of goserelin, administration of ZOLADEX every 28 days resulted in testosterone levels that were suppressed to and maintained in the range normally seen in surgically castrated men. There is no significant evidence of drug accumulation in patients with normal renal and hepatic function. However, in clinical trials the C_{min} levels of a few patients were increased. These levels can be attributed to interpatient variation. In patients treated for up to 3 years, no antibodies to ZOLADEX have been detected.

In clinical trials with the solution formulation of ZOLADEX, subjects with impaired renal function (creatinine clearance less than 20 mL/min) had a serum elimination half-life of 12.1 hours compared to 4.2 hours for subjects with normal renal function (creatinine clearance greater than 70 mL/min). However, in clinical trials with the monthly formulation of ZOLADEX, the incidence of adverse events was not increased in patients with impaired renal function. No data are available on human metabolism.

INDICATIONS AND USAGE

ZOLADEX is indicated in the palliative treatment of advanced carcinoma of the prostate. ZOLADEX offers an alternative treatment of prostatic cancer when orchiectomy or estrogen administration are either not indicated or unacceptable to the patient.

In controlled studies of patients with advanced prostatic cancer comparing ZOLADEX to orchiectomy, the long-term endocrine responses and objective responses were similar between the two treatment arms. Additionally, duration of survival was similar between the two treatment arms in a major comparative trial.

CONTRAINDICATIONS

ZOLADEX is contraindicated in women who are or may become pregnant while receiving the drug. In studies in rats and rabbits, ZOLADEX increased preimplantation loss, resorptions, and abortions (see Pregnancy section). In rats and dogs, ZOLADEX suppressed ovarian function, decreased ovarian weight and size, and led to atrophic changes in secondary sex organs. Further evidence suggests that fertility was reduced in female rats that became pregnant after ZOLADEX was stopped. These effects are an expected consequence of the hormonal alterations produced by ZOLADEX in humans. If this drug is used during pregnancy, or if pregnancy occurs while taking this drug, the patient should be apprised of the potential hazard to the fetus.

A report of anaphylactic reaction to synthetic LHRH (Factrel) has been reported in the medical literature.[1]

WARNINGS

Initially, ZOLADEX, like other LHRH agonists, transiently increases serum levels of testosterone. Transient worsening of symptoms, or the occurrence of additional signs and symptoms of prostatic cancer, may occasionally develop during the first few weeks of ZOLADEX treatment. A small number of patients may experience a temporary increase in bone pain, which can be managed symptomatically. As with other LHRH agonists, isolated cases of ureteral obstruction and spinal cord compression have been observed. If spinal cord compression or renal impairment due to ureteral obstruction develops, standard treatment of these complications should be instituted, and in extreme cases an immediate orchiectomy considered.

PRECAUTIONS

General: The use of ZOLADEX in patients at particular risk of developing ureteral obstruction or spinal cord compression should be considered carefully and the patients monitored closely during the first month of therapy. Patients with ureteral obstruction or spinal cord compression should have appropriate treatment prior to initiation of ZOLADEX therapy.

Carcinogenesis, Mutagenesis, Impairment of Fertility: After subcutaneous implant injections once every 4 weeks for 1 year at two dose levels to male and female rats equivalent to 31.5 and 62.4 times and 21.5 and 42.4 times the recommended monthly dose for a 70 kg human, respectively, an increased incidence of benign pituitary macroadenomas was found. No increase in pituitary adenomas was seen in mice receiving injections of ZOLADEX every 3 weeks for 2 years at doses up to 2,400 µg/kg/day (1,200 times the recommended human dose). An increased incidence of histiocytic sarcomas of the bone marrow in vertebral column and femur were observed at both doses in mice. No evidence of pituitary adenomas was seen in a 1 year study in dogs at doses up to 100 times the human dose or in a 6 month study in monkeys at doses up to 200 times the human dose. The relevance of rat pituitary tumors to humans has not been established.

Mutagenicity tests using bacterial and mammalian systems for point mutations and cytogenetic effects have provided no evidence for mutagenic potential.

Administration of ZOLADEX led to changes that were consistent with gonadal suppression in both male and female rats as a result of its endocrine action. In male rats treated at 30–60 times the recommended monthly dose for a 70 kg human, a decrease in weight and atrophic histological changes were observed in the testes, epididymis, seminal vesicle, and prostate gland with complete suppression of spermatogenesis. In female rats treated with 20–40 times the recommended monthly doses for a 70 kg human, suppression of ovarian function led to decreased size and weight of ovaries and secondary sex organs; follicular development was arrested at the antral stage and the corpora lutea were reduced in size and number. Except for the testes, almost complete histologic reversal of these effects in males and females was observed several weeks after dosing was stopped; however, fertility and general reproductive performance were reduced in those that became pregnant after ZOLADEX was discontinued. Fertile matings occurred within 2 weeks after cessation of dosing, even though total recovery of reproductive function may not have occurred before mating took place; and, the ovulation rate, the corresponding implantation rate, and number of live fetuses were reduced.

In male and female dogs, the suppression of fertility was fully reversible when drug treatment was stopped after continuous administration for 1 year at 100 times the recommended monthly dose.

Pregnancy, Teratogenic Effects: Pregnancy Category X. See CONTRAINDICATIONS section. Studies in both rats and rabbits at doses of 2, 10, 20, and 50 µg/kg/day and 20, 250, and 1,000 µg/kg/day, respectively (up to 25 times and 500 times the maximum recommended dose to a 70 kg human), have confirmed that ZOLADEX will increase pregnancy loss in a dose-related manner. In both rats and rabbits using the same doses, there was no evidence that ZOLADEX possessed the potential to cause teratogenicity.

Nursing Mothers: It is not known if this drug is excreted in human milk. Because many drugs are excreted in human milk and because of the potential for serious adverse reactions in nursing infants from ZOLADEX, a decision should be made whether to discontinue nursing or delay use of the drug, taking into account the importance of the drug to the mother.

Pediatric Use: Safety and effectiveness in patients below the age of 18 have not been established.

ADVERSE REACTIONS

ZOLADEX has been found to be generally well tolerated in clinical trials. Adverse reactions reported in these trials were rarely severe enough to result in the patients' withdrawal from ZOLADEX treatment. As seen with other hormonal therapies, the most commonly observed adverse events during ZOLADEX therapy were due to the expected physiological effects from decreased testosterone levels. These included hot flashes, sexual dysfunction and decreased erections.

Initially, ZOLADEX, like other LHRH agonists, transiently increases serum levels of testosterone. A small percentage of patients experienced a temporary worsening of signs and symptoms (see WARNINGS section), usually manifested by an increase in cancer-related pain which was managed symptomatically. Isolated cases of exacerbation of disease symptoms, either ureteral obstruction or spinal cord compression, occurred at similar rates in controlled clinical trials with both ZOLADEX and orchiectomy. The relationship of these events to therapy is uncertain.

As with other endocrine therapies, hypercalcemia (increased calcium) has rarely been reported in cancer patients with bone metastases following initiation of treatment with ZOLADEX or other LHRH agonists.

In the controlled clinical trials of ZOLADEX versus orchiectomy, the following events were reported as adverse reactions in greater than 5% of the patients.

	TREATMENT RECEIVED	
	ZOLADEX (n=242)	ORCHIECTOMY (n=254)
Adverse Event	%	%
Hot Flashes	62	53
Sexual Dysfunction	21	15
Decreased Erections	18	16
Lower Urinary Tract Symptoms	13	8
Lethargy	8	4
Pain (worsened in the first 30 days)	8	3
Edema	7	8
Upper Respiratory Infection	7	2
Rash	6	1
Sweating	6	4
Anorexia	5	2
Chronic Obstructive Pulmonary Disease	5	3
Congestive Heart Failure	5	1
Dizziness	5	4
Insomnia	5	1
Nausea	5	2
Complications of Surgery	0	18*

*Complications related to surgery were reported in 18% of the orchiectomy patients, while only 3% of ZOLADEX patients reported adverse reactions at the injection site. The surgical complications included scrotal infection (5.9%), groin pain (4.7%), wound seepage (3.1%), scrotal hematoma (2.8%), incisional discomfort (1.6%) and skin necrosis (1.2%).

The following additional adverse reactions were reported in greater than 1% but less than 5% of the patients treated with ZOLADEX: CARDIOVASCULAR—arrhythmia, cerebrovascular accident, hypertension, myocardial infarction, peripheral vascular disorder, chest pain; CENTRAL NERVOUS SYSTEM—anxiety, depression, headache; GASTROINTESTINAL—constipation, diarrhea, ulcer, vomiting; HEMATOLOGIC—anemia; METABOLIC/NUTRITIONAL—gout, hyperglycemia, weight increase; MISCELLANEOUS—chills, fever; UROGENITAL—renal insufficiency, urinary obstruction, urinary tract infection, breast swelling and tenderness.

OVERDOSAGE

The pharmacologic properties of ZOLADEX and its mode of administration make accidental or intentional overdosage unlikely. There is no experience of overdosage from clinical trials. Animal studies indicate that no increased pharmacologic effect occurred at higher doses or more frequent administration. Subcutaneous doses of the drug as high as 1 mg/kg/day in rats and dogs did not produce any nonendocrine related sequelae; this dose is greater than 400 times that proposed for human use. If overdosage occurs, it should be managed symptomatically.

DOSAGE AND ADMINISTRATION

ZOLADEX, at a dose of 3.6 mg, should be administered subcutaneously every 28 days into the upper abdominal wall using sterile technique under the supervision of a physician. At the physician's option, local anesthesia may be used prior to injection.

While a delay of a few days is permissible, every effort should be made to adhere to the 28-day schedule.

Administration Technique: The proper method of administration of ZOLADEX is described in the instructions that follow.

Continued on next page

ICI Pharma—Cont.

1. The package should be inspected for damage prior to opening. If the package is damaged, the syringe should not be used. Do not remove the sterile syringe from the package until immediately before use. Examine the syringe for damage, and check that ZOLADEX is visible in the translucent chamber.
2. Grasp red plastic safety clip tab, pull out and away from needle, and discard immediately. Then remove needle cover.
3. After cleaning with an alcohol swab, an area of skin on the upper abdominal wall may be anesthetized at the physician's option with a local anesthetic in the normal fashion.
4. Using an aseptic technique, stretch the patient's skin with one hand, and grip the needle with your fingers around the barrel of the syringe. Insert the hypodermic needle into the subcutaneous fat.

NOTE: The ZOLADEX syringe cannot be used for aspiration. If the hypodermic needle penetrates a large vessel, blood will be seen instantly in the syringe chamber. If a vessel is penetrated, withdraw the needle and inject with a new syringe elsewhere.

5. Change the direction of the needle so it parallels the abdominal wall. Push the needle in until the barrel hub touches the patient's skin. Withdraw the needle one centimeter to create a space to discharge ZOLADEX. Fully depress the plunger to discharge ZOLADEX.
6. Withdraw the needle. Then bandage the site. Confirm discharge of ZOLADEX by ensuring tip of the plunger is visible within the tip of the needle. Dispose of the used needle and syringe in a safe manner.

NOTE: In the unlikely event of the need to surgically remove ZOLADEX, it can be localized by ultrasound.

HOW SUPPLIED

ZOLADEX is supplied as a sterile and totally biodegradable D,L-lactic and glycolic acids copolymer (13.3–14.3 mg/dose) impregnated with goserelin acetate equivalent to 3.6 mg of goserelin in a disposable syringe device fitted with a 16 gauge hypodermic needle (NDC 0310-0960). The unit is sterile and comes in a sealed, light and moisture proof, aluminum foil laminate pouch containing a desiccant capsule. Store at room temperature (do not exceed 25°C).

---

[1] MacLeod TL, et al. 1987. Anaphylactic reaction to synthetic luteinizing hormone-releasing hormone. *Fertil Steril.* Sept;48(3);500–502.

Made in United Kingdom
Manufactured for
ICI Pharma
A business unit of ICI Americas Inc.
Wilmington, DE 19897 USA
Rev J 02/92

Shown in Product Identification Section, page 412

ICN Pharmaceuticals, Inc.
ICN PLAZA
3300 HYLAND AVENUE
COSTA MESA, CA 92626

ANDROID–10® Ⓒ℞
Methyltestosterone Tablets (Oral) USP, 10 mg

ANDROID–25® Ⓒ℞
Methyltestosterone Tablets (Oral) USP, 25 mg

DESCRIPTION

ANDROID 10 mg or 25 mg Tablets contain methyltestosterone, USP, a synthetic androgen. Androgens are steroids that develop and maintain primary and secondary male sex characteristics. ANDROID Tablets are to be taken orally.

Androgens are derivatives of cyclopentanoperhydrophenanthrene. Endogenous androgens are C-19 steriods with a side chain at C-17, and with two angular methyl groups. Testosterone is the primary endogenous androgen. In their active form, all drugs in the class have a 17-beta-hydroxy group. 17-alpha alkylation (methyltestosterone) increases the pharmacologic activity per unit weight compared to testosterone when given orally.

Methyltestosterone is the 17α-methyl derivative of testosterone, the true testicular hormone. Chemically, methyltestosterone is 17β-hydroxy-17-methylandrost-4-en-3-one, with the empirical formula $C_{20}H_{30}O_2$, a molecular weight of 302.5, and the following structural formula:

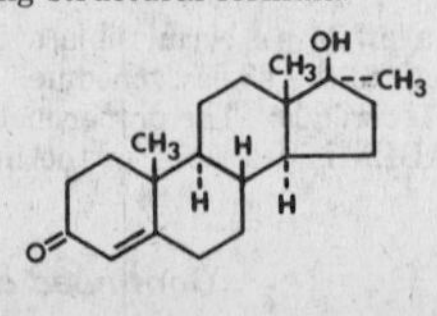

Methyltestosterone is a white or creamy white, odorless, and slightly hygroscopic powder. It is practically insoluble in water, and is soluble in alcohol, and other organic solvents. ANDROID Tablets contain 10 mg or 25 mg methyltestosterone, USP, and corn starch, lactose and magnesium stearate.

CLINICAL PHARMACOLOGY

Endogenous androgens are responsible for the normal growth and development of the male sex organs and for maintenance of secondary sex characteristics. These effects include the growth and maturation of prostate, seminal vesicles, penis and scrotum; the development of male hair distribution, such as beard, pubic, chest, and axillary hair; laryngeal enlargement, vocal chord thickening, alterations in body musculature and fat distribution. Drugs in this class also cause retention of nitrogen, sodium, potassium, phosphorus, and decreased urinary excretion of calcium. Androgens have been reported to increase protein anabolism and decrease protein catabolism. Nitrogen balance is improved only when there is sufficient intake of calories and protein.

Androgens are responsible for the growth spurt of adolescence and for the eventual termination of linear growth which is brought about by fusion of the epiphyseal growth centers. In children, exogenous androgens accelerate linear growth rates, but may cause a disproportionate advancement in bone maturation. Use over long periods may result in fusion of the epiphyseal growth centers and termination of growth process. Androgens have been reported to stimulate the production of red blood cells by enhancing the production of erythropoietic stimulating factor.

During exogenous administration of androgens, endogenous testosterone release is inhibited through feedback inhibition of pituitary luteinizing hormone (LH). With large doses of exogenous androgens, spermatogenesis may also be suppressed through feedback inhibition of pituitary follicle stimulating hormone (FSH).

There is a lack of substantial evidence that androgens are effective in fractures, surgery, convalescence, and functional uterine bleeding.

Pharmacokinetics: Testosterone given orally is metabolized by the gut and 44% is cleared by the liver in the first pass. Oral doses as high as 400 mg per day are needed to achieve clinically effective blood levels for full replacement therapy. The synthetic androgen (methyltestosterone) is less extensively metabolized by the liver and has a longer half-life. It is more suitable than testosterone for oral administration.

Testosterone in plasma is 98% bound to a specific testosterone-estradiol binding globulin, and about 2% is free. Generally, the amount of this sex-hormone binding globulin in the plasma will determine the distribution of testosterone between free and bound forms, and the free testosterone concentration will determine its half-life.

About 90% of a dose of testosterone is excreted in the urine as glucuronic and sulfuric acid conjugates of testosterone and its metabolites; about 6% of a dose is excreted in the feces, mostly in the unconjugated form. Inactivation of testosterone occurs primarily in the liver. Testosterone is metabolized to various 17-keto steroids through two different pathways. As reported in the literature, the half-life of testosterone varies considerably, ranging from 10 to 100 minutes.

In many tissues the activity of testosterone appears to depend on reduction to dihydrotestosterone, which binds to cytosol receptor proteins. The steroid-receptor complex is transported to the nucleus where it initiates transcription events and cellular changes related to androgen action.

INDICATIONS AND USAGE

In the Male: ANDROID Tablets are indicated for replacement therapy in conditions associated with a deficiency or absence of endogenous testosterone:

Primary Hypogonadism (congenital or acquired): Testicular failure due to cryptorchidism, bilateral torsion, orchitis, vanishing testis syndrome or orchidectomy.

Hypogonadotropic Hypogonadism (congenital or acquired): Idiopathic gonadotropin or LHRH deficiency, or pituitary-hypothalamic injury from tumors, trauma or radiation.

If the above conditions occur prior to puberty, androgen replacement therapy will be needed during the adolescent years for development of secondary sexual characteristics. Prolonged androgen treatment will be required to maintain sexual characteristics in these and other males who develop testosterone deficiency after puberty.

Androgens may be used to stimulate puberty in carefully selected males with clearly delayed puberty. These patients usually have a familial pattern of delayed puberty that is not secondary to a pathological disorder; puberty is expected to occur spontaneously at a relatively late date. Brief treatment with conservative doses may occasionally be justified in these patients if they do not respond to psychological support. The potential adverse effect on bone maturation should be discussed with the patient and parents prior to androgen administration. An X-ray of the hand and wrist to determine bone age should be obtained every 6 months to assess the effect of treatment on the epiphyseal centers (See **WARNINGS.**)

In the Female: ANDROID Tablets may be used secondarily in women with advancing inoperable metastatic (skeletal) breast cancer who are 1 to 5 years postmenopausal. Primary goals of therapy in these women include ablation of the ovaries. Other methods of counteracting estrogen activity are adrenalectomy, hypophysectomy, and/or anti-estrogen therapy. This treatment has also been used in premenopausal women with breast cancer who have benefited from oophorectomy and are considered to have a hormone-responsive tumor. Judgment concerning androgen therapy should be made by an oncologist with expertise in this field.

CONTRAINDICATIONS

ANDROID Tablets are contraindicated for use in men with carcinomas of the breast or with known or suspected carcinomas of the prostate, and in women who are or may become pregnant.

When administered to pregnant women, androgens cause virilization of the external genitalia of the female fetus. This virilization includes clitoromegaly, abnormal vaginal development, and fusion of genital folds to form a scrotal-like structure. The degree of masculinization is related to the amount of drug given and the age of the fetus, and is most likely to occur in the female fetus when the drugs are given in the first trimester. If the patient becomes pregnant while taking these drugs, she should be apprised of the potential hazard to the fetus.

WARNINGS

In patients with breast cancer, androgen therapy may cause hypercalcemia by stimulating osteolysis. In this case, the drug should be discontinued.

Prolonged use of high doses of androgens has been associated with the development of peliosis hepatis and hepatic neoplasms including hepatocellular carcinoma. (see **PRECAUTIONS: Carcinogenesis, Mutagenesis, Impairment of Fertility.**) Peliosis hepatis can be a life-threatening or fatal complication.

Cholestatic hepatitis and jaundice occur with 17-alpha-alkylandrogens (such as methyltestosterone) at a relatively low dose. If cholestatic hepatitis with jaundice appears or if liver function tests become abnormal, the androgen should be discontinued and the etiology should be determined. Drug-induced jaundice is reversible when the medication is discontinued.

Geriatric patients treated with androgens may be at an increased risk for the development of prostatic hypertropy and prostatic carcinoma.

Edema with or without congestive heart failure may be a serious complication in patients with pre-existing cardiac, renal or hepatic disease. In addition to discontinuation of the drug, diuretic therapy may be required.

Gynecomastia frequently develops and occasionally persists in patients being treated for hypogonadism.

Androgen therapy should be used cautiously in healthy males with delayed puberty. The effect on bone maturation should be monitored by assessing bone age of the wrist and hand every 6 months. In children, androgen treatment may accelerate bone maturation without producing compensatory gain in linear growth. This adverse effect may result in compromised adult stature. The younger the child the greater the risk of compromising final mature height.

This drug has not been shown to be safe and effective for the enhancement of athletic performance. Because of the potential risk of serious adverse health effects, this drug should not be used for such purpose.

PRECAUTIONS

General: Women should be observed for signs of virilization (deepening of the voice, hirsutism, acne, clitoromegaly and menstrual irregularities). Discontinuation of drug therapy at the time of evidence of mild virilism is necessary to prevent irreversible virilization. Such virilization is usual following androgen use at high doses. A decision may be made by the patient and the physician that some virilization will be tolerated during treatment for breast carcinoma.

Priapism or excessive sexual stimulation may develop. Males, especially the elderly, may become overstimulated. In treating males for symptoms of climacteric, avoid stimulation to the point of increasing the nervous, mental, and physical activities beyond the patient's cardiovascular capacity.

Oligospermia and reduced ejaculatory volume may occur after prolonged administration of excessive dosage.

Information for Patients: The physician should instruct patients to report any of the following side effects of androgens:

Adult or Adolescent Males: Too frequent or persistent erections of the penis.

Women: Hoarseness, acne, changes in menstrual periods, or more hair on the face.

All Patients: Any nausea, vomiting, changes in skin color or ankle swelling.

Any male adolescent patient receiving androgens for delayed puberty should have bone development checked every 6 months.

Laboratory Tests: Women with disseminated breast carcinomas should have frequent determination of urine and serum calcium levels during the course of androgen therapy. (See **WARNINGS.**)

Because of the hepatotoxicity associated with the use of 17-alpha-alkylated androgens, liver function tests should be obtained periodically.

Periodic (every 6 months) x-ray examinations of bone age should be made during treatment of pre-pubertal males to determine the rate of bone maturation and the effects of androgen therapy on the epiphyseal centers.

Hemoglobin and hematocrit should be checked periodically for polycythemia in patients who are receiving high doses of androgens.

DRUG INTERACTIONS

Anticoagulants: C-17 substituted derivatives of testosterone, such as methandrostenolone, have been reported to decrease the anticoagulant requirements of patients receiving oral anticoagulants. Patients receiving oral anticoagulant therapy require close monitoring, especially when androgens are started or stopped.

Oxyphenbutazone: Concurrent administration of oxyphenbutazone and androgens may result in elevated serum levels of oxyphenbutazone.

Insulin: In diabetic patients the metabolic effects of androgens may decrease blood glucose and insulin requirements.

Drug/Laboratory Test Interferences: Androgens may decrease levels of thyroxine-binding globulin, resulting in decreased total T_4 serum levels and increased resin uptake of T_3 and T_4. Free thyroid hormone levels remain unchanged, however, and there is no clinical evidence of thyroid dysfunction.

Carcinogenesis, Mutagenesis, Impairment of Fertility: *Animal Data:* Testosterone has been tested by subcutaneous injection and implantation in mice and rats. The implant induced cervical-uterine tumors in mice, which metastasized in some cases. There is suggestive evidence that injection of testosterone into some strains of female mice increases their susceptibility to hepatoma. Testosterone is also known to increase the number of tumors and decrease the degree of differentiation of chemically induced carcinomas of the liver in rats.

Human Data: There are rare reports of hepatocellular carcinoma in patients receiving long-term therapy with androgens in high doses. Withdrawal of the drugs did not lead to regression of the tumors in all cases.

Geriatric patients treated with androgens may be at an increased risk for the development of prostatic hypertrophy and prostatic carcinoma.

Information of mutagenesis is unknown.

Pregnancy: ***Teratogenic Effects—Pregnancy Category X:*** See **CONTRAINDICATIONS.**

Nursing Mothers: It is not known whether androgens are excreted in human milk. Because many drugs are excreted in human milk and because of the potential for serious adverse reactions in nursing infants from androgens, a decision should be made whether to discontinue nursing or to discontinue the drug, taking into account the importance of the drug to the mother.

Pediatric Use: Androgen therapy should be used very cautiously in children and only by specialists who are aware of the adverse effects on bone maturation. Skeletal maturation must be monitored every six months by an x-ray of the hand and wrist. (See **INDICATIONS AND USAGE** and **WARNINGS.**)

ADVERSE REACTIONS

Endocrine and Urogenital: *Female:* The most common side effects of androgen therapy are amenorrhea and other menstrual irregularities, inhibition of gonadotropin secretion, and virilization, including deepening of the voice and clitoral enlargement. The latter usually is not reversible after androgens are discontinued. When administered to a pregnant woman, androgens cause virilization of external genitalia of the female fetus.

Male: Gynecomastia, and excessive frequency and duration of penile erections. Oligospermia may occur at high dosages (See **CLINICAL PHARMACOLOGY.**)

Skin and Appendages: Hirsutism, male pattern of baldness, and acne.

Fluid and Electrolyte Disturbances: Retention of sodium, chloride, water, potassium, calcium, and inorganic phosphates.

Gastrointestinal: Nausea, cholestatic jaundice, alterations in liver function tests, rarely hepatocellular neoplasms and peliosis hepatis. (See **WARNINGS.**)

Hematologic: Suppression of clotting factors, II, V, VII, and X, bleeding in patients on concomitant anticoagulant therapy, and polycythemia.

Nervous System: Increased or decreased libido, headache, anxiety, depression, and generalized paresthesia.

Metabolic: Increased serum cholesterol.

Miscellaneous: Rarely anaphylactoid reactions.

DRUG ABUSE AND DEPENDENCE

Controlled Substance Class: ANDROID Tablets are classified as controlled substances under the Anabolic Steroids Control Act of 1990 and have been assigned to Schedule III.

OVERDOSAGE

Overdose of medication may be reflected in the occurrence of the signs and symptoms associated with testosterone-anabolic drugs. Nausea and appearance of the early manifestations of edema should be looked for. However, there has been no report of acute overdosage with androgens.

DOSAGE AND ADMINISTRATION

Dosage must be strictly individualized. The suggested dosage for androgens varies depending on the age, sex, and diagnosis of the individual patient. Adjustments and duration of dosage will depend upon the patient's response and the appearance of adverse reactions.

Males: In the androgen-deficient male the following guideline for replacement therapy indicates the usual initial dosages.

	Route	Dose	Frequency
ANDROID Tablets	Oral	10–50 mg	Daily

Various dosage regimens have been used to induce pubertal changes in hypogonadal males; some experts have advocated lower dosages initially, gradually increasing the dose as puberty progresses, with or without a decrease to maintenance levels. Other experts emphasize that higher dosages are needed to induce pubertal changes and lower dosages can be used for maintenance after puberty. The chronological and skeletal ages must be taken into consideration, both in determining the initial dose and in adjusting the dose.

Dosages used in delayed puberty generally are in the lower ranges of those given above, and are for limited duration, for example, 4 to 6 months.

Females: Women with metastatic breast carcinoma must be followed closely because androgen therapy occasionally appears to accelerate the disease. Thus, many experts prefer to use the shorter acting androgen preparations rather than those with prolonged activity for treating breast carcinoma particularly during the early stages of androgen therapy.

Guideline dosages and adrogens for use in the palliative treatment of women with metastatic breast cancer:

	Route	Dose	Frequency
ANDROID Tablets breast cancer	oral	50–200 mg	daily

HOW SUPPLIED

ANDROID Tablets, 10 mg compressed, white, round tablets impressed with the ICN trademark and product identification number 311; bottle of 100 (NDC-0187-0311-06).

ANDROID Tablets, 25 mg compressed peach colored, round tablets impressed with the ICN trademark and product identification number 499; bottle of 100 (NDC-0187-0499-06).

Revised 4/92

BENOQUIN® ℞

[*ben'ō-kwin*]

(Monobenzone USP 20% Cream)

FEDERAL (U.S.A.) LAW PROHIBITS DISPENSING WITHOUT PRESCRIPTION.

DESCRIPTION

Each gram of Benoquin Cream contains 200 mg of monobenzone, USP, in a water-washable base consisting of purified water, cetyl alcohol, propylene glycol, sodium lauryl sulfate and beeswax.

CLINICAL PHARMACOLOGY

The mechanism of action of Benoquin is not fully understood. Denton et al. suggested that Benoquin may be converted to hydroquinone, which they found to inhibit the enzymatic oxidation of tyrosine to DOPA.

Iijima and Watanabe suggested a direct action on tyrosinase. Another suggestion by Denton and his group was that Benoquin acts as an anti-oxidant to prevent SH-group oxidation so that more SH groups are available to inhibit tyrosinase. The primary role of inflammation in the depigmentation process was studied by Becker and Spencer who suggested that increased cell permeability allows Benoquin to enter the melanocyte to form an antigenic substance which attached to the melanin granule enters the dermis where antibodies are produced, remote positive patch-testing may result.

INDICATIONS AND USAGE

Benoquin Cream is indicated for final depigmentation in extensive vitiligo.

Benoquin Cream is not recommended for freckling, hyperpigmentation due to photosensitization following use of certain perfumes (berlock dermatitis), melasma (chloasma) of pregnancy, and hyperpigmentation following inflammation of the skin. Benoquin Cream is of no value in the treatment of cafe-au-lait spots, pigmented nevi, malignant melanoma, or pigment resulting from pigments other than melanin, including bile, silver, and artificial pigments.

CONTRAINDICATIONS

Prior history of sensitivity or allergic reaction to this product or any of its ingredients. The safety of topical monobenzone use during pregnancy or in children (12 years and under) has not been established.

WARNINGS

A. Benoquin Cream is a potent depigmenting agent, not a mild cosmetic bleach. Do not use except for final depigmentation in extensive vitiligo.
B. Keep this and all medication out of the reach of children. In case of accidental ingestion, call a physician or a poison control center immediately.

PRECAUTIONS

See Warnings.

A. Pregnancy Category C. Animal reproduction studies have not been conducted with topical monobenzone. It is also not known whether monobenzone can cause fetal harm when used topically on a pregnant woman or affect reproductive capacity. It is not known to what degree, if any, topical monobenzone is absorbed systemically. Topical monobenzone should be used in pregnant women only when clearly indicated.
B. Nursing mothers. It is not known whether topical monobenzone is absorbed or excreted in human milk. Caution is advised when topical monobenzone is used by a nursing mother.
C. Pediatric usage. Safety and effectiveness in children below the age of 12 years have not been established.

ADVERSE REACTIONS

Occasional irritation, a burning sensation, or dermatitis may occur in which case medication should be discontinued and the physician notified immediately.

DOSAGE AND ADMINISTRATION

Benoquin should be applied to the pigmented area and rubbed in well two or three times daily or as directed by physician. There is no recommended dosage for children under 12 years of age except under the advice and supervision of a physician.

NOTE

Depigmentation is usually observed after one to four months of therapy. If satisfactory results have not been obtained within four months, treatment should be discontinued.

HOW SUPPLIED

BENOQUIN Cream, 20% in $1\frac{1}{4}$ oz. tubes (NDC 0187-0380-34).

BENOQUIN Cream should be stored at room temperature (15-30°C) (59-86°F)

ELDECORT® Cream 1.0%, 2.5% ℞

(Hydrocortisone Cream USP, 1.0%, 2.5%)

FEDERAL (U.S.A.) LAW PROHIBITS DISPENSING WITHOUT PRESCRIPTION.

DESCRIPTION

Eldecort contains hydrocortisone in a water-washable cream base of stearic acid, glyceryl monostearate, mineral oil light, squalene, propylene glycol, polyoxyl 40 stearate, polyoxyethylene 25 propylene glycol stearate, citric acid, potassium sorbate, allantoin, and water.

The content of hydrocortisone in milligrams per gram of cream is as follows:

% Hydrocortisone	mg Hydrocortisone/gm Cream
1.0	10
$2\frac{1}{2}$	25

The topical corticosteroids, including hydrocortisone, constitute a class of primary synthetic steroids used as anti-inflammatory and antipruritic agents.

CLINICAL PHARMACOLOGY

Topical corticosteroids share anti-inflammatory, anti-pruritic and vasoconstrictive actions.

The mechanism of anti-inflammatory activity of the topical corticosteroids is unclear. Various laboratory methods, including vasoconstrictor assays, are used to compare and predict potencies and/or clinical efficacies of the topical corticosteroids. There is some evidence to suggest that a recognizable correlation exists between vasoconstrictor potency and therapeutic efficacy in man.

Pharmacokinetics—The extent of percutaneous absorption of topical corticosteroids is determined by many factors including the vehicle, the integrity of the epidermal barrier, and the use of occlusive dressings.

Topical corticosteroids can be absorbed from normal intact skin, inflammation and/or other disease processes in the skin increase percutaneous absorption. Occlusive dressings substantially increase the percutaneous absorption of topi-

Continued on next page

ICN—Cont.

cal corticosteroids. Thus occlusive dressings may be a valuable therapeutic adjunct for treatment of resistant dermatoses. (See DOSAGE AND ADMINISTRATION.)

Once absorbed through the skin, topical corticosteroids are handled through pharmacokinetic pathways similar to systemically administered corticosteroids. Corticosteroids are bound to plasma proteins in varying degrees. Corticosteroids are metabolized primarily in the liver and are then excreted by the kidneys. Some of the topical corticosteroids and their metabolites are also excreted into the bile.

INDICATIONS AND USAGE

Eldecort is indicated for the relief of inflammatory and pruritic manifestations of corticosteroid responsive dermatoses.

CONTRAINDICATIONS

Eldecort is contraindicated in those patients with a history of hypersensitivity to any of the components of the preparation.

PRECAUTIONS

General —Systemic absorption of topical corticosteroids has produced reversible hypothalamic-pituitary-adrenal (HPA) axis suppression, manifestations of Cushing's syndrome, hyperglycemia, and glucosuria in some patients.

Conditions which augment systemic absorption include the application of the more potent steroids, use over large surface areas, prolonged use, and the addition of occlusive dressing.

Therefore, patients receiving a large dose of potent topical steroid applied to a large surface area or under an occlusive dressing should be evaluated periodically for evidence of HPA axis suppression by using the urinary free cortisol and ACTH stimulation tests. If HPA axis suppression is noted, an attempt should be made to withdraw the drug, to reduce the frequency of application, or to substitute a less potent steroid.

Recovery of HPA axis function is generally prompt and complete upon discontinuation of the drug. Infrequently, signs and symptoms of steroid withdrawal may occur, requiring supplemental systemic corticosteroids.

Children may absorb proportionally larger amounts of topical corticosteroids, and thus be more susceptible to systemic toxicity. (See PRECAUTIONS—PEDIATRIC USE.)

If irritation develops, topical corticosteroids should be discontinued and appropriate therapy instituted.

In the presence of dermatological infections, the use of an appropriate antifungal or antibacterial agent should be instituted. If a favorable response does not occur promptly, the corticosteroid should be discontinued until the infection has been adequately controlled.

Information for the Patient —Patients using topical corticosteroids should receive the following information and instructions:

1. This medication is to be used as directed by the physician. It is for external use only. Avoid contact with the eyes.
2. Patients should be advised not to use this medication for any disorder other than for which it was prescribed.
3. The treated skin areas should not be bandaged or otherwise covered or wrapped as to be occlusive unless directed by the physician.
4. Patients should report any signs of local adverse reactions especially under occlusive dressing.
5. Parents of pediatric patients should be advised not to use tight-fitting diapers or plastic pants on a child being treated in the diaper area, as these garments may constitute occlusive dressings.

Laboratory Tests —The following tests may be helpful in evaluating the HPA axis suppression: urinary free cortisol test; ACTH stimulation test.

Carcinogenesis, Mutagenesis, and Impairment of Fertility —Long-term animal studies have not been performed to evaluate the carcinogenic potential or the effect on fertility of topical corticosteroids.

Studies to determine mutagenicity with prednisolone and hydrocortisone have revealed negative results.

Pregnancy—Category C —Corticosteroids are generally teratogenic in laboratory animals when administered systemically at relatively low dosage levels. The more potent corticosteroids have been shown to be teratogenic after dermal application in laboratory animals. There are no adequate and well-controlled studies in pregnant women on teratogenic effects from topically applied corticosteroids. Therefore, topical corticosteroids should be used during pregnancy only if the potential benefit justifies the potential risk to the fetus. Drugs of this class should not be used extensively on pregnant patients, in large amounts, or for prolonged periods of time.

Nursing Mothers —It is not known whether topical administration of corticosteroids could result in sufficient systemic absorption to produce detectable quantities in breast milk. Systemically administered corticosteroids are secreted into breast milk in quantities not likely to have a deleterious effect on the infant. Nevertheless, caution should be exercised

when topical costicosteroids are administered to a nursing woman.

Pediatric Use—Pediatric patients may demonstrate greater susceptibiliy to topical corticosteroid-induced HPA axis suppression and Cushing's syndrome than mature patients because of a larger skin surface area to body weight ratio.

Hypothalamic-pituitary-adrenal (HPA) axis suppression, Cushing's syndrome, and intracranial hypertension have been reported in children receiving topical corticosteroids. Manifestations of adrenal suppression in children include linear growth retardation, delayed weight gain, low plasma cortisol levels, and absence of response to ACTH stimulation. Manifestations of intracranial hypertension include bulging fontanelles, headaches, and bilateral papilledema.

Adminstration of topical corticosteroids to children should be limited to the least amount compatible with an effective therapeutic regimen. Chronic corticosteroid therapy may interfere with the growth and development of children.

ADVERSE REACTIONS

The following local adverse reactions are reported infrequently with topical corticosteroids, but may occur more frequently with the use of occlusive dressings. These reactions are listed in an approximate decreasing order of occurrence: burning, itching, irritation, dryness, folliculitis, hypertrichosis, acneiform eruptions, hypopigmentation, perioral dermatitis, allergic contact dermatitis, maceration of the skin, secondary infection, skin atrophy, striae, miliaria.

OVERDOSAGE

Topically applied corticosteroids can be absorbed in sufficient amounts to produce systemic effects. (See PRECAUTIONS.)

DOSAGE AND ADMINISTRATION

Apply Eldecort to areas as a thin film from two to four times daily depending on the severity of the condition.

Occlusive dressings may be used for the management of psoriasis or recalcitrant conditions.

If an infection develops, the use of occlusive dressings should be discontinued and appropriate antimicrobial therapy instituted.

HOW SUPPLIED

Concentration	Size/Tubes	NDC Number
1%	½ ounce (15 grams)	0187-0386-35
1%	1 ounce (30 grams)	0187-0386-31
2½%	½ ounce	0187-0351-35
2½%	1 ounce	0187-0351-31

Eldecort should be stored at controlled room temperature 15°–30°C (59°–86°F).

Revised 3/90   2408-01

ELDOPAQUE Forte® 4% Cream   ℞
[él-do-pāk " for 'tā]
(Hydroquinone USP, 4%)
Skin Bleaching Cream With SunBlock

FEDERAL LAW (U.S.A.) PROHIBITS DISPENSING WITHOUT A PRESCRIPTION.
FOR EXTERNAL USE ONLY

DESCRIPTION

Each gram of Eldopaque Forte 4% Cream contains 40 mg of hydroquinone in a tinted sunblocking base of water, stearic acid, talc, PEG-40 stearate, PEG-25 propylene glycol stearate, propylene glycol, glyceryl stearate, iron oxides, mineral oil, squalane, disodium EDTA, sodium metabisulfite, and potassium sorbate.

CLINICAL PHARMACOLOGY

Topical application of hydroquinone produces a reversible depigmentation of the skin by inhibition of the enzymatic oxidation of tyrosine to 3, 4-dihydroxyphenylalanine (dopa) and suppression of other melanocyte metabolic processes. Exposure to sunlight or ultraviolet light will cause repigmentation which may be prevented by the sunblocking agents contained in Eldopaque Forte.

INDICATIONS AND USAGE

Eldopaque Forte 4% Cream is indicated for the gradual bleaching of hyperpigmented skin conditions such as chloasma, melasma, freckles, senile lentigines, and other unwanted areas of melanin hyperpigmentation.

CONTRAINDICATIONS

Prior history of sensitivity or allergic reaction to this product or any of its ingredients. The safety of topical hydroquinone use during pregnancy or in children (12 years and under) has not been established.

WARNINGS

A. CAUTION: Hydroquinone is a skin bleaching agent which may produce unwanted cosmetic effects if not used as directed. The physician should be familiar with the contents of this insert before prescribing or dispensing this medication.

B. Test for skin sensitivity before using Eldopaque Forte 4% Cream by applying a small amount to an unbroken patch of skin and check in 24 hours. Minor redness is not a contraindication, but where there is itching or vesicle formation or excessive inflammatory response, further treatment is not advised. Close patient supervision is recommended.

Contact with the eyes should be avoided. If no bleaching or lightening effect is noted after 2 months of treatment use, Eldopaque Forte 4% Cream should be discontinued. Eldopaque Forte 4% Cream is formulated for use as a skin bleaching agent and should not be used for the prevention of sunburn.

C. Sunscreen use is an essential aspect of hydroquinone therapy because even minimal sunlight exposure sustains melanocytic activity. The sunscreens in Eldopaque Forte 4% Cream provide the necessary sun protection during skin bleaching therapy. After clearing and during maintenance therapy, sun exposure should be avoided on bleached skin by application of a sunscreen or sunblock agent, or protective clothing to prevent repigmentation.

D. Keep this and all medications out of the reach of children. In case of accidental ingestion, call a physician or a poison control center immediately.

E. WARNING: Contains sodium metabisulfite, a sulfite that may cause serious allergic type reactions (e.g. hives, itching, wheezing, anaphylaxis, severe asthma attacks) in certain susceptible persons.

PRECAUTIONS
SEE WARNINGS.

A. Pregnancy Category C. Animal reproduction studies have not been conducted with topical hydroquinone. It is also not known whether hydroquinone can cause fetal harm when used topically on a pregnant woman or affect reproductive capacity. It is not known to what degree, if any, topical hydroquinone is absorbed systemically. Topical hydroquinone should be used in women only when clearly indicated.

B. Nursing mothers. It is not known whether topical hydroquinone is absorbed or excreted in human milk. Caution is advised when topical hydroquinone is used by a nursing mother.

C. Pediatric usage. Safety and effectiveness in children below the age of 12 years have not been established.

ADVERSE REACTIONS

No systemic adverse reactions have been reported. Occasional hypersensitivity (localized contact dermatitis) may occur in which case the medication should be discontinued and the physician notified immediately.

OVERDOSAGE

There have been no systemic reactions from the use of topical hydroquinone or the sunblockers in Eldopaque Forte 4% Cream. However, treatment should be limited to relatively small areas of the body at one time since some patients experience a transient skin reddening and a mild burning sensation which does not preclude treatment.

DRUG DOSAGE AND ADMINISTRATION

A thin application of Eldopaque Forte 4% Cream should be applied to the affected area twice daily or as directed by a physician. Do not rub in. There is no recommendation for children under 12 years of age except under the advice and supervision of a physician.

HOW SUPPLIED

Eldopaque Forte 4% Cream is available as follows:

Size	NDC Number
½ ounce tube (15 grams)	0187-0395-35
1 ounce tube (30 grams)	0187-0395-31

Available without prescription for maintenance therapy: Eldopaque® (2% Hydroquinone) in ½ ounce (NDC 0187-0518-35) and 1 ounce (NDC 0187-0518-31) tubes.

Eldopaque Forte 4% Cream should be stored at room temperature (15-30°C) (59-86°F).

ELDOQUIN Forte® 4% Cream   ℞
[el '-dō-kwin " for 'tā]
(Hydroquinone USP, 4%)
Skin Bleaching Cream

FEDERAL LAW (U.S.A.) PROHIBITS DISPENSING WITHOUT A PRESCRIPTION.
FOR EXTERNAL USE ONLY

DESCRIPTION

Each gram of Eldoquin Forte contains 40 mg of hydroquinone in a vanishing cream base of purified water, stearic acid, propylene glycol, poloxyl 40 stearate, propylene glycol monostearate, glyceryl monostearate, mineral oil, squalane, propylparaben and sodium metabisulfite.

CLINICAL PHARMACOLOGY

Topical application of hydroquinone produces a reversible depigmentation of the skin by inhibition of the enzymatic oxidation of tyrosine to 3, 4-dihydroxyphenylalanine (dopa) and suppression of the other melanocyte metabolic processes. Exposure to sunlight or ultraviolet light will cause repigmentation of the bleached areas.

INDICATIONS AND USAGE

Eldoquin Forte 4% Cream is indicated for the gradual bleaching of hyperpigmented skin conditions such as chloasma, melasma, freckles, senile lentigines, and other unwanted areas of melanin hyperpigmentation. It is intended for night-time use only since it contains no sunblocking agents. For daytime usage, Solaquin Forte™ 4% Cream or Eldopaque Forte® 4% Cream should be prescribed.

CONTRAINDICATIONS

Prior history of sensitivity or allergic reaction to this product or any of its ingredients. The safety of topical hydroquinone use during pregnancy or in children (12 years and under) has not been established.

WARNINGS

A. CAUTION: Hydroquinone is a skin bleaching agent which may produce unwanted cosmetic effects if not used as directed. The physician should be familiar with the contents of this insert before prescribing or dispensing this medication.

B. Test for skin sensitivity before using Eldoquin Forte 4% Cream by applying a small amount to an unbroken patch of skin and check in 24 hours. Minor redness is not a contraindication, but where there is itching or vesicle formation or excessive inflammatory response, further treatment is not advised. Close patient supervision is recommended.

Contact with the eyes should be avoided. If no bleaching or lightening effect is noted after 2 months of treatment, the medication should be discontinued.

C. There are no sunblocking or sunscreening agents in Eldoquin Forte 4% Cream and since minimal sunlight exposure may reverse the bleaching effect of this preparation, it should be used only at night or on areas of the body covered by protective clothing. During the daytime, sunblocking or broad spectrum sunscreen preparations or protective clothing should be used to prevent the bleached areas from repigmentation. For daytime bleaching of unwanted pigmented areas, the use of Solaquin Forte™ 4% Cream or Eldopaque Forte® 4% Cream should be considered.

D. Keep this and all medication out of the reach of children. In case of accidental ingestion, call a physician or a poison control center immediately.

E. WARNING: Contains sodium metabisulfite, a sulfite that may cause serious allergic type reactions (e.g. hives, itching, wheezing, anaphylaxis, serious asthma attacks) in certain susceptible persons.

PRECAUTIONS

SEE WARNINGS.

A. Pregnancy Category C. Animal reproduction studies have not been conducted with topical hydroquinone. It is also not known whether hydroquinone can cause fetal harm when used topically on a pregnant woman or affect reproductive capacity. It is not known to what degree, if any, topical hydroquinone is absorbed systemically. Topical hydroquinone should be used in women only when clearly indicated.

B. Nursing mothers. It is not known whether topical hydroquinone is absorbed or excreted in human milk. Caution is advised when topical hydroquinone is used by a nursing mother.

C. Pediatric usage. Safety and effectiveness in children below the age of 12 years have not been established.

ADVERSE REACTIONS

No systemic adverse reactions have been reported. Occasional hypersensitivity (localized contact dermatitis) may occur in which case the medication should be discontinued and the physician notified immediately.

OVERDOSAGE

There have been no systemic reactions from the use of topical hydroquinone in Eldoquin Forte 4% Cream. However, treatment should be limited to relatively small areas of the body at one time since some patients experience a transient skin reddening and a mild burning sensation which does not preclude treatment.

DRUG DOSAGE AND ADMINISTRATION

Eldoquin Forte 4% Cream should be applied to the affected area and rubbed in well twice daily or as directed by a physician. There is no recommended dosage for children under 12 years of age except under the advice and supervision of a physician.

HOW SUPPLIED

ELDOQUIN FORTE 4% Cream is available as follows:

Size	NDC Number
½ ounce tube (15 grams)	0187-0394-35
1 ounce tube (30 grams)	0187-0394-31

Available without prescription for maintenance therapy: Eldoquin® (2% Hydroquinone) in ½ ounce (NDC 0187-0382-35) and 1 ounce tubes (NDC 0187-0382-31); Eldoquin Lotion (2% Hydroquinone) in ½ ounce bottles (NDC 0187-0423-35).

Eldoquin Forte 4% Cream should be stored at room temperature (15–30°C) (59–86°F).

FLUONEX™ ℞

[flū ′-ō-nex]

(FLUOCINONIDE CREAM USP, 0.05%)

DESCRIPTION

The topical corticosteroids constitute a class of primarily synthetic steroids used as anti-inflammatory and anti-pruritic agents. The steroids in this class include fluocinonide. Fluocinonide is designated chemically as pregna-1,4-diene-3,20-dione,21-(acetyloxy)-6,9-difluoro-11-hydroxy-16, 17-[(1-methylethylidene)bis(oxy)]-,(6α, 11β, 16α)-. It has the following chemical structure:

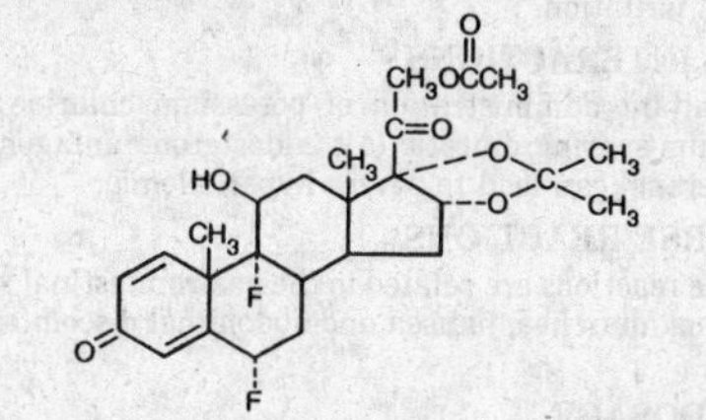

$C_{26}H_{32}F_2O_7$ M.W. 494.53

Each gram of Fluonex contains 0.5 mg. of Fluocinonide in PGEA™ cream base, a specially formulated cream base consisting of ethoxylated alcohol (Beheneth-20), polyethylene glycol 8000, sorbitan monostearate, stearic acid, propylene glycol and citric acid, anhydrous.

The cream is white, non-staining greaseless, anhydrous and water washable.

CLINCICAL PHARMACOLOGY

Topical corticosteroids share anti-inflammatory, anti-pruritic and vasoconstrictive actions.

The mechanism of anti-inflammatory activity of the topical corticosteroids is unclear. Various laboratory methods, including vasoconstrictor assays, are used to compare and predict potencies and/or clinical efficacies of the topical corticosteroids. There is some evidence to suggest that a recognizable correlation exists between vasoconstrictor potency and therapeutic efficacy in man.

Pharmacokinetics

The extent of percutaneous absorption of topical corticosteroids is determined by many factors including the vehicle, the integrity of the epidermal barrier, and the use of occlusive dressings.

Topical corticosteroids can be absorbed from normal intact skin. Inflammation and/or other disease processes in the skin increase percutaneous absorption. Occlusive dressings substantially increase the percutaneous absorption of topical corticosteroids. Thus, occlusive dressings may be a valuable therapeutic adjunct for treatment of resistant dermatoses. (See *DOSAGE AND ADMINISTRATION*).

Once absorbed through the skin, topical corticosteroids are handled through pharmacokinetic pathways similar to systemtically administered corticosteroids. Corticosteroids are bound to plasma proteins in varying degrees. Corticosteroids are metabolized primarily in the liver and are then excreted by the kidneys. Some of the topical corticosteroids and their metabolites are also excreted into the bile.

INDICATIONS AND USAGE

Relief of the inflammatory and pruritic manifestations of corticosteroid-responsive dermatoses.

CONTRAINDICATIONS

Topical corticosteroids are contraindicated in those patients with a history of hypersensitivity to any of the components of the preparation.

PRECAUTIONS

General

Systemic absorption of topical corticosteroids has produced reversible hypothalamic-pituitary-adrenal (HPA) axis suppression, manifestations of Cushing's syndrome, hyperglycemia, and glucosuria in some patients.

Conditions which augment systemic absorption include the application of the more potent steroids, use over large surface areas, prolonged use, the addition of occlusive dressings, and dosage form.

Therefore, patients receiving a large dose of a potent topical steroid applied to a large surface area or under an occlusive dressing should be evaluated periodically for evidence of HPA axis suppression by using the urinary free cortisol and ACTH stimulation tests. If HPA axis suppression is noted, an attempt should be made to withdraw the drug, to reduce the frequency of application, or to substitute a less potent steroid.

Recovery of HPA axis function is generally prompt and complete upon discontinuation of the drug. Infrequently, signs and symptoms of steroid withdrawal may occur, requiring supplemental systemic corticosteroids.

Children may absorb proportionally larger amounts of topical corticosteroids and thus be more susceptible to systemic toxicity. (See *PRECAUTIONS —Pediatric Use*).

Not for ophthalmic use. Severe irritation is possible if fluocinonide solution contacts the eye. If that should occur, immediate flushing of the eye with a large volume of water is recommended.

If irritation develops, topical corticosteroids should be discontinued and appropriate therapy instituted.

In the presence of dermatological infections, the use of an appropriate antifungal or antibacterial agent should be instituted. If a favorable response does not occur promptly, the corticosteroid should be discontinued until the infection has been adequately controlled.

Information for the Patient

Patients using topical corticosteroids should receive the following information and instructions:

1. This medication is to be used as directed by the physician. It is for external use only. Avoid contact with the eyes.
2. Patients should be advised not to use this medication for any disorder other than for which it was prescribed.
3. The treated skin area should not be bandaged or otherwise covered or wrapped as to be occlusive unless directed by the physician.
4. Patients should report any signs of local adverse reactions especially under occlusive dressing.
5. Parents of pediatric patients should be advised not to use tight-fitting diapers or plastic pants on a child being treated in the diaper area, as these garments may constitute occlusive dressings.

Laboratory Tests

The following tests may be helpful in evaluating the HPA axis suppression:

Urninary free cortisol test

ACTH stimulation test

Carcinogenesis, Mutagenesis, and Impairment of Fertility

Long-term animal studies have not been performed to evaluate the carcinogenic potential or the effect on fertility of topical corticosteroids.

Studies to determine mutagenicity with prednisolone and hydrocortisone have revealed negative results.

Pregnancy Category C

Corticosteroids are generally teratogenic in laboratory animals when administered systemically at relatively low dosage levels. The more potent corticosteroids have been shown to be teratogenic after dermal application in laboratory animals. There are no adequate and well-controlled studies in pregnant women on teratogenic effects from topically applied corticosteroids. Therefore, topical corticosteroids should be used during pregnancy only if the potential benefit justifies the potential risk to the fetus. Drugs of this class should not be used extensively on pregnant patients, in large amounts, or for prolonged periods of time.

Nursing Mothers

It is not known whether topical administration of corticosteroids could result in sufficient systemtic absorption to produce detectable quantities in breast milk. Systemically administered corticosteroids are secreted into breast milk in quantities *not* likely to have a deleterious effect on the infant. Nevertheless, caution should be exercised when topical corticosteroids are administered to a nursing woman.

Pediatric Use

Pediatric patients may demonstrate greater susceptibility to topical corticosteroid-induced HPA axis suppression and Cushing's syndrome than mature patients because of a larger skin surface area to body weight ratio.

Hypothalamic-pituitary-adrenal (HPA) axis suppression, Cushing's syndrome, and intracranial hypertension have been reported in children receiving topical corticosteroids. Manifestations of adrenal suppression in children include linear growth retardation, delayed weight gain, low plasma cortisol levels, and absence of response to ACTH stimulation. Manifestations of intracranial hypertension including bulging fontanelles, headaches, and bilateral papilledema.

Administration of topical corticosteroids to children should be limited to the least amount compatible with an effective therapeutic regimen. Chronic corticosteroid therapy may interfere with the growth and development of children.

ADVERSE REACTIONS

The following local adverse reactions are reported infrequently with topical corticosteroids, but may occur more

Continued on next page

ICN—Cont.

frequently with the use of occlusive dressings. These reactions are listed in an approximate decreasing order of occurrence beginning with column 1:

Burning	Perioral dermatitis
Itching	Allergic contact dermatitis
Irritation	Maceration of the skin
Dryness	Secondary infection
Folliculitis	Skin atrophy
Hypertrichosis	Striae
Acneiform eruptions	Miliaria
Hypopigmentation	

OVERDOSAGE
Topically applied corticosteroids can be absorbed in sufficient amounts to produce systemic effects (See *PRECAUTIONS*).

DOSAGE AND ADMINISTRATION
A small amount should be applied to the affected area two to four times daily depending on the severity of the condition.
Occlusive dressings may be used for the management of psoriasis or recalcitrant conditions.
If infection develops, the use of occlusive dressings should be discontinued and appropriate antimicrobial therapy instituted.

HOW SUPPLIED
Fluonex
15 g Tube — NDC 0187-0537-35
30 g Tube — NDC 0187-0537-31
Store at controlled room temperature 15°-30°C (59°-86°F).
Protect from freezing.

CAUTION: FEDERAL LAW PROHIBITS DISPENSING WITHOUT PRESCRIPTION.

Distributed by
ICN Pharmaceuticals, Inc.
3300 Hyland Ave.
Costa Mesa, CA 92626

Aug. 91
2472-00

KATO® ℞
[*kay'tō*]
(potassium chloride for oral solution)
20 mEq (1.5 g. KCl)

DESCRIPTION
KATO® (potassium chloride for oral solution) is a pleasantly flavored spray-dried tomato powder containing 20 mEq potassium (equivalent to 1.5 g KCl) per 5.7-grams of powder (one dose). KATO® is a potassium replacement product. Each daily dose (2 packets) contains approximately 0.5 mEq sodium.

CLINICAL PHARMACOLOGY
As the principal intracellular cation of most body tissues, potassium is instrumental in physiological processes such as maintenance of intracellular tonicity, contractility of cardiac, skeletal, and smooth muscles, maintenance of renal function and transmission of nervous impulses.
Potassium depletion may occur when potassium intake is insufficient to compensate for potassium loss from the G.I. tract or via renal excretion. Such loss may slowly develop during prolonged oral diuretic therapy, in hyperaldosteronism, diabetic ketoacidosis, severe diarrhea, or where potassium intake is inadequate in patients receiving prolonged parenteral nutrition.
The potassium deficit is usually accompanied by chloride depletion and is manifested by hypokalemia and a hypochloremic metabolic alkalosis. Clinical symptoms and signs include weakness, fatigue, disturbances of cardiac rhythmicity (primarily ectopic beats), EKG changes (prominent U waves) and, in severe cases, flaccid paralysis and/or impaired urinary concentration.
Potassium chloride is therefore regarded as the appropriate potassium salt for use in correcting potassium depletion states associated with metabolic alkalosis.

INDICATIONS AND USAGE
KATO® is indicated for the treatment or prevention of potassium deficit, particularly when accompanied by hypochloremic alkalosis in conjunction with thiazide diuretic therapy, in digitalis intoxication, or as a result of long-term corticosteroid therapy, low dietary intake of potassium, or excessive vomiting or diarrhea.

CONTRAINDICATION
Potassium is contraindicated in patients with: severe renal impairment involving oliguria, anuria or azotemia, untreated Addison's disease, familial periodic paralysis, acute dehydration, heat cramps, and hyperkalemia from any cause.

WARNINGS
Potassium intoxication may result from overdosage or from the usual therapeutic dose in patients for whom the drug is contraindicated. Hyperkalemia, when detected, must be treated immediately because lethal levels can be reached in a few hours. (See Overdosage for treatment of hyperkalemia).

PRECAUTIONS
General: Patients receiving potassium supplementation should be monitored with periodic checks of plasma potassium levels.
A high plasma concentration of potassium ion may cause death through cardiac depression, arrhythmias or arrest. Therefore, the drug should be used with caution in patients with cardiac disease.
The drug should not be used in patients with low urinary output or renal decompensation because of the heightened likelihood of overdosage.
In rare circumstances (e.g. patients with renal tubular acidosis) potassium depletion may be associated with a hyperchloremic metabolic acidosis. In such patients, potassium depletion is appropriately corrected using potassium salts other than the chloride.
As with other concentrated potassium supplements, KATO® must be reconstituted with the proper amount of water (2 oz. for 1 packet) to avoid the possibility of gastrointestinal irritation.

DRUG INTERACTIONS
Concomitant administration of potassium chloride and a potassium-sparing diuretic (e.g. aldosterone antagonists or triamterene) can lead to severe hyperkalemia.

ADVERSE REACTIONS
Adverse reactions are related to the gastrointestinal system. Vomiting, diarrhea, nausea and abdominal discomfort may occur.

OVERDOSAGE
The symptoms and signs of potassium intoxication include paresthesias of the extremities, flaccid paralysis, listlessness, mental confusion, weakness and heaviness of the legs, fall in blood pressure, cardiac arrhythmias and heart block. Hyperkalemia may be associated with the following electrocardiographic abnormalities: disappearance of the P wave, widening and slurring of QRS complex, changes of the S-T segment and tall peaked T waves.
The drug is dialyzable.
Treatment of hyperkalemia includes: 1. Elimination of potassium-containing foods and medicaments. 2. Dextrose solution 10% or 25% containing 10 units of crystalline insulin per 20 g dextrose, given i.v. with a dose of 300 cc to 500 cc in an hour. 3. Adsorption and exchange of potassium using sodium or ammonium cycle cation exchange resin, orally or as retention enema. 4. Hemodialysis or peritonial dialysis.
Warning: Digitalis toxicity can be precipitated by lowering the plasma potassium concentration too rapidly in digitalized patients.

DOSAGE AND ADMINISTRATION
The usual adult dose is 1 packet of KATO® (20 mEq potassium) mixed with 2 ounces of cold water twice daily. If possible it should stand for 15 minutes to allow the tomato powder to absorb moisture. The preparation should be taken with meals, if convenient. If not, drink ½ glass of water immediately after taking the medication. Larger doses may be required, but should be administered under close supervision because of the possibility of potassium intoxication.
The appropriate dosage of potassium for pediatric use may be calculated from the adult dosage according to relative total body weight.

HOW SUPPLIED
KATO® is available in cartons of 30 (NDC 0187-0112-03) and 120 (NDC 0187-0112-12) 5.7-gram unit dose packets (20 mEq potassium each). Store away from heat.
CAUTION: Federal (U.S.A.) law prohibits dispensing without prescription.

Rev. 6/85

MESTINON® INJECTABLE ℞
[*mes'tin-on*]
(pyridostigmine bromide)

DESCRIPTION
Mestinon (pyridostigmine bromide) Injectable is an active cholinesterase inhibitor. Chemically, pyridostigmine bromide is 3-hydroxy-1-methylpyridinium bromide dimethylcarbamate. Its structural formula is:
[See chemical structure at top of next column.]
Each ml contains 5 mg pyridostigmine bromide compounded with 0.2% parabens (methyl and propyl) as preservatives, 0.02% sodium citrate and pH adjusted to approximately 5.0 with citric acid and, if necessary, sodium hydroxide.

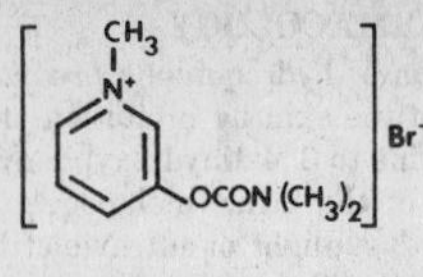

ACTIONS
Mestinon facilitates the transmission of impulses across the myoneural junction by inhibiting the destruction of acetylcholine by cholinesterase. Pyridostigmine is an analog of neostigmine (Prostigmin®) but differs from it clinically by having fewer side effects. Currently available data indicate that pyridostigmine may have a significantly lower degree and incidence of bradycardia, salivation and gastrointestinal stimulation. Animal studies using the injectable form of pyridostigmine and human studies using the oral preparation have indicated that pyridostigmine has a longer duration of action than does neostigmine measured under similar circumstances.

INDICATIONS
Mestinon Injectable is useful in the treatment of myasthenia gravis and as a reversal agent or antagonist to nondepolarizing muscle relaxants such as curariform drugs and gallamine triethiodide.

CONTRAINDICATIONS
Known hypersensitivity to anticholinesterase agents; intestinal and urinary obstructions of mechanical type.

WARNINGS
Mestinon Injectable should be used with particular caution in patients with bronchial asthma or cardiac dysrhythmias. Transient bradycardia may occur and be relieved by atropine sulfate. Atropine should also be used with caution in patients with cardiac dysrhythmias. When large doses of Mestinon are administered, as during reversal of muscle relaxants, the prior or simultaneous injection of atropine sulfate is advisable. Because of the possibility of hypersensitivity in an occasional patient, atropine and antishock medication should always be readily available.
As is true of all cholinergic drugs, overdosage of Mestinon may result in cholinergic crisis, a state characterized by increasing muscle weakness which, through involvement of the muscles of respiration, may lead to death. Myasthenic crisis due to an increase in the severity of the disease is also accompanied by extreme muscle weakness and thus may be difficult to distinguish from cholinergic crisis on a symptomatic basis. Such differentiation is extremely important, since increases in doses of Mestinon or other drugs in this class in the presence of cholinergic crisis or of a refractory or "insensitive" state could have grave consequences. Osserman and Genkins[1] indicate that the two types of crisis may be differentiated by the use of Tensilon® (edrophonium chloride) as well as by clinical judgment. The treatment of the two conditions obviously differs radically. Whereas the presence of *myasthenic crisis* requires more intensive anticholinesterase therapy, *cholinergic crisis*, according to Osserman and Genkins,[1] calls for the prompt withdrawal of all drugs of this type. The immediate use of atropine in cholinergic crisis is also recommended. A syringe containing 1 mg of atropine sulfate should be immediately available to be given in aliquots intravenously to counteract severe cholinergic reactions.
Atropine may also be used to abolish or obtund gastrointestinal side effects or other muscarinic reactions; but such use, by masking signs of overdosage, can lead to inadvertent induction of cholinergic crisis.
For detailed information on the management of patients with myasthenia gravis, the physician is referred to one of the excellent reviews such as those by Osserman and Genkins,[2] Grob[3] or Schwab.[4,5]
When used as an antagonist to nondepolarizing muscle relaxants, adequate recovery of voluntary respiration and neuromuscular transmission must be obtained prior to discontinuation of respiratory assistance and there should be continuous patient observation. Satisfactory recovery may be defined by a combination of clinical judgment, respiratory measurements and observation of the effects of peripheral nerve stimulation. If there is any doubt concerning the adequacy of recovery from the effects of the nondepolarizing muscle relaxant, artificial ventilation should be continued until all doubt has been removed.
Usage in Pregnancy: The safety of Mestinon during pregnancy or lactation in humans has not been established. Therefore, use of Mestinon in women who may become pregnant requires weighing the drug's potential benefits against its possible hazards to mother and child.

ADVERSE REACTIONS
The side effects of Mestinon are most commonly related to overdosage and generally are of two varieties, muscarinic and nicotinic. Among those in the former group are nausea, vomiting, diarrhea, abdominal cramps, increased peristalsis, increased salivation, increased bronchial secretions, miosis and diaphoresis. Nicotinic side effects are comprised chiefly

of muscle cramps, fasciculation and weakness. Muscarinic side effects can usually be counteracted by atropine, but for reasons shown in the preceding section the expedient is not without danger. As with any compound containing the bromide radical, a skin rash may be seen in an occasional patient. Such reactions usually subside promptly upon discontinuance of the medication. Thrombophlebitis has been reported subsequent to intravenous administration.

DOSAGE AND ADMINISTRATION

For Myasthenia Gravis—To supplement oral dosage, pre- and postoperatively, during labor and postpartum, during myasthenic crisis, or whenever oral therapy is impractical, approximately 1/30th of the oral dose of Mestinon may be given parenterally, either by intramuscular or *very slow* intravenous injection. *The patient must be closely observed for cholinergic reactions, particularly if the intravenous route is used.*

For details regarding the management of myasthenic patients who are to undergo major surgical procedures, see the article by Foldes.[6]

Neonates of myasthenic mothers may have transient difficulty in swallowing, sucking and breathing. Injectable Mestinon may be indicated—by symptomatology and use of the Tensilon® (edrophonium chloride) test—until Mestinon Syrup can be taken. To date the world literature consists of less than 100 neonate patients.[7] Of these only 5 were treated with injectable pyridostigmine, with the vast majority of the remaining neonates receiving neostigmine. Dosage requirements of Mestinon Injectable are minute, ranging from 0.05 mg to 0.15 mg/kg of body weight given intramuscularly. It is important to differentiate between cholinergic and myasthenic crises in neonates. (See **WARNINGS.**)

Mestinon given parenterally one hour before completion of second stage labor enables patients to have adequate strength during labor and provides protection to infants in the immediate postnatal state. For further information on the use of Mestinon Injectable in neonates of myasthenic mothers, see the article by Namba.[7]

NOTE: For information on a diagnostic test for myasthenia gravis, and on the evaluation and stabilization of therapy, please see product information on Tensilon® (edrophonium chloride).

For Reversal of Nondepolarizing Muscle Relaxants: When Mestinon Injectable is given intravenously to reverse the action of muscle relaxant drugs, it is recommended that atropine sulfate (0.6 to 1.2 mg) also be given intravenously immediately prior to the Mestinon. Side effects, notably excessive secretions and bradycardia, are thereby minimized. Usually 10 or 20 mg of Mestinon will be sufficient for antagonism of the effects of the nondepolarizing muscle relaxants. Although full recovery may occur within 15 minutes in most patients, others may require a half hour or more. Satisfactory reversal can be evident by adequate voluntary respiration, respiratory measurements and use of a peripheral nerve stimulator device. It is recommended that the patient be well ventilated and a patent airway maintained until complete recovery of normal respiration is assured. Once satisfactory reversal has been attained, recurarization has not been reported. For additional information on the use of Mestinon for antagonism of nondepolarizing muscle relaxants see the article by Katz[8] and McNall.[9]

Failure of Mestinon Injectable to provide prompt (within 30 minutes) reversal may occur, *e.g.,* in the presence of extreme debilitation, carcinomatosis, or with concomitant use of certain broad spectrum antibiotics or anesthetic agents, notably ether. Under these circumstances ventilation must be supported by artificial means until the patient has resumed control of his respiration.

HOW SUPPLIED

Mestinon is available in 2-ml ampuls (boxes of 10) (NDC 0187-3011-10).

REFERENCES

1. K. E. Osserman and G. Genkins, *J.A.M.A., 183:* 97, 1963.
2. K. E. Osserman and G. Genkins, *New York State J. Med., 61:* 2076, 1961.
3. D. Grob, *Arch. Intern. Med., 108:* 615, 1961.
4. R. S. Schwab, *New Eng. J. Med., 268:* 596, 1963.
5. R. S. Schwab, *New Eng. J. Med., 268:* 717, 1963.
6. F. F. Foldes and P. McNall, *Anesthesiology, 23:* 837, 1962.
7. T. Namba *et al., Pediatrics, 45:* 488, 1970.
8. R. L. Katz, *Anesthesiology, 28:* 528, 1967.
9. P. McNall *et al., Anesthesia and Analgesia, 48:* 1026, 1969.

Manufactured for ICN Pharmaceuticals, Inc.
Costa Mesa, CA 92626
by Hoffmann-La Roche Inc.
Nutley, N.J. 07110
Rev. 3/89

MESTINON® ℞

[mes'tin-on]
(pyridostigmine bromide)
TABLETS, SYRUP and TIMESPAN® TABLETS

DESCRIPTION

Mestinon (pyridostigmine bromide) is an orally active cholinesterase inhibitor. Chemically, pyridostigmine bromide is 3-hydroxy-1-methylpyridinium bromide dimethylcarbamate. Mestinon is available in the following forms: Syrup containing 60 mg pyridostigmine bromide per teaspoonful in a vehicle containing 5% alcohol, glycerin, lactic acid, sodium benzoate, sorbitol, sucrose, FD&C Red No. 40, FD&C Blue No. 1, flavors and water. *Tablets* containing 60 mg pyridostigmine bromide; each tablet also contains lactose, silicon dioxide and stearic acid. *Timespan Tablets* containing 180 mg pyridostigmine bromide; each tablet also contains carnauba wax, corn-derived proteins, magnesium stearate, silica gel and tribasic calcium phosphate.

ACTIONS

Mestinon inhibits the destruction of acetylcholine by cholinesterase and thereby permits freer transmission of nerve impulses across the neuromuscular junction. Pyridostigmine is an analog of neostigmine (Prostigmin®), but differs from it in certain clinically significant respects; for example, pyridostigmine is characterized by a longer duration of action and fewer gastrointestinal side effects.

INDICATION

Mestinon is useful in the treatment of myasthenia gravis.

CONTRAINDICATIONS

Mestinon is contraindicated in mechanical intestinal or urinary obstruction, and particular caution should be used in its administration to patients with bronchial asthma. Care should be observed in the use of atropine for counteracting side effects, as discussed below.

WARNINGS

Although failure of patients to show clinical improvement may reflect underdosage, it can also be indicative of overdosage. As is true of all cholinergic drugs, overdosage of Mestinon may result in cholinergic crisis, a state characterized by increasing muscle weakness which, through involvement of the muscles of respiration, may lead to death. Myasthenic crisis due to an increase in the severity of the disease is also accompanied by extreme muscle weakness, and thus may be difficult to distinguish from cholinergic crisis on a symptomatic basis. Such differentiation is extremely important, since increases in doses of Mestinon or other drugs of this class in the presence of cholinergic crisis or of a refractory or "insensitive" state could have grave consequences. Osserman and Genkins[1] indicate that the differential diagnosis of the two types of crisis may require the use of Tensilon® (edrophonium chloride) as well as clinical judgment. The treatment of the two conditions obviously differs radically. Whereas the presence of myasthenic crisis suggests the need for more intensive anticholinesterase therapy, the diagnosis of cholinergic crisis, according to Osserman and Genkins,[1] calls for the prompt *withdrawal* of all drugs of this type. The immediate use of atropine in cholinergic crisis is also recommended. Atropine may also be used to abolish or obtund gastrointestinal side effects or other muscarinic reactions; but such use, by masking signs of overdosage, can lead to inadvertent induction of cholinergic crisis.

For detailed information on the management of patients with myasthenia gravis, the physician is referred to one of the excellent reviews such as those by Osserman and Genkins,[2] Grob[3] or Schwab.[4,5]

Usage in Pregnancy: The safety of Mestinon during pregnancy or lactation in humans has not been established. Therefore, use of Mestinon in women who may become pregnant requires weighing the drug's potential benefits against its possible hazards to mother and child.

ADVERSE REACTIONS

The side effects of Mestinon are most commonly related to overdosage and generally are of two varieties, muscarinic and nicotinic. Among those in the former group are nausea, vomiting, diarrhea, abdominal cramps, increased peristalsis, increased salivation, increased bronchial secretions, miosis and diaphoresis. Nicotinic side effects are comprised chiefly of muscle cramps, fasciculation and weakness. Muscarinic side effects can usually be counteracted by atropine, but for reasons shown in the preceding section the expedient is not without danger. As with any compound containing the bromide radical, a skin rash may be seen in an occasional patient. Such reactions usually subside promptly upon discontinuance of the medication.

DOSAGE AND ADMINISTRATION

Mestinon is available in three dosage forms:

Syrup—raspberry-flavored, containing 60 mg pyridostigmine bromide per teaspoonful (5 ml). This form permits accurate dosage adjustment for children and "brittle" myasthenic patients who require fractions of 60-mg doses. It is more easily swallowed, especially in the morning, by patients with bulbar involvement.

Conventional tablets—each containing 60 mg pyridostigmine bromide.

Timespan tablets—each containing 180 mg pyridostigmine bromide. This form provides uniformly slow release, hence prolonged duration of drug action; it facilitates control of myasthenic symptoms with fewer individual doses daily. The immediate effect of a 180-mg Timespan tablet is about equal to that of a 60-mg conventional tablet; however, its duration of effectiveness, although varying in individual patients, averages 2½ times that of a 60-mg dose.

Dosage: The size and frequency of the dosage must be adjusted to the needs of the individual patient.

Syrup and conventional tablets—The average dose is ten 60-mg tablets or ten 5-ml teaspoonfuls daily, spaced to provide maximum relief when maximum strength is needed. In severe cases as many as 25 tablets or teaspoonfuls a day may be required, while in mild cases one to six tablets or teaspoonfuls a day may suffice.

Timespan tablets—One to three 180-mg tablets, once or twice daily, will usually be sufficient to control symptoms; however, the needs of certain individuals may vary markedly from this average. The interval between doses should be at least six hours. For optimum control, it may be necessary to use the more rapidly acting regular tablets or syrup in conjunction with Timespan therapy.

Note: For information on a diagnostic test for myasthenia gravis, and for the evaluation and stabilization of therapy, please see product literature on Tensilon® (edrophonium chloride).

HOW SUPPLIED

Syrup, 60 mg pyridostigmine bromide per teaspoonful (5 ml) and 5% alcohol—bottles of 16 fluid ounces (1 pint) (NDC 0187-3012-20).

Tablets, scored, 60 mg pyridostigmine bromide each—bottles of 100 (NDC 0187-3010-30) and 500 (NDC 0187-3010-40).

Timespan tablets, scored, 180 mg pyridostigmine bromide each—bottles of 100 (NDC 0187-3013-50).

Note: Because of the hygroscopic nature of the Timespan tablets, mottling may occur. This does not affect their efficacy.

REFERENCES

1. K. E. Osserman and G. Genkins, *J.A.M.A., 183:* 97, 1963.
2. K. E. Osserman and G. Genkins, *New York State J. Med., 61*:2076, 1961.
3. D. Grob, *Arch. Intern. Med., 108*:615, 1961.
4. R. S. Schwab, *New England J. Med., 268*:596, 1963.
5. R. S. Schwab, *New England J. Med., 268*:717, 1963.

Manufactured for ICN Pharmaceuticals, Inc.
Costa Mesa, CA 92626
by Hoffmann-La Roche Inc.
Nutley, N.J. 07110
Rev. 3/89

OXSORALEN® LOTION 1% ℞

[ox'sore"a-len]
(methoxsalen USP, 1%)

FEDERAL (U.S.A.) LAW PROHIBITS DISPENSING WITHOUT A PRESCRIPTION.
CAUTION: METHOXSALEN LOTION IS A POTENT TOPICAL DRUG. READ ENTIRE BROCHURE BEFORE PRESCRIBING OR USING THIS MEDICATION.

WARNING: METHOXSALEN LOTION IS A POTENT DRUG CAPABLE OF PRODUCING SEVERE BURNS IF IMPROPERLY USED. IT SHOULD BE APPLIED ONLY BY A PHYSICIAN UNDER CONTROLLED CONDITIONS FOR LIGHT EXPOSURE AND SUBSEQUENT LIGHT SHIELDING.

<u>THIS PREPARATION SHOULD NEVER BE DISPENSED TO A PATIENT</u>.

DESCRIPTION

Each ml of Oxsoralen Lotion contains 10 mg methoxsalen in an inert vehicle containing alcohol (71% v/v), propylene glycol, acetone, and purified water.

Methoxsalen is a naturally occurring substance found in the seeds of the Ammi majus (Umbelliferae) plant; it belongs to a group of compounds known as psoralens or furocoumarins. The chemical name of methoxsalen is 9-methoxy-7H-furo(3, 2g) (1)-benzopyran-7-one. It has the following structure:

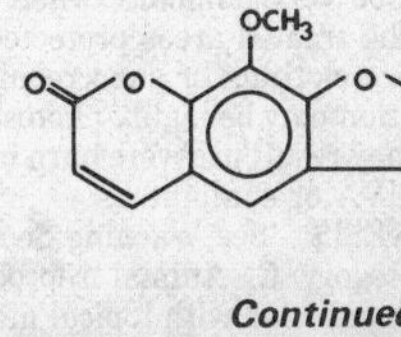

Continued on next page

ICN—Cont.

CLINICAL PHARMACOLOGY

The exact mechanism of action of methoxsalen with the epidermal melanocytes and keratinocytes is not known. Psoralens given orally are preferentially taken up by epidermal cells (Artuc et al, 1979). The best known biochemical reaction of methoxsalen is with DNA. Methoxsalen, upon photoactivation, conjugates and forms covalent bonds with DNA which leads to the formation of both monofunctional (addition to a single strand of DNA) and bifunctional adducts (crosslinking of psoralen to both strands of DNA) (Dall'Acqua et al, 1971). Reactions with proteins have also been described (Yoshikawa et al, 1979).

Methoxsalen acts as a photosensitizer. Topical application of this drug and subsequent exposure to UVA, whether artificial or sunlight, can cause cell injury. If sufficient cell injury occurs in the skin an inflammatory reaction will result. The most obvious manifestation of this reaction is delayed erythema which may not begin for several hours and may not peak for 2 to 3 days or longer. It is crucial to realize that the length of time the skin remains sensitized or when the maximum erythema will occur is quite variable from person to person. The erythematous reaction is followed over several days or weeks by repair which is manifested by increased melanization of the epidermis and thickening of the stratum corneum. The exact mechanics are unknown but it has been suggested melanocytes in the hair follicles are stimulated to move up the follicle and to repopulate the epidermis. (Ortonne, et al, 1979)

INDICATIONS AND USAGE

As a topical repigmenting agent in vitiligo in conjunction with controlled doses of ultraviolet A (320–400 nm) or sunlight.

CONTRAINDICATIONS

A. Patients exhibiting idiosyncratic reactions to psoralen compounds or a history of sensitivity reactions to them.
B. Patients exhibiting melanoma or with a history of melanoma.
C. Patients exhibiting invasive skin carcinoma generally.
D. Patients with photosensitivity diseases such as porphyria, acute lupus erythematosus, xeroderma pigmentosum, etc.
E. Children under 12 since clinical studies to determine the efficacy and safety of treatment in this age group have not been done.

WARNINGS

A. **Skin Burns**

Serious skin burns from either UVA or sunlight (even through window glass) can result if recommended exposure schedule is exceeded and/or protective covering or sunscreens are not used. The blistering of the skin sometimes encountered after UVA exposure generally heals without complication or scarring. (Farrington Daniels, Jr, M.D., personal communication). Suitable covering of the area of application or a topical sunblock should follow the therapeutic UVA exposure.

B. **Carcinogenicity**

1. Animal Studies. Topical methoxsalen has been reported to be a potent photocarcinogen in certain strains of mice. (Pathak et al 1959).
2. Human Studies. None of our clinical investigators reported skin cancers as a complication of topical treatment for vitiligo. However, it is recommended that caution be exercised when the patient is fair-skinned or has a history of prior coal tar UVA treatment, or has had ionizing radiation or taken arsenical compounds. Such patients who subsequently have oral psoralen—UVA treatment (PUVA) are at increased risk for developing skin cancer.

C. **Concomitant Therapy**

Special care should be exercised in treating patients who are receiving concomitant therapy (either topically or systemically) with known photosensitizing agents such as anthralin, coal tar or coal tar derivatives, griseofulvin, phenothiazines, nalidixic acid, halogenated salicylanilides (bacteriostatic soaps), sulfonamides, tetracyclines, thiazides, and certain organic staining dyes such as methylene blue, toluidine blue, rose bengal, and methyl orange.

PRECAUTIONS

A. This product should be applied only in small well defined lesions and preferably on lesions which can be protected by clothing or a sunscreen from subsequent exposure to radiant UVA. If this product is used to treat vitiligo of face or hands, be very emphatic when instructing patient to keep the treated areas protected from light by use of protective clothing or sunscreening agents. The area of application may be highly photosensitive for several days and may result in severe burn injury if exposed to additional UVA or sunlight.
B. CARCINOGENESIS: See Warning Section
C. Pregnancy Category C. Animal reproduction studies have not been conducted with topical methoxsalen. It is also not known whether methoxsalen can cause fetal harm when used topically on a pregnant woman or affect reproductive capacity. It is not known to what degree, if any, topical methoxsalen is absorbed systemically. Topical methoxsalen should be used in pregnant women only when clearly indicated.
D. Nursing Mothers. It is not known whether topical methoxsalen is absorbed or excreted in human milk. Caution is advised when topical methoxsalen is used in a nursing mother.
E. Pediatric Usage. Safety and effectiveness in children below the age of 12 years have not been established.

ADVERSE REACTIONS

Systemic adverse reactions have not been reported. The most common adverse reaction is severe burns of the treated area from overexposure to UVA, including sunlight. TREATMENT MUST BE INDIVIDUALIZED. Minor blistering of the skin is not a contraindication to further treatment and generally heals without incident. Treatment would be the standard for burn therapy. Since 1953, many studies have demonstrated the safety and effectiveness of topical methoxsalen and UVA for the treatment of vitiligo when used as directed. (Lerner, A.B., et al, 1953) (Fitzpatrick, T.B., et al, 1966) (Fulton, James F. et al, 1969)

OVERDOSAGE

This does not apply to topical usage. In the unlikely event that the lotion is ingested, standard procedures for poisoning should be followed, including gastric lavage. Protection from UVA or daylight for hours or days would also be necessary and the patient kept in a darkened room.

ADMINISTRATION

The OXSORALEN® Lotion is applied to a well-defined area of vitiligo by the physician and the area is then exposed to a suitable source of UVA. Initial exposure time should be conservative and not exceed that which is predicted to be one-half the minimal erythema dose. Treatment intervals should be regulated by the erythema response; generally once a week is recommended or less often depending on the results. The hands and fingers of the person applying the medication should be protected by gloves or finger cots to avoid photosensitization and possible burns.

Pigmentation may begin after a few weeks but significant repigmentation may require up to 6 to 9 months of treatment. Periodic re-treatment may be necessary to retain all of the new pigment. Idiopathic vitiligo is reversible but not equally reversible in every patient. Treatment must be individualized. Repigmentation will vary in completeness, time of onset, and duration. Repigmentation occurs more rapidly in fleshy areas such as face, abdomen, and buttocks and less rapidly over less fleshy areas such as the dorsum of the hands or feet.

HOW SUPPLIED

Oxsoralen Lotion containing 1% methoxsalen (8-methoxypsoralen) packaged in 1 ounce (30 ml) amber glass bottles (NDC 0187-0402-31).

Oxsoralen Lotion 1% should be stored at room temperature (15–30°C) (59–86°F).

OXSORALEN–ULTRA® CAPSULES ℞

[*ox ′-sore ″a-len*]

(Methoxsalen, 10 mg)

FEDERAL LAW PROHIBITS DISPENSING WITHOUT PRESCRIPTION.

CAUTION: METHOXSALEN IS A POTENT DRUG, READ ENTIRE BROCHURE PRIOR TO PRESCRIBING OR DISPENSING THIS MEDICATION.

> Methoxsalen with UV radiation should be used only by physicians who have special competence in the diagnosis and treatment of psoriasis and who have special training and experience in photochemotherapy. The use of Psoralen and ultraviolet radiation therapy should be under constant supervision of such a physician. For the treatment of patients with psoriasis, photochemotherapy should be restricted to patients with severe, recalcitrant, disabling psoriasis which is not adequately responsive to other forms of therapy, and only when the diagnosis has been supported by biopsy. Because of the possibilities of ocular damage, aging of the skin, and skin cancer (including melanoma), the patient should be fully informed by the physician of the risks inherent in this therapy.

> CAUTION: Oxsoralen-Ultra® should not be used interchangeably with regular Oxsoralen®. This new dosage form of methoxsalen exhibits significantly greater bioavailability and earlier photosensitization onset time than previous methoxsalen dosage forms. Patients should be treated in accordance with the dosimetry specifically recommended for this product. The minimum phototoxic dose (MPD) and phototoxic peak time after drug administration prior to onset of photochemotherapy with this dosage form should be determined.

DESCRIPTION

Oxsoralen-Ultra (methoxsalen, 8-methoxypsoralen) Capsules, 10mg Methoxsalen is a naturally occurring photoactive substance found in the seeds of the **Ammi majus** (Umbelliferae) plant. It belongs to a group of compounds known as psoralens, or furocoumarins. The chemical name of methoxsalen is 9-methoxy-7H-furo [3,2-g] [1]benzopyran-7-one; it has the following structure:

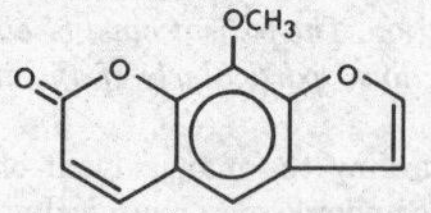

CLINICAL PHARMACOLOGY

The combination treatment regimen of psoralen (P) and ultraviolet radiation of 320–400 nm wavelength commonly referred to as UVA is known by the acronym, PUVA. Skin reactivity to UVA (320–400nm) radiation is markedly enhanced by the ingestion of methoxsalen. In a well controlled bioavailability study, Oxsoralen-Ultra Capsules reached peak drug levels in the blood of test subjects between 0.5 and 4 hours (Mean = 1.8 hours) as compared to between 1.5 and 6 hours (Mean = 3.0 hours) for regular Oxsoralen when administered with 8 ounces of milk. Peak drug levels were 2 to 3 fold greater when the overall extent of drug absorption was approximately two fold greater for Oxsoralen-Ultra Capsules as compared to regular Oxsoralen Capsules. Detectable methoxsalen levels were observed up to 12 hours post dose. The drug half-life is approximately 2 hours. Photosensitivity studies demonstrate a shorter time of peak photosensitivity of 1.5 to 2.1 hours vs. 3.9 to 4.25 hours for regular Oxsoralen capsules. In addition, the mean minimal erythema dose (MED), J/cm^2, for the Oxsoralen-Ultra Capsules is substantially less than that required for regular Oxsoralen Capsules (Levins et al., 1984 and private communication[1]).

Methoxsalen is reversibly bound to serum albumin and is also preferentially taken up by epidermal cells (Artuc et al., 1979[2]). At a dose which is six times larger than that used in humans, it induces mixed function oxidases in the liver of mice (Mandula et al., 1978[3]). In both mice and man, methoxsalen is rapidly metabolized. Approximately 95% of the drug is excreted as a series of metabolites in the urine within 24 hours (Pathak et al., 1977[4]). The exact mechanism of action of methoxsalen with the epidermal melanocytes and keratinocytes is not known. The best known biochemical reaction of methoxsalen is with DNA. Methoxsalen, upon photoactivation, conjugates and forms covalent bonds with DNA which leads to the formation of both monofunctional (addition to a single strand of DNA) and bifunctional (crosslinking of psoralen to both strands of DNA) adducts (Dall' Acqua et al., 1971[5]; Cole, 1970[6]; Musajo et al., 1974[7]; Dall' Acqua et al., 1979[8]). Reactions with proteins have also been described (Yoshikawa, et al., 1979[9]).

Methoxsalen acts as a photosensitizer. Administration of the drug and subsequent exposure to UVA can lead to cell injury. Orally administered methoxsalen reaches the skin via the blood and UVA penetrates well into the skin. If sufficient cell injury occurs in the skin, an inflammatory reaction occurs. The most obvious manifestation of this reaction is delayed erythema, which may not begin for several hours and peaks at 48–72 hours. The inflammation is followed, over several days to weeks, by repair which is manifested by increased melanization of the epidermis and thickening of the stratum corneum. The mechanisms of therapy are not known. In the treatment of psoriasis, the mechanism is most often assumed to be DNA photodamage and resulting decrease in cell proliferation but other vascular, leukocyte, or cell regulatory mechanisms may also be playing some role. Psoriasis is a hyper-proliferative disorder and other agents known to be therapeutic for psoriasis are known to inhibit DNA systhesis.

INDICATIONS AND USAGE

Photochemotherapy (methoxsalen with long wave UVA radiation) is indicated for the symptomatic control of severe, recalcitrant, disabling psoriasis not adequately responsive to other forms of therapy and when the diagnosis has been supported by biopsy. Methoxsalen is intended to be administered only in conjunction with a schedule of controlled doses of long wave ultraviolet radiation.

CONTRAINDICATIONS

A. Patients exhibiting idiosyncratic reactions to psoralen compounds.
B. Patients possessing a specific history of light sensitive disease states should not initiate methoxsalen therapy except under special circumstances. Diseases associated

with photosensitivity include lupus erythematosus, porphyria cutanea tarda, erythropoietic protoporphyria, variegate porphyria, xeroderma pigmentosum, and albinism.

C. Patients with melanoma or with a history of melanoma.

D. Patients with invasive squamous cell carcinomas.

E. Patients with aphakia, because of the significantly increased risk of retinal damage due to the absence of lenses.

WARNINGS—GENERAL

A. SKIN BURNING: Serious burns from either UVA or sunlight (even through window glass) can result if the recommended dosage of the drug and/or exposure schedules are exeeded.

B. CARCINOGENICITY:

1. ANIMAL STUDIES: Topical or intraperitoneal methoxsalen has been reported to be a potent photocarcinogen in albino mice and hairless mice (Hakim et al., 1960[10]). However, methoxsalen given by the oral route to Swiss albino mice suggests this agent exerts a protective effect against ultraviolet carcinogenesis; mice given 8-methoxypsoralen in their diet showed 38% ear tumors 180 days after the start of ultraviolet therapy compared to 62% for controls (O'Neal et al., 1957[11]).

2. HUMAN STUDIES: A 5.7 year prospective study of 1380 psoriasis patients treated with oral methoxsalen and ultraviolet A photochemotherapy (PUVA) demonstrated that the risk of cutaneous squamous-cell carcinoma developing at least 22 months following the first PUVA exposure was approximately 12.8 times higher in the high dose patients than in the low dose patients (Stern et al., 1979[12], Stern et al., 1980[13], and Stern et al., 1984[14]). The substantial dose-dependent increase was observed in patients with neither a prior history of skin cancer nor significant exposure to cutaneous carcinogens. Reduction in PUVA dosage significantly reduces the risk. No substantial dose related increase was noted for basal cell carcinoma according to Stern et al., 1984[14]. Increases appear greatest in patients who have pre-PUVA exposure to 1) prolonged tar and UVB treatment, 2) ionizing radiation, or 3) arsenic.

Roenigk et al., 1980[15], studied 690 patients for up to 4 years and found no increase in the risk of non-melanoma skin cancer, although patients in this cohort had significantly less exposure to PUVA than in the Stern et al. study. After 5 years, two of 1380 patients in the Stern et al. PUVA study have developed malignant melanoma. In addition, more than 1/5 of the patients in this cohort have developed macular pigmented lesions on the buttocks. While there is no evidence that an increased risk of melanoma exists in PUVA treated patients, these observations indicate the need for continued evaluation of melanoma risk of PUVA treated patients.

In a study in Indian patients treated for 4 years for vitiligo, 12 percent developed keratoses, but not cancer, in the depigmented, vitiliginous areas (Mosher, 1980[16]). Clinically, the keratoses were keratotic papules, actinic keratosis-like macules, nonscaling dome-shaped papules, and lichenoid porokeratotic-like papules.

C. CATARACTOGENICITY:

1. ANIMAL STUDIES: Exposure to large doses of UVA causes cataracts in animals, and this effect is enhanced by the administration of methoxsalen (Cloud et al, 1960[17]; Cloud et al, 1961[18]; Freeman et al, 1969[19]).

2. HUMAN STUDIES: It has been found that the concentration of methoxsalen in the lens is proportional to the serum level. If the lens is exposed to UVA during the time methoxsalen is present in the lens, photochemical action may lead to irreversible binding of methoxsalen to proteins and the DNA components of the lens (Lerman et al, 1980[20]). However, if the lens is shielded from UVA, the methoxsalen will diffuse out of the lens in a 24 hour period (Lerman et al., 1980[20]). Patients should be told emphatically to wear UVA-absorbing, wrap-around sunglasses for the twenty-four (24) hour period following ingestion of methoxsalen, whether exposed to direct or indirect sunlight in the open or through a window glass. Among patients using proper eye protection, there is no evidence for a significantly increased risk of cataracts in association with PUVA therapy. (Stern et al., 1979[12]). Thirty-five of 1380 patients have developed cataracts in the five years since their first PUVA treatment. This incidence is comparable to that expected in a population of this size and age distribution. No relationship between PUVA dose and cataract risk in this group has been noted.

D. ACTINIC DEGENERATION: Exposure to sunlight and/or ultraviolet radiation may result in "premature aging" of the skin.

E. BASAL CELL CARCINOMAS: Patients exhibiting multiple basal cell carcinomas or having a history of basal cell carcinomas should be diligently observed and treated.

F. RADIATION THERAPY: Patients having a history of previous x-ray therapy or grenz ray therapy should be diligently observed for signs of carcinoma.

G. ARSENIC THERAPY: Patients having a history of previous arsenic therapy should be diligently observed for signs of carcinoma.

H. HEPATIC DISEASES: Patients with hepatic insufficiency should be treated with caution since hepatic biotransformation is necessary for drug urinary excretion.

I. CARDIAC DISEASES: Patients with cardiac diseases or others who may be unable to tolerate prolonged standing or exposure to heat stress should not be treated in a vertical UVA chamber.

J. TOTAL DOSAGE: The total cumulative dose of UVA that can be given over long periods of time with safety has not as yet been established.

K. CONCOMITANT THERAPY: Special care should be exercised in treating patients who are receiving concomitant therapy (either topically or systemically) with known photosensitizing agents such as anthralin, coal tar or coal tar derivatives, griseofulvin, phenothiazines, nalidixic acid, halogenated salicylanilides (bacteriostatic soaps), sulfonamides, tetracyclines, thiazides and certain organic staining dyes such as methylene blue, toluidine blue, rose bengal, and methyl orange.

PRECAUTIONS

A. GENERAL—APPLICABLE TO PSORIASIS TREATMENT

1. BEFORE METHOXSALEN INGESTION
Patients must not sunbathe during the 24 hours prior to methoxsalen ingestion and UV exposure. The presence of a sunburn may prevent an accurate evaluation of the patient's response to photochemotherapy.

2. AFTER METHOXSALEN INGESTION
a. UVA-absorbing wrap-around sunglasses should be worn during daylight for 24 hours after methoxsalen ingestion. The protective eyewear must be designed to prevent entry of stray radiation to the eyes, including that which may enter from the sides of the eyewear. The protective eyewear is used to prevent the irreversible binding of methoxsalen to the proteins and DNA components of the lens. Cataracts form when enough of the binding occurs. Visual discrimination should be permitted by the eyewear for patient well-being and comfort.
b. Patients must avoid sun exposure, even through window glass or cloud cover, for at least 8 hours after methoxsalen ingestion. If sun exposure cannot be avoided, the patient should wear protective devices such as a hat and gloves, and/or apply sunscreens which contain ingredients that filter out UVA radiation (e.g. sunscreens containing benzophenone and/or PABA esters which exhibit a sun protective factor equal to or greater than 15). These chemical sunscreens should be applied to all areas that might be exposed to the sun (including lips). Sunscreens should not be applied to areas affected by psoriasis until after the patient has been treated in the UVA chamber.

3. DURING PUVA THERAPY
a. Total UVA-absorbing/blocking goggles mechanically designed to give maximal ocular protection must be worn. Failure to do so may increase the risk of cataract formation. A reliable radiometer can be used to verify elimination of UVA transmission through the goggles.
b. Abdominal skin, breasts, genitalia, and other sensitive areas should be protected for approximately 1/3 of the initial exposure time until tanning occurs.
c. Unless affected by disease, male genitalia should be shielded.

4. AFTER COMBINED METHOXSALEN/UVA THERAPY
a. UVA-absorbing wrap-around sunglasses should be worn during daylight for 24 hours after combined methoxsalen/UVA therapy.
b. Patients should not sunbathe for 48 hours after therapy. Erythema and/or burning due to photochemotherapy and sunburn due to sun exposure are additive.

B. INFORMATION FOR PATIENTS: See accompanying Patient Package Insert.

C. LABORATORY TESTS:

1. Patients should have an ophthalmologic examination prior to start of therapy, and thence yearly.
2. Patients should have routine laboratory tests prior to the start of therapy and at regular periods thereafter if patients are on extended treatments.

D. DRUG INTERACTIONS: See Warnings Section.

E. CARCINOGENESIS: See Warnings Section.

F. PREGNANCY:
Pregnancy Category C. Animal reproduction studies have not been conducted with methoxsalen. It is also not known whether methoxsalen can cause fetal harm when administered to a pregnant woman or can affect reproduction capacity. Methoxsalen should be given to a woman with reproductive capacity only if clearly needed.

G. NURSING MOTHERS:
It is not known whether this drug is excreted in human milk. Because many drugs are excreted in human milk, either methoxsalen ingestion or nursing should be discontinued.

H. PEDIATRIC USE:
Safety in children has not been established. Potential hazards of long-term therapy include the possibilities of carcinogenicity and cataractogenicity as described in the Warnings Section as well as the probability of actinic degeneration which is also described in the Warnings Section.

ADVERSE REACTIONS

A. METHOXSALEN:
The most commonly reported side effect of methoxsalen alone is nausea, which occurs with approximately 10% of all patients. This effect may be minimized or avoided by instructing the patient to take methoxsalen with milk or food, or to divide the dose into two portions, taken approximately one-half hour apart. Other effects include nervousness, insomnia, and psychological depression.

B. COMBINED METHOXSALEN/UVA THERAPY:

1. PRURITUS: This adverse reaction occurs with approximately 10% of all patients. In most cases, pruritus can be alleviated with frequent application of bland emollients or other topical agents; severe pruritus may require systemic treatment. If pruritus is unresponsive to these measures, shield pruritic areas from further UVA exposure until the condition resolves. If intractable pruritus is generalized, UVA treatment should be discontinued until the pruritus disappears.

2. ERYTHEMA: Mild, transient erythema at 24–48 hours after PUVA therapy is an expected reaction and indicates that a therapeutic interaction between methoxsalen and UVA occurred. Any area showing moderate erythema (greater than Grade 2—See Table 1 for grades of erythema) should be shielded during subsequent UVA exposures until the erythema has resolved. Erythema greater than Grade 2 which appears within 24 hours after UVA treatment may signal a potentially severe burn. Erythema may become progressively worse over the next 24 hours, since the peak erythemal reaction characteristically occurs 48 hours or later after methoxsalen ingestion. The patient should be protected from further UVA exposures and sunlight, and should be monitored closely.

3. IMPORTANT DIFFERENCES BETWEEN PUVA ERYTHEMA AND SUNBURN: PUVA-induced inflammation differs from sunburn or UVB phototherapy in several ways. The percent transmission of UVB varies between 0% to 34% through skin whereas UVA varies between 1% to 80% transmission; thus, UVA is transmitted to a larger percent through the skin. (Diffey, 1982[21]). The DNA lesions induced by PUVA are very different from UV-induced thymine dimers and may lead to a DNA crosslink. This DNA lesion may be more problematic to the cell because crosslinks are more lethal and psoralen-DNA photoproducts may be "new" or unfamiliar substrates for DNA repair enzymes. DNA synthesis is also suppressed longer after PUVA. The time course of delayed erythema is different with PUVA and may not involve the usual mediators seen in sunburn. PUVA-induced redness may be just beginning at 24 hours, when UVB erythema has already passed its peak. The erythema dose-response curve is also steeper for PUVA. Compared to equally erythemogenic doses of UVB, the histologic alterations induced by PUVA show more dermal vessel damage and longer duration of epidermal and dermal abnormalities.

4. OTHER ADVERSE REACTIONS: Those reported include edema, dizziness, headache, malaise, depression, hypopigmentation, vesiculation and bullae formation, non-specific rash, herpes simplex, miliaria, urticaria, folliculitis, gastrointestinal disturbances, cutaneous tenderness, leg cramps, hypotension, and extension of psoriasis.

OVERDOSAGE

In the event of methoxsalen overdosage, induce emesis and keep the patient in a darkened room for at least 24 hours. Emesis is most beneficial within the first 2 to 3 hours after ingestion of methoxsalen, since maximum blood levels are reached by this time.

DRUG DOSAGE AND ADMINISTRATION

CAUTION: Oxsoralen-Ultra represents a new dose form of methoxsalen. This new dosage form of methoxsalen exhibits significantly greater bioavailability and earlier photosensitization onset time than previous methoxsalen dosage forms. Each patient should be evaluated by determining the minimum phototoxic dose (MPD) and phototoxic peak time after drug administration prior to onset of photochemotherapy with this dos-

Continued on next page

ICN—Cont.

age form. Human bioavailability studies have indicated the following drug dosage and administration directions are to be used as a guideline only.

PSORIASIS THERAPY

1. DRUG DOSAGE-INITIAL THERAPY: The methoxsalen capsules should be taken 1½ to 2 hours before UVA exposure with some low fat food or milk according to the following table:

Patient's Weight		Dose
(kg)	(lbs)	(mg)
<30	<65	10
30–50	65–100	20
51–65	101–145	30
66–80	146–175	40
81–90	176–200	50
91–115	201–250	60
>115	>250	70

2. INITIAL EXPOSURE: The initial UVA exposure energy level and corresponding time of exposure is determined by the patient's skin characteristics for sunburning and tanning as follows:

Skin Type	History	Recommended Joules/cm²
I	Always burn, never tan (patients with erythrodermic psoriasis are to be classed as Type I for determination of UVA dosage.)	0.5 J/cm²
II	Always burn, but sometimes tan	1.0 J/cm²
III	Sometimes burn, but always tan	1.5 J/cm²
IV	Never burn, always tan	2.0 J/cm²

Skin Type	Physician Examination	Joules/cm²
V*	Moderately pigmented	2.5 J/cm²
VI*	Blacks	3.0 J/cm²

(*Patients with natural pigmentation of these types should be classified into a lower skin type category if the sunburning history so indicates.)

If the MPD is done, start at ½ MPD.

Additional drug dosage directions are as follows:

a. Weight Change: In the event that the weight of a patient changes during treatment such that he/she falls into an adjacent weight range/dose category, no change in the dose of methoxsalen is usually required. If, in the physician's opinion, however, a weight change is sufficiently great to modify the drug dose, then an adjustment in the time of exposure to UVA should be made.

b. Dose/Week: The number of doses per week of methoxsalen capsules will be determined by the patient's schedule of UVA exposures. In no case should treatments be given more often than once every other day because the full extent of phototoxic reactions may not be evident until 48 hours after each exposure.

c. Dosage Increase: Dosage may be increased by 10 mg after the fifteenth treatment under the conditions outlined under PUVA treatment protocol, clearing phase, miscellaneous situations.

UVA RADIATION SOURCE SPECIFICATIONS & INFORMATION

A. IRRADIANCE UNIFORMITY:

The following specifications should be met with the window of the detector held in a vertical plane:

1. Vertical variation: For readings taken at any point along the vertical center axis of the chamber (to within 15 cm from the top and bottom), the lowest reading should not be less than 70 percent of the highest reading.

2. Horizontal variation: Throughout any specific horizontal plane, the lowest reading must be at least 80 percent of the highest reading, excluding the peripheral 3 cm of the patient treatment space.

B. PATIENT SAFETY FEATURES:

The following safety features should be present: (1) Protection from electrical hazard: All units should be grounded and conform to applicable electrical codes. The patient or operator should not be able to touch any live electrical parts. There should be ground fault protection. (2) Protective shielding of lamps: The patient should not be able to come in contact with the bare lamps. In the event of lamp breakage, the patient should not be exposed to broken lamp components. (3) Hand rails and hand holds: Appropriate supports should be available to the patient. (4) Patient viewing window: A window which blocks UV should be provided for viewing the patient during treatment. (5) Door and latches: Patients should be able to open the door from the inside with only slight pressure to the door. (6) Non-skid floor: The floor should be of a non-skid nature. (7) Thermoregulation: Sufficient air flow should be provided for patient safety and comfort, limiting temperature within the UVA radiator cabi-

net to approximately less than 100°F. (8) Timer: The irradiator should be equipped with an automatic timer which terminates the exposure at the conclusion of a pre-set time interval. (9) Patient alarm device: An alarm device within the UVA irradiator chamber should be accessible to the patient for emergency activation. (10) Danger label: The unit should have a label prominently displayed which reads as follows:

DANGER—Ultraviolet Radiation—Follow your physicians instructions—Failure to use protective eyewear may result in eye injury.

C. UVA EXPOSURE DOSIMETRY MEASUREMENTS:

The maximum radiant exposure or irradiance (within $\pm$ 15 percent) of UVA (320–400 nm) delivered to the patient should be determined by using an appropriate radiometer calibrated to be read in Joules/cm² or mW/cm². In the absence of a standard measuring technique approved by the National Bureau of Standards, the system should use a detector corrected to a cosine spatial response. The use and recalibration frequency of such a radiometer for a specific UVA irradiator chamber should be specified by the manufacturer because the UVA dose (exposure) is determined by the design of the irradiator, the number of lamps, and the age of the lamps. If irradiance is measured, the radiometer reading in mW/cm² is used to calculate the exposure time in minutes to deliver the required UVA in Joules/cm² to a patient in the UVA irradiator cabinet. The equation is:

$$\text{Exposure Time (minutes)} = \frac{\text{Desired UVA Dose (J/cm}^2)}{0.06 \times \text{Irradiance (mW/cm}^2)}.$$

Overexposure due to human error should be minimized by using an accurate automatic timing device, which is set by the operator and controlled by energizing and de-energizing the UVA irradiator lamp. The timing device calibration interval should be specified by the manufacturer. Safety systems should be included to minimize the possibility of delivering a UVA exposure which exceeds the prescribed dose, in the event the timer or radiometer should malfunction.

D. UVA SPECTRAL OUTPUT DISTRIBUTION:

The spectral distributions of the lamps should meet the following specifications:

Wavelength band (nanometers)	Output[1]
<310	<1
310 to 320	1 to 3
320 to 330	4 to 8
330 to 340	11 to 17
340 to 350	18 to 25
350 to 360	19 to 28
360 to 370	15 to 23
370 to 380	8 to 12
380 to 390	3 to 7
390 to 400	1 to 3

[1] As a percentage of total irradiance between 320 and 400 nanometers.

PUVA TREATMENT PROTOCOL

INTRODUCTION:

The Oxsoralen-Ultra® Capsules reach their maximum bioavailability in 1½ to 2 hours after ingestion.

On average, the serum level achieved with Oxsoralen-Ultra is twice that obtained with regular Oxsoralen® and reach their peak concentration in less than ½ the time of the regular capsules.

As a result the mean MED J/cm² for the Oxsoralen-Ultra Capsules is substantially less than that required for regular Oxsoralen Capsules (Levins et al., 1984 and private communication[1]).

Photosensitivity studies demonstrate a shorter time of peak photosensitivity of 1.5 to 2.1 hours vs. 3.9 to 4.25 hours for regular methoxsalen capsules.

A. INITIAL EXPOSURE: The initial UVA exposures should be conducted according to the guidelines presented previously under Drug Dosage & Administration—Initial Therapy and Exposure.

B. CLEARING PHASE: Specific recommendations for patient treatment are as follows:

1. SKIN TYPES I, II, & III. Patients with skin types I, II, and III may be treated 2 or 3 times per week. UVA exposure may be held constant or increased by up to 1.0 Joule/cm² at each treatment, according to the patient's response. If erythema occurs, however, do not increase exposure time until erythema resolves. The severity and extent of the patient's erythema may be used to determine whether the next exposure should be shortened, omitted, or maintained at the previous dosage. See Adverse Reactions section for additional information.

2. SKIN TYPES IV, V, & VI. Patients with skin types IV, V, and VI may be treated 2 or 3 times per week. UVA exposure may be held constant or increased by up to 1.5 Joules/cm² at each treatment unless erythema occurs. If erythema occurs, follow instructions outlined above in the procedures for patients with skin types I, II, and III.

3. ERYTHRODERMIC PSORIASIS. Patients with erythrodermic psoriasis should be treated with special attention because pre-existing erythema may obscure observa-

tions of possible treatment-related phototoxic erythema. These patients may be treated 2 or 3 times per week, as a Type I patient.

4. MISCELLANEOUS SITUATIONS:

a. If there is no response after a total of 10 treatments, the exposure of UVA energy may be increased by an additional 0.5-1.0 Joules/cm² above the prior incremental increases for each treatment. (Example: a patient whose exposure dose is being increased by 1.0 Joule/cm² may now have all subsequent doses increased by 1.5-2.0 Joules/cm².)

b. If there is no response, or only minimal response, after 15 treatments, the dosage of methoxsalen may be increased by 10 mg (a one-time increase in dosage). This increased dosage may be continued for the remainder of the course of treatment but should not be exceeded.

c. If a patient misses a treatment, the UVA exposure time of the next treatment should not be increased. If more than one treatment is missed, reduce the exposure by 0.5 Joule/cm² for each treatment missed.

d. If the lower extremities are not responding as well as the rest of the body and do not show erythema, cover all other body areas and give 25 percent of the present exposure dose as an additional exposure to the lower extremities. This additional exposure to the lower extremities should be terminated if erythema develops on these areas.

e. Non-responsive psoriasis: If a patient's generalized psoriasis is not responding, or if the condition appears to be worsening during treatment, the possibility of a generalized phototoxic reaction should be considered. This may be confirmed by the improvement of the condition following temporary discontinuance of this therapy for two weeks. If no improvement occurs during the interruption of treatment, this patient may be considered a treatment failure.

C. ALTERNATIVE EXPOSURE SCHEDULE:

As an alternative to increasing the UVA exposure at each treatment, the following schedule may be followed; this schedule may reduce the total number of Joules/cm² received by the patient over the entire course of therapy.

1. Incremental increases in UVA exposure for all patients may range from 0.5 to 1.5 Joules/cm², according to the patient's response to therapy.

2. Once Grade 2 clearing (see Table 2) has been reached and the patient is progressing adequately, UVA dosage is held constant. The dosage is maintained until Grade 4 clearing is reached.

3. If the rate of clearing significantly decreases, exposure dosage may be increased at each treatment (0.1–1.5 Joules/cm²) until Grade 3 clearing and a satisfactory progress rate is attained. The UVA exposure will be held constant again until Grade 4 clearing is attained. These increases may be used also if the rate of clearing significantly decreases between Grade 3 and Grade 4 response. However, the possibility of a phototoxic reaction should be considered; see Non-responsive Psoriasis, above.

4. In summary, this schedule raises slightly the increments (Joules/cm²) of UVA dosage, but limits these increases to those periods when the patient is not responding adequately. Otherwise, the UVA exposure is held at the lowest effective dose.

D. MAINTENANCE PHASE:

The goal of maintenance treatment is to keep the patient symptom-free as possible with the least amount of UVA exposure.

1. SCHEDULE OF EXPOSURES: When patients have achieved 95 percent clearing, or Grade 4 response (Table 2), they may be placed on the following maintenance schedules (M_1–M_4), in sequence. It is recommended that each maintenance schedule be adhered to for at least 2 treatments (unless erythema or psoriatic flare occurs, in which case see (2a) and (2b) below).

Maintenance Schedules
M_1—once/week
M_2—once/2 weeks
M_3—once/3 weeks
M_4—p.r.n. (i.e. for flares)

2. LENGTH OF EXPOSURE: The UVA exposure for the first maintenance treatment of any schedule (except M_4 as noted below) is the same as that of the patient's last treatment under the previous schedule. For skin types I–IV, however, it is recommended that the maximum UVA dosage during maintenance treatments not exceed the following:

Skin Types	Joules/cm²/treatment
I	12
II	14
III	18
IV	22

If the patient develops erythema or new lesions of psoriasis, proceed as follows:

a. Erythema: During maintenance therapy, the patient's tan and threshold dose for erythema may gradually decrease. If maintenance treatments produce sig-

nificant erythema, the exposure to UVA should be decreased by 25 percent until further treatments no longer produce erythema.

b. Psoriasis: If the patient develops new areas of psoriasis during maintenance therapy (but still is classified as having a Grade 4 response), the exposure to UVA may be increased by 0.5–1.5 Joules/cm^2 at each treatment; this is appropriate for all types of patients. These increases are continued until the psoriasis is brought under control and the patient is again clear. The exposure being administered when this clearing is reached should be used for further maintenance treatment.

3. FLARES DURING MAINTENANCE: If the patient flares during maintenance treatment (i.e., develops psoriasis on more than 5 percent of the originally involved areas of the body) his maintenance treatment schedule may be changed to the preceding maintenance or clearing schedule. The patient may be kept on his schedule until again 95 percent clear. If the original maintenance treatment schedule is unable to control the psoriasis, the schedule may be changed to a more frequent regimen. If a flare occurs less than 6 weeks after the last treatment, 25 percent of the maximum exposure received during the clearing phase, with the clearing schedule received during the clearing phase, may be used and then proceed with the clearing schedule previously followed for this patient. (At 95 percent clearing, follow regular maintenance until the optimum maintenance schedule is determined for the patient.) If more than 6 weeks have elapsed since the last treatment was given, treat patients as if they were beginning therapy insofar as exposure dosages are concerned, since their threshold for erythema may have decreased.

Table 1. Grades of Erythema

Grades	Erythema
0	No erythema
1	Minimally perceptible erythema—faint pink
2	Marked erythema but with no edema
3	Fiery erythema with edema
4	Fiery erythema with edema and blistering

Table 2. Response to Therapy

Grade	Criteria	Percent Improvement (compared to original extent of disease)
−1	Psoriasis worse	0
0	No change	0
1	Minimal improvement—slightly less scale and/or erythema	5–20
2	Definite improvement—partial flattening of all plaques—less scaling and less erythema	20–50
3	Considerable improvement—nearly complete flattening of all plaques but borders of plaques still palpable	50–95
4	Clearing; complete flattening of plaques including borders; plaques may be outlined by pigmentation	95

HOW SUPPLIED

Oxsoralen-Ultra Capsules, each containing 10 mg of methoxsalen (8-methoxypsoralen) in a soft gelatin capsule packaged in amber glass bottles are available as follows:

Unit Count	NDC Number
50	NDC 0187-0650-42

Copyright October, 1986

ICN Pharmaceuticals, Inc. March, 1987
Costa Mesa, Ca 92626
Manufactured for ICN Pharmaceuticals, Inc.

BIBLIOGRAPHY

1. Levins, P.C., Gauge, R.W., Momtaz-T.K., Parrish, J.A., and Fitzpatrick, T.B.: A New Liquid Formulation of 8-Methoxypsoralen: Bioactivity and Effect of Diet: JID, *82*, No. 2, pp. 185–187 (1984) and private communication.
2. Artuc, M., Stuettgen, G. Schalla, W., Schaefer, H., and Gazith, J.: Reversible binding of 5- and 8-methoxypsoralen to human serum proteins (albumin) and to epidermis in vitro: Brit. J. Dermat. *101*, pp. 669–677 (1979).
3. Mandula, B.B., Pathak, M.A., Nakayama, T., and Davidson, S.J.: Induction of mixed-function oxidases in mouse liver by psoralens., Ibid, *99*, pp. 687–692 (1978).
4. Pathak, M.A., Fitzpatrick, T.B., Parrish, J.A.: PSORIASIS, Proceedings of the Second International Symposium. Edited by E.M. Farber, A.J. Cox, Yorke Medical Books, pp. 262–265 (1977).
5. Dall'Acqua, F., Marciani, S., Ciavatta, L., Rodighiero, G.: Formation on interstrand cross-linkings of the photoreactions between furocoumarins and DNA; Z Naturforsch (B), *26*, pp. 561–569 (1971).
6. Cole, R.S.: Light-induced cross-linkings of DNA in the presence of a furocoumarin (psoralen), Biochem. Biophys. Acta, *217*, pp. 30–39 (1970).
7. Musajo, L, Rodighiero, G., Caporale, G., Dall'Acqua, F, Marciani, S., Bordin, F., Baccichetti, F., Bevilacqua, R.: Photoreactions between Skin-Photosentizing Furocoumarins and Nucleic Acids, *Sunlight and Man;* Normal and Abnormal Photobiologic Responses. Edited by M.A. Pathak, LC. Harber, M. Seiji et al. University of Tokyo Press, pp. 369–387 (1974).
8. Dall'Acqua, F., Vedaldi, D., Bordin, F., and Rodighiero, G.: New studies in the interaction between 8-methoxypsoralen and DNA *in vitro:* JID, *73*, pp. 191–197 (1979).
9. Yoshikawa, K., Mori, N., Sakakibara, S., Mizuno, N. Song, P.: Photo Conjugation of 8-methoxypsoralen with Proteins; Photochem. & Photobiol. *29*, pp. 1127–1133 (1979).
10. Hakim, R.D., Griffin, A.C.: Knox, J.M.: Erythema and tumor formation in methoxsalen treated mice exposed to fluorescent light; Arch. Dermatol. *82*, pp. 572–577 (1960).
11. O'Neal, M.A., Griffin, A.C.: The Effect of Oxypsoralen upon Ultraviolet Carcinogenesis in Albino Mice, Cancer Res., *17*, pp. 911–916 (1957).
12. Stern, R.S., Unpublished personal communication.
13. Stern, R.S., Parrish, J.A., Zierler, S.: Skin Carcinoma in Patients with Psoriasis Treated with Topical Tar and Artificial Ultraviolet Radiation. Lancet, *1*, pp. 732–735 (1980).
14. Stern, R.S., Laird, N., Melski, J. Parrish, J.A., Fitzpatrick, T.B., Bleich, H.L.: Cutaneous Squamous-Cell Carcinoma in Patients Treated with PUVA: NEJM, *310*, No. 18, pp. 1156–1161 (1984).
15. Roenigk, Jr., H.H., and 12 Cooperating Investigators: Skin Cancer in the PUVA-48 Cooperative Study of Psoriasis. Program for Forty-First Annual Meeting for The Society of Investigative Dermatology, Inc., Sheraton Washington Hotel, Washington, D.C., May 12, 13, and 14, 1980). Abstracts JID, *74*, No. 4, p. 250 (April, 1980).
16. Mosher, D.B., Pathak, M.A., Harris, T.J., Fitzpatrick, T.B.: Development of Cutaneous Lesions in Vitiligo During Long-Term PUVA Therapy. Program for Forty-First Annual Meeting for the Society for Investigative Dermatology, Inc., Sheraton Washington Hotel, Washington, D.C., May 12, 13, and 14, 1980. Abstracts JID, *74*, No. 4, p 259 (April, 1980).
17. Cloud, T.M. Hakim, R., Griffin, A.C.: Photosensitization of the eye with methoxsalen. I. Acute effects; Arch. Ophthalmol. *64*, pp. 346–352 (1960).
18. Cloud, T.M. Hakim, R., Griffin, A.C.: Photosensitization of the eye with methoxsalen. II. Chronic effects, Ibid, *66*, pp. 689–694 (1961).
19. Freeman, R.G., Troll, D.: Photosensitization of the eye by 8-methoxypsoralen, JID, *53*, pp. 449–453 (1969).
20. Lerman, S., Megaw, J., Willis, I.:Potential ocular complications from PUVA therapy and their prevention; JID, *74*, pp. 197–199 (1980).
21. Diffey, B.L., Medical Physics Handbook 11, Ultraviolet Radiation in Medicine, Adam Hilger, Ltd., Bristol, p. 86 (1982).

Shown in Product Identification Section, page 412

PROSTIGMIN® ℞

[*pro-stig'min*]
(neostigmine methylsulfate)
INJECTABLE

DESCRIPTION

Prostigmin (neostigmine methylsulfate) Injectable, an anticholinesterase agent, is a sterile aqueous solution intended for intramuscular, intravenous or subcutaneous administration.

Prostigmin Injectable is available in the following concentrations:

Prostigmin 1:2000 Ampuls — each ml contains 0.5 mg neostigmine methylsulfate compounded with 0.2% parabens (methyl and propyl) as preservatives and sodium hydroxide to adjust pH to approximately 5.9.

Prostigmin 1:4000 Ampuls — each ml contains 0.25 mg neostigmine methylsulfate compounded with 0.2% parabens (methyl and propyl) as preservatives and sodium hydroxide to adjust pH to approximately 5.9.

Prostigmin 1:1000 Multiple Dose Vials — each ml contains 1 mg neostigmine methylsulfate compounded with 0.45% phenol as preservative, 0.2 mg sodium acetate, and acetic acid and sodium hydroxide to adjust pH to approximately 5.9.

Prostigmin 1:2000 Multiple Dose Vials — each ml contains 0.5 mg neostigmine methylsulfate compounded with 0.45% phenol as preservative, 0.2 mg sodium acetate, and acetic acid and sodium hydroxide to adjust pH to approximately 5.9.

Chemically, neostigmine methylsulfate is (*m*-hydroxyphenyl)trimethylammonium methylsulfate dimethylcarbamate. It has a molecular weight of 334.39 and the following structural formula:

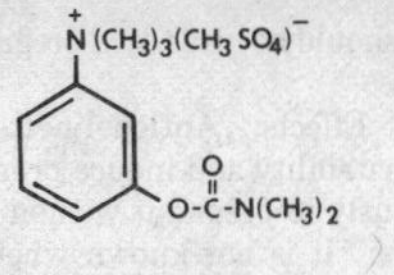

CLINICAL PHARMACOLOGY

Neostigmine inhibits the hydrolysis of acetylcholine by competing with acetylcholine for attachment to acetylcholinesterase at sites of cholinergic transmission. It enhances cholinergic action by facilitating the transmission of impulses across neuromuscular junctions. It also has a direct cholinomimetic effect on skeletal muscle and possibly on autonomic ganglion cells and neurons of the central nervous system. Neostigmine undergoes hydrolysis by cholinesterase and is also metabolized by microsomal enzymes in the liver. Protein binding to human serum albumin ranges from 15 to 25 percent.

Following intramuscular administration, neostigmine is rapidly absorbed and eliminated. In a study of five patients with myasthenia gravis, peak plasma levels were observed at 30 minutes, and the half-life ranged from 51 to 90 minutes. Approximately 80 percent of the drug was eliminated in urine within 24 hours; approximately 50% as the unchanged drug, and 30 percent as metabolites. Following intravenous administration, plasma half-life ranges from 47 to 60 minutes have been reported with a mean half-life of 53 minutes.

The clinical effects of neostigmine usually begin within 20 to 30 minutes after intramuscular injection and last from 2.5 to 4 hours.

INDICATIONS AND USAGE

Prostigmin is indicated for:

—the symptomatic control of myasthenia gravis when oral therapy is impractical.

—the prevention and treatment of postoperative distention and urinary retention after mechanical obstruction has been excluded.

—reversal of effects of nondepolarizing neuromuscular blocking agents (*e.g.,* tubocurarine, metocurine, gallamine, or pancuronium) after surgery.

CONTRAINDICATIONS

Prostigmin is contraindicated in patients with known hypersensitivity to the drug. It is also contraindicated in patients with peritonitis or mechanical obstruction of the intestinal or urinary tract.

WARNINGS

Prostigmin should be used with caution in patients with epilepsy, bronchial asthma, bradycardia, recent coronary occlusion, vagotonia, hyperthyroidism, cardiac arrhythmias or peptic ulcer. When large doses of Prostigmin are administered, the prior or simultaneous injection of atropine sulfate may be advisable. Separate syringes should be used for the Prostigmin and atropine. Because of the possibility of hypersensitivity in an occasional patient, atropine and antishock medication should always be readily available.

PRECAUTIONS

General: It is important to differentiate between myasthenic crisis and cholinergic crisis caused by overdosage of Prostigmin. Both conditions result in extreme muscle weakness but require radically different treatment. (See OVERDOSAGE section.)

Drug Interactions: Prostigmin does not antagonize, and may in fact prolong, the Phase I block of *depolarizing* muscle relaxants such as succinylcholine or decamethonium. Certain antibiotics, especially neomycin, streptomycin and kanamycin, have a mild but definite nondepolarizing blocking action which may accentuate neuromuscular block. These antibiotics should be used in the myasthenic patient only where definitely indicated, and then careful adjustment should be made of the anticholinesterase dosage. Local and some general anesthetics, antiarrhythmic agents and other drugs that interfere with neuromuscular transmission should be used cautiously, if at all, in patients with myasthenia gravis; the dose of Prostigmin may have to be increased accordingly.

Carcinogenesis, Mutagenesis and Impairment of Fertility: There have been no studies with Prostigmin which would permit an evaluation of its carcinogenic or mutagenic potential. Studies on the effect of Prostigmin on fertility and reproduction have not been performed.

Pregnancy:

Teratogenic Effects: Pregnancy Category C. There are no adequate or well-controlled studies of Prostigmin in either laboratory animals or in pregnant women. It is not known whether Prostigmin can cause fetal harm when administered to a pregnant woman or can affect reproductive capac-

Continued on next page

ICN—Cont.

ity. Prostigmin should be given to a pregnant woman only if clearly needed.
Nonteratogenic Effects: Anticholinesterase drugs may cause uterine irritability and induce premature labor when given intravenously to pregnant women near term.
Nursing Mothers: It is not known whether Prostigmin is excreted in human milk. Because many drugs are excreted in human milk and because of the potential for serious adverse reactions from Prostigmin in nursing infants, a decision should be made whether to discontinue nursing or to discontinue the drug, taking into account the importance of the drug to the mother.
Pediatric Use: Safety and effectiveness in children have not been established.

ADVERSE REACTIONS

Side effects are generally due to an exaggeration of pharmacological effects of which salivation and fasciculation are the most common. Bowel cramps and diarrhea may also occur. The following additional adverse reactions have been reported following the use of either neostigmine bromide or neostigmine methylsulfate:
Allergic: Allergic reactions and anaphylaxis.
Neurologic: Dizziness, convulsions, loss of consciousness, drowsiness, headache, dysarthria, miosis and visual changes.
Cardiovascular: Cardiac arrhythmias (including bradycardia, tachycardia, A-V block and nodal rhythm) and nonspecific EKG changes have been reported, as well as cardiac arrest, syncope and hypotension. These have been predominantly noted following the use of the injectable form of Prostigmin.
Respiratory: Increased oral, pharyngeal and bronchial secretions, dyspnea, respiratory depression, respiratory arrest and bronchospasm.
Dermatologic: Rash and urticaria.
Gastrointestinal: Nausea, emesis, flatulence and increased peristalsis.
Genitourinary: Urinary frequency.
Musculoskeletal: Muscle cramps and spasms, arthralgia.
Miscellaneous: Diaphoresis, flushing and weakness.

OVERDOSAGE

Overdosage of Prostigmin can cause cholinergic crisis, which is characterized by increasing muscle weakness, and through involvement of the muscles of respiration, may result in death. Myasthenic crisis, due to an increase in the severity of the disease, is also accompanied by extreme muscle weakness and may be difficult to distinguish from cholinergic crisis on a symptomatic basis. However, such differentiation is extremely important because increases in the dose of Prostigmin or other drugs in this class, in the presence of cholinergic crisis or of a refractory or "insensitive" state, could have grave consequences. The two types of crises may be differentiated by the use of Tensilon® (edrophonium chloride) as well as by clinical judgment.
Treatment of the two conditions differs radically. Whereas the presence of *myasthenic crisis* requires more intensive anticholinesterase therapy, *cholinergic crisis* calls for the prompt withdrawal of all drugs of this type. The immediate use of atropine in cholinergic crisis is also recommended.
Atropine may also be used to abolish or minimize gastrointestinal side effects or other muscarinic reactions; but such use, by masking signs of overdosage, can lead to inadvertent induction of cholinergic crisis.
The LD_{50} of neostigmine methylsulfate in mice is 0.3 ± 0.02 mg/kg intravenously, 0.54 ± 0.03 mg/kg subcutaneously, and 0.395 ± 0.025 mg/kg intramuscularly; in rats the LD_{50} is 0.315 ± 0.019 mg/kg intravenously, 0.445 ± 0.032 mg/kg subcutaneously, and 0.423 ± 0.032 mg/kg intramuscularly.

DOSAGE AND ADMINISTRATION

Symptomatic control of myasthenia gravis: One ml of the 1:2000 solution (0.5 mg) subcutaneously or intramuscularly. Subsequent doses should be based on the individual patient's response. In most patients, however, oral treatment with Prostigmin (neostigmine bromide) tablets, 15 mg each, is adequate for control of symptoms.
Prevention of postoperative distention and urinary retention: One ml of the 1:4000 solution (0.25 mg) subcutaneously or intramuscularly as soon as possible after operation; repeat every 4 to 6 hours for two or three days.
Treatment of postoperative distention: One ml of the 1:2000 solution (0.5 mg) subcutaneously or intramuscularly, as required.
Treatment of urinary retention: One ml of the 1:2000 solution (0.5 mg) subcutaneously or intramuscularly. If urination does not occur within an hour, the patient should be catheterized. After the patient has voided, or the bladder has been emptied, continue the 0.5 mg injections every three hours for at least 5 injections.
Reversal of Effects of Nondepolarizing Neuromuscular Blocking Agents: When Prostigmin is administered intravenously, it is recommended that atropine sulfate (0.6 to 1.2 mg) also be given intravenously using separate syringes. Some authorities have recommended that the atropine be injected several minutes before the Prostigmin rather than concomitantly. The usual dose is 0.5 to 2 mg Prostigmin given by *slow* intravenous injection, repeated as required. Only in exceptional cases should the total dose of Prostigmin exceed 5 mg. It is recommended that the patient be well ventilated and a patent airway maintained until complete recovery of normal respiration is assured. The optimum time for administration of the drug is during hyperventilation when the carbon dioxide level of the blood is low. It should never be administered in the presence of high concentrations of halothane or cyclopropane. In cardiac cases and severely ill patients, it is advisable to titrate the exact dose of Prostigmin required, using a peripheral nerve stimulator device. In the presence of bradycardia, the pulse rate should be increased to about 80/minute with atropine before administering Prostigmin.
Parenteral drug products should be inspected visually for particulate matter and discoloration prior to administration, whenever solution and container permit.

HOW SUPPLIED

Prostigmin 1:2000 (0.5 mg neostigmine methylsulfate/ml), 1-ml ampuls — boxes of 10 (NDC 0187-3100-30).
Prostigmin 1:4000 (0.25 mg neostigmine methylsulfate/ml), 1-ml ampuls — boxes of 10 (NDC 0187-3100-40).
Prostigmin 1:1000 (1 mg neostigmine methylsulfate/ml), 10-ml multiple dose vials — boxes of 10 (NDC 0187-3100-50).
Prostigmin 1:2000 (0.5 mg neostigmine methylsulfate/ml), 10-ml multiple dose vials — boxes of 10 (NDC 0187-3100-60).
Manufactured for ICN Pharmaceuticals, Inc.
Costa Mesa, CA 92626
by Hoffmann-La Roche Inc.
Nutley, N.J. 07110
Rev. 3/89

PROSTIGMIN® ℞
[*pro-stig'min*]
(neostigmine bromide)
TABLETS

DESCRIPTION

Prostigmin (neostigmine bromide), an anticholinesterase agent, is available for oral administration in 15-mg tablets. Each tablet also contains gelatin, lactose, corn starch, stearic acid, sugar and talc.
Chemically, neostigmine bromide is (*m*-hydroxyphenyl) trimethylammonium bromide dimethylcarbamate. It is a white, crystalline, bitter powder, soluble 1:1 in water, with a molecular weight of 303.20 and the following structural formula:

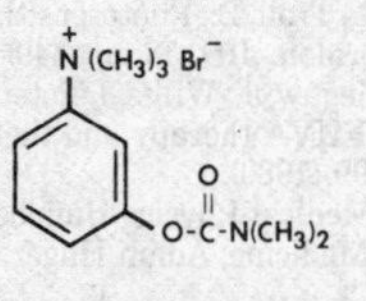

CLINICAL PHARMACOLOGY

Neostigmine inhibits the hydrolysis of acetylcholine by competing with acetylcholine for attachment to acetylcholinesterase at sites of cholinergic transmission. It enhances cholinergic action by facilitating the transmission of impulses across neuromuscular junctions. It also has a direct cholinomimetic effect on skeletal muscle and possibly on autonomic ganglion cells and neurons of the central nervous system. Neostigmine undergoes hydrolysis by cholinesterase and is also metabolized by microsomal enzymes in the liver. Protein binding to human serum albumin ranges from 15 to 25 percent.
Neostigmine bromide is poorly absorbed from the gastrointestinal tract following oral administration. As a rule, 15 mg of neostigmine bromide orally is equivalent to 0.5 mg of neostigmine methylsulfate parenterally, due to poor absorption of the tablet from the intestinal tract. In a study in fasting myasthenic patients, the extent of absorption was estimated to be 1 to 2 percent of the ingested 30-mg single oral dose. Peak concentrations in plasma occurred 1 to 2 hours following drug ingestion, with considerable individual variations. The half-life ranged from 42 to 60 minutes with a mean half-life of 52 minutes.

INDICATIONS AND USAGE

Prostigmin is indicated for the symptomatic treatment of myasthenia gravis. Its greatest usefulness is in prolonged therapy where no difficulty in swallowing is present. In acute myasthenic crisis where difficulty in breathing and swallowing is present, the parenteral form (neostigmine methylsulfate) should be used. The patient can be transferred to the oral form as soon as it can be tolerated.

CONTRAINDICATIONS

Prostigmin is contraindicated in patients with known hypersensitivity to the drug. Because of the presence of the bromide ion, it should not be used in patients with a previous history of reaction to bromides. It is contraindicated in patients with peritonitis or mechanical obstruction of the intestinal or urinary tract.

WARNINGS

Prostigmin should be used with caution in patients with epilepsy, bronchial asthma, bradycardia, recent coronary occlusion, vagotonia, hyperthyroidism, cardiac arrhythmias or peptic ulcer. As a rule, 15 mg of neostigmine bromide orally is equivalent to 0.5 mg of neostigmine methylsulfate parenterally, due to poor absorption of the tablet from the intestinal tract. Large doses should be avoided in situations where there might be an increased absorption rate from the intestinal tract. It should be used with caution when co-administered with anticholinergic drugs, in order to avoid reduction of intestinal motility.

PRECAUTIONS

General: It is important to differentiate between myasthenic crisis and cholinergic crisis caused by overdosage of Prostigmin. Both conditions result in extreme muscle weakness but require radically different treatment. (See OVERDOSAGE section.)
Drug Interactions: Certain antibiotics, especially neomycin, streptomycin and kanamycin, have a mild but definite nondepolarizing blocking action which may accentuate neuromuscular block. These antibiotics should be used in the myasthenic patient only where definitely indicated, and then careful adjustment should be made of adjunctive anticholinesterase dosage.
Local and some general anesthetics, antiarrhythmic agents and other drugs that interfere with neuromuscular transmission should be used cautiously, if at all, in patients with myasthenia gravis; the dose of Prostigmin may have to be increased accordingly.
Carcinogenesis, Mutagenesis and Impairment of Fertility: There have been no studies with Prostigmin which would permit an evaluation of its carcinogenic or mutagenic potential. Studies on the effect of Prostigmin on fertility and reproduction have not been performed.
Pregnancy:
Teratogenic Effects: Pregnancy Category C. There are no adequate or well-controlled studies of Prostigmin in either laboratory animals or in pregnant women. It is not known whether Prostigmin can cause fetal harm when administered to a pregnant woman or can affect reproductive capacity. Prostigmin should be given to a pregnant woman only if clearly needed.
Nonteratogenic Effects: Anticholinesterase drugs may cause uterine irritability and induce premature labor when given intravenously to pregnant women near term.
Nursing Mothers: It is not known whether Prostigmin is excreted in human milk. Because many drugs are excreted in human milk and because of the potential for serious adverse reactions from Prostigmin in nursing infants, a decision should be made whether to discontinue nursing or to discontinue the drug, taking into account the importance of the drug to the mother.
Pediatric Use: Safety and effectiveness in children have not been established.

ADVERSE REACTIONS

Side effects are generally due to an exaggeration of pharmacological effects of which salivation and fasciculation are the most common. Bowel cramps and diarrhea may also occur. The following additional adverse reactions have been reported following the use of either neostigmine bromide or neostigmine methylsulfate:
Allergic: Allergic reactions and anaphylaxis.
Neurologic: Dizziness, convulsions, loss of consciousness, drowsiness, headache, dysarthria, miosis and visual changes.
Cardiovascular: Cardiac arrhythmias (including bradycardia, tachycardia, A-V block and nodal rhythm) and nonspecific EKG changes have been reported, as well as cardiac arrest, syncope and hypotension. These have been predominantly noted following the use of the injectable form of Prostigmin.
Respiratory: Increased oral, pharyngeal and bronchial secretions, and dyspnea. Respiratory depression, respiratory arrest and bronchospasm have been reported following the use of the injectable form of Prostigmin.
Dermatologic: Rash and urticaria.
Gastrointestinal: Nausea, emesis, flatulence and increased peristalsis.
Genitourinary: Urinary frequency.
Musculoskeletal: Muscle cramps and spasms, arthralgia.
Miscellaneous: Diaphoresis, flushing and weakness.

OVERDOSAGE

Overdosage of Prostigmin can cause cholinergic crisis, which is characterized by increasing muscle weakness, and through involvement of the muscles of respiration, may result in death. Myasthenic crisis, due to an increase in the severity of the disease, is also accompanied by extreme muscle weakness and may be difficult to distinguish from cholinergic crisis on a symptomatic basis. However, such differentiation

is extremely important because increases in the dose of Prostigmin or other drugs in this class, in the presence of cholinergic crisis or of a refractory or "insensitive" state, could have grave consequences. The two types of crises may be differentiated by the use of Tensilon® (edrophonium chloride) as well as by clinical judgment.
Treatment of the two conditions differs radically. Whereas the presence of *myasthenic crisis* requires more intensive anticholinesterase therapy, *cholinergic crisis* calls for the prompt withdrawal of all drugs of this type. The immediate use of atropine in cholinergic crisis is also recommended.
Atropine may also be used to abolish or minimize gastrointestinal side effects or other muscarinic reactions; but such use, by masking signs of overdosage, can lead to inadvertent induction of cholinergic crisis.
The LD_{50} of neostigmine methylsulfate in mice is 0.3 ± 0.02 mg/kg intravenously, 0.54 ± 0.03 mg/kg subcutaneously, and 0.395 ± 0.025 mg/kg intramuscularly; in rats the LD_{50} is 0.315 ± 0.019 mg/kg intravenously, 0.445 ± 0.032 mg/kg subcutaneously, and 0.423 ± 0.032 mg/kg intramuscularly.

DOSAGE AND ADMINISTRATION

The onset of action of Prostigmin given orally is slower than when given parenterally, but the duration of action is longer and the intensity of action more uniform. Dosage requirements for optimal results vary from 15 mg to 375 mg per day. In some instances it may be necessary to exceed these dosages, but the possibility of cholinergic crisis must be recognized. The average dose is 10 tablets (150 mg) administered over a 24-hour period. The interval between doses is of paramount importance. The dosage schedule should be adjusted for each patient and changed as the need arises. Frequently, therapy is required day and night. Larger portions of the total daily dose may be given at times when the patient is more prone to fatigue (afternoon, mealtimes, etc.). The patient should be encouraged to keep a daily record of his or her condition to assist the physician in determining an optimal therapeutic regimen.

HOW SUPPLIED

Scored, white tablets containing 15 mg neostigmine bromide — bottles of 100 (NDC 0187-3100-10). Imprint on tablets: (front) PROSTIGMIN; (back) ICN.
Manufactured for ICN Pharmaceuticals, Inc.
Costa Mesa, CA 92626
by Hoffmann-La Roche Inc.
Nutley, N.J. 07110
Rev. 3/89

PSORION® Cream 0.05% ℞
(Betamethasone Dipropionate USP, 0.05%)
(potency expressed as betamethasone)

FEDERAL (U.S.A.) LAW PROHIBITS DISPENSING WITHOUT PRESCRIPTION.

DESCRIPTION

The topical corticosteroids constitute a class of primarily synthetic steroids used as anti-inflammatory and anti-pruritic agents. Betamethasone dipropionate is included in this class of synthetic corticosteroids. Betamethasone, an analog of prednisolone, has high corticosteroid activity and slight mineralocorticoid activity.
Chemically, betamethasone dipropionate is Pregna-1,4-diene-3,20-dione, 9-fluoro-11hydroxy-16-methyl-17,21-bis (1-oxopropoxy)-(11β, 16β)-. The structural formula:

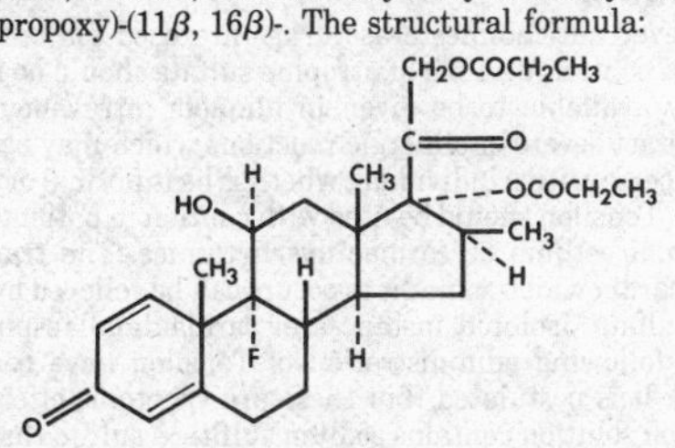

MOL. WT. 504.59 $C_{28}H_{37}FO_7$

Psorion cream, 0.05% (betamethasone dipropionate USP equivalent to 0.5 mg of betamethasone) in a base containing purified water, mineral oil, white petrolatum, polyethylene glycol 1000 monocetyl ether, cetostearyl alcohol, monobasic sodium phosphate, phosphoric acid, 4-chloro-*m*-cresol and propylene glycol.

CLINICAL PHARMACOLOGY

Topical corticosteroids share anti-inflammatory, anti-pruritic and vasoconstrictive actions.
The mechanisms of anti-inflammatory activity of the topical corticosteroids is unclear. Various laboratory methods, including vasoconstrictor assays, are used to compare the predicted potencies and/or clinical efficacies of the topical corticosteroids. There is some evidence to suggest that a recognizable correlation exists between vasoconstrictor potency and therapeutic efficacy in man.
Pharmacokinetics—The extent of percutaneous absorption of topical corticosteroids is determined by many factors including the vehicle, the integrity of the epidermal barrier, and the use of occlusive dressings. (See DOSAGE AND ADMINISTRATION.)
Topical corticosteroids can be absorbed from normal intact skin. Inflammation and/or disease processes in the skin increase percutaneous absorption. Occlusive dressings substantially increase the percutaneous absorption of topical corticosteroids. (See DOSAGE AND ADMINISTRATION.)
Once absorbed through the skin, topical corticosteroids are handled through pharmacokinetic pathways similar to systemically administered corticosteroids. Corticosteroids are bound to plasma proteins in varying degrees. Corticosteroids are metabolized primarily in the liver and are then excreted by the kindneys. Some of the topical corticosteroids and their metabolites are also excreted into the bile.

INDICATIONS AND USAGE

Topical corticosteroids are indicated for the relief of the inflammatory and pruritic manifestations of corticosteroid-responsive dermatoses.

CONTRAINDICATIONS

Topical corticosteroids are contraindicated in those patients with a history of hypersensitivity to any of the components of the preparation.

PRECAUTIONS

General—Systemic absorption of topical corticosteroids has produced reversible hypothalamic-pituitary-adrenal (HPA) axis suppression, manifestations of Cushing's syndrome, hyperglycemia, and glucosuria in some patients.
Conditions which augment systemic absorption include the application of the more potent steroids, use over large surface areas, prolonged use, and the addition of occlusive dressings. (See DOSAGE AND ADMINISTRATION.)
Therefore, patients receiving a large dose of a potent topical steroid applied to a large surface area should be evaluated periodically for evidence of HPA axis suppression by using the urinary free cortisol and ACTH stimulation tests. If HPA axis suppression is noted, an attempt should be made to withdraw the drug, to reduce the frequency of application, or to substitute a less potent steroid.
Recovery of HPA axis function is generally prompt and complete upon discontinuation of the drug. Infrequently, signs and symptoms of steroid withdrawal may occur, requiring supplemental systemic corticosteroids.
Children may absorb proportionally large amounts of topical corticosteroids and thus be more susceptible to systemic toxicity. (See PRECAUTIONS—PEDIATRIC USE.)
If irritation develops, topical corticosteroids should be discontinued and appropriate therapy instituted.
In the presence of dermatological infections, the use of an appropriate antifungal of antibacterial agent should be instituted. If a favorable response does not occur promptly, the corticosteroid should be discontinued until the infection has been adequately controlled.
Information for the Patient—Patients using topical corticosteroids should receive the following information and instructions:

1. This medication is to be used as directed by the physician. It is for external use only. Avoid contact with the eyes.
2. Patients should be advised not to use this medication for any disorder other than for which it was prescribed.
3. The treated skin area should not be bandaged or otherwise covered or wrapped as to be occlusive. (See DOSAGE AND ADMINISTRATION.)
4. Patients should report any signs of local adverse reactions.
5. Parents of pediatric patients should be advised not to use tight-fitting diapers or plastic pants on a child being treated in the diaper area, as these garments may constitute occlusive dressings. (See DOSAGE AND ADMINISTRATION.)

Laboratory Tests—The following tests may be helpful in evaluating the HPA axis suppression: urinary free cortisol test; ACTH stimulation test.
Carcinogenesis, Mutagenesis, and Impairment of Fertility—Long-term animal studies have not been performed to evaluate the carcinogenic potential or the effect on fertility of topical corticosteroids.
Studies to determine mutagenicity with prednisolone and hydrocortisone have revealed negative results.
Pregnancy—Category C—Corticosteroids are generally teratogenic in laboratory animals when administered systemically at relatively low dosage levels. The more potent corticosteroids have been shown to be teratogenic after dermal application in laboratory animals. There are no adequate and well-controlled studies in pregnant women on teratogenic effects from topically applied corticosteroids. Therefore, topical corticosteroids should be used during pregnancy only if the potential benefit justifies the potential risk to the fetus. Drugs of this class should not be used extensively on pregnant patients, in large amounts, or for prolonged periods of time.
Nursing Mothers—It is *not* known whether topical administration of corticosteroids could result in sufficient systemic absorption to produce detectable quantities in breast milk. Systemically administered corticosteroids are secreted into breast milk in quantities not likely to have a deleterious effect on the infant. Nevertheless, caution should be exercised when topical corticosteroids are administered to a nursing woman.
Pediatric Use—*Pediatric patients may demonstrate greater susceptibility to topical corticosteroid-induced HPA axis suppression and Cushing's syndrome than mature patients because of a larger skin surface area to body weight ratio.*
Hypothalamic-pituitary-adrenal (HPA) axis suppression, Cushing's syndrome, and intracranial hypertension have been reported in children receiving topical corticosteroids. Manifestations of adrenal suppression in children include linear growth retardation, delayed weight gain, low plasma cortisol levels, and absence of response to ACTH stimulation. Manifestations of intracranial hypertension include bulging fontanelles, headaches, and bilateral papilledema.
Administration of topical corticosteroids to children should be limited to the least amount compatible with an effective therapeutic regimen. Chronic corticosteroid therapy may interfere with the growth and development of children.

ADVERSE REACTIONS

The following local adverse reactions are reported infrequently when betamethasone dipropionate products are used as recommended in the DOSAGE AND ADMINISTRATION section. These reactions are listed in an approximate decreasing order of occurrence: burning, itching, irritation, dryness, folliculitis, hypertrichosis, acneiform eruptions, hypopigmentation, perioral dermatitis, allergic contact dermatitis, maceration of the skin, secondary infection, skin atrophy, striae, miliaria.
Systemic absorption of topical corticosteroids has produced reversible hypothalamic-pituitary-adrenal (HPA) axis suppression, manifestations of Cushing's syndrome, hyperglycemia, and glucosuria in some patients.

OVERDOSAGE

Topically applied corticosteroids can be absorbed in sufficient amounts to produce system effects. (See PRECAUTIONS.)

DOSAGE AND ADMINISTRATION

Psorion cream, 0.05% is generally applied to the affected area as a thin film once daily. In some cases, twice daily dosage may be necessary.
Betamethasone dipropionate products are not to be used with occlusive dressings.
If an infection develops, appropriate antimicrobial therapy should be instituted.

HOW SUPPLIED

0.05% cream in ½ ounce (15 g) (NDC 0187-0528-35), and 1½ ounce (45 g) (NDC 0187-0528-39) tubes.
Store at controlled room temperature 15°–30°C (59°–86°F).
Protect from freezing.

SOLAQUIN FORTE® 4% Cream ℞
[*sōl 'a-kwin " for 'tā*]
(HYDROQUINONE USP, 4%)
Skin Bleaching Cream with Sunscreens

FEDERAL (U.S.A.) LAW PROHIBITS DISPENSING WITHOUT PRESCRIPTION.
FOR EXTERNAL USE ONLY.

DESCRIPTION

Each gram of Solaquin Forte contains 40 mg hydroquinone, 80 mg octyl dimethyl-p-aminobenzoate, 30 mg dioxybenzone USP and 20 mg oxybenzone USP in a vanishing cream base of purified water, glyceryl monostearate, octyldodecyl stearoyl stearate, glyceryl dilaurate, quaternium-26, coceth-6, stearyl alcohol, diethylaminoethyl stearate, dimethicone, polysorbate-80, lactic acid, ascorbic acid, hydroxyethylcellulose, quaternium-14, myristylkonium chloride, disodium EDTA, and sodium metabisulfite.

CLINICAL PHARMACOLOGY

Topical application of hydroquinone produces a reversible depigmentation of the skin by inhibition of the enzymatic oxidation of tyrosine to 3, 4-dihydroxyphenylalanine (dopa) and suppression of other melanocyte metabolic processes. Exposure to sunlight or ultraviolet light will cause repigmentation which may be prevented by the broad spectrum sunscreen agents contained in Solaquin Forte.

INDICATIONS AND USAGE

Solaquin Forte 4% Cream is indicated for the gradual bleaching of hyperpigmented skin conditions such as chloasma, melasma, freckles, senile lentigines, and other unwanted areas of melanin hyperpigmentation.

Continued on next page

ICN—Cont.

CONTRAINDICATIONS
Prior history of sensitivity or allergic reaction to this product or any of its ingredients. The safety of topical hydroquinone use during pregnancy or in children (12 years and under) has not been established.

WARNINGS

A. CAUTION: Hydroquinone is a skin bleaching agent which may produce unwanted cosmetic effects if not used as directed. The physician should be familiar with the contents of this insert before prescribing or dispensing this medication.
B. Test for skin sensitivity before using Solaquin Forte 4% Cream by applying a small amount to an unbroken patch of skin and check in 24 hours. Minor redness is not a contraindication, but where there is itching or vesicle formation or excessive inflammatory response further treatment is not advised. Close patient supervision is recommended. Contact with the eyes should be avoided. If no bleaching or lightening effect is noted after 2 months of treatment use, Solaquin Forte 4% Cream should be discontinued. Solaquin Forte 4% Cream is formulated for use as a skin bleaching agent and should not be used for the prevention of sunburn.
C. Sunscreen use is an essential aspect of hydroquinone therapy because even minimal sunlight exposure sustains melanocytic activity. The sunscreens in Solaquin Forte 4% Cream provide the necessary sun protection during skin bleaching therapy. After clearing and during maintenance therapy, sun exposure should be avoided on bleached skin by application of a sunscreen or sunblock agent or protective clothing to prevent repigmentation.
D. Keep this and all medication out of the reach of children. In case of accidental ingestion, call a physician or a poison control center immediately.
E. Warning: Contains sodium metabisulfite, a sulfite that may cause serious allergic type reactions (e.g. hives, itching, wheezing, anaphylaxis, severe asthma attack) in certain susceptible persons.

PRECAUTIONS
SEE WARNINGS.

A. Pregnancy Category C. Animal reproduction studies have not been conducted with topical hydroquinone. It is also not known whether hydroquinone can cause fetal harm when used topically on a pregnant woman or affect reproductive capacity. It is not known to what degree, if any, topical hydroquinone is absorbed systemically. Topical hydroquinone should be used in pregnant women only when clearly indicated.
B. Nursing mothers. It is not known whether topical hydroquinone is absorbed or excreted in human milk. Caution is advised when topical hydroquinone is used by a nursing mother.
C. Pediatric usage. Safety and effectiveness in children below the age of 12 years have not been established.

ADVERSE REACTIONS
No systemic adverse reactions have been reported. Occasional hypersensitivity (localized contact dermatitis) may occur in which case the medication should be discontinued and the physician notified immediately.

OVERDOSAGE
There have been no systemic reactions from the use of topical hydroquinone in Solaquin Forte. However, treatment should be limited to relatively small areas of the body at one time since some patients experience a transient skin reddening and a mild burning sensation which does not preclude treatment.

DRUG DOSAGE AND ADMINISTRATION
Solaquin Forte 4% Cream should be applied to the affected area and rubbed in well twice daily or as directed by a physician. There is no recommended dosage for children under 12 years of age except under the advice and supervision of a physician.

HOW SUPPLIED
SOLAQUIN FORTE 4% Cream is available as follows:

Size	NDC Number
½ ounce tube (15 grams)	0187-0396-35
1 ounce tube (30 grams)	0187-0396-31

Available without prescription for maintenance therapy: Solaquin (2% Hydroquinone) in 1 ounce tubes (NDC 0187-0372-31).
Solaquin Forte 4% Cream should be stored at room temperature (15–30°C) (59–86°F).

SOLAQUIN FORTE® 4% GEL ℞
[*sōl 'a-kwĭn for 'tā*]
(Hydroquinone USP, 4%)
Skin Bleaching Gel with Sunscreens

FEDERAL (U.S.A.) LAW PROHIBITS DISPENSING WITHOUT A PRESCRIPTION.
FOR EXTERNAL USE ONLY

DESCRIPTION
Each gram of Solaquin Forte 4% Gel contains 40 mg of Hydroquinone, 50 mg octyl dimethyl-p-aminobenzoate and 30 mg Dioxybenzone in a hydroalcoholic base of alcohol, purified water, propylene glycol, tetrahydroxypropyl ethylenediamine, carbomer 940, disodium EDTA and sodium metabisulfite.

CLINICAL PHARMACOLOGY
Topical application of hydroquinone produces a reversible depigmentation of the skin by inhibition of the enzymatic oxidation of tyrosine to 3,4-dihydroxyphenylalanine (dopa) and suppression of other melanocyte metabolic processes. Exposure to sunlight or ultraviolet light will cause repigmentation which may be prevented by the broad spectrum sunscreen agents contained in Solaquin Forte 4% Gel.

INDICATIONS AND USAGE
Solaquin Forte 4% Gel is indicated for the gradual bleaching of hyperpigmented skin conditions such as chloasma, melasma, freckles, senile lentigines and other unwanted areas of melanin hyperpigmentation.

CONTRAINDICATIONS
Prior history of sensitivity or allergic reaction to this product or any of its ingredients. The safety of topical hydroquinone use during pregnancy or in children (12 years and under) has not been established.

WARNINGS

A. CAUTION: Hydroquinone is a skin bleaching agent which may produce unwanted cosmetic effects if not used as directed. The physician should be familiar with the contents of this insert before prescribing or dispensing this medication.
B. Test for skin sensitivity before using Solaquin Forte 4% Gel by applying a small amount to an unbroken patch of skin and check in 24 hours. Minor redness is not a contraindication, but where there is itching or vesicle formation or excessive inflammatory response further treatment is not advised. Close patient supervision is recommended. Contact with the eyes should be avoided. If no bleaching or lightening effect is noted after 2 months of treatment use, Solaquin Forte 4% Gel should be discontinued. Solaquin Forte 4% Gel is formulated for use as a skin bleaching agent and should not be used for the prevention of sunburn.
C. Sunscreen use is an essential aspect of hydroquinone therapy because even minimal sunlight sustains melanocytic activity. The sunscreens in Solaquin Forte 4% Gel provide the necessary sun protection during skin bleaching therapy. After clearing and during maintenance therapy, sun exposure should be avoided on bleached skin by application of a sunscreen or sunblock agent or protective clothing to prevent repigmentation.
D. Keep this and all medication out of the reach of children. In case of accidental ingestion, call a physician or a poison control center immediately.
E. Warning: Contains sodium metabisulfite, a sulfite that may cause serious allergic type reactions (e.g. hives, itching, wheezing, anaphylaxis) in certain susceptible persons.

PRECAUTIONS
SEE WARNINGS

A. Pregnancy Category C. Animal reproduction studies have not been conducted with topical hydroquinone. It is also not known whether hydroquinone can cause fetal harm when used topically on a pregnant woman or affect reproductive capacity. It is not known to what degree, if any, topical hydroquinone is absorbed systemically. Topical hydroquinone should be used in pregnant women only when clearly indicated.
B. Nursing mothers. It is not known whether topical hydroquinone is absorbed or excreted in human milk. Caution is advised when topical hydroquinone is used by a nursing mother.
C. Pediatric usage. Safety and effectiveness in children below the age of 12 years have not been established.

ADVERSE REACTIONS
No systemic adverse reactions have been reported. Occasional hypersensitivity (localized contact dermatitis) may occur in which case the medication should be discontinued and the physician notified immediately.

OVERDOSAGE
There have been no systemic reactions from the use of topical hydroquinone in Solaquin Forte 4% Gel. However, treatment should be limited to relatively small areas of the body at one time since some patients experience a transient skin reddening and a mild burning sensation which does not preclude treatment.

DRUG DOSAGE AND ADMINISTRATION
Solaquin Forte 4% Gel should be applied to the affected area and rubbed in well twice daily or as directed by a physician. There is no recommended dosage for children under 12 years of age except under the advice and supervision of a physician.

HOW SUPPLIED
SOLAQUIN FORTE 4% Gel is available as follows:

Size	NDC Number
½ ounce tube (15 grams)	0187-0523-35
1 ounce tube (30 grams)	0187-0523-31

Solaquin Forte 4% Gel should be stored at room temperature (15–30°C) (59–86°F).

TENSILON® ℞
[*ten 'sil-on*]
(edrophonium chloride)
Injectable Solution
ampuls • vials

DESCRIPTION
Tensilon is a short and rapid-acting cholinergic drug. Chemically, edrophonium chloride is ethyl (*m*-hydroxyphenyl)-dimethylammonium chloride.
10-ml vials: Each ml contains, in a sterile solution, 10 mg edrophonium chloride compounded with 0.45% phenol and 0.2% sodium sulfite as preservatives, buffered with sodium citrate and citric acid, and pH adjusted to approximately 5.4.
1-ml ampuls: Each ml contains, in a sterile solution, 10 mg edrophonium chloride compounded with 0.2% sodium sulfite, buffered with sodium citrate and citric acid, and pH adjusted to approximately 5.4.

ACTIONS
Tensilon is an anticholinesterase drug. Its pharmacological action is due primarily to the inhibition or inactivation of acetylcholinesterase at sites of cholinergic transmission. Its effect is manifest within 30 to 60 seconds after injection and lasts an average of 10 minutes.

INDICATIONS
Tensilon is recommended for the differential diagnosis of myasthenia gravis and as an adjunct in the evaluation of treatment requirements in this disease. It may also be used for evaluating emergency treatment in myasthenic crises. Because of its brief duration of action, it is not recommended for maintenance therapy in myasthenia gravis.
Tensilon is also useful whenever a curare antagonist is needed to reverse the neuromuscular block produced by curare, tubocurarine, gallamine triethiodide or dimethyl-tubocurarine. It is *not* effective against decamethonium bromide and succinylcholine chloride. It may be used adjunctively in the treatment of respiratory depression caused by curare overdosage.

CONTRAINDICATIONS
Known hypersensitivity to anticholinesterase agents; intestinal and urinary obstructions of mechanical type.

WARNINGS
Whenever anticholinesterase drugs are used for testing, a syringe containing 1 mg of atropine sulfate should be immediately available to be given in aliquots intravenously to counteract severe cholinergic reactions which may occur in the hypersensitive individual, whether he is normal or myasthenic. Tensilon should be used with caution in patients with bronchial asthma or cardiac dysrhythmias. The transient bradycardia which sometimes occurs can be relieved by atropine sulfate. Isolated instances of cardiac and respiratory arrest following administration of Tensilon have been reported. It is postulated that these are vagotonic effects.
Tensilon solution contains sodium sulfite, a sulfite that may cause allergic-type reactions, including anaphylactic symptoms and life-threatening or less severe asthmatic episodes in certain susceptible people. The overall prevalence of sulfite sensitivity in the general population is unknown and probably low. Sulfite sensitivity is seen more frequently in asthmatic than in nonasthmatic people.
Usage in Pregnancy: The safety of Tensilon during pregnancy or lactation in humans has not been established. Therefore, use of Tensilon in women who may become pregnant requires weighing the drug's potential benefits against its possible hazards to mother and child.

PRECAUTIONS
Patients may develop "anticholinesterase insensitivity" for brief or prolonged periods. During these periods the patients should be carefully monitored and may need respiratory assistance. Dosages of anticholinesterase drugs should be reduced or withheld until patients again become sensitive to them.

	Myasthenic*	Adequate†	Cholinergic‡
Muscle Strength (ptosis, diplopia, dysphonia, dysphagia, dysarthria, respiration, limb strength)	Increased	No change	Decreased
Fasciculations (orbicularis oculi, facial muscles, limb muscles)	Absent	Present or absent	Present or absent
Side reactions (lacrimation, diaphoresis, salivation, abdominal cramps, nausea, vomiting, diarrhea)	Absent	Minimal	Severe

* Myasthenic Response—occurs in untreated myasthenics and may serve to establish diagnosis; in patients under treatment, indicates that therapy is inadequate.
† Adequate Response—observed in treated patients when therapy is stabilized; a typical response in normal individuals. In addition to this response in nonmyasthenics, the phenomenon of forced lid closure is often observed in psychoneurotics.[1]
‡ Cholinergic Response—seen in myasthenics who have been overtreated with anticholinesterase drugs.

ADVERSE REACTIONS

Careful observation should be made for severe cholinergic reactions in the hyperreactive individual. The myasthenic patient in crisis who is being tested with Tensilon should be observed for bradycardia or cardiac standstill and cholinergic reactions if an overdose is given. The following reactions common to anticholinesterase agents may occur, although not all of these reactions have been reported with the administration of Tensilon, probably because of its short duration of action and limited indications: **Eye:** Increased lacrimation, pupillary constriction, spasm of accommodation, diplopia, conjunctival hyperemia. **CNS:** Convulsions, dysarthria, dysphonia, dysphagia. **Respiratory:** Increased tracheobronchial secretions, laryngospasm, bronchiolar constriction, paralysis of muscles of respiration, central respiratory paralysis. **Cardiac:** Arrhythmias (especially bradycardia), fall in cardiac output leading to hypotension. **G.I.:** Increased salivary, gastric and intestinal secretion, nausea, vomiting, increased peristalsis, diarrhea, abdominal cramps. **Skeletal Muscle:** Weakness, fasciculations. **Miscellaneous:** Increased urinary frequency and incontinence, diaphoresis.

DOSAGE AND ADMINISTRATION

Tensilon Test in the Differential Diagnosis of Myasthenia Gravis:[1–8]

Intravenous Dosage (Adults): A tuberculin syringe containing 1 ml (10 mg) of Tensilon is prepared with an intravenous needle, and 0.2 ml (2 mg) is injected intravenously within 15 to 30 seconds. The needle is left *in situ. Only* if no reaction occurs after 45 seconds is the remaining 0.8 ml (8 mg) injected. If a cholinergic reaction (muscarinic side effects, skeletal muscle fasciculations and increased muscle weakness) occurs after injection of 0.2 ml (2 mg), the test is discontinued and atropine sulfate 0.4 mg to 0.5 mg is administered intravenously. After one-half hour the test may be repeated.

Intramuscular Dosage (Adults): In adults with inaccessible veins, dosage for intramuscular injection is 1 ml (10 mg) of Tensilon. Subjects who demonstrate hyperreactivity to this injection (cholinergic reaction), should be retested after one-half hour with 0.2 ml (2 mg) of Tensilon intramuscularly to rule out false-negative reactions.

Dosage (Children): The intravenous testing dose of Tensilon in children weighing up to 75 lbs is 0.1 ml (1 mg); above this weight, the dose is 0.2 ml (2 mg). If there is no response after 45 seconds, it may be titrated up to 0.5 ml (5 mg) in children under 75 lbs, given in increments of 0.1 ml (1 mg) every 30 to 45 seconds and up to 1 ml (10 mg) in heavier children. In infants, the recommended dose is 0.05 ml (0.5 mg). Because of technical difficulty with intravenous injection in children, the intramuscular route may be used. In children weighing up to 75 lbs, 0.2 ml (2 mg) is injected intramuscularly. In children weighing more than 75 lbs, 0.5 ml (5 mg) is injected intramuscularly. All signs which would appear with the intravenous test appear with the intramuscular test except that there is a delay of two to ten minutes before a reaction is noted.

Tensilon Test for Evaluation of Treatment Requirements in Myasthenia Gravis: The recommended dose is 0.1 ml to 0.2 ml (1 mg to 2 mg) of Tensilon, administered intravenously one hour after oral intake of the drug being used in treatment.[1–5] Response will be myasthenic in the undertreated patient, adequate in the controlled patient, and cholinergic in the overtreated patient. Responses to Tensilon in myasthenic and nonmyasthenic individuals are summarized in the accompanying chart:[2] [See table above.]

Tensilon Test in Crisis: The term *crisis* is applied to the myasthenic whenever severe respiratory distress with objective ventilatory inadequacy occurs and the response to medication is not predictable. This state may be secondary to a sudden increase in severity of myasthenia gravis (myasthenic crisis), or to overtreatment with anticholinesterase drugs (cholinergic crisis).

When a patient is apneic, controlled ventilation must be secured immediately in order to avoid cardiac arrest and irreversible central nervous system damage. No attempt is made to test with Tensilon until respiratory exchange is adequate. *Dosage used at this time is most important:* If the patient is cholinergic, Tensilon will cause increased oropharyngeal secretions and further weakness in the muscles of respiration. If the crisis is myasthenic, the test clearly improves respiration and the patient can be treated with longer-acting intravenous anticholinesterase medication. When the test is performed, there should not be more than 0.2 ml (2 mg) Tensilon in the syringe. An intravenous dose of 0.1 ml (1 mg) is given initially. The patient's heart action is carefully observed. If, after an interval of one minute, this dose does not further impair the patient, the remaining 0.1 ml (1 mg) can be injected. If no clear improvement of respiration occurs after 0.2 ml (2 mg) dose, it is usually wisest to discontinue all anticholinesterase drug therapy and secure controlled ventilation by tracheostomy with assisted respiration.[5]

For Use as a Curare Antagonist: Tensilon should be administered by intravenous injection in 1 ml (10 mg) doses given slowly over a period of 30 to 45 seconds so that the onset of cholinergic reaction can be detected. This dosage may be repeated whenever necessary. The maximal dose for any one patient should be 4 ml (40 mg). Because of its brief effect, Tensilon should not be given prior to the administration of curare, tubocurarine, gallamine triethiodide or dimethyltubocurarine; it should be used at the time when its effect is needed. When given to counteract curare overdosage, the effect of each dose on the respiration should be carefully observed before it is repeated, and assisted ventilation should always be employed.

DRUG INTERACTIONS

Care should be given when administering this drug to patients with symptoms of myasthenic weakness who are also on anticholinesterase drugs. Since symptoms of anticholinesterase overdose (cholinergic crisis) may mimic underdosage (myasthenic weakness), their condition may be worsened by the use of this drug. (See OVERDOSAGE section for treatment.)

OVERDOSAGE

With drugs of this type, muscarine-like symptoms (nausea, vomiting, diarrhea, sweating, increased bronchial and salivary secretions and bradycardia) often appear with overdosage (cholinergic crisis). An important complication that can arise is obstruction of the airway by bronchial secretions. These may be managed with suction (especially if tracheostomy has been performed) and by the use of atropine. Many experts have advocated a wide range of dosages of atropine *(for Tensilon, see atropine dosage below)*, but if there are copious secretions, up to 1.2 mg intravenously may be given initially and repeated every 20 minutes until secretions are controlled. Signs of atropine overdosage such as dry mouth, flush and tachycardia should be avoided as tenacious secretions and bronchial plugs may form. A total dose of atropine of 5 to 10 mg or even more may be required. The following steps should be taken in the management of overdosage of Tensilon:

1. Adequate respiratory exchange should be maintained by assuring an open airway, and the use of assisted respiration augmented by oxygen.
2. Cardiac function should be monitored until complete stabilization has been achieved.
3. Atropine sulfate in doses of 0.4 to 0.5 mg should be administered intravenously. This may be repeated every 3 to 10 minutes. Because of the short duration of action of Tensilon the total dose required will seldom exceed 2 mg.
4. Pralidoxime chloride (a cholinesterase reactivator) may be given intravenously at the rate of 50 to 100 mg per minute; usually the total dose does not exceed 1000 mg. Extreme caution should be exercised in the use of pralidoxime chloride when the cholinergic symptoms are induced by double-bond phosphorous anticholinesterase drugs.[9]
5. If convulsions or shock is present, appropriate measures should be instituted.

HOW SUPPLIED

Multiple Dose Vials, 10 ml, boxes of 10 (NDC 0187-3200-20).
Ampuls, 1 ml, boxes of 10 (NDC 0187-3200-10).

REFERENCES

1. Osserman, K.E. and Kaplan, L.I., *J.A.M.A., 150:* 265, 1952.
2. Osserman, K.E., Kaplan, L.I. and Besson, G., *J. Mt. Sinai Hosp., 20:* 165, 1953.
3. Osserman, K.E. and Kaplan, L.I., *Arch. Neurol. & Psychiat., 70:* 385, 1953.
4. Osserman, K.E. and Teng, P., *J.A.M.A., 160:* 153, 1956.
5. Osserman, K.E. and Genkins, G., *Ann. N.Y. Acad. Sci., 135:* 312, 1966.
6. Tether, J.E., Second International Symposium Proceedings, Myasthenia Gravis, 1961, p. 444.
7. Tether, J.E., in H.F. Conn: *Current Therapy 1960,* Philadelphia, W. B. Saunders Company, p. 551.
8. Tether, J.E., in H.F. Conn: *Current Therapy 1965,* Philadelphia, W. B. Saunders Company, p. 556.
9. Grob, D. and Johns, R.J., *J.A.M.A., 166:* 1855, 1958.

Manufactured for ICN Pharmaceuticals, Inc.
Costa Mesa, CA 92626
by Hoffman-La Roche Inc.
Nutley, NJ 07110
Rev. 3/89

TESTRED® Ⓒ℞

Methyltestosterone Capsules, USP 10 mg

DESCRIPTION

The androgens are steroids that develop and maintain primary and secondary male sex characteristics. Androgens are derivatives of cyclopentanoperhydrophenanthrene. Endogenous androgens are C-19 steroids with a side chain at C-17, and with two angular methyl groups. Testosterone is the primary endogenous androgen. In their active form, all drugs in the class have a 17-beta-hydroxy group. 17-alpha alkylation (methyltestosterone) increases the pharmacologic activity per unit weight compared to testosterone when given orally. Methyltestosterone, a synthetic derivative of testosterone, is an androgenic preparation given by the oral route in a capsule form. Each capsule contains 10 mg of methyltestosterone USP, which has the following formula:

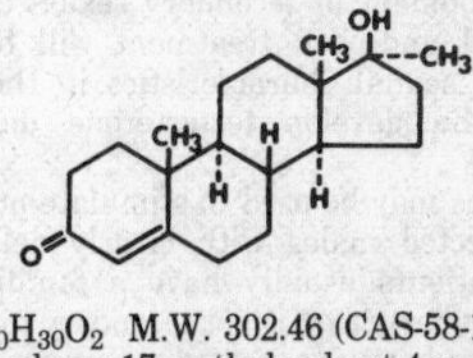

$C_{20}H_{30}O_2$ M.W. 302.46 (CAS-58-18-4)
17β-hydroxy-17-methylandrost-4-en-3-one

Methyltestosterone occurs as white or creamy white crystals or powder, which is soluble in various organic solvents but is practically insoluble in water.

CLINICAL PHARMACOLOGY

Endogenous androgens are responsible for the normal growth and development of the male sex organs and for maintenance of secondary sex characteristics. These effects include the growth and maturation of prostate, seminal vesicles, penis, and scrotum. The development of male hair distribution, such as beard, pubic, chest, and axillary hair; laryngeal enlargement, vocal chord thickening, alterations in body musculature and fat distribution. Drugs in this class also cause retention of nitrogen, sodium, potassium, phosphorus, and decreased urinary excretion of calcium. Androgens have been reported to increase protein anabolism and decrease protein catabolism. Nitrogen balance is improved only when there is sufficient intake of calories and protein.

Androgens are responsible for the growth spurt of adolescence and for the eventual termination of linear growth which is brought about by fusion of the epiphyseal growth centers. In children, exogenous androgens accelerate linear growth rates, but may cause a disproportionate advancement in bone maturation. Use over long periods may result in fusion of the epiphyseal growth centers and termination of growth process. Androgens have been reported to stimulate the production of red blood cells by enhancing the production of erythropoietic stimulating factor.

During exogenous administration of androgens, endogenous testosterone release is inhibited through feedback inhibition of pituitary luteinizing hormone (LH). At large doses of exogenous androgens, spermatogenesis may also be suppressed through feedback inhibition of pituitary follicle stimulating hormone (FSH).

There is a lack of substantial evidence that androgens are effective in fractures, surgery, convalescence and functional uterine bleeding.

Pharmacokinetics

Testosterone given orally is metabolized by the gut and 44 percent is cleared by the liver in the first pass. Oral doses as high as 400 mg per day are needed to achieve clinically effective blood levels for full replacement therapy. The synthetic androgen methyltestosterone is less extensively metabolized by the liver and has a longer half-life. It is more suitable than testosterone for oral administration.

Continued on next page

ICN—Cont.

Testosterone in plasma is 98 percent bound to a specific testosterone-estradiol binding globulin, and about 2 percent is free. Generally, the amount of this sex-hormone binding globulin in the plasma will determine the distribution of testosterone between free and bound forms, and the free testosterone concentration will determine its half-life.

About 90 percent of a dose of testosterone is excreted in the urine as glucuronic and sulfuric acid conjugates of testosterone and its metabolites; about 6 percent of a dose is excreted in the feces, mostly in the unconjugated form. Inactivation of testosterone occurs primarily in the liver. Testosterone is metabolized to various 17-keto steroids through two different pathways. There are considerable variations of the half-life of testosterone as reported in the literature, ranging from 10 to 100 minutes.

In many tissues the activity of testosterone appears to depend on reduction to dihydrotestosterone, which binds to cytosol receptor proteins. The steroid-receptor complex is transported to the nucleus where it initiates transcription events and cellular changes related to androgen action.

INDICATIONS AND USAGE

1. Males

Androgens are indicated for replacement therapy in conditions associated with a deficiency or absence of endogenous testosterone;

  a. Primary hypogonadism (congenital or acquired)—testicular failure due to cryptorchidism, bilateral torsion, orchitis, vanishing testis syndrome or orchidectomy.
  b. Hypogonadotropic hypogonadism (congenital or acquired)—idiopathic gonadotropin or LHRH deficiency, or pituitary-hypothalamic injury from tumors, trauma or radiation.
  If the above conditions occur prior to puberty, androgen therapy will be needed during the adolescent years for development of secondary sexual characteristics. Prolonged androgen treatment will be required to maintain sexual characteristics in these and other males who develop testosterone deficiency after puberty.
  c. Androgens may be used to stimulate puberty in carefully selected males with clearly delayed puberty. These patients usually have a familial pattern of delayed puberty that is not secondary to a pathological disorder; puberty is expected to occur spontaneously at a relatively late date. Brief treatment with conservative doses may occasionally be justified to these patients if they do not respond to psychological support. The potential adverse effect on bone maturation should be discussed with the patient and parents prior to androgen adminstration. An X-ray of the hand and wrist to determine bone age should be obtained every 6 months to assess the effect of treatment on the epiphyseal centers (see WARNINGS).

2. Females

Androgens may be used secondarily in women with advancing inoperable metastatic (skeletal) mammary cancer who are 1 to 5 years postmenopausal. Primary goals of therapy in these women include ablation of the ovaries. Other methods of counteracting estrogen activity are adrenalectomy, hypophysectomy, and/or antiestrogen therapy. This treatment has also been used in premenopausal women with breast cancer who have benefited from oophorectomy and are considered to have a hormone-responsive tumor. Judgment concerning androgen therapy should be made by an oncologist with expertise in this field.

CONTRAINDICATIONS

Androgens are contraindicated in men with carcinomas of the breast or with known or suspected carcinomas of the prostate, and in women who are or may become pregnant. When administered to pregnant women, androgens cause virilization of the external genitalia of the female fetus. This virilization includes clitoromegaly, abnormal vaginal development, and fusion of genital folds to form a scrotal-like structure. The degree of masculinization is related to the amount of drug given and the age of the fetus, and is most likely to occur in the female fetus when the drugs are given in the first trimester. If the patient becomes pregnant while taking these drugs, she should be apprised of the potential hazard to the fetus.

WARNINGS

In patients with breast cancer, androgen therapy may cause hypercalcemia by stimulating osteolysis. In this case, the drug should be discontinued.

Prolonged use of high doses of androgens has been associated with the development of peliosis hepatis and hepatic neoplasms including hepatocellular carcinoma. (See PRECAUTIONS-Carcinogenesis). Peliosis hepatis can be a life-threatening or fatal complication.

Cholestatic hepatitis and jaundice occur with 17-alpha-alkylandrogens at a relatively low dose. If cholestatic hepatitis with jaundice appears or if liver function tests become abnormal, the androgen should be discontinued and the etiology should be determined. Drug-induced jaundice is reversible when the medication is discontinued.

Geriatric patients treated with androgens may be at an increased risk for the development of prostatic hypertrophy and prostatic carcinoma.

Edema with or without congestive heart failure may be a serious complication in patients with preexisting cardiac, renal, or hepatic disease. In addition to discontinuation of the drug, diuretic therapy may be required.

Gynecomastia frequently develops and occasionally persists in patients being treated for hypogonadism. Androgen therapy should be used cautiously in healthy males with delayed puberty. The effect on bone maturation should be monitored by assessing bone age of the wrist and hand every 6 months. In children, androgen treatment may accelerate bone maturation without producing compensatory gain in linear growth. This adverse effect may result in compromised adult stature. The younger the child the greater the risk of compromising final mature height.

This drug has not been shown to be safe and effective for the enhancement of athletic performance. Because of the potential risk of serious adverse health effects, this drug should not be used for such purpose.

PRECAUTIONS

General

Women should be observed for signs of virilization (deepening of the voice, hirsutism, acne, clitoromegaly and menstrual irregularities). Discontinuation of drug therapy at the time of evidence of mild virilism is necessary to prevent irreversible virilization. Such virilization is usual following androgen use at high doses. A decision may be made by the patient and the physician that some virilization will be tolerated during treatment for breast carcinoma.

Information for the Patient

The physician should instruct patients to report any of the following side effects of androgens:

Adult or Adolescent Males:	Too frequent or persistent erections of the penis. Any male adolescent patient receiving androgens for delayed puberty should have bone development checked every six months.
Women:	Hoarseness, acne, changes in menstrual periods, or more hair on the face.
All Patients:	Any nausea, vomiting, changes in skin color or ankle swelling.

Laboratory Tests

1. Women with disseminated breast carcinoma should have frequent determination of urine and serum calcium levels during the course of androgen therapy. (See WARNINGS).
2. Because of the hepatotoxicity associated with the use of 17-alpha-alkylated androgens, liver function tests should be obtained periodically.
3. Periodic (every 6 months) x-ray examinations of bone age should be made during treatment of prepubertal males to determine the rate of bone maturation and the effects of androgen therapy on the epiphyseal centers.
4. Hemoglobin and hematocrit should be checked periodically for polycythemia in patients who are receiving high doses of androgens.

Drug Interactions

1. **Anticoagulants:** C-17 substituted derivatives of testosterone, such as methandrostenolone, have been reported to decrease the anticoagulant requirements of patients receiving oral anticoagulants. Patients receiving oral anticoagulant therapy require close monitoring, especially when androgens are started or stopped.
2. **Oxyphenbutazone:** Concurrent administration of oxyphenbutazone and androgens may result in elevated serum levels of oxyphenbutazone.
3. **Insulin:** In diabetic patients the metabolic effects of androgens may decrease blood glucose and insulin requirements.

Drug/Laboratory Test Interferences

Androgens may decrease levels of thyroxine-binding globulin, resulting in decreased total T4 serum levels and increased resin uptake of T3 and T4. Free thyroid hormone levels remain unchanged, however, and there is no clinical evidence of thyroid dysfunction.

Carcinogenesis

Animal Data

Testosterone has been tested by subcutaneous injection and implantation in mice and rats. The implant induced cervical-uterine tumors in mice, which metastasized in some cases. There is suggestive evidence that injection of testosterone into some strains of female mice increases their susceptibility to hepatoma. Testosterone is also known to increase the number of tumors and decrease the degree of differentiation of chemically induced carcinomas of the liver in rats.

Human Data

There are rare reports of hepatocellular carcinoma in patients receiving long-term therapy with androgens in high doses. Withdrawal of the drugs did not lead to regression of the tumors in all cases.

Geriatric patients treated with androgens may be at an increased risk for the development of prostatic hypertrophy and prostatic carcinoma.

Pregnancy

Teratogenic effects. Pregnancy Category X (See CONTRAINDICATIONS).

Nursing Mothers

It is not known whether androgens are excreted in human milk. Because many drugs are excreted in human milk and because of the potential for serious adverse reactions in nursing infants from androgens, a decision should be made whether to discontinue nursing or to discontinue the drug, taking into account the importance of the drug to the mother.

Pediatric Use

Androgen therapy should be used very cautiously in children and only by specialists who are aware of the adverse effects on bone maturation. Skeletal maturation must be monitored every six months by an x-ray of hand and wrist (See INDICATIONS AND USAGE and WARNINGS).

ADVERSE REACTIONS

Endocrine and Urogenital

Female: The most common side effects of androgen therapy are amenorrhea and other menstrual irregularities, inhibition of gonadotropin secretion, and virilization, including deepening of the voice and clitoral enlargement. The latter usually is not reversible after androgens are discontinued. When administered to a pregnant woman androgens cause virilization of external genitalia of the female fetus.

Male: Gynecomastia, and excessive frequency and duration of penile erections. Oligospermia may occur at high dosages (see CLINICAL PHARMACOLOGY).

Skin and appendages: Hirsutism, male pattern of baldness, and acne.

Fluid and Electrolyte Disturbances: Retention of sodium, chloride, water, potassium, calcium, and inorganic phosphates.

Gastrointestinal: Nausea, cholestatic jaundice, alterations in liver function tests, rarely hepatocellular neoplasms and peliosis hepatis (see WARNINGS).

Hematologic: Suppression of clotting factors II, V, VII, and X, bleeding in patients on concomitant anticoagulant therapy, and polycythemia.

Nervous System: Increased or decreased libido, headache, anxiety, depression, and generalized paresthesia.

Metabolic: Increased serum cholesterol.

Miscellaneous: Rarely anaphylactoid reactions.

DRUG ABUSE AND DEPENDENCE

Testred Capsules are classified as a schedule III Controlled Substance under the Anabolic Steroids Act of 1990.

OVERDOSAGE

There have been no reports of acute overdosage with the androgens.

DOSAGE AND ADMINISTRATION

Methyltestosterone capsules are administered orally. The suggested dosage for androgens varies depending on the age, sex, and diagnosis of the individual patient. Dosage is adjusted according to the patient's response and the appearance of adverse reactions.

Replacement therapy in androgen-deficient males is 10 to 50 mg of methyltestosterone daily. Various dosage regimens have been used to induce pubertal changes in hypogonadal males; some experts have advocated lower dosages initially, gradually increasing the dose as puberty progresses, with or without a decrease to maintenance levels. Other experts emphasize that higher dosages are needed to induce pubertal changes and lower dosages can be used for maintenance after puberty. The chronological and skeletal ages must be taken into consideration, both in determining the initial dose and in adjusting the dose.

Doses used in delayed puberty generally are in the range of that given above, and for a limited duration, for example, 4 to 6 months.

Women with metastatic breast carcinoma must be followed closely because androgen therapy occasionally appears to accelerate the disease. Thus, many experts prefer to use the shorter acting androgen preparations rather than those with prolonged activity for treating breast carcinoma, particularly during the early stages of androgen therapy. The dosage of methyltestosterone for androgen therapy in breast carcinoma in females is from 50–200 mg daily.

HOW SUPPLIED

Methyltestosterone capsules USP 10 mg are red capsules imprinted "ICN 0901" on both sections. They are available in bottles of 100.

CAUTION: Federal (U.S.A.) law prohibits dispensing without prescription.

Revision April 1992

Shown in Product Identification Section, page 412

TRISORALEN® * ℞

[*trī'sore "a-len*]
(Trioxsalen USP, 5 mg)

To facilitate repigmentation in vitiligo, increase tolerance to solar exposure and enhance pigmentation.
CAUTION: THIS IS A POTENT DRUG.
CAUTION: Federal (U.S.A.) law prohibits dispensing without prescription.

DESCRIPTION

Trisoralen Tablets 5 mg.
TRISORALEN (TRIOXSALEN) is the first synthetic psoralen compound made available to the medical profession. It possesses greater activity than Methoxsalen (1) (2) (3) (4), yet the LD 50 of (TRIOXSALEN) is six times that of Methoxsalen.

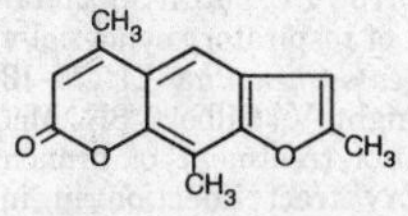

(4, 5', 8-Trimethylpsoralen)

ACTIONS

Pigment formation with TRISORALEN (TRIOXSALEN)
The normal pigmentation of the skin is due to melanin which is produced in the cytoplasm of the melanocytes located in the basal layers of the epidermis at its junction with the dermis. Melanin is formed by the oxidation of tyrosine to DOPA (Dihydroxyphenylalanine) with tyrosinase as catalyst. This enzymatic reaction, however, must be activated by radiant energy in the form of ultraviolet light, preferably between 2900 and 3800 angstroms (black light) (10).
The exact mechanism of the action of psoralens in the process of melanogenesis is not known. One group of investigators feel that the psoralens have a specific effect on the epidermis or, more specifically, on the melanocytes. Another group feels that the primary response to the psoralens is an inflammatory one and that the process of melanogenesis is secondary.

INDICATIONS

TRISORALEN (TRIOXSALEN), taken approximately two hours before measured periods of exposure to ultraviolet facilitates:

1. **Repigmentation of idiopathic vitiligo.** (12) (13) (14) Repigmentation, not equally reversible in every patient, will vary in completeness, time of onset, and duration. The rate of completeness of pigmentation with respect to locations of lesions, occurs more rapidly on fleshy regions, such as the face, abdomen, and buttocks, and less rapidly over bony areas such as the dorsum of the hands and feet. Repigmentation may begin after a few weeks; however, significant results may take as long as six to nine months, and repigmentation, at the optimum level, may, in some cases, require maintenance dosage to retain the new pigment. If follicular repigmentation is not apparent after three months of daily treatment, treatment should be discontinued as a failure.
2. **Increasing tolerance to sunlight.** (14) In blond persons and those with fair complexions who suffer painful reactions when exposed to sunlight, TRISORALEN (TRIOXSALEN) aids in increasing resistance to solar damage. Certain persons who are allergic to sunlight or exhibit sun sensitivity may be benefited by the protective action of TRISORALEN (TRIOXSALEN) (5). In albinism, TRISORALEN (TRIOXSALEN) will increase the tolerance of the skin to sunlight, although no pigment is formed (6) (7) (8). This protective action seems to be related to the thickening of the horny layer and retention of melanin which produced a thickened, melanized stratum corneum and formation of a stratum lucidum (9) (10).
3. **Enhancing pigmentation** (3) (4). The use of TRISORALEN (TRIOXSALEN) accelerates pigmentation only when the administration of the drug is followed by exposure of the skin to sunlight or ultraviolet irradiation. The increase in pigmentation is not immediate but occurs gradually within a few days of repeated exposure and may become equivalent in a degree to that achieved by a full summer of sun exposure. Since sufficient pigment will have been formed within two weeks of continuous therapy, the use of TRISORALEN (TRIOXSALEN) should not be continued beyond this period. Pigmentation can be maintained by periodic exposure to sunlight.

CONTRAINDICATIONS

In those diseases associated with photosensitivity, such as porphyria, acute lupus erythematosus, or leukoderma of infectious origin. To date, the safety of this drug in young persons (12 and under), has not been established and is, therefore contraindicated. No preparation with any photosensitizing capacity, internal or external should be used concomitantly with TRISORALEN (TRIOXSALEN) therapy.

*U.S. Patent 3,201,421

WARNINGS

TRISORALEN IS A POTENT DRUG.
Read entire brochure before prescribing or dispensing this medication. The dosage of this medication should not be increased. The dosage of TRISORALEN (TRIOXSALEN) and exposure time should not be increased. Overdosage and/or overexposure may result in serious burning and blistering. When used to increase tolerance to sunlight or accelerate tanning, TRISORALEN (TRIOXSALEN) total dosage should not exceed 28 tablets, taken in daily single doses of two tablets on a continuous or interrupted regimen. To prevent harmful effects, the physician should carefully instruct the patient to adhere to the prescribed dosage schedule and procedure.

PRECAUTIONS

ACCIDENTAL OVERDOSAGE:
If an overdose of TRISORALEN (TRIOXSALEN) or ultraviolet light has been taken, emesis should be encouraged. The individual should be kept in a darkened room for eight hours or until cutaneous reactions subside. The treatment for severe reactions resulting from overdosage or over-exposure should follow accepted procedures for treatment of severe burns. There have not been any clinical reports or tests to verify that more severe reactions may result from the concomitant ingestion of furocoumarin-containing food while on TRISORALEN (TRIOXSALEN) therapy; but the physician should warn the patient that taking limes, figs, parsley, parsnips, mustard, carrots and celery, might be dangerous.

ADVERSE REACTIONS AND SIDE EFFECTS

Severe burns can result from excessive sunlight or sun lamp ultraviolet exposure. Occasionally, there may occur gastric discomfort; to minimize this gastric effect, the tablets may be taken with milk or after a meal. Some patients who are unable to tolerate 10 mg. will tolerate 5 mg. This dosage produces the same therapeutic effect but more slowly.

DOSAGE

(Adults and children over 12 years of age)
VITILIGO: Two tablets daily, taken two to four hours before measured periods of ultraviolet exposure or fluorescent black light (10). (See suggested sun exposure guide.)
To increase tolerance to sunlight and/or enhance pigmentation: Two tablets daily, taken two hours before measured periods of exposure to sun or ultraviolet irradiation. Not to be continued for longer than 14 days. The dosage should **NOT** be increased, as severe burning may occur. (See suggested sun exposure guide.)

SUGGESTED SUN EXPOSURE GUIDE

The exposure time to sunlight should be limited according to the following plan:

	Basic Skin Color	
	Light	**Medium**
Initial Exposure	15 min.	20 min.
Second Exposure	20 min.	25 min.
Third Exposure	25 min.	30 min.
Fourth Exposure	30 min.	35 min.

Subsequent Exposure: Gradually increase exposure based on erythema and tenderness.

Sunglasses should be worn during exposure and the lips protected with a light-screening lipstick (10).

SUN-LAMP EXPOSURE: Should be initiated according to directions of the sun-lamp manufacturer.

HOW SUPPLIED

TRISORALEN Tablets 5 mg.

UNIT COUNT	NDC NO.
28	0187-0303-28
100	0187-0303-01

Shown in Product Identification Section, page 412

VIRAZOLE® ℞

[*vira'zahl'*]
(Ribavirin)
lyophilized for aerosol administration

WARNING:
RIBAVIRIN AEROSOL SHOULD NOT BE USED FOR INFANTS REQUIRING ASSISTED VENTILATION BECAUSE PRECIPITATION OF THE DRUG IN THE RESPIRATORY EQUIPMENT MAY INTERFERE WITH SAFE AND EFFECTIVE VENTILATION OF THE PATIENT. Conditions for safe use with a ventilator are still in development.
Deterioration of respiratory function has been associated with ribavirin use in infants, and in adults with chronic obstructive lung disease or asthma. Respiratory function should be carefully monitored during treatment. If initiation of ribavirin aerosol treatment appears to produce sudden deterioration of respiratory function, treatment should be stopped and re-instituted only with extreme caution and continuous monitoring.
Although ribavirin is not indicated in adults, the physician should be aware that it is teratogenic in animals (see CONTRAINDICATIONS).

DESCRIPTION

Virazole® (ribavirin) Aerosol, an antiviral drug, is a sterile, lyophilized powder to be reconstituted for aerosol administration. Each 100 ml glass vial contains 6 grams of ribavirin, and when reconstituted to the recommended volume of 300 ml with sterile water for injection or sterile water for inhalation (no preservatives added), will contain 20 mg/ml ribavirin, pH approximately 5.5. Aerosolization is to be carried out in a SPAG-2 nebulizer only.
Ribavirin is 1-beta-D-ribofuranosyl-1,2,4-triazole-3-carboxamide, with the following structural formula:

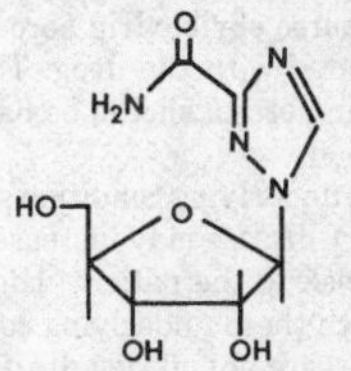

Ribavirin, a synthetic nucleoside, is a stable, white, crystalline compound with a maximum solubility in water of 142 mg/ml at 25°C and with only a slight solubility in ethanol. The empirical formula is $C_8H_{12}N_4O_5$ and the molecular weight is 244.2 Daltons.

CLINICAL PHARMACOLOGY

Antiviral effects: Ribavirin has antiviral inhibitory activity *in vitro* against respiratory syncytial virus,[1] influenza virus, and herpes simplex virus. Ribavirin is also active against respiratory syncytial virus (RSV) in experimentally infected cotton rats.[2]
In cell cultures, the inhibitory activity of ribavirin for RSV is selective. The mechanism of action is unknown. Reversal of the *in vitro* antiviral activity by guanosine or xanthosine suggests ribavirin may act as an analogue of these cellular metabolites.
Immunologic effects: Neutralizing antibody responses to RSV were decreased in ribavirin treated compared to placebo treated infants.[3] The clinical significance of this observation is unknown. In rats, ribavirin resulted in lymphoid atrophy of thymus, spleen, and lymph nodes. Humoral immunity was reduced in guinea pigs and ferrets. Cellular immunity was also mildly depressed in animal studies.
Microbiology: Several clinical isolates of RSV were evaluated for ribavirin susceptibility by plaque reduction in tissue culture. Plaques were reduced 85–98% by 16μg/ml; however, plaque reduction varies with the test system. The clinical significance of these data is unknown.
Pharmacokinetics: Assay for ribavirin in human materials is by a radioimmunoassay which detects ribavirin and at least one metabolite.
Ribavirin administered by aerosol is absorbed systemically. Four pediatric patients inhaling ribavirin aerosol administered by face mask for 2.5 hours each day for 3 days had plasma concentrations ranging from 0.44 to 1.55 μM, with a mean concentration of 0.76 μM. The plasma half-life was reported to be 9.5 hours. Three pediatric patients inhaling ribavirin aerosol administered by face mask or mist tent for 20 hours each day for 5 days had plasma concentrations ranging from 1.5 to 14.3 μM, with a mean concentration of 6.8 μM.
It is likely that the concentration of ribavirin in respiratory tract secretions is much higher than plasma concentrations in view of the route of administration.
The bioavailability of ribavirin aerosol is unknown and may depend on the mode of aerosol delivery. After aerosol treatment, peak plasma concentrations are less than the concentration that reduced RSV plaque formation in tissue culture by 85 to 98%. After aerosol treatment, respiratory tract secretions are likely to contain ribavirin in concentrations many fold higher than those required to reduce plaque formation. However, RSV is an intracellular virus and serum concentrations may better reflect intracellular concentrations in the respiratory tract than respiratory secretion concentrations.
In man, rats, and rhesus monkeys, accumulation of ribavirin and/or metabolites in the red blood cells has been noted, plateauing in red cells in man in about 4 days and gradually declining with an apparent half-life of 40 days. The extent of

Continued on next page

ICN—Cont.

accumulation of ribavirin following inhalation therapy is not well defined.

INDICATIONS AND USAGE

Ribavirin aerosol is indicated in the treatment of hospitalized infants and young children with severe lower respiratory tract infections due to respiratory syncytial virus (RSV). In two placebo controlled trials in infants hospitalized with RSV lower respiratory tract infection, ribavirin aerosol treatment had a therapeutic effect, as judged by the reduction by treatment day 3 of severity of clinical manifestations of disease.[3,4] Virus titers in respiratory secretions were also significantly reduced with ribavirin in one of these studies.[4] Only severe RSV lower respiratory tract infection is to be treated with ribavirin aerosol. The vast majority of infants and children with RSV infection have no lower respiratory tract disease or have disease that is mild, self-limited, and does not require hospitalization or antiviral treatment. Many children with mild lower respiratory tract involvement will require shorter hospitalization than would be required for a full course of ribavirin aerosol (3 to 7 days) and should not be treated with the drug. Thus the decision to treat with ribavirin aerosol should be based on the severity of the RSV infection.

The presence of an underlying condition such as prematurity or cardiopulmonary disease may increase the severity of the infection and its risk to the patient. High risk infants and young children with these underlying conditions may benefit from ribavirin treatment, although efficacy has been evaluated in only a small number of such patients.

Ribavirin aerosol treatment must be accompanied by and does not replace standard supportive respiratory and fluid management for infants and children with severe respiratory tract infection.

Diagnosis: RSV infection should be documented by a rapid diagnostic method such as demonstration of viral antigen in respiratory tract secretions by immunofluorescence[3,4] or ELISA[5] before or during the first 24 hours of treatment. Ribavirin aerosol is indicated only for lower respiratory tract infection due to RSV. Treatment may be initiated while awaiting rapid diagnostic test results. However, treatment should not be continued without documentation of RSV infection.

CONTRAINDICATIONS

Ribavirin is contraindicated in women or girls who are or may become pregnant during exposure to the drug. Ribavirin may cause fetal harm and respiratory syncytial virus infection is self-limited in this population. Ribavirin is not completely cleared from human blood even four weeks after administration. Although there are no pertinent human data, ribavirin has been found to be teratogenic and/or embryolethal in nearly all species in which it has been tested. Teratogenicity was evident after a single oral dose of 2.5 mg/kg in the hamster and after daily oral doses of 10 mg/kg in the rat. Malformations of skull, palate, eye, jaw, skeleton, and gastrointestinal tract were noted in animal studies. Survival of fetuses and offspring was reduced. The drug causes embryolethality in the rabbit at daily oral dose levels as low as 1 mg/kg.

WARNINGS

Ribavirin administered by aerosol produced cardiac lesions in mice and rats after 30 and 36 mg/kg, respectively, for 4 weeks, and after oral administration in monkeys at 120 and rats at 154 to 200 mg/kg for 1 to 6 months. Ribavirin aerosol administered to developing ferrets at 60 mg/kg for 10 or 30 days resulted in inflammatory and possibly emphysematous changes in the lungs. Proliferative changes were seen at 131 mg/kg for 30 days. The significance of these findings to human administration is unknown.

Ribavirin lyophilized in 6 gram vials is intended for use as an aerosol only.

PRECAUTIONS

General: Patients with lower respiratory tract infection due to respiratory syncytial virus require optimum monitoring and attention to respiratory and fluid status.

Drug Interactions: Interactions of ribavirin with other drugs such as digoxin, bronchodilators, other antiviral agents, antibiotics, or anti-metabolites has not been evaluated. Interference by ribavirin with laboratory tests has not been evaluated.

Carcinogenesis, mutagenesis, impairment of fertility: Ribavirin induces cell transformation in an *in vitro* mammalian system (Balb/C 3T3 cell line). However, *in vivo* carcinogenicity studies are incomplete. Results thus far, though inconclusive, suggest that chronic feeding of ribavirin to rats at dose levels in the range of 16–60 mg/kg body weight can induce benign mammary, pancreatic, pituitary and adrenal tumors. Ribavirin is mutagenic to mammalian (L5178Y) cells in culture. Results of microbial mutagenicity assays and a dominant lethal assay (mouse) were negative.

Ribavirin causes testicular lesions (tubular atrophy) in adult rats at oral dose levels as low as 16 mg/kg/day (lower doses not tested), but fertility of ribavirin-treated animals (male or female) has not been adequately investigated.

Pregnancy: Teratogenic Effects: Pregnancy Category X. See "Contraindications" section.

Nursing Mothers: Use of ribavirin aerosol in nursing mothers is not indicated because RSV infection is self-limited in this population. Ribavirin is toxic to lactating animals and their offspring. It is not known whether the drug is excreted in human milk.

ADVERSE REACTIONS

Approximately 200 patients have been treated with ribavirin aerosol in controlled or uncontrolled clinical studies. Pulmonary function significantly deteriorated during ribavirin aerosol treatment in six of six adults with chronic obstructive lung disease and in four of six asthmatic adults. Dyspnea and chest soreness were also reported in the latter group. Minor abnormalities in pulmonary function were also seen in healthy adult volunteers.

Several serious adverse events occurred in severely ill infants with life-threatening underlying diseases, many of whom required assisted ventilation. The role of ribavirin aerosol in these events is indeterminate. The following events were associated with ribavirin use:

<u>Pulmonary:</u> Worsening of respiratory status, bacterial pneumonia, pneumothorax, apnea, and ventilator dependence.

<u>Cardiovascular:</u> Cardiac arrest, hypotension, and digitalis toxicity.

There were 7 deaths during or shortly after treatment with ribavirin aerosol. No death was attributed to ribavirin aerosol by the investigators.

Some subjects requiring assisted ventilation have experienced serious difficulties, which may jeopardize adequate ventilation and gas exchange. Precipitation of drug within the ventilatory apparatus, including the endotracheal tube, has resulted in increased positive end expiratory pressure and increased positive inspiratory pressure. Accumulation of fluid in tubing ("rain out") has also been noted.

Although anemia has not been reported with use of the aerosol, it occurs frequently with oral and intravenous ribavirin, and most infants treated with the aerosol have not been evaluated 1 to 2 weeks post-treatment when anemia is likely to occur. Reticulocytosis has been reported with aerosol use. Rash and conjunctivitis have been associated with the use of ribavirin aerosol.

Overdosage: No overdosage with ribavirin by aerosol administration has been reported in the human. The LD₅₀ in mice is 2 gm orally. Hypoactivity and gastrointestinal symptoms occurred. In man, ribavirin is sequestered in red blood cells for weeks after dosing.

DOSAGE AND ADMINISTRATION

Before use, read thoroughly the Viratek Small Particle Aerosol Generator (SPAG) Model SPAG-2 Operator's Manual for small particle aerosol generator operating instructions. Treatment was effective when instituted within the first 3 days of respiratory syncytial virus lower respiratory tract infection.[3] Treatment early in the course of severe lower respiratory tract infection may be necessary to achieve efficacy.

Treatment is carried out for 12–18 hours per day for at least 3 and no more than 7 days, and is part of a total treatment program. The aerosol is delivered to an infant oxygen hood from the SPAG-2 aerosol generator. Administration by face mask or oxygen tent may be necessary if a hood cannot be employed (see SPAG-2 manual). However, the volume of distribution and condensation area are larger in a tent and efficacy of this method of administering the drug has been evaluated in only a small number of patients. Ribavirin aerosol is not to be administered with any other aerosol generating device or together with other aerosolized medications. Ribavirin aerosol should not be used for patients requiring simultaneous assisted ventilation (see Boxed Warnings).

Virazole is supplied as 6 grams of lyophilized drug per 100 ml vial for aerosol administration only. By sterile technique, solubilize drug with sterile USP water for injection or inhalation in the 100 ml vial. Transfer to the clean, sterilized 500 ml wide-mouth Erlenmeyer flask (SPAG-2 Reservoir) and further dilute to a final volume of 300 ml with sterile USP water for injection or inhalation. The final concentration should be 20 mg/ml. **Important:** This water should not have had any antimicrobial agent or other substance added. The solution should be inspected visually for particulate matter and discoloration prior to administration. Solutions that have been placed in the SPAG-2 unit should be discarded at least every 24 hours and when the liquid level is low before adding newly reconstituted solutions.

Using the recommended drug concentration of 20 mg/ml ribavirin as the starting solution in the drug reservoir of the SPAG unit, the average aerosol concentration for a 12 hour period would be 190 micrograms/liter (0.19 mg/l) of air.

HOW SUPPLIED

Virazole (ribavirin) Aerosol is supplied in 100 ml glass vials with 6 grams of sterile, lyophilized drug which is to be reconstituted with 300 ml sterile water for injection or sterile water for inhalation (no preservatives added) and administered only by a small particle aerosol generator (SPAG-2). Vials containing the lyophilized drug powder should be stored in a dry place at 15–25°C (59–78°F). Reconstituted solutions may be stored, under sterile conditions, at room temperature (20–30°C, 68–86°F) for 24 hours. Solutions which have been placed in the SPAG-2 unit should be discarded at least every 24 hours.

REFERENCES

1. Hruska JF, Bernstein JM, Douglas Jr., RG, and Hall CB. Effects of ribavirin on respiratory syncytial virus in vitro. *Antimicrob Agents Chemother* 17:770–775, 1, 1980.
2. Hruska JF, Morrow PE, Suffin SC, and Douglas Jr., RG. *In vivo* inhibition of respiratory syncytial virus by ribavirin. *Antimicrob Agents Chemother* 21:125–130, 1982.
3. Taber LH, Knight V, Gilbert BE, McClung HW et al. Ribavirin aerosol treatment of bronchiolitis associated with respiratory tract infection in infants. *Pediatrics* 72:613–618, 1983.
4. Hall CB, McBride JT, Walsh EE, Bell DM et al. Aerosolized ribavirin treatment of infants with respiratory syncytial viral infection. *N Engl J Med* 308:1443–7, 1983.
5. Hendry RM, McIntosh K, Fahnestock ML, and Pierik LT. Enzyme-linked immunosorbent assay for detection of respiratory syncytial virus infection. *J Clin Microbiol* 16:329–33, 1982.

Jan. 1991

Immunex Corporation
51 UNIVERSITY STREET
SEATTLE, WA 98101

HYDREA®   ℞
[hī″drē'ah]
(hydroxyurea capsules, USP)

DESCRIPTION

Hydrea (hydroxyurea capsules, USP) is an antineoplastic agent, available for oral use as capsules providing 500 mg hydroxyurea. Inactive ingredients: citric acid, colorants (D&C Yellow No. 10; FD&C Blue No. 1 and Red No. 3), gelatin, lactose, magnesium stearate, sodium phosphate, and titanium dioxide.

Hydroxyurea occurs as an essentially tasteless, white crystalline powder. Its structural formula is:

$$H_2N-\overset{\overset{\displaystyle O}{\displaystyle \|}}{C}-NH-OH$$

ACTIONS

Mechanism of Action

The precise mechanism by which hydroxyurea produces its cytotoxic effects cannot, at present, be described. However, the reports of various studies in tissue culture in rats and man lend support to the hypothesis that hydroxyurea causes an immediate inhibition of DNA synthesis without interfering with the synthesis of ribonucleic acid or of protein. This hypothesis explains why, under certain conditions, hydroxyurea may induce teratogenic effects.

Three mechanisms of action have been postulated for the increased effectiveness of concomitant use of hydroxyurea therapy with irradiation on squamous cell (epidermoid) carcinomas of the head and neck. *In vitro* studies utilizing Chinese hamster cells suggest that hydroxyurea (1) is lethal to normally radioresistant S-stage cells, and (2) holds other cells of the cell cycle in the G1 or pre-DNA synthesis stage where they are most susceptible to the effects of irradiation. The third mechanism of action has been theorized on the basis of *in vitro* studies of HeLa cells: it appears that hydroxyurea, by inhibition of DNA synthesis, hinders the normal repair process of cells damaged but not killed by irradiation, thereby decreasing their survival rate; RNA and protein syntheses have shown no alteration.

Absorption, Metabolism, Fate and Excretion

After oral administration in man, hydroxyurea is readily absorbed from the gastrointestinal tract. The drug reaches peak serum concentrations within 2 hours; by 24 hours the concentration in the serum is essentially zero. Approximately 80% of an oral or intravenous dose of 7 to 30 mg/kg may be recovered in the urine within 12 hours.

Animal Pharmacology and Toxicology

The oral LD₅₀ of hydroxyurea is 7330 mg/kg in mice and 5780 mg/kg in rats, given as a single dose.

In subacute and chronic toxicity studies in the rat, the most consistent pathological findings were an apparent dose-related mild to moderate bone marrow hypoplasia as well as pulmonary congestion and mottling of the lungs. At the

highest dosage levels (1260 mg/kg/day for 37 days then 2520 mg/kg/day for 40 days), testicular atrophy with absence of spermatogenesis occurred; in several animals, hepatic cell damage with fatty metamorphosis was noted. In the dog, mild to marked bone marrow depression was a consistent finding except at the lower dosage levels. Additionally, at the higher dose levels (140 to 420 mg or 140 to 1260 mg/kg/week given 3 or 7 days weekly for 12 weeks), growth retardation, slightly increased blood glucose values, and hemosiderosis of the liver or spleen were found; reversible spermatogenic arrest was noted. In the monkey, bone marrow depression, lymphoid atrophy of the spleen, and degenerative changes in the epithelium of the small and large intestines were found. At the higher, often lethal, doses (400 to 800 mg/kg/day for 7 to 15 days), hemorrhage and congestion were found in the lungs, brain and urinary tract. Cardiovascular effects (changes in heart rate, blood pressure, orthostatic hypotension, EKG changes) and hematological changes (slight hemolysis, slight methemoglobinemia) were observed in some species of laboratory animals at doses exceeding clinical levels.

INDICATIONS AND USAGE

Significant tumor response to HYDREA (hydroxyurea capsules, USP) has been demonstrated in melanoma, resistant chronic myelocytic leukemia, and recurrent, metastatic, or inoperable carcinoma of the ovary.

Hydrea used concomitantly with irradiation therapy is intended for use in the local control of primary squamous cell (epidermoid) carcinomas of the head and neck, excluding the lip.

CONTRAINDICATIONS

Hydroxyurea is contraindicated in patients with marked bone marrow depression, ie, leukopenia (< 2500 WBC) or thrombocytopenia (< 100,000), or severe anemia.

WARNINGS

Treatment with hydroxyurea should not be initiated if bone marrow function is markedly depressed (—see CONTRAINDICATIONS). Bone marrow suppression may occur, and leukopenia is generally its first and most common manifestation. Thrombocytopenia and anemia occur less often, and are seldom seen without a preceding leukopenia. However, the recovery from myelosuppression is rapid when therapy is interrupted. It should be borne in mind that bone marrow depression is more likely in patients who have previously received radiotherapy or cytotoxic cancer chemotherapeutic agents; hydroxyurea should be used cautiously in such patients.

Patients who have received irradiation therapy in the past may have an exacerbation of postirradiation erythema.

Severe anemia must be corrected with whole blood replacement before initiating therapy with hydroxyurea.

Erythrocytic abnormalities: megaloblastic erythropoiesis, which is self-limiting, is often seen early in the course of hydroxyurea therapy. The morphologic change resembles pernicious anemia, but is not related to vitamin B_{12} or folic acid deficiency. Hydroxyurea may also delay plasma iron clearance and reduce the rate of iron utilization by erythrocytes, but it does not appear to alter the red blood cell survival time.

Hydroxyurea should be used with caution in patients with marked renal dysfunction.

Elderly patients may be more sensitive to the effects of hydroxyurea, and may require a lower dose regimen.

Usage In Pregnancy

Drugs which affect DNA synthesis, such as hydroxyurea, may be potential mutagenic agents. The physician should carefully consider this possibility before administering this drug to male or female patients who may contemplate conception.

Hydrea is a known teratogenic agent in animals. Therefore, hydroxyurea should not be used in women who are or may become pregnant unless in the judgment of the physician the potential benefits outweigh the possible hazards.

PRECAUTIONS

Therapy with hydroxyurea requires close supervision. The complete status of the blood, including bone marrow examination, if indicated, as well as kidney function and liver function should be determined prior to, and repeatedly during, treatment. The determination of the hemoglobin level, total leukocyte counts, and platelet counts should be performed at least once a week throughout the course of hydroxyurea therapy. If the white blood cell count decreases to less than $2500/mm^3$, or the platelet count to less than $100,000/mm^3$, therapy should be interrupted until the values rise significantly toward normal levels. Anemia, if it occurs, should be managed with whole blood replacement, without interrupting hydroxyurea therapy.

ADVERSE REACTIONS

Adverse reactions have been primarily bone marrow depression (leukopenia, anemia, and occasionally thrombocytopenia), and less frequently gastrointestinal symptoms (stomatitis, anorexia, nausea, vomiting, diarrhea, and constipation), and dermatological reactions such as maculopapular rash

and facial erythema. Dysuria and alopecia occur very rarely. Large doses may produce moderate drowsiness. Neurological disturbances have occurred extremely rarely and were limited to headache, dizziness, disorientation, hallucinations, and convulsions. Hydroxyurea occasionally may cause temporary impairment of renal tubular function accompanied by elevations in serum uric acid, BUN, and creatinine levels. Abnormal BSP retention has been reported. Fever, chills, malaise, and elevation of hepatic enzymes have also been reported.

Adverse reactions observed with combined hydroxyurea and irradiation therapy are similar to those reported with the use of hydroxyurea alone. These effects primarily include bone marrow depression (anemia and leukopenia), and gastric irritation. Almost all patients receiving an adequate course of combined hydroxyurea and irradiation therapy will demonstrate concurrent leukopenia. Platelet depression (less than $100,000$ cells/mm^3) has occurred rarely and only in the presence of marked leukopenia. Gastric distress has also been reported with irradiation alone and in combination with hydroxyurea therapy.

It should be borne in mind that therapeutic doses of irradiation alone produce the same adverse reactions as hydroxyurea; combined therapy may cause an increase in the incidence and severity of these side effects.

Although inflammation of the mucous membranes at the irradiated site (mucositis) is attributed to irradiation alone, some investigators believe that the more severe cases are due to combination therapy.

DOSAGE AND ADMINISTRATION

Procedures for proper handling and disposal of antineoplastic drugs should be considered. Several guidelines on this subject have been published.[1–6] There is no general agreement that all of the procedures recommended in the guidelines are necessary or appropriate.

Because of the rarity of melanoma, resistant chronic myelocytic leukemia, carcinoma of the ovary, and carcinomas of the head and neck in children, dosage regimens have not been established.

All dosage should be based on the patient's actual or ideal weight, whichever is less.

NOTE: If the patient prefers, or is unable to swallow capsules, the contents of the capsules may be emptied into a glass of water and taken immediately. Some inert material used as a vehicle in the capsule may not dissolve, and may float on the surface.

SOLID TUMORS

Intermittent Therapy

80 mg/kg administered orally as a *single* dose every *third* day

Continuous Therapy

20 to 30 mg/kg administered orally as a *single* dose *daily*. The intermittent dosage schedule offers the advantage of reduced toxicity since patients on this dosage regimen have rarely required complete discontinuance of therapy because of toxicity.

Concomitant Therapy with Irradiation

(Carcinoma of the head and neck)

80 mg/kg administered orally as a *single* dose every *third* day

Administration of Hydrea (hydroxyurea capsules, USP) should be begun at least 7 days before initiation of irradiation and continued during radiotherapy as well as indefinitely afterwards provided that the patient may be kept under adequate observation and evidences no unusual or severe reactions.

Irradiation should be given at the maximum dose considered appropriate for the particular therapeutic situation; adjustment of irradiation dosage is not usually necessary when Hydrea is used concomitantly.

RESISTANT CHRONIC MYELOCYTIC LEUKEMIA

Until the intermittent therapy regimen has been evaluated, CONTINUOUS therapy (20 to 30 mg/kg administered orally as a *single* dose *daily*) is recommended.

An adequate trial period for determining the antineoplastic effectiveness of Hydrea (hydroxyurea capsules, USP) is 6 weeks of therapy. When there is regression in tumor size or arrest in tumor growth, therapy should be continued indefinitely. Therapy should be interrupted if the white blood cell count drops below $2500/mm^3$, or the platelet count below $100,000/mm^3$. In these cases, the counts should be rechecked after 3 days, and therapy resumed when the counts rise significantly toward normal values. Since the hematopoietic rebound is prompt, it is usually necessary to omit only a few doses. If prompt rebound has not occurred during combined hydroxyurea and irradiation therapy, irradiation may also be interrupted. However, the need for postponement of irradiation has been rare; radiotherapy has usually been continued using the recommended dosage and technique. Anemia, if it occurs, should be corrected with whole blood replacement, without interrupting hydroxyurea therapy. Because hematopoiesis may be compromised by extensive irradiation or by other antineoplastic agents, it is recommended that Hydrea be administered cautiously to patients who have

recently received extensive radiation therapy or chemotherapy with other cytotoxic drugs.

Pain or discomfort from inflammation of the mucous membranes at the irradiated site (mucositis) is usually controlled by measures such as topical anesthetics and orally administered analgesics. If the reaction is severe, hydroxyurea therapy may be temporarily interrupted; if it is extremely severe, irradiation dosage may, in addition, be temporarily postponed. However, it has rarely been necessary to terminate these therapies.

Severe gastric distress, such as nausea, vomiting, and anorexia, resulting from combined therapy may usually be controlled by temporary interruption of Hydrea (Hydroxyurea Capsules USP) administration; rarely has the additional interruption of irradiation been necessary.

HOW SUPPLIED

500 mg capsules in bottles of 100 (NDC 0003-0830-50). Capsule identification number: 830.

Storage

Store at room temperature; avoid excessive heat. Keep bottle tightly closed. Dispense in tight containers.

REFERENCES

1. Recommendations for the Safe Handling of Parenteral Antineoplastic Drugs. NIH Publication No. 83-2621. Available from Superintendent of Documents, US Government Printing Office, Washington, DC 20402
2. AMA Council Report: Guidelines for Handling Parenteral Antineoplastics. *JAMA.* 1985; 253:1590–1592.
3. National Study Commission on Cytotoxic Exposure: Recommendations for Handling Cytotoxic Agents. Available from Louis P. Jeffrey, ScD, Director of Pharmacy Services, Rhode Island Hospital, 593 Eddy Street, Providence, RI 02902.
4. Clinical Oncological Society of Australia: Guidelines and Recommendations for Safe Handling of Antineoplastic Agents. *Med J Australia.* 1983; 1:426–428.
5. Jones RB, et al: Safe handling of chemotherapeutic agents: A report from the Mount Sinai Medical Center. *CA—A Cancer J for Clinicians.* 1983; 133:258–263.
6. American Society of Hospital Pharmacists Technical Assistance Bulletin on Handling Cytotoxic Drugs in Hospitals. *Am J Hosp Pharm.* 1985; 42:131–137.

LEUKINE™   ℞
Sargramostim

DESCRIPTION

LEUKINE™ (Sargramostim) is a recombinant human granulocyte-macrophage colony stimulating factor (rhu GM-CSF) produced by recombinant DNA technology in a yeast (*S. cerevisiae*) expression system. GM-CSF is a hematopoietic growth factor which stimulates proliferation and differentiation of hematopoietic progenitor cells. LEUKINE is a glycoprotein of 127 amino acids characterized by 3 primary molecular species having molecular masses of 19,500, 16,800, and 15,500 daltons. The amino acid sequence of LEUKINE differs from the natural human GM-CSF by a substitution of leucine at position 23, and the carbohydrate moiety may be different from the native protein. Sargramostim has been selected as the proper name for yeast-derived rhu GM-CSF. LEUKINE is formulated as a sterile, white, preservative-free, lyophilized powder and is intended for IV infusion following reconstitution with 1 ml Sterile Water for Injection, USP. Each single-use vial of LEUKINE contains either 250 mcg or 500 mcg Sargramostim; 40 mg Mannitol, USP; 10 mg Sucrose, NF; and 1.2 mg Tromethamine, USP. The pH of the reconstituted, isotonic solution is 7.4 ± 0.3. The specific activity of LEUKINE is approximately 5×10^7 colony forming units per mg in a normal human bone marrow colony formation assay.

CLINICAL PHARMACOLOGY

General

Granulocyte-macrophage colony stimulating factor belongs to a group of growth factors termed colony stimulating factors which support survival, clonal expansion, and differentiation of hematopoietic progenitor cells. GM-CSF induces partially committed progenitor cells to divide and differentiate in the granulocyte-macrophage pathways.

GM-CSF is also capable of activating mature granulocytes and macrophages. GM-CSF is a multilineage factor and, in addition to dose-dependent effects on the myelomonocytic lineage, can promote the proliferation of megakaryocytic and erythroid progenitors.[1] However, other factors are required to induce complete maturation in these two lineages. The various cellular responses (i.e., division, maturation, activation) are induced through GM-CSF binding to specific receptors expressed on the cell surface of target cells.[2]

LEUKINE™ is a trademark of Immunex Corporation, Seattle, WA 98101

Continued on next page

Immunex—Cont.

***In vitro* Studies of LEUKINE in Human Cells**

The biological activity of GM-CSF is species-specific. Consequently, *in vitro* studies have been performed on human cells to characterize the pharmacological activity of LEUKINE. *In vitro* exposure of human bone marrow cells to LEUKINE at concentrations ranging from 1–100 ng/ml results in the proliferation of hematopoietic progenitors and in the formation of pure granulocyte, pure macrophage, and mixed granulocyte-macrophage colonies.[3] Chemotactic, anti-fungal, and antiparasitic[4] activities of granulocytes and monocytes are increased by exposure to LEUKINE in vitro. LEUKINE increases the cytotoxicity of monocytes toward certain neoplastic cell lines[3] and activates polymorphonuclear neutrophils to inhibit the growth of tumor cells.

***In vivo* Primate Studies of LEUKINE**

Pharmacology/toxicology studies of LEUKINE were performed in cynomolgus monkeys. An acute toxicity study revealed an absence of treatment-related toxicity following a single IV bolus injection at a dose of 300 mcg/kg. Two subacute studies were performed using IV injection (maximum dose 200 mcg/kg/day × 14 days) and subcutaneous injection (maximum dose 200 mcg/kg/day × 28 days). No major visceral organ toxicity was documented. Notable histopathology findings included increased cellularity in hematologic organs, heart, and lung tissues. A dose-dependent increase in leukocyte count occurred during the dosing period which consisted primarily of segmented neutrophils; increases in monocytes, basophils, eosinophils, and lymphocytes were also noted. Leukocyte counts decreased to pretreatment values over a 1–2 week recovery period.

Pharmacokinetics

Pharmacokinetic profiles have been analyzed in patients with various neoplastic diseases following intravenous administration of LEUKINE. In 2 patients receiving 250 mcg/m^2 of LEUKINE by 2 hour IV infusion, serum concentration ranged from 22,000 pg/ml to 23,000 pg/ml at the termination of the infusion. The pharmacokinetic profile, calculated on samples from 5 patients receiving 500–750 mcg/m^2 of LEUKINE by 2 hour IV infusion, revealed a rapid initial decline in GM-CSF serum concentration ($t_{1/2\alpha}$~12 to 17 minutes) followed by a slower decrease ($t_{1/2\beta}$~2 hours). In four patients treated with LEUKINE by subcutaneous injection (125 mcg/m^2 every 12 hours), LEUKINE was detected in the serum within 5 minutes after administration (range 55–450 pg/ml). Peak levels were observed 2 hours after injection (range 350–3,900 pg/ml), and LEUKINE remained at detectable levels 6 hours following injection (range 150–2,700 pg/ml).[5]

Antibody Formation

Serum samples collected before and after LEUKINE treatment from 165 patients with a variety of underlying diseases have been examined for the presence of antibodies. Neutralizing antibodies were detected in 5 of 165 patients (3.0%) after receiving LEUKINE by continuous IV infusion (3 patients) or subcutaneous injection (2 patients) for 28 to 84 days in multiple courses. All 5 patients had impaired hematopoiesis before the administration of LEUKINE and consequently the effect of the development of anti-GM-CSF antibodies on normal hematopoiesis could not be assessed. Drug-induced neutropenia, neutralization of endogenous GM-CSF activity, and diminution of the therapeutic effect of LEUKINE secondary to formation of neutralizing antibody remain a theoretical possibility. A systematic screening program to evaluate antibody formation is ongoing for patients enrolled in clinical trials.

INDICATIONS AND USAGE

Use in Myeloid Reconstitution after Autologous Bone Marrow Transplantation

LEUKINE is indicated for acceleration of myeloid recovery in patients with non-Hodgkin's lymphoma (NHL), acute lymphoblastic leukemia (ALL), and Hodgkin's disease undergoing autologous bone marrow transplantation (BMT). After autologous BMT in patients with NHL, ALL, or Hodgkin's disease, LEUKINE has been found to be safe and effective in accelerating myeloid engraftment, decreasing median duration of antibiotic administration, reducing the median duration of infectious episodes and shortening the median duration of hospitalization. Hematologic response to LEUKINE can be detected by complete blood count (CBC) with differential performed twice per week.

Insufficient data are presently available to support the efficacy of LEUKINE in accelerating myeloid recovery following peripheral blood stem cell transplantation.

Clinical Experience

Use in Bone Marrow Transplantation Failure or Engraftment Delay

LEUKINE is indicated in patients who have undergone allogeneic or autologous bone marrow transplantation *(BMT)* in whom engraftment is delayed or has failed. LEUKINE has been found to be safe and effective in prolonging survival of patients who are experiencing graft failure or engraftment delay, in the presence or absence of infection, following autologous or allogeneic BMT. Survival benefit may be relatively greater in those patients who demonstrate one or more of the following characteristics: autologous BMT failure or engraftment delay, no previous total body irradiation, malignancy other than leukemia or a multiple organ failure (MOF) score ≤2 (See CLINICAL EXPERIENCE). Hematologic response to LEUKINE can be detected by complete blood count (CBC) with differential performed twice per week.

Effects on Myeloid Reconstitution after Autologous Bone Marrow Transplantation.[6] Following a dose-ranging Phase I/II trial in patients undergoing autologous BMT for lymphoid malignancies,[7,8] three single-center, randomized, placebo-controlled and double-blinded studies were conducted to evaluate the safety and efficacy of LEUKINE for promoting hematopoietic reconstitution following autologous BMT. A total of 128 patients (65 LEUKINE, 63 placebo) were enrolled in these 3 studies. The majority of the patients had lymphoid malignancy (87 NHL, 17 ALL), 23 patients had Hodgkin's disease, and 1 patient had acute myeloblastic leukemia (AML). In 72 subjects with NHL or ALL, the bone marrow harvest was purged prior to storage with one of several monoclonal antibodies. No chemical agent was used for *in vitro* treatment of the bone marrow. Preparative regimens in the 3 studies included cylophosphamide (total dose 120–150 mg/kg) and total body irradiation (total dose 1,200–1,575 rads). Other regimens used in patients with Hodgkin's disease and NHL without radiotherapy consisted of 3 or more of the following in combination (expressed as total dose): cytosine arabinoside (400 mg/m^2) and carmustine (300 mg/m^2), cyclophosphamide (140–150 mg/kg), hydroxyurea (4.5 gm/m^2), and etoposide (375–450 mg/m^2).

Compared to placebo, administration of LEUKINE in 2 studies (n=44 and 47) significantly improved the following hematologic and clinical endpoints: time to neutrophil engraftment, duration of hospitalization, and infection experience or antibacterial usage. In the third study (n=37) there was a positive trend toward earlier myeloid engraftment in favor of LEUKINE. This latter study differed from the other 2 in having enrolled a large number of patients with Hodgkin's disease who had also received extensive radiation and chemotherapy prior to harvest of autologous bone marrow. A subgroup analysis of the data from all three studies revealed that the median time to engraftment for patients with Hodgkin's disease, regardless of treatment, was 6 days longer when compared to patients with NHL and ALL, but that the overall beneficial LEUKINE treatment effect was the same. In the following combined analysis of the 3 studies, these 2 subgroups (NHL and ALL vs. Hodgkin's disease) are presented separately.

Patients with Lymphoid Malignancy (Non-Hodgkin's Lymphoma and Acute Lymphoblastic Leukemia) Myeloid engraftment (absolute neutrophil count [ANC]≥500 cells/mm^3) in 54 patients receiving LEUKINE (Sargramostim) was observed 6 days earlier than in 50 patients treated with placebo (see table below). Accelerated myeloid engraftment was associated with significant clinical benefits. The median duration of hospitalization was 6 days shorter for the LEUKINE group than for the placebo group. Median duration of infectious episodes (defined as fever and neutropenia; or 2 positive cultures of the same organism; or fever > 38°C and 1 positive blood culture; or clinical evidence of infection) was 3 days less in the group treated with LEUKINE. The median duration of antibacterial administration in the post-transplantation period was 4 days shorter for the patients treated with LEUKINE than for placebo-treated patients. The study was unable to detect a significant difference between the treatment groups in rate of disease relapse 24 months post-transplantation. As a group, leukemic subjects receiving LEUKINE derived less benefit than NHL subjects. However, both the leukemic and NHL groups receiving LEUKINE engrafted earlier than controls. [See table above.]

Autologous BMT: Combined Analysis from Placebo-Controlled Clinical Trials of Responses in Patients with NHL and ALL

Median Values (days)

	ANC ≥500/mm^3	ANC ≥1000/mm^3	Duration of Hospitalization	Duration of Infection	Duration of Antibacterial Therapy
LEUKINE (n=54)	18*#	24*#	25*	1*	21*
Placebo (n =50)	24	32	31	4	25

* p<0.05 Wilcoxon or CMH ridit chi-squared #p<0.05 Log rank

Note: The single AML patient was not included

Patients with Hodgkin's Disease If patients with Hodgkin's disease are analyzed separately, a trend toward earlier myeloid engraftment was noted. LEUKINE-treated patients engrafted earlier (by 5 days) than the placebo-treated subjects (p=0.189, Wilcoxon) but the number of subjects was small (n=22); 1 patient (#23) from one site was noncontrolled and was excluded from the analysis. Studies are in progress to confirm statistically the trend toward earlier engraftment of LEUKINE in patients with Hodgkin's disease.

Effects in Bone Marrow Transplantation Failure or Engraftment Delay

A historically-controlled study was conducted in patients experiencing graft failure following allogeneic or autologous BMT to determine whether LEUKINE improved survival after BMT failure.

Three categories of patients were eligible for this study:

1) patients displaying a delay in engraftment (ANC ≤100 cells/mm^3 by day 28 post-transplantation);
2) patients displaying a delay in engraftment (ANC ≤100 cells/mm^3 by day 21 post-transplantation) and who had evidence of an active infection; and
3) patients who lost their marrow graft after a transient engraftment (manifested by an average of ANC ≥500 cells/mm^3 for at least one week followed by loss of engraftment with ANC <500 cells/mm^3 for at least one week beyond day 21 post-transplantation).

A total of 140 eligible patients from 35 institutions treated with LEUKINE were evaluated in comparison to 103 historical control patients from a single institution. One hundred sixty-three patients had lymphoid or myeloid leukemia, 24 patients had non-Hodgkin's lymphoma, 19 patients had Hodgkin's disease and 37 patients had other diseases, such as aplastic anemia, myelodysplasia or non-hematologic malignancy. The majority of patients (223 out of 243) had received prior chemotherapy with or without radiotherapy and/or immunotherapy prior to preparation for transplantation.

One hundred day survival was improved in favor of the patients treated with LEUKINE after graft failure following either autologous or allogeneic BMT. In addition, the median survival was improved by greater than 2-fold. The median survival of patients treated with LEUKINE after autologous failure was 474 days versus 161 days for the historical patients. Similarly, after allogeneic failure, the median survival was 97 days with LEUKINE treatment and 35 days for the historical controls. Improvement in survival was better in patients with fewer impaired organs. [See table below.]

The MOF score is a simple clinical and laboratory assessment of 7 major organ systems: cardiovascular, respiratory, gastrointestinal, hematologic, renal, hepatic and neurologic.[9] Assessment of the MOF score is recommended as an additional method of determining the need to initiate treatment with LEUKINE in patients with graft failure or delay in engraftment following autologous or allogeneic BMT.

Factors that Contribute to Survival: The probability of survival was relatively greater for patients with any one of the following characteristics: autologous BMT failure or delay in engraftment, exclusion of total body irradiation from the preparative regimen, a non-leukemic malignancy or MOF score ≤2 (0, 1 or 2 dysfunctional organ systems). Leukemic subjects derived less benefit than other subjects.

CONTRAINDICATIONS

LEUKINE is contraindicated in patients with:

1) excessive leukemic myeloid blasts in the bone marrow or peripheral blood (≥10%).
2) known hypersensitivity to GM-CSF, yeast-derived products, or any component of the product.

WARNINGS

Fluid Retention

Peripheral edema, capillary leak syndrome, pleural and/or pericardial effusion have been reported in patients after LEUKINE administration. In 156 patients enrolled in pla-

Median Survival by Multiple Organ Failure (MOF) Category

Median Survival (days)

	MOF ≤2 Organs	MOF >2 Organs	MOF (Composite of Both Groups)
Autologous BMT			
LEUKINE	474 (n=58)	78.5 (n=10)	474 (n=68)
Historical	165 (n=14)	39 (n=3)	161 (n=17)
Allogeneic BMT			
LEUKINE	174 (n=50)	27 (n=22)	97 (n=72)
Historical	52.5 (n=60)	15.5 (n=26)	35 (n=86)

cebo-controlled studies using LEUKINE at a dose of 250 mcg/m²/day by 2 hour IV infusion, the reported incidences of fluid retention (LEUKINE vs. placebo) were as follows: peripheral edema, 11% vs. 7%; pleural effusion, 1% vs. 0%; and pericardial effusion, 4% vs. 1%. Capillary leak syndrome was not observed in this limited number of studies; based on other uncontrolled studies and post-marketing reports, the incidence is estimated to be less than 1%. In patients with preexisting pleural and pericardial effusions, administration of LEUKINE may aggravate fluid retention; however, fluid retention associated with or worsened by LEUKINE has been reversible after interruption or dose reduction of LEUKINE with or without diuretic therapy. LEUKINE should be used with caution in patients with preexisting fluid retention, pulmonary infiltrates, or congestive heart failure.

Respiratory Symptoms

Sequestration of granulocytes in the pulmonary circulation has been documented following LEUKINE infusion,[10] and dyspnea has been reported occasionally in patients treated with LEUKINE. Special attention should be given to respiratory symptoms during or immediately following LEUKINE infusion, especially in patients with preexisting lung disease. In patients displaying dyspnea during LEUKINE administration, the rate of infusion should be reduced by half. If respiratory symptoms worsen despite infusion rate reduction, infusion should be discontinued. Subsequent IV infusions may be administered following the standard dose schedule with careful monitoring. LEUKINE should be administered with caution in patients with hypoxia.

Cardiovascular Symptoms

Occasional transient supraventricular arrhythmia has been reported in uncontrolled studies during LEUKINE administration, particularly in patients with a previous history of cardiac arrhythmia. However, these arrhythmias have been reversible after discontinuation of LEUKINE. LEUKINE should be used with caution in patients with preexisting cardiac disease.

Renal and Hepatic Dysfunction

In some patients with preexisting renal or hepatic dysfunction enrolled in uncontrolled clinical trials, administration of LEUKINE (Sargramostim) has induced elevation of serum creatinine or bilirubin and hepatic enzymes. Dose reduction or interruption of LEUKINE administration has resulted in a decrease in pretreatment values. However, in controlled clinical trials the incidences of renal and hepatic dysfunction were comparable between LEUKINE (250 mcg/m²/day by 2 hour IV infusion) and placebo-treated patients. Monitoring of renal and hepatic function in patients displaying renal or hepatic dysfunction prior to initiation of treatment is recommended during LEUKINE administration.

PRECAUTIONS

General

Parenteral administration of recombinant proteins should be attended by appropriate precautions in case an allergic or untoward reaction occurs. Transient rashes and local injection site reactions have occasionally been observed concomitantly with LEUKINE treatment. Serious allergic or anaphylactic reactions have been reported rarely. If any serious allergic or anaphylactoid reaction occurs, LEUKINE therapy should immediately be discontinued and appropriate therapy initiated (see WARNINGS).

Rarely, hypotension with flushing and syncope has been reported following the first administration of LEUKINE. These signs have resolved with symptomatic treatment and have not recurred with subsequent doses in the same cycle of treatment.

Stimulation of marrow precursors with LEUKINE may result in a rapid rise in white blood cell (WBC) count. If the ANC exceeds 20,000 cells/mm³ or if the platelet count exceeds 500,000/mm³, LEUKINE administration should be interrupted or the dose reduced by half. The decision to reduce the dose or interrupt treatment should be based on the clinical condition of the patient. Excessive blood counts have returned to normal or baseline levels within 3 to 7 days following cessation of LEUKINE therapy. Twice weekly monitoring of CBC with differential (including examination for the presence of blast cells) should be performed to preclude development of excessive counts.

Growth Factor Potential

LEUKINE is a growth factor that primarily stimulates normal myeloid precursors. However, the possibility that LEUKINE can act as a growth factor for any tumor type, particularly myeloid malignancies, cannot be excluded. Because of the possibility of tumor growth potentiation, precaution should be exercised when using this drug in any malignancy with myeloid characteristics.

LEUKINE has been administered to patients with AML and myelodysplastic syndromes (MDS) in uncontrolled studies without evidence of increased relapse rates.[11,12,13] Controlled studies have not been performed in patients with AML or MDS. LEUKINE may be administered to those patients with AML or MDS who experience graft failure or delay in engraftment after bone marrow ablation and transplantation.

PERCENT OF PATIENTS REPORTING EVENT

Events by Body System	LEUKINE (n=79)	Placebo (n=77)
Body, General		
Fever	95	96
Mucous membrane disorder	75	78
Asthenia	66	51
Malaise	57	51
Sepsis	11	14
Digestive System		
Nausea	90	96
Diarrhea	89	82
Vomiting	85	90
Anorexia	54	58
GI disorder	37	47
GI hemorrhage	27	33
Stomatitis	24	29
Liver damage	13	14
Skin and Appendages		
Alopecia	73	74
Rash	44	38
Metabolic/Nutritional Disorder		
Edema	34	35
Peripheral edema	11	7
Respiratory System		
Dyspnea	28	31
Lung disorder	20	23
Hemic and Lymphatic System		
Blood dyscrasis	25	27
Cardiovascular System		
Hemorrhage	23	30
Urogenital System		
Urinary tract disorder	14	13
Kidney function abnormal	8	10
Nervous System		
CNS disorder	11	16

Progression of the underlying neoplastic disease (NHL, ALL, or Hodgkin's disease) was not observed during LEUKINE administration in clinical trials; however, should disease progression be detected during LEUKINE treatment, LEUKINE therapy should be discontinued. In controlled studies, the 24 month relapse rate was comparable in patients treated with LEUKINE or placebo.

Use in Patients Receiving Purged Bone Marrow

LEUKINE is effective in accelerating myeloid recovery in patients receiving bone marrow purged by anti-B lymphocyte monoclonal antibodies. Data obtained from uncontrolled studies suggest that if *in vitro* marrow purging with chemical agents causes a significant decrease in the number of responsive hematopoietic progenitors, the patient may not respond to LEUKINE. When the bone marrow purging process preserves a sufficient number of progenitors (71.2×10^4/kg), a beneficial effect of LEUKINE on myeloid engraftment has been reported.[14]

Use in Patients Previously Exposed to Intensive Chemotherapy/Radiotherapy

In patients who before autologous BMT, have received extensive radiotherapy to hematopoietic sites for the treatment of primary disease in the abdomen or chest, or have been exposed to multiple myelotoxic agents (alkylating agents, anthracycline antibiotics, and antimetabolites), the effect of LEUKINE on myeloid reconstitution may be limited.

Patient Monitoring

LEUKINE can induce variable increases in WBC and/or platelet counts. In order to avoid potential complications of excessive leukocytosis (WBC >50,000 cells/mm³; ANC >20,000 cells/mm³), a CBC is recommended twice per week during LEUKINE therapy. Monitoring of renal and hepatic function in patients displaying renal or hepatic dysfunction prior to initiation of treatment is recommended at least *biweekly* during LEUKINE administration. Body weight and hydration status should be carefully monitored during LEUKINE administration.

Drug Interaction

Interactions between LEUKINE and other drugs have not been fully evaluated. Drugs which may potentiate the myeloproliferative effects of LEUKINE, such as lithium and corticosteroids, should be used with caution.

Concomitant Use with Chemotherapy and Radiotherapy

The safety and efficacy of LEUKINE given simultaneously with cytotoxic chemotherapy or radiotherapy have not been established. Because of potential sensitivity of rapidly dividing hematopoietic progenitor cells to cytotoxic chemotherapeutic or radiologic therapies, LEUKINE should not be administered within 24 hours preceding or following chemotherapy, or within 12 hours preceding or following radiotherapy.

Carcinogenesis, Mutagenesis, Impairment of Fertility

Animal studies have not been conducted with LEUKINE to evaluate the carinogenic potential or the effect on fertility.

Pregnancy (Category C)

Animal reproduction studies have not been conducted with LEUKINE. It is not known whether LEUKINE can cause fetal harm when administered to a pregnant woman or can affect reproductive capability. LEUKINE should be given to a pregnant woman only if clearly needed.

Nursing Mothers

It is not known whether LEUKINE is excreted in human milk. Because many drugs are excreted in human milk, LEUKINE should be administered to a nursing woman only if clearly needed.

Pediatric Use

Safety and effectiveness in children have not been established; however, available safety data indicate that LEUKINE does not exhibit any greater toxicity in children than adults. A total of 113 pediatric subjects between the ages of 4 months and 18 years have been treated with LEUKINE in clinical trials at doses ranging from 60–1,000 mcg/m²/day intravenously and 4–1,500 mcg/m²/day subcutaneously. In 53 pediatric patients enrolled in controlled studies at a dose of 250 mcg/m²/day by 2 hour IV infusion, the type and frequency of adverse events were comparable to those reported for the adult population.

ADVERSE REACTIONS

LEUKINE is generally well tolerated. In 3 placebo-controlled studies enrolling a total of 156 patients after autologous BMT or peripheral stem cell transplantation, events reported in at least 10% of patients in LEUKINE or placebo groups were:

[See table above.]

The frequency and type of adverse events were similar between LEUKINE and placebo control groups. Diarrhea, asthenia, rash, and malaise were the only events observed for 5% more subjects in the LEUKINE group than in the placebo group.

No significant differences were observed between LEUKINE and placebo-treated patients in the type or frequency of laboratory abnormalities, including renal and hepatic parameters. In some patients with preexisting renal or hepatic dysfunction enrolled in uncontrolled clinical trials, administration of LEUKINE has induced elevation of serum creatinine or bilirubin and hepatic enzymes (see WARNINGS). In addition, there was no significant difference in relapse rate and 24 month survival between the LEUKINE and placebo-treated patients.

Adverse events observed for the patients treated with LEUKINE (Sargramostim) in the historically controlled BMT failure study were similar to those reported in the placebo-controlled studies. In addition, headache (26%), pericardial effusion (25%), arthralgia (21%) and myalgia (18%) were also reported in patients treated with LEUKINE in the graft failure study.

In uncontrolled Phase I/II studies with LEUKINE in 215 patients, the most frequent adverse events were fever, asthenia, headache, bone pain, chills, and myalgia. These systemic events were generally mild or moderate and were usually prevented or reversed by the administration of analgesics and antipyretics such as acetaminophen. In these uncontolled trials, other infrequent events reported were dyspnea, peripheral edema, and rash.

In patients with preexisting peripheral edema, capillary leak syndrome, pleural and/or pericardial effusion, administration of LEUKINE may aggravate fluid retention (see WARNINGS). Body weight and hydration status should be carefully monitored during LEUKINE administration.

Adverse events observed in pediatric patients in controlled studies were comparable to those observed in adult patients.

Overdosage

The maximum amount of LEUKINE that can be safely administered in single or multiple doses has not been determined. Doses up to 100 mcg/kg/day (4,000 mcg/m²/day or 16 times the recommended dose) were administered to 4 patients in a Phase I uncontrolled clinical study by continuous IV infusion for 7 to 18 days. Increases in WBC up to 200,000 cells/mm³ were observed. Adverse events reported were: dyspnea, malaise, nausea, fever, rash, sinus tachycardia, headache, and chills. All these events were reversible after discontinuation of LEUKINE.

In case of overdosage, LEUKINE therapy should be discontinued and the patient carefully monitored for WBC increase and respiratory symptoms.

DOSAGE AND ADMINISTRATION

Myeloid Reconstitution after Autologous Bone Marrow Transplantation

The recommended dose is 250 mcg/m²/day for 21 days as a 2 hour IV infusion beginning 2 to 4 hours after the autologous bone marrow infusion, and not less than 24 hours after the

Continued on next page

Immunex—Cont.

last dose of chemotherapy and 12 hours after the last dose of radiotherapy. If a severe adverse reaction occurs, the dose can be reduced or temporarily discontinued until the reaction abates. If blast cells appear or disease progression occurs, the treatment should be discontinued.

In order to avoid potential complications of excessive leukocytosis (WBC > 50,000 cells/mm^3; ANC > 20,000 cells/mm^3), a CBC with differential is recommended twice per week during LEUKINE therapy. LEUKINE treatment should be interrupted or the dose reduced by half if the ANC exceeds 20,000 cells/mm^3.

Bone Marrow Transplantation Failure or Engraftment Delay
The recommended dose is 250 mcg/m^2/day for 14 days as a 2 hour IV infusion. The dose can be repeated after 7 days off therapy if engraftment has not occurred. If engraftment still has not occurred, a third course of 500 mcg/m^2/day for 14 days may be tried after another 7 days off therapy. If there is still no improvement, it is unlikely that further dose escalation will be beneficial. If a severe adverse reaction occurs, the dose can be reduced or temporarily discontinued until the reaction abates. If blast cells appear or disease progression occurs, the treatment should be discontinued.

In order to avoid potential complications of excessive leukocytosis (WBC > 50,000 cells/mm^3, ANC > 20,000 cells/mm^3) a CBC with differential is recommended twice per week during LEUKINE therapy. LEUKINE treatment should be interrupted or the dose reduced by half if the ANC exceeds 20,000 cells/mm^3.

Preparation of LEUKINE
1. LEUKINE is a sterile, white, preservative-free, lyophilized powder suitable for IV infusion upon reconstitution. LEUKINE (250 mcg or 500 mcg vials) should be reconstituted aseptically with 1.0 ml Sterile Water for Injection, USP (without preservative). The reconstituted LEUKINE solutions are clear, colorless, isotonic with a pH of 7.4±0.3, and contain 250 or 500mcg/ml of Sargramostim. The single-use vial should not be re-entered or reused. Do not save any unused portion for later administration.
2. During reconstitution the Sterile Water for Injection, USP should be directed at the side of the vial and the contents gently swirled to avoid foaming during dissolution. Avoid excessive or vigorous agitation; do not shake.
3. Dilution for IV infusion should be performed in 0.9% Sodium Chloride Injection, USP. If the final concentration of LEUKINE is below 10 mcg/ml, Albumin (Human) at a final concentration of 0.1% should be added to the saline prior to addition of LEUKINE to prevent adsorption to the components of the drug delivery system. To obtain a final concentration of 0.1% Albumin (Human), add 1 mg Albumin (Human) per 1 ml 0.9% Sodium Chloride Injection, USP (e.g. use 1 ml 5% Albumin [Human] in 50 ml 0.9%Sodium Chloride Injection, USP).
4. An in-line membrane filler should not be used for intravenous infusion of LEUKINE.
5. LEUKINE contains no antibacterial preservative and therefore should be administered as soon as possible, and within 6 hours following reconstitution and/or dilution for IV infusion. Store LEUKINE solutions under refrigeration at 2–8°C (36–46°F); do not freeze. LEUKINE vials are intended for single use only; discard any unused solution after 6 hours.
6. In the absence of compatibility and stability information, no other medication should be added to infusion solutions containing LEUKINE. Use only 0.9% Sodium Chloride Injection, USP to prepare IV infusion solutions.
7. Aseptic technique should be employed in the preparation of all LEUKINE solutions. To assure correct concentration following reconstitution, care should be exercised to eliminate any air bubbles from the needle hub of the syringe used to prepare the diluent. Parenteral drug products should be inspected visually for particulate matter and discoloration prior to administration whenever solution and container permit.

HOW SUPPLIED
LEUKINE is available as a sterile, white, preservative-free, lyophilized powder in vials containing 250 mcg Sargramostim (1.25×10^7 units; NDC58406-002-01) or 500 mcg Sargramostim (2.50×10^7 units; NDC 58406-001-01); 40 mg Mannitol, USP; 10 mg Sucrose, NF; and 1.2 mg Tromethamine, USP. Each dosage form is supplied packaged individually or in cartons of 10 single-use vials.

STORAGE
The sterile powder, the reconstituted solution, and the diluted solution for injection should be refrigerated at 2–8°C (36–46°F). Do not freeze or shake. Do not use beyond the expiration date printed on the vial.

REFERENCES
1. Metcalf D. The molecular biology and functions of the granulocyte-macrophage colony-stimulating factors. Blood 1986; 67(2):257–267.
2. Park LS, Friend D, Gillis S, Urdal DL. Characterization of the cell surface receptor for human granulocyte/macrophage colony stimulating factor. J Exp Med 1986; 164:251–262.
3. Grabstein KH, Urdal DL, Tushinski RJ, et al. Induction of macrophage tumoricidal activity by granulocyte-macrophage colony stimulating factors. Science 1986; 232:506–508.
4. Reed SG, Nathan CF, Pihl DL, et al. Recombinant granulocyte/macrophage colony-stimulating factor activates macrophages to inhibit *Trypanosoma cruzi* and release hydrogen peroxide. J Exp Med 1987; 166:1734–1746.
5. Shadduck RK, Waheed A, Evans C, et al. Serum and urinary levels of recombinant human granulocyte-macrophage colony stimulating factor: Assessment after intravenous infusion and subcutaneous injection. Exp Hem 1990; 18:601.
6. Nemunaitis J, Rabinowe SN, Singer JW, et al. Recombinant human granulocyte-macrophage colony-stimulating factor after autologous bone marrow transplantation for lymphoid malignancy: Pooled results of a randomized, double-blind, placebo controlled trial. NEJM 1991; 324(25):1773–1778.
7. Nemunaitis J, Singer JW, Buckner CD, et al. Use of recombinant human granulocyte-macrophage colony stimulating factor in autologous bone marrow transplantation for lymphoid malignancies. Blood 1988; 72(2):834–836.
8. Nemunaitis J, Singer JW, Buckner CD, et al. Long-term follow-up of patients who received recombinant human granulocyte-macrophage colony stimulating factor after autologous bone marrow transplantation for lymphoid malignancy. BMT 1991; 7:49–52.
9. Goris RJA, Boekhorst TPA, Nuytinck JKS, et al. Multiple organ failure: Generalized auto-destructive inflammation? Arch Surg 1985; 120:1109–1115.
10. Herrmann F, Schulz G, Lindemann A, et al. Yeast-expressed granulocyte-macrophage colony-stimulating factor in cancer patients: A phase lb clinical study. In Behring Institute Research Communications, Colony Stimulating Factors-CSF. International Symposium, Garmisch-Partenkirchen, West Germany. 1988; 83:107–118.
11. Estey EH, Dixon D, Kantarjian H, et al. Treatment of poor-prognosis, newly diagnosed acute myeloid leukemia with Ara-C and recombinant human granulocyte-macrophage colony-stimulating factor. Blood 1990; 75(9):1766–1769.
12. Vadhan-Raj S, Keating M, LeMaistre A, et al. Effects of recombinant human granulocyte-macrophage colony-stimulating factor in patients with myelodysplastic syndromes. NEJM 1987; 317:1545–1552.
13. Buchner T, Hiddemann W, Koenigsmann M, et al. Recombinant human granulocyte-macrophage colony stimulating factor after chemotherapy in patients with acute myeloid leukemia at higher age or after relapse. Blood 1991; 78(5):1190–1197.
14. Blazar BR, Kersey JH, McGlave PB, et al. In vivo administration of recombinant human granulocyte/macrophage colony-stimulating factor in acute lymphoblastic leukemia patients receiving purged autografts. Blood 1989; 73(3):849–857.

SA-001   Rev 02   Issued 3/14/91

immunex®
Immunex Corporation
Seattle, WA 98101

RUBEX®
(Doxorubicin Hydrochloride for Injection, USP)   ℞

DESCRIPTION
Doxorubicin is a cytotoxic anthracycline antibiotic isolated from cultures of **Streptomyces peucetius** var. **caesius**.

HOW SUPPLIED
Rubex (Doxorubicin hydrochloride for injection, USP) is for intravenous use only and is available as follows:
- **10 mg**—Each single-dose vial contains 10 mg of doxorubicin HCL, USP as a sterile red-orange lyophilized powder, NDC 0015-3351-22. Available as one individually cartoned vial.
- **50 mg**—Each single-dose vial contains 50 mg of doxorubicin HCL, USP as a sterile red-orange lyophilized powder, NDC 0015-3352-22. Available as one individually cartoned vial.
- **100 mg**—Each single-dose vial contains 100 mg of doxorubicin HCL, USP as a sterile red-orange lyophilized powder, NDC 0015-3353-22. Available as one individually cartoned vial.

Store dry powder at controlled room temperature 15°–30°C (59°–86°F). The reconstituted solution is stable for 24 hours at room temperature or 48 hours under refrigeration 2°–8°C (36°–46°F).
Protect from exposure to sunlight. Retain in carton until time of use.

Immuno-U.S., Inc.
1200 PARKDALE ROAD
ROCHESTER, MI 48307-1744

ALBUMIN (HUMAN) 5%   ℞

10 bottles per case.
50 mL w/o admin. set	NDC 54129-218-05
250 mL w/admin. set	NDC 54129-218-25
500 mL w/admin. set	NDC 54129-218-50

ALBUMIN (HUMAN) 25%   ℞

10 bottles per case.
20 mL w/o admin. set	NDC 54129-228-02
50 mL w/admin. set	NDC 54129-228-05
100 mL w/admin. set	NDC 54129-228-10

FEIBA® VH IMMUNO   ℞
Anti-Inhibitor Coagulant Complex, Vapor Heated

1 Vial   NDC 54129-222-04
A sterile freeze-dried human plasma fraction with Factor VIII inhibitor bypassing activity. In vitro, FEIBA® VH IMMUNO shortens the activated partial thromboplastin time (APTT) of plasma containing Factor VIII inhibitor. Factor VIII inhibitor bypassing activity is expressed in arbitrary units. One IMMUNO Unit of activity is defined as that amount of Anti-Inhibitor Coagulant Complex, Vapor Heated, FEIBA® VH IMMUNO which shortens the APTT of a high titer Factor VIII inhibitor reference plasma to 50% of the blank value. The product is intended for intravenous administration.

IVEEGAM®   ℞
Immune Globulin Intravenous (Human)

1 gm w/20 mL Recon.	NDC 54129-233-10
2.5 gm w/50 mL Recon.	NDC 54129-233-25
5 gm w/100 mL Recon.	NDC 54129-233-50
A sterile freeze-dried concentrate of immunoglobulin G (IgG). Reconstitution of the freeze-dried powder with the accompanying quantity of Sterile Water For Injection U.S.P., gives a 5% protein solution suitable for intravenous administration. This final solution contains, per mL, 50 ±5 mg of IgG, 50 mg of glucose as a stabilizer, and 3 mg of sodium chloride. Trace amounts of IgM and IgA are also present. The reconstituted solution is clear, colorless, and free of detectable aggregates. It contains no preservative.

Telephone: 1-800-346-6866

International Ethical Labs.
AVE. AMERICO MIRANDA #1021
REPARTO METROPOLITANO
RIO PIEDRAS, PR 00921

BIOCEF ℞
CEPHALEXIN Orange Color Capsule
CAPSULES USP
500mg.

Shown in Product Identification Section, page 412

BIOCEF Oral Suspension 125mg. ℞
BIOCEF Oral Suspension 250mg. ℞
BIO-TAB ℞ 50 Tabs. in boxes U/D
DOXYCYCLINE HYCLATE 100 mg.
DESPEC™ ℞ bottle of 100 Caps.
CAPSULES
Each capsule contains:
Phenylpropanolamine HCl (controlled release) 75mg.
Guaifenesin 400mg.

Shown in Product Identification Section, page 412

DESPEC™ ℞
LIQUID
Each 5ml. (one teaspoonful) contains:
Guaifenesin 100mg.
Phenylpropanolamine HCl 20mg.
Phenylephrine HCl 5mg.
Alcohol 5%

MIO-REL ℞ boxes of 25 amps.
Injectable
Orphenadrine Citrate 60mg. per 2cc ampules

MOXILIN 250mg. Cap. × 100	Amoxicillin ℞
MOXILIN 500mg. Cap. × 100	Amoxicillin ℞
MOXILIN OIS 250mg. 100ml.	Amoxicillin ℞
MOXILIN OIS 250mg. 150ml.	Amoxicillin ℞

NEUROFORTE-R — Vitamin B-12
Vial 10cc

NEUROFORTE-SIX — Vitamin B Complex
Monovial 10cc   B-12 and Vitamin C

REMULAR-500
(Muscle Relaxant)
Chlorzoxazone 500mg ℞ Bottle of 100 and 500 Caplets

REMULAR-S
(Muscle Relaxant)
Chlorzoxazone 250mg. ℞ bottle of 100

TENCON ℞ bottles of 100
Capsules
Butalbital 50mg.
Acetaminophen 650mg.
Shown in Product Identification Section, page 412

Inwood Laboratories, Inc.
Subsidiary of Forest Laboratories, Inc.
300 PROSPECT STREET
INWOOD, NY 11696

PRODUCT Generic Name Colors(s)	IDENTIFICATION CODE (Front/Back*)
CARBAMAZEPINE Tablets, USP, 200mg ℞ White	IL 3587/Blank
INDOMETHACIN E.R. Capsules, USP, 75mg ℞ Lavender/Clear	IL 3607/Blank
ISOSORBIDE DINITRATE E.R. Tablets, USP, 40mg ℞ Peach	IL 3549/Blank
PROPRANOLOL HYDROCHLORIDE E.R. Capsules, USP, 60mg ℞ Opaque Brown/Clear	IL 3609/Blank
PROPRANOLOL HYDROCHLORIDE E.R. Capsules, USP, 80mg ℞ Opaque Blue/Clear	IL 3610/Blank
PROPRANOLOL HYDROCHLORIDE E.R. Capsules, USP, 120mg ℞ Opaque Blue/Clear	IL 3611/Blank
PROPRANOLOL HYDROCHLORIDE E.R. Capsules, USP, 160mg ℞ Opaque Blue/Clear	IL 3612/Blank
THEOCHRON Tablets, 300mg ℞ White/Scored	IL 3581/Blank
THEOCHRON Tablets, 200mg ℞ White/Scored	IL 3583/Blank
THEOCHRON Tablets, 100mg ℞ White/Scored	IL 3584/Blank

*Front/Back for tablets or left and right side for capsules
Theochron Shown in Product Identification Section, page 409

Ion Laboratories, Inc.
7431 PEBBLE DR.
FORT WORTH, TEXAS 76118

RESCON Capsules   ℞

DESCRIPTION
Each timed-release, imprinted capsule contains Pseudoephedrine HCl 120 mg. and Chlorpheniramine Maleate 12 mg.
HOW SUPPLIED
100's.

RESCON Liquid   OTC
Sugar, Dye, Alcohol Free

DESCRIPTION
Each 5 ml contains Phenylpropanolamine HCl 12.5 mg. and Chlorpheniramine Maleate 2 mg.
HOW SUPPLIED
4 oz.

RESCON-DM Liquid   OTC
(Sugar, Dye, Alcohol Free)

DESCRIPTION
Each 5 ml contains Dextromethorphan Hdr. 10 mg, Pseudoephedrine HCl 30 mg and Chlorpheniramine Maleate 2 mg.
HOW SUPPLIED
4 oz.

RESCON-ED Capsules   ℞

DESCRIPTION
Each timed-release, imprinted capsule contains Pseudoephedrine HCl 120 mg. and Chlorpheniramine Maleate 8 mg.
HOW SUPPLIED
100's.

RESCON-GG Liquid   OTC
(Sugar, Dye, Alcohol Free)

DESCRIPTION
Each 5 ml contains Phenylephrine HCl 5 mg. and Guaifenesin 100 mg.
HOW SUPPLIED
4 oz.

RESCON JR Capsules   ℞

DESCRIPTION
Each timed-release, imprinted capsule contains Pseudoephedrine HCl 60 mg. and Chlorpheniramine Maleate 8 mg.
HOW SUPPLIED
100's.

SINUPAN Capsules   ℞

DESCRIPTION
Each timed-release, imprinted capsule contains Phenylephrine HCl 40 mg. and Guaifenesin 200 mg.
HOW SUPPLIED
100's.

Jacobus Pharmaceutical Co., Inc.
37 CLEVELAND LANE
P.O. BOX 5290
PRINCETON, NJ 08540

DAPSONE USP   ℞
[*dap'sōne*]
25 mg. & 100 mg.

PRODUCT OVERVIEW
KEY FACTS
Dapsone is a sulfone for the primary treatment of Dermatitis herpetiformis and an antibacterial drug for susceptible cases of leprosy.

MAJOR USES
Dapsone is used to control the dermatologic symptoms of Dermatitis herpetiformis. Dapsone is used alone or in combination with other anti-leprosy drugs for leprosy.

SAFETY INFORMATION
Dapsone is contraindicated in patients with Dapsone hypersensitivity. Complete blood counts and laboratory monitoring should be done frequently. See labeling.

PRODUCT INFORMATION
DAPSONE USP   ℞
[*dap'sōne*]
25 mg. & 100 mg.
DESCRIPTION
Dapsone-USP, 4–4' diaminodiphenylsulfone (DDS) is a primary treatment for Dermatitis herpetiformis. It is an antibacterial drug for susceptible cases of leprosy. It is a white,

---

odorless crystalline powder, practically insoluble in water and insoluble in fixed and vegetable oils.
Inactive Ingredients: Colloidal silicone dioxide, magnesium stearate, microcrystalline cellulose, and corn starch. Dapsone is issued on prescription in tablets of 25 and 100 mg. for oral use.

$$NH_2 \text{—} \bigcirc \text{—} SO_2 \text{—} \bigcirc \text{—} NH_2$$

CLINICAL PHARMACOLOGY
Actions: The mechanism of action in Dermatitis herpetiformis has not been established. By the kinetic method in mice, Dapsone is bactericidal as well as bacteriostatic against *Mycobacterium leprae*.
Absorption and Excretion: Dapsone, when given orally, is rapidly and almost completely absorbed. About 85 percent of the daily intake is recoverable from the urine mainly in the form of water-soluble metabolites. Excretion of the drug is slow and a constant blood level can be maintained with the usual dosage.
Blood Levels: Detected a few minutes after ingestion, the drug reaches peak concentration in 4–8 hours. Daily administration for at least eight days is necessary to achieve a plateau level. With doses of 200 mg. daily, this level averaged 2.3 μg/ml with a range of 0.1–7.0 μg/ml. The half-life in the plasma in different individuals varies from ten hours to fifty hours and averages twenty-eight hours. Repeat tests in the same individual are constant. Daily administration (50–100 mg.) in leprosy patients will provide blood levels in excess of the usual minimum inhibitory concentration even for patients with a short Dapsone half-life.

INDICATIONS AND USAGE
Dermatitis herpetiformis (D.H.) All forms of leprosy except for cases of proven Dapsone resistance.

CONTRAINDICATION
Hypersensitivity to Dapsone and/or its derivatives.

WARNINGS
The patient should be warned to respond to the presence of clinical signs such as sore throat, fever, pallor, purpura or jaundice. Deaths associated with the administration of Dapsone have been reported from agranulocytosis, aplastic anemia and other blood dyscrasias. Complete blood counts should be done frequently in patients receiving Dapsone. The FDA Dermatology Advisory Committee recommended that, when feasible counts should be done weekly for the first month, monthly for six months and semi-annually thereafter. If a significant reduction in leucocytes, platelets or hemopoiesis is noted, Dapsone should be discontinued and the patient followed intensively. Folic acid antagonists have similar effects and may increase the incidence of hematologic reactions; if co-administered with Dapsone the patient should be monitored more frequently. Patients on weekly Pyrimethamine and Dapsone have developed agranulocytosis during the second and third month of therapy.
Severe anemia should be treated prior to initiation of therapy and hemoglobin monitored. Hemolysis and methemoglobin may be poorly tolerated by patients with severe cardiopulmonary disease.
Carcinogenesis, mutagenesis: Dapsone has been found carcinogenic (sarcomagenic) for male rats and female mice causing mesenchymal tumors in the spleen and peritoneum, and thyroid carcinoma in female rats. Dapsone is not mutagenic with or without microsomal activation in *S. typhimurium* tester strains 1535, 1537, 1538, 98, or 100.
Cutaneous reactions, especially bullous, include exfoliative dermatitis and are probably one of the most serious, though rare, complications of sulfone therapy. They are directly due to drug sensitization. Such reactions include toxic erythema, erythema multiforme, toxic epidermal necrolysis, morbilliform and scariatiniform reactions, urticaria and erythema nodosum. If new or toxic dermatologic reactions occur, sulfone therapy must be promptly discontinued and appropriate therapy instituted.
Leprosy reactional states, including cutaneous, are not hypersensitivity reactions to Dapsone and do not require discontinuation. See special section.

PRECAUTIONS
General: Hemolysis and Heinz body formation may be exaggerated in individuals with a glucose-6-phosphate dehydrogenase (G6PD) deficiency, or methemoglobin reductase deficiency, or hemoglobin M. This reaction is frequently dose-related. Dapsone should be given with caution to these patients or if the patient is exposed to other agents or conditions such as infection or diabetic ketosis capable of producing hemolysis. Drugs or chemicals which have produced significant hemolysis in G6PD or methemoglobin reductase deficient patients include Dapsone, sulfanilamide, nitrite, aniline, phenylhydrazine, napthalene, niridazole, nitrofurantoin and 8-amino-antimalarials such as primaquine.

Continued on next page

Jacobus—Cont.

Toxic hepatitis and cholestatic jaundice have been reported early in therapy. Hyperbilirubinemia may occur more often in G6PD deficient patients. When feasible, baseline and subsequent monitoring of liver function is recommended. If abnormal, Dapsone should be discontinued until the source of the abnormality is established.

Drug Interactions: Rifampin lowers Dapsone levels 7 to 10-fold by accelerating plasma clearance; in leprosy this reduction has not required a change in dosage.

Folic acid antagonists such as pyrimethamine may increase the likelihood of hematologic reactions.

Pregnancy Category C: Animal reproduction studies have not been conducted with Dapsone. Extensive, but uncontrolled experience and two published surveys on the use of Dapsone in pregnant women have not shown that Dapsone increases the risk of fetal abnormalities if administered during all trimesters of pregnancy or can affect reproduction capacity. Because of the lack of animal studies or controlled human experience, Dapsone should be given to a pregnant woman only if clearly needed. In general, for leprosy, USPHS at Carville recommends maintenance of Dapsone. Dapsone has been important for the management of some pregnant D.H. patients.

Nursing Mothers: Dapsone is excreted in breast milk in substantial amounts. Hemolytic reactions can occur in neonates. See section on hemolysis. Because of the potential for tumorgenicity shown for Dapsone in animal studies a decision should be made whether to discontinue nursing or discontinue the drug taking into account the importance of the drug to the mother.

Pediatric Use: Children are treated on the same schedule as adults but with correspondingly smaller doses. Dapsone is generally not considered to have an effect on the later growth, development and functional development of the child.

ADVERSE REACTIONS

In addition to the warnings listed above, the following syndromes and serious reactions have been reported in patients on Dapsone.

Hematologic Effects: Dose-related hemolysis is the most common adverse effect and is seen in patients with or without G6PD deficiency. Almost all patients demonstrate the interrelated changes of a loss of 1–2g of HB, an increase in the reticulocytes (2–12%), a shortened red cell life span and a rise in methemoglobin. G6PD deficient patients have greater responses.

Nervous System Effects: Peripheral neuropathy is a definite but unusual complication of Dapsone therapy in non-leprosy patients. Motor loss is predominent. If muscle weakness appears, Dapsone should be withdrawn. Recovery on withdrawal is usually substantially complete. The mechanism of recovery is reportedly by axonal regeneration. Some recovered patients have tolerated retreatment at reduced dosage. In leprosy this complication may be difficult to distinguish from a leprosy reactional state.

Body As A Whole: In addition to the warnings and adverse effects reported above, additional adverse reactions include: nausea, vomiting, abdominal pains, vertigo, blurred vision, tinnitus, insomnia, fever, headache, psychosis, phototoxicity, tachycardia, albuminuria, the nephrotic syndrome, hypoalbuminemia without proteinuria, renal papillary necrosis, male infertility, drug-induced Lupus erythematosus and an infectious mononucleosis-like syndrome. In general, with the exception of the complications of severe anoxia from overdosage (retinal and optic nerve damage, etc.) these adverse reactions have regressed off drug.

OVERDOSAGE

Nausea, vomiting, hyperexcitability can appear a few minutes up to 24 hours after ingestion or an overdose. Methemoglobin induced depression, convulsions and severe cyanosis requires prompt treatment. In normal and methemoglobin reductase deficient patients, methylene blue, 1–2 mg/kg of body weight, given slowly intravenously is the treatment of choice. The effect is complete in 30 minutes, but may have to be repeated if methemoglobin reaccumulates. For non-emergencies, if treatment is needed, methylene blue may be given orally in doses of 3–5 mg/kg every 4–6 hours.

Methylene blue reduction depends on G6PD and should not be given to fully expressed G6PD deficient patients.

DOSAGE AND ADMINISTRATION

Dermatitis herpetiformis: The dosage should be individually titrated starting in adults with 50 mg. daily and correspondingly smaller doses in children. If full control is not achieved within the range of 50–300 mg. daily, higher doses may be tried. Dosage should be reduced to a minimum maintenance level as soon as possible. In responsive patients there is a prompt reduction in pruritus followed by clearance of skin lesions. There is no effect on the gastro-intestinal component of the disease.

Dapsone levels are influenced by acetylation rates. Patients with high acetylation rates, or who are receiving treatment affecting acetylation may require an adjustment in dosage.

A strict gluten free diet is an option for the patient to elect, permitting many to reduce or eliminate the need for Dapsone; the average time for dosage reduction is 8 months with a range of 4 months to 2½ years and for dosage elimination 29 months with a range of 6 months to 9 years.

Leprosy: In order to reduce secondary Dapsone resistance, the WHO Expert Committee on Leprosy and the USPHS at Carville, LA, recommend that Dapsone should be commenced in combination with one or more anti-leprosy drugs. In the multi-drug program Dapsone should be maintained at the full dosage of 100 mg. daily without interruption (with correspondingly smaller doses for children) and provided to all patients who have sensitive organisms with new or recrudescent disease or who have not yet completed a two year course of Dapsone monotherapy. For advice and other drugs, the USPHS at Carville, LA, (1 800-642-2477) should be contacted. Before using other drugs consult appropriate product labeling.

In bacteriologically negative tuberculoid and indeterminate disease, the recommendation is the coadministration of Dapsone 100 mg. daily with six months of Rifampin 600 mg. daily. Under WHO, daily Rifampin may be replaced by 600 mg. Rifampin monthly, if supervised. The Dapsone is continued until all signs of clinical activity are controlled—usually after an additional six months. Then Dapsone should be continued for an additional three years for tuberculoid and indeterminate patients and for five years for borderline tuberculoid patients.

In lepromatous and borderline lepromatous patients, the recommendation is the coadministration of Dapsone 100 mg. daily with two years of Rifampin 600 mg. daily. Under WHO, daily Rifampin may be replaced by 600 mg. Rifampin monthly, if supervised. One may elect the concurrent administration of a third anti-leprosy drug, usually either Clofazamine 50–100mg. daily or Ethionamide 250–500 mg. daily. Dapsone 100 mg. daily is continued 3–10 years until all signs of clinical activity are controlled with skin scrapings and biopsies negative for one year. Dapsone should then be continued for an additional 10 years for borderline patients and for life for lepromatous patients.

Secondary Dapsone resistance should be suspected whenever a lepromatous or borderline lepromatous patient receiving Dapsone treatment relapses clinically and bacteriologically, solid staining bacilli being found in the smears taken from the new active lesions. If such cases show no response to regular and supervised Dapsone therapy within three to six months or good compliance for the past 3–6 months can be assured, Dapsone resistance should be considered confirmed clinically. Determination of drug sensitivity using the mouse footpad method is recommended and, after prior arrangement, is available without charge from the USPHS, Carville, LA. Patients with proven Dapsone resistance should be treated with other drugs.

Leprosy Reactional States: Abrupt changes in clinical activity occur in leprosy with any effective treatment and are known as reactional states. The majority can be classified into two groups.

The "Reversal" reaction (Type 1) may occur in borderline or tuberculoid leprosy patients often soon after chemotherapy is started. The mechanism is presumed to result from a reduction in the antigenic load: the patient is able to mount an enhanced delayed hypersensitivity response to residual infection leading to swelling ("Reversal") of existing skin and nerve lesions. If severe, or if neuritis is present, large doses of steroids should always be used. If severe, the patient should be hospitalized. In general anti-leprosy treatment is continued and therapy to suppress the reaction is indicated such as analgesics, steroids, or surgical decompression of swollen nerve trunks. USPHS at Carville, LA should be contacted for advice in management.

Erythema nodosum leprosum (ENL) (lepromatous lepra reaction) (Type 2 reaction) occurs mainly in lepromatous patients and small numbers of borderline patients. Approximately 50% of treated patients show this reaction in the first year. The principal clinical features are fever and tender erythematous skin nodules sometimes associated with malaise, neuritis, orchitis, albuminuria, joint swelling, iritis, epistaxis or depression. Skin lesions can become pustular and/or ulcerate. Histologically there is a vasculitis with an intense polymorphonuclear infiltrate. Elevated circulating immune complexes are considered to be the mechanism of the reaction. If severe, patients should be hospitalized. In general, anti-leprosy treatment is continued. Analgesics, steroids, and other agents available from USPHS, Carville, LA, are used to suppress the reaction.

HOW SUPPLIED

Rx: Dapsone 25 mg, round white scored tablet, debossed "25" above and "102" below the score and on the obverse "Jacobus" in light and child-resistant bottles, of 100, NDC 49938-102-01.

Dapsone 100 mg, round white scored tablet, debossed "100" above and "101" below the score and on the obverse "Jacobus" in light and child-resistant bottles of 100, NDC 49938-101-01.

Store at controlled room temperature, (59–86°F).

Protect from light.

CAUTION: Federal law prohibits dispensing without prescription.

Dispense this product in a well-closed child-resistant container.

JACOBUS PHARMACEUTICAL CO., INC.
P.O. Box 5290
Princeton, NJ 08540

7F FEBRUARY, 1991

Jamol Laboratories Inc.
13 ACKERMAN AVENUE
EMERSON, NEW JERSEY 07630

PONARIS **OTC**
Nasal Mucosal Emollient

COMPOSITION

Essential oils of Pine, Eucalyptus, Peppermint, Cajeput, and Cottonseed as specially prepared iodized organic oils. Total Iodine 0.5%–0.7%. Assimilable hence NON-lipoid potential.

INDICATIONS AND USES

For relief of nasal congestion due to colds, nasal irritations, Atrophic Rhinitis, (dry, inflamed nasal passages), nasal mucosal encrustations, and allergy manifestations (Rose and Hay Fever).

Nasal intubations and sterile gauze impregnated for epistaxis packing.

ADMINISTRATION AND DOSAGE

Half dropperful each application as needed or as directed by a physician. May be used in a compressed air nebulizer or a DeVilbiss nebulizer No. 15.

Children's Dosage: As directed by physician.

HOW SUPPLIED

One ounce bottle with dropper.

Janssen Pharmaceutica Inc.
1125 TRENTON-HARBOURTON ROAD
P.O. BOX 200
TITUSVILLE, NJ 08560-0200

ALFENTA® Ⓒ℞
[ăl-fĕn´tă]
(alfentanil hydrochloride)
Injection

CAUTION: Federal Law Prohibits Dispensing Without Prescription

DESCRIPTION

ALFENTA (alfentanil hydrochloride) Injection is an opioid analgesic chemically designated as N-[1-[2-(4-ethyl-4, 5-dihydro-5-oxo-1H-tetrazol-1-yl) ethyl] -4-(methoxymethyl)-4-piperidinyl]-N-phenylpropanamide monohydrochloride (1:1) with a molecular weight of 452.98.

ALFENTA is a sterile, non-pyrogenic, preservative free aqueous solution containing alfentanil hydrochloride equivalent to 500 μg per ml of alfentanil base for intravenous injection. The solution, which contains sodium chloride for isotonicity, has a pH range of 4.0–6.0.

CLINICAL PHARMACOLOGY

ALFENTA (alfentanil hydrochloride) is an opioid analgesic with a rapid onset of action.

At doses of 8–40 μg/kg for surgical procedures lasting up to 30 minutes, ALFENTA provides analgesic protection against hemodynamic responses to surgical stress with recovery times generally comparable to those seen with equipotent fentanyl dosages. For longer procedures, doses of up to 75 μg/kg attenuate hemodynamic responses to laryngoscopy, intubation and incision, with recovery time comparable to fentanyl. At doses of 50–75 μg/kg followed by a continuous infusion of 0.5–3.0 μg/kg/min, ALFENTA attenuates the catecholamine response with more rapid recovery and reduced need for postoperative analgesics as compared to patients administered enflurane. High intrasubject and intersubject variability in the pharmacokinetic disposition of ALFENTA has been reported.

The pharmacokinetics of ALFENTA as determined in 11 patients given single bolus injections of 50 or 125 μg/kg, can be described as a three-compartment model; distribution half-life ranged from 0.4–3.1 minutes; redistribution half-life ranged from 4.6–21.6 minutes; and terminal elimination half-life ranged from 64.1–129.3 minutes (as compared to a terminal elimination half-life of approximately 219 minutes

for fentanyl and approximately 164 minutes for sufentanil). Linear kinetics have been described only with plasma concentrations up to 1000 ng/ml. Repeated or continuous administration of ALFENTA produces increasing plasma concentration and an accumulation of the drug, particularly in patients with reduced plasma clearance. The liver is the major site of biotransformation.

ALFENTA has an apparent volume of distribution of 0.6–1.0 L/kg, which is approximately one-fourth that of fentanyl, with a plasma clearance range of 1.7–17.6 ml/kg/min as compared to approximately 12.6 ml/kg/min for fentanyl. Approximately 81% of the administered dose is excreted within 24 hours and only 0.2% of the dose is eliminated as unchanged drug; urinary excretion is the major route of elimination of metabolites. Plasma protein binding of ALFENTA is approximately 92%.

In one study involving 15 patients administered ALFENTA with nitrous oxide/oxygen, a narrow range of plasma ALFENTA concentrations, approximately 310–340 ng/ml, was shown to provide adequate anesthesia for intra-abdominal surgery, while lower concentrations, approximately 190 ng/ml, blocked responses to skin closure. Plasma concentrations between 100–200 ng/ml provided adequate anesthesia for superficial surgery.

ALFENTA has an immediate onset of action. At dosages of approximately 105 µg/kg, ALFENTA produces hypnosis as determined by EEG patterns; an anesthetic ED_{90} of 182 µg/kg for ALFENTA in unpremedicated patients has been determined, based upon the ability to block response to placement of a nasopharyngeal airway. Based on clinical trials, induction dosage requirements range from 130–245 µg/kg. For procedures lasting 30–60 minutes, loading dosages of up to 50 µg/kg produce the hemodynamic responses to endotracheal intubation and skin incision comparable to those from fentanyl. A pre-intubation loading dose of 50–75 µg/kg prior to a continuous infusion attenuates the response to laryngoscopy, intubation and incision. Subsequent administration of ALFENTA infusion administered at a rate of 0.5–3.0 µg/kg/min with nitrous oxide/oxygen attenuates sympathetic responses to surgical stress with more rapid recovery than enflurane.

Requirements for volatile inhalation anesthetics were reduced by thirty to fifty percent during the first 60 minutes of maintenance in patients administered anesthetic doses (above 130 µg/kg) of ALFENTA as compared to patients given doses of 4–5 mg/kg thiopental for anesthetic induction. At anesthetic induction dosages, ALFENTA provides a deep level of anesthesia during the first hour of anesthetic maintenance and provides attenuation of the hemodynamic response during intubation and incision.

Following an anesthetic induction dose of ALFENTA, requirements for ALFENTA infusion are reduced by 30 to 50% for the first hour of maintenance.

Patients with compromised liver function and those over 65 years of age have been found to have reduced plasma clearance and extended terminal elimination for ALFENTA, which may prolong postoperative recovery.

Bradycardia may be seen in patients administered ALFENTA. The incidence and degree of bradycardia may be more pronounced when ALFENTA is administered in conjunction with non-vagolytic neuromuscular blocking agents or in the absence of anticholinergic agents such as atropine. Administration of intravenous diazepam immediately prior to or following high doses of ALFENTA has been shown to produce decreases in blood pressure that may be secondary to vasodilation; recovery may also be prolonged.

Patients administered doses up to 200 µg/kg of ALFENTA have shown no significant increase in histamine levels and no clinical evidence of histamine release.

Skeletal muscle rigidity is related to the dose and speed of administration of ALFENTA. Muscular rigidity will occur with an immediate onset following anesthetic induction dosages. Preventative measures (see WARNINGS) may reduce the rate and severity.

The duration and degree of respiratory depression and increased airway resistance usually increase with dose, but have also been observed at lower doses. Although higher doses may produce apnea and a longer duration of respiratory depression, apnea may also occur at low doses.

INDICATIONS AND USAGE

ALFENTA (alfentanil hydrochloride) is indicated:
   as an analgesic adjunct given in incremental doses in the maintenance of anesthesia with barbiturate/nitrous oxide/oxygen.
   as an analgesic administered by continuous infusion with nitrous oxide/oxygen in the maintenance of general anesthesia.
   as a primary anesthetic agent for the induction of anesthesia in patients undergoing general surgery in which endotracheal intubation and mechanical ventilation are required.

SEE DOSAGE CHART FOR MORE COMPLETE INFORMATION ON THE USE OF ALFENTA.

CONTRAINDICATIONS

ALFENTA (alfentanil hydrochloride) is contraindicated in patients with known hypersensitivity to the drug.

WARNINGS

ALFENTA SHOULD BE ADMINISTERED ONLY BY PERSONS SPECIFICALLY TRAINED IN THE USE OF INTRAVENOUS AND GENERAL ANESTHETIC AGENTS AND IN THE MANAGEMENT OF RESPIRATORY EFFECTS OF POTENT OPIOIDS.

AN OPIOID ANTAGONIST, RESUSCITATIVE AND INTUBATION EQUIPMENT AND OXYGEN SHOULD BE READILY AVAILABLE.

BECAUSE OF THE POSSIBILITY OF DELAYED RESPIRATORY DEPRESSION, MONITORING OF THE PATIENT MUST CONTINUE WELL AFTER SURGERY.

ALFENTA (alfentanil hydrochloride) administered in initial dosages up to 20 µg/kg may cause skeletal muscle rigidity, particularly of the truncal muscles. The incidence and severity of muscle rigidity is usually dose-related. Administration of ALFENTA at anesthetic induction dosages (above 130 µg/kg) will consistently produce muscular rigidity with an immediate onset. The onset of muscular rigidity occurs earlier than with other opioids. ALFENTA may produce muscular rigidity that involves all skeletal muscles, including those of the neck and extremities. The incidence may be reduced by: 1) routine methods of administration of neuromuscular blocking agents for balanced opioid anesthesia; 2) administration of up to ¼ of the full paralyzing dose of a neuromuscular blocking agent just prior to administration of ALFENTA at dosages up to 130 µg/kg; following loss of consciousness, a full paralyzing dose of a neuromuscular blocking agent should be administered; or 3) simultaneous administration of ALFENTA and a full paralyzing dose of a neuromuscular blocking agent when ALFENTA is used in rapidly administered anesthetic dosages (above 130 µg/kg).

The neuromuscular blocking agent used should be appropriate for the patient's cardiovascular status. Adequate facilities should be available for postoperative monitoring and ventilation of patients administered ALFENTA. It is essential that these facilities be fully equipped to handle all degrees of respiratory depression.

PRECAUTIONS

DELAYED RESPIRATORY DEPRESSION, RESPIRATORY ARREST, BRADYCARDIA, ASYSTOLE, ARRHYTHMIAS AND HYPOTENSION HAVE ALSO BEEN REPORTED. THEREFORE, VITAL SIGNS MUST BE MONITORED CONTINUOUSLY.

General: The initial dose of ALFENTA (alfentanil hydrochloride) should be appropriately reduced in elderly and debilitated patients. The effect of the initial dose should be considered in determining supplemental doses. In obese patients (more than 20% above ideal total body weight), the dosage of ALFENTA should be determined on the basis of lean body weight.

In one clinical trial, the dose of ALFENTA required to produce anesthesia, as determined by appearance of delta waves in EEG, was 40% lower in geriatric patients than that needed in healthy young patients.

In patients with compromised liver function and in geriatric patients, the plasma clearance of ALFENTA may be reduced and postoperative recovery may be prolonged.

Induction doses of ALFENTA should be administered slowly (over three minutes). Administration may produce loss of vascular tone and hypotension. Consideration should be given to fluid replacement prior to induction.

Diazepam administered immediately prior to or in conjunction with high doses of ALFENTA may produce vasodilation, hypotension and result in delayed recovery.

Bradycardia produced by ALFENTA may be treated with atropine. Severe bradycardia and asystole have been successfully treated with atropine and conventional resuscitative methods.

The hemodynamic effects of a particular muscle relaxant and the degree of skeletal muscle relaxation required should be considered in the selection of a neuromuscular blocking agent.

Following an anesthetic induction dose of ALFENTA, requirements for volatile inhalation anesthetics or ALFENTA infusion are reduced by 30 to 50% for the first hour of maintenance.

Administration of ALFENTA infusion should be discontinued at least 10–15 minutes prior to the end of surgery.

Respiratory depression caused by opioid analgesics can be reversed by opioid antagonists such as naloxone. Because the duration of respiratory depression produced by ALFENTA may last longer than the duration of the opioid antagonist action, appropriate surveillance should be maintained. As with all potent opioids, profound analgesia is accompanied by respiratory depression and diminished sensitivity to CO_2 stimulation which may persist into or recur in the postoperative period. Intraoperative hyperventilation may further alter postoperative response to CO_2. Appropriate postoperative monitoring should be employed, particularly after infu-

sions and large doses of ALFENTA, to ensure that adequate spontaneous breathing is established and maintained in the absence of stimulation prior to discharging the patient from the recovery area.

Head Injuries: ALFENTA may obscure the clinical course of patients with head injuries.

Impaired Respiration: ALFENTA should be used with caution in patients with pulmonary disease, decreased respiratory reserve or potentially compromised respiration. In such patients, opioids may additionally decrease respiratory drive and increase airway resistance. During anesthesia, this can be managed by assisted or controlled respiration.

Impaired Hepatic or Renal Fuction: In patients with liver or kidney dysfunction, ALFENTA should be administered with caution due to the importance of these organs in the metabolism and excretion of ALFENTA.

Drug Interactions: Both the magnitude and duration of central nervous system and cardiovascular effects may be enhanced when ALFENTA is administered in combination with other CNS depressants such as barbiturates, tranquilizers, opioids, or inhalation general anesthetics. Postoperative respiratory depression may be enhanced or prolonged by these agents. In such cases of combined treatment, the dose of one or both agents should be reduced. Limited clinical experience indicates that requirements for volatile inhalation anesthetics are reduced by 30 to 50% for the first sixty (60) minutes following ALFENTA induction.

The concomitant use of erythromycin with ALFENTA can significantly inhibit ALFENTA clearance and may increase the risk of prolonged or delayed respiratory depression.

Perioperative administration of drugs affecting hepatic blood flow or enzyme function may reduce plasma clearance and prolong recovery.

Carcinogenesis, Mutagenesis and Impairment of Fertility: No long-term animal studies of ALFENTA have been performed to evaluate carcinogenic potential. The micronucleus test in female rats and the dominant lethal test in female and male mice revealed that single intravenous doses of ALFENTA as high as 20 mg/kg (approximately 40 times the upper human dose) produced no structural chromosome mutations or induction of dominant lethal mutations. The Ames *Salmonella typhimurium* metabolic activating test also revealed no mutagenic activity.

Pregnancy Category C: ALFENTA has been shown to have an embryocidal effect in rats and rabbits when given in doses 2.5 times the upper human dose for a period of 10 days to over 30 days. These effects could have been due to maternal toxicity (decreased food consumption with increased mortality) following prolonged administration of the drug.

No evidence of teratogenic effects has been observed after administration of ALFENTA in rats or rabbits.

There are no adequate and well-controlled studies in pregnant women. ALFENTA should be used during pregnancy only if the potential benefit justifies the potential risk to the fetus.

Labor and Delivery: There are insufficient data to support the use of ALFENTA in labor and delivery. Placental transfer of the drug has been reported; therefore, use in labor and delivery is not recommended.

Nursing Mothers: In one study of nine women undergoing post-partum tubal ligation, significant levels of ALFENTA were detected in colostrum four hours after adminstration of 60 µg/kg of ALFENTA, with no detectable levels present after 28 hours. Caution should be exercised when ALFENTA is administered to a nursing woman.

Pediatric Use: Adequate data to support the use of ALFENTA in children under 12 years of age are not presently available.

ADVERSE REACTIONS

The most common adverse reactions, respiratory depression and skeletal muscle rigidity, are extensions of known pharmacological effects of opioids. See CLINICAL PHARMACOLOGY, WARNINGS and PRECAUTIONS on the management of respiratory depression and skeletal muscle rigidity.

Delayed respiratory depression, respiratory arrest, bradycardia, asystole, arrhythmias and hypotension have also been reported.

The reported incidences of adverse reactions listed in the following table are derived from controlled and open clinical trials involving 1183 patients, of whom 785 received ALFENTA. The controlled trials involved treatment comparisons with fentanyl, thiopental sodium, enflurane, saline placebo and halothane. Incidences are based on disturbing and nondisturbing adverse reactions reported. The comparative incidence of certain side effects is influenced by the type of use, e.g., chest wall rigidity has a higher reported incidence in clinical trials of alfentanil induction, and by the type of surgery, e.g., nausea and vomiting have a higher incidence in patients undergoing gynecologic surgery.
[See table on next page.]

Continued on next page

Janssen Pharmaceutica—Cont.

In addition, other adverse reactions less frequently reported (1% or less) were:
Laryngospasm, bronchospasm, postoperative confusion, headache, shivering, postoperative euphoria, hypercarbia, pain on injection, urticaria, and itching.
Some degree of skeletal muscle rigidity should be expected with induction doses of ALFENTA.

DRUG ABUSE AND DEPENDENCE

ALFENTA (alfentanil hydrochloride) is a Schedule II controlled drug substance that can produce drug dependence of the morphine type and therefore has the potential for being abused.

OVERDOSAGE

Overdosage would be manifested by extension of the pharmacological actions of ALFENTA (alfentanil hydrochloride) (see CLINICAL PHARMACOLOGY) as with other potent opioid analgesics. No experience of overdosage with ALFENTA was reported during clinical trials. The intravenous LD_{50} of ALFENTA is 43.0–50.9 mg/kg in rats, 72.2–73.6 mg/kg in mice, 71.8–81.9 mg/kg in guinea pigs and 59.5–87.5 mg/kg in dogs. Intravenous administration of an opioid antagonist such as naloxone should be employed as a specific antidote to manage respiratory depression.

The duration of respiratory depression following overdosage with ALFENTA may be longer than the duration of action of the opioid antagonist. Administration of an opioid antagonist should not preclude immediate establishment of a patent airway, administration of oxygen, and assisted or controlled ventilation as indicated for hypoventilation or apnea. If respiratory depression is associated with muscular rigidity, a neuromuscular blocking agent may be required to facilitate assisted or controlled ventilation. Intravenous fluids and vasoactive agents may be required to manage hemodynamic instability.

DOSAGE AND ADMINISTRATION

The dosage of ALFENTA (alfentanil hydrochloride) should be individualized in each patient according to body weight, physical status, underlying pathological condition, use of other drugs, and type and duration of surgical procedure and anesthesia. In obese patients (more than 20% above ideal total body weight), the dosage of ALFENTA should be determined on the basis of lean body weight. The dose of ALFENTA should be reduced in elderly or debilitated patients (see PRECAUTIONS).
Vital signs should be monitored routinely.

See Dosage Chart for the use of ALFENTA: 1) by incremental injection as an analgesic adjunct to anesthesia with barbiturate/nitrous oxide/oxygen for short surgical procedures (expected duration of less than one hour); 2) by continuous infusion as a maintenance analgesic with nitrous oxide/oxygen for general surgical procedures; and 3) by intravenous injection in anesthetic doses for the induction of anesthesia for general surgical procedures with a minimum expected duration of 45 minutes.

Usage in Children: Clinical data to support the use of ALFENTA in patients under 12 years of age are not presently available. Therefore, such use is not recommended.
Premedication: The selection of preanesthetic medications should be based upon the needs of the individual patient.
Neuromuscular Blocking Agents: The neuromuscular blocking agent selected should be compatible with the patient's condition, taking into account the hemodynamic effects of a particular muscle relaxant and the degree of skeletal muscle relaxation required (see CLINICAL PHARMACOLOGY, WARNINGS and PRECAUTIONS sections).

In patients administered anesthetic (induction) dosages of ALFENTA, it is essential that qualified personnel and adequate facilities are available for the management of intraoperative and postoperative respiratory depression.
Also see WARNINGS and PRECAUTIONS sections.

For purposes of administering small volumes of ALFENTA accurately, the use of a tuberculin syringe or equivalent is recommended.

The physical and chemical compatibility of ALFENTA have been demonstrated in solution with normal saline, 5% dextrose in normal saline, 5% dextrose in water and Lactated Ringers. Clinical studies of ALFENTA infusion have been conducted with ALFENTA diluted to a concentration range of 25 μg/ml to 80 μg/ml.

As an example of the preparation of ALFENTA for infusion, 20 ml of ALFENTA added to 230 ml of diluent provides a 40 μg/ml solution of ALFENTA.

Parenteral drug products should be inspected visually for particulate matter and discoloration prior to administration, whenever solution and container permit.

[See second table above.]

	ALFENTA (N = 785) %	Fentanyl (N = 243) %	Thiopental Sodium (N = 66) %	Enflurane (N = 55) %	Halothane (N = 18) %	Saline Placebo* (N = 18) %
Gastrointestinal						
Nausea	28	44	14	5	0	22
Vomiting	18	31	11	9	13	17
Cardiovascular						
Bradycardia	14	7	8	0	0	0
Tachycardia	12	12	39	36	31	11
Hypotension	10	8	7	7	0	0
Hypertension	18	13	30	20	6	0
Arrhythmia	2	2	5	4	6	0
Musculoskeletal						
Chest Wall Rigidity	17	12	0	0	0	0
Skeletal Muscle Movements	6	2	6	2	0	0
Respiratory						
Apnea	7	0	0	0	0	0
Postoperative Respiratory Depression	2	2	0	0	0	0
CNS						
Dizziness	3	5	0	0	0	0
Sleepiness/ Postoperative Sedation	2	8	2	0	0	6
Blurred Vision	2	2	0	0	0	0

* From two clinical trials, one involving supplemented balanced barbiturate/nitrous oxide anesthesia and one in healthy volunteers who did not undergo surgery.

DOSAGE RANGE CHART

Indication	Approximate Duration of Anesthesia	Induction Period (Initial Dose)	Maintenance Period (Increments/ Infusion)	Total Dose	Effects
Incremental Injection	≤ 30 mins	8–20 μg/kg	3–5 μg/kg or 0.5–1 μg/kg/min	8–40 μg/kg	Spontaneously breathing or assisted ventilation when required.
Incremental Injection	30–60 mins	20–50 μg/kg	5–15 μg/kg	up to 75 μg/kg	Assisted or controlled ventilation required. Attenuation of response to laryngoscopy and intubation.
Continuous Infusion **See Guidelines Below**	> 45 mins	50–75 μg/kg	0.5–3.0 μg/kg/min Average Infusion Rate 1–1.5 μg/kg/min	dependent on duration of procedure	Assisted or controlled ventilation required. Some attenuation of response to intubation and incision, with intraoperative stability.
Anesthetic Induction	> 45 mins	130–245 μg/kg	0.5 to 1.5 μg/kg/min or general anesthetic	dependent on duration of procedure	Assisted or controlled ventilation required. Administer slowly (over three minutes). Concentration of inhalation agents reduced by 30–50% for initial hour.

INFUSION DOSAGE

Continuous Infusion: 0.5–3.0 μg/kg/min administered with nitrous oxide/oxygen in patients undergoing general surgery. Following an anesthetic induction dose of ALFENTA, infusion rate requirements are reduced by 30–50% for the first hour of maintenance.

Changes in vital signs that indicate a response to surgical stress or lightening of anesthesia may be controlled by increasing the rate up to a maximum of 4.0 μg/kg/min and/or administration of bolus doses of 7 μg/kg. If changes are not controlled after three bolus doses given over a five minute period, a barbiturate, vasodilator, and/or inhalation agent should be used. Infusion rates should always be adjusted downward in the absence of these signs until there is some response to surgical stimulation.

Rather than an increase in infusion rate, 7 μg/kg bolus doses of ALFENTA or a potent inhalation agent should be administered in response to signs of lightening of anesthesia within the last 15 minutes of surgery. Administration of ALFENTA infusion should be discontinued at least 10–15 minutes prior to the end of surgery.

HOW SUPPLIED

Each ml of ALFENTA (alfentanil hydrochloride) Injection for intravenous use contains alfentanil hydrochloride equiv-

alent to 500 μg of alfentanil base. ALFENTA Injection is available as:
NDC 50458-060-02, 2 ml ampoules in packages of 10
NDC 50458-060-05, 5 ml ampoules in packages of 10
NDC 50458-060-10, 10 ml ampoules in packages of 5
NDC 50458-060-20, 20 ml ampoules in packages of 5
Protect from light. Store at room temperature 15°–30°C (59°–86°F).
U.S. Patent No. 4,167,574
March, 1987, April 1988
JANSSEN PHARMACEUTICA INC.
Titusville, NJ 08560-0200
Shown in Product Identification Section, page 412

DURAGESIC™   ℂ ℞
[dūr-a-jē 'sik]
(fentanyl transdermal system)

WARNING: May be habit forming.

DESCRIPTION

DURAGESIC is a transdermal system providing continuous systemic delivery of fentanyl, a potent opioid analgesic, for 72 hours. The chemical name is N-phenyl-N-(1-2-phenylethyl-4-piperidyl) propanamide.
The molecular weight of fentanyl base is 336.5, and the empirical formula is $C_{29}H_{28}N_2O$. The n-octanol:water partition coefficient is 860:1. The pKa is 8.4

System Components and Structure

The amount of fentanyl released from each system per hour is proportional to the surface area (25 μg/h per 10 cm^2). The composition per unit area of all system sizes is identical. Each system also contains 0.1 mL of alcohol USP per 10 cm^2.

Dose* (μg/h)	Size (cm^2)	Fentanyl Content (mg)
25	10	2.5
50**	20	5
75**	30	7.5
100**	40	10

*Nominal delivery rate per hour

**FOR USE ONLY IN OPIOID TOLERANT PATIENTS

DURAGESIC is a rectangular transparent unit comprising a protective liner and four functional layers. Proceeding from the outer surface toward the surface adhering to skin, these layers are:
1) a backing layer of polyester film; 2) a drug reservoir of fentanyl and alcohol USP gelled with hydroxyethyl cellulose; 3) an ethylene-vinyl acetate copolymer membrane that controls the rate of fentanyl delivery to the skin surface; and 4) a fentanyl containing silicone adhesive. Before use, a protective liner covering the adhesive layer is removed and discarded.

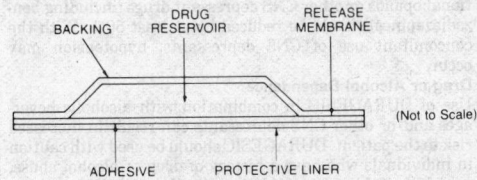

The active component of the system is fentanyl. The remaining components are pharmacologically inactive. Less than 0.2 mL of alcohol is also released from the system during use.

CLINICAL PHARMACOLOGY

Pharmacology

Fentanyl is an opioid analgesic. Fentanyl interacts predominately with the opioid μ-receptor. These μ-binding sites are discretely distributed in the human brain, spinal cord, and other tissues.

In clinical settings, fentanyl exerts its principal pharmacologic effects on the central nervous system. Its primary actions of therapeutic value are analgesia and sedation. Fentanyl may increase the patient's tolerance for pain and decrease the perception of suffering, although the presence of the pain itself may still be recognized.

In addition to analgesia, alterations in mood, euphoria and dysphoria, and drowsiness commonly occur. Fentanyl depresses the respiratory centers, depresses the cough reflex, and constricts the pupils. Analgesic blood levels of fentanyl may cause nausea and vomiting directly by stimulating the chemoreceptor trigger zone, but nausea and vomiting are significantly more common in ambulatory than in recumbent patients, as is postural syncope.

Opioids increase the tone and decrease the propulsive contractions of the smooth muscle of the gastrointestinal tract. The resultant prolongation in gastrointestinal transit time may be responsible for the constipating effect of fentanyl. Because opioids may increase biliary tract pressure, some patients with biliary colic may experience worsening rather than relief of pain.

While opioids generally increase the tone of urinary tract smooth muscle, the net effect tends to be variable, in some cases producing urinary urgency, in others, difficulty in urination.

At therapeutic dosages, fentanyl usually does not exert major effects on the cardiovascular system. However, some patients may exhibit orthostatic hypotension and fainting.

Histamine assays and skin wheal testing in man indicate that clinically significant histamine release rarely occurs with fentanyl administration. Assays in man show no clinically significant histamine release in dosages up to 50 μg/kg.

Pharmacokinetics (see table and graph)

DURAGESIC releases fentanyl from the reservoir at a nearly constant amount per unit time. The concentration gradient existing between the saturated solution of drug in the reservoir and the lower concentration in the skin drives drug release. Fentanyl moves in the direction of the lower concentration at a rate determined by the copolymer release membrane and the diffusion of fentanyl through the skin layers. While the actual rate of fentanyl delivery to the skin varies over the 72 hour application period, each system is labeled with a nominal flux which represents the average amount of drug delivered to the systemic circulation per hour across average skin.

While there is variation in dose delivered among patients, the nominal flux of the systems (25, 50, 75, and 100 μg of fentanyl per hour) are sufficiently accurate as to allow individual titration of dosage for a given patient. The small amount of alcohol which has been incorporated into the system enhances the rate of drug flux through the rate-limiting copolymer membrane and increases the permeability of the skin to fentanyl.

Following initial DURAGESIC application, the skin under the system absorbs fentanyl, and a depot of fentanyl concentrates in the upper skin layers. Fentanyl then becomes available to the systemic circulation. Serum fentanyl concentrations increase gradually following DURAGESIC application, generally leveling off between 12 and 24 hours and remaining relatively constant, with some fluctuation, for the remainder of the 72 hour application period. Peak serum levels of fentanyl generally occurred between 24 and 72 hours after a single application. Serum fentanyl concentrations achieved are proportional to the DURAGESIC delivery rate. After several sequential 72-hour applications, patients reach a steady state serum concentration that is determined by individual variation in skin permeability and body clearance of fentanyl (see graph and Table A).

After system removal, serum fentanyl concentrations decline gradually, falling about 50% in approximately 17 (range 13–22) hours. Continued absorption of fentanyl from the skin accounts for a slower disappearance of the drug from the serum than is seen after an IV infusion, where the apparent half-life ranges from 3–12 hours.

[See graph below.]
[See table above.]

Fentanyl plasma protein binding capacity increases with increasing ionization of the drug. Alterations in pH may affect its distribution between plasma and the central nervous system. Fentanyl accumulates in the skeletal muscle and fat and is released slowly into the blood.

The average volume of distribution for fentanyl is 6 L/kg (range 3–8, N=8). The average clearance in patients undergoing various surgical procedures is 46 L/h (range 27–75, N=8). The kinetics of fentanyl in geriatric patients has not been well studied, but in geriatric patients the clearance of IV fentanyl may be reduced and the terminal half-life greatly prolonged (see PRECAUTIONS).

Fentanyl is metabolized primarily in the liver. In humans the drug appears to be metabolized primarily by N-dealkylation to norfentanyl and other inactive metabolites that do not contribute materially to the observed activity of the drug. Within 72 hours of IV fentanyl administration, approximately 75% of the dose is excreted in urine, mostly as metabolites with less than 10% representing unchanged drug. Approximately 9% of the dose is recovered in the feces, primarily as metabolites. Mean values for unbound fractions of fentanyl in plasma are estimated to be between 13 and 21%. Skin does not appear to metabolize fentanyl delivered transdermally. This was determined in a human keratinocyte cell assay and in clinical studies in which 92% of the dose delivered from the system was accounted for as unchanged fentanyl that appeared in the systemic circulation.

Pharmacodynamics

Analgesia

DURAGESIC is a strong opioid analgesic. The approximate analgesic potency of transdermally administered fentanyl to parenteral morphine ranges from 1:20 to 1:30 in non opioid-tolerant patients in acute pain.

TABLE A
RANGE OF PHARMACOKINETIC PARAMETERS OF FENTANYL IN PATIENTS

	Clearance (L/h) Range (70 kg)	Volume of Distribution V_{SS} (L/kg) Range	Half Life $t_{1/2}$ (h) Range	Maximal Concentration C_{max} (ng/mL) Range	Time to Maximal Concentration (h) Range
IV Fentanyl					
Surgical Patients	27–75	3–8	3–12		
Hepatically Impaired Patients	3–80†	0.8–8†	4–12†		
Renally Impaired Patients	30–78				
DURAGESIC 25 μg/h			*	0.3–1.2	26–78
DURAGESIC 50 μg/h			*	0.6–1.8†	24–72†
DURAGESIC 75 μg/h			*	1.1–2.6	24–48
DURAGESIC 100 μg/h			*	1.9–3.8	25–72

†Estimated
* After system removal there is continued systemic absorption from residual fentanyl in the skin so that serum concentrations fall 50%, on average, in 17 hours.

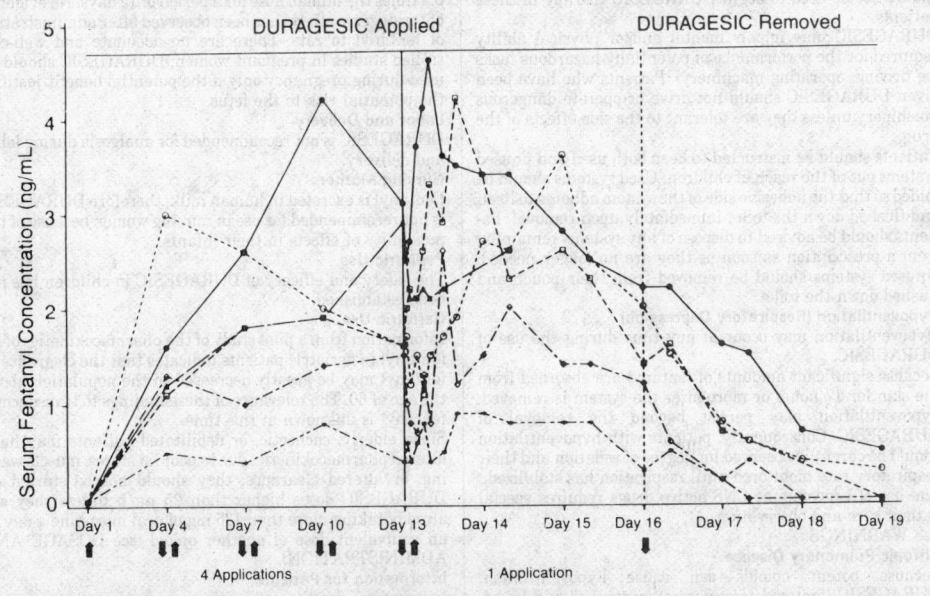

Serum Fentanyl Concentrations Following Multiple Applications of DURAGESIC 100 μg/h

Continued on next page

Janssen Pharmaceutica—Cont.

Minimum effective analgesic serum concentrations of fentanyl in opioid naive patients range from 0.2 to 1.2 ng/mL; side effects increase in frequency at serum levels above 2 ng/mL. Both the minimum effective concentration and the concentration at which toxicity occurs rise with increasing tolerance. The rate of development of tolerance varies widely among individuals.

Respiratory Effects
At equivalent analgesic serum concentrations, fentanyl and morphine produce a similar degree of hypoventilation. A small number of patients have experienced clinically significant hypoventilation with DURAGESIC. Hypoventilation was manifest by respiratory rates of less than 8 breaths/minute or a pCO_2 greater than 55 mm Hg. In clinical trials of 357 nontolerant patients using DURAGESIC, 13 patients experienced hypoventilation. As a consequence, 10 of 13 nontolerant patients received naloxone, two patients had their dose reduced and one patient required no treatment beyond verbal stimulation. Of the 13 events, seven were associated with DURAGESIC 100 μg/h and six were associated with DURAGESIC 75 μg/h. The incidence of hypoventilation was higher in nontolerant women (10) than in men (3) and in patients weighing less than 63 kg (9 of 13). Although patients with impaired respiration were not common in the trials, they had higher rates of hypoventilation.

While most patients using DURAGESIC chronically develop tolerance to fentanyl induced hypoventilation, episodes of slowed respirations may occur at any time during therapy; medical intervention generally was not required in these instances.

Hypoventilation can occur throughout the therapeutic range of fentanyl serum concentrations. However, the risk of hypoventilation increases at serum fentanyl concentrations greater than 2 ng/mL in non opioid-tolerant patients, especially for patients who have an underlying pulmonary condition or who receive usual doses of opioids or other CNS drugs associated with hypoventilation in addition to DURAGESIC. The use of DURAGESIC should be monitored by clinical evaluation. As with other drug level measurements, serum fentanyl concentrations may be useful clinically, although they do not reflect patient sensitivity to fentanyl and should not be used by physicians as a sole indicator of effectiveness or toxicity.

See WARNINGS, PRECAUTIONS, and OVERDOSAGE for additional information on hypoventilation.

Cardiovascular Effects
Intravenous fentanyl may infrequently produce bradycardia. The incidence of bradycardia in clinical trials with DURAGESIC was less than 1%.

CNS Effects
In opioid naive patients, central nervous system effects increase when serum fentanyl concentrations are greater than 3 ng/mL.

CLINICAL TRIALS
DURAGESIC was studied in patients with acute and chronic pain (postoperative and cancer pain models).

The analgesic efficacy of DURAGESIC was demonstrated in an acute pain model with surgical procedures expected to produce various intensities of pain (eg hysterectomy, major orthopedic surgery). Clinical use and safety was evaluated in patients experiencing chronic pain due to malignancy. Based on the results of these trials, DURAGESIC was determined to be effective in both populations, but safe only for use in opioid tolerant patients. Because of the risk of hypoventilation (4% incidence) in non opioid-tolerant patients, DURAGESIC should not be used for postoperative analgesia (see PRECAUTIONS).

DURAGESIC as therapy for pain due to cancer has been studied in 153 patients. In this patient population, DURAGESIC has been administered in doses of 25 μg/h to 600 μg/h. Individual patients have used DURAGESIC continuously for up to 866 days. At one month after initiation of DURAGESIC therapy, patients generally reported lower pain intensity scores as compared to a prestudy analgesic regimen of oral morphine (see graph [See next column]).

INDICATIONS AND USAGE
DURAGESIC is indicated in the management of chronic pain in patients requiring opioid analgesia.

DURAGESIC is not recommended in the management of postoperative pain because it has not been adequately studied in these patients and because of the interpatient variability in absorption and disposition of fentanyl seen in the controlled clinical trials. Based on the information available, it is not possible to identify factors to be used to select a dose which will be safe and effective in individual postoperative patients.

In patients with chronic pain, it is possible to individually titrate the dose of the transdermal system to minimize the risk of adverse effects while providing analgesia. For the

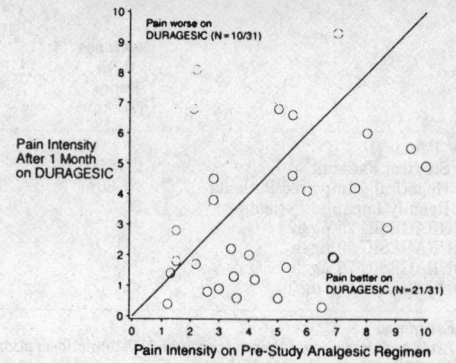

Visual Analogue Score of Pain Intensity Ratings at Entry in the Study and After One Month of DURAGESIC Use

majority of these patients DURAGESIC is a safe and effective alternative to other opioid regimens (See DOSAGE AND ADMINISTRATION).

CONTRAINDICATIONS
DURAGESIC is contraindicated in patients with known hypersensitivity to fentanyl or adhesives.

WARNINGS
PATIENTS WHO HAVE EXPERIENCED ADVERSE EVENTS SHOULD BE MONITORED FOR AT LEAST 12 HOURS AFTER DURAGESIC REMOVAL SINCE SERUM FENTANYL CONCENTRATIONS DECLINE GRADUALLY AND REACH AN APPROXIMATE 50% REDUCTION IN SERUM CONCENTRATIONS 17 HOURS AFTER SYSTEM REMOVAL.

DURAGESIC SHOULD BE PRESCRIBED ONLY BY PERSONS KNOWLEDGEABLE IN THE CONTINUOUS ADMINISTRATION OF POTENT OPIOIDS, IN THE MANAGEMENT OF PATIENTS RECEIVING POTENT OPIOIDS FOR TREATMENT OF PAIN, AND IN THE DETECTION AND MANAGEMENT OF HYPOVENTILATION INCLUDING THE USE OF OPIOID ANTAGONISTS.

THE CONCOMITANT USE OF OTHER CENTRAL NERVOUS SYSTEM DEPRESSANTS, INCLUDING OTHER OPIOIDS, SEDATIVES OR HYPNOTICS, GENERAL ANESTHETICS, PHENOTHIAZINES, TRANQUILIZERS, SKELETAL MUSCLE RELAXANTS, SEDATING ANTIHISTAMINES, AND ALCOHOLIC BEVERAGES MAY PRODUCE ADDITIVE DEPRESSANT EFFECTS. HYPOVENTILATION, HYPOTENSION AND PROFOUND SEDATION OR COMA MAY OCCUR. WHEN SUCH COMBINED THERAPY IS CONTEMPLATED, THE DOSE OF ONE OR BOTH AGENTS SHOULD BE REDUCED BY AT LEAST 50%.

PRECAUTIONS
General
DURAGESIC doses greater than 25 μg/h are too high for initiation of therapy in non opioid-tolerant patients and should not be used to begin DURAGESIC therapy in these patients.

DURAGESIC may impair mental and/or physical ability required for the performance of potentially hazardous tasks (eg driving, operating machinery). Patients who have been given DURAGESIC should not drive or operate dangerous machinery unless they are tolerant to the side effects of the drug.

Patients should be instructed to keep both used and unused systems out of the reach of children. Used systems should be folded so that the adhesive side of the system adheres to itself and flushed down the toilet immediately upon removal. Patients should be advised to dispose of any systems remaining from a prescription as soon as they are no longer needed. Unused systems should be removed from their pouch and flushed down the toilet.

Hypoventilation (Respiratory Depression)
Hypoventilation may occur at any time during the use of DURAGESIC.

Because significant amounts of fentanyl are absorbed from the skin for 17 hours or more after the system is removed, hypoventilation may persist beyond the removal of DURAGESIC. Consequently, patients with hypoventilation should be carefully observed for degree of sedation and their respiratory rate monitored until respiration has stabilized. The use of concomitant CNS active drugs requires special patient care and observation.

See WARNINGS.

Chronic Pulmonary Disease
Because potent opioids can cause hypoventilation, DURAGESIC (fentanyl transdermal system) should be administered with caution to patients with preexisting medical conditions predisposing them to hypoventilation. In such patients, normal analgesic doses of opioids may further decrease respiratory drive to the point of respiratory failure.

Head Injuries and Increased Intracranial Pressure
DURAGESIC should not be used in patients who may be particularly susceptible to the intracranial effects of CO_2 retention such as those with evidence of increased intracranial pressure, impaired consciousness, or coma. Opioids may obscure the clinical course of patients with head injury. DURAGESIC should be used with caution in patients with brain tumors.

Cardiac Disease
Intravenous fentanyl may produce bradycardia. Fentanyl should be administered with caution to patients with bradyarrhythmias.

Hepatic or Renal Disease
At the present time insufficient information exists to make recommendations regarding the use of DURAGESIC in patients with impaired renal or hepatic function. If the drug is used in these patients, it should be used with caution because of the hepatic metabolism and renal excretion of fentanyl.

Patients with Fever
Based on a pharmacokinetic model, serum fentanyl concentrations could theoretically increase by approximately one third for patients with a body temperature of 40°C (102°F) due to temperature-dependent increases in fentanyl release from the system and increased skin permeability. Therefore, patients wearing DURAGESIC systems who develop fever should be monitored for opioid side effects and the DURAGESIC dose should be adjusted if necessary.

Central Nervous System Depressants
When patients are receiving DURAGESIC, the dose of additional opioids or other CNS depressant drugs (including benzodiazepines) should be reduced by at least 50%. With the concomitant use of CNS depressants, hypotension may occur.

Drug or Alcohol Dependence
Use of DURAGESIC in combination with alcoholic beverages and/or other CNS depressants can result in increased risk to the patient. DURAGESIC should be used with caution in individuals who have a history of drug or alcohol abuse, especially if they are outside a medically controlled environment.

Ambulatory Patients
Strong opioid analgesics impair the mental or physical abilities required for the performance of potentially dangerous tasks such as driving a car or operating machinery. Patients who have been given DURAGESIC should not drive or operate dangerous machinery unless they are tolerant to the effects of the drug.

Carcinogenesis, Mutagenesis, and Impairment of Fertility
Because long-term animal studies have not been conducted, the potential carcinogenic effects of DURAGESIC are unknown. There was no evidence of mutagenicity in the Ames Salmonella mutagenicity assay, the primary rat hepatocyte unscheduled DNA synthesis assay, the BALB/c-3T3 transformation test, and the human lymphocyte and CHO chromosomal aberration in-vitro assays.

In the mouse lymphoma assay, fentanyl concentrations 2000 times greater than those seen with chronic DURAGESIC use were only mutagenic in the presence of metabolic activation.

Pregnancy —Pregnancy Category C
Fentanyl has been shown to impair fertility and to have an embryocidal effect in rats when given in intravenous doses 0.3 times the human dose for a period of 12 days. No evidence of teratogenic effects has been observed after administration of fentanyl to rats. There are no adequate and well-controlled studies in pregnant women. DURAGESIC should be used during pregnancy only if the potential benefit justifies the potential risk to the fetus.

Labor and Delivery
DURAGESIC is not recommended for analgesia during labor and delivery.

Nursing Mothers
Fentanyl is excreted in human milk; therefore DURAGESIC is not recommended for use in nursing women because of the possibility of effects in their infants.

Pediatric Use
The safety and efficacy of DURAGESIC in children has not been established.

Geriatric Use
Information from a pilot study of the pharmacokinetics of IV fentanyl in geriatric patients indicates that the clearance of fentanyl may be greatly decreased in the population above the age of 60. The relevance of these findings to transdermal fentanyl is unknown at this time.

Since elderly, cachectic, or debilitated patients may have altered pharmacokinetics due to poor fat stores, muscle wasting, or altered clearance, they should not be started on DURAGESIC doses higher than 25 μg/h unless they are already taking more than 135 mg of oral morphine a day or an equivalent dose of another opioid (see DOSAGE AND ADMINISTRATION).

Information for Patients
Instructions for the application, removal, and disposal of DURAGESIC are provided in each carton.

Disposal of DURAGESIC
DURAGESIC should be kept out of the reach of children. DURAGESIC systems should be folded so that the adhesive

side of the system adheres to itself, then the system should be flushed down the toilet immediately upon removal. Patients should dispose of any systems remaining from a prescription as soon as they are no longer needed. Unused systems should be removed from their pouch and flushed down the toilet. If the gel from the drug reservoir accidentally contacts the skin, the area should be washed with clear water.

ADVERSE REACTIONS

The safety of DURAGESIC has been evaluated in 357 postoperative patients and 153 cancer patients for a total of 510 patients. Patients with acute pain used DURAGESIC for 1 to 3 days. The duration of DURAGESIC use varied in cancer patients; 56% of patients used DURAGESIC for over 30 days, 28% continued treatment for more than 4 months, and 10% used DURAGESIC for more than 1 year.

Hypoventilation was the most serious adverse reaction observed in 13 (4%) postoperative patients and in 3 (2%) of the cancer patients. Hypotension and hypertension were observed in 11 (3%) and 4 (1%) of the opioid-naive patients.

Various adverse events were reported; a causal relationship to DURAGESIC was not always determined. The frequencies presented here reflect the actual frequency of each adverse effect in patients who received DURAGESIC. There has been no attempt to correct for a placebo effect, concomitant use of other opioids, or to subtract the frequencies reported by placebo-treated patients in controlled trials.

The following adverse reactions were reported in 153 cancer patients at a frequency of 1% or greater; similar reactions were seen in the 357 postoperative patients studied.

Body as a Whole: abdominal pain*, headache*

Cardiovascular: arrhythmia, chest pain

Digestive: nausea**, vomiting**, constipation**, dry mouth**, anorexia*, diarrhea*, dyspepsia*, flatulence

Nervous: somnolence**, confusion**, asthenia**, dizziness*, nervousness*, hallucinations*, anxiety*, depression*, euphoria*, tremor, abnormal coordination, speech disorder, abnormal thinking, abnormal gait, abnormal dreams, agitation, paresthesia, amnesia, syncope, paranoid reaction

Respiratory: dyspnea*, hypoventilation*, apnea*, hemoptysis, pharyngitis, hiccups

Skin and Appendages: sweating**, pruritus*, rash, application site reaction - erythema, papules, itching, edema

Urogenital: urinary retention*

The following adverse effects have been reported in less than 1% of the 510 postoperative and cancer patients studied; the association between these events and DURAGESIC administration is unknown. This information is listed to serve as alerting information for the physician.

Digestive: abdominal distention

Nervous: aphasia, hypertonia, vertigo, stupor, hypotonia, depersonalization, hostility

Respiratory: stertorous breathing, asthma, respiratory disorder

Skin and Appendages, General: exfoliative dermatitis, pustules

Special Senses: amblyopia

Urogenital: bladder pain, oliguria, urinary frequency

DRUG ABUSE AND DEPENDENCE

Fentanyl is a Schedule II controlled substance and can produce drug dependence similar to that produced by morphine. DURAGESIC therefore has the potential for abuse. Tolerance, physical and psychological dependence may develop upon repeated administration of opioids. Iatrogenic addiction following opioid administration is relatively rare. Physicians should not let concerns of physical dependence deter them from using adequate amounts of opioids in the management of severe pain when such use is indicated.

OVERDOSAGE

Clinical Presentation

The manifestations of fentanyl overdosage are an extension of its pharmacologic actions with the most serious significant effect being hypoventilation.

Treatment

For the management of hypoventilation immediate countermeasures include removing the DURAGESIC system and physically or verbally stimulating the patient. These actions can be followed by administration of a specific narcotic antagonist such as naloxone. The duration of hypoventilation following an overdose may be longer than the effects of the narcotic antagonist's action (the half-life of naloxone ranges from 30 to 81 minutes). The interval between IV antagonist doses should be carefully chosen because of the possibility of re-narcotization after system removal; repeated administration of naloxone may be necessary. Reversal of the narcotic effect may result in acute onset of pain and the release of catecholamines.

If the clinical situation warrants, ensure a patent airway is established and maintained, administer oxygen and assist or control respiration as indicated and use an oropharyngeal airway or endotracheal tube if necessary. Adequate body temperature and fluid intake should be maintained.

*Reactions occurring in 3%–10% of DURAGESIC patients

**Reactions occurring in 10% or more of DURAGESIC patients

If severe or persistent hypotension occurs, the possibility of hypovolemia should be considered and managed with appropriate parenteral fluid therapy.

DOSAGE AND ADMINISTRATION

As with all opioids, dosage should be individualized. The most important factor to be considered in determining the appropriate dose is the extent of preexisting opioid tolerance. Initial doses should be reduced in elderly or debilitated patients (see PRECAUTIONS).

DURAGESIC should be applied to non-irritated and non-irradiated skin on a flat surface of the upper torso. Hair at the application site should be clipped (not shaved) prior to system application. If the site of DURAGESIC application must be cleansed prior to application of the system, do so with clear water. Do not use soaps, oils, lotions, alcohol, or any other agents that might irritate the skin or alter its characteristics. Allow the skin to dry completely prior to system application.

DURAGESIC should be applied immediately upon removal from the sealed package. The transdermal system should be pressed firmly in place with the palm of the hand for 10-20 seconds, making sure the contact is complete, especially around the edges.

Each DURAGESIC may be worn continuously for 72 hours. If analgesia for more than 72 hours is required, a new system should be applied to a different skin site after removal of the previous transdermal system.

DURAGESIC should be kept out of the reach of children. Used systems should be folded so that the adhesive side of the system adheres to itself, then the system should be flushed down the toilet immediately upon removal. Patients should dispose of any systems remaining from a prescription as soon as they are no longer needed. Unused systems should be removed from their pouch and flushed down the toilet.

Dose Selection

DOSES MUST BE INDIVIDUALIZED BASED UPON THE STATUS OF EACH PATIENT AND SHOULD BE ASSESSED AT REGULAR INTERVALS AFTER DURAGESIC APPLICATION. REDUCED DOSES OF DURAGESIC ARE SUGGESTED FOR THE ELDERLY AND OTHER GROUPS DISCUSSED IN PRECAUTIONS.

In selecting an initial DURAGESIC dose, attention should be given to 1) the daily dose, potency, and characteristics of the opioid the patient has been taking previously (eg whether it is a pure agonist or mixed agonist-antagonist), 2) the reliability of the relative potency estimates used to calculate the DURAGESIC dose needed (potency estimates may vary with the route of administration), 3) the degree of opioid tolerance, if any, and 4) the general condition and medical status of the patient. Each patient should be maintained at the lowest dose providing acceptable pain control.

Initial DURAGESIC Dose Selection

There has been no systematic evaluation of DURAGESIC as an initial opioid analgesic in the management of chronic pain, since most patients in the clinical trials were converted to DURAGESIC from other narcotics. Therefore, unless the patient has preexisting opioid tolerance, the lowest DURAGESIC dose, 25 μg/h, should be used as the initial dose.

To convert patients from oral or parenteral opioids to DURAGESIC use the following methodology:

1. Calculate the previous 24-hour analgesic requirement.
2. Convert this amount to the equianalgesic oral morphine dose using Table B. [See table above.]
3. Table C displays the range of 24-hour oral and IM morphine doses that are approximately equivalent to each DURAGESIC dose. Use this table to find the calculated 24-hour morphine dose and the corresponding DURAGESIC dose. Initiate DURAGESIC treatment using the recommended dose and titrate patients upwards (no more frequently than every 3 days after the initial dose or than every 6 days thereafter) until analgesic efficacy is attained. For delivery rates in excess of 100 μg/h, multiple systems may be used.

NOTE: The analgesic activity ratio of 10 mg IM morphine to 100 μg IV fentanyl was used to derive the equivalence of morphine to DURAGESIC. A 10 mg IM or 60 mg oral dose of morphine every 4 hours for 24 hours (total of 60 mg/day IM or 360 mg/day orally) was considered approximately equivalent to DURAGESIC 100 μg/h.

The majority of patients are adequately maintained with DURAGESIC administered every 72 hours. A small number of patients may require systems to be applied every 48 hours. Because of the increase in serum fentanyl concentration over the first 24 hours following initial system application, the initial evaluation of the maximum analgesic effect of DURAGESIC cannot be made before 24 hours of wearing. The initial DURAGESIC dosage may be increased after 3 days (see Dose Titration).

During the initial application of DURAGESIC, patients should use short acting analgesics for the first 24 hours as needed until analgesic efficacy with DURAGESIC is attained. Thereafter, some patients still may require periodic supplemental doses of other short-acting analgesics for 'break-through' pain.

TABLE B
EQUIANALGESIC POTENCY CONVERSION

Name	Equianalgesic Dose (mg) IMa	PO
morphine	10	60
Hydromorphone (Dilaudid®)	1.5	7.5
methadone (Dolophine®)	10	20
oxycodone (Percocet®)	15	30
levorphanol (Levo-Dromoran®)	2	4
oxymorphone (Numorphan®)	1	10 (PR)
heroin	5	60
meperidine (Demerol®)	75	—
codeine	130	200

Note: All IM and PO doses in this chart are considered equivalent to 10 mg of IM morphine in analgesic effect. IM denotes intramuscular, PO oral, and PR rectal.

[a] Based on single-dose studies in which an intramuscular dose of each drug listed was compared with morphine to establish the relative potency. Oral doses are those recommended when changing from parenteral to an oral route.

Reference: Foley, K.M. (1985) The treatment of cancer pain. NEJM 313(2):84–95.

TABLE C
DURAGESIC DOSE PRESCRIPTION BASED UPON DAILY MORPHINE EQUIVALENCE DOSE

Oral 24-hour Morphine (mg/day)	IM 24-hour Morphine (mg/day)	DURAGESIC Dose (μg/h)
45–134	8–22	25
135–224	23–37	50
225–314	38–52	75
315–404	53–67	100
405–494	68–82	125
495–584	83–97	150
585–674	98–112	175
675–764	113–127	200
765–854	128–142	225
855–944	143–157	250
945–1034	158–172	275
1035–1124	173–187	300

Dose Titration

The conversion ratio from oral morphine to DURAGESIC is conservative, and 50% of patients are likely to require a dose increase after initial application of DURAGESIC. The initial DURAGESIC dosage may be increased after 3 days, based on the daily dose of supplemental analgesics required by the patient in the second or third day of the initial application. Physicians are advised that it may take up to 6 days after increasing the dose of DURAGESIC for the patient to reach equilibrium on the new dose (see graph in CLINICAL PHARMACOLOGY). Therefore, patients should wear a higher dose through two applications before any further increase in dosage is made on the basis of the average daily use of a supplemental analgesic.

Appropriate dosage increments should be based on the daily dose of supplementary opioids, using the ratio of 90 mg/24 hours of oral morphine to a 25 μg/h increase in DURAGESIC dose.

Discontinuation of DURAGESIC

Some patients will require a change to other methods of opioid administration when the DURAGESIC dose exceeds 300 μg/h. To convert patients to another opioid, remove DURAGESIC and initiate treatment with half the equianalgesic dose of the new opioid 12 to 18 hours later (it takes 17 hours or more for the fentanyl serum concentration to fall by 50% after system removal). Titrate the dose of the new analgesic based upon the patient's report of pain until adequate analgesia has been attained. For patients requiring discontinuation of opioids, a gradual downward titration is recommended since it is not known at what dose level the opioid may be discontinued without producing the signs and symptoms of abrupt withdrawal.

HOW SUPPLIED

DURAGESIC is supplied in cartons containing 5 individually packaged systems. See chart for information regarding individual systems.

Continued on next page

Janssen Pharmaceutica—Cont.

DURAGESIC Dose (μg/h)	System Size (cm^2)	Fentanyl Content (mg)	NDC Number
DURAGESIC-25	10	2.5	50458-033-05
DURAGESIC-50*	20	5	50458-034-05
DURAGESIC-75*	30	7.5	50458-035-05
DURAGESIC-100*	40	10	50458-036-05

*FOR USE ONLY IN OPIOID TOLERANT PATIENTS.

Safety and Handling

DURAGESIC is supplied in sealed transdermal systems which pose little risk of exposure to health care workers. If the gel from the drug reservoir accidentally contacts the skin, the area should be washed with copious amounts of water. Do not use soap, alcohol, or other solvents to remove the gel because they may enhance the drug's ability to penetrate the skin.

Do not store above 86°F (30°C). Apply immediately after removal from individually sealed package.

Do not use if the seal is broken. **For transdermal use only.**

CAUTION: Federal law prohibits dispensing without prescription

DEA order form required. A schedule CII narcotic.

Manufactured by:
ALZA Corporation
Palo Alto, CA 94304
Distributed by:
JANSSEN
PHARMACEUTICA
Titusville, NJ 08560-0200
June 1991, April 1992

Shown in the Product Identification Section, page 412

ERGAMISOL® ℞
(levamisole hydrochloride)
Tablets

DESCRIPTION

ERGAMISOL (levamisole hydrochloride) is an immunomodulator available in tablets for oral administration containing the equivalent of 50 mg as levamisole base. Fifty-nine (59) mg of levamisole HCl is equivalent to 50 mg of levamisole base. Inactive ingredients are colloidal silicon dioxide, hydrogenated vegetable oil, hydroxypropyl methylcellulose, lactose, microcystalline cellulose, polyethylene glycol 6000, polysorbate 80, and talc.

Levamisole hydrochloride is (-)-(S)-2,3,5,6-tetrahydro-6-phenylimidazo [2,1-b] thiazole monohydrochloride.

Levamisole hydrochloride is a white to pale cream colored crystalline powder which is almost odorless and is freely soluble in water. It is quite stable in acid aqueous media but hydrolyzes in alkaline or neutral solutions. It has a molecular weight of 240.75.

CLINICAL PHARMACOLOGY

Two clinical trials having essentially the same design have demonstrated an increase in survival and a reduction in recurrence rate in the subset of patients with resected Dukes' C colon cancer treated with a regimen of ERGAMISOL (levamisole hydrochloride) plus fluorouracil[1,2]. After surgery, patients were randomized to no further therapy, ERGAMISOL alone, or ERGAMISOL plus fluorouracil.

In one clinical trial in which 408 Dukes' B and C colorectal cancer patients were studied, 262 Dukes' C patients were evaluated for a minimum follow-up of five years[1]. A subset analysis of these Dukes' C patients showed the estimated reduction in death rate was 27% for ERGAMISOL plus fluorouracil ($p = 0.11$) and 28% for ERGAMISOL alone ($p = 0.11$)[3]. The estimated reduction in recurrence rate was 36% for ERGAMISOL plus fluorouracil ($p = 0.025$) and 28% for ERGAMISOL alone ($p = 0.11$)[3]. In another clinical trial designed to confirm the above results, 929 Dukes' C colon cancer patients were evaluated for a minimum follow-up of 2 years[2]. The estimated reduction in death rate was 33% for ERGAMISOL plus fluorouracil ($p = 0.006$). The estimated reduction in recurrence rate was 41% for ERGAMISOL plus fluorouracil ($p < 0.0001$). The ERGAMISOL alone group did not show advantage over no treatment on improving recurrence or survival rates. There are presently insufficient data to evaluate the effect of the combination of ERGAMISOL plus fluorouracil in Dukes' B patients. There are also insufficient data to evaluate the effect of ERGAMISOL plus fluorouracil in patients with rectal cancer because only 12 patients with rectal cancer were treated with the combination in the first study and none in the second study.

The mechanism of action of ERGAMISOL in combination with fluorouracil is unknown. The effects of levamisole on the immune system are complex. The drug appears to restore depressed immune function rather than to stimulate response to above-normal levels. Levamisole can stimulate formation of antibodies to various antigens, enhance T-cell responses by stimulating T-cell activation and proliferation, potentiate monocyte and macrophage functions including phagocytosis and chemotaxis, and increase neutrophil mobility, adherence, and chemotaxis. Other drugs have similar short-term effects and the clinical relevance is unclear.

Besides its immunomodulatory function, levamisole has other mammalian pharmacologic activities, including inhibition of alkaline phosphatase, and cholinergic activity.

The pharmacokinetics of ERGAMISOL have not been studied in the dosage regimen recommended with fluorouracil nor in patients with hepatic insufficiency. After administration of a single oral dose of 50 mg of a research formulation of ERGAMISOL, it appears that levamisole is rapidly absorbed from the gastrointestinal tract. Mean peak plasma concentrations of 0.13 mcg/ml are attained within 1.5 to 2 hours. The plasma elimination half-life of levamisole is between 3-4 hours. Following a 150-mg radio-labelled dose, levamisole is extensively metabolized by the liver in humans and the metabolities excreted mainly by the kidneys (70% over 3 days). The elimination half-life of metabolite excretion is 16 hours. Approximately 5% is excreted in the feces. Less than 5% is excreted unchanged in the urine and less than 0.2% in the feces. Approximately 12% is recovered in the urine as the glucuronide of p-hydroxy-levamisole. The clinical significance of these data are unknown since a 150-mg dose may not be proportional to a 50-mg dose.

INDICATIONS AND USAGE

ERGAMISOL (levamisole hydrochloride) is only indicated as adjuvant treatment in combination with fluorouracil after surgical resection in patients with Dukes' stage C colon cancer.

CONTRAINDICATIONS

ERGAMISOL (levamisole hydrochloride) is contraindicated in patients with a known hypersensitivity to the drug or its components.

WARNINGS

ERGAMISOL (levamisole hydrochloride) has been associated with agranulocytosis, sometimes fatal. The onset of agranulocytosis is frequently accompanied by a flu-like syndrome (fever, chills, etc.); however, in a small number of patients it is asymptomatic. A flu-like syndrome may also occur in the absence of agranulocytosis. It is essential that appropriate hematological monitoring be done routinely during therapy with ERGAMISOL and fluorouracil. Neutropenia is usually reversible following discontinuation of therapy. Patients should be instructed to report immediately any flu-like symptoms.

Higher than recommended doses of ERGAMISOL may be associated with an increased incidence of agranulocytosis, so the recommended dose should not be exceeded.

The combination of ERGAMISOL and fluorouracil has been associated with frequent neutropenia, anemia and thrombocytopenia.

PRECAUTIONS

Before beginning this combination adjuvant treatment, the physician should become familiar with the labeling for fluorouracil.

Information for Patients: The patient should be informed that if flu-like symptoms or malaise occurs, the physician should be notified immediately.

Drug Interactions: ERGAMISOL (levamisole hydrochloride) has been reported to produce "ANTABUSE®"-like side effects when given concomitantly with alcohol. Concomitant administration of phenytoin and ERGAMISOL plus fluorouracil has led to increased plasma levels of phenytoin. The physician is advised to monitor plasma levels of phenytoin and to decrease the dose if necessary.

Because of reports of prolongation of the prothrombin time beyond the therapeutic range in patients taking concurrent levamisole and coumarin-like drugs, it is suggested that the prothrombin time be monitored carefully, and the dose of coumarin-like drugs adjusted accordingly, in patients taking both drugs.

Laboratory Tests: On the first day of therapy with ERGAMISOL/fluorouracil, patients should have a CBC with differential and platelets, electrolytes and liver function tests performed. Thereafter, a CBC with differential and platelets should be performed weekly prior to each treatment with fluorouracil with electrolytes and liver function tests peformed every 3 months for a total of one year. Dosage modifications should be instituted as follows: If WBC is 2500-3500/mm^3 defer the fluorouracil dose until WBC is $>$ 3500/mm^3. If WBC is $<$ 2500/mm^3, defer the fluorouracil dose until WBC is $>$ 3500/mm^3; then resume the fluorouracil dose reduced by 20%. If WBC remains $<$ 2500/mm^3 for over 10 days despite deferring fluorouracil, discontinue administration of ERGAMISOL. Both drugs should be deferred unless enough platelets are present ($\geq$ 100,000/mm^3).

Carcinogensis, Mutagenesis, Impairment of Fertility: Adequate animal carcinogenicity studies have not been conducted with levamisole. Studies of levamisole administered in drinking water at 5, 20, and 80 mg/kg/day to mice for up to 18 months or adminstered to rats in the diet at 5, 20, and 80 mg/kg/day for 24 months showed no evidence of neoplastic effects. These studies were not conducted at the maximum tolerated dose, therefore the animals may not have been exposed to a reasonable drug challenge. No mutagenic effects were demonstrated in dominant lethal studies in male and female mice, in an Ames test, and in a study to detect chromosomal aberrations in cultured peripheral human lymphocytes.

Adverse effects were not observed on male or female fertility when levamisole was administered to rats in the diet at doses of 2.5, 10, 40, and 160 mg/kg. In a rat gavage study at doses of 20, 60, and 180 mg/kg, the copulation period was increased, the duration of pregnancy was slightly increased, and fertility, pup viability and weight, lactation index, and number of fetuses were decreased at 60 mg/kg. No negative reproductive effects were present when the offspring were allowed to mate and litter.

Pregnancy: Pregnancy Category C: Teratogenicity studies have been performed in rats and rabbits at oral doses up to 180 mg/kg. Fetal malformations were not observed. In rats, embryotoxicity was present at 160 mg/kg and in rabbits, significant embryotoxicity was observed at 180 mg/kg. There are no adequate and well-controlled studies in pregnant women and ERGAMISOL should not be administered unless the potential benefits outweigh the risks. Women taking the combination of ERGAMISOL and fluorouracil should be advised not to become pregnant.

Nursing Mothers: It is not known whether ERGAMISOL is excreted in human milk; it is excreted in cows' milk. Because of the potential for serious adverse reactions in nursing infants from ERGAMISOL, a decision should be made whether to discontinue nursing or to discontinue the drug, taking into account the importance of the drug to the mother.

Pediatric Use: Safety and effectiveness of ERGAMISOL in children have not been established.

ADVERSE REACTIONS

Almost all patients receiving ERGAMISOL (levamisole hydrochloride) and fluorouracil reported adverse experiences. Tabulated below is the incidence of adverse experiences that occurred in at least 1% of patients enrolled in two clinical trials who were adjuvantly treated with either ERGAMISOL or ERGAMISOL plus fluorouracil following colon surgery. In the larger clinical trial, 66 of 463 patients (14%) discontinued the combination of ERGAMISOL plus fluorouracil because of adverse reactions. Forty-three of these patients (9%) developed isolated or a combination of gastrointestinal toxicities. (e.g., nausea, vomiting, diarrhea, stomatitis and anorexia). Ten patients developed rash and/or pruritus. Five patients discontinued therapy because of flu-like symptoms or fever with chills; ten patients developed central nervous system symptoms such as dizziness, ataxia, depression, confusion, memory loss, weakness, inability to concentrate, and headache; two patients developed reversible neutropenia and sepsis; one patient because of thrombocytopenia; one patient because of hyperbilirubinemia. One patient in the ERGAMISOL plus fluorouracil group developed agranulocytosis and sepsis and died.

In the ERGAMISOL alone arm of the trial, 15 of 310 patients (4.8%) discontinued therapy because of adverse experiences. Six of these (2%) discontinued because of rash, six because of arthralgia/myalgia, and one each for fever and neutropenia, urinary infection, and cough.

[See table on next page.]

In worldwide experience with ERGAMISOL, less frequent adverse experiences included exfoliative dermatitis, periorbital edema, vaginal bleeding, anaphylaxis, confusion, convulsions, hallucinations, impaired concentration, renal failure, hyperlipidemia, elevated serum creatinine, and increased alkaline phosphatase.

Cases of an encephalopathy—like syndrome associated with demyelination have been reported in patients treated with ERGAMISOL. Worldwide postmarketing experience with the combination therapy of ERGAMISOL and fluorouracil has also included several reports of neurological changes associated with demyelination. The onset of symptoms and the clinical presentation in these cases are quite varied. Symptoms may include confusion, speech disturbances, muscle weakness, lethargy, and paresthesia. If an acute neurological syndrome occurs, immediate discontinuation of ERGAMISOL and fluorouracil therapy should be considered.

The following additional adverse experiences have been reported for fluorouracil alone: esophagopharyngitis, pancytopenia, myocardial ischemia, angina, gastrointestinal ulceration and bleeding, anaphylaxis and generalized allergic reactions, acute cerebellar syndrome, nystagmus, dry skin, fissuring, photosensitivity, lacrimal duct stenosis, photophobia, euphoria, thrombophlebitis, and nail changes.

OVERDOSAGE

Fatalities have been reported in a three-year-old child who ingested 15 mg/kg and in an adult who ingested 32 mg/kg. No further clinical information is available. In cases of over-

Adverse experience	ERGAMISOL N = 440 %	ERGAMISOL plus fluorouracil N = 599 %
Gastrointestinal		
Nausea	22	65
Diarrhea	13	52
Stomatitis	3	39
Vomiting	6	20
Anorexia	2	6
Abdominal pain	2	5
Constipation	2	3
Flatulence	<1	2
Dyspepsia	<1	1
Hematological		
Leukopenia		
<2000/mm^3	<1	1
≥2000 to <4000/mm^3	4	19
≥4000/mm^3	2	33
unscored category	0	<1
Thrombocytopenia		
<50,000/mm^3	0	0
≥50,000 to <130,000/mm^3	1	8
≥130,000/mm^3	1	10
Anemia	0	6
Granulocytopenia	<1	2
Epistaxis	0	1
Skin and Appendages		
Dermatitis	8	23
Alopecia	3	22
Pruritus	1	2
Skin discoloration	0	2
Urticaria	<1	0
Body as a Whole		
Fatigue	6	11
Fever	3	5
Rigors	3	5
Chest pain	<1	1
Edema	1	1
Resistance Mechanisms		
Infection	5	12
Special Senses		
Taste Perversion	8	8
Altered sense of smell	1	1
Musculoskeletal System		
Arthralgia	5	4
Myalgia	3	2
Central and peripheral nervous system		
Dizziness	3	4
Headache	3	4
Paresthesia	2	3
Ataxia	0	2
Psychiatric		
Somnolence	3	2
Depression	1	2
Nervousness	1	2
Insomnia	1	1
Anxiety	1	1
Forgetfulness	0	1
Vision		
Abnormal tearing	0	4
Blurred vision	1	2
Conjunctivitis	<1	2
Liver and biliary system		
Hyperbilirubinemia	<1	1

dosage, gastric lavage is recommended together with symptomatic and supportive measures.

DOSAGE AND ADMINISTRATION

The adjuvant use of ERGAMISOL (levamisole hydrochloride) and fluorouracil is limited to the following dosage schedule:

Initial Therapy:
ERGAMISOL: 50 mg p.o. (starting 7–30 days q8h for 3 days post-surgery)
fluorouracil: 450 mg/m^2/day (starting 21–34 days IV for 5 days post-surgery) concomitant with a 3-day course of ERGAMISOL

Maintenance:
ERGAMISOL: 50 mg p.o. q8h for 3 days every 2 weeks.
fluorouracil: 450 mg/m^2/day IV once a week beginning 28 days after the initiation of the 5-day course.

Treatment: ERGAMISOL, administered orally, should be initiated no earlier than 7 and no later than 30 days post surgery at a dose of 50 mg q8h × 3 days repeated every 14 days for 1 year. Fluorouracil therapy should be initiated no earlier than 21 days and no later than 35 days after surgery providing the patient is out of the hospital, ambulatory, maintaining normal oral nutrition, has well-healed wounds, and is fully recovered from any postoperative complications. If ERGAMISOL has been initiated from 7 to 20 days after surgery, initiation of fluorouracil therapy should be coincident with the second course of ERGAMISOL, i.e., at 21 to 34 days. If ERGAMISOL is initiated from 21 to 30 days after surgery, fluorouracil should be initiated simultaneously with the first course of ERGAMISOL.

Fluorouracil should be administered by rapid IV push at a dosage of 450 mg/m^2/day for 5 consecutive days. Dosage calculation is based on actual weight (estimated dry weight if there is evidence of fluid retention). *This course should be discontinued before the full 5 doses are administered if the patient develops any stomatitis or diarrhea* (5 or more loose stools). Twenty-eight days after initiation of this course, weekly fluorouracil should be instituted at a dosage of 450 mg/m^2/week and continued for a total treatment time of 1 year. If stomatitis or diarrhea develop during weekly therapy, the next dose of fluorouracil should be deferred until these side effects have subsided. If these side effects are moderate to severe, the fluorouracil dose should be reduced 20% when it is resumed.

Dosage modifications should be instituted as follows: If WBC is 2500-3500/mm^3 defer the fluorouracil dose until WBC is >3500/mm^3. If WBC is <2500/mm^3, defer the fluorouracil dose until WBC is >3500/mm^3; then resume the fluorouracil dose reduced by 20%. If WBC remains <2500/mm^3 for over 10 days despite deferring fluorouracil, discontinue administration of ERGAMISOL. Both drugs should be deferred unless platelets are adequate (≥100,000/mm^3).

ERGAMISOL should not be used at doses exceeding the recommended dose or frequency. Clinical studies suggest a relationship between ERGAMISOL adverse experiences and increasing dose, and since some of these, e.g. agranulocytosis, may be life-threatening, the recommended dosage regimen should not be exceeded (see "WARNINGS").

Before beginning this combination adjuvant treatment, the physician should become familiar with the labeling for fluorouracil.

HOW SUPPLIED

ERGAMISOL (levamisole hydrochloride) is available in white, coated tablets containing the equivalent of 50 mg of levamisole base, debossed "JANSSEN"and "L"/"50".

They are supplied in blister packages of 36 tablets (NDC 50458-270-36).

Store at room temperature, 15°–30°C (59°–86°F).

Protect from moisture.

REFERENCES

1. Laurie JA, Moertel CG, Fleming TR, et al. Surgical adjuvant therapy of large-bowel carcinoma: An evaluation of levamisole and the combination of levamisole and fluorouracil. *J Clin Oncol.* 1989; 7:1447–1456.
2. Moertel CG, Fleming TR, Macdonald JS, et al. Levamisole and fluorouracil for adjuvant therapy of resected colon carcinoma. *New Engl J Med.* 1990; 322:352–358.
3. Data on file, Janssen Pharmaceutica Inc.

Manufactured by:
Janssen Pharmaceutica, nv
Beerse, Belgium
Distributed by:
Janssen Pharmaceutica Inc.
Titusville, NJ 08560
November 1991, February 1992
U.S. Patent Number 4,584,305
Shown in Product Identification Section, page 412

HISMANAL®   ℞
[his'ma-nal]
(astemizole) Tablets

DESCRIPTION

HISMANAL® (astemizole) is a histamine H$_1$-receptor antagonist available in scored white tablets for oral use. Each tablet contains 10 mg of astemizole, and, as inactive ingredients: lactose, cornstarch, microcrystalline cellulose, pregelatinized starch, povidone K90, magnesium stearate, colloidal silicon dioxide, and sodium lauryl sulfate. Astemizole is chemically designated as 1-[(4-fluorophenyl)methyl]-N-[1-[2-(4-methoxyphenyl)ethyl] -4- piperidinyl]-1H-benzimidazol-2-amine, with a molecular weight of 458.58. The empirical formula is $C_{28}H_{31}FN_4O$.

Astemizole is a white to slightly off-white powder; it is insoluble in water, slightly soluble in ethanol and soluble in chloroform and methanol.

CLINICAL PHARMACOLOGY

HISMANAL is a long-acting, selective histamine H$_1$-receptor antagonist. Receptor binding studies in animals demonstrated that at pharmacological doses, HISMANAL occupies peripheral H$_1$-receptors but does not reach H$_1$-receptors in the brain. Whole body autoradiographic studies in rats, radiolabel tissue distribution studies in dogs and radioligand binding studies of guinea pig brain H$_1$-receptors have shown that HISMANAL does not readily cross the blood-brain barrier. Screening studies in rats at effective antihistaminic doses showed no anticholinergic effects. Studies in humans using the recommended dosage regimens have not been performed to determine whether HISMANAL is associated with a different frequency of anticholinergic effects than therapeutic doses of other antihistamines.

The absorption of HISMANAL is reduced by 60% when taken with meals. In single oral dose studies, HISMANAL was rapidly absorbed from the gastrointestinal tract; peak plasma concentrations of unchanged HISMANAL were reached within one hour. Due to extensive first pass metabolism and significant tissue distribution, plasma concentrations of unchanged drug were low. Elimination of unchanged HISMANAL occurred with a half-life of approximately one day. Elimination of HISMANAL plus hydroxylated metabolites, considered together to represent the pharmacologically active fraction in plasma, was biphasic with half-lives of 20 hours for the distribution phase and 7-11 days for the elimination phase. The pharmacokinetics of HISMANAL plus hydroxylated metabolites are dose proportional following single doses of 10 to 30 mg.

Following chronic administration, steady state plasma concentrations of HISMANAL plus hydroxylated metabolites (mainly desmethylastemizole) were reached within four to

Continued on next page

Janssen Pharmaceutica—Cont.

eight weeks; HISMANAL plus hydroxylated metabolites decayed biphasically with an initial half-life of 7–9 days, with plasma concentrations being reduced by 75% within this phase, and with a terminal half-life of about 19 days. The initial phase ($t_{1/2}$ = 7–9 days) appears to determine the time to reach steady state plasma concentrations of HISMANAL plus hydroxylated metabolites. Steady state plasma concentrations of unchanged HISMANAL were reached by 6 days (with a range of 6–9 days); unchanged HISMANAL was eliminated from plasma with a half-life of approximately 2 days (with a range of 1–2.5 days).

Excretion and metabolism studies with ^{14}C-labeled HISMANAL in volunteers demonstrated that the drug is almost completely metabolized in the liver and primarily excreted in the feces.

Interpatient variability in pharmacokinetic parameters may be greater in patients with liver disease as compared to normal subjects.

The in-vitro plasma protein binding of unchanged HISMANAL (100 ng/ml) was 96.7% with 2.3% being found as free drug in the plasma water. In human blood with an astemizole concentration of 100 ng/ml, 61.5% of astemizole was bound to the plasma proteins, with 36.2% being distributed to the blood cell fraction. The concentration of astemizole found in the blood was the same as that found in the plasma fraction of the blood. Binding studies for the astemizole metabolite(s) which achieve much higher concentrations than astemizole under chronic dosing conditions have not been conducted.

INDICATIONS AND USAGE

HISMANAL tablets are indicated for the relief of symptoms associated with seasonal allergic rhinitis and chronic idiopathic urticaria. Clinical trials have not been conducted to show whether HISMANAL is effective for short courses of therapy.

CONTRAINDICATIONS

HISMANAL is contraindicated in patients with known hypersensitivity to astemizole or any of the inactive ingredients.

PRECAUTIONS

General: Caution should be given to potential anticholinergic (drying) effects in patients with lower airway diseases, including asthma.

Caution should be used in patients with cirrhosis or other liver diseases (See Clinical Pharmacology section).

HISMANAL does not appear to be dialyzable.

Caution should also be used when treating patients with renal impairment.

Information for Patients: Patients taking HISMANAL should receive the following information and instructions. Antihistamines are prescribed to reduce allergic symptoms. Patients should be questioned about pregnancy or lactation before starting HISMANAL therapy, since the drug should be used in pregnancy or lactation only if the potential benefit justifies the potential risk to fetus or baby (see Pregnancy subsection). Patients should be instructed 1) to take HISMANAL only as needed, 2) not to exceed the prescribed dose, and 3) to take HISMANAL on an empty stomach, e.g., at least 2 hours after a meal. No additional food should be

taken for at least 1 hour post-dosing. Patients should also be instructed to store this medication in a tightly closed container in a cool, dry place, away from heat or direct sunlight, and away from children.

Carcinogenesis, Mutagenesis, Impairment of Fertility: Carcinogenic potential has not been revealed in rats given 260× the recommended human dose of astemizole for 24 months, or in mice given 400× the recommended human dose for 18 months. Micronucleus, dominant lethal, sister chromatid exchange and Ames tests of astemizole have not revealed mutagenic activity.

Impairment of fertility was not observed in male or female rats given 200× the recommended human dose.

Pregnancy: Pregnancy Category C: Teratogenic effects were not observed in rats administered 200× the recommended human dose or in rabbits given 200× the recommended human dose. Maternal toxicity was seen in rabbits administered 200× the recommended human dose. Embryocidal effects accompanied by maternal toxicity were observed at 100× the recommended human dose in rats. Embryotoxicity or maternal toxicity was not observed in rats or rabbits administered 50× the recommended human dose. There are no adequate and well controlled studies in pregnant women. HISMANAL should be used during pregnancy only if the potential benefit justifies the potential risk to the fetus. Metabolites may remain in the body for as long as 4 months after the end of dosing, calculated on the basis of 6 times the terminal half-life (See Clinical Pharmacology section).

Nursing Mothers: It is not known whether this drug is excreted in human milk. Because certain drugs are known to be excreted in human milk, caution should be exercised when HISMANAL is administered to a nursing woman. HISMANAL is excreted in the milk of dogs.

Pediatric Use: Safety and efficacy in children under 12 years of age has not been demonstrated.

ADVERSE REACTIONS

The reported incidences of adverse reactions listed in the following table are derived from controlled clinical studies in adults. In these studies the usual maintenance dose of HISMANAL® (astemizole) was 10 mg once daily.
[See table below.]

Adverse reaction information has been obtained from more than 7500 patients in all clinical trials. Weight gain has been reported in 3.6% of astemizole treated patients involved in controlled studies, with an average treatment duration of 53 days. In 46 of the 59 patients for whom actual weight gain data was available, the average weight gain was 3.2 kg.

Less frequently occurring adverse experiences reported in clinical trials or spontaneously from marketing experience with HISMANAL include: angioedema, asymptomatic liver enzyme elevations, bronchospasm, depression, edema, epistaxis, hepatitis, myalgia, palpitation, paresthesia, photosensitivity, pruritus, and rash.

Marketing experiences include isolated cases of convulsions. A causal relationship with HISMANAL has not been established.

OVERDOSAGE

In the event of overdosage, supportive measures including gastric lavage and emesis should be employed. Cases of overdose have been reported from foreign marketing experience. Although overdoses of up to 500 mg have been reported with no ill effects, cases of serious ventricular arrhythmias, in-

cluding Torsades de pointes following overdoses have been reported. Patients should be carefully observed and ECG monitoring is recommended in cases of suspected overdose. An appropriate antiarrhythmic treatment may be needed. HISMANAL does not appear to be dialyzable.

Care should be taken not to exceed dosing recommended in the DOSAGE AND ADMINISTRATION section.

Oral LD_{50} values for HISMANAL were 2052 mg/kg in mice and 3154 mg/kg in rats. In neonatal rats, the oral LD_{50} was 905 mg/kg in males and 1235 mg/kg in females.

DOSAGE AND ADMINISTRATION

The recommended maintenance dosage for adults and children 12 years of age and older is 10 mg (1 tablet) once daily. HISMANAL pharmacokinetics are dose proportional following single doses of 10 to 30 mg. To reduce the time to steady state concentration, a single dose of 30 mg (three 10 mg tablets) may be administered on the first day, 20 mg (two 10 mg tablets) on the second day of therapy, followed by the recommended 10 mg daily dose.

HISMANAL should be taken on an empty stomach, e.g., at least two hours before a meal. There should be no additional food intake for at least one hour post-dosing.

HOW SUPPLIED

HISMANAL is available as white, scored tablets containing 10 mg of astemizole debossed "JANSSEN" and on the reverse side debossed "AST"/₁₀.
NDC 50458-510-10
(100 tablets)
Store tablets at room temperature (59°–86°F) (15°–30°C). Protect from moisture.
U.S. Patent 4,219,559
December 1988, February 1992
JANSSEN PHARMACEUTICA INC.
Titusville, New Jersey 08560
Shown in Product Identification Section, page 412

IMODIUM®   ℞
(loperamide HCl) Capsules

DESCRIPTION

IMODIUM (loperamide hydrochloride), 4-(p-chlorophenyl)-4-hydroxy-N, N-dimethyl-α,α-diphenyl-1-piperidinebutyramide monohydrochloride, is a synthetic antidiarrheal for oral use.

IMODIUM is available in 2 mg capsules.
The inactive ingredients are:
Lactose, cornstarch, talc, and magnesium stearate.
IMODIUM capsules contain F D & C Yellow No. 6.

CLINICAL PHARMACOLOGY

In vitro and animal studies show that IMODIUM acts by slowing intestinal motility and by affecting water and electrolyte movement through the bowel. IMODIUM inhibits peristaltic activity by a direct effect on the circular and longitudinal muscles of the intestinal wall.

In man, IMODIUM prolongs the transit time of the intestinal contents. It reduces the daily fecal volume, increases the viscosity and bulk density, and diminishes the loss of fluid and electrolytes. Tolerance to the antidiarrheal effect has not been observed.

Clinical studies have indicated that the apparent elimination half-life of loperamide in man is 10.8 hours with a range of 9.1–14.4 hours. Plasma levels of unchanged drug remain below 2 nanograms per ml after the intake of a 2 mg capsule of IMODIUM. Plasma levels are highest approximately five hours after administration of the capsule and 2.5 hours after the liquid. The peak plasma levels of loperamide were similar for both formulations. Of the total excreted in urine and feces, most of the administered drug was excreted in feces. In those patients in whom biochemical and hematological parameters were monitored during clinical trials, no trends toward abnormality during IMODIUM therapy were noted. Similarly, urinalyses, EKG and clinical ophthalmological examinations did not show trends toward abnormality.

INDICATIONS AND USAGE

IMODIUM is indicated for the control and symptomatic relief of acute nonspecific diarrhea and of chronic diarrhea associated with inflammatory bowel disease. IMODIUM is also indicated for reducing the volume of discharge from ileostomies.

CONTRAINDICATIONS

IMODIUM is contraindicated in patients with known hypersensitivity to the drug and in those in whom constipation must be avoided.

WARNINGS

IMODIUM should not be used in the case of acute dysentery, which is characterized by blood in stools and elevated temperatures.

Fluid and electrolyte depletion may occur in patients who have diarrhea. The use of IMODIUM does not preclude the administration of appropriate fluid and electrolyte therapy.

Percent of Patients Reporting

Controlled Studies*

ADVERSE EVENT	Hismanal (N = 1630) %	Placebo (N = 1109) %	Classical** (N = 304) %
Central Nervous System			
Drowsiness	7.1	6.4	22.0
Headache	6.7	9.2	3.3
Fatigue	4.2	1.6	11.8
Appetite increase	3.9	1.4	0.0
Weight increase	3.6	0.7	1.0
Nervousness	2.1	1.2	0.3
Dizzy	2.0	1.8	1.0
Gastrointestinal System			
Nausea	2.5	2.9	1.3
Diarrhea	1.8	2.0	0.7
Abdominal pain	1.4	1.2	0.7
Eye, Ear, Nose, and Throat			
Mouth dry	5.2	3.8	7.9
Pharyngitis	1.7	2.3	0.3
Conjunctivitis	1.2	1.2	0.7
Other			
Arthralgia	1.2	1.6	0.0

*Duration of treatment in Controlled Studies ranged from 7 to 182 Days
**Classical Drugs: Clemastine (N = 137); Chlorpheniramine (N = 100); Pheniramine Maleate (N = 47); d-Chlorpheniramine (N = 20)

In some patients with acute ulcerative colitis, and in pseudomembranous colitis associated with broad-spectrum antibiotics, agents which inhibit intestinal motility or delay intestinal transit time have been reported to induce toxic megacolon. IMODIUM therapy should be discontinued promptly if abdominal distention occurs or if other untoward symptoms develop in patients with acute ulcerative colitis.
IMODIUM should be used with special caution in young children because of the greater variability of response in this age group. Dehydration, particularly in younger children, may further influence the variability of response to IMODIUM.

PRECAUTIONS

General: In acute diarrhea, if clinical improvement is not observed in 48 hours, the administration of IMODIUM should be discontinued.
Patients with hepatic dysfunction should be monitored closely for signs of CNS toxicity because of the apparent large first pass biotransformation.
Information for Patients: Patients should be advised to check with their physician if their diarrhea doesn't stop after a few days or if they develop a fever.
Drug Interactions: There was no evidence in clinical trials of drug interactions with concurrent medications.
Carcinogenesis, mutagenesis, impairment of fertility: In an 18-month rat study with doses up to 133 times the maximum human dose (on a mg/kg basis), there was no evidence of carcinogenesis. Mutagenicity studies were not conducted. Reproduction studies in rats indicated that high doses (150–200 times the human dose) could cause marked female infertility and reduced male fertility.
Pregnancy
Teratogenic Effects
Pregnancy Category B: Reproduction studies in rats and rabbits have revealed no evidence of impaired fertility or harm to the fetus at doses up to 30 times the human dose. Higher doses impaired the survival of mothers and nursing young. The studies offered no evidence of teratogenic activity. There are, however, no adequate and well controlled studies in pregnant women. Because animal reproduction studies are not always predictive of human response, this drug should be used during pregnancy only if clearly needed.
Nursing Mothers: It is not known whether this drug is excreted in human milk. Because many drugs are excreted in human milk, caution should be exercised when IMODIUM is administered to a nursing woman.
Pediatric Use: See the "Warnings" Section for information on the greater variability of response in this age group.
In case of accidental overdosage of IMODIUM by children, see "Overdosage" Section for suggested treatment.

ADVERSE REACTIONS

The adverse effects reported during clinical investigations of IMODIUM are difficult to distinguish from symptoms associated with the diarrheal syndrome. Adverse experiences recorded during clinical studies with IMODIUM were generally of a minor and self-limiting nature. They were more commonly observed during the treatment of chronic diarrhea.
The following patient complaints have been reported and are listed in decreasing order of frequency with the exception of hypersensitivity reactions which is listed first since it may be the most serious.

- Hypersensitivity reactions (including skin rash) have been reported with IMODIUM use.
- Abdominal pain, distention or discomfort
- Nausea and vomiting
- Constipation
- Tiredness
- Drowsiness or dizziness
- Dry mouth

DRUG ABUSE AND DEPENDENCE

Abuse: A specific clinical study designed to assess the abuse potential of loperamide at high doses resulted in a finding of extremely low abuse potential. Additionally, after years of extensive use there has been no evidence of abuse or dependence.
Dependence: Physical dependence to IMODIUM in humans has not been observed. However, studies in morphine-dependent monkeys demonstrated that loperamide hydrochloride at doses above those recommended for humans prevented signs of morphine withdrawal. However, in humans, the naloxone challenge pupil test, which when positive indicates opiate-like effects, performed after a single high dose, or after more than two years of therapeutic use of IMODIUM, was negative. Orally administered IMODIUM (loperamide formulated with magnesium stearate) is both highly insoluble and penetrates the CNS poorly.

OVERDOSAGE

Animal pharmacological and toxicological data indicate that overdosage in man may result in constipation, CNS depression and gastrointestinal irritation. Clinical trials have demonstrated that a slurry of activated charcoal administered promptly after ingestion of loperamide hydrochloride can reduce the amount of drug which is absorbed into the systemic circulation by as much as ninefold. If vomiting occurs spontaneously upon ingestion, a slurry of 100 gms of activated charcoal should be administered orally as soon as fluids can be retained.
If vomiting has not occurred, gastric lavage should be performed followed by administration of 100 gms of the activated charcoal slurry through the gastric tube. In the event of overdosage, patients should be monitored for signs of CNS depression for at least 24 hours. Children may be more sensitive to central nervous system effects than adults. If CNS depression is observed, naloxone may be administered. If responsive to naloxone, vital signs must be monitored carefully for recurrence of symptoms of drug overdose for at least 24 hours after the last dose of naloxone.
In view of the prolonged action of loperamide and the short duration (one to three hours) of naloxone, the patient must be monitored closely and treated repeatedly with naloxone as indicated. Since relatively little drug is excreted in the urine, forced diuresis is not expected to be effective for IMODIUM overdosage.
In clinical trials an adult who took three 20 mg doses within a 24 hour period was nauseated after the second dose and vomited after the third dose. In studies designed to examine the potential for side effects, intentional ingestion of up to 60 mg of loperamide hydrochloride in a single dose to healthy subjects resulted in no significant adverse effects.

DOSAGE AND ADMINISTRATION

(1 capsule = 2 mg.)
Acute Diarrhea
Adults: The recommended initial dose is 4 mg (two capsules) followed by 2 mg (one capsule) after each unformed stool. Daily dosage should not exceed 16 mg (eight capsules). Clinical improvement is usually observed within 48 hours.
Children: IMODIUM use is not recommended for children under 2 years of age. In children 2 to 5 years of age (20 kg or less), the non-prescription liquid formulation (IMODIUM A-D 1 mg/5 ml) should be used; for ages 6 to 12, either IMODIUM Capsules or IMODIUM A-D Liquid may be used. For children 2 to 12 years of age, the following schedule for capsules or liquid will usually fulfill initial dosage requirements:

Recommended First Day Dosage Schedule

Two to five years:	1 mg t.i.d.
(13 to 20 kg)	(3 mg daily dose)
Six to eight years:	2 mg b.i.d.
(20 to 30 kg)	(4 mg daily dose)
Eight to twelve years:	2 mg t.i.d.
(greater than 30 kg)	(6 mg daily dose)

Recommended Subsequent Daily Dosage
Following the first treatment day, it is recommended that subsequent IMODIUM doses (1 mg/10 kg body weight) be administered only after a loose stool. Total daily dosage should not exceed recommended dosages for the first day.
Chronic Diarrhea
Children: Although IMODIUM has been studied in a limited number of children with chronic diarrhea, the therapeutic dose for the treatment of chronic diarrhea in a pediatric population has not been established.
Adults: The recommended initial dose is 4 mg (two capsules) followed by 2 mg (one capsule) after each unformed stool until diarrhea is controlled, after which the dosage of IMODIUM should be reduced to meet individual requirements. When the optimal daily dosage has been established, this amount may then be administered as a single dose or in divided doses.
The average daily maintenance dosage in clinical trials was 4 to 8 mg (two to four capsules). A dosage of 16 mg (eight capsules) was rarely exceeded. If clinical improvement is not observed after treatment with 16 mg per day for at least 10 days, symptoms are unlikely to be controlled by further administration. IMODIUM administration may be continued if diarrhea cannot be adequately controlled with diet or specific treatment.

HOW SUPPLIED

Capsules—each capsule contains 2 mg of loperamide hydrochloride. The capsules have a light green body and a dark green cap with "JANSSEN" imprinted on one segment and "IMODIUM" on the other segment. IMODIUM capsules are supplied in bottles of 100 and 500 and in blister packs of 10 × 10 capsules.
NDC 50458-400-01
(10 × 10 capsules—blister)
NDC 50458-400-10
(100 capsules)
NDC 50458-400-50
(500 capsules)
Store at room temperature 15°–30°C (59°–86°F)
Revised May 1989, October 1990
CAUTION: FEDERAL LAW PROHIBITS DISPENSING WITHOUT A PRESCRIPTION
JANSSEN PHARMACEUTICA INC.
Titusville, New Jersey 08560-0200
U.S. Patent 3,714,159
Shown in Product Identification Section, page 412

INAPSINE® ℞

[ĭn-ăp-sēn]
(droperidol) Injection
FOR INTRAVENOUS OR INTRAMUSCULAR USE ONLY

DESCRIPTION

INAPSINE (droperidol) is a neuroleptic (tranquilizer) agent available in ampoules and vials. Each milliliter contains 2.5 mg. of droperidol in an aqueous solution adjusted to pH 3.4 ± 0.4 with lactic acid. INAPSINE in 10 ml multidose vials also contains 1.8 mg of methylparaben and 0.2 mg propylparaben. Droperidol is chemically identified as 1-(1-[3-(p-fluorobenzoyl) propyl]-1,2,3,6-tetrahydro-4-pyridyl)-2-benzimidazolinone with a molecular weight of 379.43.
INAPSINE is a sterile, non-pyrogenic aqueous solution for intravenous or intramuscular injection.

CLINICAL PHARMACOLOGY

INAPSINE (droperidol) produces marked tranquilization and sedation. It allays apprehension and provides a state of mental detachment and indifference while maintaining a state of reflex alertness.
INAPSINE produces an antiemetic effect as evidenced by the antagonism of apomorphine in dogs. It lowers the incidence of nausea and vomiting during surgical procedures and provides antiemetic protection in the postoperative period.
INAPSINE potentiates other CNS depressants. It produces mild alpha-adrenergic blockade, peripheral vascular dilatation and reduction of the pressor effect of epinephrine. It can produce hypotension and decreased peripheral vascular resistance and may decrease pulmonary arterial pressure (particularly if it is abnormally high). It may reduce the incidence of epinephrine-induced arrhythmias, but it does not prevent other cardiac arrhythmias.
The onset of action of single intramuscular and intravenous doses is from three to ten minutes following administration, although the peak effect may not be apparent for up to thirty minutes. The duration of the tranquilizing and sedative effects generally is two to four hours, although alteration of alertness may persist for as long as twelve hours.

INDICATIONS AND USAGE

INAPSINE (droperidol) is indicated:

- to produce tranquilization and to reduce the incidence of nausea and vomiting in surgical and diagnostic procedures.
- for premedication, induction, and as an adjunct in the maintenance of general and regional anesthesia.
- in neuroleptanalgesia in which INAPSINE is given concurrently with an opioid analgesic, such as SUBLIMAZE (fentanyl citrate) Injection, to aid in producing tranquility and decreasing anxiety and pain.

CONTRAINDICATIONS

INAPSINE (droperidol) is contraindicated in patients with known hypersensitivity to the drug.

WARNINGS

FLUIDS AND OTHER COUNTERMEASURES TO MANAGE HYPOTENSION SHOULD BE READILY AVAILABLE.
As with other CNS depressant drugs, patients who have received INAPSINE (droperidol) should have appropriate surveillance.
It is recommended that opioids, when required, initially be used in reduced doses.

PRECAUTIONS

General: The initial dose of INAPSINE (droperidol) should be appropriately reduced in elderly, debilitated and other poor-risk patients. The effect of the initial dose should be considered in determining incremental doses.
Certain forms of conduction anesthesia, such as spinal anesthesia and some peridural anesthetics, can alter respiration by blocking intercostal nerves and can cause peripheral vasodilatation and hypotension because of sympathetic blockade. Through other mechanisms (see CLINICAL PHARMACOLOGY), INAPSINE can also alter circulation. Therefore, when INAPSINE is used to supplement these forms of anesthesia, the anesthetist should be familiar with the physiological alterations involved, and be prepared to manage them in the patients elected for these forms of anesthesia.
If hypotension occurs, the possibility of hypovolemia should be considered and managed with appropriate parenteral fluid therapy. Repositioning the patient to improve venous return to the heart should be considered when operative conditions permit. It should be noted that in spinal and peridural anesthesia, tilting the patient into a head-down position may result in a higher level of anesthesia than is desir-

Continued on next page

Janssen Pharmaceutica—Cont.

able, as well as impair venous return to the heart. Care should be exercised in moving and positioning of patients because of a possibility of orthostatic hypotension. If volume expansion with fluids plus these other countermeasures do not correct the hypotension, then the administration of pressor agents other than epinephrine should be considered. Epinephrine may paradoxically decrease the blood pressure in patients treated with INAPSINE due to the alpha-adrenergic blocking action of INAPSINE.

Since INAPSINE may decrease pulmonary arterial pressure, this fact should be considered by those who conduct diagnostic or surgical procedures where interpretation of pulmonary arterial pressure measurements might determine final management of the patient.

Vital signs should be monitored routinely.

When the EEG is used for postoperative monitoring, it may be found that the EEG pattern returns to normal slowly.

Impaired Hepatic or Renal Function: INAPSINE should be administered with caution to patients with liver and kidney dysfunction because of the importance of these organs in the metabolism and excretion of drugs.

Drug Interactions: Other CNS depressant drugs (e.g. barbiturates, tranquilizers, opioids and general anesthetics) have additive or potentiating effects with INAPSINE. When patients have received such drugs, the dose of INAPSINE required will be less than usual. Following the administration of INAPSINE, the dose of other CNS depressant drugs should be reduced.

Carcinogenesis, Mutagenesis, Impairment of Fertility: No carcinogenicity studies have been carried out with INAPSINE. The micronucleus test in female rats revealed no mutagenic effects in single oral doses as high as 160 mg/kg. An oral study in rats (Segment I) revealed no impairment of fertility in either male or females at 0.63, 2.5 and 10 mg/kg doses (approximately 2, 9 and 36 times maximum recommended human iv/im dosage).

Pregnancy—Category C: INAPSINE administered intravenously has been shown to cause a slight increase in mortality of the newborn rat at 4.4 times the upper human dose. At 44 times the upper human dose, mortality rate was comparable to that for control animals. Following intramuscular administration, increased mortality of the offspring at 1.8 times the upper human dose is attributed to CNS depression in the dams who neglected to remove placentae from their offspring. INAPSINE has not been shown to be teratogenic in animals. There are no adequate and well-controlled studies in pregnant women. INAPSINE should be used during pregnancy only if the potential benefit justifies the potential risk to the fetus.

Labor and Delivery: There are insufficient data to support the use of INAPSINE in labor and delivery. Therefore, such use is not recommended.

Nursing Mothers: It is not known whether INAPSINE is excreted in human milk. Because many drugs are excreted in human milk, caution should be exercised when INAPSINE is administered to a nursing mother.

Pediatric Use: The safety of INAPSINE in children younger than two years of age has not been established.

ADVERSE REACTIONS

The most common adverse reactions reported to occur with INAPSINE (droperidol) are mild to moderate hypotension and tachycardia, but these effects usually subside without treatment. If hypotension occurs and is severe or persists, the possibility of hypovolemia should be considered and managed with appropriate parenteral fluid therapy. Postoperative drowsiness is also frequently reported.

Extrapyramidal symptoms (dystonia, akathisia, and oculogyric crisis) have been observed following administration of INAPSINE. Restlessness, hyperactivity and anxiety which can be either the result of inadequate dosage of INAPSINE or a part of the symptom complex of akathisia may occur. When extrapyramidal symptoms occur, they can usually be controlled with antiparkinson agents.

Other adverse reactions that have been reported are dizziness, chills and/or shivering, laryngospasm, bronchospasm and postoperative hallucinatory episodes (sometimes associated with transient periods of mental depression).

Elevated blood pressure, with or without pre-existing hypertension, has been reported following administration of INAPSINE combined with SUBLIMAZE (fentanyl citrate) or other parenteral analgesics. This might be due to unexplained alterations in sympathetic activity following large doses; however, it is also frequently attributed to anesthetic or surgical stimulation during light anesthesia.

OVERDOSAGE

Manifestations: The manifestations of INAPSINE (droperidol) overdosage are an extension of its pharmacologic actions.

Treatment: In the presence of hypoventilation or apnea, oxygen should be administered and respiration should be assisted or controlled as indicated. A patent airway must be maintained; an oropharyngeal airway or endotracheal tube might be indicated. The patient should be carefully observed for 24 hours; body warmth and adequate fluid intake should be maintained. If hypotension occurs and is severe or persists, the possibility of hypovolemia should be considered and managed with appropriate parenteral fluid therapy. (See PRECAUTIONS).

The intravenous LD_{50} of INAPSINE is 20–43 mg/kg in mice; 30 mg/kg in rats; 25 mg/kg in dogs and 11–13 mg/kg in rabbits. The intramuscular LD_{50} of INAPSINE is 195 mg/kg in mice; 104–110 mg/kg in rats; 97 mg/kg in rabbits and 200 mg/kg in guinea pigs.

DOSAGE AND ADMINISTRATION

Dosage should be individualized. Some of the factors to be considered in determining the dose are age, body weight, physical status, underlying pathological condition, use of other drugs, type of anesthesia to be used and the surgical procedure involved.

Vital signs should be monitored routinely.

Usual Adult Dosage

I. **Premedication**—(to be appropriately modified in the elderly, debilitated and those who have received other depressant drugs) 2.5 to 10 mg (1 to 4 ml) may be administered intramuscularly 30 to 60 minutes preoperatively.

II. **Adjunct to General Anesthesia—**
Induction—2.5 mg (1 ml) per 20 to 25 pounds may be administered (usually intravenously) along with an analgesic and/or general anesthetic. Smaller doses may be adequate. The total amount of INAPSINE (droperidol) administered should be titrated to obtain the desired effect based on the individual patient's response.
Maintenance—1.25 to 2.5 mg (0.5 to 1 ml) usually intravenously.

III. *Use without a general anesthetic in diagnostic procedures*—Administer the usual I.M. premedication 2.5 to 10 mg (1 to 4 ml) 30 to 60 minutes before the procedure. Additional 1.25 to 2.5 mg (0.5 to 1 ml) amounts of INAPSINE may be administered, usually intravenously.
NOTE: When INAPSINE is used in certain procedures, such as bronchoscopy, appropriate topical anesthesia is still necessary.

IV. *Adjunct to regional anesthesia*—2.5 to 5 mg (1 to 2 ml) may be administered intramuscularly or slowly intravenously when additional sedation is required.

Usual Children's Dosage

For children two to 12 years of age, a reduced dose as low as 1.0 to 1.5 mg (0.4 to 0.6 ml) per 20 to 25 pounds is recommended for premedication or for induction of anesthesia.

See WARNINGS and PRECAUTIONS for use of INAPSINE with other CNS depressants and in patients with altered response.

Parenteral drug products should be inspected visually for particulate matter and discoloration prior to administration, whenever solution and container permit. If such abnormalities are observed, the drug should not be administered.

HOW SUPPLIED

INAPSINE (droperidol) Injection is available as:
NDC 50458-010-01, 2.5 mg/ml, 1 ml ampoules in packages of 10
NDC 50458-010-02, 2.5 mg/ml, 2 ml ampoules in packages of 10
NDC 50458-010-05, 2.5 mg/ml, 5 ml ampoules in packages of 10
NDC 50458-010-10, 2.5 mg/ml, 10 ml multiple-dose vials in packages of 10.

PROTECT FROM LIGHT. STORE AT ROOM TEMPERATURE 15°C–30°C (59°F–86°F).

Manufactured by TAYLOR PHARMACAL CO. for
JANSSEN PHARMACEUTICA INC.
Titusville, NJ 08560-0200
U.S. Patent No. 3,161,645
Revised July 1986, November 1986

Shown in Product Identification Section, page 412

INNOVAR® INJECTION ℂ℞

[*ĭn 'nō-văr*]
(fentanyl citrate/droperidol)
FOR INTRAVENOUS OR INTRAMUSCULAR USE ONLY

> The two components of INNOVAR Injection, fentanyl citrate and droperidol, have different pharmacologic actions. Before administering INNOVAR Injection, the user should become familiar with the special properties of each drug, particularly the widely differing durations of action.

DESCRIPTION

INNOVAR is a potent opioid analgesic (fentanyl citrate) and a neuroleptic (tranquilizer) agent (droperidol). Each milliliter contains (in a 1:50 ratio) fentanyl citrate equivalent to 50 μg of fentanyl base and 2.5 mg of droperidol in a solution adjusted to pH 3.5 ± 0.3 with lactic acid.

The chemical names and molecular weights of the two components of INNOVAR are: Fentanyl citrate N- (1-phenethyl-4-piperidyl) propionanilide citrate (1:1). Molecular weight: 528.60

Droperidol 1-[1-[3-(p-fluorobenzoyl)propyl] -1,2,3,6-tetrahydro-4-pyridyl]-2- benzimidazolinone. Molecular weight: 379.43

INNOVAR is a sterile, preservative free aqueous solution for intravenous or intramuscular injection.

CLINICAL PHARMACOLOGY

INNOVAR (fentanyl citrate/droperidol) is a combination drug containing an opioid analgesic, fentanyl citrate, and a neuroleptic (major tranquilizer), droperidol. The combined effect, sometimes referred to as neuroleptanalgesia, is characterized by general quiescence, reduced motor activity, and profound analgesia; complete loss of consciousness usually does not occur from use of INNOVAR Injection alone. The incidence of early postoperative pain and emesis may be reduced.

A. Fentanyl citrate is an opioid analgesic. A dose of 100 μg (0.1 mg) (2.0 ml), is approximately equivalent in analgesic activity to 10 mg of morphine or 75 mg of meperidine. The principal actions of therapeutic value are analgesia and sedation. Alterations in respiratory rate and alveolar ventilation, associated with opioid analgesics, may last longer than the analgesic effect. As the dose of opioid is increased, the decrease in pulmonary exchange becomes greater. Large doses may produce apnea. Fentanyl citrate appears to have less emetic activity than either morphine or meperidine. Histamine assays and skin wheal testing in man indicate that clinically significant histamine release rarely occurs with fentanyl citrate. Assays in man show no clinically significant histamine release in dosages up to 50 μg/kg (0.05 mg/kg) (1 ml/kg).
The pharmacokinetics of fentanyl citrate can be described as a three-compartment model, with a distribution time of 1.7 minutes, redistribution of 13 minutes and a terminal elimination half-life of 219 minutes. The volume of distribution for fentanyl citrate is 4 L/kg.
Fentanyl citrate plasma protein binding capacity increases with increasing ionization of the drug. Alterations in pH may affect its distribution between plasma and the central nervous system. It accumulates in skeletal muscle and fat, and is released slowly into the blood. Fentanyl citrate, which is primarily transformed in the liver, demonstrates a high first pass clearance and releases approximately 75% of an intravenous dose in urine, mostly as metabolites with less than 10% representing the unchanged drug. Approximately 9% of the dose is recovered in the feces, primarily as metabolites.
The onset of action of fentanyl citrate is almost immediate when the drug is given intravenously; however, the maximal analgesic and respiratory depressant effect may not be noted for several minutes. The usual duration of action of the analgesic effect is 30 to 60 minutes after a single intravenous dose of up to 100 μg (0.1 mg) (2.0 ml).
Following intramuscular administration, the onset of action is from seven to eight minutes, and the duration of action is one to two hours. As with longer acting opioid analgesics, the duration of the respiratory depressant effect of fentanyl citrate may be longer than the analgesic effect. The following observations have been reported concerning altered respiratory response to CO_2 stimulation following administration of fentanyl citrate to man:
   1. DIMINISHED SENSITIVITY TO CO_2 STIMULATION MAY PERSIST LONGER THAN DEPRESSION OF RESPIRATORY RATE. [Altered sensitivity to CO_2 stimulation has been demonstrated for up to four hours following a single dose of 600 μg (0.6 mg) (12 ml) fentanyl citrate to healthy volunteers.] Fentanyl citrate frequently slows the respiratory rate, duration and degree of respiratory depression being dose related.
   2. The peak respiratory depressant effect of a single intravenous dose of fentanyl citrate is noted 5 to 15 minutes following injection. See also WARNINGS and PRECAUTIONS concerning respiratory depression.

B. Droperidol produces marked tranquilization and sedation. Droperidol allays apprehension and provides a state of mental detachment and indifference while maintaining a state of reflex alertness.
Droperidol also produces an antiemetic effect as evidenced by the antagonism of apomorphine in dogs. It lowers the incidence of nausea and vomiting during surgical procedures and provides antiemetic protection in the postoperative period.
Droperidol potentiates other CNS depressants. It produces mild alpha-adrenergic blockade, peripheral vascular dilatation and reduction of the pressor effect of epinephrine. It can produce hypotension and decreased peripheral vascular resistance and may decrease pulmonary arterial pressure (particularly if it is abnormally high). It may reduce the incidence of epinephrine-induced

arrhythmias, but does not prevent other cardiac arrhythmias.

The onset of action of single intramuscular and intravenous doses of droperidol is from three to ten minutes following administration, although the peak effect may not be apparent for up to thirty minutes. The duration of the tranquilizing and sedative effects generally is two to four hours, although alteration of consciousness may persist for as long as twelve hours. This is in contrast to the much shorter duration of fentanyl citrate.

INDICATIONS AND USAGE

INNOVAR (fentanyl citrate/droperidol) is indicated to produce tranquilization and analgesia for surgical and diagnostic procedures. It may be used as an anesthetic premedication, as an adjunct to the induction of anesthesia, and as an adjunct in the maintenance of general and regional anesthesia. If the supplementation of analgesia is necessary, SUBLIMAZE (fentanyl citrate) alone rather than the combination drug, INNOVAR, should usually be used, see DOSAGE AND ADMINISTRATION section.

CONTRAINDICATIONS

INNOVAR (fentanyl citrate/droperidol) is contraindicated in patients with known hypersensitivity to either component.

WARNINGS

INNOVAR (fentanyl citrate/droperidol) SHOULD BE ADMINISTERED ONLY BY PERSONS SPECIFICALLY TRAINED IN THE USE OF INTRAVENOUS ANESTHETICS AND MANAGEMENT OF THE RESPIRATORY EFFECTS OF POTENT OPIOIDS.
AN OPIOID ANTAGONIST, RESUSCITATIVE AND INTUBATION EQUIPMENT AND OXYGEN SHOULD BE READILY AVAILABLE.
See also discussion of opioid antagonists in PRECAUTIONS and OVERDOSAGE sections.
FLUIDS AND OTHER COUNTERMEASURES TO MANAGE HYPOTENSION SHOULD ALSO BE AVAILABLE.
The respiratory depressant effect of opioids persists longer than the measured analgesic effect. When used with INNOVAR, the total dose of all opioid analgesics administered should be considered by the practitioner before ordering opioid analgesics during recovery from anesthesia. It is recommended that opioids, when required, be used in reduced doses initially, as low as $\frac{1}{4}$ to $\frac{1}{3}$ those usually recommended.

INNOVAR may cause muscle rigidity, particularly involving the muscles of respiration. This effect is due to the fentanyl citrate component and is related to the dose and speed of injection. Its incidence can be reduced by the use of slow intravenous injection. Once the effect occurs, it is managed by the use of assisted or controlled respiration and, if necessary, by a neuromuscular blocking agent compatible with the patient's condition.

Head Injuries and Increased Intracranial Pressure: INNOVAR should be used with caution in patients who may be particularly susceptible to respiratory depression such as comatose patients who may have a head injury or brain tumor. In addition, INNOVAR may obscure the clinical course of patients with head injury.

PRECAUTIONS

General: The initial dose of INNOVAR (fentanyl citrate/droperidol) should be appropriately reduced in elderly, debilitated and other poor-risk patients. The effect of the initial dose should be considered in determining incremental doses. Certain forms of conduction anesthesia, such as spinal anesthesia and some peridural anesthetics, can alter respiration by blocking intercostal nerves and can cause peripheral vasodilation and hypotension because of sympathetic blockade. Through other mechanisms (see CLINICAL PHARMACOLOGY) fentanyl citrate and droperidol can also depress respiration and blood pressure. Therefore, when INNOVAR is used to supplement these forms of anesthesia, the anesthetist should be familiar with the physiological alterations involved, and be prepared to manage them in the patients selected for these forms of anesthesia.

The droperidol component of INNOVAR may decrease pulmonary arterial pressure. This fact should be considered by those who conduct diagnostic or surgical procedures where interpretation of pulmonary arterial pressure measurements might determine final management of the patient.

Vital signs should be monitored routinely.

When the EEG is used for postoperative monitoring, it may be found that the EEG pattern returns to normal slowly.

Hypotension: If hypotension occurs, the possibility of hypovolemia should be considered and managed with appropriate parenteral fluid therapy. Repositioning the patient to improve venous return to the heart should be considered when operative conditions permit. It should be noted that in spinal and peridural anesthesia, tilting the patient into a head down position may result in a higher level of anesthesia than is desirable, as well as impair venous return to the heart. Care should be exercised in the moving and positioning of

patients because of a possibility of orthostatic hypotension. If volume expansion with fluids plus these other countermeasures do not correct the hypotension, then the administration of pressor agents other than epinephrine should be considered. Epinephrine may paradoxically decrease the blood pressure in patients treated with INNOVAR due to the alpha-adrenergic blocking action of droperidol.

Impaired Respiration: INNOVAR and SUBLIMAZE (fentanyl citrate) should be used with caution in patients with chronic obstructive pulmonary disease, patients with decreased respiratory reserve and others with potentially compromised ventilation. In such patients opioids may additionally decrease respiratory drive and increase airway resistance. During anesthesia, this can be managed by assisted or controlled respiration. Respiratory depression caused by opioid analgesics can be reversed by opioid antagonists. Appropriate surveillance should be maintained because the duration of respiratory depression of doses of fentanyl citrate (as SUBLIMAZE (fentanyl citrate) or INNOVAR) employed during anesthesia may be longer than the duration of the opioid antagonist action. Consult individual prescribing information (levallorphan, nalorphine and naloxone) before employing opioid antagonists.

Impaired Hepatic or Renal Function: INNOVAR should be administered with caution to patients with liver and kidney dysfunction because of the importance of these organs in the metabolism and excretion of drugs.

Cardiovascular Effects: The fentanyl citrate component may produce bradycardia, which may be treated with atropine. INNOVAR should be used with caution in patients with cardiac bradyarrhythmias.

Drug Interactions: Other CNS depressant drugs (e.g. barbiturates, tranquilizers, opioids and general anesthetics) have additive or potentiating effects with INNOVAR. When patients have received such drugs, the dose of INNOVAR required will be less than usual. Following the administration of INNOVAR, the dose of other CNS depressant drugs should be reduced.

Carcinogenesis, Mutagenesis, Impairment of Fertility: No carcinogenicity studies have been conducted with INNOVAR or its components, SUBLIMAZE and INAPSINE. A subcutaneous study of INNOVAR in female rats revealed no impairment of fertility at doses 9 times the upper human dose. An intravenous study revealed no effects on fertility at 2 times the upper human dose (highest dosage level tested).

Pregnancy — Category C: INNOVAR had no embryotoxic effects in rats at intravenous doses approximately 2 times the upper human dose. A subcutaneous study of INNOVAR in female rats showed increased fetal resorptions at 18 times the upper human dose. No teratogenic effects were revealed at 36 times the upper human dose. In rabbits, increased resorptions and decreased litter size were found at intravenous doses approximately 2 times the upper human dose. Maternal mortality occurred at 7 times the upper human dose.

INNOVAR has not been shown to be teratogenic in animals. There are no adequate and well-controlled studies in pregnant women. INNOVAR should be used during pregnancy only if the potential benefit justifies the potential risk to the fetus.

Labor and Delivery: There are insufficient data to support the use of INNOVAR in labor and delivery. Therefore, such use is not recommended.

Nursing Mothers: It is not known whether fentanyl citrate or droperidol are excreted in human milk. Because many drugs are excreted in human milk, caution should be exercised when INNOVAR is administered to a nursing woman.

Pediatric Use: The safety and efficacy of INNOVAR in children under two years of age has not been established.

ADVERSE REACTIONS

The most common serious adverse reactions reported to occur with INNOVAR (fentanyl citrate/droperidol) are respiratory depression, apnea, muscular rigidity and hypotension; if these remain untreated, respiratory arrest, circulatory depression or cardiac arrest could occur.

Extrapyramidal symptoms (dystonia, akathisia and oculogyric crisis) have been observed following administration of INNOVAR. Restlessness, hyperactivity and anxiety which can be either the result of inadequate tranquilization or part of the symptom complex of akathisia may occur. When extrapyramidal symptoms occur, they can usually be controlled with anti-Parkinson agents.

Elevated blood pressure, with and without pre-existing hypertension, has been reported following administration of INNOVAR. This might be due to unexplained alterations of sympathetic activity following large doses; however, it is also frequently attributed to anesthetic or surgical stimulation during light anesthesia.

Postoperative drowsiness is also frequently reported.

Other adverse reactions that have been reported are dizziness, chills and/or shivering, twitching, blurred vision, laryngospasm, bronchospasm, bradycardia, tachycardia, nausea and emesis, diaphoresis, emergence delirium, and postoperative hallucinatory episodes (sometimes associated with transient periods of mental depression).

DRUG ABUSE AND DEPENDENCE

The fentanyl citrate component of INNOVAR (fentanyl citrate/droperidol) is a Schedule II opioid that can produce drug dependence of the morphine type and, therefore, has the potential for being abused.

OVERDOSAGE

MANIFESTATIONS: The manifestations of INNOVAR (fentanyl citrate/droperidol) overdosage are an extension of its pharmacologic actions.

TREATMENT: In the presence of hypoventilation or apnea, oxygen should be administered and respiration should be assisted or controlled as indicated. A patent airway must be maintained; an oropharyngeal airway or endotracheal tube might be indicated. If depressed respiration is associated with muscular rigidity, an intravenous neuromuscular blocking agent might be required to facilitate assisted or controlled respiration. The patient should be carefully observed for 24 hours; body warmth and adequate fluid intake should be maintained. If hypotension occurs and is severe or persists, the possibility of hypovolemia should be considered and managed with appropriate parenteral fluid therapy (See PRECAUTIONS). A specific opioid antagonist such as nalorphine, levallorphan or naloxone should be available for use as indicated to manage respiratory depression caused by the opioid component fentanyl citrate. This does not preclude the use of more immediate countermeasures. The duration of respiratory depression following overdosage of fentanyl citrate may be longer than the duration of opioid antagonist action. Consult the package inserts of the individual opioid antagonists for details about use.

The LD_{50} values after intravenous administration were 4.1–5.27 mg/kg for the rat and the rabbit and 17 mg/kg or more for the mouse and the dog. After intramuscular administration LD_{50} determinations were 6.7–14.5 mg/kg for the rabbit and 75 mg/kg for the mouse.

DOSAGE AND ADMINISTRATION

Dosage should be individualized. Some of the factors to be considered in determining dose are age, body weight, physical status, underlying pathological condition, use of other drugs, the type of anesthesia to be used and the surgical procedure involved.

Vital signs should be monitored routinely.

Most patients who have received INNOVAR (fentanyl citrate/droperidol) do not require opioid analgesics during the immediate postoperative period. It is recommended that opioid analgesics, when required, be used initially in reduced doses, as low as $\frac{1}{4}$ to $\frac{1}{3}$ those usually recommended.

USUAL ADULT DOSAGE:

I. **Premedication**—(to be appropriately modified in the elderly, debilitated and those who have received other depressant drugs)—0.5 to 2.0 ml may be administered **intramuscularly** 45 to 60 minutes prior to surgery with or without atropine.

II. **Adjunct to General Anesthesia**—
   Induction—1 ml per 20 to 25 pounds of body weight may be slowly administered intravenously. Smaller doses may be adequate.
   The total amount of INNOVAR administered should be carefully titrated to obtain the desired effect based on the individual patient's response.
   There are several methods of administration of INNOVAR Injection for induction of anesthesia.
   A. Intravenous injection—To allow for the variable needs of patients INNOVAR may be administered intravenously in fractional parts of the calculated dose. With the onset of somnolence, the general anesthetic may be administered.
   B. Intravenous drip—10 ml of INNOVAR are added to 250 ml of 5% dextrose in water and the drip given rapidly until the onset of somnolence. At that time, the drip may be either slowed or stopped and the general anesthetic administered.
   Maintenance—INNOVAR is not indicated as the sole agent for the maintenance of surgical anesthesia. It is customarily used in combination with other measures such as nitrous oxide-oxygen, other inhalation anesthetics and/or topical or regional anesthesia.
   To prevent the possibility of excessive accumulation of the relatively long-acting droperidol component, SUBLIMAZE (fentanyl citrate) alone should be used in increments of 25 to 50 µg (0.025 to 0.05 mg) (0.5 to 1.0 ml) for the maintenance of analgesia in patients initially given INNOVAR as an adjunct to general anesthesia. (See SUBLIMAZE (fentanyl citrate) package insert for additional prescribing information.) However, in prolonged operations, additional 0.5 to 1.0 ml amounts of INNOVAR may be administered with caution intravenously if changes in the patient's condition indicate lightening of tranquilization and analgesia.

III. **Use Without a General Anesthetic in Diagnostic Procedures**—Administer the usual intramuscular pre-

Continued on next page

Janssen Pharmaceutica—Cont.

medication (0.5 to 2.0 ml) 45 to 60 minutes before the procedure. To prevent the possibility of excessive accumulation of the relatively long-acting droperidol component, SUBLIMAZE (fentanyl citrate) alone should be used in increments of 25 to 50 μg (0.025 to 0.05 mg) (0.5 to 1.0 ml) for the maintenance of analgesia in patients initially given INNOVAR Injection. See SUBLIMAZE (fentanyl citrate) package insert for additional information. However, in prolonged operations, additional 0.5 to 1.0 ml amounts of INNOVAR may be administered with caution intravenously if changes in the patient's condition indicate lightening of tranquilization and analgesia. Note: When INNOVAR is used in certain procedures such as bronchoscopy, appropriate topical anesthesia is still necessary.

IV. **Adjunct to Regional Anesthesia**—1 to 2 ml may be administered intramuscularly or slowly intravenously when additional sedation and analgesia are required.

USUAL CHILDREN'S DOSAGE:

For premedication and as an adjunct to general anesthesia in children over 2 years of age (see PRECAUTIONS):

I. **Premedication**—0.25 ml per 20 lbs. body weight administered **intramuscularly** 45 to 60 minutes prior to surgery with or without atropine.

II. **Adjunct to General Anesthesia**—The total combined dose for induction and maintenance averages 0.5 ml per 20 lbs. body weight. Following induction with INNOVAR Injection, SUBLIMAZE (fentanyl citrate) alone in a dose of 1/4 to 1/3 that recommended in the adult dosage section should usually be used when indicated to avoid the possibility of excessive accumulation of droperidol. However, in prolonged operations, additional increments of INNOVAR may be administered with caution when changes in the patient's condition indicate lightening of tranquilization and analgesia.

See WARNINGS and PRECAUTIONS for use of INNOVAR with other CNS depressants, and in patients with altered response.

Parenteral drug products should be inspected visually for particulate matter and discoloration prior to administration, whenever solution and container permit. If such abnormalities are observed, the drug should not be administered.

HOW SUPPLIED

INNOVAR (fentanyl citrate/droperidol) Injection is available as:
NDC 50458-020-02, 2 ml ampoules in packages of 10
NDC 50458-020-05, 5 ml ampoules in packages of 10
containing fentanyl citrate equivalent to 50 μg/ml of fentanyl base and 2.5 mg/ml of droperidol.
(FOR INTRAVENOUS USE BY HOSPITAL PERSONNEL SPECIFICALLY TRAINED IN THE USE OF OPIOID ANALGESICS.)
PROTECT FROM LIGHT. STORE AT ROOM TEMPERATURE 15°–30°C (59°–86°F).
JANSSEN PHARMACEUTICA INC.
Titusville, NJ 08560-0200
U.S. Patent No. 3,141,823
Revised December 1986, January 1988

Shown in Product Identification Section, page 412

MONISTAT i.v.™ ℞

[*mŏn-ĭ-stăt*]
(miconazole)
10 mg/ml sterile solution

FOR INTRAVENOUS INFUSION

DESCRIPTION

MONISTAT i.v. (miconazole), 1-[2-(2,4-dichlorophenyl)-2-[(2,4-dichlorophenyl) methoxyl] ethyl]-1H-imidazole, is a synthetic antifungal agent supplied as a sterile solution for intravenous infusion. Each ml of this solution contains 10 mg of miconazole with 0.115 ml PEG 40 castor oil, 1.0 mg lactic acid USP, 0.5 mg methylparaben USP, 0.05 mg propylparaben USP in water for injection. Miconazole i.v. is a clear, colorless to slightly yellow solution having a pH of 3.7 to 5.7.

CLINICAL PHARMACOLOGY

MONISTAT i.v. is rapidly metabolized in the liver and about 14% to 22% of the administered dose is excreted in the urine, mainly as inactive metabolites. The pharmacokinetic profile fits a three compartment open model with the following biologic half life: 0.4, 2.1, and 24.1 hours for each phase respectively. The pharmacokinetic profile of MONISTAT i.v. is unaltered in patients with renal insufficiency, including those patients on hemodialysis. The in vitro antifungal activity of MONISTAT i.v. is very broad. Clinical efficacy has been demonstrated in patients with the following species of fungi: *Coccidioides immitis, Candida albicans, Cryptococcus neoformans, Pseudoallescheria boydii (Petriellidium boydii; Allescheria boydii),* and *Paracoccidioides brasiliensis.*

Recommended doses of MONISTAT i.v. produce serum concentrations of drug which exceed the in vitro minimum inhibitory concentration (MIC) values listed below.

Median Minimal Inhibitory Concentrations of Miconazole in mcg/ml

Clinical Isolates	Median	Range
Coccidioides immitis	0.4	0.1–1.6
Candida albicans	0.2	0.1–0.8
Cryptococcus neoformans	0.8	0.4–1.3
Paracoccidioides brasiliensis	0.24	0.16–0.31
Pseudoallescheria boydii (Petriellidium boydii)	1.0	0.16–10

Doses above 9 mg/kg of MONISTAT i.v. produce peak blood levels above 1 mcg/ml in most cases. The drug penetrates into joints.

INDICATIONS AND USAGE

MONISTAT i.v. is indicated for the treatment of the following severe systemic fungal infections, based on data derived from open clinical trials: coccidioidomycosis (N=52*), candidiasis (N=151), cryptococcosis (N=13), pseudallescheriosis (petriellidiosis; allescheriosis) (N=12), paracoccidioidomycosis (N=12), and for the treatment of chronic mucocutaneous candidiasis (N=16).

*Represents treatment courses, as some patients were treated more than once.

However, in the treatment of fungal meningitis and *Candida* urinary bladder infections an intravenous infusion alone is inadequate. It must be supplemented with intrathecal administration or bladder irrigation. Appropriate diagnostic procedures should be performed and MIC's should be measured to determine if the organism is susceptible to MONISTAT.

MONISTAT i.v. should only be used to treat severe systemic fungal diseases.

CONTRAINDICATIONS

MONISTAT i.v. is contraindicated in those patients who have shown hypersensitivity to it, or to its components.

WARNINGS

There have been several reports of cardiorespiratory arrest and/or anaphylaxis in patients receiving MONISTAT i.v. Excessively rapid administration of the drug may have been responsible in some cases. Rapid injection of undiluted MONISTAT i.v. may produce transient tachycardia or dysrhythmia. (See DOSAGE AND ADMINISTRATION.)

MONISTAT i.v. should only be used to treat severe systemic fungal diseases.

PRECAUTIONS

General: Before a treatment course of MONISTAT i.v. is started, the physician should ascertain insofar as possible that the patient is not hypersensitive to the drug product. MONISTAT i.v. should be given by intravenous infusion. The treatment should be started under stringent conditions of hospitalization but subsequently may be administered to suitable patients under ambulatory conditions with close clinical monitoring. It is recommended that an initial dose of 200 mg be administered with the physician in attendance. It is also recommended that clinical laboratory monitoring including hemoglobin, hematocrit, electrolytes and lipids be performed.

It should be borne in mind that systemic fungal mycoses may be complications of chronic underlying conditions which in themselves may require appropriate measures.

Since *Pseudoallescheria boydii* is difficult to distinguish histologically from species of Aspergillus, it is strongly recommended that cultures be planted.

Drug Interactions: Drugs containing cremophor type vehicles are known to cause electrophoretic abnormalities of the lipoprotein; for example, the values and/or patterns may be altered. These effects are reversible upon discontinuation of treatment but are usually not an indication that treatment should be discontinued.

Interaction with oral and i.v. anticoagulant drugs, resulting in an enhancement of the anticoagulant effect, may occur. However, this has only been reported with oral (coumadin) administration. In cases of simultaneous treatment with MONISTAT i.v. and anticoagulant drugs, the anticoagulant effect should be carefully titrated since reductions of the anticoagulant doses may be indicated.

Interactions between oral miconazole and oral hypoglycemic agents leading to severe hypoglycemia have been reported.

Since concomitant administration of rifampin and ketoconazole (an imidazole) reduces the blood levels of the latter, the concurrent administration of MONISTAT i.v. (an imidazole) and rifampin should be avoided.

Ketoconazole (an imidazole) increases the blood level of cyclosporine; therefore, there is the possibility of a similar drug interaction involving cyclosporine and MONISTAT i.v. (an imidazole). Blood levels of cyclosporine should be monitored if the two drugs must be given concurrently.

Concomitant administration of miconazole with CNS-active drugs such as carbamazepine or phenytoin may alter the metabolism of one or both of the drugs. Therefore, consideration should be given to the advisability of monitoring plasma levels of these drugs. It is not known whether miconazole may affect the metabolism of other CNS-active drugs.

Pregnancy Category C: Reproduction studies using MONISTAT i.v. (miconazole) were performed in rats and rabbits. At intravenous doses of 40 mg/kg in the rat and 20 mg/kg in the rabbit, no evidence of impaired fertility or harm to the fetus appeared. There are no adequate and well-controlled studies using MONISTAT i.v. in pregnant women. MONISTAT i.v. should be given to a pregnant woman only if clearly needed.

Pediatric Use: The safety of miconazole i.v. in children under one year has not been extensively studied. However, reports in the literature describe the treatment of 21 neonates for periods ranging from 1 to 56 days at doses ranging from 3 to 50 mg/kg per day in 3 or 4 divided doses. No unanticipated adverse events occurred in children who received these doses. The majority of use was a daily dose in the 15 to 30 mg/kg range. Seven of the eleven evaluable children recovered or improved.

ADVERSE REACTIONS

Adverse reactions which have been observed with MONISTAT i.v. therapy include phlebitis, pruritus, rash, nausea, vomiting, febrile reactions, drowsiness, diarrhea, anorexia and flushes. In the U.S. studies, 29% of 209 patients studied had phlebitis, 21% pruritus, 18% nausea, 10% fever and chills, 9% rash, and 7% emesis. Transient decreases in hematocrit and serum sodium values have been observed following infusion of MONISTAT i.v.

In rare cases, anaphylaxis has occurred.

Thrombocytopenia has also been reported. No serious renal or hepatic toxicity has been reported. If pruritus and skin rashes are severe, discontinuation of treatment may be necessary. Nausea and vomiting can be lessened with antihistaminic or antiemetic drugs given prior to MONISTAT i.v. infusion, or by reducing the dose, slowing the rate of infusion, or avoiding administration with foods.

Aggregation of erythrocytes or rouleau formation on blood smears has been reported. Hyperlipemia has occurred in patients and is reported to be due to the vehicle, Cremophor EL (PEG 40 castor oil).

DOSAGE AND ADMINISTRATION

Dosage

Adults: Doses may vary from 200 to 1200 mg per infusion depending on severity of infection and sensitivity of the organism. The following daily doses, which may be divided over 3 infusions, are recommended:

[See table below.]

Organism	Dosage Range*	Duration of Successful Therapy (weeks)
Candidiasis	600 to 1800 mg per day	1 to > 20
Cryptococcosis	1200 to 2400 mg per day	3 to > 12
Coccidioidomycosis	1800 to 3600 mg per day	3 to > 20
Pseudoallescheriosis (Petriellidiosis; Allescheriosis)	600 to 3000 mg per day	5 to > 20
Paracoccidioidomycosis	200 to 1200 mg per day	2 to > 16

*May be divided over 3 infusions

Repeated courses may be necessitated by relapse or reinfection.

Children:

Children under one year: Total daily doses of 15 to 30 mg/kg have been used (See Pediatric Use.).

Children 1 to 12 years: Total daily doses of 20 to 40 mg/kg have generally been adequate.

However, a dose of 15 mg/kg body weight per infusion should not be exceeded.

Administration

For daily doses of up to 2400 mg, MONISTAT i.v. should be diluted in at least 200 ml of diluent per ampoule and should be administered at a rate of approximately 2 hours per ampoule. For daily doses higher than 2400 mg adjust the rate of

infusion and the diluent in terms of patient tolerability (see WARNINGS).

It is recommended that 0.9% Sodium Chloride Injection be used as the diluent to minimize the possibility of transient hyponatremia following an infusion of MONISTAT i.v. Alternatively, if clinically indicated, 5% Dextrose Injection may be used.

Generally, treatment should be continued until all clinical and laboratory tests no longer indicate that active fungal infection is present. Inadequate periods of treatment may yield poor response and lead to early recurrence of clinical symptoms. The dosing intervals and sites and the duration of treatment vary from patient to patient and depend on the causative organism.

Other Modes of Administration

Intrathecal: Administration of the undiluted injectable solution of MONISTAT i.v. by the various intrathecal routes (20 mg per dose) is indicated as an adjunct to intravenous treatment in fungal meningitis. Succeeding intrathecal injections may be alternated between lumbar, cervical, and cisternal punctures every 3 to 7 days. Bladder instillation: 200 mg of miconazole in a diluted solution is indicated in the treatment of *Candida* of the urinary bladder.

HOW SUPPLIED

MONISTAT i.v. is supplied in 20 ml (200 mg) ampoules.
Store at controlled room temperature. (15° to 30° C/59° to 86°F)
NDC 50458-200-20
U.S. Patent No. 3,717,655; 3,839,574
Rev. Nov. 1988, June 1989
Janssen Pharmaceutica
Titusville, NJ 08560-0200

Shown in Product Identification Section, page 412

NIZORAL® ℞
[nī'zōr-ăl]
(ketoconazole) 2% Cream

DESCRIPTION

NIZORAL® (ketoconazole) 2% Cream contains the broad-spectrum synthetic antifungal agent, ketoconazole 2%, formulated in an aqueous cream vehicle consisting of propylene glycol, stearyl and cetyl alcohols, sorbitan monostearate, polysorbate 60, isopropyl myristate, sodium sulfite anhydrous, polysorbate 80 and purified water.

Ketoconazole is *cis*-1-acetyl-4-[4-[[2-(2,4-dichlorophenyl)-2-(1*H*-imidazol-1-ylmethyl)-1,3-dioxolan-4-yl] methoxy] phenyl]piperazine.

CLINICAL PHARMACOLOGY

When NIZORAL® (ketoconazole) 2% Cream was applied dermally to intact or abraded skin of Beagle dogs for 28 consecutive days at a dose of 80 mg, there were no detectable plasma levels using an assay method having a lower detection limit of 2 ng/ml.

After a single topical application to the chest, back and arms of normal volunteers, systemic absorption of ketoconazole was not detected at the 5 ng/ml level in blood over a 72-hour period.

Two dermal irritancy studies, a human sensitization test, a phototoxicity study and a photoallergy study conducted in 38 male and 62 female volunteers showed no contact sensitization of the delayed hypersensitivity type, no irritation, no phototoxicity and no photoallergenic potential due to NIZORAL® (ketoconazole) 2% Cream.

Microbiology: Ketoconazole is a broad spectrum synthetic antifungal agent which inhibits the *in vitro* growth of the following common dermatophytes and yeasts by altering the permeability of the cell membrane: dermatophytes: *Trichophyton rubrum, T. mentagrophytes, T. tonsurans, Microsporum canis, M. audouini, M. gypseum* and *Epidermophyton floccosum;* yeasts: *Candida albicans, Malassezia ovale* (*Pityrosporum ovale*) and *C. tropicalis;* and the organism responsible for tinea versicolor, *Malassezia furfur* (*Pityrosporum orbiculare*). Only those organisms listed in the INDICATIONS AND USAGE Section have been proven to be clinically affected. Development of resistance to ketoconazole has not been reported.

Mode of Action: *In vitro* studies suggest that ketoconazole impairs the synthesis of ergosterol, which is a vital component of fungal cell membranes. It is postulated that the therapeutic effect of ketoconazole in seborrheic dermatitis is due to the reduction of M. ovale, but this has not been proven.

INDICATIONS AND USAGE

NIZORAL® (ketoconazole) 2% Cream is indicated for the topical treatment of tinea corporis and tinea cruris caused by *Trichophyton rubrum, T. mentagrophytes** and *Epidermophyton floccosum;* in the treatment of tinea (pityriasis) versicolor caused by *Malassezia furfur (Pityrosporum orbiculare);* in the treatment of cutaneous candidiasis caused by *Candida spp.* and in the treatment of seborrheic dermatitis.

*Efficacy for this organism in this organ system was studied in fewer than ten infections.

CONTRAINDICATIONS

NIZORAL® (ketoconazole) 2% Cream is contraindicated in persons who have shown hypersensitivity to the active or excipient ingredients of this formulation.

WARNINGS

NIZORAL® (ketoconazole) 2% Cream is not for ophthalmic use.

NIZORAL® (ketoconazole) 2% Cream contains sodium sulfite anhydrous, a sulfite that may cause allergic-type reactions including anaphylactic symptoms and life-threatening or less severe asthmatic episodes in certain susceptible people. The overall prevalence of sulfite sensitivity in the general population is unknown and probably low. Sulfite sensitivity is seen more frequently in asthmatic than in nonasthmatic people.

PRECAUTIONS

General: If a reaction suggesting sensitivity or chemical irritation should occur, use of the medication should be discontinued. Hepatitis (1:10,000 reported incidence) and, at high doses, lowered testosterone and ACTH induced corticosteroid serum levels have been seen with orally administered ketoconazole; these effects have not been seen with topical ketoconazole.

Carcinogenesis, Mutagenesis, Impairment of Fertility: A long-term feeding study in Swiss Albino mice and in Wistar rats showed no evidence of oncogenic activity. The dominant lethal mutation test in male and female mice revealed that single oral doses of ketoconazole as high as 80 mg/kg produced no mutation in any stage of germ cell development. The Ames' *Salmonella* microsomal activator assay was also negative.

Pregnancy: Teratogenic effects: Pregnancy Category C: Ketoconazole has been shown to be teratogenic (syndactylia and oligodactylia) in the rat when given orally in the diet at 80 mg/kg/day, (10 times the maximum recommended human oral dose). However, these effects may be related to maternal toxicity, which was seen at this and higher dose levels.

There are no adequate and well-controlled studies in pregnant women. Ketoconazole should be used during pregnancy only if the potential benefit justifies the potential risk to the fetus.

Nursing Mothers: It is not known whether NIZORAL® (ketoconazole) 2% Cream administered topically could result in sufficient systemic absorption to produce detectable quantities in breast milk. Nevertheless, a decision should be made whether to discontinue nursing or discontinue the drug, taking into account the importance of the drug to the mother.

Pediatric Use: Safety and effectiveness in children have not been established.

ADVERSE REACTIONS

During clinical trials 45 (5.0%) of 905 patients treated with NIZORAL® (ketoconazole) 2% Cream and 5 (2.4%) of 208 patients treated with placebo reported side effects consisting mainly of severe irritation, pruritus and stinging. One of the patients treated with NIZORAL Cream developed a painful allergic reaction.

DOSAGE AND ADMINISTRATION

Cutaneous candidiasis, tinea corporis, tinea cruris, and *tinea (pityriasis) versicolor:* It is recommended that NIZORAL® (ketoconazole) 2% Cream be applied once daily to cover the affected and immediate surrounding area. Clinical improvement may be seen fairly soon after treatment is begun; however, candidal infections and tinea cruris and corporis should be treated for two weeks in order to reduce the possibility of recurrence. Patients with tinea versicolor usually require two weeks of treatment.

Seborrheic dermatitis: NIZORAL® (ketoconazole) 2% Cream should be applied to the affected area twice daily for four weeks or until clinical clearing.

If a patient shows no clinical improvement after the treatment period, the diagnosis should be redetermined.

HOW SUPPLIED

NIZORAL® (ketoconazole) 2% Cream is supplied in 15 (NDC 50458-221-15), 30 (NDC 50458-221-30) and 60 (NDC 50458-221-60) gm tubes.
Rev. Feb. 1988, April 1992
U.S. Patent No. 4,335,125
Manufactured by:
ALTANA, INC.
Melville, N.Y. 11747
Distributed by:
JANSSEN PHARMACEUTICA INC.
Titusville, NJ 08560-0200

Shown in Product Identification Section, page 412

NIZORAL® ℞
[nī'zōr-ăl]
(ketoconazole) 2% Shampoo

DESCRIPTION

NIZORAL® (ketoconazole) 2% Shampoo is a pink liquid for topical application, containing the broad-spectrum synthetic antifungal agent ketoconazole in a concentration of 2% in an aqueous suspension. It also contains: coconut fatty acid diethanolamide, disodium monolauryl ether sulphosuccinate, F.D. & C. Red No. 40, hydrochloric acid, imidurea, laurdimonium hydrolyzed animal collagen, macrogol 120 methyl glucose dioleate, perfume bouquet, purified water, and sodium lauryl ether sulphate.

Ketoconazole is cis-1-acetyl-4-[4-[[2-(2,4-dichlorophenyl)-2-(1H-imidazol-1-ylmethyl)-1,3-dioxolan-4-yl] methoxy]-phenyl]piperazine

CLINICAL PHARMACOLOGY

When ketoconazole 2% shampoo was applied dermally to intact or abraded skin of rabbits for 28 days at doses up to 50 mg/kg and allowed to remain one hour before being washed away, there were no detectable plasma ketoconazole levels using an assay method having a lower detection limit of 5 ng/ml. NIZORAL® (ketoconazole) was not detected in plasma in 39 patients who shampooed 4–10 times per week for 6 months or in 33 patients who shampooed 2–3 times per week for 3–26 months (mean: 16 months).

Twelve hours after a single shampoo, hair samples taken from six patients showed that high amounts of ketoconazole were present on the hair but only about 5% had penetrated into the hair keratin. Chronic shampooing (twice weekly for two months) increased the ketoconazole levels in the hair keratin to 20%, but did not increase levels on the hair. There were no detectable plasma levels.

An exaggerated use washing test on the sensitive antecubital skin of 10 subjects twice daily for five consecutive days showed that the irritancy potential of ketoconazole 2% shampoo was significantly less than that of 2.5% selenium sulfide shampoo.

A human sensitization test, a phototoxicity study, and a photallergy study conducted in 38 male and 22 female volunteers showed no contact sensitization of the delayed hypersensitivity type, no phototoxicity and no photoallergenic potential due to NIZORAL® (ketoconazole) 2% Shampoo.

Mode of Action: Interpretations of *in vitro* studies suggest that ketoconazole impairs the synthesis of ergosterol, which is a vital component of fungal cell membranes. It is postulated that the therapeutic effect of ketoconazole in dandruff is due to the reduction of *Pityrosporum ovale (Malassezia ovale)*, but this has not been proven. Support for this hypothesis comes from a 4-week double-blind, placebo-controlled clinical trial, in which the decrease in *P. ovale* on the scalp was significantly greater with ketoconazole (36 patients) than with placebo (20 patients) and was comparable to that with selenium sulfide (42 patients). In the same study, ketoconazole and selenium sulfide reduced the severity of adherent dandruff significantly more than the placebo did. Ketoconazole produced significantly higher proportions of patients with at least 50% reductions in adherent dandruff (50% vs. 15%) and in loose dandruff (67% vs. 15%) than did the placebo.

Microbiology: NIZORAL® (ketoconazole) is a broad-spectrum synthetic antifungal agent which inhibits the growth of the following common dermatophytes and yeasts by altering the permeability of the cell membrane: dermatophytes: *Trichophyton rubrum, T. mentagrophytes, T. tonsurans, Microsporum canis, M. audouini, M. gypseum* and *Epidermophyton floccosum;* yeasts: *Candida albicans, C. tropicalis, Pityrosporum ovale (Malassezia ovale)* and *Pityrosporum orbiculare (M. furfur).* Development of resistance by these microorganisms to ketoconazole has not been reported.

INDICATIONS AND USAGE

NIZORAL® (ketoconazole) 2% Shampoo is indicated for the reduction of scaling due to dandruff.

CONTRAINDICATIONS

NIZORAL® (ketoconazole) 2% Shampoo is contraindicated in persons who have shown hypersensitivity to the active ingredient or excipients of this formulation.

PRECAUTIONS

General: If a reaction suggesting sensitivity or chemical irritation should occur, use of the medication should be discontinued.

Information for Patients: May be irritating to mucous membranes of the eyes and contact with this area should be avoided.

There have been reports that use of the shampoo resulted in removal of the curl from permanently waved hair.

Carcinogenesis, Mutagenesis, Impairment of Fertility: The dominant lethal mutation test in male and female mice revealed that single oral doses of ketoconazole as high as 80 mg/kg produced no mutation in any stage of germ cell devel-

Continued on next page

Janssen Pharmaceutica—Cont.

opment. The Ames Salmonella microsomal activator assay was also negative. A long-term feeding study of ketoconazole in Swiss Albino mice and in Wistar rats showed no evidence of oncogenic activity.

Pregnancy: Teratogenic effects: Pregnancy Category C: Ketoconazole is not detected in plasma after chronic shampooing. Ketoconazole has been shown to be teratogenic (syndactylia and oligodactylia) in the rat when given orally in the diet at 80 mg/kg/day (10 times the maximum recommended human oral dose). However, these effects may be related to maternal toxicity, which was seen at this and higher dose levels.

There are no adequate and well-controlled studies in pregnant women. Ketoconazole should be used during pregnancy only if the potential benefit justifies the potential risk to the fetus.

Nursing mothers: Ketoconazole is not detected in plasma after chronic shampooing. Nevertheless, caution should be exercised when NIZORAL® (ketoconazole) 2% Shampoo is administered to a nursing woman.

Pediatric Use: Safety and effectiveness in children have not been established.

ADVERSE REACTIONS

In 11 double-blind trials in 264 patients using ketoconazole 2% shampoo, an increase in normal hair loss and irritation occurred in less than 1% of patients. In three open-label safety trials in which 41 patients shampooed 4–10 times weekly for six months, the following adverse experiences each occurred once: abnormal hair texture, scalp pustules, mild dryness of the skin, and itching. As with other shampoos, oiliness and dryness of hair and scalp have been reported.

OVERDOSAGE

NIZORAL® (ketoconazole) 2% Shampoo is intended for external use only. In the event of ingestion, supportive measures, including gastric lavage with sodium bicarbonate, should be employed.

DOSAGE AND ADMINISTRATION

1. Moisten hair and scalp thoroughly with water.
2. Apply sufficient shampoo to produce enough lather to wash the scalp and hair and gently massage it over the entire scalp area for approximately 1 minute.
3. Rinse the hair thoroughly with warm water.
4. Repeat, leaving the shampoo on the scalp for an additional 3 minutes.
5. After the second thorough rinse, dry the hair with a towel or warm air flow.

Shampoo twice a week for four weeks with at least three days between each shampooing the then intermittently as needed to maintain control.

HOW SUPPLIED

NIZORAL® (ketoconazole) 2% Shampoo is a pink liquid supplied in a 4-fluid ounce nonbreakable plastic bottle (NDC 50458-223-04).

Storage conditions: Store at a temperature not above 25°C (77°F). Protect from light.

Manufactured by:
Janssen Pharmaceutica n.v.
Beerse, Belgium
Distributed by:
Janssen Pharmaceutica Inc.
Titusville, NJ 08560-0200
Printed June 1990
U.S. Patent No. 4,335,125

Shown in Product Identification Section, page 412

NIZORAL® ℞
[*nī ′zōr-ăl*]
(ketoconazole)
Tablets

> **WARNING:** Ketoconazole has been associated with hepatic toxicity, including some fatalities. Patients receiving this drug should be informed by the physician of the risk and should be closely monitored. See WARNINGS and PRECAUTIONS sections.
>
> QT interval prolongation/ventricular dysrhythmia: When taken in combination with ketoconazole tablets, terfenadine has been associated with QT interval prolongation and ventricular dysrhythmia. Cases of severe cardiovascular adverse events, including death, cardiac arrest, torsades de pointes and other ventricular dysrhythmias have been observed in patients taking ketoconazole tablets concomitantly with terfenadine due to increased terfenadine concentrations induced by ketoconazole tablets. Coadministration of ketoconazole tablets and terfenadine is contraindicated. See WARNINGS and PRECAUTIONS sections.

DESCRIPTION

NIZORAL® (ketoconazole) is a synthetic broad-spectrum antifungal agent available in scored white tablets, each containing 200 mg ketoconazole base for oral administration. Inactive ingredients are colloidal silicon dioxide, corn starch, lactose, magnesium stearate, microcrystalline cellulose, and povidone. Ketoconazole is cis-1-acetyl-4-[4-[[2-(2,4-dichlorophenyl) -2- (1H-imidazol-1-ylmethyl)-1,3-dioxolan-4-yl] methoxyl]phenyl]piperazine.

Ketoconazole is a white to slightly beige, odorless powder, soluble in acids, with a molecular weight of 531.44.

CLINICAL PHARMACOLOGY

Mean peak plasma levels of approximately 3.5 μg/mL are reached within 1 to 2 hours, following oral administration of a single 200 mg dose taken with a meal. Subsequent plasma elimination is biphasic with a half life of 2 hours during the first 10 hours and 8 hours thereafter. Following absorption from the gastrointestinal tract, NIZORAL (ketoconazole) is converted into several inactive metabolites. The major identified metabolic pathways are oxidation and degradation of the imidazole and piperazine rings, oxidative O-dealkylation and aromatic hydroxylation. About 13% of the dose is excreted in the urine, of which 2 to 4% is unchanged drug. The major route of excretion is through the bile into the intestinal tract. *In vitro,* the plasma protein binding is about 99%, mainly to the albumin fraction. Only a negligible proportion of NIZORAL reaches the cerebral-spinal fluid. NIZORAL is a weak dibasic agent and thus requires acidity for dissolution and absorption.

NIZORAL is active against clinical infections with *Blastomyces dermatitidis, Candida spp., Coccidioides immitis, Histoplasma capsulatum, Paracoccidioides brasiliensis,* and *Phialophora spp.* It is also active against *Trichophyton spp., Epidermophyton spp.,* and *Microsporum spp.* NIZORAL is active *in vitro* against a variety of fungi and yeast. In animal models, activity has been demonstrated against *Candida spp., Blastomyces dermatitidis, Histoplasma capsulatum, Malassezia furfur, Coccidioides immitis,* and *Cryptococcus neoformans.*

Mode of Action: In vitro studies suggest that NIZORAL impairs the synthesis of ergosterol, which is a vital component of fungal cell membranes.

INDICATIONS AND USAGE

NIZORAL (ketoconazole) is indicated for the treatment of the following systemic fungal infections: candidiasis, chronic mucocutaneous candidiasis, oral thrush, candiduria, blastomycosis, coccidioidomycosis, histoplasmosis, chromomycosis, and paracoccidioidomycosis. NIZORAL should not be used for fungal meningitis because it penetrates poorly into the cerebral-spinal fluid.

NIZORAL is also indicated for the treatment of patients with severe recalcitrant cutaneous dermatophyte infections who have not responded to topical therapy or oral griseofulvin, or who are unable to take griseofulvin.

CONTRAINDICATIONS

NIZORAL is contraindicated in patients who have shown hypersensitivity to the drug.

WARNINGS

Hepatotoxicity, primarily of the hepatocellular type, has been associated with the use of NIZORAL (ketoconazole), including rare fatalities. The reported incidence of hepatotoxicity has been about 1:10,000 exposed patients, but this probably represents some degree of under-reporting, as is the case for most reported adverse reactions to drugs. The median duration of ketoconazole therapy in patients who developed symptomatic hepatotoxicity was about 28 days, although the range extended to as low as 3 days. The hepatic injury has usually, but not always, been reversible upon discontinuation of NIZORAL (ketoconazole) treatment. Several cases of hepatitis have been reported in children.

Prompt recognition of liver injury is essential. Liver function tests (such as SGGT, alkaline phosphatase, SGPT, SGOT and bilirubin) should be measured before starting treatment and at frequent intervals during treatment. Patients receiving ketoconazole concurrently with other potentially hepatotoxic drugs should be carefully monitored, particularly those patients requiring prolonged therapy or those who have had a history of liver disease.

Most of the reported cases of hepatic toxicity have to date been in patients treated for onychomycosis. Of 180 patients worldwide developing idiosyncratic liver dysfunction during ketoconazole therapy, 61.3% had onychomycosis and 16.8% had chronic recalcitrant dermatophytoses.

Transient minor elevations in liver enzymes have occurred during ketoconazole treatment. The drug should be discontinued if these persist, if the abnormalities worsen, or if the abnormalities become accompanied by symptoms of possible liver injury.

In rare cases anaphylaxis has been reported after the first dose. Several cases of hypersensitivity reactions including urticaria have also been reported.

Coadministration of ketoconazole tablets and terfenadine has led to elevated plasma concentrations of terfenadine which may prolong QT intervals, sometimes resulting in life-threatening cardiac dysrhythmias. Cases of torsades de pointes and other serious ventricular dysrhythmias, in rare cases leading to fatality, have been reported among patients taking terfenadine concurrently with ketoconazole tablets. Coadministration of ketoconazole tablets and terfenadine is contraindicated.

In European clinical trials involving 350 patients with metastatic prostatic cancer, eleven deaths were reported within two weeks of starting treatment with high doses of ketoconazole (1200 mg/day). It is not possible to ascertain from the information available whether death was related to ketoconazole therapy in these patients with serious underlying disease. However, high doses of ketoconazole are known to suppress adrenal corticosteroid secretion.

In female rats treated three to six months with ketoconazole at dose levels of 80 mg/kg and higher, increased fragility of long bones, in some cases leading to fracture, was seen. The maximum "no-effect" dose level in these studies was 20 mg/kg (2.5 times the maximum recommended human dose). The mechanism responsible for this phenomenon is obscure. Limited studies in dogs failed to demonstrate such an effect on the metacarpals and ribs.

PRECAUTIONS

General: NIZORAL (ketoconazole) has been demonstrated to lower serum testosterone. Once therapy with NIZORAL has been discontinued, serum testosterone levels return to baseline values. Testosterone levels are impaired with doses of 800 mg per day and abolished by 1600 mg per day. NIZORAL also decreases ACTH induced corticosteroid serum levels at similar high doses. The recommended dose of 200 mg–400 mg daily should be followed closely.

In four subjects with drug-induced achlorhydria, a marked reduction in NIZORAL (ketoconazole) absorption was observed. NIZORAL requires acidity for dissolution. If concomitant antacids, anticholinergics, and H_2-blockers are needed, they should be given at least two hours after NIZORAL administration. In cases of achlorhydria, the patients should be instructed to dissolve each tablet in 4 mL aqueous solution of 0.2 N HCl. For ingesting the resulting mixture, they should use a drinking straw so as to avoid contact with the teeth. This administration should be followed with a cup of tap water.

Information for patients: Patients should be instructed to report any signs and symptoms which may suggest liver dysfunction so that appropriate biochemical testing can be done. Such signs and symptoms may include unusual fatigue, anorexia, nausea and/or vomiting, jaundice, dark urine or pale stools (see WARNINGS).

Drug interactions: Imidazole compounds like ketoconazole may enhance the anticoagulant effect of coumarin-like drugs. In simultaneous treatment with imidazole drugs and coumarin drugs, the anticoagulant effect should be carefully titrated and monitored.

Concomitant administration of rifampin with ketoconazole reduces the blood levels of the latter. INH (Isoniazid) is also reported to affect ketoconazole concentrations adversely. These drugs should not be given concomitantly.

Ketoconazole increases the blood level of cyclosporin A. Blood levels of cyclosporin A should be monitored if the two drugs are given concomitantly.

Concomitant administration of ketoconazole with phenytoin may alter the metabolism of one or both of the drugs. It is suggested to monitor both ketoconazole and phenytoin.

Because severe hypoglycemia has been reported in patients concomitantly receiving oral miconazole (an imidazole) and oral hypoglycemic agents, such a potential interaction involving the latter agents when used concomitantly with ketoconazole (an imidazole) can not be ruled out.

Ketoconazole tablets inhibits the metabolism of terfenadine, resulting in an increased plasma concentration of terfenadine and a delay in the elimination of its acid metabolite. The increased plasma concentration of terfenadine or its metabolite may result in prolonged QT intervals (see WARNINGS).

Carcinogenesis, Mutagenesis, Impairment of Fertility: The dominant lethal mutation test in male and female mice revealed that single oral doses of NIZORAL (ketoconazole) as high as 80 mg/kg produced no mutation in any stage of germ cell development. The *Ames Salmonella* microsomal activator assay was also negative. A long term feeding study in Swiss Albino mice and in Wistar rats showed no evidence of oncogenic activity.

Pregnancy: Teratogenic effects: *Pregnancy Category C.* NIZORAL (ketoconazole) has been shown to be teratogenic (syndactylia and oligodactylia) in the rat when given in the diet at 80 mg/kg/day, (10 times the maximum recommended human dose). However, these effects may be related to maternal toxicity, evidence of which also was seen at this and higher dose levels.

There are no adequate and well controlled studies in pregnant women. NIZORAL should be used during pregnancy

only if the potential benefit justifies the potential risk to the fetus.

Nonteratogenic effects: NIZORAL has also been found to be embryotoxic in the rat when given in the diet at doses higher than 80 mg/kg during the first trimester of gestation. In addition, dystocia (difficult labor) was noted in rats administered NIZORAL during the third trimester of gestation. This occurred when NIZORAL was administered at doses higher than 10 mg/kg (higher than 1.25 times the maximum human dose).

It is likely that both the malformations and the embryotoxicity resulting from the administration of NIZORAL (ketoconazole) during gestation are a reflection of the particular sensitivity of the female rat to this drug. For example, the oral LD_{50} of NIZORAL given by gavage to the female rat is 166 mg/kg whereas in the male rat the oral LD_{50} is 287 mg/kg.

Nursing Mothers: Since NIZORAL is probably excreted in the milk, mothers who are under treatment should not breast feed.

Pediatric Use: NIZORAL has not been systematically studied in children of any age, and essentially no information is available on children under 2 years. NIZORAL should not be used in pediatric patients unless the potential benefit outweighs the risks.

ADVERSE REACTIONS

In rare cases anaphylaxis has been reported after the first dose. Several cases of hypersensitivity reactions including urticaria have also been reported. However, the most frequent adverse reactions were nausea and/or vomiting in approximately 3%, abdominal pain in 1.2%, pruritus in 1.5%, and the following in less than 1% of the patients: headache, dizziness, somnolence, fever and chills, photophobia, diarrhea, gynecomastia, impotence, thrombocytopenia, leukopenia, hemolytic anemia, and bulging fontanelles. Oligospermia has been reported in investigational studies with the drug at dosages above those currently approved. Although oligospermia has not been reported at dosages up to 400 mg daily, sperm counts have been obtained infrequently in patients treated with these dosages. Most of these reactions were mild and transient and rarely required discontinuation of NIZORAL (ketoconazole). In contrast, the rare occurrences of hepatic dysfunction require special attention (see WARNINGS).

Neuropsychiatric disturbances, including suicidal tendencies and severe depression have occurred rarely in patients using NIZORAL.

Ventricular dysrhythmias (prolonged QT intervals) have occurred with the concomitant use of terfenadine with ketoconazole tablets (see WARNINGS).

OVERDOSAGE

In the event of accidental overdosage, supportive measures, including gastric lavage with sodium bicarbonate, should be employed.

DOSAGE AND ADMINISTRATION

Adults: The recommended starting dose of NIZORAL is a single daily administration of 200 mg (one tablet). In very serious infections or if clinical responsiveness is insufficient within the expected time, the dose of NIZORAL may be increased to 400 mg (two tablets) once daily.

Children: In small numbers of children over 2 years of age, a single daily dose of 3.3 to 6.6 mg/kg has been used. NIZORAL (ketoconazole) has not been studied in children under 2 years of age.

There should be laboratory as well as clinical documentation of infection prior to starting ketoconazole therapy. Treatment should be continued until tests indicate that active fungal infection has subsided. Inadequate periods of treatment may yield poor response and lead to early recurrence of clinical symptoms. Minimum treatment for candidiasis is one or two weeks. Patients with chronic mucocutaneous candidiasis usually require maintenance therapy. Minimum treatment for the other indicated systemic mycoses is six months.

Minimum treatment for recalcitrant dermatophyte infections is four weeks in cases involving glabrous skin. Palmar and plantar infections may respond more slowly. Apparent cures may subsequently recur after discontinuation of therapy in some cases.

HOW SUPPLIED

NIZORAL (ketoconazole) is available as white, scored tablets containing 200 mg of ketoconazole debossed "JANSSEN" and on the reverse side debossed "NIZORAL". They are supplied in bottles of 100 tablets (NDC 50458-220-10) and in blister packs of 10×10 tablets (NDC 50458-220-01).

Store at room temperature 15°–30°C (59°–86°F).

U.S. Patent 4,335,125

Rev. April 1991, July 1992

Janssen Pharmaceutica Inc.

Titusville, NJ 08560-0200

USA

Shown in Product Identification Section, page 412

SUBLIMAZE®   ℂ ℞

[sa 'blĭ-māz]

(fentanyl citrate) Injection

CAUTION: Federal Law Prohibits Dispensing Without Prescription

DESCRIPTION

SUBLIMAZE (fentanyl citrate) Injection is a potent narcotic analgesic. Each milliliter of solution contains fentanyl citrate equivalent to 50 µg of fentanyl base, adjusted to pH 4.0 –7.5 with sodium hydroxide. SUBLIMAZE is chemically identified as N-(1-phenethyl-4-piperidyl) propionanilide citrate (1:1) with a molecular weight of 528.60. The empirical formula is $C_{22}H_{28}N_2O\cdot C_6H_8O_7$.

SUBLIMAZE is a sterile, non-pyrogenic, preservative free aqueous solution for intravenous or intramuscular injection.

CLINICAL PHARMACOLOGY

SUBLIMAZE (fentanyl citrate) is a narcotic analgesic. A dose of 100 µg (0.1 mg) (2.0 ml) is approximately equivalent in analgesic activity to 10 mg of morphine or 75 mg of meperidine. The principal actions of therapeutic value are analgesia and sedation. Alterations in respiratory rate and alveolar ventilation, associated with narcotic analgesics, may last longer than the analgesic effect. As the dose of narcotic is increased, the decrease in pulmonary exchange becomes greater. Large doses may produce apnea. SUBLIMAZE appears to have less emetic activity than either morphine or meperidine. Histamine assays and skin wheal testing in man indicate that clinically significant histamine release rarely occurs with SUBLIMAZE. Recent assays in man show no clinically significant histamine release in dosages up to 50 µg/kg (0.05 mg/kg) (1 ml/kg). SUBLIMAZE preserves cardiac stability, and blunts stress-related hormonal changes at higher doses.

The pharmacokinetics of SUBLIMAZE can be described as a three-compartment model, with a distribution time of 1.7 minutes, redistribution of 13 minutes and a terminal elimination half life of 219 minutes. The volume of distribution for SUBLIMAZE is 4 L/kg.

SUBLIMAZE plasma protein binding capacity decreases with increasing ionization of the drug. Alterations in pH may affect its distribution between plasma and the central nervous system. It accumulates in skeletal muscle and fat, and is released slowly into the blood. SUBLIMAZE, which is primarily transformed in the liver, demonstrates a high first pass clearance and releases approximately 75% of an intravenous dose in urine, mostly as metabolites with less than 10% representing the unchanged drug. Approximately 9% of the dose is recovered in the feces, primarily as metabolites. The onset of action of SUBLIMAZE is almost immediate when the drug is given intravenously; however, the maximal analgesic and respiratory depressant effect may not be noted for several minutes. The usual duration of action of the analgesic effect is 30 to 60 minutes after a single intravenous dose of up to 100 µg (0.1 mg) (2.0 ml). Following intramuscular administration, the onset of action is from seven to eight minutes, and the duration of action is one to two hours. As with longer acting narcotic analgesics, the duration of the respiratory depressant effect of SUBLIMAZE may be longer than the analgesic effect. The following observations have been reported concerning altered respiratory response to CO_2 stimulation following administration of SUBLIMAZE to man.

1. DIMINISHED SENSITIVITY TO CO_2 STIMULATION MAY PERSIST LONGER THAN DEPRESSION OF RESPIRATORY RATE. (Altered sensitivity to CO_2 stimulation has been demonstrated for up to four hours following a single dose of 600 µg (0.6 mg) (12 ml) SUBLIMAZE to healthy volunteers.) SUBLIMAZE frequently slows the respiratory rate, duration and degree of respiratory depression being dose related.
2. The peak respiratory depressant effect of a single intravenous dose of SUBLIMAZE is noted 5 to 15 minutes following injection. See also WARNINGS and PRECAUTIONS concerning respiratory depression.

INDICATIONS AND USAGE

SUBLIMAZE (fentanyl citrate) is indicated:

—for analgesic action of short duration during the anesthetic periods, premedication, induction and maintenance, and in the immediate postoperative period (recovery room) as the need arises.

—for use as a narcotic analgesic supplement in general or regional anesthesia.

—for administration with a neuroleptic such as INAPSINE® (droperidol) Injection as an anesthetic premedication, for the induction of anesthesia and as an adjunct in the maintenance of general and regional anesthesia.

—for use as an anesthetic agent with oxygen in selected high risk patients, such as those undergoing open heart surgery or certain complicated neurological or orthopedic procedures.

CONTRAINDICATIONS

SUBLIMAZE (fentanyl citrate) is contraindicated in patients with known intolerance to the drug.

WARNINGS

SUBLIMAZE (fentanyl citrate) SHOULD BE ADMINISTERED ONLY BY PERSONS SPECIFICALLY TRAINED IN THE USE OF INTRAVENOUS ANESTHETICS AND MANAGEMENT OF THE RESPIRATORY EFFECTS OF POTENT OPIOIDS.

AN OPIOID ANTAGONIST, RESUSCITATIVE AND INTUBATION EQUIPMENT AND OXYGEN SHOULD BE READILY AVAILABLE.

See also discussion of narcotic antagonists in PRECAUTIONS and OVERDOSAGE.

If SUBLIMAZE is administered with a tranquilizer such as INAPSINE (droperidol), the user should become familiar with the special properties of each drug, particularly the widely differing duration of action. In addition, when such a combination is used, fluids and other countermeasures to manage hypotension should be available.

As with other potent narcotics, the respiratory depressant effect of SUBLIMAZE may persist longer than the measured analgesic effect. The total dose of all narcotic analgesics administered should be considered by the practitioner before ordering narcotic analgesics during recovery from anesthesia. It is recommended that narcotics, when required, should be used in reduced doses initially, as low as $\frac{1}{4}$ to $\frac{1}{3}$ those usually recommended.

SUBLIMAZE may cause muscle rigidity, particularly involving the muscles of respiration. This rigidity has been reported to occur or recur infrequently in the extended postoperative period usually following high dose administration. In addition, skeletal muscle movements of various groups in the extremities, neck and external eye have been reported during induction of anesthesia with fentanyl; these reported movements have, on rare occasions, been strong enough to pose patient management problems. This effect is related to the dose and speed of injection and its incidence can be reduced by: 1) administration of up to $\frac{1}{4}$ of the full paralyzing dose of a non-depolarizing neuromuscular blocking agent just prior to administration of SUBLIMAZE; 2) administration of a full paralyzing dose of a neuromuscular blocking agent following loss of eyelash reflex when SUBLIMAZE is used in anesthetic doses titrated by slow intravenous infusion; or, 3) simultaneous administration of SUBLIMAZE and a full paralyzing dose of a neuromuscular blocking agent when SUBLIMAZE is used in rapidly administered anesthetic dosages. The neuromuscular blocking agent used should be compatible with the patient's cardiovascular status.

Adequate facilities should be available for postoperative monitoring and ventilation of patients administered anesthetic doses of SUBLIMAZE. Where moderate or high doses are used (above 10 µg/kg), there must be adequate facilities for postoperative observation, and ventilation if necessary, of patients who have received SUBLIMAZE. It is essential that these facilities be fully equipped to handle all degrees of respiratory depression.

SUBLIMAZE may also produce other signs and symptoms characteristic of narcotic analgesics including euphoria, miosis, bradycardia and bronchoconstriction.

Severe and unpredictable potentiation by MAO inhibitors has been reported for other narcotic analgesics. Although this has not been reported for fentanyl, there are insufficient data to establish that this does not occur with fentanyl. Therefore, when fentanyl is administered to patients who have received MAO inhibitors within 14 days, appropriate monitoring and ready availability of vasodilators and beta-blockers for the treatment of hypertension is indicated.

Head Injuries and Increased Intracranial Pressure— SUBLIMAZE should be used with caution in patients who may be particularly susceptible to respiratory depression, such as comatose patients who may have a head injury or brain tumor. In addition, SUBLIMAZE may obscure the clinical course of patients with head injury.

PRECAUTIONS

General: The initial dose of SUBLIMAZE (fentanyl citrate) should be appropriately reduced in elderly and debilitated patients. The effect of the initial dose should be considered in determining incremental doses.

Nitrous oxide has been reported to produce cardiovascular depression when given with higher doses of SUBLIMAZE. Certain forms of conduction anesthesia, such as spinal anesthesia and some peridural anesthetics, can alter respiration by blocking intercostal nerves. Through other mechanisms (see CLINICAL PHARMACOLOGY) SUBLIMAZE can also alter respiration. Therefore, when SUBLIMAZE is used to supplement these forms of anesthesia, the anesthetist should be familiar with the physiological alterations involved, and be prepared to manage them in the patients selected for these forms of anesthesia.

Continued on next page

Janssen Pharmaceutica—Cont.

When a tranquilizer such as INAPSINE (droperidol) is used with SUBLIMAZE, pulmonary arterial pressure may be decreased. This fact should be considered by those who conduct diagnostic and surgical procedures where interpretation of pulmonary arterial pressure measurements might determine final management of the patient. When high dose or anesthetic dosages of SUBLIMAZE are employed, even relatively small dosages of diazepam may cause cardiovascular depression.

When SUBLIMAZE is used with a tranquilizer such as INAPSINE (droperidol), hypotension can occur. If it occurs, the possibility of hypovolemia should also be considered and managed with appropriate parenteral fluid therapy. Repositioning the patient to improve venous return to the heart should be considered when operative conditions permit. Care should be exercised in moving and positioning of patients because of the possibility of orthostatic hypotension. If volume expansion with fluids plus other countermeasures do not correct hypotension, the administration of pressor agents other than epinephrine should be considered. Because of the alpha-adrenergic blocking action of INAPSINE (droperidol), epinephrine may paradoxically decrease the blood pressure in patients treated with INAPSINE (droperidol).

Elevated blood pressure, with and without pre-existing hypertension, has been reported following administration of SUBLIMAZE combined with INAPSINE (droperidol). This might be due to unexplained alterations in sympathetic activity following large doses; however, it is also frequently attributed to anesthetic and surgical stimulation during light anesthesia.

When INAPSINE (droperidol) is used with SUBLIMAZE and the EEG is used for postoperative monitoring, it may be found that the EEG pattern returns to normal slowly.

Vital signs should be monitored routinely.

Respiratory depression caused by opioid analgesics can be reversed by opioid antagonists such as naloxone. Because the duration of respiratory depression produced by SUBLIMAZE may last longer than the duration of the opioid antagonist action, appropriate surveillance should be maintained. As with all potent opioids, profound analgesia is accompanied by respiratory depression and diminished sensitivity to CO_2 stimulation which may persist into or recur in the postoperative period. Respiratory depression secondary to chest wall rigidity has been reported in the postoperative period. Intraoperative hyperventilation may further alter postoperative response to CO_2. Appropriate postoperative monitoring should be employed to ensure that adequate spontaneous breathing is established and maintained in the absence of stimulation prior to discharging the patient from the recovery area.

Impaired Respiration: SUBLIMAZE should be used with caution in patients with chronic obstructive pulmonary disease, patients with decreased respiratory reserve, and others with potentially compromised respiration. In such patients, narcotics may additionally decrease respiratory drive and increase airway resistance. During anesthesia, this can be managed by assisted or controlled respiration.

Impaired Hepatic or Renal Function: SUBLIMAZE should be administered with caution to patients with liver and kidney dysfunction because of the importance of these organs in the metabolism and excretion of drugs.

Cardiovascular Effects: SUBLIMAZE may produce bradycardia, which may be treated with atropine. SUBLIMAZE should be used with caution in patients with cardiac bradyarrhythmias.

Drug Interactions: Other CNS depressant drugs (e.g. barbiturates, tranquilizers, narcotics and general anesthetics) will have additive or potentiating effects with SUBLIMAZE. When patients have received such drugs, the dose of SUBLIMAZE required will be less than usual. Following the administration of SUBLIMAZE, the dose of other CNS depressant drugs should be reduced.

Carcinogenesis, Mutagenesis, Impairment of Fertility: No carcinogenicity or mutagenicity studies have been conducted with SUBLIMAZE. Reproduction studies in rats revealed a significant decrease in the pregnancy rate of all experimental groups. This decrease was most pronounced in the high dosed group (1.25 mg/kg—12.5X human dose) in which one of twenty animals became pregnant.

Pregnancy—Category C: SUBLIMAZE has been shown to impair fertility and to have an embryocidal effect in rats when given in doses 0.3 times the upper human dose for a period of 12 days. No evidence of teratogenic effects have been observed after administration of SUBLIMAZE to rats. There are no adequate and well-controlled studies in pregnant women. SUBLIMAZE should be used during pregnancy only if the potential benefit justifies the potential risk to the fetus.

Labor and Delivery: There are insufficient data to support the use of SUBLIMAZE in labor and delivery. Therefore, such use is not recommended.

Nursing Mothers: It is not known whether this drug is excreted in human milk. Because many drugs are excreted in human milk, caution should be exercised when SUBLIMAZE is administered to a nursing woman.

Pediatric Use: The safety and efficacy of SUBLIMAZE in children under two years of age has not been established. Rare cases of unexplained clinically significant methemoglobinemia have been reported in premature neonates undergoing emergency anesthesia and surgery which included combined use of fentanyl, pancuronium and atropine. A direct cause and effect relationship between the combined use of these drugs and the reported cases of methemoglobinemia has not been established.

ADVERSE REACTIONS

As with other narcotic analgesics, the most common serious adverse reactions reported to occur with SUBLIMAZE (fentanyl citrate) are respiratory depression, apnea, rigidity, and bradycardia; if these remain untreated, respiratory arrest, circulatory depression or cardiac arrest could occur. Other adverse reactions that have been reported are hypertension, hypotension, dizziness, blurred vision, nausea, emesis, laryngospasm, and diaphoresis.

It has been reported that secondary rebound respiratory depression may occasionally occur postoperatively. Patients should be monitored for this possibility and appropriate countermeasures taken as necessary.

When a tranquilizer such as INAPSINE (droperidol) is used with SUBLIMAZE, the following adverse reactions can occur: chills and/or shivering, restlessness, and postoperative hallucinatory episodes (sometimes associated with transient periods of mental depression); extrapyramidal symptoms (dystonia, akathisia, and oculogyric crisis) have been observed up to 24 hours postoperatively. When they occur,

extrapyramidal symptoms can usually be controlled with anti-parkinson agents. Postoperative drowsiness is also frequently reported following the use of INAPSINE (droperidol).

DRUG ABUSE AND DEPENDENCE

SUBLIMAZE (fentanyl citrate) is a Schedule II controlled drug substance that can produce drug dependence of the morphine type and therefore has the potential for being abused.

OVERDOSAGE

Manifestations: The manifestations of SUBLIMAZE (fentanyl citrate) overdosage are an extension of its pharmacologic actions (see CLINICAL PHARMACOLOGY) as with other opioid analgesics. The intravenous LD_{50} of SUBLIMAZE is 3 mg/kg in rats, 1 mg/kg in cats, 14 mg/kg in dogs and 0.03 mg/kg in monkeys.

Treatment: In the presence of hypoventilation or apnea, oxygen should be administered and respiration should be assisted or controlled as indicated. A patent airway must be maintained; an oropharyngeal airway or endotracheal tube might be indicated. If depressed respiration is associated with muscular rigidity, an intravenous neuromuscular blocking agent might be required to facilitate assisted or controlled respiration. The patient should be carefully observed for 24 hours; body warmth and adequate fluid intake should be maintained. If hypotension occurs and is severe or persists, the possibility of hypovolemia should be considered and managed with appropriate parenteral fluid therapy. A specific narcotic antagonist such as nalorphine, levallorphan or naloxone should be available for use as indicated to manage respiratory depression. This does not preclude the use of more immediate countermeasures. The duration of respiratory depression following overdosage of SUBLIMAZE may be longer than the duration of narcotic antagonist action. Consult the package insert of the individual narcotic antagonists for details about use.

DOSAGE AND ADMINISTRATION

$$50 \ \mu g = 0.05 \ mg = 1 \ ml$$

Dosage should be individualized. Some of the factors to be considered in determining the dose are age, body weight, physical status, underlying pathological condition, use of other drugs, type of anesthesia to be used and the surgical procedure involved. Dosage should be reduced in elderly or debilitated patients (see PRECAUTIONS).

Vital signs should be monitored routinely.

I. Premedication—Premedication (to be appropriately modified in the elderly, debilitated and those who have received other depressant drugs)—50 to 100 μg (0.05 to 0.1 mg) (1 to 2 ml) may be administered intramuscularly 30 to 60 minutes prior to surgery.

II. Adjunct to General Anesthesia—See Dosage Range Chart

III. Adjunct to Regional Anesthesia—50 to 100 μg (0.05 to 0.1 mg) (1 to 2 ml) may be administered intramuscularly or slowly intravenously, over one to two minutes, when additional analgesia is required.

IV. Postoperatively (recovery room)—50 to 100 μg (0.05 to 0.1 mg) (1 to 2 ml) may be administered intramuscularly for the control of pain, tachypnea and emergence delirium. The dose may be repeated in one to two hours as needed.

Usage in Children: For induction and maintenance in children 2 to 12 years of age, a reduced dose as low as 2 to 3 μg/kg is recommended. [See table below.]

SUBLIMAZE®

DOSAGE RANGE CHART

TOTAL DOSAGE

Low Dose—2 μg/kg (0.002 mg/kg) (0.04 ml/kg) SUBLIMAZE. SUBLIMAZE in small doses is most useful for minor, but painful, surgical procedures. In addition to the analgesia during surgery, SUBLIMAZE may also provide some pain relief in the immediate postoperative period.	**Moderate Dose**—2-20 μg/kg (0.002–0.02 mg/kg) (0.04 –0.4 ml/kg) SUBLIMAZE. Where surgery becomes more major, a larger dose is required. With this dose, in addition to adequate analgesia, one would expect to see some abolition of the stress response. However, respiratory depression will be such that artificial ventilation during anesthesia is necessary and careful observation of ventilation postoperatively is essential.	**High Dose**—20-50 μg/kg (0.02 –0.05 mg/kg) (0.4–1 ml/kg) SUBLIMAZE. During open heart surgery and certain more complicated neurosurgical and orthopedic procedures where surgery is more prolonged, and in the opinion of the anesthesiologist, the stress response to surgery would be detrimental to the well being of the patient, dosages of 20–50 μg/kg (0.02–0.05 mg) (0.4–1 ml) of SUBLIMAZE with nitrous oxide/oxygen have been shown to attenuate the	stress response as defined by increased levels of circulating growth hormone, catecholamine, ADH and prolactin. When dosages in this range have been used during surgery, postoperative ventilation and observation are essential due to extended postoperative respiratory depression. The main objective of this technique would be to produce "stress free" anesthesia.

SUBLIMAZE® — DOSAGE RANGE CHART

MAINTENANCE DOSE

Low Dose —2 µg/kg (0.002 mg/kg) (0.04 ml/kg) SUBLIMAZE. Additional dosages of SUBLIMAZE are infrequently needed in these minor procedures.	Moderate Dose —2–20 µg/kg (0.002–0.02 mg/kg) (0.04–0.4 ml/kg) SUBLIMAZE. 25 to 100 µg (0.025–0.1 mg) (0.5–2.0 ml) may be administered intravenously or intramuscularly when movement and/or changes in vital signs indicate surgical stress or lightening of analgesia.	High Dose —20–50 µg/kg (0.02–0.05 mg/kg) (0.4–1.0 ml/kg) SUBLIMAZE. Maintenance dosage (ranging from 25 µg (0.025 mg) (0.5 ml) to one half the initial loading dose) will be dictated by the changes in vital signs which indicate stress and lightening of analgesia. However, the additional dosage selected must be individualized especially if the anticipated remaining operative time is short.

[See table above.]

As a General Anesthetic

When attenuation of the responses to surgical stress is especially important, doses of 50 to 100 µg/kg (0.05 to 0.1 mg/kg) (1 to 2 ml/kg) may be administered with oxygen and a muscle relaxant. This technique has been reported to provide anesthesia without the use of additional anesthetic agents. In certain cases, doses up to 150 µg/kg (0.15 mg/kg) (3 ml/kg) may be necessary to produce this anesthetic effect. It has been used for open heart surgery and certain other major surgical procedures in patients for whom protection of the myocardium from excess oxygen demand is particularly indicated, and for certain complicated neurological and orthopedic procedures.

As noted above, it is essential that qualified personnel and adequate facilities be available for the management of respiratory depression.

See WARNINGS and PRECAUTIONS for use of SUBLIMAZE (fentanyl citrate) with other CNS depressants, and in patients with altered response.

Parenteral drug products should be inspected visually for particulate matter and discoloration prior to administration, whenever solution and container permit.

HOW SUPPLIED

SUBLIMAZE (fentanyl citrate) Injection is available as:
NDC 50458-030-02 50 µg/ml of fentanyl base, 2 ml ampoules in packages of 10
NDC 50458-030-05 50 µg/ml of fentanyl base, 5 ml ampoules in packages of 10
NDC 50458-030-10 50 µg/ml of fentanyl base, 10 ml ampoules in packages of 5
NDC 50458-030-20 50 µg/ml of fentanyl base, 20 ml ampoules in packages of 5
PROTECT FROM LIGHT. STORE AT ROOM TEMPERATURE 15°C–30°C (59°F–86°F).
JANSSEN PHARMACEUTICA INC.
Titusville, NJ 08560-0200
U.S. Patent No. 3,164,600
Revised December 1989, July 1991
Shown in Product Identification Section, page 412

SUFENTA®   Ⅽ Ⅱ R

[su-fĕn'ta]
(sufentanil citrate)
Injection

CAUTION: Federal Law Prohibits Dispensing Without Prescription

DESCRIPTION

SUFENTA® (sufentanil citrate) is a potent opioid analgesic chemically designated as N-[4-(methoxymethyl)-1-[2-(2-thienyl) ethyl]-4-piperidinyl]-N-phenylpropanamide 2-hydroxy-1,2,3-propanetricarboxylate (1:1) with a molecular weight of 578.68.

SUFENTA is a sterile, preservative free, aqueous solution containing sufentanil citrate equivalent to 50 µg per ml of sufentanil base for intravenous injection. The solution has a pH range of 3.5–6.0.

CLINICAL PHARMACOLOGY

SUFENTA is an opioid analgesic. When used in balanced general anesthesia, SUFENTA has been reported to be as much as 10 times as potent as fentanyl. When administered as a primary anesthetic agent with 100% oxygen, SUFENTA is approximately 5 to 7 times as potent as fentanyl. (See dosage chart for more complete information on the use of SUFENTA). At doses of up to 8 µg/kg, SUFENTA provides profound analgesia; at doses ≥ 8 µg/kg, SUFENTA produces a deep level of anesthesia. SUFENTA produces a dose related attenuation of catecholamine release, particularly norepinephrine.

The pharmacokinetics of SUFENTA can be described as a three-compartment model, with a distribution time of 1.4 minutes, redistribution of 17.1 minutes and an elimination half-life of 164 minutes. The liver and small intestine are the major sites of biotransformation. Approximately 80% of the administered dose is excreted within 24 hours and only 2% of the dose is eliminated as unchanged drug. Plasma protein binding of SUFENTA is approximately 92.5%.

SUFENTA has an immediate onset of action, with relatively limited accumulation. Rapid elimination from tissue storage sites allows for relatively more rapid recovery as compared with equipotent dosages of fentanyl. At dosages of SUFENTA of 1–2 µg/kg, recovery times are comparable to those observed with fentanyl; at dosages of > 2–6 µg/kg, recovery times are comparable to enflurane, isoflurane and fentanyl. Within the anesthetic dosage range of 8–30 µg/kg of SUFENTA, recovery times are more rapid compared to equipotent fentanyl dosages.

At dosages of ≥ 8 µg/kg, SUFENTA produces hypnosis and anesthesia without the use of additional anesthetic agents. A deep level of anesthesia is maintained at these dosages, as demonstrated by EEG patterns. Dosages of up to 25 µg/kg attenuate the sympathetic response to surgical stress. The catecholamine response, particularly norepinephrine, is further attenuated at doses of SUFENTA of 25–30 µg/kg, with hemodynamic stability and preservation of favorable myocardial oxygen balance.

The vagolytic effects of pancuronium may produce a dose dependent elevation in heart rate during SUFENTA-oxygen anesthesia. The use of moderate doses of pancuronium or of a less vagolytic neuromuscular blocking agent may be used to maintain a stable lower heart rate and blood pressure during SUFENTA-oxygen anesthesia. The vagolytic effect of pancuronium may be reduced in patients administered nitrous oxide with SUFENTA.

Preliminary data suggest that in patients administered high doses of SUFENTA, initial dosage requirements for neuromuscular blocking agents are generally lower as compared to patients given fentanyl or halothane, and comparable to patients given enflurane.

Bradycardia is infrequently seen in patients administered SUFENTA-oxygen anesthesia. The use of nitrous oxide with high doses of SUFENTA may decrease mean arterial pressure, heart rate and cardiac output.

Assays of histamine in patients administered SUFENTA have shown no elevation in plasma histamine levels and no indication of histamine release.

SUFENTA at 20 µg/kg has been shown to provide more adequate reduction in intracranial volume than equivalent doses of fentanyl, based upon requirements for furosemide and anesthesia supplementation in one study of patients undergoing craniotomy. During carotid endarterectomy, SUFENTA-nitrous oxide/oxygen produced reductions in cerebral blood flow comparable to those of enflurane-nitrous oxide/oxygen. During cardiovascular surgery, SUFENTA-oxygen produced EEG patterns similar to fentanyl-oxygen; these EEG changes were judged to be compatible with adequate general anesthesia.

The intraoperative use of SUFENTA at anesthetic dosages maintains cardiac output, with a slight reduction in systemic vascular resistance during the initial postoperative period. The incidence of postoperative hypertension, need for vasoactive agents and requirements for postoperative analgesics are generally reduced in patients administered moderate or high doses of SUFENTA as compared to patients given inhalation agents.

Skeletal muscle rigidity is related to the dose and speed of administration of SUFENTA. This muscular rigidity may occur unless preventative measures are taken (see WARNINGS).

Decreased respiratory drive and increased airway resistance occur with SUFENTA. The duration and degree of respiratory depression are dose related when SUFENTA is used at sub-anesthetic dosages. At high doses, a pronounced decrease in pulmonary exchange and apnea may be produced.

INDICATIONS AND USAGE

SUFENTA (sufentanil citrate) is indicated:
as an analgesic adjunct in the maintenance of balanced general anesthesia in patients who are intubated and ventilated.
as a primary anesthetic agent for the induction and maintenance of anesthesia with 100% oxygen in patients undergoing major surgical procedures, in patients who are intubated and ventilated, such as cardiovascular surgery or neurosurgical procedures in the sitting position, to provide favorable myocardial and cerebral oxygen balance or when extended postoperative ventilation is anticipated.
SEE DOSAGE CHART FOR MORE COMPLETE INFORMATION ON THE USE OF SUFENTA.

CONTRAINDICATIONS

SUFENTA is contraindicated in patients with known hypersensitivity to the drug.

WARNINGS

SUFENTA should be administered only by persons specifically trained in the use of intravenous anesthetics and management of the respiratory effects of potent opioids.
An opioid antagonist, resuscitative and intubation equipment and oxygen should be readily available.
SUFENTA may cause skeletal muscle rigidity, particularly of the truncal muscles. The incidence and severity of muscle rigidity is dose related. Administration of SUFENTA may produce muscular rigidity with a more rapid onset than that seen with fentanyl. SUFENTA may produce muscular rigidity that involves the skeletal muscles of the neck and extremities. As with fentanyl, muscular rigidity has been reported to occur or recur infrequently in the extended postoperative period. The incidence can be reduced by: 1) administration of up to ¼ of the full paralyzing dose of a non-depolarizing neuromuscular blocking agent just prior to administration of SUFENTA at dosages of up to 8 µg/kg, 2) administration of a full paralyzing dose of a neuromuscular blocking agent following loss of consciousness when SUFENTA is used in anesthetic dosages (above 8 µg/kg) titrated by slow intravenous infusion, or, 3) simultaneous administration of SUFENTA and a full paralyzing dose of a neuromuscular blocking agent when SUFENTA is used in rapidly administered anesthetic dosages (above 8 µg/kg).
The neuromuscular blocking agent used should be compatible with the patient's cardiovascular status. Adequate facilities should be available for postoperative monitoring and ventilation of patients administered SUFENTA. It is essential that these facilities be fully equipped to handle all degrees of respiratory depression.

PRECAUTIONS

General: The initial dose of SUFENTA should be appropriately reduced in elderly and debilitated patients. The effect of the initial dose should be considered in determining supplemental doses.
Vital signs should be monitored routinely.
Nitrous oxide may produce cardiovascular depression when given with high doses of SUFENTA (see CLINICAL PHARMACOLOGY).
Bradycardia has been reported infrequently with SUFENTA-oxygen anesthesia and has been responsive to atropine.
Respiratory depression caused by opioid analgesics can be reversed by opioid antagonists such as naloxone. Because the duration of respiratory depression produced by SUFENTA may last longer than the duration of the opioid antagonist action, appropriate surveillance should be maintained. As with all potent opioids, profound analgesia is accompanied by respiratory depression and diminished sensitivity to CO_2 stimulation which may persist into or recur in the postoperative period. Respiratory depression may be enhanced when SUFENTA is administered in combination with volatile inhalational agents and/or other central nervous system depressants such as barbiturates, tranquilizers, and other opioids. Appropriate postoperative monitoring should be employed to ensure that adequate spontaneous breathing is established and maintained prior to discharging the patient from the recovery area.
Neuromuscular Blocking Agents: The hemodynamic effects and degree of skeletal muscle relaxation required should be considered in the selection of a neuromuscular blocking agent. High doses of pancuronium may produce increases in heart rate during SUFENTA-oxygen anesthesia. Bradycardia and hypotension have been reported with other muscle relaxants during SUFENTA-oxygen anesthesia; this effect may be more pronounced in the presence of calcium channel and/or beta-blockers. Muscle relaxants with no clinically

Continued on next page

Janssen Pharmaceutica—Cont.

significant effect on heart rate (at recommended doses) would not counteract the vagotonic effect of SUFENTA, therefore a lower heart rate would be expected. Rare reports of bradycardia associated with the concomitant use of succinylcholine and SUFENTA have been reported.

Interaction with Other Central Nervous System Depressants: Both the magnitude and duration of central nervous system and cardiovascular effects may be enhanced when SUFENTA is administered to patients receiving barbiturates, tranquilizers, other opioids, general anesthetics or other CNS depressants. In such cases of combined treatment, the dose of SUFENTA and/or these agents should be reduced.

The use of benzodiazepines with SUFENTA during induction may result in a decrease in mean arterial pressure and systemic vascular resistance.

Interaction with Calcium Channel and Beta Blockers: The incidence and degree of bradycardia and hypotension during induction with SUFENTA may be greater in patients on chronic calcium channel and beta blocker therapy. (See Neuromuscular Blocking Agents).

Head Injuries: SUFENTA may obscure the clinical course of patients with head injuries.

Impaired Respiration: SUFENTA should be used with caution in patients with pulmonary disease, decreased respiratory reserve or potentially compromised respiration. In such patients, opioids may additionally decrease respiratory drive and increase airway resistance. During anesthesia, this can be managed by assisted or controlled respiration.

Impaired Hepatic or Renal Function: In patients with liver or kidney dysfunction, SUFENTA should be administered with caution due to the importance of these organs in the metabolism and excretion of SUFENTA.

Carcinogenesis, Mutagenesis and Impairment of Fertility: No long-term animal studies of SUFENTA have been performed to evaluate carcinogenic potential. The micronucleus test in female rats revealed that single intravenous doses of SUFENTA as high as 80 μg/kg (approximately 2.5 times the upper human dose) produced no structural chromosome mutations. The Ames *Salmonella typhimurium* metabolic activating test also revealed no mutagenic activity. See Animal Toxicology for reproduction studies in rats and rabbits.

Pregnancy Category C: SUFENTA has been shown to have an embryocidal effect in rats and rabbits when given in doses 2.5 times the upper human dose for a period of 10 days to over 30 days. These effects were most probably due to maternal toxicity (decreased food consumption with increased mortality) following prolonged administration of the drug. No evidence of teratogenic effects have been observed after administration of SUFENTA in rats or rabbits.

There are no adequate and well-controlled studies in pregnant women. SUFENTA should be used during pregnancy only if the potential benefit justifies the potential risk to the fetus.

Labor and Delivery: There are insufficient data to support the use of SUFENTA in labor and delivery. Therefore, such use is not recommended.

Nursing Mothers: It is not known whether this drug is excreted in human milk. Because many drugs are excreted in human milk, caution should be exercised when SUFENTA is administered to a nursing woman.

Pediatric Use: The safety and efficacy of SUFENTA in children under two years of age undergoing cardiovascular surgery has been documented in a limited number of cases.

Animal Toxicology: The intravenous LD_{50} of SUFENTA is 16.8 to 18.0 mg/kg in mice, 11.8 to 13.0 mg/kg in guinea pigs and 10.1 to 19.5 mg/kg in dogs. Reproduction studies performed in rats and rabbits given doses of up to 2.5 times the upper human dose for a period of 10 to over 30 days revealed high maternal mortality rates due to decreased food consumption and anoxia, which preclude any meaningful interpretation of the results.

ADVERSE REACTIONS

The most common adverse reactions of opioids are respiratory depression and skeletal muscle rigidity. See CLINICAL PHARMACOLOGY, WARNINGS and PRECAUTIONS on the management of respiratory depression and skeletal muscle rigidity.

The most frequent adverse reactions in clinical trials involving 320 patients administered SUFENTA were: hypotension (7%), hypertension (3%), chest wall rigidity (3%) and bradycardia (3%).

Other adverse reactions with a reported incidence of less than 1% were:

Cardiovascular: tachycardia, arrhythmia
Gastrointestinal: nausea, vomiting
Respiratory: apnea, postoperative respiratory depression, bronchospasm
Dermatological: itching, erythema
Central Nervous System: chills
Miscellaneous: intraoperative muscle movement

ADULT DOSAGE RANGE CHART

TOTAL DOSAGE	MAINTENANCE DOSAGE

ANALGESIC DOSAGES
●TOTAL DOSAGE REQUIREMENTS OF 1 μG/KG/HR OR LESS ARE RECOMMENDED

Incremental or Infusion

1–2 μg/kg (expected duration of anesthesia 1–2 hours). Approximately 75% or more of the total calculated SUFENTA dosage may be administered prior to intubation by either slow injection or infusion titrated to individual patient response. Dosages in this range are generally administered with nitrous oxide/oxygen in patients undergoing general surgery in which endotracheal intubation and mechanical ventilation are required.

Incremental

10–25 μg (0.2–0.5 ml) may be administered in increments as needed when movement and/or changes in vital signs indicate surgical stress or lightening of analgesia. Supplemental dosages should be individualized and adjusted to remaining operative time anticipated.

Infusion

SUFENTA may be administered as an intermittent or continuous infusion as needed in response to signs of lightening of analgesia. In absence of signs of lightening of analgesia infusion rates should always be adjusted downward until there is some response to surgical stimulation. Maintenance infusion rates should be adjusted based upon the induction dose of SUFENTA so that the total dose does not exceed 1 μg/kg/hr of expected surgical time. Dosage should be individualized and adjusted to remaining operative time anticipated.

2–8 μg/kg (expected duration of anesthesia 2–8 hours). Approximately 75% or less of the total calculated SUFENTA dosage may be administered by slow injection or infusion prior to intubation, titrated to individual patient response. Dosages in this range are generally administered with nitrous oxide/oxygen in patients undergoing more complicated major surgical procedures in which endotracheal intubation and mechanical ventilation are required. At dosages in this range, SUFENTA has been shown to provide some attenuation of sympathetic reflex activity in response to surgical stimuli, provide hemodynamic stability, and provide relatively rapid recovery.

10–50 μg (0.2–1 ml) may be administered in increments as needed when movement and/or changes in vital signs indicate surgical stress or lightening of analgesia. Supplemental dosages should be individualized and adjusted to remaining operative time anticipated.

Infusion

SUFENTA may be administered as an intermittent or continuous infusion as needed in response to signs of lightening of analgesia. In the absence of signs of lightening of analgesia, infusion rates should always be adjusted downward until there is some response to surgical stimulation. Maintenance infusion rates should be adjusted based upon the induction dose of SUFENTA so that the total dose does not exceed 1 μg/kg/hr of expected surgical time. Dosage should be individualized and adjusted to remaining operative time anticipated.

ANESTHETIC DOSAGES

Incremental or Infusion

8–30 μg/kg (anesthetic doses). At this anesthetic dosage range SUFENTA is generally administered as a slow injection, as an infusion, or as an injection followed by an infusion. SUFENTA with 100% oxygen and a muscle relaxant has been found to produce sleep at dosages ≥ 8 μg/kg and to maintain a deep level of anesthesia without the use of additional anesthetic agents. The addition of N_2O to these dosages will reduce systolic blood pressure. At dosages in this range of up to 25 μg/kg, catecholamine release is attenuated. Dosages of 25–30 μg/kg have been shown to block sympathetic responses including catecholamine release. High doses are indicated in patients undergoing major surgical procedures, in which endotracheal intubation and mechanical ventilation are required, such as cardiovascular surgery and neurosurgery in the sitting position with maintenance of favorable myocardial and cerebral oxygen balance. Postoperative observation is essential and postoperative mechanical ventilation may be required at the higher dosage range due to extended postoperative respiratory depression. Dosage should be titrated to individual patient response.

Incremental

Depending on the initial dose, maintenance doses of 0.5–10 μg/kg may be administered by slow injection in anticipation of surgical stress such as incision, sternotomy or cardiopulmonary bypass.

Infusion

SUFENTA may be administered by continuous or intermittent infusion as needed in response to signs of lightening of anesthesia. In the absence of lightening of anesthesia, infusion rates should always be adjusted downward until there is some response to surgical stimulation. The maintenance infusion rate for SUFENTA should be based upon the induction dose so that the total dose for the procedure does not exceed 30 μg/kg.

DRUG ABUSE AND DEPENDENCE

SUFENTA (sufentanil citrate) is a Schedule II controlled drug substance that can produce drug dependence of the morphine type and therefore has the potential for being abused.

OVERDOSAGE

Overdosage would be manifested by an extension of the pharmacological actions of SUFENTA (see CLINICAL PHARMACOLOGY) as with other potent opioid analgesics. However, no experiences of overdosage with SUFENTA have been established during clinical trials. The intravenous LD_{50} of SUFENTA in male rats is 9.34 to 12.5 mg/kg (see Animal Toxicology for LD_{50}s in other species). Intravenous administration of an opioid antagonist such as naloxone should be employed as a specific antidote to manage respiratory depression. The duration of respiratory depression following overdosage with SUFENTA may be longer than the duration of action of the opioid antagonist. Administration of an opioid antagonist should not preclude more immediate countermeasures. In the event of overdosage, oxygen should be administered and ventilation assisted or controlled as indicated for hypoventilation or apnea. A patent airway must be maintained, and a nasopharyngeal airway or endotracheal tube may be indicated. If depressed respiration is associated with muscular rigidity, a neuromuscular blocking agent may be required to facilitate assisted or controlled respiration. Intravenous fluids and vasopressors for the treatment of hypotension and other supportive measures may be employed.

DOSAGE AND ADMINISTRATION

The dosage of SUFENTA should be individualized in each case according to body weight, physical status, underlying pathological condition, use of other drugs, and type of surgical procedure and anesthesia. In obese patients (more than 20% above ideal total body weight), the dosage of SUFENTA should be determined on the basis of lean body weight. Dosage should be reduced in elderly and debilitated patients (see PRECAUTIONS).

Vital signs should be monitored routinely.

SUFENTA may be administered intravenously by slow injection or infusion 1) in doses of up to 8 μg/kg as an analgesic adjunct to general anesthesia, and 2) in doses ≥ 8 μg/kg as a primary anesthetic agent for induction and maintenance of anesthesia (see Dosage Range Chart). If benzodiazepines,

barbiturates, inhalation agents, other opioids or other central nervous system depressants are used concomitantly, the dose of SUFENTA and/or these agents should be reduced (see PRECAUTIONS). In all cases dosage should be titrated to individual patient response.

Usage in Children: For induction and maintenance of anesthesia in children less than 12 years of age undergoing cardiovascular surgery, an anesthetic dose of 10–25 μg/kg administered with 100% oxygen is generally recommended. Supplemental dosages of up to 25–50 μg are recommended for maintenance, based on response to initial dose and as determined by changes in vital signs indicating surgical stress or lightening of anesthesia.

Premedication: The selection of preanesthetic medications should be based upon the needs of the individual patient.

Neuromuscular Blocking Agents: The neuromuscular blocking agent selected should be compatible with the patient's condition, taking into account the hemodynamic effects of a particular muscle relaxant and the degree of skeletal muscle relaxation required (see CLINICAL PHARMACOLOGY, WARNINGS and PRECAUTIONS).

[See tables on preceding page.]

In patients administered high doses of SUFENTA, it is essential that qualified personnel and adequate facilities are available for the management of postoperative respiratory depression.

Also see WARNINGS and PRECAUTIONS sections.

For purposes of administering small volumes of SUFENTA accurately, the use of a tuberculin syringe or equivalent is recommended.

Parenteral drug products should be inspected visually for particulate matter and discoloration prior to administration, whenever solution and container permit.

HOW SUPPLIED

SUFENTA (sufentanil citrate) Injection for intravenous use is available as:

NDC 50458-050-01 50 μg/ml sufentanil base, 1 ml ampoules in packages of 10

NDC 50458-050-02 50 μg/ml sufentanil base, 2 ml ampoules in packages of 10

NDC 50458-050-05 50 μg/ml sufentanil base, 5 ml ampoules in packages of 10

Protect from light. Store at room temperature 15°–30°C (59°–86°F).

U.S. Patent No. 3,998,834

December 1989, February 1990

Shown in Product Identification Section, page 413

VERMOX® ℞

[vĕr´mŏx]

(mebendazole)

Chewable Tablets

DESCRIPTION

VERMOX® (mebendazole) is a (synthetic) broad-spectrum anthelmintic available as chewable tablets, each containing 100 mg of mebendazole. Inactive ingredients are: colloidal silicon dioxide, corn starch, hydrogenated vegetable oil, magnesium stearate, microcrystalline cellulose, sodium lauryl sulfate, sodium saccharin, sodium starch glycolate, talc, tetrarome orange, and FD&C yellow No. 6.

Mebendazole is methyl 5-benzoylbenzimidazole-2-carbamate.

Mebendazole is a white to slightly yellow powder with a molecular weight of 295.29. It is less than 0.05% soluble in water, dilute mineral acid solutions, alcohol, ether and chloroform, but is soluble in formic acid.

CLINICAL PHARMACOLOGY

Following administration of 100 mg twice daily for three consecutive days, plasma levels of VERMOX® and its primary metabolite, the 2-amine, do not exceed 0.03 μg/ml and 0.09 μg/ml, respectively. All metabolites are devoid of anthelmintic activity. In man, approximately 2% of administered VERMOX® is excreted in urine and the remainder in the feces as unchanged drug or a primary metabolite.

Vermox®	Pinworm (enterobiasis)	Whipworm (trichuriasis)	Common Roundworm (ascariasis)	Hookworm
Cure rates mean	95%	68%	98%	96%
Egg reduction mean	—	93%	99%	99%

Vermox®	Pinworm (enterobiasis)	Whipworm (trichuriasis)	Common Roundworm (ascariasis)	Hookworm
Dose	1 tablet, once	1 tablet morning and evening for 3 consecutive days.	1 tablet morning and evening for 3 consecutive days.	1 tablet morning and evening for 3 consecutive days.

Mode of Action: VERMOX® inhibits the formation of the worms' microtubules and causes the worms' glucose depletion.

INDICATIONS AND USAGE

VERMOX® is indicated for the treatment of *Enterobius vermicularis* (pinworm), *Trichuris trichiura* (whipworm), *Ascaris lumbricoides* (common roundworm), *Ancylostoma duodenale* (common hookworm), *Necator americanus* (American hookworm) in single or mixed infections.

Efficacy varies as a function of such factors as pre-existing diarrhea and gastrointestinal transit time, degree of infection, and helminth strains. Efficacy rates derived from various studies are shown in the table below:

CONTRAINDICATIONS

VERMOX® is contraindicated in persons who have shown hypersensitivity to the drug.

WARNINGS

There is no evidence that VERMOX®, even at high doses, is effective for hydatid disease.

PRECAUTIONS

Information for Patients: Patients should be informed of the potential risk to the fetus in women taking VERMOX® during pregnancy, especially during the first trimester (see Use in Pregnancy).

Patients should also be informed that cleanliness is important to prevent reinfection and transmission of the infection.

Carcinogenesis, Mutagenesis: In carcinogenicity tests of VERMOX® in mice and rats, no carcinogenic effects were seen at doses as high as 40 mg/kg given daily over two years. Dominant lethal mutation tests in mice showed no mutagenicity at single doses as high as 640 mg/kg. Neither the spermatocyte test, the F_1 translocation test, nor the Ames test indicated mutagenic properties.

Impairment of Fertility: Doses up to 40 mg/kg in mice, given to males for 60 days and to females for 14 days prior to gestation, had no effect upon fetuses and offspring, though there was slight maternal toxicity.

Use in Pregnancy: Pregnancy Category C. VERMOX® has shown embryotoxic and teratogenic activity in pregnant rats at single oral doses as low as 10 mg/kg. In view of these findings the use of VERMOX® is not recommended in pregnant women. In humans, a post-marketing survey has been done of a limited number of women who inadvertently had consumed VERMOX® during the first trimester of pregnancy. The incidence of spontaneous abortion and malformation did not exceed that in the general population. In 170 deliveries on term, no teratogenic risk of VERMOX® was identified. During pregnancy, especially during the first trimester, VERMOX® should be used only if the potential benefit justifies the potential risk to the fetus.

Nursing Mothers: It is not known whether VERMOX® is excreted in human milk. Because many drugs are excreted in human milk, caution should be exercised when VERMOX® is administered to a nursing woman.

Pediatric Use: The drug has not been extensively studied in children under two years; therefore, in the treatment of children under two years the relative benefit/risk should be considered.

ADVERSE REACTIONS

Transient symptoms of abdominal pain and diarrhea have occurred in cases of massive infection and expulsion of worms.

OVERDOSAGE

In the event of accidental overdosage gastrointestinal complaints lasting up to a few hours may occur. Vomiting and purging should be induced.

DOSAGE AND ADMINISTRATION

The same dosage schedule applies to children and adults. The tablet may be chewed, swallowed, or crushed and mixed with food.

[See table above.]

If the patient is not cured three weeks after treatment, a second course of treatment is advised. No special procedures, such as fasting or purging, are required.

HOW SUPPLIED

VERMOX® is available as chewable tablets, each containing 100 mg of mebendazole, and is supplied in boxes of thirty-six tablets.

Store at room temperature 15°–30°C (59°–86°F).

NDC 50458-110-30 (36 tablets-blister)

JANSSEN PHARMACEUTICA INC.

Titusville, NJ 08560-0200

Rev. Sept 1986, Sept 1988

U.S. Patent 3,657,267

Shown in Product Identification Section, page 413

Johnson & Johnson Medical, Inc.

P.O. BOX 130

ARLINGTON, TEXAS 76004-0130

INSTAT® ℞

[in´stat]

collagen absorbable

hemostat

DESCRIPTION

INSTAT® Collagen Absorbable Hemostat is a purified and lyophilized bovine dermal collagen. The material, prepared as a sponge-like pad, is lightly cross-linked, sterile, non-pyrogenic, and absorbable. Hemostatic activity, which is an inherent property of collagen, is largely dependent on the basic helical structure of this protein. The helical structure of native collagen is preserved during the manufacture of INSTAT Hemostat. When collagen comes into contact with blood, platelets aggregate on the collagen and release coagulation factors which, together with plasma factors result in the formation of fibrin, and finally in the formation of a clot.

INDICATIONS

INSTAT Collagen Absorbable Hemostat is indicated in surgical procedures (other than in neurosurgical, and ophthalmological surgery) for use as an adjunct to hemostasis when control of bleeding by ligature or other conventional methods is ineffective or impractical.

CONTRAINDICATIONS

INSTAT Collagen Absorbable Hemostat should not be used in the closure of skin incisions as it may interfere with the healing of skin edges. This interference is due to simple mechanical interposition of dry collagen and not due to any intrinsic interference with wound healing. It has been reported with another absorbable collagen hemostat that, in filling porosities of cancellous bone, collagen may reduce the bonding strength of methylmethacrylate. Therefore, INSTAT Hemostat should not be applied on bone surfaces to which prosthetic materials are to be attached with methylmethacrylate adhesives.

WARNINGS

INSTAT Collagen Absorbable Hemostat is inactivated by autoclaving. It should not be resterilized. As with any foreign substance, use in contaminated wounds may enhance infection.

INSTAT Hemostat should not be used in instances of pumping arterial hemorrhage.

INSTAT Hemostat should not be used where blood or other fluids have pooled or in cases where the point of hemorrhage is submerged. INSTAT Hemostat will not act as a tampon or plug in a bleeding site nor will it close off an area of blood collecting behind a tampon.

Only the amount of INSTAT Hemostat necessary to provide hemostasis should be used. The long-term effects of leaving INSTAT Hemostat in situ are unknown. Opened, unused INSTAT Hemostat should be discarded because it cannot be resterilized.

Continued on next page

Johnson & Johnson Medical—Cont.

PRECAUTIONS

As with other hemostatic agents, it is not recommended that INSTAT Collagen Absorbable Hemostat be left in an infected or contaminated space, nor is it recommended for use in persons known to be sensitive to materials of bovine origin. When placed into cavities or closed spaces, care should be exercised to avoid overpacking INSTAT Hemostat as it may absorb fluid and expand and press against neighboring structures. In urological procedures, INSTAT Hemostat should not be left in the renal pelvis or ureters to eliminate the potential foci for calculus formation.

Safety of this product has not been established in children and pregnant women; therefore, INSTAT Hemostat should only be used when benefit to risk clearly warrants its use. INSTAT Hemostat is not intended to be used to treat systemic coagulation disorders.

ADVERSE REACTIONS

INSTAT Collagen Absorbable Hemostat is a collagen product. Although several types of post-operative complications were observed in patients treated with INSTAT Hemostat, none were attributed to INSTAT Hemostat except one case of fibrotic reaction where INSTAT Hemostat involvement could not be ruled out. Adverse reactions reported for other collagen hemostats include hematoma, potentiation of infection, wound dehiscence, inflammation and edema. Other reported adverse reactions that may be related to the use of collagen hemostats include adhesion formation, allergic reaction, foreign body reaction and subgaleal seroma (in a single case). The use of microfibrillar collagen in dental extraction sockets has been reported to increase the incidence of alveolalgia. The possibility that all of the above reactions may occur with INSTAT Hemostat cannot be excluded.

ADMINISTRATION

INSTAT Collagen Absorbable Hemostat is applied directly to the bleeding surface with pressure. INSTAT Hemostat can be cut to size. The amount needed and the period of time necessary to apply pressure will vary with the type and amount of bleeding to be controlled. Hemostasis time depends upon the type of surgery and degree of pretreatment bleeding. It usually occurred between 2 to 5 minutes with INSTAT Hemostat.

INSTAT Hemostat maintains its integrity in the presence of blood and is not dispersed when wet. It is easily removed from the site following hemostasis. It is most effective when used dry.

INSTAT Hemostat may be left **in situ** whenever necessary. However, the surgeon, at his discretion, should remove any excess of INSTAT Hemostat prior to wound closure. Animal implant studies have demonstrated that absorption and tissue reaction to INSTAT Hemostat are similar to those observed with another absorbable collagen hemostatic agent. In these studies, on visual examination, most of INSTAT Hemostat was found to be absorbed in 8 to 10 weeks after implantation.

CLINICAL STUDIES

The safety, effectiveness and handling characteristics of INSTAT Collagen Absorbable Hemostat were evaluated in a variety of surgical procedures. The median time to hemostasis for INSTAT Hemostat was 3 minutes. Passive Hemagglutination Assay (PHA) and Enzyme- Linked Immunoabsorbent Assay (ELISA) methods have been used to evaluate the immunologic potential for INSTAT Hemostat to produce antibodies in patients. These assays revealed mild elevation of antibody titers in both INSTAT Hemostat treated patients and patients treated with a collagen control hemostat, confirming that INSTAT Hemostat, like other collagen hemostats, is a weak antigen.

HOW SUPPLIED

INSTAT Collagen Absorbable Hemostat is supplied in a sponge-like form in peelable plastic envelopes in the following sizes:

1 in. × 2 in. (2.5 cm × 5.1 cm) code 1981
3 in. × 4 in. (7.6 cm × 10.2 cm) code 1983
The sterility of the product is guaranteed unless the individual envelope is damaged or opened.

STORAGE

Store at controlled room temperature 15°–30°C (59°–86°F).

CAUTION

Federal law restricts this device to sale, distribution, and use by or on the order of a physician.

MATERIALS AVAILABLE

Free samples and clinical literature available to physicians, INSTAT is a registered trademark of Johnson & Johnson. Call 800-433-5009.
Johnson & Johnson Medical, Inc.
Arlington, Texas 76004-0130
©Johnson & Johnson Medical, Inc., 1990

SURGICEL® and SURGICEL   ℞
NU-KNIT® Absorbable Hemostats
[ser'ji-sel]
(oxidized regenerated cellulose)

For surgical use
(For dental application of this product, reference should be made to the package insert for dental use.)

DESCRIPTION

SURGICEL Absorbable Hemostat is a sterile absorbable knitted fabric prepared by the controlled oxidation of regenerated cellulose. The fabric is white with a pale yellow cast and has a faint, caramel-like aroma. It is strong and can be sutured or cut without fraying. It is stable and can be stored at controlled room temperature. A slight discoloration may occur with age, but this does not affect performance.

ACTIONS

The mechanism of action whereby SURGICEL Hemostat accelerates clotting is not completely understood, but it appears to be a physical effect rather than any alteration of the normal physiologic clotting mechanism. After SURGICEL Hemostat has been saturated with blood, it swells into a brownish or black gelatinous mass which aids in the formation of a clot, thereby serving as a hemostatic adjunct in the control of local hemorrhage. When used properly in minimal amounts, SURGICEL Hemostat is absorbed from the sites of implantation with practically no tissue reaction. Absorption depends upon several factors including the amount used, degree of saturation with blood, and the tissue bed.

In addition to its local hemostatic properties, SURGICEL Hemostat is bactericidal **in vitro** against a wide range of gram positive and gram negative organisms including aerobes and anaerobes. SURGICEL Hemostat is bactericidal **in vitro** against strains of species including those of:

Staphylococcus aureus
Staphylococcus epidermidis
Micrococcus luteus
Streptococcus pyogenes Group A
Streptococcus pyogenes Group B
Bacillus subtilis
Proteus vulgaris
Corynebacterium xerosis
Mycobacterium phlei
Clostridium tetani
Streptococcus salivarius
Branhamella catarrhalis
Escherichia coli
Klebsiella aerogenes
Lactobacillus sp.
Salmonella enteritidis
Shigella dysenteriae
Serratia marscescens
Clostridium perfringens
Bacteroides fragilis
Enterococcus
Enterobacter cloacae
Pseudomonas aeruginosa
Pseudomonas stutzeri
Proteus mirabilis
Studies conducted in animals show that SURGICEL Hemostat in contrast to other hemostatic agents does not tend to enhance experimental infection. (1–4)

INDICATIONS

SURGICEL Absorbable Hemostat (oxidized regenerated cellulose) is used adjunctively in surgical procedures to assist in the control of capillary, venous, and small arterial hemorrhage when ligation or other conventional methods of control are impractical or ineffective.

CONTRAINDICATIONS

Although packing or wadding sometimes is medically necessary, SURGICEL Hemostat should not be used in this manner unless it is to be removed after hemostasis is achieved. (See WARNINGS and PRECAUTIONS)

SURGICEL Hemostat should not be used for implantation in bone defects, such as fractures, since there is a possibility of interference with callus formation and a theoretical chance of cyst formation.

When SUGICEL Hemostat is used to help achieve hemostasis in, around, or in proximity to foramina in bone, areas of bony confine, the spinal cord, or the optic nerve and chiasm, it must always be removed once hemostasis is achieved since it will swell and could exert unwanted pressure.

SURGICEL Hemostat should not be used to control hemorrhage from large arteries.

SURGICEL Hemostat should not be used on non-hemorrhagic serous oozing surfaces, since body fluids other than whole blood, such as serum, do not react with SURGICEL Hemostat to produce satisfactory hemostatic effect.

SURGICEL is an absorbable hemostat and should not be used as an absorbable adhesion prevention product.

WARNINGS

SURGICEL Hemostat is supplied sterile and as the material is not compatible with autoclaving or ethylene oxide sterilization SURGICEL Hemostat should not be resterilized.

SURGICEL Hemostat is not intended as a substitute for careful surgery and the proper use of sutures and ligatures. Closing SURGICEL Hemostat in a contaminated wound without drainage may lead to complications and should be avoided.

The hemostatic effect of SURGICEL Hemostat is greater when it is applied dry; therefore it should not be moistened with water or saline.

SURGICEL Hemostat should not be impregnated with anti-infective agents or with other materials such as buffering or hemostatic substances. Its hemostatic effect is not enhanced by the addition of thrombin, the activity of which is destroyed by the low pH of the product.

Although SURGICEL Hemostat may be left *in situ* when necessary, it is advisable to remove it once hemostasis is achieved. It must *always* be removed from the site of application when used in, around, or in proximity to foramina in bone, areas of bony confine, the spinal cord, and/or the optic nerve and chiasm regardless of the type of surgical procedure because SURGICEL Hemostat, by swelling, may exert pressure resulting in paralysis and/or nerve damage. Dislodgement of SURGICEL Hemostat could possibly occur by means such as repaking, further intraoperative manipulation, lavage, exaggerated respiration, etc.

There have been reports that in procedures such as lobectomy, laminectomy and repair of a frontal skull fracture and lacerated lobe that SURGICEL Hemostat, when left in the patient after closure, migrated from the site of application into foramina in bone around spinal cord resulting in paralysis and, in another case, the left orbit of the eye, causing blindness. While these reports cannot be confirmed, special care must be taken by physicians, **regardless of the type of surgical procedure,** to consider the advisability of removing SURGICEL Absorbable Hemostat after hemostasis is achieved.

Although SURGICEL Hemostat is bactericidal against a wide range of pathogenic microorganisms, it is not intended as a substitute for systemically administered therapeutic or prophylactic antimicrobial agents to control or prevent post-operative infections.

PRECAUTIONS

Use only as much SURGICEL Hemostat as is necessary for hemostasis, holdinig it firmly in place until bleeding stops. Remove any excess before surgical closure in order to facilitate absorption and minimize the possibility of foreign body reaction.

In urological procedures, minimal amounts of SURGICEL Hemostat should be used and care must be exercised to prevent plugging of the urethra, ureter, or a catheter by dislodged portions of the product.

Since absorption of SURGICEL Hemostat could be prevented in chemically cauterized areas, its use should not be preceded by application of silver nitrate or any other escharotic chemicals.

If SURGICEL Hemostat is used temporarily to line the cavity of large open wounds, it should be placed so as not to overlap the skin edges. It should also be removed from open wounds by forceps or by irrigation with sterile water or saline solution after bleeding has stopped.

Precautions should be taken in otorhinolaryngologic surgery to assure that none of the material is aspirated by the patient. (Examples: controlling hemorrhage after tonsillectomy and controlling epistaxis.)

Care should be taken not to apply SURGICEL Hemostat too tightly when it is used as a wrap during vascular surgery (See "ADVERSE REACTIONS" section).

ADVERSE REACTIONS

"Encapsulation" of fluid and foreign body reactions have been reported.

There have been reports of stenotic effect when SURGICEL Hemostat has been applied as a wrap during vascular surgery. Although it has not been established that the stenosis was directly related to the use of SURGICEL Hemostat, it is important to be cautious and avoid applying the material tightly as a wrapping.

Paralysis and nerve damage have been reported when SURGICEL Hemostat was used around, in, or in proximity to foramina in bone, areas of bony confine, the spinal cord, and/or the optic nerve and chiasm. While most of these reports have been in connection with laminectomy, reports of paralysis have also been received in connection with other procedures. Blindness has been reported in connection with surgical repair of a lacerated left frontal lobe when SURGICEL Hemostat was placed in the anterior cranial fossa (5) (See WARNINGS and PRECAUTIONS).

Possible prolongation of drainage in cholecystectomies and difficulty passing urine per urethra after prostatectomy have been reported. There has been one report of a blocked ureter after kidney resection, in which postoperative catheterization was required.

Occasional reports of "burning" and "stinging" sensations and sneezing when SURGICEL Absorbable Hemostat has been used as packing in epistaxis, are believed due to the low pH of the product.

Burning has been reported when SURGICEL Hemostat was applied after nasal polyp removal and after hemorrhoidectomy. Headache, burning, stinging, and sneezing in epistaxis and other rhinological procedures, and stinging when SURGICEL Hemostat was applied on surface wounds (varicose ulcerations, dermabrasions, and donor sites) also have been reported.

DOSAGE AND ADMINISTRATION

Sterile technique should be observed in removing SURGICEL Hemostat from its envelope. Minimal amounts of SURGICEL Hemostat in appropriate size are laid on the bleeding site or held firmly against the tissues until hemostasis is obtained.

Opened, unused SURGICEL Hemostat should be discarded, because it cannot be resterilized.

HOW SUPPLIED

Sterile SURGICEL Hemostat (oxidized regenerated cellulose) is supplied as knitted fabric strips in envelopes in the following sizes:

Code No. 1951 2 in. × 14 in. (28 sq. in.) (5.1 cm. × 35.6 cm.) (180.6 sq. cm.)

Code 1952 4 in. × 8 in. (32 sq. in.) (10.2 cm. × 20.3 cm.) (206.5 sq. cm.)

Code 1953 2 in. × 3 in. (6 sq. in.) (5.1 cm. × 7.6 cm.) (38.7 sq. cm.)

Code 1955 ½ in. × 2 in. (1 sq. in.) (1.3 cm. × 5.1 cm.) (6.5 sq. cm.)

SURGICEL NU-KNIT

Code 1940 1 in. × 1 in. (1 sq. in.) (2.5 cm. × 2.5 cm.) (6.5 sq. cm.)

Code 1943 3 in. ×4 in. (12 sq. in.) (7.6 cm. × 10.2 cm.) (77.5 sq. cm.)

Code 1946 6 in. ×9 in. (54 sq. in.) (15.2 × 22.9 cm.)

STORAGE

Store at controlled room temperature 15°–30°C (59°–86°F).

CAUTION

Federal law restricts this device to sale by or on the order of a physician.

CLINICAL STUDIES

SURGICEL Hemostat (oxidized regenerated cellulose) has been found useful in helping to control capillary or venous bleeding in a variety of surgical applications, including abdominal, thoracic, neurosurgical, and orthopedic, as well as in otorhinolaryngologic procedures. Examples include gallbladder surgery, partial hepatectomy, hemorrhoidectomy, resections or injuries of the pancreas, spleen, kidney, prostate, bowel, breast or thyroid, and in amputations. (6,8)

SURGICEL Hemostat has been applied as a surface dressing on donor sites and superficial open wounds, controlling bleeding adequately, and causing no delay in healing or interference with epithelization (9,11). It also has been applied after dermabrasion, punch biopsy, excision biopsy, curettage, finger and toenail removal, and to traumatic wounds. In the foregoing applications, bleeding was controlled and the SURGICEL Hemostat was absorbed from the sites where it was applied. (10)

In cardiovascular surgery, investigators have found SURGICEL Hemostat useful in helping to control bleeding from implanted textile grafts, including those of the abdominal aorta. (7,12) Such grafts may leak or weep considerably, even when pre-clotted, but this seepage can be controlled by covering the graft with a layer or two of SURGICEL Hemostat after the graft is in place and before releasing the proximal and distal clamps. When the flow has been reestablished and all the bleeding controlled, the fabric either can be removed or left in situ, since absorption of SURGICEL Absorbable Hemostat has been shown to occur without constriction of the graft or other untoward incident when proper wrapping technique is employed.

Otorhinolaryngologic experience with SURGICEL Hemostat includes adjunctive use in controlling bleeding resulting from epistaxis, tonsillectomy, adenoidectomy, removal of nasal polyps, repair of deviated septum, tympanoplasty, stapes surgery, surgery for sinusitis, and removal of tumors. (13,14)

SURGICEL Hemostat has been reported useful as a hemostatic adjunct in such gynecologic procedures as oophorectomy, hysterectomy, conization of the cervix, and repair of cystorectocele. (6,15)

ANIMAL PHARMACOLOGY

The effects of SURGICEL Hemostat, absorbable gelatin sponge, and microfibrillar collagen hemostat were compared in a standardized infection model consisting of intra-abdominal and intrahepatic abscesses in mice. This infection mimics the common characteristics of human infection with non-spore-forming anaerobic bacteria, including a chronic and progressive course. SURGICEL Hemostat did not increase the infectivity of normally subinfectious inocula of mixed

anaerobic species in mice. With the other hemostatic agents, microfibrillar collagen hemostat and absorbable gelatin sponge, an enhancement of infectivity of anaerobic mixtures has been shown. SURGICEL Hemostat, in contrast to these hemostatic agents, did not enhance or provide a site for bacterial growth.

It was also found that aerobic pathogens did not grow in the presence of SURGICEL Hemostat. In these studies (1), SURGICEL Hemostat was placed in contaminated incisions of guinea pigs and markedly reduced bacterial growth of three different strains of common pathogens.

In a dog model (2), it was shown that bacterial contamination of implanted teflon patches in the aorta could be reduced by wrapping the area of the patch with SURGICEL Hemostat prior to pathogen challenge. Also, in another study (3), SURGICEL Hemostat and an absorbable gelatin sponge were placed in two splenotomy sites in large mongrel dogs and the animals were then challenged intravenously and the number of organisms from the splenotomy sites were measured over a period of time. The number of organisms at the site of SURGICEL Hemostat were significantly lower than that in the control, or the absorbable gelatin sponge site.

REFERENCES

1. Dineen, P.: Antibacterial activity of oxidized regenerated cellulose. *Surgery, Gynecology and Obstetrics* 142:481–486, 1976.
2. Dineen, P.: The effect of oxidized regenerated cellulose on experimental intravascular infection. *Surgery* 82:576–579, 1977.
3. Dineen, P.: The effect of oxidized regenerated cellulose on experimental infected splenotomies. *Journal of Surgical Research* 23:114–116, 1977.
4. Kuchta, N. and Dineen, P.: Effects of absorbable hemostats on intra-abdominal sepsis. *Infections in Surgery* 2:441–444, June 1983.
5. Dutton, J., Tse, D., and Anderson, R.: Compressive optic neuropathy following use of intra-cranial oxidized cellulose hemostat. *Ophthalmic Surgery* 14(6):487–490, June 1983.
6. Degenshein, G., Hurwitz, A., and Ribacoff, S.: Experience with regenerated oxidized cellulose. *New York State Journal of Medicine* 63(18):2639–2643, 1963.
7. Hurwitt, E.: A new absorbable hemostatic packing. *Bulletin de la Societe Internationale de Chirurgie* XXI (3):237–242, 1962.
8. Venn, R.: Reduction of postsurgical blood-replacement needs with SURGICEL® hemostasis. *Medical Times* 93(10):1113–1116, 1965.
9. Miller, J., Ginsberg, M., McElfatrick, G., and Johnson, H.: Clinical experience with oxidized regenerated cellulose. *Experimental Medicine and Surgery* 19(2-3):202–206, (June–Sept.) 1961.
10. Blau, S., Kanof, N., and Simonson, L.: Absorbable hemostatic gauze SURGICEL® in dermabrasions and dermatologic surgery. *Acta Dermato-Venereologica* 40:358–361, 1960.
11. Shea, P., Jr.: Management of the donor site: a new dressing technic. *Journal of the Medical Association of Georgia* 51(9):437–440, 1962.
12. Denck, H.: Use of resorbable oxycellulose in surgery. *Chirurg* 33(11): 486–488, 1962.
13. Tibbels, E., Jr.: Evaluation of a new method of epistaxis management. *Laryngoscope* LXXIII (30):306–314, 1963.
14. Huggins, S.: Control of hemorrhage in otorhinolaryngologic surgery with oxidized regenerated cellulose. *Eye, Ear, Nose and Throat Monthly* 48(7):(July) 1969.
15. Crisp, W.E., Shalauta, H., and Bennett, W.A.: Shallow conization of the cervix. *Obstetrics and Gynecology* 31(6):755–758, 1968.

Materials Available: Free samples and clinical literature available to physicians. Call (800)433-5009.

JOHNSON & JOHNSON MEDICAL, INC.
ARLINGTON, TEXAS 76004-0130
© **JOHNSON & JOHNSON MEDICAL, INC. 1990**

THROMBIN,   ℞
TOPICAL USP
THROMBOGEN™
[throm' bo-jen]
(bovine origin)

Thrombin, Topical USP **THROMBOGEN** must not be injected! Apply on the surface of bleeding tissue as a solution or powder.

DESCRIPTION

THROMBOGEN Thrombin is a protein substance produced through a conversion reaction in which prothrombin of bovine origin is activated by tissue thromboplastin in the presence of calcium chloride. It is supplied as a sterile powder that has been freeze-dried in the final container. Also contained in this preparation are calcium chloride, sodium chloride, aminoacetic acid (glycine) and benzethonium chloride. Glycine is included to make the dried product friable and

more readily soluble, and benzethonium chloride as a preservative at 0.2 mg./vial.

This product is prepared under rigid assay control. The unit is defined by the U.S. standard and is approximately equal to the stated unitage. A U.S. unit is defined as the amount required to clot 1 ml of standardized fibrinogen solution in 15 seconds. Approximately 2 U.S. units are required to clot 1 ml in oxalated human plasma in the same period of time.

CLINICAL PHARMACOLOGY

THROMBOGEN Thrombin requires no intermediate physiological agent for its action. It clots the fibrinogen of the blood directly. Failure to clot blood occurs in the rare cases where the primary clotting defect is the absence of fibrinogen itself. The speed with which thrombin clots blood is dependent upon its concentration.

INDICATIONS AND USAGE

THROMBOGEN Thrombin is indicated as an aid in hemostasis wherever oozing blood from capillaries and small venules is accessible.

In various types of surgery, solutions of THROMBOGEN Thrombin may be used in conjunction with Absorbable Gelatin Sponge, USP for hemostasis.

CONTRAINDICATIONS

THROMBOGEN Thrombin is contraindicated in persons known to be sensitive to any of its components and/or to material of bovine origin.

WARNING

Because of its action in the clotting mechanism, THROMBOGEN Thrombin must not be injected or otherwise allowed to enter large blood vessels. Extensive intravascular clotting and even death may result. THROMBOGEN Thrombin is an antigenic substance and has caused sensitivity and allergic reactions when injected into animals.

PRECAUTIONS

General—Consult the Absorbable Gelatin Sponge, USP product labeling for complete information for use prior to utilizing the thrombin-saturated sponge procedure.

Pregnancy—Category C—Animal reproduction studies have not been conducted with Thrombin, Topical USP (Bovine origin). It is also not known whether Thrombin, Topical USP (Bovine origin) can cause fetal harm when administered to a pregnant woman or can affect reproduction capacity. Thrombin, Topical USP (Bovine origin) should be given to a pregnant woman only if clearly indicated.

Pediatric Use—Safety and effectiveness in children have not been established.

ADVERSE REACTIONS

Allergic reactions may be encountered in persons known to be sensitive to bovine materials.

DOSAGE AND ADMINISTRATION

Solutions of THROMBOGEN Thrombin may be prepared in sterile distilled water or isotonic saline. The intended use determines the strength of the solution to prepare. For general use in plastic surgery, dental extractions, skin grafting, neurosurgery, etc. solutions containing approximately 100 units per ml are frequently used. For this, 10 ml of diluent added to the 1000 unit package is suitable. Where bleeding is profuse, as from abraded surfaces of liver and spleen, concentrations as high as 1000 to 2000 units per ml may be required. Intermediate strengths to suit the needs of the case may be prepared by selecting the proper strength package and dissolving the contents in an appropriate volume of diluent. In many situations, it may be advantageous to use THROMBOGEN Thrombin in dry form on oozing surfaces.

Caution: Solutions should be used immediately upon reconstitution. However, the solution may be refrigerated at 2–8°C for up to three hours.

The following techniques are suggested for the topical application of THROMBOGEN Thrombin .

1. The recipient surface should be sponged (not wiped) free of blood BEFORE THROMBOGEN THROMBIN IS APPLIED.
2. A spray may be used or the surface may be flooded using a sterile syringe and small gauge needle. The most effective hemostasis results when the THROMBOGEN Thrombin mixes freely with the blood as soon as it reaches the surface.
3. In instances where a concentration of approximately 1,000 units per ml is desired, the contents of the vial of sterile isotonic saline diluent may be easily transferred into the vial of THROMBOGEN Thrombin with a sterile syringe or a sterile transfer needle. If the transfer needle method is utilized, transfer the diluent as follows:
   (a) Flip plastic cover off of diluent vial.
   (b) Remove clear plastic cover from the transfer needle by twisting to break the seal.
   (c) Insert the exposed needle into the diluent.
   (d) Flip the plastic cover up on the THROMBOGEN Thrombin vial. **DO NOT REMOVE THE COVER AND ALUMINUM SEAL.**

Continued on next page

Johnson & Johnson Medical—Cont.

(e) Remove the pink plastic cap from the transfer needle exposing the needle.

(f) Invert the vial of diluent and insert the exposed needle into the THROMBOGEN Thrombin vial.

(g) Allow the vacuum to draw the complete contents of the diluent vial into the THROMBOGEN Thrombin vial.

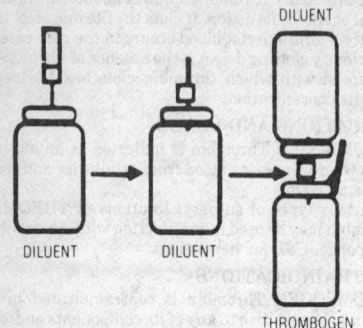

IMPORTANT

- Insert needle in DILUENT first.
- Do not remove the cover and aluminum seal on the THROMBOGEN Thrombin vial.

4. In instances where THROMBOGEN Thrombin in dry form is needed, the vial is opened by removing the metal ring by flipping up the metal tab and tearing counterclockwise. The rubber-diaphragm cap may be easily removed and the dried THROMBOGEN Thrombin is then broken up into a powder by means of a sterile glass rod or other suitable sterile instrument.

5. Sponging of treated surfaces should be avoided in order that the clot remain securely in place.

THROMBOGEN Thrombin may be used in conjunction with Absorbable Gelatin Sponge, USP as follows:

1. Prepare THROMBOGEN Thrombin solution of the desired strength.

2. Immerse sponge strips of the desired size in the THROMBOGEN Thrombin solution. Knead the sponge strips vigorously with moistened fingers to remove trapped air, thereby facilitating saturation of the sponge.

3. Apply saturated sponge to the bleeding area. Hold in place for 10 to 15 seconds with a pledget of cotton or a small gauze pad.

THROMBIN, TOPICAL USP THROMBOGEN SPRAY KIT

The THROMBOGEN Spray Kit contains one sterile vial of THROMBOGEN Thrombin, one sterile vial of isotonic saline diluent, one sterile disposable syringe and one sterile syringe spray tip. The kit may be used as follows:

OPENING THE PACKAGE

1. Remove the Tyvek† blister lid from the outermost tray by pulling up at the indicated corner. The sterile inner tray can then be lifted out or introduced into the sterile field.

2. Remove the Tyvek blister lid from the inner tray to expose the sterile contents.

PREPARING THE SOLUTION

1. Using the sterile syringe equipped with the needle, draw the desired amount of saline diluent from the vial into the syringe.

2. Inject the saline diluent into the THROMBOGEN Thrombin vial from the syringe to reconstitute the THROMBOGEN Thrombin powder.

3. When the THROMBOGEN Thrombin is completely dissolved, draw the THROMBOGEN Thrombin solution into the syringe.

ATTACHING THE SPRAY TIP

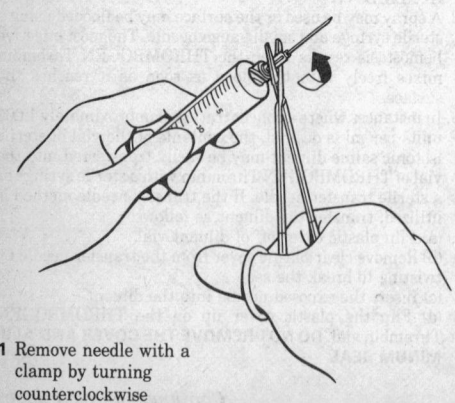

1 Remove needle with a clamp by turning counterclockwise

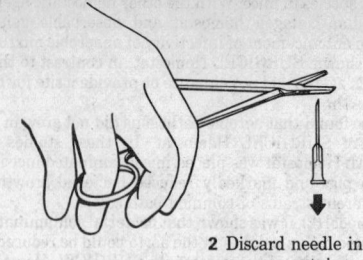

2 Discard needle in proper container

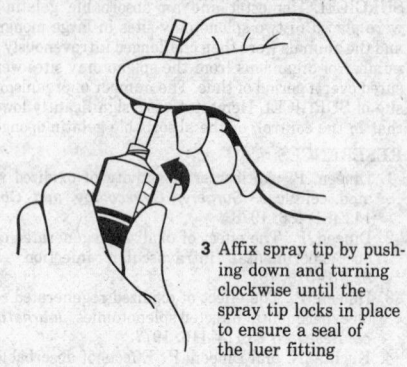

3 Affix spray tip by pushing down and turning clockwise until the spray tip locks in place to ensure a seal of the luer fitting

SPRAYING THE SOLUTION

1. Depress the syringe plunger in a normal fashion to dispense the THROMBOGEN Thrombin solution through the tip in a fine spray.

2. Alternatively, to facilitate using the THROMBOGEN Thrombin with an Absorbable Gelatin Sponge, USP, the THROMBOGEN Thrombin solution may be dispensed directly from the syringe into a sterile container vs. attaching the spray tip.

HOW SUPPLIED

THROMBOGEN Thrombin is supplied as:

NDC 56091-019-10	Package contains one 1,000 unit vial of THROMBIN, TOPICAL USP THROMBOGEN
NDC 56091-019-11	Package contains one 5,000 unit vial of THROMBIN, TOPICAL USP THROMBOGEN with one 5 ml vial of isotonic saline diluent and a transfer needle
NDC 56091-019-12	Package contains one 10,000 unit vial of THROMBIN, TOPICAL USP THROMBOGEN with one 10 ml vial of isotonic saline diluent and a transfer needle
NDC 56091-019-13	Package contains one 20,000 unit vial of THROMBIN, TOPICAL USP THROMBOGEN with one 20 ml vial of isotonic saline diluent and a transfer needle
NDC 56091-019-14	Kit contains one sterile 10,000 unit vial of THROMBIN, TOPICAL USP THROMBOGEN, one sterile 10 ml vial of isotonic saline diluent, one sterile disposable syringe and one sterile syringe spray tip in a sterile tray with a Tyvek lid
NDC 56091-019-15	Kit contains one sterile 20,000 unit vial of THROMBIN, TOPICAL USP THROMBOGEN, one sterile 20 ml vial of isotonic saline diluent, one sterile disposable syringe and one sterile syringe spray tip in a sterile tray with a Tyvek lid

STORAGE

Store at normal, controlled room temperature, except 1,000 unit vial of THROMBIN, TOPICAL USP THROMBOGEN must be stored between 2°–8°C (36°–46°F).

CAUTION

Federal law prohibits dispensing without prescription.
Manufactured by:
GENTRAC INC.
MIDDLETON, WI 53562
Distributed by:
JOHNSON & JOHNSON MEDICAL, INC.
ARLINGTON, TEXAS 76004-0130
© JOHNSON & JOHNSON MEDICAL, INC. 1990
† TYVEK IS A TRADEMARK OF DUPONT
For product information call, 1-800-433-5009
THROMBOGEN is a registered trademark of Johnson & Johnson.

Johnson & Johnson o MERCK Consumer Pharmaceuticals Co.
CAMP HILL ROAD
FORT WASHINGTON, PA 19034

ALternaGEL™   OTC
[al-tern'a-jel]
Liquid
High-Potency Aluminum Hydroxide Antacid

DESCRIPTION

ALternaGEL is available as a white, pleasant-tasting, high-potency aluminum hydroxide liquid antacid.

INGREDIENTS

Each 5 mL teaspoonful contains: Active: 600 mg aluminum hydroxide (equivalent to dried gel, USP) providing 16 milliequivalents (mEq) of acid-neutralizing capacity (ANC), and less than 2.5 mg (0.109 mEq) of sodium and no sugar. Inactive: butylparaben, flavors, propylparaben, purified water, simethicone, and other ingredients.

INDICATIONS

ALternaGEL is indicated for the symptomatic relief of hyperacidity associated with peptic ulcer, gastritis, peptic esophagitis, gastric hyperacidity, hiatal hernia, and heartburn.

ALternaGEL will be of special value to those patients for whom magnesium-containing antacids are undesirable, such as patients with renal insufficiency, patients requiring control of attendant GI complications resulting from steroid or other drug therapy, and patients experiencing the laxation which may result from magnesium or combination antacid regimens.

DIRECTIONS

One to two teaspoonfuls, as needed, between meals and at bedtime, or as directed by a physician: May be followed by a sip of water if desired. Concentrated product. Shake well before using. Keep tightly closed.

WARNINGS

Keep this and all drugs out of the reach of children. ALternaGEL may cause constipation.

Except under the advice and supervision of a physician: do not take more than 18 teaspoonfuls in a 24-hour period, or use the maximum dose of ALternaGEL for more than two weeks. ALternaGEL may cause constipation.

Prolonged use of aluminum-containing antacids in patients with renal failure may result in or worsen dialysis osteomalacia. Elevated tissue aluminum levels contribute to the development of the dialysis encephalopathy and osteomalacia syndromes. Small amounts of aluminum are absorbed from the gastrointestinal tract and renal excretion of aluminum is impaired in renal failure. Aluminum is not well removed by dialysis because it is bound to albumin and transferrin, which do not cross dialysis membranes. As a result, aluminum is deposited in bone, and dialysis osteomalacia may develop when large amounts of aluminum are ingested orally by patients with impaired renal function.

Aluminum forms insoluble complexes with phosphate in the gastrointestinal tract, thus decreasing phosphate absorption. Prolonged use of aluminum-containing antacids by normophosphatemic patients may result in hypophosphatemia if phosphate intake is not adequate. In its more severe forms, hypophosphatemia can lead to anorexia, malaise, muscle weakness, and osteomalacia.

DRUG INTERACTION PRECAUTION

Do not use this product for any patient receiving a prescription antibiotic containing any form of tetracycline.

HOW SUPPLIED

ALternaGEL is available in bottles of 12 fluid ounces and 5 fluid ounces, and 1 fluid ounce hospital unit doses. NDC 16837-860.

Shown in Product Identification Section, page 413

DIALOSE® Tablets   OTC
[di'a-lose]
Stool Softener Laxative

DESCRIPTION

DIALOSE is a very low sodium, nonhabit forming, stool softener containing 100 mg docusate sodium per tablet.

The docusate in DIALOSE is a highly efficient surfactant which facilitates absorption of water by the stool to form a soft, easily evacuated mass. Unlike stimulant laxatives, DIALOSE does not interfere with normal peristalsis, neither does it cause griping nor sensations of urgency.

INGREDIENTS

Active: docusate sodium, 100 mg per tablet
Inactive: Acacia, Calcium Carbonate, Calcium Sulfate, Carnauba Wax, Powdered Cellulose, Croscarmellose Sodium, D & C Red #27 Al. Lake, Diacetylated Monoglycerides, FD & C Yellow #6 Al. Lake. Gelatin, Hydroxypropyl Methylcellulose, Kaolin, Lactose, Magnesium Stearate, Pharmaceutical Glaze, Povidone. Colloidal Silicon Dioxide, Sodium Benzoate, Sodium Starch Glycolate, Pregelatinized Starch, Stearic Acid, Sugar, Talc, Titanium Dioxide, White Wax

INDICATIONS

DIALOSE is indicated for the relief of occasional constipation (irregularity).
DIALOSE is an effective aid to soften or prevent formation of hard stools in a wide range of conditions that may lead to constipation. DIALOSE helps to eliminate straining associated with obstetric, geriatric, cardiac, surgical, anorectal, or proctologic conditions. In cases of mild constipation, the fecal softening action of DIALOSE can prevent constipation from progressing and relieve painful defecation.

DIRECTIONS

Adults: One tablet, one to three times daily; adjust dosage as needed.
Children 6 to under 12 years: One tablet daily or as directed by physician.
Children under 6 years: As directed by physician.
It is helpful to increase the daily intake of fluids by taking a glass of water with each dose.

WARNINGS

Unless directed by a physician: Do not use when abdominal pain, nausea, or vomiting are present. Do not use for a period longer than one week. Do not take this product if you are presently taking a prescription drug or mineral oil.
As with any drug, if you are pregnant or nursing a baby, seek the advice of a health professional before using this product. Keep out of the reach of children.

HOW SUPPLIED

Bottles of 36 and 100 pink tablets. Also available in 100 tablet unit dose boxes (10 strips of 10 tablets each). NDC-16837-870.

Shown in Product Identification Section, page 413

DIALOSE® PLUS Tablets   OTC
[di'a-lose Plus]
Stool Softener/Stimulant Laxative

DESCRIPTION

DIALOSE PLUS provides a very low sodium tablet formulation of 100 mg docusate sodium and 65 mg yellow phenolphthalein.

INGREDIENTS

Each tablet contains: Actives: docusate sodium, 100 mg., yellow phenolphthalein, 65 mg.
Inactives: Acacia, Calcium Carbonate, Calcium Sulfate, Carnauba Wax, Powdered Cellulose, Croscarmellose Sodium, D & C Yellow #10 Al. Lake, Diacetylated Monoglycerides, FD & C Yellow #6 Al. Lake. Gelatin, Hydroxypropyl Methylcellulose, Kaolin, Magnesium Stearate, Pharmaceutical Glaze, Povidone, Colloidal Silicon Dioxide, Sodium Benzoate, Sodium Starch Glycolate, Pregelatinized Starch, Stearic Acid, Sugar, Talc, Titanium Dioxide, White Wax

INDICATIONS

DIALOSE PLUS is indicated for the treatment of constipation characterized by lack of moisture in the intestinal contents, resulting in hardness of stool and decreased intestinal motility.
DIALOSE PLUS combines the advantages of the stool softener, docusate sodium, with the peristaltic activating effect of yellow phenolphthalein.

DIRECTIONS

Adults: One or two tablets daily as needed, at bedtime or on arising
Children 6 to under 12 years: One tablet daily as needed
Children under 6 years: As directed by physician.
It is helpful to increase the daily intake of fluids by taking a glass of water with each dose.

WARNINGS

Unless directed by a physician: Do not use when abdominal pain, nausea, or vomiting are present. Do not use for a period longer than one week. If skin rash appears do not use this product or any other preparation containing phenolphthalein. Frequent or prolonged use may result in dependence on laxatives. Do not take this product if you are presently taking a prescription drug or mineral oil.

As with any drug, if you are pregnant or nursing a baby, seek the advice of a health professional before using this Keep out of the reach of children.

HOW SUPPLIED

Bottles of 36 and 100 yellow tablets Also available in 100 capsule unit dose boxes (10 strips of 10 capsules each). NDC 16837-871.

Shown in Product Identification Section, page 413

EFFER-SYLLIUM®   OTC
[ef'fer-sil'lium]
Natural Fiber Bulking Agent

DESCRIPTION

EFFER-SYLLIUM is an effervescent granular powder. Each rounded teaspoonful, or individual packet (7 g) contains psyllium hydrocolloid, 3 g.

INGREDIENTS

Active: psyllium hydrocolloid. Inactive: citric acid, ethyl vanillin, lemon and lime flavors, potassium bicarbonate, potassium citrate, saccharin calcium, starch, sucrose.
EFFER-SYLLIUM contains less than 5 mg sodium per rounded teaspoonful and is considered dietetically sodium free.

INDICATIONS

EFFER-SYLLIUM is indicated to restore normal bowel habits in chronic constipation, to promote normal elimination in irritable bowel syndrome, and to ease passage of stools in presence of anorectal disorders. EFFER-SYLLIUM produces a soft, lubricating bulk which promotes natural elimination. EFFER-SYLLIUM is not a one-dose, fast-acting bowel regulator. Administration for several days may be needed to establish regularity.

DIRECTIONS

Adults: One rounded teaspoonful, or one packet, in a glass of water one to three times a day, or as directed by physician.
Children, 6 years and over: One level teaspoonful, or one-half packet (3.5 g) in one-half glass of water at bedtime, or as directed by physician. *Children, under 6 years:* As directed by physician.

INSTRUCTIONS

Pour EFFER-SYLLIUM into a *dry* glass, add approximately 8 oz. of water and stir briskly. Drink immediately. To avoid caking, always use a *dry* spoon to remove EFFER-SYLLIUM from its container. Replace cap tightly. Keep in a dry place.

WARNING

Avoid inhalation. May cause a potentially severe reaction when inhaled by persons sensitive to psyllium powder or suffering from respiratory disorders. As with all medications, keep out of the reach of children.

HOW SUPPLIED

Bottles of 9 oz and 16 oz tan, granular instant mix powder. Convenient pouch package (7 g per packet) in boxes of 24. NDC 16837-440.

Shown in Product Identification Section, page 413

FERANCEE®   OTC
[fer'an-see]
Chewable Hematinic

INGREDIENTS
TWO TABLETS DAILY PROVIDE:

	US RDA*	
Iron	744%	134 mg
Vitamin C	500%	300 mg

*Percentage of US Recommended Daily Allowances for adults and children 4 or more years of age.
Active: ferrous fumarate, sodium ascorbate, ascorbic acid.
Inactive: confectioner's sugar, flavors, magnesium stearate, mannitol, povidone, saccharin calcium, starch, Yellow 5 (tartrazine), Yellow 6.

INDICATIONS

A pleasant-tasting hematinic for iron deficiency anemias, well-tolerated FERANCEE is particularly useful when chronic blood loss, onset of menses, or pregnancy create additional demands for iron supplementation. Available information indicates a low incidence of staining of the teeth by ferrous fumarate, alone or in combination with ascorbic acid. The peach-cherry flavored chewable tablets dissolve quickly in the mouth and may be either chewed or swallowed.

DIRECTIONS

Adults: Two tablets daily, or as directed by physician.
Children over 6 years of age: One tablet daily, or as directed by physician.

Children under 6 years of age: As directed by physician.
IMPORTANT: KEEP IN DRY PLACE. REPLACE CAP TIGHTLY.

WARNINGS

As with any drug, if you are pregnant or nursing a baby, seek the advice of a health professional before using this product. Keep out of the reach of children. In case of accidental overdose, seek professional assistance or contact a Poison Control Center immediately.

HOW SUPPLIED

FERANCEE is supplied in bottles of 100 brown and yellow, two-layer tablets. A child-resistant cap is standard on each bottle as a safeguard against accidental ingestion by children. Keep in a dry place. Replace cap tightly. NDC 16837-650.

Shown in Product Identification Section, page 413

FERANCEE®-HP Tablets   OTC
[fer'an-see-hp]
High Potency Hematinic

INGREDIENTS
ONE TABLET DAILY PROVIDES:

	US RDA*	
Iron	611%	110 mg
Vitamin C	1000%	600 mg

*Percentage of US Recommended Daily Allowances for adults and children 4 or more years of age.
Active: ascorbic acid, ferrous fumarate, sodium ascorbate.
Inactive: flavor, hydrogenated vegetable oil, microcrystalline cellulose, povidone, Red 40, and other ingredients.

INDICATIONS

FERANCEE-HP is a high potency formulation of iron and vitamin C and is intended for use as either:
(1) a maintenance hematinic for those patients needing a daily iron supplement to maintain normal hemoglobin levels, or
(2) intensive therapy for the acute and/or severe iron deficiency anemia where a high intake of elemental iron is required.
The use of well-tolerated ferrous fumarate provides high levels of elemental iron with a low incidence of gastric distress. The inclusion of 600 mg of vitamin C per tablet serves to maintain more of the iron in the absorbable ferrous state.

PRECAUTIONS

Because FERANCEE-HP contains 110 mg of elemental iron per tablet, it is recommended that its use be limited to adults i.e., not less than 12 years of age.

DIRECTIONS

One tablet per day taken after a meal or as directed by a physician, should be sufficient to maintain normal hemoglobin levels in most patients with a history of recurring iron deficiency anemia. Not recommended for children under 12 years of age.
For acute and/or severe iron deficiency anemia, two or three tablets per day taken one tablet per dose after meals. (Each tablet provides 110 mg elemental iron).

WARNINGS

As with all medications, keep out of the reach of children. In case of accidental overdose, seek professional assistance or contact a Poison Control Center immediately.

HOW SUPPLIED

FERANCEE-HP is supplied in bottles of 60 red, film-coated, oval-shaped tablets.
NDC 16837-863.
Note: A child-resistant safety cap is standard on each bottle of 60 tablets as a safeguard against accidental ingestion by children.

Shown in Product Identification Section, page 413

MYLANTA®   OTC
[my-lan'ta]
Alumina, Magnesia and Simethicone
Liquid and Tablets
Antacid/Anti-Gas

DESCRIPTION

MYLANTA is a well-balanced, pleasant-tasting antacid/ anti-gas medication that provides consistent, effective relief of symptoms associated with gastric hyperacidity and excess gas. Non-constipating and dietetically sodium-free, MYLANTA contains two proven antacids, magnesium hydroxide and aluminum hydroxide, plus simethicone for gas relief.

Continued on next page

Johnson & Johnson o Merck—Cont.

INGREDIENTS

Each 5mL (one teaspoonful) of liquid suspension or each chewable tablet contains: **Active:** Magnesium hydroxide 200 mg, Aluminum hydroxide (Dried Gel, USP in tablet and equiv. to Dried Gel USP in liquid) 200 mg and Simethicone 20 mg. **Inactive:** Tablets: Colliodal silicon dioxide, dextrates, flavors, magnesium stearate, mannitol, sodium saccharin,- sorbitol, Yellow 10. Liquid: Butylparaben, carboxymethylcellulose sodium, flavors, hydroxypropyl methylcellulose, microcrystalline cellulose, propylparaben, purified water, saccharin sodium and sorbitol.

Sodium Content: MYLANTA contains an insignificant amount of sodium per daily dose and is considered dietetically sodium-free. Typical values are 0.68 mg (0.03 mEq) sodium per 5 mL teaspoonful of liquid and 0.77 mg (0.03 mEq) per tablet.

Acid Neutralizing Capacity: Two teaspoonfuls of MYLANTA liquid has an acid neutralizing capacity, as measured in laboratory testing, of 25.4 mEq. Two MYLANTA tablets have an acid neutralizing capacity of 23.0 mEq.

INDICATIONS

As an antacid for symptomatic relief of hyperacidity associated with the diagnosis of peptic ulcer, gastritis, peptic esophagitis, heartburn and hiatal hernia. As an antiflatulent to alleviate the symptoms of mucus-entrapped gas, including postoperative gas pain.

ADVANTAGES

MYLANTA is homogenized for a smooth, creamy taste. The choice of two pleasant-tasting liquid flavors and the non-constipating formula encourage patient acceptance, thereby minimizing the skipping of prescribed doses. MYLANTA is also available in tablets, and both the liquid and tablet forms are sodium-free. MYLANTA provides consistent relief in patients suffering from distress associated with hyperacidity, mucus-entrapped gas, or swallowed air.

DIRECTIONS

Liquid: Shake well. 2–4 teaspoonfuls between meals and at bedtime or as directed by a physician.

Tablets: 2–4 tablets, well chewed, between meals and at bedtime or as directed by a physician.

WARNINGS

Keep this and all other drugs out of the reach of children. Do not take more than 24 tsps/tablets in a 24 hour period or use the maximum dose of this product for more than two weeks, except under the advice and supervision of a physician. Do not use this product if you have kidney disease.

Prolonged use of aluminum-containing antacids in patients with renal failure may result in or worsen dialysis osteomalacia. Elevated tissue aluminum levels contribute to the development of the dialysis encephalopathy and osteomalacia syndromes. Small amounts of aluminum are absorbed from the gastrointestinal tract and renal excretion of aluminum is impaired in renal failure. Aluminum is not well removed by dialysis because it is bound to albumin and transferrin, which do not cross dialysis membranes. As a result, aluminum is deposited in bone, and dialysis osteomalacia may develop when large amounts of aluminum are ingested orally by patients with impaired renal function.

Aluminum forms insoluble complexes with phosphate in the gastrointestinal tract, thus decreasing phosphate absorption. Prolonged use of aluminum-containing antcids by normophosphatemic patients may result in hypophosphatemia if phosphate intake is not adequate. In its more severe forms, hypophosphatemia can lead to anorexia, malaise, muscle weakness, and osteomalacia.

DRUG INTERACTION PRECAUTION

Do not use this product for any patient receiving a prescription antibiotic containing any form of tetracycline.

HOW SUPPLIED

MYLANTA is available as a white liquid suspension in three pleasant-tasting flavors, Original, Cherry Creme, and Cool Mint Creme, and as a two-layer green and white chewable Cool Mint Creme flavored tablet, as well as a two-layer pink and white Cherry Creme flavored tablet, identified on white layer "Mylanta." Liquid supplied in bottles of 5 oz., 12 oz., and 24 oz. Tablets supplied in bottles of 48 and 100 count sizes and in 12 tablet roll packs. Also available for hospital use in liquid unit dose bottles of 1 oz. and bottles of 5 oz.

NDC 16837-610 (original liquid). NDC 16837-620 (cool mint creme tablets). NDC 16837-621 (cherry creme liquid). NDC 16837-628 (cherry creme tablets). NDC 16837-629 (original liquid).

Shown in Product Identification Section, page 413

MYLANTA® GELCAPS ANTACID OTC

[*mīlăntă*]

Antacid

DESCRIPTION

MYLANTA® GELCAPS are a tasteless, non-chalky, easy to swallow antacid. The better way to get potent antacid relief.

INGREDIENTS

Each MYLANTA® GELCAP contains:

Active: Calcium carbonate 311 mg, magnesium carbonate 232 mg.

Inactives: Benzyl alcohol, butylparaben, castor oil, D&C yellow 10, disodium calcium edetate, FD&C blue 1, gelatin, hydroxypropyl cellulose, magnesium stearate, methylparaben, microcrystalline cellulose, propylparaben, sodium croscarmellose, sodium lauryl sulfate, sodium propionate, titanium dioxide.

Acid Neutralizing Capacity: Two MYLANTA ® GELCAPS have an acid neutralizing capacity of 23.0 Meq.

INDICATIONS

For the relief of acid indigestion, heartburn, sour stomach and upset stomach associated with these symptoms.

DIRECTIONS

Take 2–4 gelcaps as needed or as directed by a physician.

WARNINGS

Keep this and all other drugs out of the reach of children. Do not take more than 24 gelcaps in a 24 hour period or use the maximum dosage for more than two weeks or use if you have kidney disease, except under the advice and supervision of a physician.

HOW SUPPLIED

MYLANTA® GELCAPS are available as a swallowable blue and white gelcap identified "MYLANTA GELCAP." Supplied in bottles of 50 and boxes of 24 individual blisterpacks.

NDC 16837-850

Shown in Product Identification Section, page 413

MYLANTA® DOUBLE STRENGTH OTC

[*my-lan'ta*]

Alumina, Magnesia and Simethicone
Liquid and Tablets
Double-Strength Antacid/Anti-Gas

DESCRIPTION

MYLANTA DOUBLE STRENGTH is a well-balanced, high-potency antacid/anti-gas medication that provides rapid, effective, and long-lasting relief of symptoms associated with gastric hyperacidity and excess gas. Pleasant-tasting, non-constipating and dietetically sodium-free, MYLANTA DOUBLE STRENGTH contains two proven antacids, magnesium hydroxide and aluminum hydroxide, plus simethicone for gas relief.

INGREDIENTS

Each 5mL (one teaspoonful) of liquid suspension or each chewable tablet contains: Active: Magnesium hydroxide 400 mg, Aluminum hydroxide (Dried Gel, USP in tablet and equiv. to Dried Gel USP in liquid) 400 mg and Simethicone 40 mg. Inactive: Tablets: Blue 1, colliodal silicon dioxide, dextrates, flavors, magnesium stearate, mannitol, sodium saccharin, sorbitol, Yellow 10. Liquid: Butylparaben, carboxymethylcellulose sodium, flavors, hydroxypropyl methylcellulose, microcrystalline cellulose, potassium citrate, propylparaben, purified water, saccharin sodium and sorbitol.

Sodium Content: MYLANTA DOUBLE STRENGTH contains an insignficant amount of sodium per daily dose. Typical values are 1.14 mg (0.05 mEq) sodium per 5 mL teaspoonful of liquid and 1.3 mg (0.06 mEq) per tablet.

Acid Neutralizing Capacity: Two teaspoonfuls of MYLANTA DOUBLE STRENGTH liquid has an acid neutralizing capacity of 50.8 mEq, as measured in laboratory testing. Two MYLANTA DOUBLE STRENGTH tablets have an acid neutralizing capacity of 46.0 mEq.

INDICATIONS

As an antacid for symptomatic relief of hyperacidity associated with the diagnosis of peptic ulcer, gastritis, peptic esophagitis, heartburn and hiatal hernia. As an antiflatulent to alleviate the symptoms of mucus-entrapped gas, including postoperative gas pain.

ADVANTAGES

MYLANTA DOUBLE STRENGTH is homogenized for a smooth, creamy taste. The choice of three pleasant-tasting liquid flavors and the non-constipating formula encourage patient acceptance, thereby minimizing the skipping of prescribed doses. MYLANTA DOUBLE STRENGTH is also available in tablets, and both the liquid and tablet forms are sodium-free. The high potency of MYLANTA DOUBLE STRENGTH is achieved through greater concentration of two proven antacid ingredients, plus simethicone. MYLANTA DOUBLE STRENGTH provides rapid, consistent and long-lasting relief in patients suffering from distress associated with hyperacidity, mucus-entrapped gas, or swallowed air.

DIRECTIONS

Liquid: Shake well. 2–4 teaspoonfuls between meals and at bedtime, or as directed by a physician.

Tablets: 2–4 tablets, well chewed, between meals and at bedtime, or as directed by a physician.

Because patients with peptic ulcer vary greatly in both acid output and gastric emptying time, the amount and schedule of dosages should be varied accordingly.

WARNINGS

Keep this an all drugs out of the reach of children. Do not take more than 12 tsps/tablets in a 24-hour period or use the maximum dose of this product for more than two weeks, except under advice and supervision of a physician. Do not use this product if you have kidney disease.

Prolonged use of aluminum-containing antacids in patients with renal failure may result in or worsen dialysis osteomalacia. Elevated tissue aluminum levels contribute to the development of the dialysis encephalopahty and osteomalacia syndromes. Small amounts of aluminum are absorbed from the gastrointestinal tract and renal excretion of aluminum is impaired in renal failure. Aluminum is not well removed by dialysis because it is bound to albumin and transferrin, which do not cross dialysis membranes. As a result, aluminum is deposited in bone, and dialysis osteomalacia may develop when large amounts of aluminum are ingested orally by patients with impaired renal function.

Aluminum forms insoluble complexes with phosphate in the gastrointestinal tract, thus decreasing phosphate absorption. Prolonged use of aluminum-containing antacids by normophosphatemic patients may result in hypophosphatemia if phosphate intake is not adequate. In its more severe forms, hypophosphatemia can lead to anorexia, malaise, muscle weakness, and osteomalacia.

DRUG INTERACTION PRECAUTION

Do not use this product for any patient receiving a prescription antibiotic containing any form of tetracycline.

HOW SUPPLIED

MYLANTA DOUBLE STRENGTH is available as a white liquid suspension in three pleasant-tasting flavors, Original, Cherry Creme, and Cool Mint Creme, and as a two-layer green and white chewable Cool Mint Creme flavored tablet, as well as a two-layer pink and white Cherry Creme flavored tablet identified on white layer "MYLANTA DS." Liquid supplied in 5 oz., 12 oz., and 24 oz. bottles. Tablets supplied in bottles of 30 and 60 count sizes, and 8 tablet rollpacks. Also available for hospital use in liquid unit dose bottles of 1 oz., and bottles of 5 oz.

NDC 16837-652 (original liquid). NDC 16837-651 (cool mint creme tablets). NDC 16837-624 (cool mint creme liquid). NDC 16837-622 (cherry creme liquid). NDC 16837-627 (cherry creme tablets).

Professional Labeling

INDICATIONS

Stress-induced upper gastrointestinal hemorrhage: MYLANTA DOUBLE STRENGTH is indicated for the prevention of stress-induced upper gatrointestinal hemorrhage.

Hyperacidic conditions: As an antacid, for the symptomatic relief of hyperacidity associated with the diagnosis of peptic ulcer and other gastrointestinal conditions where a high degree of acid neutralization is desired.

DIRECTIONS

Prevention of stress-induced upper gastrointestinal hemorrhage: 1) Aspirate stomach via nasogastric tube* and record pH. 2) Instill 10 mL of MYLANTA DOUBLE STRENGTH followed by 30 mL of water via nasogastric tube. Clamp tube. 3) Wait one hour. Aspirate stomach and record pH. 4a) If pH equals or exceeds 4.0, apply drainage or intermittent suction for one hour, then repeat the cycle. 4b) If pH is less than 4.0, instill double (20 mL) MYLANTA DOUBLE STRENGTH followed by 30 mL of water. Clamp tube. 5) Wait one hour. If pH equals or exceeds 4.0, see number 7, if pH is still less than 4.0, instill double (40 mL) MYLANTA DOUBLE STRENGTH followed by 30 mL of water. Clamp tube. 6) Wait one hour. If pH equals or exceeds 4.0, see number 7. If pH is still less than 4.0, instill double (80 mL)† MYLANTA DOUBLE STRENGTH followed by 30 mL of water. 7) Drain for one hour and repeat cycle with the effective dosage of MYLANTA DOUBLE STRENGTH.

In hyperacid states for symptomatic relief: One or two teaspoonfuls as needed between meals and at bedtime or as directed by a physician. Higher dosage regimens may be employed under the direct supervision of a physician in the treatment of active peptic ulcer disease.

---

*If nasogastric tube is not in place, administer 20 mL of MYLANTA DOUBLE STRENGTH orally q2h.

† In a recent clinical study[1] 20 mL of MYLANTA DOUBLE STRENGTH, q2h, was sufficient in more than 85 percent of the patients. No patient studied required more than 80 mL of MYLANTA DOUBLE STRENGTH q2h.

PRECAUTION

Aluminum-magnesium hydroxide containing antacids should be used with caution in patients with renal impairment.

ADVERSE EFFECTS

Occasional regurgitation and mild diarrhea have been reported with the dosage recommended for the prevention of stress-induced upper gastrointestinal hemorrhage.

References: 1. Zinner MJ, Zuidema GD, Smigh PL, Mignosa M: The prevention of upper gastrointestinal tract bleeding in patients in an intensive care unit. *Surg Gynecol Obster* 153:214–220, 1981. 2. Lucas CE, Sugawa C, Riddle J, et al.: Natural history and surgical dilemma of "stress" gastric bleeding. *Arch Surg* 102:266–273, 1971. 3. Hastings PR, Skillman JJ, Bushnell LS, Silen W: Antacid titration in the prevention of acute gastrointestinal bleeding: a controlled, randomized trial in 100 critically ill patients. *N Engl J Med* 298:1042–1045, 1978. 4. Day SB, MacMillan BG, Altemeier WA: *Curling's Ulcer, An Experience of Nature.* Springfield, IL, Charles C Thomas Co., 1972, p. 205. 5. Skillman JJ, Bushnell LS, Goldman H, Silen W: Respiratory failure, hypotension, sepsis, and jaundice. A clinical syndrome associated with lethal hemorrhage from acute stress ulceration of the stomach. *Am J Surg* 117:523–530, 1969. 6. Priebe HJ, Skillman J, Bushnell LS, et al. Antacid versus cimetidine in preventing acute gastrointestinal bleeding. *N Engl J Med* 302:426–430, 1980. 7. Silen W: The prevention and management of stress ulcers. *Hosp Pract* 15:93–97, 1980. 8. Herrmann V, Kaminski DL: Evaluation of intragastric pH in acutely ill patients. *Arch Surg* 114:511–514, 1979. 9. Martin LF, Staloch DK, Simonowitz DA, et al.: Failure of cimetidine prophylaxis in the critically ill. *Arch Surg* 114:492–496, 1979. 10. Zinner MJ, Turtinen L, Gurll NJ, Reynolds DG: The effect of metiamide on gastric mucosal injury in rat restraint. *Clin Res* 23:484A, 1975. 11. Zinner M, Turtinen BA, Gurll NJ: The role of acid and ischemia in production of stress ulcers during canine hemorrhagic shock. *Surgery* 77:807–816, 1975. 12. Winans CS: Prevention and treatment of stress ulcer bleeding: Antacids or cimetidine? *Drug Ther Bull* (hospital) 12:37–45, 1981.

Shown in Product Identification Section, page 413

MYLANTA® GAS Tablets   OTC
[my'li-con]
High-Capacity Antiflatulent

INGREDIENTS

Each tablet contains:
Active: simethicone, 80 mg.
Inactive: dextrates, flavor, sorbitol, stearic acid, tricalcium phosphate.

INDICATIONS

For relief of the painful symptoms of excess gas in the digestive tract. Such gas is frequently caused by excessive swallowing of air or by eating foods that disagree. MYLANTA® GAS is a high capacity antiflatulent for adjunctive treatment of many conditions in which the retention of gas may be a problem, such as the following: air swallowing, postoperative gaseous distention, peptic ulcer, spastic or irritable colon, diverticulosis. If condition persists, consult your physician.

MYLANTA® GAS has a defoaming action that relieves flatulence by dispersing and preventing the formation of mucus-surrounded gas pockets in the gastrointestinal tract. MYLANTA® GAS acts in the stomach and intestines to change the surface tension of gas bubbles enabling them to coalesce; thus, the gas is freed and is eliminated more easily by belching or passing flatus.

DIRECTIONS

One tablet four times daily after meals and at bedtime. May also be taken as needed up to 6 tablets daily or as directed by a physician. TABLETS SHOULD BE CHEWED THOROUGHLY.

WARNINGS

Keep this and all drugs out of the reach of children.

HOW SUPPLIED

Economical bottles of 100 and convenience packages of individually wrapped 12 and 48 pink, scored, chewable tablets identified MYL GAS 80. Also available in 100 tablet unit dose boxes (10 strips of 10 tablets each).
NDC 16837-858.

Shown in Product Identification Section, page 413

Maximum Strength   OTC
MYLANTA® GAS Tablets
[my'li-con]
Maximum Strength Antiflatulent

INGREDIENTS

Each tablet contains:
Active: simethicone, 125 mg.
Inactive: dextrates, flavor, sorbitol, stearic acid, tricalcium phosphate.

INDICATIONS

Maximum Strength MYLANTA® GAS is useful for relief of the painful symptoms of excess gas in the digestive tract. Such gas is frequently caused by excessive swallowing of air or by eating foods that disagree. Maximum Strength MYLANTA® GAS is the strongest possible antiflatulent for adjunctive treatment of many conditions in which the retention of gas may be a problem, such as the following: air swallowing, postoperative gaseous distention, peptic ulcer, spastic or irritable colon, diverticulosis. If condition persists, consult your physician.

Maximum Strength MYLANTA® GAS has a defoaming action that relieves flatulence by dispersing and preventing the formation of mucus-surrounded gas pockets in the gastrointestinal tract. Maximum Strength MYLANTA® GAS acts in the stomach and intestines to change the surface tension of gas bubbles enabling them to coalesce; thus, the gas is freed and is eliminated more easily by belching or passing flatus.

DIRECTIONS

One tablet four times daily after meals and at bedtime or as directed by physician. TABLETS SHOULD BE CHEWED THOROUGHLY.

WARNINGS

Keep this and all drugs out of the reach of children.

HOW SUPPLIED

Convenience packages of individually wrapped 12 and 60 white, scored, chewable tablets, identified MYL GAS. NDC 16837-455.

Shown in Product Identification Section, page 413

MYLANTA® GAS—40 mg Tablets   OTC
MYLICON® Drops
[my'li-con]
Antiflatulent

INGREDIENTS

Each tablet or 0.6 mL of drops contains: Active: simethicone, 40 mg. Inactive: Tablets: calcium silicate, lactose, povidone, saccharin calcium. Drops: carbomer 934P, citric acid, flavors, hydroxypropyl methylcellulose, purified water, Red 3, saccharin calcium, sodium benzoate, sodium citrate.

INDICATIONS

Adults and children: For relief of the painful symptoms of excess gas in the digestive tract. Such gas is frequently caused by excessive swallowing of air or by eating foods that disagree. MYLANTA Gas-40 is a valuable adjunct in the treatment of many conditions in which the retention of gas may be a problem, such as: postoperative gaseous distention, air swallowing, peptic ulcer, spastic or irritable colon, diverticulosis. If condition persists, consult your physician.

Infants: MYLICON drops are also useful for relieve of the painful symptoms of excess gas associated with excessive swallowing of air or food intolerance.

The defoaming action of MYLICON relieves flatulence by dispersing and preventing the formation of mucus-surrounded gas pockets in the gastrointestinal tract. MYLICON acts in the stomach and intestines to change the surface tension of gas bubbles enabling them to coalesce; thus the gas is freed and is eliminated more easily by belching or passing flatus.

DIRECTIONS

Tablets—One or two tablets four times daily after meals and at bedtime. May also be taken as needed up to 12 tablets daily or as directed by a physician. TABLETS SHOULD BE CHEWED THOROUGHLY.

Drops—Adults and Children: 0.6 mL four times daily after meals and at bedtime or as directed by a physician. Shake well before using.

Infants (under 2 years): Initially, 0.3 mL four times daily, after meals and at bedtime, or as directed by a physician. The dosage can also be mixed with 1 oz of cool water, infant formula, or other suitable liquids to ease administration.

WARNINGS

Do not exceed 12 doses per day except under the advice and supervision of a physician. Keep this and all drugs out of the reach of chldren.

HOW SUPPLIED

Bottles of 100 white, scored, chewable tablets, identified MYL GAS 40, and dropper bottles of 15 mL (0.5 fl. oz) and 30 mL (1 fl. oz.) pink, pleasant tasting liquid. Also available in 100 tablet unit dose boxes (10 strips of 10 tablets each).
NDC 16837-450 (tablets).
NDC 16837-630 (drops).

Shown in Product Identification Section, page 413

THE STUART FORMULA® Tablets   OTC
Multivitamin/Multimineral Supplement

ONE TABLET DAILY PROVIDES:

VITAMINS:	US RDA*		
A	100%		5,000 IU
D	100%		400 IU
E	50%		15 IU
C	100%		60 mg
Folic Acid	100%		0.4 mg
B₁ (thiamin)	80%		1.2 mg
B₂ (riboflavin)	100%		1.7 mg
Niacin	100%		20 mg
B₆ (pyridoxine hydrochloride)	100%		2 mg
B₁₂ (cyanocobalamin)	100%		6 mcg
MINERALS:	**US RDA**		
Calcium	16%		160 mg
Phosphorus	12%		125 mg
Iodine	100%		150 mcg
Iron	100%		18 mg
Magnesium	25%		100 mg

*Percentage of US Recommended Daily Allowances for adults and children 4 or more years of age.

INGREDIENTS

Active: dibasic calcium phosphate, magnesium oxide, ascorbic acid, ferrous fumarate, dl-alpha tocopheryl acetate, folic acid, niacinamide, vitamin A palmitate, cyanocobalamin, pyridoxine hydrochloride, riboflavin, thiamin mononitrate, ergocalciferol, potassium iodide. Inactive: calcium sulfate, carnauba wax, pharmaceutical glaze, povidone, sodium starch glycolate, starch, sucrose, titanium dioxide, white wax.

INDICATIONS

The STUART FORMULA tablet provides a well-balanced multivitamin/multimineral formula intended for use as a daily dietary supplement for adults and children over age four.

DIRECTIONS

One tablet daily or as directed by physician.

WARNINGS

Keep this and all drugs out of the reach of children. In case of accidental overdose, seek professional assistance or contact a Poison Control Center immediately.

HOW SUPPLIED

Bottles of 100 and 250 white, round tablets. Child-resistant safety caps are standard on both bottles as a safeguard against accidental ingestion by children.
NDC 16837-866.

Shown in Product Identification Section, page 413

STUARTINIC® Tablets   OTC
[stu"are-tin'ic]
Hematinic

ONE TABLET DAILY PROVIDES:

	US RDA*		
Iron	556%		100 mg
VITAMINS:			
C	833%		500 mg
Thiamin	327%		4.9 mg
Riboflavin	353%		6 mg
Niacin	100%		20 mg
B₆	40%		0.8 mg
B₁₂	417%		25 mcg
Pantothenic Acid	92%		9.2 mg

*Percentage of US Recommended Daily Allowances for adults and children 4 or more years of age.

INGREDIENTS

Active: ferrous fumarate, ascorbic acid, sodium ascorbate, niacinamide, calcium pantothenate, thiamin mononitrate, riboflavin, pyridoxine hydrochloride, cyanocobalamin.
Inactive: flavor, hydrogenated vegetable oil, microcrystalline cellulose, povidone, Yellow 6, Yellow 10, and other ingredients.

Continued on next page

Johnson & Johnson o Merck—Cont.

INDICATIONS

STUARTINIC is a complete hematinic for patients with history of iron deficiency anemia who also lack proper amounts of vitamin C and B-complex vitamins due to inadequate diet.

The use of well-tolerated ferrous fumarate in STUARTINIC provides a high level of elemental iron with a low incidence of gastric distress. The inclusion of 500 mg of vitamin C per tablet serves to maintain more of the iron in the absorbable ferrous state. The B-complex vitamins improve nutrition where B-complex deficient diets contribute to the anemia.

WARNINGS

As with any drug, if you are pregnant or nursing a baby, seek the advice of a health professional before using this product. Keep out of the reach of children. In case of accidental overdose, seek professional assistance or contact a Poison Control Center immediately.

DOSAGE

One tablet daily taken after a meal or as directed by physician. Because of the high amount of iron per tablet, STUARTINIC is not recommended for children under 12 years of age.

HOW SUPPLIED

STUARTINIC is supplied in bottles of 60 yellow, film-coated, oval-shaped tablets. NDC 16837-862.

Note: A child-resistant safety cap is standard on each 60 tablet bottle as a safeguard against accidental ingestion by children.

Shown in Product Identification Section, page 413

Kabi Pharmacia

800 CENTENNIAL AVENUE
P.O. BOX 1327
PISCATAWAY, NJ 08855-1327

AZULFIDINE EN-tabs® ℞
(sulfasalazine delayed release tablets, USP)
(enteric-coated)
AZULFIDINE® Tablets ℞
(sulfasalazine tablets, USP)

DESCRIPTION

Azulfidine EN-tabs®, 500 mg enteric-coated tablets for Oral Administration

Azulfidine EN-tabs are film coated with cellulose acetate phthalate to prevent disintegration of the tablet in the stomach and thus reduce possible irritation of the gastric mucosa.

Azulfidine® Tablets, 500 mg for Oral Administration

Therapeutic classification: Anti-inflammatory agent.

Chemical designation: 5-([p-(2-Pyridylsulfamoyl) phenyl] azo) salicylic acid.

Chemical structure:

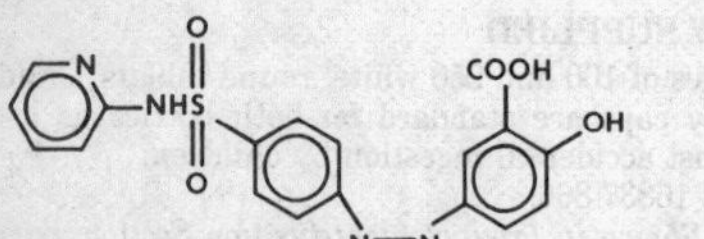

$C_{18}H_{14}N_4O_5S$

CLINICAL PHARMACOLOGY

After oral administration, AZULFIDINE is partially absorbed and extensively metabolized as described below.

About one-third of a given dose of sulfasalazine (SS) is absorbed from the small intestine. The remaining two-thirds pass to the colon where the compound is split (presumably by intestinal bacteria) into its components, 5-aminosalicylic acid (5-ASA) and sulfapyridine (SP). Most of the SP thus liberated is absorbed whereas only about one-third of the 5-ASA is absorbed, the remainder being excreted in the feces. The distribution metabolism and excretion of SS and its two components are as follows:

AZULFIDINE EN-tabs (enteric-coated tablets)

Sulfasalazine (SS): Detectable serum concentrations of SS have been found in healthy subjects within 90 minutes after the ingestion of a single 2 g dose of AZULFIDINE EN-tabs. Maximum concentrations of SS occur between 3 and 12 hours, with the mean peak concentration (6 mcg/ml) occurring at 6 hours. Small amounts of SS are excreted unchanged in the urine.

Sulfapyridine (SP): Following absorption and distribution, SP is acetylated and hydroxylated in the liver, and then conjugated with glucuronic acid. After ingestion of a single 2 g dose of AZULFIDINE EN-tabs by healthy subjects, peak concentrations of SP and its various metabolites appear in the serum between 12 and 24 hours, with the peak concentration (13 mcg/ml) occurring at 12 and lasting until 24 hours. The total recovery of SS and its SP metabolites from the urine of healthy subjects 3 days after the administration of a single 2 g dose of AZULFIDINE EN-tabs averaged 81%.

5-Aminosalicylic Acid (5-ASA): The serum concentration of 5-ASA in patients with ulcerative colitis was found to range from 0 to 4 mcg/ml, and to exist mainly in the form of acetyl-5-ASA. The urinary recovery of this compound was mostly in the acetylated form.

AZULFIDINE Tablets:

Sulfasalazine (SS): Detectable serum concentrations of SS have been found in healthy subjects within 90 minutes after the ingestion of a single 2 g dose of AZULFIDINE Tablets. Maximum concentrations of SS occur between 1.5 and 6 hours, with the mean peak concentration (14 mcg/ml) occurring at 3 hours. Small amounts of SS are excreted unchanged in the urine.

Sulfapyridine (SP): Following absorption and distribution, SP is acetylated and hydroxylated in the liver, and then conjugated with glucuronic acid. After ingestion of a single 2 g dose of AZULFIDINE Tablets by healthy subjects, SP and its various metabolites appear in the serum within 3 to 6 hours. Maximum concentrations of total SP occur between 6 and 24 hours, with the mean peak concentration (21 mcg/ml) occurring at 12 hours. The total recovery of SS and its SP metabolites from the urine of healthy subjects 3 days after the administration of a single 2 g dose of AZULFIDINE Tablets averaged 91%.

5-Aminosalicylic Acid (5-ASA): The serum concentration of 5-ASA in patients with ulcerative colitis was found to range from 0 to 4 mcg/ml, and to exist mainly in the form of acetyl-5-ASA. The urinary recovery of this compound was mostly in the acetylated form.

Mean serum concentrations of total SP, i.e. SP and its metabolites, tend to be significantly greater in patients with a slow acetylator phenotype than in those with a fast acetylator phenotype. Total serum sulfapyridine concentrations greater than 50 mcg/ml appear to be associated with an increased incidence of adverse reactions.

The mode of action of AZULFIDINE is still under investigation. It may be related to the immunosuppressant properties that have been observed in animal and **in vitro** models, to its affinity for connective tissue, and/or to the relatively high concentration it reaches in serous fluids, the liver and intestinal walls, as demonstrated in autoradiographic studies in animals. AZULFIDINE has also been described as a highly efficient vehicle for carrying its principal metabolites, SP and 5-ASA, to the colon, where a local action for both of them has been postulated. Recent clinical studies utilizing rectal administration of SS, SP, and 5-ASA have indicated that the major therapeutic action may reside in the 5-ASA moiety.

INDICATIONS AND USAGE

AZULFIDINE is indicated:

a. in the treatment of mild to moderate ulcerative colitis, and as adjunctive therapy in severe ulcerative colitis.
b. for the prolongation of the remission period between acute attacks of ulcerative colitis.

AZULFIDINE EN-tabs are particularly indicated in patients who cannot take the regular AZULFIDINE tablet because of gastrointestinal intolerance, and in whom there is evidence that this intolerance is not primarily due to high blood levels of sulfapyridine and its metabolites, e.g. patients experiencing nausea, vomiting, etc., when taking the first few doses of the drug or patients in whom a reduction in dosage does not alleviate the gastrointestinal side effects.

CONTRAINDICATIONS

Hypersensitivity to sulfasalazine, its metabolites, sulfonamides or salicylates. In infants under 2 years of age. Intestinal and urinary obstruction. Patients with porphyria should not receive sulfonamides as these drugs have been reported to precipitate an acute attack.

WARNINGS

Only after critical appraisal should AZULFIDINE be used in patients with hepatic or renal damage or blood dyscrasias. Deaths associated with the administration of AZULFIDINE have been reported from hypersensitivity reactions, agranulocytosis, aplastic anemia, other blood dyscrasias, renal and liver damage, irreversible neuromuscular and CNS changes, and fibrosing alveolitis. The presence of clinical signs such as sore throat, fever, pallor, purpura, or jaundice may be indications of serious blood disorders. Complete blood counts as well as urinalysis with careful microscopic examination should be done frequently in patients receiving AZULFIDINE. Oligospermia and infertility have been observed in men treated with AZULFIDINE. Withdrawal of the drug appears to reverse these effects.

PRECAUTIONS

General: AZULFIDINE should be given with caution to patients with severe allergy or bronchial asthma. Adequate fluid intake must be maintained in order to prevent crystalluria and stone formation. Patients with glucose-6-phosphate dehydrogenase deficiency should be observed closely for signs of hemolytic anemia. This reaction is frequently dose related. If toxic or hypersensitivity reactions occur, the drug should be discontinued immediately.

Isolated instances have been reported when AZULFIDINE EN-tabs have passed undisintegrated. This may be due to a lack of intestinal esterases in these patients. If this is observed, the administration of AZULFIDINE EN-tabs should be discontinued immediately.

Information for Patients: Patients should be informed of the possibility of adverse reactions and of the need for careful medical supervision. They should also be made aware that ulcerative colitis rarely remits completely, and that the risk of relapse can be substantially reduced by continued administration of AZULFIDINE (at a maintenance dosage). Patients should be instructed to take AZULFIDINE in evenly divided doses preferably after meals. Additionally, patients should be advised that AZULFIDINE may produce an orange-yellow discoloration of the urine or skin.

Laboratory Tests: The progress of the disease during treatment can be evaluated by clinical criteria, including the presence of fever, weight changes, degree and frequency of diarrhea and bleeding as well as by sigmoidoscopy and the evaluation of biopsy samples. The determination of serum sulfapyridine levels may be useful since concentrations greater than 50 mcg/ml appear to be associated with an increased incidence of adverse reactions. Complete blood counts, as well as a urinalysis with careful microscopic examination should be done frequently in patients receiving AZULFIDINE.

Drug Interactions: Reduced absorption of folic acid and digoxin have been reported when administered concomitantly with AZULFIDINE.

Drug/Laboratory Test Interactions: The presence of AZULFIDINE or its metabolites in body fluids has not been reported to interfere with laboratory test procedures.

Carcinogenesis, Mutagenesis, Impairment of Fertility: There have been no long-term studies of the carcinogenic or mutagenic potential of AZULFIDINE. Impairment of male fertility was observed in reproductive studies performed in rats and rabbits at doses up to six times the human dose. Oligospermia and infertility have been described in men treated with AZULFIDINE. Withdrawal of the drug appears to reverse these effects (see "**WARNINGS**").

Pregnancy:

Teratogenic Effects:

Pregnancy Category B: Reproduction studies have been performed in rats and rabbits at doses up to 6 times the human dose and have revealed no evidence of impaired female fertility or harm to the fetus due to AZULFIDINE.

There are, however, no adequate and well-controlled studies in pregnant women. Because animal reproduction studies are not always predictive of human response, this drug should be used during pregnancy only if clearly needed. A national survey evaluated the outcome of pregnancies associated with inflammatory bowel disease (IBD). In a group of 186 women treated with AZULFIDINE alone or AZULFIDINE and concomitant steroid therapy, the incidence of fetal morbidity and mortality was comparable to that for 245 untreated IBD pregnancies as well as with population data from the National Center for Health Statistics[1]. Another study of 1,445 pregnancies associated with exposure to sulfonamides in which AZULFIDINE was included indicated that this group of drugs appeared to be devoid of any association with fetal malformation[2]. A review of the medical literature covering 1,155 pregnancies which occurred in women having ulcerative colitis suggested that the outcome was similar to what was expected in the general population[3].

No clinical studies have been performed which indicate the effect of AZULFIDINE on the later growth development and functional maturation of children whose mothers received the drug during pregnancy.

Nonteratogenic Effects: AZULFIDINE and sulfapyridine pass the placental barrier. Although sulfapyridine has been shown to have a poor bilirubin displacing capacity, the potential for kernicterus in newborns should be kept in mind.

A case of agranulocytosis has been reported in an infant whose mother was taking both AZULFIDINE and prednisone throughout pregnancy.

Nursing Mothers: Caution should be exercised when AZULFIDINE is administered to a nursing woman. Sulfonamides are excreted in the milk. In the newborn, they compete with bilirubin for binding sites on the plasma proteins and may thus cause kernicterus. Insignificant amounts of uncleaved sulfasalazine have been found in milk, whereas the sulfapyridine levels in milk are about 30–60 per cent of those in the serum. Sulfapyridine has been shown to have a poor bilirubin displacing capacity.

Pediatric Use: Safety and effectiveness in children below the age of two years have not been established.

ADVERSE REACTIONS

The most common adverse reactions associated with AZULFIDINE are anorexia, headache, nausea, vomiting, gastric distress and apparently reversible oligospermia. These occur in about one-third of the patients. Less frequent adverse reactions are skin rash, pruritus, urticaria, fever, Heinz body anemia, hemolytic anemia and cyanosis which may occur at

a frequency of one in every thirty patients or less. Experience suggests that with a daily dosage of 4 g or more, or total serum sulfapyridine levels above 50 mcg/ml, the incidence of adverse reactions tends to increase.

Although the listing which follows includes a few adverse reactions which have not been reported with this specific drug, the pharmacological similarities among the sulfonamides require that each of these reactions be considered when AZULFIDINE is administered.

Other adverse reactions which occur rarely, in approximately 1 in 1000 patients or less are:

Blood dyscrasias: aplastic anemia, agranulocytosis, leukopenia, megaloblastic (macrocytic) anemia, purpura, thrombocytopenia, hypoprothrombinemia and methemoglobinemia, and congenital neutropenia.

Hypersensitivity reactions: erythema multiforme (Stevens Johnson syndrome), exfoliative dermatitis, epidermal necrolysis (Lyell's syndrome) with corneal damage, anaphylaxis, serum sickness syndrome, pneumonitis with or without eosinophilia, vasculitis, fibrosing alveolitis, pleuritis, pericarditis with or without tamponade, allergic myocarditis, polyartenitis nodosa, L.E. syndrome, hepatitis and hepatic necrosis with or without immune complexes, parapsoriasis varioliformis acuta (Mucha Haberman syndrome), rhabdomyolysis, photosensitization, arthralgia, periorbital edema, conjuctival and scleral injection and alopecia.

Gastrointestinal reactions: hepatitis, pancreatitis, bloody diarrhea, impaired folic acid absorption, impaired digoxin absorption, stomatitis, diarrhea and abdominal pains.

CNS reactions: transverse myelitis, convulsions, meningitis, transient lesions of the posterior spinal column, cauda equina syndrome, Guillain-Barre syndrome, peripheral neuropathy, mental depression, vertigo, hearing loss, insomnia, ataxia, hallucinations, tinnitus and drowsiness.

Renal reactions: toxic nephrosis with oliguria and anuria, nephritis, nephrotic syndrome, hematuria, crystalluria and proteinuria.

Other reactions: urine discoloration and skin discoloration.

The sulfonamides bear certain chemical similarities to some goitrogens, diuretics, (acetazolamide and the thiazides), and oral hypoglycemic agents. Goiter production, diuresis, and hypoglycemia have occurred rarely in patients receiving sulfonamides. Cross-sensitivity may exist with these agents.

Rats appear to be especially susceptible to the goitrogenic effects of sulfonamides and long-term administration has produced thyroid malignancies in this species.

DRUG ABUSE AND DEPENDENCE

None reported.

Overdosage: There is evidence that the incidence and severity of toxicity are directly related to the total serum sulfapyridine concentration. Symptoms of overdosage may include nausea, vomiting, gastric distress and abdominal pains. In more advanced cases, CNS symptoms such as drowsiness, convulsions, etc. may be observed. Serum sulfapyridine concentrations may be used to monitor the progress of recovery from overdosage.

Experience suggests that with a daily dosage of 4 g or more or total serum sulfapyridine levels above 50 mcg/ml the incidence of adverse reactions tends to increase. There are no documented reports of deaths due to ingestion of large single doses of AZULFIDINE.

It has not been possible to determine the oral LD_{50} in laboratory animals such as mice, since the highest daily oral dose which can be given (12 g/kg) is not lethal. Doses of AZULFIDINE of 16 g per day have been given to patients without mortality.

Instructions for overdosage: Gastric lavage or emesis plus catharsis as indicated. Alkalinize urine. If kidney function is normal, force fluids. If anuria is present, restrict fluids and salt, and treat appropriately. Catheterization of the ureters may be indicated for complete renal blockage by crystals. The low molecular weight of AZULFIDINE and its metabolites may facilitate their removal by dialysis. For agranulocytosis, discontinue the drug immediately, hospitalize the patient and institute appropriate therapy.

For hypersensitivity reactions, discontinue treatment immediately. Such reactions may be controlled with antihistamines and, if necessary, systemic corticosteroids.

When in the physician's opinion, reinstitution of AZULFIDINE is warranted, regimens modeled upon desensitization procedures may be attempted approximately two weeks after AZULFIDINE has been discontinued and symptoms have disappeared (see "**Dosage and Administration**").

DOSAGE AND ADMINISTRATION

Dosage should be adjusted to each individual's response and tolerance. The drug should be given in evenly divided doses over each 24-hour period; intervals between nighttime doses should not exceed 8 hours, with administration after meals recommended when feasible. Experience suggests that with daily dosages of 4 g or more, the incidence of adverse reactions tends to increase; hence, patients receiving these dosages should be instructed about and carefully observed for the appearance of adverse effects.

Various desensitization-like regimens have been reported to be effective in 34 of 53 patients[4], 7 of 8 patients[5] and 19 of 20 patients[6]. Upon reinstituting AZULFIDINE, such regimens comprise a total daily dose of 50 to 250 mg which, every 4 to 7 days thereafter, is doubled until the desired therapeutic level is achieved. If the symptoms of sensitivity recur, AZULFIDINE should be discontinued. Desensitization should not be attempted in patients who have a history of agranulocytosis or who have experienced an anaphylactoid reaction while on a previous course of AZULFIDINE therapy.

USUAL DOSAGE

AZULFIDINE Tablets and AZULFIDINE EN-tabs (enteric-coated tablets)

Initial therapy: ADULTS: 3-4 g daily in evenly divided doses. In some cases it is advisable to initiate therapy with a small dosage, e.g. 1-2 g daily, to lessen adverse gastrointestinal effects. If daily doses exceeding 4 g are required to achieve desired effects, the increased risk of toxicity should be kept in mind. CHILDREN TWO YEARS OF AGE AND OLDER: 40-60 mg per kg body weight in each 24-hour period, divided into 3-6 doses.

Maintenance therapy: ADULTS: 2 g daily. CHILDREN TWO YEARS OF AGE AND OLDER: 30 mg per kg body weight in each 24-hour period, divided into 4 doses.

Response to therapy and adjustment of dosage should be determined by periodic examination. It is often necessary to continue medication, even when clinical symptoms, including diarrhea, have been controlled. When endoscopic examination confirms satisfactory improvement, dosage is reduced to a maintenance level. If symptoms of gastric intolerance (anorexia, nausea, vomiting, etc.) occur after the first few doses of AZULFIDINE, they are probably due to mucosal irritation and may be alleviated by distributing the total daily dose more evenly over the day or by giving enteric-coated EN-tabs. If diarrhea recurs, dosage should be increased to previous effective levels. If such symptoms occur after the first few days of treatment with AZULFIDINE, they are probably due to increased serum levels of total sulfapyridine, and may be alleviated by halving the dose and subsequently increasing it gradually over several days. If symptoms continue, the drug should be stopped for 5–7 days, then reinstituted at a lower daily dose.

HOW SUPPLIED

AZULFIDINE Tablets are round, gold-colored, scored tablets, monogrammed "101" in the following package sizes:

AZULFIDINE Tablets 500 mg 100's—NDC No. 0016-0101-01
AZULFIDINE Tablets 500 mg 500's—NDC No. 0016-0101-05
AZULFIDINE Unit Dose Tablets
500 mg 100's—NDC No. 0016-0101-11
AZULFIDINE Unit Dose Tablets
500 mg 10 × 100's—NDC No. 0016-0101-10

AZULFIDINE EN-tabs are eliptical, gold colored, film enteric coated tablets, monogrammed "102" in the following package sizes.

AZULFIDINE EN-tabs 500 mg 100's—NDC No. 0016-0102-01
AZULFIDINE EN-tabs 500 mg 500's —NDC No. 0016-0102-05

Storage: Room temperature (15–30°C/59–86°F).

References:

1. Mogadam M, et al: Pregnancy in inflammatory bowel disease: Effect of sulfasalazine and corticosteroids on fetal outcome *Gastroenterol* 80:72–76, 1981.
2. Kaufman D W (ed): *Birth Defects and Drugs in Pregnancy.* Littleton, MA, Publishing Sciences Group, Inc. 1977, pp 296–313.
3. Jarnerot G: Fertility, sterility and pregnancy in chronic inflammatory bowel disease. *Scand J Gastroenterol* 17:1–4, 1982.
4. Korelitz BI, et al: *Gastroenterol* 82:1104, 1982.
5. Holdsworth C G: *Brit Med J* 282:110, 1981.
6. Taffet S L, Das K M: *Amer J Med* 73:520–524, 1982.

CAUTION

Federal law prohibits dispensing without prescription.

Kabi Pharmacia Inc.
800 Centennial Avenue
P.O. Box 1327
Piscataway, New Jersey 08855-1327

© 1990, Kabi Pharmacia; Revised July 1991

Shown in Product Identification Section, page 413

CYKLOKAPRON® ℞

Tablets and Injection
(Tranexamic acid)
Antifibrinolytic Agent

DESCRIPTION

Each tablet contains 500 mg of tranexamic acid.

Each ml of the sterile solution for intravenous injection contains 100 mg tranexamic acid and Water for Injection to 1 mL.

FORMULATION

Chemical Name: trans-4-(aminomethyl)cyclohexanecarboxylic acid.

Structural Formula:

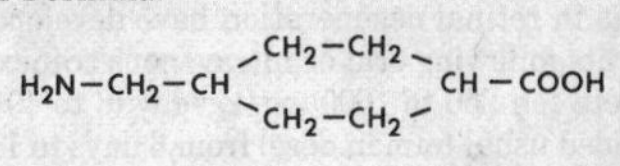
H2N–CH2–CH
CH2–CH2
CH2–CH2
CH–COOH

Empirical Formula: $C_8H_{15}NO_2$ Molecular Weight: 157.2

Tranexamic acid is a white crystalline powder. Inert ingredients in the tablets are microcrystalline cellulose, talc, magnesium stearate, silicon dioxide and povidone. The aqueous solution for injection has a pH of 6.5–7.5

CLINICAL PHARMACOLOGY

Tranexamic acid is a competitive inhibitor of plasminogen activation, and at much higher concentrations, a noncompetitive inhibitor of plasmin, actions similar to aminocaproic acid. Tranexamic acid is about 10 times more potent *in vitro* than aminocaproic acid.

Tranexamic acid binds more strongly than aminocaproic acid to both the strong and weak receptor sites of the plasminogen molecule in a ratio corresponding to the difference in potency between the compounds.

Tranexamic acid in a concentration of 1 mg per mL does not aggregate platelets *in vitro.* Tranexamic acid in concentrations up to 10 mg per mL blood has no influence on the platelet count, the coagulation time or various coagulation factors in whole blood or citrated blood from normal subjects. On the other hand, tranexamic acid in concentrations of 10 mg and 1 mg per mL blood prolongs the thrombin time.

The plasma protein binding of tranexamic acid is about 3 per cent at therapeutic plasma levels and seems to be fully accounted for by its binding to plasminogen. Tranexamic acid does not bind to serum albumin.

Absorption of tranexamic acid after oral administration in humans represents approximately 30–50% of the ingested dose and bioavailability is not affected by food intake.

After an intravenous dose of 1 g, the plasma concentration time curve shows a triexponential decay with a half-life of about 2 hours for the terminal elimination phase. The initial volume of distribution is about 9–12 liters. Urinary excretion is the main route of elimination via glomerular filtration. Overall renal clearance is equal to overall plasma clearance (110–116 mL/min) and more than 95% of the dose is excreted in the urine as the unchanged drug. Excretion of tranexamine acid is about 90 per cent at 24 hours after intravenous administration of 10 mg per kg body weight. After oral administration of 10–15 mg per kg body weight, the cumulative urinary excretion at 24 hours is 39 per cent and at 48 hours, 41 per cent of the ingested dose or 78% and 82% of the absorbed material. Only a small fraction of the drug is metabolized. After oral administration, 1 per cent of the dicarboxylic acid and 0.5 per cent of the acetylated compound are excreted.

The plasma peak level after 1 g orally is 8 mg per L and after 2 g, 15 mg per L, both obtained three hours after dosing.

An antifibrinolytic concentration of tranexamic acid remains in different tissues for about 17 hours, and in the serum, up to seven or eight hours.

Tranexamic acid passes through the placenta. The concentration in cord blood after an intravenous injection of 10 mg per kg to pregnant women is about 30 mg per L, as high as in the maternal blood. Tranexamic acid diffuses rapidly into joint fluid and the synovial membrane. In the joint fluid the same concentration is obtained in the serum. The biological half-life of tranexamic acid in the joint fluid is about three hours.

The concentration of tranexamic acid in a number of other tissues is lower than in blood. In breast milk the concentration is about one hundredth of the serum peak concentration obtained. Tranexamic acid concentration in cerebrospinal fluid is about one tenth of that of the plasma. The drug passes into the aqueous humor, the concentration being about one tenth of the plasma concentration.

Tranexamic acid has been detected in semen where it inhibits fibrinolytic activity but does not influence sperm migration.

INDICATIONS AND USAGE

Cyklokapron® is indicated in patients with hemophilia for short term use (two to eight days) to reduce or prevent hemorrhage and reduce the need for replacement therapy during and following tooth extraction.

CONTRAINDICATIONS

Cyklokapron® is contraindicated:

1. In patients with acquired defective color vision, since this prohibits measuring one endpoint that should be followed as a measure of toxicity (see WARNINGS).
2. In patients with subarachnoid hemorrhage. Anecdotal experience indicates that cerebral edema and cerebral infarction may be caused by Cyklokapron® in such patients.

Continued on next page

Kabi Pharmacia—Cont.

WARNINGS

Focal areas in retinal degeneration have developed in cats, dogs and rats following oral or intravenous tranexamic acid at doses between 250 to 1600 mg/kg/day (6 to 40 times the recommended usual human dose) from 6 days to 1 year. The incidence of such lesions has varied from 25% to 100% of animals treated and was dose-related. At lower doses some lesions have appeared to be reversible.

Limited data in cats and rabbits showed retinal changes in some animals with doses as low as 126 mg/kg/day (only about 3 times the recommended human dose) administered for several days to two weeks.

No retinal changes have been reported or noted in eye examinations in patients treated with tranexamic acid for weeks to months in clinical trials.

However, visual abnormalities, often poorly characterized, represent the most frequently reported postmarketing adverse reaction in Sweden. For patients who are to be treated continually for longer than several days, an ophthalmological examination, including visual acuity, color vision, eyeground and visual fields, is advised, before commencing and at regular intervals during the course of treatment. Tranexamic acid should be discontinued if changes in examination results are found.

PRECAUTIONS

General The dose of Cyklokapron® should be reduced in patients with renal insufficiency because of the risk of accumulation. See DOSAGE AND ADMINISTRATION.

Carcinogenesis, mutagenesis, impairment of fertility An increased incidence of leukemia in male mice receiving tranexamic acid in food at the concentration of 4.8% (equivalent to doses as high as 5 g/kg/day) may have been related to treatment. Female mice were not included in this experiment.

Hyperplasia of the bilary tract and cholangioma and adenocarcinoma of the intrahepatic biliary system have been reported in one strain of rats after dietary administration of doses exceeding the maximum tolerated dose for 22 months. Hyperplastic, but not neoplastic, lesions were reported at lower doses. Subsequent long term dietary administration studies in a different strain of rat, each with an exposure level equal to the maximum level employed in the earlier experiment, have failed to show such hyperplastic/neoplastic changes in the liver. No mutagenic activity has been demonstrated in several *in vitro* and *in vivo* test systems.

Pregnancy (Category B) Reproduction studies performed in mice, rats, and rabbits have not revealed any evidence of impaired fertility or adverse effects on the fetus due to tranexamic acid.

There are no adequate and well-controlled studies in pregnant women. However, tranexamic acid is known to pass the placenta and appears in cord blood at concentrations approximately equal to maternal concentration. Because animal reproduction studies are not alway predictive of human response, this drug should be used during pregnancy only if clearly needed.

Labor and Delivery See above under Pregnancy.

Nursing Mothers Tranexamic acid is present in the mother's milk at a concentration of about a hundredth of the corresponding serum levels. Caution should be exercised when Cyklokapron® is administered to a nursing woman.

Pediatric Use The drug has had limited use in children, principally in connection with tooth extraction. The limited data suggest that dosing instructions for adults can be used for children needing Cyklokapron® therapy.

ADVERSE REACTIONS

Gastrointestinal disturbances (nausea, vomiting, diarrhea) may occur but disappear when the dosage is reduced. Giddiness and hypotension have been reported occasionally. Hypotension has been observed when intravenous injection is too rapid. To avoid this response, the solution should not be injected more rapidly than 1 mL per minute. This adverse reaction has not been reported with oral administration.

OVERDOSAGE

There is no known case of overdosage of Cyklokapron.® Symptoms of overdosage may be nausea, vomiting, orthostatic symptoms and/or hypotension.

DOSAGE AND ADMINISTRATION

For dental extraction in patients with hemophilia: Immediately before surgery, substitution therapy is given together with tranexamic acid, 10 mg per kg body weight IV. After surgery, 25 mg per kg body weight are given orally three to four times daily for two to eight days.

Alternatively, tranexamic acid can be administered entirely orally, 25 mg per kg body weight 3 to 4 times a day beginning one day prior to surgery.

Parenteral therapy, 10 mg per kg body weight 3 to 4 times daily can be used for patients unable to take oral medication.

Note: For patients with moderate to severe impaired renal function, the following dosages are recommended:

Serum Creatinine (μmol/L)	Tranexamic Acid Dosage IV Dose	Tablets
120–250 (1.36–2.83 mg/dL)	10 mg/kg BID	15 mg/kg BID
250–500 (2.83–5.66 mg/dL)	10 mg/kg daily	15 mg/kg daily
> 500 (> 5.66 mg/dL)	10 mg/kg every 48 hours or 5 mg/kg every 24 hours	15 mg/kg every 48 hours or 7.5 mg/kg every 24 hours

For intravenous infusion, Cyklokapron® solution for injection may be mixed with most solutions for infusion such as electrolyte solutions, carbohydrate solutions, amino acid solutions and Dextran solutions. The mixture should be prepared the same day the solution is to be used. Heparin may be added to Cyklokapron® solution for injection. Cyklokapron® solutions for injection should NOT be mixed with blood. The drug is a synthetic amino acid, and should NOT be mixed with solutions containing penicillin.

HOW SUPPLIED

Tablets 500 mg (flat, white, round with bevelled edges, arcs above and below the letters CY): 100 tablets.
(NCD No. 0016-0114-00)
Ampules 100 mg/mL, 10 × 10 mL
(NCD No. 0016-1114-08)

STORAGE

Store Cyklokapron® tablets and injection at room temperature (15—30°C).
Revised October 1991

DIPENTUM® Capsules ℞
[di-pent 'um]
(olsalazine sodium)

DESCRIPTION

The active ingredient in Dipentum® (olsalazine sodium) Capsules is a sodium salt of a salicylate, disodium 3, 3'-azobis (6-hydroxybenzoate) a compound that is effectively bioconverted to 5-aminosalicylic acid (5-ASA), which has anti-inflammatory activity in ulcerative colitis. Its empirical formula is $C_{14}H_8N_2Na_2O_6$ with a molecular weight of 346.21. The structural formula is:

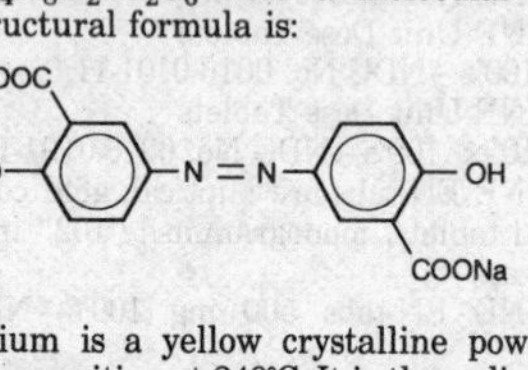

Olsalazine sodium is a yellow crystalline powder which melts with decomposition at 240°C. It is the sodium salt of a weak acid, soluble in water and DMSO, and practically insoluble in ethanol, chloroform and ether. Olsalazine sodium has acceptable stability under acidic or basic conditions.

Dipentum® is supplied in hard gelatin capsules for oral administration. The inert ingredient in each 250 mg capsule of olsalazine sodium is magnesium stearate. The capsule shell has the following inactive ingredients: black iron oxide, caramel, gelatin, and titanium dioxide.

CLINICAL PHARMACOLOGY

After oral administration, olsalazine has limited systemic bioavailability. Based on oral and intravenous dosing studies, approximately 2.4% of a single 1.0 g oral dose is absorbed. Less than 1% of olsalazine is recovered in the urine. The remaining 98–99% of an oral dose will reach the colon where each molecule is rapidly converted into two molecules of 5-aminosalicylic acid (5-ASA) by colonic bacteria and the low prevailing redox potential found in this environment. The liberated 5-ASA is absorbed slowly resulting in very high local concentrations in the colon.

The conversion of olsalazine to mesalamine (5-ASA) in the colon is similar to that of sulfasalazine, which is converted into sulfapyridine and mesalamine. It is thought that the mesalamine component is therapeutically active in ulcerative colitis (A.K. Azad-Kahn et al, *LANCET,* 2: 892–895, 1977). The usual dose of sulfasalazine for maintenance of remission in patients with ulcerative colitis is 2 grams daily, which would provide approximately 0.8 gram of mesalamine to the colon. More than 0.9 gram of mesalamine would usually be made available in the colon from 1 gram of olsalazine.

The mechanism of action of mesalamine (and sulfasalazine) is unknown, but appears to be topical rather than systemic. Mucosal production of arachidonic acid (AA) metabolites, both through the cyclooxygenase pathways, i.e., prostanoids, and through the lipoxygenase pathways, i.e., leukotrienes (LTs) and hydroxyeicosatetraenoic acids (HETEs) is increased in patients with chronic inflammatory bowel disease, and it is possible that mesalamine diminishes inflammation by blocking cyclooxygenase and inhibiting prostaglandin (PG) production in the colon.

__Pharmacokinetics__

The pharmacokinetics of olsalazine are similar in both healthy volunteers and in patients with ulcerative colitis. Maximum serum concentrations of olsalazine appear after approximately 1 hour, and even after a 1.0 g single dose are low, e.g., 1.6–6.2 μmol/L. Olsalazine, has a very short serum half-life, approximately 0.9 hours. Olsalazine is more than 99% bound to plasma proteins. It does not interfere with protein binding of warfarin. The urinary recovery of olsalazine is below 1%. Total recovery of oral 14C-labeled olsalazine in animals and humans ranges from 90 to 97%.

Approximately 0.1% of an oral dose of olsalazine is metabolized in the liver to olsalazine-O-sulfate (olsalazine-S). Olsalazine-S, in contrast to olsalazine has a half-life of 7 days. Olsalazine-S accumulates to steady state within 2-3 weeks. Patients on daily doses of 1.0 g olsalazine for 2–4 years show a stable plasma concentration of olsalazine-S (3.3–12.4 μmol/L). Olsalazine-S is more than 99% bound to plasma proteins. Its long half-life is mainly due to slow dissociation from the protein binding site. Less than 1% of both olsalazine and olsalazine-S appears undissociated in plasma.

5-aminosalicylic acid (5-ASA): Serum concentrations of 5-ASA are detected after 4–8 hours. The peak levels of 5-ASA after an oral dose of 1.0 g olsalazine are low, i.e., 0-4.3 μmol/L. Of the total 5-ASA found in the urine, more than 90% is in the form of N-acetyl-5-ASA (Ac-5-ASA). Only small amounts of 5-ASA are detected.

N-acetyl-5-ASA (Ac-5-ASA), the major metabolite of 5-ASA found in plasma and urine, is acetylated (deactivated) in at least two sites, the colonic epithelium and the liver. Ac-5-ASA is found in the serum, with peak values of 1.7–8.7 μmol/L after a single 1.0 g dose. Approximately 20% of the total 5-ASA is recovered in the urine, where it is found almost exclusively as Ac-5-ASA. The remaining 5-ASA is partially acetylated and is excreted in the feces. From fecal dialysis, the concentration of 5-ASA in the colon following olsalazine has been calculated to be 18–49 mmol/L.

No accumulation of 5-ASA or Ac-5-ASA in plasma has been detected. 5-ASA and Ac-5-ASA are 74 and 81%, respectively, bound to plasma proteins.

ANIMAL TOXICOLOGY

Preclinical subacute and chronic toxicity studies in rats have shown the kidney to be the major target organ of olsalazine toxicity. At an oral daily dose of 400 mg/kg or higher, olsalazine treatment produced nephritis and tubular necrosis in a 4-week study; interstitial nephritis and tubular calcinosis in a 6-month study; and renal fibrosis, mineralization and transitional cell hyperplasia in a 1 year study.

CLINICAL STUDIES

Two controlled studies have demonstrated the efficacy of olsalazine as maintenance therapy in patients with ulcerative colitis. In the first, ulcerative colitis patients in remission were randomized to olsalazine 500 mg B.I.D. or placebo, and relapse rates for a six month period of time were compared. For the 52 patients randomized to olsalazine, 12 relapses occurred, while for the 49 placebo patients, 22 relapses occurred. This difference in relapse rates was significant ($p < .02$).

In the second study, 164 ulcerative colitis patients in remission were randomized to olsalazine 500 mg B.I.D. or sulfasalazine 1 gram B.I.D., and relapse rates were compared after six months. The relapse rate for olsalazine was 19.5% while that for sulfasalazine was 12.2%, a non-significant difference.

INDICATIONS AND USAGE

Olsalazine is indicated for the maintenance of remission of ulcerative colitis in patients who are intolerant of sulfasalazine.

CONTRAINDICATIONS:

Hypersensitivity to salicylates.

PRECAUTIONS

__General__

Overall, approximately 17% of subjects receiving olsalazine in clinical studies reported diarrhea sometime during therapy. This diarrhea resulted in withdrawal of treatment in 6% of patients. This diarrhea appears to be dose related, although it may be difficult to distinguish from the underlying symptoms of the disease.

Exacerbation of the symptoms of colitis thought to have been caused by mesalamine or sulfasalazine has been noted.

Although renal abnormalities were not reported in clinical trials with olsalazine, the possibility of renal tubular damage due to absorbed mesalamine or its n-acetylated metabolite, as noted in the *Animal Toxicology* section, must be kept in mind, particularly for patients with pre-existing renal disease. In these patients, monitoring with urinalysis, BUN and creatinine determinations is advised.

__*Information for Patients*__

Patients should be instructed to take olsalazine with food. The drug should be taken in evenly divided doses. Patients should be informed that about 17% of subjects receiving

olsalazine during clinical studies reported diarrhea some time during therapy. If diarrhea occurs, patients should contact their physician.

Drug interactions. Increased prothrombin time in patients taking concomitant warfarin has been reported.

Drug/laboratory test interactions. None known.

Carcinogenesis, Mutagenesis, Impairment of Fertility

In a two year oral rat carcinogenicity study, olsalazine was tested in male and female Wistar rats at daily doses of 200, 400 and 800 mg/kg/day (approximately 10 to 40 times the human maintenance dose, based on a patient weight of 50 kg and a human dose of 1 g). Urinary bladder transitional cell carcinomas were found in three male rats (6%, p=0.022, exact trend test) receiving 40 times the human dose and were not found in untreated male controls. In the same study, urinary bladder transitional cell carcinoma and papilloma occurred in 2 untreated control female rats (2%). No such tumors were found in any of the female rats treated at doses of 40 times the human dose.

In an eighteen month oral mouse carcinogenicity study, olsalazine was tested in male and female CD-1 mice at daily doses of 500, 1000 and 2000 mg/kg/day (approximately 25 to 100 times the human maintenance dose). Liver hemangiosarcomata were found in two male mice (4%) receiving olsalazine at 100 times the human dose, while no such tumor occurred in the other treated male mice groups or any of the treated female mice. The observed incidence of this tumor is within the 4% incidence in historical controls.

Olsalazine was not mutagenic in *in vitro* Ames tests, mouse lymphoma cell mutation assays, human lymphocyte chromosomal aberration tests and the *in vivo* rat bone marrow cell chromosomal aberration test.

Olsalazine in a dose range of 100 to 400 mg/kg/day (approximately 5 to 20 times the human maintenance dose) did not influence the fertility of male or female rats. The oligospermia and infertility in men associated with sulfasalazine have not been reported with olsalazine.

Pregnancy: Teratogenic effects. Pregnancy Category C

Olsalazine has been shown to produce fetal developmental toxicity as indicated by reduced fetal weights, retarded ossifications and immaturity of the fetal visceral organs when given during organogenesis to pregnant rats in doses 5 to 20 times the human dose (100 to 400 mg/kg). There are no adequate and well-controlled studies in pregnant women. Olsalazine should be used during pregnancy only if the potential benefit justifies the potential risk to the fetus.

Nursing Mothers

Oral administration of olsalazine to lactating rats in doses 5 to 20 times the human dose produced growth retardation in their pups. It is not known whether this drug is excreted in human milk. Because many drugs are excreted in human milk, caution should be exercised when olsalazine is administered to a nursing woman.

Pediatric Use

Safety and effectiveness in a pediatric population have not been established.

ADVERSE REACTIONS

Olsalazine has been evaluated in ulcerative colitis patients in remission as well as those with acute disease. Both sulfasalazine-tolerant and intolerant patients have been studied in controlled clinical trials. Overall, 10.4% of patients discontinued olsalazine because of an adverse experience compared with 6.7% of placebo patients. The most commonly reported adverse reactions leading to treatment withdrawal were diarrhea or loose stools (olsalazine 5.9%; placebo 4.8%), abdominal pain and rash or itching (slightly more than 1% of patients receiving olsalazine). Other adverse reactions to olsalazine leading to withdrawal occurred in fewer than 1% of patients (Table 1).

TABLE 1:
Adverse Reactions Resulting in Withdrawal
From Controlled Studies

	Total	
	Olsalazine (N=441)	Placebo (N=208)
Diarrhea/Loose Stools	26 (5.9%)	10 (4.8%)
Nausea	3	2
Abdominal Pain	5 (1.1%)	0
Rash/Itching	5 (1.1%)	0
Headache	3	0
Heartburn	2	0
Rectal Bleeding	1	0
Insomnia	1	0
Dizziness	1	0
Anorexia	1	0
Light Headedness	1	0
Depression	1	0
Miscellaneous	4 (0.9%)	3 (1.4%)
Total Number of Patients Withdrawn	46 (10.4%)	14 (6.7%)

For these controlled studies, the comparative incidences of adverse reactions reported in 1% or more patients treated with olsalazine or placebo are provided in Table 2.

[See top of next column.]

TABLE 2: COMPARATIVE INCIDENCE (%)
OF ADVERSE EFFECTS REPORTED BY
ONE PERCENT OR MORE OF ULCERATIVE
COLITIS PATIENTS TREATED WITH
OLSALAZINE OR PLACEBO IN
DOUBLE BLIND CONTROLLED STUDIES

	OLSALAZINE (N=441)	PLACEBO (N=208)
	%	%
ADVERSE EVENT		
Digestive System		
Diarrhea	11.1	6.7
Abdominal Pain/ Cramps	10.1	7.2
Nausea	5.0	3.9
Dyspepsia	4.0	4.3
Bloating	1.5	1.4
Anorexia	1.3	1.9
Vomiting	1.0	—
Stomatitis	1.0	—
Increased Blood in Stool	—	3.4
CNS/Psychiatric		
Headache	5.0	4.8
Fatigue/Drowsiness/ Lethargy	1.8	2.9
Depression	1.5	—
Vertigo/Dizziness	1.0	—
Insomnia	—	2.4
Skin		
Rash	2.3	1.4
Itching	1.3	—
Musculoskeletal		
Arthralgia/Joint Pain	4.0	2.9
Miscellaneous		
Upper Respiratory Infection	1.5	—

Over 2,500 patients have been treated with olsalazine in various programs. In the uncontrolled studies, olsalazine was administered mainly to patients intolerant to sulfasalazine. The adverse effects related to olsalazine in these uncontrolled studies were similar to those seen in the controlled clinical trials. In addition, there were rare reports of the following adverse effects in patients receiving olsalazine. These were often difficult to distinguish from possible symptoms of the underlying disease and a causal relationship to the drug has not been demonstrated for some of these reactions.

Digestive: Pancreatitis, diarrhea with dehydration, increased blood in stool, rectal bleeding, flare in symptoms, rectal discomfort, epigastric discomfort, vomiting, flatulence.

Rare cases of granulomatous hepatitis and nonspecific, reactive hepatitis have been reported in patients receiving olsalazine. Additionally, a patient developed mild cholestatic hepatitis during treatment with sulfasalazine and experienced the same symptoms two weeks later after the treatment was changed to olsalazine. Withdrawal of olsalazine led to complete recovery in these cases.

Neurologic: Paresthesia, tremors, insomnia, mood swings, irritability, fever, chills.

Dermatologic: Erythema nodosum, photosensitivity, erythema, hot flashes, alopecia.

Musculoskeletal: Muscle cramps.

Cardiovascular/Pulmonary: Pericarditis, second degree heart block, interstitial pulmonary disease, hypertension, orthostatic hypotension, peripheral edema, chest pains, tachycardia, palpitations, bronchospasm, shortness of breath.

Genitourinary: Frequency, dysuria, hematuria, proteinuria, impotence, menorrhagia.

Hematologic: Leukopenia, neutropenia, lymphopenia, eosinophilia, thrombocytopenia, anemia, reticulocytosis.

Laboratory: ALT (SGPT) or AST (SGOT) elevated beyond the normal range.

Special senses: Dry mouth, dry eyes, watery eyes, blurred vision.

DRUG ABUSE AND DEPENDENCY

Abuse:

None reported.

Dependence:

Drug dependence has not been reported with chronic administration of olsalazine.

OVERDOSAGE

No overdosage has been reported in humans. Maximum single oral doses of 5 g/kg in mice and rats and 2 g/kg in dogs were not lethal. Symptoms of acute toxicity were decreased motor activity and diarrhea in all species tested and in addition, vomiting in dogs.

DOSAGE AND ADMINISTRATION

The usual dosage in adults for maintenance of remission is 1.0 g/day in two divided doses.

HOW SUPPLIED

Beige colored capsules, containing 250 mg olsalazine sodium imprinted with "DIPENTUM® 250 mg" on the capsule shell.

Packaged in bottles of 100 (NDC #0016-0105-01) and bottles of 500 (NDC #0016-0105-05).

Storage

Controlled Room Temperature (15–30°C/59–86°F)

Federal law prohibits dispensing without prescription.

Manufactured by: Kabi Pharmacia AB
Uppsala, Sweden
for: Kabi Pharmacia Inc.
Piscataway, N.J. 08855

11-B-077-02
March 1991
Shown in Product Identification Section, page 413

EMCYT® ℞

[em 'sit]

(estramustine phosphate sodium/Pharmacia)
CAPSULES

DESCRIPTION

Estramustine phosphate sodium, an antineoplastic agent, is an off-white powder readily soluble in water. Emcyt is available as white opaque capsules, each containing estramustine phosphate sodium as the disodium salt monohydrate equivalent to 140 mg estramustine phosphate, for oral administration. Each capsule also contains magnesium stearate, silicon dioxide, sodium lauryl sulfate and talc. Gelatin capsule shells contain the following pigment: titanium dioxide.

Chemically, estramustine phosphate sodium is estra-1,3,5(10)-triene-3,17-diol(17β)-,3-[bis(2-chloroethyl) carbamate] 17-(dihydrogen phosphate), disodium salt, monohydrate. It is also referred to as estradiol 3-[bis(2-chloroethyl) carbamate 17-(dihydrogen phosphate), disodium salt, monohydrate. Estramustine phosphate sodium has an empiric formula of $C_{23}H_{30}Cl_2NNa_2O_6P \cdot H_2O$ and a calculated molecular weight of 582.4.

CLINICAL PHARMACOLOGY

Estramustine phosphate is a molecule combining estradiol and nornitrogen mustard by a carbamate link. The molecule is phosphorylated to make it water soluble.

Estramustine phosphate taken orally is readily dephosphorylated during absorption, and the major metabolites in plasma are estramustine, the estrone analog, estradiol and estrone.

Prolonged treatment with estramustine phosphate produces elevated total plasma concentrations of estradiol that fall within ranges similar to the elevated estradiol levels found in prostatic cancer patients given conventional estradiol therapy. Estrogenic effects, as demonstrated by changes in circulating levels of steroids and pituitary hormones, are similar in patients treated with either estramustine phosphate or conventional estradiol.

The metabolic urinary patterns of the estradiol moiety of estramustine phosphate and estradiol itself are very similar, although the metabolites derived from estramustine phosphate are excreted at a slower rate.

INDICATIONS AND USAGE

Emcyt is indicated in the palliative treatment of patients with metastatic and/or progressive carcinoma of the prostate.

CONTRAINDICATIONS

Emcyt should not be used in patients with any of the following conditions:

1) Known hypersensitivity to either estradiol or to nitrogen mustard.

2) Active thrombophlebitis or thromboembolic disorders, except in those cases where the actual tumor mass is the cause of the thromboembolic phenomenon and the physician feels the benefits of therapy may outweigh the risks.

WARNINGS

It has been shown that there is an increased risk of thrombosis, including nonfatal myocardial infarction, in men receiving estrogens for prostatic cancer. Emcyt should be used with caution in patients with a history of thrombophlebitis, thrombosis or thromboembolic disorders, especially if they were associated with estrogen therapy. Caution should also be used in patients with cerebral vascular or coronary artery disease.

Glucose Tolerance—Because glucose tolerance may be decreased, diabetic patients should be carefully observed while receiving Emcyt.

Elevated Blood Pressure—Because hypertension may occur, blood pressure should be monitored periodically.

Continued on next page

Kabi Pharmacia—Cont.

PRECAUTIONS

General: Fluid Retention—Exacerbation of preexisting or incipient peripheral edema or congestive heart disease has been seen in some patients receiving Emcyt therapy. Other conditions which might be influenced by fluid retention, such as epilepsy, migraine or renal dysfunction, require careful observation.

Emcyt may be poorly metabolized in patients with impaired liver function and should be administered with caution in such patients.

Because Emcyt may influence the metabolism of calcium and phosphorus, it should be used with caution in patients with metabolic bone diseases that are associated with hypercalcemia or in patients with renal insufficiency.

Information for the Patient: Because of the possibility of mutagenic effects, patients should be advised to use contraceptive measures.

Laboratory Tests: Certain endocrine and liver function tests may be affected by estrogen-containing drugs. Abnormalities of hepatic enzymes and of bilirubin have occurred in patients receiving Emcyt, but have seldom been severe enough to require cessation of therapy. Such tests should be done at appropriate intervals during therapy and repeated after the drug has been withdrawn for two months.

Food/Drug Interaction: Milk, milk products and calcium-rich foods or drugs may impair the absorption of Emcyt.

Carcinogenesis, Mutagenesis, Impairment of Fertility: Long-term continuous administration of estrogen in certain animal species increases the frequency of carcinomas of the breast and liver. Compounds structurally similar to Emcyt are carcinogenic in mice. Carcinogenic studies of Emcyt have not been conducted in man. Although testing by the Ames method failed to demonstrate mutagenicity for estramustine phosphate sodium, it is known that both estradiol and nitrogen mustard are mutagenic. For this reason and because some patients who had been impotent while on estrogen therapy have regained potency while taking Emcyt, the patient should be advised to use contraceptive measures.

ADVERSE REACTIONS

In a randomized, double-blind trial comparing therapy with Emcyt in 93 patients (11.5 to 15.9 mg/kg/day) or diethylstilbestrol (DES) in 93 patients (3.0 mg/day), the following adverse effects were reported: [See table at right.]

OVERDOSAGE

Although there has been no experience with overdosage to date, it is reasonable to expect that such episodes may produce pronounced manifestations of the known adverse reactions. In the event of overdosage, the gastric contents should be evacuated by gastric lavage and symptomatic therapy should be initiated. Hematologic and hepatic parameters should be monitored for at least six weeks after overdosage of Emcyt.

DOSAGE AND ADMINISTRATION

The recommended daily dose is 14 mg per kg of body weight (*i.e.,* one 140 mg capsule for each 10 kg or 22 lb of body weight), given in 3 or 4 divided doses. Most patients in studies in the United States have been treated at a dosage range of 10 to 16 mg per kg per day.

Patients should be instructed to take Emcyt at least one hour before or two hours after meals. Emcyt should be swallowed with water. Milk, milk products and calcium-rich foods or drugs (such as calcium-containing antacids) must not be taken simultaneously with Emcyt.

Patients should be treated for 30 to 90 days before the physician determines the possible benefits of continued therapy. Therapy should be continued as long as the favorable response lasts. Some patients have been maintained on therapy for more than three years at doses ranging from 10 to 16 mg per kg of body weight per day.

Procedures for proper handling and disposal of anticancer drugs should be considered. Several guidelines on this subject have been published.[1-6] There is no general agreement that all of the procedures recommended in the guidelines are necessary or appropriate.

HOW SUPPLIED

White opaque capsules, each containing estramustine phosphate sodium as the disodium salt monohydrate equivalent to 140 mg estramustine phosphate—bottles of 100 (NDC 0016-0132-02).

Note: Emcyt should be stored in the refrigerator at 36° to 46°F (2° to 8°C).

REFERENCES

1. Recommendations for the safe handling of parenteral antineoplastic drugs. Washington, DC, U.S. Government Printing Office (NIH Publication No. 83-2621). 2. AMA Council Report. Guidelines for handling parenteral antineoplastics. *JAMA* 253:1590–1592, Mar. 15, 1985. 3. National Study Commission on Cytotoxic Exposure: Recommendations for handling cytotoxic agents. Available from Louis P. Jeffrey,

	EMCYT n=93	DES n=93
CARDIOVASCULAR–RESPIRATORY		
Cardiac Arrest	0	2
Cerebrovascular Accident	2	0
Myocardial Infarction	3	1
Thrombophlebitis	3	7
Pulmonary Emboli	2	5
Congestive Heart Failure	3	2
Edema	19	17
Dyspnea	11	3
Leg Cramps	8	11
Upper Respiratory Discharge	1	1
Hoarseness	1	0
GASTROINTESTINAL		
Nausea	15	8
Diarrhea	12	11
Minor Gastrointestinal Upset	11	6
Anorexia	4	3
Flatulence	2	0
Vomiting	1	1
Gastrointestinal Bleeding	1	0
Burning Throat	1	0
Thirst	1	0
INTEGUMENTARY		
Rash	1	4
Pruritus	2	2
Dry Skin	2	0
Pigment Changes	0	3
Easy Bruising	3	0
Flushing	1	0
Night Sweats	0	1
Fingertip—Peeling Skin	1	0
Thinning Hair	1	1
BREAST CHANGES		
Tenderness	66	64
Enlargement		
Mild	60	54
Moderate	10	16
Marked	0	5
MISCELLANEOUS		
Lethargy Alone	4	3
Depression	0	2
Emotional Lability	2	0
Insomnia	3	0
Headache	1	1
Anxiety	1	0
Chest Pain	1	1
Hot Flashes	0	1
Pain in Eyes	0	1
Tearing of Eyes	1	0
Tinnitus	0	1
LABORATORY ABNORMALITIES		
Hematologic		
Leukopenia	4	2
Thrombopenia	1	2
Hepatic		
Bilirubin Alone	1	5
Bilirubin and LDH	0	1
Bilirubin and SGOT	2	1
Bilirubin, LDH and SGOT	2	0
LDH and/or SGOT	31	28
Miscellaneous		
Hypercalcemia—Transient	0	1

ScD, Director of Pharmacy Services, Rhode Island Hospital, 593 Eddy Street, Providence, Rhode Island 02902. 4. Clinical Oncological Society of Australia: Guidelines and recommendations for safe handling of antineoplastic agents. *Med J Aust 1*:426–428, Apr. 30, 1983. 5. Jones RB, Frank R, Mass T: Safe handling of chemotherapeutic agents: a report from the Mount Sinai Medical Center, *CA 33*:258–263, Sept-Oct 1983. 6. ASHP technical assistance bulletin on handling cytotoxic drugs in hospitals. *Am J Hosp Pharm 42*:131–137, Jan 1985.

© 1988, Kabi Pharmacia text issued January 1988

Shown in Product Identification Section, page 413

HYSKON® Hysteroscopy Fluid   ℞
[*his'kon*]
32% (W/V) dextran-70 in dextrose

DESCRIPTION

HYSKON® Hysteroscopy Fluid is a clear, viscid, sterile, non-pyrogenic solution of dextran-70 (32% W/V) in dextrose (10% W/V). Dextran-70 is that fraction of dextran, a branched polysaccharide composed of glucose units, having a weight average molecular weight of 70,000. The fluid is electrolyte-free and non-conductive. At room temperature HYSKON® Hysteroscopy Fluid has a viscosity of 220 cS. HYSKON® has a tendency to crystalize when subjected to temperature variations or when stored for long periods. If flakes of dextran are present, heat at 100°–110° C until complete dissolution is achieved.

INDICATIONS

HYSKON® Hysteroscopy Fluid is indicated for use with the hysteroscope as an aid in distending the uterine cavity and in irrigating and visualizing its surfaces.

CONTRAINDICATIONS

HYSKON® Hysteroscopy Fluid should not be instilled in patients known to be hypersensitive to dextran. All other contraindications are those related to the hysteroscopic procedure itself, such as pregnancy, endometrial carcinoma, etc.

WARNINGS

It is possible that during hysteroscopy dextran may leak into the peritoneal cavity, the precise amount depending on the volume of HYSKON® used and the infusion pressure. Slow absorption from the peritoneal cavity (peak blood levels are reached in 3–4 days) (1) may result in systemic effects varying from simple plasma volume expansion or a transient prolongation of the bleeding time, to severe, fatal anaphylactic reactions. It is also reported that dextran may enter the pleural cavity through a pathway that has yet to be defined (2). When HYSKON® is employed during diagnostic hysteroscopy adverse effects are rare. In hysteroscopic surgery greater volumes of HYSKON® are infused over a longer period of time and the exposed blood vessels of the freshly traumatized endometrium allow the dextran direct access to the systemic circulation.

There is, therefore, the potential for these patients to rapidly develop adverse systemic effects, in particular pulmonary edema (3). Patients are considered at increased risk of developing pulmonary edema if:

1. They undergo a surgical procedure lasting more than 45 minutes when HYSKON® is being used to distend the uterus.
2. Greater than 500 ml of HYSKON® are infused.
3. Large areas of endometrium are traumatized during surgery.

ADVERSE REACTIONS

The following adverse reactions, although rare, have been reported for HYSKON®: fatal anaphylactic reaction, generalized itching, macular rash, urticaria, nasal congestion, flushing, hypotension, dyspnea, tightness of chest, cyanosis, wheezing, coughing, peripheral edema, pulmonary edema, pleural effusion, ascites, nausea, vomiting, fever, joint pains, oliguria, convulsions and increased clotting time.

DOSAGE AND ADMINISTRATION

The amount of HYSKON® Hysteroscopy Fluid required depends on a number of factors, including the type and length of the procedure and whether manipulation or surgery is performed. Usually, the amount of HYSKON® instilled into the uterus will be between 50 ml and 100 ml. HYSKON® should be introduced into the uterine cavity through the cannula of a hysteroscope under low pressure (approximately 100 mm Hg) until the uterus is sufficiently distended to permit adequate visualization. During the hysteroscopic examination, HYSKON® should be infused at a rate that keeps the cavity suitably distended. To avoid injection of the fluid into the tissues of the uterus and parametria and to prevent unnecessary amounts of the fluid leaking into the peritoneal cavity and backwards along the side of the hysteroscope, infusion pressures should not exceed 150 mm Hg.

HOW SUPPLIED

HYSKON® Hysteroscopy Fluid (32% W/V dextran-70 in 10% W/V dextrose) is available as a sterile, nonpyrogenic solution in 100 ml bottles packed 12 to a carton.
          (NDC No. 0016-0231-61)
and 250 ml bottles packed 6 to a carton
          (NDC No. 0016-0231-62)
Store at 20–25°C (68–77°F). Protect from cold.

CAUTION

Federal law restricts this device to sale by or on the order of a physician.

REFERENCES

1. Cleary R.E., Howard T., diZerega G.S.: Plasma dextran levels after abdominal instillation of 32% dextran 70: Evidence for prolonged intraperitoneal retention. Submitted for publication, 1984.
2. Adoni A., Adatto-Levy R., Mogle P., Palti Z.: Post-operative pleural effusion caused by dextran. Int J Gyn Obs 18:243, 1980.
3. Flores E., Neuwirth R.S.: Acute pulmonary edema occurring after a hysteroscopic surgical procedure using HYSKON® as the distending medium. Submitted for publication, 1984.

Revised November 1987

KABIKINASE®   ℞
[kah 'be-ki ''nas]
(Streptokinase)

DESCRIPTION
KABIKINASE (streptokinase) is a purified preparation of a bacterial protein elaborated by group C B-hemolytic streptococci. It is supplied as a water soluble white lyophilized powder for intravenous infusion following reconstitution and dilution. KABIKINASE (streptokinase) contains 11.0 mg Sodium L-Glutamate and 13 mg Albumin Human per 100,000 IU of streptokinase as stabilizers.

HOW SUPPLIED
KABIKINASE (streptokinase) is supplied as a lyophilized powder in 8 ml vials containing 250,000, 600,000, or 750,000 IU per vial of purified streptokinase or in a 10 ml vial containing 1,500,000 IU per vial of purified streptokinase, and shipped in cartons containing 10 vials.
250,000 IU NDC 0016-0110-59 Color Code Blue
600,000 IU NDC 0016-1110-67 Color Code Yellow
750,000 IU NDC 0016-0119-35 Color Code Pink
1,500,000 IU NDC 0016-0111-75 Color Code Green

MACRODEX®   ℞
[mak 'ro-dex]
(Plasma Volume Expander)

6% Dextran 70 in 0.9% Sodium Chloride Injection. 500 ml.

RHEOMACRODEX®   ℞
[re ''o-mak 'ro-dex]
(Plasma Volume Expander)

10% Dextran 40 in 5% Dextrose Injection. 500 ml.
10% Dextran 40 in 0.9% Sodium Chloride Injection. 500 ml.

Kenwood Laboratories
a division of
BRADLEY PHARMACEUTICALS, INC.
383 ROUTE 46 WEST
FAIRFIELD, NJ 07004-2402

APATATE® Liquid/Tablets   OTC
[ăp 'ah-tāt]
Vitamins B_1, B_6, B_{12}

COMPOSITION
Each teaspoonful (5 cc) or tablet contains: Vitamin B_1 (thiamine), 15 mg; Vitamin B_{12} (cyanocobalamin), 25 mcg; Vitamin B_6 pyridoxine, 0.5 mg.

HOW SUPPLIED
Liquid	Bottles of 4 fl. oz.	NDC 0482-0130-13
	Bottles of 8 fl. oz.	NDC 0482-0130-14
Tablets	Bottles of 50	NDC 0482-0135-18

APATATE® Liquid with Fluoride   ℞
[ăp 'ah-tāt]
Vitamins B_1, B_6, B_{12} with 0.5 mg flouride

COMPOSITION
Each teaspoonful (5 ml) contains: Vitamin B_1 (thiamine), 15 mg; Vitamin B_6 (pyridoxine), 0.5 mg; Vitamin B_{12} (cyanocobalamin), 25 mcg; 0.5 mg fluoride as sodium fluoride.

HOW SUPPLIED
Liquid Bottles of 4 fl. oz.   NDC 0482-0140-13

DUADACIN® COLD AND ALLERGY CAPSULES   OTC
[dū-ah 'dah-sĭn]
Multiple Symptom Relief

COMPOSITION
Each capsule contains acetaminophen USP, 325 mg; chlorpheniramine maleate USP, 2mg; phenylpropanolamine HCl USP, 12.5 mg.

HOW SUPPLIED
Bottles of 100 capsules   NDC 0482-0722-10
Bottles of 1000 capsules   NDC 0482-0722-70

GLUTOFAC® Caplets   OTC
[glū 'tō-făc]
High-Potency Metabolic Supplement To Restore Depleted Vitamin/Mineral Reserves

COMPOSITION
Each caplet contains: beta-carotene (vitamin A, 5,000 I.U.); vitamin E (dl-tocopherol), 30 I.U.; vitamin C (ascorbic acid), 300 mg; vitamin B_1 (thiamine hydrochloride), 15 mg; vitamin B_2 (riboflavin), 10 mg; niacinamide, 50 mg; vitamin B_6 (pyridoxine hydrochloride), 50 mg; pantothenic acid, 20 mg; zinc, elemental (zinc sulfate), 5 mg; copper, 1 mg; magnesium oxide, 133 mg; selenium, 25 mcg; chromium, (chromium picolinate), 50 mcg. In addition to label content, GLUTOFAC® Caplets contain calcium 50 mg, phosphorus 40 mg, and the following elements in trace amounts: manganese, potassium and iron. FREE OF SUGAR, STARCH, YEAST.

HOW SUPPLIED
Bottles of 90   NDC 0482-0154-90

I●L●X® B12 Elixir   OTC
Crystalline

I●L●X® B12 Sugar Free Elixir   OTC
Crystalline
Iron, Liver and B Vitamins

COMPOSITION
Each three teaspoonfuls (15 ml) contains: elemental iron (from iron ammonium citrate, brown), 102 mg; liver fraction 1, 98 mg; thiamine hydrochloride (vitamin B_1), 5 mg; riboflavin (vitamin B_2), 2 mg; nicotinamide, 10 mg; cyanocobalamin (vitamin B_{12} crystalline), 10 mcg; alcohol 8% by volume.

HOW SUPPLIED
ILX® B_{12} Elixir
Bottles of 8 fl. oz.   NDC 0482-0106-14
ILX® B_{12} Sugar Free Elixir
Bottles of 8 fl. oz.   NDC 0482-0107-14

I●L●X® B12 Caplets   OTC
Crystalline
Iron, Liver and B Vitamins

COMPOSITION
Each caplet contains: elemental iron (micronized iron from Ferronyl®, Carbonyl Iron), 37.5 mg; liver (dessicated), 130 mg; Vitamin C, 120 mg; thiamine hydrochloride (Vitamin B_1), 2 mg; riboflavin (Vitamin B_2), 2 mg; niacinamide, 20 mg; cyanocobalamin (Vitamin B_{12} crystalline), 12 mcg.

HOW SUPPLIED
Bottles of 100   NDC 0482-0110-23

IRCON® Tablets   OTC
[ir 'kŏn]
Iron

COMPOSITION
Each tablet contains ferrous fumarate, 200 mg.

HOW SUPPLIED
Bottles of 100   NDC 0482-0628-01

IRCON®–FA Tablets   OTC
[ir 'kŏn]
Iron and Folic Acid

COMPOSITION
Each tablet contains ferrous fumarate, 250 mg and folic acid, 0.8 mg.

HOW SUPPLIED
Bottles of 100   NDC 0482-0932-01

KENWOOD THERAPEUTIC LIQUID   OTC
High-Potency Multivitamin/Mineral Formulation

COMPOSITION
Each 3 teaspoonfuls (15 cc) contains: Vitamin A (Palmitate), 10,000 I.U.; Vitamin D (Ergocalciferol), 400 I.U.; Vitamin E (dl-alpha Tocopherol Acetate), 4.5 I.U.; Vitamin C (Ascorbic Acid), 150 mg; Vitamin B_1, (Thiamine Hydrochloride), 6 mg; Vitamin B_2 (Riboflavin 5-Phosphate Sodium), 3 mg; Niacinamide, 60 mg; Vitamin B_6 (Pyridoxine Hydrochloride), 1 mg;

Calcium Pantothenate, 6 mg; Calcium (Calcium Glycerophosphate), 38 mg; Phosphorus (Calcium Glycerophosphate), 29 mg; Magnesium (Magnesium Gluconate), 6 mg; Manganese (Manganese Gluconate), 1 mg; Potassium (Potassium Citrate), 5 mg.

HOW SUPPLIED
Bottles of 8 fl. oz.   NDC 0482-0116-14

NEOLOID® EMULSIFIED CASTOR OIL   OTC
[nē-ō-loid]

COMPOSITION
Castor Oil USP 36.4% (w/w) with 0.1% (w/w) Sodium Benzoate and 0.2% (w/w) Potassium Sorbate added as preservatives, emulsifying and flavoring agents in water. Does not contain sugar.

HOW SUPPLIED
Bottles of 4 fl. oz.   NDC 0482-5442-58

NITROGLYN® Extended-Release Capsules   ℞
[nĭ' trō-glĭn]
nitroglycerin

COMPOSITION
Each extended-release capsule contains nitroglycerin in one of four available dosage forms; 2.5 mg; 6.5 mg; 9 mg; 13 mg. The capsules are not sublingual or chewable.

HOW SUPPLIED
Bottles of 100
2.5 mg   NDC 0482-1025-01
6.5 mg   NDC 0482-1065-01
9 mg   NDC 0482-1090-01
13 mg   NDC 0482-1130-01
For full prescribing information, please see package insert.

TYZINE®   ℞
[tĭ' zēn]
tetrahydrozoline hydrochloride
Nasal Solution/Nasal Spray/Pediatric Nasal Drops

DESCRIPTION
Each ml of TYZINE Nasal Solution and TYZINE Nasal Spray contains 1.0 mg of tetrahydrozoline hydrochloride (0.1%) with sodium chloride, sodium citrate, disodium edetate, and 0.02% benzalkonium chloride as a preservative; in aqueous solution adjusted to optimum pH with hydrochloric acid. Each ml of Tyzine Pediatric Nasal Drops contains 0.5 mg of tetrahydrozoline hydrochloride (0.05%) with sodium chloride, sodium citrate, disodium edetate, and 0.02% benzalkonium chloride as a preservative, in aqueous solution adjusted to optimum pH with hydrochloric acid.

HOW SUPPLIED
Nasal Solution: Bottle of 30 ml (1 fl. oz.) with dropper
NDC 0482-4760-30
Nasal Spray: Spray bottle of 15 ml (½ fl. oz.)
NDC 0482-4760-15
Pediatric Nasal Drops: Bottle of 15 ml (½ fl. oz.) with dropper NDC 0482-4770-15
For full prescribing information, please see package insert.

The following are additional KENWOOD LABORATORIES products for which literature is available upon request:

Product Name	How Supplied	NDC
I●L●X® Elixir	8 oz. bottles	0482-0105-14
(High-potency hematinic; formulated with iron, liver and vitamins)		
IPSATOL® Cough Formula	4 oz. bottles	0482-0650-04
(Pleasant-tasting, nonalcoholic cough syrup)		

Products are cross-indexed
by product classifications
in the
BLUE SECTION.

Key Pharmaceuticals, Inc.
GALLOPING HILL ROAD
KENILWORTH, NJ 07033

K-DUR® ℞
[*kay-dur*]
Microburst Release System®
(potassium chloride) USP
Extended Release Tablets

DESCRIPTION

K-DUR® 20 is an immediately dispersing extended release oral dosage form of potassium chloride containing 1500 mg of microencapsulated potassium chloride USP equivalent to 20 mEq of potassium in a tablet.
K-DUR® 10 is an immediately dispersing extended release oral dosage form of potassium chloride containing 750 mg of microencapsulated potassium chloride USP equivalent to 10 mEq of potassium in a tablet.
These formulations are intended to slow the release of potassium so that the likelihood of a high localized concentration of potassium chloride within the gastrointestinal tract is reduced.
K-DUR is an electrolyte replenisher. The chemical name of the active ingredient is potassium chloride, and the structural formula is KCl. Potassium chloride USP occurs as a white, granular powder or as colorless crystals. It is odorless and has a saline taste. Its solutions are neutral to litmus. It is freely soluble in water and insoluble in alcohol.
K-DUR is a tablet formulation (not enteric coated or wax matrix) containing individually microencapsulated potassium chloride crystals which disperse upon tablet disintegration. In simulated gastric fluid at 37°C and in the absence of outside agitation, K-DUR begins disintegrating into microencapsulated crystals within seconds and completely disintegrates within one minute. The microencapsulated crystals are formulated to provide an extended release of potassium chloride.
Inactive Ingredients: Crospovidone, Ethylcellulose, Hydroxypropyl Cellulose, Magnesium Stearate, and Microcrystalline Cellulose.

CLINICAL PHARMACOLOGY

Potassium ion is the principal intracellular cation of most body tissues. Potassium ions participate in a number of essential physiological processes including the maintenance of intracellular tonicity, the transmission of nerve impulses, the contraction of cardiac, skeletal and smooth muscle and the maintenance of normal renal function.
The intracellular concentration of potassium is approximately 150 to 160 mEq per liter. The normal adult plasma concentration is 3.5 to 5 mEq per liter. An active ion transport system maintains this gradient across the plasma membrane.
Potassium is a normal dietary constituent and under steady state conditions the amount of potassium absorbed from the gastrointestinal tract is equal to the amount excreted in the urine. The usual dietary intake of potassium is 50 to 100 mEq per day.
Potassium depletion will occur whenever the rate of potassium loss through renal excretion and/or loss from the gastrointestinal tract exceeds the rate of potassium intake. Such depletion usually develops slowly as a consequence of therapy with diuretics, primary or secondary hyperaldosteronism, diabetic ketoacidosis, or inadequate replacement of potassium in patients on prolonged parenteral nutrition. Depletion can develop rapidly with severe diarrhea, especially if associated with vomiting. Potassium depletion due to these causes is usually accompanied by a concomitant loss of chloride and is manifested by hypokalemia and metabolic alkalosis. Potassium depletion may produce weakness, fatigue, disturbances of cardiac rhythm (primarily ectopic beats), prominent U-waves in the electrocardiogram, and in advanced cases, flaccid paralysis and/or impaired ability to concentrate urine.
If potassium depletion associated with metabolic alkalosis cannot be managed by correcting the fundamental cause of the deficiency, e.g., where the patient requires long term diuretic therapy, supplemental potassium in the form of high potassium food or potassium chloride may be able to restore normal potassium levels. In rare circumstances (e.g., patients with renal tubular acidosis) potassium depletion may be associated with metabolic acidosis and hyperchloremia. In such patients potassium replacement should be accomplished with potassium salts other than the chloride, such as potassium bicarbonate, potassium citrate, potassium acetate, or potassium gluconate.

INDICATIONS AND USAGE

BECAUSE OF REPORTS OF INTESTINAL AND GASTRIC ULCERATION AND BLEEDING WITH CONTROLLED RELEASE POTASSIUM CHLORIDE PREPARATIONS, THESE DRUGS SHOULD BE RESERVED FOR THOSE PATIENTS WHO CANNOT TOLERATE OR REFUSE TO TAKE LIQUID OR EFFERVESCENT POTASSIUM PREPARATIONS OR FOR PATIENTS IN WHOM THERE IS A PROBLEM OF COMPLIANCE WITH THESE PREPARATIONS.

1. For the treatment of patients with hypokalemia with or without metabolic alkalosis, in digitalis intoxication and in patients with hypokalemic familial periodic paralysis. If hypokalemia is the result of diuretic therapy, consideration should be given to the use of a lower dose of diuretic, which may be sufficient without leading to hypokalemia.
2. For the prevention of hypokalemia in patients who would be at particular risk if hypokalemia were to develop, e.g., digitalized patients or patients with significant cardiac arrhythmias.

The use of potassium salts in patients receiving diuretics for uncomplicated essential hypertension is often unnecessary when such patients have a normal dietary pattern and when low doses of the diuretic are used. Serum potassium should be checked periodically, however, and if hypokalemia occurs, dietary supplementation with potassium-containing foods may be adequate to control milder cases. In more severe cases, and if dose adjustment of the diuretic is ineffective or unwarranted, supplementation with potassium salts may be indicated.

CONTRAINDICATIONS

Potassium supplements are contraindicated in patients with hyperkalemia since a further increase in serum potassium concentration in such patients can produce cardiac arrest. Hyperkalemia may complicate any of the following conditions: chronic renal failure, systemic acidosis such as diabetic acidosis, acute dehydration, extensive tissue breakdown as in severe burns, adrenal insufficiency, or the administration of a potassium-sparing diuretic (e.g., spironolactone, triamterene, amiloride) (see **OVERDOSAGE**).
Controlled release formulations of potassium chloride have produced esophageal ulceration in certain cardiac patients with esophageal compression due to enlarged left atrium. Potassium supplementation, when indicated in such patients, should be given as a liquid preparation or as an aqueous (water) suspension of K-DUR (see **PRECAUTIONS; Information for Patients,** and **DOSAGE AND ADMINISTRATION** sections).
All solid oral dosage forms of potassium chloride are contraindicated in any patient in whom there is structural, pathological (e.g., diabetic gastroparesis) or pharmacologic (use of anticholinergic agents or other agents with anticholinergic properties at sufficient doses to exert anticholinergic effects) cause for arrest or delay in tablet passage through the gastrointestinal tract.

WARNINGS

Hyperkalemia (see **OVERDOSAGE**) In patients with impaired mechanisms for excreting potassium, the administration of potassium salts can produce hyperkalemia and cardiac arrest. This occurs most commonly in patients given potassium by the intravenous route but may also occur in patients given potassium orally. Potentially fatal hyperkalemia can develop rapidly and be asymptomatic. The use of potassium salts in patients with chronic renal disease, or any other condition which impairs potassium excretion, requires particularly careful monitoring of the serum potassium concentration and appropriate dosage adjustment.
Interaction with Potassium Sparing Diuretics—Hypokalemia should not be treated by the concomitant administration of potassium salts and a potassium-sparing diuretic (e.g., spironolactone, triamterene or amiloride) since the simultaneous administration of these agents can produce severe hyperkalemia.
Interaction with Angiotensin Converting Enzyme Inhibitors—Angiotensin converting enzyme (ACE) inhibitors (e.g., captopril, enalapril) will produce some potassium retention by inhibiting aldosterone production. Potassium supplements should be given to patients receiving ACE inhibitors only with close monitoring.
Gastrointestinal Lesions—Solid oral dosage forms of potassium chloride can produce ulcerative and/or stenotic lesions of the gastrointestinal tract. Based on spontaneous adverse reaction reports, enteric coated preparations of potassium chloride are associated with an increased frequency of small bowel lesions (40–50 per 100,000 patient years) compared to sustained release wax matrix formulations (less than one per 100,000 patient years). Because of the lack of extensive marketing experience with microencapsulated products, a comparison between such products and wax matrix or enteric coated products is not available. K-DUR is a tablet formulated to provide a controlled rate of release of microencapsulated potassium chloride and thus to minimize the possibility of a high local concetration of potassium near the gastrointestinal wall.
Prospective trials have been conducted in normal human volunteers in which the upper gastrointestinal tract was evaluated by endoscopic inspection before and after one week of solid oral potassium chloride therapy. The ability of this model to predict events occurring in usual clinical practice is unknown. Trials which approximated usual clinical practice did not reveal any clear differences between the wax matrix and microencapsulated dosage forms. In contrast, there was a higher incidence of gastric and duodenal lesions in subjects receiving a high dose of a wax matrix controlled release formulation under conditions which did not resemble usual or recommended clinical practice (i.e., 96 mEq per day in divided doses of potassium chloride administered to fasted patients, in the presence of an anticholinergic drug to delay gastric emptying). The upper gastrointestinal lesions observed by endoscopy were asymptomatic and were not accompanied by evidence of bleeding (Hemoccult testing). The relevance of these findings to the usual conditions (i.e., non-fasting, no anticholinergic agent, smaller doses) under which controlled release potassium chloride products are used is uncertain; epidemiologic studies have not identified an elevated risk, compared to microencapsulated products, for upper gastrointestinal lesions in patients receiving wax matrix formulations. K-DUR should be discontinued immediately and the possibility of ulceration, obstruction or perforation considered if severe vomiting, abdominal pain, distention, or gastrointestinal bleeding occurs.
Metabolic Acidosis—Hypokalemia in patients with metabolic acidosis should be treated with an alkalinizing potassium salt such as potassium bicarbonate, potassium citrate, potassium acetate, or potassium gluconate.

PRECAUTIONS

General: The diagnosis of potassium depletion is ordinarily made by demonstrating hypokalemia in a patient with a clinical history suggesting some cause for potassium depletion. In interpreting the serum potassium level, the physician should bear in mind that acute alkalosis per se can produce hypokalemia in the absence of a deficit in total body potassium while acute acidosis per se can increase the serum potassium concentration into the normal range even in the presence of a reduced total body potassium. The treatment of potassium depletion, particularly in the presence of cardiac disease, renal disease, or acidosis requires careful attention to acid-base balance and appropriate monitoring of serum electrolytes, the electrocardiogram, and the clinical status of the patient.
Information for Patients: Physicians should consider reminding the patient of the following:
To take each dose with meals and with a full glass of water or other liquid.
To take each dose without crushing, chewing, or sucking the tablets. If those patients are having difficulty swallowing whole tablets, they may try one of the following alternate methods of administration:

a. Break the tablet in half, and take each half separately with a glass of water.
b. Prepare an aqueous (water) suspension as follows:
   1. Place the whole tablet(s) in approximately one-half glass of water (4 fluid ounces).
   2. Allow approximately 2 minutes for the tablet(s) to disintegrate.
   3. Stir for about half a minute after the tablet(s) has disintegrated.
   4. Swirl the suspension and consume the entire contents of the glass immediately by drinking or by the use of a straw.
   5. Add another one fluid ounce of water, swirl, and consume immediately.
   6. Then, add an additional one fluid ounce of water, swirl, and consume immediately.

Aqueous suspension of K-DUR tablets that is not taken immediately should be discarded. The use of other liquids for suspending K-DUR tablets is not recommended.
To take this medicine following the frequency and amount prescribed by the physician. This is especially important if the patient is also taking diuretics and/or digitalis preparations.
To check with the physician at once if tarry stools or other evidence of gastrointestional bleeding is noticed.
Laboratory Tests: When blood is drawn for analysis of plasma potassium it is important to recognize that artifactual elevations can occur after improper venipuncture technique or as a result of in-vitro hemolysis of the sample.
Drug Interactions: Potassium-sparing diuretics, angiotensin converting enzyme inhibitors (see **WARNINGS**).
Carcinogenesis, Mutagenesis, Impairment of Fertility: Carcinogenicity, mutagenicity and fertility studies in animals have not been performed. Potassium is a normal dietary constituent.
Pregnancy Category C: Animal reproduction studies have not been conducted with K-DUR. It is unlikely that potassium supplementation that does not lead to hyperkalemia would have an adverse effect on the fetus or would affect reproductive capacity.
Nursing Mothers: The normal potassium ion content of human milk is about 13 mEq per liter. Since oral potassium becomes part of the body potassium pool, so long as body potassium is not excessive, the contribution of potassium chloride supplementation should have little or no effect on the level in human milk.
Pediatric Use: Safety and effectiveness in children have not been established.

ADVERSE REACTIONS

One of the most severe adverse effects is hyperkalemia (see CONTRAINDICATIONS, WARNINGS, and OVERDOSAGE). There have also been reports of upper and lower gastrointestinal conditions including obstruction, bleeding, ulceration, and perforation (see CONTRAINDICATIONS and WARNINGS).

The most common adverse reactions to oral potassium salts are nausea, vomiting, flatulence, abdominal discomfort, and diarrhea. These symptoms are due to irritation of the gastrointestinal tract and are best managed by diluting the preparation further, taking the dose with meals or reducing the amount taken at one time.

OVERDOSAGE

The administration of oral potassium salts to persons with normal excretory mechanisms for potassium rarely causes serious hyperkalemia. However, if excretory mechanisms are impaired or if potassium is administered too rapidly intravenously, potentially fatal hyperkalemia can result (see CONTRAINDICATIONS and WARNINGS). It is important to recognize that hyperkalemia is usually asymptomatic and may be manifested only by an increased serum potassium concentration (6.5–8.0 mEq/L) and characteristic electrocardiographic changes (peaking of T-waves, loss of P-waves, depression of S-T segment, and prolongation of the QT-interval). Late manifestations include muscle-paralysis and cardiovascular collapse from cardiac arrest. (9–12 mEq/L).

Treatment measures for hyperkalemia include the following:

1. Elimination of foods and medications containing potassium and of any agents with potassium-sparing properties.
2. Intravenous administration of 300 to 500 mL/hr of 10% dextrose solution containing 10–20 units of crystalline insulin per 1,000 mL.
3. Correction of acidosis, if present, with intravenous sodium bicarbonate.
4. Use of exchange resins, hemodialysis, or peritoneal dialysis.

In treating hyperkalemia, it should be recalled that in patients who have been stabilized on digitalis, too rapid a lowering of the serum potassium concentration can produce digitalis toxicity.

DOSAGE AND ADMINISTRATION

The usual dietary intake of potassium by the average adult is 50 to 100 mEq per day.

Potassium depletion sufficient to cause hypokalemia usually requires the loss of 200 or more mEq of potassium from the total body store.

Dosage must be adjusted to the individual needs of each patient. The dose for the prevention of hypokalemia is typically in the range of 20 mEq per day. Doses of 40–100 mEq per day or more are used for the treatment of potassium depletion. Dosage should be divided if more than 20mEq per day is given such that no more than 20 mEq is given in a single dose.

Each K-DUR 20 tablet provides 20 mEq of potassium chloride.

Each K-DUR 10 tablet provides 10 mEq of potassium chloride.

K-DUR tablets should be taken with meals and with a glass of water or other liquid. This product should not be taken on an empty stomach because of its potential for gastric irritation (see **WARNINGS**).

Patients having difficulty swallowing whole tablets may try one of the following alternate methods of administration:
a. Break the tablet in half, and take each half separately with a glass of water.
b. Prepare an aqueous (water) suspension as follows:
 1. Place the whole tablet(s) in approximately one-half glass of water (4 fluid ounces).
 2. Allow approximately 2 minutes for the tablet(s) to disintegrate.
 3. Stir for about half a minute after the tablet(s) has disintegrated.
 4. Swirl the suspension and consume the entire contents of the glass immediately by drinking or by the use of a straw.
 5. Add another one fluid ounce of water, swirl, and consume immediately.
 6. Then, add an additional one fluid ounce of water, swirl, and consume immediately.

Aqueous suspension of K-DUR tablets that is not taken immediately should be discarded. The use of other liquids for suspending K-DUR tablets is not recommended.

HOW SUPPLIED

K-DUR 20 mEq Extended Release Tablets are available in bottles of 100 (NDC 0085-0787-01); bottles of 500 (NDC 0085-0787-06); bottles of 1000 (NDC 0085-0787-10) and boxes of 100 for unit dose dispensing (NDC 0085-0787-81). K-DUR 20 mEq tablets are white, oblong, imprinted K-DUR 20 and scored for flexibility of dosing.

K-DUR 10 mEq Extended Release Tablets are available in bottles of 100 (NDC 0085-0263-01) and boxes of 100 for unit dose dispensing (NDC 0085-0263-81). K-DUR 10 mEq tablets are white, oblong, imprinted K-DUR 10.

STORAGE CONDITIONS

Keep tightly closed. Store at controlled room temperature 15–30°C (59–86°F).

CAUTION

Federal law prohibits dispensing without prescription.
Rev. 4/90   16237620
Shown in Product Identification Section, page 413

NITRO–DUR®   ℞
[nī'tra-dur]
(nitroglycerin)
Transdermal Infusion System

DESCRIPTION

Nitroglycerin is 1,2,3-propanetriol trinitrate, an organic nitrate whose structural formula is:

$$H_2CONO_2$$
$$|$$
$$HCONO_2$$
$$|$$
$$H_2CONO_2$$

and whose molecular weight is 227.09. The organic nitrates are vasodilators, active on both arteries and veins.

The NITRO-DUR (nitroglycerin) Transdermal Infusion System is a flat unit designed to provide continuous controlled release of nitroglycerin through intact skin. The rate of release of nitroglycerin is linearly dependent upon the area of the applied system; each cm² of applied system delivers approximately 0.02 mg of nitroglycerin per hour. Thus, the 5-, 10-, 15-, 20-, and 30-cm² systems deliver approximately 0.1, 0.2, 0.3, 0.4 and 0.6 mg of nitroglycerin per hour, respectively.

The remainder of the nitroglycerin in each system serves as a reservoir and is not delivered in normal use.

After 12 hours, for example, each system has delivered approximately 6% of its original content of nitroglycerin.

The NITRO-DUR transdermal system contains nitroglycerin in acrylic-based polymer adhesives with a resinous cross-linking agent to provide a continuous source of active ingredient. Each unit is sealed in a paper polyethylene-foil pouch.

Cross section of the system:

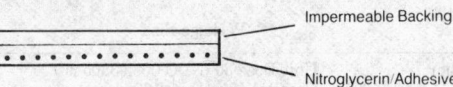

Impermeable Backing

Nitroglycerin/Adhesive

CLINICAL PHARMACOLOGY

The principal pharmacological action of nitroglycerin is relaxation of vascular smooth muscle and consequent dilatation of peripheral arteries and veins, especially the latter. Dilatation of the veins promotes peripheral pooling of blood and decreases venous return to the heart, thereby reducing left ventricular end-diastolic pressure and pulmonary capillary wedge pressure (preload). Arteriolar relaxation reduces systemic vascular resistance, systolic arterial pressure, and mean arterial pressure (afterload). Dilatation of the coronary arteries also occurs. The relative importance of preload reduction, afterload reduction, and coronary dilatation remains undefined.

Dosing regimens for most chronically used drugs are designed to provide plasma concentrations that are continuously greater than a minimally effective concentration. This strategy is inappropriate for organic nitrates. Several well-controlled clinical trials have used exercise testing to assess the anti-anginal efficacy of continuously-delivered nitrates. In the large majority of these trials, active agents were indistinguishable from placebo after 24 hours (or less) of continuous therapy. Attempts to overcome nitrate tolerance by dose escalation, even to doses far in excess of those used acutely, have consistently failed. Only after nitrates have been absent from the body for several hours has their anti-anginal efficacy restored.

Pharmacokinetics: The volume of distribution of nitroglycerin is about 3 L/kg, and nitroglycerin is cleared from this volume at extremely rapid rates, with a resulting serum half-life of about 3 minutes. The observed clearance rates (close to 1 L/kg/min) greatly exceed hepatic blood flow; known sites of extrahepatic metabolism include red blood cells and vascular walls.

The first products in the metabolism of nitroglycerin are inorganic nitrate and the 1,2- and 1,3-dinitroglycerols. The dinitrates are less effective vasodilators than nitroglycerin, but they are longer-lived in the serum, and their net contribution to the overall effect of chronic nitroglycerin regimens is not known. The dinitrates are further metabolized to (non-vasoactive) mononitrates and, ultimately, to glycerol and carbon dioxide.

To avoid development of tolerance to nitroglycerin, drug-free intervals of 10–12 hours are known to be sufficient; shorter intervals have not been well studied. In one well-controlled clinical trial, subjects receiving nitroglycerin appeared to exhibit a rebound or withdrawal effect, so that their exercise tolerance at the end of the daily drug-free interval was *less* than that exhibited by the parallel group receiving placebo.

In the healthy volunteers, steady-state plasma concentrations of nitroglycerin are reached by about 2 hours after application of a patch and are maintained for the duration of wearing the system (observations have been limited to 24 hours). Upon removal of the patch, the plasma concentration declines with a half-life of about an hour.

Clinical trials: Regimens in which nitroglycerin patches were worn for 12 hours daily have been studied in well-controlled trials up to 4 weeks in duration. Starting about 2 hours after application and continuing until 10–12 hours after application, patches that deliver at least 0.4 mg of nitroglycerin per hour have consistently demonstrated greater anti-anginal activity than placebo. Lower-dose patches have not been as well studied, but in one large, well-controlled trial in which higher-dose patches were also studied, patches delivering 0.2 mg/hr had significantly *less* anti-anginal activity than placebo.

It is reasonable to believe that the rate of nitroglycerin absorption from patches may vary with the site of application, but this relationship has not been adequately studied.

The onset of action of transdermal nitroglycerin is not sufficiently rapid for this product to be useful in aborting an acute anginal episode.

INDICATIONS AND USAGE

This drug product has been conditionally approved by the FDA for the prevention of angina pectoris due to coronary artery disease. Tolerance to the antianginal effects of nitrates (measured by exercise stress testing) has been shown to be a major factor limiting efficacy when transdermal nitrates are used continuously for longer than 12 hours each day. The development of tolerance can be altered (prevented or attenuated) by use of a noncontinuous (intermittent) dosing schedule with a nitrate-free interval of 10–12 hours.

Controlled clinical trial data suggest that the intermittent use of nitrates is associated with decreased exercise tolerance, in comparison to placebo, during the last part of the nitrate-free interval; the clinical relevance of this observation is unknown, but the possibility of increased frequency or severity of angina during the nitrate-free interval should be considered. Further investigations of the tolerance phenomenon and best regimen are ongoing. A final evaluation of the effectiveness of the product will be announced by the FDA.

CONTRAINDICATIONS

Allergic reactions to organic nitrates are extremely rare, but they do occur. Nitroglycerin is contraindicated in patients who are allergic to it. Allergy to the adhesives used in nitroglycerin patches has also been reported, and it similarly constitutes a contraindication to the use of this product.

WARNINGS

The benefits of transdermal nitroglycerin in patients with acute myocardial infarction or congestive heart failure have not been established. If one elects to use nitroglycerin in these conditions, careful clinical or hemodynamic monitoring must be used to avoid the hazards of hypotension and tachycardia.

A cardiovertor/defibrillator should not be discharged through a paddle electrode that overlies a NITRO-DUR patch. The arcing that may be seen in this situation is harmless in itself, but it may be associated with local current concentration that can cause damage to the paddles and burns to the patient.

PRECAUTIONS

General: Severe hypotension, particularly with upright posture, may occur with even small doses of nitroglycerin. This drug should therefore be used with caution in patients who may be volume depleted or who, for whatever reason, are already hypotensive. Hypotension induced by nitroglycerin may be accompanied by paradoxical bradycardia and increased angina pectoris.

Nitrate therapy may aggravate the angina caused by hypertrophic cardiomyopathy.

As tolerance to other forms of nitroglycerin develops, the effects of sublingual nitroglycerin on exercise tolerance, although still observable, is somewhat blunted.

Continued on next page

Key—Cont.

In industrial workers who have had long-term exposure to unknown (presumably high) doses of organic nitrates, tolerance clearly occurs. Chest pain, acute myocardial infarction, and even sudden death have occurred during temporary withdrawal of nitrates from these workers, demonstrating the existence of true physical dependence.

Several clinical trials in patients with angina pectoris have evaluated nitroglycerin regimens which incorporated a 10-to-12 hour, nitrate-free interval. In some of these trials, an increase in the frequency of anginal attacks during the nitrate-free interval was observed in a small number of patients. In one trial, patients had decreased exercise tolerance at the end of the nitrate-free interval. Hemodynamic rebound has been observed only rarely; on the other hand, few studies were so designed that rebound, if it had occurred, would have been detected. The importance of these observations to the routine, clinical use of transdermal nitroglycerin is unknown.

Information for Patients: Daily headaches sometimes accompany treatment with nitroglycerin. In patients who get these headaches, the headaches may be a marker of the activity of the drug. Patients should resist the temptation to avoid headaches by altering the schedule of their treatment with nitroglycerin, since loss of headache may be associated with simultaneous loss of antianginal efficacy.

Treatment with nitroglycerin may be associated with lightheadedness on standing, especially just after rising from a recumbent or seated position. This effect may be more frequent in patients who have also consumed alcohol.

After normal use, there is enough residual nitroglycerin in discarded patches that they are a potential hazard to children and pets.

A patient leaflet is supplied with the systems.

Drug Interactions: The vasodilating effects of nitroglycerin may be additive with those of other vasodilators. Alcohol, in particular, has been found to exhibit additive effects of this variety.

Carcinogenesis, Mutagenesis, Impairment of Fertility: No long-term animal studies have examined the carcinogenic or mutagenic potential of nitroglycerin. Nitroglycerin's effect upon reproductive capacity is similarly unknown.

Pregnancy Category C: Animal reproduction studies have not been conducted with nitroglycerin. It is also not known whether nitroglycerin can cause fetal harm when administered to a pregnant woman or whether it can affect reproductive capacity. Nitroglycerin should be given to a pregnant woman only if clearly needed.

Nursing Mothers: It is not known whether nitroglycerin is excreted in human milk. Because many drugs are excreted in human milk, caution should be exercised when nitroglycerin is administered to a nursing woman.

Pediatric Use: Safety and effectiveness in children have not been established.

ADVERSE REACTIONS

Adverse reactions to nitroglycerin are generally dose-related, and almost all of these reactions are the result of nitroglycerin's activity as a vasodilator. Headache, which may be severe, is the most commonly reported side effect. Headache may be recurrent with each daily dose, especially at higher doses. Transient episodes of lightheadedness, occasionally related to blood pressure changes, may also occur. Hypotension occurs infrequently, but in some patients it may be severe enough to warrant discontinuation of therapy. Syncope, crescendo angina, and rebound hypertension have been reported but are uncommon.

Extremely rarely, ordinary doses of organic nitrates have caused methemoglobinemia in normal-seeming patients. Methemoglobinemia is so infrequent at these doses that further discussion of its diagnosis and treatment is deferred (see **OVERDOSAGE**).

Application-site irritation may occur but is rarely severe.

In two placebo-controlled trials of intermittent therapy with nitroglycerin patches at 0.2 to 0.8 mg/hr, the most frequent adverse reactions among 307 subjects were as follows:

	placebo	patch
headache	18%	63%
lightheadedness	4%	6%
hypotension, and/or syncope	0%	4%
increased angina	2%	2%

OVERDOSAGE

Hemodynamic Effects: The ill effects of nitroglycerin overdose are generally the results of nitroglycerin's capacity to induce vasodilatation, venous pooling, reduced cardiac output, and hypotension. These hemodynamic changes may have protean manifestations, including increased intracranial pressure, with any or all of persistent throbbing headache, confusion, and moderate fever; vertigo; palpitations; visual disturbances; nausea and vomting (possibly with colic and even bloody diarrhea); syncope (especially in the upright posture); air hunger and dyspnea, later followed by reduced ventilatory effort, diaphoresis, with the skin either flushed or cold and clammy; heart block and bradycardia; paralysis; coma; seizures; and death.

Laboratory determinations of serum levels of nitroglycerin and its metabolites are not widely available, and such determinations have, in any event, no established role in the management of nitroglycerin overdose.

No data are available to suggest physiological maneuvers (e.g., maneuvers to change the pH of the urine) that might accelerate elimination of nitroglycerin and its active metabolites. Similarly, it is not known which—if any—of these substances can usefully be removed from the body by hemodialysis.

No specific antagonist to the vasodilator effects of nitroglycerin is known, and no intervention has been subject to controlled study as a therapy of nitroglycerin overdose. Because the hypotension associated with nitroglycerin overdose is the result of venodilatation and arterial hypovolemia, prudent therapy in this situation should be directed toward increase in central fluid volume. Passive elevation of the patient's legs may be sufficient, but intravenous infusion of normal saline or similar fluid may also be necessary.

The use of epinephrine or other arterial vasoconstrictors in this setting is likely to do more harm than good.

In patients with renal disease or congestive heart failure, therapy resulting in central volume expansion is not without hazard. Treatment of nitroglycerin overdose in these patients may be subtle and difficult, and invasive monitoring may be required.

Methemoglobinemia: Nitrate ions liberated during metabolism of nitroglycerin can oxidize hemoglobin into methemoglobin. Even in patients totally without cytochrome b_5 reductase activity, however, and even assuming that the nitrate moieties of nitroglycerin are quantitatively applied to oxidation of hemoglobin, about 1 mg/kg of nitroglycerin should be required before any of these patients manifests clinically significant ($\geq 10\%$) methemoglobinemia. In patients with normal reductase function, significant production of methemoglobin should require even larger doses of nitroglycerin. In one study in which 36 patients received 2–4 weeks of continuous nitroglycerin therapy at 3.1 to 4.4 mg/hr, the average methemoglobin level measured was 0.2%; this was comparable to that observed in parallel patients who received placebo.

Notwithstanding these observations, there are case reports of significant methemoglobinemia in association with moderate overdoses of organic nitrates. None of the affected patients had been thought to be unusually susceptible.

Methemoglobin levels are available from most clinical laboratories. The diagnosis should be suspected in patients who exhibit signs of impaired oxygen delivery despite adequate cardiac output and adequate arterial pO_2. Classically, methemoglobinemic blood is described as chocolate brown, without color change on exposure to air.

When methemoglobinemia is diagnosed, the treatment of choice is methylene blue, 1–2 mg/kg intravenously.

DOSAGE AND ADMINISTRATION

The suggested starting dose is between 0.2 mg/hr*, and 0.4 mg/hr*. Doses between 0.4 mg/hr* and 0.8 mg/hr* have shown continued effectiveness for 10–12 hours daily for at least one month (the longest period studied) of intermittent administration. Although the minimum nitrate-free interval has not been defined, data show that a nitrate-free interval of 10–12 hours is sufficient (see **CLINICAL PHARMACOLOGY**). Thus, an appropriate dosing schedule for nitroglycerin patches would include a daily patch-on period of 12–14 hours and a daily patch-off period of 10–12 hours.

Although some well controlled clinical trials using exercise tolerance testing have shown maintenance of effectiveness when patches are worn continuously, the large majority of such controlled trials have shown the development of tolerance (i.e., complete loss of effect) within the first 24 hours after therapy was initiated. Dose adjustment even to levels much higher than generally used, did not restore efficacy.

HOW SUPPLIED
[See table at left.]

CAUTION: Federal Law prohibits dispensing without prescription.

Key Pharmaceuticals, Inc.
Kenilworth, NJ 07033 USA
Revised 8/90   B-14362339
Copyright © 1987, 1989, 1990 Key Pharmaceuticals, Inc. All Rights Reserved.

*Release rates were formerly described in terms of drug delivered per 24 hours. In these terms, the supplied NITRO-DUR systems would be rated at 2.5 mg/24 hours (0.1 mg/hour), 5 mg/24 hours (0.2 mg/hour), 7.5 mg/24 hours (0.3 mg/hour), 10 mg/24 hours (0.4 mg/hour), and 15 mg/24 hours (0.6 mg/hour).

Shown in Product Identification Section, page 413

THEO-DUR®   ℞
Theophylline
Extended-Release Tablets

DESCRIPTION

THEO-DUR® Extended-Release Tablets contain anhydrous theophylline, a bronchodilator structurally classified as a xanthine derivative. THEO-DUR is available in an extended-release formulation for oral administration which allows a 12-hour dosing interval for a majority of patients and a 24-hour dosing interval for selected patients (see **DOSAGE AND ADMINISTRATION** for a description of appropriate

Nitro-Dur System Rated Release In Vivo*	Total Nitroglycerin Content	System Size	Package Size
0.1 mg/hr	20 mg	5 cm²	Unit Dose 30 (NDC 0085-3305-30) Hospital Unit Dose 100 (NDC 0085-3305-01) Institutional Package 30 (NDC 0085-3305-35) Institutional Package 100 (NDC 0085-3305-10)
0.2 mg/hr	40 mg	10 cm²	Unit Dose 30 (NDC 0085-3310-30) Hospital Unit Dose 100 (NDC 0085-3310-01) Institutional Package 30 (NDC 0085-3310-35) Institutional Package 100 (NDC 0085-3310-10)
0.3 mg/hr	60 mg	15 cm²	Unit Dose 30 (NDC 0085-3315-30) Hospital Unit Dose 100 (NDC 0085-3315-01) Institutional Package 30 (NDC 0085-3315-35) Institutional Package 100 (NDC 0085-3315-10)
0.4 mg/hr	80 mg	20 cm²	Unit Dose 30 (NDC 0085-3320-30) Hospital Unit Dose 100 (NDC 0085-3320-01) Institutional Package 30 (NDC 0085-3320-35) Institutional Package 100 (NDC 0085-3320-10)
0.6 mg/hr	120 mg	30 cm²	Unit Dose 30 (NDC 0085-3330-30) Hospital Unit Dose 100 (NDC 0085-3330-01) Institutional Package 30 (NDC 0085-3330-35) Institutional Package 100 (NDC 0085-3330-10)

*Release rates were formerly described in terms of drug delivered per 24 hours. In these terms, the supplied NITRO-DUR Systems would be rated at 2.5 mg/24 hours (0.1 mg/hour), 5 mg/24 hours (0.2 mg/hour), 7.5 mg/24 hours (0.3 mg/hour), 10 mg/24 hours (0.4 mg/hour), and 15 mg/24 hours (0.6 mg/hour).

patient populations). THEO-DUR Extended-Release Tablets contain no color additives and are available in four strengths: 100 mg, 200 mg, 300 mg, and 450 mg.

The inactive ingredients for THEO-DUR 100 mg Extended-Release Tablets include: Acacia NF, Acetone USP, Alcohol, Cellulose Acetate Phthalate, NF, Cetyl Alcohol NF, Chloroform NF, Confectioner's Sugar 6X NF, Corn Starch NF, Diethyl Phthalate (Ethyl Phthalate), Ethyl Acetate NF, Glyceryl Monostearate NF (Atmul 84), Isopropyl Alcohol USP, Lactose Hydrous Spray Dried USP, Magnesium Stearate NF, Myristyl Alcohol, Non-Pareil Seeds 18-20 Mesh, Purified Water USP, Sodium Lauryl Sulfate NF (Dupanol C), Talc USP, White Wax NF.

The inactive ingredients for THEO-DUR 200 mg, 300 mg and 450 mg Extended-Release Tablets include: Acetone USP, Cellulose Acetate Phthalate NF, Cetyl Alcohol NF, Diethyl Phthalate (Ethyl Phthalate), Glyceryl Monostearate NF (Atmul 84), Hydroxypropyl Methylcellulose 2910 USP (Methocel E-50). Isopropyl Alcohol USP, Lactose Anhydrous USP Crystalline, Magnesium Stearate NF, Myristyl Alcohol Non-Pareil Seeds 18-20 Mesh, Purified Water USP, White Wax NF.

The structural formula of theophylline, 1H-Purine-2, 6-dione, 3, 7-dihydro-1, 3-dimethyl-is:

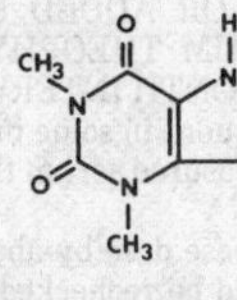

Anhydrous theophylline is a white, odorless, crystalline powder having a bitter taste.

CLINICAL PHARMACOLOGY

Theophylline directly relaxes the smooth muscle of the bronchial airways and pulmonary blood vessels, thus acting mainly as a bronchodilator and smooth muscle relaxant. It has also been demonstrated that aminophylline has a potent effect on diaphragmatic contractility in normal persons and may then be capable of reducing fatigability and thereby improve contractility in patients with chronic obstructive airways disease. The exact mode of action remains unsettled. Although theophylline does cause inhibition of phosphodiesterase with a resultant increase in intracellular cyclic AMP, other agents similarly inhibit the enzyme producing a rise of cyclic AMP but are unassociated with any demonstrable bronchodilation. Other mechanisms proposed include an effect on translocation of intracellular calcium; prostaglandin antagonism; stimulation of catecholamines endogenously; inhibition of cyclic guanosine monophosphate metabolism and adenosine receptor antagonism. None of these mechanisms has been proved, however.

In vitro, theophylline has been shown to act synergistically with beta agonists and there are now available data which demonstrate an additive effect *in vivo* with combined use.

Pharmacokinetics: The half-life of theophylline is influenced by a number of known variables. It may be prolonged in chronic alcoholics, particularly those with liver disease (cirrhosis or alcoholic liver disease) or in patients with congestive heart failure and in patients taking certain other drugs (see **PRECAUTIONS, Drug Interactions**).

Newborns and neonates have extremely slow clearance rates compared to older infants and children (i.e. those over 1 year of age). Older children have rapid clearance rates while most non-smoking adults have clearance rates between these two extremes. In premature neonates the decreased clearance is related to metabolic pathways that have yet to be established.

THEOPHYLLINE ELIMINATION CHARACTERISTICS

	Range	Mean
Children	1–9	3.7
Adults	3–15	7.7

In cigarette smokers (1–2 packs/day) the mean half-life is 4–5 hours, much shorter than in non-smokers. The increase in clearance associated with smoking is presumably due to stimulation of the hepatic metabolic pathway by components of cigarette smoke. The duration of this effect after cessation of smoking is unknown but may require 6 months to 2 years before the rate approaches that of the non-smokers.

THEO-DUR (100, 200, 300 and 450 mg) Extended-Release Tablets: In single dose studies with 18 normal fasting subjects, THEO-DUR at 8 mg/kg body weight (300–700 mg/dose) produced mean peak theophylline plasma levels of 7.5 ± 1.9 mcg/mL at 9.2 ± 1.9 hours following administration. In multiple dose, steady-state, 3 and 5 day studies with 12 normal subjects, THEO-DUR administered at 8 mg/kg (300–600 mg/dose) twice daily, achieved an average peak-trough difference of 4 mcg/mL. The Cmax and Cmin were 13.9 ± 6.9 and 9.9 ± 6.0, respectively. The mean % fluctuation ± S.D. of the plasma concentration at steady state [% fluctuation = 100 (Cmax-Cmin)/Cmin] was 54.2±45.7%. These pharmacokinetic parameters were measured under fasting conditions.

THEO-DUR (200, 300 and 450 mg) Extended-Release Tablets: In a multiple dose (300–500 mg BID) steady-state, 5 day study involving 14 normal, nonfasting subjects with theophylline half-lives between 5.8 and 12.3 hours (mean 8.0 ± 1.8 hours), THEO-DUR, dosed twice daily, produced mean Cmax and Cmin levels of 12.2 ± 2.0 and 10.2 ± 1.6 mcg/mL, respectively, over the a.m. dosing interval and Cmax and Cmin of 11.6 ± 1.6 and 8.7 ± 1.8 mcg/mL, respectively, over the p.m. dosing interval. The mean % fluctuation ± S.D. over the a.m. dosing interval was 30.4 ± 12.9% and 33.7 ± 13.1% over the p.m. dosing interval. In the same subjects, THEO-DUR given once daily, in the morning, in doses ranging from 600–1000 mg (same daily dose as for BID, above) produced a mean Cmax and Cmin of 14.4 ± 2.2 and 5.5 ± 2.0, respectively and a mean % fluctuation ± S.D. of 195.8 ± 106.0%. Average peak-through differences over 24 hours were 8.9 ± 1.3 and 3.7 ± 1.2 mcg/mL when THEO-DUR was given once or twice daily, respectively. In both the twice daily and once daily dosing regimens, THEO-DUR exhibited complete bioavailability when compared to an immediate release product.

THEO-DUR (200, 300 and 450 mg) Extended-Release Tablets: In a single-dose bioavailability study in eleven subjects, 1000 mg of THEO-DUR was administered under fasting conditions and immediately following a high fat content (62 g) breakfast of approximately 1100 kcal. The rate and extent of absorption of theophylline from THEO-DUR administered in fasting and fed conditions were similar.

INDICATIONS AND USAGE

For relief and/or prevention of symptoms from asthma and reversible bronchospasm associated with chronic bronchitis and emphysema.

CONTRAINDICATIONS

This product is contraindicated in individuals who have shown hypersensitivity to its components. It is also contraindicated in patients with active peptic ulcer disease, and in individuals with underlying seizure disorders (unless receiving appropriate anticonvulsant medication).

WARNINGS

Serum levels above 20 mcg/mL are rarely found after appropriate administration of recommended doses. However, in individuals in whom theophylline plasma clearance is reduced *for any reason*, even conventional doses may result in increased serum levels and potential toxicity. Reduced theophylline clearance has been documented in the following readily identifiable groups: 1) patients with impaired liver function, 2) patients over 55 years of age, particularly males and those with chronic lung disease; 3) those with cardiac failure from any cause; 4) patients with sustained high fever; 5) neonates and infants under 1 year of age; 6) those patients taking certain drugs (see **PRECAUTIONS, Drug Interactions**). Frequently, such patients have markedly prolonged theophylline serum levels following discontinuation of the drug.

Reduction of dosage and laboratory monitoring is especially appropriate in the above individuals.

Serious side effects such as ventricular arrhythmias, convulsions or even death may appear as the first sign of toxicity without any previous warning. Less serious signs of theophylline toxicity (i.e. nausea and restlessness) may occur frequently when initiating therapy, but are usually transient; when signs are persistent during maintenance therapy, they are often associated with serum concentrations above 20 mcg/mL. Stated differently: *serious toxicity is not reliably preceded by less severe side effects.* Serum concentration measurements may contribute significant information towards predicting potential life-threatening toxicity.

Many patients who require theophylline may exhibit tachycardia due to their underlying disease process so that the cause/effect relationship to elevated serum theophylline concentrations may not be appreciated.

Theophylline products may cause or worsen arrhythmias and any pre-existing arrhythmias, and any significant change in rate and/or rhythm warrants monitoring and further investigation.

Studies in laboratory animals (minipigs, rodents, and dogs) recorded the occurrence of cardiac arrhythmias and sudden death (with histologic evidence of myocardial necrosis) when beta-agonists and methylxanthines were administered concurrently. The significance of these findings when applied to humans is currently unknown.

PRECAUTIONS

THEO-DUR TABLETS SHOULD NOT BE CHEWED OR CRUSHED.

General: On the average, theophylline half-life is shorter in cigarette and marijuana smokers than in non-smokers, but smokers can have half-lives as long as non-smokers. Theophylline should not be administered concurrently with other xanthines medication. Use with caution in patients with hypoxemia, hypertension or those with a history of peptic ulcer. Theophylline may occasionally act as a local irritant to the G.I. tract although gastrointestinal symptoms are more commonly centrally mediated and associated with serum drug concentrations over 20 mcg/mL.

Information for Patients: This information is intended to aid in the safe and effective use of this medication. It is not a disclosure of all possible adverse or intended effects.

The physician should reinforce the importance of taking only the prescribed dose and time interval between doses. THEO-DUR Extended-Release Tablets should not be chewed or crushed. When dosing THEO-DUR Extended-Release Tablets on a once daily (q24h) basis, tablets should be taken whole and not split. As with any controlled-release theophylline product, the patient should alert the physician if symptoms occur repeatedly, especially near the end of the dosing interval.

Laboratory Tests: Serum theophylline levels should be monitored periodically to assure achievement of optimal levels for safety and efficacy. For such measurements, the serum sample should be obtained at the time of peak concentration, 4 to 8 hours when medication is taken every 12 hours or 8 hours when taken once daily. It is important that the patient has not missed or taken additional doses during the previous 48 hours and that dosing intervals were reasonably equally spaced. DOSAGE ADJUSTMENT BASED ON SERUM THEOPHYLLINE MEASUREMENTS WHEN THESE INSTRUCTIONS HAVE NOT BEEN FOLLOWED MAY RESULT IN RECOMMENDATIONS THAT PRESENT RISK OF TOXICITY TO THE PATIENT.

Drug Interactions: Toxic synergism with ephedrine has been documented and may occur with some other sympathomimetic bronchodilators. In addition, the following drug interactions have been demonstrated:

Theophylline with:	
Allopurinol (high dose)	Increased serum theophylline levels
Cimetidine	Increased serum theophylline levels
Ciprofloxacin	Increased serum theophylline levels
Erythromycin, Troleandomycin	Increased serum theophylline levels
Lithium carbonate	Increased renal excretion of lithium
Oral contraceptives	Increased serum theophylline levels
Phenytoin	Decreased theophylline and phenytoin serum levels
Propranolol	Increased serum theophylline levels
Rifampin	Decreased serum theophylline levels

Drug-Food Interactions: *THEO-DUR 100 mg Extended-Release Tablets* have not been adequately studied to determine whether their bioavailability is altered when given with food. Available data suggest that drug administration at the time of food ingestion may influence the absorption characteristics of theophylline controlled-release products resulting in serum values different from those found after administration in the fasting state.

A drug-food effect, if any, would likely have its greatest clinical significance when high theophylline serum levels are being maintained and/or when large single doses (greater than 13 mg/kg or 900 mg) of a controlled-release theophylline product are given.

THEO-DUR (200, 300 and 450 mg) Extended-Release Tablets: The rate and extent of absorption of theophylline from THEO-DUR 200 mg, 300 mg, and 450 mg tablets are similar when administered fasting or immediately after a high fat content breakfast such as 8 oz. whole milk, egg/cheese/bacon on muffin, 1 blueberry muffin with margarine, and 1 serving of hash brown potatoes (about 1100 kcal, including approximately 62 g of fat). (See **CLINICAL PHARMACOLOGY, Pharmacokinetics.)**

Drug—Laboratory Test Interactions: Currently available analytical methods, including high pressure liquid chromatography and immunoassay techniques, for measuring serum theoophylline levels are specific. Metabolites and other drugs generally do not affect the results. Other new analytic methods are also now in use. The physician should be aware of the laboratory method used and whether other drugs will interfere with the assay for theophylline.

Carcinogenesis, Mutagenesis, and Impairment of Fertility: Long-term carcinogenicity studies have not been performed with theophylline.

Chromosome-breaking activity was detected in human cell cultures at concentrations of theophylline up to 50 times the therapeutic serum concentration in humans. Theophylline was not mutagenic in the dominant lethal assay in male mice given theophylline intraperitoneally in doses up to 30 times the maximum daily human oral dose.

Studies to determine the effects on fertility have not been performed with theophylline.

Pregnancy: Category C Animal reproduction studies have not been conducted with theophylline. It is not known

Continued on next page

Key—Cont.

whether theophylline can cause fetal harm when administered to a pregnant woman or can affect reproduction capacity. Xanthines should be given to a pregnant woman only if clearly needed.

Nursing Mothers: Theophylline is distributed into breast milk and may cause irritability or other signs of toxicity in nursing infants. Because of the potential for serious adverse reactions in nursing infants from theophylline, a decision should be made whether to discontinue nursing or to discontinue the drug, taking into account the importance of the drug to the mother.

Pediatric Use: Safety and effectiveness of THEO-DUR Extended-Release Tablets administered:

1. Every 24 hours in children under 12 years of age, have not been established.
2. Every 12 hours in children under 6 years of age, have not been established.

ADVERSE REACTIONS

The following adverse actions have been observed, but there has not been enough systemic collection of data to support an estimate of their frequency.

1. *Gastrointestinal:* nausea, vomiting, epigastric pain, hematemesis, diarrhea.
2. *Central Nervous System:* headaches, irritability, restlessness, insomnia, reflex hyperexcitability, muscle twitching, clonic and tonic generalized convulsions.
3. *Cardiovascular:* palpitation, tachycardia, extrasystole, flushing, hypotension, circulatory failure, ventricular arrhythmia.
4. *Respiratory:* tachypnea.
5. *Renal:* potentiation of diuresis.
6. *Others:* alopecia, hyperglycemia, inappropriate ADH syndrome, rash.

OVERDOSAGE

Management: It is suggested that the management principles (consistent with the clinical status of the patient when first seen) outlined below be instituted and that simultaneous contact with a Regional Poison Control Center be established. In this way both updated information and individualization regarding the required therapy may be provided.

1. When potential oral overdose is established and seizure has not occurred:
   a) If patient is alert and seen within the early hours after ingestion, induction of emesis may be of value. Gastric lavage has been demonstrated to be of no value in influencing outcome in patients who present more than 1 hour after ingestion.
   b) Administer a cathartic. Sorbitol solution is reported to be of value.
   c) Administer repeated doses of activated charcoal and monitor theophylline serum levels.
   d) Prophylactic administration of phenobarbital has been shown to elevate the seizure threshold in laboratory animals, and administration of this drug can be considered.
2. If patient presents with a seizure:
   a) Establish an airway.
   b) Administer oxygen.
   c) Treat the seizure with intravenous diazepam, 0.1 to 0.3 mg/kg up to 10 mg. If seizures cannot be controlled, the use of general anesthesia should be considered.
   d) Monitor vital signs, maintain blood pressure and provide adequate hydration.
3. If post-seizure coma is present:
   a) Maintain airway and oxygenation.
   b) If result of oral medication, follow above recommendations to prevent absorption of the drug, but intubation and lavage will have to be performed instead of inducing emesis, and the cathartic and charcoal will need to be introduced via a large bore gastric lavage tube.
   c) Continue to provide full supportive care and adequate hydration until the drug is metabolized. In general drug metabolism is sufficiently rapid so as not to warrant dialysis. If repeated oral activated charcoal is ineffective (as noted by stable or rising serum levels) charcoal hemoperfusion may be indicated.

DOSAGE and ADMINISTRATION

THEO-DUR (200, 300 and 450 mg) Extended-Release Tablets: The rate and extent of absorption of theophylline from THEO-DUR 200, 300 and 450 mg tablets when administered fasting or immediately after a high fat content breakfast are similar (see **CLINICAL PHARMACOLOGY, Pharmacokinetics**).

THEO-DUR 100 mg Extended-Release Tablets have not been adequately studied for their bioavailability when administered with food (see **PRECAUTIONS, Drug—Food Interactions**).

Effective use of theophylline (i.e., the concentration of drug in the serum associated with optimal benefit and minimal risk of toxicity) is considered to occur when the theophylline concentration is maintained from 10 to 20 mcg/mL. The early studies from which these levels were derived were carried out in patients immediately or shortly after recovery from acute exacerbations of their disease (some hospitalized with status asthmaticus).

Although the 20 mcg/mL remains appropriate as a critical value (above which toxicity is more likely to occur) for safety purposes, additional data are now available which indicate that the serum theophylline concentrations required to produce maximum physiologic benefit may, in fact, fluctuate with the degree of bronchospasm present and are variable. Therefore, the physician should individualize the range appropriate to the patient's requirements, based on both symptomatic response and improvement in pulmonary function.

It should be stressed that serum theophylline concentrations maintained at the upper level of the 10 to 20 mcg/mL range may be associated with potential toxicity when factors known to reduce theophylline clearance are operative (see **WARNINGS**).

If it is not possible to obtain serum level determinations, restriction of the daily dose (in otherwise healthy adults) to not greater than 13 mg/kg/day, to a maximum of 900 mg of theophylline will result in relatively few patients exceeding serum levels of 20 mcg/mL and the resultant greater risk of toxicity.

Caution should be exercised for younger children who cannot complain of minor side effects. Older adults, particularly those with cor pulmonale, congestive heart failure, and/or liver disease may have unusually low dosage requirements and thus may experience toxicity at the maximal dosage recommended below.

Theophylline does not distribute into fatty tissue. Dosage should be calculated on the basis of lean (ideal) body weight where mg/kg doses are presented.

Frequency of Dosing: When immediate release products with rapid absorption are used, dosing to maintain serum levels generally requires administration every 6 hours. This is particularly true in children, but dosing intervals up to 8 hours may be satisfactory in adults since they eliminate the drug at a slower rate. Some children, and adults requiring higher than average doses (those having rapid rates of clearance, e.g. half-lives of under 6 hours) may benefit and be more effectively controlled during chronic therapy when given products with extended-release characteristics since these provide longer dosing intervals and/or less fluctuation in serum concentration between dosing.

Dosage guidelines are approximations only and the wide range of theophylline clearance between individuals (particularly those with concomitant disease) makes indiscriminate usage hazardous.

DOSAGE GUIDELINES

WARNING: DO NOT ATTEMPT TO MAINTAIN ANY DOSE THAT IS NOT TOLERATED.

It is recommended that dosing be considered in two stages: initiation of therapy with THEO-DUR, and titration, adjustment, and chronic maintenance.

Initiation of Therapy:

It is recommended that the appropriate dosage be established using an immediate-release preparation. Slow clinical titration is generally preferred to help assure acceptance and safety of the medication, and to allow the patient to develop tolerance to the transient caffeine-like side effects. Then, if the total 24 hour dose can be given by use of the available strengths of this product, the patient can usually be switched to THEO-DUR giving one-half of the daily dose at 12 hour intervals. However, certain patients, such as the young, smokers and some non-smoking adults are likely to metabolize theophylline rapidly and require dosing at 8 hour intervals. Such patients can generally be identified as having trough serum concentrations lower than desired or repeatedly exhibiting symptoms near the end of a dosing interval.

Alternatively, therapy can be initiated with THEO-DUR since it is available in dosage forms/strengths which permit titration and adjustment in dosage as outlined in the following dosing guidelines. It is recommended that for children under 25 kg, proper dosage be established with a liquid preparation to permit titration in small increments.

THE AVERAGE INITIAL ADULT AND CHILDREN'S (over 25 kg) DOSE IS ONE THEO-DUR 200 mg TABLET q12h.

Titration and Adjustment and Chronic Maintenance:

If the desired response is not achieved with the above AVERAGE INITIAL DOSE recommendations, there are no adverse reactions and the serum theophylline level cannot be measured, dosage adjustment should proceed by increasing the dose in approximately 25% increments at three day intervals. Following each adjustment, the clinical response should be assessed. If the clinical response is satisfactory, then that dosage level should be maintained. Dosage increases may be made in this manner up to the following: [See table top right.]

It is important that no patient be maintained on any dosage that is not tolerated. In instructing patients to increase dosage according to the schedule above, they should be instructed not to take a subsequent dose if apparent side effects occur and to resume therapy at a lower dose once adverse effects have disappeared.

MAXIMUM DOSE WITHOUT MEASUREMENT OF SERUM CONCENTRATION

	Dose Per Interval
Children (25–35 kg)	250 mg q12h
Adults and Children (35–70 kg)	300 mg q12h
Adults (over 70 kg)	450 mg q12h

If an increased dose is not tolerated because of headaches or stomach upset (nausea, vomiting, diarrhea, etc.), decrease dose to previous tolerated level. Do not exceed the above recommended doses unless serum theophylline levels can be measured.

If serum theophylline levels can be measured and the concentration is between 10 and 20 mcg/ml, maintain dose if tolerated. CHECK SERUM CONCENTRATION AT APPROXIMATELY 8 HOURS AFTER A DOSE WHEN NONE HAVE BEEN MISSED OR ADDED FOR AT LEAST 3 DAYS. RECHECK SERUM THEOPHYLLINE CONCENTRATION AT 6 TO 12 MONTH INTERVALS. This interval may need to be more frequent in some individuals. Take the following action if the measured serum theophylline concentration is too high.

20 to 25 mcg/mL—Decrease dose by about 10% and serum theophylline levels should be rechecked after 3 days*.

25 to 30 mcg/mL—Skip next dose and decrease subsequent doses by 25% and serum theophylline levels should be rechecked after 3 days.

Over 30 mcg/mL—Skip next 2 doses and decrease subsequent doses by 50% and serum theophylline levels should be rechecked after 3 days.

Take the following action if the measured serum theophylline concentration is too low.

7.5 to 10 mcg/mL—Increase dose by 25%**.

5 to 7.5 mcg/mL—Increase dose by 25%.

RECHECK SERUM THEOPHYLLINE FOR GUIDANCE IN FURTHER DOSAGE ADJUSTMENT.

DOSAGE ADJUSTMENT BASED ON SERUM THEOPHYLLINE CONCENTRATION MEASUREMENTS WHEN THESE INSTRUCTIONS HAVE NOT BEEN FOLLOWED MAY RESULT IN RECOMMENDATIONS THAT PRESENT RISK OF TOXICITY TO THE PATIENT.

Once-Daily Dosing:

The slow absorption rate of this preparation may allow once-daily administration in adult non-smokers with appropriate total body clearance and other patients with low dosage requirements. Once-daily dosing should be considered only after the patient has been gradually and satisfactorily titrated to therapeutic levels with q12h dosing. Once-daily dosing should be based on twice the q12h dose and should be initiated at the end of the last q12h dosing interval. The trough concentration (Cmin) obtained following conversion to once-daily dosing may be lower (especially in high clearance patients) and the peak concentration (Cmax) may be higher (especially in low clearance patients) than that obtained with q12h dosing. If symptoms recur, or signs of toxicity appear during the once-daily dosing interval, dosing on the q12h basis should be reinstituted.

It is essential that serum theophylline concentrations be monitored before and after transfer to once-daily dosing.

Food and posture, along with changes associated with circadian rhythm, may influence the rate of absorption and/or clearance rates of theophylline from controlled-release dosage forms administered at night. The exact relationship of these and other factors to nighttime serum concentrations and the clinical significance of such findings require additional study. Therefore, it is not recommended that THEO-DUR, when used as a once-a-day product, be administered at night. THEO-DUR, when used as a once-a-day product, must be taken whole and not broken.

HOW SUPPLIED

THEO-DUR 100 mg, 200 mg, and 300 mg Extended-Release Tablets are available in bottles of 100, 500, 1000 and 5000, and in unit dose packages of 100. THEO-DUR 450 mg Extended-Release Tablets are available in bottles of 100, and unit dose packages of 100.

100 mg tablet: NDC 0085-0487: round, white to off-white, debossed THEO-DUR 100 on one side and scored on the other side.

200 mg tablet: NDC 0085-0933: oval, white to off-white, debossed THEO-DUR 200 on one side and scored on the other side.

*Finer adjustments in dosage may be needed for some patients.

**Dividing the daily dosage into 3 doses administered at 8 hour intervals may be indicated if symptoms occur repeatedly at the end of a dosing interval.

300 mg tablet: NDC 0085-0584: capsule shaped, white to off-white, debossed THEO-DUR 300 on one side and scored on the other side.
450 mg tablet: NDC 0085-0806: capsule shaped, white to off-white, scored, debossed THEO-DUR 450 on one side.

STORAGE CONDITIONS

Keep tightly closed. Store at controlled room temperature 15-30°C (59-86°F).

CAUTION

Federal law prohibits dispensing without prescription.

Key Pharmaceuticals, Inc.
Kenilworth, NJ 07033 USA

Revised 10/89 B-16087416
1080319

Shown in Product Identification Section, page 413

THEO-DUR® SPRINKLE ℞

[*thē-a-dur*]
Theophylline (anhydrous)
Sustained Action Capsules

DESCRIPTION

THEO-DUR® SPRINKLE Sustained Action Capsules contain 50 mg, 75 mg, 125 mg or 200 mg theophylline anhydrous in the form of long acting, microencapsulated beads within a hard gelatin capsule and are intended for oral administration.
The theophylline has been microencapsulated in a proprietary coating of polymers to mask the bitter taste associated with the drug, while providing a prolonged effect. The entire contents of a THEO-DUR SPRINKLE capsule is intended to be sprinkled on a small amount of soft food immediately prior to ingestion, or may be swallowed whole. SUBDIVIDING THE CONTENTS OF A CAPSULE IS NOT RECOMMENDED. Each capsule is oversized to allow ease of opening.
Theophylline is a bronchodilator and is a member of the xanthine class of chemical compounds related to both theobromine and caffeine. Theophylline is a white, odorless, crystalline powder having a bitter taste. Theophylline is 3,7-dihydro-1,3-dimethyl-1*H*-purine-2,6-dione represented by the following structural formula:

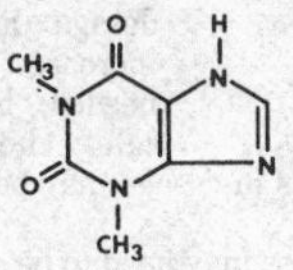

CLINICAL PHARMACOLOGY

Theophylline directly relaxes the smooth muscle of the bronchial airways and pulmonary blood vessels, thus acting mainly as a bronchodilator and smooth muscle relaxant. The drug also produces other actions typical of the xanthine derivatives: cardiac stimulation, coronary vasodilation, stimulation of skeletal muscles, cerebral stimulation, and diuresis. The actions of theophylline may be mediated through inhibition of phosphodiesterase and a resultant increase in intracellular cyclic AMP.
In vitro theophylline has been shown to act synergistically with beta agonists that increase intracellular cyclic AMP through the stimulation of adenyl cyclase, but synergism has not been demonstrated in patient studies. More data are needed to determine if theophylline and beta agonists have a clinically important additive effect *in vivo*. Apparently, no development of tolerance occurs with chronic use of theophylline.
Pharmacokinetics: The half-life of theophylline is influenced by a number of known variables. It is prolonged in patients suffering from chronic alcoholism, impaired hepatic or renal function, congestive heart failure, and in patients receiving macrolide antibiotics and cimetidine. Older adults (over age 55) and patients with chronic obstructive pulmonary disease, with or without cor pulmonale, may also have much slower clearance rates. For such patients, the theophylline half-life may exceed 24 hours.
Newborns and neonates have extremely slow clearance rates compared to older infants (over 6 months) and children, and may also have a theophylline half-life of over 24 hours. High fever for prolonged periods may also reduce the rate of theophylline elimination.

THEOPHYLLINE ELIMINATION CHARACTERISTICS

Theophylline Clearance Rates (mean±S.D.)	Half-Life Average (mean±S.D.)
Children (over 6 months of age)	
1.45±0.58 ml/kg/min	3.7±1.1 hrs
Adult non-smokers uncomplicated asthma	
0.65±0.19 ml/kg/min	8.7±2.2 hrs

The half-life of theophylline in smokers (1 to 2 packs/day) averages 4–5 hours, much shorter than the half-life in non-smokers which averages 7–9 hours. The increase in theophylline clearance caused by smoking is probably the result of induction of drug-metabolizing enzymes that do not readily normalize after cessation of smoking. It appears that between 3 months and 2 years may be necessary for normalization of the effect of smoking on theophylline pharmacokinetics.
In two separate single dose studies utilizing different subjects, the following bioavailability parameters were observed. THEO-DUR SPRINKLE administered in a 500 mg dose as pellets on applesauce to 6 healthy adults produced mean peak theophylline serum levels of 9.03 ±2.59 mcg/ml at 8.67 ±1.03 hours following administration. Administration of two lots of THEO-DUR SPRINKLE as intact capsules in a 600 mg dose to 6 healthy adults produced mean peak theophylline serum levels of 9.08 ±1.30 mcg/ml and 7.60 ±0.95 mcg/ml at 8.33 ±1.50 and 8.67 ±3.01 hours after administration respectively. In these studies THEO-DUR SPRINKLE exhibited complete bioavailability when compared to an immediate release product. In both of these studies, the subjects fasted for 10 hours prior to dosing and for 4 hours after dosing.
In a multiple dose, two-way, crossover study with 18 healthy, normal adults, the bioavailability from THEO-DUR SPRINKLE administered as intact capsules was evaluated using THEO-DUR Sustained Action Tablets as the reference product. Fifteen subjects received 400 mg at 7:00 AM and 7:00 PM while three subjects received 200 mg because of low theophylline clearance. All meals and snacks were provided to the subjects during the course of this study, with breakfast at 9:00 AM, lunch at 12:30 PM a snack at 3:00 PM, and dinner at 9:00 PM. THEO-DUR SPRINKLE produced mean Cmax and Cmin levels of 10.4 ±2.6 and 6.9 ±1.8 mcg/ml as compared to a Cmax and Cmin of 10.5 ±2.8 and 7.5 ±2.7 mcg/ml for THEO-DUR tablets. The mean percent fluctuation normalized to Css was 38.8±8.5% for THEO-DUR SPRINKLE and 33.4±9.7% for THEO-DUR tablets [100(Cmax-Cmin)/Css where Css = AUC_{0-12}/dosing interval]. The mean percent fluctuation when normalized to Cmin was 51.9±15.4% for THEO-DUR SPRINKLE and 43.9±17.4% for THEO-DUR tablets [% fluctuation = 100 (Cmax-Cmin)/Cmin]. The average peak-trough differences over 12 hours for THEO-DUR SPRINKLE and THEO-DUR tablets were 3.5±1.2 and 3.0 ±0.7 mcg/ml respectively. The AUC for THEO-DUR SPRINKLE was 108.4±26.0 while that for THEO-DUR tablets was 112.1±32.5 mcg-hr/ml. In a separate study, THEO-DUR exhibited complete bioavailability when compared to an immediate release product. This would suggest that bioavailability from THEO-DUR SPRINKLE was complete and not statistically different from that of the THEO-DUR tablets.

INDICATIONS AND USE

For relief and/or prevention of symptoms of asthma and for reversible bronchospasm associated with chronic bronchitis and emphysema.

CONTRAINDICATIONS

THEO-DUR SPRINKLE is contraindicated in individuals who have shown hypersensitivity to theophylline or any of the capsule components.

WARNINGS

Status asthmaticus should be considered a medical emergency and is defined as that degree of bronchospasm which is not rapidly responsive to usual doses of conventional bronchodilators. Optimal therapy for such patients frequently requires both *additional medication*, parenterally administered, and *close monitoring*, preferably in an intensive care setting. Although increasing the dose of theophylline may bring about relief, such treatment may be associated with toxicity. The likelihood of such toxicity developing increases significantly when the serum theophylline concentration exceeds 20 mcg/ml. Therefore, determination of serum theophylline levels is recommended to assure maximal benefit without excessive risk.
Serum levels above 20 mcg/ml are rarely found after appropriate administration of the recommended doses. However, in individuals in whom theophylline plasma clearance is reduced for any reason, even conventional doses may result in increased serum levels and potential toxicity. Reduced theophylline clearance has been documented in the following readily identifiable groups: 1) patients with impaired renal or liver function; 2) patients over 55 years of age, particularly males and those with chronic lung disease; 3) those with cardiac failure from any cause; 4) neonates; and 5) those patients taking certain drugs (macrolide antibiotics and cimetidine). Decreased clearance of theophylline may be associated with either influenza immunization or active infection with influenza.
Reduction of dosage and laboratory monitoring is especially appropriate in the above individuals.
Less serious signs of theophylline toxicity (i.e., nausea and restlessness) may occur frequently when initiating therapy, but are usually transient; when such signs are persistent during maintenance therapy, they are often associated with serum concentrations above 20 mcg/ml.
Unfortunately, however, serious side effects such as ventricular arrhythmias, convulsions or even death may appear as the first sign of toxicity without any previous warning. *Stated differently; serious toxicity is not reliably preceded by less severe side effects.*
Many patients who require theophylline may exhibit tachycardia due to their underlying disease process so that the cause/effect relationship to elevated serum theophylline concentrations may not be appreciated.
Theophylline products may cause dysrhythmia and/or worsen pre-existing arrhythmias and any significant change in rate and/or rhythm warrants monitoring and futher investigation.
The occurrence of arrhythmias and sudden death (with histological evidence of necrosis of the myocardium) has been recorded in laboratory animals (minipigs, rodents and dogs) when theophylline and beta agonists were administered concomitantly, although not when either was administered alone. The significance of these findings when applied to human usage is currently unknown.

PRECAUTIONS

THE CONTENTS OF THE THEO-DUR SPRINKLE CAPSULE SHOULD NOT BE CHEWED OR CRUSHED.
General: Mean half-life in smokers is shorter than non-smokers. Therefore, smokers may require larger or more frequent doses of theophylline. Morphine and curare should be used with caution in patients with airway obstruction as they may suppress respiration and stimulate histamine release. Alternative drugs should be used when possible.
Theophylline should not be administered concurrently with other xanthine preparations. Use with caution in patients with severe cardiac disease, severe hypoxemia, hypertension, hyperthyroidism, acute myocardial injury, cor pulmonale, congestive heart failure, alcoholism, liver disease and in the elderly, especially males, and in neonates. Great caution should be used in giving theophylline to patients with congestive heart failure. Frequently, such patients have shown markedly prolonged theophylline blood levels with theophylline persisting in serum for long periods following discontinuation of the drug. Use theophylline cautiously in patients with a history of peptic ulcer. Theophylline may occasionally act as a local gastrointestinal irritant although G.I. symptoms are more commonly centrally mediated and associated with serum drug concentrations over 20 mcg/ml.
Information for Patients: The physician should reinforce the importance of taking only the prescribed dose at the prescribed time intervals. The patient should alert the physician if symptoms occur repeatedly, especially near the end of a dosing interval.
When prescribing administration by the sprinkle method, details of the proper technique should be explained to the patient (see DOSAGE AND ADMINISTRATION Sprinkling Contents on Food).
Patients should be informed of the need to take this drug in the fasting state, and that drug administration should be one hour before, or two hours after meals (see PRECAUTIONS, Drug-Food Interactions and DOSAGE AND ADMINISTRATION).
Drug Interactions:
Drug-Drug: Toxic synergism with ephedrine has been documented and may occur with some other sympathomimetic bronchodilators. In addition, the following drug interactions have been demonstrated.

Drug	Effect
Theophylline with lithium carbonate	Increased excretion of lithium carbonate
Theophylline with propranolol	Increased theophylline serum concentrations
	Antagonism of propranolol effect
Theophylline with troleandomycin or erythromycin	Increased theophylline serum concentrations
Theophylline with Cimetidine	Increased theophylline serum concentrations

Drug-Food: THEO-DUR SPRINKLE has not been adequately studied to determine the extent of alteration of bioavailability when it is given with food as compared to the fasting state.

Continued on next page

Key—Cont.

However, there is data to indicate that drug administration at the time of food ingestion will result in significantly lower peak serum concentrations and reduced extent of absorption (bioavailability).
The influence of the type and amount of food as well as the time interval between drug and food, on performance of THEO-DUR SPRINKLE is under study.

Drug/Laboratory Test Interactions: When plasma levels of theophylline are measured by spectrophotometric methods, coffee, tea, cola beverages, chocolate, and acetaminophen contribute falsely high values.

Carcinogenesis, Mutagenesis, and Impairment of Fertility: Long-term animal studies have not been performed to evaluate the carcinogenic potential, mutagenic potential, or the effect on fertility of xanthine compounds.

Pregnancy: Pregnancy Category C: Animal reproduction studies have not been conducted with theophylline. It is not known whether theophylline can cause fetal harm when administered to a pregnant woman or can affect reproduction capacity. Theophylline should be give to a pregnant woman only if clearly needed.

Nursing Mothers: It has been reported that theophylline distributes readily into breast milk and may cause adverse effects in the infant. Caution must be used if prescribing xanthines to a mother who is nursing, taking into account the risk-benefit of this therapy.

Pediatric Use: Safety and effectiveness in children under 6 years of age have not been established with this product.

ADVERSE REACTIONS

The most consistent adverse reactions are usually due to overdose and are:

Gastrointestinal: Nausea, vomiting, epigastric pain, hematemesis, diarrhea.

Central nervous system: headaches, irritability, restlessness, insomnia, reflex hyperexcitability, muscle twitching, clonic and tonic generalized convulsions.

Cardiovascular: palpitation, tachycardia, extrasystoles, flushing, hypotension, circulatory failure, ventricular arrhythmias.

Respiratory: tachypnea.

Renal: albuminuria, increased excretion of renal tubular cells and red blood cells, potentiation of diuresis.

Other: hyperglycemia and inappropriate ADH syndrome and rash.

OVERDOSAGE

Management:

A. If potential oral overdose is established and seizure has not occurred:
1. Induce vomiting.
2. Administer a cathartic (this is particulary important if sustained-released preparations have been taken).
3. Administer activated charcoal.
4. Monitor vital signs, maintain blood pressure and provide adequate hydration.

B. If patient is having a seizure:
1. Establish an airway.
2. Administer oxygen.
3. Treat the seiure with intravenous diazepam, 0.1 to 0.3 mg/kg up to a total dose of 10 mg.
4. Monitor vital signs, maintain blood pressure and provide adequate hydration.

C. Post Seizure Coma:
1. Maintain airway and oxygenation.
2. If a result of oral medication, follow above recommendations to prevent absorption of the drug, but intubation and lavage will have to be performed instead of inducing emesis, and the cathartic and charcoal will need to be introduced via a large bore gastric lavage tube.
3. Continue to provide full supportive care and adequate hydration while waiting for drug to be metabolized. In general, the drug is metabolized sufficiently rapidly so as to not warrant consideration of dialysis. However, if serum levels exceed 50 mcg/ml, charcoal hemoperfusion may be indicated.

DOSAGE AND ADMINISTRATION

There is data to indicate that administration of THEO-DUR SPRINKLE at the time of food ingestion will result in significantly lower peak serum concentrations and reduced extent of absorption (bioavailability).
Therefore, the patient should be instructed to take this medication at least one hour before or two hours after a meal (see PRECAUTIONS, Drug-Food Interactions).
For most patients, effective use of theophylline, i.e. associated with optimal likelihood of benefit combined with minimal risk of toxicity, is considered to occur when serum levels are maintained between 10 and 20 mcg/ml. Levels above 20 mcg/ml may produce toxicity and in a small number of patients, toxicity may even be seen with serum levels between 15–20 mcg/ml, particularly during initation of therapy.
There is considerable variation from patient to patient in the dosage required to achieve and maintain therapeutic and safe levels, primarily due to variable rates of elimination. Therefore, it is essential that not only must dosage be individualized but titration and monitoring of serum levels be utilized where available. When serum concentrations cannot be obtained, restriction of dosage to the amounts and intervals recommended in the guidelines listed below becomes essential. Dosage should be calculated on the basis of lean (ideal) body weight where mg/kg doses are presented. Theophylline does not distribute into fatty tissue.
As a practical consideration, it is not always possible to obtain serum level determinations. Under such conditions, restriction of the daily dose (in otherwise healthy adults) to not greater than 13 mg/kg/day of anhydrous theophylline in divided doses will result in relatively few patients exceeding serum levels of 20 mcg/ml and the resultant risk of toxicity.

Sprinkling Contents on Food: *THEO-DUR SPRINKLE may be administered by carefully opening the capsule and sprinkling the beaded contents on a spoonful of soft food such as applesauce or pudding. The soft food should be swallowed immediately without chewing and followed with a glass of cool water or juice to ensure complete swallowing of the beads. It is recommended that the food used should not be hot and should be soft enough to be swallowed without chewing. Any bead/food mixture should be used immediately and not stored for future use. The small amount of food (one spoonful) used to administer the dose will not alter the bioavailablity of THEO-DUR SPRINKLE, however, the dosing should be at least one hour before or two hours after a meal. SUBDIVIDING THE CONTENTS OF A CAPSULE IS NOT RECOMMENDED.*

Dosage Guidelines: Because administration of Theo-Dur Sprinkle at the time of food ingestion has been shown to result in significantly lower peak serum concentrations and reduced extent of absorption (bioavailability), patients should be instructed to take this medication at least one hour before or two hours after a meal (see PRECAUTIONS, Drug-Food Interactions).
Taking THEO-DUR SPRINKLE at 12 hour intervals under the above restrictive recommendations in regard to food ingestion may be difficult for the patient to follow. Under such circumstances, consideration should be given to prescribing this drug every 8 hours (giving one third of the 24 hour dosage requirement with each dose), if this regimen would more easily permit dosing under fasting conditions.

I. Acute Symptoms: THEO-DUR SPRINKLE is not intended for patients experiencing an acute episode of bronchospasm (associated with asthma, chronic bronchitis, or emphysema). Such patients require rapid relief of symptoms and should be treated with an immediate-release or intravenous theophylline preparation (or other bronchodilators) and not with controlled release products.

II. Chronic Therapy:

A. Initating Therapy with an Immediate-Release Product: It is recommended that the appropriate dosage be established using an immediate-release preparation. Children weighing less than 25 kg should have their daily dosage requirements established with a liquid preparation to permit small dosage increments. Slow clinical titration is generally preferred to help assure acceptance and safety of the medication, and to allow the patient to develop tolerance to transient caffeine-like side effects. Then, if the total 24 hour dose can be given by use of the sustained release product, the patient can usually be switched to THEO-DUR SPRINKLE giving one-half of the daily dose at 12 hour intervals. Patients who metabolize theophylline rapidly such as the young, smokers, and some non-smoking adults are the most likely candidates for dosing at 8-hour intervals. Such patients can generally be identified as having trough serum concentrations lower than desired or repeatedly exhibiting symptoms near the end of a dosing interval.

B. Initating Therapy with THEO-DUR SPRINKLE: Alternatively, therapy can be initiated with THEO-DUR SPRINKLE since it is available in dosage strengths which permit titration and adjustments of dosage in adults and older children:

Initial Dose	16 mg/kg/24 hours or 400 mg/24 hours (whichever is less) of anhydrous theophylline in 2 divided doses 12-hour intervals.
Increasing Dose	The above dosage may be increased in approximately 25 percent increments at 3-day intervals so long as the drug is tolerated; until clinical reponse is satisfactory or the maximum dose as indicated in section III (below) is reached. The serum concentration may be checked at these intervals, but at a minimum, should be determined at the end of this adjustment period.

III. Maintenance Dose of Theophylline where the Serum Concentration is not Measured:
WARNING: DO NOT ATTEMPT TO MAINTAIN ANY DOSE THAT IS NOT TOLERATED.

Not to exceed the following:

			Dose per 12 hours
Age	6–9 years	24 mg/kg/day	12.0 mg/kg
Age	9–12 years	20 mg/kg/day	10.0 mg/kg
Age	12–16 years	18 mg/kg/day	9.0 mg/kg
Age	Over 16 years	13 mg/kg/day or 900 mg	6.5 mg/kg

(WHICHEVER IS LESS)

IV. Measurement of Serum Theophylline Concentrations During Chronic Therapy: If the above maximum doses are to be maintained or exceeded, serum theophylline measurement is recommended. The serum sample should be obtained at the time of peak absorption: 1 to 2 hours after administration for immediate-release products and 5 to 10 hours after dosing for THEO-DUR SPRINKLE. It is important that the patient will have missed no doses during the previous 48 hours and that the dosing intervals will have been reasonably typical with no added doses during that period of time. DOSAGE ADJUSTMENT BASED ON SERUM THEOPHYLLINE CONCENTRATION MEASUREMENTS WHEN THESE INSTRUCTIONS HAVE NOT BEEN FOLLOWED MAY RESULT IN RECOMMENDATIONS THAT PRESENT RISK OF TOXICITY TO THE PATIENT.

V. Final Adjustment of Dosage (see Table 1)

Table 1—Dosage adjustment after serum theophylline measurement

If serum theophylline is:		Directions:
Within normal Limits	10 to 20 mcg/ml	Maintain dosage if tolerated. Recheck serum theophylline concentration at 6- to 12-month intervals*
Too high	20 to 25 mcg/ml	Decrease doses by about 10%. Recheck serum theophylline concentration at 6- to 12-month intervals*
	25 to 30 mcg/ml	Skip next dose and decrease subsequent doses by about 25%.
	over 30 mcg/ml	Skip next 2 doses and decrease subsequent doses by 50%. Recheck serum theophylline.
Too low	7.5 to 10 mcg/ml	Increase dose by about 25%.** Recheck serum theophylline concentration at 6- to 12-month intervals.*
	5 to 7.5 mcg/ml	Increase dose by about 25% to the nearest dose increment and recheck serum theophylline for guidance in further dosage adjustment (another increase will probably be needed, but this provides a safety check).

*Finer adjustments in dosage may be needed for some patients.
**The total daily dose may need to be administered at more frequent intervals if symptoms occur repeatedly at the end of a dosing interval.

From the Journal of Respiratory Diseases 2(7):16,1981.
Caution should be exercised for younger children who cannot complain of minor side effects. Those with cor pulmonale, congestive heart failure, and/or liver disease may have unusually low dosage requirements and thus may experience toxicity at the maximal dosage recommended above. It is important that no patient be maintained on any dosage that is not tolerated. In instructing patients to increase dosage according to the schedule above, they should be instructed not to take a subsequent dose if apparent side effects occur and to resume therapy at a lower dose once adverse effects have disappeared.

HOW SUPPLIED

THEO-DUR SPRINKLE 50, 75, 125 and 200 mg Sustained Action Capsules are available in bottles of 100.
50 mg capsule: NDC 0085-0928: white opaque capsule body with clear cap embossed in black. THIS END UP THEO-DUR® SPRINKLE 50 mg
75 mg capsule: NDC 0085-0875: white opaque capsule body with clear cap embossed in green. THIS END UP THEO-DUR® SPRINKLE 75 mg
125 mg capsule: NDC 0085-0381: white opaque capsule body with clear cap embossed in red. THIS END UP THEO-DUR® SPRINKLE 125 mg
200 mg capsule: NDC 0085-0620: white opaque capsule body with clear cap embossed in blue. THIS END UP THEO-DUR® SPRINKLE 200 mg

STORAGE CONDITIONS

Keep tightly closed. Store at controlled room temperature 15–30°C (59–86°F).

CAUTION

Federal law prohibits dispensing without prescription.
Keep this and all medications out of the reach of children.
Rev. 3/87

KEY PHARMACEUTICALS, INC.

Shown in Product Identification Section, page 413

TRINALIN® ℞

[trin 'a-lin]
brand of azatadine maleate, USP and pseudoephedrine sulfate, USP
Long-Acting Antihistamine/Decongestant REPETABS® Tablets

DESCRIPTION

TRINALIN Long-Acting Antihistamine/Decongestant REPETABS (brand of repeat-action tablets) Tablets contain 1 mg azatadine maleate, USP in the tablet coating and 120 mg pseudoephedrine sulfate, USP, equally distributed between the tablet coating and the barrier-coated core. Following ingestion, the two active components in the coating are quickly liberated; release of the decongestant in the core is delayed for several hours.

Azatadine maleate is an antihistamine having the empirical formula, $C_{20}H_{22}N_2 \cdot 2C_4H_4O_4$, the chemical name, 6,11-Dihydro-11-(1-methyl-4-piperidylidene)-5*H*-benzo [5,6] cyclohepta [1,2-*b*] pyridine maleate (1:2).

The molecular weight of azatadine maleate is 522.54. Azatadine maleate is a white to off-white powder and is very soluble in water and soluble in alcohol.

Pseudoephedrine sulfate, a sympathomimetic amine, is a salt of pseudoephedrine, one of the naturally occurring alkaloids obtained from various species of the plant *Ephedra.* The empirical formula for pseudoephedrine sulfate is $(C_{10}H_{15}NO)_2 \cdot H_2SO_4$; the chemical name is Benzenemethanol, α-[1-(methylamino)ethyl]-, [*S*-(*R**, *R**)]-, sulfate (2:1) (salt).

The molecular weight of pseudoephedrine sulfate is 428.56. It is a white to off-white crystal or powder, very soluble in water, freely soluble in alcohol, and sparingly soluble in chloroform.

The inactive ingredients for TRINALIN REPETABS Tablets are: Acacia, Butylparaben, Calcium Sulfate, Carnauba Wax, Corn Starch, D&C Red No. 30 Al Lake, FD&C Yellow No. 6 Al Lake, Gelatin, Lactose, Magnesium Stearate, Neutral Soap, Oleic Acid, Povidone, Rosin, Sugar, Talc, White Wax, and Zein.

CLINICAL PHARMACOLOGY

Azatadine maleate is an antihistamine, related to cyproheptadine, with antiserotonin, anticholinergic (drying), and sedative effects. Antihistamines appear to compete with histamine for histamine H_1-receptor sites on effector cells. The antihistamines antagonize those pharmacological effects of histamine which are mediated through activation of H_1-receptor sites and thereby reduce the intensity of allergic reactions and tissue injury response involving histamine release. Antihistamines antagonize the vasodilator effect of endogenously released histamine, especially in small vessels, and mitigate the effect of histamine which results in increased capillary permeability and edema formation. As consequences of these actions, antihistamines antagonize the physiological manifestations of histamine release in the nose following antigen-antibody interaction, such as congestion related to vascular engorgement, mucosal edema, and profuse, watery secretion, and irritation and sneezing resulting from histamine action on afferent nerve terminals.

Pseudoephedrine sulfate (d-isoephedrine sulfate) is an orally effective nasal decongestant which appears to exert its sympathomimetic effect indirectly, predominantly through release of adrenergic mediators from post-ganglionic nerve terminals. In effective recommended oral dosage, pseudoephedrine sulfate produces minimal other sympathomimetic effects, such as pressor activity and CNS stimulation. Use of an orally administered vasoconstrictor for shrinkage of congested nasal mucosa has several advantages: a) it produces a gradual but sustained decongestant effect, causing little, if any "rebound" congestion; b) it facilitates shrinkage of swollen mucosa in upper respiratory areas that are relatively inaccessible to topically applied sprays or drops; c) it relieves nasal obstruction without the additional irritation that may result from local medication.

Pseudoephedrine passes through the blood-brain and placental barriers. While the antihistamines have not been studied systematically for passage through these barriers, the occurrence of pharmacologic effects in the central nervous system and in newborns indicate presence of the drug.

Following administration of the two drugs to normal volunteers in either a single TRINALIN REPETABS Tablet or similar doses in two conventional pseudoephedrine sulfate tablets and a conventional tablet of azatadine maleate, the blood levels of pseudoephedrine and the urinary excretion of azatadine showed that the TRINALIN REPETABS Tablets are bioequivalent to the conventional dosage forms. The apparent elimination half-life of pseudoephedrine in TRINALIN REPETABS Tablets was approximately 6½ hours. The apparent elimination of half-life of azatadine maleate (available from the outer layer of the TRINALIN REPETABS Tablets or from the conventional azatadine maleate tablet) was approximately 12 hours.

INDICATIONS AND USAGE

TRINALIN Long-Acting Antihistamine/Decongestant REPETABS Tablets are indicated for the relief of the symptoms of upper respiratory mucosal congestion in perennial and allergic rhinitis, and for the relief of nasal congestion and eustachian tube congestion. Analgesics, antibiotics, or both may be administered concurrently, when indicated.

CONTRAINDICATIONS

Antihistamines should not be used to treat lower respiratory tract symptoms, including asthma.

This product is contraindicated in patients with narrow-angle glaucoma or urinary retention, and in patients receiving monoamine oxidase (MAO) inhibitor therapy or within ten days of stopping such treatment. (See Drug Interactions section.) It is also contraindicated in patients with severe hypertension, severe coronary artery disease, hyperthyroidism, and in those who have shown hypersensitivity or idiosyncrasy to its components, to adrenergic agents, or to other drugs of similar chemical structures. Manifestations of patient idiosyncrasy to adrenergic agents include: insomnia, dizziness, weakness, tremor, or arrhythmias.

WARNINGS

TRINALIN REPETABS Tablets should be used with considerable caution in patients with: stenosing peptic ulcer, pyloroduodenal obstruction, urinary bladder obstruction due to symptomatic prostatic hypertrophy, or narrowing of the bladder neck. It should also be administered with caution to patients with cardiovascular disease, including hypertension or ischemic heart disease; increased intraocular pressure (See CONTRAINDICATIONS); diabetes mellitus, or in patients receiving digitalis or oral anticoagulants.

Central nervous system stimulation and convulsions or cardiovascular collapse with accompanying hypotension may be produced by sympathomimetics.

Do not exceed recommended dosage.

Use in Activities Requiring Mental Alertness: Patients should be warned about engaging in activities requiring mental alertness, such as driving a car or operating appliances, machinery, etc.

Use in Patients Approximately 60 Years and Older: Antihistamines are more likely to cause dizziness, sedation, and hypotension in patients over 60 years of age. In these patients, sympathomimetics are also more likely to cause adverse reactions, such as confusion, hallucinations, convulsions, CNS depression, and death. For this reason, before considering the use of a repeat-action formulation, the safe use of a short-acting sympathomimetic in that particular patient should be demonstrated.

PRECAUTIONS

General: Because of the atropine-like action of antihistamines, this product should be used with caution in patients with a history of bronchial asthma.

Information for Patients:

1. Products containing antihistamines may cause drowsiness.
2. Patients should not engage in activities requiring mental alertness, such as driving or operating machinery or appliances.
3. Alcohol or other sedative drugs may enhance the drowsiness caused by antihistamines.
4. Patients should not take TRINALIN REPETABS Tablets if they are receiving a monoamine oxidase inhibitor or within 10 days of stopping such treatment, or if they are receiving oral anticoagulants.
5. This medication should not be given to children less than 12 years of age.

Drug Interactions: MAO inhibitors prolong and intensify the effects of antihistamines. Concomitant use of antihistamines with alcohol, tricyclic antidepressants, barbiturates, or other central nervous system depressants may have an additive effect.

When sympathomimetic drugs are given to patients receiving monoamine oxidase inhibitors, hypertensive reactions, including hypertensive crises, may occur. The antihypertensive effects of methyldopa, mecamylamine, reserpine, and veratrum alkaloids may be reduced by sympathomimetics. Beta-adrenergic blocking agents may also interact with sympathomimetics. Increased ectopic pacemaker activity can occur when pseudoephedrine is used concomitantly with digitalis. Antacids increase the rate of absorption of pseudoephedrine, while kaolin decreases it.

Drug/Laboratory Test Interactions: The *in vitro* addition of pseudoephedrine to sera containing the cardiac isoenzyme MB of serum creatine phosphokinase progressively inhibits the activity of the enzyme. The inhibition becomes complete over six hours.

Carcinogenesis, Mutagenesis, and Impairment of Fertility: There is no animal or laboratory study of the mixture of azatadine maleate and pseudoephedrine sulfate to evaluate carcinogenesis or mutagenesis. Reproduction studies of this mixture in rats showed no evidence of impaired fertility.

Pregnancy Category C: Retarded fetal development and the presence of angulated hyoid wings were seen in the offspring of pregnant rabbits administered TRINALIN at about 12.5 times and 5 times the recommended human dosage, respectively; increased resorption was noted at about 25 times the human dosage. A decreased survival rate at day 21 was seen in rat pups born of mothers given TRINALIN during pregnancy at a dose about 12.5 times the human dosage. There are no adequate and well-controlled studies in pregnant women. TRINALIN REPETABS Tablets should be used during pregnancy only if the potential benefits to the mother justify the potential risks to the infant. (See Nonteratogenic Effects.)

Nonteratogenic Effects: Antihistamines should not be used in the third trimester of pregnancy, because newborns and premature infants may have severe reactions to them such as convulsions.

Nursing Mothers: It is not known whether these drugs are excreted in human milk. However, certain antihistamines and sympathomimetics are known to be excreted in human milk. Because of the higher risks of antihistamines for infants generally and for newborns and prematures in particular, a decision should be made whether to discontinue nursing or to discontinue the drug, taking into account the importance of the drug to the mother.

There is a report of irritability, excessive crying and disturbed sleeping patterns in a nursing infant whose mother had taken a product containing an antihistamine and pseudoephedrine.

Pediatric use: Safety and effectiveness in children below the age of 12 years have not been established.

ADVERSE REACTIONS

The following adverse reactions are associated with antihistamine and sympathomimetic drugs. (Those adverse reactions which occur most frequently with the antihistamines are underlined.)

General: Urticaria, drug rash, anaphylactic shock, photosensitivity, excessive perspiration, chills, dryness of mouth, nose, and throat.

Cardiovascular: Hypertension (see CONTRAINDICATIONS and WARNINGS), hypotension, arrhythmias and cardiovascular collapse, headache, palpitations, extrasystoles, tachycardia, angina.

Hematologic: Hemolytic anemia, hypoplastic anemia, thrombocytopenia, agranulocytosis.

Central Nervous System: Sedation, sleepiness, dizziness, vertigo, tinnitus, acute labyrinthitis, disturbed coordination, fatigue, mydriasis, confusion, restlessness, excitation, nervousness, tension, tremor, irritability, insomnia, euphoria, paresthesias, blurred vision, hysteria, neuritis, convulsions, fear, anxiety, hallucinations, CNS depression, weakness, pallor.

Gastrointestinal: Epigastric distress, anorexia, nausea, vomiting, diarrhea, constipation, abdominal cramps.

Genitourinary: Urinary frequency, urinary retention, dysuria, early menses.

Respiratory: Thickening of bronchial secretions, tightness of chest and wheezing, nasal stuffiness, respiratory difficulty.

DRUG ABUSE AND DEPENDENCE

There is no information to indicate that abuse or dependency occurs with azatadine maleate.

Pseudoephedrine, like other central nervous system stimulants, has been abused. At high doses, subjects commonly experience an elevation of mood, a sense of increased energy and alertness, and decreased appetite. Some individuals become anxious, irritable, and loquacious. In addition to the marked euphoria, the user experiences a sense of markedly enhanced physical strength and mental capacity. With continued use, tolerance develops, the user increases the dose, and toxic signs and symptoms appear. Depression may follow rapid withdrawal.

OVERDOSAGE

In the event of overdosage, emergency treatment should be started immediately.

Manifestations of overdosage may vary from central nervous system depression (sedation, apnea, diminished mental alertness, cyanosis, coma, cardiovascular collapse) to stimulation (insomnia, hallucinations, tremors, or convulsions) to death. Other signs and symptoms may be euphoria, excitement, tachycardia, palpitations, thirst, perspiration, nausea, dizziness, tinnitus, ataxia, blurred vision, and hypertension or hypotension. Stimulation is particularly likely in children, as are atropine-like signs and symptoms (dry mouth; fixed, dilated pupils, flushing; hyperthermia; and gastrointestinal symptoms).

In large doses sympathomimetics may give rise to giddiness, headache, nausea, vomiting, sweating, thirst, tachycardia, precordial pain, palpitations, difficulty in micturition, muscular weakness and tenseness, anxiety, restlessness, and

Continued on next page

Key—Cont.

insomnia. Many patients can present a toxic psychosis with delusions and hallucinations. Some may develop cardiac arrhythmias, circulatory collapse, convulsions, coma, and respiratory failure.

The oral LD_{50} of the mixture of the two drugs in mature rats and mice was greater than 1700 mg/kg and 600 mg/kg, respectively.

Treatment—The patient should be induced to vomit, even if emesis has occurred spontaneously. Pharmacologically induced vomiting by the administration of ipecac syrup is a preferred method. However, vomiting should not be induced in patients with impaired consciousness. The action of ipecac is facilitated by physical activity and by the administration of eight to twelve fluid ounces of water. If emesis does not occur within fifteen minutes, the dose of ipecac should be repeated. Precautions against aspiration must be taken, especially in infants and children. Following emesis, any drug remaining in the stomach may be adsorbed by activated charcoal administered as a slurry with water. If vomiting is unsuccessful or contraindicated, gastric lavage should be performed. Isotonic and one-half isotonic saline are the lavage solutions of choice. Saline cathartics, such as milk of magnesia, draw water into the bowel by osmosis and therefore may be valuable for their action in rapid dilution of bowel content. Dialysis is of little value in antihistamine poisoning. After emergency treatment the patient should continue to be medically monitored.

Treatment of the signs and symptoms of overdosage is symptomatic and supportive. Stimulants (analeptic agents) should <u>not</u> be used. Vasopressors may be used to treat hypotension. Short-acting barbiturates, diazepam, or paraldehyde may be administered to control seizures. Hyperpyrexia, especially in children, may require treatment with tepid water sponge baths or a hypothermic blanket. Apnea is treated with ventilatory support.

DOSAGE AND ADMINISTRATION

TRINALIN REPETABS Tablets ARE NOT INTENDED FOR USE IN CHILDREN UNDER 12 YEARS OF AGE. The usual adult dosage is one tablet twice a day.

HOW SUPPLIED

TRINALIN REPETABS Tablets contain 1 mg azatadine maleate and 120 mg pseudoephedrine sulfate. TRINALIN REPETABS Tablets are coral-colored, sugar-coated tablets branded in black with the product name TRINALIN and product identification numbers, 703; bottle of 100 (NDC-0085-0703-04).

Store between 2° and 30°C (36° and 86°F).

Copyright © 1981, 1985, 1987, 1988, 1991 Key Pharmaceuticals, Inc., USA. All rights reserved.

Revised 2/91   14276424

Shown in Product Identification Section, page 413

Knoll Pharmaceuticals
A Unit of BASF K&F Corporation
WHIPPANY, NJ 07981

BASF Group

AKINETON® TABLETS AND AMPULES   ℞
[ā-kĭn'ĕ-ton]
biperiden hydrochloride and biperiden lactate

DESCRIPTION

Each AKINETON® Tablet for oral administration contains 2 mg biperiden hydrochloride. Other ingredients may include corn syrup, lactose, magnesium stearate, potato starch and talc. Each 1 mL AKINETON Ampule for intramuscular or intravenous administration contains 5 mg biperiden lactate in an aqueous 1.4 percent sodium lactate solution. No added preservative. AKINETON is an anticholinergic agent. Biperiden is α-5-Norbornen-2-yl-α-phenyl-1-piperidine-propanol. It is a white, crystalline, odorless powder, slightly soluble in water and alcohol. It is stable in air at normal temperatures. Biperiden may be represented by the following structural formula:

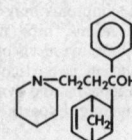

CLINICAL PHARMACOLOGY

AKINETON is a weak peripheral anticholinergic agent. It has, therefore, some antisecretory, antispasmodic and mydriatic effects. In addition, AKINETON possesses nicotino-

lytic activity. Parkinsonism is thought to result from an imbalance between the excitatory (cholinergic) and inhibitory (dopaminergic) systems in the corpus striatum. The mechanism of action of centrally active anticholinergic drugs such as AKINETON is considered to relate to competitive antagonism of acetylcholine at cholinergic receptors in the corpus striatum, which then restores the balance.

The parenteral form of AKINETON is an effective and reliable agent for the treatment of acute episodes of extrapyramidal disturbances sometimes seen during treatment with neuroleptic agents. Akathisia, akinesia, dyskinetic tremors, rigor, oculogyric crisis, spasmodic torticollis, and profuse sweating are markedly reduced or eliminated. With parenteral AKINETON, these drug-induced disturbances are rapidly brought under control. Subsequently, this can usually be maintained with oral doses which may be given with tranquilizer therapy in psychotic and other conditions requiring an uninterrupted therapeutic program.

Pharmacokinetics and Metabolism: Only limited pharmacokinetic studies of biperiden in humans are available The serum concentration at 1 to 1.5 hours following a single, 4 mg oral dose was 4–5 ng/mL. Plasma levels (0.1–0.2 ng/mL) could be determined up to 48 hours after dosing. Six hours after an oral dose of 250 mg/kg in rats, 87% of the drug had been absorbed. The metabolism of AKINETON is also incompletely understood, but does involve hydroxylation. In normal volunteers a single 10 mg intravenous dose of biperiden seemed to cause a transient rise in plasma cortisol and prolactin. No change in GH, LH, FSH, or TSH levels were seen. Biperiden lactate (10 mg/mL) was not irritating to the tissue of rabbits when injected intramuscularly (1.0 mL) into the sacrospinalis muscles and intradermally (0.25 mL) and subcutaneously (0.5 mL) into the shaved abdominal skin.

INDICATIONS AND USAGE

● As an adjunct in the therapy of all forms of parkinsonism (idiopathic, postencephalitic, arteriosclerotic)
● Control of extrapyramidal disorders secondary to neuroleptic drug therapy (e.g., phenothiazines)

CONTRAINDICATIONS

1) Hypersensitivity to biperiden 2) Narrow angle glaucoma 3) Bowel obstruction 4) Megacolon

WARNINGS

Isolated instances of mental confusion, euphoria, agitation and disturbed behavior have been reported in susceptible patients. Also, the central anticholinergic syndrome can occur as an adverse reaction to properly prescribed anticholinergic medication, although it is more frequently due to overdosage. It may also result from concomitant administration of an anticholinergic agent and a drug that has secondary anticholinergic actions (see Drug Interactions and Overdosage sections). Caution should be observed in patients with manifest glaucoma, though no prohibitive rise in intraocular pressure has been noted following either oral or parenteral administration. Patients with prostatism, epilepsy or cardiac arrhythmia should be given this drug with caution. Occasionally, drowsiness may occur, and patients who drive a car or operate any other potentially dangerous machinery should be warned of this possibility. As with other drugs acting on the central nervous system, the consumption of alcohol should be avoided during AKINETON therapy.

PRECAUTIONS

Drug Interactions: The central anticholinergic syndrome can occur when anticholinergic agents such as AKINETON are administered concomitantly with drugs that have secondary anticholinergic actions, e.g., certain narcotic analgesics such as meperidine, the phenothiazines and other antipsychotics, tricyclic antidepressants, certain antiarrhythmics such as the quinidine salts, and antihistamines. See Overdosage section for signs and symptoms of the central anticholinergic syndrome, and for treatment.

Pregnancy: Pregnancy Category C. Animal reproduction studies have not been conducted with AKINETON. It is also not known whether AKINETON can cause fetal harm when administered to a pregnant woman or can affect reproduction capacity. AKINETON should be given to a pregnant woman only if clearly needed.

Nursing Mothers: It is not known whether this drug is excreted in human milk. Because many drugs are excreted in human milk, caution should be exercised when AKINETON is administered to a nursing woman.

Pediatric Use: Safety and effectiveness in children have not been established.

ADVERSE REACTIONS

Atropine-like side effects such as dry mouth; blurred vision; drowsiness; euphoria or disorientation; urinary retention; postural hypotension; constipation; agitation; disturbed behavior may be seen. There usually are no significant changes in blood pressure or heart rate in patients who have been given the parenteral form of AKINETON. Mild transient postural hypotension and bradycardia may occur. These side effects can be minimized or avoided by slow intravenous administration. No local tissue reactions have been reported following intramuscular injection. If gastric irritation oc-

curs following oral administration, it can be avoided by administering the drug during or after meals.

The central anticholinergic syndrome can occur as an adverse reaction to properly prescribed anticholinergic medication. See Overdosage section for signs and symptoms of the central anticholinergic syndrome, and for treatment.

OVERDOSAGE

Signs and Symptoms: Overdosage with AKINETON produces typical central symptoms of atropine intoxication (the central anticholinergic syndrome). Correct diagnosis depends upon recognition of the peripheral signs of parasympathetic blockade including dilated and sluggish pupils; warm, dry skin; facial flushing; decreased secretions of the mouth, pharynx, nose, and bronchi; foul-smelling breath; elevated temperature, tachycardia, cardiac arrhythmias, decreased bowel sounds, and urinary retention. Neuropsychiatric signs such as delirium, disorientation, anxiety, hallucinations, illusions, confusion, incoherence, agitation, hyperactivity, ataxia, loss of memory, paranoia, combativeness, and seizures may be present. The condition can progress to stupor, coma, paralysis, and cardiac and respiratory arrest and death.

Treatment: Treatment of acute overdose revolves around symptomatic and supportive therapy. If AKINETON was administered orally, gastric lavage or other measures to limit absorption should be instituted. A small dose of diazepam or a short acting barbiturate may be administered if CNS excitation is observed. Phenothiazines are contraindicated because the toxicity may be intensified due to their antimuscarinic action, causing coma. Respiratory support, artificial respiration or vasopressor agents may be necessary. Hyperpyrexia must be reversed, fluid volume replaced and acid-base balance maintained. Urinary catheterization may be necessary.

Routine use of physostigmine for overdose is controversial. Delirium, hallucinations, coma, and supraventricular tachycardia (not ventricular tachycardias or conduction defects) seem to respond. If indicated, 1 mg (half this amount for children or the elderly) may be given intramuscularly or by slow intravenous infusion. If there is no response within 20 minutes, an additional 1 mg dose may be given; this may be repeated until a total of 4 mg has been administered, a reversal of the toxic effects occur or excessive cholinergic signs are seen. Frequent monitoring of clinical signs should be done. Since physostigmine is rapidly destroyed, additional injections may be required every one or two hours to maintain control. The relapse intervals tend to lengthen as the toxic anticholinergic agent is metabolized, so the patient should be carefully observed for 8 to 12 hours following the last relapse.

Toxicity in Animals: The LD_{50} of biperiden in the white mouse is 545 mg/kg orally, 195 mg/kg subcutaneously, and 56 mg/kg intravenously. The acute oral toxicity (LD_{50}) in rats is 750 mg/kg. The intraperitoneal toxicity (LD_{50}) of biperiden lactate in rats was 270 mg/kg and the intravenous toxicity (LD_{50}) in dogs is 222 mg/kg. In dogs under general anesthesia, respiratory arrest occurred at 33 mg/kg (intravenous) and circulatory standstill at 45 mg/kg (intravenous). The oral LD_{50} in dogs was 340 mg/kg. Chronic toxicity studies in both rat and dog have been reported.

DOSAGE AND ADMINISTRATION

Drug-Induced Extrapyramidal Symptoms:
Parenteral: The average adult dose is 2 mg intramuscularly or intravenously. May be repeated every half-hour until there is resolution of symptoms, but not more than four consecutive doses should be given in a 24-hour period.

Note: Parenteral drug products should be inspected visually for particulate matter and discoloration prior to administration, whenever solution and container permit.

Oral: One tablet one to three times daily.

Parkinson's Disease: Oral: The usual beginning dose is one tablet three or four times daily. The dosage should be individualized with the dose titrated upward to a maximum of 8 tablets (16 mg) per 24 hours.

HOW SUPPLIED

AKINETON Tablets, 2 mg each, white, embossed on one face with a triangle, bisected on the reverse and imprinted with the number "11."

Bottles of 100—NDC #0044-0120-02.
Bottles of 1000—NDC #0044-0120-04.
AKINETON Ampules, 1 mL each containing 5 mg biperiden lactate per mL.
Boxes of 10—NDC #0044-0110-01.
Storage: All dosage forms of AKINETON should be stored at 59°–86°F (15°–30°C).
Dispense in tight, light-resistant container as defined in USP.
MR 1987/5427
Revised June, 1987   5427

Shown in Product Identification Section, page 413

COLLAGENASE SANTYL® Ointment   ℞
[săn'til]
(collagenase)

DESCRIPTION
SANTYL® OINTMENT is a sterile enzymatic debriding ointment which contains 250 collagenase units per gram of white petrolatum USP. The enzyme collagenase is derived from the fermentation by *Clostridium histolyticum*. It possesses the unique ability to digest native and denatured collagen in necrotic tissue.

CLINICAL PHARMACOLOGY
Since collagen accounts for 75% of the dry weight of skin tissue, the ability of collagenase to digest collagen in the physiological pH range and temperature makes it particularly effective in the removal of detritus.[1] Collagenase thus contributes towards the formation of granulation tissue and subsequent epithelization of dermal ulcers and severely burned areas.[2,3,4,5,6] Collagen in healthy tissue or in newly formed granulation tissue is not attacked.[2,3,4,5,6,7,8]

INDICATIONS
Santyl Ointment is indicated for debriding chronic dermal ulcers[2,3,4,5,6,8,9,10,11,12,13,14,15,16,17,18] and severely burned areas.[3,4,5,7,16,19,20,21]

CONTRAINDICATIONS
Santyl Ointment is contraindicated in patients who have shown local or systemic hypersensitivity to collagenase.

PRECAUTIONS
The optimal pH range of collagenase is 6 to 8. Higher or lower pH conditions will decrease the enzyme's activity and appropriate precautions should be taken. The enzymatic activity is also adversely affected by detergents, hexachlorophene and heavy metal ions such as mercury and silver which are used in some antiseptics. When it is suspected such materials have been used, the site should be carefully cleansed by repeated washings with normal saline before Santyl Ointment is applied. Soaks containing metal ions or acidic solutions such as Burow's solution should be avoided because of the metal ion and low pH. Cleansing materials such as hydrogen peroxide, Dakin's solution, and sterile saline are compatible with Santyl Ointment.
Debilitated patients should be closely monitored for systemic bacterial infections because of the theoretical possibility that debriding enzymes may increase the risk of bacteremia. A slight transient erythema has been noted occasionally in the surrounding tissue, particularly when Santyl Ointment was not confined to the lesion. Therefore, the ointment should be applied carefully within the area of the lesion.

ADVERSE REACTIONS
No allergic sensitivity or toxic reactions have been noted in the recorded clinical investigations. However, one case of systemic manifestations of hypersensitivity to collagenase in a patient treated for more than one year with a combination of collagenase and cortisone has been reported to us.

OVERDOSAGE
Action of the enzyme may be stopped, should this be desired, by the application of Burow's solution USP (pH 3.6–4.4) to the lesion.

DOSAGE AND ADMINISTRATION
Santyl Ointment should be applied once daily (or more frequently if the dressing becomes soiled, as from incontinence) in the following manner:
(1) Prior to application the lesion should be cleansed of debris and digested material by gently rubbing with a gauze pad saturated with hydrogen peroxide or Dakin's solution followed by sterile normal saline.
(2) Whenever infection is present it is desirable to use an appropriate topical antibiotic powder. The antibiotic should be applied to the lesion prior to the application of Santyl Ointment. Should the infection not respond, therapy with Santyl Ointment should be discontinued until remission of the infection.
(3) Santyl Ointment should be applied directly to deep lesions with a wooden tongue depressor or spatula. For shallow lesions, Santyl Ointment may be applied to a sterile gauze pad which is then applied to the wound and properly secured.
(4) Crosshatching thick eschar with a #10 blade allows collagenase more surface contact with necrotic debris. It is also desirable to remove, with forceps and scissors, as much loosened detritus as can be done readily.
(5) All excess ointment should be removed each time dressing is changed.
(6) Use of Santyl Ointment should be terminated when debridement of necrotic tissue is complete and granulation tissue is well established.

HOW SUPPLIED
Santyl Ointment contains 250 units of collagenase enzyme per gram of white petrolatum USP. The potency assay of collagenase is based on the digestion of undenatured collagen (from bovine Achilles tendon) at pH 7.2 and 37°C for 24 hours. The number of peptide bonds cleaved are measured by reaction with ninhydrin. Amino groups released by a trypsin digestion control are subtracted. One net collagenase unit will solubilize ninhydrin reactive material equivalent to 4 micromoles of leucine.
Collagenase Santyl Ointment 15g
   NDC# 0044-5270-02
Collagenase Santyl Ointment 30g
   NDC# 0044-5270-03

REFERENCES
1—Mandl, I., Adv. Enzymol. 23:163, 1961.
2—Boxer, A.M., Gotteman, N., Bernstein, H., & Mandl, I., Geriatrics 24:75, 1969.
3—Mazurek, I., Med. Welt 22:150, 1971.
4—Zimmerman, W.E., in "Collagenase," I. Mandl, ed., Gordon & Breach, Science Publishers, New York, 1971, p. 131, p. 185.
5—Vetra, H., & Whittaker, D., Geriatrics 30:53, 1975.
6—Rao, D.B., Sane, P.G., & Georgiev, E.L., J. Am. Geriatrics Soc. 23:22, 1975.
7—Vrabec, R., Moserova, J., Konickova, Z., Behounkova, E., & Blaha, J., J. Hyg. Epidemiol. Microbiol. Immunol. 18:496, 1974.
8—Lippmann, H.I., Arch. Phys. Med. Rehabil. 54:588, 1973.
9—German, F.M., in "Collagenase," I. Mandl, ed. Gordon & Breach, Science Publishers, New York, 1971, p. 165.
10—Haimovici, H. & Strauch, B., in "Collagenase," I. Mandl, ed., Gordon & Breach, Science Publishers, New York, 1971, p. 177.
11—Lee, L.K., & Ambrus, J.L., Geriatrics 30:91, 1975.
12—Locke, R.K., & Heifitz, N.M., J. Am. Pod. Assoc. 65:242, 1975.
13—Varma, A.O., Bugatch, E., & German, F.M., Surg. Gynecol. Obstet. 136:281, 1973.
14—Barrett, D., Jr., & Klibanski, A., Am. J. Nurs. 73:849, 1973.
15—Bardfeld, L.A., J. Pod. Ed. 1:41, 1970.
16—Blum, G., Schweiz. Rundschau Med. Praxis 62:820, 1973. Abstr. in Dermatology Digest, Feb. 1974, p. 36.
17—Zaruba, F., Lettl, A., Brozkova, L., Skrdlantova, H., & Krs, V., J. Hyg. Epidemiol. Microbiol. Immunol. 18:499, 1974.
18—Altman, M.I., Goldstein, L., Horowitz, S., J. Am. Pod. Assoc. 68:11, 1978.
19—Rehn, V.J., Med. Klin. 58:799, 1963.
20—Krauss, H., Koslowski, L., & Zimmermann, W.E., Langenbecks Arch. Klin. Chir. 303:23, 1963.
21—Gruenagel, H.H., Med. Klin. 58:442, 1963.

Manufactured by
ADVANCE BIOFACTURES CORP.
35 Wilbur Street
Lynbrook, New York 11563
Distributed by
Knoll Pharmaceuticals
A Unit of BASF K & F Corporation
30 North Jefferson Road
Whippany, New Jersey 07981
Revised: November, 1987   6103
Shown in Product Identification Section, page 414

DILAUDID®   © ℞
[dī"law'dĭd]
(hydromorphone hydrochloride)

DESCRIPTION
DILAUDID (hydromorphone hydrochloride) (WARNING: May be habit forming), a hydrogenated ketone of morphine, is a narcotic analgesic. It is available in:
Ampules (for parenteral administration) containing: 1 mg, 2 mg, and 4 mg hydromorphone hydrochloride per mL with 0.2% sodium citrate, 0.2% citric acid solution. DILAUDID ampules are sterile.
Multiple Dose Vials (for parenteral administration) containing 20 mL of solution. Each mL contains 2 mg hydromorphone hydrochloride and 0.5 mg edetate disodium with 1.8 mg methylparaben and 0.2 mg propylparaben as preservatives. Sodium hydroxide or hydrochloric acid is used for pH adjustment. DILAUDID multiple dose vials are sterile.
Color Coded Tablets (for oral administration) containing:
  1 mg hydromorphone hydrochloride (green tablet) and FD&C blue #1 Lake dye, D&C yellow #10 Lake dye, lactose, and magnesium stearate.
  2 mg hydromorphone hydrochloride (orange tablet) and D&C red #30 Lake dye, D&C yellow #10 Lake dye, lactose, and magnesium stearate.
  3 mg hydromorphone hydrochloride (pink tablet) and D&C red #30 Lake dye, lactose, and magnesium stearate.
  4 mg hydromorphone hydrochloride (yellow tablet) and D&C yellow #10 Lake dye, lactose, and magnesium stearate.
Suppositories (for rectal administration) containing 3 mg hydromorphone hydrochloride in a cocoa butter base with silicon dioxide.

Non-Sterile Powder (for prescription compounding) containing hydromorphone hydrochloride.
The structural formula of DILAUDID (hydromorphone hydrochloride) is:

CLINICAL PHARMACOLOGY
DILAUDID is a narcotic analgesic; its principal therapeutic effect is relief of pain. The precise mechanism of action of DILAUDID and other opiates is not known, although it is believed to relate to the existence of opiate receptors in the central nervous system. There is no intrinsic limit to the analgesic effect of DILAUDID; like morphine, adequate doses will relieve even the most severe pain. Clinically, however, dosage limitations are imposed by the adverse effects, primarily respiratory depression, nausea, and vomiting, which can result from high doses.
DILAUDID has diverse additional actions. It may produce drowsiness, changes in mood and mental clouding, depress the respiratory center and the cough center, stimulate the vomiting center, produce pinpoint constriction of the pupil, enhance parasympathetic activity, elevate cerebrospinal fluid pressure, increase biliary pressure, produce transient hyperglycemia.
Generally, the analgesic action of parenterally administered DILAUDID is apparent within 15 minutes and usually remains in effect for more than five hours. The onset of action of oral DILAUDID is somewhat slower, with measurable analgesia occurring within 30 minutes.
In human plasma the half-life of a DILAUDID 4 mg tablet is 2.6 hours. In a random crossover study in six subjects, 4 mg of *oral* DILAUDID produced a mean concentration/time curve similar to that of 2 mg DILAUDID I.V., after the first hours.

INDICATIONS AND USAGE
DILAUDID is indicated for the relief of moderate to severe pain such as that due to:
  Surgery
  Cancer
  Trauma (soft tissue & bone)
  Biliary Colic
  Myocardial Infarction
  Burns
  Renal Colic

CONTRAINDICATIONS
DILAUDID is contraindicated in patients with a known hypersensitivity to hydromorphone; in the presence of an intracranial lesion associated with increased intracranial pressure; and whenever ventilatory function is depressed (chronic obstructive pulmonary disease, cor pulmonale, emphysema, kyphoscoliosis, status asthmaticus).

WARNINGS
Respiratory Depression: DILAUDID produces dose-related respiratory depression by acting directly on brain stem respiratory centers. DILAUDID also affects centers that control respiratory rhythm, and may produce irregular and periodic breathing.
Head Injury and Increased Intracranial Pressure: The respiratory depressant effects of narcotics and their capacity to elevate cerebrospinal fluid pressure may be markedly exaggerated in the presence of head injury, other intracranial lesions or a preexisting increase in intracranial pressure. Furthermore, narcotics produce effects which may obscure the clinical course of patients with head injuries.
Acute Abdominal Conditions: The administration of narcotics may obscure the diagnosis or clinical course of patients with acute abdominal conditions.

PRECAUTIONS
Special Risk Patients: DILAUDID should be used with caution in elderly or debilitated patients and those with impaired renal or hepatic function, hypothyroidism, Addison's disease, prostatic hypertrophy or urethral stricture. As with any narcotic analgesic agent, the usual precautions should be observed and the possibility of respiratory depression should be kept in mind.
Cough Reflex: DILAUDID suppresses the cough reflex; as with all narcotics, caution should be exercised when DILAUDID is used postoperatively and in patients with pulmonary disease.
Usage in Ambulatory Patients: Narcotics may impair the mental and/or physical abilities required for the performance of potentially hazardous tasks such as driving a

Continued on next page

Knoll—Cont.

car or operating machinery; patients should be cautioned accordingly.

Drug Interactions: Patients receiving other narcotic analgesics, general anesthetics, phenothiazines, tranquilizers, sedative-hypnotics, tricyclic antidepressants or other CNS depressants (including alcohol) concomitantly with DILAUDID may exhibit an additive CNS depression. When such combined therapy is contemplated, the dose of one or both agents should be reduced.

Parenteral Administration: The parenteral form of DILAUDID may be given intravenously, but the injection should be given very slowly. Rapid intravenous injection of narcotic analgesics increases the possibility of side effects such as hypotension and respiratory depression.

Pregnancy: Pregnancy Category C. DILAUDID has been shown to be teratogenic in hamsters when given in doses 600 times the human dose. There are no adequate and well-controlled studies in pregnant women. DILAUDID should be used during pregnancy only if the potential benefit justifies the potential risk to the fetus.

Nonteratogenic effects: Babies born to mothers who have been taking opioids regularly prior to delivery will be physically dependent. The withdrawal signs include irritability and excessive crying, tremors, hyperactive reflexes, increased respiratory rate, increased stools, sneezing, yawning, vomiting, and fever. The intensity of the syndrome does not always correlate with the duration of maternal opioid use or dose. There is no consensus on the best method of managing withdrawal. Chlorpromazine 0.7 to 1.0 mg/kg q6h, phenobarbital 2 mg/kg q6h, and paregoric 2 to 4 drops/kg q4h, have been used to treat withdrawal symptoms in infants. The duration of therapy is 4 to 28 days, with the dosages decreased as tolerated.

Labor and Delivery: As with all narcotics, administration of DILAUDID to the mother shortly before delivery may result in some degree of respiratory depression in the newborn, especially if higher doses are used.

Nursing Mothers: It is not known whether this drug is excreted in human milk. Because many drugs are excreted in human milk and because of the potential for serious adverse reactions in nursing infants from DILAUDID, a decision should be made whether to discontinue nursing or to discontinue the drug, taking into account the importance of the drug to the mother.

Pediatric Use: Safety and effectiveness in children have not been established.

ADVERSE REACTIONS

Central Nervous System: Sedation, drowsiness, mental clouding, lethargy, impairment of mental and physical performance, anxiety, fear, dysphoria, dizziness, psychic dependence, mood changes.

Gastrointestinal System: Nausea and vomiting occur infrequently; they are more frequent in ambulatory than in recumbent patients. The antiemetic phenothiazines are useful in suppressing these effects; however, some phenothiazine derivatives seem to be antianalgesic and to increase the amount of narcotic required to produce pain relief, while other phenothiazines reduce the amount of narcotic required to produce a given level of analgesia. Prolonged administration of DILAUDID may produce constipation. Opiate agonist-induced increase in intraluminal pressure may endanger surgical anastomosis.

Cardiovascular System: Circulatory depression, peripheral circulatory collapse and cardiac arrest have occurred after rapid intravenous injection. Orthostatic hypotension and fainting may occur if a patient stands up suddenly after receiving an injection of DILAUDID.

Genitourinary System: Ureteral spasm, spasm of vesical sphincters and urinary retention have been reported.

Respiratory Depression: DILAUDID produces dose-related respiratory depression by acting directly on brain stem respiratory centers. DILAUDID also affects centers that control respiratory rhythm, and may produce irregular and periodic breathing. If significant respiratory depression occurs, it may be antagonized by the use of naloxone hydrochloride. The usual adult dose of 0.4 to 0.8 mg given *intramuscularly* or *intravenously,* promptly reverses the effects of morphine-like opioid agonists such as DILAUDID. In patients who are physically dependent, small doses of naloxone may be sufficient not only to antagonize respiratory depression, but also to precipitate withdrawal phenomena. The dose of naloxone should therefore be adjusted accordingly in such patients. Since the duration of action of DILAUDID may exceed that of the antagonist, the patient should be kept under continued surveillance; repeated doses of the antagonist may be required to maintain adequate respiration. Apply other supportive measures when indicated.

DRUG ABUSE AND DEPENDENCE

DILAUDID is a Schedule CII narcotic. Psychic dependence, physical dependence, and tolerance may develop upon repeated administration of narcotics; therefore, DILAUDID should be prescribed and administered with caution. However, psychic dependence is unlikely to develop when DILAUDID is used for a short time for the treatment of pain. Physical dependence, the condition in which continued administration of the drug is required to prevent the appearance of a withdrawal syndrome, usually assumes clinically significant proportions only after several weeks of continued narcotic use, although some mild degree of physical dependence may develop after a few days of narcotic therapy. Tolerance, in which increasingly large doses are required in order to produce the same degree of analgesia, is manifested initially by a shortened duration of analgesic effect, and subsequently by decreases in the intensity of analgesia. The rate of development of tolerance varies among patients.

OVERDOSAGE

Signs and Symptoms: Serious overdosage with DILAUDID is characterized by respiratory depression (a decrease in respiratory rate and/or tidal volume, Cheyne-Stokes respiration, cyanosis), extreme somnolence progressing to stupor or coma, skeletal muscle flaccidity, cold and clammy skin, and sometimes bradycardia and hypotension. In severe overdosage, particularly by the intravenous route, apnea, circulatory collapse, cardiac arrest, and death may occur.

Treatment: Primary attention should be given to the reestablishment of adequate respiratory exchange through provision of a patent airway and institution of assisted or controlled ventilation. The narcotic antagonist naloxone hydrochloride is a specific antidote against respiratory depression which may result from overdosage or unusual sensitivity to narcotics, including DILAUDID. Therefore, naloxone hydrochloride should be administered as described under *Adverse Reactions* (see *Respiratory Depression*) in conjunction with ventilatory assistance.

Since the duration of action of DILAUDID may exceed that of the antagonist, the patient should be kept under continued surveillance; repeated doses of the antagonist may be required to maintain adequate respiration. An antagonist should not be administered in the absence of clinically significant respiratory or cardiovascular depression. Oxygen, intravenous fluids, vasopressors, and other supportive measures should be employed as indicated.

In cases of overdosage with oral DILAUDID, gastric lavage or induced emesis may be useful in removing unabsorbed drug from conscious patients.

DOSAGE AND ADMINISTRATION

Parenteral: The usual starting dose is 1–2 mg *subcutaneously* or *intramuscularly* every 4 to 6 hours as necessary for pain control. The dose should be adjusted according to the severity of pain, as well as the patient's underlying disease, age, and size. Patients with terminal cancer may be tolerant to narcotic analgesics and may, therefore, require higher doses for adequate pain relief. Intravenous or subcutaneous administration is usually not painful. Should intravenous administration be necessary, the injection should be given *slowly,* over at least 2 to 3 minutes, depending on the dose. A gradual increase in dose may be required if analgesia is inadequate, tolerance occurs, or if pain severity increases. The first sign of tolerance is usually a reduced duration of effect.

NOTE: Parenteral drug products should be inspected visually for particulate matter and discoloration prior to administration, whenever solution and container permit. A slight yellowish discoloration may develop in DILAUDID ampules and multiple dose vials. No loss of potency has been demonstrated.

Oral: The usual oral dose is 2 mg every 4 to 6 hours as necessary. The dose must be individually adjusted according to severity of pain, patient response and patient size. More severe pain may require 4 mg or more every 4 to 6 hours. If the pain increases in severity, analgesia is not adequate or tolerance occurs, a gradual increase in dosage may be required. If pain is exceedingly severe, or if prompt response is desired, parenteral DILAUDID should be used initially in adequate amounts to control the pain.

Rectal: DILAUDID suppositories (3 mg) may provide longer duration of relief which could obviate additional medication during the sleeping hours. The usual adult dose is one (1) suppository inserted rectally every 6 to 8 hours or as directed by physician.

HOW SUPPLIED

Ampules: (One mL sterile solution for parenteral administration)

1 mg/mL ampules—Boxes of 10—
NDC# 0044-1011-01.

2 mg/mL ampules—Boxes of 10—
NDC# 0044-1012-01.
Boxes of 25—NDC# 0044-1012-09.

4 mg/mL ampules—Boxes of 10—
NDC# 0044-1014-01.

Multiple Dose Vials: (20 mL sterile solution for parenteral administration)

2 mg/mL—20 mL multiple dose vials
NDC# 0044-1062-05.

Oral Color Coded Tablets: (NOT FOR INJECTION)

1 mg tablet (green)—Bottles of 100—
NDC# 0044-1021-02.

2 mg tablet (orange)—Bottles of 100—
NDC# 0044-1022-02.
Unit Dose of 100 (4 × 25)—
NDC# 0044-1022-45
Bottles of 500—NDC# 0044-1022-03.

3 mg tablet (pink)—Bottles of 100—
NDC# 0044-1023-02.

4 mg tablet (yellow)—Bottles of 100—
NDC# 0044-1024-02.
Unit Dose of 100 (4 × 25)—
NDC# 0044-1024-45
Bottles of 500—NDC# 0044-1024-03.

Rectal Suppositories: 3 mg suppositories—
Boxes of 6—NDC# 0044-1053-01.

Non-Sterile Powder: For prescription compounding.
15 grain vial—NDC# 0044-1040-01.

Storage: Parenteral and oral dosage forms of DILAUDID should be stored at 59°–86°F (15°–30°C).

Protect from light. DILAUDID suppositories should be stored in a refrigerator.

A Schedule CII Narcotic.
DEA order form required.

Parenteral Products
Manufactured for
Knoll Pharmaceuticals
Whippany, NJ 07981
by Sterling Drug, Inc.
McPherson, KS 67460
RE-1m/Dil6738D/1-9-92
Revised January 1992 6738D

Shown in Product Identification Section, page 413

DILAUDID® COUGH SYRUP CII ℞

[dī″law′dĭd]
(hydromorphone hydrochloride)

DESCRIPTION

Each 5 mL (1 teaspoonful) contains 1 mg DILAUDID (hydromorphone HCl) (**WARNING:** May be habit forming) and 100 mg guaifenesin in a peach-flavored syrup containing 5% alcohol. DILAUDID is a hydrogenated ketone of morphine; it is a narcotic analgesic and antitussive.

The structural formula of DILAUDID (hydromorphone hydrochloride) is:

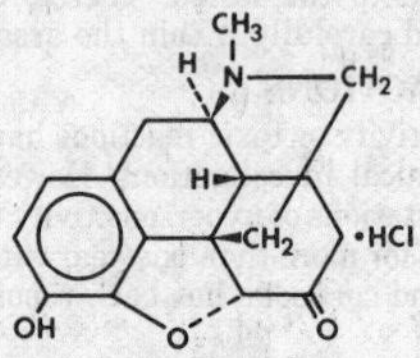

CLINICAL PHARMACOLOGY

DILAUDID (hydromorphone HCl) is a centrally acting narcotic antitussive which acts directly on the cough reflex center.

DILAUDID is also a narcotic analgesic; its principal therapeutic effect is relief of pain. The precise mechanism of action of DILAUDID and other opiates is not known, although it is believed to relate to the existence of opiate receptors in the central nervous system. There is no intrinsic limit to the analgesic effect of DILAUDID; like morphine, adequate doses will relieve even the most severe pain. Clinically, however, dosage limitations are imposed by the adverse effects, primarily respiratory depression, nausea, and vomiting, which can result from high doses.

DILAUDID has diverse additional actions. It produces drowsiness, changes in mood and mental clouding, depresses the respiratory center and the cough center, stimulates the vomiting center, produces pinpoint constriction of the pupil, enhances parasympathetic activity, elevates cerebrospinal fluid pressure, increases biliary pressure, produces transient hyperglycemia.

Generally, the analgesic action of parenterally administered DILAUDID is apparent within 15 minutes and usually remains in effect for more than five hours. The onset of action of oral DILAUDID is somewhat slower, with measurable analgesia occurring within 30 minutes.

Radioimmunoassay techniques have recently been developed for the analysis of DILAUDID in human plasma. In humans the half-life of a DILAUDID 4 mg tablet is 2.6 hours. In a random crossover study in six subjects, 4 mg of oral DILAUDID produced a mean concentration/time curve similar to that of 2 mg DILAUDID I.V., after the first hour.

Guaifenesin (glyceryl guaiacolate) reduces the viscosity of secretions, thereby increasing the efficiency of the cough reflex and of ciliary action in removing accumulated secretions from the trachea and bronchi. Unlike many other expectorants, guaifenesin rarely causes gastric irritation.

INDICATIONS AND USAGE

DILAUDID Cough Syrup is indicated for the control of persistent, exhausting cough or dry, non-productive cough.

CONTRAINDICATIONS

DILAUDID Cough Syrup is contraindicated in patients known to have a hypersensitivity to hydromorphone; in the presence of an intracranial lesion associated with increased intracranial pressure; and whenever ventilatory function is depressed (chronic obstructive pulmonary disease, cor pulmonale, emphysema, kyphoscoliosis, status asthmaticus).

WARNINGS

Respiratory Depression: DILAUDID produces dose-related respiratory depression by acting directly on brain stem respiratory centers. DILAUDID also affects centers that control respiratory rhythm and may produce irregular and periodic breathing.

Head Injury and Increased Intracranial Pressure: The respiratory depressant effects of narcotics and their capacity to elevate cerebrospinal fluid pressure may be markedly exaggerated in the presence of head injury, other intracranial lesions or a preexisting increase in intracranial pressure. Furthermore, narcotics produce adverse effects which may obscure the clinical course of patients with head injuries.

Acute Abdominal Conditions: The administration of narcotics may obscure the diagnosis or clinical course of patients with acute abdominal conditions.

PRECAUTIONS

Special Risk Patients: DILAUDID Cough Syrup should be used with caution in elderly or debilitated patients and those with impaired renal or hepatic function, hypothyroidism, Addison's disease, prostatic hypertrophy or urethral stricture. As with any narcotic analgesic agent, the usual precautions should be observed and the possibility of respiratory depression should be kept in mind.

Cough Reflex: DILAUDID Cough Syrup suppresses the cough reflex; as with all narcotics, caution should be exercised when DILAUDID Cough Syrup is used postoperatively and in patients with pulmonary disease.

Usage in Ambulatory Patients: Narcotics may impair the mental and/or physical abilities required for the performance of potentially hazardous tasks such as driving a car or operating machinery; patients should be cautioned accordingly.

Drug Interactions: Patients receiving other narcotic analgesics, general anesthetics, phenothiazines, tranquilizers, sedative-hypnotics, tricyclic antidepressants or other CNS depressants (including alcohol) concomitantly with DILAUDID Cough Syrup may exhibit an additive CNS depression. When such combined therapy is contemplated, the dose of one or both agents should be reduced.

Usage in Pregnancy: Pregnancy Category C. DILAUDID has been shown to be teratogenic in hamsters when given in doses 600 times the human dose. There are no adequate and well-controlled studies in pregnant women. DILAUDID Cough Syrup should be used during pregnancy only if the potential benefit justifies the potential risk to the fetus.

Nonteratogenic effects: Babies born to mothers who have been taking opioids regularly prior to delivery will be physically dependent. The withdrawal signs include irritability and excessive crying, tremors, hyperactive reflexes, increased respiratory rate, increased stools, sneezing, yawning, vomiting, and fever. The intensity of the syndrome does not always correlate with the duration of maternal opioid use or dose. There is no consensus on the best method of managing withdrawal. Chlorpromazine 0.7 to 1.0 mg/kg q6h, phenobarbital 2 mg/kg q6h, and paregoric 2 to 4 drops/kg q4h, have been used to treat withdrawal symptoms in infants. The duration of therapy is 4 to 28 days, with the dosage decreased as tolerated.

Labor and Delivery: As with all narcotics, administration of DILAUDID Cough Syrup to the mother shortly before delivery may result in some degree of respiratory depression in the newborn, especially if higher doses are used.

Nursing Mothers: It is not known whether this drug is excreted in human milk. Because many drugs are excreted in human milk and because of the potential for serious adverse reactions in nursing infants from DILAUDID Cough Syrup, a decision should be made whether to discontinue nursing or to discontinue the drug, taking into account the importance of the drug to the mother.

Pediatric Use: Safety and effectiveness in children have not been established.

FD&C Yellow No. 5: DILAUDID Cough Syrup contains FD&C Yellow No. 5 (tartrazine) dye which may cause allergic-type reactions (including bronchial asthma) in certain susceptible individuals. Although the overall incidence of FD&C Yellow No. 5 (tartrazine) dye sensitivity in the general population is low, it is frequently seen in patients who also have aspirin hypersensitivity.

ADVERSE REACTIONS

Central Nervous System: Sedation, drowsiness, mental clouding, lethargy, impairment of mental and physical performance, anxiety, fear, dysphoria, dizziness, psychic dependence, mood changes.

Gastrointestinal System: Nausea and vomiting occur more frequently in ambulatory than in recumbent patients. The antiemetic phenothiazines are useful in suppressing these effects. Prolonged administration of DILAUDID may produce constipation. Opiate agonist-induced increase in intraluminal pressure may endanger surgical anastomosis.

Genitourinary System: Ureteral spasm, spasm of vesical sphincters and urinary retention have been reported.

Respiratory Depression: DILAUDID produces dose-related respiratory depression by acting directly on brain stem respiratory centers. DILAUDID also affects centers that control respiratory rhythm, and may produce irregular and periodic breathing. If significant respiratory depression occurs, it may be antagonized by the use of naloxone hydrochloride. The usual adult dose of 0.4 to 0.8 mg given intramuscularly or intravenously, promptly reverses the effects of morphine-like opioid agonists such as DILAUDID. In patients who are physically dependent, small doses of naloxone may be sufficient not only to antagonize respiratory depression, but also to precipitate withdrawal phenomena. The dose of naloxone should therefore be adjusted accordingly in such patients. Since the duration of action of DILAUDID may exceed that of the antagonist, the patient should be kept under continued surveillance; repeated doses of the antagonist may be required to maintain adequate respiration. Apply other supportive measures when indicated.

DRUG ABUSE AND DEPENDENCE

DILAUDID is a Schedule CII narcotic. Psychic dependence, physical dependence, and tolerance may develop upon repeated administration of narcotics; therefore, DILAUDID should be prescribed and administered with caution. However, psychic dependence is unlikely to develop when DILAUDID Cough Syrup is used for a short time as indicated. Physical dependence, the condition in which continued administration of the drug is required to prevent the appearance of a withdrawal syndrome, usually assumes clinically significant proportions only after several weeks of continued narcotic use, although some mild degree of physical dependence may develop after few days of narcotic therapy.

OVERDOSAGE

Signs and Symptoms: Serious overdosage with DILAUDID is characterized by respiratory depression (a decrease in respiratory rate and/or tidal volume, Cheyne-Stokes respiration, cyanosis), extreme somnolence progressing to stupor or coma, skeletal muscle flaccidity, cold and clammy skin, and sometimes bradycardia and hypotension. In severe overdosage particularly by the intravenous route, apnea, circulatory collapse, cardiac arrest and death may occur.

Treatment: Primary attention should be given to the reestablishment of adequate respiratory exchange through provision of a patent airway and the institution of assisted or controlled ventilation. The narcotic antagonist naloxone hydrochloride is a specific antidote against respiratory depression which may result from overdosage or unusual sensitivity to narcotics, including DILAUDID. Therefore, naloxone hydrochloride should be administered as described under ADVERSE REACTIONS (see Respiratory Depression) in conjunction with ventilatory assistance.

Since the duration of action of Dilaudid may exceed that of the antagonist, the patient should be kept under continued surveillance; repeated doses of the antagonist may be required to maintain adequate respiration. An antagonist should not be administered in the absence of clinically significant respiratory or cardiovascular depression. Oxygen, intravenous fluids, vasopressors and other supportive measures should be employed as indicated.

In cases of overdosage with oral DILAUDID, gastric lavage or induced emesis may be useful in removing unabsorbed drug from conscious patients.

DOSAGE AND ADMINISTRATION

The usual adult dose of DILAUDID Cough Syrup is one teaspoonful (5 mL) every 3 to 4 hours.

HOW SUPPLIED

Bottles of 1 pint (473 mL)—NDC #0044-1080-01.
Storage: Store at 59°–86°F (15°–30°C).
A Schedule CII Narcotic.
DEA order form required.
Revised September 1986 8074

DILAUDID-HP® INJECTION CII ℞

[*dī"law'did*]
10 mg/mL
(hydromorphone hydrochloride)

PRODUCT OVERVIEW

KEY FACTS

Dilaudid-HP is a narcotic analgesic, containing 10 mg of hydromorphone per ml; it is administered by intravenous, subcutaneous and intramuscular injection. Because of its highly concentrated solution, a smaller injection volume can be used than with other parenteral narcotic formulations, thereby avoiding the discomfort associated with the intramuscular or subcutaneous injection of an unusually large volume of solution.

MAJOR USE

This high-potency hydromorphone formulation is used to relieve moderate-to severe pain in narcotic-tolerant patients who require abnormally high doses of narcotic analgesics for adequate pain relief. Usually these are patients who have already been treated with other narcotic analgesics.

SAFETY INFORMATION

Is contraindicated in: patients who are not already receiving large amounts of parenteral narcotics, patients with known hypersensitivity to the drug, patients with respiratory depression in the absence of resuscitative equipment, patients with status asthmaticus, and for use in obstetrical analgesia. Similar to other narcotic analgesics, the major adverse reactions include respiratory depression and apnea, and, to a lesser extent, circulatory depression, respiratory arrest, shock and cardiac arrest.

PRESCRIBING INFORMATION

DILAUDID-HP® INJECTION CII ℞

[*dī"law'did*]
10 mg/mL
(hydromorphone hydrochloride)

WARNING

DILAUDID-HP® (HIGH POTENCY) IS A HIGHLY CONCENTRATED SOLUTION OF HYDROMORPHONE INTENDED FOR USE IN NARCOTIC-TOLERANT PATIENTS. DO NOT CONFUSE DILAUDID-HP WITH STANDARD PARENTERAL FORMULATIONS OF DILAUDID OR OTHER NARCOTICS. OVERDOSE AND DEATH COULD RESULT.

DESCRIPTION

DILAUDID (hydromorphone hydrochloride) (WARNING: May be habit forming), a hydrogenated ketone of morphine, is a narcotic analgesic, ***HIGH POTENCY*** DILAUDID is available in AMBER ampules or single dose vials for intravenous (IV) subcutaneous (SC) or intramuscular (IM) administration. Each 1 mL of sterile solution contains 10 mg hydromorphone hydrochloride with 0.2% sodium citrate, 0.2% citric acid solution.

The structural formula of DILAUDID (hydromorphone hydrochloride) is:

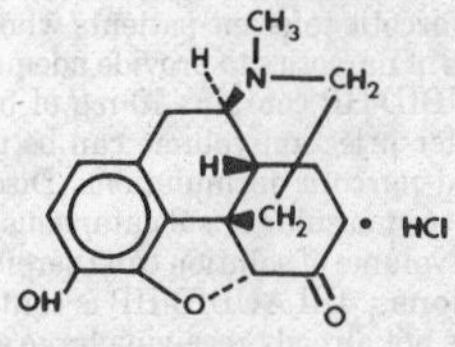

CLINICAL PHARMACOLOGY

Many of the effects described below are common to the class of narcotic analgesics. In some instances, data may not exist to demonstrate that DILAUDID-HP possesses similar or different effects than those observed with other narcotic analgesics. However, in the absence of data to the contrary, it is assumed that DILAUDID-HP would possess these effects.

Central Nervous System: Narcotic analgesics have multiple actions but exert their primary effects on the central nervous system and organs containing smooth muscle. The principal actions of therapeutic value are analgesia and sedation. A significant feature of the analgesia is that it occurs without loss of consciousness. Narcotic analgesics also suppress the cough reflex and cause respiratory depression, mood changes, mental clouding, euphoria, dysphoria, nausea, vomiting and electroencephalographic changes. The precise mode of analgesic action of narcotic analgesics is unknown. However, specific CNS opiate receptors have been identified. Narcotics are believed to express their pharmacological effects by combining with these receptors.

Narcotics depress the cough reflex by direct effect on the cough center in the medulla.

Narcotics produce respiratory depression by direct effect on brain stem respiratory centers. The mechanism of respiratory depression also involves a reduction in the responsiveness of the brain stem respiratory centers to increases in carbon dioxide tension.

Narcotics cause miosis. Pinpoint pupils are a common sign of narcotic overdose but are not pathognomonic (e.g., pontine lesions of hemorrhagic or ischemic origin may produce similar findings) and marked mydriasis occurs when asphyxia intervenes.

Gastrointestinal Tract and Other Smooth Muscle: Gastric, biliary and pancreatic secretions are decreased by narcotics. Narcotics cause a reduction in motility associated with an

Continued on next page

Knoll—Cont.

increase in tone in the antrum portion of the stomach and duodenum. Digestion of food in the small intestine is delayed and propulsive contractions are decreased. Propulsive peristaltic waves in the colon are decreased, and tone may be increased to the point of spasm. The end result is constipation. Narcotics can cause a marked increase in biliary tract pressure as a result of spasm of the sphincter of Oddi.

Cardiovascular System: Certain narcotics produce peripheral vasodilation which may result in orthostatic hypotension. Release of histamine may occur with narcotics and may contribute to narcotic-induced hypotension. Other manifestations of histamine release and/or peripheral vasodilation may include pruritis, flushing, and red eyes.

Effects on the myocardium after i.v. administration of narcotics are not significant in normal persons, vary with different narcotic analgesic agents and vary with the hemodynamic state of the patient, state of hydration and sympathetic drive.

Pharmacokinetics: In normal human volunteers hydromorphone is metabolized primarily in the liver. It is excreted primarily as the glucuronidated conjugate, with small amounts of parent drug and minor amounts of 6-hydroxy reduction metabolites.

Following intravenous administration of DILAUDID to normal volunteers, the mean half-life of elimination was 2.64 +/− 0.88 hours. The mean volume of distribution was 91.5 liters, suggesting extensive tissue uptake. DILAUDID is rapidly removed from the blood stream and distributed to skeletal muscle, kidneys, liver, intestinal tract, lungs, spleen and brain. DILAUDID also crosses the placental membranes.

In terms of area under the analgesic time-effect curve, hydromorphone is approximately 8 times more potent than morphine (i.e., 1.3 mg of hydromorphone produces analgesia equal to that produced by 10 mg of morphine). After intramuscular administration, hydromorphone has a slightly more rapid onset and slightly shorter duration of action than morphine. The duration of DILAUDID analgesia in the non-tolerant patient with usual doses may be up to 4–5 hours. However, in tolerant subjects, duration will vary substantially depending on tolerance and dose. Dose should be adjusted so that 3–4 hours of pain relief may be achieved.

INDICATIONS AND USAGE

DILAUDID-HP is indicated for the relief of moderate-to-severe pain in narcotic-tolerant patients who require larger than usual doses of narcotics to provide adequate pain relief. Because DILAUDID-HP contains 10 mg of hydromorphone per mL, a smaller injection volume can be used than with other parenteral narcotic formulations. Discomfort associated with the intramuscular or subcutaneous injection of an unusually large volume of solution can therefore be avoided.

Contraindications: DILAUDID-HP is contraindicated in: patients who are not already receiving large amounts of parenteral narcotics, patients with known hypersensitivity to the drug, patients with respiratory depression in the absence of resuscitative equipment, and in patients with status asthmaticus. DILAUDID-HP is also contraindicated for use in obstetrical analgesia.

Warnings—Drug Dependence: DILAUDID-HP can produce drug dependence of the morphine type and therefore has the potential for being abused. Psychic dependence, physical dependence and tolerance may develop upon repeated administration of DILAUDID-HP, and it should be prescribed and administered with the same degree of caution appropriate for the use of morphine. Since DILAUDID-HP is indicated for use in patients who are already tolerant to and hence physically dependent on narcotics, abrupt discontinuance in the administration of DILAUDID-HP is likely to result in a withdrawal syndrome. (See ***Drug Abuse and Dependence***).

Infants born to mothers physically dependent on DILAUDID-HP will also be physically dependent and may exhibit respiratory difficulties and withdrawal symptoms (see ***Drug Abuse and Dependence***).

Impaired Respiration: Respiratory depression is the chief hazard of DILAUDID-HP. Respiratory depression occurs most frequently in the elderly, in the debilitated, and in those suffering from conditions accompanied by hypoxia or hypercapnia when even moderate therapeutic doses may dangerously decrease pulmonary ventilation.

DILAUDID-HP should be used with extreme caution in patients with chronic obstructive pulmonary disease or cor pulmonale, patients having a substantially decreased respiratory reserve, hypoxia, hypercapnia, or preexisting respiratory depression. In such patients even usual therapeutic doses of narcotic analgesics may decrease respiratory drive while simultaneously increasing airway resistance to the point of apnea.

Head Injury and Increased Intracranial Pressure: The respiratory depressant effects of DILAUDID-HP with carbon dioxide retention and secondary elevation of cerebrospinal fluid pressure may be markedly exaggerated in the presence of head injury, other intracranial lesions, or preexisting increase in intracranial pressure. Narcotic analgesics including DILAUDID-HP may produce effects which can obscure the clinical course and neurologic signs of further increase in pressure in patients with head injuries.

Hypotensive Effect: Narcotic analgesics, including DILAUDID-HP, may cause severe hypotension in an individual whose ability to maintain his blood pressure has already been compromised by a depleted blood volume, or a concurrent administration of drugs such as phenothiazines or general anesthetics (see also ***Precautions—Drug Interactions***). DILAUDID-HP may produce orthostatic hypotension in ambulatory patients.

DILAUDID-HP should be administered with caution to patients in circulatory shock, since vasodilation produced by the drug may further reduce cardiac output and blood pressure.

PRECAUTIONS

General: Because of its high concentration, the delivery of precise doses of DILAUDID-HP may be difficult if low doses of hydromorphone are required. Therefore, DILAUDID-HP should be used only if the amount of hydromorphone required can be delivered accurately with this formulation.

In general, narcotics should be given with caution and the initial dose should be reduced in the elderly or debilitated and those with severe impairment of hepatic, pulmonary or renal function; myxedema or hypothyroidism; adrenocortical insufficiency (e.g., Addison's Disease); CNS depression or coma; toxic psychoses; prostatic hypertrophy or urethral stricture; gallbladder disease; acute alcoholism; delirium tremens; or kyphoscoliosis.

In the case of DILAUDID-HP, however, the patient is presumed to be receiving a narcotic to which he or she exhibits tolerance and the initial dose of DILAUDID-HP selected should be estimated based on the relative potency of hydromorphone and the narcotic previously used by the patient. See ***(Dosage and Administration)*** section.

The administration of narcotic analgesics including DILAUDID-HP may obscure the diagnosis or clinical course in patients with acute abdominal conditions and may aggravate preexisting convulsions in patients with convulsive disorders.

Narcotic analgesics including DILAUDID-HP should also be used with caution in patients about to undergo surgery of the biliary tract since it may cause spasm of the sphincter of Oddi.

Drug Interactions: The concomitant use of other central nervous system depressants including sedatives or hypnotics, general anesthetics, phenothiazines, tranquilizers and alcohol may produce additive depressant effects. Respiratory depression, hypotension and profound sedation or coma may occur. When such combined therapy is contemplated, the dose of one or both agents should be reduced. Narcotic analgesics, including DILAUDID-HP, may enhance the action of neuromuscular blocking agents and produce an increased degree of respiratory depression.

Pregnancy—Category C:

Human: Adequate animal studies on reproduction have not been performed to determine whether hydromorphone affects fertility in males or females. There are no well-controlled studies in women. Reports based on marketing experience do not identify any specific teratogenic risks following routine (short-term) clinical use. Although there is no clearly defined risk, such reports do not exclude the possibility of infrequent or subtle damage to the human fetus. DILAUDID-HP should be used in pregnant women only when clearly needed (see ***Labor and Delivery*** and ***Drug Abuse and Dependence***).

Animal: Literature reports of hydromorphone hydrochloride administration to pregnant Syrian hamsters show that DILAUDID is teratogenic at a dose of 20 mg/kg which is 600 times the human dose. A maximal teratogenic effect (50% of fetuses affected) in the Syrian hamster was observed at a dose of 125 mg/kg.

Labor and Delivery: DILAUDID-HP is contraindicated in Labor and Delivery (see ***Contraindications*** section).

Nursing Mothers: Low levels of narcotic analgesics have been detected in human milk. As a general rule, nursing should not be undertaken while a patient is receiving DILAUDID-HP since it, and other drugs in this class, may be excreted in the milk.

Pediatric Use: Safety and effectiveness in children have not been established.

ADVERSE REACTIONS

The adverse effects of DILAUDID-HP are similar to those of other narcotic analgesics, and represent established pharmacological effects of the drug class. The major hazards include respiratory depression and apnea. To a lesser degree, circulatory depression, respiratory arrest, shock and cardiac arrest have occurred.

The most frequently observed adverse effects are lightheadedness, dizziness, sedation, nausea, vomiting, and sweating. These effects seem to be more prominent in ambulatory patients and in those not experiencing severe pain. Some adverse reactions in ambulatory patients may be alleviated if the patient lies down.

Less Frequently Observed With Narcotic Analgesics:

General and CNS: Dysphoria, euphoria, weakness, headache, agitation, tremor, uncoordinated muscle movements, alterations of mood (nervousness, apprehension, depression, floating feelings, dreams), muscle rigidity, paresthesia, muscle tremor, blurred vision, nystagmus, diplopia and miosis, transient hallucinations* and disorientation, visual disturbances, insomnia and increased intracranial pressure may occur.

Cardiovascular: Flushing of the face, chills, tachycardia, bradycardia, palpitation, faintness, syncope, hypotension and hypertension have been reported.

Respiratory: Bronchospasm and laryngospasm have been known to occur.

Gastrointestinal: Dry mouth, constipation, biliary tract spasm, anorexia, diarrhea, cramps and taste alterations have been reported.

Genitourinary: Urinary retention or hesitancy, and antidiuretic effects have been reported.

Dermatologic: Pruritis, urticaria, other skin rashes, wheal and flare over the vein with intravenous injection, and diaphoresis have been reported with narcotic analgesics.

Other: In clinical trials, neither local tissue irritation nor induration was observed at the site of subcutaneous injection of DILAUDID-HP; pain at the injection site was rarely observed. However, local irritation and induration have been seen following parenteral injection of other narcotic drug products.

DRUG ABUSE AND DEPENDENCE

Narcotic analgesics may cause psychological and physical dependence (see ***Warnings***). Physical dependence results in withdrawal symptoms in patients who abruptly discontinue the drug. Withdrawal symptoms also may be precipitated in the patient with physical dependence by the administration of a drug with narcotic antagonist activity, e.g., naloxone (see also ***Overdosage***). Physical dependence usually does not occur to a clinically significant degree until after several weeks of continued narcotic usage. Tolerance, in which increasingly large doses are required in order to produce the same degree of analgesia, is initially manifested by a shortened duration of analgesic effect, and subsequently, by decreases in the intensity of analgesia. In chronic pain patients, and in narcotic-tolerant cancer patients, the dose of DILAUDID-HP should be guided by the degree of tolerance manifested.

In chronic pain patients in whom narcotic analgesics including DILAUDID-HP are abruptly discontinued, a severe abstinence syndrome should be anticipated. This may be similar to the abstinence syndrome noted in patients who withdraw from heroin. The latter abstinence syndrome may be characterized by restlessness, lacrimation, rhinorrhea, yawning, perspiration, gooseflesh, restless sleep or "yen" and mydriasis during the first 24 hours. These symptoms may increase in severity and over the next 72 hours may be accompanied by increasing irritability, anxiety, weakness, twitching and spasms of muscles, kicking movements, severe backache, abdominal and leg pains, abdominal and muscle cramps, hot and cold flashes, insomnia, nausea, anorexia, vomiting, intestinal spasm, diarrhea, coryza and repetitive sneezing, increase in body temperature, blood pressure, respiratory rate and heart rate.

Because of excessive loss of fluids through sweating, or vomiting and diarrhea, there is usually marked weight loss, dehydration, ketosis, and disturbances in acid-base balance. Cardiovascular collapse can occur. Without treatment most observable symptoms disappear in 5–14 days; however, there appears to be a phase of secondary or chronic abstinence which may last for 2–6 months characterized by insomnia, irritability, muscular aches, and autonomic instability.

In the treatment of physical dependence on DILAUDID-HP, the patient may be detoxified by gradual reduction of the dosage, although this is unlikely to be necessary in the terminal cancer patient. If abstinence symptoms become severe, the patient may be given methadone. Temporary administration of tranquilizers and sedatives may aid in reducing patient anxiety. Gastrointestinal disturbances or dehydration should be treated accordingly.

OVERDOSAGE

Serious overdosage with DILAUDID-HP is characterized by respiratory depression, somnolence progressing to stupor or coma, skeletal muscle flaccidity, cold and clammy skin, constricted pupils, and sometimes bradycardia and hypotension. In serious overdosage, particularly following intravenous injection, apnea, circulatory collapse, cardiac arrest and death may occur.

* Hallucinations, although unusual with pure agonist narcotics, have been observed in one patient following both a 6 mg and a 4 mg DILAUDID-HP dose. However, the patient was receiving several concomitant medications during the second episode and a causal relationship cannot be established.

In the treatment of overdosage primary attention should be given to the reestablishment of adequate respiratory exchange through provision of a patent airway and institution of assisted or controlled ventilation.

NARCOTIC-TOLERANT PATIENT: Since tolerance to the respiratory and CNS depressant effects of narcotics develops concomitantly with tolerance to their analgesic effects, serious respiratory depression due to an acute overdose is unlikely to be seen in narcotic-tolerant patients receiving DILAUDID-HP for chronic pain.

NOTE: In such an individual who is physically dependent on narcotics, administration of the usual dose of the antagonist will precipitate an acute withdrawal syndrome. The severity will depend on the degree of physical dependence and the dose of the antagonist administered. Use of a narcotic antagonist in such a person should be avoided. If necessary to treat serious respiratory depression in the physically-dependent patient, the antagonist should be administered with extreme care and by titration with smaller than usual doses of the antagonist.

NON-TOLERANT PATIENT: The narcotic antagonist, naloxone, is a specific antidote against respiratory depression which may result from overdosage, or unusual sensitivity to DILAUDID-HP. A dose of naloxone (usually 0.4 to 2.0 mg) should be administered intravenously, if possible, simultaneously with respiratory resuscitation. The dose can be repeated in 3 minutes. Naloxone should not be administered in the absence of clinically significant respiratory or circulatory depression. Naloxone should be administered cautiously to persons who are known, or suspected to be physically dependent on DILAUDID-HP. In such cases, an abrupt or complete reversal of narcotic effects may precipitate an acute abstinence syndrome.

Since the duration of action of DILAUDID may exceed that of the antagonist, the patient should be kept under continued surveillance; repeated doses of the antagonist may be required to maintain adequate respiration. Apply other supportive measures when indicated.

Supportive measures (including oxygen, vasopressors) should be employed in the management of circulatory shock and pulmonary edema accompanying overdose as indicated. Cardiac arrest or arrhythmias may require cardiac massage or defibrillation.

DOSAGE AND ADMINISTRATION

Parenteral: **DILAUDID-HP SHOULD BE GIVEN ONLY TO PATIENTS WHO ARE ALREADY RECEIVING LARGE DOSES OF NARCOTICS.** DILAUDID-HP is indicated for relief of moderate-to-severe pain in narcotic-tolerant patients. Thus, these patients will already have been treated with other narcotic analgesics. If the patient is being changed from regular DILAUDID to DILAUDID-HP, similar doses should be used, depending on the patient's clinical response to the drug. If DILAUDID-HP is substituted for a different narcotic analgesic, the following equivalency table should be used as a guide to determine the appropriate starting dose of DILAUDID-HP (hydromorphone hydrochloride). [See table above.]

In open clinical trials with DILAUDID-HP in patients with terminal cancer, doses ranged from 1–14 mg subcutaneously or intramuscularly; one patient received 30 mg subcutaneously on two occasions. In these trials, both subcutaneous and intramuscular injections of DILAUDID-HP were well-tolerated, with minimal pain and/or burning at the injection site. Mild erythema was rarely noted after intramuscular injection. There was no induration after either intramuscular or subcutaneous administration of DILAUDID-HP. Subcutaneous injections of DILAUDID-HP were particularly well accepted when administered with a short, 30-gauge needle.

Experience with administration of DILAUDID-HP by the intravenous route is limited. Should intravenous administration be necessary, the injection should be given slowly, over at least 2 to 3 minutes. The intravenous route is usually painless.

A gradual increase in dose may be required if analgesia is inadequate, tolerance occurs, or if pain severity increases. The first sign of tolerance is usually a reduced duration of effect.

NOTE: Parenteral drug products should be inspected visually for particulate matter and discoloration prior to administration, whenever solution and container permit. A slight yellowish discoloration may develop in DILAUDID-HP ampules. No loss of potency has been demonstrated. Dilaudid injection is physically compatible and chemically stable for at least 24 hours at 25°C protected from light in most common large volume parenteral solutions.

500mg/50mL Vial: To use this single dose presentation, do not penetrate the stopper with a syringe. Instead, remove both the aluminum flipseal and rubber stopper in a suitable work area such as under a laminar flow hood (or equivalent clean air compounding area). The contents may then be withdrawn for preparation of a single, large volume parenteral solution. Any unused portion should be discarded in an appropriate manner.

STRONG ANALGESICS AND STRUCTURALLY RELATED DRUGS USED IN THE TREATMENT OF CANCER PAIN*

IM or SC Administration

Nonproprietary (Trade) Names	Dose, mg Equianalgesic to 10 mg of IM Morphine†	Duration Compared With Morphine
Morphine sulfate	10	Same
Papaveretum (Pantopon)	20	Same
Hydromorphone hydrochloride (DILAUDID)	1.3	Slightly shorter
Oxymorphone hydrochloride (Numorphan)	1.1	Slightly shorter
Nalbuphine hydrochloride (Nubain)	12	Same
Heroin, diamorphine hydrochloride (NA in U.S.)	4–5	Slightly shorter
Levorphanol tartrate (Levo-Dromoran)	2.3	Same
Butorphanol tartrate (Stadol)	1.5–2.5	Same
Pentazocine lactate or hydrochloride (Talwin)	60	Shorter
Meperidine, pethidine hydrochloride (Demerol)	80	Shorter
Methadone hydrochloride (Dolophine)	10	Same

*From Beaver WT. Management of cancer pain with parenteral medication. J. Am. Med. Assoc. 244:2653–2657 (1980).
†(In terms of the area under the analgesic time-effect curve.)

HOW SUPPLIED

DILAUDID-HP _amber_ ampules contain 10 mg hydromorphone hydrochloride per mL with 0.2% sodium citrate and 0.2% citric acid solution. No added preservative.

NOTE: DILAUDID-HP ampules are _amber_ in color and marked with a distinctive identification band.

HIGH POTENCY

10 mg/mL—Box of 10 ampules
      NDC 0044 1017-10
*50 mg/5 mL—Box of 10 ampules
      NDC 0044 1017-25
*500 mg/50 mL
Single Dose Vial NDC 0044-1017-06

*FOR USE IN THE PREPARATION OF LARGE VOLUME PARENTERAL SOLUTIONS

STORAGE

Parenteral forms of DILAUDID should be stored at 59°–86°F, (15–30°C). Protect from light.

DEA Order Form Required
A Schedule Ⓒ Narcotic.
August 1991   6750A

Manufactured for
Knoll Pharmaceuticals
A Unit of BASF K & F Corporation
Whippany, NJ 07981
By Sterling Drug, Inc.
McPherson, KS 67460
Shown in Product Identification Section, page 413

ISOPTIN®   ℞
[ī-sŏp "tĭn]
(verapamil hydrochloride)
Intravenous Injection

DESCRIPTION

ISOPTIN® (verapamil hydrochloride) is a calcium antagonist or slow channel inhibitor. ISOPTIN is available in 5 mg/2 mL and 10 mg/4 mL ampules, 5 mg/2 mL and 10 mg/4 mL single dose vials (for intravenous administration). Each 1 mL of solution contains 2.5 mg verapamil HCl and 8.5 mg sodium chloride in water for injection. Hydrochloric acid and/or sodium hydroxide is used for pH adjustment. The pH of the solution is between 4.1 and 6.0. Protect contents from light. ISOPTIN ampules, and vials are sterile. The structural formula of verapamil HCl is given below:

$C_{27}H_{38}N_2O_4 \cdot$ HCl   M.W. = 491.08
Benzeneacetonitrile, α-[3-[[2-(3,4-dimethoxyphenyl) ethyl] methylamino]propyl]-3,4-dimethoxy-α-(1-methylethyl) hydrochloride

Verapamil HCl is an almost white, crystalline powder, practically free of odor, with a bitter taste. It is soluble in water, chloroform and methanol. Verapamil HCl is not chemically related to other antiarrhythmic drugs.

CLINICAL PHARMACOLOGY

Mechanism of Action: ISOPTIN (verapamil HCl) inhibits the calcium ion (and possibly sodium ion) influx through slow channels into conductile and contractile myocardial cells and vascular smooth muscle cells. The antiarrhythmic effect of ISOPTIN appears to be due to its effect on the slow channel in cells of the cardiac conduction system. The vasodilatory effect of ISOPTIN appears to be due to its effect on blockade of calcium channels as well as α-receptors.

In the isolated rabbit heart, concentrations of ISOPTIN that markedly affect SA nodal fibers or fibers in the upper and middle regions of the AV node, have very little effect on fibers in the lower AV node (NH region) and no effect on atrial action potentials or His bundle fibers.

Electrical activity in the SA and AV nodes depends, to a large degree, upon calcium influx through the slow channel. By inhibiting this influx, ISOPTIN slows AV conduction and prolongs the effective refractory period within the AV node in a rate-related manner. This effect results in a reduction of the ventricular rate in patients with atrial flutter and/or atrial fibrillation and a rapid ventricular response.

By interrupting reentry at the AV node, ISOPTIN can restore normal sinus rhythm in patients with paroxysmal supraventricular tachycardias (PSVT), including PSVT associated with Wolff-Parkinson-White syndrome.

ISOPTIN does not induce peripheral arterial spasm.

ISOPTIN has a local anesthetic action that is 1.6 times that of procaine on an equimolar basis. It is not known whether this action is important at the doses used in man.

ISOPTIN does not alter total serum calcium levels.

Hemodynamics: ISOPTIN (verapamil HCl) reduces afterload and myocardial contractility. The commonly used intravenous doses of 5–10 mg ISOPTIN produce transient, usually asymptomatic, reduction in normal systemic arterial pressure, systemic vascular resistance and contractility; left ventricular filling pressure is slightly increased. In most patients, including those with organic cardiac disease, the negative inotropic action of ISOPTIN is countered by reduction of afterload, and cardiac index is usually not reduced. However, in patients with moderately severe to severe cardiac dysfunction (pulmonary wedge pressure above 20 mm Hg, ejection fraction less than 30%), acute worsening of heart failure may be seen. Peak therapeutic effects occur within 3 to 5 minutes after a bolus injection.

Pharmacokinetics: Intravenously administered ISOPTIN (verapamil HCl) has been shown to be rapidly metabolized. Following intravenous infusion in man, verapamil is eliminated biexponentially, with a rapid early distribution phase (half-life about 4 minutes) and a slower terminal elimination phase (half-life 2–5 hours). In healthy men, orally administered ISOPTIN undergoes extensive metabolism in the liver; 12 metabolites having been identified, most in only trace amounts. The major metabolites have been identified as

Continued on next page

Knoll—Cont.

various N- and O-dealkylated products of ISOPTIN. Approximately 70% of an administered dose is excreted in the urine and 16% or more in the feces within 5 days. About 3–4% is excreted as unchanged drug.
Aging may affect the pharmacokinetics of verapamil given to hypertensive patients. Elimination half-life may be prolonged in the elderly.

INDICATIONS AND USAGE

ISOPTIN (verapamil HCl) is indicated for the following:

- Rapid conversion to sinus rhythm of paroxysmal supraventricular tachycardias, including those associated with accessory bypass tracts (Wolff-Parkinson-White [W-P-W] and Lown-Ganong-Levine [L-G-L] syndromes). When clinically advisable, appropriate vagal maneuvers (e.g. Valsalva maneuver) should be attempted prior to ISOPTIN administration.
- Temporary control of rapid ventricular rate in atrial flutter or atrial fibrillation **except** when the atrial flutter and/or atrial fibrillation are associated with accessory bypass tracts (Wolff-Parkinson-White [W-P-W] and Lown-Ganong-Levine [L-G-L] syndromes).

In controlled studies in the United States, about 60% of patients with supraventricular tachycardia converted to normal sinus rhythm within 10 minutes after intravenous ISOPTIN. Uncontrolled studies reported in the world literature describe a conversion rate of about 80%. About 70% of patients with atrial flutter and/or fibrillation with a fast ventricular rate respond with a decrease in ventricular rate of at least 20%. Conversion of atrial flutter or fibrillation to sinus rhythm is uncommon (about 10%) after ISOPTIN and may reflect the spontaneous conversion rate, since the conversion rate after placebo was similar. Slowing of the ventricular rate in patients with atrial fibrillation/flutter lasts 30–60 minutes after a single injection.

Because a small fraction (< 1.0%) of patients treated with ISOPTIN respond with life-threatening adverse responses (rapid ventricular rate in atrial flutter/fibrillation and an accessory bypass tract, marked hypotension, or extreme bradycardia/asystole—see Contraindications and Warnings), the initial use of intravenous ISOPTIN should, if possible, be in a treatment setting with monitoring and resuscitation facilities, including DC-cardioversion capability (see Suggested Treatment of Acute Cardiovascular Adverse Reactions). As familiarity with the patient's response is gained, use in an office setting may be acceptable.

Cardioversion has been used safely and effectively after intravenous ISOPTIN.

CONTRAINDICATIONS

ISOPTIN (verapamil HCl) is contraindicated in:

1. Severe hypotension or cardiogenic shock
2. Second- or third-degree AV block (except in patients with a functioning artificial ventricular pacemaker)
3. Sick sinus syndrome (except in patients with a functioning artificial ventricular pacemaker)
4. Severe congestive heart failure (unless secondary to a supraventricular tachycardia amenable to verapamil therapy)
5. Patients receiving **intravenous** beta adrenergic blocking drugs (e.g., propranolol). **Intravenous** verapamil and **intravenous** beta adrenergic blocking drugs should not be administered in close proximity to each other (within a few hours), since both may have a depressant effect on myocardial contractility and AV conduction.
6. Patients with atrial flutter or atrial fibrillation and an accessory bypass tract (e.g. Wolff-Parkinson-White, Lown-Ganong-Levine syndromes) are at risk to develop ventricular tachyarrhythmia including ventricular fibrillation if verapamil is administered. Therefore the use of verapamil in these patients is contraindicated.
7. Ventricular Tachycardia. Administration of intravenous verapamil to patients with wide-complex ventricular tachycardia (QRS ≥0.12 sec) can result in marked hemodynamic deterioration and ventricular fibrillation. Proper pre-therapy diagnosis and differentiation from wide complex supraventricular tachycardia is imperative in the emergency room setting.
8. Known hypersensitivity to verapamil hydrochloride.

WARNINGS

ISOPTIN SHOULD BE GIVEN AS A SLOW INTRAVENOUS INJECTION OVER AT LEAST A TWO MINUTE PERIOD OF TIME. (See Dosage and Administration)

Hypotension: Intravenous ISOPTIN (verapamil HCl) often produces a decrease in blood pressure below baseline levels that is usually transient and asymptomatic but may result in dizziness. Administration of intravenous calcium chloride prior to intravenous administration of verapamil may prevent this hemodynamic response. Systolic pressure less than 90 mm Hg and/or diastolic pressure less than 60 mm Hg was seen in 5–10% of patients in controlled U.S. trials in supraventricular tachycardia and in about 10% of the patients with atrial flutter/fibrillation. The incidence of symptomatic hypotension observed in studies conducted in the U.S. was approximately 1.5%. Three of the five symptomatic patients required intravenous pharmacologic treatment (levarterenol bitartrate, metaraminol bitartrate, or 10% calcium gluconate). All recovered without sequelae.

Extreme Bradycardia/Asystole: ISOPTIN (verapamil HCl) affects the AV and SA nodes and rarely may produce second- or third-degree AV block, bradycardia and, in extreme cases, asystole. This is more likely to occur in patients with a sick sinus syndrome (SA nodal disease), which is more common in older patients. Bradycardia associated with sick sinus syndrome was reported in 0.3% of the patients treated in controlled double-blind trials in the United States. The total incidence of bradycardia (ventricular rate less than 60 beats/min) was 1.2% in these studies. Asystole in patients other than those with sick sinus syndrome is usually of short duration (few seconds or less), with spontaneous return to AV nodal or normal sinus rhythm. If this does not occur promptly, appropriate treatment should be initiated immediately. (See Adverse Reactions and Treatment of Adverse Reactions.)

Heart Failure: When heart failure is not severe or rate related, it should be controlled with digitalis glycosides and diuretics, as appropriate, before ISOPTIN is used. In patients with moderately severe to severe cardiac dysfunction (pulmonary wedge pressure above 20 mm Hg, ejection fraction less than 30%), acute worsening of heart failure may be seen.

Concomitant Antiarrhythmic Therapy:

Digitalis: Intravenous verapamil has been used concomitantly with digitalis preparations without the occurrence of serious adverse effects. However, since both drugs slow AV conduction, patients should be monitored for AV block or excessive bradycardia.

Procainamide: Intravenous verapamil has been administered to a small number of patients receiving oral procainamide without the occurrence of serious adverse effects.

Quinidine: Intravenous verapamil has been administered to a small number of patients receiving oral Quinidine without the occurrence of serious adverse effects. However, three patients have been described in whom the combination resulted in an exaggerated hypotensive response presumably from the combined ability of both drugs to antagonize the effects of catecholamines on α-adrenergic receptors. Caution should therefore be used when employing this combination of drugs.

Beta Adrenergic Blocking Drugs: Intravenous verapamil has been administered to patients receiving oral beta blockers without the development of serious adverse effects. However, since both drugs may depress myocardial contractility or AV conduction, the possibility of detrimental interactions should be considered. The concomitant administration of **intravenous** beta blockers and **intravenous** verapamil has resulted in serious adverse reactions (see Contraindications), especially in patients with severe cardiomyopathy, congestive heart failure or recent myocardial infarction.

Disopyramide: Until data on possible interactions between verapamil and all forms of disopyramide phosphate are obtained, disopyramide should not be administered within 48 hours before or 24 hours after verapamil administration.

Flecainide: A study in healthy volunteers showed that the concomitant administration of flecainide and verapamil have additive effects on myocardial contractility, AV conduction, and repolarization. Concomitant therapy with flecainide and verapamil may result in additive negative inotropic effect and prolongation of atrioventricular conduction.

Heart Block: ISOPTIN (verapamil HCl) prolongs AV conduction time. While high degree AV block has not been observed in controlled clinical trials in the U.S., a low percentage (less than 0.5%) has been reported in the world literature. Development of second- or third-degree AV block or unifascicular, bifascicular or trifascicular bundle branch block requires reduction in subsequent doses or discontinuation of verapamil and institution of appropriate therapy, if needed. (See Treatment of Acute Cardiovascular Adverse Reactions.)

Hepatic and Renal Failure: Significant hepatic and renal failure should not increase the effects of a single intravenous dose of ISOPTIN (verapamil HCl) but may prolong its duration. Repeated injections of intravenous ISOPTIN in such patients may lead to accumulation and an excessive pharmacologic effect of the drug. There is no experience to guide use of multiple doses in such patients and this generally should be avoided. If repeated injections are essential, blood pressure and PR interval should be closely monitored and smaller repeat doses should be utilized. Verapamil cannot be removed by hemodialysis.

Premature Ventricular Contractions: During conversion to normal sinus rhythm, or marked reduction in ventricular rate, a few benign complexes of unusual appearance (sometimes resembling premature ventricular contractions) may be seen after treatment with ISOPTIN (verapamil HCl). Similar complexes are seen during spontaneous conversion of supraventricular tachycardias, after DC-cardioversion and other pharmacologic therapy. These complexes appear to have no clinical significance.

Duchenne's Muscular Dystrophy: Intravenous ISOPTIN (verapamil HCl) can precipitate respiratory muscle failure in these patients and should, therefore, be used with caution.

Increased Intracranial Pressure: Intravenous ISOPTIN (verapamil HCl) has been seen to increase intracranial pressure in patients with supratentorial tumors at the time of anesthesia induction. Caution should be taken and appropriate monitoring performed.

PRECAUTIONS

Drug Interactions: (See Warnings: Concomitant Antiarrhythmic Therapy) Intravenous ISOPTIN (verapamil HCl) has been used concomitantly with other cardioactive drugs (especially digitalis) without evidence of serious negative drug interactions. In rare instances, when patients with severe cardiomyopathy, congestive heart failure or recent myocardial infarction were given **intravenous** beta-adrenergic blocking agents or disopyramide concomitantly with intravenous verapamil, serious adverse effects have occurred. Concomitant use of ISOPTIN with α-adrenergic blockers may result in an exaggerated hypotensive response. Such an effect was observed in one study following the concomitant administrtation of verapamil and prazosin. As verapamil is highly bound to plasma proteins, it should be administered with caution to patients receiving other highly protein bound drugs.

Other

Cimetidine: The interaction between cimetidine and chronically administered verapamil has not been studied. Variable results on clearance have been obtained in acute studies of healthy volunteers; clearance of verapamil was either reduced or unchanged.

Lithium: Pharmacokinetic and pharmacodynamic interactions between oral verapamil and lithium have been reported. The former may result in a lowering of serum lithium levels in patients receiving chronic stable oral lithium therapy. The latter may result in an increased sensitivity to the effects of lithium. Patients receiving both drugs must be monitored carefully.

Carbamazephine: Verapamil therapy may increase carbamazepine concentrations during combined therapy. This may produce carbamazepine side effects such as diplopia, headache, ataxia, or dizziness.

Rifampin: Therapy with rifampin may markedly reduce oral verapamil bioavailability.

Phenobarbital: Phenobarbital therapy may increase verapamil clearance.

Cyclosporin: Verapamil therapy may increase serum levels of cyclosporin.

Inhalation Anesthetics: Animal experiments have shown that inhalation anesthetics depress cardiovascular activity by decreasing the inward movement of calcium ions. When used concomitantly, inhalation anesthetics and calcium antagonists, such as verapamil, should be titrated carefully to avoid excessive cardiovascular depression.

Neuromuscular Blocking Agents: Clinical data and animal studies suggested that verapamil may potentiate the activity of neuromuscular blocking agents (curare-like and depolarizing). It may be necessary to decrease the dose of verapamil and/or the dose of neuromuscular blocking agent when the drugs are used concomitantly.

Dantrolene: Two animal studies suggest concomitant use of intravenous verapamil and intravenous dantrolene sodium may result in cardiovascular collapse. There has been one report of hyperkalemia and myocardial depression following the coadministration of oral verapamil and intravenous dantrolene.

Pregnancy: Pregnancy Category C. Reproduction studies have been performed in rabbits and rats at oral verapamil doses up to 1.5 (15 mg/kg/day) and 6 (60 mg/kg/day) times the human oral daily dose, respectively, and have revealed no evidence of teratogenicity. In the rat, however, this multiple of the human dose was embryocidal and retarded fetal growth and development, probably because of adverse maternal effects reflected in reduced weight gains of the dams. This oral dose has also been shown to cause hypotension in rats. There are no adequate and well-controlled studies in pregnant women. Because animal reproduction studies are not always predictive of human response, this drug should be used during pregnancy only if clearly needed.

Labor and Delivery: There have been few controlled studies to determine whether the use of verapamil during labor or delivery has immediate or delayed adverse effects on the fetus, or whether it prolongs the duration of labor or increases the need for forceps delivery or other obstetric intervention. Such adverse experiences have not been reported in the literature, despite a long history of use of intravenous ISOPTIN in Europe in the treatment of cardiac side effects of beta-adrenergic agonist agents used to treat premature labor.

Nursing Mothers: ISOPTIN crosses the placental barrier and can be detected in umbilical vein blood at delivery. Also, ISOPTIN is excreted in human milk. Because of the potential for adverse reactions in nursing infants from verapamil,

Suggested Treatment of Acute Cardiovascular Adverse Reactions*
The frequency of these adverse reactions was quite low and experience with their treatment has been limited.

Adverse Reaction	Proven Effective Treatment	Supportive Treatment
1. Symptomatic hypotension requiring treatment	Calcium chloride (IV) Levarterenol bitartrate (IV) Metaraminol bitartrate (IV) Isoproterenol HCl (IV) Dopamine (IV)	Intravenous fluids Trendelenburg position
2. Bradycardia, AV block, Asystole	Isoproterenol HCl (IV) Calcium chloride (IV) Cardiac pacing Levarterenol bitartrate (IV) Atropine (IV)	Intravenous fluids (slow drip)
3. Rapid ventricular rate (due to antegrade conduction in flutter/fibrillation with W-P-W or L-G-L syndromes)	DC-cardioversion (high energy may be required) Procainamide (IV) Lidocaine (IV)	Intravenous fluids (slow drip)

* Actual treatment and dosage should depend on the severity of the clinical situation and the judgment and experience of the treating physician.

nursing should be discontinued while verapamil is administered.

Pediatrics: Controlled studies with verapamil have not been conducted in pediatric patients, but uncontrolled experience with intravenous administration in more than 250 patients, about half under 12 months of age and about 25% newborn, indicates that results of treatment are similar to those in adults. **However, in rare instances, severe hemodynamic side effects have occurred, which can be fatal, following the intravenous administration of verapamil in neonates and infants. Caution should therefore be used when administering verapamil to this group of pediatric patients.**

The most commonly used single doses in patients up to 12 months of age have ranged from 0.1 to 0.2 mg/kg of body weight, while in patients aged 1 to 15 years, the most commonly used single doses ranged from 0.1 to 0.3 mg/kg of body weight. Most of the patients received the lower dose of 0.1 mg/kg once but, in some cases, the dose was repeated once or twice every 10 to 30 minutes.

ADVERSE REACTIONS
The following reactions were reported with intravenous ISOPTIN (verapamil HCl) use in controlled U.S. clinical trials involving 324 patients:

Cardiovascular: Symptomatic hypotension (1.5%); bradycardia (1.2%); severe tachycardia (1.0%). The worldwide experience in open clinical trials in more than 7,900 patients was similar.

Central Nervous System Effects: Dizziness (1.2%); headache (1.2%). Occasional cases of seizures during verapamil injection have been reported.

Gastrointestinal: Nausea (0.9%); abdominal discomfort (0.6%).

In rare cases of hypersensitive patients, broncho/laryngeal spasm accompanied by itch and urticaria have been reported.

The following reactions were reported in a few patients: emotional depression, rotary nystagmus, sleepiness, vertigo, muscle fatigue, diaphoresis or respiratory failure.
[See table above.]

OVERDOSAGE
Treatment of overdosage should be supportive and individualized. Beta-adrenergic stimulation and/or parenteral administration of calcium solutions may increase calcium ion flux across the slow channel, and have been effectively used in treatment of deliberate overdosage with oral ISOPTIN (verapamil HCL). Verapamil cannot be removed by hemodialysis. Clinically significant hypotensive reactions or high degree AV block should be treated with vasopressor agents or cardiac pacing, respectively. Asystole should be handled by the usual measures including isoproterenol hydrochloride, other vasopressor agents or cardiopulmonary resuscitation. (See Treatment of Cardiovascular Adverse Reactions.)

DOSAGE AND ADMINISTRATION
(For Intravenous Use Only): ISOPTIN SHOULD BE GIVEN AS A SLOW INTRAVENOUS INJECTION OVER AT LEAST A TWO MINUTE PERIOD OF TIME UNDER CONTINUOUS ELECTROCARDIOGRAPHIC AND BLOOD PRESSURE MONITORING.
The recommended intravenous doses of ISOPTIN are as follows:
ADULT: Initial dose: 5–10 mg (0.075–0.15 mg/kg body weight) given as an intravenous bolus over at least 2 minutes.
Repeat dose: 10 mg (0.15 mg/kg body weight) 30 minutes after the first dose if the initial response is not adequate.

An optimal interval for subsequent I.V. doses has not been determined, and should be individualized for each patient.
Older Patients: The dose should be administered over at least 3 minutes to minimize the risk of untoward drug effects.
PEDIATRIC: Initial dose:
0–1 year: 0.1–0.2 mg/kg body weight (usual single dose range 0.75–2 mg) should be administered as an intravenous bolus over at least 2 minutes **under continuous ECG monitoring.**
1–15 years: 0.1–0.3 mg/kg body weight (usual single dose range 2–5 mg) should be administered as an intravenous bolus over at least 2 minutes. **Do not exceed 5 mg.**
Repeat dose:
0–1 year: 0.1–0.2 mg/kg body weight (usual single dose range 0.75–2 mg) 30 minutes after the first dose if the initial response is not adequate **(under continuous ECG monitoring).** An optimal interval for subsequent I.V. doses has not been determined, and should be individualized for each patient.
1–15 years: 0.1–0.3 mg/kg body weight (usual single dose range 2–5 mg) 30 minutes after the first dose if the initial response is not adequate. **Do not exceed 10 mg as a single dose.** An optimal interval for subsequent I.V. doses has not been determined, and should be individualized for each patient.

NOTE
Parenteral drug products should be inspected visually for particulate matter and discoloration prior to administration, whenever solution and container permit. ISOPTIN is physically compatible and chemically stable for at least 24 hours at 25°C protected from light in most common large volume parenteral solutions. Admixing ISOPTIN with albumin, amphotericin B, hydralazine HCl and trimethoprim with sulfamethoxazole should be avoided. ISOPTIN will precipitate in any solution with a pH above 6.0.

HOW SUPPLIED
Each 1 mL of sterile solution contains 2.5 mg verapamil HCl and 8.5 mg sodium chloride. pH adjusted with hydrochloric acid and/or sodium hydroxide.
5 mg/2 mL ampule—Individual unit carton—NDC 0044-1815-01
  Space saver pack of 10 ampules—NDC 0044-1815-05
5 mg/2 mL vial—Single dose. No preservative. Individual unit carton—NDC 0044-1816-21
10 mg/4 mL ampule—Individual unit carton—NDC 0044-1815-11
  Space saver pack of 10 ampules—NDC 0044-1815-15
10 mg/4 mL vial—Single dose. No preservative. Individual unit carton—NDC 0044-1816-41
Storage: 59°–86°F (15°–30°C). Protect from light.
MR 1988/1207
RE-4m/Iso 1212B-1213B/11-14-90
Revised May, 1990   1212
Shown in Product Identification Section, pages 413 and 414

ISOPTIN®   ℞
[ĭ-sŏp″tĭn]
(verapamil hydrochloride)
Oral Tablets

DESCRIPTION
ISOPTIN (verapamil hydrochloride) is a calcium ion influx inhibitor (slow channel blocker or calcium ion antagonist). ISOPTIN is available for oral administration as round, scored, film-coated tablets containing 40 mg, 80 mg or 120 mg of verapamil hydrochloride.

The structural formula of verapamil HCl is given below:

$C_{27}H_{38}N_2O_4 \cdot HCl$ M.W. = 491.08
Benzeneacetonitrile,
α-[3-[[2-(3,4-dimethoxyphenyl) ethyl] methylamino]
propyl]-3,4-dimethoxy-α-(1-methylethyl) hydrochloride

Verapamil HCl is an almost white, crystalline powder, practically free of odor, with a bitter taste. It is soluble in water, chloroform and methanol. Verapamil HCl is not chemically related to other cardioactive drugs.
In addition to verapamil HCl, ISOPTIN tablets may contain: colloidal silicon dioxide, corn starch, dibasic calcium phosphate, lactose, gelatin, microcrystalline cellulose, sodium carboxymethylcellulose, talc, and magnesium stearate. The film coating used for ISOPTIN 40mg, 80mg and 120mg tablets contains hydroxypropyl methylcellulose, polyethylene glycol, propylene glycol, titanium dioxide and polysorbate 80. The ISOPTIN 80mg tablets also contain D&C yellow #10 Lake dye. The ISOPTIN 40mg tablet contains FD&C blue #2 Aluminum Lake dye.

CLINICAL PHARMACOLOGY
ISOPTIN is a calcium ion influx inhibitor (slow channel blocker or calcium ion antagonist) that exerts its pharmacologic effects by modulating the influx of ionic calcium across the cell membrane of the arterial smooth muscle as well as in conductile and contractile myocardial cells.
Mechanism of Action
Angina
The precise mechanism of action of ISOPTIN as an antianginal agent remains to be fully determined, but includes the following two mechanisms:
1. **Relaxation and prevention of coronary artery spasm**
   ISOPTIN dilates the main coronary arteries and coronary arterioles, both in normal and ischemic regions, and is a potent inhibitor of coronary artery spasm, whether spontaneous or ergonovine-induced. This property increases myocardial oxygen delivery in patients with coronary artery spasm, and is responsible for the effectiveness of ISOPTIN in vasospastic (Prinzmetal's or variant) as well as unstable angina at rest. Whether this effect plays any role in classical effort angina is not clear, but studies of exercise tolerance have not shown an increase in the maximum exercise rate-pressure product, a widely accepted measure of oxygen utilization. This suggests that, in general, relief of spasm or dilation of coronary arteries is not an important factor in classical angina.
2. **Reduction of oxygen utilization**
   ISOPTIN regularly reduces the total peripheral resistance (afterload) against which the heart works both at rest and at a given level of exercise by dilating peripheral arterioles. This unloading of the heart reduces myocardial energy consumption and oxygen requirements and probably accounts for the effectiveness of ISOPTIN in chronic stable effort angina.

Arrhythmia
Electrical activity through the AV node depends, to a significant degree, upon calcium influx through the slow channel. By decreasing the influx of calcium, ISOPTIN prolongs the effective refractory period within the AV node and slows AV conduction in a rate-related manner. This property accounts for the ability of ISOPTIN to slow the ventricular rate in patients with chronic atrial flutter or atrial fibrillation. Normal sinus rhythm is usually not affected, but in patients with sick sinus syndrome, ISOPTIN may interfere with sinus node impulse generation and may induce sinus arrest, or sinoatrial block. Atrioventricular block can occur in patients without preexisting conduction defects (see WARNINGS). ISOPTIN decreases the frequency of episodes of paroxysmal supraventricular tachycardia.
ISOPTIN does not alter the normal atrial action potential or intraventricular conduction time, but in depressed atrial fibers it decreases amplitude, velocity of depolarization and conduction velocity. ISOPTIN may shorten the antegrade effective refractory period of accessory bypass tracts. Acceleration of ventricular rate and/or ventricular fibrillation has been reported in patients with atrial flutter or atrial fibrillation and a coexisting accessory AV pathway following administration of verapamil (see WARNINGS).
ISOPTIN has a local anesthetic action that is 1.6 times that of procaine on an equimolar basis. It is not known whether this action is important at the doses used in man.

Continued on next page

Knoll—Cont.

Essential Hypertension

ISOPTIN exerts antihypertensive effects by decreasing systemic vascular resistance usually without orthostatic decreases in blood pressure or reflex tachycardia; bradycardia (rate less than 50 beats/min) is uncommon (1.4%). During isometric or dynamic exercise ISOPTIN does not alter systolic cardiac function in patients with normal ventricular function.

ISOPTIN does not alter total serum calcium levels. However, one report suggested that calcium levels above the normal range may alter the therapeutic effect of ISOPTIN.

Pharmacokinetics and Metabolism: More than 90% of the orally administered dose of ISOPTIN is absorbed. Because of rapid biotransformation of verapamil during its first pass through the portal circulation, bioavailability ranges from 20% to 35%. Peak plasma concentrations are reached between 1 and 2 hours after oral administration. Chronic oral administration of 120 mg of ISOPTIN every 6 hours resulted in plasma levels of verapamil ranging from 125 to 400 ng/mL with higher values reported occasionally. A nonlinear correlation between the verapamil dose administered and verapamil plasma levels does exist.

In early dose titration with verapamil a relationship exists between verapamil plasma concentrations and the prolongation of the PR interval. However, during chronic administration this relationship may disappear. The mean elimination half-life in single dose studies ranged from 2.8 to 7.4 hours. In these same studies, after repetitive dosing, the half-life increased to a range from 4.5 to 12.0 hours (after less than 10 consecutive doses given 6 hours apart). Half-life of verapamil may increase during titration. Aging may affect the pharmacokinetics of verapamil. Elimination half-life may be prolonged in the elderly.

In healthy men, orally administered ISOPTIN undergoes extensive metabolism in the liver. Twelve metabolites have been identified in plasma; all except norverapamil are present in trace amounts only. Norverapamil can reach steady-state plasma concentrations approximately equal to those of verapamil itself. The cardiovascular activity of norverapamil appears to be approximately 20% that of verapamil. Approximately 70% of an administered dose is excreted as metabolites in the urine and 16% or more in the feces within 5 days. About 3% to 4% is excreted in the urine as unchanged drug. Approximately 90% is bound to plasma proteins. In patients with hepatic insufficiency, metabolism is delayed and elimination half-life prolonged up to 14 to 16 hours (see PRECAUTIONS); the volume of distribution is increased and plasma clearance reduced to about 30% of normal. Verapamil clearance values suggest that patients with liver dysfunction may attain therapeutic verapamil plasma concentrations with one-third of the oral daily dose required for patients with normal liver function.

After four weeks of oral dosing (120 mg q.i.d.), verapamil and norverapamil levels were noted in the cerebrospinal fluid with estimated partition coefficient of 0.06 for verapamil and 0.04 for norverapamil.

Hemodynamics and Myocardial Metabolism: ISOPTIN reduces afterload and myocardial contractility. Improved left ventricular diastolic function in patients with IHSS and those with coronary heart disease has also been observed with ISOPTIN therapy. In most patients, including those with organic cardiac disease, the negative inotropic action of ISOPTIN is countered by reduction of afterload and cardiac index is usually not reduced. However, in patients with severe left ventricular dysfunction (e.g., pulmonary wedge pressure above 20 mmHg or ejection fraction lower than 30%), or in patients on beta-adrenergic blocking agents or other cardiodepressant drugs, deterioration of ventricular function may occur (see DRUG INTERACTIONS).

Pulmonary Function: ISOPTIN does not induce bronchoconstriction and hence, does not impair ventilatory function.

INDICATIONS AND USAGE

ISOPTIN tablets are indicated for the treatment of the following:

Angina
1. Angina at rest including:
   - Vasospastic (Prinzmetal's, variant) angina
   - Unstable (crescendo, pre-infarction) angina
2. Chronic stable angina (classic effort-associated angina)

Arrhythmias
1. In association with digitalis, for the control of ventricular rate at rest and during stress in patients with chronic atrial flutter and/or atrial fibrillation (see WARNINGS: Accessory Bypass Tract)
2. Prophylaxis of repetitive paroxysmal supraventricular tachycardia

Essential Hypertension

CONTRAINDICATIONS

Verapamil HCl tablets are contraindicated in:
1. Severe left ventricular dysfunction (see WARNINGS)

2. Hypotension (systolic pressure less than 90 mmHg) or cardiogenic shock
3. Sick sinus syndrome (except in patients with a functioning artificial ventricular pacemaker)
4. Second- or third-degree AV block (except in patients with a functioning artificial ventricular pacemaker)
5. Patients with atrial flutter or atrial fibrillation and an accessory bypass tract (e.g., Wolff-Parkinson-White, Lown-Ganong-Levine syndromes) (see Warnings)
6. Patients with known hypersensitivity to verapamil hydrochloride

WARNINGS

Heart Failure: Verapamil has a negative inotropic effect which, in most patients, is compensated by its afterload reduction (decreased systemic vascular resistance) properties without a net impairment of ventricular performance. In clinical experience with 4,954 patients, 87 (1.8%) developed congestive heart failure or pulmonary edema. Verapamil should be avoided in patients with severe left ventricular dysfunction (e.g., pulmonary wedge pressure above 20 mmHg or ejection fraction less than 30%) or moderate to severe symptoms of cardiac failure and in patients with any degree of ventricular dysfunction if they are receiving a beta adrenergic blocker (see DRUG INTERACTIONS). Patients with milder ventricular dysfunction should, if possible, be controlled with optimum doses of digitalis and/or diuretics before verapamil treatment (Note interactions with digoxin under: PRECAUTIONS).

Hypotension: Occasionally, the pharmacologic action of verapamil may produce a decrease in blood pressure below normal levels which may result in dizziness or symptomatic hypotension. The incidence of hypotension observed in 4,954 patients enrolled in clinical trials was 2.5%. In hypertensive patients, decreases in blood pressure below normal are unusual. Tilt table testing (60 degrees) was not able to induce orthostatic hypotension.

Elevated Liver Enzymes: Elevations of transaminases with and without concomitant elevations in alkaline phosphatase and bilirubin have been reported. Such elevations have sometimes been transient and may disappear even with continued verapamil treatment. Several cases of hepatocellular injury related to verapamil have been proven by rechallenge; half of these cases had clinical symptoms (malaise, fever, and/or right upper quadrant pain) in addition to elevations of SGOT, SGPT and alkaline phosphatase. Periodic monitoring of liver function in patients receiving verapamil is therefore prudent.

Accessory Bypass Tract (Wolff-Parkinson-White or Lown-Ganong-Levine): Some patients with paroxysmal and/or chronic atrial fibrillation or atrial flutter and a coexisting accessory AV pathway have developed increased antegrade conduction across the accessory pathway bypassing the AV node, producing a very rapid ventricular response or ventricular fibrillation after receiving intravenous verapamil (or digitalis). Although a risk of this occurring with oral verapamil has not been established, such patients receiving oral verapamil may be at risk and its use in these patients is contraindicated (see CONTRAINDICATIONS).

Treatment is usually DC-cardioversion. Cardioversion has been used safely and effectively after oral ISOPTIN.

Atrioventricular Block: The effect of verapamil on AV conduction and the SA node may cause asymptomatic first-degree AV block and transient bradycardia, sometimes accompanied by nodal escape rhythms. PR interval prolongation is correlated with verapamil plasma concentrations, especially during the early titration phase of therapy. Higher degrees of AV block, however, were infrequently (0.8%) observed. Marked first-degree block or progressive development to second- or third-degree AV block requires a reduction in dosage or, in rare instances, discontinuation of verapamil HCl and institution of appropriate therapy depending upon the clinical situation.

Patients with Hypertrophic Cardiomyopathy (IHSS): In 120 patients with hypertrophic cardiomyopathy (most of them refractory or intolerant to propranolol) who received therapy with verapamil at doses up to 720 mg/day, a variety of serious adverse effects were seen. Three patients died in pulmonary edema; all had severe left ventricular outflow obstruction and a past history of left ventricular dysfunction. Eight other patients had pulmonary edema and/or severe hypotension; abnormally high (greater than 20 mmHg) pulmonary wedge pressure and a marked left ventricular outflow obstruction were present in most of these patients. Concomitant administration of quinidine (See DRUG INTERACTIONS) preceded the severe hypotension in 3 of the 8 patients (2 of whom developed pulmonary edema). Sinus bradycardia occurred in 11% of the patients, second-degree AV block in 4% and sinus arrest in 2%. It must be appreciated that this group of patients had a serious disease with a high mortality rate. Most adverse effects responded well to dose reduction and only rarely did verapamil have to be discontinued.

PRECAUTIONS

General

Use in Patients with Impaired Hepatic Function: Since verapamil is highly metabolized by the liver, it should be administered cautiously to patients with impaired hepatic function. Severe liver dysfunction prolongs the elimination half-life of verapamil to about 14 to 16 hours; hence, approximately 30% of the dose given to patients with normal liver function should be administered to these patients. Careful monitoring for abnormal prolongation of the PR interval or other signs of excessive pharmacologic effects (See OVERDOSAGE) should be carried out.

Use in Patients with Attenuated (decreased) Neuromuscular Transmission: It has been reported that verapamil decreases neuromuscular transmission in patients with Duchenne's muscular dystrophy, and that verapamil prolongs recovery from the neuromuscular blocking agent vecuronium. It may be necessary to decrease the dosage of verapamil when it is administered to patients with attenuated neuromuscular transmission.

Use in Patients with Impaired Renal Function: About 70% of an administered dose of verapamil is excreted as metabolites in the urine. Verapamil is not removed by hemodialysis. Until further data are available, verapamil should be administered cautiously to patients with impaired renal function. These patients should be carefully monitored for abnormal prolongation of the PR interval or other signs of overdosage (see OVERDOSAGE).

Drug Interactions

Beta Blockers: Controlled studies in small numbers of patients suggest that the concomitant use of ISOPTIN and oral beta-adrenergic blocking agents may be beneficial in certain patients with chronic stable angina or hypertension, but available information is not sufficient to predict with confidence the effects of concurrent treatment in patients with left ventricular dysfunction or cardiac conduction abnormalities. Concomitant therapy with beta-adrenergic blockers and verapamil may result in additive negative effects on heart rate, atrioventricular conduction and/or cardiac contractility.

In one study involving 15 patients treated with high doses of propranolol (median dose: 480 mg/day, range 160 to 1280 mg/day) for severe angina, with preserved left ventricular function (ejection fraction greater than 35%), the hemodynamic effects of additional therapy with verapamil HCl were assessed using invasive methods. The addition of verapamil to high-dose beta blockers induced modest negative inotropic and chronotropic effects which were not severe enough to limit short-term (48 hours) combination therapy in this study. These modest cardiodepressant effects persisted for greater than 6, but less than 30 hours after abrupt withdrawal of beta blockers and were closely related to plasma levels of propranolol. The primary verapamil/beta-blocker interaction in this study appeared to be hemodynamic rather than electrophysiologic.

In other studies, verapamil did not generally induce significant negative inotropic, chronotropic, or dromotropic effects in patients with preserved left ventricular function receiving low or moderate doses of propranolol (less than or equal to 320 mg/day); in some patients, however, combined therapy did produce such effects. Therefore, if combined therapy is used, close surveillance of clinical status should be carried out. Combined therapy should usually be avoided in patients with atrioventricular conduction abnormalities and those with depressed left ventricular function.

Asymptomatic bradycardia (36 beats/min) with a wandering atrial pacemaker has been observed in a patient receiving concomitant timolol (a beta-adrenergic blocker) eyedrops and oral verapamil.

A decrease in metoprolol clearance has been observed when verapamil and metoprolol were administered together. A similar effect has not been seen when verapamil and atenolol were given together.

Digitalis: Clinical use of verapamil in digitalized patients has shown the combination to be well tolerated if digoxin doses are properly adjusted. However, chronic verapamil treatment can increase serum digoxin levels by 50% to 75% during the first week of therapy, and this can result in digitalis toxicity. In patients with hepatic cirrhosis the influence of verapamil on digoxin kinetics is magnified. Verapamil may reduce total body clearance and extrarenal clearance of digitoxin by 27% and 29%, respectively. Maintenance and digitalization doses should be reduced when verapamil is administered, and the patient should be reassessed to avoid over- or underdigitalization. Whenever overdigitalization is suspected, the daily dose of digitalis should be reduced or temporarily discontinued. Upon discontinuation of ISOPTIN (verapamil HCl), the patient should be reassessed to avoid underdigitalization.

Antihypertensive Agents: Verapamil administered concomitantly with oral antihypertensive agents (e.g., vasodilators, angiotensin-converting enzyme inhibitors, diuretics, beta blockers) will usually have an additive effect on lowering blood pressure. Patients receiving these combinations should be appropriately monitored. Concomitant use of

agents that attenuate alpha-adrenergic function with verapamil may result in a reduction in blood pressure that is excessive in some patients. Such an effect was observed in one study following the concomitant administration of verapamil and prazosin.

Antiarrhythmic Agents

Disopyramide: Until data on possible interactions between verapamil and disopyramide are obtained, disopyramide should not be administered within 48 hours before or 24 hours after verapamil administration.

Flecainide: A study in healthy volunteers showed that the concomitant administration of flecainide and verapamil may have additive effects on myocardial contractility, AV conduction, and repolarization. Concomitant therapy with flecainide and verapamil may result in additive negative inotropic effect and prolongation of atrioventricular conduction.

Quinidine: In a small number of patients with hypertrophic cardiomyopathy (IHSS), concomitant use of verapamil and quinidine resulted in significant hypotension. Until further data are obtained, combined therapy of verapamil and quinidine in patients with hypertrophic cardiomyopathy should probably be avoided.

The electrophysiological effects of quinidine and verapamil on AV conduction were studied in 8 patients. Verapamil significantly counteracted the effects of quinidine on AV conduction. There has been a report of increased quinidine levels during verapamil therapy.

Other

Nitrates: Verapamil has been given concomitantly with short- and long-acting nitrates without any undesirable drug interactions. The pharmacologic profile of both drugs and the clinical experience suggest beneficial interactions.

Cimetidine: The interaction between cimetidine and chronically administered verapamil has not been studied. Variable results on clearance have been obtained in acute studies of healthy volunteers; clearance of verapamil was either reduced or unchanged.

Lithium: Pharmacokinetic and pharmacodynamic interactions between oral verapamil and lithium have been reported. The former may result in a lowering of serum lithium levels in patients receiving chronic stable oral lithium therapy. The latter may result in an increased sensitivity to the effects of lithium. Patients receiving both drugs must be monitored carefully.

Carbamazepine: Verapamil therapy may increase carbamazepine concentrations during combined therapy. This may produce carbamazepine side effects such as diplopia, headache, ataxia, or dizziness.

Rifampin: Therapy with rifampin may markedly reduce oral verapamil bioavailability.

Phenobarbital: Phenobarbital therapy may increase verapamil clearance.

Cyclosporin: Verapamil therapy may increase serum levels of cyclosporin.

Inhalation Anesthetics: Animal experiments have shown that inhalation anesthetics depress cardiovascular activity by decreasing the inward movement of calcium ions. When used concomitantly, inhalation anesthetics and calcium antagonists, such as verapamil, should each be titrated carefully to avoid excessive cardiovascular depression.

Neuromuscular Blocking Agents: Clinical data and animal studies suggest that verapamil may potentiate the activity of neuromuscular blocking agents (curare-like and depolarizing). It may be necessary to decrease the dose of verapamil and/or the dose of the neuromuscular blocking agent when the drugs are used concomitantly.

Carcinogenesis, Mutagenesis, Impairment of Fertility: An 18-month toxicity study in rats, at a low multiple (6 fold) of the maximum recommended human dose, and not the maximum tolerated dose, did not suggest a tumorigenic potential. There was no evidence of a carcinogenic potential of verapamil administered in the diet of rats for two years at doses of 10, 35 and 120 mg/kg per day or approximately 1x, 3.5x and 12x, respectively, the maximum recommended human daily dose (480 mg per day or 9.6 mg/kg/day).

Verapamil was not mutagenic in the Ames test in 5 test strains at 3 mg per plate, with or without metabolic activation.

Studies in female rats at daily dietary doses up to 5.5 times (55 mg/kg/day) the maximum recommended human dose did not show impaired fertility. Effects on male fertility have not been determined.

Pregnancy: Pregnancy Category C. Reproduction studies have been performed in rabbits and rats at oral doses up to 1.5 (15 mg/kg/day) and 6 (60 mg/kg/day) times the human oral daily dose, respectively, and have revealed no evidence of teratogenicity. In the rat, however, this multiple of the human dose was embryocidal and retarded fetal growth and development, probably because of adverse maternal effects reflected in the reduced weight gains of the dams. This oral dose has also been shown to cause hypotension in rats. There are no adequate and well-controlled studies in pregnant women. Because animal reproduction studies are not always predictive of human response, this drug should be used during pregnancy only if clearly needed.

Verapamil crosses the placental barrier and can be detected in umbilical vein blood at delivery.

Labor and Delivery: It is not known whether the use of verapamil during labor or delivery has immediate or delayed adverse effects on the fetus, or whether it prolongs the duration of labor or increases the need for forceps delivery or other obstetric intervention. Such adverse experiences have not been reported in the literature, despite a long history of use of verapamil in Europe in the treatment of cardiac side effects of beta-adrenergic agonist agents used to treat premature labor.

Nursing Mothers: Verapamil is excreted in human milk. Because of the potential for adverse reactions in nursing infants from verapamil, nursing should be discontinued while verapamil is administered.

Pediatric Use: Safety and efficacy of ISOPTIN in children below the age of 18 years have not been established.

Animal Pharmacology and/or Animal Toxicology: In chronic animal toxicology studies verapamil caused lenticular and/or suture line changes at 30 mg/kg/day or greater and frank cataracts at 62.5 mg/kg/day or greater in the beagle dog but not the rat. Development of cataracts due to verapamil has not been reported in man.

ADVERSE REACTIONS

Serious adverse reactions are uncommon when ISOPTIN therapy is initiated with upward dose titration within the recommended single and total daily dose. See WARNINGS for discussion of heart failure, hypotension, elevated liver enzymes, AV block and rapid ventricular response. The following reactions to orally administered verapamil occurred at rates greater than 1.0% or occurred at lower rates but appeared clearly drug-related in clinical trials in 4,954 patients.

Constipation	7.3%	Fatigue	1.7%
Dizziness	3.3%	Dyspnea	1.4%
Nausea	2.7%	Bradycardia (HR $<$ 50/min)	1.4%
Hypotension	2.5%	AV block—total 1°, 2°, 3°	1.2%
Headache	2.2%	2° and 3°	0.8%
Edema	1.9%	Rash	1.2%
CHF, Pulmonary Edema	1.8%	Flushing	0.6%

Elevated Liver Enzymes (see WARNINGS)

In clinical trials related to the control of ventricular response in digitalized patients who had atrial fibrillation or flutter, ventricular rate below 50 at rest occurred in 15% of patients and asymptomatic hypotension occurred in 5% of patients.

The following reactions, reported in 1.0% or less of patients, occurred under conditions (open trials, marketing experience) where a causal relationship is uncertain; they are listed to alert the physician to a possible relationship:

Cardiovascular: angina pectoris, atrioventricular dissociation, chest pain, claudication, myocardial infarction, palpitations, purpura (vasculitis), syncope.

Digestive System: diarrhea, dry mouth, gastrointestinal distress, gingival hyperplasia.

Hemic and Lymphatic: ecchymosis or bruising.

Nervous System: cerebrovascular accident, confusion, equilibrium disorders, insomnia, muscle cramps, paresthesia, psychotic symptoms, shakiness, somnolence.

Skin: arthralgia and rash, exanthema, hair loss, hyperkeratosis, maculae, sweating, urticaria, Stevens-Johnson syndrome, erythema multiforme.

Special Senses: blurred vision.

Urogenital: gynecomastia, increased urination, spotty menstruation, impotence.

Treatment of Acute Cardiovascular Adverse Reactions: The frequency of cardiovascular adverse reactions which require therapy is rare; hence, experience with their treatment is limited. Whenever severe hypotension or complete AV block occur following oral administration of verapamil, the appropriate emergency measures should be applied immediately, e.g., intravenously administered norepinephrine bitartrate, atropine sulfate, isoproterenol HCl (all in the usual doses), or calcium gluconate (10% solution). In patients with hypertrophic cardiomyopathy (IHSS), alpha-adrenergic agents (phenylephrine HCl, metaraminol bitartrate or methoxamine HCl) should be used to maintain blood pressure, and isoproterenol and norepinephrine should be avoided. If further support is necessary, dopamine HCl or dobutamine HCl may be administered. Actual treatment and dosage should depend on the severity and the clinical situation and the judgment and experience of the treating physician.

OVERDOSAGE

Treatment of overdosage should be supportive. Beta-adrenergic stimulation or parenteral administration of calcium solutions may increase calcium ion flux across the slow channel, and have been used effectively in treatment of deliberate overdosage with verapamil. Verapamil cannot be removed by hemodialysis. Clinically significant hypotensive reactions or fixed high degree AV block should be treated with vasopressor agents or cardiac pacing, respectively. Asystole should be handled by the usual measures including cardiopulmonary resuscitation.

DOSAGE AND ADMINISTRATION

The dose of verapamil must be individualized by titration. ISOPTIN is available in 40 mg, 80 mg, and 120 mg tablets. The usefulness and safety of dosages exceeding 480 mg/day have not been established; therefore, this daily dosage should not be exceeded. Since the half-life of verapamil increases during chronic dosing, maximum response may be delayed.

Angina: Clinical trials show that the usual dose is 80 mg to 120 mg three times a day. However, 40 mg three times a day may be warranted in patients who may have an increased response to verapamil (e.g., decreased hepatic function, elderly, etc.). Upward titration should be based on therapeutic efficacy and safety evaluated approximately eight hours after dosing. Dosage may be increased at daily (e.g., patients with unstable angina) or weekly intervals until optimum clinical response is obtained.

Arrhythmias: The dosage in digitalized patients with chronic atrial fibrillation (see PRECAUTIONS) ranges from 240 to 320 mg per day in divided (t.i.d. or q.i.d.) doses. The dosage for prophylaxis of PSVT (non-digitalized patients) ranges from 240 to 480 mg in divided (t.i.d. or q.i.d.) doses. In general, maximum effects for any given dosage will be apparent during the first 48 hours of therapy.

Essential Hypertension: Dose should be individualized by titration. The usual initial monotherapy dose in clinical trials was 80 mg three times a day (240 mg). Daily dosages of 360 and 480 mg have been used but there is no evidence that doses beyond 360 mg provide added effect. Consideration should be given to beginning titration at 40 mg, three times per day in patients who might respond to lower doses, such as the elderly or people of small stature. The antihypertensive effects of ISOPTIN are evident within the first week of therapy. Upward titration should be based on therapeutic efficacy, assessed at the end of the dosing interval.

HOW SUPPLIED

ISOPTIN (verapamil HCl) tablets are supplied as round, scored, film-coated tablets containing either 40 mg, 80 mg or 120 mg of verapamil hydrochloride. The 80 mg and 120 mg tablets are embossed with "ISOPTIN 80" or "ISOPTIN 120" on one side and "Knoll" on the reverse side. The 40 mg tablet is embossed on one side with the number "40" surrounded by the Knoll triangle.

40 mg (lt. blue)—
- Bottle of 100—NDC #0044-1821-02
- Hospital Unit Dose (100 tablets-Strips of 10)—NDC #0044-1821-10

80 mg (yellow)—
- Bottle of 100—NDC #0044-1822-02
- Bottle of 500—NDC #0044-1822-05
- Bottle of 1000—NDC #0044-1822-04
- Hospital Unit Dose (100 tablets—Strips of 10)—NDC #0044-1822-10

120 mg (white)—
- Bottle of 100—NDC #0044-1823-02
- Bottle of 500—NDC #0044-1823-05
- Bottle of 1000—NDC #0044-1823-04
- Hospital Unit Dose (100 tablets—Strips of 10)—NDC #0044-1823-10

Storage: 59° to 86°F (15° to 30°C).

Dispense in a tight, light-resistant container as defined in the USP.

MR 1988/ 2636

Revised September 1988 2659

Shown in Product Identification Section, page 414

ISOPTIN® SR ℞
(verapamil HCl)
Sustained Release Oral Tablets

DESCRIPTION

ISOPTIN SR (verapamil hydrochloride) is a calcium ion influx inhibitor (slow channel blocker or calcium ion antagonist). ISOPTIN SR is available for oral administration as light green, capsule shaped, scored, film-coated tablets containing 240 mg verapamil hydrochloride, as light pink, oval shaped, scored, film-coated tablets containing 180 mg verapamil hydrochloride, and as light violet, oval shaped, film-coated tablets containing 120 mg verapamil hydrochloride. The tablets are designed for sustained release of the drug in the gastrointestinal tract; sustained release characteristics are not altered when the tablet is divided in half.

The structural formula of verapamil HCl is given [on next page.]

Verapamil HCl is an almost white, crystalline powder, practically free of odor, with a bitter taste. It is soluble in water, chloroform and methanol. Verapamil HCl is not chemically related to other cardioactive drugs.

In addition to verapamil HCl, the ISOPTIN SR tablet contains the following ingredients: alginate, hydroxypropyl

Continued on next page

Knoll—Cont.

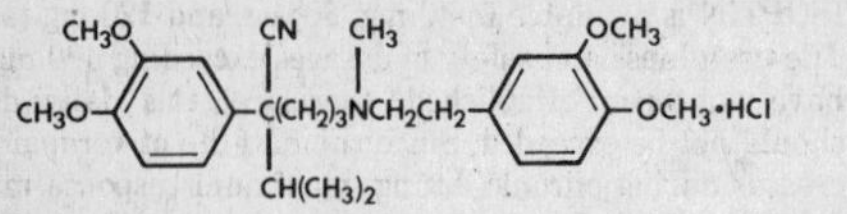

$C_{27}H_{38}N_2O_4 \cdot HCl$ M.W. = 491.08

Benzeneacetonitrile,
α[3-[[2-(3,4-dimethoxyphenyl) ethyl]
methylamino]
propyl]-3,4-dimethoxy-α-(1-methylethyl) hydrochloride

methylcellulose, magnesium stearate, microcrystalline cellulose, polyethylene glycol, polyvinyl pyrrolidone, talc, and titanium dioxide. The following are the color additives per tablet strength:

Strength (mg)	Color Additive(s)
120	Iron Oxide
180	Iron Oxide
240	D&C yellow #10 Lake dye, and FD&C blue #2 Lake dye.

CLINICAL PHARMACOLOGY

ISOPTIN is a calcium ion influx inhibitor (slow channel blocker or calcium ion antagonist) which exerts its pharmacologic effects by modulating the influx of ionic calcium across the cell membrane of the arterial smooth muscle as well as in conductile and contractile myocardial cells.

Mechanism of Action

Essential Hypertension

ISOPTIN exerts antihypertensive effects by decreasing systemic vascular resistance, usually without orthostatic decreases in blood pressure or reflex tachycardia; bradycardia (rate less than 50 beats/min) is uncommon (1.4%). During isometric or dynamic exercise ISOPTIN does not alter systolic cardiac function in patients with normal ventricular function.

ISOPTIN does not alter total serum calcium levels. However, one report suggested that calcium levels above the normal range may alter the therapeutic effect of ISOPTIN.

Other Pharmacological Actions of ISOPTIN include the Following

ISOPTIN (verapamil HCl) dilates the main coronary arteries and coronary arterioles, both in normal and ischemic regions, and is a potent inhibitor of coronary artery spasm, whether spontaneous or ergonovine-induced. This property increases myocardial oxygen delivery in patients with coronary artery spasm, and is responsible for the effectiveness of ISOPTIN in vasospastic (Prinzmetal's or variant) as well as unstable angina at rest. Whether this effect plays any role in classical effort angina is not clear, but studies of exercise tolerance have not shown an increase in the maximum exercise rate-pressure product, a widely accepted measure of oxygen utilization. This suggests that, in general, relief of spasm of dilation of coronary arteries is not an important factor in classical angina.

ISOPTIN regularly reduces the total systemic resistance (afterload) against which the heart works both at rest and at a given level of exercise by dilating peripheral arterioles.

Electrical activity through the AV node depends, to a significant degree, upon calcium influx through the slow channel. By decreasing the influx of calcium, ISOPTIN prolongs the effective refractory period within the AV node and slows AV conduction in a rate-related manner.

Normal sinus rhythm is usually not affected, but in patients with sick sinus syndrome, ISOPTIN may interfere with sinus node impulse generation and may induce sinus arrest or sinoatrial block. Atrioventricular block can occur in patients without preexisting conduction defects (see WARNINGS).

ISOPTIN does not alter the normal atrial action potential or intraventricular conduction time, but depresses amplitude, velocity of depolarization and conduction in depressed atrial fibers. ISOPTIN may shorten the antegrade effective refractory period of accessory bypass tracts. Acceleration of ventricular rate and/or ventricular fibrillation has been reported in patients with atrial flutter or atrial fibrillation and a coexisting accessory AV pathway following administration of verapamil (see WARNINGS).

ISOPTIN has a local anesthetic action that is 1.6 times that of procaine on an equimolar basis. It is not known whether this action is important at the doses used in man.

Pharmacokinetics and Metabolism: With the immediate release formulation, more than 90% of the orally administered dose of ISOPTIN is absorbed. Because of rapid biotransformation of verapamil during its first pass through the portal circulation, bioavailability ranges from 20% to 35%. Peak plasma concentrations are reached between 1 and 2 hours after oral administration. Chronic oral administration of 120 mg of ISOPTIN every 6 hours resulted in plasma levels of verapamil ranging from 125 to 400 mg/mL with higher values reported occasionally. A nonlinear correlation between the verapamil dose administered and verapamil plasma levels does exist. No relationship has been established between the plasma concentration of verapamil and a reduction in blood pressure.

In early dose titration with verapamil a relationship exists between verapamil plasma concentrations and the prolongation of the PR interval. However, during chronic administration this relationship may disappear. The mean elimination half-life in single dose studies ranged from 2.8 to 7.4 hours. In these same studies, after repetitive dosing, the half-life increased to a range from 4.5 to 12.0 hours (after less than 10 consecutive doses given 6 hours apart). Half-life of verapamil may increase during titration.

Aging may affect the pharmacokinetics of verapamil. Elimination half-life may be prolonged in the elderly.

In multiple dose studies under fasting conditions the bioavailability measured by AUC of ISOPTIN SR was similar to ISOPTIN immediate release; rates of absorption were, of course, different. In a randomized, single-dose, crossover study using healthy volunteers, administration of 240 mg ISOPTIN SR with food produced peak plasma verapamil concentrations of 79 ng/mL, time to peak plasma verapamil concentration of 7.71 hours, and AUC (0–24 hr) of 841 ng-hr/mL. When ISOPTIN SR was administered to fasting subjects, peak plasma verapamil concentration was 164 ng/mL; time to peak plasma verapamil concentration was 5.21 hours; and AUC (0–24 hr) was 1,478 ng-hr/mL. Similar results were demonstrated for plasma norverapamil. Food thus produces decreased bioavailability (AUC) but a narrower peak to trough ratio. Good correlation of dose and response is not available, but controlled studies of ISOPTIN SR have shown effectiveness of doses similar to the effective doses of ISOPTIN (immediate release).

In healthy man, orally administered ISOPTIN undergoes extensive metabolism in the liver. Twelve metabolites have been identified in plasma; all except norverapamil are present in trace amounts only. Norverapamil can reach steady-state plasma concentrations approximately equal to those of verapamil itself. The cardiovascular activity of norverapamil appears to be approximately 20% that of verapamil. Approximately 70% of an administered dose is excreted as metabolites in the urine and 16% or more in the feces within 5 days. About 3% to 4% is excreted in the urine as unchanged drug. Approximately 90% is bound to plasma proteins. In patients with hepatic insufficiency, metabolism of immediate release verapamil is delayed and elimination half-life prolonged up to 14 to 16 hours (see PRECAUTIONS); the volume of distribution is increased and plasma clearance reduced to about 30% of normal. Verapamil clearance values suggest that patients with liver dysfunction may attain therapeutic verapamil plasma concentrations with one-third of the oral daily dose required for patients with normal liver function.

After four weeks of oral dosing (120 mg q.i.d.), verapamil and norverapamil levels were noted in the cerebrospinal fluid with estimated partition coefficient of 0.06 for verapamil and 0.04 for norverapamil.

Hemodynamics and Myocardial Metabolism: ISOPTIN reduces afterload and myocardial contractility. Improved left ventricular diastolic function in patients with IHSS and those with coronary heart disease has also been observed with ISOPTIN therapy. In most patients, including those with organic cardiac disease, the negative inotropic action of ISOPTIN is countered by reduction of afterload and cardiac index is usually not reduced. In patients with severe left ventricular dysfunction however, (e.g., pulmonary wedge pressure above 20 mmHg or ejection fraction lower than 30%), or in patients on beta-adrenergic blocking agents or other cardiodepressant drugs, deterioration of ventricular function may occur (see DRUG INTERACTIONS).

Pulmonary Function: ISOPTIN does not induce bronchoconstriction and hence, does not impair ventilatory function.

INDICATIONS AND USAGE

ISOPTIN SR (verapamil HCl) is indicated for the management of essential hypertension.

CONTRAINDICATIONS

Verapamil HCl is contraindicated in:

1. Severe left ventricular dysfunction (see WARNINGS).
2. Hypotension (less than 90 mmHg systolic pressure) or cardiogenic shock.
3. Sick sinus syndrome (except in patients with a functioning artificial ventricular pacemaker).
4. Second- or third-degree AV block (except in patients with a functioning artificial ventricular pacemaker).
5. Patients with atrial flutter or atrial fibrillation and an accessory bypass tract (e.g., Wolff-Parkinson-White, Lown-Ganong-Levine syndromes). (see WARNINGS).
6. Patients with known hypersensitivity to verapamil hydrochloride.

WARNINGS

Heart Failure: Verapamil has a negative inotropic effect which, in most patients, is compensated by its afterload reduction (decreased systemic vascular resistance) properties without a net impairment of ventricular performance. In clinical experience with 4,954 patients, 87 (1.8%) developed congestive heart failure or pulmonary edema. Verapamil should be avoided in patients with severe left ventricular dysfunction (e.g., ejection fraction less than 30%, pulmonary wedge pressure above 20 mm Hg, or severe symptoms of cardiac failure) and in patients with any degree of ventricular dysfunction if they are receiving a beta adrenergic blocker (see DRUG INTERACTIONS). Patients with milder ventricular dysfunction should, if possible, be controlled with optimum doses of digitalis and/or diuretics before verapamil treatment (*Note interactions with digoxin under: PRECAUTIONS*).

Hypotension: Occasionally, the pharmacologic action of verapamil may produce a decrease in blood pressure below normal levels which may result in dizziness or symptomatic hypotension. The incidence of hypotension observed in 4,954 patients enrolled in clinical trials was 2.5%. In hypertensive patients, decreases in blood pressure below normal are unusual. Tilt table testing (60 degrees) was not able to induce orthostatic hypotension.

Elevated Liver Enzymes: Elevations of transaminases with and without concomitant elevations in alkaline phosphatase and bilirubin have been reported. Such elevations have sometimes been transient and may disappear even in the face of continued verapamil treatment. Several cases of hepatocellular injury related to verapamil have been proven by rechallenge; half of these had clinical symptoms (malaise, fever, and/or right upper quadrant pain) in addition to elevations of SGOT, SGPT and alkaline phosphatase. Periodic monitoring of liver function in patients receiving verapamil is therefore prudent.

Accessory Bypass Tract (Wolff-Parkinson-White or Lown-Ganong-Levine): Some patients with paroxysmal and/or chronic atrial fibrillation or atrial flutter and a coexisting accessory AV pathway have developed increased antegrade conduction across the accessory pathway bypassing the AV node, producing a very rapid ventricular response or ventricular fibrillation after receiving intravenous verapamil (or digitalis). Although a risk of this occurring with oral verapamil has not been established, such patients receiving oral verapamil may be at risk and its use in these patients is contraindicated (see CONTRAINDICATIONS).

Treatment is usually DC-cardioversion. Cardioversion has been used safely and effectively after oral ISOPTIN.

Atrioventricular Block: The effect of verapamil on AV conduction and the SA node may lead to asymptomatic first-degree AV block and transient bradycardia, sometimes accompanied by nodal escape rhythms. PR interval prolongation is correlated with verapamil plasma concentrations, especially during the early titration phases of therapy. Higher degrees of AV block, however, were infrequently (0.8%) observed. Marked first-degree block or progressive development to second- or third-degree AV block requires a reduction in dosage or, in rare instances, discontinuation of verapamil HCl and institution of appropriate therapy depending upon the clinical situation.

Patients with Hypertrophic Cardiomyopathy (IHSS): In 120 patients with hypertrophic cardiomyopathy (most of them refractory or intolerant to propranolol) who received therapy with verapamil at doses up to 720 mg/day, a variety of serious adverse effects were seen. Three patients died in pulmonary edema; all had severe left ventricular outflow obstruction and a past history of left ventricular dysfunction. Eight other patients had pulmonary edema and/or severe hypotension; abnormally high (over 20 mmHg) capillary wedge pressure and a marked left ventricular outflow obstruction were present in most of these patients. Concomitant administration of quinidine (see DRUG INTERACTIONS) preceded the severe hypotension in 3 of the 8 patients (2 of whom developed pulmonary edema). Sinus bradycardia occurred in 11% of the patients, second-degree AV block in 4% and sinus arrest in 2%. It must be appreciated that this group of patients had a serious disease with a high mortality rate. Most adverse effects responded well to dose reduction and only rarely did verapamil have to be discontinued.

PRECAUTIONS

General

Use in Patients with Impaired Hepatic Function: Since verapamil is highly metabolized by the liver, it should be administered cautiously to patients with impaired hepatic function. Severe liver dysfunction prolongs the elimination half-life of immediate release verapamil to about 14 to 16 hours; hence, approximately 30% of the dose given to patients with normal liver function should be administered to these patients. Careful monitoring for abnormal prolongation of the PR interval or other signs of excessive pharmacologic effects (see OVERDOSAGE) should be carried out.

Use in Patients with Attenuated (Decreased) Neuromuscular Transmission: It has been reported that verapamil decreases neuromuscular transmission in patients with Duchenne's muscular dystrophy, and that verapamil prolongs recovery from the neuromuscular blocking agent vecuronium. It may be necessary to decrease the dosage of verapamil when it is administered to patients with attenuated neuromuscular transmission.

Use in Patients with Impaired Renal Function: About 70% of an administered dose of verapamil is excreted as metabolites in the urine. Verapamil is not removed by hemodialysis. Until further data are available, verapamil should be administered cautiously to patients with impaired renal function. These patients should be carefully monitored for abnormal prolongation of the PR interval or other signs of overdosage (see OVERDOSAGE).

Drug Interactions

Beta Blockers: Concomitant therapy with beta-adrenergic blockers and verapamil may result in additive negative effects on heart rate, atrioventricular conduction, and/or cardiac contractility. The combination of sustained-release verapamil and beta-adrenergic blocking agents has not been studied. However, there have been reports of excessive bradycardia and AV block, including complete heart block, when the combination has been used for the treatment of hypertension. For hypertensive patients, the risks of combined therapy may outweigh the potential benefits. The combination should be used only with caution and close monitoring.

Asymptomatic bradycardia (36 beats/min) with a wandering atrial pacemaker has been observed in a patient receiving concomitant timolol (a beta-adrenergic blocker) eyedrops and oral verapamil.

A decrease in metoprolol and propranolol clearance has been observed when either drug is administered concomitantly with verapamil. A variable effect has been seen when verapamil and atenolol are given together.

Digitalis: Clinical use of verapamil in digitalized patients has shown the combination to be well tolerated if digoxin doses are properly adjusted. Chronic verapamil treatment can increase serum digoxin levels by 50 to 75% during the first week of therapy, and this can result in digitalis toxicity. In patients with hepatic cirrhosis the influence of verapamil on digoxin kinetics is magnified. Verapamil may reduce total body clearance and extrarenal clearance of digitoxin by 27% and 29%, respectively. Maintenance digitalis doses should be reduced when verapamil is administered, and the patient should be carefully monitored to avoid over- or underdigitalization. Whenever overdigitalization is suspected, the daily dose of digitalis should be reduced or temporarily discontinued. Upon discontinuation of ISOPTIN (verapamil HCl), the patient should be reassessed to avoid underdigitalization.

Antihypertensive Agents: Verapamil administered concomitantly with oral antihypertensive agents (e.g., vasodilators, angiotensin-converting enzyme inhibitors, diuretics, beta blockers) will usually have an additive effect on lowering blood pressure. Patients receiving these combinations should be appropriately monitored. Concomitant use of agents that attenuate alpha-adrenergic function with verapamil may result in a reduction in blood pressure that is excessive in some patients. Such an effect was observed in one study following the concomitant administration of verapamil and prazosin.

Antiarrhythmic Agents

Disopyramide: Until data on possible interactions between verapamil and disopyramide phosphate are obtained, disopyramide should not be administered within 48 hours before or 24 hours after verapamil administration.

Flecainide: A study in healthy volunteers showed that the concomitant administration of flecainide and verapamil may have additive effects on myocardial contractility, AV conduction, and repolarization. Concomitant therapy with flecainide and verapamil may result in additive negative inotropic effect and prolongation of atrioventricular conduction.

Quinidine: In a small number of patients with hypertrophic cardiomyopathy (IHSS), concomitant use of verapamil and quinidine resulted in significant hypotension. Until further data are obtained, combined therapy of verapamil and quinidine in patients with hypertrophic cardiomyopathy should probably be avoided.

The electrophysiological effects of quinidine and verapamil on AV conduction were studied in 8 patients. Verapamil significantly counteracted the effects of quinidine on AV conduction. There has been a report of increased quinidine levels during verapamil therapy.

Nitrates: Verapamil has been given concomitantly with short- and long-acting nitrates without any undesirable drug interactions. The pharmacologic profile of both drugs and the clinical experience suggest beneficial interactions.

Other

Cimetidine: The interaction between cimetidine and chronically administered verapamil has not been studied. Variable results on clearance have been obtained in acute studies of healthy volunteers; clearance of verapamil was either reduced or unchanged.

Lithium: Increased sensitivity to the effects of lithium (neurotoxocity) has been reported during concomitant verapamil-lithium therapy with either no change or an increase in serum lithium levels. However, the addition of verapamil has also resulted in the lowering of serum lithium levels in patients receiving chronic stable oral lithium. Patients receiving both drugs must be monitored carefully.

Carbamazepine: Verapamil therapy may increase carbamazepine concentrations during combined therapy. This may produce carbamazepine side effects such as diplopia, headache, ataxia, or dizziness.

Rifampin: Therapy with rifampin may markedly reduce oral verapamil bioavailability.

Phenobarbital: Phenobarbital therapy may increase verapamil clearance.

Cyclosporin: Verapamil therapy may increase serum levels of cyclosporin.

Theophylline: Verapamil may inhibit the clearance and increase the plasma levels of theophylline.

Inhalation Anesthetics: Animal experiments have shown that inhalation anesthetics depress cardiovascular activity by decreasing the inward movement of calcium ions. When used concomitantly, inhalation anesthetics and calcium antagonists, such as verapamil, should be titrated carefully to avoid excessive cardiovascular depression.

Neuromuscular Blocking Agents: Clinical data and animal studies suggest that verapamil may potentiate the activity of neuromuscular blocking agents (curare-like and depolarizing). It may be necessary to decrease the dose of verapamil and/or the dose of the neuromuscular blocking agent when the drugs are used concomitantly.

Carcinogenesis, Mutagenesis, Impairment of Fertility: An 18-month toxicity study in rats, at a low multiple (6 fold) of the maximum recommended human dose, and not the maximum tolerated dose, did not suggest a tumorigenic potential. There was no evidence of a carcinogenic potential of verapamil administered in the diet of rats for two years at doses of 10, 35, and 120 mg/kg per day or approximately 1x, 3.5x, and 12x, respectively, the maximum recommended human daily dose (480 mg per day or 9.6 mg/kg/day).

Verapamil was not mutagenic in the Ames test in 5 test strains at 3 mg per plate, with or without metabolic activation.

Studies in female rats at daily dietary doses up to 5.5 times (55 mg/kg/day) the maximum recommended human dose did not show impaired fertility. Effects on male fertility have not been determined.

Pregnancy: Pregnancy Category C. Reproduction studies have been performed in rabbits and rats at oral doses up to 1.5 (15 mg/kg/day) and 6 (60 mg/kg/day) times the human oral daily dose, respectively, and have revealed no evidence of teratogenicity. In the rat, however, this multiple of the human dose was embryocidal and retarded fetal growth and development, probably because of adverse maternal effects reflected in the reduced weight gains of the dams. This oral dose has also been shown to cause hypotension in rats. There are no adequate and well-controlled studies in pregnant women. Because animal reproduction studies are not always predictive of human response, this drug should be used during pregnancy only if clearly needed. ISOPTIN (verapamil HCl) crosses the placental barrier and can be detected in umbilical vein blood at delivery.

Labor and Delivery: It is not known whether the use of verapamil during labor or delivery has immediate or delayed adverse effects on the fetus, or whether it prolongs the duration of labor or increases the need for forceps delivery or other obstetric intervention. Such adverse experiences have not been reported in the literature, despite a long history of use of ISOPTIN in Europe in the treatment of cardiac side effects of beta-adrenergic agonist agents used to treat premature labor.

Nursing Mothers: ISOPTIN is excreted in human milk. Because of the potential for adverse reactions in nursing infants from verapamil, nursing should be discontinued while verapamil is administered.

Pediatric Use: Safety and efficacy of ISOPTIN in children below the age of 18 years have not been established.

Animal Pharmacology and/or Animal Toxicology: In chronic animal toxicology studies verapamil caused lenticular and/or suture line changes at 30 mg/kg/day or greater and frank cataracts at 62.5 mg/kg/day or greater in the beagle dog but not the rat. Development of cataracts due to verapamil has not been reported in man.

ADVERSE REACTIONS

Serious adverse reactions are uncommon when ISOPTIN (verapamil HCl) therapy is initiated with upward dose titration within the recommended single and total daily dose. See WARNINGS for discussion of heart failure, hypotension, elevated liver enzymes, AV block, and rapid ventricular response.

Reversible (upon discontinuation of verapamil) non-obstructive, paralytic, ileus has been infrequently reported in association with the use of verapamil. The following reactions to orally administered ISOPTIN occurred at rates greater than 1.0% or occurred at lower rates but appeared clearly drug-related in clinical trials in 4,954 patients.

[See table above.]

In clinical trials related to the control of ventricular response in digitalized patients who had atrial fibrillation or atrial flutter, ventricular rates below 50/min at rest occurred in 15% of patients and asymptomatic hypotension occurred in 5% of patients.

Constipation	7.3%	Fatigue	1.7%
Dizziness	3.3%	Dyspnea	1.4%
Nausea	2.7%	Bradycardia (HR < 50/min)	1.4%
Hypotension	2.5%	AV Block—total 1°, 2°, 3°	1.2%
Headache	2.2%	2° and 3°	0.8%
Edema	1.9%	Rash	1.2%
CHF/Pulmonary Edema	1.8%	Flushing	0.6%

Elevated Liver Enzymes (see WARNING)

The following reactions, reported in 1.0% or less of patients, occurred under conditions (open trials, marketing experience) where a causal relationship is uncertain; they are listed to alert the physician to a possible relationship:

Cardiovascular: angina pectoris, atrioventricular dissociation, chest pain, claudication, myocardial infarction, palpitations, purpura (vasculitis), syncope.

Digestive System: diarrhea, dry mouth, gastrointestinal distress, gingival hyperplasia.

Hemic and Lymphatic: ecchymosis or bruising.

Nervous System: cerebrovascular accident, confusion, equilibrium disorders, insomnia, muscle cramps, parathesia, psychotic symptoms, shakiness, somnolence.

Skin: arthralgia and rash, exanthema, hair loss, hyperkeratosis, maculae, sweating, urticaria, Stevens-Johnson syndrome, erythema multiforme.

Special Senses: blurred vision.

Urogenital: gynecomastia, impotence, galactorrhea/hyperprolactinemia, increased urination, spotty menstruation.

Treatment of Acute Cardiovascular Adverse Reactions: The frequency of cardiovascular adverse reactions which require therapy is rare; hence, experience with their treatment is limited. Whenever severe hypotension or complete AV block occur following oral administration of verapamil, the appropriate emergency measures should be applied immediately, e.g., intravenously administered isoproterenol HCl, levarterenol bitartrate, atropine (all in the usual doses), or calcium gluconate (10% solution). In patients with hypertrophic cardiomyopathy (IHSS), alpha-adrenergic agents (phenylephrine, metaraminol bitartrate or methoxamine) should be used to maintain blood pressure, and isoproterenol and levarterenol should be avoided. If further support is necessary, inotropic agents (dopamine or dobutamine) may be administered. Actual treatment and dosage should depend on the severity and the clinical situation and the judgment and experience of the treating physician.

OVERDOSAGE

Treat all verapamil overdoses as serious and maintain observation for at least 48 hours (especially Isoptin SR), preferably under continuous hospital care. Delayed pharmacodynamic consequences may occur with the sustained released formulation. Verapamil is known to decrease gastrointestinal transit time.

Treatment of overdosage should be supportive. Beta-adrenergic stimulation or parenteral administration of calcium solutions may increase calcium ion flux across the slow channel, and have been used effectively in treatment of deliberate overdosage with verapamil. Verapamil cannot be removed by hemodialysis. Clinically significant hypotensive reactions or high degree AV block should be treated with vasopressor agents or cardiac pacing, respectively. Asystole should be handled by the usual measures including cardiopulmonary resuscitation.

DOSAGE AND ADMINISTRATION

Essential Hypertension

The dose of ISOPTIN SR should be individualized by titration and the drug should be administered with food. Initiate therapy with 180 mg of sustained-release verapamil HCl, ISOPTIN SR, given in the morning. Lower, initial doses of 120 mg a day may be warranted in patients who may have an increased response to verapamil (e.g., the elderly or small people etc.). Upward titration should be based on therapeutic efficacy and safety evaluated weekly and approximately 24 hours after the previous dose. The antihypertensive effects of ISOPTIN SR are evident within the first week of therapy.

If adequate response is not obtained with 180 mg of ISOPTIN SR, the dose may be titrated upward in the following manner:

a) 240 mg each morning,

b) 180 mg each morning plus 180 mg each evening, or 240 mg each morning plus 120 mg each evening

c) 240 mg every twelve hours.

When switching from immediate release ISOPTIN to ISOPTIN SR, the total daily dose in milligrams may remain the same.

HOW SUPPLIED

ISOPTIN® SR 240 mg tablets are supplied as light green, capsule shaped, scored, film-coated tablets containing 240 mg of verapamil hydrochloride. The tablet is embossed with a double Knoll triangle on one side and "ISOPTIN SR" on the other side. ISOPTIN® SR 180 mg tablets are supplied as light pink, oval shaped, scored, film-coated tablets contain-

Continued on next page

Knoll—Cont.

ing 180 mg of verapamil hydrochloride. The tablet is embossed with "ISOPTIN SR" on one side, and "180 mg" on the other side. The Isoptin® SR 120 mg tablets are supplied as light violet, oval shaped, film-coated tablets containing 120 mg of verapamil hydrochloride. The tablet is embossed with "KNOLL" on one side and "120 SR" on the other side.

240 mg (light green)
 Bottle of 30-NDC #0044-1826-93
 Bottle of 100-HDC #0044-1826-02
 Hospital Unit Dose (100 Tablets-Strips of 10)-
  NDC #0044-1826-10
180 mg (light pink)
 Bottle of 100-NDC #0044-1825-02
 Hospital Unit Dose (100 Tablets-Strips of 10)-
  NDC #0044-1825-12
120 mg (light violet)
 Bottle of 100-NDC #0044-1827-02
 Hospital Unit Dose (100 Tablets-Strips of 10)-
  NDC #0044-1827-12

Storage: 59° to 86°F (15° to 30°C).
Protect from light and moisture
Dispense in a tight, light-resistant container as defined in the USP.

Knoll Pharmaceuticals
A Unit of BASF K&F Corporation
30 North Jefferson Road
Whippany, New Jersey 07981
BASF Group
RE-6/IsoSR2808/1-16-91   2816
Revised December 1991
Shown in Product Identification Section, page 414

QUADRINAL™ Tablets   ℞
[kwă'drĭ-nawl]

DESCRIPTION
Each QUADRINAL™ Tablet contains ephedrine hydrochloride 24 mg; phenobarbital 24 mg [Warning: May be habit forming]; theophylline calcium salicylate 130 mg (equivalent to 65 mg anhydrous theophylline); potassium iodide 320 mg. Other ingredients include magnesium stearate, potato starch, sodium thiosulfate and talc.
QUADRINAL contains two bronchodilators, theophylline and ephedrine. Phenobarbital serves as a mild sedative to help counteract central nervous system stimulation which may be caused by ephedrine. Wheezing and coughing are relieved by improved bronchodilation while the expectorant action of potassium iodide helps to remove secretions from the bronchial tree. Dyspnea is thus relieved or prevented and acute episodes of bronchospasm are often eliminated with consequent lessening of apprehension and distress.

CLINICAL PHARMACOLOGY
Theophylline directly relaxes the smooth muscle of the bronchial airways and pulmonary blood vessels, thus acting mainly as a bronchodilator, pulmonary vasodilator and smooth muscle relaxant. It also possesses other actions typical of the xanthine derivatives: coronary vasodilator, diuretic, and cardiac, cerebral, and skeletal muscle stimulant. The actions of theophylline may be mediated through inhibition of phosphodiesterase and a resultant increase in intracellular cyclic AMP which could mediate smooth muscle relaxation.
In vitro, theophylline has been shown to react synergistically with beta agonists (such as isoproterenol) that increase intracellular cyclic AMP through the stimulation of adenyl cyclase, but synergism has not been demonstrated in clinical studies and more data are needed to determine if theophylline and beta agonists have clinically important additive effects *in vivo*.
Apparently, tolerance does not develop with chronic use of theophylline.
The half-life is shortened with cigarette smoking. The half-life of theophylline in smokers (1 to 2 packs/day) averaged 4 to 5 hours in various studies, much shorter than the 7 to 9 hour half-life in nonsmokers. The increase in theophylline clearance caused by smoking is probably the result of induction of drug-metabolizing enzymes that do not readily normalize after cessation of smoking. It appears that between 3 months and 2 years may be necessary for normalization of the effect of smoking on theophylline pharmacokinetics.
The half-life is prolonged in alcoholism, reduced hepatic or renal function, congestive heart failure, and in patients receiving cimetidine or antibiotics such as troleandomycin (TAO, Cyclamycin), erythromycin, lincomycin and clindamycin. High fever for prolonged periods may decrease theophylline elimination.
Newborn infants have extremely slow clearances with half-lives exceeding 24 hours. These approach those seen for older children after about 3-6 months.
Older adults with chronic obstructive pulmonary disease, patients with cor pulmonale or other causes of heart failure,

and patients with liver pathology may have much lower clearances with half-lives that may exceed 24 hours.

Theophylline Elimination Characteristics

	Theophylline Clearance Rates (mean ± S.D.)	Half-life Average (mean ± S.D.)
Children (over 6 months of age)	1.45 ± .58 mL/kg/min	3.7 ± 1.1 hours
Adult non-smokers with uncomplicated asthma	0.65 ± .19 mL/kg/min	8.7 ± 2.2 hours

INDICATIONS
For chronic respiratory disease in which tenacious mucus and bronchospasm are dominant symptoms, such as bronchial asthma, chronic bronchitis and pulmonary emphysema.

CONTRAINDICATIONS
Use of QUADRINAL is contraindicated in patients with enlarged thyroid or goiter or with known sensitivity to theophylline, potassium iodide, ephedrine or sympathomimetics, or barbiturates.
The iodide in QUADRINAL can cause fetal harm when administered to a pregnant woman. Development of goiter has been reported in infants whose mothers received iodide-containing medications during pregnancy. A few neonatal deaths resulting from tracheal obstruction due to congenital goiters have been reported. Use of barbiturates during pregnancy may cause physical dependence with resulting withdrawal symptoms in the neonate; may cause birth defects; may be associated with neonatal hemorrhage due to reduction in levels of vitamin K-dependent clotting factors in the neonate; may cause respiratory depression in the neonate. QUADRINAL is contraindicated in women who are or may become pregnant. If this drug is used during pregnancy, or if the patient becomes pregnant while taking this drug, the patient should be apprised of the potential hazard to the fetus.

WARNINGS
QUADRINAL contains thiosulfate, a sulfite that may cause allergic-type reactions including anaphylactic symptoms and life-threatening or less severe asthmatic episodes in certain susceptible people. The overall prevalence of sulfite sensitivity in the general population is unknown and probably low. Sulfite sensitivity is seen more frequently in asthmatic than non-asthmatic people.
QUADRINAL contains theophylline calcium salicylate. Salicylates have been reported to be associated with the develop-

ment of Reye's syndrome in children and teenagers with chicken pox or flu.
Excessive theophylline doses may be associated with toxicity; determination of serum theophylline levels is recommended to assure maximal benefit without excessive risk. Incidence of toxicity increases at serum levels greater than 20 mcg/mL. Because of the theophylline content of QUADRINAL, it is unlikely that toxic levels of theophylline would be reached unless a serious overdosage occurs.
Morphine, curare, and stilbamidine should be used with caution in patients with airflow obstruction since they stimulate histamine release and can induce asthmatic attacks. They may also suppress respiration leading to respiratory failure. Alternative drugs should be chosen whenever possible.
There is an excellent correlation between clinical manifestations of toxicity and high blood levels of theophylline resulting from conventional doses in patients with lowered body plasma clearances (due to transient cardiac decompensation), patients with liver dysfunction or chronic obstructive lung disease, and patients who are older than 55 years of age, particularly males. In about 50% of patients, nausea and restlessness precede more severe manifestations of toxicity. In other patients, ventricular arrhythmias or seizures may be the first signs of toxicity. These more serious side effects are more likely to occur after intravenous administration of theophylline. Many patients who have high theophylline serum levels exhibit a tachycardia, and theophylline may worsen preexisting arrhythmias.

PRECAUTIONS
Mean half-life in smokers is shorter than in nonsmokers; therefore, smokers may require larger doses of theophylline. QUADRINAL, like all theophylline products, should not be administered concurrently with other xanthine medications. Use with caution in patients with severe cardiac disease, severe hypoxemia, hypertension, hyperthyroidism, acute myocardial injury, cor pulmonale, congestive heart failure, liver disease, peptic ulcer and in the elderly (especially males) and in neonates. Great caution should be used especially in giving theophylline to patients in congestive heart failure; such patients have shown markedly prolonged theophylline blood level curves with theophylline persisting in serum for long periods following discontinuation of the drug.
Theophylline may occasionally act as a local irritant to the G.I. tract although gastrointestinal symptoms are more commonly central in origin and associated with serum concentrations over 20 mcg/mL.
Ephedrine-containing medications should be used with caution in patients with cardiovascular disease, diabetes mellitus, predisposition to glaucoma, hypertension, hyperthyroidism, or prostatic hypertrophy.
Potassium iodide may aggravate acne in adolescents and adults.

Drug	Effect
Aminophylline with lithium carbonate	Increased excretion of lithium carbonate
Potassium iodide with lithium	Increased hypothyroid and goiterogenic effects
Aminophylline with propranolol	Antagonism of propranolol effect
Theophylline with furosemide	Increased diuresis
Theophylline with hexamethonium	Decreased hexamethonium induced chronotropic effect
Theophylline with reserpine	Reserpine-induced tachycardia
Theophylline with chlordiazepoxide	Chlordiazepoxide-induced fatty acid mobilization
Theophylline with troleandomycin (TAO, Cyclamycin), erythromycin, lincomycin, clindamycin	Increased theophylline plasma levels
Theophylline with phenytoin	Decreased phenytoin levels
Theophylline with cimetidine	Increased theophylline blood levels
Ephedrine with digitalis glycosides or anesthetics	May cause cardiac arrhythmias
Ephedrine with ergonovine, methylergonovine or oxytocin	Hypertension
Ephedrine with guanethidine	Decreased hypotensive effect
Ephedrine with MAO inhibitors	Potentiation of pressor effect of ephedrine
Ephedrine with reserpine	Decreased pressor effect of ephedrine
Ephedrine with other sympatho-mimetics	Increased effects of either medication
Ephedrine with tricyclic antidepressants	May antagonize the pressor action of ephedrine
Phenobarbital with alcohol, general anesthetics, other CNS depressants, or MAO inhibitors	Increased effects of either medication
Phenobarbital with oral anticoagulants	Decreased anticoagulant effects
Phenobarbital with corticosteroids, digitalis, digitoxin, doxycycline, tricyclic antidepressants, griseofulvin or phenytoin	Decreased effects of these drugs

Phenobarbital should be used with caution in patients with a history of drug abuse or dependence, impaired renal or hepatic function, hyperkinesis, uncontrolled pain, or history of porphyria.

Usage in Pregnancy: Pregnancy Category X. See "Contraindications" section.

Nursing Mothers: Because of the potential for serious adverse reactions in nursing infants from the potassium iodide, ephedrine and phenobarbital in QUADRINAL, a decision should be made whether to discontinue nursing or to discontinue the drug, taking into account the importance of the drug to the mother.

Pediatric Use: QUADRINAL is indicated for use in children on a short term basis. Chronic use should be reserved for patients in whom other expectorants have not been effective. If QUADRINAL is used chronically in children, the patient should be observed for signs of thyroid enlargement and worsening of acne.

Geriatric Patients: Geriatric patients may be more sensitive to the effects of ephedrine.

ADVERSE REACTIONS

The most frequent adverse reactions to theophylline are usually due to overdose (serum levels in excess of 20 mcg/mL) and are: nausea, vomiting, epigastric pain, hematemesis, diarrhea, headaches, irritability, restlessness, insomnia, reflex hyperexcitability, muscle twitching, clonic and tonic generalized convulsions, palpitations, tachycardia, extra systoles, flushing, hypotension, circulatory failure, ventricular arrhythmias, tachypnea, albuminuria, increased excretion of renal tubular cells and red blood cells, potentiation of diuresis, hyperglycemia and inappropriate ADH syndrome.

Thyroid adenoma, goiter and myxedema are possible side effects of potassium iodide.

Hypersensitivity to iodides may be manifested by angioneurotic edema, cutaneous and mucosal hemorrhages, and symptoms resembling serum sickness, such as fever, arthralgia, lymph node enlargement and eosinophilia.

Chronic ingestion of iodides may result in chronic iodide poisoning, or iodism. Initial symptoms include an unpleasant brassy taste, burning in the mouth and throat, soreness of the teeth and gums, increased salivation, coryza, sneezing, irritation of the eyes with swelling of the eyelids, headache, cough, skin lesions, diarrhea, gastric irritation, anorexia, fever and depression. The symptoms of iodism disappear spontaneously within a few days after stopping the administration of iodide. Therefore, treatment consists of stopping QUADRINAL therapy and providing supportive measures as indicated by the symptoms. Abundant fluid and sodium chloride intake may hasten iodide elimination. In severe cases, the use of mannitol to establish an osmotic diuresis may be appropriate. Potassium iodide may produce hyperkalemia and, if ingested chronically, may lead to goiter.

Adverse reactions to ephedrine include nervousness, restlessness, trouble in sleeping, irregular heartbeat, difficult or painful urination, dizziness or light-headedness, headache, loss of appetite, nausea or vomiting, trembling, troubled breathing, unusual increase in sweating, unusual paleness, feeling of warmth, and weakness. Tolerance to ephedrine may develop with prolonged or excessive use.

Adverse reactions to phenobarbital include mental confusion or depression, shortness of breath or troubled breathing, skin rash, hives, swelling of eyelids, face or lips, wheezing or tightness in chest, sore throat and fever, unusual bleeding or bruising, unusual excitement, tiredness or weakness, unusually slow heartbeat, yellowing of eyes or skin.

DRUG INTERACTIONS

Toxic synergism of theophylline with ephedrine has been documented and may occur with some other sympathomimetic bronchodilators. [See table on preceding page.]

OVERDOSAGE

A. If potential overdose is established and seizure has not occurred and patient is conscious:
   1) Induce vomiting.
   2) Administer a cathartic.
   3) Administer activated charcoal.
B. If patient is having a seizure:
   1) Establish an airway.
   2) Administer O_2.
   3) Treat the seizure with intravenous diazepam, 0.1 to 0.3 mg/kg up to 10 mg.
   4) Monitor vital signs, maintain blood pressure and provide adequate hydration.
C. Post-seizure coma:
   1) Maintain airway and oxygenation.
   2) Following above recommendations to prevent absorption of drug, but intubation and lavage will have to be performed instead of inducing emesis, and introduce the cathartic and charcoal via a large bore gastric lavage tube.
   3) Continue to provide full supportive care and adequate hydration while waiting for drug to be metabolized. In general, the drug is metabolized sufficiently rapidly so as not to require dialysis.

DOSAGE AND ADMINISTRATION

When rapidly absorbed products such as uncoated tablets with rapid dissolution are used, dosing to maintain "around the clock" blood levels generally requires administration every 6 hours in children; dosing intervals up to 8 hours may be satisfactory for adults because of their slower elimination rate.

Pulmonary function measurements before and after a period of treatment permit an objective assessment of response to QUADRINAL.

Usual dose:

Adults—One tablet 3 or 4 times daily; if needed, an additional one tablet upon retiring for nighttime relief. In severe attacks, the usual dose may be increased by one half.

Children 6 to 12 years—one half tablet three times daily.

Children under 6 years—dose is proportionately less.

HOW SUPPLIED

QUADRINAL Tablets— white, round, bi-convex tablets, engraved with a triangle on one side, bisected on the other side and imprinted with the number "14".

Bottles of 100—NDC #0044-4520-02.

STORAGE

Store at 59°–86°F (15°–30°C).

Dispense in tight, light-resistant container as defined in USP.

MR 1987/8448

Revised May, 1987 8449

Shown in Product Identification Section, page 414

RYTHMOL® TABLETS ℞
(propafenone hydrochloride)

DESCRIPTION

RYTHMOL (propafenone hydrochloride) is an antiarrhythmic drug supplied in scored, film-coated tablets of 150 and 300 mg for oral administration. Propafenone has some structural similarities to beta-blocking agents.

The structural formula of propafenone hydrochloride is given below:

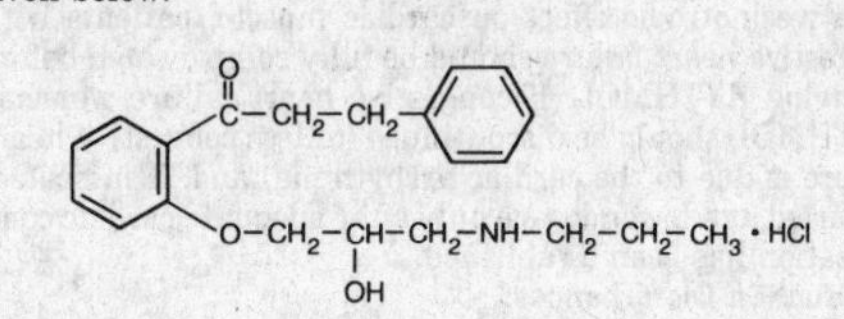

$C_{21}H_{27}NO_3 \cdot HCl$ M.W.=377.92

2′-[2-Hydroxy-3-(propylamino)-propoxy]-3-phenylpropiophenone hydrochloride

Propafenone hydrochloride occurs as colorless crystals or white crystalline powder with a very bitter taste. It is slightly soluble in water (20°C), chloroform and ethanol. The following inactive ingredients are contained in the tablet: corn starch, hydroxypropyl methyl cellulose, magnesium stearate, polyethylene glycol, polysorbate, povidone, propylene glycol, sodium starch glycolate and titanium dioxide.

CLINICAL PHARMACOLOGY

Mechanism of Action:

RYTHMOL (propafenone HCl) is a Class IC antiarrhythmic drug with local anesthetic effects, and a direct stabilizing action on myocardial membranes. The electrophysiological effect of RYTHMOL manifests itself in a reduction of upstroke velocity (Phase 0) of the monophasic action potential. In Purkinje fibers, and to a lesser extent myocardial fibers, RYTHMOL reduces the fast inward current carried by sodium ions. Diastolic excitability threshold is increased and effective refractory period prolonged. Propafenone reduces spontaneous automaticity and depresses triggered activity.

Studies in anesthetized dogs and isolated organ preparations show that RYTHMOL has beta-sympatholytic activity at about $\frac{1}{50}$ the potency of propranolol. Clinical studies employing isoproterenol challenge and exercise testing after single doses of propafenone indicate a beta-adrenergic blocking potency (per mg) about $\frac{1}{40}$ that of propranolol in man. In clinical trials, resting heart rate decreases of about 8% were noted at the higher end of the therapeutic plasma concentration range. At very high concentrations in vitro, propafenone can inhibit the slow inward current carried by calcium but this calcium antagonist effect probably does not contribute to antiarrhythmic efficacy. Propafenone has local anesthetic activity approximately equal to procaine.

Electrophysiology:

Electrophysiology studies in patients with ventricular tachycardia have shown that RYTHMOL prolongs atrioventricular conduction while having little or no effect on sinus node function. Both AV nodal conduction time (AH interval) and His-Purkinje conduction time (HV interval) are prolonged. Propafenone has little or no effect on the atrial functional refractory period, but AV nodal functional and effective refractory periods are prolonged. In patients with WPW, RYTHMOL reduces conduction and increases the effective refractory period of the accessory pathway in both directions. Propafenone slows conduction and consequently produces dose-related changes in the PR interval and QRS duration. QT_c interval does not change.

[See table below.]

In any individual patient, the above ECG changes cannot be readily used to predict either efficacy or plasma concentration.

RYTHMOL causes a dose-related and concentration-related decrease in the rate of single and multiple PVCs and can suppress recurrence of ventricular tachycardia. Based on the percent of patients attaining substantial (80–90%) suppression of ventricular ectopic activity, it appears that trough plasma levels of 0.2 to 1.5 μg/mL can provide good suppression, with higher concentrations giving a greater rate of good response.

Hemodynamics:

Sympathetic stimulation may be a vital component supporting circulatory function in patients with congestive heart failure, and its inhibition by the beta blockade produced by RYTHMOL may in itself aggravate congestive heart failure. Additionally, like other Class IC antiarrhythmic drugs, studies in humans have shown that RYTHMOL exerts a negative inotropic effect on the myocardium. Cardiac catheterization studies in patients with moderately impaired ventricular function (mean C.I.=2.61 L/min/m^2) utilizing intravenous propafenone infusions (2 mg/kg over 10 min + 2 mg/min for 30 min) that gave mean plasma concentrations of 3.0 μg/mL (well above the therapeutic range of 0.2–1.5 μg/mL) showed significant increases in pulmonary capillary wedge pressure, systemic and pulmonary vascular resistances and depression of cardiac output and cardiac index.

Pharmacokinetics and Metabolism:

RYTHMOL is nearly completely absorbed after oral administration with peak plasma levels occurring approximately 3.5 hours after administration in most individuals. Propafenone exhibits extensive saturable presystemic biotransformation (first pass effect) resulting in a dose dependent and dosage form dependent absolute bioavailability; e.g., a 150 mg tablet had absolute bioavailability of 3.4%, while a 300 mg tablet had absolute bioavailability of 10.6%. A 300 mg solution which was rapidly absorbed, had absolute bioavailability of 21.4%. At still larger doses, above those recommended, bioavailability increases still further. Decreased liver function also increases bioavailability; bioavailability is inversely related to indocyanine green clearance reaching 60–70% at clearances of 7 mL/min and below. The clearance of propafenone is reduced and the elimination half-life increased in patients with significant hepatic dysfunction (see PRECAUTIONS).

RYTHMOL follows a nonlinear pharmacokinetic disposition presumably due to saturation of first pass hepatic metabolism as the liver is exposed to higher concentrations of pro-

Mean Changes in ECG Intervals*
Total Daily Dose (mg)

	337.5 mg		450 mg		675 mg		900 mg	
Interval	msec	(%)	msec	(%)	msec	(%)	msec	(%)
RR	−14.5	−1.8	30.6	3.8	31.5	3.9	41.7	5.1
PR	3.6	2.1	19.1	11.6	28.9	17.8	35.6	21.9
QRS	5.6	6.4	5.5	6.1	7.7	8.4	15.6	17.3
QT_c	2.7	0.7	−7.5	−1.8	5.0	1.2	14.7	3.7

*Change and percent change based on mean baseline values for each treatment group.

Continued on next page

Knoll—Cont.

pafenone and shows a very high degree of interindividual variability. For example, for a three-fold increase in daily dose from 300 to 900 mg/day there is a ten-fold increase in steady-state plasma concentration. The top 25% of patients given 375 mg/day, however, had a mean concentration of propafenone larger than the bottom 25%, and about equal to the second 25%, of patients given a dose of 900 mg. Although food increased peak blood level and bioavailability in a single dose study, during multiple dose administration of propafenone to healthy volunteers food did not change bioavailability significantly.

There are two genetically determined patterns of propafenone metabolism. In over 90% of patients, the drug is rapidly and extensively metabolized with an elimination half-life from 2–10 hours. These patients metabolize propafenone into two active metabolites: 5-hydroxypropafenone and N-depropylpropafenone. In vitro preparations have shown these two metabolites to have antiarrhythmic activity comparable to propafenone, but in man they both are usually present in concentrations less than 20% of propafenone. Nine additional metabolites have been identified, most in only trace amounts. It is the saturable hydroxylation pathway that is responsible for the nonlinear pharmacokinetic disposition.

In less than 10% of patients (and in any patient also receiving quinidine, see PRECAUTIONS), metabolism of propafenone is slower because the 5-hydroxy metabolite is not formed or is minimally formed. The estimated propafenone elimination half-life ranges from 10–32 hours. Decreased ability to form the 5-hydroxy metabolite of propafenone is associated with a diminished ability to metabolize debrisoquine and a variety of other drugs (encainide, metoprolol, dextromethorphan). In these patients, the N-depropylpropafenone occurs in quantities comparable to the levels occurring in extensive metabolizers. In slow metabolizers propafenone pharmacokinetics are linear.

There are significant differences in plasma concentrations of propafenone in slow and extensive metabolizers, the former achieving concentrations 1.5 to 2.0 times those of the extensive metabolizers at daily doses of 675–900 mg/day. At low doses the differences are greater, with slow metabolizers attaining concentrations more than five times that of extensive metabolizers. Because the difference decreases at high doses and is mitigated by the lack of the active 5-hydroxy metabolite in the slow metabolizers, and because steady-state conditions are achieved after 4–5 days of dosing in all patients, the recommended dosing regimen is the same for all patients. The greater variability in blood levels require that the drug be titrated carefully in all patients with close attention to clinical and ECG evidence of toxicity (see DOSAGE AND ADMINISTRATION).

INDICATIONS AND USAGE

RYTHMOL (propafenone HCL) is indicated for the treatment of documented ventricular arrhythmias, such as sustained ventricular tachycardia, that, in the judgment of the physician are life-threatening. Because of the proarrhythmic effects of RYTHMOL, its use with lesser arrhythmias is generally not recommended. Treatment of patients with asymptomatic ventricular premature contractions should be avoided.

Initiation of RYTHMOL treatment, as with other antiarrhythmic agents used to treat life-threatening arrhythmias, should be carried out in the hospital.

Antiarrhythmic drugs have not been shown to enhance survival in patients with ventricular arrhythmias.

CONTRAINDICATIONS

RYTHMOL (propafenone HCl) is contraindicated in the presence of uncontrolled congestive heart failure, cardiogenic shock, sinoatrial, atrioventricular and intraventricular disorders of impulse generation and/or conduction (e.g., sick sinus node syndrome, atrioventricular block) in the absence of an artificial pacemaker, bradycardia, marked hypotension, bronchospastic disorders, manifest electrolyte imbalance, and known hypersensitivity to the drug.

WARNINGS

Mortality:

In the National Heart, Lung and Blood Institute's Cardiac Arrhythmia Suppression Trial (CAST), a long-term, multicentered, randomized, double-blind study in patients with asymptomatic non-life-threatening arrhythmias who had had myocardial infarctions more than six days but less than two years previously, an excessive mortality or non-fatal cardiac arrest rate was seen in patients treated with encainide or flecainide (56/730) compared with that seen in patients assigned to matched placebo-treated groups (22/725). The average duration of treatment with encainide or flecainide in this study was ten months.

The applicability of these results to other populations (e.g., those without recent myocardial infarctions) or to other antiarrhythmic drugs is uncertain, but at present it is prudent to consider any antiarrhythmic agent to have a significant risk in patients with structural heart disease.

Proarrhythmic Effects

RYTHMOL (propafenone HCl), like other antiarrhythmic agents, may cause new or worsened arrhythmias. Such proarrhythmic effects range from an increase in frequency of PVCs to the development of more severe ventricular tachycardia, ventricular fibrillation or torsade de pointes; i.e., tachycardia that is more sustained or more rapid which may lead to fatal consequences. It is therefore essential that each patient given RYTHMOL be evaluated electrocardiographically and clinically prior to, and during therapy to determine whether the response to RYTHMOL supports continued treatment.

Overall in clinical trials with propafenone, 4.7% of all patients had new or worsened ventricular arrhythmia possibly representing a proarrhythmic event (0.7% was an increase in PVCs; 4.0% a worsening, or new appearance, of VT or VF). Of the patients who had a worsening of VT (4%), 92% had a history of VT and/or VT/VF, 71% had coronary artery disease, and 68% had a prior myocardial infarction. The incidence of proarrhythmia in patients with less serious or benign arrhythmias, which include patients with an increase in frequency of PVCs, was 1.6%. Although most proarrhythmic events occurred during the first week of therapy, late events also were seen and the CAST study (see above) suggests that an increased risk is present throughout treatment.

Nonallergic Bronchospasm (e.g., chronic bronchitis, emphysema):

PATIENTS WITH BRONCHOSPASTIC DISEASE SHOULD IN GENERAL NOT RECEIVE PROPAFENONE or other agents with beta-adrenergic-blocking activity.

Congestive Heart Failure:

During treatment with oral propafenone in patients with depressed baseline function (mean EF=33.5%), no significant decreases in ejection fraction were seen. In clinical trial experience, new or worsened CHF has been reported in 3.7% of patients; of those 0.9% were considered probably or definitely related to RYTHMOL. Of the patients with congestive heart failure probably related to propafenone, 80% had preexisting heart failure and 85% had coronary artery disease. CHF attributable to RYTHMOL developed rarely (<0.2%) in patients who had no previous history of CHF.

As RYTHMOL exerts both beta blockade and a (dose-related) negative inotropic effect on cardiac muscle, patients with congestive heart failure should be fully compensated before receiving RYTHMOL. If congestive heart failure worsens, RYTHMOL should be discontinued (unless congestive heart failure is due to the cardiac arrhythmia) and, if indicated, restarted at a lower dosage only after adequate cardiac compensation has been established.

Conduction Disturbances:

RYTHMOL slows atrioventricular conduction and also causes first degree AV block. Average PR interval prolongation and increases in QRS duration are closely correlated with dosage increases and concomitant increases in propafenone plasma concentrations. The incidence of first degree, second degree, and third degree AV block observed in 2,127 patients was 2.5%, 0.6%, and 0.2%, respectively. Development of second or third degree AV block requires a reduction in dosage or discontinuation of RYTHMOL. Bundle branch block (1.2%) and intraventricular conduction delay (1.1%) have been reported in patients receiving propafenone. Bradycardia has also been reported (1.5%). Experience in patients with sick sinus node syndrome is limited and these patients should not be treated with propafenone.

Effects on Pacemaker Threshold:

RYTHMOL may alter both pacing and sensing thresholds of artificial pacemakers. Pacemakers should be monitored and programmed accordingly during therapy.

Hematologic Disturbances:

One case of agranulocytosis with fever and sepsis, probably related to the use of propafenone, was seen in U.S. clinical trials. The agranulocytosis appeared after 8 weeks of therapy. Propafenone therapy was stopped and the white count had normalized by 14 days. The patient recovered. In the course of over 800,000 patient years of exposure during marketing outside the U.S. since 1978, seven additional cases have been reported. In one of these, concomitant captopril, a drug known to cause agranulocytosis, was used. Unexplained fever and/or decrease in white cell count, particularly during the first three months of therapy, warrant consideration of possible agranulocytosis/granulocytopenia. Patients should be instructed to promptly report the development of any signs of infection such as fever, sore throat, or chills.

PRECAUTIONS

Hepatic Dysfunction:

Propafenone is highly metabolized by the liver and should, therefore, be administered cautiously to patients with impaired hepatic function. Severe liver dysfunction increases the bioavailability of propafenone to approximately 70% compared to 3–40% for patients with normal liver function. In eight patients with moderate to severe liver disease, the mean half-life was approximately 9 hours. As a result, the dose of propafenone given to patients with impaired hepatic function should be approximately 20–30% of the dose given to patients with normal hepatic function (see DOSAGE AND ADMINISTRATION). Careful monitoring for excessive pharmacological effects (see OVERDOSAGE) should be carried out.

Renal Dysfunction:

A considerable percentage of propafenone metabolites (18.5%–38% of the dose/48 hours) are excreted in the urine. Until further data are available, RYTHMOL (propafenone HCl) should be administered cautiously to patients with impaired renal function. These patients should be carefully monitored for signs of overdosage (see OVERDOSAGE).

Elevated ANA Titers:

Positive ANA titers have been reported in patients receiving propafenone. They have been reversible upon cessation of treatment and may disappear even in the face of continued propafenone therapy. These laboratory findings were usually not associated with clinical symptoms, but there is one published case of drug-induced lupus erythematosus (positive rechallenge); it resolved completely upon discontinuation of therapy. Patients who develop an abnormal ANA test should be carefully evaluated and, if persistent or worsening elevation of ANA titers is detected, consideration should be given to discontinuing therapy.

Impaired Spermatogenesis:

Reversible disorders of spermatogenesis have been demonstrated in monkeys, dogs and rabbits after high dose intravenous administration. Evaluation of the effects of short-term propafenone administration on spermatogenesis in 11 normal subjects suggests that propafenone produced a reversible, short-term drop (within normal range) in sperm count. Subsequent evaluation in 11 patients receiving propafenone chronically have suggested no effect of propafenone on sperm count.

Drug Interactions:

Quinidine: Small doses of quinidine completely inhibit the hydroxylation metabolic pathway, making all patients, in effect, slow metabolizers (see CLINICAL PHARMACOLOGY). There is, as yet, too little information to recommend concomitant use of propafenone and quinidine.

Local Anesthetics: Concomitant use of local anesthetics (i.e., during pacemaker implantations, surgery, or dental use) may increase the risks of central nervous system side effects.

Digitalis: RYTHMOL produces dose-related increases in serum digoxin levels ranging from about 35% at 450 mg/day to 85% at 900 mg/day of propafenone without affecting digoxin renal clearance. These elevations of digoxin levels were maintained for up to 16 months during concomitant administration. Plasma digoxin levels of patients on concomitant therapy should be measured, and digoxin dosage should ordinarily be reduced when propafenone is started, especially if a relatively large digoxin dose is used or if plasma concentrations are relatively high.

Beta-Antagonists: In a study involving healthy subjects, concomitant administration of propafenone and propranolol has resulted in substantial increases in propranolol plasma concentration and elimination half-life with no change in propafenone plasma levels from control values. Similar observations have been reported with metoprolol. Propafenone appears to inhibit the hydroxylation pathway for the two beta-antagonists (just as quinidine inhibits propafenone metabolism). Increased plasma concentrations of metoprolol could overcome its relative cardioselectivity. In propafenone clinical trials, patients who were receiving beta-blockers concurrently did not experience an increased incidence of side effects. While the therapeutic range for beta-blockers is wide, a reduction in dosage may be necessary during concomitant administration with propafenone.

Warfarin: In a study of eight healthy subjects receiving propafenone and warfarin concomitantly, mean steady-state warfarin plasma concentrations increased 39% with a corresponding increase in prothrombin times of approximately 25%. It is therefore recommended that prothrombin times be routinely monitored and the dose of warfarin be adjusted if necessary.

Cimetidine: Concomitant administration of propafenone and cimetidine in 12 healthy subjects resulted in a 20% increase in steady-state plasma concentrations of propafenone with no detectable changes in electrocardiographic parameters beyond that measured on propafenone alone.

Other: Limited experience with propafenone combined with calcium antagonists and diuretics has been reported without evidence of clinically significant adverse reactions.

Carcinogenesis, Mutagenesis, Impairment of Fertility:

Lifetime maximally tolerated oral dose studies in mice (up to 360 mg/kg/day) and rats (up to 270 mg/kg/day) provided no evidence of a carcinogenic potential for propafenone.

RYTHMOL was not mutagenic when assayed for genotoxicity in 1) mouse Dominant Lethal test, 2) rat bone marrow Chromosome Analysis, 3) Chinese hamster bone marrow and spermatogonia chromosome analysis, 4) Chinese hamster micronucleus test, and 5) Ames bacterial test.

Propafenone administered intravenously to rabbits, dogs, and monkeys has been shown to decrease spermatogenesis. These effects were reversible, were not found following oral dosing of propafenone, were seen only at lethal or sublethal

dose levels and were not seen in rats treated either orally or intravenously (see PRECAUTIONS, Impaired Spermatogenesis). Propafenone did not affect either male or female fertility rates when administered intravenously to rats and rabbits at dose levels up to 18 times the maximum recommended daily human dose of 900 mg (based on 60 kg human body weight).

Pregnancy-Teratogenic Effects:
Pregnancy Category C:
Propafenone has been shown to be embryotoxic in rabbits and rats when given in doses 10 and 40 times, respectively, the maximum recommended human dose. No teratogenic potential was apparent in either species. There are no adequate and well-controlled studies in pregnant women. Propafenone should be used during pregnancy only if the potential benefit justifies the potential risk to the fetus.

Pregnancy-Nonteratogenic Effects:
In a perinatal and postnatal study in rats, propafenone, at dose levels of 6 or more times the maximum recommended human dose, produced dose dependent increases in maternal and neonatal mortality, decreased maternal and pup body weight gain and reduced neonatal physiologic development.

Labor and Delivery:
It is not known whether the use of propafenone during labor or delivery has immediate or delayed adverse effects on the fetus, or whether it prolongs the duration of labor or increases the need for forceps delivery or other obstetrical intervention.

Nursing Mothers:
It is not known whether this drug is excreted in human milk. Because many drugs are excreted in human milk and because of the potential for serious adverse reactions in nursing infants from RYTHMOL, a decision should be made whether to discontinue nursing or to discontinue the drug, taking into account the importance of the drug to the mother.

Pediatric Use:
The safety and efficacy of RYTHMOL in children has not been established.

Geriatric Use:
There do not appear to be any age-related differences in adverse reaction rates in the most commonly reported adverse reactions. Because of the possible increased risk of impaired hepatic or renal function in this age group, RYTHMOL should be used with caution. The effective dose may be lower in these patients.

Animal Toxicology:
Renal changes have been observed in the rat following 6 months of oral administration of propafenone at doses of 180 and 360 mg/kg/day (12–24 times the maximum recommended human dose) but not 90 mg/kg/day. Both inflammatory and noninflammatory changes in the renal tubules with accompanying interstitial nephritis were observed. These lesions were reversible in that they were not found in rats treated at these dosage levels and allowed to recover for 6 weeks. Fatty degenerative changes of the liver were found in rats following chronic administration of propafenone at dose levels 19 times the maximum recommended human dose.

ADVERSE REACTIONS

Adverse reactions associated with RYTHMOL (propafenone HCl) occur most frequently in the gastrointestinal, cardiovascular, and central nervous systems. About 20% of patients discontinued due to adverse reactions. Results of controlled trials comparing adverse reaction rates on propafenone and placebo, and on propafenone and quinidine are shown in the following table. Adverse reactions appearing in the table were reported for ≥ 1% of the patients receiving propafenone. The most common events were dizziness, unusual taste, first degree AV block, intraventricular conduction delay, nausea and/or vomiting, and constipation. Headache was relatively common also, but was not increased compared to placebo.
[See table above.]
Adverse reactions reported for ≥ 1% of 2127 patients who received propafenone in U.S. clinical trials are presented in the following table by propafenone daily dose. The most common adverse reactions in controlled clinical trials appeared dose related (but note that most patients spent more time at the larger doses), especially dizziness, nausea and/or vomiting, unusual taste, constipation, and blurred vision. Some less common reactions may also have been dose related such as first degree AV block, congestive heart failure, dyspepsia, and weakness. The principal causes of discontinuation were the most common events and are shown in the table.
[See table on next page.]
In addition, the following adverse reactions were reported less frequently than 1% either in clinical trials or in marketing experience (*adverse events for marketing experience are given in italics*). Causality and relationship to propafenone therapy cannot necessarily be judged from these events.
Cardiovascular System: Atrial flutter, AV dissociation, cardiac arrest, flushing, hot flashes, sick sinus syndrome, sinus pause or arrest, supraventricular tachycardia

Adverse Reactions Reported for ≥ 1% of the Patients				
	Prop./Placebo Trials		Prop./Quinidine Trial	
	Prop. (N=247)	Placebo (N=111)	Prop. (N=53)	Quinidine (N=52)
Unusual Taste	7.3%	0.9%	22.6%	0.0%
Dizziness	6.5%	5.4%	15.1%	9.6%
First Degree AV Block	4.5%	0.9%	1.9%	0.0%
Headache(s)	4.5%	4.5%	1.9%	7.7%
Constipation	4.0%	0.0%	5.7%	1.9%
Intraventricular Conduction Delay	4.0%	0.0%	—	—
Nausea and/or Vomiting	2.8%	0.9%	5.7%	15.4%
Fatigue	—	—	3.8%	1.9%
Palpitations	2.4%	0.9%	—	—
Blurred Vision	2.0%	0.9%	5.7%	1.9%
Dry Mouth	2.0%	0.9%	5.7%	5.8%
Dyspnea	2.0%	2.7%	3.8%	0.0%
Abdominal Pain/Cramps	—	—	1.9%	7.7%
Dyspepsia	—	—	1.9%	7.7%
Congestive Heart Failure	—	—	1.9%	0.0%
Fever	—	—	1.9%	9.6%
Tinnitus	—	—	1.9%	1.9%
Vision Abnormal	—	—	1.9%	1.9%
Esophagitis	—	—	1.9%	0.0%
Gastroenteritis	—	—	1.9%	0.0%
Anxiety	2.0%	1.8%	—	—
Anorexia	1.6%	0.9%	—	1.9%
Proarrhythmia	1.2%	0.0%	1.9%	1.9%
Flatulence	1.2%	0.0%	1.9%	0.0%
Angina	1.2%	0.0%	1.9%	3.8%
Second Degree AV Block	1.2%	0.0%	—	—
Bundle Branch Block	1.2%	0.0%	1.9%	1.9%
Loss of Balance	1.2%	0.0%	—	—
Diarrhea	1.2%	0.9%	5.7%	38.5%

Nervous System: Abnormal dreams, abnormal speech, abnormal vision, *apnea, coma,* confusion, depression, memory loss, numbness, paresthesias, psychosis/mania, seizures (0.3%), tinnitus, unusual smell sensation, vertigo
Gastrointestinal: A number of patients with liver abnormalities associated with propafenone therapy have been reported in foreign post-marketing experience. Some appeared due to hepatocellular injury, some were cholestatic and some showed a mixed picture. Some of these reports were simply discovered through clinical chemistries, others because of clinical symptoms. One case was rechallenged with a positive outcome.
Cholestasis (0.1%), elevated liver enzymes (alkaline phosphatase, serum transaminases) (0.2%), gastroenteritis, hepatitis (0.03%)
Hematologic: Agranulocytosis, anemia, bruising, granulocytopenia, *increased bleeding time,* leukopenia, purpura, thrombocytopenia
Other: Alopecia, eye irritation, *hyponatremia/inappropriate ADH secretion,* impotence, increased glucose, *kidney failure,* positive ANA (0.7%), *lupus erythematosus,* muscle cramps, muscle weakness, nephrotic syndrome, pain, pruritus

OVERDOSAGE
The symptoms of overdosage, which are usually most severe within 3 hours of ingestion, may include hypotension, somnolence, bradycardia, intra-atrial and intraventricular conduction disturbances, and rarely convulsions and high grade ventricular arrhythmias. Defibrillation as well as infusion of dopamine and isoproterenol have been effective in controlling rhythm and blood pressure. Convulsions have been alleviated with intravenous diazepam. General supportive measures such as mechanical respiratory assistance and external cardiac massage may be necessary.

DOSAGE AND ADMINISTRATION
The dose of RYTHMOL (propafenone HCl) must be individually titrated on the basis of response and tolerance. It is recommended that therapy be initiated with 150 mg propafenone given every eight hours (450 mg/day). Dosage may be increased at a minimum of 3 to 4 day intervals to 225 mg every 8 hours (675 mg/day) and, if necessary, to 300 mg every 8 hours (900 mg/day). The usefulness and safety of dosages exceeding 900 mg per day have not been established. In those patients in whom significant widening of the QRS complex or second or third degree AV block occurs, dose reduction should be considered.
As with other antiarrhythmic agents, in the elderly or in patients with marked previous myocardial damage, the dose of RYTHMOL should be increased more gradually during the initial phase of treatment.

HOW SUPPLIED
RYTHMOL (propafenone HCl) tables are supplied as white, scored, round, film-coated tablets containing either 150 mg or 300 mg of propafenone hydrochloride and embossed with 150 or 300 and an arched triangle on the same side.
150 mg (white)—Bottle of 100—NDC #0044-5022-02
—Hospital Unit Dose (100 tablets—strips of 10)—NDC #0044-5022-10
300 mg (white)—Bottle of 100—NDC #0044-5023-02
—Hospital Unit Dose (100 tablets—strips of 10)—NDC #0044-5023-10

Continued on next page

Knoll—Cont.

Storage: Store at controlled room temperature. 59° to 86°F (15°–30°C). Dispense in tight, light-resistant container as defined in U.S.P.
RE-3/Ry4869/1-15-90

Knoll Pharmaceuticals
A Unit of BASF K&F Corporation
30 North Jefferson Road
Whippany, New Jersey 07981
BASF Group
Shown in Product Identification Section, page 414

ADVERSE REACTIONS REPORTED FOR ≥ 1% OF THE PATIENTS
N=2127

	Incidence by Total Daily Dose			Total Incidence (N=2127)	% of Pts. Who Discont.
	450 mg (N=1430)	600 mg (N=1337)	≥ 900 mg (N=1333)		
Dizziness	3.6%	6.6%	11.0%	12.5%	2.4%
Nausea and/or Vomiting	2.4%	6.1%	8.9%	10.7%	3.4%
Unusual Taste	2.5%	4.9%	6.3%	8.8%	0.7%
Constipation	2.0%	4.1%	5.3%	7.2%	0.5%
Fatigue	1.8%	2.8%	4.1%	6.0%	1.0%
Dyspnea	2.2%	2.3%	3.6%	5.3%	1.6%
Proarrhythmia	2.0%	2.1%	2.9%	4.7%	4.7%
Angina	1.7%	2.1%	3.2%	4.6%	0.5%
Headache(s)	1.5%	2.5%	2.8%	4.5%	1.0%
Blurred Vision	0.6%	2.4%	3.1%	3.8%	0.8%
CHF	0.8%	2.2%	2.6%	3.7%	1.4%
Ventricular Tachycardia	1.4%	1.6%	2.9%	3.4%	1.2%
Dyspepsia	1.3%	1.7%	2.5%	3.4%	0.9%
Palpitations	0.6%	1.6%	2.6%	3.4%	0.5%
Rash	0.6%	1.4%	1.9%	2.6%	0.8%
AV Block, First Degree	0.8%	1.2%	2.1%	2.5%	0.3%
Diarrhea	0.5%	1.6%	1.7%	2.5%	0.6%
Weakness	0.6%	1.6%	1.7%	2.4%	0.7%
Dry Mouth	0.9%	1.0%	1.4%	2.4%	0.2%
Syncope/Near Syncope	0.8%	1.3%	1.4%	2.2%	0.7%
QRS Duration, Increased	0.5%	0.9%	1.7%	1.9%	0.5%
Chest Pain	0.5%	0.7%	1.4%	1.8%	0.2%
Anorexia	0.5%	0.7%	1.6%	1.7%	0.4%
Abdominal Pain/Cramps	0.8%	0.9%	1.1%	1.7%	0.4%
Ataxia	0.3%	0.6%	1.5%	1.6%	0.2%
Insomnia	0.3%	1.3%	0.7%	1.5%	0.3%
Premature Ventricular Contraction(s)	0.6%	0.6%	1.1%	1.5%	0.1%
Bradycardia	0.5%	0.6%	1.1%	1.5%	0.5%
Anxiety	0.7%	0.5%	0.9%	1.5%	0.6%
Edema	0.6%	0.4%	1.0%	1.4%	0.2%
Tremor(s)	0.3%	0.8%	1.1%	1.4%	0.3%
Diaphoresis	0.6%	0.4%	1.1%	1.4%	0.3%
Bundle Branch Block	0.3%	0.7%	1.0%	1.2%	0.5%
Drowsiness	0.6%	0.5%	0.7%	1.2%	0.2%
Atrial Fibrillation	0.7%	0.7%	0.5%	1.2%	0.4%
Flatulence	0.3%	0.7%	0.9%	1.2%	0.1%
Hypotension	0.1%	0.5%	1.0%	1.1%	0.4%
Intraventricular Conduction Delay	0.2%	0.7%	0.9%	1.1%	0.1%
Pain, Joint(s)	0.2%	0.4%	0.9%	1.0%	0.1%

VICODIN® TABLETS   Ⓒ Ⓡ
[vĭ'kō-dĭn]

DESCRIPTION
Each VICODIN® tablet contains:
Hydrocodone Bitartrate .... 5 mg
      (WARNING: May be habit forming.)
Acetaminophen .... 500 mg
Other ingredients include colloidal silicon dioxide, corn starch, croscarmellose sodium Type A, dibasic calcium phosphate, magnesium stearate, microcrystalline cellulose, povidone, stearic acid and sodium metabisulfite.
Hydrocodone bitartrate is an opioid analgesic and antitussive and occurs as fine, white crystals or as a crystalline powder. It is affected by light. The chemical name is 4,5α-epoxy-3-methoxy-17-methylmorphinan-6-one tartrate (1:1) hydrate (2:5).
Its structure is as follows:

$C_{18}H_{21}NO_3 \cdot C_4H_6O_6 \cdot 2\tfrac{1}{2}H_2O$ M.W. 494.50

Acetaminophen, 4'-hydroxyacetanilide, is a non-opiate, non-salicylate analgesic and antipyretic which occurs as a white, odorless, crystalline powder possessing a slightly bitter taste. Its structure is as follows:

$C_8H_9NO_2$ M.W. 151.16

CLINICAL PHARMACOLOGY
Hydrocodone is a semisynthetic narcotic analgesic and antitussive with multiple actions qualitatively similar to those of codeine. Most of these involve the central nervous system and smooth muscle. The precise mechanism of action of hydrocodone and other opiates is not known, although it is believed to relate to the existence of opiate receptors in the central nervous system. In addition to analgesia, narcotics may produce drowsiness, changes in mood and mental clouding.
Radioimmunoassay techniques have recently been developed for the analysis of hydrocodone in human plasma. After a 10 mg oral dose of hydrocodone bitartrate, a mean peak serum drug level of 23.6 ng/mL and an elimination half-life of 3.8 hours were found.
The analgesic action of acetaminophen involves peripheral and central influences, but the specific mechanism is as yet undetermined. Antipyretic activity is mediated through hypothalamic heat regulating centers. Acetaminophen inhibits prostaglandin synthetase. Therapeutic doses of acetaminophen have negligible effects on the cardiovascular or respiratory systems; however, toxic doses may cause circulatory failure and rapid, shallow breathing. Acetaminophen is rapidly and almost completely absorbed from the gastrointestinal tract, producing maximum serum concentrations within 30 minutes to one hour. The plasma half-life in adults and children ranges from 0.90 hours to 3.25 hours with an average of approximately 2 hours. The drug distributes uniformly in most body fluids and is approximately 25% protein bound. Acetaminophen is conjugated in the liver, with less than 3% of the dose excreted unchanged in 24 hours. The primary metabolic pathway is conjugation to sulfate and glucuronide by-products. A minor oxidative pathway forms cysteine and mercapturic acid. These compounds are subsequently excreted by the kidneys into the urine.

INDICATIONS AND USAGE
For the relief of moderate to moderately severe pain.

CONTRAINDICATIONS
Hypersensitivity to acetaminophen or hydrocodone.

WARNINGS

Allergic-Type Reaction: VICODIN Tablets contain sodium metabisulfite, a sulfite that may cause allergic-type reactions including anaphylactic symptoms and life-threatening or less severe asthmatic episodes in certain susceptible people. The overall prevalence of sulfite sensitivity in the general population is unknown and probably low. Sulfite sensitivity is seen more frequently in asthmatic than non-asthmatic people.

Respiratory Depression: At high doses or in sensitive patients, hydrocodone may produce dose-related respiratory depression by acting directly on brain stem respiratory centers. Hydrocodone also affects the center that controls respiratory rhythm, and may produce irregular and periodic breathing.

Head Injury and Increased Intracranial Pressure: The respiratory depressant effects of narcotics and their capacity to elevate cerebrospinal fluid pressure may be markedly exaggerated in the presence of head injury, other intracranial lesions or a preexisting increase in intracranial pressure. Furthermore, narcotics produce adverse reactions which may obscure the clinical course of patients with head injuries.

Acute Abdominal Conditions: The administration of narcotics may obscure the diagnosis or clinical course of patients with acute abdominal conditions.

PRECAUTIONS

Special Risk Patients: As with any narcotic analgesic agent, VICODIN Tablets should be used with caution in elderly or debilitated patients and those with severe impairment of hepatic or renal function, hypothyroidism, Addison's disease, prostatic hypertrophy or urethral stricture. The usual precautions should be observed and the possibility of respiratory depression should be kept in mind.

Information for Patients: VICODIN Tablets, like all narcotics, may impair the mental and/or physical abilities required for the performance of potentially hazardous tasks such as driving a car or operating machinery; patients should be cautioned accordingly.

Cough Reflex: Hydrocodone suppresses the cough reflex; as with all narcotics, caution should be exercised when VICODIN Tablets are used postoperatively and in patients with pulmonary disease.

Drug Interactions: Patients receiving other narcotic analgesics, antipsychotics, antianxiety agents, or other CNS depressants (including alcohol) concomitantly with VICODIN Tablets may exhibit an additive CNS depression. When combined therapy is contemplated, the dose of one or both agents should be reduced.

The use of MAO inhibitors or tricyclic antidepressants with hydrocodone preparations may increase the effect of either the antidepressant or hydrocodone.

The concurrent use of anticholinergics with hydrocodone may produce paralytic ileus.

Usage in Pregnancy:

Teratogenic Effects: Pregnancy Category C. Hydrocodone has been shown to be teratogenic in hamsters when given in doses 700 times the human dose. There are no adequate and well-controlled studies in pregnant women. VICODIN Tablets should be used during pregnancy only if the potential benefit justifies the potential risk to the fetus.

Nonteratogenic Effects: Babies born to mothers who have been taking opioids regularly prior to delivery will be physically dependent. The withdrawal signs include irritability and excessive crying, tremors, hyperactive reflexes, increased respiratory rate, increased stools, sneezing, yawning, vomiting, and fever. The intensity of the syndrome does not always correlate with the duration of maternal opioid use or dose. There is no consensus on the best method of managing withdrawal. Chlorpromazine 0.7 to 1.0 mg/kg q6h, and paregoric 2 to 4 drops/kg q4h, have been used to treat withdrawal symptoms in infants. The duration of therapy is 4 to 28 days, with the dosage decreased as tolerated.

Labor and Delivery: As with all narcotics, administration of VICODIN Tablets to the mother shortly before delivery may result in some degree of respiratory depression in the newborn, especially if higher doses are used.

Nursing Mothers: It is not known whether this drug is excreted in human milk. Because many drugs are excreted in human milk and because of the potential for serious adverse reactions in nursing infants from VICODIN Tablets, a decision should be made whether to discontinue nursing or to discontinue the drug, taking into account the importance of the drug to the mother.

Pediatric Use: Safety and effectiveness in children have not been established.

ADVERSE REACTIONS

The most frequently observed adverse reactions include lightheadedness, dizziness, sedation, nausea and vomiting. These effects seem to be more prominent in ambulatory than in nonambulatory patients and some of these adverse reactions may be alleviated if the patient lies down.

Other adverse reactions include:

Central Nervous System: Drowsiness, mental clouding, lethargy, impairment of mental and physical performance, anxiety, fear, dysphoria, psychic dependence, mood changes.

Gastrointestinal System: The antiemetic phenothiazines are useful in suppressing the nausea and vomiting which may occur (see above) however, some phenothiazine derivatives seem to be antianalgesic and to increase the amount of narcotic required to produce pain relief, while other phenothiazines reduce the amount of narcotic required to produce a given level of analgesia. Prolonged administration of VICODIN Tablets may produce constipation.

Genitourinary System: Ureteral spasm, spasm of vesical sphincters and urinary retention have been reported.

Respiratory Depression: Hydrocodone bitartrate may produce dose-related respiratory depression by acting directly on brain stem respiratory centers. Hydrocodone also affects centers that controls respiratory rhythm, and may produce irregular and periodic breathing. If significant respiratory depression occurs, it may be antagonized by the use of naloxone hydrochloride. Apply other supportive measures when indicated.

DRUG ABUSE AND DEPENDENCE

VICODIN Tablets are subject to the Federal Controlled Substances Act (Schedule Ⓒ III).

Psychic dependence, physical dependence, and tolerance may develop upon repeated administration of narcotics; therefore, VICODIN Tablets should be prescribed and administered with caution. However, psychic dependence is unlikely to develop when VICODIN Tablets are used for a short time for the treatment of pain.

Physical dependence, the condition in which continued administration of the drug is required to prevent the appearance of a withdrawal syndrome, assumes clinically significant proportions only after several weeks of continued narcotic use, although some mild degree of physical dependence may develop after a few days of narcotic therapy. Tolerance, in which increasingly large doses are required in order to produce the same degree of analgesia, is manifested initially by a shortened duration of analgesic effect, and subsequently by decreases in the intensity of analgesia. The rate of development of tolerance varies among patients.

OVERDOSAGE

Acetaminophen:

Signs and Symptoms: In acute acetaminophen overdosage, dose-dependent, potentially fatal hepatic necrosis is the most serious adverse effect. Renal tubular necrosis, hypoglycemic coma, and thrombocytopenia may also occur.

In adults, hepatic toxicity has rarely been reported with acute overdoses of less than 10 grams and fatalities with less than 15 grams. Importantly, young children seem to be more resistant than adults to the hepatotoxic effect of an acetaminophen overdosage. Despite this, the measures outlined below should be initiated in any adult or child suspected of having ingested an acetaminophen overdose.

Early symptoms following a potentially hepatotoxic overdose may include: nausea, vomiting, diaphoresis and general malaise. Clinical and laboratory evidence of hepatic toxicity may not be apparent until 48 to 72 hours post-ingestion.

Treatment: The stomach should be emptied promptly by lavage or by induction of emesis with syrup of ipecac. Patients' estimates of the quantity of a drug ingested are notoriously unreliable. Therefore, if an acetaminophen overdose is suspected, a serum acetaminophen assay should be obtained as early as possible, but no sooner than four hours following ingestion. Liver function studies should be obtained initially and repeated at 24-hours intervals.

The antidote, N-acetylcysteine, should be administered as early as possible, preferably within 16 hours of the overdose ingestion for optimal results, but in any case, within 24 hours. Following recovery, there are no residual, structural or functional hepatic abnormalities.

Hydrocodone:

Signs and Symptoms: Serious overdose with hydrocodone is characterized by respiratory depression (a decrease in respiratory rate and/or tidal volume, Cheyne-Stokes respiration, cyanosis), extreme somnolence progressing to stupor or coma, skeletal muscle flaccidity, cold and clammy skin, and sometimes bradycardia and hypotension. In severe overdosage, apnea, circulatory collapse, cardiac arrest and death may occur.

Treatment: Primary attention should be given to the reestablishment of adequate respiratory exchange through provision of a patent airway and the institution of assisted or controlled ventilation. The narcotic antagonist naloxone is a specific antidote against respiratory depression which may result from overdosage or unusual sensitivity to narcotics, including hydrocodone. Therefore, an appropriate dose of naloxone hydrochloride (see package insert) should be administered, preferably by the intravenous route, and simultaneously with efforts at respiratory resuscitation. Since the duration of action of hydrocodone may exceed that of the antagonist, the patient should be kept under continued surveillance and repeated doses of the antagonist should be administered as needed to maintain adequate respiration.

An antagonist should not be administered in the absence of clinically significant respiratory or cardovascular depression. Oxygen, intravenous fluids, vasopressors and other supportive measures should be employed as indicated.

Gastric emptying may be useful in removing unabsorbed drug.

DOSAGE AND ADMINISTRATION

Dosage should be adjusted according to the severity of the pain and the response of the patient. However, it should be kept in mind that tolerance to hydrocodone can develop with continued use and the incidence of untoward effects is dose related.

The usual adult dosage is one or two tablets every four to six hours as needed for pain. The total 24 hour dose should not exceed 8 tablets.

HOW SUPPLIED

White, capsule shaped tablet bisected on one side and imprinted with "VICODIN" on the other side.

Bottles of 100—NDC #0044-0727-02.

Bottles of 500—NDC #0044-0727-03

Hospital Unit Dose Package—100 tablets (4×25 tablets)—NDC #0044-0727-41.

Storage: Store at controlled room temperature 15°–30°C (59°–86°F).

Dispense in a tight, light-resistant container as defined in the USP.

A Schedule Ⓒ III Narcotic.

Knoll Pharmaceuticals
a Unit of BASF K & F Corporation
Whippany, New Jersey 07981
MR 1987/5809
Revised February, 1988 5828
BASF Group

Shown in Product Identification Section, page 414

VICODIN ES® TABLETS Ⓒ III ℞

(hydrocodone bitartrate 7.5 mg
[Warning: May be habit forming]
and acetaminophen 750 mg)

DESCRIPTION

Each VICODIN ES® tablet contains: Hydrocodone Bitartrate 7.5 mg (**WARNING:** May be habit forming) and Acetaminophen 750 mg

Other ingredients include colloidal silicon dioxide, corn starch, croscarmellose sodium, magnesium stearate, povidone, and stearic acid.

Hydrocodone bitartrate is an opioid analgesic and antitussive and occurs as fine, white crystals or as a crystalline powder. It is affected by light. The chemical name is: 4,5α-epoxy-3-methoxy-17-methylmorphinan-6-one tartrate (1:1) hydrate (2:5). Its structure is as follows:

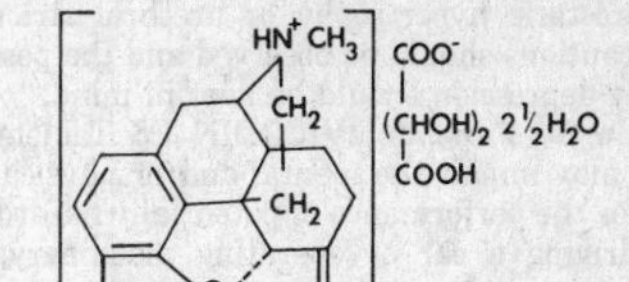

$C_{18}H_{21}NO_3 \cdot C_4H_6O_6 \cdot 2\frac{1}{2}\ H_2O$ M.W. 494.50

Acetaminophen, 4'-hydroxyacetanilide, is a non-opiate, non-salicylate analgesic and antipyretic which occurs as a white, odorless crystalline powder possessing a slightly bitter taste. Its structure is as follows:

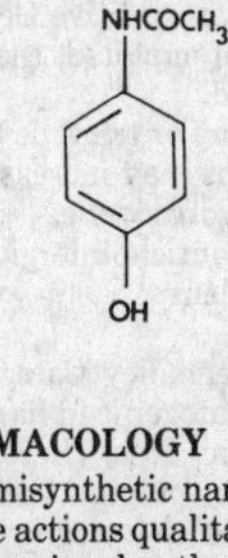

$C_8H_9NO_2$ M.W.151.16

CLINICAL PHARMACOLOGY

Hydrocodone is a semisynthetic narcotic analgesic and antitussive with multiple actions qualitatively similar to those of codeine. Most of these involve the central nervous system and smooth muscle. The precise mechanism of action of hydrocodone and other opiates is not known, although it is believed to relate to the existence of opiate receptors in the central nervous system. In addition to analgesia, narcotics may produce drowsiness, changes in mood and mental clouding.

Continued on next page

Knoll—Cont.

Radioimmunoassay techniques have recently been developed for the analysis of hydrocodone in human plasma. After a 10 mg oral dose of hydrocodone bitartrate, a mean peak serum drug level of 23.6 ng/mL and an elimination half life of 3.8 hours were found.
The analgesic action of acetaminophen involves peripheral and central influences, but the specific mechanism is as yet undetermined. Antipyretic activity is mediated through hypothalamic heat regulating centers. Acetaminophen inhibits prostaglandin synthetase. Therapeutic doses of acetaminophen have negligible effects on the cardiovascular or respiratory systems; however, toxic doses may cause circulatory failure and rapid, shallow breathing. Acetaminophen is rapidly and almost completely absorbed from the gastrointestinal tract, producing maximum serum concentrations within 30 minutes to one hour. The plasma half-life in adults and children ranges from 0.90 hours to 3.25 hours with an average of approximately 2 hours. The drug distributes uniformly in most body fluids and is approximately 25% protein bound. Acetaminophen is conjugated in the liver, with less than 3% of the dose excreted unchanged in 24 hours. The primary metabolic pathway is conjugation to sulfate and glucuronide by-products. A minor oxidative pathway forms cysteine and mercapturic acid. These compounds are subsequently excreted by the kidneys into the urine.

INDICATIONS AND USAGE

For the relief of moderate to moderately severe pain.

CONTRAINDICATIONS

Hypersensitivity to acetaminophen or hydrocodone.

WARNINGS

Respiratory Depression: At high doses or in sensitive patients, hydrocodone may produce dose-related respiratory depression by acting directly on the brain stem respiratory center. Hydrocodone also affects the center that controls respiratory rhythm, and may produce irregular and periodic breathing.
Head Injury and Increased Intracranial Pressure: The respiratory depressant effects of narcotics and their capacity to elevate cerebrospinal fluid pressure may be markedly exaggerated in the presence of head injury, other intracranial lesions or a preexisting increase in intracranial pressure. Furthermore, narcotics produce adverse reactions which may obscure the clinical course of patients with head injuries.
Acute Abdominal Conditions: The administration of narcotics may obscure the diagnosis or clinical course of patients with acute abdominal conditions.

PRECAUTIONS

Special Risk Patients: As with any narcotic analgesic agent, VICODIN ES Tablets should be used with caution in elderly or debilitated patients and those with severe impairment of hepatic or renal function, hypothyroidism, Addison's disease, prostatic hypertrophy or urethral stricture. The usual precautions should be observed and the possibility of respiratory depression should be kept in mind.
Information for Patients: VICODIN ES Tablets, like all narcotics, may impair the mental and/or physical abilities required for the performance of potentially hazardous tasks such as driving a car or operating machinery; patients should be cautioned accordingly.
Cough Reflex: Hydrocodone suppresses the cough reflex; as with all narcotics, caution should be exercised when VICODIN ES Tablets are used postoperatively and in patients with pulmonary disease.
Drug Interactions: Patients receiving other narcotic analgesics, antipsychotics, antianxiety agents, or other CNS depressants (including alcohol) concomitantly with VICODIN ES Tablets may exhibit an additive CNS depression. When combined therapy is contemplated, the dose of one or both agents should be reduced.
The use of MAO inhibitors or tricyclic antidepressants with hydrocodone preparations may increase the effect of either the antidepressant or hydrocodone.
The concurrent use of anticholinergics with hydrocodone may produce paralytic ileus.
Usage in Pregnancy:
Teratogenic Effects: Pregnancy Category C. Hydrocodone has been shown to be teratogenic in hamsters when given in doses 700 times the human dose. There are no adequate and well-controlled studies in pregnant women. VICODIN ES Tablets should be used during pregnancy only if the potential benefit justifies the potential risk to the fetus.
Nonteratogenic Effects: Babies born to mothers who have been taking opioids regularly prior to delivery will be physically dependent. The withdrawal signs include irritability and excessive crying, tremors, hyperactive reflexes, increased respiratory rate, increased stools, sneezing, yawning, vomiting, and fever. The intensity of the syndrome does not always correlate with the duration of maternal opioid use or dose. There is no consensus on the best method of managing withdrawal. Chlorpromazine 0.7 to 1 mg/kg q6h, and paregoric 2 to 4 drops/kg q4h, have been used to treat withdrawal symptoms in infants. The duration of therapy is 4 to 28 days, with the dosage decreased as tolerated.
Labor and Delivery: As with all narcotics, administration of VICODIN ES Tablets to the mother shortly before delivery may result in some degree of respiratory depression in the newborn, especially if higher doses are used.
Nursing Mothers: It is not known whether this drug is excreted in human milk. Because many drugs are excreted in human milk and because of the potential for serious adverse reactions in nursing infants from VICODIN ES Tablets, a decision should be made whether to discontinue nursing or to discontinue the drug, taking into account the importance of the drug to the mother.
Pediatric Use: Safety and effectiveness in children have not been established.

ADVERSE REACTIONS

The most frequently observed adverse reactions include lightheadedness, dizziness, sedation, nausea and vomiting. These effects seem to be more prominent in ambulatory than in nonambulatory patients and some of these adverse reactions may be alleviated if the patient lies down.
Other adverse reactions include:
Central Nervous System: Drowsiness, mental clouding, lethargy, impairment of mental and physical performance, anxiety, fear, dysphoria, psychic dependence, mood changes.
Gastrointestinal System: The antiemetic phenothiazines are useful in suppressing the nausea and vomiting which may occur (see above); however, some phenothiazine derivatives seem to be antianalgesic and to increase the amount of narcotic required to produce pain relief, while other phenothiazines reduce the amount of narcotic required to produce a given level of analgesia. Prolonged administration of VICODIN ES Tablets may produce constipation.
Genitourinary System: Ureteral spasm, spasm of vesical sphincters and urinary retention have been reported.
Respiratory Depression: Hydrocodone bitartrate may produce dose-related respiratory depression by acting directly on the brain stem respiratory center. Hydrocodone also affects the center that controls respiratory rhythm, and may produce irregular and periodic breathing.
If significant respiratory depression occurs, it may be antagonized by the use of naloxone hydrochloride. Apply other supportive measures when indicated.

DRUG ABUSE AND DEPENDENCE

VICODIN ES Tablets are subject to the Federal Controlled Substance Act (Schedule CIII)
Psychic dependence, physical dependence, and tolerance may develop upon repeated administration of narcotics; therefore, VICODIN ES Tablets should be prescribed and administered with caution. However, psychic dependence is unlikely to develop when VICODIN ES Tablets are used for a short time for the treatment of pain.
Physical dependence, the condition in which continued administration of the drug is required to prevent the appearance of a withdrawal syndrome, assumes clinically significant proportions only after several weeks of continued narcotic use, although some mild degree of physical dependence may develop after a few days of narcotic therapy. Tolerance, in which increasingly large doses are required in order to produce the same degree of analgesia, is manifested initially by a shortened duration of analgesic effect, and subsequently by decreases in the intensity of analgesia. The rate of development of tolerance varies among patients.

OVERDOSAGE

Acetaminophen:
Signs and Symptoms: In acute acetaminophen overdosage, dose-dependent, potentially fatal hepatic necrosis is the most serious adverse effect. Renal tubular necrosis, hypoglycemic coma, and thrombocytopenia may also occur.
In adults, hepatic toxicity has rarely been reported with acute overdoses of less than 10 grams and fatalities with less than 15 grams. Importantly, young children seem to be more resistant than adults to the hepatotoxic effect of an acetaminophen overdose. Despite this, the measures outlined below should be initiated in any adult or child suspected of having ingested an acetaminophen overdose.
Early symptoms following a potentially hepatotoxic overdose may include: nausea, vomiting, diaphoresis and general malaise. Clinical and laboratory evidence of hepatic toxicity may not be apparent until 48 to 72 hours post-ingestion.
Treatment: The stomach should be emptied promptly by lavage or by induction of emesis with syrup of ipecac. Patients' estimates of the quantity of a drug ingested are notoriously unreliable. Therefore, if an acetaminophen overdose is suspected, a serum acetaminophen assay should be obtained as early as possible, but no sooner than four hours following ingestion. Liver function studies should be obtained initially and repeated at 24-hour intervals.
The antidote, N-acetylcysteine, should be administered as early as possible, preferably within 16 hours of the overdose ingestion for optimal results, but in any case, within 24 hours. Following recovery, there are no residual, structural or functional hepatic abnormalities.
Hydrocodone:
Signs and Symptoms: Serious overdose with hydrocodone is characterized by respiratory depression (a decrease in respiratory rate and/or tidal volume, Cheyne-Stokes respiration, cyanosis), extreme somnolence progressing to stupor or coma, skeletal muscle flaccidity, cold and clammy skin, and sometimes bradycardia and hypotension. In severe overdosage, apnea, circulatory collapse, cardiac arrest and death may occur.
Treatment: Primary attention should be given to the reestablishment of adequate respiratory exchange through provision of a patent airway and the institution of assisted or controlled ventilation. The narcotic antagonist naloxone is a specific antidote against respiratory depression which may result from overdosage or unusual sensitivity to narcotics, including hydrocodone. Therefore, an appropriate dose of naloxone hydrochloride (see package insert) should be administered, preferably by the intravenous route, and simultaneously with efforts at respiratory resuscitation. Since the duration of action of hydrocodone may exceed that of the antagonist, the patient should be kept under continued surveillance and repeated doses of the antagonist should be administered as needed to maintain adequate respiration.
An antagonist should not be administered in the absence of clinically significant respiratory or cardiovascular depression. Oxygen, intravenous fluids, vasopressors and other supportive measures should be employed as indicated.
Gastric emptying may be useful in removing unabsorbed drug.

DOSAGE AND ADMINISTRATION

Dosage should be adjusted according to the severity of the pain and the response of the patient. However, it should be kept in mind that tolerance to hydrocodone can develop with continued use and that the incidence of untoward effects is dose related.
The usual adult dosage is one tablet every four to six hours as needed for pain. The total 24 hour dose should not exceed 5 tablets.

HOW SUPPLIED

VICODIN ES is supplied as a white, oval-shaped, faceted edged tablet containing 7.5 mg hydrocodone bitartrate and 750 mg acetaminophen, bisected on one side and imprinted with "VICODIN ES" on the other side. Bottles of 100—NDC #0044-0728-02. Bottles of 500—NDC #0044-0728-03.
Hospital Unit Dose Package—100 tablets (4×25 tablets)—NDC #0044-0728-41.
Storage: Store at controlled room temperature 15°–30°C (59°–86°F).
Dispense in a tight, light-resistant container as defined in the USP.
A Schedule CIII Narcotic.
Knoll Pharmaceuticals
A Unit of BASF K&F Corporation
Whippany, New Jersey 07981
RE-5/VicES5852/10-10-89
Revised September 1989 5852
BASF Group

Shown in Product Identification Section, page 414

EDUCATIONAL MATERIAL

Continuing Education Booklets
"Calcium in Cardiac Metabolism" (3 credits)
Home Study Module—Pharmacists
"Cardiac Arrhythmias" (2 credits)
Home Study Module—Pharmacists
"Angina Pectoris" (2 credits)
Home Study Module—Pharmacists
"Oral, Controlled-Release Dosage Products: New Developments and Implications" (3 credits)
Home Study Module—Pharmacists
"Treatment of Ventricular Arrhythmias" (3 credits)
Home Study Module—Pharmacists
"Treatment of Ventricular Arrhythmias" (3 credits)
Home Study Module—Nurses
"Cancer Pain Management" (3 credits)
Home Study Module—Pharmacists

Products are cross-indexed by generic and chemical names in the **YELLOW SECTION.**

Kramer Laboratories, Inc.
8778 S.W. 8TH STREET
MIAMI, FL 33174

CHARCOAL PLUS®   OTC
Antiflatulent/Antidiarrheal

DESCRIPTION
Each dosage of two, two phase tablets contains simethicone, 80 mg., in the layer for immediate release in the stomach and activated charcoal, 400 mg. USP, in an enteric-coated core for release in the small intestine.

INDICATIONS
For the relief of the symptoms of gas distress. CHARCOAL PLUS has a two-fold action on the painful symptoms of gas distress: simethicone acts in the stomach to neutralize and prevent the formation of gas pockets and provides for the relief of the pain and pressure symptoms of excess gas: activated charcoal is an adsorbent, detoxicant and soothing agent which provides for the relief of the symptoms of intestinal gas, diarrhea, and gastrointestinal distress associated with indigestion.

DIRECTIONS
Two tablets, four times daily, after meals and at bedtime. May also be taken as needed, up to 8 tablets daily, or as directed by a physician.

WARNING
Keep this and all medications out of the reach of children.

HOW SUPPLIED
Pink, round tablets in bottles of 120 and 36 tablets. (NDC 55505-105-16)

FUNGI-NAIL™   OTC
[fun'gi-nāl]
Tincture

DESCRIPTION
FUNGI-NAIL™ is a topical antifungal compound indicated for treatment of fungal nail infections. The composition of Fungi-Nail is:
Undecylenic Acid 10%
Salicylic Acid 5%
Isopropyl Alcohol .... 70% v/v
In a base of acetic acid, hydroxypropyl methylcellulose, propylene glycol and purified water. May also contain other ingredients.
Salicylic Acid is a keratolytic which occurs as white crystals, usually in fine needles, or as a fluffy white crystalline powder.
Undecylenic Acid is a monounsaturated fatty acid with a chain length of 11 carbon atoms. Typically, it is prepared from castor oil. Undecylenic Acid has been used for a number of years as a topical treatment for fungal infections of the skin and hair.
Isopropyl Alcohol is an antiseptic and solvent which occurs as a transparent, colorless, mobile, volatile liquid, having a characteristic odor.

CLINICAL PHARMACOLOGY
Fungi-Nail is a topical liquid antifungal compound which is indicated for the treatment of fungal (ringworm) nail infections. Fungi-Nail contains a keratolytic agent, Salicylic Acid which will promote peeling of the skin around the nail and allow the fungicidal ingredient, Undecylenic Acid, to reach the infected areas.

INDICATIONS AND USAGE
For the topical treatment of ringworm infections of the finger and toenails. Symptoms are thickened, lusterless and scaly nails (Tinea unguium or onchomycosis).

CONTRAINDICATIONS
Hypersensitivity to any of the ingredients.

DOSAGE AND ADMINISTATION
Wash and dry infected nails and surrounding tissue morning and evening. Then apply Fungi-Nail to affected nails and cutical area twice daily (morning and evening) using the brush applicator. TREATMENT SHOULD BE CONTINUED FOR AT LEAST 6 MONTHS, SINCE IT TAKES AN AVERAGE NAIL THIS LONG TO GROW OUT.

HOW SUPPLIED
Fungi-Nail is supplied in a 1 fluid ounce bottle with a brush applicator.

YOHIMEX™ Tablets   ℞
[yō-him'eks]

DESCRIPTION
Each tablet for oral administration contains yohimbine hydrochloride, 5.4 mg. (¹/₁₂ grain). Yohimbine is an indoalkylamine alkaloid with chemical similarity to reserpine. It is the principal alkaloid of the bark of the West African Corynanthe yohimbe tree and is also found in Rauwolfia Serpentina (L) Benth.

ACTIONS
Yohimbine is primarily an alpha-2 adrenergic blocker, which blocks presynaptic alpha-2-adrenoreceptors.
PHARMACOLOGY: Its peripheral autonomic nervous system effect is to increase parasympathetic (cholinergic) and decrease sympathetic (adrenergic) activity. In male sexual performance, erection is linked to cholinergic activity which theoretically results in increased penile blood inflow, decreased penile blood outflow or both, causing erectile stimulation without increasing sexual desire. Yohimbine exerts a stimulating action on mood and may increase anxiety. Such actions are not adequately studied, although they appear to require high doses. Yohimbine has a mild antidiuretic action, probably via stimulation of hypothalmic centers and release of posterior pituitary hormone. Its action on peripheral blood vessels resembles that of reserpine, though it is weaker and of short duration. The drug reportedly exerts no significant influence on cardiac stimulation and other effects mediated by beta-adrenergic receptors.

INDICATIONS
Sympathicolytic and mydriatic agent. Impotence has been successfully treated with yohimbine in male patients with vascular or diabetic origins and psychogenic origins (18 mg./day). Urologists have used yohimbine experimentally for the treatment and the diagnostic classification of certain types of male erectile impotence.

CONTRAINDICATIONS
In patients with renal disease; hypersensitivity to any component.

WARNINGS
Not for use in geriatric patients, psychiatric patients or cardio-renal patients with a history of gastric or duodenal ulcer. Generally not for use in females.
USAGE IN PREGNANCY: Do not use during pregnancy.
USAGE IN CHILDREN: Do not use in children.

DRUG INTERACTIONS
Do not use yohimbine with antidepressants and other mood-modifying drugs.

ADVERSE REACTIONS
CNS: Yohimbine readily penetrates the CNS and produces a complex pattern of responses in doses lower than those required to produce peripheral alpha-adrenergic blockade. These include: antidiuresis and central excitation including elevated blood pressure and heart rate, increased motor activity, nervousness, irritability and tremor. Dizziness, headache and skin flushing have been reported.

OVERDOSAGE
Daily doses of 20–30 mg. may produce increases in heart rate and blood pressure, piloerection and rhinorrhea. More severe symptoms may include paresthesias, incoordination, tremulousness and a dissociative state with higher doses.

DOSAGE AND ADMINISTRATION
USUAL ADULT DOSE: One tablet taken 3 times daily. If side effects occur, the dosage is to be reduced to ½ tablet 3 times a day followed by gradual increase to 1 tablet 3 times a day. The therapy reported is not more than 10 weeks.

HOW SUPPLIED
Pink, round tablets in bottles of 100 tablets (NDC 55505-100-15)

Kremers Urban Company
See SCHWARZ PHARMA

Lactaid, Inc.
PLEASANTVILLE, NJ 08232

LACTAID® Caplets   OTC
(lactase enzyme)

PRODUCT OVERVIEW
KEY FACTS
Lactaid® lactase enzyme hydrolyzes lactose into two digestible simple sugars: glucose and galactose. Lactaid Caplets are taken orally for *in vivo* hydrolysis of lactose.

MAJOR USES
Lactase insufficiency, suspected from gastrointestinal discomfort (ie, gas, bloating, flatulence, cramps, and diarrhea) after the ingestion of milk or lactose-containing products.

PRESCRIBING INFORMATION
DESCRIPTION
Each Caplet contains 3300 FCC (Food Chemical Codex) units of lactase enzyme (derived from *Aspergillus oryzae*).

ACTION
Lactase enzyme hydrolyzes the lactose sugar (a double sugar) into its simple sugar components, glucose and galactose.

INDICATIONS
Lactase insufficiency, suspected from gastrointestinal discomfort (ie, gas, bloating, flatulence, cramps, and diarrhea) after the ingestion of milk or lactose-containing products.

USUAL DOSAGE
These convenient, portable caplets are easy to swallow or chew and can be used with milk or any dairy food. We recommend taking 2 or 3 caplets with the first bite of any meal containing dairy. Take no more than 6 caplets at a time. Don't be discouraged if at first Lactaid does not work to your satisfaction. Because the degree of enzyme deficiency naturally varies from person to person and from food to food, you may have to adjust the number of caplets up or down to find your own level of comfort. Lactaid Caplets are nonhabit-forming, and because they work only on the food as you eat it, use them every time you enjoy dairy foods.

WARNING
If you experience any discomfort which is unusual or seems unrelated to the condition for which you took this product, consult a doctor before taking any more of it. Do not use if carton is opened or if printed plastic neckwrap is broken.

INACTIVE INGREDIENTS
Dextrates, Dibasic Calcium Phosphate, Microcrystalline Cellulose, Croscarmellose Sodium, Hydrogenated Vegetable Oil and Cornstarch.

NUTRITIONAL INFORMATION
Serving size: 2 Caplets; Calories: 2; Protein: 0g; Carbohydrate: 0g; Fat: 0g; Sodium: 0 mg;. Percentage of U.S. Recommended Daily Allowances (U.S.RDA): Contains less than 2% of the U.S. RDA of Protein, Vitamin A, Vitamin C and Thiamine.

HOW SUPPLIED
Lactaid Caplets are available in bottles of 12, 50, and 100 counts. Store at or below room temperature (below 77°F) but do not refrigerate. Keep away from heat.
Shown in Product Identification Section, page 414

LACTAID® Drops   OTC
(lactase enzyme)

PRODUCT OVERVIEW
KEY FACTS
Lactaid® lactase enzyme hydrolyzes lactose into two digestible simple sugars: glucose and galactose. Lactaid Drops are added to milk for *in vitro* hydrolysis of lactose.

MAJOR USES
Lactase insufficiency, suspected from gastrointestinal discomfort (ie, gas, bloating, flatulence, cramps, and diarrhea) after the ingestion of milk.

PRESCRIBING INFORMATION
DESCRIPTION
Each 5 drop dosage contains sufficient lactase enzyme (derived from *Kluyveromyces lactis*) to hydrolyze 70% of lactose from a quart of milk.

Continued on next page

Lactaid—Cont.

ACTION
The lactase enzyme hydrolyzes the lactose sugar (a double sugar) into its simple sugar components, glucose and galactose.

INDICATIONS
Lactase insufficiency, suspected from gastrointestinal discomfort (ie, gas, bloating, flatulence, cramps, and diarrhea) after the ingestion of milk.

USUAL DOSAGE
Lactaid drops are a liquid form of the natural lactase enzyme that makes milk more digestible. To use, add 5 drops of Lactaid in a quart of milk, shake gently and refrigerate for 24 hours. This makes 70% of the lactose digestible. Most people need only 5 drops per quart of milk, but because sensitivity to lactose can vary, you may have to adjust the number of drops you use. For greater lactose reduction: Use 10 drops per quart of milk for 90% reduction or 15 drops for 99+% lactose removal. Lactaid can be used with any kind of milk: whole, 1%, 2%, non-fat, skim, powdered and chocolate milk.

WARNING
If you experience any discomfort which is unusual or seems unrelated to the condition for which you took this product, consult a doctor before taking any more of it. Do not use if carton is opened or if printed plastic neckwrap is broken.

INACTIVE INGREDIENTS
Glycerin, Water

NUTRITIONAL INFORMATION
Serving size: 5 drops; Calories: 0; Protein: 0g; Carbohydrate: 0g; Fat: 0g; Sodium: 0 mg. Percentage of U.S. Recommended Daily Allowances (U.S. RDA): Contains less than 2% of the U.S. RDA of Protein, Vitamin A, Vitamin C and Thiamine.

HOW SUPPLIED
Lactaid Drops are available in .09 fl. oz. (12 quart supply), .22 fl. oz. (30 quart supply), and .53 fl. oz. (75 quart supply). Store at or below room temperature (below 77°F). Refrigerate after opening.

Shown in Product Identification Section, page 414

Laser, Inc.
2000 N. MAIN ST.
P.O. BOX 905
CROWN POINT, IN 46307

DALLERGY® SYRUP, TABLETS, CAPSULES   ℞

Each 5 mL of grape-flavored Syrup contains: Chlorpheniramine Maleate 2 mg, Phenylephrine Hydrochloride 10 mg, Methscopolamine Nitrate 0.625 mg. Each Tablet contains: Chlorpheniramine Maleate 4 mg, Phenylephrine Hydrochloride 10 mg, Methscopolamine Nitrate 1.25 mg. Each Extended-Release Capsule* contains: Chlorpheniramine Maleate 8 mg, Phenylephrine Hydrochloride 20 mg, Methscopolamine Nitrate 2.5 mg.

*In a specially prepared base to provide prolonged action.

DALLERGY® –JR. CAPSULES   ℞

Each Extended-Release Capsule* contains: Brompheniramine Maleate 6 mg, Pseudoephedrine Hydrochloride 60 mg.

*In a specially prepared base to provide prolonged action.

DONATUSSIN DC SYRUP   ©℞

Each 5 mL contains: Hydrocodone Bitartrate* 2.5 mg *(WARNING: May be habit forming), Phenylephrine Hydrochloride 7.5 mg, Guaifenesin 50 mg. Red Syrup.

DONATUSSIN DROPS   ℞

Each mL contains: Chlorpheniramine Maleate 1 mg, Phenylephrine Hydrochloride 2 mg, Guaifenesin 20 mg. Peach-flavored, orange color.

LACTOCAL–F TABLETS   ℞

Multivitamin, Multimineral supplement for pregnant or lactating women. White coated dye free tablet.

RESPAIRE®–SR CAPSULES 60 & 120   ℞

Each Extended-Release RESPAIRE-60 SR Capsule contains: Pseudoephedrine Hydrochloride* 60 mg and Guaifenesin 200 mg. Each Extended-Release RESPAIRE-120 SR Capsule contains: Pseudoephrine Hydrochloride* 120 mg and Guaifenesin 250 mg.

*In a specially prepared base to provide prolonged action.

THEOSTAT® 80 SYRUP   ℞
(theophylline anhydrous)

Each 15 mL contains: Theophylline anhydrous 80 mg, alcohol 1%. Dye-free cherry-vanilla flavor.

Lederle Laboratories
A Division of American Cyanamid Co.
ONE CYANAMID PLAZA
WAYNE, NJ 07470

Lederle Parenterals, Inc.
CAROLINA, PUERTO RICO 00630

Lederle Piperacillin, Inc.
CAROLINA, PUERTO RICO 00630

LEDERLE PRODUCTS

The following list of Lederle products includes the alphanumeric LEDERMARK® codes which provide quick and positive identification of Lederle capsules and tablets:

Product Identity Code No.	Product
	ACEL-IMUNE® Diphtheria and Tetanus Toxoids and Acellular Pertussis Vaccine Adsorbed
—	ACHROMYCIN® Ointment 3%
—	ACHROMYCIN® Ophthalmic Ointment 1%, 10mg/gm
—	ACHROMYCIN® Ophthalmic Suspension 1%
A3	ACHROMYCIN® V Caps., 250mg
A5	ACHROMYCIN® V Caps., 500mg
—	ACHROMYCIN® Oral Suspension, 125mg/5mL
A9	ARTANE® SEQUELS®, 5mg
A10	AMICAR® Tabs., 500mg
—	AMICAR® IV, 250mg/mL
—	AMICAR® Syrup, 25%
A11	ARTANE® Tabs., 2mg
A12	ARTANE® Tabs., 5mg
—	ARTANE® Elixir, 2mg/5mL
A13	ASENDIN® Tabs., 25mg
A15	ASENDIN® Tabs., 50mg
A17	ASENDIN® Tabs., 100mg
A18	ASENDIN® Tabs., 150mg
A31	Ampicillin Trihydrate Capsules, USP, 250mg
A32	Ampicillin Trihydrate Capsules, USP, 500mg
—	Ampicillin Trihydrate for Oral Suspension, USP, 125mg/5mL
—	Ampicillin Trihydrate for Oral Suspension, USP, 250mg/5mL
A33	Amoxicillin Capsules, USP, 250mg
A34	Amoxicillin Capsules, USP, 500mg
—	Amoxicillin for Oral Suspension, USP, 125mg/5mL
—	Amoxicillin for Oral Suspension, USP, 250mg/5mL
A45	Albuterol Sulfate Tablets, 2mg
A46	Albuterol Sulfate Tablets, 4mg
A7	Atenolol Tablets, 25mg
A49	Atenolol Tablets, 50mg
A71	Atenolol Tablets, 100mg
—	AUREOMYCIN® Ointment 3%, 30mg/g
—	AUREOMYCIN® Ointment (Ophthalmic) 1%, 10mg/g
B10	Benztropine Mesylate Tablets, USP, 1mg
B11	Benztropine Mesylate Tablets, USP, 2mg
C1	CENTRUM® Tabs.
C2	CENTRUM, JR.® + Iron Tabs.
C12	Leucovorin Calcium Tabs., 10mg
C31	Cloxacillin Sodium Capsules, USP, 500mg
—	Clindamycin Phosphate Injection, USP, 150mg/mL, 2mL vial
—	Clindamycin Phosphate Injection, USP, 150mg/mL, 4mL vial
—	Clindamycin Phosphate Injection, USP, 150mg/mL, 6mL vial
—	Clindamycin Phosphate Injection, USP, 150mg/mL, 60 mL vial
C33	Leucovorin Calcium Tabs., 5mg
C35	Leucovorin Calcium Tabs., 15mg
—	Leucovorin Calcium IM, 50mg vial, 100mg vial
C39	CENTRUM, JR.® Extra C Tabs.
C40	CALTRATE® 600 + Vit. D Tabs.
C42	Clonidine HCl Tablets, USP, 0.1mg
C43	Clonidine HCl Tablets, USP, 0.2mg
C44	Clonidine HCl Tablets, USP, 0.3mg
C45	CALTRATE® 600 + Iron Tabs.
C55	Clorazepate Dipotassium Capsules, USP, 3.75mg
C56	Clorazepate Dipotassium Capsules, USP, 7.5mg
C57	Clorazepate Dipotassium Capsules, USP, 15mg
C60	CENTRUM, JR.® + Extra Calcium Tabs.
C61	Cephradine Capsules, USP, 250mg
C62	Cephradine Capsules, USP, 500mg
C64	Cephalexin Capsules, USP, 250mg
C65	Cephalexin Capsules, USP, 500mg
C69	Clorazepate Dipotassium Tablets, USP, 3.75mg
C70	Clorazepate Dipotassium Tablets, USP, 7.5mg
C71	Clorazepate Dipotassium Tablets, USP, 15mg
C81	Cephalexin Tablets, USP, 250mg
C82	Cephalexin Tablets, USP, 500mg
—	Cephalexin for Oral Suspension, USP, 125mg/5mL
—	Cephalexin for Oral Suspension, USP, 250mg/5mL
C600	CALTRATE® 600 Tabs.
CS11	CENTRUM SILVER®
D1	DIAMOX® Tabs., 125mg
D2	DIAMOX® Tabs., 250mg
D3	DIAMOX® SEQUELS®, 500mg
—	DIAMOX® PARENTERAL, 500mg
D11	DECLOMYCIN® Tabs., 150mg
D12	DECLOMYCIN® Tabs., 300mg
—	Diazepam Injection, USP, 5mg/mL, 2mL disposable syringe
D16	Dicloxacillin Sodium Capsules, USP, 250mg
D17	Dicloxacillin Sodium Capsules, USP, 500mg
—	Diphtheria & Tetanus Toxoids Adsorbed PUROGENATED®
—	Diphtheria & Tetanus Toxoids & Pertussis Vaccine Adsorbed TRI-IMMUNOL®
D25	Doxycycline Hyclate Capsules, USP, 100mg
D32	Docusate Sodium Capsules, USP, 100mg
D34	Docusate Sodium w/Casanthranol Capsules, 100mg/30mg
D41	Doxycycline Hyclate Tablets, USP, 100mg
D44	Dipyridamole Tablets, 25mg
D45	Dipyridamole Tablets, 50mg
D46	Dipyridamole Tablets, 75mg
D47	Doxepin HCl Capsules, USP, 25mg
D48	Doxepin HCl Capsules, USP, 50mg
D49	Doxepin HCl Capsules, USP, 75mg
D50	Doxepin HCl Capsules, USP, 10mg
D51	Diazepam Tablets, USP, 2mg
D52	Diazepam Tablets, USP, 5mg
D53	Diazepam Tablets, USP, 10mg
D54	Doxepin HCl Capsules, USP, 100mg
D55	Doxepin HCl Capsules, USP, 150mg
D62	Disopyramide Phosphate Capsules, USP, 100mg
—	Erythromycin Estolate for Oral Suspension, USP, 125mg/5mL
—	Erythromycin Estolate for Oral Suspension, USP, 250mg/5mL
—	Erythromycin Ethylsuccinate for Oral Suspension, USP, 200mg/5mL
—	Erythromycin Ethylsuccinate for Oral Suspension, USP, 400mg/5mL
—	Erythromycin Ethylsuccinate/Sulfisoxazole Acetyl for Oral Suspension, 200mg/5mL
—	Sterile Erythromycin Lactobionate for Injection, USP, 500mg/5 x 10mL vials
—	Sterile Erythromycin Lactobionate for Injection, USP, 1000mg/5 x 20mL vials
—	FOLVITE® Solution, 5mg/mL
F1	Folic Acid Tablets, 1mg
F2	FERRO-SEQUELS®
F4	FILIBON® Tabs.
F5	FILIBON® F.A. Tabs.
F6	FILIBON® FORTE Tabs.
—	FLU-IMUNE® Influenza Virus Vaccine
F11	Furosemide Tablets, USP, 20mg
F12	Furosemide Tablets, USP 40mg
F13	Furosemide Tablets, USP, 80mg
F21	Ferrous Gluconate Iron Supplement Tablets, 300mg

F22	Fenoprofen Calcium Tablets, USP, 600mg
F66	FIBERCON® Tabs., 625mg
G2	GEVRAL® T Tabs.
—	GEVRABON® Vitamin-Mineral Supplement 16 fl. oz.
—	HibTITER® Haemophilus b Conjugate Vaccine
H1	HYDROMOX® Tabs., 50mg
H11	Hydralazine HCl Tablets, USP, 25mg
H12	Hydralazine HCl Tablets, USP, 50mg
H14	Hydrochlorothiazide Tablets, USP, 25mg
H15	Hydrochlorothiazide Tablets, USP, 50mg
—	INCREMIN® w/Iron Syrup 4 fl. oz.
—	INCREMIN® w/Iron Syrup 16 fl. oz.
I19	Indomethacin Capsules, USP, 25mg
I20	Indomethacin Capsules, USP, 50mg
L1	LOXITANE® Caps., 5mg
L2	LOXITANE® Caps., 10mg
L3	LOXITANE® Caps., 25mg
L4	LOXITANE® Caps., 50mg
—	LOXITANE® IM, 50mg base/mL
—	LOXITANE® C Oral Concentrate, 25mg/mL
L9	LEDERCILLIN® VK, Tablets, USP, 500mg
L10	LEDERCILLIN® VK, Tablets, USP, 250mg
—	LEDERCILLIN® VK, for Oral Solution, 125mg/5mL
—	LEDERCILLIN® VK, for Oral Solution, 250mg/5mL
—	LEVO-T™ Tablets, USP, 25mcg
—	LEVO-T™ Tablets, USP, 50mcg
—	LEVO-T™ Tablets, USP, 75mcg
—	LEVO-T™ Tablets, USP, 100mcg
—	LEVO-T™ Tablets, USP, 125mcg
—	LEVO-T™ Tablets, USP, 150mcg
—	LEVO-T™ Tablets, USP, 200mcg
—	LEVO-T™ Tablets, USP, 300mcg
M1	Methotrexate Tabs., 2.5mg
—	Methotrexate Sodium Parenteral, 5mg, 20mg, 50mg, 100mg, 250mg, 1g
—	Methotrexate LFP® Sodium Parenteral, 50mg, 100mg, 200mg, 250mg
M1	RHEUMATREX® Tabs., 2.5mg
M3	Minocycline HCl Tablets, 50mg
M5	Minocycline HCl Tablets, 100mg
M6	MYAMBUTOL® Tabs., 100mg
M7	MYAMBUTOL® Tabs., 400mg
M8	MAXZIDE® Tabs., 75/50mg
M9	MAXZIDE®-25 MG Tabs., 37.5/25mg
M19	Methocarbamol Tablets, USP, 500mg
M20	Methocarbamol Tablets, USP, 750mg
M21	Methyldopa Tablets, USP, 125mg
M22	Methyldopa Tablets, USP, 250mg
M23	Methyldopa Tablets, USP, 500mg
M26	Metronidazole Tablets, USP, 250mg
M27	Metronidazole Tablets, USP, 500mg
M28	Metoclopramide Tablets, 10mg
M36	Methyldopa and Hydrochlorothiazide Tablets, USP, 250mg/15mg
M37	Methyldopa and Hydrochlorothiazide Tablets, USP, 250mg/25mg
M40	MATERNA® Tabs.
M45	MINOCIN® Pellet-Filled Caps., 50mg
M46	MINOCIN® Pellet-Filled Caps., 100mg
—	MINOCIN® IV, 100mg vial
—	MINOCIN® Oral Suspension, 50mg/5mL
N1	NEPTAZANE® Tabs., 50mg
N2	NEPTAZANE® Tabs., 25mg
—	NILSTAT® Oral Suspension, 100,000 units/mL
—	NILSTAT® Powder, USP
N21	Nitroglycerin SR Capsules, 6.5mg
—	NOVANTRONE® 20mg/mL, 10mL vial
—	NOVANTRONE® 25mg/mL, 12.5mL vial
—	NOVANTRONE® 30mg/mL, 15mL vial
—	OCCUCOAT®
O4	OCUVITE® Tabs.
—	ORIMUNE® Poliovirus Vaccine Live Oral Trivalent
—	PIPRACIL® 2gm
—	PIPRACIL® 3gm
—	PIPRACIL® 4gm
—	PIPRACIL® 40gm
—	PNU-IMUNE® 23 Pneumococcal Vaccine Polyvalent
P9	PRONEMIA® Caps.
P33	Propylthiouracil Tablets, USP, 50mg
—	PROSTEP$_{TM}$ nicotine transdermal system, 11mg,
—	PROSTEP$_{TM}$ nicotine transdermal system, 22mg
P36	Pyrazinamide Tablets, 500mg
P44	Propranolol HCl Tablets, USP, 10mg
P45	Propranolol HCl Tablets, USP, 20mg
P46	Propranolol HCl Tablets, USP, 40mg
P47	Propranolol HCl Tablets, USP, 80mg
P48	Procainamide HCl SR Tablets, 250mg
P65	Propranolol HCl Tablets, USP, 60mg
P69	Prazosin HCl Capsules, 1mg
P70	Prazosin HCl Capsules, 2mg
P71	Prazosin HCl Capsules, 5mg
Q11	Quinidine Sulfate Tablets, USP, 200mg
S1	STRESSTABS®
S2	STRESSTABS® w/Iron
S3	STRESSTABS® w/Zinc
—	Sulfamethoxazole and Trimethoprim Pediatric Suspension, USP, 200mg/40mg per 5mL
S14	Sulfasalazine Tablets, USP, 0.5g
S16	Sulindac Tablets, USP, 150mg
S17	Sulindac Tablets, USP, 200mg
S200	SUPRAX® Tablets, 200mg
S400	SUPRAX® Tablets, 400mg
—	SUPRAX® Powder for oral suspension
—	Tetanus Toxoid Adsorbed PUROGENATED®
—	Tetanus and Diphtheria Toxoids, Adsorbed PUROGENATED®
—	Thiotepa Parenteral, 15mg vial
—	Tobramycin Sulfate Injection, USP, 40mg/mL
—	TRI-IMMUNOL® Diphtheria and Tetanus Toxoids and Pertussis Vaccine, Adsorbed
—	Tuberculin, OLD, TINE TEST®
—	Tuberculin Purified Protein Derivative TINE TEST® (PPD)
T1	TriHEMIC® 600 Tabs.
T13	Sulfamethoxazole and Trimethoprim Tablets, USP, 400mg/80mg
T16	Sulfamethoxazole and Trimethoprim Tablets, USP, 800mg/160mg
T29	Trazodone HCl Tablets, 50mg
T30	Trazodone HCl Tablets, 100mg
T31	Trazodone HCl Tablets, 150mg
—	VANCOLED® Sterile Vancomycin HCl, USP, 500mg vial
—	VANCOLED® Sterile Vancomycin HCl, USP, 1g vial
—	VANCOLED® Sterile Vancomycin HCl, USP, 5g vial
V4	Verapamil HCl Tablets, 80mg
V5	Verapamil HCl Tablets, 120mg
V7	VERELAN® Caps., 180mg
V8	VERELAN® Caps., 120mg
V9	VERELAN® Caps., 240mg
	ZINCON®

DIPHTHERIA and TETANUS TOXOIDS and ACELLULAR PERTUSSIS VACCINE ADSORBED ACEL–IMUNE® ℞

DESCRIPTION

Diphtheria and Tetanus Toxoids and Acellular Pertussis Vaccine Adsorbed, ACEL-IMUNE, is a sterile combination of PUROGENATED® Diphtheria Toxoid, PUROGENATED Tetanus Toxoid, and Acellular Pertussis Vaccine, which is adsorbed to an aluminum salt. ACEL-IMUNE is for intramuscular use only. After shaking, the vaccine is a homogeneous white suspension.

The *Corynebacterium diphtheriae* and *Clostridium tetani* organisms are grown in media according to the method of Mueller and Miller[1,2] and are detoxified by use of formaldehyde. The diphtheria and tetanus toxoids are refined by the Pillemer alcohol fractionation method[3] and are diluted with a solution containing phosphate buffer, glycine, and thimerosal (mercury derivative) as a preservative. The acellular pertussis vaccine component is prepared by growing Phase I *Bordetella pertussis* in Stainer-Scholte defined medium and harvesting the culture fluid. Purification of the acellular pertussis vaccine component is accomplished by ammonium sulfate fractionation steps and a final sucrose density gradient centrifugation. The acellular pertussis vaccine component is detoxified with formaldehyde and thimerosal (mercury derivative) is added as a preservative.

The Diphtheria Toxoid, Tetanus Toxoid, and Acellular Pertussis Vaccine are combined, diluted in phosphate buffered saline (PBS), and adsorbed to aluminum. The aluminum adjuvant content by assay is ≤0.85 mg aluminum per 0.5 mL dose and is present as aluminum hydroxide and aluminum phosphate. The residual free formaldehyde content by assay is ≤0.02%. Thimerosal (mercury derivative) is present in a final concentration of 1:10,000. The final product may also contain gelatin and polysorbate 80 which are used in early stages of the process.

Each 0.5 mL dose is formulated to contain 7.5 Lf of diphtheria toxoid and 5.0 Lf of tetanus toxoid (both toxoids induce not less than 2 units of antitoxin per mL in the guinea pig potency test) and 300 hemagglutinating (HA) units of Acellular Pertussis Vaccine. A hemagglutination unit is that amount of material which completely agglutinates chicken red blood cells as measured by the HA assay.[4] The acellular pertussis vaccine component contains approximately 40 μg (but not more than 60 μg) of pertussis antigens per 0.5 mL dose with approximately 86% filamentous hemagglutinin (FHA), approximately 8% lymphocytosis promoting factor (LPF), approximately 4% per dose 69-kilodalton (69kd) outer membrane protein, and approximately 2% type 2 fimbriae (pertussis-specific agglutinogen).

The potency of the pertussis component is evaluated by measurement of ELISA titers in immunized mice against FHA, LPF, and 69kd and fimbriae.

The acellular pertussis vaccine component is produced by Takeda Chemical Industries, Ltd., Osaka, Japan and is combined with diphtheria and tetanus toxoids manufactured by Lederle Laboratories. The bulk vaccine is prepared by Lederle Laboratories. ACEL-IMUNE is filled, labeled, packaged and released by Lederle Laboratories.

CLINICAL PHARMACOLOGY

Simultaneous immunization against diphtheria, tetanus, and pertussis (whooping cough) during infancy and childhood has been a routine practice in the US since the late 1940s. It has played a major role in markedly reducing the incidence of cases and deaths from each of these diseases.

Diphtheria is primarily a localized and generalized intoxication caused by diphtheria toxin, an extracellular protein metabolite of toxinogenic strains of *Corynebacterium diphtheriae.* While the incidence of diphtheria in the US has decreased from over 200,000 cases reported in 1921, before the general use of diphtheria toxoid, to only 15 cases reported from 1980 to 1983,[5] case fatality rate has remained constant at about 5% to 10%.

The highest case fatality rates are in the very young and in the elderly.

Following adequate immunization with diphtheria toxoid, it is thought that protection lasts for at least 10 years.[5] Antitoxin levels of at least 0.01 antitoxin units/mL are generally regarded as protective.[6] This significantly reduces both the risk of developing diphtheria and the severity of clinical illness. It does not, however, eliminate carriage of *C diphtheriae* in the pharynx or on the skin.[5]

Tetanus is an intoxication manifested primarily by neuromuscular dysfunction caused by a potent exotoxin elaborated by *Clostridium tetani.* The incidence of tetanus in the US has dropped dramatically with the routine use of tetanus toxoid, remaining relatively constant over the last decade at about 90 cases reported annually. Spores of *C tetani* are ubiquitous, and there is essentially no natural immunity to tetanus toxin.

Thus, universal primary immunization with tetanus toxoid with subsequent maintenance of adequate antitoxin levels, by means of timed boosters, is necessary to protect all age groups.[5] Tetanus toxoid is a highly effective antigen, and a completed primary series generally induces serum antitoxin levels of at least 0.01 antitoxin units, a level which has been reported to be protective.[7] It is thought that protection persists for at least 10 years.[5]

Pertussis (whooping cough) is a highly communicable disease of the respiratory tract that has an attack rate in unimmunized household contacts of over 90%.[5] Since immunization against pertussis (whooping cough) became widespread, the number of reported cases and associated mortality in the US has declined from about 120,000 cases and 1,100 deaths in 1950,[8] to an annual average of about 3,500 cases and 10 fatalities in recent years.[5,9] Precise data do not exist, since bacteriological confirmation of pertussis can be obtained in less than half of the suspected cases. Most reported illness from *B pertussis* occurs in infants and young children; two thirds of reported deaths occur in children less than 1 year old. Older children and adults, in whom classic signs are often absent, may go undiagnosed and serve as reservoirs of disease.[5]

Pertussis disease (whooping cough) is caused by a gram-negative coccobacillus, *B pertussis.* Several antigens which are thought to play a role in protective immunity have been isolated from cultures of *B pertussis.* These include filamentous hemagglutinin (FHA), lymphocytosis promoting factor (LPF), also known as pertussis toxin (PT), a 69-kilodalton (69kd) outer membrane protein, and fimbriae (pertussis-specific agglutinogens).[10–12] Another biologically active component, endotoxin, may contribute to reactogenicity of pertussis vaccines.[13] The Takeda acellular pertussis vaccine component used in Diphtheria and Tetanus Toxoids and Acellular Pertussis Vaccine Adsorbed, ACEL-IMUNE contains inactivated LPF, FHA, 69kd outer membrane protein

Continued on next page

Information on Lederle products listed on these pages is the full prescribing information from product literature or package inserts effective in August 1992. Information concerning all Lederle products may be obtained from the Professional Services Department, Lederle Laboratories, Pearl River, New York 10965.

Lederle—Cont.

and type 2 fimbriae (pertussis-specific agglutinogen), with minimal endotoxin compared to that in whole-cell pertussis vaccine. The pertussis component induces immunity against pertussis (whooping cough).

Acellular pertussis vaccines have been used in Japan since 1981, mostly in 2-year-old children. Evidence for the efficacy of these vaccines, as a group, is demonstrated by the decline in pertussis disease with their routine use in that country.[14,15] In addition, a review of epidemiological studies of the Japanese acellular pertussis vaccines estimated that these vaccines, as a group, were 88% efficacious in protecting against clinical pertussis on household exposure, with a 95% confidence interval of 79% to 93%.[16] In three Japanese household contact studies which employed retrospective case ascertainment and nonstandard case definitions, the vaccine-specific efficacy of the Takeda vaccine ranged between 89% and 94% but confidence intervals were wide, due to the small number of children in each study.[16,18,19,20] Although there were differences in study methods, these estimates of efficacy are quite comparable to that for whole-cell pertussis vaccine in the United States.[17]

Efficacy of the DTP vaccine containing the Takeda acellular pertussis vaccine component was examined, in particular, in a nonblinded household contact study, conducted by Lederle Laboratories that included both retrospective and prospective case evaluation.[21] As a consequence of the immunization schedule in Japan at the time of study, none of the vaccinated contacts were less than 2 years of age while some of the unvaccinated contacts were less than 2 years of age. When analysis of results was limited to vaccinated and unvaccinated household contacts 2 years of age and over, efficacy was established to be 79% (95% confidence interval, 60% to 89%) for physician-diagnosed pertussis disease. This included respiratory illnesses that may have been mild pertussis. When cases were restricted to disease diagnosed as typical pertussis, omitting mild suspect cases, efficacy was estimated to be 97% (95% confidence interval, 82% to 99%). When unvaccinated household contacts under 2 years of age are also included in the analysis, efficacy was estimated to be 81% (95% confidence interval, 64% to 90%) against pertussis disease (including mild suspect cases) and 98% (95% confidence interval, 84% to 99%) against typical pertussis. While there is some uncertainty with regard to the absolute magnitude of these estimates, the data as a whole demonstrate the efficacy of the Takeda Pertussis Vaccine.

Immunogenicity of ACEL-IMUNE compared with whole-cell DTP was studied in approximately 1,000 US children receiving these vaccines as a fourth or fifth dose at 17 to 24 months or 4 to 6 years of age. Antibody response following ACEL-IMUNE was similar to whole-cell DTP for LPF, 69kd protein, and agglutinins, and higher than DTP for FHA (the DTP used in these comparative studies was manufactured by Lederle Laboratories). All children achieved protective antibody levels to diphtheria and tetanus toxoids. A serologic correlate to protection against pertussis disease has not been established.[22] ACEL-IMUNE was less reactogenic than the whole-cell DTP vaccine (manufactured by Lederle Laboratories) in these studies[23,24,25] with regard to local reactions including less pain/tenderness, erythema, induration and warmth at the injection site. In addition, there was less drowsiness, fretfulness, fever and antipyretic use following ACEL-IMUNE as compared with DTP. The relative frequency of rare events that may be associated with immunization can only be determined in large postmarketing surveillance studies.

INDICATIONS AND USAGE

Diphtheria and Tetanus Toxoids and Acellular Pertussis Vaccine Adsorbed, ACEL-IMUNE, is indicated as a fourth and/or fifth dose for children from 17 months of age up to age 7 years (prior to seventh birthday) who have previously been immunized against diphtheria, tetanus, and pertussis with three or four doses of whole-cell DTP vaccine. The administration of ACEL-IMUNE may be considered for children as young as 15 months of age when it is expected that the child will not return at 18 months to receive the fourth dose in this immunization series although studies in this age group have not been completed.

THIS PRODUCT IS NOT RECOMMENDED FOR USE IN CHILDREN BELOW THE AGE OF 15 MONTHS.

Children who have recovered from culture-confirmed pertussis need not receive further doses of a pertussis-containing vaccine.[5] This vaccine is intended for active immunization against diphtheria, tetanus and pertussis, and is not to be used for treatment of actual infection.

If a contraindication to the pertussis vaccine component occurs, Diphtheria and Tetanus Toxoids, Adsorbed for pediatric use (DT) should be substituted for each of the remaining doses.

As with any vaccine, ACEL-IMUNE may not protect 100% of individuals receiving the vaccine.

CONTRAINDICATIONS

HYPERSENSITIVITY TO ANY COMPONENT OF THE VACCINE, INCLUDING THIMEROSAL, A MERCURY DERIVATIVE, IS A CONTRAINDICATION.

IMMUNIZATION SHOULD BE DEFERRED DURING THE COURSE OF ANY FEBRILE ILLNESS OR ACUTE INFECTION. A MINOR AFEBRILE ILLNESS SUCH AS A MILD UPPER RESPIRATORY INFECTION IS NOT USUALLY REASON TO DEFER IMMUNIZATION.[5,26]

DATA ON THE USE OF ACEL-IMUNE IN CHILDREN FOR WHOM WHOLE-CELL PERTUSSIS VACCINE IS CONTRAINDICATED ARE NOT AVAILABLE. UNTIL SUCH DATA ARE AVAILABLE, IT WOULD BE PRUDENT TO CONSIDER THE IMMUNIZATION PRACTICES ADVISORY COMMITTEE (ACIP) AND AMERICAN ACADEMY OF PEDIATRICS (AAP) CONTRAINDICATIONS TO WHOLE-CELL PERTUSSIS VACCINE AS CONTRAINDICATIONS TO ACEL-IMUNE.

IMMUNIZATION WITH ACEL-IMUNE IS CONTRAINDICATED IF THE CHILD HAS EXPERIENCED ANY EVENT FOLLOWING PREVIOUS IMMUNIZATION WITH PERTUSSIS VACCINE (DTP or acellular pertussis-containing vaccine), WHICH IS CONSIDERED BY THE AAP OR ACIP TO BE A CONTRAINDICATION TO FURTHER DOSES OF PERTUSSIS VACCINE.

THE ACIP STATES THAT "IF ANY OF THE FOLLOWING EVENTS OCCUR IN TEMPORAL RELATION TO RECEIPT OF DTP, THE DECISION TO GIVE SUBSEQUENT DOSES OF VACCINE CONTAINING THE PERTUSSIS COMPONENT SHOULD BE CAREFULLY CONSIDERED...

CONTRAINDICATIONS AND PRECAUTIONS TO FURTHER DTP VACCINATION

CONTRAINDICATIONS

AN IMMEDIATE ANAPHYLACTIC REACTION.

ENCEPHALOPATHY OCCURRING WITHIN 7 DAYS FOLLOWING DTP VACCINATION.

PRECAUTIONS

TEMPERATURE OF $\geq 40.5°$ C (105° F) WITHIN 48 HOURS NOT DUE TO ANOTHER IDENTIFIABLE CAUSE.

COLLAPSE OR SHOCK-LIKE STATE (HYPOTONIC-HYPORESPONSIVE EPISODE) WITHIN 48 HOURS.

PERSISTENT, INCONSOLABLE CRYING LASTING ≥ 3 HOURS, OCCURRING WITHIN 48 HOURS.

CONVULSIONS WITH OR WITHOUT FEVER OCCURRING WITHIN 3 DAYS.

ALTHOUGH THESE EVENTS WERE CONSIDERED ABSOLUTE CONTRAINDICATIONS IN PREVIOUS ACIP RECOMMENDATIONS, THERE MAY BE CIRCUMSTANCES, SUCH AS A HIGH INCIDENCE OF PERTUSSIS, IN WHICH THE POTENTIAL BENEFITS OUTWEIGH POSSIBLE RISKS, PARTICULARLY BECAUSE THESE EVENTS ARE NOT ASSOCIATED WITH PERMANENT SEQUELAE."[5]

The occurrence of any type of neurological symptoms or signs, including one or more convulsions (seizures) following administration of Diphtheria and Tetanus Toxoids and Acellular Pertussis Vaccine Adsorbed, ACEL-IMUNE or whole-cell DTP vaccine is generally a contraindication to further use. The presence of any evolving or changing disorder affecting the central nervous system is a contraindication to administration of pertussis vaccine regardless of whether the suspected neurological disorder is associated with occurrence of seizure activity of any type.[5,26]

The ACIP and the AAP recognize certain circumstances in which children with stable central nervous system disorders, including well-controlled seizures or satisfactorily explained single seizures, may receive pertussis vaccine. The ACIP and AAP do not consider a family history of seizures to be a contraindication to pertussis vaccine.[5,26,27]

The decision to administer a pertussis-containing vaccine to such children must be made by the physician on an individual basis, with consideration of all relevant factors, and assessment of potential risks and benefits for that individual. The physician should review the full text of ACIP and AAP guidelines prior to considering vaccination for such children.[5,26,27] The parent or guardian should be advised of the potential increased risk involved.

There are no data on whether the prophylactic use of antipyretics can decrease the risk of febrile convulsions. However, data suggest that acetaminophen will reduce the incidence of postvaccination fever. The ACIP and AAP suggest administering acetaminophen at age-appropriate doses at the time of vaccination and every 4 to 6 hours to children at higher risk for seizures than the general population.[5,26,27]

The clinical judgment of the attending physician should prevail at all times.

WARNINGS

THIS PRODUCT IS NOT RECOMMENDED FOR USE IN CHILDREN BELOW THE AGE OF 15 MONTHS. STUDIES IN CHILDREN 15-17 MONTHS OF AGE HAVE NOT BEEN COMPLETED.

NO DETERMINATION OF EFFICACY IN INFANTS HAS BEEN MADE TO DATE. STUDIES DESIGNED TO EVAL-UATE EFFICACY IN INFANTS ARE ONGOING BUT ARE NOT YET COMPLETE. IN ONE IMMUNOGENICITY STUDY, INFANTS RECEIVING ACEL-IMUNE EXHIBITED REDUCED RESPONSES TO LPF AND AGGLUTINOGENS, SIMILAR RESPONSES TO 69kd PROTEIN AND HIGHER SEROLOGICAL RESPONSES TO FHA, COMPARED TO THOSE RECEIVING LEDERLE WHOLE-CELL DTP VACCINE.[22] THE ROLE OF SERUM ANTIBODIES TO PERTUSSIS ANTIGENS IN PROTECTION AGAINST PERTUSSIS DISEASE IS UNKNOWN.

THIS PRODUCT IS NOT RECOMMENDED FOR IMMUNIZING PERSONS ON OR AFTER THEIR SEVENTH BIRTHDAY.

DATA ON THE USE OF ACEL-IMUNE IN CHILDREN FOR WHOM WHOLE-CELL PERTUSSIS VACCINE IS CONTRAINDICATED ARE NOT AVAILABLE. UNTIL SUCH DATA ARE AVAILABLE IT WOULD BE PRUDENT TO CONSIDER ACIP AND AAP CONTRAINDICATIONS TO WHOLE-CELL PERTUSSIS VACCINE AS CONTRAINDICATIONS TO ACEL-IMUNE. (See **CONTRAINDICATIONS.**)

Diphtheria and Tetanus Toxoids and Acellular Pertussis Vaccine Adsorbed, ACEL-IMUNE should be given with caution to children with thrombocytopenia or any coagulation disorder that would contraindicate intramuscular injection. (See **Drug Interactions.**)

Routine immunization should be deferred during an outbreak of poliomyelitis, providing the patient has not sustained an injury that increases the risk of tetanus and providing an outbreak of diphtheria or pertussis does not occur simultaneously.

PRECAUTIONS

General

1. PREVIOUS IMMUNIZATION HISTORY SHOULD BE ASCERTAINED TO CONFIRM THAT AT LEAST THREE DOSES OF WHOLE-CELL DTP VACCINE HAVE BEEN GIVEN.

2. PRIOR TO ADMINISTRATION OF ANY DOSE OF ACEL-IMUNE, THE PARENT OR GUARDIAN SHOULD BE ASKED ABOUT THE PERSONAL HISTORY, FAMILY HISTORY, AND RECENT HEALTH STATUS. THE PHYSICIAN SHOULD ASCERTAIN PREVIOUS IMMUNIZATION HISTORY, CURRENT HEALTH STATUS AND OCCURRENCE OF ANY SYMPTOMS AND/OR SIGNS OF AN ADVERSE EVENT AFTER PREVIOUS IMMUNIZATIONS IN THE CHILD TO BE IMMUNIZED, IN ORDER TO DETERMINE THE EXISTENCE OF ANY CONTRAINDICATION TO IMMUNIZATION WITH ACEL-IMUNE AND TO ALLOW AN ASSESSMENT OF BENEFITS AND RISKS.

3. BEFORE THE INJECTION OF ANY BIOLOGICAL, THE PHYSICIAN SHOULD TAKE ALL PRECAUTIONS KNOWN FOR THE PREVENTION OF ALLERGIC OR ANY OTHER SIDE REACTIONS. This should include: a review of the patient's history regarding possible sensitivity; the ready availability of epinephrine 1:1000 and other appropriate agents used for control of immediate allergic reactions; and a knowledge of the recent literature pertaining to use of the biological concerned, including the nature of side effects and adverse reactions that may follow its use.

4. Children with impaired immune responsiveness, whether due to the use of immunosuppressive therapy (including irradiation, corticosteroids, antimetabolites, alkylating agents, and cytotoxic agents), a genetic defect, human immunodeficiency virus (HIV) infection, or other causes, may have reduced antibody response to active immunization procedures.[5,26,28] Deferral of administration of vaccine may be considered in individuals receiving immunosuppressive therapy.[5,26] Other groups should receive this vaccine according to the usual recommended schedule.[5,26,28,29] (See **Drug Interactions.**)

5. This product is not contraindicated for use in individuals with HIV.

6. *Since this product is a suspension containing an adjuvant, shake vigorously to obtain a uniform suspension prior to withdrawing each dose from the multiple dose vial.*

7. A separate sterile syringe and needle or a sterile disposable unit should be used for each individual patient to prevent transmission of hepatitis or other infectious agents from one person to another. Needles should be disposed of properly and should not be recapped.

8. Special care should be taken to prevent injection into a blood vessel.

National Childhood Vaccine Injury Act: This Act requires that the manufacturer and lot number of the vaccine administered be recorded by the health care provider in the vaccine recipient's permanent medical record, along with the date of administration of the vaccine and the name, address, and title of the person administering the vaccine.

The Act further requires the health care provider to report to a health department or to the FDA the occurrence following immunization of any event set forth in the Vaccine Injury Table including: anaphylaxis or anaphylactic shock within 24 hours, encephalopathy or encephalitis within 7

days, shock-collapse or hypotonic-hyporesponsive collapse within 7 days, residual seizure disorder, any acute complication or sequelae (including death) of above events, or any event that would contraindicate further doses of vaccine, according to this Diphtheria and Tetanus Toxoids and Acellular Pertussis Vaccine Adsorbed, ACEL-IMUNE package insert.[30]

The U.S. Department of Health and Human Services has established a new Vaccine Adverse Event Reporting System (VAERS) to accept all reports of suspected adverse events after the administration of any vaccine, including but not limited to the reporting of events required by the National Childhood Vaccine Injury Act of 1986.[30] The VAERS toll-free number for VAERS forms and information is 800-822-7967.

Information for Patient: PRIOR TO ADMINISTRATION OF THIS VACCINE, HEALTH CARE PERSONNEL SHOULD INFORM THE PARENT, GUARDIAN, OR OTHER RESPONSIBLE ADULT OF THE RECOMMENDED IMMUNIZATION SCHEDULE FOR PROTECTION AGAINST DIPHTHERIA, TETANUS AND PERTUSSIS AND THE BENEFITS AND RISKS TO THE CHILD RECEIVING A VACCINE CONTAINING AN ACELLULAR PERTUSSIS COMPONENT. GUIDANCE SHOULD BE PROVIDED ON MEASURES TO BE TAKEN SHOULD ADVERSE EVENTS OCCUR, SUCH AS, ANTIPYRETIC MEASURES FOR ELEVATED TEMPERATURES AND THE NEED TO REPORT ADVERSE EVENTS TO THE HEALTH CARE PROVIDER. PARENTS SHOULD BE PROVIDED WITH VACCINE INFORMATION SHEETS (WHEN AVAILABLE FROM THE CENTERS FOR DISEASE CONTROL) AT THE TIME OF EACH VACCINATION, AS STATED IN THE NATIONAL CHILDHOOD VACCINE INJURY ACT.[30]

Drug Interactions: Children receiving immunosuppressive therapy may have a reduced response to active immunization procedures.[5,26,28]

As with other intramuscular injections, ACEL-IMUNE should be given with caution to children on anticoagulant therapy.

Carcinogenesis, Mutagenesis, Impairment of Fertility: Diphtheria and Tetanus Toxoids and Acellular Pertussis Vaccine Adsorbed, ACEL-IMUNE has not been evaluated for its carcinogenic, mutagenic potentials or impairment of fertility.

Pediatric Use: This product is not recommended for use in children below the age of 15 months. Studies in children under 15–17 months of age have not been completed.

No determination of efficacy in infants has been made to date. Studies designed to evaluate efficacy in infants are ongoing but are not yet complete. In one immunogenicity study infants receiving ACEL-IMUNE exhibited reduced responses to LPF and agglutinogens, similar responses to 69kd protein, and higher serological responses to FHA, compared to those receiving Lederle Laboratories' whole-cell DTP vaccine.[22] The role of serum antibodies to pertussis antigens in protection against pertussis disease is unknown. The vaccine is not recommended for use as a primary series in children of any age.

For immunization of children 7 years of age and older, Tetanus and Diphtheria Toxoids, Adsorbed for Adult Use (Td) is recommended.[5,26]

If a contraindication to the pertussis component exists, Diphtheria and Tetanus Toxoids Adsorbed for pediatric use (DT) should be substituted.

ADVERSE REACTIONS

Adverse reactions associated with ACEL-IMUNE have been evaluated in 911 children receiving this vaccine as the fourth or fifth dose in the DTP series. The percent of children experiencing common symptoms at any time within 72 hours following immunization is summarized below.[25]

Symptom	% of children* reporting symptoms within 72 hours of immunization (n=911)
Tenderness	26
Erythema (≥ 2 cm)	10
Induration (≥ 2 cm)	7
Injection site temp	17
Fever ≥38°C (100.4°F)	19
>39°C (102.2°F)	1.5
Drowsiness	6
Fretfulness	17
Vomiting	2

*Children age groups 17–24 months and 4–6 years of age (fourth and fifth doses) are included.

During a 72-hour period following immunization, the most frequently reported adverse events, excluding those listed above, in decreasing order of frequency were: upper respiratory infection/rhinitis (6%), diarrhea/loose stools (3.5%), rash (1.2%). One child experienced a febrile seizure 78 hours after immunization.[25] A cause and effect relationship be-

tween these latter events and vaccination has not been established.

In investigational studies in 2,041 infants administered a total of 5,719 doses of ACEL-IMUNE the combined frequency of common symptoms, at any time within 72 hours following any dose was as follows: erythema ≥ 2 cm, 4%; induration ≥ 2 cm, 1.5%; fever ≥ 38°C (100.4°F), 7%; drowsiness, 12%; fretfulness, 20%; vomiting, 3%. During this period, events judged by the investigators to contraindicate further doses of vaccine occurred in the indicated number of children: persistent or unusual cry (11); fever ≥ 40.5°C (104.9°F) (1); possible seizure (1); hypotonic-hyporesponsive episode (1); lethargy (1); injection site rash (1). One child died suddenly 6 weeks after immunization following apparent recovery from an enteroviral meningitis[25]; however, a causal relationship with Diphtheria and Tetanus Toxoids and Acellular Pertussis Vaccine Adsorbed, ACEL-IMUNE has not been established.

As with other aluminum-containing vaccines,[31] a nodule may occasionally be palpable at the injection site for several weeks. Although not seen in studies with ACEL-IMUNE, sterile abscess formation or subcutaneous atrophy at the injection site may also occur.

As with any vaccine, there is the possibility that broad use of ACEL-IMUNE could reveal adverse reactions not observed in clinical trials. Events have been reported following administration of other vaccines containing diphtheria, tetanus, and/or pertussis antigens. These include those listed below. Urticaria, erythema multiforme or other rash, arthralgias[32] and more rarely, a severe anaphylactic reaction (eg, urticaria with swelling of the mouth, difficulty breathing, hypotension, or shock) have been reported following administration of preparations containing diphtheria, tetanus, and/or pertussis antigens.

Neurological complications,[33] such as convulsions,[32] encephalopathy[32,34] and various mono- and polyneuropathies,[34–40] including Guillain-Barre syndrome[41,42] have been reported following administration of preparations containing diphtheria, tetanus, and/or pertussis antigens.

Permanent neurological disability and death have been reported rarely in temporal relation to immunization with vaccines containing pertussis antigens.

DOSAGE AND ADMINISTRATION

The dose is 0.5 mL to be given intramuscularly only.

A fourth and/or fifth dose with ACEL-IMUNE is indicated for children who have previously been immunized with at least three doses of whole-cell DTP vaccine.

The fourth dose consists of 0.5 mL of ACEL-IMUNE administered at approximately 18 months of age, and at least 6 months following the third DTP immunization.

A fifth dose consists of 0.5 mL of Diphtheria and Tetanus Toxoids and Acellular Pertussis Vaccine Adsorbed, ACEL-IMUNE and is indicated at 4 to 6 years of age, preferably prior to entrance into kindergarten or elementary school. However, if the fourth dose of the basic immunizing series was administered after the fourth birthday, a booster prior to school entry is not considered necessary.[5]

Shake vigorously to obtain a uniform suspension prior to withdrawing each dose from the multiple dose vial. The vaccine should not be used if it cannot be resuspended.

Parenteral drug products should be inspected visually for particulate matter and discoloration prior to administration whenever solution and container permit. (See **DESCRIPTION.**)

The vaccine should be injected intramuscularly. The preferred sites are the anterolateral aspect of the thigh or the deltoid muscle of the upper arm. The vaccine should not be injected in the gluteal area or areas where there may be a major nerve trunk. Before injection, the skin at the injection site should be cleansed and prepared with a suitable germicide.

After insertion of the needle, aspirate to help avoid inadvertent injection into a blood vessel.

If a contraindication to the pertussis vaccine component occurs, Diphtheria and Tetanus Toxoids, Adsorbed for pediatric use (DT) should be substituted for each of the remaining doses.

For either primary or booster immunization against tetanus and diphtheria of individuals 7 years of age or older, the use of Tetanus and Diphtheria Toxoids Adsorbed for Adult Use (Td) is recommended.[5,26]

HOW SUPPLIED

NDC 0005-1950-31 5.0 mL vial
NSN 6505-01-356-1193 5.0 mL vial

STORAGE

DO NOT FREEZE. STORE REFRIGERATED, AWAY FROM FREEZER COMPARTMENT, AT 2°C TO 8°C (36°F TO 46°F).

REFERENCES

1. Mueller JH, Miller PA. Production of diphtheria toxin of high potency (100 Lf) on a reproducible medium. *J Immunol* 1941;40:21–32.

2. Mueller JH, Miller PA. Factors influencing the production of tetanus toxin. *J Immunol* 1947; 56;143–147.

3. Pillemer L, Grossberg DB, Wittler RG. The immunochemistry of toxins and toxoids. II. The preparation of immunologic evaluation of purified tetanal toxoid. *J Immunol* 1946; 54:213–224.

4. Arai H, Sato Y. Separation and characterization of two distinct hemagglutinins contained in purified leukocytosis promoter factor from Bordetella pertussis. *Biochimica et Biophysica Acta* 1976;444:765–782.

5. Diphtheria, tetanus and pertussis: Recommendations for vaccine use and other preventive measures—Recommendations of the Immunization Practices Advisory Committee (ACIP). *MMWR* 1991; Vol. 40/No. RR-10.

6. Ipsen J. Immunization of adults against diphtheria and tetanus. *N Engl J Med* 1954; 251:459–466.

7. *Fed. Reg.* Vol. 50, No. 240, Dec. 13, 1985.

8. Reported incidence of notifiable diseases in the United States. *MMWR* 1970; 19(53):44.

9. Pertussis Surveillance—United States, 1986–1988. *MMWR* 1990; 39(4);57–66.

10. Cowell JL, Oda M, Burstyn DG, et al. Prospective protective antigens and animal models for pertussis. In: Leive L and Schlessinger D, eds. *Microbiology—1984.* Washington, DC: American Society for Microbiology; 1984: 172–175.

11. Shahin RD, Brennan MJ, Li ZM, et al. Characterization of the protective capacity and immunogenicity of the 69 K Da outer membrane protein of *Bordetella pertussis*. *J Exper Med* 1990; 171 (1):63–73.

12. Novotny P, Kobisch M, Cownley K, et al. Evaluation of *Bordetella bronchiseptica* vaccines in specific-pathogen-free piglets with bacterial cell surface antigens in enzyme linked immunosorbent assay. *Infect Immun* 1985; 50:190–198.

13. Manclark CR, Cowell JL. Pertussis. In: Germanier R. ed. *Bacterial Vaccines.* Orlando, Fl.: Academic Press, Inc.; 1984: 69–106.

14. Report of the Task Force on Pertussis and Pertussis Immunization—1988. *Pediatrics* Vol. 81, No. 6, Part 2, 939–984.

15. Kimura M, Kuno-Sakai H. Developments in pertussis immunisation in Japan. *Lancet* 1990; 30–32.

16. Noble GR, Bernier RH, Esber EC, et al. Acellular and whole-cell pertussis vaccines in Japan. *JAMA* 1987; 257:1351–1356.

17. Pertussis—United States, 1982 and 1983. *MMWR* 1984; 33(40):573–575.

18. Isomura S, Suzuki S, Sato Y. Clinical efficacy of the Japanese acellular pertussis vaccine after intrafamiliar exposure to pertussis patients. Proceedings of the Fourth International Symposium on Pertussis, Joint IABS/WHO Meeting, Geneva, Switzerland, 1984. *Dev. Biol. Standard.* Vol. 61: 531–537 (S. Karger, Basel, 1985).

19. Aoyama T, Murase Y, Gonda T, Iwata T. Type-specific efficacy of acellular pertussis vaccine. *AJDC* 1988; 142:40–42.

20. Kato T, Goshima T, Nakajima N, Kaku H, Arimoto Y, Hayashi F. Protection against pertussis by acellular pertussis vaccines (Takeda, Japan): Household contact studies in Kawasaki City, Japan. *Acta Paediatr Jpn* 1989; 31:698–701.

21. Mortimer EA, Kimura M, Cherry JD, et al. Protective efficacy of the Takeda Acellular Pertussis Vaccine combined with diphtheria and tetanus toxoids following household exposure of Japanese children. *AJDC* 1990; 144:899–904.

22. Blumberg DA, Mink CM, Cherry JD, et al. Comparison of acellular and whole-cell pertussis-component diphtheria-tetanus-pertussis vaccines in infants. *J. Pediatr* 1991; 119:194–204.

23. Morgan CM, Blumberg DA, Cherry JD, et al. Comparison of acellular and whole-cell pertussis-component DTP vaccines. *AJDC* 1990; 144:41–45.

24. Blumberg DA, Mink CM, Cherry JD, et al. Comparison of an acellular pertussis-component DTP vaccine with a whole-cell pertussis-component DTP vaccine in 17- to 24-month-old children, with measurement of 69-kilodalton outer membrane protein antibody. *J Pediatr* 1990; 117:46–51.

25. Data on file, Lederle Laboratories, Pearl River, NY.

26. American Academy of Pediatrics: *Report of the Committee on Infectious Diseases.* 22nd ed. Elk Grove Village, IL: American Academy of Pediatrics; 1991.

Continued on next page

Information on Lederle products listed on these pages is the full prescribing information from product literature or package inserts effective in August 1992. Information concerning all Lederle products may be obtained from the Professional Services Department, Lederle Laboratories, Pearl River, New York 10965.

Lederle—Cont.

27. Pertussis immunization: family history of convulsions and use of antipyretics—supplementary ACIP statement. *MMWR* 1987; 36(18):281–282.
28. Recommendation of the ACIP: immunization of children infected with Human T-Lymphotropic Virus Type III/Lymphadenopathy-associated virus. *MMWR* 1986; 35(38):595–606.
29. Immunization of children infected with Human Immunodeficiency Virus—Supplementary ACIP statement. *MMWR* 1988; 37(12):181–183.
30. National Childhood Vaccine Injury Act: Requirements for permanent vaccination records and for reporting of selected events after vaccination. *MMWR* 1988; 37(13):197–200.
31. Fawcett HA, Smith NP. Injection-site granuloma due to aluminum. *Arch Dermatol* 1984; 120:1318–1322.
32. Adverse events following immunization. *MMWR* 1985; 34(3):43–47.
33. Rutledge SL, Snead OC. Neurological complications of immunizations. *J Pediatr* 1986; 109:917–924.
34. Schlenska GK. Unusual neurological complications following tetanus toxoid administration. *J Neurol* 1977; 215:299–302.
35. Blumstein GI, Kreithen H. Peripheral neuropathy following tetanus toxoid administration. *JAMA* 1966; 198:1030–1031.
36. Reinstein L, Pargament JM, Goodman JS. Peripheral neuropathy after multiple tetanus toxoid injections. *Arch Phys Med Rehabil* 1982; 63:332–334.
37. Tsairis P, Dyck PJ, Mulder DW. Natural history of brachial plexus neuropathy. *Arch Neurol* 1972; 27:109–117.
38. Quast U, Hennessen W, Widmark RM. Mono- and polyneuritis after tetanus vaccination. *Devel Biol Stand* 1979; 43:25–32.
39. Holliday PL, Bauer RB. Polyradiculoneuritis secondary to immunization with tetanus and diphtheria toxoids. *Arch Neurol* 1983; 40:56–57.
40. Fenichel GM. Neurological complications of tetanus toxoid. *Arch Neurol* 1983; 40:390.
41. Pollard JD, Selby G. Relapsing neuropathy due to tetanus toxoid. *J Neurol Sci* 1978; 37:113–125.
42. Newton N, Janati A. Guillain-Barre syndrome after vaccination with purified tetanus toxoid. *S Med J* 1987; 80:1053–1054.

LEDERLE LABORATORIES DIVISION
American Cyanamid Company, Pearl River, NY 10965

20249-92
Rev. 2/92

Shown in Product Identification Section, page 414

ACHROMYCIN® ℞
[a-krō-mī-cin]
tetracycline hydrochloride
Ophthalmic Suspension, USP, 1% Sterile

(See PDR For Ophthalmology.)
Shown in Product Identification Section, page 414

ACHROMYCIN® V ℞
[a-krō-mī-cin]
tetracycline HCl
for ORAL USE

DESCRIPTION
ACHROMYCIN V is an antibiotic isolated from *Streptomyces aureofaciens*. Chemically it is the monohydrochloride of [4S-(4α,4aα,5aα,6β,12aα,)] -4- (Dimethylamino)-1,4,4a,5,5a,6,11,12a-octahydro-3, 6, 10, 12, 12a-pentahydroxy-6-methyl-1, 11-dioxo-2-naphthacenecarboxamide.

ACHROMYCIN V oral dosage forms contain the following inactive ingredients:

Capsules: Blue 1, FD&C Yellow No. 6, Gelatin, Lactose, Magnesium Stearate, Red 28, Titanium Dioxide, Yellow 10 and other ingredients.

CLINICAL PHARMACOLOGY
The tetracyclines are primarily bacteriostatic and are thought to exert their antimicrobial effect by the inhibition of protein synthesis. Tetracyclines are active against a wide range of gram-negative and gram-positive organisms. The drugs in the tetracycline class have closely similar antimicrobial spectra, and cross-resistance among them is common. Microorganisms may be considered susceptible if the MIC (minimum inhibitory concentration) is not more than 4 mcg/mL and intermediate if the MIC is 4 to 12.5 mcg/mL. Susceptibility plate testing: A tetracycline disc may be used to determine microbial susceptibility to drugs in the tetracycline class. If the Kirby-Bauer method of disc susceptibility testing is used, a 30 mcg tetracycline HCl disc should give a

zone of at least 19 mm when tested against a tetracycline-susceptible bacterial strain.

Tetracyclines are readily absorbed and are bound to plasma proteins in varying degrees. They are concentrated by the liver in the bile and excreted in the urine and feces at high concentrations and in a biologically active form.

INDICATIONS
ACHROMYCIN V is indicated in infections caused by the following microorganisms.

Rickettsiae: (Rocky Mountain spotted fever, typhus fever, and the typhus group, Q fever, rickettsialpox, tick fevers).

Mycoplasma pneumoniae (PPLO, Eaton agent).

Agents of psittacosis and ornithosis.

Agents of lymphogranuloma venereum and granuloma inguinale.

The spirochetal agent of relapsing fever (*Borrelia recurrentis*).

The following gram-negative microorganisms:

Haemophilus ducreyi (chancroid),

Yersinia pestis and *Francisella tularensis*, formerly *Pasteurella pestis* and *Pasteurella tularensis*,

Bartonella bacilliformis,

Bacteroides species,

Vibrio comma and *Vibrio fetus*,

Brucella species (in conjunction with streptomycin).

Because many strains of the following groups of microorganisms have been shown to be resistant to tetracyclines, culture and susceptibility testing are recommended.

ACHROMYCIN is indicated for treatment of infections caused by the following gram-negative microorganisms, when bacteriologic testing indicates appropriate susceptibility to the drug:

Escherichia coli,

Enterobacter aerogenes (formerly *Aerobacter aerogenes*),

Shigella species,

Mima species and *Herellea* species,

Haemophilus influenzae (respiratory infections),

Klebsiella species (respiratory and urinary infections).

ACHROMYCIN *tetracycline HCl* is indicated for treatment of infections caused by the following gram-positive microorganisms when bacteriologic testing indicates appropriate susceptibility to the drug:

Streptococcus species:

Up to 44% of strains of *Streptococcus pyogenes* and 74% of *Streptococcus faecalis* have been found to be resistant to tetracycline drugs. Therefore, tetracyclines should not be used for streptococcal disease unless the organism has been demonstrated to be sensitive.

For upper respiratory infections due to Group A beta-hemolytic streptococci, penicillin is the usual drug of choice, including prophylaxis of rheumatic fever.

Streptococcus pneumoniae,

Staphylococcus aureus, skin and soft tissue infections.

Tetracyclines are not the drug of choice in the treatment of any type of staphylococcal infection.

When penicillin is contraindicated, tetracyclines are alternative drugs in the treatment of infections due to:

Neisseria gonorrhoeae,

Treponema pallidum and *Treponema pertenue* (syphilis and yaws),

Listeria monocytogenes,

Clostridium species,

Bacillus anthracis,

Fusobacterium fusiforme (Vincent's infection),

Actinomyces species.

In acute intestinal amebiasis, the tetracyclines may be a useful adjunct to amebicides.

In severe acne, the tetracyclines may be useful adjunctive therapy.

ACHROMYCIN V is indicated in the treatment of trachoma, although the infectious agent is not always eliminated, as judged by immunofluorescence.

Inclusion conjunctivitis may be treated with oral tetracyclines or with a combination of oral and topical agents.

ACHROMYCIN is indicated for the treatment of uncomplicated urethral, endocervical or rectal infections in adults caused by *Chlamydia trachomatis*.[1]

CONTRAINDICATIONS
This drug is contraindicated in persons who have shown hypersensitivity to any of the tetracyclines.

WARNINGS
THE USE OF DRUGS OF THE TETRACYCLINE CLASS DURING TOOTH DEVELOPMENT (LAST HALF OF PREGNANCY, INFANCY AND CHILDHOOD TO THE AGE OF 8 YEARS) MAY CAUSE PERMANENT DISCOLORATION OF THE TEETH (YELLOW-GRAY-BROWN).

This adverse reaction is more common during long-term use of the drugs but has been observed following repeated short-term courses. Enamel hypoplasia has also been reported. TETRACYCLINE DRUGS, THEREFORE, SHOULD NOT BE USED IN THIS AGE GROUP UNLESS OTHER DRUGS ARE NOT LIKELY TO BE EFFECTIVE OR ARE CONTRAINDICATED.

If renal impairment exists, even usual oral or parenteral doses may lead to excessive systemic accumulation of the drug and possible liver toxicity. Under such conditions, lower than usual total doses are indicated and, if therapy is prolonged, serum level determinations of the drug may be advisable.

Photosensitivity manifested by an exaggerated sunburn reaction has been observed in some individuals taking tetracyclines. Patients apt to be exposed to direct sunlight or ultraviolet light should be advised that this reaction can occur with tetracycline drugs, and treatment should be discontinued at the first evidence of skin erythema.

The anti-anabolic action of the tetracyclines may cause an increase in BUN. While this is not a problem in those with normal renal function, in patients with significantly impaired function, higher serum levels of tetracycline may lead to azotemia, hyperphosphatemia, and acidosis.

Usage in Pregnancy: (See above **WARNINGS** about use during tooth development.) Results of animal studies indicate that tetracyclines cross the placenta, are found in fetal tissues and can have toxic effects on the developing fetus (often related to retardation of skeletal development). Evidence of embryotoxicity has also been noted in animals treated early in pregnancy.

Usage in Newborns, Infants, and Children: (See above **WARNINGS** about use during tooth development.)

All tetracyclines form a stable calcium complex in any bone-forming tissue. A decrease in the fibula growth rate has been observed in prematures given oral tetracycline in doses of 25 mg/kg every 6 hours. This reaction was shown to be reversible when the drug was discontinued.

Tetracyclines are present in the milk of lactating women who are taking a drug in this class.

PRECAUTIONS
General: Pseudotumor cerebri (benign intracranial hypertension) in adults has been associated with the use of tetracyclines. The usual clinical manifestations are headache and blurred vision. Bulging fontanels have been associated with the use of tetracyclines in infants. While both of these conditions and related symptoms usually resolve soon after discontinuation of the tetracycline, the possibility for permanent sequelae exists.

As with other antibiotic preparations, use of this drug may result in overgrowth of nonsusceptible organisms, including fungi. If superinfection occurs, the antibiotic should be discontinued and appropriate therapy should be instituted.

In venereal diseases when coexistent syphilis is suspected, darkfield examination should be done before treatment is started and the blood serology repeated monthly for at least 4 months.

In long-term therapy, periodic laboratory evaluation of organ systems, including hematopoietic, renal and hepatic studies should be performed.

All infections due to Group A beta-hemolytic streptococci should be treated for at least 10 days.

Drug Interactions: Because tetracyclines have been shown to depress plasma prothrombin activity, patients who are on anticoagulant therapy may require downward adjustment of their anticoagulant dosage.

Since bacteriostatic drugs, such as the tetracycline class of antibiotics, may interfere with the bactericidal action of penicillins, it is not advisable to administer these drugs concomitantly.

Concurrent use of tetracyclines with oral contraceptives may render oral contraceptives less effective. Breakthrough bleeding has been reported.

ADVERSE REACTIONS
Gastrointestinal: Anorexia, nausea, vomiting, diarrhea, glossitis, dysphagia, enterocolitis, pancreatitis, and inflammatory lesions (with monilial overgrowth) in the anogenital region, increases in liver enzymes, and hepatic toxicity have been reported rarely. Rare instances of esophagitis and esophageal ulcerations have been reported in patients taking the tetracycline-class antibiotics in capsule and tablet form. Most of these patients took the medication immediately before going to bed (see **DOSAGE AND ADMINISTRATION**).

Skin: Maculopapular and erythematous rashes. Exfoliative dermatitis has been reported but is uncommon. Photosensitivity is discussed above. (See **WARNINGS**.)

Renal toxicity: Rise in BUN has been reported and is apparently dose related. (See **WARNINGS**.)

Hypersensitivity reactions: Urticaria, angioneurotic edema, anaphylaxis, anaphylactoid purpura, pericarditis and exacerbation of systemic lupus erythematosus.

Blood: Hemolytic anemia, thrombocytopenia, neutropenia and eosinophilia have been reported.

CNS: Pseudotumor cerebri (benign intracranial hypertension) in adults and bulging fontanels in infants. (See **PRECAUTIONS—General**. Dizziness, tinnitus, and visual disturbances have been reported. Myasthenic syndrome has been reported rarely.

Other: When given over prolonged periods, tetracyclines have been reported to produce brown-black microscopic dis-

coloration of thyroid glands. No abnormalities of thyroid function studies are known to occur.

DOSAGE AND ADMINISTRATION

Therapy should be continued for at least 24 to 48 hours after symptoms and fever have subsided.

Concomitant therapy: Antacids containing aluminum, calcium, or magnesium impair absorption and should not be given to patients taking oral tetracycline.

Foods and some dairy products also interfere with absorption. Oral forms of tetracycline should be given 1 hour before or 2 hours after meals.

In patients with renal impairment: (See **WARNINGS**.) Total dosage should be decreased by reduction of recommended individual doses and/or by extending time intervals between doses.

In the treatment of streptococcal infections, a therapeutic dose of tetracycline should be administered for at least 10 days.

Adults: Usual daily dose, 1 to 2 grams divided in two or four equal doses, depending on the severity of the infection.

For children above 8 years of age: Usual daily dose, 10 to 20 mg (25 to 50 mg/kg) per pound of body weight divided in two or four equal doses.

For treatment of brucellosis, 500 mg tetracycline four times daily for 3 weeks should be accompanied by streptomycin, 1 gram intramuscularly twice daily the first week and once daily the second week.

For treatment of syphilis, a total of 30 to 40 grams in equally divided doses over a period of 10 to 15 days should be given. Close follow-up, including laboratory tests, is recommended.

Gonorrhea patients sensitive to pencillin may be treated with tetracycline, administered as an initial oral dose of 1.5 grams followed by 0.5 gram every 6 hours for 4 days to a total dosage of 9 grams.

Uncomplicated urethral, endocervical, or rectal infection in adults caused by *Chlamydia trachomatis:* 500 mg, by mouth, 4 times a day for at least 7 days.[1]

HOW SUPPLIED

ACHROMYCIN V *tetracycline HCl* oral dosage forms are available as follows:

CAPSULES

500 mg - Two-piece, hard shell, elongated, opaque capsules with a blue cap and a yellow body, printed with Lederle over A5 on one half and Lederle over 500 mg on the other in gray ink, supplied as follows:
NDC 0005-4875-23—Bottle of 100
NDC 0005-4875-34—Bottle of 1,000

250 mg - Two-piece, hard shell, opaque capsules with a blue cap and yellow body, printed with Lederle over A3 on one half and Lederle over 250 mg on the other in gray ink, supplied as follows:
NDC 0005-4880-23—Bottle of 100
NDC 0005-4880-34—Bottle of 1,000
NDC 0005-4880-61—Unit of Issue 12 × 40s
NDC 0005-4880-65—Unit of Issue 12 × 100s

Military Depots:
NSN 6505-01-059-8997—250 mg, Bottle of 40
NSN 6505-00-655-8355—250 mg, Bottle of 100
NSN 6505-00-963-4924—250 mg, Bottle of 1,000

Store at Controlled Room Temperature 15°–30°C (59°–86°F).

Reference: 1. CDC Sexually Transmitted Diseases Treatment Guidelines 1982.

LEDERLE LABORATORIES DIVISION
American Cyanamid Company
Pearl River, NY 10965 Rev. 7/91
10783-91

Shown in Product Identification Section, page 414

ACHROMYCIN® ℞
tetracycline

is also supplied in a number of other dosage forms and combinations for special purposes (for details of indications, dosage, administration and precautions, see circular in package).

ACHROMYCIN® ℞
tetracycline HCl
Ophthalmic Ointment, USP, 1% sterile

1/8 oz tube—NDC 0005-3501-51
(See PDR For Ophthalmology.)

ACHROMYCIN ® OTC
tetracycline HCl
3% Ointment
(For topical use)

1 oz tube—NDC 0005-4796-55
℞ not required

AMICAR® ℞
Aminocaproic Acid
Syrup, Tablets, and Injection, USP

DESCRIPTION

AMICAR, USP, is 6-aminohexanoic acid, which acts as an inhibitor of fibrinolysis.

Its chemical formula is $C_6H_{13}NO_2$. Its molecular weight is 131.17.

AMICAR is soluble in water, acids, and alkalies; it is sparingly soluble in methanol and practically insoluble in chloroform.

AMICAR Injection, USP, for intravenous administration, is a sterile pyrogen free solution containing 250 mg/mL of Aminocaproic Acid with Benzyl Alcohol 0.9% as preservative and Water for Injection qs 100%. Hydrochloric acid may be added to adjust pH to approximately 6.8 during manufacture.

AMICAR Syrup, USP 25%, for oral administration, contains 250 mg/mL of Aminocaproic Acid with Potassium Sorbate 0.2% and Sodium Benzoate 0.1% as preservatives and the following inactive ingredients: Citric Acid, Flavorings, Sodium Saccharin and Sorbitol.

Each AMICAR Tablet, USP, for oral administration, contains 500 mg of Aminocaproic Acid and the following inactive ingredients: Magnesium Stearate, Stearic Acid, and Povidone.

CLINICAL PHARMACOLOGY

The fibrinolysis-inhibitory effects of AMICAR appear to be exerted principally via inhibition of plasminogen activators and to a lesser degree through antiplasmin activity.

In adults, oral absorption appears to be a zero-order process with an absorption rate of 5.2 g/hr. The mean lag time in absorption is 10 minutes. After a single oral dose of 5 g, absorption was complete (F=1). Mean ± SD peak plasma concentrations (164 ± 28 mcg/mL) were reached within 1.2 ± 0.45 hours.

After oral administration, the apparent volume of distribution was estimated to be 23.1 ± 6.6 L (mean ± SD). Correspondingly, the volume of distribution after intravenous administration has been reported to be 30.0 ± 8.2 L. After prolonged administration, AMICAR has been found to distribute throughout extravascular and intravascular compartments of the body, penetrating human red blood cells as well as other tissue cells.

Renal excretion is the primary route of elimination, whether AMICAR is administered orally or intravenously. Sixty-five percent of the dose is recovered in the urine as unchanged drug and 11% of the dose appears as the metabolite adipic acid. Renal clearance (116 mL/min) approximates endogenous creatinine clearance. The total body clearance is 169 mL/min. The terminal elimination half-life for AMICAR is approximately 2 hours.

INDICATIONS AND USAGE

AMICAR is useful in enhancing hemostasis when fibrinolysis contributes to bleeding. In life-threatening situations, fresh whole blood transfusions, fibrinogen infusions, and other emergency measures may be required.

Fibrinolytic bleeding may frequently be associated with surgical complications following heart surgery (with or without cardiac bypass procedures) and portacaval shunt; hematological disorders such as aplastic anemia, abruptio placentae, hepatic cirrhosis, neoplastic disease such as carcinoma of the prostate, lung, stomach, and cervix.

Urinary fibrinolysis, usually a normal physiological phenomenon, may frequently be associated with life-threatening complications following severe trauma, anoxia, and shock. Symptomatic of such complications is surgical hematuria (following prostatectomy and nephrectomy) or nonsurgical hematuria (accompanying polycystic or neoplastic diseases of the genitourinary system). (See **WARNINGS**.)

CONTRAINDICATIONS

AMICAR should not be used when there is evidence of an active intravascular clotting process.

When there is uncertainty as to whether the cause of bleeding is primary fibrinolysis or disseminated intravascular coagulation (DIC), this distinction must be made before administering AMICAR *aminocaproic acid.*

The following tests can be applied to differentiate the two conditions:

- Platelet count is usually decreased in DIC but normal in primary fibrinolysis.
- Protamine paracoagulation test is positive in DIC; a precipitate forms when protamine sulphate is dropped into citrated plasma. The test is negative in the presence of primary fibrinolysis.
- The euglobulin clot lysis test is abnormal in primary fibrinolysis but normal in DIC.

AMICAR must not be used in the presence of DIC without concomitant heparin.

WARNINGS

In patients with upper urinary tract bleeding, AMICAR administration has been known to cause intrarenal obstruction in the form of glomerular capillary thrombosis, or clots in the renal pelvis and ureters. For this reason, AMICAR should not be used in hematuria of upper urinary tract origin, unless the possible benefits outweigh the risk.

Subendocardial hemorrhages have been observed in dogs given intravenous infusions of 0.2 times the maximum human therapeutic dose of AMICAR and in monkeys given eight times the maximum human therapeutic dose of AMICAR.

Fatty degeneration of the myocardium has been reported in dogs given intravenous doses of AMICAR at 0.8 to 3.3 times the maximum human therapeutic dose and in monkeys given intravenous doses of AMICAR at six times the maximum human therapeutic dose.

Rarely, skeletal muscle weakness with necrosis of muscle fibers has been reported following prolonged administration. Clinical presentation may range from mild myalgias with weakness and fatigue to a severe proximal myopathy with rhabdomyolysis, myoglobinuria, and acute renal failure. Muscle enzymes, especially creatine phosphokinase (CPK) are elevated. CPK levels should be monitored in patients on long-term therapy. AMICAR administration should be stopped if a rise in CPK is noted. Resolution follows discontinuation of AMICAR; however, the syndrome may recur if AMICAR is restarted.

The possibility of cardiac muscle damage should also be considered when skeletal myopathy occurs. One case of *cardiac* and *hepatic lesions* observed in man has been reported. The patient received 2 g of aminocaproic acid every 6 hours for a total dose of 26 g. Death was due to continued cerebrovascular hemorrhage. Necrotic changes in the heart and liver were noted at autopsy.

PRECAUTIONS

General: AMICAR *aminocaproic acid* inhibits both the action of plasminogen activators and, to a lesser degree, plasmin activity. The drug should NOT be administered without a definite diagnosis, and/or laboratory finding indicative of hyperfibrinolysis (hyperplasminemia).*

Rapid intravenous administration of the drug should be avoided since this may induce hypotension, bradycardia, and/or arrhythmia.

Inhibition of fibrinolysis by aminocaproic acid may theoretically result in clotting or thrombosis. However, there is no definite evidence that administration of aminocaproic acid has been responsible for the few reported cases of intravascular clotting which followed this treatment. Rather, it appears that such *intravascular clotting* was most likely due to the patient's preexisting clinical condition, eg, the presence of DIC. It has been postulated that *extravascular clots* formed *in vivo* may not undergo spontaneous lysis as do normal clots.

Reports have appeared in the literature of an increased incidence of certain neurological deficits such as hydrocephalus, cerebral ischemia, or cerebral vasospasm associated with the use of antifibrinolytic agents in the treatment of subarachnoid hemorrhage (SAH). All of these events have also been described as part of the natural course of SAH, or as a consequence of diagnostic procedures such as angiography. Drug relatedness remains unclear.

Thrombophlebitis, a possibility with all intravenous therapy, should be guarded against by strict attention to the proper insertion of the needle and the fixing of its position.

Laboratory Tests: The use of AMICAR should be accompanied by tests designed to determine the amount of fibrinolysis present. There are presently available (a) general tests such as those for the determination of the lysis of a clot of blood or plasma and (b) more specific tests for the study of various phases of fibrinolytic mechanisms. These latter tests include both semiquantitative and quantitative techniques for the determination of profibrinolysin, fibrinolysin, and antifibrinolysin.

Drug/Laboratory Test Interactions: Prolongation of the template bleeding time has been reported during continuous intravenous infusion of AMICAR at dosages exceeding 24 g/day. Platelet function studies in these patients have not demonstrated any significant platelet dysfunction. However, *in vitro* studies have shown that at high concentrations (7.4 mMol/L or 0.97 mg/mL and greater) EACA inhibits ADP and collagen-induced platelet aggregation, the release of ATP and serotonin, and the binding of fibrinogen to the platelets in a concentration-response manner. Following a 10 g bolus of AMICAR, transient peak plasma concentrations of 4.6 mMol/L or 0.60 mg/mL have been obtained. The

*Stefanini, M, Dameshek, W: The Hemorrhagic Disorders, Ed. 2, New York, Grune and Stratton. 1962; pp. 510–514.

Continued on next page

Information on Lederle products listed on these pages is the full prescribing information from product literature or package inserts effective in August 1992. Information concerning all Lederle products may be obtained from the Professional Services Department, Lederle Laboratories, Pearl River, New York 10965.

Lederle—Cont.

concentration of AMICAR necessary to maintain inhibition of fibrinolysis is 0.99 mMol/L or 0.13 mg/mL. Administration of a 5 g bolus followed by 1 to 1.25 g/hr should achieve and sustain plasma levels of 0.13 mg/mL. Thus, concentrations which have been obtained *in vivo* clinically in patients with normal renal function are considerably lower than the *in vitro* concentrations found to induce abnormalities in platelet function tests. However, higher plasma concentrations of AMICAR may occur in patients with severe renal failure.

Carcinogenesis, Mutagenesis, Impairment of Fertility: Long-term studies in animals to evaluate the carcinogenic potential of AMICAR and studies to evaluate its mutagenic potential have not been conducted. Dietary administration of an equivalent of the maximum human therapeutic dose of AMICAR to rats of both sexes impaired fertility as evidenced by decreased implantations, litter sizes and number of pups born.

Pregnancy: *Pregnancy Category C.* Animal teratological studies have not been conducted with AMICAR. It is also not known whether AMICAR can cause fetal harm when administered to a pregnant woman or can affect reproduction capacity. AMICAR *aminocaproic acid* should be given to a pregnant woman only if clearly needed.

Nursing Mothers: It is not known whether this drug is excreted in human milk. Because many drugs are excreted in human milk, caution should be exercised when AMICAR is administered to a nursing woman.

Pediatric Use: Safety and effectiveness in children have not been established.

ADVERSE REACTIONS

Occasionally nausea, cramps, diarrhea, hypotension, dizziness, tinnitus, malaise, conjunctival suffusion, nasal stuffiness, headache, and skin rash have been reported as results of the administration of aminocaproic acid. Only rarely has it been necessary to discontinue or reduce medication because of one or more of these effects. Myopathy (see **WARNINGS**) may be accompanied by general weakness, fatigue, and elevated serum enzymes. Rarely, rhabdomyolysis with myoglobinuria and renal failure may occur.

There have also been some reports of dry ejaculation during the period of AMICAR treatment. These have been reported to date only in hemophilia patients who received the drug after undergoing dental surgical procedures. However, this symptom resolved in all patients within 24 to 48 hours of completion of therapy.

Two cases of convulsions have been reported to occur following intravenous administration of AMICAR.

OVERDOSAGE

Signs, symptoms, laboratory findings, and complications have not been reported in association with acute overdosage of AMICAR. Concentrations of AMICAR in biologic fluids related to toxicity and/or death in humans are not known. Further, the single dose of AMICAR causing symptoms of overdosage or considered to be life-threatening is unknown.

The intravenous and oral LD_{50} of AMICAR were 3.0 and 12.0 g/kg, respectively in the mouse and 3.2 and 16.4 g/kg, respectively in the rat. An intravenous infusion dose of 2.3 g/kg was lethal in the dog. On intravenous administration, tonic-clonic convulsions were observed in dogs and mice.

No treatment for overdosage is known, although evidence exists that AMICAR is removed by hemodialysis and may be removed by peritoneal dialysis.

DOSAGE AND ADMINISTRATION

Intravenous: AMICAR Injection is administered by infusion, utilizing the usual compatible intravenous vehicles (eg, Sterile Water for Injection, Sodium Chloride for Injection, 5% Dextrose or Ringer's Injection). Although Sterile Water for Injection is compatible for intravenous injection the resultant solution is hypo-osmolar. RAPID INJECTION OF AMICAR INJECTION UNDILUTED INTO A VEIN IS NOT RECOMMENDED.

For the treatment of *acute* bleeding syndromes due to elevated fibrinolytic activity, it is suggested that 16 to 20 mL (4 to 5 g) of AMICAR *aminocaproic acid* Injection in 250 mL of diluent be administered by infusion during the first hour of treatment, followed by a continuing infusion at the rate of 4 mL (1 g) per hour in 50 mL of diluent. This method of treatment would ordinarily be continued for about 8 hours or until the bleeding situation has been controlled.

Parenteral drug products should be inspected visually for particulate matter and discoloration prior to administration, whenever solution and container permit.

Oral Therapy: If the patient is able to take medication by mouth, an identical dosage regimen may be followed by administering AMICAR Tablets or AMICAR Syrup 25% as follows: For the treatment of acute bleeding syndromes due to elevated fibrinolytic activity, it is suggested that 10 tablets (5 g) or 4 teaspoonfuls of syrup (5 g) of AMICAR be administered during the first hour of treatment, followed by a continuing rate of 2 tablets (1 g) or 1 teaspoonful of syrup (1.25 g) per hour. This method of treatment would ordinarily be continued for about 8 hours or until the bleeding situation has been controlled.

HOW SUPPLIED

AMICAR Injection, USP, supplied as follows:
Each 20 mL vial contains 5 g of aminocaproic acid (250 mg/mL) as an aqueous solution, with benzyl alcohol 0.9% as preservative.
20 mL vial—NDC 0205-4668-37.
Each 96 mL piggyback infusion vial for single use contains 24 g of aminocaproic acid (250 mg/mL) as an aqueous solution, with benzyl alcohol 0.9% as preservative.
96 mL vial—NDC 0205-4668-73.
Store at Controlled Room Temperature 15°–30°C (59°–86°F).
DO NOT FREEZE.
LEDERLE PARENTERALS, INC.
Carolina, Puerto Rico 00630
AMICAR Syrup, USP 25%, supplied as follows:
Each mL of raspberry-flavored syrup contains 250 mg of aminocaproic acid.
16 fl oz (473 mL) Bottle—NDC 0005-4667-65.
Store at Controlled Room Temperature 15°–30°C (59°–86°F).
Dispense in tight containers.
DO NOT FREEZE.
AMICAR Tablets, USP, supplied as follows:
Each round, white tablet, engraved with LL on one side and scored on the other with A to the left of the score and 10 on the right, contains 500 mg of aminocaproic acid.
Bottle of 100—NDC 0005-4665-23.
Store at Controlled Room Temperature 15°–30°C (59°–86°F).
Dispense in tight containers.

Military Depots:
Tablets, 500 mg NSN 6505-01-147-9535, 100s
Syrup, 25% NSN 6505-01-202-2232, 16 oz

LEDERLE LABORATORIES DIVISION
American Cyanamid Company
Pearl River, NY 10965
REFERENCES

10771-91
Rev. 4/91

Shown in Product Identification Section, page 414

ARTANE® ℞
[*ar-tāne*]
trihexyphenidyl HCl
For Oral Use

DESCRIPTION

ARTANE is a synthetic antispasmodic drug available in the following forms:
TABLETS: Containing 2 mg and 5 mg ARTANE, each strength also containing as inactive ingredients Corn Starch, Dibasic Calcium Phosphate, Magnesium Stearate and Modified Starch.
ELIXIR: Containing 2 mg/5 mL ARTANE in a clear, colorless, lime-mint flavored preparation, also containing as inactive ingredients Alcohol, Citric Acid, Flavorings, Methylparaben, Propylparaben, Sodium Chloride and Sorbitol.
SEQUELS: Containing 5 mg ARTANE as Sustained Release soft shell capsules, also containing as inactive ingredients Beeswax, Benzoin Gum, Blue 1, Colloidal Silicon Dioxide, Dibasic Calcium Phosphate, Ethyl Cellulose, Ethyl Vanillin, Gelatin, Glycerin, Glyceryl Stearate, Magnesium Stearate, Methylparaben, Mineral Oil, Non-pareil Seeds, Propylene Glycol, Propylparaben, Sucrose, Talc and Terpene Resin.

ACTIONS

ARTANE is the substituted piperidine salt, 3-(1-piperidyl)-1-phenyl-cyclohexyl-1-propanol hydrochloride, which exerts a direct inhibitory effect upon the parasympathetic nervous system. It also has a relaxing effect on smooth musculature; exerted both directly upon the muscle tissue itself and indirectly through an inhibitory effect upon the parasympathetic nervous system. Its therapeutic properties are similar to those of atropine, although undesirable side effects are ordinarily less frequent and severe than with the latter.

INDICATIONS

This drug is indicated as an adjunct in the treatment of all forms of parkinsonism (postencephalitic, arteriosclerotic, and idiopathic). It is often useful as adjuvant therapy when treating these forms of parkinsonism with levodopa. Additionally, it is indicated for the control of extrapyramidal disorders caused by central nervous system drugs such as the dibenzoxazepines, phenothiazines, thioxanthenes, and butyrophenones.
SEQUELS—For maintenance therapy after patients have been stabilized on trihexyphenidyl hydrochloride in conventional dosage forms (tablets or elixir).

WARNING

Patients to be treated with ARTANE should have a gonioscope evaluation and close monitoring of intraocular pressures at regular periodic intervals.

PRECAUTIONS

Although trihexyphenidyl HCl is not contraindicated for patients with cardiac, liver, or kidney disorders, or with hypertension, such patients should be maintained under close observation.

Since the use of trihexyphenidyl HCl may in some cases continue indefinitely and since it has atropine-like properties, patients should be subjected to constant and careful long-term observation to avoid allergic and other untoward reactions. Inasmuch as trihexyphenidyl HCl possesses some parasympatholytic activity, it should be used with caution in patients with glaucoma, obstructive disease of the gastrointestinal or genitourinary tracts, and in elderly males with possible prostatic hypertrophy. Geriatric patients, particularly over the age of 60, frequently develop increased sensitivity to the actions of drugs of this type, and hence, require strict dosage regulation. Incipient glaucoma may be precipitated by parasympatholytic drugs such as trihexyphenidyl HCl.

Tardive dyskinesia may appear in some patients on long-term therapy with antipsychotic drugs or may occur after therapy with these drugs has been discontinued. Antiparkinsonism agents do not alleviate the symptoms of tardive dyskinesia, and in some instances may aggravate them. However, parkinsonism and tardive dyskinesia often coexist in patients receiving chronic neuroleptic treatment, and anticholinergic therapy with ARTANE may relieve some of these parkinsonism symptoms.

ADVERSE REACTIONS

Minor side effects, such as dryness of the mouth, blurring of vision, dizziness, mild nausea or nervousness, will be experienced by 30 to 50 percent of all patients. These sensations, however, are much less troublesome with ARTANE *trihexyphenidyl HCl* than with belladonna alkaloids and are usually less disturbing than unalleviated parkinsonism. Such reactions tend to become less pronounced, and even to disappear, as treatment continues. Even before these reactions have remitted spontaneously, they may often be controlled by careful adjustment of dosage form, amount of drug, or interval between doses.

Isolated instances of suppurative parotitis secondary to excessive dryness of the mouth, skin rashes, dilatation of the colon, paralytic ileus, and certain psychiatric manifestations such as delusions and hallucinations, plus one doubtful case of paranoia all of which may occur with any of the atropine-like drugs, have been reported rarely with ARTANE.

Patients with arteriosclerosis or with a history of idiosyncrasy to other drugs may exhibit reactions of mental confusion, agitation, disturbed behavior, or nausea and vomiting. Such patients should be allowed to develop a tolerance through the initial administration of a small dose and gradual increase in dose until an effective level is reached. If a severe reaction should occur, administration of the drug should be discontinued for a few days and then resumed at a lower dosage. Psychiatric disturbances can result from indiscriminate use (leading to overdosage) to sustain continued euphoria.

Potential side effects associated with the use of any atropine-like drugs include constipation, drowsiness, urinary hesitancy or retention, tachycardia, dilation of the pupil, increased intraocular tension, weakness, vomiting, and headache.

The occurrence of angle-closure glaucoma due to long-term treatment with trihexyphenidyl hydrochloride has been reported.

DOSAGE AND ADMINISTRATION

Dosage should be individualized. The initial dose should be low and then increased gradually, especially in patients over 60 years of age. Whether ARTANE may best be given before or after meals should be determined by the way the patient reacts. Postencephalitic patients, who are usually more prone to excessive salivation, may prefer to take it after meals and may, in addition, require small amounts of atropine which, under such circumstances, is sometimes an effective adjuvant. If ARTANE *trihexyphenidyl HCl* tends to dry the mouth excessively, it may be better to take it before meals, unless it causes nausea. If taken after meals, the thirst sometimes induced can be allayed by mint candies, chewing gum or water.

ARTANE in Idiopathic Parkinsonism: As initial therapy for parkinsonism, 1 mg of ARTANE in tablet or elixir form may be administered the first day. The dose may then be increased by 2 mg increments at intervals of 3 to 5 days, until a total of 6 to 10 mg is given daily. The total daily dose will depend upon what is found to be the optimal level. Many patients derive maximum benefit from this daily total of 6 to 10 mg, but some patients, chiefly those in the postencephalitic group, may require a total daily dose of 12 to 15 mg.

ARTANE in Drug-Induced Parkinsonism: The size and frequency of dose of ARTANE needed to control extrapyramidal reactions to commonly employed tranquilizers, notably the phenothiazines, thioxanthenes, and butyrophenones, must be determined empirically. The total daily dosage usually ranges between 5 and 15 mg although, in some cases, these reactions have been satisfactorily controlled on as little as 1 mg daily. It may be advisable to commence therapy with a single 1 mg dose. If the extrapyramidal manifestations are not controlled in a few hours, the subsequent doses may be progressively increased until satisfactory control is achieved. Satisfactory control may sometimes be more rapidly achieved by temporarily reducing the dosage of the tranquilizer on instituting ARTANE therapy and then adjusting dosage of both drugs until the desired ataractic effect is retained without onset of extrapyramidal reactions.

It is sometimes possible to maintain the patient on a reduced ARTANE dosage after the reactions have remained under control for several days. Instances have been reported in which these reactions have remained in remission for long periods after ARTANE therapy was discontinued.

Concomitant Use of ARTANE with Levodopa: When ARTANE is used concomitantly with levodopa, the usual dose of each may need to be reduced. Careful adjustment is necessary, depending on side effects and degree of symptom control. ARTANE dosage of 3 to 6 mg daily, in divided doses, is usually adequate.

Concomitant Use of ARTANE with Other Parasympathetic Inhibitors: ARTANE may be substituted, in whole or in part, for other parasympathetic inhibitors. The usual technique is partial substitution initially, with progressive reduction in the other medication as the dose of trihexyphenidyl HCl is increased.

ARTANE TABLETS and ELIXIR—The total daily intake of ARTANE tablets or elixir is tolerated best if divided into three doses and taken at mealtimes. High doses (>10 mg daily) may be divided into four parts, with three doses administered at mealtimes and the fourth at bedtime.

ARTANE SEQUELS—Because of the relatively high dosage in each controlled release capsule, this dosage form should not be used for initial therapy. After patients are stabilized on trihexyphenidyl HCl in conventional dosage forms (tablet or elixir), for convenience of administration they may be switched to the controlled release capsules on a milligram per milligram total daily dose basis, as a single dose after breakfast or in two divided doses 12 hours apart. Most patients will be adequately maintained on the controlled release form, but some may develop an exacerbation of parkinsonism and have to be returned to the conventional form.

HOW SUPPLIED

ARTANE *trihexyphenidyl HCl* is available as follows:
TABLETS: 2 mg—round, flat, scored, white tablets; engraved ARTANE above 2 on one side and LL above A11 below the score on the other side, supplied as follows:

NDC 0005-4434-23—Bottle of 100
NDC 0005-4434-34—Bottle of 1000
NDC 0005-4434-60—Unit Dose 10 (2 × 5) Strips

5 mg—round, flat, scored, white tablets; engraved ARTANE above 5 on one side and LL above A12 below the score on the other side, supplied as follows:

NDC 0005-4436-23—Bottle of 100
NDC 0005-4436-34—Bottle of 1000
NDC 0005-4436-60—Unit Dose 10 (2 × 5) Strips

Store at Controlled Room Temperature 15°-30°C (59°-86°F).
ELIXIR: 2 mg/5 mL—NDC 0005-4440-65—Bottle of 16 fl oz
Store at Controlled Room Temperature 15°-30°C (59°-86°F).
DO NOT FREEZE.
SEQUELS SUSTAINED RELEASE CAPSULES: 5 mg—soft shell, oval shaped, clear blue, printed A9L, supplied as follows:

NDC 0005-4438-32—Unit-of-Issue 60s with CRC

Store at Controlled Room Temperature 15°-30° C (59°-86° F).

LEDERLE LABORATORIES DIVISION
American Cyanamid Company
Pearl River, NY 10965 Rev. 1/92
20893-92

Shown in Product Identification Section, page 414

ASENDIN® ℞

[*a-sen-din*]
amoxapine tablets

DESCRIPTION

ASENDIN is an antidepressant of the dibenzoxazepine class, chemically distinct from the dibenzazepines, dibenzocycloheptenes, and dibenzoxepines.

It is designated chemically as 2-chloro-11-(1-piperazinyl) dibenz-[*b,f*][1,4]oxazepine. The molecular weight is 313.8. The empirical formula is $C_{17}H_{16}ClN_3O$.

ASENDIN is supplied for oral administration as 25 mg, 50 mg, 100 mg, and 150 mg tablets.

Inactive Ingredients: All tablets contain Corn Starch, Dibasic Calcium Phosphate, Magnesium Stearate, Pregelatinized Starch, and Stearic Acid. Additionally, the 50 and 150 mg tablets contain Yellow No. 6 and the 100 mg tablet contains Blue 2.

CLINICAL PHARMACOLOGY

ASENDIN is an antidepressant with a mild sedative component to its action. The mechanism of its clinical action in man is not well understood. In animals, amoxapine reduced the uptake of norepinephrine and serotonin and blocked the response of dopamine receptors to dopamine. Amoxapine is not a monoamine oxidase inhibitor.

ASENDIN is absorbed rapidly and reaches peak blood levels approximately 90 minutes after ingestion. It is almost completely metabolized. The main route of excretion is the kidney. *In vitro* tests show that amoxapine binding to human serum is approximately 90%.

In man, amoxapine serum concentration declines with a half-life of 8 hours. However, the major metabolite, 8-hydroxyamoxapine, has a biologic half-life of 30 hours. Metabolites are excreted in the urine in conjugated form as glucuronides.

Clinical studies have demonstrated that ASENDIN has a more rapid onset of action than either amitriptyline or imipramine. The initial clinical effect may occur within 4 to 7 days and occurs within 2 weeks in over 80% of responders.

INDICATIONS AND USAGE

ASENDIN is indicated for the relief of symptoms of depression in patients with neurotic or reactive depressive disorders as well as endogenous and psychotic depressions. It is indicated for depression accompanied by anxiety or agitation.

CONTRAINDICATIONS

ASENDIN is contraindicated in patients who have shown prior hypersensitivity to dibenzoxazepine compounds. It should not be given concomitantly with monoamine oxidase inhibitors. Hyperpyretic crises, severe convulsions, and deaths have occurred in patients receiving tricyclic antidepressants and monoamine oxidase inhibitors simultaneously. When it is desired to replace a monoamine oxidase inhibitor with ASENDIN, a minimum of 14 days should be allowed to elapse after the former is discontinued. ASENDIN should then be initiated cautiously with gradual increase in dosage until optimum response is achieved. The drug is not recommended for use during the acute recovery phase following myocardial infarction.

WARNINGS

Tardive Dyskinesia: Tardive dyskinesia, a syndrome consisting of potentially irreversible, involuntary, dyskinetic movements may develop in patients treated with neuroleptic (ie, antipsychotic) drugs. (Amoxapine is not an antipsychotic, but it has substantive neuroleptic activity.) Although the prevalence of the syndrome appears to be highest among the elderly, especially elderly women, it is impossible to rely upon prevalence estimates to predict, at the inception of neuroleptic treatment, which patients are likely to develop the syndrome. Whether neuroleptic drug products differ in their potential to cause tardive dyskinesia is unknown.

Both the risk of developing the syndrome and the likelihood that it will become irreversible are believed to increase as the duration of treatment and the total cumulative dose of neuroleptic drugs administered to the patient increase. However, the syndrome can develop, although much less commonly, after relatively brief treatment periods at low doses.

There is no known treatment for established cases of tardive dyskinesia, although the syndrome may remit, partially or completely, if neuroleptic treatment is withdrawn. Neuroleptic treatment itself, however, may suppress (or partially suppress) the signs and symptoms of the syndrome and thereby may possibly mask the underlying disease process. The effect that symptomatic suppression has upon the long-term course of the syndrome is unknown.

Given these considerations, neuroleptics should be prescribed in a manner that is most likely to minimize the occurrence of tardive dyskinesia. Chronic neuroleptic treatment should generally be reserved for patients who suffer from a chronic illness that 1) is known to respond to neuroleptic drugs, and 2) for whom alternative, equally effective, but potentially less harmful treatments are not available or appropriate. In patients who do require chronic treatment, the smallest dose and the shortest duration of treatment producing a satisfactory clinical response should be sought. The need for continued treatment should be reassessed periodically.

If signs and symptoms of tardive dyskinesia appear in a patient on neuroleptics, drug discontinuation should be considered. However, some patients may require treatment despite the presence of the syndrome.

(For further information about the description of tardive dyskinesia and its clinical detection, please refer to the sections on **Information for the Patient** and **ADVERSE REACTIONS.**)

Neuroleptic Malignant Syndrome (NMS): A potentially fatal symptom complex sometimes referred to as Neuroleptic Malignant Syndrome (NMS) has been reported in association with antipsychotic drugs and with amoxapine. Clinical manifestations of NMS are hyperpyrexia, muscle rigidity, altered mental status and evidence of autonomic instability (irregular pulse or blood pressure, tachycardia, diaphoresis, and cardiac dysrhythmias).

The diagnostic evaluation of patients with this syndrome is complicated. In arriving at a diagnosis, it is important to identify cases where the clinical presentation includes both serious medical illness (eg, pneumonia, systemic infection, etc) and untreated or inadequately treated extrapyramidal signs and symptoms (EPS). Other important considerations in the differential diagnosis include central anticholinergic toxicity, heat stroke, drug fever, and primary central nervous system (CNS) pathology.

The management of NMS should include 1) immediate discontinuation of antipsychotic drugs and other drugs not essential to concurrent therapy, 2) intensive symptomatic treatment and medical monitoring, and 3) treatment of any concomitant serious medical problems for which specific treatments are available. There is no general agreement about specific pharmacological treatment regimens for uncomplicated NMS.

If a patient requires antipsychotic drug treatment after recovery from NMS, the potential reintroduction of drug therapy should be carefully considered. The patient should be carefully monitored since recurrences of NMS have been reported.

ASENDIN *amoxapine* should be used with caution in patients with a history of urinary retention, angle-closure glaucoma, or increased intraocular pressure. Patients with cardiovascular disorders should be watched closely. Tricyclic antidepressant drugs, particularly when given in high doses, can induce sinus tachycardia, changes in conduction time, and arrhythmias. Myocardial infarction and stroke have been reported with drugs of this class.

Extreme caution should be used in treating patients with a history of convulsive disorder or those with overt or latent seizure disorders.

PRECAUTIONS

General: In prescribing the drug it should be borne in mind that the possibility of suicide is inherent in any severe depression, and persists until a significant remission occurs; the drug should be dispensed in the smallest suitable amount. Manic depressive patients may experience a shift to the manic phase. Schizophrenic patients may develop increased symptoms of psychosis; patients with paranoid symptomatology may have an exaggeration of such symptoms. This may require reduction of dosage or the addition of a major tranquilizer to the therapeutic regimen. Antidepressant drugs can cause skin rashes and/or "drug fever" in susceptible individuals. These allergic reactions may, in rare cases, be severe. They are more likely to occur during the first few days of treatment, but may also occur later. ASENDIN should be discontinued if rash and/or fever develop. Amoxapine possesses a degree of dopamine-blocking activity which may cause extrapyramidal symptoms in <1% of patients. Rarely, symptoms indicative of tardive dyskinesia have been reported.

Information for the Patient: Given the likelihood that some patients exposed chronically to neuroleptics will develop tardive dyskinesia, it is advised that all patients in whom chronic use is contemplated be given, if possible, full information about this risk. The decision to inform patients and/or their guardians must obviously take into account the clinical circumstances and the competency of the patient to understand the information provided.

Patients should be warned of the possibility of drowsiness that may impair performance of potentially hazardous tasks such as driving an automobile or operating machinery.

Drug Interactions: See **CONTRAINDICATIONS** about concurrent usage of tricyclic antidepressants and monoamine oxidase inhibitors. Paralytic ileus may occur in patients taking tricyclic antidepressants in combination with anticholinergic drugs. ASENDIN may enhance the response to alcohol and the effects of barbiturates and other CNS depressants. Serum levels of several tricyclic antidepressants have been reported to be significantly increased when cimetidine is administered concurrently. Although such an interaction has not been reported to date with ASENDIN, specific interaction studies have not been done, and the possibility should be considered.

Continued on next page

Information on Lederle products listed on these pages is the full prescribing information from product literature or package inserts effective in August 1992. Information concerning all Lederle products may be obtained from the Professional Services Department, Lederle Laboratories, Pearl River, New York 10965.

Lederle—Cont.

Therapeutic Interactions: Concurrent administration with electroshock therapy may increase the hazards associated with such therapy.

Carcinogenesis, Impairment of Fertility: In a 21-month toxicity study at three dose levels in rats, pancreatic islet cell hyperplasia occurred with slightly increased incidence at doses 5 to 10 times the human dose. Pancreatic adenocarcinoma was detected in low incidence in the mid-dose group only, and may possibly have resulted from endocrine-mediated organ hyperfunction. The significance of these findings to man is not known.

Treatment of male rats with 5 to 10 times the human dose resulted in a slight decrease in the number of fertile matings. Female rats receiving oral doses within the therapeutic range displayed a reversible increase in estrous cycle length.

Pregnancy: *Pregnancy Category C:* Studies performed in mice, rats, and rabbits have demonstrated no evidence of teratogenic effect due to ASENDIN. Embryotoxicity was seen in rats and rabbits given oral doses approximating the human dose. Fetotoxic effects (intrauterine death, stillbirth, decreased birth weight) were seen in animals studied at oral doses 3 to 10 times the human dose. Decreased postnatal survival (between days 0 to 4) was demonstrated in the offspring of rats at 5 to 10 times the human dose. There are no adequate and well-controlled studies in pregnant women. ASENDIN *amoxapine* should be used during pregnancy only if the potential benefit justifies the potential risk to the fetus.

Nursing Mothers: ASENDIN, like many other systemic drugs, is excreted in human milk. Because effects of the drug on infants are unknown, caution should be exercised when ASENDIN is administered to nursing women.

Pediatric Use: Safety and effectiveness in children below the age of 16 have not been established.

ADVERSE REACTIONS

Adverse reactions reported in controlled studies in the United States are categorized with respect to incidence below. Following this is a listing of reactions known to occur with other antidepressant drugs of this class but not reported to date with ASENDIN.

INCIDENCE GREATER THAN 1%

The most frequent types of adverse reactions occurring with ASENDIN in controlled clinical trials were sedative and anticholinergic: these included drowsiness (14%), dry mouth (14%), constipation (12%), and blurred vision (7%).

Less frequently reported reactions are:

CNS and Neuromuscular: anxiety, insomnia, restlessness, nervousness, palpitations, tremors, confusion, excitement, nightmares, ataxia, alterations in EEG patterns.

Allergic: edema, skin rash.

Endocrine: elevation of prolactin levels.

Gastrointestinal: nausea.

Other: dizziness, headache, fatigue, weakness, excessive appetite, increased perspiration.

INCIDENCE LESS THAN 1%

Anticholinergic: disturbances of accommodation, mydriasis, delayed micturition, urinary retention, nasal stuffiness.

Cardiovascular: hypotension, hypertension, syncope, tachycardia.

Allergic: drug fever, urticaria, photosensitization, pruritus, rarely vasculitis, hepatitis.

CNS and Neuromuscular: tingling, paresthesias of the extremities, tinnitus, disorientation, seizures, hypomania, numbness, incoordination, disturbed concentration, hyperthermia, extrapyramidal symptoms, including, rarely, tardive dyskinesia. Neuroleptic malignant syndrome has been reported. (See **WARNINGS.**)

Hematologic: leukopenia, agranulocytosis.

Gastrointestinal: epigastric distress, vomiting, flatulence, abdominal pain, peculiar taste, diarrhea.

Endocrine: increased or decreased libido, impotence, menstrual irregularity, breast enlargement and galactorrhea in the female, syndrome of inappropriate antidiuretic hormone secretion.

Other: lacrimation, weight gain or loss, altered liver function, painful ejaculation.

DRUG RELATIONSHIP UNKNOWN

The following reactions have been reported very rarely, and occurred under uncontrolled circumstances where a drug relationship was difficult to assess. These observations are listed to serve as alerting information to physicians.

Anticholinergic: paralytic ileus.

Cardiovascular: atrial arrhythmias (including atrial fibrillation), myocardial infarction, stroke, heart block.

CNS and Neuromuscular: hallucinations.

Hematologic: thrombocytopenia, eosinophilia, purpura, petechiae.

Gastrointestinal: parotid swelling.

Endocrine: change in blood glucose levels.

Other: pancreatitis, hepatitis, jaundice, urinary frequency, testicular swelling, anorexia, alopecia.

ADDITIONAL ADVERSE REACTIONS

The following reactions have been reported with other antidepressant drugs, but not with ASENDIN *amoxapine*.

Anticholinergic: sublingual adenitis, dilation of the urinary tract.

CNS and Neuromuscular: delusions.

Gastrointestinal: stomatitis, black tongue.

Endocrine: gynecomastia.

OVERDOSAGE

Signs and Symptoms: Toxic manifestations of ASENDIN overdosage differ significantly from those of other tricyclic antidepressants. Serious cardiovascular effects are seldom if ever observed. However, CNS effects—particularly grand mal convulsions—occur frequently, and treatment should be directed primarily toward prevention or control of seizures. Status epilepticus may develop and constitutes a neurologic emergency. Coma and acidosis are other serious complications of substantial ASENDIN overdosage in some cases. Renal failure may develop 2 to 5 days after toxic overdosage in patients who may appear otherwise recovered. Acute tubular necrosis with rhabdomyolysis and myoglobinuria is the most common renal complication in such cases. This reaction probably occurs in less than 5% of overdose cases, and typically in those who have experienced multiple seizures.

Treatment: Treatment of ASENDIN overdosage should be symptomatic and supportive, but with special attention to prevention or control of seizures. If the patient is conscious, induced emesis followed by gastric lavage with appropriate precautions to prevent pulmonary aspiration should be accomplished as soon as possible. Following lavage, activated charcoal may be administered to reduce absorption, and repeated administrations may facilitate drug elimination. An adequate airway should be established in comatose patients and assisted ventilation instituted if necessary. Seizures may respond to standard anticonvulsant therapy such as intravenous diazepam and/or phenytoin. The value of physostigmine appears less certain. Status epilepticus, should it develop, requires vigorous treatment such as that described by Delgado-Escueta et al (*N Engl J Med* 1982; 306:1337-1340).

Convulsions, when they occur, typically begin within 12 hours after ingestion. Because seizures may occur precipitously in some overdosage patients who appear otherwise relatively asymptomatic, the treating physician may wish to consider prophylactic administration of anticonvulsant medication during this period.

Treatment of renal impairment, should it occur, is the same as that for nondrug-induced renal dysfunction.

Serious cardiovascular effects are remarkably rare following ASENDIN *amoxapine* overdosage, and the ECG typically remains within normal limits except for sinus tachycardia. Hence, prolongation of the QRS interval beyond 100 milliseconds within the first 24 hours is *not* a useful guide to the severity of overdosage with this drug.

Fatalities and, rarely, neurologic sequelae have resulted from prolonged status epilepticus in ASENDIN overdosage patients. While the lethal dose appears higher than that of other tricyclic antidepressants (80% of lethal ASENDIN overdosages have involved ingestion of 3 grams or more), many factors other than amount ingested are important in assessing probability of survival. These include age and physical condition of the patient, concomitant ingestion of other drugs, and especially the interval between drug ingestion and initiation of emergency treatment.

DOSAGE AND ADMINISTRATION

Effective dosage of ASENDIN may vary from one patient to another. Usual effective dosage is 200 to 300 mg daily. Three weeks constitutes an adequate period of trial providing dosage has reached 300 mg daily (or lower level of tolerance) for at least 2 weeks. If no response is seen at 300 mg, dosage may be increased, depending upon tolerance, up to 400 mg daily. Hospitalized patients who have been refractory to antidepressant therapy and who have no history of convulsive seizures may have dosage raised cautiously up to 600 mg daily in divided doses.

ASENDIN may be given in a single daily dose, not to exceed 300 mg, preferably at bedtime. If the total daily dosage exceeds 300 mg, it should be given in divided doses.

Initial Dosage for Adults: Usual starting dosage is 50 mg two or three times daily. Depending upon tolerance, dosage may be increased to 100 mg two or three times daily by the end of the first week. (Initial dosage of 300 mg daily may be given, but notable sedation may occur in some patients during the first few days of therapy at this level.) Increases above 300 mg daily should be made only if 300 mg daily has been ineffective during a trial period of at least 2 weeks. When effective dosage is established, the drug may be given in a single dose (not to exceed 300 mg) at bedtime.

Elderly Patients: In general, lower dosages are recommended for these patients. Recommended starting dosage of ASENDIN is 25 mg two or three times daily. If no intolerance is observed, dosage may be increased by the end of the first week to 50 mg two or three times daily. Although 100 to 150 mg daily may be adequate for many elderly patients,

some may require higher dosage. Careful increases up to 300 mg daily are indicated in such cases.

Once an effective dosage is established, ASENDIN may conveniently be given in a single bedtime dose, not to exceed 300 mg.

Maintenance: Recommended maintenance dosage of ASENDIN is the lowest dose that will maintain remission. If symptoms reappear, dosage should be increased to the earlier level until they are controlled.

For maintenance therapy at dosages of 300 mg or less, a single dose at bedtime is recommended.

HOW SUPPLIED

ASENDIN *amoxapine* Tablets are supplied as follows:

25 mg—White, heptagon-shaped tablets, engraved on one side with LL above 25 and with A13 on the other scored side.
  NDC 0005-5389-23—Bottle of 100

50 mg—Orange, heptagon-shaped tablets, engraved on one side with LL above 50 and with A15 on the other scored side.
  NDC 0005-5390-23—Bottle of 100
  NDC 0005-5390-31—Bottle of 500
  NDC 0005-5390-60—10 (2 × 5) strips

100 mg—Blue, heptagon-shaped tablets, engraved on one side with LL above 100 and with A17 on the other scored side.
  NDC 0005-5391-23—Bottle of 100
  NDC 0005-5391-60—10 (2 × 5) strips

150 mg—Peach, heptagon-shaped tablets, engraved on one side with LL above 150 and with A18 on the other scored side.
  NDC 0005-5392-38—Bottle of 30 with CRC

Store at Controlled Room Temperature 15°–30° C (59°–86° F).

Military and VA Depots:
NSN 6505-01-111-3195 50 mg—(100s)
NSN 6505-01-111-3194 100 mg—(100s)

LEDERLE LABORATORIES DIVISION
American Cyanamid Company
Pearl River, NY 10965   Rev. 2/90
                                           27278

Shown in Product Identification Section, page 414

CALTRATE® 600   OTC
[*căl-trāte*]
High Potency Calcium Supplement
Nature's Most Concentrated Form of Calcium™
No Sugar, No Salt, No Lactose, No Cholesterol, No Preservatives, Film-Coated for Easy Swallowing

INACTIVE INGREDIENTS

Croscarmellose Sodium, Hydroxypropyl Methylcellulose, Magnesium Stearate, Microcrystalline Cellulose, PVPP, Sodium Lauryl Sulfate, and Titanium Dioxide.

TWO TABLETS DAILY PROVIDE:

	Adults— % U.S. RDA
3000 mg Calcium Carbonate which provides 1200 mg elemental calcium	120%

RECOMMENDED INTAKE

One or two tablets daily or as directed by the physician.

WARNINGS

Keep out of the reach of children.

HOW SUPPLIED

Bottle of 60—
NDC 0005-5510-19
Store at Room Temperature.

                                       11643-91
                                            D15

Shown in Product Identification Section, page 414

CALTRATE® 600 + Vitamin D   OTC
[*căl-trāte*]
High Potency Calcium Supplement
Nature's Most Concentrated Form of Calcium™
No Sugar, No Salt, No Lactose, No Cholesterol, Film-Coated for Easy Swallowing

INACTIVE INGREDIENTS

Blue 2, Croscarmellose Sodium, FD&C Yellow No. 6, Hydroxypropyl Methylcellulose, Magnesium Stearate, Microcrystalline Cellulose, Povidone, PVPP, Red 40, Sodium Lauryl Sulfate, and Titanium Dioxide.

TWO TABLETS DAILY PROVIDE:

	Adults— % U.S. RDA
3000 mg Calcium Carbonate which provides 1200 mg elemental calcium	120%
Vitamin D 250 IU	62%

RECOMMENDED INTAKE

One or two tablets daily or as directed by the physician.

WARNINGS

Keep out of the reach of children.

HOW SUPPLIED

Bottle of 60—
NDC 0005-5509-19
Store at Room Temperature.

11642-91
D12

Shown in Product Identification Section, page 414

CALTRATE® 600 + Iron & Vitamin D   OTC

[căl-trāte]
High Potency Calcium Supplement
Nature's Most Concentrated Form of Calcium™
No Sugar, No Salt, No Lactose, No Cholesterol, Film-Coated for Easy Swallowing

ONE TABLET DAILY CONTAINS:

	Adults—% U.S. RDA
1500 mg Calcium Carbonate which provides 600 mg elemental calcium	60%
18 mg elemental Iron in the Optisorb® Time-Release System (as ferrous fumarate)	100%
125 IU Vitamin D	31%

INACTIVE INGREDIENTS

Blue 2, Croscarmellose Sodium, Hydroxypropyl Cellulose, Magnesium Stearate, Microcrystalline Cellulose, Polysorbate 80, Povidone, PVPP, Red 40, Sodium Lauryl Sulfate, Titanium Dioxide, and Triethyl Citrate.
* CALTRATE + Iron contains pure calcium and time-release iron for diets deficient in both minerals
* Plus Vitamin D to help absorb calcium

RECOMMENDED INTAKE

One or two tablets daily or as directed by the physician.

WARNINGS

Keep out of the reach of children.

HOW SUPPLIED

Bottle of 60—
NDC-0005-5523-19
Store at Room Temperature.

11602-91
D9

Shown in Product Identification Section, page 414

Advanced Formula
CENTRUM®   OTC
[sĕn-trŭm]
High Potency
Multivitamin-Multimineral Formula

(See PDR For Nonprescription Drugs.)

Children's Chewable
CENTRUM, JR.®   OTC
[sĕn-trŭm]
Vitamin/Mineral Formula + Iron

(See PDR For Nonprescription Drugs.)

Children's Chewable
CENTRUM, JR.®   OTC
[sĕn-trŭm]
Vitamin/Mineral Formula + Extra C

(See PDR For Nonprescription Drugs.)

Children's Chewable
CENTRUM, JR.®   OTC
[sĕn-trŭm]
Vitamin/Mineral Formula +
Extra Calcium

(See PDR For Nonprescription Drugs.)

DECLOMYCIN®   ℞

[dĕk-lō-mī-sĭn]
Demeclocycline Hydrochloride
For Oral Use

DESCRIPTION

DECLOMYCIN is an antibiotic isolated from a mutant strain of *Streptomyces aureofaciens*. Chemically it is [4S-(4α,4aα,5aα,6β,12aα)]-7-Chloro-4-dimethylamino)-1,4,4a,5,5a,6,11,12a-octahydro- 3,6,10,12,12a- pentahydroxy- 1,11-dioxo -2- naphthacenecarboxamide monohydrochloride.
DECLOMYCIN tablets contain the following inactive ingredients: Alginic Acid, Corn Starch, Ethylcellulose, Hydroxypropyl Methylcellulose, Magnesium Stearate, Red 7, Sorbitol, Titanium Dioxide, Yellow 10 and other ingredients. May also contain Sodium Lauryl Sulfate.

CLINICAL PHARMACOLOGY

The tetracyclines are primarily bacteriostatic and are thought to exert their antimicrobial effect by the inhibition of protein synthesis. Tetracyclines are active against a wide range of gram-negative and gram-positive organisms.
The drugs in the tetracycline class have closely similar antimicrobial spectra, and cross-resistance among them is common. Microorganisms may be considered susceptible if the MIC (minimum inhibitory concentration) is not more than 4 mcg/mL and intermediate if the MIC is 4 to 12.5 mcg/mL. Susceptibility plate testing: A tetracycline disc may be used to determine microbial susceptibility to drugs in the tetracycline class. If the Kirby-Bauer method of disc susceptibility testing is used, a 30 mcg tetracycline disc should give a zone of at least 19 mm when tested against a tetracycline-susceptible bacterial strain.
Tetracyclines are readily absorbed and are bound to plasma proteins in varying degrees. They are concentrated by the liver in the bile and excreted in the urine and feces at high concentrations and in a biologically active form.

INDICATIONS AND USAGE

DECLOMYCIN is indicated in infections caused by the following microorganisms:
Rickettsiae: (Rocky Mountain spotted fever, typhus fever and the typhus group, Q fever, rickettsialpox, tick fevers).
Mycoplasma pneumoniae (PPLO, Eaton agent).
Agents of psittacosis and ornithosis.
Agents of lymphogranuloma venereum and granuloma inguinale.
The spirochetal agent of relapsing fever (*Borrelia recurrentis*).
The following gram-negative microorganisms:
Haemophilus ducreyi (chancroid),
Yersinia pestis and *Francisella tularensis*, formerly *Pasteurella pestis* and *Pasteurella tularensis*,
Bartonella bacilliformis,
Bacteroides species,
Vibrio comma and *Vibrio fetus*.
Brucella species (in conjunction with streptomycin).
Because many strains of the following groups of microorganisms have been shown to be resistant to tetracyclines, culture and susceptibility testing is recommended.
Demeclocycline is indicated for treatment of infections caused by the following gram-negative microorganisms, when bacteriologic testing indicates appropriate susceptibility to the drug:
Escherichia coli,
Enterobacter aerogenes (formerly *Aerobacter aerogenes*),
Shigella species,
Mima species and *Herellea* species,
Haemophilus influenzae (respiratory infections),
Klebsiella species (respiratory and urinary infections).
DECLOMYCIN *demeclocycline hydrochloride* is indicated for treatment of infections caused by the following gram-positive microorganisms when bacteriologic testing indicates appropriate susceptibility to the drug:
Streptococcus species:
Up to 44% of strains of *Streptococcus pyogenes* and 74% of *Streptococcus faecalis* have been found to be resistant to tetracycline drugs. Therefore, tetracyclines should not be used for streptococcal disease unless the organism has been demonstrated to be sensitive.
For upper respiratory infections due to Group A beta-hemolytic streptococci, penicillin is the usual drug of choice, including prophylaxis of rheumatic fever.
Streptococcus pneumoniae,
Staphylococcus aureus, skin and soft tissue infections. Tetracyclines are not the drugs of choice in the treatment of any type of staphylococcal infection.
When penicillin is contraindicated, tetracyclines are alternative drugs in the treatment of infections due to:
Neisseria gonorrhoeae,
Treponema pallidum and *Treponema pertenue* (syphilis and yaws),
Listeria monocytogenes,
Clostridium species,
Bacillus anthracis,

Fusobacterium fusiforme (Vincent's infection),
Actinomyces species.
In acute intestinal amebiasis, the tetracyclines may be a useful adjunct to amebicides.
DECLOMYCIN is indicated in the treatment of trachoma, although the infectious agent is not always eliminated, as judged by immunofluorescence.
Inclusion conjunctivitis may be treated with oral tetracyclines or with a combination of oral and topical agents.

CONTRAINDICATIONS

This drug is contraindicated in persons who have shown hypersensitivity to any of the tetracyclines.

WARNINGS

THE USE OF DRUGS OF THE TETRACYCLINE CLASS DURING TOOTH DEVELOPMENT (LAST HALF OF PREGNANCY, INFANCY, AND CHILDHOOD TO THE AGE OF 8 YEARS) MAY CAUSE PERMANENT DISCOLORATION OF THE TEETH (YELLOW-GRAY-BROWN).
This adverse reaction is more common during long-term use of the drugs but has been observed following repeated short-term courses. Enamel hypoplasia has also been reported. TETRACYCLINE DRUGS, THEREFORE, SHOULD NOT BE USED IN THIS AGE GROUP UNLESS OTHER DRUGS ARE NOT LIKELY TO BE EFFECTIVE OR ARE CONTRAINDICATED.
If renal impairment exists, even usual oral or parenteral doses may lead to excessive systemic accumulation of the drug and possible liver toxicity. Under such conditions, lower than usual total doses are indicated and, if therapy is prolonged, serum level determinations of the drug may be advisable.
Phototoxic reactions can occur in individuals taking demeclocycline, and are characterized by severe burns of exposed surfaces resulting from direct exposure of patients to sunlight during therapy with moderate or large doses of demeclocycline. Patients apt to be exposed to direct sunlight or ultraviolet light should be advised that this reaction can occur, and treatment should be discontinued at the first evidence of skin erythema.
The anti-anabolic action of the tetracyclines may cause an increase in BUN. While this is not a problem in those with normal renal function, in patients with significantly impaired function, higher serum levels of tetracycline may lead to azotemia, hyperphosphatemia, and acidosis.
Administration of DECLOMYCIN *demeclocycline hydrochloride* has resulted in appearance of the diabetes insipidus syndrome (polyuria, polydipsia, and weakness) in some patients on long-term therapy. The syndrome has been shown to be nephrogenic, dose-dependent, and reversible on discontinuance of therapy.
Usage in pregnancy: (See above **WARNINGS** about use during tooth development.) Results of animal studies indicate that tetracyclines cross the placenta, are found in fetal tissues and can have toxic effects on the developing fetus (often related to retardation of skeletal development). Evidence of embryotoxicity has also been noted in animals treated early in pregnancy.
Usage in newborns, infants, and children: (See above **WARNINGS** about use during tooth development.)
All tetracyclines form a stable calcium complex in any bone forming tissue. A decrease in the fibula growth rate has been observed in prematures given oral tetracycline in doses of 25 mg/kg every 6 hours. This reaction was shown to be reversible when the drug was discontinued.
Tetracyclines are present in the milk of lactating women who are taking a drug in this class.

PRECAUTIONS

General: Pseudotumor cerebri (benign intracranial hypertension) in adults has been associated with the use of tetracyclines. The usual clinical manifestations are headache and blurred vision. Bulging fontanels have been associated with the use of tetracyclines in infants. While both of these conditions and related symptoms usually resolve soon after discontinuation of the tetracycline, the possibility for permanent sequelae exists.
As with other antibiotic preparations, use of this drug may result in overgrowth of nonsusceptible organisms, including fungi. If superinfection occurs, the antibiotic should be discontinued and appropriate therapy should be instituted.
In venereal diseases when coexistent syphilis is suspected, darkfield examination should be done before treatment is started and the blood serology repeated monthly for at least 4 months.

Continued on next page

Information on Lederle products listed on these pages is the full prescribing information from product literature or package inserts effective in August 1992. Information concerning all Lederle products may be obtained from the Professional Services Department, Lederle Laboratories, Pearl River, New York 10965.

Lederle—Cont.

In long-term therapy, periodic laboratory evaluation of organ systems, including hematopoietic, renal and hepatic studies should be performed.

All infections due to Group A beta-hemolytic streptococci should be treated for at least 10 days.

Interpretation of Bacteriologic Studies: Following a course of therapy, persistence for several days in both urine and blood of bacterio-suppressive levels of demeclocycline may interfere with culture studies. These levels should not be considered therapeutic.

Drug Interactions: Because the tetracyclines have been shown to depress plasma prothrombin activity, patients who are on anticoagulant therapy may require downward adjustment of their anticoagulant dosage.

Since bacteriostatic drugs, such as the tetracycline class of antibiotics, may interfere with the bactericidal action of penicillins, it is not advisable to administer these drugs concomitantly.

Concurrent use of tetracyclines with oral contraceptives may render oral contraceptives less effective. Breakthrough bleeding has been reported.

ADVERSE REACTIONS

Gastrointestinal: Anorexia, nausea, vomiting, diarrhea, glossitis, dysphagia, enterocolitis, pancreatitis, and inflammatory lesions (with monilial overgrowth) in the anogenital region, increases in liver enzymes, and hepatic toxicity has been reported rarely. Rare instances of esophagitis and esophageal ulcerations have been reported in patients taking the tetracycline-class antibiotics in capsule and tablet form. Most of these patients took the medication immediately before going to bed. (See **DOSAGE AND ADMINISTRATION.**)

Skin: Maculopapular and erythematous rashes. Exfoliative dermatitis has been reported but is uncommon. Photosensitivity is discussed above. (See **WARNINGS.**)

Renal Toxicity: Rise in BUN has been reported and is apparently dose related. Nephrogenic diabetes insipidus. (See **WARNINGS.**)

Hypersensitivity Reactions: Urticaria, angioneurotic edema, anaphylaxis, anaphylactoid purpura, pericarditis, and exacerbation of systemic lupus erythematosus.

Blood: Hemolytic anemia, thrombocytopenia, neutropenia, and eosinophilia have been reported.

CNS: Pseudotumor cerebri (benign intracranial hypertension) in adults and bulging fontanels in infants (see **PRECAUTIONS—General**). Dizziness, tinnitus, and visual disturbances have been reported. Myasthenic syndrome has been reported rarely.

Other: When given over prolonged periods, tetracyclines have been reported to produce brown-black microscopic discoloration of thyroid glands. No abnormalities of thyroid function studies are known to occur.

DOSAGE AND ADMINISTRATION

Therapy should be continued for at least 24 to 48 hours after symptoms and fever have subsided.

Concomitant therapy: Antacids containing aluminum, calcium, or magnesium impair absorption and should not be given to patients taking oral tetracycline.

Foods and some dairy products also interfere with absorption. Oral forms of tetracycline should be given 1 hour before or 2 hours after meals.

In patients with renal impairment: (See **WARNINGS.**) Total dosage should be decreased by reduction of recommended individual doses and/or by extending time intervals between doses.

In the treatment of streptococcal infections, a therapeutic dose of demeclocycline should be administered for at least 10 days.

Adults: Usual daily dose—Four divided doses of 150 mg each or two divided doses of 300 mg each.

For children above 8 years of age: Usual daily dose, 3 to 6 mg per pound body weight per day, depending upon the severity of the disease, divided into two to four doses.

Gonorrhea patients sensitive to penicillin may be treated with demeclocycline administered as an initial oral dose of 600 mg followed by 300 mg every 12 hours for 4 days to a total of 3 grams.

HOW SUPPLIED

DECLOMYCIN *demeclocycline hydrochloride* Tablets, 150 mg are round, convex, red, film coated tablets, engraved with LL on one side and D11 on the other, supplied as follows:

NDC 0005-9218-23—Bottle of 100

DECLOMYCIN Tablets, 300 mg are round, convex, red, film coated tablets, engraved with LL on one side and D12 on the other, supplied as follows:

NDC 0005-9270-29—Bottle of 48

Store at Controlled Room Temperature 15°–30°C (59°–86°F).

LEDERLE LABORATORIES DIVISION
American Cyanamid Company
Pearl River, NY 10965   Rev. 7/91
10785-91

Shown in Product Identification Section, page 414

DIAMOX®   ℞
Acetazolamide Tablets USP
and
DIAMOX®
Sterile Acetazolamide Sodium USP
Intravenous

DESCRIPTION

DIAMOX, an inhibitor of the enzyme carbonic anhydrase is a white to faintly yellowish white crystalline, odorless powder, weakly acidic, very slightly soluble in water and slightly soluble in alcohol. The chemical name for DIAMOX is N-(5-Sulfamoyl-1,3,4-thiadiazol-2yl)-acetamide. Its molecular weight is 222.24. Its chemical formula is $C_4H_6N_4O_3S_2$.

DIAMOX is available as oral tablets containing 125 mg and 250 mg of acetazolamide, respectively, and the following inactive ingredients: Corn Starch, Dibasic Calcium Phosphate, Magnesium Stearate, Povidone, and Sodium Starch Glycolate.

DIAMOX is also available for intravenous use, and is supplied as a sterile powder requiring reconstitution. Each vial contains an amount of acetazolamide sodium equivalent to 500 mg of acetazolamide. The bulk solution is adjusted to pH 9.2 using sodium hydroxide and, if necessary, hydrochloric acid prior to lyophilization.

CLINICAL PHARMACOLOGY

DIAMOX is a potent carbonic anhydrase inhibitor, effective in the control of fluid secretion (eg, some types of glaucoma), in the treatment of certain convulsive disorders (eg, epilepsy) and in the promotion of diuresis in instances of abnormal fluid retention (eg, cardiac edema).

DIAMOX is not a mercurial diuretic. Rather, it is a nonbacteriostatic sulfonamide possessing a chemical structure and pharmacological activity distinctly different from the bacteriostatic sulfonamides.

DIAMOX is an enzyme inhibitor that acts specifically on carbonic anhydrase, the enzyme that catalyzes the reversible reaction involving the hydration of carbon dioxide and the dehydration of carbonic acid. In the eye, this inhibitory action of acetazolamide decreases the secretion of aqueous humor and results in a drop in intraocular pressure, a reaction considered desirable in cases of glaucoma and even in certain nonglaucomatous conditions. Evidence seems to indicate that DIAMOX has utility as an adjuvant in the treatment of certain dysfunctions of the central nervous system (eg, epilepsy). Inhibition of carbonic anhydrase in this area appears to retard abnormal, paroxysmal, excessive discharge from central nervous system neurons. The diuretic effect of DIAMOX is due to its action in the kidney on the reversible reaction involving hydration of carbon dioxide and dehydration of carbonic acid. The result is renal loss of HCO_3 ion, which carries out sodium, water, and potassium. Alkalinization of the urine and promotion of diuresis are thus effected. Alteration in ammonia metabolism occurs due to increased reabsorption of ammonia by the renal tubules as a result of urinary alkalinization.

Placebo-controlled clinical trials have shown that prophylactic administration of DIAMOX at a dose of 250 mg every 8 to 12 hours (or a 500 mg controlled-release capsule once daily) before and during rapid ascent to altitude results in fewer and/or less severe symptoms (such as headache, nausea, shortness of breath, dizziness, drowsiness, and fatigue) of acute mountain sickness (AMS). Pulmonary function (eg, minute ventilation, expired vital capacity, and peak flow) is greater in the DIAMOX treated group, both in subjects with AMS and asymptomatic subjects. The DIAMOX treated climbers also had less difficulty in sleeping.

INDICATIONS AND USAGE

For adjunctive treatment of: edema due to congestive heart failure; drug-induced edema; centrencephalic epilepsies (petit mal, unlocalized seizures); chronic simple (open-angle) glaucoma, secondary glaucoma, and preoperatively in acute angle-closure glaucoma where delay of surgery is desired in order to lower intraocular pressure. DIAMOX is also indicated for the prevention or amelioration of symptoms associated with acute mountain sickness in climbers attempting rapid ascent and in those who are very susceptible to acute mountain sickness despite gradual ascent.

CONTRAINDICATIONS

DIAMOX therapy is contraindicated in situations in which sodium and/or potassium blood serum levels are depressed, in cases of marked kidney and liver disease or dysfunction, in suprarenal gland failure, and in hyperchloremic acidosis. It is contraindicated in patients with cirrhosis because of the risk of development of hepatic encephalopathy.

Long-term administration of DIAMOX is contraindicated in patients with chronic noncongestive angle-closure glaucoma since it may permit organic closure of the angle to occur while the worsening glaucoma is masked by lowered intraocular pressure.

WARNINGS

Fatalities have occurred, although rarely, due to severe reactions to sulfonamides including Stevens-Johnson syndrome, toxic epidermal necrolysis, fulminant hepatic necrosis, agranulocytosis, aplastic anemia, and other blood dyscrasias. Sensitizations may recur when a sulfonamide is readministered irrespective of the route of administration. If signs of hypersensitivity or other serious reactions occur, discontinue use of this drug.

Caution is advised for patients receiving concomitant high-dose aspirin and DIAMOX *acetazolamide*, as anorexia, tachypnea, lethargy, coma and death have been reported.

PRECAUTIONS

General: Increasing the dose does not increase the diuresis and may increase the incidence of drowsiness and/or paresthesia. Increasing the dose often results in a decrease in diuresis. Under certain circumstances, however, very large doses have been given in conjunction with other diuretics in order to secure diuresis in complete refractory failure.

Information for Patients:

Adverse reactions common to all sulfonamide derivatives may occur: anaphylaxis, fever, rash (including erythema multiforme, Stevens-Johnson syndrome, toxic epidermal necrolysis), crystalluria, renal calculus, bone marrow depression, thrombocytopenic purpura, hemolytic anemia, leukopenia, pancytopenia and agranulocytosis. Precaution is advised for early detection of such reactions and the drug should be discontinued and appropriate therapy instituted.

In patients with pulmonary obstruction or emphysema where alveolar ventilation may be impaired, DIAMOX *acetazolamide* which may precipitate or aggravate acidosis, should be used with caution.

Gradual ascent is desirable to try to avoid acute mountain sickness. If rapid ascent is undertaken and DIAMOX is used, it should be noted that such use does not obviate the need for prompt descent if severe forms of high altitude sickness occur, ie, high altitude pulmonary edema (HAPE) or high-altitude cerebral edema.

Caution is advised for patients receiving concomitant high-dose aspirin and DIAMOX, as anorexia, tachypnea, lethargy, coma and death have been reported (see **WARNINGS**).

Laboratory Tests: To monitor for hematologic reactions common to all sulfonamides, it is recommended that a baseline CBC and platelet count be obtained on patients prior to initiating DIAMOX therapy and at regular intervals during therapy. If significant changes occur, early discontinuance and institution of appropriate therapy are important. Periodic monitoring of serum electrolytes is recommended.

Carcinogenesis, Mutagenesis, Impairment of Fertility: Long-term studies in animals to evaluate the carcinogenic potential of DIAMOX have not been conducted. In a bacterial mutagenicity assay, DIAMOX was not mutagenic when evaluated with and without metabolic activation.

The drug had no effect on fertility when administered in the diet to male and female rats at a daily intake of up to four times the recommended human dose of 1000 mg in a 50 kg individual.

Pregnancy: Pregnancy Category C: Acetazolamide, administered orally or parenterally, has been shown to be teratogenic (defects of the limbs) in mice, rats, hamsters, and rabbits. There are no adequate and well-controlled studies in pregnant women. Acetazolamide should be used in pregnancy only if the potential benefit justifies the potential risk to the fetus.

Nursing Mothers: Because of the potential for serious adverse reaction in nursing infants from DIAMOX, a decision should be made whether to discontinue nursing or to discontinue the drug, taking into account the importance of the drug to the mother.

Pediatric Use: The safety and effectiveness of DIAMOX in children have not been established.

ADVERSE REACTIONS

Adverse reactions, occurring most often early in therapy, include paresthesias, particularly a "tingling" feeling in the extremities, hearing dysfunction or tinnitus, loss of appetite, taste alteration and gastrointestinal disturbances such as nausea, vomiting and diarrhea; polyuria, and occasional instances of drowsiness and confusion.

Metabolic acidosis and electrolyte imbalance may occur.

Transient myopia has been reported. This condition invariably subsides upon diminution or discontinuance of the medication.

Other occasional adverse reactions include urticaria, melena, hematuria, glycosuria, hepatic insufficiency, flaccid paralysis, photosensitivity and convulsions. Also see **PRECAUTIONS: Information for Patients** for possible reactions common to sulfonamide derivatives. Fatalities have occurred although rarely, due to severe reactions to sulfonamides including Stevens-Johnson syndrome, toxic epidermal

necrolysis, fulminant hepatic necrosis, agranulocytosis, aplastic anemia and other blood dyscrasias (see **WARNINGS**).

OVERDOSAGE

No data are available regarding DIAMOX *acetazolamide* overdosage in humans as no cases of acute poisoning with this drug have been reported. Animal data suggest that DIAMOX is remarkably nontoxic. No specific antidote is known. Treatment should be symptomatic and supportive.
Electrolyte imbalance, development of an acidotic state, and central nervous effects might be expected to occur. Serum electrolyte levels (particularly potassium) and blood pH levels should be monitored.
Supportive measures are required to restore electrolyte and pH balance. The acidotic state can usually be corrected by the administration of bicarbonate.
Despite its high intraerythrocytic distribution and plasma protein binding properties, DIAMOX may be dialyzable. This may be particularly important in the management of DIAMOX overdosage when complicated by the presence of renal failure.

DOSAGE AND ADMINISTRATION

Preparation and Storage of Parenteral Solution: Each 500 mg vial containing DIAMOX sterile acetazolamide sodium parenteral should be reconstituted with at least 5 mL of Sterile Water for Injection prior to use. Reconstituted solutions retain potency for 1 week if refrigerated. Since this product contains no preservative, use within 24 hours of reconstitution is strongly recommended. The direct intravenous route of administration is preferred. Intramuscular administration is not recommended.
Glaucoma: DIAMOX should be used as an adjunct to the usual therapy. The dosage employed in the treatment of *chronic simple (open-angle) glaucoma* ranges from 250 mg to 1 g of DIAMOX per 24 hours, usually in divided doses for amounts over 250 mg. It has usually been found that a dosage in excess of 1 g per 24 hours does not produce an increased effect. In all cases, the dosage should be adjusted with careful individual attention both to symptomatology and ocular tension. Continuous supervision by a physician is advisable.
In treatment of secondary glaucoma and in the preoperative treatment of some cases of *acute congestive (closed-angle) glaucoma*, the preferred dosage is 250 mg every 4 hours, although some cases have responded to 250 mg twice daily on short-term therapy. In some acute cases, it may be more satisfactory to administer an initial dose of 500 mg followed by 125 or 250 mg every 4 hours depending on the individual case. Intravenous therapy may be used for rapid relief of ocular tension in acute cases. A complementary effect has been noted when DIAMOX has been used in conjunction with miotics or mydriatics as the case demanded.
Epilepsy: It is not clearly known whether the beneficial effects observed in epilepsy are due to direct inhibition of carbonic anhydrase in the central nervous system or whether they are due to the slight degree of acidosis produced by the divided dosage. The best results to date have been seen in petit mal in children. Good results, however, have been seen in patients, both children and adult, in other types of seizures such as grand mal, mixed seizure patterns, myoclonic jerk patterns, etc. The suggested total daily dose is 8 to 30 mg per kg in divided doses. Although some patients respond to a low dose, the optimum range appears to be from 375 to 1000 mg daily. However, some investigators feel that daily doses in excess of 1 g do not produce any better results than a 1 g dose. When DIAMOX is given in combination with other anticonvulsants, it is suggested that the starting dose should be 250 mg once daily in addition to the existing medications. This can be increased to levels as indicated above. The change from other medications to DIAMOX should be gradual and in accordance with usual practice in epilepsy therapy.
Congestive Heart Failure: For diuresis in congestive heart failure, the starting dose is usually 250 to 375 mg once daily in the morning (5 mg/kg). If, after an initial response, the patient fails to continue to lose edema fluid, do not increase the dose but allow for kidney recovery by skipping medication for a day. DIAMOX *acetazolamide* yields best diuretic results when given on alternate days, or for 2 days alternating with a day of rest.
Failures in therapy may be due to overdosage or too frequent dosage. The use of DIAMOX does not eliminate the need for other therapy such as digitalis, bed rest, and salt restriction.
Drug-Induced Edema: Recommended dosage is 250 to 375 mg of DIAMOX once a day for 1 or 2 days, alternating with a day of rest.
Acute Mountain Sickness: Dosage is 500 mg to 1000 mg daily, in divided doses using tablets or sustained-release capsules as appropriate. In circumstances of rapid ascent, such as in rescue or military operations, the higher dose level of 1000 mg is recommended. It is preferable to initiate dosing 24 to 48 hours before ascent and to continue for 48 hours while at high altitude, or longer as necessary to control symptoms.
Note: The dosage recommendations for glaucoma and epilepsy differ considerably from those for congestive heart failure, since the first two conditions are not dependent upon carbonic anhydrase inhibition in the kidney which requires intermittent dosage if it is to recover from the inhibitory effect of the therapeutic agent.
Parenteral drug products should be inspected visually for particulate matter and discoloration prior to administration, whenever solution and container permit.

HOW SUPPLIED

Tablets:
125 mg—Round, flat-faced, beveled, white tablets engraved with DIAMOX and 125 on one side and scored in half on the other side. Engraved with LL on the right of the score and D1 on the left, are supplied as follows:
NDC 57706-754-23—Bottle of 100
250 mg—Round, convex, white tablets engraved with DIAMOX and 250 on one side and scored in quarters on the other side. Engraved with LL in the upper right quadrant and D2 in the lower left quadrant, are supplied as follows:
NDC 57706-755-23—Bottle of 100
NDC 57706-755-34—Bottle of 1000
NDC 57706-755-60—Unit Dose 10 × 10s
Store at Controlled Room Temperature 15°–30°C (59°–86°F).
Manufactured for
STORZ OPHTHALMICS, INC.
St. Louis, MO 63122
by
LEDERLE LABORATORIES DIVISION
American Cyanamid Company, Pearl River, NY 10965
Intravenous:
Sterile intravenous (lyophilized) powder.
NDC 57706-762-96—500 mg Vial
Store at Controlled Room Temperature 15°–30°C (59°–86°F).
Manufactured for
STORZ OPHTHALMICS, INC.
St. Louis, MO 63122
by
LEDERLE PARENTERALS, INC.
Carolina, Puerto Rico 00630 10248-91
Rev. 3/91

Shown in Product Identification Section, page 414

DIAMOX® ℞
Acetazolamide
SEQUELS®
Sustained-Release Capsules

DESCRIPTION

DIAMOX is an inhibitor of the enzyme carbonic anhydrase.
DIAMOX is a white to faintly yellowish white crystalline, odorless powder, weakly acidic, very slightly soluble in water and slightly soluble in alcohol. The chemical name for DIAMOX is *N*-(5-Sulfamoyl-1,3,4-thiadiazol-2yl)-acetamide. The molecular weight of DIAMOX is 222.24. Its chemical formula is $C_4H_6N_4O_3S_2$.
DIAMOX SEQUELS are sustained-release capsules, for oral administration, each containing 500 mg of acetazolamide and the following inactive ingredients: Beeswax, Benzoin Gum, Corn Starch, Ethylcellulose, FD&C Blue No. 1, FD&C Yellow No. 6, Gelatin, Glycerin, Magnesium Stearate, Methylparaben, Mineral Oil, Mono- and Diglycerides, Propylene Glycol, Propylparaben, Silica, Sucrose, Talc, Terpene Resin, and Vanillin.

CLINICAL PHARMACOLOGY

DIAMOX is a potent carbonic anhydrase inhibitor, effective in the control of fluid secretion (eg, some types of glaucoma), in the treatment of certain convulsive disorders (eg, epilepsy), and in the promotion of diuresis in instances of abnormal fluid retention (eg, cardiac edema).
DIAMOX is not a mercurial diuretic. Rather, it is a nonbacteriostatic sulfonamide possessing a chemical structure and pharmacological activity distinctly different from the bacteriostatic sulfonamides.
DIAMOX is an enzyme inhibitor that acts specifically on carbonic anhydrase, the enzyme that catalyzes the reversible reaction involving the hydration of carbon dioxide and the dehydration of carbonic acid. In the eye, this inhibitory action of acetazolamide decreases the secretion of aqueous humor and results in a drop in intraocular pressure, a reaction considered desirable in cases of glaucoma and even in certain nonglaucomatous conditions. Evidence seems to indicate that DIAMOX has utility as an adjuvant in the treatment of certain dysfunctions of the central nervous system (eg, epilepsy). Inhibition of carbonic anhydrase in this area appears to retard abnormal, paroxysmal, excessive discharge from central nervous system neurons. The diuretic effect of DIAMOX is due to its action in the kidney on the reversible reaction involving hydration of carbon dioxide and dehydration of carbonic acid. The result is renal loss of HCO_3 ion, which carries out sodium, water, and potassium. Alkalinization of the urine and promotion of diuresis are thus effected. Alteration in ammonia metabolism occurs due to increased reabsorption of ammonia by the renal tubules as a result of urinary alkalinization.
DIAMOX SEQUELS sustained-release capsules provide prolonged action to inhibit aqueous humor secretion for 18 to 24 hours after each dose, whereas tablets act for only 8 to 12 hours. The prolonged continuous effect of SEQUELS permits a reduction in dosage frequency.
Plasma concentrations of acetazolamide peak between 3 to 6 hours after administration of DIAMOX SEQUELS, compared to 1 to 4 hours with tablets.
Placebo-controlled clinical trials have shown that prophylactic administration of DIAMOX at a dose of 250 mg every 8 to 12 hours (or a 500 mg controlled-release capsule once daily) before and during rapid ascent to altitude results in fewer and/or less severe symptoms (such as headache, nausea, shortness of breath, dizziness, drowsiness, and fatigue) of acute mountain sickness (AMS). Pulmonary function (eg, minute ventilation, expired vital capacity, and peak flow) is greater in the DIAMOX treated group, both in subjects with AMS and asymptomatic subjects. The DIAMOX treated climbers also had less difficulty in sleeping.

INDICATIONS AND USAGE

For adjunctive treatment of: chronic simple (open-angle) glaucoma, secondary glaucoma, and preoperatively in acute angle-closure glaucoma where delay of surgery is desired in order to lower intraocular pressure. DIAMOX is also indicated for the prevention or amelioration of symptoms associated with acute mountain sickness in climbers attempting rapid ascent and in those who are very susceptible to acute mountain sickness despite gradual ascent.

CONTRAINDICATIONS

Acetazolamide therapy is contraindicated in situations in which sodium and/or potassium blood serum levels are depressed, in cases of marked kidney and liver disease or dysfunction, in suprarenal gland failure, and in hyperchloremic acidosis. It is contraindicated in patients with cirrhosis because of the risk of development of hepatic encephalopathy.
Long-term administration of DIAMOX *acetazolamide* is contraindicated in patients with chronic noncongestive angle-closure glaucoma since it may permit organic closure of the angle to occur while the worsening glaucoma is masked by lowered intraocular pressure.

WARNINGS

Fatalities have occurred, although rarely, due to severe reactions to sulfonamides including Stevens-Johnson syndrome, toxic epidermal necrolysis, fulminant hepatic necrosis, agranulocytosis, aplastic anemia, and other blood dyscrasias.
Sensitizations may recur when a sulfonamide is readministered irrespective of the route of administration. If signs of hypersensitivity or other serious reactions occur, discontinue use of this drug.
Caution is advised for patients receiving concomitant high-dose aspirin and DIAMOX, as anorexia, tachypnea, lethargy, coma and death have been reported.

PRECAUTIONS

General: Increasing the dose does not increase the diuresis and may increase the incidence of drowsiness and/or paresthesia. Increasing the dose often results in a decrease in diuresis. Under certain circumstances, however, very large doses have been given in conjunction with other diuretics in order to secure diuresis in complete refractory failure.
Information for Patients: Adverse reactions common to all sulfonamide derivatives may occur: anaphylaxis, fever, rash (including erythema multiforme, Stevens-Johnson syndrome, toxic epidermal necrolysis), crystalluria, renal calculus, bone marrow depression, thrombocytopenic purpura, hemolytic anemia, leukopenia, pancytopenia and agranulocytosis. Precaution is advised for early detection of such reactions and the drug should be discontinued and appropriate therapy instituted.
In patients with pulmonary obstruction or emphysema where alveolar ventilation may be impaired, DIAMOX, which may aggravate acidosis, should be used with caution.
Gradual ascent is desirable to try to avoid acute mountain sickness. If rapid ascent is undertaken and DIAMOX is used, it should be noted that such use does not obviate the need for prompt descent if severe forms of high altitude sickness occur, ie, high altitude pulmonary edema (HAPE) or high altitude cerebral edema.
Caution is advised for patients receiving concomitant high-dose aspirin and DIAMOX *acetazolamide*, as anorexia, tachypnea, lethargy, coma and death have been reported (see **WARNINGS**).

Continued on next page

Information on Lederle products listed on these pages is the full prescribing information from product literature or package inserts effective in August 1992. Information concerning all Lederle products may be obtained from the Professional Services Department, Lederle Laboratories, Pearl River, New York 10965.

Lederle—Cont.

Laboratory Tests: To monitor for hematologic reactions common to all sulfonamides, it is recommended that a baseline CBC and platelet count be obtained on patients prior to initiating DIAMOX therapy and at regular intervals during therapy. If significant changes occur, early discontinuance and institution of appropriate therapy are important. Periodic monitoring of serum electrolytes is recommended.

Carcinogenesis, Mutagenesis, Impairment of Fertility: Long-term studies in animals to evaluate the carcinogenic potential of DIAMOX have not been conducted. In a bacterial mutagenicity assay, DIAMOX was not mutagenic when evaluated with and without metabolic activation. The drug had no effect on fertility when administered in the diet to male and female rats at a daily intake of up to four times the maximum recommended human dose of 1000 mg in a 50 kg individual.

Pregnancy Category C: Acetazolamide, administered orally or parenterally, has been shown to be teratogenic (defects of the limbs) in mice, rats, hamsters, and rabbits. There are no adequate and well-controlled studies in pregnant women. Acetazolamide should be used in pregnancy only if the potential benefit justifies the potential risk to the fetus.

Nursing Mothers: Because of the potential for serious adverse reactions in nursing infants from DIAMOX, a decision should be made whether to discontinue nursing or to discontinue the drug, taking into account the importance of the drug to the mother.

Pediatric Use: The safety and effectiveness of DIAMOX in children have not been established.

ADVERSE REACTIONS

Adverse reactions, occurring most often early in therapy, include paresthesias, particularly a "tingling" feeling in the extremities, hearing dysfunction or tinnitus, loss of appetite, taste alteration and gastrointestinal disturbances such as nausea, vomiting and diarrhea; polyuria, and occasional instances of drowsiness and confusion.

Metabolic acidosis and electrolyte imbalance may occur.

Transient myopia has been reported. This condition invariably subsides upon diminution or discontinuance of the medication.

Other occasional adverse reactions include urticaria, melena, hematuria, glycosuria, hepatic insufficiency, flaccid paralysis, photosensitivity, and convulsions. Also see **PRECAUTIONS: Information for Patients** for possible reactions common to sulfonamide derivatives. Fatalities have occurred, although rarely, due to severe reactions to sulfonamides including Stevens-Johnson syndrome, toxic epidermal necrolysis, fulminant hepatic necrosis, agranulocytosis, aplastic anemia, and other blood dyscrasias (see **WARNINGS**).

OVERDOSAGE

No data are available regarding DIAMOX overdosage in humans as no cases of acute poisoning with this drug have been reported. Animal data suggest that DIAMOX is remarkably nontoxic. No specific antidote is known. Treatment should be symptomatic and supportive.

Electrolyte imbalance, development of an acidotic state, and central nervous system effects might be expected to occur. Serum electrolyte levels (particularly potassium) and blood pH levels should be monitored.

Supportive measures are required to restore electrolyte and pH balance. The acidotic state can usually be corrected by the administration of bicarbonate.

Despite its high intraerythrocytic distribution and plasma protein binding properties, DIAMOX may be dialyzable. This may be particularly important in the management of DIAMOX overdosage when complicated by the presence of renal failure.

DOSAGE AND ADMINISTRATION

Glaucoma: The recommended dosage is one capsule (500 mg) two times a day. Usually one capsule is administered in the morning and one capsule in the evening. It may be necessary to adjust the dose, but it has usually been found that dosage in excess of two capsules (1 g) does not produce an increased effect. The dosage should be adjusted with careful individual attention both to symptomatology and intraocular tension. In all cases, continuous supervision by a physician is advisable.

In those unusual instances where adequate control is not obtained by the twice-a-day administration of DIAMOX *acetazolamide* SEQUELS sustained-release capsules the desired control may be established by means of DIAMOX (tablets or parenteral). Use tablets or parenteral in accordance with the more frequent dosage schedules recommended for these dosage forms, such as 250 mg every 4 hours, or an initial dose of 500 mg followed by 250 mg or 125 mg every 4 hours, depending on the case in question.

Acute Mountain Sickness: Dosage is 500 mg to 1000 mg daily, in divided doses using tablets or sustained-release capsules as appropriate. In circumstances of rapid ascent, such as in rescue or military operations, the higher dose level of

1000 mg is recommended. It is preferable to initiate dosing 24 to 48 hours before ascent and to continue for 48 hours while at high altitude, or longer as necessary to control symptoms.

HOW SUPPLIED

DIAMOX SEQUELS, 500 mg orange capsules printed with DIAMOX over D3 are supplied as follows:
NDC 57706-753-13—Bottle of 30
NDC 57706-753-23—Bottle of 100
Store at Controlled Room Temperature 15°–30°C (59°–86°F).

Manufactured for
STORZ OPHTHALMICS, INC.
St. Louis, MO 63122
by
LEDERLE LABORATORIES DIVISION
American Cyanamid Company
Pearl River, NY 10965

28463
Rev. 11/90
Shown in Product Identification Section, page 414

DIPHTHERIA AND TETANUS   ℞
TOXOIDS ADSORBED
Aluminum Phosphate-Adsorbed PUROGENATED®
For Pediatric Use

DESCRIPTION

Diphtheria and Tetanus Toxoids Adsorbed, aluminum phosphate-adsorbed PUROGENATED is a sterile combination of refined diphtheria and tetanus toxoids for intramuscular use only. After shaking, the vaccine is a homogeneous white suspension.

The diphtheria and tetanus toxins are produced according to the method of Mueller and Miller[1,2] and are detoxified by use of formaldehyde. The toxoids are refined by the Pillemer alcohol fractionation method[3] and are diluted with a solution containing sodium phosphate monobasic, sodium phosphate dibasic, aluminum phosphate, glycine and thimerosal (mercury derivative) as a preservative. The final concentration of thimerosal in the combined vaccine is 1:10,000. The aluminum content of the final product does not exceed 0.80 mg per 0.5 mL dose.

Each 0.5 mL dose is formulated to contain 12.5 Lf units of diphtheria toxoid, and 5 Lf units of tetanus toxoid.

CLINICAL PHARMACOLOGY

Diphtheria is primarily a localized and generalized intoxication caused by diphtheria toxin, an extracellular protein metabolite of toxinogenic strains of *Corynebacterium diphtheriae*. While the incidence of diphtheria in the U.S. has decreased from over 200,000 cases reported in 1921 before the general use of diphtheria toxoid, to only 15 cases reported from 1980 through 1983, the ratio of fatalities to attack rate has remained constant at about 5% to 10%.[4] The highest case fatality rates are in the very young and the elderly.

Following adequate immunization with diphtheria toxoid, which induces antitoxin, it is thought that protection lasts for at least 10 years.[4] This significantly reduces both the risk of developing diphtheria and the severity of clinical illness. It does not, however, eliminate carriage of *C diphtheriae* in the pharynx or on the skin.[4]

Tetanus is an intoxication manifested primarily by neuromuscular dysfunction, caused by a potent exotoxin elaborated by *Clostridium tetani*. The incidence of tetanus in the U.S. has dropped dramatically with the routine use of tetanus toxoid, remaining relatively constant over the last decade at about 90 cases reported annually.[4] Spores of *C tetani* are ubiquitous, and there is essentially no natural immunity to tetanus toxin. Thus, universal primary immunization with tetanus toxoid, and subsequent maintenance of adequate antitoxin levels by means of timed boosters, is necessary to protect all age groups.[4,6] Tetanus toxoid is a highly effective antigen, and a completed primary series generally induces protective levels of serum antitoxin that persist for at least 10 years.[4]

INDICATIONS AND USAGE

Diphtheria and Tetanus Toxoids Adsorbed is indicated for active immunization of infants and children from 2 months of age up to their seventh birthday both for routine protection and as a preventive measure against diphtheria and tetanus, in circumstances in which the use of a combined triple vaccine containing pertussis antigen is contraindicated.[4,5]

Tetanus or diphtheria infection may not confer immunity; therefore, initiation or completion of active immunization is indicated at the time of recovery from these infections.[4]

CONTRAINDICATIONS

HYPERSENSITIVITY TO ANY COMPONENT OF THE VACCINE, INCLUDING THIMEROSAL, A MERCURY DERIVATIVE, IS A CONTRAINDICATION.

THE OCCURRENCE OF ANY NEUROLOGICAL SYMPTOMS OR SIGNS FOLLOWING ADMINISTRATION OF THIS PRODUCT IS A CONTRAINDICATION TO FURTHER USE.

IMMUNIZATION SHOULD BE DEFERRED DURING THE COURSE OF ANY FEBRILE ILLNESS OR ACUTE INFECTION. A MINOR AFEBRILE ILLNESS SUCH AS A MILD UPPER RESPIRATORY INFECTION IS NOT USUALLY REASON TO DEFER IMMUNIZATION.[4,5]

The clinical judgment of the attending physician should prevail at all times.

Routine immunization should be deferred during an outbreak of poliomyelitis, providing the patient has not sustained an injury that increases the risk of tetanus and providing an outbreak of diphtheria does not occur simultaneously.

WARNINGS

THIS PRODUCT IS NOT RECOMMENDED FOR IMMUNIZING PERSONS ON OR AFTER THEIR SEVENTH BIRTHDAY. For individuals 7 years of age or older, Tetanus and Diphtheria Toxoids Adsorbed For Adult Use (Td) should be used instead of Diphtheria and Tetanus Toxoids Adsorbed For Pediatric Use (DT). The concentration of diphtheria toxoid in preparations intended for use in persons 7 years of age or older is lower than that of the pediatric formulation; a lower dosage of diphtheria toxoid is recommended for persons 7 years of age or older because adverse reactions to the diphtheria component are thought to be related to both dose and age.[4]

THE OCCURRENCE OF A NEUROLOGICAL OR SEVERE HYPERSENSITIVITY REACTION FOLLOWING A PREVIOUS DOSE IS A CONTRAINDICATION TO FURTHER USE OF THIS PRODUCT.[4]

DT should not be given to infants or children with thrombocytopenia or any coagulation disorder that would contraindicate intramuscular injection unless the potential benefits clearly outweigh the risk of administration.

Patients with impaired immune responsiveness, whether due to the use of immunosuppressive therapy (including irradiation, corticosteroids, antimetabolites, alkylating agents, and cytotoxic agents), a genetic defect, human immunodeficiency virus (HIV) infection, or other causes, may have a reduced antibody response to active immunization procedures.[4,5,6] Deferral of administration of DT may be considered in individuals receiving immunosuppressive therapy.[4,5] Other groups should generally receive this vaccine according to the usual recommended schedule.[4–7]

Special care should be taken to prevent injection into a blood vessel.

PRECAUTIONS

General:
1. THIS PRODUCT SHOULD BE USED FOR THE AGE GROUP BETWEEN 2 MONTHS AND THE SEVENTH BIRTHDAY.
2. PRIOR TO ADMINISTRATION OF ANY DOSE OF DT, THE PARENT OR GUARDIAN SHOULD BE ASKED ABOUT THE RECENT HEALTH STATUS OF THE INFANT OR CHILD TO BE IMMUNIZED IN ORDER TO DETERMINE THE EXISTENCE OF ANY CONTRAINDICATION TO IMMUNIZATION WITH DT (SEE CONTRAINDICATIONS, WARNINGS).
3. WHEN AN INFANT OR CHILD RETURNS FOR THE NEXT DOSE IN A SERIES, THE PARENT OR GUARDIAN SHOULD BE QUESTIONED CONCERNING OCCURRENCE OF ANY SYMPTOM AND/OR SIGN OF AN ADVERSE REACTION AFTER THE PREVIOUS DOSE (SEE CONTRAINDICATIONS, ADVERSE REACTIONS).
4. BEFORE THE INJECTION OF ANY BIOLOGICAL, THE PHYSICIAN SHOULD TAKE ALL PRECAUTIONS KNOWN FOR PREVENTION OF ALLERGIC OR ANY OTHER SIDE REACTIONS. This should include: a review of the patient's history regarding possible sensitivity; the ready availability of epinephrine 1:1,000 and other appropriate agents used for control of immediate allergic reactions; and a knowledge of the recent literature pertaining to use of the biological concerned, including the nature of side effects and adverse reactions that may follow its use.
5. A separate sterile syringe and needle or a sterile disposable unit should be used for each individual patient to prevent transmission of hepatitis or other infectious agents from one person to another.
6. **Shake vigorously before withdrawing each dose to resuspend the contents of the vial.**
7. NATIONAL CHILDHOOD VACCINE INJURY ACT OF 1986 (AS AMENDED IN 1987)
   This Act requires that the manufacturer and lot number of the vaccine administered be recorded by the health care provider in the vaccine recipient's permanent medical record, along with the date of administration of the vaccine and the name, address and title of the person administering the vaccine.
   The Act further requires the health care provider to report to a health department or to the FDA the occurrence

following immunization of any event set forth in the Vaccine Injury Table including: anaphylaxis or anaphylactic shock within 24 hours, encephalopathy or encephalitis within 7 days, residual seizure disorder, any acute complication or sequelae (including death) of above events, or any event that would contraindicate further doses of vaccine, according to this package insert.[8]

Information for the Patient: PRIOR TO THE ADMINISTRATION OF THIS VACCINE, HEALTH CARE PERSONNEL SHOULD INFORM THE PARENT, GUARDIAN, OR OTHER RESPONSIBLE ADULT OF THE BENEFITS AND RISKS TO THE CHILD OF VACCINATION AGAINST DIPHTHERIA AND TETANUS.

Use in Pregnancy: This product is not recommended for administration to females of child-bearing age.

ADVERSE REACTIONS

Local reactions, manifested by varying degrees of erythema, induration, and tenderness, may occur after administration of DT.[9,10] Such local reactions are usually self-limited and require no therapy. Nodule,[11] sterile abscess formation, or subcutaneous atrophy may occur at the site of injection. Systemic symptoms, including drowsiness, fretfulness, vomiting, anorexia, and persistent crying have been described following DT immunization.[9,10]

In one study, fever $\geq 38°C$ (100.4°F) was reported in 9.3% of DT recipients, and fever $\geq 39°C$ (102.2°F) was reported in 0.7% of recipients.[9]

Pallor, coldness, and hyporesponsiveness have been reported in a child receiving a DT vaccine.[10]

NEUROLOGICAL COMPLICATIONS,[12] SUCH AS CONVULSIONS,[13] ENCEPHALOPATHY,[13,14] AND VARIOUS MONO- AND POLYNEUROPATHIES,[14-20] INCLUDING GUILLAIN-BARRE SYNDROME,[21,22] HAVE BEEN REPORTED FOLLOWING ADMINISTRATION OF PREPARATIONS CONTAINING DIPHTHERIA AND/OR TETANUS ANTIGENS.

URTICARIA, ERYTHEMA MULTIFORME OR OTHER RASH, ARTHRALGIAS[13] AND, MORE RARELY, A SEVERE ANAPHYLACTIC REACTION (IE, URTICARIA WITH SWELLING OF THE MOUTH, DIFFICULTY BREATHING, HYPOTENSION, OR SHOCK) HAVE BEEN REPORTED FOLLOWING ADMINISTRATION OF PREPARATIONS CONTAINING DIPHTHERIA, AND/OR TETANUS ANTIGENS.

DOSAGE AND ADMINISTRATION

For Intramuscular Use Only: Shake vigorously before withdrawing each dose to resuspend the contents of the vial. Parenteral drug products should be inspected visually for particulate matter and discoloration prior to administration. (See DESCRIPTION.)

The vaccine should be injected intramuscularly, preferably into the midlateral muscles of the thigh or deltoid, with care to avoid major peripheral nerve trunks.

Before injection, the skin at the injection site should be cleansed and prepared with a suitable germicide.

After insertion of the needle, aspirate to help avoid inadvertent injection into a blood vessel.

This combined preparation against both diphtheria and tetanus is designed particularly to meet the need of children less than 7 years of age for whom the use of a combined triple vaccine containing pertussis antigen is contraindicated.

It is recommended that active immunization against diphtheria and tetanus be started at 2 months of age.

Unimmunized infants and children less than 1 year of age for whom vaccine containing pertussis antigen is contraindicated should receive three doses of 0.5 mL each of DT at 4 to 8 week intervals, followed by a fourth (reinforcing) dose of 0.5 mL, 6 to 12 months after the third dose, for the primary series.

Unimmunized children 1 year of age or older for whom vaccine containing pertussis antigen is contraindicated should receive two doses of 0.5 mL each of DT, 4 to 8 weeks apart, followed by a third (reinforcing) dose 6 to 12 months later, for the primary series.

If after beginning a DTP series, further doses of vaccine containing pertussis antigen become contraindicated, DT should be substituted for each of the remaining doses.[4,5]

The reinforcing dose is an integral part of the primary immunizing series.

Interruption of the recommended schedule with a delay between doses does not interfere with the final immunity achieved, nor does it necessitate starting the series over again, regardless of the length of time elapsed between doses.[4,5]

A booster dose of 0.5 mL is indicated at age 4 to 6 years, preferably prior to entrance into kindergarten or elementary school. However, if the last dose of the primary immunizing series was administered after the fourth birthday, a booster prior to school entry is not considered necessary.[4,5]

For either primary or booster immunization against tetanus and diphtheria of individuals 7 years of age and older, the use of Tetanus and Diphtheria Toxoids Adsorbed For Adult Use is recommended.[4,5]

Diphtheria Prophylaxis for Case Contacts: All case contacts, household and others, who have previously received fewer than three doses of diphtheria toxoid should receive an immediate dose of an appropriate diphtheria toxoid-containing preparation and should complete the series according to schedule. Case contacts who previously received three or more doses, but who have not received a dose of a preparation containing diphtheria toxoid within the previous 5 years, should receive a dose of a diphtheria toxoid-containing preparation appropriate for their age. This combined preparation against both diphtheria and tetanus is designed particularly to meet the need of children less than 7 years of age for whom the use of a combined triple vaccine containing pertussis antigen is contraindicated.

Tetanus Prophylaxis in Wound Management: For routine wound management of children under 7 years of age who are not completely immunized, DT should be used instead of single-antigen tetanus toxoid (if pertussis antigen is contraindicated or individual circumstances are such that potential febrile reactions following DTP might confound the management of the patient).[4] Completion of primary vaccination thereafter should be ensured.

For tetanus-prone wounds in children who have had fewer than three, or an unknown number of immunizations with a tetanus-toxoid containing product, passive immunization with human Tetanus-Immune Globulin (TIG) is also recommended.[4] A separate syringe and site of injection should be used.

HOW SUPPLIED

NDC 0005-1858-31 5.0 mL vial

STORAGE

DO NOT FREEZE. STORE REFRIGERATED, AWAY FROM FREEZER COMPARTMENT, AT 2°C to 8°C (36°F to 46°F).

REFERENCES

1. Mueller JH, Miller PA: Production of diphtheria toxin of high potency (100Lf) on a reproducible medium. *J Immunol* 1941;40:21–32.
2. Mueller JH, Miller PA: Factors influencing the production of tetanal toxin. *J Immunol* 1947;56:143–147.
3. Pillemer L, Grossberg DB, Wittler RG: The immunochemistry of toxins and toxoids. II. The preparation and immunological evaluation of purified tetanal toxoid. *J Immunol* 1946;54:213–224.
4. Recommendation of the Immunization Practices Advisory Committee (ACIP): Diphtheria, tetanus and pertussis: Guidelines for vaccine prophylaxis and other preventive measures. *MMWR* 1985;34:405–426.
5. American Academy of Pediatrics: Report of the Committee on Infectious Diseases, ed 20. Elk Grove Village, IL, American Academy of Pediatrics, 1986.
6. Recommendation of the ACIP: Immunization of children infected with Human T-Lymphotrophic Virus Type III/ Lymphadenopathy associated virus. *MMWR* 1986; 35(38):595–606.
7. Immunization of children infected with Human Immunodeficiency Virus—Supplementary ACIP statement. *MMWR* 1988;37(12):181–183.
8. National Childhood Vaccine Injury Act: Requirements for permanent vaccination records and for reporting of selected events after vaccination. *MMWR* 1988;37(13):197–200.
9. Cody C, et al: Nature and rates of adverse reactions associated with DTP and DT immunizations in infants and children. *Pediatrics* 1981;68:650–660.
10. Feery BJ: Incidence and type of reactions to triple antigen (DTP) and DT (CDT) vaccines. *Med Jour of Australia* 1982;2:511–515.
11. Fawcett HA, Smith NP: Injection-site granuloma due to aluminum. *Arch Dermatol* 1984;120:1318–1322.
12. Rutledge SL, Snead OC: Neurological complications of immunizations. *J Pediatr* 1986;109:917–924.
13. Adverse Events Following Immunization. *MMWR* 1985;34(3):43–47.
14. Schlenska GK: Unusual neurological complications following tetanus toxoid administration. *J Neurol* 1977;215:299–302.
15. Blumstein GI, Kreithen H: Peripheral neuropathy following tetanus toxoid administration. *JAMA* 1966;198:1030–1031.
16. Reinstein L, Pargament JM, Goodman JS: Peripheral neuropathy after multiple tetanus toxoid injections. *Arch Phys Med Rehabil* 1982;63:332–334.
17. Tsairis P, Duck PJ, Mulder DW: Natural history of brachial plexus neuropathy. *Arch Neurol* 1972;27:109–117.
18. Quast U, Hennessen W, Widmark RM: Mono- and polyneuritis after tetanus vaccination. *Devel Bio Stand* 1979;43:25–32.
19. Holliday PL, Bauer RB: Polyradiculoneuritis secondary to immunization with tetanus and diphtheria toxoids. *Arch Neurol* 1983;40:56–57.
20. Fenichel GM: Neurological complications of tetanus toxoid. *Arch Neurol* 1983;40:390.
21. Pollard JD, Selby G: Relapsing neuropathy due to tetanus toxoid. *J Neurol Sci* 1978;37:113–125.
22. Newton N, Janati A: Guillain-Barre syndrome after vaccination with purified tetanus toxoid. *S Med J* 1987;80:1053–1054.

LEDERLE LABORATORIES DIVISION
American Cyanamid Company
Pearl River, NY 10965

Rev. 5/88
23590

FERRO–SEQUELS®   OTC

[fĕrrō-sē-quls]
High potency, time-release iron supplement

DESCRIPTION

Each FERRO-SEQUELS tablet contains 150 mg of ferrous fumarate, equivalent to 50 mg of elemental iron and 100 mg of docusate sodium (DSS). FERRO-SEQUELS is a high potency iron supplement that employs a time release system to deliver iron slowly to maximize absorption, and to reduce the irritation associated with iron tablets.

Inactive Ingredients: Blue 1, Corn Starch, Crospovidone, Hydroxypropyl Methylcellulose, Lactose, Magnesium Stearate, Microcrystalline Cellulose, Modified Food Starch, Povidone, Silica Gel, Sodium Lauryl Sulfate, Titanium Dioxide, and Yellow 10.

INDICATIONS

For the treatment of simple iron deficiency and iron deficiency anemia.

RECOMMENDED INTAKE

One tablet, once or twice daily, or as prescribed by the physician.

WARNING

As with any drug, if you are pregnant or nursing a baby, seek the advice of a health professional before using this product. Keep this and all medications out of the reach of children. In case of accidental overdose, seek professional assistance or contact a Poison Control Center immediately.

HOW SUPPLIED

Box of 30 tablets, NDC 0005-5267-68
Bottle of 30 tablets, NDC 0005-5267-13
Bottle of 100 tablets, NDC 0005-5267-23
Unit Dose Package 10 × 10, NDC 0005-5267-60
Bottle of 1,000 tablets, NDC 0005-5267-34
Store at Controlled Room Temperature 15°–30°C (59°–86°F).
LEDERLE LABORATORIES DIVISION
American Cyanamid Company
Pearl River, NY 10965
MADE IN USA

6/90
27533

Shown in Product Identification Section, page 414

FIBERCON®   OTC

[fī-ber-con]
Calcium polycarbophil
Bulk-forming fiber laxative
Concentrated fiber laxative

DESCRIPTION

Each FIBERCON tablet contains 625 mg calcium polycarbophil equivalent to 500 mg polycarbophil. FIBERCON promotes normal function of the bowel by increasing bulk volume and water content of the stool. Contains no chemical stimulants and is not habit forming.

Inactive Ingredients: Calcium Carbonate, Caramel, Crospovidone, Hydroxypropyl Methylcellulose, Magnesium Stearate, Microcrystalline Cellulose, Povidone, and Silica Gel.

INDICATIONS

FIBERCON may be used to help restore and maintain regularity; relieve constipation; and promote normal function of the bowel. FIBERCON works naturally so continued use for 1 to 3 days is normally required to provide full benefit.

RECOMMENDED INTAKE

Dosage will vary according to diet, exercise, previous laxative use, or severity of constipation. Recommended adult starting dose: Two or four tablets daily. May be increased up to eight tablets daily.

Continued on next page

Information on Lederle products listed on these pages is the full prescribing information from product literature or package inserts effective in August 1992. Information concerning all Lederle products may be obtained from the Professional Services Department, Lederle Laboratories, Pearl River, New York 10965.

Lederle—Cont.

Adults and children 12 years and older: swallow two tablets one to four times a day. Children 6 to 12 years: swallow one tablet one to three times a day. Children under 6 years: consult a physician.

A full glass (8 fl. oz.) of liquid should be taken with each dose. See package insert for additional information.

WARNING

Any sudden change in bowel habits may indicate a more serious condition than constipation. Consult your physician if symptoms such as nausea, vomiting, abdominal pain, or rectal bleeding occur or if this product has no effect within 1 week.

For chronic or continued constipation, consult your physician.

Interaction Precaution: Contains calcium. If you are taking any form of tetracycline antibiotic, FIBERCON should be taken at least 1 hour before or 2 hours after you have taken the antibiotic. Keep this and all medicines out of the reach of children.

HOW SUPPLIED

Film coated tablets, scored, engraved LL and F66.
Package of 36 tablets, NDC 0005-2500-02
Package of 60 tablets, NDC 0005-2500-86
Package of 90 tablets, NDC 0005-2500-33
Bottle of 500 tablets, NDC 0005-2500-31
Unit Dose Pkg, 10 × 20's, NDC 0005-2500-28
Store at Controlled Room Temperature 15°–30° C (59°–86° F).
Protect contents from moisture.   Rev. 8/91
                                                    10995-91

LEDERLE LABORATORIES DIVISION
American Cyanamid Company
Pearl River, NY 10965
Shown in Product Identification Section, page 414

FILIBON®   ℞
[fil-ă-bŏn]
prenatal tablets

Each Tablet Contains		For Pregnant or Lactating Women Percentage of US Recommended Daily Allowance (US RDA)
Vitamin A (as Acetate)	5000 IU	(63%)
Vitamin D₂	400 IU	(100%)
Vitamin E (as dl-Alpha Tocopheryl Acetate)	30 IU	(100%)
Vitamin C (Ascorbic Acid)	60 mg	(100%)
Folic Acid	0.4 mg	(50%)
Vitamin B₁ (as Thiamine Mononitrate)	1.5 mg	(88%)
Vitamin B₂ (as Riboflavin)	1.7 mg	(85%)
Niacinamide	20 mg	(100%)
Vitamin B₆	2 mg	(80%)
Vitamin B₁₂ (Cyanocobalamin)	6 mcg	(75%)
Calcium (as Calcium Carbonate)	125 mg	(10%)
Iodine (as Potassium Iodide)	150 mcg	(100%)
Iron (as Ferrous Fumarate)	18 mg	(100%)
Magnesium (as Magnesium Oxide)	100 mg	(22%)

Inactive Ingredients: Ethylcellulose, Hydroxypropyl Methylcellulose, Lactose, Magnesium Stearate, Microcrystalline Cellulose, Povidone, Pregelatinized Starch, Red 40, Silicon Dioxide, Sodium Lauryl Sulfate, Sodium Starch Glycolate, Titanium Dioxide and Stearic Acid.

DESCRIPTION
Multivitamin-Multimineral Supplement for pregnant or lactating women. A Phosphorus-Free Vitamin and Mineral Dietary Supplement for use in prenatal care and lactation.

RECOMMENDED INTAKE
1 daily, or as prescribed by the physician.

HOW SUPPLIED
Pink, capsule-shaped, film-coated tablets engraved LL-F4.
Bottles of 100 NDC 0005-4294-23
LEDERLE LABORATORIES DIVISION
American Cyanamid Company
Pearl River, N.Y. 10965   7/91
Shown in Product Identification Section, page 414

FILIBON® F.A.   ℞
[fil-ă-bŏn]
prenatal tablets

Each Tablet Contains		For Pregnant or Lactating Women Percentage of US Recommended Daily Allowance (US RDA)
Vitamin A (as Acetate)	8000 IU	(100%)
Vitamin D	400 IU	(100%)
Vitamin E (as dl-Alpha Tocopheryl Acetate)	30 IU	(100%)
Vitamin C (Ascorbic Acid)	60 mg	(100%)
Folic Acid	1 mg	(125%)
Vitamin B₁ (as Thiamine Mononitrate)	1.7 mg	(100%)
Vitamin B₂ (as Riboflavin)	2 mg	(100%)
Niacinamide	20 mg	(100%)
Vitamin B₆	4 mg	(160%)
Vitamin B₁₂ (Cyanocobalamin)	8 mcg	(100%)
Calcium (as Calcium Carbonate)	250 mg	(19%)
Iodine (as Potassium Iodide)	150 mcg	(100%)
Iron (as Ferrous Fumarate)	45 mg	(250%)
Magnesium (as Magnesium Oxide)	100 mg	(22%)

Inactive Ingredients: Colloidal Silicon Dioxide, Ethylcellulose, Hydroxypropyl Methylcellulose, Lactose, Magnesium Stearate, Microcrystalline Cellulose, Povidone, Pregelatinized Starch, Red 40, Sodium Lauryl Sulfate, Sodium Starch Glycolate and Titanium Dioxide.

DESCRIPTION
Multivitamin-Multimineral Supplement for pregnant or lactating women. A Phosphorus-Free Vitamin and Mineral Dietary Supplement for use in prenatal care and lactation.

RECOMMENDED INTAKE
1 tablet daily.

CAUTION
Federal law prohibits dispensing without prescription.

PRECAUTION
Folic acid may obscure pernicious anemia in that the peripheral blood picture may revert to normal while neurological manifestations remain progressive.

HOW SUPPLIED
Capsule-shaped tablets (film-coated, pink) engraved LL-F5—bottles of 100 NDC 0005-4225-23.
Store at Controlled Room Temperature 15°–30°C (59°–86°F).
LEDERLE LABORATORIES DIVISION
American Cyanamid Company
Pearl River, N.Y. 10965   5/91
Shown in Product Identification Section, page 414

FILIBON® FORTE   ℞
[fil-ă-bŏn for-tā]
prenatal tablets

Each Tablet Contains		For Pregnant or Lactating Women Percentage of US Recommended Daily Allowance (US RDA)
Vitamin A (as Acetate)	8000 IU	(100%)
Vitamin D₂	400 IU	(100%)
Vitamin E (as dl-Alpha Tocopheryl Acetate)	45 IU	(150%)
Vitamin C (Ascorbic Acid)	90 mg	(150%)
Folic Acid	1 mg	(125%)
Vitamin B₁ (as Thiamine Mononitrate)	2 mg	(118%)
Vitamin B₂ (as Riboflavin)	2.5 mg	(125%)
Niacinamide	30 mg	(150%)
Vitamin B₆	3 mg	(120%)
Vitamin B₁₂ (Cyanocobalamin)	12 mcg	(150%)
Calcium (as Calcium Carbonate)	300 mg	(23%)
Iodine (as Potassium Iodide)	200 mcg	(133%)
Iron (as Ferrous Fumarate)	45 mg	(250%)
Magnesium (as Magnesium Oxide)	100 mg	(22%)

Inactive Ingredients: Ethylcellulose, Hydroxypropyl Methylcellulose, Magnesium Stearate, Povidone, Red 30, Silicon Dioxide, Sodium Lauryl Sulfate, Sodium Starch Glycolate, Titanium Dioxide and Stearic Acid.

DESCRIPTION
Multivitamin-Multimineral Supplement for pregnant or lactating women. A Phosphorus-Free Vitamin and Mineral Dietary Supplement for use in prenatal care and lactation.

RECOMMENDED INTAKE
1 tablet daily. This dosage provides 23% and 22% of the Recommended Daily Allowance of calcium and magnesium, respectively; therefore, supplementation of the diet by milk or other sources of calcium may be advisable.

CAUTION
Federal law prohibits dispensing without prescription.

PRECAUTION
Folic Acid may obscure pernicious anemia in that the peripheral blood picture may revert to normal while neurological manifestations remain progressive.

HOW SUPPLIED
Pink, capsule-shaped, film-coated tablets engraved LL-F6.
Bottles of 100—NDC 0005-4226-23.
Store at Controlled Room Temperature 15°–30°C (59°–86°F).
LEDERLE LABORATORIES DIVISION
American Cyanamid Company
Pearl River, N.Y. 10965   2/92
Shown in Product Identification Section, page 414

INFLUENZA VIRUS VACCINE   ℞
FLU-IMUNE®*
Purified Surface Antigen Vaccine, Trivalent, Types A and B
For six months of age and older
1992–1993 Formula

DESCRIPTION
Influenza Virus Vaccine, FLU-IMUNE, Types A and B (Surface Antigen) is a sterile parenteral for intramuscular use only. The vaccine is a slightly opalescent liquid.

FLU-IMUNE, a purified surface antigen vaccine, is prepared from the extraembryonic fluid of embryonated chicken eggs inoculated with a specific type of influenza virus containing neomycin and polymyxin. The fluid containing the virus is harvested and clarified by centrifugation and filtration prior to inactivation with betapropiolactone. The inactivated virus is concentrated and purified by zonal centrifugation.

The surface antigens, hemagglutinin and neuraminidase, are obtained from the influenza virus particle by further centrifugation in the presence of Triton®† N101, a process which removes most of the internal proteins. The Triton N101 is removed from the surface antigen preparation and the antigens are suspended in 0.01M phosphate buffered saline. The hemagglutinin content is standardized according to current US Public Health Service requirements. Each dose (0.5 mL) contains the recommended ratio of not less than 15 μg of hemagglutinin of each strain similar to: A/Texas/36/91 (H₁N₁), A/Beijing/353/89 (H₃N₂), and B/Panama/45/90.

Thimerosal (mercury derivative) 0.01% is added as a preservative. Polymyxin, neomycin, and betapropiolactone cannot be detected in the final product by current assay procedures. This vaccine is produced and filled by Evans Medical Limited; it is labeled, packaged, and released by Lederle Laboratories under a divided manufacturing arrangement.

CLINICAL PHARMACOLOGY
Influenza A viruses are classified into subtypes on the basis of two surface antigens: hemagglutinin (H) and neuraminidase (N). Three subtypes of hemagglutinin (H₁, H₂, and H₃) and two subtypes of neuraminidase (N₁, N₂) are recognized among influenza A viruses that have caused widespread human disease. Immunity to these antigens, especially the hemagglutinin, reduces the likelihood of infection and lessens the severity of the disease if infection occurs. Infection with a virus of one subtype confers little or no protection against viruses of other subtypes. Furthermore, over time, antigenic variation (antigenic drift) within a subtype may be so marked that infection or immunization with one strain may not induce immunity to distantly related strains of the same subtype. Although influenza B viruses have shown more antigenic stability than influenza A viruses, antigenic variation does occur. For these reasons major epidemics of respiratory disease caused by new variants of influenza continue to occur. The antigenic characteristics of strains currently circulating provide the basis for selecting the virus strains included in each year's vaccine.[1]

Typical influenza illness is characterized by abrupt onset of fever, myalgia, sore throat, and nonproductive cough. Unlike other common respiratory infections, influenza can cause severe malaise lasting several days. More severe illness can result if primary influenza pneumonia or secondary bacterial pneumonia occurs. During influenza epidemics, high attack rates of acute illness result in increased numbers of visits to physicians' offices, walk-in clinics, and emergency rooms and increased hospitalization for management of lower respiratory tract complications.[1]

Elderly persons and persons with underlying health problems are at increased risk of complications from influenza infection. If infected, such high-risk persons or groups (listed as "groups at increased risk for influenza-related complications" under Target Groups for Special Vaccination Programs) are more likely than the general population to require hospitalization. During major epidemics, hospitaliza-

---

*FLU-IMMUNE is a registered tradename of Lederle Laboratories

†Triton is a registered trademark of Rohm & Haas Corporation.

tion rates for high-risk persons may increase two to fivefold, depending on the age group. Previously healthy children and young adults may also require hospitalization for influenza-related complications, but the relative increase in their hospitalization rates is less than for persons who belong to high-risk groups.[1]

An increase in mortality further indicates the impact of influenza epidemics. Increased mortality results not only from pneumonia but also cardiopulmonary and other chronic diseases that can be exacerbated by influenza infection. It is estimated that more than 10,000 excess deaths occurred during each of 7 different US epidemics in the period 1977 to 1988, and more than 40,000 excess deaths occurred during each of two of these epidemics. Approximately 80% to 90% of the excess deaths attributed to pneumonia and influenza were among persons 65 years of age or older.[1] However, during major epidemics, influenza-associated deaths also occur among children and previously healthy adults under 65 years of age.

Because the proportion of elderly persons in the United States population is increasing and because age and its associated chronic diseases are risk factors for severe influenza illness, the toll from influenza can be expected to increase unless control measures are used more vigorously. The number of younger persons at increased risk for influenza-related complications is also increasing for various reasons, such as the success of neonatal intensive care units, better management of diseases such as cystic fibrosis, acquired immunodeficiency syndrome (AIDS), and better survival rates for organ transplant recipients.[1]

Reye's syndrome has been associated primarily with influenza B, but also with influenza A infection.[2]

Clinical studies have demonstrated that influenza vaccines give between 70% and 80% protection when the vaccine strain and infecting strain are related. Lower levels of protection occur when the infecting virus is antigenically different from the vaccine virus.[2]

Based upon epidemiological studies of circulating influenza virus strains, the Public Health Service has recommended that the 1992–1993 vaccine will be trivalent and contain 15 μg of hemagglutinin of each strain similar to: A/Texas/36/91 (H_1N_1), A/Beijing/353/89 (H_3N_2), and B/Panama/45/90.[1]

INDICATIONS AND USAGE

Influenza Virus Vaccine, FLU-IMUNE, Types A and B (Surface Antigen) is indicated for immunization against influenza viruses containing antigens related to those in the vaccine.

Influenza vaccine is strongly recommended for persons 6 months of age or older who, by virtue of age or underlying medical condition, are at increased risk of complications from influenza. Health care workers and others (including household members) in close contact with high-risk persons should also be immunized. In addition, influenza vaccine may be given to any person who wishes to reduce the chances of becoming infected with influenza. Guidelines for the use of vaccine among different groups follow.[1]

Although the current Influenza Virus Vaccine can contain one or more antigens used in previous years, annual immunization using the current vaccine is necessary because immunity declines in the year following immunization.[1] **Because the 1992-1993 vaccine differs from the 1991-1992 vaccine, supplies of 1991-1992 vaccine should not be used to provide protection for the 1992-1993 influenza season.[1]**

Two doses given at least one month apart may be required for a satisfactory response among previously unvaccinated children less than 9 years of age; however, studies with vaccines similar to those in current use have shown little or no improvement in antibody responses when a second dose is given to adults during the same season.[1]

Target Groups for Special Immunization Programs

To maximize protection of high-risk persons, they and their close contacts should be targeted for organized immunization programs.

Groups at increased medical risk of influenza-related complications.

1. Persons 65 years of age or older[1] (regardless of health status).
2. Residents of nursing homes and other chronic-care facilities housing persons of any age with chronic medical conditions.[1]
3. Adults and children with chronic disorders of the pulmonary or cardiovascular systems, including children with asthma.[1]
4. Adults and children who have required regular medical follow-up or hospitalization during the preceding year because of chronic metabolic diseases (including diabetes mellitus), renal dysfunction, hemoglobinopathies, or immunosuppression (including immunosuppression caused by medication).[1]
5. Children and teenagers (6 months through 18 years of age) who are receiving long-term aspirin therapy and, therefore, may be at risk of developing Reye's syndrome following influenza infection.[1]

Groups that can transmit influenza to high-risk persons:
Persons who are clinically or subclinically infected and who attend or live with high-risk persons can transmit influenza virus to them. Some high-risk persons (eg, the elderly, transplant recipients, or persons with acquired immunodeficiency syndrome [AIDS]) can have low antibody responses to influenza vaccine. Efforts to protect these high-risk persons against influenza may be improved by reducing the chances of exposure to influenza from their care providers. Therefore, the following groups should be immunized[1]:

1. Physicians, nurses, and other personnel in both hospital and outpatient care settings who have contact with high-risk persons among all age groups, including infants.[1]
2. Employees of nursing homes and chronic-care facilities who have contact with patients or residents.[1]
3. Providers of home care to high-risk persons (eg, visiting nurses, volunteer workers).[1]
4. Household members (including children) of high-risk persons.[1]

Immunization of Other Groups

General Population: Physicians should administer influenza vaccine to any person who wishes to reduce their chances of acquiring influenza infection. Persons who provide essential community services may be considered for immunization to minimize disruption of essential activities during influenza outbreaks. Similarly, students or other persons in institutional settings such as those who reside in dormitories may be considered for immunization to minimize the disruption of routine activities during epidemics.[1]

Pregnant Women: Influenza-associated excess mortality among pregnant women has not been documented, except in the largest pandemics of 1918–1919 and 1957–1958. However, the Immunization Practices Advisory Committee (ACIP) of the US Public Health Service recommends that pregnant women who have other medical conditions that increase their risk for complications from influenza should be immunized, as the vaccine is considered safe for pregnant women. The ACIP has stated that administering the vaccine after the first trimester is a reasonable precaution to minimize any concern over the theoretical possibility of teratogenicity. The ACIP has also stated however that it may be undesirable to delay immunization of pregnant women with high-risk conditions who will still be in the first trimester of pregnancy when the influenza season begins.[1] **The clinical judgment of the attending physician should prevail at all times in determining whether to administer the vaccine to a pregnant woman (see PRECAUTIONS, Use in Pregnancy).**

Persons Infected with Human Immunodeficiency Virus (HIV):
Recent reports suggest that symptoms of influenza may be prolonged and the risk of complications increased in this high-risk group.[1]

Because influenza may result in serious illness and complications in some HIV-infected persons, immunization is a prudent precaution and will result in protective antibody levels in many recipients.[1] However, the antibody response to vaccine may be low in persons with advanced HIV-related illnesses; a booster dose of vaccine has not improved the immune response in these individuals.[1]

Foreign Travelers:
Increasingly, the elderly and persons with high-risk medical conditions are embarking on international travel. The risk of exposure to influenza during foreign travel varies, depending on the season and destination. Influenza can occur throughout the year in the tropics; the season of greatest influenza activity in the Southern Hemisphere is April–September. Because of the short incubation period for influenza, exposure to the virus during travel can result in clinical illness that also begins during travel, an inconvenient or potentially dangerous situation, especially for those at increased risk for complications. Persons preparing to travel to the tropics at any time of year or to the Southern Hemisphere during April–September should review their influenza immunization histories. If they were not immunized the previous fall/winter, they should be considered for influenza immunization prior to travel. The most current available vaccine should be used. High-risk persons given the previous season's vaccine prior to travel should be reimmunized in the fall/winter with current vaccine.[1]

Timing of Immunization:
Beginning each September, when vaccine for the upcoming influenza season becomes available, high-risk persons who are seen by health-care providers for routine care or as a result of hospitalization should be offered influenza vaccine. Opportunities to vaccinate persons at high-risk for complications of influenza should not be missed.

The optimal time for organized vaccination campaigns for high-risk persons usually is the period between mid-October and mid-November. In the United States influenza activity generally peaks between late December and early March, and high levels of influenza activity infrequently occur in the contiguous 48 states before December. It is particularly important to avoid administering vaccine too far in advance of the influenza season in facilities such as nursing homes because antibody levels may begin to decline within a few months of vaccination. Vaccination programs may be undertaken as soon as current vaccine is available if regional influenza activity is expected to begin earlier than December.[1]

Children under 9 years of age who have not been immunized previously require two doses with at least one month between doses. The second dose should be given before December, if possible. Vaccine can be given to both children and adults up to the time influenza virus activity is documented in a region, and even thereafter, which may be as late as April in some areas.[1]

CONTRAINDICATIONS

INFLUENZA VIRUS IS PROPAGATED IN EGGS FOR THE PREPARATION OF INFLUENZA VIRUS VACCINE. THUS, THIS VACCINE SHOULD NOT BE ADMINISTERED TO ANYONE WITH A HISTORY OF HYPERSENSITIVITY (ALLERGY) TO CHICKEN EGGS.[1] THE VACCINE IS ALSO CONTRAINDICATED IN INDIVIDUALS HYPERSENSITIVE TO ANY COMPONENT OF THE VACCINE INCLUDING THIMEROSAL (A MERCURY DERIVATIVE) (see **ADVERSE REACTIONS**). EPINEPHRINE INJECTION (1:1000) MUST BE IMMEDIATELY AVAILABLE SHOULD AN ACUTE ANAPHYLACTIC REACTION OCCUR DUE TO ANY COMPONENT OF THE VACCINE.

IMMUNIZATION SHOULD BE DELAYED IN PERSONS WITH AN ACTIVE NEUROLOGICAL DISORDER CHARACTERIZED BY CHANGING NEUROLOGICAL FINDINGS, BUT SHOULD BE CONSIDERED WHEN THE DISEASE PROCESS HAS BEEN STABILIZED.

THE OCCURRENCE OF ANY NEUROLOGICAL SYMPTOMS OR SIGNS FOLLOWING ADMINISTRATION OF THIS PRODUCT IS A CONTRAINDICATION TO FURTHER USE.

THE VACCINE SHOULD NOT BE ADMINISTERED TO PERSONS WITH ACUTE FEBRILE ILLNESSES UNTIL THEIR TEMPORARY SYMPTOMS HAVE ABATED.[1]

The clinical judgment of the attending physician should prevail at all times.

WARNINGS

Influenza Virus Vaccine should not be given to individuals with thrombocytopenia or any coagulation disorder that would contraindicate intramuscular injection unless, in the judgment of the physician, the potential benefits clearly outweigh the risk of administration.

Patients with impaired immune responsiveness, whether due to the use of immunosuppressive therapy (including irradiation, corticosteroids, antimetabolites, alkylating agents, and cytotoxic agents), a genetic defect, human immunodeficiency virus (HIV) infection, or other causes, may have a reduced antibody response to active immunization procedures.

Because of the lower potential for causing febrile reactions, only split-virus vaccines should be used for children. These vaccines may be labeled as "split," "subvirion," or "purified-surface-antigen" vaccine. For adults, immunogenicity and side effects of split- and whole-virus vaccines are comparable when the vaccines are used at the recommended dosage.[1]

Since the likelihood of febrile convulsions from any cause is greater in children between 6 and 35 months, special care should be taken in weighing the relative risks and benefits of immunization in this age group.

As with any vaccine, immunization with Influenza Virus Vaccine may not result in seroconversion of all individuals given the vaccine.

PRECAUTIONS

General:

1. PRIOR TO ADMINISTRATION OF ANY DOSE OF INFLUENZA VIRUS VACCINE, THE PARENT, GUARDIAN, OR ADULT PATIENT SHOULD BE ASKED ABOUT THE RECENT HEALTH STATUS, MEDICAL AND IMMUNIZATION HISTORY OF THE PATIENT TO BE IMMUNIZED IN ORDER TO DETERMINE THE EXISTENCE OF ANY CONTRAINDICATION TO IMMUNIZATION WITH INFLUENZA VIRUS VACCINE (see **CONTRAINDICATIONS, WARNINGS**).
2. BEFORE ADMINISTRATION OF ANY BIOLOGICAL, THE PHYSICIAN SHOULD TAKE ALL PRECAUTIONS KNOWN FOR PREVENTION OF ALLERGIC OR ANY OTHER SIDE REACTIONS. This should include: a review of the patient's history regarding possible sensitivity, the ready availability of epinephrine 1:1000 and other appropriate agents used for control of immediate allergic reactions, and a knowledge of the recent literature pertaining

Continued on next page

Information on Lederle products listed on these pages is the full prescribing information from product literature or package inserts effective in August 1992. Information concerning all Lederle products may be obtained from the Professional Services Department, Lederle Laboratories, Pearl River, New York 10965.

Lederle—Cont.

to use of the biological concerned, including the nature of side effects and adverse reactions that may follow its use.
3. A separate sterile syringe and needle or a sterile disposable unit should be used for each individual patient to prevent transmission of infectious agents from one person to another.
4. Special care should be taken to prevent injection into a blood vessel.

Information for the Patient: PRIOR TO ADMINISTRATION OF THIS VACCINE, HEALTH CARE PERSONNEL SHOULD INFORM THE PARENT, GUARDIAN, OR ADULT PATIENT OF THE BENEFITS AND RISKS OF IMMUNIZATION AGAINST INFLUENZA.

Drug Interactions: Although influenza immunization can inhibit the clearance of warfarin and theophylline, studies have failed to show any adverse clinical effects attributable to these drugs in patients receiving influenza vaccine.[1] Individuals receiving immunosuppressive therapy (including irradiation, corticosteroids, antimetabolites, alkylating agents, and cytotoxic agents) may have a reduced antibody response to immunization with Influenza Virus Vaccine.

Use in Pregnancy: *Pregnancy Category C:* Animal reproduction studies have not been conducted with Influenza Virus Vaccine. It is also not known whether Influenza Virus Vaccine can cause fetal harm when administered to a pregnant woman or can affect reproductive capacity. Influenza Virus Vaccine should therefore be given to a pregnant woman ONLY if clearly needed. The ACIP has clearly stated that administering the vaccine after the first trimester is a reasonable precaution to minimize any concern over the theoretical possibility of teratogenicity. The ACIP has also stated however that it may be undesirable to delay immunization of pregnant women with high-risk conditions who will still be in the first trimester of pregnancy when the influenza season begins[1] (see **INDICATIONS AND USAGE, Pregnant Women**).

The clinical judgment of the attending physician should prevail at all times in determining whether to administer Influenza Virus Vaccine to a pregnant woman.

ADVERSE REACTIONS

Because influenza vaccine contains only noninfectious purified viral proteins, it cannot cause influenza. Occasional cases of respiratory disease following immunization represent coincidental illnesses unrelated to influenza immunization.[1]

Vaccine Adverse Event Reporting System: The US Department of Health and Human Services has established a new Vaccine Adverse Event Reporting System (VAERS) to accept all reports of suspected adverse events after the administration of any vaccine, including, but not limited to the reporting of events required by the National Childhood Vaccine Injury Act of 1986.[3] The VAERS toll-free number for VAERS forms and information is 1-800-822-7967.[4]

Local Symptoms: Slight tenderness, redness or induration at the site of injection lasting for 1 or 2 days may occur in less than one third of recipients.[1]

Systemic Symptoms: Fever, malaise, myalgia, and other systemic symptoms occur infrequently and most often affect persons who have had no exposure to the influenza virus antigens in the vaccine (eg, young children). These reactions begin 6 to 12 hours after immunization and can persist for 1 or 2 days.[1]

Immediate, presumably allergic, reactions such as hives, angioedema, allergic asthma, or systemic anaphylaxis occur rarely after influenza immunization. These reactions probably result from hypersensitivity to some vaccine component—most likely residual egg protein. Although current influenza vaccines contain only a small quantity of egg protein, this protein is presumed capable of inducing immediate hypersensitivity reactions in persons with severe egg allergy, and such persons should not be given influenza vaccine. This includes persons who develop hives, have swelling of the lips or tongue, or experience acute respiratory distress or collapse after eating eggs. Persons with a documented immunoglobulin E (IgE)-mediated hypersensitivity to eggs, including those who have experienced occupational asthma or other allergic responses from occupational exposure to egg protein, may also be at increased risk of reactions from influenza vaccine[1] (see **CONTRAINDICATIONS**).

Unlike the 1976 swine influenza vaccine, subsequent vaccines that have been prepared from other virus strains have not been clearly associated with an increased frequency of Guillain-Barre syndrome (GBS).[1,2,5–8] Candidates for Influenza Virus Vaccine should be made aware of the benefits and possible risks of vaccine administration. Other neurological disorders, including encephalopathies not defined as GBS, have been temporally associated with influenza immunization, but no causal link has been established.[9,10]

DOSAGE AND ADMINISTRATION

For Intramuscular Use Only: Shake well before withdrawing each dose. DO NOT INJECT INTRAVENOUSLY.

Parenteral drug products should be inspected visually for particulate matter and discoloration prior to administration whenever solution and container permit (see **DESCRIPTION**).

Remaining 1991–1992 influenza vaccine should not be used.

Although Influenza Virus Vaccine often contains one or more antigens used in previous years, immunity declines during the year following immunization. Therefore, a history of immunization in any previous year with a vaccine containing one or more antigens included in the current vaccine does NOT preclude the need for reimmunization for the 1992–1993 influenza season in order to provide optimal protection.

See **INDICATIONS AND USAGE** section for information regarding the optimal time of administration of this vaccine.

During the past decade, data on influenza vaccine immunogenicity and side effects have generally been obtained when vaccine has been administered intramuscularly. Because there has been no adequate evaluation of recent influenza vaccines administered by other routes, the intramuscular route should be used. Adults and older children should be immunized in the deltoid muscle; infants and young children in the anterolateral aspect of the thigh.

Before immunization, the skin over the site to be injected should be cleansed with a suitable germicide. After insertion of the needle, aspirate to help avoid inadvertent injection into a blood vessel.

Because of the lower potential for causing febrile reactions, only split-virus vaccines should be used for children. These vaccines may be labeled as "split," "subvirion," or "purified-surface-antigen" vaccine. For adults, immunogenicity and side effects of split- and whole-virus vaccines are comparable when vaccines are used at the recommended dosage.[1]

[See table below.]

Two doses given at least one month apart are recommended for children under 9 years of age who are receiving influenza vaccine for the first time. With the two-dose regimen, allow four weeks or more between doses.[1,2]

Simultaneous Administration with Other Vaccines

The target groups for influenza and pneumococcal immunization overlap considerably. Both vaccines may be given at the same time at different sites without increasing side effects. However, influenza vaccine is given annually, **while it is currently recommended that, with few exceptions, pneumococcal vaccine be given only once.** Detailed immunization records should be provided to each patient to record the date when pneumococcal vaccine was administered.[1,11]

The ACIP state that children at high-risk of influenza complications may receive influenza vaccine at the same time as mumps-measles-rubella, Haemophilus b, pneumococcal, and oral polio vaccine. Vaccines should be given at different sites.[1]

The American Academy of Pediatrics suggest that since influenza vaccine and pertussis-containing vaccine may produce febrile reactions in children, it may be prudent not to administer these vaccines simultaneously.[1,2]

IMPORTANT INFORMATION for Group Immunization Programs:

If this vaccine is to be used in an immunization program sponsored by any organization WHERE A TRADITIONAL PHYSICIAN/PATIENT RELATIONSHIP DOES NOT EXIST, each recipient (or legal guardian) must be made aware of the benefits and risks of immunization. These are summarized in the current labeling, and informed consent should be obtained from the recipient (or legal guardian) before immunization. PLEASE CONTACT YOUR LOCAL LEDERLE REPRESENTATIVE for copies of the CDC Important Information about Influenza and Influenza Consent Form.

HOW SUPPLIED

NDC 0005-2060-31 5.0 mL Vial

STORAGE

DO NOT FREEZE. STORE REFRIGERATED, AWAY FROM FREEZER COMPARTMENT, AT 2°C to 8°C (36°F to 46°F).

REFERENCES

1. Prevention and control of influenza. Recommendations of the Immunization Practices Advisory Committee (ACIP). *MMWR.* 1992; 41 RR-9:1–17.
2. American Academy of Pediatrics: *Report of the Committee on Infectious Diseases,* ed. 22. Elk Grove Village, IL: American Academy of Pediatrics; 1991.
3. National Childhood Vaccine Injury Act: Requirements for permanent vaccination records and for reporting of selected events after vaccination. *MMWR.* 1988; 37(13):197–200.
4. Vaccine Adverse Event Reporting System—United States. *MMWR.* 1990; 39(41):730–733.
5. Schonberger L, *et al:* Guillain-Barre syndrome: Its epidemiology and associations with influenza vaccination. *Ann Neurol.* 1981; 9 (Suppl 31).
6. Hurwitz E, *et al:* Guillain-Barre syndrome and the 1978–1979 influenza vaccine. *New Eng. J Med.* 1981; 304:1557–1561.
7. Kaplan J, *et al:* Guillain-Barre syndrome in the United States, 1979–1980 and 1980–1981. Lack of association with influenza vaccination. *JAMA.* 1982; 248:689–700.
8. Safranek TJ, *et al:* Reassessment of the association between Guillain-Barre syndrome and receipt of swine influenza vaccine in 1976–1977: Results of a two-state study. *Am J Epidemiol.* 1991; 133(9):940–951.
9. Centers for Disease Control: December 1986; Adverse events following immunization: Report No. 2, 1982–1984.
10. Retailliou H, *et al:* Illness after influenza vaccination reported through a nation-wide surveillance system, 1976–1977. *Am J Epidemiol.* 1980; 111:270–278.
11. Recommendations of the Immunization Practices Advisory Committee. Pneumococcal polysaccharide vaccine. *MMWR.* 1989; 38(5):64-8, 73-6.

Manufactured by:
EVANS MEDICAL LIMITED
Langhurst, Horsham
West Sussex RH12 4QD, England
and
LEDERLE LABORATORIES DIVISION
American Cyanamid Company
Pearl River, NY 10965

Rev. 6/92
20488-92

Influenza Vaccine Dosage, by Age Group, 1992–1993 Season

Age Group	Product	Dose	No. of Doses (see below for details)
6–35 months	Split virus only	0.25 mL	1 or 2 Doses
3–8 years	Split virus only	0.50 mL	1 or 2 Doses
9–12 years	Split virus only	0.50 mL	1 Dose
13 years and older	Whole or Split virus	0.50 mL	1 Dose

GEVRABON® OTC
[jĕv-ra-bŏn]
Vitamin-Mineral Supplement

(See PDR For Nonprescription Drugs.)

GEVRAL® T OTC
[jĕv-ral]
High Potency
Multivitamin and Multimineral Supplement Tablets

(See PDR For Nonprescription Drugs.)

HibTITER® ℞
HAEMOPHILUS b CONJUGATE VACCINE
(Diphtheria CRM_{197} Protein Conjugate)

DESCRIPTION

HibTITER is a sterile solution of a conjugate of oligosaccharides of the capsular antigen of *Haemophilus influenzae* type b (Haemophilus b) and diphtheria CRM_{197} protein (CRM_{197}) dissolved in 0.9% sodium chloride. The oligosaccharides are derived from highly purified capsular polysaccharide, polyribosylribitol phosphate, isolated from Haemophilus b strain Eagan grown in a chemically defined medium, and coupled by reductive amination directly to highly purified CRM_{197}. CRM_{197} is a nontoxic variant of diphtheria toxin isolated from cultures of *Corynebacterium diphtheriae* C7 (β197) grown in a casamino acids and yeast extract based medium that is ultrafiltered before use. The conjugate is purified to remove unreacted protein, oligosaccharides, and reagents; sterilized by filtration; and filled into vials. HibTITER is intended for intramuscular use.

The vaccine is a clear, colorless solution. Each single dose of 0.5 mL is formulated to contain 10 μg of purified Haemophi-

lus b saccharide and approximately 25 μg of CRM_{197} protein. Multidose vials contain thimerosal (mercurial derivative) 1:10,000 as a preservative.

CLINICAL PHARMACOLOGY

Haemophilus influenzae type b (Haemophilus b) is the most common cause of invasive bacterial disease, including meningitis, in young children in the United States. Although nonencapsulated *Haemophilus influenzae* are common and six capsular polysaccharide types are known, strains with the type b capsule cause most of the invasive Haemophilus diseases.[1]

Haemophilus b diseases occur primarily in children under 5 years of age. In the United States, the cumulative risk of developing invasive Haemophilus b disease during the first 5 years of life is about 1 in 200. Approximately 60% of cases are meningitis. Cellulitis, epiglottitis, pericarditis, pneumonia, sepsis or septic arthritis make up the remaining 40%. An estimated 12,000 cases of Haemophilus b meningitis occurred annually prior to the routine use of conjugate vaccines in toddlers.[1,2] The mortality rate can be 5%, and neurologic sequelae have been observed in up to 38% of survivors.[3]

The incidence of invasive Haemophilus b disease peaks between 6 months and 1 year of age, and approximately 55% of disease occurs between 6 and 18 months of age.[1] Interpersonal transmission of Haemophilus b occurs, and risk of invasive disease is increased in children younger than 4 years of age who are exposed in the household to a primary case of disease. Clusters of cases in children in day care have been reported, and recent studies suggest that the rate of secondary cases may also be increased among children exposed to a primary case in the day-care setting.[1,4]

The incidence of invasive Haemophilus b disease is increased in certain children, such as those who are native Americans, black, or from lower socioeconomic status and those with medical conditions such as asplenia, sickle-cell disease, malignancies associated with immunosuppression, and antibody deficiency syndromes.[1,2,4]

The protective activity of antibody to Haemophilus b polysaccharide was (1) inferred from the protection produced by antibody passively administered to animals before challenge with Haemophilus b and to children with agammaglobulinemia or with Haemophilus b disease,[5] and (2) demonstrated by the efficacy of Haemophilus b Polysaccharide (HbPs) Vaccine.[6] A controlled trial of highly purified HbPs Vaccine was conducted in Finland in 1974. Approximately 98,000 children were studied, about half of whom received the vaccine. Among children of 18 to 71 months of age, the protective efficacy in preventing invasive Haemophilus b disease through a 4-year follow-up was 90% (95% confidence limits, 55% to 98%).[6] Data from passive antibody studies indicate that a preexisting titer of antibody to HbPs of 0.15 μg/mL correlates with protection.[7] Data from the Finnish field trial indicate that a titer of ≥1.0 μg/mL 3 weeks after vaccination is associated with long-term protection.[8]

HbPs vaccine was licensed for use in toddlers of 18 months to 5 years of age in April 1985. Post-licensure studies conducted in the U.S. indicated that the HbPs vaccine is quite safe; four of five studies documented efficacy rates of 41 to 88%.[1] A fifth study showed higher rates of disease among vaccinated children than control children.[1] Vaccination was associated with significant decline in the age-related incidence of Haemophilus b disease in studies of certain areas of the country,[1] and the benefits were generally accepted.

Studies on the immunogenicity of HbPs indicated that, although the vaccine promotes an antibody response in older children, it does not induce an antibody response in infants, and it does not induce immunologic memory.[1]

The characteristics of an immune response depend on the type of cells producing the response and the antigens stimulating the process. Certain antigens, such as proteins, induce B lymphocytes to produce antibody aided by thymus-derived lymphocytes called T helper (T_H) cells.[9] These antigens are called thymus dependent or TD antigens. The immune response is potentially boostable, and IgG antibody predominates.[10] In contrast, polysaccharide antigens stimulate B cells without T-cell help, producing a nonboostable response of both IgG and IgM antibodies. These antigens are known as thymus independent or TI antigens. Linkage of Haemophilus b saccharides to a protein such as CRM_{197} can convert the TI saccharide to a TD antigen, and result in an enhanced antibody response to the saccharide that is boostable and predominantly of the IgG isotype.[11] Laboratory evidence indicates that the native state of the CRM_{197} protein and the use of oligosaccharides in the formulation of HibTITER Haemophilus b Conjugate Vaccine (Diphtheria CRM_{197} Protein Conjugate) enhances its T_H potential and thus its immunogenicity.[12–14] Conjugate vaccines with other carrier proteins will be recognized differently by the immune system. No data are available to support the interchangeability of HibTITER and other Haemophilus b conjugate vaccines with one another.

The immunogenicity of HibTITER was evaluated in infants vaccinated initially at 1 to 6 months of age in 10 centers in the United States.[15] Infants received three doses at approximately 2-month intervals. Total anti-Haemophilus b polysaccharide (HbPs) antibody levels were determined by a radioimmunoassay in one laboratory whose results correlate with the assay used by the National Public Health Institute of Finland.[8,15,16] Anti-HbPs antibody levels ≥1 μg/mL were attained by more than 90% of infants of all ages after two doses and by more than 98% after three doses. One month after the third vaccination, the geometric mean antibody levels were 16.8, 26.8, and 30.0 in infants initially vaccinated at 1 to 2, 3 to 4, and 5 to 6 months of age, respectively.[15,16] In infants vaccinated initially at 1 to 6 months of age, the percentage with levels ≥1 μg/mL were 27.9, 90.3, and 99.2% after the first, second, and third dose of vaccine, respectively (Table 1). Long-term persistence of the antibody response was observed. More than 80% of 235 infants who received three doses of vaccine had an anti-HbPs antibody level ≥1 μg/mL at 2 years of age.[16]

TABLE 1
Immunogenicity of HibTITER Vaccine[a]

Age at Initial[b] Vacc. (Mos.)	No. of Doses	No.[c]	GM μg/mL				% ≥ 1 μg/mL			
			Pre	Post 1	Post 2	Post 3	Pre	Post 1	Post 2	Post 3
1–6[d]	3	423	0.18	0.45	8.49	22.4	8.7	27.9	90.3	99.2
1–2	3	186	0.20	0.30	5.11	16.8	11.3	15.1	83.8	98.2
3–4	3	194	0.18	0.53	11.70	26.8	7.7	33.0	94.8	100.0
5–6	3	43	0.12	1.21	17.80	30.0	2.3	60.5	97.6	100.0
7–11	2	273	0.11	3.23	27.93	—	0.0	80.7	99.5	—
12–14	2	159	0.12	6.45	32.66	—	0.0	89.9	100.0	—
15–23	1	377	0.14	11.40	—	—	0.0	97.6	—	—

[a] Only subjects with preimmunization titers ≤0.6 μg/mL were included in the analysis. Values used in calculations of GMT: lower limit ≤0.1 = 0.1; upper limit ≥40 = 40. Antibody activities are from sera drawn immediately before the initial dose of vaccine, 2 months after dose 1 or 2 and 1 month after dose 3.

[b] Infants initially vaccinated at 1 to 6 or 7 to 14 months of age received three or two doses, respectively, at approximately 2-month intervals.

[c] Number of children receiving at least one immunization in the age group.

[d] Represents the sum of groups initially vaccinated at 1 to 2, 3 to 4, and 5 to 6 months of age.

The vaccine generated an immune response characteristic of a protein antigen: IgG anti-HbPs antibodies of IgG_1 subclass predominated and the immune system was primed for a booster response to HibTITER Haemophilus b Conjugate Vaccine (Diphtheria CRM_{197} Protein Conjugate), and there is some evidence suggesting natural increases in antibody levels over time after vaccination.[16]

When evaluated in an *in vitro*, complement-mediated bactericidal assay, none of the prevaccination sera of the 1 to 6 month old infants killed *H influenzae* type b. Two months after the second dose of vaccine, 95% of the infants' sera had bactericidal activity; and 1 month after the third dose, 98% of the sera had bactericidal activity.[15,16]

One month after the second dose, 99.5% of the infants vaccinated at 7 to 11 and 100% of the infants vaccinated at 12 to 14 months of age responded with anti-HbPs antibody levels ≥1 μg/mL, and the geometric mean antibody levels were 27.93 and 32.66, respectively (Table 1); 100% of the infants' sera had bactericidal activity.[16]

These data may be compared to the response to a single dose of HibTITER administered to 377 children 15 to 23 months of age: a geometric mean antibody level of 11.35 μg/mL was generated, and more than 97% had anti-HbPs antibody levels ≥1 μg/mL (Table 1); 92.2% of the infants' sera had bactericidal activity.[16] [See table above.]

In one study, immunogenicity of HibTITER Haemophilus b Conjugate Vaccine (Diphtheria CRM_{197} Protein Conjugate) was evaluated in 26 children 22 months to 5 years of age who had not responded to earlier vaccination with Haemophilus b Polysaccharide Vaccine. One dose of HibTITER was immunogenic in all 26 children and generated titers of ≥1 μg/mL in 25 of the 26 infants.[16] HibTITER has been found to be immunogenic in children with sickle-cell disease, a condition which may cause increased susceptibility to Haemophilus b disease. In 20 of these infants aged 2 to 6 months, three doses of HibTITER given at 2-month intervals generated a geometric mean anti-HbPs antibody level of 22.1 μg/mL and 100% of the subjects had a level ≥1 μg/mL 1 month after the third dose. Ninety percent of the infants had a level ≥1 μg/mL 18 months after the initial vaccination.[17] HibTITER has also been shown to be immunogenic in native American infants, such as the group of 50 studied in Alaska who received three doses at 2, 4, and 6 months of age. One month after the third vaccination, the geometric mean was 15.1 μg/mL and 95% of infants had levels ≥1 μg/mL. Antibody levels ≥1 μg/mL were observed in 71% of these infants at 15 to 18 months of age.[16] These levels are comparable to those seen in healthy U.S. infants who received their first dose at 1 to 2 months of age and subsequent doses at 4 and 6 months of age.[15,16]

The efficacy of HibTITER has been evaluated in a large-scale controlled clinical trial in northern California.[16] The multiethnic composition of those in the California study was representative of the general population in northern California. The study was conducted from February 1988 through June 1990. 30,884 infants less than 6 months of age were vaccinated with HibTITER, of whom 22,124 received three doses at about 2, 4, and 6 months of age simultaneously with DTP but at a separate injection site. A control group of 30,558 infants received DTP alone. After more than 24,000 person years of follow up (average 7 months of follow up per infant), there have been no (0) vaccine failures in infants who received three doses of HibTITER and 12 cases of Haemophilus b disease (6 cases of meningitis) in the control group. The incidence of Haemophilus b disease was 0 and 105 per 100,000 in the vaccinated and control infants, respectively. The estimate of efficacy is 100% (p=0.0002); 95% Confidence Intervals (C.I.), 2 tailed, 68%, 100%. When the data was corrected for age and seasonality, there were 0 cases among vaccinated infants, 18 cases in the control group. Efficacy is 100% (p=0.0001); 95% C.I., 71%, 100%. There have also been 5,445 person years of follow up among infants after two doses of vaccine which is predominantly time between the second and third doses. There have been no (0) cases of Haemophilus b disease in this group whereas, among similar aged control subjects, there were eight cases; the rates of disease were therefore 0 and 149 cases/100,000 in vaccinees and controls, respectively. There has been one case of Haemophilus b disease after one dose of HibTITER Haemophilus b Conjugate Vaccine (Diphtheria CRM_{197} Protein Conjugate) (defined as occurring >21 days after immunization; two other cases occurred <21 days after immunization). There were five cases among similar aged control subjects. The rates of disease were therefore 21 and 123 cases per 100,000 in the vaccinated and control populations, respectively.

A comparative clinical trial was performed in Finland where approximately 53,000 infants received HibTITER at 4 and 6 months of age and a booster dose at 14 months in a trial conducted from January 1988 through June 1990. Only two children developed Haemophilus b disease after receiving the 2-dose primary vaccination schedule. One child became ill at 15 months of age and the other at 18 months of age; neither child received the scheduled booster at 14 months of age. No vaccine failure has been reported in children who received the 2-dose primary series and the booster dose at 14 months of age. Based on more than 32,000 person years of follow-up time, the estimate of efficacy is about 95% when compared to historical control groups followed between 1985 and 1988.[16] Historical controls were used since all infants recieved one of two Haemophilus b conjugate vaccines during the period of the trial.

HibTITER will not protect against *H influenzae* other than type b strains or other microorganisms that cause meningitis or septic disease.

No impairment of the antibody response to the individual antigens was demonstrated when HibTITER was given at the same time but at separate sites as Diphtheria and Tetanus Toxoid and Pertussis Vaccine Adsorbed (DTP) plus Oral Polio Vaccine (OPV) to children 2 to 20 months of age or Measles, Mumps and Rubella Vaccine (MMR) to children 15 ± 1 month of age.[16]

Continued on next page

Information on Lederle products listed on these pages is the full prescribing information from product literature or package inserts effective in August 1992. Information concerning all Lederle products may be obtained from the Professional Services Department, Lederle Laboratories, Pearl River, New York 10965.

Lederle—Cont.

INDICATIONS AND USAGE

HibTITER is indicated for the immunization of children 2 months to 5 years of age against invasive diseases caused by *Haemophilus influenzae* type b.

CONTRAINDICATIONS

Hypersensitivity to any component of the vaccine, including diphtheria toxoid or thimerosal in the multidose presentation, is a contraindication to use of HibTITER.

WARNINGS

If the vaccine is used in persons deficient in producing antibody, whether due to genetic defect or to immunosuppressive therapy, the expected immune response may not be obtained.

As with any vaccine, HibTITER may not protect 100% of individuals receiving the vaccine.

PRECAUTIONS

GENERAL

Prior to an injection of any vaccine, all reasonable precautions should be taken to prevent adverse reactions. Any febrile illness or acute infection is reason for delaying use of HibTITER Haemophilus b Conjugate Vaccine (Diphtheria CRM_{197} Protein Conjugate). A minor afebrile illness such as a mild upper respiratory infection is not usually reason to defer immunization.

As with the injection of any biological material, Epinephrine Injection (1:1000) should be available for immediate use should an anaphylactic or other allergic reaction occur.

As reported with Haemophilus b Polysaccharide Vaccine, cases of Haemophilus b disease may occur prior to the onset of the protective effects of the vaccine.[1,18]

Antigenuria has been detected following receipt of Haemophilus b Conjugate Vaccine,[19] and therefore antigen detection may not have diagnostic value in suspected Haemophilus b disease within 2 weeks of immunization.

The vaccine should not be injected intradermally or intravenously, since the safety and immunogenicity of these routes have not been evaluated. The vaccine should be given intramuscularly. Special care should be taken to ensure that the injection does not enter a blood vessel.

A separate, sterile syringe and needle or a sterile disposable unit should be used for each patient to prevent transmission of infectious agents from one person to another.

ALTHOUGH SOME ANTIBODY RESPONSE TO DIPHTHERIA TOXIN OCCURS, IMMUNIZATION WITH HibTITER DOES NOT SUBSTITUTE FOR ROUTINE DIPHTHERIA IMMUNIZATION.

CARCINOGENESIS, MUTAGENESIS, IMPAIRMENT OF FERTILITY

HibTITER has not been evaluated for its carcinogenic, mutagenic potential, or impairment of fertility.

PREGNANCY

REPRODUCTIVE STUDIES—PREGNANCY CATEGORY C

Animal reproduction studies have not been conducted with HibTITER. It is also not known whether HibTITER can cause fetal harm when administered to a pregnant woman or can affect reproduction capacity. HibTITER is NOT recommended for use in a pregnant woman.

ADVERSE REACTIONS

Adverse reactions associated with HibTITER Haemophilus b Conjugate Vaccine (Diphtheria CRM $_{197}$ Protein Conjugate) have been evaluated in 401 infants vaccinated initially at 1 to 6 months of age given 1,118 doses independent of DTP vaccine. Observations were made during the day of vaccination and days 1 and 2 postvaccination. A temperature > 38.3°C was recorded at least once during the observation period following 2% of the vaccinations. Local erythema, warmth, or swelling (≥ 2 cm) was observed following 3.3% of vaccinations. The incidence of temperature > 38.3°C was greater during the first postvaccination day than during the day of vaccination or the second postvaccination day. The incidence of local erythema, warmth, or swelling was similar during the day of vaccination and the first postvaccination day; it was lower during the second postvaccination day. All side effects have been infrequent, mild, and transient with no serious sequelae (Table 2). No difference in the rates of these complaints was reported after dose 1, 2, or 3.

[See table at top right.]

Additional safety data with HibTITER Haemophilus b Conjugate Vaccine (Diphtheria CRM $_{197}$ Protein Conjugate) are available from the efficacy studies conducted in young infants.[16] 79,483 doses were given to 30,844 infants at approximately 2, 4, and 6 months of age in California usually at the same time as DTP (but at a separate injection site) and oral polio vaccine; approximately 100,000 doses have been given to 53,000 infants at 4 and 6 months in Finland at the same time as a combined DTP and inactivated polio (IPV) vaccine but at a separate injection site. The rate and type of reactions associated with the vaccinations were no different from those seen when DTP or DTP-IPV was administered alone. These included fever, local reactions, rash and one hyporesponsive episode with a single seizure. The safety of HibTITER was also evaluated in the California study by direct phone questioning of the parents or guardians of 6,887 vaccine recipients. The incidence and type of side effects reported within 24 hours of vaccination were similar to those cited in Table 2. In addition, analysis of emergency room (ER) visits within 30 days and hospitalization within 60 days after receipt of 23,800 doses of HibTITER showed no increase in the rates of any type of ER visit or hospitalization.

Table 3 details the side effects associated with a single vaccination of HibTITER given (without DTP) to infants of 15 to 23 months of age.

Similar results have been observed in the analysis of 2,285 subjects of 18 to 60 months of age, vaccinated as part of a post-marketing safety study of HibTITER.[16] This data was collected by telephone survey 24 to 48 hours postvaccination. Additional observations included irritability, restless sleep and GI symptoms (diarrhea, vomiting, and loss of appetite) in the group that received HibTITER alone. A cause and effect relationship between these observations and the vaccinations has not been established.

TABLE 2
Number of Subjects (Percent) Manifesting
Side Effects Associated with HibTITER
Administered Independently from DTP*
(Infants Vaccinated Initially at 1 to 6 Months of Age)

Symptoms	Dose 1 n = 401			Dose 2 n = 383			Dose 3 n = 334		
	Same Day As Vacc.	+1 Day	+2 Days	Same Day As Vacc.	+1 Day	+2 Days	Same Day As Vacc.	+1 Day	+2 Days
Temp > 38.3°C	0 —	2 <1%	2 <1%	2 <1%	3 <1%	2 <1%	2 <1%	6 1.8%	5 1.5%
Redness ≥ 2 cm	1 <1%	0 —	0	1 1%	6 1.6%	0 —	6 1.5%	4 1.2%	0
Warmth ≥ 2 cm	1 <1%	1 <1%	0 —	2 <1%	1 <1%	0 —	1 <1%	6 1.8%	0 —
Swelling ≥ 2 cm	5 1.2%	1 <1%	0 —	2 <1%	2 <1%	0 —	1 <1%	0	0

* DTP and HibTITER given 2 weeks apart with DTP having been given first.
The following complaints were also reported after 1,118 vaccinations with HibTITER: irritability (133), sleepiness (91), prolonged crying [≥ 4 hours] (38), appetite loss (23), vomiting (9), diarrhea (2), and rash (1).

TABLE 3
Selected Adverse Reactions* in
Children of 15 to 23 Months of Age
Following Vaccination with HibTITER
Haemophilus b Conjugate Vaccine
(Diphtheria CRM $_{197}$ Protein Conjugate)

Adverse Reaction	No. of Subjects	Reaction % Post Vaccination Within 24 Hrs.	At 48 Hrs.
Fever > 38.3°C	354	1.4	0.6
Erythema	354	2.0	—
Swelling	354	1.7	—
Tenderness	354	3.7	0.3

* The following complaints were reported after vaccination of these 354 children in the indicated number of children: diarrhea (9), vomiting (5), prolonged crying [> 4 hours] (4), and rashes (2).

Following the use of Haemophilus b Polysaccharide Vaccine and another Haemophilus b Conjugate Vaccine, reports of the following types of associated adverse reactions were recorded by passive reporting and postmarketing surveillance methods: fever > 38.3°C, local erythema, swelling, and tenderness.[20]

Rash, hives, convulsions,[20] vomiting/diarrhea,[20] and Guillain-Barre syndrome[21] have been observed. A cause and effect relationship among any of these events and the vaccination has not been established.

DOSAGE AND ADMINISTRATION

HibTITER Haemophilus b Conjugate Vaccine (Diphtheria CRM $_{197}$ Protein Conjugate) is for intramuscular use only. Any parenteral drug product should be inspected visually for extraneous particulate matter and/or discoloration prior to administration whenever solution and container permit. If these conditions exist, HibTITER should not be administered.

HibTITER is indicated for children 2 months to 5 years of age for the prevention of invasive Haemophilus b disease. For infants 2 to 6 months of age, the immunizing dose is three separate injections of 0.5 mL given at approximately 2-month intervals intramuscularly, preferably in the outer aspect of the vastus lateralis (mid-thigh). Previously unvaccinated infants from 7 through 11 months of age should receive two separate intramuscular injections as described approximately 2 months apart. Children from 12 through 14 months of age who have not been vaccinated previously receive one intramuscular injection. All vaccinated children receive a single booster dose at 15 months of age or older, but not less than 2 months after the previous dose. Previously unvaccinated children 15 to 60 months of age receive a single intramuscular injection of HibTITER as described or in the deltoid muscle.

Age at First Immunization (Mos.)	No. of Doses	Booster
2–6	3	Yes
7–11	2	Yes
12–14	1	Yes
15 and Over	1	No

NO DATA ARE AVAILABLE TO SUPPORT THE INTERCHANGEABILITY OF HibTITER OR OTHER HAEMOPHILUS b CONJUGATE VACCINES WITH ONE ANOTHER. THEREFORE, IT IS RECOMMENDED THAT THE SAME CONJUGATE VACCINE BE USED THROUGHOUT EACH IMMUNIZATION SCHEDULE, CONSISTENT WITH THE DATA SUPPORTING APPROVAL AND LICENSURE OF THE VACCINE.

The current recommendation of the Immunization Practices Advisory Committee (ACIP) is for routine vaccination of children at 15 months of age.[22] The ACIP has not yet reviewed the new indication for children less than 15 months of age.

Each dose of 0.5 mL is formulated to contain 10 μg of purified Haemophilus b saccharide and approximately 25 μg of CRM $_{197}$ protein.

Before injection, the skin over the site to be injected should be cleansed with a suitable germicide. After insertion of the needle, aspirate to ensure that the needle has not entered a blood vessel.

DO NOT INJECT INTRAVENOUSLY.

STORAGE

Stability studies indicate that HibTITER Haemophilus b Conjugate Vaccine (Diphtheria CRM $_{197}$ Protein Conjugate) can be shipped at ambient temperatures and stored at 2°–8°C (35°–46°F). DO NOT FREEZE.

HOW SUPPLIED

Vial, 1 Dose (4 per package)—Product No. 53124-104-41	
Vial, 5 Dose	—Product No. 53124-201-05
Vial, 10 Dose	—Product No. 53124-201-10

Military Depots
Vial, 10 Dose—NSN 6505-01-315-4767

REFERENCES

1. Wenger JD, et al. Prevention of *Haemophilus influenzae* type b disease: vaccines and passive prophylaxis. In: Remington JS and Schwartz MN eds. *Current Clinical Topics in Infectious Diseases.* 1989; 10:306–339.
2. Recommendation of the Immunization Practices Advisory Committee (ACIP): Polysaccharide vaccine for prevention of *Haemophilus influenzae* type b disease. *MMWR.* 1985; 34:201–205.
3. Sell SH. Long term sequelae of bacterial meningitis in children. *Pediatr Infect Dis J.* 1983; 2:90–93.
4. Broome CV. Epidemiology of *Haemophilus influenzae* type b infections in the United States. *Pediatr Infect Dis J.* 1987; 6:779–782.

5. Alexander HE. The productive or curative element in type b *H. influenzae* rabbit serum. *Yale J Biol Med.* 1944; 16:425–434.
6. Peltola H. *Haemophilus influenzae* type b capsular polysaccharide vaccine in children: A double-blind field study of 100,000 vaccinees 3 months to 5 years of age in Finland. *Pediatrics.* 1977; 60:730–737.
7. Robbins JB. Quantitative measurement of "natural" and immunization-induced *Haemophilus influenzae* type b capsular polysaccharide antibodies. *Pediatr Res.* 1973; 7:103–110.
8. Kayhty H. Serum antibodies after vaccination with *Haemophilus influenzae* type b capsular polysaccharide and responses to reimmunization: No evidence of immunologic tolerance or memory. *Pediatrics.* 1984; 74:857–865.
9. Roitt IM. The cellular basis of immunological responses. *Lancet II:* 367–371, 1969.
10. Ovary Z, et al. Immunological specificity of the secondary response with dinitrophenylated proteins. *Proc Soc Exp Biol Med.* 1963; 114:72–76.
11. Weinberg GA, Granoff DM. Polysaccharide-protein conjugate vaccines for the prevention of *Haemophilus influenzae* type b disease. *J. Pediatr.* 1988; 113:621–631.
12. Makela O, et al. Immunogenic properties of α (1–6) dextran, its protein conjugates, and conjugates of its breakdown products in mice. *Scand J Immunol.* 1984; 19:541–550.
13. Anderson P. Immunogens consisting of oligosaccharides from *Haemophilus influenzae* type b coupled to diphtheria toxoid or the toxin protein CRM_{197}. *J Clin Invest.* 1985; 76:52–59.
14. Madore DV, et al. Immune response of young children vaccinated with *Haemophilus influenzae* type b conjugate vaccines. In: Cruse JM and Lewis RE eds. *Contributions to Microbiology and Immunology: Conjugate Vaccines.* 1989; 10:125–150.
15. Madore DV, Phipps DC, Eby R, et al. Safety and immunologic response to *Haemophilus influenzae* type b Oligosaccharide-CRM_{197} Conjugate Vaccine in 1- to 6-month-old infants. *Pediatrics.* 1990; 85:331–337.
16. Unpublished data available from Praxis Biologics, Inc.
17. Gigliotti F, et al. Immunization of young infants with sickle cell disease with a *Haemophilus influenzae* type b saccharide-diphtheria CRM_{197} protein conjugate vaccine. *J Pediatr.* 1989; 114:1006–1010.
18. Mortimer EA. Efficacy of Haemophilus b polysaccharide vaccine: An engima. *JAMA.* 1988; 260:1454–1455.
19. Scheifele D, et al. Antigenuria after receipt of Haemophilus b Diphtheria Toxoid Conjugate Vaccine. *Pediatr Infect Dis J.* 1989; 8:887–888.
20. Milstien JB, et al. Adverse reactions reported following receipt of *Haemophilus influenzae* type b vaccine: An analysis after one year of marketing. *Pediatrics.* 1987; 80:270–274.
21. D'Cruz OF, et al. Acute inflammatory demyelinating polyradiculoneuropathy (Guillain-Barre syndrome) after immunization with *Haemophilus influenzae* type b conjugate vaccine. *J Pediatr.* 1989; 115:743–746.
22. Recommendation of the Immunization Practices Advisory Committee (ACIP). Supplementary statement: change in administration schedule for Haemophilus b conjugate vaccines. *MMWR.* 1990; 39:225–241.

Manufactured by:
PRAXIS BIOLOGICS INC.
Rochester, NY 14623 USA
A Subsidiary of American Cyanamid Company
Distributed by LEDERLE-PRAXIS BIOLOGICALS
A Cyanamid Business Unit.

10120-91
Rev. 12/91

Shown in Product Identification Section, page 414

HYDROMOX® ℞

[*hū-drō-mŏx*]
quinethazone
Tablets

DESCRIPTION

Chemistry: HYDROMOX is a quinazoline derivative, in which a cyclic carbamyl group replaces the cyclic sulfamyl group present in the thiazide derivatives.
Quinethazone is 7-chloro-2- ethyl-1, 2, 3, 4-tetrahydro-4-oxo-6-quinazolinesulfonamide.
HYDROMOX tablets contain the following inactive ingredients: Corn Starch, Dibasic Calcium Phosphate, Magnesium Stearate, Modified Food Starch.

ACTIONS

HYDROMOX produces urinary excretion of sodium and chloride in approximately equivalent amounts (saluresis), while potassium is excreted to a much lesser degree. The saluretic effect of HYDROMOX is rapid and relatively prolonged, beginning within 2 hours after administration, reaching a peak at 6 hours, and lasting for 18 to 24 hours. While HYDROMOX is chemically different, it is pharmacologically genetic to the benzothiadiazine group of drugs.
The dominant action of quinethazone is to increase the renal excretion of sodium and chloride and an accompanying volume of water. This results from inhibition of the tubular mechanism of electrolyte reabsorption. The renal effect is virtually independent of alterations in acid-base balance.
HYDROMOX, like other drugs in this class, inhibits the proximal reabsorption of sodium and chloride. The excretion of potassium results from increased potassium secretion by the distal tubule where potassium is exchanged for sodium.
HYDROMOX may exert its antihypertensive effect by diuresis and sodium loss and/or on vascular function to reduce peripheral resistance.

INDICATIONS

HYDROMOX, a nonmercurial oral diuretic agent, is indicated as adjunctive therapy in edema associated with congestive heart failure, hepatic cirrhosis and corticosteroid and estrogen therapy.
HYDROMOX has also been found useful in edema due to various forms of renal dysfunction such as: nephrotic syndrome; acute glomerulonephritis; and chronic renal failure.
HYDROMOX is indicated in the management of hypertension either as the sole therapeutic agent or to enhance the effectiveness of other antihypertensive drugs in the more severe forms of hypertension.
Usage in Pregnancy: The routine use of diuretics in an otherwise healthy woman is inappropriate and exposes mother and fetus to unnecessary hazard. Diuretics do not prevent development of toxemia of pregnancy, and there is no satisfactory evidence that they are useful in the treatment of developed toxemia.
Edema during pregnancy may arise from pathological causes or from the physiologic and mechanical consequences of pregnancy. Diuretics are indicated in pregnancy when edema is due to pathologic causes, just as they are in the absence of pregnancy (however, see **WARNINGS**, below). Dependent edema in pregnancy, resulting from restriction of venous return by the expanded uterus, is properly treated through elevation of the lower extremities and use of support hose; use of diuretics to lower intravascular volume in this case is illogical and unnecessary. There is hypervolemia during normal pregnancy which is harmful to neither the fetus nor the mother (in the absence of cardiovascular disease), but which is associated with edema, including generalized edema, in the majority of pregnant women. If this edema produces discomfort, increased recumbency will often provide relief. In rare instances, this edema may cause extreme discomfort which is not relieved by rest. In these cases, a short course of diuretics may provide relief and may be appropriate.

CONTRAINDICATIONS

A. Anuria.
B. Hypersensitivity to this or other sulfonamide derived drugs.

WARNINGS

Diuretics should be used with caution in severe renal disease. In patients with renal disease, diuretics may precipitate azotemia. Cumulative effects of the drug may develop in patients with impaired renal function.
Diuretics should be used with caution in patients with impaired hepatic function or progressive liver disease, since minor alterations of fluid and electrolyte balance may precipitate hepatic coma.
Quinethazone may add to or potentiate the action of other antihypertensive drugs. Potentiation occurs with ganglionic or peripheral adrenergic blocking drugs.
Sensitivity reactions may occur in patients with a history of allergy or bronchial asthma.
The possibility of exacerbation or activation of systemic lupus erythematosus has been reported.
Usage in Pregnancy: HYDROMOX *quinethazone* crosses the placental barrier and appears in cord blood. The use of quinethazone in pregnant women requires that the anticipated benefit be weighed against possible hazards to the fetus. These hazards include fetal or neonatal jaundice, thrombocytopenia, and possible other adverse reactions which have occurred in the adult.
Nursing Mothers: HYDROMOX appears in breast milk. If use of the drug is deemed essential, the patient should stop nursing.

PRECAUTIONS

(1) HYDROMOX should be used with caution in patients with impaired hepatic function or progressive liver disease, since minor alterations of fluid and electrolyte balance may precipitate hepatic coma.
(2) Whereas electrolyte abnormalities are often present in such conditions as heart failure and cirrhosis as a result of underlying disease process, they may also be aggravated or may be produced independently by any potent diuretic affecting electrolyte excretion. Caution is especially important during prolonged or intensive therapy and when salt intake is restricted or during concomitant use of steroids or ACTH. Hypokalemia attributable to HYDROMOX therapy has been mild and infrequent, and other electrolyte abnormalities have been rare.
The possibility of potassium depletion and its toxic sequelae must be kept in mind, particularly in cirrhotics and patients receiving digitalis. As a preventive measure the use of foods rich in potassium, such as orange juice, or supplements of potassium chloride may be desirable.
(3) In patients with impaired renal function, azotemia and/or excessive drug accumulation may develop.
(4) As with other potent diuretics, when HYDROMOX is added to a regimen that includes ganglionic-blocking agents, the dosage of these latter preparations should be reduced to avoid a sudden drop in blood pressure. Reduction of dosage is also necessary when one or more of these antihypertensive agents is added to an established HYDROMOX regimen.
(5) As with the thiazide diuretics, increases of serum uric acid may occur but precipitation of gout has been rare.
(6) A decreased glucose tolerance as evidenced by hyperglycemia and glycosuria thus aggravating or provoking diabetes mellitus has occurred.
(7) HYDROMOX *quinethazone* may decrease arterial responsiveness to norepinephrine and therefore should be withdrawn 48 hours before elective surgery. If emergency surgery is indicated, preanesthetic and anesthetic agents should be administered in reduced dosage. Quinethazone may also increase the responsiveness to tubocurarine. The antihypertensive effects of the drug may be enhanced in the postsympathectomy patient.
(8) Sensitivity reactions may be more likely to occur in patients with a history of allergy or bronchial asthma.
(9) The possibility of exacerbation or activation of systemic lupus erythematosus has been suggested for sulfonamide derived drugs.

ADVERSE REACTIONS

The following adverse reactions have been reported with the diuretic drugs, some of which may be expected to occur with quinethazone:

A. Gastrointestinal System Reactions
 1. anorexia
 2. gastric irritation
 3. nausea
 4. vomiting
 5. cramping
 6. diarrhea
 7. constipation
 8. jaundice (intrahepatic cholestatic jaundice)
 9. pancreatitis
 10. hyperglycemia
 11. glycosuria
B. Central Nervous System Reactions
 1. dizziness
 2. vertigo
 3. paresthesias
 4. headache
 5. xanthopsia
C. Hematologic Reactions
 1. leukopenia
 2. thrombocytopenia
 3. agranulocytosis
 4. aplastic anemia
D. Dermatologic—Hypersensitivity Reactions
 1. purpura
 2. photosensitivity
 3. rash
 4. urticaria
 5. necrotizing angiitis (vasculitis) (cutaneous vasculitis)
E. Cardiovascular Reactions
 1. orthostatic hypotension may occur and may be potentiated by alcohol, barbiturates, or narcotics
F. Miscellaneous
 1. muscle spasm
 2. weakness
 3. restlessness

Whenever adverse reactions are moderate or severe, thiazide dosage should be reduced or therapy withdrawn.

DOSAGE AND ADMINISTRATION

Average Adult Dosage: One or two 50 mg tablets, orally, once a day. Because of its relatively prolonged duration of activity, a single daily dose is generally sufficient. Occasionally, one tablet (50 mg) is administered twice a day. Infrequently, a total daily dose of three to four tablets (150 to 200 mg) may be necessary. The dosage employed depends upon the severity of the condition being treated and the responsiveness of

Continued on next page

Information on Lederle products listed on these pages is the full prescribing information from product literature or package inserts effective in August 1992. Information concerning all Lederle products may be obtained from the Professional Services Department, Lederle Laboratories, Pearl River, New York 10965.

Lederle—Cont.

the patient, and often must be adjusted at the beginning or during the course of therapy. When HYDROMOX is used in combination with other antihypertensive agents, the dosage of each drug may often be reduced because of potentiation. (See under **PRECAUTIONS** concerning the necessity for dosage adjustment when one or more of these drugs is added to an already established therapeutic regime.)

HOW SUPPLIED

HYDROMOX *quinethazone* Tablets, are round, white, flat-faced, scored, beveled, engraved with H above and 1 below the score on one side and LL on the other side, supplied as follows:

NDC 0005-4458-23—Bottle of 100
Store at Controlled Room Temperature 15°–30° C (59°–86° F).
LEDERLE LABORATORIES DIVISION
American Cyanamid Company
Pearl River, NY 10965

Rev. 12/85
17404

Shown in Product Identification Section, page 414

INCREMIN®   **OTC**
[ĭn-cre-mĭn]
WITH IRON SYRUP
(Vitamins B$_1$, B$_6$, B$_{12}$-Lysine-Iron)
Dietary Supplement
For the prevention of iron deficiency anemia in children and adults.

(See PDR For Nonprescription Drugs.)

LEUCOVORIN CALCIUM FOR INJECTION   ℞
[lu-cō-vor-ĭn căl-sēē-um]

DESCRIPTION

Leucovorin is one of several active, chemically reduced derivatives of folic acid. It is useful as an antidote to drugs which act as folic acid antagonists.

Also known as folinic acid, Citrovorum factor, or 5-formyl-5,6,7,8-tetrahydrofolic acid, this compound has the chemical designation of Calcium *N*-[4-[[(2-amino-5-formyl-1,4,5,6,7,8-hexahydro-4-oxo-6-pteridinyl)-methyl]amino]benzoyl]-*L*-Glutamic acid (1:1). The formula weight is 511.51.

Leucovorin Calcium for Injection: Leucovorin Calcium for Injection is indicated for intravenous or intramuscular administration and is supplied as a sterile cryodesiccated powder. The 50, 100, and 350 mg vials are preservative free. The inactive ingredient is sodium chloride 40 mg/vial for the 50 mg vial, 80 mg/vial for the 100 mg vial, and 140 mg/vial for the 350 mg vial. Sodium hydroxide and/or hydrochloric acid are used to adjust the pH to approximately 8.1 during manufacture. There is 0.004 mEq of calcium per mg of leucovorin in each dosage form.

CLINICAL PHARMACOLOGY

Leucovorin is a mixture of the diastereoisomers of the 5-formyl derivative of tetrahydrofolic acid (THF). The biologically active compound of the mixture is the (-)-*l*-isomer, known as Citrovorum factor or (-)-folinic acid. Leucovorin does not require reduction by the enzyme dihydrofolate reductase in order to participate in reactions utilizing folates as a source of "one-carbon" moieties. *l*-Leucovorin (*l*-5-formyltetrahydrofolate) is rapidly metabolized (via 5, 10-methenyltetrahydrofolate then 5,10-methylenetetrahydrofolate) to *l*-5-methyltetrahydrofolate. *l*-5-Methyltetrahydrofolate can in turn be metabolized via other pathways back to 5,10-methylenetetrahydrofolate, which is converted to 5-methyltetrahydrofolate by an irreversible, enzyme catalyzed reduction using the cofactors FADH$_2$ and NADPH.

Administration of leucovorin can counteract the therapeutic and toxic effects of folic acid antagonists such as methotrexate, which act by inhibiting dihydrofolate reductase.

In contrast, leucovorin can enhance the therapeutic and toxic effects of fluoropyrimidines used in cancer therapy, such as 5-fluorouracil. Concurrent administration of leucovorin does not appear to alter the plasma pharmacokinetics of 5-fluorouracil. 5-Fluorouracil is metabolized to fluorodeoxyuridylic acid, which binds to and inhibits the enzyme thymidylate synthase (an enzyme important in DNA repair and replication).

Leucovorin is readily converted to another reduced folate, 5,10-methylenetetrahydrofolate, which acts to stabilize the binding of fluorodeoxyuridylic acid to thymidylate synthase and thereby enhances the inhibition of this enzyme.

The pharmacokinetics after intravenous, intramuscular, and oral administration of a 25 mg dose of leucovorin were studied in male volunteers. After intravenous administration, serum total reduced folates (as measured by *Lactobacillus casei* assay) reached a mean peak of 1259 ng/mL (range

897 ng/mL to 1625 ng/mL). The mean time to peak was 10 minutes. This initial rise in total reduced folates was primarily due to the parent compound 5-formyl-THF (measured by *Streptococcus faecalis* assay) which rose to 1206 ng/mL at 10 minutes. A sharp drop in parent compound followed and coincided with the appearance of the active metabolite 5-methyl-THF which became the predominant circulating form of the drug.

The mean peak of 5-methyl-THF was 258 ng/mL and occurred at 1.3 hours. The terminal half-life for total reduced folates was 6.2 hours. The area under the concentration versus time curves (AUCs) for *l*-leucovorin, *d*-leucovorin and 5-methyltetrahydrofolate were 28.4 ± 3.5, 956 ± 97 and 129 ± 12 (mg.min/L ± S.E.). When a higher dose of *d,l*-leucovorin (200 mg/m^2) was used, similar results were obtained. The *d*-isomer persisted in plasma at concentrations greatly exceeding those of the *l*-isomer.

After intramuscular injection, the mean peak of serum total reduced folates was 436 ng/mL (range 240 ng/mL to 725 ng/mL) and occurred at 52 minutes. Similar to IV administration, the initial sharp rise was due to the parent compound. The mean peak of 5-formyl-THF was 360 ng/mL and occurred at 28 minutes. The level of the metabolite 5-methyl-THF increased subsequently over time until at 1.5 hours it represented 50% of the circulating total folates. The mean peak of 5-methyl-THF was 226 ng/mL at 2.8 hours. The terminal half-life of total reduced folates was 6.2 hours. There was no difference of statistical significance between IM and IV administration in the AUC for total reduced folates, 5-formyl-THF, or 5-methyl-THF.

After oral administration of leucovorin reconstituted with aromatic elixir, the mean peak concentration of serum total reduced folates was 393 ng/mL (range 160 ng/mL to 550 ng/mL). The mean time to peak was 2.3 hours and the terminal half-life was 5.7 hours. The major component was the metabolite 5-methyltetrahydrofolate to which leucovorin is primarily converted in the intestinal mucosa. The mean peak of 5-methyl-THF was 367 ng/mL at 2.4 hours. The peak level of the parent compound was 51 ng/mL at 1.2 hours. The AUC of total reduced folates after oral administration of the 25 mg dose was 92% of the AUC after intravenous administration.

Following oral administration, leucovorin is rapidly absorbed and expands the serum pool of reduced folates. At a dose of 25 mg, almost 100% of the *l*-isomer but only 20% of the *d*-isomer is absorbed. Oral absorption of leucovorin is saturable at doses above 25 mg. The apparent bioavailability of leucovorin was 97% for 25 mg, 75% for 50 mg, and 37% for 100 mg.

In a randomized clinical study conducted by the Mayo Clinic and the North Central Cancer Treatment Group (Mayo/NCCTG) in patients with advanced metastatic colorectal cancer three treatment regimens were compared: Leucovorin (LV) 200 mg/m^2 and 5-fluorouracil (5-FU) 370 mg/m^2 versus LV 20 mg/m^2 and 5-FU 425 mg/m^2 versus 5-FU 500 mg/m^2. All drugs were by slow intravenous infusion daily for 5 days repeated every 28 to 35 days. Response rates were 26% (P = 0.04 versus 5-FU alone), 43% (P =0.001 versus 5-FU alone), and 10% for the high-dose leucovorin, low-dose leucovorin and 5-FU alone groups, respectively. Respective median survival times were 12.2 months (P = 0.037), 12 months (P = 0.050), and 7.7 months. The low-dose LV regimen gave a statistically significant improvement in weight gain of more than 5%, relief of symptoms, and improvement in performance status. The high-dose LV regimen gave a statistically significant improvement in performance status and trended toward improvement in weight gain and in relief of symptoms but these were not statistically significant.[1]

In a second Mayo/NCCTG randomized clinical study the 5-FU alone arm was replaced by a regimen of sequentially administered methotrexate (MTX), 5-FU, and LV. Response rates with LV 200 mg/m^2 and 5-FU 370 mg/m^2 versus LV 20 mg/m^2 and 5-FU 425 mg/m^2 versus sequential MTX and 5-FU and LV were, respectively, 31% (P = <.01), 42% (P = <.01), and 14%. Respective median survival times were 12.7 months (P = <.04), 12.7 months (P = <.01), and 8.4 months. No statistically significant difference in weight gain of more than 5% or in improvement in performance status was seen between the treatment arms.[2]

INDICATIONS AND USAGE

Leucovorin calcium rescue is indicated after high-dose methotrexate therapy in osteosarcoma. Leucovorin calcium is also indicated to diminish the toxicity and counteract the effects of impaired methotrexate elimination and of inadvertent overdosages of folic acid antagonists.

Leucovorin calcium is indicated in the treatment of megaloblastic anemias due to folic acid deficiency when oral therapy is not feasible.

Leucovorin is also indicated for use in combination with 5-fluorouracil to prolong survival in the palliative treatment of patients with advanced colorectal cancer.

CONTRAINDICATIONS

Leucovorin is improper therapy for pernicious anemia and other megaloblastic anemias secondary to the lack of vitamin B$_{12}$. A hematologic remission may occur while neurologic manifestations continue to progress.

WARNINGS

In the treatment of accidental overdosages of folic acid antagonists, leucovorin should be administered as promptly as possible. As the time interval between antifolate administration [eg, methotrexate (MTX)] and leucovorin rescue increases, leucovorin's effectiveness in counteracting toxicity decreases.

Monitoring of the serum MTX concentration is essential in determining the optimal dose and duration of treatment with leucovorin.

Delayed MTX excretion may be caused by a third space fluid accumulation (ie, ascites, pleural effusion), renal insufficiency, or inadequate hydration. Under such circumstances, higher doses of leucovorin or prolonged administration may be indicated. Doses higher than those recommended for oral use must be given intravenously.

Because of the benzyl alcohol contained in certain diluents used for Leucovorin Calcium for Injection, when doses greater than 10 mg/m^2 are administered, Leucovorin Calcium for Injection should be reconstituted with Sterile Water for Injection, USP, and used immediately (see **DOSAGE AND ADMINISTRATION**).

Because of the calcium content of the leucovorin solution, no more than 160 mg of leucovorin should be injected intravenously per minute (16 mL of a 10 mg/mL, or 8 mL of a 20 mg/mL solution per minute).

Leucovorin enhances the toxicity of 5-fluorouracil. When these drugs are administered concurrently in the palliative therapy of advanced colorectal cancer, the dosage of 5-fluorouracil must be lower than usually administered. Although the toxicities observed in patients treated with the combination of leucovorin plus 5-fluorouracil are qualitatively similar to those observed in patients treated with 5-fluorouracil alone, gastrointestinal toxicities (particularly stomatitis and diarrhea) are observed more commonly and may be more severe and of prolonged duration in patients treated with the combination.

In the first Mayo/NCCTG controlled trial, toxicity, primarily gastrointestinal, resulted in 7% of patients requiring hospitalization when treated with 5-fluorouracil alone or 5-fluorouracil in combination with 200 mg/m^2 of leucovorin and 20% when treated with 5-fluorouracil in combination with 20 mg/m^2 of leucovorin. In the second Mayo/NCCTG trial, hospitalizations related to treatment toxicity also appeared to occur more often in patients treated with the low-dose leucovorin/5-fluorouracil combination than in patients treated with the high-dose combination—11% versus 3%. Therapy with leucovorin/5-fluorouracil must not be initiated or continued in patients who have symptoms of gastrointestinal toxicity of any severity, until those symptoms have completely resolved. Patients with diarrhea must be monitored with particular care until the diarrhea has resolved, as rapid clinical deterioration leading to death can occur. In an additional study utilizing higher weekly doses of 5-FU and leucovorin, elderly and/or debilitated patients were found to be at greater risk for severe gastrointestinal toxicity.[3]

PRECAUTIONS

General: Parenteral administration is preferable to oral dosing if there is a possibility that the patient may vomit or not absorb the leucovorin. Leucovorin has no effect on nonhematologic toxicities of MTX such as the nephrotoxicity resulting from drug and/or metabolite precipitation in the kidney.

Since leucovorin enhances the toxicity of fluorouracil, leucovorin/5-fluorouracil combination therapy for advanced colorectal cancer should be administered under the supervision of a physician experienced in the use of antimetabolite cancer chemotherapy. Particular care should be taken in the treatment of elderly or debilitated colorectal cancer patients, as these patients may be at increased risk of severe toxicity.

Laboratory Tests: Patients being treated with the leucovorin/5-fluorouracil combination should have a CBC with differential and platelets prior to each treatment. During the first two courses a CBC with differential and platelets has to be repeated weekly and thereafter once each cycle at the time of anticipated WBC nadir. Electrolytes and liver function tests should be performed prior to each treatment for the first three cycles, then prior to every other cycle. Dosage modifications of fluorouracil should be instituted as follows, based on the most severe toxicities:

Diarrhea and/or Stomatitis	WBC/mm^3 Nadir	Platelets/mm^3 Nadir	5-FU Dose
Moderate	1,000–1,900	25–75,000	decrease 20%
Severe	<1,000	<25,000	decrease 30%

If no toxicity occurs, the 5-fluorouracil dose may increase 10%.

Treatment should be deferred until WBCs are 4,000/mm³ and platelets 130,000/mm³. If blood counts do not reach these levels within 2 weeks, treatment should be discontinued. Patients should be followed up with physical examination prior to each treatment course and appropriate radiological examination as needed. Treatment should be discontinued when there is clear evidence of tumor progression.

Drug Interactions: Folic acid in large amounts may counteract the antiepileptic effect of phenobarbital, phenytoin, and primidone, and increase the frequency of seizures in susceptible children.

Preliminary animal and human studies have shown that small quantities of systemically administered leucovorin enter the CSF primarily as 5-methyltetrahydrofolate and, in humans, remain 1 to 3 orders of magnitude lower than the usual methotrexate concentrations following intrathecal administration. However, high doses of leucovorin may reduce the efficacy of intrathecally administered methotrexate.

Leucovorin may enhance the toxicity of 5-fluorouracil (see **WARNINGS**).

Pregnancy: *Teratogenic Effects:* Pregnancy Category C. Adequate animal reproduction studies have not been conducted with leucovorin. It is also not known whether leucovorin can cause fetal harm when administered to a pregnant woman or can affect reproduction capacity. Leucovorin should be given to a pregnant woman only if clearly needed.

Nursing Mothers: It is not known whether this drug is excreted in human milk. Because many drugs are excreted in human milk, caution should be exercised when leucovorin is administered to a nursing mother.

Pediatric Use: See **Drug Interactions.**

ADVERSE REACTIONS

Allergic sensitization, including anaphylactoid reactions and urticaria, has been reported following the administration of both oral and parenteral leucovorin. No other adverse reactions have been attributed to the use of leucovorin *per se.* The following table summarizes significant adverse events occurring in 316 patients treated with the leucovorin-5-fluorouracil combinations compared against 70 patients treated with 5-fluorouracil alone for advanced colorectal carcinoma. These data are taken from the Mayo/NCCTG large multicenter prospective trial evaluating the efficacy and safety of the combination regimen.

[See table below.]

OVERDOSAGE

Excessive amounts of leucovorin may nullify the chemotherapeutic effect of folic acid antagonists.

DOSAGE AND ADMINISTRATION

Advanced Colorectal Cancer: Either of the following two regimens is recommended:

1. Leucovorin is administered at 200 mg/m² by slow intravenous injection over a minimum of 3 minutes, followed by 5-fluorouracil at 370 mg/m² by intravenous injection.
2. Leucovorin is administered at 20 mg/m² by intravenous injection followed by 5-fluorouracil at 425 mg/m² by intravenous injection.

Treatment is repeated daily for 5 days. This 5-day treatment course may be repeated at 4-week (28 day) intervals, for two

GUIDELINES FOR LEUCOVORIN DOSAGE AND ADMINISTRATION

Clinical Situation	Laboratory Findings	Leucovorin Dosage and Duration
Normal Methotrexate Elimination	Serum methotrexate level approximately 10 micromolar at 24 hours after administration, 1 micromolar at 48 hours, and less than 0.2 micromolar at 72 hours.	15 mg PO, IM, or IV q 6 hours for 60 hours (10 doses starting at 24 hours after start of methotrexate infusion).
Delayed Late Methotrexate Elimination	Serum methotrexate level remaining above 0.2 micromolar at 72 hours, and more than 0.05 micromolar at 96 hours after administration.	Continue 15 mg PO, IM, or IV q 6 hours, until methotrexate level is less than 0.05 micromolar.
Delayed Early Methotrexate Elimination and/or Evidence of Acute Renal Injury	Serum methotrexate level of 50 micromolar or more at 24 hours, or 5 micromolar or more at 48 hours after administration, OR; a 100% or greater increase in serum creatinine level at 24 hours after methotrexate administration (eg, an increase from 0.5 mg/dL to a level of 1 mg/dL or more).	150 mg IV q 3 hours, until methotrexate level is less than 1 micromolar; then 15 mg IV q 3 hours, until methotrexate level is less than 0.05 micromolar.

courses and then repeated at 4- to 5-week (28- to 35-day) intervals provided that the patient has completely recovered from the toxic effects of the prior treatment course.

In subsequent treatment courses, the dosage of 5-fluorouracil should be adjusted based on patient tolerance of the prior treatment course. The daily dosage of 5-fluorouracil should be reduced by 20% for patients who experienced moderate hematologic or gastrointestinal toxicity in the prior treatment course, and by 30% for patients who experienced severe toxicity (see **PRECAUTIONS: Laboratory Tests**). For patients who experienced no toxicity in the prior treatment course, 5-fluorouracil dosage may be increased by 10%. Leucovorin dosages are not adjusted for toxicity.

Several other doses and schedules of leucovorin/5-fluorouracil therapy have also been evaluated in patients with advanced colorectal cancer; some of these alternative regimens may also have efficacy in the treatment of this disease. However, further clinical research will be required to confirm the safety and effectiveness of these alternative leucovorin/5-fluorouracil treatment regimens.

Leucovorin Rescue After High-Dose Methotrexate Therapy: The recommendations for leucovorin rescue are based on a methotrexate dose of 12 to 15 grams/m² administered by intravenous infusion over 4 hours (see methotrexate package insert for full Prescribing Information).[4] Leucovorin rescue at a dose of 15 mg (approximately 10 mg/m²) every 6

hours for 10 doses starts 24 hours after the beginning of the methotrexate infusion. In the presence of gastrointestinal toxicity, nausea, or vomiting, leucovorin should be administered parenterally.

Serum creatinine and methotrexate levels should be determined at least once daily. Leucovorin administration, hydration, and urinary alkalinization (pH of 7.0 or greater) should be continued until the methotrexate level is below 5×10^{-8} M (0.05 micromolar). The leucovorin dose should be adjusted or leucovorin rescue extended based on the following guidelines:

[See table above.]

Patients who experience delayed early methotrexate elimination are likely to develop reversible renal failure. In addition to appropriate leucovorin therapy, these patients require continuing hydration and urinary alkalinization, and close monitoring of fluid and electrolyte status, until the serum methotrexate level has fallen to below 0.05 micromolar and the renal failure has resolved.

Some patients will have abnormalities in methotrexate elimination or renal function following methotrexate administration, which are significant but less severe than the abnormalities described in the table above. These abnormalities may or may not be associated with significant clinical toxicity. If significant clinical toxicity is observed, leucovorin rescue should be extended for an additional 24 hours (total of 14 doses over 84 hours) in subsequent courses of therapy. The possibility that the patient is taking other medications which interact with methotrexate (eg, medications which may interfere with methotrexate elimination or binding to serum albumin) should always be reconsidered when laboratory abnormalities or clinical toxicities are observed.

Impaired Methotrexate Elimination or Inadvertent Overdosage: Leucovorin rescue should begin as soon as possible after an inadvertent overdosage and within 24 hours of methotrexate administration when there is delayed excretion (see **WARNINGS**). Leucovorin 10 mg/m² should be administered IV, IM, or PO every 6 hours until the serum methotrexate level is less than 10^{-8} M. In the presence of gastrointestinal toxicity, nausea, or vomiting, leucovorin should be administered parenterally.

Serum creatinine and methotrexate levels should be determined at 24-hour intervals. If the 24-hour serum creatinine has increased 50% over baseline or if the 24-hour methotrexate level is greater than 5×10^{-6} M or the 48-hour level is greater than 9×10^{-7} M, the dose of leucovorin should be

Continued on next page

PERCENTAGE OF PATIENTS TREATED WITH LEUCOVORIN/FLUOROURACIL FOR ADVANCED COLORECTAL CARCINOMA REPORTING ADVERSE EXPERIENCES OR HOSPITALIZED FOR TOXICITY

	(High LV)/5-FU (N = 155)		(Low LV)/5-FU (N = 161)		5-FU Alone (N = 70)	
	Any (%)	Grade 3+ (%)	Any (%)	Grade 3+ (%)	Any (%)	Grade 3+ (%)
Leukopenia	69	14	83	23	93	48
Thrombocytopenia	8	2	8	1	18	3
Infection	8	1	3	1	7	2
Nausea	74	10	80	9	60	6
Vomiting	46	8	44	9	40	7
Diarrhea	66	18	67	14	43	11
Stomatitis	75	27	84	29	59	16
Constipation	3	0	4	0	1	—
Lethargy/Malaise/ Fatigue	13	3	12	2	6	3
Alopecia	42	5	43	6	37	7
Dermatitis	21	2	25	1	13	—
Anorexia	14	1	22	4	14	—
Hospitalization for Toxicity	5%		15%		7%	

High LV = Leucovorin 200 mg/m², Low LV = Leucovorin 20 mg/m²
Any = percentage of patients reporting toxicity of any severity
Grade 3 + = percentage of patients reporting toxicity of Grade 3 or higher

Information on Lederle products listed on these pages is the full prescribing information from product literature and package inserts effective in August 1992. Information concerning all Lederle products may be obtained from the Professional Services Department, Lederle Laboratories, Pearl River, New York 10965.

Lederle—Cont.

increased to 100 mg/m^2 IV every 3 hours until the methotrexate level is less than 10^{-8} M.

Hydration (3 L/d) and urinary alkalinization with sodium bicarbonate solution should be employed concomitantly. The bicarbonate dose should be adjusted to maintain the urine pH at 7.0 or greater.

Megaloblastic Anemia Due to Folic Acid Deficiency: Up to 1 mg daily. There is no evidence that doses greater than 1 mg/day have greater efficacy than those of 1 mg; additionally, loss of folate in urine becomes roughly logarithmic as the amount administered exceeds 1 mg.

Each 50 mg and 100 mg vial of Leucovorin Calcium for Injection when reconstituted with 5 mL and 10 mL, respectively, of sterile diluent yields a leucovorin concentration of 10 mg per mL. Each 350 mg vial of Leucovorin Calcium for Injection when reconstituted with 17 mL of sterile diluent yields a leucovorin concentration of 20 mg leucovorin per mL. Leucovorin Calcium for Injection contains no preservative. Reconstitute with Bacteriostatic Water for Injection, USP, which contains benzyl alcohol, or with Sterile Water for Injection, USP. When reconstituted with Bacteriostatic Water for Injection, USP, the resulting solution must be used within 7 days. If the product is reconstituted with Sterile Water for Injection, USP, it must be used immediately. Because of the benzyl alcohol contained in Bacteriostatic Water for Injection, USP, when doses greater than 10 mg/m^2 are administered Leucovorin Calcium for Injection should be reconstituted with Sterile Water for Injection, USP, and used immediately (see **DOSAGE AND ADMINISTRATION**). Because of the calcium content of the leucovorin solution, no more than 160 mg of leucovorin should be injected intravenously per minute (16 mL of a 10 mg/mL, or 8 mL of a 20 mg/mL solution per minute).

Parenteral drug products should be inspected visually for particulate matter and discoloration prior to administration, whenever solution and container permit.

HOW SUPPLIED

Leucovorin Calcium for Injection:
50 mg Vial of cryodesiccated powder—NDC 0205-5330-92
50 mg Vial of cryodesiccated powder—Box of 25—NDC 0205-5330-19
100 mg Vial of cryodesiccated powder—NDC 0205-4646-94
350 mg Vial of cryodesiccated powder—NDC 0205-4645-77
Store between 15°C (59°F) and 25°C (77°F).
Protect from Light.

REFERENCES

1. Poon MA, et al. Biochemical modulation of fluorouracil: evidence of significant improvement of survival and quality of life in patients with advanced colorectal carcinoma. *J Clin Oncol.* 1989; 7:1407–1418.
2. Poon MA, et al. Biochemical modulation of fluorouracil with leucovorin: confirmatory evidence of improved therapeutic efficacy in advanced colorectal cancer. *J Clin Oncol.* 1991; 9:1967–1972.
3. Grem JL, Shoemaker DD, Petrelli NJ, et al. Severe and fatal toxic effects observed in treatment with high- and low-dose leucovorin plus 5-fluorouracil for colorectal carcinoma. *Cancer Treat Rep.* 1987; 71:1122.
4. Link MP, Goorin AM, Miser AW, et al. The effect of adjuvant chemotherapy on relapse-free survival in patients with osteosarcoma of the extremity. *N Engl J Med.* 1986; 314:1600–1606.

LEDERLE PARENTERALS, INC.
Carolina, Puerto Rico 00987

Rev. 8/92
21844-92

Shown in Product Identification Section, page 415

LEUCOVORIN CALCIUM TABLETS ℞
[lu-có-vor-ĭn căl-sēē-um]

DESCRIPTION

Leucovorin is one of several active, chemically reduced derivatives of folic acid. It is useful as an antidote to drugs which act as folic acid antagonists. Also known as folinic acid, Citrovorum factor, or 5-formyl-5,6,7,8-tetrahydrofolic acid, this compound has the chemical designation of L-Glutamic acid, N-[4-[[(2-amino-5-formyl-1,4,5,6,7,8-hexahydro-4-oxo-6-pteridinyl)methyl] amino] benzoyl]-, calcium salt (1:1). The formula weight is 511.51.

Leucovorin Calcium Tablets, 5 mg, contain 5 mg of leucovorin (equivalent to 5.40 mg of anhydrous leucovorin calcium) and the following inactive ingredients: Corn Starch, Dibasic Calcium Phosphate, Magnesium Stearate, and Pregelatinized Starch.

Leucovorin Calcium Tablets, 10 mg, contain 10 mg of leucovorin (equivalent to 10.80 mg of anhydrous leucovorin calcium) and the following inactive ingredients: Lactose,

Magnesium Stearate, Microcrystalline Cellulose, Pregelatinized Starch, and Sodium Starch Glycolate.

Leucovorin Calcium Tablets, 15 mg, contain 15 mg of leucovorin (equivalent to 16.20 mg of anhydrous leucovorin calcium) and the following inactive ingredients: Lactose, Magnesium Stearate, Microcrystalline Cellulose, Pregelatinized Starch, and Sodium Starch Glycolate.

Leucovorin Calcium Tablets are indicated for oral administration only.

CLINICAL PHARMACOLOGY

Leucovorin is a mixture of the diastereoisomers of the 5-formyl derivative of tetrahydrofolic acid. The biologically active component of the mixture is the (-)-L-isomer, known as Citrovorum factor, or (-)-folinic acid. Leucovorin does not require reduction by the enzyme dihydrofolate reductase in order to participate in reactions utilizing folates as a source of "one-carbon" moieties. Following oral administration, leucovorin is rapidly absorbed and enters the general body pool of reduced folates.

The increase in plasma and serum reduced folate activity (determined microbiologically with *Lactobacillus casei*) seen after oral administration of leucovorin is predominantly due to 5-methyltetrahydrofolate.

Following a 20 mg dose of leucovorin calcium, the mean maximum serum total reduced folate concentrations were:

Tablet	364±12.1 ng/mL at	2.0±0.07 hours
Oral Solution	375±12.8 ng/mL at	2.1±0.11 hours
Parenteral	355±17.2 ng/mL at	0.96±0.10 hours

The half-life of plasma 5-formyltetrahydrofolate was 1.5 ± 0.08 hours and that of the 5-methyltetrahydrofolate was 3.0 ± 0.09 hours.

Oral tablets produced equivalent bioavailability (8% difference) when compared to the parenteral administration. The parenteral solution also provided equal bioavailability to the tablets when administered orally (2% difference). Oral absorption of leucovorin is saturable at doses above 25 mg. The apparent bioavailability of leucovorin was 97% for 25 mg, 75% for 50 mg, and 37% for 100 mg.

INDICATIONS

Leucovorin calcium rescue is indicated after high-dose methotrexate therapy in osteosarcoma. Leucovorin is also indicated to diminish the toxicity and counteract the effects of impaired methotrexate elimination and of inadvertent overdosages of folic acid antagonists.

CONTRAINDICATIONS

Leucovorin is improper therapy for pernicious anemia and other megaloblastic anemias secondary to the lack of vitamin B$_{12}$. A hematologic remission may occur while neurologic manifestations remain progressive.

WARNINGS

In the treatment of accidental overdosages of folic acid antagonists, leucovorin should be administered as promptly as possible. As the time interval between antifolate administration [eg, methotrexate (MTX)] and leucovorin rescue increases, leucovorin's effectiveness in counteracting toxicity diminishes.

Monitoring of serum MTX concentration is essential in determining the optimal dose and duration of treatment with leucovorin.

Delayed MTX excretion may be caused by a third-space fluid accumulation (ie, ascites, pleural effusion), renal insufficiency, or inadequate hydration. Under such circumstances, higher doses of leucovorin or prolonged administration may be indicated. Doses higher than those recommended for oral use must be given intravenously.

Leucovorin may enhance the toxicity of fluorouracil. Deaths from severe enterocolitis, diarrhea, and dehydration have been reported in elderly patients receiving weekly leucovorin and fluorouracil.[1] Concomitant granulocytopenia and fever were present in some but not all of the patients.

PRECAUTIONS

General: Parenteral administration is preferable to oral dosing if there is a possibility that the patient may vomit or not absorb the leucovorin. Leucovorin has no effect on other established toxicities of MTX such as the nephrotoxicity resulting from drug and/or metabolite precipitation in the kidney.

Drug Interactions: Folic acid in large amounts may counteract the antiepileptic effect of phenobarbital, phenytoin, and primidone, and increase the frequency of seizures in susceptible children.

Preliminary animal and human studies have shown that small quantities of systemically administered leucovorin enter the CSF primarily as 5-methyltetrahydrofolate and, in humans, remain 1 to 3 orders of magnitude lower than the usual methotrexate concentrations following intrathecal administration. However, high doses of leucovorin may reduce the efficacy of intrathecally administered methotrexate.

Leucovorin may enhance the toxicity of fluorouracil (see **WARNINGS**).

Pregnancy: *Teratogenic Effects:* Pregnancy Category C. Animal reproduction studies have not been conducted with

leucovorin. It is also not known whether leucovorin can cause fetal harm when administered to a pregnant woman or can affect reproduction capacity. Leucovorin should be given to a pregnant woman only if clearly needed.

Nursing Mothers: It is not known whether this drug is excreted in human milk. Because many drugs are excreted in human milk, caution should be exercised when leucovorin is administered to a nursing mother.

Pediatric Use: See **Drug Interactions.**

ADVERSE REACTIONS

Allergic sensitization, including anaphylactoid reactions and urticaria, has been reported following the administration of both oral and parenteral leucovorin.

OVERDOSAGE

Excessive amounts of leucovorin may nullify the chemotherapeutic effect of folic acid antagonists.

DOSAGE AND ADMINISTRATION

Leucovorin Calcium Tablets are intended for oral administration. Because absorption is saturable, oral administration of doses greater than 25 mg is not recommended.

Leucovorin Rescue After High-Dose Methotrexate Therapy: The recommendations for leucovorin rescue are based on a methotrexate dose of 12 to 15 grams/m^2 administered by intravenous infusion over 4 hours (see methotrexate package insert for full Prescribing Information).[2] Leucovorin rescue at a dose of 15 mg (approximately 10 mg/m^2) every 6 hours for 10 doses starts 24 hours after the beginning of the methotrexate infusion. In the presence of gastrointestinal toxicity, nausea or vomiting, leucovorin should be administered parenterally.

Serum creatinine and methotrexate levels should be determined at least once daily. Leucovorin administration, hydration, and urinary alkalinization (pH of 7.0 or greater) should be continued until the methotrexate level is below 5×10^{-8} M (0.05 micromolar). The leucovorin dose should be adjusted or leucovorin rescue extended based on the following guidelines:

[See table on next page.]

Patients who experience delayed early methotrexate elimination are likely to develop reversible renal failure. In addition to appropriate leucovorin therapy, these patients require continuing hydration and urinary alkalinization, and close monitoring of fluid and electrolyte status, until the serum methotrexate level has fallen to below 0.05 micromolar and the renal failure has resolved.

Some patients will have abnormalities in methotrexate elimination or renal function following methotrexate administration, which are significant but less severe than the abnormalities described in the table above. These abnormalities may or may not be associated with significant clinical toxicity. If significant clinical toxicity is observed, leucovorin rescue should be extended for an additional 24 hours (total of 14 doses over 84 hours) in subsequent courses of therapy. The possibility that the patient is taking other medications which interact with methotrexate (eg, medications which may interfere with methotrexate elimination or binding to serum albumin) should always be reconsidered when laboratory abnormalities or clinical toxicities are observed.

Impaired Methotrexate Elimination or Inadvertent Overdosage: The same dosage and administration guidelines may be used. However, leucovorin administration should begin as soon as possible after an inadvertent overdosage is recognized.

HOW SUPPLIED

Leucovorin Calcium Tablets, 5 mg, are round, convex, yellowish-white, engraved LL above 5 on one side, scored in half on the other side, and engraved C above the score and 33 below, each containing 5 mg of leucovorin as the calcium salt, supplied as follows:
NDC 0005-4536-38—Bottle of 30 with CRC
NDC 0005-4536-23—Bottle of 100
NDC 0005-4536-40—Unit Dose 10 × 5s
Leucovorin Calcium Tablets, 10 mg, are square with rounded corners, convex, yellowish-white, engraved LL above 10 on one side and scored in half on the other side with C above the score and 12 below, containing 10 mg of leucovorin as the calcium salt, supplied as follows:
NDC 0005-4525-83—Bottle of 12 with CRC
NDC 0005-4525-90—Bottle of 24 with CRC
NDC 0005-4525-64—Unit Dose 5 × 10s
Leucovorin Calcium Tablets, 15 mg, are oval, convex, yellowish-white, engraved LL on left and 15 on right on one side, scored in half on the other side, and engraved C to the left of the score and 35 to the right, each containing 15 mg of leucovorin as the calcium salt, supplied as follows:
NDC 0005-4501-83—Bottle of 12 with CRC
NDC 0005-4501-90—Bottle of 24 with CRC
NDC 0005-4501-64—Unit Dose 5 × 10s
Store at Controlled Room Temperature 15°–30°C (59°–86°F).
Protect From Light.

REFERENCES

1. Grem JL, Shoemaker DD, Petrelli NJ, et al. Severe and fatal toxic effects observed in treatment with high- and

GUIDELINES FOR LEUCOVORIN DOSAGE AND ADMINISTRATION

Clinical Situation	Laboratory Findings	Leucovorin Dosage and Duration
Normal Methotrexate Elimination	Serum methotrexate level approximately 10 micromolar at 24 hours after administration, 1 micromolar at 48 hours, and less than 0.2 micromolar at 72 hours.	15 mg PO, IM, or IV q6h for 60 hours (10 doses starting at 24 hours after start of methotrexate infusion).
Delayed Late Methotrexate Elimination	Serum methotrexate level remaining above 0.2 micromolar at 72 hours, and more than 0.05 micromolar at 96 hours after administration.	Continue 15 mg PO, IM, or IV q6h, until methotrexate level is less than 0.05 micromolar.
Delayed Early Methotrexate Elimination and/or Evidence of Acute Renal Injury	Serum methotrexate level of 50 micromolar or more at 24 hours, or 5 micromolar or more at 48 hours after administration, OR; a 100% or greater increase in serum creatinine level at 24 hours after methotrexate administration (eg, an increase from 0.5 mg/dL to a level of 1 mg/dL or more).	150 mg IV q3h, until methotrexate level is less than 1 micromolar; then 15 mg IV q3h until methotrexate level is less than 0.05 micromolar.

low-dose leucovorin plus 5-fluorouracil for colorectal carcinoma. *Cancer Treat Rep.* 1987; 71:1122.
2. Link MP, Goorin AM, Miser AW, et al: The effect of adjuvant chemotherapy on relapse-free survival in patients with osteosarcoma of the extremity. *N Engl J Med.* 1986; 314:1600–1606.

LEDERLE LABORATORIES DIVISION
American Cyanamid Company, Pearl River, NY 10965

Rev. 3/91
10715-91

Shown in Product Identification Section, page 414

LOXITANE®   ℞
[lŏks-ĭ-tāne]
Loxapine Succinate
Capsules
LOXITANE® C   ℞
Loxapine Hydrochloride
Oral Concentrate
For Oral Use
LOXITANE® IM   ℞
Loxapine Hydrochloride
For Intramuscular Use Only

DESCRIPTION

LOXITANE, a dibenzoxazepine compound, represents a new subclass of tricyclic antipsychotic agent, chemically distinct from the thioxanthenes, butyrophenones, and phenothiazines. Chemically, it is 2-chloro-11-(4-methyl-1-piperazinyl)-dibenz[b,f][1,4]oxazepine. It is present in capsules as the succinate salt, and in the concentrate and parenteral primarily as the hydrochloride salt.

CAPSULES

Each capsule contains loxapine succinate equivalent to 5, 10, 25, or 50 mg of loxapine base and the following inactive ingredients: Blue 1, Gelatin, Lactose, Magnesium Stearate, Titanium Dioxide, and Yellow 10. Additionally, the 5 mg capsule contains Red 33, the 10 mg capsule contains Red 28 and Red 33, and the 25 mg capsule contains FD&C Yellow No. 6.

ORAL CONCENTRATE

Each mL contains loxapine hydrochloride equivalent to 25 mg of loxapine base and propylene glycol as an inactive ingredient.

Hydrochloric acid and, if necessary, sodium hydroxide are used to adjust pH to approximately 5.8 during manufacture.

INTRAMUSCULAR (Sterile)

Not for Intravenous Use—Each mL contains loxapine hydrochloride equivalent to 50 mg of loxapine base. Inactive Ingredients: Polysorbate 80 NF 5% w/v, Propylene Glycol 70% v/v, and Water for Injection qs ad 100% v.

Hydrochloric acid and, if necessary, sodium hydroxide are used to adjust pH to approximately 5.8 during manufacture.

CLINICAL PHARMACOLOGY

Pharmacodynamics: Pharmacologically, loxapine is a tranquilizer for which the exact mode of action has not been established. However, changes in the level of excitability of subcortical inhibitory areas have been observed in several animal species in association with such manifestations of tranquilization as calming effects and suppression of aggressive behavior.

In normal human volunteers, signs of sedation were seen within 20 to 30 minutes after administration, were most pronounced within $1\frac{1}{2}$ to 3 hours, and lasted through 12 hours. Similar timing of primary pharmacologic effects was seen in animals.

Absorption, Distribution, Metabolism, and Excretion: After administration of LOXITANE as an oral solution, systemic bioavailability of the parent drug was only about one third that after an equivalent intramuscular dose (25 mg base) in male volunteers. C_{max} for the parent drug was similar for the IM and oral administrations, whereas T_{max} was significantly longer for the IM administration than the oral administration (approximately 5 v 1 hour). The lower systemic availability of the parent drug after oral administration as compared to the IM administration may be due to first pass metabolism of the oral form. This is supported by the finding that two metabolites found in serum (8-hydroxyloxapine and 8-hydroxydesmethylloxapine) were formed to a lesser extent after IM administration of loxapine as compared to oral administration.

The apparent half-life of loxapine after oral and IM administration is approximately 4 hours (range, 1 to 14 hours) and 12 hours (range, 8 to 23 hours), respectively. The extended half-life for the IM administration as compared to the oral administration may be explained by prolonged absorption of loxapine from the muscle during the concurrent elimination process.

Loxapine is extensively metabolized, and urinary recovery over 48 hours resulted in recoveries of approximately 30% and 40% of an IM and orally administered loxapine dose as five metabolites.

INDICATIONS

LOXITANE is indicated for the management of the manifestations of psychotic disorders. The antipsychotic efficacy of LOXITANE *loxapine* was established in clinical studies which enrolled newly hospitalized and chronically hospitalized acutely ill schizophrenic patients as subjects.

CONTRAINDICATIONS

LOXITANE is contraindicated in comatose or severe drug-induced depressed states (alcohol, barbiturates, narcotics, etc).

LOXITANE is contraindicated in individuals with known hypersensitivity to dibenzoxazepines.

WARNINGS

Tardive Dyskinesia: Tardive dyskinesia, a syndrome consisting of potentially irreversible, involuntary, dyskinetic movements, may develop in patients treated with neuroleptic (antipsychotic) drugs. Although the prevalence of the syndrome appears to be highest among the elderly, especially elderly women, it is impossible to rely upon prevalence estimates to predict, at the inception of neuroleptic treatment, which patients are likely to develop the syndrome. Whether neuroleptic drug products differ in their potential to cause tardive dyskinesia is unknown.

Both the risk of developing the syndrome and the likelihood that it will become irreversible are believed to increase as the duration of treatment and the total cumulative dose of neuroleptic drugs administered to the patient increase. However, the syndrome can develop, although much less commonly, after relatively brief treatment periods at low doses. There is no known treatment for established cases of tardive dyskinesia, although the syndrome may remit, partially or completely, if neuroleptic treatment is withdrawn. Neuroleptic treatment, itself, however, may suppress (or partially suppress) the signs and symptoms of the syndrome, and thereby may possibly mask the underlying disease process. The effect that symptomatic suppression has upon the long-term course of the syndrome is unknown.

Given these considerations, neuroleptics should be prescribed in a manner that is most likely to minimize the occurrence of tardive dyskinesia. Chronic neuroleptic treatment should generally be reserved for patients who suffer from a chronic illness that (1) is known to respond to neuroleptic drugs, and (2) for whom alternative, equally effective, but potentially less harmful treatments are *not* available or appropriate. In patients who do require chronic treatment, the smallest dose and the shortest duration of treatment producing a satisfactory clinical response should be sought. The need for continued treatment should be reassessed periodically.

If signs and symptoms of tardive dyskinesia appear in a patient on neuroleptics, drug discontinuation should be considered. However, some patients may require treatment despite the presence of the syndrome. (See **ADVERSE REACTIONS** and **Information for Patients** sections.)

Neuroleptic Malignant Syndrome (NMS): A potentially fatal symptom complex sometimes referred to as Neuroleptic Malignant Syndrome (NMS) has been reported in association with antipsychotic drugs. Clinical manifestations of NMS are hyperpyrexia, muscle rigidity, altered mental status and evidence of autonomic instability (irregular pulse or blood pressure, tachycardia, diaphoresis, and cardiac dysrhythmias).

The diagnostic evaluation of patients with this syndrome is complicated. In arriving at a diagnosis, it is important to identify cases where the clinical presentation includes both serious medical illness (eg, pneumonia, systemic infection, etc) and untreated or inadequately treated extrapyramidal signs and symptoms (EPS). Other important considerations in the differential diagnosis include central anticholinergic toxicity, heat stroke, drug fever and primary central nervous system (CNS) pathology.

The management of NMS should include: (1) immediate discontinuation of antipsychotic drugs and other drugs not essential to concurrent therapy, (2) intensive symptomatic treatment and medical monitoring, and (3) treatment of any concomitant serious medical problems for which specific treatments are available. There is no general agreement about specific pharmacological treatment regimens for uncomplicated NMS.

If a patient requires antipsychotic drug treatment after recovery from NMS, the potential reintroduction of drug therapy should be carefully considered. The patient should be

Continued on next page

Lederle—Cont.

carefully monitored, since recurrences of NMS have been reported.
LOXITANE, like other tranquilizers, may impair mental and/or physical abilities, especially during the first few days of therapy. Therefore, ambulatory patients should be warned about activities requiring alertness (eg, operating vehicles or machinery) and about concomitant use of alcohol and other CNS depressants.
LOXITANE has not been evaluated for the management of behavioral complications in patients with mental retardation, and therefore, it cannot be recommended.

PRECAUTIONS

General: LOXITANE *loxapine* should be used with extreme caution in patients with a history of convulsive disorders since it lowers the convulsive threshold. Seizures have been reported in patients receiving LOXITANE at antipsychotic dose levels, and may occur in epileptic patients even with maintenance of routine anticonvulsant drug therapy.
LOXITANE has an antiemetic effect in animals. Since this effect may also occur in man, LOXITANE may mask signs of overdosage of toxic drugs and may obscure conditions such as intestinal obstruction and brain tumor.
LOXITANE should be used with caution in patients with cardiovascular disease. Increased pulse rates have been reported in the majority of patients receiving antipsychotic doses; transient hypotension has been reported. In the presence of severe hypotension requiring vasopressor therapy, the preferred drugs may be norepinephrine and angiotensin. Usual doses of epinephrine may be ineffective because of inhibition of its vasopressor effect by LOXITANE.
The possibility of ocular toxicity from loxapine cannot be excluded at this time. Therefore, careful observation should be made for pigmentary retinopathy and lenticular pigmentation, since these have been observed in some patients receiving certain other antipsychotic drugs for prolonged periods.
Because of possible anticholinergic action, the drug should be used cautiously in patients with glaucoma or a tendency to urinary retention, particularly with concomitant administration of anticholinergic-type antiparkinson medication.
Experience to date indicates the possibility of a slightly higher incidence of extrapyramidal effects following intramuscular administration than normally anticipated with oral formulations. The increase may be attributable to higher plasma levels following intramuscular injection.
Neuroleptic drugs elevate prolactin levels; the elevation persists during chronic administration. Tissue culture experiments indicate that approximately one third of human breast cancers are prolactin-dependent *in vitro*, a factor of potential importance if the prescription of these drugs is contemplated in a patient with a previously detected breast cancer. Although disturbances such as galactorrhea, amenorrhea, gynecomastia, and impotence have been reported, the clinical significance of elevated serum prolactin levels is unknown for most patients. An increase in mammary neoplasms has been found in rodents after chronic administration of neuroleptic drugs. Neither clinical studies nor epidemiologic studies conducted to date, however, have shown an association between chronic administration of these drugs and mammary tumorigenesis; the available evidence is considered too limited to be conclusive at this time.
Information for Patients: Given the likelihood that some patients exposed chronically to neuroleptics will develop tardive dyskinesia, it is advised that all patients in whom chronic use is contemplated be given, if possible, full information about this risk. The decision to inform patients and/or their guardians must obviously take into account the clinical circumstances and the competency of the patient to understand the information provided.
Usage in Pregnancy: Safe use of LOXITANE *loxapine* during pregnancy or lactation has not been established; therefore, its use in pregnancy, in nursing mothers, or in women of childbearing potential requires that the benefits of treatment be weighed against the possible risks to mother and child. No embryotoxicity or teratogenicity was observed in studies in rats, rabbits, or dogs, although, with the exception of one rabbit study, the highest dosage was only two times the maximum recommended human dose and in some studies it was below this dose. Perinatal studies have shown renal papillary abnormalities in offspring of rats treated from midpregnancy with doses of 0.6 and 1.8 mg/kg, doses which approximate the usual human dose, but which are considerably below the maximum recommended human dose.
Nursing Mothers: The extent of the excretion of LOXITANE or its metabolites in human milk is not known. However, LOXITANE and its metabolites have been shown to be transported into the milk of lactating dogs. LOXITANE *loxapine* administration to nursing women should be avoided if clinically possible.
Usage in Children: Studies have not been performed in children; therefore, this drug is not recommended for use in children below the age of 16.

ADVERSE REACTIONS

CNS Effects: Manifestations of adverse effects on the central nervous system, other than extrapyramidal effects, have been seen infrequently. Drowsiness, usually mild, may occur at the beginning of therapy or when dosage is increased. It usually subsides with continued LOXITANE therapy. The incidence of sedation has been less than that of certain aliphatic phenothiazines and slightly more than the piperazine phenothiazines. Dizziness, faintness, staggering gait, shuffling gait, muscle twitching, weakness, insomnia, agitation, tension, seizures, akinesia, slurred speech, numbness and confusional states have been reported. Neuroleptic malignant syndrome (NMS) has been reported (see **WARNINGS**).
Extrapyramidal Reactions: Neuromuscular (extrapyramidal) reactions during the administration of LOXITANE *loxapine* have been reported frequently, often during the first few days of treatment. In most patients, these reactions involved parkinsonian-like symptoms such as tremor, rigidity, excessive salivation, and masked facies. Akathisia (motor restlessness) also has been reported relatively frequently. These symptoms are usually not severe and can be controlled by reduction of LOXITANE dosage or by administration of antiparkinson drugs in usual dosage. Dystonic and dyskinetic reactions have occurred less frequently, but may be more severe. Dystonias include spasms of muscles of the neck and face, tongue protrusion, and oculogyric movement. Dyskinetic reactions have been described in the form of choreoathetoid movements. These reactions sometimes require reduction or temporary withdrawal of loxapine dosage in addition to appropriate counteractive drugs.
Persistent Tardive Dyskinesia: As with all antipsychotic agents, tardive dyskinesia may appear in some patients on long-term therapy or may appear after drug therapy has been discontinued. The risk appears to be greater in elderly patients on high-dose therapy, especially females. The symptoms are persistent and in some patients appear to be irreversible. The syndrome is characterized by rhythmical involuntary movement of the tongue, face, mouth, or jaw (eg, protrusion of tongue, puffing of cheeks, puckering of mouth, chewing movements). Sometimes these may be accompanied by involuntary movements of extremities.
There is no known effective treatment for tardive dyskinesia; antiparkinson agents usually do not alleviate the symptoms of this syndrome. It is suggested that all antipsychotic agents be discontinued if these symptoms appear. Should it be necessary to reinstitute treatment, or increase the dosage of the agent, or switch to a different antipsychotic agent, the syndrome may be masked. It has been suggested that fine vermicular movements of the tongue may be an early sign of the syndrome, and if the medication is stopped at that time the syndrome may not develop.
Cardiovascular Effects: Tachycardia, hypotension, hypertension, orthostatic hypotension, lightheadedness, and syncope have been reported.
A few cases of ECG changes similar to those seen with phenothiazines have been reported. It is not known whether these were related to LOXITANE *loxapine* administration.
Hematologic: Rarely, agranulocytosis, thrombocytopenia, leukopenia.
Skin: Dermatitis, edema (puffiness of face), pruritus, rash, alopecia and seborrhea have been reported with loxapine.
Anticholinergic Effects: Dry mouth, nasal congestion, constipation, blurred vision, urinary retention and paralytic ileus have occurred.
Gastrointestinal: Nausea and vomiting have been reported in some patients. Hepatocellular injury (ie, SGOT/SGPT elevation) has been reported in association with loxapine administration and, rarely, jaundice and/or hepatitis questionably related to LOXITANE treatment.
Other Adverse Reactions: Weight gain, weight loss, dyspnea, ptosis, hyperpyrexia, flushed facies, headache, paresthesia, and polydipsia have been reported in some patients. Rarely, galactorrhea, amenorrhea, gynecomastia and menstrual irregularity of uncertain etiology have been reported.

DOSAGE AND ADMINISTRATION

LOXITANE is administered, usually in divided doses, two to four times a day. Daily dosage (in terms of base equivalents) should be adjusted to the individual patient's needs as assessed by the severity of symptoms and previous history of response to antipsychotic drugs.
Oral Administration: Initial dosage of 10 mg twice daily is recommended, although in severely disturbed patients initial dosage up to a total of 50 mg daily may be desirable. Dosage should then be increased fairly rapidly over the first 7 to 10 days until there is effective control of psychotic symptoms. The usual therapeutic and maintenance range is 60 to 100 mg daily. However, as with other antipsychotic drugs, some patients respond to lower dosage and others require higher dosage for optimal benefit. Daily dosage higher than 250 mg is not recommended.
LOXITANE C Oral Concentrate should be mixed with orange or grapefruit juice shortly before administration. Use only the enclosed calibrated (10 mg, 15 mg, 25 mg, 50 mg) dropper for dosage.
Maintenance Therapy: For maintenance therapy, dosage should be reduced to the lowest level compatible with symptom control; many patients have been maintained satisfactorily at dosages in the range of 20 to 60 mg daily.
Intramuscular Administration: LOXITANE IM is utilized for prompt symptomatic control in the acutely agitated patient and in patients whose symptoms render oral medication temporarily impractical. During clinical trial there were only rare reports of significant local tissue reaction.
LOXITANE IM is administered by intramuscular (not intravenous) injection in doses of 12.5 mg ($\frac{1}{4}$ mL) to 50 mg (1 mL) at intervals of 4 to 6 hours or longer, both dose and interval depending on patient response. Many patients have responded satisfactorily to twice-daily dosage. As described above for oral administration, attention is directed to the necessity for dosage adjustment on an individual basis over the early days of loxapine administration.
Once the desired symptomatic control is achieved and the patient is able to take medication orally, loxapine should be administered in capsule or oral concentrate form. Usually this should occur within 5 days.

OVERDOSAGE

Signs and symptoms of overdosage will depend on the amount ingested and individual patient tolerance. As would be expected from the pharmacologic actions of the drug, the clinical findings may range from mild depression of the CNS and cardiovascular systems to profound hypotension, respiratory depression, and unconsciousness. The possibility of occurrence of extrapyramidal symptoms and/or convulsive seizures should be kept in mind. Renal failure following loxapine overdosage has also been reported.
The treatment of overdosage is essentially symptomatic and supportive. Early gastric lavage and extended dialysis might be expected to be beneficial. Centrally acting emetics may have little effect because of the antiemetic action of loxapine. In addition, emesis should be avoided because of the possibility of aspiration of vomitus. Avoid analeptics, such as pentylenetetrazol, which may cause convulsions. Severe hypotension might be expected to respond to the administration of levarterenol or phenylephrine. EPINEPHRINE SHOULD NOT BE USED SINCE ITS USE IN A PATIENT WITH PARTIAL ADRENERGIC BLOCKADE MAY FURTHER LOWER THE BLOOD PRESSURE. Severe extrapyramidal reactions should be treated with anticholinergic antiparkinson agents or diphenhydramine hydrochloride, and anticonvulsant therapy should be initiated as indicated. Additional measures include oxygen and intravenous fluids.

HOW SUPPLIED

LOXITANE *loxapine succinate* capsules are available in the following base equivalent strengths:
5 mg—Hard shell, opaque, dark green capsules, printed with Lederle over L1 on one half and 5 mg on the other, are supplied as follows:
NDC 0005-5359-23—Bottle of 100
NDC 0005-5359-60—Unit Dose 10 (2 × 5) strips
10 mg—Hard shell, opaque, with yellow body and a dark green cap, printed with Lederle over L2 on one half and 10 mg on the other, are supplied as follows:
NDC 0005-5360-23—Bottle of 100
NDC 0005-5360-34—Bottle of 1000
NDC 0005-5360-60—Unit Dose 10 (2 × 5) strips
25 mg—Hard shell, opaque, with a light green body and a dark green cap, printed with Lederle over L3 on one half and 25 mg on the other, are supplied as follows:
NDC 0005-5361-23—Bottle of 100
NDC 0005-5361-34—Bottle of 1000
NDC 0005-5361-60—Unit Dose 10 (2 × 5) strips
50 mg—Hard shell, opaque, with a blue body and a dark green cap, printed with Lederle over L4 on one half and 50 mg on the other, are supplied as follows:
NDC 0005-5362-23—Bottle of 100
NDC 0005-5362-34—Bottle of 1000
NDC 0005-5362-60—Unit Dose 10 (2 × 5) strips
Store at Controlled Room Temperature 15°–30° C (59°–86° F).
LOXITANE C *loxapine hydrochloride* Oral Concentrate is supplied as follows:
NDC 0005-5387-58—4 fl oz (120 mL) with calibrated dropper. Each mL contains loxapine HCl equivalent to 25 mg of loxapine base.
Store at Controlled Room Temperature 15°–30° C (59°–86° F).
DO NOT FREEZE.
LOXITANE loxapine succinate Capsules
VA Depot:
NSN 6505-01-048-3719—25 mg (1000s)
NSN 6505-01-048-3718—50 mg (1000s)
LOXITANE C loxapine hydrochloride Oral Concentrate For Oral Use
VA Depot:
NSN 6505-01-026-0101—25 mg/mL (4 oz)
LEDERLE LABORATORIES DIVISION
American Cyanamid Company
Pearl River, NY 10965
LOXITANE IM for Intramuscular use only is supplied as follows:

NDC 0205-5385-55—sterile 10—1 mL ampul
NDC 0205-5385-34—10 mL multidose vial
Each mL contains loxapine HCl equivalent to 50 mg of loxapine base.
Keep package closed to protect from light. Intensification of the straw color to a light amber will not alter potency or therapeutic efficacy; if noticeably discolored, ampul or vial should not be used.
Store at Controlled Room Temperature 15°-30° C (59°-86° F).
DO NOT FREEZE.
LEDERLE PARENTERALS, INC.
Carolina, Puerto Rico 00630 Rev. 1/90
23012

Shown in Product Identification Section, page 415

MATERNA® ℞
[*ma-ter-na*]
Enhanced Formula
Prenatal Vitamin and
Mineral Tablets

Each tablet contains:	For Pregnant or Lactating Women Percentage of U.S. Recommended Daily Allowance (U.S. RDA)	
Vitamin A (as Acetate)	5,000 I.U.	(62.5%)
Vitamin D	400 I.U.	(100%)
Vitamin E (as *dl*-Alpha Tocopheryl Acetate)	30 I.U.	(100%)
Vitamin C (Ascorbic Acid)	100 mg	(167%)
Folic Acid	1 mg	(125%)
Vitamin B_1 (as Thiamine Mononitrate)	3 mg	(224%)
Vitamin B_2 (as Riboflavin)	3.4 mg	(170%)
Vitamin B_6 (as Pyridoxine Hydrochloride)	10 mg	(400%)
Niacinamide	20 mg	(100%)
Vitamin B_{12} (Cyanocobalamin)	12 mcg	(150%)
Biotin	30 mcg	(10%)
Pantothenic Acid (as Calcium Pantothenate)	10 mg	(100%)
Calcium (as Calcium Carbonate)	250 mg	(19%)
Iodine (as Potassium Iodide)	150 mcg	(100%)
Iron (as Ferrous Fumarate)	60 mg	(333%)
Magnesium (as Magnesium Oxide)	25 mg	(6%)
Copper (as Cupric Oxide)	2 mg	(100%)
Zinc (as Zinc Oxide)	25 mg	(167%)
Chromium (as Chromium Chloride)	25 mcg*	
Molybdenum (as Sodium Molybdate)	25 mcg*	
Manganese (as Manganese Sulfate)	5 mg*	

*Recognized as essential in human nutrition, but no U.S. RDA established.

Inactive Ingredients: Gelatin, Hydrolyzed Protein, Hydroxypropyl Methylcellulose, Lactose, Magnesium Stearate, Methylparaben, Modified Food Starch, Mono- and Di-glycerides, Polacrilin, Potassium Sorbate, Povidone, Propylparaben, Silica Gel, Sodium Benzoate, Sodium Lauryl Sulfate, Sodium Starch Glycolate, Sorbic Acid, Stearic Acid, Sucrose, and Titanium Dioxide.
Contains no Color or Dyes from Artificial Sources.
CAUTION: Federal law prohibits dispensing without prescription.
RECOMMENDED INTAKE: 1 daily with or without food or as prescribed by physician.
WARNING: Keep out of the reach of children.
Notice: Contact with moisture may produce surface discoloration or erosion of the tablet.
PRECAUTION: Folic Acid may obscure pernicious anemia in that the peripheral blood picture may revert to normal while neurological manifestations remain progressive.
Allergic sensitization has been reported following both oral and parenteral administration of Folic Acid.
Store at Controlled Room Temperature 15°-30°C (59°-86°F).

HOW SUPPLIED
Bottles of 100.
NDC 0005-5560-23
PATENTED Made in USA
U.S. Pat. No. 4,431,634
©1986
LEDERLE LABORATORIES DIVISION
American Cyanamid Company
Pearl River, NY 10965
Rev. 11/88
23967

Shown in Product Identification Section, page 415

MAXZIDE® and MAXZIDE®-25 MG Tablets ℞
Triamterene/Hydrochlorothiazide

PRODUCT OVERVIEW

KEY FACTS

MAXZIDE is a potassium-sparing diuretic, antihypertensive product. MAXZIDE delivers optimally bioavailable doses of both hydrochlorothiazide and triamterene in an optimal ratio of HCTZ to TMT for potassium-sparing action.

MAJOR USES

This fixed combination drug is indicated for the following: (1) the treatment of hypertension or edema in patients who develop hypokalemia on hydrochlorothiazide alone; (2) those patients who require a thiazide diuretic and in whom the development of hypokalemia cannot be risked.
MAXZIDE may be used alone or in combination with other antihypertensive drugs such as beta blockers. Since MAXZIDE may enhance the actions of these drugs, dosage adjustments may be necessary.
Use caution when used concomitantly with ACE inhibitors due to the possibility of hyperkalemia. (See **SAFETY INFORMATION.**)

SAFETY INFORMATION

MAXZIDE should not be used in the presence of elevated serum potassium levels (greater than or equal to 5.5 mEq/liter). Hyperkalemia is more likely to occur in patients with renal impairment, diabetes (even without evidence of renal impairment), and elderly or severely ill patients. Since uncorrected hyperkalemia may be fatal, serum potassium levels must be monitored at frequent intervals, especially in patients first receiving MAXZIDE, when dosages are changed, or with any illness that may influence renal function. Avoid potassium-conserving therapy in severely ill patients in whom respiratory or metabolic acidosis may occur. Acidosis may be associated with rapid elevations in serum potassium levels. If MAXZIDE is employed, frequent evaluation of acid balance and serum electrolytes are necessary. (See full **PRESCRIBING INFORMATION.**) If hyperkalemia develops, discontinue drug and substitute a thiazide alone. MAXZIDE should not be given to patients receiving other potassium-conserving agents, potassium containing salt substitutes, or potassium-enriched diets. Because of the potassium-sparing properties of angiotensin-converting enzyme (ACE) inhibitors, use MAXZIDE cautiously, if at all, with these agents.

PRESCRIBING INFORMATION

MAXZIDE® and MAXZIDE®-25 MG Tablets
Triamterene/Hydrochlorothiazide

DESCRIPTION

MAXZIDE combines triamterene, a potassium-conserving diuretic, with the natriuretic agent, hydrochlorothiazide. Each MAXZIDE tablet contains triamterene, USP, 75 mg and hydrochlorothiazide, USP, 50 mg. Each MAXZIDE-25 MG tablet contains triamterene, USP, 37.5 mg and hydrochlorothiazide, USP, 25 mg.
MAXZIDE and MAXZIDE-25 MG tablets for oral administration contain the following inactive ingredients: Colloidal Silicon Dioxide, Croscarmellose Sodium, Magnesium Stearate, Microcrystalline Cellulose, Powdered Cellulose, Sodium Lauryl Sulfate, and D&C Yellow #10. MAXZIDE-25 MG tablets also contain FD&C Blue #1.
Triamterene is 2,4,7-triamino-6-phenylpteridine. Triamterene is practically insoluble in water, benzene, chloroform, ether and dilute alkali hydroxides. It is soluble in formic acid and sparingly soluble in methoxyethanol. Triamterene is very slightly soluble in acetic acid, alcohol and dilute mineral acids. Its molecular weight is 253.27.
Hydrochlorothiazide is 6-chloro-3,4-dihydro-2*H*-1,2,4, benzothiadiazine-7-sulfonamide 1, 1-dioxide. Hydrochlorothiazide is slightly soluble in water and freely soluble in sodium hydroxide solution, n-butylamine and dimethylformamide. It is sparingly soluble in methanol and insoluble in ether, chloroform and dilute mineral acids. Its molecular weight is 297.73.

CLINICAL PHARMACOLOGY

MAXZIDE *triamterene/hydrochlorothiazide* is a diuretic, antihypertensive drug product, principally due to its hydrochlorothiazide component; the triamterene component of MAXZIDE reduces the excessive potassium loss which may occur with hydrochlorothiazide use.
Hydrochlorothiazide: Hydrochlorothiazide is a diuretic and antihypertensive agent. It blocks the renal tubular absorption of sodium and chloride ions. This natriuresis and diuresis is accompanied by a secondary loss of potassium and bicarbonate. Onset of hydrochlorothiazide's diuretic effect occurs within 2 hours and the peak action takes place in 4 hours. Diuretic activity persists for approximately 6 to 12 hours.
The exact mechanism of hydrochlorothiazide's antihypertensive action is not known although it may relate to the excretion and redistribution of body sodium. Hydrochlorothiazide does not affect normal blood pressure.
Following oral administration, peak hydrochlorothiazide plasma levels are attained in approximately 2 hours. It is excreted rapidly and unchanged in the urine.
Well-controlled studies have demonstrated that doses of hydrochlorothiazide as low as 25 mg given once daily are effective in treating hypertension, but the dose response has not been clearly established.
Triamterene: Triamterene is a potassium-conserving (antikaliuretic) diuretic with relatively weak natriuretic properties. It exerts its diuretic effect on the distal renal tubule to inhibit the reabsorption of sodium in exchange for potassium and hydrogen. With this action, triamterene increases sodium excretion and reduces the excessive loss of potassium and hydrogen associated with hydrochlorothiazide. Triamterene is not a competitive antagonist of the mineralocorticoids and its potassium-conserving effect is observed in patients with Addison's disease, ie, without aldosterone. Triamterene's onset and duration of activity is similar to hydrochlorothiazide. No predictable antihypertensive effect has been demonstrated with triamterene.
Triamterene is rapidly absorbed following oral administration. Peak plasma levels are achieved within 1 hour after dosing. Triamterene is primarily metabolized to the sulfate conjugate of hydroxytriamterene. Both the plasma and urine levels of this metabolite greatly exceed triamterene levels.
The amount of triamterene added to 50 mg of hydrochlorothiazide in MAXZIDE tablets was determined from steady-state dose response evaluations in which various doses of liquid preparations of triamterene were administered to hypertensive persons who developed hypokalemia with hydrochlorothiazide (50 mg given once daily). Single daily doses of 75 mg triamterene resulted in greater increases in serum potassium than lower doses (25 mg and 50 mg), while doses greater than 75 mg of triamterene resulted in no additional elevations in serum potassium levels. The amount of triamterene added to the 25 mg of hydrochlorothiazide in MAXZIDE-25 MG tablets was also determined from steady-state dose response evaluations in which various doses of liquid preparations of triamterene were administered to hypertensive persons who developed hypokalemia with hydrochlorothiazide (25 mg given once daily). Single daily doses of 37.5 mg triamterene resulted in greater increases in serum potassium than a lower dose (25 mg), while doses greater than 37.5 mg of triamterene, ie, 75 mg and 100 mg, resulted in no additional elevations in serum potassium levels. The dose response relationship of triamterene was also evaluated in patients rendered hypokalemic by hydrochlorothiazide given 25 mg twice daily. Triamterene given twice daily increased serum potassium levels in a dose-related fashion. However, the combination of triamterene and hydrochlorothiazide given twice daily also appeared to produce an increased frequency of elevation in serum BUN and creatinine levels. The largest increases in serum potassium, BUN and creatinine in this study were observed with 50 mg of triamterene given twice daily, the largest dose tested. Ordinarily, triamterene does not entirely compensate for the kaliuretic effect of hydrochlorothiazide and some patients may remain hypokalemic while receiving triamterene and hydrochlorothiazide. In some individuals, however, it may induce hyperkalemia (see **WARNINGS**).
The triamterene and hydrochlorothiazide components of MAXZIDE and MAXZIDE-25 MG are well absorbed and are bioequivalent to liquid preparations of the individual components administered orally. Food does not influence the absorption of triamterene or hydrochlorothiazide from MAXZIDE or MAXZIDE-25 MG tablets. The hydrochlorothiazide component of MAXZIDE is bioequivalent to single-entity hydrochlorothiazide tablet formulations.

INDICATIONS AND USAGE

This fixed combination drug is not indicated for the initial therapy of edema or hypertension except in individuals in whom the development of hypokalemia cannot be risked.

1. MAXZIDE *triamterene/hydrochlorothiazide* is indicated for the treatment of hypertension or edema in patients who develop hypokalemia on hydrochlorothiazide alone.
2. MAXZIDE is also indicated for those patients who require a thiazide diuretic and in whom the development of hypokalemia cannot be risked (eg, patients on concomitant digitalis preparations, or with a history of cardiac arrhythmias, etc).

MAXZIDE may be used alone or in combination with other antihypertensive drugs such as beta blockers. Since

Continued on next page

Information on Lederle products listed on these pages is the full prescribing information from product literature or package inserts effective in August 1992. Information concerning all Lederle products may be obtained from the Professional Services Department, Lederle Laboratories, Pearl River, New York 10965.

Lederle—Cont.

MAXZIDE may enhance the actions of these drugs, dosage adjustments may be necessary.

Usage in Pregnancy: The routine use of diuretics in an otherwise healthy woman is inappropriate and exposes mother and fetus to unnecessary hazard. Diuretics do not prevent development of toxemia of pregnancy, and there is no satisfactory evidence that they are useful in the treatment of developed toxemia.

Edema during pregnancy may arise from pathological causes or from the physiologic and mechanical consequences of pregnancy. Thiazides are indicated in pregnancy when edema is due to pathologic causes, just as they are in absence of pregnancy. Dependent edema in pregnancy, resulting from restriction of venous return by the expanded uterus, is properly treated through elevation of the lower extremities and use of support hose; use of diuretics to lower intravascular volume in this case is illogical and unnecessary. There is hypervolemia during normal pregnancy which is harmful to neither the fetus nor the mother (in the absence of cardiovascular disease), but which is associated with edema, including generalized edema, in the majority of pregnant women. If this edema produces discomfort, increased recumbency will often provide relief. In rare instances, this edema may cause extreme discomfort which is not relieved by rest. In these cases, a short course of diuretics may provide relief and may be appropriate.

CONTRAINDICATIONS

Hyperkalemia: MAXZIDE *triamterene/hydrochlorothiazide* should not be used in the presence of elevated serum potassium levels (greater than or equal to 5.5 mEq/liter). If hyperkalemia develops, this drug should be discontinued and a thiazide alone should be substituted.

Antikaliuretic Therapy or Potassium Supplementation: MAXZIDE should not be given to patients receiving other potassium-conserving agents such as spironolactone, amiloride HCl or other formulations containing triamterene. Concomitant potassium supplementation in the form of medication, potassium-containing salt substitute or potassium-enriched diets should also not be used.

Impaired Renal Function: MAXZIDE is contraindicated in patients with anuria, acute and chronic renal insufficiency or significant renal impairment.

Hypersensitivity: MAXZIDE should not be used in patients who are hypersensitive to triamterene or hydrochlorothiazide or other sulfonamide-derived drugs.

WARNINGS

Hyperkalemia: Abnormal elevation of serum potassium levels (greater than or equal to 5.5 mEq/liter) can occur with all potassium-conserving diuretic combinations, including MAXZIDE. Hyperkalemia is more likely to occur in patients with renal impairment, diabetes (even without evidence of renal impairment), or elderly or severely ill patients. Since uncorrected hyperkalemia may be fatal, serum potassium levels must be monitored at frequent intervals, especially in patients first receiving MAXZIDE, when dosages are changed, or with any illness that may influence renal function.

If hyperkalemia is suspected (warning signs include paresthesias, muscular weakness, fatigue, flaccid paralysis of the extremities, bradycardia, and shock), an electrocardiogram (ECG) should be obtained. However, it is important to monitor serum potassium levels because mild hyperkalemia may not be associated with ECG changes.

If hyperkalemia is present, MAXZIDE should be discontinued immediately and a thiazide alone should be substituted. If the serum potassium exceeds 6.5 mEq/liter, more vigorous therapy is required. The clinical situation dictates the procedures to be employed. These include the intravenous administration of calcium chloride solution, sodium bicarbonate solution and/or the oral or parenteral administration of glucose with a rapid-acting insulin preparation. Cationic exchange resins such as sodium polystyrene sulfonate may be orally or rectally administered. Persistent hyperkalemia may require dialysis.

The development of hyperkalemia associated with potassium-sparing diuretics is accentuated in the presence of renal impairment (see **CONTRAINDICATIONS**). Patients with mild renal functional impairment should not receive this drug without frequent and continuing monitoring of serum electrolytes. Cumulative drug effects may be observed in patients with impaired renal function. The renal clearances of hydrochlorothiazide and the pharmacologically active metabolite of triamterene, the sulfate ester of hydroxytriamterene, have been shown to be reduced and the plasma levels increased following MAXZIDE administration to elderly patients and patients with impaired renal function.

Hyperkalemia has been reported in diabetic patients with the use of potassium-conserving agents even in the ab-

---

sence of apparent renal impairment. Accordingly, MAXZIDE *triamterene/hydrochlorothiazide* should be avoided in diabetic patients. If it is employed, serum electrolytes must be frequently monitored.

Because of the potassium-sparing properties of angiotensin-converting enzyme (ACE) inhibitors, MAXZIDE should be used cautiously, if at all, with these agents (see **PRECAUTIONS, Drug Interactions**).

Metabolic or Respiratory Acidosis: Potassium-conserving therapy should also be avoided in severely ill patients in whom respiratory or metabolic acidosis may occur. Acidosis may be associated with rapid elevations in serum potassium levels. If MAXZIDE is employed, frequent evaluations of acid/base balance and serum electrolytes are necessary.

PRECAUTIONS

General: Electrolyte Imbalance and BUN Increases: Patients receiving MAXZIDE should be carefully monitored for fluid or electrolyte imbalances, ie, hyponatremia, hypochloremic alkalosis, hypokalemia, and hypomagnesemia. Determination of serum electrolytes to detect possible electrolyte imbalance should be performed at appropriate intervals. Serum and urine electrolyte determinations are especially important and should be frequently performed when the patient is vomiting or receiving parenteral fluids. Warning signs or symptoms of fluid and electrolyte imbalance include: dryness of mouth, thirst, weakness, lethargy, drowsiness, restlessness, muscle pains or cramps, muscular fatigue, hypotension, oliguria, tachycardia and gastrointestinal disturbances such as nausea and vomiting.

Any chloride deficit during thiazide therapy is generally mild and usually does not require any specific treatment except under extraordinary circumstances (as in liver disease or renal disease). Dilutional hyponatremia may occur in edematous patients in hot weather; appropriate therapy is water restriction, rather than administration of salt, except in rare instances when the hyponatremia is life threatening. In actual salt depletion, appropriate replacement is the therapy of choice.

Hypokalemia may develop with thiazide therapy, especially with brisk diuresis, when severe cirrhosis is present, or during concomitant use of corticosteroids, ACTH, amphotericin B or after prolonged thiazide therapy. However, hypokalemia of this type is usually prevented by the triamterene component of MAXZIDE.

Interference with adequate oral electrolyte intake will also contribute to hypokalemia. Hypokalemia can sensitize or exaggerate the response of the heart to the toxic effects of digitalis (eg, increased ventricular irritability).

MAXZIDE *triamterene/hydrochlorothiazide* may produce an elevated blood urea nitrogen level (BUN), creatinine level or both. This is probably not the result of renal toxicity but is secondary to a reversible reduction of the glomerular filtration rate or a depletion of the intravascular fluid volume. Elevations in BUN and creatinine levels may be more frequent in patients receiving divided dose diuretic therapy. Periodic BUN and creatinine determinations should be made especially in elderly patients, patients with suspected or confirmed hepatic disease or renal insufficiencies. If azotemia increases, MAXZIDE should be discontinued.

Thiazide diuretics have been shown to increase the urinary excretion of magnesium; this may result in hypomagnesemia.

Hepatic Coma: MAXZIDE should be used with caution in patients with impaired hepatic function or progressive liver disease, since minor alterations of fluid and electrolyte balance may precipitate hepatic coma.

Renal Stones: Triamterene has been reported in renal stones in association with other calculus components. MAXZIDE should be used with caution in patients with histories of renal lithiasis.

Folic Acid Deficiency: Triamterene is a weak folic acid antagonist and may contribute to the appearance of megaloblastosis in instances where folic acid stores are decreased. In such patients, periodic blood evaluations are recommended.

Hyperuricemia: Hyperuricemia may occur or acute gout may be precipitated in certain patients receiving thiazide therapy.

Metabolic and Endocrine Effects: The thiazides may decrease serum PBI levels without signs of thyroid disturbance.

Calcium excretion is decreased by thiazides. Pathological changes in the parathyroid gland with hypercalcemia and hypophosphatemia have been observed in a few patients on prolonged thiazide therapy. The common complications of hyperparathyroidism such as renal lithiasis, bone resorption, and peptic ulceration have not been seen. Thiazides should be discontinued before carrying out tests for parathyroid function.

Insulin requirements in diabetic patients may be increased, decreased or unchanged. Diabetes mellitus which has been latent may become manifest during thiazide administration.

Hypersensitivity: Sensitivity reactions to thiazides may occur in patients with or without a history of allergy or bronchial asthma.

Possible exacerbation or activation of systemic lupus erythematosus by thiazides has been reported.

Drug Interactions: Thiazides may add to or potentiate the action of other antihypertensive drugs.

The thiazides may decrease arterial responsiveness to norepinephrine. This diminution is not sufficient to preclude effectiveness of the pressor agent for therapeutic use. Thiazides have also been shown to increase responsiveness to tubocurarine.

Lithium generally should not be given with diuretics because they reduce its renal clearance and add a high risk of lithium toxicity. Refer to the package insert on lithium before use of such concomitant therapy.

Acute renal failure has been reported in a few patients receiving indomethacin and formulations containing triamterene and hydrochlorothiazide. Caution is therefore advised when administering nonsteroidal anti-inflammatory agents with MAXZIDE *triamterene/hydrochlorothiazide.*

Potassium-sparing agents should be used very cautiously, if at all, in conjunction with angiotensin-converting enzyme (ACE) inhibitors due to a greatly increased risk of hyperkalemia. Serum potassium should be monitored frequently.

Drug/Laboratory Test Interactions: Triamterene and quinidine have similar fluorescence spectra; thus MAXZIDE may interfere with the measurement of quinidine.

Carcinogenesis, Mutagenesis, Impairment of Fertility
Studies have not been performed to evaluate the mutagenic or carcinogenic potential of MAXZIDE.

Hydrochlorothiazide
Two-year feeding studies in mice and rats conducted under the auspices of the National Toxicology Program (NTP) uncovered no evidence of a carcinogenic potential of hydrochlorothiazide in female mice (at doses of up to approximately 600 mg/kg/day) or in male and female rats (at doses of up to approximately 100 mg/kg/day). The NTP, however, found equivocal evidence for hepatocarcinogenicity in male mice. Hydrochlorothiazide was not genotoxic in *in vitro* assays using strains TA 98, TA 100, TA 1535, TA 1537 and TA 1538 of *Salmonella typhimurium* (Ames assay) and in the Chinese Hamster Ovary (CHO) test for chromosomal aberrations, or in *in vivo* assays using mouse germinal cell chromosomes, Chinese hamster bone marrow chromosomes, and the *Drosophila* sex-linked recessive lethal trait gene. Positive test results were obtained only in the *in vitro* CHO Sister Chromatid Exchange (clastogenicity) and in the Mouse Lymphoma Cell (mutagenicity) assays, using concentrations of hydrochlorothiazide from 43 to 1300 µg/mL, and in the *Aspergillus nidulans* non-disjunction assay at an unspecified concentration.

Hydrochlorothiazide had no adverse effects on the fertility of mice and rats of either sex in studies wherein these species were exposed, via their diet, to doses of up to 100 and 4 mg/kg, respectively, prior to conception and throughout gestation.

Triamterene
Studies have not been performed to determine the carcinogenic or mutagenic potential of triamterene. Reproductive studies have been performed in rats at doses up to 30 times the human dose and have revealed no evidence of impaired fertility.

Pregnancy Category C
Teratogenic Effects—Animal reproduction studies have not been conducted with MAXZIDE. It is also not known if MAXZIDE can cause fetal harm when administered to a pregnant woman.

Hydrochlorothiazide
Studies in which hydrochlorothiazide was orally administered to pregnant mice and rats during their respective periods of major organogenesis at doses up to 3000 and 1000 mg hydrochlorothiazide/kg, respectively, provided no evidence of harm to the fetus. There are, however, no adequate and well-controlled studies in pregnant women.

Triamterene
Reproduction studies have been performed in rats at doses up to 30 times the human dose and have revealed no evidence of harm to the fetus due to triamterene. There are, however, no adequate and well-controlled studies in pregnant women.

Because animal reproduction studies are not always predictive of human response, MAXZIDE should be used during pregnancy only if clearly needed.

Nonteratogenic Effects
Thiazides and triamterene cross the placental barrier and appear in cord blood of animals. The use of MAXZIDE in pregnant women requires that the anticipated benefit be weighed against possible hazards to the fetus. These hazards include fetal or neonatal jaundice, thrombocytopenia following thiazides and possible other adverse reactions that have occurred in the adults.

Nursing Mothers
Thiazides appear and triamterene may appear in breast milk. If use of the drug product is deemed essential the patient should stop nursing.

Pediatric Use: The safety and effectiveness of MAXZIDE in children have not been established.

ADVERSE REACTIONS

Side effects observed in association with the use of MAXZIDE, other combination products containing triamterene/hydrochlorothiazide, and products containing triamterene or hydrochlorothiazide include the following:

Gastrointestinal: jaundice (intrahepatic cholestatic jaundice), pancreatitis, nausea, appetite disturbance, taste alteration, vomiting, diarrhea, constipation, anorexia, gastric irritation, cramping.

Central Nervous System: drowsiness and fatigue, insomnia, headache, dizziness, dry mouth, depression, anxiety, vertigo, restlessness, paresthesias.

Cardiovascular: tachycardia, shortness of breath and chest pain, orthostatic hypotension (may be aggravated by alcohol, barbiturates or narcotics).

Renal: acute renal failure, acute interstitial nephritis, renal stones composed of triamterene in association with other calculus materials, urine discoloration.

Hematologic: leukopenia, agranulocytosis, thrombocytopenia, aplastic anemia, hemolytic anemia and megaloblastosis.

Ophthalmic: xanthopsia, transient blurred vision.

Hypersensitivity: anaphylaxis, photosensitivity, rash, urticaria, purpura, necrotizing angiitis (vasculitis, cutaneous vasculitis), fever, respiratory distress including pneumonitis.

Other: muscle cramps and weakness, decreased sexual performance and sialadenitis.

Whenever adverse reactions are moderate to severe, therapy should be reduced or withdrawn.

Altered Laboratory Findings:

Serum Electrolytes: hyperkalemia, hypokalemia, hyponatremia, hypomagnesemia, hypochloremia (see **WARNINGS, PRECAUTIONS**).

Creatinine, Blood Urea Nitrogen: Reversible elevations in BUN and serum creatinine have been observed in hypertensive patients treated with MAXZIDE.

Glucose: hyperglycemia, glycosuria and diabetes mellitus (see **PRECAUTIONS**).

Serum Uric Acid, PBI and Calcium: (see **PRECAUTIONS**).

Other: Elevated liver enzymes have been reported in patients receiving MAXZIDE.

OVERDOSAGE

No specific data are available regarding MAXZIDE *triamterene/hydrochlorothiazide* overdosage in humans and no specific antidote is available.

Fluid and electrolyte imbalances are the most important concern. Excessive doses of the triamterene component may elicit hyperkalemia, dehydration, nausea, vomiting and weakness and possibly hypotension. Overdosing with hydrochlorothiazide has been associated with hypokalemia, hypochloremia, hyponatremia, dehydration, lethargy (may progress to coma) and gastrointestinal irritation. Treatment is symptomatic and supportive. Therapy with MAXZIDE should be discontinued. Induce emesis or institute gastric lavage. Monitor serum electrolyte levels and fluid balance. Institute supportive measures as required to maintain hydration, electrolyte balance, respiratory, cardiovascular and renal function.

DOSAGE AND ADMINISTRATION

The usual dose of MAXZIDE-25 MG is one or two tablets daily, given as a single dose, with appropriate monitoring of serum potassium (see **WARNINGS**). The usual dose of MAXZIDE is one tablet daily, with appropriate monitoring of serum potassium (see **WARNINGS**). There is no experience with the use of more than one MAXZIDE tablet daily or more than two MAXZIDE-25 MG tablets daily. Clinical experience with the administration of two MAXZIDE-25 MG tablets daily in divided doses (rather than as a single dose) suggests an increased risk of electrolyte imbalance and renal dysfunction.

Patients receiving 50 mg of hydrochlorothiazide who become hypokalemic may be transferred to MAXZIDE directly. Patients receiving 25 mg hydrochlorothiazide who become hypokalemic may be transferred to MAXZIDE-25 MG (37.5 mg triamterene/25 mg hydrochlorothiazide) directly.

In patients requiring hydrochlorothiazide therapy and in whom hypokalemia cannot be risked, therapy may be initiated with MAXZIDE-25 MG. If an optimal blood pressure response is not obtained with MAXZIDE-25 MG, the dose should be increased to two MAXZIDE-25 MG tablets daily as a single dose, or one MAXZIDE tablet daily. If blood pressure still is not controlled, another antihypertensive agent may be added (see **PRECAUTIONS, Drug Interactions**).

Clinical studies have shown that patients taking less bioavailable formulations of triamterene and hydrochlorothiazide in daily doses of 25 to 50 mg hydrochlorothiazide and 50 to 100 mg triamterene may be safely changed to one MAXZIDE-25 MG tablet daily. All patients changed from less bioavailable formulations to MAXZIDE should be monitored clinically and for serum potassium after the transfer.

HOW SUPPLIED

MAXZIDE *triamterene/hydrochlorothiazide* tablets are bowtie-shaped, flat-faced beveled, light yellow tablets, engraved with MAXZIDE on one side and scored on the other with LL on the left and M8 on the right of the score. Each tablet contains 75 mg of triamterene, USP and 50 mg of hydrochlorothiazide, USP. They are supplied as follows:

NDC 0005-4460-43—Bottle of 100 with CRC
NDC 0005-4460-31—Bottle of 500
NDC 0005-4460-60—Unit Dose 10 × 10s

MAXZIDE-25 MG tablets are bowtie-shaped, flat-faced beveled, light green tablets, engraved with MAXZIDE on one side and scored on the other with LL on the left and M9 on the right of the score. Each tablet contains 37.5 mg of triamterene, USP and 25 mg hydrochlorothiazide, USP. They are supplied as follows:

NDC 0005-4464-43—Bottle of 100 with CRC
NDC 0005-4464-60—Unit Dose 10 × 10s

Store at Controlled Room Temperature 15°–30°C (59°–86°F). Protect From Light.

Dispense in a tight, light-resistant, child-resistant container.

Triamterene 37.5 mg/Hydrochlorothiazide 25 mg
Military Depot:
NSN 6505-01-290-2999—(100s)
Manufactured for
LEDERLE LABORATORIES DIVISION
American Cyanamid Company, Pearl River, NY 10965
by
MYLAN PHARMACEUTICALS, INC.
Morgantown, WV 26505

Rev. 7/92
22157-92

Shown in Product Identification Section, page 415

METHOTREXATE Sodium Tablets℞
METHOTREXATE Sodium for Injection℞
METHOTREXATE LPF® Sodium (METHOTREXATE Sodium Injection) and℞
METHOTREXATE Sodium Injection℞

WARNINGS

METHOTREXATE SHOULD BE USED ONLY BY PHYSICIANS WHOSE KNOWLEDGE AND EXPERIENCE INCLUDES THE USE OF ANTIMETABOLITE THERAPY.

THE USE OF METHOTREXATE HIGH-DOSE REGIMENS RECOMMENDED FOR OSTEOSARCOMA REQUIRES METICULOUS CARE (see **DOSAGE AND ADMINISTRATION**). HIGH-DOSAGE REGIMENS FOR OTHER NEOPLASTIC DISEASES ARE INVESTIGATIONAL AND A THERAPEUTIC ADVANTAGE HAS NOT BEEN ESTABLISHED.

BECAUSE OF THE POSSIBILITY OF SERIOUS TOXIC REACTIONS, THE PATIENT SHOULD BE INFORMED BY THE PHYSICIAN OF THE RISKS INVOLVED AND SHOULD BE UNDER A PHYSICIAN'S CONSTANT SUPERVISION.

DEATHS HAVE BEEN REPORTED WITH THE USE OF METHOTREXATE IN THE TREATMENT OF MALIGNANCY, PSORIASIS, AND RHEUMATOID ARTHRITIS.

IN THE TREATMENT OF PSORIASIS OR RHEUMATOID ARTHRITIS, METHOTREXATE USE SHOULD BE RESTRICTED TO PATIENTS WITH SEVERE, RECALCITRANT, DISABLING DISEASE, WHICH IS NOT ADEQUATELY RESPONSIVE TO OTHER FORMS OF THERAPY, AND ONLY WHEN THE DIAGNOSIS HAS BEEN ESTABLISHED AND AFTER APPROPRIATE CONSULTATION.

1. Methotrexate has been reported to cause fetal death and/or congenital anomalies. Therefore, it is not recommended for women of childbearing potential unless there is clear medical evidence that the benefits can be expected to outweigh the considered risks. Pregnant patients with psoriasis or rheumatoid arthritis should not receive methotrexate. (See **CONTRAINDICATIONS**.)

2. Periodic monitoring for toxicity, including CBC with differential and platelet counts, and liver and renal function tests is a mandatory part of methotrexate therapy. Periodic liver biopsies may be indicated in some situations. Patients at increased risk for impaired methotrexate elimination (eg, renal dysfunction, pleural effusions, or ascites) should be monitored more frequently. (See **PRECAUTIONS**.)

3. Methotrexate causes hepatotoxicity, fibrosis, and cirrhosis, but generally only after prolonged use. Acutely, liver enzyme elevations are frequently seen; these are usually transient and asymptomatic, and also do not appear predictive of subsequent hepatic disease. Liver biopsy after sustained use often shows histologic changes, and fibrosis and cirrhosis have been reported; these latter lesions often are not preceded by symptoms or abnormal liver function tests. (See **PRECAUTIONS**.)

4. Methotrexate-induced lung disease is a potentially dangerous lesion, which may occur acutely at any time during therapy and which has been reported at doses as low as 7.5 mg/week. It is not always fully reversible. Pulmonary symptoms (especially a dry, nonproductive cough) may require interruption of treatment and careful investigation.

5. Methotrexate may produce marked bone marrow depression, with resultant anemia, leukopenia, and/or thrombocytopenia.

6. Diarrhea and ulcerative stomatitis require interruption of therapy; otherwise, hemorrhagic enteritis and death from intestinal perforation may occur.

7. Methotrexate therapy in patients with impaired renal function should be undertaken with extreme caution, and at reduced dosages, because renal dysfunction will prolong methotrexate elimination.

8. Unexpectedly severe (sometimes fatal) marrow suppression and gastrointestinal toxicity have been reported with concomitant administration of methotrexate (usually in high dosage) along with some nonsteroidal anti-inflammatory drugs (NSAIDs). (See **PRECAUTIONS, Drug Interactions**.)

METHOTREXATE FORMULATIONS AND DILUENTS CONTAINING PRESERVATIVES MUST NOT BE USED FOR INTRATHECAL OR HIGH-DOSE METHOTREXATE THERAPY.

DESCRIPTION

Methotrexate (formerly Amethopterin) is an antimetabolite used in the treatment of certain neoplastic diseases, severe psoriasis, and adult rheumatoid arthritis.

Chemically methotrexate is N-[4-[[(2,4-diamino-6-pteridinyl)-methyl]methylamino]benzoyl]-L-glutamic acid.

Methotrexate Sodium Tablets for oral administration are available in bottles of 100 and in a packaging system designated as the RHEUMATREX® Methotrexate Sodium Dose Pack for therapy with a weekly dosing schedule of 5 mg, 7.5 mg, 10 mg, 12.5 mg, and 15 mg. Methotrexate Sodium Tablets contain an amount of methotrexate sodium equivalent to 2.5 mg of methotrexate and the following inactive ingredients: Lactose, Magnesium Stearate and Pregelatinized Starch. May also contain Corn Starch.

Methotrexate Sodium Injection and for Injection products are sterile and nonpyrogenic and may be given by the intramuscular, intravenous, intra-arterial or intrathecal route. (See **DOSAGE AND ADMINISTRATION**.) However, the preservative formulation contains Benzyl Alcohol and must not be used for intrathecal or high-dose therapy.

Methotrexate Sodium Injection, Isotonic Liquid, Preservative Protected, is available in 25 mg/mL, 2 mL (50 mg), and 10 mL (250 mg) vials.

Each 25 mg/mL, 2 mL, and 10 mL vial contains methotrexate sodium equivalent to 50 mg and 250 mg methotrexate, respectively, 0.90% w/v of Benzyl Alcohol as a preservative, and the following inactive ingredients: Sodium Chloride 0.260% w/v and Water for Injection qs ad 100% v. Sodium Hydroxide and, if necessary, Hydrochloric Acid are added to adjust the pH to approximately 8.5.

Methotrexate LPF® **Sodium (methotrexate sodium injection), Isotonic Liquid, Preservative Free,** for single use only, is available in 25 mg/mL, 2 mL (50 mg), 4 mL (100 mg), 8 mL (200 mg), and 10 mL (250 mg) vials.

Each 25 mg/mL, 2 mL, 4 mL, 8 mL, and 10 mL vial contains methotrexate sodium equivalent to 50 mg, 100 mg, 200 mg, and 250 mg methotrexate, respectively, and the following inactive ingredients: Sodium Chloride 0.490% w/v and Water for Injection qs ad 100% v. Sodium Hydroxide and, if necessary, Hydrochloric Acid are added to adjust the pH to approximately 8.5. The 2 mL, 4 mL, 8 mL, and 10 mL solutions contain approximately 0.43 mEq, 0.86 mEq, 1.72 mEq, and 2.15 mEq of Sodium per vial, respectively, and are isotonic solutions.

Methotrexate Sodium for Injection, Freeze Dried, Preservative Free, Low Sodium, for single use only, is available in 20 mg, 50 mg, and 1 gram vials.

Each low sodium 20 mg, 50 mg, and 1 g vial of cryodesiccated powder contains methotrexate sodium equivalent to 20 mg, 50 mg, and 1 g methotrexate, respectively. Contains no preservative. Sodium Hydroxide and, if necessary, Hydrochloric Acid are added during manufacture to adjust the pH. The 20 mg vial contains approximately 0.14 mEq of Sodium, the 50 mg vial contains approximately 0.33 mEq of Sodium, and the 1 g vial contains approximately 7 mEq Sodium.

Continued on next page

Information on Lederle products listed on these pages is the full prescribing information from product literature or package inserts effective in August 1992. Information concerning all Lederle products may be obtained from the Professional Services Department, Lederle Laboratories, Pearl River, New York 10965.

Lederle—Cont.

CLINICAL PHARMACOLOGY

Methotrexate inhibits dihydrofolic acid reductase. Dihydrofolates must be reduced to tetrahydrofolates by this enzyme before they can be utilized as carriers of one-carbon groups in the synthesis of purine nucleotides and thymidylate. Therefore, methotrexate interferes with DNA synthesis, repair, and cellular replication. Actively proliferating tissues such as malignant cells, bone marrow, fetal cells, buccal and intestinal mucosa, and cells of the urinary bladder are in general more sensitive to this effect of methotrexate. When cellular proliferation in malignant tissues is greater than in most normal tissues, methotrexate may impair malignant growth without irreversible damage to normal tissues.

The mechanism of action in rheumatoid arthritis is unknown; it may affect immune function. Two reports describe *in vitro* methotrexate inhibition of DNA precursor uptake by stimulated mononuclear cells, and another describes, in animal polyarthritis, partial correction by methotrexate of spleen cell hyporesponsiveness and suppressed IL 2 production. Other laboratories, however, have been unable to demonstrate similar effects. Clarification of methotrexate's effect on immune activity and its relation to rheumatoid immunopathogenesis await further studies.

In patients with rheumatoid arthritis, effects of methotrexate on articular swelling and tenderness can be seen as early as 3 to 6 weeks. Although methotrexate clearly ameliorates symptoms of inflammation (pain, swelling, stiffness), there is no evidence that it induces remission of rheumatoid arthritis nor has a beneficial effect been demonstrated on bone erosions and other radiologic changes which result in impaired joint use, functional disability, and deformity.

Most studies of methotrexate in patients with rheumatoid arthritis are relatively short term (3 to 6 months). Limited data from long-term studies indicate that an initial clinical improvement is maintained for at least 2 years with continued therapy.

In psoriasis, the rate of production of epithelial cells in the skin is greatly increased over normal skin. This differential in proliferation rates is the basis for the use of methotrexate to control the psoriatic process.

Methotrexate in high doses, followed by leucovorin rescue, is used as a part of the treatment of patients with nonmetastatic osteosarcoma. The original rationale for high-dose methotrexate therapy was based on the concept of selective rescue of normal tissues by leucovorin. More recent evidence suggests that high-dose methotrexate may also overcome methotrexate resistance caused by impaired active transport, decreased affinity of dihydrofolic acid reductase for methotrexate, increased levels of dihydrofolic acid reductase resulting from gene amplification, or decreased polyglutamation of methotrexate. The actual mechanism of action is unknown.

Two Pediatric Oncology Group studies (one randomized and one nonrandomized) demonstrated a significant improvement in relapse-free survival in patients with nonmetastatic osteosarcoma, when high-dose methotrexate with leucovorin rescue was used in combination with other chemotherapeutic agents following surgical resection of the primary tumor. These studies were not designed to demonstrate the specific contribution of high-dose methotrexate/leucovorin rescue therapy to the efficacy of the combination. However, a contribution can be inferred from the reports of objective responses to this therapy in patients with metastatic osteosarcoma, and from reports of extensive tumor necrosis following preoperative administration of this therapy to patients with nonmetastatic osteosarcoma.

Pharmacokinetics: *Absorption:* In adults, oral absorption appears to be dose dependent. Peak serum levels are reached within 1 to 2 hours. At doses of 30 mg/m^2 or less, methotrexate is generally well absorbed with a mean bioavailability of about 60%. The absorption of doses greater than 80 mg/m^2 is significantly less, possibly due to a saturation effect.

In leukemic children, oral absorption has been reported to vary widely (23% to 95%). A twentyfold difference between highest and lowest peak levels (C_{max}: 0.11 to 2.3 micromolar after a 20 mg/m^2 dose) has been reported. Significant interindividual variability has also been noted in time to peak concentration (T_{max}: 0.67 to 4h after a 15 mg/m^2 dose) and fraction of dose absorbed. Food has been shown to delay absorption and reduce peak concentration.

Methotrexate is generally completely absorbed from parenteral routes of injection. After intramuscular injection, peak serum concentrations occur in 30 to 60 minutes.

Distribution: After intravenous administration, the initial volume of distribution is approximately 0.18 L/kg (18% of body weight) and steady-state volume of distribution is approximately 0.4 to 0.8 L/kg (40% to 80% of body weight). Methotrexate competes with reduced folates for active transport across cell membranes by means of a single carrier-mediated active transport process. At serum concentrations greater than 100 micromolar, passive diffusion becomes a major pathway by which effective intracellular concentrations can be achieved. Methotrexate in serum is approximately 50% protein bound. Laboratory studies demonstrate that it may be displaced from plasma albumin by various compounds including sulfonamides, salicylates, tetracyclines, chloramphenicol, and phenytoin.

Methotrexate does not penetrate the blood-cerebrospinal fluid barrier in therapeutic amounts when given orally or parenterally. High CSF concentrations of the drug may be attained by intrathecal administration.

In dogs, synovial fluid concentrations after oral dosing were higher in inflamed than uninflamed joints. Although salicylates did not interfere with this penetration, prior prednisone treatment reduced penetration into inflamed joints to the level of normal joints.

Metabolism: After absorption, methotrexate undergoes hepatic and intracellular metabolism to polyglutamated forms which can be converted back to methotrexate by hydrolase enzymes. These polyglutamates act as inhibitors of dihydrofolate reductase and thymidylate synthetase. Small amounts of methotrexate polyglutamates may remain in tissues for extended periods. The retention and prolonged drug action of these active metabolites vary among different cells, tissues, and tumors. A small amount of metabolism to 7-hydroxymethotrexate may occur at doses commonly prescribed. Accumulation of this metabolite may become significant at the high doses used in osteogenic sarcoma. The aqueous solubility of 7-hydroxymethotrexate is three- to fivefold lower than the parent compound. Methotrexate is partially metabolized by intestinal flora after oral administration.

Half-Life: The terminal half-life reported for methotrexate is approximately 3 to 10 hours for patients receiving treatment for psoriasis, or rheumatoid arthritis or low-dose antineoplastic therapy (less than 30 mg/m^2). For patients receiving high doses of methotrexate, the terminal half-life is 8 to 15 hours.

Excretion: Renal excretion is the primary route of elimination and is dependent upon dosage and route of administration. With IV administration, 80% to 90% of the administered dose is excreted unchanged in the urine within 24 hours. There is limited biliary excretion amounting to 10% or less of the administered dose. Enterohepatic recirculation of methotrexate has been proposed.

Renal excretion occurs by glomerular filtration and active tubular secretion. Nonlinear elimination due to saturation of renal tubular reabsorption has been observed in psoriatic patients at doses between 7.5 and 30 mg. Impaired renal function, as well as concurrent use of drugs such as weak organic acids that also undergo tubular secretion, can markedly increase methotrexate serum levels. Excellent correlation has been reported between methotrexate clearance and endogenous creatinine clearance.

Methotrexate clearance rates vary widely and are generally decreased at higher doses. Delayed drug clearance has been identified as one of the major factors responsible for methotrexate toxicity. It has been postulated that the toxicity of methotrexate for normal tissues is more dependent upon the duration of exposure to the drug rather than the peak level achieved. When a patient has delayed drug elimination due to compromised renal function, a third-space effusion, or other causes, methotrexate serum concentrations may remain elevated for prolonged periods.

The potential for toxicity from high-dose regimens or delayed excretion is reduced by the administration of leucovorin calcium during the final phase of methotrexate plasma elimination. Pharmacokinetic monitoring of methotrexate serum concentrations may help identify those patients at high risk for methotrexate toxicity and aid in proper adjustment of leucovorin dosing. Guidelines for monitoring serum methotrexate levels, and for adjustment of leucovorin dosing to reduce the risk of methotrexate toxicity, are provided below in **DOSAGE AND ADMINISTRATION.**

Methotrexate has been detected in human breast milk. The highest breast milk to plasma concentration ratio reached was 0.08:1.

INDICATIONS AND USAGE

Neoplastic Diseases: Methotrexate is indicated in the treatment of gestational choriocarcinoma, chorioadenoma destruens, and hydatidiform mole.

In acute lymphocytic leukemia, methotrexate is indicated in the prophylaxis of meningeal leukemia and is used in maintenance therapy in combination with other chemotherapeutic agents. Methotrexate is also indicated in the treatment of meningeal leukemia.

Methotrexate is used alone or in combination with other anticancer agents in the treatment of breast cancer, epidermoid cancers of the head and neck, advanced mycosis fungoides, and lung cancer, particularly squamous cell and small cell types. Methotrexate is also used in combination with other chemotherapeutic agents in the treatment of advanced stage non-Hodgkin's lymphomas.

Methotrexate in high doses followed by leucovorin rescue in combination with other chemotherapeutic agents is effective in prolonging relapse-free survival in patients with nonmetastatic osteosarcoma who have undergone surgical resection or amputation for the primary tumor.

Psoriasis: Methotrexate is indicated in the symptomatic control of severe, recalcitrant, disabling psoriasis that is not adequately responsive to other forms of therapy, *but only when the diagnosis has been established, as by biopsy and/or after dermatologic consultation.* It is important to ensure that a psoriasis "flare" is not due to an undiagnosed concomitant disease affecting immune responses.

Rheumatoid Arthritis: Methotrexate is indicated in the management of selected adults with severe, active, classical, or definite rheumatoid arthritis (ARA criteria) who have had an insufficient therapeutic response to, or are intolerant of, an adequate trial of first-line therapy including full dose NSAIDs and usually a trial of at least one or more disease-modifying antirheumatic drugs.

Aspirin, nonsteroidal anti-inflammatory agents, and/or low-dose steroids may be continued, although the possibility of increased toxicity with concomitant use of NSAIDs including salicylates has not been fully explored (see **PRECAUTIONS, Drug Interactions**). Steroids may be reduced gradually in patients who respond to methotrexate. Combined use of methotrexate with gold, penicillamine, hydroxychloroquine, sulfasalazine, or cytotoxic agents, has not been studied and may increase the incidence of adverse effects. Rest and physiotherapy as indicated should be continued.

CONTRAINDICATIONS

Methotrexate can cause fetal death or teratogenic effects when administered to a pregnant woman. Methotrexate is contraindicated in pregnant patients with psoriasis or rheumatoid arthritis and should be used in the treatment of neoplastic diseases only when the potential benefit outweighs the risk to the fetus. Women of childbearing potential should not be started on methotrexate until pregnancy is excluded and should be fully counseled on the serious risk to the fetus (see **PRECAUTIONS**) should they become pregnant while undergoing treatment. Pregnancy should be avoided if either partner is receiving methotrexate; during and for a minimum of 3 months after therapy for male patients, and during and for at least one ovulatory cycle after therapy for female patients. (See Boxed **WARNINGS.**)

Because of the potential for serious adverse reactions from methotrexate in breast fed infants, it is contraindicated in nursing mothers.

Patients with psoriasis or rheumatoid arthritis with alcoholism, alcoholic liver disease, or other chronic liver disease should not receive methotrexate.

Patients with psoriasis or rheumatoid arthritis who have overt or laboratory evidence of immunodeficiency syndromes should not receive methotrexate.

Patients with psoriasis or rheumatoid arthritis who have preexisting blood dyscrasias, such as bone marrow hypoplasia, leukopenia, thrombocytopenia, or significant anemia, should not receive methotrexate.

Patients with a known hypersensitivity to methotrexate should not receive the drug.

WARNINGS—SEE BOXED WARNINGS.

PRECAUTIONS

General: Methotrexate has the potential for serious toxicity (see Boxed **WARNINGS**). Toxic effects may be related in frequency and severity to dose or frequency of administration but have been seen at all doses. Because they can occur at any time during therapy, it is necessary to follow patients on methotrexate closely. Most adverse reactions are reversible if detected early. When such reactions do occur, the drug should be reduced in dosage or discontinued and appropriate corrective measures should be taken. If necessary, this could include the use of leucovorin calcium (see **OVERDOSAGE**). If methotrexate therapy is reinstituted, it should be carried out with caution, with adequate consideration of further need for the drug, and with increased alertness as to possible recurrence of toxicity.

The clinical pharmacology of methotrexate has not been well studied in older individuals. Due to diminished hepatic and renal function as well as decreased folate stores in this population, relatively low doses should be considered, and these patients should be closely monitored for early signs of toxicity.

Information for Patients: Patients should be informed of the early signs and symptoms of toxicity, of the need to see their physician promptly if they occur, and the need for close follow-up, including periodic laboratory tests to monitor toxicity.

Both the physician and pharmacist should emphasize to the patient that the recommended dose is taken weekly in rheumatoid arthritis and psoriasis, and that mistaken daily use of the recommended dose has led to fatal toxicity. Patients should be encouraged to read the Patient Instructions sheet within the Dose Pack. Prescriptions should not be written or refilled on a PRN basis.

Patients should be informed of the potential benefit and risk in the use of methotrexate. The risk of effects on reproduc-

tion should be discussed with both male and female patients taking methotrexate.

Laboratory Tests: Patients undergoing methotrexate therapy should be closely monitored so that toxic effects are detected promptly. Baseline assessment should include a complete blood count with differential and platelet counts, hepatic enzymes, renal function tests, and a chest X-ray. During therapy of rheumatoid arthritis and psoriasis, monitoring of these parameters is recommended: hematology at least monthly, and liver and renal function every 1 to 3 months. More frequent monitoring is usually indicated during antineoplastic therapy. *During initial or changing doses,* or during periods of increased risk of elevated methotrexate blood levels (eg, dehydration), more frequent monitoring may also be indicated.

A relationship between abnormal liver function tests and fibrosis or cirrhosis of the liver has not been established. Transient liver function test abnormalities are observed frequently after methotrexate administration and are usually not cause for modification of methotrexate therapy. Persistent liver function test abnormalities just prior to dosing and/or depression of serum albumin may be indicators of serious liver toxicity and require evaluation.

Pulmonary function tests may be useful if methotrexate-induced lung disease is suspected, especially if baseline measurements are available.

Drug Interactions: Nonsteroidal anti-inflammatory drugs should not be administered prior to or concomitantly with the high doses of methotrexate used in the treatment of osteosarcoma. Concomitant administration of some NSAIDs with high-dose methotrexate therapy has been reported to elevate and prolong serum methotrexate levels, resulting in deaths from severe hematologic and gastrointestinal toxicity.

Caution should be used when NSAIDs and salicylates are administered concomitantly with lower doses of methotrexate. These drugs have been reported to reduce the tubular secretion of methotrexate in an animal model and may enhance its toxicity.

Despite the potential interactions, studies of methotrexate in patients with rheumatoid arthritis have usually included concurrent use of constant dosage regimens of NSAIDs, without apparent problems. It should be appreciated however, that the doses used in rheumatoid arthritis (7.5 to 15 mg/week) are somewhat lower than those used in psoriasis and that larger doses could lead to unexpected toxicity.

Methotrexate is partially bound to serum albumin, and toxicity may be increased because of displacement by certain drugs, such as salicylates, phenylbutazone, phenytoin, and sulfonamides. Renal tubular transport is also diminished by probenecid; use of methotrexate with this drug should be carefully monitored.

In the treatment of patients with osteosarcoma, caution must be exercised if high-dose methotrexate is administered in combination with a potentially nephrotoxic chemotherapeutic agent (eg, cisplatin).

Oral antibiotics such as tetracycline, chloramphenicol, and nonabsorbable broad-spectrum antibiotics, may decrease intestinal absorption of methotrexate or interfere with the enterohepatic circulation by inhibiting bowel flora and suppressing metabolism of the drug by bacteria.

Vitamin preparations containing folic acid or its derivatives may decrease responses to systemically administered methotrexate. Preliminary animal and human studies have shown that small quantities of intravenously administered leucovorin enter the CSF primarily as 5-methyltetrahydrofolate and, in humans, remain 1 to 3 orders of magnitude lower than the usual methotrexate concentrations following intrathecal administration. However, high doses of leucovorin may reduce the efficacy of intrathecally administered methotrexate.

Folate deficiency states may increase methotrexate toxicity. Trimethoprim/sulfamethoxazole has been reported rarely to increase bone marrow suppression in patients receiving methotrexate, probably by an additive antifolate effect.

Carcinogenesis, Mutagenesis, and Impairment of Fertility: No controlled human data exist regarding the risk of neoplasia with methotrexate. Methotrexate has been evaluated in a number of animal studies for carcinogenic potential with inconclusive results. Although there is evidence that methotrexate causes chromosomal damage to animal somatic cells and human bone marrow cells, the clinical significance remains uncertain. Assessment of the carcinogenic potential of methotrexate is complicated by conflicting evidence of an increased risk of certain tumors in rheumatoid arthritis. Benefit should be weighed against this potential risk before using methotrexate alone or in combination with other drugs, especially in children or young adults. Methotrexate causes embryotoxicity, abortion, and fetal defects in humans. It has also been reported to cause impairment of fertility, oligospermia, and menstrual dysfunction in humans, during and for a short period after cessation of therapy.

Pregnancy: Psoriasis and rheumatoid arthritis: Methotrexate is in Pregnancy Category X. See **CONTRAINDICATIONS.**

Nursing Mothers: See **CONTRAINDICATIONS.**

Pediatric Use: Safety and effectiveness in children have not been established, other than in cancer chemotherapy.

Organ System Toxicity: *Gastrointestinal:* If vomiting, diarrhea, or stomatitis occur, which may result in dehydration, methotrexate should be discontinued until recovery occurs. Methotrexate should be used with extreme caution in the presence of peptic ulcer disease or ulcerative colitis.

Hematologic: Methotrexate can suppress hematopoiesis and cause anemia, leukopenia, and/or thrombocytopenia. In patients with malignancy and preexisting hematopoietic impairment, the drug should be used with caution, if at all. In controlled clinical trials in rheumatoid arthritis (n = 128), leukopenia (WBC <3000/mm^3) was seen in two patients, thrombocytopenia (platelets <100,000/mm^3) in six patients, and pancytopenia in two patients.

In psoriasis and rheumatoid arthritis, methotrexate should be stopped immediately if there is a significant drop in blood counts. In the treatment of neoplastic diseases, methotrexate should be continued only if the potential benefit warrants the risk of severe myelosuppression. Patients with profound granulocytopenia and fever should be evaluated immediately and usually require parenteral broad-spectrum antibiotic therapy.

Hepatic: Methotrexate has the potential for acute (elevated transaminases) and chronic (fibrosis and cirrhosis) hepatotoxicity. Chronic toxicity is potentially fatal; it generally has occurred after prolonged use (generally 2 years or more) and after a total dose of at least 1.5 grams. In studies in psoriatic patients, hepatotoxicity appeared to be a function of total cumulative dose and appeared to be enhanced by alcoholism, obesity, diabetes, and advanced age. An accurate incidence rate has not been determined; the rate of progression and reversibility of lesions is not known. Special caution is indicated in the presence of preexisting liver damage or impaired hepatic function.

Liver function tests, including serum albumin, should be performed periodically prior to dosing but are often normal in the face of developing fibrosis or cirrhosis. These lesions may be detectable only by biopsy.

In psoriasis, the usual recommendation is to obtain a liver biopsy at a total cumulative dose of 1.5 grams. Moderate fibrosis or any cirrhosis normally leads to discontinuation of the drug; mild fibrosis normally suggests a repeat biopsy in 6 months. Milder histologic findings, such as fatty change and low grade portal inflammation, are relatively common pretherapy. Although these mild changes are usually not a reason to avoid or discontinue methotrexate therapy, the drug should be used with caution.

Clinical experience with liver disease in rheumatoid arthritis is limited, but the same risk factors would be anticipated. Liver function tests are also usually not reliable predictors of histological changes in this population.

When to perform a liver biopsy in rheumatoid arthritis patients has not been established, either in terms of cumulative methotrexate dose or duration of therapy. There is a combined reported experience in 217 rheumatoid arthritis patients with liver biopsies both before and during treatment (after a cumulative dose of at least 1500 mg) and in 714 patients with a biopsy only during treatment. There are 64 (7%) cases of fibrosis and 1 (0.1%) case of cirrhosis. Of the 64 cases of fibrosis, 60 were deemed mild. The reticulin stain is more sensitive for early fibrosis and its use may increase these figures. It is unknown whether even longer use will increase these risks.

Infection or Immunologic States: Methotrexate should be used with extreme caution in the presence of active infection, and is usually contraindicated in patients with overt or laboratory evidence of immunodeficiency syndromes. Immunization may be ineffective when given during methotrexate therapy. Immunization with live virus vaccines is generally not recommended. There have been reports of disseminated vaccinia infections after smallpox immunization in patients receiving methotrexate therapy. Hypogammaglobulinemia has been reported rarely.

Neurologic: There have been reports of leukoencephalopathy following intravenous administration of methotrexate to patients who have had craniospinal irradiation. Chronic leukoencephalopathy has also been reported in patients with osteosarcoma who received repeated doses of high-dose methotrexate with leucovorin rescue even without cranial irradiation. Discontinuation of methotrexate does not always result in complete recovery.

A transient acute neurologic syndrome has been observed in patients treated with high-dosage regimens. Manifestations of this neurologic disorder may include behavioral abnormalities, focal sensorimotor signs, and abnormal reflexes. The exact cause is unknown.

After the intrathecal use of methotrexate, the central nervous system toxicity which may occur can be classified as follows: chemical arachnoiditis manifested by such symptoms as headache, back pain, nuchal rigidity, and fever; paresis, usually transient, manifested by paraplegia associated with involvement with one or more spinal nerve roots; leukoencephalopathy manifested by confusion, irritability,

somnolence, ataxia, dementia, and occasionally major convulsions.

Pulmonary: Pulmonary symptoms (especially a dry, nonproductive cough) or a nonspecific pneumonitis occurring during methotrexate therapy may be indicative of a potentially dangerous lesion and require interruption of treatment and careful investigation. Although clinically variable, the typical patient with methotrexate-induced lung disease presents with fever, cough, dyspnea, hypoxemia, and an infiltrate on chest X-ray; infection needs to be excluded. This lesion can occur at all dosages.

Renal: High doses of methotrexate used in the treatment of osteosarcoma may cause renal damage leading to acute renal failure. Nephrotoxicity is due primarily to the precipitation of methotrexate and 7-hydroxymethotrexate in the renal tubules. Close attention to renal function including adequate hydration, urine alkalinization and measurement of serum methotrexate and creatinine levels are essential for safe administration.

Other Precautions: Methotrexate should be used with extreme caution in the presence of debility.

Methotrexate exits slowly from third-space compartments (eg, pleural effusions or ascites). This results in a prolonged terminal plasma half-life and unexpected toxicity. In patients with significant third-space accumulations, it is advisable to evacuate the fluid before treatment and to monitor plasma methotrexate levels.

Lesions of psoriasis may be aggravated by concomitant exposure to ultraviolet radiation. Radiation dermatitis and sunburn may be "recalled" by the use of methotrexate.

ADVERSE REACTIONS

IN GENERAL, THE INCIDENCE AND SEVERITY OF ACUTE SIDE EFFECTS ARE RELATED TO DOSE AND FREQUENCY OF ADMINISTRATION. THE MOST SERIOUS REACTIONS ARE DISCUSSED ABOVE UNDER ORGAN SYSTEM TOXICITY IN THE PRECAUTIONS SECTION. THAT SECTION SHOULD ALSO BE CONSULTED WHEN LOOKING FOR INFORMATION ABOUT ADVERSE REACTIONS WITH METHOTREXATE.

The most frequently reported adverse reactions include ulcerative stomatitis, leukopenia, nausea, and abdominal distress. Other frequently reported adverse effects are malaise, undue fatigue, chills and fever, dizziness, and decreased resistance to infection.

Other adverse reactions that have been reported with methotrexate are listed below by organ system. In the oncology setting, concomitant treatment and the underlying disease make specific attribution of a reaction to methotrexate difficult.

Alimentary System: Gingivitis, pharyngitis, stomatitis, anorexia, nausea, vomiting, diarrhea, hematemesis, melena, gastrointestinal ulceration and bleeding, enteritis.

Central Nervous System: Headaches, drowsiness, blurred vision. Aphasia, hemiparesis, paresis, and convulsions have also occurred following administration of methotrexate. Following low doses, occasional patients have reported transient subtle cognitive dysfunction, mood alteration, or unusual cranial sensations.

Pulmonary System: Interstitial pneumonitis deaths have been reported, and chronic interstitial obstructive pulmonary disease has occasionally occurred.

Skin: Erythematous rashes, pruritus, urticaria, photosensitivity, pigmentary changes, alopecia, ecchymosis, telangiectasia, acne, furunculosis.

Urogenital System: Severe nephropathy or renal failure, azotemia, cystitis, hematuria; defective oogenesis or spermatogenesis, transient oligospermia, menstrual dysfunction and vaginal discharge; infertility, abortion, fetal defects.

Other rarer reactions related to or attributed to the use of methotrexate such as opportunistic infection, arthralgia/myalgia, loss of libido/impotence, diabetes, osteoporosis, and sudden death. A few cases of anaphylactoid reactions have been reported.

Adverse Reactions in Double-Blind Rheumatoid Arthritis Studies: The approximate incidences of methotrexate-attributed (ie, placebo rate subtracted) adverse reactions in 12- to 18-week double-blind studies of patients (n = 128) with rheumatoid arthritis treated with low-dose oral (7.5 to 15 mg/week) pulse methotrexate, are listed below. Virtually all of these patients were on concomitant nonsteroidal anti-inflammatory drugs and some were also taking low dosages of corticosteroids.

Incidence greater than 10%: Elevated liver function tests 15%, nausea/vomiting 10%.

Continued on next page

Information on Lederle products listed on these pages is the full prescribing information from product literature or package inserts effective in August 1992. Information concerning all Lederle products may be obtained from the Professional Services Department, Lederle Laboratories, Pearl River, New York 10965.

Lederle—Cont.

Incidence 3% to 10%: Stomatitis, thrombocytopenia (platelet count less than 100,000/mm^3).
Incidence 1% to 3%: Rash/pruritus/dermatitis, diarrhea, alopecia, leukopenia (WBC <3000/mm^3), pancytopenia, dizziness.
No pulmonary toxicity was seen in these two trials. Thus, the incidence is probably less than 2.5% (95% C.L.). Hepatic histology was not examined in these short-term studies (see **PRECAUTIONS**).
Other less common reactions included decreased hematocrit, headache, upper respiratory infection, anorexia, arthralgias, chest pain, coughing, dysuria, eye discomfort, epistaxis, fever, infection, sweating, tinnitus, and vaginal discharge.
Adverse Reactions in Psoriasis: There are no recent placebo-controlled trials in patients with psoriasis. There are two literature reports (Roenigk, 1969 and Nyfors, 1978) describing large series (n = 204, 248) of psoriasis patients treated with methotrexate. Dosages ranged up to 25 mg per week, and treatment was administered for up to 4 years. With the exception of alopecia, photosensitivity, and "burning of skin lesions" (each 3% to 10%), the adverse reaction rates in these reports were very similar to those in the rheumatoid arthritis studies.

OVERDOSAGE

Leucovorin is indicated to diminish the toxicity and counteract the effect of inadvertently administered overdosages of methotrexate. Leucovorin administration should begin as promptly as possible. As the time interval between methotrexate administration and leucovorin initiation increases, the effectiveness of leucovorin in counteracting toxicity decreases. Monitoring of the serum methotrexate concentration is essential in determining the optimal dose and duration of treatment with leucovorin.
In cases of massive overdosage, hydration and urinary alkalinization may be necessary to prevent the precipitation of methotrexate and/or its metabolites in the renal tubules. Neither hemodialysis nor peritoneal dialysis has been shown to improve methotrexate elimination.

DOSAGE AND ADMINISTRATION

Neoplastic Diseases: Oral administration in tablet form is often preferred when low doses are being administered since absorption is rapid and effective serum levels are obtained. Methotrexate sodium parenteral may be given by the intramuscular, intravenous, intra-arterial, or intrathecal route. However, the preserved formulation contains Benzyl Alcohol and must not be used for intrathecal or high-dose therapy. Parenteral drug products should be inspected visually for particulate matter and discoloration prior to administration, whenever solution and container permit.
Choriocarcinoma and Similar Trophoblastic Diseases: Methotrexate is administered orally or intramuscularly in doses of 15 to 30 mg daily for a 5-day course. Such courses are usually repeated for three to five times as required, with rest periods of 1 or more weeks interposed between courses, until any manifesting toxic symptoms subside. The effectiveness of therapy is ordinarily evaluated by 24-hour quantitative analysis of urinary chorionic gonadotropin (hCG), which should return to normal or less than 50 IU/24h usually after the third or fourth course and usually be followed by a complete resolution of measurable lesions in 4 to 6 weeks. One to two courses of methotrexate after normalization of hCG is usually recommended. Before each course of the drug careful clinical assessment is essential. Cyclic combination therapy of methotrexate with other antitumor drugs has been reported as being useful.
Since hydatidiform mole may precede choriocarcinoma, prophylactic chemotherapy with methotrexate has been recommended.
Chorioadenoma destruens is considered to be an invasive form of hydatidiform mole. Methotrexate is administered in these disease states in doses similar to those recommended for choriocarcinoma.
Leukemia: Acute lymphoblastic leukemia in children and young adolescents is the most responsive to present-day chemotherapy. In young adults and older patients, clinical remission is more difficult to obtain and early relapse is more common.
Methotrexate alone or in combination with steroids was used initially for induction of remission in acute lymphoblastic leukemias. More recently corticosteroid therapy, in combination with other antileukemic drugs or in cyclic combinations with methotrexate included, has appeared to produce rapid and effective remissions. When used for induction, methotrexate in doses of 3.3 mg/m^2 in combination with 60 mg/m^2 of prednisone, given daily, produced remissions in 50% of patients treated, usually within a period of 4 to 6 weeks. Methotrexate in combination with other agents appears to be the drug of choice for securing maintenance of drug-induced remissions. When remission is achieved and supportive care has produced general clinical improvement, maintenance therapy is initiated, as follows: Methotrexate is administered two times weekly either by mouth or intramuscularly in total weekly doses of 30 mg/m^2. It has also been given in doses of 2.5 mg/kg intravenously every 14 days. If and when relapse does occur, reinduction of remission can again usually be obtained by repeating the initial induction regimen.
A variety of combination chemotherapy regimens have been used for both induction and maintenance therapy in acute lymphoblastic leukemia. The physician should be familiar with the new advances in antileukemic therapy.
Meningeal Leukemia: In the treatment or prophylaxis of meningeal leukemia, methotrexate must be administered intrathecally. Preservative-free methotrexate is diluted to a concentration of 1 mg/mL in an appropriate sterile, preservative-free medium such as 0.9% Sodium Chloride Injection, USP.
The cerebrospinal fluid volume is dependent on age and not on body surface area. The CSF is at 40% of the adult volume at birth and reaches the adult volume in several years.
Intrathecal methotrexate administration at a dose of 12 mg/m^2 (maximum 15 mg) has been reported to result in low CSF methotrexate concentrations and reduced efficacy in children and high concentrations and neurotoxicity in adults. The following dosage regimen is based on age instead of body surface area:

Age (years)	Dose (mg)
<1	6
1	8
2	10
3 or older	12

In one study in patients under the age of 40, this dosage regimen appeared to result in more consistent CSF methotrexate concentrations and less neurotoxicity. Another study in children with acute lymphocytic leukemia compared this regimen to a dose of 12 mg/m^2 (maximum 15 mg). A significant reduction in the rate of CNS relapse was observed in the group whose dose was based on age.
Because the CSF volume and turnover may decrease with age, a dose reduction may be indicated in elderly patients.
For the treatment of meningeal leukemia, intrathecal methotrexate may be given at intervals of 2 to 5 days. However, administration at intervals of less than 1 week may result in increased subacute toxicity. Methotrexate is administered until the cell count of the cerebrospinal fluid returns to normal. At this point one additional dose is advisable. For prophylaxis against meningeal leukemia, the dosage is the same as for treatment except for the intervals of administration. On this subject, it is advisable for the physician to consult the medical literature.
Untoward side effects may occur with any given intrathecal injection and are commonly neurological in character. Large doses may cause convulsions. Methotrexate given by the intrathecal route appears significantly in the systemic circulation and may cause systemic methotrexate toxicity. Therefore, systemic antileukemic therapy with the drug should be appropriately adjusted, reduced, or discontinued. Focal leukemic involvement of the CNS may not respond to intrathecal chemotherapy and is best treated with radiotherapy.
Lymphomas: In Burkitt's tumor, Stages I to II, methotrexate has produced prolonged remissions in some cases. Recommended dosage is 10 to 25 mg/day orally for 4 to 8 days. In Stage III, methotrexate is commonly given concomitantly with other antitumor agents. Treatment in all stages usually consists of several courses of the drug interposed with 7- to 10-day rest periods. Lymphosarcomas in Stage III may respond to combined drug therapy with methotrexate given in doses of 0.625 to 2.5 mg/kg daily.
Mycosis fungoides: Therapy with methotrexate appears to produce clinical remissions in one half of the cases treated. Dosage is usually 2.5 to 10 mg daily by mouth for weeks or months. Dose levels of drug and adjustment of dose regimen by reduction or cessation of drug are guided by patient response and hematologic monitoring. Methotrexate has also been given intramuscularly in doses of 50 mg once weekly or 25 mg two times weekly.
Osteosarcoma: An effective adjuvant chemotherapy regimen requires the administration of several cytotoxic chemotherapeutic agents. In addition to high-dose methotrexate with leucovorin rescue, these agents may include doxorubicin, cisplatin, and the combination of bleomycin, cyclophosphamide and dactinomycin (BCD) in the doses and schedule shown in the table below. The starting dose for high-dose methotrexate treatment is 12 grams/m^2. If this dose is not sufficient to produce a peak serum methotrexate concentration of 1,000 micromolar (10^{-3} mol/L) at the end of the methotrexate infusion, the dose may be escalated to 15 grams/m^2 in subsequent treatments. If the patient is vomiting or is unable to tolerate oral medication, leucovorin is given IV or IM at the same dose and schedule.
[See table below.]

Drug*	Dose*	Treatment Week After Surgery
Methotrexate	12 g/m^2 IV as 4 hour infusion (starting dose)	4, 5, 6, 7, 11, 12, 15, 16, 29, 30, 44, 45
Leucovorin	15 mg orally every 6 hours for 10 doses starting at 24 hours after start of methotrexate infusion.	
Doxorubicin† as a single drug	30 mg/m^2/day IV × 3 days	8, 17
Doxorubicin†	50 mg/m^2 IV	20, 23, 33, 36
Cisplatin†	100 mg/m^2 IV	20, 23, 33, 36
Bleomycin†	15 units/m^2 IV × 2 days	2, 13, 26, 39, 42
Cyclophosphamide†	600 mg/m^2 IV × 2 days	2, 13, 26, 39, 42
Dactinomycin†	0.6 mg/m^2 IV × 2 days	2, 13, 26, 39, 42

* Link MP, Goorin AM, Miser AW, et al: The effect of adjuvant chemotherapy on relapse-free survival in patients with osteosarcoma of the extremity. *N Engl J Med* 1986; 314(no.25):1600–1606.
† See each respective package insert for full Prescribing Information. Dosage modifications may be necessary because of drug-induced toxicity.

When these higher doses of methotrexate are to be administered, the following safety guidelines should be closely observed.

GUIDELINES FOR METHOTREXATE THERAPY WITH LEUCOVORIN RESCUE

1. Administration of methotrexate should be delayed until recovery if:
   - the WBC count is < 1500/microliter
   - the neutrophil count is < 200/microliter
   - the platelet count is < 75,000/microliter
   - the serum bilirubin level is >1.2 mg/dL
   - the SGPT level is > 450 U
   - mucositis is present, until there is evidence of healing
   - persistent pleural effusion is present; this should be drained dry prior to infusion.
2. Adequate renal function must be documented.
   a. Serum creatinine must be normal, and creatinine clearance must be greater than 60 mL/min, before initiation of therapy.
   b. Serum creatinine must be measured prior to each subsequent course of therapy. If serum creatinine has increased by 50% or more compared to a prior value, the creatinine clearance must be measured and documented to be greater than 60 mL/min (even if the serum creatinine is still within the normal range).
3. Patients must be well hydrated, and must be treated with sodium bicarbonate for urinary alkalinization.
   a. Administer 1,000 mL/m^2 of intravenous fluid over 6 hours prior to initiation of the methotrexate infusion. Continue hydration at 125 mL/m^2/hr (3 liters/m^2/day) during the methotrexate infusion, and for 2 days after the infusion has been completed.
   b. Alkalinize urine to maintain pH above 7.0 during methotrexate infusion and leucovorin calcium therapy. This can be accomplished by the administration of sodium bicarbonate orally or by incorporation into a separate intravenous solution.
4. Repeat serum creatinine and serum methotrexate 24 hours after starting methotrexate and at least once daily until the methotrexate level is below 5×10^{-8} mol/L (0.05 micromolar).
5. The table below provides guidelines for leucovorin calcium dosage based upon serum methotrexate levels. (See table on next page.‡)

Patients who experience delayed early methotrexate elimination are likely to develop nonreversible oliguric renal failure. In addition to appropriate leucovorin therapy, these patients require continuing hydration and urinary alkalinization, and close monitoring of fluid and electrolyte status, until the serum methotrexate level has fallen to below 0.05 micromolar and the renal failure has resolved.

6. Some patients will have abnormalities in methotrexate elimination, or abnormalities in renal function following methotrexate administration, which are significant but less severe than the abnormalities described in the table below. These abnormalities may or may not be associated with significant clinical toxicity. If significant clinical toxicity is observed, leucovorin rescue should be extended for an additional 24 hours (total 14 doses over 84 hours) in subsequent courses of therapy. The possibility that the patient is taking other medications which interact with methotrexate (eg, medications which may interfere with methotrexate binding to serum albumin, or elimination) should always be reconsidered when laboratory abnormalities or clinical toxicities are observed.

Psoriasis and Rheumatoid Arthritis: *The patient should be fully informed of the risks involved and should be under constant supervision of the physician.* (See **Information for Patients** under **PRECAUTIONS**.) Assessment of hematologic, hepatic, renal, and pulmonary function should be made by history, physical examination, and laboratory tests before beginning, periodically during, and before reinstituting methotrexate therapy (see **PRECAUTIONS**). Appropriate steps should be taken to avoid conception during methotrexate therapy. (See **PRECAUTIONS** and **CONTRAINDICATIONS**.)

Weekly therapy may be instituted with the RHEUMATREX® Methotrexate 2.5 mg Tablet Dose Packs which are designed to provide doses over a range of 5 mg to 15 mg administered as a single weekly dose. The dose packs are not recommended for administration of methotrexate in weekly doses greater than 15 mg. All schedules should be continually tailored to the individual patient. An initial test dose may be given prior to the regular dosing schedule to detect any extreme sensitivity to adverse effects (see **ADVERSE REACTIONS**). Maximal myelosuppression usually occurs in 7 to 10 days.

Psoriasis: Recommended Starting Dose Schedules
1. Weekly single oral, IM, or IV dose schedule: 10 to 25 mg per week until adequate response is achieved.
2. Divided oral dose schedule: 2.5 mg at 12-hour intervals for three doses.

Dosages in each schedule may be gradually adjusted to achieve optimal clinical response; 30 mg/week should not ordinarily be exceeded.

Once optimal clinical response has been achieved, each dosage schedule should be reduced to the lowest possible amount of drug and to the longest possible rest period. The use of methotrexate may permit the return to conventional topical therapy, which should be encouraged.

Rheumatoid Arthritis: Recommended Starting Dosage Schedules
1. Single oral doses of 7.5 mg once weekly.
2. Divided oral dosages of 2.5 mg at 12-hour intervals for three doses given as a course once weekly.

Dosages in each schedule may be adjusted gradually to achieve an optimal response, but not ordinarily to exceed a total weekly dose of 20 mg. Limited experience shows a significant increase in the incidence and severity of serious toxic reactions, especially bone marrow suppression, at doses greater than 20 mg/wk.

Once response has been achieved, each schedule should be reduced, if possible, to the lowest possible effective dose.

Therapeutic response usually begins within 3 to 6 weeks and the patient may continue to improve for another 12 weeks or more.

The optimal duration of therapy is unknown. Limited data available from long-term studies indicate that the initial clinical improvement is maintained for at least 2 years with continued therapy. When methotrexate is discontinued, the arthritis usually worsens within 3 to 6 weeks.

HANDLING AND DISPOSAL

Procedures for proper handling and disposal of anticancer drugs should be considered. Several guidelines on this subject have been published.[1-6] There is no general agreement that all of the procedures recommended in the guidelines are necessary or appropriate.

RECONSTITUTION OF LOW SODIUM CRYODESICCATED POWDERS

Reconstitute immediately prior to use.

Methotrexate Sodium for Injection should be reconstituted with an appropriate sterile, preservative-free medium such as 5% Dextrose Solution, USP, or Sodium Chloride Injection, USP. Reconstitute the 20 mg and 50 mg vials to a concentration no greater than 25 mg/mL. **The 1 gram vial should be reconstituted with 19.4 mL to a concentration of 50 mg/mL.**

‡LEUCOVORIN RESCUE SCHEDULES FOLLOWING TREATMENT WITH HIGHER DOSES OF METHOTREXATE

Clinical Situation	Laboratory Findings	Leucovorin Dosage and Duration
Normal Methotrexate Elimination	Serum methotrexate level approximately 10 micromolar at 24 hours after administration, 1 micromolar at 48 hours, and less than 0.2 micromolar at 72 hours.	15 mg PO, IM, or IV q6h for 60 hours (10 doses starting at 24 hours after start of methotrexate infusion).
Delayed Late Methotrexate Elimination	Serum methotrexate level remaining above 0.2 micromolar at 72 hours, and more than 0.05 micromolar at 96 hours after administration.	Continue 15 mg PO, IM, or IV q6h, until methotrexate level is less than 0.05 micromolar.
Delayed Early Methotrexate Elimination and/or Evidence of Acute Renal Injury	Serum methotrexate level of 50 micromolar or more at 24 hours, or 5 micromolar or more at 48 hours after administration, OR; a 100% or greater increase in serum creatinine level at 24 hours after methotrexate administration (eg, an increase from 0.5 mg/dL to a level of 1.0 mg/dL or more).	150 mg IV q3h, until methotrexate level is less than 1 micromolar; then 15 mg IV q3h, until methotrexate level is less than 0.05 micromolar.

When high doses of methotrexate are administered by IV infusion, the total dose is diluted in 5% Dextrose Solution. For intrathecal injection, reconstitute to a concentration of 1 mg/mL with an appropriate sterile, preservative-free medium such as Sodium Chloride Injection, USP.

DILUTION INSTRUCTIONS FOR LIQUID METHOTREXATE SODIUM INJECTION PRODUCTS

Methotrexate Sodium Injection, Preservative Protected: If desired, the solution may be further diluted with a compatible medium such as Sodium Chloride Injection, USP. Storage for 24 hours at a temperature of 21° to 25°C results in a product which is within 90% of label potency.

Methotrexate LPF® Sodium (methotrexate sodium injection), Isotonic, Preservative Free, for Single Use Only: If desired, the solution may be further diluted immediately prior to use with an appropriate sterile, preservative-free medium such as 5% Dextrose Solution, USP or Sodium Chloride Injection, USP.

HOW SUPPLIED

Parenteral:
Methotrexate Sodium for Injection, Freeze Dried, Preservative Free, Low Sodium, for Single Use Only. Each low sodium 20 mg, 50 mg, and 1 g vial of cryodesiccated powder contains methotrexate sodium equivalent to 20 mg, 50 mg, and 1 g methotrexate, respectively.
   NDC 0205-4654-90 (Dark Blue Cap)—20 mg Vial
   NDC 0205-9337-92 (Violet Cap)—50 mg Vial
   NDC 0205-4653-02 (Red Cap)—1 g Vial
Methotrexate LPF® Sodium (methotrexate sodium injection), Isotonic Liquid, Preservative Free, for Single Use Only. Each 25 mg/mL, 2 mL, 4 mL, and 10 mL vial contains methotrexate sodium equivalent to 50 mg, 100 mg, 200 mg, and 250 mg methotrexate, respectively.
   NDC 0205-5325-26 (Brown Cap)—50 mg (25 mg/mL)—2 mL Vial
   NDC 0205-5326-18 (Light Blue Cap)—100 mg (25 mg/mL)—4 mL Vial
   NDC 0205-5327-30 (Orange Cap)—200 mg (25 mg/mL)—8 mL Vial
   NDC 0205-5337-34 (Violet Cap)—250 mg (25 mg/mL)—10 mL Vial
   NDC 0205-5337-98 (Violet Cap)—250 mg (25 mg/mL)—10 mL Vial—25 vials per box
Methotrexate Sodium Injection, Isotonic Liquid, Preservative Protected. Each 25 mg/mL, 2 mL, and 10 mL vial contains methotrexate sodium equivalent to 50 mg and 250 mg methotrexate, respectively.
   NDC 0205-4556-26 (Red Cap)—50 mg (25 mg/mL)—2 mL Vial
   NDC 0205-5338-34 (Brown Cap)—250 mg (25 mg/mL)—10 mL Vial
Storage between 15°C (59°F) and 25°C (77°F) is recommended. Protect From Light.
LEDERLE PARENTERALS, INC.
Carolina, Puerto Rico 00630

Oral: Description: Methotrexate Sodium Tablets contain an amount of methotrexate sodium equivalent to 2.5 mg of methotrexate and are round, convex, yellow tablets, engraved with LL on one side, scored in half on the other side, and engraved with M above the score, and 1 below.
NDC 0005-4507-23—Bottle of 100
RHEUMATREX® Methotrexate Sodium Tablet 2.5 mg Dose Packs—(each tablet equivalent to 2.5 mg of methotrexate).

NDC 0005-4507-04—RHEUMATREX® Methotrexate Sodium Tablets Dose Pack—4 cards each containing two 2.5 mg tablets, ie, 5 mg per week.
NDC 0005-4507-05—RHEUMATREX® Methotrexate Sodium Tablets Dose Pack—4 cards each containing three 2.5 mg tablets, ie, 7.5 mg per week.
NDC 0005-4507-07—RHEUMATREX® Methotrexate Sodium Tablets Dose Pack—4 cards each containing four 2.5 mg tablets, ie, 10 mg per week.
NDC 0005-4507-09—RHEUMATREX® Methotrexate Sodium Tablets Dose Pack—4 cards each containing five 2.5 mg tablets, ie, 12.5 mg per week.
NDC 0005-4507-91—RHEUMATREX® Methotrexate Sodium Tablets Dose Pack—4 cards each containing six 2.5 mg tablets, ie, 15 mg per week.

Military Depot:
NSN 6505-00-963-5353—Bottle of 100
Store at Controlled Room Temperature 15°–30°C (59°–86°F). Protect From Light.
LEDERLE LABORATORIES DIVISION
American Cyanamid Company, Pearl River, NY 10965
© 1991   Rev. 2/92
                                                 20878-92

REFERENCES

1. Recommendations for the Safe Handling of Parenteral Antineoplastic Drugs. NIH Publication No. 83–2621. For sale by the Superintendent of Documents, U.S. Government Printing Office, Washington, D.C. 20402.
2. AMA Council Report. Guidelines for Handling Parenteral Antineoplastics. *JAMA*, March 15, 1985.
3. National Study Commission on Cytotoxic Exposure-Recommendations for Handling Cytotoxic Agents. Available from Louis P. Jeffrey, ScD, Director of Pharmacy Services, Rhode Island Hospital, 593 Eddy Street, Providence, Rhode Island 02902.
4. Clinical Oncological Society of Australia: Guidelines and recommendations for safe handling of antineoplastic agents. *Med J Australia* 1983;1:426–428.
5. Jones RB, et al. Safe handling of chemotherapeutic agents: A report from the Mount Sinai Medical Center. *CA: A Cancer Journal for Clinicians* Sept/Oct, 1983; 258–263.
6. American Society of Hospital Pharmacists. Technical assistance bulletin on handling cytotoxic drugs in hospitals. *Am J Hosp Pharm* 1985;42:131–137.

   Shown in Product Identification Section, page 415

Continued on next page

Information on Lederle products listed on these pages is the full prescribing information from product literature or package inserts effective in August 1992. Information concerning all Lederle products may be obtained from the Professional Services Department, Lederle Laboratories, Pearl River, New York 10965.

Lederle—Cont.

MINOCIN® ℞
[mī-nō-sĭn]
Sterile
Minocycline Hydrochloride
Intravenous
100 mg/Vial

DESCRIPTION

MINOCIN, a semisynthetic derivative of tetracycline, is named [4S-(4α,4aα,5aα,12aα)]-4,7-bis(dimethylamino)-1,4,4a, 5,5a,6,11,12a-octahydro-3, 10, 12, 12a-tetrahydroxy-1, 11-dioxo-2-naphthacenecarboxamide monohydrochloride.

Each vial, dried by cryodesiccation, contains sterile minocycline HCl equivalent to 100 mg minocycline. When reconstituted with 5 mL of Sterile Water for Injection, the pH ranges from 2.0 to 2.8.

ACTIONS

Microbiology: The tetracyclines are primarily bacteriostatic and are thought to exert their antimicrobial effect by the inhibition of protein synthesis. Minocycline HCl is a tetracycline with antibacterial activity comparable to other tetracyclines with activity against a wide range of gram-negative and gram-positive organisms.

Tube dilution testing: Microorganisms may be considered susceptible (likely to respond to minocycline therapy) if the minimum inhibitory concentration (MIC) is not more than 4 mcg/mL. Microorganisms may be considered intermediate (harboring partial resistance) if the MIC is 4 to 12.5 mcg/mL and resistant (not likely to respond to minocycline therapy) if the MIC is greater than 12.5 mcg/mL.

Susceptibility plate testing: If the Kirby-Bauer method of susceptibility testing (using a 30 mcg tetracycline disc) gives a zone of 18 mm or greater, the bacterial strain is considered to be susceptible to any tetracycline. Minocycline shows moderate *in vitro* activity against certain strains of staphylococci which have been found resistant to other tetracyclines. For such strains, minocycline susceptibility powder may be used for additional susceptibility testing.

Human Pharmacology: Following a single dose of 200 mg administered intravenously to 10 healthy male volunteers, serum levels ranged from 2.52 to 6.63 mcg/mL (average 4.18), after 12 hours they ranged from 0.82 to 2.64 mcg/mL (average 1.38). In a group of five healthy male volunteers, serum levels of 1.4 to 1.8 mcg/mL were maintained at 12 and 24 hours with doses of 100 mg every 12 hours for 3 days. When given 200 mg once daily for 3 days, the serum levels had fallen to approximately 1 mcg/mL at 24 hours. The serum half-life following IV doses of 100 mg every 12 hours or 200 mg once daily did not differ significantly and ranged from 15 to 23 hours. The serum half-life following a single 200 mg oral dose in 12 essentially normal volunteers ranged from 11 to 17 hours, in 7 patients with hepatic dysfunction ranged from 11 to 16 hours, and in 5 patients with renal dysfunction from 18 to 69 hours.

Intravenously administered minocycline appears similar to oral doses in excretion. The urinary and fecal recovery of oral minocycline when administered to 12 normal volunteers is one-half to one-third that of other tetracyclines.

INDICATIONS

MINOCIN *minocycline HCl* is indicated in infections caused by the following microorganisms:

Rickettsiae: (Rocky Mountain spotted fever, typhus fever and the typhus group, Q fever, rickettsialpox, tick fevers).

Mycoplasma pneumoniae (PPLO, Eaton agent).

Agents of psittacosis and ornithosis.

Agents of lymphogranuloma venereum and granuloma inguinale.

The spirochetal agent of relapsing fever (*Borrelia recurrentis*).

The following gram-negative microorganisms:

Haemophilus ducreyi (chancroid), *Yersinia pestis* and *Francisella tularensis,* formerly *Pasteurella pestis* and *Pasteurella tularensis, Bartonella bacilliformis, Bacteroides* species, *Vibrio comma* and *Vibrio fetus, Brucella* species (in conjunction with streptomycin).

Because many strains of the following groups of microorganisms have been shown to be resistant to tetracyclines, culture and susceptibility testing are recommended.

MINOCIN is indicated for treatment of infections caused by the following gram-negative microorganisms, when bacteriologic testing indicates appropriate susceptibility to the drug:

Escherichia coli, Enterobacter aerogenes (formerly *Aerobacter aerogenes*), *Shigella* species, *Mima* species and *Herellea* species, *Haemophilus influenzae* (respiratory infections), *Klebsiella* species (respiratory and urinary infections).

MINOCIN is indicated for treatment of infections caused by the following gram-positive microorganisms when bacteriologic testing indicates appropriate susceptibility to the drug:

Streptococcus species: Up to 44% of strains of *Streptococcus pyogenes* and 74% of *Streptococcus faecalis* have been found to be resistant to tetracycline drugs. Therefore, tetracyclines should not be used for streptococcal disease unless the organism has been demonstrated to be sensitive.

For upper respiratory infections due to Group A beta-hemolytic streptococci, penicillin is the usual drug of choice, including prophylaxis of rheumatic fever.

Streptococcus pneumoniae, Staphylococcus aureus, skin and soft tissue infections.

Tetracyclines are not the drugs of choice in the treatment of any type of staphylococcal infection.

When penicillin is contraindicated, tetracyclines are alternative drugs in the treatment of infections due to:

Neisseria gonorrhoeae, and *Neisseria meningitidis, Treponema pallidum* and *Treponema pertenue* (syphilis and yaws), *Listeria monocytogenes, Clostridium* species, *Bacillus anthracis, Fusobacterium fusiforme* (Vincent's infection), *Actinomyces* species.

In acute intestinal amebiasis, the tetracyclines may be a useful adjunct to amebicides.

MINOCIN is indicated in the treatment of trachoma, although the infectious agent is not always eliminated, as judged by immunofluorescence.

Inclusion conjunctivitis may be treated with oral tetracyclines or with a combination of oral and topical agents.

CONTRAINDICATIONS

This drug is contraindicated in persons who have shown hypersensitivity to any of the tetracyclines.

WARNINGS

In the presence of renal dysfunction, particularly in pregnancy, intravenous tetracycline therapy in daily doses exceeding 2 g has been associated with deaths through liver failure.

When the need for intensive treatment outweighs its potential dangers (mostly during pregnancy or in individuals with known or suspected renal or liver impairment), it is advisable to perform renal and liver function tests before and during therapy. Also, tetracycline serum concentrations should be followed.

If renal impairment exists, even usual oral or parenteral doses may lead to excessive systemic accumulation of the drug and possible liver toxicity. Under such conditions, lower than usual total doses are indicated, and if therapy is prolonged, serum level determinations of the drug may be advisable. This hazard is of particular importance in the parenteral administration of tetracyclines to pregnant or postpartum patients with pyelonephritis. When used under these circumstances, the blood level should not exceed 15 mcg/mL and liver function tests should be made at frequent intervals. Other potentially hepatotoxic drugs should not be prescribed concomitantly.

THE USE OF TETRACYCLINES DURING TOOTH DEVELOPMENT (LAST HALF OF PREGNANCY, INFANCY, AND CHILDHOOD TO THE AGE OF 8 YEARS) MAY CAUSE PERMANENT DISCOLORATION OF THE TEETH (YELLOW-GRAY-BROWN). This adverse reaction is more common during long-term use of the drugs but has been observed following repeated short-term courses. Enamel hypoplasia has also been reported. TETRACYCLINES, THEREFORE, SHOULD NOT BE USED IN THIS AGE GROUP UNLESS OTHER DRUGS ARE NOT LIKELY TO BE EFFECTIVE OR ARE CONTRAINDICATED.

Photosensitivity manifested by an exaggerated sunburn reaction has been observed in some individuals taking tetracyclines. Patients apt to be exposed to direct sunlight or ultraviolet light should be advised that this reaction can occur with tetracycline drugs, and treatment should be discontinued at the first evidence of skin erythema. Studies to date indicate that photosensitivity is rarely reported with MINOCIN *minocycline HCl.*

The anti-anabolic action of the tetracyclines may cause an increase in BUN. While this is not a problem in those with normal renal function, in patients with significantly impaired function, higher serum levels of tetracycline may lead to azotemia, hyperphosphatemia, and acidosis.

CNS side effects including lightheadedness, dizziness or vertigo have been reported. Patients who experience these symptoms should be cautioned about driving vehicles or using hazardous machinery while on minocycline therapy. These symptoms may disappear during therapy and usually disappear rapidly when the drug is discontinued.

Usage in Pregnancy: (See above **WARNINGS** about use during tooth development.)

Results of animal studies indicate that tetracyclines cross the placenta, are found in fetal tissues and can have toxic effects on the developing fetus (often related to retardation of skeletal development). Evidence of embryotoxicity has also been noted in animals treated early in pregnancy.

The safety of MINOCIN *minocycline HCl* for use during pregnancy has not been established.

Usage in Newborns, Infants, and Children: (See above **WARNINGS** about use during tooth development.)

All tetracyclines form a stable calcium complex in any bone-forming tissue. A decrease in the fibula growth rate has been observed in prematures given oral tetracycline in doses of 25 mg/kg every 6 hours. This reaction was shown to be reversible when the drug was discontinued.

Tetracyclines are present in the milk of lactating women who are taking a drug in this class.

PRECAUTIONS

General: Pseudotumor cerebri (benign intracranial hypertension) in adults has been associated with the use of tetracyclines. The usual clinical manifestations are headache and blurred vision. Bulging fontanels have been associated with the use of tetracyclines in infants. While both of these conditions and related symptoms usually resolve soon after discontinuation of the tetracycline, the possibility for permanent sequelae exists.

As with other antibiotic preparations, use of this drug may result in overgrowth of nonsusceptible organisms, including fungi. If superinfection occurs, the antibiotic should be discontinued and appropriate therapy should be instituted.

In venereal diseases when coexistent syphilis is suspected, darkfield examination should be done before treatment is started and the blood serology repeated monthly for at least 4 months.

In long-term therapy, periodic laboratory evaluation of organ systems, including hematopoietic, renal, and hepatic studies should be performed.

All infections due to Group A beta-hemolytic streptococci should be treated for at least 10 days.

Drug Interactions: Because tetracyclines have been shown to depress plasma prothrombin activity, patients who are on anticoagulant therapy may require downward adjustment of their anticoagulant dosage.

Since bacteriostatic drugs may interfere with the bactericidal action of penicillin, it is advisable to avoid giving tetracycline in conjunction with penicillin.

Concurrent use of tetracyclines may render oral contraceptives less effective. Breakthrough bleeding has been reported.

ADVERSE REACTIONS

Gastrointestinal: Anorexia, nausea, vomiting, diarrhea, glossitis, dysphagia, enterocolitis, pancreatitis, and inflammatory lesions (with monilial overgrowth) in the anogenital region, and increases in liver enzymes and, rarely, hepatitis. These reactions have been caused by both the oral and parenteral administration of tetracyclines.

Skin: Maculopapular and erythematous rashes. Exfoliative dermatitis has been reported but is uncommon. Erythema multiforme and rarely Stevens-Johnson syndrome have been reported. Photosensitivity is discussed above. (See **WARNINGS.**)

Pigmentation of the skin and mucous membranes has been reported.

Tooth discoloration has been reported, rarely, in adults.

Renal Toxicity: Rise in BUN has been reported and is apparently dose related. (See **WARNINGS.**)

Hypersensitivity Reactions: Urticaria, angioneurotic edema, polyarthralgia, anaphylaxis, anaphylactoid purpura, pericarditis, exacerbation of systemic lupus erythematosus, and rarely, pulmonary infiltrates with eosinophilia.

Blood: Hemolytic anemia, thrombocytopenia, neutropenia, and eosinophilia have been reported.

CNS: (See **WARNINGS.**) Pseudotumor cerebri (benign intracranial hypertension) in adults and bulging fontanels in infants. (See **PRECAUTIONS—General.**) Headache has also been reported.

Other: When given over prolonged periods, tetracyclines have been reported to produce brown-black microscopic discoloration of thyroid glands. No abnormalities of thyroid function studies are known to occur.

DOSAGE AND ADMINISTRATION

Note: Rapid administration is to be avoided. Parenteral therapy is indicated only when oral therapy is not adequate or tolerated. Oral therapy should be instituted as soon as possible. If intravenous therapy is given over prolonged periods of time, thrombophlebitis may result.

Adults: Usual adult dose: 200 mg followed by 100 mg every 12 hours and should not exceed 400 mg in 24 hours. The drug should be initially dissolved and then further diluted to 500 mL to 1,000 mL with either Sodium Chloride Injection USP, Dextrose Injection USP, Dextrose and Sodium Chloride Injection USP, Ringer's Injection USP, or Lactated Ringer's Injection USP but not in other solutions containing calcium (a precipitate may form).

The reconstituted solutions are stable at room temperature for 24 hours without a significant loss of potency. Any unused portions must be discarded after that period. The final dilution for administration should be administered immediately.

For children above 8 years of age: Usual pediatric dosage: 4 mg/kg followed by 2 mg/kg every 12 hours.

In patients with renal impairment: (See **WARNINGS.**) Total dosage should be decreased by reduction of recommended individual doses and/or extending time intervals between doses.

Parenteral drug products should be inspected visually for particulate matter and discoloration prior to administration, whenever solution and container permit.

HOW SUPPLIED

MINOCIN *minocycline HCl* Intravenous is supplied as 100 mg vials of sterile cryodesiccated powder.
Product No. NDC 0205-5305-94
Store at Controlled Room Temperature 15°–30°C (59°–86°F).
LEDERLE PARENTERALS, INC.
Carolina, Puerto Rico 00630   Rev. 7/91
                                        10787-91
Shown in Product Identification Section, page 415

MINOCIN®   ℞
Minocycline Hydrochloride
Pellet-Filled Capsules

DESCRIPTION

MINOCIN, a semisynthetic derivative of tetracycline, is [4S-(4α,4aα,5aα,12aα)] -4,7-bis(dimethylamino)-1,4,4a,5,5a,6,11,-12a-octahydro-3, 10,12,12a-tetrahydroxy-1,11-dioxo-2-naphthacenecarboxamide monohydrochloride.
MINOCIN pellet-filled capsules for oral administration contain pellets of minocycline HCl equivalent to 50 mg or 100 mg of minocycline in microcrystalline cellulose.
The capsule shells contain the following inactive ingredients: Blue 1, Gelatin, Titanium Dioxide, and Yellow 10. The 50 mg capsule shells also contain Black and Yellow Iron Oxides.

CLINICAL PHARMACOLOGY

MINOCIN pellet-filled capsules are rapidly absorbed from the gastrointestinal tract following oral administration. Following a single dose of two 100 mg pellet-filled capsules of MINOCIN administered to 18 normal fasting adult volunteers, maximum serum concentrations were attained in 1 to 4 hours (average 2.1 hours) and ranged from 2.1 to 5.1 mcg/mL (average 3.5 mcg/mL). The serum half-life in the normal volunteers ranged from 11.1 to 22.1 hours (average 15.5 hours).
When MINOCIN pellet-filled capsules were given concomitantly with a meal which included dairy products, the extent of absorption of MINOCIN pellet-filled capsules was not noticeably influenced. The peak plasma concentrations were slightly decreased (11.2%) and delayed by 1 hour when administered with food, compared to dosing under fasting conditions.
In previous studies with other minocycline dosage forms, the minocycline serum half-life ranged from 11 to 16 hours in 7 patients with hepatic dysfunction, and from 18 to 69 hours in 5 patients with renal dysfunction. The urinary and fecal recovery of minocycline when administered to 12 normal volunteers is one-half to one-third that of other tetracyclines.
Microbiology: The tetracyclines are primarily bacteriostatic and are thought to exert their antimicrobial effect by the inhibition of protein synthesis. The tetracyclines, including minocycline, have similar antimicrobial spectra of activity against a wide range of gram-positive and gram-negative organisms. Cross-resistance of these organisms to tetracyclines is common.
While *in vitro* studies have demonstrated the susceptibility of most strains of the following microorganisms, clinical efficacy for infections other than those included in the **INDICATIONS AND USAGE** section has not been documented.
Gram-Negative Bacteria:
  Bartonella bacilliformis
  Brucella species
  Campylobacter fetus
  Francisella tularensis
  Haemophilus ducreyi
  Haemophilus influenzae
  Listeria monocytogenes
  Neisseria gonorrhoeae
  Vibrio cholerae
  Yersinia pestis
Because many strains of the following groups of gram-negative microorganisms have been shown to be resistant to tetracyclines, culture and susceptibility tests are especially recommended:
  Acinetobacter species
  Bacteroides species
  Enterobacter aerogenes
  Escherichia coli
  Klebsiella species
  Shigella species
Gram-Positive Bacteria: Because many strains of the following groups of gram-positive microorganisms have been shown to be resistant to tetracyclines, culture and susceptibility testing are especially recommended. Up to 44 percent of *Streptococcus pyogenes* strains have been found to be resistant to tetracycline drugs. Therefore, tetracyclines should not be used for streptococcal disease unless the organism has been demonstrated to be susceptible.

Alpha-hemolytic streptococci (viridans group)
  Streptococcus pneumoniae
  Streptococcus pyogenes
Other Microorganisms:
  Actinomyces species
  Bacillus anthracis
  Balantidium coli
  Borrelia recurrentis
  Chlamydia psittaci
  Chlamydia trachomatis
  Clostridium species
  Entamoeba species
  Fusobacterium fusiforme
  Propionibacterium acnes
  Treponema pallidum
  Treponema pertenue
  Ureaplasma urealyticum
Susceptibility Tests: *Diffusion Techniques:* The use of antibiotic disk susceptibility test methods which measure zone diameter gives an accurate estimation of susceptibility of microorganisms to MINOCIN *minocycline HCl pellet-filled capsules*. One such standard procedure[1] has been recommended for use with disks for testing antimicrobials. Either the 30 mcg tetracycline-class disk or the 30 mcg minocycline disk should be used for the determination of the susceptibility of microorganisms to minocycline.
With this type of procedure a report of "susceptible" from the laboratory indicates that the infecting organism is likely to respond to therapy. A report of "intermediate susceptibility" suggests that the organism would be susceptible if a high dosage is used or if the infection is confined to tissues and fluids (eg, urine) in which high antibiotic levels are attained. A report of "resistant" indicates that the infecting organism is not likely to respond to therapy. With either the tetracycline-class disk or the minocycline disk, zone sizes of 19 mm or greater indicate susceptibility, zone sizes of 14 mm or less indicate resistance, and zone sizes of 15 to 18 mm indicate intermediate susceptibility.
Standardized procedures require the use of laboratory control organisms. The 30 mcg tetracycline disk should give zone diameters between 19 and 28 mm for *Staphylococcus aureus* ATCC 25923 and between 18 and 25 mm for *Escherichia coli* ATCC 25922. The 30 mcg minocycline disk should give zone diameters between 25 and 30 mm for *S aureus* ATCC 25923 and between 19 and 25 mm for *E coli* ATCC 25922.
Dilution Techniques: When using the NCCLS agar dilution or broth dilution (including microdilution) method[2] or equivalent, a bacterial isolate may be considered susceptible if the MIC (minimal inhibitory concentration) of minocycline is 4 mcg/mL or less. Organisms are considered resistant if the MIC is 16 mcg/mL or greater. Organisms with an MIC value of less than 16 mcg/mL but greater than 4 mcg/mL are expected to be susceptible if a high dosage is used or if the infection is confined to tissues and fluids (eg, urine) in which high antibiotic levels are attained.
As with standard diffusion methods, dilution procedures require the use of laboratory control organisms. Standard tetracycline or minocycline powder should give MIC values of 0.25 mcg/mL to 1.0 mcg/mL for *S aureus* ATCC 25923, and 1.0 mcg/mL to 4.0 mcg/mL for *E coli* ATCC 25922.

INDICATIONS AND USAGE

MINOCIN *minocycline HCl pellet-filled capsules* are indicated in the treatment of the following infections due to susceptible strains of the designated microorganisms:
  Rocky Mountain spotted fever, typhus fever and the typhus group, Q fever, rickettsialpox and tick fevers caused by Rickettsiae
  Respiratory tract infections caused by *Mycoplasma pneumoniae*
  Lymphogranuloma venereum caused by *Chlamydia trachomatis*
  Psittacosis (Ornithosis) due to *Chlamydia psittaci*
  Trachoma caused by *Chlamydia trachomatis*, although the infectious agent is not always eliminated, as judged by immunofluorescence
  Inclusion conjunctivitis caused by *Chlamydia trachomatis*
  Nongonococcal urethritis in adults caused by *Ureaplasma urealyticum* or *Chlamydia trachomatis*
  Relapsing fever due to *Borrelia recurrentis*
  Chancroid caused by *Haemophilus ducreyi*
  Plague due to *Yersinia pestis*
  Tularemia due to *Francisella tularensis*
  Cholera caused by *Vibrio cholerae*
  Campylobacter fetus infections caused by *Campylobacter fetus*
  Brucellosis due to *Brucella* species (in conjunction with streptomycin)
  Bartonellosis due to *Bartonella bacilliformis*
  Granuloma inguinale caused by *Calymmatobacterium granulomatis*
Minocycline is indicated for treatment of infections caused by the following gram-negative microorganisms, when bacteriologic testing indicates appropriate susceptibility to the drug:

  Escherichia coli
  Enterobacter aerogenes
  Shigella species
  Acinetobacter species
  Respiratory tract infections caused by *Haemophilus influenzae*
  Respiratory tract and urinary tract infections caused by *Klebsiella* species
MINOCIN *minocycline HCl pellet-filled capsules* are indicated for the treatment of infections caused by the following gram-positive microorganisms when bacteriologic testing indicates appropriate susceptibility to the drug:
  Upper respiratory tract infections caused by *Streptococcus pneumoniae*
  Skin and skin structure infections caused by *Staphylococcus aureus*. (Note: Minocycline is not the drug of choice in the treatment of any type of staphylococcal infection.)
  Uncomplicated urethritis in men due to *Neisseria gonorrhoeae* and for the treatment of other gonococcal infections when penicillin is contraindicated.
When penicillin is contraindicated, minocycline is an alternative drug in the treatment of the following infections:
  Infections in women caused by *Neisseria gonorrhoeae*
  Syphilis caused by *Treponema pallidum*
  Yaws caused by *Treponema pertenue*
  Listeriosis due to *Listeria monocytogenes*
  Anthrax due to *Bacillus anthracis*
  Vincent's infection caused by *Fusobacterium fusiforme*
  Actinomycosis caused by *Actinomyces israelii*
  Infections caused by *Clostridium* species
In *acute intestinal amebiasis,* minocycline may be a useful adjunct to amebicides.
In severe *acne,* minocycline may be useful adjunctive therapy.
Oral minocycline is indicated in the treatment of asymptomatic carriers of *Neisseria meningitidis* to eliminate meningococci from the nasopharynx. In order to preserve the usefulness of minocycline in the treatment of asymptomatic meningococcal carrier, diagnostic laboratory procedures, including serotyping and susceptibility testing, should be performed to establish the carrier state and the correct treatment. It is recommended that the prophylactic use of minocycline be reserved for situations in which the risk of meningococcal meningitis is high.
Oral minocycline is not indicated for the treatment of meningococcal infection.
Although no controlled clinical efficacy studies have been conducted, limited clinical data show that oral minocycline hydrochloride has been used successfully in the treatment of infections caused by *Mycobacterium marinum.*

CONTRAINDICATIONS

This drug is contraindicated in persons who have shown hypersensitivity to any of the tetracyclines.

WARNINGS

MINOCIN PELLET-FILLED CAPSULES, LIKE OTHER TETRACYCLINE-CLASS ANTIBIOTICS, CAN CAUSE FETAL HARM WHEN ADMINISTERED TO A PREGNANT WOMAN. IF ANY TETRACYCLINE IS USED DURING PREGNANCY OR IF THE PATIENT BECOMES PREGNANT WHILE TAKING THESE DRUGS, THE PATIENT SHOULD BE APPRISED OF THE POTENTIAL HAZARD TO THE FETUS. THE USE OF DRUGS OF THE TETRACYCLINE CLASS DURING TOOTH DEVELOPMENT (LAST HALF OF PREGNANCY, INFANCY, AND CHILDHOOD TO THE AGE OF 8 YEARS) MAY CAUSE PERMANENT DISCOLORATION OF THE TEETH (YELLOW-GRAY-BROWN).
This adverse reaction is more common during long-term use of the drug but has been observed following repeated short-term courses. Enamel hypoplasia has also been reported. TETRACYCLINE DRUGS, THEREFORE, SHOULD NOT BE USED DURING TOOTH DEVELOPMENT UNLESS OTHER DRUGS ARE NOT LIKELY TO BE EFFECTIVE OR ARE CONTRAINDICATED.
All tetracyclines form a stable calcium complex in any bone-forming tissue. A decrease in fibula growth rate has been observed in young animals (rats and rabbits) given oral tetracycline in doses of 25 mg/kg every 6 hours. This reaction was shown to be reversible when the drug was discontinued.
Results of animal studies indicate that tetracyclines cross the placenta, are found in fetal tissues, and can have toxic effects on the developing fetus (often related to retardation of skeletal development). Evidence of embryotoxicity has been noted in animals treated early in pregnancy.

Continued on next page

Lederle—Cont.

The anti-anabolic action of the tetracyclines may cause an increase in BUN. While this is not a problem in those with normal renal function, in patients with significantly impaired function, higher serum levels of tetracycline may lead to azotemia, hyperphosphatemia, and acidosis. If renal impairment exists, even usual oral or parenteral doses may lead to excessive systemic accumulations of the drug and possible liver toxicity. Under such conditions, lower than usual total doses are indicated, and if therapy is prolonged, serum level determinations of the drug may be advisable.
Photosensitivity manifested by an exaggerated sunburn reaction has been observed in some individuals taking tetracyclines. This has been reported rarely with minocycline. Central nervous system side effects including lightheadedness, dizziness, or vertigo have been reported with minocycline therapy. Patients who experience these symptoms should be cautioned about driving vehicles or using hazardous machinery while on minocycline therapy. These symptoms may disappear during therapy and usually disappear rapidly when the drug is discontinued.

PRECAUTIONS

General: As with other antibiotic preparations, use of this drug may result in overgrowth of nonsusceptible organisms, including fungi. If superinfection occurs, the antibiotic should be discontinued and appropriate therapy instituted. Pseudotumor cerebri (benign intracranial hypertension) in adults has been associated with the use of tetracyclines. The usual clinical manifestations are headache and blurred vision. Bulging fontanels have been associated with the use of tetracyclines in infants. While both of these conditions and related symptoms usually resolve after discontinuation of tetracycline, the possibility for permanent sequelae exists. Incision and drainage or other surgical procedures should be performed in conjunction with antibiotic therapy when indicated.
Information for Patients: Photosensitivity manifested by an exaggerated sunburn reaction has been observed in some individuals taking tetracyclines. Patients apt to be exposed to direct sunlight or ultraviolet light should be advised that this reaction can occur with tetracycline drugs, and treatment should be discontinued at the first evidence of skin erythema. This reaction has been reported rarely with use of minocycline.
Patients who experience central nervous system symptoms (see **WARNINGS**) should be cautioned about driving vehicles or using hazardous machinery while on minocycline therapy.
Concurrent use of tetracycline may render oral contraceptives less effective (see **Drug Interactions**).
Laboratory Tests: In venereal disease when coexistent syphilis is suspected, a darkfield examination should be done before treatment is started and the blood serology repeated monthly for at least 4 months.
In long-term therapy, periodic laboratory evaluations of organ systems, including hematopoietic, renal, and hepatic studies should be performed.
Drug Interactions: Because tetracyclines have been shown to depress plasma prothrombin activity, patients who are on anticoagulant therapy may require downward adjustment of their anticoagulant dosage.
Since bacteriostatic drugs may interfere with the bactericidal action of penicillin, it is advisable to avoid giving tetracycline-class drugs in conjunction with penicillin.
Absorption of tetracyclines is impaired by antacids containing aluminum, calcium or magnesium, and iron-containing preparations.
The concurrent use of tetracycline and methoxyflurane has been reported to result in fatal renal toxicity.
Concurrent use of tetracyclines may render oral contraceptives less effective. Breakthrough bleeding has been reported.
Drug/Laboratory Test Interactions: False elevations of urinary catecholamine levels may occur due to interference with the fluorescence test.
Carcinogenesis, Mutagenesis, Impairment of Fertility: Dietary administration of minocycline in long-term tumorigenicity studies in rats resulted in evidence of thyroid tumor production. Minocycline has also been found to produce thyroid hyperplasia in rats and dogs. In addition, there has been evidence of oncogenic activity in rats in studies with a related antibiotic, oxytetracycline (ie, adrenal and pituitary tumors). Likewise, although mutagenicity studies of minocycline have not been conducted, positive results in *in vitro* mammalian cell assays (ie, mouse lymphoma and Chinese hamster lung cells) have been reported for related antibiotics (tetracycline hydrochloride and oxytetracycline). Segment I (fertility and general reproduction) studies have provided evidence that minocycline impairs fertility in male rats.
Teratogenic Effects: *Pregnancy:* Pregnancy Category D (see **WARNINGS**).
Labor and Delivery: The effect of tetracyclines on labor and delivery is unknown.

Nursing Mothers: Tetracyclines are excreted in human milk. Because of the potential for serious adverse reactions in nursing infants from the tetracyclines, a decision should be made whether to discontinue nursing or discontinue the drug, taking into account the importance of the drug to the mother (see **WARNINGS**).
Pediatric Use: (See **WARNINGS**).

ADVERSE REACTIONS

Due to oral minocycline's virtually complete absorption, side effects to the lower bowel, particularly diarrhea, have been infrequent. The following adverse reactions have been observed in patients receiving tetracyclines.
Gastrointestinal: Anorexia, nausea, vomiting, diarrhea, glossitis, dysphagia, enterocolitis, pancreatitis, and inflammatory lesions (with monilial overgrowth) in the anogenital region, increases in liver enzymes, and rarely hepatitis have been reported. Rare instances of esophagitis and esophageal ulcerations have been reported in patients taking the tetracycline-class antibiotics in capsule and tablet form. Most of these patients took the medication immediately before going to bed (see **DOSAGE AND ADMINISTRATION**).
Skin: Maculopapular and erythematous rashes. Exfoliative dermatitis has been reported but is uncommon. Erythema multiforme and rarely Stevens-Johnson syndrome have been reported. Photosensitivity is discussed above (see **WARNINGS**). Pigmentation of the skin and mucous membranes has been reported.
Renal Toxicity: Elevations in BUN have been reported and are apparently dose related (see **WARNINGS**).
Hypersensitivity Reactions: Urticaria, angioneurotic edema, polyarthralgia, anaphylaxis, anaphylactoid purpura, pericarditis, exacerbation of systemic lupus erythematosus and rarely pulmonary infiltrates with eosinophilia have been reported.
Blood: Hemolytic anemia, thrombocytopenia, neutropenia, and eosinophilia have been reported.
Central Nervous System: Bulging fontanels in infants and benign intracranial hypertension (Pseudotumor cerebri) in adults (see **PRECAUTIONS—General**) have been reported. Headache has also been reported.
Other: When given over prolonged periods, tetracyclines have been reported to produce brown-black microscopic discoloration of the thyroid glands. No abnormalities of thyroid function are known to occur in man.
Tooth discoloration in children less than 8 years of age (see **WARNINGS**) and also, rarely, in adults have been reported.

OVERDOSAGE

In case of overdosage, discontinue medication, treat symptomatically, and institute supportive measures.

DOSAGE AND ADMINISTRATION

THE USUAL DOSAGE AND FREQUENCY OF ADMINISTRATION OF MINOCYCLINE DIFFERS FROM THAT OF THE OTHER TETRACYCLINES. EXCEEDING THE RECOMMENDED DOSAGE MAY RESULT IN AN INCREASED INCIDENCE OF SIDE EFFECTS.
MINOCIN pellet-filled capsules may be taken with or without food (see **CLINICAL PHARMACOLOGY**).
ADULTS: The usual dosage of MINOCIN pellet-filled capsules is 200 mg initially followed by 100 mg every 12 hours. Alternatively, if more frequent doses are preferred, two or four 50 mg pellet-filled capsules may be given initially followed by one 50 mg capsule four times daily.
For children above 8 years of age: The usual dosage of MINOCIN *minocycline HCl pellet-filled capsules* is 4 mg/kg initially followed by 2 mg/kg every 12 hours.
Uncomplicated gonococcal infections other than urethritis and anorectal infections in men: 200 mg initially, followed by 100 mg every 12 hours for a minimum of 4 days, with post-therapy cultures within 2 to 3 days.
In the treatment of uncomplicated gonococcal urethritis in men, 100 mg every 12 hours for 5 days is recommended.
For the treatment of syphilis, the usual dosage of MINOCIN pellet-filled capsules should be administered over a period of 10 to 15 days. Close follow-up, including laboratory tests, is recommended.
In the treatment of meningococcal carrier state, the recommended dosage is 100 mg every 12 hours for 5 days.
Mycobacterium marinum infections: Although optimal doses have not been established, 100 mg every 12 hours for 6 to 8 weeks have been used successfully in a limited number of cases.
Uncomplicated nongonococcal urethral infection in adults caused by *Chlamydia trachomatis* or *Ureaplasma urealyticum:* 100 mg orally, every 12 hours for at least 7 days.
Ingestion of adequate amounts of fluids along with capsule and tablet forms of drugs in the tetracycline-class is recommended to reduce the risk of esophageal irritation and ulceration.
In patients with renal impairment (see **WARNINGS**), the total dosage should be decreased by either reducing the recommended individual doses and/or by extending the time intervals between doses.

HOW SUPPLIED

MINOCIN *minocycline HCl pellet-filled capsules* are supplied as capsules containing minocycline hydrochloride equivalent to 100 mg and 50 mg minocycline.
100 mg, two-piece, hard-shell capsule with an opaque light green cap and a transparent green body, printed in white ink with Lederle over M46 on one half and Lederle over 100 mg on the other half. Each capsule contains pellets of minocycline HCl equivalent to 100 mg of minocycline, supplied as follows:
NDC 0005-5344-18—Bottle of 50
50 mg, two-piece, hard-shell capsule with an opaque yellow cap and a transparent green body, printed in black ink with Lederle over M45 on one half and Lederle over 50 mg on the other half. Each capsule contains pellets of minocycline HCl equivalent to 50 mg of minocycline, supplied as follows:
NDC 0005-5343-23—Bottle of 100
Military Depots:
NSN 6505-01-015-4147—50 mg (100s)
NSN 6505-00-003-5112—100 mg (50s)
V.A. Depots:
NSN 6505-01-015-4147—50 mg (100s)
NSN 6505-01-108-9040—100 mg (100s)
Store at Controlled Room Temperature 15°–30°C (59°–86°F). Protect from light, moisture, and excessive heat.

ANIMAL PHARMACOLOGY AND TOXICOLOGY

MINOCIN has been observed to cause a dark discoloration of the thyroid in experimental animals (rats, minipigs, dogs, and monkeys). In the rat, chronic treatment with MINOCIN has resulted in goiter accompanied by elevated radioactive iodine uptake, and evidence of thyroid tumor production. MINOCIN has also been found to produce thyroid hyperplasia in rats and dogs.

REFERENCES

1. National Committee for Clinical Laboratory Standards, Approved Standard: *Performance Standards for Antimicrobial Disk Susceptibility Tests,* 3rd Edition, Vol. 4(16):M2–A3, Villanova, PA, December 1984.
2. National Committee for Clinical Laboratory Standards, Approved Standard: *Methods for Dilution Antimicrobial Susceptibility Tests for Bacteria that Grow Aerobically,* 2nd Edition, Vol. 5(22):M7–A, Villanova, PA, December 1985.
©1990
LEDERLE LABORATORIES DIVISION
American Cyanamid Company, Pearl River, NY 10965
Rev. 7/91
10799-91
Shown in Product Identification Section, page 415

MINOCIN®   ℞
] [mĭ-nō-sĭn]
Minocycline Hydrochloride
Oral Suspension

DESCRIPTION

MINOCIN, a semisynthetic derivative of tetracycline, is named [4S-(4α,4aα,5aα,12aα)]-4,7-bis(dimethylamino)-1,4,4a,5,5a,6,11,12a-octahydro- 3,10,12,12a-tetrahydroxy-1, 11-dioxo-2-naphthacenecarboxamide monohydrochloride.
MINOCIN Oral Suspension contains minocycline HCl equivalent to 50 mg of minocycline per 5 mL (10 mg/mL) and the following inactive ingredients: Alcohol, Butylparaben, Calcium Hydroxide, Cellulose, Decaglyceryl Tetraoleate, Edetate Calcium Disodium, Glycol, Guar Gum, Polysorbate 80, Propylparaben, Propylene Glycol, Sodium Saccharin, Sodium Sulfite (see **WARNINGS**) and Sorbitol.

ACTIONS

Microbiology: The tetracyclines are primarily bacteriostatic and are thought to exert their antimicrobial effect by the inhibition of protein synthesis. Minocycline HCl is a tetracycline with antibacterial activity comparable to other tetracyclines with activity against a wide range of gram-negative and gram-positive organisms.
Tube dilution testing: Microorganisms may be considered susceptible (likely to respond to minocycline therapy) if the minimum inhibitory concentration (MIC) is not more than 4 mcg/mL. Microorganisms may be considered intermediate (harboring partial resistance) if the MIC is 4 to 12.5 mcg/mL and resistant (not likely to respond to minocycline therapy) if the MIC is greater than 12.5 mcg/mL.
Susceptibility plate testing: If the Kirby-Bauer method of susceptibility testing (using a 30 mcg tetracycline disc) gives a zone of 18 mm or greater, the bacterial strain is considered to be susceptible to any tetracycline. Minocycline shows moderate *in vitro* activity against certain strains of staphylococci which have been found resistant to other tetracyclines. For such strains minocycline susceptibility powder may be used for additional susceptibility testing.
Human Pharmacology: Following a single dose of two 100 mg minocycline HCl capsules administered to 10 normal adult volunteers, serum levels ranged from 0.74 to 4.45 mcg/mL in

1 hour (average 2.24), after 12 hours, they ranged from 0.34 to 2.36 mcg/mL (average 1.25). The serum half-life following a single 200 mg dose in 12 essentially normal volunteers ranged from 11 to 17 hours. In seven patients with hepatic dysfunction it ranged from 11 to 16 hours, and in five patients with renal dysfunction from 18 to 69 hours. The urinary and fecal recovery of minocycline when administered to 12 normal volunteers is one half to one third that of other tetracyclines.

INDICATIONS

MINOCIN *minocycline HCl* is indicated in infections caused by the following microorganisms:

Rickettsiae: (Rocky Mountain spotted fever, typhus fever and the typhus group, Q fever, rickettsialpox, tick fevers).

Mycoplasma pneumoniae (PPLO, Eaton agent).

Agents of psittacosis and ornithosis.

Agents of lymphogranuloma venereum and granuloma inguinale.

The spirochetal agent of relapsing fever (*Borrelia recurrentis*).

The following gram-negative microorganisms:

Haemophilus ducreyi (chancroid),

Yersinia pestis and *Francisella tularensis* (formerly *Pasteurella pestis* and *Pasteurella tularensis),*

Bartonella bacilliformis,

Bacteroides species,

Vibrio comma and *Vibrio fetus,*

Brucella species (in conjunction with streptomycin).

Because many strains of the following groups of microorganisms have been shown to be resistant to tetracyclines, culture and susceptibility testing are recommended.

MINOCIN *minocycline HCl* is indicated for treatment of infections caused by the following gram-negative microorganisms when bacteriologic testing indicates appropriate susceptibility to the drug:

Escherichia coli,

Enterobacter aerogenes (formerly *Aerobacter aerogenes*),

Shigella species,

Acinetobacter calcoaceticus (formerly *Herellea, Mima*),

Haemophilus influenzae (respiratory infections),

Klebsiella species (respiratory and urinary infections).

MINOCIN is indicated for treatment of infections caused by the following gram-positive microorganisms when bacteriologic testing indicates appropriate susceptibility to the drug:

Streptococcus species:

Up to 44% of strains of *Streptococcus pyogenes* and 74% of *Streptococcus faecalis* have been found to be resistant to tetracycline drugs. Therefore, tetracyclines should not be used for streptococcal disease unless the organism has been demonstrated to be sensitive.

For upper respiratory infections due to Group A beta-hemolytic streptococci, penicillin is the usual drug of choice, including prophylaxis of rheumatic fever.

Streptococcus pneumoniae (formerly *Diplococcus pneumoniae),*

Staphylococcus aureus, skin and soft tissue infections.

Tetracyclines are not the drugs of choice in the treatment of any type of staphylococcal infection.

MINOCIN is indicated for the treatment of uncomplicated gonococcal urethritis in men due to *Neisseria gonorrhoeae.* When penicillin is contraindicated, tetracyclines are alternative drugs in the treatment of infections due to:

Neisseria gonorrhoeae (in women),

Treponema pallidum and *Treponema pertenue* (syphilis and yaws),

Listeria monocytogenes,

Clostridium species,

Bacillus anthracis,

Fusobacterium fusiforme (Vincent's infection),

Actinomyces species.

In acute intestinal amebiasis, the tetracyclines may be a useful adjunct to amebicides.

In severe acne, the tetracyclines may be useful adjunctive therapy.

MINOCIN is indicated in the treatment of trachoma, although the infectious agent is not always eliminated, as judged by immunofluorescence.

MINOCIN *minocycline HCl* is indicated for the treatment of uncomplicated urethral, endocervical, or rectal infections in adults caused by *Chlamydia trachomatis* or *Ureaplasma urealyticum.*[1]

Inclusion conjunctivitis may be treated with oral tetracyclines or with a combination of oral and topical agents.

MINOCIN is indicated in the treatment of asymptomatic carriers of *Neisseria meningitidis* to eliminate meningococci from the nasopharynx.

In order to preserve the usefulness of MINOCIN in the treatment of asymptomatic meningococcal carriers, diagnostic laboratory procedures, including serotyping and susceptibility testing, should be performed to establish the carrier state and the correct treatment. It is recommended that the drug be reserved for situations in which the risk of meningococcal meningitis is high.

MINOCIN by oral administration is not indicated for the treatment of meningococcal infection.

Although no controlled clinical efficacy studies have been conducted, limited clinical data show that oral MINOCIN has been used successfully in the treatment of infections caused by Mycobacterium marinum.

CONTRAINDICATIONS

This drug is contraindicated in persons who have shown hypersensitivity to any of the tetracyclines.

WARNINGS

THE USE OF DRUGS OF THE TETRACYCLINE CLASS DURING TOOTH DEVELOPMENT (LAST HALF OF PREGNANCY, INFANCY, AND CHILDHOOD TO THE AGE OF 8 YEARS) MAY CAUSE PERMANENT DISCOLORATION OF THE TEETH (YELLOW-GRAY-BROWN). This adverse reaction is more common during long-term use of the drugs but has been observed following repeated short-term courses. Enamel hypoplasia has also been reported. TETRACYCLINE DRUGS, THEREFORE, SHOULD NOT BE USED IN THIS AGE GROUP UNLESS OTHER DRUGS ARE NOT LIKELY TO BE EFFECTIVE OR ARE CONTRAINDICATED.

If renal impairment exists, even usual oral or parenteral doses may lead to excessive systemic accumulations of the drug and possible liver toxicity. Under such conditions, lower-than-usual total doses are indicated, and if therapy is prolonged, serum level determinations of the drug may be advisable.

Photosensitivity manifested by an exaggerated sunburn reaction has been observed in some individuals taking tetracyclines. Patients apt to be exposed to direct sunlight or ultraviolet light should be advised that this reaction can occur with tetracycline drugs, and treatment should be discontinued at the first evidence of skin erythema. Studies to date indicate that photosensitivity is rarely reported with MINOCIN *minocycline HCl.*

The anti-anabolic action of the tetracyclines may cause an increase in BUN. While this is not a problem in those with normal renal function, in patients with significantly impaired function, higher serum levels of tetracycline may lead to azotemia, hyperphosphatemia, and acidosis.

CNS side effects including lightheadedness, dizziness, or vertigo have been reported. Patients who experience these symptoms should be cautioned about driving vehicles or using hazardous machinery while on minocycline therapy. These symptoms may disappear during therapy and usually disappear rapidly when the drug is discontinued.

MINOCIN *minocycline HCl* Oral Suspension contains sodium sulfite, a sulfite that may cause allergic-type reactions including anaphylactic symptoms and life-threatening or less severe asthmatic episodes in certain susceptible people. The overall prevalence of sulfite sensitivity in the general population is unknown and probably low. Sulfite sensitivity is seen more frequently in asthmatic than in nonasthmatic people.

Usage in pregnancy: (See above WARNINGS about use during tooth development.) Results of animal studies indicate that tetracyclines cross the placenta, are found in fetal tissues, and can have toxic effects on the developing fetus (often related to retardation of skeletal development). Evidence of embryotoxicity has also been noted in animals treated early in pregnancy.

The safety of MINOCIN for use during pregnancy has not been established.

Usage in newborns, infants, and children: (See above WARNINGS about use during tooth development.)

All tetracyclines form a stable calcium complex in any bone-forming tissue. A decrease in the fibula growth rate has been observed in prematures given oral tetracycline in doses of 25 mg/kg every 6 hours. This reaction was shown to be reversible when the drug was discontinued.

Tetracyclines are present in the milk of lactating women who are taking a drug in this class.

PRECAUTIONS

General: Pseudotumor cerebri (benign intracranial hypertension) in adults has been associated with the use of tetracyclines. The usual clinical manifestations are headache and blurred vision. Bulging fontanels have been associated with the use of tetracyclines in infants. While both of these conditions and related symptoms usually resolve soon after discontinuation of the tetracycline, the possibility for permanent sequelae exists.

As with other antibiotic preparations, use of this drug may result in overgrowth of nonsusceptible organisms, including fungi. If superinfection occurs, the antibiotic should be discontinued and appropriate therapy should be instituted.

In venereal diseases when coexistent syphilis is suspected, darkfield examination should be done before treatment is started and the blood serology repeated monthly for at least 4 months.

In long-term therapy, periodic laboratory evaluation of organ systems, including hematopoietic, renal, and hepatic studies should be performed.

All infections due to Group A beta-hemolytic streptococci should be treated for at least 10 days.

Drug Interactions: Because tetracyclines have been shown to depress plasma prothrombin activity, patients who are on anticoagulant therapy may require downward adjustment of their anticoagulant dosage.

Since bacteriostatic drugs may interfere with the bactericidal action of penicillin, it is advisable to avoid giving tetracycline in conjunction with penicillin.

Concurrent use of tetracyclines may render oral contraceptives less effective. Breakthrough bleeding has been reported.

ADVERSE REACTIONS

Gastrointestinal: Anorexia, nausea, vomiting, diarrhea, glossitis, dysphagia, enterocolitis, pancreatitis, and inflammatory lesions (with monilial overgrowth) in the anogenital region, increases in liver enzymes and, rarely, hepatitis.

These reactions have been caused by both the oral and parenteral administration of tetracyclines.

Skin: Maculopapular and erythematous rashes. Exfoliative dermatitis has been reported but is uncommon. Erythema multiforme and rarely Stevens-Johnson syndrome have been reported. Photosensitivity is discussed above. (See WARNINGS.)

Pigmentation of the skin and mucous membranes has been reported.

Tooth discoloration has been reported rarely in adults.

Renal toxicity: Rise in BUN has been reported and is apparently dose related. (See WARNINGS.)

Hypersensitivity reactions: Urticaria, angioneurotic edema, polyarthralgia, anaphylaxis, anaphylactoid purpura, pericarditis, exacerbation of systemic lupus erythematosus and, rarely, pulmonary infiltrates with eosinophilia.

Blood: Hemolytic anemia, thrombocytopenia, neutropenia, and eosinophilia have been reported.

CNS: (See WARNINGS.) Pseudotumor cerebri (benign intracranial hypertension) in adults and bulging fontanels in infants. (See PRECAUTIONS—General.) Headache has also been reported.

Other: When given over prolonged periods, tetracyclines have been reported to produce brown-black microscopic discoloration of thyroid glands. No abnormalities of thyroid function studies are known to occur.

DOSAGE AND ADMINISTRATION

Therapy should be continued for at least 24 to 48 hours after symptoms and fever have subsided.

Concomitant therapy: Antacids containing aluminum, calcium, or magnesium impair absorption and should not be given to patients taking oral tetracycline.

Studies to date have indicated that the absorption of MINOCIN is not notably influenced by foods and dairy products.

In patients with renal impairment: (See WARNINGS.) Total dosage should be decreased by reduction of recommended individual doses and/or extending time intervals between doses.

In the treatment of streptococcal infections, a therapeutic dosage of tetracycline should be administered for at least 10 days.

ADULTS: The usual dosage of MINOCIN *minocycline HCl* is 200 mg initially followed by 100 mg every 12 hours.

For children above 8 years of age: The usual dosage of MINOCIN is 4 mg/kg initially followed by 2 mg/kg every 12 hours.

For treatment of syphilis, the usual dosage of MINOCIN should be administered over a period of 10 to 15 days. Close follow-up, including laboratory tests, is recommended.

Gonorrhea patients sensitive to penicillin may be treated with MINOCIN, administered as 200 mg initially, followed by 100 mg every 12 hours for a minimum of 4 days, with post-therapy cultures within 2 to 3 days.

In the treatment of meningococcal carrier state, recommended dosage is 100 mg every 12 hours for 5 days.

Mycobacterium marinum infections: Although optimal doses have not been established, 100 mg twice a day for 6 to 8 weeks have been used successfully in a limited number of cases.

Uncomplicated urethral, endocervical, or rectal infection in adults caused by *Chlamydia trachomatis* or *Ureaplasma urealyticum:* 100 mg, by mouth, two times a day for at least 7 days.[1]

In the treatment of uncomplicated gonococcal urethritis in men, 100 mg twice a day orally for 5 days is recommended.

Continued on next page

Information on Lederle products listed on these pages is the full prescribing information from product literature or package inserts effective in August 1992. Information concerning all Lederle products may be obtained from the Professional Services Department, Lederle Laboratories, Pearl River, New York 10965.

Lederle—Cont.

HOW SUPPLIED

ORAL SUSPENSION

MINOCIN Oral Suspension contains minocycline hydrochloride equivalent to 50 mg minocycline per teaspoonful (5 mL). Preserved with propylparaben 0.10% and butylparaben 0.06% with Alcohol USP 5% v/v, Custard-flavored.

NDC 0005-5313-56 Bottle 2 fl oz (60 mL)

Store at Controlled Room Temperature 15°-30° C (59°-86° F). DO NOT FREEZE.

ANIMAL PHARMACOLOGY AND TOXICOLOGY

MINOCIN *minocycline HCl* has been found to produce high blood concentrations following oral dosage to various animal species and to be extensively distributed to all tissues examined in ^{14}C-labeled drug studies in dogs. MINOCIN has been found experimentally to produce discoloration of the thyroid glands. This finding has been observed in rats and dogs. Changes in thyroid function have also been found in these animal species. However, no change in thyroid function has been observed in humans.

Reference: 1. CDC Sexually Transmitted Diseases Treatment Guidelines 1982.

LEDERLE LABORATORIES DIVISION
American Cyanamid Company
Pearl River, NY 10965 Rev. 7/91
10793-91

Shown in Product Identification Section, page 415

MYAMBUTOL® ℞

[*mī-am-bū-tōl*]
Ethambutol Hydrochloride
Tablets

DESCRIPTION

MYAMBUTOL is an oral chemotherapeutic agent which is specifically effective against actively growing microorganisms of the genus *Mycobacterium,* including *M tuberculosis.*

MYAMBUTOL 100 mg and 400 mg tablets contain the following inactive ingredients: Gelatin, Hydroxypropyl Methylcellulose, Magnesium Stearate, Sodium Lauryl Sulfate, Sorbitol, Stearic Acid, Sucrose, Titanium Dioxide, and other ingredients.

ACTION

MYAMBUTOL, following a single oral dose of 25 mg/kg of body weight, attains a peak of 2 to 5 micrograms/mL in serum 2 to 4 hours after administration. When the drug is administered daily for longer periods of time at this dose, serum levels are similar. The serum level of MYAMBUTOL falls to undetectable levels by 24 hours after the last dose except in some patients with abnormal renal function. The intracellular concentrations of erythrocytes reach peak values approximately twice those of plasma and maintain this ratio throughout the 24 hours.

During the 24-hour period following oral administration of MYAMBUTOL, approximately 50% of the initial dose is excreted unchanged in the urine, while an additional 8% to 15% appears in the form of metabolites. The main path of metabolism appears to be an initial oxidation of the alcohol to an aldehydic intermediate, followed by conversion to a dicarboxylic acid. From 20% to 22% of the initial dose is excreted in the feces as unchanged drug. No drug accumulation has been observed with consecutive single daily doses of 25 mg/kg in patients with normal kidney function, although marked accumulation has been demonstrated in patients with renal insufficiency.

MYAMBUTOL diffuses into actively growing *mycobacterium* cells such as tubercle bacilli. MYAMBUTOL appears to inhibit the synthesis of one or more metabolites, thus causing impairment of cell metabolism, arrest of multiplication, and cell death. No cross resistance with other available antimycobacterial agents has been demonstrated.

MYAMBUTOL has been shown to be effective against strains of *Mycobacterium tuberculosis* but does not seem to be active against fungi, viruses, or other bacteria. *Mycobacterium tuberculosis* strains previously unexposed to MYAMBUTOL have been uniformly sensitive to concentrations of 8 or less micrograms/mL, depending on the nature of the culture media. When MYAMBUTOL has been used alone for treatment of tuberculosis, tubercle bacilli from these patients have developed resistance to MYAMBUTOL by *in vitro* susceptibility tests; the development of resistance has been unpredictable and appears to occur in a step-like manner. No cross resistance between MYAMBUTOL and other antituberculous drugs has been reported. MYAMBUTOL has reduced the incidence of the emergence of mycobacterial resistance to isoniazid when both drugs have been used concurrently.

An agar diffusion microbiologic assay, based upon inhibition of *Mycobacterium smegmatis* (ATCC 607) may be used to determine concentrations of MYAMBUTOL in serum and urine. This technique has not been published, but further information can be obtained upon inquiry to Lederle Laboratories.

ANIMAL PHARMACOLOGY

Toxicological studies in dogs on high prolonged doses produced evidence of myocardial damage and failure, and depigmentation of the tapetum lucidum of the eyes, the significance of which is not known. Degenerative changes in the central nervous system, apparently not dose-related, have also been noted in dogs receiving ethambutol hydrochloride over a prolonged period.

In the rhesus monkey, neurological signs appeared after treatment with high doses given daily over a period of several months. These were correlated with specific serum levels of ethambutol hydrochloride and with definite neuroanatomical changes in the central nervous system. Focal interstitial carditis was also noted in monkeys which received ethambutol hydrochloride in high doses for a prolonged period.

When pregnant mice or rabbits were treated with high doses of ethambutol hydrochloride, fetal mortality was slightly but not significantly ($P > 0.05$) increased. Female rats treated with ethambutol hydrochloride displayed slight but insignificant ($P > 0.05$) decreases in fertility and litter size.

In fetuses born of mice treated with high doses of MYAMBUTOL during pregnancy, a low incidence of cleft palate, exencephaly and abnormality of the vertebral column were observed. Minor abnormalities of the cervical vertebra were seen in the newborn of rats treated with high doses of MYAMBUTOL during pregnancy. Rabbits receiving high doses of MYAMBUTOL during pregnancy gave birth to two fetuses with monophthalmia, one with a shortened right forearm accompanied by bilateral wrist-joint contracture and one with hare lip and cleft palate.

INDICATIONS

MYAMBUTOL *ethambutol hydrochloride* is indicated for the treatment of pulmonary tuberculosis. It should not be used as the sole antituberculous drug, but should be used in conjunction with at least one other antituberculous drug. Selection of the companion drug should be based on clinical experience, considerations of comparative safety and appropriate *in vitro* susceptibility studies. In patients who have not received previous antituberculous therapy, ie, initial treatment, the most frequently used regimens have been the following:

MYAMBUTOL plus isoniazid
MYAMBUTOL plus isoniazid plus streptomycin.

In patients who have received previous antituberculous therapy, mycobacterial resistance to other drugs used in initial therapy is frequent. Consequently, in such retreatment patients, MYAMBUTOL should be combined with at least one of the second line drugs not previously administered to the patient and to which bacterial susceptibility has been indicated by appropriate *in vitro* studies. Antituberculous drugs used with MYAMBUTOL have included cycloserine, ethionamide, pyrazinamide, viomycin, and other drugs. Isoniazid, aminosalicylic acid, and streptomycin have also been used in multiple drug regimens. Alternating drug regimens have also been utilized.

CONTRAINDICATIONS

MYAMBUTOL *ethambutol hydrochloride* is contraindicated in patients who are known to be hypersensitive to this drug. It is also contraindicated in patients with known optic neuritis unless clinical judgment determines that it may be used.

PRECAUTIONS

The effects of combinations of MYAMBUTOL with other antituberculous drugs on the fetus is not known. While administration of this drug to pregnant human patients has produced no detectable effect upon the fetus, the possible teratogenic potential in women capable of bearing children should be weighed carefully against the benefits of therapy.

There are published reports of five women who received the drug during pregnancy without apparent adverse effect upon the fetus.

MYAMBUTOL is not recommended for use in children under 13 years of age since safe conditions for use have not been established.

Patients with decreased renal function need the dosage reduced as determined by serum levels of MYAMBUTOL, since the main path of excretion of this drug is by the kidneys.

Because this drug may have adverse effects on vision, physical examination should include ophthalmoscopy, finger perimetry, and testing of color discrimination. In patients with visual defects such as cataracts, recurrent inflammatory conditions of the eye, optic neuritis, and diabetic retinopathy, the evaluation of changes in visual acuity is more difficult, and care should be taken to be sure the variations in vision are not due to the underlying disease conditions. In such patients, consideration should be given to relationship between benefits expected and possible visual deterioration since evaluation of visual changes is difficult. (For recommended procedures, see next paragraphs under **ADVERSE REACTIONS.**)

As with any potent drug, periodic assessment of organ system functions, including renal, hepatic, and hematopoietic, should be made during long-term therapy.

ADVERSE REACTIONS

MYAMBUTOL may produce decreases in visual acuity which appear to be due to optic neuritis and to be related to dose and duration of treatment. The effects are generally reversible when administration of the drug is discontinued promptly. In rare cases recovery may be delayed for up to 1 year or more and the effect may possibly be irreversible in these cases.

Patients should be advised to report promptly to their physician any change of visual acuity.

The change in visual acuity may be unilateral or bilateral and hence *each eye must be tested separately and both eyes tested together.* Testing of visual acuity should be performed before beginning MYAMBUTOL therapy and periodically during drug administration, except that it should be done monthly when a patient is on a dosage of more than 15 mg per kilogram per day. Snellen eye charts are recommended for testing of visual acuity. Studies have shown that there are definite fluctuations of one or two lines of the Snellen chart in the visual acuity of many tuberculous patients *not* receiving MYAMBUTOL.

The following table may be useful in interpreting possible changes in visual acuity attributable to MYAMBUTOL.

[See table below.]

Initial Snellen Reading	Reading Indicating Significant Decrease	Significant Number of Lines	Decrease Number of Points
20/13	20/25	3	12
20/15	20/25	2	10
20/20	20/30	2	10
20/25	20/40	2	15
20/30	20/50	2	20
20/40	20/70	2	30
20/50	20/70	1	20

In general, changes in visual acuity less than those indicated under "Significant Number of Lines" and "Decrease-Number of Points," may be due to chance variation, limitations of the testing method or physiologic variability. Conversely, changes in visual acuity equaling or exceeding those under "Significant Number of Lines" and "Decrease-Number of Points" indicate need for retesting and careful evaluation of the patient's visual status. If careful evaluation confirms the magnitude of visual change and fails to reveal another cause, MYAMBUTOL should be discontinued and the patient reevaluated at frequent intervals. Progressive decreases in visual acuity during therapy must be considered to be due to MYAMBUTOL *ethambutol hydrochloride.*

If corrective glasses are used prior to treatment, these must be worn during visual acuity testing. During 1 to 2 years of therapy, a refractive error may develop which must be corrected in order to obtain accurate test results. Testing the visual acuity through a pinhole eliminates refractive error.

Patients developing visual abnormality during MYAMBUTOL treatment may show subjective visual symptoms before, or simultaneously with, the demonstration of decreases in visual acuity, and all patients receiving MYAMBUTOL should be questioned periodically about blurred vision and other subjective eye symptoms.

Recovery of visual acuity generally occurs over a period of weeks to months after the drug has been discontinued. Patients have then received MYAMBUTOL again without recurrence of loss of visual acuity.

Other adverse reactions reported include: anaphylactoid reactions, dermatitis pruritus and joint pain; anorexia, nausea, vomiting, gastrointestinal upset, abdominal pain; fever, malaise, headache, and dizziness; mental confusion, disorientation and possible hallucinations. Numbness and tingling of the extremities due to peripheral neuritis have been reported infrequently.

Elevated serum uric acid levels occur and precipitation of acute gout has been reported. Transient impairment of liver function as indicated by abnormal liver function tests is not an unusual finding. Since MYAMBUTOL is recommended for therapy in conjunction with one or more other antituberculous drugs, these changes may be related to the concurrent therapy.

DOSAGE AND ADMINISTRATION

MYAMBUTOL should not be used alone, in initial treatment or in retreatment. MYAMBUTOL should be administered on a once every 24-hour basis only. Absorption is not significantly altered by administration with food. Therapy, in general, should be continued until bacteriological conversion has become permanent and maximal clinical improvement has occurred.

MYAMBUTOL *ethambutol hydrochloride* is not recommended for use in children under 13 years of age since safe conditions for use have not been established.

Initial Treatment: In patients who have not received previous antituberculous therapy, administer MYAMBUTOL 15 mg per kilogram (7 mg per pound) of body weight, as a single oral dose once every 24 hours. In the more recent studies, isoniazid has been administered concurrently in a single, daily, oral dose.

Retreatment: In patients who have received previous antituberculous therapy, administer MYAMBUTOL 25 mg per kilogram (11 mg per pound) of body weight, as a single oral dose once every 24 hours. Concurrently administer at least one other antituberculous drug to which the organisms have been demonstrated to be susceptible by appropriate *in vitro* tests. Suitable drugs usually consist of those not previously used in the treatment of the patient. After 60 days of MYAMBUTOL administration, decrease the dose to 15 mg per kilogram (7 mg per pound) of body weight, and administer as a single oral dose once every 24 hours.

During the period when a patient is on a daily dose of 25 mg/kg, monthly eye examinations are advised.

See Table for easy selection of proper weight-dose tablet(s).

Weight-Dose Table
15 mg/kg (7 mg/lb) Schedule

Weight Range		Daily Dose
Pounds	Kilograms	In mg
Under 85 lbs	Under 37 kg	500
85–94.5	37–43	600
95–109.5	43–50	700
110–124.5	50–57	800
125–139.5	57–64	900
140–154.5	64–71	1000
155–169.5	71–79	1100
170–184.5	79–84	1200
185–199.5	84–90	1300
200–214.5	90–97	1400
215 and Over	Over 97	1500

25 mg/kg (11 mg/lb) Schedule

Under 85 lbs	Under 38 kg	900
85–92.5	38–42	1000
93–101.5	42–45.5	1100
102–109.5	45.5–50	1200
110–118.5	50–54	1300
119–128.5	54–58	1400
129–136.5	58–62	1500
137–146.5	62–67	1600
147–155.5	67–71	1700
156–164.5	71–75	1800
165–173.5	75–79	1900
174–182.5	79–83	2000
183–191.5	83–87	2100
192–199.5	87–91	2200
200–209.5	91–95	2300
210–218.5	95–99	2400
219 and Over	Over 99	2500

HOW SUPPLIED

MYAMBUTOL *ethambutol hydrochloride* Tablets
100 mg—round, convex, white, coated tablets engraved M6 on one side and LL on the other, are supplied as follows:
  NDC 0005-5015-23 - Bottle of 100
400 mg—round, convex, white, scored, film-coated tablets engraved with LL on one side and M to the left and 7 to the right of the score on the other side, are supplied as follows:
  NDC 0005-5084-62 - Unit-of-Issue 100s with CRC
  NDC 0005-5084-34 - Bottle of 1000
  NDC 0005-5084-60 - Unit Dose 10 (2 × 5) Strips
Store at Controlled Room Temperature 15°–30°C (59°–86°F).
Military Depot:
Tablets, 100 mg NSN 6505-00-403-7645, 100s
Tablets, 400 mg NSN 6505-00-812-2579, 100s
VA Depot:
Tablets, 400 mg NSN 6505-00-812-2543, 1000s
LEDERLE LABORATORIES DIVISION
American Cyanamid Company
Pearl River, NY 10965   Rev. 1/90
           23016

Shown in Product Identification Section, page 415

NEPTAZANE®   ℞

[*nĕp-ta-zāne*]
methazolamide
Tablets, USP

DESCRIPTION

NEPTAZANE, a sulfonamide derivative, is a white crystalline powder, weakly acidic, slightly soluble in water, alcohol and acetone. The chemical name for methazolamide is: *N*-[5-(aminosulfonyl)-3-methyl-1,3,4-thiadiazol-2(3H)-ylidene]-acetamide.

NEPTAZANE is available for oral administration as 25 mg and 50 mg tablets containing the following inactive ingredients: Acacia, Alginic Acid, Corn Starch, Dibasic Calcium Phosphate, Gelatin, and Magnesium Stearate.

CLINICAL PHARMACOLOGY

NEPTAZANE is a potent inhibitor of carbonic anhydrase. NEPTAZANE is well absorbed from the gastrointestinal tract. Peak plasma concentrations are observed 1 to 2 hours after dosing. In a multiple-dose, pharmacokinetic study, administration of NEPTAZANE 25 mg bid, 50 mg bid, and 100 mg bid demonstrated a linear relationship between plasma methazolamide levels and NEPTAZANE dose. Peak plasma concentrations (C_{max}) for the 25 mg, 50 mg, and 100 mg bid regimens were 2.5 mcg/mL, 5.1 mcg/mL, and 10.7 mcg/mL, respectively. The area under the plasma concentration-time curves (AUC) was 1130 mcg.min/mL, 2571 mcg.min/mL, and 5418 mcg.min/mL for the 25 mg, 50 mg, and 100 mg dosage regimens, respectively. NEPTAZANE is distributed throughout the body including the plasma, cerebrospinal fluid, aqueous humor of the eye, red blood cells, bile and extracellular fluid. The mean apparent volume of distribution (V_{area}/F) ranges from 17 L to 23 L. Approximately 55% is bound to plasma proteins. The steady-state NEPTAZANE red blood cell: plasma ratio varies with dose and was found to be 27:1, 16:1, and 10:1 following the administration of NEPTAZANE 25 mg bid, 50 mg bid, and 100 mg bid, respectively.

The mean steady-state plasma elimination half-life for NEPTAZANE is approximately 14 hours. At steady state approximately 25% of the dose is recovered unchanged in the urine over the dosing interval. Renal clearance accounts for 20% to 25% of the total clearance of drug. After repeated bid-tid dosing, NEPTAZANE accumulates to steady-state concentrations in 7 days.

Methazolamide's inhibitory action on carbonic anhydrase decreases the secretion of aqueous humor and results in a decrease in intraocular pressure. The onset of the decrease in intraocular pressure generally occurs within 2 to 4 hours, has a peak effect in 6 to 8 hours, and a total duration of 10 to 18 hours.

NEPTAZANE is a sulfonamide derivative; however, it does not have any clinically significant antimicrobial properties. Although NEPTAZANE achieves a high concentration in the cerebrospinal fluid, it is not considered an effective anticonvulsant.

NEPTAZANE has a weak and transient diuretic effect, therefore use results in an increase in urinary volume, with excretion of sodium, potassium, and chloride. The drug should not be used as a diuretic. Inhibition of renal bicarbonate reabsorption produces an alkaline urine. Plasma bicarbonate decreases, and a relative, transient metabolic acidosis may occur due to a disequilibrium in carbon dioxide transport in the red cell. Urinary citrate excretion is decreased by approximately 40% after doses of 100 mg every 8 hours. Uric acid output has been shown to decrease 36% in the first 24 hour period.

INDICATIONS AND USAGE

NEPTAZANE is indicated in the treatment of ocular conditions where lowering intraocular pressure is likely to be of therapeutic benefit, such as chronic open-angle glaucoma, secondary glaucoma, and preoperatively in acute angle-closure glaucoma where lowering the intraocular pressure is desired before surgery.

CONTRAINDICATIONS

NEPTAZANE therapy is contraindicated in situations in which sodium and/or potassium serum levels are depressed, in cases of marked kidney or liver disease or dysfunction, in adrenal gland failure, and in hyperchloremic acidosis. In patients with cirrhosis, use may precipitate the development of hepatic encephalopathy.

Long-term administration of NEPTAZANE is contraindicated in patients with angle-closure glaucoma, since organic closure of the angle may occur in spite of lowered intraocular pressure.

WARNINGS

Fatalities have occurred, although rarely, due to severe reactions to sulfonamides including Stevens-Johnson syndrome, toxic epidermal necrolysis, fulminant hepatic necrosis, agranulocytosis, aplastic anemia, and other blood dyscrasias. Hypersensitivity reactions may recur when a sulfonamide is readministered, irrespective of the route of administration.

If hypersensitivity or other serious reactions occur, the use of this drug should be discontinued.

Caution is advised for patients receiving high-dose aspirin and NEPTAZANE concomitantly, as anorexia, tachypnea, lethargy, coma, and death have been reported with concomitant use of high-dose aspirin and carbonic anhydrase inhibitors.

PRECAUTIONS

General: Potassium excretion is increased initially upon administration of NEPTAZANE and in patients with cirrhosis or hepatic insufficiency could precipitate a hepatic coma. In patients with pulmonary obstruction or emphysema, where alveolar ventilation may be impaired, NEPTAZANE should be used with caution because it may precipitate or aggravate acidosis.

Information for Patients: Adverse reactions common to all sulfonamide derivatives may occur: anaphylaxis, fever, rash (including erythema multiforme, Stevens-Johnson syndrome, toxic epidermal necrolysis), crystalluria, renal calculus, bone marrow depression, thrombocytopenic purpura, hemolytic anemia, leukopenia, pancytopenia, and agranulocytosis. Precaution is advised for early detection of such reactions, and the drug should be discontinued and appropriate therapy instituted.

Caution is advised for patients receiving high-dose aspirin and NEPTAZANE concomitantly.

Laboratory Tests: To monitor for hematologic reactions common to all sulfonamides, it is recommended that a baseline CBC and platelet count be obtained on patients prior to initiating NEPTAZANE therapy and at regular intervals during therapy. If significant changes occur, early discontinuance and institution of appropriate therapy are important. Periodic monitoring of serum electrolytes is also recommended.

Drug Interactions: NEPTAZANE should be used with caution in patients on steroid therapy because of the potential for developing hypokalemia.

Caution is advised for patients receiving high-dose aspirin and NEPTAZANE concomitantly, as anorexia, tachypnea, lethargy, coma, and death have been reported with concomitant use of high-dose aspirin and carbonic anhydrase inhibitors (see **WARNINGS**).

Carcinogenesis, Mutagenesis, Impairment of Fertility: Long-term studies in animals to evaluate the carcinogenic potential of NEPTAZANE and its effect on fertility have not been conducted. NEPTAZANE was not mutagenic in the Ames bacterial test.

Pregnancy: *Teratogenic effects.* Pregnancy Category C. NEPTAZANE has been shown to be teratogenic (skeletal anomalies) in rats when given in doses approximately 40 times the human dose. There are no adequate and well-controlled studies in pregnant women. NEPTAZANE should be used during pregnancy only if the potential benefit justifies the potential risk to the fetus.

Nursing Mothers: It is not known whether this drug is excreted in human milk. Because many drugs are excreted in human milk and because of the potential for serious adverse reactions in nursing infants from NEPTAZANE, a decision should be made whether to discontinue nursing or to discontinue the drug, taking into account the importance of the drug to the mother.

Pediatric Use: The safety and effectiveness of NEPTAZANE in children have not been established.

ADVERSE REACTIONS

Adverse reactions, occurring most often early in therapy, include paresthesias, particularly a "tingling" feeling in the extremities; hearing dysfunction or tinnitus; fatigue; malaise; loss of appetite; taste alteration; gastrointestinal disturbances such as nausea, vomiting, and diarrhea; polyuria; and occasional instances of drowsiness and confusion.

Metabolic acidosis and electrolyte imbalance may occur. Transient myopia has been reported. This condition invariably subsides upon diminution or discontinuance of the medication.

Other occasional adverse reactions include urticaria, melena, hematuria, glycosuria, hepatic insufficiency, flaccid paralysis, photosensitivity, convulsions, and, rarely, crystalluria and renal calculi. Also see **PRECAUTIONS: Information for Patients** for possible reactions common to sulfonamide derivatives. Fatalities have occurred, although rarely, due to severe reactions to sulfonamides including Stevens-Johnson syndrome, toxic epidermal necrolysis, fulminant hepatic necrosis, agranulocytosis, aplastic anemia, and other blood dyscrasias (see **WARNINGS**).

Continued on next page

Information on Lederle products listed on these pages is the full prescribing information from product literature or package inserts effective in August 1992. Information concerning all Lederle products may be obtained from the Professional Services Department, Lederle Laboratories, Pearl River, New York 10965.

Lederle—Cont.

OVERDOSAGE

No data are available regarding NEPTAZANE overdosage in humans as no cases of acute poisoning with this drug have been reported. Animal data suggest that even a high dose of NEPTAZANE is nontoxic. No specific antidote is known. Treatment should be symptomatic and supportive.

Electrolyte imbalance, development of an acidotic state, and central nervous system effects might be expected to occur. Serum electrolyte levels (particularly potassium) and blood pH levels should be monitored.

Supportive measures may be required to restore electrolyte and pH balance.

DOSAGE AND ADMINISTRATION

The effective therapeutic dose administered varies from 50 mg to 100 mg two to three times daily. The drug may be used concomitantly with miotic and osmotic agents.

HOW SUPPLIED

NEPTAZANE *methazolamide* Tablets, USP, 25 mg, are square white tablets with engraved N2 on one side and embossed large N on the other side, supplied as follows:

NDC 57706-756-23—Bottle of 100

NEPTAZANE Tablets, USP, 50 mg, are round white scored tablets engraved with LL on one side and N above and 1 below the score on the other side, supplied as follows:

NDC 57706-757-23—Bottle of 100

NEPTAZANE is not available for parenteral use.

Store at Controlled Room Temperature 15° to 30°C (59° to 86°F).

Military and VA Depots:

NSN 6505-00-065-4205—50 mg (100s)

Manufactured for

STORZ OPHTHALMICS, INC.

St. Louis, MO 63122

by

LEDERLE LABORATORIES DIVISION

American Cyanamid Company

Pearl River, NY 10965   Rev. 1/92

     20218-92

NOVANTRONE®   ℞

[nō-văn-trōne]

Mitoxantrone for Injection Concentrate

PRODUCT OVERVIEW

KEY FACTS

NOVANTRONE is a synthetic antineoplastic anthracenedione for intravenous use. The precise mechanism of action by which NOVANTRONE exerts its tumoricidal effect has not been fully defined. It is believed to be associated with the inhibition of nucleic acid synthesis, resulting in cell death. Several studies have demonstrated that NOVANTRONE inhibits both RNA and DNA synthesis.

MAJOR USES

NOVANTRONE, in combination with other approved drugs, is indicated for initial therapy of acute nonlymphocytic leukemia (ANLL) in adults, including myelogenous, promelocytic, monocytic, and erythroid acute leukemias.

SAFETY INFORMATION

NOVANTRONE is intended for intravenous use only. The nonvesicant properties of NOVANTRONE minimize the likelihood of severe local reaction. When NOVANTRONE is used as indicated for leukemia, severe myelosuppression will occur as expected. It is, therefore, recommended that NOVANTRONE be administered by physicians experienced in the chemotherapy of this disease. Therapy with NOVANTRONE should be accompanied by close and frequent monitoring of hematologic and chemical laboratory parameters, as well as frequent patient observation.

PRESCRIBING INFORMATION

NOVANTRONE®   ℞

[nō-văn-trōne]

Mitoxantrone for Injection Concentrate

DESCRIPTION

NOVANTRONE is a synthetic antineoplastic anthracenedione for intravenous use. Its molecular formula is $C_{22}H_{28}N_4O_6 \cdot 2HCl$ and its molecular weight is 517.41. It is supplied as a concentrate which **MUST BE DILUTED PRIOR TO INJECTION**. The concentrate is a sterile, nonpyrogenic, dark blue aqueous solution containing mitoxantrone hydrochloride equivalent to 2 mg/mL mitoxantrone free base, with sodium chloride (0.80% w/v), sodium acetate (0.005% w/v), and acetic acid (0.046% w/v) as inactive ingredients. The solution has a pH of 3.0 to 4.5 and contains 0.14 mEq of sodium per mL. The product does not contain preservatives. Its chemical name is: 1,4-Dihydroxy-5,

8-bis [[2-[(2-hydroxyethyl) amino] ethyl] amino]-9, 10-anthracenedione dihydrochloride.

CLINICAL PHARMACOLOGY

Although its mechanism of action is not fully elucidated, NOVANTRONE is a DNA-reactive agent. It has a cytocidal effect on both proliferating and nonproliferating cultured human cells, suggesting lack of cell cycle phase specificity. Pharmacokinetic studies have not been performed in humans receiving multiple daily doses. Pharmacokinetic studies in adult patients following a single intravenous administration of NOVANTRONE have demonstrated multi-exponential plasma clearance. Distribution to tissues is rapid and extensive. Distribution to the brain, spinal cord, eye, and spinal fluid in the monkey is low. The apparent steady-state volume of distribution exceeds $1000L/m^2$. Elimination of drug is slow with an apparent mean terminal plasma half-life of 5.8 days (range 2.3 to 13.0). The half-life in tissues may be longer. Multiple intravenous doses in dogs daily for 5 days resulted in significant accumulation in plasma and tissue. The extent of accumulation was fourfold. NOVANTRONE is 78% bound to plasma proteins in the observed concentration range of 26 to 455 ng/mL. This binding is independent of concentration and was not affected by the presence of diphenylhydantoin, doxorubicin, methotrexate, prednisone, prednisolone, heparin, or acetylsalicylic acid.

NOVANTRONE is excreted via the renal and hepatobiliary systems. Renal excretion is limited; only 6% to 11% of the dose is recovered in the urine within 5 days after drug administration. Of the material recovered in the urine, 65% is unchanged drug; the remaining 35% is comprised primarily of two inactive metabolites and their glucuronide conjugates. The metabolites are mono- and dicarboxylic acid derivatives. Hepatobiliary elimination of drug appears to be of greater significance with as much as 25% of the dose recovered in the feces within 5 days of intravenous dosing. No significant difference in the pharmacokinetics of NOVANTRONE was observed in seven patients with moderately impaired liver function (serum bilirubin 1.3 to 3.4 mg/dL) as compared with 16 patients without hepatic dysfunction. Results of pharmacokinetic studies on four patients with severe hepatic dysfunction (bilirubin greater than 3.4 mg/dL) suggest that these patients have a lower total body clearance and a larger Area Under Curve than other patients at a comparable NOVANTRONE dose.

In two large randomized multicenter trials, remission induction therapy for ANLL with NOVANTRONE *mitoxantrone for Injection Concentrate* 12 mg/m² daily for 3 days as a 10-minute intravenous infusion and cytosine arabinoside 100 mg/m² for 7 days given as a continuous 24-hour infusion was compared with daunorubicin 45 mg/m² daily by intravenous infusion for 3 days plus the same dose and schedule of cytosine arabinoside used with NOVANTRONE. Patients who had an incomplete antileukemic response received a second induction course in which NOVANTRONE or daunorubicin was given for 2 days and cytosine arabinoside for 5 days using the same daily dosage schedule. Response rates and median survival information for both the US and international multicenter trials are given in the following table:

Trial	% Complete Response (CR)		Median Time to CR (days)		Median Survival (days)	
	NOV	DAUN	NOV	DAUN	NOV	DAUN
US	63 (62/98)	53 (54/102)	35	42	312	237
Foreign	50 (56/112)	51 (62/123)	36	42	192	230

NOV = NOVANTRONE + Cytosine arabinoside
DAUN = Daunorubicin + Cytosine arabinoside

In these studies, two consolidation courses were administered to complete responders on each arm. Consolidation therapy consisted of the same drug and daily dosage used for remission induction, but only 5 days of cytosine arabinoside and 2 days of NOVANTRONE *mitoxantrone for Injection Concentrate* or daunorubicin were given. The first consolidation course was administered 6 weeks after the start of the final induction course if the patient achieved a complete remission. The second consolidation course was generally administered 4 weeks later. Full hematologic recovery was necessary for patients to receive consolidation therapy. For the US trial, median granulocyte nadirs for patients receiving NOVANTRONE + cytosine arabinoside for consolidation courses 1 and 2 were 10/mm³ for both courses, and for those patients receiving daunorubicin + cytosine arabinoside were 170/mm³ and 260/mm³, respectively. Median platelet nadirs for patients who received NOVANTRONE + cytosine arabinoside for consolidation courses 1 and 2 were 17,000/mm³ and 14,000/mm³, respectively, and were 33,000/mm³ and 22,000/mm³ in courses 1 and 2 for those patients who received daunorubicin + cytosine arabinoside. The benefit of consolidation therapy in ANLL patients who

achieve a complete remission remains controversial. However, in the only well-controlled prospective, randomized multicenter trials with NOVANTRONE in ANLL, consolidation therapy was given to all patients who achieved a complete remission. During consolidation in the US study, two myelosuppression-related deaths occurred on the NOVANTRONE arm and one on the daunorubicin arm. However, in the foreign study there were eight deaths on the NOVANTRONE arm during consolidation which were related to the myelosuppression and none on the daunorubicin arm where less myelosuppression occurred.

INDICATIONS AND USAGE

NOVANTRONE in combination with other approved drug(s) is indicated in the initial therapy of acute nonlymphocytic leukemia (ANLL) in adults. This category includes myelogenous, promyelocytic, monocytic, and erythroid acute leukemias.

CONTRAINDICATIONS

NOVANTRONE is contraindicated in patients who have demonstrated prior hypersensitivity to it.

WARNINGS

WHEN NOVANTRONE IS USED IN DOSES INDICATED FOR THE TREATMENT OF LEUKEMIA, SEVERE MYELOSUPPRESSION WILL OCCUR. THEREFORE, IT IS RECOMMENDED THAT NOVANTRONE BE ADMINISTERED ONLY BY PHYSICIANS EXPERIENCED IN THE CHEMOTHERAPY OF THIS DISEASE. LABORATORY AND SUPPORTIVE SERVICES MUST BE AVAILABLE FOR HEMATOLOGIC AND CHEMISTRY MONITORING AND ADJUNCTIVE THERAPIES, INCLUDING ANTIBIOTICS: BLOOD AND BLOOD PRODUCTS MUST BE AVAILABLE TO SUPPORT PATIENTS DURING THE EXPECTED PERIOD OF MEDULLARY HYPOPLASIA AND SEVERE MYELOSUPPRESSION. PARTICULAR CARE SHOULD BE GIVEN TO ASSURING FULL HEMATOLOGIC RECOVERY BEFORE UNDERTAKING CONSOLIDATION THERAPY (IF THIS TREATMENT IS USED) AND PATIENTS SHOULD BE MONITORED CLOSELY DURING THIS PHASE.

Patients with preexisting myelosuppression as the result of prior drug therapy should not receive NOVANTRONE unless it is felt that the possible benefit from such treatment warrants the risk of further medullary suppression. Because of the possible danger of cardiac effects in patients previously treated with daunorubicin or doxorubicin, the benefit-to-risk ratio of NOVANTRONE therapy in such patients should be determined before starting therapy.

The safety of NOVANTRONE in patients with hepatic insufficiency is not established. (See **CLINICAL PHARMACOLOGY**.)

Cardiac Effects: *General:* Functional cardiac changes including congestive heart failure and decreases in left ventricular ejection fraction (LVEF) occur with NOVANTRONE. Cardiac toxicity may be more common in patients with prior treatment with anthracyclines, prior mediastinal radiotherapy, or with preexisting cardiovascular disease. Such patients should have regular cardiac monitoring of LVEF from the initiation of therapy. In investigational trials of intermittent single doses in other tumor types, patients who received up to the cumulative dose of 140 mg/m² had a cumulative 2.6% probability of clinical congestive heart failure. The overall cumulative probability rate of moderate or serious decreases in LVEF at this dose was 13% in comparative trials.

Leukemia: Acute CHF may occasionally occur in patients treated with NOVANTRONE for ANLL. In first-line comparative trials of NOVANTRONE + cytosine arabinoside v daunorubicin + cytosine arabinoside in adult patients with previously untreated ANLL, therapy was associated with congestive heart failure in 6.5% of patients on each arm. A causal relationship between drug therapy and cardiac effects is difficult to establish in this setting since myocardial function is frequently depressed by the anemia, fever and infection, and hemorrhage, which often accompany the underlying disease.

Pregnancy Category D: NOVANTRONE *mitoxantrone for Injection Concentrate* may cause fetal harm when administered to a pregnant woman. In treated rats, low fetal birth weight and retarded development of the fetal kidney were seen in greater frequency. In rabbits an increased incidence of premature delivery was observed. NOVANTRONE was not teratogenic in rabbits. There are no adequate and well-controlled studies in pregnant women. If this drug is used during pregnancy, or if the patient becomes pregnant while taking this drug, the patient should be apprised of the potential hazard to the fetus. Women of childbearing potential should be advised to avoid becoming pregnant.

Safety for use by routes other than intravenous administration has not been established.

PRECAUTIONS

General: Therapy with NOVANTRONE should be accompanied by close and frequent monitoring of hematologic and

chemical laboratory parameters, as well as frequent patient observation.

Hyperuricemia may occur as a result of rapid lysis of tumor cells by NOVANTRONE. Serum uric acid levels should be monitored and hypouricemic therapy instituted prior to the initiation of antileukemic therapy.

Systemic infections should be treated concomitantly with or just prior to commencing therapy with NOVANTRONE.

Information for Patients: NOVANTRONE may impart a blue-green color to the urine for 24 hours after administration, and patients should be advised to expect this during therapy. Bluish discoloration of the sclera may also occur. Patients should be advised of the signs and symptoms of myelosuppression.

Laboratory Tests: Serial complete blood counts and liver function tests are necessary for appropriate dose adjustments. (See **DOSAGE AND ADMINISTRATION**.)

Carcinogenesis, Mutagenesis: NOVANTRONE *mitoxantrone for Injection Concentrate* can result in chromosomal aberrations in animals and it is mutagenic in bacterial systems. NOVANTRONE caused DNA damage and sister chromatid exchanges *in vitro*.

Pregnancy Category D: (See **WARNINGS**.)

Nursing Mothers: It is not known whether NOVANTRONE is excreted in human milk. Because of the potential for serious adverse reactions in infants from NOVANTRONE, breast feeding should be discontinued before starting treatment.

Pediatric Use: Safety and effectiveness in children have not been established.

ADVERSE REACTIONS

NOVANTRONE has been studied in approximately 600 patients with acute nonlymphocytic leukemia. The table below represents the adverse reaction experience in the large US comparative study of mitoxantrone + cytosine arabinoside *v* daunorubicin + cytosine arabinoside. Experience in the large foreign study was similar. A much wider experience in a variety of other tumor types revealed no additional important reactions other than cardiomyopathy (see **WARNINGS**.) It should be appreciated that the listed adverse reaction categories include overlapping clinical symptoms related to the same condition, eg, dyspnea, cough, and pneumonia. In addition, the listed adverse reactions cannot all necessarily be attributed to chemotherapy as it is often impossible to distinguish effects of the drug and effects of the underlying disease. It is clear, however, that the combination of NOVANTRONE + cytosine arabinoside was responsible for nausea and vomiting, alopecia, mucositis/stomatitis, and myelosuppression.

The following table summarizes adverse reactions occurring in patients treated with NOVANTRONE + cytosine arabinoside in comparison with those who received daunorubicin + cytosine arabinoside for therapy of ANLL in a large, multicenter, randomized prospective US trial. Adverse reactions are presented as major categories and selected examples of clinically significant subcategories.

[See table above.]

Allergic Reaction: Hypotension, urticaria, dyspnea, and rashes have been reported occasionally.

Cutaneous: Phlebitis has been reported infrequently at the site of infusion. There have been rare reports of tissue necrosis following extravasation.

Hematologic: Myelosuppression is rapid in onset and is consistent with the requirement to produce significant marrow hypoplasia in order to achieve a response. The incidences of infection and bleeding seen in the US trial are consistent with those reported for other standard induction regimens.

Gastrointestinal: Nausea and vomiting occurred acutely in most patients, but were generally mild to moderate and could be controlled through the use of antiemetics. Stomatitis/mucositis occurs within 1 week of therapy.

Cardiovascular: Congestive heart failure, tachycardia, EKG changes including arrhythmias, chest pain, and asymptomatic decreases in left ventricular ejection fraction have occurred (see **WARNINGS**).

OVERDOSAGE

There is no known specific antidote for NOVANTRONE *mitoxantrone for Injection Concentrate*. Accidental overdoses have been reported. Four patients receiving 140 to 180 mg/m^2 as a single bolus injection died as a result of severe leukopenia with infection. Hematologic support and antimicrobial therapy may be required during prolonged periods of medullary hypoplasia.

Although patients with severe renal failure have not been studied, NOVANTRONE is extensively tissue bound and it is unlikely that the therapeutic effect or toxicity would be mitigated by peritoneal or hemodialysis.

DOSAGE AND ADMINISTRATION
(See **WARNINGS**.)

NOVANTRONE SOLUTION MUST BE DILUTED PRIOR TO USE.

Combination Initial Therapy for ANLL in Adults: For induction, the recommended dosage is 12 mg/m^2 of

	ALL INDUCTION (percentage of pts entering induction)		ALL CONSOLIDATION (percentage of pts entering consolidation)	
	NOV N=102	DAUN N=102	NOV N=55	DAUN N=49
Cardiovascular	26	28	11	24
CHF	5	6	0	0
Arrhythmias	3	3	4	4
Bleeding	37	41	20	6
GI	16	12	2	2
Petechiae/Ecchymoses	7	9	11	2
Gastrointestinal	88	85	58	51
Nausea/Vomiting	72	67	31	31
Diarrhea	47	47	18	8
Abdominal Pain	15	9	9	4
Mucositis/Stomatitis	29	33	18	8
Hepatic	10	11	14	2
Jaundice	3	8	7	0
Infections	66	73	60	43
UTI	7	2	7	2
Pneumonia	9	7	9	0
Sepsis	34	36	31	18
Fungal Infections	15	13	9	6
Renal Failure	8	6	0	2
Fever	78	71	24	18
Alopecia	37	40	22	16
Pulmonary	43	43	24	14
Cough	13	9	9	2
Dyspnea	18	20	6	0
CNS	30	30	34	35
Seizures	4	4	2	8
Headache	10	9	13	8
Eye	7	6	2	4
Conjunctivitis	1	1	0	0

NOVANTRONE daily on days 1 to 3 given as an intravenous infusion, and 100 mg/m^2 cytosine arabinoside for 7 days given as a continuous 24-hour infusion on days 1 to 7.

Most complete remissions will occur following the initial course of induction therapy. In the event of an incomplete antileukemic response, a second induction course may be given. NOVANTRONE *mitoxantrone for Injection Concentrate* should be given for 2 days and cytosine arabinoside for 5 days using the same daily dosage levels.

If severe or life-threatening nonhematologic toxicity is observed during the first induction course, the second induction course should be withheld until toxicity clears.

Consolidation therapy which was used in two large, randomized, multicenter trials consisted of NOVANTRONE 12 mg/m^2 given by intravenous infusion daily for days 1 and 2 and cytosine arabinoside 100 mg/m^2 for 5 days given as a continuous 24-hour infusion on days 1 to 5. The first course was given approximately 6 weeks after the final induction course; the second was generally administered 4 weeks after the first. Severe myelosuppression occurred. (See **CLINICAL PHARMACOLOGY**.)

The dose of NOVANTRONE should be diluted to at least 50 mL with either 0.9% Sodium Chloride Injection (USP) or 5% Dextrose Injection (USP). This solution should be introduced slowly into the tubing as a freely running intravenous infusion of 0.9% Sodium Chloride Injection (USP) or 5% Dextrose Injection (USP) over a period of not less than 3 minutes. Unused infusion solutions should be discarded in an appropriate fashion. In the case of multidose use, the remaining portion of the undiluted NOVANTRONE concentrate should be stored not longer than 7 days between 15°C (59°F) and 25°C (77°F) or 14 days under refrigeration. If extravasation occurs, the administration should be stopped immediately and restarted in another vein. The nonvesicant properties of NOVANTRONE minimize the possibility of severe local reactions following extravasation. However, care should be taken to avoid extravasation at the infusion site and to avoid contact of NOVANTRONE with the skin, mucous membranes, or eyes.

Skin accidentally exposed to NOVANTRONE should be rinsed copiously with warm water and if the eyes are involved, standard irrigation techniques should be used immediately. The use of goggles, gloves, and protective gowns is recommended during preparation and administration of the drug. Spills on equipment and environmental surfaces may be cleaned using an aqueous solution of calcium hypochlorite (5.5 parts calcium hypochlorite in 13 parts by weight of water for each 1 part of NOVANTRONE). Absorb the solution with gauze or towels and dispose of these in a safe manner. Appropriate safety equipment such as goggles and gloves should be worn while working with calcium hypochlorite.

NOVANTRONE should not be mixed in the same infusion as heparin since a precipitate may form. Because specific compatibility data are not available, it is recommended that NOVANTRONE not be mixed in the same infusion with other drugs.

Procedures for proper handling and disposal of anticancer drugs should be considered. Several guidelines on this subject have been published.[1-6] There is no general agreement that all of the procedures recommended in the guidelines are necessary or appropriate.

REFERENCES

1. Recommendations for the Safe Handling of Parenteral Antineoplastic Drugs. NIH Publication No. 83-2621. For sale by the Superintendent of Documents, U.S. Government Printing Office, Washington, D.C. 20402.
2. AMA Council Report. Guidelines for Handling Parenteral Antineoplastics. *JAMA*. March 15, 1985.
3. National Study Commission on Cytotoxic Exposure—Recommendations for Handling Cytotoxic Agents. Available from Louis P. Jeffrey, Sc. D., Director of Pharmacy Services, Rhode Island Hospital, 593 Eddy Street, Providence, Rhode Island 02902.
4. Clinical Oncological Society of Australia: Guidelines and recommendations for safe handling of antineoplastic agents. *Med J Australia*. 1983; 1:426–428.
5. Jones RB, et al. Safe handling of chemotherapeutic agents: A report from the Mount Sinai Medical Center. *Ca—A Cancer Journal for Clinicians*. Sept/Oct. 1983; 258–263.
6. American Society of Hospital Pharmacists: Technical assistance bulletin on handling cytotoxic drugs in hospitals. *Am J Hosp Pharm*. 1985; 42:131–137.

NOVANTRONE may be further diluted into Dextrose 5% in Water, Normal Saline or Dextrose 5% with Normal Saline and used immediately. DO NOT FREEZE.

Parenteral drug products should be inspected visually for particulate matter and discoloration prior to administration whenever solution and container permit.

HOW SUPPLIED

NOVANTRONE *mitoxantrone for Injection Concentrate* is a sterile aqueous solution containing mitoxantrone hydrochloride at a concentration equivalent to 2 mg mitoxantrone free base per mL supplied in vials for single dose use as follows:

NDC 0205-9393-34—10 mL/multidose vial (20 mg)
NDC 0205-9393-72—12.5 mL/multidose vial (25 mg)
NDC 0205-9393-36—15 mL/multidose vial (30 mg)

NOVANTRONE should be stored between 15°C (59°F) and 25°C (77°F). DO NOT FREEZE.

After the penetration of the stopper, the remaining portion of NOVANTRONE may be stored no longer than 7 days between 15°C (59°F) and 25°C (77°F) or 14 days under refrigeration. CONTAINS NO PRESERVATIVE.

Rev. 2/92
21827-92

LEDERLE PARENTERALS
Carolina, Puerto Rico 00630

Shown in Product Identification Section, page 415

Continued on next page

Lederle—Cont.

OCCUCOAT®
2% Hydroxypropylmethylcellulose

(See PDR For Ophthalmology.)

ORIMUNE® ℞
[or-ĭ-mune]
POLIOVIRUS VACCINE
LIVE ORAL TRIVALENT
0.5 mL Dose Contains Sorbitol
SABIN STRAINS TYPES 1, 2 and 3
FOR ORAL ADMINISTRATION—
NOT FOR INJECTION

DESCRIPTION
Manufacture and Composition: ORIMUNE is a mixture of three types of attenuated polioviruses that have been propagated in monkey kidney cell culture. The cells are grown in the presence of Eagle's basal medium consisting of Earle's balanced salt solution containing amino acids, antibiotics, and calf serum. After cell growth, the medium is removed and replaced with fresh medium containing the inoculating virus but no calf serum. The final vaccine is diluted with a modified cell-culture maintenance medium containing sorbitol. Each dose (0.5 mL) contains less than 25 micrograms of each of the antibiotics, streptomycin and neomycin.
Potency of the vaccine is expressed in terms of the amount of virus (log_{10}) contained in the recommended dose as tissue culture infective doses ($TCID_{50}$). The human dose of vaccine containing all three virus types shall be constituted to have infectivity titers in the final container material of $10^{5.4}$ to $10^{6.4}$ for Type 1, $10^{4.5}$ to $10^{5.5}$ for Type 2, and $10^{5.2}$ to $10^{6.2}$ for Type 3, when the primary monkey kidney tube titration method is used.[1] If the more sensitive Hep-2 microtitration procedure is employed to determine the infectivity titers in each human dose, then equivalent vaccine is achieved with numerical infectivity titers of $10^{6.0}$ to $10^{7.0}$ for Type 1, $10^{5.1}$ to $10^{6.1}$ for Type 2, and $10^{5.8}$ to $10^{6.8}$ for Type 3.[2]

CLINICAL PHARMACOLOGY
Administration of attenuated, live oral poliovirus vaccine (OPV) simulates natural infection, inducing active mucosal and systemic immunity without producing symptoms of disease. For optimal mucosal immunity to occur, it is necessary for the viruses to multiply in the intestinal tract. A primary series of trivalent vaccine is designed to produce an antibody response to poliovirus Types 1, 2, and 3. This response is comparable to the immunity induced by the natural disease. The antibodies thus formed help protect the individual against clinical poliomyelitis infection by any of the three types of poliovirus. Multiple sequential doses of OPV are administered to ensure that immunity to all three types of poliovirus has been achieved.[3] When used in the prescribed manner for immunization, type-specific neutralizing antibodies will be induced in 95% or more of susceptibles.[4]

INDICATIONS AND USAGE
This vaccine is indicated for use in the prevention of poliomyelitis caused by poliovirus Types 1, 2, and 3.
Infants from 6 to 12 weeks of age, *all unimmunized children*, and *adolescents* up to age 18 are the usual candidates for routine prophylaxis.
The Immunization Practices Advisory Committee (ACIP) of the Public Health Service states that trivalent oral poliovirus vaccine (OPV) and inactivated poliovirus vaccine (IPV) are both effective in preventing poliomyelitis.
The choice of OPV as the preferred poliovirus vaccine for primary administration to children in the United States has been made by the ACIP, the Committee on Infectious Diseases of the American Academy of Pediatrics, and a special expert committee of the Institute of Medicine, National Academy of Science.[3–6] OPV is preferred because it induces intestinal immunity, is simple to administer, is well accepted by patients, results in immunization of some contacts of vaccinated persons, and has a record of having essentially eliminated disease associated with wild poliovirus in this country.[4] OPV is also recommended for control of epidemic poliomyelitis.[3,5]
IPV is specifically indicated for use in immunodeficient individuals, their household contacts, or in certain adults (see **CONTRAINDICATIONS** and **INDICATIONS AND USAGE: Use in Adults** for details).[6]
Prior to immunization, the parent, guardian, or adult patient should be informed of the two types of poliovirus vaccines available, the risks and benefits of each to the individual and to the community, and the reasons why recommendations are made for giving specific vaccines under certain circumstances.
Past history of clinical poliomyelitis or prior vaccination with IPV in otherwise healthy individuals does not preclude the administration of OPV when otherwise indicated.

The simultaneous administration of OPV, diphtheria and tetanus toxoids and pertussis vaccine (DTP), and/or measles-mumps-rubella vaccine (MMR), has resulted in seroconversion rates and rates of side effects similar to those observed when the vaccines are administered separately.[7]
Administration of Immune Globulin (IG), if necessary, within 7 days prior to immunization with OPV does not reduce the antibody response to OPV based on a study conducted in Peace Corps volunteers.[8]
Use in Adults: Routine primary poliovirus immunization of adults (generally those 18 years of age or older), residing in the United States, is not recommended by the Immunization Practices Advisory Committee (ACIP). Immunization *is* recommended by the ACIP for certain adults who are at greater risk of exposure to wild polioviruses than the general population, including travelers to areas where poliomyelitis is endemic or epidemic, members of communities or specific population groups with disease caused by wild polioviruses, laboratory workers handling specimens that may contain polioviruses, and health care workers in close contact with patients who might be excreting polioviruses as follows:
Unimmunized adults - primary immunization with enhanced-potency IPV is recommended. However, if less than 1 month is available before protection is needed, a single dose of either OPV or enhanced-potency IPV is recommended, with the remaining doses given later if the person remains at increased risk. *Incompletely immunized adults* who have had (1) at least one dose of OPV, (2) fewer than three doses of conventional IPV, or (3) a combination of conventional IPV and OPV totaling fewer than three doses, should receive at least one dose of OPV or enhanced-potency IPV. Additional doses needed to complete a primary series should be given prior to exposure, if time permits. *Adults who have completed a primary series* with any one or a combination of polio vaccines may be given a dose of OPV or enhanced-potency IPV.[6]
Immunization with IPV may be undertaken in unimmunized or inadequately immunized adults in households in which children are to be given OPV (see **ADVERSE REACTIONS**).[3,6]
Epidemic Control: Poliovirus Vaccine Live Oral Trivalent has been recommended for epidemic control. Within an epidemic area, OPV should be provided for all persons over 6 weeks of age who have not been completely immunized or whose immunization status is unknown, with the exceptions noted under immunodeficiency.[3,5] (See **CONTRAINDICATIONS**.)
In certain tropical endemic areas, where poliomyelitis has been increasing in recent years, the physician may wish to administer OPV to the infant at birth. Because successful immunization is less likely in newborn infants, a complete series of OPV should follow the neonatal dose beginning when the infants are 2 months old.[3] If the physician elects to immunize the infant at birth, it may be prudent to wait until the child is 3 days old, and to recommend abstention from breast-feeding for 2 to 3 hours before and after oral immunization to minimize exposure of the vaccine viruses to colostrum and to permit the establishment of the vaccine viruses in the gut.[9]

CONTRAINDICATIONS
Under no circumstances should this vaccine be administered parenterally.
Poliovirus vaccine live oral trivalent ORIMUNE *must not* be administered to patients with immune deficiency diseases such as combined immunodeficiency, hypogammaglobulinemia and agammaglobulinemia. Further, ORIMUNE *must not* be administered to patients with altered immune states, such as those occurring in human immunodeficiency virus (HIV) infection, thymic abnormalities, leukemia, lymphoma, generalized malignancy, or advanced debilitating conditions, or by lowered resistance from therapy with corticosteroids, alkylating drugs, antimetabolites, or radiation. Because vaccine viruses are excreted by the vaccinee, and may spread to contacts, ORIMUNE should not be used in families with immunodeficient members.[3,4]
Recipients of the vaccine should avoid close household-type contact with all persons with altered immune status for at least 6 to 8 weeks.
Because of the possibility of immunodeficiency in other children born to a family in which there has been one such case, OPV should not be given to a member of a household in which there is a family history of immunodeficiency until the immune status of the intended recipient and other children in the family is determined to be normal.[4]
Immunization of all persons in the above described circumstances should be with IPV.

WARNINGS
Under no circumstances should this vaccine be administered parenterally.
Immunization should be deferred during the course of any febrile illness or acute infection. In addition, immunization should be deferred in the presence of persistent vomiting or diarrhea, or suspected gastroenteritis infection. Other

viruses (including poliovirus and other enteroviruses) may compromise the desired response to this vaccine, since their presence in the intestinal tract may interfere with replication of the attenuated strains of poliovirus.

PRECAUTIONS
The vaccine is not effective in modifying or preventing cases of existing and/or incubating poliomyelitis.

Records Required by the National Childhood Vaccine Injury Act: This Act requires that the manufacturer and lot number of the vaccine administered be recorded by the health care provider in the vaccine recipient's permanent record, along with the date of administration of the vaccine and the name, address, and title of the person administering the vaccine.
The Act further requires that the health care provider report to a health department or to the FDA the occurrence, following immunization, of any event set forth in the Vaccine Injury Table including: paralytic poliomyelitis—in a nonimmunodeficient recipient within 30 days of vaccination,—in an immunodeficient recipient within 6 months of vaccination; any vaccine-associated community case of paralytic poliomyelitis; or any acute complication or sequela (including death) of above events.[10]

Use in Pregnancy: *Pregnancy Category C:* Animal reproduction studies have not been conducted with Poliovirus Vaccine Live Oral Trivalent. It is also not known whether OPV can cause fetal harm when administered to a pregnant woman or can affect reproduction capacity.
Although there is no convincing evidence documenting adverse effects of either OPV or IPV on the developing fetus or pregnant women, it is prudent on theoretical grounds to avoid vaccinating pregnant women. However, if immediate protection against poliomyelitis is needed, OPV is recommended.[3,6] (See **CONTRAINDICATIONS** and **ADVERSE REACTIONS**.)

ADVERSE REACTIONS
Paralytic disease following the ingestion of live poliovirus vaccines has been, on rare occasion, reported in individuals receiving the vaccine, and in persons who were in close contact with vaccinees.[3,4,11,12] The vaccine viruses are shed in the vaccinee's stools up to 6 to 8 weeks as well as via the pharyngeal route. Most reports of paralytic disease following ingestion of the vaccine or contact with a recent vaccinee are based on epidemiological analysis and temporal association between vaccination or contact and the onset of symptoms and most authorities believe that a causal relationship exists.[2,5,10,11,12]
A retrospective study of a large population given OPV suggests that this vaccine may also be temporally associated with Guillain-Barre syndrome.[13] A causal relationship has not been established.
Prior to administration of the vaccine, the attending physician should warn or specifically direct personnel acting under their authority to convey the warnings to the vaccinee, parent, guardian, or other responsible person of the possibility of vaccine-associated paralysis, particularly to the recipient, susceptible family members and other close personal contacts.[3,4]
The Centers for Disease Control report that during the years 1973 through 1984 approximately 274.1 million OPV doses were distributed in the United States. During this same period, 105 vaccine-associated cases were reported (1 case per 2.6 million doses distributed). Of these 105 cases, 35 occurred in vaccine recipients (1 case per 7.8 million doses distributed), 50 occurred in household and nonhousehold contacts of vaccinees (1 case per 5.5 million doses distributed), 14 occurred in immunodeficient recipients or contacts, and 6 occurred in persons with no history of vaccine exposure, from whom vaccine-like viruses were isolated.[11] Thirty-three (94%) of the recipient cases, 41 (82%) of the contact cases, and 5 (36%) of the immune deficient cases were associated with the recipient's first dose of OPV. Because most cases of vaccine-associated paralysis have occurred in association with the first dose, the CDC has estimated the likelihood of paralysis in association with first *v* subsequent doses of OPV, using the number of births during 1973–1984 to estimate the number of first doses distributed, and subtracting this from the total distribution to estimate the number of subsequent doses distributed. This method estimates a frequency of paralysis for recipients of one case per 1.2 million first doses *v* one case per 116.5 million subsequent doses; for contacts, one case per 1 million first doses *v* one case per 25.9 million subsequent doses; with an overall frequency of 1 case per 520,000 first doses *v* one case per 12.3 million subsequent doses.[11]
Other methods of estimating the likelihood of paralysis in association with OPV have been described. Because the number of susceptible vaccine recipients or contacts of recipients is not known, the true risk of vaccine-associated poliomyelitis is impossible to determine precisely.[10]

When the attenuated vaccine strains are to be introduced into a household with adults who are unimmunized or whose immune status cannot be determined, the risk of vaccine-associated paralysis can be reduced by giving these adults two doses of enhanced potency IPV a month apart before the children receive *poliovirus vaccine live oral trivalent* ORIMUNE. The children may receive the first dose of ORIMUNE at the same visit that the adults receive the second dose of enhanced potency IPV. For partially immunized adult contacts, a booster dose of enhanced potency IPV can be given at the same visit that the first dose of OPV is given to the child.[3]

The responsible adult should also be informed of precautions to be taken such as handwashing after diaper changes.[14]

The ACIP states: "Because of the overriding importance of ensuring prompt and complete immunization of the child and the extreme rarity of OPV-associated disease in contacts, the Committee recommends the administration of OPV to a child regardless of the poliovirus-vaccine status of adult household contacts. This is the usual practice in the United States. The responsible adult should be informed of the small risk involved. An acceptable alternative, if there is a strong assurance that ultimate, full immunization of the child will not be jeopardized or unduly delayed, is to immunize adults... [with IPV]... before giving OPV to the child."[4]

The American Academy of Pediatrics and the American College of Physicians have made similar recommendations.[3,14]

DOSAGE AND ADMINISTRATION

Poliovirus vaccine live oral trivalent ORIMUNE is to be administered *orally, under the supervision of a physician. Under no circumstances should this vaccine be administered parenterally.* For convenience, the vaccine is supplied in a disposable pipette containing a single dose of 0.5 mL which should be administered directly into the mouth of the vaccinee. Breast feeding does not interfere with successful immunization when OPV is administered according to the following schedule.[4]

Primary Series: The primary series consists of three doses. *Infants:* The ACIP and AAP recommend that the first dose of OPV be administered when the infant is approximately 2 months (6 to 12 weeks) of age. The second dose should be given not less than 6 and preferably 8 weeks later, commonly at 4 months of age. A third dose of OPV should be given when the child is approximately 15 to 18 months of age to complete the primary series, but may be given at any time between 12 and 24 months of age.[3] In endemic areas an additional dose administered 2 months after the second dose is desirable.[3,4]

Older Children and Adolescents (up to 18 years of age): Unimmunized children and adolescents should receive two doses given not less than 6 and preferably 8 weeks apart, followed by a third dose 6 to 12 months after the second dose. If there is substantial risk of exposure to polio, the third dose should be given 6 to 8 weeks after the second dose.[3,4]

Children at any age who are unimmunized or partially immunized should receive the number of doses necessary to complete the required series of three doses. If the schedule has been interrupted, the series does not need to be reinitiated.[3,7]

Adults: See **INDICATIONS** and **ADVERSE REACTIONS.** Where OPV is given to unimmunized adults the dosage regimen is as indicated for older children and adolescents.

Supplemental Doses: *School Entry:* On entering elementary school, all children who have completed the primary series should be given a single follow-up dose of OPV[3,4] (all others should complete the primary series). The fourth supplemental dose is not required in those who received the third primary dose on or after their fourth birthday.[3,4] The ACIP and AAP do not recommend routine booster doses of vaccine beyond that given at the time of entering school.[3,4] It has been shown that over 95% of children studied 5 years after full immunization with oral polio vaccine had protective antibodies to all three types of poliovirus.[15]

Increased Risk: If an individual who has completed a primary series is subjected to a substantially increased risk because of personal contact, travel, or occupation, a single dose of OPV may be given.[3,4]

SIMULTANEOUS ADMINISTRATION WITH OTHER VACCINES

The simultaneous administration of OPV, diphtheria and tetanus toxoids and pertussis vaccine (DTP) and/or measles-mumps-rubella vaccine (MMR), has resulted in seroconversion rates and rates of side effects similar to those observed when the vaccines are administered separately.[7] The AAP states that OPV, DTP, MMR and/or Haemophilus b conjugate vaccines may be given concomitantly.[3,16]

STORAGE

To maintain the potency of *poliovirus live oral trivalent* ORIMUNE, it is necessary to store this vaccine at a temperature which will maintain ice continuously in a solid state (below 0°C or 32°F). However, since the vaccine contains sorbitol it may remain fluid at temperatures above -14°C (+7°F). Ice cubes that remain frozen continuously when stored in the same freezer compartment will confirm that the temperature is appropriate for storage of ORIMUNE. If frozen, the vaccine must be completely thawed prior to use. A container of vaccine that has been frozen and then is thawed may be carried through a maximum of 10 freeze-thaw cycles, provided the temperature does not exceed 8°C (46°F) during the periods of thaw, and provided the total cumulative duration of thaw does not exceed 24 hours. If the 24-hour period is exceeded, the vaccine must then be used within 30 days, during which time it must be stored at a temperature between 2°C to 8°C (36°F to 46°F). Ideally, an ORIMUNE DISPETTE® should be removed from the freezer and thawed immediately prior to use.

Color Change: This vaccine contains phenol red as a pH indicator. The usual color of the vaccine is pink, although some containers of vaccine, shipped or stored in dry ice, may exhibit a yellow coloration due to the very low temperature or possible absorption of carbon dioxide. The color of the vaccine prior to use (red-pink-yellow) has no effect on the virus or efficacy of the vaccine.

DIRECTIONS FOR USE: Pull off the protective cap and squeeze to expel contents into the vaccinee's mouth.

HOW SUPPLIED

NDC 0005-2084-08—10 (0.5 mL) DISPETTE
NDC 0005-2084-12—50 (0.5 mL) DISPETTE

Military Depot:
NSN 6505-01-185-8848 50 1-dose DISPETTE

REFERENCES

1. *Code of Federal Regulations.* 21 CFR:630.17[c], page 94, Revised April 1, 1989.
2. Albrecht P, Enterline JC, Boone EJ, et al. Poliovirus and polio antibody assay in Hep-2 and Vero cell cultures. *J Biol Stand.* 1983; 11:91–97.
3. *Report of the Committee on Infectious Diseases. American Academy of Pediatrics.* 21st Edition, 1988; 334–342. Elk Grove Village, IL
4. Recommendations of the Immunization Practices Advisory Committee [ACIP], Poliomyelitis Prevention. *MMWR.* 1982; 31[3]:22–34.
5. An evaluation of poliomyelitis vaccine policy options. Institute of Medicine, National Academy of Sciences, 1988. Publication No. 10M 88–04.
6. ACIP. Poliomyelitis prevention: Enhanced-Potency Inactivated Poliomyelitis Vaccine—Supplementary Statement. *MMWR.* 1987; 36[48]:795–798.
7. ACIP. General recommendations on immunization. *MMWR.* 1989; 38[13]:206–227.
8. Kaplan JE, Nelson DB, Schonberger LB, et al. The effect of immune globulin on the response to trivalent oral poliovirus and yellow fever vaccinations. *Bull WHO.* 1984; 62[4]:585–590.
9. Welsh JH, et al. Anti-infective properties of breast milk. *J Pediatr.* 1979; 94[1]:1–9.
10. National Childhood Injury Act: Requirements for permanent vaccination records and for reporting of selected events after vaccination. *MMWR.* 1988; 37[13]; 197–200.
11. Nkowane BM, Wassilak SGF, Orenstein WA, et al. Vaccine-associated paralytic poliomyelitis. United States: 1973 through 1984. *JAMA.* 1987; 257[10]:1335–1340.
12. Esteves K. Safety of oral poliomyelitis vaccine: results of a WHO enquiry. *Bull WHO.* 1988; 66[6]:739–746.
13. Kinnunen E, Farkkila M, Hovi T, et al. Incidence of Guillain-Barre syndrome during a nationwide oral poliovirus vaccine campaign. *Neurology.* 1989; 39:1034–1036.
14. Guide for Adult Immunization. American College of Physicians, 2nd Edition, 25, 1990. Philadelpia, PA.
15. Krugman RD, et al. Antibody persistence after primary immunization with trivalent oral poliovirus vaccine. *Pediatrics.* 1977; 60[1]:80–82.
16. American Academy of Pediatrics, Haemophilus Influenzae Type B Conjugate Vaccines. Immunization of children 2 to 15 months of age. *PED COMM: AAP MEMBER ALERT,* October 1990.

LEDERLE LABORATORIES DIVISION
American Cyanamid Company, Pearl River, NY 10965
Rev. 1/91
10286-91

Shown in Product Identification Section, page 415

PIPRACIL® ℞
[*pĭp-ra-sĭl*]
sterile piperacillin sodium
For Intravenous and Intramuscular Use

PRODUCT OVERVIEW

KEY FACTS

PIPRACIL is a semisynthetic broad-spectrum penicillin antibiotic for parenteral administration. PIPRACIL is bactericidal against a wide range of gram-negative and gram-positive pathogens, including aerobic and anaerobic strains. PIPRACIL has demonstrated excellent activity against *Pseudomonas aeruginosa,* with little development of resistance. It is particularly useful for treating mixed infections and for presumptive therapy prior to identifying the causative organisms.

MAJOR USES

PIPRACIL has been proven effective for treatment of serious infections, including bacteremia, caused by susceptible strains of microorganisms. (See full Prescribing Information.) PIPRACIL may be administered as a single drug in some situations where two antibiotics might otherwise be employed. It has also been used successfully with aminoglycosides. Before initiating therapy, obtain cultures for susceptibility testing; once results are known, adjust therapy, if necessary.

SAFETY INFORMATION

PIPRACIL is contraindicated in patients with a history of hypersensitivity reaction to any of the penicillins and/or cephalosporins. While PIPRACIL possesses the characteristic low toxicity of the penicillin group of antibiotics, periodic assessment of organ system functions, including renal, hepatic, and hematopoietic, is advisable during prolonged therapy.

PRESCRIBING INFORMATION

PIPRACIL® ℞
[*pĭp-ra-sĭl*]
sterile piperacillin sodium
For Intravenous and Intramuscular Use

DESCRIPTION

PIPRACIL is a semisynthetic broad-spectrum penicillin for parenteral use derived from D(-)α-aminobenzylpenicillin. The chemical name of piperacillin sodium is [2S-[2α,5α,6β(S*)]]-6-[[[[(4-ethyl-2,3-dioxo-1-piperazinyl) carbonyl]amino]phenylacetyl]amino]-3,3-dimethyl-7-oxo-4-thia-1-azabicyclo[3.2.0]heptane-2-carboxylic acid, monosodium salt.

PIPRACIL is a white to off-white hygroscopic cryodesiccated crystalline powder which is readily soluble in water and gives a colorless to pale-yellow solution. The pH of the aqueous solution is 5.5 to 7.5. One gram contains 1.85 mEq (42.5 mg) of sodium (Na^+).

CLINICAL PHARMACOLOGY

Intravenous Administration: In healthy adult volunteers, mean serum levels immediately after a 2 to 3 minute intravenous injection of 2, 4, or 6 g were 305, 412, and 775 mcg/mL. Serum levels lack dose proportionality.

[See table on next page.]

Intramuscular Administration: PIPRACIL *sterile piperacillin sodium* is rapidly absorbed after intramuscular injection. In healthy volunteers, the mean peak serum concentration occurs approximately 30 minutes after a single dose of 2 g and is about 36 mcg/mL. The oral administration of 1 g probenecid before injection produces an increase in piperacillin peak serum level of about 30%. The area under the curve (AUC) is increased by approximately 60%.

General: PIPRACIL is not absorbed when given orally. Peak serum concentrations are attained approximately 30 minutes after intramuscular injections and immediately after completion of intravenous injection or infusion. The serum half-life in healthy volunteers ranges from 36 minutes to 1 hour and 12 minutes. The mean elimination half-life of PIPRACIL in healthy adult volunteers is 54 minutes following administration of 2 g and 63 minutes following 6 g. As with other penicillins, PIPRACIL is eliminated primarily by glomerular filtration and tubular secretion; it is excreted rapidly as unchanged drug in high concentrations in the urine. Approximately 60% to 80% of the administered dose is excreted in the urine in the first 24 hours. Piperacillin urine concentrations, determined by microbioassay, were as high as 14,100 mcg/mL following a 6 g intravenous dose and 8,500 mcg/mL following a 4 g intravenous dose. These urine drug concentrations remained well above 1,000 mcg/mL throughout the dosing interval. The elimination half-life is increased twofold in mild-to-moderate renal impairment and fivefold to sixfold in severe impairment.

PIPRACIL binding to human serum proteins is 16%. The drug is widely distributed in human tissues and body fluids, including bone, prostate, and heart, and reaches high concentrations in bile. After a 4 g bolus, maximum biliary concentrations averaged 3,205 mcg/mL. It penetrates into the cerebrospinal fluid in the presence of inflamed meninges. Because PIPRACIL is excreted by the biliary route as well as by the renal route, it can be used safely in appropriate dosage (see **DOSAGE AND ADMINISTRATION**) in patients with

Continued on next page

Information on Lederle products listed on these pages is the full prescribing information from product literature or package inserts effective in August 1992. Information concerning all Lederle products may be obtained from the Professional Services Department, Lederle Laboratories, Pearl River, New York 10965.

Lederle—Cont.

severely restricted kidney function, and can be used effectively in treatment of hepatobiliary infections.

Microbiology: PIPRACIL *sterile piperacillin sodium* is an antibiotic which exerts its bactericidal activity by inhibiting both septum and cell wall synthesis. It is active against a variety of gram-positive and gram-negative aerobic and anaerobic bacteria. *In vitro*, piperacillin is active against most strains of clinical isolates of the following microorganisms:

Aerobic and facultatively anaerobic organisms:

Gram-negative bacteria:
Escherichia coli
Proteus mirabilis
Proteus vulgaris
Morganella morganii (formerly *Proteus morganii*)
Providencia rettgeri (formerly *Proteus rettgeri*)
Serratia species including *S marcescens* and *S liquefaciens*
Klebsiella pneumoniae
Klebsiella species
Enterobacter species including *E aerogenes* and *E cloacae*
Citrobacter species including *C freundii* and *C diversus*
Salmonella species*
Shigella species*
Pseudomonas aeruginosa
Pseudomonas species including *P cepacia*,* *P maltophilia*,* and *P fluorescens*
Acinetobacter species (formerly *Mima-Herellea*)
Haemophilus influenzae (non-β-lactamase-producing strains)
Neisseria gonorrhoeae
Neisseria meningitidis
Moraxella species*
Yersinia species* (formerly *Pasteurella*)

Gram-positive bacteria:
Group D streptococci including
   Enterococci (*Streptococcus faecalis, S faecium*)
   Non-enterococci*
β-hemolytic streptococci including
   Group A *Streptococcus* (*S pyogenes*)
   Group B *Streptococcus* (*S agalactiae*)
Streptococcus pneumoniae
Streptococcus viridans
Staphylococcus aureus (non-penicillinase-producing)*
Staphylococcus epidermidis (non-penicillinase-producing)*

Anaerobic bacteria:
Actinomyces species*
Bacteroides species including
   B fragilis group (*B fragilis, B vulgatus*)
   Non-*B fragilis* group (*B melaninogenicus*)
   B asaccharolyticus
Clostridium species including
   C perfringens and *C difficile*
Eubacterium species
Fusobacterium species including
   F nucleatum and *F necrophorum*
Peptococcus species
Peptostreptococcus species
Veillonella species

In vitro, PIPRACIL *sterile piperacillin sodium* is inactivated by staphylococcal β-lactamases, and β-lactamases produced by gram-negative bacteria. However, it is active against β-lactamase-producing gonococci.

Many strains of gram-negative organisms resistant to certain antibiotics have been found to be susceptible to PIPRACIL.

PIPRACIL has excellent activity against gram-positive organisms, including enterococci (*S faecalis*). It is active

---

*Piperacillin has been shown to be active *in vitro* against these organisms; however, clinical efficacy has not yet been established.

---

against obligate anaerobes such as *Bacteroides* species and also against *C difficile* (which has been associated with pseudomembranous colitis).

Piperacillin is active against many gram-negative bacteria including *Enterobacteriaceae, Klebsiella, Serratia, Pseudomonas, E coli, Proteus*, and *Citrobacter*, and, in addition, it is active against anaerobes and enterococci.

In vitro tests show piperacillin to act synergistically with aminoglycoside antibiotics against most isolates of *P aeruginosa*.

Susceptibility Testing: The use of a 100 mcg piperacillin antibiotic disk with susceptibility test methods which measure zone diameter gives an accurate estimation of susceptibility of organisms to PIPRACIL. The following standard procedure† has been recommended for use with disks for testing antimicrobials.

With this type of procedure, a report of "susceptible" from the laboratory indicates that the infecting organism is likely to respond to therapy. A report of "intermediate susceptibility" suggests that the organism would be susceptible if high dosage is used or if the infection is confined to tissue and fluids (eg, urine) in which high antibiotic levels are obtained. A report of "resistant" indicates that the infecting organism is not likely to respond to therapy. With the piperacillin disk, a zone of 18 mm or greater indicates susceptibility, zone sizes of 14 mm or less indicate resistance, and zone sizes of 15 to 17 mm indicate intermediate susceptibility.

Haemophilus and *Neisseria* species which give zones of ≥ 29 mm are susceptible; resistant strains give zones of ≤ 28 mm. The above interpretive criteria are based on the use of the standardized procedure. Antibiotic susceptibility testing requires carefully prescribed procedures. Susceptibility tests are biased to a considerable degree when different methods are used.

The standardized procedure requires the use of control organisms. The 100 mcg piperacillin disk should give zone diameters between 24 and 30 mm for *E coli* ATCC No. 25922 and between 25 and 33 mm for *Pseudomonas aeruginosa* ATCC No. 27853.

Dilution methods such as those described in the International Collaborative Study‡ have been used to determine susceptibility of organisms to PIPRACIL.

Enterobacteriaceae, Pseudomonas species and *Acinetobacter* sp are considered susceptible if the minimal inhibitory concentration (MIC) of piperacillin is no greater than 64 mcg/mL and are considered resistant if the MIC is greater than 128 mcg/mL.

Haemophilus and *Neisseria* species are considered susceptible if the MIC of piperacillin is ≤ 1 mcg/mL.

When anaerobic organisms are isolated from infection sites, it is recommended that other tests such as the modified Broth-Disk Method§ be used to determine the antibiotic susceptibility of these slowly growing organisms.

INDICATIONS AND USAGE

Therapeutic: PIPRACIL is indicated for the treatment of serious infections caused by susceptible strains of the designated organisms in the conditions as listed below.

Intra-abdominal Infections including hepatobiliary and surgical infections caused by *E coli, P aeruginosa*, enterococci, *Clostridium* sp, anaerobic cocci, and *Bacteroides* sp, including *B fragilis*.

---

†NCCLS Approved Standard; M2-A2 (Formerly ASM-2) Performance Standards for Antimicrobic Disk Susceptibility Tests, Second Edition, available from the National Committee of Clinical Laboratory Standards.

‡*Acta Pathol Microbiol Scand* [B] 1971; (suppl) 217.

§ Wilkins TD and Thiel T: *Antimicrob Agents Chemother* 1973; 3:350–356.

Urinary Tract Infections caused by *E coli, Klebsiella* sp, *P aeruginosa, Proteus* sp, including *P mirabilis*, and enterococci.

Gynecologic Infections including endometritis, pelvic inflammatory disease, pelvic cellulitis caused by *Bacteroides* sp including *B fragilis*, anaerobic cocci, *Neisseria gonorrhoeae*, and enterococci (*S faecalis*).

Septicemia including bacteremia caused by *E coli, Klebsiella* sp, *Enterobacter* sp, *Serratia* sp, *P mirabilis, S pneumoniae*, enterococci, *P aeruginosa, Bacteroides* sp, and anaerobic cocci.

Lower Respiratory Tract Infections caused by *E coli, Klebsiella* sp, *Enterobacter* sp, *Pseudomonas aeruginosa, Serratia* sp, *H influenzae, Bacteroides* sp, and anaerobic cocci. Although improvement has been noted in patients with cystic fibrosis, lasting bacterial eradication may not necessarily be achieved.

Skin and Skin Structure Infections caused by *E coli, Klebsiella* sp, *Serratia* sp, *Acinetobacter* sp, *Enterobacter* sp, *Pseudomonas aeruginosa*, indole-positive *Proteus* sp, *Proteus mirabilis, Bacteroides* sp, including *B fragilis*, anaerobic cocci, and enterococci.

Bone and Joint Infections caused by *P aeruginosa*, enterococci, *Bacteroides* sp, and anaerobic cocci.

Gonococcal Infections: PIPRACIL has been effective in the treatment of uncomplicated gonococcal urethritis.

PIPRACIL *sterile piperacillin sodium* has also been shown to be clinically effective for the treatment of infections at various sites caused by *Streptococcus* species including Group A β-hemolytic *Streptococcus* and *S pneumoniae*; however, infections caused by these organisms are ordinarily treated with more narrow spectrum penicillins. Because of its broad spectrum of bactericidal activity against gram-positive and gram-negative aerobic and anaerobic bacteria, PIPRACIL is particularly useful for the treatment of mixed infections and presumptive therapy prior to the identification of the causative organisms.

Also, PIPRACIL may be administered as single drug therapy in some situations where normally two antibiotics might be employed.

Piperacillin has been successfully used with aminoglycosides, especially in patients with impaired host defenses. Both drugs should be used in full therapeutic doses.

Appropriate cultures should be made for susceptibility testing before initiating therapy and therapy adjusted, if appropriate, once the results are known.

Prophylaxis: PIPRACIL is indicated for prophylactic use in surgery including intra-abdominal (gastrointestinal and biliary) procedures, vaginal hysterectomy, abdominal hysterectomy, and cesarean section. Effective prophylactic use depends on the time of administration, and PIPRACIL *sterile piperacillin sodium* should be given one-half to 1 hour before the operation so that effective levels can be achieved in the site prior to the procedure.

The prophylactic use of piperacillin should be stopped within 24 hours, since continuing administration of any antibiotic increases the possibility of adverse reactions, but in the majority of surgical procedures, does not reduce the incidence of subsequent infections. If there are signs of infection, specimens for culture should be obtained for identification of the causative organism so that appropriate therapy can be instituted.

CONTRAINDICATIONS

A history of allergic reactions to any of the penicillins and/or cephalosporins.

WARNINGS

Serious and occasionally fatal hypersensitivity (anaphylactic) reactions have been reported in patients receiving therapy with penicillins. These reactions are more apt to occur in persons with a history of sensitivity to multiple allergens. There have been reports of patients with a history of penicillin hypersensitivity who have experienced severe hypersensitivity reactions when treated with a cephalosporin. Before

---

PIPERACILLIN SERUM LEVELS IN ADULTS (mcg/mL) AFTER A TWO- TO THREE-MINUTE IV INJECTION

DOSE	0	10 min	20 min	30 min	1 h	1.5 h	2 h	3 h	4 h	6 h	8 h
2	305	202	156	67	40	24	20	8	3	2	—
	(159–615)	(164–225)	(52–165)	(41–88)	(25–57)	(18–31)	(14–24)	(3–11)	(2–4)	(<0.6–3)	
4	412	344	295	117	93	60	36	20	8	4	0.9
	(389–484)	(315–379)	(269–330)	(98–138)	(78–110)	(50–67)	(26–51)	(17–24)	(7–11)	(3.7–4.1)	(0.7–1)
6	775	609	563	325	208	138	90	38	33	8	3.2
	(695–849)	(530–670)	(492–630)	(292–363)	(180–239)	(115–175)	(71–113)	(29–53)	(25–44)	(3–19)	(<2–6)

PIPERACILLIN SERUM LEVELS IN ADULTS (mcg/mL) AFTER A 30-MINUTE IV INFUSION

DOSE	0	5 min	10 min	15 min	30 min	45 min	1 h	1.5 h	2 h	4 h	6 h	7.5 h
4	244	215	186	177	141	146	105	72	53	15	4	2
	(155–298)	(169–247)	(140–209)	(142–213)	(122–156)	(110–265)	(85–133)	(53–105)	(36–69)	(6–24)	(1–9)	(0.5–3)
6	353	298	298	272	229	180	149	104	73	22	16	—
	(324–371)	(242–339)	(232–331)	(219–314)	(185–249)	(144–209)	(117–171)	(89–113)	(66–94)	(12–39)	(5–49)	—

A 30-minute infusion of 6 g every 6 h gave, on the fourth day, a mean peak serum concentration of 420 mcg/mL.

initiating therapy with PIPRACIL, careful inquiry should be made concerning previous hypersensitivity reactions to penicillins, cephalosporins, and other allergens. If an allergic reaction occurs during therapy with PIPRACIL, the antibiotic should be discontinued. The usual agents (antihistamines, pressor amines, and corticosteroids) should be readily available. SERIOUS ANAPHYLACTOID REACTIONS REQUIRE IMMEDIATE EMERGENCY TREATMENT WITH EPINEPHRINE. OXYGEN AND INTRAVENOUS CORTICOSTEROIDS AND AIRWAY MANAGEMENT INCLUDING INTUBATION SHOULD ALSO BE ADMINISTERED AS NECESSARY.

PRECAUTIONS

General: While piperacillin possesses the characteristic low toxicity of the penicillin group of antibiotics, periodic assessment of organ system functions, including renal, hepatic, and hematopoietic, during prolonged therapy is advisable. Bleeding manifestations have occurred in some patients receiving β-lactam antibiotics, including piperacillin. These reactions have sometimes been associated with abnormalities of coagulation tests such as clotting time, platelet aggregation and prothrombin time and are more likely to occur in patients with renal failure.

If bleeding manifestations occur, the antibiotic should be discontinued and appropriate therapy instituted.

The possibility of the emergence of resistant organisms which might cause superinfections should be kept in mind, particularly during prolonged treatment. If this occurs, appropriate measures should be taken.

As with other penicillins, patients may experience neuromuscular excitability or convulsions if higher than recommended doses are given intravenously.

PIPRACIL *sterile piperacillin sodium* is a monosodium salt containing 1.85 mEq of Na⁺ per g. This should be considered when treating patients requiring restricted salt intake. Periodic electrolyte determinations should be made in patients with low potassium reserves, and the possibility of hypokalemia should be kept in mind with patients who have potentially low potassium reserves and who are receiving cytotoxic therapy or diuretics.

Antimicrobials used in high doses for short periods to treat gonorrhea may mask or delay the symptoms of incubating syphilis. Therefore, prior to treatment, patients with gonorrhea should also be evaluated for syphilis. Specimens for darkfield examination should be obtained from patients with any suspected primary lesion, and serologic tests should be performed. In all cases where concomitant syphilis is suspected, monthly serological tests should be made for a minimum of 4 months.

As with other semisynthetic penicillins, PIPRACIL therapy has been associated with an increased incidence of fever and rash in cystic fibrosis patients.

Drug Interactions: The mixing of piperacillin with an aminoglycoside *in vitro* can result in substantial inactivation of the aminoglycosides.

Pregnancy: *Pregnancy Category B:* Although reproduction studies in mice and rats performed at doses up to four times the human dose have shown no evidence of impaired fertility or harm to the fetus, safety of PIPRACIL use in pregnant women has not been determined by adequate and well-controlled studies. Because animal reproduction studies are not always predictive of human response, this drug should be used during pregnancy only if clearly needed. It has been found to cross the placenta in rats.

Nursing Mothers: Caution should be exercised when PIPRACIL is administered to nursing mothers. It is excreted in low concentrations in milk.

Pediatric Use: Dosages for children under the age of 12 have not been established. The safety of PIPRACIL in neonates is not known. In dog neonates, dilated renal tubules and peritubular hyalinization occurred following administration of PIPRACIL.

ADVERSE EFFECTS

PIPRACIL is generally well tolerated. The most common adverse reactions have been local in nature, following intravenous or intramuscular injection. The following adverse reactions may occur.

Local Reactions: In clinical trials thrombophlebitis was noted in 4% of patients. Pain, erythema, and/or induration at the injection site occurred in 2% of patients. Less frequent reactions including ecchymosis, deep vein thrombosis, and hematomas have also occurred.

Gastrointestinal: Diarrhea and loose stools were noted in 2% of patients. Other less frequent reactions included vomiting, nausea, increases in liver enzymes (LDH, SGOT, SGPT), hyperbilirubinemia, cholestatic hepatitis, bloody diarrhea, and, rarely, pseudomembranous colitis.

Hypersensitivity Reactions: Anaphylactoid reactions, see WARNINGS.

Rash was noted in 1% of patients. Other less frequent findings included pruritus, vesicular eruptions, positive Coombs tests.

Other dermatologic manifestations such as erythema multiforme and Stevens-Johnson syndrome have been reported rarely.

Renal: Elevations of creatinine or BUN, and, rarely, interstitial nephritis.

Central Nervous System: Headache, dizziness, fatigue.

Hemic and Lymphatic: Reversible leukopenia, neutropenia, thrombocytopenia, and/or eosinophilia have been reported. As with other β-lactam antibiotics, reversible leukopenia (neutropenia) is more apt to occur in patients receiving prolonged therapy at high dosages or in association with drugs known to cause this reaction.

Serum Electrolytes: Individuals with liver disease or individuals receiving cytotoxic therapy or diuretics were reported rarely to demonstrate a decrease in serum potassium concentrations with high doses of piperacillin.

Skeletal: Rarely, prolonged muscle relaxation.

Other: Superinfection, including candidiasis. Hemorrhagic manifestations.

DOSAGE AND ADMINISTRATION

PIPRACIL may be administered by the intramuscular route (see Note) or intravenously or given in a 3- to 5-minute intravenous injection. The usual dosage of PIPRACIL *sterile piperacillin sodium* for serious infections is 3 to 4 g given every 4 to 6 hours as a 20- to 30-minute infusion. For serious infections, the intravenous route should be used.

PIPRACIL should not be mixed with an aminoglycoside in a syringe or infusion bottle since this can result in inactivation of the aminoglycoside.

The maximum daily dose for adults is usually 24 g/day, although higher doses have been used.

Intramuscular injections (see Note) should be limited to 2 g per injection site. This route of administration has been used primarily in the treatment of patients with uncomplicated gonorrhea and urinary tract infections.

NOTE: THE ADD-Vantage VIAL IS NOT FOR IM USE.

DOSAGE RECOMMENDATIONS

Type of Infection	Usual Total Daily Dose
Serious infections such as septicemia, nosocomial pneumonia, intra-abdominal infections, aerobic and anaerobic gynecologic infections, and skin and soft tissue infections	12 to 18 g/d IV (200 to 300 mg/kg/d) in divided doses every 4 to 6 h
Complicated urinary tract infections	8 to 16 g/d IV (125 to 200 mg/kg/d) in divided doses every 6 to 8 h
Uncomplicated urinary tract infections and most community-acquired pneumonia	6 to 8 g/d IM or IV (100 to 125 mg/kg/d) in divided doses every 6 to 12 h
Uncomplicated gonorrhea infections	2 g IM″ as a one-time dose

″ One gram of probenecid given orally one-half hour prior to injection.

The average duration of PIPRACIL *sterile piperacillin sodium* treatment is from 7 to 10 days, except in the treatment of gynecologic infections, in which it is from 3 to 10 days; the duration should be guided by the patient's clinical and bacteriological progress. For most acute infections, treatment should be continued for at least 48 to 72 hours after the patient becomes asymptomatic. Antibiotic therapy for Group A β-hemolytic streptococcal infections should be maintained for at least 10 days to reduce the risk of rheumatic fever or glomerulonephritis.

When PIPRACIL is given concurrently with aminoglycosides, both drugs should be used in full therapeutic doses.

Renal Impairment:

Dosage in Renal Impairment

Creatinine Clearance mL/min	Urinary Tract Infection (uncomplicated)	Urinary Tract Infection (complicated)	Serious Systemic Infection
>40	No dosage adjustment necessary		
20 to 40	No dosage adjustment necessary	9 g/day 3 g every 8 h	12 g/day 4 g every 8 h
<20	6 g/day 3 g every 12 h	6 g/day 3 g every 12 h	8 g/day 4 g every 12 h

For patients on hemodialysis, the maximum daily dose is 6 g/day (2 g every 8 h). In addition, because hemodialysis removes 30% to 50% of piperacillin in 4 hours, 1 g additional dose should be administered following each dialysis period. For patients with renal failure and hepatic insufficiency, measurement of serum levels of PIPRACIL will provide additional guidance for adjusting dosage.

Prophylaxis: When possible, PIPRACIL should be administered as a 20- to 30-minute infusion just prior to anesthesia. Administration while the patient is awake will facilitate identification of possible adverse reactions during drug infusion.

INDICATION	1st Dose	2nd Dose	3rd Dose
Intra-abdominal Surgery	2 g IV just prior to surgery	2 g during surgery	2 g every 6 h postop for no more than 24 h
Vaginal Hysterectomy	2 g IV just prior to surgery	2 g 6 h after 1st dose	2 g 12 h after 1st dose
Cesarean Section	2 g IV after cord is clamped	2 g 4 h after 1st dose	2 g 8 h after 1st dose
Abdominal Hysterectomy	2 g IV just prior to surgery	2 g on return to recovery room	2 g after 6 h

Infants and Children: Dosages in infants and children under 12 years of age have not been established.

PRODUCT RECONSTITUTION/DOSAGE PREPARATION

Conventional Vials:
Diluents for Reconstitution
Sterile Water for Injection
Bacteriostatic£ Water for Injection
Sodium Chloride Injection
Bacteriostatic£ Sodium Chloride Injection
Dextrose 5% in Water
Dextrose 5% and 0.9% Sodium Chloride
Lidocaine HCl 0.5% to 1% (without epinephrine) #
Conventional Vials:
Intravenous Solutions
Dextrose 5% in Water
0.9% Sodium Chloride
Dextrose 5% and 0.9% Sodium Chloride
Lactated Ringer's Injection
Dextran 6% in 0.9% Sodium Chloride
Intravenous Admixtures
Normal Saline [+ KCl 40 mEq]
5% Dextrose in Water [+ KCl 40 mEq]
5% Dextrose/Normal Saline [+ KCl 40 mEq]
Ringer's Injection [+ KCl 40 mEq]
Lactated Ringer's Injection [+ KCl 40 mEq]
ADD-Vantage Vials:**
ADD-Vantage System Admixtures
Dextrose 5% in Water (50 or 100 mL)
0.9% Sodium Chloride (50 or 100 mL)

INTRAVENOUS ADMINISTRATION:
Reconstitution Directions for Conventional Vials: Reconstitute each gram of PIPRACIL *sterile piperacillin sodium* with at least 5 mL of a suitable diluent (except Lidocaine HCl 0.5% to 1% without epinephrine) listed above. Shake well until dissolved. Reconstituted solution may be further diluted to the desired volume (eg, 50 or 100 mL) in the above listed intravenous solutions and admixtures.
Reconstitution Directions for ADD-Vantage Vials: See Instruction Sheet provided in box.

£ Either Parabens or Benzyl Alcohol
For Intramuscular Use Only. Lidocaine is contraindicated in patients with a known history of hypersensitivity to local anesthetics of the amide type.

** (ADD-Vantage is the registered trademark of Abbott Laboratories.)

Continued on next page

Lederle—Cont.

Reconstitution Directions for PHARMACY BULK VIAL: Reconstitute the 40 g vial with 172 mL of a suitable diluent (except Lidocaine HCl 0.5% to 1% without epinephrine) listed above to achieve a concentration of 1 g per 5 mL.

Directions for Administration: *Intermittent IV Infusion* — Infuse diluted solution over period of about 30 minutes. During infusion it is desirable to discontinue the primary intravenous solution.

Intravenous Injection (Bolus) — Reconstituted solution should be injected slowly over a 3- to 5-minute period to help avoid vein irritation.

INTRAMUSCULAR ADMINISTRATION (CONVENTIONAL VIALS ONLY):

Reconstitution Directions: Reconstitute each gram of PIPRACIL with 2 mL of a suitable diluent listed above to achieve a concentration of 1 g per 2.5 mL. Shake well until dissolved.

Directions for Administration: When indicated by clinical and bacteriological findings, intramuscular administration of 6 to 8 g daily of PIPRACIL, in divided doses, may be utilized for initiation of therapy. In addition, intramuscular administration of the drug may be considered for maintenance therapy after clinical and bacteriologic improvement has been obtained with intravenous piperacillin sodium treatment. Intramuscular administration should not exceed 2 g per injection at any one site.

The preferred site is the upper outer quadrant of the buttock (ie, gluteus maximus).

The deltoid area should be used only if well-developed, and then only with caution to avoid radial nerve injury. Intramuscular injections should not be made into the lower or mid-third of the upper arm.

STABILITY OF PIPRACIL FOLLOWING RECONSTITUTION:

PIPRACIL is stable in both glass and plastic containers when reconstituted with recommended diluents and when diluted with the intravenous solutions and intravenous admixtures indicated above.

Extensive stability studies have demonstrated chemical stability (potency, pH, and clarity) through 24 hours at room temperature, up to 1 week refrigerated, and up to 1 month frozen (−10° to −20°C). (Note: The 40 g Pharmacy Bulk Vial should not be frozen after reconstitution.) Appropriate consideration of aseptic technique and individual hospital policy, however, may recommend discarding unused portions after storage for 48 hours under refrigeration and discarding after 24 hours storage at room temperature.

ADD-Vantage System:

Stability studies with the ad-mixed ADD-Vantage system have demonstrated chemical stability (potency, pH, and clarity) through 24 hours at room temperature. (Note: The admixed ADD-Vantage should not be refrigerated or frozen after reconstitution.)

Additional stability data available upon request.

HOW SUPPLIED

PIPRACIL *sterile piperacillin sodium* is available in vials containing sterile freeze-dried piperacillin sodium powder equivalent to 2, 3, 4 and 40 g of piperacillin. One gram of piperacillin (as a monosodium salt) contains 1.85 mEq (42.5 mg) of sodium.

Product Numbers:

NDC 0206-3879-16—2 gram/Vial (10s)
NDC 0206-3882-55—3 gram/Vial (10s)
NDC 0206-3880-25—4 gram/Vial (10s)
NDC 0206-3879-47—2 gram infusion Bottle (10s)
NDC 0206-3882-65—3 gram infusion Bottle (10s)
NDC 0206-3880-66—4 gram infusion Bottle (10s)
NDC 0206-3879-27—2 gram ADD-Vantage Vial (10s)
NDC 0206-3882-28—3 gram ADD-Vantage Vial (10s)
NDC 0206-3880-29—4 gram ADD-Vantage Vial (10s)
NDC 0206-3877-60—40 gram Pharmacy Bulk Vial

Military Depot:

NSN 6505-01-137-0039—3 g infusion bottle (10s)

Military and VA Depots:

NSN 6505-01-280-2317—3 g vial (10s)
NSN 6505-01-280-2318—4 g vial (10s)

Store at Controlled Room Temperature 15°–30°C (59°–86°F).

LEDERLE PIPERACILLIN, INC. Rev. 7/88
Carolina, Puerto Rico 00630 24378

Shown in Product Identification Section, page 415

PNU-IMUNE® 23 ℞

[*new-ī-mune*]
Pneumococcal Vaccine, Polyvalent

DESCRIPTION

Pneumococcal Vaccine Polyvalent, PNU-IMUNE 23 is a sterile preparation intended for intramuscular or subcutaneous use. PNU-IMUNE 23 is indicated for immunization against infections caused by the 23 most prevalent types of *Streptococcus pneumoniae* (pneumococci) which are responsible for approximately 90% of serious pneumococcal disease in the United States and worldwide.[1–5] PNU-IMUNE 23 consists of a mixture of purified capsular polysaccharides from types of *S pneumoniae.* [See table below.]

Each of the pneumococcal polysaccharide types is produced separately to assure a high degree of purity. After an individual pneumococcal type is grown, the polysaccharide is separated from the cell and purified by a series of steps including ethanol fractionation. The vaccine is formulated to contain 25 μg of each of the 23 purified polysaccharide types per 0.5 mL dose of vaccine. Thimerosal (a mercury derivative) at a final concentration of 0.01% is added as a preservative. The vaccine is a clear, colorless liquid.

CLINICAL PHARMACOLOGY

Disease caused by *S pneumoniae* remains an important cause of morbidity and mortality in the United States, particularly in the very young, the elderly, and persons with certain high-risk conditions. Pneumococcal pneumonia accounts for 10% to 25% of all pneumonias and an estimated 40,000 deaths annually.[2]

Studies suggest annual rates of bacteremia of 15 to 19/100,000 for the total population, and 50/100,000 for persons 65 and older. Certain population groups, eg, Native Americans may have considerably higher disease rates.[2]

Mortality from pneumococcal disease is highest in patients with bacteremia or meningitis, patients with underlying medical conditions, and older persons. In some high-risk patients, mortality has been reported to be over 40% for bacteremic disease and 55% for meningitis, despite appropriate antimicrobial therapy.[2]

In addition to the very young and persons 65 years of age or older, patients with certain chronic conditions are at increased risk of developing pneumococcal infection and severe pneumococcal illness. Patients with chronic cardiovascular or pulmonary disease, diabetes mellitus, alcoholism, and cirrhosis are generally immunocompetent but have increased risk. Other patients at greater risk because of decreased responsiveness to polysaccharide antigens or more rapid decline in serum antibody include those with functional or anatomic asplenia (eg, sickle-cell disease or splenectomy), Hodgkin's disease, lymphoma, multiple myeloma, chronic renal failure, nephrotic syndrome, and organ transplantation. Studies indicate that patients with acquired immunodeficiency syndrome (AIDS) are also at increased risk of pneumococcal disease.[6,7] Recurrent pneumococcal meningitis may occur in patients with cerebrospinal fluid leakage that complicates skull fractures or neurologic procedures.

The polysaccharide capsules of pneumococci give these organisms resistance to the phagocytic action of polymorphonuclear leukocytes and monocytes. However, type-specific antibody facilitates their destruction in the body by the mechanism of complement-mediated lysis.

Most healthy adults, including the elderly, demonstrate at least a twofold rise in type-specific antibodies within 2 to 3 weeks of immunization. Similar antibody responses have been reported in patients with alcoholic cirrhosis and diabetes mellitus. In contrast, elderly individuals with chronic pulmonary disease failed to mount a comparable immune response.[26] In immunocompromised patients, the response to immunization may also be lower. Children under 2 years of age respond poorly to most capsular polysaccharide types. Further, response to some pneumococcal types (eg, 6A and 14) important in pediatric infection is decreased in children less than 5 years of age.[8]

In clinical studies with PNU-IMUNE 23 *pneumococcal vaccine, polyvalent* more than 90% of all adults showed twofold or greater increase in geometric mean antibody titer for each capsular type contained in the vaccine.[9]

Patients over the age of 2 years with anatomical or functional asplenia and otherwise intact lymphoid function generally respond to pneumococcal vaccines with a serological conversion comparable to that observed in healthy individuals of the same age.[10]

Patients with acquired immunodeficiency syndrome (AIDS) may have an impaired antibody response to pneumococcal vaccine.[7,11] However, asymptomatic human immunodeficiency virus (HIV)-infected patients, or those with generalized lymphadenopathy, respond to the 23-valent pneumococcal vaccine.[12]

Following immunization of healthy adults, antibody levels remain elevated for at least 5 years, but in some individuals these may fall to preimmunization levels within 10 years.[13,14] A more rapid decline in antibodies may occur in children, particularly those who have undergone a splenectomy and those with sickle-cell disease, in whom antibodies for some types can fall to preimmunization levels 3 to 5 years after immunization.[15,16] Similar rates of decline can occur in children with nephrotic syndrome.[17]

Controlled clinical trials in South Africa involving 12,000 gold miners have shown a 6-valent and a 13-valent pneumococcal vaccine to be 78.5% effective in preventing type-specific pneumococcal pneumonia and 82.3% effective in preventing pneumococcal bacteremia with the types contained in the vaccine.[18] In a preliminary study of an 8-valent polysaccharide vaccine in a group consisting of 77 patients with sickle-cell disease and 19 asplenic persons, there were no pneumococcal infections in the immunized patients within 2 years of immunization. There were eight cases of pneumococcal infection in 106 unimmunized, age-matched patients with sickle-cell disease. Antibody response of the asplenic patients was comparable to that of normal controls.[19]

In a study carried out by Austrian and colleagues with 13-valent pneumococcal vaccines prepared for the National Institute of Allergy and Infectious Disease, the reduction in pneumonias caused by the capsular types present in the vaccines was 79%. Reduction in type-specific pneumococcal bacteremia was 82%.[18]

In a double-blind study of a 14-valent pneumococcal vaccine carried out in Papua, New Guinea, pneumococcal infection was 84% lower in the immunized group and mortality from pneumonia 44% lower.[20] Five case-control studies in the US have evaluated the efficacy of pneumococcal vaccine in the prevention of serious pneumococcal disease. Four of these studies showed the vaccine to be efficacious, with point estimates of efficacy ranging from 61% to 70%.[21–24] One study failed to show efficacy in preventing pneumococcal bacteremia.[25] This study was judged inadequate in determination of vaccination status, and the selection of controls was considered potentially biased.[2]

A prospective study failed to demonstrate efficacy against pneumococcal pneumonia and bronchitis;[26] this study has been criticized for methodological flaws.[2] In contrast, a prospective French study found pneumococcal vaccine to be 77% effective in reducing the incidence of pneumonia among nursing home residents.[27]

Despite conflicting findings, the data continue to support the use of pneumococcal vaccine for certain well-defined groups at risk.[2]

INDICATIONS AND USAGE

PNU-IMUNE 23 *pneumococcal vaccine, polyvalent* is indicated for immunization against pneumococcal disease caused by those pneumococcal types included in the vaccine.

Adults:

1. All adults 65 or older,[2] with emphasis on immunization of the older adult while in good health.
2. Immunocompetent adults who are at increased risk of pneumococcal disease or its complications because of chronic illnesses (eg, cardiovascular or pulmonary disease, diabetes mellitus, alcoholism, cirrhosis, or cerebrospinal fluid leaks).[2]
3. Immunocompromised adults at increased risk of pneumococcal disease or its complications (eg, splenic dysfunction or anatomic asplenia, Hodgkin's disease, lymphoma, multiple myeloma, chronic renal failure, nephrotic syndrome, or conditions such as organ transplantation associated with immunosuppression).[2]

Children:

1. Children 2 years of age or older with chronic illnesses specifically associated with increased risk of pneumococcal disease or its complications (eg, anatomic or functional asplenia [including sickle-cell disease], nephrotic syndrome, cerebrospinal fluid leaks, and conditions associated with immunosuppression).[2]

Special Groups:

1. Persons living in special environments or social settings with an identified increased risk of pneumococcal disease or its complications.[2]
2. Patients with acquired immunodeficiency syndrome (AIDS) have been shown to have an impaired antibody response to pneumococcal vaccine. However, asymptomatic or symptomatic human immunodeficiency virus (HIV)-infected patients or those with persistent generalized lymphadenopathy respond to the 23-valent vaccine.[2]

Timing of Immunization: When elective splenectomy is being considered, pneumococcal vaccine should be given at least 2 weeks before surgery, if possible.[2]

For planning cancer chemotherapy or other immunosuppressive therapy, the interval between immunization and

Nomenclature	Pneumococcal Types																						
Danish	1	2	3	4	5	6B	7F	8	9N	9V	10A	11A	12F	14	15B	17F	18C	19F	19A	20	22F	23F	33F
U.S.	1	2	3	4	5	26	51	8	9	68	34	43	12	14	54	17	56	19	57	20	22	23	70

initiation of chemotherapy or immunosuppression should be at least 2 weeks.[2]

CONTRAINDICATIONS

HYPERSENSITIVITY TO ANY COMPONENT OF THE VACCINE, INCLUDING THIMEROSAL, A MERCURY DERIVATIVE, IS A CONTRAINDICATION TO THE USE OF THE PRODUCT.

THE OCCURRENCE OF ANY TYPE OF NEUROLOGICAL SYMPTOMS OR SIGNS FOLLOWING ADMINISTRATION OF THIS PRODUCT IS A CONTRAINDICATION TO FURTHER USE.

THE VACCINE SHOULD NOT BE ADMINISTERED TO PERSONS WITH ACUTE FEBRILE ILLNESSES UNTIL THEIR TEMPORARY SYMPTOMS AND/OR SIGNS HAVE ABATED.

The clinical judgment of the attending physician should prevail at all times.

WARNINGS

PNU-IMUNE 23 *pneumococcal vaccine, polyvalent* is not an effective agent for prophylaxis against pneumococcal disease caused by types not present in the vaccine.

PNU-IMUNE 23 is not indicated for children under 2 years of age, since antibody response to most capsular polysaccharide types is poor in this age group.[2]

Patients with impaired immune responsiveness whether due to the use of immunosuppressive therapy, a genetic defect, human immunodeficiency virus (HIV) infection, or other causes may have a reduced antibody response to active immunization procedures.[2]

Patients who have received extensive chemotherapy and/or splenectomy for the treatment of Hodgkin's disease have been shown to have an impaired serum antibody response to pneumococcal vaccine.[28,29]

In one study, administration of the vaccine to patients on immunosuppressive drugs and/or irradiation for Hodgkin's disease resulted in reduction of preexisting antibody levels in several patients.[28] It is unclear whether this effect was due to the vaccine or to the effects of irradiation and/or chemotherapy.

At least 2 weeks should elapse between immunization and the initiation of chemotherapy or immunosuppressive therapy.[2]

Routine reimmunization with this vaccine is not recommended. For reimmunization recommendations (including recommendations regarding reimmunization of individuals at highest risk of fatal pneumococcal infection) see **DOSAGE AND ADMINISTRATION.**

In one study, local reactions after reimmunization were more severe than after initial immunization when the interval between immunizations was 13 months.[30]

Patients who have had episodes of pneumococcal pneumonia or other pneumococcal infection may have high levels of preexisting pneumococcal antibodies that may result in increased reactions to PNU-IMUNE 23 *pneumococcal vaccine, polyvalent,* mostly local, but occasionally systemic.[31] Caution should be exercised if such patients are considered for immunization with PNU-IMUNE 23.

Do not administer the vaccine intradermally since severe reactions may occur.

PRECAUTIONS

General:

1. This product should not be used in children under 2 years of age.
2. PRIOR TO ADMINISTRATION OF ANY DOSE OF PNU-IMUNE 23, THE PARENT, GUARDIAN, OR ADULT PATIENT SHOULD BE ASKED ABOUT THE RECENT HEALTH STATUS, MEDICAL AND IMMUNIZATION HISTORY OF THE PATIENT TO BE IMMUNIZED TO DETERMINE THE EXISTENCE OF ANY CONTRAINDICATION TO IMMUNIZATION WITH PNEUMOCOCCAL VACCINE (SEE **CONTRAINDICATIONS, WARNINGS**).
3. BEFORE ADMINISTRATION OF ANY BIOLOGICAL, THE PHYSICIAN SHOULD TAKE ALL KNOWN PRECAUTIONS FOR PREVENTION OF ALLERGIC OR ANY OTHER REACTIONS. This includes: a review of the patient's history regarding possible sensitivity, the ready availability of epinephrine 1:1,000 and other appropriate agents used for control of immediate allergic reactions, and a knowledge of the recent literature pertaining to use of the biological concerned, including the nature of side effects and adverse reactions that may follow its use.
4. A separate sterile syringe and needle or a sterile disposable unit should be used for each individual patient to prevent transmission of infectious agents from one person to another.

PRIOR TO ADMINISTRATION OF THIS VACCINE, HEALTH CARE PERSONNEL SHOULD INFORM THE PATIENT, GUARDIAN, OR ADULT PATIENT OF THE BENEFITS AND RISKS OF IMMUNIZATION WITH PNEUMOCOCCAL VACCINE.

Pregnancy Category C: Animal reproduction studies have not been conducted with PNU-IMUNE 23. It is also not known whether PNU-IMUNE 23 can cause fetal harm when administered to a pregnant woman or affect reproduction capacity. PNU-IMUNE 23 is not recommended for use in pregnant women.

It is not known whether the drug is excreted in human milk. Because many drugs are excreted in human milk, caution should be exercised when PNU-IMUNE 23 is administered to a nursing woman.

ADVERSE REACTIONS

PNU-IMUNE 23 is associated with a relatively low incidence of adverse reactions. The adverse reactivity observed in clinical studies was of short duration and not serious.

In a study of 32 individuals who received PNU-IMUNE 23 *pneumococcal vaccine, polyvalent,* 23 (72%) experienced local reaction characterized by soreness at the injection site within 3 days after immunization.[9]

Low grade fever (less than 100°F) and mild myalgia occur occasionally and are usually confined to the 24-hour period following immunization. Rash and arthralgia have been reported infrequently.

Although rare, fever over 102°F and marked local swelling have been reported with pneumococcal polysaccharide vaccine. Rash, urticaria, arthritis, arthralgia, and adenitis have been reported rarely.

Patients with otherwise stabilized idiopathic thrombocytopenic purpura have, on rare occasions, experienced a relapse in their thrombocytopenia, occurring 2 to 14 days after immunization, and lasting up to 2 weeks.[32]

Reactions of greater severity, or extent are unusual. Rarely, anaphylactoid reactions have been reported.

Temporal association of neurological disorders such as paresthesias and acute radiculoneuropathy, including Guillain-Barre syndrome, have been reported following parenteral injections of biological products including pneumococcal vaccine.

DOSAGE AND ADMINISTRATION

The immunization schedule consists of a single 0.5 mL dose given intramuscularly or subcutaneously. Intradermal administration should be avoided. **Do not inject intravenously.** Parenteral drug products should be inspected visually for particulate matter and discoloration prior to administration (see **DESCRIPTION**).

Before injection, the skin at the injection site should be cleansed with a suitable germicide. After insertion of the needle, aspirate to help avoid inadvertent injection into a blood vessel.

Simultaneous Administration With Other Vaccines: Many patients who receive pneumococcal vaccine should also be immunized with influenza vaccine which may be given simultaneously at a different site. In contrast to pneumococcal vaccine, influenza vaccine is recommended annually.[2]

Reimmunization: The incidence of local reactions after reimmunization were found to be more severe than after initial immunization when the interval between immunizations was 13 months.[29] Reports of reimmunization after longer intervals in children and adults, including a large group of elderly persons reimmunized at least 4 years after primary immunization, suggest a similar incidence of such reactions.[2]

The Immunization Practices Advisory Committee (ACIP) recommendations regarding reimmunization are as follows: Persons who receive the 14-valent vaccine should not *routinely* be reimmunized with the 23-valent vaccine. However, reimmunization with 23-valent vaccine should be strongly considered for persons who received the 14-valent vaccine *if they are at highest risk* of fatal pneumococcal infection (eg, asplenic patients). Reimmunization should also be carefully considered for adults at highest risk who received the 23-valent vaccine more than 6 years before and for those shown to have a rapid decline in antibody levels (eg, patients with nephrotic syndrome, renal failure, or transplant patients). Reimmunization should be carefully considered after 3 to 5 years for children with nephrotic syndrome, asplenia, or sickle-cell anemia who would be 10 years old or younger at the time of reimmunization.[2]

HOW SUPPLIED

PNU-IMUNE 23 *pneumococcal vaccine, polyvalent* is supplied as follows:

NDC 0005 2309-31 2.5 mL Vial, for use with syringe only.

NDC 0005 2309-33 5 × One Dose (0.5 mL) LEDERJECT® Disposable Syringes.

STORAGE

DO NOT FREEZE. STORE REFRIGERATED, AWAY FROM FREEZER COMPARTMENT AT 2°C TO 8°C (36°F TO 46°F).

Directions for Use of the LEDERJECT® Disposable Syringe:

1. Twist the plunger rod clockwise to be sure the rod is secure to rubber plunger base.
2. Hold needle shield in place with index finger and thumb of one hand while, with the other thumb, exert light pressure on plunger rod until the plunger base has been freed and demonstrates slight movement when pressure is applied.
3. Grasp the rubber needle shield at its base; twist and pull to remove.
4. To prevent needle-stick injuries, needles should not be recapped, purposely bent, or broken by hand.

REFERENCES

1. Austrian R. Surveillance of pneumococcal infection for field trials of polyvalent vaccines. *Annual Contract Prog Report to the Nat Inst of Allerg and Inf Dis* 1975; Update to Dec. 1977, personal communication.
2. Recommendations of the Immunization Practices Advisory Committee Pneumococcal Polysaccharide Vaccine *MMWR* Feb. 10, 1989; 38(5):64–76. Recommendations also published in: *JAMA* March 3, 1989; 261(9):1265–1267.
3. Lund E. Distribution of pneumococcal types at different times and different areas. In *Bayer Symposium III Bacterial Infections.* Finland M, Marget W, Bartman K (eds). Berlin, Springer-Verlag, 1971:49.
4. Mufson MA, Kruss DM, et al. Capsular types and outcome of bacteremic pneumococcal disease in the antibiotic era. *Arch Int Med* 1974; 134:505–510.
5. Robbins JB, Austrian R, Lee CJ, et al. Consideration for formulating the second generation pneumococcal capsular polysaccharide vaccine with emphasis on the cross-reactive types within groups. *J Infec Dis* 1983; 148(6):1136–1159.
6. Lane CH, Masur H, Edgar LC, et al. Abnormalities of B-cell activation and immunoregulation in patients with the acquired immunodeficiency syndrome. *N Engl J Med* 1983; 309:453–458.
7. Ammann AJ, Schiffman G, Abrams D, et al. B-cell immunodeficiency in acquired immune deficiency syndrome. *JAMA* 1984; 251:1447–1449.
8. Douglas RM, Paton JC, et al. Antibody response to pneumococcal vaccination in children younger than five years of age. *J Infect Dis* 1983; 148:131–137.
9. Data on file, Lederle Laboratories.
10. Sullivan JL, Ochs HD, Schiffman G, et al. Immune response after splenectomy. *Lancet* 1978; 1:178–181.
11. Ballet J-J, Sulcebe G, Couderc L-J, et al. Impaired anti-pneumococcal antibody response in patients with AIDS-related persistent generalized lymphadenopathy. *Clin Exp Immunol* 1987; 68:479–487.
12. Huang K-L, Ruben FL, Rinaldo CR Jr, et al. Antibody responses after influenza and pneumococcal immunization in HIV-infected homosexual men. *JAMA* 1987; 257:2047–2050.
13. Mufson MA, Krause HE, et al. Long term persistence of antibodies following immunization with pneumococcal polysaccharide vaccine. *Proc Soc Exp Bio Med* 1983; 173:270–275.
14. Mufson MA, Krause HE, et al. Pneumococcal antibody levels one decade after immunization of healthy adults. *Am J Med Sci* 1987; 293:279–284.
15. Giebiuk GS, Le CT, Schiffman G. Decline of serum antibody in splenectomized children after vaccination with pneumococcal capsular polysaccharides. *J Pediatr* 1984; 105:576–584.
16. Weintrub PS, Schiffman G, Addiego JE Jr, et al. Long-term follow-up and booster immunization with polyvalent pneumococcal polysaccharide in patient with sickle cell anemia. *J Pediatr* 1984; 105:261–263.
17. Spika JS, Halsey NA, Le CT, et al. Decline of vaccine-induced antipneumococcal antibody in children with nephrotic syndrome. *Am J Kidney Dis* 1986; 7:466–470.
18. Austrian R, Douglas RM, Schiffman G, et al. Prevention of pneumococcal pneumonia by vaccination. *Trans Assoc Am Physicians* 1976; 89:184–194.
19. Ammann AJ, Addiego K, Wara DW, et al. Polyvalent pneumococcal-polysaccharide immunization of patients with sickle-cell anemia and patients with splenectomy. *N Engl J Med* 1977; 297:897–900.
20. Riley ID, Tarr PI, Andrews M, et al. Immunisation with a polyvalent pneumococcal vaccine: reduction of adult respiratory mortality in a New Guinea Highlands community. *Lancet* 1977; 1(8023):1338–1341.
21. Shapiro ED, Clemens JD. A controlled evaluation of the protective efficacy of pneumococcal vaccine for patients at high risk of serious pneumococcal infections. *Ann Intern Med* 1984; 101:325–330.
22. Shapiro ED, Austrian R, Adair RK, et al. The protective efficacy of pneumococcal vaccine (Abstract). *Clin Res* 1988; 36:470A.
23. Sims RV, Steinmann WC, McConville JH, et al. The clinical effectiveness of pneumococcal vaccine in the elderly. *Ann Intern Med* 1988; 108:653–657.

Continued on next page

Information on Lederle products listed on these pages is the full prescribing information from product literature or package inserts effective in August 1992. Information concerning all Lederle products may be obtained from the Professional Services Department, Lederle Laboratories, Pearl River, New York 10965.

Lederle—Cont.

24. Bolan G, Broome CV, Facklam RR, et al. Pneumococcal vaccine efficacy in selected populations in the United States. *Ann Intern Med* 1986; 104:1–6.
25. Forrester HL, Jahnigen DW, LaForce FM. Inefficacy of pneumococcal vaccine in a high-risk population. *Am J Med* 1987; 83:425–430.
26. Simberkoff MS, Cross AP, Al-Ibrahim M, et al. Efficacy of pneumococcal vaccine in high-risk patients: results of a Veterans Administration cooperative study. *N Engl J Med* 1986; 315:1318–27.
27. Gaillat J, Zmirou D, Mallaret MR, et al. Essai clinique du vaccin antipneumococcique chez des personnes agees vivant en institution. *Rev Epidemiol Sante Publique* 1985; 33:437–444.
28. Siber GR, Weitzman SA, Aisenberg AC, et al. Impaired antibody response to pneumococcal vaccine after treatment for Hodgkin's disease. *N Engl J Med* 1978; 299:442–448.
29. Siber GR, Gorham C, Martin P, et al. Antibody response to pretreatment immunization and post-treatment boosting with bacterial polysaccharide vaccines in patients with Hodgkin's disease. *Ann Intern Med* 1986; 104:467–475.
30. Borgono JM, McLean AA, Vella PP, et al. Vaccination and revaccination with polyvalent pneumococcal polysaccharide vaccines in adults and infants. *Proc Soc Exper Biol Med* 1978; 157:148–154.
31. Ponka A, Leinonen M: Adverse reactions to polyvalent pneumococcal vaccine. *Scand J Infect Dis* 1982; 14:67–71.
32. Kelton JG: Vaccination-associated relapse of immune thrombocytopenia. *JAMA* 1981; 245(4):369–371.

LEDERLE LABORATORIES DIVISION
American Cyanamid Company   27781
Pearl River, NY 10965   Rev. 8/90
Shown in Product Identification Section, page 415

PROSTEP™   ℞
(nicotine transdermal system)
Systemic delivery of 22 or 11 mg/day over 24 hours

DESCRIPTION

PROSTEP is a transdermal system that provides systemic delivery of nicotine following its application to intact skin. Nicotine is a tertiary amine composed of a pyridine and a pyrrolidine ring. It is a colorless to pale yellow, freely water-soluble, strongly alkaline, oily, volatile, hygroscopic liquid obtained from the tobacco plant. Nicotine has a characteristic pungent odor and turns brown on exposure to air or light. Of its two stereoisomers, S (-)-nicotine is the more active. It is the prevalent form in tobacco, and is the form in the PROSTEP system. The free alkaloid is absorbed rapidly through the skin and respiratory tract.

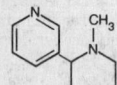

Chemical Name:
S - 3 - (1-methyl-2-pyrrolidinyl) pyridine
Molecular Formula: $C_{10}H_{14}N_2$
Molecular Weight: 162.23
Ionization Contents: pK_{a1}=7.84, pK_{a2}=3.04
Octanol-Water Partition Coefficient: 15.1 at pH 7

The PROSTEP system is a round, flat, adhesive pad with a round well in the center containing nicotine (the active agent) in a hydrogel matrix. Proceeding from the visible outer surface toward the inner surface attached to the skin are: (1) a beige-colored foam tape and pressure-sensitive acrylate adhesive; (2) backing foil, gelatin and low-density polyethylene; (3) nicotine-gel matrix; (4) protective foil with well and (5) release liner which overlies the adhesive layer and must be removed prior to use. PROSTEP systems are packaged in child-resistant pouches. [See illustration at top of next column.]

Nicotine is the active ingredient; other components of the system are pharmacologically inactive.
The amount of nicotine delivered to the patient from each system (130 mcg/cm²-h) is proportional to the surface area of the nicotine-gel matrix. About 27% of the total amount of nicotine remains in the system 24 hours after application. PROSTEP (nicotine transdermal system) systems are labelled with the average dose absorbed by the patient. The dose of nicotine absorbed from a PROSTEP system represents 98% of the amount released from the system in 24 hours.
[See table at right.]

Dose Absorbed in 24 Hours (mg/day)	System Surface Area (cm²)	Total Nicotine Content (mg)	Residual Nicotine After 24 Hours (mg)
22	7	30	8
11	3.5	15	4

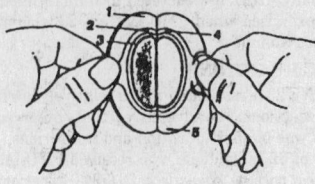

STICKY SIDE: APPLY TO SKIN	NONSTICKY SIDE: DISCARD

1— FOAM TAPE AND ACRYLATE ADHESIVE
2— BACKING FOIL, GELATIN AND LOW-DENSITY POLYETHYLENE COATING
3— NICOTINE-GEL MATRIX
4— PROTECTIVE FOIL WITH WELL
5— RELEASE LINER

CLINICAL PHARMACOLOGY

Pharmacologic Action: Nicotine, the chief alkaloid in tobacco products, binds stereoselectively to acetylcholine receptors at the autonomic ganglia, in the adrenal medulla, at neuromuscular junctions, and in the brain. Two types of central nervous system effects are believed to be the basis of nicotine's positively reinforcing properties. A stimulating effect, exerted mainly in the cortex via the locus ceruleus, produces increased alertness and cognitive performance. A "reward" effect via the "pleasure system" in the brain is exerted in the limbic system. At low doses the stimulant effects predominate while at high doses the reward effects predominate. Intermittent intravenous administration of nicotine activates neurohormonal pathways, releasing acetylcholine, norepinephrine, dopamine, serotonin, vasopressin, beta-endorphin, growth hormone, and ACTH.

Pharmacodynamics: The cardiovascular effects of nicotine include peripheral vasoconstriction, tachycardia, and elevated blood pressure. Acute and chronic tolerance to nicotine develops from smoking tobacco or ingesting nicotine preparations. Acute tolerance (a reduction in response for a given dose) develops rapidly (less than 1 hour) but not at the same rate for different physiologic effects (skin temperature, heart rate, subjective effects). Withdrawal symptoms, such as cigarette craving, can be reduced in some individuals by plasma-nicotine levels lower than those from smoking.
Withdrawal from nicotine in addicted individuals is characterized by craving, nervousness, restlessness, irritability, mood lability, anxiety, drowsiness, sleep disturbances, impaired concentration, increased appetite, minor somatic complaints (headache, myalgia, constipation, fatigue), and weight gain. Nicotine toxicity is characterized by nausea, abdominal pain, vomiting, diarrhea, diaphoresis, flushing, dizziness, disturbed hearing and vision, confusion, weakness, palpitations, altered respirations, and hypotension.
The cardiovascular effects of PROSTEP 22 mg/day systems include slight increase in heart rate and blood pressure. The cardiovascular effects of applying one or two PROSTEP 22 mg/day systems used continuously for 24 hours were compared to placebo for 7 days. Changes in heart rate (increased 4 beats/min), systolic blood pressure (increased 4 mmHg) and diastolic blood pressure (increased 3 mmHg) were observed.
Both smoking and nicotine can increase circulating cortisol and catecholamines, and tolerance does not develop to the catecholamine-releasing effects of nicotine. Changes in the response to a concomitantly administered adrenergic agonist or antagonist should be watched for when nicotine intake is altered during nicotine replacement therapy with PROSTEP (nicotine transdermal system) systems (see **Drug Interactions**).

Pharmacokinetics: Following application of the PROSTEP system to the upper body or upper outer arm, virtually all of the nicotine released from the system enters the systemic circulation. All PROSTEP systems are labelled as to the average amount of nicotine absorbed by patients. The volume of distribution following IV administration of nicotine is approximately 2 to 3 L/kg and the half-life ranges from 1 to 2 hours. The major eliminating organ is the liver, and average plasma clearance is about 1.2 L/min; the kidney and lung also metabolize nicotine. There is no significant

---

skin metabolism of nicotine. More than 20 metabolites of nicotine have been identified, all of which are believed to be less active than the parent compound. The primary metabolite of nicotine in plasma, cotinine, has a half-life of 15 to 20 hours and concentrations that exceed nicotine by tenfold. Plasma-protein binding of nicotine is <5%. Therefore, changes in nicotine binding from use of concomitant drugs or alterations of plasma proteins by disease states would not be expected to have significant effects on nicotine kinetics.
The primary urinary metabolites are cotinine (15% of the dose) and trans-3-hydroxycotinine (45% of the dose). Usually about 10% of nicotine is excreted unchanged in the urine. As much as 30% may be excreted unchanged in the urine with high urine flow rates and acidification below pH 5.
The pharmacokinetic model which best fits the plasma nicotine concentrations from PROSTEP systems is an open, two-compartment model with a skin depot through which nicotine enters the central disposition compartment.
The PROSTEP system gel matrix contacts the skin directly and acts as a reservoir from which nicotine is absorbed slowly over the 24 hours.

Steady-State Plasma-Nictone Concentrations for Two Consecutive Applications of PROSTEP 22 mg/day (Mean ± 2 SD, N=22)

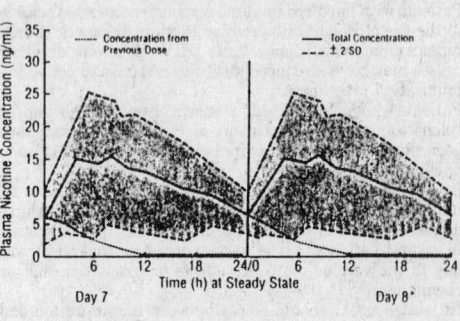

*Day 8 is a reproduction of Day 7 data to represent steady-state dosing

---

Following application of a system, nicotine concentrations increase to a peak between 4 and 12 hours and then decrease gradually (see graph). Steady state for nicotine is attained within 2 days of initiating PROSTEP (nicotine transdermal system) treatment and plasma nicotine concentrations average 23% higher compared to single-dose application. Plasma nicotine concentrations are proportional to dose (ie, linear kinetics are observed) for the two dosages of PROSTEP systems. Nicotine kinetics are similar for all sites of application on the upper torso and upper outer arm.
Following removal of PROSTEP systems, plasma nicotine concentrations decline in an exponential fashion with an apparent mean half-life of 3 to 4 hours due to continued absorption from the skin depot (see dotted line in figure) in contrast to a half-life of 1 to 2 hours following IV administration. Most nonsmoking patients will have nondetectable nicotine concentrations in 10 to 12 hours after patch removal.

Steady-State Nicotine Pharmacokinetic Parameters for 22 mg/day PROSTEP Systems (mean, std dev, range)

Parameter (units)	22 mg/day (N=22)		
	Mean	SD	Range
C_{max} (ng/mL)	16	6	7–31
C_{avg} (ng/mL)	11	3	6–17
C_{min} (ng/mL)	5	1	3–9
T_{max} (h)	9	5	4–24

C_{max}: maximum observed plasma concentration
C_{avg}: average plasma concentration
C_{min}: minimum observed plasma concentration
T_{max}: time of maximum plasma concentration

CLINICAL TRIALS

The efficacy of PROSTEP treatment as an aid to smoking cessation was demonstrated in two placebo-controlled, double-blind trials in otherwise healthy patients smoking at least one pack per day (N=516). In one of these trials, PROSTEP therapy was combined with concomitant individual patient counseling (10 minutes each visit) and in the other trial PROSTEP therapy was used with group counseling (1 hour each visit). In both trials, patients were treated for 8 weeks with a fixed dosage of 22 mg/day or placebo followed by abrupt cessation of PROSTEP treatment and decrease in support therapy. Patients in these two trials received prestudy counseling at two visits before beginning

treatment. Two earlier trials (N=409) were carried out without prestudy counseling with treatment for 6 weeks and weaning to the 11 mg/day patch in one of them (N=329). In all four trials quitting was defined as total abstinence from smoking as measured by patient diary and verified by expired carbon monoxide. The "quit rates" are the proportions of all persons initially enrolled who abstained after week 2.

Quit Rates by Treatment After Week 2
(range by clinics)*

Nicotine Treatment	Number of Patients	After 6 Weeks	After 6 Months
PROSTEP (22 mg/day)	259	10%–57%	0%–37%
Placebo	257	3%–30%	0%–20%

*Trial involved 7 clinics, number of patients per treatment ranged from 29 to 60.

The two trials with prestudy counseling demonstrated that with concomitant support, fixed-dosage therapy with PROSTEP therapy was more effective than placebo after 6 weeks and data from these two studies are combined in the quit rate table. At 8 weeks, just prior to abrupt termination of PROSTEP treatment (no weaning), quit rates were 6% to 50%. At follow-up, 3 to 5 days later, quit rates were 3% to 50%. In the two other studies without prestudy counseling, quit rates of 0% to 46% with PROSTEP 22 mg/day and 3% to 31% with placebo were observed at 6 weeks. In each of the four studies, there was a large variation in quit rates among clinics for each treatment.

Patients using PROSTEP systems dropped out of the trials significantly less frequently than did patients receiving placebo (26% vs 34%). The quit rate for 30 patients over age 60 was comparable to the quit rate for 486 patients aged 60 and under.

Patients who used the 22 mg/day PROSTEP treatment in clinical trials had a significant reduction in craving for cigarettes (desire to smoke), a major nicotine withdrawal symptom, as compared to placebo-treated patients (see figure). Reduction in craving, as with quit rate, is quite variable. This variability from clinic to clinic is presumed to be due to inherent differences in patient populations, eg, patient motivation, concomitant illnesses, number of cigarettes smoked per day, number of years smoking, exposure to other smokers, socioeconomic status, etc, as well as differences among the clinics.

Severity of Craving by Treatment From Clinical Trials
(N=516)

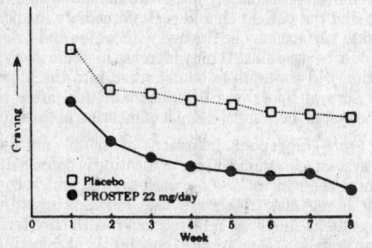

□ Placebo
● PROSTEP 22 mg/day

Individualization of Dosage: It is important to make sure that patients read the instructions made available to them and have their questions answered. They should clearly understand the directions for applying and disposing of PROSTEP (nicotine transdermal system) systems. They should be instructed to stop smoking completely when the first PROSTEP system is applied.

The success or failure of smoking cessation depends heavily on the quality, intensity, and frequency of supportive care. Patients are more likely to quit smoking if they are seen frequently and participate in formal smoking-cessation programs.

The goal of PROSTEP therapy is complete abstinence. Significant health benefits have not been demonstrated for reduction of smoking. If a patient is unable to stop smoking by the fourth week of therapy, treatment should probably be discontinued. Patients who have not stopped smoking after 4 weeks of PROSTEP therapy are unlikely to quit on that attempt.

Patients who fail to quit on any attempt may benefit from interventions to improve their chances for success on subsequent attempts. Patients who were unsuccessful should be counseled to determine why they failed. Patients should then probably be given a "therapy holiday" before the next attempt. A new quit attempt should be encouraged when the factors that contributed to failure can be eliminated or reduced, and conditions are more favorable.

Based on the clinical trials, a reasonable approach to assisting patients in their attempt to quit smoking is to initiate therapy with PROSTEP 22 mg/day except for small patients less than 100 pounds (see **DOSING SCHEDULE** below). The need for dose adjustment should be assessed during the first 2 weeks. The symptoms of nicotine withdrawal and toxicity overlap (see **Pharmacodynamics** and **ADVERSE REACTIONS** sections). Since patients using PROSTEP (nicotine transdermal systems) treatment may also smoke intermittently, it may be difficult to determine if patients are experiencing nicotine withdrawal or nicotine excess.

The controlled clinical trials using PROSTEP therapy suggest that sweating, abdominal pain, and somnolence are more often symptoms of nicotine excess while irritability is more often a symptom of nicotine withdrawal.

Patients should continue the dose selected with counseling and support over the following month. Those who have successfully stopped smoking during that time can stop PROSTEP treatment or may be weaned (reduction to 11 mg/day) over 4 weeks, after which treatment should be terminated.

DOSING SCHEDULE

	Patients ≥ 100 lbs	Patients < 100 lbs
Initial/Starting Dose	22 mg/day	11 mg/day
Duration of Treatment	4–8 weeks	4–8 weeks
Optional Weaning Dose	11 mg/day	off
Duration of Treatment	2–4 weeks	

INDICATIONS AND USAGE

PROSTEP treatment is indicated as an aid to smoking cessation for the relief of nicotine withdrawal symptoms. PROSTEP treatment should be used as a part of a comprehensive behavioral smoking-cessation program.

The use of PROSTEP systems for longer than 3 months has not been studied.

CONTRAINDICATIONS

Use of PROSTEP (nicotine transdermal system) systems is contraindicated in patients with hypersensitivity or allergy to nicotine or to any of the components of the therapeutic system.

WARNINGS

Nicotine from any source can be toxic and addictive. Smoking causes lung cancer, heart disease, emphysema, and may adversely affect the fetus and the pregnant woman. For any smoker, with or without concomitant disease or pregnancy, the risk of nicotine replacement in a smoking-cessation program should be weighed against the hazard of continued smoking while using PROSTEP systems, and the likelihood of achieving cessation of smoking without nicotine replacement.

Pregnancy Warning: Tobacco smoke, which has been shown to be harmful to the fetus, contains nicotine, hydrogen cyanide, and carbon monoxide. Nicotine has been shown in animal studies to cause fetal harm. It is therefore presumed that PROSTEP treatment can cause fetal harm when administered to a pregnant woman. The effect of nicotine delivery by PROSTEP systems has not been examined in pregnancy (see **PRECAUTIONS**). Therefore, pregnant smokers should be encouraged to attempt cessation using educational and behavioral interventions before using pharmacological approaches. If PROSTEP therapy is used during pregnancy, or if the patient becomes pregnant while using PROSTEP treatment, the patient should be apprised of the potential hazard to the fetus.

Safety Note Concerning Children: The amounts of nicotine that are tolerated by adult smokers can produce symptoms of poisoning and could prove fatal if PROSTEP systems are applied or ingested by children or pets. Used 22 mg/day systems contain about 27% (8 mg) of their initial drug content. Therefore, patients should be cautioned to keep both used and unused PROSTEP systems out of the reach of children and pets.

PRECAUTIONS

The patient should be urged to stop smoking completely when initiating PROSTEP therapy (see **DOSAGE AND ADMINISTRATION**). Patients should be informed that if they continue to smoke while using PROSTEP systems, they may experience adverse effects due to peak nicotine levels higher than those experienced from smoking alone. If there is a clinically significant increase in cardiovascular or other effects attributable to nicotine, the PROSTEP dose should be reduced or PROSTEP treatment discontinued (see **WARNINGS**). Physicians should anticipate that concomitant medications may need dosage adjustment (see **Drug Interactions**). The use of PROSTEP systems beyond 3 months by patients who stop smoking should be discouraged because the chronic consumption of nicotine by any route can be harmful and addicting.

Allergic Reactions: In a 3-week open-label dermal irritation and sensitization study of PROSTEP systems, 16 of 205 patients (8%) exhibited definite erythema at 24 hours after system removal. None of those patients exhibited contact allergy. In the first 4 weeks of the efficacy trials, moderate erythema following system removal was seen in 22% of patients, some edema in 8%, and dropouts due to skin reactions occurred in 7% of 459 patients using the 22 mg/day system. Patients who develop contact sensitization should be cautioned that a serious reaction could occur from exposure to other nicotine-containing products or smoking.

Patients should be instructed to promptly discontinue the PROSTEP treatment and contact their physician if they experience severe or persistent local skin reactions at the site of application (eg, severe erythema, pruritus, or edema) or a generalized skin reaction (eg, urticaria, hives, or generalized rash).

Skin Disease: PROSTEP systems are usually well tolerated by patients with normal skin, but may be irritating for patients with some skin disorders (atopic or eczematous dermatitis).

Cardiovascular or Peripheral Vascular Diseases: The risks of nicotine replacement in patients with certain cardiovascular and peripheral vascular diseases should be weighed against the benefits of including nicotine replacement in a smoking-cessation program for them. Specifically, patients with coronary heart disease (history of myocardial infarction and/or angina pectoris), serious cardiac arrhythmias, or vasospastic diseases (Buerger's disease, Prinzmetal's variant angina) should be carefully screened and evaluated before nicotine replacement is prescribed.

Tachycardia occurring in association with the use of PROSTEP treatment was reported occasionally. If serious cardiovascular symptoms occur with PROSTEP treatment, it should be discontinued.

PROSTEP treatment should generally not be used in patients during the immediate postmyocardial infarction period, patients with serious arrhythmias, and patients with severe or worsening angina pectoris.

Renal or Hepatic Insufficiency: The pharmacokinetics of nicotine have not been studied in the elderly or patients with renal or hepatic impairment. However, given that nicotine is extensively metabolized and that its total system clearance is dependent on liver blood flow, some influence of hepatic impairment on drug kinetics (reduced clearance) should be anticipated. Only severe renal impairment would be expected to affect the clearance of nicotine or its metabolites from the circulation (see **Pharmacokinetics**).

Endocrine Diseases: PROSTEP (nicotine transdermal system) treatment should be used with caution in patients with hyperthyroidism, pheochromocytoma, or insulin-dependent diabetes since nicotine causes the release of catecholamines by the adrenal medulla.

Peptic Ulcer Disease: Nicotine delays healing in peptic ulcer disease; therefore, PROSTEP treatment should be used with caution in patients with active peptic ulcers and only when the benefits of including nicotine replacement in a smoking-cessation program outweigh the risks.

Accelerated Hypertension: Nicotine constitutes a risk factor for development of malignant hypertension in patients with accelerated hypertension; therefore, PROSTEP treatment should be used with caution in these patients and only when the benefits of including nicotine replacement in a smoking-cessation program outweigh the risks.

Information for Patient: A patient instruction sheet is included in the package of PROSTEP systems dispensed to the patient. It contains important information and instructions on how to use and dispose of PROSTEP systems properly. Patients should be encouraged to ask questions of the physician and pharmacist.

Patients must be advised to keep both used and unused systems out of the reach of children and pets.

Drug Interactions: Smoking cessation, with or without nicotine replacement, may alter the pharmacokinetics of certain concomitant medications.

[See table on next page.]

Carcinogenesis, Mutagenesis, Impairment of Fertility: Nicotine itself does not appear to be a carcinogen in laboratory animals. However, nicotine and its metabolites increased the incidences of tumors in the cheek pouches of hamsters and forestomach of F344 rats, respectively, when given in combination with tumor-initiators. One study, which could not be replicated, suggested that cotinine, the primary metabolite of nicotine, may cause lymphoreticular sarcoma in the large intestine in rats.

Continued on next page

Information on Lederle products listed on these pages is the full prescribing information from product literature or package inserts effective in August 1992. Information concerning all Lederle products may be obtained from the Professional Services Department, Lederle Laboratories, Pearl River, New York 10965.

Lederle—Cont.

Neither nicotine nor cotinine were mutagenic in the Ames *Salmonella* test. Nicotine-induced repairable DNA damage in an *Escherichia coli* test system. Nicotine was shown to be genotoxic in a test system using Chinese hamster ovary cells. In rats and rabbits, implantation can be delayed or inhibited by a reduction in DNA synthesis that appears to be caused by nicotine. Studies have shown a decrease in litter size in rats treated with nicotine during gestation.

PREGNANCY

Pregnancy Category D (see **WARNINGS** section): The harmful effects of cigarette smoking on maternal and fetal health are clearly established. These include low birth weight, an increased risk of spontaneous abortion, and increased perinatal mortality. The specific effects of PROSTEP treatment on fetal development are unknown. Therefore, pregnant smokers should be encouraged to attempt cessation using educational and behavioral interventions before using pharmacological approaches.

Spontaneous abortion during nicotine replacement therapy has been reported; as with smoking, nicotine as a contributing factor cannot be excluded.

PROSTEP treatment should be used during pregnancy only if the likelihood of smoking cessation justifies the potential risk of use of nicotine replacement by the patient, who may continue to smoke.

Teratogenicity: *Animal Studies:* Nicotine was shown to produce skeletal abnormalities in the offspring of mice when given doses toxic to the dams (25 mg/kg IP or SC).

Human Studies: Nicotine teratogenicity has not been studied in humans except as a component of cigarette smoke (each cigarette smoked delivers about 1 mg of nicotine). It has not been possible to conclude whether cigarette smoking is teratogenic to humans.

Other Effects: *Animal Studies:* A nicotine bolus (up to 2 mg/kg) to pregnant rhesus monkeys caused acidosis, hypercarbia, and hypotension (fetal and maternal concentrations were about 20 times those achieved after smoking one cigarette in 5 minutes). Fetal breathing movements were reduced in the fetal lamb after intravenous injection of 0.25 mg/kg nicotine to the ewe (equivalent to smoking one cigarette every 20 seconds for 5 minutes). Uterine blood flow was reduced about 30% after infusion of 0.1 mg/kg/min nicotine for 20 minutes to pregnant rhesus monkeys (equivalent to smoking about six cigarettes every minute for 20 minutes).

Human Experience: Cigarette smoking during pregnancy is associated with an increased risk of spontaneous abortion, low birth weight infants and perinatal mortality. Nicotine and carbon monoxide are considered the most likely mediators of these outcomes. The effects of cigarette smoking on fetal cardiovascular parameters have been studied near term. Cigarettes increased fetal aortic blood flow and heart rate and decreased uterine blood flow and fetal breathing movements. PROSTEP (nicotine transdermal system) treatment has not been studied in pregnant humans.

Labor and Delivery: PROSTEP systems are not recommended to be left on during labor and delivery. The effects of nicotine on the mother or the fetus during labor are unknown.

Use in Nursing Mothers: Caution should be exercised when PROSTEP therapy is administered to nursing women. The safety of PROSTEP treatment in nursing infants has not been examined. Nicotine passes freely into breast milk; the milk-to-plasma ratio averages 2.9. Nicotine is absorbed orally. An infant has the ability to clear nicotine by hepatic first-pass clearance; however, the efficiency of removal is probably lowest at birth. The nicotine concentrations in milk can be expected to be lower with PROSTEP treatment when used as directed than with cigarette smoking, as maternal plasma nicotine concentrations are generally reduced with nicotine replacement. The risk of exposure of the infant to nicotine from PROSTEP systems should be weighed against the risks associated with the infant's exposure to nicotine from continued smoking by the mother (passive smoke exposure and contamination of breast milk with other components of tobacco smoke) and from PROSTEP systems alone or in combination with continued smoking.

Pediatric Use: PROSTEP systems are not recommended for use in children because the safety and effectiveness of PROSTEP treatment in children and adolescents who smoke have not been evaluated.

Geriatric Use: Thirty patients over the age of 60 participated in clinical trials of PROSTEP therapy. PROSTEP therapy appeared to be as effective in this age group as in younger smokers.

ADVERSE REACTIONS

Assessment of adverse events in the 903 patients who participated in controlled clinical trials is complicated by the occurrence of GI and CNS effects of nicotine withdrawal as well as nicotine excess. The actual incidences of both are confounded by concurrent smoking by many of the patients. In the trials, when reporting adverse events, the investigators did not attempt to identify the cause of the symptom.

May Require a Decrease in Dose at Cessation of Smoking	Possible Mechanism
Acetaminophen, caffeine, imipramine, oxazepam, pentazocine, propranolol, theophylline	Deinduction of hepatic enzymes on smoking cessation
Insulin	Increase of subcutaneous insulin absorption with smoking cessation
Adrenergic antagonists (eg, prazosin, labetalol)	Decrease in circulating catecholamines with smoking cessation

May Require an Increase in Dose at Cessation of Smoking	Possible Mechanism
Adrenergic agonists (eg, isoproterenol, phenylephrine)	Decrease in circulating catecholamines with smoking cessation

Topical Adverse Events: The most common adverse event associated with topical nicotine is a mild short-lived erythema, pruritus, or burning at the application site, which was seen at least once in 54% of patients (N=459) on PROSTEP treatment in the 6- to 8-week clinical trials. Local erythema after system removal was noted at least once in 22% of patients and local edema in 8%. Erythema generally resolved within 24 hours. Cutaneous hypersensitivity (contact sensitization) occurred in 3% of patients on PROSTEP treatment (see **PRECAUTIONS, Allergic Reactions**).

Probably Causally Related: The following adverse events were reported more frequently in PROSTEP treated patients than in placebo-treated patients or exhibited a dose response in clinical trials. The reports of awakening at night were collected as one of the expected withdrawal symptoms.

Digestive system—Abdominal pain†
Nervous system—Somnolence*
Skin—Rash,† sweating†

Frequencies for 22 mg/day system
* Reported in 3% to 9% of patients
† Reported in 1% to 3% of patients
Unmarked if reported in <1% of patients

Causal Relationship UNKNOWN: Adverse events reported in PROSTEP (nicotine transdermal system) and placebo-treated patients at about the same frequency in clinical trials are listed below. The clinical significance of the association between PROSTEP treatment and these events is unknown, but they are reported as alerting information for the clinician.

Body as a whole—Back pain,† pain*
Digestive system—Constipation,† dyspepsia, nausea†
Musculoskeletal system—Myalgia†
Nervous system—Dizziness,† headache (11%), insomnia*
Respiratory system—Pharyngitis,* sinusitis*
Urogenital system—Dysmenorrhea†

Frequencies for 22 mg/day system
* Reported in 3% to 9% of patients
† Reported in 1% to 3% of patients
Unmarked if reported in <1% of patients

DRUG ABUSE AND DEPENDENCE

PROSTEP systems are likely to have a low abuse potential based on differences between it and cigarettes in four characteristics commonly considered important in contributing to abuse: much slower absorption, much smaller fluctuations in blood levels, lower blood levels of nicotine, and less frequent use (ie, once daily).

The abuse potential of PROSTEP systems was examined in a prospective, randomized trial of 10 smokers (five drug abusers and five nonabusers). "Liking" scores for either one (22 mg/day) or two systems (44 mg/day) were no different from placebo. No abuse potential was observed in that study.

Dependence on nicotine polacrilex chewing gum replacement therapy has been reported and such dependence might also occur from transference to PROSTEP systems of tobacco-based nicotine dependence. The use of the system beyond 3 months has not been evaluated and should be discouraged.

PROSTEP therapy has been evaluated in both a gradual and abrupt discontinuation of treatment. If gradual withdrawal is desirable, patients using the 22 mg/day PROSTEP treatment should use the 11 mg/day dosage for 2 to 4 weeks (see **Individualization of Dosage** and **DOSAGE AND ADMINISTRATION**).

OVERDOSAGE

The effects of applying several PROSTEP systems simultaneously or of swallowing unused PROSTEP systems are unknown (see **WARNINGS, Safety Note Concerning Children**).

The oral LD_{50} for nicotine in rodents varies with the species but is in excess of 24 mg/kg; death is due to respiratory paralysis. The oral minimum lethal dose of nicotine in dogs is greater than 5 mg/kg. The oral minimum acute lethal dose for nicotine in human adults is reported to be 40 to 60 mg (<1 mg/kg).

PROSTEP gels containing 8 mg of nicotine were ingested by 12 adult smokers with an average weight of 74 kg (range 62 to 93 kg). Peak nicotine serum levels were 9.5 ng/mL (range 3 to 18 ng/mL) and occurred at 2 hours (1 to 2 hours) and declined to baseline levels by 8 hours after ingestion. Some gastrointestinal effects (burning on ingestion and nausea) were reported.

Signs and symptoms of an overdose of PROSTEP (nicotine transdermal system) systems would be expected to be the same as those of acute nicotine poisoning including: pallor, cold sweat, nausea, salivation, vomiting, abdominal pain, diarrhea, headache, dizziness, disturbed hearing and vision, tremor, mental confusion, and weakness. Prostration, hypotension, and respiratory failure may ensue with large overdoses. Lethal doses produce convulsions quickly and death follows as a result of peripheral or central respiratory paralysis or, less frequently, cardiac failure.

Overdose From Topical Exposure: The PROSTEP system should be removed immediately if the patient shows signs of overdosage and the patient should seek immediate medical care. The skin surface may be flushed with water and dried. No soap should be used since it may increase nicotine absorption. Nicotine will continue to be delivered into the bloodstream for several hours (see **Pharmacokinetics**) after removal of the system because of a depot of nicotine in the skin.

Overdose From Ingestion: Ingestion of a 22 mg/day PROSTEP system containing 30 mg of nicotine is potentially more harmful than ingestion of a used system which contains about 8 mg after 24 hours use. Persons ingesting PROSTEP systems should be referred to a health care facility for management. Due to the possibility of nicotine-induced seizures, activated charcoal should be administered. In unconscious patients with a secure airway, instill activated charcoal via nasogastric tube. A saline cathartic or sorbitol added to the first dose of activated charcoal may speed gastrointestinal passage of the system. Repeated doses of activated charcoal should be administered as long as the system remains in the gastrointestinal tract since it will continue to release nicotine for many hours.

Management of Nicotine Poisoning: Other supportive measures include diazepam or barbiturates for seizures, atropine for excessive bronchial secretions or diarrhea, respiratory support for respiratory failure, and vigorous fluid support for hypotension and cardiovascular collapse.

DOSAGE AND ADMINISTRATION

Patients must desire to stop smoking and should be instructed to *stop smoking immediately* as they begin using PROSTEP (nicotine transdermal system) therapy. The patient should read the patient instruction sheet on PROSTEP treatment and be encouraged to ask any questions. Treatment should be initiated with PROSTEP 22 mg/day except for patients who weigh less than 100 pounds. They may start with PROSTEP 11 mg/day and the dose increased as appropriate (see **Individualization of Dosage**). Once the appropriate dosage is selected the patient should begin 4 to 8 weeks of therapy at that dosage. The patient should stop smoking cigarettes completely during this period. If the patient is unable to stop cigarette smoking within 4 weeks,

Nicotine Delivery Rate (in vivo)	Nicotine in System	System Size	Package Size	NDC Number
22 mg/day	30 mg	7.0 cm^2	7 systems	0005-2402-90
11 mg/day	15 mg	3.5 cm^2	7 systems	0005-2401-90

PROSTEP should probably be stopped, since few additional patients in clinical trials were able to quit after this time. Those who have successfully stopped smoking during that time may have PROSTEP therapy discontinued. If a gradual reduction is desired, patients may be treated for an additional 2 to 4 weeks, after which treatment should be terminated.

The entire course of nicotine substitution should take 6 to 12 weeks. The use of PROSTEP systems beyond 3 months has not been studied and should be discouraged.

The PROSTEP system should be applied promptly upon its removal from the protective pouch to prevent evaporative loss of nicotine from the system. PROSTEP systems should be used only when the pouch is intact to assure that the product has not been tampered with.

PROSTEP systems should be applied only once a day to a nonhairy, clean, and dry skin site on the upper trunk or upper outer arm. After 24 hours, the used PROSTEP system should be removed and a new system applied to an alternate skin site. Skin sites should not be reused for at least a week. Patients should be cautioned not to continue to use the same system for more than 24 hours.

SAFETY AND HANDLING

PROSTEP systems can be a dermal irritant and can cause contact sensitization. Although exposure of health care workers to nicotine from PROSTEP (nicotine transdermal system) systems should be minimal, care should be taken to avoid unnecessary contact with active systems. If you do handle active systems, wash with water alone, since soap may increase nicotine absorption. Do not touch your eyes.

Disposal: When the used system is removed from the skin, it should be folded over with the adhesive sides together and placed in the protective pouch which contained the new system. The used system should be immediately disposed of in such a way as to prevent its access by children or pets. See patient information for further directions for handling and disposal.

HOW SUPPLIED

[See table above.]

How to Store: Do not store above 30°C (86°F) because PROSTEP systems are sensitive to heat. A slight discoloration of the system is not significant.

Do not store unpouched. Once removed from the protective pouch, PROSTEP systems should be applied promptly since nicotine is volatile and the system may lose strength.

CAUTION

Federal law prohibits dispensing without prescription.
© 1992
Manufactured for
Advantus Pharmaceuticals and
LEDERLE LABORATORIES DIVISION
American Cyanamid Company
Pearl River, New York 10965
by
élan pharma Ltd.
Athlone, County Westmeath
Ireland
                            Rev. 6/92
                            21469-92

Shown in Product Identification Section, page 415

PYRAZINAMIDE TABLETS, USP   ℞
500 mg

DESCRIPTION

Pyrazinamide, the pyrazine analogue of nicotinamide, is an antituberculous agent. It is a white crystalline powder, stable at room temperature, and sparingly soluble in water. Pyrazinamide has the following molecular weight; 123.11. Each Pyrazinamide tablet for oral administration contains 500 mg of pyrazinamide and the following inactive ingredients: corn starch, magnesium stearate, modified food starch and stearic acid.

CLINICAL PHARMACOLOGY

Pyrazinamide is well absorbed from the GI tract and attains peak plasma concentrations within 2 hours. Plasma concentrations generally range from 30 to 50 mcg/mL with doses of 20 to 25 mg/kg. It is widely distributed in body tissues and fluids including the liver, lungs and cerebrospinal fluid (CSF). The CSF concentration is approximately equal to concurrent steady-state plasma concentrations in patients with inflamed meninges.[1] Pyrazinamide is approximately 10% bound to plasma proteins.[2]

The half-life (t1/2) of pyrazinamide is 9 to 10 hours in patients with normal renal and hepatic function. The plasma half-life may be prolonged in patients with impaired renal or hepatic function. Pyrazinamide is hydrolyzed in the liver to its major active metabolite, pyrazinoic acid. Pyrazinoic acid is hydroxylated to the main excretory product, 5-hydroxy-pyrazinoic acid.[3]

Approximately 70% of an oral dose is excreted in urine, mainly by glomerular filtration within 24 hours.[3]

Pyrazinamide may be bacteriostatic or bactericidal against *Mycobacterium tuberculosis* depending on the concentration of the drug attained at the site of infection. The mechanism of action is unknown. *In vitro* and *in vivo* the drug is active only at a slightly acidic pH.

INDICATIONS AND USAGE

Pyrazinamide is indicated for the initial treatment of active tuberculosis in adults and children when combined with other antituberculous agents. (The current recommendation of the CDC for drug-susceptible disease is to use a six-month regimen for initial treatment of active tuberculosis, consisting of isoniazid, rifampin and pyrazinamide given for 2 months, followed by isoniazid and rifampin for 4 months.*[4])

(Patients with drug-resistant disease should be treated with regimens individualized to their situation. Pyrazinamide frequently will be an important component of such therapy.) (In patients with concomitant HIV infection, the physician should be aware of current recommendations of CDC. It is possible these patients may require a longer course of treatment.)

It is also indicated after treatment failure with other primary drugs in any form of active tuberculosis.

Pyrazinamide should only be used in conjunction with other effective antituberculous agents.

CONTRAINDICATIONS

Pyrazinamide is contraindicated in persons:
• with severe hepatic damage.
• who have shown hypersensitivity to it.
• with acute gout.

WARNINGS

Patients started on pyrazinamide should have baseline serum uric acid and liver function determinations. Those patients with preexisting liver disease or those at increased risk for drug related hepatitis (e.g., alcohol abusers) should be followed closely.

Pyrazinamide should be discontinued and not be resumed if signs of hepatocellular damage or hyperuricemia accompanied by an acute gouty arthritis appear.

PRECAUTIONS

General: Pyrazinamide inhibits renal excretion of urates, frequently resulting in hyperuricemia which is usually asymptomatic. If hyperuricemia is accompanied by acute gouty arthritis, pyrazinamide should be discontinued.

Pyrazinamide should be used with caution in patients with a history of diabetes mellitus, as management may be more difficult.

Primary resistance of *M. tuberculosis* to pyrazinamide is uncommon. In cases with known or suspected drug resistance, *in vitro* susceptibility tests with recent cultures of *M. tuberculosis* against pyrazinamide and the usual primary drugs should be performed. There are few reliable *in vitro* tests for pyrazinamide resistance. A reference laboratory capable of performing these studies must be employed.

Information for Patients: Patients should be instructed to notify their physicians promptly if they experience any of the following: fever, loss of appetite, malaise, nausea and vomiting, darkened urine, yellowish discoloration of the skin and eyes, pain or swelling of the joints.

Compliance with the full course of therapy must be emphasized, and the importance of not missing any doses must be stressed.

Laboratory Tests: Baseline liver function studies [especially ALT (SGPT), AST (SGOT) determinations] and uric acid levels should be determined prior to therapy. Appropriate laboratory testing should be performed at periodic intervals and if any clinical signs or symptoms occur during therapy.

Drug/Laboratory Test Interactions: Pyrazinamide has been reported to interfere with ACETEST® and KETOSTIX® urine tests to produce a pink-brown color.[5]

Carcinogenicity, Mutagenicity, Impairment of Fertility[6,7,8]: In lifetime bioassays in rats and mice, pyrazinamide was administered in the diet at concentrations of up to 10,000 ppm. This resulted in estimated daily doses for the mouse of 2 g/kg, or 40 times the maximum human dose, and for the rat of 0.5 g/kg, or 10 times the maximum human dose. Pyrazinamide was not carcinogenic in rats or male mice and no conclusion was possible for female mice due to insufficient numbers of surviving control mice.

Pyrazinamide was not mutagenic in the Ames bacterial test, but induced chromosomal aberrations in human lymphocyte cell cultures.

Pregnancy: Teratogenic Effects—Pregnancy Category C: Animal reproduction studies have not been conducted with pyrazinamide. It is also not known whether pyrazinamide can cause fetal harm when administered to a pregnant woman or can affect reproduction capacity. Pyrazinamide should be given to a pregnant woman only if clearly needed.

Nursing Mothers: Pyrazinamide has been found in small amounts in breast milk. Therefore, it is advised the pyrazinamide be used with caution in nursing mothers taking into account the risk-benefit of this therapy.[9]

Usage in Children: Pyrazinamide regimens employed in adults are probably equally effective in children.[4,10,11] Pyrazinamide appears to be well tolerated in children.

Geriatric Use[12]: Clinical studies of pyrazinamide did not include sufficient numbers of patients aged 65 and over to determine whether they respond differently from younger patients. Other reported clinical experience has not identified differences in responses between the elderly and younger patients. In general, dose selection for an elderly patient should be cautious, usually starting at the low end of the dosing range, reflecting the greater frequency of decreased hepatic or renal function, and of concomitant disease or other drug therapy.

It does not appear that patients with impaired renal function require a reduction in dose. It may be prudent to select doses at the low end of the dosing range, however.[13]

ADVERSE REACTIONS

General: Fever, porphyria and dysuria have rarely been reported. Gout (see PRECAUTIONS).

Gastrointestinal: The principal adverse effect is a hepatic reaction (see WARNINGS). Hepatotoxicity appears to be dose related, and may appear at any time during therapy. GI disturbances including nausea, vomiting and anorexia have also been reported.

Hematologic and Lymphatic: Thrombocytopenia and sideroblastic anemia with erythroid hyperplasia, vacuolation of erythrocytes and increased serum iron concentration have occurred rarely with this drug. Adverse effects on blood clotting mechanisms have also been rarely reported.

Other: Mild arthralgia and myalgia have been reported frequently. Hypersensitivity reactions including rashes, urticaria, and pruritus have been reported. Fever, acne, photosensitivity, porphyria, dysuria and interstitial nephritis have been reported rarely.

OVERDOSAGE

Overdosage experience is limited. In one case report of overdose, abnormal liver function tests developed. These spontaneously reverted to normal when the drug was stopped. Clinical monitoring and supportive therapy should be employed. Pyrazinamide is dialyzable.[13]

DOSAGE AND ADMINISTRATION

Pyrazinamide should always be administered with other effective antituberculous drugs. It is administered for the initial 2 months of a 6-month or longer treatment regimen for drug-susceptible patients. Patients who are known or suspected to have drug-resistant disease should be treated with regimens individualized to their situation. Pyrazinamide frequently will be an important component of such therapy.

Patients with concomitant HIV infection may require longer courses of therapy. Physicians treating such patients should be alert to any revised recommendations from CDC for this group of patients.

Usual dose: Pyrazinamide is administered orally, 15 to 30 mg/kg once daily. Older regimens employed 3 to 4 divided doses daily, but most current recommendations are for once a day. Three grams per day should not be exceeded. The CDC recommendations do not exceed 2 g per day when given as a daily regimen (see table).

Alternatively, a twice weekly dosing regimen (50 to 70 mg/kg twice weekly based on lean body weight) has been developed to promote patient compliance with a regimen on an outpatient basis. In studies evaluating the twice weekly regimen, doses of pyrazinamide in excess of 3 g twice weekly have been administered. This exceeds the recommended maximum 3 g/daily dose. However, an increased incidence of adverse reactions has not been reported.

Continued on next page

---

* See recommendations of Centers for Disease Control (CDC) and American Thoracic Society for complete regimen and dosage recommendations.[4]

Information on Lederle products listed on these pages is the full prescribing information from product literature or package inserts effective in August 1992. Information concerning all Lederle products may be obtained from the Professional Services Department, Lederle Laboratories, Pearl River, New York 10965.

Lederle—Cont.

Recommended Drugs for the Initial Treatment of Tuberculosis in Children and Adults

Drug	Daily Dose* Children	Daily Dose* Adults	Maximal Daily Dose in Children and Adults	Twice Weekly Dose Children	Twice Weekly Dose Adults
Isoniazid	10 to 20 mg/kg PO or IM	5 mg/kg PO or IM	300 mg	20 to 40 mg/kg Max. 900 mg	15 mg/kg Max. 900 mg
Rifampin	10 to 20 mg/kg PO	10 mg/kg PO	600 mg	10 to 20 mg/kg Max. 600 mg	10 mg/kg Max. 600 mg
Pyrazinamide	15 to 30 mg/kg PO	15 to 30 mg/kg PO	2 g	50 to 70 mg/kg	50 to 70 mg/kg
Streptomycin	20 to 40 mg/kg IM	15 mg/kg** IM	1 g**	25 to 30 mg/kg IM	25 to 30 mg/kg IM
Ethambutol	15 to 25 mg/kg PO	15 to 25 mg/kg PO	2.5 g	50 mg/kg	50 mg/kg

Definition of abbreviations: PO = perorally; IM = intramuscularly.
*Doses based on weight should be adjusted as weight changes
**In persons older than 60 yr of age the daily dose of streptomycin should be limited to 10 mg/kg with a maximal dose of 750 mg.

The table is taken from the CDC-American Thoracic Society joint recommendations:[4]
[See table above.]

HOW SUPPLIED
Pyrazinamide Tablets, USP 500 mg are round, white, scored tablets, engraved P36 on the scored side, and LL on the other side, supplied as:
NDC 0005-5093-23 - Bottle of 100
NDC 0005-5093-31 - Bottle of 500
Store in a well-closed container at controlled room temperature 15°–30°C (59°–86°F).
Caution: Federal law prohibits dispensing without prescription.
LEDERLE LABORATORIES DIVISION
American Cyanamid Company, Pearl River, NY 10965
Rev. 3/92
20929-92

REFERENCES
1. *Drug Information, American Hospital Formulary Service.* American Society of Hospital Pharmacists. Bethesda, Md. 1991.
2. *USPDI, Drug Information for the Health Care Professional.* United States Pharmacopeial Convention, Inc. Rockville, Md. 1991:1B:2226–2227.
3. Goodman-Gilman A, Rall TW, Nies AS, Taylor P. *The Pharmacological Basis of Therapeutics,* ed 8. New York, Pergamon Press. 1990;1154.
4. Treatment of tuberculosis and tuberculosis infection in adults and children. *Am Rev Respir Dis.* 1986;134:363–368.
5. Reynolds JEF, Parfitt K, Parsons AV, Sweetman SC. *Martindale The Extra Pharmacopoeia,* ed 29. London, The Pharmaceutical Press. 1989;569-570.
6. Bioassay of pyrazinamide for possible carcinogenicity. National Cancer Institute Carcinogenesis Technical Report Series No. 48, 1978.
7. Zerger E, Anderson B, Haworth S, Lawlor T, Mortelmans K, Speck W. Salmonella mutagenicity tests: III. Results from the testing of 255 chemicals. *Environ Mutagen.* 1987;9(Suppl 9):1–109.
8. Roman IC, Georgian L. Cytogenetic effects of some antituberculosis drugs in vitro. *Mutation Research.* 1977;48:215–224.
9. Holdiness M. Antituberculosis drugs and breast-feeding. *Arch Intern Med.* 1984;144:1888.
10. Turcios N, Evans H. Preventing and managing tuberculosis in children. *J Resp Dis.* 1989;10(6)(Jun):23.
11. Starke JR. Multidrug therapy for tuberculosis in children. *Pediatr Infec Dis J.* 1990;9:785–793.
12. Specific requirements on content and format of labeling for human prescription drugs; proposed addition of "geriatric use" subsection in the labeling. *Federal Register.* 1990;55(212) (Nov 1):46134–46137.
13. Stamathakis G, Montes C, Trouvin JH, et al. Pyrazinamide and pyrazinoic acid pharmacokinetics in patients with chronic renal failure. *Clinical Nephrology.* 1988;30:230–234.

Shown in Product Identification Section, page 415

RHEUMATREX® Dose Pack   ℞
Methotrexate 2.5 mg Tablets

PRODUCT OVERVIEW
KEY FACTS
RHEUMATREX is a folic acid antagonist given orally in second-line therapy for adult rheumatoid arthritis. While it has not been shown to modify the disease process,

RHEUMATREX reduces articular swelling and tenderness and ameliorates signs and symptoms of inflammation (pain, swelling, stiffness). Clinical improvement may begin as early as 3 to 6 weeks and is maintained with continued therapy. Tablets are supplied in a Dose Pack in weekly doses of 5 mg, 7.5 mg, 10 mg, 12.5 mg, and 15 mg.

MAJOR USES
RHEUMATREX is used in the treatment of selected adults with active, rheumatoid arthritis (ARA Criteria).

SAFETY INFORMATION
There is a potential for severe toxic reactions. Physicians should monitor patients closely. Patients should be informed of early signs of toxicity plus the need to see their physicians promptly if these signs occur, and of the need for regular follow-up, including periodic lab tests. Physician and pharmacist should emphasize that the recommended dose is taken weekly and that mistaken daily use has led to fatal toxicity. (See box **Warnings, Precautions,** and **Adverse Reactions** sections in full PRESCRIBING INFORMATION for Methotrexate).

PRESCRIBING INFORMATION
Please see page 1245 for full Prescribing Information for Methotrexate.
Shown in Product Identification Section, page 415

STRESSTABS®   OTC
[strĕs-tabs]
High Potency
Stress Formula Vitamins

(See PDR For Nonprescription Drugs.)

STRESSTABS® with IRON   OTC
[strĕs-tabs]
High Potency
Stress Formula Vitamins

(See PDR For Nonprescription Drugs.)

STRESSTABS® with ZINC   OTC
[strĕs-tabs]
High Potency
Stress Formula Vitamins

(See PDR For Nonprescription Drugs.)

SUPRAX®   ℞
Cefixime
Oral

PRODUCT OVERVIEW
KEY FACTS
SUPRAX is a semisynthetic, third-generation cephalosporin antibiotic for oral administration. The bactericidal action of SUPRAX results from inhibition of cell-wall synthesis. SUPRAX is highly beta-lactamase stable and, as a result, many organisms resistant to penicillins and some cephalosporins, due to the presence of beta-lactamases, may be susceptible to SUPRAX.
SUPRAX has been shown to be active against most strains of gram-negative and gram-positive organisms, both *in vitro* and in clinical studies. (See full **PRESCRIBING INFORMATION.**) The serum half-life of SUPRAX averages 3.0 to 4.0 hours, but may range up to 9 hours in some normal volunteers.

MAJOR USES
SUPRAX is indicated for the treatment of the following infections caused by susceptible strains of the designated microorganisms: otitis media caused by *Haemophilus influenzae* (beta-lactamase positive and negative strains), *Branhamella catarrhalis* (most of which are beta-lactamase positive), and *Streptococcus pyogenes* (see CLINICAL STUDIES section of full PRESCRIBING INFORMATION for information on *Streptococcus pneumoniae*); pharyngitis and tonsillitis caused by *S pyogenes;* acute bronchitis, caused by *S pneumoniae* and *H influenzae* (beta-lactamase positive and negative strains); uncomplicated urinary tract infections caused by *Escherichia coli* and *Proteus mirabilis.*

SAFETY INFORMATION
SUPRAX is contraindicated in patients with known allergy to the cephalosporin group of antibiotics. In patients with renal impairment, dosage adjustment is necessary. Prescribe with caution in patients with a history of gastrointestinal disease, particularly colitis.

PRESCRIBING INFORMATION
SUPRAX®   ℞
Cefixime
Oral

DESCRIPTION
SUPRAX is a semisynthetic, cephalosporin antibiotic for oral administration. Chemically, it is (6R, 7R)-7-[2-(2-Amino-4-thiazolyl) gloxylamido] -8- oxo-3-vinyl-5-thia -1- azabicyclo [4.2.0]oct-2-ene-2-carboxylic acid, 7^2-(Z)-[O-(carboxymethyl) oxime]-trihydrate. Molecular weight = 507.50 as the trihydrate.
SUPRAX is available in scored 200 mg and 400 mg film-coated tablets and in a powder for oral suspension which, when reconstituted, provides 100 mg/5 mL.
Inactive ingredients contained in the 200 mg and 400 mg tablets are: dibasic calcium phosphate, hydroxypropyl methylcellulose 2910, light mineral oil, magnesium stearate, microcrystalline cellulose, pregelatinized starch, sodium lauryl sulfate, and titanium dioxide. The powder for oral suspension is strawberry flavored and contains sodium benzoate, sucrose, and xanthan gum.

CLINICAL PHARMACOLOGY
SUPRAX *cefixime,* given orally, is about 40% to 50% absorbed whether administered with or without food; however, time to maximal absorption is increased approximately 0.8 hours when administered with food. A single 200 mg tablet of SUPRAX produces an average peak serum concentration of approximately 2 mcg/mL (range 1 to 4 mcg/mL); a single 400 mg tablet produces an average peak concentration of approximately 3.7 mcg/mL (range 1.3 to 7.7 mcg/mL). The oral suspension produces average peak concentrations approximately 25% to 50% higher than the tablets. Two hundred milligram and 400 mg doses of oral suspension produce average peak concentrations of 3 mcg/mL (range 1 to 4.5 mcg/mL) and 4.6 mcg/mL (range 1.9 to 7.7 mcg/mL), respectively. The area under the time versus concentration curve is greater by approximately 10% to 25% with the oral suspension than with the tablet after doses of 100 mg to 400 mg. This increased absorption should be taken into consideration if the oral suspension is to be substituted for the tablet. Because of the lack of bioequivalence, tablets should not be substituted for oral suspension in the treatment of otitis media. (See DOSAGE AND ADMINISTRATION.) Peak serum concentrations occur between 2 and 6 hours following oral administration of a single 200 mg tablet, a single 400 mg tablet, or 400 mg of suspension of SUPRAX. Peak serum concentrations occur between 2 and 5 hours following a single administration of 200 mg of suspension.

Serum Levels of Cefixime
After Administration of Tablets (mcg/mL)

DOSE	1h	2h	4h	6h	8h	12h	24h
100 mg	0.3	0.8	1.0	0.7	0.4	0.2	0.02
200 mg	0.7	1.4	2.0	1.5	1.0	0.4	0.03
400 mg	1.2	2.5	3.5	2.7	1.7	0.6	0.04

Serum Levels of Cefixime
After Administration of Oral Suspension (mcg/mL)

DOSE	1h	2h	4h	6h	8h	12h	24h
100 mg	0.7	1.1	1.3	0.9	0.6	0.2	0.02
200 mg	1.2	2.1	2.8	2.0	1.3	0.5	0.07
400 mg	1.8	3.3	4.4	3.3	2.2	0.8	0.07

Approximately 50% of the absorbed dose is excreted unchanged in the urine in 24 hours. In animal studies, it was noted that cefixime is also excreted in the bile in excess of 10% of the administered dose. Serum protein binding is concentration-independent with a bound fraction of approxi-

mately 65%. In a multiple dose study conducted with a research formulation which is less bioavailable than the tablet or suspension, there was little accumulation of drug in serum or urine after dosing for 14 days.
The serum half-life of cefixime in healthy subjects is independent of dosage form and averages 3.0 to 4.0 hours but may range up to 9 hours in some normal volunteers. Average AUCs at steady state in elderly patients are approximately 40% higher than average AUCs in other healthy adults.
In subjects with moderate impairment of renal function (20 to 40 mL/min creatinine clearance), the average serum half-life of cefixime is prolonged to 6.4 hours. In severe renal impairment (5 to 20 mL/min creatinine clearance), the half-life increased to an average of 11.5 hours. The drug is not cleared significantly from the blood by hemodialysis or peritoneal dialysis. However, a study indicated that with doses of 400 mg, patients undergoing hemodialysis have similar blood profiles as subjects with creatinine clearances of 21 to 60 mL/min. There is no evidence of metabolism of cefixime *in vivo*.
Adequate data on CSF levels of cefixime are not available.
Microbiology: As with other cephalosporins, bactericidal action of SUPRAX *cefixime* results from inhibition of cell-wall synthesis. SUPRAX is highly stable in the presence of beta-lactamase enzymes. As a result, many organisms resistant to penicillins and some cephalosporins, due to the presence of beta-lactamases, may be susceptible to cefixime.
SUPRAX has been shown to be active against most strains of the following organisms both *in vitro* and in clinical infections (see **INDICATIONS AND USAGE**):

Gram-positive Organisms
Streptococcus pneumoniae
Streptococcus pyogenes

Gram-negative Organisms
Haemophilus influenzae (beta-lactamase positive and negative strains)
Moraxella (Branhamella) catarrhalis (most of which are beta-lactamase positive)
Escherichia coli
Proteus mirabilis

SUPRAX has been shown to be active *in vitro* against most strains of the following organisms; however, clinical efficacy has not been established.

Gram-positive Organisms
Streptococcus agalactiae

Gram-negative Organisms
Neisseria gonorrhoeae (beta-lactamase positive and negative strains)
Haemophilus parainfluenzae (beta-lactamase positive and negative strains)
Proteus vulgaris
Klebsiella pneumoniae
Klebsiella oxytoca
Pasteurella multocida
Providencia species
Salmonella species
Shigella species
Citrobacter amalonaticus
Citrobacter diversus
Serratia marcescens

Note: *Pseudomonas* species, strains of group D streptococci (including enterococci), *Listeria monocytogenes*, most strains of staphylococci (including methicillin-resistant strains) and most strains of *Enterobacter* are resistant to SUPRAX. In addition, most strains of *Bacteroides fragilis* and clostridia are resistant to SUPRAX.

SUSCEPTIBILITY TESTING

Susceptibility Tests: *Diffusion Techniques:* Quantitative methods that require measurement of zone diameters give an estimate of antibiotic susceptibility. One such procedure[1–3] has been recommended for use with disks to test susceptibility to cefixime. Interpretation involves correlation of the diameters obtained in the disk test with minimum inhibitory concentration (MIC) for cefixime.
Reports from the laboratory giving results of the standard single-disk susceptibility test with a 5-mcg cefixime disk should be interpreted according to the following criteria:

Zone diameter (mm)	Interpretation
≥ 19	(S) Susceptible
16–18	(MS) Moderately Susceptible
≤ 15	(R) Resistant

A report of "Susceptible" indicates that the pathogen is likely to be inhibited by generally achievable blood levels. A report of "Moderately Susceptible" indicates that inhibitory concentrations of the antibiotic may well be achieved if high dosage is used or if the infection is confined to tissues and fluids (eg, urine) in which high antibiotic levels are attained. A report of "Resistant" indicates that achievable concentrations of the antibiotic are unlikely to be inhibitory and other therapy should be selected.

Bacteriological Outcome of Otitis Media at Two- to Four-Weeks Posttherapy
Based on Repeat Middle Ear Fluid Culture or
Extrapolation From Clinical Outcome

Organism	Cefixime[a] 4 mg/kg bid	Cefixime[a] 8 mg/kg qd	Control[a] drugs
Streptococcus pneumoniae	48/70 (69%)	18/22 (82%)	82/100 (82%)
Haemophilus influenzae beta-lactamase negative	24/34 (71%)	13/17 (76%)	23/34 (68%)
Haemophilus influenzae beta-lactamase positive	17/22 (77%)	9/12 (75%)	1/1[b]
Moraxella (Branhamella) catarrhalis	26/31 (84%)	5/5	18/24 (75%)
Streptococcus pyogenes	5/5	3/3	6/7
All Isolates	120/162 (74%)	48/59 (81%)	130/166 (78%)

[a] Number eradicated/number isolated.
[b] An additional 20 beta-lactamase positive strains of *Haemophilus influenzae* were isolated, but were excluded from this analysis because they were resistant to the control antibiotic. In 19 of these, the clinical course could be assessed and a favorable outcome occurred in 10. When these cases are included in the overall bacteriological evaluation of therapy with the control drugs, 140/185 (76%) of pathogens were considered to be eradicated.

Standardized procedures require the use of laboratory control organisms. The 5-mcg disk should give the following zone diameter:

Organism	Zone diameter (mm)
E coli ATCC 25922	23–27

The class disk for cephalosporin susceptibility testing (the cephalothin disk) is not appropriate because of spectrum differences with cefixime. The 5-mcg cefixime disk should be used for all *in vitro* testing of isolates.
Dilution Techniques: In other susceptibility testing procedures, eg, ICS agar dilution or equivalent, a bacterial isolate may be considered susceptible if the MIC value for cefixime is 1 mcg/mL or less. Organisms are considered resistant to cefixime if the MIC is equal to or greater than 4 mcg/mL. Organisms having an MIC of 2 mcg/mL are moderately susceptible.
As with standard diffusion methods, dilution procedures require the use of laboratory control organisms. Standard cefixime powder should give MIC values in the range of 0.25 to 1 mcg/mL for *E coli* ATCC 25922 and in the range of 8 to 32 mcg/mL for *S aureus* ATCC 29213.

INDICATIONS AND USAGE

SUPRAX *cefixime* is indicated in the treatment of the following infections when caused by susceptible strains of the designated microorganisms:
Uncomplicated Urinary Tract Infections caused by *Escherichia coli* and *Proteus mirabilis.*
Otitis Media caused by *Haemophilus influenzae* (beta-lactamase positive and negative strains), *Moraxella (Branhamella) catarrhalis* (most of which are beta-lactamase positive), and *Streptococcus pyogenes.**
Note: For information on otitis media caused by *Streptococcus pneumoniae,* see **CLINICAL STUDIES** section.
Pharyngitis and Tonsillitis, caused by *Streptococcus pyogenes.*
Note: Penicillin is the usual drug of choice in the treatment of *Streptococcus pyogenes* infections, including the prophylaxis of rheumatic fever. SUPRAX *cefixime* is generally effective in the eradication of *Streptococcus pyogenes* from the nasopharynx; however, data establishing the efficacy of SUPRAX in the subsequent prevention of rheumatic fever are not available.
Acute Bronchitis and Acute Exacerbations of Chronic Bronchitis, caused by *Streptococcus pneumoniae* and *Haemophilus influenzae* (beta-lactamase positive and negative strains).
Appropriate cultures and susceptibility studies should be performed to determine the causative organism and its susceptibility to SUPRAX; however, therapy may be started while awaiting the results of these studies. Therapy should be adjusted, if necessary, once these results are known.

CLINICAL STUDIES

In clinical trials of otitis media in nearly 400 children between the ages of 6 months to 10 years, *Streptococcus pneumoniae* was isolated from 47% of the patients, *Haemophilus influenzae* from 34%, *Moraxella (Branhamella) catarrhalis* from 15%, and *Streptococcus pyogenes* from 4%.
The overall response rate of *Streptococcus pneumoniae* to cefixime was approximately 10% lower and that of *Haemophilus influenzae* or *Moraxella (Branhamella) catarrhalis* approximately 7% higher (12% when beta-lactamase positive strains of *H influenzae* are included) than the response rates of these organisms to the active control drugs.
In these studies, patients were randomized and treated with either cefixime at dose regimens of 4 mg/kg bid or 8 mg/kg qd, or with a standard antibiotic regimen. Sixty-nine to 70% of the patients in each group had resolution of signs and symptoms of otitis media when evaluated 2 to 4 weeks post-treatment, but persistent effusion was found in 15% of the patients. When evaluated at the completion of therapy, 17% of patients receiving cefixime and 14% of patients receiving effective comparative drugs (18% including those patients who had *Haemophilus influenzae* resistant to the control drug and who received the control antibiotic) were considered to be treatment failures. By the 2- to 4-week follow-up, a total of 30% to 31% of patients had evidence of either treatment failure or recurrent disease.
[See table above.]

*Efficacy for this organism in this organ system was studied in fewer than 10 infections.

CONTRAINDICATIONS

SUPRAX is contraindicated in patients with known allergy to the cephalosporin group of antibiotics.

WARNINGS

BEFORE THERAPY WITH SUPRAX IS INSTITUTED, CAREFUL INQUIRY SHOULD BE MADE TO DETERMINE WHETHER THE PATIENT HAS HAD PREVIOUS HYPERSENSITIVITY REACTIONS TO CEPHALOSPORINS, PENICILLINS, OR OTHER DRUGS. IF THIS PRODUCT IS TO BE GIVEN TO PENICILLIN-SENSITIVE PATIENTS, CAUTION SHOULD BE EXERCISED BECAUSE CROSS HYPERSENSITIVITY AMONG BETA-LACTAM ANTIBIOTICS HAS BEEN CLEARLY DOCUMENTED AND MAY OCCUR IN UP TO 10% OF PATIENTS WITH A HISTORY OF PENICILLIN ALLERGY. IF AN ALLERGIC REACTION TO SUPRAX OCCURS, DISCONTINUE THE DRUG. SERIOUS ACUTE HYPERSENSITIVITY REACTIONS MAY REQUIRE TREATMENT WITH EPINEPHRINE AND OTHER EMERGENCY MEASURES, INCLUDING OXYGEN, INTRAVENOUS FLUIDS, INTRAVENOUS ANTIHISTAMINES, CORTICOSTEROIDS, PRESSOR AMINES AND AIRWAY MANAGEMENT, AS CLINICALLY INDICATED.
Antibiotics, including SUPRAX, should be administered cautiously to any patient who has demonstrated some form of allergy, particularly to drugs.
Treatment with broad-spectrum antibiotics, including SUPRAX, alters the normal flora of the colon and may permit overgrowth of clostridia. Studies indicate that a toxin produced by *Clostridium difficile* is a primary cause of severe antibiotic-associated diarrhea including pseudomembranous colitis.
Pseudomembranous colitis has been reported with the use of SUPRAX *cefixime* and other broad-spectrum antibiotics (including macrolides, semisynthetic penicillins, and cephalosporins); therefore, it is important to consider this diagnosis in patients who develop diarrhea in association with the use of antibiotics. Symptoms of pseudomembranous colitis may occur during or after antibiotic treatment and may range in severity from mild to life threatening. Mild cases of pseudomembranous colitis usually respond to drug discontinuation alone. In moderate-to-severe cases, management should include fluids, electrolytes, and protein supplementation. If the colitis does not improve after the drug has been discontinued, or if the symptoms are severe, oral vancomycin is the drug of choice for antibiotic-associated pseudomembranous colitis produced by *C difficile.* Other causes of colitis should be excluded.

Continued on next page

Information on Lederle products listed on these pages is the full prescribing information from product literature or package inserts effective in August 1992. Information concerning all Lederle products may be obtained from the Professional Services Department, Lederle Laboratories, Pearl River, New York 10965.

Lederle—Cont.

PRECAUTIONS

General: The possibility of the emergence of resistant organisms which might result in overgrowth should be kept in mind, particularly during prolonged treatment. In such use, careful observation of the patient is essential. If superinfection occurs during therapy, appropriate measures should be taken.

The dose of SUPRAX should be adjusted in patients with renal impairment as well as those undergoing continuous ambulatory peritoneal dialysis (CAPD) and hemodialysis (HD). Patients on dialysis should be monitored carefully. (See **DOSAGE AND ADMINISTRATION**.)

SUPRAX should be prescribed with caution in individuals with a history of gastrointestinal disease, particularly colitis.

Drug Interactions: No significant drug interactions have been reported to date.

Drug/Laboratory Test Interactions: A false-positive reaction for ketones in the urine may occur with tests using nitroprusside but not with those using nitroferricyanide.

The administration of SUPRAX may result in a false-positive reaction for glucose in the urine using Clinitest®,** Benedict's solution, or Fehling's solution. It is recommended that glucose tests based on enzymatic glucose oxidase reactions (such as Clinistix®** or Tes-Tape®**) be used.

A false-positive direct Coombs test has been reported during treatment with other cephalosporin antibiotics; therefore, it should be recognized that a positive Coombs test may be due to the drug.

Carcinogenesis, Mutagenesis, Impairment of Fertility: Lifetime studies in animals to evaluate carcinogenic potential have not been conducted. SUPRAX did not cause point mutations in bacteria or mammalian cells, DNA damage, or chromosome damage *in vitro* and did not exhibit clastogenic potential *in vivo* in the mouse micronucleus test. In rats, fertility and reproductive performance were not affected by cefixime at doses up to 125 times the adult therapeutic dose.

Usage in Pregnancy: *Pregnancy Category B:* Reproduction studies have been performed in mice and rats at doses up to 400 times the human dose and have revealed no evidence of harm to the fetus due to SUPRAX. There are no adequate and well-controlled studies in pregnant women. Because animal reproduction studies are not always predictive of human response, this drug should be used during pregnancy only if clearly needed.

Labor and Delivery: SUPRAX *cefixime* has not been studied for use during labor and delivery. Treatment should only be given if clearly needed.

Nursing Mothers: It is not known whether SUPRAX is excreted in human milk. Consideration should be given to discontinuing nursing temporarily during treatment with this drug.

Pediatric Use: Safety and effectiveness of SUPRAX in children aged less than 6 months old have not been established.

The incidence of gastrointestinal adverse reactions, including diarrhea and loose stools, in the pediatric patients receiving the suspension, was comparable to the incidence seen in adult patients receiving tablets.

ADVERSE REACTIONS

Most of the adverse reactions observed in clinical trials were of a mild and transient nature. Five percent (5%) of patients in the US trials discontinued therapy because of drug-related adverse reactions. The most commonly seen adverse reactions in US trials of the tablet formulation were gastrointestinal events, which were reported in 30% of adult patients on either the bid or the qd regimen. Clinically mild gastrointestinal side effects occurred in 20% of all patients, moderate events occurred in 9% of all patients, and severe adverse reactions occurred in 2% of all patients. Individual event rates included diarrhea 16%, loose or frequent stools 6%, abdominal pain 3%, nausea 7%, dyspepsia 3%, and flatulence 4%. The incidence of gastrointestinal adverse reactions, including diarrhea and loose stools in pediatric patients receiving the suspension was comparable to the incidence seen in adult patients receiving tablets.

These symptoms usually responded to symptomatic therapy or ceased when SUPRAX was discontinued.

Several patients developed severe diarrhea and/or documented pseudomembranous colitis, and a few required hospitalization.

The following adverse reactions have been reported following the use of SUPRAX. Incidence rates were less than 1 in 50 (less than 2%), except as noted above for gastrointestinal events.

Gastrointestinal: (SEE ABOVE): Diarrhea, loose stools, abdominal pain, dyspepsia, nausea, and vomiting. Several cases of documented pseudomembranous colitis were identified during the studies. The onset of pseudomembranous colitis symptoms may occur during or after therapy.

Hypersensitivity Reactions: Skin rashes, urticaria, drug fever, and pruritus. Erythema multiforme, Stevens-Johnson syndrome, and serum sickness-like reactions have been reported.

Hepatic: Transient elevations in SGPT, SGOT, and alkaline phosphatase.

Renal: Transient elevations in BUN or creatinine.

Central Nervous System: Headaches or dizziness.

Hemic and Lymphatic Systems: Transient thrombocytopenia, leukopenia, and eosinophilia. Prolongation in prothrombin time was seen rarely.

Other: Genital pruritus, vaginitis, candidiasis.

In addition to the adverse reactions listed above, which have been observed in patients treated with SUPRAX, the following adverse reactions and altered laboratory tests have been reported for cephalosporin-class antibiotics:

Adverse Reactions: Allergic reactions including anaphylaxis, toxic epidermal necrolysis, superinfection, renal dysfunction, toxic nephropathy, hepatic dysfunction including cholestasis, aplastic anemia, hemolytic anemia, hemorrhage, and colitis.

Several cephalosporins have been implicated in triggering seizures, particularly in patients with renal impairment when the dosage was not reduced (see **DOSAGE AND ADMINISTRATION** and **OVERDOSAGE**). If seizures associated with drug therapy occur, the drug should be discontinued. Anticonvulsant therapy can be given if clinically indicated.

Abnormal Laboratory Tests: Positive direct Coombs test, elevated bilirubin, elevated LDH, pancytopenia, neutropenia, agranulocytosis.

OVERDOSAGE

Gastric lavage may be indicated; otherwise, no specific antidote exists. Cefixime is not removed in significant quantities from the circulation by hemodialysis or peritoneal dialysis. Adverse reactions in small numbers of healthy adult volunteers receiving single doses up to 2 g of SUPRAX did not differ from the profile seen in patients treated at the recommended doses.

DOSAGE AND ADMINISTRATION

Adults: The recommended dose of SUPRAX *cefixime* is 400 mg daily. This may be given as a 400 mg tablet daily or as a 200 mg tablet every 12 hours.

Children: The recommended dose is 8 mg/kg/day of the suspension. This may be administered as a single daily dose or may be given in two divided doses, as 4 mg/kg every 12 hours.

PEDIATRIC DOSAGE CHART

Patient Weight kg	Dose/Day mg	Dose/Day mL	Dose/Day tsp of suspension
6.25	50	2.5	½
12.5	100	5.0	1
18.75	150	7.5	1½
25.0	200	10.0	2
31.25	250	12.5	2½
37.5	300	15.0	3

Children weighing more than 50 kg or older than 12 years should be treated with the recommended adult dose.

Otitis media should be treated with the suspension. Clinical studies of otitis media were conducted with the suspension, and the suspension results in higher peak blood levels than the tablet when administered at the same dose. Therefore, the tablet should not be substituted for the suspension in the treatment of otitis media (see **CLINICAL PHARMACOLOGY**).

Efficacy and safety in infants aged less than 6 months have not been established.

In the treatment of infections due to *S pyogenes*, a therapeutic dosage of SUPRAX *cefixime* should be administered for at least 10 days.

Renal Impairment: SUPRAX may be administered in the presence of impaired renal function. Normal dose and schedule may be employed in patients with creatinine clearances of 60 mL/min or greater. Patients whose clearance is between 21 and 60 mL/min or patients who are on renal hemodialysis may be given 75% of the standard dosage at the standard dosing interval (ie, 300 mg daily). Patients whose clearance is < 20 mL/min, or patients who are on continuous ambulatory peritoneal dialysis may be given half the standard dosage at the standard dosing interval (ie, 200 mg daily). Neither hemodialysis nor peritoneal dialysis remove significant amounts of drug from the body.

[See table top of next column.]

After reconstitution, the suspension may be kept for 14 days either at room temperature, or under refrigeration, without significant loss of potency. Keep tightly closed. Shake well before using. Discard unused portion after 14 days.

Reconstitution Directions for Oral Suspension

Bottle Size	Reconstitution Directions
100 mL	To reconstitute, suspend with 69 mL water. Method: Tap the bottle several times to loosen powder contents prior to reconstitution. Add approximately half the total amount of water for reconstitution and shake well. Add the remainder of water and shake well.
75 mL	To reconstitute, suspend with 52 mL water. Method: Tap the bottle several times to loosen powder contents prior to reconstitution. Add approximately half the total amount of water for reconstitution and shake well. Add the remainder of water and shake well.
50 mL	To reconstitute, suspend with 36 mL water. Method: Tap the bottle several times to loosen powder contents prior to reconstitution. Add approximately half the total amount of water for reconstitution and shake well. Add the remainder of water and shake well.

HOW SUPPLIED

SUPRAX *cefixime* Tablets, 200 mg, are convex, rectangular, white, film-coated tablets with rounded corners and beveled edges and a divided break line on each side, engraved with SUPRAX across one side and LL to the left and 200 to the right on the other side, supplied as follows:

NDC 0005-3899-23—Bottle of 100

Store at Controlled Room Temperature 15°-30°C (59°-86°F).

SUPRAX Tablets, 400 mg, are convex, rectangular, white, film-coated tablets with rounded corners and beveled edges and a divided break line on each side, engraved with SUPRAX across one side and LL to the left and 400 to the right on the other side, supplied as follows:

NDC 0005-3897-94—Unit of Issue 10s with CRC
NDC 0005-3897-18—Bottle of 50
NDC 0005-3897-23—Bottle of 100
NDC 0005-3897-60—10 (2 × 5) Strips

Store at Controlled Room Temperature 15°-30°C (59°-86°F).

SUPRAX Powder for Oral Suspension is an off-white to cream-colored powder which when reconstituted as directed contains cefixime 100 mg/5 mL, supplied as follows:

NDC 0005-3898-40—50 mL Bottle
NDC 0005-3898-42—75 mL Bottle
NDC 0005-3898-46—100 mL Bottle

Military Depots:
Powder for Oral Suspension 100 mg/5 mL
NSN 6505-01-310-4160–50 mL Bottle
NSN 6505-01-310-4161–100 mL Bottle

Prior to Reconstitution: Store at Controlled Room Temperature 15°-30°C (59°-86°F).

REFERENCES

1. Bauer AW, Kirby WMM, Sherris JC, et al: Antibiotic susceptibility testing by a standard single disk method. *Am J Clin Pathol* 1966; 45: 493.
2. National Committee for Clinical Laboratory Standards, Approved Standard: Performance Standards for Antimicrobial Disk Susceptibility Tests (M2-A3), December 1984.
3. Standardized disk susceptibility test. Federal Register 1974; 39 (May 30): 19182–19184.

Manufactured for
LEDERLE LABORATORIES DIVISION
American Cyanamid Company, Pearl River, NY 10965
By
BIOCRAFT LABORATORIES, INC.
Elmwood Park, NJ 07407
Under License of
Fujisawa Pharmaceutical Co., Ltd.
Osaka, Japan

Rev. 4/92
21406-92

Shown in Product Identification Section, page 416

TETANUS AND DIPHTHERIA TOXOIDS ADSORBED ℞
FOR ADULT USE
Aluminum Phosphate-Adsorbed
PUROGENATED®

DESCRIPTION

Tetanus and Diphtheria Toxoids Adsorbed, For Adult Use, aluminum phosphate-adsorbed PUROGENATED is a sterile combination of refined tetanus and diphtheria toxoids for intramuscular use only. After shaking, the vaccine is a homogeneous white suspension.

**Clinitest® and Clinistix® are registered trademarks of Ames Division, Miles Laboratories, Inc. Tes-Tape® is a registered trademark of Eli Lilly and Company.

The tetanus and diphtheria toxins are produced according to the method of Mueller and Miller,[1,2] and are detoxified by use of formaldehyde. The toxoids are refined by the Pillemer alcohol fractionation method[3] and are diluted with a solution containing sodium phosphate monobasic, sodium phosphate dibasic, aluminum phosphate, glycine and thimerosal (mercury derivative) as a preservative. The final concentration of thimerosal in the combined vaccine is 1:10,000. The aluminum content of the final product does not exceed 0.80 mg per 0.5 mL dose.

Each 0.5 mL dose is formulated to contain 5 Lf units of tetanus toxoid and 2 Lf units of diphtheria toxoid.

CLINICAL PHARMACOLOGY

Tetanus is an intoxication manifested primarily by neuromuscular dysfunction, caused by a potent exotoxin elaborated by *Clostridium tetani.* The incidence of tetanus in the U.S. has dropped dramatically with the routine use of tetanus toxoid, remaining relatively constant over the last decade at about 90 cases reported annually.[4] Spores of *C tetani* are ubiquitous, and there is essentially no natural immunity to tetanus toxin. Thus, universal primary immunization with tetanus toxoid, and subsequent maintenance of adequate antitoxin levels by means of timed boosters, is necessary to protect all age groups.[4] Tetanus toxoid is a highly effective antigen, and a completed primary series generally induces protective levels of serum antitoxin that persist for at least 10 years.[4]

Diphtheria is primarily a localized and generalized intoxication caused by diphtheria toxin, an extracellular protein metabolite of toxinogenic strains of *Corynebacterium diphtheriae.* While the incidence of diphtheria in the U.S. has decreased from over 200,000 cases reported in 1921 before the general use of diphtheria toxoid to only 15 cases reported from 1980 to 1983, the ratio of fatalities to attack rate has remained constant at about 5% to 10%.[4] The highest case fatality rates are in the very young and the elderly.

Following adequate immunization with diphtheria toxoid, which induces antitoxin, it is thought that protection lasts for at least 10 years.[4] This significantly reduces both the risk of developing diphtheria and the severity of clinical illness. It does not, however, eliminate carriage of *C diphtheriae* in the pharynx or on the skin.[4]

INDICATIONS AND USAGE

Tetanus and Diphtheria Toxoids For Adult Use, aluminum phosphate-adsorbed PUROGENATED (Td) is indicated for active immunization against tetanus and diphtheria in adults and children 7 years of age and older.[4,5]

The Immunization Practices Advisory Committee (ACIP) of the U.S. Public Health Service recommends the use of the combined toxoids vaccine rather than single component vaccines for both primary and booster injections, including active tetanus immunization in wound management.[4]

Persons recovering from tetanus or diphtheria: Tetanus or diphtheria infection may not confer immunity; therefore, initiation or completion of active immunization is indicated at the time of recovery from these infections.[4]

Neonatal tetanus prevention: There is no evidence that tetanus and diphtheria toxoids are teratogenic. A previously unimmunized pregnant woman, who may deliver her child under nonhygienic circumstances and/or surroundings, should receive two properly spaced doses of Td before delivery, preferably during the last two trimesters. Incompletely immunized pregnant women should complete the three-dose series. Those immunized more than 10 years previously should have a booster dose.[4] (See also pregnancy information under **PRECAUTIONS.)**

CONTRAINDICATIONS

HYPERSENSITIVITY TO ANY COMPONENT OF THE VACCINE, INCLUDING THIMEROSAL, A MERCURY DERIVATIVE, IS A CONTRAINDICATION.

THE OCCURRENCE OF ANY NEUROLOGICAL SYMPTOMS OR SIGNS FOLLOWING ADMINISTRATION OF THIS PRODUCT IS A CONTRAINDICATION TO FURTHER USE.

IMMUNIZATION SHOULD BE DEFERRED DURING THE COURSE OF ANY FEBRILE ILLNESS OR ACUTE INFECTION. A MINOR AFEBRILE ILLNESS SUCH AS A MILD UPPER RESPIRATORY INFECTION IS NOT USUALLY REASON TO DEFER IMMUNIZATION.[4]

The clinical judgment of the attending physician should prevail at all times.

Routine immunization should be deferred during an outbreak of poliomyelitis, providing the patient has not sustained an injury that increases the risk of tetanus and providing an outbreak of diphtheria does not occur simultaneously.

WARNINGS

THIS PRODUCT IS NOT RECOMMENDED FOR IMMUNIZING PERSONS LESS THAN 7 YEARS OF AGE. The concentration of diphtheria toxoid in preparations intended for use in persons 7 years of age or older is lower than that of the pediatric formulation (Diphtheria and Tetanus Toxoids Adsorbed, for pediatric use, [DT]): a lower dosage of diphtheria toxoid is recommended for persons 7 years of age or older because adverse reactions to the diphtheria component are thought to be related to both dose and age.[4]

THE OCCURRENCE OF A NEUROLOGICAL OR SEVERE HYPERSENSITIVITY REACTION FOLLOWING A PREVIOUS DOSE IS A CONTRAINDICATION TO FURTHER USE OF THIS PRODUCT.[4]

THE ADMINISTRATION OF BOOSTER DOSES MORE FREQUENTLY THAN RECOMMENDED (see **DOSAGE AND ADMINISTRATION**) MAY BE ASSOCIATED WITH INCREASED INCIDENCE AND SEVERITY OF REACTIONS.[4]

Persons who experience Arthus-type hypersensitivity reactions or temperature greater than 39.4°C (103°F), after a previous dose of tetanus toxoid usually have very high serum tetanus antitoxin levels and should not be given even emergency doses of Td more frequently than every 10 years, even if they have a wound that is neither clean nor minor.[4]

If a contraindication to using tetanus toxoid-containing preparations exists in a person who has not completed a primary immunizing course of tetanus toxoid, and other than a clean, minor wound is sustained, only passive immunization should be given using human Tetanus Immune Globulin (TIG).[4]

Td should not be given to individuals with thrombocytopenia or any coagulation disorder that would contraindicate intramuscular injection unless the potential benefits clearly outweigh the risk of administration.

Patients with impaired immune responsiveness, whether due to the use of immunosuppressive therapy (including irradiation, corticosteroids, antimetabolites, alkylating agents, and cytotoxic agents), a genetic defect, human immunodeficiency virus (HIV) infection, or other causes, may have a reduced antibody response to active immunization procedures.[4–6] Deferral of administration of vaccine may be considered in individuals receiving immunosuppressive therapy.[4,5]

Special care should be taken to prevent injection into a blood vessel.

PRECAUTIONS

General:

1. **THIS PRODUCT SHOULD BE USED FOR INDIVIDUALS 7 YEARS OF AGE OR OLDER.**
2. PRIOR TO ADMINISTRATION OF ANY DOSE OF Td, THE PARENT, GUARDIAN, OR ADULT PATIENT SHOULD BE ASKED ABOUT THE RECENT HEALTH STATUS AND IMMUNIZATION HISTORY OF THE PATIENT TO BE IMMUNIZED IN ORDER TO DETERMINE THE EXISTENCE OF ANY CONTRAINDICATION TO IMMUNIZATION WITH Td (SEE **CONTRAINDICATIONS, WARNINGS**).
3. WHEN THE PATIENT RETURNS FOR THE NEXT DOSE IN A SERIES, THE PARENT, GUARDIAN, OR ADULT PATIENT SHOULD BE QUESTIONED CONCERNING OCCURRENCE OF ANY SYMPTOM AND/OR SIGN OF AN ADVERSE REACTION AFTER THE PREVIOUS DOSE (SEE **CONTRAINDICATIONS, ADVERSE REACTIONS**).
4. BEFORE THE INJECTION OF ANY BIOLOGICAL, THE PHYSICIAN SHOULD TAKE ALL PRECAUTIONS KNOWN FOR PREVENTION OF ALLERGIC OR ANY OTHER SIDE REACTIONS. This should include: a review of the patient's history regarding possible sensitivity; the ready availability of epinephrine 1:1,000 and other appropriate agents used for control of immediate allergic reactions; and a knowledge of the recent literature pertaining to use of the biological concerned, including the nature of side effects and adverse reactions that may follow its use.
5. A separate sterile syringe and needle or a sterile disposable unit should be used for each individual patient to prevent transmission of hepatitis or other infectious agents from one person to another.
6. **Shake vigorously before withdrawing each dose to resuspend the contents of the vial or syringe.**
7. NATIONAL CHILDHOOD VACCINE INJURY ACT OF 1986 (AS AMENDED IN 1987)

   This Act requires that the manufacturer and lot number of the vaccine administered be recorded by the health care provider in the vaccine recipient's permanent medical record, along with the date of administration of the vaccine and the name, address and title of the person administering the vaccine.

   The Act further requires the health care provider to report to a health department or to the FDA the occurrence following immunization of any event set forth in the Vaccine Injury Table including: anaphylaxis or anaphylactic shock within 24 hours, encephalopathy or encephalitis within 7 days, residual seizure disorder, any acute complication or sequelae (including death) of above events, or any event that would contraindicate further doses of vaccine, according to this package insert.[7]

Information for the Patient: PRIOR TO THE ADMINISTRATION OF THIS VACCINE, HEALTH CARE PERSONNEL SHOULD INFORM THE PARENT, GUARDIAN, OR ADULT PATIENT OF THE BENEFITS AND RISKS OF VACCINATION AGAINST TETANUS AND DIPHTHERIA.

Use in Pregnancy: *Pregnancy Category C:* Animal reproductive studies have not been conducted with this product. There is no evidence that tetanus and diphtheria toxoids are teratogenic. Td should be given to inadequately immunized pregnant women because it affords protection against neonatal tetanus.[8] Waiting until the second trimester is a reasonable precaution to minimize any theoretical concern.[4] Maintenance of adequate immunization by routine boosters in nonpregnant women of childbearing age (see **DOSAGE AND ADMINISTRATION**) can obviate the need to vaccinate women during pregnancy.

ADVERSE REACTIONS

Local reactions, such as erythema, induration, and tenderness, are common after the administration of Td.[9–12] Such local reactions are usually self-limited and require no therapy. Nodule,[13] sterile abscess formation, or subcutaneous atrophy may occur at the site of injection. Systemic reactions, such as fever, chills, myalgias, and headaches also may occur.[9–12]

Arthus-type hypersensitivity reactions, or high fever, may occur in persons who have very high serum antitoxin antibodies due to overly frequent injections of toxoid (see **WARNINGS**).

NEUROLOGICAL COMPLICATIONS,[14] SUCH AS CONVULSIONS,[15] ENCEPHALOPATHY,[15,16] AND VARIOUS MONO- AND POLYNEUROPATHIES,[16–22] INCLUDING GUILLAIN-BARRE SYNDROME,[23,24] HAVE BEEN REPORTED FOLLOWING ADMINISTRATION OF PREPARATIONS CONTAINING TETANUS AND/OR DIPHTHERIA ANTIGENS.

URTICARIA, ERYTHEMA MULTIFORME OR OTHER RASH, ARTHRALGIAS,[15] AND, MORE RARELY, A SEVERE ANAPHYLACTIC REACTION (IE, URTICARIA WITH SWELLING OF THE MOUTH, DIFFICULTY BREATHING, HYPOTENSION, OR SHOCK) HAVE BEEN REPORTED FOLLOWING ADMINISTRATION OF PREPARATIONS CONTAINING TETANUS AND/OR DIPHTHERIA ANTIGENS.

DOSAGE AND ADMINISTRATION

For Intramuscular Use Only: Shake vigorously before withdrawing each dose to resuspend the contents of the vial or syringe.

Parenteral drug products should be inspected visually for particulate matter and discoloration prior to administration. (See **DESCRIPTION.)**

The vaccine should be injected intramuscularly, preferably into the deltoid muscle, with care to avoid major peripheral nerve trunks. Before injection, the skin at the injection site should be cleansed and prepared with a suitable germicide. After insertion of the needle, aspirate to help avoid inadvertent injection into a blood vessel.

The primary immunizing course for unimmunized individuals 7 years of age or older consists of two doses of 0.5 mL each, 4 to 8 weeks apart, followed by a third (reinforcing) dose of 0.5 mL 6 to 12 months after the second dose. The reinforcing dose is an integral part of the primary immunizing course.[4] Interruption of the recommended schedule with a delay between doses does not interfere with the final immunity achieved, nor does it necessitate starting the series over again, regardless of the length of time elapsed between doses.[4]

A booster dose of 0.5 mL of Td is given 10 years after completion of primary immunization and every 10 years thereafter. If a dose is given sooner than 10 years, as part of wound management or on exposure to diphtheria, the next booster is not needed for 10 years thereafter. MORE FREQUENT BOOSTER DOSES ARE NOT INDICATED AND MAY BE ASSOCIATED WITH INCREASED INCIDENCE AND SEVERITY OF REACTIONS.[4] (See **WARNINGS.)**

Diphtheria Prophylaxis for Case Contacts: All case contacts, household and others, who have previously received fewer than three doses of diphtheria toxoid, should receive an immediate dose of an appropriate diphtheria toxoid-containing preparation and should complete the series according to schedule. Case contacts who previously received three or more doses, but who have not received a dose of a preparation containing diphtheria toxoid within the previous 5 years, should receive a booster dose of a diphtheria toxoid-containing preparation appropriate for their age.[4] Td is an appropriate preparation in these circumstances for persons 7 years of age or older.

Continued on next page

Information on Lederle products listed on these pages is the full prescribing information from product literature or package inserts effective in August 1992. Information concerning all Lederle products may be obtained from the Professional Services Department, Lederle Laboratories, Pearl River, New York 10965.

Lederle—Cont.

Tetanus Prophylaxis in Wound Management: The need for active immunization with a tetanus toxoid-containing preparation, with or without passive immunization with human Tetanus Immune Globulin (TIG) depends on both the condition of the wound and the patient's immunization history. Tetanus has rarely occurred among persons with a documented primary series of tetanus toxoid injections. A thorough attempt must be made to determine whether a patient has completed primary immunization.[4]

Individuals who have completed primary immunization against tetanus, and who sustain wounds which are minor and uncontaminated, should receive a booster dose of a tetanus-toxoid preparation only if they have not received tetanus toxoid within the preceding 10 years. For other wounds, a booster is appropriate if the patient has not received tetanus toxoid within the preceding 5 years. Antitoxin antibodies develop rapidly in persons who have previously received at least two doses of tetanus toxoid.[4]

Individuals who have not completed primary immunization against tetanus, or whose immunization history is unknown or uncertain, should be immunized with a tetanus toxoid-containing product. Completion of primary immunization thereafter should be ensured. In addition, if these individuals have sustained a tetanus-prone wound, the use of human Tetanus Immune Globulin (TIG) is recommended. A separate syringe and site of administration should be used.[4]

Summary guide to tetanus prophylaxis in routine wound management[4]*

History of tetanus toxoid (doses)	Clean, minor wounds		All other wounds†	
	Td	TIG	Td	TIG
Unknown <three	Yes	No	Yes	Yes
≥three‡	No§	No	No″	No

* Important details are in the text.
† Such as, but not limited to, wounds contaminated with dirt, feces, soil, saliva, etc; puncture wounds; avulsions; and wounds resulting from missiles, crushing, burns, and frostbite.
‡ If only three doses of **fluid** toxoid have been received, a fourth dose of toxoid, preferably an adsorbed toxoid, should be given.
§ Yes, if more than 10 years since last dose.
″ Yes, if more than 5 years since last dose. (More frequent boosters are not needed and can accentuate side effects.)

Td is the preferred preparation for active tetanus immunization in wound management of patients 7 years of age or older. This is to enhance diphtheria protection, since a large proportion of adults are susceptible. Thus, by taking advantage of acute health care visits for wound management, some patients can be protected who otherwise would remain susceptible.[4]

HOW SUPPLIED

NDC 0005-1875-31   5.0 mL vial
NDC 0005-1875-47   10 (0.5 mL) LEDERJECT® disposable syringes. For directions on use of LEDERJECT® disposable syringe, please see package insert accompanying product.

STORAGE

DO NOT FREEZE. STORE REFRIGERATED, AWAY FROM FREEZER COMPARTMENT, AT 2℃ to 8℃ (36℉ to 46℉).

REFERENCES

1. Mueller JH, Miller PA: Factors influencing the production of tetanal toxin. *J Immunol* 1947;56:143–147.
2. Mueller JH, Miller PA: Production of diphtheria toxin of high potency (100Lf) on a reproducible medium. *J Immunol* 1941;40:21–32.
3. Pillemer L, Grossberg DB, Wittler RG: The immunochemistry of toxins and toxoids. II. The preparation and immunological evaluation of purified tetanal toxoid. *J Immunol* 1946;54:213–224.
4. Recommendation of the Immunization Practices Advisory Committee (ACIP): Diphtheria, tetanus and pertussis: Guidelines for vaccine prophylaxis and other preventive measures. *MMWR* 1985;34:405–426.
5. Committee on Immunization, Council of Medical Societies American College of Physicians: Guide for Adult Immunization, 1st Edition 1985; Philadelphia, PA.
6. Recommendation of the ACIP: Immunization of children infected with Human T-Lymphotrophic Virus Type III/Lymphadenopathy associated virus. *MMWR* 1986;35(38):595–606.
7. National Childhood Vaccine Injury Act: Requirements for permanent vaccination records and for reporting of selected events after vaccination. *MMWR* 1988;37(13):197–200.
8. Recommendations of the ACIP: General recommendations on immunization. *MMWR* 1983;32(1):1–17.
9. Deacon SP, et al: A comparative clinical study of adsorbed tetanus vaccine and adult-type tetanus-diphtheria vaccine. *J Hyg (Cambridge)* 1982;89:513–519.
10. Macko MB, Powell CE: Comparison of the morbidity of tetanus toxoid boosters with tetanus-diphtheria toxoid boosters. *Ann Emerg Med* 1985;14:(1):33–35.
11. Myers MG, et al: Primary immunization with tetanus and diphtheria toxoids. *JAMA* 1982;248:(19):2478–2480.
12. Sisk CW, et al: Reactions to tetanus-diphtheria toxoid (adult). *Arch Environ Health* 1965;11:34–36.
13. Fawcett HA, Smith NP: Injection-site granuloma due to aluminum. *Arch Dermatol* 1984;120:1318–1322.
14. Rutledge SL, Snead OC: Neurological complications of immunizations. *J Pediatr* 1986;109:917–924.
15. Adverse Events Following Immunization. *MMWR* 1985;34(3):43–47.
16. Schlenska GK: Unusual neurological complications following tetanus toxoid administration. *J Neurol* 1977;215:299–302.
17. Blumstein GI, Kreithen H: Peripheral neuropathy following tetanus toxoid administration. *JAMA* 1966;198:1030–1031.
18. Reinstein L, Pargament JM, Goodman JS: Peripheral neuropathy after multiple tetanus toxoid injections. *Arch Phys Med Rehabil* 1982;63:332–334.
19. Tsairis P, Duck PJ, Mulder DW: Natural history of brachial plexus neuropathy. *Arch Neurol* 1972;27:109–117.
20. Quast U, Hennessen W, Widmark RM: Mono- and polyneuritis after tetanus vaccination. *Devel Bio Stand* 1979;43:25–32.
21. Holliday PL, Bauer RB: Polyradiculoneuritis secondary to immunization with tetanus and diphtheria toxoids. *Arch Neurol* 1983;40:56–67.
22. Fenichel GM: Neurological complications of tetanus toxoid. *Arch Neurol* 1983;40:390.
23. Pollard JD, Selby G: Relapsing neuropathy due to tetanus toxoid. *J Neurol Sci* 1978;37:113–125.
24. Newton N, Janati A: Guillain-Barre syndrome after vaccination with purified tetanus toxoid. *S Med J* 1987;80:1053–1054.

LEDERLE LABORATORIES DIVISION
American Cyanamid Company
Pearl River, NY 10965

Rev. 5/88
23591

TETANUS TOXOID ADSORBED   ℞
Tetanus Toxoid Aluminum Phosphate-Adsorbed
Purogenated®

DESCRIPTION

Tetanus Toxoid Adsorbed, aluminum phosphate-adsorbed, PUROGENATED is a sterile preparation of refined tetanus toxoid for intramuscular use only. After shaking, the product is a homogeneous white suspension.

The tetanus toxin is produced according to the method of Mueller and Miller[1] and is detoxified by use of formaldehyde. The toxoid is refined by the Pillemer alcohol fractionation method[2] and is diluted with a solution containing sodium phosphate dibasic, sodium phosphate monobasic, glycine, sodium chloride and thimerosal (mercury derivative) in a final concentration of 1:10,000 as a preservative and aluminum phosphate as adjuvant. The aluminum content does not exceed 0.80 mg per 0.5 mL dose.

Each 0.5 mL dose is formulated to contain 5 Lf units of tetanus toxoid.

CLINICAL PHARMACOLOGY

Tetanus is an intoxication manifested primarily by neuromuscular dysfunction, caused by a potent exotoxin elaborated by *Clostridium tetani.* The incidence of tetanus in the U.S. has dropped dramatically with the routine use of tetanus toxoid, remaining relatively constant over the last decade at about 90 cases reported annually.[3] Spores of *C tetani* are ubiquitous, and there is essentially no natural immunity to tetanus toxin. Thus, universal primary immunization with tetanus toxoid, and subsequent maintenance of adequate antitoxin levels by means of timed boosters, is necessary to protect all age groups.[3] Tetanus toxoid is a highly effective antigen, and a completed primary series generally induces protective levels of serum antitoxin that persist for at least 10 years.[3]

INDICATIONS AND USAGE

Tetanus Toxoid Adsorbed is indicated for active immunization against tetanus in adults and children 2 months of age or older.

Immunization of persons 7 years of age or older may be accomplished by the use of Tetanus and Diphtheria Toxoids Adsorbed, for Adult Use (Td), Tetanus Toxoid Adsorbed, or Tetanus Toxoid Fluid. The Immunization Practices Advisory Committee (ACIP) of the U.S. Public Health Service recommends the use of the combined toxoids vaccine rather than single component vaccines for both primary and booster injections, including active tetanus immunization in wound management.[3] Individuals for whom the use of a vaccine containing diphtheria toxoid is contraindicated should receive a single-component tetanus toxoid-containing vaccine. Immunization of infants and children 2 months of age up to the seventh birthday is usually accomplished by the use of Diphtheria and Tetanus Toxoids and Pertussis Vaccine Adsorbed (DTP) or Diphtheria and Tetanus Toxoids Adsorbed, for pediatric use (DT). Tetanus Toxoid Adsorbed may be used for immunizing infants and children for whom the use of a vaccine containing diphtheria toxoid and pertussis antigen is contraindicated.

Comparative tests have shown that the adsorbed toxoids are superior to the fluid toxoids in antibody titers produced and in the durability of protection achieved. The promptness of antibody response to booster doses of either fluid or adsorbed toxoid is not sufficiently different to be of clinical importance. When Tetanus Immune Globulin (TIG) is to be administered at the same visit as tetanus toxoid, the adsorbed toxoid should be used. [3,4]

Persons Recovering from Tetanus: Tetanus infection may not confer immunity; therefore, initiation or completion of active immunization is indicated at the time of recovery from this infection.[3]

Neonatal Tetanus Prevention: There is no evidence that tetanus toxoid is teratogenic. A previously unimmunized pregnant woman, who may deliver her child under nonhygienic circumstances and/or surroundings, should receive two properly spaced doses of a tetanus toxoid-containing preparation before delivery, preferably during the last two trimesters. Incompletely immunized pregnant women should complete the three-dose series. Those immunized more than 10 years previously should have a booster dose.[3] (See also pregnancy information under **PRECAUTIONS**).

CONTRAINDICATIONS

HYPERSENSITIVITY TO ANY COMPONENT OF THE VACCINE, INCLUDING THIMEROSAL, A MERCURY DERIVATIVE, IS A CONTRAINDICATION.

THE OCCURRENCE OF ANY TYPE OF NEUROLOGICAL SYMPTOMS OR SIGNS FOLLOWING ADMINISTRATION OF THIS PRODUCT IS A CONTRAINDICATION TO FURTHER USE.

IMMUNIZATION SHOULD BE DEFERRED DURING THE COURSE OF ANY FEBRILE ILLNESS OR ACUTE INFECTION. A MINOR AFEBRILE ILLNESS SUCH AS A MILD UPPER RESPIRATORY INFECTION IS NOT USUALLY REASON TO DEFER IMMUNIZATION.[3]

The clinical judgment of the attending physician should prevail at all times.

Routine immunization should be deferred during an outbreak of poliomyelitis, providing the patient has not sustained an injury that increases the risk of tetanus.

WARNINGS

THE OCCURRENCE OF A NEUROLOGICAL OR SEVERE HYPERSENSITIVITY REACTION FOLLOWING A PREVIOUS DOSE IS A CONTRAINDICATION TO FURTHER USE OF THIS PRODUCT.[3]

THE ADMINISTRATION OF BOOSTER DOSES MORE FREQUENTLY THAN RECOMMENDED (see **DOSAGE AND ADMINISTRATION**) MAY BE ASSOCIATED WITH INCREASED INCIDENCE AND SEVERITY OF REACTIONS.[3]

Persons who experience Arthus-type hypersensitivity reactions or temperature greater than 39.4℃ (103℉) after a previous dose of tetanus toxoid usually have very high serum tetanus antitoxin levels and should not be given even emergency doses of tetanus toxoid more frequently than every 10 years, even if they have a wound that is neither clean nor minor.[3]

If a contraindication to using tetanus toxoid exists in a person who has not completed a primary immunizing course of tetanus toxoid, and other than a clean, minor wound is sustained, only passive immunization should be given using human Tetanus Immune Globulin (TIG).[3]

Tetanus Toxoid Adsorbed should not be given to individuals with thrombocytopenia or any coagulation disorder that would contraindicate intramuscular injection, unless the potential benefit clearly outweighs the risk of administration.

Patients with impaired immune responsiveness, whether due to the use of immunosuppressive therapy (including irradiation, corticosteroids, antimetabolites, alkylating agents, and cytotoxic agents), a genetic defect, human immunodeficiency virus (HIV) infection, or other causes, may have a reduced antibody response to active immunization procedures.[3–5] Deferral of administration of vaccine may be considered in individuals receiving immunosuppressive therapy.[3,4]

Special care should be taken to prevent injection into a blood vessel.

PRECAUTIONS

General:

1. PRIOR TO ADMINISTRATION OF ANY DOSE OF VACCINE THE PARENT, GUARDIAN, OR ADULT PATIENT SHOULD BE ASKED ABOUT THE RECENT HEALTH STATUS AND IMMUNIZATION HISTORY OF THE PATIENT TO BE IMMUNIZED IN ORDER TO DETERMINE THE EXISTENCE OF ANY CONTRAINDICATIONS TO IMMUNIZATION (SEE **CONTRAINDICATIONS, WARNINGS**).
2. WHEN THE PATIENT RETURNS FOR THE NEXT DOSE IN A SERIES, THE PARENT, GUARDIAN, OR ADULT PATIENT SHOULD BE QUESTIONED CONCERNING OCCURRENCE OF ANY SYMPTOM AND/OR SIGN OF AN ADVERSE REACTION AFTER THE PREVIOUS DOSE (SEE **CONTRAINDICATIONS, ADVERSE REACTIONS**).
3. BEFORE THE INJECTION OF ANY BIOLOGICAL, THE PHYSICIAN SHOULD TAKE ALL PRECAUTIONS KNOWN FOR PREVENTION OF ALLERGIC OR ANY OTHER SIDE REACTIONS. This should include: a review of the patient's history regarding possible sensitivity; the ready availability of epinephrine 1:1,000 and other appropriate agents used for control of immediate allergic reactions; and a knowledge of the recent literature pertaining to use of the biological concerned, including the nature of side effects and adverse reactions that may follow its use.
4. A separate sterile syringe and needle or a sterile disposable unit should be used for each individual patient to prevent transmission of hepatitis or other infectious agents from one person to another.
5. *Shake vigorously before withdrawing each dose to resuspend the contents of the vial.*
6. NATIONAL CHILDHOOD VACCINE INJURY ACT OF 1986 (AS AMENDED IN 1987)

   This Act requires that the manufacturer and lot number of the vaccine administered be recorded by the health care provider in the vaccine recipient's permanent record, along with the date of administration of the vaccine and the name, address and title of the person administering the vaccine.

   The Act further requires the health care provider to report to a health department or to the FDA the occurrence following immunization of any event set forth in the Vaccine Injury Table including: anaphylaxis or anaphylactic shock within 24 hours, encephalopathy or encephalitis within 7 days, residual seizure disorder, any acute complication or sequelae (including death) of above events, or any event that would contraindicate further doses of vaccine, according to this package insert.[6]

Information for the Patient: PRIOR TO ADMINISTRATION OF THIS VACCINE, HEALTH CARE PERSONNEL SHOULD INFORM THE PARENT, GUARDIAN, OR ADULT PATIENT OF THE BENEFITS AND RISKS OF VACCINATION AGAINST TETANUS.

Use in Pregnancy: *Pregnancy Category C:* Animal reproductive studies have not been conducted with this product. There is no evidence that tetanus toxoid is teratogenic. An appropriate tetanus toxoid-containing preparation (usually Td) should be given to inadequately immunized women because it affords protection against neonatal tetanus.[7] Waiting until the second trimester is a reasonable precaution to minimize any theoretical concern.[4] Maintenance of adequate immunization by routine boosters in non-pregnant women of child-bearing age (see **DOSAGE AND ADMINISTRATION**) can obviate the need to vaccinate women during pregnancy.

ADVERSE REACTIONS

Local reactions, such as erythema, induration, and tenderness, are common after the administration of tetanus toxoid.[8–10] Such local reactions are usually self-limiting and require no therapy. Nodule,[11] sterile abscess formation, or subcutaneous atrophy may occur at the site of injection. Systemic reactions, such as fever, chills, myalgia, and headaches also may occur.[8–10]

Arthus-type hypersensitivity reactions, or high fever, may occur in persons who have very high serum antitoxin antibodies due to overly frequent injections of toxoid.[3] (See **WARNINGS**.)

NEUROLOGICAL COMPLICATIONS,[12] SUCH AS CONVULSIONS,[13] ENCEPHALOPATHY,[13,14] AND VARIOUS MONO- AND POLYNEUROPATHIES,[14–20] INCLUDING GUILLAIN-BARRE SYNDROME,[21,22] HAVE BEEN REPORTED FOLLOWING ADMINISTRATION OF PREPARATIONS CONTAINING TETANUS ANTIGEN.

URTICARIA, ERYTHEMA MULTIFORME OR OTHER RASH, ARTHRALGIAS[13] AND, MORE RARELY, A SEVERE ANAPHYLACTIC REACTION (IE, URTICARIA WITH SWELLING OF THE MOUTH, DIFFICULTY BREATHING, HYPOTENSION, OR SHOCK) HAVE BEEN REPORTED FOLLOWING ADMINISTRATION OF PREPARATIONS CONTAINING TETANUS ANTIGEN.

DOSAGE AND ADMINISTRATION

For Intramuscular Use Only: *Shake vigorously before withdrawing each dose to resuspend the contents of the vial or syringe.*

Parenteral drug products should be inspected visually for particulate matter and discoloration prior to administration. (See **DESCRIPTION.**)

Preferred injection sites for intramuscular injection include the anterolateral aspect of the upper thigh and the deltoid area of the upper arm. Care should be taken to avoid major peripheral nerve trunks.

Before injection, the skin at the injection site should be cleansed and prepared with a suitable germicide.

After insertion of the needle, aspirate to help avoid inadvertent injection into a blood vessel.

The primary immunizing course for unimmunized individuals 1 year of age or older consists of **two** doses of 0.5 mL each, 4 to 8 weeks apart, followed by a **third** (reinforcing) dose of 0.5 mL, 6 to 12 months after the second dose. The reinforcing dose is an integral part of the primary immunizing course.

If, after beginning combined immunization against diphtheria, tetanus, and pertussis, further doses of vaccine containing pertussis and diphtheria antigens become contraindicated, Tetanus Toxoid Adsorbed may be substituted for each of the remaining doses.

When immunization with Tetanus Toxoid Adsorbed is begun in the first year of life, the primary series consists of **three** doses of 0.5 mL each, 4 to 8 weeks apart, followed by a **fourth** (reinforcing) dose of 0.5 mL, 6 to 12 months after the third dose.

Interruption of the recommended schedule with a delay between doses does not interfere with the final immunity achieved with Tetanus Toxoid Adsorbed. There is no need to start the series over again, regardless of the length of time elapsed between doses.[3]

Booster Doses: A single injection of 0.5 mL of Tetanus Toxoid Adsorbed is given 10 years after completion of primary immunization and every 10 years thereafter. If a dose is given sooner as part of wound management, the next booster is not needed for 10 years thereafter. MORE FREQUENT BOOSTER DOSES ARE NOT INDICATED AND MAY BE ASSOCIATED WITH INCREASED INCIDENCE AND SEVERITY OF REACTIONS.[3]

Tetanus Prophylaxis in Wound Management: The need for active immunization with a tetanus toxoid-containing preparation, with or without passive immunization with human Tetanus Immune Globulin (TIG) depends on both the condition of the wound and the patient's immunization history. Tetanus has rarely occurred among persons with a documented primary series of toxoid injections. A thorough attempt must be made to determine whether a patient has completed primary immunization.[3]

Individuals who have completed primary immunization against tetanus, and who sustain wounds which are minor and uncontaminated, should receive a booster dose of the appropriate tetanus toxoid-containing preparation (see **INDICATIONS AND USAGE**) only if they have not received tetanus toxoid within the preceding 10 years. For other wounds, a booster is appropriate if the patient has not received tetanus toxoid within the preceding 5 years. Antitoxin antibodies develop rapidly in persons who have previously received at least two doses of tetanus toxoid.[3]

Individuals who have not completed primary immunization against tetanus, or whose immunization history is unknown or uncertain, should be immunized with the appropriate tetanus toxoid-containing product (see **INDICATIONS AND USAGE**). Completion of primary immunization thereafter should be ensured. In addition, if these individuals have sustained a tetanus-prone wound, the use of human Tetanus Immune Globulin (TIG) is recommended. A separate syringe and site of administration should be used. When TIG is to be administered at the same visit as tetanus toxoid, an adsorbed tetanus toxoid-containing preparation should be used.[3]

[See table at top of next column.]

In order to enhance diphtheria protection in the population, the ACIP recommends Tetanus and Diphtheria Toxoid For Adult Use as the preferred preparation for active tetanus immunization in wound management of patients 7 years of age or older.[3]

HOW SUPPLIED

NDC 0005-1938-31 5.0 mL vial

NDC 0005-1938-47 10×0.5 mL LEDERJECT® disposable syringe. For directions on use of LEDERJECT® disposable syringe, please see package insert accompanying product.

STORAGE

DO NOT FREEZE. STORE REFRIGERATED, AWAY FROM FREEZER COMPARTMENT, AT 2°C TO 8°C (36°F to 46°F).

REFERENCES

1. Mueller JH, Miller PA: Factors influencing the production of tetanal toxin. *J Immunol* 1947;56:143–147.

§ If only three doses of **fluid** toxoid have been received, a fourth dose of toxoid, preferably an adsorbed toxoid, should be given.

″ Yes, if more than 10 years since last dose.

£ Yes, if more than 5 years since last dose. (More frequent boosters are not needed and can accentuate side effects.)

SUMMARY GUIDE TO TETANUS PROPHYLAXIS IN ROUTINE WOUND MANAGEMENT[3]*

History of tetanus toxoid (doses)	Clean, minor wounds		All other wounds†	
	Td‡	TIG	Td‡	TIG
Unknown or < three	Yes	No	Yes	Yes
≥ three§	No″	No	No£	No

* Important details are in the text.

† Such as, but not limited to, wounds contaminated with dirt, feces, soil, saliva, etc; puncture wounds; avulsions; and wounds resulting from missiles, crushing, burns and frostbite.

‡ For children under 7 years old DTP (DT, if pertussis vaccine is contraindicated) is preferred to tetanus toxoid alone. For persons 7 years and older, Td is preferred to tetanus toxoid alone.

2. Pillemer L, Grossberg DB, Wittler RG: The immunochemistry of toxins and toxoids. II. The preparation and immunological evaluation of purified tetanal toxoid. *J Immunol* 1946;54:213–224.
3. Recommendation of the Immunization Practices Advisory Committee (ACIP): Diphtheria, tetanus and pertussis: Guidelines for vaccine prophylaxis and other preventive measures. *MMWR* 1985;34:405–426.
4. Committee on Immunization, Council of Medical Societies, American College of Physicians: Guide for Adult Immunization, 1st Edition 1985; Philadelphia, PA.
5. Recommendation of the ACIP: Immunization of children infected with Human T-Lymphotrophic Virus Type III/Lymphadenopathy associated virus. *MMWR* 1986;35(38):595–606.
6. National Childhood Vaccine Injury Act: Requirements for permanent vaccination records and for reporting of selected events after vaccination. *MMWR* 1988;37(13):197–200.
7. Recommendations of the ACIP: General recommendations on immunization. *MMWR* 1983;32(1):1–17.
8. Macko MB, Powell CE: Comparison of the morbidity of tetanus toxoid boosters with tetanus-diphtheria toxoid boosters. *Ann Emerg Med* 1985;14:(1):33–35.
9. Deacon SP, et al: A comparative clinical study of adsorbed tetanus vaccine and adult-type tetanus-diphtheria vaccine. *J Hyg (Cambridge)* 1982;89:513–519.
10. Jacobs RL, et al: Adverse reactions to tetanus toxoid. *JAMA* 1982: 247;(1):40–42.
11. Fawcett HA, Smith N: Injection-site granuloma due to aluminum. *Arch Dermatol* 1984;120:1318–1322.
12. Rutledge SL, Snead OC: Neurologic complications of immunizations. *J Pediatr* 1986;109:917–924.
13. Adverse Events Following Immunization. *MMWR* 1985;34(3):43–47.
14. Schlenska GK: Unusual neurological complications following tetanus toxoid administration. *J Neurol* 1977;215:299–302.
15. Blumstein GI, Kreithen H: Peripheral neuropathy following tetanus toxoid administration. *JAMA* 1966;198:1030–1031.
16. Reinstein L, Pargament JM, Goodman JS: Peripheral neuropathy after multiple tetanus toxoid injections. *Arch Phys Med Rehabil* 1982;63:332–334.
17. Tsairis P, Duck PJ, Mulder DW: Natural history of brachial plexus neuropathy. *Arch Neurol* 1972;27:109–117.
18. Quast U, Hennessen W, Widmark RM: Mono- and polyneuritis after tetanus vaccination. *Devel Bio Stand* 1979;43:25–32.
19. Holliday PL, Bauer RB: Polyradiculoneuritis secondary to immunization with tetanus and diphtheria toxoids. *Arch Neurol* 1983;40:56–57.
20. Fenichel GM: Neurological complications of tetanus toxoid. *Arch Neurol* 1983;40:390.
21. Pollard JD, Selby G: Relapsing neuropathy due to tetanus toxoid. *J Neurol Sci* 1978;37:113–125.
22. Newton N, Janati A: Guillain-Barre syndrome after vaccination with purified tetanus toxoid. *S Med J* 1987;80:1053–1054.

Continued on next page

Information on Lederle products listed on these pages is the full prescribing information from product literature or package inserts effective in August 1992. Information concerning all Lederle products may be obtained from the Professional Services Department, Lederle Laboratories, Pearl River, New York 10965.

Lederle—Cont.

LEDERLE LABORATORIES DIVISION
American Cyanamid Company
Pearl River, NY 10965

Rev. 5/88
23588

THIOTEPA ℞
[*thī̆ō-tē̆pa*]
For Injection
Sterile
15 mg/Vial

THIOTEPA is a polyfunctional alkylating agent used in the chemotherapy of certain neoplastic diseases.

DESCRIPTION

Thiotepa is an ethylenimine-type compound, 1,1′,1″-phosphinothioylidynetris-aziridine available in powder form in vials which contain a sterile mixture of 15 mg Thiotepa, 80 mg NaCl, and 50 mg $NaHCO_3$. Thiotepa has also been known as TESPA and TSPA and is not the same as TEPA. Thiotepa is stable in alkaline medium and unstable in acid medium. When reconstituted with Sterile Water for Injection, the resulting solution has a pH of approximately 7.6.

ACTION

Thiotepa is a cytotoxic agent of the polyfunctional alkylating type (more than one reactive ethylenimine group) related chemically and pharmacologically to nitrogen mustard. Its radiomimetic action is believed to occur through the release of ethylenimine radicals which, like irradiation, disrupt the bonds of DNA. One of the principal bond disruptions is initiated by alkylation of guanine at the N-7 position, which severs the linkage between the purine base and the sugar and liberates alkylated guanines.

On the basis of tissue concentration studies, it is reported that Thiotepa has no differential affinity for neoplasms. Most of the drug appears to be excreted unchanged in the urine.

INDICATIONS

Thiotepa has been tried with varying results in the palliation of a wide variety of neoplastic diseases. However, the most consistent results have been seen in the following tumors:

1. Adenocarcinoma of the breast.
2. Adenocarcinoma of the ovary.
3. For controlling intracavitary effusions secondary to diffuse or localized neoplastic disease of various serosal cavities.
4. For the treatment of superficial papillary carcinoma of the urinary bladder.

While now largely superseded by other treatments, Thiotepa has been effective against other lymphomas, such as lymphosarcoma and Hodgkin's disease.

CONTRAINDICATIONS

Therapy is probably contraindicated in cases of existing hepatic, renal, or bone marrow damage. However, if the need outweighs the risk in such patients, Thiotepa may be used in low dosage, and accompanied by hepatic, renal, and hemopoietic function tests.

Thiotepa is contraindicated in patients with a known hypersensitivity (allergy) to this preparation.

WARNINGS

The administration of Thiotepa to pregnant women is not recommended except in cases where the benefit to be gained outweighs the risk of teratogenicity involved.

Thiotepa is highly toxic to the hematopoietic system. A rapidly falling white blood cell or platelet count indicates the necessity for discontinuing or reducing the dosage of Thiotepa. Weekly blood and platelet counts are recommended during therapy and for at least 3 weeks after therapy has been discontinued.

Thiotepa is a polyfunctional alkylating agent, capable of cross-linking the DNA within a cell and changing its nature. The replication of the cell is, therefore, altered, and Thiotepa may be described as mutagenic. An *in vitro* study has shown that it causes chromosomal aberrations of the chromatid type and that the frequency of induced aberrations increases with the age of the subject.

Like all alkylating agents, Thiotepa is carcinogenic. Carcinogenicity is shown most clearly in mouse studies, but there is strong circumstantial evidence of carcinogenicity in man.

PRECAUTIONS

The serious complication of excessive Thiotepa therapy, or sensitivity to the effects of Thiotepa, is bone marrow depression. If proper precautions are not observed, Thiotepa may cause leukopenia, thrombocytopenia, and anemia. Death from septicemia and hemorrhage has occurred as a direct result of hematopoietic depression by Thiotepa.

It is not advisable to combine, simultaneously or sequentially, cancer chemotherapeutic agents or a cancer chemotherapeutic agent and a therapeutic modality having the same mechanism of action. Therefore, Thiotepa combined with other alkylating agents such as nitrogen mustard or cyclophosphamide or Thiotepa combined with irradiation would serve to intensify toxicity rather than to enhance therapeutic response. If these agents must follow each other, it is important that recovery from the first agent, as indicated by white blood cell count, be complete before therapy with the second agent is instituted.

The most reliable guide to Thiotepa toxicity is the white blood cell count. If this falls to 3000 or less, the dose should be discontinued. Another good index of Thiotepa toxicity is the platelet count; if this falls to 150,000, therapy should be discontinued. Red blood cell count is a less accurate indicator of Thiotepa toxicity.

Other drugs which are known to produce bone marrow depression should be avoided.

There is no known antidote for overdosage with Thiotepa. Transfusions of whole blood or platelets or leukocytes have proved beneficial to the patient in combating hematopoietic toxicity.

ADVERSE REACTIONS

Apart from its effect on the blood-forming elements, Thiotepa may cause other adverse reactions. These include pain at the site of injection, nausea, vomiting, anorexia, dizziness, headache, amenorrhea, and interference with spermatogenesis.

Febrile reaction and weeping from a subcutaneous lesion may occur as the result of breakdown of tumor tissue.

Allergic reactions are rare, but hives and skin rash have been noted occasionally. One case of alopecia has been reported. In addition, a patient who has received Thiotepa and other anticancer agents experienced prolonged apnea after succinylcholine was administered prior to surgery. It was theorized that this was caused by decrease of pseudocholinesterase activity caused by the anticancer drugs.

There have been rare reports of chemical cystitis or hemorrhagic cystitis following intravesical, but not parenteral administration of Thiotepa.

DOSAGE

Parenteral routes of administration are most reliable since absorption of Thiotepa from the gastrointestinal tract is variable.

Since Thiotepa is nonvesicant, intravenous doses may be given directly and rapidly without need for slow drip or large volumes of diluent. Some physicians prefer to give Thiotepa directly into the tumor mass. This may be effected transrectally, transvaginally, or intracerebrally. The technique is discussed in the appropriate section which follows. For the control of malignant effusions, Thiotepa is instilled directly into the cavity involved.

Dosage must be carefully individualized. A slow response to Thiotepa may be deceptive and may occasion unwarranted frequency of administration with subsequent signs of toxicity. After maximum benefit is obtained by initial therapy, it is necessary to continue patient on maintenance therapy (1- to 4-week intervals). In order to continue optimal effect, maintenance doses should be no more frequent than weekly in order to preserve correlation between dose and blood counts.

Initial and Maintenance Doses: Initially the higher dose in the given range is commonly administered. The maintenance dose should be adjusted weekly on the basis of pretreatment control blood counts and subsequent blood counts.

Intravenous Administration: Thiotepa may be given by rapid intravenous administration in doses of 0.3 to 0.4 mg/kg. Doses should be given at 1- to 4-week intervals.

For conversion of mg/kg of body weight to mg/M^2 of body surface or the reverse, a ratio of 1:30 is given as a guideline. The conversion factor varies between 1:20 and 1:40 depending on age and body build.

Intratumor Administration: Thiotepa in initial doses of 0.6 to 0.8 mg/kg may be injected directly into a tumor by means of a 22-gauge needle. A small amount of local anesthetic is injected first; then the syringe is removed and the Thiotepa solution is injected through the same needle. The drug is diluted in Sterile Water for Injection, 10 mg per 1 mL. Maintenance doses at 1- to 4-week intervals range from 0.07 mg/kg to 0.8 mg/kg depending on the condition of the patient.

Intracavitary Administration: The dosage recommended is 0.6 to 0.8 mg/kg. Administration is usually effected through the same tubing which is used to remove the fluid from the cavity involved.

Intravesical Administration: Patients with papillary carcinoma of the bladder are dehydrated for 8 to 12 hours prior to treatment. Then 60 mg of Thiotepa in 30 to 60 mL of Sterile Water for Injection is instilled into the bladder by catheter. For maximum effect, the solution should be retained for 2 hours. If the patient finds it impossible to retain 60 mL for 2 hours, the dose may be given in a volume of 30 mL. If desired, the patient may be positioned every 15 minutes for maximum area contact. The usual course of treatment is once a week for 4 weeks. The course may be repeated if necessary, but second and third courses must be given with caution since bone marrow depression may be increased. Deaths have occurred after intravesical administration, caused by bone marrow depression from systemically absorbed drug.

Preparation of Solution: The powder should be reconstituted preferably in Sterile Water for Injection. The amount of diluent most often used is 1.5 mL resulting in a drug concentration of 5 mg in each 0.5 mL of solution. Larger volumes are usually employed for intracavitary use, intravenous drip, or perfusion therapy. The 1.5 mL reconstituted preparation may be added to larger volumes of other diluents: Sodium Chloride Injection USP, Dextrose Injection USP, Dextrose and Sodium Chloride Injection USP, Ringer's Injection USP, or Lactated Ringer's Injection USP. Reconstituted solutions should be clear to slightly opaque but solutions that are grossly opaque or precipitated should not be used.

Since the original powder form contains 15 mg Thiotepa, 80 mg NaCl, and 50 mg $NaHCO_3$, reconstitution and further dilution of the powder with Sterile Water for Injection to a concentration of approximately 1 mg/mL produces an isotonic solution. Reconstitution and further dilution with other diluents may result in hypertonic solutions, which may cause mild to moderate discomfort on injection.

For local use into single or multiple sites, Thiotepa may be mixed with procaine HCl 2%, epinephrine HCl 1:1000, or both.

Procedures for proper handling and disposal of anti-cancer drugs should be considered. Several guidelines on this subject have been published.[1–6] There is no general agreement that all of the procedures recommended in the guidelines are necessary or appropriate.

HOW SUPPLIED

15 mg Vial, Sterile, for parenteral use—NDC 0005-4650-91.

Whether in its original powder form or in reconstituted solution, Thiotepa must be stored in the refrigerator at 2°–8° C. (36°–46° F.) Reconstituted solutions may be kept for 5 days in a refrigerator without substantial loss of potency.

REFERENCES

1. Recommendations for the Safe Handling of Parenteral Antineoplastic Drugs. NIH Publication No. 83-2621. For sale by the Superintendent of Documents, U.S. Government Printing Office, Washington, D.C. 20402.
2. AMA Council Report. Guidelines for Handling Parenteral Antineoplastics. *JAMA,* March 15, 1985.
3. National Study Commission on Cytotoxic Exposure—Recommendations for Handling Cytotoxic Agents. Available from Louis P. Jeffrey, ScD, Director of Pharmacy Services, Rhode Island Hospital, 593 Eddy Street, Providence, Rhode Island 02902.
4. Clinical Oncological Society of Australia: Guidelines and recommendations for safe handling of antineoplastic agents. *Med J Australia.* 1983; 1: 426–428.
5. Jones, RB, et al. Safe handling of chemotherapeutic agents: A report from the Mount Sinai Medical Center. *Ca—A Cancer Journal for Clinicians* Sept/Oct 1983; 258–263.
6. American Society of Hospital Pharmacists technical assistance bulletin on handling cytotoxic drugs in hospitals. *Am J Hosp Pharm.* 1985; 42:131–137.

LEDERLE LABORATORIES DIVISION
American Cyanamid Company
Pearl River, NY 10965 Rev. 11/90
27924

Shown in Product Identification Section, page 415

TRI-IMMUNOL® ℞
Diphtheria and Tetanus Toxoids and Pertussis Vaccine Adsorbed

DESCRIPTION

Diphtheria and Tetanus Toxoids and Pertussis Vaccine Adsorbed (DTP), TRI-IMMUNOL, is a sterile combination of PUROGENATED® Diphtheria Toxoid aluminum phosphate-adsorbed, PUROGENATED Tetanus Toxoid aluminum phosphate-adsorbed, and Pertussis Vaccine for intramuscular use only. After shaking, the vaccine is a homogeneous white suspension.

The diphtheria and tetanus toxins are produced according to the method of Mueller and Miller[1,2] and are detoxified by use of formaldehyde. The toxoids are refined by the Pillemer alcohol fractionation method[3] and are diluted with a solution containing sodium phosphate monobasic, sodium phosphate dibasic, glycine, and thimerosal (mercury derivative) as a preservative. Pertussis Vaccine is prepared by growing Phase I *Bordetella pertussis* in a modified Cohen-Wheeler broth containing acid hydrolysate of casein. The *B pertussis* culture is harvested, inactivated, and then suspended in a solution containing potassium phosphate monobasic, sodium phosphate dibasic, aluminum phosphate, sodium chloride, and thimerosal as a preservative and is then combined with the refined Diphtheria and Tetanus

Toxoids in physiological saline diluent containing thimerosal as a preservative. The final concentration of thimerosal (mercury derivative) in the combined vaccine is 1:10,000. The aluminum content of the final product does not exceed 0.80 mg per 0.5 mL dose.

Each 0.5 mL dose is formulated to contain 12.5 Lf of diphtheria toxoid, and 5 Lf of tetanus toxoid. The total human immunizing dose (the first three 0.5 mL doses given) contains an estimate of 12 units of pertussis vaccine. Each component of the vaccine—diphtheria, tetanus, and pertussis—meets the required potency standards.

The primary immunization against diphtheria, tetanus, and pertussis consists of four 0.5 mL doses when administered as recommended.[4,5]

CLINICAL PHARMACOLOGY

Simultaneous immunization against diphtheria, tetanus, and pertussis during infancy and childhood has been a routine practice in the United States since the late 1940s. It has played a major role in markedly reducing the incidence of cases and deaths from each of these diseases.

Diphtheria is primarily a localized and generalized intoxication caused by diphtheria toxin, an extracellular protein metabolite of toxinogenic strains of *Corynebacterium diphtheriae.* While the incidence of diphtheria in the U.S. has decreased from over 200,000 cases reported in 1921, before the general use of diphtheria toxoid, to only 15 cases reported from 1980 to 1983,[4] the ratio of fatalities to attack rate has remained constant at about 5% to 10%. The highest case fatality rates are in the very young and in the elderly. Following adequate immunization with diphtheria toxoid, which induces antitoxin, it is thought that protection lasts for at least 10 years.[4] This significantly reduces both the risk of developing diphtheria and the severity of clinical illness. It does not, however, eliminate carriage of *C diphtheriae* in the pharynx or on the skin.[4]

Tetanus is an intoxication manifested primarily by neuromuscular dysfunction caused by a potent exotoxin elaborated by *Clostridium tetani.* The incidence of tetanus in the U.S. has dropped dramatically with the routine use of tetanus toxoid, remaining relatively constant over the last decade at about 90 cases reported annually. Spores of *C tetani* are ubiquitous, and there is essentially no natural immunity to tetanus toxin. Thus, universal primary immunization with tetanus toxoid with subsequent maintenance of adequate antitoxin levels, by means of timed boosters, is necessary to protect all age groups.[4] Tetanus toxoid is a highly effective antigen and a completed primary series generally induces protective levels of serum antitoxin that persist for at least 10 years.[4]

Pertussis is a disease of the respiratory tract caused by *B pertussis.* This Gram-negative coccobacillus produces a variety of active components including endotoxin and a number of other substances that have been defined primarily on the basis of their biological activity in animals. These active components have been associated with a number of effects, such as lymphocytosis, leukocytosis, sensitivity to histamine, changes in glucose and/or insulin levels, possible neurological effects and adjuvant activity.[6] The role of each of the different components in either the pathogenesis of, or immunity to, pertussis is not well understood.

Pertussis is a highly communicable disease which has an attack rate in unimmunized populations of over 90%.[4] Since pertussis vaccine has come into widespread use, the number of reported cases and associated mortality in the U.S. has declined from about 120,000 cases and 1,100 deaths in 1950,[7] to an annual average of about 2,000 cases and 10 fatalities over the last 10 years.[4] Accurate data do not exist, as bacteriological confirmation of pertussis can be obtained in less than half of the suspected cases. Most reported illnesses from *B pertussis* occur in infants and young children; two thirds of reported deaths occur in children less than 1 year old. Older children and adults, in whom classic signs are often absent, may go undiagnosed and serve as reservoirs of disease.[4]

Evidence of the efficacy of pertussis vaccine can be provided by the recent British experience, where a reduction in the number of immunized individuals from 79% in 1973, to 31% in 1978 resulted in an epidemic of 102,500 pertussis cases and 36 deaths between late 1977 and 1980, and 1,440 cases per week reported during the winter of 1981 to 1982. A similar situation occurred in Japan.[7]

Because the severity of pertussis decreases with age, and the vaccine may cause side effects and adverse reactions, routine pertussis immunization is not recommended for persons 7 years of age or older.[4]

INDICATIONS AND USAGE

Diphtheria and Tetanus Toxoids and Pertussis Vaccine Adsorbed TRI-IMMUNOL is indicated for active immunization of infants and children from 2 months of age up to their seventh birthday against diphtheria, tetanus, and pertussis.[4,5] Children who have recovered from culture-confirmed pertussis need not receive further doses of a vaccine containing pertussis.[4]

CONTRAINDICATIONS

HYPERSENSITIVITY TO ANY COMPONENT OF THE VACCINE, INCLUDING THIMEROSAL, A MERCURY DERIVATIVE, IS A CONTRAINDICATION.

IMMUNIZATION SHOULD BE DEFERRED DURING THE COURSE OF ANY FEBRILE ILLNESS OR ACUTE INFECTION. A MINOR AFEBRILE ILLNESS SUCH AS A MILD UPPER RESPIRATORY INFECTION IS NOT USUALLY REASON TO DEFER IMMUNIZATION.[4,5]

THE OCCURRENCE OF ANY TYPE OF NEUROLOGICAL SYMPTOMS OR SIGNS, INCLUDING ONE OR MORE CONVULSIONS (SEIZURES) FOLLOWING ADMINISTRATION OF THIS PRODUCT IS A CONTRAINDICATION TO FURTHER USE. USE OF THIS PRODUCT IS ALSO CONTRAINDICATED IF THE CHILD HAS A PERSONAL HISTORY OF SEIZURES (SEE FOLLOWING DISCUSSION FOR INFORMATION REGARDING CHILDREN WITH A FAMILY HISTORY OF SEIZURES). THE PRESENCE OF ANY EVOLVING OR CHANGING DISORDER AFFECTING THE CENTRAL NERVOUS SYSTEM IS A CONTRAINDICATION TO ADMINISTRATION OF DTP REGARDLESS OF WHETHER THE SUSPECTED NEUROLOGICAL DISORDER IS ASSOCIATED WITH OCCURRENCE OF SEIZURE ACTIVITY OF ANY TYPE.

STUDIES HAVE INDICATED THAT A PERSONAL OR FAMILY HISTORY OF SEIZURES IS ASSOCIATED WITH INCREASED FREQUENCY OF SEIZURES FOLLOWING PERTUSSIS IMMUNIZATION.[8–10]

Personal History: THE IMMUNIZATION PRACTICES ADVISORY COMMITTEE (ACIP) OF THE U.S. PUBLIC HEALTH SERVICE STATES: "THE PRESENCE OF A NEUROLOGIC CONDITION CHARACTERIZED BY CHANGING DEVELOPMENTAL OR NEUROLOGIC FINDINGS, REGARDLESS OF WHETHER A DEFINITIVE DIAGNOSIS HAS BEEN MADE, IS . . . CONSIDERED A CONTRAINDICATION TO RECEIPT OF PERTUSSIS VACCINE, BECAUSE ADMINISTRATION OF DTP MAY COINCIDE WITH OR POSSIBLY EVEN AGGRAVATE MANIFESTATIONS OF THE DISEASE. SUCH DISORDERS INCLUDE UNCONTROLLED EPILEPSY, INFANTILE SPASMS, AND PROGRESSIVE ENCEPHALOPATHY."[4]

THE IMMUNIZATION PRACTICES ADVISORY COMMITTEE (ACIP) AND THE AMERICAN ACADEMY OF PEDIATRICS (AAP) RECOGNIZE CERTAIN CIRCUMSTANCES IN WHICH CHILDREN WITH STABLE CENTRAL NERVOUS SYSTEM DISORDERS, INCLUDING WELL-CONTROLLED SEIZURES OR SATISFACTORILY EXPLAINED SINGLE SEIZURES, MAY RECEIVE PERTUSSIS VACCINE. THE DECISION TO ADMINISTER VACCINE TO SUCH CHILDREN MUST BE MADE BY THE PHYSICIAN ON AN INDIVIDUAL BASIS, WITH CONSIDERATION OF ALL RELEVANT FACTORS, TO ALLOW AN ACCURATE ASSESSMENT OF RISKS AND BENEFITS FOR THAT INDIVIDUAL. THE PHYSICIAN SHOULD REVIEW THE FULL TEXT OF THE ACIP AND AAP GUIDELINES PRIOR TO CONSIDERING VACCINATION FOR SUCH CHILDREN.[4,5,8] THE PARENT OR GUARDIAN SHOULD BE ADVISED OF THE INCREASED RISK INVOLVED.

Family History: **THE ACIP AND AAP DO NOT CONSIDER A FAMILY HISTORY OF SEIZURES TO BE A CONTRAINDICATION TO PERTUSSIS VACCINE.**[4,5,8] DESPITE THE INCREASED RISK OF SEIZURES IN THESE INDIVIDUALS. THE DECISION TO ADMINISTER VACCINE TO SUCH CHILDREN MUST BE MADE BY THE PHYSICIAN ON AN INDIVIDUAL BASIS, WITH CONSIDERATION OF ALL RELEVANT FACTORS, TO ALLOW AN ACCURATE ASSESSMENT OF RISKS AND BENEFITS FOR THAT INDIVIDUAL. THE PARENT OR GUARDIAN SHOULD BE ADVISED OF THE INCREASED RISK INVOLVED.

THE ACIP STATES: "THERE ARE NO DATA ON WHETHER THE PROPHYLACTIC USE OF ANTIPYRETICS CAN DECREASE THE RISK OF FEBRILE CONVULSIONS. HOWEVER, PRELIMINARY DATA SUGGEST THAT ACETAMINOPHEN. . . WILL REDUCE THE INCIDENCE OF POSTVACCINATION FEVER. THUS, IT IS REASONABLE TO CONSIDER ADMINISTERING. . . ACETAMINOPHEN AT AGE-APPROPRIATE DOSES AT THE TIME OF VACCINATION AND EVERY 4 TO 6 HOURS FOR 48 TO 72 HOURS TO CHILDREN AT HIGHER RISK FOR SEIZURES THAN THE GENERAL POPULATION."[8]

Adverse Events Following Previous Immunization: THE ACIP AND AAP CONSIDER THE OCCURRENCE OF ANY OF THE FOLLOWING EVENTS AFTER VACCINATION WITH PERTUSSIS-CONTAINING VACCINE TO BE AN ABSOLUTE CONTRAINDICATION TO FURTHER PERTUSSIS VACCINATION:

1. ALLERGIC HYPERSENSITIVITY TO ANY COMPONENT OF THE VACCINE
2. FEVER OF 40.5°C (105°F) OR GREATER WITHIN 48 HOURS
3. COLLAPSE OR SHOCK-LIKE STATE (HYPOTONIC-HYPORESPONSIVE EPISODE) WITHIN 48 HOURS
4. PERSISTING, INCONSOLABLE CRYING LASTING 3 HOURS OR MORE, OR AN UNUSUAL HIGH-PITCHED CRY OCCURRING WITHIN 48 HOURS
5. CONVULSION(S) WITH OR WITHOUT FEVER OCCURRING WITHIN 3 DAYS. (For convulsions occurring beyond 3 days, see discussion in **CONTRAINDICATIONS** section and in references 4 and 5 concerning children with a personal history of convulsions.)
6. ENCEPHALOPATHY OCCURRING WITHIN 7 DAYS; THIS INCLUDES SEVERE ALTERATIONS IN CONSCIOUSNESS WITH GENERALIZED OR FOCAL NEUROLOGIC SIGNS.[4,5]

The clinical judgment of the attending physician should prevail at all times.

Routine immunization should be deferred during an outbreak of poliomyelitis, providing the patient has not sustained an injury that increases the risk of tetanus and providing an outbreak of diphtheria or pertussis does not occur simultaneously.

WARNINGS

THIS PRODUCT IS NOT RECOMMENDED FOR IMMUNIZING PERSONS ON OR AFTER THEIR SEVENTH BIRTHDAY. DO NOT ATTEMPT IMMUNIZATION IF THE CHILD HAS OR IS SUSPECTED TO HAVE AN EVOLVING NEUROLOGICAL DISORDER. STUDIES HAVE INDICATED THAT A PERSONAL OR FAMILY HISTORY OF SEIZURES IS ASSOCIATED WITH INCREASED FREQUENCY OF SEIZURES FOLLOWING PERTUSSIS IMMUNIZATION.[8–10] (SEE DISCUSSION IN **CONTRAINDICATIONS** SECTION.)

SHOULD ANY SYMPTOMATOLOGY RELATED TO NEUROLOGICAL DISORDERS DEVELOP FOLLOWING ADMINISTRATION, DO NOT ATTEMPT FURTHER ADMINISTRATION OF PERTUSSIS VACCINE. THE OCCURRENCE OF ENCEPHALOPATHY (INCLUDING SEVERE ALTERATIONS IN CONSCIOUSNESS WITH GENERALIZED OR FOCAL NEUROLOGICAL SIGNS), CONVULSION, PERSISTING INCONSOLABLE CRYING FOR 3 OR MORE HOURS' DURATION, AN UNUSUAL HIGH-PITCHED CRY, COLLAPSE OR SHOCK-LIKE STATE, FEVER OF 40.5°C (105°F) OR GREATER, AND ALLERGIC REACTIONS AFTER ADMINISTRATION ARE CONTRAINDICATIONS FOR ANY FURTHER USE OF PERTUSSIS-CONTAINING VACCINE. (SEE **CONTRAINDICATIONS** SECTION.)

If a contraindication to pertussis is found, the infant or child should be given Diphtheria and Tetanus Toxoids, Adsorbed, for pediatric use (DT) instead of DTP. **Unimmunized children less than 1 year of age** should receive three doses of DT at 4 to 8 week intervals, followed by a fourth dose 6 to 12 months after the third dose, for the primary series. **Unimmunized children 1 year of age or older** should receive two doses of DT 4 to 8 weeks apart, followed by a third dose 6 to 12 months after the second dose for the primary series. **If, after beginning a DTP series, further doses of vaccine containing pertussis antigen become contraindicated, DT should be substituted for each of the remaining doses.**[4,5]

PARTIAL DOSES OF DTP VACCINE SHOULD NOT BE GIVEN.[4,5] Neither the efficacy of such practice in reducing the frequency of associated serious adverse events, nor the resulting protection against disease has been determined.

The occurrence of sudden infant death syndrome (SIDS) has been reported following administration of DTP.[11–13] However, a large case-control study in the U.S. revealed no causal relationship between receipt of DTP vaccine and SIDS.[14]

Onset of infantile spasms has occurred in infants who have recently received DTP or DT. Analysis of data from the National Childhood Encephalopathy Study on children with infantile spasms showed that receipt of DTP or DT was not causally related to infantile spasms.[15] The incidence of onset of infantile spasms increases at 3 to 9 months of age, the time period in which the second and third doses of DTP are generally given. Therefore, some cases of infantile spasms can be expected to be related by chance alone to recent receipt of DTP.[4]

DTP should not be given to infants or children with thrombocytopenia or any coagulation disorder that would contraindicate intramuscular injection unless the potential benefit clearly outweighs the risk of administration.

Patients with impaired immune responsiveness, whether due to the use of immunosuppressive therapy (including irradiation, corticosteroids, antimetabolites, alkylating agents, and cytotoxic agents), a genetic defect, human immunodeficiency virus (HIV) infection, or other causes, may have a reduced antibody response to active immunization

Continued on next page

Information on Lederle products listed on these pages is the full prescribing information from product literature or package inserts effective in August 1992. Information concerning all Lederle products may be obtained from the Professional Services Department, Lederle Laboratories, Pearl River, New York 10965.

Lederle—Cont.

procedures.[4,5,16] Deferral of administration of vaccine may be considered in individuals receiving immunosuppressive therapy.[4,5] Other groups should receive this vaccine according to the usual recommended schedule.[4,5,16,17]

Special care should be taken to prevent injection into a blood vessel.

PRECAUTIONS

General

1. THIS PRODUCT SHOULD BE USED FOR THE AGE GROUP BETWEEN 2 MONTHS AND THE SEVENTH BIRTHDAY.
2. PRIOR TO ADMINISTRATION OF ANY DOSE OF DTP, THE PARENT OR GUARDIAN SHOULD BE ASKED ABOUT THE PERSONAL AND FAMILY HISTORY AND THE RECENT HEALTH STATUS OF THE INFANT OR CHILD TO BE IMMUNIZED IN ORDER TO DETERMINE THE EXISTENCE OF ANY CONTRAINDICATION TO IMMUNIZATION WITH DTP AND TO ALLOW AN ACCURATE ASSESSMENT OF BENEFITS AND RISKS. (SEE **CONTRAINDICATIONS; WARNINGS**.)
3. WHEN AN INFANT OR CHILD RETURNS FOR THE NEXT DOSE IN THE SERIES, THE PARENT OR GUARDIAN SHOULD BE QUESTIONED CONCERNING OCCURRENCE OF ANY SYMPTOM AND/OR SIGNS OF AN ADVERSE REACTION AFTER THE PREVIOUS DOSE (SEE **CONTRAINDICATIONS, ADVERSE REACTIONS**.)
4. BEFORE THE INJECTION OF ANY BIOLOGICAL, THE PHYSICIAN SHOULD TAKE ALL PRECAUTIONS KNOWN FOR PREVENTION OF ALLERGIC OR ANY OTHER SIDE REACTIONS. This should include: a review of the patient's history regarding possible sensitivity; the ready availability of epinephrine 1:1,000 and other appropriate agents used for control of immediate allergic reactions; and a knowledge of the recent literature pertaining to use of the biological concerned, including the nature of side effects and adverse reactions that may follow its use.
5. Since this product contains both a bacterial suspension and an adjuvant, shake vigorously before withdrawing each dose from multiple dose vials.
6. A separate sterile syringe and needle or a sterile disposable unit should be used for each individual patient to prevent transmission of hepatitis or other infectious agents from one person to another.
7. NATIONAL CHILDHOOD VACCINE INJURY ACT OF 1986 (AS AMENDED IN 1987). This Act requires that the manufacturer and lot number of the vaccine administered be recorded by the health care provider in the vaccine recipient's permanent medical record, along with the date of administration of the vaccine and the name, address and title of the person administering the vaccine.

The Act further requires the health care provider to report to a health department or to the FDA the occurrence following immunization of any event set forth in the Vaccine Injury Table including: anaphylaxis or anaphylactic shock within 24 hours, encephalopathy or encephalitis within 7 days, shock-collapse or hypotonic-hyporesponsive collapse within 7 days, residual seizure disorder, any acute complication or sequelae (including death) of above events, or any event that would contraindicate further doses of vaccine, according to this package insert.[18]

Information for Patient: PRIOR TO ADMINISTRATION OF THIS VACCINE, HEALTH CARE PERSONNEL SHOULD INFORM THE PARENT, GUARDIAN, OR OTHER RESPONSIBLE ADULT OF THE BENEFITS AND RISKS TO THE CHILD OF DTP VACCINE. GUIDANCE SHOULD BE PROVIDED ON MEASURES TO BE TAKEN SHOULD ADVERSE EVENTS OCCUR, eg, ANTIPYRETIC MEASURES FOR ELEVATED TEMPERATURES.

ADVERSE REACTIONS

Local reactions are common after administration of DTP, occurring in 35% to 50% of recipients[19] and are manifested by varying degrees of erythema, induration, and tenderness which may occasionally be severe. Such local reactions are usually self-limited and require no therapy. A nodule may be palpable at the injection site for a few weeks. Sterile abscess formation,[20] or subcutaneous atrophy at the site of injection has been reported. Cervical lymphadenopathy has been reported following DTP injections into the arm.[21]

Temperature elevations, fretfulness, drowsiness, vomiting, and anorexia frequently follow DTP administration.[19,22,23] Approximately 50% of DTP recipients will develop temperature elevations > 38°C (100.4°F) after one or more doses of the series; approximately 6% > 39°C (102.2°F);[20] and approximately 0.3% ≥ 40.5°C (105°F).[4] Some data suggest that febrile reactions are more likely to occur in those who have experienced such responses after prior doses.[22]

SIGNIFICANT REACTIONS ATTRIBUTED TO THE PERTUSSIS VACCINE COMPONENT HAVE BEEN: HIGH FEVER OF 40.5°C (105°F), A TRANSIENT SHOCK-LIKE EPISODE, EXCESSIVE SCREAMING (PERSISTENT CRYING OR SCREAMING FOR 3 OR MORE HOURS' DURATION), AN UNUSUAL HIGH-PITCHED CRY, AND CONVULSIONS.

ENCEPHALOPATHY HAS BEEN REPORTED FOLLOWING PERTUSSIS VACCINATION; ONE STUDY SUGGESTS THE INCIDENCE OF ENCEPHALOPATHY OCCURRING WITHIN 7 DAYS OF VACCINATION MAY BE 1 PER 140,000 DOSES, WITH ENCEPHALOPATHY RESULTING IN DEATH OR PERMANENT DAMAGE TO THE CENTRAL NERVOUS SYSTEM ESTIMATED TO OCCUR IN 1 PER 330,000 DOSES.[24] (SEE **CONTRAINDICATIONS** AND **WARNINGS**.)

THE INCIDENCE OF CONVULSION OR TRANSIENT SHOCK-LIKE EPISODE OCCURRING WITHIN 48 HOURS OF VACCINATION HAS BEEN ESTIMATED TO BE 1 PER 1,750 DOSES.[19]

BULGING FONTANEL[25-27] HAS BEEN REPORTED AFTER DTP IMMUNIZATION, ALTHOUGH NO CAUSE AND EFFECT RELATIONSHIP HAS BEEN ESTABLISHED.

CARDIAC EFFECTS[28-30] AND RESPIRATORY DIFFICULTIES, INCLUDING APNEA HAVE BEEN REPORTED RARELY.

PERTUSSIS VACCINE HAS BEEN ASSOCIATED WITH A GREATER PROPORTION OF ADVERSE REACTIONS THAN MANY OTHER CHILDHOOD IMMUNIZATIONS.[31] SHOULD SYMPTOMATOLOGY REFERABLE TO THE CENTRAL NERVOUS SYSTEM DEVELOP WITHIN 7 DAYS FOLLOWING ADMINISTRATION, FURTHER IMMUNIZATION WITH THIS PRODUCT IS CONTRAINDICATED. (SEE **CONTRAINDICATIONS**.)

NEUROLOGICAL COMPLICATIONS,[32] SUCH AS CONVULSIONS,[19,31] ENCEPHALOPATHY,[24,33] AND VARIOUS MONO- AND POLYNEUROPATHIES,[32-39] INCLUDING GUILLAIN-BARRE SYNDROME,[40,41] HAVE BEEN REPORTED FOLLOWING ADMINISTRATION OF PREPARATIONS CONTAINING DIPHTHERIA, TETANUS, AND/OR PERTUSSIS ANTIGENS.

URTICARIA, ERYTHEMA MULTIFORME OR OTHER RASH, ARTHRALGIAS[31] AND RARELY, A SEVERE ANAPHYLACTIC REACTION (eg, URTICARIA WITH SWELLING OF THE MOUTH, DIFFICULTY BREATHING, HYPOTENSION OR SHOCK) HAVE BEEN REPORTED FOLLOWING ADMINISTRATION OF PREPARATIONS CONTAINING DIPHTHERIA, TETANUS, AND/OR PERTUSSIS ANTIGENS.

DOSAGE AND ADMINISTRATION

For Intramuscular Use Only: *Shake vigorously before withdrawing each dose from the multiple dose vials.*

Parenteral drug products should be inspected visually for particulate matter and discoloration prior to administration. (See **DESCRIPTION**.)

The vaccine should be injected intramuscularly. Preferred sites are the anterolateral aspect of the thigh and the deltoid muscle of the upper arm. Care should be taken to avoid major peripheral nerve trunks.

Before injection, the skin at the injection site should be cleansed and prepared with a suitable germicide.

After insertion of the needle, aspirate to help avoid inadvertent injection into a blood vessel.

The primary immunizing course for infants and children from 2 months of age up to their seventh birthday consists of three doses of 0.5 mL each at 4 to 8 week intervals, followed by a fourth dose of 0.5 mL 6 to 12 months after the third dose.[4,5]

If a contraindication to the pertussis component occurs, Diphtheria and Tetanus Toxoids, Adsorbed for pediatric use (DT) should be substituted for the remaining doses, according to the schedule discussed under **WARNINGS**.

The simultaneous administration of DTP, oral poliovirus vaccine (OPV), and/or measles-mumps-rubella vaccine (MMR) has resulted in seroconversion rates and rates of side effects similar to those observed when the vaccines are administered separately.[4]

The simultaneous administration of DTP and *Haemophilus* b Conjugate Vaccine has resulted in antibody responses to the individual antigens and rates of side effects similar to those observed when the vaccines are administered separately.[42]

The AAP and ACIP recommend that DTP may be administered simultaneously (at separate sites) with other routine childhood vaccines such as *Haemophilus* b Conjugate Vaccine, OPV, and/or MMR.[43,44]

The American Academy of Pediatrics recommends that Influenza Virus Vaccine should not be administered within 3 days of immunization with a pertussis-containing vaccine.[5]

Premature infants may be immunized with DTP at the usual chronological age.[5]

Interruption of the recommended schedule with a delay between doses does not interfere with the final immunity achieved; nor does it necessitate starting the series over again, regardless of the length of time elapsed between doses.[4,5]

A booster dose of 0.5 mL is indicated at age 4 to 6 years, preferably prior to entrance into kindergarten or elementary school. (Substitute DT when contraindication to pertussis-containing vaccine exists.) (See **CONTRAINDICATIONS** and **WARNINGS** sections.) However, if the fourth dose of the basic immunizing series was administered after the fourth birthday a booster prior to school entry is not considered necessary.[4]

For either primary or booster immunization against tetanus and diphtheria of individuals 7 years of age and older, the use of Tetanus and Diphtheria Toxoids Adsorbed For Adult Use is recommended.[4,5]

HOW SUPPLIED

NDC 0005-1948-33   7.5 mL vial

STORAGE

DO NOT FREEZE. STORE REFRIGERATED, AWAY FROM FREEZER COMPARTMENT, AT 2°C TO 8°C (36°F TO 46°F).

REFERENCES

1. Mueller JH, Miller PA: Production of diphtheria toxin of high potency (100Lf) on a reproducible medium. *J Immunol* 1941;40:21–32.
2. Mueller JH, Miller PA: Factors influencing the production of tetanal toxin. *J Immunol* 1947;56:143–147.
3. Pillemer L, Grossberg DB, Wittler RG: The immunochemistry of toxins and toxoids. II. The preparation and immunological evaluation of purified tetanal toxoid. *J Immunol* 1946;54:213–224.
4. Diphtheria, tetanus and pertussis: Guidelines for vaccine prophylaxis and other preventive measures—recommendation of the Immunization Practices Advisory Committee (ACIP). *MMWR* 1985;34(27):405–426.
5. American Academy of Pediatrics: Report of the Committee on Infectious Diseases, ed 21. Elk Grove Village, IL, American Academy of Pediatrics, 1988.
6. Manclark CR, Cowell JL: Pertussis vaccine, in Germanier R. (ed): Bacterial Vaccines. New York, Academic Press Inc, 1984;69–106.
7. Reported incidence of notifiable diseases in the United States. *MMWR* 1970;19(53):44.
8. Pertussis immunization: family history of convulsions and use of antipyretics—supplementary ACIP statement. *MMWR* 1987;36(18):281–282.
9. Stetler HC, et al: History of convulsions and use of pertussis vaccine. *J Pediatr* 1985;107(2):175–179.
10. Hirtz DG, et al: Seizures following childhood immunizations. *J Pediatr* 1983;102(1):14–18.
11. Bernier R, et al: Diphtheria-tetanus toxoids, pertussis vaccination and sudden infant deaths in Tennessee. *J Pediatr* 1982;101:419–421.
12. Baraff L, et al: Possible temporal association between diphtheria-tetanus toxoid, pertussis vaccination and sudden infant death syndrome. *Pediatr Inf Dis* 1983;2:7–11.
13. Walker AM, et al: Diphtheria-tetanus-pertussis immunization and sudden infant death syndrome. *AJPH* 1987;77(8):945–951.
14. Hoffman HJ, et al: Diphtheria-tetanus-pertussis immunization and sudden infant death; results of the National Institute of Child Health and Human Development cooperative study of sudden infant death syndrome risk factors. *Pediatrics* 1987;79(4):598–611.
15. Bellman MH, et al: Infantile spasms and pertussis immunization. *Lancet* 1983;1:1031–1034.
16. Recommendation of the ACIP: Immunization of children infected with Human T-Lymphotrophic Virus Type III/Lymphadenopathy-associated virus. *MMWR* 1986;35(38):595–606.
17. Immunization of children infected with Human Immunodeficiency Virus—Supplementary ACIP statement. *MMWR* 1988;37(12):181–183.
18. National Childhood Vaccine Injury Act: Requirements for permanent vaccination records and for reporting of selected events after vaccination. *MMWR* 1988; 37(13):197–200.
19. Cody C, et al: Nature and rates of adverse reactions associated with DTP and DT immunizations in infants and children. *Pediatrics* 1981;68:650–660.
20. Bernier R, et al: Abscesses complicating DTP vaccination. *Am J Dis Child* 1981;135:826–828.
21. Omokoku B, Castells S: Post-DPT inoculation-caused lymphadenitis in children. *NY State J Med* 1981;81:1667–1668.
22. Baraff L, et al: DTP-associated reactions: An analysis by injection site, manufacturer, prior reactions and dose. *Pediatrics* 1984;73:31–36.
23. Barkin R, Pichichero M: Diphtheria-pertussis-tetanus vaccine: Reactogenicity of commercial products. *Pediatrics* 1979;63:256–260.
24. Miller DL, et al: Pertussis vaccine and whooping cough as risk factors in acute neurological illness and death in young children. *Dev Biol Stand* 1985;61:389–394.
25. Mathur et al: Bulging fontanel following triple vaccine (letter). *Indian Pediatrics* 1981;18(6):417–418.
26. Shendurnikar et al: Bulging fontanel following DTP vaccine (letter). *Indian Pediatrics* 1986;23(11):960.

27. Jacob et al: Increased intracranial pressure after diphtheria, tetanus, and pertussis immunization. *Am J Dis Child* 1979;133:217–218.
28. Leung A: Congenital heart disease and DTP vaccination. *Can Med Assoc J* 1984;131:541.
29. Park JM, et al: Paroxysmal supraventricular tachycardia precipitated by pertussis vaccine. *Pediatrics* 1983;102(6):883–885.
30. Amsel SG, et al: Myocarditis after triple immunization. *Arch Dis Child* 1986;61:403–404.
31. Adverse events following immunization. *MMWR* 1985;34:43–47.
32. Rutledge SL, Snead OC: Neurologic complications of immunizations. *J Pediatr* 1986;109:917–924.
33. Schlenska GK: Unusual neurological complications following tetanus toxoid administration. *J Neurol* 1977;215:299–302.
34. Blumstein GI, Kreithen H: Peripheral neuropathy following tetanus toxoid administration. *JAMA* 1966;198:1030–1031.
35. Reinstein L, Pargament JM, Goodman JS: Peripheral neuropathy after multiple tetanus toxoid injections. *Arch Phys Med Rehabil* 1982;63:332–334.
36. Tsairis P, Dyck PJ, Mulder DW: Natural history of brachial plexus neuropathy. *Arch Neurol* 1972;27:109–117.
37. Quast U, Hennessen W, Widmark RM: Mono- and polyneuritis after tetanus vaccination. *Devel Bio Stand* 1979;43:25–32.
38. Holliday PL, Bauer RB: Polyradiculoneuritis secondary to immunization with tetanus and diphtheria toxoids. *Arch Neurol* 1983;40:56–67.
39. Fenichel GM: Neurological complications of tetanus toxoid. *Arch Neurol* 1983;40:390.
40. Pollard JD, Selby G: Relapsing neuropathy due to tetanus toxoid. *J Neurol Sci* 1978;37:113–125.
41. Newton N, Janati A: Guillain-Barre syndrome after vaccination with purified tetanus toxoid. *S Med J* 1987;80:1053–1054.
42. Unpublished data, Praxis Biologics, Inc., Rochester, New York 14623, USA.
43. Recommendation of the AAP: *Haemophilus influenzae* Type b Conjugate Vaccines: Recommendations for Immunization of Infants and Children 2 Months of Age and Older: Update. *Pediatrics.* In Press.
44. Recommendation of the ACIP: *Haemophilus b* Conjugate Vaccines for Prevention of *Haemophilus influenzae* Type b Disease Among Infants and Children Two Months of Age and Older. *MMWR* 1991; 40:1–7.

LEDERLE LABORATORIES DIVISION
American Cyanamid Company
Pearl River, NY 10965

Rev. 8/91
11088-91

Shown in Product Identification Section, page 415

VERELAN® ℞
Verapamil HCl
Sustained-Release Pellet-Filled Capsules

PRODUCT OVERVIEW

KEY FACTS

VERELAN, a calcium influx inhibitor (slow channel blocker or calcium ion antagonist), provides a sustained-release of the drug in the gastrointestinal tract. Food does not affect the extent or rate of the controlled absorption of verapamil from the VERELAN Capsule. VERELAN exerts antihypertensive effects by decreasing systemic vascular resistance, usually without orthostatic decreases in blood pressure or reflex tachycardia.

MAJOR USES

VERELAN is indicated for the management of essential hypertension.

SAFETY INFORMATION

See complete safety information set forth below.

PRESCRIBING INFORMATION

VERELAN® ℞
Verapamil HCl
Sustained-Release Pellet-Filled Capsules

DESCRIPTION

VERELAN is a calcium influx inhibitor (slow channel blocker or calcium ion antagonist). VERELAN is available for oral administration as a 240 mg hard gelatin capsule (dark blue cap/yellow body), a 180 mg hard gelatin capsule (light grey cap/yellow body), and a 120 mg hard gelatin capsule (yellow cap/yellow body). These pellet-filled capsules provide a sustained-release of the drug in the gastrointestinal tract.

Chemical name: Benzeneacetonitrile, α-[3-[[2-(3,4-dimethoxyphenyl)-ethyl]methylamino]propyl]-3,4-dimethoxy-α-(1-methylethyl) monohydrochloride.

Verapamil HCl is an almost white, crystalline powder, practically free of odor, with a bitter taste. It is soluble in water, chloroform, and methanol. Verapamil HCl is not structurally related to other cardioactive drugs.

In addition to verapamil HCl, the VERELAN capsule contains the following inactive ingredients: fumaric acid, talc, sugar spheres, povidone, shellac, gelatin, FD&C red #40, yellow iron oxide, titanium dioxide, methylparaben, propylparaben, silicon dioxide, and sodium lauryl sulfate. In addition the VERELAN 240 mg capsule contains FD&C blue #1 and D&C red #28; and the VERELAN 180 mg capsule contains black iron oxide.

CLINICAL PHARMACOLOGY

VERELAN is a calcium ion influx inhibitor (slow channel blocker or calcium ion antagonist) which exerts its pharmacologic effects by modulating the influx of ionic calcium across the cell membrane of the arterial smooth muscle as well as in conductile and contractile myocardial cells.

Normal sinus rhythm is usually not affected by verapamil HCl. However in patients with sick sinus syndrome, verapamil HCl may interfere with sinus node impulse generation and may induce sinus arrest or sinoatrial block. Atrioventricular block can occur in patients without preexisting condition defects (see **WARNINGS**). Verapamil HCl does not alter the normal atrial action potential or intraventricular conduction time, but depresses amplitude, velocity of depolarization and conduction in depressed atrial fibers. Verapamil HCl may shorten the antegrade effective refractory period of accessory bypass tracts. Acceleration of ventricular rate and/or ventricular fibrillation has been reported in patients with atrial flutter or atrial fibrillation and a coexisting accessory AV pathway following administration of verapamil (see **WARNINGS**).

Verapamil HCl has a local anesthetic action that is 1.6 times that of procaine on an equimolar basis. It is not known whether this action is important at the doses used in man.

Mechanism of Action: *Essential Hypertension:* Verapamil HCl exerts antihypertensive effects by decreasing systemic vascular resistance, usually without orthostatic decreases in blood pressure or reflex tachycardia; bradycardia (rate less than 50 beats/minute is uncommon). Verapamil HCl regularly reduces arterial pressure at rest and at a given level of exercise by dilating peripheral arterioles and reducing the total peripheral resistance (afterload) against which the heart works.

Pharmacokinetics and Metabolism: With the immediate release formulations, more than 90% of the orally administered dose is absorbed, and peak plasma concentrations of verapamil are observed 1 to 2 hours after dosing. Because of rapid biotransformation of verapamil during its first pass through the portal circulation, the absolute bioavailability ranges from 20% to 35%. Chronic oral administration of the highest recommended dose (120 mg every 6 hours) resulted in plasma verapamil levels ranging from 125 to 400 ng/mL with higher values reported occasionally. A nonlinear correlation between the verapamil HCl dose administered and verapamil plasma levels does exist.

During initial dose titration with verapamil, a relationship exists between verapamil plasma concentrations and the prolongation of the PR interval. However, during chronic administration this relationship may disappear. The quantitative relationship between plasma verapamil concentrations and blood pressure reduction has not been fully characterized.

In a multiple dose pharmacokinetic study, peak concentrations for a single daily dose of VERELAN *verapamil HCl* 240 mg were approximately 65% of those obtained with an 80 mg tid dose of the conventional immediate release tablets, and the 24-hour post-dose concentrations were approximately 30% higher. At a total daily dose of 240 mg, VERELAN was shown to have a similar extent of verapamil bioavailability based on the AUC-24 as that obtained with the conventional immediate release tablets. In this same study, VERELAN doses of 120 mg, 240 mg, and 360 mg once daily were compared after multiple doses. The ratios of the verapamil and norverapamil AUCs for the VERELAN 120 mg, 240 mg, and 360 mg once daily doses are 1 (565 ng·hr/mL):3 (1660 ng·hr/mL):5 (2729 ng·hr/mL) and 1 (621 ng·hr/mL):3 (1614 ng·hr/mL):4 (2535 ng·hr/mL), respectively, indicating that the AUC increased nonproportionately with increasing doses.

Food does not affect the extent or rate of the absorption of verapamil from the controlled release VERELAN capsule. The VERELAN 240 mg capsule when administered with food had a C_{max} of 77 ng/mL which occurred 9.0 hours after dosing, and an AUC(O-inf) of 1387 ng·hr/mL. VERELAN 240 mg under fasting conditions had a C_{max} of 77 ng/mL which occurred 9.8 hours after dosing, and an AUC(O-inf) of 1541 ng·hr/mL.

The time to reach maximum verapamil concentrations (T_{max}) with VERELAN *verapamil HCl* has been found to be approximately 7 to 9 hours in each of the single dose (fasting), single dose (fed), the multiple dose (steady state) studies, and dose proportionality pharmacokinetic studies. Similarly, the apparent half-life ($t_{1/2}$) has been found to be approximately 12 hours independent of dose. Aging may affect the pharmacokinetics of verapamil. Elimination half-life may be prolonged in the elderly.

In healthy man, orally administered verapamil HCl undergoes extensive metabolism in the liver. Twelve metabolites have been identified in plasma; all except norverapamil are present in trace amounts only. Norverapamil can reach steady-state plasma concentrations approximately equal to those of verapamil itself. The biologic activity of norverapamil appears to be approximately 20% that of verapamil.

Approximately 70% of an administered dose of verapamil HCl is excreted as metabolites in the urine and 16% or more in the feces within 5 days. About 3% to 4% is excreted in the urine as unchanged drug. Approximately 90% is bound to plasma proteins. In patients with hepatic insufficiency, metabolism is delayed and elimination half-life prolonged up to 14 to 16 hours (see **PRECAUTIONS**), the volume of distribution is increased, and plasma clearance reduced to about 30% of normal. Verapamil clearance values suggest that patients with liver dysfunction may attain therapeutic verapamil plasma concentrations with one third of the oral daily dose required for patients with normal liver function.

After 4 weeks of oral dosing (120 mg qid), verapamil and norverapamil levels were noted in the cerebrospinal fluid with estimated partition coefficient of 0.06 for verapamil and 0.04 for norverapamil.

Hemodynamics and Myocardial Metabolism: Verapamil HCl reduces afterload and myocardial contractility. Improved left ventricular diastolic function in patients with IHSS and those with coronary heart disease has also been observed with verapamil HCl therapy. In most patients, including those with organic cardiac disease, the negative inotropic action of verapamil HCl is countered by reduction of afterload and cardiac index is usually not reduced. In patients with severe left ventricular dysfuntion however (eg, pulmonary wedge pressure above 20 mmHg or ejection fraction lower than 30%), or in patients on beta-adrenergic blocking agents or other cardiodepressant drugs, deterioration of ventricular function may occur (see **DRUG INTERACTIONS**).

Pulmonary Function: Verapamil HCl does not induce broncho-constriction and hence, does not impair ventilatory function.

INDICATIONS AND USAGE

VERELAN is indicated for the management of essential hypertension.

CONTRAINDICATIONS

Verapamil HCl is contraindicated in:

1. Severe left ventricular dysfunction (see **WARNINGS**).
2. Hypotension (less than 90 mmHg systolic pressure) or cardiogenic shock.
3. Sick sinus syndrome (except in patients with a functioning artificial ventricular pacemaker).
4. Second- or third-degree AV block (except in patients with a functioning artificial ventricular pacemaker).
5. Patients with atrial flutter or atrial fibrillation and an accessory bypass tract (eg, Wolff-Parkinson-White, Lown-Ganong-Levine syndromes) (see **WARNINGS**).
6. Patients with known hypersensitivity to verapamil HCl.

WARNINGS

Heart Failure: Verapamil has a negative inotropic effect which, in most patients, is compensated by its afterload reduction (decreased systemic vascular resistance) properties without a net impairment of ventricular performance. In clinical experience with 4,954 patients, 87 (1.8%) developed congestive heart failure or pulmonary edema. Verapamil should be avoided in patients with severe left ventricular dysfunction (eg, ejection fraction less than 30% or moderate to severe symptoms of cardiac failure) and in patients with any degree of ventricular dysfunction if they are receiving a beta-adrenergic blocker (see **DRUG INTERACTIONS**). Patients with milder ventricular dysfunction should, if possible, be controlled with optimum doses of digitalis and/or diuretics before verapamil treatment (note interactions with digoxin under **PRECAUTIONS**).

Hypotension: Occasionally, the pharmacologic action of verapamil may produce a decrease in blood pressure below normal levels which may result in dizziness or symptomatic hypotension. The incidence of hypotension observed in 4,954 patients enrolled in clinical trials was 2.5%. In hypertensive patients, decreases in blood pressure below normal are unusual. Tilt table testing (60 degrees) was not able to induce orthostatic hypotension.

Continued on next page

Information on Lederle products listed on these pages is the full prescribing information from product literature or package inserts effective in August 1992. Information concerning all Lederle products may be obtained from the Professional Services Department, Lederle Laboratories, Pearl River, New York 10965.

Lederle—Cont.

Elevated Liver Enzymes: Elevations of transaminases with and without concomitant elevations in alkaline phosphatase and bilirubin have been reported. Such elevations have sometimes been transient and may disappear even in the face of continued verapamil treatment. Several cases of hepatocellular injury related to verapamil have been proven by rechallenge; half of these had clinical symptoms (malaise, fever, and/or right upper quadrant pain) in addition to elevations of SGOT, SGPT, and alkaline phosphatase. Periodic monitoring of liver function in patients receiving verapamil is therefore prudent.

Accessory Bypass Tract (Wolff-Parkinson-White or Lown-Ganong-Levine): Some patients with paroxysmal and/or chronic atrial flutter or atrial fibrillation and a coexisting accessory AV pathway have developed increased antegrade conduction across the accessory pathway bypassing the AV node, producing a very rapid ventricular response or ventricular fibrillation after receiving intravenous verapamil (or digitalis). Although a risk of this occurring with oral verapamil has not been established, such patients receiving oral verapamil may be at risk and its use in these patients is contraindicated (see **CONTRAINDICATIONS**).

Treatment is usually DC-cardioversion. Cardioversion has been used safely and effectively after oral verapamil.

Atrioventricular Block: The effect of verapamil on AV conduction and the SA node may lead to asymptomatic first-degree AV block and transient bradycardia, sometimes accompanied by nodal escape rhythms. PR interval prolongation is correlated with verapamil plasma concentrations, especially during the early titration phase of therapy. Higher degrees of AV block, however, were infrequently (0.8%) observed.

Marked first-degree block or progressive development to second- or third-degree AV block requires a reduction in dosage or, in rare instances, discontinuation of verapamil HCl and institution of appropriate therapy depending upon the clinical situation.

Patients with Hypertrophic Cardiomyopathy (IHSS): In 120 patients with hypertrophic cardiomyopathy (most of them refractory or intolerant to propranolol) who received therapy with verapamil at doses up to 720 mg/day, a variety of serious adverse effects were seen. Three patients died in pulmonary edema; all had severe left ventricular outflow obstruction and a past history of left ventricular dysfunction. Eight other patients had pulmonary edema and/or severe hypotension; abnormally high (over 20 mmHg) capillary wedge pressure and a marked left ventricular outflow obstruction were present in most of these patients. Concomitant administration of quinidine (see **DRUG INTERACTIONS**) preceded the severe hypotension in three of the eight patients (two of whom developed pulmonary edema). Sinus bradycardia occurred in 11% of the patients, second-degree AV block in 4% and sinus arrest in 2%. It must be appreciated that this group of patients had a serious disease with a high mortality rate. Most adverse effects responded well to dose reduction and only rarely did verapamil have to be discontinued.

PRECAUTIONS

General: *Use in Patients with Impaired Hepatic Function:* Since verapamil is highly metabolized by the liver, it should be administered cautiously to patients with impaired hepatic function. Severe liver dysfunction prolongs the elimination half-life of immediate release verapamil to about 14 to 16 hours; hence, approximately 30% of the dose given to patients with normal liver function should be administered to these patients. Careful monitoring for abnormal prolongation of the PR interval or other signs of excessive pharmacologic effects (see **OVERDOSAGE**) should be carried out.

Use in Patients with Attenuated (Decreased) Neuromuscular Transmission: It has been reported that verapamil decreases neuromuscular transmission in patients with Duchenne's muscular dystrophy, and that verapamil prolongs recovery from the neuromuscular blocking agent vecuronium. It may be necessary to decrease the dosage of verapamil when it is administered to patients with attenuated neuromuscular transmission.

Use in Patients with Impaired Renal Function: About 70% of an administered dose of verapamil is excreted as metabolites in the urine. Until further data are available, verapamil should be administered cautiously to patients with impaired renal function. These patients should be carefully monitored for abnormal prolongation of the PR interval or other signs of overdosage (see **OVERDOSAGE**).

Drug Interactions: *Beta Blockers:* Concomitant therapy with beta-adrenergic blockers and verapamil may result in additive negative effects on heart rate, atrioventricular conduction, and/or cardiac contractility. The combination of sustained-release verapamil and beta-adrenergic blocking agents has not been studied. However, there have been reports of excess bradycardia and AV block, including complete heart block, when the combination has been used for the treatment of hypertension. For hypertensive patients, the risk of combined therapy may outweigh the potential benefits. The combination should be used only with caution and close monitoring.

Asymptomatic bradycardia (36 beats/min) with a wandering atrial pacemaker has been observed in a patient receiving concomitant timolol (a beta-adrenergic blocker) eyedrops and oral verapamil.

A decrease in metoprolol clearance has been reported when verapamil and metoprolol were administered together. A similar effect has not been observed when verapamil and atenolol are given together.

Digitalis: Clinical use of verapamil in digitalized patients has shown the combination to be well tolerated if digoxin doses are properly adjusted. Chronic verapamil treatment can increase serum digoxin levels by 50% to 75% during the first week of therapy, and this can result in digitalis toxicity. In patients with hepatic cirrhosis the influence of verapamil on digoxin kinetics is magnified. Maintenance digitalis doses should be reduced when verapamil is administered, and the patient should be carefully monitored to avoid over- or underdigitalization. Whenever overdigitalization is suspected, the daily dose of digoxin should be reduced or temporarily discontinued. Upon discontinuation of verapamil HCl, the patient should be reassessed to avoid underdigitalization.

Antihypertensive Agents: Verapamil administered concomitantly with oral antihypertensive agents (eg, vasodilators, angiotensin-converting enzyme inhibitors, diuretics, beta blockers) will usually have an additive effect on lowering blood pressure. Patients receiving these combinations should be appropriately monitored. Concomitant use of agents that attenuate alpha-adrenergic function with verapamil may result in reduction in blood pressure that is excessive in some patients. Such an effect was observed in one study following the concomitant administration of verapamil and prazosin.

Antiarrhythmic Agents: Disopyramide: Until data on possible interactions between verapamil and disopyramide phosphate are obtained, disopyramide should not be administered within 48 hours before or 24 hours after verapamil administration.

Flecainide: A study in healthy volunteers showed that the concomitant administration of flecainide and verapamil may have additive effects on myocardial contractility, AV conduction, and repolarization. Concomitant therapy with flecainide and verapamil may result in additive negative inotropic effect and prolongation of atrioventricular conduction.

Quinidine: In a small number of patients with hypertrophic cardiomyopathy (IHSS), concomitant use of verapamil and quinidine resulted in significant hypotension. Until further data are obtained, combined therapy of verapamil and quinidine in patients with hypertrophic cardiomyopathy should probably be avoided.

The electrophysiological effects of quinidine and verapamil on AV conduction were studied in eight patients. Verapamil significantly counteracted the effects of quinidine on AV conduction. There has been a report of increased quinidine levels during verapamil therapy.

Nitrates: Verapamil has been given concomitantly with short- and long-acting nitrates without any undesirable drug interactions. The pharmacologic profile of both drugs and the clinical experience suggest beneficial interactions.

Other: Cimetidine: The interaction between cimetidine and chronically administered verapamil has not been studied. Variable results on clearance have been obtained in acute studies of healthy volunteers; clearance of verapamil was either reduced or unchanged.

Lithium: Pharmacokinetic and pharmacodynamic interactions between oral verapamil and lithium have been reported. The former may result in a lowering of serum lithium levels in patients receiving chronic stable oral lithium therapy. The latter may result in an increased sensitivity to the effects of lithium. Patients receiving both drugs must be monitored carefully.

Carbamazepine: Verapamil therapy may increase carbamazepine concentrations during combined therapy. This may produce carbamazepine side effects such as diplopia, headache, ataxia, or dizziness.

Rifampin: Therapy with rifampin may markedly reduce oral verapamil bioavailability.

Phenobarbital: Phenobarbital therapy may increase verapamil clearance.

Cyclosporine: Verapamil therapy may increase serum levels of cyclosporine.

Inhalation Anesthetics: Animal experiments have shown that inhalation anesthetics depress cardiovascular activity by decreasing the inward movement of calcium ions. When used concomitantly, inhalation anesthetics and calcium antagonists, such as verapamil, should be titrated carefully to avoid excessive cardiovascular depression.

Neuromuscular Blocking Agents: Clinical data and animal studies suggest that verapamil may potentiate the activity of neuromuscular blocking agents (curare-like and depolarizing). It may be necessary to decrease the dose of verapamil and/or the dose of the neuromuscular blocking agent when the drugs are used concomitantly.

Carcinogenesis, Mutagenesis, Impairment of Fertility: An 18-month toxicity study in rats, at a low multiple (sixfold) of the maximum recommended human dose, and not the maximum tolerated dose, did not suggest a tumorigenic potential. There was no evidence of a carcinogenic potential of verapamil administered in the diet of rats for 2 years at doses of 10, 35, and 120 mg/kg per day or approximately 1x, 3.5x, and 12x, respectively, the maximum recommended human daily dose (480 mg per day or 9.6 mg/kg/day).

Verapamil was not mutagenic in the Ames test in five test strains at 3 mg per plate, with or without metabolic activation.

Studies in female rats at daily dietary doses up to 5.5 times (55 mg/kg/day) the maximum recommended human dose did not show impaired fertility. Effects on male fertility have not been determined.

Pregnancy: *Pregnancy Category C:* Reproduction studies have been performed in rabbits and rats at oral doses up to 1.5 (15 mg/kg/day) and 6 (60 mg/kg/day) times the maximum recommended human daily dose, respectively, and have revealed no evidence of teratogenicity. In the rat, however, this multiple of the human dose was embryocidal and retarded fetal growth and development, probably because of adverse maternal effects reflected in reduced weight gains of the dams. This oral dose has also been shown to cause hypotension in rats. There are no adequate and well-controlled studies in pregnant women. Because animal reproduction studies are not always predictive of human response, this drug should be used during pregnancy only if clearly needed. Verapamil crosses the placental barrier and can be detected in umbilical vein blood at delivery.

Labor and Delivery: It is not known whether the use of verapamil during labor or delivery has immediate or delayed adverse effects on the fetus, or whether it prolongs the duration of labor or increases the need for forceps delivery or other obstetric intervention. Such adverse experiences have not been reported in the literature, despite a long history of use of verapamil HCl in Europe in the treatment of cardiac side effects of beta-adrenergic agonist agents used to treat premature labor.

Nursing Mothers: Verapamil is excreted in human milk. Because of the potential for adverse reactions in nursing infants from verapamil, nursing should be discontinued while verapamil is administered.

Pediatric Use: Safety and efficacy of verapamil in children below the age of 18 years have not been established.

Animal Pharmacology and/or Animal Toxicology: In chronic animal toxicology studies verapamil causes lenticular and/or suture line changes at 30 mg/kg/day or greater and frank cataracts at 62.5 mg/kg/day or greater in the beagle dog but not the rat. Development of cataracts due to verapamil has not been reported in man.

ADVERSE REACTIONS

Serious adverse reactions are uncommon when verapamil HCl therapy is initiated with upward dose titration within the recommended single and total daily dose. See **WARNINGS** for discussion of heart failure, hypotension, elevated liver enzymes, AV block, and rapid ventricular response.

Reversible (upon discontinuation of verapamil) nonobstructive, paralytic ileus has been infrequently reported in association with the use of verapamil.

In clinical trials involving 285 hypertensive patients on VERELAN *verapamil HCl* for greater than 1 week the following adverse reactions were reported in greater than 1.0% of the patients: Constipation 7.4%, Headache 5.3%, Dizziness 4.2%, Lethargy 3.2%, Dyspepsia 2.5%, Rash 1.4%, Ankle Edema 1.4%, Sleep Disturbance 1.4%, Myalgia 1.1%.

In clinical trials of other formulations of verapamil HCl (N=4,954) the following reactions have occurred at rates greater than 1.0%: Constipation 7.3%, Dizziness 3.3%, Nausea 2.7%, Hypotension 2.5%, Edema 1.9%, Headache 2.2%, Rash 1.2%, CHF/Pulmonary Edema 1.8%, Fatigue 1.7%, Bradycardia (HR<50/min) 1.4%, AV block-total 1°, 2°, 3° 1.2%, 2° and 3° 0.8%, Flushing 0.6%, Elevated Liver Enzymes (see **WARNINGS**).

In clinical trials related to the control of ventricular response in digitalized patients who had atrial fibrillation or atrial flutter, ventricular rate below 50/min at rest occurred in 15% of patients and asymptomatic hypotension occurred in 5% of patients.

The following reactions, reported in 1.0% or less of patients, occurred under conditions (open trials, marketing experience) where a causal relationship is uncertain; they are listed to alert the physician to a possible relationship:

Cardiovascular: angina pectoris, atrioventricular dissociation, chest pain, claudication, myocardial infarction, palpitations, purpura (vasculitis), syncope.

Digestive System: diarrhea, dry mouth, gastrointestinal distress, gingival hyperplasia.

Hemic and Lymphatic: ecchymosis or bruising.

Nervous System: cerebrovascular accident, confusion, equilibrium disorders, insomnia, muscle cramps, paresthesia, psychotic symptoms, shakiness, somnolence.

Respiratory: dyspnea.

Skin: arthralgia and rash, exanthema, hair loss, hyperkeratosis, maculae, sweating, urticaria, Stevens-Johnson syndrome, erythema multiforme.

Special Senses: blurred vision.

Urogenital: gynecomastia, impotence, increased urination, spotty menstruation.

Treatment of Acute Cardiovascular Adverse Reactions: The frequency of cardiovascular adverse reactions which require therapy is rare; hence, experience with their treatment is limited. Whenever severe hypotension or complete AV block occur following oral administration of verapamil, the appropriate emergency measures should be applied immediately, eg, intravenously administered isoproterenol HCl, levarterenol bitartrate, atropine (all in the usual doses), or calcium gluconate (10% solution). In patients with hypertrophic cardiomyopathy (IHSS), alpha-adrenergic agents (phenylephrine, metaraminol bitartrate or methoxamine) should be used to maintain blood pressure, and isoproterenol and levarterenol should be avoided. If further support is necessary, inotropic agents (dopamine or dobutamine) may be administered. Actual treatment and dosage should depend on the severity and the clinical situation and the judgment and experience of the treating physician.

OVERDOSAGE

Treatment of overdosage should be supportive. Beta-adrenergic stimulation or parenteral administration of calcium solutions may increase calcium ion flux across the slow channel, and have been used effectively in treatment of deliberate overdosage with verapamil. Verapamil cannot be removed by hemodialysis. Clinically significant hypotensive reactions or high degree AV block should be treated with vasopressor agents or cardiac pacing, respectively. Asystole should be handled by the usual measures including cardiopulmonary resuscitation.

DOSAGE AND ADMINISTRATION

Essential Hypertension: The dose of VERELAN *verapamil HCl* should be individualized by titration. The usual daily dose of sustained-release verapamil, VERELAN, in clinical trials has been 240 mg given by mouth once daily in the morning. However, initial doses of 120 mg a day may be warranted in patients who may have an increased response to verapamil (eg, elderly, small people, etc). Upward titration should be based on therapeutic efficacy and safety evaluated approximately 24 hours after dosing. The antihypertensive effects of VERELAN are evident within the first week of therapy.

If adequate response is not obtained with 120 mg of VERELAN, the dose may be titrated upward in the following manner: (a) 180 mg in the morning, (b) 240 mg in the morning, (c) 360 mg in the morning, (d) 480 mg in the morning. VERELAN sustained-release capsules are for once-a-day administration. When switching from immediate-release verapamil to VERELAN capsules, the same total daily dose of VERELAN capsules can be used.

As with immediate-release verapamil, dosages of VERELAN capsules should be individualized and titration may be needed in some patients.

HOW SUPPLIED

VERELAN *verapamil HCl sustained-release pellet-filled capsules* are supplied in three dosage strengths:

120 mg—Two-piece, size 2 hard gelatin capsule (yellow cap/yellow body), printed with Lederle above V8 on left and VERELAN above 120 mg on right side of the capsule in black ink, supplied as follows:

NDC 0005-2490-23—Bottle of 100s

180 mg—Two-piece, size 1 elongated hard gelatin capsule (light grey cap/yellow body), printed with Lederle above V7 on left and VERELAN above 180 mg on right side of the capsule in black ink, supplied as follows:

NDC 0005-2489-23—Bottle of 100s

240 mg—Two-piece, size 0 hard gelatin capsule (dark blue cap/yellow body), printed with Lederle above V9 on left and VERELAN above 240 mg on right side of the capsule in black ink, supplied as follows:

NDC 0005-2491-23—Bottle of 100s

STORE AT CONTROLLED ROOM TEMPERATURE 15°–30°C (59°–86°F), PROTECTED FROM MOISTURE. Dispense in tight, light-resistant container as defined in USP.

Manufactured for
LEDERLE LABORATORIES DIVISION
American Cyanamid Company
Pearl River, NY 10965
by
ELAN PHARMACEUTICAL RESEARCH CORP.
Gainesville, GA 30501

Rev. 1/92
20801-92

Shown in Product Identification Section, page 416

ZINCON® Pyrithione Zinc 1%   OTC
[*zink'on*]
Dandruff Shampoo

(See PDR For Nonprescription Drugs.)

EDUCATIONAL MATERIAL

Brochures
Product: FiberCon® Bulk-Forming Fiber Laxative
Patient Information Brochure
For consumer information on *Digestive Regularity*, write to:
    Lederle Promotional Center
    Bradley Corporate Park
    2200 Bradley Hill Road
    Blauvelt, NY 10913
Slide Lecture Kits
Product: MAXZIDE® *75 triamterene/50 mg hydrochlorothiazide*
Practical Considerations in Hypertension
Electrolytes in Cardiovascular Disease: Focus on Magnesium
Free Samples available for MAXZIDE
Call: 800-L-E-D-E-R-L-E—between the hours of 8:30 am and 4:30 pm

---

Lemmon Company
See GATE Pharmaceuticals

Eli Lilly and Company
LILLY CORPORATE CENTER
INDIANAPOLIS, IN 46285

LEGEND

ADD-Vantage®—*Vials and Diluent Containers, Abbott*
Disket®—*Dispersible Tablet, Lilly*
Enseal®—*Enteric-Release Tablet, Lilly*
Faspak®—*Flexible Plastic Bag, Lilly*
Gelseal®—*Filled Elastic Capsule, Lilly*
Identi-Code®—*Formula Identification Code, Lilly*
Identi-Dose®—*Unit Dose Medication, Lilly*
Pulvule®—*Filled Gelatin Capsule, Lilly*
Redi Vial®—*Dual Compartment Vial, Lilly*
℞Pak—*Prescription Package, Lilly*
Solvet®—*Soluble Tablet, Lilly*
Traypak™—*Multivial Carton, Lilly*

IDENTI-CODE® Index
(formula identification code, Lilly)
Provides Positive Product Identification
A letter-number symbol, a 4-digit number, the name of the product, the strength of the product, or a combination of these appears on each Lilly capsule and most tablets and on each label of pediatric liquids, powders for oral suspension, and suppositories. The letter/number or 4-digit number identifies the product.

Identi-Code®	Product Name

Coated Tablets

C51   **Darvocet-N® 50**
Composition (Each Coated Tablet): Propoxyphene napsylate, 50 mg; acetaminophen, 325 mg (USP)

C53   **Darvon-N®**
Composition (Each Coated Tablet): Propoxyphene Napsylate, USP, 100 mg

C63   **Darvocet-N® 100**
Composition (Each Coated Tablet): Propoxyphene napsylate, 100 mg; acetaminophen, 650 mg (USP)

Pulvules®

F04   **Seromycin®**
Composition (Each Pulvule®): Cycloserine, USP, 250 mg

F40   **Seconal® Sodium**
Composition (Each Pulvule®): Secobarbital Sodium, USP, 100 mg

F65   **Tuinal®**
Composition (Each Pulvule®): Secobarbital sodium, 50 mg; amobarbital sodium, 50 mg (USP)

F66   **Tuinal®**
Composition (Each Pulvule®): Secobarbital sodium, 100 mg; amobarbital sodium, 100 mg (USP)

H03   **Darvon®**
Composition (Each Pulvule®): Propoxyphene Hydrochloride, USP, 65 mg

H17   **Aventyl® HCl**
Composition (Each Pulvule®): Nortriptyline Hydrochloride, USP, 10 mg (equiv. to base)

H19   **Aventyl® HCl**
Composition (Each Pulvule®): Nortriptyline Hydrochloride, USP, 25 mg (equiv. to base)

3061   **Ceclor®**
Composition (Each Pulvule®): Cefaclor, USP, 250 mg

3062   **Ceclor®**
Composition (Each Pulvule®): Cefaclor, USP, 500 mg

3111   **Darvon® Compound-65**
Composition (Each Pulvule®): Propoxyphene hydrochloride, 65 mg; aspirin, 389 mg; caffeine, 32.4 mg

3125   **Vancocin® HCl**
Composition (Each Pulvule®): Vancomycin hydrochloride, 125 mg

3126   **Vancocin® HCl**
Composition (Each Pulvule®): Vancomycin hydrochloride, 250 mg

3144   **Axid®**
Composition (Each Pulvule®): Nizatidine, 150 mg

3145   **Axid®**
Composition (Each Pulvule®): Nizatidine, 300 mg

3170   **Lorabid™**
Composition (Each Pulvule®): Loracarbef, 200 mg

Compressed Tablets

J10   **Codeine Sulfate**
Composition (Each Compressed Tablet): Codeine Sulfate, USP, 30 mg

J11   **Codeine Sulfate**
Composition (Each Compressed Tablet): Codeine Sulfate, USP, 60 mg

J31   **Phenobarbital**
Composition (Each Compressed Tablet): Phenobarbital, USP, 15 mg

J32   **Phenobarbital**
Composition (Each Compressed Tablet): Phenobarbital, USP, 30 mg

J33   **Phenobarbital**
Composition (Each Compressed Tablet): Phenobarbital, USP, 100 mg

J37   **Phenobarbital**
Composition (Each Compressed Tablet): Phenobarbital, USP, 60 mg

J52   **Diethylstilbestrol**
Composition (Each Compressed Tablet): Diethylstilbestrol, USP, 1 mg

J54   **Diethylstilbestrol**
Composition (Each Compressed Tablet): Diethylstilbestrol, USP, 5 mg

J60   **Crystodigin®**
Composition (Each Compressed Tablet): Digitoxin, USP, 0.1 mg

J64   **Dolophine® Hydrochloride**
Composition (Each Compressed Tablet): Methadone Hydrochloride, USP, 5 mg

J72   **Dolophine® Hydrochloride**
Composition (Each Compressed Tablet): Methadone Hydrochloride, USP, 10 mg

J94   **Tapazole®**
Composition (Each Compressed Tablet): Methimazole, USP, 5 mg

J95   **Tapazole®**
Composition (Each Compressed Tablet): Methimazole, USP, 10 mg

T23   **Sodium Chloride**
Composition (Each Compressed Tablet): Sodium Chloride, USP, 2.25 g

T24   **Sodium Chloride**
Composition (Each Compressed Tablet): Sodium Chloride, USP, 1 g

Continued on next page

---

* **Identi-Code® symbol. This product information was prepared in June 1992. Current information on these and other products of Eli Lilly and Company may be obtained by direct inquiry to Lilly Research Laboratories, Lilly Corporate Center, Indianapolis, Indiana 46285, (317) 276-3714.**

Lilly—Cont.

T29	**Sodium Bicarbonate**	Composition (Each Compressed Tablet): Sodium Bicarbonate, USP, 10 grs (648 mg)
T35	**Calcium Carbonate**	Composition (Each Compressed Tablet): Calcium Carbonate, USP, Aromatic, 10 grs (648 mg)
U03	**Dymelor®**	Composition (Each Compressed Tablet): Acetohexamide, USP, 250 mg
U07	**Dymelor®**	Composition (Each Compressed Tablet): Acetohexamide, USP, 500 mg
U53	**Methadone Hydrochloride**	Composition (Each Disket®): Methadone Hydrochloride, USP, 40 mg
4131	**Permax®**	Composition (Each Compressed Tablet): Pergolide mesylate, 0.05 mg
4133	**Permax®**	Composition (Each Compressed Tablet): Pergolide mesylate, 0.25 mg
4135	**Permax®**	Composition (Each Compressed Tablet): Pergolide mesylate, 1 mg

UNIT-DOSE PACKAGING

Identi-Dose® (unit dose medication, Lilly)
Reverse-Numbered Package
Closed-circuit control of medication from pharmacy to nurse to patient and return. Simplifies counting and dispensing whether in single-unit or prescription-size quantities. Fits into any dispensing system for ready identification and legibility, better inventory control, protection from contamination, easier handling and recording under Medicare, prevention of drug loss through pilferage or spilling, better control of Federal Controlled Substances, and less chance of medication errors.
The following products are available through normal channels of supply:

Identi-Dose® (ID100)
Pulvules®
No.
ℂ 365 Darvon®, 65 mg
ℂ 369 Darvon® Compound-65
387 Aventyl® HCl, 10 mg
389 Aventyl® HCl, 25 mg
3061 Ceclor®, 250 mg
3062 Ceclor®, 500 mg
Tablets
No.
ℂ 1883 Darvon-N®, 100 mg
ℂ 1890 Darvocet-N® 50
ℂ 1893 Darvocet-N® 100

Reverse-Numbered Package (RN500)
Pulvules®
No.
Tablets
No.
ℂ 1893 Darvocet-N® 100

Single-Cut Identi-Dose® (ID500)
Tablets
No.
ℂ 1893 Darvocet-N® 100

ℂ, ℂ, ℂ Federal Controlled Substances.

AXID®   ℞
[ak'sid]
(nizatidine capsules USP)
PULVULES®

DESCRIPTION

Axid® (Nizatidine, USP, Lilly) is a histamine H_2-receptor antagonist. Chemically, it is N-[2-[[[2-[(dimethylamino)methyl]-4-thiazolyl] methyl] thio]-ethyl]-N'-methyl-2-nitro-1,1-ethenediamine.
The structural formula is as follows:

O₂NCH=C with NHCH₃ group and NHCH₂CH₂SCH₂ group connected to thiazole ring with CH₂N(CH₃)₂ substituent

Nizatidine

Nizatidine has the empirical formula $C_{12}H_{21}N_5O_2S_2$ representing a molecular weight of 331.45. It is an off-white to buff crystalline solid that is soluble in water. Nizatidine has a bitter taste and mild sulfur-like odor. Each Pulvule® (capsule) contains for oral administration gelatin, pregelatinized starch, silicone, starch, titanium dioxide, yellow iron oxide, 150 mg (0.45 mmol) or 300 mg (0.91 mmol) of nizatidine, and other inactive ingredients. The 150-mg Pulvule also contains magnesium stearate, and the 300-mg Pulvule also contains carboxymethylcellulose sodium, povidone, red iron oxide, and talc.

CLINICAL PHARMACOLOGY

Axid® (Nizatidine, Lilly) is a competitive, reversible inhibitor of histamine at the histamine H_2 receptors, particularly those in the gastric parietal cells.
Antisecretory Activity—1. Effects on Acid Secretion: Axid significantly inhibited nocturnal gastric acid secretion for up to 12 hours. Axid also significantly inhibited gastric acid secretion stimulated by food, caffeine, betazole, and pentagastrin (Table 1).

Table 1
Effect of Oral Axid on Gastric Acid Secretion

Time After Dose (h)	% Inhibition of Gastric Acid Output by Dose (mg)				
	20–50	75	100	150	300
Nocturnal	Up to 10	57		73		90
Betazole	Up to 3		93		100	99
Pentagastrin	Up to 6		25		64	67
Meal	Up to 4	41	64		98	97
Caffeine	Up to 3		73		85	96

2. Effects on Other Gastrointestinal Secretions—Pepsin: Oral administration of 75 to 300 mg of Axid did not affect pepsin activity in gastric secretions. Total pepsin output was reduced in proportion to the reduced volume of gastric secretions.
Intrinsic Factor: Oral administration of 75 to 300 mg of Axid increased betazole-stimulated secretion of intrinsic factor.
Serum Gastrin: Axid had no effect on basal serum gastrin. No rebound of gastrin secretion was observed when food was ingested 12 hours after administration of Axid.
3. Other Pharmacologic Actions:
a. Hormones: Axid was not shown to affect the serum concentrations of gonadotropins, prolactin, growth hormone, antidiuretic hormone, cortisol, triiodothyronine, thyroxin, testosterone, 5α-dihydrotestosterone, androstenedione, or estradiol.
b. Axid had no demonstrable antiandrogenic action.
4. Pharmacokinetics—The absolute oral bioavailability of nizatidine exceeds 70%. Peak plasma concentrations (700 to 1,800 µg/L for a 150-mg dose and 1,400 to 3,600 µg/L for a 300-mg dose) occur from 0.5 to 3 hours following the dose. A concentration of 1,000 µg/L is equivalent to 3 µmol/L; a dose of 300 mg is equivalent to 905 µmoles. Plasma concentrations 12 hours after administration are less than 10 µg/L. The elimination half-life is 1 to 2 hours, plasma clearance is 40 to 60 L/h, and the volume of distribution is 0.8 to 1.5 L/kg. Because of the short half-life and rapid clearance of nizatidine, accumulation of the drug would not be expected in individuals with normal renal function who take either 300 mg once daily at bedtime or 150 mg twice daily. Axid exhibits dose proportionality over the recommended dose range.
The oral bioavailability of nizatidine is unaffected by concomitant ingestion of propantheline. Antacids consisting of aluminum and magnesium hydroxides with simethicone decrease the absorption of nizatidine by about 10%. With food, the AUC and C_{max} increase by approximately 10%.
In humans, less than 7% of an oral dose is metabolized as N2-monodesmethylnizatidine, an H_2-receptor antagonist, which is the principal metabolite excreted in the urine. Other

likely metabolites are the N2-oxide (less than 5% of the dose) and the S-oxide (less than 6% of the dose).
More than 90% of an oral dose of nizatidine is excreted in the urine within 12 hours. About 60% of an oral dose is excreted as unchanged drug. Renal clearance is about 500 mL/min, which indicates excretion by active tubular secretion. Less than 6% of an administered dose is eliminated in the feces. Moderate to severe renal impairment significantly prolongs the half-life and decreases the clearance of nizatidine. In individuals who are functionally anephric, the half-life is 3.5 to 11 hours, and the plasma clearance is 7 to 14 L/h. To avoid accumulation of the drug in individuals with clinically significant renal impairment, the amount and/or frequency of doses of Axid should be reduced in proportion to the severity of dysfunction (see Dosage and Administration).
Approximately 35% of nizatidine is bound to plasma protein, mainly to α_1-acid glycoprotein. Warfarin, diazepam, acetaminophen, propantheline, phenobarbital, and propranolol did not affect plasma protein binding of nizatidine in vitro.
Clinical Trials—1. Active Duodenal Ulcer: In multicenter, double-blind, placebo-controlled studies in the United States, endoscopically diagnosed duodenal ulcers healed more rapidly following administration of Axid, 300 mg h.s. or 150 mg b.i.d., than with placebo (Table 2). Lower doses, such as 100 mg h.s., had slightly lower effectiveness. [See table below.]
2. Maintenance of Healed Duodenal Ulcer:
Treatment with a reduced dose of Axid has been shown to be effective as maintenance therapy following healing of active duodenal ulcers. In multicenter, double-blind, placebo-controlled studies conducted in the United States, 150 mg of Axid taken at bedtime resulted in a significantly lower incidence of duodenal ulcer recurrence in patients treated for up to 1 year (Table 3).

Table 3
Percentage of Ulcers Recurring by 3, 6, and 12 Months in Double-Blind Studies Conducted in the United States

Month	Axid, 150 mg h.s.	Placebo
3	13% (28/208)*	40% (82/204)
6	24% (45/188)*	57% (106/187)
12	34% (57/166)*	64% (112/175)

*$P < 0.001$ as compared with placebo.
3. Gastroesophageal Reflux Disease (GERD):
In 2 multicenter, double-blind, placebo-controlled clinical trials performed in the United States and Canada, Axid was more effective than placebo in improving endoscopically diagnosed esophagitis and in healing erosive and ulcerative esophagitis.
In patients with erosive or ulcerative esophagitis, 150 mg b.i.d. of Axid given to 88 patients compared with placebo in 98 patients in Study 1 yielded a higher healing rate at 3 weeks (16% vs 7%) and at 6 weeks (32% vs 16%, $P < 0.05$). Of 99 patients on Axid and 94 patients on placebo, Study 2 at the same dosage yielded similar results at 6 weeks (21% vs 11%, $P < 0.05$) and at 12 weeks (29% vs 13%, $P < 0.01$).
In addition, relief of associated heartburn was greater in patients treated with Axid. Patients treated with Axid consumed fewer antacids than did patients treated with placebo.

INDICATIONS AND USAGE

Axid® (Nizatidine, Lilly) is indicated for up to 8 weeks for the treatment of active duodenal ulcer. In most patients, the ulcer will heal within 4 weeks.
Axid is indicated for maintenance therapy for duodenal ulcer patients, at a reduced dosage of 150 mg h.s. after healing of an active duodenal ulcer. The consequences of continuous therapy with Axid for longer than 1 year are not known.
Axid is indicated for up to 12 weeks for the treatment of endoscopically diagnosed esophagitis, including erosive and ulcerative esophagitis, and associated heartburn due to GERD.

CONTRAINDICATION

Axid® (Nizatidine, Lilly) is contraindicated in patients with known hypersensitivity to the drug. Because cross sensitiv-

Table 2
Healing Response of Ulcers to Axid® (Nizatidine, Lilly)

	Axid						Placebo	
	300 mg h.s.			150 mg b.i.d.				
	Number Entered	Healed/ Evaluable		Number Entered	Healed/ Evaluable		Number Entered	Healed/ Evaluable
STUDY 1								
Week 2				276	93/265	(35%)*	279	55/260 (21%)
Week 4					198/259	(76%)*		95/243 (39%)
STUDY 2								
Week 2	108	24/103	(23%)*	106	27/101	(27%)*	101	9/93 (10%)
Week 4		65/97	(67%)*		66/97	(68%)*		24/84 (29%)
STUDY 3								
Week 2	92	22/90	(24%)†				98	13/92 (14%)
Week 4		52/85	(61%)*					29/88 (33%)
Week 8		68/83	(82%)*					39/79 (49%)

* $P < 0.01$ as compared with placebo.
† $P < 0.05$ as compared with placebo.

ity in this class of compounds has been observed, H_2-receptor antagonists, including Axid, should not be administered to patients with a history of hypersensitivity to other H_2-receptor antagonists.

PRECAUTIONS

General—1. Symptomatic response to nizatidine therapy does not preclude the presence of gastric malignancy.
2. Because nizatidine is excreted primarily by the kidney, dosage should be reduced in patients with moderate to severe renal insufficiency (*see* Dosage and Administration).
3. Pharmacokinetic studies in patients with hepatorenal syndrome have not been done. Part of the dose of nizatidine is metabolized in the liver. In patients with normal renal function and uncomplicated hepatic dysfunction, the disposition of nizatidine is similar to that in normal subjects.
Laboratory Tests—False-positive tests for urobilinogen with Multistix® may occur during therapy with nizatidine.
Drug Interactions—No interactions have been observed between Axid® (Nizatidine, Lilly) and theophylline, chlordiazepoxide, lorazepam, lidocaine, phenytoin, and warfarin. Axid does not inhibit the cytochrome P-450-linked drug-metabolizing enzyme system; therefore, drug interactions mediated by inhibition of hepatic metabolism are not expected to occur. In patients given very high doses (3,900 mg) of aspirin daily, increases in serum salicylate levels were seen when nizatidine, 150 mg b.i.d., was administered concurrently.
Carcinogenesis, Mutagenesis, Impairment of Fertility—A 2-year oral carcinogenicity study in rats with doses as high as 500 mg/kg/day (about 80 times the recommended daily therapeutic dose) showed no evidence of a carcinogenic effect. There was a dose-related increase in the density of enterochromaffin-like (ECL) cells in the gastric oxyntic mucosa. In a 2-year study in mice, there was no evidence of a carcinogenic effect in male mice, although hyperplastic nodules of the liver were increased in the high-dose males as compared with placebo. Female mice given the high dose of Axid (2,000 mg/kg/day, about 330 times the human dose) showed marginally statistically significant increases in hepatic carcinoma and hepatic nodular hyperplasia with no numerical increase seen in any of the other dose groups. The rate of hepatic carcinoma in the high-dose animals was within the historical control limits seen for the strain of mice used. The female mice were given a dose larger than the maximum tolerated dose, as indicated by excessive (30%) weight decrement as compared with concurrent controls and evidence of mild liver injury (transaminase elevations). The occurrence of a marginal finding at high dose only in animals given an excessive and somewhat hepatotoxic dose, with no evidence of a carcinogenic effect in rats, male mice, and female mice (given up to 360 mg/kg/day, about 60 times the human dose), and a negative mutagenicity battery are not considered evidence of a carcinogenic potential for Axid.
Axid was not mutagenic in a battery of tests performed to evaluate its potential genetic toxicity, including bacterial mutation tests, unscheduled DNA synthesis, sister chromatid exchange, the mouse lymphoma assay, chromosome aberration tests, and a micronucleus test.
In a 2-generation, perinatal and postnatal fertility study in rats, doses of nizatidine up to 650 mg/kg/day produced no adverse effects on the reproductive performance of parental animals or their progeny.
Pregnancy—Teratogenic Effects—Pregnancy Category C—Oral reproduction studies in rats at doses up to 300 times the human dose and in Dutch Belted rabbits at doses up to 55 times the human dose revealed no evidence of impaired fertility or teratogenic effect; but, at a dose equivalent to 300 times the human dose, treated rabbits had abortions, decreased number of live fetuses, and depressed fetal weights. On intravenous administration to pregnant New Zealand White rabbits, nizatidine at 20 mg/kg produced cardiac enlargement, coarctation of the aortic arch, and cutaneous edema in 1 fetus, and at 50 mg/kg, it produced ventricular anomaly, distended abdomen, spina bifida, hydrocephaly, and enlarged heart in 1 fetus. There are, however, no adequate and well-controlled studies in pregnant women. It is also not known whether nizatidine can cause fetal harm when administered to a pregnant woman or can affect reproduction capacity. Nizatidine should be used during pregnancy only if the potential benefit justifies the potential risk to the fetus.
Nursing Mothers—Studies conducted in lactating women have shown that 0.1% of the administered oral dose of nizatidine is secreted in human milk in proportion to plasma concentrations. Because of the growth depression in pups reared by lactating rats treated with nizatidine, a decision should be made whether to discontinue nursing or discontinue the drug, taking into account the importance of the drug to the mother.
Pediatric Use—Safety and effectiveness in children have not been established.
Use in Elderly Patients—Ulcer healing rates in elderly patients are similar to those in younger age groups. The incidence rates of adverse events and laboratory test abnormalities are also similar to those seen in other age groups. Age alone may not be an important factor in the disposition of

nizatidine. Elderly patients may have reduced renal function (*see* Dosage and Administration).

ADVERSE REACTIONS

Worldwide, controlled clinical trials of nizatidine included over 6,000 patients given nizatidine in studies of varying durations. Placebo-controlled trials in the United States and Canada included over 2,600 patients given nizatidine and over 1,700 given placebo. Among the adverse events in these placebo-controlled trials, anemia (0.2% vs 0%) and urticaria (0.5% vs 0.1%) were significantly more common in the nizatidine group.
Incidence in Placebo-Controlled Clinical Trials in the United States and Canada—Table 4 lists adverse events that occurred at a frequency of 1% or more among nizatidine-treated patients who participated in placebo-controlled trials. The cited figures provide some basis for estimating the relative contribution of drug and nondrug factors to the side effect incidence rate in the population studied.

Table 4
INCIDENCE OF TREATMENT-EMERGENT
ADVERSE EVENTS IN PLACEBO-CONTROLLED
CLINICAL TRIALS
IN THE UNITED STATES AND CANADA

System/Adverse Event*	Percentage of Patients Reporting Event	
	Nizatidine (N=2,694)	Placebo (N=1,729)
Body as a Whole		
Headache	16.6	15.6
Abdominal pain	7.5	12.5
Pain	4.2	3.8
Asthenia	3.1	2.9
Back pain	2.4	2.6
Chest pain	2.3	2.1
Infection	1.7	1.1
Fever	1.6	2.3
Surgical procedure	1.4	1.5
Injury, accident	1.2	0.9
Digestive		
Diarrhea	7.2	6.9
Nausea	5.4	7.4
Flatulence	4.9	5.4
Vomiting	3.6	5.6
Dyspepsia	3.6	4.4
Constipation	2.5	3.8
Dry mouth	1.4	1.3
Nausea and vomiting	1.2	1.9
Anorexia	1.2	1.6
Gastrointestinal disorder	1.1	1.2
Tooth disorder	1.0	0.8
Musculoskeletal		
Myalgia	1.7	1.5
Nervous		
Dizziness	4.6	3.8
Insomnia	2.7	3.4
Abnormal dreams	1.9	1.9
Somnolence	1.9	1.6
Anxiety	1.6	1.4
Nervousness	1.1	0.8
Respiratory		
Rhinitis	9.8	9.6
Pharyngitis	3.3	3.1
Sinusitis	2.4	2.1
Cough, increased	2.0	2.0
Skin and Appendages		
Rash	1.9	2.1
Pruritus	1.7	1.3
Special Senses		
Amblyopia	1.0	0.9

* Events reported by at least 1% of nizatidine-treated patients are included.

A variety of less common events were also reported; it was not possible to determine whether these were caused by nizatidine.
Hepatic—Hepatocellular injury, evidenced by elevated liver enzyme tests (SGOT [AST], SGPT [ALT], or alkaline phosphatase), occurred in some patients and was possibly or probably related to nizatidine. In some cases there was marked elevation of SGOT/SGPT enzymes (greater than 500 IU/L) and, in a single instance, SGPT was greater than 2,000 IU/L. The overall rate of occurrences of elevated liver enzymes and elevations to 3 times the upper limit of normal, however, did not significantly differ from the rate of liver enzyme abnormalities in placebo-treated patients. All abnormalities were reversible after discontinuation of Axid® (Nizatidine, Lilly). Since market introduction, hepatitis and jaundice have been reported. Rare cases of cholestatic or mixed hepatocellular and cholestatic injury with jaundice have been reported with reversal of the abnormalities after discontinuation of Axid.

Cardiovascular—In clinical pharmacology studies, short episodes of asymptomatic ventricular tachycardia occurred in 2 individuals administered Axid and in 3 untreated subjects.
CNS—Rare cases of reversible mental confusion have been reported.
Endocrine—Clinical pharmacology studies and controlled clinical trials showed no evidence of antiandrogenic activity due to Axid. Impotence and decreased libido were reported with similar frequency by patients who received Axid and by those given placebo. Rare reports of gynecomastia occurred.
Hematologic—Anemia was reported significantly more frequently in nizatidine- than in placebo-treated patients. Fatal thrombocytopenia was reported in a patient who was treated with Axid and another H_2-receptor antagonist. On previous occasions, this patient had experienced thrombocytopenia while taking other drugs. Rare cases of thrombocytopenic purpura have been reported.
Integumental—Urticaria was reported significantly more frequently in nizatidine- than in placebo-treated patients. Rash and exfoliative dermatitis were also reported.
Hypersensitivity—As with other H_2-receptor antagonists, rare cases of anaphylaxis following administration of nizatidine have been reported. Rare episodes of hypersensitivity reactions (eg, bronchospasm, laryngeal edema, rash, and eosinophilia) have been reported.
Other—Hyperuricemia unassociated with gout or nephrolithiasis was reported. Eosinophilia, fever, and nausea related to nizatidine administration have been reported.

OVERDOSAGE

Overdoses of Axid® (Nizatidine, Lilly) have been reported rarely. The following is provided to serve as a guide should such an overdose be encountered.
Signs and Symptoms—There is little clinical experience with overdosage of Axid in humans. Test animals that received large doses of nizatidine have exhibited cholinergic-type effects, including lacrimation, salivation, emesis, miosis, and diarrhea. Single oral doses of 800 mg/kg in dogs and of 1,200 mg/kg in monkeys were not lethal. Intravenous median lethal doses in the rat and mouse were 301 mg/kg and 232 mg/kg respectively.
Treatment—To obtain up-to-date information about the treatment of overdose, a good resource is your certified Regional Poison Control Center. Telephone numbers of certified poison control centers are listed in the *Physicians' Desk Reference (PDR)*. In managing overdosage, consider the possibility of multiple drug overdoses, interaction among drugs, and unusual drug kinetics in your patient.
If overdosage occurs, use of activated charcoal, emesis, or lavage should be considered along with clinical monitoring and supportive therapy. The ability of hemodialysis to remove nizatidine from the body has not been conclusively demonstrated; however, due to its large volume of distribution, nizatidine is not expected to be efficiently removed from the body by this method.

DOSAGE AND ADMINISTRATION

Active Duodenal Ulcer—The recommended oral dosage for adults is 300 mg once daily at bedtime. An alternative dosage regimen is 150 mg twice daily.
Maintenance of Healed Duodenal Ulcer—The recommended oral dosage for adults is 150 mg once daily at bedtime.
Gastroesophageal Reflux Disease—The recommended oral dosage in adults for the treatment of erosions, ulcerations, and associated heartburn is 150 mg twice daily.
Dosage Adjustment for Patients With Moderate to Severe Renal Insufficiency—The dose for patients with renal dysfunction should be reduced as follows:

Active Duodenal Ulcer or GERD

Ccr	Dose
20–50 mL/min	150 mg daily
< 20 mL/min	150 mg every other day

Maintenance Therapy

Ccr	Dose
20–50 mL/min	150 mg every other day
< 20 mL/min	150 mg every 3 days

Some elderly patients may have creatinine clearances of less than 50 mL/min, and, based on pharmacokinetic data in patients with renal impairment, the dose for such patients should be reduced accordingly. The clinical effects of this dosage reduction in patients with renal failure have not been evaluated.

Continued on next page

• Identi-Code® symbol. This product information was prepared in June 1992. Current information on these and other products of Eli Lilly and Company may be obtained by direct inquiry to Lilly Research Laboratories, Lilly Corporate Center, Indianapolis, Indiana 46285, (317) 276-3714.

Lilly—Cont.

HOW SUPPLIED

℞Pulvules*:

150 mg, pale yellow and dark yellow (No. 3144)—(RxPak† of 60) NDC 0002-3144-60

300 mg, pale yellow and brown (No. 3145)—(Rx Pak of 30) NDC 0002-3145-30

* Pulvules® (filled gelatin capsules, Lilly)

† Rx Pak (prescription package, Lilly)

Store at controlled room temperature, 59° to 86°F (15° to 30°C).

[101591]

Shown in Product Identification Section, page 416

BREVITAL® SODIUM ©

[*brĕv 'ĭ-tăl sō 'dĭ-ŭm*]

(methohexital sodium)

For Injection, USP

For Intravenous Use

> **WARNING**
>
> **This drug should be administered by persons qualified in the use of intravenous anesthetics. Cardiac life support equipment must be immediately available during use of methohexital.**

DESCRIPTION

Brevital® Sodium (Methohexital Sodium for Injection, USP, Lilly) is 2,4,6 (1H,3H,5H)-Pyrimidinetrione, 1-methyl-5- (1-methyl-2-pentynyl) -5- (2-propenyl)-,(±)-, monosodium salt.

Methohexital sodium for injection is a freeze-dried, sterile, nonpyrogenic mixture of methohexital sodium and anhydrous sodium carbonate added as a buffer,which is prepared from an aqueous solution of methohexital, sodium hydroxide, and sodium carbonate. It contains not less than 90% and not more than 110% of the labeled amount of $C_{14}H_{17}N_2NaO_3$. This mixture is ordinarily intended to be reconstituted so as to contain 1% methohexital sodium in Sterile Water for Injection for direct intravenous injection or 0.2% methohexital sodium in 5% dextrose injection (or 0.9% sodium chloride injection) for administration by continuous intravenous drip. The pH of the 1% solution is between 10 and 11; the pH of the 0.2% solution in 5% dextrose is between 9.5 and 10.5

Methohexital sodium is a rapid, ultrashort-acting barbiturate anesthetic. It occurs as a white, crystalline powder that is freely soluble in water.

CLINICAL PHARMACOLOGY

Compared with thiamylal and thiopental, methohexital is at least twice as potent on a weight basis, and its duration of action is only about half as long. Although the metabolic fate of methohexital in the body is not clear, the drug does not appear to concentrate in fat depots to the extent that other barbiturate anesthetics do. Thus, cumulative effects are fewer and recovery is more rapid with methohexital than with thiobarbiturates. In experimental animals, the drug cannot be detected in the blood 24 hours after administration.

Methohexital differs chemically from the established barbiturate anesthetics in that it contains no sulfur. Little analgesia is conferred by barbiturates; their use in the presence of pain may result in excitation.

Intravenous administration of methohexital results in rapid uptake by the brain (within 30 seconds) and rapid induction of sleep. With single doses, the rate of redistribution determines duration of pharmacologic effect. Metabolism occurs in the liver through demethylation and oxidation. Side-chain oxidation is the most important biotransformation involved in termination of biologic activity. Excretion occurs via the kidneys through glomerular filtration.

INDICATIONS AND USAGE

Brevital® Sodium (Methohexital Sodium for Injection, USP, Lilly) can be used as follows:

1. For intravenous induction of anesthesia prior to the use of other general anesthetic agents.
2. For intravenous induction of anesthesia and as an adjunct to subpotent inhalational anesthetic agents (such as nitrous oxide in oxygen) for short surgical procedures; Brevital Sodium may be given by infusion or intermittent injection.
3. For use along with other parenteral agents, usually narcotic analgesics, to supplement subpotent inhalational anesthetic agents (such as nitrous oxide in oxygen) for longer surgical procedures.
4. As intravenous anesthesia for short surgical, diagnostic, or therapeutic procedures associated with minimal painful stimuli (*see* Precautions).
5. As an agent for inducing a hypnotic state.

CONTRAINDICATIONS

Brevital® Sodium (Methohexital Sodium for Injection, USP, Lilly) is contraindicated in patients in whom general anesthesia is contraindicated, in those with latent or manifest porphyria, or in patients with a known hypersensitivity to barbiturates.

WARNINGS

See boxed Warning.

AS WITH ALL POTENT ANESTHETIC AGENTS AND ADJUNCTS, THIS DRUG SHOULD BE ADMINISTERED ONLY BY THOSE TRAINED IN THE ADMINISTRATION OF GENERAL ANESTHESIA, THE MAINTENANCE OF A PATENT AIRWAY AND VENTILATION, AND THE MANAGEMENT OF CARDIOVASCULAR DEPRESSION ENCOUNTERED DURING ANESTHESIA AND SURGERY.

Because the liver is involved in demethylation and oxidation of methohexital and because barbiturates may enhance preexisting circulatory depression, severe hepatic dysfunction, severe cardiovascular instability, or a shock-like condition may be reason for selecting another induction agent.

Psychomotor seizures may be elicited in susceptible individuals.[1]

Prolonged administration may result in cumulative effects, including extended somnolence, protracted unconsciousness, and respiratory and cardiovascular depression. Respiratory depression in the presence of an impaired airway may lead to hypoxia, cardiac arrest, and death.

The CNS-depressant effect of Brevital® Sodium (Methohexital Sodium for Injection, USP, Lilly) may be additive with that of other CNS depressants, including ethyl alcohol and propylene glycol.

DANGER OF INTRA-ARTERIAL INJECTION—Unintended intra-arterial injection of barbiturate solutions may be followed by the production of platelet aggregates and thrombosis, starting in arterioles distal to the site of injection. The resulting necrosis may lead to gangrene, which may require amputation. The first sign in conscious patients may be a complaint of fiery burning that roughly follows the distribution path of the injected artery; if noted, the injection should be stopped immediately and the situation reevaluated. Transient blanching may or may not be noted very early; blotchy cyanosis and dark discoloration may then be the first sign in anesthetized patients. There is no established treatment other than prevention. The following should be considered prior to injection.

1. The extent of injury is related to concentration. Concentrations of 1% methohexital will usually suffice; higher concentrations should ordinarily be avoided.
2. Check the infusion to ensure that the catheter is in the lumen of a vein before injection. Injection through a running intravenous infusion may enhance the possibility of detecting arterial placement; however, it should be remembered that the characteristic bright-red color of arterial blood is often altered by contact with drugs. The possibility of aberrant arteries should always be considered.

Postinjury arterial injection of vasodilators and/or arterial infusion of parenteral fluids are generally regarded to be of no value in altering outcome. Animal experiments and published individual case reports concerned with a variety of arteriolar irritants, including barbiturates, suggest that 1 or more of the following may be of benefit in reducing the area of necrosis:

1. Arterial injection of heparin at the site of injury, followed by systemic anticoagulation.
2. Sympathetic blockade (or brachial plexus blockade in the arm).
3. Intra-arterial glucocorticoid injection at the site of injury, followed by systemic steroids.
4. A recent case report (nonbarbiturate injury) suggests that intra-arterial urokinase may promote fibrinolysis, even if administered late in treatment.

If extravasation is noted during injection of methohexital, the injection should be discontinued until the situation is remedied. Local irritation may result from extravasation; subcutaneous swelling may also serve as a sign of arterial or periarterial placement of the catheter.

PRECAUTIONS

General—Maintenance of a patent airway and adequacy of ventilation must be ensured during induction and maintenance of anesthesia with methohexital sodium solution. Laryngospasm is common during induction with all barbiturates and may be due to a combination of secretions and accentuated reflexes following induction or may result from painful stimuli during light anesthesia. Transient apnea may be noted during induction, which may impair pulmonary ventilation; the duration of apnea may be longer than that produced by other barbiturate anesthetics. Cardiorespiratory arrest may occur. Intravenous administration of Brevital® Sodium (Methohexital Sodium for Injection, USP, Lilly) is often associated with hiccups, coughing, and/or muscle twitching, which may also impair pulmonary ventilation.

Following induction, temporary hypotension and tachycardia may occur.

Recovery from methohexital anesthesia is rapid and smooth. The incidence of postoperative nausea and vomting is low if the drug is administered to fasting patients. Postanesthetic shivering has occurred in a few instances.

The usual precautions taken with any barbiturate anesthetic should be observed with Brevital Sodium. The drug should be used with caution in patients with asthma, obstructive pulmonary disease, severe hypertension or hypotension, myocardial disease, congestive heart failure, severe anemia, or extreme obesity.

Methohexital sodium should be used with extreme caution in patients in status asthmaticus.

Caution should be exercised in debilitated patients or in those with impaired function of respiratory, circulatory, renal, hepatic, or endocrine systems.

Information for Patients—When appropriate, patients should be instructed as to the hazards of drowsiness that may follow use of Brevital® Sodium (Methohexital Sodium for Injection, USP, Lilly). Outpatients should be released in the company of another individual, and no skilled activities, such as operating machinery or driving a motor vehicle, should be engaged in for 8 to 12 hours.

Laboratory Tests—BSP and liver function studies may be influenced by administration of a single dose of barbiturates.

Drug Interactions—Barbiturates may influence the absorption and elimination of other concomitantly used drugs, such as diphenylhydantoin, halothane, anticoagulants, corticosteroids, ethyl alcohol,[2] and propylene glycol-containing solutions.

Carcinogenesis, Mutagenesis, Impairment of Fertility—Studies in animals to evaluate the carcinogenic and mutagenic potential of Brevital Sodium have not been conducted. Reproduction studies in animals have revealed no evidence of impaired fertility.[3]

Usage in Pregnancy—*Pregnancy Category B*—Reproduction studies have been performed in rabbits and rats at doses up to 4 and 7 times the human dose respectively and have revealed no evidence of harm to the fetus due to methohexital sodium.[3] There are, however, no adequate and well-controlled studies in pregnant women. Because animal reproduction studies are not always predictive of human response, this drug should be used during pregnancy only if clearly needed.

Labor and Delivery—Brevital Sodium has been used in cesarean section delivery but, because of its solubility and lack of protein binding, it readily and rapidly traverses the placenta.

Nursing Mothers—Caution should be exercised when Brevital Sodium is administered to a nursing woman.

Usage in Children—Safety and effectiveness in children have not been established.

ADVERSE REACTIONS

Side effects associated with Brevital® Sodium (Methohexital Sodium for Injection, USP, Lilly) are extensions of pharmacologic effects and include:

Cardiovascular—Circulatory depression, thrombophlebitis, hypotension, peripheral vascular collapse, and convulsions in association with cardiorespiratory arrest

Respiratory—Respiratory depression (including apnea), cardiorespiratory arrest, laryngospasm, bronchospasm, hiccups, and dyspnea

Neurologic—Skeletal muscle hyperactivity (twitching), injury to nerves adjacent to injection site, and seizures

Psychiatric—Emergence delirium, restlessness, and anxiety may occur, especially in the presence of postoperative pain

Gastrointestinal—Nausea, emesis, and abdominal pain

Allergic—Erythema, pruritus, urticaria, and cases of anaphylaxis have been reported

Other—Other adverse reactions include pain at injection site, salivation, headache, and rhinitis

DRUG ABUSE AND DEPENDENCE

Controlled Substance—Brevital® Sodium (Methohexital Sodium for Injection, USP, Lilly) is a Schedule IV drug. Brevital Sodium may be habit-forming.

OVERDOSAGE

Signs and Symptoms—The onset of toxicity following an overdose of intravenously administered methohexital will be within seconds of the infusion. If methohexital is administered rectally or is ingested, the onset of toxicity may be delayed. The manifestations of an ultrashort-acting barbiturate in overdose include central nervous system depression,

1. Rockoff MA, Goudsouzian NG: Seizures induced by methohexital. *Anesthesiology* 1981; 54:333.

2. Hansten PD: *Drug Interactions,* ed 4. Philadelphia, Lea & Febiger, 1979, p 224.

3. Gibson, WR, et al: Reproduction and teratology studies in rats and rabbits using sodium methohexital, Lilly Toxicology Laboratories, Eli Lilly and Company, Greenfield, Indiana 46140, unpublished manuscript, August 1970.

Preparation of Solutions of Brevital® Sodium (Methohexital Sodium for Injection, USP)

Preparation of Solution —FOLLOW DILUTING INSTRUCTIONS EXACTLY.
Diluents —DO NOT USE DILUENTS CONTAINING BACTERIOSTATS.
Sterile Water for Injection is the preferred diluent.
Five percent Dextrose Injection or 0.9% Sodium Chloride Injection may be used.
(Brevital Sodium is not compatible with Lactated Ringer's Injection.)
Dilution Instructions —For a 1% solution (10 mg/mL), contents of vials should be diluted as follows:
Vials No. 660 (500 mg)—add 50 mL of diluent
Vials No. 760 (500 mg)—add 50 mL of accompanying diluent

Vial No.	Amount of Diluent to Be Added to the Vial	For 1% Solution Dilute to
663 (2.5 g)	15 mL	250 mL
659 (5 g)	30 mL	500 mL

When the first dilution is made with Vials No. 663 or No. 659, the solution in the vial will be yellow. When further diluted to make a 1% solution, it must be *clear and colorless* or should not be used.
Solutions of Brevital Sodium should be freshly prepared and used promptly. Reconstituted solutions of Brevital Sodium are chemically stable at room temperature for 24 hours.

respiratory depression, hypotension, loss of peripheral vascular resistance, and muscular hyperactivity ranging from twitching to convulsive-like movements. Other findings may include convulsions and allergic reactions. Following massive exposure to any barbiturate, pulmonary edema, circulatory collapse with loss of peripheral vascular tone, and cardiac arrest may occur.

Treatment—To obtain up-to-date information about the treatment of overdose, a good resource is your certified Regional Poison Control Center. Telephone numbers of certified poison control centers are listed in the *Physicians' Desk Reference (PDR)*. In managing overdosage, consider the possibility of multiple drug overdoses, interaction among drugs, and unusual drug kinetics in your patient.

Establish an airway and ensure oxygenation and ventilation. Resuscitative measures should be initiated promptly. For hypotension, intravenous fluids should be administered and the patient's legs raised. If desirable increase in blood pressure is not obtained, vasopressor and/or inotropic drugs may be used as dictated by the clinical situation.

For convulsions, diazepam intravenously and phenytoin may be required. If the seizures are refractory to diazepam and phenytoin, general anesthesia and paralysis with a neuromuscular blocking agent may be necessary.

Protect the patient's airway and support ventilation and perfusion. Meticulously monitor and maintain, within acceptable limits, the patient's vital signs, blood gases, serum electrolytes, etc. Absorption of drugs from the gastrointestinal tract may be decreased by giving activated charcoal, which, in many cases, is more effective than emesis or lavage; consider charcoal instead of or in addition to gastric emptying. Repeated doses of charcoal over time may hasten elimination of some drugs that have been absorbed. Safeguard the patient's airway when employing gastric emptying or charcoal.

DOSAGE AND ADMINISTRATION

Preanesthetic medication is generally advisable. Brevital® Sodium (Methohexital Sodium for Injection, USP, Lilly) may be used with any of the recognized preanesthetic medications, but the phenothiazines are less satisfactory than the combination of an opiate and a belladonna derivative.

Facilities for assisting respiration and administering oxygen are necessary adjuncts for intravenous anesthesia. Since cardiorespiratory arrest may occur, patients should be observed carefully during and after use of Brevital Sodium. Resuscitative equipment (ie, intubation and cardioversion equipment, oxygen, suction, and a secure intravenous line) and personnel qualified in its use must be immediately available. [See table above.]

For continuous drip anesthesia, prepare a 0.2% solution by adding 500 mg of Brevital Sodium to 250 mL of diluent. For this dilution, either 5% glucose solution or isotonic (0.9%) sodium chloride solution is recommended instead of distilled water in order to avoid extreme hypotonicity.

Administration—Brevital® Sodium (Methohexital Sodium for Injection, USP, Lilly) is administered intravenously in a concentration of no higher than 1%. Higher concentrations markedly increase the incidence of muscular movements and irregularities in respiration and blood pressure. Dosage is highly individualized; the drug should be administered only by those completely familiar with its quantitative differences from other barbiturate anesthetics.

Brevital Sodium may be dissolved in Sterile Water for Injection, 5% Dextrose Injection, or Sodium Chloride Injection. For induction of anesthesia, a 1% solution is administered at a rate of about 1 mL/5 seconds. Gaseous anesthetics and/or skeletal muscle relaxants may be administered concomitantly. The dose required for induction may range from 50 to 120 mg or more but averages about 70 mg. The induction dose usually provides anesthesia for 5 to 7 minutes.

The usual dosage in adults ranges from 1 to 1.5 mg/kg. Data on dosage requirements in children are not available.

Maintenance of anesthesia may be accomplished by intermittent injections of the 1% solution or, more easily, by continuous intravenous drip of a 0.2% solution. Intermittent injections of about 20 to 40 mg (2 to 4 mL of a 1% solution) may be given as required, usually every 4 to 7 minutes. For continuous drip, the average rate of administration is about 3 mL of a 0.2% solution/minute (1 drop/second). The rate of flow must be individualized for each patient. For longer surgical procedures, gradual reduction in the rate of administration is recommended (*see* discussion of prolonged administration in Warnings). Other parenteral agents, usually narcotic analgesics, are ordinarily employed along with Brevital Sodium during longer procedures.

Parenteral drug products should be inspected visually for particulate matter and discoloration prior to administration, whenever solution and container permit.

COMPATIBILITY INFORMATION

Solutions of Brevital® Sodium (Methohexital Sodium for Injection, USP, Lilly) should not be mixed in the same syringe or administered simultaneously during intravenous infusion through the same needle with acid solutions, such as atropine sulfate, Metubine® Iodide (Metocurine Iodide Injection, USP, Lilly), and succinylcholine chloride. Alteration of pH may cause free barbituric acid to be precipitated. Solubility of the soluble sodium salts of barbiturates, including Brevital Sodium, is maintained only at a relatively high (basic) pH.

Because of numerous requests from anesthesiologists for information regarding the chemical compatibility of these mixtures, the following chart contains information obtained from compatibility studies in which a 1% solution of Brevital Sodium was mixed with therapeutic amounts of agents whose solutions have a low (acid) pH. [See table below.]

Solutions of Brevital Sodium are incompatible with silicone and should not be allowed to come in contact with rubber stoppers or parts of disposable syringes that have been treated with silicone.

Compatibility of Brevital® Sodium (Methohexital Sodium for Injection, USP) with Solutions Having a Low pH

Active Ingredient	Potency per mL	Volume Used	Physical Change: Immediate	15 min	30 min	1 h
Brevital Sodium	10 mg	10 mL			CONTROL	
Atropine sulfate	1/150 gr	1 mL	None	Haze		
Atropine sulfate	1/100 gr	1 mL	None	Ppt	Ppt	
Succinylcholine chloride	0.5 mg	4 mL	None	None	Haze	
Succinylcholine chloride	1 mg	4 mL	None	None	Haze	
Metocurine iodide	0.5 mg	4 mL	None	None	Ppt	
Metocurine iodide	1 mg	4 mL	None	None	Ppt	
Scopolamine hydrobromide	1/120 gr	1 mL	None	None	None	Haze
Tubocurarine chloride	3 mg	4 mL	None	Haze		

HOW SUPPLIED

The vials may be stored at room temperature, 77°F (25°C or below). The expiration period for the vials is 2 years.

(Ⓒ) *Vials* Brevital® Sodium (Methohexital Sodium for Injection, USP)* are supplied as follows:

500 mg (with 30 mg anhydrous sodium carbonate), 50-mL size, multiple dose (No. 660)—(1s) NDC 0002-1446-01; (25s) NDC 0002-1446-25

500 mg (with 30 mg anhydrous sodium carbonate), 50-mL size, multiple dose, with one 50-mL vial Sterile Water for Injection (No. 760)—(1s) NDC 0002-1465-01

2.5 g (with 150 mg anhydrous sodium carbonate) (No. 663)—NDC 0002-1448-25

5 g (with 300 mg anhydrous sodium carbonate) (No. 659)—(1s) NDC 0002-1445-01

*In crystalline form.

[020392]

CAPASTAT® SULFATE ℞

[*kăp'a-stăt sŭl'fāt*]
(capreomycin sulfate)
Sterile, USP
Not for Pediatric Use

Warnings

This preparation is for intramuscular use only.

The use of Capastat® Sulfate (Sterile Capreomycin Sulfate, USP, Lilly) in patients with renal insufficiency or preexisting auditory impairment must be undertaken with great caution, and the risk of additional cranial nerve VIII impairment or renal injury should be weighed against the benefits to be derived from therapy. *Refer to* Animal Pharmacology *for additional information.*

Since other parenteral antituberculosis agents (streptomycin, viomycin) also have similar and sometimes irreversible toxic effects, particularly on cranial nerve VIII and renal function, simultaneous administration of these agents with Capastat Sulfate is not recommended. Use with nonantituberculosis drugs (polymyxin A sulfate, colistin sulfate, amikacin, gentamicin, tobramycin, vancomycin, kanamycin, and neomycin) having ototoxic or nephrotoxic potential should be undertaken only with great caution.

Usage in Pregnancy—The safety of the use of Capastat Sulfate in pregnancy has not been determined.

Pediatric Usage—Safety of the use of Capastat Sulfate in infants and children has not been established.

DESCRIPTION

Capastat® Sulfate (Sterile Capreomycin Sulfate, USP, Lilly) is a polypeptide antibiotic isolated from *Streptomyces capreolus*. It is a complex of 4 microbiologically active components, which have been characterized in part; however, complete structural determination of all the components has not been established.

Capreomycin is supplied as the disulfate salt and is soluble in water. In complete solution, it is almost colorless.

Each vial contains the equivalent of 1 g capreomycin activity.

CLINICAL PHARMACOLOGY

Human Pharmacology—Capreomycin is not absorbed in significant quantities from the gastrointestinal tract and must be administered parenterally. In 2 studies of 10 patients each, peak serum concentrations following 1 g of capreomycin given intramuscularly were achieved 1 to 2 hours after administration, and average peak levels reached were 28 and 32 μg/mL respectively (range, 20 to 47 μg/mL). Low serum concentrations were present at 24 hours. However, 1 g of capreomycin daily for 30 days or more produced no significant accumulation in subjects with normal renal function. Two patients with marked reduction of renal function had high serum concentrations 24 hours after administration of the drug. When a 1-g dose of capreomycin was given intramuscularly to normal volunteers, 52% was excreted in the urine within 12 hours.

Paper chromatographic studies indicated that capreomycin is excreted essentially unaltered. Urine concentrations averaged 1.68 μg/mL (average urine volume, 228 mL) during the 6 hours following a 1-g dose.

Continued on next page

*** Identi-Code® symbol. This product information was prepared in June 1992. Current information on these and other products of Eli Lilly and Company may be obtained by direct inquiry to Lilly Research Laboratories, Lilly Corporate Center, Indianapolis, Indiana 46285, (317) 276-3714.**

Lilly—Cont.

Microbiology—Capreomycin is active against strains of *Mycobacterium tuberculosis* found in humans.

Susceptibility Tests—The in vitro susceptibility of strains of *M. tuberculosis* to capreomycin varies with the media and techniques employed. In general, the minimum inhibitory concentrations for *M. tuberculosis* are lowest in liquid media that are free of egg protein (7H10 or Dubos) and range from 1 to 5 μg/mL when the indirect method is used. Comparable inhibitory concentrations are obtained when 7H10 agar is used for direct susceptibility testing. When indirect susceptibility tests are performed on standard tube slants with 7H10 media, susceptible strains are inhibited by 10 to 25 μg/mL capreomycin. Egg-containing media, such as Löwenstein-Jensen or ATS, require concentrations of 25 to 50 μg/mL to inhibit susceptible strains.

Cross-Resistance—Frequent cross-resistance occurs between capreomycin and viomycin. Varying degrees of cross-resistance between capreomycin and kanamycin and neomycin have been reported. No cross-resistance has been observed between capreomycin and isoniazid, aminosalicylic acid, cycloserine, streptomycin, ethionamide, or ethambutol.

INDICATIONS AND USAGE

Capastat® Sulfate (Sterile Capreomycin Sulfate, USP, Lilly), which is to be used concomitantly with other appropriate antituberculosis agents, is indicated in pulmonary infections caused by capreomycin-susceptible strains of *M. tuberculosis* when the primary agents (isoniazid, rifampin, ethambutol, aminosalicylic acid, and streptomycin) have been ineffective or cannot be used because of toxicity or the presence of resistant tubercle bacilli.

Susceptibility studies should be performed to determine the presence of a capreomycin-susceptible strain of *M. tuberculosis.*

CONTRAINDICATION

Capastat® Sulfate (Sterile Capreomycin Sulfate, USP, Lilly) is contraindicated in patients who are hypersensitive to it.

PRECAUTIONS

General—Audiometric measurements and assessment of vestibular function should be performed prior to initiation of therapy with Capastat® Sulfate (Sterile Capreomycin Sulfate, USP, Lilly) and at regular intervals during treatment. Renal injury, with tubular necrosis, elevation of the blood urea nitrogen (BUN) or serum creatinine, and abnormal urinary sediment, has been noted. Slight elevation of the BUN and serum creatinine has been observed in a significant number of patients receiving prolonged therapy. The appearance of casts, red cells, and white cells in the urine has been noted in a high percentage of these cases. Elevation of the BUN above 30 mg/100 mL or any other evidence of decreasing renal function with or without a rise in BUN levels calls for careful evaluation of the patient, and the dosage should be reduced or the drug completely withdrawn. The clinical significance of abnormal urine sediment and slight elevation in the BUN (or serum creatinine) observed during long-term therapy with Capastat Sulfate has not been established.

The peripheral neuromuscular blocking action that has been attributed to other polypeptide antibiotics (colistin sulfate, polymyxin A sulfate, paromomycin, and viomycin) and to aminoglycoside antibiotics (streptomycin, dihydrostreptomycin, neomycin, and kanamycin) has been studied with Capastat Sulfate. A partial neuromuscular blockade was demonstrated after large intravenous doses of Capastat Sulfate. This action was enhanced by ether anesthesia (as has been reported for neomycin) and was antagonized by neostigmine.

Caution should be exercised in the administration of antibiotics, including Capastat Sulfate, to any patient who has demonstrated some form of allergy, particularly to drugs.

Laboratory Tests—Regular tests of renal function should be made throughout the period of treatment, and reduced dosage should be employed in patients with known or suspected renal impairment.

Renal function studies should be made both before therapy with Capastat Sulfate is started and on a weekly basis during treatment.

Since hypokalemia may occur during therapy, serum potassium levels should be determined frequently.

Drug Interactions—For neuromuscular blocking action of this drug, see Precautions, General.

Carcinogenesis, Mutagenesis, Impairment of Fertility—Studies have not been performed to determine potential for carcinogenicity, mutagenicity, or impairment of fertility.

Usage in Pregnancy—Pregnancy Category C—Capastat Sulfate has been shown to be teratogenic in rats when given in doses 3½ times the human dose. There are no adequate and well-controlled studies in pregnant women. Capastat Sulfate should be used during pregnancy only if the potential benefit justifies the potential risk to the fetus (see boxed Warnings and Animal Pharmacology).

DILUTION TABLE FOR CAPASTAT® SULFATE (Sterile Capreomycin Sulfate, USP)

Diluent Added to 1-g, 10-mL Vial	Volume of Capastat Sulfate Solution	Concentration (Approx)
2.15 mL	2.85 mL	350 mg*/mL
2.63 mL	3.33 mL	300 mg*/mL
3.3 mL	4 mL	250 mg*/mL
4.3 mL	5 mL	200 mg*/mL

*Equivalent to capreomycin activity.

Nursing Mothers—It is not known whether this drug is excreted in human milk. Because many drugs are excreted in human milk, caution should be exercised when Capastat Sulfate is administered to a nursing woman.

Pediatric Use—Safety and effectiveness in children have not been established (*see boxed* Warnings).

ADVERSE REACTIONS

Nephrotoxicity—In 36% of 722 patients treated with Capastat® Sulfate (Sterile Capreomycin Sulfate, USP, Lilly), elevation of the BUN above 20 mg/100 mL has been observed. In many instances, there was also depression of PSP excretion and abnormal urine sediment. In 10% of this series, the BUN elevation exceeded 30 mg/100 mL.

Toxic nephritis was reported in 1 patient with tuberculosis and portal cirrhosis who was treated with Capastat Sulfate (1 g) and aminosalicylic acid daily for 1 month. This patient developed renal insufficiency and oliguria and died. Autopsy showed subsiding acute tubular necrosis.

Electrolyte disturbances resembling Bartter's syndrome have been reported in 1 patient.

Ototoxicity—Subclinical auditory loss was noted in approximately 11% of 722 patients undergoing treatment with Capastat Sulfate. This was a 5- to 10-decibel loss in the 4,000- to 8,000-CPS range. Clinically apparent hearing loss occurred in 3% of the 722 subjects. Some audiometric changes were reversible. Other cases with permanent loss were not progressive following withdrawal of Capastat Sulfate.

Tinnitus and vertigo have occurred.

Liver—Serial tests of liver function have demonstrated a decrease in BSP excretion without change in AST (SGOT) or ALT (SGPT) in the presence of preexisting liver disease. Abnormal results in liver function tests have occurred in many persons receiving Capastat Sulfate in combination with other antituberculosis agents that also are known to cause changes in hepatic function. The role of Capastat Sulfate in producing these abnormalities is not clear; however, periodic determinations of liver function are recommended.

Blood—Leukocytosis and leukopenia have been observed. The majority of patients treated have had eosinophilia exceeding 5% while receiving daily injections of Capastat Sulfate. This has subsided with reduction of the dosage of Capastat Sulfate to 2 or 3 g weekly.

Pain and induration at the injection site have been observed. Excessive bleeding at the injection site has been reported. Sterile abscesses have been noted. Rare cases of thrombocytopenia have been reported.

Hypersensitivity—Urticaria and maculopapular skin rashes associated in some cases with febrile reactions have been reported when Capastat Sulfate and other antituberculosis drugs were given concomitantly.

OVERDOSAGE

Signs and Symptoms—Nephrotoxicity following the parenteral administration of Capastat® Sulfate (Sterile Capreomycin Sulfate, USP, Lilly) is most closely related to the area under the curve of the serum concentration versus time graph. The elderly patient, patients with abnormal renal function or dehydration, and patients receiving other nephrotoxic drugs are at much greater risk for developing acute tubular necrosis.

Damage to the auditory and vestibular divisions of cranial nerve VIII has been associated with Capastat Sulfate given to patients with abnormal renal function or dehydration and in those receiving medications with additive auditory toxicities. These patients often experience dizziness, tinnitus, vertigo, and a loss of high-tone acuity.

Neuromuscular blockage or respiratory paralysis may occur following rapid intravenous administration.

If capreomycin is ingested, toxicity would be unlikely because it is poorly absorbed (less then 1%) from an intact gastrointestinal system.

Hypokalemia, hypocalcemia, hypomagnesemia, and an electrolyte disturbance resembling Bartter's syndrome have been reported to occur in patients with capreomycin toxicity. The subcutaneous median lethal dose in mice was 514 mg/kg.

Treatment—To obtain up-to-date information about the treatment of overdose, a good resource is your certified Regional Poison Control Center. Telephone numbers of certified poison control centers are listed in the *Physicians' Desk Reference (PDR)*. In managing overdosage, consider the possibility of multiple drug overdoses, interaction among drugs, and unusual drug kinetics in your patient.

Protect the patient's airway and support ventilation and perfusion. Meticulously monitor and maintain, within acceptable limits, the patient's vital signs, blood gases, serum electrolytes, etc. Absorption of drugs from the gastrointestinal tract may be decreased by giving activated charcoal, which, in many cases, is more effective than emesis or lavage; consider charcoal instead of or in addition to gastric emptying. Repeated doses of charcoal over time may hasten elimination of some drugs that have been absorbed. Safeguard the patient's airway when employing gastric emptying or charcoal.

Patients who have received an overdose of capreomycin and have normal renal function should be carefully hydrated to maintain a urine output of 3 to 5 mL/kg/h. Fluid balance, electrolytes, and creatinine clearance should be carefully monitored.

Hemodialysis may be effectively used to remove capreomycin in patients with significant renal disease.

DOSAGE AND ADMINISTRATION

Capastat® Sulfate (Sterile Capromycin Sulfate, USP, Lilly) is for intramuscular use only.

Capastat Sulfate should be given by deep intramuscular injection into a large muscle mass, since superficial injection may be associated with increased pain and the development of sterile abscesses.

Capastat Sulfate should be dissolved in 2 mL of 0.9% Sodium Chloride Injection or Sterile Water for Injection. Two to 3 minutes should be allowed for complete dissolution. For administration of a 1-g dose, the entire contents of the vial should be given. For dosages lower than 1 g, the accompanying dilution table may be used. [See table above.]

The solution may acquire a pale straw color and darken with time, but this is not associated with loss of potency or the development of toxicity. After reconstitution, solutions of Capastat Sulfate may be stored for 48 hours at room temperature and up to 14 days under refrigeration.

Capreomycin is always administered in combination with at least 1 other antituberculosis agent to which the patient's strain of tubercle bacilli is susceptible. The usual dose is 1 g daily (not to exceed 20 mg/kg/day) given intramuscularly for

Table 1. Estimated Dosages to Attain Mean Steady-State Serum Capreomycin Concentration of 10 μg/mL (Based on Creatinine Clearance)

CrCl (mL/min)	Capreomycin Clearance (L/kg/h × 10⁻²)	Half-life (hours)	Dose[a] (mg/kg) for the Following Dosing Intervals 24h	48h	72h
0	0.54	55.5	1.29	2.58	3.87
10	1.01	29.4	2.43	4.87	7.30
20	1.49	20.0	3.58	7.16	10.7
30	1.97	15.1	4.72	9.45	14.2
40	2.45	12.2	5.87	11.7	
50	2.92	10.2	7.01	14.0	
60	3.40	8.8	8.16		
80	4.35	6.8	10.4[b]		
100	5.31	5.6	12.7[b]		
110	5.78	5.2	13.9[b]		

a—For patients with renal impairment, initial maintenance dose estimates are given for optional dosing intervals; longer dosing intervals are expected to provide greater peak and lower trough serum capreomycin levels than shorter dosing intervals.

b—The usual dosage for patients with *normal* renal function is 1,000 mg daily, not to exceed 20 mg/kg/day, for 60 to 120 days, then 1,000 mg 2 to 3 times weekly.

60 to 120 days, followed by 1 g intramuscularly 2 or 3 times weekly. (*Note*—Therapy for tuberculosis should be maintained for 12 to 24 months. If facilities for administering injectable medication are not available, a change to appropriate oral therapy is indicated on the patient's release from the hospital.)

Patients with reduced renal function should have dosage reduction based on creatinine clearance using the guidelines included in Table 1. These dosages are designed to achieve a mean steady-state capreomycin level of 10 μg/mL.

[See table on preceding page.]

HOW SUPPLIED

(℞) Vials:

1g,* 10-mL size (No. 718)—(1s) NDC 0002-1485-01

ANIMAL PHARMACOLOGY

In addition to renal and cranial nerve VIII toxicity demonstrated in animal toxicology studies, cataracts developed in 2 dogs on doses of 62 mg/kg and 100 mg/kg for prolonged periods.

In teratology studies, a low incidence of "wavy ribs" was noted in litters of female rats treated with daily doses of 50 mg/kg or more of capreomycin.

[030392]

* Equivalent to capreomycin activity.

CECLOR® ℞

[sē'klôr]

(cefaclor)

USP

DESCRIPTION

Ceclor® (Cefaclor, USP, Lilly) is a semisynthetic cephalosporin antibiotic for oral administration. It is chemically designated as 3-chloro-7-D-(2-phenylglycinamido)-3-cephem-4-carboxylic acid monohydrate.

Each Pulvule® contains cefaclor monohydrate equivalent to 250 mg (0.68 mmol) or 500 mg (1.36 mmol) cefaclor. The Pulvules also contain cornstarch, FD&C Blue No. 1, FD&C Red No. 3, gelatin, magnesium stearate, silicone, titanium dioxide, and other inactive ingredients. The 500-mg Pulvule also contains iron oxide.

After mixing, each 5 mL of Ceclor for Oral Suspension will contain cefaclor monohydrate equivalent to 125 mg (0.34 mmol), 187 mg (0.51 mmol), 250 mg (0.68 mmol), or 375 mg (1.0 mmol) cefaclor. The suspensions also contain cellulose, cornstarch, FD&C Red No. 40, flavors, silicone, sodium lauryl sulfate, sucrose, and xanthan gum.

CLINICAL PHARMACOLOGY

Cefaclor is well absorbed after oral administration to fasting subjects. Total absorption is the same whether the drug is given with or without food; however, when it is taken with food, the peak concentration achieved is 50% to 75% of that observed when the drug is administered to fasting subjects and generally appears from three fourths to 1 hour later. Following administration of 250-mg, 500-mg, and 1-g doses to fasting subjects, average peak serum levels of approximately 7, 13, and 23 μg/mL respectively were obtained within 30 to 60 minutes. Approximately 60% to 85% of the drug is excreted unchanged in the urine within 8 hours, the greater portion being excreted within the first 2 hours. During this 8-hour period, peak urine concentrations following the 250-mg, 500-mg, and 1-g doses were approximately 600, 900, and 1,900 μg/mL respectively. The serum half-life in normal subjects is 0.6 to 0.9 hour. In patients with reduced renal function, the serum half-life of cefaclor is slightly prolonged. In those with complete absence of renal function, the plasma half-life of the intact molecule is 2.3 to 2.8 hours. Excretion pathways in patients with markedly impaired renal function have not been determined. Hemodialysis shortens the half-life by 25% to 30%.

Microbiology—In vitro tests demonstrate that the bactericidal action of the cephalosporins results from inhibition of cell-wall synthesis. Cefaclor is active in vitro against most strains of clinical isolates of the following organisms:

Staphylococci, including coagulase-positive, coagulase-negative, and penicillinase-producing strains (when tested by in vitro methods), exhibit cross-resistance between cefaclor and methicillin

Streptococcus pyogenes (group A β-hemolytic streptococci)

Streptococcus pneumoniae

Moraxella (Branhamella) catarrhalis

Haemophilus influenzae, including β-lactamase-producing ampicillin-resistant strains

Escherichia coli

Proteus mirabilis

Klebsiella sp

Citrobacter diversus

Neisseria gonorrhoeae

Propionibacterium acnes and *Bacteroides* sp (excluding *Bacteroides fragilis*)

Peptococci

Peptostreptococci

Note: Pseudomonas sp, *Acinetobacter calcoaceticus* (formerly *Mima* sp and *Herellea* sp), and most strains of enterococci (*Enterococcus faecalis* [formerly *Streptococcus faecalis*], group D streptococci), *Enterobacter* sp, indole-positive *Proteus*, and *Serratia* sp are resistant to cefaclor. When tested by in vitro methods, staphylococci exhibit cross-resistance between cefaclor and methicillin-type antibiotics.

Disk Susceptibility Tests—Quantitative methods that require measurement of zone diameters give the most precise estimates of antibiotic susceptibility. One such procedure[1] has been recommended for use with disks for testing susceptibility to cephalothin. The currently accepted zone diameter interpretative criteria for the cephalothin disk are appropriate for determining bacterial susceptibility to cefaclor. With this procedure, a report from the laboratory of "resistant" indicates that the infecting organism is not likely to respond to therapy. A report of "intermediate susceptibility" suggests that the organism would be susceptible if the infection is confined to tissues and fluids (eg, urine) in which high antibiotic levels can be obtained or if high dosage is used.

INDICATIONS AND USAGE

Ceclor® (Cefaclor, USP, Lilly) is indicated in the treatment of the following infections when caused by susceptible strains of the designated microorganisms:

Otitis media caused by *S. pneumoniae, H. influenzae*, staphylococci, and *S. pyogenes* (group A β-hemolytic streptococci)

Lower respiratory infections, including pneumonia, caused by *S. pneumoniae, H. influenzae*, and *S. pyogenes* (group A β-hemolytic streptococci)

Upper respiratory infections, including pharyngitis and tonsillitis, caused by *S. pyogenes* (group A β-hemolytic streptococci)

Note: Penicillin is the usual drug of choice in the treatment and prevention of streptococcal infections, including the prophylaxis of rheumatic fever. Ceclor is generally effective in the eradication of streptococci from the nasopharynx; however, substantial data establishing the efficacy of Ceclor in the subsequent prevention of rheumatic fever are not available at present.

Urinary tract infections, including pyelonephritis and cystitis, caused by *E. coli, P. mirabilis, Klebsiella* sp, and coagulase-negative staphylococci

Skin and skin structure infections caused by *Staphylococcus aureus* and *S. pyogenes* (group A β-hemolytic streptococci)

Appropriate culture and susceptibility studies should be performed to determine susceptibility of the causative organism to Ceclor.

CONTRAINDICATION

Ceclor® (Cefaclor, USP, Lilly) is contraindicated in patients with known allergy to the cephalosporin group of antibiotics.

WARNINGS

IN PENICILLIN-SENSITIVE PATIENTS, CEPHALOSPORIN ANTIBIOTICS SHOULD BE ADMINISTERED CAUTIOUSLY. THERE IS CLINICAL AND LABORATORY EVIDENCE OF PARTIAL CROSS-ALLERGENICITY OF THE PENICILLINS AND THE CEPHALOSPORINS, AND THERE ARE INSTANCES IN WHICH PATIENTS HAVE HAD REACTIONS, INCLUDING ANAPHYLAXIS, TO BOTH DRUG CLASSES.

Antibiotics, including Ceclor® (Cefaclor, USP, Lilly), should be administered cautiously to any patient who has demonstrated some form of allergy, particularly to drugs.

Pseudomembranous colitis has been reported with virtually all broad-spectrum antibiotics (including macrolides, semisynthetic penicillins, and cephalosporins); therefore, it is important to consider its diagnosis in patients who develop diarrhea in association with the use of antibiotics. Such colitis may range in severity from mild to life threatening.

Treatment with broad-spectrum antibiotics alters the normal flora of the colon and may permit overgrowth of clostridia. Studies indicate that a toxin produced by *Clostridium difficile* is a primary cause of antibiotic-associated colitis.

Mild cases of pseudomembranous colitis usually respond to drug discontinuance alone. In moderate to severe cases, management should include sigmoidoscopy, appropriate bacteriologic studies, and fluid, electrolyte, and protein supplementation. When the colitis does not improve after the drug has been discontinued, or when it is severe, oral vancomycin is the drug of choice for antibiotic-associated pseudomembranous colitis produced by *C. difficile*. Other causes of colitis should be ruled out.

PRECAUTIONS

General—If an allergic reaction to Ceclor® (Cefaclor, USP, Lilly) occurs, the drug should be discontinued, and, if necessary, the patient should be treated with appropriate agents, eg, pressor amines, antihistamines, or corticosteroids.

Prolonged use of Ceclor may result in the overgrowth of nonsusceptible organisms. Careful observation of the patient is essential. If superinfection occurs during therapy, appropriate measures should be taken.

1. *Am J Clin Pathol* 1966;45:493; *Federal Register* 1974;39:19182–19184.

Positive direct Coombs' tests have been reported during treatment with the cephalosporin antibiotics. In hematologic studies or in transfusion cross-matching procedures when antiglobulin tests are performed on the minor side or in Coombs' testing of newborns whose mothers have received cephalosporin antibiotics before parturition, it should be recognized that a positive Coombs' test may be due to the drug.

Ceclor should be administered with caution in the presence of markedly impaired renal function. Since the half-life of cefaclor in anuria is 2.3 to 2.8 hours, dosage adjustments for patients with moderate or severe renal impairment are usually not required. Clinical experience with cefaclor under such conditions is limited; therefore, careful clinical observation and laboratory studies should be made.

As a result of administration of Ceclor, a false-positive reaction for glucose in the urine may occur. This has been observed with Benedict's and Fehling's solutions and also with Clinitest® tablets but not with Tes-Tape® (Glucose Enzymatic Test Strip, USP, Lilly).

Broad-spectrum antibiotics should be prescribed with caution in individuals with a history of gastrointestinal disease, particularly colitis.

Usage in Pregnancy—Pregnancy Category B—Reproduction studies have been performed in mice and rats at doses up to 12 times the human dose and in ferrets given 3 times the maximum human dose and have revealed no evidence of impaired fertility or harm to the fetus due to Ceclor. There are, however, no adequate and well-controlled studies in pregnant women. Because animal reproduction studies are not always predictive of human response, this drug should be used during pregnancy only if clearly needed.

Nursing Mothers—Small amounts of Ceclor have been detected in mother's milk following administration of single 500-mg doses. Average levels were 0.18, 0.20, 0.21, and 0.16 μg/mL at 2, 3, 4, and 5 hours respectively. Trace amounts were detected at 1 hour. The effect on nursing infants is not known. Caution should be exercised when Ceclor is administered to a nursing woman.

Usage in Children—Safety and effectiveness of this product for use in infants less than 1 month of age have not been established.

ADVERSE REACTIONS

Adverse effects considered related to therapy with Ceclor® (Cefaclor, USP, Lilly) are listed below:

Hypersensitivity reactions have been reported in about 1.5% of patients and include morbilliform eruptions (1 in 100). Pruritus, urticaria, and positive Coombs' tests each occur in less than 1 in 200 patients.

Cases of **serum-sickness-like** reactions have been reported with the use of Ceclor. These are characterized by findings of erythema multiforme, rashes, and other skin manifestations accompanied by arthritis/arthralgia, with or without fever, and differ from classic serum sickness in that there is infrequently associated lymphadenopathy and proteinuria, no circulating immune complexes, and no evidence to date of sequelae of the reaction. While further investigation is ongoing, **serum-sickness-like** reactions appear to be due to hypersensitivity and more often occur during or following a second (or subsequent) course of therapy with Ceclor. Such reactions have been reported more frequently in children than in adults with an overall occurrence ranging from 1 in 200 (0.5%) in one focused trial to 2 in 8,346 (0.024%) in overall clinical trials (with an incidence in children in clinical trials of 0.055%) to 1 in 38,000 (0.003%) in spontaneous event reports. Signs and symptoms usually occur a few days after initiation of therapy and subside within a few days after cessation of therapy; occasionally these reactions have resulted in hospitalization, usually of short duration (median hospitalization = two to three days, based on postmarketing surveillance studies). In those requiring hospitalization, the symptoms have ranged from mild to severe at the time of admission with more of the severe reactions occurring in children. Antihistamines and glucocorticoids appear to enhance resolution of the signs and symptoms. No serious sequelae have been reported.

More severe hypersensitivity reactions, including Stevens-Johnson syndrome, toxic epidermal necrolysis, and anaphylaxis, have been reported rarely. Anaphylaxis may be more common in patients with a history of penicillin allergy.

Continued on next page

• **Identi-Code® symbol. This product information was prepared in June 1992. Current information on these and other products of Eli Lilly and Company may be obtained by direct inquiry to Lilly Research Laboratories, Lilly Corporate Center, Indianapolis, Indiana 46285, (317) 276-3714.**

Lilly—Cont.

Gastrointestinal symptoms occur in about 2.5% of patients and include diarrhea (1 in 70).

Symptoms of pseudomembranous colitis may appear either during or after antibiotic treatment. Nausea and vomiting have been reported rarely. As with some penicillins and some other cephalosporins, transient hepatitis and cholestatic jaundice have been reported rarely.

Other effects considered related to therapy included eosinophilia (1 in 50 patients), genital pruritus or vaginitis (less than 1 in 100 patients), and, rarely, thrombocytopenia or reversible interstitial nephritis.

Causal Relationship Uncertain —CNS —Rarely, reversible hyperactivity, nervousness, insomnia, confusion, hypertonia, dizziness, and somnolence have been reported.

Transitory abnormalities in clinical laboratory test results have been reported. Although they were of uncertain etiology, they are listed below to serve as alerting information for the physician.

Hepatic —Slight elevations of AST (SGOT), ALT (SGPT), or alkaline phosphatase values (1 in 40).

Hematopoietic —As has also been reported with other β-lactam antibiotics, transient lymphocytosis, leukopenia, and, rarely, hemolytic anemia and reversible neutropenia of possible clinical significance.

There have been rare reports of increased prothrombin time with or without clinical bleeding in patients receiving Ceclor and Coumadin concomitantly.

Renal —Slight elevations in BUN or serum creatinine (less than 1 in 500) or abnormal urinalysis (less than 1 in 200).

OVERDOSAGE

Signs and Symptoms —The toxic symptoms following an overdose of cefaclor may include nausea, vomiting, epigastric distress, and diarrhea. The severity of the epigastric distress and the diarrhea are dose related. If other symptoms are present, it is probable that they are secondary to an underlying disease state, an allergic reaction, or the effects of other intoxication.

Treatment —To obtain up-to-date information about the treatment of overdose, a good resource is your certified Regional Poison Control Center. Telephone numbers of certified poison control centers are listed in the *Physicians' Desk Reference* (*PDR*). In managing overdosage, consider the possibility of multiple drug overdoses, interaction among drugs, and unusual drug kinetics in your patient.

Unless 5 times the normal dose of cefaclor has been ingested, gastrointestinal decontamination will not be necessary.

Protect the patient's airway and support ventilation and perfusion. Meticulously monitor and maintain, within acceptable limits, the patient's vital signs, blood gases, serum electrolytes, etc. Absorption of drugs from the gastrointestinal tract may be decreased by giving activated charcoal, which, in many cases, is more effective than emesis or lavage; consider charcoal instead of or in addition to gastric emptying. Repeated doses of charcoal over time may hasten elimination of some drugs that have been absorbed. Safeguard the patient's airway when employing gastric emptying or charcoal.

Forced diuresis, peritoneal dialysis, hemodialysis, or charcoal hemoperfusion have not been established as beneficial for an overdose of cefaclor.

DOSAGE AND ADMINISTRATION

Ceclor® (Cefaclor, USP, Lilly) is administered orally.

Adults —The usual adult dosage is 250 mg every 8 hours. For more severe infections (such as pneumonia) or those caused by less susceptible organisms, doses may be doubled.

Children —The usual recommended daily dosage for children is 20 mg/kg/day in divided doses every 8 hours.

In more serious infections, otitis media, and infections caused by less susceptible organisms, 40 mg/kg/day are recommended, with a maximum dosage of 1 g/day.

Ceclor Suspension

Child's Weight	125 mg/5 mL	250 mg/5 mL
20 mg/kg/day		
9 kg	½ tsp t.i.d.	
18 kg	1 tsp t.i.d.	½ tsp t.i.d.
40 mg/kg/day		
9 kg	1 tsp t.i.d.	½ tsp t.i.d.
18 kg		1 tsp t.i.d.

B.I.D. Treatment Option—For the treatment of otitis media and pharyngitis, the total daily dosage may be divided and administered every 12 hours.

[See table top of next column.]

Ceclor may be administered in the presence of impaired renal function. Under such a condition, the dosage usually is unchanged (*see* Precautions).

Ceclor Suspension

Child's Weight	187 mg/5 mL	375 mg/5 mL
20 mg/kg/day (Pharyngitis)		
9 kg	½ tsp b.i.d.	
18 kg	1 tsp b.i.d.	½ tsp b.i.d.
40 mg/kg/day (Otitis Media)		
9 kg	1 tsp b.i.d.	½ tsp b.i.d.
18 kg		1 tsp b.i.d.

In the treatment of β-hemolytic streptococcal infections, a therapeutic dosage of Ceclor should be administered for at least 10 days.

HOW SUPPLIED

℞ Pulvules:

250 mg, purple and white (No. 3061)—(RxPak* of 15) NDC 0002-3061-15; (100s) NDC 0002-3061-02; (ID†100) NDC 0002-3061-33

500 mg, purple and gray (No. 3062)—(RxPak of 15) NDC 0002-3062-15; (100s) NDC 0002-3062-02; (ID100) NDC 0002-3062-33

℞ For Oral Suspension:

125 mg/5 mL, strawberry flavor (M-5057‡)—(75-mL size) NDC 0002-5057-18; (150-mL size) NDC 0002-5057-68

187 mg/5 mL, strawberry flavor (M-5130‡)—(50-mL size) NDC 0002-5130-87; (100-mL size) NDC 0002-5130-48

250 mg/5 mL, strawberry flavor (M-5058‡)—(75-mL size) NDC 0002-5058-18; (150-mL size) NDC 0002-5058-68

375 mg/5 mL, strawberry flavor (M-5132‡)—(50-mL size) NDC 0002-5132-87; (100-mL size) NDC 0002-5132-48

Store at controlled room temperature, 59° to 86°F (15° to 30°C).

M-5057—150 mL
M-5058—75 mL
M-5058—150 mL
Pulvules® No. 3061—100s

* All RxPaks (prescription packages, Lilly) have safety closures.

† Identi-Dose® (unit dose medication, Lilly)

‡ After mixing, store in a refrigerator. Shake well before using. Keep tightly closed. The mixture may be kept for 14 days without significant loss of potency. Discard unused portion after 14 days.

[030392]

Shown in Product Identification Section, page 416

CEFACLOR, *see* Ceclor® (Cefaclor, USP, Lilly).

CEFAMANDOLE NAFATE, *see* Mandol® (Cefamandole Nafate, USP, Lilly).

CEFAZOLIN SODIUM, *see* Kefzol® (Cefazolin Sodium, USP, Lilly).

CEFTAZIDIME, *see* Tazidime® (Ceftazidime, USP, Lilly).

CEFUROXIME SODIUM, *see* Kefurox® (Cefuroxime Sodium, USP, Lilly).

COLCHICINE ℞

[*kōl 'chă-sēn*]

Injection, USP

This product is to be used by or under the direction of a physician.

DESCRIPTION

A phenanthrene derivative, colchicine is the active alkaloidal principle derived from various species of *Colchicum;* it appears as pale-yellow amorphous scales or powder that darkens on exposure to light. One g dissolves in 25 mL of water and in 220 mL of ether. Colchicine is freely soluble in alcohol and chloroform.

Chemically, it is Acetamide, *N*-(5,6,7,9-tetrahydro- 1,2,3,10-tetramethoxy-9-oxobenzo[*a*]heptalen-7-yl)- , (*S*)-. The molecular weight is 399.44, the empirical formula is $C_{22}H_{25}NO_6$, and the structure is as follows:

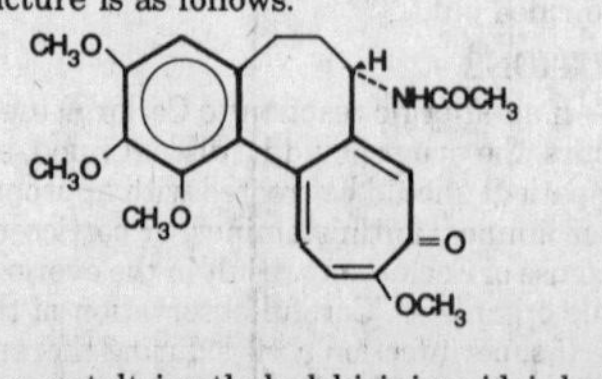

Colchicine, an acetyltrimethylcolchicinic acid, is hydrolyzed in the presence of dilute acids or alkalies, with cleavage of a methyl group as methanol and formation of *colchiceine,* which has very little therapeutic activity. On hydrolysis with strong acids, colchicine is converted to trimethylcolchicinic acid.

Ampoules Colchicine Injection, USP, provide a sterile aqueous solution of colchicine for intravenous use. Each ampoule contains 1 mg (2.5 μmol) of colchicine in 2 mL of solution. Sodium hydroxide may have been added during manufacture to adjust the pH.

CLINICAL PHARMACOLOGY

The mechanism of the relief afforded by colchicine in acute attacks of gouty arthritis is not completely known, but studies on the processes involved in precipitation of an acute attack have helped elucidate how this drug may exert its effects. The drug is not an analgesic, does not relieve other types of pain or inflammation, and is of no value in other types of arthritis. It is not a diuretic and does not influence the renal excretion of uric acid or its level in the blood or the magnitude of the "miscible pool" of uric acid. It also does not alter the solubility of urate in the plasma.

Colchicine is not a uricosuric agent. An acute attack of gout apparently occurs as a result of an inflammatory reaction to crystals of monosodium urate that are deposited in the joint tissue from hyperuric body fluids; the reaction is aggravated as more urate crystals accumulate. The initial inflammatory response involves local infiltration of granulocytes that phagocytize the urate crystals. Interference with these processes will prevent the development of an acute attack. Colchicine apparently exerts its effect by reducing the inflammatory response to the deposited crystals and also by diminishing phagocytosis. The deposition of uric acid is favored by an acid pH. In synovial tissues and in leukocytes associated with inflammatory processes, lactic acid production is high; this favors a local decrease in pH that enhances uric acid deposition. Colchicine diminishes lactic acid production by leukocytes both directly and by diminishing phagocytosis, thereby interrupting the cycle of urate crystal deposition and inflammatory response that sustains the acute attack. The oxidation of glucose in phagocytizing as well as in nonphagocytizing leukocytes in vitro is suppressed by colchicine; this suppression may explain the diminished lactic acid production. The precise biochemical step that is affected by colchicine is not yet known. The antimitotic activity of colchicine is unrelated to its effectiveness in the treatment of acute gout, as indicated by the fact that trimethylcolchicinic acid, an analog of colchicine, has no antimitotic activity except in extremely high doses.

INDICATIONS AND USAGE

Colchicine is indicated for the treatment of gout. It is effective in relieving the pain of acute attacks, especially if therapy is begun early in the attack and in adequate dosage. Many therapists use colchicine as interval therapy to prevent acute attacks of gout. It has no effect on nongouty arthritis or on uric acid metabolism.

The intravenous use of colchicine is advantageous when a rapid response is desired or when gastrointestinal side effects interfere with oral administration of the medication. Occasionally, intravenous colchicine is effective when the oral preparation is not. After the acute attack has subsided, the patient can usually be given colchicine tablets by mouth.

CONTRAINDICATIONS

Colchicine is contraindicated in patients with gout who also have serious gastrointestinal, renal, hepatic, or cardiac disorders. Colchicine should not be given in the presence of combined renal and hepatic disease.

WARNINGS

Colchicine can cause fetal harm when administered to a pregnant woman. If this drug is used during pregnancy, or if the patient becomes pregnant while taking it, the woman should be apprised of the potential hazard to the fetus.

***Mortality Related to Overdosage*—Cumulative intravenous doses of colchicine above 4 mg have resulted in irreversible multiple organ failure and death (*see* Overdosage *and* Dosage and Administration).**

PRECAUTIONS

General —Reduction in dosage is indicated if weakness, anorexia, nausea, vomiting, or diarrhea occurs. Rarely, thrombophlebitis occurs at the site of injection. Colchicine should be administered with great caution to aged and debilitated patients, especially those with renal, hepatic, gastrointestinal, or heart disease.

Drug Interactions —Colchicine has been shown to induce reversible malabsorption of vitamin B_{12}, apparently by altering the function of ileal mucosa. The possibility that colchicine may increase response to central nervous system depressants and to sympathomimetic agents is suggested by the results of experiments on animals.

Usage in Pregnancy —Pregnancy Category D —See Warnings.

Nursing Mothers —It is not known whether this drug is excreted in human milk. Because many drugs are excreted in human milk, caution should be exercised when colchicine is administered to a nursing woman.

Usage in Children —Safety and effectiveness in children have not been established.

ADVERSE REACTIONS

These are usually gastrointestinal in nature and consist of abdominal pain, nausea, vomiting, and diarrhea. The diarrhea may be severe. The gastrointestinal symptoms may occur even though the drug is given intravenously; however, such symptoms are unusual unless the recommended dose is exceeded.

Prolonged administration may cause bone marrow depression, with agranulocytosis, thrombocytopenia, and aplastic anemia. Peripheral neuritis and depilation have also been reported.

Myopathy may occur in patients on usual maintenance doses, especially in the presence of renal impairment.

OVERDOSAGE

Signs and Symptoms—Symptoms, the onset of which may be delayed, include nausea, vomiting, diarrhea, abdominal pain, hemorrhagic gastroenteritis, and burning pain in the throat, stomach, and skin. Fluid extravasation may lead to shock. Myocardial injury may be accompanied by ST-segment elevation, decreased contractility, and profound shock. Muscle weakness or paralysis may occur and progress to respiratory failure. Hepatocellular damage, renal failure, and lung parenchymal infiltrates may occur and, by the fifth day after overdose, leukopenia, thrombocytopenia, and coagulopathy may also occur. If the patient survives, alopecia and stomatitis may be experienced. There is no clear separation of nontoxic, toxic, and lethal doses of colchicine. The lethal dose of colchicine has been estimated to be 65 mg; however, **death has resulted from intravenous doses as small as 7 mg acutely (*see* Warnings *and* Dosage and Administration).** Serum concentrations that may be toxic or lethal are not defined. The intravenous median lethal dose in rats is 1.7 mg/kg.

Treatment—To obtain up-to-date information about the treatment of overdose, a good resource is your certified Regional Poison Control Center. Telephone numbers of certified poison control centers are listed in the *Physicians' Desk Reference (PDR).* In managing overdosage, consider the possibility of multiple drug overdoses, interaction among drugs, and unusual drug kinetics in your patient.

Protect the patient's airway and support ventilation and perfusion. Meticulously monitor and maintain, within acceptable limits, the patient's vital signs, blood gases, serum electrolytes, etc. If colchicine was recently ingested and vomiting has not occurred, perform gastric lavage once the patient is stabilized. Absorption of drugs from the gastrointestinal tract may be decreased by giving activated charcoal, which, in many cases, is more effective than emesis or lavage; consider charcoal instead of or in addition to gastric emptying. Repeated doses of charcoal over time may hasten elimination of some drugs that have been absorbed. Safeguard the patient's airway when employing gastric emptying or charcoal.

Forced diuresis, peritoneal dialysis, hemodialysis, or charcoal hemoperfusion have not been established as beneficial for an overdose of colchicine.

DOSAGE AND ADMINISTRATION

Colchicine Injection is for intravenous use only. Severe local irritation occurs if it is administered subcutaneously or intramuscularly.

It is extremely important that the needle be properly positioned in the vein before colchicine is injected. If leakage into surrounding tissue or outside the vein along its course should occur during intravenous administration, considerable irritation and possible tissue damage may follow. There is no specific antidote for the prevention of this irritation. Local application of heat or cold, as well as the administration of analgesics, may afford relief.

The injection should take 2 to 5 minutes for completion. To minimize the risk of extravasation, it is recommended that the injection be made into an established intravenous line into a large vein using normal saline as the intravenous fluid. Colchicine Injection should not be diluted with 5% Dextrose in Water. If a decrease in concentration of colchicine in solution is required, 0.9% Sodium Chloride Injection, which does not contain a bacteriostatic agent, should be used. Solutions that become turbid should not be used.

In the treatment of acute gouty arthritis, the average initial dose of Colchicine Injection is 2 mg (4 mL). This may be followed by 0.5 mg (1 mL) every 6 hours until a satisfactory response is achieved. In general, the total dosage for the first 24-hour period should not exceed 4 mg (8 mL). Cumulative doses of colchicine above 4 mg have resulted in irreversible multiple organ failure and death. The total dosage for a single course of treatment should not exceed 4 mg. Some clinicians recommend a single intravenous dose of 3 mg, whereas others recommend an initial dose of not more than 1 mg of colchicine intravenously, followed by 0.5 mg once or twice daily if needed.

If pain recurs, it may be necessary to administer a daily dose of 1 to 2 mg (2 to 4 mL) for several days; however, **no more colchicine should be given *by any route* for at least 7 days after a full course of IV therapy (4 mg).**[1,2] Many patients can be transferred to oral colchicine at a dosage similar to that being given intravenously.

In the prophylactic or maintenance therapy of recurrent or chronic gouty arthritis, a dosage of 0.5 to 1 mg (1 to 2 mL) once or twice daily may be used. However, in these cases, oral administration of colchicine is preferable, usually taken in conjunction with a uricosuric agent. If an acute attack of gout occurs while the patient is taking colchicine as maintenance therapy, an alternative drug should be instituted in preference to increasing the dose of colchicine.

Parenteral drug products should be inspected visually for particulate matter and discoloration prior to administration, whenever solution and container permit.

HOW SUPPLIED

(℞) Ampoules:

1 mg, 2 mL (No. 656)—(6s) NDC 0002-1443-16

Store at controlled room temperature, 59° to 86°F (15° to 30°C).

REFERENCES

1. Wallace SL, Singer JZ: Review: Systemic toxicity associated with the intravenous administration of colchicine—guidelines for use. *J Rheumatol 1988;* 15:495–499.
2. Simons RJ, Kingma DW: Fatal colchicine toxicity. *Am J Med* 1989; 86:356–357.

[043090]

CRYSTODIGIN® ℞

[*krĭs-tō-dĭj'ĭn*]

(digitoxin)

Tablets, USP

DESCRIPTION

Crystodigin® (Digitoxin Tablets, USP, Lilly) is a crystalline-pure single cardiac glycoside obtained from *Digitalis purpurea* and is identical in pharmacologic action with whole-leaf digitalis.

Digitoxin is the most slowly excreted of all digitalis compounds (excretion time is 14 to 21 days). It is most useful in patients with impaired renal function, since excretion and metabolism are independent of renal function.

Crystodigin is noted for its uniform potency, complete absorption, and lack of gastrointestinal irritation. It permits accurate dosage adjustments to produce maximum therapeutic effect smoothly and dependably.

Crystodigin, for oral administration, is available in tablets containing 0.05 mg (0.07 μmol) or 0.1 mg (0.13 μmol) crystalline digitoxin. The tablets also contain cornstarch, lactose, magnesium stearate, and povidone. The 0.05-mg tablet also contains FD&C Yellow No. 6, and the 0.1-mg tablet also contains FD&C Red No. 40.

Digitoxin is a cardiotonic glycoside. The chemical name is card-20 (22) - enolide,3-[(*O* -2,6-dideoxy-*β*- D-*ribo*-hexopyranosyl-(1→4)-*O* -2,6 - dideoxy-*β*- D - *ribo* -hexopyranosyl- (1→4) - 2,6- dideoxy- *β*-D- *ribo*- hexopyranosyl) oxy]-14-hydroxy, (3*β*,5*β*) -. The empirical formula of digitoxin is $C_{41}H_{64}O_{13}$.

CLINICAL PHARMACOLOGY

The cellular basis for the inotropic effects of digitalis is probably enhancement of excitation-contraction coupling, that process by which chemical energy is converted into mechanical energy when triggered by membrane depolarization. Most evidence relates this process to the entry of calcium ions into the cell during depolarization of the membrane and/or to the release of calcium from intracellular binding sites on the sarcoplasmic reticulum. The free calcium ion mediates the interaction of actin and myosin, resulting in contraction.

The amount of glycoside absorbed depends largely on its polarity, which is a function of the net electronic charge on the molecule. The more nonpolar or lipid soluble, the better is the absorption, because of the greater permeability of lipid membrane of the intestinal mucosa for lipid-soluble substances. The nonpolar, lipophilic digitoxin is completely absorbed. Other glycosides are not as well absorbed.

Nonpolar digitoxin is over 90% bound to tissue proteins. The firm binding of digitoxin to protein is responsible for its long half-life (7 to 9 days).

Digitoxin differs from other commonly used glycosides not only in its firm binding to protein but also because it is metabolized in the liver, with the only active metabolite being digoxin, which represents only a small fraction of the total metabolites. All other metabolites are inert and are probably excreted as such in the urine. The portion of digitoxin that is not metabolized is excreted in the bile to the intestines and recycled to the liver until it is completely metabolized. The portion of digitoxin that is bound to protein is in equilibrium with free digitoxin in the serum. Thus, as more and more of the free digitoxin is metabolized after a single dose, there is proportionately less bound digitoxin.

INDICATIONS AND USAGE

Crystodigin® (Digitoxin Tablets, USP, Lilly) is indicated in the treatment of heart failure, atrial flutter, atrial fibrillation, and supraventricular tachycardia.

CONTRAINDICATIONS

If the indications are carefully observed, there are few contraindications to digitalis therapy except toxic response or idiosyncrasy to digitalis, ventricular tachycardia, beriberi, heart disease, and some instances of the hypersensitive carotid sinus syndrome.

Patients already taking digitalis preparations must not be given the rapid digitalizing dose of Crystodigin® (Digitoxin Tablets, USP, Lilly) or parenteral calcium.

WARNINGS

Many of the arrhythmias for which digitalis is advised are identical with those reflecting digitalis intoxication. When the possibility of digitalis intoxication cannot be excluded, cardiac glycosides should be withheld temporarily if the clinical situation permits.

The patient with congestive heart failure may complain of nausea and vomiting. Since these symptoms may also be associated with digitalis intoxication, a clinical determination of their cause must be attempted before further administration of the drug.

Cases of idiopathic hypertrophic subaortic stenosis must be managed with extreme care. Unless cardiac failure is severe, it is doubtful whether digitalis should be employed.

NOTE: Digitalis glycosides are an important cause of accidental poisoning in children.

PRECAUTIONS

General—When the risk of digitalis intoxication is great, the use of a short-acting, rapidly eliminated glycoside, such as digoxin, is advisable. Although intoxication cannot always be prevented by the selection of one glycoside over another, certain glycosides may be preferred in patients who have fixed disabilities (eg, liver impairment, drug intolerance). However, digitoxin can be used in patients with impaired renal function.

Special care must be exercised in elderly patients receiving digitalis, because their body mass tends to be small and renal clearance is likely to be reduced. Frequent electrocardiographic monitoring is important in these patients. In addition, digitalis must be used cautiously in the presence of active heart disease, such as acute myocardial infarction or acute myocarditis. In patients with acute or unstable chronic atrial fibrillation, digitalis may not normalize the ventricular rate even when the serum concentration exceeds the usual therapeutic level. Although these patients may be less sensitive to the toxic effects of digitalis than are patients with normal sinus rhythm, dosage should not be increased to potentially toxic levels.

Hypokalemia predisposes to digitalis toxicity, and even a moderate decrease in the concentration of serum potassium can precipitate serious arrhythmias.

Impaired liver function may necessitate reduction in dosage of any digitalis preparation, including digitoxin.

Sensitive radioimmunoassay techniques have been developed for measuring serum levels of digitoxin, and these procedures can be instituted in almost any hospital. Serum levels must, however, be evaluated in conjunction with clinical history and the results of the electrocardiogram and other laboratory tests. A therapeutic serum level for one patient may be excessive or inadequate for another patient.

Drug Interactions—The synthesis of microsomal enzymes that metabolize digitoxin in the liver is subject to stimulation by a number of drugs, such as antihistamines, anticonvulsants, barbiturates, oral hypoglycemic agents, and others.

When digitoxin is the glycoside used for digitalis maintenance, drugs that are liver-microsomal-enzyme inducers should not be used at the same time. Phenobarbital, phenylbutazone, and diphenylhydantoin will increase the rate of metabolism of digitoxin. In patients receiving 60 mg of phenobarbital 3 times a day for 12 weeks, the steady-state concentration of digitoxin in plasma fell approximately 50% when the drugs were administered concurrently and returned to previous levels when phenobarbital was discontinued.

When drugs that increase the rate of metabolism of digitoxin in the liver are discontinued, toxicity may occur.

Hypokalemia is most frequently encountered in patients receiving concomitant diuretic therapy, because the most widely used and most effective diuretics (ie, thiazides and furosemide) increase the urinary loss of potassium. Prescrib-

Continued on next page

• Identi-Code® symbol. This product information was prepared in June 1992. Current information on these and other products of Eli Lilly and Company may be obtained by direct inquiry to Lilly Research Laboratories, Lilly Corporate Center, Indianapolis, Indiana 46285, (317) 276-3714.

Lilly—Cont.

ing a potassium-sparing agent (spironolactone or triamterene) together with the potassium-wasting diuretic is a reliable means for maintaining the serum potassium level. Alternately, potassium chloride supplements may be prescribed.

Mineralocorticoids (eg, prednisone) and, rarely, certain antibiotics (eg, amphotericin B) may also cause increased excretion of potassium.

Usage in Pregnancy —Pregnancy Category C —Animal reproduction studies have not been conducted with Crystodigin® (Digitoxin Tablets, USP, Lilly). It is also not known whether this drug can cause fetal harm when administered to a pregnant woman or can affect reproduction capacity. Crystodigin should be given to a pregnant woman only if clearly needed.

Labor and Delivery —No information is available concerning the use of Crystodigin in labor and delivery.

Nursing Mothers —It is not known whether this drug is excreted in human breast milk. Because many drugs are excreted in human breast milk, caution should be exercised when Crystodigin is administered to a nursing woman.

ADVERSE REACTIONS

Anorexia, nausea, and vomiting have been reported. These effects are central in origin, but following large oral doses, there is also a local emetic action. Abdominal discomfort or pain and diarrhea may also occur.

OVERDOSAGE

Signs and Symptoms —Symptoms may include alterations in mental status, nausea, vomiting, bradycardia, visual disturbances, heart block, and all known cardiac arrhythmias. Hyperkalemia may be present following acute overdose, whereas hypokalemia is associated with chronic overdose. Peak toxic effects following acute overdose may be delayed up to 12 hours.

Older patients, particularly those with coronary insufficiency, are more susceptible to dysrhythmias. Ventricular fibrillation is the most common cause of death from digitalis poisoning. There is insufficient information to accurately determine the minimum toxic or lethal dose in humans. Death from ventricular fibrillation was reported 24 hours after admission in a patient with a plasma concentration of 124 ng/mL shortly before death.

Treatment —To obtain up-to-date information about the treatment of overdose, a good resource is your certified Regional Poison Control Center. Telephone numbers of certified poison control centers are listed in the *Physicians' Desk Reference (PDR)*. In managing overdosage, consider the possibility of multiple drug overdoses, interaction among drugs, and unusual drug kinetics in your patient.

Continuous ECG monitoring is necessary. For any suspected digitoxin-induced dysrhythmia, discontinue the drug. Monitor potassium and digitoxin concentrations. Severe hyperkalemia may require administration of sodium bicarbonate, glucose, and regular insulin.

Protect the patient's airway and support ventilation and perfusion. Meticulously monitor and maintain, within acceptable limits, the patient's vital signs, blood gases, serum electrolytes, etc. Absorption of drugs from the gastrointestinal tract may be decreased by giving activated charcoal, which, in many cases, is more effective than emesis or lavage; consider charcoal instead of or in addition to gastric emptying. Repeated doses of charcoal over time may hasten elimination of some drugs that have been absorbed. Safeguard the patient's airway when employing gastric emptying or charcoal.

Atropine or a pacemaker may be used for bradycardia and heart block. Phenytoin (15 mg/kg), at a rate not to exceed 50 mg/min, may be useful for treating ventricular dysrhythmias and to improve atrioventricular conduction. Lidocaine may also be used, but impaired AV conduction may require a pacemaker. Consider use of digitalis-specific Fab fragments.

Forced diuresis, peritoneal dialysis, hemodialysis, or charcoal hemoperfusion have not been established as beneficial for an overdose of Crystodigin® (Digitoxin Tablets, USP, Lilly).

DOSAGE AND ADMINISTRATION

Adults: *Slow Digitalization* —0.2 mg twice daily for a period of 4 days, followed by maintenance dosage.

Rapid Digitalization —Preferably 0.6 mg initially, followed by 0.4 mg and then 0.2 mg at intervals of 4 to 6 hours.

Maintenance Dosage —Ranges from 0.05 to 0.3 mg daily, the most common dose being 0.15 mg daily.

HOW SUPPLIED

(℞) Tablets (scored):
0.05 mg. orange (No. 1736)—(100s) NDC 0002-1075-02
0.1 mg, pink (No. 1703)—(100s) NDC 0002-1060-02
Protect from light. Store at controlled room temperature, 59° to 86°F (15° to 30°C).

[060590]

CYCLOSERINE, *see* Seromycin® (Cycloserine, USP, Lilly).

DARVOCET-N® 50   ℅
[*där 'vō-sĕt ĕn*]
and
DARVOCET-N® 100
(propoxyphene napsylate
and acetaminophen tablets)
USP

DARVON-N®
[*där 'vŏn ĕn*]
(propoxyphene napsylate)
USP

DESCRIPTION

Darvon-N® (Propoxyphene Napsylate, USP) is an odorless, white crystalline powder with a bitter taste. It is very slightly soluble in water and soluble in methanol, ethanol, chloroform, and acetone. Chemically, it is $(\alpha S,1R)$-α-[2-(Dimethylamino)-1-methylethyl]-α-phenylphenethyl propionate compound with 2-naphthalenesulfonic acid (1:1) monohydrate. Its molecular weight is 565.72.

Propoxyphene napsylate differs from propoxyphene hydrochloride in that it allows more stable liquid dosage forms and tablet formulations. Because of differences in molecular weight, a dose of 100 mg (176.8 μmol) of propoxyphene napsylate is required to supply an amount of propoxyphene equivalent to that present in 65 mg (172.9 μmol) of propoxyphene hydrochloride.

Each tablet of Darvocet-N 50 contains 50 mg (88.4 μmol) propoxyphene napsylate and 325 mg (2,150 μmol) acetaminophen.

Each tablet of Darvocet-N 100 contains 100 mg (176.8 μmol) propopoxyphene napsylate and 650 mg (4,300 μmol) acetaminophen.

Tablets Darvocet-N 50 and Darvocet-N 100 also contain amberlite, cellulose, cornstarch, F D & C Yellow No. 6, magnesium stearate, stearic acid, titanium dioxide, and other inactive ingredients.

Each tablet of Darvon-N contains 100 mg (176.8 μmol) propoxyphene napsylate. The tablet also contain cellulose, cornstarch, iron oxides, lactose, magnesium stearate, silicon dioxide, stearic acid, and titanium dioxide.

Each 5 mL of Suspension Darvon-N contains 50 mg (88.4 μmol) propoxyphene napsylate. The suspension also contains butylparaben, D&C Yellow No. 10, FD&C Yellow No. 6, flavors, glucose, hydroxypropyl methylcellulose, methylparaben, propylparaben, saccharin, silicone, sodium-2-naphthalene sulfonate, sucrose, and other inactive ingredients.

CLINICAL PHARMACOLOGY

Propoxyphene is a centrally acting narcotic analgesic agent. Equimolar doses of propoxyphene hydrochloride or napsylate provide similar plasma concentrations. Following administration of 65, 130, or 195 mg of propoxyphene hydrochloride, the bioavailability of propoxyphene is equivalent to that of 100, 200, or 300 mg respectively of propoxyphene napsylate. Peak plasma concentrations of propoxyphene are reached in 2 to 2 ½ hours. After a 100-mg oral dose of propoxyphene napsylate, peak plasma levels of 0.05 to 0.1 μg/mL are achieved. As shown in Figure 1, the napsylate salt tends to be absorbed more slowly than the hydrochloride. At or near therapeutic doses, this absorption difference is small when compared with that among subjects and among doses. (See Figure 1 [top of next column])

Because of this several hundredfold difference in solubility, the absorption rate of very large doses of the napsylate salt is significantly lower than that of equimolar doses of the hydrochloride.

Repeated doses of propoxyphene at 6-hour intervals lead to increasing plasma concentrations, with a plateau after the ninth dose at 48 hours.

Propoxyphene is metabolized in the liver to yield norpropoxyphene. Propoxyphene has a half-life of 6 to 12 hours, whereas that of norpropoxyphene is 30 to 36 hours.

Norpropoxyphene has substantially less central-nervous-system-depressant effect than propoxyphene but a greater local anesthetic effect, which is similar to that of amitriptyline and antiarrhythmic agents, such as lidocaine and quinidine.

In animal studies in which propoxyphene and norpropoxyphene were continuously infused in large amounts, intracardiac conduction time (PR and QRS intervals) was prolonged. Any intracardiac conduction delay attributable to high concentrations of norpropoxyphene may be of relatively long duration.

ACTIONS

Propoxyphene is a mild narcotic analgesic structurally related to methadone. The potency of propoxyphene napsylate is from two-thirds to equal that of codeine.

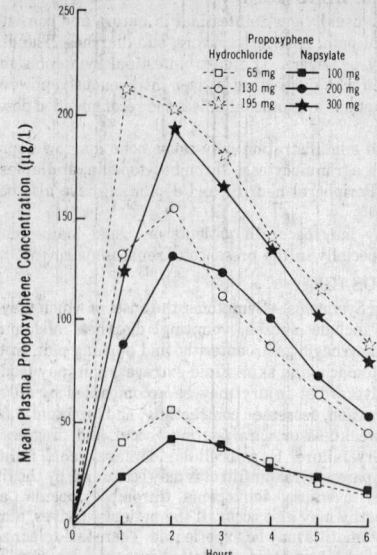

Figure 1. Mean plasma concentrations of propoxyphene in 8 human subjects following oral administration of 65 and 130 mg of the hydrochloride salt and 100 and 200 mg of the napsylate salt and in 7 given 195 mg of the hydrochloride and 300 mg of the napsylate salt

---

Darvocet-N 50 and Darvocet-N 100 provide the analgesic activity of propoxyphene napsylate and the antipyretic-analgesic activity of acetaminophen.

The combination of propoxyphene and acetaminophen produces greater analgesia than that produced by either propoxyphene or acetaminophen administered alone.

INDICATIONS

Darvocet-N® 50 and Darvocet-N® 100 (propoxyphene napsylate and acetaminophen tablets, USP, Lilly) are indicated for the relief of mild to moderate pain, either when pain is present alone or when it is accompanied by fever.

Darvon-N® (propoxyphene napsylate, Lilly) is indicated for the relief of mild to moderate pain.

CONTRAINDICATIONS

Hypersensitivity to propoxyphene or acetaminophen.

> **WARNINGS**
> - **Do not prescribe propoxyphene for patients who are suicidal or addiction-prone.**
> - **Prescribe propoxyphene with caution for patients taking tranquilizers or antidepressant drugs and patients who use alcohol in excess.**
> - **Tell your patients not to exceed the recommended dose and to limit their intake of alcohol.**
>
> Propoxyphene products in excessive doses, either alone or in combination with other CNS depressants, including alcohol, are a major cause of drug-related deaths. Fatalities within the first hour of overdosage are not uncommon. In a survey of deaths due to overdose conducted in 1975, in approximately 20% of the fatal cases, death occurred within the first hour (5% occurred within 15 minutes). Propoxyphene should not be taken in doses higher than those recommended by the physician. The judicious prescribing of propoxyphene is essential to the safe use of this drug. With patients who are depressed or suicidal, consideration should be given to the use of non-narcotic analgesics. Patients should be cautioned about the concomitant use of propoxyphene products and alcohol because of potentially serious CNS-additive effects of these agents. Because of its added depressant effects, propoxyphene should be prescribed with caution for those patients whose medical condition requires the concomitant administration of sedatives, tranquilizers, muscle relaxants, antidepressants, or other CNS-depressant drugs. Patients should be advised of the additive depressant effects of these combinations.
>
> Many of the propoxyphene-related deaths have occurred in patients with previous histories of emotional disturbances or suicidal ideation or attempts as well as histories of misuse of tranquilizers, alcohol, and other CNS-active drugs. Some deaths have occurred as a consequence of the accidental ingestion of excessive quantities of propoxyphene alone or in combination with other drugs. Patients taking propoxyphene should be warned not to exceed the dosage recommended by the physician.

Drug Dependence—Propoxyphene, when taken in higher-than-recommended doses over long periods of time, can produce drug dependence characterized by psychic dependence and, less frequently, physical dependence and tolerance. Propoxyphene will only partially suppress the withdrawal syndrome in individuals physically dependent on morphine or other narcotics. The abuse liability of propoxyphene is qualitatively similar to that of codeine although quantitatively less, and propoxyphene should be prescribed with the same degree of caution appropriate to the use of codeine.

Usage in Ambulatory Patients—Propoxyphene may impair the mental and/or physical abilities required for the performance of potentially hazardous tasks, such as driving a car or operating machinery. The patient should be cautioned accordingly.

PRECAUTIONS

General—Propoxyphene should be administered with caution to patients with hepatic or renal impairment, since higher serum concentrations or delayed elimination may occur.

Drug Interactions—The CNS-depressant effect of propoxyphene is additive with that of other CNS depressants, including alcohol.

As is the case with many medicinal agents, propoxyphene may slow the metabolism of a concomitantly administered drug. Should this occur, the higher serum concentrations of that drug may result in increased phamacologic or adverse effects of that drug. Such occurrences have been reported when propoxyphene was administered to patients on antidepressants, anticonvulsants, or warfarin-like drugs. Severe neurologic signs, including coma, have occurred with concurrent use of carbamazepine.

Usage in Pregnancy—Safe use in pregnancy has not been established relative to possible adverse effects on fetal development. Instances of withdrawal symptoms in the neonate have been reported following usage during pregnancy. Therefore, propoxyphene should not be used in pregnant women unless, in the judgment of the physician, the potential benefits outweigh the possible hazards.

Usage in Nursing Mothers—Low levels of propoxyphene have been detected in human milk. In postpartum studies involving nursing mothers who were given propoxyphene, no adverse effects were noted in infants receiving mother's milk.

Usage in Children—Propoxyphene is not recommended for use in children, because documented clinical experience has been insufficient to establish safety and a suitable dosage regimen in the pediatric age group.

Usage in the Elderly—The rate of propoxyphene metabolism may be reduced in some patients. Increased dosing interval should be considered.

A Patient Information Sheet is available for these products. See text following "How Supplied" section below.

ADVERSE REACTIONS

In a survey conducted in hospitalized patients, less than 1% of patients taking propoxyphene hydrochloride at recommended doses experienced side effects. The most frequently reported were dizziness, sedation, nausea, and vomiting. Some of these adverse reactions may be alleviated if the patient lies down.

Other adverse reactions include constipation, abdominal pain, skin rashes, lightheadedness, headache, weakness, euphoria, dysphoria, hallucinations, and minor visual disturbances.

Liver dysfunction has been reported in association with both active components of Darvocet-N® 50 and Darvocet-N® 100 (propoxyphene napsylate and acetaminophen tablets, USP, Lilly).

Propoxyphene therapy has been associated with abnormal liver function tests and, more rarely, with instances of reversible jaundice (including cholestatic jaundice). Hepatic necrosis may result from acute overdose of acetaminophen (*see* Management of Overdosage). In chronic ethanol abusers, this has been reported rarely with short-term use of acetaminophen doses of 2.5 to 10 g/day. Fatalities have occurred.

Renal papillary necrosis may result from chronic acetaminophen use, particularly when the dosage is greater than recommended and when combined with aspirin.

Subacute painful myopathy has occurred following chronic propoxyphene overdosage.

DOSAGE AND ADMINISTRATION

These products are given orally. The usual dosage of Darvocet-N® 50 or Darvocet-N® 100 (propoxyphene napsylate and acetaminophen tablets, USP, Lilly) is 100 mg propoxyphene napsylate and 650 mg acetaminophen every 4 hours as needed for pain.

The maximum recommended dose of propoxyphene napsylate is 600 mg/day.

Consideration should be given to a reduced total daily dosage in patients with hepatic or renal impairment.

MANAGEMENT OF OVERDOSAGE

In all cases of suspected overdosage, call your regional Poison Control Center to obtain the most up-to-date information about the treatment of overdose. This recommendation is made because, in general, information regarding the treatment of overdosage may change more rapidly than do package inserts.

Initial consideration should be given to the management of the CNS effects of propoxyphene overdosage. Resuscitative measures should be initiated promptly.

Symptoms of Propoxyphene Overdosage—The manifestations of acute overdosage with propoxyphene are those of narcotic overdosage. The patient is usually somnolent but may be stuporous or comatose and convulsing. Respiratory depression is characteristic. The ventilatory rate and/or tidal volume is decreased, which results in cyanosis and hypoxia. Pupils, initially pinpoint, may become dilated as hypoxia increases. Cheyne-Stokes respiration and apnea may occur. Blood pressure and heart rate are usually normal initially, but blood pressure falls and cardiac performance deteriorates, which ultimately results in pulmonary edema and circulatory collapse, unless the respiratory depression is corrected and adequate ventilation is restored promptly. Cardiac arrhythmias and conduction delay may be present. A combined respiratory-metabolic acidosis occurs owing to retained CO_2 (hypercapnia) and to lactic acid formed during anaerobic glycolysis. Acidosis may be severe if large amounts of salicylates have also been ingested. Death may occur.

Treatment of Propoxyphene Overdosage—Attention should be directed first to establishing a patent airway and to restoring ventilation. Mechanically assisted ventilation, with or without oxygen, may be required, and positive pressure respiration may be desirable if pulmonary edema is present. The narcotic antagonist naloxone will markedly reduce the degree of respiratory depression, and 0.4 to 2 mg should be administered promptly, preferably intravenously. If the desired degree of counteraction with improvement in respiratory functions is not obtained, naloxone should be repeated at 2- to 3-minute intervals. The duration of action of the antagonist may be brief. If no response is observed after 10 mg of naloxone have been administered, the diagnosis of propoxyphene toxicity should be questioned. Naloxone may also be administered by continuous intravenous infusion.

Treatment of Propoxyphene Overdosage in Children—The usual inital dose of naloxone in children is 0.01 mg/kg body weight given intravenously. If this dose does not result in the desired degree of clinical improvement, a subsequent increased dose of 0.1 mg/kg body weight may be administered. If an IV route of administration is not available, naloxone may be administered IM or subcutaneously in divided doses. If necessary, naloxone can be diluted with Sterile Water for Injection.

Blood gases, pH, and electrolytes should be monitored in order that acidosis and any electrolyte disturbance present may be corrected promptly. Acidosis, hypoxia, and generalized CNS depression predispose to the development of cardiac arrhythmias. Ventricular fibrillation or cardiac arrest may occur and necessitate the full complement of cardiopulmonary resuscitation (CPR) measures. Respiratory acidosis rapidly subsides as ventilation is restored and hypercapnia eliminated, but lactic acidosis may require intravenous bicarbonate for prompt correction.

Electrocardiographic monitoring is essential. Prompt correction of hypoxia, acidosis, and electrolyte disturbance (when present) will help prevent these cardiac complications and will increase the effectiveness of agents administered to restore normal cardiac function.

In addition to the use of a narcotic antagonist, the patient may require careful titration with an anticonvulsant to control convulsions. Analeptic drugs (for example, caffeine or amphetamine) should not be used because of their tendency to precipitate convulsions.

General supportive measures, in addition to oxygen, include, when necessary, intravenous fluids, vasopressor-inotropic compounds, and, when infection is likely, anti-infective agents. Gastric lavage may be useful, and activated charcoal can adsorb a significant amount of ingested propoxyphene. Dialysis is of little value in poisoning due to propoxyphene. Efforts should be made to determine whether other agents, such as alcohol, barbiturates, tranquilizers, or other CNS depressants, were also ingested, since these increase CNS depression as well as cause specific toxic effects.

Symptoms of Acetaminophen Overdosage—Shortly after oral ingestion of an overdose of acetaminophen and for the next 24 hours, anorexia, nausea, vomiting, diaphoresis, general malaise, and abdominal pain have been noted. The patient may then present no symptoms, but evidence of liver dysfunction may become apparent up to 72 hours after ingestion, with elevated serum transaminase and lactic dehydrogenase levels, an increase in serum bilirubin concentrations, and a prolonged prothrombin time. Death from hepatic failure may result 3 to 7 days after overdosage.

Acute renal failure may accompany the hepatic dysfunction and has been noted in patients who do not exhibit signs of fulminant hepatic failure. Typically, renal impairment is more apparent 6 to 9 days after ingestion of the overdose.

Treatment of Acetaminophen Overdosage—Acetaminophen in massive overdosage may cause hepatic toxicity in some patients. *In all cases of suspected overdose, immediately call your regional poison center or the Rocky Mountain Poison Center's toll-free number* (800-525-6115) for assistance in diagnosis and for directions in the use of N-acetylcysteine as an antidote.

In adults, hepatic toxicity has rarely been reported with acute overdoses of less than 10 g and fatalities with less than 15 g. Importantly, young children seem to be more resistant than adults to the hepatotoxic effect of an acetaminophen overdose. Despite this, the measures outlined below should be initiated in any adult or child suspected of having ingested an acetaminophen overdose.

Because clinical and laboratory evidence of hepatic toxicity may not be apparent until 48 to 72 hours postingestion, liver function studies should be obtained initially and repeated at 24-hour intervals.

Consider emptying the stomach promptly by lavage or by induction of emesis with syrup of ipecac. Patients' estimates of the quantity of a drug ingested are notoriously unreliable. Therefore, if an acetaminophen overdose is suspected, a serum acetaminophen assay should be obtained as early as possible, but no sooner than 4 hours following ingestion. The antidote, N-acetylcysteine, should be administered as early as possible, and within 16 hours of the overdose ingestion for optimal results. Following recovery, there are no residual, structural, or functional hepatic abnormalities.

ANIMAL TOXICOLOGY

The acute lethal doses of the hydrochloride and napsylate salts of propoxyphene were determined in 4 species. The results shown in Figure 2 indicate that, on a molar basis, the napsylate salt is less toxic than the hydrochloride. This may be due to the relative insolubility and retarded absorption of propoxyphene napsylate.

Figure 2. Acute oral toxicity of propoxyphene

LD_{50} (mg/kg) ± SE / LD_{50} (mmol/kg)

Species	Propoxyphene Hydrochloride	Propoxyphene Napsylate
Mouse	282 ± 39 / 0.75	915 ± 163 / 1.62
Rat	230 ± 44 / 0.61	647 ± 95 / 1.14
Rabbit	*ca.* 82 / 0.22	>183 / >0.32
Dog	*ca.* 100 / 0.27	>183 / >0.32

Some indication of the relative insolubility and retarded absorption of propoxyphene napsylate was obtained by measuring plasma propoxyphene levels in 2 groups of 4 dogs following oral administration of equimolar doses of the 2 salts. As shown in Figure 3, the peak plasma concentration observed with propoxyphene hydrochloride was much higher than that obtained after administration of the napsylate salt.

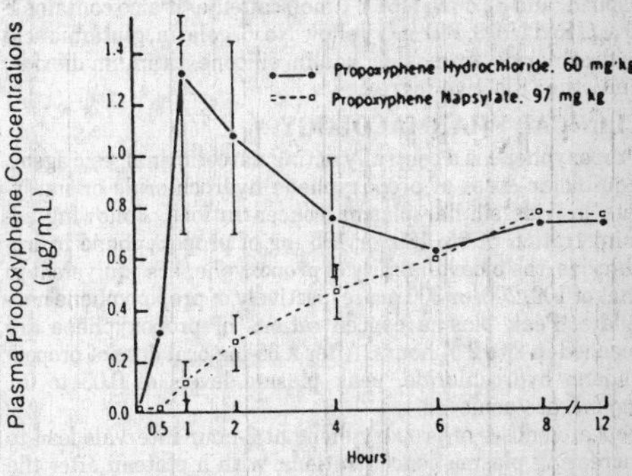

Figure 3. Plasma propoxyphene concentrations in dogs following large doses of the hydrochloride and napsylate salts

Continued on next page

*** Identi-Code® symbol. This product information was prepared in June 1992. Current information on these and other products of Eli Lilly and Company may be obtained by direct inquiry to Lilly Research Laboratories, Lilly Corporate Center, Indianapolis, Indiana 46285, (317) 276-3714.**

Lilly—Cont.

Although none of the animals in this experiment died, 3 of the 4 dogs given propoxyphene hydrochloride exhibited convulsive seizures during the time interval corresponding to the peak plasma levels. The 4 animals receiving the napsylate salt were mildly ataxic but not acutely ill.

HOW SUPPLIED

(CIV) Tablets:

Darvocet-N 50, dark orange (No. 1890)—(RxPak* of 100) NDC 0002-0351-02; (ID†100) NDC 0002-0351-33; (500s) NDC 0002-0351-03

Darvocet-N 100, dark orange (No. 1893)—(RxPak of 100) NDC 0002-0363-02; (ID100) NDC 0002-0363-33; (500s) NDC 0002-0363-03; (ID500) NDC 0002-0363-43; (RN‡500) NDC 0002-0363-46

Darvon-N, 100 mg, buff (No. 1883)—(RxPak of 100) NDC 0002-0353-02; (ID100) NDC 0002-0353-33; (500s) NDC 0002-0353-03

(CIV) Darvon-N, Suspension§, 50 mg/5 mL (No. M-135)—(16 fl oz) NDC 0002-2371-05

Store at controlled room temperature, 59° to 86°F (15° to 30°C).

* All RxPaks (prescription packages, Lilly) have safety closures.

† Identi-Dose® (unit dose medication, Lilly).

‡ Reverse-numbered package.

§ Shake well before using. Avoid freezing. Keep tightly closed.

[032992]

Shown in Product Identification Section, page 416

Patient information, including illustrations of dosage forms and the maximum daily dosage of each, is available to patients receiving Darvon (propoxyphene) products (*see under* Darvon®.)

DARVON® (CIV)
[*där'von*]
(propoxyphene hydrochloride)
Capsules, USP

DARVON® COMPOUND-65
(propoxyphene hydrochloride, aspirin, and caffeine)
[*där'vŏn kŏm'pound*]

DESCRIPTION

Darvon® (Propoxyphene Hydrochloride, USP, Lilly) is an odorless, white crystalline powder with a bitter taste. It is freely soluble in water. Chemically, it is (2S, 3R)-(+)-4-(Dimethylamino)-3-methyl- 1,2-diphenyl-2-butanol propionate (ester) hydrochloride. Its molecular weight is 375.94.

Each Pulvule® Darvon contains 65 mg (172.9 μmol) (No. 365) propoxyphene hydrochloride. It also contains D & C Red No. 33, F D & C Yellow No. 6, gelatin, magnesium stearate, silicone, starch, titanium dioxide, and other inactive ingredients.

Each Pulvule Darvon Compound-65 contains 65 mg (172.9 μmol) propoxyphene hydrochloride, 389 mg (2,159 μmol) aspirin, and 32.4 mg (166.8 μmol) caffeine. It also contains F D & C Red No. 3, F D & C Yellow No. 6, gelatin, glutamic acid hydrochloride, iron oxide, kaolin, silicone, titanium dioxide, and other inactive ingredients.

CLINICAL PHARMACOLOGY

Propoxyphene is a centrally acting narcotic analgesic agent. Equimolar doses of propoxyphene hydrochloride or napsylate provide similar plasma concentrations. Following administration of 65, 130, or 195 mg of propoxyphene hydrochloride, the bioavailability of propoxyphene is equivalent to that of 100, 200, or 300 mg respectively of propoxyphene napsylate. Peak plasma concentrations of propoxyphene are reached in 2 to 2 ½ hours. After a 65-mg oral dose of propoxyphene hydrochloride, peak plasma levels of 0.05 to 0.1 μg/mL are achieved.

Repeated doses of propoxyphene at 6-hour intervals lead to increasing plasma concentrations, with a plateau after the ninth dose at 48 hours.

Propoxyphene is metabolized in the liver to yield norpropoxyphene. Propoxyphene has a half-life of 6 to 12 hours, whereas that of norpropoxyphene is 30 to 36 hours.

Norpropoxyphene has substantially less central-nervous-system-depressant effect than propoxyphene but a greater local anesthetic effect, which is similar to that of amitriptyline and antiarrhythmic agents, such as lidocaine and quinidine.

In animal studies in which propoxyphene and norpropoxyphene were continuously infused in large amounts, intracardiac conduction time (PR and QRS intervals) was prolonged. Any intracardiac conduction delay attributable to high concentrations of norpropoxyphene may be of relatively long duration.

ACTIONS

Propoxyphene is a mild narcotic analgesic structurally related to methadone. The potency of propoxyphene hydrochloride is from two-thirds to equal that of codeine.

The combination of propoxyphene with a mixture of aspirin and caffeine produces greater analgesia than that produced by either propoxyphene or aspirin and caffeine administered alone.

INDICATIONS

Darvon® (propoxyphene hydrochloride, Lilly) is indicated for the relief of mild to moderate pain.

Darvon Compound-65 is indicated for the relief of mild to moderate pain, either when pain is present alone or when it is accompanied by fever.

CONTRAINDICATION

Hypersensitivity to propoxyphene, aspirin, or caffeine.

WARNINGS

- **Do not prescribe propoxyphene for patients who are suicidal or addiction-prone.**
- **Prescribe propoxyphene with caution for patients taking tranquilizers or antidepressant drugs and patients who use alcohol in excess.**
- **Tell your patients not to exceed the recommended dose and to limit their intake of alcohol.**

Propoxyphene products in excessive doses, either alone or in combination with other CNS depressants, including alcohol, are a major cause of drug-related deaths. Fatalities within the first hour of overdosage are not uncommon. In a survey of deaths due to overdosage conducted in 1975, in approximately 20% of the fatal cases, death occurred within the first hour (5% occurred within 15 minutes). Propoxyphene should not be taken in doses higher than those recommended by the physician. The judicious prescribing of propoxyphene is essential to the safe use of this drug. With patients who are depressed or suicidal, consideration should be given to the use of non-narcotic analgesics. Patients should be cautioned about the concomitant use of propoxyphene products and alcohol because of potentially serious CNS-additive effects of these agents. Because of its added depressant effects, propoxyphene should be prescribed with caution for those patients whose medical condition requires the concomitant administration of sedatives, tranquilizers, muscle relaxants, antidepressants, or other CNS-depressant drugs. Patients should be advised of the additive depressant effects of these combinations.

Many of the propoxyphene-related deaths have occurred in patients with previous histories of emotional disturbances or suicidal ideation or attempts as well as histories of misuse of tranquilizers, alcohol, and other CNS-active drugs. Some deaths have occurred as a consequence of the accidental ingestion of excessive quantities of propoxyphene alone or in combination with other drugs. Patients taking propoxyphene should be warned not to exceed the dosage recommended by the physician.

Drug Dependence—Propoxyphene, when taken in higher-than-recommended doses over long periods of time, can produce drug dependence characterized by psychic dependence and, less frequently, physical dependence and tolerance. Propoxyphene will only partially suppress the withdrawal syndrome in individuals physically dependent on morphine or other narcotics. The abuse liability of propoxyphene is qualitatively similar to that of codeine although quantitatively less, and propoxyphene should be prescribed with the same degree of caution appropriate to the use of codeine.

Usage in Ambulatory Patients—Propoxyphene may impair the mental and/or physical abilities required for the performance of potentially hazardous tasks, such as driving a car or operating machinery. The patient should be cautioned accordingly.

Warning—Reye syndrome is a rare but serious disease which can follow flu or chickenpox in children and teenagers. Although the cause of Reye syndrome is unknown, some reports claim aspirin (or salicylates) may increase the risk of developing this disease.

PRECAUTIONS

General—Salicylates should be used with extreme caution in the presence of peptic ulcer or coagulation abnormalities. Propoxyphene should be administered with caution to patients with hepatic or renal impairment since higher serum concentrations or delayed elimination may occur.

Drug Interactions—The CNS-depressant effect of propoxyphene is additive with that of other CNS depressants, including alcohol.

Salicylates may enhance the effect of anticoagulants and inhibit the uricosuric effect of uricosuric agents.

As is the case with medicinal agents, propoxyphene may slow the metabolism of a concomitantly administered drug. Should this occur, the higher serum concentrations of that drug may result in increased pharmacologic or adverse effects of that drug. Such occurrences have been reported when propoxyphene was administered to patients on antidepressants, anticonvulsants, or warfarin-like drugs. Severe neurologic signs, including coma, have occurred with concurrent use of carbamazepine.

Usage in Pregnancy—Safe use in pregnancy has not been established relative to possible adverse effects on fetal development. Instances of withdrawal symptoms in the neonate have been reported following usage during pregnancy. Therefore, propoxyphene should not be used in pregnant women unless, in the judgment of the physician, the potential benefits outweigh the possible hazards. Aspirin does not appear to have teratogenic effects. However, prolonged pregnancy and labor with increased bleeding before and after delivery, decreased birth weight, and increased rate of stillbirth were reported with high blood salicylate levels. Because of possible adverse effects on the neonate and the potential for increased maternal blood loss, aspirin should be avoided during the last 3 months of pregnancy.

Usage in Nursing Mothers—Low levels of propoxyphene have been detected in human milk. In postpartum studies involving nursing mothers who were given propoxyphene, no adverse effects were noted in infants receiving mother's milk.

Usage in Children—Propoxyphene is not recommended for use in children, because documented clinical experience has been insufficient to establish safety and a suitable dosage regimen in the pediatric age group.

Usage in the Elderly—The rate of propoxyphene metabolism may be reduced in some patients. Increased dosing interval should be considered.

A Patient Information Sheet is available for this product. See text following "How Supplied" section below.

ADVERSE REACTIONS

In a survey conducted in hospitalized patients, less than 1% of patients taking propoxyphene hydrochloride at recommended doses experienced side effects. The most frequently reported were dizziness, sedation, nausea, and vomiting. Some of these adverse reactions may be alleviated if the patient lies down.

Other adverse reactions include constipation, abdominal pain, skin rashes, lightheadedness, headache, weakness, euphoria, dysphoria, hallucinations, and minor visual disturbances.

Propoxyphene therapy has been associated with abnormal liver function tests and, more rarely, with instances of reversible jaundice (including cholestatic jaundice).

Renal papillary necrosis may result from chronic aspirin use, particularly when the dosage is greater than recommended and when combined with acetaminophen.

Subacute painful myopathy has occurred following chronic propoxyphene overdosage.

DOSAGE AND ADMINISTRATION

These products are given orally. The usual dosage of Darvon® (propoxyphene hydrochloride, Lilly) is 65 mg every 4 hours as needed for pain.

The usual dosage of Darvon Compound-65 is 65 mg propoxyphene hydrochloride, 389 mg aspirin, and 32.4 mg caffeine every 4 hours as needed for pain.

The maximum recommended dose of propoxyphene hydrochloride is 390 mg/day.

Consideration should be given to a reduced total daily dosage in patients with hepatic or renal impairment.

MANAGEMENT OF OVERDOSAGE

In all cases of suspected overdosage, call your regional Poison Control Center to obtain the most up-to-date information about the treatment of overdose. This recommendation is made because, in general, information regarding the treatment of overdosage may change more rapidly than do package inserts.

Initial consideration should be given to the management of the CNS effects of propoxyphene overdosage. Resuscitative measures should be initiated promptly.

Symptoms of Propoxyphene Overdosage—The manifestations of acute overdosage with propoxyphene are those of narcotic overdosage. The patient is usually somnolent but may be stuporous or comatose and convulsing. Respiratory depression is characteristic. The ventilatory rate and/or tidal volume is decreased, which results in cyanosis and hypoxia. Pupils, initially pinpoint, may become dilated as hypoxia increases. Cheyne-Stokes respiration and apnea may occur. Blood pressure and heart rate are usually normal initially, but blood pressure falls and cardiac performance deteriorates, which ultimately results in pulmonary edema and circulatory collapse, unless the respiratory depression is corrected and adequate ventilation is restored promptly. Cardiac arrhythmias and conduction delay may be present. A combined respiratory-metabolic acidosis occurs owing to retained CO_2 (hypercapnia) and to lactic acid formed during

anaerobic glycolysis. Acidosis may be severe if large amounts of salicylates have also been ingested. Death may occur.

Treatment of Propoxyphene Overdosage—Attention should be directed first to establishing a patent airway and to restoring ventilation. Mechanically assisted ventilation, with or without oxygen, may be required, and positive pressure respiration may be desirable if pulmonary edema is present. The narcotic antagonist naloxone will markedly reduce the degree of respiratory depression, and 0.4 to 2 mg should be administered promptly, preferably intravenously. If the desired degree of counteraction with improvement in respiratory functions is not obtained, naloxone should be repeated at 2- to 3-minute intervals. The duration of action of the antagonist may be brief. If no response is observed after 10 mg of naloxone have been administered, the diagnosis of propoxyphene toxicity should be questioned. Naloxone may also be administered by continuous intravenous infusion.

Treatment of Propoxyphene Overdosage in Children—The usual initial dose of naloxone in children is 0.01 mg/kg body weight given intravenously. If this dose does not result in the desired degree of clinical improvement, a subsequent increased dose of 0.1 mg/kg body weight may be administered. If an IV route of administration is not available, naloxone may be administered IM or subcutaneously in divided doses. If necessary, naloxone can be diluted with Sterile Water for Injection.

Blood gases, pH, and electrolytes should be monitored in order that acidosis and any electrolyte disturbance present may be corrected promptly. Acidosis, hypoxia, and generalized CNS depression predispose to the development of cardiac arrhythmias. Ventricular fibrillation or cardiac arrest may occur and necessitate the full complement of cardiopulmonary resuscitation (CPR) measures. Respiratory acidosis rapidly subsides as ventilation is restored and hypercapnia eliminated, but lactic acidosis may require intravenous bicarbonate for prompt correction.

Electrocardiographic monitoring is essential. Prompt correction of hypoxia, acidosis, and electrolyte disturbance (when present) will help prevent these cardiac complications and will increase the effectiveness of agents administered to restore normal cardiac function.

In addition to the use of a narcotic antagonist, the patient may require careful titration with an anticonvulsant to control convulsions. Analeptic drugs (for example, caffeine or amphetamine) should not be used because of their tendency to precipitate convulsions.

General supportive measures, in addition to oxygen, include, when necessary, intravenous fluids, vasopressor-inotropic compounds, and, when infection is likely, anti-infective agents. Gastric lavage may be useful and activated charcoal can adsorb a significant amount of ingested propoxyphene. Dialysis is of little value in poisoning due to propoxyphene. Efforts should be made to determine whether other agents, such as alcohol, barbiturates, tranquilizers, or other CNS depressants, were also ingested, since these increase CNS depression as well as cause specific toxic effects.

Symptoms of Salicylate Overdosage—Such symptoms include central nausea and vomiting, tinnitus and deafness, vertigo and headaches, mental dullness and confusion, diaphoresis, rapid pulse, and increased respiration and respiratory alkalosis.

Treatment of Salicylate Overdosage—When Darvon Compound-65 has been ingested, the clinical picture may be complicated by salicylism.

The treatment of acute salicylate intoxication includes minimizing drug absorption, promoting elimination through the kidneys, and correcting metabolic derangements affecting body temperature, hydration, acid-base balance, and electrolyte balance. The technique to be employed for eliminating salicylate from the bloodstream depends on the degree of drug intoxication.

If the patient is seen within 4 hours of ingestion, the stomach should be emptied by inducing vomiting or by gastric lavage as soon as possible.

The nomogram of Done is a useful prognostic guide in which the expected severity of salicylate intoxication is based on serum salicylate levels and the time interval between ingestion and taking the blood sample.

Exchange transfusion is most feasible for a small infant. Intermittent peritoneal dialysis is useful for cases of moderate severity in adults. Intravenous fluids alkalinized by the addition of sodium bicarbonate or potassium citrate are helpful. Hemodialysis with the artificial kidney is the most effective means of removing salicylate and is indicated for the very severe cases of salicylate intoxication.

HOW SUPPLIED

(Ⓒ) Pulvules:

Darvon, 65 mg, pink (No. 365)—(RxPak* of 100) NDC 0002-0803-02; (ID†100) NDC 0002-0803-33; (500s) NDC 0002-0803-03

Darvon Compound-65, red and gray (No. 369)—(RxPak of 100) NDC 0002-3111-02; (ID100) NDC 0002-3111-33; (500s) NDC 0002-3111-03

Store at controlled room temperature, 59° to 86°F (15° to 30°C).

[032992]

Shown in Product Identification Section, page 416

The following information, including illustrations of dosage forms and the maximum daily dosage of each, is available to patients receiving Darvon products.

Patient Information Sheet

YOUR PRESCRIPTION FOR A DARVON® (PROPOXYPHENE) PRODUCT Ⓒ

Summary: Products containing Darvon are used to relieve pain.

LIMIT YOUR INTAKE OF ALCOHOL WHILE TAKING THIS DRUG. Make sure your doctor knows if you are taking tranquilizers, sleep aids, antidepressants, antihistamines, or any other drugs that make you sleepy. Combining propoxyphene with alcohol or these drugs in excessive doses is dangerous.

Use care while driving a car or using machines until you see how the drug affects you, because propoxyphene can make you sleepy. Do not take more of the drug than your doctor prescribed. Dependence has occurred when patients have taken propoxyphene for a long period of time at doses greater than recommended.

The rest of this leaflet gives you more information about propoxyphene. Please read it and keep it for future use.

Uses of Darvon: Products containing Darvon are used for the relief of mild to moderate pain. Products that contain Darvon plus aspirin or acetaminophen are prescribed for the relief of pain or pain associated with fever.

Before Taking Darvon: Make sure your doctor knows if you have ever had an allergic reaction to propoxyphene, aspirin, or acetaminophen. Some forms of propoxyphene products contain aspirin to help relieve the pain. Your doctor should be advised if you have a history of ulcers or if you are taking an anticoagulant ("blood thinner"). The aspirin may irritate the stomach lining and may cause bleeding, particularly if an ulcer is present. Also, bleeding may occur if you are taking an anticoagulant. In a small group of people, aspirin may cause an asthma attack. If you are one of these people, be sure your drug does not contain aspirin.

The effect of propoxyphene in children under 12 has not been studied. Therefore, use of the drug in this age group is not recommended.

Also, due to the possible association between aspirin and Reye syndrome, those propoxyphene products containing aspirin should not be given to children, including teenagers, with chickenpox or flu unless prescribed by a physician. The following propoxyphene product contains aspirin:

Darvon® Compound-65 (Propoxyphene Hydrochloride, Aspirin, and Caffeine, USP, Lilly)

How to Take Darvon: Follow your doctor's directions exactly. Do not increase the amount you take without your doctor's approval. If you miss a dose of the drug, do not take twice as much the next time.

Pregnancy: Do not take propoxyphene during pregnancy unless your doctor knows you are pregnant and specifically recommends its use. Cases of temporary dependence in the newborn have occurred when the mother has taken propoxyphene consistently in the weeks before delivery. As a general principle, no drug should be taken during pregnancy unless it is clearly necessary. **IT IS ESPECIALLY IMPORTANT NOT TO USE DARVON COMPOUND-65 DURING THE LAST 3 MONTHS OF PREGNANCY UNLESS SPECIFICALLY DIRECTED TO DO SO BY A DOCTOR BECAUSE ASPIRIN MAY CAUSE PROBLEMS IN THE UNBORN CHILD OR COMPLICATIONS DURING DELIVERY.**

General Cautions: Heavy use of alcohol with propoxyphene is hazardous and may lead to overdosage symptoms (see "Overdose" below). THEREFORE, LIMIT YOUR INTAKE OF ALCOHOL WHILE TAKING PROPOXYPHENE.

Combinations of excessive doses of propoxyphene, alcohol, and tranquilizers are dangerous. Make sure your doctor knows if you are taking tranquilizers, sleep aids, antidepressant drugs, antihistamines, or any other drugs that make you sleepy. The use of these drugs with propoxyphene increases their sedative effects and may lead to overdosage symptoms, including death (*see* "Overdose" below).

Propoxyphene may cause drowsiness or impair your mental and/or physical abilities; therefore, use caution when driving a vehicle or operating dangerous machinery. DO NOT perform any hazardous task until you have seen your response to this drug.

Propoxyphene may increase the concentration in the body of medications, such as anticoagulants ("blood thinners"), antidepressants, or drugs used for epilepsy. The result may be excessive or adverse effects of these medications. Make sure your doctor knows if you are taking any of these medications.

Dependence: You can become dependent on propoxyphene if you take it in higher than recommended doses over a long period of time. Dependence is a feeling of need for the drug and a feeling that you cannot perform normally without it.

Overdose: An overdose of Darvon, alone or in combination with other drugs, including alcohol, may cause weakness, difficulty in breathing, confusion, anxiety, and more severe drowsiness and dizziness. Extreme overdosage may lead to unconsciousness and death.

If the propoxyphene product contains acetaminophen, the overdosage symptoms include nausea, vomiting, lack of appetite, and abdominal pain. Liver damage may occur even after symptoms disappear. Death can occur days later.

When the propoxyphene product contains aspirin, symptoms of taking too much of the drug are headache, dizziness, ringing in the ears, difficulty in hearing, dim vision, confusion, drowsiness, sweating, thirst, rapid breathing, nausea, vomiting, and, occasionally, diarrhea.

In any suspected overdosage situation, contact your doctor or nearest hospital emergency room. GET EMERGENCY HELP IMMEDIATELY.

KEEP THIS DRUG AND ALL DRUGS OUT OF THE REACH OF CHILDREN.

Possible Side Effects: When propoxyphene is taken as directed, side effects are infrequent. Among those reported are drowsiness, dizziness, nausea, and vomiting. If these effects occur, it may help if you lie down and rest.

Less frequently reported side effects are constipation, abdominal pain, skin rashes, lightheadedness, headache, weakness, hallucinations, minor visual disturbances, and feelings of elation or discomfort.

If side effects occur and concern you, contact your doctor.

Other Information: The safe and effective use of propoxyphene depends on your taking it exactly as directed. This drug has been prescribed specifically for you and your present condition. Do not give this drug to others who may have similar symptoms. Do not use it for any other reason.

If you would like more information about propoxyphene, ask your doctor or pharmacist. They have a more technical leaflet (professional labeling) you may read.

Prescription Vial Sticker

Tell your doctor if you are taking tranquilizers, antidepressant drugs, or sleep aids. LIMIT alcohol use with Darvon-N® (propoxyphene napsylate) and Darvon® (propoxyphene hydrochloride) products.

[032992]

DIETHYLSTILBESTROL ℞

[*dī-eth 'il-stil-bĕs 'trōl*]

USP

1. USE OF ESTROGENS HAS BEEN REPORTED TO INCREASE THE RISK OF ENDOMETRIAL CARCINOMA

Three independent case-control studies have reported an increased risk of endometrial cancer in postmenopausal women exposed to exogenous estrogens for more than 1 year. This risk was independent of other known risk factors for endometrial cancer. These studies are further supported by the finding that, since 1969, the incidence rate of endometrial cancer has increased sharply in 8 different areas of the United States which have population-based cancer reporting systems.

The 3 case-control studies reported that the risk of endometrial cancer in estrogen users was about 4.5 to 13.9 times greater than in nonusers. The risk appears to depend on both the duration of treatment and the dose of estrogen. In view of these findings, the lowest dose that will control symptoms should be utilized when estrogens are used for the treatment of menopausal symptoms, and medication should be discontinued as soon as possible. When prolonged treatment is medically indicated, a reassessment should be made on at least a semiannual basis to determine the need for continued therapy. Although the evidence must be considered preliminary, 1 study suggests that cyclic administration of low doses of estrogen may carry less risk than does continuous administration; it therefore appears prudent to utilize such a regimen.

Close clinical surveillance of all women taking estrogens is important. In all cases of undiagnosed persistent or recurring abnormal vaginal bleeding, adequate di-

Continued on next page

* All RxPaks (prescription packages, Lilly) have safety closures.

† Identi-Dose® (unit dose medication, Lilly).

*** Identi-Code® symbol. This product information was prepared in June 1992. Current information on these and other products of Eli Lilly and Company may be obtained by direct inquiry to Lilly Research Laboratories, Lilly Corporate Center, Indianapolis, Indiana 46285, (317) 276-3714.**

Lilly—Cont.

agnostic measures should be undertaken to rule out malignancy.

At present, there is no evidence that "natural" estrogens are more or less hazardous than "synthetic" estrogens at equivalent estrogenic doses.

2. *ESTROGENS SHOULD NOT BE USED DURING PREGNANCY*

The use of female sex hormones, both estrogens and progestogens, during early pregnancy may affect the offspring. It has been reported that females exposed *in utero* to diethylstilbestrol, a nonsteroidal estrogen, may have an increased risk of developing later in life a rare form of vaginal or cervical cancer. This risk has been estimated to be 0.14 to 1.4 per 1,000 exposures. Furthermore, from 30% to 90% of such exposed women have been found to have vaginal adenosis and epithelial changes of the vagina and cervix. Although these changes are histologically benign, it is not known whether they are precursors of malignancy. Even though similar data are not available with the use of other estrogens, it cannot be presumed that they would not induce similar changes.

Several reports suggest that there is an association between intrauterine exposure to female sex hormones and congenital anomalies, including congenital heart defects and limb-reduction defects. One case-control study estimated a 4.7-fold increased risk of limb-reduction defects in infants exposed *in utero* to sex hormones (oral contraceptives, hormone withdrawal tests for pregnancy, or attempted treatment for threatened abortion). Some of these exposures were very short and involved only a few days of treatment. The data suggest that the risk of limb-reduction defects in exposed fetuses is somewhat less than 1 per 1,000.

In the past, female sex hormones have been used during pregnancy in an attempt to treat threatened or habitual abortion; however, their efficacy was never conclusively proved or disproved.

If diethylstilbestrol is administered during pregnancy, or if the patient becomes pregnant while taking this drug, she should be apprised of the potential risks to the fetus and of the advisability of pregnancy continuation.

THIS DRUG PRODUCT SHOULD NOT BE USED AS A POSTCOITAL CONTRACEPTIVE

DESCRIPTION

Diethylstilbestrol is a crystalline synthetic estrogenic substance capable of producing all the pharmacologic and therapeutic responses attributed to natural estrogens. Diethylstilbestrol may be administered orally (in the form of Enseals® [enteric-release tablets, Lilly] and tablets). Chemically, diethylstilbestrol is α,α'-diethyl-4,4′-stilbenediol.

The Enseals contain cornstarch, FD&C Blue No. 2, FD&C Red No. 3, FD&C Yellow No. 6, lactose, magnesium stearate, sucrose, talc, titanium dioxide, and other inactive ingredients.

The tablets contain cornstarch, lactose, magnesium stearate, and talc.

INDICATIONS AND USAGE

Diethylstilbestrol is indicated in the treatment of:

1. Breast cancer (for palliation only) in appropriately selected women and men with metastatic disease
2. Prostatic carcinoma—palliative therapy of advanced disease

DIETHYLSTILBESTROL SHOULD NOT BE USED FOR ANY PURPOSE DURING PREGNANCY. ITS USE MAY CAUSE SEVERE HARM TO THE FETUS (SEE BOXED WARNING).

CONTRAINDICATIONS

Estrogens should not be used in women (or men) with any of the following conditions:

1. Known or suspected cancer of the breast, except in appropriately selected patients being treated for metastatic disease
2. Known or suspected estrogen-dependent neoplasia
3. Known or suspected pregnancy (*see* boxed Warning)
4. Undiagnosed abnormal genital bleeding
5. Active thrombophlebitis or thromboembolic disorders
6. A past history of thrombophlebitis, thrombosis, or thromboembolic disorders associated with previous use of estrogen (except when used in treatment of breast or prostatic malignancy)

WARNINGS

1. *Induction of Malignant Neoplasms*—In certain animal species, long-term continuous administration of natural and synthetic estrogens increases the frequency of carcinomas of the breast, cervix, vagina, kidney, and liver. There are now reports that prolonged use of estrogens increases the risk of carcinoma of the endometrium in humans (*see* boxed Warning).

At the present time, there is no satisfactory evidence that administration of estrogens to postmenopausal women increases the risk of cancer of the breast. This possibility, however, has been raised by a recent long-term follow-up of 1 physician's practice. Because of the animal data, there is a need for caution in prescribing estrogens for women with a family history of breast cancer or for women who have breast nodules, fibrocystic disease, or abnormal mammograms.

2. *Gallbladder Disease*—A recent study reported a 2-to-3-fold increase in the risk of gallbladder disease occurring in women receiving postmenopausal estrogen therapy, similar to the 2-fold increased risk previously noted in women using oral contraceptives. In the case of oral contraceptives, this increased risk appeared after 2 years of use.

3. *Effects Similar to Those Caused by Estrogen-Progestogen Oral Contraceptives*—There are several serious adverse effects associated with the use of oral contraceptives; however, most of these adverse effects have not as yet been documented as consequences of postmenopausal estrogen therapy. This may reflect the comparatively low doses of estrogen used in postmenopausal women. It would be expected that these adverse effects are more likely to occur following administration of the larger doses of estrogen used for treating prostatic or breast cancer. It has, in fact, been shown that there is an increased risk of thrombosis with the administration of estrogens for prostatic cancer in men and for postpartum breast engorgement in women.

a. *Thromboembolic Disease*—It is now well established that women taking oral contraceptives run an increased risk of various thromboembolic and thrombotic vascular diseases, such as thrombophlebitis, pulmonary embolism, stroke, and myocardial infarction. Cases of retinal thrombosis, mesenteric thrombosis, and optic neuritis have been reported in users of oral contraceptives. There is evidence that the risk of several of these adverse reactions is related to the dose of the drug. An increased risk of postsurgical thromboembolic complications has also been reported in users of oral contraceptives. If feasible, estrogen therapy should be discontinued at least 4 weeks before surgery such as that associated with an increased risk of thromboembolism, or that requiring periods of prolonged immobilization.

Although an increased rate of thromboembolic and thrombotic disease has not been noted in postmenopausal users of estrogen, this does not rule out the possibility that such an increase may be present or that it exists in subgroups of women who have underlying risk factors or who are receiving relatively large doses of estrogens. Therefore, estrogens should not be used in persons with active thrombophlebitis or thromboembolic disorders, nor should they be used (except in treatment of malignancy) in persons with a history of such disorders associated with estrogen therapy. Estrogens should be administered cautiously to patients with cerebral vascular or coronary artery disease and only when such therapy is clearly needed.

In a large prospective clinical trial in men, large doses of estrogen (5 mg of conjugated estrogens per day), comparable to those used to treat cancer of the prostate and breast, have been shown to increase the risk of nonfatal myocardial infarction, pulmonary embolism, and thrombophlebitis. When such large doses of estrogen are used, any of the thromboembolic and thrombotic adverse effects associated with the use of oral contraceptives should be considered a clear risk.

b. *Hepatic Adenoma*—Benign hepatic adenomas appear to be associated with the use of oral contraceptives. Although these adenomas are benign and rare, they may rupture and may cause death by intra-abdominal hemorrhage. Such lesions have not yet been reported in association with the administration of other estrogen or progestogen preparations, but they should be considered when abdominal pain and tenderness, abdominal mass, or hypovolemic shock occurs in persons receiving estrogen therapy. Hepatocellular carcinoma has also been reported in women taking estrogen-containing oral contraceptives. The relationship of this malignancy to these drugs is not known at this time.

c. *Elevated Blood Pressure*—Increased blood pressure is not uncommon in women taking oral contraceptives. There is now 1 report that this may occur with use of estrogens in the menopause, and blood pressure should be monitored during estrogen therapy, especially if high doses are used.

d. *Glucose Tolerance*—A decrease in glucose tolerance has been observed in a significant percentage of patients on estrogen-containing oral contraceptives. For this reason, diabetic patients should be carefully observed while receiving estrogen.

4. *Hypercalcemia*—Administration of estrogens may lead to severe hypercalcemia in patients with breast cancer and bone metastases. If this occurs, the drug should be stopped and appropriate measures taken to reduce the serum calcium level.

PRECAUTIONS

General—1. A complete medical and family history should be taken prior to initiation of any estrogen therapy. In the pretreatment and periodic physical examinations, special consideration should be given to blood pressure, breasts, abdomen, and pelvic organs, and a Papanicolaou smear should be performed. As a general rule, estrogen should not be prescribed for over a year without another physical examination.

2. Fluid retention—Because estrogens may cause some degree of fluid retention, conditions which might be influenced by this factor, such as epilepsy, migraine, and cardiac or renal dysfunction, require careful observation.

3. Certain patients may develop undesirable manifestations of excessive estrogenic stimulation, such as abnormal or excessive uterine bleeding, mastodynia, etc.

4. Oral contraceptives appear to be associated with an increased incidence of mental depression. Although it is not clear whether this is due to the estrogenic or progestogenic component of the contraceptive agent, patients with a history of depression should be carefully observed.

5. Preexisting uterine leiomyomata may increase in size with administration of estrogens.

6. The pathologist should be advised of estrogen therapy when relevant specimens are submitted.

7. Patients with a past history of jaundice during pregnancy run an increased risk of recurrence of jaundice while receiving estrogen-containing oral contraceptive therapy. If jaundice develops in any patient receiving estrogen, the medication should be discontinued while the cause is investigated.

8. Estrogens may be poorly metabolized in patients with impaired liver function, and they should therefore be administered with caution in such patients.

9. Because estrogens influence the metabolism of calcium and phosphorus, they should be used with caution in patients with metabolic bone diseases associated with hypercalcemia or in patients with renal insufficiency.

10. Because of the effects of estrogens on epiphyseal closure, they should be used judiciously in young patients in whom bone growth is not complete.

11. Certain endocrine and liver function tests may be affected by estrogen-containing oral contraceptives. The following similar changes may be expected with larger doses of estrogen:

a. Increased sulfobromophthalein retention

b. Increased prothrombin and factors VII, VIII, IX, and X; decreased antithrombin 3; increased norepinephrine-induced platelet aggregability

c. Increased thyroid-binding globulin (TBG) leading to increased circulating total thyroid hormone, as measured by PBI, T4 by column, or T4 by radioimmunoassay. Free T3 resin uptake is decreased, reflecting the elevated TBG; free T4 concentration is unaltered

d. Impaired glucose tolerance

e. Decreased pregnanediol excretion

f. Reduced response to metyrapone test

g. Reduced serum folate concentration

h. Increased serum triglyceride and phospholipid concentration

Information for the Patient—*See* text of Patient Package Insert.

Pregnancy Category X—*See* Contraindications *and* boxed Warning.

Nursing Mothers—As a general principle, the administration of any drug to nursing mothers should be done only when clearly necessary, since many drugs are excreted in human milk.

ADVERSE REACTIONS

(*See* Warnings regarding induction of neoplasia, adverse effects on the fetus, increased incidence of gallbladder disease, and adverse effects similar to those of oral contraceptives, including thromboembolism.) The following additional adverse reactions have been reported with estrogenic therapy, including oral contraceptives:

1. *Genitourinary System*
   - Breakthrough bleeding, spotting, change in menstrual flow
   - Dysmenorrhea
   - Premenstrual-like syndrome
   - Amenorrhea during and after treatment
   - Increase in size of uterine fibromyomata
   - Vaginal candidiasis
   - Change in cervical eversion and in degree of cervical secretion
   - Cystitis-like syndrome
2. *Breasts*
   - Tenderness, enlargement, secretion
3. *Gastrointestinal*
   - Nausea, vomiting
   - Abdominal cramps, bloating
   - Cholestatic jaundice
4. *Skin*
   - Chloasma or melasma, which may persist when drug is discontinued
   - Erythema multiforme
   - Erythema nodosum
   - Hemorrhagic eruption
   - Loss of scalp hair
   - Hirsutism

5. *Eyes*
   Steepening of corneal curvature
   Intolerance to contact lenses
6. *CNS*
   Headache, migraine, dizziness
   Mental depression
   Chorea
7. *Miscellaneous*
   Increase or decrease in weight
   Reduced carbohydrate tolerance
   Aggravation of porphyria
   Edema
   Changes in libido

OVERDOSAGE

Signs and Symptoms—Symptoms of acute overdose include anorexia, nausea, vomiting, abdominal cramps, and diarrhea. Withdrawal vaginal bleeding may follow large doses. Chronic toxicity may include salt and water retention, edema, headache, vertigo, leg cramps, gynecomastia, chloasma, and porphyria cutanea tarda. Polydipsia, polyuria, fatigue, and an abnormal glucose tolerance may occur in some patients with preclinical diabetes mellitus.

No information is available on the following: LD_{50}, concentration of diethylstilbestrol in biologic fluids associated with toxicity and/or death, the amount of drug in a single dose usually associated with symptoms of overdosage, or the amount of diethylstilbestrol in a single dose likely to be life threatening.

Treatment—Chronic diethylstilbestrol toxicity should be treated by discontinuing all estrogenic medications and providing supportive care for any symptoms that may be present.

To obtain up-to-date information about the treatment of overdose, a good resource is your certified Regional Poison Control Center. Telephone numbers of certified poison control centers are listed in the *Physicians' Desk Reference (PDR)*. In managing overdosage, consider the possibility of multiple drug overdoses, interaction among drugs, and unusual drug kinetics in your patient.

In treating acute overdose, protect the patient's airway and support ventilation and perfusion. Meticulously monitor and maintain, within acceptable limits, the patient's vital signs, blood gases, serum electrolytes, etc. Absorption of drugs from the gastrointestinal tract may be decreased by giving activated charcoal, which, in many cases, is more effective than emesis or lavage; consider charcoal instead of or in addition to gastric emptying. Repeated doses of charcoal over time may hasten elimination of some drugs that have been absorbed. Safeguard the patient's airway when employing gastric emptying or charcoal.

Forced diuresis, peritoneal dialysis, hemodialysis, or charcoal hemoperfusion have not been established as beneficial for an overdose of diethylstilbestrol.

DOSAGE AND ADMINISTRATION

Given Chronically:

Inoperable progressing prostatic cancer

1 to 3 mg daily initially, increased in advanced cases; the dosage may later be reduced to an average of 1 mg daily.

Inoperable progressing breast cancer in appropriately selected men and postmenopausal women (*see* Indications)

15 mg daily

Patients with an intact uterus should be closely monitored for signs of endometrial cancer, and appropriate diagnostic measures should be taken to rule out malignancy in the event of persistent or recurring abnormal vaginal bleeding.

HOW SUPPLIED

(℞) Diethylstilbestrol, USP, is supplied in the following forms:

Enseals:

1 mg (No. 49)—(100s) NDC 0002-0122-02; (1000s) NDC 0002-0122-04

5 mg (No. 85)—(100s) NDC 0002-0133-02

Tablets:

1 mg (No. 1649)—(100s) NDC 0002-1052-02; (1000s) NDC 0002-1052-04

5 mg (No. 1685)—(100s) NDC 0002-1054-02 [083188]

DOBUTREX® SOLUTION ℞

[dō'bū-trĕks]

(dobutamine hydrochloride)

Injection

DESCRIPTION

Dobutrex® Solution (Dobutamine Hydrochloride Injection, Lilly) is 1,2-benzenediol, 4-[2-[[3-(4-hydroxyphenyl)-1-methylpropyl]amino]ethyl]-, hydrochloride, (±)-. It is a synthetic catecholamine.

Molecular Formula: $C_{18}H_{23}NO_3 \cdot HCl$

Molecular Weight: 337.85

The clinical formulation is supplied in a sterile form for intravenous use only. Each mL contains 12.5 mg (41.5 μmol) dobutamine, 0.24 mg sodium bisulfite (added during manufacture), and water for injection, q.s. Hydrochloric acid and/or sodium hydroxide may have been added during manufacture to adjust the pH.

CLINICAL PHARMACOLOGY

Dobutrex® Solution (Dobutamine Hydrochloride Injection, Lilly) is a direct-acting inotropic agent whose primary activity results from stimulation of the β receptors of the heart while producing comparatively mild chronotropic, hypertensive, arrhythmogenic, and vasodilative effects. It does not cause the release of endogenous norepinephrine, as does dopamine. In animal studies, dobutamine produces less increase in heart rate and less decrease in peripheral vascular resistance for a given inotropic effect than does isoproterenol.

In patients with depressed cardiac function, both dobutamine and isoproterenol increase the cardiac output to a similar degree. In the case of dobutamine, this increase is usually not accompanied by marked increases in heart rate (although tachycardia is occasionally observed), and the cardiac stroke volume is usually increased. In contrast, isoproterenol increases the cardiac index primarily by increasing the heart rate while stroke volume changes little or declines.

Facilitation of atrioventricular conduction has been observed in human electrophysiologic studies and in patients with atrial fibrillation.

Systemic vascular resistance is usually decreased with administration of dobutamine. Occasionally, minimum vasoconstriction has been observed.

Most clinical experience with dobutamine is short-term—not more than several hours in duration. In the limited number of patients who were studied for 24, 48, and 72 hours, a persistent increase in cardiac output occurred in some, whereas output returned toward baseline values in others.

The onset of action of Dobutrex Solution is within 1 to 2 minutes; however, as much as 10 minutes may be required to obtain the peak effect of a particular infusion rate.

The plasma half-life of dobutamine in humans is 2 minutes. The principal routes of metabolism are methylation of the catechol and conjugation. In human urine, the major excretion products are the conjugates of dobutamine and 3-O-methyl dobutamine. The 3-O-methyl derivative of dobutamine is inactive.

Alteration of synaptic concentrations of catecholamines with either reserpine or tricyclic antidepressants does not alter the actions of dobutamine in animals, which indicates that the actions of dobutamine are not dependent on presynaptic mechanisms.

INDICATIONS AND USAGE

Dobutrex® Solution (Dobutamine Hydrochloride Injection, Lilly) is indicated when parenteral therapy is necessary for inotropic support in the short-term treatment of adults with cardiac decompensation due to depressed contractility resulting either from organic heart disease or from cardiac surgical procedures.

In patients who have atrial fibrillation with rapid ventricular response, a digitalis preparation should be used prior to institution of therapy with Dobutrex Solution.

CONTRAINDICATIONS

Dobutrex® Solution (Dobutamine Hydrochloride Injection, Lilly) is contraindicated in patients with idiopathic hypertrophic subaortic stenosis and in patients who have shown previous manifestations of hypersensitivity to Dobutrex Solution.

WARNINGS

1. *Increase in Heart Rate or Blood Pressure*—Dobutrex® Solution (Dobutamine Hydrochloride Injection, Lilly) may cause a marked increase in heart rate or blood pressure, especially systolic pressure. Approximately 10% of patients in clinical studies have had rate increases of 30 beats/minute or more, and about 7.5% have had a 50 mm Hg or greater increase in systolic pressure. Usually, reduction of dosage promptly reverses these effects. Because dobutamine facilitates atrioventricular conduction, patients with atrial fibrillation are at risk of developing rapid ventricular response. Patients with preexisting hypertension appear to face an increased risk of developing an exaggerated pressor response.
2. *Ectopic Activity*—Dobutrex Solution may precipitate or exacerbate ventricular ectopic activity, but it rarely has caused ventricular tachycardia.
3. *Hypersensitivity*—Reactions suggestive of hypersensitivity associated with administration of Dobutrex Solution, including skin rash, fever, eosinophilia, and bronchospasm, have been reported occasionally.
4. Dobutrex Solution contains sodium bisulfite, a sulfite that may cause allergic-type reactions, including anaphylactic symptoms and life-threatening or less severe asthmatic episodes, in certain susceptible people. The overall prevalence of sulfite sensitivity in the general population is unknown and probably low. Sulfite sensitivity is seen more frequently in asthmatic than in nonasthmatic people.

PRECAUTIONS

1. During the administration of Dobutrex® Solution (Dobutamine Hydrochloride Injection, Lilly), as with any adrenergic agent, ECG and blood pressure should be continuously monitored. In addition, pulmonary wedge pressure and cardiac output should be monitored whenever possible to aid in the safe and effective infusion of Dobutrex Solution.

2. Hypovolemia should be corrected with suitable volume expanders before treatment with Dobutrex Solution is instituted.

3. Animal studies indicate that dobutamine may be ineffective if the patient has recently received a β-blocking drug. In such a case, the peripheral vascular resistance may increase.

4. No improvement may be observed in the presence of marked mechanical obstruction, such as severe valvular aortic stenosis.

5. Dobutamine, like other β_2-agonists, can produce a mild reduction in serum potassium concentration, rarely to hypokalemic levels. Accordingly, consideration should be given to monitoring serum potassium.

Usage Following Acute Myocardial Infarction—Clinical experience with Dobutrex Solution following myocardial infarction has been insufficient to establish the safety of the drug for this use. There is concern that any agent that increases contractile force and heart rate may increase the size of an infarction by intensifying ischemia, but it is not known whether dobutamine does so.

Usage in Pregnancy—Reproduction studies performed in rats and rabbits have revealed no evidence of impaired fertility, harm to the fetus, or teratogenic effects due to dobutamine. However, the drug has not been administered to pregnant women and should be used only when the expected benefits clearly outweigh the potential risks to the fetus.

Pediatric Use—The safety and effectiveness of Dobutrex Solution for use in children have not been studied.

Drug Interactions—There was no evidence of drug interactions in clinical studies in which Dobutrex Solution was administered concurrently with other drugs, including digitalis preparations, furosemide, spironolactone, lidocaine, glyceryl trinitrate, isosorbide dinitrate, morphine, atropine, heparin, protamine, potassium chloride, folic acid, and acetaminophen. Preliminary studies indicate that the concomitant use of dobutamine and nitroprusside results in a higher cardiac output and, usually, a lower pulmonary wedge pressure than when either drug is used alone.

ADVERSE REACTIONS

Increased Heart Rate, Blood Pressure, and Ventricular Ectopic Activity—A 10- to 20-mm increase in systolic blood pressure and an increase in heart rate of 5 to 15 beats/minute have been noted in most patients (*see* Warnings regarding exaggerated chronotropic and pressor effects). Approximately 5% of patients have had increased premature ventricular beats during infusions. These effects are dose related.

Hypotension—Precipitous decreases in blood pressure have occasionally been described in association with dobutamine therapy. Decreasing the dose or discontinuing the infusion typically results in rapid return of blood pressure to baseline values. In rare cases, however, intervention may be required and reversibility may not be immediate.

Reactions at Sites of Intravenous Infusion—Phlebitis has occasionally been reported. Local inflammatory changes have been described following inadvertent infiltration.

Miscellaneous Uncommon Effects—The following adverse effects have been reported in 1% to 3% of patients: nausea, headache, anginal pain, nonspecific chest pain, palpitations, and shortness of breath.

Administration of Dobutrex® Solution (Dobutamine Hydrochloride Injection, Lilly), like other catecholamines, can produce a mild reduction in serum potassium concentration, rarely to hypokalemic levels (*see* Precautions).

Longer-Term Safety—Infusions of up to 72 hours have revealed no adverse effects other than those seen with shorter infusions.

OVERDOSAGE

Overdoses of dobutamine have been reported rarely. The following is provided to serve as a guide if such an overdose is encountered.

Signs and Symptoms—Toxicity from dobutamine hydrochloride is usually due to excessive cardiac β-receptor stimulation. The duration of action of dobutamine hydrochloride is generally short ($T_{1/2}$ = 2 minutes) because it is rapidly metabolized by catechol-O-methyltransferase. The symptoms of

Continued on next page

• Identi-Code® symbol. This product information was prepared in June 1992. Current information on these and other products of Eli Lilly and Company may be obtained by direct inquiry to Lilly Research Laboratories, Lilly Corporate Center, Indianapolis, Indiana 46285, (317) 276-3714.

Lilly—Cont.

Dobutrex® Solution (Dobutamine Hydrochloride Injection, Lilly)—Rates of Infusion for Concentrations of 250, 500, and 1,000 µg/mL

Drug Delivery Rate (µg/kg/min)	Infusion Delivery Rate		
	250 µg/mL* (mL/kg/min)	500 µg/mL† (mL/kg/min)	1,000 µg/mL‡ (mL/kg/min)
2.5	0.01	0.005	0.0025
5	0.02	0.01	0.005
7.5	0.03	0.015	0.0075
10	0.04	0.02	0.01
12.5	0.05	0.025	0.0125
15	0.06	0.03	0.015

*250 µg/mL of diluent
†500 µg/mL or 250 mg/500 mL of diluent
‡1,000 µg/mL or 250 mg/250 mL of diluent

toxicity may include anorexia, nausea, vomiting, tremor, anxiety, palpitations, headache, shortness of breath, and anginal and nonspecific chest pain. The positive inotropic and chronotropic effects of dobutamine on the myocardium may cause hypertension, tachyarrhythmias, myocardial ischemia, and ventricular fibrillation. Hypotension may result from vasodilation.

If the product is ingested, unpredictable absorption may occur from the mouth and the gastrointestinal tract.

Treatment —To obtain up-to-date information about the treatment of overdose, a good resource is your certified Regional Poison Control Center. Telephone numbers of certified poison control centers are listed in the *Physicians' Desk Reference (PDR)*. In managing overdosage, consider the possibility of multiple drug overdoses, interaction among drugs, and unusual drug kinetics in your patient.

The initial actions to be taken in a dobutamine hydrochloride overdose are discontinuing administration, establishing an airway, and ensuring oxygenation and ventilation. Resuscitative measures should be initiated promptly. Severe ventricular tachyarrhythmias may be successfully treated with propranolol or lidocaine. Hypertension usually responds to a reduction in dose or discontinuation of therapy.

Protect the patient's airway and support ventilation and perfusion. If needed, meticulously monitor and maintain, within acceptable limits, the patient's vital signs, blood gases, serum electrolytes, etc. Absorption of drugs from the gastrointestinal tract may be decreased by giving activated charcoal, which, in many cases, is more effective than emesis or lavage; consider charcoal instead of or in addition to gastric emptying. Repeated doses of charcoal over time may hasten elimination of some drugs that have been absorbed. Safeguard the patient's airway when employing gastric emptying or charcoal.

Forced diuresis, peritoneal dialysis, hemodialysis, or charcoal hemoperfusion have not been established as beneficial for an overdose of dobutamine hydrochloride.

DOSAGE AND ADMINISTRATION

Note —Do not add Dobutrex® Solution (Dobutamine Hydrochloride Injection, Lilly) to 5% Sodium Bicarbonate Injection or to any other strongly alkaline solution. Because of potential physical incompatibilities, it is recommended that Dobutrex Solution not be mixed with other drugs in the same solution. Dobutrex Solution should not be used in conjunction with other agents or diluents containing both sodium bisulfite and ethanol.

Reconstitution and Stability —At the time of administration, Dobutrex Solution must be further diluted in an IV container to at least a 50-mL solution using 1 of the following intravenous solutions as a diluent: 5% Dextrose Injection, 5% Dextrose and 0.45% Sodium Chloride Injection, 5% Dextrose and 0.9% Sodium Chloride Injection, 10% Dextrose Injection, Isolyte® M with 5% Dextrose Injection, Lactated Ringer's Injection, 5% Dextrose in Lactated Ringer's Injection, Normosol®-M in D5-W, 20% Osmitrol® in Water for Injection, 0.9% Sodium Chloride Injection, or Sodium Lactate Injection. Intravenous solutions should be used within 24 hours.

Solutions containing Dobutrex Solution may exhibit a pink color that, if present, will increase with time. This color change is due to slight oxidation of the drug, but there is no significant loss of potency during the reconstitution time period stated above.

Recommended Dosage —The rate of infusion needed to increase cardiac output usually ranged from 2.5 to 10 µg/kg/min (see table). On rare occasions, infusion rates up to 40 µg/kg/min have been required to obtain the desired effect. [See table above.]

The rate of administration and the duration of therapy should be adjusted according to the patient's response as determined by heart rate, presence of ectopic activity, blood pressure, urine flow, and, whenever possible, measurement of central venous or pulmonary wedge pressure and cardiac output.

Concentrations up to 5,000 µg/mL have been administered to humans (250 mg/50 mL). The final volume administered should be determined by the fluid requirements of the patient.

HOW SUPPLIED

(℞) Vials:
250 mg,* 20-mL size (No. 7175)—(1s) NDC 0002-7175-01; (Traypak† of 10) NDC 0002-7175-10

Store at controlled room temperature, 59° to 86°F (15° to 30°C).

* Equivalent to dobutamine.
† Traypak™(multivial carton, Lilly)

[112691]

DOLOPHINE® HYDROCHLORIDE   Ⓒ
[dō′lō-fēn hī-drō-klō′rīd]
(methadone hydrochloride)
Injection, USP

AMPOULES AND VIALS

CONDITIONS FOR DISTRIBUTION AND USE OF METHADONE PRODUCTS:
Code of Federal Regulations,
Title 21, Sec. 291.505

METHADONE PRODUCTS, WHEN USED FOR THE TREATMENT OF NARCOTIC ADDICTION IN DETOXIFICATION OR MAINTENANCE PROGRAMS, SHALL BE DISPENSED ONLY BY APPROVED HOSPITAL PHARMACIES, APPROVED COMMUNITY PHARMACIES, AND MAINTENANCE PROGRAMS APPROVED BY THE FOOD AND DRUG ADMINISTRATION AND THE DESIGNATED STATE AUTHORITY.
APPROVED MAINTENANCE PROGRAMS SHALL DISPENSE AND USE METHADONE IN ORAL FORM ONLY AND ACCORDING TO THE TREATMENT REQUIREMENTS STIPULATED IN THE FEDERAL METHADONE REGULATIONS (21 CFR 291.505).
FAILURE TO ABIDE BY THE REQUIREMENTS IN THESE REGULATIONS MAY RESULT IN CRIMINAL PROSECUTION, SEIZURE OF THE DRUG SUPPLY, REVOCATION OF THE PROGRAM APPROVAL, AND INJUNCTION PRECLUDING OPERATION OF THE PROGRAM.
A METHADONE PRODUCT, WHEN USED AS AN ANALGESIC, MAY BE DISPENSED IN ANY LICENSED PHARMACY.

DESCRIPTION

Dolophine® Hydrochloride (Methadone Hydrochloride, USP, Lilly) (3-heptanone, 6-(dimethylamino)-4,4-diphenyl-,hydrochloride), is a white, crystalline material that is water soluble. Its molecular weight is 345.91.

Each mL contains methadone hydrochloride, 10 mg (0.029 mmol), and sodium chloride, 0.9%. Sodium hydroxide and/or hydrochloric acid may have been added during manufacture to adjust the pH. The 20-mL vials also contain chlorobutanol (chloroform derivative), 0.5%, as a preservative.

ACTIONS

Methadone hydrochloride is a synthetic narcotic analgesic with multiple actions quantitatively similar to those of morphine, the most prominent of which involve the central nervous system and organs composed of smooth muscle. The principal actions of therapeutic value are analgesia and sedation and detoxification or temporary maintenance in narcotic addiction. The methadone abstinence syndrome, although qualitatively similar to that of morphine, differs in

that the onset is slower, the course is more prolonged, and the symptoms are less severe.

A parenteral dose of 8 to 10 mg of methadone is approximately equivalent in analgesic effect to 10 mg of morphine. With single-dose administration, the onset and duration of analgesic action of the 2 drugs are similar.

When administered orally, methadone is approximately one-half as potent as when given parenterally. Oral administration results in a delay of the onset, a lowering of the peak, and an increase in the duration of analgesic effect.

INDICATIONS

(See boxed Note.)
For relief of severe pain.
For detoxification treatment of narcotic addiction.
For temporary maintenance treatment of narcotic addiction.

NOTE

If methadone is administered for treatment of heroin dependence for more than 3 weeks, the procedure passes from treatment of the acute withdrawal syndrome (detoxification) to maintenance therapy. Maintenance treatment is permitted to be undertaken only by approved methadone programs. This does not preclude the maintenance treatment of an addict who is hospitalized for medical conditions other than addiction and who requires temporary maintenance during the critical period of his/her stay or whose enrollment has been verified in a program approved for maintenance treatment with methadone.

CONTRAINDICATION

Hypersensitivity to methadone.

WARNINGS

Methadone hydrochloride, a narcotic, is a Schedule II controlled substance under the Federal Controlled Substances Act. Appropriate security measures should be taken to safeguard stocks of methadone against diversion.

DRUG DEPENDENCE—METHADONE CAN PRODUCE DRUG DEPENDENCE OF THE MORPHINE TYPE AND, THEREFORE, HAS THE POTENTIAL FOR BEING ABUSED. PSYCHIC DEPENDENCE, PHYSICAL DEPENDENCE, AND TOLERANCE MAY DEVELOP ON REPEATED ADMINISTRATION OF METHADONE, AND IT SHOULD BE PRESCRIBED AND ADMINISTERED WITH THE SAME DEGREE OF CAUTION APPROPRIATE TO THE USE OF MORPHINE.

Interaction With Other Central Nervous System Depressants —Methadone should be used with caution and in reduced dosage in patients who are concurrently receiving other narcotic analgesics, general anesthetics, phenothiazines, other tranquilizers, sedative-hypnotics, tricyclic antidepressants, and other CNS depressants (including alcohol). Respiratory depression, hypotension, and profound sedation or coma may result.

Anxiety —Since methadone, as used by tolerant subjects at a constant maintenance dosage, is not a tranquilizer, patients who are maintained on this drug will react to life problems and stresses with the same symptoms of anxiety as do other individuals. The physician should not confuse such symptoms with those of narcotic abstinence and should not attempt to treat anxiety by increasing the dosage of methadone. The action of methadone in maintenance treatment is limited to the control of narcotic symptoms and is ineffective for relief of general anxiety.

Head Injury and Increased Intracranial Pressure —The respiratory depressant effects of methadone and its capacity to elevate cerebrospinal-fluid pressure may be markedly exaggerated in the presence of increased intracranial pressure. Furthermore, narcotics produce side effects that may obscure the clinical course of patients with head injuries. In such patients, methadone must be used with caution and only if it is deemed essential.

Asthma and Other Respiratory Conditions — Methadone should be used with caution in patients having an acute asthmatic attack, in those with chronic obstructive pulmonary disease or cor pulmonale, and in individuals with a substantially decreased respiratory reserve, preexisting respiratory depression, hypoxia, or hypercapnia. In such patients, even usual therapeutic doses of narcotics may decrease respiratory drive while simultaneously increasing airway resistance to the point of apnea.

Hypotensive Effect —The administration of methadone may result in severe hypotension in an individual whose ability to maintain normal blood pressure has already been compromised by a depleted blood volume or concurrent administration of such drugs as the phenothiazines or certain anesthetics.

Use in Ambulatory Patients —Methadone may impair the mental and/or physical abilities required for the performance of potentially hazardous tasks, such as driving a car or operating machinery. The patient should be cautioned accordingly.

Methadone, like other narcotics, may produce orthostatic hypotension in ambulatory patients.

Use in Pregnancy—Safe use in pregnancy has not been established in relation to possible adverse effects on fetal development. Therefore, methadone should not be used in pregnant women unless, in the judgment of the physician, the potential benefits outweigh the possible hazards.

Methadone is not recommended for obstetric analgesia because its long duration of action increases the probability of respiratory depression in the newborn.

Use in Children—Methadone is not recommended for use as an analgesic in children, since documented clinical experience has been insufficient to establish a suitable dosage regimen for the pediatric age group.

PRECAUTIONS

Drug Interactions:

Pentazocine—**Patients who are addicted to heroin or who are on the methadone maintenance program may experience withdrawal symptoms when given an opioid agonist-antagonist, such as pentazocine.**

Rifampin—The concurrent administration of rifampin may possibly reduce the blood concentration of methadone to a degree sufficient to produce withdrawal symptoms. The mechanism by which rifampin may decrease blood concentrations of methadone is not fully understood, although enhanced microsomal drug-metabolized enzymes may influence drug disposition.

Monoamine Oxidase (MAO) Inhibitors—Therapeutic doses of meperidine have precipitated severe reactions in patients concurrently receiving monoamine oxidase inhibitors or those who have received such agents within 14 days. Similar reactions thus far have not been reported with methadone; but if the use of methadone is necessary in such patients, a sensitivity test should be performed in which repeated small incremental doses are administered over the course of several hours while the patient's condition and vital signs are under careful observation.

Desipramine—Blood levels of desipramine have increased with concurrent methadone therapy.

Special-Risk Patients—Methadone should be given with caution and the initial dose should be reduced in certain patients, such as the elderly or debilitated and those with severe impairment of hepatic or renal function, hypothyroidism, Addison's disease, prostatic hypertrophy, or urethral stricture.

Acute Abdominal Conditions—The administration of methadone or other narcotics may obscure the diagnosis or clinical course in patients with acute abdominal conditions.

ADVERSE REACTIONS

THE MAJOR HAZARDS OF METHADONE, AS OF OTHER NARCOTIC ANALGESICS, ARE RESPIRATORY DEPRESSION AND, TO A LESSER DEGREE, CIRCULATORY DEPRESSION. RESPIRATORY ARREST, SHOCK, AND CARDIAC ARREST HAVE OCCURRED.

The most frequently observed adverse reactions include lightheadedness, dizziness, sedation, nausea, vomiting, and sweating. These effects seem to be more prominent in ambulatory patients and in those who are not suffering severe pain. In such individuals, lower doses are advisable. Some adverse reactions may be alleviated if the ambulatory patient lies down.

Other adverse reactions include the following:

Central Nervous System—Euphoria, dysphoria, weakness, headache, insomnia, agitation, disorientation, and visual disturbances.

Gastrointestinal—Dry mouth, anorexia, constipation, and biliary tract spasm.

Cardiovascular—Flushing of the face, bradycardia, palpitation, faintness, and syncope.

Genitourinary—Urinary retention or hesitancy, antidiuretic effect, and reduced libido and/or potency.

Allergic—Pruritus, urticaria, other skin rashes, edema, and, rarely, hemorrhagic urticaria.

Hematologic—Reversible thrombocytopenia has been described in a narcotics addict with chronic hepatitis.

In addition, pain at injection site; local tissue irritation and induration following subcutaneous injection, particularly when repeated.

OVERDOSAGE

Signs and Symptoms—Methadone is an opioid and produces effects similar to those of morphine. Symptoms of overdose begin within seconds after intravenous administration and within minutes of nasal, oral, or rectal administration. Prominent symptoms are miosis, respiratory depression, somnolence, coma, cool clammy skin, skeletal muscle flaccidity that may progress to hypotension, apnea, bradycardia, and death. Noncardiac pulmonary edema may occur and monitoring of heart filling pressures may be helpful.

Treatment—To obtain up-to-date information about the treatment of overdose, a good resource is your certified Regional Poison Control Center. Telephone numbers of certified poison control centers are listed in the *Physicians' Desk Reference (PDR)*. In managing overdosage, consider the possibility of multiple drug overdoses, interaction among drugs, and unusual drug kinetics in your patient.

Initial management of opioid overdose should include establishment of a secure airway and support of ventilation and perfusion. Naloxone may be given to antagonize opioid effects, but the airway must be secured as vomiting may ensue. **The duration of methadone effect is much longer (36 to 48 hours) than the duration of naloxone effect (1 to 3 hours) and repeated doses (or continuous intravenous infusion) of naloxone may be required.**

If the patient has chronically abused opioids, administration of naloxone may precipitate a withdrawal syndrome that may include yawning, tearing, restlessness, sweating, dilated pupils, piloerection, vomiting, diarrhea, and abdominal cramps. If these symptoms develop, they should abate quickly as the effects of naloxone dissipate.

If methadone has been taken by mouth, protect the patient's airway and support ventilation and perfusion. Meticulously monitor and maintain, within acceptable limits, the patient's vital signs, blood gases, serum electrolytes, etc. Absorption of drugs from the gastrointestinal tract may be decreased by giving activated charcoal, which, in many cases, is more effective than emesis or lavage; consider charcoal instead of or in addition to gastric emptying. Repeated doses of charcoal over time may hasten elimination of some drugs that have been absorbed. Safeguard the patient's airway when employing gastric emptying or charcoal.

Forced diuresis, pertoneal dialysis, hemodialysis, or charcoal hemoperfusion have not been established as beneficial for an overdose of methadone.

> NOTE: IN AN INDIVIDUAL PHYSICALLY DEPENDENT ON NARCOTICS, THE ADMINISTRATION OF THE USUAL DOSE OF A NARCOTIC ANTAGONIST WILL PRECIPITATE AN ACUTE WITHDRAWAL SYNDROME. THE SEVERITY OF THIS SYNDROME WILL DEPEND ON THE DEGREE OF PHYSICAL DEPENDENCE AND THE DOSE OF THE ANTAGONIST ADMINISTERED. THE USE OF A NARCOTIC ANTAGONIST IN SUCH A PERSON SHOULD BE AVOIDED IF POSSIBLE. IF IT MUST BE USED TO TREAT SERIOUS RESPIRATORY DEPRESSION IN THE PHYSICALLY DEPENDENT PATIENT, THE ANTAGONIST SHOULD BE ADMINISTERED WITH EXTREME CARE AND BY TITRATION WITH SMALLER THAN USUAL DOSES OF THE ANTAGONIST.

DOSAGE AND ADMINISTRATION

For Relief of Pain—Dosage should be adjusted according to the severity of the pain and the response of the patient. Occasionally, it may be necessary to exceed the usual dosage recommended in cases of exceptionally severe pain or in those patients who have become tolerant to the analgesic effect of narcotics.

Although subcutaneous administration is suitable for occasional use, intramuscular injection is preferred when repeated doses are required.

The usual adult dosage is 2.5 to 10 mg intramuscularly or subcutaneously every 3 or 4 hours as necessary.

For Detoxification Treatment—THE DRUG SHALL BE ADMINISTERED DAILY UNDER CLOSE SUPERVISION AS FOLLOWS:

A detoxification treatment course shall not exceed 21 days and may not be repeated earlier than 4 weeks after completion of the preceding course.

The oral form of administration is preferred. However, if the patient is unable to ingest oral medication, parenteral administration may be substituted.

In detoxification, the patient may receive methadone when there are significant symptoms of withdrawal. The dosage schedules indicated below are recommended but could be varied in accordance with clinical judgment. Initially, a single dose of 15 to 20 mg of methadone will often be sufficient to suppress withdrawal symptoms. Additional methadone may be provided if withdrawal symptoms are not suppressed or if symptoms reappear. When patients are physically dependent on high doses, it may be necessary to exceed these levels. Forty mg/day in single or divided doses will usually constitute an adequate stabilizing dosage level. Stabilization can be continued for 2 to 3 days, and then the amount of methadone normally will be gradually decreased. The rate at which methadone is decreased will be determined separately for each patient. The dose of methadone can be decreased on a daily basis or at 2-day intervals, but the amount of intake shall always be sufficient to keep withdrawal symptoms at a tolerable level. In hospitalized patients, a daily reduction of 20% of the total daily dose may be tolerated and may cause little discomfort. In ambulatory patients, a somewhat slower schedule may be needed. If methadone is administered for more than 3 weeks, the procedure is considered to have progressed from detoxification or treatment of the acute withdrawal syndrome to maintenance treatment, even though the goal and intent may be eventual total withdrawal.

HOW SUPPLIED

(Ⓒ) Ampoules:

10 mg, 1 mL (No. 456)—(12s) NDC 0002-1687-12; (100s) NDC 0002-1687-02

(Ⓒ) Multiple-Dose Vials:

10 mg/mL, 20 mL (No. 435)—(1s) NDC 0002-1682-01; (25s) NDC 0002-1682-25

Store at controlled room temperature, 59° to 86°F (15° to 30°C).

[052891]

DOLOPHINE® HYDROCHLORIDE Ⓒ

[*dō'lō-fēn hī-drō-klō'rīd*]

(methadone hydrochloride)

Tablets, USP

> CONDITIONS FOR DISTRIBUTION AND USE OF METHADONE PRODUCTS:
> Code of Federal Regulations, Title 21, Sec. 291.505
> METHADONE PRODUCTS, WHEN USED FOR THE TREATMENT OF NARCOTIC ADDICTION IN DETOXIFICATION OR MAINTENANCE PROGRAMS, SHALL BE DISPENSED ONLY BY APPROVED HOSPITAL PHARMACIES, APPROVED COMMUNITY PHARMACIES, AND MAINTENANCE PROGRAMS APPROVED BY THE FOOD AND DRUG ADMINISTRATION AND THE DESIGNATED STATE AUTHORITY.
> APPROVED MAINTENANCE PROGRAMS SHALL DISPENSE AND USE METHADONE IN ORAL FORM ONLY AND ACCORDING TO THE TREATMENT REQUIREMENTS STIPULATED IN THE FEDERAL METHADONE REGULATIONS (21 CFR 291.505).
> FAILURE TO ABIDE BY THE REQUIREMENTS IN THESE REGULATIONS MAY RESULT IN CRIMINAL PROSECUTION, SEIZURE OF THE DRUG SUPPLY, REVOCATION OF THE PROGRAM APPROVAL, AND INJUNCTION PRECLUDING OPERATION OF THE PROGRAM.
> A METHADONE PRODUCT, WHEN USED AS AN ANALGESIC, MAY BE DISPENSED IN ANY LICENSED PHARMACY.

DESCRIPTION

Dolophine ® Hydrochloride (Methadone Hydrochloride Tablets, USP, Lilly) (3-heptanone, 6-(dimethylamino)-4,4-diphenyl-,hydrochloride), is a white, crystalline material that is water soluble. Its molecular weight is 345.91.

Each tablet contains 5 mg (0.015 mmol, No. 1712) or 10 mg (0.029 mmol, No. 1730) methadone hydrochloride. The tablets also contain cellulose, cornstarch, lactose, magnesium stearate, sucrose, and talc. The 10-mg tablet also contains acacia.

ACTIONS

Methadone hydrochloride is a synthetic narcotic analgesic with multiple actions quantitatively similar to those of morphine, the most prominent of which involve the central nervous system and organs composed of smooth muscle. The principal actions of therapeutic value are analgesia and sedation and detoxification or temporary maintenance in narcotic addiction. The methadone abstinence syndrome, although qualitatively similar to that of morphine, differs in that the onset is slower, the course is more prolonged, and the symptoms are less severe.

A parenteral dose of 8 to 10 mg of methadone is approximately equivalent in analgesic effect to 10 mg of morphine. With single-dose administration, the onset and duration of analgesic action of the 2 drugs are similar.

When administered orally, methadone is approximately one half as potent as when given parenterally. Oral administration results in a delay of the onset, a lowering of the peak, and an increase in the duration of analgesic effect.

INDICATIONS (See boxed Note)

For relief of severe pain.

For detoxification treatment of narcotic addiction.

For temporary maintenance treatment of narcotic addiction.

> **NOTE**
> If methadone is administered for treatment of heroin dependence for more than 3 weeks, the procedure passes from treatment of the acute withdrawal syndrome (de-

Continued on next page

• **Identi-Code® symbol. This product information was prepared in June 1992. Current information on these and other products of Eli Lilly and Company may be obtained by direct inquiry to Lilly Research Laboratories, Lilly Corporate Center, Indianapolis, Indiana 46285, (317) 276-3714.**

Lilly—Cont.

toxification) to maintenance therapy. Maintenance treatment is permitted to be undertaken only by approved methadone programs. This does not preclude the maintenance treatment of an addict who is hospitalized for medical conditions other than addiction and who requires temporary maintenance during the critical period of his/her stay or whose enrollment has been verified in a program approved for maintenance treatment with methadone.

CONTRAINDICATION

Hypersensitivity to methadone.

WARNINGS

Tablets Dolophine® Hydrochloride (Methadone Hydrochloride, USP, Lilly) are for oral administration only and *must not* be used for injection. It is recommended that Tablets Dolophine Hydrochloride, if dispensed, be packaged in child-resistant containers and kept out of the reach of children to prevent accidental ingestion.

Methadone hydrochloride, a narcotic, is a Schedule II controlled substance under the Federal Controlled Substances Act. Appropriate security measures should be taken to safeguard stocks of methadone against diversion.

DRUG DEPENDENCE—METHADONE CAN PRODUCE DRUG DEPENDENCE OF THE MORPHINE TYPE AND, THEREFORE, HAS THE POTENTIAL FOR BEING ABUSED. PSYCHIC DEPENDENCE, PHYSICAL DEPENDENCE, AND TOLERANCE MAY DEVELOP ON REPEATED ADMINISTRATION OF METHADONE, AND IT SHOULD BE PRESCRIBED AND ADMINISTERED WITH THE SAME DEGREE OF CAUTION APPROPRIATE TO THE USE OF MORPHINE.

Interaction With Other Central Nervous System Depressants —Methadone should be used with caution and in reduced dosage in patients who are concurrently receiving other narcotic analgesics, general anesthetics, phenothiazines, other tranquilizers, sedative-hypnotics, tricyclic antidepressants, and other CNS depressants (including alcohol). Respiratory depression, hypotension, and profound sedation or coma may result.

Anxiety —Since methadone, as used by tolerant subjects at a constant maintenance dosage, is not a tranquilizer, patients who are maintained on this drug will react to life problems and stresses with the same symptoms of anxiety as do other individuals. The physician should not confuse such symptoms with those of narcotic abstinence and should not attempt to treat anxiety by increasing the dosage of methadone. The action of methadone in maintenance treatment is limited to the control of narcotic symptoms and is ineffective for relief of general anxiety.

Head Injury and Increased Intracranial Pressure —The respiratory depressant effects of methadone and its capacity to elevate cerebrospinal-fluid pressure may be markedly exaggerated in the presence of increased intracranial pressure. Furthermore, narcotics produce side effects that may obscure the clinical course of patients with head injuries. In such patients, methadone must be used with caution and only if it is deemed essential.

Asthma and Other Respiratory Conditions —Methadone should be used with caution in patients having an acute asthmatic attack, in those with chronic obstructive pulmonary disease or cor pulmonale, and in individuals with a substantially decreased respiratory reserve, preexisting respiratory depression, hypoxia, or hypercapnia. In such patients, even usual therapeutic doses of narcotics may decrease respiratory drive while simultaneously increasing airway resistance to the point of apnea.

Hypotensive Effect —The administration of methadone may result in severe hypotension in an individual whose ability to maintain normal blood pressure has already been compromised by a depleted blood volume or concurrent administration of such drugs as the phenothiazines or certain anesthetics.

Use in Ambulatory Patients —Methadone may impair the mental and/or physical abilities required for the performance of potentially hazardous tasks, such as driving a car or operating machinery. The patient should be cautioned accordingly.

Methadone, like other narcotics, may produce orthostatic hypotension in ambulatory patients.

Use in Pregnancy —Safe use in pregnancy has not been established in relation to possible adverse effects on fetal development. Therefore, methadone should not be used in pregnant women unless, in the judgment of the physician, the potential benefits outweigh the possible hazards.

Methadone is not recommended for obstetric analgesia because its long duration of action increases the probability of respiratory depression in the newborn.

Use in Children —Methadone is not recommended for use as an analgesic in children, since documented clinical experience has been insufficient to establish a suitable dosage regimen for the pediatric age group.

PRECAUTIONS

Drug Interactions:

Pentazocine—**Patients who are addicted to heroin or who are on the methadone maintenance program may experience withdrawal symptoms when given an opioid agonist-antagonist, such as pentazocine.**

Rifampin—The concurrent administration of rifampin may possibly reduce the blood concentration of methadone to a degree sufficient to produce withdrawal symptoms. The mechanism by which rifampin may decrease blood concentrations of methadone is not fully understood, although enhanced microsomal drug-metabolized enzymes may influence drug disposition.

Monoamine Oxidase (MAO) Inhibitors—Therapeutic doses of meperidine have precipitated severe reactions in patients concurrently receiving monoamine oxidase inhibitors or those who have received such agents within 14 days. Similar reactions thus far have not been reported with methadone; but if the use of methadone is necessary in such patients, a sensitivity test should be performed in which repeated small incremental doses are administered over the course of several hours while the patient's condition and vital signs are under careful observation.

Desipramine—Blood levels of desipramine have increased with concurrent methadone therapy.

Special-Risk Patients —Methadone should be given with caution and the initial dose should be reduced in certain patients, such as the elderly or debilitated and those with severe impairment of hepatic or renal function, hypothyroidism, Addison's disease, prostatic hypertrophy, or urethral stricture.

Acute Abdominal Conditions —The administration of methadone or other narcotics may obscure the diagnosis or clinical course in patients with acute abdominal conditions.

ADVERSE REACTIONS

THE MAJOR HAZARDS OF METHADONE, AS OF OTHER NARCOTIC ANALGESICS, ARE RESPIRATORY DEPRESSION AND, TO A LESSER DEGREE, CIRCULATORY DEPRESSION, RESPIRATORY ARREST, SHOCK, AND CARDIAC ARREST HAVE OCCURRED.

The most frequently observed adverse reactions include lightheadedness, dizziness, sedation, nausea, vomiting, and sweating. These effects seem to be more prominent in ambulatory patients and in those who are not suffering severe pain. In such individuals, lower doses are advisable. Some adverse reactions may be alleviated if the ambulatory patient lies down.

Other adverse reactions include the following:

Central Nervous System —Euphoria, dysphoria, weakness, headache, insomnia, agitation, disorientation, and visual disturbances.

Gastrointestinal —Dry mouth, anorexia, constipation, and biliary tract spasm.

Cardiovascular —Flushing of the face, bradycardia, palpitation, faintness, and syncope.

Genitourinary —Urinary retention or hesitancy, antidiuretic effect, and reduced libido and/or potency.

Allergic —Pruritus, urticaria, other skin rashes, edema, and, rarely, hemorrhagic urticaria.

Hematologic —Reversible thrombocytopenia has been described in a narcotics addict with chronic hepatitis.

OVERDOSAGE

Signs and Symptoms —Methadone is an opioid and produces effects similar to those of morphine. Symptoms of overdose begin within seconds after intravenous administration and within minutes of nasal, oral, or rectal administration. Prominent symptoms are miosis, respiratory depression, somnolence, coma, cool clammy skin, skeletal muscle flaccidity that may progress to hypotension, apnea, bradycardia, and death. Noncardiac pulmonary edema may occur and monitoring of heart filling pressures may be helpful.

Treatment —To obtain up-to-date information about the treatment of overdose, a good resource is your certified Regional Poison Center. Telephone numbers of certified poison control centers are listed in the *Physicians' Desk Reference (PDR).* In managing overdosage, consider the possibility of multiple drug overdoses, interaction among drugs, and unusual drug kinetics in your patient.

Initial management of opioid overdose should include establishment of a secure airway and support of ventilation and perfusion. Naloxone may be given to antagonize opioid effects, but the airway must be secured as vomiting may ensue. **The duration of methadone effect is much longer (36 to 48 hours) than the duration of naloxone effect (1 to 3 hours) and repeated doses (or continuous intravenous infusion) of naloxone may be required.**

If the patient has chronically abused opioids, administration of naloxone may precipitate a withdrawal syndrome that may include yawning, tearing, restlessness, sweating, dilated pupils, piloerection, vomiting, diarrhea, and abdominal cramps. If these symptoms develop, they should abate quickly as the effects of naloxone dissipate.

If methadone has been taken by mouth, protect the patient's airway and support ventilation and perfusion. Meticulously monitor and maintain, within acceptable limits, the patient's vital signs, blood gases, serum electrolytes, etc. Absorption of drugs from the gastrointestinal tract may be decreased by giving activated charcoal, which, in many cases, is more effective than emesis or lavage; consider charcoal instead of or in addition to gastric emptying. Repeated doses of charcoal over time may hasten elimination of some drugs that have been absorbed. Safeguard the patient's airway when employing gastric emptying or charcoal.

Forced diuresis, peritoneal dialysis, hemodialysis, or charcoal hemoperfusion have not been established as beneficial for an overdose of methadone.

NOTE: IN AN INDIVIDUAL PHYSICALLY DEPENDENT ON NARCOTICS, THE ADMINISTRATION OF THE USUAL DOSE OF A NARCOTIC ANTAGONIST WILL PRECIPITATE AN ACUTE WITHDRAWAL SYNDROME. THE SEVERITY OF THIS SYNDROME WILL DEPEND ON THE DEGREE OF PHYSICAL DEPENDENCE AND THE DOSE OF THE ANTAGONIST ADMINISTERED. THE USE OF A NARCOTIC ANTAGONIST IN SUCH A PERSON SHOULD BE AVOIDED IF POSSIBLE. IF IT MUST BE USED TO TREAT SERIOUS RESPIRATORY DEPRESSION IN THE PHYSICALLY DEPENDENT PATIENT, THE ANTAGONIST SHOULD BE ADMINISTERED WITH EXTREME CARE AND BY TITRATION WITH SMALLER THAN USUAL DOSES OF THE ANTAGONIST.

DOSAGE AND ADMINISTRATION

For Relief of Pain —Dosage should be adjusted according to the severity of the pain and the response of the patient. Occasionally, it may be necessary to exceed the usual dosage recommended in cases of exceptionally severe pain or in those patients who have become tolerant to the analgesic effect of narcotics.

The usual adult dosage is 2.5 to 10 mg every 3 or 4 hours as necessary.

For Detoxification Treatment —THE DRUG SHALL BE ADMINISTERED DAILY UNDER CLOSE SUPERVISION AS FOLLOWS:

A detoxification treatment course shall not exceed 21 days and may not be repeated earlier than 4 weeks after completion of the preceding course.

In detoxification, the patient may receive methadone when there are significant symptoms of withdrawal. The dosage schedules indicated below are recommended but could be varied in accordance with clinical judgment. Initially, a single oral dose of 15 to 20 mg of methadone will often be sufficient to suppress withdrawal symptoms. Additional methadone may be provided if withdrawal symptoms are not suppressed or if symptoms reappear. When patients are physically dependent on high doses, it may be necessary to exceed these levels. Forty mg/day in single or divided doses will usually constitute an adequate stabilizing dosage level. Stabilization can be continued for 2 to 3 days, and then the amount of methadone normally will be gradually decreased. The rate at which methadone is decreased will be determined separately for each patient. The dose of methadone can be decreased on a daily basis or at 2-day intervals, but the amount of intake shall always be sufficient to keep withdrawal symptoms at a tolerable level. In hospitalized patients, a daily reduction of 20% of the total daily dose may be tolerated and may cause little discomfort. In ambulatory patients, a somewhat slower schedule may be needed. If methadone is administered for more than 3 weeks, the procedure is considered to have progressed from detoxification or treatment of the acute withdrawal syndrome to maintenance treatment, even though the goal and intent may be eventual total withdrawal.

If the patient is unable to ingest oral medication, parenteral administration may be substituted.

HOW SUPPLIED

(CII) Tablets:

5 mg (No. 1712)—(100s) NDC 0002-1064-02

10 mg (No. 1730)—(100s) NDC 0002-1072-02

Store at controlled room temperature, 59° to 86°F (15° to 30°C).

[052891]

ERGOTRATE® MALEATE ℞
[*ŭr'gō-trāt măl'ē-āt*]
(ergonovine maleate)
Injection, USP
This product is to be used by or under the direction of a physician.

DESCRIPTION

Ergonovine is the hydroxyisopropylamide of lysergic acid. It is somewhat soluble in water, and its salts are readily soluble. It is obtained from ergot and has been shown to possess all of the desirable oxytocic activity of ergot.
Each ampoule contains 0.2 mg (0.45 μmol) of the active ingredient, ergonovine maleate, with ethyl lactate, 0.1%, lactic acid, 0.1%, and phenol, 0.25%, as a preservative.
The empirical formula of ergonovine maleate is $C_{19}H_{23}N_3O_2 \cdot C_4H_4O_4$. Chemically, it is 9,10-didehydro-*N*-[(*S*)-2-hydroxy-1-methylethyl]-6-methylergoline-8β-carboxamide maleate (1:1) salt.

CLINICAL PHARMACOLOGY

Injection Ergotrate® Maleate (Ergonovine Maleate Injection, USP, Lilly) produces a firm contraction of the uterus. Superimposed upon the initial tetanic contraction is a succession of minor relaxations and contractions. The extent of relaxation gradually increases over a period of about 1½ hours, but vigorous rhythmic contractions continue for a period of 3 or more hours after injection. The prolonged initial contraction is the type necessary to control uterine hemorrhage.

INDICATIONS AND USAGE

Ergotrate Maleate is indicated for the prevention and treatment of postpartum and postabortal hemorrhage due to uterine atony.

CONTRAINDICATIONS

Ergotrate Maleate is contraindicated for the induction of labor and in cases of threatened spontaneous abortion. It should not be administered to those patients who have shown allergic or idiosyncratic reactions to it.

WARNINGS

All oxytocic agents are potentially dangerous. Mothers and infants have been injured, and some have died because of their injudicious use. Hyperstimulation of the uterus during labor may lead to uterine tetany with marked impairment of the uteroplacental blood flow, uterine rupture, cervical and perineal lacerations, amniotic fluid embolism, and trauma to the infant (eg, hypoxia, intracranial hemorrhage). Because of these hazards, which result from overdosage, oxytocic agents must be administered under conditions of meticulous observation.

PRECAUTIONS

General—Because of the high uterine tone produced, Ergotrate® Maleate (Ergonovine Maleate Injection, USP, Lilly) is not recommended for routine use prior to the delivery of the placenta unless the operator is versed in the technique described by Davis[1,2] and others and unless adequate facilities and personnel are available.
As is the case with all ergot preparations, prolonged use of Ergotrate Maleate is to be avoided. Discontinue Ergotrate Maleate if symptoms of ergotism appear.
Ergotrate Maleate should be used cautiously in patients with hypertension, heart disease, venoatrial shunts, mitral-valve stenosis, obliterative vascular disease, sepsis, or hepatic or renal impairment
The character and amount of vaginal bleeding should be observed. Hypocalcemia may affect patient response to the drug. If the patient is not also taking digitalis, cautious administration of calcium gluconate IV may produce the desired oxytocic action.
Laboratory Tests—Blood pressure, pulse, and uterine response should be monitored. Sudden changes in vital signs or frequent periods of uterine relaxation should be noted.

ADVERSE REACTIONS

Nausea and vomiting may occur, but they are uncommon. Allergic phenomena, including shock, have been reported. Ergotism has also been reported. Elevation of blood pressure (sometimes extreme) may appear in a small percentage of patients, mostly frequently in association with regional anesthesia (caudal or spinal), previous administration of a vasoconstrictor, or the intravenous route of administration of an oxytocic. The mechanism of such hypertension is obscure, since it may occur in the absence of anesthesia, vasoconstrictors, and oxytocics. These elevations are no more frequent with Ergotrate® Maleate (Ergonovine Maleate Injection, USP, Lilly) than with other oxytocics. They usually subside promptly following intravenous administration of 15 mg of chlorpromazine.
Postpartum use of ergotrates has been associated with rare cases of myocardial infarction.

OVERDOSAGE

Signs and Symptoms—Symptoms may begin within minutes of overdosage of ergot compounds and may include nausea, vomiting, headache, diarrhea, and, in women, uterine cramping. A neonate was reported to have respiratory depression, cyanosis, and convulsions. The vasoconstriction prominent with ergotamine, other ergots, and "Saint Anthony's Fire" is much less common with ergonovine. Severe chest pain, cardiac ischemia, myocardial infarction, and death may occur in patients with coronary artery disease.
Toxicity may be seen with doses of 3 mg or more. Death was reported in a 14-month old following a dose of 12 mg. Twenty-five mg given over several days proved fatal in 1 case. Toxicity and serum concentrations do not correlate well. No median lethal dose information is available.
Treatment—To obtain up-to-date information about the treatment of overdose, a good resource is your certified Regional Poison Control Center. Telephone numbers of certified poison control centers are listed in the *Physicians' Desk Reference (PDR)*. In managing overdosage, consider the possibility of multiple drug overdoses, interaction among drugs, and unusual drug kinetics in your patient.
Patients with ergot overdose should be monitored closely. A secure airway should be established and electrocardiograms monitored to assess cardiac ischemia and rhythm. Cardiac ischemia may be treated with nitroglycerin. Seizures may respond to diazepam or phenytoin. If peripheral vasoconstriction is a problem, sodium nitroprusside or phentolamine may be useful.
Protect the patient's airway and support ventilation and perfusion. Meticulously monitor and maintain, within acceptable limits, the patient's vital signs, blood gases, serum electrolytes, etc. If ergonovine was recently ingested and vomiting has not occurred, absorption of drugs from the gastrointestinal tract may be decreased by giving activated charcoal, which, in many cases, is more effective than emesis or lavage; consider charcoal instead of or in addition to gastric emptying. Repeated doses of charcoal over time may hasten elimination of some drugs that have been absorbed. Safeguard the patient's airway when employing gastric emptying or charcoal.
Forced diuresis, peritoneal dialysis, hemodialysis, or charcoal hemoperfusion have not been established as beneficial for an overdose of ergonovine.

DOSAGE AND ADMINISTRATION

Ergotrate® Maleate (Ergonovine Maleate Injection, USP, Lilly) is intended primarily for routine intramuscular injection in obstetric practice. By this route, it usually produces a firm contraction of the uterus within a few minutes.
Intravenous administration leads to a quicker response. However, because of the higher incidence of nausea and other side effects, it is recommended that the intravenous route be confined to emergencies such as excessive uterine bleeding.
The usual intramuscular (or emergency intravenous) dose of Ergotrate Maleate is 0.2 mg, 1 ampoule. Severe uterine bleeding may call for repeated doses, but injection will rarely be required more often than once in 2 to 4 hours.
In some calcium-deficient patients, the uterus may fail to respond to Ergotrate Maleate. In such instances, responsiveness can be immediately restored by the cautious intravenous injection of calcium salts. Calcium should not be given intravenously to patients under the influence of digitalis.
Tablets Ergotrate Maleate are available for oral administration.
Storage—Ampoules Ergotrate Maleate should be stored in a cold place (below 46°F). However, delivery-room stock may be kept at room temperature (although periods of more than 60 days at room temperature prior to use are not recommended).

HOW SUPPLIED

(℞) Ampoules:
0.2 mg, 1 mL (No. 302)—(6s) NDC 0002-1629-16; (100s) NDC 0002-1629-02

REFERENCES

1. Davis ME: Postpartum hemorrhage. *Am J Surg* 1940;48:154.
2. Davis ME, Boynton MW: The use of ergonovine in the placental stage of labor. *Am J Obstet Gynecol* 1942;43:775.

[101190]

FLUOXETINE HYDROCHLORIDE, *see* Prozac® (Fluoxetine Hydrochloride, Dista).

GLUCAGON FOR INJECTION ℞
[*glōō'ka-gŏn*]
USP

DESCRIPTION

Glucagon, manufactured by Eli Lilly and Company, is extracted from beef and pork pancreas.
Chemically unrelated to insulin, glucagon is a single-chain polypeptide containing 29 amino acid residues and having a molecular weight of 3,483.
The empirical formula is $C_{153}H_{225}N_{43}O_{49}S$. The structure of glucagon is shown below.

His-Ser-Gln-Gly-Thr-Phe-Thr-Ser-Asp-Tyr-Ser-Lys-Tyr-Leu-Asp-Ser-
1 2 3 4 5 6 7 8 9 10 11 12 13 14 15 16

Arg-Arg-Ala-Gln-Asp-Phe-Val-Gln-Trp-Leu-Met-Asn-Thr
17 18 19 20 21 22 23 24 25 26 27 28 29

Crystalline glucagon is a white powder containing less than 0.05% zinc. It is relatively insoluble in water but is soluble at a pH of less than 3 or more than 9.5. Glucagon is stable in lyophilized form at room temperatures.
Glucagon for Injection, USP, contains glucagon as the hydrochloride. The 1-mg vials contain 1 mg (1 unit) of glucagon and 49 mg of lactose. The 10-mg vial contains 10 mg (10 units) of glucagon and 140 mg of lactose. One USP unit of glucagon is equivalent to 1 International Unit of glucagon and also to about 1 mg of glucagon.[1] The diluent contains glycerin, 1.6%, with 0.2% phenol as a preservative. Sodium hydroxide and/or hydrochloric acid may have been added during manufacture to adjust the pH.

CLINICAL PHARMACOLOGY

Glucagon causes an increase in blood glucose concentration and is used in the treatment of hypoglycemia. It is effective in small doses, and no evidence of toxicity has been reported with its use. Glucagon acts only on liver glycogen, converting it to glucose.
Parenteral administration of glucagon produces relaxation of the smooth muscle of the stomach, duodenum, small bowel, and colon.
The half-life of glucagon in plasma is approximately 3 to 6 minutes, which is similar to that of insulin.

INDICATIONS AND USAGE

For the treatment of hypoglycemia: Glucagon is useful in counteracting severe hypoglycemic reactions.
The patient with type I diabetes does not have as great a response in blood glucose levels as does the type II stable patient. Therefore, supplementary carbohydrate should be given as soon as possible, especially to the child or adolescent patient.
For use as a diagnostic aid: Glucagon is indicated as a diagnostic aid in the radiologic examination of the stomach, duodenum, small bowel, and colon when a hypotonic state would be advantageous.
Glucagon is as effective for this examination as are the anticholinergic drugs, but it has fewer side effects. When glucagon is administered concomitantly with an anticholinergic agent, the response is not significantly greater than when either drug is used alone. However, the addition of the anticholinergic agent results in increased side effects.

CONTRAINDICATIONS

Glucagon is contraindicated in patients with known hypersensitivity to it or in patients with pheochromocytoma.

WARNINGS

Glucagon should be administered cautiously to patients with a history suggestive of insulinoma and/or pheochromocytoma. In patients with insulinoma, intravenous administration of glucagon will produce an initial increase in blood glucose; however, because of glucagon's insulin-releasing effect, it may cause the insulinoma to release its insulin and subsequently cause hypoglycemia. A patient developing symptoms of hypoglycemia after a dose of glucagon should be given glucose orally, intravenously, or by gavage, whichever is more appropriate.
Exogenous glucagon also stimulates the release of catecholamines. In the presence of pheochromocytoma, glucagon can cause the tumor to release catecholamines, which results in a sudden and marked increase in blood pressure. If a patient suddenly develops a marked increase in blood pressure, 5 to 10 mg of phentolamine mesylate may be administered intravenously in an attempt to control the blood pressure.
Generalized allergic reactions, including urticaria, respiratory distress, and hypotension, have been reported in patients who received glucagon by injection.

PRECAUTIONS

General—Glucagon is helpful in hypoglycemia only if liver glycogen is available. Because glucagon is of little or no help in states of starvation, adrenal insufficiency, or chronic hypoglycemia, glucose should be considered for the treatment of hypoglycemia.

1. *Drug Information for the Health Care Professional.* 11th ed. Rockville, MD: The United States Pharmacopeial Convention, Inc; 1991; IA: 1380.

Continued on next page

*** Identi-Code® symbol. This product information was prepared in June 1992. Current information on these and other products of Eli Lilly and Company may be obtained by direct inquiry to Lilly Research Laboratories, Lilly Corporate Center, Indianapolis, Indiana 46285, (317) 276-3714.**

Lilly—Cont.

Laboratory Tests—Blood glucose determinations may be obtained to follow the patient in hypoglycemic shock until he or she is asymptomatic.

Carcinogenesis, Mutagenesis, Impairment of Fertility—Because glucagon is usually given in a single dose and has a very short half-life (3 to 6 minutes), no studies have been done regarding carcinogenesis.

Reproduction studies have been performed in rats at doses up to 2 mg/kg b.i.d. (up 120 times the human dose) and have revealed no evidence of impaired fertility.

Usage in Pregnancy—Pregnancy Category B—Reproduction studies have been performed in rats at doses up to 2 mg/kg b.i.d. (up to 120 times the human dose), and have revealed no evidence of harm to the fetus due to glucagon. There are, however, no adequate and well-controlled studies in pregnant women. Because animal reproduction studies are not always predictive of human response, this drug should be used during pregnancy only if clearly needed.

Nursing Mothers—It is not known whether this drug is excreted in human milk. Because many drugs are excreted in human milk, caution should be exercised when glucagon is administered to a nursing woman. If the drug is excreted in human milk during its short half-life, it will be handled like any other polypeptide, ie, it will be hydrolyzed and absorbed. Glucagon is not active when taken orally because it is destroyed in the gastrointestinal tract before it can be absorbed.

ADVERSE REACTIONS

Glucagon is relatively free of adverse reactions except for occasional nausea and vomiting, which may also occur with hypoglycemia. Generalized allergic reactions have been reported (*see* Warnings).

OVERDOSAGE

Signs and Symptoms—No cases of human overdosage of glucagon have been reported. Glucagon is generally well tolerated. If overdosage occurred, it would not be expected to cause consequential toxicity but would be expected to be associated with nausea, vomiting, gastric hypotonicity, and diarrhea.

Intravenous administration of glucagon has been shown to have a positive inotropic and chronotropic effect. A transient increment in both blood pressure and pulse rate may occur following the administration of glucagon. Patients taking β-blockers might be expected to have a greater increment in both pulse and blood pressure. This increase will be transient because of glucagon's short half-life. The increase in blood pressure and pulse rate may require therapy in patients with pheochromocytoma or coronary artery disease.

When glucagon was given in large doses to cardiac patients, investigators reported a positive inotropic effect. These investigators administered glucagon in doses of 0.5 to 16 mg/hour by continuous infusion for periods of 5 to 166 hours. Total doses ranged from 25 to 996 mg, and a 21-month child received approximately 8.25 mg in 165 hours. Side effects included nausea, vomiting, and decreasing serum potassium concentration. Serum potassium concentration could be maintained within normal limits with supplemental potassium.

The intravenous median lethal dose for glucagon in mice is approximately 300 mg/kg.

Because glucagon is a polypeptide, it would be rapidly destroyed in the gastrointestinal tract if it were to be accidentally ingested.

Treatment—To obtain up-to-date information about the treatment of overdose, a good resource is your certified Regional Poison Control Center. Telephone numbers of certified poison control centers are listed in the *Physicians' Desk Reference (PDR)*. In managing overdosage, consider the possibility of multiple drug overdoses, interaction among drugs, and unusual drug kinetics in your patient.

In view of the extremely short half-life of glucagon and its prompt destruction and excretion, the treatment of overdosage is symptomatic, primarily for nausea, vomiting, and possible hypokalemia.

If the patient develops a dramatic increase in blood pressure, 5 mg to 10 mg of phentolamine has been shown to be effecitve in lowering blood pressure for the short time that control would be needed.

Forced diuresis, peritoneal dialysis, hemodialysis, or charcoal hemoperfusion have not been established as beneficial for an overdose of glucagon; it is extremely unlikely that one of these procedures would ever be indicated.

DOSAGE AND ADMINISTRATION

For the treatment of hypoglycemia: The diluent is provided for use only in the preparation of glucagon for *intermittent* parenteral injection and for no other use.

If glucagon is to be given at doses higher than 2 mg, it should be reconstituted with Sterile Water for Injection instead of the supplied diluting solution and used immediately.

Directions for Use of Glucagon—1. Dissolve the lyophilized glucagon in the accompanying diluent.

2. Glucagon should not be used at concentrations greater than 1 mg (1 unit/mL).

3. Glucagon solutions should not be used unless they are clear and of a water-like consistency.

4. Give 0.5 to 1 mg (0.5 to 1 unit) of glucagon by subcutaneous, intramuscular, or intravenous injection.

5. The patient will usually awaken within 15 minutes. If the response is delayed, there is no contraindication to the administration of 1 or 2 additional doses of glucagon; however, in view of the deleterious effects of cerebral hypoglycemia and depending on the duration and depth of coma, the use of parenteral glucose *must* be considered by the physician.

6. Intravenous glucose *must* be given if the patient fails to respond to glucagon.

7. When the patient responds, give supplemental carbohydrate to restore the liver glycogen and prevent secondary hypoglycemia.

General Management of Hypoglycemia—The following are helpful measures in the prevention of hypoglycemic reactions due to insulin:

1. Reasonable uniformity from day to day with regard to diet, insulin, and exercise.

2. Careful adjustment of the insulin program so that the type (or types) of insulin, dose, and time (or times) of administration are suited to the individual patient.

3. Frequent testing of the blood or urine so that a change in insulin requirements can be foreseen.

4. Routine carrying of sugar, candy, or other readily absorbable carbohydrate by the patient so that it may be taken at the first warning of an oncoming reaction.

If the patient is unaware of the symptoms of hypoglycemia, he/she may lapse into insulin shock; therefore, the physician should instruct the patient in this regard when feasible.

It is important that the patient be aroused as quickly as possible, because prolonged hypoglycemic reactions may result in cortical damage. Glucagon or intravenous glucose will awaken the patient sufficiently so that oral carbohydrates may be taken.

Instructions to the Family—Instructions describing the method of using this preparation are included in the literature that accompanies the patient's package. It is advisable for the patient and family members to become familiar with the technique of preparing Glucagon for Injection before an emergency arises. Patient instructions include the use of 0.5 mg (0.5 units) for small children if recommended by the physician.

CAUTION—Although the patient may use glucagon for the treatment of hypoglycemia during an emergency, the physician must still be notified when hypoglycemic reactions occur so that the dose of insulin may be adjusted if necessary.

For use as a diagnostic aid: Dissolve the lyophilized glucagon in the accompanying diluting solution.

Glucagon should not be used at concentrations greater than 1 mg (1 unit/mL).

The following doses may be administered for relaxation of the stomach, duodenum, and small bowel, depending on the time of onset of action and the duration of effect required for the examination. Since the stomach is less sensitive to the effect of glucagon, 0.5 mg (0.5 units) IV or 2 mg (2 units) IM are recommended.

[See table below.]

For examination of the colon, it is recommended that a 2-mg (2 units) dose be administered intramuscularly approximately 10 minutes prior to initiation of the procedure. Relaxation of the colon and reduction of discomfort to the patient will allow the radiologist to perform a more satisfactory examination.

Stability and Storage:

Before Reconstitution—Vials of Glucagon as well as the Diluting Solution for Glucagon for Injection, USP, may be stored at controlled room temperature, 59° to 86°F (15° to 30°C).

After Reconstitution—Glucagon in 1-mL vials or Hyporets should be used immediately. Glucagon reconstituted with the Diluting Solution for Glucagon for Injection in multiple-dose vials may be stored at 41°F (5°C) for up to 48 hours if necessary. Glucagon reconstituted with Sterile Water for Injection should be used immediately.

Dose	Route of Administration	Time of Onset of Action	Approximate Duration of Effect
0.25–0.5 mg	IV	1 minute	9–17 minutes
1 mg	IM	8–10 minutes	12–27 minutes
2 mg*	IV	1 minute	22–25 minutes
2 mg*	IM	4–7 minutes	21–32 minutes

* Administration of 2-mg (2 units) doses produces a higher incidence of nausea and vomiting than do lower doses.

HOW SUPPLIED

(℞) Vials:

1 mg (1 unit)—(No. 666), with 1-mL vial of diluting solution (No. 667) (1s) NDC 0002-1450-01

10 mg (10 units)—(No. 668), multiple dose, with 10-mL vials of diluting solution (No. 669) (1s) NDC 0002-1451-01

(℞) Glucagon Emergency Kit (M-8030): 1 mg (1 unit)—(No. 7286), with 1-mL of diluting solution (Hyporet* No. 7287) (1s) NDC 0002-8030-01

* Hyporet® (disposable syringe, Lilly)

[040792]

HEPARIN SODIUM ℞

[*hĕp'ă-rŭn sō'dē-ŭm*]

Injection, USP

WARNING—This is a potent drug, and serious consequences may result if used without constant medical supervision.

DESCRIPTION

Heparin is a heterogenous group of straight-chain anionic mucopolysaccharides, called glycosaminoglycans, having anticoagulant properties. Although others may be present, the main sugars in heparin are: (1) α-L-iduronic acid 2-sulfate, (2) 2-deoxy-2-sulfamino-α-glucose 6-sulfate, (3) β-D-glucuronic acid, (4) 2-acetamido-2-deoxy-α-D-glucose, and (5) α-L-iduronic acid. These sugars are present in decreasing amounts, usually in the order (2) > (1) > (4) > (3) > (5), and are joined by glycosidic linkages, forming polymers of varying sizes. Heparin is strongly acidic because of its covalently linked sulfate and carboxylic acid groups. In heparin sodium, the acidic protons of the sulfate units are partially replaced by sodium ions.

Structure of Heparin Sodium (representative subunits):

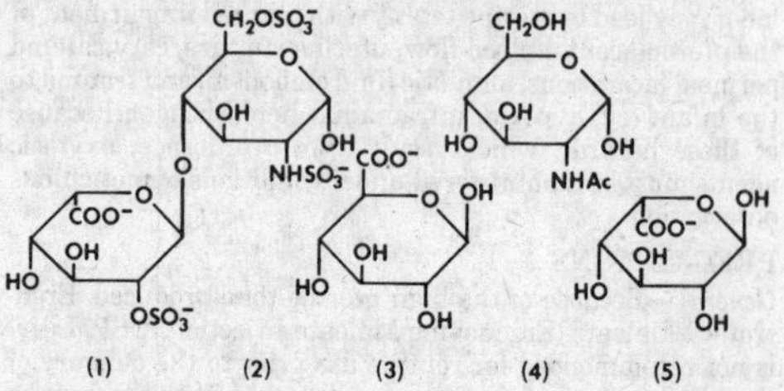

(1) (2) (3) (4) (5)

Heparin Sodium Injection, USP, is a sterile solution of heparin sodium derived from porcine intestinal mucosa, which is standardized for anticoagulant activity. It is to be administered by intravenous or deep subcutaneous routes. The potency is determined by a biological assay using a USP reference standard based on units of heparin activity per milligram.

Each mL of Vial No. 520 contains 10,000 USP heparin units (derived from porcine intestinal mucosa) and sodium chloride, 0.1%.

During manufacture, 1% benzyl alcohol is added as a preservative to each vial of heparin sodium. Sodium hydroxide and/or hydrochloric acid may be added during manufacture to adjust the pH.

CLINICAL PHARMACOLOGY

Heparin inhibits reactions that lead to the clotting of blood and the formation of fibrin clots both in vitro and in vivo. Heparin acts at multiple sites in the normal coagulation system. Small amounts of heparin in combination with antithrombin III (heparin cofactor) can inhibit thrombosis by inactivating activated Factor X and inhibiting the conversion of prothrombin to thrombin. Once active thrombosis has developed, larger amounts of heparin can inhibit further coagulation by inactivating thrombin and preventing the conversion of fibrinogen to fibrin. Heparin also prevents the formation of a stable fibrin clot by inhibiting the activation of the fibrin stabilizing factor.

Bleeding time is usually unaffected by heparin. Clotting time is prolonged by full therapeutic doses of heparin; in most cases, it is not measurably affected by low doses.

Peak plasma levels of heparin are achieved 2 to 4 hours following subcutaneous administration, although there are considerable individual variations. Log linear plots of heparin plasma concentrations with time for a wide range of dose levels are linear, which suggests the absence of zero order processes. The liver and the reticuloendothelial system are the sites of biotransformation. The biphasic elimination

curve, a rapidly declining α phase ($t_{1/2} = 10'$) and, after the age of 40, a slower β phase indicate uptake in organs. The absence of a relationship between anticoagulant half-life and concentration half-life may reflect factors such as protein binding of heparin.

Heparin does not have fibrinolytic activity; therefore, it will not lyse existing clots.

INDICATIONS AND USAGE

Heparin sodium is indicated for:

Anticoagulant therapy in prophylaxis and treatment of venous thrombosis and its extension.

Prevention (in a low-dose regimen) of postoperative deep venous thrombosis and pulmonary embolism in patients undergoing major abdominothoracic surgery or who, for other reasons, are at risk of developing thromboembolic disease (see Dosage and Administration)

Prophylaxis and treatment of pulmonary embolism

Atrial fibrillation with embolization

Diagnosis and treatment of acute and chronic consumption coagulopathies (eg, disseminated intravascular coagulation)

Prevention of clotting in arterial and heart surgery

Prophylaxis and treatment of peripheral arterial embolism

As an anticoagulant in blood transfusions, extracorporeal circulation, and dialysis procedures and in blood samples for laboratory purposes

CONTRAINDICATIONS

Heparin sodium should not be used in patients with severe thrombocytopenia or patients for whom suitable blood coagulation tests (eg, tests for whole-blood clotting time and partial thromboplastin time) cannot be performed at appropriate intervals. (This restriction refers to full-dose administration of heparin; it is usually unnecessary to monitor coagulation parameters in patients receiving low-dose heparin). In addition, heparin sodium should not be administered to patients in an uncontrollable active bleeding state (see Warnings), except when this condition is the result of disseminated intravascular coagulation.

WARNINGS

Heparin is not intended for intramuscular use.

Hypersensitivity—Patients with documented hypersensitivity to heparin should be given the drug only in clearly life-threatening situations.

Hemorrhage—Hemorrhage can occur at virtually any site in patients receiving heparin. An unexplained fall in hematocrit, a fall in blood pressure, or any other unexplained symptom warrants consideration of a hemorrhagic event.

Heparin sodium should be used with extreme caution in disease states in which there is increased danger of hemorrhage. Some of the conditions in which this danger exists are as follows:

Cardiovascular—Subacute bacterial endocarditis. Severe hypertension.

Surgical—During and immediately following (a) a spinal tap or spinal anesthesia or (b) major surgery, especially involving the brain, spinal cord, or eye.

Hematologic—Conditions associated with increased bleeding tendencies, such as hemophilia, thrombocytopenia, and some vascular purpuras.

Gastrointestinal—Ulcerative lesions and continuous tube drainage of the stomach or small intestine.

Other—Menstruation and liver disease with impaired hemostasis.

Coagulation Testing—When heparin sodium is administered in therapeutic amounts, its dosage should be regulated by frequent blood coagulation tests. If the coagulation test result is unduly prolonged or if hemorrhage occurs, heparin sodium should be discontinued promptly (see Overdosage).

Thrombocytopenia—Thrombocytopenia occurs in patients receiving heparin with a reported incidence of 0% to 30%. Mild thrombocytopenia (count greater than 100,000/mm^3) may remain stable or reverse, even if heparin is continued. However, thrombocytopenia of any degree should be monitored closely. If the count falls below 100,000/mm^3 or if recurrent thrombosis develops (see Precautions, *White-Clot Syndrome*), the heparin product should be discontinued. If continued heparin therapy is essential, utilize heparin from a different organ source and reinstitute therapy with caution.

Miscellaneous—This product contains benzyl alcohol as a preservative. Benzyl alcohol has been reported to be associated with a fatal "gasping syndrome" in premature infants.

PRECAUTIONS

General—White-Clot Syndrome—It has been reported that patients taking heparin may develop new thrombus formation in association with thrombocytopenia. This development is the result of the irreversible aggregation of platelets induced by heparin, ie, the so-called "white-clot syndrome." The process may lead to severe thromboembolic complications such as skin necrosis, gangrene of the extremities that may lead to amputation, myocardial infarction, pulmonary embolism, stroke, and possibly death. Therefore, heparin administration should be promptly discontinued if a patient

develops new thrombosis in association with thrombocytopenia.

Heparin Resistance—Increased resistance to heparin is frequently encountered in cases involving fever, thrombosis, thrombophlebitis, infections with thrombosing tendencies, myocardial infarction, and cancer. Increased resistance can also occur in postsurgical patients.

Increased Risk in Older Women—A higher incidence of bleeding has been reported in women over 60 years of age.

Laboratory Tests—Periodic platelet counts, hematocrit determinations, and tests for occult blood in the stool are recommended during the entire course of heparin therapy, regardless of the route of administration (see Dosage and Administration).

Drug Interactions—Oral anticoagulants: Heparin sodium may prolong the one-stage prothrombin time. Therefore, if a valid prothrombin time is to be obtained when heparin sodium is given with dicumarol or warfarin sodium, a period of at least 5 hours after the last intravenous dose or 24 hours after the last subcutaneous dose should elapse before blood is drawn.

Platelet inhibitors: Drugs such as acetylsalicylic acid, dextran, phenylbutazone, ibuprofen, indomethacin, dipyridamole, hydroxychloroquine, and others that interfere with platelet-aggregation reactions (the main hemostatic defense of heparinized patients) may induce bleeding and should be used with caution in patients receiving heparin sodium.

Other interactions: Digitalis, tetracyclines, nicotine, or antihistamines may partially counteract the anticoagulant action of heparin sodium.

Intravenous nitroglycerin administered to heparinized patients may result in a decrease of the partial thromboplastin time with subsequent rebound effect upon discontinuation of nitroglycerin. Careful monitoring of partial thromboplastin time and adjustment of heparin dosage are recommended during coadministration of heparin and intravenous nitroglycerin.

When clinical circumstances require reversal heparinization, consult the labeling of Protamine Sulfate Injection, USP.

Drug/Laboratory Test Interactions—Hyperaminotransferasemia. Significant elevations of aminotransferase (SGOT and SGPT) levels have occurred in a high percentage of patients (and healthy subjects) who have received heparin. Since aminotransferase determinations are important in the differential diagnosis of myocardial infarction, liver disease, and pulmonary emboli, increases that might be caused by drugs (eg, heparin) should be interpreted with caution.

Carcinogenesis, Mutagenesis, Impairment of Fertility—No long-term studies in animals have been performed to evaluate the carcinogenic potential of heparin. Also, no reproduction studies in animals have been performed concerning mutagenesis or impairment of fertility.

Pregnancy—Teratogenic Effects: Pregnancy Category C—Animal reproduction studies have not been conducted with heparin sodium. It is also not known whether heparin sodium can cause fetal harm when administered to a pregnant woman or can affect reproduction capacity. Heparin sodium should be given to a pregnant woman only if clearly needed.

Nonteratogenic Effects: Heparin does not cross the placental barrier.

Nursing Mothers—Heparin is not excreted in human milk.

Pediatric Use—See Dosage and Administration.

ADVERSE REACTIONS

Hemorrhage—Hemorrhage is the chief complication that may result from heparin therapy (see Warnings). An overly prolonged clotting time or minor bleeding during therapy can usually be controlled by withdrawing the drug (see Overdosage). *Gastrointestinal or urinary tract bleeding during anticoagulant therapy may indicate the presence of an underlying occult lesion.* Bleeding can occur at any site, but certain specific hemorrhagic complications may be difficult to detect:

Adrenal hemorrhage, with resultant acute adrenal insufficiency, has occurred during anticoagulant therapy. Therefore, such treatment should be discontinued in patients who develop signs and symptoms of acute adrenal hemorrhage and insufficiency. Initiation of corrective therapy should not be delayed for laboratory confirmation of the diagnosis, since any delay in an acute situation may result in the patient's death.

Ovarian (corpus luteum) hemorrhage developed in a number of women of reproductive age receiving short- or long-term anticoagulant therapy. If unrecognized, this complication may be fatal.

Retroperitoneal hemorrhage has occurred.

Local Irritation—Local irritation, erythema, mild pain, hematoma, or ulceration may follow deep subcutaneous (intrafat) injection of heparin sodium. These complications are much more common after intramuscular use; therefore, such use is not recommended.

Hypersensitivity—Generalized hypersensitivity reactions have been reported, with chills, fever, and urticaria as the most common manifestations; asthma, rhinitis, lacrimation,

headache, nausea and vomiting, and anaphylactoid reactions (including shock) have occurred more rarely. Itching and burning, especially on the plantar site of the feet, may occur.

The occurrence of thrombocytopenia has been reported in patients receiving heparin, with an incidence of 0% to 30%. Although often mild and of no obvious clinical significance, such thrombocytopenia can be accompanied by severe thromboembolic complications, such as skin necrosis, gangrene of the extremities that may lead to amputation, myocardial infarction, pulmonary embolism, stroke, and possibly death (see Warnings and Precautions).

Certain episodes of painful, ischemic, and cyanosed limbs have, in the past, been attributed to allergic vasospastic reactions. Whether these are, in fact, identical to the thrombocytopenia-associated complications remains to be determined.

Miscellaneous—Osteoporosis following long-term administration of high doses of heparin, cutaneous necrosis after systemic administration, suppression of aldosterone synthesis, delayed transient alopecia, priapism, and rebound hyperlipemia occurring after discontinuation of heparin sodium have also been reported.

Significant elevations of aminotransferase (SGOT and SGPT) levels have occurred in a high percentage of patients (and healthy subjects) who have received heparin.

OVERDOSAGE

Signs and Symptoms—Overdose of heparin may follow parenteral administration, but oral heparin has little systemic effect. Bleeding is the chief sign of heparin overdosage. Excessive heparin effect also increases whole-blood clotting time and activated partial thromboplastin time (APTT). The half-life of heparin ranges from 0.5 to 2.5 hours and may vary widely in cases involving an overdose.

The intravenous median lethal dose in mice is 1,500 mg/kg.

Treatment—To obtain up-to-date information about the treatment of overdose, a good resource is your certified Regional Poison Control Center. Telephone numbers of certified poison control centers are listed in the *Physicians' Desk Reference (PDR)*. In managing overdosage, consider the possibility of multiple drug overdoses, interaction among drugs, and unusual drug kinetics in your patient.

Minor bleeding occurring during therapy with heparin can often be treated by reducing the dose or increasing the dosing interval.

For major bleeding episodes, heparin may be neutralized by protamine; 1 mg of protamine will neutralize approximately 115 units of heparin of porcine intestinal mucosal origin. Protamine dosage may be guided by determining the amount of time by which clotting is shortened in vitro or by the results of other hematologic tests. Note that protamine may cause anaphylactoid reactions that may be life threatening. (See the protamine label for additional information.) The administration of whole blood or fresh frozen plasma should be considered for patients with significant blood losses. Vitamin K will not reverse the activity of heparin.

DOSAGE AND ADMINISTRATION

Parenteral drug products should be inspected visually for particulate matter and discoloration prior to administration if solution and container permit. Slight discoloration does not alter potency.

When heparin is added to an infusion solution for continuous intravenous administration, the container should be inverted at least 6 times to ensure adequate mixing and prevent pooling of the heparin in the solution.

Heparin sodium is not effective by oral administration and should be given by intermittent intravenous injection, intravenous infusion, or deep subcutaneous (intrafat, ie, above the iliac crest or abdominal fat layer) injection. *The intramuscular route of administration should be avoided because of frequent occurrence of hematoma at the injection site.*

The dosage of heparin sodium should be adjusted according to the patient's coagulation test results. When heparin is given by continuous intravenous infusion, the coagulation time should be determined approximately every 4 hours in the early stages of treatment. When the drug is administered intermittently by intravenous injection, coagulation tests should be performed before each injection during the early stages of treatment and at appropriate intervals thereafter. Dosage is considered adequate when the APTT is 1.5 to 2 times normal or when the whole-blood clotting time is elevated approximately 2.5 to 3 times the control value. After deep subcutaneous (intrafat) injections, tests for adequacy of dosage are best performed on samples drawn 4 to 6 hours after the injections.

Continued on next page

• Identi-Code® symbol. This product information was prepared in June 1992. Current information on these and other products of Eli Lilly and Company may be obtained by direct inquiry to Lilly Research Laboratories, Lilly Corporate Center, Indianapolis, Indiana 46285, (317) 276-3714.

Lilly—Cont.

Method of Administration	Frequency	Recommended Dose*
Deep Subcutaneous (Intrafat) Injection (A different site should be used for each injection to prevent the development of massive hematoma)	Initial dose	5,000 units by IV injection, followed by 10,000–20,000 units of a concentrated solution, subcutaneously
	Every 8 hours or	8,000–10,000 units of a concentrated solution
	Every 12 hours	15,000–20,000 units of a concentrated solution
Intermittent Intravenous Injection	Initial dose	10,000 units, either undiluted or in 50–100 mL of 0.9% Sodium Chloride Injection, USP
	Every 4 to 6 hours	5,000–10,000 units, either undiluted or in 50–100 mL of 0.9% Sodium Chloride Injection, USP
Continuous Intravenous infusion	Initial dose	5,000 units by IV injection
	Continuous Infusion	20,000–40,000 units/24 hours in 1,000 mL of 0.9% Sodium-Chloride Injection, USP (or in any compatible solution) for infusion

*Based on 150-lb (68-kg) patient.

Periodic platelet counts, hematocrit determinations, and tests for occult blood in the stool are recommended during the entire course of heparin therapy, regardless of the route of administration.

Converting to Oral Anticoagulant—When an oral anticoagulant of the coumarin (or similar) type is to be administered in patients already receiving heparin sodium, baseline and subsequent tests of prothrombin activity must be determined at times during which heparin activity is too low to affect the prothrombin time. Such a time usually occurs about 5 hours after the last IV bolus and 24 hours after the last subcutaneous dose. If heparin is continuously infused by IV, prothrombin time can usually be measured at any time. In converting from heparin to an oral anticoagulant, the oral anticoagulant should be given in the usual initial amount; thereafter, prothrombin time should be determined at the usual intervals. To ensure continuous anticoagulation, it is advisable to continue full heparin therapy for several days after the prothrombin time has reached the limit of the therapeutic range. Heparin therapy may then be discontinued without tapering.

Therapeutic Anticoagulant Effect With Full-Dose Heparin—Although dosage must be adjusted for the individual patient according to the results of appropriate laboratory tests, the following dosage schedule may be used as a guideline: [See table above.]

Pediatric Use—Follow recommendations of appropriate pediatric reference texts.

In general, the following dosage schedule may be used as a guideline:

Initial Dose: 50 units/kg (IV, drip)

Maintenance Dose: 100 units/kg (IV, drip) every 4 hours, or 20,000 units/m^2/24 hours, infused continuously

Surgery of the Heart and Blood Vessels—Patients undergoing total body perfusion for open heart surgery should receive an initial dose of not less than 150 units of heparin sodium per kg of body weight. Frequently, a dose of 300 units/kg is used for procedures estimated to last less than 60 minutes; a dose of 400 units/kg is often used for those procedures likely to last longer than 60 minutes.

Low-Dose Prophylaxis of Postoperative Thromboembolism—A number of well-controlled clinical trials have demonstrated that low-dose heparin prophylaxis, given prior to and after surgery, will reduce the incidences of postoperative deep-vein thrombosis in the legs (as measured by the I-125 fibrinogen technique and venography) and of clinical pulmonary embolism. The most widely used dosage is 5,000 units given 2 hours before surgery and 5,000 units given every 8 to 12 hours thereafter for 7 days or until the patient is fully ambulatory, whichever is longer. The heparin is given by deep subcutaneous (intrafat, ie, above the iliac crest or abdominal fat layer, arm, or thigh) injection with a fine (25- to 26-gauge) needle to minimize tissue trauma. A concentrated solution of heparin sodium is recommended. Such prophylaxis should be reserved for patients over the age of 40 who are undergoing major surgery. Patients with bleeding disorders and those having brain or spinal-cord surgery, spinal anesthesia, eye surgery, or potentially sanguineous operations should be excluded from this treatment, as should patients receiving oral anticoagulants or platelet-active drugs (*see* Warnings). The value of such prophylaxis in hip surgery has not been established. The possibility of increased bleeding during surgery or postoperatively should be borne in mind. If such bleeding occurs, discontinuance of heparin and neutralization with protamine sulfate are advisable. If clinical evidence of thromboembolism develops despite low-dose prophylaxis, full therapeutic doses of anticoagulants should be given unless contraindicated. Prior to initiating heparinization, the physician should rule out the probability of bleeding disorders by taking a thorough history and performing the appropriate laboratory tests. Appropriate coagulation tests should be repeated just prior to surgery. Coagulation test values should be normal or only slightly elevated at these times.

Extracorporeal Dialysis—Follow equipment manufacturers' operating directions carefully.

Blood Transfusion—The addition of 400 to 600 USP units to each 100 mL of whole blood for transfusion is usually employed to prevent coagulation. Usually, 7,500 USP units of heparin sodium are mixed with 100 mL of 0.9% Sodium Chloride Injection, USP (or 75,000 USP units/1,000 mL of 0.9% Sodium Chloride Injection, USP); 6 to 8 mL of this sterile solution is then added to each 100 mL of whole blood used.

Laboratory Samples—70 to 150 units of heparin sodium are usually added per 10- to 20-mL sample of whole blood to prevent coagulation of the sample. Leukocyte counts should be performed on heparinized blood within 2 hours after the addition of the heparin. Heparinized blood should not be used for isoagglutinin, complement, or erythrocyte fragility tests or for taking platelet counts.

Clearing Intermittent Infusion (Heparin Lock) Sets—To prevent clot formation in a heparin lock set following its proper insertion, dilute heparin solution (*see* USP monograph for Heparin Lock Flush Solution, USP) should be injected via the injection hub in a quantity sufficient to fill the entire set to the needle tip. This solution should be replaced each time the heparin lock is used. Aspirate before administering any solution via the lock in order to confirm the patency and location of the needle or catheter tip. If the drug to be administered is incompatible with heparin, the entire heparin lock set should be flushed with sterile water or normal saline before and after the medication is administered; following the second cleansing flush, the dilute heparin solution may be reinstilled in the set. The set manufacturer's instructions should be consulted for specifics concerning the heparin lock set being used at a given time.

NOTE: Since repeated injections of small doses of heparin can alter tests for activated partial thromboplastin time (APTT), a baseline value for APTT should be obtained prior to insertion of a heparin lock set.

HOW SUPPLIED

(℞) Multiple-Dose Vials:

10,000 USP heparin units/mL, 5 mL (No. 520)—(1s) NDC 0002-7217-01

Protect from light. Store at controlled room temperature, 59° to 86°F (15° to 30°C).

[040292]

HUMATROPE® ℞

[*hū ′ma-trōp*]

(somatropin (rDNA origin) for injection)

DESCRIPTION

Humatrope® (Somatropin, rDNA Origin, for Injection, Lilly) is a polypeptide hormone of recombinant DNA origin. Humatrope has 191 amino acid residues and a molecular weight of about 22,125 daltons. The amino acid sequence of the product is identical to that of human growth hormone of pituitary origin. Humatrope is synthesized in a strain of *Escherichia coli* that has been modified by the addition of the gene for human growth hormone.

Humatrope is a sterile, white, lyophilized powder intended for subcutaneous or intramuscular administration after reconstitution. Each vial of Humatrope contains 5 mg somatropin (approximately 13 IU or 225 picomoles); 25 mg mannitol; 5 mg glycine; and 1.13 mg dibasic sodium phosphate. Phosphoric acid and/or sodium hydroxide may have been added at the time of manufacture to adjust the pH. Each vial is supplied in a combination package with an accompanying 5-mL vial of diluting solution. The diluent contains water for injection with 0.3% *m*-cresol as a preservative and 1.7% glycerin added at the time of manufacture.

Humatrope is a highly purified preparation. The 1.7% glycerin content makes the reconstituted product nearly isotonic at a concentration of 2 mg of Humatrope/mL diluent. Reconstituted solutions have a pH of approximately 7.5.

CLINICAL PHARMACOLOGY

Linear Growth—Humatrope® (Somatropin, rDNA Origin, for Injection, Lilly) stimulates linear growth in children who lack adequate normal endogenous growth hormone. In vitro, preclinical, and clinical testing have demonstrated that Humatrope is therapeutically equivalent to human growth hormone of pituitary origin and achieves equivalent pharmacokinetic profiles in normal adults. Treatment of growth-hormone-deficient children with Humatrope produces increased growth rate and IGF-1 (Insulin-like Growth Factor/Somatomedin-C) concentrations similar to those seen after therapy with human growth hormone of pituitary origin.

In addition, the following actions have been demonstrated for Humatrope and/or human growth hormone of pituitary origin.

A. Tissue Growth—1. Skeletal Growth: Humatrope stimulates skeletal growth in patients with growth hormone deficiency. The measurable increase in body length after administration of either Humatrope or human growth hormone of pituitary origin results from an effect on the growth plates of long bones. Concentrations of IGF-1, which may play a role in skeletal growth, are low in the serum of growth-hormone-deficient children but increase during treatment with Humatrope. Elevations in mean serum alkaline phosphatase concentrations are also seen. 2. Cell Growth: It has been shown that there are fewer skeletal muscle cells in short-statured children who lack endogenous growth hormone as compared with normal children. Treatment with human growth hormone of pituitary origin results in an increase in both the number and size of muscle cells.

B. Protein Metabolism—Linear growth is facilitated in part by increased cellular protein synthesis. Nitrogen retention, as demonstrated by decreased urinary nitrogen excretion and serum urea nitrogen, follows the initiation of therapy with human growth hormone of pituitary origin. Treatment with Humatrope results in a similar decrease in serum urea nitrogen.

C. Carbohydrate Metabolism—Children with hypopituitarism sometimes experience fasting hypoglycemia that is improved by treatment with Humatrope. Large doses of human growth hormone may impair glucose tolerance.

D. Lipid Metabolism—In growth-hormone-deficient patients, administration of human growth hormone of pituitary origin has resulted in lipid mobilization, reduction in body fat stores, and increased plasma fatty acids.

E. Mineral Metabolism—Retention of sodium, potassium, and phosphorus is induced by human growth hormone of pituitary origin. Serum concentrations of inorganic phosphate increased in patients with growth hormone deficiency after therapy with Humatrope or human growth hormone of pituitary origin. Serum calcium is not significantly altered in patients with either human growth hormone of pituitary origin or Humatrope.

INDICATION AND USAGE

Humatrope® (Somatropin, rDNA Origin, for Injection, Lilly) is indicated only for the long-term treatment of children who have growth failure due to an inadequate secretion of normal endogenous growth hormone.

CONTRAINDICATIONS

Humatrope® (Somatropin, rDNA Origin, for Injection, Lilly) should not be used in subjects with closed epiphyses. Humatrope should not be used when there is any evidence of activity of a tumor. Intracranial lesions must be inactive and antitumor therapy complete prior to the institution of therapy. Humatrope should be discontinued if there is evidence of tumor growth.

Humatrope should not be reconstituted with the supplied Diluent for Humatrope by patients with a known sensitivity to either *m*-cresol or glycerin.

WARNING

If sensitivity to the diluent should occur, the vials may be reconstituted with Sterile Water for Injection, USP. When Humatrope® (Somatropin, rDNA Origin, for Injection, Lilly) is reconstituted in this manner, (1) use only 1 reconstituted dose per vial, (2) refrigerate the solution (36° to 46°F [2° to 8°C]) if it is not used immediately after reconstitution, (3) use the reconstituted dose within 24 hours, and (4) discard the unused portion.

PRECAUTIONS

Therapy with Humatrope® (Somatropin, rDNA Origin, for Injection, Lilly) should be directed by physicians who are experienced in the diagnosis and management of patients with growth hormone deficiency.

Patients with growth hormone deficiency secondary to an intracranial lesion should be examined frequently for progression or recurrence of the underlying disease process.

Because human growth hormone may induce a state of insulin resistance, patients should be observed for evidence of glucose intolerance.

Excessive glucocorticoid therapy will inhibit the growth-promoting effect of human growth hormone. Patients with coexisting ACTH deficiency should have their glucocorticoid replacement dose carefully adjusted to avoid an inhibitory effect on growth.

Hypothyroidism may develop during treatment with human growth hormone, and inadequate treatment of hypothyroidism may prevent optimal response to human growth hormone. Therefore, patients should have periodic thyroid function tests and be treated with thyroid hormone when indicated.

Patients with endocrine disorders, including growth hormone deficiency, may develop slipped capital epiphyses more frequently. Any child with the onset of a limp during growth hormone therapy should be evaluated.

Carcinogenesis, Mutagenesis, Impairment of Fertility—Long-term animal studies for carcinogenicity and impairment of fertility with this human growth hormone (Humatrope) have not been performed. There has been no evidence to date of Humatrope-induced mutagenicity.

Pregnancy—Pregnancy Category C—Animal reproduction studies have not been conducted with Humatrope. It is not known whether Humatrope can cause fetal harm when administered to a pregnant woman or can affect reproduction capacity. Humatrope should be given to a pregnant woman only if clearly needed.

Nursing Mothers—There have been no studies conducted with Humatrope in nursing mothers. It is not known whether this drug is excreted in human milk. Because many drugs are excreted in human milk, caution should be exercised when Humatrope is administered to a nursing woman.

ADVERSE REACTIONS

Approximately 2% of 481 naive and previously treated clinical trial patients treated with Humatrope® (Somatropin, rDNA Origin, for Injection, Lilly) have developed antibodies to growth hormone, as demonstrated by a binding capacity determination threshold ≥ 0.02 μg/mL. Nevertheless, even these patients experienced increases in linear growth and other salutary effects of Humatrope and did not experience any unusual adverse events. Although growth-limiting antibodies have been observed with other growth hormone preparations (including products of pituitary origin), antibodies in patients treated with Humatrope have not limited growth. The long-term implications of antibody development are uncertain at this time.

Of the 232 naive and previously treated clinical trial patients receiving Humatrope for 6 months or more, 4.7% had serum binding of radiolabeled growth hormone in excess of twice the binding observed in control sera when the serum samples were assayed at a tenfold dilution. Among these patients were 160 naive patients, of whom 6.9% had positive serum binding. In comparison, 74.5% of 106 naive patients treated for 6 months or more with somatrem (produced by Lilly) in a similar clinical trial had serum binding of radiolabeled growth hormone of at least twice the binding observed in control sera.

In addition to an evaluation of compliance with the treatment program and of thyroid status, testing for antibodies to human growth hormone should be carried out in any patient who fails to respond to therapy.

In clinical studies in which high doses of Humatrope were administered to healthy adult volunteers, the following events have occurred infrequently: headache, localized muscle pain, weakness, mild hyperglycemia, and glucosuria. In studies with growth-hormone-deficient children, injection site pain was reported infrequently. A mild and transient edema, which appeared in 2.5% of patients, was observed early during the course of treatment.

Leukemia has been reported in a small number of children who have been treated with growth hormone, including growth hormone of pituitary origin as well as of recombinant DNA origin (somatrem and somatropin). The relationship, if any, between leukemia and growth hormone therapy is uncertain.

OVERDOSAGE

The recommended dosage is up to 0.06 mg/kg (0.16 IU/kg) of body weight 3 times per week. Acute overdosage could lead initially to hypoglycemia and subsequently to hyperglycemia. Long-term overdosage could result in signs and symptoms of acromegaly consistent with the known effects of excess human growth hormone.

DOSAGE AND ADMINISTRATION

A dosage of up to 0.06 mg/kg (0.16 IU/kg) of body weight administered 3 times per week by subcutaneous or intramuscular injection is recommended. The dosage and administration schedule for Humatrope® (Somatropin, rDNA Origin, for Injection, Lilly) should be individualized for each patient. Each 5-mg vial of Humatrope should be reconstituted with 1.5 to 5 mL of Diluent for Humatrope. The diluent should be injected into the vial of Humatrope by aiming the stream of liquid against the glass wall. Following reconstitution, the vial should be swirled with a GENTLE rotary motion until the contents are completely dissolved. DO NOT SHAKE. The resulting solution should be clear, without particulate matter. If the solution is cloudy or contains particulate matter, the contents MUST NOT be injected.

Before and after injection, the septum of the vial should be wiped with rubbing alcohol or an alcoholic antiseptic solution to prevent contamination of the contents by repeated needle insertions. Sterile disposable syringes and/or needles should be used for administration of Humatrope. The volume of the syringe should be small enough so that the prescribed dose can be withdrawn from the vial with reasonable accuracy.

STABILITY AND STORAGE

Before Reconstitution—Vials of Humatrope® (Somatropin, rDNA Origin, for Injection, Lilly) as well as the Diluent for Humatrope are stable when refrigerated (36° to 46°F [2° to 8°C]). Avoid freezing Diluent for Humatrope. Expiration dates are stated on the labels.

After Reconstitution—Vials of Humatrope are stable for up to 14 days when reconstituted with Diluent for Humatrope and stored in a refrigerator at 36° to 46°F (2° to 8°C). Avoid freezing the reconstituted Vial of Humatrope.

HOW SUPPLIED

℞ Vials:

5 mg (No. 7335)—(6s) NDC 0002-7335-16, and 5-mL vial of Diluent for Humatrope (No. 7336)

[041692]

HUMULIN® 50/50® OTC

[*hū′mū-lĭn*]

(50% Human Insulin Isophane Suspension and 50% Human Insulin Injection [Recombinant DNA Origin])

INFORMATION FOR THE PATIENT

WARNINGS

THIS LILLY HUMAN INSULIN PRODUCT DIFFERS FROM ANIMAL-SOURCE INSULINS BECAUSE IT IS STRUCTURALLY IDENTICAL TO THE INSULIN PRODUCED BY YOUR BODY'S PANCREAS AND BECAUSE OF ITS UNIQUE MANUFACTURING PROCESS.

ANY CHANGE OF INSULIN SHOULD BE MADE CAUTIOUSLY AND ONLY UNDER MEDICAL SUPERVISION. CHANGES IN PURITY, STRENGTH, BRAND (MANUFACTURER), TYPE (REGULAR, NPH, LENTE®, ETC), SPECIES (BEEF, PORK, BEEF-PORK, HUMAN), AND/OR METHOD OF MANUFACTURE (RECOMBINANT DNA VERSUS ANIMAL-SOURCE INSULIN) MAY RESULT IN THE NEED FOR A CHANGE IN DOSAGE.

SOME PATIENTS TAKING HUMULIN® (HUMAN INSULIN, RECOMBINANT DNA ORIGIN, LILLY) MAY REQUIRE A CHANGE IN DOSAGE FROM THAT USED WITH ANIMAL-SOURCE INSULINS. IF AN ADJUSTMENT IS NEEDED, IT MAY OCCUR WITH THE FIRST DOSE OR DURING THE FIRST SEVERAL WEEKS OR MONTHS.

DIABETES

Insulin is a hormone produced by the pancreas, a large gland that lies near the stomach. This hormone is necessary for the body's correct use of food, especially sugar. Diabetes occurs when the pancreas does not make enough insulin to meet your body's needs.

To control your diabetes, your doctor has prescribed injections of insulin to keep your blood glucose at a nearly normal level. Proper control of your diabetes requires close and constant cooperation with your doctor. In spite of diabetes, you can lead an active, healthy, and useful life if you eat a balanced diet daily, exercise regularly, and take your insulin injections as prescribed.

You have been instructed to test your blood and/or your urine regularly for glucose. If your blood tests consistently show above- or below-normal glucose levels or your urine tests consistently show the presence of glucose, your diabetes is not properly controlled and you must let your doctor know.

Always keep an extra supply of insulin as well as a spare syringe and needle on hand. Always wear diabetic identification so that appropriate treatment can be given if complications occur away from home.

50/50 HUMAN INSULIN

Description

Humulin is synthesized in a non-disease-producing special laboratory strain of *Escherichia coli* bacteria that has been genetically altered by the addition of the gene for human insulin production. Humulin 50/50 is a mixture of 50% Human Insulin Isophane Suspension and 50% Human Insulin Injection. It is an intermediate-acting insulin combined with the more rapid onset of action of regular insulin. The duration of activity may last up to 24 hours following injection. The time course of action of any insulin may vary considerably in different individuals or at different times in the same individual. As with all insulin preparations, the duration of action of Humulin 50/50 is dependent on dose, site of injection, blood supply, temperature, and physical activity. Humulin 50/50 is a sterile suspension and is for subcutaneous injection only. It should not be used intravenously or intramuscularly. The concentration of Humulin 50/50 is 100 units/mL (U-100).

Identification

Human insulin manufactured by Eli Lilly and Company has the trademark Humulin and is available in 7 formulations—Regular (**R**), Buffered Regular (**BR**), NPH (**N**), Lente (**L**), Ultralente® (**U**), 50% Human Insulin Isophane Suspension [NPH]/50% Human Insulin Injection [buffered regular] (**50/50**) and 70% Human Insulin Isophane Suspension [NPH]/30% Human Insulin Injection [buffered regular] (**70/30**). Your doctor has prescribed the type of insulin that he/she believes is best for you. **DO NOT USE ANY OTHER INSULIN EXCEPT ON HIS/HER ADVICE AND DIRECTION.**

Always check the carton and the bottle label for the name and letter designation of the insulin you receive from your pharmacy to make sure it is the same as that your doctor has prescribed. (*See illustration under* Humulin® L.)

Always examine the appearance of your bottle of insulin before withdrawing each dose. A bottle of Humulin 50/50 must be carefully shaken or rotated before each injection so that the contents are uniformly mixed. Humulin 50/50 should look uniformly cloudy or milky after mixing. Do not use it if the insulin substance (the white material) remains at the bottom of the bottle after mixing. Do not use a bottle of Humulin 50/50 if there are clumps in the insulin after mixing (*See Figure 1 under* Humulin® N.) Do not use a bottle of Humulin 50/50 if solid white particles stick to the bottom or wall of the bottle, giving it a frosted appearance (*See Figure 2 under* Humulin® N.) Always check the appearance of your bottle of insulin before using, and if you note anything unusual in the appearance of your insulin or notice your insulin requirements changing markedly, consult your doctor.

Storage

Insulin should be stored in a refrigerator but not in the freezer. If refrigeration is not possible, the bottle of insulin that you are currently using can be kept unrefrigerated as long as it is kept as cool as possible (below 86°F [30°C]) and away from heat and light. Do not use insulin if it has been frozen. Do not use a bottle of insulin after the expiration date stamped on the label.

INJECTION PROCEDURES

Correct Syringe

Doses of insulin are measured in **units.** U-100 insulin contains 100 units/mL (1 mL = 1 cc). With Humulin 50/50, it is important to use a syringe that is marked for U-100 insulin preparations. Failure to use the proper syringe can lead to a mistake in dosage, causing serious problems for you, such as a blood glucose level that is too low or too high.

Syringe Use

To help avoid contamination and possible infection, follow these instructions exactly.

Disposable syringes and needles should be used only once and then discarded.

NEEDLES AND SYRINGES MUST NOT BE SHARED.

Reusable syringes and needles must be sterilized before each injection. **Follow the package directions supplied with your syringe.** Described below are 2 methods of sterilizing.

Boiling

1. Put syringe, plunger, and needle in strainer, place in saucepan, and cover with water. Boil for 5 minutes.
2. Remove articles from water. When they have cooled, insert plunger into barrel, and fasten needle to syringe with a slight twist.
3. Push plunger in and out several times until water is completely removed.

Isopropyl Alcohol

If the syringe, plunger, and needle cannot be boiled, as when you are traveling, they may be sterilized by immersion for at least 5 minutes in Isopropyl Alcohol, 91%. Do not use bathing, rubbing, or medicated alcohol for this sterilization. If the syringe is sterilized with alcohol, it must be absolutely dry before use.

Preparing the Dose

1. Wash your hands.
2. Carefully shake or rotate the insulin bottle several times to completely mix the insulin.
3. Inspect the insulin. Humulin 50/50 should look uniformly cloudy or milky. Do not use it if you notice anything unusual in the appearance.
4. If using a new bottle, flip off the plastic protective cap, but **do not** remove the stopper. When using a new bottle, wipe the top of the bottle with an alcohol swab.

Continued on next page

• Identi-Code® symbol. This product information was prepared in June 1992. Current information on these and other products of Eli Lilly and Company may be obtained by direct inquiry to Lilly Research Laboratories, Lilly Corporate Center, Indianapolis, Indiana 46285, (317) 276-3714.

Lilly—Cont.

5. Draw air into the syringe equal to your insulin dose. Put the needle through rubber top of the insulin bottle and inject the air into the bottle.
6. Turn the bottle and syringe upside down. Hold the bottle and syringe firmly in 1 hand and shake gently.
7. Making sure the tip of the needle is in the insulin, withdraw the correct dose of insulin into the syringe.
8. Before removing the needle from the bottle, check your syringe for air bubbles which reduce the amount of insulin in it. If bubbles are present, hold the syringe straight up and tap its side until the bubbles float to the top. Push them out with the plunger and withdraw the correct dose.
9. Remove the needle from the bottle and lay the syringe down so that the needle does not touch anything.

Injection
Cleanse the skin with alcohol where the injection is to be made. Stabilize the skin by spreading it or pinching up a large area. Insert the needle as instructed by your doctor. Push the plunger in as far as it will go. Pull the needle out and apply gentle pressure over the injection site for several seconds. **Do not rub the area.** To avoid tissue damage, give the next injection at a site at least ½" from the previous site.

DOSAGE
Your doctor has told you which insulin to use, how much, and when and how often to inject it. Because each patient's case of diabetes is different, this schedule has been individualized for you.
Your usual insulin dose may be affected by changes in your food, activity, or work schedule. Carefully follow your doctor's instructions to allow for these changes. Other things that may affect your insulin dose are:

Illness
Illness, especially with nausea and vomiting, may cause your insulin requirements to change. Even if you are not eating, you will still require insulin. You and your doctor should establish a sick day plan for you to use in case of illness. When you are sick, test your blood/urine frequently and call your doctor as instructed.

Pregnancy
Good control of diabetes is especially important for you and your unborn baby. Pregnancy may make managing your diabetes more difficult. If you are planning to have a baby, are pregnant, or are nursing a baby, consult your doctor.

Medication
Insulin requirements may be increased if you are taking other drugs with hyperglycemic activity, such as oral contraceptives, corticosteroids, or thyroid replacement therapy. Insulin requirements may be reduced in the presence of drugs with hypoglycemic activity, such as oral hypoglycemics, salicylates (for example, aspirin), sulfa antibiotics, and certain antidepressants. Always discuss any medications you are taking with your doctor.

Exercise
Exercise may lower your body's need for insulin during and for some time after the activity. Exercise may also speed up the effect of an insulin dose, especially if the exercise involves the area of injection site (for example, the leg should not be used for injection just prior to running). Discuss with your doctor how you should adjust your regimen to accommodate exercise.

Travel
Persons traveling across more than 2 time zones should consult their doctor concerning adjustments in their insulin schedule.

COMMON PROBLEMS OF DIABETES

Hypoglycemia (Insulin Reactions)
Hypoglycemia (too little glucose in the blood) is one of the most frequent adverse events experienced by insulin users. It can be brought about by:
1. Taking too much insulin
2. Missing or delaying meals
3. Exercising or working more than usual
4. An infection or illness (especially with diarrhea or vomiting)
5. A change in the body's need for insulin
6. Diseases of the adrenal, pituitary, or thyroid gland, or progression of kidney or liver disease
7. Interactions with other drugs that lower blood glucose, such as oral hypoglycemics, salicylates (for example, aspirin), sulfa antibiotics, and certain antidepressants
8. Consumption of alcoholic beverages

Symptoms of mild to moderate hypoglycemia may occur suddenly and can include:
- sweating
- dizziness
- palpitation
- tremor
- hunger
- restlessness
- tingling in the hands, feet, lips, or tongue
- lightheadedness
- inability to concentrate
- headache
- drowsiness
- sleep disturbances
- anxiety
- blurred vision
- slurred speech
- depressive mood
- irritability
- abnormal behavior
- unsteady movement
- personality changes

Signs of severe hypoglycemia can include:
- disorientation
- unconsciousness
- seizures
- death

Therefore, it is important that assistance be obtained immediately.
Early warning symptoms of hypoglycemia may be different or less pronounced under certain conditions, such as long duration of diabetes, diabetic nerve disease, medications such as beta-blockers, change in insulin preparations, or intensified control (3 or more insulin injections per day) of diabetes.
A few patients who have experienced hypoglycemic reactions after transfer from animal-source insulin to human insulin have reported that the early warning symptoms of hypoglycemia were less pronounced or different from those experienced with their previous insulin.
Without recognition of early warning symptoms, you may not be able to take steps to avoid more serious hypoglycemia. Be alert for all of the various types of symptoms that may indicate hypoglycemia. Patients who experience hypoglycemia without early warning symptoms should monitor their blood glucose frequently, especially prior to activities such as driving. If the blood glucose is below your normal fasting glucose, you should consider eating or drinking sugar-containing foods to treat your hypoglycemia.
Mild to moderate hypoglycemia may be treated by eating foods or drinks that contain sugar. Patients should always carry a quick source of sugar, such as candy mints or glucose tablets. More severe hypoglycemia may require the assistance of another person. Patients who are unable to take sugar orally or who are unconscious require an injection of glucagon or should be treated with intravenous administration of glucose at a medical facility.
You should learn to recognize your own symptoms of hypoglycemia. If you are uncertain about these symptoms, you should monitor your blood glucose frequently to help you learn to recognize the symptoms that you experience with hypoglycemia.
If you have frequent episodes of hypoglycemia or experience difficulty in recognizing the symptoms, you should consult your doctor to discuss possible changes in therapy, meal plans, and/or exercise programs to help you avoid hypoglycemia.

Hyperglycemia and Diabetic Acidosis
Hyperglycemia (too much glucose in the blood) may develop if your body has too little insulin. Hyperglycemia can be brought about by:
1. Omitting your insulin or taking less than the doctor has prescribed
2. Eating significantly more than your meal plan suggests
3. Developing a fever or infection

In patients with insulin-dependent diabetes, prolonged hyperglycemia can result in diabetic acidosis. The first symptoms of diabetic acidosis usually come on gradually, over a period of hours or days, and include a drowsy feeling, flushed face, thirst, loss of appetite, and fruity odor on the breath. With acidosis, urine tests show large amounts of glucose and acetone. Heavy breathing and a rapid pulse are more severe symptoms. If uncorrected, prolonged hyperglycemia or diabetic acidosis can result in loss of consciousness or death. Therefore, it is important that you obtain medical assistance immediately.

Lipodystrophy
Rarely, administration of insulin subcutaneously can result in lipoatrophy (depression in the skin) or lipohypertrophy (enlargement or thickening of tissue). If you notice either of these conditions, consult your doctor. A change in your injection technique may help alleviate the problem.

Allergy to Insulin
Local Allergy—Patients occasionally experience redness, swelling, and itching at the site of injection of insulin. This condition, called local allergy, usually clears up in a few days to a few weeks. In some instances, this condition may be related to factors other than insulin, such as irritants in the skin cleansing agent or poor injection technique. If you have local reactions, contact your doctor.
Systemic Allergy—Less common, but potentially more serious, is generalized allergy to insulin, which may cause rash over the whole body, shortness of breath, wheezing, reduction in blood pressure, fast pulse, or sweating. Severe cases of generalized allergy may be life threatening. If you think you are having a generalized allergic reaction to insulin, notify a doctor immediately.

HOW SUPPLIED
Vials, U-100, 100 units/mL, 10 mL (No. HI-1510) (1's), NDC 0002-9515-01

[031292]

HUMULIN® 70/30 OTC
[*hū 'mŭ-lĭn*]
(70% Human Insulin Isophane Suspension and 30% Human Insulin Injection [Recombinant DNA origin])

INFORMATION FOR THE PATIENT

WARNINGS

THIS LILLY HUMAN INSULIN PRODUCT DIFFERS FROM ANIMAL-SOURCE INSULINS, BECAUSE IT IS STRUCTURALLY IDENTICAL TO THE INSULIN PRODUCED BY YOUR BODY'S PANCREAS AND BECAUSE OF ITS UNIQUE MANUFACTURING PROCESS.
ANY CHANGE OF INSULIN SHOULD BE MADE CAUTIOUSLY AND ONLY UNDER MEDICAL SUPERVISION. CHANGES IN PURITY, STRENGTH, BRAND (MANUFACTURER), TYPE (REGULAR, NPH, LENTE®, ETC), SPECIES (BEEF, PORK, BEEF-PORK, HUMAN), AND/OR METHOD OF MANUFACTURE (RECOMBINANT DNA VERSUS ANIMAL-SOURCE INSULIN) MAY RESULT IN THE NEED FOR A CHANGE IN DOSAGE.
SOME PATIENTS TAKING HUMULIN® (HUMAN INSULIN, RECOMBINANT DNA ORIGIN, LILLY) MAY REQUIRE A CHANGE IN DOSAGE FROM THAT USED WITH ANIMAL-SOURCE INSULINS. IF AN ADJUSTMENT IS NEEDED, IT MAY OCCUR WITH THE FIRST DOSE OR DURING THE FIRST SEVERAL WEEKS OR MONTHS.

DIABETES
Insulin is a hormone produced by the pancreas, a large gland that lies near the stomach. This hormone is necessary for the body's correct use of food, especially sugar. Diabetes occurs when the pancreas does not make enough insulin to meet your body's needs.
To control your diabetes, your doctor has prescribed injections of insulin to keep your blood glucose at a nearly normal level. Proper control of your diabetes requires close and constant cooperation with your doctor. In spite of diabetes, you can lead an active, healthy, and useful life if you eat a balanced diet daily, exercise regularly, and take your insulin injections as prescribed.
You have been instructed to test your blood and/or your urine regularly for glucose. If your blood tests consistently show above- or below-normal glucose levels or your urine tests consistently show the presence of glucose, your diabetes is not properly controlled and you must let your doctor know. Always keep an extra supply of insulin as well as spare syringe and needle on hand. Always wear diabetic identification so that appropriate treatment can be given if complications occur away from home.

70/30 HUMAN INSULIN

Description
Humulin is synthesized in a non-disease-producing special laboratory strain of *Escherichia coli* bacteria that has been genetically altered by the addition of the gene for human insulin production. Humulin 70/30 is a mixture of 70% Human Insulin Isophane Suspension and 30% Human Insulin Injection. It is an intermediate-acting insulin combined with the more rapid onset of action of regular insulin. The duration of activity may last up to 24 hours following injection. The time course of action of any insulin may vary considerably in different individuals or at different times in the same individual. As with all insulin preparations, the duration of action of Humulin 70/30 is dependent on dose, site of injection, blood supply, temperature, and physical activity. Humulin 70/30 is a sterile suspension and is for subcutaneous injection only. It should not be used intravenously or intramuscularly. The concentration of Humulin 70/30 is 100 units/mL (U-100).

Identification
Human insulin manufactured by Eli Lilly and Company has the trademark Humulin and is available in 7 formulations—Regular (**R**), Buffered Regular (**BR**), NPH (**N**), Lente (**L**), Ultralente® (**U**), 50% Human Insulin Isophane Suspension [NPH]/50% Human Insulin Injection [buffered regular] (**50/50**), and 70% Human Insulin Isophane Suspension [NPH]/30% Human Insulin Injection [buffered regular] (**70/30**). Your doctor has prescribed the type of insulin that he/she believes is best for you. **DO NOT USE ANY OTHER INSULIN EXCEPT ON HIS/HER ADVICE AND DIRECTION.**
Always check the carton and the bottle label for the name and letter designation of the insulin you receive from your pharmacy to make sure it is the same as that your doctor has prescribed (*See illustration under* Humulin® L.)
Always examine the appearance of your bottle of insulin before withdrawing each dose. A bottle of Humulin 70/30 must be carefully shaken or rotated before each injection so

that the contents are uniformly mixed. Humulin 70/30 should look uniformly cloudy or milky after mixing. Do not use it if the insulin substance (the white material) remains at the bottom of the bottle after mixing. Do not use a bottle of Humulin 70/30 if there are clumps in the insulin after mixing (*See Figure 1 under* Humulin® N). Do not use a bottle of Humulin 70/30 if solid white particles stick to the bottom or wall of the bottle, giving it a frosted appearance (*See Figure 2 under* Humulin® N). Always check the appearance of your bottle of insulin before using, and if you note anything unusual in the appearance of your insulin or notice your insulin requirements changing markedly, consult your doctor.

Storage

Insulin should be stored in a refrigerator but not in the freezer. If refrigeration is not possible, the bottle of insulin that you are currently using can be kept unrefrigerated as long as it is kept as cool as possible (below 86°F [30°C]) and away from heat and light. Do not use insulin if it has been frozen. Do not use a bottle of insulin after the expiration date stamped on the label.

INJECTION PROCEDURES

Correct Syringe

Doses of insulin are measured in **units.** U-100 insulin contains 100 units/mL (1 mL=1 cc). With Humulin 70/30, it is important to use a syringe that is marked for U-100 insulin preparations. Failure to use the proper syringe can lead to a mistake in dosage, causing serious problems for you, such as a blood glucose level that is too low or too high.

Syringe Use

To help avoid contamination and possible infection, follow these instructions exactly.

Disposable syringes and needles should be used only once and then discarded.

NEEDLES AND SYRINGES MUST NOT BE SHARED.
Reusable syringes and needles must be sterilized before each injection. **Follow the package directions supplied with your syringe.** Described below are 2 methods of sterilizing.

Boiling

1. Put syringe, plunger, and needle in strainer, place in saucepan, and cover with water. Boil for 5 minutes.
2. Remove articles from water. When they have cooled, insert plunger into barrel, and fasten needle to syringe with a slight twist.
3. Push plunger in and out several times until water is completely removed.

Isopropyl Alcohol

If the syringe, plunger, and needle cannot be boiled, as when you are traveling, they may be sterilized by immersion for at least 5 minutes in Isopropyl Alcohol, 91%. Do not use bathing, rubbing, or medicated alcohol for this sterilization. If the syringe is sterilized with alcohol, it must be absolutely dry before use.

Preparing the Dose

1. Wash your hands.
2. Carefully shake or rotate the insulin bottle several times to completely mix the insulin.
3. Inspect the insulin. Humulin 70/30 should look uniformly cloudy or milky. Do not use it if you notice anything unusual in the appearance.
4. If using a new bottle, flip off the plastic protective cap, but **do not** remove the stopper. When using a new bottle, wipe the top of the bottle with an alcohol swab.
5. Draw air into the syringe equal to your insulin dose. Put the needle through rubber top of the insulin bottle and inject the air into the bottle.
6. Turn the bottle and syringe upside down. Hold the bottle and syringe firmly in 1 hand and shake gently.
7. Making sure the tip of the needle is in the insulin, withdraw the correct dose of insulin into the syringe.
8. Before removing the needle from the bottle, check your syringe for air bubbles which reduce the amount of insulin in it. If bubbles are present, hold the syringe straight up and tap its side until the bubbles float to the top. Push them out with the plunger and withdraw the correct dose.
9. Remove the needle from the bottle and lay the syringe down so that the needle does not touch anything.

Injection

Cleanse the skin with alcohol where the injection is to be made. Stabilize the skin by spreading it or pinching up a large area. Insert the needle as instructed by your doctor. Push the plunger in as far as it will go. Pull the needle out and apply gentle pressure over the injection site for several seconds. **Do not rub the area.** To avoid tissue damage, give the next injection at a site at least ½″ from the previous site.

DOSAGE

Your doctor has told you which insulin to use, how much, and when and how often to inject it. Because each patient's case of diabetes is different, this schedule has been individualized for you.

Your usual insulin dose may be affected by changes in your food, activity, or work schedule. Carefully follow your doctor's instructions to allow for these changes. Other things that may affect your insulin dose are:

Illness

Illness, especially with nausea and vomiting, may cause your insulin requirements to change. Even if you are not eating, you will still require insulin. You and your doctor should establish a sick day plan for you to use in case of illness. When you are sick, test your blood/urine frequently and call your doctor as instructed.

Pregnancy

Good control of diabetes is especially important for you and your unborn baby. Pregnancy may make managing your diabetes more difficult. If you are planning to have a baby, are pregnant, or are nursing a baby, consult your doctor.

Medication

Insulin requirements may be increased if you are taking other drugs with hyperglycemic activity, such as oral contraceptives, corticosteroids, or thyroid replacement therapy. Insulin requirements may be reduced in the presence of drugs with hypoglycemic activity, such as oral hypoglycemics, salicylates (for example, aspirin), sulfa antibiotics, and certain antidepressants. Always discuss any medications you are taking with your doctor.

Exercise

Exercise may lower your body's need for insulin during and for some time after the activity. Exercise may also speed up the effect of an insulin dose, especially if the exercise involves the area of injection site (for example, the leg should not be used for injection just prior to running). Discuss with your doctor how you should adjust your regimen to accommodate exercise.

Travel

Persons traveling across more than 2 time zones should consult their doctor concerning adjustments in their insulin schedule.

COMMON PROBLEMS OF DIABETES

Hypoglycemia (Insulin Reaction)

Hypoglycemia (too little glucose in the blood) is one of the most frequent adverse events experienced by insulin users. It can be brought about by:

1. Taking too much insulin
2. Missing or delaying meals
3. Exercising or working more than usual
4. An infection or illness (especially with diarrhea or vomiting)
5. A change in the body's need for insulin
6. Diseases of the adrenal, pituitary, or thyroid gland, or progression of kidney or liver disease
7. Interactions with other drugs that lower blood glucose, such as oral hypoglycemics, salicylates (for example, aspirin), sulfa antibiotics, and certain antidepressants
8. Consumption of alcoholic beverages

Symptoms of mild to moderate hypoglycemia may occur suddenly and can include:

- sweating
- dizziness
- palpitation
- tremor
- hunger
- restlessness
- tingling in the hands, feet, lips, or tongue
- lightheadedness
- inability to concentrate
- headache
- drowsiness
- sleep disturbances
- anxiety
- blurred vision
- slurred speech
- depressive mood
- irritability
- abnormal behavior
- unsteady movement
- personality changes

Signs of severe hypoglycemia can include:

- disorientation
- unconsciousness
- seizures
- death

Therefore, it is important that assistance be obtained immediately.

Early warning symptoms of hypoglycemia may be different or less pronounced under certain conditions, such as long duration of diabetes, diabetic nerve disease, medications such as beta-blockers, change in insulin preparations, or intensified control (3 or more insulin injections per day) of diabetes.

A few patients who have experienced hypoglycemic reactions after transfer from animal-source insulin to human insulin have reported that the early warning symptoms of hypoglycemia were less pronounced or different from those experienced with their previous insulin.

Without recognition of early warning symptoms, you may not be able to take steps to avoid more serious hypoglycemia. Be alert for all of the various types of symptoms that may indicate hypoglycemia. Patients who experience hypoglycemia without early warning symptoms should monitor their

blood glucose frequently, especially prior to activities such as driving. If the blood glucose is below your normal fasting glucose, you should consider eating or drinking sugar-containing foods to treat your hypoglycemia.

Mild to moderate hypoglycemia may be treated by eating foods or drinks that contain sugar. Patients should always carry a quick source of sugar, such as candy mints or glucose tablets. More severe hypoglycemia may require the assistance of another person. Patients who are unable to take sugar orally or who are unconscious require an injection of glucagon or should be treated with intravenous administration of glucose at a medical facility.

You should learn to recognize your own symptoms of hypoglycemia. If you are uncertain about these symptoms, you should monitor your blood glucose frequently to help you learn to recognize the symptoms that you experience with hypoglycemia.

If you have frequent episodes of hypoglycemia or experience difficulty in recognizing the symptoms, you should consult your doctor to discuss possible changes in therapy, meal plans, and/or exercise programs to help you avoid hypoglycemia.

Hyperglycemia and Diabetic Acidosis

Hyperglycemia (too much glucose in the blood) may develop if your body has too little insulin. Hyperglycemia can be brought about by:

1. Omitting your insulin or taking less than the doctor has prescribed
2. Eating significantly more than your meal plan suggests
3. Developing a fever or infection

In patients with insulin-dependent diabetes, prolonged hyperglycemia can result in diabetic acidosis. The first symptoms of diabetic acidosis usually come on gradually, over a period of hours or days, and include a drowsy feeling, flushed face, thirst, loss of appetite, and fruity odor on the breath. With acidosis, urine tests show large amounts of glucose and acetone. Heavy breathing and a rapid pulse are more severe symptoms. If uncorrected, prolonged hyperglycemia or diabetic acidosis can result in loss of consciousness or death. Therefore, it is important that you obtain medical assistance immediately.

Lipodystrophy

Rarely, administration of insulin subcutaneously can result in lipoatrophy (depression in the skin) or lipohypertrophy (enlargement or thickening of tissue). If you notice either of these conditions, consult your doctor. A change in your injection technique may help alleviate the problem.

Allergy to Insulin

Local Allergy—Patients occasionally experience redness, swelling, and itching at the site of injection of insulin. This condition, called local allergy, usually clears up in a few days to a few weeks. In some instances, this condition may be related to factors other than insulin, such as irritants in the skin cleansing agent or poor injection technique. If you have local reactions, contact your doctor.

Systemic Allergy—Less common, but potentially more serious, is generalized allergy to insulin, which may cause rash over the whole body, shortness of breath, wheezing, reduction in blood pressure, fast pulse, or sweating. Severe cases of generalized allergy may be life threatening. If you think you are having a generalized allergic reaction to insulin, notify a doctor immediately.

ADDITIONAL INFORMATION

Additional information about diabetes may be obtained from your diabetes educator.

DIABETES FORECAST is a national magazine designed especially for patients with diabetes and their families and is available by subscription from the American Diabetes Association, National Service Center, 1660 Duke Street, Alexandria, Virginia 22314.

Another publication, **DIABETES COUNTDOWN,** is available from the Juvenile Diabetes Foundation, 432 Park Avenue South, New York, New York 10016-8013.

HOW SUPPLIED

Vials, U-100, 100 units/mL, 10 mL (No. HI-710) (1's), NDC 0002-8715-01

[060592]

Continued on next page

• Identi-Code® symbol. This product information was prepared in June 1992. Current information on these and other products of Eli Lilly and Company may be obtained by direct inquiry to Lilly Research Laboratories, Lilly Corporate Center, Indianapolis, Indiana 46285, (317) 276-3714.

Lilly—Cont.

HUMULIN® BR   OTC
[hū'mŭ-lĭn bē är]
Buffered Regular
(insulin human injection, USP
[recombinant DNA origin])
FOR EXTERNAL INSULIN PUMPS ONLY

INFORMATION FOR THE PATIENT
WARNINGS
FOR USE ONLY IN EXTERNAL INSULIN PUMPS.
DO NOT MIX WITH OTHER INSULIN PRODUCTS.
HUMULIN BR SHOULD NOT BE MIXED WITH OTHER IN-
SULINS BECAUSE THE BUFFERING INGREDIENT COULD
INTERACT WITH OTHER INSULINS AND CHANGE THEIR
ACTIVITY. THIS COULD LEAD TO AN UNDESIRED EF-
FECT ON BLOOD GLUCOSE, SUCH AS HYPOGLYCEMIA
(LOW BLOOD GLUCOSE).
HUMULIN BR HAS BEEN TESTED ONLY IN CARDIAC
PACEMAKERS, INC, SERIES 9100 AND 9200 INFUSION
DEVICES. PATIENTS PARTICIPATING IN THE STUDY
CHANGED THE INSULIN IN THE RESERVOIR (SYRINGE)
EVERY 24 HOURS.
THIS LILLY HUMAN INSULIN PRODUCT DIFFERS FROM
ANIMAL-SOURCE INSULINS BECAUSE IT IS STRUCTUR-
ALLY IDENTICAL TO THE INSULIN PRODUCED BY YOUR
BODY'S PANCREAS AND BECAUSE OF ITS UNIQUE MAN-
UFACTURING PROCESS.
ANY CHANGE OF INSULIN SHOULD BE MADE CAU-
TIOUSLY AND ONLY UNDER MEDICAL SUPERVISION.
CHANGES IN PURITY, STRENGTH, BRAND (MANUFAC-
TURER), TYPE (REGULAR, NPH, LENTE®, ETC), SPECIES
(BEEF, PORK, BEEF-PORK, HUMAN), AND/
OR METHOD OF MANUFACTURE (RECOMBINANT DNA
VERSUS ANIMAL-SOURCE INSULIN) MAY RESULT IN THE
NEED FOR A CHANGE IN DOSAGE.
SOME PATIENTS TAKING HUMULIN® (HUMAN INSULIN,
RECOMBINANT DNA ORIGIN, LILLY) MAY REQUIRE A
CHANGE IN DOSAGE FROM THAT USED WITH ANIMAL-
SOURCE INSULINS. IF AN ADJUSTMENT IS NEEDED, IT
MAY OCCUR WITH THE FIRST DOSE OR DURING THE
FIRST SEVERAL WEEKS OR MONTHS.

BUFFERED REGULAR HUMAN INSULIN
Description
Humulin is synthesized in a special non-disease-producing
laboratory strain of *Escherichia coli* bacteria that has been
genetically altered by the addition of the gene for human
insulin production. Humulin BR consists of zinc-insulin crystals dissolved in a clear fluid containing disodium phosphate
buffer. Humulin BR has had nothing added to change the
speed or length of its action. It takes effect rapidly and has a
relatively short duration of activity (4 to 12 hours) as compared with other insulins. The time course of action of any
insulin may vary considerably in different individuals or at
different times in the same individual. As with all insulin
preparations, the duration of action of Humulin BR is dependent on dose, site of injection, blood supply, temperature,
and physical activity. Humulin BR is a sterile solution and is
for subcutaneous injection. It should not be used intramuscularly. The concentration of Humulin BR is 100 units/mL
(U-100).
Identification
Human insulin manufactured by Eli Lilly and Company has
the trademark Humulin and is available in 7 formulations—Regular (**R**), Buffered Regular (**BR**), NPH (**N**), Lente
(**L**), Ultralente® (**U**), 50% Human Insulin Isophane Suspension [NPH]/50% Human Insulin Injection [buffered regular]
(**50/50**), and 70% Human Insulin Isophane Suspension
[NPH]/30% Human Insulin Injection [buffered regular]
(**70/30**). Your doctor has prescribed the type of insulin that
he/she believes is best for you. **DO NOT USE ANY OTHER
INSULIN EXCEPT ON HIS/HER ADVICE AND DIRECTION.**
Always check the carton and the bottle label for the name
and letter designation of the insulin you receive from your
pharmacy to make sure it is the same as that your doctor has
prescribed. (*See illustration under* Humulin® L.)
Always examine the appearance of your bottle of insulin
before withdrawing each dose. Humulin BR is a clear and
colorless liquid with a water-like appearance and consistency. Do not use if it appears cloudy, thickened, or slightly
colored or if solid particles are visible. Always check the appearance of your bottle of insulin before using, and if you
note anything unusual in the appearance of your insulin or
notice your insulin requirements changing markedly, consult your doctor.
In some individuals who use insulin infusion pumps, the
catheters tend to become clogged with insulin crystals. The
phosphate buffer in this preparation may prevent this type
of blockage. During menses, there may still be a tendency
toward insulin-related catheter obstruction. This may be
treated by changing catheter sets more frequently or by minimizing direct contact of the catheter with the skin.

USE THE CORRECT SYRINGE/RESERVOIR FOR
THE PUMP THAT YOU ARE USING
Doses of insulin are measured in units. U-100 insulin contains 100 units/mL (1 mL = 1 cc). The number of units in
each milliliter (mL) is clearly stated on the package. **It is important to follow the instructions from the manufacturer of
the pump that you are using regarding loading the syringe or
reservoir. Failure to do so can lead to a mistake in dosage,
and you may receive too little or too much insulin. This can
cause serious problems for you, such as a blood glucose level
that is too low or too high.**

HOW SUPPLIED
Vials, U-100, 100 units/mL, 10 mL (No. HI-211) (1's), NDC
0002-8216-01

[060592]

HUMULIN® L   OTC
[hū'mŭ-lĭn ĕl]
Lente
(human insulin [recombinant DNA origin]
zinc suspension)

INFORMATION FOR THE PATIENT
WARNINGS
THIS LILLY HUMAN INSULIN PRODUCT DIFFERS FROM
ANIMAL-SOURCE INSULINS BECAUSE IT IS STRUCTUR-
ALLY IDENTICAL TO THE INSULIN PRODUCED BY YOUR
BODY'S PANCREAS AND BECAUSE OF ITS UNIQUE MAN-
UFACTURING PROCESS.
ANY CHANGE OF INSULIN SHOULD BE MADE CAU-
TIOUSLY AND ONLY UNDER MEDICAL SUPERVISION.
CHANGES IN PURITY, STRENGTH, BRAND (MANUFAC-
TURER), TYPE (REGULAR, NPH, LENTE®, ETC), SPECIES
(BEEF, PORK, BEEF-PORK, HUMAN), AND/OR METHOD OF
MANUFACTURE (RECOMBINANT DNA VERSUS ANIMAL-
SOURCE INSULIN) MAY RESULT IN THE NEED FOR A
CHANGE IN DOSAGE.
SOME PATIENTS TAKING HUMULIN® (HUMAN INSULIN,
RECOMBINANT DNA ORIGIN, LILLY) MAY REQUIRE A
CHANGE IN DOSAGE FROM THAT USED WITH ANIMAL-
SOURCE INSULINS. IF AN ADJUSTMENT IS NEEDED, IT
MAY OCCUR WITH THE FIRST DOSE OR DURING THE
FIRST SEVERAL WEEKS OR MONTHS.

DIABETES
Insulin is a hormone produced by the pancreas, a large gland
that lies near the stomach. This hormone is necessary for the
body's correct use of food, especially sugar. Diabetes occurs
when the pancreas does not make enough insulin to meet
your body's needs.
To control your diabetes, your doctor has prescribed injections of insulin to keep your blood glucose at a nearly normal
level. Proper control of your diabetes requires close and constant cooperation with your doctor. In spite of diabetes, you
can lead an active, healthy, and useful life if you eat a balanced diet daily, exercise regularly, and take your insulin
injections as prescribed.
You have been instructed to test your blood and/or your
urine regularly for glucose. If your blood tests consistently
show above- or below-normal glucose levels or your urine
tests consistently show the presence of glucose, your diabetes
is not properly controlled and you must let your doctor know.
Always keep an extra supply of insulin as well as spare syringe and needle on hand. Always wear diabetic identification so that appropriate treatment can be given if complications occur away from home.

LENTE HUMAN INSULIN
Description
Humulin is synthesized in a special non-disease-producing
laboratory strain of *Escherichia coli* bacteria that has been
genetically altered by the addition of the gene for human
insulin production. Humulin L is an amorphous and crystalline suspension of human insulin with zinc providing an intermediate-acting insulin with a slower onset and a longer
duration of activity (up to 24 hours) than regular insulin. The
time course of action of any insulin may vary considerably in
different individuals or at different times in the same individual. As with all insulin preparations, the duration of action of Humulin L is dependent on dose, site of injection,
blood supply, temperature, and physical activity. Humulin L
is a sterile suspension and is for subcutaneous injection only.
It should not be used intravenously or intramuscularly. The
concentration of Humulin L is 100 units/mL (U-100).

Identification
Human insulin manufactured by Eli Lilly and Company has
the trademark Humulin and is available in 7 formulations—Regular (**R**), Buffered Regular (**BR**), NPH (**N**), Lente
(**L**), Ultralente® (**U**), 50% Human Insulin Isophane Suspension [NPH]/50% Human Insulin Injection [buffered regular]
(**50/50**), and 70% Human Insulin Isophane Suspension
[NPH]/30% Human Insulin Injection [buffered regular]
(**70/30**). Your doctor has prescribed the type of insulin that
he/she believes is best for you. **DO NOT USE ANY OTHER
INSULIN EXCEPT ON HIS/HER ADVICE AND DIRECTION.**
Always check the carton and the bottle label for the name
and letter designation of the insulin you receive from your
pharmacy to make sure it is the same as that your doctor has
prescribed. Humulin L can be identified as follows:
[See illustration below.]
Always examine the appearance of your bottle of insulin
before withdrawing each dose. A bottle of Humulin L must
be carefully shaken or rotated before each injection so that
the contents are uniformly mixed. Humulin L should look
uniformly cloudy or milky after mixing. Do not use it if the
insulin substance (the white material) remains at the bottom
of the bottle after mixing (*See Figure 1 under* Humulin® N).
Do not use a bottle of Humulin L if there are clumps in the
insulin after mixing (*See Figure 2 under* Humulin® N). Always check the appearance of your bottle of insulin before
using, and if you note anything unusual in the appearance of
your insulin or notice your insulin requirements changing
markedly, consult your doctor.
Storage
Insulin should be stored in a refrigerator but not in the
freezer. If refrigeration is not possible, the bottle of insulin
that you are currently using can be kept unrefrigerated as
long as it is kept as cool as possible (below 86°F [30°C]) and
away from heat and light. Do not use insulin if it has been
frozen. Do not use a bottle of insulin after the expiration date
stamped on the label.

INJECTION PROCEDURES
Correct Syringe
Doses of insulin are measured in **units**. U-100 insulin contains 100 units/mL (1 mL = 1 cc). With Humulin L, it is important to use a syringe that is marked for U-100 insulin
preparations. Failure to use the proper syringe can lead to a
mistake in dosage, causing serious problems for you, such as
a blood glucose level that is too low or too high.
Syringe Use
To help avoid contamination and possible infection, follow
these instructions exactly. Disposable syringes and needles
should be used only once and then discarded. **NEEDLES AND
SYRINGES MUST NOT BE SHARED.**
Reusable syringes and needles must be sterilized before each
injection. **Follow the package directions supplied with your
syringe.** Described below are 2 methods of sterilizing.

Boiling
1. Put syringe, plunger, and needle in strainer, place in
saucepan, and cover with water. Boil for 5 minutes.
2. Remove articles from water. When they have cooled,
insert plunger into barrel, and fasten needle to syringe
with a slight twist.

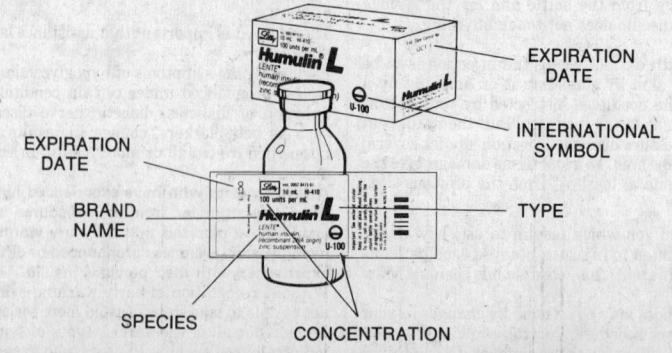

EXPIRATION DATE — INTERNATIONAL SYMBOL — EXPIRATION DATE — BRAND NAME — TYPE — SPECIES — CONCENTRATION

3. Push plunger in and out several times until water is completely removed.

Isopropyl Alcohol
If the syringe, plunger, and needle cannot be boiled, as when you are traveling, they may be sterilized by immersion for at least 5 minutes in Isopropyl Alcohol, 91%. Do not use bathing, rubbing, or medicated alcohol for this sterilization. If the syringe is sterilized with alcohol, it must be absolutely dry before use.

Preparing the Dose
1. Wash your hands.
2. Carefully shake or rotate the insulin bottle several times to completely mix the insulin.
3. Inspect the insulin. Humulin L should look uniformly cloudy or milky. Do not use it if you notice anything unusual in the appearance.
4. If using a new bottle, flip off the plastic protective cap, but **do not** remove the stopper. When using a new bottle, wipe the top of the bottle witth an alcohol swab.
5. If you are mixing insulins, refer to the instructions for mixing that follow.
6. Draw air into the syringe equal to your insulin dose. Put the needle through rubber top of the insulin bottle and inject the air into the bottle.
7. Turn the bottle and syringe upside down. Hold the bottle and syringe firmly in 1 hand and shake gently.
8. Making sure the tip of the needle is in the insulin, withdraw the correct dose of insulin into the syringe.
9. Before removing the needle from the bottle, check your syringe for air bubbles which reduce the amount of insulin in it. If bubbles are present, hold the syringe straight up and tap its side until the bubbles float to the top. Push them out with the plunger and withdraw the correct dose.
10. Remove the needle from the bottle and lay the syringe down so that the needle does not touch anything.

Mixing Humulin L with Regular or Ultralente Human Insulin
1. Lente human insulin should be mixed with regular or Ultralente human insulin only on the advice of your doctor.
2. Draw air into your syringe equal to the amount of Humulin L you are taking. Insert the needle into the Humulin L bottle and inject the air. Withdraw the needle.
3. Now inject air into your regular or Ultralente human insulin bottle in the same manner, but **do not** withdraw the needle.
4. Turn the bottle and syringe upside down.
5. Making sure the tip of the needle is in the insulin, withdraw the correct dose of regular or Ultralente insulin into the syringe.
6. Before removing the needle from the bottle, check your syringe for air bubbles which reduce the amount of insulin in it. If bubbles are present, hold the syringe straight up and tap its side until the bubbles float to the top. Push them out with the plunger and withdraw the correct dose.
7. Remove the needle from the bottle of regular or Ultralente insulin and insert it into the bottle of Humulin L. Turn the bottle and syringe upside down. Hold the bottle and syringe firmly in 1 hand and shake gently. Making sure the tip of the needle is in the insulin, withdraw your dose of Humulin L.
8. Remove the needle and lay the syringe down so that the needle does not touch anything.

Follow your doctor's instructions on whether to mix your insulins ahead of time or just before giving your injection. It is important to be consistent in your method.

Syringes from different manufacturers may vary in the amount of space between the bottom line and the needle. Because of this, do not change:
• the sequence of mixing, or
• the model and brand of syringe or needle that the doctor has prescribed.

Injection
Cleanse the skin with alcohol where the injection is to be made. Stabilize the skin by spreading it or pinching up a large area. Insert the needle as instructed by your doctor. Push the plunger in as far as it will go. Pull the needle out and apply gentle pressure over the injection site for several seconds. **Do not rub the area.** To avoid tissue damage, give the next injection at a site at least ½" from the previous site.

DOSAGE
Your doctor has told you which insulin to use, how much, and when and how often to inject it. Because each patient's case of diabetes is different, this schedule has been individualized for you.
Your usual insulin dose may be affected by changes in your food, activity, or work schedule. Carefully follow your doctor's instructions to allow for these changes. Other things that may affect your insulin dose are:

Illness
Illness, especially with nausea and vomiting, may cause your insulin requirements to change. Even if you are not eating, you will still require insulin. You and your doctor should

establish a sick day plan for you to use in case of illness. When you are sick, test your blood/urine frequently and call your doctor as instructed.

Pregnancy
Good control of diabetes is especially important for you and your unborn baby. Pregnancy may make managing your diabetes more difficult. If you are planning to have a baby, are pregnant, or are nursing a baby, consult your doctor.

Medication
Insulin requirements may be increased if you are taking other drugs with hyperglycemic activity, such as oral contraceptives, corticosteroids, or thyroid replacement therapy. Insulin requirements may be reduced in the presence of drugs with hypoglycemic activity, such as oral hypoglycemics, salicylates (for example, aspirin), sulfa antibiotics, and certain antidepressants. Always discuss any medications you are taking with your doctor.

Exercise
Exercise may lower your body's need for insulin during and for some time after the activity. Exercise may also speed up the effect of an insulin dose, especially if the exercise involves the area of injection site (for example, the leg should not be used for injection just prior to running). Discuss with your doctor how you should adjust your regimen to accommodate exercise.

Travel
Persons traveling across more than 2 time zones should consult their doctor concerning adjustments in their insulin schedule.

COMMON PROBLEMS OF DIABETES
Hypoglycemia (Insulin Reaction)
Hypoglycemia (too little glucose in the blood) is one of the most frequent adverse events experienced by insulin users. It can be brought about by:
1. Taking too much insulin
2. Missing or delaying meals
3. Exercising or working more than usual
4. An infection or illness (especially with diarrhea or vomiting)
5. A change in the body's need for insulin
6. Diseases of the adrenal, pituitary, or thyroid gland, or progression of kidney or liver disease
7. Interactions with other drugs that lower blood glucose, such as oral hypoglycemics, salicylates (for example, aspirin), sulfa antibiotics, and certain antidepressants
8. Consumption of alcoholic beverages
Symptoms of mild to moderate hypoglycemia may occur suddenly and can include:
• sweating
• dizziness
• palpitation
• tremor
• hunger
• restlessness
• tingling in the hands, feet, lips, or tongue
• lightheadedness
• inability to concentrate
• headache
• drowsiness
• sleep disturbances
• anxiety
• blurred vision
• slurred speech
• depressive mood
• irritability
• abnormal behavior
• unsteady movement
• personality changes
Signs of severe hypoglycemia can include:
• disorientation
• unconsciousness
• seizures
• death
Therefore, it is important that assistance be obtained immediately.
Early warning symptoms of hypoglycemia may be different or less pronounced under certain conditions, such as long duration of diabetes, diabetic nerve disease, medications such as beta-blockers, change in insulin preparations, or intensified control (3 or more insulin injections per day) of diabetes.
A few patients who experienced hypoglycemic reactions after transfer from animal-source insulin to human insulin have reported that the early warning symptoms of hypoglycemia were less pronounced or different from those experienced with their previous insulin.
Without recognition of early warning symptoms, you may not be able to take steps to avoid more serious hypoglycemia. Be alert for all of the various types of symptoms that may indicate hypoglycemia. Patients who experience hypoglycemia without early warning symptoms should monitor their blood glucose frequently, especially prior to activities such as driving. If the blood glucose is below your normal fasting glucose, you should consider eating or drinking sugar-containing foods to treat your hypoglycemia.

Mild to moderate hypoglycemia may be treated by eating foods or drinks that contain sugar. Patients should always carry a quick source of sugar, such as candy mints or glucose tablets. More severe hypoglycemia may require the assistance of another person. Patients who are unable to take sugar orally or who are unconscious require an injection of glucagon or should be treated with intravenous administration of glucose at a medical facility.
You should learn to recognize your own symptoms of hypoglycemia. If you are uncertain about these symptoms, you should monitor your blood glucose frequently to help you learn to recognize the symptoms that you experience with hypoglycemia.
If you have frequent episodes of hypoglycemia or experience difficulty in recognizing the symptoms, you should consult your doctor to discuss possible changes in therapy, meal plans, and/or exercise programs to help you avoid hypoglycemia.

Hyperglycemia and Diabetic Acidosis
Hyperglycemia (too much glucose in the blood) may develop if your body has too little insulin. Hyperglycemia can be brought about by:
1. Omitting your insulin or taking less than the doctor has prescribed
2. Eating significantly more than your meal plan suggests
3. Developing a fever or infection
In patients with insulin-dependent diabetes, prolonged hyperglycemia can result in diabetic acidosis. The first symptoms of diabetic acidosis usually come on gradually, over a period of hours or days, and include a drowsy feeling, flushed face, thirst, loss of appetite, and fruity odor on the breath. With acidosis, urine tests show large amounts of glucose and acetone. Heavy breathing and a rapid pulse are more severe symptoms. If uncorrected, prolonged hyperglycemia or diabetic acidosis can result in loss of consciousness or death. Therefore, it is important that you obtain medical assistance immediately.

Lipodystrophy
Rarely, administration of insulin subcutaneously can result in lipoatrophy (depression in the skin) or lipohypertrophy (enlargement or thickening of tissue). If you notice either of these conditions, consult your doctor. A change in your injection technique may help alleviate the problem.

Allergy to Insulin
Local Allergy—Patients occasionally experience redness, swelling, and itching at the site of injection of insulin. This condition, called local allergy, usually clears up in a few days to a few weeks. In some instances, this condition may be related to factors other than insulin, such as irritants in the skin cleansing agent or poor injection technique. If you have local reactions, contact your doctor.
Systemic Allergy—Less common, but potentially more serious, is generalized allergy to insulin, which may cause rash over the whole body, shortness of breath, wheezing, reduction in blood pressure, fast pulse, or sweating. Severe cases of generalized allergy may be life threatening. If you think you are having a generalized allergic reaction to insulin, notify a doctor immediately.

HOW SUPPLIED
Vials, U-100, 100 units/mL, 10 mL (No. HI-410) (1's), NDC 0002-8415-01

[060592]

HUMULIN® N   OTC
[hū'mŭ-lĭn ĕn]
NPH
(human insulin [recombinant DNA origin]
isophane suspension)

INFORMATION FOR THE PATIENT
WARNINGS
THIS LILLY HUMAN INSULIN PRODUCT DIFFERS FROM ANIMAL-SOURCE INSULINS BECAUSE IT IS STRUCTURALLY IDENTICAL TO THE INSULIN PRODUCED BY YOUR BODY'S PANCREAS AND BECAUSE OF ITS UNIQUE MANUFACTURING PROCESS.
ANY CHANGE OF INSULIN SHOULD BE MADE CAUTIOUSLY AND ONLY UNDER MEDICAL SUPERVISION. CHANGES IN PURITY, STRENGTH, BRAND (MANUFACTURER), TYPE (REGULAR, NPH, LENTE®, ETC), SPECIES (BEEF, PORK, BEEF-PORK, HUMAN), AND/OR METHOD OF MANUFACTURE (RECOMBINANT DNA VERSUS ANIMAL-SOURCE INSULIN) MAY RESULT IN THE NEED FOR A CHANGE IN DOSAGE.

Continued on next page

• Identi-Code® symbol. This product information was prepared in June 1992. Current information on these and other products of Eli Lilly and Company may be obtained by direct inquiry to Lilly Research Laboratories, Lilly Corporate Center, Indianapolis, Indiana 46285, (317) 276-3714.

Lilly—Cont.

SOME PATIENTS TAKING HUMULIN® (HUMAN INSULIN, RECOMBINANT DNA ORIGIN, LILLY) MAY REQUIRE A CHANGE IN DOSAGE FROM THAT USED WITH ANIMAL-SOURCE INSULINS. IF AN ADJUSTMENT IS NEEDED, IT MAY OCCUR WITH THE FIRST DOSE OR DURING THE FIRST SEVERAL WEEKS OR MONTHS.

DIABETES

Insulin is a hormone produced by the pancreas, a large gland that lies near the stomach. This hormone is necessary for the body's correct use of food, especially sugar. Diabetes occurs when the pancreas does not make enough insulin to meet your body's needs.

To control your diabetes, your doctor has prescribed injections of insulin to keep your blood glucose at a nearly normal level. Proper control of your diabetes requires close and constant cooperation with your doctor. In spite of diabetes, you can lead an active, healthy, and useful life if you eat a balanced diet daily, exercise regularly, and take your insulin injections as prescribed.

You have been instructed to test your blood and/or your urine regularly for glucose. If your blood tests consistently show above- or below-normal glucose levels or your urine tests consistently show the presence of glucose, your diabetes is not properly controlled and you must let your doctor know. Always keep an extra supply of insulin as well as a spare syringe and needle on hand. Always wear diabetic identification so that appropriate treatment can be given if complications occur away from home.

NPH HUMAN INSULIN
Description

Humulin is synthesized in a special non-disease-producing laboratory strain of *Escherichia coli* bacteria that has been genetically altered by the addition of the gene for human insulin production. Humulin N is a crystalline suspension of human insulin with protamine and zinc providing an intermediate-acting insulin with a slower onset of action and a longer duration of activity (up to 24 hours) than that of regular insulin. The time course of action of any insulin may vary considerably in different individuals or at different times in the same individual. As with all insulin preparations, the duration of action of Humulin N is dependent on dose, site of injection, blood supply, temperature, and physical activity. Humulin N is a sterile suspension and is for subcutaneous injection only. It should not be used intravenously or intramuscularly. The concentration of Humulin N is 100 units/mL (U-100).

Identification

Human insulin manufactured by Eli Lilly and Company has the trademark Humulin and is available in 7 formulations—Regular (**R**), Buffered Regular (**BR**), NPH (**N**), Lente (**L**), Ultralente® (**U**), 50% Human Insulin Isophane Suspension [NPH]/50% Human Insulin Injection [buffered regular] (**50/50**), and 70% Human Insulin Isophane Suspension [NPH]/30% Human Insulin Injection [buffered regular] (**70/30**). Your doctor has prescribed the type of insulin that he/she believes is best for you. **DO NOT USE ANY OTHER INSULIN EXCEPT ON HIS/HER ADVICE AND DIRECTION.**

Always check the carton and the bottle label for the name and letter designation of the insulin you receive from your pharmacy to make sure it is the same as that your doctor has prescribed. (*See illustration under* Humulin® L.)

Always examine the appearance of your bottle of insulin before withdrawing each dose. A bottle of Humulin N must be carefully shaken or rotated before each injection so that the contents are uniformly mixed. Humulin N should look uniformly cloudy or milky after mixing. Do not use it if the insulin substance (the white material) remains at the bottom of the bottle after mixing. Do not use a bottle of Humulin N if there are clumps in the insulin after mixing (Figure 1). Do not use a bottle of Humulin N if solid white particles stick to the bottom or wall of the bottle, giving it a frosted appearance (Figure 2). Always check the appearance of your bottle of insulin before using, and if you note anything unusual in the appearance of your insulin or notice your insulin requirements changing markedly, consult your doctor.

Storage

Insulin should be stored in a refrigerator but not in the freezer. If refrigeration is not possible, the bottle of insulin that you are currently using can be kept unrefrigerated as long as it is kept as cool as possible (below 86°F [30°C]) and away from heat and light. Do not use insulin if it has been frozen. Do not use a bottle of insulin after the expiration date stamped on the label.

INJECTION PROCEDURES
Correct Syringe

Doses of insulin are measured in *units*. U-100 insulin contains 100 units/mL (1 mL = 1 cc). With Humulin N, it is important to use a syringe that is marked for U-100 insulin

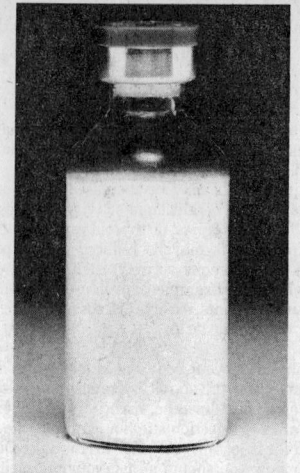

Fig. 1.—Do not use if there are clumps in the insulin after mixing.

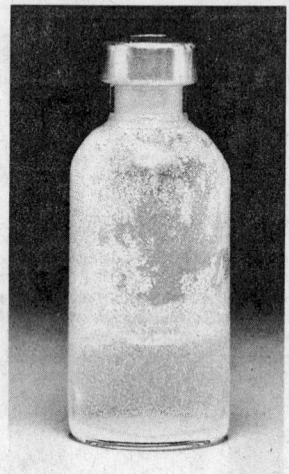

Fig. 2.—Do not use if particles on the bottom or wall give the bottle a frosted appearance.

preparations. Failure to use the proper syringe can lead to a mistake in dosage, causing serious problems for you, such as a blood glucose level that is too low or too high.

Syringe Use

To help avoid contamination and possible infection, follow these instructions exactly.

Disposable syringes and needles should be used only once and then discarded. **NEEDLES AND SYRINGES MUST NOT BE SHARED.**

Reusable syringes and needles must be sterilized before each injection. **Follow the package directions supplied with your syringe.** Described below are 2 methods of sterilizing.

Boiling

1. Put syringe, plunger, and needle in strainer, place in saucepan, and cover with water. Boil for 5 minutes.
2. Remove articles from water. When they have cooled, insert plunger into barrel, and fasten needle to syringe with a slight twist.
3. Push plunger in and out several times until water is completely removed.

Isopropyl Alcohol

If the syringe, plunger, and needle cannot be boiled, as when you are traveling, they may be sterilized by immersion for at least 5 minutes in Isopropyl Alcohol, 91%. Do not use bathing, rubbing, or medicated alcohol for this sterilization. If the syringe is sterilized with alcohol, it must be absolutely dry before use.

Preparing the Dose

1. Wash your hands.
2. Carefully shake or rotate the insulin bottle several times to completely mix the insulin.
3. Inspect the insulin. Humulin N should look uniformly cloudy or milky. Do not use it if you notice anything unusual in the appearance.
4. If using a new bottle, flip off the plastic protective cap, but **do not** remove the stopper. When using a new bottle, wipe the top of the bottle with an alcohol swab.

5. If you are mixing insulins, refer to the instructions for mixing that follow.
6. Draw air into the syringe equal to your insulin dose. Put the needle through rubber top of the insulin bottle and inject the air into the bottle.
7. Turn the bottle and syringe upside down. Hold the bottle and syringe firmly in 1 hand and shake gently.
8. Making sure the tip of the needle is in the insulin, withdraw the correct dose of insulin into the syringe.
9. Before removing the needle from the bottle, check your syringe for air bubbles which reduce the amount of insulin in it. If bubbles are present, hold the syringe straight up and tap its side until the bubbles float to the top. Push them out with the plunger and withdraw the correct dose.
10. Remove the needle from the bottle and lay the syringe down so that the needle does not touch anything.

Mixing Humulin N and Regular Human Insulin

1. NPH human insulin should be mixed only with regular human insulin.
2. Draw air into your syringe equal to the amount of Humulin N you are taking. Insert the needle into the Humulin N bottle and inject the air. Withdraw the needle.
3. Now inject air into your regular human insulin bottle in the same manner, but **do not** withdraw the needle.
4. Turn the bottle and syringe upside down.
5. Making sure the tip of the needle is in the insulin, withdraw the correct dose of regular insulin into the syringe.
6. Before removing the needle from the bottle, check your syringe for air bubbles which reduce the amount of insulin in it. If bubbles are present, hold the syringe straight up and tap its side until the bubbles float to the top. Push them out with the plunger and withdraw the correct dose.
7. Remove the needle from the bottle of regular insulin and insert it into the bottle of Humulin N. Turn the bottle and syringe upside down. Hold the bottle and syringe firmly in 1 hand and shake gently. Making sure the tip of the needle is in the insulin, withdraw your dose of Humulin N.
8. Remove the needle and lay the syringe down so that the needle does not touch anything.

Follow your doctor's instructions on whether to mix your insulins ahead of time or just before giving your injection. It is important to be consistent in your method.

Syringes from different manufacturers may vary in the amount of space between the bottom line and the needle. Because of this, do not change:

- the sequence of mixing, or
- the model and brand of syringe or needle that the doctor has prescribed.

Injection

Cleanse the skin with alcohol where the injection is to be made. Stabilize the skin by spreading it or pinching up a large area. Insert the needle as instructed by your doctor. Push the plunger in as far as it will go. Pull the needle out and apply gentle pressure over the injection site for several seconds. **Do not rub the area.** To avoid tissue damage, give the next injection at a site at least ½″ from the previous site.

DOSAGE

Your doctor has told you which insulin to use, how much, and when and how often to inject it. Because each patient's case of diabetes is different, this schedule has been individualized for you.

Your usual insulin dose may be affected by changes in your food, activity, or work schedule. Carefully follow your doctor's instructions to allow for these changes. Other things that may affect your insulin dose are:

Illness

Illness, especially with nausea and vomiting, may cause your insulin requirements to change. Even if you are not eating, you will still require insulin. You and your doctor should establish a sick day plan for you to use in case of illness. When you are sick, test your blood/urine frequently and call your doctor as instructed.

Pregnancy

Good control of diabetes is especially important for you and your unborn baby. Pregnancy may make managing your diabetes more difficult. If you are planning to have a baby, are pregnant, or are nursing a baby, consult your doctor.

Medication

Insulin requirements may be increased if you are taking other drugs with hyperglycemic activity, such as oral contraceptives, corticosteroids, or thyroid replacement therapy. Insulin requirements may be reduced in the presence of drugs with hypoglycemic activity, such as oral hypoglycemics, salicylates (for example, aspirin), sulfa antibiotics, and certain antidepressants. Always discuss any medications you are taking with your doctor.

Exercise

Exercise may lower your body's need for insulin during and for some time after the activity. Exercise may also speed up the effect of an insulin dose, especially if the exercise involves the area of injection site (for example, the leg should not be used for injection just prior to running). Discuss with your doctor how you should adjust your regimen to accommodate exercise.

Travel

Persons traveling across more than 2 time zones should consult their doctor concerning adjustments in their insulin schedule.

COMMON PROBLEMS OF DIABETES

Hypoglycemia (Insulin Reaction)

Hypoglycemia (too little glucose in the blood) is one of the most frequent adverse events experienced by insulin users. It can be brought about by:

1. Taking too much insulin
2. Missing or delaying meals
3. Exercising or working more than usual
4. An infection or illness (especially with diarrhea or vomiting)
5. A change in the body's need for insulin
6. Diseases of the adrenal, pituitary, or thyroid gland, or progression of kidney or liver disease
7. Interactions with other drugs that lower blood glucose, such as oral hypoglycemics, salicylates (for example, aspirin), sulfa antibiotics, and certain antidepressants
8. Consumption of alcoholic beverages

Symptoms of mild to moderate hypoglycemia may occur suddenly and can include:

- sweating
- dizziness
- palpitation
- tremor
- hunger
- restlessness
- tingling in the hands, feet, lips, or tongue
- lightheadedness
- inability to concentrate
- headache
- drowsiness
- sleep disturbances
- anxiety
- blurred vision
- slurred speech
- depressive mood
- irritability
- abnormal behavior
- unsteady movement
- personality changes

Signs of severe hypoglycemia can include:

- disorientation
- unconsciousness
- seizures
- death

Therefore, it is important that assistance be obtained immediately.

Early warning symptoms of hypoglycemia may be different or less pronounced under certain conditions, such as long duration of diabetes, diabetic nerve disease, medications such as beta-blockers, change in insulin preparations, or intensified control (3 or more insulin injections per day) of diabetes.

A few patients who have experienced hypoglycemic reactions after transfer from animal-source insulin to human insulin have reported that the early warning symptoms of hypoglycemia were less pronounced or different from those experienced with their previous insulin.

Without recognition of early warning symptoms, you may not be able to take steps to avoid more serious hypoglycemia. Be alert for all of the various types of symptoms that may indicate hypoglycemia. Patients who experience hypoglycemia without early warning symptoms should monitor their blood glucose frequently, especially prior to activities such as driving. If the blood glucose is below your normal fasting glucose, you should consider eating or drinking sugar-containing foods to treat your hypoglycemia.

Mild to moderate hypoglycemia may be treated by eating foods or drinks that contain sugar. Patients should always carry a quick source of sugar, such as candy mints or glucose tablets. More severe hypoglycemia may require the assistance of another person. Patients who are unable to take sugar orally or who are unconscious require an injection of glucagon or should be treated with intravenous administration of glucose at a medical facility.

You should learn to recognize your own symptoms of hypoglycemia. If you are uncertain about these symptoms, you should monitor your blood glucose frequently to help you learn to recognize the symptoms that you experience with hypoglycemia.

If you have frequent episodes of hypoglycemia or experience difficulty in recognizing the symptoms, you should consult your doctor to discuss possible changes in therapy, meal plans, and/or exercise programs to help you avoid hypoglycemia.

Hyperglycemia and Diabetic Acidosis

Hyperglycemia (too much glucose in the blood) may develop if your body has too little insulin. Hyperglycemia can be brought about by:

1. Omitting your insulin or taking less than the doctor has prescribed

2. Eating significantly more than your meal plan suggests
3. Developing a fever or infection

In patients with insulin-dependent diabetes, prolonged hyperglycemia can result in diabetic acidosis. The first symptoms of diabetic acidosis usually come on gradually, over a period of hours or days, and include a drowsy feeling, flushed face, thirst, loss of appetite, and fruity odor on the breath. With acidosis, urine tests show large amounts of glucose and acetone. Heavy breathing and a rapid pulse are more severe symptoms. If uncorrected, prolonged hyperglycemia or diabetic acidosis can result in loss of consciousness or death. Therefore, it is important that you obtain medical assistance immediately.

Lipodystrophy

Rarely, administration of insulin subcutaneously can result in lipoatrophy (depression in the skin) or lipohypertrophy (enlargement or thickening of tissue). If you notice either of these conditions, consult your doctor. A change in your injection technique may help alleviate the problem.

Allergy to Insulin

Local Allergy—Patients occasionally experience redness, swelling, and itching at the site of injection of insulin. This condition, called local allergy, usually clears up in a few days to a few weeks. In some instances, this condition may be related to factors other than insulin, such as irritants in the skin cleansing agent or poor injection technique. If you have local reactions, contact your doctor.

Systemic Allergy—Less common, but potentially more serious, is generalized allergy to insulin, which may cause rash over the whole body, shortness of breath, wheezing, reduction in blood pressure, fast pulse, or sweating. Severe cases of generalized allergy may be life threatening. If you think you are having a generalized allergic reaction to insulin, notify a doctor immediately.

HOW SUPPLIED

Vials, U-100, 100 units/mL, 10 mL (No. HI-310)(1's) NDC 0002-8315-01

[060592]

HUMULIN® R   OTC
[hū 'mŭ-lĭn är]

Regular
(insulin human injection, USP [recombinant DNA origin])

INFORMATION FOR THE PATIENT
WARNINGS

THIS LILLY HUMAN INSULIN PRODUCT DIFFERS FROM ANIMAL-SOURCE INSULINS BECAUSE IT IS STRUCTURALLY IDENTICAL TO THE INSULIN PRODUCED BY YOUR BODY'S PANCREAS AND BECAUSE OF ITS UNIQUE MANUFACTURING PROCESS.

ANY CHANGE OF INSULIN SHOULD BE MADE CAUTIOUSLY AND ONLY UNDER MEDICAL SUPERVISION. CHANGES IN PURITY, STRENGTH, BRAND (MANUFACTURER), TYPE (REGULAR, NPH, LENTE®, ETC), SPECIES (BEEF, PORK, BEEF-PORK, HUMAN), AND/OR METHOD OF MANUFACTURE (RECOMBINANT DNA VERSUS ANIMAL-SOURCE INSULIN) MAY RESULT IN THE NEED FOR A CHANGE IN DOSAGE.

SOME PATIENTS TAKING HUMULIN® (HUMAN INSULIN, RECOMBINANT DNA ORIGIN, LILLY) MAY REQUIRE A CHANGE IN DOSAGE FROM THAT USED WITH ANIMAL-SOURCE INSULINS. IF AN ADJUSTMENT IS NEEDED, IT MAY OCCUR WITH THE FIRST DOSE OR DURING THE FIRST SEVERAL WEEKS OR MONTHS.

REGULAR HUMAN INSULIN

Description

Humulin is synthesized in a special non-disease-producing special laboratory strain of *Escherichia coli* bacteria that has been genetically altered by the addition of the gene for human insulin production. Humulin R consists of zinc-insulin crystals dissolved in a clear fluid. Humulin R has had nothing added to change the speed or length of its action. It takes effect rapidly and has a relatively short duration of activity (4 to 12 hours) as compared with other insulins. The time course of action of any insulin may vary considerably in different individuals or at different times in the same individual. As with all insulin preparations, the duration of action of Humulin R is dependent on dose, site of injection, blood supply, temperature, and physical activity. Humulin R is a sterile solution and is for subcutaneous injection. It should not be used intramuscularly. The concentration of Humulin R is 100 units/mL (U-100).

Identification

Human insulin manufactured by Eli Lilly and Company has the trademark Humulin and is available in 7 formulations—Regular (**R**), Buffered Regular (**BR**), NPH (**N**), Lente (**L**), Ultralente® (**U**), 50% Human Insulin Isophane Suspension [NPH]/50% Human Insulin Injection [buffered regular] (**50/50**), and 70% Human Insulin Isophane Suspension [NPH]/30% Human Insulin Injection [buffered regular] (**70/30**). Your doctor has prescribed the type of insulin that

he/she believes is best for you. **DO NOT USE ANY OTHER INSULIN EXCEPT ON HIS/HER ADVICE AND DIRECTION.** Always check the carton and the bottle label for the name and letter designation of the insulin you receive from your pharmacy to make sure it is the same as that your doctor has prescribed. (*See illustration under* Humulin® L.)

Always examine the appearance of your bottle of insulin before withdrawing each dose. Humulin R is a clear and colorless liquid with a water-like appearance and consistency. Do not use if it appears cloudy, thickened, or slightly colored or if solid particles are visible. Always check the appearance of your bottle of insulin before using, and if you note anything unusual in the appearance of your insulin or notice your insulin requirements changing markedly, consult your doctor.

INJECTION PROCEDURES

See under Humulin® L, *except:* Do not rotate or shake the insulin bottle.

HOW SUPPLIED

Vials, U-100, 100 units/mL, 10 mL (No. HI-210) (1's), NDC 0002-8215-01

[060592]

HUMULIN® U   OTC
[hū 'mŭ-lĭn ū]

Ultralente
(human Insulin [recombinant DNA origin] extended zinc suspension)

INFORMATION FOR THE PATIENT
WARNINGS

THIS LILLY HUMAN INSULIN PRODUCT DIFFERS FROM ANIMAL-SOURCE INSULINS BECAUSE IT IS STRUCTURALLY IDENTICAL TO THE INSULIN PRODUCED BY YOUR BODY'S PANCREAS AND BECAUSE OF ITS UNIQUE MANUFACTURING PROCESS.

ANY CHANGE OF INSULIN SHOULD BE MADE CAUTIOUSLY AND ONLY UNDER MEDICAL SUPERVISION. CHANGES IN PURITY, STRENGTH, BRAND (MANUFACTURER), TYPE (REGULAR, NPH, LENTE®, ETC), SPECIES (BEEF, PORK, BEEF-PORK, HUMAN), AND/OR METHOD OF MANUFACTURE (RECOMBINANT DNA VERSUS ANIMAL-SOURCE INSULIN) MAY RESULT IN THE NEED FOR A CHANGE IN DOSAGE.

SOME PATIENTS TAKING HUMULIN® (HUMAN INSULIN, RECOMBINANT DNA ORIGIN, LILLY) MAY REQUIRE A CHANGE IN DOSAGE FROM THAT USED WITH ANIMAL-SOURCE INSULINS. IF AN ADJUSTMENT IS NEEDED, IT MAY OCCUR WITH THE FIRST DOSE OR DURING THE FIRST SEVERAL WEEKS OR MONTHS.

ULTRALENTE HUMAN INSULIN

Description

Humulin is synthesized in a special non-disease-producing laboratory strain of *Escherichia coli* bacteria that has been genetically altered by the addition of the gene for human insulin production. Humulin U is a crystalline suspension of human insulin with zinc providing a slower onset and a longer and less intense duration of activity (up to 28 hours) than regular insulin or the intermediate-acting insulins (NPH and Lente). The time course of action of any insulin may vary considerably in different individuals or at different times in the same individual. As with all insulin preparations, the duration of action of Humulin U is dependent on dose, site of injection, blood supply, temperature, and physical activity. Humulin U is a sterile suspension and is for subcutaneous injection only. It should not be used intravenously or intramuscularly. The concentration of Humulin U is 100 units/mL (U-100).

Identification

Human insulin manufactured by Eli Lilly and Company has the trademark Humulin and is available in 7 formulations—Regular (**R**), Buffered Regular (**BR**), NPH (**N**), Lente (**L**), Ultralente (**U**), 50% Human Insulin Isophane Suspension [NPH]/50% Human Insulin Injection [buffered regular] (**50/50**), and 70% Human Insulin Isophane Suspension [NPH]/30% Human Insulin Injection [buffered regular] (**70/30**). Your doctor has prescribed the type of insulin that he/she believes is best for you. **DO NOT USE ANY OTHER INSULIN EXCEPT ON HIS/HER ADVICE AND DIRECTION.** Always check the carton and the bottle label for the name and letter designation of the insulin you receive from your pharmacy to make sure it is the same as that your doctor has prescribed. (*See illustration under* Humulin® L.)

Continued on next page

• Identi-Code® symbol. This product information was prepared in June 1992. Current information on these and other products of Eli Lilly and Company may be obtained by direct inquiry to Lilly Research Laboratories, Lilly Corporate Center, Indianapolis, Indiana 46285, (317) 276-3714.

Lilly—Cont.

Always examine the appearance of your bottle of insulin before withdrawing each dose. A bottle of Humulin U must be carefully shaken or rotated before each injection so that the contents are uniformly mixed. Humulin U should look uniformly cloudy or milky after mixing. Do not use it if the insulin substance (the white material) remains at the bottom of the bottle after mixing (See Figure 1 under Humulin® N). Do not use a bottle of Humulin U if there are clumps in the insulin after mixing (See Figure 2 under Humulin® N). Always check the appearance of your bottle of insulin before using, and if you note anything unusual in the appearance of your insulin or notice your insulin requirements changing markedly, consult your doctor.

INJECTION PROCEDURES
See under Humulin® L.

HOW SUPPLIED
Vials, U-100, 100 units/mL, 10 mL (No. HI-610) (1's), NDC 0002-8615-01

[060592]

LENTE® ILETIN® I   OTC
[lĕn-ta ī-lĕ-tĭn]
(Insulin Zinc Suspension, USP, beef-pork)

SEMILENTE® ILETIN® I   OTC
[sĕm'ĭ-lĕn'tā ī'lĕ-tĭn]
(Prompt Insulin Zinc Suspension, USP, beef-pork)

ULTRALENTE® ILETIN® I   OTC
[ŭl'trā-lĕn'tā ī'lĕ-tĭn]
(Extended Insulin Zinc Suspension, USP, beef-pork)

INFORMATION FOR THE PATIENT
WARNINGS and Diabetes: See under Regular Iletin® I.

LENTE BEEF-PORK INSULIN
Description
Lente beef-pork insulin is obtained from beef and pork pancreas.
Lente® Iletin® I (insulin, Lilly) is an amorphous and crystalline suspension of insulin with zinc providing an intermediate-acting insulin with a slower onset and a longer duration of activity (slightly more than 24 hours) than regular insulin. The time course of action of any insulin may vary considerably in different individuals or at different times in the same individual. As with all insulin preparations, the duration of action of Lente Iletin I is dependent on dose, site of injection, blood supply, temperature, and physical activity. Lente Iletin I is a sterile suspension and is for subcutaneous injection only. It should not be used intravenously or intramuscularly. The concentration of Lente Iletin I is 100 units/mL (U-100).
Identification
This insulin, manufactured by Eli Lilly and Company, has the trademark Iletin I and is available in various types—Regular, NPH, Lente, Semilente®, and Ultralente®. Your doctor has prescribed the type of insulin that he/she believes is best for you. DO NOT USE ANY OTHER INSULIN EXCEPT ON HIS/HER ADVICE AND DIRECTION.
Always check the carton and the bottle label for the name and letter designation of the insulin you receive from your pharmacy to make sure it is the same as that your doctor has prescribed.
Always examine the appearance of your bottle of insulin before withdrawing each dose. A bottle of Lente Iletin I must be carefully shaken or rotated before each injection so that the contents are uniformly mixed. Lente Iletin I should look uniformly cloudy or milky after mixing. Do not use it if the insulin substance (the white material) remains at the bottom of the bottle after mixing. Do not use a bottle of Lente Iletin I if there are clumps in the insulin after mixing. Always check the appearance of your bottle of insulin before using, and if you note anything unusual in the appearance of your insulin or notice your insulin requirements changing markedly, consult your doctor.

SEMILENTE BEEF-PORK INSULIN
Description
Semilente beef-pork insulin is obtained from beef and pork pancreas.
Semilente® Iletin® I (insulin, Lilly) is an amorphous and crystalline suspension of insulin with zinc providing an intermediate-acting insulin. Semilente Iletin I has an onset of action similar to regular insulin but has a longer duration of activity (approximately 12 to 16 hours). The time course of action of any insulin may vary considerably in different individuals or at different times in the same individual. As with all insulin preparations, the duration of action of Semilente Iletin I is dependent on dose, site of injection, blood supply, temperature, and physical activity. Semilente Iletin I is a

sterile suspension and is for subcutaneous injection only. It should not be used intravenously or intramuscularly. The concentration of Semilente Iletin I is 100 units/mL (U-100).
Identification
This insulin, manufactured by Eli Lilly and Company, has the trademark Iletin I and is available in various types—Regular, NPH, Lente, Semilente®, and Ultralente®. Your doctor has prescribed the type of insulin that he/she believes is best for you. DO NOT USE ANY OTHER INSULIN EXCEPT ON HIS/HER ADVICE AND DIRECTION.
Always check the carton and the bottle label for the name and letter designation of the insulin you receive from your pharmacy to make sure it is the same as that your doctor has prescribed.
Always examine the appearance of your bottle of insulin before withdrawing each dose. A bottle of Semilente Iletin I must be carefully shaken or rotated before each injection so that the contents are uniformly mixed. Semilente Iletin I should look uniformly cloudy or milky after mixing. Do not use it if the insulin substance (the white material) remains at the bottom of the bottle after mixing. Do not use a bottle of Semilente Iletin I if there are clumps in the insulin after mixing. Always check the appearance of your bottle of insulin before using, and if you note anything unusual in the appearance of your insulin or notice your insulin requirements changing markedly, consult your doctor.

ULTRALENTE BEEF-PORK INSULIN
Description
Ultralente beef-pork insulin is obtained from beef and pork pancreas.
Ultralente® Iletin® I (insulin, Lilly) is a crystalline suspension of insulin with zinc providing a slower onset and a longer and less intense duration of activity (slightly more than 28 hours) than regular insulin or the intermediate-acting insulins (NPH and Lente). The time course of action of any insulin may vary considerably in different individuals or at different times in the same individual. As with all insulin preparations, the duration of action of Ultralente Iletin I is dependent on dose, site of injection, blood supply, temperature, and physical activity. Ultralente Iletin I is a sterile suspension and is for subcutaneous injection only. It should not be used intravenously or intramuscularly. The concentration of Ultralente Iletin I is 100 units/mL (U-100).
Identification
This insulin, manufactured by Eli Lilly and Company, has the trademark Iletin I and is available in various types—Regular, NPH, Lente, Semilente®, and Ultralente®. Your doctor has prescribed the type of insulin that he/she believes is best for you. DO NOT USE ANY OTHER INSULIN EXCEPT ON HIS/HER ADVICE AND DIRECTION.
Always check the carton and the bottle label for the name and letter designation of the insulin you receive from your pharmacy to make sure it is the same as that your doctor has prescribed.
Always examine the appearance of your bottle of insulin before withdrawing each dose. A bottle of Ultralente Iletin I must be carefully shaken or rotated before each injection so that the contents are uniformly mixed. Ultralente Iletin I should look uniformly cloudy or milky after mixing. Do not use it if the insulin substance (the white material) remains at the bottom of the bottle after mixing. Do not use a bottle of Ultralente Iletin I if there are clumps in the insulin after mixing. Always check the appearance of your bottle of insulin before using, and if you note anything unusual in the appearance of your insulin or notice your insulin requirements changing markedly, consult your doctor.

Storage, Injection Procedures, additional Warnings, Dosage, and Common Problems of Diabetes: See under Regular Iletin® I.

HOW SUPPLIED
Vials, U-100, 100 units/mL, 10 mL:
Lente® Iletin® I (Insulin Zinc Suspension, USP)
(No. CP-410) (1's), NDC 0002-8410-01
Semilente® Iletin® I (Prompt Insulin Zinc Suspension, USP)
(No. CP-510) (1's), NDC 0002-8510-01
Ultralente® Iletin® I (Extended Insulin Zinc Suspension, USP)
(No. CP-610) (1's), NDC 0002-8610-01

[060592]

NPH ILETIN® I   OTC
[ĕn'pē-āch ī'lĕ-tĭn]
(Isophane Insulin Suspension, USP, beef-pork)

INFORMATION FOR THE PATIENT
WARNINGS and Diabetes: See under Regular Iletin® I.

NPH BEEF-PORK INSULIN
Description
NPH beef-pork insulin is obtained from beef and pork pancreas.

NPH Iletin® I (insulin, Lilly) is a crystalline suspension of insulin with protamine and zinc providing an intermediate-acting insulin with a slower onset of action and a longer duration of activity (slightly more than 24 hours) than that of regular insulin. The time course of action of any insulin may vary considerably in different individuals or at different times in the same individual. As with all insulin preparations, the duration of action of NPH Iletin I is dependent on dose, site of injection, blood supply, temperature, and physical activity. NPH Iletin I is a sterile suspension and is for subcutaneous injection only. It should not be used intravenously or intramuscularly. The concentration of NPH Iletin I is 100 units/mL (U-100).
Identification
This insulin, manufactured by Eli Lilly and Company, has the trademark Iletin I and is available in various types—Regular, NPH, Lente, Semilente®, and Ultralente®. Your doctor has prescribed the type of insulin that he/she believes is best for you. DO NOT USE ANY OTHER INSULIN EXCEPT ON HIS/HER ADVICE AND DIRECTION.
Always check the carton and the bottle label for the name and letter designation of the insulin you receive from your pharmacy to make sure it is the same as that your doctor has prescribed.
Always examine the appearance of your bottle of insulin before withdrawing each dose. A bottle of NPH Iletin I must be carefully shaken or rotated before each injection so that the contents are uniformly mixed. NPH Iletin I should look uniformly cloudy or milky after mixing. Do not use it if the insulin substance (the white material) remains at the bottom of the bottle after mixing. Do not use a bottle of NPH Iletin I if there are clumps in the insulin after mixing. Always check the appearance of your bottle of insulin before using, and if you note anything unusual in the appearance of your insulin or notice your insulin requirements changing markedly, consult your doctor.

Storage, Injection Procedures, additional Warnings, Dosage, and Common Problems of Diabetes: See under Regular Iletin® I.

HOW SUPPLIED
Vials, U-100, 100 units/mL, 10 mL (No. CP-310) (1's), NDC 0002-8310-01

[031392]

ILETIN® (INSULIN, LILLY)—   OTC
[ī'lĕ-tĭn]
REGULAR AND MODIFIED
INSULIN PRODUCTS

REGULAR ILETIN® I   OTC
[rĕg'ū-lĕr ī'lĕ-tĭn]
(Insulin Injection, USP, beef-pork)

INFORMATION FOR THE PATIENT

WARNINGS
ANY CHANGE OF INSULIN SHOULD BE MADE CAUTIOUSLY AND ONLY UNDER MEDICAL SUPERVISION. CHANGES IN PURITY, STRENGTH, BRAND (MANUFACTURER), TYPE (REGULAR, NPH, LENTE®, ETC), SPECIES (BEEF, PORK, BEEF-PORK, HUMAN), AND/OR METHOD OF MANUFACTURE (RECOMBINANT DNA VERSUS ANIMAL-SOURCE INSULIN) MAY RESULT IN THE NEED FOR A CHANGE IN DOSAGE. IF AN ADJUSTMENT IS NEEDED, IT MAY OCCUR WITH THE FIRST DOSE OR DURING THE FIRST SEVERAL WEEKS OR MONTHS.

DIABETES
Insulin is a hormone produced by the pancreas, a large gland that lies near the stomach. This hormone is necessary for the body's correct use of food, especially sugar. Diabetes occurs when the pancreas does not make enough insulin to meet your body's needs.
To control your diabetes, your doctor has prescribed injections of insulin to keep your blood glucose at a nearly normal level. Proper control of your diabetes requires close and constant cooperation with your doctor. In spite of diabetes, you can lead an active, healthy, and useful life if you eat a balanced diet daily, exercise regularly, and take your insulin injections as prescribed.
You have been instructed to test your blood and/or your urine regularly for glucose. If your blood tests consistently show above- or below-normal glucose levels or your urine tests consistently show the presence of glucose, your diabetes is not properly controlled and you must let your doctor know. Always keep an extra supply of insulin as well as a spare syringe and needle on hand. Always wear diabetic identification so that appropriate treatment can be given if complications occur away from home.

REGULAR BEEF-PORK INSULIN

Description

Regular beef-pork insulin is obtained from beef and pork pancreas.

Regular Iletin® I (insulin, Lilly) consists of zinc-insulin crystals dissolved in a clear fluid. Regular Iletin I has had nothing added to change the speed or length of its action. It takes effect rapidly and has a relatively short duration of activity (4 to 12 hours) as compared with other insulins. The time course of action of any insulin may vary considerably in different individuals or at different times in the same individual. As with all insulin preparations, the duration of action of Regular Iletin I is dependent on dose, site of injection, blood supply, temperature, and physical activity. Regular Iletin I is a sterile solution and is for subcutaneous injection. It should not be used intramuscularly. The concentration of Regular Iletin I is 100 units/mL (U-100).

Identification

This insulin, manufactured by Eli Lilly and Company, has the trademark Iletin I and is available in various types— Regular, NPH, Lente, Semilente®, and Ultralente®. Your doctor has prescribed the type of insulin that he/she believes is best for you. DO NOT USE ANY OTHER INSULIN EXCEPT ON HIS/HER ADVICE AND DIRECTION.

Always check the carton and the bottle label for the name and letter designation of the insulin you receive from your pharmacy to make sure it is the same as that your doctor has prescribed.

Always examine the appearance of your bottle of insulin before withdrawing each dose. Regular Iletin I is a clear and colorless liquid with a water-like appearance and consistency. Do not use if it appears cloudy, thickened, or slightly colored or if solid particles are visible. Always check the appearance of your bottle of insulin before using, and if you note anything unusual in the appearance of your insulin or notice your insulin requirements changing markedly, consult your doctor.

Storage

Insulin should be stored in a refrigerator but not in the freezer. If refrigeration is not possible, the bottle of insulin that you are currently using can be kept unrefrigerated as long as it is kept as cool as possible (below 86°F [30°C]) and away from heat and light. Do not use insulin if it has been frozen. Do not use a bottle of insulin after the expiration date stamped on the label.

INJECTION PROCEDURES

Correct Syringe

Doses of insulin are measured in **units.** U-100 insulin contains 100 units/mL (1 mL = 1 cc). With Regular Iletin I, it is important to use a syringe that is marked for U-100 insulin preparations. Failure to use the proper syringe can lead to a mistake in dosage, causing serious problems for you, such as a blood glucose level that is too low or too high.

Syringe Use

To help avoid contamination and possible infection, follow these instructions exactly.

Disposable syringes and needles should be used only once and then discarded. NEEDLES AND SYRINGES MUST NOT BE SHARED.

Reusable syringes and needles must be sterilized before each injection. Follow the package directions supplied with your syringe. Described below are 2 methods of sterilizing.

Boiling

1. Put syringe, plunger, and needle in strainer, place in saucepan, and cover with water. Boil for 5 minutes.
2. Remove articles from water. When they have cooled, insert plunger into barrel, and fasten needle to syringe with a slight twist.
3. Push plunger in and out several times until water is completely removed.

Isopropyl Alcohol

If the syringe, plunger, and needle cannot be boiled, as when you are traveling, they may be sterilized by immersion for at least 5 minutes in Isopropyl Alcohol, 91%. Do not use bathing, rubbing, or medicated alcohol for this sterilization. If the syringe is sterilized with alcohol, it must be absolutely dry before use.

Preparing the Dose

1. Wash your hands.
2. Inspect the insulin. Regular Iletin I should look clear and colorless. Do not use Regular Iletin I if it appears cloudy, thickened, or slightly colored or if solid particles are visible.
3. If using a new bottle, flip off the plastic protective cap, but do not remove the stopper. When using a new bottle, wipe the top of the bottle with an alcohol swab.
4. If you are mixing insulins, refer to the Warnings below.
5. Draw air into the syringe equal to your insulin dose. Put the needle through rubber top of the insulin bottle and inject the air into the bottle.
6. Turn the bottle and syringe upside down. Hold the bottle and syringe firmly in 1 hand.
7. Making sure the tip of the needle is in the insulin, withdraw the correct dose of insulin into the syringe.

8. Before removing the needle from the bottle, check your syringe for air bubbles which reduce the amount of insulin in it. If bubbles are present, hold the syringe straight up and tap its side until the bubbles float to the top. Push them out with the plunger and withdraw the correct dose.
9. Remove the needle from the bottle and lay the syringe down so that the needle does not touch anything.

WARNINGS—SEE ADDITIONAL WARNINGS ABOVE

Patients who have been directed by their doctors to mix 2 types of insulin should be aware that insulin hypodermic syringes of different manufacturers may vary in the amount of space between the bottom line and the needle.

Because of this, do not change:
1. The order of mixing that the doctor has prescribed or
2. The model and brand of syringe or needle without first consulting your doctor.

The mixing should be done immediately prior to injection. Failure to heed this warning could result in a dosage error.

Injection

Cleanse the skin with alcohol where the injection is to be made. Stabilize the skin by spreading it or pinching up a large area. Insert the needle as instructed by your doctor. Push the plunger in as far as it will go. Pull the needle out and apply gentle pressure over the injection site for several seconds. Do not rub the area. To avoid tissue damage, give the next injection at a site at least ½" from the previous site.

DOSAGE

Your doctor has told you which insulin to use, how much, and when and how often to inject it. Because each patient's case of diabetes is different, this schedule has been individualized for you.

Your usual insulin dose may be affected by changes in your food, activity, or work schedule. Carefully follow your doctor's instructions to allow for these changes. Other things that may affect your insulin dose are:

Illness

Illness, especially with nausea and vomiting, may cause your insulin requirements to change. Even if you are not eating, you will still require insulin. You and your doctor should establish a sick day plan for you to use in case of illness. When you are sick, test your blood/urine frequently and call your doctor as instructed.

Pregnancy

Good control of diabetes is especially important for you and your unborn baby. Pregnancy may make managing your diabetes more difficult. If you are planning to have a baby, are pregnant, or are nursing a baby, consult your doctor.

Medication

Insulin requirements may be increased if you are taking other drugs with hyperglycemic activity, such as oral contraceptives, corticosteroids, or thyroid replacement therapy. Insulin requirements may be reduced in the presence of drugs with hypoglycemic activity, such as oral hypoglycemics, salicylates (for example, aspirin), sulfa antibiotics, and certain antidepressants. Always discuss any medications you are taking with your doctor.

Exercise

Exercise may lower your body's need for insulin during and for some time after the activity. Exercise may also speed up the effect of an insulin dose, especially if the exercise involves the area of injection site (for example, the leg should not be used for injection just prior to running). Discuss with your doctor how you should adjust your regimen to accommodate exercise.

Travel

Persons traveling across more than 2 time zones should consult their doctor concerning adjustments in their insulin schedule.

COMMON PROBLEMS OF DIABETES

Hypoglycemia (Insulin Reaction)

Hypoglycemia (too little glucose in the blood) is one of the most frequent adverse events experienced by insulin users. It can be brought about by:
1. Taking too much insulin
2. Missing or delaying meals
3. Exercising or working more than usual
4. An infection or illness (especially with diarrhea or vomiting)
5. A change in the body's need for insulin
6. Diseases of the adrenal, pituitary, or thyroid gland, or progression of kidney or liver disease
7. Interactions with other drugs that lower blood glucose, such as oral hypoglycemics, salicylates (for example, aspirin), sulfa antibiotics, and certain antidepressants
8. Consumption of alcoholic beverages

Symptoms of mild to moderate hypoglycemia may occur suddenly and can include:
- sweating
- dizziness
- palpitation
- tremor
- hunger
- restlessness
- tingling in the hands, feet, lips, or tongue

- lightheadedness
- inability to concentrate
- headache
- drowsiness
- sleep disturbances
- anxiety
- blurred vision
- slurred speech
- depressive mood
- irritability
- abnormal behavior
- unsteady movement
- personality changes

Signs of severe hypoglycemia can include:
- disorientation
- unconsciousness
- seizures
- death

Therefore, it is important that assistance be obtained immediately.

Early warning symptoms of hypoglycemia may be different or less pronounced under certain conditions, such as long duration of diabetes, diabetic nerve disease, medications such as beta-blockers, change in insulin preparations, or intensified control (3 or more insulin injections per day) of diabetes.

Without recognition of early warning symptoms, you may not be able to take steps to avoid more serious hypoglycemia. Be alert for all of the various types of symptoms that may indicate hypoglycemia. Patients who experience hypoglycemia without early warning symptoms should monitor their blood glucose frequently, especially prior to activities such as driving. If the blood glucose is below your normal fasting glucose, you should consider eating or drinking sugar-containing foods to treat your hypoglycemia.

Mild to moderate hypoglycemia may be treated by eating foods or drinks that contain sugar. Patients should always carry a quick source of sugar, such as candy mints or glucose tablets. More severe hypoglycemia may require the assistance of another person. Patients who are unable to take sugar orally or who are unconscious require an injection of glucagon or should be treated with intravenous administration of glucose at a medical facility.

You should learn to recognize your own symptoms of hypoglycemia. If you are uncertain about these symptoms, you should monitor your blood glucose frequently to help you learn to recognize the symptoms that you experience with hypoglycemia.

If you have frequent episodes of hypoglycemia or experience difficulty in recognizing the symptoms, you should consult your doctor to discuss possible changes in therapy, meal plans, and/or exercise programs to help you avoid hypoglycemia.

Hyperglycemia and Diabetic Acidosis

Hyperglycemia (too much glucose in the blood) may develop if your body has too little insulin. Hyperglycemia can be brought about by:
1. Omitting your insulin or taking less than the doctor has prescribed
2. Eating significantly more than your meal plan suggests
3. Developing a fever or infection

In patients with insulin-dependent diabetes, prolonged hyperglycemia can result in diabetic acidosis. The first symptoms of diabetic acidosis usually come on gradually, over a period of hours or days, and include a drowsy feeling, flushed face, thirst, loss of appetite, and fruity odor on the breath. With acidosis, urine tests show large amounts of glucose and acetone. Heavy breathing and a rapid pulse are more severe symptoms. If uncorrected, prolonged hyperglycemia or diabetic acidosis can result in loss of consciousness or death. Therefore, it is important that you obtain medical assistance immediately.

Lipodystrophy

Rarely, administration of insulin subcutaneously can result in lipoatrophy (depression in the skin) or lipohypertrophy (enlargement or thickening of tissue). If you notice either of these conditions, consult your doctor. A change in your injection technique may help alleviate the problem.

Allergy to Insulin

Local Allergy—Patients occasionally experience redness, swelling, and itching at the site of injection of insulin. This condition, called local allergy, usually clears up in a few days to a few weeks. In some instances, this condition may be related to factors other than insulin, such as irritants in the skin cleansing agent or poor injection technique. If you have local reactions, contact your doctor.

Continued on next page

* Identi-Code® symbol. This product information was prepared in June 1992. Current information on these and other products of Eli Lilly and Company may be obtained by direct inquiry to Lilly Research Laboratories, Lilly Corporate Center, Indianapolis, Indiana 46285, (317) 276-3714.

Lilly—Cont.

Systemic Allergy—Less common, but potentially more serious, is generalized allergy to insulin, which may cause rash over the whole body, shortness of breath, wheezing, reduction in blood pressure, fast pulse, or sweating. Severe cases of generalized allergy may be life threatening. If you think you are having a generalized allergic reaction to insulin, notify a doctor immediately.

ADDITIONAL INFORMATION
Additional information about diabetes may be obtained from your diabetes educator.

DIABETES FORECAST is a national magazine designed especially for patients with diabetes and their families and is available by subscription from the American Diabetes Association, National Service Center, 1660 Duke Street, Alexandria, Virginia 22314.
Another publication, **DIABETES COUNTDOWN, is** available from the Juvenile Diabetes Foundation, 432 Park Avenue South, New York, New York 10016-8013.

HOW SUPPLIED
Vials, U-100, 100 units/mL, 10 mL (No. CP-210) (1's), NDC 0002-8210-01

[031392]

LENTE® ILETIN® II (Beef) OTC
[lĕn-tā ī'lĕ-tĭn]
(Insulin Zinc Suspension, USP, purified beef)

INFORMATION FOR THE PATIENT
WARNINGS and Diabetes: *See under* Regular Iletin® II (Pork).

LENTE BEEF INSULIN
Description
Lente beef insulin is obtained from beef pancreas.
Lente® Iletin® II (purified insulin, Lilly) is an amorphous and crystalline suspension of human insulin with zinc providing an intermediate-acting insulin with a slower onset and a longer duration of activity (slightly more than 24 hours) than regular insulin. The time course of action of any insulin may vary considerably in different individuals or at different times in the same individual. As with all insulin preparations, the duration of action of Lente Iletin II is dependent on dose, site of injection, blood supply, temperature, and physical activity. Lente Iletin II is a sterile suspension and is for subcutaneous injection only. It should not be used intravenously or intramuscularly. The concentration of Lente Iletin II is 100 units/mL (U-100).
Identification
This insulin, manufactured by Eli Lilly and Company, has the trademark Iletin II and is available in various types—Regular, NPH, and Lente. Your doctor has prescribed the type of insulin that he/she believes is best for you. **DO NOT USE ANY OTHER INSULIN EXCEPT ON HIS/HER ADVICE AND DIRECTION.**
Always check the carton and the bottle label for the name and letter designation of the insulin you receive from your pharmacy to make sure it is the same as that your doctor has prescribed.
Always examine the appearance of your bottle of insulin before withdrawing each dose. A bottle of Lente Iletin II must be carefully shaken or rotated before each injection so that the contents are uniformly mixed. Lente Iletin II should look uniformly cloudy or milky after mixing. Do not use it if the insulin substance (the white material) remains at the bottom of the bottle after mixing. Do not use a bottle of Lente Iletin II if there are clumps in the insulin after mixing. Always check the appearance of your bottle of insulin before using, and if you note anything unusual in the appearance of your insulin or notice your insulin requirements changing markedly, consult your doctor.
Storage, Injection Procedures, additional Warnings, Dosage, and Common Problems of Diabetes: *See under* Regular Iletin® II (Pork).

HOW SUPPLIED
Vials, U-100, 100 units/mL, 10 mL (No. CP-410S) (1's), NDC 0002-8412-01

[051192]

NPH ILETIN® II (BEEF) OTC
[ĕn'pē-āch ī'lĕ-tĭn]
(Isophane Insulin Suspension, USP, purified beef)

INFORMATION FOR THE PATIENT
WARNINGS and Diabetes: *See under* Regular Iletin® II (Pork).

NPH BEEF INSULIN
Description
NPH beef insulin is obtained from beef pancreas.
NPH Iletin® II (purified insulin, Lilly) is a crystalline suspension of insulin with protamine and zinc providing an intermediate-acting insulin with a slower onset of action and a longer duration of activity (slightly more than 24 hours) than that of regular insulin. The time course of action of any insulin may vary considerably in different individuals or at different times in the same individual. As with all insulin preparations, the duration of action of NPH Iletin II is dependent on dose, site of injection, blood supply, temperature, and physical activity. NPH Iletin II is a sterile suspension and is for subcutaneous injection only. It should not be used intravenously or intramuscularly. The concentration of NPH Iletin II is 100 units/mL (U-100).
Identification
This insulin, manufactured by Eli Lilly and Company, has the trademark Iletin II and is available in various types—Regular, NPH, and Lente. Your doctor has prescribed the type of insulin that he/she believes is best for you. **DO NOT USE ANY OTHER INSULIN EXCEPT ON HIS/HER ADVICE AND DIRECTION.**
Always check the carton and the bottle label for the name and letter designation of the insulin you receive from your pharmacy to make sure it is the same as that your doctor has prescribed.
Always examine the appearance of your bottle of insulin before withdrawing each dose. A bottle of NPH Iletin II must be carefully shaken or rotated before each injection so that the contents are uniformly mixed. NPH Iletin II should look uniformly cloudy or milky after mixing. Do not use it if the insulin substance (the white material) remains at the bottom of the bottle after mixing. Do not use a bottle of NPH Iletin II if there are clumps in the insulin after mixing. Always check the appearance of your bottle of insulin before using, and if you note anything unusual in the appearance of your insulin or notice your insulin requirements changing markedly, consult your doctor.
Storage, Injection Procedures, additional Warnings, Dosage, and Common Problems of Diabetes: *See under* Regular Iletin® II (Pork).

HOW SUPPLIED
Vials, U-100, 100 units/mL, 10 mL (No. CP-310S) (1's), NDC 0002-8312-01

[051192]

REGULAR ILETIN® II (BEEF) OTC
[rĕg-ū-lĕr ī'lĕ-tĭn]
(Insulin Injection, USP, purified beef)

INFORMATION FOR THE PATIENT
WARNINGS and Diabetes: *See under* Regular Iletin® II (Pork).

REGULAR BEEF INSULIN
Description
Regular beef insulin is obtained from beef pancreas.
Regular Iletin® II (purified insulin, Lilly) consists of zinc-insulin crystals dissolved in a clear fluid. Regular Iletin II has had nothing added to change the speed or length of its action. It takes effect rapidly and has a relatively short duration of activity (4 to 12 hours) as compared with other insulins. The time course of action of any insulin may vary considerably in different individuals or at different times in the same individual. As with all insulin preparations, the duration of action of Regular Iletin II is dependent on dose, site of injection, blood supply, temperature, and physical activity. Regular Iletin II is a sterile solution and is for subcutaneous injection. It should not be used intramuscularly. The concentration of Regular Iletin II is 100 units/mL (U-100).
Identification
This insulin, manufactured by Eli Lilly and Company, has the trademark Iletin II and is available in various types—Regular, NPH, and Lente. Your doctor has prescribed the type of insulin that he/she believes is best for you. **DO NOT USE ANY OTHER INSULIN EXCEPT ON HIS/HER ADVICE AND DIRECTION.**
Always check the carton and the bottle label for the name and letter designation of the insulin you receive from your pharmacy to make sure it is the same as that your doctor has prescribed.
Always examine the appearance of your bottle of insulin before withdrawing each dose. Regular Iletin II is a clear and colorless liquid with a water-like appearance and consistency. Do not use if it appears cloudy, thickened, or slightly colored or if solid particles are visible. Always check the appearance of your bottle of insulin before using, and if you note anything unusual in the appearance of your insulin or notice your insulin requirements changing markedly, consult your doctor.

Storage, Injection Procedures, additional Warnings, Dosage, and Common Problems of Diabetes: *See under* Regular Iletin® II (Pork).

HOW SUPPLIED
Vials, U-100, 100 units/mL, 10 mL (No. CP-210S) (1's), NDC 0002-8212-01

[051192]

LENTE® ILETIN® II (PORK) OTC
[lĕn-tā ī'lĕ-tĭn]
(Insulin Zinc Suspension, USP, purified pork)

INFORMATION FOR THE PATIENT
WARNINGS and Diabetes: *See under* Regular Iletin® II (Pork).

LENTE PORK INSULIN
Description
Lente pork insulin is obtained from pork pancreas.
Lente® Iletin® II (purified insulin, Lilly) is an amorphous and crystalline suspension of a human insulin with zinc providing an intermediate-acting insulin with a slower onset and a longer duration of activity (slightly more than 24 hours) than regular insulin. The time course of action of any insulin may vary considerably in different individuals or at different times in the same individual. As with all insulin preparations, the duration of action of Lente Iletin II is dependent on dose, site of injection, blood supply, temperature, and physical activity. Lente Iletin II is a sterile suspension and is for subcutaneous injection only. It should not be used intravenously or intramuscularly. The concentration of Lente Iletin II is 100 units/mL (U-100).
Identification
This insulin, manufactured by Eli Lilly and Company, has the trademark Iletin II and is available in various types—Regular, NPH, and Lente. Your doctor has prescribed the type of insulin that he/she believes is best for you. **DO NOT USE ANY OTHER INSULIN EXCEPT ON HIS/HER ADVICE AND DIRECTION.**
Always check the carton and the bottle label for the name and letter designation of the insulin you receive from your pharmacy to make sure it is the same as that your doctor has prescribed.
Always examine the appearance of your bottle of insulin before withdrawing each dose. A bottle of Lente Iletin II must be carefully shaken or rotated before each injection so that the contents are uniformly mixed. Lente Iletin II should look uniformly cloudy or milky after mixing. Do not use it if the insulin substance (the white material) remains at the bottom of the bottle after mixing. Do not use a bottle of Lente Iletin II if there are clumps in the insulin after mixing. Always check the appearance of your bottle of insulin before using, and if you note anything unusual in the appearance of your insulin or notice your insulin requirements changing markedly, consult your doctor.
Storage, Injection Procedures, additional Warnings, Dosage, and Common Problems of Diabetes: *See under* Regular Iletin® II (Pork).

HOW SUPPLIED
Vials, U-100, 100 units/mL, 10 mL (No. CP-410P) (1's), NDC 0002-8411-01

[051192]

NPH ILETIN® II (PORK) OTC
[ĕn'pē-āch ī'lĕ-tĭn]
(Isophane Insulin Suspension, USP, purified pork)

INFORMATION FOR THE PATIENT
WARNINGS and Diabetes: *See under* Regular Iletin® II (Pork).

NPH PORK INSULIN
Description
NPH pork insulin is obtained from pork pancreas.
NPH Iletin® II (purified insulin, Lilly) is a crystalline suspension of insulin with protamine and zinc providing an intermediate-acting insulin with a slower onset of action and a longer duration of activity (slightly more than 24 hours) than that of regular insulin. The time course of action of any insulin may vary considerably in different individuals or at different times in the same individual. As with all insulin preparations, the duration of action of NPH Iletin II is dependent on dose, site of injection, blood supply, temperature, and physical activity. NPH Iletin II is a sterile suspension and is for subcutaneous injection only. It should not be used intravenously or intramuscularly. The concentration of NPH Iletin II is 100 units/mL (U-100).
Identification
This insulin, manufactured by Eli Lilly and Company, has the trademark Iletin II and is available in various types—Regular, NPH, and Lente. Your doctor has prescribed the

type of insulin that he/she believes is best for you. **DO NOT USE ANY OTHER INSULIN EXCEPT ON HIS/HER ADVICE AND DIRECTION.**

Always check the carton and the bottle label for the name and letter designation of the insulin you receive from your pharmacy to make sure it is the same as that your doctor has prescribed.

Always examine the appearance of your bottle of insulin before withdrawing each dose. A bottle of NPH Iletin II must be carefully shaken or rotated before each injection so that the contents are uniformly mixed. NPH Iletin II should look uniformly cloudy or milky after mixing. Do not use it if the insulin substance (the white material) remains at the bottom of the bottle after mixing. Do not use a bottle of NPH Iletin II if there are clumps in the insulin after mixing. Always check the appearance of your bottle of insulin before using, and if you note anything unusual in the appearance of your insulin or notice your insulin requirements changing markedly, consult your doctor.

Storage, Injection Procedures, additional Warnings, Dosage, and Common Problems of Diabetes: *See under* Regular Iletin® II (Pork).

HOW SUPPLIED

Vials, U-100, 100 units/mL, 10 mL (No. CP-310P) (1's), NDC 0002-8311-01

[051192]

REGULAR ILETIN® II (PORK) OTC

[*rĕg-ū-lĕr ī'lĕ-tĭn*]

(Insulin Injection, USP, purified pork)

INFORMATION FOR THE PATIENT

WARNINGS

ANY CHANGE OF INSULIN SHOULD BE MADE CAUTIOUSLY AND ONLY UNDER MEDICAL SUPERVISION. CHANGES IN PURITY, STRENGTH, BRAND (MANUFACTURER), TYPE (REGULAR, NPH, LENTE®, ETC), SPECIES (BEEF, PORK, BEEF-PORK, HUMAN), AND/OR METHOD OF MANUFACTURE (RECOMBINANT DNA VERSUS ANIMAL-SOURCE INSULIN) MAY RESULT IN THE NEED FOR A CHANGE IN DOSAGE. IF AN ADJUSTMENT IS NEEDED, IT MAY OCCUR WITH THE FIRST DOSE OR DURING THE FIRST SEVERAL WEEKS OR MONTHS.

DIABETES

Insulin is a hormone produced by the pancreas, a large gland that lies near the stomach. This hormone is necessary for the body's correct use of food, especially sugar. Diabetes occurs when the pancreas does not make enough insulin to meet your body's needs.

To control your diabetes, your doctor has prescribed injections of insulin to keep your blood glucose at a nearly normal level. Proper control of your diabetes requires close and constant cooperation with your doctor. In spite of diabetes, you can lead an active, healthy, and useful life if you eat a balanced diet daily, exercise regularly, and take your insulin injections as prescribed.

You have been instructed to test your blood and/or your urine regularly for glucose. If your blood tests consistently show above- or below-normal glucose levels or your urine tests consistently show the presence of glucose, your diabetes is not properly controlled and you must let your doctor know.

Always keep an extra supply of insulin as well as a spare syringe and needle on hand. Always wear diabetic identification so that appropriate treatment can be given if complications occur away from home.

REGULAR PORK INSULIN

Description

Regular pork insulin is obtained from pork pancreas.

Regular Iletin® II (purified insulin, Lilly) consists of zinc-insulin crystals dissolved in a clear fluid. Regular Iletin II has had nothing added to change the speed or length of its action. It takes effect rapidly and has a relatively short duration of activity (4 to 12 hours) as compared with other insulins. The time course of action of any insulin may vary considerably in different individuals or at different times in the same individual. As with all insulin preparations, the duration of action of Regular Iletin II is dependent on dose, site of injection, blood supply, temperature, and physical activity.

Regular Iletin II is a sterile solution and is for subcutaneous injection. It should not be used intramuscularly. The concentration of Regular Iletin II is 100 units/mL (U-100).

Identification

This insulin, manufactured by Eli Lilly and Company, has the trademark Iletin II and is available in various types—Regular, NPH, and Lente. Your doctor has prescribed the type of insulin that he/she believes is best for you. **DO NOT USE ANY OTHER INSULIN EXCEPT ON HIS/HER ADVICE AND DIRECTION.**

Always check the carton and the bottle label for the name and letter designation of the insulin you receive from your pharmacy to make sure it is the same as that your doctor has prescribed.

Always examine the appearance of your bottle of insulin before withdrawing each dose. Regular Iletin II is a clear and colorless liquid with a water-like appearance and consistency. Do not use if it appears cloudy, thickened, or slightly colored or if solid particles are visible. Always check the appearance of your bottle of insulin before using, and if you note anything unusual in the appearance of your insulin or notice your insulin requirements changing markedly, consult your doctor.

Storage

Insulin should be stored in a refrigerator but not in the freezer. If refrigeration is not possible, the bottle of insulin that you are currently using can be kept unrefrigerated as long as it is kept as cool as possible (below 86°F [30°C]) and away from heat and light. Do not use insulin if it has been frozen. Do not use a bottle of insulin after the expiration date stamped on the label.

INJECTION PROCEDURES

Correct Syringe

Doses of insulin are measured in **units.** U-100 insulin contains 100 units/mL (1 mL = 1 cc). With Regular Iletin II, it is important to use a syringe that is marked for U-100 insulin preparations. Failure to use the proper syringe can lead to a mistake in dosage, causing serious problems for you, such as a blood glucose level that is too low or too high.

Syringe Use

To help avoid contamination and possible infection, follow these instructions exactly.

Disposable syringes and needles should be used only once and then discarded. **NEEDLES AND SYRINGES MUST NOT BE SHARED.**

Reusable syringes and needles must be sterilized before each injection. **Follow the package directions supplied with your syringe.** Described below are 2 methods of sterilizing.

Boiling

1. Put syringe, plunger, and needle in strainer, place in saucepan, and cover with water. Boil for 5 minutes.
2. Remove articles from water. When they have cooled, insert plunger into barrel, and fasten needle to syringe with a slight twist.
3. Push plunger in and out several times until water is completely removed.

Isopropyl Alcohol

If the syringe, plunger, and needle cannot be boiled, as when you are traveling, they may be sterilized by immersion for at least 5 minutes in Isopropyl Alcohol, 91%. Do not use bathing, rubbing, or medicated alcohol for this sterilization. If the syringe is sterilized with alcohol, it must be absolutely dry before use.

Preparing the Dose

1. Wash your hands.
2. Inspect the insulin. Regular Iletin II should look clear and colorless. Do not use Regular Iletin II if it appears cloudy, thickened, or slightly colored or if solid particles are visible.
3. If using a new bottle, flip off the plastic protective cap, but **do not** remove the stopper. When using a new bottle, wipe the top of the bottle with an alcohol swab.
4. If you are mixing insulins, refer to the Warnings below.
5. Draw air into the syringe equal to your insulin dose. Put the needle through rubber top of the insulin bottle and inject the air into the bottle.
6. Turn the bottle and syringe upside down. Hold the bottle and syringe firmly in 1 hand.
7. Making sure the tip of the needle is in the insulin, withdraw the correct dose of insulin into the syringe.
8. Before removing the needle from the bottle, check your syringe for air bubbles which reduce the amount of insulin in it. If bubbles are present, hold the syringe straight up and tap its side until the bubbles float to the top. Push them out with the plunger and withdraw the correct dose.
9. Remove the needle from the bottle and lay the syringe down so that the needle does not touch anything.

WARNINGS—SEE ADDITIONAL WARNINGS ABOVE

Patients who have been directed by their doctors to mix 2 types of insulin should be aware that insulin hypodermic syringes of different manufacturers may vary in the amount of space between the bottom line and the needle.

Because of this, do not change:

1. The order of mixing that the doctor has prescribed or
2. The model and brand of syringe or needle without first consulting your doctor.

The mixing should be done immediately prior to injection. Failure to heed this warning could result in a dosage error.

Injection

Cleanse the skin with alcohol where the injection is to be made. Stabilize the skin by spreading it or pinching up a large area. Insert the needle as instructed by your doctor. Push the plunger in as far as it will go. Pull the needle out and apply gentle pressure over the injection site for several seconds. **Do not rub the area.** To avoid tissue damage, give the next injection at a site at least ½″ from the previous site.

DOSAGE

Your doctor has told you which insulin to use, how much, and when and how often to inject it. Because each patient's case of diabetes is different, this schedule has been individualized for you.

Your usual insulin dose may be affected by changes in your food, activity, or work schedule. Carefully follow your doctor's instructions to allow for these changes. Other things that may affect your insulin dose are:

Illness

Illness, especially with nausea and vomiting, may cause your insulin requirements to change. Even if you are not eating, you will still require insulin. You and your doctor should establish a sick day plan for you to use in case of illness. When you are sick, test your blood/urine frequently and call your doctor as instructed.

Pregnancy

Good control of diabetes is especially important for you and your unborn baby. Pregnancy may make managing your diabetes more difficult. If you are planning to have a baby, are pregnant, or are nursing a baby, consult your doctor.

Medication

Insulin requirements may be increased if you are taking other drugs with hyperglycemic activity, such as oral contraceptives, corticosteroids, or thyroid replacement therapy. Insulin requirements may be reduced in the presence of drugs with hypoglycemic activity, such as oral hypoglycemics, salicylates (for example, aspirin), sulfa antibiotics, and certain antidepressants. Always discuss any medications you are taking with your doctor.

Exercise

Exercise may lower your body's need for insulin during and for some time after the activity. Exercise may also speed up the effect of an insulin dose, especially if the exercise involves the area of injection site (for example, the leg should not be used for injection just prior to running). Discuss with your doctor how you should adjust your regimen to accommodate exercise.

Travel

Persons traveling across more than 2 time zones should consult their doctor concerning adjustments in their insulin schedule.

COMMON PROBLEMS OF DIABETES

Hypoglycemia (Insulin Reaction)

Hypoglycemia (too little glucose in the blood) is one of the most frequent adverse events experienced by insulin users. It can be brought about by:

1. Taking too much insulin
2. Missing or delaying meals
3. Exercising or working more than usual
4. An infection or illness (especially with diarrhea or vomiting)
5. A change in the body's need for insulin
6. Diseases of the adrenal, pituitary, or thyroid gland, or progression of kidney or liver disease
7. Interactions with other drugs that lower blood glucose, such as oral hypoglycemics, salicylates (for example, aspirin), sulfa antibiotics, and certain antidepressants
8. Consumption of alcoholic beverages

Symptoms of mild to moderate hypoglycemia may occur suddenly and can include:

- sweating
- dizziness
- palpitation
- tremor
- hunger
- restlessness
- tingling in the hands, feet, lips, or tongue
- lightheadedness
- inability to concentrate
- headache
- drowsiness
- sleep disturbances
- anxiety
- blurred vision
- slurred speech
- depressive mood
- irritability
- abnormal behavior
- unsteady movement
- personality changes

Signs of severe hypoglycemia can include:

- disorientation
- unconsciousness
- seizures
- death

Continued on next page

*** Identi-Code® symbol. This product information was prepared in June 1992. Current information on these and other products of Eli Lilly and Company may be obtained by direct inquiry to Lilly Research Laboratories, Lilly Corporate Center, Indianapolis, Indiana 46285, (317) 276-3714.**

Lilly—Cont.

Therefore, it is important that assistance be obtained immediately.

Early warning symptoms of hypoglycemia may be different or less pronounced under certain conditions, such as long duration of diabetes, diabetic nerve disease, medications such as beta-blockers, change in insulin preparations, or intensified control (3 or more insulin injections per day) of diabetes.

Without recognition of early warning symptoms, you may not be able to take steps to avoid more serious hypoglycemia. Be alert for all of the various types of symptoms that may indicate hypoglycemia. Patients who experience hypoglycemia without early warning symptoms should monitor their blood glucose frequently, especially prior to activities such as driving. If the blood glucose is below your normal fasting glucose, you should consider eating or drinking sugar-containing foods to treat your hypoglycemia.

Mild to moderate hypoglycemia may be treated by eating foods or drinks that contain sugar. Patients should always carry a quick source of sugar, such as candy mints or glucose tablets. More severe hypoglycemia may require the assistance of another person. Patients who are unable to take sugar orally or who are unconscious require an injection of glucagon or should be treated with intravenous administration of glucose at a medical facility.

You should learn to recognize your own symptoms of hypoglycemia. If you are uncertain about these symptoms, you should monitor your blood glucose frequently to help you learn to recognize the symptoms that you experience with hypoglycemia.

If you have frequent episodes of hypoglycemia or experience difficulty in recognizing the symptoms, you should consult your doctor to discuss possible changes in therapy, meal plans, and/or exercise programs to help you avoid hypoglycemia.

Hyperglycemia and Diabetic Acidosis

Hyperglycemia (too much glucose in the blood) may develop if your body has too little insulin. Hyperglycemia can be brought about by:
1. Omitting your insulin or taking less than the doctor has prescribed
2. Eating significantly more than your meal plan suggests
3. Developing a fever or infection

In patients with insulin-dependent diabetes, prolonged hyperglycemia can result in diabetic acidosis. The first symptoms of diabetic acidosis usually come on gradually, over a period of hours or days, and include a drowsy feeling, flushed face, thirst, loss of appetite, and fruity odor on the breath. With acidosis, urine tests show large amounts of glucose and acetone. Heavy breathing and a rapid pulse are more severe symptoms. If uncorrected, prolonged hyperglycemia or diabetic acidosis can result in loss of consciousness or death. Therefore, it is important that you obtain medical assistance immediately.

Lipodystrophy

Rarely, administration of insulin subcutaneously can result in lipoatrophy (depression in the skin) or lipohypertrophy (enlargement or thickening of tissue). If you notice either of these conditions, consult your doctor. A change in your injection technique may help alleviate the problem.

Allergy to Insulin

Local Allergy —Patients occasionally experience redness, swelling, and itching at the site of injection of insulin. This condition, called local allergy, usually clears up in a few days to a few weeks. In some instances, this condition may be related to factors other than insulin, such as irritants in the skin cleansing agent or poor injection technique. If you have local reactions, contact your doctor.

Systemic Allergy —Less common, but potentially serious, is generalized allergy to insulin, which may cause rash over the whole body, shortness of breath, wheezing, reduction in blood pressure, fast pulse, or sweating. Severe cases of generalized allergy may be life threatening. If you think you are having a generalized allergic reaction to insulin, notify a doctor immediately.

HOW SUPPLIED

Vials, U-100, 100 units/mL, 10 mL (No. CP-210P) (1's), NDC 0002-8211-01

[051192]

REGULAR (CONCENTRATED)   ℞
ILETIN® II, U-500
[rĕg-ū-lĕr ī'lĕ-tĭn]
(Insulin Injection, USP, purified pork)

WARNINGS
ANY CHANGE OF INSULIN SHOULD BE MADE CAUTIOUSLY AND ONLY UNDER MEDICAL SUPERVISION.

CHANGES IN PURITY, STRENGTH (U-100), BRAND (MANUFACTURER), TYPE (LENTE®, NPH, REGULAR, ETC.), AND/OR SPECIES SOURCE (BEEF, PORK, BEEF-PORK, OR HUMAN) MAY RESULT IN THE NEED FOR A CHANGE IN DOSAGE. SEE BELOW.

IT IS NOT POSSIBLE TO IDENTIFY WHICH PATIENTS WILL REQUIRE A REDUCTION IN DOSE TO AVOID HYPOGLYCEMIA WHEN USING THIS INSULIN. HOWEVER, IT IS KNOWN THAT A SMALL NUMBER OF PATIENTS MAY REQUIRE A SIGNIFICANT CHANGE.

ADJUSTMENT MAY BE NEEDED WITH THE FIRST DOSE OR OCCUR OVER A PERIOD OF SEVERAL WEEKS. BE AWARE OF THE POSSIBILITY OF SYMPTOMS OF EITHER HYPOGLYCEMIA OR HYPERGLYCEMIA.

This insulin is prepared from pork pancreas only. The dose of pork insulin for patients with insulin resistance due to antibodies to beef insulin may be only a fraction of that of beef insulin.

This insulin preparation contains 500 units of insulin in each milliliter. Extreme caution must be observed in the measurement of dosage because inadvertent overdose may result in irreversible insulin shock. Serious consequences may result if it is used other than under constant medical supervision.

DESCRIPTION

This Lilly pork insulin product differs from previous pork insulin preparations because it has undergone additional steps of chromatographic purification.

Regular (Concentrated) Iletin® II (insulin injection, USP, purified pork, Lilly), U-500, is an aqueous solution made from the antidiabetic principle of pork pancreas as stated on the label. Each milliliter contains 500 units of regular (unmodified) insulin and approximately 1.6% glycerin (w/v), with approximately 0.25% m-cresol (w/v) as a preservative. Sodium hydroxide and hydrochloric acid are added during manufacture to adjust the pH. All preparations of Iletin® II (insulin purified pork, Lilly) are made from zinc-insulin crystals.

CLINICAL PHARMACOLOGY

Adequate insulin dosage permits the diabetic patient to utilize carbohydrates and fats in a comparatively satisfactory manner. Regardless of concentration, the action of insulin is basically the same: to enable carbohydrate metabolism to occur and thus to prevent the production of ketone bodies by the liver. Although, under usual circumstances, diabetes can be controlled with doses in the vicinity of 40 to 60 units or less, an occasional patient develops such resistance or becomes so unresponsive to the effect of insulin that daily doses of several hundred, or even several thousand, units are required. Patients who require doses in excess of 300 to 500 units daily usually have impaired receptor function.

Occasionally, a cause of the insulin resistance can be found (such as hemochromatosis, cirrhosis of the liver, some complicating disease of the endocrine glands other than the pancreas, allergy, or infection), but in other cases, no cause of the high insulin requirement can be determined.

Iletin II, U-500, is unmodified by any agent that might prolong its action; however, clinical experience has shown that it frequently has a time action similar to a repository insulin preparation and that a single dose may show activity over a 24-hour period. This effect has been credited to the high concentration of the preparation.

INDICATIONS AND USAGE

Iletin® II (insulin injection, purified pork, Lilly), U-500, is especially useful for the treatment of diabetic patients with marked insulin resistance (daily requirements more than 200 units), since a large dose may be administered subcutaneously in a reasonable volume.

CONTRAINDICATIONS

Patients with a history of systemic allergic reactions to pork or mixed beef/pork insulin should not receive the insulin formulation unless they have been successfully desensitized.

PRECAUTIONS

General —Every patient exhibiting insulin resistance who requires Iletin® II (insulin injection, purified pork, Lilly), U-500, for control of diabetes should be under close observation until dosage is established. The response will vary among patients. Some can be controlled with a single dose daily; others may require 2 or 3 injections per day. Most patients will show a "tolerance" to insulin, so that minor variations in dosage can occur without the development of untoward symptoms of insulin shock.

Insulin resistance is frequently self-limited; after several weeks or months during which high dosage is required, responsiveness to the pharmacologic effect of insulin may be regained and dosage can be reduced.

Patients with immunologic insulin resistance to beef insulin (this diagnosis is usually confirmed by the finding of increased serum antibody titers) may require an immediate dosage reduction of 20 to 50% when treated with pork insulin.

Information for Patients —Patients should be instructed regarding their dosage and should be reminded that this

formulation requires the administration of a smaller volume of solution than is the case with less concentrated formulations.

Laboratory Tests —Blood and urine glucose, glycohemoglobin, and urine ketones should be monitored frequently.

Drug Interactions —The concurrent use of oral hypoglycemic agents with Iletin II, U-500, is not recommended since there are no data to support such use.

Pregnancy—Teratogenic Effects —No reproduction studies have been conducted in animals, and there are no adequate and well-controlled studies in pregnant women. It would be anticipated that the benefits of this insulin preparation would outweigh any risk to the developing fetus.

Nonteratogenic Effects —Insulin does not cross the placenta as does glucose.

Labor and Delivery —Careful monitoring of the patient is required, since the insulin requirement may decrease following delivery.

Nursing Mothers —It is not known whether insulin is excreted in significant amounts in human milk. Because many drugs are excreted in human milk, caution should be exercised when Iletin II, U-500, insulin injection is administered to a nursing woman.

Pediatric Use —There are no special precautions relating to the use of this insulin formulation in the pediatric age group.

ADVERSE REACTIONS

As with other insulin preparations, hypoglycemic reactions may be associated with the administration of Iletin® II (insulin injection, purified pork, Lilly), U-500. However, deep secondary hypoglycemic reactions may develop 18 to 24 hours after the original injection of Iletin II, U-500. Consequently, patients should be carefully observed, and prompt treatment of such reactions should be initiated with glucagon injections and/or with glucose by intravenous injection or gavage.

ALLERGIC REACTIONS

Erythema, swelling, or pruritus may occur at injection sites. Such localized allergic manifestations usually resolve within a few days to a few weeks.

Less common, but potentially more serious, is systemic allergy to insulin, manifested by generalized urticaria, dyspnea, and wheezing, which may progress to anaphylaxis. If a severe allergic reaction occurs, the drug should be discontinued and the patient treated with the usual agents (eg, epinephrine, antihistamines, or corticosteroids). Patients who have experienced severe systemic allergic reactions to insulin (eg, generalized urticaria, angioedema, anaphylaxis) should be skin-tested with each new preparation to be used before starting therapy with that preparation. Desensitization procedures may permit resumption of insulin administration.

DOSAGE AND ADMINISTRATION

Iletin® II (insulin injection, purified pork, Lilly), U-500, can be administered by both the subcutaneous and the intramuscular routes. It is inadvisable to inject Iletin II, U-500, intravenously because of the possible development of allergic or anaphylactoid reactions.

It is recommended that a tuberculin type of syringe be utilized for the measurement of dosage. Variations in dosage are frequently possible in the insulin-resistant patient, since the individual is unresponsive to the pharmacologic effect of the insulin. Nevertheless, accuracy of measurement is to be encouraged because of the potential danger of the preparation.

HOW SUPPLIED

Insulin should be kept in a cold place, preferably in a refrigerator, but must not be frozen.

Do not inject insulin that is not water-clear. Discoloration, turbidity, or unusual viscosity indicates deterioration or contamination.

Use of a package of insulin should not be started after the expiration date stamped on it.

(℞) Vials, U-500, 500 units/mL, 20 mL (No. CP-2500) (1's), NDC 0002-8500-01

[022192]

KEFUROX®   ℞
[kĕf'yū-rŏeks]
(sterile cefuroxime sodium)
USP

DESCRIPTION

Kefurox® (Sterile Cefuroxime Sodium, USP, Lilly) is a semisynthetic, broad-spectrum cephalosporin antibiotic for parenteral administration. Chemically, it is sodium (6R,7R)-7-[2-(2-furyl) glyoxylamido]-3-(hydroxymethyl)-8-oxo-5-thia-1-azabicyclo [4.2.0] oct-2-ene-2-carboxylate, 7^2-(Z)-(O-methyloxime), carbamate (ester). The chemical formula is $C_{16}H_{15}N_4NaO_8S$, and the molecular weight is 446.37. Kefurox contains approximately 54.2 mg (2.4 mEq) of sodium per gram of cefuroxime activity. Solutions of Kefurox range

from light yellow to amber, depending on the concentration and diluent used. The pH of freshly reconstituted solutions usually ranges from 6.0 to 8.5.

CLINICAL PHARMACOLOGY

After intramuscular injection of a 750-mg dose of cefuroxime to normal volunteers, the mean peak serum concentration was 27 μg/mL. The peak occurred at approximately 45 minutes (range 15–60 minutes). Following intravenous doses of 750 mg and 1.5 g, serum concentrations were approximately 50 μg/mL and 100 μg/mL respectively at 15 minutes. Therapeutic serum concentrations of approximately 2 μg/mL or more were maintained for 5.3 hours and 8 hours or more respectively. There was no evidence of accumulation of cefuroxime in the serum following intravenous administration of 1.5-g doses every 8 hours to normal volunteers. The serum half-life after either intramuscular or intravenous injections is approximately 80 minutes.

Approximately 89% of a dose of cefuroxime is excreted by the kidneys over an 8-hour period, resulting in high urinary concentrations.

Following the intramuscular administration of a 750-mg single dose, urinary concentrations averaged 1,300 μg/mL during the first 8 hours. Intravenous doses of 750 mg and 1.5 g produced urinary levels averaging 1,150 μg/mL and 2,500 μg/mL respectively during the first 8-hour period.

The concomitant oral administration of probenecid with cefuroxime slows tubular secretion, decreases renal clearance by approximately 40%, increases the peak serum level by approximately 30%, and increases the serum half-life by approximately 30%. Kefurox® (Sterile Cefuroxime Sodium, USP, Lilly) is detectable in therapeutic concentrations in pleural fluid, joint fluid, bile, sputum, bone, cerebrospinal fluid (in patients with meningitis), and aqueous humor.

Cefuroxime is approximately 50% bound to serum protein.

Microbiology—Cefuroxime has in vitro activity against a wide range of gram-positive and gram-negative organisms, and it is highly stable in the presence of β-lactamases of certain gram-negative bacteria. The bactericidal action of cefuroxime results from inhibition of cell-wall synthesis.

Cefuroxime is usually active against the following organisms in vitro.

Gram-Negative—*Haemophilus influenzae* (including ampicillin-resistant strains), *Haemophilus parainfluenzae, Neisseria gonorrhoeae* (including penicillinase- and non-penicillinase-producing strains), *Neisseria meningitidis, Escherichia coli, Klebsiella* sp. (including *Klebsiella pneumoniae*), *Enterobacter* sp., *Citrobacter* sp., *Salmonella* sp., *Shigella* sp., *Proteus mirabilis, Proteus inconstans* (formerly *Providencia inconstans*), *Providencia rettgeri* (formerly *Proteus rettgeri*), *Morganella morganii* (formerly *Proteus morganii*).

Some strains of *M. morganii, Enterobacter cloacae,* and *Citrobacter* sp. have been shown by in vitro tests to be resistant to cefuroxime and other cephalosporins.

Gram-Positive—*Staphyloccus aureus* (including penicillinase- and non-penicillinase-producing strains), *Staphylococcus epidermidis,* and certain strains of streptococci, eg, *Streptococcus pyogenes* and *Streptococcus pneumoniae.*

Certain strains of enterococci, eg, *Enterococcus faecalis* (formerly *Streptococcus faecalis*), are resistant.

Anaerobic Organisms—Gram-positive and gram-negative cocci (including *Peptococcus* and *Peptostreptococcus* sp.), gram-positive bacilli (including *Clostridium* sp.), gram-negative bacilli (including *Bacteroides* and *Fusobacterium* sp.). Most strains of *Bacteroides fragilis* are resistant.

Pseudomonas and *Campylobacter* sp., *Acinetobacter calcoaceticus* (formerly *Mima* and *Herellea* sp.), and most strains of *Serratia* sp. and *Proteus vulgaris* are resistant to cephalosporins. Methicillin-resistant staphylococci, *Clostridium difficile,* and *Listeria monocytogenes* are resistant to cefuroxime.

Susceptibility Tests—Diffusion Techniques—Quantitative methods that require measurement of zone diameters give the most precise estimates of antibiotic susceptibility. One such procedure[1] has been recommended for use with disks to test susceptibility to cefuroxime. Interpretation involves correlation of the diameters obtained in the disk test with minimum inhibitory concentration (MIC) values for cefuroxime.

Reports from the laboratory giving results of the standardized single-disk susceptibility test[1] using a 30- μg cefuroxime disk should be interpreted according to the following criteria:

Susceptible organisms produce zones of ≥ 18 mm, indicating that the tested organism is likely to respond to therapy.

Organisms that produce zones of 15 to 17 mm are expected to be susceptible if high dosage is used or if the infection is confined to tissues and fluids (eg, urine) in which high antibiotic levels are attained.

Resistant organisms produce zones of ≤ 14 mm, indicating that other therapy should be selected.

For gram-positive isolates, the test may be performed with either the cephalosporin-class disk (30 μg cephalothin) or the cefuroxime disk (30 μg cefuroxime) and a zone of ≥ 18 mm indicates a cefuroxime-susceptible organism.

Gram-negative organisms should be tested with the cefuroxime disk (using the above criteria) because cefuroxime has been shown by in vitro tests to have activity against certain strains of *Enterobacteriaceae* found to be resistant when tested with the cephalosporin-class disk. When using the cephalothin disk, gram-negative organisms with zone diameters < 18 mm do not necessarily indicate either intermediate susceptibility or resistance to cefuroxime.

The cefuroxime disk should not be used for testing susceptibility to other cephalosporins.

Standardized procedures require the use of laboratory control organisms. The 30-μg cefuroxime disk should give zone diameters from 27 to 35 mm for *S. aureus* ATCC 25923. For *E. coli* ATCC 25922, the zone diameters should range from 20 to 26 mm.

Dilution Techniques—A bacterial isolate may be considered susceptible if the MIC value for cefuroxime is ≤ 16 μg/mL. Organisms are considered resistant if the MIC is > 32 μg/mL.

As with standard diffusion methods, dilution procedures require the use of laboratory control organisms. Standard cefuroxime powder should give MIC values that range from 0.5 μg/mL to 2 μg/mL for *S. aureus* ATCC 25923. For *E. coli* ATCC 25922, MIC should range from 2 μg/mL to 8 μg/mL.

1. Bauer AW, Kirby WMM, Sherris JC, Turck M: Antibiotic susceptibility testing by a standardized single disk method. *Am J Clin Pathol* 1966; 45:493. Standardized disk susceptibility test. *Federal Register* 1974; 39:19182–19184. National Committee for Clinical Laboratory Standards, Approved Standard: M2-A3 Performance Standards for Antimicrobial Disk Susceptibility Tests,—Third Edition, December, 1984.

INDICATIONS AND USAGE

Kefurox® (Sterile Cefuroxime Sodium, USP, Lilly) is indicated for the treatment of infections caused by susceptible strains of the designated microorganisms in the diseases listed below:

Lower Respiratory Infections, including pneumonia caused by *S. pneumoniae, H. influenzae* (including ampicillin-resistant strains), *Klebsiella* sp., *S. aureus* (penicillinase- and non-penicillinase-producing), *S. pyogenes,* and *E. coli.*

Urinary Tract Infections caused by *E. coli* and *Klebsiella* sp.

Skin and Skin Structure Infections caused by *S. aureus* (penicillinase- and non-penicillinase-producing), *S. pyogenes, E. coli, Klebsiella* sp., and *Enterobacter* sp.

Septicemia caused by *S. aureus* (penicillinase-and non-penicillinase-producing), *S. pneumoniae, E. coli, H. influenzae* (including ampicillin-resistant strains), and *Klebsiella* sp.

Meningitis caused by *S. pneumoniae, H. influenzae* (including ampicillin-resistant strains), *N. meningitidis,* and *S. aureus* (penicillinase- and non-penicillinase-producing). (*See* Adverse Reactions regarding further information on the use of Kefurox in childhood meningitis.)

Gonorrhea—Uncomplicated and disseminated gonococcal infections due to *N. gonorrhoeae* (penicillinase- and non-penicillinase-producing strains) in both males and females.

Bone and Joint Infections—Caused by *S. aureus* (including penicillinase- and non-penicillinase-producing strains).

Clinical microbiologic studies in skin and skin structure infections frequently reveal the growth of susceptible strains of both aerobic and anaerobic organisms. Kefurox has been used successfully in these mixed infections in which several organisms have been isolated. Appropriate cultures and susceptibility studies should be performed to determine the susceptibility of the causative organisms to Kefurox.

Therapy may be started while awaiting the results of these studies; however, once these results become available, the antibiotic treatment should be adjusted accordingly. In certain cases of confirmed or suspected gram-positive or gram-negative sepsis or in patients with other serious infections in which the causative organism has not been identified, Kefurox may be used concomitantly with an aminoglycoside (*see* Precautions *and* Dosage and Administration). If warranted by the severity of the infection and the patient's condition, the recommended doses of both antibiotics may be given.

Prevention: The preoperative prophylactic administration of Kefurox® (Sterile Cefuroxime Sodium, USP, Lilly) may prevent the growth of susceptible disease-causing bacteria and, thereby, may reduce the incidence of certain postoperative infections in patients undergoing surgical procedures (eg, vaginal hysterectomy) that are classified as clean-contaminated or potentially contaminated procedures. Effective prophylactic use of antibiotics in surgery depends on the time of administration. Kefurox should usually be given ½ to 1 hour before the operation to allow sufficient time to achieve effective antibiotic concentrations in the wound tissues during the procedure. The dose should be repeated intraoperatively if the surgical procedure is lengthy. Prophylactic administration is usually not required after the surgical procedure ends and should be stopped within 24 hours. In the majority of surgical procedures, continuing prophylactic administration of any antibiotic does not reduce the incidence of subsequent infections but will increase the possibility of adverse reactions and the development of bacterial resistance. The perioperative use of Kefurox has also been effective during open heart surgery for surgical patients in whom infections at the operative site would present a serious risk. For these patients, it is recommended that therapy with Kefurox be continued for at least 48 hours after the surgical procedure ends. If an infection is present, specimens for culture should be obtained for the identification of the causative organism and appropriate antimicrobial therapy should be instituted.

CONTRAINDICATION

Kefurox® (Sterile Cefuroxime Sodium, USP, Lilly) is contraindicated in patients with known allergy to the cephalosporin group of antibiotics.

WARNINGS

BEFORE THERAPY WITH KEFUROX® (STERILE CEFUROXIME SODIUM, USP, LILLY) IS INSTITUTED, CAREFUL INQUIRY SHOULD BE MADE TO DETERMINE WHETHER THE PATIENT HAS HAD PREVIOUS HYPERSENSITIVITY REACTIONS TO CEPHALOSPORINS, PENICILLINS, OR OTHER DRUGS. THIS PRODUCT SHOULD BE GIVEN CAUTIOUSLY TO PENICILLIN-SENSITIVE PATIENTS. ANTIBIOTICS SHOULD BE ADMINISTERED WITH CAUTION TO ANY PATIENT WHO HAS DEMONSTRATED SOME FORM OF ALLERGY, PARTICULARLY TO DRUGS. IF AN ALLERGIC REACTION TO KEFUROX OCCURS, DISCONTINUE THE DRUG. SERIOUS ACUTE HYPERSENSITIVITY REACTIONS MAY REQUIRE EPINEPHRINE AND OTHER EMERGENCY MEASURES.

Pseudomembranous colitis has been reported with the use of cephalosporins (and other broad-spectrum antibiotics); therefore, it is important to consider its diagnosis in patients who develop diarrhea in association with antibiotic use.

Treatment with broad-spectrum antibiotics alters normal flora of the colon and may permit overgrowth of clostridia. Studies indicate a toxin produced by *C. difficile* is one primary cause of antibiotic-associated colitis. Cholestyramine and colestipol resins have been shown to bind the toxin in vitro.

Mild cases of colitis may respond to drug discontinuance alone. Moderate to severe cases should be managed with fluid, electrolyte, and protein supplementation as indicated.

When the colitis is not relieved by drug discontinuance or when it is severe, oral vancomycin is the treatment of choice for antibiotic-associated pseudomembranous colitis produced by *C. difficile.* Other causes of colitis should also be considered.

PRECAUTIONS

Although Kefurox® (Sterile Cefuroxime Sodium, USP, Lilly) rarely produces alterations in kidney function, evaluation of renal status during therapy is recommended, especially in seriously ill patients receiving the maximum doses. Cephalosporins should be given with caution to patients receiving concurrent treatment with potent diuretics as these regimens are suspected of adversely affecting renal function. The total daily dose of Kefurox should be reduced in patients with transient or persistent renal insufficiency (*see* Dosage and Administration) because high and prolonged serum antibiotic concentrations can occur in such individuals from usual doses.

As with other antibiotics, prolonged use of Kefurox may result in overgrowth of nonsusceptible organisms. Careful observation of the patient is essential. If superinfection does occur during therapy, appropriate measures should be taken.

Broad-spectrum antibiotics should be prescribed with caution in individuals with a history of gastrointestinal disease, particularly colitis.

Nephrotoxicity has been reported following concomitant administration of aminoglycoside antibiotics and cephalosporins.

Interference with Laboratory Tests—A false-positive reaction for glucose in the urine may occur with copper reduction tests (Benedict's or Fehling's solution or with Clinitest® tablets), but not with enzyme-based tests for glycosuria (eg, Tes-Tape®). A false-negative reaction may occur in the ferricyanide test for blood glucose.

Cefuroxime does not interfere with the assay of serum and urine creatinine by the the alkaline picrate method.

Carcinogenesis, Mutagenesis, and Impairment of Fertility—Although no long-term studies in animals have been performed to evaluate carcinogenic potential, no mutagenic potential of cefuroxime was found in standard laboratory tests.

Reproductive studies revealed no impairment of fertility in animals.

Continued on next page

*** Identi-Code® symbol. This product information was prepared in June 1992. Current information on these and other products of Eli Lilly and Company may be obtained by direct inquiry to Lilly Research Laboratories, Lilly Corporate Center, Indianapolis, Indiana 46285, (317) 276-3714.**

Lilly—Cont.

*Usage in Pregnancy—Pregnancy Category B —*Reproduction studies have been performed in mice and rabbits at doses up to 60 times the human dose and have revealed no evidence of impaired fertility or harm to the fetus due to cefuroxime. There are, however, no adequate, well-controlled studies in pregnant women. Because animal reproduction studies are not always predictive of human response, this drug should be used during pregnancy only if clearly needed.

*Nursing Mothers —*Since Kefurox is excreted in human milk, caution should be exercised when Kefurox is administered to a nursing woman.

*Pediatric Use —*Safety and effectiveness in children below the age of 3 months have not been established. Accumulation of other members of the cephalosporin class in newborn infants (with resulting prolongation of drug half-life) has been reported.

ADVERSE REACTIONS

Kefurox® (Sterile Cefuroxime Sodium, USP, Lilly) is generally well tolerated. The most common adverse effects have been local reactions following intravenous administration. Other adverse reactions have been encountered only rarely.

*Local Reactions —*Thrombophlebitis has occurred with intravenous administration in 1 in 60 patients.

*Gastrointestinal —*Gastrointestinal symptoms occurred in 1 in 150 patients and included diarrhea (1 in 220 patients) and nausea (1 in 440 patients). Symptoms of pseudomembranous colitis can appear during or after antibiotic treatment. Vomiting has been reported.

*Hypersensitivity Reactions —*Hypersensitivity reactions have been reported in less than 1% of the patients treated with Kefurox and include rash (1 in 125). Pruritus and urticaria and positive Coombs' test each occurred in less than 1 in 250 patients, and, as with other cephalosporins, cases of anaphylaxis have occurred rarely. Erythema multiforme and Stevens-Johnson syndrome have occurred.

*Blood —*A decrease in hemoglobin and hematocrit has been observed in 1 in 10 patients and transient eosinophilia in 1 in 14 patients. Less common reactions seen were transient neutropenia (less than 1 in 100 patients) and leukopenia (1 in 750 patients). A similar pattern and incidence were seen with other cephalosporins used in controlled studies. Hemolysis, aplastic anemia, agranulocytosis, pancytopenia, prolonged prothrombin time, and thrombocytopenia have been reported.

*Hepatic —*Transient rise in SGOT and SGPT (1 in 25 patients), alkaline phosphatase (1 in 50 patients), LDH (1 in 75 patients), and bilirubin (1 in 500 patients) levels has been noted.

*Kidney —*Elevations in serum creatinine and/or blood urea nitrogen and a decreased creatinine clearance have been observed, but their relationship to cefuroxime is unknown.

*Other —*Delayed sterilization of cerebrospinal fluid has been reported in occasional children treated with cefuroxime for bacterial meningitis. Moderate to severe hearing impairment has occurred as a complication of meningitis in occasional children treated with cefuroxime for bacterial meningitis. Fever has been reported.

OVERDOSAGE

*Signs and Symptoms —*Experience with overdose of cefuroxime sodium in humans is limited. The administration of inappropriately large doses of parenteral cephalosporins may cause seizures, particularly in patients with renal failure in whom accumulation is likely to occur.

The oral median lethal dose in the adult mouse was > 10 g/kg, representing 83 times the routine maximum adult dose. In animals, doses up to 5 g/kg produced no tissue toxicity. With chronic doses greater than 5 g/kg, tubular necrosis was seen in animals.

*Treatment —*To obtain up-to-date information about the treatment of overdose, a good resource is your certified Regional Poison Control Center. Telephone numbers of certified poison control centers are listed in the *Physicians' Desk Reference (PDR).* In managing overdosage, consider the possibility of multiple drug overdoses, interaction among drugs, and unusual drug kinetics in your patient.

Protect the patient's airway and support ventilation and perfusion. Meticulously monitor and maintain, within acceptable limits, the patient's vital signs, blood gases, serum electrolytes, etc. If the patient develops convulsions, the drug should be promptly discontinued; anticonvulsant therapy may be administered if clinically indicated. The use of hemodialysis in the treatment of cefuroxime overdose has not been established.

DOSAGE AND ADMINISTRATION

*Adults —*The usual adult dosage range for Kefurox® (Sterile Cefuroxime Sodium, USP, Lilly) is 750 mg to 1.5 g every 8 hours, usually for 5 to 10 days. In uncomplicated urinary tract infections, skin and skin structure infections, disseminated gonococcal infections, and uncomplicated pneumonia, a 750-mg dose every 8 hours is recommended. In severe or complicated infections, a 1.5-g dose every 8 hours is recommended.

In bone and joint infections, a dosage of 1.5 g every 8 hours is recommended. In clinical trials, surgical intervention was performed, when indicated, as an adjunct to therapy with Kefurox. A course of oral antibiotic therapy was administered when appropriate following the completion of parenteral administration of Kefurox.

In life-threatening infections or infections due to less susceptible organisms, 1.5 g every 6 hours may be required. In bacterial meningitis, the dose should not exceed 3.0 g every 8 hours. The recommended dose for uncomplicated gonococcal infection is 1.5 g intramuscularly given as a single dose at two different sites together with 1.0 g of oral probenecid. For preventive use for clean-contaminated or potentially contaminated surgical procedures, a 1.5-g dose administered intravenously just prior to surgery (approximately ½ to 1 hour before the initial incision) is recommended. Thereafter, give 750 mg intravenously or intramuscularly every 8 hours when the procedure is prolonged.

For preventive use during open heart surgery, a 1.5-g dose administered intravenously at the induction of anesthesia and every 12 hours thereafter for a total of 6.0 g is recommended.

*Impaired Renal Function —*When renal function is impaired, a reduced dosage must be employed. Dosage should be determined by the degree of renal impairment and the susceptibility of the causative organism (see Table 1).

TABLE 1: Dosage of Kefurox® (Sterile Cefuroxime Sodium, USP) in Adults With Reduced Renal Function

Creatinine Clearance (mL/min)	Dose	Frequency
> 20	750 mg–1.5 g	Every 8 hours
10–20	750 mg	Every 12 hours
< 10	750 mg	Every 24 hours*

*Since Kefurox is dialyzable, patients on hemodialysis should be given a further dose at the end of the dialysis.

When only serum creatinine is available, the following formula (based on sex, weight, and age of the patient) may be used to convert this value into creatinine clearance. The serum creatinine should represent a steady state of renal function.

Males: $\dfrac{\text{Weight (kg)} \times (140 - \text{age})}{72 \times \text{serum creatinine (mg/100 mL)}}$

Females: 0.9 ×above value

Note: As with antibiotic therapy in general, administration of Kefurox should be continued for a minimum of 48 to 72 hours after the patient becomes asymptomatic or after evidence of bacterial eradication has been obtained; a minimum of 10 days of treatment is recommended in infections caused by *S. pyogenes* in order to guard against the risk of rheumatic fever or glomerulonephritis; frequent bacteriologic and clinical appraisal is necessary during therapy of chronic urinary tract infection and may be required for several months after therapy has been completed; persistent infections may require treatment for several weeks; and doses smaller than those indicated above should not be used. In staphylococcal and other infections involving a collection of pus, surgical drainage should be carried out when indicated.

*Infants and Children Above 3 Months of Age —*Administration of 50 to 100 mg/kg/day in equally divided doses, every 6 to 8 hours, has been successful for most infections susceptible to cefuroxime. The higher dose of 100 mg/kg/day (not to exceed the maximum adult dose) should be used for the more severe or serious infections.

In cases of bacterial meningitis, larger doses of Kefurox are recommended, initially 200 to 240 mg/kg/day intravenously in divided doses every 6 to 8 hours.

In children with renal insufficiency, the frequency of dosage should be modified consistent with the recommendations for adults.

*Preparation of Solution and Suspension —*The directions for preparing Kefurox for both intravenous and intramuscular use are summarized in Table 2.

*For Intramuscular Use —*Each 750-mg/10 mL vial of Kefurox should be reconstituted with 3.6 mL of Sterile Water for Injection. Shake gently to disperse and withdraw 3.6 mL of the resulting suspension for injection.

*For Intravenous Use —*Each 750-mg/10 mL vial should be reconstituted with 9.0 mL of Sterile Water for Injection. Withdraw 8.0 mL of the resulting solution for injection. Each 1.5-g/20 mL vial should be reconstituted with 14.0 mL of Sterile Water for Injection and the solution completely withdrawn for injection.

For infusion, each 750-mg or 1.5-g dose should be reconstituted with 50 to 100 mL of Sterile Water for Injection, 5% Dextrose Injection, 0.9% Sodium Chloride Injection, or any of the solutions listed under the Intravenous portion of the Compatibility and Stability section. If Sterile Water for Injection is used as the diluent, reconstitute with approximately 20 mL/g to avoid a hypotonic solution. [See table below.]

*Administration —*After reconstitution, Kefurox® (Sterile Cefuroxime Sodium, USP, Lilly) may be given intravenously or by deep intramuscular injection into a large muscle mass (such as the gluteus or lateral part of the thigh). Prior to injecting intramuscularly, aspiration is necessary to avoid inadvertent injection into a blood vessel.

*Intravenous Administration —*The intravenous route may be preferable for patients with bacterial septicemia or other severe or life-threatening infections or for patients who may be poor risks because of decreased resistance, particularly if shock is present or impending.

*For Direct Intermittent Intravenous Administration —*Slowly inject the solution into a vein over a period of 3 to 5 minutes or give it through the tubing system by which the patient is also receiving other intravenous solutions.

*For Intermittent Intravenous Infusion with a Y-Type Administration Set —*Dosing can be accomplished through the tubing system by which the patient may be receiving other intravenous solutions. However, during infusion of the solution containing Kefurox, it is advisable to temporarily discontinue administration of any other solutions at the same site.

*For Continuous Intravenous Infusion —*A solution of Kefurox may be added to an intravenous bottle containing 1 of the following fluids:

0.9% Sodium Chloride Injection, 5% Dextrose Injection, 10% Dextrose Injection, 5% Dextrose and 0.9% Sodium Chloride Injection, 5% Dextrose and 0.45% Sodium Chloride Injection, and M/6 Sodium Lactate Injection

Solutions of Kefurox, like those of most β-lactam antibiotics, should not be added to solutions of aminglycoside antibiotics because of potential interaction. However, if concurrent therapy with Kefurox and an aminoglycoside is indicated, each of these antibiotics can be administered separately to the same patient.

*Compatibility and Stability —*Intramuscular—When reconstituted as directed with Sterile Water for Injection, suspensions of Kefurox® (Sterile Cefuroxime Sodium, USP, Lilly)

TABLE 2
Preparation of Solution and Suspension
(Glass Vials, ADD-Vantage®, and Faspak)

Strength	Amount of Diluent to Be Added (mL)		Volume to Be Withdrawn (mL)	Approximate Concentration (mg/mL)
750 mg/10 mL vial	3.6	(IM)	3.6*	220
750 mg/10 mL vial	9	(IV)	8	100
1.5 g/20 mL vial	14	(IV)	Total	100
750 mg/100 mL bottle	50	(IV)	—	15
750 mg/100 mL bottle	100	(IV)	—	7.5
1.5 g/100 mL bottle	50	(IV)	—	30
1.5 g/100 mL bottle	100	(IV)	—	15
750 mg/Faspak	50	(IV)	—	15
750 mg/Faspak	100	(IV)	—	7.5
1.5 g/Faspak	50	(IV)	—	30
1.5 g/Faspak	100	(IV)	—	15
750 mg/ADD-Vantage†	50	(IV)	—	15
750 mg/ADD-Vantage†	100	(IV)	—	7.5
1.5 g/ADD-Vantage†	50	(IV)	—	30
1.5 g/ADD-Vantage†	100	(IV)	—	15

* KEFUROX® (Sterile Cefuroxime Sodium, USP, Lilly) is a suspension at IM concentrations.
† Instructions for use of the ADD-Vantage Vials are enclosed in the package.

for intramuscular injection maintain satisfactory potency for 24 hours at room temperature and for 48 hours under refrigeration (5°C).
After the periods mentioned above, any unused suspensions should be discarded.
Intravenous—When the 750-mg and 1.5-g vials are reconstituted as directed with Sterile Water for Injection, the solutions of Kefurox for intravenous administration maintain satisfactory potency for 24 hours at room temperature and for 48 hours under refrigeration (5°C). More dilute solutions, such as 750 mg or 1.5 g reconstituted with 50 to 100 mL of Sterile Water for Injection, 5% Dextrose Injection, or 0.9% Sodium Chloride Injection, maintain satisfactory potency for 24 hours at room temperature and for 7 days under refrigeration.
These solutions may be further diluted to concentrations of between 1 mg/mL and 30 mg/mL in the following solutions and will lose not more than 10% activity for 24 hours at room temperature or for at least 7 days under refrigeration: 0.9% Sodium Chloride Injection, M/6 Sodium Lactate Injection, Ringer's Injection USP, Lactated Ringer's Injection USP, 5% Dextrose and 0.9% Sodium Chloride Injection, 5% Dextrose Injection, 5% Dextrose and 0.45% Sodium Chloride Injection, 5% Dextrose and 0.225% Sodium Chloride Injection, 10% Dextrose Injection, or 10% Invert Sugar in Water for Injection.
Unused solutions should be discarded after the time periods mentioned above.
Kefurox has also been found compatible for 24 hours at room temperature when admixed in intravenous infusion with the following: Heparin (10 and 50 units/mL) in 0.9% Sodium Chloride Injection, or Potassium Chloride (10 and 40 mEq/L) in 0.9% Sodium Chloride Injection.
Note: Prior to administration, parenteral drug products should be inspected visually for particulate matter and discoloration whenever solution and container permit.
As with other cephalosporins, however, cefuroxime powder as well as solutions and suspensions tend to darken depending on storage conditions without adversely affecting product potency.
Protect from light. Prior to reconstitution, store at controlled room temperature, 59° to 86°F (15° to 30°C).

HOW SUPPLIED

(℞) Vials:
750 mg,* 10-mL size (No. 7271)—(Traypak† of 25) NDC 0002-7271-25
1.5 g,* 20-mL size (No. 7272)—(Traypak of 10) NDC 0002-7272-10
750 mg,* 100-mL size (No. 7273)—(Traypak of 10) NDC 0002-7273-10
1.5 g,* 100-mL size (No. 7274)—(Traypak of 10) NDC 0002-7274-10
(℞) Faspak‡:
750 mg (No. 7276)—(24s) NDC 0002-7276-24
1.5 g (No. 7277)—(24s) NDC 0002-7277-24
(℞) ADD-Vantage§ Vials:
750 mg,* (No. 7278)—(Tray pak of 25) NDC 0002-7278-25
1.5 g,* (No. 7279)—(Traypak of 10) NDC 0002-7279-10
The above ADD-Vantage Vials are to be used with Abbott Laboratories' ADD-Vantage Antibiotic Diluent Container. Instructions for use of the ADD-Vantage Vials are enclosed in the package.
Also available:
(℞) Pharmacy Bulk Package;
7.5 g,* 100-mL size (No. 7275)—(Traypak of 6) NDC 0002-7275-16

* Equivalent to cefuroxime.
† Traypak™ (multivial carton, Lilly)
‡ Faspak® (flexible plastic bag, Lilly)
§ ADD-Vantage® (vials and diluent containers, Abbott).
[030591]

KEFZOL® ℞
[kĕf'zōl]
(cefazolin sodium)
Sterile, USP

DESCRIPTION

Kefzol® (cefazolin sodium, Lilly) is a sterile, semisynthetic cephalosporin for intramuscular or intravenous administration. It is 5-Thia-1-azabicyclo[4.2.0]oct-2-ene-2-carboxylic acid, 3-[[(5-methyl-1,3,4-thiadiazol-2-yl)thio]methyl]-8-oxo-7-[[(1*H*-tetrazol-1-yl) acetyl]amino]-, monosodium salt (6*R*-*trans*). The sodium content is 48.3 mg/g of cefazolin sodium. In addition to cefazolin sodium, the Faspak® and the ADD-Vantage® System vial also contain 0.04% polysorbate 80. The molecular formula is $C_{14}H_{13}N_8NaO_4S_3$. The molecular weight is 476.5.
The pH of the reconstituted solution is between 4.5 and 6.

CLINICAL PHARMACOLOGY

Human Pharmacology—Table 1 demonstrates the blood levels and duration of cefazolin following intramuscular administration.

TABLE 1. SERUM CONCENTRATIONS AFTER INTRAMUSCULAR ADMINISTRATION

	Serum Concentrations (μg/mL)					
Dose	½ h	1 h	2 h	4 h	6 h	8 h
250 mg	15.5	17	13	5.1	2.5	
500 mg	36.2	36.8	37.9	15.5	6.3	3
1 g*	60.1	63.8	54.3	29.3	13.2	7.1

*Average of 2 studies

Clinical pharmacology studies in patients hospitalized with infections indicate that cefazolin produces mean peak serum levels approximately equivalent to those seen in normal volunteers.
In a study (using normal volunteers) of constant intravenous infusion with dosages of 3.5 mg/kg for 1 hour (approximately 250 mg) and 1.5 mg/kg the next 2 hours (approximately 100 mg), cefazolin produced a steady serum level at the 3rd hour of approximately 28 μg/mL. Table 2 shows the average serum concentrations after IV injection of a single 1-g dose; average half-life was 1.4 hours.

TABLE 2. SERUM CONCENTRATIONS AFTER 1-G INTRAVENOUS DOSE

Serum Concentrations (μg/mL)					
5 min	15 min	30 min	1 h	2 h	4 h
188.4	135.8	106.8	73.7	45.6	16.5

Controlled studies on adult normal volunteers receiving 1 g 4 times a day for 10 days, monitoring CBC, AST (SGOT), ALT (SGPT), bilirubin, alkaline phosphatase, BUN, creatinine, and urinalysis, indicated no clinically significant changes attributed to cefazolin.
Cefazolin is excreted unchanged in the urine, primarily by glomerular filtration and, to a lesser degree, by tubular secretion. Following intramuscular injection of 500 mg, 56% to 89% of the administered dose is recovered within 6 hours and 80% to nearly 100% in 24 hours. Cefazolin achieves peak urine concentrations greater than 1,000 μg/mL and 4,000 μg/mL respectively following 500-mg and 1-g intramuscular doses.
In patients undergoing peritoneal dialysis (2 L/h), mean serum levels of cefazolin were approximately 10 and 30 μg/mL after 24 hours' instillation of a dialyzing solution containing 50 μg/mL and 150 μg/mL respectively. Mean peak levels were 29 μg/mL (range 13-44 μg/mL) with 50 μg/mL (3 patients) and 72 μg/mL (range 26-142 μg/mL) with 150 μg/mL (6 patients). Intraperitoneal administration of cefazolin is usually well tolerated.
When cefazolin is administered to patients with unobstructed biliary tracts, high concentrations well over serum levels occur in the gallbladder tissue and bile. In the presence of obstruction, however, concentration of the antibiotic is considerably lower in bile than in serum.
Cefazolin readily crosses an inflamed synovial membrane, and the concentration of the antibiotic achieved in the joint space is comparable to levels measured in the serum.
Cefazolin readily crosses the placental barrier into the cord blood and amniotic fluid. It is present in very low concentrations in the milk of nursing mothers.
Microbiology—In vitro tests demonstrate that the bactericidal action of cephalosporins results from inhibition of cell-wall synthesis. Kefzol® (cefazolin sodium, Lilly) is active against the following organisms in vitro and in clinical infections.

Staphylococcus aureus (including penicillinase-producing strains)
Staphylococcus epidermidis
Methicillin-resistant staphylococci are uniformly resistant to cefazolin.
Group A β-hemolytic streptococci and other strains of streptococci (many strains of enterococci are resistant)
Streptococcus pneumoniae
Escherichia coli
Proteus mirabilis
Klebsiella sp.
Enterobacter aerogenes
Haemophilus influenzae

Most strains of indole-positive *Proteus* (*Proteus vulgaris*), *Enterobacter cloacae, Morganella morganii,* and *Providencia rettgeri* are resistant. *Serratia, Pseudomonas,* and *Acinetobacter calcoaceticus* (formerly *Mima* and *Herellea* sp.) are almost uniformly resistant to cefazolin.
Disk Susceptibility Tests—Quantitative methods that require measurement of zone diameters give the most precise estimates of antibiotic susceptibility. One such procedure* has been recommended for use with disks for testing susceptibility to cefazolin. With this procedure, a report from the laboratory of "susceptible" indicates that the infecting organism is likely to respond to therapy. A report of "resistant" indicates that the infecting organism is not likely to respond to therapy. A report of "moderately susceptible" suggests that the organism would be susceptible if high dosage is used or if the infection were confined to tissues and fluids (eg, urine) in which high antibiotic levels are attained.
For gram-positive isolates, a zone of 18 mm is indicative of a cefazolin-susceptible organism when tested with either the cephalosporin-class disk (30 μg cephalothin) or the cefazolin disk (30 μg cefazolin).
Gram-negative organisms should be tested with the cefazolin disk (using the above criteria) because cefazolin has been shown by in vitro tests to have activity against certain strains of *Enterobacteriaceae* found to be resistant when tested with the cephalothin disk. When using the cephalothin disk, gram-negative organisms with zone diameters ≥ 18 mm may be considered susceptible to cefazolin; however, organisms with zone diameters less than 18 mm are not necessarily resistant or moderately susceptible to cefazolin.
The cefazolin disk should not be used for testing susceptibility to other cephalosporins.
Dilution Techniques—A bacterial isolate may be considered susceptible if the minimal inhibitory concentration (MIC) for cefazolin is ≤ 16 μg/mL. Organisms are considered resistant if the MIC is ≥ 64 μg/mL.

INDICATIONS AND USAGE

Kefzol® (cefazolin sodium, Lilly) is indicated in the treatment of the following serious infections due to susceptible organisms:
Respiratory tract infections due to *S. pneumoniae, Klebsiella* sp., *H. influenzae, S. aureus* (including penicillinase-producing strains), and group A β-hemolytic streptococci
Injectable penicillin G benzathine is considered to be the drug of choice in the treatment and prevention of streptococcal infections, including the prophylaxis of rheumatic fever. Kefzol is effective in the eradication of streptococci from the nasopharynx; however, data establishing the efficacy of Kefzol in the subsequent prevention of rheumatic fever are not available at present.
Genitourinary tract infections due to *E. coli, P. mirabilis, Klebsiella* sp., and some strains of *Enterobacter* and enterococci
Skin and skin structure infections due to *S. aureus* (including penicillinase-producing strains) and group A β-hemolytic streptococci and other strains of streptococci
Biliary tract infections due to *E. coli*, various strains of streptococci, *P. mirabilis, Klebsiella* sp., and *S. aureus*
Bone and joint infections due to *S. aureus*
Septicemia due to *S. pneumoniae, S. aureus* (penicillin-susceptible and penicillin-resistant), *P. mirabilis, E. coli,* and *Klebsiella* sp.
Endocarditis due to *S. aureus* (penicillin-susceptible and penicillin-resistant) and group A β-hemolytic streptococci
Appropriate culture and susceptibility studies should be performed to determine susceptibility of the causative organism to Kefzol.
Perioperative prophylaxis—The prophylactic administration of Kefzol preoperatively, intraoperatively, and postoperatively may reduce the incidence of certain postoperative infections in patients undergoing surgical procedures that are classified as contaminated or potentially contaminated (eg, vaginal hysterectomy or cholecystectomy in high-risk patients such as those over 70 years of age who have acute cholecystitis, obstructive jaundice, or common-bile-duct stones).
The perioperative use of Kefzol also may be effective in surgical patients in whom infection at the operative site would present a serious risk (eg, during open-heart surgery and prosthetic arthroplasty).
The prophylactic administration of Kefzol should usually be discontinued within a 24-hour period after the surgical procedure. For surgery in which the occurrence of infection may be particularly devastating (eg, open-heart surgery and prosthetic arthroplasty), the prophylactic administration of Kefzol may be continued for 3 to 5 days following the completion of surgery. If there are signs of infection, specimens for cul-

*National Committee for Clinical Laboratory Standards (NCCLS), 1984. Performance Standards for Antimicrobial Disk Susceptibility Tests, Approved Standard, M2-A3, NCCLS, Villanova, PA 19085.

Continued on next page

*** Identi-Code® symbol. This product information was prepared in June 1992. Current information on these and other products of Eli Lilly and Company may be obtained by direct inquiry to Lilly Research Laboratories, Lilly Corporate Center, Indianapolis, Indiana 46285, (317) 276-3714.**

Lilly—Cont.

ture should be obtained for the identification of the causative organism so that appropriate therapy may be instituted. (*See* DOSAGE AND ADMINISTRATION.)

CONTRAINDICATION

Kefzol® (cefazolin sodium, Lilly) is contraindicated in patients with known allergy to the cephalosporin group of antibiotics.

WARNINGS

BEFORE CEFAZOLIN THERAPY IS INSTITUTED, CAREFUL INQUIRY SHOULD BE MADE CONCERNING PREVIOUS HYPERSENSITIVITY REACTIONS TO CEPHALOSPORINS AND PENICILLIN. CEPHALOSPORIN C DERIVATIVES SHOULD BE GIVEN CAUTIOUSLY TO PENICILLIN-SENSITIVE PATIENTS.

SERIOUS ACUTE HYPERSENSITIVITY REACTIONS MAY REQUIRE EPINEPHRINE AND OTHER EMERGENCY MEASURES.

There is some clinical and laboratory evidence of partial cross-allergenicity of the penicillins and the cephalosporins. Patients have been reported to have had severe reactions (including anaphylaxis) to both drugs.

Antibiotics, including Kefzol® (cefazolin sodium, Lilly), should be administered cautiously to any patient who has demonstrated some form of allergy, particularly to drugs.

Pseudomembranous colitis has been reported with virtually all broad-spectrum antibiotics (including macrolides, semisynthetic penicillins, and cephalosporins); therefore, it is important to consider its diagnosis in patients who develop diarrhea in association with the use of antibiotics. Such colitis may range in severity from mild to life threatening.

Treatment with broad-spectrum antibiotics alters the normal flora of the colon and may permit overgrowth of clostridia. Studies indicate that a toxin produced by *Clostridium difficile* is a primary cause of antibiotic-associated colitis. Cholestyramine and colestipol resins have been shown to bind the toxin in vitro.

Mild cases of pseudomembranous colitis usually respond to drug discontinuance alone. In moderate to severe cases, management should include sigmoidoscopy, appropriate bacteriologic studies, and fluid, electrolyte, and protein supplementation. When the colitis does not improve after the drug has been discontinued, or when it is severe, oral vancomycin is the drug of choice for antibiotic-associated pseudomembranous colitis produced by *C. difficile.* Other causes of colitis should be considered.

Usage in Infants—Safety for use in prematures and infants under 1 month of age has not been established.

PRECAUTIONS

General—If an allergic reaction to Kefzol® (cefazolin sodium, Lilly) occurs, the drug should be discontinued and the patient treated with the usual agents (eg, epinephrine or other pressor amines, antihistamines, or corticosteroids).

Prolonged use of Kefzol may result in the overgrowth of nonsusceptible organisms. Careful clinical observation of the patient is essential. If superinfection occurs during therapy, appropriate measures should be taken.

When Kefzol is administered to patients with low urinary output because of impaired renal function, lower daily dosage is required (*see* Dosage and Administration).

Drug Interactions—Used concurrently, probenecid may decrease renal tubular secretion of cephalosporins, resulting in increased and more prolonged cephalosporin blood levels.

Drug/Laboratory Test Interactions—A false-positive reaction for glucose in the urine may occur with Benedict's solution, Fehling's solution, or Clinitest® tablets but not with enzyme-based tests, such as Clinistix® and Tes-Tape® (Glucose Enzymatic Test Strip, USP, Lilly).

Positive direct and indirect antiglobulin (Coombs') tests have occurred; these may also occur in neonates whose mothers received cephalosporins before delivery.

Broad-spectrum antibiotics should be prescribed with caution in individuals with a history of gastrointestinal disease, particularly colitis.

Carcinogenesis, Mutagenesis, Impairment of Fertility—Mutagenicity studies and long-term studies in animals to determine the carcinogenic potential of cefazolin have not been performed. Studies performed in rats have revealed no evidence of impaired fertility.

Pregnancy: Teratogenic Effects: Pregnancy Category B—Reproduction studies have been performed in rats given doses of 500 mg or 1 g of cefazolin/kg and have revealed no harm to the fetus due to Kefzol. There are, however, no adequate and well-controlled studies in pregnant women. Because animal reproduction studies are not always predictive of human response, this drug should be used during pregnancy only if clearly needed.

Labor and Delivery—When cefazolin has been administered prior to cesarean section, drug levels in cord blood have been approximately one fourth to one third of maternal drug levels. The drug appears to have no adverse effect on the fetus.

Nursing Mothers—Cefazolin is present in very low concentrations in the milk of nursing mothers. Caution should be exercised when cefazolin is administered to a nursing woman.

ADVERSE REACTIONS

The following reactions have been reported:

Hypersensitivity—Drug fever, skin rash, vulvar pruritus, eosinophilia, and anaphylaxis have occurred.

Blood—Neutropenia, leukopenia, thrombocythemia, and positive direct and indirect Coombs' tests have occurred.

Renal—Transient rise in BUN levels has been observed without clinical evidence of renal impairment. Interstitial nephritis and other renal disorders have been reported rarely. Most patients experiencing these reactions have been seriously ill and were receiving multiple drug therapies. The role of Kefzol® (cefazolin sodium, Lilly) in the development of nephropathies has not been determined.

Hepatic—Transient rise in AST, ALT, and alkaline phosphatase levels has been observed rarely. As with some penicillins and some other cephalosporins, transient hepatitis and cholestatic jaundice have been reported rarely.

Gastrointestinal—Symptoms of pseudomembranous colitis may appear either during or after antibiotic treatment. Nausea and vomiting have been reported rarely. Anorexia, diarrhea, and oral candidiasis (oral thrush) have been reported.

Other—Pain on intramuscular injection, sometimes with induration, has occurred infrequently. Phlebitis at the site of injection has been noted. Other reactions have included genital and anal pruritus, genital moniliasis, and vaginitis.

OVERDOSAGE

Signs and Symptoms—Toxic signs and symptoms following an overdose of cefazolin may include pain, inflammation, and phlebitis at the injection site.

The administration of inappropriately large doses of parenteral cephalosporins may cause dizziness, paresthesias, and headaches. Seizures may occur following overdosage with some cephalosporins, particularly in patients with renal impairment in whom accumulation is likely to occur.

Laboratory abnormalities that may occur after an overdose include elevations in creatinine, BUN, liver enzymes and bilirubin, a positive Coombs' test, thrombocytosis, thrombocytopenia, eosinophilia, leukopenia, and prolongation of the prothrombin time.

Treatment—To obtain up-to-date information about the treatment of overdose, a good resource is your certified Regional Poison Control Center. Telephone numbers of certified poison control centers are listed in the *Physicians' Desk Reference (PDR).* In managing overdosage, consider the possibility of multiple drug overdoses, interaction among drugs, and unusual drug kinetics in your patient.

If seizures occur, the drug should be discontinued promptly; anticonvulsant therapy may be administered if clinically indicated. Protect the patient's airway and support ventilation and perfusion. Meticulously monitor and maintain, within acceptable limits, the patient's vital signs, blood gases, serum electrolytes, etc.

In cases of severe overdosage, especially in a patient with renal failure, combined hemodialysis and hemoperfusion may be considered if response to more conservative therapy fails. However, no data supporting such therapy are available.

DOSAGE AND ADMINISTRATION

Kefzol® (cefazolin sodium, Lilly) may be administered intramuscularly or intravenously after reconstitution. Total daily dosages are the same for either route of administration.

Intramuscular Administration—Reconstitute 1-g vial as directed by Table 3 with Sterile Water for Injection. Shake well until dissolved. Kefzol should be injected into a large muscle mass. Pain on injection is infrequent with Kefzol. (NOTE: ADD-VANTAGE VIALS ARE NOT TO BE USED IN THIS MANNER.)

[See table below.]

Intravenous Administration—Kefzol® (cefazolin sodium, Lilly) may be administered by intravenous injection or by continuous or intermittent infusion.

TABLE 3. DILUTION TABLE FOR KEFZOL® (CEFAZOLIN SODIUM, LILLY)

Vial Size	Diluent to Be Added	Approximate Available Volume	Approximate Average Concentration
1 g	2.5 mL	3 mL	330 mg/mL

Intermittent intravenous infusion: Kefzol can be administered along with primary intravenous fluid management programs in a volume control set or in a separate, secondary IV bottle. Reconstituted 1 g of Kefzol may be diluted in 50 to 100 mL of 1 of the following intravenous solutions: 0.9% Sodium Chloride Injection, 5% or 10% Dextrose Injection, 5% Dextrose in Lactated Ringer's Injection, 5% Dextrose and 0.9% Sodium Chloride Injection (also may be used with 5% Dextrose and 0.45% or 0.2% Sodium Chloride Injection), Lactated Ringer's Injection, 5% or 10% Invert Sugar in Sterile Water for Injection, Ringer's Injection, Normosol®-M in D5-W, Ionosol® B with Dextrose 5%, or Plasma-Lyte® with 5% Dextrose.

ADD-Vantage Vials of Kefzol are to be reconstituted *only* with 0.9% Sodium Chloride Injection or 5% Dextrose Injection in the 50-mL or 100-mL Flexible Diluent Containers.

Intravenous injection (Administer solution directly into vein or though tubing): Dilute the reconstituted 1 g of Kefzol in a minimum of 10 mL of Sterile Water for Injection. Inject solution slowly over 3 to 5 minutes. Do not inject in less than 3 minutes. (NOTE: ADD-VANTAGE VIALS ARE NOT TO BE USED IN THIS MANNER.)

Dosage—The usual adult dosages are given in Table 4.

TABLE 4. USUAL ADULT DOSAGE OF KEFZOL® (CEFAZOLIN SODIUM, LILLY)

Type of Infection	Dose	Frequency
Pneumococcal pneumonia	500 mg	q12h
Mild infections caused by susceptible gram-positive cocci	250 to 500 mg	q8h
Acute uncomplicated urinary tract infections	1 g	q12h
Moderate to severe infections	500 mg to 1 g	q6 to 8h
Severe, life-threatening infections (eg, endocarditis, septicemia)*	1 g to 1.5 g	q6h

* In rare instances, doses up to 12 g of cefazolin per day have been used.

Dosage Adjustment for Patients With Reduced Renal Function—Kefzol may be used in patients with reduced renal function with the following dosage adjustments: Patients with a creatinine clearance of ≥ 55 mL/min or a serum creatinine of ≤ 1.5 mg % can be given full doses. Patients with creatinine clearance rates of 35 to 54 mL/min or serum creatinine of 1.6 to 3.0 mg % can also be given full doses, but dosage should be restricted to at least 8-hour intervals. Patients with creatinine clearance rates of 11 to 34 mL/min or serum creatinine of 3.1 to 4.5 mg % should be given one half the usual dose every 12 hours. Patients with creatinine clearance rates of ≤ 10 mL/min or serum creatinine of ≥ 4.6 mg % should be given one half the usual dose every 18 to 24 hours. All reduced dosage recommendations apply after an initial loading dose appropriate to the severity of the infection. For information about peritoneal dialysis, see *Human Pharmacology.*

Perioperative Prophylactic Use—To prevent postoperative infection in contaminated or potentially contaminated surgery, the recommended doses are as follows:

a. 1 g IV or IM administered one half to 1 hour prior to the start of surgery.
b. For lengthy operative procedures (eg, 2 hours or longer), 0.5 to 1 g IV or IM during surgery (administration modified according to the duration of the operative procedure).
c. 0.5 to 1 g IV or IM every 6 to 8 hours for 24 hours postoperatively.

It is important that (1) the preoperative dose be given just prior (one half to 1 hour) to the start of surgery so that adequate antibiotic levels are present in the serum and tissues at the time of the initial surgical incision and (2) if exposure to infectious organisms is likely, Kefzol be administered at appropriate intervals during surgery in order that sufficient levels of the antibiotic be present when needed.

In surgery in which infection may be particularly devastating (eg, open-heart surgery and prosthetic arthroplasty), the prophylactic administration of Kefzol may be continued for 3 to 5 days following the completion of surgery.

In children, a total daily dosage of 25 to 50 mg/kg (approximately 10 to 20 mg/lb) of body weight, divided into 3 or 4 equal doses, is effective for most mild to moderately severe

infections (Table 5). Total daily dosage may be increased to 100 mg/kg (45 mg/lb) of body weight for severe infections.

TABLE 5. PEDIATRIC DOSAGE GUIDE FOR KEFZOL® (CEFAZOLIN SODIUM, LILLY)

Weight		25 mg/kg/Day Divided into 3 Doses		25 mg/kg/Day Divided into 4 Doses	
lb	kg	Approximate Single Dose (mg q8h)	Vol (mL) Needed with Dilution of 125 mg/mL	Approximate Single Dose (mg q6h)	Vol (mL) Needed with Dilution of 125 mg/mL
10	4.5	40 mg	0.35 mL	30 mg	0.25 mL
20	9	75 mg	0.6 mL	55 mg	0.45 mL
30	13.6	115 mg	0.9 mL	85 mg	0.7 mL
40	18.1	150 mg	1.2 mL	115 mg	0.9 mL
50	22.7	190 mg	1.5 mL	140 mg	1.1 mL

Weight		50 mg/kg/Day Divided into 3 Doses		50 mg/kg/Day Divided into 4 Doses	
lb	kg	Approximate Single Dose (mg q8h)	Vol (mL) Needed with Dilution of 225 mg/mL	Approximate Single Dose (mg q6h)	Vol (mL) Needed with Dilution of 225 mg/mL
10	4.5	75 mg	0.35 mL	55 mg	0.25 mL
20	9	150 mg	0.7 mL	110 mg	0.5 mL
30	13.6	225 mg	1 mL	170 mg	0.75 mL
40	18.1	300 mg	1.35 mL	225 mg	1 mL
50	22.7	375 mg	1.7 mL	285 mg	1.25 mL

In children with mild to moderate renal impairment (creatinine clearance of 70 to 40 mL/min), 60% of the normal daily dosage given in divided doses every 12 hours should be sufficient. In children with moderate impairment (creatinine clearance of 40 to 20 mL/min), 25% of the normal daily dosage given in divided doses every 12 hours should be sufficient. In children with severe impairment (creatinine clearance of 20 to 5 mL/min), 10% of the normal daily dosage given every 24 hours should be adequate. All dosage recommendations apply after an initial loading dose is administered.

Since safety for use in premature infants and in infants under 1 month of age has not been established, the use of Kefzol in these patients is not recommended.

STABILITY
In those situations in which the drug and diluent have been mixed, but not immediately administered to the patient, the admixture may be stored under the following conditions:

Vials and Faspak Containers—Reconstituted Kefzol® (cefozolin sodium, Lilly) diluted in Sterile Water for Injection, 5% Dextrose Injection, or 0.9% Sodium Chloride Injection, is stable for 24 hours at room temperature and for 10 days if stored under refrigeration, 2° to 8°C (36° to 46°F).

Solutions of Kefzol in Sterile Water for Injection, 5% Dextrose Injection, or 0.9% Sodium Chloride Injection that are frozen immediately after reconstitution in the original vials or Faspak containers are stable for as long as 12 weeks if stored at −20°C. Once thawed, these solutions are stable for 24 hours at room temperature and for 10 days if stored under refrigeration, 2° to 8°C (36° to 46° F). If the product is warmed, care should be taken to avoid heating it after the thawing is complete. Once thawed, the solution should not be refrozen.

Secondary Diluents—Solutions of Kefzol for infusion in 10% Dextrose Injection, 5% Dextrose in Lactated Ringer's Injection, 5% Dextrose and 0.9% Sodium Chloride Injection (also may be used with 5% Dextrose and 0.45% or 0.2% Sodium Chloride Injection), Lactated Ringer's Injection, 5% or 10% Invert Sugar in Sterile Water for Injection, Ringer's Injection, Normosol®-M in D5-W, Ionosol®-B with Dextrose 5%, or Plasma-Lyte with 5% Dextrose should be used within 24 hours after dilution if stored at room temperature or within 96 hours if stored under refrigeration, 2° to 8° C (36° to 46° F). (DO NOT FREEZE KEFZOL DILUTED WITH THE ABOVE DILUENTS.)

ADD-Vantage Vials—Only 0.9% Sodium Chloride Injection and 5% Dextrose Injection in the 50-mL or 100-mL Flexible Diluent Containers are approved for reconstituting ADD-Vantage Kefzol. Ordinarily, ADD-Vantage vials should be reconstituted only when it is certain that the patient is ready to receive the drug. However, reconstituted Kefzol diluted in 5% Dextrose Injection and 0.9% Sodium Chloride Injection is stable of 24 hours at room temperature. (DO NOT RE-

FRIGERATE OR FREEZE KEFZOL IN ADD-VANTAGE VIALS.)

Prior to administration, parenteral drug products should be inspected visually for particulate matter and discoloration whenever solution and container permit.

HOW SUPPLIED
℞ Vials:
1 g,* 10-mL size (No. 768)—(1s) NDC 0002-1498-01; (Traypak† of 25) NDC 0002-1498-25
℞ Faspak‡:
1 g* (No. 7202)§—(Faspak of 96) NDC 0002-7202-74
℞ ADD-Vantage‖ Vials:
500 mg* (No. 7265)—(Traypak of 25) NDC 0002-7265-25
1 g* (No. 7266)—(Traypak of 25) NDC 0002-7266-25
The above ADD-Vantage Vials are to be used *only* with Abbott Laboratories' 50-mL or 100-mL Flexible Diluent Containers containing 0.9% Sodium Chloride Injection or 5% Dextrose Injection.
Instructions for use of the ADD-Vantage Vials are enclosed in the package.
Also available:
℞ Pharmacy Bulk Package:
10 g,* 100-mL size (No. 7014)—(Traypak of 6) NDC 0002-7014-16

---

* Equivalent to cefazolin.
† Traypak™ (multivial carton, Lilly).
‡ Faspak® (flexible plastic bag, Lilly).
§For IV use.
‖ ADD-Vantage® (vials and diluent containers, Abbott).
[052092]

LENTE® ILETIN® I AND II   OTC
(insulin zinc suspension, Lilly) *See under* Iletin® (insulin, Lilly)

LORABID™   ℞
[*lŏr ′ă-bĭd*]
(Loracarbef)

DESCRIPTION
LORABID™ (Loracarbef) is a synthetic β-lactam antibiotic of the carbacephem class for oral administration. Chemically, carbacephems differ from cephalosporin-class antibiotics in the dihydrothiazine ring where a methylene group has been substituted for a sulfur atom.
The chemical name for loracarbef is (6R, 7S)-7-[(R)-2-amino-2-phenylacetamido]-3-chloro-8-oxo-1-azabicyclo[4.2.0] oct-2-ene-2-carboxylic acid, monohydrate. It is a white crystalline compound with a molecular weight of 367.8. The empirical formula is $C_{16}O_4N_3H_{16}Cl \cdot H_2O$. The structural formula is:

Lorabid Pulvules® and Lorabid for Oral Suspension are intended for oral administration only.
Each Pulvule contains loracarbef equivalent to 200 mg (0.57 mmol) anhydrous loracarbef activity. They also contain cornstarch, dimethicone, F D & C Blue No. 2, gelatin, iron oxides, magnesium stearate, titanium dioxide, and other inactive ingredients.
After reconstitution, each 5 mL of Lorabid for Oral Suspension contains loracarbef equivalent to 100 mg (0.286 mmol) or 200 mg (0.57 mmol) anhydrous loracarbef activity. The suspensions also contain cellulose, F D & C Red No. 40, flavors, methylparaben, propylparaben, sodium carboxymethylcellulose, silicone, sucrose, and xanthan gum.

CLINICAL PHARMACOLOGY
Loracarbef, after oral administration, was approximately 90% absorbed from the gastrointestinal tract. When capsules were taken with food, peak plasma concentrations were 50% to 60% of those achieved when the drug was administered to fasting subjects and occurred from 30 to 60 minutes later. Total absorption, as measured by urinary recovery and area under the plasma concentration versus time curve (AUC), was unchanged. The effect of food on the rate and extent of absorption of the suspension formulation has not been studied to date.
The pharmacokinetics of loracarbef were linear over the recommended dosage range of 200 to 400 mg, with no accumulation of the drug noted when it was given twice daily.

Average peak plasma concentrations after administration of 200-mg or 400-mg single doses of loracarbef as capsules to fasting subjects were approximately 8 and 14 μg/mL, respectively, and were obtained within 1.2 hours after dosing. The average peak plasma concentration in adults following a 400-mg single dose of suspension was 17 μg/mL and was obtained within 0.8 hour after dosing (*see* Table).

Dosage (mg)	Mean Plasma Loracarbef Concentrations (μg/mL)	
	Peak Cmax	Time to Peak Tmax
Capsule (single dose)		
200 mg	8	1.2 h
400 mg	14	1.2 h
Suspension (single dose)		
400 mg (adult)	17	0.8 h
7.5 mg/kg (pediatric)	13	0.8 h
15 mg/kg (pediatric)	19	0.8 h

Following administration of 7.5 and 15 mg/kg single doses of oral suspension to children, average peak plasma concentrations were 13 and 19 μg/mL, respectively, and were obtained within 40 to 60 minutes.
This increased rate of absorption (suspension > capsule) should be taken into consideration if the oral suspension is to be substituted for the capsule, and capsules should not be substituted for the oral suspension in the treatment of otitis media (*see* Dosage and Administration).
The elimination half-life was an average of 1.0 h in patients with normal renal function. Concomitant administration of probenecid decreased the rate of urinary excretion and increased the half-life to 1.5 hours.
In subjects with moderate impairment of renal function (creatinine clearance 10 to 50 mL/min/1.73 m²), following a single 400-mg dose, the plasma half-life was prolonged to approximately 5.6 hours. In subjects with severe renal impairment (creatinine clearance < 10 mL/min/1.73 m²), the half-life was increased to approximately 32 hours. During hemodialysis the half-life was approximately 4 hours. In patients with severe renal impairment, the C_{max} increased from 15.4 μg/mL to 23 μg/mL (*see* Precautions *and* Dosage and Administration).
In single-dose studies, plasma half-life and AUC were not significantly altered in healthy elderly subjects with normal renal function.
There is no evidence of metabolism of loracarbef in humans. Approximately 25% of circulating loracarbef is bound to plasma proteins.
Middle-ear fluid concentrations of loracarbef were approximately 48% of the plasma concentration 2 hours after drug administration in children. The peak concentration of loracarbef in blister fluid was approximately half that obtained in plasma. Adequate data on CSF levels of loracarbef are not available.
Microbiology—Loracarbef exerts its bactericidal action by binding to essential target proteins of the bacterial cell wall, leading to inhibition of cell-wall synthesis. It is stable in the presence of some bacterial β-lactamases. Loracarbef has been shown to be active against most strains of the following organisms both *in vitro* and in clinical infections (*see* Indications and Usage):
Gram-positive aerobes:
  Staphylococcus aureus (including penicillinase-producing strains)
    NOTE: Loracarbef (like most β-lactam antimicrobials) is inactive against methicillin-resistant staphylococci.
  Staphylococcus saprophyticus
  Streptococcus pneumoniae
  Streptococcus pyogenes
Gram-negative aerobes:
  Escherichia coli
  Haemophilus influenzae (including β-lactamase-producing strains)
  Moraxella (Branhamella) catarrhalis (including β-lactamase-producing strains)
The following *in vitro* data are available: however, their clinical significance is unknown.
Loracarbef exhibits *in vitro* minimum inhibitory concentrations (MIC) of 8 μg/mL or less against most strains of the following organisms; however, the safety and efficacy of loracarbef in treating clinical infections due to these organisms have not been established in adequate and well-controlled trials.

Continued on next page

Lilly—Cont.

Gram-positive aerobes:
Staphylococcus epidermidis
Streptococcus agalactiae (group B streptococci)
Streptococcus bovis
Streptococci, groups C, F, and G
viridans group streptococci

Gram-negative aerobes:
Citrobacter diversus
Haemophilus parainfluenzae
Klebsiella pneumoniae
Neisseria gonorrhoeae (including penicillinase-producing strains)
Pasteurella multocida
Proteus mirabilis
Salmonella species
Shigella species
Yersinia enterocolitica

NOTE: Loracarbef is inactive against most strains of *Acinetobacter, Enterobacter, Morganella morganii, Proteus vulgaris, Providencia, Pseudomonas,* and *Serratia.*

Anaerobic organisms:
Clostridium perfringens
Fusobacterium necrophorum
Peptococcus niger
Peptostreptococcus intermedius
Propionibacterium acnes

Susceptibility Testing

Diffusion Techniques—Quantitative methods that require measurement of zone diameters give the most precise estimate of the susceptibility of bacteria to antimicrobial agents. One such standardized method[1] has been recommended for use with the 30-μg loracarbef disk. Interpretation involves the correlation of the diameter obtained in the disk test with MIC for loracarbef.

Reports from the laboratory giving results of the standard single-disk susceptibility test with a 30-μg loracarbef disk should be interpreted according to the following criteria:

Zone Diameter (mm)	Interpretation
≥ 18	(S) Susceptible
15–17	(MS) Moderately Susceptible
≤ 14	(R) Resistant

A report of "susceptible" implies that the pathogen is likely to be inhibited by generally achievable blood concentrations. A report of "moderately susceptible" indicates that inhibitory concentrations of the antibiotic may be achieved if high dosage is used or if the infection is confined to tissues and fluids (eg, urine) in which high antibiotic concentrations are attained. A report of "resistant" indicates that achievable concentrations of the antibiotic are unlikely to be inhibitory and other therapy should be selected.

Standardized procedures require the use of laboratory control organisms. The 30-μg loracarbef disk should give the following zone diameters with the NCCLS approved procedure:

Organism	Zone Diameter (mm)
E. coli ATCC 25922	23–29
S. aureus ATCC 25923	23–31

Dilution Techniques—Use a standardized dilution method[2] (broth, agar, or microdilution) or equivalent with loracarbef powder. The MIC values obtained should be interpreted according to the following criteria:

MIC (μg/mL)	Interpretation
≤8	(S) Susceptible
16	(MS) Moderately Susceptible
≥32	(R) Resistant

As with standard diffusion methods, dilution procedures require the use of laboratory control organisms. Standard loracarbef powder should give the following MIC values with the NCCLS approved procedure:

Organism	MIC Range (μg/mL)
E. coli ATCC 25922	0.5–2
S. aureus ATCC 29213	0.5–2

INDICATIONS AND USAGE

Lorabid™ (loracarbef) is indicated in the treatment of patients with mild to moderate infections caused by susceptible strains of the designated microorganisms in the conditions listed below. (As recommended dosages, durations of therapy, and applicable patient populations vary among these infections, please see Dosage and Administration for specific recommendations.)

Lower Respiratory Tract

Secondary Bacterial Infection of Acute Bronchitis caused by *S. pneumoniae, H. influenzae* (including β-lactamase-producing strains), or *M. catarrhalis* (including β-lactamase-producing strains).

Acute Bacterial Exacerbations of Chronic Bronchitis caused by *S. pneumoniae, H. influenzae* (including β-lactamase-producing strains), or *M. catarrhalis* (including β-lactamase-producing strains).

Pneumonia caused by *S. pneumoniae or H. influenzae* (non-β-lactamase-producing strains only). Data are insufficient at this time to establish efficacy in patients with pneumonia caused by β-lactamase-producing strains of *H. influenzae.*

Upper Respiratory Tract

Otitis Media* caused by *S. pneumoniae, H. influenzae* (including β-lactamase-producing strains), *M. catarrhalis* (including β-lactamase-producing strains), or *S. pyogenes.*

Acute Maxillary Sinusitis* caused by *S. pneumoniae, H. influenzae* (non-β-lactamase-producing strains only), or *M. catarrhalis* (including β-lactamase-producing strains). Data are insufficient at this time to establish efficacy in patients with acute maxillary sinusitis caused by β-lactamase-producing strains of *H. influenzae.*

* In a patient population with significant numbers of β-lactamase-producing organisms, loracarbef's clinical cure and bacteriological eradication rates were somewhat less than those observed with a product containing a β-lactamase inhibitor. Lorabid's decreased potential for toxicity compared to products containing β-lactamase inhibitors along with the susceptibility patterns of the common microbes in a given geographic area should be taken into account when considering the use of an antimicrobial (*see* Clinical Studies section).

Pharyngitis and Tonsillitis caused by *S. pyogenes.* (The usual drug of choice in the treatment and prevention of streptococcal infections, including the prophylaxis of rheumatic fever, is penicillin administered by the intramuscular route. Lorabid is generally effective in the eradication of *S. pyogenes* from the nasopharynx; however, data establishing the efficacy of Lorabid in the subsequent prevention of rheumatic fever are not available at present.)

Skin and Skin Structure

Uncomplicated Skin and Skin Structure Infections caused by *S. aureus* (including penicillinase-producing strains) or *S. pyogenes.* Abscesses should be surgically drained as clinically indicated.

Urinary Tract

Uncomplicated Urinary Tract Infections (cystitis) caused by *E. coli* or *S. saprophyticus**.

NOTE: In considering the use of Lorabid in the treatment of cystitis, Lorabid's lower bacterial eradication rates and lower potential for toxicity should be weighed against the increased eradication rates and increased potential for toxicity demonstrated by some other classes of approved agents (*see* Clinical Studies section).

Uncomplicated Pyelonephritis caused by *E. coli.*

Culture and susceptibility testing should be performed when appropriate to determine the causative organism and its susceptibility to loracarbef. Therapy may be started while awaiting the results of these studies. Once these results become available, antimicrobial therapy should be adjusted accordingly.

CONTRAINDICATION

Lorabid™ (loracarbef) is contraindicated in patients with known allergy to loracarbef or cephalosporin-class antibiotics.

WARNINGS

BEFORE THERAPY WITH LORABID IS INSTITUTED, CAREFUL INQUIRY SHOULD BE MADE TO DETERMINE WHETHER THE PATIENT HAS HAD PREVIOUS HYPERSENSITIVITY REACTIONS TO LORACARBEF, CEPHALOSPORINS, PENICILLINS, OR OTHER DRUGS. IF THIS PRODUCT IS TO BE GIVEN TO PENICILLIN-SENSITIVE PATIENTS, CAUTION SHOULD BE EXERCISED BECAUSE CROSS-HYPERSENSITIVITY AMONG β-LACTAM ANTIBIOTICS HAS BEEN CLEARLY DOCUMENTED AND MAY OCCUR IN UP TO 10% OF PATIENTS WITH A HISTORY OF PENICILLIN ALLERGY. IF AN ALLERGIC REACTION TO LORABID OCCURS, DISCONTINUE THE DRUG. SERIOUS ACUTE HYPERSENSITIVITY REACTIONS MAY REQUIRE THE USE OF EPINEPHRINE AND OTHER EMERGENCY MEASURES, INCLUDING OXYGEN, INTRAVENOUS FLUIDS, INTRAVENOUS ANTIHISTAMINES, CORTICOSTEROIDS, PRESSOR AMINES, AND AIRWAY MANAGEMENT, AS CLINICALLY INDICATED.

Pseudomembranous colitis has been reported with nearly all antibacterial agents and may range from mild to life-threatening. Therefore, it is important to consider this diagnosis in patients who present with diarrhea subsequent to the administration of antibacterial agents.

Treatment with broad-spectrum antibiotics alters the normal flora of the colon and may permit overgrowth of clostridia. Studies indicate that a toxin produced by *Clostridium difficile* is a primary cause of "antibiotic-associated colitis." After the diagnosis of pseudomembranous colitis has been established, therapeutic measures should be initiated. Mild cases of pseudomembranous colitis usually respond to discontinuation of drug alone. In moderate to severe cases, consideration should be given to management with fluids and electrolytes, protein supplementation, and treatment with an antibacterial drug effective against *C. difficile* -associated colitis.

*Although treatment of infections due to this organism in this organ system demonstrated a clinically acceptable overall outcome, efficacy was studied in fewer than 10 infections.

PRECAUTIONS

General —In patients with known or suspected renal impairment (*see* Dosage and Administration), careful clinical observation and appropriate laboratory studies should be performed prior to and during therapy. The total daily dose of loracarbef should be reduced in these patients because high and/or prolonged plasma antibiotic concentrations can occur in such individuals administered the usual doses. Loracarbef, like cephalosporins, should be given with caution to patients receiving concurrent treatment with potent diuretics because these diuretics are suspected of adversely affecting renal function.

As with other broad-spectrum antimicrobials, prolonged use of loracarbef may result in the overgrowth of nonsusceptible organisms. Careful observation of the patient is essential. If superinfection occurs during therapy, appropriate measures should be taken.

Loracarbef, as with other broad-spectrum antimicrobials, should be prescribed with caution in individuals with a history of colitis.

Information for Patients —Lorabid™ (loracarbef) should be taken either at least 1 hour prior to eating or at least 2 hours after eating a meal.

Drug Interactions —

Probenecid: As with other β-lactam antibiotics, renal excretion of loracarbef is inhibited by probenecid and resulted in an approximate 80% increase in the AUC for loracarbef (*see* Clinical Pharmacology).

Carcinogenesis, Mutagenesis, Impairment of Fertility —Although lifetime studies in animals have not been performed to evaluate carcinogenic potential, no mutagenic potential was found for loracarbef in standard tests of genotoxicity, which included bacterial mutation tests and *in vitro* and *in vivo* mammalian systems. In rats, fertility and reproductive performance were not affected by loracarbef at doses up to 33 times the maximum human exposure in mg/kg (10 times the exposure based on mg/m^2).

Usage in Pregnancy—Pregnancy Category B —Reproduction studies have been performed in mice, rats, and rabbits at doses up to 33 times the maximum human exposure in mg/kg (4, 10, and 4 times the exposure, respectively, based on mg/m^2) and have revealed no evidence of impaired fertility or harm to the fetus due to loracarbef. There are, however, no adequate and well-controlled studies in pregnant women. Because animal reproduction studies are not always predictive of human response, this drug should be used during pregnancy only if clearly needed.

Labor and Delivery —Lorabid has not been studied for use during labor and delivery. Treatment should be given only if clearly needed.

Nursing Mothers —It is not known whether this drug is excreted in human milk. Because many drugs are excreted in human milk, caution should be exercised when Lorabid is administered to a nursing woman.

Pediatric Use —Efficacy and safety in infants less than 6 months of age have not been established.

Geriatric Use —Healthy geriatric volunteers (≥65 years old) with normal renal function who received a single 400-mg dose of loracarbef had no significant differences in AUC or clearance when compared to healthy adult volunteers 20 to 40 years of age. In clinical studies, when geriatric patients received the usual recommended adult doses, clinical efficacy and safety were comparable to results in nongeriatric adult patients. Because significant numbers of elderly patients have decreased renal function, evaluation of renal function in this population is recommended (*see* Dosage and Administration).

ADVERSE REACTIONS

The nature of adverse reactions to loracarbef are similar to those observed with orally administered β-lactam antimicrobials. The majority of adverse reactions observed in clinical trials were of a mild and transient nature; 1.5% of patients discontinued therapy because of drug-related adverse reactions. No one reaction requiring discontinuation accounted for >0.03% of the total patient population; however, of those reactions resulting in discontinuation, gastrointestinal events (diarrhea and abdominal pain) and skin rashes predominated.

All Patients

The following adverse events, irrespective of relationship to drug, have been reported following the use of Lorabid in clinical trials. Incidence rates (combined for all dosing regimens and dosage forms) were less than 1% for the total patient population, except as otherwise noted:

Gastrointestinal: The most commonly observed adverse reactions were related to the gastrointestinal system. The incidence of gastrointestinal adverse reactions increased in patients treated with higher doses. Individual event rates included diarrhea, 4.1%; nausea, 1.9%; vomiting, 1.4%; abdominal pain, 1.4%; and anorexia.

Population/Infection	Dosage (mg)	Duration (days)
ADULTS (13 years and older)		
Lower Respiratory Tract		
Secondary Bacterial Infection of Acute Bronchitis	200–400 q12h	7
Acute Bacterial Exacerbation of Chronic Bronchitis	400 q12h	7
Pneumonia	400 q12h	14
Upper Respiratory Tract		
Pharyngitis/Tonsillitis	200 q12h	10*
Sinusitis	400 q12h	10
(See Clinical Studies and Indications and Usage for further information.)		
Skin and Skin Structure		
Uncomplicated Skin and Skin Structure Infections	200 q12h	7
Urinary Tract		
Uncomplicated cystitis	200 q24h	7
(See Clinical Studies and Indications and Usage for further information.)		
Uncomplicated pyelonephritis	400 q12h	14
INFANTS AND CHILDREN (6 months to 12 years)		
Upper Respiratory Tract		
Acute Otitis Media**	30 mg/kg/day in divided doses q12h	10
(See Clinical Studies and Indications and Usage for further information.)		
Pharyngitis/Tonsillitis	15 mg/kg/day in divided doses q12h	10*
Skin and Skin Structure		
Impetigo	15 mg/kg/day in divided doses q12h	7

*In the treatment of infections due to S. pyogenes, Lorabid should be administered for at least 10 days.

**Otitis media should be treated with the suspension. Clinical studies of otitis media were conducted with the suspension formulation only. The suspension is more rapidly absorbed than the capsules, resulting in higher peak plasma concentrations when administered at the same dose. Therefore, the capsule should not be substituted for the suspension in the treatment of otitis media (see Clinical Pharmacology). [See tables above.]

Hypersensitivity: Hypersensitivity reactions including, skin rashes (1.2%), urticaria, pruritus, and erythema multiforme.

Central Nervous System: Headache (2.9%), somnolence, nervousness, insomnia, and dizziness.

Hemic and Lymphatic Systems: Transient thrombocytopenia, leukopenia, and eosinophilia.

Hepatic: Transient elevations in SGPT, SGOT, and alkaline phosphatase.

Renal: Transient elevations in BUN and creatinine.

Cardiovascular System: Vasodilatation.

Genitourinary: Vaginitis (1.3%), vaginal moniliasis (1.1%).

Pediatric Patients

The incidences of several adverse events, irrespective of relationship to drug, following treatment with Lorabid™ (loracarbef) were significantly different in the pediatric population and the adult population as follows:

Event	Pediatric	Adult
Diarrhea	5.8%	3.6%
Headache	0.9%	3.2%
Rhinitis	6.3%	1.6%
Nausea	0.0%	2.5%
Rash	2.9%	0.7%
Vomiting	3.3%	0.5%
Somnolence	2.1%	0.4%
Anorexia	2.3%	0.3%

β-Lactam Antimicrobial Class Labeling:

Although not observed in patients treated with Lorabid in clinical trials, the following adverse reactions and altered laboratory test results have been reported in patients treated with β-lactam antibiotics:

Adverse Reactions—Allergic reactions including anaphylaxis, Stevens-Johnson syndrome, serum sickness-like reactions, aplastic anemia, hemolytic anemia, hemorrhage, agranulocytosis, toxic epidermal necrolysis, renal dysfunction, toxic nephropathy, and hepatic dysfunction including cholestasis.

Several β-lactam antibiotics have been implicated in triggering seizures, particularly in patients with renal impairment when the dosage was not reduced. If seizures associated with drug therapy should occur, the drug should be discontinued. Anticonvulsant therapy can be given if clinically indicated.

Altered Laboratory Tests—Increased prothrombin time, positive direct Coombs' test, elevated LDH, pancytopenia, and neutropenia.

PEDIATRIC DOSAGE CHART FOR LORABID™ (loracarbef) DAILY DOSE 15 mg/kg/day

		100 mg/5 mL Suspension		200 mg/5 mL Suspension	
Weight		Dose given twice daily		Dose given twice daily	
lb	kg	mL	tsp	mL	tsp
15	7	2.6	0.5	—	—
29	13	4.9	1.0	2.5	0.5
44	20	7.5	1.5	3.8	0.75
57	26	9.8	2.0	4.9	1.0

PEDIATRIC DOSAGE CHART DAILY DOSE 30 mg/kg/day

		100 mg/5 mL Suspension		200 mg/5 mL Suspension	
Weight		Dose given twice daily		Dose given twice daily	
lb	kg	mL	tsp	mL	tsp
15	7	5.2	1.0	2.6	0.5
29	13	9.8	2.0	4.9	1.0
44	20	—	—	7.5	1.5
57	26	—	—	9.8	2.0

OVERDOSAGE

Signs and Symptoms—The toxic symptoms following an overdose of β-lactams may include nausea, vomiting, epigastric distress, and diarrhea.

Loarcarbef is eliminated primarily by the kidneys. Forced diuresis, peritoneal dialysis, hemodialysis, or hemoperfusion have not been established as beneficial for an overdose of loracarbef. Hemodialysis has been shown to be effective in hastening the elimination of loracarbef from plasma in patients with chronic renal failure.

DOSAGE AND ADMINISTRATION

Lorabid is administered orally either at least 1 hour prior to eating or at least 2 hours after eating. The recommended dosages, durations of treatment, and applicable patient populations are described in the following chart:

[See table at top left.]

Renal Impairment: Lorabid™ (loracarbef) may be administered to patients with impaired renal function. The usual dose and schedule may be employed in patients with creatinine clearance levels of 50 mL/min or greater. Patients with creatinine clearance between 10 and 49 mL/min may be given half of the recommended dose at the usual dosage interval, or the normal recommended dose at twice the usual dosage interval. Patients with creatinine clearance levels less than 10 mL/min may be treated with the recommended dose given every 3 to 5 days; patients on hemodialysis should receive another dose following dialysis.

When only the serum creatinine is available, the following formula (based on sex, weight, and age of the patient) may be used to convert this value into creatinine clearance (CL_{cr}, mL/min). The equation assumes the patient's renal function is stable.

$$\text{Males} = \frac{(\text{weight in kg}) \times (140 - \text{age})}{(72) \times \text{serum creatinine (mg/100 mL)}}$$

$$\text{Females} = (0.85) \times (\text{above value})$$

Reconstitution Directions for Oral Suspension

Bottle Size	Reconstitution Directions
100 mL	Add 60 mL of water in 2 portions to the dry mixture in the bottle. Shake well after each addition.
50 mL	Add 30 mL of water in 2 portions to the dry mixture in the bottle. Shake well after each addition.

After mixing, the suspension may be kept at room temperature, 59°F to 86°F (15° to 30°C), for 14 days without significant loss of potency. Keep tightly closed. Discard unused portion after 14 days.

HOW SUPPLIED

Pulvules:

200 mg, (blue and gray) (No. 3170) (Identi-Code* 3170) (30s) NDC 0002-3170-30

Keep tightly closed. Store at controlled room temperature, 59° to 86°F (15° to 30°C). Protect from heat.

For Oral Suspension (strawberry bubble gum flavor):

100 mg/5 mL, (M-5135) (50-mL size) NDC 0002-5135-87; (100-mL size) NDC 0002-5135-48

200 mg/5 mL, (M-5136) (50-mL size) NDC 0002-5136-87; (100-mL size) NDC 0002-5136-48

Clinical Studies:

US Acute Otitis Media Study
Loracarbef (L) vs β-lactamase inhibitor-containing control drug (C)

Efficacy: In a controlled study of acute otitis media performed in the United States where significant rates of β-lactamase-producing organisms were found, loracarbef was

*Identi-Code® (formula identification code, Lilly).

compared to an oral antimicrobial agent that contained a specific β-lactamase inhibitor. In this study, using very strict evaluability criteria and microbiologic and clinical response criteria at the 10- to 16-day posttherapy follow-up, the following presumptive bacterial eradication/clinical cure outcomes (ie, clinical success) and safety results were obtained:

	% of Cases With	
Pathogen	Pathogens (n=204)	Success Rate
S. pneumoniae	42.6%	L equivalent to C
H. influenzae	30.4%	L 9% less than C
M. catarrhalis	20.6%	L 19% less than C
S. pyogenes	6.4%	L equivalent to C
Overall	100.0%	L 12% less than C

Safety: The incidences of the following adverse events were clinically and statistically significantly higher in the control arm versus the loracarbef arm.

Event	Loracarbef	Control
Diarrhea	15%	26%
Rash*	8%	15%

*The majority of these involved the diaper area in young children.

European Acute Otitis Media Study
Loracarbef (L) vs Amoxicillin (A)

Efficacy: In a controlled clinical study of acute otitis media performed in Europe, loracarbef was compared to amoxicillin. As expected in a European population, this study population had a lower incidence of β-lactamase-producing organisms than usually seen in US trials. In this study, using very strict evaluability criteria and microbiologic and clinical response criteria at the 10- to 16-day posttherapy follow-up, the following presumptive bacterial eradication/clinical cure outcomes (ie, clinical success) were obtained:

	% of Cases With	
Pathogen	Pathogens (n=291)	Success Rate
S. pneumoniae	51.5%	L equivalent to A
H. influenzae	29.2%	L 14% greater than A
M. catarrhalis	15.8%	L 31% greater than A
S. pyogenes	3.4%	L equivalent to A
Overall	100.0%	L equivalent to A

European Acute Maxilliary Sinusitis Study
Loracarbef (L) vs Doxycycline (D)

Efficacy: In a controlled clinical study of acute maxillary sinusitis performed in Europe, loracarbef was compared to doxycycline. In this study, there were 210 sinus-puncture evaluable patients. As expected in a European population, this study population had a lower incidence of β-lactamase-producing organisms than usually seen in US trials. In this study, using very strict evaluability criteria and microbiologic and clinical response criteria at the 1- to 2-week posttherapy follow-up, the following presumptive bacterial eradication/clinical cure outcomes (ie, clinical success) were obtained:

	% of Cases With	
Pathogen	Pathogens (n=210)	Success Rate
S. pneumoniae	47.6%	L equivalent to D
H. influenzae	41.4%	L equivalent to D
M. catarrhalis	11.0%	L equivalent to D
Overall	100.0%	L equivalent to D

Continued on next page

* Identi-Code® symbol. This product information was prepared in June 1992. Current information on these and other products of Eli Lilly and Company may be obtained by direct inquiry to Lilly Research Laboratories, Lilly Corporate Center, Indianapolis, Indiana 46285, (317) 276-3714.

Lilly—Cont.

US Uncomplicated Cystitis Study
Loracarbef (L) vs Cefaclor (C)

Efficacy: In a controlled clinical study of cystitis performed in the United States, loracarbef was compared to cefaclor. In this study, using very strict evaluability criteria and microbiologic and clinical response criteria at the 5- to 9-day posttherapy follow-up, the following bacterial eradication rates were obtained:

Pathogen	% of Cases With Pathogens (n=186)	Eradication Rate
E. coli	77.4%	L 4% greater than C (L = 80%)
Other major *Enterobacteriaceae*	12.5%	L equivalent to C (L = 61%)
S. saprophyticus	3.8%	L equivalent to C

European Uncomplicated Cystitis Study
Loracarbef (L) vs Quinolone (Q)

Efficacy: In a second controlled clinical study of cystitis, performed in Europe, loracarbef was compared to an oral quinolone. In this study, using very strict evaluability criteria and microbiologic and clinical response criteria at the 5- to 9-day posttherapy follow-up, the following bacterial eradication rates were obtained:

Pathogen	% of Cases With Pathogens (n=189)	Eradication Rate
E. coli	82.0%	L 7% less than Q (L = 81%)
Other major *Enterobacteriaceae*	10.1%	L 32% less than Q (L = 50%)

REFERENCES

1. National Committee for Clinical Laboratory Standards, M2-A4 performance standards for antimicrobial disk susceptibility tests, ed 4, Villanova, PA, April, 1990.
2. National Committee for Clinical Laboratory Standards, M7-A2 methods for dilution antimicrobial susceptibility tests for bacteria that grow aerobically, ed 2, Villanova, PA, April, 1990.

Shown in Product Identification Section, page 416

[032592]

MANDOL® ℞

[*măn'dōl*]
(Cefamandole Nafate for Injection, USP)

DESCRIPTION

Mandol® (Cefamandole Nafate for Injection, USP, Lilly) is a semisynthetic broad-spectrum cephalosporin antibiotic for parenteral administration. It is 5-Thia-1-azabicyclo[4.2.0]oct-2-ene-2-carboxylic acid, 7-[[(formyloxy)phenylacetyl]amino]-3-[[(1-methyl-1*H*-tetrazol-5-yl)thio]methyl]-8-oxo-, monosodium salt, [6*R*-[6α,7β(*R* *)]]. Cefamandole has the empirical formula $C_{19}H_{17}N_6NaO_6S_2$ representing a molecular weight of 512.49. Mandol also contains 63 mg sodium carbonate/g of cefamandole activity. The total sodium content is approximately 77 mg (3.3 mEq sodium ion) per g of cefamandole activity. After addition of diluent, cefamandole nafate rapidly hydrolyzes to cefamandole, and both compounds have microbiologic activity in vivo. Solutions of Mandol range from light-yellow to amber, depending on concentration and diluent used. The pH of freshly reconstituted solutions usually ranges from 6.0 to 8.5.

CLINICAL PHARMACOLOGY

After intramuscular administration of a 500-mg dose of cefamandole to normal volunteers, the mean peak serum concentration was 13 μg/mL. After a 1-g dose, the mean peak concentration was 25 μg/mL. These peaks occurred at 30 to 120 minutes. Following intravenous doses of 1, 2, and 3 g, serum concentrations were 139, 240, and 533 μg/mL respectively at 10 minutes. These concentrations declined to 0.8, 2.2, and 2.9 μg/mL at 4 hours. Intravenous administration of 4-g doses every 6 hours produced no evidence of accumulation in the serum. The half-life after an intravenous dose is 32 minutes; after intramuscular administration, the half-life is 60 minutes.

Sixty-five to 85% of cefamandole is excreted by the kidneys over an 8-hour period, resulting in high urinary concentrations. Following intramuscular doses of 500 mg and 1 g, urinary concentrations averaged 254 and 1,357 μg/mL respectively. Intravenous doses of 1 and 2 g produced urinary levels averaging 750 and 1,380 μg/mL respectively. Probenecid slows tubular excretion and doubles the peak serum level and the duration of measurable serum concentrations.

The antibiotic reaches therapeutic levels in pleural and joint fluids and in bile and bone.

Microbiology—The bactericidal action of cefamandole results from inhibition of cell-wall synthesis. Cephalosporins have in vitro activity against a wide range of gram-positive and gram-negative organisms. Cefamandole is usually active against the following organisms in vitro and in clinical infections:

Gram-positive
- *Staphylococcus aureus*, including penicillinase- and non-penicillinase-producing strains
- *Staphylococcus epidermidis*
- β-hemolytic and other streptococci (Most strains of enterococci, eg, *Enterococcus faecalis* [formerly *Streptococcus faecalis*], are resistant.)
- *Streptococcus pneumoniae*

Gram-negative
- *Escherichia coli*
- *Klebsiella* sp
- *Enterobacter* sp (Initially susceptible organisms occasionally may become resistant during therapy.)
- *Haemophilus influenzae*
- *Proteus mirabilis*
- *Providencia rettgeri* (formerly *Proteus rettgeri*)
- *Morganella morganii* (formerly *Proteus morganii*)
- *Proteus vulgaris* (Some strains of *P. vulgaris* have been shown by in vitro tests to be resistant to cefamandole and other cephalosporins.)

Anaerobic organisms
- Gram-positive and gram-negative cocci (including *Peptococcus* and *Peptostreptococcus* sp)
- Gram-positive bacilli (including *Clostridium* sp)
- Gram-negative bacilli (including *Bacteroides* and *Fusobacterium* sp). Most strains of *Bacteroides fragilis* are resistant.

Pseudomonas, Acinetobacter calcoaceticus (formerly *Mima* and *Herellea* sp), and most *Serratia* strains are resistant to cefamandole and certain other cephalosporins. Cefamandole is resistant to degradation by β-lactamases from certain members of the *Enterobacteriaceae*.

Susceptibility Tests—Quantitative methods that require measurement of zone diameters give the most precise estimates of antibiotic susceptibility. One such procedure[1] has been recommended for use with disks to test susceptibility to cefamandole. Interpretation involves correlation of the diameters obtained in the disk test with minimal inhibitory concentration (MIC) values for cefamandole.

Reports from the laboratory giving results of the standardized single-disk susceptibility test[1] using a 30-μg cefamandole disk should be interpreted according to the following criteria:

Susceptible organisms produce zones of 18 mm or greater, indicating that the tested organism is likely to respond to therapy.

Organisms of intermediate susceptibility produce zones of 15 to 17 mm, indicating that the tested organism would be susceptible if high dosage is used or if the infection is confined to tissues and fluids (eg, urine) in which high antibiotic levels are attained.

Resistant organisms produce zones of 14 mm or less, indicating that other therapy should be selected.

For gram-positive isolates, the test may be performed with either the cephalosporin-class disk (30 μg cephalothin) or the cefamandole disk (30 μg cefamandole), and a zone of 18 mm is indicative of a cefamandole-susceptible organism.

Gram-negative organisms should be tested with the cefamandole disk (using the above criteria), since cefamandole has been shown by in vitro tests to have activity against certain strains of *Enterobacteriaceae* found resistant when tested with the cephalosporin-class disk. Gram-negative organisms having zones of less than 18 mm around the cephalothin disk are not necessarily of intermediate susceptibility or resistant to cefamandole.

The cefamandole disk should not be used for testing susceptibility to other cephalosporins.

A bacterial isolate may be considered susceptible if the MIC value for cefamandole[2] is not more than 16 μg/mL. Organisms are considered resistant if the MIC is greater than 32 μg/mL.

INDICATIONS AND USAGE

Mandol® (Cefamandole Nafate, USP, Lilly) is indicated for the treatment of serious infections caused by susceptible strains of the designated microorganisms in the diseases listed below:

Lower respiratory infections, including pneumonia, caused by *S. pneumoniae, H. influenzae, Klebsiella* sp, *S. aureus* (penicillinase- and non-penicillinase-producing), β-hemolytic streptococci, and *P. mirabilis*

Urinary tract infections caused by *E. coli, Proteus* sp (both indole-negative and indole-positive), *Enterobacter* sp, *Klebsiella* sp, group D streptococci (*Note:* Most enterococci, eg, *E. faecalis*, are resistant), and *S. epidermidis*

Peritonitis caused by *E. coli* and *Enterobacter* sp.

Septicemia caused by *E. coli, S. aureus* (penicillinase- and non-penicillinase-producing), *S. pneumoniae, S. pyogenes* (group A β-hemolytic streptococci), *H. influenzae*, and *Klebsiella* sp

Skin and skin structure infections caused by *S. aureus* (penicillinase- and non-penicillinase-producing), *S. pyogenes* (group A β-hemolytic streptococci), *H. influenzae, E. coli, Enterobacter* sp, and *P. mirabilis*

Bone and joint infections caused by *S. aureus* (penicillinase- and non-penicillinase-producing)

Clinical microbiologic studies in nongonococcal pelvic inflammatory disease in females, lower respiratory infections, and skin infections frequently reveal the growth of susceptible strains of both aerobic and anaerobic organisms. Mandol has been used successfully in those infections in which several organisms have been isolated. Most strains of *B. fragilis* are resistant in vitro; however, infections caused by susceptible strains have been treated successfully.

Specimens for bacteriologic cultures should be obtained in order to isolate and identify causative organisms and to determine their susceptibilities to cefamandole. Therapy may be instituted before results of susceptibility studies are known; however, once these results become available, the antibiotic treatment should be adjusted accordingly.

In certain cases of confirmed or suspected gram-positive or gram-negative sepsis or in patients with other serious infections in which the causative organism has not been identified, Mandol may be used concomitantly with an aminoglycoside (*see* Precautions). The recommended doses of both antibiotics may be given, depending on the severity of the infection and the patient's condition. The renal function of the patient should be carefully monitored, especially if higher dosages of the antibiotics are to be administered.

Antibiotic therapy of β-hemolytic streptococcal infections should continue for at least 10 days.

Preventive Therapy—The administration of Mandol preoperatively, intraoperatively, and postoperatively may reduce the incidence of certain postoperative infections in patients undergoing surgical procedures that are classified as contaminated or potentially contaminated (eg, gastrointestinal surgery, cesarean section, vaginal hysterectomy, or cholecystectomy in high-risk patients such as those with acute cholecystitis, obstructive jaundice, or common-bile-duct stones).

In major surgery in which the risk of postoperative infection is low but serious (cardiovascular surgery, neurosurgery, or prosthetic arthroplasty), Mandol may be effective in preventing such infections.

The perioperative use of Mandol should be discontinued after 48 hours; however, in prosthetic arthroplasty, it is recommended that administration be continued for 72 hours. If signs of infection occur, specimens for culture should be obtained for identification of the causative organism so that appropriate antibiotic therapy may be instituted.

CONTRAINDICATION

Mandol® (Cefamandole Nafate, USP, Lilly) is contraindicated in patients with known allergy to the cephalosporin group of antibiotics.

WARNINGS

BEFORE THERAPY WITH MANDOL® (Cefamandole Nafate, USP, Lilly) IS INSTITUTED, CAREFUL INQUIRY SHOULD BE MADE TO DETERMINE WHETHER THE PATIENT HAS HAD PREVIOUS HYPERSENSITIVITY REACTIONS TO CEPHALOSPORINS, PENICILLINS, OR OTHER DRUGS. THIS PRODUCT SHOULD BE GIVEN CAUTIOUSLY TO PENICILLIN-SENSITIVE PATIENTS. ANTIBIOTICS SHOULD BE ADMINISTERED WITH CAUTION TO ANY PATIENT WHO HAS DEMONSTRATED SOME FORM OF ALLERGY, PARTICULARLY TO DRUGS. SERIOUS ACUTE HYPERSENSITIVITY REACTIONS MAY REQUIRE EPINEPHRINE AND OTHER EMERGENCY MEASURES.

In newborn infants, accumulation of other cephalosporin-class antibiotics (with resulting prolongation of drug half-life) has been reported.

Pseudomembranous colitis has been reported with virtually all broad-spectrum antibiotics (including macrolides, semisynthetic penicillins, and cephalosporins); therefore, it is important to consider its diagnosis in patients who develop diarrhea in association with the use of antibiotics. Such colitis may range in severity from mild to life threatening.

Treatment with broad-spectrum antibiotics alters the normal flora of the colon and may permit overgrowth of clostridia. Studies indicate that a toxin produced by *Clostridium difficile* is a primary cause of antibiotic-associated colitis.

---

1. Bauer AW, Kirby WMM, et al: Antibiotic susceptibility testing by a standardized single disk method. *Am J Clin Pathol* 1966;45:493. Standardized disk susceptibility test. *Federal Register* 1974;39:19182–19184. National Committee for Clinical Laboratory Standards. Approved Standard: M2-A3 Performance standards for antimicrobial disk susceptibility tests—Fourth Edition, December, 1988.
2. Determined by the ICS agar-dilution method (Ericsson HM, Sherris JC: *Acta Pathol Microbiol Scand* 1971;[suppl 217]: B), or any other method that has been shown to give equivalent results.

Mild cases of pseudomembranous colitis usually respond to drug discontinuance alone. In moderate to severe cases, management should include sigmoidoscopy, appropriate bacteriologic studies, and fluid, electrolyte, and protein supplementation. When the colitis does not improve after the drug has been discontinued, or when it is severe, oral vancomycin is the drug of choice for antibiotic-associated pseudomembranous colitis produced by *C. difficile.* Other causes of colitis should be ruled out.

PRECAUTIONS

General —Although Mandol® (Cefamandole Nafate, USP, Lilly) rarely produces alteration in kidney function, evaluation of renal status is recommended, especially in seriously ill patients receiving maximum doses.

Prolonged use of Mandol may result in the overgrowth of nonsusceptible organisms. Careful observation of the patient is essential. If superinfection occurs during therapy, appropriate measures should be taken.

Nephrotoxicity has been reported following concomitant administration of aminoglycoside antibiotics and cephalosporins.

A false-positive reaction for glucose in the urine may occur with Benedict's or Fehling's solution or with Clinitest® tablets but not with Tes-Tape® (Glucose Enzymatic Test Strip, USP, Lilly). There may be a false-positive test for proteinuria with acid and denaturization-precipitation tests.

As with other broad-spectrum antibiotics, hypoprothrombinemia, with or without bleeding, has been reported rarely, but it has been promptly reversed by administration of vitamin K. Such episodes usually have occurred in elderly, debilitated, or otherwise compromised patients with deficient stores of vitamin K. Treatment of such individuals with antibiotics possessing significant gram-negative and/or anaerobic activity is thought to alter the number and/or type of intestinal bacterial flora, with consequent reduction in synthesis of vitamin K. Prophylactic administration of vitamin K may be indicated in such patients, especially when intestinal sterilization and surgical procedures are performed.

In a few patients receiving Mandol, nausea, vomiting, and vasomotor instability with hypotension and peripheral vasodilatation occurred following the ingestion of ethanol. Cefamandole inhibits the enzyme acetaldehyde dehydrogenase in laboratory animals. This causes accumulation of acetaldehyde when ethanol is administered concomitantly. Broad-spectrum antibiotics should be prescribed with caution in individuals with a history of gastrointestinal disease, particularly colitis.

Carcinogenesis, Mutagenesis, Impairment of Fertility —Certain β-lactam antibiotics containing the N-methylthiotetrazole side chain have been reported to cause delayed maturity of the testicular germinal epithelium when given to neonatal rats during initial spermatogenic development (6 to 36 days of age). In animals that were treated from 6 to 36 days of age with 1,000 mg/kg/day of cefamandole (approximately 5 times the maximum clinical dose), the delayed maturity was pronounced and was associated with decreased testicular weights and a reduced number of germinal cells in the leading waves of spermatogenic development. The effect was slight in rats given 50 or 100 mg/kg/day. Some animals that were given 1,000 mg/kg/day during days 6 to 36 were infertile after becoming sexually mature. No adverse effects have been observed in rats exposed in utero, in neonatal rats (4 days of age or younger) treated prior to the initiation of spermatogenesis, or in older rats (more than 36 days of age) after exposure for up to 6 months. The significance to man of these findings in rats is unknown because of differences in the time of initiation of spermatogenesis, rate of spermatogenic development, and duration of puberty.

Usage in Pregnancy —*Pregnancy Category B* —Reproduction studies have been performed in rats given doses of 500 or 1,000 mg/kg/day and have revealed no evidence of impaired fertility or harm to the fetus due to Mandol. There are, however, no adequate and well-controlled studies in pregnant women. Because animal reproduction studies are not always predictive of human response, this drug should be used during pregnancy only if clearly needed.

Nursing Mothers —Caution should be exercised when Mandol is administered to a nursing woman.

Usage in Infancy —Mandol has been effectively used in this age group, but all laboratory parameters have not been extensively studied in infants between 1 and 6 months of age; safety of this product has not been established in prematures and infants under 1 month of age. Therefore, if Mandol is administered to infants, the physician should determine whether the potential benefits outweigh the possible risks involved.

ADVERSE REACTIONS

Gastrointestinal —Symptoms of pseudomembranous colitis may appear either during or after antibiotic treatment. Nausea and vomiting have been reported rarely. As with some

MANDOL® (CEFAMANDOLE NAFATE)—MAINTENANCE DOSAGE GUIDE FOR PATIENTS WITH RENAL IMPAIRMENT

Creatinine Clearance (mL/min/1.73 m^2)	Renal Function	Life-Threatening Infections— Maximum Dosage	Less Severe Infections
>80	Normal	2 g q4h	1–2 g q6h
80–50	Mild Impairment	1.5 g q4h OR 2 g q6h	0.75–1.5 g q6h
50–25	Moderate Impairment	1.5 g q6h OR 2 g q8h	0.75–1.5 g q8h
25–10	Severe Impairment	1 g q6h OR 1.25 g q8h	0.5–1 g q8h
10–2	Marked Impairment	0.67 g q8h OR 1 g q12h	0.5–0.75 g q12h
<2	None	0.5 g q8h OR 0.75 g q12h	0.25–0.5 g q12h

penicillins and some other cephalosporins, transient hepatitis and cholestatic jaundice have been reported rarely.

Hypersensitivity —Anaphylaxis, maculopapular rash, urticaria, eosinophilia, and drug fever have been reported. These reactions are more likely to occur in patients with a history of allergy, particularly to penicillin.

Blood —Thrombocytopenia has been reported rarely. Neutropenia has been reported, especially in long courses of treatment. Some individuals have developed positive direct Coombs' tests during treatment with the cephalosporin antibiotics.

Liver —Transient rise in SGOT, SGPT, and alkaline phosphatase levels has been noted.

Kidney —Decreased creatinine clearance has been reported in patients with prior renal impairment. As with some other cephalosporins, transitory elevations of BUN have occasionally been observed with Mandol® (Cefamandole Nafate, USP, Lilly); their frequency increases in patients over 50 years of age. In some of these cases, there was also a mild increase in serum creatinine.

Local Reactions —Pain on intramuscular injection is infrequent. Thrombophlebitis occurs rarely.

OVERDOSAGE

The administration of inappropriately large doses of parenteral cephalosporins may cause seizures, particularly in patients with renal impairment. Dosage reduction is necessary when renal function is impaired (*see* Dosage and Administration). If seizures occur, the drug should be promptly discontinued; anticonvulsant therapy may be administered if clinically indicated. Hemodialysis may be considered in cases of overwhelming overdosage.

DOSAGE AND ADMINISTRATION

Dosage—Adults: The usual dosage range for cefamandole is 500 mg to 1 g every 4 to 8 hours.

In infections of skin structures and in uncomplicated pneumonia, a dosage of 500 mg every 6 hours is adequate.

In uncomplicated urinary tract infections, a dosage of 500 mg every 8 hours is sufficient. In more serious urinary tract infections, a dosage of 1 g every 8 hours may be needed.

In severe infections, 1-g doses may be given at 4 to 6-hour intervals.

In life-threatening infections or infections due to less susceptible organisms, doses up to 2 g every 4 hours (ie, 12 g/day) may be needed.

Infants and Children: Administration of 50 to 100 mg/kg/day in equally divided doses every 4 to 8 hours has been effective for most infections susceptible to Mandol® (Cefamandole Nafate, USP, Lilly). This may be increased to a total daily dose of 150 mg/kg (not to exceed the maximum adult dose) for severe infections. (*See* recommendations regarding this age group in Warnings *and* Precautions.)

Note: As with antibiotic therapy in general, administration of Mandol should be continued for a minimum of 48 to 72 hours after the patient becomes asymptomatic or after evidence of bacterial eradication has been obtained; a minimum of 10 days of treatment is recommended in infections caused by group A β-hemolytic streptococci in order to guard against the risk of rheumatic fever or glomerulonephritis; frequent bacteriologic and clinical appraisal is necessary during therapy of chronic urinary tract infection and may be

required for several months after therapy has been completed; persistent infections may require treatment for several weeks; and doses smaller than those indicated above should not be used.

For perioperative use of Mandol, the following dosages are recommended:

Adults —1 or 2 g intravenously or intramuscularly ½ to 1 hour prior to the surgical incision followed by 1 or 2 g every 6 hours for 24 to 48 hours.

Children (3 months of age and older) —50 to 100 mg/kg/day in equally divided doses by the routes and schedule designated above.

Note: In patients undergoing prosthetic arthroplasty, administration is recommended for as long as 72 hours.

In patients undergoing cesarean section, the initial dose may be administered just prior to surgery or immediately after the cord has been clamped.

Impaired Renal Function —When renal function is impaired, a reduced dosage must be employed and the serum levels closely monitored. After an initial dose of 1 to 2 g (depending on the severity of infection), a maintenance dosage schedule should be followed (see chart). Continued dosage should be determined by degree of renal impairment, severity of infection, and susceptibility of the causative organism. [See table above.]

When only serum creatinine is available, the following formula (based on sex, weight, and age of the patient) may be used to convert this value into creatinine clearance. The serum creatinine should represent a steady state of renal function.

$$\text{Males:} \quad \frac{\text{Weight (kg)} \times (140 - \text{age})}{72 \times \text{serum creatinine}}$$

Females: 0.9 × above value

Modes of Administration —Mandol® (Cefamandole Nafate, USP, Lilly) may be given intravenously or by deep intramuscular injection into a large muscle mass (such as the gluteus or lateral part of the thigh) to minimize pain.

Intramuscular Administration —Each g of Mandol should be diluted with 3 mL of 1 of the following diluents: Sterile Water for Injection, Bacteriostatic Water for Injection, 0.9% Sodium Chloride Injection, or Bacteriostatic Sodium Chloride Injection. Shake well until dissolved.

Intravenous Administration —The intravenous route may be preferable for patients with bacterial septicemia, localized parenchymal abscesses (such as intra-abdominal abscess), peritonitis, or other severe or life-threatening infections when they may be poor risks because of lowered resistance. In those with normal renal function, the intravenous dosage for such infections is 3 to 12 g of Mandol daily. In conditions such as bacterial septicemia, 6 to 12 g/day may be given initially by the intravenous route for several days, and dosage may then be gradually reduced according to clinical response and laboratory findings.

Continued on next page

* Identi-Code® symbol. This product information was prepared in June 1992. Current information on these and other products of Eli Lilly and Company may be obtained by direct inquiry to Lilly Research Laboratories, Lilly Corporate Center, Indianapolis, Indiana 46285, (317) 276-3714.

Lilly—Cont.

If combination therapy with Mandol and an aminoglycoside is indicated, each of these antibiotics should be administered in different sites. *Do not mix an aminoglycoside with Mandol in the same intravenous fluid container.*

A SOLUTION OF 1 G OF MANDOL IN 22 ML OF STERILE WATER FOR INJECTION IS ISOTONIC.

The choice of saline, dextrose, or electrolyte solution and the volume to be employed are dictated by fluid and electrolyte management.

For direct intermittent intravenous administration, each g of cefamandole should be reconstituted with 10 mL of Sterile Water for Injection, 5% Dextrose Injection, or 0.9% Sodium Chloride Injection. Slowly inject the solution into the vein over a period of 3 to 5 minutes, or give it through the tubing of an administration set while the patient is also receiving one of the following intravenous fluids: 0.9% Sodium Chloride Injection; 5% Dextrose Injection; 10% Dextrose Injection; 5% Dextrose and 0.9% Sodium Chloride Injection; 5% Dextrose and 0.45% Sodium Chloride Injection; 5% Dextrose and 0.2% Sodium Chloride Injection; or Sodium Lactate Injection (M/6).

Intermittent intravenous infusion with a Y-type administration set or volume control set can also be accomplished while any of the above-mentioned intravenous fluids are being infused. However, during infusion of the solution containing Mandol, it is desirable to discontinue the other solution. When this technique is employed, careful attention should be paid to the volume of the solution containing Mandol so that the calculated dose will be infused. When a Y-tube hookup is used, 100 mL of the appropriate diluent should be added to the 1- or 2-g piggyback (100-mL) vial. If Sterile Water for Injection is used as the diluent, reconstitute with approximately 20 mL/g to avoid a hypotonic solution.

For continuous intravenous infusion, each g of cefamandole should be diluted with 10 mL of Sterile Water for Injection. An appropriate quantity of the resulting solution may be added to an IV bottle containing 1 of the following fluids: 0.9% Sodium Chloride Injection; 5% Dextrose Injection; 10% Dextrose Injection; 5% Dextrose and 0.9% Sodium Chloride Injection; 5% Dextrose and 0.45% Sodium Chloride Injection; 5% Dextrose and 0.2% Sodium Chloride Injection; or Sodium Lactate Injection (M/6).

STABILITY

Reconstituted Mandol® (Cefamandole Nafate, USP, Lilly) is stable for 24 hours at room temperature (25°C) and for 96 hours if stored under refrigeration (5°C). *During storage at room temperature, carbon dioxide develops inside the vial after reconstitution. This pressure may be dissipated prior to withdrawal of the vial contents, or it may be used to aid withdrawal if the vial is inverted over the syringe needle and the contents are allowed to flow into the syringe.*

Solutions of Mandol in Sterile Water for Injection, 5% Dextrose Injection, or 0.9% Sodium Chloride Injection that are frozen immediately after reconstitution in Faspak containers and the conventional vials in which the drugs are supplied are stable for 6 months when stored at −20°C. **If the product is warmed (to a maximum of 37°C), care should be taken to avoid heating it after the thawing is complete. Once thawed, the solution should not be refrozen.**

HOW SUPPLIED

(℞) Vials (Dry Powder):
500 mg,* 10-mL size (No. 7060)—(Traypak† of 25) NDC 0002-7060-25
1 g,* 10-mL size (No. 7061)—(Traypak of 25) NDC 0002-7061-25
1 g,* 100-mL size (No. 7068)—(Traypak of 10) NDC 0002-7068-10
2 g,* 20-mL (No. 7064)—(Traypak of 10) NDC 0002-7064-10
2 g,* 100-mL size (No. 7069)—(Traypak of 10) NDC 0002-7069-10
(℞) Faspak‡:
1 g* (No. 7208)—(Faspak of 96) NDC 0002-7208-74
2 g* (No. 7209)—(Faspak of 96) NDC 0002-7209-74
(℞) ADD-Vantage§ Vials:
1 g* (No. 7268)—(Traypak of 25) NDC 0002-7268-25
2 g* (No. 7269)—(Traypak of 10) NDC 0002-7269-10

The above ADD-Vantage Vials are to be used only with Abbott Laboratories' ADD-Vantage Diluent Containers. Instructions for use of the ADD-Vantage Vials are enclosed in the package.

Also Available:
(℞) Pharmacy Bulk Package:
10 g,* 100-mL size (No. 7072)—(Traypak of 6) NDC 0002-7072-16

---

*Equivalent to cefamandole activity.
†Traypak™ (multivial carton, Lilly).
‡Faspak® (flexible plastic bag, Lilly).
§ADD-Vantage® (vials and diluent containers, Abbott).

[031390]

METHADONE HYDROCHLORIDE Ⓒ

[mĕth 'ă-dōn hī-drō- klō-rīd]
DISKETS® (dispersible tablets, Lilly)
Tablets, USP
(See also **Dolophine® Hydrochloride)**

CONDITIONS FOR DISTRIBUTION AND USE OF METHADONE PRODUCTS:
Code of Federal Regulations,
Title 21, Sec. 291.505

METHADONE PRODUCTS, WHEN USED FOR THE TREATMENT OF NARCOTIC ADDICTION IN DETOXIFICATION OR MAINTENANCE PROGRAMS, SHALL BE DISPENSED ONLY BY APPROVED HOSPITAL PHARMACIES, APPROVED COMMUNITY PHARMACIES, AND MAINTENANCE PROGRAMS APPROVED BY THE FOOD AND DRUG ADMINISTRATION AND THE DESIGNATED STATE AUTHORITY.

APPROVED MAINTENANCE PROGRAMS SHALL DISPENSE AND USE METHADONE IN ORAL FORM ONLY AND ACCORDING TO THE TREATMENT REQUIREMENTS STIPULATED IN THE FEDERAL METHADONE REGULATIONS (21 CFR 291.505).

FAILURE TO ABIDE BY THE REQUIREMENTS IN THESE REGULATIONS MAY RESULT IN CRIMINAL PROSECUTION, SEIZURE OF THE DRUG SUPPLY, REVOCATION OF THE PROGRAM APPROVAL, AND INJUNCTION PRECLUDING OPERATION OF THE PROGRAM.

DESCRIPTION

Methadone Hydrochloride, USP, Lilly, (3-heptanone, 6-(dimethylamino)-4,4-diphenyl-, hydrochloride), is a white, crystalline material that is water soluble. However, the Disket® preparation of methadone hydrochloride has been specially formulated with insoluble excipients to deter the use of this drug by injection. Its molecular weight is 345.91.

Each Disket contains 40 mg (0.116 mmol) methadone hydrochloride. Each tablet also contains cellulose, FD&C Yellow No. 6, flavors, magnesium stearate, potassium phosphate, silicon dioxide, cornstarch, and stearic acid.

ACTIONS

Methadone hydrochloride is a synthetic narcotic analgesic with multiple actions quantitatively similar to those of morphine, the most prominent of which involve the central nervous system and organs composed of smooth muscle. The principal actions of therapeutic value are analgesia and sedation and detoxification or maintenance in narcotic addiction. The methadone abstinence syndrome, although qualitatively similar to that of morphine, differs in that the onset is slower, the course is more prolonged, and the symptoms are less severe.

When administered orally, methadone is approximately one-half as potent as when given parenterally. Oral administration results in a delay of the onset, a lowering of the peak, and an increase in the duration of analgesic effect.

INDICATIONS

1. Detoxification treatment of narcotic addiction (heroin or other morphine-like drugs).
2. Maintenance treatment of narcotic addiction (heroin or other morphine-like drugs), in conjunction with appropriate social and medical services.

NOTE

If methadone is administered for treatment of heroin dependence for more than 3 weeks, the procedure passes from treatment of the acute withdrawal syndrome (detoxification) to maintenance therapy. Maintenance treatment is permitted to be undertaken only by approved methadone programs. This does not preclude the maintenance treatment of an addict who is hospitalized for medical conditions other than addiction and who requires temporary maintenance during the critical period of his/her stay or whose enrollment has been verified in a program approved for maintenance treatment with methadone.

CONTRAINDICATION

Hypersensitivity to methadone.

WARNINGS

Diskets Methadone Hydrochloride are for oral administration only. This preparation contains insoluble excipients and therefore *must not* be injected. It is recommended that Diskets Methadone Hydrochloride, if dispensed, be packaged in child-resistant containers and kept out of the reach of children to prevent accidental ingestion.

Methadone hydrochloride, a narcotic, is a Schedule II controlled substance under the Federal Controlled Substances Act. Appropriate security measures should be taken to safeguard stocks of methadone against diversion.

DRUG DEPENDENCE—**METHADONE CAN PRODUCE DRUG DEPENDENCE OF THE MORPHINE TYPE AND, THEREFORE, HAS THE POTENTIAL FOR BEING ABUSED. PSYCHIC DEPENDENCE, PHYSICAL DEPENDENCE, AND TOLERANCE MAY DEVELOP ON REPEATED ADMINISTRATION OF METHADONE, AND IT SHOULD BE PRESCRIBED AND ADMINISTERED WITH THE SAME DEGREE OF CAUTION APPROPRIATE TO THE USE OF MORPHINE.**

Interaction With Other Central Nervous-System Depressants—Methadone should be used with caution and in reduced dosage in patients who are concurrently receiving other narcotic analgesics, general anesthetics, phenothiazines, other tranquilizers, sedative-hypnotics, tricyclic antidepressants, and other CNS depressants (including alcohol). Respiratory depression, hypotension, and profound sedation or coma may result.

Anxiety—Since methadone, as used by tolerant subjects at a constant maintenance dosage, is not a tranquilizer, patients who are maintained on this drug will react to life problems and stresses with the same symptoms of anxiety as do other individuals. The physician should not confuse such symptoms with those of narcotic abstinence and should not attempt to treat anxiety by increasing the dosage of methadone. The action of methadone in maintenance treatment is limited to the control of narcotic symptoms and is ineffective for relief of general anxiety.

Head Injury and Increased Intracranial Pressure—The respiratory depressant effects of methadone and its capacity to elevate cerebrospinal-fluid pressure may be markedly exaggerated in the presence of increased intracranial pressure. Furthermore, narcotics produce side effects that may obscure the clinical course of patients with head injuries. In such patients, methadone must be used with caution and only if it is deemed essential.

Asthma and Other Respiratory Conditions—Methadone should be used with caution in patients having an acute asthmatic attack, in those with chronic obstructive pulmonary disease or cor pulmonale, and in individuals with a substantially decreased respiratory reserve, preexisting respiratory depression, hypoxia, or hypercapnia. In such patients, even usual therapeutic doses of narcotics may decrease respiratory drive while simultaneously increasing airway resistance to the point of apnea.

Hypotensive Effect—The administration of methadone may result in severe hypotension in an individual whose ability to maintain normal blood pressure has already been compromised by a depleted blood volume or concurrent administration of such drugs as the phenothiazines or certain anesthetics.

Use in Ambulatory Patients—Methadone may impair the mental and/or physical abilities required for the performance of potentially hazardous tasks, such as driving a car or operating machinery. The patient should be cautioned accordingly.

Methadone, like other narcotics, may produce orthostatic hypotension in ambulatory patients.

Use in Pregnancy—Safe use in pregnancy has not been established in relation to possible adverse effects on fetal development. Therefore, methadone should not be used in pregnant women unless, in the judgment of the physician, the potential benefits outweigh the possible hazards.

PRECAUTIONS

Drug Interactions:

Pentazocine—**Patients who are addicted to heroin or who are on the methadone maintenance program may experience withdrawal symptoms when given an opioid agonist-antagonist, such as pentazocine.**

Rifampin—The concurrent administration of rifampin may possibly reduce the blood concentration of methadone to a degree sufficient to produce withdrawal symptoms. The mechanism by which rifampin may decrease blood concentrations of methadone is not fully understood, although enhanced microsomal drug-metabolized enzymes may influence drug disposition.

Monoamine Oxidase (MAO) Inhibitors—Therapeutic doses of meperidine have precipitated severe reactions in patients concurrently receiving monoamine oxidase inhibitors or those who have received such agents within 14 days. Similar reactions thus far have not been reported with methadone; but if the use of methadone is necessary in such patients, a sensitivity test should be performed in which repeated small incremental doses are administered over the course of several hours while the patient's condition and vital signs are under careful observation.

Desipramine—Blood levels of desipramine have increased with concurrent methadone therapy.

Special-Risk Patients—Methadone should be given with caution and the initial dose should be reduced in certain patients, such as the elderly or debilitated and those with severe impairment of hepatic or renal function, hypothyroid-

ism, Addison's disease, prostatic hypertrophy, or urethral stricture.
Acute Abdominal Conditions—The administration of methadone or other narcotics may obscure the diagnosis or clinical course in patients with acute abdominal conditions.

ADVERSE REACTIONS

Heroin Withdrawal—During the induction phase of methadone maintenance treatment, patients are being withdrawn from heroin and may therefore show typical withdrawal symptoms, which should be differentiated from methadone-induced side effects. They may exhibit some or all of the following symptoms associated with acute withdrawal from heroin or other opiates: lacrimation, rhinorrhea, sneezing, yawning, excessive perspiration, goose-flesh, fever, chilliness alternating with flushing, restlessness, irritability, "sleepy yen," weakness, anxiety, depression, dilated pupils, tremors, tachycardia, abdominal cramps, body aches, involuntary twitching and kicking movements, anorexia, nausea, vomiting, diarrhea, intestinal spasms, and weight loss.
Initial Administration—Initially, the dosage of methadone should be carefully titrated to the individual. Induction too rapid for the patient's sensitivity is more likely to produce the following effects.
THE MAJOR HAZARDS OF METHADONE, AS OF OTHER NARCOTIC ANALGESICS, ARE RESPIRATORY DEPRESSION AND, TO A LESSER DEGREE, CIRCULATORY DEPRESSION. RESPIRATORY ARREST, SHOCK, AND CARDIAC ARREST HAVE OCCURRED.
The most frequently observed adverse reactions include lightheadedness, dizziness, sedation, nausea, vomiting, and sweating. These effects seem to be more prominent in ambulatory patients and in those who are not suffering severe pain. In such individuals, lower doses are advisable. Some adverse reactions may be alleviated if the ambulatory patient lies down.
Other adverse reactions include the following:
Central Nervous System—Euphoria, dysphoria, weakness, headache, insomnia, agitation, disorientation, and visual disturbances.
Gastrointestinal—Dry mouth, anorexia, constipation, and biliary tract spasm.
Cardiovascular—Flushing of the face, bradycardia, palpitation, faintness, and syncope.
Genitourinary—Urinary retention or hesitancy, antidiuretic effect, and reduced libido and/or potency.
Allergic—Pruritus, urticaria, other skin rashes, edema, and, rarely, hemorrhagic urticaria.
Hematologic—Reversible thrombocytopenia has been described in a narcotics addict with chronic hepatitis.
Maintenance on a Stabilized Dose—During prolonged administration of methadone, as in a methadone maintenance treatment program, there is a gradual, yet progressive, disappearance of side effects over a period of several weeks. However, constipation and sweating often persist.

OVERDOSAGE

Signs and Symptoms—Methadone is an opioid and produces effects similar to those of morphine. Symptoms of overdose begin within seconds after intravenous administration and within minutes of nasal, oral, or rectal administration. Prominent symptoms are miosis, respiratory depression, somnolence, coma, cool clammy skin, skeletal muscle flaccidity that may progress to hypotension, apnea, bradycardia, and death. Noncardiac pulmonary edema may occur and monitoring of heart filling pressures may be helpful.
Treatment—To obtain up-to-date information about the treatment of overdose, a good resource is your certified Regional Poison Control Center. Telephone numbers of certified poison control centers are listed in the *Physicians' Desk Reference (PDR)*. In managing overdosage, consider the possibility of multiple drug overdoses, interaction among drugs, and unusual drug kinetics in your patient.
Initial management of opioid overdose should include establishment of a secure airway and support of ventilation and perfusion. Naloxone may be given to antagonize opioid effects, but the airway must be secured as vomiting may ensue. **The duration of methadone effect is much longer (36 to 48 hours) than the duration of naloxone effect (1 to 3 hours), and repeated doses (or continuous intravenous infusion) of naloxone may be required.**
If the patient has chronically abused opioids, administration of naloxone may precipitate a withdrawal syndrome that may include yawning, tearing, restlessness, sweating, dilated pupils, piloerection, vomiting, diarrhea, and abdominal cramps. If these symptoms develop, they should abate quickly as the effects of naloxone dissipate.
If methadone has been taken by mouth, protect the patient's airway and support ventilation and perfusion. Meticulously monitor and maintain, within acceptable limits, the patient's vital signs, blood gases, serum electrolytes, etc. Absorption of drugs from the gastrointestinal tract may be decreased by giving activated charcoal, which, in many cases, is more effective than emesis or lavage; consider charcoal instead of or in addition to gastric emptying. Repeated doses of charcoal over time may hasten elimination of some drugs that have been absorbed. Safeguard the patient's airway when employing gastric emptying or charcoal.
Forced diuresis, peritoneal dialysis, hemodialysis, or charcoal hemoperfusion have not been established as beneficial for an overdose of methadone.

> NOTE: IN AN INDIVIDUAL PHYSICALLY DEPENDENT ON NARCOTICS, THE ADMINISTRATION OF THE USUAL DOSE OF A NARCOTIC ANTAGONIST WILL PRECIPITATE AN ACUTE WITHDRAWAL SYNDROME. THE SEVERITY OF THIS SYNDROME WILL DEPEND ON THE DEGREE OF PHYSICAL DEPENDENCE AND THE DOSE OF THE ANTAGONIST ADMINISTERED. THE USE OF A NARCOTIC ANTAGONIST IN SUCH A PERSON SHOULD BE AVOIDED IF POSSIBLE. IF IT MUST BE USED TO TREAT SERIOUS RESPIRATORY DEPRESSION IN THE PHYSICALLY DEPENDENT PATIENT, THE ANTAGONIST SHOULD BE ADMINISTERED WITH EXTREME CARE AND BY TITRATION WITH SMALLER THAN USUAL DOSES OF THE ANTAGONIST.

DOSAGE AND ADMINISTRATION

For Detoxification Treatment—THE DRUG SHALL BE ADMINISTERED DAILY UNDER CLOSE SUPERVISION AS FOLLOWS:
A detoxification treatment course shall not exceed 21 days and may not be repeated earlier than 4 weeks after completion of the preceding course.
In detoxification, the patient may receive methadone when there are significant symptoms of withdrawal. The dosage schedules indicated below are recommended but could be varied in accordance with clinical judgment. Initially, a single oral dose of 15 to 20 mg of methadone will often be sufficient to suppress withdrawal symptoms. Additional methadone may be provided if withdrawal symptoms are not suppressed or if symptoms reappear. When patients are physically dependent on high doses, it may be necessary to exceed these levels. Forty mg/day in single or divided doses will usually constitute an adequate stabilizing dosage level. Stabilization can be continued for 2 to 3 days, and then the amount of methadone normally will be gradually decreased. The rate at which methadone is decreased will be determined separately for each patient. The dose of methadone can be decreased on a daily basis or at 2-day intervals, but the amount of intake shall always be sufficient to keep withdrawal symptoms at a tolerable level. In hospitalized patients, a daily reduction of 20% of the total daily dose may be tolerated and may cause little discomfort. In ambulatory patients, a somewhat slower schedule may be needed. If methadone is administered for more than 3 weeks, the procedure is considered to have progressed from detoxification or treatment of the acute withdrawal syndrome to maintenance treatment, even though the goal and intent may be eventual total withdrawal.
For Maintenance Treatment—In maintenance treatment, the initial dosage of methadone should control the abstinence symptoms that follow withdrawal of narcotic drugs but should not be so great as to cause sedation, respiratory depression, or other effects of acute intoxication. It is important that the initial dosage be adjusted on an individual basis to the narcotic tolerance of the new patient. If such a patient has been a heavy user of heroin up to the day of admission, he/she may be given 20 mg 4 to 8 hours later or 40 mg in a single oral dose. If the patient enters treatment with little or no narcotic tolerance (eg, if he/she has recently been released from jail or other confinement), the initial dosage may be one half these quantities. When there is any doubt, the smaller dose should be used initially. The patient should then be kept under observation, and, if symptoms of abstinence are distressing, additional 10-mg doses may be administered as needed. Subsequently, the dosage should be adjusted individually, as tolerated and required, up to a level of 120 mg daily. The patient will initially ingest the drug under observation daily, or at least 6 days a week, for the first 3 months. After demonstrating satisfactory adherence to the program regulations for at least 3 months, the patient may be permitted to reduce to 3 times weekly the occasions when he/she must ingest the drug under observation. The patient shall receive no more than a 2-day take-home supply. With continuing adherence to the program's requirements for at least 2 years, he/she may then be permitted twice-weekly visits to the program for drug ingestion under observation, with a 3-day take-home supply. A daily dose of 120 mg or more shall be justified in the medical record. Prior approval from state authority and the Food and Drug Administration is required for any dose above 120 mg administered at the clinic and for any dose above 100 mg to be taken at home. A regular review of dosage level should be made by the responsible physician, with careful consideration given to reduction of dosage as indicated on an individual basis. A new dosage level is only a test level until stability is achieved.
Special Considerations for a Pregnant Patient—Caution shall be taken in the maintenance treatment of pregnant patients. Dosage levels shall be kept as low as possible if continued methadone treatment is deemed necessary. It is the responsibility of the program sponsor to assure that each female patient be fully informed concerning the possible risks to a pregnant woman or her unborn child from the use of methadone.
Special Limitations—
Treatment of Patients under Age 18
1. The safety and effectiveness of methadone for use in the treatment of adolescents have not been proved by adequate clinical study. Special procedures are therefore necessary to assure that patients under age 16 will not be admitted to a program and that patients between 16 and 18 years of age will be admitted to maintenance treatment only under limited conditions.
2. Patients between 16 and 18 years of age who were enrolled and under treatment in approved programs on December 15, 1972, may continue in maintenance treatment. No new patients between 16 and 18 years of age may be admitted to a maintenance treatment program after March 15, 1973, unless a parent, legal guardian, or responsible adult designated by the state authority completes and signs Form FD 2635, "Consent for Methadone Treatment."
Methadone treatment of new patients between the ages of 16 and 18 years will be permitted after December 15, 1972, only with a documented history of 2 or more unsuccessful attempts at detoxification and a documented history of dependence on heroin or other morphine-like drugs beginning 2 years or more prior to application for treatment. No patient under age 16 may be continued or started on methadone treatment after December 15, 1972, but these patients may be detoxified and retained in the program in a drug-free state for follow-up and aftercare.
3. Patients under age 18 who are not placed on maintenance treatment may be detoxified. Detoxification may not exceed 3 weeks. A repeat episode of detoxification may not be initiated until 4 weeks after the completion of the previous detoxification.

HOW SUPPLIED

(Ⓒ) Diskets*:
40 mg (peach-colored, cross-scored) (No. 1)—(100s) NDC 0002-2153-02
Store at controlled room temperature, 59° to 86°F (15° to 30°C).

*Diskets® (dispersible tablets, Lilly)

[052891]

Shown in Product Identification Section, page 416

METUBINE® IODIDE ℞

[*mĕ-tū′bēn ī-ō-dīd*]
(Metocurine Iodide Injection, USP)

THIS DRUG SHOULD BE ADMINISTERED ONLY BY ADEQUATELY TRAINED INDIVIDUALS WHO ARE FAMILIAR WITH ITS ACTIONS, CHARACTERISTICS, AND HAZARDS.

DESCRIPTION

Metubine® Iodide (Metocurine Iodide Injection, USP, Lilly) is a nondepolarizing muscle relaxant and is presented as a sterile isotonic solution for intravenous injection. It is (+)-*O*, *O′*-dimethylchondrocurarine diiodide.
The empirical formula is $C_{40}H_{48}I_2N_2O_6$, and the molecular weight is 906.64.
Each mL contains 2 mg (2.2 μmol) metocurine iodide and sodium chloride, 0.9%, with 0.5% phenol as a preservative. Sodium carbonate and/or hydrochloric acid may have been added during manufacture to adjust the pH in the range of 4 to 4.3.

CLINICAL PHARMACOLOGY

Metubine® Iodide (Metocurine Iodide Injection, USP, Lilly) is a methyl analogue of tubocurarine which produces nondepolarizing (competitive) neuromuscular blockade at the myoneural junction. Recent animal studies suggest that Metubine Iodide does not produce the autonomic ganglionic blockade seen with other nondepolarizing muscle relaxants. Recent clinical findings suggest that Metubine Iodide reaches the neuromuscular junction more rapidly than does tubocurarine. After intravenous injection, there is rapid onset (1 to 4 minutes) of muscle relaxation with maximum twitch inhibition (96%) in 1.5 to 10 minutes. The maximum effect lasts 35 to 60 minutes. The time for recovery to 50% of control twitch response is in excess of 3 hours.
Following bolus injection of 0.05 mg/kg, the mean terminal half-life of Metubine Iodide was 3.6 hours (217 minutes). Approximately 50% of the dose was excreted as unchanged drug in the urine over 48 hours, and 2% was excreted un-

Continued on next page

*** Identi-Code® symbol. This product information was prepared in June 1992. Current information on these and other products of Eli Lilly and Company may be obtained by direct inquiry to Lilly Research Laboratories, Lilly Corporate Center, Indianapolis, Indiana 46285, (317) 276-3714.**

Lilly—Cont.

changed in the bile. Approximately 35% is protein bound, mainly to the beta and gamma globulins.

The use of repeated doses may be accompanied by a cumulative effect. The duration of action and degree of muscle relaxation may be altered by dehydration, body temperature changes, hypocalcemia, excess magnesium, or acid-base imbalance. Concurrently administered general anesthetics, certain antibiotics, and neuromuscular disease may potentiate the neuromuscular blocking action of Metubine Iodide. Histamine release with Metubine Iodide occurs less frequently than with d-tubocurarine and is related to dosage and rapidity of administration. Effects on the cardiovascular system (eg, changes in pulse rate, hypotension) are less than those reported with equipotent doses of d-tubocurarine and gallamine.

Because the main excretory pathway for Metubine Iodide is through the kidneys, severe renal disease or conditions associated with poor renal perfusion (shock states) may result in prolonged neuromuscular blockade.

Following intravenous injection in the mother, placental transfer of Metubine Iodide occurs rapidly, and, after 6 minutes, the fetal plasma concentration is approximately one-tenth the maternal level.

INDICATIONS AND USAGE

Metubine® Iodide (Metocurine Iodide Injection, USP, Lilly) is indicated as an adjunct to anesthesia to induce skeletal-muscle relaxation. It may be employed to reduce the intensity of muscle contractions in pharmacologically or electrically induced convulsions. It may also be employed to facilitate the management of patients undergoing mechanical ventilation.

CONTRAINDICATIONS

Metubine® Iodide (Metocurine Iodide Injection, USP, Lilly) is contraindicated in those persons with known hypersensitivity to the drug or to its iodide content.

WARNINGS

METUBINE® IODIDE (METOCURINE IODIDE INJECTION, USP, LILLY) SHOULD BE ADMINISTERED IN CAREFULLY ADJUSTED DOSES BY OR UNDER THE SUPERVISION OF EXPERIENCED CLINICIANS WHO ARE FAMILIAR WITH THE COMPLICATIONS WHICH MAY OCCUR WITH THE USE OF THIS DRUG. Metubine Iodide should not be administered unless facilities for intubation, artificial ventilation, oxygen therapy, and reversal agents are immediately available. The clinician must be prepared to assist or control respiration.

Metubine Iodide should be used with extreme caution in patients with myasthenia gravis. In such patients, a peripheral nerve stimulator may be valuable in assessing the effects of administration.

PRECAUTIONS

General—Metubine® Iodide (Metocurine Iodide Injection, USP, Lilly) should be used with caution in patients with poor renal perfusion or severe renal disease (see Clinical Pharmacology).

Rapid administration of large doses of Metubine Iodide may produce changes in blood pressure or heart rate or signs of histamine release.

Metubine Iodide has no effect on consciousness, pain threshold, or cerebration; therefore, it should be used with adequate anesthesia.

Drug Interactions—Synergistic or antagonistic effects may result when depolarizing and nondepolarizing muscle relaxants are administered simultaneously or sequentially.

Parenteral administration of high doses of certain antibiotics may intensify or resemble the neuroblocking action of muscle relaxants. These include neomycin, streptomycin, bacitracin, kanamycin, gentamicin, dihydrostreptomycin, polymyxin B, colistin, sodium colistimethate, and tetracyclines. If muscle relaxants and antibiotics must be administered simultaneously, the patient should be observed closely for any unexpected prolongation of respiratory depression.

Certain general anesthetics have a synergistic action with neuromuscular blocking agents. Diethyl ether, halothane, and isoflurane potentiate the neuromuscular blocking action of other nondepolarizing agents and may be presumed to do so with Metubine Iodide.

Administration of quinidine shortly after recovery may produce recurrent paralysis.

The effect of diazepam on neuromuscular blockade by Metubine Iodide is not clear. Until more information is available, patients should be carefully monitored for unexpected drug response and prolongation of action.

The use of magnesium sulfate in preeclamptic patients potentiates the effects of both depolarizing and nondepolarizing muscle relaxants.

Usage in Pregnancy—Pregnancy Category C—Intrauterine growth retardation and limb deformities resembling club-foot were produced by d-tubocurarine chloride and succinylcholine chloride when administered to the rat fetus between the 16th and 19th days of gestation or when injected in chick embryos from the 5th to the 15th day of incubation. When d-tubocurarine was injected intramuscularly into the interscapular region of the fetuses on the 16th to the 19th day of gestation, the incidence of growth retardation and limb deformity ranged from 21 to 23% and 7 to 8% respectively. There are no adequate and well-controlled studies of Metubine Iodide in pregnant women. Metubine Iodide should be used during pregnancy only if the potential benefit justifies the risk to the fetus.

Labor and Delivery—It is not known whether the use of muscle relaxants during labor or delivery has immediate or delayed adverse effects on the fetus, prolongs the duration of labor, or increases the likelihood that forceps delivery, obstetric intervention, or resuscitation of the newborn will be necessary.

Nursing Mothers—It is not known whether Metubine Iodide is excreted in human milk. Because many drugs are excreted in human milk, caution should be exercised when Metubine Iodide is administered to a nursing woman.

Usage in Children—A clinical study has shown that Metubine Iodide is twice as potent as d-tubocurarine in children, but the rate of recovery is the same. There may be a slight increase in heart rate, but no change occurs in blood pressure or ECG. Doses calculated on the basis of body weight or body surface area may be applicable when the advantages of nondepolarizing neuromuscular blockade are desired.

ADVERSE REACTIONS

The most frequently noted adverse reaction is prolongation of the drug's pharmacologic action. Neuromuscular effects may range from skeletal-muscle weakness to a profound relaxation that produces respiratory insufficiency or apnea. Possible adverse reactions include allergic or hypersensitivity reactions to the drug or its iodide content and histamine release when large doses are administered rapidly. Signs of histamine release include erythema, edema, flushing, tachycardia, arterial hypotension, bronchospasm, and circulatory collapse.

Prolonged apnea and respiratory depression have occurred following the use of muscle relaxants. Many physiologic factors, drug interactions, and individual sensitivities may contribute to the development of respiratory paralysis (see Clinical Pharmacology and Precautions).

OVERDOSAGE

To obtain up-to-date information about the treatment of overdose, a good resource is your certified Regional Poison Control Center. Telephone numbers of certified poison control centers are listed in the *Physicians' Desk Reference (PDR)*. In managing overdosage, consider the possibility of multiple drug overdoses, interaction among drugs, and unusual drug kinetics in your patient.

An overdose of Metubine® Iodide (Metocurine Iodide Injection, USP, Lilly) may result in prolonged apnea, cardiovascular collapse, and sudden release of histamine.

Massive doses of metocurarine are not reversible by the antagonists edrophonium or neostigmine and atropine.

Overdosage may be avoided by the careful monitoring of response by means of a peripheral nerve stimulator.

The primary treatment for residual neuromuscular blockade with respiratory paralysis or inadequate ventilation is maintenance of the patient's airway and manual or mechanical ventilation.

Accompanying derangements of blood pressure, electrolyte imbalance, or circulating blood volume should be determined and corrected by appropriate fluid and electrolyte therapy.

Residual neuromuscular blockade following surgery may be reversed by the use of anticholinesterase inhibitors such as neostigmine or pyridostigmine bromide and atropine. Prescribing information should be consulted for the appropriate drug selection based on dosage and desired duration of action.

DOSAGE AND ADMINISTRATION

Metubine® Iodide (Metocurine Iodide Injection, USP, Lilly) should be administered intravenously as a sustained injection over a period of 30 to 60 seconds. INTRAMUSCULAR ADMINISTRATION OF METUBINE IODIDE IS NOT RECOMMENDED. Care must be taken to avoid overdosage. The use of a peripheral nerve stimulator to monitor response will minimize the risk of overdosage. The type of anesthetic used and nature of the surgical procedure will influence the amount of Metubine Iodide required. Doses of 0.2 to 0.4 mg/kg have been found satisfactory for endotracheal intubation. Relaxation following the initial dose may be expected to be effective for periods of 25 to 90 minutes, with an average of approximately 60 minutes. Supplemental administration may be made as indicated to provide needed surgical relaxation. Supplemental doses average 0.5 to 1 mg. The use of strong anesthetics that potentiate the effect of neuromuscular blocking drugs such as halothane, diethyl ether, isoflurane, or enflurane reduces the requirement for Metubine Iodide. Incremental doses should be reduced by approximately one-third to one-half.

Recommended Doses for Use During Electroshock Therapy—Doses required for satisfactory relaxation range from 1.75 to 5.5 mg. When the patient is treated for the 1st time, the drug is administered slowly by the intravenous route as a sustained injection until a head-drop response ensues. After dosage has been established, subsequent injections are completed in 15 to 50 seconds. The average dose ranges from 2 to 3 mg.

Drug Incompatibilities—Metubine Iodide is unstable in alkaline solutions. When it is combined with barbiturate solutions, precipitation may occur. Solutions of barbiturates, meperidine, and morphine sulfate should not be administered from the same syringe.

Parenteral drug products should be inspected visually for particulate matter and discoloration prior to administration, whenever solution and container permit.

HOW SUPPLIED

(℞) Multiple-Dose Vials:
2 mg/mL, 20 mL (No. 586) (1s), NDC 0002-1421-01
Store at controlled room temperature, 59° to 86°F (15° to 30°C).
Metubine Iodide is a clear, colorless solution.

[032690]

NEBCIN®   ℞
[*nĕb'sĭn*]
(Tobramycin Sulfate Injection, USP)

> ### WARNINGS
> Patients treated with Nebcin® (Tobramycin Sulfate Injection, USP, Lilly) and other aminoglycosides should be under close clinical observation, because these drugs have an inherent potential for causing ototoxicity and nephrotoxicity.
>
> Neurotoxicity, manifested as both auditory and vestibular ototoxicity, can occur. The auditory changes are irreversible, are usually bilateral, and may be partial or total. Eighth-nerve impairment and nephrotoxicity may develop, primarily in patients having preexisting renal damage and in those with normal renal function to whom aminoglycosides are administered for longer periods or in higher doses than those recommended. Other manifestations of neurotoxicity may include numbness, skin tingling, muscle twitching, and convulsions. The risk of aminoglycoside-induced hearing loss increases with the degree of exposure to either high peak or high trough serum concentrations. Patients who develop cochlear damage may not have symptoms during therapy to warn them of eighth-nerve toxicity, and partial or total irreversible bilateral deafness may continue to develop after the drug has been discontinued.
>
> Rarely, nephrotoxicity may not become apparent until the first few days after cessation of therapy. Aminoglycoside-induced nephrotoxicity usually is reversible. Renal and eighth-nerve function should be closely monitored in patients with known or suspected renal impairment and also in those whose renal function is initially normal but who develop signs of renal dysfunction during therapy. Peak and trough serum concentrations of aminoglycosides should be monitored periodically during therapy to assure adequate levels and to avoid potentially toxic levels. Prolonged serum concentrations above 12 μg/mL should be avoided. Rising trough levels (above 2 μg/mL) may indicate tissue accumulation. Such accumulation, excessive peak concentrations, advanced age, and cumulative dose may contribute to ototoxicity and nephrotoxicity (see Precautions). Urine should be examined for decreased specific gravity and increased excretion of protein, cells, and casts. Blood urea nitrogen, serum creatinine, and creatinine clearance should be measured periodically. When feasible, it is recommended that serial audiograms be obtained in patients old enough to be tested, particularly high-risk patients. Evidence of impairment of renal, vestibular, or auditory function requires discontinuation of the drug or dosage adjustment.
>
> Nebcin should be used with caution in premature and neonatal infants because of their renal immaturity and the resulting prolongation of serum half-life of the drug. Concurrent and sequential use of other neurotoxic and/or nephrotoxic antibiotics, particularly other aminoglycosides (eg, amikacin, streptomycin, neomycin, kanamycin, gentamicin, and paromomycin), cephaloridine, viomycin, polymyxin B, colistin, cisplatin, and vancomycin, should be avoided. Other factors that may increase patient risk are advanced age and dehydration. Aminoglycosides should not be given concurrently with potent diuretics, such as ethacrynic acid and furosemide. Some diuretics themselves cause ototoxicity, and intravenously administered diuretics enhance aminoglycoside toxicity by altering antibiotic concentrations in serum and tissue.
>
> Aminoglycosides can cause fetal harm when administered to a pregnant woman (see Precautions).

DESCRIPTION

Tobramycin sulfate, a water-soluble antibiotic of the aminoglycoside group, is derived from the actinomycete *Streptomyces tenebrarius*. Nebcin® (Tobramycin Sulfate, USP, Lilly), Injection, is a clear and colorless sterile aqueous solution for parenteral administration.

Tobramycin sulfate is D-streptamine, *O*-3-amino-3-deoxy-α-D-glucopyranosyl-(1→6)-*O*-[2,6-diamino-2,3,6-trideoxy-α-D-*ribo*-hexopyranosyl-(1→4)]-2-deoxy-, sulfate (2:5)(salt) and has the chemical formula $(C_{18}H_{37}N_5O_9)_2 \cdot 5H_2SO_4$. The molecular weight is 1,425.39.

Each mL also contains phenol as a preservative (5 mg, multiple-dose vials; 1.25 mg, ADD-Vantage® vials), sodium bisulfite (3.2 mg, multiple-dose vials; 1.6 mg, ADD-Vantage vials), 0.1 mg edetate disodium, and water for injection, qs. Sulfuric acid and/or sodium hydroxide may have been added to adjust the pH.

CLINICAL PHARMACOLOGY

Tobramycin is rapidly absorbed following intramuscular administration. Peak serum concentrations of tobramycin occur between 30 and 90 minutes after intramuscular administration. Following an intramuscular dose of 1 mg/kg of body weight, maximum serum concentrations reach about 4 μg/mL, and measurable levels persist for as long as 8 hours. Therapeutic serum levels are generally considered to range from 4 to 6 μg/mL. When Nebcin® (Tobramycin Sulfate, USP, Lilly) is administered by intravenous infusion over a 1-hour period, the serum concentrations are similar to those obtained by intramuscular administration. Nebcin is poorly absorbed from the gastrointestinal tract.

In patients with normal renal function, except neonates, Nebcin administered every 8 hours does not accumulate in the serum. However, in those patients with reduced renal function and in neonates, the serum concentration of the antibiotic is usually higher and can be measured for longer periods of time than in normal adults. Dosage for such patients must, therefore, be adjusted accordingly (*see* Dosage and Administration).

Following parenteral administration, little, if any, metabolic transformation occurs, and tobramycin is eliminated almost exclusively by glomerular filtration. Renal clearance is similar to that of endogenous creatinine. Ultrafiltration studies demonstrate that practically no serum protein binding occurs. In patients with normal renal function, up to 84% of the dose is recoverable from the urine in 8 hours and up to 93% in 24 hours.

Peak urine concentrations ranging from 75 to 100 μg/mL have been observed following the intramuscular injection of a single dose of 1 mg/kg. After several days of treatment, the amount of tobramycin excreted in the urine approaches the daily dose administered. When renal function is impaired, excretion of Nebcin is slowed, and accumulation of the drug may cause toxic blood levels.

The serum half-life in normal individuals is 2 hours. An inverse relationship exists between serum half-life and creatinine clearance, and the dosage schedule should be adjusted according to the degree of renal impairment (*see* Dosage and Administration). In patients undergoing dialysis, 25% to 70% of the administered dose may be removed, depending on the duration and type of dialysis.

Tobramycin can be detected in tissues and body fluids after parenteral administration. Concentrations in bile and stools ordinarily have been low, which suggests minimum biliary excretion. Tobramycin has appeared in low concentration in the cerebrospinal fluid following parenteral administration, and concentrations are dependent on dose, rate of penetration, and degree of meningeal inflammation. It has also been found in sputum, peritoneal fluid, synovial fluid, and abscess fluids, and it crosses the placental membranes. Concentrations in the renal cortex are several times higher than the usual serum levels.

Probenecid does not affect the renal tubular transport of tobramycin.

Microbiology—In vitro tests demonstrate that tobramycin is bactericidal and that it acts by inhibiting the synthesis of protein in bacterial cells.

Tobramycin is usually active against most strains of the following organisms in vitro and in clinical infections:

- *Pseudomonas aeruginosa*
- *Proteus* sp (indole-positive and indole-negative), including *Proteus mirabilis, Morganella morganii,* and *Proteus vulgaris*
- *Escherichia coli*
- *Klebsiella-Enterobacter-Serratia* group
- *Citrobacter* sp
- *Providencia* sp, including *Providencia rettgeri* (formerly *Proteus rettgeri*)
- Staphylococci, including *Staphylococcus aureus* (coagulase-positive and coagulase-negative)

Aminoglycosides have a low order of activity against most gram-positive organisms, including *Streptococcus pyogenes, Streptococcus pneumoniae,* and enterococci.

Although most strains of enterococci demonstrate in vitro resistance, some strains in this group are susceptible. In vitro studies have shown that an aminoglycoside combined with an antibiotic that interferes with cell-wall synthesis affects some enterococcal strains synergistically. The combination of penicillin G and tobramycin results in a synergistic bactericidal effect in vitro against certain strains of *Enterococcus (Streptococcus) faecalis*. However, this combination is not synergistic against other closely related organisms, eg, *Enterococcus (Streptococcus) faecium.* Speciation of enterococci alone cannot be used to predict susceptibility. Susceptibility testing and tests for antibiotic synergism are emphasized.

Cross-resistance between aminoglycosides occurs and depends largely on inactivation by bacterial enzymes.

Susceptibility Tests—If the FDA Standardized Disk Test method (formerly the Bauer-Kirby-Sherris-Turck method) of disk susceptibility testing is used, a disk containing 10 μg tobramycin should give a zone of at least 15 mm when tested against a tobramycin-susceptible bacterial strain, a zone of 13 to 14 mm against strains of intermediate susceptibility, and a zone of 12 mm or less against resistant organisms. The minimum inhibitory concentration correlates are ≤4 μg/mL for susceptibility and ≥ 8 μg/mL for resistance.

INDICATIONS AND USAGE

Nebcin® (Tobramycin Sulfate, USP, Lilly) is indicated for the treatment of serious bacterial infections caused by susceptible strains of the designated microorganisms in the diseases listed below:

Septicemia in the neonate, child, and adult caused by *P. aeruginosa, E. coli,* and *Klebsiella* sp

Lower respiratory tract infections caused by *P. aeruginosa, Klebsiella* sp, *Enterobacter* sp, *Serratia* sp, *E. coli,* and *S. aureus* (penicillinase- and non-penicillinase-producing strains)

Serious central-nervous-system infections (meningitis) caused by susceptible organisms

Intra-abdominal infections, including peritonitis, caused by *E. coli, Klebsiella* sp, and *Enterobacter* sp

Skin, bone, and skin structure infections caused by *P. aeruginosa, Proteus* sp, *E. coli, Klebsiella* sp, *Enterobacter* sp, and *S. aureus*

Complicated and recurrent urinary tract infections caused by *P. aeruginosa, Proteus* sp (indole-positive and indole-negative), *E. coli, Klebsiella* sp, *Enterobacter* sp, *Serratia* sp, *S. aureus, Providencia* sp, and *Citrobacter* sp

Aminoglycosides, including Nebcin, are not indicated in uncomplicated initial episodes of urinary tract infections unless the causative organisms are not susceptible to antibiotics having less potential toxicity. Nebcin may be considered in serious staphylococcal infections when penicillin or other potentially less toxic drugs are contraindicated and when bacterial susceptibility testing and clinical judgment indicate its use.

Bacterial cultures should be obtained prior to and during treatment to isolate and identify etiologic organisms and to test their susceptibility to tobramycin. If susceptibility tests show that the causative organisms are resistant to tobramycin, other appropriate therapy should be instituted. In patients in whom a serious life-threatening gram-negative infection is suspected, including those in whom concurrent therapy with a penicillin or cephalosporin and an aminoglycoside may be indicated, treatment with Nebcin may be initiated before the results of susceptibility studies are obtained. The decision to continue therapy with Nebcin should be based on the results of susceptibility studies, the severity of the infection, and the important additional concepts discussed in the WARNINGS box above.

CONTRAINDICATIONS

A hypersensitivity to any aminoglycoside is a contraindication to the use of tobramycin. A history of hypersensitivity or serious toxic reactions to aminoglycosides may also contraindicate the use of any other aminoglycoside because of the known cross-sensitivity of patients to drugs in this class.

WARNINGS

See WARNINGS box above.

Nebcin® (Tobramycin Sulfate, USP, Lilly) contains sodium bisulfite, a sulfite that may cause allergic-type reactions, including anaphylactic symptoms and life-threatening or less severe asthmatic episodes, in certain susceptible people. The overall prevalence of sulfite sensitivity in the general population is unknown and probably low. Sulfite sensitivity is seen more frequently in asthmatic than in nonasthmatic people.

PRECAUTIONS

Serum and urine specimens for examination should be collected during therapy, as recommended in the WARNINGS box. Serum calcium, magnesium, and sodium should be monitored.

Peak and trough serum levels should be measured periodically during therapy. Prolonged concentrations above 12 μg/mL should be avoided. Rising trough levels (above 2 μg/mL) may indicate tissue accumulation. Such accumulation, advanced age, and cumulative dosage may contribute to ototoxicity and nephrotoxicity. It is particularly important to monitor serum levels closely in patients with known renal impairment.

A useful guideline would be to perform serum level assays after 2 or 3 doses, so that the dosage could be adjusted if necessary, and at 3- to 4-day intervals during therapy. In the event of changing renal function, more frequent serum levels should be obtained and the dosage or dosage interval adjusted according to the guidelines provided in the Dosage and Administration section.

In order to measure the peak level, a serum sample should be drawn about 30 minutes following intravenous infusion or 1 hour after an intramuscular injection. Trough levels are measured by obtaining serum samples at 8 hours or just prior to the next dose of Nebcin®(Tobramycin Sulfate, USP, Lilly). These suggested time intervals are intended only as guidelines and may vary according to institutional practices. It is important, however, that there be consistency within the individual patient program unless computerized pharmacokinetic dosing programs are available in the institution. These serum-level assays may be especially useful for monitoring the treatment of severely ill patients with changing renal function or of those infected with less susceptible organisms or those receiving maximum dosage.

Neuromuscular blockade and respiratory paralysis have been reported in cats receiving very high doses of tobramycin (40 mg/kg). The possibility of prolonged or secondary apnea should be considered if tobramycin is administered to anesthetized patients who are also receiving neuromuscular blocking agents, such as succinylcholine, tubocurarine, or decamethonium, or to patients receiving massive transfusions of citrated blood. If neuromuscular blockade occurs, it may be reversed by the administration of calcium salts.

Cross-allergenicity among aminoglycosides has been demonstrated.

In patients with extensive burns, altered pharmacokinetics may result in reduced serum concentrations of aminoglycosides. In such patients treated with Nebcin, measurement of serum concentration is especially recommended as a basis for determination of appropriate dosage.

Elderly patients may have reduced renal function that may not be evident in the results of routine screening tests, such as BUN or serum creatinine. A creatinine clearance determination may be more useful. Monitoring of renal function during treatment with aminoglycosides is particularly important in such patients.

An increased incidence of nephrotoxicity has been reported following concomitant administration of aminoglycoside antibiotics and cephalosporins.

Aminoglycosides should be used with caution in patients with muscular disorders, such as myasthenia gravis or parkinsonism, since these drugs may aggravate muscle weakness because of their potential curare-like effect on neuromuscular function.

Aminoglycosides may be absorbed in significant quantities from body surfaces after local irrigation or application and may cause neurotoxicity and nephrotoxicity.

Although not indicated for intraocular and/or subconjunctival use, there have been reports of macular necrosis following this type of injection of aminoglycosides, including tobramycin.

See WARNINGS box regarding concurrent use of potent diuretics and concurrent and sequential use of other neurotoxic or nephrotoxic drugs.

The inactivation of tobramycin and other aminoglycosides by β-lactam-type antibiotics (penicillins or cephalosporins) has been demonstrated in vitro and in patients with severe renal impairment. Such inactivation has not been found in patients with normal renal function who have been given the drugs by separate routes of administration.

Therapy with tobramycin may result in overgrowth of nonsusceptible organisms. If overgrowth of nonsusceptible organisms occurs, appropriate therapy should be initiated.

Pregnancy Category D—Aminoglycosides can cause fetal harm when administered to a pregnant woman. Aminoglycoside antibiotics cross the placenta, and there have been several reports of total irreversible bilateral congenital deafness in children whose mothers received streptomycin during pregnancy. Serious side effects to mother, fetus, or newborn have not been reported in the treatment of pregnant women with other aminoglycosides. If tobramycin is used during pregnancy or if the patient becomes pregnant while taking tobramycin, she should be apprised of the potential hazard to the fetus.

Usage in Children—*See* Indications and Usage *and* Dosage and Administration.

Continued on next page

*** Identi-Code® symbol. This product information was prepared in June 1992. Current information on these and other products of Eli Lilly and Company may be obtained by direct inquiry to Lilly Research Laboratories, Lilly Corporate Center, Indianapolis, Indiana 46285, (317) 276-3714.**

Lilly—Cont.

ADVERSE REACTIONS

Neurotoxicity—Adverse effects on both the vestibular and auditory branches of the eighth nerve have been noted, especially in patients receiving high doses or prolonged therapy, in those given previous courses of therapy with an ototoxin, and in cases of dehydration. Symptoms include dizziness, vertigo, tinnitus, roaring in the ears, and hearing loss. Hearing loss is usually irreversible and is manifested initially by diminution of high-tone acuity. Tobramycin and gentamicin sulfates closely parallel each other in regard to ototoxic potential.

Nephrotoxicity—Renal function changes, as shown by rising BUN, NPN, and serum creatinine and by oliguria, cylindruria, and increased proteinuria, have been reported, especially in patients with a history of renal impairment who are treated for longer periods or with higher doses than those recommended. Adverse renal effects can occur in patients with initially normal renal function.

Clinical studies and studies in experimental animals have been conducted to compare the nephrotoxic potential of tobramycin and gentamicin. In some of the clinical studies and in the animal studies, tobramycin caused nephrotoxicity significantly less frequently than gentamicin. In some other clinical studies, no significant difference in the incidence of nephrotoxicity between tobramycin and gentamicin was found.

Other reported adverse reactions possibly related to Nebcin® (Tobramycin Sulfate, USP, Lilly) include anemia, granulocytopenia, and thrombocytopenia; and fever, rash, itching, urticaria, nausea, vomiting, diarrhea, headache, lethargy, pain at the injection site, mental confusion, and disorientation. Laboratory abnormalities possibly related to Nebcin include increased serum transaminases (SGOT, SGPT); increased serum LDH and bilirubin; decreased serum calcium, magnesium, sodium, and potassium; and leukopenia, leukocytosis, and eosinophilia.

OVERDOSAGE

Signs and Symptoms—The severity of the signs and symptoms following a tobramycin overdose are dependent on the dose administered, the patient's renal function, state of hydration, and age and whether or not other medications with similar toxicities are being administered concurrently. Toxicity may occur in patients treated more than 10 days, in adults given more than 5 mg/kg/day, in children given more than 7.5 mg/kg/day, or in patients with reduced renal function where dose has not been appropriately adjusted.

Nephrotoxicity following the parenteral administration of an aminoglycoside is most closely related to the area under the curve of the serum concentration versus time graph. Nephrotoxicity is more likely if trough blood concentrations fail to fall below 2 μg/mL and is also proportional to the average blood concentration. Patients who are elderly, have abnormal renal function, are receiving other nephrotoxic drugs, or are volume depleted are at greater risk for developing acute tubular necrosis. Auditory and vestibular toxicities have been associated with aminoglycoside overdose. These

toxicities occur in patients treated longer than 10 days, in patients with abnormal renal function, in dehydrated patients, or in patients receiving medications with additive auditory toxicities. These patients may not have signs or symptoms or may experience dizziness, tinnitus, vertigo, and a loss of high-tone acuity as ototoxicity progresses. Ototoxicity signs and symptoms may not begin to occur until long after the drug has been discontinued.

Neuromuscular blockade or respiratory paralysis may occur following administration of aminoglycosides. Neuromuscular blockade, respiratory failure, and prolonged respiratory paralysis may occur more commonly in patients with myasthenia gravis or Parkinson's disease. Prolonged respiratory paralysis may also occur in patients receiving decamethonium, tubocurarine, or succinylcholine. If neuromuscular blockade occurs, it may be reversed by the administration of calcium salts but mechanical assistance may be necessary. If tobramycin were ingested, toxicity would be less likely because aminoglycosides are poorly absorbed from an intact gastrointestinal tract.

Treatment—In all cases of suspected overdosage, call your Regional Poison Control Center to obtain the most up-to-date information about the treatment of overdose. This recommendation is made because, in general, information regarding the treatment of overdose may change more rapidly than the package insert. In managing overdosage, consider the possibility of multiple drug overdoses, interaction among drugs, and unusual drug kinetics in your patient.

The initial intervention in a tobramycin overdose is to establish an airway and ensure oxygenation and ventilation. Resuscitative measures should be initiated promptly if respiratory paralysis occurs.

Patients who have received an overdose of tobramycin and who have normal renal function should be adequately hydrated to maintain a urine output of 3 to 5 mL/kg/hr. Fluid balance, creatinine clearance, and tobramycin plasma levels should be carefully monitored until the serum tobramycin level falls below 2 μg/mL.

Patients in whom the elimination half-life is greater than 2 hours or whose renal function is abnormal may require more aggressive therapy. In such patients, hemodialysis may be beneficial.

DOSAGE AND ADMINISTRATION

Nebcin® (Tobramycin Sulfate, USP, Lilly) may be given intramuscularly or intravenously. ADD-Vantage vials are not for intramuscular administration. Recommended dosages are the same for both routes. The patient's pretreatment body weight should be obtained for calculation of correct dosage. It is desirable to measure both peak and trough serum concentrations (see WARNINGS box *and* Precautions).

Administration for Patients With Normal Renal Function —Adults With Serious Infections: 3 mg/kg/day in 3 equal doses every 8 hours (see Table 1).

Adults With Life-Threatening Infections: Up to 5 mg/kg/day may be administered in 3 or 4 equal doses (see Table 1). The dosage should be reduced to 3 mg/kg/day as soon as clinically indicated. To prevent increased toxicity due to excessive blood levels, dosage should not exceed 5 mg/kg/day un-

less serum levels are monitored (see WARNINGS box *and* Precautions).

Children: 6 to 7.5 mg/kg/day in 3 or 4 equally divided doses (2 to 2.5 mg/kg every 8 hours or 1.5 to 1.89 mg/kg every 6 hours).

Premature or Full-Term Neonates 1 Week of Age or Less: Up to 4 mg/kg/day may be administered in 2 equal doses every 12 hours.

It is desirable to limit treatment to a short term. The usual duration of treatment is 7 to 10 days. A longer course of therapy may be necessary in difficult and complicated infections. In such cases, monitoring of renal, auditory, and vestibular functions is advised, because neurotoxicity is more likely to occur when treatment is extended longer than 10 days.

Administration for Patients With Impaired Renal Function—Whenever possible, serum tobramycin concentrations should be monitored during therapy.

Following a loading dose of 1 mg/kg, subsequent dosage in these patients must be adjusted, either with reduced doses administered at 8-hour intervals or with normal doses given at prolonged intervals. Both of these methods are suggested as guides to be used when serum levels of tobramycin cannot be measured directly. They are based on either the creatinine clearance level or the serum creatinine level of the patient because these values correlate with the half-life of tobramycin. The dosage schedule derived from either method should be used in conjunction with careful clinical and laboratory observations of the patient and should be modified as necessary. Neither method should be used when dialysis is being performed.

<u>Reduced dosage at 8-hour intervals:</u> When the creatinine clearance rate is 70 mL or less per minute or when the serum creatinine value is known, the amount of the reduced dose can be determined by multiplying the normal dose from Table 1 by the percent of normal dose from the accompanying nomogram.

REDUCED DOSAGE NOMOGRAM*
Creatinine Clearance (mL/min/1.73 m²)

Serum Creatinine
(mg/100 mL)
*Scales have been adjusted to
facilitate dosage calculations.

An alternate rough guide for determining reduced dosage at 8-hour intervals (for patients whose steady-state serum creatinine values are known) is to divide the normally recommended dose by the patient's serum creatinine.

<u>Normal dosage at prolonged intervals:</u> If the creatinine clearance rate is not available and the patient's condition is stable, a dosage frequency *in hours* for the dosage given in Table 1 can be determined by multiplying the patient's serum creatinine by 6.

Dosage in Obese Patients—The appropriate dose may be calculated by using the patient's estimated lean body weight plus 40% of the excess as the basic weight on which to figure mg/kg.

Intramuscular Administration—Nebcin may be administered by withdrawing the appropriate dose directly from a vial or by using a prefilled Hyporet®. ADD-Vantage vials are not for intramuscular administration.

Intravenous Administration—For intravenous administration, the usual volume of diluent (0.9% Sodium Chloride Injection or 5% Dextrose Injection) is 50 to 100 mL for adult doses. For children, the volume of diluent should be proportionately less than that for adults. The diluted solution usually should be infused over a period of 20 to 60 minutes. Infusion periods of less than 20 minutes are not recommended, because peak serum levels may exceed 12 μg/mL (see WARNINGS box).

Use of ADD-Vantage Nebcin Vials—ADD-Vantage Nebcin vials are not intended for multiple use and should not be used with a syringe in the conventional way. These products are intended for use only with Abbott ADD-Vantage diluent containers and in those instances in which the physician's order specified 60-mg or 80-mg doses. Use within 24 hours after activation.

TABLE 1. DOSAGE SCHEDULE GUIDE FOR NEBCIN® (TOBRAMYCIN SULFATE, USP) IN ADULTS WITH NORMAL RENAL FUNCTION
(Dosage at 8-Hour Intervals)

For Patient Weighing		Usual Dose for Serious Infections 1 mg/kg q8h (Total, 3 mg/kg/day)			Maximum Dose for Life-Threatening Infections (Reduce as soon as possible) 1.66 mg/kg q8h (Total, 5 mg/kg/day)		
kg	lb	mg/dose	mL/dose* q8h		mg/dose	mL/dose* q8h	
120	264	120 mg	3	mL	200 mg	5	mL
115	253	115 mg	2.9	mL	191 mg	4.75	mL
110	242	110 mg	2.75	mL	183 mg	4.5	mL
105	231	105 mg	2.6	mL	175 mg	4.4	mL
100	220	100 mg	2.5	mL	166 mg	4.2	mL
95	209	95 mg	2.4	mL	158 mg	4	mL
90	198	90 mg	2.25	mL	150 mg	3.75	mL
85	187	85 mg	2.1	mL	141 mg	3.5	mL
80	176	80 mg	2	mL	133 mg	3.3	mL
75	165	75 mg	1.9	mL	125 mg	3.1	mL
70	154	70 mg	1.75	mL	116 mg	2.9	mL
65	143	65 mg	1.6	mL	108 mg	2.7	mL
60	132	60 mg	1.5	mL	100 mg	2.5	mL
55	121	55 mg	1.4	mL	91 mg	2.25	mL
50	110	50 mg	1.25	mL	83 mg	2.1	mL
45	99	45 mg	1.1	mL	75 mg	1.9	mL
40	88	40 mg	1	mL	66 mg	1.6	mL

*Applicable to all product forms except Nebcin, Pediatric, Injection (see How Supplied).

Nebcin® (Tobramycin Sulfate, USP, Lilly) should not be physically premixed with other drugs but should be administered separately according to the recommended dose and route.

Prior to administration, parenteral drug products should be inspected visually for particulate matter and discoloration whenever solution and container permit.

HOW SUPPLIED

(℞) Multiple-Dose Vials:

80 mg*/2 mL, 2 mL (No. 781)—(1s) NDC 0002-1499-01; (Traypak† of 25) NDC 0002-1499-25

Pediatric, 20 mg*/2 mL, 2 mL (No. 782)—(1s) NDC 0002-0501-01

40 mg*/mL, 1.2 g/30 mL (No. 7090)—(Traypak of 6) NDC 0002-7090-16

(℞) Hyporets®,‡ each scored with a 10-mg (0.25-mL) fractional dose scale:

60 mg*/1.5 mL, 1.5 mL (No. 55)—(24s) NDC 0002-0509-24

80 mg*/2 mL, 2 mL (No. 42)—(24s) NDC 0002-0503-24

(℞) ADD-Vantage§ Vials:

60 mg*/6 mL, 6 mL (No. 7293)—(Traypak of 25) NDC 0002-7293-25

80 mg*/8 mL, 8 mL (No. 7294)—(Traypak of 25) NDC 0002-7294-25

The above ADD-Vantage vials are to be used only with Abbott Laboratories' diluent containers.

Instructions for the use of ADD-Vantage vials are enclosed in the package.

Also Available:

(℞) Pharmacy Bulk Vial:

1.2 g* (Dry Powder) (40-mL size) (No. 7040)—(Traypak of 6) NDC 0002-7040-16

* Equivalent to tobramycin.

† Traypak™ (multivial carton, Lilly).

‡ Hyporet® (disposable syringe, Lilly).

§ ADD-Vantage® (vials and diluent containers, Abbott).

[031292]

NPH ILETIN® I AND II OTC

(isophane insulin suspension, Lilly) *See Under* Iletin® (insulin, Lilly)

ONCOVIN® ℞

[ŏn 'kō-vĭn]

(Vincristine Sulfate Injection, USP)

Solution

> **WARNINGS**
>
> *Caution—This preparation should be administered by individuals experienced in the administration of Oncovin. It is extremely important that the intravenous needle or catheter be properly positioned before any vincristine is injected. Leakage into surrounding tissue during intravenous administration of Oncovin may cause considerable irritation. If extravasation occurs, the injection should be discontinued immediately, and any remaining portion of the dose should then be introduced into another vein. Local injection of hyaluronidase and the application of moderate heat to the area of leakage help disperse the drug and are thought to minimize discomfort and the possibility of cellulitis.*
>
> *FATAL IF GIVEN INTRATHECALLY. FOR INTRAVENOUS USE ONLY. See Warnings section for the treatment of patients given intrathecal Oncovin.*

DESCRIPTION

Oncovin® (Vincristine Sulfate, USP, Lilly) is the salt of an alkaloid obtained from a common flowering herb, the periwinkle plant (*Vinca rosea* Linn). Originally known as leurocristine, it has also been referred to as LCR and VCR. The empirical formula for vincristine sulfate is $C_{46}H_{56}N_4O_{10} \cdot H_2SO_4$. It has a molecular weight of 923.04.

Vincristine sulfate is a white to off-white powder. It is soluble in methanol, freely soluble in water, but only slightly soluble in 95% ethanol. In 98% ethanol, vincristine sulfate has an ultraviolet spectrum with maxima at 221 nm (E + 47,100).

Each mL contains vincristine sulfate, 1 mg (1.08 μmol); mannitol, 100 mg; methylparaben, 1.3 mg; propylparaben, 0.2 mg; and water for injection, qs. Acetic acid and sodium acetate have been added for pH control. The pH of Oncovin Solution ranges from 3.5 to 5.5. This product is a sterile solution for cancer/oncolytic use.

CLINICAL PHARMACOLOGY

The mechanisms of action of Oncovin® (Vincristine Sulfate, USP, Lilly) remain under investigation. The mechanism of action of Oncovin has been related to the inhibition of microtubule formation in the mitotic spindle, resulting in an arrest of dividing cells at the metaphase stage.

Central-nervous-system leukemia has been reported in patients undergoing otherwise successful therapy with Oncovin. This suggests that Oncovin does not penetrate well into the cerebrospinal fluid.

Pharmacokinetic studies in patients with cancer have shown a triphasic serum decay pattern following rapid intravenous injection. The initial, middle, and terminal half-lives are 5 minutes, 2.3 hours, and 85 hours respectively; however, the range of the terminal half-life in humans is from 19 to 155 hours. The liver is the major excretory organ in humans and animals; about 80% of an injected dose of Oncovin appears in the feces and 10% to 20% can be found in the urine. Within 15 to 30 minutes after injection, over 90% of the drug is distributed from the blood into tissue, where it remains tightly, but not irreversibly, bound.

Current principles of cancer chemotherapy involve the simultaneous use of several agents. Generally, each agent used has a unique toxicity and mechanism of action so that therapeutic enhancement occurs without additive toxicity. It is rarely possible to achieve equally good results with single-agent methods of treatment. Thus, Oncovin is often chosen as part of polychemotherapy because of lack of significant bone-marrow suppression (at recommended doses) and of unique clinical toxicity (neuropathy). *See* Dosage and Administration for possible increased toxicity when used in combination therapy.

INDICATIONS AND USAGE

Oncovin® (Vincristine Sulfate, USP, Lilly) is indicated in acute leukemia.

Oncovin has also been shown to be useful in combination with other oncolytic agents in Hodgkin's disease, non-Hodgkin's malignant lymphomas (lymphocytic, mixed-cell, histiocytic, undifferentiated, nodular, and diffuse types), rhabdomyosarcoma, neuroblastoma, and Wilms' tumor.

CONTRAINDICATIONS

Patients with the demyelinating form of Charcot-Marie-Tooth syndrome should not be given Oncovin® (Vincristine Sulfate, USP, Lilly). Careful attention should be given to those conditions listed under Warnings *and* Precautions.

WARNINGS

> *This preparation is for intravenous use only. It should be administered by individuals experienced in the administration of Oncovin. The intrathecal administration of Oncovin usually results in death. Syringes containing this product should be labeled "WARNING—FOR IV USE ONLY."*
>
> Extemporaneously prepared syringes containing this product must be packaged in an overwrap which is labeled "FATAL IF GIVEN INTRATHECALLY. FOR INTRAVENOUS USE ONLY."
>
> Treatment of patients following intrathecal administration of Oncovin has included immediate removal of spinal fluid and flushing with Lactated Ringer's, as well as other solutions and has not prevented ascending paralysis and death. In one case, progressive paralysis in an adult was arrested by the following treatment **initiated immediately after the intrathecal injection:**
>
> 1. As much spinal fluid was removed as could be safely done through lumbar access.
> 2. The subarachnoid space was flushed with Lactated Ringer's solution infused continuously through a catheter in a cerebral lateral ventricle at the rate of 150 mL/h. The fluid was removed through a lumbar access.
> 3. As soon as fresh frozen plasma became available, the fresh frozen plasma, 25 mL, diluted in 1 L of Lactated Ringer's solution was infused through the cerebral ventricular catheter at the rate of 75 mL/h with removal through the lumbar access. The rate of infusion was adjusted to maintain a protein level in the spinal fluid of 150 mg/dL.
> 4. Glutamic acid, 10 g, was given intravenously over 24 hours followed by 500 mg 3 times daily by mouth for 1 month or until neurological dysfunction stabilized. The role of glutamic acid in this treatment is not certain and may not be essential.

Pregnancy Category D—Oncovin can cause fetal harm when administered to a pregnant woman. When pregnant mice and hamsters were given doses of Oncovin that caused the resorption of 23% to 85% of fetuses, fetal malformations were produced in those that survived. Five monkeys were given single doses of Oncovin between days 27 and 34 of their pregnancies; 3 of the fetuses were normal at term, and 2 viable fetuses had grossly evident malformations at term. In several animal species, Oncovin can induce teratogenesis as well as embryo death at doses that are nontoxic to the pregnant animal. There are no adequate and well-controlled studies in pregnant women. If this drug is used during pregnancy or if the patient becomes pregnant while receiving this drug, she should be apprised of the potential hazard to the fetus. Women of childbearing potential should be advised to avoid becoming pregnant.

PRECAUTIONS

General—Acute uric acid nephropathy, which may occur after the administration of oncolytic agents, has also been reported with Oncovin® (Vincristine Sulfate, USP, Lilly). In the presence of leukopenia or a complicating infection, administration of the next dose of Oncovin warrants careful consideration.

If central-nervous-system leukemia is diagnosed, additional agents may be required, because Oncovin does not appear to cross the blood-brain barrier in adequate amounts.

Particular attention should be given to dosage and neurologic side effects if Oncovin is administered to patients with preexisting neuromuscular disease and when other drugs with neurotoxic potential are also being used.

Acute shortness of breath and severe bronchospasm have been reported following the administration of vinca alkaloids. These reactions have been encountered most frequently when the vinca alkaloid was used in combination with mitomycin-C and may require aggressive treatment, particularly when there is preexisting pulmonary dysfunction. The onset of these reactions may occur minutes to several hours after the vinca alkaloid is injected and may occur up to 2 weeks following the dose of mitomycin. Progressive dyspnea requiring chronic therapy may occur. Oncovin should not be readministered.

Care must be taken to avoid contamination of the eye with concentrations of Oncovin used clinically. If accidental contamination occurs, severe irritation (or, if the drug was delivered under pressure, even corneal ulceration) may result. The eye should be washed immediately and thoroughly.

Laboratory Tests—Because dose-limiting clinical toxicity is manifested as neurotoxicity, clinical evaluation (eg, history, physical examination) is necessary to detect the need for dosage modification. Following administration of Oncovin, some individuals may have a fall in the white-blood-cell count or platelet count, particularly when previous therapy or the disease itself has reduced bone-marrow function. Therefore, a complete blood count should be done before administration of each dose. Acute elevation of serum uric acid may also occur during induction of remission in acute leukemia; thus, such levels should be determined frequently during the first 3 to 4 weeks of treatment or appropriate measures taken to prevent uric acid nephropathy. The laboratory performing these tests should be consulted for its range of normal values.

Drug Interaction—The simultaneous oral or intravenous administration of phenytoin and antineoplastic chemotherapy combinations that included vincristine sulfate has been reported to reduce blood levels of the anticonvulsant and to increase seizure activity. Dosage adjustment should be based on serial blood level monitoring. The contribution of vincristine sulfate to this interaction is not certain. The interaction may result from reduced absorption of phenytoin and an increase in the rate of its metabolism and elimination.

Carcinogenesis, Mutagenesis, Impairment of Fertility—Neither in vivo nor in vitro laboratory tests have conclusively demonstrated the mutagenicity of this product. Fertility following treatment with Oncovin alone for malignant disease has not been studied in humans. Clinical reports of both male and female patients who received multiple-agent chemotherapy that included Oncovin indicate that azoospermia and amenorrhea can occur in postpubertal patients. Recovery occurred many months after completion of chemotherapy in some but not all patients. When the same treatment is administered to prepubertal patients, permanent azoospermia and amenorrhea are much less likely.

Patients who received chemotherapy with Oncovin in combination with anticancer drugs known to be carcinogenic have developed second malignancies. The contributing role of Oncovin in this development has not been determined. No evidence of carcinogenicity was found following intraperitoneal administration of Oncovin in rats and mice, although this study was limited.

Usage in Pregnancy—*Pregnancy Category D*—*See* Warnings.

Nursing Mothers—It is not known whether this drug is excreted in human milk. Because many drugs are excreted in human milk and because of the potential for serious adverse reactions due to Oncovin in nursing infants, a decision should be made either to discontinue nursing or the drug, taking into account the importance of the drug to the mother.

Continued on next page

*** Identi-Code® symbol. This product information was prepared in June 1992. Current information on these and other products of Eli Lilly and Company may be obtained by direct inquiry to Lilly Research Laboratories, Lilly Corporate Center, Indianapolis, Indiana 46285, (317) 276-3714.**

Lilly—Cont.

ADVERSE REACTIONS

Prior to the use of this drug, patients and/or their parents/guardian should be advised of the possibility of untoward symptoms.

In general, adverse reactions are reversible and are related to dosage. The most common adverse reaction is hair loss; the most troublesome adverse reactions are neuromuscular in origin.

When single, weekly doses of the drug are employed, the adverse reactions of leukopenia, neuritic pain, and constipation occur but are usually of short duration (ie, less than 7 days). When the dosage is reduced, these reactions may lessen or disappear. The severity of such reactions seems to increase when the calculated amount of drug is given in divided doses. Other adverse reactions, such as hair loss, sensory loss, paresthesia, difficulty in walking, slapping gait, loss of deep-tendon reflexes, and muscle wasting, may persist for at least as long as therapy is continued. Generalized sensorimotor dysfunction may become progressively more severe with continued treatment. Although most such symptoms usually disappear by about the sixth week after discontinuance of treatment, some neuromuscular difficulties may persist for prolonged periods in some patients. Regrowth of hair may occur while maintenance therapy continues.

The following adverse reactions have been reported:

Hypersensitivity—Rare cases of allergic-type reactions, such as anaphylaxis, rash, and edema, that are temporally related to vincristine therapy have been reported in patients receiving vincristine as a part of multidrug chemotherapy regimens.

Gastrointestinal—Constipation, abdominal cramps, weight loss, nausea, vomiting, oral ulceration, diarrhea, paralytic ileus, intestinal necrosis and/or perforation, and anorexia have occurred. Constipation may take the form of upper-colon impaction, and, on physical examination, the rectum may be empty. Colicky abdominal pain coupled with an empty rectum may mislead the physician. A flat film of the abdomen is useful in demonstrating this condition. All cases have responded to high enemas and laxatives. A routine prophylactic regimen against constipation is recommended for all patients receiving Oncovin® (Vincristine Sulfate, USP, Lilly).

Paralytic ileus (which mimics the "surgical abdomen") may occur, particularly in young children. The ileus will reverse itself with temporary discontinuance of Oncovin and with symptomatic care.

Genitourinary—Polyuria, dysuria, and urinary retention due to bladder atony have occurred. Other drugs known to cause urinary retention (particularly in the elderly) should, if possible, be discontinued for the first few days following administration of Oncovin.

Cardiovascular—Hypertension and hypotension have occurred. Chemotherapy combinations that have included vincristine sulfate, when given to patients previously treated with mediastinal radiation, have been associated with coronary artery disease and myocardial infarction. Causality has not been established.

Neurologic—Frequently, there is a sequence to the development of neuromuscular side effects. Initially, only sensory impairment and paresthesia may be encountered. With continued treatment, neuritic pain and, later, motor difficulties may occur. There have been no reports made of any agent that can reverse the neuromuscular manifestations that may accompany therapy with Oncovin.

Loss of deep-tendon reflexes, foot drop, ataxia, and paralysis have been reported with continued administration. Cranial nerve manifestations, including isolated paresis and/or paralysis of muscles controlled by cranial motor nerves, may occur in the absence of motor impairment elsewhere; extraocular and laryngeal muscles are those most commonly involved. Jaw pain, pharyngeal pain, parotid gland pain, bone pain, back pain, limb pain, and myalgias have been reported; pain in these areas may be severe. Convulsions, frequently with hypertension, have been reported in a few patients receiving Oncovin. Several instances of convulsions followed by coma have been reported in children. Transient cortical blindness and optic atrophy with blindness have been reported.

Pulmonary—*See* Precautions.

Endocrine—Rare occurrences of a syndrome attributable to inappropriate antidiuretic hormone secretion have been observed in patients treated with Oncovin. This syndrome is characterized by high urinary sodium excretion in the presence of hyponatremia; renal or adrenal disease, hypotension, dehydration, azotemia, and clinical edema are absent. With fluid deprivation, improvement occurs in the hyponatremia and in the renal loss of sodium.

Hematologic—Oncovin does not appear to have any constant or significant effect on platelets or red blood cells. Serious bone-marrow depression is usually not a major dose-limiting event. However, anemia, leukopenia, and thrombocytopenia have been reported. Thrombocytopenia, if present when therapy with Oncovin is begun, may actually improve before the appearance of marrow remission.

Skin—Alopecia and rash have been reported.

Other—Fever and headache have occurred.

OVERDOSAGE

Side effects following the use of Oncovin® (Vincristine Sulfate, USP, Lilly) are dose related. In children under 13 years of age, death has occurred following doses of Oncovin that were 10 times those recommended for therapy. Severe symptoms may occur in this patient group following dosages of 3 to 4 mg/m^2. Adults can be expected to experience severe symptoms after single doses of 3 mg/m^2 or more (*see* Adverse Reactions). Therefore, following administration of doses higher than those recommended, patients can be expected to experience exaggerated side effects. Supportive care should include the following: (1) prevention of side effects resulting from the syndrome of inappropriate antidiuretic hormone secretion (preventive treatment would include restriction of fluid intake and perhaps the administration of a diuretic affecting the function of Henle's loop and the distal tubule); (2) administration of anticonvulsants; (3) use of enemas or cathartics to prevent ileus (in some instances, decompression of the gastrointestinal tract may be necessary); (4) monitoring the cardiovascular system; and (5) determining daily blood counts for guidance in transfusion requirements.

Folinic acid has been observed to have a protective effect in normal mice that were administered lethal doses of Oncovin (*Cancer Res* 1963, 23:1390). Isolated case reports suggest that folinic acid may be helpful in treating humans who have received an overdose of Oncovin. It is suggested that 100 mg of folinic acid be administered intravenously every 3 hours for 24 hours and then every 6 hours for at least 48 hours. Theoretically (based on pharmacokinetic data), tissue levels of Oncovin can be expected to remain significantly elevated for at least 72 hours. Treatment with folinic acid does not eliminate the need for the above-mentioned supportive measures.

Most of an intravenous dose of Oncovin is excreted into the bile after rapid tissue binding (*see* Clinical Pharmacology). Because only very small amounts of the drug appear in dialysate, hemodialysis is not likely to be helpful in cases of overdosage. An increase in the severity of side effects may be experienced by patients with liver disease that is severe enough to decrease biliary excretion.

Enhanced fecal excretion of parenterally administered vincristine has been demonstrated in dogs pretreated with cholestyramine. There are no published clinical data on the use of cholestyramine as an antidote in humans.

There are no published clinical data on the consequences of oral ingestion of vincristine. Should oral ingestion occur, the stomach should be evacuated. Evacuation should be followed by oral administration of activated charcoal and a cathartic.

DOSAGE AND ADMINISTRATION

This preparation is for intravenous use only (see Warnings).

Neurotoxicity appears to be dose related. Extreme care must be used in calculating and administering the dose of Oncovin® (Vincristine Sulfate, USP, Lilly), since overdosage may have a very serious or fatal outcome.

The concentration of vincristine contained in all vials and Hyporets® of Oncovin is 1 mg/mL. Do not add extra fluid to the vial prior to removal of the dose. Withdraw the solution of Oncovin into an accurate dry syringe, measuring the dose carefully. Do not add extra fluid to the vial in an attempt to empty it completely.

Caution—It is extremely important that the intravenous needle or catheter be properly positioned before any vincristine is injected. Leakage into surrounding tissue during intravenous administration of Oncovin may cause considerable irritation. If extravasation occurs, the injection should be discontinued immediately, and any remaining portion of the dose should then be introduced into another vein. Local injection of hyaluronidase and the application of moderate heat to the area of leakage will help disperse the drug and may minimize discomfort and the possibility of cellulitis.

Oncovin must be administered via an intact, free-flowing intravenous needle or catheter. Care should be taken that there is no leakage or swelling occurring during administration (*see* boxed Warnings).

The solution may be injected either directly into a vein or into the tubing of a running intravenous infusion (*see* Drug Interactions below). Injection of Oncovin should be accomplished within 1 minute.

The drug is administered intravenously *at weekly intervals.*

The usual dose of Oncovin for children is 2 mg/m^2. For children weighing 10 kg or less, the starting dose should be 0.05 mg/kg, administered once a week. The usual dose of Oncovin for adults is 1.4 mg/m^2. A 50% reduction in the dose of Oncovin is recommended for patients having a direct serum bilirubin value above 3 mg/100 mL.

Oncovin should not be given to patients while they are receiving radiation therapy through ports that include the liver.

When Oncovin is used in combination with L-asparaginase, Oncovin should be given 12 to 24 hours before administration of the enzyme in order to minimize toxicity; administering L-asparaginase before Oncovin may reduce hepatic clearance of Oncovin.

Drug Interactions—Oncovin should not be diluted in solutions that raise or lower the pH outside the range of 3.5 to 5.5. It should not be mixed with anything other than normal saline or glucose in water.

Whenever solution and container permit, parenteral drug products should be inspected visually for particulate matter and discoloration prior to administration.

Procedures for proper handling and disposal of anticancer drugs should be considered. Several guidelines on this subject have been published. There is no general agreement that all of the procedures recommended in the guidelines are necessary or appropriate.

Special Dispensing Information—When dispensing Oncovin in other than the original container, eg, a syringe containing a specific dose, it is imperative that it be packaged in an overwrap bearing the statement: "DO NOT REMOVE COVERING UNTIL MOMENT OF INJECTION. FATAL IF GIVEN INTRATHECALLY. FOR INTRAVENOUS USE ONLY (*see* Warnings).

See package insert for references.

HOW SUPPLIED

(℞) Multiple-Dose Vials:

1 mg/1 mL, 1 mL (No. 7194)—(1s) NDC 0002-7194-01

2 mg/2 mL, 2 mL (No. 7195)—(1s) NDC 0002-7195-01

5 mg/5 mL, 5 mL (No. 7196)—(1s) NDC 0002-7196-01

(℞) Hyporets® (disposable syringes, Lilly), each marked with a 0.1-mg (0.1-mL) fractional dose scale:

1 mg/1 mL, 1 mL (No. 7198)—(3s) NDC 0002-7198-09

2 mg/2 mL, 2 mL (No. 7199)—(3s) NDC 0002-7199-09

This product should be refrigerated.

[020692]

PAPAVERINE HYDROCHLORIDE ℞

[*pă-păv 'ŭr-ēn hī 'drō-klōr-īd*]

Injection, USP

This product is to be used by or under the direction of a physician.

Each ampoule or vial contains a sufficient amount to permit withdrawal and administration of the volume specified on the label.

DESCRIPTION

Papaverine hydrochloride is the hydrochloride of an alkaloid obtained from opium or prepared synthetically. It belongs to the benzylisoquinoline group of alkaloids. It does not contain a phenanthrene group as do morphine and codeine.

Papaverine hydrochloride is 6,7-dimethoxy-1-veratrylisoquinoline hydrochloride and contains, on the dried basis, not less than 98.5% of $C_{20}H_{21}NO_4 \cdot HCl$. The molecular weight is 375.85.

Papaverine hydrochloride occurs as white crystals or white crystalline powder. One g dissolves in about 30 mL of water and in 120 mL of alcohol. It is soluble in chloroform and practically insoluble in ether.

Papaverine Hydrochloride Injection, USP, is a clear, colorless to pale-yellow solution.

Papaverine hydrochloride, for parenteral administration, is a smooth-muscle relaxant that is available in ampoules or vials containing 30 mg/mL (88.4 μmol/L) of papaverine base. Each ampoule or vial also contains edetate disodium, 0.005%. Sodium hydroxide may have been added during manufacture to adjust the pH.

CLINICAL PHARMACOLOGY

The most characteristic effect of papaverine is relaxation of the tonus of all smooth muscle, especially when it has been spasmodically contracted. Papaverine hydrochloride apparently acts directly on the muscle itself. This relaxation is noted in the *vascular system* and *bronchial musculature* and in the *gastrointestinal, biliary,* and *urinary tracts.*

The main actions of papaverine are exerted on cardiac and smooth muscle. Papaverine relaxes various smooth muscles, especially those of larger arteries; this relaxation may be prominent if spasm exists. The antispasmodic effect is a direct one and unrelated to muscle innervation, and the muscle still responds to drugs and other stimuli causing contraction. Papaverine has minimal actions on the central nervous system, although very large doses tend to produce some sedation and sleepiness in some patients. In certain circumstances, mild respiratory stimulation can be observed, but this is therapeutically inconsequential. Papaverine stimulates respiration by acting on carotid and aortic body chemoreceptors.

Papaverine relaxes the smooth musculature of the larger blood vessels, including the coronary, cerebral, peripheral, and pulmonary arteries. This action is particularly evident when such vessels are in spasm, induced reflexly or by drugs, and it provides the basis for the clinical use of papaverine in peripheral or pulmonary arterial embolism.

Experimentally in dogs, the alkaloid has been shown to cause fairly marked and long-lasting coronary vasodilata-

tion and an increase in coronary blood flow. However, it also appears to have a direct inotropic effect and, when increased mechanical activity coincides with decreased systemic pressure, increases in coronary blood flow may not be sufficient to prevent brief periods of hypoxic myocardial depression.
Papaverine is effective by all routes of administration. A considerable fraction of the drug localizes in fat depots and in the liver, with the remainder being distributed throughout the body. It is metabolized in the liver. About 90% of the drug is bound to plasma protein. Although estimates of its biologic half-life vary widely, reasonably constant plasma levels can be maintained with oral administration at 6-hour intervals. The drug is excreted in the urine in an inactive form.

INDICATIONS AND USAGE

Papaverine is recommended in various conditions accompanied by spasm of smooth muscle, such as *vascular spasm* associated with acute myocardial infarction (coronary occlusion), angina pectoris, peripheral and pulmonary embolism, peripheral vascular disease in which there is a vasospastic element, or certain cerebral angiospastic states; and *visceral spasm*, as in ureteral, biliary, or gastrointestinal colic.

CONTRAINDICATIONS

Intravenous injection of papaverine is contraindicated in the presence of complete atrioventricular heart block. When conduction is depressed, the drug may produce transient ectopic rhythms of ventricular origin, either premature beats or paroxysmal tachycardia.
Papaverine hydrochloride is not indicated for the treatment of impotence by intracorporeal injection. The intracorporeal injection of papaverine hydrochloride has been reported to have resulted in persistent priapism requiring medical and surgical intervention.

PRECAUTIONS

General—Papaverine Hydrochloride Injection, USP, should not be added to Lactated Ringer's Injection, because precipitation would result.
Papaverine hydrochloride should be used with caution in patients with glaucoma. The medication should be discontinued if hepatic hypersensitivity with gastrointestinal symptoms, jaundice, or eosinophilia becomes evident or if liver function test values become altered.
Usage in Pregnancy—Pregnancy Category C—No teratogenic effects were observed in rats when papaverine hydrochloride was administered subcutaneously as a single agent. It is not known whether papaverine can cause fetal harm when administered to a pregnant woman or can affect reproduction capacity. Papaverine hydrochloride should be given to a pregnant woman only if clearly needed.
Nursing Mothers—It is not known whether this drug is excreted in human milk. Because many drugs are excreted in human milk, caution should be exercised when papaverine hydrochloride is administered to a nursing woman.
Usage in Children—Safety and effectiveness in children have not been established.

ADVERSE REACTIONS

The following side effects have been reported: general discomfort, nausea, abdominal discomfort, anorexia, constipation or diarrhea, skin rash, malaise, vertigo, headache, intensive flushing of the face, perspiration, increase in the depth of respiration, increase in heart rate, a slight rise in blood pressure, and excessive sedation.
Hepatitis, probably related to an immune mechanism, has been reported infrequently. Rarely, this has progressed to cirrhosis.

DRUG ABUSE AND DEPENDENCE

Drug dependence resulting from the abuse of many of the selective depressants, including papaverine hydrochloride, has been reported.

OVERDOSAGE

Signs and Symptoms—The symptoms of toxicity from papaverine hydrochloride often result from vasomotor instability and include nausea, vomiting, weakness, central nervous system depression, nystagmus, diplopia, diaphoresis, flushing, dizziness, and sinus tachycardia. In large overdoses, papaverine is a potent inhibitor of cellular respiration and a weak calcium antagonist. Following an oral overdose of 15 g, metabolic acidosis with hyperventilation, hyperglycemia, and hypokalemia have been reported. No information on toxic serum concentrations is available.
Following intravenous overdosing in animals, seizures, tachyarrhythmias, and ventricular fibrillation have been reported. The oral median lethal dose in rats is 360 mg/kg.
Treatment—To obtain up-to-date information about the treatment of overdose, a good resource is your certified Regional Poison Control Center. Telephone numbers of certified poison control centers are listed in the *Physicians' Desk Reference (PDR)*. In managing overdosage, consider the possibility of multiple drug overdoses, interaction among drugs, and unusual drug kinetics in your patient.
Protect the patient's airway and support ventilation and perfusion. Meticulously monitor vital signs, blood gases, blood chemistry values, and other variables.
If convulsions occur, consider diazepam, phenytoin, or phenobarbital. If the seizures are refractory, general anesthesia with thiopental or halothane and paralysis with a neuromuscular blocking agent may be necessary.
For hypotension, consider intravenous fluids, elevation of the legs, and an inotropic vasopressor, such as dopamine or levarterenol. Theoretically, calcium gluconate may be helpful in treating some of the toxic cardiovascular effects of papaverine; monitor the ECG and plasma calcium concentrations.
Forced diuresis, peritoneal dialysis, hemodialysis, or charcoal hemoperfusion have not been established as beneficial for an overdose of papaverine hydrochloride.

DOSAGE AND ADMINISTRATION

Papaverine hydrochloride may be administered intravenously or intramuscularly. The intravenous route is recommended when an immediate effect is desired, but the drug *must* be injected *slowly* over the course of 1 or 2 minutes to avoid uncomfortable or alarming side effects.
Parenteral administration of papaverine hydrochloride in doses of 1 to 4 mL is repeated every 3 hours as indicated. In the treatment of cardiac extrasystoles, 2 doses may be given 10 minutes apart.

HOW SUPPLIED

(℞) Multiple-Dose Vials:
30 mg/mL, 10 mL, with 0.5% chlorobutanol (chloroform derivative) (No. 423)—(1s) NDC 0002-1676-01; (25s) NDC 0002-1676-25
(℞) Ampoules:
60 mg in 2 mL (No. 396)—(12s) NDC 0002-1664-12; (100s) NDC 0002-1664-02

[100290]

PERMAX® ℞
[pĕr′măks]
(pergolide mesylate)

DESCRIPTION

Permax® (Pergolide Mesylate, Lilly) is an ergot derivative dopamine receptor agonist at both D_1 and D_2 receptor sites. Pergolide mesylate is chemically designated as 8β-[(Methylthio)methyl]-6-propylergoline monomethanesulfonate; the structural formula is as follows:

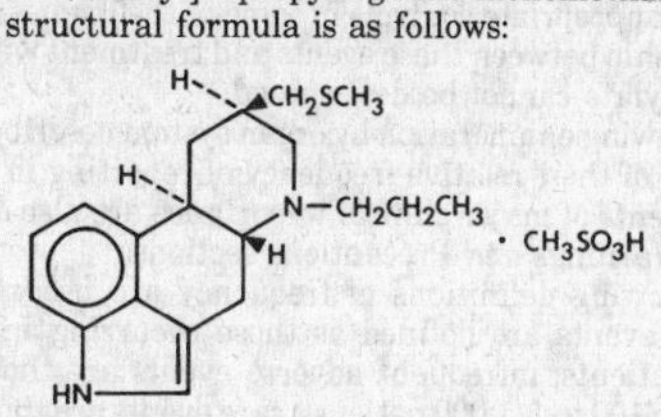

The formula weight of the base is 314.5; 1 mg of base corresponds to 3.18 μmol.
Permax is provided for oral administration in tablets containing 0.05 mg (0.159 μmol), 0.25 mg (0.795 μmol), or 1 mg (3.18 μmol) pergolide as the base. The tablets also contain croscarmellose sodium, iron oxide, lactose, magnesium stearate, and povidone. The 0.05-mg tablet also contains methionine, and the 0.25-mg tablet also contains F D & C Blue No. 2.

CLINICAL PHARMACOLOGY

Pharmacodynamic Information—Pergolide mesylate is a potent dopamine receptor agonist. Pergolide is 10 to 1,000 times more potent than bromocriptine on a milligram per milligram basis in various in vitro and in vivo test systems. Pergolide mesylate inhibits the secretion of prolactin in humans; it causes a transient rise in serum concentrations of growth hormone and a decrease in serum concentrations of luteinizing hormone. In Parkinson's disease, pergolide mesylate is believed to exert its therapeutic effect by directly stimulating postsynaptic dopamine receptors in the nigrostriatal system.
Pharmacokinetic Information (Absorption, Distribution, Metabolism, and Elimination)—Information on oral systemic bioavailability of pergolide mesylate is unavailable because of the lack of a sufficiently sensitive assay to detect the drug after the administration of a single dose. However, following oral administration of ^{14}C radiolabeled pergolide mesylate, approximately 55% of the administered radioactivity can be recovered from the urine and 5% from expired CO_2, suggesting that a significant fraction is absorbed. Nothing can be concluded about the extent of presystemic clearance, if any.
Data on postabsorption distribution of pergolide are unavailable.
At least 10 metabolites have been detected, including N-despropylpergolide, pergolide sulfoxide, and pergolide sulfone. Pergolide sulfoxide and pergolide sulfone are dopamine agonists in animals. The other detected metabolites have not been identified, and it is not known whether any other metabolites are active pharmacologically.
The major route of excretion is the kidney.
Pergolide is approximately 90% bound to plasma proteins. This extent of protein binding may be important to consider when pergolide mesylate is coadministered with other drugs known to affect protein binding.

INDICATIONS AND USAGE

Permax is indicated as adjunctive treatment to levodopa/carbidopa in the management of the signs and symptoms of Parkinson's disease.
Evidence to support the efficacy of pergolide mesylate as an antiparkinsonian adjunct was obtained in a multicenter study enrolling 376 patients with mild to moderate Parkinson's disease who were intolerant to *l*-dopa/carbidopa as manifested by moderate to severe dyskinesia and/or on-off phenomena. On average, the patients evaluated had been on *l*-dopa/carbidopa for 3.9 years (range, 2 days to 16.8 years).
The administration of pergolide mesylate permitted a 5% to 30% reduction in the daily dose of *l*-dopa. On average these patients treated with pergolide mesylate maintained an equivalent or better clinical status than they exhibited at baseline.

CONTRAINDICATIONS

Pergolide mesylate is contraindicated in patients who are hypersensitive to this drug or other ergot derivatives.

WARNINGS

Symptomatic Hypotension—In clinical trials, approximately 10% of patients taking pergolide mesylate with *l*-dopa versus 7% taking placebo with *l*-dopa experienced symptomatic orthostatic and/or sustained hypotension, especially during initial treatment. With gradual dosage titration, tolerance to the hypotension usually develops. It is therefore important to warn patients of the risk, to begin therapy with low doses, and to increase the dosage in carefully adjusted increments over a period of 3 to 4 weeks (*see* Dosage and Administration).
Hallucinosis—In controlled trials, pergolide mesylate with *l*-dopa caused hallucinosis in about 14% of patients as opposed to 3% taking placebo with *l*-dopa. This was of sufficient severity to cause discontinuation of treatment in about 3% of those enrolled; tolerance to this untoward effect was not observed.
Fatalities—In the placebo-controlled trial, 2 of 187 patients treated with placebo died as compared with 1 of 189 patients treated with pergolide mesylate. Of the 2,299 patients treated with pergolide mesylate in premarketing studies evaluated as of October 1988, 143 died while on the drug or shortly after discontinuing it. Because the patient population under evaluation was elderly, ill, and at high risk for death, it seems unlikely that pergolide mesylate played any role in these deaths, but the possibility that pergolide shortens survival of patients cannot be excluded with absolute certainty.
In particular, a case-by-case review of the clinical course of the patients who died failed to disclose any unique set of signs, symptoms, or laboratory results that would suggest that treatment with pergolide caused their deaths. Sixty-eight percent (68%) of the patients who died were 65 years of age or older. No death (other than a suicide) occurred within the first month of treatment; most of the patients who died had been on pergolide for years. A relative frequency of the causes of death by organ system are: Pulmonary failure/Pneumonia, 35%; Cardiovascular, 30%; Cancer, 11%; Unknown, 8.4%; Infection, 3.5%; Extrapyramidal syndrome, 3.5%; Stroke, 2.1%; Dysphagia, 2.1%; Injury, 1.4%; Suicide, 1.4%; Dehydration, 0.7%; Glomerulonephritis, 0.7%.

PRECAUTIONS

General—Caution should be exercised when administering pergolide mesylate to patients prone to cardiac dysrhythmias.
In a study comparing pergolide mesylate and placebo, patients taking pergolide mesylate were found to have significantly more episodes of atrial premature contractions (APCs) and sinus tachycardia.
The use of pergolide mesylate in patients on *l*-dopa may cause and/or exacerbate preexisting states of confusion and hallucinations (*see* Warnings) and preexisting dyskinesia.
Also, the abrupt discontinuation of pergolide mesylate in patients receiving it chronically as an adjunct to *l*-dopa may precipitate the onset of hallucinations and confusion; these may occur within a span of several days. Discontinuation of pergolide should be undertaken gradually whenever possible, even if the patient is to remain on *l*-dopa.

Continued on next page

• Identi-Code® symbol. This product information was prepared in June 1992. Current information on these and other products of Eli Lilly and Company may be obtained by direct inquiry to Lilly Research Laboratories, Lilly Corporate Center, Indianapolis, Indiana 46285, (317) 276-3714.

Lilly—Cont.

Information for Patients—Patients and their families should be informed of the common adverse consequences of the use of pergolide mesylate (*see* Adverse Reactions) and the risk of hypotension (*see* Warnings).

Patients should be advised to notify their physician if they become pregnant or intend to become pregnant during therapy.

Patients should be advised to notify their physician if they are breast-feeding an infant.

Laboratory Tests—No specific laboratory tests are deemed essential for the management of patients on Permax® (Pergolide Mesylate, Lilly). Periodic routine evaluation of all patients, however, is appropriate.

Drug Interactions—Dopamine antagonists, such as the neuroleptics (phenothiazines, butyrophenones, thioxanthines) or metoclopramide, ordinarily should not be administered concurrently with Permax (a dopamine agonist); these agents may diminish the effectiveness of Permax.

Because pergolide mesylate is approximately 90% bound to plasma proteins, caution should be exercised if pergolide mesylate is coadministered with other drugs known to affect protein binding.

Carcinogenesis, Mutagenesis, and Impairment of Fertility—A 2-year carcinogenicity study was conducted in mice using dietary levels of pergolide mesylate equivalent to oral doses of 0.6, 3.7, and 36.4 mg/kg/day in males and 0.6, 4.4, and 40.8 mg/kg/day in females. A 2-year study in rats was conducted using dietary levels equivalent to oral doses of 0.04, 0.18, and 0.88 mg/kg/day in males and 0.05, 0.28, and 1.42 mg/kg/day in females. The highest doses tested in the mice and rats were approximately 340 and 12 times the maximum human oral dose administered in controlled clinical trials (6 mg/day equivalent to 0.12 mg/kg/day).

A low incidence of uterine neoplasms occurred in both rats and mice. Endometrial adenomas and carcinomas were observed in rats. Endometrial sarcomas were observed in mice. The occurrence of these neoplasms is probably attributable to the high estrogen/progesterone ratio that would occur in rodents as a result of the prolactin-inhibiting action of pergolide mesylate. The endocrine mechanisms believed to be involved in the rodents are not present in humans. However, even though there is no known correlation between uterine malignancies occurring in pergolide-treated rodents and human risk, there are no human data to substantiate this conclusion.

Pergolide mesylate was evaluated for mutagenic potential in a battery of tests that included an Ames bacterial mutation assay, a DNA repair assay in cultured rat hepatocytes, an in vitro mammalian cell-point-mutation assay in cultured L5178Y cells, and a determination of chromosome alteration in bone marrow cells of Chinese hamsters. A weak mutagenic response was noted in the mammalian cell-point-mutation assay only after metabolic activation with rat liver microsomes. No mutagenic effects were obtained in the 2 other in vitro assays and in the vivo assay. The relevance of these findings in humans is unknown.

A fertility study in male and female mice showed that fertility was maintained at 0.6 and 1.7 mg/kg/day but decreased at 5.6 mg/kg/day. Prolactin has been reported to be involved in stimulating and maintaining progesterone levels required for implantation in mice, and, therefore, the impaired fertility at the high dose may have occurred because of depressed prolactin levels.

Usage in Pregnancy—*Pregnancy Category B*—Reproduction studies were conducted in mice at doses of 5, 16, and 45 mg/kg/day and in rabbits at doses of 2, 6, and 16 mg/kg/day. The highest doses tested in mice and rabbits were 375 and 133 times the 6 mg/day maximum human dose administered in controlled clinical trials. In these studies, there was no evidence of harm to the fetus due to pergolide mesylate.

There are, however, no adequate and well-controlled studies in pregnant women. Among women who received pergolide mesylate for endocrine disorders in premarketing studies, there were 33 pregnancies that resulted in healthy babies and 5 pregnancies that resulted in congential abnormalities (2 major, 3 minor); a causal relationship has not been established. Because human data are limited and because animal reproduction studies are not always predictive of human response, this drug should be used during pregnancy only if clearly needed.

Nursing Mothers—It is not known whether this drug is excreted in human milk. The pharmacologic action of pergolide mesylate suggests that it may interfere with lactation. Because many drugs are excreted in human milk and because of the potential for serious adverse reactions to pergolide mesylate in nursing infants, a decision should be made whether to discontinue nursing or to discontinue the drug, taking into account the importance of the drug to the mother.

Pediatric Use—Safety and effectiveness in children have not been established.

ADVERSE REACTIONS

Commonly Observed—In premarketing clinical trials, the most commonly observed adverse events associated with use of pergolide mesylate which were not seen at an equivalent incidence among placebo-treated patients were: nervous system complaints, including dyskinesia, hallucinations, somnolence, insomnia; digestive complaints, including nausea, constipation, diarrhea, dyspepsia; and respiratory system complaints, including rhinitis.

Associated With Discontinuation of Treatment—Twenty-seven percent (27%) of approximately 1,200 patients receiving pergolide mesylate for treatment of Parkinson's disease in premarketing clinical trials in the US and Canada discontinued treatment due to adverse reactions. The events most commonly causing discontinuation were related to the nervous system (15.5%), primarily hallucinations (7.8%) and confusion (1.8%).

Fatalities—*See* Warnings.

Incidence in Controlled Clinical Trials—The table that follows enumerates adverse events that occurred at a frequency of 1% or more among patients taking pergolide mesylate who participated in the premarketing controlled clinical trials comparing pergolide mesylate with placebo. In a double-blind, controlled study of 6 months' duration, patients with Parkinson's disease were continued on *l*-dopa/carbidopa and were randomly assigned to receive either pergolide mesylate or placebo as additional therapy.

The prescriber should be aware that these figures cannot be used to predict the incidence of side effects in the course of usual medical practice where patient characteristics and other factors differ from those which prevailed in the clinical trials. Similarly, the cited frequencies cannot be compared with figures obtained from other clinical investigations involving different treatments, uses, and investigators. The cited figures, however, do provide the prescribing physician with some basis for estimating the relative contribution of drug and nondrug factors to the side-effect incidence rate in the population studied.

[See table on next page.]

Events Observed During the Premarketing Evaluation of Permax® (Pergolide Mesylate, Lilly)—This section reports event frequencies evaluated as of October 1988 for adverse events occurring in a group of approximately 1,800 patients who took multiple doses of pergolide mesylate. The conditions and duration of exposure to pergolide mesylate varied greatly, involving well-controlled studies as well as experience in open and uncontrolled clinical settings. In the absence of appropriate controls in some of the studies, a causal relationship between these events and treatment with pergolide mesylate cannot be determined.

The following enumeration by organ system describes events in terms of their relative frequency of reporting in the data base. Events of major clinical importance are also described in the Warnings *and* Precautions sections.

The following definitions of frequency are used: frequent adverse events are defined as those occurring in at least 1/100 patients; infrequent adverse events are those occurring in 1/100 to 1/1,000 patients; rare events are those occurring in fewer than 1/1,000 patients.

Body as a Whole—*Frequent:* headache, asthenia, accidental injury, abdominal pain, chest pain, back pain, flu syndrome, neck pain, fever; *Infrequent:* facial edema, chills, enlarged abdomen, malaise, neoplasm, hernia, pelvic pain, sepsis, cellulitis, moniliasis, abscess, jaw pain, hypothermia; *Rare:* acute abdominal syndrome, LE syndrome

Cardiovascular System—*Frequent:* postural hypotension, syncope, hypertension, palpitations, vasodilatations, congestive heart failure; *Infrequent:* myocardial infarction, tachycardia, heart arrest, abnormal electrocardiogram, angina pectoris, thrombophlebitis, bradycardia, ventricular extrasystoles, cerebrovascular accident, ventricular tachycardia, cerebral ischemia, atrial fibrillation, varicose vein, pulmonary embolus, AV block, shock; *Rare:* vasculitis, pulmonary hypertension, pericarditis, migraine, heart block, cerebral hemorrhage

Digestive System—*Frequent:* nausea, vomiting, dyspepsia, diarrhea, constipation, dry mouth, dysphagia; *Infrequent:* flatulence, abnormal liver function tests, increased appetite, salivary gland enlargement, thirst, gastroenteritis, gastritis, periodontal abscess, intestinal obstruction, nausea and vomiting, gingivitis, esophagitis, cholelithiasis, tooth caries, hepatitis, stomach ulcer, melena, hepatomegaly, hematemesis, eructation; *Rare:* sialadenitis, peptic ulcer, pancreatitis, jaundice, glossitis, fecal incontinence, duodenitis, colitis, cholecystitis, aphthous stomatitis, esophageal ulcer

Endocrine System—*Infrequent:* hypothyroidism, adenoma, diabetes mellitus, ADH inappropriate; *Rare:* endocrine disorder, thyroid adenoma

Hemic and Lymphatic System—*Frequent:* anemia; *Infrequent:* leukopenia, lymphadenopathy, leukocytosis, thrombocytopenia, petechia, megaloblastic anemia, cyanosis; *Rare:* purpura, lymphocytosis, eosinophilia, thrombocythemia, acute lymphoblastic leukemia, polycythemia, splenomegaly

Metabolic and Nutritional System—*Frequent:* peripheral edema, weight loss, weight gain; *Infrequent:* dehydration, hypokalemia, hypoglycemia, iron deficiency anemia, hyperglycemia, gout, hypercholesteremia; *Rare:* electrolyte imbalance, cachexia, acidosis, hyperuricemia

Musculoskeletal System—*Frequent:* twitching, myalgia, arthralgia; *Infrequent:* bone pain, tenosynovitis, myositis, bone sarcoma, arthritis; *Rare:* osteoporosis, muscle atrophy, osteomyelitis

Nervous System—*Frequent:* dyskinesia, dizziness, hallucinations, confusion, somnolence, insomnia, dystonia, paresthesia, depression, anxiety, tremor, akinesia, extrapyramidal syndrome, abnormal gait, abnormal dreams, incoordination, psychosis, personality disorder, nervousness, choreoathetosis, amnesia, paranoid reaction, abnormal thinking; *Infrequent:* akathisia, neuropathy, neuralgia, hypertonia, delusions, convulsion, libido increased, euphoria, emotional lability, libido decreased, vertigo, myoclonus, coma, apathy, paralysis, neurosis, hyperkinesia, ataxia, acute brain syndrome, torticollis, meningitis, manic reaction, hypokinesia, hostility, agitation, hypotonia; *Rare:* stupor, neuritis, intracranial hypertension, hemiplegia, facial paralysis, brain edema, myelitis, hallucinations and confusion after abrupt discontinuation

Respiratory System—*Frequent:* rhinitis, dyspnea, pneumonia, pharyngitis, cough increased; *Infrequent:* epistaxis, hiccup, sinusitis, bronchitis, voice alteration, hemoptysis, asthma, lung edema, pleural effusion, laryngitis, emphysema, apnea, hyperventilation; *Rare:* pneumothorax, lung fibrosis, larynx edema, hypoxia, hypoventilation, hemothorax, carcinoma of lung

Skin and Appendages System—*Frequent:* sweating, rash; *Infrequent:* skin discoloration, pruritus, acne, skin ulcer, alopecia, dry skin, skin carcinoma, seborrhea, hirsutism, herpes simplex, eczema, fungal dermatitis, herpes zoster; *Rare:* vesiculobullous rash, subcutaneous nodule, skin nodule, skin benign neoplasm, lichenoid dermatitis

Special Senses System—*Frequent:* diplopia; *Infrequent:* otitis media, conjunctivitis, tinnitus, deafness, taste perversion, ear pain, eye pain, glaucoma, eye hemorrhage, photophobia, visual field defect; *Rare:* blindness, cataract, retinal detachment, retinal vascular disorder

Urogenital System—*Frequent:* urinary tract infection, urinary frequency, urinary incontinence, hematuria, dysmenorrhea; *Infrequent:* dysuria, breast pain, menorrhagia, impotence, cystitis, urinary retention, abortion, vaginal hemorrhage, vaginitis, priapism, kidney calculus, fibrocystic breast, lactation, uterine hemorrhage, urolithiasis, salpingitis, pyuria, metrorrhagia, menopause, kidney failure, breast carcinoma, cervical carcinoma; *Rare:* amenorrhea, bladder carcinoma, breast engorgement, epididymitis, hypogonadism, leukorrhea, nephrosis, pyelonephritis, urethral pain, uricaciduria, withdrawal bleeding

OVERDOSAGE

There is no clinical experience with massive overdosage. The largest overdose involved a young hospitalized adult patient who was not being treated with pergolide mesylate but who intentionally took 60 mg of the drug. He experienced vomiting, hypotension, and agitation. Another patient receiving a daily dosage of 7 mg of pergolide mesylate unintentionally took 19 mg/day for 3 days, after which his vital signs were normal but he experienced severe hallucinations. Within 36 hours of resumption of the prescribed dosage level, the hallucinations stopped. One patient unintentionally took 14 mg/day for 23 days instead of her prescribed 1.4 mg/day dosage. She experienced severe involuntary movements and tingling in her arms and legs. Another patient who inadvertently received 7 mg instead of the prescribed 0.7 mg experienced palpitations, hypotension, and ventricular extrasystoles. The highest total daily dose (prescribed for several patients with refractory Parkinson's disease) has exceeded 30 mg.

Symptoms—Animal studies indicate that the manifestations of overdosage in man might include nausea, vomiting, convulsions, decreased blood pressure, and CNS stimulation. The oral median lethal doses in mice and rats were 54 and 15 mg/kg respectively.

Treatment—To obtain up-to-date information about the treatment of overdose, a good resource is your certified Regional Poison Control Center. Telephone numbers of certified poison control centers are listed in the *Physicians' Desk Reference (PDR)*. In managing overdosage, consider the possibility of multiple drug overdoses, interaction among drugs, and unusual drug kinetics in your patient.

Management of overdosage may require supportive measures to maintain arterial blood pressure. Cardiac function should be monitored; an antiarrhythmic agent may be necessary. If signs of CNS stimulation are present, a phenothiazine or other butyrophenone neuroleptic agent may be indicated; the efficacy of such drugs in reversing the effects of overdose has not been assessed.

Protect the patient's airway and support ventilation and perfusion. Meticulously monitor and maintain, within acceptable limits, the patient's vital signs, blood gases, serum electrolytes, etc. Absorption of drugs from the gastrointestinal tract may be decreased by giving activated charcoal,

Incidence of Treatment-Emergent Adverse Experiences in the Placebo-Controlled Clinical Trial
Percentage of Patients Reporting Events

Body System/ Adverse Event*	Pergolide Mesylate N = 189	Placebo N = 187
Body as a Whole		
Pain	7.0	2.1
Abdominal pain	5.8	2.1
Injury, accident	5.8	7.0
Headache	5.3	6.4
Asthenia	4.2	4.8
Chest pain	3.7	2.1
Flu syndrome	3.2	2.1
Neck pain	2.7	1.6
Back pain	1.6	2.1
Surgical procedure	1.6	<1
Chills	1.1	0
Face edema	1.1	0
Infection	1.1	0
Cardiovascular		
Postural hypotension	9.0	7.0
Vasodilatation	3.2	<1
Palpitation	2.1	<1
Hypotension	2.1	<1
Syncope	2.1	1.1
Hypertension	1.6	1.1
Arrhythmia	1.1	<1
Myocardial infarction	1.1	<1
Digestive		
Nausea	24.3	12.8
Constipation	10.6	5.9
Diarrhea	6.4	2.7
Dyspepsia	6.4	2.1
Anorexia	4.8	2.7
Dry mouth	3.7	<1
Vomiting	2.7	1.6
Hemic and Lymphatic		
Anemia	1.1	<1
Metabolic and Nutritional		
Peripheral edema	7.4	4.3
Edema	1.6	0
Weight gain	1.6	0
Musculoskeletal		
Arthralgia	1.6	2.1
Bursitis	1.6	<1
Myalgia	1.1	<1
Twitching	1.1	0
Nervous System		
Dyskinesia	62.4	24.6
Dizziness	19.1	13.9
Hallucinations	13.8	3.2
Dystonia	11.6	8.0
Confusion	11.1	9.6
Somnolence	10.1	3.7
Insomnia	7.9	3.2
Anxiety	6.4	4.3
Tremor	4.2	7.5
Depression	3.2	5.4
Abnormal dreams	2.7	4.3
Personality disorder	2.1	<1
Psychosis	2.1	0
Abnormal gait	1.6	1.6
Akathisia	1.6	0
Extrapyramidal syndrome	1.6	1.1
Incoordination	1.6	<1
Paresthesia	1.6	3.2
Akinesia	1.1	1.1
Hypertonia	1.1	0
Neuralgia	1.1	<1
Speech disorder	1.1	1.6
Respiratory System		
Rhinitis	12.2	5.4
Dyspnea	4.8	1.1
Epistaxis	1.6	<1
Hiccup	1.1	0
Skin and Appendages		
Rash	3.2	2.1
Sweating	2.1	2.7
Special Senses		
Abnormal vision	5.8	5.4
Diplopia	2.1	0
Taste perversion	1.6	0
Eye disorder	1.1	0
Urogenital System		
Urinary frequency	2.7	6.4
Urinary tract infection	2.7	3.7
Hematuria	1.1	<1

*Events reported by at least 1% of patients receiving pergolide mesylate are included.

which, in many cases, is more effective than emesis or lavage; consider charcoal instead of or in addition to gastric emptying. Repeated doses of charcoal over time may hasten elimination of some drugs that have been absorbed. Safeguard the patient's airway when employing gastric emptying or charcoal.

There is no experience with dialysis or hemoperfusion, and these procedures are unlikely to be of benefit.

DOSAGE AND ADMINISTRATION

Administration of Permax® (Pergolide Mesylate, Lilly) should be initiated with a daily dosage of 0.05 mg for the first 2 days. The dosage should then be gradually increased by 0.1 or 0.15 mg/day every third day over the next 12 days of therapy. The dosage may then be increased by 0.25 mg/day every third day until an optimal therapeutic dosage is achieved. Permax is usually administered in divided doses 3 times per day. During dosage titration, the dosage of concurrent *l*-dopa/carbidopa may be cautiously decreased.

In clinical studies, the mean therapeutic daily dosage of Permax was 3 mg/day. The average concurrent daily dosage of *l*-dopa/carbidopa (expressed as *l*-dopa) was approximately 650 mg/day. The efficacy of Permax at doses above 5 mg/day has not been systematically evaluated.

HOW SUPPLIED

(R) *Permax® (Pergolide Mesylate, Lilly)*
Tablets (scored):
0.05 mg, ivory (No. 4131)—(RxPak* of 30) NDC 0002-4131-30
0.25 mg, green (No. 4133)—(RxPak of 100) NDC 0002-4133-02
1 mg, pink (No. 4135)—(RxPak of 100) NDC 0002-4135-02
Store at controlled room temperature, 59° to 86°F (15° to 30°C).

*All RxPaks (prescription packages, Lilly) have safety closures.

[022691]

Shown in Product Identification Section, page 416

PHENOBARBITAL   ℂ
[fē 'nō-bär 'bĭ-tăl]
Elixir & Tablets, USP

WARNING: MAY BE HABIT-FORMING
DESCRIPTION

The barbiturates are nonselective central nervous system (CNS) depressants that are primarily used as sedative-hypnotics. In subhypnotic doses, they are also used as anticonvulsants. The barbiturates and their sodium salts are subject to control under the Federal Controlled Substances Act.

Phenobarbital is a barbituric acid derivative and occurs as white, odorless, small crystals or crystalline powder that is very slightly soluble in water; soluble in alcohol, in ether, and in solutions of fixed alkali hydroxides and carbonates; sparingly soluble in chloroform. Phenobarbital is 5-ethyl-5-phenylbarbituric acid and has the empirical formula $C_{12}H_{12}N_2O_3$ Its molecular weight is 232.24.

Phenobarbital is a substituted pyrimidine derivative in which the basic structure is barbituric acid, a substance that has no CNS activity. CNS activity is obtained by substituting alkyl, alkenyl, or aryl groups on the pyrimidine ring.

Each 5 mL of the elixir contains 20 mg (0.086 mmol) phenobarbital. The elixir also contains FD & C Red No. 40, flavors, glycerin, sucrose, water, and alcohol, 14%.

The tablets contain 15 mg (0.064 mmol), 30 mg (0.129 mmol), 60 mg (0.258 mmol), or 100 mg (0.431 mmol) phenobarbital. The tablets also contain cornstarch, lactose, magnesium stearate, and talc.

CLINICAL PHARMACOLOGY

Barbiturates are capable of producing all levels of CNS mood alteration, from excitation to mild sedation, hypnosis, and deep coma. Overdosage can produce death. In high enough therapeutic doses, barbiturates induce anesthesia.

Barbiturates depress the sensory cortex, decrease motor activity, alter cerebellar function, and produce drowsiness, sedation, and hypnosis.

Barbiturate-induced sleep differs from physiologic sleep. Sleep laboratory studies have demonstrated that barbiturates reduce the amount of time spent in the rapid eye movement (REM) phase of sleep or the dreaming stage. Also, Stages III and IV sleep are decreased. Following abrupt cessation of barbiturates used regularly, patients may experience markedly increased dreaming, nightmares, and/or insomnia. Therefore, withdrawal of a single therapeutic dose over 5 or 6 days has been recommended to lessen the REM rebound and disturbed sleep that contribute to the drug withdrawal syndrome (for example, the dose should be decreased from 3 to 2 doses/day for 1 week).

In studies, secobarbital sodium and pentobarbital sodium have been found to lose most of their effectiveness for both inducing and maintaining sleep by the end of 2 weeks of con-

Continued on next page

* Identi-Code® symbol. This product information was prepared in June 1992. Current information on these and other products of Eli Lilly and Company may be obtained by direct inquiry to Lilly Research Laboratories, Lilly Corporate Center, Indianapolis, Indiana 46285, (317) 276-3714.

Lilly—Cont.

tinued drug administration even with the use of multiple doses. As with secobarbital sodium and pentobarbital sodium, other barbiturates (including amobarbital) might be expected to lose their effectiveness for inducing and maintaining sleep after about 2 weeks. The short-, intermediate-, and to a lesser degree, long-acting barbiturates have been widely prescribed for treating insomnia. Although the clinical literature abounds with claims that the short-acting barbiturates are superior for producing sleep whereas the intermediate-acting compounds are more effective in maintaining sleep, controlled studies have failed to demonstrate these differential effects. Therefore, as sleep medications, the barbiturates are of limited value beyond short-term use.

Barbiturates have little analgesic action at subanesthetic doses. Rather, in subanesthetic doses, these drugs may increase the reaction to painful stimuli. All barbiturates exhibit anticonvulsant activity in anesthetic doses. However, of the drugs in this class, only phenobarbital, mephobarbital, and metharbital are effective as oral anticonvulsants in subhypnotic doses.

Barbiturates are respiratory depressants, and the degree of respiratory depression is dependent upon the dose. With hypnotic doses, respiratory depression produced by barbiturates is similar to that which occurs during physiologic sleep and is accompanied by a slight decrease in blood pressure and heart rate.

Studies in laboratory animals have shown that barbiturates cause reduction in the tone and contractility of the uterus, ureters, and urinary bladder. However, concentrations of the drugs required to produce this effect in humans are not reached with sedative-hypnotic doses.

Barbiturates do not impair normal hepatic function but have been shown to induce liver microsomal enzymes, thus increasing and/or altering the metabolism of barbiturates and other drugs (*see* Drug Interactions *under* Precautions).

Pharmacokinetics—Barbiturates are absorbed in varying degrees following oral or parenteral administration. The salts are more rapidly absorbed than are the acids. The rate of absorption is increased if the sodium salt is ingested as a dilute solution or taken on an empty stomach.

Duration of action, which is related to the rate at which the barbiturates are redistributed throughout the body, varies among persons and in the same person from time to time.

Phenobarbital is classified as a long-acting barbiturate when taken orally. Its onset of action is 1 hour or longer, and its duration of action ranges from 10 to 12 hours.

Barbiturates are weak acids that are absorbed and rapidly distributed to all tissues and fluids, with high concentrations in the brain, liver, and kidneys. Lipid solubility of the barbiturates is the dominant factor in their distribution within the body. The more lipid soluble the barbiturate, the more rapidly it penetrates all tissues of the body. Barbiturates are bound to plasma and tissue proteins to a varying degree with the degree of binding increasing directly as a function of lipid solubility.

Phenobarbital has the lowest lipid solubility, lowest plasma binding, lowest brain protein binding, the longest delay in onset activity, and the longest duration of action. The plasma half-life for phenobarbital in adults ranges between 53 and 118 hours with a mean of 79 hours. The plasma half-life for phenobarbital in children and newborns (less than 48 hours old) ranges between 60 to 180 hours with a mean of 110 hours.

Barbiturates are metabolized primarily by the hepatic microsomal enzyme system, and the metabolic products are excreted in the urine and, less commonly, in the feces. Approximately 25% to 50% of a dose of phenobarbital is eliminated unchanged in the urine. The excretion of unmetabolized barbiturate is one feature that distinguishes the long-acting category from those belonging to other categories, which are almost entirely metabolized. The inactive metabolities of the barbiturates are excreted as conjugates of glucuronic acid.

INDICATIONS AND USAGE

A. Sedative
B. Anticonvulsant—For the treatment of generalized and partial seizures.

CONTRAINDICATIONS

Phenobarbital is contraindicated in patients who are hypersensitive to barbiturates, in patients with a history of manifest or latent porphyria, and in patients with marked impairment of liver function or respiratory disease in which dyspnea or obstruction is evident.

WARNINGS

1. *Habit Forming*—Phenobarbital may be habit forming. Tolerance and psychological and physical dependence may occur with continued use (*see* Drug Abuse and Dependence *and* Pharmacokinetics *under* Clinical Pharmacology). Patients who have psychologic dependence on barbiturates may increase the dosage or decrease the dosage interval without consulting a physician and may subsequently develop a physical dependence on barbiturates. In order to minimize the possibility of overdosage or the development of dependence, the prescribing and dispensing of sedative-hypnotic barbiturates should be limited to the amount required for the interval until the next appointment. Abrupt cessation after prolonged use in a person who is dependent on the drug may result in withdrawal symptoms, including delirium, convulsions, and possibly death. Barbiturates should be withdrawn gradually from any patient known to be taking excessive doses over long periods of time (*see* Drug Abuse and Dependence).

2. *Acute or Chronic Pain*—Caution should be exercised when barbiturates are administered to patients with acute or chronic pain, because paradoxical excitement could be induced or important symptoms could be masked. However, the use of barbiturates as sedatives in the postoperative surgical period and as adjuncts to cancer chemotherapy is well established.

3. *Usage in Pregnancy*—Barbiturates can cause fetal damage when administered to a pregnant woman. Retrospective, case-controlled studies have suggested a connection between the maternal consumption of barbiturates and a higher than expected incidence of fetal abnormalities. Barbiturates readily cross the placental barrier and are distributed throughout fetal tissues; the highest concentrations are found in the placenta, fetal liver, and brain. Fetal blood levels approach maternal blood levels following parenteral administration.

Withdrawal symptoms occur in infants born to women who receive barbiturates throughout the last trimester of pregnancy (*see* Drug Abuse and Dependence).

If phenobarbital is used during pregnancy or if the patient becomes pregnant while taking this drug, the patient should be apprised of the potential hazard to the fetus.

4. *Usage in Children*—Phenobarbital has been reported to be associated with cognitive deficits in children taking it for complicated febrile seizures.

5. *Synergistic Effects*—The concomitant use of alcohol or other CNS depressants may produce additive CNS depressant effects.

PRECAUTIONS

General—Barbiturates may be habit forming. Tolerance and psychological and physical dependence may occur with continued use (*see* Drug Abuse and Dependence).

Barbiturates should be administered with caution, if at all, to patients who are mentally depressed, have suicidal tendencies, or have a history of drug abuse.

Elderly or debilitated patients may react to barbiturates with marked excitement, depression, or confusion. In some persons, especially children, barbiturates repeatedly produce excitement rather than depression.

In patients with hepatic damage, barbiturates should be administered with caution and initially in reduced doses. Barbiturates should not be administered to patients showing the premonitory signs of hepatic coma.

The systemic effects of exogenous and endogenous corticosteroids may be diminished by phenobarbital. Thus, this product should be administered with caution to patients with borderline hypoadrenal function, regardless of whether it is of pituitary or of primary adrenal origin.

Information for Patients—The following information and instructions should be given to patients receiving barbiturates.

1. The use of barbiturates carries with it an associated risk of psychological and/or physical dependence. The patient should be warned against increasing the dose of the drug without consulting a physician.
2. Barbiturates may impair the mental and/or physical abilities required for the performance of potentially hazardous tasks, such as driving a car or operating machinery. The patient should be cautioned accordingly.
3. Alcohol should not be consumed while taking barbiturates. The concurrent use of the barbiturates with other CNS depressants (eg, alcohol, narcotics, tranquilizers, and antihistamines) may result in additional CNS-depressant effects.

Laboratory Tests—Prolonged therapy with barbiturates should be accompanied by periodic laboratory evaluation of organ systems, including hematopoietic, renal, and hepatic systems (*see* General *under* Precautions *and* Adverse Reactions).

Drug Interactions—Most reports of clinically significant drug interactions occurring with the barbiturates have involved phenobarbital. However, the application of these data to other barbiturates appears valid and warrants serial blood level determinations of the relevant drugs when there are multiple therapies.

1. *Anticoagulants*—Phenobarbital lowers the plasma levels of dicumarol and causes a decrease in anticoagulant activity as measured by the prothrombin time. Barbiturates can induce hepatic microsomal enzymes resulting in increased metabolism and decreased anticoagulant response of oral anticoagulants (eg, warfarin, acenocoumarol, dicumarol, and phenprocoumon). Patients stabilized on anticoagulant therapy may require dosage adjustments if barbiturates are added to or withdrawn from their dosage regimen.
2. *Corticosteroids*—Barbiturates appear to enhance the metabolism of exogenous corticosteroids, probably through the induction of hepatic microsomal enzymes. Patients stabilized on corticosteroid therapy may require dosage adjustments if barbiturates are added to or withdrawn from their dosage regimen.
3. *Griseofulvin*—Phenobarbital appears to interfere with the absorption of orally administered griseofulvin, thus decreasing its blood level. The effect of the resultant decreased blood levels of griseofulvin on therapeutic response has not been established. However, it would be preferable to avoid concomitant administration of these drugs.
4. *Doxycycline*—Phenobarbital has been shown to shorten the half-life of doxycycline for as long as 2 weeks after barbiturate therapy is discontinued. This mechanism is probably through the induction of hepatic microsomal enzymes that metabolize the antibiotic. If phenobarbital and doxycycline are administered concurrently, the clinical response to doxycycline should be monitored closely.
5. *Phenytoin, Sodium Valproate, Valproic Acid*—The effect of barbiturates on the metabolism of phenytoin appears to be variable. Some investigators report an accelerating effect, whereas others report no effect. Because the effect of barbiturates on the metabolism of phenytoin is not predictable, phenytoin and barbiturate blood levels should be monitored more frequently if these drugs are given concurrently. Sodium valproate and valproic acid increase the phenobarbital serum levels; therefore, phenobarbital blood levels should be closely monitored and appropriate dosage adjustments made as clinically indicated.
6. *CNS Depressants*—The concomitant use of other CNS depressants, including other sedatives or hypnotics, antihistamines, tranquilizers, or alcohol, may produce additive depressant effects.
7. *Monoamine Oxidase Inhibitors (MAOIs)*—MAOIs prolong the effects of barbiturates, probably because metabolism of the barbiturate is inhibited.
8. *Estradiol, Estrone, Progesterone, and Other Steroidal Hormones*—Pretreatment with or concurrent administration of phenobarbital may decrease the effect of estradiol by increasing its metabolism. There have been reports of patients treated with antiepileptic drugs (eg, phenobarbital) who become pregnant while taking oral contraceptives. An alternate contraceptive method might be suggested to women taking phenobarbital.

Carcinogenesis—1. *Animal Data.* Phenobarbital sodium is carcinogenic in mice and rats after lifetime administration. In mice, it produced benign and malignant liver cell tumors. In rats, benign liver cell tumors were observed very late in life.

2. *Human Data*—In a 29-year epidemiologic study of 9,136 patients who were treated on an anticonvulsant protocol that included phenobarbital, results indicated a higher than normal incidence of hepatic carcinoma. Previously, some of these patients had been treated with thorotrast, a drug which is known to produce hepatic carcinomas. Thus, this study did not provide sufficient evidence that phenobarbital sodium is carcinogenic in humans.

A retrospective study of 84 children with brain tumors matched to 73 normal controls and 78 cancer controls (malignant disease other than brain tumors) suggested an association between exposure to barbiturates prenatally and an increased incidence of brain tumors.

Usage in Pregnancy—*1. Teratogenic Effects. Pregnancy Category D*—*See* Usage in Pregnancy *under* Warnings.

2. *Nonteratogenic Effects*—Reports of infants suffering from long-term barbiturate exposure in utero included the acute withdrawal syndrome of seizures and hyperirritability from birth to a delayed onset of up to 14 days (*see* Drug Abuse and Dependence).

Labor and Delivery—Hypnotic doses of barbiturates do not appear to impair uterine activity significantly during labor. Full anesthetic doses of barbiturates decrease the force and frequency of uterine contractions. Administration of sedative-hypnotic barbiturates to the mother during labor may result in respiratory depression in the newborn. Premature infants are particularly susceptible to the depressant effects of barbiturates. If barbiturates are used during labor and delivery, resuscitation equipment should be available.

Data are not available to evaluate the effect of barbiturates when forceps delivery or other intervention is necessary or to determine the effect of barbiturates on the later growth, development, and functional maturation of the child.

Nursing Mothers—Caution should be exercised when phenobarbital is administered to a nursing woman, because small amounts of barbiturates are excreted in the milk.

ADVERSE REACTIONS

The following adverse reactions have been reported:

CNS Depression—Residual sedation or "hangover," drowsiness, lethargy, and vertigo. Emotional disturbances and phobias may be accentuated. In some persons, barbiturates such as phenobarbital repeatedly produce excitement rather

than depression, and the patient may appear to be inebriated. Irritability and hyperactivity can occur in children. Like other nonanalgesic hypnotic drugs, barbiturates such as phenobarbital, when given in the presence of pain, may cause restlessness, excitement, and even delirium. Rarely, the use of barbiturates results in localized or diffuse myalgic, neuralgic, or arthritic pain, especially in psychoneurotic patients with insomnia. The pain may appear in paroxysms, is most intense in the early morning hours, and is most frequently located in the region of the neck, shoulder girdle, and upper limbs. Symptoms may last for days after the drug is discontinued.

Respiratory/Circulatory —Respiratory depression, apnea, circulatory collapse.

Allergic —Acquired hypersensitivity to barbiturates consists chiefly in allergic reactions that occur especially in persons who tend to have asthma, urticaria, angioedema, and similar conditions. Hypersensitivity reactions in this category include localized swelling, particularly of the eyelids, cheeks, or lips, and erythematous dermatitis. Rarely, exfoliative dermatitis (eg, Stevens-Johnson syndrome and toxic epidermal necrolysis) may be caused by phenobarbital and can prove fatal. The skin eruption may be associated with fever, delirium, and marked degenerative changes in the liver and other parenchymatous organs. In a few cases, megaloblastic anemia has been associated with the chronic use of phenobarbital.

Other —Nausea and vomiting; headache, osteomalacia.

The following adverse reactions and their incidence were compiled from surveillance of thousands of hospitalized patients who received barbiturates. Because such patients may be less aware of the milder adverse effects of barbiturates, the incidence of these reactions may be somewhat higher in fully ambulatory patients.

More than 1 in 100 Patients

The most common adverse reaction, estimated to occur at a rate of 1 to 3 patients per 100, is:

Nervous System: Somnolence

Less than 1 in 100 Patients

Adverse reactions estimated to occur at a rate of less than 1 in 100 patients are listed below, grouped by organ system and by decreasing order of occurrence:

Nervous System: Agitation, confusion, hyperkinesia, ataxia, CNS depression, nightmares, nervousness, psychiatric disturbance, hallucinations, insomnia, anxiety, dizziness, abnormality in thinking

Respiratory System: Hypoventilation, apnea

Cardiovascular System: Bradycardia, hypotension, syncope

Digestive System: Nausea, vomiting, constipation

Other Reported Reactions: Headache, injection site reactions, hypersensitivity reactions (angioedema, skin rashes, exfoliative dermatitis), fever, liver damage, megaloblastic anemia following chronic phenobarbital use

DRUG ABUSE AND DEPENDENCE

Controlled Substance —Phenobarbital is a Schedule IV drug.

Dependence —Barbiturates may be habit forming. Tolerance, psychological dependence, and physical dependence may occur, especially following prolonged use of high doses of barbiturates. Daily administration in excess of 400 mg of pentobarbital or secobarbital for approximately 90 days is likely to produce some degreee of physical dependence. A dosage of 600 to 800 mg taken for at least 35 days is sufficient to produce withdrawal seizures. The average daily dose for the barbiturate addict is usually about 1.5 g. As tolerance to barbiturates develops, the amount needed to maintain the same level of intoxication increases; tolerance to a fatal dosage, however, does not increase more than twofold. As this occurs, the margin between intoxicating dosage and fatal dosage becomes smaller.

Symptoms of acute intoxication with barbiturates include unsteady gait, slurred speech, and sustained nystagmus. Mental signs of chronic intoxication include confusion, poor judgment, irritability, insomnia, and somatic complaints. Symptoms of barbiturate dependence are similar to those of chronic alcoholism. If an individual appears to be intoxicated with alcohol to a degree that is radically disproportionate to the amount of alcohol in his or her blood, the use of barbiturates should be suspected. The lethal dose of a barbiturate is far less if alcohol is also ingested.

The symptoms of barbiturate withdrawal can be severe and may cause death. Minor withdrawal symptoms may appear 8 to 12 hours after the last dose of a barbiturate. These symptoms usually appear in the following order: anxiety, muscle twitching, tremor of hands and fingers, progressive weakness, dizziness, distortion in visual perception, nausea, vomiting, insomnia, and orthostatic hypotension. Major withdrawal symptoms (convulsions and delirium) may occur within 16 hours and last up to 5 days after abrupt cessation of barbiturates. The intensity of withdrawal symptoms gradually declines over a period of approximately 15 days. Individuals susceptible to barbiturate abuse and dependence include alcoholics and opiate abusers as well as other sedative-hypnotic and amphetamine abusers.

Drug dependence on barbiturates arises from repeated administration of a barbiturate or agent with barbiturate-like effect on a continuous basis, generally in amounts exceeding therapeutic dose levels. The characteristics of drug dependence on barbiturates include: (a) a strong desire or need to continue taking the drug; (b) a tendency to increase the dose; (c) a psychic dependence on the effects of the drug related to subjective and individual appreciation of those effects; and (d) a physical dependence on the effects of the drug, requiring its presence for maintenance of homeostasis and resulting in a definite, characteristic, and self-limited abstinence syndrome when the drug is withdrawn.

Treatment of barbiturate dependence consists of cautious and gradual withdrawal of the drug. Barbiturate-dependent patients can be withdrawn by using a number of different withdrawal regimens. In all cases, withdrawal requires an extended period of time. One method involves substituting a 30-mg dose of phenobarbital for each 100- to 200-mg dose of barbiturate that the patient has been taking. The total daily amount of phenobarbital is then administered in 3 or 4 divided doses, not to exceed 600 mg daily. If signs of withdrawal occur on the first day of treatment, a loading dose of 100 to 200 mg of phenobarbital may be administered IM in addition to the oral dose. After stabilization on phenobarbital, the total daily dose is decreased by 30 mg/day as long as withdrawal is proceeding smoothly. A modification of this regimen involves initiating treatment at the patient's regular dosage level and decreasing the daily dosage by 10% if tolerated by the patient.

Infants who are physically dependent on barbiturates may be given phenobarbital, 3 to 10 mg/kg/day. After withdrawal symptoms (hyperactivity, disturbed sleep, tremors, and hyperreflexia) are relieved, the dosage of phenobarbital should be gradually decreased and completely withdrawn over a 2-week period.

OVERDOSAGE

Signs and Symptoms —The onset of symptoms following a toxic oral exposure to phenobarbital may not occur until several hours following ingestion. The toxic dose of barbiturates varies considerably. In general, an oral dose of 1 g of most barbiturates produces serious poisoning in an adult. Death commonly occurs after 2 to 10 g of ingested barbiturate. The sedated, therapeutic blood levels of phenobarbital range between 5 to 40 μg/mL; the usual lethal blood level ranges from 100 to 200 μg/mL. Barbiturate intoxication may be confused with alcoholism, bromide intoxication, and various neurologic disorders. Potential tolerance must be considered when evaluating significance of dose and plasma concentration.

The manifestations of a long-acting barbiturate in overdose include nystagmus, ataxia, CNS depression, respiratory depression, hypothermia, and hypotension. Other findings may include absent or depressed reflexes and erythematous or hemorrhagic blisters (primarily at pressure points). Following massive exposure to phenobarbital, pulmonary edema, circulatory collapse with loss of peripheral vascular tone, cardiac arrest, and death may occur.

In extreme overdose, all electrical activity in the brain may cease, in which case a "flat" EEG normally equated with clinical death should not be accepted. This effect is fully reversible unless hypoxic damage occurs.

Consideration should be given to the possibility of barbiturate intoxication even in situations that appear to involve trauma.

Complications such as pneumonia, pulmonary edema, cardiac arrhythmias, congestive heart failure, and renal failure may occur. Uremia may increase CNS sensitivity to barbiturates if renal function is impaired. Differential diagnosis should include hypoglycemia, head trauma, cerebrovascular accidents, convulsive states, and diabetic coma.

Treatment —To obtain up-to-date information about the treatment of overdose, a good resource is your certified Regional Poison Control Center. Telephone numbers of certified poison control centers are listed in the *Physicians' Desk Reference (PDR)*. In managing overdosage, consider the possibility of multiple drug overdoses, interaction among drugs, and unusual drug kinetics in your patient.

Protect the patient's airway and support ventilation and perfusion. Meticulously monitor and maintain, within acceptable limits, the patient's vital signs, blood gases, serum electrolytes, etc. Absorption of drugs from the gastrointestinal tract may be decreased by giving activated charcoal, which, in many cases, is more effective than emesis or lavage; consider charcoal instead of or in addition to gastric emptying. Repeated doses of charcoal over time may hasten elimination of some drugs that have been absorbed. Safeguard the patient's airway when employing gastric emptying or charcoal.

Alkalinization of urine hastens phenobarbital excretion, but dialysis and hemoperfusion are more effective and cause less troublesome alterations in electrolyte equilibrium. If the patient has chronically abused sedatives, withdrawal reactions may be manifest following acute overdose.

DOSAGE AND ADMINISTRATION

The dose of phenobarbital must be individualized with full knowledge of its particular characteristics. Factors of consideration are the patient's age, weight, and condition.

Sedation:

For sedation, the drug may be administered in single does of 30 to 120 mg repeated at intervals: frequency will be determined by the patient's response. It is generally considered that no more than 400 mg of phenobarbital should be administered during a 24-hour period.

Adults:

Daytime Sedation: 30 to 120 mg daily in 2 to 3 divided doses

Oral Hypnotic: 100 to 200 mg.

Anticonvulsant Use —Clinical laboratory reference values should be used to determine the therapeutic anticonvulsant level of phenobarbital in the serum. To achieve the blood levels considered therapeutic in children, higher per-kilogram dosages are generally necessary for phenobarbital and most other anticonvulsants. In children and infants, phenobarbital at a loading dose of 15 to 20 mg/kg produces blood levels of about 20 μg/mL shortly after administration.

Phenobarbital has been used in the treatment and prophylaxis of febrile seizures. However, it has not been established that prevention of febrile seizures influences the subsequent development of epilepsy.

Adults: 60 to 200 mg/day.

Children: 3 to 6 mg/kg/day.

Special Patient Population —Dosage should be reduced in the elderly or debilitated because these patients may be more sensitive to barbiturates. Dosage should be reduced for patients with impaired renal function or hepatic disease.

HOW SUPPLIED

ℭ Elixir:

0.4 g/100 mL (No. 227)*—(16 fl oz) NDC 0002-2438-05

ℭ Tablets:

15 mg (No. 1544)—(100s) NDC 0002-1031-02; (1000s) NDC 0002-1031-04

30 mg (No. 1545)—(100s) NDC 0002-1032-02; (1000s) NDC 0002-1032-04

60 mg (No. 1574)—(100s) NDC 0002-1037-02; (1000s) NDC 0002-1037-04

100 mg (No. 1546)—(100s) NDC 0002-1033-02

Keep tightly closed. Store at controlled room temperature, 59° to 86°F (15° to 30°C).

*Contains alcohol, 14%.

[103091]

PROTAMINE SULFATE   ℞

[prō'ta-mĕn sŭl'fāt]

Injection, USP

DESCRIPTION

Protamines are simple proteins of low molecular weight that are rich in arginine and strongly basic. They occur in the sperm of salmon and certain other species of fish.

Protamine sulfate occurs as fine white or off-white amorphous or crystalline powder. It is sparingly soluble in water. The pH is between 6 and 7. The cationic hydrogenated protamine at a pH of 6.8 to 7.1 reacts with anionic heparin at a pH of 5.0 to 7.5 to form an inactive complex.

Protamine Sulfate Injection, USP, is a sterile, isotonic solution of protamine sulfate. It acts as a heparin antagonist. It is also a weak anticoagulant.

Each 5-mL ampoule of Protamine Sulfate Injection contains protamine sulfate equivalent to 50 mg of activity, and each 25-mL vial contains protamine sulfate equivalent to 250 mg of activity. Both products also contain 0.9% Sodium Chloride Reagent in Water for Injection, USP. Sodium phosphate and/or sulfuric acid may have been added during manufacture to adjust the pH. Contains no preservative.

Protamine sulfate is administered intravenously.

CLINICAL PHARMACOLOGY

When administered alone, protamine has an anticoagulant effect. However, when it is given in the presence of heparin (which is strongly acidic), a stable salt is formed and the anticoagulant activity of both drugs is lost.

Protamine sulfate has a rapid onset of action. Neutralization of heparin occurs within 5 minutes after intravenous administration of an appropriate dose of protamine sulfate. Although the metabolic fate of the heparin-protamine complex has not been elucidated, it has been postulated that protamine sulfate in the heparin-protamine complex may be partially metabolized or may be attacked by fibrinolysin, thus freeing heparin.

Continued on next page

---

* Identi-Code® symbol. This product information was prepared in June 1992. Current information on these and other products of Eli Lilly and Company may be obtained by direct inquiry to Lilly Research Laboratories, Lilly Corporate Center, Indianapolis, Indiana 46285, (317) 276-3714.

Lilly—Cont.

INDICATIONS AND USAGE
Protamine sulfate is indicated in the treatment of heparin overdosage.

CONTRAINDICATION
Protamine sulfate is contraindicated in patients who have shown previous intolerance to the drug.

WARNINGS
Hyperheparinemia or bleeding has been reported in experimental animals and in some patients 30 minutes to 18 hours after cardiac surgery (under cardiopulmonary bypass) in spite of complete neutralization of heparin by adequate doses of protamine sulfate at the end of the operation. It is important to keep the patient under close observation after cardiac surgery. Additional doses of protamine sulfate should be administered if indicated by coagulation studies, such as the heparin titration test with protamine and the determination of plasma thrombin time.
Too-rapid administration of protamine sulfate can cause severe hypotensive and anaphylactoid reactions (*see* Dosage and Administration). Facilities to treat shock should be available.

PRECAUTIONS
General—**Because of the anticoagulant effect of protamine, it is unwise to give more than 100 mg over a short period unless a larger dose is clearly needed.**
Patients with a history of allergy to fish may develop hypersensitivity reactions to protamine, although to date no relationship has been established between allergic reactions to protamine and fish allergy.
Previous exposure to protamine through use of protamine-containing insulins or during heparin neutralization may predispose susceptible individuals to the development of untoward reactions from the subsequent use of this drug.
Reports of the presence of antiprotamine antibodies in the serums of infertile or vasectomized men suggest that some of these individuals may react to use of protamine sulfate.
Fatal anaphylaxis has been reported in one patient with no prior history of allergies.
Drug Interactions—Protamine sulfate has been shown to be incompatible with certain antibiotics, including several of the cephalosporins and penicillins (*see* Dosage and Administration).
Carcinogenesis, Mutagenesis, Impairment of Fertility—Studies have not been performed to determine potential for carcinogenicity, mutagenicity, or impairment of fertility.
Usage in Pregnancy—Pregnancy Category C—Animal reproduction studies have not been conducted with protamine sulfate. It is also not known whether protamine sulfate can cause fetal harm when administered to a pregnant woman or can affect reproduction capacity. Protamine sulfate should be given to a pregnant woman only if clearly needed.
Nursing Mothers—It is not known whether this drug is excreted in human milk. Because many drugs are excreted in human milk, caution should be exercised when protamine sulfate is administered to a nursing woman.
Pediatric Use—Safety and effectiveness in children have not been established.

ADVERSE REACTIONS
The intravenous administration of protamine sulfate may cause a sudden fall in blood pressure and bradycardia. Other reactions include transitory flushing and feeling of warmth, dyspnea, nausea, vomiting, and lassitude. Back pain has been reported in conscious patients undergoing such procedures as cardiac catheterization.
Severe adverse reactions have been reported including: (1) Anaphylaxis that resulted in severe respiratory distress, circulatory collapse, and capillary leak (*see* Precautions). Fatal anaphylaxis has been reported in one patient with no prior history of allergies; (2) Anaphylactoid reactions with circulatory collapse, capillary leak, and noncardiogenic pulmonary edema; acute pulmonary hypertension.
Complement activation by the heparin-protamine complexes, release of lysosomal enzymes from neutrophils, and prostaglandin and thromboxane generation have been associated with the development of anaphylactoid reactions.
Severe and potentially irreversible circulatory collapse associated with myocardial failure and reduced cardiac output can also occur. The mechanism(s) of this reaction and the role played by concurrent factors are unclear.
High-protein, noncardiogenic pulmonary edema associated with the use of protamine has been reported in patients on cardiopulmonary bypass who are undergoing cardiovascular surgery. The etiologic role of protamine in the pathogenesis of this condition is uncertain, and multiple factors have been present in most cases. The condition has been reported in association with administration of certain blood products, other drugs, cardiopulmonary bypass alone, and other etiologic factors. It is difficult to treat, and it can be life threatening. Because fatal anaphylactic and anaphylactoid reactions have been reported after the administration of protamine sulfate, the drug should be given only when resuscitation techniques and treatment of anaphylactic and anaphylactoid shock are readily available.

OVERDOSAGE
Signs and Symptoms—Overdose of protamine sulfate may cause bleeding. Protamine has a weak anticoagulant effect due to an interaction with platelets and with many proteins including fibrinogen. This effect should be distinguished from the rebound anticoagulation that may occur 30 minutes to 18 hours following the reversal of heparin with protamine.
Rapid administration of protamine is more likely to result in bradycardia, dyspnea, a sensation of warmth, flushing, and severe hypotension. Hypertension has also occurred.
The median lethal dose of protamine sulfate is 100 mg/kg in mice. Serum concentrations of protamine sulfate are not clinically useful. Information is not available on the amount of drug in a single dose that is associated with overdosage or is likely to be life threatening.
Treatment—To obtain up-to-date information about the treatment of overdose, a good resource is your certified Regional Poison Control Center. Telephone numbers of certified poison control centers are listed in the *Physicians' Desk Reference (PDR)*. In managing overdosage, consider the possibility of multiple drug overdoses, interaction among drugs, and unusual drug kinetics in your patient.
Replace blood loss with blood transfusions or fresh frozen plasma.
If the patient is hypotensive, consider fluids, epinephrine, dobutamine, or dopamine.

DOSAGE AND ADMINISTRATION
Each mg of protamine sulfate neutralizes approximately 90 USP units of heparin activity derived from lung tissue or about 115 USP units of heparin activity derived from intestinal mucosa.
Protamine Sulfate Injection should be given by very slow intravenous injection over a 10-minute period in doses not to exceed 50 mg (*see* Warnings).
Protamine sulfate is intended for injection without further dilution; however, if further dilution is desired, D5-W or normal saline may be used. Diluted solutions should not be stored since they contain no preservative.
Protamine sulfate should not be mixed with other drugs without knowledge of their compatibility, because protamine sulfate has been shown to be incompatible with certain antibiotics, including several of the cephalosporins and penicillins.
Because heparin disappears rapidly from the circulation, the dose of protamine sulfate required also decreases rapidly with the time elapsed following intravenous injection of heparin. For example, if the protamine sulfate is administered 30 minutes after the heparin, one half the usual dose may be sufficient.
The dosage of protamine sulfate should be guided by blood coagulation studies (*see* Warnings).
Parenteral drug products should be inspected visually for particulate matter and discoloration prior to administration whenever solution and container permit.

HOW SUPPLIED
(℞) Ampoules:
5 mL (No. 473)—(6s) NDC 0002-1691-16; (25s) NDC 0002-1691-25
(℞) Vials:
25 mL (No. 735)—(1s) NDC 0002-1462-01
Ampoules and vials should be stored in the refrigerator between 2° and 8°C (35.6° and 46.4°F).
CAUTION—The total dose of protamine sulfate contained in Vials No. 735 (250 mg of activity in 25 mL) is 5 times greater than that in Ampoules No. 473 (50 mg of activity in 5 mL).
The large-size vials (No. 735) are designed for antiheparin treatment only when large doses of heparin have been given during surgery and are to be neutralized by large doses of protamine sulfate after surgical procedures.

[100590]

REGULAR ILETIN® I AND II OTC
(insulin injection, Lilly) *See under* Iletin® (insulin, Lilly)

SEMILENTE® ILETIN® I OTC
(prompt insulin zinc suspension, Lilly) *See under* Iletin® (insulin, Lilly)

SECONAL® SODIUM Ⓒ
[*sĕk'ō-năl sō'dē-ŭm*]
(secobarbital sodium)
Capsules, USP
WARNING: MAY BE HABIT-FORMING

DESCRIPTION
The barbiturates are nonselective central nervous system (CNS) depressants that are primarily used as sedative-hypnotics. In subhypnotic doses, they are also used as anticonvulsants. The barbiturates and their sodium salts are subject to control under the Federal Controlled Substances Act.
Seconal® Sodium (Secobarbital Sodium, USP, Lilly) is a barbituric acid derivative and occurs as a white, odorless, bitter powder that is very soluble in water, soluble in alcohol, and practically insoluble in ether. Chemically, the drug is sodium 5-allyl-5-(1-methylbutyl)barbiturate, with the empirical formula $C_{12}H_{17}N_2NaO_3$. Its molecular weight is 260.27.
Each Pulvule® contains 100 mg (0.38 mmol) of secobarbital sodium. It also contains cornstarch, D & C Yellow No. 10, F D & C Red No. 3, gelatin, magnesium stearate, silicone, and other inactive ingredients.

CLINICAL PHARMACOLOGY
Barbiturates are capable of producing all levels of CNS mood alteration, from excitation to mild sedation, hypnosis, and deep coma. Overdosage can produce death. In high enough therapeutic doses, barbiturates induce anesthesia. Barbiturates depress the sensory cortex, decrease motor activity, alter cerebellar function, and produce drowsiness, sedation, and hypnosis.
Barbiturate-induced sleep differs from physiologic sleep. Sleep laboratory studies have demonstrated that barbiturates reduce the amount of time spent in the rapid eye movement (REM) phase, or dreaming stage of sleep. Also, Stages III and IV sleep are decreased. Following abrupt cessation of regularly used barbiturates, patients may experience markedly increased dreaming, nightmares, and/or insomnia. Therefore, withdrawal of a single therapeutic dose over 5 or 6 days has been recommended to lessen the REM rebound and disturbed sleep that contribute to drug withdrawal syndrome (for example, decreasing the dose from 3 to 2 doses a day for 1 week).
In studies, secobarbital sodium and pentobarbital sodium have been found to lose most of their effectiveness for both inducing and maintaining sleep by the end of 2 weeks of continued drug administration, even with the use of multiple doses. As with secobarbital sodium and pentobarbital sodium, other barbiturates (including amobarbital) might be expected to lose their effectiveness for inducing and maintaining sleep after about 2 weeks. The short-, intermediate-, and to a lesser degree, long-acting barbiturates have been widely prescribed for treating insomnia. Although the clinical literature abounds with claims that the short-acting barbiturates are superior for producing sleep whereas the intermediate-acting compounds are more effective in maintaining sleep, controlled studies have failed to demonstrate these differential effects. Therefore, as sleep medications, the barbiturates are of limited value beyond short-term use.
Barbiturates have little analgesic action at subanesthetic doses. Rather, in subanesthetic doses, these drugs may increase the reaction to painful stimuli. All barbiturates exhibit anticonvulsant activity in anesthetic doses. However, of the drugs in this class, only phenobarbital, mephobarbital, and metharbital are effective as oral anticonvulsants in subhypnotic doses.
Barbiturates are respiratory depressants, and the degree of depression is dependent on the dose. With hypnotic doses, respiratory depression is similar to that which occurs during physiologic sleep accompanied by a slight decrease in blood pressure and heart rate.
Studies in laboratory animals have shown that barbiturates cause reduction in the tone and contractility of the uterus, ureters, and urinary bladder. However, concentrations of the drugs required to produce this effect in humans are not reached with sedative-hypnotic doses.
Barbiturates do not impair normal hepatic function, but have been shown to induce liver microsomal enzymes, thus increasing and/or altering the metabolism of barbiturates and other drugs (*see* Drug Interactions *under* Precautions).
Pharmacokinetics—Barbiturates are absorbed in varying degrees following oral or parenteral administration. The salts are more rapidly absorbed than are the acids. The rate of absorption is increased if the sodium salt is ingested as a dilute solution or taken on an empty stomach.
Duration of action, which is related to the rate at which the barbiturates are redistributed throughout the body, varies among persons and in the same person from time to time.
Seconal® Sodium (Secobarbital Sodium, USP, Lilly) is classified as a short-acting barbiturate when taken orally. Its onset of action is 10 to 15 minutes and its duration of action ranges from 3 to 4 hours.
Barbiturates are weak acids that are absorbed and rapidly distributed to all tissues and fluids, with high concentrations in the brain, liver, and kidneys. Lipid solubility of the bar-

biturates is the dominant factor in their distribution within the body. The more lipid soluble the barbiturate, the more rapidly it penetrates all tissues of the body. Barbiturates are bound to plasma and tissue proteins to a varying degree, with the degree of binding increasing directly as a function of lipid solubility.

Phenobarbital has the lowest lipid solubility, lowest plasma binding, lowest brain protein binding, the longest delay in onset of activity, and the longest duration of action. At the opposite extreme is secobarbital, which has the highest lipid solubility, highest plasma protein binding, highest brain protein binding, the shortest delay in onset of activity, and the shortest duration of action. The plasma half-life for secobarbital sodium in adults ranges between 15 to 40 hours, with a mean of 28 hours. No data are available for children and newborns.

Barbiturates are metabolized primarily by the hepatic microsomal enzyme system, and the metabolic products are excreted in the urine and, less commonly, in the feces. The excretion of unmetabolized barbiturate is one feature that distinguishes the long-acting category from those belonging to other categories, which are almost entirely metabolized. The inactive metabolites of the barbiturates are excreted as conjugates of glucuronic acid.

INDICATIONS AND USAGE

A. Hypnotic, for the short-term treatment of insomnia, since it appears to lose its effectiveness for sleep induction and sleep maintenance after 2 weeks (see Clinical Pharmacology).
B. Preanesthetic

CONTRAINDICATIONS

Seconal® Sodium (Secobarbital Sodium, USP, Lilly) is contraindicated in patients who are hypersensitive to barbiturates. It is also contraindicated in patients with a history of manifest or latent porphyria, marked impairment of liver function, or respiratory disease in which dyspnea or obstruction is evident.

WARNINGS

1. *Habit-Forming*—Seconal Sodium may be habit-forming. Tolerance and psychological and physical dependence may occur with continued use (see Drug Abuse and Dependence and Pharmacokinetics under Clinical Pharmacology). Patients who have psychological dependence on barbiturates may increase the dosage or decrease the dosage interval without consulting a physician and subsequently may develop a physical dependence on barbiturates. To minimize the possibility of overdosage or development of dependence, the prescribing and dispensing of sedative-hypnotic barbiturates should be limited to the amount required for the interval until the next appointment. The abrupt cessation after prolonged use in a person who is dependent on the drug may result in withdrawal symptoms, including delirium, convulsions, and possibly death. Barbiturates should be withdrawn gradually from any patient known to be taking excessive doses over long periods of time (see Drug Abuse and Dependence).

2. *Acute or Chronic Pain*—Caution should be exercised when barbiturates are administered to patients with acute or chronic pain, because paradoxical excitement could be induced or important symptoms could be masked.

3. *Usage in Pregnancy*—Barbiturates can cause fetal harm when administered to a pregnant woman. Retrospective, case-controlled studies have suggested that there may be a connection between the maternal consumption of barbiturates and a higher than expected incidence of fetal abnormalities. Barbiturates readily cross the placental barrier and are distributed throughout fetal tissues; the highest concentrations are found in the placenta, fetal liver, and brain. Fetal blood levels approach maternal blood levels following parenteral administration.

Withdrawal symptoms occur in infants born to women who receive barbiturates throughout the last trimester of pregnancy (see Drug Abuse and Dependence). If Seconal® Sodium (Secobarbital Sodium, USP, Lilly) is used during pregnancy or if the patient becomes pregnant while taking this drug, the patient should be apprised of the potential hazard to the fetus.

4. *Synergistic Effects*—The concomitant use of alcohol or other CNS depressants may produce additive CNS-depressant effects.

PRECAUTIONS

General—Barbiturates may be habit-forming. Tolerance and psychological and physical dependence may occur with continuing use (see Drug Abuse and Dependence). Barbiturates should be administered with caution, if at all, to patients who are mentally depressed, have suicidal tendencies, or have a history of drug abuse.

Elderly or debilitated patients may react to barbiturates with marked excitement, depression, or confusion. In some persons, especially children, barbiturates repeatedly produce excitement rather than depression.

In patients with hepatic damage, barbiturates should be administered with caution and initially in reduced doses.

Barbiturates should not be administered to patients showing the premonitory signs of hepatic coma.

Information for Patients—The following information should be given to patients receiving Seconal Sodium:
1. The use of Seconal® Sodium (Secobarbital Sodium, USP, Lilly) carries with it an associated risk of psychological and/or physical dependence. The patient should be warned against increasing the dose of the drug without consulting a physician.
2. Seconal Sodium may impair the mental and/or physical abilities required for the performance of potentially hazardous tasks, such as driving a car or operating machinery. The patient should be cautioned accordingly.
3. Alcohol should not be consumed while taking Seconal Sodium. The concurrent use of Seconal Sodium with other CNS depressants (eg, alcohol, narcotics, tranquilizers, and antihistamines) may result in additional CNS-depressant effects.

Laboratory Tests—Prolonged therapy with barbiturates should be accompanied by periodic laboratory evaluation of organic systems, including hematopoietic, renal, and hepatic systems (see General under Precautions and Adverse Reactions).

Drug Interactions—Most reports of clinically significant drug interactions occurring with the barbiturates have involved phenobarbital. However, the application of these data to other barbiturates appears valid and warrants serial blood level determinations of the relevant drugs when there are multiple therapies.
1. *Anticoagulants*—Phenobarbital lowers the plasma levels of dicumarol and causes a decrease in anticoagulant activity as measured by the prothrombin time. Barbiturates can induce hepatic microsomal enzymes, resulting in increased metabolism and decreased anticoagulant response of oral anticoagulants (eg, warfarin, acenocoumarol, dicumarol, and phenprocoumon). Patients stabilized on anticoagulant therapy may require dosage adjustments if barbiturates are added to or withdrawn from their dosage regimen.
2. *Corticosteroids*—Barbiturates appear to enhance the metabolism of exogenous corticosteroids, probably through the induction of hepatic microsomal enzymes. Patients stabilized on corticosteroid therapy may require dosage adjustments if barbiturates are added to or withdrawn from their dosage regimen.
3. *Griseofulvin*—Phenobarbital appears to interfere with the absorption of orally administered griseofulvin, thus decreasing its blood level. The effect of the resultant decreased blood levels of griseofulvin on therapeutic response has not been established. However, it would be preferable to avoid concomitant administration of these drugs.
4. *Doxycycline*—Phenobarbital has been shown to shorten the half-life of doxycycline for as long as 2 weeks after barbiturate therapy is discontinued.
This mechanism is probably through the induction of hepatic microsomal enzymes that metabolize the antibiotic. If barbiturates and doxycycline are administered concurrently, the clinical response to doxycycline should be monitored closely.
5. *Phenytoin, Sodium Valproate, Valproic Acid*—The effect of barbiturates on the metabolism of phenytoin appears to be variable. Some investigators report an accelerating effect, whereas others report no effect. Because the effect of barbiturates on the metabolism of phenytoin is not predictable, phenytoin and barbiturate blood levels should be monitored more frequently if these drugs are given concurrently. Sodium valproate and valproic acid increase secobarbital sodium serum levels; therefore, secobarbital sodium blood levels should be monitored closely and appropriate dosage adjustment made as clinically indicated.
6. *CNS Depressants*—The concomitant use of other CNS depressants, including other sedatives or hypnotics, antihistamines, tranquilizers, or alcohol, may produce additive depressant effects.
7. *Monoamine Oxidase Inhibitors (MAOIs)*—MAOIs prolong the effects of barbiturates, probably because metabolism of the barbiturate is inhibited.
8. *Estradiol, Estrone, Progesterone, and Other Steroidal Hormones*—Pretreatment with or concurrent administration of phenobarbital may decrease the effect of estradiol by increasing its metabolism. There have been reports of patients treated with antiepileptic drugs (eg, phenobarbital) who become pregnant while taking oral contraceptives. An alternate contraceptive method might be suggested to women taking barbiturates.
Carcinogenesis—1. *Animal Data.* Phenobarbital sodium is carcinogenic in mice and rats after lifetime administration. In mice, it produced benign and malignant liver cell tumors. In rats, benign liver cell tumors were observed very late in life.
2. *Human Data*—In a 29-year epidemiologic study of 9,136 patients who were treated on an anticonvulsant protocol that included phenobarbital, results indicated a higher than normal incidence of hepatic carcinoma. Previously, some of these patients had been treated with thorotrast, a

drug that is known to produce hepatic carcinomas. Thus, this study did not provide sufficient evidence that phenobarbital sodium is carcinogenic in humans.

A retrospective study of 84 children with brain tumors matched to 73 normal controls and 78 cancer controls (malignant disease other than brain tumors) suggested an association between exposure to barbiturates prenatally and an increased incidence of brain tumors.

Usage in Pregnancy—1. *Teratogenic Effects. Pregnancy Category D. See* Usage in Pregnancy *under* Warnings.
2. *Nonteratogenic Effects.* Reports of infants suffering from long-term barbiturate exposure in utero included the acute withdrawal syndrome of seizures and hyperirritability from birth to a delayed onset of up to 14 days (see Drug Abuse and Dependence).

Labor and Delivery—Hypnotic doses of barbiturates do not appear to impair uterine activity significantly during labor. Full anesthetic doses of barbiturates decrease the force and frequency of uterine contractions. Administration of sedative-hypnotic barbiturates to the mother during labor may result in respiratory depression in the newborn. Premature infants are particularly susceptible to the depressant effects of barbiturates. If barbiturates are used during labor and delivery, resuscitation equipment should be available.

Data are not available to evaluate the effect of barbiturates when forceps delivery or other intervention is necessary or to determine the effect of barbiturates on the later growth, development, and functional maturity of the child.

Nursing Mothers—Caution should be exercised when Seconal® Sodium (Secobarbital Sodium, USP, Lilly) is administered to a nursing woman, because small amounts of barbiturates are excreted in the milk.

ADVERSE REACTIONS

The following adverse reactions and their incidences were compiled from surveillance of thousands of hospitalized patients who received barbiturates. Because such patients may be less aware of some of the milder adverse effects of barbiturates, the incidence of these reactions may be somewhat higher in fully ambulatory patients.

More than 1 in 100 Patients
The most common adverse reaction estimated to occur at a rate of 1 to 3 patients per 100 is the following:
Nervous System: Somnolence
Less than 1 in 100 Patients
Adverse reactions estimated to occur at a rate of less than 1 in 100 patients are listed below, grouped by organ system and by decreasing order of occurrence:
Nervous System: Agitation, confusion, hyperkinesia, ataxia, CNS depression, nightmares, nervousness, psychiatric disturbance, hallucinations, insomnia, anxiety, dizziness, abnormality in thinking
Respiratory System: Hypoventilation, apnea
Cardiovascular System: Bradycardia, hypotension, syncope
Digestive System: Nausea, vomiting, constipation
Other Reported Reactions: Headache, injection site reactions, hypersensitivity reactions (angioedema, skin rashes, exfoliative dermatitis), fever, liver damage, megaloblastic anemia following chronic phenobarbital use.

DRUG ABUSE AND DEPENDENCE

Controlled Substance—Seconal® Sodium Capsules (Secobarbital Sodium, USP, Lilly) are a Schedule II drug.
Dependence—Barbiturates may be habit-forming; tolerance, psychological dependence, and physical dependence may occur, especially following prolonged use of high doses of barbiturates. Daily administration in excess of 400 mg of secobarbital for approximately 90 days is likely to produce some degree of physical dependence. A dosage of 600 to 800 mg for at least 35 days is sufficient to produce withdrawal seizures. The average daily dose for the barbiturate addict is usually about 1.5 g. As tolerance to barbiturates develops, the amount needed to maintain the same level of intoxication increases; tolerance to a fatal dosage, however, does not increase more than twofold. As this occurs, the margin between intoxicating dosage and fatal dosage becomes smaller. Symptoms of acute intoxication with barbiturates include unsteady gait, slurred speech, and sustained nystagmus. Mental signs of chronic intoxication include confusion, poor judgment, irritability, insomnia, and somatic complaints. Symptoms of barbiturate dependence are similar to those of chronic alcoholism. If an individual appears to be intoxicated with alcohol to a degree that is radically disproportionate to the amount of alcohol in his or her blood, the use of barbiturates should be suspected. The lethal dose of a barbiturate is far less if alcohol is also ingested.

Continued on next page

---

* Identi-Code® symbol. This product information was prepared in June 1992. Current information on these and other products of Eli Lilly and Company may be obtained by direct inquiry to Lilly Research Laboratories, Lilly Corporate Center, Indianapolis, Indiana 46285, (317) 276-3714.

Lilly—Cont.

The symptoms of barbiturate withdrawal can be severe and may cause death. Minor withdrawal symptoms may appear 8 to 12 hours after the last dose of a barbiturate. These symptoms usually appear in the following order: anxiety, muscle twitching, tremor of hands and fingers, progressive weakness, dizziness, distortion in visual perception, nausea, vomiting, insomnia, and orthostatic hypotension. Major withdrawal symptoms (convulsions and delirium) may occur within 16 hours and last up to 5 days after abrupt cessation of barbiturates. Intensity of withdrawal symptoms gradually declines over a period of approximately 15 days. Individuals susceptible to barbiturate abuse and dependence include alcoholics and opiate abusers, as well as other sedative-hypnotic and amphetamine abusers.
Drug dependence on barbiturates arises from repeated administration on a continuous basis, generally in amounts exceeding therapeutic dose levels. The characteristics of drug dependence on barbiturates include the following: (a) a strong desire or need to continue taking the drug; (b) a tendency to increase the dose; (c) a psychic dependence on the effects of the drug related to subjective and individual appreciation of those effects; and (d) a physical dependence on the effects of the drug, requiring its presence for maintenance of homeostasis and resulting in a definite, characteristic, and self-limited abstinence syndrome when the drug is withdrawn.
Treatment of barbiturate dependence consists of cautious and gradual withdrawal of the drug. Barbiturate-dependent patients can be withdrawn by using a number of withdrawal regimens. In all cases, withdrawal takes an extended period. One method involves substituting a 30-mg dose of phenobarbital for each 100- to 200-mg dose of barbiturate that the patient has been taking. The total daily amount of phenobarbital is then administered in 3 or 4 divided doses, not to exceed 600 mg daily. Should signs of withdrawal occur on the first day of treatment, a loading dose of 100 to 200 mg of phenobarbital may be administered IM in addition to the oral dose. After stabilization on phenobarbital, the total daily dose is decreased by 30 mg a day as long as withdrawal is proceeding smoothly. A modification of this regimen involves initiating treatment at the patient's regular dosage level and decreasing the daily dosage by 10% as tolerated by the patient.
Infants that are physically dependent on barbiturates may be given phenobarbital, 3 to 10 mg/kg/day. After withdrawal symptoms (hyperactivity, disturbed sleep, tremors, and hyperreflexia) are relieved, the dosage of phenobarbital should be gradually decreased and completely withdrawn over a 2-week period.

OVERDOSAGE

The toxic dose of barbiturates varies considerably. In general, an oral dose of 1 g of most barbiturates produces serious poisoning in an adult. Death commonly occurs after 2 to 10 g of ingested barbiturate. The sedated, therapeutic blood levels of secobarbital range between 0.5 to 5 μg/mL; the usual lethal blood level ranges from 15 to 40 μg/mL. Barbiturate intoxication may be confused with alcoholism, bromide intoxication, and various neurologic disorders. Potential tolerance must be considered when evaluating significance of dose and plasma concentration.
Signs and Symptoms—Symptoms of oral overdose may occur within 15 minutes and begin with central nervous system depression, underventilation, hypotension, and hypothermia, which may progress to pulmonary edema and death. Hemorrhagic blisters may develop, especially at pressure points.
In extreme overdose, all electrical activity in the brain may cease, in which case a "flat" EEG normally equated with clinical death cannot be accepted as indicative of brain death. This effect is fully reversible unless hypoxic damage occurs. Consideration should be given to the possibility of barbiturate intoxication even in situations that appear to involve trauma.
Complications such as pneumonia, pulmonary edema, cardiac arrhythmias, congestive heart failure, and renal failure may occur. Uremia may increase CNS sensitivity to barbiturates if renal function is impaired. Differential diagnosis should include hypoglycemia, head trauma, cerebrovascular accidents, convulsive states, and diabetic coma.
Treatment—To obtain up-to-date information about the treatment of overdose, a good resource is your certified Regional Poison Control Center. Telephone numbers of certified poison control centers are listed in the *Physicians' Desk Reference (PDR)*. In managing overdosage, consider the possibility of multiple drug overdoses, interaction among drugs, and unusual drug kinetics in your patient.
Protect the patient's airway and support ventilation and perfusion. Meticulously monitor and maintain, within acceptable limits, the patient's vital signs, blood gases, serum electrolytes, etc. Absorption of drugs from the gastrointestinal tract may be decreased by giving activated charcoal, which, in many cases, is more effective than emesis or lavage; consider charcoal instead of or in addition to gastric emptying. Repeated doses of charcoal over time may hasten elimination of some drugs that have been absorbed. Safeguard the patient's airway when employing gastric emptying or charcoal.
Diuresis and peritoneal dialysis are of little value; hemodialysis and hemoperfusion enhance drug clearance and should be considered in serious poisoning. If the patient has chronically abused sedatives, withdrawal reactions may be manifest following acute overdose.

DOSAGE AND ADMINISTRATION

Dosages of barbiturates must be individualized with full knowledge of their particular characteristics. Factors of consideration are the patient's age, weight, and condition.
Adults—As a hypnotic, 100 mg at bedtime. Preoperatively, 200 to 300 mg 1 to 2 hours before surgery.
Children—Preoperatively, 2 to 6 mg/kg, with a maximum dosage of 100 mg.
Special patient population—Dosage should be reduced in the elderly or debilitated because these patients may be more sensitive to barbiturates. Dosage should be reduced for patients with impaired renal function or hepatic disease.

HOW SUPPLIED

Ⓒ Pulvules Seconal Sodium (capsules) (orange):
100 mg (No. 240) (Identi-Code* F40)—(100s) NDC 0002-0640-02; (ID† 100) NDC 0002-0640-33
Store at controlled room temperature, 15° to 30°C (59° to 86°F). Dispense in a tight container.

*Identi-Code® (formula identification code, Lilly)
†Identi-Dose (unit dose medication, Lilly)

[010891]

SEROMYCIN® ℞
[sĕr-ō-mī'sĭn]
(Cycloserine)
Capsules, USP

DESCRIPTION

Seromycin® (Cycloserine Capsules, USP, Lilly), 3-isoxazolidinone, 4-amino-, (R)-, is a broad-spectrum antibiotic that is produced by a strain of *Streptomyces orchidaceus* and has also been synthesized. Cycloserine is a white to off-white powder that is soluble in water and stable in alkaline solution. It is rapidly destroyed at a neutral or acid pH.
Cycloserine has a pH between 5.5 and 6.5 in a solution containing 100 mg/mL. The molecular weight of cycloserine is 102.09, and it has an empirical formula of $C_3H_6N_2O_2$.
Each Pulvule® contains cycloserine, 250 mg (2.45 mmol); D & C Yellow No. 10, F D & C Blue No. 1, F D & C Red No. 3, F D & C Yellow No. 6, gelatin, iron oxide, talc, titanium dioxide, and other inactive ingredients.

CLINICAL PHARMACOLOGY

After oral administration, cycloserine is readily absorbed from the gastrointestinal tract, with peak blood levels occurring in 4 to 8 hours. Blood levels of 25 to 30 μg/mL can generally be maintained with the usual dosage of 250 mg twice a day, although the relationship of plasma levels to dosage is not always consistent. Concentrations in the cerebrospinal fluid, pleural fluid, fetal blood, and mother's milk approach those found in the serum. Detectable amounts are found in ascitic fluid, bile, sputum, amniotic fluid, and lung and lymph tissues. Approximately 65% of a single dose of cycloserine can be recovered in the urine within 72 hours after oral administration. The remaining 35% is apparently metabolized to unknown substances. The maximum excretion rate occurs 2 to 6 hours after administration, with 50% of the drug eliminated in 12 hours.
Microbiology—Cycloserine inhibits cell-wall synthesis in susceptible strains of gram-positive and gram-negative bacteria and in *Mycobacterium tuberculosis*.
Susceptibility Tests—Cycloserine clinical laboratory standard powder is available for both direct and indirect methods[1] of determining the susceptibility of strains of mycobacteria. Cycloserine MICs for susceptible strains are 25 μg/mL or lower.

INDICATIONS AND USAGE

Seromycin® (Cycloserine Capsules, USP, Lilly) is indicated in the treatment of active pulmonary and extrapulmonary tuberculosis (including renal disease) when the causative organisms are susceptible to this drug and when treatment with the primary medications (streptomycin, isoniazid, rifampin, and ethambutol) has proved inadequate. Like all antituberculosis drugs, Seromycin should be administered in conjunction with other effective chemotherapy and not as the sole therapeutic agent.
Seromycin may be effective in the treatment of acute urinary tract infections caused by susceptible strains of gram-positive and gram-negative bacteria, especially *Enterobacter* sp and *Escherichia coli*. It is generally no more and is usually less effective than other antimicrobial agents in the treatment of urinary tract infections caused by bacteria other than mycobacteria. Use of Seromycin in these infections should be considered only when more conventional therapy has failed and when the organism has been demonstrated to be susceptible to the drug.

CONTRAINDICATIONS

Administration is contraindicated in patients with any of the following:
- Hypersensitivity to cycloserine
- Epilepsy
- Depression, severe anxiety, or psychosis
- Severe renal insufficiency
- Excessive concurrent use of alcoholic beverages

WARNINGS

Administration of Seromycin® (Cycloserine Capsules, USP, Lilly) should be discontinued or the dosage reduced if the patient develops allergic dermatitis or symptoms of CNS toxicity, such as convulsions, psychosis, somnolence, depression, confusion, hyperreflexia, headache, tremor, vertigo, paresis, or dysarthria.
The toxicity of Seromycin is closely related to excessive blood levels (above 30 μg/mL), as determined by high dosage or inadequate renal clearance. The ratio of toxic dose to effective dose in tuberculosis is small.
The risk of convulsions is increased in chronic alcoholics.
Patients should be monitored by hematologic, renal excretion, blood level, and liver function studies.

PRECAUTIONS

General—Before treatment with Seromycin® (Cycloserine Capsules, USP, Lilly) is initiated, cultures should be taken and the organism's susceptibility to the drug should be established. In tuberculous infections, the organism's susceptibility to the other antituberculosis agents in the regimen should also be demonstrated.
Anticonvulsant drugs or sedatives may be effective in controlling symptoms of CNS toxicity, such as convulsions, anxiety, and tremor. Patients receiving more than 500 mg of Seromycin daily should be closely observed for such symptoms. The value of pyridoxine in preventing CNS toxicity from Seromycin has not been proved.
Administration of Seromycin and other antituberculosis drugs has been associated in a few instances with vitamin B_{12} and/or folic acid deficiency, megaloblastic anemia, and sideroblastic anemia. If evidence of anemia develops during treatment, appropriate studies and therapy should be instituted.
Laboratory Tests—Blood levels should be determined at least weekly for patients with reduced renal function, for individuals receiving a daily dosage of more than 500 mg, and for those showing signs and symptoms suggestive of toxicity. The dosage should be adjusted to keep the blood level below 30 μg/mL.
Drug Interactions—Concurrent administration of ethionamide has been reported to potentiate neurotoxic side effects.
Alcohol and Seromycin are incompatible, especially during a regimen calling for large doses of the latter. Alcohol increases the possibility and risk of epileptic episodes.
Concurrent administration of isoniazid may result in increased incidence of CNS effects, such as dizziness or drowsiness. Dosage adjustments may be necessary and patients should be monitored closely for signs of CNS toxicity.
Carcinogenesis, Mutagenicity, and Impairment of Fertility—Studies have not been performed to determine potential for carcinogenicity. The Ames test and unscheduled DNA repair test were negative. A study in 2 generations of rats showed no impairment of fertility relative to controls for the first mating but somewhat lower fertility in the second mating.
Pregnancy Category C—A study in 2 generations of rats given doses up to 100 mg/kg/day demonstrated no teratogenic effect in offspring. It is not known whether Seromycin can cause fetal harm when administered to a pregnant woman or can affect reproduction capacity. Seromycin should be given to a pregnant woman only if clearly needed.
Nursing Mothers—Because of the potential for serious adverse reactions in nursing infants from Seromycin, a decision should be made whether to discontinue nursing or to discontinue the drug, taking into account the importance of the drug to the mother.
Usage in Children—Safety and dosage have not been established for pediatric use.

ADVERSE REACTIONS

Most adverse reactions occurring during therapy with Seromycin® (Cycloserine Capsules, USP, Lilly) involve the nervous system or are manifestations of drug hypersensitivity. The following side effects have been observed in patients receiving Seromycin:

Nervous system symptoms (which appear to be related to higher dosages of the drug, ie, more than 500 mg daily)
- Convulsions
- Drowsiness and somnolence
- Headache
- Tremor
- Dysarthria
- Vertigo

Confusion and disorientation with loss of memory
Psychoses, possibly with suicidal tendencies
Character changes
Hyperirritability
Aggression
Paresis
Hyperreflexia
Paresthesia
Major and minor (localized) clonic seizures
Coma

Cardiovascular
Sudden development of congestive heart failure in patients receiving 1 to 1.5 g of Seromycin daily has been reported.

Allergy (apparently not related to dosage)
Skin rash
Miscellaneous
Elevated serum transaminase, especially in patients with preexisting liver disease

OVERDOSAGE

Signs and Symptoms—Acute toxicity from cycloserine can occur if more than 1 g is ingested by an adult. Chronic toxicity from cycloserine is dose related and can occur if more than 500 mg is administered daily. Patients with renal impairment will accumulate cycloserine and may develop toxicity if the dosing regimen is not modified. Patients with severe renal impairment should not receive the drug. The central nervous system is the most common organ system involved with toxicity. Toxic effects may include headache, vertigo, confusion, drowsiness, hyperirritability, paresthesias, dysarthria, and psychosis. Following larger ingestions, paresis, convulsions, and coma often occur. Ethyl alcohol may increase the risk of seizures in patients receiving cycloserine.
The oral median lethal dose in mice is 5,290 mg/kg.
Treatment—To obtain up-to-date information about the treatment of overdose, a good resource is your certified Regional Poison Control Center. Telephone numbers of certified poison control centers are listed in the *Physicians' Desk Reference (PDR).* In managing overdosage, consider the possibility of multiple drug overdoses, interaction among drugs, and unusual drug kinetics in your patient.
Overdoses of cycloserine have been reported rarely. The following is provided to serve as a guide should such an overdose be encountered.
Protect the patient's airway and support ventilation and perfusion. Meticulously monitor and maintain, within acceptable limits, the patient's vital signs, blood gases, serum electrolytes, etc. Absorption of drugs from the gastrointestinal tract may be decreased by giving activated charcoal, which, in many cases, is more effective than emesis or lavage; consider charcoal instead of or in addition to gastric emptying. Repeated doses of charcoal over time may hasten elimination of some drugs that have been absorbed. Safeguard the patient's airway when employing gastric emptying or charcoal.
In adults, many of the neurotoxic effects of cycloserine can be both treated and prevented with the administration of 200 to 300 mg of pyridoxine daily.
The use of hemodialysis has been shown to remove cycloserine from the bloodstream. This procedure should be reserved for patients with life-threatening toxicity that is unresponsive to less invasive therapy.

DOSAGE AND ADMINISTRATION

Seromycin® (Cycloserine Capsules, USP, Lilly) is effective orally and is currently administered only by this route. The usual dosage is 500 mg to 1 g daily in divided doses monitored by blood levels.[2] The initial adult dosage most frequently given is 250 mg twice daily at 12-hour intervals for the first 2 weeks. A daily dosage of 1 g should not be exceeded.

REFERENCES

1. Kubica GP, Dye WE: Laboratory methods for clinical and public health—mycobacteriology. US Department of Health, Education and Welfare, Public Health Service, 1967, pp. 47–55, 66–70.
2. Jones LR: Colorimetric determination of cycloserine, a new antibiotic. *Anal Chem* 1956; 28:39.

HOW SUPPLIED

(℞) Pulvules, 250 mg (No. 12)—(40s) NDC 0002-0604-40
Store at controlled room temperature, 59° to 86°F (15° to 30°C).
[122491]

TAPAZOLE® ℞

[*tăp'ă-zōl*]
(methimazole)
Tablets, USP

DESCRIPTION

Tapazole® (Methimazole Tablets, USP, Lilly) (1-methylimidazole-2-thiol) is a white, crystalline substance that is freely soluble in water. It differs chemically from the drugs of the thiouracil series primarily because it has a 5- instead of a 6-membered ring.
Each tablet contains 5 or 10 mg (43.8 or 87.6 μmol) methimazole, an orally administered antithyroid drug.
Each tablet also contains lactose, magnesium stearate, starch, and talc.
The molecular weight is 114.16, and the empirical formula is $C_4H_6N_2S$.

CLINICAL PHARMACOLOGY

Methimazole inhibits the synthesis of thyroid hormones and thus is effective in the treatment of hyperthyroidism. The drug does not inactivate existing thyroxine and triiodothyronine that are stored in the thyroid or circulating in the blood nor does it interfere with the effectiveness of thyroid hormones given by mouth or by injection.
The actions and use of methimazole are similar to those of propylthiouracil. On a weight basis, the drug is at least 10 times as potent as propylthiouracil, but methimazole may be less consistent in action.
Methimazole is readily absorbed from the gastrointestinal tract. It is metabolized rapidly and requires frequent administration. Methimazole is excreted in the urine.
In laboratory animals, various regimens that continuously suppress thyroid function and thereby increase TSH secretion result in thyroid tissue hypertrophy. Under such conditions, the appearance of thyroid and pituitary neoplasms has also been reported. Regimens that have been studied in this regard include antithyroid agents, such as methimazole, as well as dietary iodine deficiency, subtotal thyroidectomy, implantation of autonomous thyrotropic hormone-secreting pituitary tumors, and administration of chemical goitrogens.

INDICATIONS AND USAGE

Tapazole® (Methimazole Tablets, USP, Lilly) is indicated in the medical treatment of hyperthyroidism. Long-term therapy may lead to remission of the disease. Tapazole may be used to ameliorate hyperthyroidism in preparation for subtotal thyroidectomy or radioactive iodine therapy. Tapazole is also used when thyroidectomy is contraindicated or not advisable.

CONTRAINDICATIONS

Tapazole is contraindicated in the presence of hypersensitivity to the drug and in nursing mothers because the drug is excreted in milk.

WARNINGS

Agranulocytosis is potentially a serious side effect. Patients should be instructed to report to their physicians any symptoms of agranulocytosis, such as fever or sore throat. Leukopenia, thrombocytopenia, and aplastic anemia (pancytopenia) may also occur. The drug should be discontinued in the presence of agranulocytosis, aplastic anemia (pancytopenia), hepatitis, or exfoliative dermatitis. The patient's bone marrow function should be monitored.
Due to the similar hepatic toxicity profiles of Tapazole and propylthiouracil, attention is drawn to the severe hepatic reactions which have occurred with both drugs. There have been rare reports of fulminant hepatitis, hepatic necrosis, encephalopathy, and death. Symptoms suggestive of hepatic dysfunction (anorexia, pruritus, right upper quadrant pain, etc) should prompt evaluation of liver function. Drug treatment should be discontinued promptly in the event of clinically significant evidence of liver abnormality including hepatic transaminase values exceeding 3 times the upper limit of normal.
Tapazole can cause fetal harm when administered to a pregnant woman. Tapazole readily crosses the placental membranes and can induce goiter and even cretinism in the developing fetus. In addition, rare instances of aplasia cutis, as manifested by scalp defects, have occurred in infants born to mothers who received Tapazole during pregnancy. If Tapazole is used during pregnancy or if the patient becomes pregnant while taking this drug, the patient should be warned of the potential hazard to the fetus.
Since scalp defects have not been reported in offspring of patients treated with propylthiouracil, that agent may be preferable to Tapazole in pregnant women requiring treatment with antithyroid drugs.
Postpartum patients receiving Tapazole should not nurse their babies.

PRECAUTIONS

General—Patients who receive Tapazole® (Methimazole Tablets, USP, Lilly) should be under close surveillance and should be cautioned to report immediately any evidence of illness, particularly sore throat, skin eruptions, fever, headache, or general malaise. In such cases, white-blood-cell and differential counts should be made to determine whether agranulocytosis has developed. Particular care should be exercised with patients who are receiving additional drugs known to cause agranulocytosis.
Laboratory Tests—Because Tapazole may cause hypoprothrombinemia and bleeding, prothrombin time should be monitored during therapy with the drug, especially before surgical procedures (*see* General *under* Precautions).
Periodic monitoring of thyroid function is warranted, and the finding of an elevated TSH warrants a decrease in the dosage of Tapazole.
Drug Interactions—The activity of anticoagulants may be potentiated by anti-vitamin-K activity attributed to Tapazole.
Carcinogenesis, Mutagenesis, Impairment of Fertility—Rats treated for 2 years with methimazole demonstrated thyroid hyperplasia and thyroid adenoma and carcinoma formation. Such findings are seen with continuous suppression of thyroid function by sufficient doses of a variety of antithyroid agents. Pituitary adenomas have also been observed (*see* Clinical Pharmacology)
Pregnancy Category D—*See* Warnings—Tapazole used judiciously is an effective drug in hyperthyroidism complicated by pregnancy. In many pregnant women, the thyroid dysfunction diminishes as the pregnancy proceeds; consequently, a reduction in dosage may be possible. In some instances, use of Tapazole can be discontinued 2 or 3 weeks before delivery.
Nursing Mothers—The drug appears in human breast milk and its use is contraindicated in nursing mothers (*see* Warnings).
Usage in Children—*See* Dosage and Administration.

ADVERSE REACTIONS

Major adverse reactions (which occur with much less frequency than the minor adverse reactions) include inhibition of myelopoiesis (agranulocytosis, granulocytopenia, and thrombocytopenia), aplastic anemia, drug fever, a lupuslike syndrome, insulin autoimmune syndrome (which can result in hypoglycemic coma), hepatitis (jaundice may persist for several weeks after discontinuation of the drug), periarteritis, and hypoprothrombinemia. Nephritis occurs very rarely.
Minor adverse reactions include skin rash, urticaria, nausea, vomiting, epigastric distress, arthralgia, paresthesia, loss of taste, abnormal loss of hair, myalgia, headache, pruritus, drowsiness, neuritis, edema, vertigo, skin pigmentation, jaundice, sialadenopathy, and lymphadenopathy.
It should be noted that about 10% of patients with untreated hyperthyroidism have leukopenia (white-blood-cell count of less than 4,000/mm^3), often with relative granulopenia.

OVERDOSAGE

Signs and Symptoms—Symptoms may include nausea, vomiting, epigastric distress, headache, fever, joint pain, pruritus, and edema. Aplastic anemia (pancytopenia) or agranulocytosis may be manifested in hours to days. Less frequent events are hepatitis, nephrotic syndrome, exfoliative dermatitis, neuropathies, and CNS stimulation or depression. Although not well studied, methimazole-induced agranulocytosis is generally associated with doses of 40 mg or more in patients older than 40 years of age.
No information is available on the median lethal dose of the drug or the concentration of methimazole in biologic fluids associated with toxicity and/or death.
Treatment—To obtain up-to-date information about the treatment of overdose, a good resource is your certified Regional Poison Control Center. Telephone numbers of certified poison control centers are listed in the *Physicians' Desk Reference (PDR).* In managing overdosage, consider the possibility of multiple drug overdoses, interaction among drugs, and unusual drug kinetics in your patient.
Protect the patient's airway and support ventilation and perfusion. Meticulously monitor and maintain, within acceptable limits, the patient's vital signs, blood gases, serum electrolytes, etc. The patient's bone marrow function should be monitored. Absorption of drugs from the gastrointestinal tract may be decreased by giving activated charcoal, which, in many cases, is more effective than emesis or lavage; consider charcoal instead of or in addition to gastric emptying. Repeated doses of charcoal over time may hasten elimination of some drugs that have been absorbed. Safeguard the patient's airway when employing gastric emptying or charcoal.
Forced diuresis, peritoneal dialysis, hemodialysis, or charcoal hemoperfusion have not been established as beneficial for an overdose of methimazole.

DOSAGE AND ADMINISTRATION

Tapazole® (Methimazole Tablets, USP, Lilly) is administered orally. It is usually given in 3 equal doses at approximately 8-hour intervals.
Adult—The initial daily dosage is 15 mg for mild hyperthyroidism, 30 to 40 mg for moderately severe hyperthyroidism, and 60 mg for severe hyperthyroidism, divided into 3 doses at 8-hour intervals. The maintenance dosage is 5 to 15 mg daily.

Continued on next page

*** Identi-Code® symbol. This product information was prepared in June 1992. Current information on these and other products of Eli Lilly and Company may be obtained by direct inquiry to Lilly Research Laboratories, Lilly Corporate Center, Indianapolis, Indiana 46285, (317) 276-3714.**

Lilly—Cont.

Pediatric—Initially, the daily dosage is 0.4 mg/kg of body weight divided into 3 doses and given at 8-hour intervals. The maintenance dosage is approximately ½ of the initial dose.

HOW SUPPLIED

(℞) Tablets:
5 mg, white (scored) (No.1765)—(100s) NDC 0002-1094-02
10 mg, white (scored) (No. 1770)—(100s) NDC 0002-1095-02
Store at controlled room temperature, 59° to 86°F (15° to 30°C).

[111991]

TAZIDIME® ℞

[*tă´zĭ-dĕm*]
(ceftazidime)
for injection
USP

DESCRIPTION

Tazidime® (Ceftazidime, USP, Lilly) is a semisynthetic, broad-spectrum β-lactam antibiotic for parenteral administration. It is the pentahydrate of pyridinium, 1-[[7-[[(2-amino-4-thiazolyl) [(1-carboxy-1-methylethoxy) imino] acetyl]amino]-2-carboxy -8- oxo-5-thia -1-azabicyclo[4.2.0]oct -2-en-3-yl]methyl]-, hydroxide, inner salt, [6R-[6α,7β(Z)]]. The molecular formula is $C_{22}H_{22}N_6O_7S_2 \cdot 5H_2O$ and the molecular weight is 636.6.

Tazidime is a sterile, dry powder. Tazidime contains 118 mg (18.5 mmol) sodium carbonate/g of ceftazidime activity. The total sodium content of the mixture is approximately 54 mg (2.3 mEq)/g of ceftazidime activity. Solutions of Tazidime range from light yellow to amber, depending on the diluent and concentration. The pH of freshly reconstituted solutions usually ranges from 5.0 to 8.0.

CLINICAL PHARMACOLOGY

After intravenous administration of a 500-mg or a 1-g dose of ceftazidime over 5 minutes to normal adult male volunteers, mean peak serum concentrations were 45 μg/mL and 90 μg/mL respectively. Following intravenous infusion of 500-mg, 1-g, and 2-g doses of ceftazidime over 20 to 30 minutes to normal adult male volunteers, mean peak serum concentrations of 42, 69, and 170 μg/mL respectively were achieved. The average serum concentrations following intravenous infusion of 500-mg, 1-g, and 2-g doses to these volunteers over an 8-hour period are given in Table 1.

Table 1. Ceftazidime Concentrations in Serum

Ceftazidime Dosage IV	Serum Concentrations (μg/mL) ½ h	1 h	2 h	4 h	8 h
500 mg	42	25	12	6	2
1 g	60	39	23	11	3
2 g	129	75	42	13	5

The absorption and elimination of ceftazidime were directly proportional to the size of the dose. Following intravenous administration, the half-life was approximately 1.9 hours. Less than 10% of ceftazidime was protein bound. The degree of protein binding was independent of concentration. Following multiple intravenous doses of 1 g and 2 g every 8 hours for 10 days, there was no evidence of accumulation of ceftazidime in the serum in individuals with normal renal function.

Following intramuscular administration of 500-mg and 1-g doses of ceftazidime to normal adult volunteers, the mean peak serum concentrations at approximately 1 hour were 17 μg/mL and 39 μg/mL respectively. Serum concentrations remained above 4 μg/mL for 6 and 8 hours after the intramuscular administration of 500-mg and 1-g doses respectively. The half-life of ceftazidime in these volunteers was approximately 2 hours.

The presence of hepatic dysfunction had no effect on the pharmacokinetics of ceftazidime in individuals who received 2 g intravenously every 8 hours for 5 days. Therefore, dosage adjustment is not required for patients with hepatic dysfunction, unless renal function is impaired.

Approximately 80% to 90% of an intramuscular or intravenous dose of ceftazidime is excreted unchanged by the kidneys over a 24-hour period. After the intravenous administration of a single 500-mg or 1-g dose, approximately 50% of the dose appeared in the urine in the first 2 hours. An additional 20% was excreted 2 and 4 hours after administration, and approximately another 12% of the dose appeared in the urine 4 to 8 hours later. The elimination of ceftazidime by the kidneys resulted in high urinary concentrations.

The mean renal clearance of ceftazidime was approximately 100 mL/min. The calculated plasma clearance of approximately 115 mL/min indicated almost complete elimination of ceftazidime by the renal route. The administration of probenecid prior to administration of ceftazidime had no effect on the elimination kinetics of ceftazidime. This suggested that ceftazidime is eliminated by glomerular filtration and is not actively secreted by renal tubular mechanisms.

Since ceftazidime is eliminated almost solely by the kidneys, its serum half-life is significantly prolonged in patients with impaired renal function. Consequently, dosage for such patients must be adjusted (*see* Dosage and Administration).

Therapeutic concentrations of ceftazidime are achieved in tissues and body fluids as listed in Table 2.

Microbiology—In vitro tests demonstrate that ceftazidime is bactericidal, exerting its effect by inhibition of enzymes responsible for cell-wall synthesis. Ceftazidime has in vitro activity against a wide range of gram-negative organisms, including strains resistant to gentamicin and other aminoglycosides. In addition, ceftazidime has been shown to be active against gram-positive organisms. It is highly stable to most clinically important β-lactamases, plasmid or chromosomal, that are produced by gram-negative or gram-positive organisms and consequently is active against many strains resistant to ampicillin and other cephalosporins.

Ceftazidime has been shown to be active against the following organisms both in vitro and in clinical infections:

Gram-Negative—*Pseudomonas* sp (including *Pseudomonas aeruginosa*); *Klebsiella* sp (including *Klebsiella pneumoniae*); *Proteus mirabilis; Proteus vulgaris; Escherichia coli; Enterobacter* sp (including *Enterobacter cloacae* and *Enterobacter aerogenes*); *Citrobacter* sp (including *Citrobacter freundii* and *Citrobacter diversus*); *Serratia* sp; *Haemophilus influenzae*, including ampicillin-resistant strains; and *Neisseria meningitidis*

Gram-Positive—*Staphylococcus aureus*, including penicillinase- and non-penicillinase-producing strains; *Streptococcus pyogenes* (group A β-hemolytic streptococci); *Streptococcus agalactiae* (group B streptococci); and *Streptococcus pneumoniae*

Anaerobic Organisms—*Bacteroides* sp (NOTE: most strains of *Bacteroides fragilis* are resistant.)

Although clinical efficacy has not been established, ceftazidime has also been shown to demonstrate in vitro activity against the following microorganisms:

Staphylococcus epidermidis; Morganella morganii (formerly *Proteus morganii*); *Providencia* sp (including *Providencia rettgeri*, formerly *Proteus rettgeri*); *Acinetobacter* sp; *Salmonella* sp; *Clostridium* sp (not including *Clostridium difficile*); *Peptococcus* sp; *Peptostreptococcus* sp; *Neisseria gonorrhoeae; Haemophilus parainfluenzae; Yersinia enterocolitica;* and *Shigella* sp

Ceftazidime and the aminoglycosides have been shown to be synergistic in vitro against some strains of *P. aeruginosa* and the *Enterobacteriaceae*. Ceftazidime and carbenicillin have also been shown to be synergistic in vitro against *P. aeruginosa*.

Ceftazidime is not active in vitro against methicillin-resistant staphylococci; *Enterococcus faecalis* (formerly *Streptococcus faecalis*) and many other enterococci; *Listeria monocytogenes; Campylobacter* sp.; or *C. difficile*.

Disk Susceptibility Tests—Quantitative methods that require measurement of zone diameters give the most precise estimates of antibiotic susceptibility. One such procedure[1–3] has been recommended for use with disks to test susceptibility to ceftazidime.

Reports from the laboratory giving results of the standardized single-disk susceptibility test using a 30-μg ceftazidime disk should be interpreted according to the following criteria:

Susceptible organisms produce zones of 18 mm or greater, indicating that the tested organism is likely to respond to therapy.

Organisms of moderate susceptibility produce zones of 15 mm to 17 mm, indicating that the tested organism would be susceptible if high dosage is used or if the infection is confined to tissues and fluids (eg, urine) in which high antibiotic levels are attained.

Resistant organisms produce zones of ≤ 14 mm, indicating that other therapy should be selected.

Organisms should be tested with the ceftazidime disk, because ceftazidime has been shown by in vitro tests to have activity against certain strains found to be resistant when tested with other β-lactam disks.

Standardized procedures require the use of laboratory control organisms. The 30-μg ceftazidime disk should give zone diameters between 25 mm and 32 mm for *E. coli* ATCC 25922, between 22 mm and 29 mm for *P. aeruginosa* ATCC 27853, and between 16 mm and 20 mm for *S. aureus* ATCC 25923.

In other susceptibility testing procedures (eg, ICS agar dilution or its equivalent), a bacterial isolate may be considered susceptible if the MIC value for ceftazidime is not > 16 μg/mL. Organisms are considered resistant if the MIC is ≥ 64 μg/mL. Organisms having an MIC value of < 64 μg/mL but > 16 μg/mL are expected to be susceptible if high dosage is used or if the infection is confined to tissues and fluids (eg, urine) in which high antibiotic levels are attained.

As with standard diffusion methods, dilution procedures require the use of laboratory control organisms. Standard ceftazidime powder should give MIC values of 4 μg/mL to 16 μg/mL for *S. aureus* ATCC 29213, 0.125 μg/mL to 0.5 μg/mL for *E. coli* ATCC 25922, and 0.5 μg/mL to 2 μg/mL for *P. aeruginosa* ATCC 27853.

Table 2: Ceftazidime Concentration in Tissues and Body Fluids

Tissue or Fluid	Dose/ Route	No. of Patients	Time of Sample Post-Dose	Average Tissue or Fluid Level (μg/mL)
Urine	500 mg IM	6	0–2 h	2,100
	2 g IV	6	0–2 h	12,000
Bile	2 g IV	3	90 min	36.4
Synovial fluid	2 g IV	13	2 h	25.6
Peritoneal fluid	2 g IV	8	2 h	48.6
Sputum	1 g IV	8	1 h	9
Cerebrospinal fluid	2 g q8h IV	5	120 min	9.8
(inflamed meninges)	2 g q8h IV	6	180 min	9.4
Aqueous humor	2 g IV	13	1–3 h	11
Blister fluid	1 g IV	7	2–3 h	19.7
Lymphatic fluid	1 g IV	7	2–3 h	23.4
Bone	2 g IV	8	0.67 h	31.1
Heart muscle	2 g IV	35	30–280 min	12.7
Skin	2 g IV	22	30–180 min	6.6
Skeletal muscle	2 g IV	35	30–280 min	9.4
Myometrium	2 g IV	31	1–2 h	18.7

INDICATIONS AND USAGE

Tazidime® (Ceftazidime, USP, Lilly) is indicated for the treatment of infections caused by susceptible strains of the designated organisms in the diseases listed below:

Lower respiratory tract infections, including pneumonia, caused by *P. aeruginosa* and other *Pseudomonas* sp., *H. influenzae* (including ampicillin-resistant strains), *Klebsiella* sp., *Enterobacter* sp., *P. mirabilis, E. coli, Serratia* sp., *Citrobacter* sp., *S. pneumoniae*, and *S. aureus* (methicillin-susceptible strains)

Skin and skin structure infections caused by *P. aeruginosa, Klebsiella* sp., *E. coli, Proteus* sp. (including *P. mirabilis* and indole-positive *Proteus*), *Enterobacter* sp., *Serratia* sp., *S. aureus* (methicillin-susceptible strains), and *S. pyogenes* (group A β-hemolytic streptococci)

Urinary tract infections, both complicated and uncomplicated, caused by *P. aeruginosa, Enterobacter* sp., *Proteus* sp. (including *P. mirabilis* and indole-positive *Proteus*), *Klebsiella* sp., and *E. coli*

Bacterial septicemia caused by *P. aeruginosa, Klebsiella* sp., *H. influenzae, E. coli, Serratia* sp., *S. pneumoniae*, and *S. aureus* (methicillin-susceptible strains)

Bone and joint infections caused by *P. aeruginosa; Klebsiella* sp., *Enterobacter* sp., and *S. aureus* (methicillin-susceptible strains)

Gynecologic infections, including endometritis, pelvic cellulitis, and other infections of the female genital tract caused by *E. coli*

Intra-abdominal infections, including peritonitis, caused by *E. coli, Klebsiella* sp., and *S. aureus* (methicillin-susceptible strains) and polymicrobial infections caused by aerobic and anaerobic organisms and *Bacteroides* sp. (NOTE: Most strains of *B. fragilis* are resistant.)

Central nervous system infections, including meningitis, caused by *H. influenzae* and *N. meningitidis*. Tazidime has also been used successfully in a limited number of cases of menigitis due to *P. aeruginosa* and *S. pneumoniae*

Specimens for bacteriologic cultures should be obtained prior to therapy in order to isolate and identify causative organisms and to determine their susceptibilities to ceftazidime. Therapy may be instituted before results of susceptibility studies are known; however, once these results become available, the antibiotic treatment should be adjusted accordingly.

Tazidime may be used alone in cases of confirmed or suspected sepsis. Tazidime has been used successfully as empiric therapy in clinical trial cases involving concomitant therapies with other antibiotics.

Tazidime may also be used concomitantly with other antibiotics, such as aminoglycosides, vancomycin, and clindamycin, in severe and life-threatening infections and in the immunocompromised patient. When such concomitant treatment is appropriate, prescribing information in the labeling for the other anitibiotics should be followed. The dose depends on the severity of the infection and the patient's condition.

CONTRAINDICATION

Tazidime® (Ceftazidime, USP, Lilly) is contraindicated in patients who have shown hypersensitivity to ceftazidime or the cephalosporin group of antibiotics.

WARNINGS

BEFORE THERAPY WITH TAZIDIME® (Ceftazidime, USP, Lilly) IS INSTITUTED, CAREFUL INQUIRY SHOULD BE MADE TO DETERMINE WHETHER THE PATIENT HAS HAD PREVIOUS HYPERSENSITIVITY REACTIONS TO CEFTAZIDIME, CEPHALOSPORINS, PENICILLINS, OR OTHER DRUGS. ANTIBIOTICS SHOULD BE ADMINISTERED WITH CAUTION TO ANY PATIENT WHO HAS DEMONSTRATED SOME FORM OF ALLERGY, PARTICULARLY TO DRUGS. THIS PRODUCT SHOULD BE GIVEN WITH CAUTION TO PATIENTS WITH TYPE I HYPERSENSITIVITY REACTIONS TO PENICILLIN. IF AN ALLERGIC REACTION TO TAZIDIME OCCURS, DISCONTINUE TREATMENT WITH THE DRUG. SERIOUS ACUTE HYPERSENSITIVITY REACTIONS MAY REQUIRE EPINEPHRINE AND OTHER EMERGENCY MEASURES.

Pseudomembranous colitis has been reported with virtually all broad-spectrum antibiotics (including macrolides, semisynthetic penicillins, and cephalosporins); therefore, it is important to consider its diagnosis in patients who develop diarrhea in association with antibiotic use.

Treatment with broad-spectrum antibiotics alters normal flora of the colon and may permit overgrowth of clostridia. Studies indicate that a toxin produced by *C. difficile* is a primary cause of antibiotic-associated colitis.

Mild cases of pseudomembraneous colitis respond to drug discontinuance alone. In moderate to severe cases, management should include fluid, electrolyte, and protein supplementation. When the colitis does not improve with drug discontinuance or when it is severe, oral vancomycin is the drug of choice for antibiotic-associated pseudomembranous colitis produced by *C. difficile*. Other causes of colitis should be ruled out.

PRECAUTIONS

General —Tazidime® (Ceftazidime, USP, Lilly) has not been shown to be nephrotoxic; however, because high and prolonged serum antibiotic concentrations can occur from usual doses in patients with transient or persistent reduction of urinary output because of renal insufficiency, the total daily dosage should be reduced when ceftazidime is administered to such patients (*see* Dosage and Administration). In such cases, dosage should be determined by degree of renal impairment, severity of infection, and susceptibility of the causative organisms.

As with other antibiotics, prolonged use of Tazidime may result in the overgrowth of nonsusceptible organisms. Repeated evaluation of the patient's condition is essential. If superinfection occurs during therapy, appropriate measures should be taken.

Tazidime should be prescribed with caution in individuals with a history of gastrointestinal disease, particularly colitis.

Drug Interactions —Nephrotoxicity has been reported following the concomitant administration of cephalosporins with aminoglycoside antibiotics or potent diuretics, such as furosemide. Renal function should be carefully monitored because of the potential nephrotoxicity and ototoxicity of aminoglycoside antibiotics, especially if higher dosages of the aminoglycosides are to be administered or if therapy is prolonged. Nephrotoxicity and ototoxicity were not noted when Tazidime was given alone in clinical trials.

Carcinogenesis, Mutagenesis, Impairment of Fertility —Long-term studies in animals have not been performed to evaluate carcinogenic potential. However, a mouse micronucleus test and an Ames test were both negative for mutagenic effects.

Usage in Pregnancy —Pregnancy Category B —Reproduction studies have been performed in mice and rats at doses up to 40 times the human dose and have revealed no evidence of impaired fertility or harm to the fetus due to Tazidime. There are, however, no adequate and well-controlled studies in pregnant women. Because animal reproduction studies

Table 3: Recommended Dosage Schedule for Ceftazidime

	Dose	Frequency
Adults		
Usual recommended dose	**1 g IV or IM**	**q8 or 12h**
Uncomplicated urinary tract infections	250 mg IV or IM	q12h
Bone and joint infections	2 g IV	q12h
Complicated urinary tract infections	500 mg IV or IM	q8 or 12h
Uncomplicated pneumonia; mild skin and skin structure infections	500 mg–1 g IV or IM	q8h
Serious gynecologic and intra-abdominal infections	2 g IV	q8h
Meningitis	2 g IV	q8h
Very severe life-threatening infections, especially in immunocompromised patients	2 g IV	q8h
Pseudomonal lung infections in patients with cystic fibrosis with normal renal function*	30–50 mg/kg IV to a maximum of 6 g/day	q8h
Neonates (0 to 4 weeks)	30 mg/kg IV	q12h
Infants and Children (1 month to 12 years of age)	30–50 mg/kg IV to a maximum of 6 g/day†	q8h

* Although clinical improvement has been shown, bacteriologic cures cannot be expected in patients with chronic respiratory disease and cystic fibrosis.
† The higher dose should be reserved for immunocompromised children or children with cystic fibrosis or meningitis.

are not always predictive of human response, this drug should be used during pregnancy only if clearly needed.

Nursing Mothers —Ceftazidime is excreted in human milk in low concentrations. Caution should be exercised when Tazidime is administered to a nursing woman.

ADVERSE REACTIONS

Tazidime® (Ceftazidime, USP, Lilly) is generally well tolerated. The incidence of adverse reactions associated with the administration of Tazidime was low in clinical trials. The most common were local reactions following intravenous injection and allergic and gastrointestinal reactions. Other adverse reactions were encountered infrequently. No disulfiram-like reactions were reported. The following adverse effects during clinical trials were considered to be either related to ceftazidime therapy or of uncertain etiology:

Local effects, reported in < 2% of patients, were phlebitis and inflammation at the site of injection (1 in 69 patients).

Hypersensitivity reactions, reported in 2% of patients, were pruritus, rash, and fever. Immediate hypersensitivity reactions occurred in 1 in 285 patients.

Gastrointestinal symptoms, reported in < 2% of patients, were diarrhea (1 in 78), nausea (1 in 156), vomiting (1 in 500), and abdominal pain (1 in 416).

Less frequent adverse events (< 1%) were candidiasis and vaginitis; central nervous system events included headache, dizziness, and paresthesia.

Laboratory test changes noted during clinical trials with Tazidime were transient and included eosinophilia (1 in 13), positive Coombs' test without hemolysis (1 in 23), thrombocytosis (1 in 45), and slight elevations in 1 or more of the hepatic enzymes: SGOT (1 in 16), SGPT (1 in 15), LDH (1 in 18), and alkaline phosphatase (1 in 23). As with some other cephalosporins, transient elevations of blood urea, blood urea nitrogen, and/or serum creatinine were observed occasionally. Transient leukopenia, neutropenia, thrombocytopenia, and lymphocytosis were seen very rarely.

OVERDOSAGE

Signs and Symptoms —Toxic signs and symptoms following an overdose of ceftazidime may include pain, inflammation, and phlebitis at the injection site.

The administration of inappropriately large doses of parenteral cephalosporins may cause dizziness, paresthesias, and headaches. Seizures may occur following overdosage with some cephalosporins, particularly in patients with renal impairment where accumulation is likely to occur.

Laboratory abnormalities that may occur after an overdose include elevations in creatinine, BUN, liver enzymes and bilirubin, a positive Coombs' test, thrombocytosis, thrombocytopenia, eosinophilia, leukopenia, and prolongation of the prothrombin time.

The subcutaneous median lethal dose in rats and mice ranged from 5.8 to 20 g/kg, and the intravenous median lethal dose in rabbits were > 2 g/kg.

Treatment —To obtain up-to-date information about the treatment of overdose, a good resource is your certified Regional Poison Control Center. Telephone numbers of certified poison control centers are listed in the *Physicians' Desk Reference (PDR)*. In managing overdosage, consider the possibility of multiple drug overdoses, interaction among drugs, and unusual drug kinetics in your patient.

If seizures occur, the drug should be discontinued promptly; anticonvulsant therapy may be administered if clinically indicated. Protect the patient's airway and support ventilation and perfusion. Meticulously monitor and maintain, within acceptable limits, the patient's vital signs, blood gases, serum electrolytes, etc.

In cases of severe overdosage, especially in a patient with renal failure, combined hemodialysis and hemoperfusion may be considered if response to more conservative therapy fails. However, no data supporting such therapy are available.

DOSAGE AND ADMINISTRATION

The usual adult dosage is 1 g administered intravenously or intramuscularly every 8 or 12 hours. The dosage and route of administration should be determined by the susceptibility of the causative organisms, the severity of infection, and the condition and renal function of the patient.

The guidelines for dosage of Tazidime® (Ceftazidime, USP, Lilly) are listed in Table 3. The following dosage schedule is recommended:

Patients With Impaired Hepatic Function —No adjustment in dosage is required for patients with hepatic dysfunction.

Patients With Impaired Renal Function —Ceftazidime is excreted by the kidneys almost exclusively by glomerular filtration. Therefore, in patients with impaired renal function (GFR < 50 mL/min), it is recommended that the dose of Tazidime be reduced to compensate for its slower excretion. In patients with suspected renal insufficiency, an initial loading dose of 1 g of Tazidime may be given. An estimate of GFR should be made to determine the appropriate maintenance dose. The recommended dosage is presented in Table 4.

Table 4. Recommended Maintenance Dosage of Tazidime® (Ceftazidime, USP, Lilly) in Patients With Renal Insufficiency

Creatinine Clearance (mL/min)	Recommended Dose of Tazidime	Frequency
50–31	1 g	q12h
30–16	1 g	q24h
15–6	500 mg	q24h
<5	500 mg	q48h

When only serum creatinine is available, the following formula (Cockcroft's equation)[4] may be used to estimate creatinine clearance. The serum creatinine should represent a steady state of renal function:

Continued on next page

Lilly—Cont.

Males:

$$\text{Creatinine Clearance} = \frac{\text{Weight (kg)} \times (140 - \text{age})}{72 \times \text{serum creatinine}}$$

(mL/min)   (mg/dL)

Females: 0.85 × above value

In patients with severe infections who would normally receive 6 g of Tazidime daily were it not for renal insufficiency, the dose given in the above table may be increased by 50% or the dosing frequency increased appropriately. Continued dosage should be determined by therapeutic monitoring, severity of the infection, and susceptibility of the causative organism.

In children, as in adults, the creatinine clearance should be adjusted for body surface area or lean body mass, and the dosing frequency should be reduced in cases of renal insufficiency.

In patients undergoing hemodialysis, a loading dose of 1 g of Tazidime is recommended, followed by 1 g after each hemodialysis period.

Tazidime can also be used in patients undergoing intraperitoneal dialysis (IPD) and continuous ambulatory peritoneal dialysis (CAPD). In such patients, a loading dose of 1 g of Tazidime may be given, followed by 500 mg every 24 hours. In addition to intravenous use, Tazidime can be incorporated in dialysis fluid at a concentration of 250 mg/2 L of dialysis fluid.

NOTE: Tazidime should generally be continued for 2 days after the signs and symptoms of infection have disappeared; however, in complicated infections, longer therapy may be required.

Administration —Tazidime® (Ceftazidime, USP, Lilly) may be given intravenously or by deep intramuscular injection into a large muscle mass (such as the upper outer quadrant of the gluteus maximus or lateral part of the thigh).

Intramuscular Administration —For intramuscular administration, Tazidime should be reconstituted with 1 of the following diluents: Sterile Water for Injection, Bacteriostatic Water for Injection, or 0.5% or 1.0% Lidocaine Hydrochloride Injection. Refer to Table 5.

Intravenous Administration —The IV route is preferable for patients with bacterial septicemia, bacterial meningitis, peritonitis, or other severe or life-threatening infections. It is also preferable for patients who may be poor risks because of lowered resistance resulting from such debilitating conditions as malnutrition, trauma, surgery, diabetes, heart failure, or malignancy, particularly if shock is present or impending.

For direct intermittent intravenous administration, reconstitute Tazidime with Sterile Water for Injection (see Table 5). Slowly inject the solution directly into the vein over a period of 3 to 5 minutes or give through the tubing of an administration set while the patient is also receiving 1 of the compatible intravenous fluids (*see* Compatibility and Stability).

For intravenous infusion, reconstitute the 1-g or 2-g piggyback (100-mL) vial with 100 mL Sterile Water for Injection or 1 of the compatible intravenous fluids listed in the Compatibility and Stability section. Alternatively, reconstitute the 500-mg, 1-g, or 2-g vial, and add an appropriate quantity of the resulting solution to an IV container with 1 of the compatible intravenous fluids.

Intermittent intravenous infusion with a Y-type administration set can be accomplished with compatible solutions. However, during infusion of a solution containing ceftazidime, it is desirable to discontinue the other solution.

ADD-Vantage® vials are to be used only with Abbott ADD-Vantage diluent bags according to the printed tray card instructions included in each Traypak of vials.

ADD-Vantage vials that have been joined to Abbott ADD-Vantage bags of diluent and activated to dissolve the drug are stable for 24 hours at room temperature. Joined vials

that have not been activated may be used within a 14-day period; this period corresponds to that for use of Abbott ADD-Vantage containers following removal of the outer packaging (overwrap).

Freezing solutions of Tazidime in the ADD-Vantage system is not recommended.

When Tazidime® (Ceftazidime, USP, Lilly) is dissolved, carbon dioxide is released and a positive pressure develops. For ease of use, please follow the recommended techniques of reconstitution described below.

Solutions of Tazidime, like those of most β-lactam antibiotics, should not be added to solutions of aminoglycoside antibiotics because of potential interaction. However, if concurrent therapy with Tazidime and an aminoglycoside is indicated, each of these antibiotics should be administered in different sites.

Instructions for Reconstitution:
For 500-mg IM/IV, 1-g IM/IV, and 2-g IV vials
1. Inject the diluent and shake well to dissolve.
2. Carbon dioxide is released as the antibiotic dissolves, generating pressure within the vial. The solution will become clear within 1 to 2 minutes.
3. Invert the vial, and completely depress the syringe plunger prior to insertion.
4. Insert the needle through the vial stopper. Be sure the needle remains within the solution, and withdraw contents of the vial in the usual manner. Pressure in the vial may aid withdrawal.
5. The withdrawn solution may contain carbon dioxide bubbles which should be expelled from the syringe before injection.

For 1-g and 2-g piggyback vials
1. Inject 10 mL of the diluent and shake to dissolve.
2. Carbon dioxide is released as the antibiotic dissolves, generating pressure within the vial. The solution will become clear within 1 to 2 minutes.
3. Insert a vent needle to release pressure before adding additional diluent to the vial. Add diluent and then remove the vent needle.
4. After storage, any additional pressure that may develop in the vial prior to administration should be released.

COMPATIBILITY AND STABILITY

Intramuscular —Vials of Tazidime® (Ceftazidime, USP, Lilly), when reconstituted as directed with Sterile Water for Injection, Bacteriostatic Water for Injection, or 0.5% or 1% Lidocaine Hydrochloride Injection, maintain satisfactory potency for 24 hours at room temperature or for 7 days under refrigeration. Solutions in Sterile Water for Injection that are frozen immediately after reconstitution in the original container are stable for 3 months when stored at −20°C. Once thawed, solutions should not be refrozen. Thawed solutions may be stored for up to 8 hours at room temperature or for 4 days in a refrigerator.

Intravenous —Vials of Tazidime, when reconstituted as directed with Sterile Water for Injection, maintain satisfactory potency for 24 hours at room temperature or for 7 days under refrigeration. Solutions in Sterile Water for Injection in the original container or in 0.9% Sodium Chloride Injection or 5% Dextrose Injection in PVC small-volume containers that are frozen immediately after reconstitution are stable for 3 months when stored at −20°C. When it is necessary to warm a large volume of the frozen product (to a maximum of 40°C), care should be taken to avoid heating it after thawing is complete. Once thawed, solutions should not be refrozen. Thawed solutions may be stored for up to 24 hours at room temperature or for 4 days in a refrigerator.

Tazidime is compatible with the more commonly used intravenous fluids. Solutions at concentrations from 1 mg/mL to 40 mg/mL in the following infusion fluids may be stored for up to 24 hours at room temperature or for 7 days if refrigerated: 0.9% Sodium Chloride Injection; M/6 Sodium Lactate Injection; Ringer's Injection, USP; Lactated Ring-

er's Injection, USP; 5% Dextrose Injection; 5% Dextrose and 0.225% Sodium Chloride Injection; 5% Dextrose and 0.45% Sodium Chloride Injection; 5% Dextrose and 0.9% Sodium Chloride Injection; 10% Dextrose Injection; 10% Invert Sugar in Water for Injection; and Normosol®-M in 5% Dextrose Injection.

When diluted with Abbott's ADD-Vantage diluents, 0.9% Sodium Chloride Injection and 5% Dextrose Injection, ADD-Vantage Tazidime may be stored for up to 24 hours at room temperature.

Tazidime is less stable in Sodium Bicarbonate Injection than in other intravenous fluids. Sodium Bicarbonate Injection is not recommended as a diluent. Solutions of Tazidime in 5% Dextrose or 0.9% Sodium Chloride Injection are stable for at least 6 hours at room temperature in plastic tubing, drip chambers, and volume control devices of common intravenous infusion sets.

At a concentration of 4 mg/mL, Tazidime has been found to be compatible for 24 hours at room temperature or for 7 days under refrigeration in 0.9% Sodium Chloride Injection or 5% Dextrose Injection when admixed with cefuroxime sodium, 3 mg/mL; heparin, 10 units/mL or 50 units/mL; or potassium chloride, 10 mEq/L or 40 mEq/L.

Note: Parenteral drug products should be inspected visually for particulate matter whenever solution and container permit.

Tazidime powder and solutions will darken under certain storage conditions. However, product potency is not adversely affected if proper storage conditions and periods are observed.

HOW SUPPLIED

(℞) Vials (Dry Powder):
   500 mg,* 10-mL size (No. 7230)—(Traypak† of 25) NDC 0002-7230
   1 g,* 20-mL size (No. 7231)—(Traypak of 25) NDC 0002-7231-25
   1 g,* 100-mL size (No. 7238)—(Traypak of 10) NDC 0002-7238-10
   2 g,* 50-mL size (No. 7234)—(Traypak of 10) NDC 0002-7234-10
   2 g,* 100-mL size (No. 7239)—(Traypak of 10) NDC 0002-7239-10
(℞) Faspak‡:
   1 g* (No. 7245)—(Faspak of 24) NDC 0002-7245-24
   2 g* (No. 7246)—(Faspak of 24) NDC 0002-7246-24
(℞) ADD-Vantage§ Vials:
   1 g* (No. 7290)—(Traypak of 25) NDC 0002-7290-25
   2 g* (No. 7291)—(Traypak of 10) NDC 0002-7291-10
The above ADD-Vantage Vials are to be used only with Abbott Laboratories' ADD-Vantage Diluent Containers. Instructions for the use of ADD-Vantage Vials are enclosed in the package.
Also available:
(℞) Pharmacy Bulk Package:
   6 g,* 100-mL size (No. 7241)—(Traypak of 6) NDC 0002-7241-16

REFERENCES

1. Bauer AW, Kirby WMM, Sherris J C, et al: Antibiotic susceptibility testing by a standardized single disk method. *Am J Clin Pathol* 1966; 45:493.
2. *Performance standards for antimicrobial disk susceptibility tests*, ed 4, Tentative Standard: M2-T4. NCCLS, Villanova, PA, 1988.
3. Standardized disk susceptibility test. *Federal Register 1974; 39* (May 30):19182–19184.
4. Cockcroft DW, Gault MH: Prediction of creatinine clearance from serum creatinine. *Nephron* 1978; 16:31–41.

*Equivalent to ceftazidime activity.
†Traypak™(multivial carton, Lilly).
‡Faspak® (flexible plastic bag, Lilly).
§ADD-Vantage® (vials and diluent containers, Abbott).

[030290]

Table 5: Preparation of Solutions of Tazidime® (Ceftazidime, USP, Lilly)

	Amount of Diluent to Be Added (mL)	Approximate Available Volume (mL)	Approximate Ceftazidime Concentration (mg/mL)
Intramuscular			
500 mg, Vial No. 7230	1.5	1.8	280
1 g, Vial No. 7231	3.0	3.6	280
Intravenous			
500 mg, Vial No. 7230	5	5.3	100
1 g, Vial No. 7231	10	10.6	100
2 g, Vial No. 7234	10	11.2	180
Piggyback (100 mL)			
1 g, Vial No. 7238	100*	100	10
2 g, Vial No. 7239	100*	100	20

*Note: Addition should be in 2 stages (*see* Instructions for Reconstitution *below*).

TOBRAMYCIN SULFATE   ℞
See Nebcin® (Tobramycin Sulfate Injection, USP, Lilly).

ULTRALENTE®ILETIN® I   OTC
(extended insulin zinc suspension, Lilly) *see under* Iletin®
(insulin, Lilly).

VANCOCIN® HCl ℞

[*văn 'kō-sĭn ăch 'sē-ĕl*]

(Sterile Vancomycin Hydrochloride, USP)

IntraVenous

DESCRIPTION

Vancocin® HCl (Sterile Vancomycin Hydrochloride, USP, Lilly), IntraVenous, is a chromatographically purified, tricyclic glycopeptide antibiotic derived from *Amycolatopsis orientalis* (formerly *Nocardia orientalis*) and has the chemical formula $C_{66}H_{75}Cl_2H_9O_{24}$·HCl. The molecular weight is 1,486; 500 mg of the base is equivalent to 0.34 mmol.

The vials contain sterile vancomycin hydrochloride equivalent to either 500 mg or 1 g vancomycin activity. Vancomycin hydrochloride is an off-white lyophilized plug. When reconstituted in water, it forms a clear solution with a pH range of 2.5 to 4.5.

CLINICAL PHARMACOLOGY

Vancomycin is poorly absorbed after oral administration; it is given intravenously for therapy of systemic infections. Intramuscular injection is painful.

In subjects with normal kidney function, multiple intravenous dosing of 1 g of vancomycin (15 mg/kg) infused over 60 minutes produces mean plasma concentrations of approximately 63 μg/mL immediately after the completion of infusion, mean plasma concentrations of approximately 23 μg/mL 2 hours after infusion, and mean plasma concentrations of approximately 8 μg/mL 11 hours after the end of the infusion. Multiple dosing of 500 mg infused over 30 minutes produces mean plasma concentrations of about 49 μg/mL at the completion of infusion, mean plasma concentrations of about 19 μg/mL 2 hours after infusion, and mean plasma concentrations of about 10 μg/mL 6 hours after infusion. The plasma concentrations during multiple dosing are similar to those after a single dose.

The mean elimination half-life of vancomycin from plasma is 4 to 6 hours in subjects with normal renal function. In the first 24 hours, about 75% of an administered dose of vancomycin is excreted in urine by glomerular filtration. Mean plasma clearance is about 0.058 L/kg/h, and mean renal clearance is about 0.048 L/kg/h. Renal dysfunction slows excretion of vancomycin. In anephric patients, the average half-life of elimination is 7.5 days. The distribution coefficient is from 0.3 to 0.43 L/kg. There is no apparent metabolism of the drug. About 60% of an intraperitoneal dose of vancomycin administered during peritoneal dialysis is absorbed systemically in 6 hours. Serum concentrations of about 10 μg/mL are achieved by intraperitoneal injection of 30 mg/kg of vancomycin. Although vancomycin is not effectively removed by either hemodialysis or peritoneal dialysis, there have been reports of increased vancomycin clearance with hemoperfusion and hemofiltration.

Total systemic and renal clearance of vancomycin may be reduced in the elderly.

Vancomycin is approximately 55% serum protein bound as measured by ultrafiltration at vancomycin serum concentrations of 10 to 100 μg/mL. After IV administration of Vancocin® HCl (Sterile Vancomycin Hydrochloride, USP, Lilly), inhibitory concentrations are present in pleural, pericardial, ascitic, and synovial fluids; in urine; in peritoneal dialysis fluid; and in atrial appendage tissue. Vancocin HCl does not readily diffuse across normal meninges into the spinal fluid; but, when the meninges are inflamed, penetration into the spinal fluid occurs.

Microbiology—The bactericidal action of vancomycin results primarily from inhibition of cell-wall biosynthesis. In addition, vancomycin alters bacterial-cell-membrane permeability and RNA synthesis. There is no cross-resistance between vancomycin and other antibiotics. Vancomycin is active against staphylococci, including *Staphylococcus aureus* and *Staphylococcus epidermidis* (including heterogeneous methicillin-resistant strains); streptococci, including *Streptococcus pyogenes, Streptococcus pneumoniae* (including penicillin-resistant strains), *Streptococcus agalactiae*, the viridans group, *Streptococcus bovis*, and enterococci (eg, *Enterococcus faecalis* [formerly *Streptococcus faecalis*]); *Clostridium difficile* (eg, toxigenic strains implicated in pseudomembranous enterocolitis); and diphtheroids. Other organisms that are susceptible to vancomycin in vitro include *Listeria monocytogenes, Lactobacillus* species, *Actinomyces* species, *Clostridium* species, and *Bacillus* species.

Vancomycin is not active in vitro against gram-negative bacilli, mycobacteria, or fungi.

Synergy—The combination of vancomycin and an aminoglycoside acts synergistically in vitro against many strains of *S. aureus*, nonenterococcal group D streptococci, enterococci, and *Streptococcus* species (viridans group).

Disk Susceptibility Tests—The standardized disk method described by the National Committee for Clinical Laboratory Standards has been recommended to test susceptibility to vancomycin. Results of standard susceptibility tests with a 30-μg vancomycin hydrochloride disk should be interpreted according to the following criteria: Susceptible organisms produce zones greater than or equal to 12 mm, indicating that the test organism is likely to respond to therapy. Organisms that produce zones of 10 or 11 mm are considered to be of intermediate susceptibility. Organisms in this category are likely to respond if the infection is confined to tissues or fluids in which high antibiotic concentrations are attained. Resistant organisms produce zones of 9 mm or less, indicating that other therapy should be selected.

Using a standardized dilution method, a bacterial isolate may be considered susceptible if the MIC value for vancomycin is 4 μg/mL or less. Organisms are considered resistant to vancomycin if the MIC is greater than or equal to 16 μg/mL. Organisms having an MIC value of less than 16 μg/mL but greater than 4 μg/mL are considered to be of intermediate susceptibility.[1–3]

Standardized procedures require the use of laboratory control organisms. The 30-μg vancomycin disk should give zone diameters between 15 and 19 mm for *S. aureus* ATCC 25923. As with the standard diffusion methods, dilution procedures require the use of laboratory control organisms. Standard vancomycin powder should give MIC values in the range of 0.5 μg/mL to 2.0 μg/mL for *S. aureus* ATCC 29213. For *E. faecalis* ATCC 29212, the MIC range should be 1.0 to 4.0 μg/mL.

INDICATIONS AND USAGE

Vancocin® HCl (Sterile Vancomycin Hydrochloride, USP, Lilly) is indicated for the treatment of serious or severe infections caused by susceptible strains of methicillin-resistant (β-lactam-resistant) staphylococci. It is indicated for penicillin-allergic patients, for patients who cannot receive or who have failed to respond to other drugs, including the penicillins or cephalosporins, and for infections caused by vancomycin-susceptible organisms that are resistant to other antimicrobial drugs. Vancocin HCl is indicated for initial therapy when methicillin-resistant staphylococci are suspected, but after susceptibility data are available, therapy should be adjusted accordingly.

Vancocin HCl is effective in the treatment of staphylococcal endocarditis. Its effectiveness has been documented in other infections due to staphylococci, including septicemia, bone infections, lower respiratory tract infections, and skin and skin structure infections. When staphylococcal infections are localized and purulent, antibiotics are used as adjuncts to appropriate surgical measures.

Vancocin HCl has been reported to be effective alone or in combination with an aminoglycoside for endocarditis caused by *Streptococcus viridans* or *S. bovis*. For endocarditis caused by enterococci (eg, *E. faecalis*), Vancocin HCl has been reported to be effective only in combination with an aminoglycoside.

Vancocin HCl has been reported to be effective for the treatment of diphtheroid endocarditis. Vancocin HCl has been used successfully in combination with either rifampin, an aminoglycoside, or both in early-onset prosthetic valve endocarditis caused by *S. epidermidis* or diphtheroids.

Specimens for bacteriologic cultures should be obtained in order to isolate and identify causative organisms and to determine their susceptibilities to Vancocin HCl.

The parenteral form of Vancocin HCl may be administered orally for treatment of antibiotic-associated pseudomembranous colitis caused by *C. difficile* and for staphylococccal enterocolitis. Parenteral administration of Vancocin HCl alone is of unproven benefit for these indications. **Vancocin HCl is not effective by the oral route for other types of infection.**

Although no controlled clinical efficacy studies have been conducted, intravenous vancomycin has been suggested by the American Heart Association and the American Dental Association as prophylaxis against bacterial endocarditis in penicillin-allergic patients who have congenital heart disease or rheumatic or other acquired valvular heart disease when these patients undergo dental procedures or surgical procedures of the upper respiratory tract.

Note: When selecting antibiotics for the prevention of bacterial endocarditis, the physician or dentist should read the full joint statement of the American Heart Association and the American Dental Association.[4]

CONTRAINDICATION

Vancocin® HCl (Sterile Vancomycin Hydrochloride, USP, Lilly) is contraindicated in patients with known hypersensitivity to this antibiotic.

WARNINGS

Rapid bolus administration (eg, over several minutes) may be associated with exaggerated hypotension, including shock, and, rarely, cardiac arrest.

Vancocin® HCl (Sterile Vancomycin Hydrochloride, USP, Lilly) should be administered in a dilute solution over a period of not less than 60 minutes to avoid rapid-infusion-related reactions. Stopping the infusion usually results in prompt cessation of these reactions.

Ototoxicity has occurred in patients receiving Vancocin HCl. It may be transient or permanent. It has been reported mostly in patients who have been given excessive doses, who have an underlying hearing loss, or who are receiving concomitant therapy with another ototoxic agent, such as an aminoglycoside. Vancomycin should be used with caution in patients with renal insufficiency because the risk of toxicity is appreciably increased by high, prolonged blood concentrations.

Dosage of Vancocin HCl must be adjusted for patients with renal dysfunction (*see* Precautions *and* Dosage and Administration).

PRECAUTIONS

General—Clinically significant serum concentrations have been reported in some patients who have taken multiple oral doses of vancomycin for active *C. difficile*- induced pseudomembranous colitis.

Prolonged use of Vancocin HCl may result in the overgrowth of nonsusceptible organisms. Careful observation of the patient is essential. If superinfection occurs during therapy, appropriate measures should be taken. In rare instances, there have been reports of pseudomembranous colitis due to *C. difficile* developing in patients who received intravenous vancomycin.

In order to minimize the risk of nephrotoxicity when treating patients with underlying renal dysfunction or patients receiving concomitant therapy with an aminoglycoside, serial monitoring of renal function should be performed and particular care should be taken in following appropriate dosing schedules (*see* Dosage and Administration).

Serial tests of auditory function may be helpful in order to minimize the risk of ototoxicity.

Reversible neutropenia has been reported in patients receiving Vancocin® HCl (Sterile Vancomycin Hydrochloride, USP, Lilly) (*see* Adverse Reactions). Patients who will undergo prolonged therapy with Vancocin HCl or those who are receiving concomitant drugs that may cause neutropenia should have periodic monitoring of the leukocyte count.

Vancocin HCl is irritating to tissue and must be given by a secure intravenous route of administration. Pain, tenderness, and necrosis occur with intramuscular injection of Vancocin HCl or with inadvertent extravasation. Thrombophlebitis may occur, the frequency and severity of which can be minimized by administering the drug slowly as a dilute solution (2.5 to 5 g/L) and by rotating the sites of infusion.

There have been reports that the frequency of infusion-related events (including hypotension, flushing, erythema, urticaria, and pruritus) increases with the concomitant administration of anesthetic agents. Infusion-related events may be minimized by the administration of Vancocin HCl as a 60-minute infusion prior to anesthetic induction.

The safety and efficacy of vancomycin administration by the intrathecal (intralumbar or intraventricular) routes have not been assessed.

Drug Interactions—Concomitant administration of vancomycin and anesthetic agents has been associated with erythema and histamine-like flushing (*see* Usage in Pediatrics *under* Precautions) and anaphylactoid reactions (*see* Adverse Reactions).

Concurrent and/or sequential systemic or topical use of other potentially neurotoxic and/or nephrotoxic drugs, such as amphotericin B, aminoglycosides, bacitracin, polymyxin B, colistin, viomycin, or cisplatin, when indicated, requires careful monitoring.

Usage in Pregnancy—Pregnancy Category C—Animal reproduction studies have not been conducted with Vancocin® HCl (Sterile Vancomycin Hydrochloride, USP, Lilly). It is not known whether Vancocin HCl can affect reproduction capacity. In a controlled clinical study, the potential ototoxic and nephrotoxic effects of Vancocin HCl on infants were evaluated when the drug was administered to pregnant women for serious staphylococcal infections complicating intravenous drug abuse. Vancocin HCl was found in cord blood. No sensorineural hearing loss or nephrotoxicity attributable to Vancocin HCl was noted. One infant whose mother received Vancocin HCl in the third trimester experienced conductive hearing loss that was not attributed to the administration of Vancocin HCl. Because the number of patients treated in this study was limited and Vancocin HCl was administered only in the second and third trimesters, it is not known whether Vancocin HCl causes fetal harm. Vancocin HCl should be given to a pregnant woman only if clearly needed.

Nursing Mothers—Vancocin HCl is excreted in human milk. Caution should be exercised when Vancocin HCl is administered to a nursing woman. Because of the potential for adverse events, a decision should be made whether to discontinue nursing or to discontinue the drug, taking into account the importance of the drug to the mother.

Usage in Pediatrics—In premature neonates and young infants, it may be appropriate to confirm desired vancomycin

Continued on next page

*** Identi-Code® symbol. This product information was prepared in June 1992. Current information on these and other products of Eli Lilly and Company may be obtained by direct inquiry to Lilly Research Laboratories, Lilly Corporate Center, Indianapolis, Indiana 46285, (317) 276-3714.**

Lilly—Cont.

serum concentrations. Concomitant administration of vancomycin and anesthetic agents has been associated with erythema and histamine-like flushing in children (see Adverse Reactions).

Geriatrics—The natural decrement of glomerular filtration with increasing age may lead to elevated vancomycin serum concentrations if dosage is not adjusted. Vancomycin dosage schedules should be adjusted in elderly patients (see Dosage and Administration).

ADVERSE REACTIONS

Infusion-Related Events—During or soon after rapid infusion of Vancocin® HCl (Sterile Vancomycin Hydrochloride, USP, Lilly), patients may develop anaphylactoid reactions, including hypotension, wheezing, dyspnea, urticaria, or pruritus. Rapid infusion may also cause flushing of the upper body ("red neck") or pain and muscle spasm of the chest and back. These reactions usually resolve within 20 minutes but may persist for several hours. In animal studies, hypotension and bradycardia occurred in animals given large doses of vancomycin at high concentrations and rates. Such events are infrequent if Vancocin HCl is given by a slow infusion over 60 minutes. In studies of normal volunteers, infusion-related events did not occur when Vancocin HCl was administered at a rate of 10 mg/min or less.

Nephrotoxicity—Rarely, renal failure, principally manifested by increased serum creatinine or BUN concentrations, especially in patients given large doses of Vancocin HCl, has been reported. Rare cases of interstitial nephritis have been reported. Most of these have occurred in patients who were given aminoglycosides concomitantly or who had preexisting kidney dysfunction. When Vancocin HCl was discontinued, azotemia resolved in most patients.

Ototoxicity—A few dozen cases of hearing loss associated with Vancocin HCl have been reported. Most of these patients had kidney dysfunction or a preexisting hearing loss or were receiving concomitant treatment with an ototoxic drug. Vertigo, dizziness, and tinnitus have been reported rarely.

Hematopoietic—Reversible neutropenia, usually starting 1 week or more after onset of therapy with Vancocin HCl or after a total dosage of more than 25 g, has been reported for several dozen patients. Neutropenia appears to be promptly reversible when Vancocin HCl is discontinued. Thrombocytopenia has rarely been reported.

Although a causal relationship has not been established, reversible agranulocytosis (granulocyte count less than 500/mm³) has been reported rarely.

Phlebitis—Inflammation at the injection site has been reported.

Miscellaneous—Infrequently, patients have been reported to have had anaphylaxis, drug fever, nausea, chills, eosinophilia, rashes (including exfoliative dermatitis), Stevens-Johnson syndrome, and rare cases of vasculitis in association with administration of Vancocin HCl.

OVERDOSAGE

Supportive care is advised, with maintenance of glomerular filtration. Vancomycin is poorly removed by dialysis. Hemofiltration and hemoperfusion with polysulfone resin have been reported to result in increased vancomycin clearance. The median lethal intravenous dose is 319 mg/kg in rats and 400 mg/kg in mice.

To obtain up-to-date information about the treatment of overdose, a good resource is your certified Regional Poison Control Center. Telephone numbers of certified poison control centers are listed in the *Physicians' Desk Reference (PDR)*. In managing overdosage, consider the possibility of multiple drug overdoses, interaction among drugs, and unusual drug kinetics in your patient.

DOSAGE AND ADMINISTRATION

Infusion-related events are related to both concentration and rate of administration of vancomycin. Concentrations of no more than 5 mg/mL and rates of no more than 10 mg/min are recommended in adults (see also age-specific recommendations). In selected patients in need of fluid restriction, a concentration up to 10 mg/mL may be used; use of such higher concentrations may increase the risk of infusion-related events. Infusion-related events may occur, however, at any rate or concentration.

Patients With Normal Renal Function

Adults—The usual daily intravenous dose is 2 g divided either as 500 mg every 6 hours or 1 g every 12 hours. Each dose should be administered at no more than 10 mg/min or over a period of at least 60 minutes, whichever is longer. Other patient factors, such as age or obesity, may call for modification of the usual intravenous daily dose.

Children—The usual intravenous dosage of Vancocin HCl is 10 mg/kg per dose given every 6 hours. Each dose should be administered over a period of at least 60 minutes.

Infants and Neonates—In neonates and young infants, the total daily intravenous dosage may be lower. In both neonates and infants, an initial dose of 15 mg/kg is suggested,

followed by 10 mg/kg every 12 hours for neonates in the 1st week of life and every 8 hours thereafter up to the age of 1 month. Each dose should be administered over 60 minutes. Close monitoring of serum concentrations of vancomycin may be warranted in these patients.

Patients With Impaired Renal Function and Elderly Patients
Dosage adjustment must be made in patients with impaired renal function. In premature infants and the elderly, greater dosage reductions than expected may be necessary because of decreased renal function. Measurement of vancomycin serum concentrations can be helpful in optimizing therapy, especially in seriously ill patients with changing renal function. Vancomycin serum concentrations can be determined by use of microbiologic assay, radioimmunoassay, fluorescence polarization immunoassay, fluorescence immunoassay, or high-pressure liquid chromatography.

If creatinine clearance can be measured or estimated accurately, the dosage for most patients with renal impairment can be calculated using the following table. The dosage of Vancocin HCl per day in mg is about 15 times the glomerular filtration rate in mL/min:

DOSAGE TABLE FOR VANCOMYCIN
IN PATIENTS WITH IMPAIRED RENAL FUNCTION
(Adapted from Moellering et al[5])

Creatinine Clearance mL/min	Vancomycin Dose mg/24 h
100	1,545
90	1,390
80	1,235
70	1,080
60	925
50	770
40	620
30	465
20	310
10	155

The initial dose should be no less than 15 mg/kg, even in patients with mild to moderate renal insufficiency.

The table is not valid for functionally anephric patients. For such patients, an initial dose of 15 mg/kg of body weight should be given to achieve prompt therapeutic serum concentrations. The dose required to maintain stable concentrations is 1.9 mg/kg/24 h. In patients with marked renal inpairment, it may be more convenient to give maintenance doses of 250 to 1,000 mg once every several days rather than administering the drug on a daily basis. In anuria, a dose of 1,000 mg every 7 to 10 days has been recommended.
When only the serum creatinine concentration is known, the following formula (based on sex, weight, and age of the patient) may be used to calculate creatinine clearance. Calculated creatinine clearances (mL/min) are only estimates. The creatinine clearance should be measured promptly.

Men: $\dfrac{\text{Weight (kg)} \times (140 - \text{age in years})}{72 \times \text{serum creatinine concentration (mg/dL)}}$

Women: $0.85 \times$ above value

The serum creatinine must represent a steady state of renal function. Otherwise, the estimated value for creatinine clearance is not valid. Such a calculated clearance is an overestimate of actual clearance in patients with conditions: (1) characterized by decreasing renal function, such as shock, severe heart failure, or oliguria; (2) in which a normal relationship between muscle mass and total body weight is not present, such as obese patients or those with liver disease, edema, or ascites; and (3) accompanied by debilitation, malnutrition, or inactivity.

The safety and efficacy of vancomycin administration by the intrathecal (intralumbar or intraventricular) routes have not been assessed.

Intermittent infusion is the recommended method of administration.

PREPARATION AND STABILITY

At the time of use, reconstitute by adding either 10 mL of Sterile Water for Injection to the 500-mg vial or 20 mL of Sterile Water for Injection to the 1-g vial of dry, sterile vancomycin powder. Vials reconstituted in this manner will give a solution of 50 mg/mL. FURTHER DILUTION IS REQUIRED.
After reconstitution, the vials may be stored in a refrigerator for 14 days without significant loss of potency. Reconstituted solutions containing 500 mg of vancomycin must be diluted with at least 100 mL of diluent. Reconstituted solutions containing 1 g of vancomycin must be diluted with at least 200 mL of diluent. The desired dose, diluted in this manner, should be administered by intermittent intravenous infusion over a period of at least 60 minutes.

Compatibility With Intravenous Fluids—Solutions that are diluted with 5% Dextrose Injection or 0.9% Sodium Chloride Injection may be stored in a refrigerator for 14 days without significant loss of potency. Solutions that are diluted with the following infusion fluids may be stored in a refrigerator for 96 hours:

5% Dextrose Injection and 0.9% Sodium Chloride Injection, USP
Lactated Ringer's Injection, USP
Lactated Ringer's and 5% Dextrose Injection
Normosol®-M and 5% Dextrose
Isolyte® E
Acetated Ringer's Injection

Vancomycin solution has a low pH and may cause chemical or physical instability when it is mixed with other compounds.
Prior to administration, parenteral drug products should be inspected visually for particulate matter and discoloration whenever solution or container permits.

For Oral Administration—Oral Vancocin HCl is used in treating antibiotic-associated pseudomembranous colitis caused by *C. difficile* and for staphylococcal enterocolitis. Vancocin HCl is not effective by the oral route for other types of infections. The usual adult total daily dosage is 500 mg to 2 g given in 3 or 4 divided doses for 7 to 10 days. The total daily dosage in children is 40 mg/kg of body weight in 3 or 4 divided doses for 7 to 10 days. The total daily dosage should not exceed 2 g. The appropriate dose may be diluted in 1 oz of water and given to the patient to drink. Common flavoring syrups may be added to the solution to improve the taste for oral administration. The diluted solution may be administered via a nasogastric tube.

HOW SUPPLIED

(℞) Vials:
500 mg,* 10-mL size (No. 657)—(1s) NDC 0002-1444-01; (Traypak† of 10) NDC 0002-1444-10
1 g,* 20-mL size (No. 7321)—(Traypak of 10) NDC 0002-7321-10

Also available:
(℞) ADD-Vantage‡ Vials:
500 mg,* 15-mL size (No. 7297)—(Traypak of 10) NDC 0002-7297-10
1 g,* 15-mL size (No. 7298)—(Traypak of 10) NDC 0002-7298-10

(℞) Pharmacy Bulk Package:
10 g,* 100-mL size (No. 7355)—(1s) NDC 0002-7355-01
Prior to reconstitution, the vials may be stored at room temperature, 59° to 86°F (15° to 30°C).

REFERENCES

1. National Committee for Clinical Laboratory Standards, 1984. Performance standards for antimicrobial disk susceptibility tests, MZ-A3, NCCLS, Villanova, PA 19805.
2. National Committee for Clinical Laboratory Standards, 1983. Methods for dilution antimicrobial susceptibility tests for bacteria that grow aerobically, M7-T, NCCLS, Villanova, PA 19805.
3. National Committee for Clinical Laboratory Standards, 1984. Reference agar dilution procedure for antimicrobial susceptibility testing of anaerobic bacteria, M11-A, NCCLS, Villanova, PA 19805.
4. Shulman ST, Amren DP, Bisno AL, et al: Prevention of bacterial endocarditis. *Circulation* 1984; 70:1123A.
5. Moellering RC, Krogstad DJ, Greenblatt DJ: Vancomycin therapy in patients with impaired renal function: A nomogram for dosage. *Ann Intern Med* 1981; 94:343.

*Equivalent to vancomycin.
†Traypak™ (multivial carton, Lilly).
‡ADD-Vantage® (vials and diluent containers, Abbott).

[052191]

VANCOCIN® HCl ℞
[văn΄kō-sĭn āch΄sē-ĕl]
(vancomycin hydrochloride)
For Oral Solution, USP

Pulvules®
Capsules, USP

This preparation for the treatment of colitis is for oral use only and is not systemically absorbed. Vancocin HCl must be given orally for treatment of staphylococcal enterocolitis and antibiotic-associated pseudomembranous colitis caused by *Clostridium difficile*. Orally administered Vancocin HCl is *not* effective for other types of infection.
Parenteral administration of Vancocin HCl is not effective for treatment of staphylococcal enterocolitis and antibiotic-associated pseudomembranous colitis caused by *C. difficile*. If parenteral vancomycin therapy is desired, use Vancocin® HCl (Sterile Vancomycin Hydrochloride, USP, Lilly), IntraVenous, and consult package insert accompanying that preparation.

DESCRIPTION

Vancocin® HCl for Oral Solution (Vancomycin Hydrochloride for Oral Solution, USP, Lilly) and Pulvules® Vancocin® HCl (Vancomycin Hydrochloride Capsules, USP, Lilly), contain chromatographically purified vancomycin hydrochloride, a tricyclic glycopeptide antibiotic derived

from *Amycolatopsis orientalis* (formerly *Nocardia orientalis*), which has the chemical formula $C_{66}H_{75}Cl_2N_9O_{24} \cdot HCl$. The molecular weight of vancomycin hydrochloride is 1,486; 500 mg of the base is equivalent to 0.34 mmol.

Vancocin HCl for Oral Solution contains vancomycin hydrochloride equivalent to 10 g (6.7 mmol) or 1 g (0.67 mmol) vancomycin. Calcium disodium edetate, 0.022%, is added at the time of manufacture. The 10-g bottle may contain up to 40 mg of ethanol per gram of vancomycin.

The Pulvules contain vancomycin hydrochloride equivalent to 125 mg (0.08 mmol) or 250 mg (0.17 mmol) vancomycin. The Pulvules also contain FD&C Blue No. 2, gelatin, iron oxide, polyethylene glycol, titanium dioxide, and other inactive ingredients.

CLINICAL PHARMACOLOGY

Vancomycin is poorly absorbed after oral administration. During multiple dosing of 250 mg every 8 hours for 7 doses, fecal concentrations of vancomycin in volunteers exceeded 100 mg/kg in the majority of samples. No blood concentrations were detected and urinary recovery did not exceed 0.76%. In anephric patients with no inflammatory bowel disease, blood concentrations of vancomycin were barely measurable (0.66 μg/mL) in 2 of 5 subjects who received 2 g of Vancocin HCl for Oral Solution daily for 16 days. No measurable blood concentrations were attained in the other 3 patients. With doses of 2 g daily, very high concentrations of drug can be found in the feces (> 3,100 mg/kg) and very low concentrations (< 1 μg/mL) can be found in the serum of patients with normal renal function who have pseudomembranous colitis. Orally administered vancomycin does not usually enter the systemic circulation even when inflammatory lesions are present. After multiple-dose oral administration of vancomycin, measurable serum concentrations may infrequently occur in patients with active *C. difficile* -induced pseudomembranous colitis, and, in the presence of renal impairment, the possibility of accumulation exists.

Microbiology —The bactericidal action of vancomycin results primarily from inhibition of cell-wall biosynthesis. In addition, vancomycin alters bacterial-cell-membrane permeability and RNA synthesis. There is no cross-resistance between vancomycin and other antibiotics. Vancomycin is active against *C. difficile* (eg, toxigenic strains implicated in pseudomembranous enterocolitis). It is also active against staphylococci, including *Staphylococcus aureus.*

For further information, see prescribing information for Vancocin HCl, IntraVenous.

Vancomycin is not active in vitro against gram-negative bacilli, mycobacteria, or fungi.

Disk Susceptibility Tests —The standardized disk and/or dilution methods described by the National Committee for Clinical Laboratory Standards have been recommended to test susceptibility to vancomycin.

INDICATIONS AND USAGE

Vancocin® HCl for Oral Solution (vancomycin hydrochloride, Lilly) and Pulvules® Vancocin® HCl (Vancomycin Hydrochloride Capsules, Lilly) are administered orally for treatment of staphylococcal enterocolitis and antibiotic-associated pseudomembranous colitis caused by *C. difficile.* Parenteral administration of Vancocin HCl is not effective for the above indications; therefore, Vancocin HCl must be given orally for these indications. **Orally administered Vancocin HCl is not effective for other types of infection.**

CONTRAINDICATION

Vancocin® HCl (vancomycin hydrochloride, Lilly) is contraindicated in patients with known hypersensitivity to this antibiotic.

PRECAUTIONS

General —Clinically significant serum concentrations have been reported in some patients who have taken multiple oral doses of vancomycin for active *C. difficile*-induced pseudomembranous colitis.

Some patients with inflammatory disorders of the intestinal mucosa may have significant systemic absorption of vancomycin and, therefore, may be at risk for the development of adverse reactions associated with the parenteral administration of vancomycin (See package insert accompanying the intravenous preparation.) The risk is greater if renal impairment is present. It should be noted that the total systemic and renal clearances of vancomycin are reduced in the elderly.

Ototoxicity has occurred in patients receiving Vancocin® HCl (vancomycin hydrochloride, Lilly). It may be transient or permanent. It has been reported mostly in patients who have been given excessive intravenous doses, who have an underlying hearing loss, or who are receiving concomitant therapy with another ototoxic agent, such as an aminoglycoside. Serial tests of auditory function may be helpful in order to minimize the risk of ototoxicity.

When patients with underlying renal dysfunction or those receiving concomitant therapy with an aminoglycoside are being treated, serial monitoring of renal function should be performed.

Usage in Pregnancy —Pregnancy Category C —Animal reproduction studies have not been conducted with Vancocin HCl. It is not known whether Vancocin HCl can affect reproduction capacity. In a controlled clinical study, the potential ototoxic and nephrotoxic effects of Vancocin HCl on infants were evaluated when the drug was administered to pregnant women for serious staphylococcal infections complicating intravenous drug abuse. Vancocin HCl was found in cord blood. No sensorineural hearing loss or nephrotoxicity attributable to Vancocin HCl was noted. One infant whose mother received Vancocin HCl in the third trimester experienced conductive hearing loss that was not attributed to the administration of Vancocin HCl. Because the number of patients treated in this study was limited and Vancocin HCl was administered only in the second and third trimesters, it is not known whether Vancocin HCl causes fetal harm. Vancocin HCl should be given to a pregnant woman only if clearly needed.

Nursing Mothers —Vancocin HCl is excreted in human milk. Caution should be exercised when Vancocin HCl is administered to a nursing woman. Because of the potential for adverse events, a decision should be made whether to discontinue nursing or discontinue the drug, taking into account the importance of the drug to the mother.

ADVERSE REACTIONS

Nephrotoxicity —Rarely, renal failure, principally manifested by increased serum creatinine or BUN concentrations, especially in patients given large doses of intravenously administered Vancocin HCl (Vancomycin Hydrochloride, Lilly) has been reported. Rare cases of interstitial nephritis have been reported. Most of these have occurred in patients who were given aminoglycosides concomitantly or who had preexisting kidney dysfunction. When Vancocin HCl (Vancomycin Hydrochloride, Lilly) was discontinued, azotemia resolved in most patients.

Ototoxicity —A few dozen cases of hearing loss associated with intravenously administered Vancocin HCl have been reported. Most of these patients had kidney dysfunction or a preexisting hearing loss or were receiving concomitant treatment with an ototoxic drug. Vertigo, dizziness, and tinnitus have been reported rarely.

Hematopoietic —Reversible neutropenia, usually starting 1 week or more after onset of intravenous therapy with Vancocin HCl or after a total dosage of more than 25 g, has been reported for several dozen patients. Neutropenia appears to be promptly reversible when Vancocin HCl is discontinued. Thrombocytopenia has rarely been reported.

Miscellaneous —Infrequently, patients have been reported to have had anaphylaxis, drug fever, chills, nausea, eosinophilia, and rashes (including exfoliative dermatitis), Stevens-Johnson syndrome, and rare cases of vasculitis in association with the administration of Vancocin HCl.

OVERDOSAGE

Supportive care is advised, with maintenance of glomerular filtration. Vancomycin is poorly removed by dialysis. Hemofiltration and hemoperfusion with polysulfone resin have been reported to result in increased vancomycin clearance.

Treatment —To obtain up-to-date information about the treatment of overdose, a good resource is your certified Regional Poison Control Center. Telephone numbers of certified poison control centers are listed in the *Physicians' Desk Reference (PDR).* In managing overdosage, consider the possibility of multiple drug overdoses, interaction among drugs, and unusual drug kinetics in your patient.

DOSAGE AND ADMINISTRATION

Adults —Oral Vancocin HCl is used in treating antibiotic-associated pseudomembranous colitis caused by *C. difficile* and staphylococcal enterocolitis. Vancocin HCl is not effective by the oral route for other types of infections. The usual adult total daily dosage is 500 mg to 2 g administered orally in 3 or 4 divided doses for 7 to 10 days.

Children —The usual daily dosage is 40 mg/kg in 3 or 4 divided doses for 7 to 10 days. The total daily dosage should not exceed 2 g.

PREPARATION AND STABILITY

Vancocin® HCl (vancomycin hydrochloride, Lilly) for Oral Solution

The contents of the 10-g bottle may be mixed with distilled or deionized water (115 mL) for oral administration. When mixed with 115 mL of water, each 6 mL provides approximately 500 mg of vancomycin. The contents of the 1-g bottle may be mixed with distilled or deionized water (20 mL). When reconstituted with 20 mL, each 5 mL contains approximately 250 mg of vancomycin. Mix thoroughly to dissolve. These mixtures may be kept for 2 weeks in a refrigerator without significant loss of potency.

The appropriate oral solution dose may be diluted in 1 oz of water and given to the patient to drink. Common flavoring syrups may be added to the solution to improve the taste for oral administration. The diluted material may be administered via nasogastric tube.

HOW SUPPLIED

℞ For Oral Solution:

10 g* (screw-cap bottle) (No. M-206)—(1s) NDC 0002-2372-37

1 g* (screw-cap bottle) (No. M-5105)—(Traypak† of 6) NDC 0002-5105-16

Prior to reconstitution, store at controlled room temperature, 59° to 86°F (15° to 30°C).

℞ Pulvules.®

125 mg,* blue and brown (No. 3125)—(ID‡20) NDC 0002-3125-42

250 mg,* blue and lavender (No. 3126)—(ID20) NDC 0002-3126-42

Store at controlled room temperature, 59° to 86°F (15° to 30°C).

*Equivalent to vancomycin.
†Traypak™ (multivial carton, Lilly).
‡Identi-Dose® (unit dose medication, Lilly).

[041091]
[040991]

VANCOMYCIN HYDROCHLORIDE ℞

See Vancocin® HCl (Vancomycin Hydrochloride, USP, Lilly).

VELBAN® ℞

[*vĕl 'băn*]
(vinblastine sulfate)
Sterile, USP

WARNINGS

Caution—This preparation should be administered by individuals experienced in the administration of Velban. It is extremely important that the needle be properly positioned in the vein before this product is injected. If leakage into surrounding tissue should occur during intravenous administration of Velban, it may cause considerable irritation. The injection should be discontinued immediately, and any remaining portion of the dose should then be introduced into another vein. Local injection of hyaluronidase and the application of moderate heat to the area of leakage help disperse the drug and are thought to minimize discomfort and the possibility of cellulitis.

FATAL IF GIVEN INTRATHECALLY. FOR INTRAVENOUS USE ONLY. *See Warnings section for the treatment of patients given intrathecal Velban.*

DESCRIPTION

Velban® (Vinblastine Sulfate, USP, Lilly) is the salt of an alkaloid extracted from *Vinca rosea* Linn, a common flowering herb known as the periwinkle (more properly known as *Catharanthus roseus* G. Don). Previously, the generic name was vincaleukoblastine, abbreviated VLB. It is a stathmokinetic oncolytic agent. When treated in vitro with this preparation, growing cells are arrested in metaphase.

Chemical and physical evidence indicate that Velban has the empirical formula $C_{46}H_{58}N_4O_9 \cdot H_2SO_4$ and that it is a dimeric alkaloid containing both indole and dihydroindole moieties.

Vials of Velban contain 10 mg (0.011 mmol) of vinblastine sulfate, in the form of a lyophilized plug, without excipients. When sodium chloride solution is added prior to injection, the pH of the resulting solution lies in the range of 3.5 to 5.

CLINICAL PHARMACOLOGY

Experimental data indicate that the action of Velban® (Vinblastine Sulfate, USP, Lilly) is different from that of other recognized antineoplastic agents. Tissue-culture studies suggest an interference with metabolic pathways of amino acids leading from glutamic acid to the citric acid cycle and to urea. In vivo experiments tend to confirm the in vitro results. A number of studies in vitro and in vivo have demonstrated that Velban produces a stathmokinetic effect and various atypical mitotic figures. The therapeutic responses, however, are not fully explained by the cytologic changes, since these changes are sometimes observed clinically and experimentally in the absence of any oncolytic effects.

Reversal of the antitumor effect of Velban by glutamic acid or tryptophan has been observed. In addition, glutamic acid and aspartic acid have protected mice from lethal doses of Velban. Aspartic acid was relatively ineffective in reversing the antitumor effect.

Continued on next page

*** Identi-Code® symbol. This product information was prepared in June 1992. Current information on these and other products of Eli Lilly and Company may be obtained by direct inquiry to Lilly Research Laboratories, Lilly Corporate Center, Indianapolis, Indiana 46285, (317) 276-3714.**

Lilly—Cont.

Other studies indicate that Velban has an effect on cell-energy production required for mitosis and interferes with nucleic acid synthesis. The mechanism of action of Velban has been related to the inhibition of microtubule formation in the mitotic spindle, resulting in an arrest of dividing cells at the metaphase stage.

Pharmacokinetic studies in patients with cancer have shown a triphasic serum decay pattern following rapid intravenous injection. The initial, middle, and terminal half-lives are 3.7 minutes, 1.6 hours, and 24.8 hours respectively. The volume of the central compartments is 70% of body weight, probably reflecting very rapid tissue binding to formed elements of the blood. Extensive reversible tissue binding occurs. Low body stores are present at 48 and 72 hours after injection. Since the major route of excretion may be through the biliary system, toxicity from this drug may be increased when there is hepatic excretory insufficiency. Following injection of tritiated vinblastine in the human cancer patient, 10% of the radioactivity was found in the feces and 14% in the urine; the remaining activity was not accounted for. Similar studies in dogs demonstrated that, over 9 days, 30% to 36% of radioactivity was found in the bile and 12% to 17% in the urine. A similar study in the rat demonstrated that the highest concentrations of radioactivity were found in the lung, liver, spleen, and kidney 2 hours after injection.

Hematologic Effects—Clinically, leukopenia is an expected effect of Velban® (Vinblastine Sulfate, USP, Lilly), and the level of the leukocyte count is an important guide to therapy with this drug. In general, the larger the dose employed, the more profound and longer lasting the leukopenia will be. The fact that the white-blood-cell count returns to normal levels after drug-induced leukopenia is an indication that the white-cell-producing mechanism is not permanently depressed. Usually, the white count has completely returned to normal after the virtual disappearance of white cells from the peripheral blood.

Following therapy with Velban, the nadir in white-blood-cell count may be expected to occur 5 to 10 days after the last day of drug administration. Recovery of the white blood count is fairly rapid thereafter and is usually complete within another 7 to 14 days. With the smaller doses employed for maintenance therapy, leukopenia may not be a problem.

Although the thrombocyte count ordinarily is not significantly lowered by therapy with Velban, patients whose bone marrow has been recently impaired by prior therapy with radiation or with other oncolytic drugs may show thrombocytopenia (less than 200,000 platelets/mm³). When other chemotherapy or radiation has not been employed previously, thrombocyte reduction below the level of 200,000/mm³ is rarely encountered, even when Velban may be causing significant leukopenia. Rapid recovery from thrombocytopenia within a few days is the rule.

The effect of Velban upon the red-cell count and hemoglobin is usually insignificant when other therapy does not complicate the picture. It should be remembered, however, that patients with malignant disease may exhibit anemia even in the absence of any therapy.

INDICATIONS AND USAGE

Vinblastine sulfate is indicated in the palliative treatment of the following:

I. *Frequently Responsive Malignancies—*
   Generalized Hodgkin's disease (Stages III and IV, Ann Arbor modification of Rye staging system)
   Lymphocytic lymphoma (nodular and diffuse, poorly and well differentiated)
   Histiocytic lymphoma
   Mycosis fungoides (advanced stages)
   Advanced carcinoma of the testis
   Kaposi's sarcoma
   Letterer-Siwe disease (histiocytosis X)

II. *Less Frequently Responsive Malignancies—*
   Choriocarcinoma resistant to other chemotherapeutic agents
   Carcinoma of the breast, unresponsive to appropriate endocrine surgery and hormonal therapy

Current principles of chemotherapy for many types of cancer include the concurrent administration of several antineoplastic agents. For enhanced therapeutic effect without additive toxicity, agents with different dose-limiting clinical toxicities and different mechanisms of action are generally selected. Therefore, although Velban® (Vinblastine Sulfate, USP, Lilly) is effective as a single agent in the aforementioned indications, it is usually administered in combination with other antineoplastic drugs. Such combination therapy produces a greater percentage of response than does a single-agent regimen. These principles have been applied, for example, in the chemotherapy of Hodgkin's disease.

Hodgkin's Disease—Velban has been shown to be one of the most effective single agents for the treatment of Hodgkin's disease. Advanced Hodgkin's disease has also been successfully treated with several multiple-drug regimens that included Velban. Patients who had relapses after treatment with the MOPP program—mechlorethamine hydrochloride (nitrogen mustard), vincristine sulfate (Oncovin® [Vincristine Sulfate Injection, USP, Lilly]), prednisone, and procarbazine—have likewise responded to combination-drug therapy that included Velban. A protocol using cyclophosphamide in place of nitrogen mustard and Velban instead of Oncovin is an alternative therapy for previously untreated patients with advanced Hodgkin's disease.

Advanced testicular germinal-cell cancers (embryonal carcinoma, teratocarcinoma, and choriocarcinoma) are sensitive to Velban alone, but better clinical results are achieved when Velban is administered concomitantly with other antineoplastic agents. The effect of bleomycin is significantly enhanced if Velban is administered 6 to 8 hours prior to the administration of bleomycin; this schedule permits more cells to be arrested during metaphase, the stage of the cell cycle in which bleomycin is active.

CONTRAINDICATIONS

Velban® (Vinblastine Sulfate, USP, Lilly) is contraindicated in patients who have significant granulocytopenia unless this is a result of the disease being treated. It should not be used in the presence of bacterial infections. Such infections must be brought under control prior to the initiation of therapy with Velban.

WARNINGS

This product is for intravenous use only. It should be administered by individuals experienced in the administration of Velban. The intrathecal administration of Velban has resulted in death. Syringes containing this product should be labeled "WARNING—FOR IV USE ONLY." Extemporaneously prepared syringes containing this product must be packaged in an overwrap that is labeled "DO NOT REMOVE COVERING UNTIL MOMENT OF INJECTION. FATAL IF GIVEN INTRATHECALLY. FOR INTRAVENOUS USE ONLY." The following treatment successfully arrested progressive paralysis in a single patient mistakenly given the related vinca alkaloid, vincristine sulfate, intrathecally. If Velban is mistakenly administered intrathecally, this treatment is recommended and should be initiated immediately after the intrathecal injection.

1. Remove as much spinal fluid as can be safely done through the lumbar access.
2. Insert a catheter in a lateral cerebral ventricle for the purpose of flushing the subarachnoid space from above with removal through a lumbar access.
3. Initiate flushing through the cerebral catheter with Lactated Ringer's solution infused at the rate of 150 mL/h.
4. As soon as fresh frozen plasma becomes available, infuse fresh frozen plasma, 25 mL, diluted in 1 L of Lactated Ringer's solution through the cerebral ventricular catheter at the rate of 75 mL/h with removal through the lumbar access. The rate of infusion should be adjusted to maintain a protein level in the spinal fluid of 150 mg/dL.
5. Administer 10 g of glutamic acid intravenously over 24 hours followed by 500 mg 3 times daily by mouth for 1 month or until neurological dysfunction stabilizes. The role of glutamic acid in this treatment is not certain and may not be essential.

The use of this treatment has not been reported following intrathecal vinblastine sulfate.

Usage in Pregnancy—Caution is necessary with the administration of all oncolytic drugs during pregnancy. Information on the use of Velban during human pregnancy is very limited. Animal studies with Velban suggest that teratogenic effects may occur. Vinblastine sulfate can cause fetal harm when administered to a pregnant woman. Laboratory animals given this drug early in pregnancy suffer resorption of the conceptus: surviving fetuses demonstrate gross deformities. There are no adequate and well-controlled studies in pregnant women. If this drug is used during pregnancy, or if the patient becomes pregnant while receiving this drug, she should be apprised of the potential hazard to the fetus. Women of childbearing potential should be advised to avoid becoming pregnant.

Aspermia has been reported in man. Animal studies show metaphase arrest and degenerative changes in germ cells. Leukopenia (granulocytopenia) may reach dangerously low levels following administration of the higher recommended doses. It is therefore important to follow the dosage technique recommended under the Dosage and Administration section. Stomatitis and neurologic toxicity, although not common or permanent, can be disabling.

PRECAUTIONS

General—Toxicity may be enhanced in the presence of hepatic insufficiency.

If leukopenia with less than 2,000 white blood cells/mm³ occurs following a dose of Velban® (Vinblastine Sulfate, USP, Lilly), the patient should be watched carefully for evidence of infection until the white-blood-cell count has returned to a safe level.

When cachexia or ulcerated areas of the skin surface are present, there may be a more profound leukopenic response to the drug; therefore, its use should be avoided in older persons suffering from either of these conditions.

In patients with malignant-cell infiltration of the bone marrow, the leukocyte and platelet counts have sometimes fallen precipitously after moderate doses of Velban. Further use of the drug in such patients is inadvisable.

Acute shortness of breath and severe bronchospasm have been reported following the administration of vinca alkaloids. These reactions have been encountered most frequently when the vinca alkaloid was used in combination with mitomycin-C and may require aggressive treatment, particularly when there is preexisting pulmonary dysfunction. The onset may be within minutes or several hours after the vinca is injected and may occur up to 2 weeks following a dose of mitomycin. Progressive dyspnea requiring chronic therapy may occur. Velban should not be readministered. *The use of small amounts of Velban daily for long periods is not advised,* even though the resulting total weekly dosage may be similar to that recommended. Little or no added therapeutic effect has been demonstrated when such regimens have been used. *Strict adherence to the recommended dosage schedule is very important.* When amounts equal to several times the recommended weekly dosage were given in 7 daily installments for long periods, convulsions, severe and permanent central-nervous-system damage, and even death occurred.

Care must be taken to avoid contamination of the eye with concentrations of Velban used clinically. If accidental contamination occurs, severe irritation (or, if the drug was delivered under pressure, even corneal ulceration) may result. The eye should be washed with water immediately and thoroughly.

It is not necessary to use preservative-containing solvents if unused portions of the remaining solutions are discarded immediately. Unused preservative-containing solutions should be refrigerated for future use.

Information for Patients—The patient should be warned to report immediately the appearance of sore throat, fever, chills, or sore mouth. Advice should be given to avoid constipation, and the patient should be made aware that alopecia may occur and that jaw pain and pain in the organs containing tumor tissue may occur. The latter is thought possibly to result from swelling of tumor tissue during its response to treatment. Scalp hair will regrow to its pretreatment extent even with continued treatment with Velban® (Vinblastine Sulfate, USP, Lilly). Nausea and vomiting, although not common, may occur. Any other serious medical event should be reported to the physician.

Laboratory Tests—Since dose-limiting clinical toxicity is the result of depression of the white-blood-cell count, it is imperative that this count be obtained just before the planned dose of Velban. Following administration of Velban, a fall in the white-blood-cell count may occur. The nadir of this fall is observed from 5 to 10 days following a dose. Recovery to pretreatment levels is usually observed from 7 to 14 days after treatment. These effects will be exaggerated when preexisting bone marrow damage is present and also with the higher recommended doses (*see* Dosage and Administration). The presence of this drug or its metabolites in blood or body tissues is not known to interfere with clinical laboratory tests.

Drug Interactions—Velban should not be diluted with solvents that raise or lower the pH of the resulting solution from between 3.5 and 5. Solutions should be made with normal saline (with or without preservative) and should not be combined in the same container with any other chemical. Unused portions of the remaining solutions that do not contain preservatives should be discarded immediately.

The simultaneous oral or intravenous administration of phenytoin and antineoplastic chemotherapy combinations that included vinblastine sulfate has been reported to have reduced blood levels of the anticonvulsant and to have increased seizure activity. Dosage adjustment should be based on serial blood level monitoring. The contribution of vinblastine sulfate to this interaction is not certain. The interaction may result from either reduced absorption of phenytoin or an increase in the rate of its metabolism and elimination.

Carcinogenesis, Mutagenesis, Impairment of Fertility— Aspermia has been reported in man. Animal studies suggest that teratogenic effects may occur. *See* Warnings regarding impaired fertility. Animal studies have shown metaphase arrest and degenerative changes in germ cells. Amenorrhea has occurred in some patients treated with the combination consisting of an alkylating agent, procarbazine, prednisone, and Velban. Its occurrence was related to the total dose of these 4 agents used. Recovery of menses was frequent. The same combination of drugs given to male patients produced azoospermia; if spermatogenesis did return, it was not likely to do so with less than 2 years of unmaintained remission. *Mutagenicity*—Tests in *Salmonella typhimurium* and with the dominant lethal assay in mice failed to demonstrate mutagenicity. Sperm abnormalities have been noted in mice. Velban has produced an increase in micronuclei formation

in bone marrow cells of mice; however, since Velban inhibits mitotic spindle formation, it cannot be concluded that this is evidence of mutagenicity. Additional studies in mice demonstrated no reduction in fertility of males. Chromosomal translocations did occur in male mice. First-generation male offspring of these mice were not heterozygous translocation carriers.

In vitro tests using hamster lung cells in culture have produced chromosomal changes, including chromatid breaks and exchanges, whereas tests using another type of hamster cell failed to demonstrate mutation. Breaks and aberrations were not observed on chromosome analysis of marrow cells from patients being treated with this drug.

It is not clear from the literature how this drug affects synthesis of DNA and RNA. Some believe that there is no interference. Others believe that vinblastine interferes with nucleic acid metabolism but may not do so by direct effect but possibly as the result of biochemical disturbance in some other part of the molecular organization of the cell. No inhibition of RNA synthesis occurred in rat hepatoma cells exposed in culture to noncytotoxic levels of vinblastine. Conflicting results have been noted by others regarding interference with DNA synthesis.

Carcinogenesis—There is no currently available evidence to indicate that Velban itself has been carcinogenic in humans since the inception of its clinical use in the late 1950s. Patients treated for Hodgkin's disease have developed leukemia following radiation therapy and administration of Velban in combination with other chemotherapy, including agents known to intercalate with DNA. It is not known to what extent Velban may have contributed to the appearance of leukemia. Available data in rats and mice have failed to demonstrate clearly evidence of carcinogenesis when the animals were treated with the maximum tolerated dose and with one half that dose for 6 months. This testing system demonstrated that other agents were clearly carcinogenic, whereas Velban was in the group of drugs causing slightly increased or the same tumor incidence as controls in one study and 1.5 to twofold increase in tumor incidence over controls in another study.

Usage in Pregnancy—Pregnancy Category D (*See* Warnings). Velban should be given to a pregnant woman only if clearly needed. Animal studies suggest that teratogenic effects may occur.

Pediatric Usage—The dosage schedule for children is indicated under Dosage and Administration.

Nursing Mothers—It is not known whether this drug is excreted in human milk. Because many drugs are excreted in human milk and because of the potential for serious adverse reactions from Velban in nursing infants, a decision should be made whether to discontinue nursing or the drug, taking into account the importance of the drug to the mother.

ADVERSE REACTIONS

Prior to the use of the drug, patients should be advised of the possibility of untoward symptoms.

In general, the incidence of adverse reactions attending the use of Velban® (Vinblastine Sulfate, USP, Lilly) appears to be related to the size of the dose employed. With the exception of epilation, leukopenia, and neurologic side effects, adverse reactions generally have not persisted for longer than 24 hours. Neurologic side effects are not common; but when they do occur, they often last for more than 24 hours. Leukopenia, the most common adverse reaction, is usually the dose-limiting factor.

The following are manifestations that have been reported as adverse reactions, in decreasing order of frequency. The most common adverse reactions are underlined:

Hematologic—Leukopenia (granulocytopenia), anemia, thrombocytopenia (myelosuppression).

Dermatologic—Alopecia is common. A single case of light sensitivity associated with this product has been reported.

Gastrointestinal—Constipation, anorexia, nausea, vomiting, abdominal pain, ileus, vesiculation of the mouth, pharyngitis, diarrhea, hemorrhagic enterocolitis, bleeding from an old peptic ulcer, rectal bleeding.

Neurologic—Numbness of digits (paresthesias), loss of deep tendon reflexes, peripheral neuritis, mental depression, headache, convulsions.

Cardiovascular—Hypertension. Cases of unexpected myocardial infarction and cerebrovascular accidents have occurred in patients undergoing combination chemotherapy with vinblastine, bleomycin, and cisplatin. Raynaud's phenomenon has also been reported with this combination.

Pulmonary—*See* Precautions.

Miscellaneous—Malaise, bone pain, weakness, pain in tumor-containing tissue, dizziness, jaw pain, skin vesiculation, hypertension, Raynaud's phenomenon when patients are being treated with Velban in combination with bleomycin and cis-platinum for testicular cancer. The syndrome of inappropriate secretion of antidiuretic hormone has occurred with higher-than-recommended doses.

Nausea and vomiting usually may be controlled with ease by antiemetic agents. When epilation develops, it frequently is not total; and, in some cases, hair regrows while maintenance therapy continues.

Extravasation during intravenous injection may lead to cellulitis and phlebitis. If the amount of extravasation is great, sloughing may occur.

OVERDOSAGE

Signs and Symptoms—Side effects following the use of Velban® (Vinblastine Sulfate, USP, Lilly) are dose related. Therefore, following administration of more than the recommended dose, patients can be expected to experience these effects in an exaggerated fashion. (*See* Clinical Pharmacology, Contraindications, Warnings, Precautions, *and* Adverse Reactions.) There is no specific antidote. In addition, neurotoxicity similar to that with Oncovin may be observed. Since the major route of excretion may be through the biliary system, toxicity from this drug may be increased when there is hepatic insufficiency.

Treatment—To obtain up-to-date information about the treatment of overdose, a good resource is your certified Regional Poison Control Center. Telephone numbers of certified poison control centers are listed in the *Physicians' Desk Reference (PDR)*. In managing overdosage, consider the possibility of multiple drug overdoses, interaction among drugs, and unusual drug kinetics in your patient. Overdoses of Velban have been reported rarely. The following is provided to serve as a guide should such an overdose be encountered.

Supportive care should include the following: (1) prevention of side effects that result from the syndrome of inappropriate secretion of antidiuretic hormone (this would include restriction of the volume of daily fluid intake to that of the urine output plus insensible loss and perhaps the administration of a diuretic affecting the function of the loop of Henle and the distal tubule); (2) administration of an anticonvulsant; (3) prevention of ileus; (4) monitoring the cardiovascular system; and (5) determining daily blood counts for guidance in transfusion requirements and assessing the risk of infection. The major effect of excessive doses of Velban will be myelosuppression, which may be life threatening. There is no information regarding the effectiveness of dialysis nor of cholestyramine for the treatment of overdosage.

Velban in the dry state is irregularly and unpredictably absorbed from the gastrointestinal tract following oral administration. Absorption of the solution has not been studied. If vinblastine is swallowed, activated charcoal in a water slurry may be given by mouth along with a cathartic. The use of cholestyramine in this situation has not been reported.

Symptoms of overdose will appear when greater-than-recommended doses are given. Any dose of Velban that results in elimination of platelets and neutrophils from blood and marrow and their precursors from marrow should be considered life threatening. The exact dose that will do this in all patients is unknown. Overdoses occurring during prolonged, consecutive-day infusions may be more toxic than the same total dose given by rapid intravenous injection. The intravenous median lethal dose in mice is 10 mg/kg body weight; in rats, it is 2.9 mg/kg. The oral median lethal dose in rats is 7 mg/kg.

Protect the patient's airway and support ventilation and perfusion. Meticulously monitor and maintain, within acceptable limits, the patient's vital signs, blood gases, serum electrolytes, etc. Absorption of drugs from the gastrointestinal tract may be decreased by giving activated charcoal, which, in many cases, is more effective than emesis or lavage; consider charcoal instead of or in addition to gastric emptying if the drug has been swallowed. Repeated doses of charcoal over time may hasten elimination of some drugs that have been absorbed. Safeguard the patient's airway when employing gastric emptying or charcoal.

DOSAGE AND ADMINISTRATION

Caution—**It is extremely important that the needle be properly positioned in the vein before this product is injected. If leakage into surrounding tissue should occur during intravenous administration of Velban® (Vinblastine Sulfate, USP, Lilly), it may cause considerable irritation. The injection should be discontinued immediately, and any remaining portion of the dose should then be introduced into another vein. Local injection of hyaluronidase and the application of moderate heat to the area of leakage help disperse the drug and are thought to minimize discomfort and the possibility of cellulitis.**

There are variations in the depth of the leukopenic response that follows therapy with Velban. For this reason, it is recommended that the drug be given no more frequently than *once every 7 days*. It is wise to initiate therapy for adults by administering a single intravenous dose of 3.7 mg/m^2 of body surface area (bsa); the initial dose for children should be 2.5 mg/m^2. Thereafter, white-blood-cell counts should be made to determine the patient's sensitivity to Velban. A reduction of 50% in the dose of Velban is recommended for patients having a direct serum bilirubin value above 3 mg/100 mL. Since metabolism and excretion are primarily hepatic, no modification is recommended for patients with impaired renal function.

A simplified and conservative incremental approach to dosage *at weekly intervals* may be outlined as follows:

	Adults	Children
First dose	3.7 mg/m^2 bsa	2.5 mg/m^2 bsa
Second dose	5.5 mg/m^2 bsa	3.75 mg/m^2 bsa
Third dose	7.4 mg/m^2 bsa	5.0 mg/m^2 bsa
Fourth dose	9.25 mg/m^2 bsa	6.25 mg/m^2 bsa
Fifth dose	11.1 mg/m^2 bsa	7.5 mg/m^2 bsa

The above-mentioned increases may be used until a maximum dose (not exceeding 18.5 mg/m^2 bsa for adults and 12.5 mg/m^2 bsa for children) is reached. The dose should not be increased after that dose which reduces the white-cell count to approximately 3,000 cells/mm^3. In some adults, 3.7 mg/m^2 bsa may produce this leukopenia; other adults may require more than 11.1 mg/m^2 bsa; and, very rarely, as much as 18.5 mg/m^2 bsa may be necessary. For most adult patients, however, the weekly dosage will prove to be 5.5 to 7.4 mg/m^2 bsa.

When the dose of Velban which will produce the above degree of leukopenia has been established, a dose of *1 increment smaller* than this should be administered at weekly intervals for maintenance. Thus, the patient is receiving the maximum dose that does not cause leukopenia. *It should be emphasized that, even though 7 days have elapsed, the next dose of Velban should not be given until the white-cell count has returned to at least 4,000/mm^3.* In some cases, oncolytic activity may be encountered before leukopenic effect. When this occurs, there is no need to increase the size of subsequent doses (*see* Precautions).

The duration of maintenance therapy varies according to the disease being treated and the combination of antineoplastic agents being used. There are differences of opinion regarding the duration of maintenance therapy with the same protocol for a particular disease; for example, various durations have been used with the MOPP program in treating Hodgkin's disease. Prolonged chemotherapy for maintaining remissions involves several risks, among which are life-threatening infectious diseases, sterility, and possibly the appearance of other cancers through suppression of immune surveillance.

In some disorders, survival following complete remission may not be as prolonged as that achieved with shorter periods of maintenance therapy. On the other hand, failure to provide maintenance therapy in some patients may lead to unnecessary relapse; complete remissions in patients with testicular cancer, unless maintained for at least 2 years, often result in early relapse.

To prepare a solution containing 1 mg of Velban/mL, add 10 mL of Sodium Chloride Injection (preserved with phenol or benzyl alcohol) to the 10 mg of Velban in the sterile vial. Other solutions are not recommended. The drug dissolves instantly to give a clear solution. After a solution has been made in this way and a portion of it has been removed from a vial, the remainder of the vial's contents may be stored in a refrigerator for future use for 30 days without significant loss of potency.

The dose of Velban (calculated to provide the desired amount) may be injected either into the tubing of a running intravenous infusion or directly into a vein. The latter procedure is readily adaptable to outpatient therapy. In either case, the injection may be completed in about 1 minute. If care is taken to insure that the needle is securely within the vein and that no solution containing Velban is spilled extravascularly, cellulitis and/or phlebitis will not occur. To minimize further the possibility of extravascular spillage, it is suggested that the syringe and needle be rinsed with venous blood before withdrawal of the needle. The dose should not be diluted in large volumes of diluent (ie, 100 to 250 mL) or given intravenously for prolonged periods (ranging from 30 to 60 minutes or more), since this frequently results in irritation of the vein and increases the chance of extravasation.

Because of the enhanced possibility of thrombosis, it is considered inadvisable to inject a solution of Velban® (Vinblastine Sulfate, USP, Lilly) into an extremity in which the circulation is impaired or potentially impaired by such conditions as compressing or invading neoplasm, phlebitis, or varicosity.

Parenteral drug products should be inspected visually for particulate matter and discoloration prior to administration, whenever solution and container permit.

It is not necessary to use preservative-containing solvents if unused portions of the remaining solutions are discarded

Continued on next page

• Identi-Code® symbol. This product information was prepared in June 1992. Current information on these and other products of Eli Lilly and Company may be obtained by direct inquiry to Lilly Research Laboratories, Lilly Corporate Center, Indianapolis, Indiana 46285, (317) 276-3714.

Lilly—Cont.

immediately. Unused preservative-containing solutions should be refrigerated for future use.

Procedures for proper handling and disposal of anticancer drugs should be considered. Several guidelines on this subject have been published. There is no general agreement that all of the procedures recommended in the guidelines are necessary or appropriate.

Special Dispensing Information —When dispensing Velban in other than the original container, eg, a syringe containing a specific dose, it is imperative that it be packaged in an overwrap bearing the statement: "DO NOT REMOVE COVERING UNTIL MOMENT OF INJECTION. FATAL IF GIVEN INTRATHECALLY. FOR INTRAVENOUS USE ONLY" (*see* Warnings).

References are available in the package insert or on request.

HOW SUPPLIED

(℞) Vials, 10 mg, 10-mL size (No. 687)—(1s) NDC 0002-1452-01.

The vials should be stored in a refrigerator (2° to 8°C, or 36° to 46°F) to assure extended stability.

[032492]

ZINC-INSULIN CRYSTALS   OTC
See under Iletin® (insulin, Lilly).

EDUCATIONAL MATERIAL

Diabetes Patient Education Materials
Managing Your Diabetes Patient Education System
- Comprehensive book on self-care
- Topical brochures (eg, complications, insulin and travel)
- Video
- Self-monitoring records
- Meal plans
- Spanish and English versions

Professional Education Materials and Services
CE programs
Speaker programs
Professional slide series
Diabetes patient management software
For information on these and other educational materials, see your Lilly sales representative.

Lotus Biochemical Corporation
P.O. BOX 126
BLAND, VA 24315

ADAPIN®   ℞
[*ad'uh-pin"*]
(doxepin HCl)

DESCRIPTION

Adapin (doxepin HCl) is an isomeric mixture of 1-Propanamine, 3-dibenz [*b,e*] oxepin-11 (*6H*) ylidene-*N,N*-dimethyl-, hydrochloride.

Other ingredients in **Adapin Capsules:** gelatin, magnesium stearate, sodium lauryl sulfate, starch, titanium dioxide. Dyes: D&C Yellow No. 10, FD&C Blue No. 1, FD&C Yellow No. 6, (10,25,50,75,100mg); D&C Red No. 33, D&C Yellow No. 10, iron oxides (150mg).

ACTIONS

Adapin has a variety of pharmacological actions with its predominant action on the central nervous system. While its mechanism of action is not known, studies have demonstrated that it is neither a monoamine oxidase inhibitor nor a primary stimulant of the central nervous system.

INDICATIONS

In controlled clinical evaluations, **Adapin** has shown marked antianxiety and significant antidepressant effects. **Adapin** has been found to be well tolerated even in elderly patients. **Adapin** is indicated for the treatment of patients with:

1. Psychoneurotic anxiety and/or depressive reactions.
2. Mixed symptoms of anxiety and depression.
3. Anxiety and/or depression associated with alcoholism.
4. Anxiety associated with organic disease.
5. Psychotic depressive disorders including involutional depression and manic-depressive reactions.

Target symptoms of psychoneurosis that respond particularly well to **Adapin** include: anxiety, tension, depression, somatic symptoms and concerns, insomnia, guilt, lack of energy, fear, apprehension and worry.

Because **Adapin** provides antidepressant as well as antianxiety effects, it is of particular value in patients in whom anxiety masks depression. Patients who have not responded to other antianxiety or antidepressant drugs may benefit from **Adapin.**

CONTRAINDICATIONS

Because **Adapin** has an anticholinergic effect, it is contraindicated in patients with glaucoma or a tendency toward urinary retention.

Use of **Adapin** is contraindicated in patients who have been found hypersensitive to it.

WARNINGS

Usage in Pregnancy
Adapin has not been evaluated in pregnant patients. Therefore, it should not be used during pregnancy unless, in the judgement of the physician, it is essential to the welfare of the patient. In animal reproduction studies of **Adapin**, gross and microscopic examination of the offspring gave no evidence drug-related teratogenic effect. Following doses of up to 25mg/kg/day for 8 to 9 months, no changes were observed in the number of live births, litter size, or lactation. A decreased rate of conception was observed when male rats were given 25mg/kg/day for prolonged periods-an effect which has occurred with other psychotropic drugs and has been attributed to drug effect on the central and/or autonomic nervous systems.

Nursing Mothers
Doxepin is excreted in human milk and has been reported to cause respiratory depression in an 8-week-old breast-fed infant. Because of the potential for adverse effects, mothers who require doxepin should not nurse.

Usage in Children
The use of **Adapin** in children under 12 years of age is not recommended, because safe conditions for its use have not been established.

MAO Inhibitors
Serious side effects and even death have been reported following the concomitant use of certain drugs with MAO inhibitors. Therefore, MAO inhibitors should be discontinued with **Adapin**. The exact length of time may vary and is dependent upon the particular MAO inhibitor being used, the length of time it has been administered, and the dosage involved.

Alcohol
In patients who may use alcohol excessively, it should be borne in mind that the potentiation may increase the danger inherent in any suicide attempt or overdosage.

PRECAUTIONS

Drowsiness may occur with **Adapin**; therefore, patients should be warned of its possible occurrence and cautioned against driving a motor vehicle or operating hazardous machinery while taking the drug.

Patients should also be cautioned that the effects of alcoholic beverages may be increased.

Since suicide is an inherent risk in depressed patients and remains a risk through the initial phases of improvement, depressed patients should be closely supervised.

Although **Adapin** (doxepin HCl) has shown effective tranquilizing activity, the possibility of activating or unmasking latent psychotic symptoms should be kept in mind.

Compounds structurally related to **Adapin** can block the effects of guanethidine and similarly acting compounds. However, at the usual clinical dosages, 75mg to 150mg per day, **Adapin** has been given concomitantly with guanethidine without blocking its antihypertensive effect. But at dosages of 300mg per day or higher, **Adapin** has exerted a significant blocking effect.

When administering cimetidine concurrently with tricyclic antidepressants, close supervision and careful adjustment of dosages are required because of the possibility of producing significant increases or decreases in the plasma concentrations of the tricyclic antidepressant.

Tolazamide: A case of severe hypoglycemia has been reported in a type II diabetic patient maintained on tolazamide (1gm/day) 11 days after the addition of doxepin (75mg/day). **Adapin**, like other structurally related psychotropic drugs, potentiates norepinephrine response in animals. But this effect has not been observed with **Adapin** in humans, which is in accord with the low incidence of tachycardia reported clinically.

ADVERSE REACTIONS

Anticholinergic Effects: Dry mouth, blurred vision and constipation have been reported. These are usually mild, and often subside as therapy is continued or dosage reduced.

Central Nervous System Effects: Drowsiness has been observed. It usually occurs early in the course of therapy and tends to subside as therapy continues.

Cardiovascular Effects: Tachycardia and hypotension have been reported infrequently.

Other infrequently reported adverse effects with tricyclic antidepressants include extrapyramidal symptoms, syndrome of inappropriate ADH (anti-diuretic hormone), secretion, gastrointestinal reactions, secretory effects such as increased sweating, weakness, dizziness, fatigue, weight gain, edema, paresthesias, flushing, chills, tinnitus, photophobia, decreased libido, rash and pruritus.

Withdrawal Symptoms: Abrupt cessation of treatment after prolonged administration may produce nausea, headache and malaise. These are not indicative of addiction.

DOSAGE AND ADMINISTRATION

In most patients with mild to moderate anxiety and/or depression: A starting dose of 25 mg t.i.d. is recommended. Decrease or increase the dosage at appropriate intervals according to individual response. Usual optimum dosage is 75mg to 150mg per day. As an alternative regimen the total daily dosage, up to 150mg, may be given at bedtime without loss of effectiveness.

In some patients with mild symptomatology or emotional symptoms accompanying organic disease, dosage as low as 25mg to 50mg per day has provided effective control.

In more severe anxiety and/or depression: 50mg t.i.d. may be required to start—if necessary, gradually increase to 300mg per day. Additional effectiveness is rarely obtained by exceeding 300mg per day.

Although optimal antidepressant response may not be evident for two to three weeks, antianxiety activity is rapidly apparent.

OVERDOSAGE

Symptoms —An increase of any of the reported adverse reactions, primarily excessive sedation and anticholinergic effects such as blurred vision and dry mouth. Other effects may be: pronounced tachycardia, hypotension and extrapyramidal symptoms. *Treatment* —Essentially symptomatic; supportive therapy in the case of hypotension and excessive sedation.

HOW SUPPLIED

Capsules: Each capsule contains doxepin hydrochloride equivalent to doxepin 10mg (NDC 59417-0356-71), 25mg (NDC 59417-0357-71), 50mg (NDC 59417-0358-71), 75mg (NDC 59417-0361-71), 100mg (NDC 59417-0359-71), which are available in bottles of 100. 150mg capsules (NDC 59417-0370-65) are available in bottles of 50. Bottles of 1000 are available for 10mg (NDC 59417-0356-90), 25mg (NDC 59417-0357-90), 50mg (NDC 59417-0358-90), 75mg (NDC 59417-0361-90).

Marketed by
LOTUS BIOCHEMICAL CORPORATION
Bland, VA 24315 USA
Mfd. by Fisons Corporation
Rochester, NY 14623
Adapin is a registered trademark of Lotus Biochemical Corporation.
©1992, Lotus Biochemical Corporation
Rev. 6/92
Shown in Product Identification Section, page 416

Lunsco, Inc.
ROUTE 2, BOX 62
PULASKI, VA 24301

DYTUSS   ℞

COMPOSITION

Each 30cc represents: Diphenhydramine HCl. 80 mg., Alcohol 5%.

SUPPLIED

Pint.

FETRIN   ℞

COMPOSITION

Each sustained-release capsule contains: Ferrous Fumarate (Equivalent to 66 mg. Elemental Iron) 200 mg., Ascorbic Acid 60 mg., Cyanocobalamin 5mcg with Intrinsic Factor.

SUPPLIED

Bottles of 100.

HYCO–PAP   ⓒ ℞

COMPOSITION
Each capsule contains: Hydrocodone Bitartrate 5 mg., (Warning: May be Habit Forming), Acetaminophen 500 mg.

SUPPLIED
Bottles of 100.

PACAPS   ℞

COMPOSITION
Each capsule represents: Butalbital 50 mg., Caffeine 40 mg., Acetaminophen 325 mg.

SUPPLIED
Bottles of 100.

PROTID   ℞

COMPOSITION
Each tablet represents: Acetaminophen 500 mg., Chlorpheniramine Maleate 8 mg., Phenylephrine HCl. 40 mg.

SUPPLIED
Bottles of 100.

MDR Fitness Corp.
MEDICAL DOCTORS' RESEARCH
5207 NW 163rd STREET
MIAMI, FL 33014

MDR FITNESS TABS FOR MEN AND WOMEN   OTC

DESCRIPTION
MDR Fitness Tabs are formulated by medical doctors based on a two tablet per day system to allow improved absorption of nutrients. The A.M. and P.M. dosage allows more absorption of the water soluble vitamins (B-complex and C) which are not readily stored by the body. The AM tablet provides more micronutrients required for energy producing reactions when physical activity is greater.

INDICATIONS AND USAGE
MDR Fitness Tabs are designed for the maintenance of good health and nutrition for men and women 11 years of age or older, whenever a multi-vitamin mineral supplement is indicated to help replace nutrients missing from the diet or lost from use of oral contraceptives, cigarettes, alcohol, antacids, physical or emotional stress, exercise, illness, or recent surgery. Daily use of MDR Fitness Tabs may also play a protective role for good health by assuring adequate intake of essential nutrients. Pregnant and lactating women may need additional supplementation.
[See table above.]

DIRECTIONS
With breakfast or lunch, take one "AM" Fitness Tab. After dinner, take one "PM" Fitness Tab. Swallow Fitness Tab with a full glass of water.

PRECAUTIONS
Not recommended for persons with severe kidney disease or those undergoing renal dialysis, unless under a physician's supervision.
Note: MDR Fitness also provides a Stress Defense supplement to be taken with MDR Fitness Tabs when higher dosages are indicated.
For Products or Order Information Call 1-800-MDR-TABS

IDENTIFICATION PROBLEM?
Consult PDR's
Product Identification Section
where you'll find over 1700
products pictured actual size
and in full color.

Each Fitness Tab Contains:

	Men		Women		U.S.RDA+	
Vitamin A (Fish Oil)	5000 I.U.		5000 I.U.		5000 I.U.	
Vitamin A (Beta Carotene)	2500 I.U.		2500 I.U.		***	
Vitamin E (d-alpha tocopherol)	60 I.U.		70 I.U.		30	I.U.
Vitamin D-3 (Colecalciferol)	400 I.U.		400 I.U.		400	I.U.
Vitamin C*	300 mg.		250 mg.		60	mg.
Vitamin B-1 (Thiamine HCL)	6 mg.		6 mg.		1.5	mg.
Vitamin B-2 (Riboflavin)	6 mg.		6 mg.		1.7	mg.
Niacin (Niacinamide)	40 mg.		40 mg.		20	mg.
Vitamin B-6 (Pyridoxine HCL)	6 mg.		8 mg.		2	mg.
Folic Acid	400 mcg.		400 mcg.		400	mcg.
Vitamin B-12	6 mcg.		6 mcg.		6	mcg.
Pantothenic Acid	20 mg.		20 mg.		10	mg.
Biotin	200 mcg.		200 mcg.		300	mcg.
Calcium (Carbonate and Ascorbate)	500 mg.		545 mg.		1000	mg.
Magnesium (Oxide)	200 mg.		200 mg.		400	mg.
Iron (Fumarate)	10 mg.		18 mg.		18	mg.
Zinc (Sulfate, Gluconate, Picolinate)	20 mg.		15 mg.		15	mg.
Manganese (Gluconate)	5 mg.		5 mg.		***	
Selenium (L-Selenomethionine)	40 mcg.		40 mcg.		***	
Chromium (Picolinate)**	100 mcg.		100 mcg.		***	
Copper (Gluconate)	0.5 mg.		0.5 mg.		2	mg.
Garlic (Odorless)	100 mg.		75 mg.		***	

Free of Sugars, Starches, Dyes, Yeast, Preservatives, Soy, Wheat, Gluten and Lactose.
*Sources of Vitamin C include Buffered Calcium Ascorbate, Ascorbic Acid (water soluble), and Ascorbyl Palmitate (fat soluble).
**Chromium Picolinate is licensed under U.S. Patent 4,315,927 of the U.S. Dept. of Agriculture.
***No U.S. RDA established.
+USRDA—Percentage of United States Recommended Daily Allowance for Adults.

MGI Pharma, Inc.
SUITE 300 E, OPUS CENTER
9900 BREN ROAD EAST
MINNEAPOLIS, MN 55343-9667

DIDRONEL® I.V. INFUSION   ℞
(etidronate disodium)
DILUTE BEFORE USE

DESCRIPTION
Didronel I.V. Infusion is a clear, colorless, sterile solution of etidronate disodium, the disodium salt of (1-hydroxyethylidene) diphosphonic acid. Each 6-ml ampule contains a 5% solution of 300 mg etidronate disodium in water for injection for slow intravenous infusion.
Etidronate disodium is a white powder, highly soluble in water, with a molecular weight of 250 and the following structural formula:

$$HO-\underset{\underset{O}{\|}}{\overset{\overset{ONa}{\|}}{P}}-\underset{\underset{CH_3}{\|}}{\overset{\overset{OH}{\|}}{C}}-\underset{\underset{O}{\|}}{\overset{\overset{ONa}{\|}}{P}}-OH$$

CLINICAL PHARMACOLOGY
Didronel acts primarily on bone. Its major pharmacologic action is the reduction of normal and abnormal bone resorption. Secondarily, its reduces bone formation since formation is coupled to resorption. This reduces bone turnover, but the reduction of bone turnover, *per se*, is not the important action in the reduction of hypercalcemia.
Didronel's reduction of abnormal bone resorption is responsible for its therapeutic benefit in hypercalcemia. The antiresorptive action of Didronel has been demonstrated under a variety of conditions, although the exact mechanism(s) is not fully understood. It may be related to the drug's inhibition of hydroxyapatite crystal dissolution and/or its action on bone resorbing cells. The number of osteoclasts in active bone turnover sites is substantially reduced after Didronel therapy is administered. Didronel also can inhibit the formation and growth of hydroxyapatite crystals and their amorphous precursors at concentrations in excess of those required to inhibit crystal dissolution.
Etidronate disodium is not metabolized. A large fraction of the infused dose is excreted rapidly and unchanged in the urine. The mean residence time in the exchangeable pool is approximately 8.7 ± 1.0 hours. The mean volume of distribution at steady-state in normal humans is 1370 ± 203 ml/kg while the plasma half-life ($t\frac{1}{2}$) is 6.0 ± 0.7 hours. In these same subjects, nonrenal clearance from the exchangeable pool amounts to 30–50% of the infused dose. This nonrenal clearance is considered to be due to uptake of the drug by bone; subsequently the drug is slowly eliminated through bone turnover. The half-life of the dose on bone is in excess of 90 days.
Hyperphosphatemia, which is often observed in association with oral Didronel medication at doses of 10–20 mg/kg/day, occurs less frequently, in association with intravenous medication of patients with hypercalcemia of malignancy.

Hyperphosphatemia is apparently due to increased tubular reabsorption of phosphate by the kidney. No adverse effects have been associated with Didronel-related hyperphosphatemia and its occurrence is not a contraindication to therapy. Serum phosphate elevations usually return to normal 2–4 weeks after medication is discontinued.
The responsiveness of animal tumors susceptible to four commonly employed classes or subclasses of chemotherapeutic agents, antitumor antibiotics (doxorubicin), a classic alkylating agent (cyclophosphamide), a nitrosourea (carmustine), and a pyrimidine antagonist (5-fluorouracil), were not adversely altered by the concurrent administration of intravenous Didronel.
Hypercalcemia of Malignancy: Hypercalcemia of malignancy is usually related to increased bone resorption associated with the presence of neoplastic tissue. It occurs in 8 to 20% of patients with malignant disease. Whereas hypercalcemia is more often seen in patients with demonstrable osteolytic, osteoblastic, or mixed metastatic tumors in bone, discrete skeletal lesions cannot be demonstrated in at least 30% of patients.
Patients with certain types of neoplasms, such as carcinoma of the breast, bronchogenic carcinoma, renal cell carcinoma, cancers of the head and neck, lymphomas, and multiple myeloma, are especially prone to developing hypercalcemia. As hypercalcemia of malignancy evolves, the renal tubules develop a diminished capacity to concentrate urine. The resultant polyuria and nocturia decrease the extracellular fluid volume. This decrease may be aggravated by vomiting and reduced fluid intake. Thus, the ability of the kidney to eliminate excess calcium is compromised. Renal impairment can eventually cause nitrogen retention, acidosis, renal failure, and future decrease in excretion of calcium. Didronel I.V. Infusion, by inhibiting excessive bone resorption, interrupts this process. Salt loading and use of "high ceiling" or "loop" diuretics may be used to promote calcium excretion, because the rate of renal calcium excretion is directly related to the rate of sodium excretion.
The physiologic derangements induced by excessive serum calcium are due to increased levels of ionized calcium. The pathophysiologic effects of excessive serum calcium are heightened by reductions in serum albumin which normally binds a fraction (about 40%) of the total serum calcium. In patients with hypercalcemia of malignancy, serum albumin is often reduced and this tends to mask the magnitude of the increase in the level of ionized calcium. By reducing the flow of calcium from resorbing bone, Didronel I.V. Infusion effectively reduces total and ionized serum calcium.
In the principal clinical study of Didronel for hypercalcemia of malignancy, patients with elevated calcium levels (10.1–17.4 mg/dl) were treated simultaneously with daily administrations of intravenous Didronel over a 3-day period and up to 3000 ml of saline and 80 mg of loop diuretic. The response to treatment for these patients was compared with that from patients treated with saline and loop diuretics alone. In terms of total serum calcium changes, 88% of patients treated with Didronel I.V. Infusion as described, had reductions of serum calcium of 1 mg/dl or more. Total serum calcium returned to normal in 63% of patients within 7 days compared to 33% of patients treated with hydration alone. Reductions in urinary calcium excretion, which accompany reductions in excessive bone resorption, became apparent after 24 hours. This was accompanied or followed by maximum decreases in serum calcium which were observed, most

Continued on next page

MGI Pharma—Cont.

frequently, 72 hours after the first infusion. The physiologically important component of serum calcium is the ionized portion. In most institutions, this cannot be measured directly. It is important to recognize that factors influencing the ratio of free and bound calcium such as serum proteins, particularly albumin, may complicate the interpretation of total serum calcium measurements. If indicated, a corrected serum calcium value should be calculated using an established algorithm.

When the total serum values are adjusted for serum albumin levels, there was a return to normocalcemia in 24% of Didronel-treated patients and in 7% of patients treated with saline infusion. Eighty-seven percent of patients receiving Didronel and 67% of patients on saline had albumin-adjusted serum calcium levels returned to normal or reduced by at least 1 mg/dl.

In the above mentioned study, a second course of Didronel I.V. Infusion was tried in a small number of patients who had a recurrence of hypercalcemia following an initial response to a 3-day infusion of the drug. All patients who received a second 3-day course of Didronel I.V. Infusion showed a decrease of total serum calcium of at least 1 mg/dl. Normalization of total serum calcium occurred in 11 out of 14 patients.

Didronel I.V. Infusion does not appear to alter renal tubular reabsorption of calcium, and does not affect hypercalcemia in patients with hyperparathyroidism where increased calcium reabsorption may be a factor in the hypercalcemia.

Limited clinical study results suggest that continuation of Didronel therapy with oral tablets may maintain clinically acceptable serum calcium levels and prolong normocalcemia.

INDICATIONS AND USAGE

Didronel I.V. Infusion, together with achievement and maintenance of adequate hydration, is indicated for the treatment of hypercalcemia of malignancy inadequately managed by dietary modification and/or oral hydration.

In the treatment of hypercalcemia of malignancy, it is important to initiate rehydration with saline together with "high ceiling" or "loop" diuretics if indicated to restore urine output. This also is intended to increase the renal excretion of calcium and initiate a reduction in serum calcium. Since increased bone resorption is usually the underlying cause of an increased flux of calcium into the vascular compartment, concurrent therapy with Didronel I.V. Infusion is recommended as soon as there is a restoration of urine output. Since Didronel is excreted by the kidney, it is important to know that renal function is adequate to handle not only the increased fluid load but also the excretion of the drug itself. (See WARNINGS.)

Didronel I.V. Infusion is also indicated for the treatment of hypercalcemia of malignancy which persists after adequate hydration has been restored. Patients with and without metastases and with a variety of tumors have been responsive to treatment with Didronel I.V. Infusion. Adequate hydration of patients should be maintained, but in aged patients and in those with cardiac failure, care must be taken to avoid overhydration.

CONTRAINDICATIONS

In patients with Class Dc and higher renal functional impairment (serum creatinine greater than 5.0 mg/dl) Didronel I.V. Infusion should be withheld.

WARNINGS

Occasional mild to moderate abnormalities in renal function (elevated BUN and/or serum creatinine) have been observed when Didronel I.V. Infusion was given as directed to patients with hypercalcemia of malignancy. These changes were reversible or remained stable, without worsening, after completion of the course of Didronel I.V. Infusion. In some patients with pre-existing renal impairment or in those who had received potentially nephrotoxic drugs, further depression of renal function was sometimes seen. This suggests that Didronel I.V. Infusion may produce or aggravate the depression of renal function in approximately 8 of 203 treatment courses when used to treat hypercalcemia of malignancy. Therefore, it is recommended that appropriate monitoring of renal function with serum creatinine and/or BUN be carried out with Didronel I.V. Infusion treatment.

The effects of Didronel I.V. Infusion administration on renal function in patients with serum creatinine greater than 2.5 mg/dl (Class Cc and higher, Classification of Renal Functional Impairment, Council on the Kidney in Cardiovascular Disease, American Heart Association, Ann. Int. Med. 75:251–52, 1971) has not been systematically examined in controlled trials.

Since Didronel is excreted by the kidney, it is important to know that renal function is adequate to handle not only the increased fluid load but also the excretion of the drug itself. Since these capacities are impaired in patients with underlying renal disease and since experience with Didronel I.V.

Infusion in patients with serum creatinine > 2.5 mg/dl is limited, the use of Didronel I.V. Infusion in such patients should occur only after a careful assessment of renal status or potential risks and potential benefits.

Reduction of the dose of Didronel I.V. Infusion, if used at all, may be advisable in Class Cc renal functional impairment (serum creatinine 2.5 to 4.9 mg/dl); and, Didronel I.V. Infusion be used only if the potential benefit of hypercalcemia correction will substantially exceed the potential for worsening of renal function. In patients with Class Dc and higher renal functional impairment (serum creatinine greater than 5.0 mg/dl) Didronel I.V. Infusion should be withheld.

PRECAUTIONS

General: Hypercalcemia may cause or exacerbate impaired renal function. In clinical trials, while elevations of serum creatinine or blood urea nitrogen were seen in patients with hypercalcemia of malignancy prior to treatment with Didronel I.V. Infusion, these measurements improved in some patients or remained unchanged in most patients. Nevertheless, elevations in serum creatinine during treatment with Didronel I.V. Infusion have been observed in approximately 10% of patients.

In animal preclinical studies, administration of Didronel I.V. Infusion in amounts or at rates in excess of those recommended produced transient hypocalcemia or induced proximal renal tubular damage.

In the principal clinical trial of Didronel I.V. Infusion, 33 of 185 patients (18%) treated one or more times with Didronel I.V. Infusion had serum calcium values below the lower limits of normal. When adjusted for levels of reduced serum albumin, less than 1% of the 185 patients are estimated to have hypocalcemic ionized serum calcium levels. No adverse effects have been traced to hypocalcemia.

The hypercalcemia of hyperparathyroidism is refractory to Didronel I.V. Infusion. It is possible for this disease to coexist in patients with malignancy.

Carcinogenesis, Mutagenesis, Impairment of Fertility: Long-term studies in rats indicate that Didronel is not carcinogenic.

Pregnancy: Teratogenic Effects: Pregnancy Category C. Animal reproduction studies have not been conducted with Didronel I.V. Infusion. It is also not known whether Didronel I.V. Infusion can cause fetal harm when administered to a pregnant woman or can affect reproduction capacity. Didronel I.V. Infusion should be given to a pregnant woman only if clearly needed.

Nursing Mothers: It is not known whether this drug is excreted in human milk. Because many drugs are excreted in human milk, caution should be exercised when Didronel I.V. Infusion is administered to a nursing woman.

Pediatric Use: Safety and effectiveness in children have not been established.

ADVERSE REACTIONS

Hypercalcemia of malignancy is frequently associated with abnormal elevations of serum creatinine and BUN. One-third of the patients participating in multiclinic trials had such elevations before receiving Didronel I.V. Infusion. In these trials, the elevations of BUN or serum creatinine improved in some patients, or remained unchanged in most patients; however, in approximately 10% of patients, occasional mild to moderate abnormalities in renal function (increases of > 0.5 mg/dl serum creatinine) were observed during or immediately after treatment. The possibility that Didronel I.V. Infusion contributed to these changes cannot be excluded (see WARNINGS).

Of patients who participated in the controlled hypercalcemia trials, 10 of 221 (5%) treatment courses reported a metallic or altered taste, or loss of taste, which usually disappeared within hours, during and/or shortly after Didronel I.V. Infusion. A few patients with Paget's Disease of bone have reported allergic skin rashes in association with oral Didronel medication.

OVERDOSAGE

Rapid intravenous administration of Didronel at doses above 27 mg/kg has produced ECG changes and bleeding problems in animals. These abnormalities are probably related to marked and/or rapid decreases in ionized calcium levels in blood and tissue fluids. They are thought to be due to chelation of calcium by massive amounts of diphosphonate. These abnormalities have been shown to be reversible in animal studies by the administration of ionizable calcium salts.

Similar problems are not expected to occur in humans treated with Didronel I.V. Infusion used as recommended (see DOSAGE AND ADMINISTRATION). Moreover, signs and symptoms of hypocalcemia such as paresthesias and carpopedal spasms have not been reported. The chelation effects of the diphosphonate, should they occur in man, should be reversible with the intravenous administration of calcium gluconate.

Administration of intravenous etidronate disodium at doses and possibly at rates in excess of those recommended has been reported to be associated with renal insufficiency.

DOSAGE AND ADMINISTRATION

Didronel I.V. Infusion: The recommended dose of Didronel I.V. Infusion is 7.5 mg/kg body weight/day for three successive days. **This daily dose must be diluted in at least 250 ml of sterile normal saline.** Stability studies show that diluted solution stored at controlled room temperature (59°F to 86°F or 15°C to 30°C) shows no loss of drug for a 48-hour period THE DILUTED DOSE OF DIDRONEL I.V. INFUSION SHOULD BE ADMINISTERED INTRAVENOUSLY OVER A PERIOD OF AT LEAST 2 HOURS. Didronel I.V. Infusion may be added to volumes of fluid greater than 250 ml when this is convenient.

REGARDLESS OF THE VOLUME OF SOLUTION IN WHICH DIDRONEL I.V. INFUSION IS DILUTED, SLOW INFUSION IS IMPORTANT TO SAFETY. The minimum infusion time of two hours at the recommended dose, or smaller doses, should be observed. The usual course of treatment is one infusion of 7.5 mg/kg body weight/day on each of 3 consecutive days but some patients have been treated for up to 7 days. When patients are treated for more than 3 days, there may be an increased possibility of producing hypocalcemia.

Retreatment with Didronel I.V. Infusion may be appropriate if hypercalcemia recurs. There should be at least a seven-day interval between courses of treatment with Didronel I.V. Infusion. The dose and manner of retreatment is the same as that for initial treatment. Retreatment for more than three days has not been adequately studied. The safety and efficacy of more than two courses of therapy with Didronel I.V. Infusion have not been studied. In the presence of renal impairment, reduction of the dose may be advisable.

Parenteral drug products should be inspected visually for particulate matter and discoloration prior to administration whenever solution and container permit.

Didronel Oral Tablets: Didronel (etidronate disodium) tablets may be started on the day following the last dose of Didronel I.V. Infusion. The recommended oral dose of Didronel for patients who have hypercalcemia is 20 mg/kg body weight/day for 30 days. If serum calcium levels remain normal or at clinically acceptable levels, treatment may be extended. Treatment for more than 90 days has not been adequately studied and is not recommended. Please consult the package insert pertaining to oral Didronel tabelts for additional prescribing information.

HOW SUPPLIED

Didronel I.V. Infusion is supplied in 6 ml ampules as a 5% solution containing 300 mg etidronate disodium.

NDC 58063-457-01 carton of 6 ampules.

Avoid excessive heat (over 104°F or 40°c) for undiluted product.

Address medical inquires to **MGI PHARMA**, Medical Department, Suite 300E, Opus Center, 9900 Bren Road East, Minneapolis, MN 55343-9667. Phone 1-800-562-5580
CAUTION: Federal law prohibits dispensing without prescription.
®Registered trademark of Norwich Eaton Pharmaceuticals, Inc.
Manufactured by
Taylor Pharmacal Company
Decatur, Illinois 62525
for **MGI PHARMA, INC.**
Minneapolis, Minneosta 55343
JAN 1991

Oratect™ Gel   **OTC**
Topical Oral Anesthetic

DESCRIPTION

Oratect Gel contains 15% benzocaine in a patent protected base that dries quickly to form a durable film for long-lasting pain relief and protection of the lesion.

INDICATION

For temporary relief of occasional minor irritation, pain and sore mouth.

WARNINGS

USE THIS PRODUCT ONLY AS DIRECTED BY YOUR DOCTOR. IF SYMPTOMS DO NOT IMPROVE IN 7 DAYS, SEE YOUR DOCTOR PROMPTLY. **DO NOT USE IN OR NEAR THE EYES.** KEEP OUT OF REACH OF CHILDREN

DIRECTIONS

Dry the affected area by gently rolling with one of the enclosed swabs. Apply Oratect Gel to the second swab and roll gently over the dry area leaving a thin coating of the product. Keep mouth open and dry for 30–60 seconds to allow gel to dry and form a protective film. A mild, temporary stinging sensation may occur when applied. Wait 20 minutes to allow peak benzocaine effect to pass prior to eating. Use up to 4 times daily or as directed by a doctor. Children under 12 years of age should be supervised in the use of this product. Do not use in children under 2 years of age.

DIRECTIONS FOR APPLICATION

For best results, it is important to thoroughly dry the affected area before applying Oratect Gel.

1. First, dry the site to be treated with one of the enclosed swabs by gently rolling the swab over the affected area.

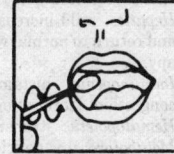

2. Second, apply a bead of Oratect Gel around a second swab. Rotate the swab, as shown, while dispensing product from the tube.

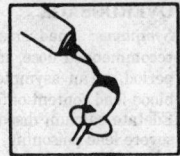

3. Third, apply Oratect Gel by rolling the second swab over the affected area, leaving a thin coating of the product in place.

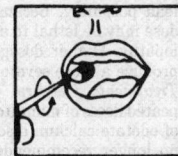

4. Keep mouth open and prevent contact with the affected area for 30 to 60 seconds to allow gel to air dry and form a protective film over the affected area. The film slowly dissipates over 6 hours, therefore, do not try to mechanically remove the Oratect Gel once it has adhered to the mucosal tissue.

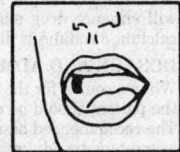

ACTIVE INGREDIENT
Benzocaine (15%), suspended in SD alcohol.

OTHER INGREDIENTS
Purified water, tannic acid, propylene glycol, salicylic acid, hydroxypropylcellulose, boric acid, wintergreen flavoring.

CONTRAINDICATION
Known sensitivity to benzocaine.

HOW SUPPLIED
Oratect Gel is supplied in a .37 oz. (10.5 gram) tube with 10 applicator packages containing two sterilized rayon swabs per package.
Address medical inquiries to MGI PHARMA, Medical Department, Suite 300E, Opus Center, 9900 Bren Road East, Minneapolis, MN 55343-9667. Phone 1-800-562-5580
Store at room temperature.
Pat. No. 4,381,296
Distributed by: MGI PHARMA, INC.   **NDC** 58063-209-01
Minneapolis, MN 55343-9667   March 1992

3M Pharmaceuticals
**275-3W-01 3M CENTER
ST. PAUL, MN 55144**

ALU-TAB™ Tablets   OTC
(aluminum hydroxide)
and
ALU-CAP™ Capsules
(aluminum hydroxide)

DESCRIPTION
Each green Alu-Tab tablet contains dried hydroxide gel equivalent to 500 mg of aluminum hydroxide. Alu-Tab tablets also contain cellulose, hydrogenated vegetable oil, hydroxpropyl methylcellulose, magnesium stearate, polyethylene glycol, polysorbate 80, propylene glycol, sodium starch glycolate, starch, talc, titanium dioxide, D&C yellow #10, FD&C blue #1, and FD&C yellow #6. Each red and green Alu-Cap capsule contains dried aluminum hydroxide gel equivalent to 400 mg of aluminum hydroxide. Alu-Cap capsules also contain cellulose, gelatin, polyethylene glycol, talc, titanium dioxide, D&C yellow #10, FD&C blue #1, FD&C green #3, FD&C red #40, and FD&C yellow #6.

ACTIONS
Antacid actions include neutralization of gastric hyperacidity and mild astringent and adsorbent properties.

The following 3M Pharmaceutical products are available in Military and Veterans Administration depots:

Military Depot Items	**National Stock Number**
Norflex Tablets 100's	6505-00-138-8462
Theolair™ 250 mg. Tablets 100's	6505-01-149-3555
Urex™ Tablets 100's	6505-00-126-3207
Norgesic™ Tablets 500's	6505-00-952-6762
Norgesic™ Forte Tablets 500's	6505-01-029-9116
Tambocor™ 100 mg Tablets 100's	6505-01-240-5767
Medihaler-Iso™ 15 ml. vial w/adapter	6505-00-023-6481
Maxair™ Inhalation Aersol 25.6 gm., 300 inhalations	6505-01-288-0526

Public Health Service	
Norgesic™ Forte Tablets 500's	6505-01-029-9116

Veterans Administration Depot Items	**National Stock Number**
Norgesic™ Tablets 500's	6505-00-952-6762
Norgesic™ Forte Tablets 500's	6505-01-029-9116
Tambocor™ 100 mg Tablets 100's	6505-01-240-5767

ACID NEUTRALIZING CAPACITY
Three Alu-Tab tablets have the capacity to neutralize 31.8 mEq of acid.
Three Alu-Cap capsules have the capacity to neutralize 25.4 mEq of acid.

INDICATIONS
Uncomplicated peptic ulcer and gastric hyperacidity.

WARNINGS
Do not take more than 9 Alu-Tab tablets or 9 Alu-Cap capsules in a 24 hour period, or use maximum dosage of this product for more than two weeks, except under the advice and supervision of a physician.
Prolonged use of aluminum-containing antacids in patients with renal failure may result in or worsen dialysis osteomalacia. Elevated tissue aluminum levels contribute to the development of the dialysis encephalopathy and osteomalacia syndromes. Small amounts of aluminum are absorbed from the gastrointestinal tract and renal excretion of aluminum is impaired in renal failure. Aluminum is not well removed by dialysis because it is bound to albumin and transferrin, which do not cross dialysis membranes. As a result, aluminum is deposited in bone, and dialysis osteomalacia may develop when large amounts of aluminum are ingested orally by patients with impaired renal function.
Aluminum forms insoluble complexes with phosphate in the gastrointestinal tract, thus decreasing phosphate absorption. Prolonged use of aluminum-containing antacids by normophosphatemic patients may result in hypophosphatemia if phosphate intake is not adequate. In its more severe forms, hypophosphatemia can lead to anorexia, malaise, muscle weakness, and osteomalacia.

PRECAUTIONS
If constipation occurs, medication should be discontinued and a physician should be consulted. Aluminum hydroxide must be given with care to patients who have recently suffered massive upper gastrointestinal hemorrhage. Do not give this product to any patient presently taking a prescription antibiotic drug containing any form of tetracycline.

DIRECTIONS FOR USE
Three Alu-Tab tablets three times a day or as directed by physician. Three Alu-Cap capsules three times a day or as directed by physician.

HOW SUPPLIED
Bottles of 250 green film-coated Alu-Tab tablets (NDC **0089-0107-25**). Bottles of 100 red and green Alu-Cap capsules (NDC **0089-0105-10**).

CALCIUM DISODIUM VERSENATE   ℞
(edetate calcium disodium injection, USP)
STERILE
Injection

> ### WARNINGS
> Calcium Disodium Versenate is capable of producing toxic effects which can be fatal. Lead encephalopathy is relatively rare in adults, but occurs more often in children in whom it may be incipient and thus overlooked. The mortality rate in these children has been high. Patients with lead encephalopathy and cerebral edema may experience a lethal increase in intracranial pressure following intravenous infusion; the intramuscular route is preferred for these patients and for young children. In cases where the intravenous route is necessary, avoid rapid infusion. The dosage schedule should be followed and at no time should the recommended daily dose be exceeded.

DESCRIPTION
Calcium Disodium Versenate (edetate calcium disodium injection, USP) is a sterile, injectable, chelating agent in concentrated solution for intravenous infusion or intramuscular injection. Each 5 ml ampul contains 1000 mg of edetate calcium disodium [equivalent to 200 mg/ml] in water for injection. Chemically, this product is called [[N,N'-1,2-ethanediylbis[N-(carboxymethyl)-glycinato]](4-)-N,N',O,O',O^N,O^N'],disodium, hydrate, (OC-6-21)-Calciate(2-).

Structural Formula:

$$NaOOCCH_2 \quad N \overset{CH_2---CH_2}{\quad} N \quad CH_2COONa$$

$$H_2C \qquad Ca \qquad CH_2 \qquad \cdot x\, H_2O$$

$$O{=}C{-}O \qquad\qquad O{-}C{=}O$$

$C_{10}H_{10}CaN_2Na_2O_8 \cdot xH_2O$
Molecular weight 374.27 (anhydrous)

CLINICAL PHARMACOLOGY
The pharmacologic effects of edetate calcium disodium are due to the formation of chelates with divalent and trivalent metals. A stable chelate will form with any metal that has the ability to displace calcium from the molecule, a feature shared by lead, zinc, cadmium, manganese, iron and mercury. The amounts of manganese and iron mobilized are not significant. Copper[1] is not mobilized and mercury is unavailable for chelation because it is too tightly bound to body ligands or it is stored in inaccessible body compartments. The excretion of calcium by the body is not increased following intravenous administration of edetate calcium disodium, but the excretion of zinc is considerably increased.[1]
Edetate calcium disodium is poorly absorbed from the gastrointestinal tract. In blood, all the drug is found in the plasma. Edetate calcium disodium does not appear to penetrate cells; it is distributed primarily in the extracellular fluid with only about 5% of the plasma concentration found in spinal fluid.
The half life of edetate calcium disodium is 20 to 60 minutes. It is excreted primarily by the kidney, with about 50% excreted in one hour and over 95% within 24 hours.[2] Almost none of the compound is metabolized.
The primary source of lead chelated by Calcium Disodium Versenate is from bone; subsequently, soft-tissue lead is redistributed to bone when chelation is stopped.[3,4] There is also some reduction in kidney lead levels following chelation therapy.
It has been shown in animals that following a single dose of Calcium Disodium Versenate urinary lead output increases, blood lead concentration decreasees, but brain lead is significantly increased due to internal redistribution of lead.[5] (See WARNINGS.) These data are in agreement with the recent results of others in experimental animals showing that after a five day course of treatment there is no net reduction in brain lead.[6]

INDICATIONS AND USAGE
Edetate calcium disodium is indicated for the reduction of blood levels and depot stores of lead in lead poisoning (acute and chronic) and lead encephalopathy, in both children and adults.
Chelation therapy should not replace effective measures to eliminate or reduce further exposure to lead.

CONTRAINDICATIONS
Edetate calcium disodium should not be given during periods of anuria, nor to patients with active renal disease or hepatitis.

WARNINGS
See boxed warning.

PRECAUTIONS
General Precautions: Edetate calcium disodium may produce the same renal damage as lead poisoning, such as pro-

Continued on next page

3M—Cont.

teinuria and microscopic hematuria. Treatment-induced nephrotoxicity is dose-dependent and may be reduced by assuring adequate diuresis before therapy begins. Urine flow must be monitored throughout therapy which must be stopped if anuria or severe olyguria develop. The proximal tubule hydropic degeneration usually recovers upon cessation of therapy. Edetate calcium disodium must be used in reduced doses in patients with pre-existing mild renal disease.

Patients should be monitored for cardiac rhythm irregularities and other ECG changes during intravenous therapy.

Information for patients: Patients should be instructed to immediately inform their physician if urine output stops for a period of 12 hours.

Laboratory Tests: Urinarlysis and urine sediment, renal and hepatic function and serum electrolyte levels should be checked before each course of therapy and then be monitored daily during therapy in severe cases, and in less serious cases after the second and fifth day of therapy. Therapy must be discontinued at the first sign of renal toxicity. The presence of large renal epithelial cells or increasing number of red blood cells in urinary sediment or greater proteinuria call for immediate stopping of edetate calcium disodium administration. Alkaline phosphatase values are frequently depressed (possibly due to decreased serum zinc levels), but return to normal within 48 hours after cessation of therapy. Elevated erythrocyte protoporphyrin levels (> 35 mcg/dl of whole blood) indicate the need to perform a venous blood lead determination. If the whole blood lead concentration is between 25–55 mcg/dl a mobilization test can be considered.[7,8] (See Diagnostic Test.) An elevation of urinary coproporphyrin (adults: > 250 mcg/day; children under 80 lbs: > 75 mcg/day) and elevation of urinary delta aminolevulinic acid (ALA) (adults: > 4 mg/day; children: > 3 mg/m^2/day) are associated with blood lead levels > 40 mcg/dl. Urinary coproporphyrin may be falsely negative in terminal patients and in severely iron-depleted children who are not regenerating heme.[9] In growing children long bone x-rays showing lead lines and abdominal x-rays showing radio-opaque material in the abdomen may be of help in estimating the level of exposure to lead.

Drug Interactions: There is no known drug interference with standard clinical laboratory tests. Steroids enhance the renal toxicity of edetate calcium disodium in animals.[7] Edetate calcium disodium interferes with the action of zinc insulin preparations by chelating the zinc.[7]

Carcinogenesis, Mutagenesis, Impairment of Fertility: Long term animal studies have not been conducted with edetate calcium disodium to evaluate its carcinogenic potential, mutagenic potential or its effect on fertility.

Pregnancy: Category B: One reproduction study was performed in rats at doses up to 13 times the human dose and revealed no evidence of impaired fertility or harm to the fetus due to Caclium Disodium Versenate.[10] Another reproduction study performed in rats at doses up to about 25 to 40 times the human dose revealed evidence of fetal malformations due to Calcium Disodium Versenate, which were prevented by simultaneous supplementation of dietary zinc.[11] There are, however, no adequate and well-controlled studies in pregnant women. Because animal reproduction studies are not always predictive of human response, this drug should be used during pregnancy only if clearly needed.

Labor and Delivery: Calcium Disodium Versenate has no recognized use during labor and delivery, and its effects during these processes are unknown.

Nursing Mothers: It is not known whether this durg is excreted in human milk. Because many drugs are excreted in human milk, caution should be exercised when Calcium Disodium Versenate is administered to a nursing woman.

Pediatric Use: Since lead poisoning occurs in children and adults but is frequently more severe in children, Calcium Disodium Versenate is used in patients of all ages.

ADVERSE REACTIONS

The following adverse effects have been associated with the use of edetate calcium disodium:

Body as a Whole: pain at intramuscular injection site, fever, chills, malaise, fatigue, myalgia, arthralgia.

Cardiovascular: hypotension, cardiac rhythm irregularities.

Renal: acute necrosis of proximal tubules (which may result in fatal nephrosis), infrequent changes in distal tubules and glomeruli.

Urinary: glycosuria, proteinuria, microscopic hematuria and large epithelial cells in urinary sediment.

Nervous System: tremors, headache, numbness, tingling.

Gastrointestinal: cheilosis, nausea, vomiting, anorexia, excessive thirst.

Hepatic: mild increases in SGOT and SGPT are common, and return to normal within 48 hours after cessation of therapy.

Immunogenic: histamine-like reactions (sneezing, nasal congestion, lacrimation), rash.

Hematopoietic: transient bone marrow depression, anemia.

Metabolic: zinc deficiency, hypercalcemia.

OVERDOSAGE

Symptoms: Inadvertent administration of 5 times the recommended dose, infused intravenously over a 24 hour period, to an asymptomatic 16 month old patient with a blood lead content of 56 mcg/dl did not cause any ill effects. Edetate calcium disodium can aggravate the symptoms of severe lead poisoning, therefore, most toxic effects (cerebral edema, renal tubular necrosis) appear to be associated with lead poisoning. Because of cerebral edema, a therapeutic dose may be lethal to an adult or a child with lead encephalopathy. Higher dosage of edetate calcium disodium may produce a more severe zinc deficiency.

Treatment: Cerebral edema should be treated with repeated doses of mannitol. Steroids enhance the renal toxicity of edetate calcium disodium in animals and, therefore, are no longer recommended.[7] Zinc levels must be monitored. Good urinary output must be maintained because diuresis will enhance drug elimination. It is not known if edetate calcium disodium is dialyzable.

DOSAGE AND ADMINISTRATION

When a source for the lead intoxication has been identified, the patient should be removed from the source, if possible.

The recommended dose of Calcium Disodium Versenate for asymptomatic adults and children whose blood lead level is < 70 mcg/dl but > 20 mcg/dl (World Health Organization recommended upper allowable level) is 1000 mg/m^2/day whether given intravenously or intramuscularly. (See Surface Area Nomogram.)

For adults with lead nephropathy, the following dosage regimen has been suggested: 500 mg/m^2 every 24 hours for 5 days for patients with serum creatinine levels of 2–3 mg/dl, every 48 hours for 3 doses for patients with creatinine levels of 3–4 mg/dl, and once weekly for patients with creatinine levels above 4 mg/dl. These regimens may be repeated at one month intervals.[12]

Calcium Disodium Versenate, used alone, may aggravate symptoms in patients with very high blood lead levels. When the blood lead level is > 70 mcg/dl or clinical symptoms consistent with lead poisoning are present, it is recommended that Calcium Disodium Versenate be used in conjunction with BAL (dimercaprol). Please consult published protocols and specialized references for dosage recommendations of combination therapy.[14–18]

Therapy of lead poisoning in adults and children with Calcium Disodium Versenate is continued over a period of five days. Therapy is then interrupted for 2 to 4 days to allow redistribution of the lead and to prevent severe depletion of zinc and other essential metals. Two courses of treatment are usually employed; however, it depends on severity of the lead toxicity and the patient's tolerance of the drug.

Calcium Disodium Versenate is equally effective whether administered intravenously or intramuscularly. The intramuscular route is used for all patients with overt lead encephalopathy and this route is recommended for young children.

Acutely ill individuals may be dehydrated from vomiting. Since edetate calcium disodium is excreted almost exclusively in the urine, it is very important to establish urine flow with intravenous fluid administration before the first dose of the chelating agent is given; however, excessive fluid must be avoided in patients with encephalopathy. Once urine flow is established, further intravenous fluid is restricted to basal water and electrolyte requirements. Administration of Calcium Disodium Versenate should be stopped whenever there is cessation of urine flow in order to avoid unduly high tissue levels of the drug. Edetate calcium disodium must be used in reduced doses in patients with pre-existing mild renal disease.

Intravenous Administration: Add the total daily dose of Calcium Disodium Versenate (1000 mg/m^2/day) to 250–500 ml of 5% dextrose or 0.9% sodium chloride injection. The total daily dose should be infused over a period of 8–12 hours. Calcium Disodium Versenate injection is incompatible with 10% dextrose, 10% invert sugar in 0.9% sodium chloride, lactate Ringer's, Ringer's, one-sixth molar sodium lactate injections, and with injectable amphotericin B and hydralazine hydrochloride.

Intramuscular Administration: The total daily dosage (1000 mg/m^2/day) should be divided into equal doses spaced 8–12 hours apart. Lidocaine or procaine should be added to the Calcium Disodium Versenate injection to minimize pain at the injection site. The final lidocaine or procaine concentra-

SURFACE AREA NOMOGRAM

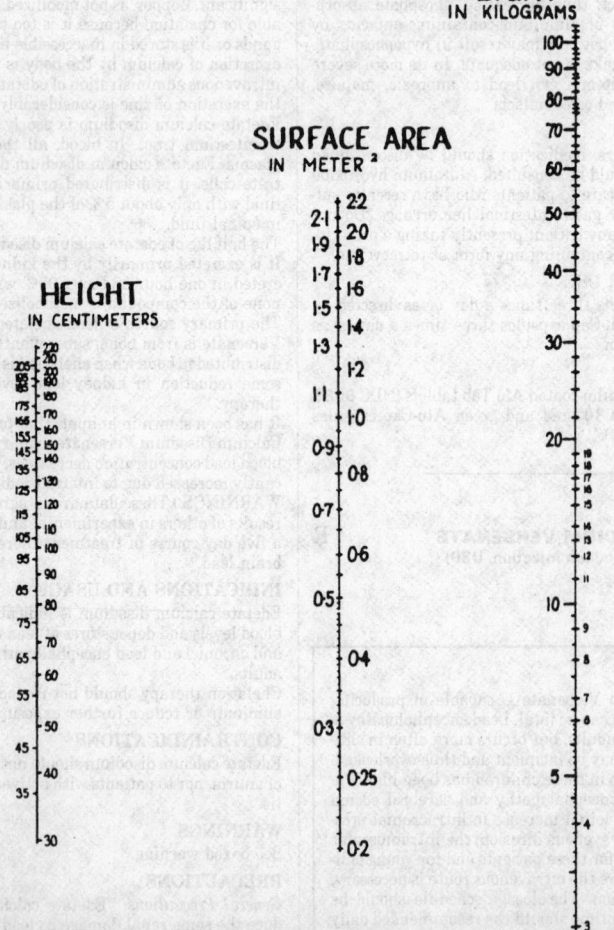

Drawn from Gehan and George, Cancer Chemotherapy Reports 54:225, 1970

tion of 5 mg/ml (0.5%) can be obtained as follows: 0.25 ml of 10% lidocaine solution per 5 ml (entire content of ampul) concentrated Calcium Disodium Versenate; 1 ml of 1% lidocaine or procaine solution per ml of concentrated Calcium Disodium Versenate. When used alone, regardless of method of administration, Calcium Disodium Versenate should not be given at doses larger than those recommended.

Diagnostic Test: Several methods have been described for lead mobilization tests using edetate calcium disodium to assess body stores.[7,9,12,13,18]

These procedures have advantages and disadvantages that should be reviewed in current references. Edetate calcium disodium mobilization test should not be performed in symptomatic patients and in patients with blood lead levels above 55 mcg/dl for whom appropriate therapy is indicated.

Parenteral drug should be inspected visually for particulate matter and discoloration prior to administration, whenever solution and container permit.

HOW SUPPLIED

Calcium Disodium Versenate injection, 5 ml ampuls containing 200 mg of edetate calcium disodium per ml (1 g per ampul), in boxes containing 6 ampuls (NDC 0089-0510-06).

Store at controlled room temperature 15–30C degrees (59–86F degrees).

CAUTION

Federal law prohibits dispensing without prescription.

REFERENCES

1. Thomas DJ, Chisolm JJ. Lead, zinc and copper decorporation during calcium disodium ethylenediamine tetraacetate treatment of lead-poisoned children. J Pharmacol Exp Therapeu 1986; 239:829-835.
2. The Pharmacological Basis of Therapeutics, 7th edition, Goodman and Gilman, editors. Macmillan Publishing Company, New York, 1985, pp. 1619–1622.
3. Hammond PB, Aronson AL, Olson WC. The mechanism of mobilization of lead by ethylenediaminetetraacetate. J Pharmacol Exp Therapeu 1967; 157:196-206.
4. Van deVyver FL, D'Haese PC, Visser WJ, et al. Bone lead in dialysis patients. Kidney Intl 1988; 33:601-607.
5. Cory-Slecta DA, Weiss B, Cox C. Mobilization and redistribution of lead over the course of calcium disodium ethylenediamine tetraacetate chelation therapy. J Pharmacol Exp Therapeu 1987; 243:804-813.
6. Chisolm JJ. Mobilization of lead by calcium disodium edetate. Am J Dis Child 1987; 141:1256-1257.
7. Drug Evaluations, 6th Edition, American Medical Association, Saunders, Philadelphia, 1986, pp. 1637–1639.
8. Centers for Disease Control: Preventing lead poisoning in young children. Atlanta, GA, Department of Health and Human Services, 1985 Jan.
9. Finberg L, Rajagopal V. Diagnosis and treatment of lead poisoning in children. J Family Med 1985 April: 3–12.
10. Schardein JL, Sakowski R, Petrere J, et al. Teratogenesis studies with EDTA and its salts in rats. Toxicol Appl Pharmacol 1981; 61:423-428.
11. Swenerton H, Hurley LS. Teratogenic effects of a chelating agent and their prevention by zinc. Science 1971; 173:62-64.
12. American Hospital Formulary Service, Drug Information, 1988, pp. 1695–1698.
13. Markowitz ME, Rosen JF. Assessment of lead stores in children: Validation of an 8-hour $CaNa_2EDTA$ (Calcium Disodium Versenate) provocative test. J Pediatrics 1984; 104:337-341.
14. Piomelli S, Rosen JF, Chisolm JJ, et al. Management of childhood lead poisoning. J Pediatrics 1984; 105:523-532.
15. Sachs HK, Blanksma LA, Murray EF, et al. Ambulatory treatment of lead poisoning: Report of 1,155 cases. Pediatrics 1970; 46:389.
16. Chisolm JJ. The use of chelating agents in the treatment of acute and chronic lead intoxication in childhood. J Pediatrics 1968; 73:1.
17. Coffin R, Phillips JL, Staples WI, et al. Treatment of lead encephalopathy in children. J Pediatrics 1966; 69: 198-206.
18. Chisolm JJ. Increased lead absorption and acute lead poisoning. Current Pediatric Therapy 12, Gillis and Kagan, editors, WB Saunders, Philadelphia, 1986, pp. 667–671.

Manufactured for
3M Pharmaceuticals
Northridge, CA 91324
By Sanofi Winthrop Pharmaceuticals
McPherson, Kansas 67460
C-161-13 April 1, 1992

DISALCID™ ℞
(salsalate)
Tablets and Capsules

DESCRIPTION

DISALCID (salsalate) is a nonsteroidal anti-inflammatory agent for oral administration. Chemically, salsalate (salicylsalicylic acid or 2-hydroxy-benzoic acid, 2-carboxyphenyl ester) is a dimer of salicylic acid; its structural formula is shown below.

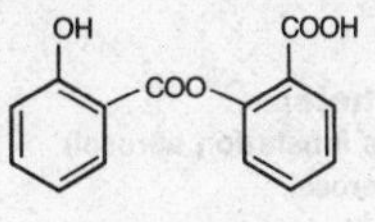

Salsalate

Each round, aqua, scored, film coated DISALCID tablet contains 500 mg salsalate.

Each aqua and white DISALCID capsule contains 500 mg salsalate. DISALCID capsules also contain: colloidal silicon dioxide, gelatin, magnesium stearate, pregelatinized starch, corn starch, titanium dioxide, FD&C blue #1, and D&C yellow #10.

Each capsule-shaped aqua, scored, film coated DISALCID tablet contains 750 mg salsalate. DISALCID tablets also contain: hydroxypropyl methylcellulose, magnesium stearate, microcrystalline cellulose, polyethylene glycol, polysorbate 80, propylene glycol, corn starch, talc, titanium dioxide, FD&C blue #1, and D&C yellow #10. (See HOW SUPPLIED).

CLINICAL PHARMACOLOGY

DISALCID is insoluble in acid gastric fluids (<0.1 mg/ml at pH 1.0), but readily soluble in the small intestine where it is partially hydrolyzed to two molecules of salicylic acid. A significant portion of the parent compound is absorbed unchanged and undergoes rapid esterase hydrolysis in the body; its half-life is about one hour. About 13% is excreted through the kidneys as a glucuronide conjugate of the parent compound, the remainder as salicylic acid and its metabolites. Thus, the amount of salicylic acid available from DISALCID is about 15% less than from aspirin, when the two drugs are administered on a salicylic acid molar equivalent basis (3.6 g salsalate/5 g aspirin). Salicylic acid biotransformation is saturated at anti-inflammatory doses of DISALCID. Such capacity-limited biotransformation results in an increase in the half-life of salicylic acid from 3.5 to 16 or more hours. Thus, dosing with DISALCID twice a day will satisfactorily maintain blood levels within the desired therapeutic range (10 to 30 mg/100 ml) throughout the 12-hour intervals. Therapeutic blood levels continue for up to 16 hours after the last dose. The parent compound does not show capacity-limited biotransformation, nor does it accumulate in the plasma on multiple dosing. Food slows the absorption of all salicylates including DISALCID.

The mode of anti-inflammatory action of DISALCID and other nonsteroidal anti-inflammatory drugs is not fully defined. Although salicylic acid (the primary metabolite of DISALCID) is a weak inhibitor of prostaglandin synthesis **in vitro**, DISALCID appears to selectively inhibit prostaglandin synthesis **in vivo**,[1] providing anti-inflammatory activity equivalent to aspirin[2] and indomethacin.[3] Unlike aspirin, DISALCID does not inhibit platelet aggregation.[4]

The usefulness of salicylic acid, the active **in vivo** product of DISALCID, in the treatment of arthritic disorders has been established.[5,6] In contrast to aspirin, DISALCID causes no greater fecal gastrointestinal blood loss than placebo.[7]

INDICATIONS AND USAGE

DISALCID is indicated for relief of the signs and symptoms of rheumatoid arthritis, osteoarthritis and related rheumatic disorders.

CONTRAINDICATIONS

DISALCID is contraindicated in patients hypersensitive to salsalate.

WARNINGS

Reye's Syndrome may develop in individuals who have chicken pox, influenza, or flu symptoms. Some studies suggest possible association between the development of Reye's Syndrome and the use of medicines containing salicylate or aspirin. DISALCID contains a salicylate and therefore is not recommended for use in patients with chicken pox, influenza, or flu symptoms.

PRECAUTIONS

General Precautions: Patients on treatment with DISALCID should be warned not to take other salicylates so as to avoid potentially toxic concentrations. Great care should be exercised when DISALCID is prescribed in the presence of chronic renal insufficiency or peptic ulcer disease. Protein binding of salicylic acid can be influenced by nutritional status, competitive binding of other drugs, and fluctuations in serum proteins caused by disease (rheumatoid arthritis, etc.).

Although cross reactivity, including bronchospasm, has been reported occasionally with non-acetylated salicylates, including salsalate, in aspirin-sensitive patients,[8,9] salsalate is less likely than aspirin to induce asthma in such patients.[10]

Laboratory Tests: Plasma salicylic acid concentrations should be periodically monitored during long-term treatment with DISALCID to aid maintenance of therapeutically effective levels: 10 to 30 mg/100 ml. Toxic manifestations are not usually seen until plasma concentrations exceed 30 mg/100 ml (see OVERDOSAGE). Urinary pH should also be regularly monitored: sudden acidification, as from pH 6.5 to 5.5, can double the plasma level, resulting in toxicity.

Drug Interactions: Salicylates antagonize the uricosuric action of drugs used to treat gout. ASPIRIN AND OTHER SALICYLATE DRUGS WILL BE ADDITIVE TO DISALCID AND MAY INCREASE PLASMA CONCENTRATIONS OF SALICYLIC ACID TO TOXIC LEVELS. Drugs and foods that raise urine pH will increase renal clearance and urinary excretion of salicylic acid, thus lowering plasma levels; acidifying drugs or foods will decrease urinary excretion and increase plasma levels. Salicylates given concomitantly with anticoagulant drugs may predispose to systemic bleeding. Salicylates may enhance the hypoglycemic effect of oral antidiabetic drugs of the sulfonylurea class. Salicylate competes with a number of drugs for protein binding sites, notably penicillin, thiopental, thyroxine, triiodothyronine, phenytoin, sulfinpyrazone, naproxen, warfarin, methotrexate, and possibly corticosteroids.

Drug/Laboratory Test Interactions: Salicylate competes with thyroid hormone for binding to plasma proteins, which may be reflected in a depressed plasma T_4 value in some patients; thyroid function and basal metabolism are unaffected.

Carcinogenesis: No long-term animal studies have been performed with DISALCID to evaluate its carcinogenic potential.

Use in Pregnancy: Pregnancy Category C: Salsalate and salicylic acid have been shown to be teratogenic and embryocidal in rats when given in doses 4 to 5 times the usual human dose. These effects were not observed at doses twice as great as the usual human dose. There are no adequate and well-controlled studies in pregnant women. DISALCID should be used during pregnancy only if the potential benefit justifies the potential risk to the fetus.

Labor and Delivery: There exist no adequate and well-controlled studies in pregnant women. Although adverse effects on mother or infant have not been reported with DISALCID use during labor, caution is advised when anti-inflammatory dosage is involved. However, other salicylates have been associated with prolonged gestation and labor, maternal and neonatal bleeding sequelae, potentiation of narcotic and barbiturate effects (respiratory or cardiac arrest in the mother), delivery problems and stillbirth.

Nursing Mothers: It is not known whether salsalate per se is excreted in human milk; salicylic acid, the primary metabolite of DISALCID, has been shown to appear in human milk in concentrations approximating the maternal blood level. Thus, the infant of a mother on DISALCID therapy might ingest in mother's milk 30 to 80% as much salicylate per kg body weight as the mother is taking. Accordingly, caution should be exercised when DISALCID is administered to a nursing woman.

Pediatric Use: Safety and effectiveness of DISALCID use in children have not been established. (See WARNINGS section.)

ADVERSE REACTIONS

In two well-controlled clinical trials, the following reversible adverse experiences characteristic of salicylates were most commonly reported with DISALCID (n = 280 pts; listed in descending order of frequency): tinnitus, nausea, hearing impairment, rash, and vertigo. These common symptoms of salicylates, i.e., tinnitus or reversible hearing impairment, are often used as a guide to therapy.

Although cause-and-effect relationships have not been established, spontaneous reports over a ten-year period have included the following additional medically significant adverse experiences: abdominal pain, abnormal hepatic function, anaphylactic shock, angioedema, bronchospasm, decreased creatinine clearance, diarrhea, G.I. bleeding, hepatitis, hypotension, nephritis and urticaria.

DRUG ABUSE AND DEPENDENCE

Drug abuse and dependence have not been reported with DISALCID.

OVERDOSAGE

Death has followed ingestion of 10 to 30 g of salicylates in adults, but much larger amounts have been ingested without fatal outcome.

Symptoms: The usual symptoms of salicylism—tinnitus, vertigo, headache, confusion, drowsiness, sweating, hyperventilation, vomiting and diarrhea—will occur. More severe intoxication will lead to disruption of electrolyte balance and blood pH, and hyperthermia and dehydration.

Continued on next page

3M—Cont.

Treatment: Further absorption of DISALCID from the G.I. tract should be prevented by emesis (syrup of ipecac), and, if necessary, by gastric lavage.
Fluid and electrolyte imbalance should be corrected by the administration of appropriate I.V. therapy. Adequate renal function should be maintained. Hemodialysis or peritoneal dialysis may be required in extreme cases.

DOSAGE AND ADMINISTRATION

Adults: The usual dosage is 3000 mg daily, given in divided doses as follows: 1) two doses of two 750 mg tablets; 2) two doses of three 500 mg tablets/capsules; or 3) three doses of two 500 mg tablets/capsules. Some patients, e.g., the elderly, may require a lower dosage to achieve therapeutic blood concentrations and to avoid the more common side affects such as auditory.
Alleviation of symptoms is gradual, and full benefit may not be evident for 3 to 4 days, when plasma salicylate levels have achieved steady state. There is no evidence for development of tissue tolerance (tachyphylaxis), but salicylate therapy may induce increased activity of metabolizing liver enzymes, causing a greater rate of salicyluric acid production and excretion, with a resultant increase in dosage requirement for maintenance of therapeutic serum salicylate levels.
Children: Dosage recommendations and indications for DISALCID use in children have not been established.

HOW SUPPLIED

750 mg tablets in bottles of 100 (NDC **0089-0151-10**)
750 mg tablets in boxes of 100 in unit-dose blister strips (NDC **0089-0151-16**)
750 mg tablets in bottles of 500 (NDC **0089-0151-50**)
500 mg tablets in bottles of 100 (NDC **0089-0149-10**)
500 mg tablets in boxes of 100 in unit-dose blister strips (NDC **0089-0149-16**)
500 mg tablets in bottles of 500 (NDC **0089-0149-50**)
500 mg capsules in bottles of 100 (NDC **0089-0148-10**)
Store at controlled room temperature 15°–30°C (59°–86°F).
CAUTION: Federal law prohibits dispensing without prescription.

REFERENCES

1. Morris HG, Sherman NA, McQuain C, et al: Effects of Salsalate (Non-Acetylated Salicylate) and Aspirin (ASA) on Serum and Prostaglandins in Humans. Ther. Drug Monit. **7**:435–438, 1985.
2. April PA, Curran NJ, Ekholm BP, et al: Multicenter Comparative Study of Salsalate (SSA) vs Aspirin (ASA) in Rheumatoid Arthritis (RA). Arthritis Rheumatism **30**(4 supplement):S93, 1987.
3. Deodhar SD, McLeod MM, Dick WC, et al: A Short-Term Comparative Trial of Salsalate and Indomethacin in Rheumatoid Arthritis. Curr. Med. Res. Opin. **5**:185–188, 1977.
4. Estes D, Kaplan K: Lack of Platelet Effect With the Aspirin Analog, Salsalate. Arthritis and Rheumatism **23**:1303–1307, 1980.
5. Dick C, Dick PH, Nuki G, et al: Effect of Anti-inflammatory Drug Therapy on Clearance of ^{133}Xe from Knee Joints of Patients with Rheumatoid Arthritis. British Med. J. **3**:278–280, 1969.
6. Dick WC, Grayson MF, Woodburn A, et al: Indices of Inflammatory Activity. Ann. of the Rheum. Dis. **29**:643–648, 1970.
7. Cohen A: Fecal Blood Loss and Plasma Salicylate Study of Salicylsalicylic Acid and Aspirin. J. Clin. Pharmacol. **19**:242–247, 1979.
8. Chudwin DS, Strub M, Golden HE, et al: Sensitivity to Non-Acetylated Salicylates in a Patient with Asthma, Nasal Polyps, and Rheumatoid Arthritis. Annals of Allergy **57**:133–134, 1986.
9. Spector SL, Wangaard CH, Farr RS: Aspirin and Concomitant Idiosyncrasies in Adult Asthmatic Patients. J. Allergy Clin. Immunol. **64**:500–506, 1979.
10. Stevenson DD, Schrank PJ, Hougham AJ, et al: Salsalate Cross Sensitivity in Aspirin-Sensitive Asthmatics. J. Allergy Clin. Immunol. **81**:181, 1988.

DSD-18 June 1991
Shown in Product Identification Section, page 416

DUO-MEDIHALER™ ℞

(isoproterenol hydrochloride and phenylephrine bitartrate)
Inhalation Aerosol

DESCRIPTION

DUO-MEDIHALER (isoproterenol hydrochloride and phenylephrine bitartrate) is an aerosol device which delivers micronized particles of isoproterenol hydrochloride and phenylephrine bitartrate. Also contains: cetylpyridinium chloride, dichlorodifluoromethane, dichlorotetrafluoroethane, sorbitan trioleate, and trichloromonofluoromethane. This drug-propellant system is contained in a hermetically sealed metal vial. Each valve actuation releases a uniform aerosolized dose of 0.16 mg. isoproterenol hydrochloride and 0.24 mg. phenylephrine bitartrate.

HOW SUPPLIED

DUO-MEDIHALER with adapter (300 doses, 15 ml.) NDC **0089-0735-21.**
DUO-MEDIHALER refill (300 doses, 15 ml.) NDC **0089-0735-11.**

MAXAIR™ Inhaler ℞

(pirbuterol acetate inhalation aerosol)
Bronchodilator Aerosol
For Inhalation Only

DESCRIPTION

The active component of MAXAIR Inhaler is α^6-{[(1,1-dimethylethyl)amino]methyl}-3-hydroxy-2,6-pyridinedimethanol monoacetate salt having the following chemical structure:

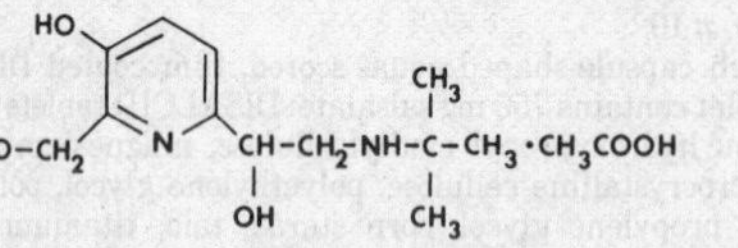

MAXAIR (pirbuterol acetate) is a white, crystalline powder, freely soluble in water, with a molecular weight of 300.3 and empirical formula of $C_{12}H_{20}N_2O_3 \cdot C_2H_4O_2$.
MAXAIR Inhaler is a metered dose aerosol unit for oral inhalation. It provides a fine-particle suspension of pirbuterol acetate in the propellant mixture of trichloromonofluoromethane and dichlorodifluoromethane, with sorbitan trioleate. Each actuation delivers from the mouthpiece pirbuterol acetate equivalent to 0.2 mg of pirbuterol with the majority of particles less than 5 microns in diameter. Each canister provides at least 300 inhalations.

CLINICAL PHARMACOLOGY

In vitro studies and *in vivo* pharmacologic studies have demonstrated that MAXAIR has a preferential effect on beta-2 adrenergic receptors compared with isoproterenol. While it is recognized that beta-2 adrenergic receptors are the predominant receptors in bronchial smooth mucle, recent data indicate that there is a population of beta-2 receptors in the human heart, existing in a concentration between 10–50%. The precise function of these, however, is not yet established (see WARNINGS section).
The pharmacologic effects of beta adrenergic agonist drugs, including MAXAIR, are at least in part attributable to stimulation through beta adrenergic receptors of intracellular adenyl cyclase, the enzyme which catalyzes the conversion of adenosine triphosphate (ATP) to cyclic-3′,5′-adenosine monophosphate (c-AMP). Increased c-AMP levels are associated with relaxation of bronchial smooth muscle and inhibition of release of mediators of immediate hypersensitivity from cells, especially from mast cells.
Bronchodilator activity of MAXAIR was manifested clinically by an improvement in various pulmonary function parameters (FEV_1, MMF, PEFR, airway resistance [RAW] and conductance [GA/V_{tg}]).
In controlled double-blind single dose clinical trials, the onset of improvement in pulmonary function occurred within 5 minutes in most patients as determined by forced expiratory volume in one second (FEV_1). FEV_1 and MMF measurements also showed that maximum improvement in pulmonary function generally occurred 30–60 minutes following one (1) or two (2) inhalations of pirbuterol (0.2–0.4 mg). The duration of action of MAXAIR is maintained for 5 hours (the time at which the last observations were made) in a substantial number of patients, based on a 15% or greater increase in FEV_1. In controlled repetitive dose studies of 12 weeks duration, 74% of 156 patients on pirbuterol and 62% of 141 patients on metaproterenol showed a clinically significant improvement based on a 15% or greater increase in FEV_1 on at least half of the days. Onset and duration were equivalent to that seen in single dose studies. Continued effectiveness was demonstrated over the 12-week period in the majority (94%) of responding patients; however, chronic dosing was associated with the development of tachyphylaxis (tolerance) to the bronchodilator effect in some patients in both treatment groups.
A placebo-controlled double-blind single dose study (24 patients per treatment group), utilizing continuous Holter monitoring for 5 hours after drug administration, showed no significant difference in ectopic activity between the placebo control group and MAXAIR at the recommended dose (0.2–0.4 mg), and twice the recommended dose (0.8 mg). As with other inhaled beta adrenergic agonists, supraventricular and ventricular ectopic beats have been seen with MAXAIR (see WARNINGS).
Recent studies in laboratory animals (minipigs, rodents, and dogs) recorded the occurrence of cardiac arrhythmias and sudden death (with histologic evidence of myocardial necrosis) when beta agonists and methylxanthines were administered concurrently. The significance of these findings when applied to humans is currently unknown.

Pharmacokinetics
As expected by extrapolation from oral data, systemic blood levels of pirbuterol are below the limit of assay sensitivity (2–5 ng/ml) following inhalation of doses up to 0.8 mg (twice the maximum recommended dose). A mean of 51% of the dose is recovered in urine as pirbuterol plus its sulfate conjugate following administration by aerosol. Pirbuterol is not metabolized by catechol-O-methyltransferase. The percent of administered dose recovered as pirbuterol plus its sulfate conjugate does not change significantly over the dose range of 0.4 mg to 0.8 mg and is not significantly different from that after oral administration of pirbuterol. The plasma half-life measured after oral administration is about two hours.

INDICATIONS AND USAGE

MAXAIR Inhaler is indicated for the prevention and reversal of bronchospasm in patients with reversible bronchospasm including asthma. It may be used with or without concurrent theophylline and/or steroid therapy.

CONTRAINDICATIONS

MAXAIR is contraindicated in patients with a history of hypersensitivity to any of its ingredients.

WARNINGS

As with other beta adrenergic aerosols, MAXAIR should not be used in excess. Controlled clinical studies and other clinical experience have shown that MAXAIR like other inhaled beta adrenergic agonists can produce a significant cardiovascular effect in some patients, as measured by pulse rate, blood pressure, symptoms, and/or ECG changes. As with other beta adrenergic aerosols, the potential for paradoxical bronchospasm (which can be life threatening) should be kept in mind. If it occurs, the preparation should be discontinued immediately and alternative therapy instituted.
Fatalities have been reported in association with excessive use of inhaled sympathomimetic drugs.
The contents of MAXAIR Inhaler are under pressure. Do not puncture. Do not use or store near heat or open flame. Exposure to temperature above 120°F may cause bursting. Never throw container into fire or incinerator. Keep out of reach of children.

PRECAUTIONS

General
Since pirbuterol is a sympathomimetic amine, it should be used with caution in patients with cardiovascular disorders, including ischemic heart disease, hypertension, or cardiac arrhythmias, in patients with hyperthyroidism or diabetes mellitus, and in patients who are unusually responsive to sympathomimetic amines or who have convulsive disorders. Significant changes in systolic and diastolic blood pressure could be expected to occur in some patients after use of any beta adrenergic aerosol bronchodilator.

Information for Patients
MAXAIR effects may last up to five hours or longer. It should not be used more often than recommended and the patient should not increase the number of inhalations or frequency of use without first asking the physician. If symptoms of asthma get worse, adverse reactions occur, or the patient does not respond to the usual dose, the patient should be instructed to contact the physician immediately. The patient should be advised to see the Illustrated Directions for Use.

Drug Interactions
Other beta adrenergic aerosol bronchodilators should not be used concomitantly with MAXAIR because they may have additive effects. Beta adrenergic agonists should be administered with caution to patients being treated with monoamine oxidase inhibitors or tricyclic antidepressants, since the action of beta adrenergic agonists on the vascular system may be potentiated.

Carcinogenesis, Mutagenesis and Impairment of Fertility
Pirbuterol hydrochloride administered in the diet to rats for 24 months and to mice for 18 months was free of carcinogenic activity at doses corresponding to 200 times the maximum human inhalation dose. In addition, the intragastric intubation of the drug at doses corresponding to 6250 times the maximum recommended human daily inhalation dose resulted in no increase in tumors in a 12-month rat study. Studies with pirbuterol revealed no evidence of mutagenesis. Reproduction studies in rats revealed no evidence of impaired fertility.

Teratogenic Effects—Pregnancy Category C
Reproduction studies have been performed in rats and rabbits by the inhalation route at doses up to 12 times (rat) and 16 times (rabbit) the maximum human inhalation dose and have revealed no significant findings. Animal reproduction studies in rats at *oral doses* up to 300 mg/kg and in rabbits at oral doses up to 100 mg/kg have shown no adverse effect on reproductive behavior, fertility, litter size, peri- and postna-

tal viability or fetal development. In rabbits at the highest dose level given, 300 mg/kg, abortions and fetal mortality were observed. There are no adequate and well controlled studies in pregnant women and MAXAIR should be used during pregnancy only if the potential benefit justifies the potential risk to the fetus.

Nursing Mothers

It is not known whether MAXAIR is excreted in human milk. Therefore, MAXAIR should be used during nursing only if the potential benefit justifies the possible risk to the newborn.

Pediatric Use

MAXAIR Inhaler is not recommended for patients under the age of 12 years because of insufficient clinical data to establish safety and effectiveness.

ADVERSE REACTIONS

The following rates of adverse reactions to pirbuterol are based on single and multiple dose clinical trials involving 761 patients, 400 of whom received multiple doses (mean duration of treatment was 2.5 months and maximum was 19 months).

The following were the adverse reactions reported more frequently than 1 in 100 patients:

CNS: nervousness (6.9%), tremor (6.0%), headache (2.0%), dizziness (1.2%).

Cardiovascular: palpitations (1.7%), tachycardia (1.2%).

Respiratory: cough (1.2%).

Gastrointestinal: nausea (1.7%).

The following adverse reactions occurred less frequently than 1 in 100 patients and there may be a causal relationship with pirbuterol:

CNS: depression, anxiety, confusion, insomnia, weakness, hyperkinesia, syncope.

Cardiovascular: hypotension, skipped beats, chest pain.

Gastrointestinal: dry mouth, glossitis, abdominal pain/cramps, anorexia, diarrhea, stomatitis, nausea and vomiting.

Ear, Nose and Throat: smell/taste changes, sore throat.

Dermatological: rash, pruritus.

Other: numbness in extremities, alopecia, bruising, fatigue, edema, weight gain, flushing.

Other adverse reactions were reported with a frequency of less than 1 in 100 patients but a causal relationship between pirbuterol and the reaction could not be determined: migraine, productive cough, wheezing, and dermatitis.

The following rates of adverse reactions during three-month controlled clinical trials involving 310 patients are noted. The table does not include mild reactions.

PERCENT OF PATIENTS WITH MODERATE TO SEVERE ADVERSE REACTIONS

Reaction	Pirbuterol N=157	Metaproterenol N=153
Central Nervous System		
tremors	1.3%	3.3%
nervousness	4.5%	2.6%
headache	1.3%	2.0%
weakness	.0%	1.3%
drowsiness	.0%	0.7%
dizziness	0.6%	.0%
Cardiovascular		
palpitations	1.3%	1.3%
tachycardia	1.3%	2.0%
Respiratory		
chest pain/tightness	1.3%	.0%
cough	.0%	0.7%
Gastrointestinal		
nausea	1.3%	2.0%
diarrhea	1.3%	0.7%
dry mouth	1.3%	1.3%
vomiting	.0%	0.7%
Dermatological		
skin reaction	.0%	0.7%
rash	.0%	1.3%
Other		
bruising	0.6%	.0%
smell/taste change	0.6%	.0%
backache	.0%	0.7%
fatigue	.0%	0.7%
hoarseness	.0%	0.7%
nasal congestion	.0%	0.7%

OVERDOSAGE

The expected symptoms with overdosage are those of excessive beta-stimulation and/or any of the symptoms listed under adverse reactions, e.g., angina, hypertension or hypotension, arrhythmias, nervousness, headache, tremor, dry mouth, palpitation, nausea, dizziness, fatigue, malaise, and insomnia.

Treatment consists of discontinuation of pirbuterol together with appropriate symptomatic therapy.

The oral acute lethal dose in male and female rats and mice was greater than 2000 mg base/kg. The aerosol acute lethal dose was not determined.

DOSAGE AND ADMINISTRATION

The usual dose for adults and children 12 years and older is two inhalations (0.4 mg) repeated every 4–6 hours. One inhalation (0.2 mg) repeated every 4–6 hours may be sufficient for some patients.

A total daily dose of 12 inhalations should not be exceeded. If a previously effective dosage regimen fails to provide the usual relief, medical advice should be sought immediately as this is often a sign of seriously worsening asthma which would require reassessment of therapy.

HOW SUPPLIED

MAXAIR Inhaler is supplied in a pressurized aluminum canister with plastic actuator. Each actuation delivers pirbuterol acetate equivalent to 0.2 mg of pirbuterol from the mouthpiece.

Net content weight 25.6 g, a minimum of 300 actuations (NDC **0089-0790-21**).

CAUTION

Federal law prohibits dispensing without prescription.

Store between 15° and 30°C (59° to 86°F).

PIR-5 April 1991

Shown in Product Identification Section, page 416

MEDIHALER-EPI™ OTC

(epinephrine bitartrate)

FOR TEMPORARY RELIEF FROM ACUTE PAROXYSMS OF BRONCHIAL ASTHMA

FOR ORAL INHALATION THERAPY ONLY

Each inhalation delivers 0.3 mg epinephrine bitartrate equivalent to 0.16 mg of epinephrine base. Also contains: cetylpyridinium chloride, dichlorodifluoromethane, dichlorotetrafluoroethane, sorbitan trioleate, and trichloromonofluoromethane.

HOW SUPPLIED

15 ml size: Available as a combination package (vial with oral adapter) or as a refill (vial only).

MEDIHALER-ISO™ ℞

(isoproterenol sulfate)

Inhalation Aerosol

DESCRIPTION

Medihaler-Iso (isoproterenol sulfate) is an aerosol device which contains a fine particle suspension of 2.0 mg per ml isoproterenol sulfate. Also contains: dichlorodifluoromethane, dichlorotetrafluoroethane, sorbitan trioleate, and trichloromonofluoromethane. Each depression of the valve delivers a measured dose of 0.08 mg isoproterenol sulfate.

HOW SUPPLIED

15-ml vial with oral adapter (300 doses). NDC **0089-0785-21**.
15-ml refill vial only (300 doses). NDC **0089-0785-11**.

MINITRAN™ ℞

(nitroglycerin)

Transdermal Delivery System

DESCRIPTION

Nitroglycerin is a 1,2,3-propanetriol trinitrate, an organic nitrate whose structural formula is

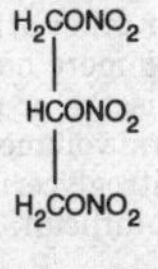

and whose molecular weight is 227.09. The organic nitrates are vasodilators, active on both arteries and veins.

The MINITRAN (nitroglycerin) Transdermal Delivery System is a unit designed to provide continuous controlled release of nitroglycerin through intact skin. The rate of release of nitroglycerin is linearly dependent upon the area of the applied system; each cm^2 of applied system delivers approximately 0.03 mg of nitroglycerin per hour. Thus, the 3.3, 6.7, 13.3 and 20 cm^2 system delivers approximately 0.1, 0.2, 0.4 and 0.6 mg of nitroglycerin per hour, respectively.

The remainder of the nitroglycerin in each system serves as a reservoir and is not delivered in normal use. After 12 hours, for example, each system has delivered about 14% of its original content of nitroglycerin.

The MINITRAN Transdermal Delivery System contains nitroglycerin in a hypoallergenic, medical grade, acrylate-based polymer adhesive. Each patch is packaged in foil/polymer film laminate.

Prior to use, a protective peel strip is removed from the adhesive surface. Following use, the patch should be discarded in a manner that prevents accidental application or ingestion by children or others.

CLINICAL PHARMACOLOGY

The principal pharmacological action of nitroglycerin is relaxation of the vascular smooth muscle and consequent dilatation of peripheral arteries and veins, especially the latter. Dilatation of the veins promotes peripheral pooling of blood and decreases venous return to the heart, thereby reducing left ventricular end-diastolic pressure and pulmonary capillary wedge pressure (preload). Arteriolar relaxation reduces systemic vascular resistance, systolic arterial pressure, and mean arterial pressure (afterload). Dilatation of the coronary arteries also occurs. The relative importance of preload reduction, afterload reduction, and coronary dilatation remains undefined.

Dosing regimens for most chronically used drugs are designed to provide plasma concentrations that are continuously greater than a minimally effective concentration. This strategy is inappropriate for organic nitrates. Several well-controlled clinical trials have used exercise testing to assess the anti-anginal efficacy of continouously-delivered nitrates. In the large majority of these trials, active agents were indistinguishable from placebo after 24 hours (or less) of continuous therapy. Attempts to overcome nitrate tolerance by dose escalation, even to doses far in excess of those used acutely, have consistently failed. Only after nitrates have been absent from the body for several hours has their anti-anginal efficacy been restored.

Pharmacokinetics: The volume of distribution of nitroglycerin is about 3 L/kg, and nitroglycerin is cleared from this volume at extremely rapid rates, with a resulting serum half-life of about 3 minutes. The observed clearance rates (close to 1 L/kg/min) greatly exceed hepatic blood flow; known sites of extrahepatic metabolism include red blood cells and vascular walls.

The first products in the metabolism of nitroglycerin are inorganic nitrate and the 1,2- and 1,3-dinitroglycerols. The dinitrates are less effective vasodilators than nitroglycerin, but they are longer-lived in the serum, and their net contribution to the overall effect of chronic nitroglycerin regimens is not known. The dinitrates are further metabolized to (non-vasoactive) mononitrates and, ultimately, to glycerol and carbon dioxide.

To avoid development of tolerance to nitroglycerin, drug-free intervals of 10–12 hours are known to be sufficient; shorter intervals have not been well studied. In one well-controlled clinical trial, subjects receiving nitroglycerin appeared to exhibit a rebound or withdrawal effect, so that their exercise tolerance at the end of the daily drug-free interval was less than that exhibited by the parallel group receiving placebo.

In healthy volunteers, steady-state plasma concentrations of nitroglycerin are reached by about two hours after application of a patch and are maintained for the duration of wearing the system (observations have been limited to 24 hours). Upon removal of the patch, the plasma concentration declines with a half-life of about an hour.

Clinical Trials: Regimens in which nitroglycerin patches were worn for 12 hours daily have been studied in well-controlled trials up to 4 weeks in duration. Starting about 2 hours after application and continuing until 10–12 hours after application, patches that deliver at least 0.4 mg of nitroglycerin per hour have consistently demonstrated greater anti-anginal activity than placebo. Lower-dose patches have not been as well studied, but in one large, well-controlled trial in which higher-dose patches were also studied, patches delivering 0.2 mg/hr had significantly less anti-anginal activity than placebo.

It is reasonable to believe that the rate of nitroglycerin absorption from patches may vary with the site of application, but this relationship has not been adequately studied.

The onset of action of transdermal nitroglycerin is not sufficiently rapid for this product to be useful in aborting an acute anginal episode.

INDICATIONS AND USAGE

This drug product has been conditionally approved by the FDA for the prevention of angina pectoris due to coronary artery disease. Tolerance to the anti-anginal effects of nitrates (measured by exercise stress testing) has been shown to be a major factor limiting efficacy when transdermal nitrates are used continuously for longer than 12 hours each day. The development of tolerance can be altered (prevented or attenuated) by use of a noncontinuous (intermittent) dosing schedule with a nitrate-free interval of 10–12 hours.

Controlled clinical trial data suggest that the intermittent use of nitrates is associated with decreased exercise tolerance, in comparison to placebo, during the last part of the nitrate-free interval; the clinical relevance of this observation is unknown, but the possibility of increased frequency or severity of angina during the nitrate-free interval should be considered. Further investigations of

Continued on next page

3M—Cont.

the tolerance phenomenon and best regimen are ongoing. A final evaluation of the effectiveness of the product will be announced by the FDA.

CONTRAINDICATIONS

Allergic reactions to organic nitrates are extremely rare, but they do occur. Nitroglycerin is contraindicated in patients who are allergic to it. Allergy to the adhesives used in nitroglycerin patches has also been reported, and it similarly constitutes a contraindication to the use of this product.

WARNINGS

The benefits of transdermal nitroglycerin in patients with acute myocardial infarction or congestive heart failure have not been established. If one elects to use nitroglycerin in these conditions, careful clinical or hemodynamic monitoring must be used to avoid the hazards of hypotension and tachycardia.

A cardiovertor/defibrillator should not be discharged through a paddle electrode that overlies a MINITRAN patch. The arcing that may be seen in this situation is harmless in itself, but it may be associated with local current concentration that can cause damage to the paddles and burns to the patient.

PRECAUTIONS

General: Severe hypotension, particularly with upright posture, may occur with even small doses of nitroglycerin. This drug should therefore be used with caution in patients who may be volume depleted or who, for whatever reason, are already hypotensive. Hypotension induced by nitroglycerin may be accompanied by paradoxical bradycardia and increased angina pectoris.

Nitrate therapy may aggravate the angina caused by hypertrophic cardiomyopathy.

As tolerance to other forms of nitroglycerin develops, the effect of sublingual nitroglycerin on exercise tolerance, although still observable, is somewhat blunted.

In industrial workers who have had long-term exposure to unknown (presumably high) doses of organic nitrates, tolerance clearly occurs. Chest pain, acute myocardial infarction, and even sudden death have occurred during temporary withdrawal of nitrates from these workers, demonstrating the existence of true physical dependence.

Several clinical trials in patients with angina pectoris have evaluated nitroglycerin regimens which incorporated a 10–12 hour nitrate-free interval. In some of these trials, an increase in the frequency of anginal attacks during the nitrate-free interval was observed in a small number of patients. In one trial, patients demonstrated decreased exercise tolerance at the end of the nitrate-free interval. Hemodynamic rebound has been observed only rarely; on the other hand, few studies were so designed that rebound, if it had occurred, would have been detected. The importance of these observations to the routine, clinical use of transdermal nitroglycerin is unknown.

Information for Patients: Daily headaches sometimes accompany treatment with nitroglycerin. In patients who get these headaches, the headaches may be a marker of the activity of the drug. Patients should resist the temptation to avoid headaches by altering the schedule of their treatment with nitroglycerin, since loss of headache may be associated with simultaneous loss of anti-anginal efficacy.

Treatment with nitroglycerin may be associated with lightheadedness on standing, especially just after rising from a recumbent or seated position. This effect may be more frequent in patients who have also consumed alcohol.

After normal use, there is enough residual nitroglycerin in discarded patches that they are a potential hazard to children and pets.

A patient leaflet is supplied with the systems.

Drug Interactions: The vasodilating effects of nitroglycerin may be additive with those of other vasodilators. Alcohol, in particular, has been found to exhibit additive effects of this variety.

Carcinogenesis, Mutagenesis, and Impairment of Fertility: No long-term animal studies have examined the carcinogenic or mutagenic potential of nitroglycerin. Nitroglycerin's effect upon reproductive capacity is similarly unknown.

Pregnancy Category C: Animal reproduction studies have not been conducted on nitroglycerin. It is also not known whether nitroglycerin can cause fetal harm when administered to a pregnant woman or whether it can affect reproductive capacity. Nitroglycerin should be given to a pregnant woman only if clearly needed.

Nursing Mothers: It is not known whether nitroglycerin is excreted in human milk. Because many drugs are excreted in human milk, caution should be exercised when nitroglycerin is administered to a nursing woman.

Pediatric Use: Safety and effectiveness in children have not been established.

ADVERSE REACTIONS

Adverse reactions to nitroglycerin are generally dose-related, and almost all of these reactions are the result of nitroglycerin's activity as a vasodilator. Headache, which may be severe, is the most commonly reported side effect. Headache may be recurrent with each daily dose, especially at higher doses. Transient episodes of lightheadedness, occasionally related to blood pressure changes, may also occur. Hypotension occurs infrequently, but in some patients it may be severe enough to warrant discontinuation of therapy. Syncope, crescendo angina, and rebound hypotension have been reported but are uncommon.

Extremely rarely, ordinary doses of organic nitrates have caused methemoglobinemia in normal-seeming patients. Methemoglobinemia is so infrequent at these doses that further discussion of its diagnosis and treatment is deferred (see **Overdosage**).

Application-site irritation may occur but is rarely severe.

In two placebo-controlled trials of intermittent therapy with nitroglycerin patches at 0.2 to 0.8 mg/hr, the most frequent adverse reactions among 307 subjects were as follows:

	placebo	patch
headache	18%	63%
lightheadedness	4%	6%
hypotension and/or syncope	0%	4%
increased angina	2%	2%

OVERDOSAGE

Hemodynamic Effects: The ill effects of nitroglycerin overdose are generally the results of nitroglycerin's capacity to induce vasodilatation, venous pooling, reduced cardiac output, and hypotension. These hemodynamic changes may have protean manifestations, including increased intracranial pressure, with any or all of persistent throbbing headache, confusion, and moderate fever; vertigo; palpitations; visual disturbances; nausea and vomiting (possibly with colic and even bloody diarrhea); syncope (especially in the upright posture); air hunger and dyspnea, later followed by reduced ventilatory effort; diaphoresis, with the skin either flushed or cold and clammy; heart block and bradycardia; paralysis; coma; seizures; and death.

Laboratory determinations of serum levels of nitroglycerin and its metabolites are not widely available, and such determinations have, in any event, no established role in the management of nitroglycerin overdose.

No data are available to suggest physiological maneuvers (e.g., maneuvers to change the pH of the urine) that might accelerate elimination of nitroglycerin and its active metabolites. Similarly, it is not known which—if any—of these substances can usefully be removed from the body by hemodialysis.

No specific antagonist to the vasodilator effects of nitroglycerin is known, and no intervention has been subject to controlled study as a therapy of nitroglycerin overdose. Because the hypotension associated with nitroglycerin overdose is the result of venodilatation and arterial hypovolemia, prudent therapy in this situation should be directed toward increase in central fluid volume. Passive elevation of the patient's legs may be sufficient, but intravenous infusion of normal saline or similar fluid may also be necessary.

The use of epinephrine or other arterial vasoconstrictors in this setting is likely to do more harm than good.

In patients with renal disease or congestive heart failure, therapy resulting in central volume expansion is not without hazard. Treatment of nitroglycerin overdose in these patients may be subtle and difficult, and invasive monitoring may be required.

Methemoglobinemia: Nitrate ions liberated during metabolism of nitroglycerin can oxidize hemoglobin into methemoglobin. Even in patients totally without cytochrome b_5 reductase activity, however, and even assuming that nitrate moieties of nitroglycerin are quantitatively applied to oxidation of hemoglobin, about 1 mg/kg of nitroglycerin should be required before any of these patients manifests clinically significant ($\geq 10\%$) methemoglobinemia. In patients with normal reductase function, significant production of methemoglobin should require even larger doses of nitroglycerin. In one study in which 36 patients received 2–4 weeks of continuous nitroglycerin therapy at 3.1 to 4.4 mg/hr, the average methemoglobin level measured was 0.2%; this was comparable to that observed in parallel patients who received placebo.

Notwithstanding these observations, there are case reports of significant methemoglobinemia in association with moderate overdoses of organic nitrates. None of the affected patients had been thought to be unusually susceptible.

Methemoglobin levels are available from most clinical laboratories. The diagnosis should be suspected in patients who exhibit signs of impaired oxygen delivery despite adequate cardiac output and adequate arterial pO_2. Classically, methemoglobinemic blood is described as chocolate brown, without color change on exposure to air.

When methemoglobinemia is diagnosed, the treatment of choice is methylene blue, 1–2 mg/kg intravenously.

DOSAGE AND ADMINISTRATION

The suggested starting dose is between 0.2 mg/hr* and 0.4 mg/hr*. Doses between 0.4 mg/hr* and 0.8 mg/hr* have shown continued effectiveness for 10–12 hours daily for at least one month (the longest period studied) of intermittent administration. Although the minimum nitrate-free interval has not been defined, data show that a nitrate-free interval of 10–12 hours is sufficient (see **Clinical Pharmacology**). Thus, an appropriate dosing schedule for nitroglycerin patches would include a daily patch-on period of 12–14 hours and a daily patch-off period of 10–12 hours.

Although some well-controlled clinical trials using exercise tolerance testing have shown maintenance of effectiveness when patches are worn continuously, the large majority of such controlled trials have shown the development of tolerance (i.e., complete loss of effect) within the first 24 hours after therapy was initiated. Dose adjustment, even to levels much higher than generally used, did not restore efficacy.

HOW SUPPLIED

[See table below.]

MINITRAN Transdermal Delivery System, 0.1 mg/hr, 0.2 mg/hr, 0.4 mg/hr, 0.6 mg/hr, is available in cartons of 33 patches.

STORAGE CONDITIONS

Store at controlled room temperature 15°–30°C (59°–86°F). Extremes of temperature and/or humidity should be avoided.

CAUTION

Federal law prohibits dispensing without prescription.

* Release rates were formerly described in terms of drug delivered per 24 hours. In these terms, the supplied MINITRAN systems would be rated at 2.5 mg/24 hours (0.1 mg/hr), 5 mg/24 hours (0.2 mg/hr), 10 mg/24 hours (0.4 mg/hr), and 15 mg/24 hours (0.6 mg/hr).

NTR-6 JUNE 1991

3M Pharmaceuticals
Northridge, CA 91324

Shown in Product Identification Section, page 416

NORFLEX™ ℞
(orphenadrine citrate)
Tablets and Injection

PRODUCT OVERVIEW

KEY FACTS

Norflex sustained-release tablets provide 12 hours relief from the pain of muscle spasm. Also available in injectable form, IV or IM, also given every 12 hours.

MAJOR USES

Norflex is indicated as an adjunct to rest, physical therapy, and other measures for the relief of discomfort associated with painful musculoskeletal disorders.

SAFETY INFORMATION

Contraindicated in patients with glaucoma, pyloric or duodenal obstruction, stenosing peptic ulcers, prostatic hypertrophy or obstruction of the bladder neck, cardiospasm (megaesophagus) and myasthenia gravis. Contraindicated in patients who have a previous sensitivity to the drug.

PRESCRIBING INFORMATION

NORFLEX™ ℞
(orphenadrine citrate)
Tablets and Injection

DESCRIPTION

Orphenadrine citrate is the citrate salt of orphenadrine (2-dimethylaminoethyl 2-methylbenzhydryl ether citrate). It occurs as a white, crystalline powder having a bitter taste. It is practically odorless; sparingly soluble in water, slightly soluble in alcohol.

Each Norflex Tablet contains 100 mg orphenadrine citrate. Norflex Tablets also contain: calcium stearate, ethylcellulose, and lactose. Norflex Injection contains 60 mg of orphen-

MINITRAN System Rated Release In Vivo	System Size	Total Nitroglycerin in System	NDC Number
0.1 mg/hr*	3.3 cm^2	9 mg	NDC-0089-0301-03
0.2 mg/hr*	6.7 cm^2	18 mg	NDC-0089-0302-03
0.4 mg/hr*	13.3 cm^2	36 mg	NDC-0089-0303-03
0.6 mg/hr*	20.0 cm^2	54 mg	NDC-0089-0304-03

adrine citrate in aqueous solution in each ampul. Norflex Injection also contains: sodium bisulfite NF, 2.0 mg; sodium chloride USP, 5.8 mg; sodium hydroxide, to adjust pH; and water for injection USP, q.s. to 2 mL.

ACTIONS

The mode of therapeutic action has not been clearly identified, but may be related to its analgesic properties. Orphenadrine citrate also possesses anticholinergic actions.

INDICATIONS

Orphenadrine citrate is indicated as an adjunct to rest, physical therapy, and other measures for the relief of discomfort associated with acute painful musculoskeletal conditions. The mode of action of the drug has not been clearly identified, but may be related to its analgesic properties. Orphenadrine citrate does not directly relax tense skeletal muscles in man.

CONTRAINDICATIONS

Contraindicated in patients with glaucoma, pyloric or duodenal obstruction, stenosing peptic ulcers, prostatic hypertrophy or obstruction of the bladder neck, cardio-spasm (megaesophagus) and myasthenia gravis. Contraindicated in patients who have demonstrated a previous hypersensitivity to the drug.

WARNINGS

Some patients may experience transient episodes of lightheadedness, dizziness or syncope. Norflex may impair the ability of the patient to engage in potentially hazardous activities such as operating machinery or driving a motor vehicle; ambulatory patients should therefore be cautioned accordingly.

Norflex Injection contains sodium bisulfite, a sulfite that may cause allergic-type reactions including anaphylactic symptoms and life-threatening or less severe asthmatic episodes in certain susceptible people. The overall prevalence of sulfite sensitivity in the general population is unknown and probably low. Sulfite sensitivity is seen more frequently in asthmatic than nonasthmatic people.

PREGNANCY

Pregnancy Category C. Animal reproduction studies have not been conducted with Norflex. It is also not known whether Norflex can cause fetal harm when administered to a pregnant woman or can affect reproduction capacity. Norflex should be given to a pregnant woman only if clearly needed.

USAGE IN CHILDREN

Safety and effectiveness in children have not been established; therefore, this drug is not recommended for use in the pediatric age group.

PRECAUTIONS

Confusion, anxiety and tremors have been reported in a few patients receiving propoxyphene and orphenadrine concomitantly. As these symptoms may be simply due to an additive effect, reduction of dosage and/or discontinuation of one or both agents is recommended in such cases.

Orphenadrine citrate should be used with caution in patients with tachycardia, cardiac decompensation, coronary insufficiency, cardiac arrhythmias.

Safety of continuous long-term therapy with orphenadrine has not been established. Therefore, if orphenadrine is prescribed for prolonged use, periodic monitoring of blood, urine and liver function values is recommended.

ADVERSE REACTIONS

Adverse reactions of orphenadrine are mainly due to the mild anticholinergic action of orphenadrine, and are usually associated with higher dosage. Dryness of the mouth is usually the first adverse effect to appear. When the daily dose is increased, possible adverse effects include: tachycardia, palpitation, urinary hesitancy or retention, blurred vision, dilatation of pupils, increased ocular tension, weakness, nausea, vomiting, headache, dizziness, constipation, drowsiness, hypersensitivity reactions, pruritus, hallucinations, agitation, tremor, gastric irritation, and rarely urticaria and other dermatoses. Infrequently, an elderly patient may experience some degree of mental confusion. These adverse reactions can usually be eliminated by reduction in dosage. Very rare cases of aplastic anemia associated with the use of orphenadrine tablets have been reported. No causal relationship has been established.

Rare instances of anaphylactic reaction have been reported associated with the intramuscular injection of Norflex Injection.

DOSAGE AND ADMINISTRATION

TABLETS: Adults—Two tablets per day; one in the morning and one in the evening.

INJECTION: Adults—One 2 mL ampul (60 mg) intravenously or intramuscularly; may be repeated every 12 hours. Relief may be maintained by 1 Norflex tablet twice daily.

HOW SUPPLIED

TABLETS: Each round, white tablet imprinted with "3M" on one side and "221" on the other. Bottles of 100 (NDC **0089-0221-10**) and 500 (NDC **0089-0221-50**). Boxes of 100 in unit dose, aluminum foil strips (NDC **0089-0221-16**). Each tablet contains 100 mg of orphenadrine citrate.

INJECTION: Boxes of 6 (NDC **0089-0540-06**) and 50 (NDC **0089-0540-50**) 2 mL ampuls, each ampul containing 60 mg of orphenadrine citrate in aqueous solution.

A.H.F.S. Category 12:08

Store at controlled room temperature, 15°–30°C (59°–86°F).

CAUTION

Federal law prohibits dispensing without prescription.

NRF-14 January 1992

Shown in Product Identification Section, page 416

NORGESIC™ ℞
and
NORGESIC™ FORTE ℞
Tablets

ACTIONS

Orphenadrine citrate is a centrally acting (brain stem) compound which in animals selectively blocks facilitatory functions of the reticular formation. Orphenadrine does not produce myoneural block, nor does it affect crossed extensor reflexes. Orphenadrine prevents nicotine-induced convulsions but not those produced by strychnine.

Chronic administration of Norgesic to dogs and rats has revealed no drug-related toxicity. No blood or urine changes were observed, nor were there any macroscopic or microscopic pathological changes detected. Extensive experience with combinations containing aspirin and caffeine has established them as safe agents. The addition of orphenadrine citrate does not alter the toxicity of aspirin and caffeine.

The mode of therapeutic action of orphenadrine has not been clearly identified, but may be related to its analgesic properties. Orphenadrine citrate also possesses anticholinergic actions.

INDICATIONS

1. Symptomatic relief of mild to moderate pain of acute musculoskeletal disorders.
2. The orphenadrine component is indicated as an adjunct to rest, physical therapy, and other measures for the relief of discomfort associated with acute painful musculoskeletal conditions.
   The mode of action of orphenadrine has not been clearly identified, but may be related to its analgesic properties. Norgesic and Norgesic Forte do not directly relax tense skeletal muscles in man.

CONTRAINDICATIONS

Because of the mild anticholinergic effect of orphenadrine, Norgesic or Norgesic Forte should not be used in patients with glaucoma, pyloric or duodenal obstruction, achalasia, prostatic hypertrophy or obstructions at the bladder neck. Norgesic or Norgesic Forte is also contraindicated in patients with myasthenia gravis and in patients known to be sensitive to aspirin or caffeine.

The drug is contraindicated in patients who have demonstrated a previous hypersensitivity to the drug.

WARNINGS

Reye Syndrome may develop in individuals who have chicken pox, influenza, or flu symptoms. Some studies suggest possible association between the development of Reye Syndrome and the use of medicines containing salicylate or aspirin. Norgesic and Norgesic Forte contain aspirin and therefore are not recommended for use in patients with chicken pox, influenza, or flu symptoms.

Norgesic Forte may impair the ability of the patient to engage in potentially hazardous activities such as operating machinery or driving a motor vehicle; ambulatory patients should therefore be cautioned accordingly.

Aspirin should be used with extreme caution in the presence of peptic ulcers and coagulation abnormalities.

USAGE IN PREGNANCY

Since safety of the use of this preparation in pregnancy, during lactation, or in the childbearing age has not been established, use of the drug in such patients requires that the potential benefits of the drug be weighed against its possible hazard to the mother and child.

USAGE IN CHILDREN

The safe and effective use of this drug in children has not been established. Usage of this drug in children under 12 years of age is not recommended.

PRECAUTIONS

Confusion, anxiety and tremors have been reported in a few patients receiving propoxyphene and orphenadrine concomitantly. As these symptoms may be simply due to an additive effect, reduction of dosage and/or discontinuation of one or both agents is recommended in such cases.

Safety of continuous long term therapy with Norgesic Forte has not been established; therefore, if Norgesic Forte is prescribed for prolonged use, periodic monitoring of blood, urine and liver function values is recommended.

ADVERSE REACTIONS

Side effects of Norgesic or Norgesic Forte are those seen with aspirin and caffeine or those usually associated with mild anticholinergic agents. These may include tachycardia, palpitation, urinary hesitancy or retention, dry mouth, blurred vision, dilatation of the pupil, increased intraocular tension, weakness, nausea, vomiting, headache, dizziness, constipation, drowsiness, and rarely, urticaria and other dermatoses. Infrequently, an elderly patient may experience some degree of confusion. Mild central excitation and occasional hallucinations may be observed. These mild side effects can usually be eliminated by reduction in dosage. One case of aplastic anemia associated with the use of Norgesic has been reported. No causal relationship has been established. Rare G.I. hemorrhage due to aspirin content may be associated with the administration of Norgesic or Norgesic Forte. Some patients may experience transient episodes of light-headedness, dizziness or syncope.

DOSAGE AND ADMINISTRATION

Norgesic: Adults 1 to 2 tablets 3 to 4 times daily.

Norgesic Forte: Adults ½ to 1 tablet 3 to 4 times daily.

HOW SUPPLIED

Norgesic tablets can be identified by their three layers colored light green, white and yellow. Each round tablet contains orphenadrine citrate (2-dimethylaminoethyl 2-methylbenzhydryl ether citrate) 25 mg, aspirin 385 mg, and caffeine 30 mg.

Norgesic Forte tablets are exactly twice the strength of Norgesic. They are identified by their scored capsule shape and by their three layers colored light green, white and yellow. Each capsule shaped tablet contains orphenadrine citrate 50 mg, aspirin 770 mg, and caffeine 60 mg.

Norgesic and Norgesic Forte also contain: lactose, polyethylene glycol, povidone, starch, sucrose, zinc stearate, D&C yellow #10, and FD&C blue #1.

Norgesic: Bottles of 100 tablets (NDC **0089-0231-10**) and 500 tablets (NDC **0089-0231-50**); Boxes of 100 in unit dose, aluminum foil strips (NDC **0089-0231-16**).

Norgesic Forte: Bottles of 100 tablets (NDC **0089-0233-10**) and 500 tablets (NDC **0089-0233-50**); Boxes of 100 in unit dose, aluminum foil strips (NDC **0089-0233-16**)

Store below 30°C (86°F).

CAUTION

Federal law prohibits dispensing without prescription.

NG-13 MARCH 1991

Shown in Product Identification Section, page 416

TAMBOCOR™ ℞
[tăm-ba-kōr]
(flecainide acetate)
Oral Tablets

DESCRIPTION

TAMBOCOR (flecainide acetate) is an antiarrhythmic drug available in tablets of 50, 100 or 150 mg for oral administration.

Flecainide acetate is benzamide, N-(2-piperidinylmethyl)-2,5-bis(2,2,2-trifluoroethoxy)-, monoacetate. The structural formula is given below.

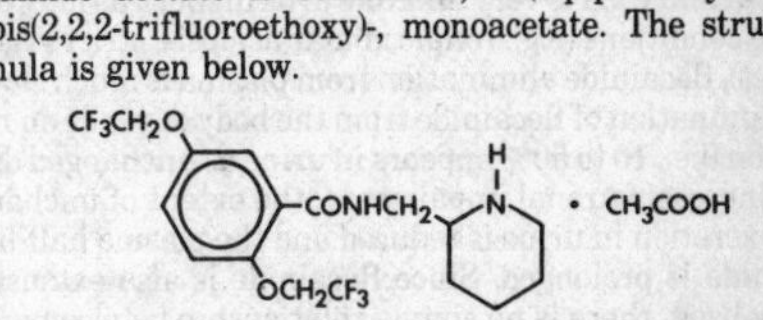
CF3CH2O
CONHCH2
H
N
• CH3COOH
OCH2CF3

Flecainide acetate is a white crystalline substance with a pK_a of 9.3. It has an aqueous solubility of 48.4 mg/mL at 37°C.

TAMBOCOR tablets also contain: croscarmellose sodium, hydrogenated vegetable oil, magnesium stearate, microcrystalline cellulose and starch.

CLINICAL PHARMACOLOGY

TAMBOCOR has local anesthetic activity and belongs to the membrane stabilizing (Class 1) group of antiarrhythmic agents; it has electrophysiologic effects characteristic of the IC class of antiarrhythmics.

Electrophysiology. In man, TAMBOCOR produces a dose-related decrease in intracardiac conduction in all parts of the heart with the greatest effect on the His-Purkinje system (H-V conduction). Effects upon atrioventricular (AV) nodal conduction time and intra-atrial conduction times, although present, are less pronounced than those on ventricular conduction velocity. Significant effects on refractory periods were observed only in the ventricle. Sinus node recovery times (corrected) following pacing and spontaneous cycle lengths are somewhat increased. This latter effect may be-

Continued on next page

3M—Cont.

come significant in patients with sinus node dysfunction. (See Warnings.)

TAMBOCOR causes a dose-related and plasma-level related decrease in single and multiple PVCs and can suppress recurrence of ventricular tachycardia. In limited studies of patients with a history of ventricular tachycardia, TAMBOCOR has been successful 30–40% of the time in fully suppressing the inducibility of arrhythmias by programmed electrical stimulation. Based on PVC suppression, it appears that plasma levels of 0.2 to 1.0 μg/mL may be needed to obtain the maximal therapeutic effect. It is more difficult to assess the dose needed to suppress serious arrhythmias, but trough plasma levels in patients successfully treated for recurrent ventricular tachycardia were between 0.2 and 1.0 μg/mL. Plasma levels above 0.7–1.0 μg/mL are associated with a higher rate of cardiac adverse experiences such as conduction defects or bradycardia. The relation of plasma levels to proarrhythmic events is not established, but dose reduction in clinical trials of patients with ventricular tachycardia appears to have led to a reduced frequency and severity of such events.

Hemodynamics. TAMBOCOR does not usually alter heart rate, although bradycardia and tachycardia have been reported occasionally.

In animals and isolated myocardium, a negative inotropic effect of flecainide has been demonstrated. Decreases in ejection fraction, consistent with a negative inotropic effect, have been observed after single administration of 200 to 250 mg of the drug in man; both increases and decreases in ejection fraction have been encountered during multidose therapy in patients at usual therapeutic dose. (See Warnings.)

Metabolism in Humans. Following oral administration, the absorption of TAMBOCOR is nearly complete. Peak plasma levels are attained at about three hours in most individuals (range, 1 to 6 hours). Flecainide does not undergo any consequential presystemic biotransformation (first-pass effect). Food or antacid do not affect absorption.

The apparent plasma half-life averages about 20 hours and is quite variable (range, 12 to 27 hours) after multiple oral doses in patients with premature ventricular contractions (PVCs). With multiple dosing, plasma levels increase because of its long half-life with steady-state levels approached in 3 to 5 days; once at steady-state, no additional (or unexpected) accumulation of drug in plasma occurs during chronic therapy. Over the usual therapeutic range, data suggest that plasma levels in an individual are approximately proportional to dose, deviating upwards from linearity only slightly (about 10 to 15% per 100 mg on average).

In healthy subjects, about 30% of a single oral dose (range, 10 to 50%) is excreted in urine as unchanged drug. The two major urinary metabolites are meta-O-dealkylated flecainide (active, but about one-fifth as potent) and the meta-O-dealkylated lactam of flecainide (non-active metabolite). These two metabolites (primarily conjugated) account for most of the remaining portion of the dose. Several minor metabolites (3% of the dose or less) are also found in urine; only 5% of an oral dose is excreted in feces. In patients, free (unconjugated) plasma levels of the two major metabolites are very low (less than 0.05 μg/mL).

When urinary pH is very alkaline (8 or higher), as may occur in rare conditions (e.g., renal tubular acidosis, strict vegetarian diet), flecainide elimination from plasma is much slower.

The elimination of flecainide from the body depends on renal function (i.e., 10 to 50% appears in urine as unchanged drug). With increasing renal impairment, the extent of unchanged drug excretion in urine is reduced and the plasma half-life of flecainide is prolonged. Since flecainide is also extensively metabolized, there is no simple relationship between creatinine clearance and the rate of flecanide elimination from plasma. (See Dosage and Administration.)

In patients with NYHA class III congestive heart failure (CFH), the rate of flecainide elimination from plasma (mean half-life, 19 hours) is moderately slower than for healthy subjects (mean half-life, 14 hours), but similar to the rate for patients with PVCs without CHF. The extent of excretion of unchanged drug in urine is also similar. (See Dosage and Administration.)

From age 20 to 80, plasma levels are only slightly higher with advancing age; flecainide elimination from plasma is somewhat slower in elderly subjects than in younger subjects. Patients up to age 80+ have been safely treated with usual dosages.

The extent of flecainide binding to human plasma proteins is about 40% and is independent of plasma drug level over the range of 0.015 to about 3.4 μg/mL. Thus, clinically significant drug interactions based on protein binding effects would not be expected.

Hemodialysis removes only about 1% of an oral dose as unchanged flecainide.

Small increases in plasma digoxin levels are seen during coadministration of TAMBOCOR with digoxin. Small increases in both flecainide and propranolol plasma levels are seen during coadministration of these two drugs. (See Precautions, Drug Interactions.)

Clinical Trials. In two randomized, crossover, placebo-controlled clinical trials of 16 weeks double-blind duration, 79% of patients with paroxysmal supraventricular tachycardia (PSVT) receiving flecainide were attack free, whereas 15% of patients receiving placebo remained attack free. The median time-before-recurrence of PSVT in patients receiving placebo was 11 to 12 days, whereas over 85% of patients receiving flecainide had no recurrence at 60 days.

In two randomized, crossover, placebo-controlled clinical trials of 16 weeks double-blind duration, 31% of patients with paroxysmal atrial fibrillation/flutter (PAF) receiving flecainide were attack free, whereas 8% receiving placebo remained attack free. The median time-before-recurrence of PAF in patients receiving placebo was about 2 to 3 days, whereas for those receiving flecainide the median time-before recurrence was 15 days.

INDICATIONS AND USAGE

In patients withou structural heart disease, TAMBOCOR is indicated for the prevention of

—paroxysmal supraventricular tachycardias (PSVT), including atrioventricular nodal reentrant tachycardia, atrioventricular reentrant tachycardia and other supraventricular tachycardias of unspecified mechanism associated with disabling symptoms

—paroxysmal atrial fibrillation/flutter (PAF) associated with disabling symptoms

TAMBOCOR is also indicated for the prevention of

—documented ventricular arrhythmias, such as sustained ventricular tachycardia (sustained VT), that in the judgment of the physician, are life-threatening.

Use of TAMBOCOR for the treatment of sustained VT, like other antiarrhythmics, should be initiated in the hospital. The use of TAMBOCOR is not recommended in patients with less severe ventricular arrhythmias even if the patients are symptomatic.

Because of the proarrhythmic effects of TAMBOCOR, its use should be reserved for patients in whom, in the opinion of the physician, the benefits of treatment outweigh the risks.

TAMBOCOR should not be used in patients with recent myocardial infarction. (See Boxed Warnings.)

Use of TAMBOCOR in chronic atrial fibrillation has not been adequately studied and is not recommended. (See Boxed Warnings.)

As is the case for other antiarrhythmic agents, there is no evidence from controlled trials that the use of TAMBOCOR favorably affects survival or the incidence of sudden death.

CONTRAINDICATIONS

TAMBOCOR is contraindicated in patients with pre-existing second- or third-degree AV block, or with right bundle branch block when associated with a left hemiblock (bifascicular block), unless a pacemaker is present to sustain the cardiac rhythm should complete heart block occur. TAMBOCOR is also contraindicated in the presence of cardiogenic shock or known hypersensitivity to the drug.

WARNINGS

Mortality. TAMBOCOR was included in the National Heart Lung and Blood Institute's Cardiac Arrhythmia Suppression Trial (CAST), a long-term, multicenter, randomized, double-blind study in patients with asymptomatic non-life-threatening ventricular arrhythmias who had a myocardial infarction more than six days, but less than two years previously. An excessive mortality or non-fatal cardiac arrest rate was seen in patients treated with TAMBOCOR compared with that seen in a carefully matched placebo-treated group. This rate was 16/315 (5.1%) for TAMBOCOR and 7/309 (2.3%) for its matched placebo. The average duration of treatment with TAMBOCOR in this study was 10 months.

Ventricular Proarrhythmic Effects in Patients with Atrial Fibrillation/Flutter. A review of the world literature revealed reports of 568 patients treated with oral TAMBOCOR for paroxysmal atrial fibrillation/flutter (PAF). Ventricular tachycardia was experienced in 0.4% (2/568) of these patients. Of 19 patients in the literature with chronic atrial fibrillation (CAF), 10.5% (2) experienced VT or VF. FLECAINIDE IS NOT RECOMMENDED FOR USE IN PATIENTS WITH CHRONIC ATRIAL FIBRILLATION. Case reports of ventricular proarrhythmic effects in patients treated with TAMBOCOR for atrial fibrillation/flutter have included increased PVCs, VT, ventricular fibrillation (VF), and death.

As with other class I agents, patients treated with TAMBOCOR for atrial flutter have been reported with 1:1 atrioventricular conduction due to slowing the atrial rate. A paradoxical increase in the ventricular rate also may occur in patients with atrial fibrillation who receive TAMBOCOR. Concomitant negative chronotropic therapy such as digoxin or beta-blockers may lower the risk of this complication.

The applicability of the CAST results to other populations (e.g., those without recent infarction) is uncertain, but at present it is prudent to consider the risks of Class IC agents, coupled with the lack of any evidence of improved survival, generally unacceptable in patients whose ventricular arrhythmias are not life-threatening, even if the patients are experiencing unpleasant, but not life-threatening, symptoms or signs.

PROARRHYTHMIC EFFECTS

TAMBOCOR, like other antiarrhythmic agents, can cause new or worsened supraventricular or ventricular arrhythmias. Ventricular proarrhythmic effects range from an increase in frequency of PVCs to the development of more severe ventricular tachycardia, e.g., tachycardia that is more sustained or more resistant to conversion to sinus rhythm, with potentially fatal consequences. In studies of ventricular arrhythmia patients treated with TAMBOCOR, three-fourths of proarrhythmic events were new or worsened ventricular tachyarrhythmias, the remainder being increased frequency of PVCs or new supraventricular arrhythmias. In patients treated with flecainide for sustained ventricular tachycardia, 80% (51/54) of proarrhythmic events occurred within 14 days of the onset of therapy. In studies of 225 patients with supraventricular arrhythmias (108 with paroxysmal supraventricular tachycardia and 117 with paroxysmal atrial fibrillation), there were 9 (4%) proarrhythmic events, 8 of them in patients with paroxysmal atrial fibrillation. Of the 9, 7 (including the one in a PSVT patient) were exacerbations of supraventricular arrhythmias (longer duration, more rapid rate, harder to reverse) while 2 were ventricular arrhythmias, including one fatal case of VT/VF and one wide complex VT (the patient showed inducible VT, however, after withdrawal of flecainide), both in patients with paroxysmal atrial fibrillation and known coronary artery disease.

It is uncertain if TAMBOCOR's risk of proarrhythmia is exaggerated in patients with chronic atrial fibrillation (CAF), high ventricular rate, and/or exercise. Wide complex tachycardia and ventricular fibrillation have been reported in two of 12 CAF patients undergoing maximal exercise tolerance testing.

In patients with complex ventricular arrhythmias, it is often difficult to distinguish a spontaneous variation in the patient's underlying rhythm disorder from drug-induced worsening, so that the following occurrence rates must be considered approximations. Their frequency appears to be related to dose and to the underlying cardiac disease.

Among patients treated for sustained VT (who frequently also had CHF, a low ejection fraction, a history of myocardial infarction and/or an episode of cardiac arrest), the incidence of proarrhythmic events was 13% when dosage was initiated at 200 mg/day with slow upward titration, and did not exceed 300 mg/day in most patients. In early studies in patients with sustained VT utilizing a higher initial dose (400 mg/day) the incidence of proarrhythmic events was 26%; moreover, in about 10% of the patients treated proarrhythmic events resulted in death, despite prompt medical attention. With lower initial doses, the incidence of proarrhythmic events resulting in death decreased to 0.5% of these patients. Accordingly, it is extremely important to follow the recommended dosage schedule. (See Dosage and Administration.)

The relatively high frequency of proarrhythmic events in patients with sustained VT and serious underlying heart disease, and the need for careful titration and monitoring, requires that therapy of patients with sustained VT be started in the hospital. (See Dosage and Administration.)

HEART FAILURE

TAMBOCOR has a negative inotropic effect and may cause or worsen CHF, particularly in patients with cardiomyopathy, preexisting severe heart failure (NYHA functional class III or IV) or low ejection fractions (less than 30%). In patients with supraventricular arrhythmias new or worsened CHF developed in 0.4% (1/225) of patients. In patients with sustained ventricular tachycardia during a mean duration of 7.9 months TAMBOCOR therapy, 6.3% (20/317) developed new CHF. In patients with sustained ventricular tachycardia and a history of CHF, during a mean duration of 5.4 months of TAMBOCOR therapy, 25.7% (78/304) developed worsened CHF. Exacerbation of preexisting CHF occurred more commonly in studies which included patients with class III or IV failure than in studies which excluded such patients. TAMBOCOR should be used cautiously in patients who are known to have a history of CHF or myocardial dysfunction. The initial dosage in such patients should be no more than 100 mg bid (see Dosage and Administration) and patients should be monitored carefully. Close attention must be given to maintenance of cardiac function, including optimization of digitalis, diuretic, or other therapy. In cases where CHF has developed or worsened during treatment with TAMBOCOR, the time of onset has ranged from a few hours to sev-

eral months after starting therapy. Some patients who develop evidence of reduced myocardial function while on TAMBOCOR can continue on TAMBOCOR with adjustment of digitalis or diuretics, others may require dosage reduction or discontinuation of TAMBOCOR. When feasible, it is recommended that plasma flecainide levels be monitored. Attempts should be made to keep trough plasma levels below 0.7 to 1.0 μg/mL.

Effects on Cardiac Conduction. TAMBOCOR slows cardiac conduction in most patients to produce dose-related increases in PR, QRS, and QT intervals.

PR interval increases on average about 25% (0.04 seconds) and as much as 118% in some patients. Approximately one-third of patients may develop new first-degree AV heart block (PR interval ≥ 0.20 seconds). The QRS complex increases on average about 25% (0.02 seconds) and as much as 150% in some patients. Many patients develop QRS complexes with a duration of 0.12 seconds or more. In one study, 4% of patients developed new bundle branch block while on TAMBOCOR. The degree of lengthening of PR and QRS intervals does not predict either efficacy or the development of cardiac adverse effects. In clinical trials, it was unusual for PR intervals to increase to 0.30 seconds or more, or for QRS intervals to increase to 0.18 seconds or more. Thus, caution should be used when such intervals occur, and dose reductions may be considered. The QT interval widens about 8%, but most of this widening (about 60% to 90%) is due to widening of the QRS duration. The JT interval (QT minus QRS) only widens about 4% on the average. Significant JT prolongation occurs in less than 2% of patients. There have been rare cases of Torsade de Pointes-type arrhythmia associated with TAMBOCOR therapy.

Clinically significant conduction changes have been observed at these rates: sinus node dysfunction such as sinus pause, sinus arrest and symptomatic bradycardia (1.2%), second-degree AV block (0.5%) and third-degree AV block (0.4%). An attempt should be made to manage the patient on the lowest effective dose in an effort to minimize these effects. (See Dosage and Administration.) If second- or third-degree AV block, or right bundle branch block associated with a left hemiblock occur, TAMBOCOR therapy should be discontinued unless a temporary or implanted ventricular pacemaker is in place to ensure an adequate ventricular rate.

Sick Sinus Syndrome (Bradycardia-Tachycardia Syndrome). TAMBOCOR should be used only with extreme caution in patients with sick sinus syndrome because it may cause sinus bradycardia, sinus pause, or sinus arrest.

Effects on Pacemaker Thresholds. TAMBOCOR is known to increase endocardial pacing thresholds and may suppress ventricular escape rhythms. These effects are reversible if flecainide is discontinued. It should be used with caution in patients with permanent pacemakers or temporary pacing electrodes and should not be administered to patients with existing poor thresholds or nonprogrammable pacemakers unless suitable pacing rescue is available.

The pacing threshold in patients with pacemakers should be determined prior to instituting therapy with TAMBOCOR, again after one week of administration and at regular intervals thereafter. Generally threshold changes are within the range of multiprogrammable pacemakers and, when these occur, a doubling of either voltage or pulse width is usually sufficient to regain capture.

Electrolyte Disturbances. Hypokalemia or hyperkalemia may alter the effects of Class I antiarrhythmic drugs. Preexisting hypokalemia or hyperkalemia should be corrected before administration of TAMBOCOR.

PRECAUTIONS

Drug Interactions. TAMBOCOR has been administered to patients receiving **digitalis** preparations or **beta-adrenergic blocking agents** without adverse effects. During administration of multiple oral doses of TAMBOCOR to healthy subjects stabilized on a maintenance dose of **digoxin**, a 13%–19% increase in plasma **digoxin** levels occurred at six hours postdose.

In a study involving healthy subjects receiving TAMBOCOR and **propranolol** concurrently, plasma flecainide levels were increased about 20% and **propranolol** levels were increased about 30% compared to control values. In this formal interaction study, TAMBOCOR and **propranolol** were each found to have negative inotropic effects; when the drugs were administered together, the effects were additive. The effects of concomitant administration of TAMBOCOR and **propranolol** on the PR interval were less than additive. In TAMBOCOR clinical trials, patients who were receiving **beta blockers** concurrently did not experience an increased incidence of side effects. Nevertheless, the possibility of additive negative inotropic effects of **beta blockers** and flecainide should be recognized.

Flecainide is not extensively bound to plasma proteins. In vitro studies with several drugs which may be administered concomitantly showed that the extent of flecainide binding to human plasma proteins is either unchanged or only slightly less. Consequently, interactions with other drugs which are highly protein bound (e.g., **anticoagulants**) would not be expected. TAMBOCOR has been used in a large number of patients receiving **diuretics** without apparent interaction. Limited data in patients receiving known enzyme inducers (**phenytoin, phenobarbital, carbamazepine**) indicate only a 30% increase in the rate of flecainide elimination. In healthy subjects receiving **cimetidine** (1 gm daily) for one week, plasma flecainide levels increased by about 30% and half-life increased by about 10%.

When **amiodarone** is added to flecainide therapy, plasma flecainide levels may increase two-fold or more in some patients, if flecainide dosage is not reduced. (See Dosage and Administration.)

There has been little experience with the coadministration of TAMBOCOR and either **disopyramide** or **verapamil**. Because both of these drugs have negative inotropic properties and the effects of coadministration with TAMBOCOR are unknown, neither **disopyramide** nor **verapamil** should be administered concurrently with TAMBOCOR unless, in the judgment of the physician, the benefits of this combination outweigh the risks. There has been too little experience with the coadministration of TAMBOCOR with **nifedipine** or **diltiazem** to recommend concomitant use.

Carcinogenesis, Mutagenesis, Impairment of Fertility. Long-term studies with flecainide in rats and mice at doses up 60 mg/kg/day have not revealed any compound-related carcinogenic effects. Mutagenicity studies (Ames test, mouse lymphoma and in vivo cytogenetics) did not reveal any mutagenic effects. A rat reproduction study at doses up to 50 mg/kg/day (seven times the usual human dose) did not reveal any adverse effect on male or female fertility.

Pregnancy. Pregnancy Category C. Flecainide has been shown to have teratogenic effects (club paws, sternebrae and vertebrae abnormalities, pale hearts with contracted ventricular septum) and an embryotoxic effect (increased resorptions) in one breed of rabbit (New Zealand White) when given doses of 30 and 35 mg/kg/day, but not in another breed of rabbit (Dutch Belted) when given up to 30 mg/kg/day. No teratogenic effects were observed in rats and mice given doses up to 50 and 80 mg/kg/day, respectively; however, delayed sternebral and vertebral ossification was observed at the high dose in rats. Because there are no adequate and well-controlled studies in pregnant women, TAMBOCOR should be used during pregnancy only if the potential benefit justifies the potential risk to the fetus.

Labor and Delivery. It is not known whether the use of TAMBOCOR during labor or delivery has immediate or delayed adverse effects on the mother or fetus, affects the duration of labor or delivery, or increases the possibility of forceps delivery or other obstetrical intervention.

Nursing Mothers. Results from a multiple dose study conducted in mothers soon after delivery indicates that flecainide is excreted in human breast milk in concentrations as high as 4 times (with average levels about 2.5 times) corresponsing plasma levels; assuming a maternal plasma level at the top of the therapeutic range (1 μg/mL), the calculated daily dose to a nursing infant (assuming about 700 mL breast milk over 24 hours) would be less than 3 mg. Because of the drug's potential for serious adverse effects in nursing infants, a decision should be made whether to discontinue nursing or discontinue the drug, taking into account the importance of the drug to the mother.

Pediatric Use. The safety and effectiveness of TAMBOCOR in children less than 18 years of age have not been established.

Hepatic Impairment. Since flecainide elimination from plasma can be markedly slower in patients with significant hepatic impairment, TAMBOCOR should not be used in such patients unless the potential benefits clearly outweigh the risks. If used, frequent and early plasma level monitoring is required to guide dosage (see Plasma Level Monitoring); dosage increases should be made very cautiously when plasma levels have plateaued (after more than four days).

ADVERSE REACTIONS

In post-myocardial infarction patients with asymptomatic PVCs and non-sustained ventricular tachycardia, TAMBOCOR therapy was found to be associated with a 5.1% rate of death and non-fatal cardiac arrest, compared with a 2.3% rate in a matched placebo group. (See Warnings.)

Adverse effects reported for TAMBOCOR, described in detail in the Warnings section, were new or worsened arrhythmias which occurred in 1% of 108 patients with PSVT and in 7% of 117 patients with PAF; and new or exacerbated ventricular arrhythmias which occurred in 7% of 1330 patients with PVCs, non-sustained or sustained VT. In patients treated with flecainide for sustained VT, 80% (51/64) of proarrhythmic events occurred within 14 days of the onset of therapy. 198 patients with sustained VT experienced a 13% incidence of new or exacerbated ventricular arrhythmias when dosage was initiated at 200 mg/day with slow upward titration, and did not exceed 300 mg/day in most patients. In some patients, TAMBOCOR treatment has been associated with episodes of unresuscitatable VT or ventricular fibrillation (cardiac arrest). (See Warnings.) New or worsened CHF occurred in 6.3% of 1046 patients with PVCs, non-sustained or sustained VT. Of 297 patients with sustained VT, 9.1% experienced new or worsened CHF. New or worsened CHF was reported in 0.4% of 225 patients with supraventricular arrhythmias. There have also been instances of second- (0.5%) or third-degree (0.4%) AV block. Patients have developed sinus bradycardia, sinus pause, or sinus arrest, about 1.2% altogether (see Warnings). The frequency of most of these serious adverse events probably increases with higher trough plasma levels, especially when these trough levels exceed 1.0 μg/mL.

There have been rare reports of isolated elevations of serum alkaline phosphatase and isolated elevations of serum transaminase levels. These elevations have been asymptomatic and no cause and effect relationship with TAMBOCOR has been established. In foreign postmarketing surveillance studies, there have been rare reports of hepatic dysfunction including reports of cholestasis and hepatic failure, and extremely rare reports of blood dyscrasias. Although no cause and effect relationship has been established, it is advisable to discontinue TAMBOCOR in patients who develop unexplained jaundice or signs of hepatic dysfunction or blood dyscrasias in order to eliminate TAMBOCOR as the possible causative agent.

Incidence figures for other adverse effects in patients with ventricular arrhythmias are based on a multicenter efficacy study, utilizing starting doses of 200 mg/day with gradual upward titration to 400 mg/day. Patients were treated for an average of 4.7 months, with some receiving up to 22 months of therapy. In this trial, 5.4% of patients discontinued due to non-cardiac adverse effects. [See table above.]

Table 1
Most Common Non-Cardiac Adverse Effects in Ventricular Arrhythmia Patients Treated with TAMBOCOR in the Multicenter Study

Adverse Effect	Incidence in All 429 Patients at Any Dose	Incidence By Dose During Upward Titration 200 mg/Day (N=426)	300 mg/Day (N=293)	400 mg/Day (N=100)
Dizziness*	18.9%	11.0%	10.6%	13.0%
Visual Disturbance†	15.9%	5.4%	12.3%	18.0%
Dyspnea	10.3%	5.2%	7.5%	4.0%
Headache	9.6%	4.5%	6.1%	9.0%
Nausea	8.9%	4.9%	4.8%	6.0%
Fatigue	7.7%	4.5%	4.4%	3.0%
Palpitation	6.1%	3.5%	2.4%	7.0%
Chest Pain	5.4%	3.1%	3.8%	1.0%
Asthenia	4.9%	2.6%	2.0%	4.0%
Tremor	4.7%	2.4%	3.4%	2.0%
Constipation	4.4%	2.8%	2.1%	1.0%
Edema	3.5%	1.9%	1.4%	2.0%
Abdominal pain	3.3%	1.9%	2.4%	1.0%

* Dizziness includes reports of dizziness, lightheadedness, faintness, unsteadiness, near syncope, etc.
† Visual disturbance includes reports of blurred vision, difficulty in focusing, spots before eyes, etc.

The following additional adverse experiences, possibly related to TAMBOCOR therapy and occurring in 1% to less than 3% of patients, have been reported in acute and chronic studies: *Body as a Whole*—malaise, fever; *Cardiovascular*—tachycardia, sinus pause or arrest; *Gastrointestinal*—vomiting, diarrhea, dyspepsia, anorexia; *Skin*—rash; *Visual*—diplopia; *Nervous System*—hypoesthesia, paresthesia, paresis, ataxia, flushing, increased sweating, vertigo, syncope, somnolence, tinnitus; *Psychiatric*—anxiety, insomnia, depression.

The following additional adverse experiences, possibly related to TAMBOCOR, have been reported in less than 1% of patients: *Body as a Whole*—swollen lips, tongue and mouth; arthralgia, bronchospasm, myalgia; *Cardiovascular*—angina pectoris, second-degree and third-degree AV block, bradycardia, hypertension, hypotension; *Gastrointestinal*—

Continued on next page

3M—Cont.

flatulence; *Urinary System*—polyuria, urinary retention; *Hematologic*—leukopenia, thrombocytopenia; *Skin*—urticaria, exfoliative dermatitis, pruritus, alopecia; *Visual*—eye pain or irritation, photophobia, nystagmus; *Nervous System*—twitching, weakness, change in taste, dry mouth, convulsions, impotence, speech disorder, stupor, neuropathy; *Psychiatric*—amnesia, confusion, decreased libido, depersonalization, euphoria, morbid dreams, apathy.

For patients with supraventricular arrhythmias, the most commonly reported noncardiac adverse experiences remain consistent with those known for patients treated with TAMBOCOR for ventricular arrhythmias. Dizziness is possibly more frequent in PAF patients.

OVERDOSAGE

No specific antidote has been identified for the treatment of TAMBOCOR overdosage. Animal studies suggest that the following events might occur with overdosage: lengthening of the PR interval; increase in the QRS duration, QT interval and amplitude of the T-wave; a reduction in myocardial rate and contractility; conduction disturbances; hypotension; and death from respiratory failure or asystole. Treatment of overdosage should be supportive and may include the following: removal of unabsorbed drug from the gastrointestinal tract, administration of inotropic agents or cardiac stimulants such as dopamine, dobutamine or isoproterenol; mechanically assisted respiration; circulatory assists such as intra-aortic balloon pumping; and transvenous pacing in the event of conduction block. Because of the long plasma half-life of flecainide (12 to 27 hours in patients receiving usual doses), and the possibility of markedly non-linear elimination kinetics at very high doses, these supportive treatments may need to be continued for extended periods of time.

Hemodialysis is not an effective means of removing flecainide from the body. Since flecainide elimination is much slower when urine is very alkaline (pH 8 or higher), theoretically, acidification of urine to promote drug excretion may be beneficial in overdose cases with very alkaline urine. There is no evidence that acidification from normal urinary pH increases excretion.

DOSAGE AND ADMINISTRATION

For patients with sustained VT, no matter what their cardiac status, TAMBOCOR, like other antiarrhythmics, should be initiated in-hospital with rhythm monitoring.

Flecainide has a long half-life (12 to 27 hours in patients). Steady-state plasma levels, in patients with normal renal and hepatic function, may not be achieved until the patient has received 3 to 5 days of therapy at a given dose. Therefore, **increases in dosage should be made no more frequently than once every four days,** since during the first 2 to 3 days of therapy the optimal effect of a given dose may not be achieved.

For patients with PSVT and patients with PAF the recommended starting dose is 50 mg every 12 hours. TAMBOCOR doses may be increased in increments of 50 mg bid every four days until efficacy is achieved. For PAF patients, a substantial increase in efficacy without a substantial increase in discontinuations for adverse experiences may be achieved by increasing the TAMBOCOR dose from 50 mg to 100 mg bid. The maximum recommended dose for patients with paroxysmal supraventricular arrhythmias is 300 mg/day.

For sustained VT the recommended starting dose is 100 mg every 12 hours. This dose may be increased in increments of 50 mg bid every four days until efficacy is achieved. Most patients with sustained VT do not require more than 150 mg every 12 hours (300 mg/day), and the maximum dose recommended is 400 mg/day.

In patients with sustained VT, the use of higher initial doses and more rapid dosage adjustments have resulted in an increased incidence of proarrhythmic events and CHF, particularly during the first few days of dosing (see Warnings). Therefore, a loading dose is not recommended.

Intravenous lidocaine has been used occasionally with TAMBOCOR while awaiting the therapeutic effect of TAMBOCOR. No adverse drug interactions were apparent. However, no formal studies have been performed to demonstrate the usefulness of this regimen.

An occasional patient not adequately controlled by (or intolerant to) a dose given at 12-hour intervals may be dosed at eight-hour intervals.

Once adequate control of the arrhythmia has been achieved, it may be possible in some patients to reduce the dose as necessary to minimize side effects or effects on conduction. In such patients, efficacy at the lower dose should be evaluated.

TAMBOCOR should be used cautiously in patients with a history of CHF or myocardial dysfunction (see Warnings).

In patients with severe renal impairment (creatinine clearance of 35 mL/min/1.73 square meters or less), the initial dosage should be 100 mg once daily (or 50 mg bid); when used in such patients, frequent plasma level monitoring is required to guide dosage adjustments (see Plasma Level Monitoring). In patients with less severe renal disease, the initial dosage should be 100 mg every 12 hours; plasma level monitoring may also be useful in these patients during dosage adjustment. In both groups of patients, dosage increases should be made very cautiously when plasma levels have plateaued (after more than four days), observing the patient closely for signs of adverse cardiac effects or other toxicity. It should be borne in mind that in these patients it may take longer than four days before a new steady-state plasma level is reached following a dosage change.

Based on theoretical considerations, rather than experimental data, the following suggestion is made: when transferring patients from another antiarrhythmic drug to TAMBOCOR allow at least two to four plasma half-lives to elapse for the drug being discontinued before starting TAMBOCOR at the usual dosage. In patients where withdrawal of a previous antiarrhythmic agent is likely to produce life-threatening arrhythmias, the physician should consider hospitalizing the patient.

When flecainide is given in the presence of amiodarone, reduce the usual flecainide dose by 50% and monitor the patient closely for adverse effects. Plasma level monitoring is strongly recommended to guide dosage with such combination therapy (see below).

Plasma Level Monitoring. The large majority of patients successfully treated with TAMBOCOR were found to have trough plasma levels between 0.2 and 1.0 μg/mL. The probability of adverse experiences, especially cardiac, may increase with higher trough plasma levels, especially when these exceed 1.0 μg/mL. Periodic monitoring of trough plasma levels may be useful in patient management. Plasma level monitoring is required in patients with severe renal failure or severe hepatic disease, since elimination of flecainide from plasma may be markedly slower. Monitoring of plasma levels is strongly recommended in patients on concurrent amiodarone therapy and may also be helpful in patients with CHF and in patients with moderate renal disease.

HOW SUPPLIED

All tablets are embossed with "3M" on one side and "TR 50", "TR 100" or "TR 150" on the other side.

Tambocor, 50 mg per white, round tablet, is available in
Bottles of 100—NDC #0089-0305-10,
Boxes of 100 in unit dose blister strips—
NDC #0089-0305-16.

Tambocor, 100 mg per white, round, scored tablet, is available in
Bottles of 100—NDC #0089-0307-10,
Boxes of 100 in unit dose blister strips—
NDC #0089-0307-16.

Tambocor, 150 mg per white, oval, scored tablet, is available in
Bottles of 100—NDC #0089-0314-10.

Store at controlled room temperature 15°-30°C (59°-86°F) in a tight, light-resistant container.

CAUTION: Federal law prohibits dispensing without prescription.

TR-11 October 1991

Shown in Product Identification Section, page 416

THEOLAIR™ ℞
(theophylline tablets USP)
TABLETS

THEOLAIR™ ℞
(theophylline oral solution)
LIQUID

DESCRIPTION

Theophylline is a bronchodilator structurally classified as a xanthine derivative. It occurs as a white, odorless, crystalline powder having a bitter taste. Theophylline anhydrous has the chemical name, 1*H*-Purine-2, 6-dione, 3,7-dihydro-1,3-dimethyl-, and is represented by the following structural formula:

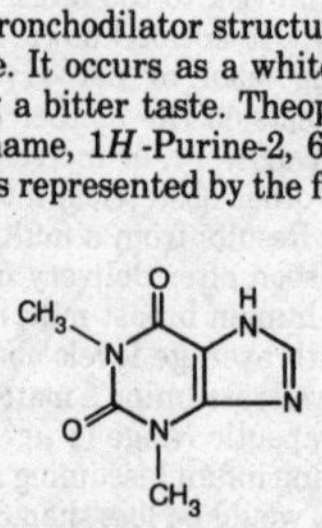

$C_7H_8N_4O_2$
Molecular Weight 180.17

THEOLAIR Tablets contain 125 mg or 250 mg of theophylline anhydrous intended for oral administration. THEOLAIR Tablets also contain: colloidal silicon dioxide, lactose, magnesium stearate, and pregelatinized starch.

THEOLAIR Liquid contains theophylline equivalent to 80 mg theophylline anhydrous per 15 ml (tablespoonful) in a nonalcoholic, clear, colorless solution intended for oral administration. THEOLAIR Liquid also contains: flavor, methylparaben and propylparaben, purified water, sorbitol, and sucrose.

CLINICAL PHARMACOLOGY

Theophylline directly relaxes the smooth muscle of the bronchial airways and pulmonary blood vessels, thus acting mainly as a bronchodilator and smooth muscle relaxant. It has also been demonstrated that aminophylline (the ethylenediamine salt of theophylline) has a potent effect on diaphragmatic contractility in normal persons and may then be capable of reducing fatigability and thereby improve contractility in patients with chronic obstructive airways disease. The exact mode of action remains unsettled. Although theophylline does cause inhibition of phosphodiesterase with a resultant increase in intracellular cyclic AMP, other agents similarly inhibit the enzyme producing a rise of cyclic AMP but are unassociated with any demonstrable bronchodilation. Other mechanisms proposed include an effect on translocation of intracellular calcium; prostaglandin antagonism; stimulation of catecholamines endogenously; inhibition of cyclic guanosine monophosphate metabolism and adenosine receptor antagonism. None of these mechanisms has been proved, however.

In vitro, theophylline has been shown to act synergistically with beta agonists and there are now available data which do demonstrate an additive effect *in vivo* with combined use.

Pharmacokinetics:

The half-life of theophylline is influenced by a number of known variables. It may be prolonged in chronic alcoholics, particularly those with liver disease (cirrhosis or alcoholic liver disease), in patients with congestive heart failure, and in those patients taking certain other drugs (see PRECAUTIONS, Drug Interactions). Newborns and neonates have extremely slow clearance rates compared to older infants and children, i.e., those over 1 year. Older children have rapid clearance rates while most nonsmoking adults have clearance rates between these two extremes. In premature neonates the decreased clearance is related to oxidative pathways that have yet to be established.

Theophylline Elimination Characteristics

	Half-Life (in hours)	
	Range	Mean
Children	1– 9	3.7
Adults	3–15	7.7

In cigarette smokers (1–2 packs/day) the mean half-life is 4–5 hours, much shorter than in nonsmokers. The increase in clearance associated with smoking is presumably due to stimulation of the hepatic metabolic pathway by components of cigarette smoke. The duration of this effect after cessation of smoking is unknown but may require 6 months to 2 years before the rate approaches that of the nonsmoker.

INDICATIONS AND USAGE

For relief and/or prevention of symptoms from asthma and reversible bronchospasm associated with chronic bronchitis and emphysema.

CONTRAINDICATIONS

This product is contraindicated in individuals who have shown hypersensitivity to its components. It is also contraindicated in patients with active peptic ulcer disease, and in individuals with underlying seizure disorders (unless receiving appropriate anticonvulsant medication).

WARNINGS

Serum levels above 20 mcg/ml are rarely found after appropriate administration of the recommended doses. However, in individuals in whom theophylline plasma clearance is reduced *for any reason,* even conventional doses may result in increased serum levels and potential toxicity. Reduced theophylline clearance has been documented in the following readily identifiable groups: 1) patients with impaired liver function; 2) patients over 55 years of age, particularly males and those with chronic lung disease; 3) those with cardiac failure from any cause; 4) patients with sustained high fever; 5) neonates and infants under 1 year of age; and 6) those patients taking certain drugs (see PRECAUTIONS, Drug Interactions). Frequently, such patients have markedly prolonged theophylline serum levels following discontinuation of the drug.

Reduction of dosage and laboratory monitoring is especially appropriate in the above individuals.

Serious side effects such as ventricular arrhythmias, convulsions or even death may appear as the first sign of toxicity without any previous warning. Less serious signs of theophylline toxicity (i.e., nausea and restlessness) may occur frequently when initiating therapy, but are usually transient; when such signs are persistent during maintenance therapy, they are often associated with serum concentrations above 20 mcg/ml.

Stated differently, *serious toxicity is not reliably preceded by less severe side effects.* A serum concentration measurement is the only reliable method of predicting potentially life-threatening toxicity.

Many patients who require theophylline exhibit tachycardia due to their underlying disease process so that the cause/effect relationship to elevated serum theophylline concentrations may not be appreciated.

Theophylline products may cause or worsen arrhythmias and any significant change in rate and/or rhythm warrants monitoring and further investigation.

Studies in laboratory animals (minipigs, rodents, and dogs) recorded the occurrence of cardiac arrhythmias and sudden death (with histologic evidence of myocardial necrosis) when beta-agonists and methylxanthines were administered concurrently. The significance of these findings when applied to humans is currently unknown.

PRECAUTIONS

General:

On the average, theophylline half-life is shorter in cigarette and marijuana smokers than in nonsmokers, but smokers can have half-lives as long as nonsmokers. Theophylline should not be administered concurrently with other xanthines. Use with caution in patients with hypoxemia, hypertension, or those with history of peptic ulcer. Theophylline may occasionally act as a local irritant to G.I. tract although gastrointestinal symptoms are more commonly centrally mediated and associated with serum drug concentrations over 20 mcg/ml.

Information for Patients:

If nausea, vomiting, restlessness, irregular heartbeat, or convulsions occur, contact a physician immediately.

Take only the amount of drug that has been prescribed. Do not take a larger dose, or take the drug more often, or for a longer time than recommended.

Do not take other medicines, especially those for pulmonary disorders, except on the advice of a physician.

Avoid drinking large amounts of coffee, tea, cocoa, or cola, or eating large quantities of chocolate while taking this medicine, since these foods may increase the side effects of theophylline.

Laboratory Tests:

Serum levels should be monitored periodically to determine the theophylline level associated with observed clinical response and as the method of predicting toxicity. For such measurements, the serum sample should be obtained at the time of peak concentration, 1 to 2 hours after administration for immediate release products. It is important that the patient will not have missed or taken additional doses during the previous 48 hours and that dosing intervals will have been reasonably equally spaced. DOSAGE ADJUSTMENTS BASED ON SERUM THEOPHYLLINE MEASUREMENTS WHEN THESE INSTRUCTIONS HAVE NOT BEEN FOLLOWED MAY RESULT IN RECOMMENDATIONS THAT PRESENT RISK OF TOXICITY TO THE PATIENT.

Drug Interactions:

Toxic synergism with ephedrine has been documented and may occur with other sympathomimetic bronchodilators. In addition, the following drug interactions have been demonstrated.

Theophylline with:	
Allopurinol (high-dose)	Increased serum theophylline levels
Cimetidine	Increased serum theophylline levels
Ciprofloxacin	Increased serum theophylline levels
Erythromycin, Troleandomycin	Increased serum theophylline levels
Lithium carbonate	Increased renal excretion of lithium
Oral Contraceptives	Increased serum theophylline levels
Phenytoin	Decreased theophylline and phenytoin serum levels
Propranolol	Increased serum theophylline levels
Rifampin	Decreased serum theophylline levels

Drug-Laboratory Test Interactions:

Currently available analytical methods, including high pressure liquid chromatography and immunoassay techniques, for measuring serum theophylline levels are specific. Metabolites and other drugs generally do not affect the results. Other new analytical methods are also now in use. The physician should be aware of the laboratory method used and whether other drugs will interfere with the assay for theophylline.

Carcinogenesis, Mutagenesis, and Impairment of Fertility:

Long-term carcinogenicity studies have not been performed with theophylline.

Chromosome-breaking activity was detected in human cell cultures at concentrations of theophylline up to 50 times the therapeutic serum concentration in humans. Theophylline was not mutagenic in the dominant lethal assay in male mice given theophylline intraperitoneally in doses up to 30 times the maximum daily oral dose.

Studies to determine the effect on fertility have not been performed with theophylline.

Pregnancy:

Category C—Animal reproduction studies have not been conducted with theophylline. It is also not known whether theophylline can cause fetal harm when administered to a pregnant woman or can affect reproduction capacity. Xanthines should be given to a pregnant woman only if clearly needed.

Nursing Mothers:

Theophylline is distributed into breast milk and may cause irritability or other signs of toxicity in nursing infants. Because of the potential for serious adverse reactions in nursing infants from theophylline, a decision should be made whether to discontinue nursing or to discontinue the drug, taking into account the importance of the drug to the mother.

Pediatric Use:

Sufficient numbers of infants under the age of 1 year have not been studied in clinical trials to support use in this age group; however, there is evidence recorded that the use of dosage recommendations for older infants and young children (16 mg/kg/24 hours) may result in the development of toxic serum levels. Such findings very probably reflect differences in the metabolic handling of the drug related to absent or undeveloped enzyme systems. Consequently, the use of the drug in this age group should carefully consider the associated benefits and risks. If used, the maintenance dose must be conservative and in accord with the following guidelines:

Initial Maintenance Dosage of Anhydrous Theophylline:

Premature Infants:

Up to 24 days postnatal age—1.0 mg/kg q 12h

Beyond 24 days postnatal age—1.5 mg/kg q 12h

Infants 6 to 52 Weeks:

$[(0.2 \times \text{age in weeks}) + 5.0] \times \text{kg body wt} = 24$ hour dose in mg. Up to 26 weeks, divide into q8h dosing intervals. From 26–52 weeks, divide into q6h dosing intervals.

Final dosage should be guided by serum concentration after a steady state (no further accumulation of drug) has been achieved.

ADVERSE REACTIONS

The following adverse reactions have been observed, but there has not been enough systematic collection of data to support an estimate of their frequency. The most consistent adverse reactions are usually due to overdosage.

1. *Gastrointestinal:* nausea, vomiting, epigastric pain, hematemesis, diarrhea.
2. *Central nervous system:* headaches, irritability, restlessness, insomnia, reflex hyperexcitability, muscle twitching, clonic and tonic generalized convulsions.
3. *Cardiovascular:* palpitation, tachycardia, extrasystoles, flushing, hypotension, circulatory failure, ventricular arrhythmias.
4. *Respiratory:* tachypnea.
5. *Renal:* potentiation of diuresis.
6. *Others:* hyperglycemia, inappropriate ADH syndrome, rash, alopecia.

OVERDOSAGE

Management:

It is suggested that the management principles (consistent with the clinical status of the patient when first seen) outlined below be instituted and that simultaneous contact with a Regional Poison Control Center be established. In this way both updated information and individualization regarding therapy may be provided.

1. When potential oral overdose is established and seizure has not occurred:
   a) If patient is alert and seen within the early hours after ingestion, induction of emesis may be of value. Gastric lavage has been demonstrated to be of no value in influencing outcome in patients who present more than 1 hour after ingestion.
   b) Administer a cathartic. Sorbitol solution is reported to be of value.
   c) Adminster repeated doses of activated charcoal and monitor theophylline serum levels.
   d) Prophylactic administration of phenobarbital has been shown to increase the seizure threshold in laboratory animals, and administration of this drug can be considered.
2. If patient presents with a seizure:
   a) Establish an airway.
   b) Administer oxygen.
   c) Treat the seizure with intravenous diazepam, 0.1 to 0.3 mg/kg up to 10 mg. If seizures cannot be controlled, the use of general anesthesia should be considered.
   d) Monitor vital signs, maintain blood pressure and provide adequate hydration.
3. If post-seizure coma is present:
   a) Maintain airway and oxygenation.
   b) If a result of oral medication, follow above recommendations to prevent absorption of the drug, but intubation and lavage will have to be performed instead of inducing emesis, and the cathartic and charcoal will need to be introduced via a large bore gastric lavage tube.
   c) Continue to provide full supportive care and adequate hydration until the drug is metabolized. In general, drug metabolism is sufficiently rapid so as not to warrant dialysis. If repeated oral activated charcoal is ineffective (as noted by stable or rising serum levels), charcoal hemoperfusion may be indicated.

DOSAGE AND ADMINISTRATION

Effective use of theophylline (i.e., the concentration of drug in the serum associated with optimal benefit and minimal risk of toxicity) is considered to occur when the theophylline concentration is maintained from 10 to 20 mcg/ml. The early studies from which these levels were derived were carried out in patients immediately or shortly after recovery from acute exacerbations of their disease (some hospitalized with status asthmaticus).

Although the 20 mcg/ml level remains appropriate as a critical value (above which toxicity is more likely to occur) for safety purposes, additional data are now available which indicate that the serum theophylline concentrations required to produce maximum physiologic benefit may, in fact, fluctuate with the degree of bronchospasm present and are variable. Therefore, the physician should individualize the range appropriate to the patient's requirements, based on both symptomatic response and improvement in pulmonary function. It should be stressed that serum theophylline concentrations maintained at the upper level of the 5 to 20 mcg/ml range may be associated with potential toxicity when factors known to reduce theophylline clearance are operative. (See Warnings.)

If it is not possible to obtain serum level determinations, restriction of the daily dose (in otherwise healthy adults) to not greater than 13 mg/kg day, to a maximum of 900 mg, in divided doses will result in relatively few patients exceeding serum level of 20 mcg/ml and the resultant greater risk of toxicity.

Caution should be exercised for younger children who cannot complain of minor side effects. Older adults, those with cor pulmonale, congestive heart failure, and/or liver disease may have unusually low dosage requirements and thus may experience toxicity at the maximal dosage recommended below.

Theophylline does not distribute into fatty tissue. Dosage should be calculated on the basis of lean (ideal) body weight where mg/kg doses are presented.

Frequency of Dosing: When immediate release products with rapid absorption are used, dosing to maintain serum levels generally requires administration every 6 hours. This is particularly true in children, but dosing intervals up to 8 hours may be satisfactory in adults since they eliminate the drug at a slower rate. Some children, and adults requiring higher than average doses (those having rapid rates of clearance, e.g., half-lives of under 6 hours) may benefit and be more effectively controlled during chronic therapy when given products with sustained-release characteristics since these provide longer dosing intervals and/or less fluctuation in serum concentration between dosing.

Dosage guidelines are appoximations only and the wide range of theophylline clearance between individuals (particularly those with concomitant disease) makes indiscriminate usage hazardous.

Dosage Guidelines:

I. Acute Symptoms of Bronchospasm Requiring Rapid Attainment of Theophylline Serum Levels for Bronchodilation:

NOTE: Status asthmaticus should be considered a medical emergency and is defined as that degree of bronchospasm which is not rapidly responsive to usual doses of conventional bronchodilators. Optimal therapy for such patients frequently requires both *additional medication*, parenterally administered, and *close monitoring*, preferably in an intensive care setting.

A. Patients not currently receiving theophylline products:

	Theophylline Dosage	
	Oral Loading	Maintenance
Children age 1 to under 9 years	5 mg/kg	4 mg/kg q 6 hours
Children age 9 to under 16 years; and smokers	5 mg/kg	3 mg/kg q 6 hours
Otherwise healthy non-smoking adults	5 mg/kg	3 mg/kg q 8 hours
Older patients and patients with cor pulmonale	5 mg/kg	2 mg/kg q 8 hours
Patients with congestive heart failure	5 mg/kg	1–2 mg/kg q 12 hours

B. Patients currently receiving theophylline products:

Determine, where possible, the time, amount, dosage form, and route of administration of the last dose the patient received.

The loading dose for theophylline is based on the principle that each 0.5 mg/kg of theophylline administered as a loading dose will result in a 1.0 mcg/ml increase in serum theophylline concentration. Ideally, the loading dose should be deferred if a serum theophylline concentration can be obtained rapidly.

Continued on next page

3M—Cont.

If this is not possible, the clinician must exercise judgment in selecting a dose based on the potential for benefit and risk. When there is sufficient respiratory distress to warrant a small risk, then 2.5 mg/kg of theophylline administered in rapidly absorbed form is likely to increase serum concentration by approximately 5 mcg/ml. If the patient is not experiencing theophylline toxicity, this is unlikely to result in dangerous adverse effects.
Subsequent to the decision regarding use of a loading dose for this group of patients, the maintenance dosage recommendations are the same as those described above.

II. Chronic Therapy:
Theophylline is a treatment for the management of reversible bronchospasm (asthma, chronic bronchitis and emphysema) to prevent symptoms and maintain patent airways. A dosage form which allows small incremental doses is desirable for initiating therapy. A liquid preparation should be considered for children to permit both greater ease of and more accurate dosage adjustment. Slow clinical titration is generally preferred to assure acceptance and safety of the medication, and to allow the patient to develop tolerance to transient caffeine-like side effects.

Initial Dose: 16 mg/kg/24 hours or 400 mg/24 hours (whichever is less) of theophylline in divided doses at 6 or 8 hour intervals.

Increasing Dose: The above dosage may be increased in approximately 25 percent increments at 3 day intervals so long as the drug is tolerated; until clinical response is satisfactory or the maximum dose as indicated in section III (below) is reached. The serum concentration may be checked at these intervals but, at a minimum, should be determined at the end of this adjustment period.
It is important that no patient be maintained on any dosage that is not tolerated. When instructing patients to increase dosage according to the schedule above, they should be told not to take a subsequent dose if apparent side effects occur and to resume therapy at a lower dose once adverse effects have disappeared.

III. Maximum Dose of Theophylline Where the Serum Concentration Is Not Measured:
WARNING: DO NOT ATTEMPT TO MAINTAIN ANY DOSE THAT IS NOT TOLERATED.
Not to exceed the following: (or 900 mg, whichever is less)

Age 1 to under 9 years	24 mg/kg/day
Age 9 to under 12 years	20 mg/kg/day
Age 12 to under 16 years	18 mg/kg/day
Age 16 years or older	13 mg/kg/day

IV. Measurement of Serum Theophylline Concentrations During Chronic Therapy:
If the above maximum doses are to be maintained, serum theophylline measurement is recommended. Serum theophylline measurement is essential if the above doses are exceeded. (See PRECAUTIONS, Laboratory Tests, for guidance.)

V. Final Adjustment of Dosage:
Dosage adjustment after serum theophylline measurement

If serum theophylline is:		Directions:
Within desired range		Maintain dosage if tolerated.
Too high	20–25 mcg/ml	Decrease doses by about 10% and recheck serum level after 3 days.
	25–30 mcg/ml	Skip the next dose and decrease subsequent doses by about 25%. Recheck serum level after 3 days.
	Over 30 mcg/ml	Skip next two doses and decrease subsequent doses by 50%. Recheck serum level after 3 days.
Too low		Increase dosage by 25% at 3 day intervals until either the desired serum concentration and/or clinical response is achieved. The total daily dose may need to be administered at more frequent intervals if symptoms occur repeatedly at the end of a dosing interval.

The serum concentration may be rechecked at appropriate intervals, but at least at the end of any adjustment period. When the patient's condition is otherwise clinically stable and none of the recognized factors which alter elimination are present, measurement of serum levels need be repeated only every 6 to 12 months.

HOW SUPPLIED

THEOLAIR™ Tablets:
125 mg tablets—Each round, white, scored tablet imprinted with "3M" on one side and "342" on the other. Bottles of 100 (NDC 0089-0342-10).
250 mg tablets—Each capsule-shaped, white, scored tablet imprinted with "3M" on one side and "THEOLAIR 250" on the other. Bottles of 100 (NDC 0089-0344-10).
STORE BELOW 30°C (86°F).

THEOLAIR™ Liquid:
1 pint bottles of clear, colorless solution. Each tablespoonful (15 ml) contains theophylline equivalent to 80 mg of theophylline anhydrous (NDC 0089-0960-16).
STORE BETWEEN 15–30°C (59–86°F).

CAUTION: Federal law prohibits dispensing without prescription.

THEO-23 MAY 1991
3M PHARMACEUTICALS
Northridge, CA 91324
Shown in Product Identification Section, page 416

THEOLAIR™-SR ℞
(anhydrous theophylline, sustained-release) TABLETS

DESCRIPTION

Theophylline is a bronchodilator structurally classified as a xanthine derivative. It occurs as a white, odorless, crystalline powder having a bitter taste. Theophylline anhydrous has the chemical name, 1H-Purine-2, 6-dione, 3,7-dihydro-1,3-dimethyl-, and is represented by the following structural formula:

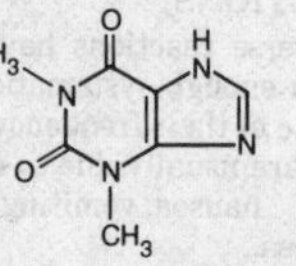

$C_7H_8N_4O_2$ Molecular Weight 180.17

THEOLAIR-SR Tablets contain 200, 250, 300, or 500 mg theophylline anhydrous, in a sustained-release formulation for oral administration. THEOLAIR-SR Tablets also contain: cellulose acetate phthalate, lactose, and magnesium stearate.

CLINICAL PHARMACOLOGY

Theophylline directly relaxes the smooth muscle of the bronchial airways and pulmonary blood vessels, thus acting mainly as a bronchodilator and smooth muscle relaxant. It has also been demonstrated that aminophylline has a potent effect on diaphragmatic contractility in normal persons and may then be capable of reducing fatigability and thereby improve contractility in patients with chronic obstructive airways disease. The exact mode of action remains unsettled. Although theophylline does cause inhibition of phosphodiesterase with a resultant increase in intracellular cyclic AMP, other agents similarly inhibit the enzyme producing a rise of cyclic AMP but are unassociated with any demonstrable bronchodilation. Other mechanisms proposed include an effect on translocation of intracellular calcium; prostaglandin antagonism; stimulation of catecholamines endogenously; inhibition of cyclic guanosine monophosphate metabolism and adenosine receptor antagonism. None of these mechanisms has been proved, however.
In vitro, theophylline has been shown to act synergistically with beta agonists and there are now available data which do demonstrate an additive effect *in vivo* with combined use.

Pharmacokinetics:
The half-life of theophylline is influenced by a number of known variables. It may be prolonged in chronic alcoholics, particularly those with liver disease (cirrhosis or alcoholic liver disease), in patients with congestive heart failure, and in those patients taking certain other drugs (see PRECAUTIONS, Drug Interactions). Newborns and neonates have extremely slow clearance rates compared to older infants and children, i.e., those over 1 year. Older children have rapid clearance rates while most nonsmoking adults have clearance rates between these two extremes. In premature neonates the decreased clearance is related to oxidative pathways that have yet to be established.

Theophylline Elimination Characteristics

	Half-Life (in Hours) Range	Mean
Children	1– 9	3.7
Adults	3–15	7.7

In cigarette smokers (1–2 packs/day) the mean half-life is 4–5 hours, much shorter than in nonsmokers. The increase in clearance associated with smoking is presumably due to stimulation of the hepatic metabolic pathway by components of cigarette smoke. The duration of this effect after cessation of smoking is unknown but may require 6 months to 2 years before the rate approaches that of the nonsmoker.
A single 500 mg dose of THEOLAIR-SR in 8 healthy male subjects fasted for 10 hours predose (overnight) through 4 hours postdose resulted in mean peak theophylline plasma levels of 9.1 ±3.8 (SD) mcg/ml occurring at 5.0 ±1.5 hours following dose administration. The extent of theophylline absorption from THEOLAIR-SR was complete in these subjects when compared with that from an immediate-release tablet. In another single dose study, comparable rates and extents of theophylline absorption were seen for the 200, 250, and 300 mg THEOLAIR-SR Tablets in 18 healthy male subjects, fasted as above.
In a five-day multiple-dose study, 18 healthy male subjects received 250 mg THEOLAIR-SR Tablets in doses ranging from 375 mg to 625 mg twice daily (mean dose of 11 mg/kg per day). Subjects were allowed to take drug with milk and were permitted their normal daily meals except for fasting from 10 hours before through 4 hours after the morning dose on day 5. Following that dose, mean minimum and maximum plasma theophylline levels were 7.3 ±2.3 mcg/ml and 10.8 ±3.1 mcg/ml, respectively. The average percent fluctuation $[(C_{max}-C_{min}/C_{min})\times 100]$ was 48%. The extent of theophylline absorption fromTHEOLAIR-SR averaged 94 ±19% of that from an immediate-release liquid given four times daily.
In other studies: A single 500 mg dose of THEOLAIR-SR was administered to 35 healthy volunteers in both a fasting state and with a high-fat content breakfast. The resultant pharmacokinetic values recorded a delay in the rate of absorption (but not the extent) for the fed group.
In a multiple-dose study involving 12 adolescent patients, the rate and extent of absorption was similar whether the drug was taken immediately after, or two hours after, a low-fat content breakfast (see PRECAUTONS, Drug/Food Interactions).

INDICATIONS AND USAGE

For relief and/or prevention of symptoms from asthma and reversible bronchospasm associated with chronic bronchitis and emphysema.

CONTRAINDICATIONS

THEOLAIR-SR Tablets are contraindicated in individuals who are hypersensitive to theophylline or any of the tablet components. It is also contraindicated in patients with active peptic ulcer disease, and in individuals with underlying seizure disorders (unless receiving appropriate anticonvulsant therapy).

WARNINGS

Serum levels above 20 mcg/ml are rarely found after appropriate administration of the recommended doses. However, in individuals in whom theophylline plasma clearance is reduced *for any reason,* even conventional doses may result in increased serum levels and potential toxicity. Reduced theophylline clearance has been documented in the following readily identifiable groups: 1) patients with impaired liver function; 2) patients over 55 years of age, particularly males and those with chronic lung disease; 3) those with cardiac failure from any cause; 4) patients with sustained high fever; 5) neonates and infants under 1 year of age; and 6) those patients taking certain drugs (see PRECAUTIONS, Drug Interactions). Frequently, such patients have markedly prolonged theophylline serum levels following discontinuation of the drug.
Reduction of dosage and laboratory monitoring is especially appropriate in the above individuals.
Serious side effects such as ventricular arrhythmias, convulsions or even death may appear as the first sign of toxicity without any previous warning. Less serious signs of theophylline toxicity (i.e., nausea and restlessness) may occur frequently when initiating therapy, but are usually transient; when such signs are persistent during maintenance therapy, they are often associated with serum concentrations above 20 mcg/ml. Stated differently, *serious toxicity is not reliably preceded by less severe side effects.* A serum concentration measurement is the only reliable method of predicting potentially life-threatening toxicity.
Many patients who require theophylline exhibit tachycardia due to their underlying disease process so that the cause/effect relationship to elevated serum theophylline concentrations may not be appreciated.
Theophylline products may cause or worsen arrhythmias and any significant change in rate and/or rhythm warrants monitoring and further investigation.
Studies in laboratory animals (minipigs, rodents, and dogs) recorded the occurrence of cardiac arrhythmias and sudden death (with histologic evidence of myocardial necrosis) when beta-agonists and methylxanthines were administered concurrently. The significance of these findings when applied to humans is currently unknown.

PRECAUTIONS

General:
On the average, theophylline half-life is shorter in cigarette and marijuana smokers than in nonsmokers, but smokers

can have half-lives as long as nonsmokers. Theophylline should not be administered concurrently with other xanthines. Use with caution in patients with hypoxemia, hypertension, or those with history of peptic ulcer. Theophylline may occasionally act as a local irritant to G.I. tract although gastrointestinal symptoms are more commonly centrally mediated and associated with serum drug concentrations over 20 mcg/ml.

Information for Patients:
If nausea, vomiting, restlessness, irregular heartbeat, or convulsions occur, contact a physician immediately.
Take only the amount of drug that has been prescribed. Do not take a larger dose, or take the drug more often, or for a longer time then recommended.
Take this drug consistently with respect to food: either with meals, or fasted (at least 2 hours pre- or 2 hours post-meals).
Do not take other medicines, especially those for pulmonary disorders, except on the advice of a physician.
Contact your physician if pulmonary symptoms occur repeatedly, especially at the end of a dosing interval.
Avoid drinking large amounts of caffeine-containing beverages, such as coffee, tea, cocoa, or cola, or eating large quantities of chocolate while taking this medicine, since these foods increase the side effects of theophylline.
THEOLAIR-SR Tablets should not be chewed or crushed.

Laboratory Tests:
Serum levels should be monitored periodically to determine the theophylline level associated with observed clinical response and as the method of predicting toxicity. For such measurements, the serum sample should be obtained four to six hours after administration of THEOLAIR-SR Tablets. It is important that the patient will not have missed or taken additional doses during the previous 48 hours and that dosing intervals will have been reasonably equally spaced. DOSAGE ADJUSTMENT BASED ON SERUM THEOPHYLLINE MEASUREMENTS WHEN THESE INSTRUCTIONS HAVE NOT BEEN FOLLOWED MAY RESULT IN RECOMMENDATIONS THAT PRESENT RISK OF TOXICITY TO THE PATIENT.

Drug Interactions:
Drug/Drug—Toxic synergism with ephedrine has been documented and may occur with other sympathomimetic bronchodilators. In addition, the following drug interactions have been demonstrated:

Theophylline with:	
Allopurinol (high-dose)	Increased serum theophylline levels
Cimetidine	Increased serum theophylline levels
Ciprofloxacin	Increased serum theophylline levels
Erythromycin, Troleandomycin	Increased serum theophylline levels
Lithium carbonate	Increased renal excretion of lithium
Oral Contraceptives	Increased serum theophylline levels
Phenytoin	Decreased theophylline and phenytoin serum levels
Propranolol	Increased serum theophylline levels
Rifampin	Decreased serum theophylline levels

Drug/Food—Administration of a single dose of THEOLAIR-SR immediately after a high-fat content breakfast (8 ounces of whole milk, 2 fried eggs, 2 bacon strips, 2 ounces of hash browns and 2 slices of buttered toast, which equates to approximately 71 grams of fat and 985 calories) to 35 healthy volunteers resulted in plasma concentration levels (for the first 8 hours) of 40–60% of those noted during the fasted state and a delay in the time to peak plasma level (T-max) of 17.1 hours in contrast to the 5.1 hours observed during the fasted state.
However, when THEOLAIR-SR was administered on an every 12 hour schedule for 5 days, no consequential effect on absorption was noted following similar high-fat content breakfast, and the time to peak concentration averaged 5.4 hours. The rate and extent of absorption seen was similar when the drug was taken immediately after, and two hours after, a low-fat content breakfast.
The effect of other types and amounts of food, and the pharmacokinetic profile following an evening meal is not presently known.

Drug-Laboratory Test Interactions:
Currently available analytical methods, including high pressure liquid chromatography and immunoassay techniques, for measuring serum theophylline levels are specific. Metabolites and other drugs generally do not affect the results. Other new analytic methods are also now in use. The physician should be aware of the laboratory method used and whether other drugs will interfere with the assay for theophylline.

Carcinogenesis, Mutagenesis, and Impairment of Fertility:
Long-term carcinogenicity studies have not been performed with theophylline.
Chromosome-breaking activity was detected in human cell cultures at concentrations of theophylline up to 50 times the therapeutic serum concentration in humans. Theophylline was not mutagenic in the dominant lethal assay in male mice given theophylline intraperitoneally in doses up to 30 times the maximum daily human oral dose.
Studies to determine the effect on fertility have not been performed with theophylline.

Pregnancy:
Category C—Animal reproduction studies have not been conducted with theophylline. It is also not known whether theophylline can cause fetal harm when administered to a pregnant woman or can affect reproduction capacity. Xanthines should be given to a pregnant woman only if clearly needed.

Nursing Mothers:
Theophylline is distributed into breast milk and may cause irritability or other signs of toxicity in nursing infants. Because of the potential for serious adverse reactions in nursing infants from theophylline, a decision should be made whether to discontinue nursing or to discontinue the drug, taking into account the importance of the drug to the mother.

Pediatric Use:
THEOLAIR-SR Tablets are not recommended for administration to children less than six years of age.

ADVERSE REACTIONS

The following adverse reactions have been observed, but there has not been enough systematic collection of data to support an estimate of their frequency. The most consistent adverse reactions are usually due to overdosage.

1. Gastrointestinal: nausea, vomiting, epigastric pain, hematemesis, diarrhea.
2. Central nervous system: headaches, irritability, restlessness, insomnia, reflex hyperexcitability, muscle twitching, clonic and tonic generalized convulsions.
3. Cardiovascular: palpitation, tachycardia, extrasystoles, flushing, hypotension, circulatory failure, ventricular arrhythmias.
4. Respiratory: tachypnea.
5. Renal: potentiation of diuresis.
6. Others: alopecia, hyperglycemia, inappropriate ADH syndrome, rash.

OVERDOSAGE

Management: It is suggested that the management principles (consistent with the clinical status of the patient when first seen) outlined below be instituted and that simultaneous contact with a Regional Poison Control Center be established. In this way both updated information and individualization regarding required therapy may be provided.

1. When potential oral overdose is established and seizure has not occurred:
a) If patient is alert and seen within the early hours after ingestion, induction of emesis may be of value. Gastric lavage has been demonstrated to be of no value in influencing outcome in patients who present more than 1 hour after ingestion.
b) Administer a cathartic. Sorbitol solution is reported to be of value.
c) Administer repeated doses of activated charcoal and monitor theophylline serum levels.
d) Prophylactic administration of phenobarbital has been shown to increase the seizure threshold in laboratory animals, and administration of this drug can be considered.

2. If patient presents with a seizure:
a) Establish an airway.
b) Administer oxygen.
c) Treat the seizure with intravenous diazepam, 0.1 to 0.3 mg/kg up to 10 mg. If seizures cannot be controlled, the use of general anesthesia should be considered.
d) Monitor vital signs, maintain blood pressure and provide adequate hydration.

3. If post-seizure coma is present:
a) Maintain airway and oxygenation.
b) If a result of oral medication, follow above recommendations to prevent absorption of the drug, but intubation and lavage will have to be performed instead of inducing emesis, and the cathartic and charcoal will need to be introduced via a large bore gastric lavage tube.
c) Continue to provide full supportive care and adequate hydration until the drug is metabolized. In general, drug metabolism is sufficiently rapid so as not to warrant dialysis. If repeated oral activated charcoal is ineffective (as noted by stable or rising serum levels) charcoal hemoperfusion may be indicated.

DOSAGE AND ADMINISTRATION

Effective use of theophylline (i.e., the concentration of drug in the serum associated with optimal benefit and minimal risk of toxicity) is considered to occur when the theophylline concentration is maintained from 10 to 20 mcg/ml. The early studies from which these levels were derived were carried out in patients immediately or shortly after recovery from acute exacerbations of their disease (some hospitalized with status asmaticus).
Although the 20 mcg/ml level remains appropriate as a critical value (above which toxicity is more likely to occur) for safety purposes, additional data are now available which indicate that the serum theophylline concentrations required to produce maximum physiologic benefit may, in fact, fluctuate with the degree of bronchospasm present and are variable. Therefore, the physician should individualize the range appropriate to the patient's requirements, based on both symptomatic response and improvement in pulmonary function. It should be stressed that serum theophylline concentrations maintained at the upper level of the 10 to 20 mcg/ml range may be associated with potential toxicity when factors known to reduce theophylline clearance are operative (see WARNINGS).
If it is not possible to obtain serum level determinations, restriction of the daily dose (in otherwise healthy adults) to not greater than 13 mg/kg/day, to a maximum of 900 mg, in divided doses, will result in relatively few patients exceeding serum levels of 20 mcg/ml and the resultant greater risk of toxicity.
Caution should be exercised for younger children who cannot complain of minor side effects. Older adults, those with cor pulmonale, congestive heart failure, and/or liver diseases may have unusually low dosage requirements and thus may experience toxicity at the maximal dosage recommended below.
Theophylline does not distribute into fatty tissue. Dosage should be calculated on the basis of lean (ideal) body weight where mg/kg doses are presented.
Dosage guidelines are approximations only and the wide range of theophylline clearance between individuals (particularly those with concomitant disease) makes indiscriminate usage hazardous.
THEOLAIR-SR Tablets Should Not Be Chewed or Crushed.

Dosage Guidelines:
There is information which shows that taking THEOLAIR-SR consistently after both high-fat and low-fat content breakfasts does not result in a decrease in peak concentration or delay in time to peak concentration that are seen when a single dose of THEOLAIR-SR is taken immediately after a high-fat content breakfast. Therefore, THEOLAIR-SR should be administered consistently with respect to food: either with meals,, or fasted (at least 2 hours pre- or 2 hours post-meals). (See PRECAUTIONS, Drug/Food Interactions.)
Status asthmaticus should be considered a medical emergency and is defined as that degree of bronchospasm which is not rapidly responsive to usual doses of conventional bronchodilators. Optimal therapy for such patients frequently requires both additional medication, parenterally administered, and close monitoring, preferably in an intensive care setting.
Acute Symptoms—THEOLAIR-SR Tablets are not intended for patients experiencing an acute episode of bronchospasm (associated with asthma, chronic bronchitis, or emphysema). Such patients require rapid relief of symptoms and should be treated with an immediate-release theophylline preparation (such as THEOLAIR Tablets or Liquid), an intravenous theophylline preparation or other bronchodilators, and not with controlled-release products.
Chronic Symptoms—Theophylline administration is a treatment for the management of reversible bronchospasm (asthma, chronic bronchitis and emphysema) to prevent symptoms and maintain patent airways. The appropriate dosage of theophylline can be established using an immediate-release preparation. Slow clinical titration is preferred to help assure acceptance and safety of the medication. When appropriate theophylline serum levels have been attained and clinical improvement has been maintained, the patient can usually be switched to THEOLAIR-SR Tablets by dividing the total daily dose of immediate-release theophylline by two and administering the appropriate THEOLAIR-SR Tablet every 12 hours (see conversion chart below). However, certain patients, such as the young, smokers, or some nonsmoking adults are likely to metabolize theophylline rapidly and require the total daily dose administered as three equal doses at eight-hour intervals. Such patients can generally be identified as having trough serum levels lower than desired or repeatedly exhibiting symptoms near the end of a dosing interval.

If the established daily dose is:	The q12 hr regimen is: number tablets:	strength:
400 mg	1	THEOLAIR-SR 200 mg
500 mg	1	THEOLAIR-SR 250 mg
600 mg	1	THEOLAIR-SR 300 mg
1000 mg	1	THEOLAIR-SR 500 mg

Alternatively, therapy can be initiated with THEOLAIR-SR since it is available in dosage strengths which permit titration and adjustment of dosage as noted above. A liquid preparation should be considered for children to permit both greater ease of and more accurate dosage adjustment.

Continued on next page

3M—Cont.

Recommended Doses for Initiating Therapy with THEO-LAIR-SR:

Initial Dose —As an initial dose, 16 mg/kg per 24 hours or 400 mg per 24 hours (whichever is less) of THEOLAIR-SR Tablets in divided doses at 8- or 12-hour intervals, as appropriate (see DOSAGE AND ADMINISTRATION).

Increasing Dose —The above dosage may be increased in approximately 25% increments at three-day intervals so long as the drug is tolerated, until clinical response is satisfactory or the maximum dose as indicated in the following section is reached. The serum concentration may be checked at these intervals, but at a minimum, should be determined at the end of this adjustment period.

IT IS IMPORTANT THAT NO PATIENT BE MAINTAINED ON ANY DOSAGE THAT IS NOT TOLERATED. In instructing patients to increase dosage, they should be instructed not to take a subsequent dose if side effects occur and to resume therapy at a lower dose once adverse effects have disappeared.

Maximum Dose Where the Serum Concentration is Not Measured:

WARNING: DO NOT ATTEMPT TO MAINTAIN ANY DOSE THAT IS NOT TOLERATED.

Do not exceed the following (or 900 mg, whichever is less):

Age 6 —under 9 years	24 mg/kg/day
Age 9 —under 12 years	20 mg/kg/day
Age 12 —under 16 years	18 mg/kg/day
Age 16 years and older	13 mg/kg/day

Measurement of Serum Theophylline Concentrations During Chronic Therapy

If the above maximum doses are to be maintained or exceeded, serum theophylline measurement is essential (see PRECAUTIONS, Laboratory Tests, for guidance).

Dosage Adjustment After Serum Theophylline Measurement:

If serum theophylline is:		Directions:
Within desired range		Maintain dosage if tolerated. Recheck serum theophylline concentration at 6- to 12- month intervals.*
Too high	20 to 25 mcg/ml	Decrease doses by about 10% and recheck serum level after 3 days.
	25 to 30 mcg/ml	Skip the next dose and decrease subsequent doses by about 25%. Recheck serum level after 3 days.
	Over 30 mcg/ml	Skip next two doses and decrease subsequent doses by 50%. Recheck serum level after 3 days.
Too low		Increase dosage by 25% at 3 day intervals until either the desired serum concentration and/or clinical response is achieved.* The total daily dose may need to be administered at more frequent intervals if symptoms occur repeatedly at the end of a dosing interval.

The serum concentration may be rechecked at appropriate intervals, but at least at the end of any adjustment period. When the patient's condition is otherwise clinically stable, and none of the recognized factors which alter elimination are present, measurement of serum levels need be repeated only every 6 to 12 months.

* Finer adjustments in dosage may be needed for some patients.

HOW SUPPLIED

THEOLAIR-SR Tablets:

200 mg sustained-release tablets—Each round, white, scored tablet imprinted with "3M" on one side and "SR 200" on the other. Bottles of 100 (NDC 0089-0341-10) and 1000 (NDC 0089-0341-80).

250 mg sustained-release tablets—Each round, white, scored tablet imprinted with "3M" on one side and "SR 250" on the other. Bottles of 100 (NDC 0089-0345-10) and 250 (NDC 0089-0345-25).

300 mg sustained-release tablets—Each oval, white, scored tablet imprinted with "3M" on one side and "SR 300" on other other. Bottles of 100 (NDC 0089-0343-10) and 1000 (NDC 0089-0343-80).

500 mg sustained-release tablets—Each capsule-shaped, white, scored tablet imprinted with "3M" on one side and "SR 500" on the other. Bottles of 100 (NDC 0089-0347-10) and 250 (NDC 0089-0347-25).

STORE AT CONTROLLED ROOM TEMPERATURE 15°–30°C (59°–86°F).

Caution: Federal law prohibits dispensing without prescription.

THSR-9   MAY 1991
3M Riker
3M Health Care
Northridge, CA 91324   3M
Shown in Product Identification Section, page 416

UREX™   ℞
(methenamine hippurate)

DESCRIPTION

Urex (methenamine hippurate) is the hippuric acid salt of methenamine (hexamethylenetetramine). Urex tablets also contain: magnesium stearate, povidone, and saccharin sodium.

HOW SUPPLIED

One gram scored, white tablets, bottles of 100 (NDC 0089-0371-10).

Macsil, Inc.
1326 FRANKFORD AVENUE
PHILADELPHIA, PA 19125

BALMEX® BABY POWDER   OTC

(See PDR For Nonprescription Drugs.)

BALMEX® EMOLLIENT LOTION   OTC

(See PDR For Nonprescription Drugs.)

BALMEX® OINTMENT   OTC

(See PDR For Nonprescription Drugs.)

Marion Merrell Dow Inc.
9300 WARD PARKWAY
MAIL: P.O. BOX 8480
KANSAS CITY, MO 64114-0480

PRODUCT IDENTIFICATION
NUMERICAL SUMMARY
SOLID ORAL DOSAGE FORMS

Marion Merrell Dow Inc.
Kansas City, MO 64114
To provide quick and positive identification of Marion Merrell Dow Inc. prescription drug products, we have imprinted an identifying number and the name MARION on the following tablets or capsules.

1375   DITROPAN® Tablets (oxybutynin chloride)
1555   PAVABID® Capsules, 150 mg (papaverine hydrochloride)*
1771   CARDIZEM® Tablets, 30 mg (diltiazem hydrochloride)
1772   CARDIZEM® Tablets, 60 mg (diltiazem hydrochloride)

BENTYL® Capsules, 10 mg (dicyclomine hydrochloride USP) is imprinted BENTYL 10.
BENTYL® Tablets, 20 mg (dicyclomine hydrochloride USP) is debossed BENTYL 20.
BRICANYL® Tablets, 2.5 mg (terbutaline sulfate USP) is debossed BRICANYL 2½.
BRICANYL® Tablets, 5 mg (terbutaline sulfate USP) is debossed BRICANYL 5.
CANTIL® Tablets, 25 mg (mepenzolate bromide USP) is debossed MERRELL 37.
CARAFATE® Tablets, 1 gm (sucralfate) is identified by the brand name CARAFATE embossed on one side and 1712 bracketed by C's imprinted on the reverse side.
CARDIZEM® Tablets, 90 mg (diltiazem hydrochloride) is imprinted with the brand name CARDIZEM on one side and 90 mg on the reverse side.
CARDIZEM® Tablets, 120 mg (diltiazem hydrochloride) is imprinted with the brand name CARDIZEM on one side and 120 mg on the reverse side.

* PAVABID Capsules, 150 mg (papaverine hydrochloride) also bear the brand name PAVABID.

CARDIZEM® SR Capsules, 60 mg (diltiazem hydrochloride) is imprinted with the Cardizem logo on one end and Cardizem SR 60 mg on the other.
CARDIZEM® SR Capsules, 90 mg (diltiazem hydrochloride) is imprinted with the Cardizem logo on one end and Cardizem SR 90 mg on the other.
CARDIZEM® SR Capsules, 120 mg (diltiazem hydrochloride) is imprinted with the Cardizem logo on one end and Cardizem SR 120 mg on the other.
CARDIZEM® CD Capsules, 180 mg (diltiazem hydrochloride) is imprinted with the Marion Merrell Dow Inc. logo on one end and 1796 and 180 mg on the other or CARDIZEM CD and 180 mg on the other.
CARDIZEM® CD Capsules, 240 mg (diltiazem hydrochloride) is imprinted with the Marion Merrell Dow Inc. logo on one end and 1797 and 240 mg on the other or CARDIZEM CD and 240 mg on the other.
CARDIZEM® CD Capsules, 300 mg (diltiazem hydrochloride) is imprinted with the Marion Merrell Dow Inc. logo on one end and 1798 and 300 mg on the other or CARDIZEM CD and 300 mg on the other.
CLOMID® Tablets, 50 mg (clomiphene citrate) is debossed CLOMID 50.
HIPREX® Tablets, 1 gm (methenamine hippurate) is debossed MERRELL 277.
LORELCO® Tablets, 250 mg (probucol) is imprinted LORELCO 250.
LORELCO® Tablets, 500 mg (probucol) is marked LORELCO 500.
NORPRAMIN® Tablets, 10 mg (desipramine hydrochloride USP) is imprinted 68-7.
NORPRAMIN® Tablets, 25 mg (desipramine hydrochloride USP) is imprinted NORPRAMIN 25.
NORPRAMIN® Tablets, 50 mg (desipramine hydrochloride USP) is imprinted NORPRAMIN 50.
NORPRAMIN® Tablets, 75 mg (desipramine hydrochloride USP) is imprinted NORPRAMIN 75.
NORPRAMIN® Tablets, 100 mg (desipramine hydrochloride USP) is imprinted NORPRAMIN 100.
NORPRAMIN® Tablets, 150 mg (desipramine hydrochloride USP) is imprinted NORPRAMIN 150.
NOVAFED® A Capsules, 120 mg pseudoephedrine hydrochloride and 8 mg chlorpheniramine maleate is imprinted NOVAFED A.
NOVAFED® Capsules, 120 mg (pseudoephedrine hydrochloride) is imprinted NOVAFED.
QUINAMM™ Tablets, 260 mg (quinine sulfate) is embossed W on one side and MERRELL 547 on the other.
RIFADIN® Capsules, 150 mg (rifampin) is imprinted RIFADIN 150.
RIFADIN® Capsules, 300 mg (rifampin) is imprinted RIFADIN 300.
RIFAMATE® Capsules, 300 mg rifampin and 150 mg isoniazid is imprinted RIFAMATE.
SELDANE® Tablets, 60 mg (terfenadine) is debossed SELDANE.
SELDANE®-D Tablets, 60 mg terfenadine and 120 mg pseudoephedrine hydrochloride is debossed SELDANE-D.
TACE® Capsules, 12 mg (chlorotrianisene USP) is imprinted MERRELL 690.
TACE® Capsules, 25 mg (chlorotrianisene USP) is imprinted MERRELL 691.
TENUATE® Tablets, 25 mg (diethylpropion hydrochloride USP) is debossed TENUATE 25.
TENUATE DOSPAN® Controlled-Release Tablets, 75 mg (diethylpropion hydrochloride USP) is debossed TENUATE 75.

AVC™   ℞
(sulfanilamide)
Cream/Suppositories

DESCRIPTION

AVC™ is a preparation for vaginal administration for the treatment of *Candida albicans* infections and available in the following forms:

AVC Cream
Each tube contains:
Sulfanilamide 15.0%
in a water-miscible, non-staining base made from lactose, propylene glycol, stearic acid, diglycol stearate, methylparaben, propylparaben, trolamine, and water; buffered with lactic acid to an acid pH of approximately 4.3.

AVC Suppositories
Each suppository contains:
Sulfanilamide .... 1.05 g
with lactose, in a base made from polyethylene glycol 400, polysorbate 80, polyethylene glycol 3350, and glycerin; buffered with lactic acid to an acid pH of approximately 4.5. AVC Suppositories have an inert, white, non-staining covering, which dissolves promptly in the vagina. The covering is composed of gelatin, glycerin, water, methylparaben, propylparaben, and coloring.

Sulfanilamide is an anti-infective agent. It is p-aminobenzenesulfonamide with the chemical structure:

H₂N—⬡—SO₂NH₂

Sulfanilamide occurs as a white odorless crystalline powder with a slightly bitter taste and sweet aftertaste. It is slightly soluble in water, alcohol, acetone, glycerin, propylene glycol, hydrochloric acid, and solutions of potassium and sodium hydroxide. It is practically insoluble in chloroform, ether, benzene, and petroleum ether.

CLINICAL PHARMACOLOGY
Sulfanilamide has been a useful ingredient of vaginal formulations for about four decades. It blocks certain metabolic processes essential for the growth of susceptible bacteria. In AVC, the sulfanilamide is in a specifically compounded base buffered to the pH (about 4.3) of the normal vagina to encourage the presence of the normally occurring Döderlein's bacilli of the vagina.
The use of AVC for the treatment of vulvovaginitis caused by *Candida albicans* is supported by three clinical investigations. The three studies show AVC with sulfanilamide to be significantly more effective (p ≤ 0.01) than placebo as follows:
In Study I, the ratio of effectiveness was 71% for the AVC with sulfanilamide versus 49% for placebo with 30 days of treatment;
In Study II, the percentages were 48% and 24%, respectively, with 15 days of treatment;
In Study III, the percentages were 66% versus 33%, respectively, with 30 days of treatment.

INDICATIONS AND USAGE
For the treatment of vulvovaginitis caused by *Candida albicans*. (See CLINICAL PHARMACOLOGY.)

CONTRAINDICATIONS
AVC should not be used in patients known to be sensitive to this product or to the sulfonamides.

PRECAUTIONS
General
Because sulfonamides are absorbed from the vaginal mucosa, the usual precautions for oral sulfonamides apply. Patients should be observed for skin rash or evidence of systemic toxicity, and if these develop, the medications should be discontinued.
Deaths associated with administration of oral sulfonamides have reportedly occurred from hypersensitivity reactions, agranulocytosis, aplastic anemia, and other blood dyscrasias. Goiter production, diuresis, and hypoglycemia have reportedly occurred rarely in patients receiving oral sulfonamides. Cross-sensitivity may exist with these agents. Rats appear to be especially susceptible to the goitrogenic effects of sulfonamides, and long-term administration has reportedly produced thyroid malignancies in this species.
Vaginal applicators or inserters should be used with caution after the seventh month of pregnancy.
Information For Patients
The doctor should advise the patient that in the event unusual local itching and burning occur, or other unusual symptoms develop, medication should be discontinued and not re-started without further consultation.
Drug Interactions
Drug interactions have not been documented with AVC.
Carcinogenesis, Mutagenesis, Impairment of Fertility
No data are available on long-term potential of AVC for carcinogenicity, mutagenicity, or impairment of fertility in animals or humans.
Pregnancy
Teratogenic Effects
Pregnancy Category C
Animal reproductive studies have been conducted with sulfonamides, including sulfanilamide (see below). It is not known whether AVC can cause fetal harm when administered to a pregnant woman or can affect reproductive capacity. AVC should be given to a pregnant woman only if clearly needed.
Sulfonamides, including sulfanilamide, readily pass through the placenta and reach fetal circulation. The concentration in the fetus is from 50–90% of that in the maternal blood and if high enough, can cause toxic effects. The safe use of sulfonamides, including sulfanilamide, in pregnancy has not been established. The teratogenic potential of most sulfonamides has not been thoroughly investigated in either animals or humans. However, a significant increase in the incidence of cleft palate and other bony abnormalities of offspring has been observed when certain sulfonamides of the short, intermediate, and long-acting types (including sulfanilamide) were given to pregnant rats and mice at high oral doses (seven to 25 times the human therapeutic oral dose).
Nursing Mothers
Sulfanilamide should be avoided in nursing mothers because absorbed sulfonamides will appear in maternal milk, and have caused kernicterus in the newborn. Because of the po-

tential for serious adverse reactions in nursing infants from sulfonamides, a decision should be made whether to discontinue nursing or to discontinue the drug.
Pediatric Use
Safety and effectiveness of AVC in children have not been established.

ADVERSE REACTIONS
Local sensitivity reactions such as increased discomfort or a burning sensation have occasionally been reported following the use of topical sulfonamides. With the use of AVC Cream, sensitivity reactions (only local) were reported for 0.2% of the investigational patients.
Treatment should be discontinued if either local or systemic manifestations of sulfonamide toxicity or sensitivity occur.

DRUG ABUSE AND DEPENDENCE
Tolerance, abuse, or dependence with AVC have not been reported.

OVERDOSAGE
There have been no reports of accidental overdosage with AVC.
The acute oral LD₅₀ of sulfanilamide is 3700–4200 mg/kg in mice.
The minimum human lethal dose of AVC has not been established.
It is not known if AVC is dialyzable.

DOSAGE AND ADMINISTRATION
One applicatorful (about 6 g) or one suppository intravaginally once or twice daily. Improvements in symptoms should occur within a few days, but treatment should be continued for a period of 30 days.
Douching with a suitable solution before insertion may be recommended for hygienic purposes.

HOW SUPPLIED
AVC *Cream*
NDC 0068-0099-04   4 oz tube with applicator
Store at room temperature, below 86°F. Protect from cold. Product darkens with age. Potency is maintained throughout labeled shelf life when stored as directed.
AVC *Suppositories*
NDC 0068-0098-16   Box of 16 white gelatin suppositories with inserter
Store at room temperature, below 86°F. Protect from excessive cold and moisture.
Product Information as of March, 1991
Merrell Dow Pharmaceuticals Inc.
Subsidiary of Marion Merrell Dow Inc.
Kansas City, MO 64114

J174D

BENTYL® ℞
[*bĕn′til*]
(dicyclomine hydrochloride USP)
Tablets, Capsules, Syrup, Injection

DESCRIPTION
Bentyl is an antispasmodic and anticholinergic (antimuscarinic) agent available in the following forms:
1. Bentyl capsules for oral use contain 10 mg dicyclomine hydrochloride USP. Bentyl 10 mg capsules also contain inactive ingredients: calcium sulfate, corn starch, FD&C Blue No. 1, FD&C Red No. 3, gelatin, lactose, magnesium stearate, pregelatinized corn starch, and titanium dioxide.
2. Bentyl tablets for oral use contain 20 mg dicyclomine hydrochloride USP. Bentyl 20 mg tablets also contain inactive ingredients: acacia, dibasic calcium phosphate, corn starch, FD&C Blue No. 1, lactose, magnesium stearate, pregelatinized corn starch, and sucrose.
3. Bentyl syrup for oral use contains 10 mg dicyclomine hydrochloride USP in each 5 mL (1 teaspoonful). Bentyl syrup also contains inactive ingredients: citric acid, D&C Red No. 33, FD&C Blue No. 1, FD&C Red No. 40, FD&C Yellow No. 6, flavors, glucose, methylparaben, propylene glycol, propylparaben, saccharin sodium, and water.
4. Bentyl Injection is a sterile, pyrogen free, aqueous solution for intramuscular injection (NOT FOR INTRAVENOUS USE).
Ampul—2 mL—Each mL contains 10 mg dicyclomine hydrochloride USP in sterile water for injection, made isotonic with sodium chloride.
Vial—10 mL—Each mL contains 10 mg dicyclomine hydrochloride USP in sterile water for injection, made isotonic with sodium chloride. A preservative containing 0.5% chlorobutanol hydrous (chloral derivative) has been added.
Chemically, Bentyl (dicyclomine hydrochloride) is [bicyclohexyl]-1-carboxylic acid, 2-(diethylamino)ethyl ester, hydrochloride with the chemical structure:
[See chemical structure at top of next column.]
Dicyclomine hydrochloride occurs as a fine, white, crystalline, practically odorless powder with a bitter taste. It is solu-

[chemical structure diagram]
•HCl

ble in water, freely soluble in alcohol and chloroform, and very slightly soluble in ether.

CLINICAL PHARMACOLOGY
Dicyclomine relieves smooth muscle spasm of the gastrointestinal tract. Animal studies indicate that this action is achieved via a dual mechanism: (1) a specific anticholinergic effect (antimuscarinic) at the acetylcholine-receptor sites with approximately ⅛ the milligram potency of atropine (*in vitro*, guinea pig ileum); and (2) a direct effect upon smooth muscle (musculotropic) as evidenced by dicyclomine's antagonism of bradykinin- and histamine-induced spasms of the isolated guinea pig ileum. Atropine did not affect responses to these two agonists. *In vivo* studies in cats and dogs showed dicyclomine to be equally potent against acetylcholine (ACh)- or barium chloride (BaCl₂)-induced intestinal spasm while atropine was at least 200 times more potent against effects of ACh than BaCl₂. Tests for mydriatic effects in mice showed that dicyclomine was approximately ¹⁄₅₀₀ as potent as atropine: antisialogogue tests in rabbits showed dicyclomine to be ¹⁄₃₀₀ as potent as atropine.
In man, dicyclomine is rapidly absorbed after oral administration, reaching peak values within 60–90 minutes. The principal route of elimination is via the urine (79.5% of the dose). Excretion also occurs in the feces, but to a lesser extent (8.4%). Mean half-life of plasma elimination in one study was determined to be approximately 1.8 hours when plasma concentrations were measured for 9 hours after a single dose. In subsequent studies, plasma concentrations were followed for up to 24 hours after a single dose, showing a secondary phase of elimination with a somewhat longer half-life. Mean volume of distribution for a 20 mg oral dose is approximately 3.65 L/kg suggesting extensive distribution in tissues.
In controlled clinical trials involving over 100 patients who received drug, 82% of patients treated for functional bowel/irritable bowel syndrome with dicyclomine hydrochloride at initial doses of 160 mg daily (40 mg q.i.d.) demonstrated a favorable clinical response compared with 55% treated with placebo. (P < .05). In these trials, most of the side effects were typically anticholinergic in nature (see table) and were reported by 61% of the patients.

Side Effect	Dicyclomine Hydrochloride (40 mg q.i.d.) %	Placebo %
Dry Mouth	33	5
Dizziness	29	2
Blurred Vision	27	2
Nausea	14	6
Light-headedness	11	3
Drowsiness	9	1
Weakness	7	1
Nervousness	6	2

Nine percent (9%) of patients were discontinued from the drug because of one or more of these side effects (compared with 2% in the placebo group). In 41% of the patients with side effects, side effects disappeared or were tolerated at the 160 mg daily dose without reduction. A dose reduction from 160 mg daily to an average daily dose of 90 mg was required in 46% of the patients with side effects who then continued to experience a favorable clinical response; their side effects either disappeared or were tolerated. (See ADVERSE REACTIONS.)

INDICATIONS AND USAGE
For the treatment of functional bowel/irritable bowel syndrome.

CONTRAINDICATIONS
1. Obstructive uropathy
2. Obstructive disease of the gastrointestinal tract
3. Severe ulcerative colitis (see PRECAUTIONS)
4. Reflux esophagitis
5. Unstable cardiovascular status in acute hemorrhage
6. Glaucoma
7. Myasthenia gravis
8. Evidence of prior hypersensitivity to dicyclomine hydrochloride or other ingredients of these formulations
9. Infants less than 6 months of age (See WARNINGS and PRECAUTIONS: *Information for Patients.*)
10. Nursing Mothers (See WARNINGS and PRECAUTIONS: *Information for Patients.*)

Continued on next page

Marion Merrell Dow—Cont.

WARNINGS

In the presence of a high environmental temperature, heat prostration can occur with drug use (fever and heat stroke due to decreased sweating). If symptoms occur, the drug should be discontinued and supportive measures instituted.

Diarrhea may be an early symptom of incomplete intestinal obstruction, especially in patients with ileostomy or colostomy. In this instance, treatment with this drug would be inappropriate and possibly harmful.

Bentyl may produce drowsiness or blurred vision. The patient should be warned not to engage in activities requiring mental alertness, such as operating a motor vehicle or other machinery or performing hazardous work while taking this drug.

Psychosis has been reported in sensitive individuals given anticholinergic drugs. CNS signs and symptoms include confusion, disorientation, short-term memory loss, hallucinations, dysarthria, ataxia, coma, euphoria, decreased anxiety, fatigue, insomnia, agitation and mannerisms, and inappropriate affect. These CNS signs and symptoms usually resolve within 12 to 24 hours after discontinuation of the drug.

There are reports that administration of dicyclomine hydrochloride syrup to infants has been followed by serious respiratory symptoms (dyspnea, shortness of breath, breathlessness, respiratory collapse, apnea, asphyxia), seizures, syncope, pulse rate fluctuations, muscular hypotonia, and coma. Death has been reported. No causal relationship between these effects observed in infants and dicyclomine administration has been established. BENTYL IS CONTRAINDICATED IN INFANTS LESS THAN 6 MONTHS OF AGE AND IN NURSING MOTHERS. (See CONTRAINDICATIONS and PRECAUTIONS: *Nursing Mothers* and *Pediatric Use.)*

Safety and efficacy of dicyclomine hydrochloride in children have not been established.

PRECAUTIONS

General

Use with caution in patients with:

1. Autonomic neuropathy
2. Hepatic or renal disease
3. Ulcerative colitis—large doses may suppress intestinal motility to the point of producing a paralytic ileus and the use of this drug may precipitate or aggravate the serious complication of toxic megacolon (see CONTRAINDICATIONS)
4. Hyperthyroidism
5. Hypertension
6. Coronary heart disease
7. Congestive heart failure
8. Cardiac tachyarrhythmia
9. Hiatal hernia (see CONTRAINDICATIONS: reflux esophagitis)
10. Known or suspected prostatic hypertrophy.

Investigate any tachycardia before administration of dicyclomine hydrochloride, since it may increase the heart rate.

With overdosage, a curare-like action may occur (i.e., neuromuscular blockade leading to muscular weakness and possible paralysis).

Information For Patients

Bentyl may produce drowsiness or blurred vision. The patient should be warned not to engage in activities requiring mental alertness, such as operating a motor vehicle or other machinery or to perform hazardous work while taking this drug.

Bentyl is contraindicated in infants less than 6 months of age and in nursing mothers. (See CONTRAINDICATIONS, WARNINGS, and PRECAUTIONS: *Nursing Mothers* and *Pediatric Use.)*

In the presence of a high environmental temperature, heat prostration can occur with drug use (fever and heat stroke due to decreased sweating). If symptoms occur, the drug should be discontinued and a physician contacted.

Drug Interactions

The following agents may increase certain actions or side effects of anticholinergic drugs: amantadine, antiarrhythmic agents of class I (e.g., quinidine), antihistamines, antipsychotic agents (e.g., phenothiazines), benzodiazepines, MAO inhibitors, narcotic analgesics (e.g., meperidine), nitrates and nitrites, sympathomimetic agents, tricyclic antidepressants, and other drugs having anticholinergic activity.

Anticholinergics antagonize the effects of antiglaucoma agents. Anticholinergic drugs in the presence of increased intraocular pressure may be hazardous when taken concurrently with agents such as corticosteroids. (See also CONTRAINDICATIONS.)

Anticholinergic agents may affect gastrointestinal absorption of various drugs, such as slowly dissolving dosage forms of digoxin; increased serum digoxin concentrations may result. Anticholinergic drugs may antagonize the effects of drugs that alter gastrointestinal motility, such as metoclopramide. Because antacids may interfere with the absorption of anticholinergic agents, simultaneous use of these drugs should be avoided.

The inhibiting effects of anticholinergic drugs on gastric hydrochloric acid secretion are antagonized by agents used to treat achlorhydria and those used to test gastric secretion.

Carcinogenesis, Mutagenesis, Impairment of Fertility

There are no known human data on long-term potential for carcinogenicity or mutagenicity.

Long-term studies in animals to determine carcinogenic potential are not known to have been conducted.

In studies in rats at doses of up to 100 mg/kg/day, Bentyl produced no deleterious effects on breeding, conception, or parturition.

Pregnancy

Tetatogenic Effects

Pregnancy Category B

Reproduction studies have been performed in rats and rabbits at doses up to 33 times the maximum recommended human dose based on 160 mg/day (3 mg/kg) and have revealed no evidence of impaired fertility or harm to the fetus due to dicyclomine. Epidemiologic studies in pregnant women with products containing dicyclomine hydrochloride (at doses up to 40 mg/day) have not shown that dicyclomine increases the risk of fetal abnormalities if administered during the first trimester of pregnancy. There are, however, no adequate and well-controlled studies in pregnant women at the recommended doses (80–160 mg/day). Because animal reproduction studies are not always predictive of human response, Bentyl as indicated for functional bowel/irritable bowel syndrome should be used during pregnancy only if clearly needed.

Nursing Mothers

Since dicyclomine hydrochloride has been reported to be excreted in human milk, BENTYL IS CONTRAINDICATED IN NURSING MOTHERS. (See CONTRAINDICATIONS, WARNINGS, PRECAUTIONS: *Pediatric Use* and ADVERSE REACTIONS.)

Pediatric Use (See CONTRAINDICATIONS, WARNINGS, and PRECAUTIONS: *Nursing Mothers.)* BENTYL IS CONTRAINDICATED IN INFANTS LESS THAN 6 MONTHS OF AGE.

Safety and effectiveness in children have not been established.

ADVERSE REACTIONS

Controlled clinical trials have provided frequency information for reported adverse effects of dicyclomine hydrochloride listed in a decreasing order of frequency. (See CLINICAL PHARMACOLOGY.)

Not all of the following adverse reactions have been reported with dicyclomine hydrochloride. Adverse reactions are included here that have been reported for pharmacologically similar drugs with anticholinergic/antispasmodic action.

Gastrointestinal: dry mouth, nausea, vomiting, constipation, bloated feeling, abdominal pain, taste loss, anorexia

Central Nervous System: dizziness, light-headedness, tingling, headache, drowsiness, weakness, nervousness, numbness, mental confusion and/or excitement (especially in elderly persons), dyskinesia, lethargy, syncope, speech disturbance, insomnia

Ophthalmologic: blurred vision, diplopia, mydriasis, cycloplegia, increased ocular tension

Dermatologic/Allergic: rash, urticaria, itching, and other dermal manifestations; severe allergic reaction or drug idiosyncrases including anaphylaxis

Genitourinary: urinary hesitancy, urinary retention

Cardiovascular: tachycardia, palpitations

Respiratory: Dyspnea, apnea, asphyxia (see WARNINGS)

Other: decreased sweating, nasal stuffiness or congestion, sneezing, throat congestion, impotence, suppression of lactation (see PRECAUTIONS: *Nursing Mothers*)

With the injectable form, there may be a temporary sensation of light-headedness. Some local irritation and focal coagulation necrosis may occur following the I.M. injection of the drug.

DRUG ABUSE AND DEPENDENCE

Tolerance, abuse, or dependence with Bentyl has not been reported.

OVERDOSAGE

Signs and Symptoms

The signs and symptoms of overdosage are headache; nausea; vomiting; blurred vision; dilated pupils; hot, dry skin; dizziness; dryness of the mouth; difficulty in swallowing; and CNS stimulation. A curare-like action may occur (i.e., neuromuscular blockade leading to muscular weakness and possible paralysis).

Oral LD_{50}

The acute oral LD_{50} of the drug is 625 mg/kg in mice.

Minimum Human Lethal Dose/Maximum Human Dose Recorded

The amount of drug in a single dose that is ordinarily associated with symptoms of overdosage or that is likely to be life threatening, has not been defined. The maximum human oral dose recorded was 600 mg by mouth in a 10-month-old child and approximately 1500 mg in an adult, each of whom survived.

In three of the infants who died following administration of dicyclomine hydrochloride (see WARNINGS), the blood concentrations of drug were 200, 220, and 505 ng/mL, respectively.

Dialysis

It is not known if Bentyl is dialyzable.

Treatment

Treatment should consist of gastric lavage, emetics, and activated charcoal. Sedatives (e.g., short-acting barbiturates, benzodiazepines) may be used for management of overt signs of excitement. If indicated, an appropriate parenteral cholinergic agent may be used as an antidote.

DOSAGE AND ADMINISTRATION

DOSAGE MUST BE ADJUSTED TO INDIVIDUAL PATIENT NEEDS. (See CLINICAL PHARMACOLOGY.)

Adults—Oral

The only oral dose clearly shown to be effective is 160 mg per day (in 4 equally divided doses). Since this dose is associated with a significant incidence of side effects, it is prudent to begin with 80 mg per day (in 4 equally divided doses). Depending upon the patient's response during the first week of therapy, the dose should be increased to 160 mg per day unless side effects limit dosage escalation.

If efficacy is not achieved within 2 weeks or side effects require doses below 80 mg per day, the drug should be discontinued. Documented safety data are not available for doses above 80 mg daily for periods longer than 2 weeks.

Adults—Intramuscular injection

NOT FOR INTRAVENOUS USE.

The intramuscular dosage form is to be used temporarily when the patient cannot take oral medication. Intramuscular injection is about twice as bioavailable as oral dosage forms; consequently, the recommended intramuscular dose is 80 mg daily (in 4 equally divided doses).

Oral dicyclomine hydrochloride should be started as soon as possible and the intramuscular form should not be used for periods longer than 1 or 2 days.

ASPIRATE THE SYRINGE BEFORE INJECTING TO AVOID INTRAVASCULAR INJECTION, SINCE THROMBOSIS MAY OCCUR IF THE DRUG IS INADVERTENTLY INJECTED INTRAVASCULARLY. Parenteral drug products should be inspected visually for particulate matter and discoloration prior to administration, whenever solution and container permit.

HOW SUPPLIED

10 mg blue capsules, imprinted BENTYL 10

NDC 0068-0120-61: bottles of 100

NDC 0068-0120-65: bottles of 500

Store at room temperature, preferably below 86°F (30°C).

20 mg compressed, light blue, round tablets, debossed BENTYL 20

NDC 0068-0123-61: bottles of 100

NDC 0068-0123-65: bottles of 500

NDC 0068-0123-71: bottles of 1000

To prevent fading, avoid exposure to direct sunlight. Store at room temperature, preferably below 86°F (30°C).

10 mg/5mL pink syrup

NDC 0068-0125-16: 16 ounce bottle

Store at room temperature, preferably below 86°F (30°C). Protect from excessive heat.

10 mg/mL injection (for intramuscular use only, NOT FOR INTRAVENOUS USE)

NDC 0068-0810-61: 10 mL multiple dose vials

Store at room temperature, preferably below 86°F (30°C). Protect from freezing.

NDC 0068-0809-23: boxes of five 2 mL ampuls

Store at room temperature, preferably below 86°F (30°C). Protect from freezing.

Product Information as of April, 1991

Injectable dosage forms manufactured by
TAYLOR PHARMACAL COMPANY
Decatur, Illinois 62525 for
Marion Merrell Dow Inc.
Kansas City, MO 64114

Shown in Product Identification Section, page 416

BRICANYL® ℞

[brĭk'ă-nĭl]

(terbutaline sulfate USP)

Subcutaneous Injection

CAUTION: Federal law prohibits dispensing without prescription.

DESCRIPTION

Bricanyl (terbutaline sulfate USP) Subcutaneous Injection is a sterile isotonic solution. Each mL of solution contains 1 mg terbutaline sulfate (equivalent to 0.82 mg free base) and 8.9 mg sodium chloride in water for injection. Hydrochloric acid is used to adjust pH to 3–5.

Terbutaline sulfate (5-[2-[(1,1-dimethylethyl)amino]-1-hydroxyethyl]-1,3-benzenediol sulfate) is a β-adrenergic agonist bronchodilator having the chemical structure:

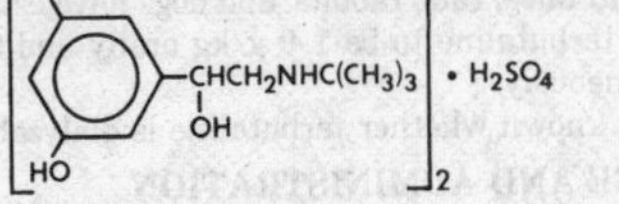

CLINICAL PHARMACOLOGY

Bricanyl is a β-adrenergic receptor agonist which has been shown by *in vitro* and *in vivo* pharmacologic studies in animals to exert a preferential effect on β_2-adrenergic receptors, such as those located in bronchial smooth muscle. However, controlled clinical studies of patients who were administered the drug have not revealed a preferential β_2-adrenergic effect.

It has been postulated that β-adrenergic agonists produce many of their pharmacologic effects by activation of adenyl cyclase, the enzyme which catalyzes the conversion of adenosine triphosphate to cyclic adenosine monophosphate.

Bricanyl Injection has been shown in controlled clinical studies to relieve acute bronchospasm in acute and chronic obstructive pulmonary disease, resulting in a clinically significant increase in pulmonary flow rates, e.g., an increase of 15% or greater in FEV_1 in some patients. Following administration of 0.25 mg by subcutaneous injection, a measurable change in flow rate is usually observed within five minutes, and a clinically significant increase in FEV_1 occurs by 15 minutes following the injection. The maximum effect usually occurs within 30–60 minutes and clinically significant bronchodilator activity has been observed to persist for 90 minutes to four hours in most patients. The duration of clinically significant improvement is comparable to that found with equimilligram doses of epinephrine.

Subcutaneously administered Bricanyl shows peak plasma concentrations 15–30 minutes after injection (0.5 mg dose, mean peak plasma level 7.6 μg/L). Approximately one-third is metabolized (inactive), the majority of the dose being excreted in urine unchanged. A half-life of 3–4 hours has been reported.

Terbutaline crosses the placenta. After single dose IV administration of terbutaline to 22 women in late pregnancy who were delivered by elective Caesarean section due to clinical reasons, umbilical blood levels of terbutaline were found to range from 11 to 48% of the maternal blood levels.

Recent studies in laboratory animals (minipigs, rodents, and dogs) recorded the occurrence of cardiac arrhythmias and sudden death (with histologic evidence of myocardial necrosis) when β agonists and methylxanthines were administered concurrently. The significance of these findings when applied to humans is currently unknown.

INDICATIONS AND USAGE

Bricanyl is indicated as a bronchodilator for the relief of reversible bronchospasm in patients with obstructive airway diseases such as asthma, bronchitis and emphysema.

CONTRAINDICATIONS

Bricanyl is contraindicated in patients with a history of hypersensitivity to any of its components or sympathomimetic amines.

WARNINGS

Usage in Labor and Delivery: Bricanyl is not indicated and should not be used for the management of preterm labor. Serious adverse reactions have been reported following administration of terbutaline sulfate to women in labor. These reports have included transient hypokalemia, pulmonary edema (sometimes after delivery) and hypoglycemia in the mother and/or the neonatal child. Maternal death has been reported with terbutaline sulfate and other drugs of this class.

There have been rare reports of seizures occurring in patients receiving terbutaline, which do not recur when the drug is discontinued and have not been explained on any other basis.

PRECAUTIONS

General

Terbutaline sulfate is a sympathomimetic amine and as such should be used with caution in patients with cardiovascular disorders (including arrhythmias, coronary insufficiency and hypertension), in patients with hyperthyroidism or diabetes mellitus, history of seizures, or in patients who are unusually responsive to sympathomimetic amines. Age-related differences in the hemodynamic response to β-adrenergic receptor stimulation have been reported.

Patients susceptible to hypokalemia should be monitored because transient early falls in serum potassium levels have been reported with β agonists.

Immediate hypersensitivity reactions and exacerbation of bronchospasm have been reported after terbutaline administration.

Preparation of Other Dosage Forms: Use of the subcutaneous injection for preparation of other dosage forms, e.g., IV infusion, is not appropriate. Sterility, stability, and accurate dosing cannot be assured if the ampuls are not used in accordance with information in DOSAGE AND ADMINISTRATION.

Large doses of intravenous terbutaline sulfate have been reported to aggravate preexisting diabetes and ketoacidosis.

Information for Patients

Patients should be advised regarding the potential adverse reactions associated with Bricanyl.

Drug Interactions

Other sympathomimetic bronchodilators or epinephrine should not be used concomitantly with terbutaline sulfate since their combined effect on the cardiovascular system may be deleterious to the patient.

Terbutaline sulfate should be administered with caution in patients being treated with monoamine oxidase (MAO) inhibitors or tricyclic antidepressants, since the action of terbutaline sulfate on the vascular system may be potentiated.

β-adrenergic receptor blocking agents not only block the pulmonary effect of terbutaline but may produce severe asthmatic attacks in asthmatic patients. Therefore, patients requiring treatment for both bronchospastic disease and hypertension should be treated with medication other than β-adrenergic blocking agents for hypertension.

Carcinogenesis, Mutagenesis, Impairment of Fertility

A two-year, oral carcinogenesis bioassay of terbutaline sulfate (50, 500, 1000, and 2000 mg/kg, corresponding to 5,000, 50,000, 100,000, and 200,000 times the recommended daily adult subcutaneous dose, respectively) in the Sprague-Dawley rat revealed drug-related changes in the female genital system. Females showed dose-related increases in leiomyomas of the mesovarium: 3 (5%) at 50 mg/kg, 17 (28%) at 500 mg/kg, 21 (35%) at 1000 mg/kg, and 23 (38%) at 2000 mg/kg, which were significant at the three highest levels. None occurred in female controls. The incidence of ovarian cysts was significantly elevated at all dose levels except at 2000 mg/kg and hyperplasia of the mesovarium was increased significantly at 500 and 2000 mg/kg. A 21-month oral study of terbutaline sulfate (5, 50 and 200 mg/kg, corresponding to 500, 5,000 and 20,000 times the recommended daily adult subcutaneous dose, respectively) in the mouse revealed no evidence of carcinogenicity.

Studies of terbutaline sulfate have not been conducted to determine mutagenic potential.

An oral reproduction study of terbutaline sulfate up to 50 mg/kg (corresponding to 5,000 times the human subcutaneous dose) in the rat revealed no adverse effects on fertility.

Pregnancy

Teratogenic Effects

Pregnancy Category B: Reproduction studies in mice (up to 1.1 mg/kg subcutaneously, corresponding to 110 times the human subcutaneous dose) and in rats and rabbits (up to 50 mg/kg orally, corresponding to 5,000 times the human subcutaneous dose) have revealed no evidence of impaired fertility or harm to the fetus due to terbutaline. There are, however, no adequate and well-controlled studies in pregnant women. Because animal reproduction studies are not always predictive of human response, this drug should be used during pregnancy only if clearly needed.

Labor and Delivery

Usage in Labor and Delivery: The safe use of Bricanyl for the management of preterm labor or for other uses during labor and delivery has not been established and the drug should not be used. (See WARNINGS.)

Nursing Mothers

Terbutaline is excreted in breast milk. Caution should be exercised when Bricanyl is administered to a nursing woman.

Pediatric Use

Safety and effectiveness in children below the age of 12 have not been established.

ADVERSE REACTIONS

The adverse reactions of terbutaline sulfate are similar to those of other sympathomimetic agents.

The most commonly observed side effects are tremor and nervousness. These occur more frequently at doses in excess of 0.25 mg. Other commonly reported reactions include increased heart rate, palpitations and dizziness. Other reported reactions include headache, drowsiness, vomiting, nausea, sweating, and muscle cramps. These reactions are generally transient and usually do not require treatment.

OVERDOSAGE

Overdosage information is limited. Excessive adrenergic-receptor stimulation may augment the signs and symptoms listed under ADVERSE REACTIONS and may be accompanied by other adrenergic effects.

Signs and symptoms of overdosage may include the following—

CARDIOVASCULAR: tachycardia of varying degrees, transient arrhythmias, and extrasystoles. A significant drop in blood pressure may occur due to peripheral vasodilation.

NEUROMUSCULAR: tremors of varying degrees, nervousness, drowsiness, muscle cramps, headache, and sweating.

GASTROINTESTINAL: nausea and vomiting.

ENDOCRINE: varying degrees of hyperglycemia and rise in insulin levels which could be followed by rebound hypoglycemia. Hypokalemia in the early stages may occur. The duration of these signs and symptoms will be dependent on the degree of overdosage.

In the case of terbutaline overdosage, the patient should be treated symptomatically for sympathomimetic overdosage with careful consideration to the appropriateness of any chosen therapy and possible effect on the patient's underlying disease state. (See also WARNINGS.)

Studies in mice, rats, rabbits, and dogs have established the LD_{50} of terbutaline to be 1–9 g/kg orally and 0.3–1.6 g/kg subcutaneously.

It is not known whether terbutaline is dialyzable.

DOSAGE AND ADMINISTRATION

Parenteral drug products should be inspected visually for particulate matter and discoloration prior to administration, whenever solution and container permit.

The usual subcutaneous dose of Bricanyl is 0.25 mg (0.25 mL, ¼ ampul contents) injected into the lateral deltoid area. If significant clinical improvement does not occur by 15–30 minutes, a second dose of 0.25 mg may be administered. A total dose of 0.5 mg should not be exceeded within a four-hour period. If a patient fails to respond to a second 0.25 mg (0.25 mL) dose within 15–30 minutes, other therapeutic measures should be considered.

HOW SUPPLIED

Each 2 mL size ampul contains 1 mL of solution (1 mg terbutaline sulfate). Note: 0.25 mL of solution will provide the usual clinical dose of 0.25 mg.

NDC 0068-0702-20: package of 10 ampuls

Solutions of terbutaline sulfate are sensitive to excessive heat and light. Ampuls should, therefore, be stored at controlled room temperature 15°–30°C (59°–86°F) in their original carton to provide protection from light until dispensed. Solutions should not be used if discolored.

Product Information as of August, 1987

Manufactured by
Astra Pharmaceutical Products, Inc.
Westborough, Mass. 01581

Shown in Product Identification Section, page 416

BRICANYL® ℞
[*brĭk'ă-nĭl*]
(terbutaline sulfate USP)
Tablets

DESCRIPTION

Bricanyl (terbutaline sulfate USP) Tablets for oral administration contain 2.5 mg or 5 mg of terbutaline sulfate (equivalent to 2.05 and 4.1 mg free base, respectively). Both the 2.5 and 5 mg tablets contain the following inactive ingredients: corn starch (or pregelatinized corn starch), lactose, magnesium stearate, microcrystalline cellulose, and povidone.

Terbutaline sulfate (5-[2-[(1,1-dimethylethyl)amino]-1-hydroxyethyl]-1,3-benzenediol sulfate) is a β-adrenergic agonist bronchodilator having the chemical structure:

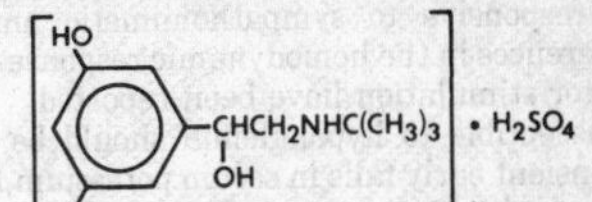

CLINICAL PHARMACOLOGY

Bricanyl is a β-adrenergic receptor agonist which has been shown by *in vitro* and *in vivo* pharmacologic studies in animals to exert a preferential effect on β_2-adrenergic receptors, such as those located in bronchial smooth muscle. However, controlled clinical studies on patients who were administered the drug have not revealed a preferential β_2-adrenergic effect.

It has been postulated that β-adrenergic agonists produce many of their pharmacologic effects by activation of adenyl cyclase, the enzyme which catalyzes the conversion of adenosine triphosphate to cyclic adenosine monophosphate.

Bricanyl Tablets have been shown in controlled clinical studies to relieve bronchospasm in chronic obstructive pulmonary disease such as asthma, chronic bronchitis and emphysema. This action was manifested by a clinically significant increase in pulmonary function as demonstrated by an increase of 15% or greater in FEV_1 in some patients. A measurable change in pulmonary function usually occurs within 30 minutes following oral administration. The maximum effect usually occurs within 120–180 minutes. There is a clinically significant decrease in airway and pulmonary resis-

Continued on next page

Marion Merrell Dow—Cont.

tance which persists for at least 4 hours or longer in most patients. Significant bronchodilator action as measured by various pulmonary function determinations (airway resistance, MMEFR, PEFR) has been demonstrated in studies for periods up to 8 hours in many patients.
Clinical studies have evaluated the effectiveness of oral Bricanyl for periods up to 12 months and the drug continued to produce significant improvement of pulmonary function throughout the period of treatment.
Orally administered terbutaline sulfate is 30–70% absorbed in the GI tract (food reduces bioavailability by one-third). Sixty percent of the absorbed oral dose is metabolized via first pass conjugation in the gut wall and liver. There are no known active metabolites. After single oral doses, peak concentrations are found 30 minutes to 5 hours after administration. Each mg of orally administered terbutaline sulfate (in fasting adults) produces an average peak serum concentration of approximately 1 μg/L. Terbutaline has a half-life of 3–4 hours and is excreted in the urine.
Terbutaline crosses the placenta. After single dose IV administration of terbutaline to 22 women in late pregnancy who were delivered by elective Caesarean section due to clinical reasons, umbilical blood levels of terbutaline were found to range from 11 to 48% of the maternal blood levels.
Recent studies in laboratory animals (minipigs, rodents, and dogs) recorded the occurrence of cardiac arrhythmias and sudden death (with histologic evidence of myocardial necrosis) when β agonist and methylxanthines were administered concurrently. The significance of these findings when applied to humans is currently unknown.

INDICATIONS AND USAGE

Bricanyl is indicated as a bronchodilator for the relief of reversible bronchospasm in patients with obstructive airway diseases such as asthma, bronchitis and emphysema.

CONTRAINDICATIONS

Bricanyl is contraindicated in patients with a history of hypersensitivity to any of its components or sympathomimetic amines.

WARNINGS

Usage in Labor and Delivery: Bricanyl is not indicated and should not be used for the management of preterm labor. Serious adverse reactions have been reported following administration of terbutaline sulfate to women in labor. These reports have included transient hypokalemia, pulmonary edema (sometimes after delivery) and hypoglycemia in the mother and/or neonatal child. Maternal death has been reported with terbutaline sulfate and other drugs of this class. There have been rare reports of seizures occurring in patients receiving terbutaline, which do not recur when the drug is discontinued and have not been explained on any other basis.

PRECAUTIONS

General
Terbutaline sulfate is a sympathomimetic amine and as such should be used with caution in patients with cardiovascular disorders (including arrhythmias, coronary insufficiency, and hypertension), in patients with hyperthyroidism or diabetes mellitus, history of seizures, or in patients who are unusually responsive to sympathomimetic amines. Age-related differences in the hemodynamic response to β-adrenergic receptor stimulation have been reported.
Patients susceptible to hypokalemia should be monitored because transient early falls in serum potassium levels have been reported with β agonists.
Large doses of intravenous terbutaline sulfate have been reported to aggravate preexisting diabetes and ketoacidosis. The relevance of this observation to the use of Bricanyl Tablets is unknown.
Immediate hypersensitivity reactions and exacerbation of bronchospasm have been reported after terbutaline administration.
Information for Patients
The patient should be advised regarding the potential adverse reactions associated with Bricanyl and that: (1) the action of Bricanyl Tablets may last up to 8 hours and, therefore should not be used more frequently than recommended. (2) the number or frequency of doses should not be increased without medical consultation, (3) medical consultation should be sought promptly if symptoms get worse, and (4) other medicines should not be used while taking Bricanyl without consulting the physician.
Drug Interactions
Other sympathomimetic bronchodilators or epinephrine should not be used concomitantly with terbutaline sulfate, since their combined effect on the cardiovascular system may be deleterious to the patient. This recommendation does not preclude the judicious use of an aerosol bronchodilator of the adrenergic stimulant type in patients receiving Bricanyl Tablets. Such concomitant use, however, should be individualized and not given on a routine basis. If regular coadministration is required, alternative therapy should be considered. Terbutaline sulfate should be administered with caution in patients being treated with monoamine oxidase (MAO) inhibitors or tricyclic antidepressants, since the action of terbutaline sulfate on the vascular system may be potentiated. β-adrenergic receptor blocking agents not only block the pulmonary effect of terbutaline but may produce severe asthmatic attacks in asthmatic patients. Therefore, patients requiring treatment for both bronchospastic disease and hypertension should be treated with medication other than β-adrenergic blocking agents for their hypertension.
Carcinogenesis, Mutagenesis, Impairment of Fertility
A two-year, oral carcinogenesis bioassay of terbutaline sulfate (50, 500, 1000 and 2000 mg/kg, corresponding to 167, 1667, 3333, and 6667 times the recommended daily adult oral dose, respectively) in the Sprague-Dawley rat revealed drug-related changes in the female genital system. Females showed dose-related increases in leiomyomas of the mesovarium: 3 (5%) at 50 mg/kg, 17 (28%) at 500 mg/kg, 21 (35%) at 1000 mg/kg, and 23 (38%) at 2000 mg/kg, which were significant at the three highest levels. None occurred in female controls. The incidence of ovarian cysts was significantly elevated at all dose levels except at 2000 mg/kg and hyperplasia of the mesovarium was increased significantly at 500 and 2000 mg/kg. A 21-month oral study of terbutaline sulfate (5, 50 and 200 mg/kg, corresponding to 17, 167 and 667 times the recommended daily adult oral dose, respectively) in the mouse revealed no evidence of carcinogenicity.
Studies of terbutaline sulfate have not been conducted to determine mutagenic potential.
An oral reproduction study of terbutaline sulfate up to 50 mg/kg (corresponding to 167 times the human oral dose) in the rat revealed no adverse effects on fertility.
Pregnancy
Teratogenic Effects
Pregnancy Category B: Reproduction studies in mice (up to 1.1 mg/kg subcutaneously, corresponding to 4 times the human oral dose) and in rats and rabbits (up to 50 mg/kg orally, corresponding to 167 times the human oral dose) have revealed no evidence of impaired fertility or harm to the fetus due to terbutaline. There are, however, no adequate and well-controlled studies in pregnant women. Because animal reproduction studies are not always predictive of human response, this drug should be used during pregnancy only if clearly needed.
Labor and Delivery
Usage in Labor and Delivery: The safe use of Bricanyl for mangement of preterm labor or for other uses during labor and delivery has not been established and the drug should not be used. (See WARNINGS.)
Nursing Mothers
Terbutaline is excreted in breast milk. Caution should be exercised when Bricanyl is administered to a nursing woman.
Pediatric Use
Safety and effectiveness in children below the age of 12 have not been established.

ADVERSE REACTIONS

The adverse reactions of terbutaline sulfate are similar to those of other sympathomimetic agents.
The most commonly observed side effects are tremor and nervousness. The frequency of these side effects appear to diminish with continued therapy. Other commonly reported reactions include increased heart rate, palpitations and dizziness. Other reported reactions include headache, drowsiness, vomiting, nausea, sweating, and muscle cramps. These reactions are generally transient and usually do not require treatment.

OVERDOSAGE

Overdosage information is limited. Excessive adrenergic-receptor stimulation may augment the signs and symptoms listed under ADVERSE REACTIONS and may be accompanied by other adrenergic effects.
Signs and symptoms of overdosage may include the following—*CARDIOVASCULAR:* tachycardia of varying degrees, transient arrhythmias, and extrasystoles. A significant drop in blood pressure may occur due to peripheral vasodilation.
NEUROMUSCULAR: tremors of varying degrees, nervousness, drowsiness, muscle cramps, headache, and sweating.
GASTROINTESTINAL: nausea and vomiting.
ENDOCRINE: varying degrees of hyperglycemia and rise in insulin levels which could be followed by rebound hypoglycemia. Hypokalemia in the early stages may occur. The duration of these signs and symptoms will be dependent on the degree of overdosage.
Treat the alert patient who has taken excessive oral medication by emptying the stomach by means of induced emesis, followed by gastric lavage. In the unconscious patient, secure the airway with a cuffed endotracheal tube before beginning lavage (do not induce emesis). Instillation of activated charcoal slurry may help reduce absorption of terbutaline sulfate. Maintain adequate respiratory exchange. Provide cardiac and respiratory support as needed. Continue observation until symptom-free. Careful consideration should be given to the appropriateness of any chosen therapy and possible effect on the patient's underlying disease state. (See also WARNINGS.)
Studies in mice, rats, rabbits, and dogs have established the LD_{50} of terbutaline to be 1–9 g/kg orally and 0.3–1.6 g/kg subcutaneously.
It is not known whether terbutaline is dialyzable.

DOSAGE AND ADMINISTRATION

ADULTS: Usual dose is 5 mg three times daily. Dosing may be initiated at 2.5 mg three or four times daily and titrated upward depending on clinical response. A total dose of 15 mg in a 24-hour period should not be exceeded.
CHILDREN (12–15 yrs): 2.5 mg three times daily.
If a previously effective dosage regimen fails to provide the usual relief, medical advice should be sought immediately as this is often a sign of seriously worsening asthma which would require reassessment of therapy.

HOW SUPPLIED

2.5 mg tablets (*round*, white, debossed "BRICANYL 2½"):
NDC 0068-0725-61: Bottle of 100
NDC 0068-0725-71: Bottle of 1000
5.0 mg tablets (*square*, white, scored, debossed "BRICANYL 5"):
NDC 0068-0750-61: Bottle of 100
NDC 0068-0750-71: Bottle of 1000
Store at controlled room temperature (15°–30°C) (59°–86°F).
Product Information as of May, 1991
Shown in Product Identification Section, page 416

CANTIL® ℞

[*kăn'tĭl*]
(mepenzolate bromide USP)
Tablets

DESCRIPTION

Cantil tablets for oral administration contain 25 mg mepenzolate bromide USP. The anticholinergic agent mepenzolate bromide USP chemically is 3-[(hydroxydiphenylacetyl)oxy]-1,1-dimethylpiperidinium bromide and has the following structure:

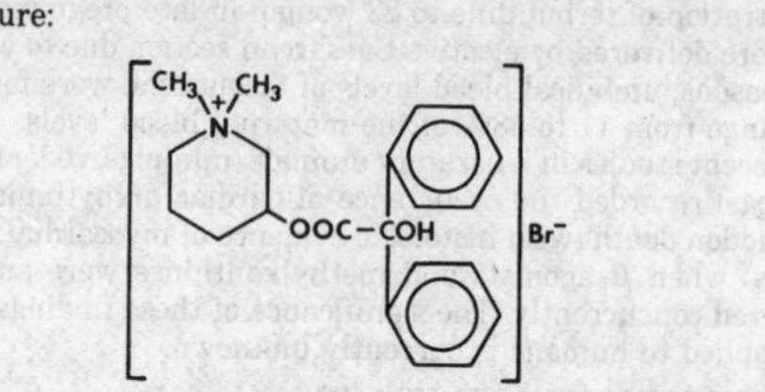

Mepenzolate bromide occurs as a white or light cream-colored powder, which is freely soluble in methanol, slightly soluble in water and chloroform, and practically insoluble in ether.
Each yellow tablet contains 25 mg mepenzolate bromide USP. This tablet also contains inactive ingredients: confectioners sugar, corn starch, corn syrup solids, FD&C Yellow No. 5 (tartrazine, See PRECAUTIONS), lactose, magnesium stearate, and microcrystalline cellulose.

CLINICAL PHARMACOLOGY

Cantil diminishes gastric acid and pepsin secretion. Cantil also suppresses spontaneous contractions of the colon. Pharmacologically, it is a post-ganglionic parasympathetic inhibitor.
Radiotracer studies in which Cantil-^{14}C was used in animals and humans indicate that absorption following oral administration, as with other quaternary ammonium compounds, is low. Between 3 and 22% of an orally administered dose is excreted in the urine over a 5-day period, with the majority of the radioactivity appearing on Day 1. The remainder appears in the next 5 days in the feces and presumably has not been absorbed.

INDICATIONS AND USAGE

Cantil is indicated for use as adjunctive therapy in the treatment of peptic ulcer. It has not been shown to be effective in contributing to the healing of peptic ulcer, decreasing the rate of recurrence or preventing complications.

CONTRAINDICATIONS

1. Glaucoma
2. Obstructive uropathy (for example, bladder neck obstruction due to prostatic hypertrophy)
3. Obstructive disease of the gastrointestinal tract (for example, pyloroduodenal stenosis, achalasia)
4. Paralytic ileus
5. Intestinal atony of the elderly or debilitated patient
6. Unstable cardiovascular status in acute gastrointestinal hemorrhage

7. Toxic megacolon complicating ulcerative colitis
8. Myasthenia gravis
9. Allergic or idiosyncratic reactions to Cantil or related compounds

WARNINGS

In the presence of high environmental temperature, heat prostration (fever and heat stroke due to decreased sweating) can occur with use of Cantil.

Diarrhea may be an early symptom of incomplete intestinal obstruction especially in patients with ileostomy or colostomy. In this instance, treatment with this drug would be inappropriate and possibly harmful.

Cantil may produce drowsiness or blurred vision. The patient should be cautioned regarding activities requiring mental alertness such as operating a motor vehicle or other machinery or performing hazardous work while taking this drug.

With overdosage, a curare-like action may occur, i.e., neuromuscular blockage leading to muscular weakness and possible paralysis.

It should be noted that the use of anticholinergic drugs in the treatment of gastric ulcer may produce a delay in gastric emptying time and may complicate such therapy (antral stasis).

Psychosis has been reported in sensitive individuals given anticholinergic drugs. CNS signs and symptoms include confusion, disorientation, short-term memory loss, hallucinations, dysarthria, ataxia, coma, euphoria, decreased anxiety, fatigue, insomnia, agitation and mannerisms and inappropriate affect. These CNS signs and symptoms usually resolve within 12 to 24 hours after discontinuation of the medication.

PRECAUTIONS

General

Use Cantil with caution in the elderly and in all patients with:

1. Autonomic neuropathy
2. Hepatic or renal disease
3. Ulcerative colitis. Large doses may suppress intestinal motility to the point of producing paralytic ileus and for this reason precipitate or aggravate "toxic megacolon," a serious complication of the disease.
4. Hiatal hernia associated with reflux esophagitis, since anticholinergic drugs may aggravate this condition.
5. Coronary heart disease
6. Congestive heart failure
7. Cardiac arrhythmias
8. Tachycardia
9. Hypertension
10. Prostatic hypertrophy
11. Hyperthyroidism

Investigate any tachycardia before giving anticholinergic (atropine-like) drugs since they may increase the heart rate. This product contains FD&C Yellow No. 5 (tartrazine), which may cause allergic-type reactions (including bronchial asthma) in certain susceptible individuals. Although the overall incidence of FD&C Yellow No. 5 (tartrazine) sensitivity in the general population is low, it is frequently seen in patients who also have aspirin sensitivity.

Information for Patients

Cantil may produce drowsiness or blurred vision. The patient should be cautioned regarding activities requiring mental alertness, such as operating a motor vehicle or other machinery or performing hazardous work while taking this drug.

Drug Interactions

The following agents may increase certain actions or side effects of anticholinergic drugs: amantadine, antiarrhythmic agents of class I (e.g., quinidine), antihistamines, antipsychotic agents (e.g., phenothiazines), benzodiazepines, MAO inhibitors, narcotic analgesics (e.g., meperidine), nitrates and nitrites, sympathomimetic agents, tricyclic antidepressants, and other drugs having anticholinergic activity. Anticholinergics antagonize the effects of antiglaucoma agents. Anticholinergic drugs in the presence of increased intraocular pressure may be hazardous when taken concurrently with agents such as corticosteroids. (See also CONTRAINDICATIONS.)

Anticholinergic agents may affect gastrointestinal absorption of various drugs, such as slowly dissolving dosage forms of digoxin; increased serum digoxin concentrations may result. Anticholinergic drugs may antagonize the effects of drugs that alter gastrointestinal motility, such as metoclopramide. Because antacids may interfere with the absorption of anticholinergic agents, simultaneous use of these drugs should be avoided.

The inhibiting effects of anticholinergic drugs on gastric hydrochloric acid secretion are antagonized by agents used to treat achlorhydria and those used to test gastric secretion.

Carcinogensis, Mutagenesis, Impairment of Fertility

No data are available on long-term potential for carcinogenicity, mutagenicity, or impairment of fertility in animals or humans.

Pregnancy

Teratogenic Effects

Pregnancy Category B

Reproduction studies have been performed in rats and rabbits at doses up to 30 times the human dose (based on 50 kg weight) and have shown no evidence of impaired fertility or harm to the animal fetus. There are, however, no adequate and well controlled studies with Cantil in pregnant women. Because animal reproduction studies are not always predictive of human response, Cantil should be used during pregnancy only if clearly needed.

Nonteratogenic Effects

No data are available on nonteratogenic effects in the fetus or newborn infant.

Nursing Mothers

It is not known whether Cantil is secreted in human milk. Because many drugs are excreted in human milk, caution should be exercised when Cantil is administered to a nursing woman.

Pediatric Use

Safety and effectiveness in children have not been established. Studies in newborn animals (rats) show that younger animals are more sensitive to the toxic effects of Cantil than are older animals.

ADVERSE REACTIONS

Precise frequency data from controlled clinical studies with Cantil are not available.

Gastrointestinal Systems: vomiting, nausea, constipation, loss of taste, bloated feeling, dry mouth

Central Nervous System: mental confusion, dizziness, weakness, drowsiness, headache, nervousness

Ophthalmologic: increased ocular tension, cycloplegia, blurred vision, dilation of the pupil

Dermatologic-Hypersensitivity: anaphylaxis, urticaria

Cardiovascular: tachycardia, palpitations

Genitourinary: urinary retention, urinary hesitancy

Miscellaneous: decreased sweating, drowsiness, insomnia, impotence, suppression of lactation

DRUG ABUSE AND DEPENDENCE

Tolerance, abuse, or dependence has not been reported with Cantil.

OVERDOSAGE

Signs and Symptoms

The signs and symptoms of overdosage are headache; nausea; vomiting; blurred vision; dilated pupils; hot, dry skin; dizziness; dryness of the mouth; difficulty in swallowing; and CNS stimulation. A curare-like action may occur (i.e., neuromuscular blockade leading to muscular weakness and possible paralysis).

Oral LD$_{50}$

The oral LD$_{50}$ is greater than 750 mg/kg in mice and greater than 1000 mg/kg in rats.

Maximum Human Dose Recorded

The maximum human dose recorded is 375 to 500 mg in a 4-year-old child (no adverse effects reported) and 500 to 750 mg in a 30-year-old adult (resulted in death).

Dialysis

It is not known if the drug is dialyzable.

Treatment

Treatment should consist of gastric lavage, emetics, and activated charcoal. Sedatives (e.g., short-acting barbiturates, benzodiazepines) may be used for management of overt signs of excitement. If indicated, an appropriate parenteral cholinergic agent may be used as an antidote.

DOSAGE AND ADMINISTRATION

The usual adult dose is 1 or 2 tablets (25 or 50 mg) 4 times a day preferably with meals and at bedtime. Begin with the lower dosage when possible and adjust subsequently according to the patient's response.

Safety and efficacy in children have not been established.

HOW SUPPLIED

25 mg mepenzolate bromide, compressed yellow tablets debossed MERRELL 37

NDC 0068-0037-01: bottles of 100

Keep tightly closed. Store at room temperature, preferably below 86°F. Protect from excessive heat. Dispense in tight containers with child-resistant closure.

Product Information as of July, 1990
Shown in Product Identification Section, page 417

CARAFATE® Tablets   ℞
[kar'afāt]
(sucralfate) 1 gm

DESCRIPTION

CARAFATE® (sucralfate) is an α-D-glucopyranoside, β-D-fructofuranosyl-, octakis-(hydrogen sulfate), aluminum complex.

[See chemical structure at top of next column.]

$$R = SO_3[Al_2(OH)_5 \cdot (H_2O)_2]$$

Tablets for oral administration contain 1 gm of sucralfate. Also contain: D&C Red #30 Lake, FD&C Blue #1 Lake, magnesium stearate, microcrystalline cellulose, and starch. Therapeutic category: antiulcer

CLINICAL PHARMACOLOGY

Sucralfate is only minimally absorbed from the gastrointestinal tract. The small amounts of the sulfated disaccharide that are absorbed are excreted primarily in the urine.

Although the mechanism of sucralfate's ability to accelerate healing of duodenal ulcers remains to be fully defined, it is known that it exerts its effect through a local, rather than systemic, action. The following observations also appear pertinent:

1. Studies in human subjects and with animal models of ulcer disease have shown that sucralfate forms an ulcer-adherent complex with proteinaceous exudate at the ulcer site.
2. In vitro, a sucralfate-albumin film provides a barrier to diffusion of hydrogen ions.
3. In human subjects, sucralfate given in doses recommended for ulcer therapy inhibits pepsin activity in gastric juice by 32%.
4. In vitro, sucralfate adsorbs bile salts.

These observations suggest that sucralfate's antiulcer activity is the result of formation of an ulcer-adherent complex that covers the ulcer site and protects it against further attack by acid, pepsin, and bile salts. There are approximately 14–16 mEq of acid-neutralizing capacity per 1-gm dose of sucralfate.

CLINICAL TRIALS

Acute Duodenal Ulcer

Over 600 patients have participated in well-controlled clinical trials worldwide. Multicenter trials conducted in the United States, both of them placebo-controlled studies with endoscopic evaluation at 2 and 4 weeks, showed:

STUDY 1

Treatment Groups	Ulcer Healing/No. Patients	
	2 wk	4 wk (Overall)
Sucralfate	37/105 (35.2%)	82/109 (75.2%)
Placebo	26/106 (24.5%)	68/107 (63.6%)

STUDY 2

Treatment Groups	Ulcer Healing/No. Patients	
	2 wk	4 wk (Overall)
Sucralfate	8/24 (33%)	22/24 (92%)
Placebo	4/31 (13%)	18/31 (58%)

The sucralfate-placebo differences were statistically significant in both studies at 4 weeks but not at 2 weeks. The poorer result in the first study may have occurred because sucralfate was given 2 hours after meals and at bedtime rather than 1 hour before meals and at bedtime, the regimen used in international studies and in the second United States study. In addition, in the first study liquid antacid was utilized as needed, whereas in the second study antacid tablets were used.

Maintenance Therapy After Healing of Duodenal Ulcer

Two double-blind randomized placebo-controlled U.S. multicenter trials have demonstrated that sucralfate (1 gm bid) is effective as maintenance therapy following healing of duodenal ulcers.

In one study, endoscopies were performed monthly for 4 months. Of the 254 patients who enrolled, 239 were analyzed in the intention-to-treat life table analysis presented below.

		Duodenal Ulcer Recurrence Rate (%)			
		Months of Therapy			
Drug	N	1	2	3	4
Carafate	122	20*	30*	38**	42**
Placebo	117	33	46	55	63

*$p < 0.05$, **$p < 0.01$
Prn antacids were not permitted in this study.

In the other study, scheduled endoscopies were performed at 6 and 12 months, but for cause endoscopies were permitted as symptoms dictated. Median symptom scores between the sucralfate and placebo groups were not significantly different. A life table intention-to-treat analysis for the 94 patients enrolled in the trial had the following results:

Continued on next page

Marion Merrell Dow—Cont.

Duodenal Ulcer Recurrence Rate (%)

Drug	N	6 months	12 months
Carafate	48	19*	27*
Placebo	46	54	65

*$p < 0.002$

Prn antacids were permitted in this study.

Data from placebo-controlled studies longer than 1 year are not available.

INDICATIONS AND USAGE

CARAFATE® (sucralfate) is indicated in:

- Short-term treatment (up to 8 weeks) of active duodenal ulcer. While healing with sucralfate may occur during the first week or two, treatment should be continued for 4 to 8 weeks unless healing has been demonstrated by x-ray or endoscopic examination.
- Maintenance therapy for duodenal ulcer patients at reduced dosage after healing of acute ulcers.

CONTRAINDICATIONS

There are no known contraindications to the use of sucralfate.

PRECAUTIONS

Duodenal ulcer is a chronic, recurrent disease. While short-term treatment with sucralfate can result in complete healing of the ulcer, a successful course of treatment with sucralfate should not be expected to alter the posthealing frequency or severity of duodenal ulceration.

Special Populations: Chronic Renal Failure and Dialysis Patients: When sucralfate is administered orally, small amounts of aluminum are absorbed from the gastrointestinal tract. Concomitant use of sucralfate with other products that contain aluminum, such as aluminum-containing antacids, may increase the total body burden of aluminum. Patients with normal renal function receiving the recommended doses of sucralfate and aluminum-containing products adequately excrete aluminum in the urine. Patients with chronic renal failure or those receiving dialysis have impaired excretion of absorbed aluminum. In addition, aluminum does not cross dialysis membranes because it is bound to albumin and transferrin plasma proteins. Aluminum accumulation and toxicity (aluminum osteodystrophy, osteomalacia, encephalopathy) have been described in patients with renal impairment. Sucralfate should be used with caution in patients with chronic renal failure.

Drug Interactions: Some studies have shown that simultaneous sucralfate administration in healthy volunteers reduced the extent of absorption (bioavailability) of single doses of the following drugs: cimetidine, ciprofloxacin, digoxin, norfloxacin, phenytoin, ranitidine, tetracycline, and theophylline. The mechanism of these interactions appears to be nonsystemic in nature, presumably resulting from sucralfate binding to the concomitant agent in the gastrointestinal tract. In all cases studied to date (cimetidine, ciprofloxacin, digoxin, and ranitidine), dosing the concomitant medication 2 hours before sucralfate eliminated the interaction. Because of the potential of CARAFATE to alter the absorption of some drugs, CARAFATE should be administered separately from other drugs when alterations in bioavailability are felt to be critical. In these cases, patients should be monitored appropriately.

Carcinogenesis, Mutagenesis, Impairment of Fertility: Chronic oral toxicity studies of 24 months' duration were conducted in mice and rats at doses up to 1 gm/kg (12 times the human dose). There was no evidence of drug-related tumorigenicity. A reproduction study in rats at doses up to 38 times the human dose did not reveal any indication of fertility impairment. Mutagenicity studies were not conducted.

Pregnancy: Teratogenic effects. Pregnancy Category B. Teratogenicity studies have been performed in mice, rats, and rabbits at doses up to 50 times the human dose and have revealed no evidence of harm to the fetus due to sucralfate. There are, however, no adequate and well-controlled studies in pregnant women. Because animal reproduction studies are not always predictive of human response, this drug should be used during pregnancy only if clearly needed.

Nursing Mothers: It is not known whether this drug is excreted in human milk. Because many drugs are excreted in human milk, caution should be exercised when sucralfate is administered to a nursing woman.

Pediatric Use: Safety and effectiveness in children have not been established.

ADVERSE REACTIONS

Adverse reactions to sucralfate in clinical trials were minor and only rarely led to discontinuation of the drug. In studies involving over 2700 patients treated with sucralfate tablets, adverse effects were reported in 129 (4.7%).

Constipation was the most frequent complaint (2%). Other adverse effects reported in less than 0.5% of the patients are listed below by body system:

Gastrointestinal:	diarrhea, nausea, vomiting, gastric discomfort, indigestion, flatulence, dry mouth
Dermatological:	pruritus, rash
Nervous system:	dizziness, sleepiness, vertigo
Other:	back pain, headache

Postmarketing reports of hypersensitivity reactions, including urticaria (hives), angioedema, respiratory difficulty, and rhinitis have been received. However, a causal relationship has not been established.

OVERDOSAGE

There is no experience in humans with overdosage. Acute oral toxicity studies in animals, however, using doses up to 12 gm/kg body weight, could not find a lethal dose. Risks associated with overdosage should, therefore, be minimal.

DOSAGE AND ADMINISTRATION

Active Duodenal Ulcer: The recommended adult oral dosage for duodenal ulcer is 1 gm four times a day on an empty stomach.

Antacids may be prescribed as needed for relief of pain but should not be taken within one-half hour before or after sucralfate.

While healing with sucralfate may occur during the first week or two, treatment should be continued for 4 to 8 weeks unless healing has been demonstrated by x-ray or endoscopic examination.

Maintenance Therapy: The recommended adult oral dosage is 1 gm twice a day.

HOW SUPPLIED

CARAFATE (sucralfate) 1-gm tablets are supplied in bottles of 100 (NDC 0088-1712-47), 120 (NDC 0088-1712-53), and 500 (NDC 0088-1712-55) and in Unit Dose Identification Paks of 100 (NDC 0088-1712-49). Light pink scored oblong tablets are embossed with CARAFATE on one side and 1712 on the other.

Issued 3/91

Shown in Product Identification Section, page 417

CARDIZEM® CD Capsules ℞

[*kar'dizem*]

(diltiazem hydrochloride)

180 mg, 240 mg, and 300 mg

DESCRIPTION

CARDIZEM® (diltiazem hydrochloride) is a calcium ion influx inhibitor (slow channel blocker or calcium antagonist). Chemically, diltiazem hydrochloride is 1,5-Benzothiazepin-4(5H)one,3-(acetyloxy)-5-[2-(dimethylamino)ethyl]-2,3-dihydro-2-(4-methoxyphenyl)-, monohydrochloride, (+)-cis-. The chemical structure is:

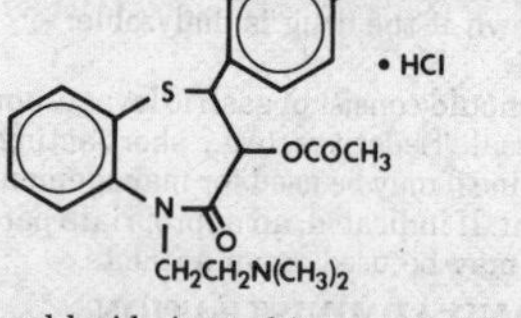

Diltiazem hydrochloride is a white to off-white crystalline powder with a bitter taste. It is soluble in water, methanol, and chloroform. It has a molecular weight of 450.98. CARDIZEM CD is formulated as a once-a-day extended release capsule containing either 180 mg, 240 mg, or 300 mg diltiazem hydrochloride.

Also contains: black iron oxide, ethylcellulose, FD&C Blue #1, fumaric acid, gelatin-NF, sucrose, starch, talc, titanium dioxide, white wax, and other ingredients.

For oral administration.

CLINICAL PHARMACOLOGY

The therapeutic effects of CARDIZEM CD are believed to be related to its ability to inhibit the influx of calcium ions during membrane depolarization of cardiac and vascular smooth muscle.

Mechanisms of Action. CARDIZEM CD produces its antihypertensive effect primarily by relaxation of vascular smooth muscle and the resultant decrease in peripheral vascular resistance. The magnitude of blood pressure reduction is related to the degree of hypertension; thus hypertensive individuals experience an antihypertensive effect, whereas there is only a modest fall in blood pressure in normotensives.

Hemodynamic and Electrophysiologic Effects. Like other calcium channel antagonists, diltiazem decreases sinoatrial and atrioventricular conduction in isolated tissues and has a negative inotropic effect in isolated preparations. In the intact animal, prolongation of the AH interval can be seen at higher doses.

In man, diltiazem prevents spontaneous and ergonovine-provoked coronary artery spasm. It causes a decrease in peripheral vascular resistance and a modest fall in blood pressure in normotensive individuals and, in exercise tolerance studies in patients with ischemic heart disease, reduces the heart rate-blood pressure product for any given work load. Studies to date, primarily in patients with good ventricular function, have not revealed evidence of a negative inotropic effect; cardiac output, ejection fraction, and left ventricular end diastolic pressure have not been affected. Such data has no predictive value with respect to effects in patients with poor ventricular function, and increased heart failure has been reported in patients with preexisting impairment of ventricular function. There are as yet few data on the interaction of diltiazem and beta-blockers in patients with poor ventricular function. Resting heart rate is usually slightly reduced by diltiazem.

CARDIZEM CD produces antihypertensive effects both in the supine and standing positions. In a double-blind, parallel, dose-response study utilizing doses ranging from 90 to 540 mg once daily, CARDIZEM CD lowered supine diastolic blood pressure in an apparent linear manner over the entire dose range studied. The changes in diastolic blood pressure, measured at trough, for placebo, 90 mg, 180 mg, 360 mg, and 540 mg were −2.9, −4.5, −6.1, −9.5, and −10.5 mm Hg, respectively. Postural hypotension is infrequently noted upon suddenly assuming an upright position. No reflex tachycardia is associated with the chronic antihypertensive effects. CARDIZEM CD decreases vascular resistance, increases cardiac output (by increasing stroke volume), and produces a slight decrease or no change in heart rate. During dynamic exercise, increases in diastolic pressure are inhibited while maximum achievable systolic pressure is usually reduced. Chronic therapy with CARDIZEM CD produces no change or an increase in plasma catecholamines. No increased activity of the renin-angiotensin-aldosterone axis has been observed. CARDIZEM CD reduces the renal and peripheral effects of angiotensin II. Hypertensive animal models respond to diltiazem with reductions in blood pressure and increased urinary output and natriuresis without a change in urinary sodium/potassium ratio.

Intravenous diltiazem in doses of 20 mg prolongs AH conduction time and AV node functional and effective refractory periods by approximately 20%. In a study involving single oral doses of 300 mg of CARDIZEM in six normal volunteers, the average maximum PR prolongation was 14% with no instances of greater than first-degree AV block. Diltiazem-associated prolongation of the AH interval is not more pronounced in patients with first-degree heart block. In patients with sick sinus syndrome, diltiazem significantly prolongs sinus cycle length (up to 50% in some cases).

Chronic oral administration of CARDIZEM to patients in doses of up to 540 mg/day has resulted in small increases in PR interval, and on occasion produces abnormal prolongation. (See WARNINGS.)

Pharmacokinetics and Metabolism. Diltiazem is well absorbed from the gastrointestinal tract and is subject to an extensive first-pass effect, giving an absolute bioavailability (compared to intravenous administration) of about 40%. CARDIZEM undergoes extensive metabolism in which only 2% to 4% of the unchanged drug appears in the urine. Drugs which induce or inhibit hepatic microsomal enzymes may alter diltiazem disposition.

Total radioactivity measurement following short IV administration in healthy volunteers suggests the presence of other unidentified metabolites which attain higher concentrations than those of diltiazem and are more slowly eliminated; half-life of total radioactivity is about 20 hours compared to 2 to 5 hours for diltiazem.

In vitro binding studies show CARDIZEM is 70% to 80% bound to plasma proteins. Competitive in vitro ligand binding studies have also shown CARDIZEM binding is not altered by therapeutic concentrations of digoxin, hydrochlorothiazide, phenylbutazone, propranolol, salicylic acid, or warfarin. The plasma elimination half-life following single or multiple drug administration is approximately 3.0 to 4.5 hours. Desacetyl diltiazem is also present in the plasma at levels of 10% to 20% of the parent drug and is 25% to 50% as potent as a coronary vasodilator as diltiazem. Minimum therapeutic plasma diltiazem concentrations appear to be in the range of 50 to 200 ng/mL. There is a departure from linearity when dose strengths are increased; the half-life is slightly increased with dose. A study that compared patients with normal hepatic function to patients with cirrhosis found an increase in half-life and a 69% increase in bioavailability in the hepatically impaired patients. A single study in patients with severely impaired renal function showed no difference in the pharmacokinetic profile of diltiazem compared to patients with normal renal function.

CARDIZEM CD Capsules. When compared to a regimen of CARDIZEM tablets at steady-state, more than 95% of drug is absorbed from the CARDIZEM CD formulation. A single 360-mg dose of the capsule results in detectable plasma levels within 2 hours and peak plasma levels between 10 and 14 hours; absorption occurs throughout the dosing interval. When CARDIZEM CD was coadministered with a high fat

content breakfast, the extent of diltiazem absorption was not affected. Dose-dumping does not occur. The apparent elimination half-life after single or multiple dosing is 5 to 8 hours. A departure from linearity similar to that seen with CARDIZEM tablets and CARDIZEM SR capsules is observed. As the dose of CARDIZEM CD capsules is increased from a daily dose of 120 mg to 240 mg, there is an increase in the area-under-the-curve of 2.7 times. When the dose is increased from 240 mg to 360 mg there is an increase in the area-under-the-curve of 1.6 times.

INDICATIONS AND USAGE

CARDIZEM CD is indicated for the treatment of hypertension. It may be used alone or in combination with other antihypertensive medications.

CONTRAINDICATIONS

CARDIZEM is contraindicated in (1) patients with sick sinus syndrome except in the presence of a functioning ventricular pacemaker, (2) patients with second- or third-degree AV block except in the presence of a functioning ventricular pacemaker, (3) patients with severe hypotension (less than 90 mm Hg systolic), (4) patients who have demonstrated hypersensitivity to the drug, and (5) patients with acute myocardial infarction and pulmonary congestion documented by x-ray on admission.

WARNINGS

1. **Cardiac Conduction.** CARDIZEM prolongs AV node refractory periods without significantly prolonging sinus node recovery time, except in patients with sick sinus syndrome. This effect may rarely result in abnormally slow heart rates (particularly in patients with sick sinus syndrome) or second- or third-degree AV block (13 of 3007 patients or 0.43%). Concomitant use of diltiazem with beta-blockers or digitalis may result in additive effects on cardiac conduction. A patient with Prinzmetal's angina developed periods of asystole (2 to 5 seconds) after a single dose of 60 mg of diltiazem.
2. **Congestive Heart Failure.** Although diltiazem has a negative inotropic effect in isolated animal tissue preparations, hemodynamic studies in humans with normal ventricular function have not shown a reduction in cardiac index nor consistent negative effects on contractility (dp/dt). An acute study of oral diltiazem in patients with impaired ventricular function (ejection fraction 24% ± 6%) showed improvement in indices of ventricular function without significant decrease in contractile function (dp/dt). Worsening of congestive heart failure has been reported in patients with preexisting impairment of ventricular function. Experience with the use of CARDIZEM (diltiazem hydrochloride) in combination with beta-blockers in patients with impaired ventricular function is limited. Caution should be exercised when using this combination.
3. **Hypotension.** Decreases in blood pressure associated with CARDIZEM therapy may occasionally result in symptomatic hypotension.
4. **Acute Hepatic Injury.** Mild elevations of transaminases with and without concomitant elevation in alkaline phosphatase and bilirubin have been observed in clinical studies. Such elevations were usually transient and frequently resolved even with continued diltiazem treatment. In rare instances, significant elevations in enzymes such as alkaline phosphatase, LDH, SGOT, and SGPT, and other phenomena consistent with acute hepatic injury have been noted. These reactions tended to occur early after therapy initiation (1 to 8 weeks) and have been reversible upon discontinuation of drug therapy. The relationship to CARDIZEM is uncertain in some cases, but probable in some. (See PRECAUTIONS.)

PRECAUTIONS

General. CARDIZEM (diltiazem hydrochloride) is extensively metabolized by the liver and excreted by the kidneys and in bile. As with any drug given over prolonged periods, laboratory parameters of renal and hepatic function should be monitored at regular intervals. The drug should be used with caution in patients with impaired renal or hepatic function. In subacute and chronic dog and rat studies designed to produce toxicity, high doses of diltiazem were associated with hepatic damage. In special subacute hepatic studies, oral doses of 125 mg/kg and higher in rats were associated with histological changes in the liver, which were reversible when the drug was discontinued. In dogs, doses of 20 mg/kg were also associated with hepatic changes; however, these changes were reversible with continued dosing.

Dermatological events (see ADVERSE REACTIONS section) may be transient and may disappear despite continued use of CARDIZEM. However, skin eruptions progressing to erythema multiforme and/or exfoliative dermatitis have also been infrequently reported. Should a dermatologic reaction persist, the drug should be discontinued.

Drug Interactions. Due to the potential for additive effects, caution and careful titration are warranted in patients receiving CARDIZEM concomitantly with other agents known to affect cardiac contractility and/or conduction. (See WARNINGS.)

Pharmacologic studies indicate that there may be additive effects in prolonging AV conduction when using beta-blockers or digitalis concomitantly with CARDIZEM. (See WARNINGS.)

As with all drugs, care should be exercised when treating patients with multiple medications. CARDIZEM undergoes biotransformation by cytochrome P-450 mixed function oxidase. Coadministration of CARDIZEM with other agents which follow the same route of biotransformation may result in the competitive inhibition of metabolism. Dosages of similarly metabolized drugs such as cyclosporin, particularly those of low therapeutic ratio or in patients with renal and/or hepatic impairment, may require adjustment when starting or stopping concomitantly administered CARDIZEM to maintain optimum therapeutic blood levels.

Beta-blockers. Controlled and uncontrolled domestic studies suggest that concomitant use of CARDIZEM and beta-blockers is usually well tolerated, but available data are not sufficient to predict the effects of concomitant treatment in patients with left ventricular dysfunction or cardiac conduction abnormalities.

Administration of CARDIZEM (diltiazem hydrochloride) concomitantly with propranolol in five normal volunteers resulted in increased propranolol levels in all subjects and bioavailability of propranolol was increased approximately 50%. If combination therapy is initiated or withdrawn in conjunction with propranolol, an adjustment in the propranolol dose may be warranted. (See WARNINGS.)

Cimetidine. A study in six healthy volunteers has shown a significant increase in peak diltiazem plasma levels (58%) and area-under-the-curve (53%) after a 1-week course of cimetidine at 1200 mg per day and a single dose of diltiazem 60 mg. Ranitidine produced smaller, nonsignificant increases. The effect may be mediated by cimetidine's known inhibition of hepatic cytochrome P-450, the enzyme system responsible for the first-pass metabolism of diltiazem. Patients currently receiving diltiazem therapy should be carefully monitored for a change in pharmacological effect when initiating and discontinuing therapy with cimetidine. An adjustment in the diltiazem dose may be warranted.

Digitalis: Administration of CARDIZEM with digoxin in 24 healthy male subjects increased plasma digoxin concentrations approximately 20%. Another investigator found no increase in digoxin levels in 12 patients with coronary artery disease. Since there have been conflicting results regarding the effect of digoxin levels, it is recommended that digoxin levels be monitored when initiating, adjusting, and discontinuing CARDIZEM therapy to avoid possible over- or under-digitalization. (See WARNINGS.)

Anesthetics: The depression of cardiac contractility, conductivity, and automaticity as well as the vascular dilation associated with anesthetics may be potentiated by calcium channel blockers. When used concomitantly, anesthetics and calcium blockers should be titrated carefully.

Carcinogenesis, Mutagenesis, Impairment of Fertility. A 24-month study in rats at oral dosage levels of up to 100 mg/kg/day, and a 21-month study in mice at oral dosage levels of up to 30 mg/kg/day showed no evidence of carcinogenicity. There was also no mutagenic response in vitro or in vivo in mammalian cell assays or in vitro in bacteria. No evidence of impaired fertility was observed in a study performed in male and female rats at oral dosages of up to 100 mg/kg/day.

Pregnancy. Category C. Reproduction studies have been conducted in mice, rats, and rabbits. Administration of doses ranging from five to ten times greater (on a mg/kg basis) than the daily recommended therapeutic dose has resulted in embryo and fetal lethality. These doses, in some studies, have been reported to cause skeletal abnormalities. In the perinatal/postnatal studies, there was an increased incidence of stillbirths at doses of 20 times the human dose or greater.

There are no well-controlled studies in pregnant women; therefore, use CARDIZEM in pregnant women only if the potential benefit justifies the potential risk to the fetus.

Nursing Mothers. Diltiazem is excreted in human milk. One report suggests that concentrations in breast milk may approximate serum levels. If use of CARDIZEM is deemed essential, an alternative method of infant feeding should be instituted.

Pediatric Use. Safety and effectiveness in children have not been established.

ADVERSE REACTIONS

Serious adverse reactions have been rare in studies carried out to date, but it should be recognized that patients with impaired ventricular function and cardiac conduction abnormalities have usually been excluded from these studies.

The following table presents the most common adverse reactions reported in placebo-controlled trials in patients receiving CARDIZEM CD up to 360 mg with rates in placebo patients shown for comparison. [See table above.]

Adverse Reaction	Cardizem CD N=324	Placebo N=175
Headache	9.0%	8.0%
Bradycardia	4.3%	2.3%
Edema	3.7%	2.3%
Dizziness	3.1%	3.4%
ECG Abnormalitiy	3.1%	2.9%
AV Block First Degree	2.2%	0.0%
Asthenia	1.9%	1.7%

In clinical trials of CARDIZEM CD Capsules, CARDIZEM Tablets, and CARDIZEM SR Capsules involving over 3000 patients, the most common events (ie, greater than 1%) were edema (4.9%), headache (4.9%), dizziness (3.5%), asthenia (2.7%), first-degree AV block (2.2%), bradycardia (1.6%), flushing (1.5%), nausea (1.4%), rash (1.3%), and dyspepsia (1.2%).

In addition, the following events were reported infrequently (less than 1%):

Cardiovascular: Angina, arrhythmia, AV block (second- or third-degree), bundle branch block, congestive heart failure, ECG abnormalities, hypotension, palpitations, syncope, tachycardia, ventricular extrasystoles.

Nervous System: Abnormal dreams, amnesia, depression, gait abnormality, hallucinations, insomnia, nervousness, paresthesia, personality change, somnolence, tinnitus, tremor.

Gastrointestinal: Anorexia, constipation, diarrhea, dry mouth, dysgeusia, mild elevations of SGOT, SGPT, LDH, and alkaline phosphatase (see hepatic warnings), thirst, vomiting, weight increase.

Dermatological: Petechiae, photosensitivity, pruritus, urticaria.

Other: Amblyopia, CPK increase, dyspnea, epistaxis, eye irritation, hyperglycemia, hyperuricemia, impotence, muscle cramps, nasal congestion, nocturia, osteoarticular pain, polyuria, sexual difficulties.

The following postmarketing events have been reported infrequently in patients receiving CARDIZEM: alopecia, erythema multiforme, exfoliative dermatitis, extrapyramidal symptoms, gingival hyperplasia, hemolytic anemia, increased bleeding time, leukopenia, purpura, retinopathy, and thrombocytopenia. In addition, events such as myocardial infarction have been observed which are not readily distinguishable from the natural history of the disease in these patients. A number of well-documented cases of generalized rash, characterized as leukocytoclastic vasculitis, have been reported. However, a definitive cause and effect relationship between these events and CARDIZEM therapy is yet to be established.

OVERDOSAGE

The oral LD_{50}'s in mice and rats range from 415 to 740 mg/kg and from 560 to 810 mg/kg, respectively. The intravenous LD_{50}'s in these species were 60 and 38 mg/kg, respectively. The oral LD_{50} in dogs is considered to be in excess of 50 mg/kg, while lethality was seen in monkeys at 360 mg/kg.

The toxic dose in man is not known. Due to extensive metabolism, blood levels after a standard dose of diltiazem can vary over tenfold, limiting the usefulness of blood levels in overdose cases.

There have been 29 reports of diltiazem overdose in doses ranging from less than 1 gm to 10.8 gm. Sixteen of these reports involved multiple drug ingestions.

Twenty-two reports indicated patients had recovered from diltiazem overdose ranging from less than 1 gm to 10.8 gm. There were seven reports with a fatal outcome; although the amount of diltiazem ingested was unknown, multiple drug ingestions were confirmed in six of the seven reports.

Events observed following diltiazem overdose included bradycardia, hypotension, heart block, and cardiac failure. Most reports of overdose described some supportive medical measure and/or drug treatment. Bradycardia frequently responded favorably to atropine as did heart block, although cardiac pacing was also frequently utilized to treat heart block. Fluids and vasopressors were used to maintain blood pressure, and in cases of cardiac failure, inotropic agents were administered. In addition, some patients received treatment with ventilatory support, gastric lavage, activated charcoal, and/or intravenous calcium. Evidence of the effectiveness of intravenous calcium administration to reverse the pharmacological effects of diltiazem overdose was conflicting.

In the event of overdose or exaggerated response, appropriate supportive measures should be employed in addition to gastrointestinal decontamination. Diltiazem does not appear to be removed by peritoneal or hemodialysis. Based on the known pharmacological effects of diltiazem and/or reported clinical experiences, the following measures may be considered:

Bradycardia: Administer atropine (0.60 to 1.0 mg). If there is no response to vagal blockade, administer isoproterenol cautiously.

High-Degree AV Block: Treat as for bradycardia above. Fixed high-degree AV block should be treated with cardiac pacing.

Cardiac Failure: Administer inotropic agents (isoproterenol, dopamine, or dobutamine) and diuretics.

Continued on next page

Marion Merrell Dow—Cont.

CARDIZEM® CD
(diltiazem hydrochloride)
Capsules

Strength	Quantity	NDC Number	Descripton
180 mg	30 btl	0088-1796-30	Light turquoise blue/blue capsule imprinted
	90 btl	0088-1796-42	with the Marion Merrell Dow Inc. logo on one
	100 UDIP®	0088-1796-49	end and 1796 and 180 mg on the other or CARDIZEM CD and 180 mg on the other.
240 mg	30 btl	0088-1797-30	Blue/blue capsule imprinted with the Marion
	90 btl	0088-1797-42	Merrell Dow Inc. logo on one end and 1797
	100 UDIP®	0088-1797-49	and 240 mg on the other or CARDIZEM CD and 240 mg on the other.
300 mg	30 btl	0088-1798-30	Light gray/blue capsule imprinted with the
	90 btl	0088-1798-42	Marion Merrell Dow Inc. logo on one end and
	100 UDIP®	0088-1798-49	1798 and 300 mg on the other or CARDIZEM CD and 300 mg on the other.

Hypotension: Vasopressors (eg, dopamine or levarterenol bitartrate).

Actual treatment and dosage should depend on the severity of the clinical situation and the judgment and experience of the treating physician.

DOSAGE AND ADMINISTRATION

Dosage needs to be adjusted by titration to individual patient needs. When used as monotherapy, reasonable starting doses are 180 to 240 mg once daily, although some patients may respond to lower doses. Maximum antihypertensive effect is usually observed by 14 days of chronic therapy; therefore, dosage adjustments should be scheduled accordingly. The usual dosage range studied in clinical trials was 240 to 360 mg once daily. There is limited clinical experience with doses above 360 mg.

Hypertensive patients controlled on diltiazem alone or in combination with other antihypertensive medications may be safely switched to CARDIZEM CD capsules at the nearest equivalent total daily dose. Subsequent titration to higher or lower doses may be necessary and should be initiated as clinically warranted.

CARDIZEM CD has an additive antihypertensive effect when used with other antihypertensive agents. Therefore, the dosage of CARDIZEM CD or the concomitant antihypertensives may need to be adjusted when adding one to the other. See WARNINGS and PRECAUTIONS regarding use with beta-blockers.

HOW SUPPLIED

[See table above.]
Storage Conditions: Store at controlled room temperature 59–86°F (15–30°C).
Avoid excessive humidity.

Product Information as of March 1992 (a)
Shown in Product Identification Section, page 417

CARDIZEM® Injectable   ℞
(diltiazem hydrochloride)

DESCRIPTION

CARDIZEM® (diltiazem hydrochloride) is a calcium ion influx inhibitor (slow channel blocker or calcium antagonist). Chemically, diltiazem hydrochloride is 1,5-benzothiazepin-4(5H)one, 3-(acetyloxy)-5-[2-(dimethylamino)ethyl]-2,3-dihydro-2-(4-methoxyphenyl)-, monohydrochloride, (+)-cis-. The chemical structure is:

Diltiazem hydrochloride is a white to off-white crystalline powder with a bitter taste. It is soluble in water, methanol, and chloroform. It has a molecular weight of 450.98.
CARDIZEM Injectable (diltiazem hydrochloride) is a clear, colorless, sterile, nonpyrogenic solution. It has a pH range of 3.7 to 4.1.
CARDIZEM Injectable is for direct intravenous bolus injection and continuous intravenous infusion.
25-mg, 5-mL vial—each sterile vial contains 25 mg diltiazem hydrochoride, 3.75 mg citric acid USP, 3.25 mg sodium citrate dihydrate USP, 357 mg sorbitol solution USP, and water for injection USP up to 5 mL. Sodium hydroxide or hydrochloric acid is used for pH adjustment.
50-mg, 10-mL vial—each sterile vial contains 50 mg diltiazem hydrochloride, 7.5 mg citric acid USP, 6.5 mg sodium citrate dihydrate USP, 714 mg sorbitol solution USP, and water for injection USP up to 10 mL. Sodium hydroxide or hydrochloric acid is used for pH adjustment.

CLINICAL PHARMACOLOGY

Mechanisms of Action. CARDIZEM inhibits the influx of calcium (Ca^{2+}) ions during membrane depolarization of cardiac and vascular smooth muscle. The therapeutic benefits of CARDIZEM in supraventricular tachycardias are related to its ability to slow AV nodal conduction time and prolong AV nodal refractoriness. CARDIZEM exhibits frequency (use) dependent effects on AV nodal conduction such that it may selectively reduce the heart rate during tachycardias involving the AV node with little or no effect on normal AV nodal conduction at normal heart rates.
CARDIZEM slows the ventricular rate in patients with a rapid ventricular response during atrial fibrillation or atrial flutter. CARDIZEM converts paroxysmal supraventricular tachycardia (PSVT) to normal sinus rhythm by interrupting the reentry circuit in AV nodal reentrant tachycardias and reciprocating tachycardias, eg, Wolff-Parkinson-White syndrome (WPW).
CARDIZEM prolongs the sinus cycle length. It has no effects on the sinus node recovery time or on the sinoatrial conduction time in patients without SA nodal dysfunction.
CARDIZEM has no significant electrophysiologic effect on tissues in the heart that are fast sodium channel dependent, eg, His-Purkinje tissue, atrial and ventricular muscle, and extranodal accessory pathways.
Like other calcium channel antagonists, because of its effect on vascular smooth muscle, CARDIZEM decreases total peripheral resistance resulting in a decrease in both systolic and diastolic blood pressure.
Hemodynamics. In patients with cardiovascular disease, CARDIZEM Injectable (diltiazem hydrochloride) administered intravenously in single bolus doses, followed in some cases by a continuous infusion, reduced blood pressure, systemic vascular resistance, the rate-pressure product, and coronary vascular resistance and increased coronary blood flow. In a limited number of studies of patients with compromised myocardium (severe congestive heart failure, acute myocardial infarction, hypertrophic cardiomyopathy), administration of intravenous diltiazem produced no significant effect on contractility, left ventricular end diastolic pressure, or pulmonary capillary wedge pressure. The mean ejection fraction and cardiac output/index remained unchanged or increased. Maximal hemodynamic effects usually occurred within 2 to 5 minutes of an injection. However, in rare instances, worsening of congestive heart failure has been reported in patients with preexisting impaired ventricular function.
Pharmacodynamics. The prolongation of PR interval correlated significantly with plasma diltiazem concentration in normal volunteers using the Sigmoidal E_{max} model. Changes in heart rate, systolic blood pressure, and diastolic blood pressure did not correlate with diltiazem plasma concentrations in normal volunteers. Reduction in mean arterial pressure correlated linearly with diltiazem plasma concentration in a group of hypertensive patients.
In patients with atrial fibrillation and atrial flutter, a significant correlation was observed between the percent reduction in HR and plasma diltiazem concentration using the Sigmoidal E_{max} model. Based on this relationship, the mean plasma diltiazem concentration required to produce a 20% decrease in heart rate was determined to be 80 ng/mL. Mean plasma diltiazem concentrations of 130 ng/mL and 300 ng/mL were determined to produce reductions in heart rate of 30% and 40%.
Pharmacokinetics and Metabolism. Following a single intravenous injection in healthy male volunteers, CARDIZEM appears to obey linear pharmacokinetics over a dose range of 10.5 to 21.0 mg. The plasma elimination half-life is approximately 3.4 hours. The apparent volume of distribution of CARDIZEM is approximately 305 L. CARDIZEM is extensively metabolized in the liver with a systemic clearance of approximately 65 L/h.
After constant rate intravenous infusion to healthy male volunteers, diltiazem exhibits nonlinear pharmacokinetics over an infusion range of 4.8 to 13.2 mg/h for 24 hours. Over this infusion range, as the dose is increased, systemic clearance decreases from 64 to 48 L/h while the plasma elimination half-life increases from 4.1 to 4.9 hours. The apparent volume of distribution remains unchanged (360 to 391 L). In patients with atrial fibrillation or atrial flutter, diltiazem systemic clearance has been found to be decreased compared to healthy volunteers. In patients administered bolus doses ranging from 2.5 mg to 38.5 mg, systemic clearance averaged 36 L/h. In patients administered continuous infusions at 10 mg/h or 15 mg/h for 24 hours, diltiazem systemic clearance averaged 42 L/h and 31 L/h, respectively.
Based on the results of pharamcokinetic studies in healthy volunteers administered different *oral* CARDIZEM formulations, constant rate intravenous infusions of CARDIZEM at 3, 5, 7, and 11 mg/h are predicted to produce steady-state plasma diltiazem concentrations equivalent to 120-, 180-, 240-, and 360-mg total daily oral doses of CARDIZEM tablets or CARDIZEM SR capsules.
After oral administration, CARDIZEM undergoes extensive metabolism in man by deacetylation, N-demethylation, and O-demethylation via cytochrome P-450 (oxidative metabolism) in addition to conjugation. Metabolites N-monodesmethyldiltiazem, desacetyldiltiazem, desacetyl-N-monodesmethyldiltiazem, desacetyl-O-desmethyldiltiazem, and desacetyl-N, O-desmethyldiltiazem have been identified in human urine. Following oral administration, 2% to 4% of the unchanged CARDIZEM appears in the urine. Drugs which induce or inhibit hepatic microsomal enzymes may alter diltiazem disposition.
Following single intravenous injection of CARDIZEM, however, plasma concentrations of N-monodesmethyldiltiazem and desacetyldiltiazem, two principal metabolities found in plasma after oral adminstration, are typically not detected. These metabolites are observed, however, following 24 hour constant rate intravenous infusion. Total radioactivity measurement following short IV administration in healthy volunteers suggests the presence of other unindentified metabolities which attain higher concentrations than those of diltiazem and are more slowly eliminated; half-life of total radioactivity is about 20 hours compared to 2 to 5 hours for diltiazem.
CARDIZEM is 70% to 80% bound to plasma proteins. In vitro studies suggest alpha$_1$-acid glycoprotein binds approximately 40% of the drug at clinically significant concentrations. Albumin appears to bind approximately 30% of the drug, while other constituents bind the remaining bound fraction. Competitive in vitro ligand binding studies have shown that CARDIZEM binding is not altered by therapeutic concentrations of digoxin, phenytoin, hydrochlorothiazide, indomethacin, phenylbutazone, propranolol, salicylic acid, tolbutamide, or warfarin.
Renal insufficiency, or even end-stage renal disease, does not appear to influence diltiazem disposition following *oral* administration. Liver cirrhosis was shown to reduce diltiazem's apparent *oral* clearance and prolong its half-life.

INDICATIONS AND USAGE

CARDIZEM Injectable (diltiazem hydrochloride) is indicated for the following:
1. **Atrial Fibrillation or Atrial Flutter.** Temporary control of rapid ventricular rate in atrial fibrillation or atrial flutter. It should not be used in patients with atrial fibrillation or atrial flutter associated with an accessory bypass tract such as in Wolff-Parkinson-White (WPW) syndrome or short PR syndrome.
2. **Paroxysmal Supraventricular Tachycardia.** Rapid conversion of paroxysmal supraventicular tachycardias (PSVT) to sinus rhythm. This includes AV nodal reentrant tachycardias and reciprocating tachycardias associated with an extranodal accessory pathway such as the WPW syn-

drome or short PR syndrome. Unless otherwise contraindicated, appropriate vagal maneuvers should be attempted prior to administration of CARDIZEM Injectable.

The use of CARDIZEM Injectable for control of ventricular response in patients with atrial fibrillation or atrial flutter or conversion to sinus rhythm in patients with PSVT should be undertaken with caution when the patient is compromised hemodynamically or is taking other drugs that decrease any or all of the following: peripheral resistance, myocardial filling, myocardial contractility, or electrical impulse propagation in the myocardium.

For either indication and particularly when employing continuous intravenous infusion, the setting should include continuous monitoring of the ECG and frequent measurement of blood pressure. A defibrillator and emergency equipment should be readily available.

In domestic controlled trials in patients with atrial fibrillation or atrial flutter, bolus administration of CARDIZEM Injectable was effective in reducing heart rate by at least 20% in 95% of patients. CARDIZEM Injectable rarely converts atrial fibrillation or atrial flutter to normal sinus rhythm. Following administration of one or two intravenous bolus doses of CARDIZEM Injectable, response usually occurs within 3 minutes and maximal heart rate reduction generally occurs in 2 to 7 minutes. Heart rate reduction may last from 1 to 3 hours. If hypotension occurs, it is generally short-lived, but may last from 1 to 3 hours.

A 24-hour continuous infusion of CARDIZEM Injectable in the treatment of atrial fibrillation or atrial flutter maintained at least a 20% heart rate reduction during the infusion in 83% of patients. Upon discontinuation of infusion, heart rate reduction may last from 0.5 hours to more than 10 hours (median duration 7 hours). Hypotension, if it occurs, may be similarly persistent.

In the controlled clinical trials, 3.2% of patients required some form of intervention (typically, use of intravenous fluids or the Trendelenburg position) for blood pressure support following CARDIZEM Injectable.

In domestic controlled trials, bolus administration of CARDIZEM Injectable was effective in converting PSVT to normal sinus rhythm in 88% of patients within 3 minutes of the first or second bolus dose.

Symptoms associated with the arrhythmia were improved in conjunction with decreased heart rate or conversion to normal sinus rhythm following administration of CARDIZEM Injectable.

CONTRAINDICATIONS

CARDIZEM Injectable is contraindicated in:

1. Patients with sick sinus syndrome except in the presence of a functioning ventricular pacemaker.
2. Patients with second- or third-degree AV block except in the presence of a functioning ventricular pacemaker.
3. Patients with severe hypotension or cardiogenic shock.
4. Patients who have demonstrated hypersensitivity to the drug.
5. Intravenous diltiazem and intravenous beta-blockers should not be administered together or in close proximity (within a few hours).
6. Patients with atrial fibrillation or atrial flutter associated with an accessory bypass tract such as in WPW syndrome or short PR syndrome.

   As with other agents which slow AV nodal conduction and do not prolong the refractoriness of the accessory pathway (eg, verapamil, digoxin), in rare instances patients in atrial fibrillation or atrial flutter associated with an accessory bypass tract may experience a potentially life-threatening increase in heart rate accompanied by hypotension when treated with CARDIZEM Injectable. As such, the initial use of CARDIZEM Injectable should be, if possible, in a setting where monitoring and resuscitation capabilities, including DC cardioversion/defibrillation, are present (see OVERDOSAGE). Once familiarity of the patient's response is established, use in an office setting may be acceptable.
7. Patients with ventricular tachycardia. Administration of other calcium channel blockers to patients with wide complex tachycardia (QRS ≥ 0.12 seconds) has resulted in hemodynamic deterioration and ventricular fibrillation. It is important that an accurate pretreatment diagnosis distinguish wide complex QRS tachycardia of supraventricular origin from that of ventricular origin prior to administration of CARDIZEM Injectable.

WARNINGS

1. **Cardiac Conduction.** Diltiazem prolongs AV nodal conduction and refractoriness that may rarely result in second- or third-degree AV block in sinus rhythm. Concomitant use of diltiazem with agents known to affect cardiac conduction may result in additive effects (see DRUG INTERACTIONS). If high-degree AV block occurs in sinus rhythm, intravenous diltiazem should be discontinued and appropriate supportive measures instituted (see OVERDOSAGE).
2. **Congestive Heart Failure.** Although diltiazem has a negative inotropic effect in isolated animal tissue preparations, hemodynamic studies in humans with normal ventricular function, and in patients with a compromised myocardium, such as severe CHF, acute MI, and hypertrophic cardiomyopathy, have not shown a reduction in cardiac index nor consistent negative effects on contractility (dp/dt). Administration of oral diltiazem in patients with acute myocardial infarction and pulmonary congestion) documented by x-ray on admission is contraindicated. Experience with the use of CARDIZEM Injectable in patients with impaired ventricular function is limited. Caution should be exercised when using the drug in such patients.
3. **Hypotension.** Decreases in blood pressure associated with CARDIZEM Injectable therapy may occasionally result in symptomatic hypotension (3.2%). The use of intravenous diltiazem for control of ventricular response in patients with supraventricular arrhythmias should be undertaken with caution when the patient is compromised hemodynamically. In addition, caution should be used in patients taking other drugs that decrease peripheral resistance, intravascular volume, myocardial contractility or conduction.
4. **Acute Hepatic Injury.** In rare instances, significant elevations in enzymes such as alkaline phosphatase, LDH, SGOT, SGPT, and other phenomena consistent with acute hepatic injury have been noted following oral diltiazem. Therefore, the potential for acute hepatic injury exists following administration of intravenous diltiazem.
5. **Ventricular Premature Beats (VPBs).** VPBs may be present on conversion of PSVT to sinus rhythm with CARDIZEM Injectable. These VPBs are transient, are typically considered to be benign, and appear to have no clinical significance. Similar ventricular complexes have been noted during cardioversion, other pharmacologic therapy, and during spontaneous conversion of PSVT to sinus rhythm.

PRECAUTIONS

General. CARDIZEM (diltiazem hydrochloride) is extensively metabolized by the liver and excreted by the kidneys and in bile. The drug should be used with caution in patients with impaired renal or hepatic function (see WARNINGS). High intravenous dosages (4.5 mg/kg tid) administered to dogs resulted in significant bradycardia and alterations in AV conduction. In subacute and chronic dog and rat studies designed to produce toxicity, high oral doses of diltiazem were associated with hepatic damage. In special subacute hepatic studies, oral doses of 125 mg/kg and higher in rats were associated with histological changes in the liver, which were reversible when the drug was discontinued. In dogs, oral doses of 20 mg/kg were also associated with hepatic changes; however, these changes were reversible with continued dosing.

Dermatological events progressing to erythema multiforme and/or exfoliative dermatitis have been infrequently reported following oral diltiazem. Therefore, the potential for these dermatologic reactions exists following exposure to intravenous diltiazem. Should a dermatologic reaction persist, the drug should be discontinued.

Drug Interactions. Due to potential for additive effects, caution is warranted in patients receiving CARDIZEM Injectable concomitantly with any agent(s) known to affect cardiac contractility and/or SA or AV node conduction (see WARNINGS).

As with all drugs, care should be exercised when treating patients with multiple medications. CARDIZEM undergoes extensive metabolism by the cytochrome P-450 mixed function oxidase system. Although specific pharmacokinetic drug-drug interaction studies havd not been conducted with single intravenous injection or constant rate intravenous infusion, coadministration of CARDIZEM Injectable with other agents which primarily undergo the same route of biotransformation may result in competitive inhibition of metabolism.

Digitalis: Intravenous diltiazem has been administered to patients receiving either intravenous or oral digitalis therapy. The combination of the two drugs was well tolerated without serious adverse effects. However, since both drugs affect AV nodal conduction, patients should be monitored for excessive slowing of the heart rate and/or AV block.

Beta-blockers: Intravenous diltiazem has been administered to patients on chronic oral beta-blocker therapy. The combination of the two drugs was generally well tolerated without serious adverse effects. If intravenous diltiazem is administered to patients receiving chronic oral beta-blocker therapy, the possibility for bradycardia, AV block, and/or depression of contractility should be considered (see CONTRAINDICATIONS). *Oral* administration of diltiazem with propranolol in five normal volunteers resulted in increased propranolol levels in all subjects and bioavailability of propranolol was increased approximately 50%. In vitro, propranolol appears to be displaced from its binding sites by diltiazem.

Anesthetics: The depression of cardiac contractility, conductivity, and automaticity as well as the vascular dilation associated with anesthetics may be potentiated by calcium channel blockers. When used concomitantly, anesthetics and calcium blockers should be titrated carefully.

Carcinogenesis, Mutagenesis, Impairment of Fertility. A 24-month study in rats at oral dosage levels of up to 100 mg/kg/day, and a 21-month study in mice at oral dosage levels of up to 30 mg/kg/day showed no evidence of carcinogenicity. There was also no mutagenic response in vitro or in vivo in mammalian cell assays or in vitro in bacteria. No evidence of impaired fertility was observed in a study performed in male and female rats at oral dosages of up to 100 mg/kg/day.

Pregnancy. Category C. Reproduction studies have been conducted in mice, rats, and rabbits. Administration of oral doses ranging from five to ten times greater (on a mg/kg basis) than the daily recommended oral antianginal therapeutic dose has resulted in embryo and fetal lethality. These doses, in some studies, have been reported to cause skeletal abnormalities. In the perinatal/postnatal studies there was some reduction in early individual pup weights and survival rates. There was an increased incidence of stillbirths at doses of 20 times the human oral antianginal dose or greater.

There are no well-controlled studies in pregnant women; therefore, use CARDIZEM in pregnant women only if the potential benefit justifies the potential risk to the fetus.

Nursing Mothers. Diltiazem is excreted in human milk. One report with oral diltiazem suggests that concentrations in breast milk may approximate serum levels. If use of CARDIZEM is deemed essential, an alternative method of infant feeding should be instituted.

Pediatric Use. Safety and effectiveness in children have not been established.

ADVERSE REACTIONS

The following adverse reaction rates are based on the use of CARDIZEM Injectable in over 400 domestic clinical trial patients with atrial fibrillation/flutter or PSVT under double-blind or open-label conditions. Worldwide experience in over 1,300 patients was similar.

Adverse events reported in controlled and uncontrolled clinical trials were generally mild and transient. Hypotension was the most commonly reported adverse event during clinical trials. Asymptomatic hypotension occurred in 4.3% of patients. Symptomatic hypotension occurred in 3.2% of patients. When treatment for hypotension was required, it generally consisted of administration of saline or placing the patient in the Trendelenburg position. Other events reported in at least 1% of the diltiazem-treated patients were injection site reactions (eg, itching, burning)—3.9%, vasodilation (flushing)—1.7%, and arrhythmia (junctional rhythm or isorhythmic dissociation)—1.0%.

In addition, the following events were reported infrequently (less than 1%):

Cardiovascular. Atrial flutter, AV block first degree, AV block second degree, bradycardia, chest pain, congestive heart failure, sinus pause, sinus node dysfunction, syncope, ventricular arrhythmia, ventricular fibrillation, ventricular tachycardia.

Dermatologic: Pruritus, sweating.

Gastrointestinal: Constipation, elevated SGOT or alkaline phosphatase, nausea, vomiting.

Nervous System: Dizziness, paresthesia.

Other: Amblyopia, asthenia, dry mouth, dyspnea, edema, headache, hyperuricemia.

Although not observed in clinical trials with CARDIZEM Injectable, other reactions associated with oral diltiazem may occur.

OVERDOSAGE

Overdosage experience is limited. In the event of overdosage or an exaggerated response, appropriate supportive measures should be employed. The following measures may be considered:

Bradycardia: Administer atropine (0.60 to 1.0 mg). If there is no response to vagal blockade, administer isoproterenol cautiously.

High-degree AV block: Treat as for bradycardia above. Fixed high-degree AV block should be treated with cardiac pacing.

Cardiac failure: Administer inotropic agents (isoproterenol, dopamine, or dobutamine) and diuretics.

Hypotension: Vasopressors (eg, dopamine or levarterenol bitartrate).

Actual treatment and dosage should depend on the severity of the clinical situation and the judgment and experience of the treating physician.

The intravenous LD_{50}'s in mice and rats were 60 and 38 mg/kg, respectively. The toxic dose in man is not known.

DOSAGE AND ADMINISTRATION

Direct Intravenous Single Injections (Bolus)

The initial dose of CARDIZEM Injectable should be 0.25 mg/kg actual body weight as a bolus administered over 2 minutes (20 mg is a reasonable dose for the average patient). If response is inadequate, a second dose may be administered after 15 minutes. The second bolus dose of CARDIZEM Injectable should be 0.35 mg/kg actual body weight adminis-

Continued on next page

Marion Merrell Dow—Cont.

tered over 2 minutes (25 mg is a reasonable dose for the average patient). Subsequent intravenous bolus doses should be individualized for each patient. Patients with low body weights should be dosed on a mg/kg basis. Some patients may respond to an initial dose of 0.15 mg/kg, although duration of action may be shorter. Experience with this dose is limited.

Continuous Intravenous Infusion
For continued reduction of the heart rate (up to 24 hours) in patients with atrial fibrillation or atrial flutter, an intravenous infusion of CARDIZEM Injectable may be administered. Immediately following bolus administration of 20 mg (0.25 mg/kg) or 25 mg (0.35 mg/kg) CARDIZEM Injectable and reduction of heart rate, begin an intravenous infusion of CARDIZEM Injectable. The recommended initial infusion rate of CARDIZEM Injectable is 10 mg/h. Some patients may maintain response to an initial rate of 5 mg/h. The infusion rate may be increased in 5 mg/h increments up to 15 mg/h as needed, if further reduction in heart rate is required. The infusion may be maintained for up to 24 hours.
Diltiazem shows dose-dependent, non-linear pharmacokinetics. Duration of infusion longer than 24 hours and infusion rates greater than 15 mg/h have not been studied. Therefore, infusion duration exceeding 24 hours and infusion rates exceeding 15 mg/h are not recommended.

Dilution: To prepare CARDIZEM Injectable for continuous intravenous infusion aseptically transfer the appropriate quantity (see chart) of CARDIZEM Injectable to the desired volume of either Normal Saline, D5W, or D5W/0.45% NaCl. Mix thoroughly. Use within 24 hours. Keep refrigerated until use.

[See table below.]

CARDIZEM Injectable was tested for compatibility with three commonly used intravenous fluids at a maximal concentration of 1 mg diltiazem hydrochloride per milliliter. CARDIZEM Injectable was found to be physically compatible and chemically stable in the following parenteral solutions for at least 24 hours when stored in glass or polyvinylchloride (PVC) bags at controlled room temperature 15–30°C (59–86°F) or under refrigeration 2–8°C (36–46°F).

- dextrose (5%) injection USP
- sodium chloride (0.9%) injection USP
- dextrose (5%) and sodium chloride (0.45%) injection USP

CARDIZEM Injectable is incompatible when mixed directly with furosemide solution.
Parenteral drug products should be inspected visually for particulate matter and discoloration prior to administration whenever solution and container permit.

Translation to Further Antiarrhythmic Therapy. Transition to other antiarrhythmic agents following administration of CARDIZEM Injectable is generally safe. However, reference should be made to the respective agent manufacturer's package insert for information relative to dosage and administration.
In controlled clinical trials, therapy with antiarrhythmic agents to maintain reduced heart rate in atrial fibrillation or atrial flutter or for prophylaxis of PSVT was generally started within 3 hours after bolus administration of CARDIZEM Injectable. These antiarrhythmic agents were intravenous or oral digoxin, Class I antiarrhythmics (eg, quinidine, procainamide), calcium channel blockers, and oral beta-blockers.
Experience in the use of antiarrhythmic agents following maintenance infusion of CARDIZEM Injectable is limited. Patients should be dosed on an individual basis and reference should be made to the respective manufacturer's package insert for information relative to dosage and administration.

HOW SUPPLIED

CARDIZEM® Injectable (diltiazem hydrochloride injection) is supplied in boxes of six 5-mL vials with each vial containing 25 mg of diltiazem hydrochloride (5 mg/mL) (NDC 0088-1790-32) and boxes of six 10-mL vials with each vial containing 50 mg diltiazem hydrochloride (5 mg/mL) (NDC 0088-1790-33).

SINGLE-USE CONTAINERS. DISCARD UNUSED PORTION.
STORE PRODUCT UNDER REFRIGERATION 2–8°C (36–46°F). DO NOT FREEZE. MAY BE STORED AT ROOM TEMPERATURE FOR UP TO 1 MONTH. DESTROY AFTER 1 MONTH AT ROOM TEMPERATURE.
Product information as of October 1991

Shown in Product Identification Section, page 416

Diluent Volume	Quantity of Cardizem Injection	Final Concentration	Administration: Dose*	Administration: Infusion Rate
100 mL	125 mg (25 mL)	10 mg/mL	10 mg/h	10 mL/h
			15 mg/h	15 mL/h
250 mL	250 mg (50 mL)	0.83 mg/mL	10 mg/h	12 mL/h
			15 mg/h	18 mL/h
500 mL	250 mg (50 mL)	0.45 mg/mL	10 mg/h	22 mL/h
			15 mg/h	33 mL/h

*5 mg/h may be appropriate for some patients

CARDIZEM® SR ℞

[kar'diz-em]
(diltiazem hydrochloride)
Sustained Release Capsules

DESCRIPTION

CARDIZEM® (diltiazem hydrochloride) is a calcium ion influx inhibitor (slow channel blocker or calcium antagonist). Chemically, diltiazem hydrochloride is 1,5-Benzothiazepin-4(5H)one,3-(acetyloxy)-5-[2-(dimethylamino)-ethyl]-2,3-dihydro-2-(4-methoxyphenyl)-, monohydrochloride, (+)-cis-. The chemical structure is:

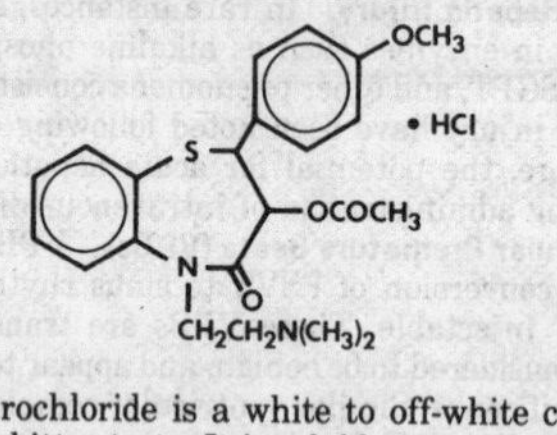

Diltiazem hydrochloride is a white to off-white crystalline powder with a bitter taste. It is soluble in water, methanol, and chloroform. It has a molecular weight of 450.98. Each CARDIZEM SR capsule contains either 60 mg, 90 mg, or 120 mg diltiazem hydrochloride.
Also contains: fumaric acid, povidone, starch, sucrose, talc, and other ingredients.
For oral administration.

CLINICAL PHARMACOLOGY

The therapeutic effects of CARDIZEM are believed to be related to its ability to inhibit the influx of calcium ions during membrane depolarization of cardiac and vascular smooth muscle.

Mechanisms of Action. CARDIZEM SR produces its antihypertensive effect primarily by relaxation of vascular smooth muscle and the resultant decrease in peripheral vascular resistance. The magnitude of blood pressure reduction is related to the degree of hypertension; thus hypertensive individuals experience an antihypertensive effect, whereas there is only a modest fall in blood pressure in normotensives.

Hemodynamic and Electrophysiologic Effects. Like other calcium antagonists, diltiazem decreases sinoatrial and atrioventricular conduction in isolated tissues and has a negative inotropic effect in isolated preparations. In the intact animal, prolongation of the AH interval can be seen at higher doses.
In man, diltiazem prevents spontaneous and ergonovine-provoked coronary artery spasm. It causes a decrease in peripheral vascular resistance and a modest fall in blood pressure in normotensive individuals and, in exercise tolerance studies in patients with ischemic heart disease, reduces the heart rate-blood pressure product for any given work load. Studies to date, primarily in patients with good ventricular function, have not revealed evidence of a negative inotropic effect; cardiac output, ejection fraction, and left ventricular end diastolic pressure have not been affected. Increased heart failure has, however, been reported in occasional patients with preexisting impairment of ventricular function. There are as yet few data on the interaction of diltiazem and beta-blockers in patients with poor ventricular function. Resting heart rate is usually slightly reduced by diltiazem.
CARDIZEM SR produces antihypertensive effects both in the supine and standing positions. Postural hypotension is infrequently noted upon suddenly assuming an upright position. No reflex tachycardia is associated with the chronic antihypertensive effects. CARDIZEM SR decreases vascular resistance, increases cardiac output (by increasing stroke volume), and produces a slight decrease or no change in heart rate. During dynamic exercise, increases in diastolic pressure are inhibited while maximum achievable systolic pressure is usually reduced. Heart rate at maximum exercise does not change or is slightly reduced. Chronic therapy with CARDIZEM produces no change or an increase in plasma catecholamines. No increased activity of the renin-angiotensin-aldosterone axis has been observed. CARDIZEM SR antagonizes the renal and peripheral effects of angiotensin II. Hypertensive animal models respond to diltiazem with reductions in blood pressure and increased urinary output and natriuresis without a change in urinary sodium/potassium ratio.
Intravenous diltiazem in doses of 20 mg prolongs AH conduction time and AV node functional and effective refractory periods approximately 20%. In a study involving single oral doses of 300 mg of CARDIZEM in six normal volunteers, the average maximum PR prolongation was 14% with no instances of greater than first-degree AV block. Diltiazem-associated prolongation of the AH interval is not more pronounced in patients with first-degree heart block. In patients with sick sinus syndrome, diltiazem significantly prolongs sinus cycle length (up to 50% in some cases).
Chronic oral administration of CARDIZEM in doses of up to 360 mg/day has resulted in small increases in PR interval, and on occasion produces abnormal prolongation. (See WARNINGS.)

Pharmacokinetics and Metabolism. Diltiazem is well absorbed from the gastrointestinal tract and is subject to an extensive first-pass effect, giving an absolute bioavailability (compared to intravenous administration) of about 40%. CARDIZEM undergoes extensive metabolism in which 2% to 4% of the unchanged drug appears in the urine. In vitro binding studies show CARDIZEM is 70% to 80% bound to plasma proteins. Competitive in vitro ligand binding studies have also shown CARDIZEM binding is not altered by therapeutic concentrations of digoxin, hydrochlorothiazide, phenylbutazone, propranolol, salicylic acid, or warfarin. The plasma elimination half-life following single or multiple drug administration is approximately 3.0 to 4.5 hours. Desacetyl diltiazem is also present in the plasma at levels of 10% to 20% of the parent drug and is 25% to 50% as potent a coronary vasodilator as diltiazem. Minimum therapeutic plasma levels of CARDIZEM appear to be in the range of 50–200 ng/mL. There is a departure from linearity when dose strengths are increased; the half-life is slightly increased with dose. A study that compared patients with normal hepatic function to patients with cirrhosis found an increase in half-life and a 69% increase in bioavailability in the hepatically impaired patients. A single study in patients with severely impaired renal function showed no difference in the pharmacokinetic profile of diltiazem compared to patients with normal renal function.

Cardizem SR Capsules. Diltiazem is absorbed from the capsule formulation to about 92% of a reference solution at steady-state. A single 120-mg dose of the capsule results in detectable plasma levels within two to three hours and peak plasma levels at six to 11 hours. The apparent elimination half-life after single or multiple dosing is five to seven hours. A departure from linearity similar to that observed with the CARDIZEM tablet is observed. As the dose of CARDIZEM SR capsules is increased from a daily dose of 120 mg (60 mg bid) to 240 mg (120 mg bid) daily, there is an increase in bioavailability of 2.6 times. When the dose is increased from 240 mg to 360 mg daily there is an increase in bioavailability of 1.8 times. The average plasma levels of the capsule dosed twice daily at steady-state are equivalent to the tablet dosed four times daily when the same total daily dose is administered.

INDICATIONS AND USAGE

CARDIZEM SR is indicated for the treatment of hypertension. It may be used alone or in combination with other antihypertensive medications, such as diuretics.

CONTRAINDICATIONS

CARDIZEM is contraindicated in (1) patients with sick sinus syndrome except in the presence of a functioning ventricular pacemaker, (2) patients with second- or third-degree AV block except in the presence of a functioning ventricular pacemaker, (3) patients with hypotension (less than 90 mm Hg systolic), (4) patients who have demonstrated hypersensitivity to the drug, and (5) patients with acute myocardial infarction and pulmonary congestion documented by x-ray on admission.

WARNINGS

1. Cardiac Conduction. CARDIZEM prolongs AV node refractory periods without significantly prolonging sinus node recovery time, except in patients with sick sinus syndrome. This effect may rarely result in abnormally slow heart rates (particularly in patients with sick sinus syndrome) or second- or third-degree AV block (nine of 2,111 patients or 0.43%). Concomitant use of diltiazem with beta-blockers or digitalis may result in additive effects on cardiac conduction. A patient with Prinzmetal's angina

developed periods of asystole (2 to 5 seconds) after a single dose of 60 mg of diltiazem.

2. **Congestive Heart Failure.** Although diltiazem has a negative inotropic effect in isolated animal tissue preparations, hemodynamic studies in humans with normal ventricular function have not shown a reduction in cardiac index nor consistent negative effects on contractility (dp/dt). An acute study of oral diltiazem in patients with impaired ventricular function (ejection fraction 24%±6%) showed improvement in indices of ventricular function without significant decrease in contractile function (dp/dt). Experience with the use of CARDIZEM (diltiazem hydrochloride) in combination with beta-blockers in patients with impaired ventricular function is limited. Caution should be exercised when using this combination.

3. **Hypotension.** Decreases in blood pressure associated with CARDIZEM therapy may occasionally result in symptomatic hypotension.

4. **Acute Hepatic Injury.** Mild elevations of transaminases with and without concomitant elevation in alkaline phosphatase and bilirubin have been observed in clinical studies. Such elevations were usually transient and frequently resolved even with continued diltiazem treatment. In rare instances, significant elevations in enzymes such as alkaline phosphatase, LDH, SGOT, SGPT, and other phenomena consistent with acute hepatic injury have been noted. These reactions tended to occur early after therapy initiation (1 to 8 weeks) and have been reversible upon discontinuation of drug therapy. The relationship to CARDIZEM is uncertain in some cases, but probable in some. (See PRECAUTIONS.)

PRECAUTIONS

General. CARDIZEM (diltiazem hydrochloride) is extensively metabolized by the liver and excreted by the kidneys and in bile. As with any drug given over prolonged periods, laboratory parameters should be monitored at regular intervals. The drug should be used with caution in patients with impaired renal or hepatic function. In subacute and chronic dog and rat studies designed to produce toxicity, high doses of diltiazem were associated with hepatic damage. In special subacute hepatic studies, oral doses of 125 mg/kg and higher in rats were associated with histological changes in the liver which were reversible when the drug was discontinued. In dogs, doses of 20 mg/kg were also associated with hepatic changes; however, these changes were reversible with continued dosing.

Dermatological events (see ADVERSE REACTIONS section) may be transient and may disappear despite continued use of CARDIZEM. However, skin eruptions progressing to erythema multiforme and/or exfoliative dermatitis have also been infrequently reported. Should a dermatologic reaction persist, the drug should be discontinued.

Drug Interaction. Due to the potential for additive effects, caution and careful titration are warranted in patients receiving CARDIZEM concomitantly with any agents known to affect cardiac contractility and/or conduction. (See WARNINGS.) Pharmacologic studies indicate that there may be additive effects in prolonging AV conduction when using beta-blockers or digitalis concomitantly with CARDIZEM. (See WARNINGS.)

As with all drugs, care should be exercised when treating patients with multiple medications. CARDIZEM undergoes biotransformation by cytochrome P-450 mixed function oxidase. Coadministration of CARDIZEM with other agents which follow the same route of biotransformation may result in the competitive inhibition of metabolism. Dosages of similarly metabolized drugs, particularly those of low therapeutic ratio or in patients with renal and/or hepatic impairment, may require adjustment when starting or stopping concomitantly administered CARDIZEM to maintain optimum therapeutic blood levels.

Beta-blockers: Controlled and uncontrolled domestic studies suggest that concomitant use of CARDIZEM and beta-blockers or digitalis is usually well tolerated, but available data are not sufficient to predict the effects of concomitant treatment in patients with left ventricular dysfunction or cardiac conduction abnormalities.

Administration of CARDIZEM (diltiazem hydrochloride) concomitantly with propranolol in five normal volunteers resulted in increased propranolol levels in all subjects and bioavailability of propranolol was increased approximately 50%. If combination therapy is initiated or withdrawn in conjunction with propranolol, an adjustment in the propranolol dose may be warranted. (See WARNINGS.)

Cimetidine: A study in six healthy volunteers has shown a significant increase in peak diltiazem plasma levels (58%) and area-under-the-curve (53%) after a 1-week course of cimetidine at 1,200 mg per day and diltiazem 60 mg per day. Ranitidine produced smaller, nonsignificant increases. The effect may be mediated by cimetidine's known inhibition of hepatic cytochrome P-450, the enzyme system probably responsible for the first-pass metabolism of diltiazem. Patients

currently receiving diltiazem therapy should be carefully monitored for a change in pharmacological effect when initiating and discontinuing therapy with cimetidine. An adjustment in the diltiazem dose may be warranted.

Digitalis: Administration of CARDIZEM with digoxin in 24 healthy male subjects increased plasma digoxin concentrations approximately 20%. Another investigator found no increase in digoxin levels in 12 patients with coronary artery disease. Since there have been conflicting results regarding the effect of digoxin levels, it is recommended that digoxin levels be monitored when initiating, adjusting, and discontinuing CARDIZEM therapy to avoid possible over- or underdigitalization. (See WARNINGS.)

Anesthetics: The depression of cardiac contractility, conductivity, and automaticity as well as the vascular dilation associated with anesthetics may be potentiated by calcium channel blockers. When used concomitantly, anesthetics and calcium blockers should be titrated carefully.

Carcinogenesis, Mutagenesis, Impairment of Fertility. A 24-month study in rats and a 21-month study in mice showed no evidence of carcinogenicity. There was also no mutagenic response in in vitro bacterial tests. No intrinsic effect on fertility was observed in rats.

Pregnancy. Category C. Reproduction studies have been conducted in mice, rats, and rabbits. Administration of doses ranging from five to ten times greater (on a mg/kg basis) than the daily recommended therapeutic dose has resulted in embryo and fetal lethality. These doses, in some studies, have been reported to cause skeletal abnormalities. In the perinatal/postnatal studies, there was some reduction in early individual pup weights and survival rates. There was an increased incidence of stillbirths at doses of 20 times the human dose or greater.

There are no well-controlled studies in pregnant women; therefore, use CARDIZEM in pregnant women only if the potential benefit justifies the potential risk to the fetus.

Nursing Mothers. Diltiazem is excreted in human milk. One report suggests that concentrations in breast milk may approximate serum levels. If use of CARDIZEM is deemed essential, an alternative method of infant feeding should be instituted.

Pediatric Use. Safety and effectiveness in children have not been established.

ADVERSE REACTIONS

Serious adverse reactions have been rare in studies carried out to date, but it should be recognized that patients with impaired ventricular function and cardiac conduction abnormalities have usually been excluded from these studies.

The adverse events described below represent events observed in clinical studies of hypertensive patients receiving either CARDIZEM Tablets or CARDIZEM SR Capsules as well as experiences observed in studies of angina and during marketing. The most common events in hypertension studies are shown in a table with rates in placebo patients shown for comparison. Less common events are listed by body system; these include any adverse reactions seen in angina studies that were not observed in hypertension studies. In all hypertensive patients studied (over 900), the most common adverse events were edema (9%), headache (8%), dizziness (6%), asthenia (5%), sinus bradycardia (3%), flushing (3%), and first degree AV block (3%). Only edema and perhaps bradycardia and dizziness were dose related. The most common events observed in clinical studies (over 2,100 patients) of angina patients and hypertensive patients receiving CARDIZEM Tablets or CARDIZEM SR Capsules were (ie, greater than 1%) edema (5.4%), headache (4.5%), dizziness (3.4%), asthenia (2.8%), first degree AV block (1.8%), flushing (1.7%), nausea (1.6%), bradycardia (1.5%), and rash (1.5%). [See table above.]

In addition, the following events were reported infrequently (less than 1%) with CARDIZEM SR Capsules or CARDIZEM Tablets or have been observed in angina or hypertension trials.

Cardiovascular: Angina, arrhythmia, second- or third degree AV block (see conduction warning), bundle branch block, congestive heart failure, syncope, tachycardia, ventricular extrasystoles.

Nervous System: Abnormal dreams, amnesia, depression, gait abnormality, hallucinations, nervousness, paresthesia, personality change, tremor.

Gastrointestinal: Anorexia, diarrhea, dry mouth, dysgeusia, mild elevations of SGOT, SGPT, and LDH (see Hepatic Warnings), thirst, vomiting, weight increase.

Dermatological: Petechiae, photosensitivity, pruritus, urticaria.

DOUBLE BLIND PLACEBO CONTROLLED HYPERTENSION TRIALS

Adverse	Diltiazem N=315 # pts (%)	Placebo N=211 # pts (%)
headache	38 (12%)	17 (8%)
AV block first degree	24 (7.6%)	4 (1.9%)
dizziness	22 (7%)	6 (2.8%)
edema	19 (6%)	2 (0.9%)
bradycardia	19 (6%)	3 (1.4%)
ECG abnormality	13 (4.1%)	3 (1.4%)
asthenia	10 (3.2%)	1 (0.5%)
constipation	5 (1.6%)	2 (0.9%)
dyspepsia	4 (1.3%)	1 (0.5%)
nausea	4 (1.3%)	2 (0.9%)
palpitations	4 (1.3%)	2 (0.9%)
polyuria	4 (1.3%)	2 (0.9%)
somnolence	4 (1.3%)	—
alk phos increase	3 (1%)	1 (0.5%)
hypotension	3 (1%)	1 (0.5%)
insomnia	3 (1%)	1 (0.5%)
rash	3 (1%)	1 (0.5%)
AV block second degree	2 (0.6%)	—

Other: Amblyopia, CPK increase, dyspnea, epistaxis, eye irritation, hyperglycemia, hyperurucemia, impotence, muscle cramps, nasal congestion, nocturia, osteoarticular pain, sexual difficulties, tinnitus.

The following postmarketing events have been reported infrequently in patients receiving CARDIZEM: alopecia, erythema multiforme, extrapyramidal symptoms, gingival hyperplasia, hemolytic anemia, increased bleeding time, leukopenia, purpura, retinopathy, and thrombocytopenia. There have been observed cases of generalized rash, characterized as leukocytoclastic vasculitis. In addition, events such as myocardial infarction have been observed which are not readily distinguishable from the natural history of the disease in these patients. A definitive cause and effect relationship between these events and CARDIZEM therapy cannot yet be established. Exfoliative dermatitis (proven by rechallenge) has also been reported.

OVERDOSAGE OR EXAGGERATED RESPONSE

The oral LD_{50}'s in mice and rats range from 415 to 740 mg/kg and from 560 to 810 mg/kg, respectively. The intravenous LD_{50}'s in these species were 60 and 38 mg/kg, respectively. The oral LD_{50} in dogs is considered to be in excess of 50 mg/kg, while lethality was seen in monkeys at 360 mg/kg.

The toxic dose in man is not known. Due to extensive metabolism, blood levels after a standard dose of diltiazem can vary over tenfold, limiting the usefulness of blood levels in overdose cases.

There have been 29 reports of diltiazem overdose in doses ranging from less than 1 g to 10.8 g. Sixteen of these reports involve multiple drug ingestions.

Twenty-two reports indicated patients had recovered from diltiazem overdose ranging from less than 1 g to 10.8 g. There were seven reports with a fatal outcome; although the amount of diltiazem ingested was unknown, multiple drug ingestions were confirmed in six of the seven reports.

Events observed following diltiazem overdose included bradycardia, hypotension, heart block, and cardiac failure. Most reports of overdose described some supportive medical measure and/or drug treatment. Bradycardia frequently responded favorably to atropine, as did heart block, although cardiac pacing was also frequently utilized to treat heart

Continued on next page

Marion Merrell Dow—Cont.

CARDIZEM® SR
(diltiazem hydrochloride)
Sustained Release Capsules

Strength	Quantity	NDC Number	Description
60 mg	100 btl 100 UDIP®	0088-1777-47 0088-1777-49	Ivory/brown capsule imprinted with CARDIZEM logo on one end and CARDIZEM SR 60 mg on the other
90 mg	100 btl 100 UDIP®	0088-1778-47 0088-1778-49	Gold/brown capsule imprinted with CARDIZEM logo on one end and CARDIZEM SR 90 mg on the other
120 mg	100 btl 100 UDIP®	0088-1779-47 0088-1779-49	Caramel/brown capsule imprinted with CARDIZEM logo on one end and CARDIZEM SR 120 mg on the other

block. Fluids and vasopressors were used to maintain blood pressure and in cases of cardiac failure inotropic agents were administered. In addition, some patients received treatment with ventilatory support, gastric lavage, activated charcoal, and/or intravenous calcium. Evidence of the effectiveness of intravenous calcium administration to reverse the pharmacological effects of diltiazem overdose was conflicting.

In the event of overdosage or exaggerated response, appropriate supportive measures should be employed in addition to gastrointestinal decontamination. Diltiazem does not appear to be removed by peritoneal or hemodialysis. Based on the known pharmacological effects of diltiazem and/or reported clinical experiences the following measures may be considered:

Bradycardia: Administer atropine (0.60 to 1.0 mg). If there is no response to vagal blockade, administer isoproterenol cautiously.

High-Degree AV Block: Treat as for bradycardia above. Fixed high-degree AV block should be treated with cardiac pacing.

Cardiac Failure: Administer inotropic agents (isoproterenol, dopamine, or dobutamine) and diuretics.

Hypotension: Vasopressors (eg, dopamine or levarterenol bitartrate).

Actual treatment and dosage should depend on the severity of the clinical situation and the judgment and experience of the treating physician.

DOSAGE AND ADMINISTRATION

Dosages must be adjusted to each patient's needs, starting with 60 to 120 mg twice daily. Maximum antihypertensive effect is usually observed by 14 days of chronic therapy; therefore, dosage adjustments should be scheduled accordingly. Although individual patients may respond to lower doses, the usual optimum dosage range in clinical trials was 240 to 360 mg/day.

CARDIZEM SR has an additive antihypertensive effect when used with other antihypertensive agents. Therefore, the dosage of CARDIZEM SR or the concomitant antihypertensives may need to be adjusted when adding one to the other. See WARNINGS and PRECAUTIONS regarding use with beta-blockers.

HOW SUPPLIED

[See table above.]
Storage Conditions: Store at controlled room temperature 59–86°F (15–30°C).

Issued 1/91

Shown in Product Identification Section, page 417

CARDIZEM® Tablets   ℞
[kar'diz-em]
(diltiazem HCl)
30 mg, 60 mg, 90 mg, and 120 mg

DESCRIPTION

CARDIZEM® (diltiazem hydrochloride) is a calcium ion influx inhibitor (slow channel blocker or calcium antagonist). Chemically, diltiazem hydrochloride is 1,5-Benzothiazepin-4(5H)one, 3-(acetyloxy)-5-[2-(dimethylamino)ethyl]-2,3-dihydro-2-(4-methoxyphenyl)-, monohydrochloride, (+)-cis-. The chemical structure is:
[See chemical structure at top of next column.]

Diltiazem hydrochloride is a white to off-white crystalline powder with a bitter taste. It is soluble in water, methanol, and chloroform. It has a molecular weight of 450.98. Each tablet of CARDIZEM contains 30 mg, 60 mg, 90 mg, or 120 mg diltiazem hydrochloride.

Also contains: D&C Yellow #10, FD&C Yellow #6 (60 mg and 120 mg), or FD&C Blue #1 (30 mg and 90 mg), hydroxypropylcellulose, hydroxypropyl methylcellulose, lactose, magnesium stearate, methylparaben, polyethylene glycol, talc, and other ingredients.

For oral administration.

CLINICAL PHARMACOLOGY

The therapeutic benefits achieved with CARDIZEM are believed to be related to its ability to inhibit the influx of calcium ions during membrane depolarization of cardiac and vascular smooth muscle.

Mechanisms of Action. Although precise mechanisms of its antianginal actions are still being delineated, CARDIZEM is believed to act in the following ways:

1. Angina Due to Coronary Artery Spasm: CARDIZEM has been shown to be a potent dilator of coronary arteries both epicardial and subendocardial. Spontaneous and ergovine-induced coronary artery spasm are inhibited by CARDIZEM.

2. Exertional Angina: CARDIZEM has been shown to produce increases in exercise tolerance, probably due to its ability to reduce myocardial oxygen demand. This is accomplished via reductions in heart rate and systemic blood pressure at submaximal and maximal exercise work loads.

In animal models, diltiazem interferes with the slow inward (depolarizing) current in excitable tissue. It causes excitation-contraction uncoupling in various myocardial tissues without changes in the configuration of the action potential. Diltiazem produces relaxation of coronary vascular smooth muscle and dilation of both large and small coronary arteries at drug levels which cause little or no negative inotropic effect. The resultant increases in coronary blood flow (epicardial and subendocardial) occur in ischemic and nonischemic models and are accompanied by dose-dependent decreases in systemic blood pressure and decreases in peripheral resistance.

Hemodynamic and Electrophysiologic Effects. Like other calcium antagonists, diltiazem decreases sinoatrial and atrioventricular conduction in isolated tissues and has a negative inotropic effect in isolated preparations. In the intact animal, prolongation of the AH interval can be seen at higher doses.

In man, diltiazem prevents spontaneous and ergonovine-provoked coronary artery spasm. It causes a decrease in peripheral vascular resistance and a modest fall in blood pressure and, in exercise tolerance studies in patients with ischemic heart disease, reduces the heart rate-blood pressure product for any given work load. Studies to date, primarily in patients with good ventricular function, have not revealed evidence of a negative inotropic effect; cardiac output, ejection fraction, and left ventricular end diastolic pressure have not been affected. There are as yet few data on the interaction of diltiazem and beta-blockers. Resting heart rate is usually unchanged or slightly reduced by diltiazem.

Intravenous diltiazem in doses of 20 mg prolongs AH conduction time and AV node functional and effective refractory

periods approximately 20%. In a study involving single oral doses of 300 mg of CARDIZEM in six normal volunteers, the average maximum PR prolongation was 14% with no instances of greater than first-degree AV block. Diltiazem-associated prolongation of the AH interval is not more pronounced in patients with first-degree heart block. In patients with sick sinus syndrome, diltiazem significantly prolongs sinus cycle length (up to 50% in some cases).

Chronic oral administration of CARDIZEM in doses of up to 240 mg/day has resulted in small increases in PR interval, but has not usually produced abnormal prolongation.

Pharmacokinetics and Metabolism. Diltiazem is absorbed from the tablet formulation to about 80% of a reference capsule and is subject to an extensive first-pass effect, giving an absolute bioavailability (compared to intravenous dosing) of about 40%. CARDIZEM undergoes extensive hepatic metabolism in which 2% to 4% of the unchanged drug appears in the urine. In vitro binding studies show CARDIZEM is 70% to 80% bound to plasma proteins. Competitive ligand binding studies have also shown CARDIZEM binding is not altered by therapeutic concentrations of digoxin, hydrochlorothiazide, phenylbutazone, propranolol, salicylic acid, or warfarin. Single oral doses of 30 to 120 mg of CARDIZEM result in detectable plasma levels within 30 to 60 minutes and peak plasma levels two to three hours after drug administration. The plasma elimination half-life following single or multiple drug administration is approximately 3.5 hours. Desacetyl diltiazem is also present in the plasma at levels of 10% to 20% of the parent drug and is 25% to 50% as potent as a coronary vasodilator as diltiazem. Therapeutic blood levels of CARDIZEM appear to be in the range of 50–200 ng/mL. There is a departure from dose-linearity when single doses above 60 mg are given; a 120-mg dose gave blood levels three times that of the 60-mg dose. There is no information about the effect of renal or hepatic impairment on excretion or metabolism of diltiazem.

INDICATIONS AND USAGE

1. **Angina Pectoris Due to Coronary Artery Spasm.** CARDIZEM is indicated in the treatment of angina pectoris due to coronary artery spasm. CARDIZEM has been shown effective in the treatment of spontaneous coronary artery spasm presenting as Prinzmetal's variant angina (resting angina with ST-segment elevation occurring during attacks).

2. **Chronic Stable Angina (Classic Effort-Associated Angina).** CARDIZEM is indicated in the management of chronic stable angina in patients who cannot tolerate therapy with beta-blockers and/or nitrates or who remain symptomatic despite adequate doses of these agents. CARDIZEM has been effective in short-term controlled trials in reducing angina frequency and increasing exercise tolerance but confirmation of sustained effectiveness is incomplete.

There are few controlled studies of the effectiveness of the concomitant use of diltiazem and beta-blockers or of the safety of this combination in patients with impaired ventricular function or conduction abnormalities.

CONTRAINDICATIONS

CARDIZEM is contraindicated in (1) patients with sick sinus syndrome except in the presence of a functioning ventricular pacemaker, (2) patients with second- or third-degree AV block except in the presence of a functioning ventricular pacemaker, (3) patients with hypotension (less than 90 mm Hg systolic), (4) patients who have demonstrated hypersensitivity to the drug, and (5) patients with acute myocardial infarction and pulmonary congestion documented by x-ray on admission.

WARNINGS

1. **Cardiac Conduction.** CARDIZEM prolongs AV node refractory periods without significantly prolonging sinus node recovery time, except in patients with sick sinus syndrome. This effect may rarely result in abnormally slow heart rates (particularly in patients with sick sinus syndrome) or second- or third-degree AV block (six of 1,243 patients for 0.48%). Concomitant use of diltiazem with beta-blockers or digitalis may result in additive effects on cardiac conduction. A patient with Prinzmetal's angina developed periods of asystole (2 to 5 seconds) after a single dose of 60 mg of diltiazem.

2. **Congestive Heart Failure.** Although diltiazem has a negative inotropic effect in isolated animal tissue preparations, hemodynamic studies in humans with normal ventricular function have not shown a reduction in cardiac index nor consistent negative effects on contractility (dp/dt). Experience with the use of CARDIZEM alone or in combination with beta-blockers in patients with impaired ventricular function is very limited. Caution should be exercised when using the drug in such patients.

3. **Hypotension.** Decreases in blood pressure associated with CARDIZEM therapy may occasionally result in symptomatic hypotension.

4. **Acute Hepatic Injury.** In rare instances, significant elevations in enzymes such as alkaline phosphatase, LDH, SGOT, SGPT, and other phenomena consistent with acute

hepatic injury have been noted. These reactions have been reversible upon discontinuation of drug therapy. The relationship to CARDIZEM is uncertain in most cases, but probable in some. (See PRECAUTIONS.)

PRECAUTIONS

General. CARDIZEM (diltiazem hydrochloride) is extensively metabolized by the liver and excreted by the kidneys and in bile. As with any drug given over prolonged periods, laboratory parameters should be monitored at regular intervals. The drug should be used with caution in patients with impaired renal or hepatic function. In subacute and chronic dog and rat studies designed to produce toxicity, high doses of diltiazem were associated with hepatic damage. In special subacute hepatic studies, oral doses of 125 mg/kg and higher in rats were associated with histological changes in the liver which were reversible when the drug was discontinued. In dogs, doses of 20 mg/kg were also associated with hepatic changes; however, these changes were reversible with continued dosing.

Dermatological events (see ADVERSE REACTIONS section) may be transient and may disappear despite continued use of CARDIZEM. However, skin eruptions progressing to erythema multiforme and/or exfoliative dermatitis have also been infrequently reported. Should a dermatologic reaction persist, the drug should be discontinued.

Drug Interaction. Due to the potential for additive effects, caution and careful titration are warranted in patients receiving CARDIZEM concomitantly with any agents known to affect cardiac contractility and/or conduction. (See WARNINGS.)

Pharmacologic studies indicate that there may be additive effects in prolonging AV conduction when using beta-blockers or digitalis concomitantly with CARDIZEM. (See WARNINGS.)

As with all drugs, care should be exercised when treating patients with multiple medications. CARDIZEM undergoes biotransformation by cytochrome P-450 mixed function oxidase. Coadministration of CARDIZEM with other agents which follow the same route of biotransformation may result in the competitive inhibition of metabolism. Dosages of similarly metabolized drugs, particularly those of low therapeutic ratio or in patients with renal and/or hepatic impairment, may require adjustment when starting or stopping concomitantly administered CARDIZEM to maintain optimum therapeutic blood levels.

Beta-blockers: Controlled and uncontrolled domestic studies suggest that concomitant use of CARDIZEM and beta-blockers or digitalis is usually well tolerated. Available data are not sufficient, however, to predict the effects of concomitant treatment, particularly in patients with left ventricular dysfunction or cardiac conduction abnormalities.

Administration of CARDIZEM (diltiazem hydrochloride) concomitantly with propranolol in five normal volunteers resulted in increased propranolol levels in all subjects and bioavailability of propranolol was increased approximately 50%. If combination therapy is initiated or withdrawn in conjunction with propranolol, an adjustment in the propranolol dose may be warranted. (See WARNINGS.)

Cimetidine: A study in six healthy volunteers has shown a significant increase in peak diltiazem plasma levels (58%) and area-under-the-curve (53%) after a 1-week course of cimetidine at 1,200 mg per day and diltiazem 60 mg per day. Ranitidine produced smaller, nonsignificant increases. The effect may be mediated by cimetidine's known inhibition of hepatic cytochrome P-450, the enzyme system probably responsible for the first-pass metabolism of diltiazem. Patients currently receiving diltiazem therapy should be carefully monitored for a change in pharmacological effect when initiating and discontinuing therapy with cimetidine. An adjustment in the diltiazem dose may be warranted.

Digitalis: Administration of CARDIZEM with digoxin in 24 healthy male subjects increased plasma digoxin concentrations approximately 20%. Another investigator found no increase in digoxin levels in 12 patients with coronary artery disease. Since there have been conflicting results regarding the effect of digoxin levels, it is recommended that digoxin levels be monitored when initiating, adjusting, and discontinuing CARDIZEM therapy to avoid possible over- or under-digitalization. (See WARNINGS.)

Anesthetics: The depression of cardiac contractility, conductivity, and automaticity as well as the vascular dilation associated with anesthetics may be potentiated by calcium channel blockers. When used concomitantly, anesthetics and calcium blockers should be titrated carefully.

Carcinogenesis, Mutagenesis, Impairment of Fertility. A 24-month study in rats and a 21-month study in mice showed no evidence of carcinogenicity. There was also no mutagenic response in in vitro bacterial tests. No intrinsic effect on fertility was observed in rats.

Pregnancy. Category C. Reproduction studies have been conducted in mice, rats, and rabbits. Administration of doses ranging from five to ten times greater (on a mg/kg basis) than the daily recommended therapeutic dose has resulted in embryo and fetal lethality. These doses, in some studies, have been reported to cause skeletal abnormalities. In the perinatal/postnatal studies, there was some reduction in early individual pup weights and survival rates. There was an increased incidence of stillbirths at doses of 20 times the human dose or greater.

There are no well-controlled studies in pregnant women; therefore, use CARDIZEM in pregnant women only if the potential benefit justifies the potential risk to the fetus.

Nursing Mothers. Diltiazem is excreted in human milk. One report suggests that concentrations in breast milk may approximate serum levels. If use of CARDIZEM is deemed essential, an alternative method of infant feeding should be instituted.

Pediatric Use. Safety and effectiveness in children have not been established.

ADVERSE REACTIONS

Serious adverse reactions have been rare in studies carried out to date, but it should be recognized that patients with impaired ventricular function and cardiac conduction abnormalities have usually been excluded.

In domestic placebo-controlled angina trials, the incidence of adverse reactions reported during CARDIZEM therapy was not greater than that reported during placebo therapy.

The following represent occurrences observed in clinical studies of angina patients. In many cases, the relationship to CARDIZEM has not been established. The most common occurrences from these studies, as well as their frequency of presentation, are: edema (2.4%), headache (2.1%), nausea (1.9%), dizziness (1.5%), rash (1.3%), asthenia (1.2%). In addition, the following events were reported infrequently (less than 1%):

Cardiovascular: Angina, arrhythmia, AV block (first degree), AV block (second or third degree—see conduction warning), bradycardia, bundle branch block, congestive heart failure, ECG abnormality, flushing, hypotension, palpitations, syncope, tachycardia, ventricular extrasystoles.

Nervous System: Abnormal dreams, amnesia, depression, gait abnormality, hallucinations, insomnia, nervousness, paresthesia, personality change, somnolence, tremor.

Gastrointestinal: Anorexia, constipation, diarrhea, dysgeusia, dyspepsia, mild elevations of alkaline phosphatase, SGOT, SGPT, and LDH (see hepatic warnings), thirst, vomiting, weight increase.

Dermatologic: Petechiae, photosensitivity, pruritus, urticaria.

Other: Amblyopia, CPK elevation, dry mouth, dyspnea, epistaxis, eye irritation, hyperglycemia, hyperuricemia, impotence, muscle cramps, nasal congestion, nocturia, osteoarticular pain, polyuria, sexual difficulties, tinnitus.

The following postmarketing events have been reported infrequently in patients receiving CARDIZEM: alopecia, erythema multiforme, extrapyramidal symptoms, gingival hyperplasia, hemolytic anemia, increased bleeding time, leukopenia, purpura, retinopathy and thrombocytopenia. There have been observed cases of a generalized rash, characterized as leukocytoclastic vasculitis. In addition, events such as myocardial infarction have been observed which are not readily distinguishable from the natural history of the disease in these patients. A definitive cause and effect relationship between these events and CARDIZEM therapy cannot yet be established. Exfoliative dermatitis (proven by rechallenge) has also been reported.

OVERDOSAGE OR EXAGGERATED RESPONSE

The oral LD_{50}'s in mice and rats range from 415 to 740 mg/kg and from 560 to 810 mg/kg, respectively. The intravenous LD_{50}'s in these species were 60 and 38 mg/kg, respectively. The oral LD_{50} in dogs is considered to be in excess of 50 mg/kg, while lethality was seen in monkeys at 360 mg/kg.

The toxic dose in man is not known. Due to extensive metabolism, blood levels after a standard dose of diltiazem can vary over tenfold, limiting the usefulness of blood levels in overdose cases.

There have been 29 reports of diltiazem overdose in doses ranging from less than 1 g to 10.8 g. Sixteen of these reports involve multiple drug ingestions.

Twenty-two reports indicated patients had recovered from diltiazem overdose ranging from less than 1 g to 10.8 g. There were seven reports with a fatal outcome; although the amount of diltiazem ingested was unknown, multiple drug ingestions were confirmed in six of the seven reports.

Events observed following diltiazem overdose included bradycardia, hypotension, heart block, and cardiac failure. Most reports of overdose described some supportive medical measure and/or drug treatment. Bradycardia frequently responded favorably to atropine, as did heart block, although cardiac pacing was also frequently utilized to treat heart block. Fluids and vasopressors were used to maintain blood pressure, and in cases of cardiac failure inotropic agents were administered. In addition, some patients received treatment with ventilatory support, gastric lavage, activated charcoal, and/or intravenous calcium. Evidence of the effectiveness of intravenous calcium administration to reverse the pharmacological effects of diltiazem overdose was conflicting.

In the event of overdosage or exaggerated response, appropriate supportive measures should be employed in addition to gastrointestinal decontamination. Diltiazem does not appear to be removed by peritoneal or hemodialysis. Based on the known pharmacological effects of diltiazem and/or reported clinical experiences the following measures may be considered:

Bradycardia: Administer atropine (0.60 to 1.0 mg). If there is no response to vagal blockade, administer isoproterenol cautiously.

High-Degree AV Block: Treat as for bradycardia above. Fixed high-degree AV block should be treated with cardiac pacing.

Cardiac Failure: Administer inotropic agents (isoproterenol, dopamine, or dobutamine) and diuretics.

Hypotension: Vasopressors (eg, dopamine or levarterenol bitartrate).

Actual treatment and dosage should depend on the severity of the clinical situation and the judgment and experience of the treating physician.

DOSAGE AND ADMINISTRATION

Exertional Angina Pectoris Due to Atherosclerotic Coronary Artery Disease or Angina Pectoris at Rest Due to Coronary Artery Spasm. Dosage must be adjusted to each patient's needs. Starting with 30 mg four times daily, before meals and at bedtime, dosage should be increased gradually (given in divided doses three or four times daily) at one- to two-day intervals until optimum response is obtained. Although individual patients may respond to any dosage level, the average optimum dosage range appears to be 180 to 360 mg/day. There are no available data concerning dosage requirements in patients with impaired renal or hepatic function. If the drug must be used in such patients, titration should be carried out with particular caution.

Concomitant Use With Other Cardiovascular Agents

1. **Sublingual NTG** may be taken as required to abort acute anginal attacks during CARDIZEM (diltiazem hydrochloride) therapy.
2. **Prophylactic Nitrate Therapy**—CARDIZEM may be safely coadministered with short- and long-acting nitrates, but there have been no controlled studies to evaluate the antianginal effectiveness of this combination.
3. **Beta-blockers.** (See WARNINGS and PRECAUTIONS.)

HOW SUPPLIED

CARDIZEM 30-mg tablets are supplied in bottles of 100 (NDC 0088-1771-47) and 500 (NDC 0088-1771-55), and in Unit Dose Identification Paks of 100 (NDC 0088-1771-49). Each green tablet is engraved with MARION on one side and 1771 engraved on the other.

CARDIZEM 60-mg scored tablets are supplied in bottles of 90 (NDC 0088-1772-42), 100 (NDC 0088-1772-47), 500 (NDC 0088-1772-55), and in Unit Dose Identification Paks of 100 (NDC 0088-1772-49). Each yellow tablet is engraved with MARION on one side and 1772 engraved on the other.

CARDIZEM 90-mg scored tablets are supplied in bottles of 90 (NDC 0088-1791-42), and 100 (NDC 0088-1791-47), and in Unit Dose Identification Paks of 100 (NDC 0088-1791-49). Each green oblong tablet is engraved with CARDIZEM on one side and 90 mg engraved on the other.

CARDIZEM 120-mg scored tablets are supplied in bottles of 90 (NDC 0088-1792-42), and 100 (NDC 0088-1792-47), and in Unit Dose Identification Paks of 100 (NDC 0088-1792-49). Each yellow oblong tablet is engraved with CARDIZEM on one side and 120 mg engraved on the other.

Store at controlled room temperature 59–86°F (15–30°C).

Issued 1/91

Shown in Product Identification Section, page 416

CĒPACOL® Anesthetic Lozenges (Troches) OTC
[*sēp'ă-cŏl*]

(See PDR For Nonprescription Drugs.)

CĒPACOL® Throat Lozenges OTC
[*sēp'ă-cŏl*]

(See PDR For Nonprescription Drugs.)

CĒPACOL® Mouthwash/Gargle OTC
[*sēp'ă-cŏl*]

(See PDR For Nonprescription Drugs.)

Continued on next page

Marion Merrell Dow—Cont.

Cherry Flavor
CĒPASTAT® Sore Throat Lozenges   OTC
[sĕp'ă-stăt]

(See PDR For Nonprescription Drugs.)

CĒPASTAT® Lozenges   OTC
[sĕp'ă-stăt]

(See PDR For Nonprescription Drugs.)

CEPHULAC® (lactulose) Syrup   ℞
[sĕf'ū-lăk]
FOR ORAL OR RECTAL ADMINISTRATION

DESCRIPTION
Cephulac (lactulose) is a synthetic disaccharide in syrup form for oral or rectal administration. Each 15 mL of Cephulac contains: 10 g lactulose (and less than 2.2 g galactose, less than 1.2 g lactose, and 1.2 g or less of other sugars). Also contains FD&C Blue No. 1, FD&C Yellow No. 6, water, and flavoring. A minimal quantity of sodium hydroxide is used to adjust pH when necessary. The pH range is 3.0 to 7.0. Cephulac is a colonic acidifier for treatment and prevention of portal-systemic encephalopathy.
The chemical name for lactulose is 4-O-β-D-galactopyranosyl-D-fructofuranose. It has the following structural formula:

The molecular weight is 342.30. It is freely soluble in water.

CLINICAL PHARMACOLOGY
Lactulose causes a decrease in blood ammonia concentration and reduces the degree of portal-systemic encephalopathy. These actions are considered to be results of the following:
Bacterial degradation of lactulose in the colon acidifies the colonic contents.
This acidification of colonic contents results in the retention of ammonia in the colon as the ammonium ion. Since the colonic contents are then more acid than the blood, ammonia can be expected to migrate from the blood into the colon to form the ammonium ion.
The acid colonic contents convert NH_3 to the ammonium ion $[NH_4]^+$, trapping it and preventing its absorption.
The laxative action of the metabolites of lactulose then expels the trapped ammonium ion from the colon.
Experimental data indicate that lactulose is poorly absorbed. Lactulose given orally to man and experimental animals resulted in only small amounts reaching the blood. Urinary excretion has been determined to be 3% or less and is essentially complete within 24 hours.
When incubated with extracts of human small intestinal mucosa, lactulose was not hydrolyzed during a 24-hour period and did not inhibit the activity of these extracts on lactose. Lactulose reaches the colon essentially unchanged. There it is metabolized by bacteria with the formation of low molecular weight acids that acidify the colon contents.

INDICATIONS AND USAGE
For the prevention and treatment of portal-systemic encephalopathy, including the stages of hepatic pre-coma and coma. Controlled studies have shown that lactulose syrup therapy reduces the blood ammonia levels by 25–50%; this is generally paralleled by an improvement in the patients' mental state and by an improvement in EEG patterns. The clinical response has been observed in about 75% of patients, which is at least as satisfactory as that resulting from neomycin therapy. An increase in patients' protein tolerance is also frequently observed with lactulose therapy. In the treatment of chronic portal-systemic encephalopathy, Cephulac has been given for over 2 years in controlled studies.

CONTRAINDICATIONS
Since Cephulac contains galactose (less than 2.2 g/15 mL), it is contraindicated in patients who require a low galactose diet.

WARNINGS
A theoretical hazard may exist for patients being treated with lactulose syrup who may be required to undergo electrocautery procedures during proctoscopy or colonoscopy. Accumulation of H_2 gas in significant concentration in the presence of an electrical spark may result in an explosive reaction. Although this complication has not been reported with lactulose, patients on lactulose therapy undergoing such procedures should have a thorough bowel cleansing with a non-fermentable solution. Insufflation of CO_2 as an additional safeguard may be pursued but is considered to be a redundant measure.

PRECAUTIONS
General
Since Cephulac contains galactose (less than 2.2 g/15 mL) and lactose (less than 1.2 g/15 mL), it should be used with caution in diabetics.
In the overall management of portal-systemic encephalopathy, it should be recognized that there is serious underlying liver disease with complications such as electrolyte disturbance (e.g., hypokalemia) for which other specific therapy may be required.
Infants receiving lactulose may develop hyponatremia and dehydration.
Drug Interactions
There have been conflicting reports about the concomitant use of neomycin and lactulose syrup. Theoretically, the elimination of certain colonic bacteria by neomycin and possibly other anti-infective agents may interfere with the desired degradation of lactulose and thus prevent the acidification of colonic contents. Thus the status of the lactulose-treated patient should be closely monitored in the event of concomitant oral anti-infective therapy.
Results of preliminary studies in humans and rats suggest that nonabsorbable antacids given concurrently with lactulose may inhibit the desired lactulose-induced drop in colonic pH. Therefore, a possible lack of desired effect of treatment should be taken into consideration before such drugs are given concomitantly with Cephulac.
Other laxatives should not be used, especially during the initial phase of therapy for portal-systemic encephalopathy, because the loose stools resulting from their use may falsely suggest that adequate Cephulac dosage has been achieved.
Carcinogenesis, Mutagenesis, Impairment of Fertility
There are no known human data on long-term potential for carcinogenicity, mutagenicity, or impairment of fertility.
There are no known animal data on long-term potential for mutagenicity.
Administration of lactulose syrup in the diet of mice for 18 months in concentrations of 3 and 10 percent (V/W) did not produce any evidence of carcinogenicity.
In studies in mice, rats, and rabbits, doses of lactulose syrup up to 6 or 12 mL/kg/day produced no deleterious effects on breeding, conception, or parturition.
Pregnancy
Teratogenic Effects
Pregnancy Category B
Reproduction studies have been performed in mice, rats, and rabbits at doses up to 2 or 4 times the usual human oral dose and have revealed no evidence of impaired fertility or harm to the fetus due to Cephulac. There are, however, no adequate and well-controlled studies in pregnant women. Because animal reproduction studies are not always predictive of human response, this drug should be used during pregnancy only if clearly needed.
Nursing Mothers
It is not known whether this drug is excreted in human milk. Because many drugs are excreted in human milk, caution should be exercised when Cephulac is administered to a nursing woman.
Pediatric Use
Very little information on the use of lactulose in young children and adolescents has been recorded. (See DOSAGE AND ADMINISTRATION.)

ADVERSE REACTIONS
Precise frequency data are not available.
Cephulac may produce gaseous distention with flatulence or belching and abdominal discomfort such as cramping in about 20% of patients. Excessive dosage can lead to diarrhea with potential complications such as loss of fluids, hypokalemia, and hypernatremia. Nausea and vomiting have been reported.

OVERDOSAGE
Signs and Symptoms
There have been no reports of accidental overdosage. In the event of overdosage, it is expected that diarrhea and abdominal cramps would be the major symptoms. Medication should be terminated.

Oral LD₅₀

Oral LD_{50}
The acute oral LD_{50} of the drug is 48.8 mL/kg in mice and greater than 30 mL/kg in rats.
Dialysis
Dialysis data are not available for lactulose. Its molecular similarity to sucrose, however, would suggest it should be dialyzable.

DOSAGE AND ADMINISTRATION
Oral
Adult: The usual adult, oral dosage is 2 to 3 tablespoonfuls (30 to 45 mL, containing 20 g to 30 g of lactulose) three or four times daily. The dosage may be adjusted every day or two to produce 2 or 3 soft stools daily.
Hourly doses of 30 to 45 mL of Cephulac may be used to induce the rapid laxation indicated in the initial phase of the therapy of portal-systemic encephalopathy. When the laxative effect has been achieved, the dose of Cephulac may then be reduced to the recommended daily dose. Improvement in the patient's condition may occur within 24 hours but may not begin before 48 hours or even later.
Continuous long-term therapy is indicated to lessen the severity and prevent the recurrence of portal-systemic encephalopathy. The dose of Cephulac for this purpose is the same as the recommended daily dose.
Pediatric: Very little information on the use of lactulose in young children and adolescents has been recorded. As with adults, the subjective goal in proper treatment is to produce 2 or 3 soft stools daily. On the basis of information available, the recommended initial daily oral dose in infants is 2.5 to 10 mL in divided doses. For older children and adolescents, the total daily dose is 40 to 90 mL. If the initial dose causes diarrhea, the dose should be reduced immediately. If diarrhea persists, lactulose should be discontinued.
Rectal
When the adult patient is in the impending coma or coma stage of portal-systemic encephalopathy and the danger of aspiration exists, or when the necessary endoscopic or intubation procedures physically interfere with the administration of the recommended oral doses, Cephulac may be given as a retention enema via a rectal balloon catheter. Cleansing enemas containing soapsuds or other alkaline agents should not be used.
Three hundred mL of Cephulac should be mixed with 700 mL of water or physiologic saline and retained for 30 to 60 minutes. Cephulac enema may be repeated every 4 to 6 hours. If the enema is inadvertently evacuated too promptly, it may be repeated immediately.
The goal of treatment is reversal of the coma stage in order that the patient may be able to take oral medication. Reversal of coma may take place within 2 hours of the first enema in some patients. Cephulac, given orally in the recommended doses, should be started before Cephulac by enema is stopped entirely.

HOW SUPPLIED
NDC 0068-0413-16
1 pint bottle
NDC 0068-0413-64
2 quart bottles
NDC 0068-0413-39
30 mL unit dose cups in trays of 10 cups
Cephulac contains lactulose 667 mg/mL (10 g/15 mL). Store at room temperature, 59°–86°F (15°–30°C).
Under recommended storage conditions, a normal darkening of color may occur. Such darkening is characteristic of sugar solutions and does not affect therapeutic action. Prolonged exposure to temperatures above 86°F (30°C) or to direct light may cause extreme darkening and turbidity which may be pharmaceutically objectionable. If this condition develops, do not use.
Prolonged exposure to freezing temperatures may cause change to a semisolid, too viscous to pour. Viscosity will return to normal upon warming to room temperature.
Product Information as of May, 1991
Shown in Product Identification Section, page 417

CHRONULAC®   ℞
[krŏn'ū-lăk]
(lactulose)
Syrup

CAUTION: Federal law prohibits dispensing without prescription.

DESCRIPTION
Chronulac (lactulose) is a synthetic disaccharide in syrup form for oral administration. Each 15 mL of Chronulac contains: 10 g lactulose (and less than 2.2 g galactose, less than 1.2 g lactose, and 1.2 g or less of other sugars). Also contains FD&C Blue No. 1, FD&C Yellow No. 6, water and flavoring. A minimal quantity of sodium hydroxide is used to adjust pH when necessary. The pH range is 3.0 to 7.0.

Chronulac is a colonic acidifier which promotes laxation. The chemical name for lactulose is 4-0-β-D-galactopyranosyl-D-fructofuranose. It has the following structural formula:

The molecular weight is 342.30. It is freely soluble in water.

CLINICAL PHARMACOLOGY

Chronulac is poorly absorbed from the gastrointestinal tract and no enzyme capable of hydrolysis of this disaccharide is present in human gastrointestinal tissue. As a result, oral doses of Chronulac reach the colon virtually unchanged. In the colon, Chronulac is broken down primarily to lactic acid, and also to small amounts of formic and acetic acids, by the action of colonic bacteria, which results in an increase in osmotic pressure and slight acidification of the colonic contents. This in turn causes an increase in stool water content and softens the stool.

Since Chronulac does not exert its effect until it reaches the colon, and since transit time through the colon may be slow, 24 to 48 hours may be required to produce the desired bowel movement.

Chronulac given orally to man and experimental animals resulted in only small amounts reaching the blood. Urinary excretion has been determined to be 3% or less and is essentially complete within 24 hours.

INDICATIONS AND USAGE

For the treatment of constipation. In patients with a history of chronic constipation, lactulose syrup (Chronulac) therapy increases the number of bowel movements per day and the number of days on which bowel movements occur.

CONTRAINDICATIONS

Since Chronulac contains galactose (less than 2.2 g/15 mL), it is contraindicated in patients who require a low galactose diet.

WARNINGS

A theoretical hazard may exist for patients being treated with lactulose syrup who may be required to undergo electrocautery procedures during proctoscopy or colonoscopy. Accumulation of H_2 gas in significant concentration in the presence of an electrical spark may result in an explosive reaction. Although this complication has not been reported with lactulose, patients on lactulose therapy undergoing such procedures should have a thorough bowel cleansing with a non-fermentable solution. Insufflation of CO_2 as an additional safeguard may be pursued but is considered to be a redundant measure.

PRECAUTIONS

General
Since Chronulac contains galactose (less than 2.2 g/15 mL) and lactose (less than 1.2 g/15 mL), it should be used with caution in diabetics.
Information for Patients
In the event that an unusual diarrheal condition occurs, contact your physician.
Laboratory Tests
Elderly, debilitated patients who receive Chronulac for more than six months should have serum electrolytes (potassium, chloride, carbon dioxide) measured periodically.
Drug Interactions
Results of preliminary studies in humans and rats suggest that nonabsorbable antacids given concurrently with lactulose may inhibit the desired lactulose-induced drop in colonic pH. Therefore, a possible lack of desired effect of treatment should be taken into consideration before such drugs are given concomitantly with Chronulac.
Carcinogenesis, Mutagenesis, Impairment of Fertility
There are no known human data on long-term potential for carcinogenicity, mutagenicity, or impairment of fertility. There are no known animal data on long-term potential for mutagenicity.
Administration of lactulose syrup in the diet of mice for 18 months in concentrations of 3 and 10 percent (V/W) did not produce any evidence of carcinogenicity.
In studies in mice, rats, and rabbits doses of lactulose syrup up to 6 or 12 mL/kg/day produced no deleterious effects in breeding, conception, or parturition.
Pregnancy
Teratogenic Effects
Pregnancy Category B
Reproduction studies have been performed in mice, rats, and rabbits at doses up to 3 or 6 times the usual human oral dose and have revealed no evidence of impaired fertility or harm to the fetus due to Chronulac. There are, however, no adequate and well-controlled studies in pregnant women.

Because animal reproduction studies are not always predictive of human response, this drug should be used during pregnancy only if clearly needed.
Nursing Mothers
It is not known whether this drug is excreted in human milk. Because many drugs are excreted in human milk, caution should be exercised when Chronulac is administered to a nursing woman.
Pediatric Use
Safety and effectiveness in children have not been established.

ADVERSE REACTIONS

Precise frequency data are not available.
Initial dosing may produce flatulence and intestinal cramps, which are usually transient. Excessive dosage can lead to diarrhea with potential complications such as loss of fluids, hypokalemia, and hypernatremia.
Nausea and vomiting have been reported.

OVERDOSAGE

Signs and Symptoms
There have been no reports of accidental overdosage. In the event of overdosage, it is expected that diarrhea and abdominal cramps would be the major symptoms. Medication should be terminated.
Oral LD₅₀
The acute oral LD_{50} of the drug is 48.8 mL/kg in mice and greater than 30 mL/kg in rats.
Dialysis
Dialysis data are not available for lactulose. Its molecular similarity to sucrose, however, would suggest that it should be dialyzable.

DOSAGE AND ADMINISTRATION

The usual dose is 1 to 2 tablespoonfuls (15 to 30 mL, containing 10 g to 20 g of lactulose) daily. The dose may be increased to 60 mL daily if necessary. Twenty-four to 48 hours may be required to produce a normal bowel movement.
Note: Some patients have found that Chronulac may be more acceptable when mixed with fruit juice, water, or milk.

HOW SUPPLIED

NDC 0068-0409-08
  8 fl oz bottles
NDC 0068-0409-30
  30 mL unit dose cups in trays of 10 cups
NDC 0068-0409-32
  1 quart bottles
Chronulac contains lactulose 667 mg/mL (10 g/15 mL).
Store at room temperature, 59°–86°F (15°–30°C).
Under recommended storage conditions, a normal darkening of color may occur. Such darkening is characteristic of sugar solutions and does not affect therapeutic action.
Prolonged exposure to temperatures above 86°F (30°C) or to direct light may cause extreme darkening and turbidity which may be pharmaceutically objectionable. If this condition develops, do not use.
Prolonged exposure to freezing temperatures may cause change to a semisolid, too viscous to pour. Viscosity will return to normal upon warming to room temperature.
Product Information as of January, 1988
Shown in Product Identification Section, page 417

CLOMID®   ℞
[*klăhm ´ĭd*]
(clomiphene citrate tablets USP)

For prescribing information, write to:
Professional Information Department
Marion Merrell Dow Inc.
Cincinnati, Ohio 45242-9553, U.S.A.
Shown in Product Identification Section, page 416

DEBROX® Drops   OTC
[*de ´brox*]

(See PDR For Nonprescription Drugs.)

DITROPAN® Tablets and Syrup   ℞
[*di ´tro-pan*]
(oxybutynin chloride)

DESCRIPTION

Each scored biconvex, engraved blue DITROPAN® Tablet contains 5 mg of oxybutynin chloride. Each 5 mL of DITROPAN® Syrup contains 5 mg of oxybutynin chloride. Chemically, oxybutynin chloride is d,l (racemic) 4-diethylamino-2-butynyl phenylcyclohexylglycolate hydrochloride. The

empirical formula of oxybutynin chloride is $C_{22}H_{31}NO_3 \cdot HCl$. The structural formula appears below:

Oxybutynin chloride is a white crystalline solid with a molecular weight of 393.9. It is readily soluble in water and acids, but relatively insoluble in alkalis.
DITROPAN® Tablets
Also contains: calcium stearate, FD&C Blue #1 Lake, lactose, and microcrystalline cellulose.
DITROPAN® Syrup
Also contains: citric acid, FD&C Green #3, glycerin, methylparaben, flavor, sodium citrate, sorbitol, sucrose, and water.
DITROPAN® Tablets and Syrup are for oral administration.
Therapeutic Category: Antispasmodic, anticholinergic.

CLINICAL PHARMACOLOGY

DITROPAN® (oxybutynin chloride) exerts direct antispasmodic effect on smooth muscle and inhibits the muscarinic action of acetylcholine on smooth muscle. DITROPAN exhibits only one fifth of the anticholinergic activity of atropine on the rabbit detrusor muscle, but four to ten times the antispasmodic activity. No blocking effects occur at skeletal neuromuscular junctions or autonomic ganglia (antinicotinic effects).
DITROPAN relaxes bladder smooth muscle. In patients with conditions characterized by involuntary bladder contractions, cystometric studies have demonstrated that DITROPAN increases bladder (vesical) capacity, diminishes the frequency of uninhibited contractions of the detrusor muscle, and delays the initial desire to void. DITROPAN thus decreases urgency and the frequency of both incontinent episodes and voluntary urination.
DITROPAN was well tolerated in patients administered the drug in controlled studies of 30 days' duration and in uncontrolled studies in which some of the patients received the drug for 2 years. Pharmacokinetic information is not currently available.

INDICATIONS AND USAGE

DITROPAN is indicated for the relief of symptoms of bladder instability associated with voiding in patients with uninhibited neurogenic or reflex neurogenic bladder (ie, urgency, frequency, urinary leakage, urge incontinence, dysuria).

CONTRAINDICATIONS

DITROPAN® (oxybutynin chloride) is contraindicated in patients with untreated angle closure glaucoma and in patients with untreated narrow anterior chamber angles since anticholinergic drugs may aggravate these conditions.
It is also contraindicated in partial or complete obstruction of the gastrointestinal tract, paralytic ileus, intestinal atony of the elderly or debilitated patient, megacolon, toxic megacolon complicating ulcerative colitis, severe colitis, and myasthenia gravis. It is contraindicated in patients with obstructive uropathy and in patients with unstable cardiovascular status in acute hemorrhage.
DITROPAN is contraindicated in patients who have demonstrated hypersensitivity to the product.

WARNINGS

DITROPAN® (oxybutynin chloride), when administered in the presence of high environmental temperature, can cause heat prostration (fever and heat stroke due to decreased sweating).
Diarrhea may be an early symptom of incomplete intestinal obstruction, especially in patients with ileostomy or colostomy. In this instance treatment with DITROPAN would be inappropriate and possibly harmful.
DITROPAN may produce drowsiness or blurred vision. The patient should be cautioned regarding activities requiring mental alertness such as operating a motor vehicle or other machinery or performing hazardous work while taking this drug.
Alcohol or other sedative drugs may enhance the drowsiness caused by DITROPAN.

PRECAUTIONS

DITROPAN® (oxybutynin chloride) should be used with caution in the elderly and in all patients with autonomic neuropathy, hepatic or renal disease. DITROPAN may aggravate the symptoms of hyperthyroidism, coronary heart disease, congestive heart failure, cardiac arrhythmias, hiatal hernia, tachycardia, hypertension, and prostatic hypertrophy. Administration of DITROPAN® (oxybutynin chloride) to patients with ulcerative colitis may suppress intestinal motility to the point of producing a paralytic ileus and pre-

Continued on next page

Marion Merrell Dow—Cont.

cipitate or aggravate toxic megacolon, a serious complication of the disease.

CARCINOGENESIS, MUTAGENESIS, IMPAIRMENT OF FERTILITY. A 24-month study in rats at dosages up to approximately 400 times the recommended human dosage showed no evidence of carcinogenicity.

DITROPAN showed no increase of mutagenic activity when tested in *Schizosaccharomyces pompholiciformis*, *Saccharomyces cerevisiae* and *Salmonella typhimurium* test systems. Reproduction studies in the hamster, rabbit, rat, and mouse have shown no definite evidence of impaired fertility.

PREGNANCY: Category B. Reproduction studies in the hamster, rabbit, rat, and mouse have shown no definite evidence of impaired fertility or harm to the animal fetus. The safety of DITROPAN administered to women who are or who may become pregnant has not been established. Therefore, DITROPAN should not be given to pregnant women unless, in the judgment of the physician, the probable clinical benefits outweigh the possible hazards.

NURSING MOTHERS. It is not known whether this drug is excreted in human milk. Because many drugs are excreted in human milk, caution should be exercised when DITROPAN is administered to a nursing woman.

PEDIATRIC USE. The safety and efficacy of DITROPAN administration have been demonstrated for children 5 years of age and older (see DOSAGE AND ADMINISTRATION). However, as there is insufficient clinical data for children under age 5, DITROPAN is not recommended for this age group.

ADVERSE REACTIONS

Following administration of DITROPAN® (oxybutynin chloride), the symptoms that can be associated with the use of other anticholinergic drugs may occur:

Cardiovascular: Palpitations, tachycardia, vasodilatation.

Dermatologic: Decreased sweating, rash.

Gastrointestinal/Genitourinary: Constipation, decreased gastrointestinal motility, dry mouth, nausea, urinary hesitance and retention.

Nervous System: Asthenia, dizziness, drowsiness, hallucinations, insomnia, restlessness.

Ophthalmic: Amblyopia, cycloplegia, decreased lacrimation, mydriasis.

Other: Impotence, suppression of lactation.

OVERDOSAGE

The symptoms of overdosage with DITROPAN® (oxybutynin chloride) may be any of those seen with other anticholinergic agents. Symptoms may include signs of central nervous system excitation (eg, restlessness, tremor, irritability, convulsions, delirium, hallucinations), flushing, fever, nausea, vomiting, tachycardia, hypotension or hypertension, respiratory failure, paralysis, and coma.

In the event of an overdose or exaggerated response, treatment should be symptomatic and supportive. Maintain respiration and induce emesis or perform gastric lavage (emesis is contraindicated in precomatose, convulsive, or psychotic state). Activated charcoal may be administered as well as a cathartic. Physostigmine may be considered to reverse symptoms of anticholinergic intoxication. Hyperpyrexia may be treated symptomatically with ice bags or other cold applications and alcohol sponges.

DOSAGE AND ADMINISTRATION

Tablets

Adults: The usual dose is one 5-mg tablet two to three times a day. The maximum recommended dose is one 5-mg tablet four times a day.

Children over 5 years of age: The usual dose is one 5-mg tablet two times a day. The maximum recommended dose is one 5-mg tablet three times a day.

Syrup

Adults: The usual dose is one teaspoon (5 mg/5 mL) syrup two to three times a day. The maximum recommended dose is one teaspoon (5 mg/5 mL) syrup four times a day.

Children over 5 years of age: The usual dose is one teaspoon (5 mg/5 mL) two times a day. The maximum recommended dose is one teaspoon (5 mg/5 mL) three times a day.

HOW SUPPLIED

DITROPAN® (oxybutynin chloride) Tablets are supplied in bottles of 100 tablets (NDC 0088-1375-47) and 1,000 tablets (NDC 0088-1375-58) and in Unit Dose Identification Paks of 100 tablets (NDC 0088-1375-49).

Blue scored tablets (5 mg) are engraved with DITROPAN on one side and 13 and 75, separated by a horizontal score, on the other side.

DITROPAN® Syrup (5 mg/5 mL) is supplied in bottles of 16 fluid ounces (473 mL) (NDC 0088-1373-18).

Pharmacist: Dispense in tight, light-resistant container as defined in the USP.

Store at controlled room temperature (59°–86°F).

Product information as of May, 1991

Shown in Product Identification Section, page 417

GAVISCON® Antacid Tablets   OTC
[gav'is-kon]

(See PDR For Nonprescription Drugs.)

GAVISCON® EXTRA STRENGTH RELIEF FORMULA Antacid Tablets   OTC
[găv'is-kŏn]

(See PDR For Nonprescription Drugs.)

GAVISCON® EXTRA STRENGTH RELIEF FORMULA Liquid Antacid   OTC
[găv'is-kŏn]

(See PDR For Nonprescription Drugs.)

GAVISCON® Liquid Antacid   OTC
[gav'is-kon]

(See PDR For Nonprescription Drugs.)

GLY–OXIDE® Liquid   OTC
[gli'ok-sīd]

(See PDR For Nonprescription Drugs.)

HIPREX®   ℞
[hĭp'rĕx]
(methenamine hippurate)

DESCRIPTION

Each yellow capsule-shaped tablet contains 1 g Methenamine Hippurate which is the Hippuric Acid Salt of Methenamine (hexamethylenetetramine). The tablet also contains inactive ingredients: FD&C Yellow No. 5 (tartrazine, See PRECAUTIONS), Magnesium Stearate, Povidone, and Saccharin Sodium.

ACTIONS

Microbiology: Hiprex (methenamine hippurate) has antibacterial activity because the methenamine component is hydrolyzed to formaldehyde in acid urine. Hippuric acid, the other component, has some antibacterial activity and also acts to keep the urine acid. The drug is generally active against *E. coli*, enterococci and staphylococci. *Enterobacter aerogenes* is generally resistant. The urine must be kept sufficiently acid for urea-splitting organisms such as *Proteus* and *Pseudomonas* to be inhibited.

Human Pharmacology: Within ½ hour after ingestion of a single 1-gram dose of Hiprex, antibacterial activity is demonstrable in the urine. Urine has continuous antibacterial activity when Hiprex is administered at the recommended dosage schedule of 1 gram twice daily. Over 90% of methenamine moiety is excreted in the urine within 24 hours after administration of a single 1-gram dose. Similarly, the hippurate moiety is rapidly absorbed and excreted, and it reaches the urine by both tubular secretion and glomerular filtration. This action may be important in older patients or in those with some degree of renal impairment.

INDICATIONS

Hiprex is indicated for prophylactic or suppressive treatment of frequently recurring urinary tract infections when long-term therapy is considered necessary. This drug should only be used after eradication of the infection by other appropriate antimicrobial agents.

CONTRAINDICATIONS

Hiprex (methenamine hippurate) is contraindicated in patients with renal insufficiency, severe hepatic insufficiency, or severe dehydration. Methenamine preparations should not be given to patients taking sulfonamides because some sulfonamides may form an insoluble precipitate with formaldehyde in the urine.

WARNING

Large doses of methenamine (8 grams daily for 3 to 4 weeks) have caused bladder irritation, painful and frequent micturition, albuminuria, and gross hematuria.

PRECAUTIONS

1. Care should be taken to maintain an acid pH of the urine, especially when treating infections due to urea-splitting organisms such as *Proteus* and strains of *Pseudomonas*.

2. In a few instances in one study, the serum transaminase levels were slightly elevated during treatment but returned to normal while the patients were still taking Hiprex. Because of this report, it is recommended that liver

---

function studies be performed periodically on patients taking the drug, especially those with liver dysfunction.

3. *Use in Pregnancy:* In early pregnancy the safe use of Hiprex is not established. In the last trimester, safety is suggested, but not definitely proved. No adverse effects on the fetus were seen in studies in pregnant rats and rabbits. Hiprex taken during pregnancy can interfere with laboratory tests of urine estriol (resulting in unmeasurably low values) when acid hydrolysis is used in the laboratory procedure. This interference is due to the presence in the urine of methenamine and/or formaldehyde. Enzymatic hydrolysis, in place of acid hydrolysis, will circumvent this problem.

4. This product contains FD&C Yellow No. 5 (tartrazine), which may cause allergic-type reactions (including bronchial asthma) in certain susceptible individuals. Although the overall incidence of FD&C Yellow No. 5 (tartrazine) sensitivity in the general population is low, it is frequently seen in patients who also have aspirin hypersensitivity.

ADVERSE REACTIONS

Minor adverse reactions have been reported in less than 3.5% of patients treated. These reactions have included nausea, upset stomach, dysuria, and rash.

DOSAGE AND ADMINISTRATION

1 tablet (1.0 g) twice daily (morning and night) for adults and children over 12 years of age.

½ to 1 tablet (0.5 to 1.0 g) twice daily (morning and night) for children 6 to 12 years of age.

Since the antibacterial activity of Hiprex is greater in acid urine, restriction of alkalinizing foods and medications is desirable. If necessary, as indicated by urinary pH and clinical response, supplemental acidification of the urine should be instituted. The efficacy of therapy should be monitored by repeated urine cultures.

HOW SUPPLIED

1-gram scored, capsule-shaped yellow tablets debossed MERRELL 277 in bottles of 100

Product Information as of May, 1991

Shown in Product Identification Section, page 417

LORELCO® Tablets   ℞
[lō-rĕl-cō]
(probucol)

CAUTION: Federal law prohibits dispensing without prescription.

DESCRIPTION

Lorelco (probucol) film-coated tablets for oral administration contain 250 mg or 500 mg of probucol per tablet. Each tablet also contains as inactive ingredients: corn starch, ethylcellulose, glycerin, hydroxypropyl cellulose, hydroxypropyl methylcellulose 2910, iron oxide, lactose, magnesium stearate, microcrystalline cellulose, polysorbate 80, talc, and titanium dioxide. Lorelco is an agent for the reduction of elevated serum cholesterol. The chemical name is 4,4'-[(1-methylethylidene)bis(thio)]bis[2,6-bis(1,1-dimethylethyl)phenol]. Its chemical structure does not resemble that of any other available cholesterol-lowering agent. It is lipophilic.

CLINICAL PHARMACOLOGY

Lorelco lowers total serum cholesterol and has relatively little effect on serum triglycerides. Patients responding to probucol exhibit a decrease in low-density lipoprotein (LDL) cholesterol. Cholesterol is reduced not only in the LDL fraction, but also in the high-density lipoprotein (HDL) fraction with proportionally greater effect on the high-density portion. Epidemiologic studies have shown that both low HDL-cholesterol and high LDL-cholesterol are independent risk factors for coronary heart disease. The risk of lowering HDL-cholesterol while lowering LDL-cholesterol remains unknown. There is little or no effect reported on very low-density lipoprotein (VLDL).

Studies on the mode of action of Lorelco indicate that it increases the fractional rate of LDL catabolism. This effect may be linked to the observed increased excretion of fecal bile acids, a final metabolic pathway for the elimination of cholesterol from the body. Lorelco also exhibits inhibition of early stages of cholesterol biosynthesis and slight inhibition of absorption of dietary cholesterol. There is no increase in the cyclic precursors of cholesterol, namely desmosterol and 7-dehydrocholesterol. On this basis, it is concluded that Lorelco does not affect the later stages of cholesterol biosynthesis.

Absorption of Lorelco from the gastrointestinal tract is limited and variable. When it is administered with food, peak blood levels are higher and less variable. With continuous administration in a dosage of 500 mg b.i.d., the blood levels of an individual gradually increase over the first three to four months and thereafter remain fairly constant. In 116 patients treated with Lorelco for periods of three months to one year, the mean blood level was 23.6 ± 17.2 mcg/mL (± S.D.) ranging to 78.3 mcg/mL. Levels observed after seven years of treatment in 40 patients yielded an average value of 21.5 ± 16.5 mcg/mL (± S.D.) ranging to 62.0 mcg/mL. In a separate study in eight patients, blood levels averaged 19.0 mcg/mL at the end of 12 months of treatment. Six weeks after cessation of therapy, the average had fallen by 60%. After six months, the average had fallen by 80%.

In December 1984, a National Institutes of Health Consensus Development Conference Panel[1] concluded that lowering definitely elevated blood cholesterol levels (specifically blood levels of LDL-cholesterol) will reduce the risk of heart attacks due to coronary heart disease. The effect of probucol-induced reduction of serum cholesterol or triglyceride levels, or reduction of HDL-cholesterol levels on morbidity or mortality due to coronary heart disease has not been established.

INDICATIONS AND USAGE

Serious animal toxicity has been encountered with probucol. See WARNINGS and ANIMAL PHARMACOLOGY AND TOXICOLOGY sections. Probucol is not an innocuous drug and strict attention should be paid to the INDICATIONS, CONTRAINDICATIONS, and WARNINGS.

Drug therapy should not be used for the routine treatment of elevated blood lipids for the prevention of coronary heart disease. Dietary therapy specific for the type of hyperlipidemia is the initial treatment of choice. Excess body weight may be an important factor and should be addressed prior to any drug therapy. Physical exercise can be an important ancillary measure. Contributory disease such as hypothyroidism or diabetes mellitus should be looked for and adequately treated. The use of drugs should be considered only when reasonable attempts have been made to obtain satisfactory results with nondrug methods. If the decision ultimately is to use drugs, the patient should be instructed that this does not reduce the importance of adhering to diet.

The selection of patients for cholesterol-lowering drug therapy should take into account other important coronary risk factors such as smoking, hypertension, and diabetes mellitus. Consideration should be given to the efficacy, safety, and compliance factors for each of the cholesterol-lowering drugs prior to selecting the one most appropriate for an individual patient.

Lorelco may be indicated for the reduction of elevated serum cholesterol in patients with primary hypercholesterolemia (Types IIa and IIb hyperlipoproteinemia),[2] whose elevated LDL-cholesterol has not responded adequately to diet, weight reduction and control of diabetes mellitus. Lorelco may be useful to lower elevated LDL-cholesterol that occurs in those patients with combined hypercholesterolemia and hypertriglyceridemia (Type IIb) due to elevation of both LDL and VLDL, but it is not indicated where hypertriglyceridemia is the abnormality of most concern. After establishing that the elevation in serum total cholesterol represents a primary lipid disorder, it should be determined that patients being considered for treatment with Lorelco have an elevated LDL-cholesterol as the cause for an elevated total serum cholesterol. This may be particularly relevant for patients with elevated triglycerides or with markedly elevated HDL-cholesterol values, where non-LDL fractions may contribute significantly to total cholesterol levels without apparent increase in cardiovascular risk. In most patients, LDL-cholesterol may be estimated according to the following equation:

LDL-cholesterol = Total cholesterol − [(0.16 × triglycerides) + HDL-cholesterol]

When total triglycerides are greater than 400 mg/dL, this equation is less accurate. In such patients, LDL-cholesterol may be obtained by ultracentrifugation.

It is not always possible to predict from the lipoprotein type or other factors which patients will exhibit favorable results. Lipid levels,including HDL-cholesterol, should be periodically assessed.

The effect of probucol-induced reduction of serum cholesterol or triglyceride levels, or reduction of HDL-cholesterol levels on morbidity or mortality due to coronary heart disease has not been established.

CONTRAINDICATIONS

(See also WARNINGS and PRECAUTIONS.) Lorelco is contraindicated in patients who are known to have a hypersensitivity to it. Lorelco is contraindicated in patients with evidence of recent or progressive myocardial damage or findings suggestive of serious ventricular arrhythmias or with unexplained syncope or syncope of cardiovascular origin. **Lorelco is contraindicated in patients with an abnormally long QT interval.**

WARNINGS

SERIOUS ANIMAL TOXICITY HAS BEEN ENCOUNTERED WITH PROBUCOL IN RHESUS MONKEYS FED AN ATHEROGENIC DIET AND IN BEAGLE DOGS. (SEE ANIMAL PHARMACOLOGY AND TOXICOLOGY SECTION.)

Prolongation of the QT interval can occur in patients on Lorelco. Serious arrhythmias have been seen in association with an abnormally long QT interval in patients on Lorelco alone and in patients on Lorelco and a concomitant antiarrhythmic drug. The following precautions are deemed prudent:

1. Patients should be advised to adhere to a low cholesterol, low fat diet at the start of treatment with Lorelco and throughout the treatment period.
2. An ECG should be done prior to starting treatment and repeated at appropriate intervals during treatment. If an abnormally long QT interval is observed, the possible benefits and risks should be carefully considered before making a decision to continue Lorelco.

Lorelco therapy should be discontinued or not started if the QT interval at an observed heart rate on a resting ECG is persistently more than one of the values listed below:

Observed Heart Rate (beats/min)	QT Interval in sec (15% above the upper limit of normal)* Males	Females
40	0.56	0.58
50	0.52	0.53
60	0.49	0.50
70	0.45	0.47
80	0.43	0.44
86	0.42	0.43
92	0.40	0.41
100	0.39	0.40
109	0.37	0.38
120	0.36	0.36
133	0.34	0.35

*Values calculated from Burch GE, Winsor T. A primer of electrocardiography. Philadelphia, PA: Lea and Febiger; 1958; p. 272 (Table 6).

3. Patients developing unexplained syncope or syncope of cardiovascular origin should have Lorelco therapy discontinued and should have ECG surveillance.
4. Drugs that prolong the QT interval are more likely to be associated with ventricular tachycardia after:
   a. An increase in the dose of the drug.
   b. Addition of a second drug that prolongs the QT interval (including tricyclic antidepressants, class I and III antiarrhythmics, and phenothiazines).
   c. Hypokalemia or hypomagnesemia.
   d. Severe bradycardia due to intrinsic heart disease or drug effects on the atrial rate (beta-blockers) or AV block (digoxin).
   e. Development of recent or acute myocardial infarction, ischemia, or inflammation.

The use of Lorelco in patients receiving any of these drugs should be based on the conclusion that alternate methods of hypocholesterolemic therapy are either ineffective or not tolerated, and the potential benefits of cholesterol lowering outweigh the risk of serious arrhythmia.

The following conditions should be resolved or corrected prior to initiation of therapy with Lorelco:

a. Hypokalemia
b. Hypomagnesemia
c. Severe bradycardia due to intrinsic heart disease or drug effects on the atrial rate (beta-blockers) or AV block (digoxin).
d. Recent or acute myocardial infarction, ischemia, or inflammation.

PRECAUTIONS

General: Before instituting therapy with Lorelco, adequate baseline studies should be performed to determine that the patient has persistently elevated total and LDL-cholesterol levels representing a primary lipid disorder, and that the increased cholesterol is not due to secondary conditions such as hypothyroidism, poorly controlled diabetes mellitus, obstructive liver disease, nephrotic syndrome, or dysproteinemias. Serum lipid levels, including HDL-cholesterol, should be determined after an overnight fast before treatment, during an adequate trial of diet and weight reduction therapy prior to addition of drug therapy, and periodically during combined diet and drug therapy, including assessment during the first several months of drug treatment. A favorable trend in lipid levels should be evident during the first three to four months of administration of Lorelco, and if satisfactory lipid alteration is not achieved, the drug should be discontinued. Lorelco lowers serum total and LDL-cholesterol, and also lowers HDL-cholesterol in most patients with elevated LDL-cholesterol. Epidemiologic studies within hypercholesterolemic populations have shown that serum HDL-cholesterol is an independent, inversely correlated, risk factor for coronary heart disease (see CLINICAL PHARMACOLOGY). Human studies which will attempt to confirm or deny the hypothesis that drug-induced alteration in HDL-cholesterol affects cardiovascular risk are currently under evaluation. It is not known whether probucol-induced reduction of serum HDL-cholesterol will affect cardiovascular risk since no long-term, controlled clinical trials of Lorelco for the prevention of coronary heart disease, similar to the LRC-CPPT (See CLINICAL STUDIES), have been performed. The probable benefits obtained from LDL-cholesterol reduction must be weighed against the possible risk of a reduction in HDL-cholesterol when assessing the response of each patient receiving Lorelco treatment. If satisfactory lipid alteration is not achieved, the drug should be discontinued.

Information for Patients: The patient should be instructed to adhere to a prudent diet. Females should be cautioned against becoming pregnant for at least six months after discontinuing Lorelco and should not breast-feed their infants during therapy with Lorelco.

Laboratory Tests: The physician should schedule periodic blood lipid determinations and periodic ECGs. (See WARNINGS.)

Elevations of the serum transaminases (SGOT, SGPT), bilirubin, alkaline phosphatase, creatine phosphokinase, uric acid, blood urea nitrogen and blood glucose above the normal range were observed on one or more occasions in various patients treated with Lorelco. Most often these were transient and/or could have been related to the patient's clinical state or other modes of therapy. Although the basis for the relationship between Lorelco and these abnormalities is not firm, the possibility that some of these are drug related cannot be excluded. In the controlled trials, the incidence of abnormal laboratory values was no higher in the patients treated with Lorelco than in the patients who received placebo. If abnormal laboratory tests persist or worsen, if clinical signs consistent with the abnormal laboratory tests develop, or if systemic manifestations occur, Lorelco should be discontinued.

Drug Interactions: The addition of clofibrate to Lorelco is not recommended, since the lowering effect on mean serum levels of either LDL or total cholesterol is generally not significantly additive and, in some patients, there may be a pronounced lowering of HDL-cholesterol.

Neither oral hypoglycemic agents nor oral anticoagulants alter the effect of Lorelco on serum cholesterol. The dosage of these agents is not usually modified when given with Lorelco.

Monkeys fed a high fat, high cholesterol diet admixed with probucol exhibited serious toxicity. (See WARNINGS and ANIMAL PHARMACOLOGY AND TOXICOLOGY sections.) Prolongation of the QT interval can occur in patients on Lorelco and serious arrhythmias have been seen in association with an abnormally long QT interval in patients on Lorelco. The addition of a second drug that prolongs the QT interval (including tricyclic antidepressants, class I and III antiarrhythmics, and phenothiazines) may increase the risk of serious arrhythmia. (See CONTRAINDICATIONS AND WARNINGS.)

Carcinogenesis, Mutagenesis, Impairment of Fertility

In chronic studies of two years' duration in rats, no toxicity or carcinogenicity was observed. These results are consistent with the lack of any adverse effect on fertility and the negative findings in tests for mutagenic activity in rats.

Pregnancy:

Teratogenic Effects

Pregnancy—Category B: Reproduction studies have been performed in rats and rabbits at doses up to 50 times the human dose, and have revealed no evidence of impaired fertility or harm to the fetus due to probucol. There are, however, no adequate and well-controlled studies in pregnant women. Because animal reproduction studies are not always predictive of human response, this drug should be used during pregnancy only if clearly needed. Furthermore, if a patient wishes to become pregnant, it is recommended that the drug be withdrawn and birth control procedures be used for at least six months because of persistence of the drug in the body for prolonged periods. (See CLINICAL PHARMACOLOGY.)

Labor and Delivery: The effect of Lorelco on human labor and delivery is unknown.

Nursing Mothers: It is not known whether this drug is excreted in human milk, but it is likely, since such excretion has been shown in animals. It is recommended that nursing not be undertaken while a patient is on Lorelco.

Pediatric Use: Safety and effectiveness in children have not been established.

ADVERSE REACTIONS

Gastrointestinal

diarrhea or loose stools, flatulence, abdominal pain, nausea, vomiting, indigestion, gastrointestinal bleeding

Cardiovascular

prolongation of the QT interval on ECG, syncope, ventricular arrhythmias (ventricular tachycardia, torsades de pointes, ventricular fibrillation), sudden death

Continued on next page

Marion Merrell Dow—Cont.

Neurologic
headache, dizziness, paresthesia, insomnia, tinnitus, peripheral neuritis

Hematologic
eosinophilia, low hemoglobin and/or hematocrit, thrombocytopenia

Dermatologic
rash, pruritus, ecchymosis, petechiae, hyperhidrosis, fetid sweat

Genitourinary
impotency, nocturia

Ophthalmic
conjunctivitis, tearing, blurred vision

Endocrine
enlargement of multinodular goiter

Idiosyncrasies
observed with initiation of therapy and characterized by dizziness, palpitations, syncope, nausea, vomiting and chest pain

Other
diminished sense of taste and smell, anorexia, angioneurotic edema

DRUG ABUSE AND DEPENDENCE
No evidence of abuse potential has been associated with Lorelco, nor is there evidence of psychological or physical dependence in humans.

OVERDOSAGE
There is a single report of a 15-kg, three-year-old, male child who ingested 5 g of probucol. Emesis was induced by ipecac. The child remained well, apart from a brief episode of loose stools and flatulence. No specific information is available on the treatment of overdosage with Lorelco and no specific antidote is available. Probucol is not dialyzable. Treatment is symptomatic and supportive. Probucol has shown no identifiable acute toxicity in mice and rats. In these animals, the LD_{50} (oral) is in excess of 5 g/kg of body weight.

DOSAGE AND ADMINISTRATION
For adult use only. The recommended and maximal dose is 1000 mg daily given in two divided doses of 500 mg each (two 250 mg tablets or one 500 mg tablet) with the morning and evening meals.

HOW SUPPLIED
250 mg round, white, film-coated tablets imprinted with either the DOW diamond trademark over the code number 51 or LORELCO 250. Bottles of 120 (NDC 0068-0051-52)
500 mg capsule-shaped, white, film-coated tablets, marked LORELCO 500. Bottles of 100 (NDC 0068-0053-61)
Keep well closed. Store in a dry place. Avoid excessive heat. Dispense in well-closed light-resistant containers with child-resistant closures.

ANIMAL PHARMACOLOGY AND TOXICOLOGY
In rhesus monkeys, administration of probucol in diets containing unusually high amounts of cholesterol and saturated fat resulted in the death of four of eight animals after several weeks. Premonitory syncope was frequently observed and was associated with a pronounced prolongation of the QT intervals (30 to 50% longer than that observed in untreated monkeys). Serum levels of probucol greater than 20 mcg/mL were generally associated with some prolongation in the QT interval in the cholesterol-fed monkey. A 75 msec or greater increase in QT interval from control values was usually seen at 40 mcg/mL and above. Blood levels in humans receiving Lorelco average approximately 20 mcg/mL and not uncommonly reach levels of 40 mcg/mL and higher. Rhesus monkeys fed normal (low fat) chow and receiving probucol three to thirty times the human dose equivalent achieved blood levels only one-third those of many human subjects. No adverse effects were detected in these monkeys over an eight-year period of continuous drug administration. In another study in rhesus monkeys, an atherogenic diet was fed for two years and daily treatment with probucol, separated in time from the atherogenic meal, was carried out during the second year. Serum probucol levels ranged 20 to 50 mcg/mL in five of ten monkeys, and less in the remaining animals. Marked prolongation of the QT_c interval in the ECG or syncopal behavior was never observed over the entire one-year treatment period. Regression of gross aortic lesions comparable to that observed in a parallel group of monkeys receiving cholestyramine was seen in animals receiving probucol. It should be emphasized that both HDL-cholesterol and LDL-cholesterol were markedly reduced in this regression study. During the performance of a two-year chronic study involving 32 probucol-treated dogs (beagles), there were 12 fatalities.
Subsequent experiments have indicated that probucol sensitizes the canine myocardium to epinephrine, resulting in ventricular fibrillation in many dogs. Among the animal species in which probucol has been studied, the dog is peculiar with respect to the phenomenon of sudden death due to the sensitization of the myocardium to epinephrine. In contrast to findings in the dog, injections of epinephrine to probucol-treated monkeys did not induce ventricular fibrillation.
In other studies, monkeys were given probucol either before and after, or only after myocardial infarction induced by coronary artery ligation. In these studies, there was no difference between probucol- and placebo-treated groups with respect to either survival or detailed blind quantitation of myocardial changes (gross and histopathologic).
Probucol has shown no identifiable toxicity in mice and rats. In these animals, the LD_{50} (oral) is in excess of 5 g/kg of body weight. In chronic studies of two years' duration in rats, no toxicity or carcinogenicity was observed.
From studies in rats, dogs, and monkeys, it is known that probucol accumulates slowly in adipose tissue. Approximately 90% of probucol administered orally is unabsorbed. For that which is absorbed, the biliary tract is the major pathway for clearance from the body and very little is excreted by way of the kidneys.
Myocardial injury was produced in various groups of rats by one of the following procedures: aortic coarctation, coronary ligation, or cobalt or isoproterenol injection. After probucol administration, no deleterious effects related to treatment occurred as measured by survival and microscopic examination of myocardial damage.
Probucol was administered to minipigs beginning ten days before ligation of coronary artery and continued for 60 days after surgery. Challenge with epinephrine at the end of 60 days failed to induce ventricular fibrillation in any of the coronary-ligated, probucol-treated minipigs.

CLINICAL STUDIES
In a multicenter, randomized, double-blind study, the LRC-CPPT[3], hypercholesterolemic patients treated with an oral bile acid sequestrant (cholestyramine) and a cholesterol-lowering diet experienced average total and LDL-cholesterol reductions greater than those obtained in the placebo group treated with diet alone. The cumulative seven-year incidence of the primary end point—combined incidence of definite CHD death and/or definite nonfatal myocardial infarction—was 7% in the cholestyramine group and 8.6% in the placebo group. This was a 19% reduction in risk (P less than 0.05, single-tail test) of the primary end point reflecting a 24% reduction in definite CHD death and a 19% reduction in nonfatal myocardial infarction.
The subjects included in the study were middle-aged men (35–59 years old) with serum cholesterol levels at least 265 mg/dL and no previous history of heart disease. It is not clear to what extent these findings can be extrapolated to other segments of the hypercholesterolemic population not studied.
The bile acid sequestrant, cholestyramine, was used in the above trial. Caution should be exercised in extrapolating these results to Lorelco since it differs from cholestyramine with regard to its mode of action, spectrum of cholesterol-lowering potency, effect on HDL-cholesterol, and possible toxicity. The effect of probucol-induced reduction of serum cholesterol levels on morbidity or mortality due to coronary heart disease has not been established.

REFERENCES
1. Consensus Development Panel. Lowering blood cholesterol to prevent heart disease. *JAMA.* 1985; 253:2080–2086.
2. Fredrickson DS, Levy RI. Lees RS. Fat transport in lipoproteins—an integrated approach to mechanisms and disorders. *N. Engl J Med.* 1967; 276:34–44.
3. The Lipid Research Clinics Program. The Lipid Research Clinics coronary primary prevention trial results: I. Reduction in incidence of coronary heart disease. *JAMA.* 1984; 251:351–364.
Product Information as of June, 1988
Shown in Product Identification Section, page 417

NICODERM®   ℞
[nĭk 'ŏ derm]
(nicotine transdermal system)
Systemic delivery of 21, 14, or 7 mg/day over 24 hours

DESCRIPTION
Nicoderm is a transdermal system that provides systemic delivery of nicotine for 24 hours following its application to intact skin.
Nicotine is a tertiary amine composed of a pyridine and a pyrrolidine ring. It is a colorless to pale yellow, freely water-soluble, strongly alkaline, oily, volatile, hygroscopic liquid obtained from the tobacco plant. Nicotine has a characteristic pungent odor and turns brown on exposure to air or light. Of its two stereoisomers, S(-)-nicotine is the more active and is the more prevalent form in tobacco. The free alkaloid is absorbed rapidly through the skin and respiratory tract.
[See chemical structure at top of next column.]

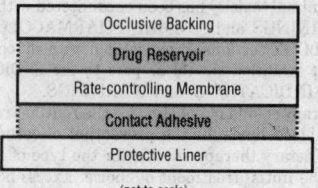

Chemical Name: S-3-(1-methyl-2-pyrrolidinyl) pyridine
Molecular Formula: $C_{10}H_{14}N_2$
Molecular Weight: 162.23
Ionization Constants: $pK_a1 = 7.84$,
$\quad\quad\quad\quad\quad\quad\quad pK_a2 = 3.04$
Octanol-Water Partition Coefficient: 15:1 at pH 7
The Nicoderm system is a multilayered rectangular film containing nicotine as the active agent. For the three doses the composition per unit area is identical. Proceeding from the visible surface toward the surface attached to the skin are (1) an occlusive backing (polyethylene/aluminum/polyester/ethylene-vinyl acetate copolymer); (2) a drug reservoir containing nicotine (in an ethylene-vinyl acetate copolymer matrix); (3) a rate-controlling membrane (polyethylene); (4) a polyisobutylene adhesive; and (5) a protective liner that covers the adhesive layer and must be removed before application to the skin.

| Occlusive Backing |
| Drug Reservoir |
| Rate-controlling Membrane |
| Contact Adhesive |
| Protective Liner |

(not to scale)

Nicotine is the active ingredient; other components of the system are pharmacologically inactive.
The rate of delivery of nicotine to the patient from each system (40 μg/cm²-h) is proportional to the surface area. About 73% of the total amount of nicotine remains in the system 24 hours after application. Nicoderm systems are labeled by the dose actually absorbed by the patient. The dose of nicotine absorbed from the Nicoderm system represents 68% of the amount released in 24 hours. The other 32% (eg, 9 mg/day for the 21 mg/day system) volatizes from the edge of the system.

Dose Absorbed in 24 Hours (mg/day)	System Area (cm²)	Total Nicotine Content (mg)
21	22	114
14	15	78
7	7	36

CLINICAL PHARMACOLOGY
Pharmacologic Action
Nicotine, the chief alkaloid in tobacco products, binds stereoselectively to acetylcholine receptors at the autonomic ganglia, in the adrenal medulla, at neuromuscular junctions, and in the brain. Two types of central nervous system effects are believed to be the basis of nicotine's positively reinforcing properties. A stimulating effect, exerted mainly in the cortex via the locus ceruleus, produces increased alertness and cognitive performance. A "reward" effect via the "pleasure system" in the brain is exerted in the limbic system. At low doses the stimulant effects predominate, while at high doses the reward effects predominate. Intermittent intravenous administration of nicotine activates neurohormonal pathways, releasing acetycholine, norepinephrine, dopamine, serotonin, vasopressin, beta-endorphin, growth hormone, and ACTH.
Pharmacodynamics
The cardiovascular effects of nicotine include peripheral vasoconstriction, tachycardia, and elevated blood pressure. Acute and chronic tolerance to nicotine develops from smoking tobacco or ingesting nicotine preparations. Acute tolerance (a reduction in response for a given dose) develops rapidly (less than 1 hour), but at distinct rates for different physiologic effects (skin temperature, heart rate, subjective effects). Withdrawal symptoms, such as cigarette craving, can be reduced in some individuals by plasma nicotine levels lower than those for smoking.
Withdrawal from nicotine in addicted indivduals is characterized by craving, nervousness, restlessness, irritability, mood lability, anxiety, drowsiness, sleep disturbances, impaired concentration, increased appetite, minor somatic complaints (headache, myalgia, constipation, fatigue), and weight gain. Nicotine toxicity is characterized by nausea, abdominal pain, vomiting, diarrhea, diaphoresis, flushing, dizziness, disturbed hearing and vision, confusion, weakness, palpitations, altered respiration, and hypotension.

The cardiovascular effects of Nicoderm 21 mg/day used continuously for 24 hours and smoking every 30 minutes during waking hours for 5 days were compared. Both regimens elevated heart rate (about 10 beats/min) and blood pressure (about 5 mm Hg) compared with an abstinence period, and these increases were similar between treatments throughout the 24-hour period, including during sleep.

The circadian pattern and release of plasma cortisol following 5 days of treatment with Nicoderm 21 mg/day did not differ from that following 5 days of nicotine abstinence. Urinary excretion of norepinephrine, epinephrine, and dopamine was also similar for Nicoderm 21 mg/day and abstinence.

Pharmacokinetics

Following application of the Nicoderm system to the upper body or upper outer arm, approximately 68% of the nicotine released from the system enters the systemic circulation (eg, 21 mg/day for the highest dose of Nicoderm). The remainder of the nicotine released from the system is lost via evaporation from the edge. All Nicoderm systems are labeled by the actual amount of nicotine absorbed by the patient.

The volume of distribution following IV administration of nicotine is approximately 2 to 3 L/kg, and the half-life of nicotine ranges from 1 to 2 hours. The major eliminating organ is the liver, and average plasma clearance is about 1.2 L/min; the kidney and lung also metabolize nicotine. There is no significant skin metabolism of nicotine. More than 20 metabolites of nicotine have been identified, all of which are believed to be less active than the parent compound. The primary metabolite of nicotine in plasma, cotinine, has a half-life of 15 to 20 hours and concentrations that exceed nicotine by 10-fold.

Plasma protein binding of nicotine is <5%. Therefore, changes in nicotine binding from use of concomitant drugs or alterations of plasma proteins by disease states would not be expected to have significant consequences.

The primary urinary metabolites are cotinine (15% of the dose) and trans-3-hydroxycotinine (45% of the dose). About 10% of nicotine is excreted unchanged in the urine. As much as 30% may be excreted in the urine with high urine flow rates and urine acidification below pH 5.

After Nicoderm application, plasma concentrations rise rapidly, plateau within 2 to 4 hours, and then slowly decline until the system is removed; after which they decline more rapidly.

The pharmacokinetic model that best fits the plasma nicotine concentrations from Nicoderm systems is an open, two-compartment disposition model with a skin depot through which nicotine enters the central circulation compartment. Nicotine in the adhesive layer is absorbed into and then through the skin, causing the initial rapid rise in plasma concentrations. The nicotine from the reservoir is released slowly through the membrane with a release rate constant approximately 20 times smaller than the skin absorption rate constant, as demonstrated *in vitro* in cadaver skin flux studies and verified by pharmacokinetic trials. Therefore, the slow decline of plasma nicotine concentrations during 4 to 24 hours (see Figure) is determined primarily by the release of nicotine from the system.

Steady-State Plasma Nicotine Concentrations for Two Consecutive Applications of Nicoderm 21 mg/day (Mean ±2 SD)

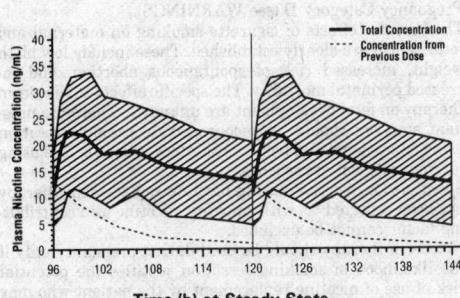

Time (h) at Steady State

Following the second daily Nicoderm system application, steady-state plasma nicotine concentrations are achieved and are on average 30% higher compared with single-dose applications. Plasma nicotine concentrations are proportional to dose (ie, linear kinetics are observed) for the three dosages of Nicoderm systems. Nicotine kinetics are similar for all sites of application on the upper body and upper outer arm. Plasma nicotine concentrations from Nicoderm 21 mg/day are the same as those from simultaneous use of Nicoderm 14 mg/day and 7 mg/day.

Following removal of the Nicoderm system, plasma nicotine concentrations decline in an exponential fashion with an apparent mean half-life of 3 to 4 hours (see dotted line in Figure) compared with 1 to 2 hours for IV administration, due to continued absorption from the skin depot. Most non-

Steady-State Nicotine Pharmacokinetic Parameters for Nicoderm Systems (Mean, SD, and Range)

| | Dose Absorbed (mg/day) | | | | | | | | |
| | **21** | | | **14** | | | **7** | | |
	Mean	SD	Range	Mean	SD	Range	Mean	SD	Range
C_{max} ng/mL	23	5	13–32	17	3	10–24	8	2	5–12
C_{avg} ng/mL	17	4	10–26	12	3	8–17	6	1	4–10
C_{min} ng/mL	11	3	6–17	7	2	4–11	4	1	3–6
T_{max} h	4	3	1–10	4	3	1–10	4	4	1–18

C_{max}:maximum observed plasma concentration
C_{avg}:average plasma concentration
C_{min}:minimum observed plasma concentration
T_{max}:time of maximum plasma concentration

smoking patients will have nondetectable nicotine concentrations in 10 to 12 hours.
[See table above.]

Half-hourly smoking of cigarettes produces average plasma nicotine concentrations of approximately 44 ng/mL. In comparison, average plasma nicotine concentrations from Nicoderm 21 mg/day are about 17 ng/mL.

There are no differences in nicotine kinetics between men and women using Nicoderm systems. Linear regression of both AUC and C_{max} vs total body weight shows the expected inverse relationship. Obese men using Nicoderm systems had significantly lower AUC and C_{max} values than normal weight men. Men and women having low body weight are expected to have higher AUC and C_{max} values.

CLINICAL STUDIES

The efficacy of Nicoderm systems as an aid to smoking cessation was demonstrated in two placebo-controlled, double-blind trials of otherwise healthy smokers (n=756) smoking at least one pack of cigarettes per day. The trials consisted of 6 weeks of active treatment, 6 weeks of weaning off Nicoderm systems, and 12 weeks of follow-up on no medication. Quitting was defined as total abstinence from smoking (as determined by patient diary and verified by expired carbon monoxide). The "quit rates" are the proportion of patients enrolled who abstained after week 2.

The two trials in otherwise healthy smokers showed that all Nicoderm doses were more effective than placebo, and that treatment with Nicoderm 21 mg/day for 6 weeks provided significantly higher quit rates than the 14 mg/day and placebo treatments at 6 weeks. Data from these two studies are combined in the Quit Rate table. Quit rates were still significantly different after an additional 6-week weaning period and at follow-up 3 months later. All patients were given weekly behavioral supportive care. As shown in the following table, the quit rates on each treatment varied 2- to 3-fold among clinics at 6 weeks.

Quit Rates After Week 2 According to Starting Dose
(N=756 smokers in 9 clinics)

Nicoderm Delivery Rate (mg/day)	Number of Patients	After 6 Weeks Range*	After Weaning Range*	All 6 Months Range*
21	249	32–92%	18–63%	3–50%
14	254	30–61%	15–52%	0–48%
Placebo	253	15–46%	0–38%	0–35%

*Range for 9 centers, number of patients per treatment ranged from 23–34

In a study of smokers with coronary artery disease, 77 patients treated with Nicoderm systems (75% on 14 mg/day and 25% on 21 mg/day) had higher quit rates than 78 placebo-treated patients at the end of the 8-week study period (5 weeks of active treatment and 3 weeks of weaning). Nicoderm systems did not affect angina frequency or the appearance of arrhythmias on Holter monitoring in these patients. Symptoms presumed related to nicotine withdrawal and the stress of smoking cessation caused more patients to terminate the study than symptoms thought to be related to nicotine substitution. Seven patients on placebo and one on Nicoderm 14 mg/day dropped out for symptoms probably related to nicotine withdrawal (7 of these 8 patients experienced cardiovascular symptoms), while only two patients dropped out for nicotine-related symptoms (one patient with severe nausea on Nicoderm 14 mg/day and one with nausea and palpitations on Nicoderm 21 mg/day).

Patients who used Nicoderm systems in clinical trials had a significant reduction in craving for cigarettes, a major nicotine withdrawal symptom, compared with placebo-treated patients (see Figure). Reduction in craving, as with quit rate, is quite variable. This variability is presumed to be due to inherent differences in patient populations (eg, patient motivation, concomitant illnesses, number of cigarettes smoked per day, number of years smoking, exposure to other smokers, socioeconomic status) as well as differences among the clinics.

Severity of Craving by Treatment From Clinical Trials (N=877)

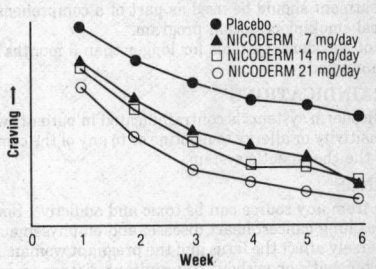

● Placebo
▲ NICODERM 7 mg/day
□ NICODERM 14 mg/day
○ NICODERM 21 mg/day

Patients using Nicoderm systems dropped out of the trials less frequently than patients receiving placebo. Quit rates for the 56 patients over age 60 were comparable to the quit rates for the 821 patients aged 60 and under.

Individualization of Dosage

It is important to make sure that patients read the instructions made available to them and have their questions answered. They should clearly understand the directions for applying and disposing of Nicoderm systems. They should be instructed to stop smoking completely when the first system is applied.

The success or failure of smoking cessation depends heavily on the quality, intensity, and frequency of supportive care. Patients are more likely to quit smoking if they are seen frequently and participate in formal smoking-cessation programs.

The goal of Nicoderm therapy is complete abstinence. Significant health benefits have not been demonstrated for reduction of smoking. If a patient is unable to stop smoking by the fourth week of therapy, treatment should probably be discontinued. Patients who have not stopped smoking after 4 weeks of Nicoderm therapy are unlikely to quit on that attempt.

Patients who fail to quit on any attempt may benefit from interventions to improve their chances for success on subsequent attempts. These patients should be counselled to determine why they failed and then probably be given a "therapy holiday" before the next attempt. A new quit attempt should be encouraged when the factors that contributed to failure can be eliminated or reduced, and conditions are more favorable.

Based on the clinical trials, a reasonable approach to assisting patients in their attempt to quit smoking is to assign their initial Nicoderm treatment using the recommended dosing schedule (see Dosing Schedule below). The need for dose adjustment should be assessed during the first 2 weeks. Patients should continue the dose selected with counselling and support over the following month. Those who have successfully stopped smoking during that time should be supported during 4 to 8 weeks of weaning, after which treatment should be terminated.

Therapy generally should begin with the Nicoderm 21 mg/day (see Dosing Schedule) except if the patient is small (less than 100 pounds), is a light smoker (less than ½ pack of cigarettes per day), or has cardiovascular disease.
[See top of next page.]

Continued on next page

Marion Merrell Dow—Cont.

Dosing Schedule

	Otherwise Healthy Patients	Other* Patients
Initial/Starting Dose	21 mg/day	14 mg/day
Duration of Treatment	4–8 weeks	4–8 weeks
First Weaning Dose	14 mg/day	7 mg/day
Duration of Treatment	2–4 weeks	2–4 weeks
Second Weaning Dose	7 mg/day	
Duration of Treatment	2–4 weeks	

* Small patient (less than 100 pounds)
  or light smoker (less than 10 cigarettes/day)
  or patient with cardiovascular disease

The symptoms of nicotine withdrawal and excess overlap (see *Pharmacodynamics* and ADVERSE REACTIONS). Since patients using Nicoderm systems may also smoke intermittently, it may be difficult to determine if patients are experiencing nicotine withdrawal or nicotine excess.
The controlled clinical trials using Nicoderm therapy suggest that abnormal dreams and insomnia are more often symptoms of nicotine excess while anxiety, somnolence, and depression are more often symptoms of nicotine withdrawal.

INDICATIONS AND USAGE

Nicoderm treatment is indicated as an aid to smoking cessation for the relief of nicotine withdrawal symptoms. Nicoderm treatment should be used as part of a comprehensive behavioral smoking-cessation program.
The use of Nicoderm systems for longer than 3 months has not been studied.

CONTRAINDICATIONS

Use of Nicoderm systems is contraindicated in patients with hypersensitivity or allergy to nicotine or to any of the components of the therapeutic system.

WARNINGS

Nicotine from any source can be toxic and addictive. Smoking causes lung cancer, heart disease, and emphysema and may adversely affect the fetus and the pregnant woman. For any smoker, with or without concomitant disease or pregnancy, the risk of nicotine replacement in a smoking-cessation program should be weighed against the hazard of continued smoking while using Nicoderm systems and the likelihood of achieving cessation of smoking without nicotine replacement.

Pregnancy Warning
Tobacco smoke, which has been shown to be harmful to the fetus, contains nicotine, hydrogen cyanide, and carbon monoxide. Nicotine has been shown in animal studies to cause fetal harm. It is therefore presumed that Nicoderm systems can cause fetal harm when administered to a pregnant woman. The effect of nicotine delivery by Nicoderm systems has not been examined in pregnancy (see PRECAUTIONS).

Therefore pregnant smokers should be encouraged to attempt cessation using educational and behavioral interventions before using pharmacological approaches. If Nicoderm systems are used during pregnancy, or if the patient becomes pregnant while using Nicoderm systems, the patient should be apprised of the potential hazard to the fetus.

Safety Note Concerning Children
The amounts of nicotine that are tolerated by adult smokers can produce symptoms of poisoning and could prove fatal if the Nicoderm system is applied or ingested by children or pets. Used 21 mg/day systems contain about 73% (83 mg) of

their initial drug content. Therefore, patients should be cautioned to keep both the used and unused Nicoderm systems out of the reach of children and pets.

PRECAUTIONS

The patient should be urged to stop smoking completely when initiating Nicoderm therapy (see DOSAGE AND ADMINISTRATION). Patients should be informed that if they continue to smoke while using Nicoderm systems, they may experience adverse effects due to peak nicotine levels higher than those experienced from smoking alone. If there is a clinically significant increase in cardiovascular or other effects attributable to nicotine, the Nicoderm dose should be reduced or Nicoderm treatment discontinued (see WARNINGS). Physicians should anticipate that concomitant medications may need dosage adjustment (see *Drug Interactions*). The use of Nicoderm systems beyond 3 months by patients who stop smoking should be discouraged, because the chronic consumption of nicotine by any route can be harmful and addicting.

Allergic Reactions
In a 6-week, open-label, dermal irritation and sensitization study of Nicoderm systems, 7 of 230 patients exhibited definite erythema at 24 hours after application. Upon rechallenge, 4 patients exhibited mild to moderate contact allergy. Patients with contact sensitization should be cautioned that a serious reaction could occur from exposure to other nicotine-containing products or smoking. In the efficacy trials, erythema following system removal was typically seen in about 14% of patients, some edema in 3%, and dropouts due to skin reactions occurred in 2% of patients.
Patients should be instructed to promptly discontinue the use of Nicoderm systems and contact their physicians, if they experience severe or persistant local skin reactions (eg, severe erythema, pruritus, or edema) at the site of application or a generalized skin reaction (eg, urticaria, hives or generalized rash).
Patients using Nicoderm therapy concurrently with other transdermal products may exhibit local reactions at both application sites. Reactions were seen in 2 of 7 patients using concomitant Estraderm® (estradiol transdermal system) in clinical trials. In such patients, use of one or both systems may have to be discontinued.

Skin Disease
Nicoderm systems are usually well tolerated by patients with normal skin, but may be irritating for patients with some skin disorders (atopic or eczematous dermatitis).

Cardiovascular or Peripheral Vascular Diseases
The risks of nicotine replacement in patients with certain cardiovascular and peripheral vascular diseases should be weighed against the benefits of including nicotine replacement in a smoking-cessation program for them. Specifically, patients with coronary heart disease (history of myocardial infarction and/or angina pectoris), serious cardiac arrhythmias, or vasospastic diseases (Buerger's disease, Prinzmetal's variant angina) should be carefully screened and evaluated before nicotine replacement is prescribed.
Tachycardia occurring in association with the use of Nicoderm therapy was reported occasionally. If serious cardiovascular symptoms occur with the use of Nicoderm therapy, it should be discontinued.
Nicoderm therapy was as well tolerated as placebo in a controlled trial in patients with coronary artery disease (see CLINICAL STUDIES). One patient on Nicoderm 21 mg/day, two on Nicoderm 14 mg/day, and eight on placebo discontinued treatment due to adverse events.
Nicoderm therapy did not affect angina frequency or the appearance of arrhythmias on Holter monitoring in these patients.

Nicoderm therapy generally should not be used in patients during the immediate post-myocardial infarction period, patients with serious arrhythmias, and patients with severe or worsening angina pectoris.

Renal or Hepatic Insufficiency
The pharmacokinetics of nicotine have not been studied in the elderly or in patients with renal or hepatic impairment. However, given that nicotine is extensively metabolized and that its total system clearance is dependent on liver blood flow, some influence of hepatic impairment on drug kinetics (reduced clearance) should be anticipated. Only severe renal impairment would be expected to affect the clearance of nicotine or its metabolites from the circulation (see *Pharmacokinetics*).

Endocrine Diseases
Nicoderm therapy should be used with caution in patients with hyperthyroidism, pheochromocytoma, or insulin-dependent diabetes, since nicotine causes the release of catecholamines by the adrenal medulla.

Peptic Ulcer Disease
Nicotine delays healing in peptic ulcer disease; therefore, Nicoderm therapy should be used with caution in patients with active peptic ulcers and only when the benefits of including nicotine replacement in a smoking-cessation program outweigh the risks.

Accelerated Hypertension
Nicotine therapy constitutes a risk factor for development of malignant hypertension in patients with accelerated hypertension; therefore, Nicoderm therapy should be used with caution in these patients and only when the benefits of including nicotine replacement in a smoking-cessation program outweigh the risks.

Information for Patient
A patient instruction booklet is included in the package of Nicoderm systems dispensed to the patient. The instruction sheet contains important information and instructions on how to properly use and dispose of Nicoderm systems. Patients should be encouraged to ask questions of the physician and pharmacist.
Patients must be advised to keep both used and unused systems out of the reach of children and pets.

Drug Interactions
Smoking cessation, with or without nicotine replacement, may alter the pharmacokinetics of certain concomitant medications.
[See table below.]

Carcinogenesis, Mutagenesis, Impairment of Fertility
Nicotine itself does not appear to be a carcinogen in laboratory animals. However, nicotine and its metabolites increased the incidences of tumors in the cheek pouches of hamsters and forestomach of F344 rats, respectively, when given in combination with tumor initiators. One study, which could not be replicated, suggested that cotinine, the primary metabolite of nicotine, may cause lymphoreticular sarcoma in the large intestine in rats.
Nicotine and cotinine were not mutagenic in the Ames *Salmonella* test. Nicotine induced repairable DNA damage in an *E. coli* test system. Nicotine was shown to be genotoxic in a test system using Chinese hamster ovary cells. In rats and rabbits, implantation can be delayed or inhibited by a reduction in DNA synthesis that appears to be caused by nicotine. Studies have shown a decrease in litter size in rats treated with nicotine during gestation.

Pregnancy
Pregnancy Category D (see WARNINGS).
The harmful effects of cigarette smoking on maternal and fetal health are clearly established. These include low birth weight, increased risk of spontaneous abortion, and increased perinatal mortality. The specific effects of Nicoderm therapy on fetal development are unknown. Therefore pregnant smokers should be encouraged to attempt cessation using educational and behavioral interventions before using pharmacological approaches.
Spontaneous abortion during nicotine replacement therapy has been reported; as with smoking, nicotine as a contributing factor cannot be excluded.
Nicoderm therapy should be used during pregnancy only if the likelihood of smoking cessation justifies the potential risk of use of nicotine replacement by the patient who may continue to smoke.

Teratogenicity
<u>Animal Studies</u>: Nicotine was shown to produce skeletal abnormalities in the offspring of mice when given doses toxic to the dams (25 mg/kg IP or SC).
<u>Human Studies</u>: Nicotine teratogenicity has not been studied in humans except as a component of cigarette smoke (each cigarette smoked delivers about 1 mg of nicotine). It has not been possible to conclude whether cigarette smoking is teratogenic to humans.

Other Effects
<u>Animal Studies</u>: A nicotine bolus (up to 2 mg/kg) to pregnant rhesus monkeys caused acidosis, hypercarbia, and hypotension (fetal and maternal concentrations were about 20 times those achieved after smoking 1 cigarette in 5 minutes). Fetal breathing movements were reduced in the fetal lamb after intravenous injection of 0.25 mg/kg nicotine to the ewe

May Require a Decrease in Dose at Cessation of Smoking	Possible Mechanism
acetaminophen, caffeine, imipramine, oxazepam, pentazocine, propranolol, theophylline	Deinduction of hepatic enzymes on smoking cessation.
Insulin	Increases in subcutaneous insulin absorption with smoking cessation.
adrenergic antagonists (eg, prazosin, labetalol)	Decrease in circulating catecholamines with smoking cessation.

May Require an Increase in Dose at Cessation of Smoking	Possible Mechanism
adrenergic agonists (eg, isoproterenol, phenylephrine)	Decrease in circulating catecholamines with smoking cessation.

(equivalent to smoking 1 cigarette every 20 seconds for 5 minutes). Uterine blood flow was reduced about 30% after infusion of 0.1 mg/kg/min nicotine for 20 minutes to pregnant rhesus monkeys (equivalent to smoking about 6 cigarettes every minute for 20 minutes).

Human Experience: Cigarette smoking during pregnancy is associated with an increased risk of spontaneous abortion, low birth weight infants, and perinatal mortality. Nicotine and carbon monoxide are considered the most likely mediators of these outcomes. The effect of cigarette smoking on fetal cardiovascular parameters has been studied near term. Cigarettes increased fetal aortic blood flow and heart rate and decreased uterine blood flow and fetal breathing movements. Nicoderm therapy has not been studied in pregnant humans.

Labor and Delivery

The Nicoderm system is not recommended to be left on during labor and delivery. The effects of nicotine on a mother or the fetus during labor are unknown.

Use in Nursing Mothers

Caution should be exercised when Nicoderm therapy is administered to nursing women. The safety of Nicoderm therapy in nursing infants has not been examined. Nicotine passes freely into breast milk; the milk to plasma ratio averages 2.9. Nicotine is absorbed orally. An infant has the ability to clear nicotine by hepatic first-pass clearance; however, the efficiency of removal is probably lowest at birth. The nicotine concentrations in milk can be expected to be lower with Nicoderm therapy, when used as directed, than with cigarette smoking, as maternal plasma nicotine concentrations are generally reduced with nicotine replacement. The risk of exposure of the infant to nicotine from Nicoderm therapy should be weighed against the risks associated with the infant's exposure to nicotine from continued smoking by the mother (passive smoke exposure and contamination of breast milk with other components of tobacco smoke) and from Nicoderm therapy alone or in combination with continued smoking.

Pediatric Use

Nicoderm therapy is not recommended for use in children, because the safety and effectiveness of Nicoderm therapy in children and adolescents who smoke have not been evaluated.

Geriatric Use

Fifty-six patients over the age of 60 participated in clinical trials of Nicoderm therapy. Nicoderm therapy appeared to be as effective in this age group as in younger smokers. However, asthenia, various body aches, and dizziness occurred slightly more often in patients over 60 years of age.

ADVERSE REACTIONS

Assessment of adverse events in the 1,131 patients who participated in controlled clinical trials is complicated by the occurrence of GI and CNS effects of nicotine withdrawal as well as nicotine excess. The actual incidences of both are confounded by concurrent smoking by many of the patients. When reporting adverse events during the trials, the investigators did not attempt to identify the cause of the symptom.

Topical Adverse Events

The most common adverse event associated with topical nicotine is a short-lived erythema, pruritus, and/or burning at the application site, which was seen at least once in 47% of patients on the Nicoderm system in the clinical trials. Local erythema after system removal was noted at least once in 14% of patients and local edema in 3%. Erythema generally resolved within 24 hours. Cutaneous hypersensitivity (contact sensitization) occurred in 2% of patients on Nicoderm systems (see PRECAUTIONS, *Allergic Reactions*).

[See table at top of next column.]

DRUG ABUSE AND DEPENDENCE

Nicoderm therapy is likely to have a low abuse potential based on differences between it and cigarettes in four characteristics commonly considered important in contributing to abuse; much slower absorption, much smaller fluctuations in blood levels, lower blood levels of nicotine, and less frequent use (ie, once daily).

Dependence on nicotine polacrilex chewing gum replacement therapy has been reported. Such dependence might also occur from transference to Nicoderm systems of tobacco-based nicotine dependence. The use of the system beyond 3 months has not been evaluated and should be discouraged. To minimize the risk of dependence, patients should be encouraged to withdraw gradually from Nicoderm treatment after 4 to 8 weeks of use. Recommended dose reduction is to progressively decrease the dose every 2 to 4 weeks (see DOSAGE AND ADMINISTRATION).

OVERDOSAGE

The effects of applying several Nicoderm systems simultaneously or swallowing Nicoderm systems are unknown (see WARNINGS, *Safety Note Concerning Children*).

The oral LD_{50} for nicotine in rodents varies with species but is in excess of 24 mg/kg; death is due to respiratory paralysis. The oral minimum lethal dose of nicotine in dogs is greater than 5 mg/kg. The oral minimum acute lethal dose for nicotine in human adults is reported to be 40 to 60 mg (<1 mg/kg).

Three dogs, each weighing 11 kg, were fed two damaged Nicoderm 14 mg/day systems. Nicotine plasma concentrations of 32 to 79 ng/mL were observed. No ill effects were apparent.

Signs and symptoms of an overdose from a Nicoderm system would be expected to be the same as those of acute nicotine poisoning, including pallor, cold sweat, nausea, salivation, vomiting, abdominal pain, diarrhea, headache, dizziness, disturbed hearing and vision, tremor, mental confusion, and weakness. Prostration, hypotension, and respiratory failure may ensue with large overdoses. Letal doses produce convulsions quickly, and death follows as a result of peripheral or central respiratory paralysis or, less frequently, cardiac failure.

Overdose From Topical Exposure

The Nicoderm system should be removed immediately if the patient shows signs of overdosage, and the patient should seek immediate medical care. The skin surface may be flushed with water and dried. No soap should be used, since it may increase nicotine absorption. Nicotine will continue to be delivered into the bloodstream for several hours (see *Pharmacokinetics*) after removal of the system because of a depot of nicotine in the skin.

Overdose From Ingestion

Persons ingesting Nicoderm systems should be referred to a health care facility for management. Due to the possibility of nicotine-induced seizures, activated charcoal should be administered. In unconscious patients with a secure airway, instill activated charcoal via a nasogastric tube. A saline cathartic or sorbitol added to the first dose of activated charcoal may speed gastrointestinal passage of the system. Repeated doses of activated charcoal should be administered as long as the system remains in the gastrointestinal tract since it will continue to release nicotine for many hours.

Management of Nicotine Poisoning

Other supportive measures include diazepam or barbiturates for seizures, atropine for excessive bronchial secretions or diarrhea; respiratory support for respiratory failure, and vigorous fluid support for hypotension and cardiovascular collapse.

Probably Causally Related

The following adverse events were reported more frequently in Nicoderm-treated patients than in placebo-treated patients or exhibited a dose response in clinical trials.

Digestive system—Diarrhea*, dyspepsia*
Mouth/Tooth disorders—Dry mouth†
Musculoskeletal system—Arthralgia†, myalgia*
Nervous system—Abnormal dreams*, insomnia (23%), nervousness*
Skin and appendages—Sweating†

Frequencies for 21 mg/day system
* Reported in 3% to 9% of patients
† Reported in 1% to 3% of patients
Unmarked if reported in <1% of patients

Causal Relationship UNKNOWN

Adverse events reported in Nicoderm- and placebo-treated patients at about the same frequency in clinical trials are listed below. The clinical significance of the association between Nicoderm systems and these events is unknown, but they are reported as alerting information for the clinician.

Body as a whole—Asthenia*, back pain*, chest pain*, pain*
Digestive system—Abdominal pain†, constipation*, nausea*, vomiting †
Nervous system—Dizziness*, headache (29%), paresthesia†
Respiratory system—Cough increased*, pharyngitis*, sinusitis†
Skin and appendages—Rash*
Special senses—Taste perversion*
Urogenital system—Dysmenorrhea*

Frequencies for 21 mg/day systems
* Reported in 3% to 9% of patients
† Reported in 1% to 3% of patients
Unmarked if reported in <1% of patients

DOSAGE AND ADMINISTRATION

Patients must desire to stop smoking and should be instructed to *stop smoking immediately* as they begin using Nicoderm therapy. The patient should read the patient instruction booklet on Nicoderm therapy and be encouraged to ask any questions. Treatment should be initiated with Nicoderm 21 mg/day or 14 mg/day systems (see *Individualization of Dosage*).

Once the appropriate dosage is selected the patient should begin 4 to 6 weeks of therapy at that dosage. The patient should stop smoking cigarettes completely during this period. If the patient is unable to stop cigarette smoking within 4 weeks, Nicoderm therapy probably should be stopped, since few additional patients in clinical trials were able to quit after this time.

Recommdended Dosing Schedule for Healthy Patients[a]
(See Individualization of Dosage)

Dose	Duration
Nicoderm 21 mg/day	First 6 Weeks
Nicoderm 14 mg/day	Next 2 Weeks[b]
Nicoderm 7 mg/day	Last 2 Weeks[c]

[a] Start with Nicoderm 14 mg/day for 6 weeks for patients who:
- have cardiovascular disease
- weigh less than 100 pounds
- smoke less than ½ a pack of cigarettes/day

Decrease dose to Nicoderm 7 mg/day for the final 2–4 weeks.

[b] Patients who have successfully abstained from smoking should have their dose of Nicoderm reduced after each 2–4 weeks of treatment until the 7 mg/day dose has been used for 2–4 weeks (see *Individualization of Dosage*).

[c] The entire course of nicotine substitution and gradual withdrawal should take 8–12 weeks, depending on the size of the initial dose. The use of Nicoderm systems beyond 3 months has not been studied.

The Nicoderm system should be applied promptly upon its removal from the protective pouch to prevent evaporative loss of nicotine from the system. Nicoderm systems should be used only when the pouch is intact to assure that the product has not been tampered with.

Nicoderm systems should be applied only once a day to a non-hairy, clean, dry skin site on the upper body or upper outer arm. After 24 hours, the used Nicoderm system should be removed and a new system applied to an alternate skin site. Skin sites should not be reused for at least a week. Patients should be cautioned not to continue to use the same system for more than 24 hours.

SAFETY AND HANDLING

The Nicoderm system can be a dermal irritant and can cause contact sensitization. Patients should be instructed in the proper use of Nicoderm systems by using demonstration systems. Although exposure of health care workers to nicotine from Nicoderm systems should be minimal, care should be taken to avoid unnecessary contact with active systems. If you do handle active systems, wash with water alone, since soap may increase nicotine absorption. Do not touch your eyes.

Disposal

When the used system is removed from the skin, it should be folded over and placed in the protective pouch that contained the new system. The used system should be immediately disposed of in such a way to prevent its access by children or pets. See patient information for further directions on handling and disposal.

HOW SUPPLIED

See DESCRIPTION for total nicotine content per unit.

NDC 0088-0050-61
Nicoderm 21 mg/day, 14 systems per box
NDC 0088-0051-61
Nicoderm 14 mg/day, 14 systems per box
NDC 0088-0052-61
Nicoderm 7 mg/day, 14 systems per box

How to Store

Do not store above 86°F (30°C) because Nicoderm systems are sensitive to heat. A slight discoloration of the system is not significant.

Do not store unpouched. Once removed from the protective pouch, Nicoderm systems should be applied promptly, since nicotine is volatile and the systems may lose strength.

CAUTION: Federal law prohibits dispensing without prescription.

Manufactured by
ALZA Corporation
Palo Alto, CA 94304 for
Marion Merrell Dow Inc.
Kansas City, MO 64114

Product Information as of January, 1992

Patient Instructions
Nicoderm®
(nicotine transdermal system)

IMPORTANT

YOUR DOCTOR HAS PRESCRIBED THIS DRUG FOR YOUR USE ONLY. DO NOT LET ANYONE ELSE USE IT. KEEP THIS MEDICINE OUT OF THE REACH OF CHILDREN AND PETS. Nicotine can be very toxic and harmful. Small amounts of nicotine can cause serious illness in children. Even used Nicoderm patches contain enough nicotine to poison children and pets. Be sure to throw away Nicoderm patches out of the reach of children and pets. If a child puts on or plays with a Nicoderm patch that is out of its sealed pouch, take it away from the child and contact a poison control center or a doctor immediately.

Women: Nicotine in any form may cause harm to your unborn baby, if you use nicotine while you are pregnant. Do not

Continued on next page

Marion Merrell Dow—Cont.

use Nicoderm patches if you are pregnant or nursing unless advised by your doctor. If you become pregnant while using Nicoderm patches, or if you think you might be pregnant, stop smoking and don't use Nicoderm patches until you have talked to your doctor.

This leaflet will provide you with general information about nicotine and specific instructions about how to use Nicoderm patches. It is important that you read it carefully and completely before you start using Nicoderm patches. Be sure to read the PRECAUTIONS section before using Nicoderm patches, because as with all drugs, Nicoderm patches have side effects. Since this leaflet is only a summary of information, be sure to ask your doctor if you have any questions or want to know more.

Marion Merrell Dow has developed "The 6-2-2 Committed Quitter's Program," which gives you useful tips on how to quit smoking while using Nicoderm patches. If you do not have a copy, please ask your doctor or pharmacist about it. They can order it for you, or you can call for it yourself at 1-800-835-5634. There is no charge for the 6-2-2 Committed Quitter's Program.

INTRODUCTION

IT IS IMPORTANT THAT YOU ARE FIRMLY COMMITTED TO GIVING UP SMOKING.

Nicoderm is a skin patch containing nicotine designed to help you quit smoking cigarettes. When you wear a Nicoderm patch, it releases nicotine through the skin into your bloodstream while you are wearing it. The nicotine that is in your skin will still be entering your bloodstream for several hours after you take the patch off.

It is the nicotine in cigarettes that causes addiction to smoking. The Nicoderm patch replaces some of the nicotine you crave when you are stopping smoking. The Nicoderm patch may also help relieve other symptoms of nicotine withdrawal that may occur when you stop smoking such as irritability, frustration, anger, anxiety, difficulty in concentration, and restessness.

There are three doses of Nicoderm patches. Your doctor has chosen the dose of the Nicoderm patch you are using and may adjust it during the first week or two. After about 6 weeks, your doctor will give you smaller Nicoderm patches approximately every 2 weeks. The smaller patches give you less nicotine. In time, you will be completely off nicotine.

INFORMATION ABOUT NICODERM PATCHES

How the Nicoderm Patch Works
Nicoderm patches contain nicotine. When you put a Nicoderm patch on your skin, nicotine passes from the patch through the skin and into your blood.

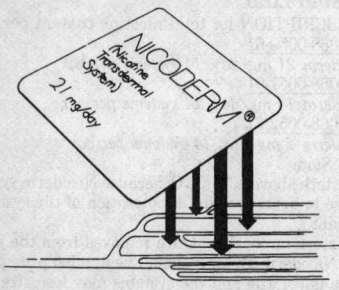

How to Apply Nicoderm Patches
Step 1.   Choose a non-hairy, clean, dry area of your front or back above the waist or the upper outer part of your arm. Do not put Nicoderm patches on skin that is burned, broken out, cut, or irritated in any way.
Step 2.   Do not remove the Nicoderm patch from its sealed protective pouch until you are ready to use it. Nicoderm patches will lose nicotine to the air if you store them out of the pouch. Before putting on the patch, tear open the pouch. Do not use scissors to open the pouch because you might accidentally cut the patch. Discard the used patch you take off by putting it in the pouch that you take the new patch out of. The used patch should be thrown away in the trash out of the reach of children and pets (see Step 7).
Step 3.   A stiff, clear, protective liner covers the sticky silver side of the Nicoderm patch—the side that will be put on your skin. The liner has a slit down the middle to help you remove it from the patch. With the silver side facing you, pull one half of the liner away from the Nicoderm patch starting at the middle slit. Hold the Nicoderm patch at one of the outside edges (touch the sticky side as little as possible), and pull off the other half of the protective liner. Throw away this liner.

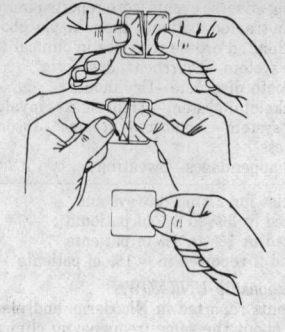

Step 4.   Immediately apply the sticky side of the Nicoderm patch to your skin. Press the patch firmly on your skin with the palm of your hand for about 10 seconds. Make sure it sticks well to your skin, especially around the edges.
Step 5.   Wash your hands when you have finished applying the Nicoderm patch. Nicotine on your hands could get into your eyes and nose and could cause stinging, redness, or more serious problems.
Step 6.   After approximately 24 hours, remove the patch you have been wearing. Choose a *different* place on your skin to apply the next Nicoderm patch and repeat Steps 1 to 5. Do not return to a previously used skin site for at least one week. Do not leave on the Nicoderm patch for more than 24 hours because it may irritate your skin and because it also loses strength after 24 hours.

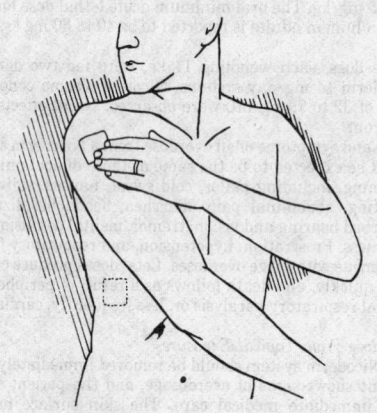

Step 7.   Fold the used Nicoderm patch in half with the silver side together. After you have put on a new patch, take its pouch and place the used folded Nicoderm patch inside of it. Throw the pouch in the trash away from children and pets.

When to Apply Nicoderm Patches
Applying the Nicoderm patch at about the same time each day will help you to remember when to put on a new Nicoderm patch. If you want to change the time when you put on your patch, you can do so. Just remove the Nicoderm patch you are wearing and put on a new one. After that, apply the Nicoderm patch at the new time each day.

If Your Nicoderm Patch Gets Wet
Water will not harm the Nicoderm patch you are wearing. You can bathe, swim, use the hot tub, or shower while you are wearing the Nicoderm patch.

If Your Nicoderm Patch Comes Off
If your Nicoderm patch falls off, put on a new one. Remove the Nicoderm patch at your regular time to keep your schedule the same or 24 hours after applying the replacement patch if you wish to change the time each day that you apply a new patch. Before putting on a new patch, make sure you select a non-hairy area that is not irritated and that is clean and dry.

Disposing of Nicoderm Patches
Fold the used patch in half with the silver side together. After you put on a new Nicoderm patch, take its opened pouch or aluminum foil and place the used folded Nicoderm patch inside of it. THROW THE POUCH IN THE TRASH AWAY FROM CHILDREN AND PETS.

Storage Instructions
Keep each Nicoderm patch in its protective pouch until you are ready to use it, because the patch will lose nicotine into the air if it's outside the pouch. Do not store Nicoderm patches above 86°F (30°C) because they are sensitive to heat.

Remember, the inside of your car can reach temperatures much higher than this in the summer.

PRECAUTIONS

What to Ask Your Doctor
Ask your doctor about possible problems with Nicoderm patches. Be sure to tell your doctor if you have had any of the following:
● a recent heart attack (myocardial infarction)
● irregular heart beat (arrhythmia)
● severe or worsening heart pain (angina pectoris)
● allergies to drugs
● rashes from adhesive tape or bandages
● skin diseases
● very high blood pressure
● stomach ulcers
● overactive thyroid
● diabetes requiring insulin
● kidney or liver disease

If You Are Taking Medicines
Nicoderm treatment, together with stopping smoking, may change the effect of other medicines. It is important to tell your doctor about all the medicines you are taking.

What to Watch For (Adverse Effects)
You should not smoke while using the Nicoderm patch. It is possible to get too much nicotine (an overdose), especially if you use the Nicoderm patch and smoke at the same time. Signs of an overdose include bad headaches, dizziness, upset stomach, drooling, vomiting, diarrhea, cold sweat, blurred vision, difficulty with hearing, mental confusion, and weakness. An overdose might cause you to faint.

If Your Skin Reacts to the Nicoderm Patch
When you first put on a Nicoderm patch, mild itching, burning, or tingling is normal and should go away within an hour. After you remove a Nicoderm patch, the skin under the patch might be somewhat red. Your skin should not stay red for more than a day. If you get a skin rash after using a Nicoderm patch, or if the skin under the patch becomes swollen or very red, call your doctor. Do not put on a new patch. You may be allergic to one of the components of the Nicoderm patch. If you do become allergic to the nicotine in the Nicoderm patch, you could get sick from using cigarettes or other nicotine-containing products.

Shown in Product Identification Section, page 417

NICORETTE®   ℞
[nĭk 'ō-rĕt ″]
(nicotine polacrilex)

CAUTION
Federal law prohibits dispensing without prescription.

DESCRIPTION
Nicorette (nicotine polacrilex) contains nicotine bound to an ion exchange resin in a sugar-free flavored chewing gum base. Nicotine is absorbed through the buccal mucosa when Nicorette is chewed. Each piece of Nicorette contains nicotine polacrilex equivalent to 2 mg nicotine and also contains flavors, glycerin, gum base, sodium bicarbonate, sodium carbonate, and sorbitol. Nicorette is to be used as an adjunct to smoking cessation programs. The chemical name for nicotine is (S)-3-(1-methyl-2-pyrrolidinyl)pyridine.

CLINICAL PHARMACOLOGY
Nicotine is an agonist at nicotinic receptors in the peripheral and central nervous systems. In man, as in animals, nicotine has been shown to produce both behavioral stimulation and depression.

Nicotine's effects are generally dose-dependent, and extremely high doses (achievable through parenteral, rectal, and perhaps percutaneous routes), can produce toxic symptoms, i.e., delirium. These effects can occur in nicotine-tolerant individuals. In nonsmokers, CNS-mediated symptoms of hiccups, nausea, and emesis are commonly associated with the use of even small doses of inhaled smoke or chewed Nicorette gum. However, in smokers these symptoms occur only with much larger doses.

Nicotine has actions at the sympathetic ganglia and on the chemoreceptors of the aorta and carotid bodies. Nicotine also affects the adrenal medulla, with the attendant release of catecholamines. The overall effect on the cardiovascular system leads to acceleration of the heart, peripheral vasoconstriction, and elevation of blood pressure with an attendant increase in the work of the heart. Nicotine may induce vasospasm and cardiac arrhythmias. Tolerance does not develop to the catecholamine-releasing effects of nicotine.

Results of cardiovascular studies comparing Nicorette with cigarettes document that each source of nicotine produces similar dose-dependent effects on cardiovascular performance (see *Biopharmaceutics and Pharmacokinetics* section). However, if Nicorette gum (2 mg/piece) is used by smokers at a rate not exceeding one piece per hour, the cardiovascular effects produced do not differ from those seen with placebo. Reinforcement of cigarette smoking behavior is considered to have both psychologic (or learned) and pharmacologic

components. Buffered nicotine-containing gum is designed to provide an alternative source of nicotine for nicotine-dependent individuals acutely withdrawing from tobacco smoking.

Biopharmaceutics and Pharmacokinetics

The nicotine in Nicorette is bound to an ion exchange resin and is released only during chewing; nicotine will not be released in significant amounts if the gum is swallowed. The blood level of nicotine obtained with Nicorette will depend upon the vigor, rapidity, and duration of chewing.

In studies comparing the nicotine blood level achieved with Nicorette to that achieved with smoking, it was found that the trough level of nicotine obtained by smoking one cigarette per hour is approximately twice that of chewing one 2 mg Nicorette per hour.

The pronounced early peak in nicotine blood levels seen with the inhalation of cigarette smoke is not observed with the chewing of Nicorette. Swallowing Nicorette does not produce clinically significant blood levels of nicotine. Nicotine is metabolized mainly by the liver, but may also be metabolized to a lesser extent by the kidney and the lung. The principal metabolites are cotinine and nicotine-1'-N-oxide. Both nicotine and its metabolites are excreted through the kidneys with about 10 to 20% of absorbed nicotine excreted unchanged in the urine. Excretion of nicotine is increased in acid urine and by high urine output. The metabolism of nicotine absorbed buccally from Nicorette is qualitatively similar to the metabolism observed when nicotine is absorbed through inhalation of cigarette smoke.

INDICATION AND USAGE

Nicorette is indicated as a temporary aid to the cigarette smoker seeking to give up his or her smoking habit while participating in a behavioral modification program under medical or dental supervision.

The efficacy of Nicorette as an aid to smoking cessation was demonstrated in clinical studies which showed that Nicorette gum, in comparison to control chewing gums, increased the likelihood of smoking cessation among participants in behavioral modification programs. As used in the context of this labeling, behavioral modification refers to supervised programs of education, counselling and psychologic support. The efficacy of Nicorette use without concomitant participation in a behavioral modification program has not been established.

In general, smokers who have a high 'physical' type of nicotine dependence are most likely to benefit from the use of Nicorette. The following subject characteristics are correlated with a 'physical' type of nicotine dependence: (1) smoke more than 15 cigarettes per day, (2) prefer brands of cigarettes with nicotine levels of greater than 0.9 mg/cigarette, (3) usually inhale the smoke frequently and deeply, (4) smoke the first cigarette within 30 minutes of arising, (5) find the first cigarette in the morning the hardest to give up, (6) smoke more frequently during the morning than the rest of the day, (7) find it difficult to refrain from smoking in places where it is forbidden, or (8) smoke even when they are so ill they are confined to bed most of the day.

The benefits of Nicorette use beyond three months have not been demonstrated.

CONTRAINDICATIONS

Nicorette is contraindicated in non-smokers.

Nicorette is contraindicated in patients during the immediate post-myocardial infarction period, patients with life-threatening arrhythmias, and patients with severe or worsening angina pectoris. (See WARNINGS.)

Also, Nicorette is contraindicated in patients with active temporomandibular joint disease.

Current medical opinion indicates that nicotine in any form may be harmful to an unborn child. Nicorette and cigarettes both contain nicotine.

Nicorette may cause fetal harm when administered to a pregnant woman.

Use of cigarettes or Nicorette during the last trimester has been associated with a decrease in fetal breathing movements. These effects may be the result of decreased placental perfusion caused by nicotine. Rare reports of miscarriages have been received, and a relationship to drug therapy as a contributing factor cannot be excluded. Studies in pregnant rhesus monkeys have shown that maternal nicotine administration produced acidosis, hypoxia and hypercarbia in the fetus.

Nicotine has been shown to be teratogenic in mice treated subcutaneously with 25 mg/kg, which is approximately 300 times the human buccal dose. Studies in rats and monkeys have not demonstrated a teratogenic effect of nicotine in doses which would occur during cigarette smoking.

Nicorette is therefore contraindicated in women who are or may become pregnant, and female patients should be advised to take adequate precautions to avoid becoming pregnant. The physician may wish to consider a pregnancy test before instituting therapy with Nicorette. If this drug is used during pregnancy, or if the patient becomes pregnant while taking this drug, the patient should be apprised of the potential hazard to the fetus.

Treatment Emergent Symptom Incidence for the 2 mg Gum

	U.S.		British	
	Drug	Placebo	Drug	Placebo
Number of Subjects Reporting	94	95	58	58
Percent of Subjects Reporting				
Autonomic				
Excess Salivation	2.1	0.0		
CNS				
Insomnia	1.1	1.1		
Dizziness/Light-headedness	2.1	2.1	19.0	13.8
Irritable/Fussy	1.1	1.1		
Headache	1.1	5.3	24.1	29.3
Gastrointestinal				
Nonspecific GI Distress	9.6	6.3		
Eructation	6.4	1.1		
Indigestion			41.4	20.7
Nausea/Vomiting	18.1	4.2	31.0	15.5
Reactions Referable to Mouth, Throat, Jaw, or Teeth				
Mouth or Throat Soreness	37.2	31.6	56.9	53.4
Jaw Muscle Ache	18.1	9.5	44.8	44.8
Others				
Anorexia	1.1	1.1		
Hiccups	14.9	0.0	22.4	3.4

WARNINGS

The risks of nicotine in patients with certain cardiovascular and endocrine diseases should be carefully weighed against the benefits of including Nicorette in a smoking cessation program in these patients. Specifically, patients with coronary heart disease (history of myocardial infarction and/or angina pectoris), serious cardiac arrhythmias, or vasospastic diseases (Buerger's disease, Prinzmetal variant angina) should be carefully screened and evaluated before Nicorette is prescribed. Occasional reports of tachyarrhythmias occurring in association with the use of Nicorette have been reported; therefore, if an increase in cardiovascular symptoms occurs with the use of Nicorette, it should be discontinued. As the action of nicotine on the adrenal medulla (release of catecholamines) does not appear to be affected by tolerance, Nicorette should be used with caution in patients with hyperthyroidism, pheochromocytoma or insulin-dependent diabetes. Cigarette smoking is felt to play a perpetuating role in hypertension and peptic ulcer disease. Therefore, Nicorette should be used in patients with systemic hypertension or peptic ulcer (active or inactive) only when the benefits of including Nicorette in a smoking cessation program outweigh the risks.

PRECAUTIONS

Nicorette should be used with caution in patients with oral or pharyngeal inflammation and in patients with a history of esophagitis or peptic ulcer.

The dosage form of Nicorette dictates that it be used with caution in patients whose dental problems might be exacerbated by chewing gum. In such patients prior dental evaluation may be advisable.

Nicorette is sugar-free and has been formulated to minimize stickiness. As with other gums, however, the degree to which Nicorette may stick to dentures, dental caps or partial bridges may depend on the materials from which they are made and other factors such as amount of saliva produced, possible interaction with denture adhesives, denture cleaning compounds, dryness of mouth due to other causes and salivary constituents. Should an excessive degree of stickiness to dental work occur, there is the possibility that as with other gums, Nicorette may damage dental work; if this should occur, the patient should discontinue its use and consult a physician or dentist.

The sustained use of Nicorette by ex-smokers is not to be encouraged because the chronic consumption of nicotine is toxic and addicting. The physician must, however, weigh the relative risks of a possible return to smoking versus continued, long-term use of the gum.

Information for Patients

The patient instruction sheet is attached at the end of the professional labeling text. It is intended for detachment by the pharmacist and inclusion in the package of Nicorette dispensed to the patient. It contains important selected information on patient selection, risks and adverse effects and instructions on how to use Nicorette properly.

Drug Interactions

Smoking cessation, with or without nicotine substitutes, may alter response to concomitant medication in ex-smokers. Smoking is considered to increase metabolism and thus lower blood levels of drugs such as phenacetin, caffeine, theophylline, imipramine and pentazocine, through enzyme induction. Cessation of smoking may result in increased levels of these drugs. Absorption of glutethimide may be decreased, and the "first pass" metabolism of propoxyphene may be decreased by smoking cessation. Other reported effects of

smoking, which do not involve enzyme induction, include reduced diuretic effects of furosemide and decreased cardiac output, and increased blood pressure with propranolol, which may also relate to the hormonal effects of nicotine. Smoking cessation may reverse these actions.

Both smoking and nicotine can increase circulating cortisol and catecholamines. Therapy with adrenergic agonists or with adrenergic blockers may need to be adjusted according to changes in nicotine therapy or smoking status.

Carcinogenesis, Mutagenesis, Impairment of Fertility

Nicotine was not mutagenic in the Ames *Salmonella* test. Literature reports indicate that nicotine is neither an initiator nor a tumor-promoter in mice. There is inconclusive evidence to suggest that cotinine, an oxidized metabolite of nicotine, may be carcinogenic in rats. Cotinine was not mutagenic in the Ames *Salmonella* test.

Studies have shown a decrease of litter size in rats treated with nicotine during the time of fertilization.

Pregnancy

Pregnancy Category X. (See CONTRAINDICATIONS.)

Nursing Mothers

Nicotine passes freely into the breast milk. Because of the potential for serious adverse reactions in nursing infants from nicotine, a decision should be made whether to discontinue nursing or to discontinue the drug, taking into account the importance of the drug to the mother.

Pediatric Use

Safety and effectiveness in children and adolescents who smoke have not been evaluated.

ADVERSE REACTIONS

Adverse reactions reported in association with the use of Nicorette include both local effects and systemic effects representing the pharmacologic action of nicotine. Rare reports of an apparent severe allergic reaction have been received.

Local side effects

Mechanical effects of gum chewing include traumatic injury to oral mucosa or teeth, jaw ache, and eructation secondary to air swallowing. These side effects may be minimized by modifying chewing technique. Oral mucosal changes such as stomatitis, glossitis, gingivitis, pharyngitis, and aphthous ulcers, in addition to changes in taste perception, can occur during smoking cessation efforts with or without the use of Nicorette.

Systemic side effects

Although the systemic effects seen in trials were generally similar, the reported frequency of adverse drug effects was highly variable, as illustrated by the variation observed in adverse event incidences estimated from the results of two well controlled studies (one performed in the United States, and the other in England) designed to evaluate the safety and efficacy of Nicorette. (See table, above.) Given this variability, the table can be used only as an indication of the relative frequency of adverse events reported in representative clinical trials. It cannot predict expected incidences of these effects during the course of usual medical practice.

The only potentially serious systemic adverse effect observed among the 152 patients evaluated in the controlled clinical trials used to support the efficacy of Nicorette was cardiac irritability: a patient displayed what may have been nicotine-induced, but reversible, atrial fibrillation. Cardiac irritability is a well known consequence of cigarette smoking. A 46-year-old male patient participating in a clinical trial of Nicorette was reported to have developed nicotine intoxica-

Continued on next page

Marion Merrell Dow—Cont.

tion requiring his hospitalization. After 4 days, he was discharged, fully recovered. He died suddenly one month later. Nicorette was not used during this one-month interval. The relationship of the patient's death to his prior treatment is undetermined.

Since the marketing of Nicorette in the U.S., reports of several other deaths and reports including myocardial infarction, congestive heart failure, cerebrovascular accident and cardiac arrest have been received. A cause and effect relationship between these reports and the use of Nicorette has not been established.

In addition to the reported effects listed above, the following events have been reported: *CARDIOVASCULAR*—edema, flushing, hypertension, palpitations, tachyarrhythmias, tachycardia; *CNS*—confusion, convulsions, depression, euphoria, numbness, paresthesia, syncope, tinnitus, weakness; *DERMATOLOGIC*—erythema, itching, rash, urticaria; *GASTROINTESTINAL*—alteration of liver function tests, constipation, diarrhea; *RESPIRATORY*—breathing difficulty, cough, hoarseness, sneezing, wheezing; *OTHER*—dry mouth, systemic nicotine intoxication.

Rare reports of miscarriages have been received, and a relationship to drug therapy as a contributing factor cannot be excluded.

DRUG ABUSE AND DEPENDENCE

Dependence on the use of Nicorette gum has been reported. Such dependence may result from transference to Nicorette of tobacco-based nicotine dependence. The use of the Nicorette beyond three months has not been demonstrated to increase the smoking cessation rate. Use beyond 3 months should be discouraged. To minimize the risk of dependence, after 3 months' usage, patients should be encouraged to gradually withdraw over the next 3 months or stop gum usage altogether. (See DOSAGE AND ADMINISTRATION.) In patients who have used the gum for longer periods, gradual withdrawal should be instituted. (See PRECAUTIONS.)

OVERDOSAGE

Overdosage could occur if many pieces were chewed simultaneously or in rapid succession. Risk of poisoning by swallowing the gum is small because absorption in the absence of chewing is slow and incomplete. The consequences of overdose will most likely be minimized by the early nausea and vomiting known to occur with excessive nicotine intake. However, toxic systemic effects may occur. Should an overdose occur, the symptoms would be those of acute nicotine poisoning. Symptoms and signs include nausea, salivation, abdominal pain, vomiting, diarrhea, cold sweat, headache, dizziness, disturbed hearing and vision, mental confusion and marked weakness. Faintness and prostration will likely ensue and hypotension may occur; breathing is difficult; the pulse may be rapid, weak and irregular; circulatory collapse may be followed by terminal convulsions. Death may result within a few minutes from respiratory failure caused by paralysis of the muscles of respiration.

The oral LD_{50} for nicotine in rodents varies with species but is in excess of 24 mg/kg. Death in rodents was due to respiratory paralysis. The oral minimum lethal dose of nicotine in dogs is greater than 5 mg/kg. The oral minimum lethal dose for nicotine in human adults is 40–60 mg.

Under no circumstances should Nicorette be used in children.

TREATMENT OF OVERDOSAGE

In view of the lack of actual experience in the treatment of Nicorette overdose, the procedures recommended are those that have been suggested for the treatment of acute nicotine poisoning.

If emesis has not occurred, it should be induced with ipecac syrup in conscious patients. A saline cathartic will speed gastrointestinal passage of the gum. In unconscious patients with a secure airway, gastric lavage with a wide-bore tube followed by suspension of activated charcoal will aid in nicotine removal. Mechanical ventilation for respiratory paralysis may be necessary in severe nicotine poisoning. Hypotension and/or cardiovascular collapse may occur and should be treated vigorously.

DOSAGE AND ADMINISTRATION

Nicorette is an adjunct to smoking cessation programs (see INDICATION AND USAGE), and dosage should be individualized. A patient who is a candidate for Nicorette therapy must desire to stop smoking and should be instructed to *stop smoking immediately*. The patient should be given an instruction sheet on Nicorette gum chewing, and be allowed to read the instruction sheet and ask any questions. The patient should arrange for follow-up visits at intervals not greater than one month. At follow-up visits the patient's progress in smoking cessation should be determined and continued usage of Nicorette reassessed; successful abstainers at three months should stop using gum or gradually withdraw from gum usage. Patients who chew gum beyond a 3-month period should be considered as possibly using Nico-

rette as a substitute source of nicotine for their nicotine dependence. (See DRUG ABUSE AND DEPENDENCE.)

At the initial office or group visit, patients should be instructed to chew one piece of gum whenever they have the urge to smoke. Each piece should be chewed slowly and intermittently for about 30 minutes. The aim of this chewing is to promote even, slow, buccal absorption of the nicotine released from the buffered gum. Chewing quickly can release the nicotine too rapidly, leading to effects similar to oversmoking; e.g., nausea, hiccups or irritation of the throat.

As the nature of adverse effects experienced by an individual patient will be primarily related to the balance between the degree of nicotine tolerance and the rate and degree of absorption of nicotine from the gum, it is important for the patient to learn to chew the gum slowly and to self-titrate the nicotine dose, in order to minimize side effects. (SEE PATIENT INSTRUCTION SHEET AT END OF PRODUCT LABELING.)

Most patients require approximately 10 to 12 pieces of gum per day during the first month of treatment. Patients should be instructed not to exceed 30 Nicorette pieces per day. Patients should be assessed after one month of treatment to determine smoking status, and the use of Nicorette as an adjunct should be reevaluated. Gradual withdrawal from Nicorette should be initiated after 3 months' usage and completed by 6 months. The use of Nicorette beyond 6 months is not recommended.

Gradual Reduction Procedures

With Nicorette, as with cigarette smoking, the abrupt cessation of nicotine may result in withdrawal symptoms which may lead to a return to smoking. Therefore, Nicorette dosing should be gradually reduced. The suggested procedures for a gradual reduction of Nicorette include, but are not limited to, the following:

1. decrease the total number of pieces of Nicorette used per day by one or more pieces every 4 to 7 days,
2. decrease the chewing time with each piece of Nicorette from the normal 30 minutes to 10 or 15 minutes for 4 to 7 days then gradually decrease the total number of pieces used per day, while continuing the 10 or 15 minute chewing time,
3. substitute one or more pieces of sugarless gum for an equal number of pieces of Nicorette. The number of pieces of sugarless gum substituted for Nicorette should be increased every 4 to 7 days.

Combination or modification of the above procedures may be adjusted to the individual patient. Nicorette dosing may be stopped when usage has been reduced to one or two pieces per day.

Most patients in Nicorette assisted programs who resumed smoking have done so within six months of treatment. If necessary, a separate course of Nicorette may be prescribed at a later time for patients who continue or resume smoking.

HOW SUPPLIED

Nicorette is available in 2 mg (beige) square chewing pieces, packaged in child-resistant blister strips of 12 chewing pieces per strip with 8 strips per box.

Each chewing piece contains nicotine polacrilex equivalent to 2 mg nicotine.

Boxes of 96 chewing pieces, 2 mg (NDC 0068-0045-55). Store at room temperature, below 86°F (30°C). Protect from light.

Product Information as of May, 1989

Manufactured by Aktiebolaget Leo, Helsingborg, Sweden

NICORETTE®
(nicotine polacrilex)

INSTRUCTIONS FOR USE
IMPORTANT!

YOU MUST READ THESE INSTRUCTIONS CAREFULLY BEFORE USING NICORETTE GUM. THE CORRECT USE OF THIS MEDICATION IS DIFFERENT FROM CHEWING OTHER GUMS.

THE FOLLOWING GIVES IMPORTANT INFORMATION ABOUT NICORETTE. IT DOES NOT GIVE ALL INFORMATION ABOUT THE DRUG. IF YOU HAVE QUESTIONS, CALL YOUR DOCTOR.

WARNINGS

—NICORETTE IS USED AS PART OF A PROGRAM TO HELP YOU STOP SMOKING. IT IS A DRUG. IT HAS BEEN PRESCRIBED FOR YOU BY YOUR DOCTOR. DO NOT LET ANYONE ELSE USE IT.

—YOU MUST BE 18 YEARS OLD OR OLDER.

—YOU MUST BE A SMOKER.

—KEEP THIS AND ALL OTHER DRUGS AWAY FROM CHILDREN.

—FEMALES: NICORETTE CONTAINS NICOTINE. NICOTINE MAY CAUSE HARM TO THE UNBORN BABY WHEN TAKEN BY A PREGNANT WOMAN. DO NOT TAKE NICORETTE IF YOU ARE PREGNANT OR NURSING A CHILD. AVOID BECOMING PREGNANT WHILE USING NICORETTE. IF YOU THINK YOU ARE

PREGNANT, STOP USING NICORETTE AT ONCE. TELL YOUR DOCTOR IMMEDIATELY.

HOW TO USE NICORETTE

READ ALL OF THE FOLLOWING STEPS BEFORE USING NICORETTE. REFER TO THESE INSTRUCTIONS OFTEN TO MAKE SURE YOU ARE USING NICORETTE CORRECTLY.

1. Starting now, you must give up smoking **completely**.
2. When you want to smoke, put 1 piece of Nicorette in your mouth. Nicorette will taste different from other gums.
3. Chew Nicorette **very slowly**.
4. **Stop chewing** when you have a peppery taste or feel a slight tingling in your mouth. (This happens after about 15 chews. The number of chews is not the same for all people.)
5. "Park" the gum. To "park" the gum, place it between the cheek and gums.
6. Start to chew **slowly** again when the taste or tingling is almost gone (about 1 minute). When the peppery taste or tingling returns, **stop chewing**.
7. "Park" the gum again **in a different part of the mouth**.
8. Repeat steps 3–7 until most of the nicotine is gone from the gum (about 30 minutes).

DO NOT USE MORE THAN 30 PIECES OF NICORETTE A DAY. MOST PEOPLE FIND THAT 10–12 PIECES OF NICORETTE A DAY WILL CONTROL THEIR URGE TO SMOKE. DO NOT USE NICORETTE FOR MORE THAN 6 MONTHS.

SOME WAYS TO STOP YOUR USE OF NICORETTE

(This is often called "weaning.")

As your urge to smoke fades, **gradually** use fewer pieces of Nicorette. This may be possible in 2–3 months.

There are many possible ways for you to reduce your use of Nicorette. Below are some plans. Choose the plan or combination of plans that works best for you.

As you reduce your use of Nicorette, you should continue proper chewing procedures. See "HOW TO USE NICORETTE"—STEPS 1–8.

—Every 4 to 7 days, **reduce by 1** the number of pieces you use each day. For example: If you are using 12 pieces of Nicorette a day, begin to use 11 pieces a day. Four to 7 days later, begin to use 10 pieces a day, and so on.

—Use some pieces of Nicorette **for only 10 or 15 minutes** instead of 30 minutes before throwing the gum away. Maintain the shorter time for each piece and also begin to gradually reduce the number of pieces used. (See the above example.)

—Use some sugarless gum in place of Nicorette. Increase the number of sugarless pieces **every 4 to 7 days.**

For example: If you are using 12 pieces of Nicorette a day, begin to use 11 pieces of Nicorette and 1 piece of sugarless gum.

Four to 7 days later, use 10 pieces of Nicorette and 2 pieces of sugarless gum.

Keep using **1 more** piece of **sugarless gum** and **1 less** piece of **Nicorette** every 4 to 7 days.

STOP USING NICORETTE WHEN YOU ARE SATISFIED WITH 1 OR 2 PIECES A DAY—UNLESS YOUR DOCTOR TELLS YOU OTHERWISE.
IF YOU HAVE TROUBLE IN REDUCING YOUR USE OF NICORETTE, CALL YOUR DOCTOR.
CARRY NICORETTE WITH YOU AT ALL TIMES IN CASE YOU FEEL THE URGE TO SMOKE AGAIN.
ONE CIGARETTE IS ENOUGH TO START YOUR SMOKING HABIT AGAIN.

SOME POSSIBLE SIDE EFFECTS

Some people find it hard to stop using Nicorette. This may occur for people who have depended on the nicotine in cigarettes. They may transfer that dependence to the nicotine in Nicorette.

—Do not chew Nicorette too fast or too hard. Doing this may cause the same effects as inhaling a cigarette for the first time or smoking too fast.

Some of these effects are:

light-headedness, nausea, vomiting, throat and mouth soreness, hiccups, and upset stomach.

—Some other effects which may occur especially during the first few days of using Nicorette include:

mouth sores, headaches, heart palpitations (flutterings), and more saliva in the mouth.

Most side effects can be controlled by chewing more slowly. Go over steps 3–7 under "HOW TO USE NICORETTE."

If you **swallow** a piece of Nicorette, you probably will have no side effects.

There are other side effects with the use of Nicorette which have been reported. Your doctor can answer questions you may have about side effects. Report any problems to your doctor.

OVERDOSE

—OVERDOSE may occur if you chew many pieces of Nicorette at one time.

—OVERDOSE may occur if you chew many pieces, one right after another.

IN CASE OF OVERDOSE
OR
IF A CHILD CHEWS OR SWALLOWS ONE OR MORE
PIECES OF NICORETTE, CONTACT YOUR DOCTOR
OR LOCAL POISON CONTROL CENTER AT ONCE!

OTHER INFORMATION

When you chew Nicorette properly, nicotine is released slowly. It is absorbed through the lining of your mouth. You may adjust the amount of nicotine you receive by changing how fast you chew Nicorette and how much time you wait before chewing another piece.

If you use cigarettes while you use Nicorette, you may not succeed in your goal to quit smoking. You are also more likely to have side effects.

PLEASE NOTE
Like other gums, chewing Nicorette may cause:
—injury to your teeth
—injury to the lining of your mouth
—jaw ache
—belching when air is swallowed
Proper use of Nicorette may reduce the chance that these effects may occur.
—Any gum may stick to your dentures, dental caps, or partial bridges.
This may depend on the materials used in the dental work and other factors.
—Nicorette is sugar-free and has been made in such a way as to reduce stickiness. If Nicorette often sticks to your dental work, there may be damage to the dental work. Stop using Nicorette, and contact your doctor or dentist.
  —Store Nicorette at room temperature, below 86°F (30°C). Remember the trunk and glove box of your car can reach temperatures much higher than this in the summer.
  —Protect Nicorette from light.

TO REMOVE GUM

 Tear off single unit.

 Peel off backing. Start at corner with loose edge.

 Push gum through foil.

Shown in Product Identification Section, page 417

NITRO–BID® IV   ℞
[ni'tro-bid]
(nitroglycerin injection, USP)
FOR INTRAVENOUS USE ONLY

FOR INTRAVENOUS USE ONLY: NOT FOR DIRECT INTRAVENOUS INJECTION (MUST BE DILUTED), NITRO-BID IV MUST BE DILUTED IN DEXTROSE 5% INJECTION, USP OR SODIUM CHLORIDE (0.9%) INJECTION, USP BEFORE INTRAVENOUS ADMINISTRATION. THE ADMINISTRATION SET USED FOR INFUSION MAY AFFECT THE AMOUNT OF NITRO-BID IV DELIVERED TO THE PATIENT. (SEE WARNINGS AND DOSAGE AND ADMINISTRATION SECTIONS.)

CAUTION

SEVERAL PREPARATIONS OF NITROGLYCERIN INJECTION, USP ARE AVAILABLE. THEY DIFFER IN CONCENTRATION AND/OR VOLUME PER VIAL. WHEN SWITCHING FROM ONE PRODUCT TO ANOTHER, ATTENTION MUST BE PAID TO THE DILUTION AND DOSAGE AND ADMINISTRATION INSTRUCTIONS.

DESCRIPTION

NITRO-BID IV (nitroglycerin injection, USP) is a clear, practically colorless additive solution for intravenous infusion after dilution. Each milliliter contains 5 mg nitroglycerin and 45 mg propylene glycol.

The solution is sterile, nonpyrogenic, and nonexplosive. NITRO-BID IV, an organic nitrate, is a vasodilator. The chemical name for nitroglycerin is 1,2,3 propanetriol trinitrate and its chemical structure is:

$$CH_2-ONO_2$$
$$|$$
$$CH-ONO_2$$
$$|$$
$$CH_2-ONO_2$$

$C_3H_5N_3O_9$ MOL WT 227.09

CLINICAL PHARMACOLOGY

Relaxation of vascular smooth muscle is the principal pharmacologic action of nitroglycerin. Although venous effects predominate, nitroglycerin produces, in a dose-related manner, dilation of both arterial and venous beds. Dilation of the postcapillary vessels, including large veins, promotes peripheral pooling of blood and decreases venous return to the heart, reducing left ventricular end-diastolic pressure (preload). Arteriolar relaxation reduces systemic vascular resistance and arterial pressure (afterload). Myocardial oxygen consumption or demand (as measured by the pressure-rate product, tension-time index, and stroke-work index) is decreased by both the arterial and venous effects of nitroglycerin, and a more favorable supply-demand ratio can be achieved.

Therapeutic doses of intravenous nitroglycerin reduce systolic, diastolic, and mean arterial blood pressures. Effective coronary perfusion pressure is usually maintained, but can be compromised if blood pressure falls excessively or increased heart rate decreases diastolic filling time.

Elevated central venous and pulmonary capillary wedge pressures, pulmonary vascular resistance, and systemic vascular resistance are also reduced by nitroglycerin therapy. Heart rate is usually slightly increased, presumably a reflex response to the fall in blood pressure. Cardiac index may be increased, decreased, or unchanged. Patients with elevated left ventricular filling pressure and systemic vascular resistance values in conjunction with a depressed cardiac index are likely to experience an improvement in cardiac index. On the other hand, when filling pressures and cardiac index are normal, cardiac index may be slightly reduced by intravenous nitroglycerin.

Nitroglycerin is widely distributed in the body with an apparent volume of distribution of approximately 200 liters in adult male subjects, and is rapidly metabolized to dinitrates and mononitrates, with a short half-life, estimated at one to four minutes. This results in a low plasma concentration after intravenous infusion. At plasma concentrations of between 50 and 500 ng/mL, the binding of nitroglycerin to plasma proteins is approximately 60%, while that of 1,2 dinitroglycerin and 1,3 dinitroglycerin is 60% and 30%, respectively. The activity and half-life of the nitroglycerin metabolites are not well characterized. The mononitrate is not active.

INDICATIONS AND USAGE

NITRO-BID IV (nitroglycerin injection, USP) is indicated for:
1. **Control of blood pressure in perioperative hypertension,** ie, hypertension associated with surgical procedures, especially cardiovascular procedures, such as the hypertension seen during intratracheal intubation, anesthesia, skin incision, sternotomy, cardiac bypass, and in the immediate postsurgical period.
2. **Congestive heart failure associated with acute myocardial infarction.**
3. **Treatment of angina pectoris** in patients who have not responded to recommended doses of organic nitrates and/or a beta-blocker.
4. **Production of controlled hypotension during surgical procedures.**

CONTRAINDICATIONS

NITRO-BID IV (nitroglycerin injection, USP) should not be administered to individuals with:
1. A known hypersensitivity to nitroglycerin or a known idiosyncratic reaction to organic nitrates.
2. Hypotension or uncorrected hypovolemia, as the use of NITRO-BID IV in such states could produce severe hypotension or shock.
3. Increased intracranial pressure (eg, head trauma or cerebral hemorrhage).
4. Inadequate cerebral circulation.
5. Constrictive pericarditis and pericardial tamponade.

WARNINGS

1. Nitroglycerin readily migrates into many plastics. To avoid absorption of nitroglycerin into plastic parenteral solution containers, the dilution of nitroglycerin injection, USP should be made only in glass parenteral solution bottles.
2. Some filters absorb nitroglycerin; they should be avoided.
3. Forty percent (40%) to eighty percent (80%) of the total amount of nitroglycerin in the final diluted solution for infusion is absorbed by the polyvinyl chloride (PVC) tubing of the intravenous administration sets currently in general use. The higher rates of absorption occur when flow rates are low, nitroglycerin concentrations are high, and tubing is long. Although the rate of loss is highest during the early phase of administration (when flow rates are lowest), the loss is neither constant nor self-limiting; consequently, no simple calculation or correction can be performed to convert the theoretical infusion rate (based on the concentration of the infusion solution) to the actual delivery rate. Because of this problem, Marion Laboratories recommends the use of the least absorptive infusion

---

tubing available (ie, non-PVC tubing) for infusions of NITRO-BID IV. DOSING INSTRUCTIONS MUST BE FOLLOWED WITH CARE. IT SHOULD BE NOTED THAT WHEN THE APPROPRIATE INFUSION SETS ARE USED, THE CALCULATED DOSE WILL BE DELIVERED TO THE PATIENT BECAUSE THE LOSS OF NITROGLYCERIN DUE TO ABSORPTION IN STANDARD PVC TUBING WILL BE KEPT TO A MINIMUM. NOTE THAT THE DOSAGES COMMONLY USED IN PUBLISHED STUDIES UTILIZED GENERAL-USE PVC INFUSION SETS, AND RECOMMENDED DOSES BASED ON THIS EXPERIENCE ARE TOO HIGH IF THE LOW ABSORBING INFUSION SETS ARE USED.

4. A potential safety problem exists with the combined use of some infusion pumps and some non-PVC infusion sets. Because the special tubing required to prevent the absorption of nitroglycerin tends to be less pliable than the conventional PVC tubing normally used with such infusion pumps, the pumps may fail to occlude the infusion sets completely. The results may be excessive flow at low infusion rate settings, causing alarms, or unregulated gravity flow when the infusion pump is stopped; this could lead to over-infusion of nitroglycerin. All infusion pumps should be tested with the infusion sets to ensure their ability to deliver nitroglycerin accurately at low flow rates, and to occlude the infusion sets properly when the infusion is stopped.

PRECAUTIONS

NITRO-BID IV (nitroglycerin injection, USP) should be used with caution in patients who have severe hepatic or renal disease.

Excessive hypotension, especially for prolonged periods of time, must be avoided because of possible deleterious effects on the brain, heart, liver, and kidney from poor perfusion and the attendant risk of ischemia, thrombosis, and altered function of these organs. Paradoxical bradycardia and increased angina pectoris may accompany nitroglycerin-induced hypotension. Patients with normal or low pulmonary capillary wedge pressure are especially sensitive to the hypotensive effects of NITRO-BID IV. If pulmonary capillary wedge pressure is being monitored, it will be noted that a fall in wedge pressure precedes the onset of arterial hypotension, and the pulmonary capillary wedge pressure is thus a useful guide to safe titration of the drug.

NITRO-BID IV contains alcohol and propylene glycol; safety for intracoronary injection has not been shown.

Carcinogenesis, Mutagenesis, Impairment of Fertility:
No long-term studies in animals were performed to evaluate carcinogenic potential of NITRO-BID IV (nitroglycerin injection, USP).

Pregnancy:
Category C. Animal reproduction studies have not been conducted with NITRO-BID IV. It is also not known whether NITRO-BID IV can cause fetal harm when administered to a pregnant woman or can affect reproduction capacity. NITRO-BID IV should be given to a pregnant woman only if clearly needed.

Nursing Mothers:
It is not known whether nitroglycerin is excreted in human milk. Because many drugs are excreted in human milk, caution should be exercised when NITRO-BID IV is administered to a nursing woman.

Pediatric Use:
The safety and effectiveness of NITRO-BID IV in children have not been established.

ADVERSE REACTIONS

The most frequent adverse reaction in patients treated with NITRO-BID IV is headache, which occurs in approximately 2% of patients. Other adverse reactions occurring in less than 1% of patients are the following: tachycardia, nausea, vomiting, apprehension, restlessness, muscle twitching, retrosternal discomfort, palpitations, dizziness, and abdominal pain.

The following additional adverse reactions have been reported with the oral and/or topical use of nitroglycerin: cutaneous flushing, weakness, and occasionally, drug rash or exfoliative dermatitis.

OVERDOSAGE

Accidental overdosage of NITRO-BID IV may result in severe hypotension and reflex tachycardia which can be treated by elevating the legs and decreasing or temporarily terminating the infusion until the patient's condition stabilizes. Since the duration of the hemodynamic effects following NITRO-BID IV administration is quite short, additional corrective measures are usually not required. However, if further therapy is indicated, administration of an intravenous alpha-adrenergic agonist (eg, methoxamine or phenylephrine) should be considered.

Continued on next page

Marion Merrell Dow—Cont.

DOSAGE AND ADMINISTRATION

NOT FOR DIRECT INTRAVENOUS INJECTION.
NITRO-BID IV (nitroglycerin injection, USP) IS A CONCENTRATED, POTENT DRUG WHICH MUST BE DILUTED IN DEXTROSE 5% INJECTION, USP OR SODIUM CHLORIDE (0.9%) INJECTION, USP PRIOR TO ITS INFUSION. NITRO-BID IV SHOULD NOT BE ADMIXED WITH OTHER DRUGS.

Initial Dilution:
Aseptically transfer the desired volume of NITRO-BID IV (see chart below) into a glass bottle containing the stated volume of either 5% dextrose injection, USP or 0.9% sodium chloride injection, USP. This yields a final concentration of 100 to 400 μg/mL (see chart below). Invert the glass parenteral bottle several times following admixture to assure uniform dilution of nitroglycerin injection.

Maintenance Dilution:
It is important to consider the fluid requirements of the patient as well as the expected duration of infusion in selecting the appropriate dilution of NITRO-BID IV.
After the initial dosage titration, the concentration of the admixture may be increased, if necessary, to limit fluids given to the patient. The concentration of the infusion solution should not exceed 400 μg/mL of nitroglycerin.
If the concentration is adjusted, it is imperative to flush or replace the infusion set before a new concentration is utilized. If the set were not flushed, or replaced, it could take minutes to hours, depending upon the flow rate and the dead space of the set, for the new concentration to reach the patient.

DILUTION TABLE

Diluent Volume	Quantity of NITRO-BID IV (5 mg/mL)	Approximate Final Concentration
100 mL	10 mg (2 mL)	100 mcg/mL
100 mL	20 mg (4 mL)	200 mcg/mL
100 mL	40 mg (8 mL)	400 mcg/mL
250 mL	25 mg (5 mL)	100 mcg/mL
250 mL	50 mg (10 mL)	200 mcg/mL
250 mL	100 mg (20 mL)	400 mcg/mL
500 mL	50 mg (10 mL)	100 mcg/mL
500 mL	100 mg (20 mL)	200 mcg/mL
500 mL	200 mg (40 mL)	400 mcg/mL

ADMINISTRATION TABLE
(60 microdrops = 1 milliliter)

Concentration (μg/mL)	100	200	400
Dose (μg/min)	Flow Rate (microdrops/min = mL/hr)		
5	3	—	—
10	6	3	—
15	9	—	—
20	12	6	3
30	18	9	—
40	24	12	6
60	36	18	9
80	48	24	12
120	72	36	18
160	96	48	24
240	—	72	36
320	—	96	48
480	—	—	72
640	—	—	96

Dosage:
Dosage is affected by the type of infusion set used (see WARNINGS). Although the usual starting adult dose range reported in clinical studies was 25 μg/min or more, those studies used PVC TUBING. **The use of nonabsorbing tubing will result in the need to use reduced doses.**
When using a nonabsorbing infusion set, initial dosage should be 5 μg/min delivered through an infusion pump capable of exact and constant delivery of the drug. Subsequent titration must be adjusted to the clinical situation, with dose increments becoming more cautious as partial response is seen. Initial titration should be in 5-μg/min increments, with increases every three to five minutes until some response is noted. If no response is seen at 20 μg/min, increments of 10 and later 20 μg/min can be used. Once a partial blood pressure response is observed, the dose increase should be reduced and the interval between increments should be lengthened. Patients with normal or low left ventricular filling pressure or pulmonary capillary wedge pressure (eg, angina patients without other complications) may be hypersensitive to the effects of NITRO-BID IV and may

respond fully to doses as small as 5 μg/min. These patients require especially careful titration and monitoring.
There is no fixed optimum dose of NITRO-BID IV. Due to variations in the responsiveness of individual patients to the drug, each patient must be titrated to the desired level of hemodynamic function. Therefore, continuous monitoring of physiologic parameters (eg, blood pressure, heart rate, and pulmonary capillary wedge pressure) MUST BE PERFORMED to achieve the correct dose. Adequate systemic blood pressure and coronary perfusion pressure must be maintained.
Parenteral drug products should be inspected visually for particulate matter and discoloration prior to administration, whenever solution and container permit.

HOW SUPPLIED
VIALS (5 mg/mL)
NITRO-BID® IV is supplied in boxes of ten 1-mL vials (NDC 0088-1800-31), each vial containing 5 mg of nitroglycerin (5 mg/mL); ten 5-mL vials (NDC 0088-1800-32), each vial containing 25 mg nitroglycerin (5 mg/mL); and five 10-mL vials (NDC 0088-1800-33), each vial containing 50 mg nitroglycerin (5 mg/mL).
PROTECT FROM LIGHT BY RETAINING PRODUCT IN CARTON UNTIL READY TO USE.
NITRO-BID IV VIALS ARE INTENDED FOR SINGLE-DOSE ONLY. PROPERLY DISCARD ANY UNUSED PORTION.
STORE AT CONTROLLED ROOM TEMPERATURE 15–30°C (59–86°F).
PROTECT FROM FREEZING.

Issued 4/89

NITRO–BID® Ointment ℞
[ni'tro-bid]
(nitroglycerin 2%)

DESCRIPTION
Nitroglycerin, an organic nitrate, is a vasodilator which has effects on both arteries and veins. The chemical name for nitroglycerin is 1,2,3-Propanetriol trinitrate. The compound has a molecular weight of 227.09. The chemical structure is:

$$CH_2—ONO_2$$
$$|$$
$$CH —ONO_2$$
$$|$$
$$CH_2—ONO_2$$

NITRO-BID® Ointment contains 2% nitroglycerin ointment and lactose in a lanolin and white petrolatum base. Each inch, as squeezed from the tube, contains approximately 15 mg nitroglycerin.

CLINICAL PHARMACOLOGY
The principal pharmacological action of nitroglycerin is relaxation of vascular smooth muscle, producing a vasodilator effect on both peripheral arteries and veins with more prominent effects on the latter. Dilation of the post-capillary vessels, including large veins, promotes peripheral pooling of blood and decreases venous return to the heart, thereby reducing left ventricular end-diastolic pressure (preload). Arteriolar relaxation reduces systemic vascular resistance and arterial pressure (afterload).
The mechanism by which nitroglycerin relieves angina pectoris is not fully understood. Myocardial oxygen consumption or demand (as measured by the pressure-rate product, tension-time index, and stroke work index) for a given level of external exercise is decreased by both the arterial and venous effects of nitroglycerin and, presumably, a more favorable supply-demand ratio is achieved. While the large epicardial coronary arteries are also dilated by nitroglycerin, the extent to which this action contributes to relief of exertional angina is unclear.
Nitroglycerin is rapidly metabolized, principally by a liver reductase to form glycerol nitrate metabolites and inorganic nitrate. Two active major metabolites, the 1, 2 and 1, 3 dinitroglycerols, the products of hydrolysis, appear to be less potent than nitroglycerin as vasodilators but have longer plasma half-lives.
The dinitrates are further metabolized to mononitrates (biologically inactive with respect to cardiovascular effects) and ultimately glycerol and carbon dioxide. There is extensive first-pass deactivation by the liver of nitroglycerin following gastrointestinal absorption.
Adequate studies defining the pharmacokinetics of NITRO-BID have not been reported. The clinical relevance of nitroglycerin blood levels has not been established, since therapeutic levels of the drug and metabolites have not been defined. In general, it appears that blood levels are proportional to surface covered, but they are also related to location (chest placement gives higher levels than extremities) and to the thickness of the applied paste. Duration of effect would be expected to depend on the total amount of nitroglycerin (thickness of paste) per unit of surface area, but this has not been well studied.
Therapeutic doses of nitroglycerin have been shown to reduce systolic and mean arterial blood pressures, especially

when the patient assumes upright posture, for as long as seven hours after a single application. Nitroglycerin ointment reduces abnormally elevated left ventricular end-diastolic pressure (LVEDP), a hemodynamic concomitant of acute episodes of angina pectoris. The onset of hemodynamic effects of nitroglycerin ointment is not sufficiently rapid to be of use in aborting an acute episode of angina pectoris.

INDICATIONS AND USAGE
NITRO-BID is indicated for the treatment and prevention of angina pectoris due to coronary artery disease. Controlled clinical trials have demonstrated that this form of nitroglycerin is effective in improving exercise tolerance in patients with exertional angina pectoris. Double-blind, placebo-controlled trials have shown significant improvement in exercise time until chest pain for up to six hours after single application of various doses of nitroglycerin ointment (mean doses ranged from 5 to 36 mg) to a 36-inch^2 area of trunk.

CONTRAINDICATIONS
Nitroglycerin is contraindicated in patients who have shown purported hypersensitivity or idiosyncrasy to it or other nitrates or nitrites.

WARNINGS
The benefits of nitroglycerin ointment during the early days of acute myocardial infarction have not been established. If one elects to use organic nitrates in early infarction, careful assessment and hemodynamic monitoring should be used because of the potential deleterious effects of hypotension.

PRECAUTIONS
General. Severe hypotensive response, particularly with upright posture, may occur even with small doses of nitroglycerin. The drug therefore should be used with caution in patients who may have volume depletion from diuretic therapy or in patients who have low systolic blood pressure (eg, below 90 mm Hg). Paradoxical bradycardia and increased angina pectoris may accompany nitroglycerin-induced hypotension.
Nitrate therapy may aggravate the angina caused by hypertrophic cardiomyopathy.
Tolerance to this drug and cross-tolerance to other nitrates and nitrites may occur. Tolerance to the vascular and antianginal effects of nitrates has been demonstrated in clinical trials, in experience through occupational exposure, and in isolated tissue experiments. The importance of tolerance to the appropriate use of nitroglycerin ointment in the management of patients with angina pectoris has not been determined. In controlled clinical trials in angina pectoris patients, sustained therapy with some nitrate preparations has resulted in significantly less improvement and a shorter duration of improvement in exercise time than had been seen when therapy was initiated. Sustained improvement in exercise tolerance has been reported in patients with angina pectoris who applied nitroglycerin ointment three times daily for 8 to 12 weeks in open studies, but there have been no controlled clinical studies involving exercise testing that have examined the efficacy of repetitive doses of NITRO-BID for the long-term treatment of angina pectoris.
In industrial workers continuously exposed to nitroglycerin, tolerance clearly occurs. Moreover, physical dependence also occurs since chest pain, acute myocardial infarction, and even sudden death have occurred during temporary withdrawal of nitroglycerin from the workers. In clinical trials in angina patients, there are reports of anginal attacks being more easily provoked and of rebound in the hemodynamic effects soon after nitrate withdrawal. The relative importance of these observations to the routine, clinical use of nitroglycerin is not known, but it seems prudent to gradually withdraw patients from nitroglycerin when the therapy is being terminated, rather than stopping the drug abruptly.
Drug Interactions. Alcohol may enhance sensitivity to the hypotensive effects of nitrates.
Nitroglycerin acts directly on vascular muscle. Therefore, any other agent that directly or indirectly acts on vascular smooth muscle may have decreased or increased effect depending upon the agent.
Marked symptomatic orthostatic hypotension has been reported when calcium channel blockers and organic nitrates were used in combination. Dose adjustments of either class of agents may be necessary.
Carcinogenesis, Mutagenesis, Impairment of Fertility. No long-term studies in animals have been performed to evaluate carcinogenic potential of NITRO-BID; neither has its mutagenic potential been studied. It is also not known whether nitroglycerin can affect reproduction capacity.
Pregnancy. Pregnancy Category C. Animal reproduction studies have not been conducted with NITRO-BID. It is also not known whether nitroglycerin can cause fetal harm when administered to a pregnant woman. Nitroglycerin should be given to a pregnant woman only if clearly needed.
Nursing Mothers. It is not known whether nitroglycerin is excreted in human milk. Because many drugs are excreted in human milk, caution should be exercised when NITRO-BID is administered to a nursing woman.

Pediatric Use. Safety and effectiveness in children have not been established.

ADVERSE REACTIONS

Adverse reactions to NITRO-BID, particularly headache and hypotension, are generally dose-related. In clinical trials at various doses of nitroglycerin, the following adverse effects have been observed.

Headache, which may be severe and persistent, is the most commonly reported side effect of nitroglycerin, with an incidence in the order of 50% in some studies. Cutaneous vasodilation with flushing may occur. Transient episodes of dizziness and weakness, as well as other signs of cerebral ischemia associated with postural hypotension may occasionally develop. An occasional individual may exhibit marked sensitivity to the hypotensive effects of nitrates and severe responses (nausea, vomiting, weakness, restlessness, pallor, perspiration, and collapse) may occur even with therapeutic doses of nitrates. Drug rash and/or exfoliative dermatitis have been reported in patients receiving nitrate therapy. Nausea and vomiting can occur, but appear to be uncommon.

OVERDOSAGE

Signs and Symptoms. Nitrate overdosage may result in: severe hypotension, persistent throbbing headache, vertigo, palpitation, visual disturbance, flushing and perspiring skin (later becoming cold and cyanotic), nausea and vomiting (possibly with colic and even bloody diarrhea), syncope (especially in the upright posture), methemoglobinemia with cyanosis and anorexia, initial hyperpnea, dyspnea and slow breathing, slow pulse (dicrotic and intermittent), heart block, increased intracranial pressure with cerebral symptoms of confusion and moderate fever, paralysis and coma followed by clonic convulsions and possibly death due to circulatory collapse.

Treatment of Overdosage. Keep the patient recumbent in a shock position and comfortably warm. Wipe the skin clean of the nitroglycerin ointment. Passive movement of the extremities may aid venous return. Administer oxygen and artificial ventilation if necessary. If methemoglobinemia is present, administration of methylene blue (1% solution), 1 to 2 mg/kg intravenously, may be required.

Methemoglobin. Case reports of clinically significant methemoglobinemia are rare at conventional doses of organic nitrates. The formation of methemoglobin is dose-related and in the case of genetic abnormalities of hemoglobin that favor methemoglobin formation, even conventional doses of organic nitrates could produce harmful concentrations of methemoglobin.

WARNINGS

Epinehprine is ineffective in reversing the severe hypotensive events associated with overdose. It and related compounds are contraindicated in this situation.

DOSAGE AND ADMINISTRATION

When applying the ointment, place the dose-determining applicator supplied with the package printed-side down and squeeze the necessary amount of ointment from the tube onto the applicator. Then place the applicator with the ointment-side down onto the desired area of skin, usually the chest or back. Several studies suggest that absorption of nitroglycerin through the skin varies with the site of application of the drug. Application of the drug to the skin of the chest is reported to give higher blood levels of nitroglycerin and greater hemodynamic effects than application to the extremities.

The amount of nitroglycerin entering the circulation varies directly with the size of skin area exposed to the drug and the amount of ointment applied. Although in major clinical trials the dose of nitroglycerin was often applied to a 6×6-inch (150×150-mm) area of skin, in clinical practice the dose is usually applied to a smaller area. The ointment should be applied in a thin, uniform layer and the dose-to-area ratio kept reasonably constant. For example: 1 inch on a 2×3-inch area; 2 inches on a 3×4-inch area; 3 inches on a 4×5-inch area. When doubling the dose, the surface area over which the ointment is placed should also be doubled.

As with all nitrates, clinical studies suggest that clinical response is variable. A suggested starting dose for NITRO-BID is ½ inch (7.5 mg) applied to a 1×3-inch area every eight hours. Response to treatment should be assessed over the next several days. If angina occurs while the ointment is in place, the dose should be increased, for example, to 1 inch on a 2×3-inch area. NITRO-BID should be titrated upward until a dose effective in controlling angina is determined or until side effects limit the dose. If angina occurs after the ointment has been in place for several hours, the frequency of dosing should be increased (eg, every six hours). Administer the smallest effective dose three to four times daily, unless clinical response suggests a different regimen. At initiation of therapy or change in dosage, blood pressure (patient standing) should be monitored. Controlled trials have been carried out for up to seven hours after dosing; therefore, it is not known whether the drug is effective in prevention of exertional angina beyond seven hours after dosing. The effectiveness of repetitive applications of nitroglycerin ointment for the chronic management of angina pectoris has not been established.

NITRO-BID is not intended for immediate relief of anginal attacks.

HOW SUPPLIED

NITRO-BID® Ointment (nitroglycerin 2%) is available in 20-gm (NDC 0088-1552-20) and 60-gm (NDC 0088-1552-60) tubes and in Unit Dose Identification Paks of 100 1-gm foil pouches (NDC 0088-1552-49).

Issued 10/86

NORPRAMIN® ℞

[*nŏr'prăm-ĭn*]

(desipramine hydrochloride tablets USP)

DESCRIPTION

Norpramin (desipramine hydrochloride USP) is an antidepressant drug of the tricyclic type, and is chemically: 5*H*-Dibenz[*b,f*]azepine-5-propanamine, 10, 11-dihydro-*N*-methyl-, monohydrochloride

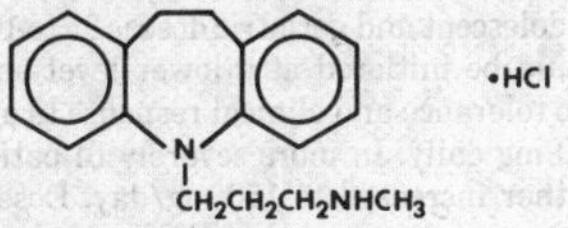

INACTIVE INGREDIENTS

The following inactive ingredients are contained in all dosage strengths: acacia, calcium carbonate, corn starch, D&C Red No. 30 and D&C Yellow No. 10 (except 10 mg and 150 mg), FD&C Blue No. 1 (except 50 mg. 75 mg. and 100 mg), hydrogenated soy oil, iron oxide, light mineral oil, magnesium stearate, mannitol, polyethylene glycol 8000, pregelatinized corn starch, sodium benzoate (except 150 mg), sucrose, talc, titanium dioxide, and other ingredients.

CLINICAL PHARMACOLOGY

Mechanism of Action

Available evidence suggests that many depressions have a biochemical basis in the form of a relative deficiency of neurotransmitters such as norepinephrine and serotonin. Norepinephrine deficiency may be associated with relatively low urinary 3-methoxy-4-hydroxyphenyl glycol (MHPG) levels, while serotonin deficiencies may be associated with low spinal fluid levels of 5-hydroxyindoleacetic acid.

While the precise mechanism of action of the tricyclic antidepressants is unknown, a leading theory suggests that they restore normal levels of neurotransmitters by blocking the re-uptake of these substances from the synapse in the central nervous system. Evidence indicates that the secondary amine tricyclic antidepressants, including Norpramin, may have greater activity in blocking the re-uptake of norepinephrine. Tertiary amine tricyclic antidepressants, such as amitriptyline, may have greater effect on serotonin re-uptake.

Norpramin (desipramine hydrochloride) is not a monoamine oxidase (MAO) inhibitor and does not act primarily as a central nervous system stimulant. It has been found in some studies to have a more rapid onset of action than imipramine. Earliest therapeutic effects may occasionally be seen in 2 to 5 days, but full treatment benefit usually requires 2 to 3 weeks to obtain.

Metabolism

Tricyclic antidepressants, such as desipramine hydrochloride, are rapidly absorbed from the gastrointestinal tract. Tricyclic antidepressants or their metabolites are to some extent excreted through the gastric mucosa and reabsorbed from the gastrointestinal tract. Desipramine is metabolized in the liver and approximately 70% is excreted in the urine.

The rate of metabolism of tricyclic antidepressants varies widely from individual to individual, chiefly on a genetically determined basis. Up to a thirty-sixfold difference in plasma level may be noted among individuals taking the same oral dose of desipramine. In general, the elderly metabolize tricyclic antidepressants more slowly than do younger adults.

Certain drugs, particularly the psychostimulants and the phenothiazines, increase plasma levels of concomitantly administered tricyclic antidepressants through competition for the same metabolic enzyme systems. Concurrent administration of cimetidine and tricyclic antidepressants can produce clinically significant increases in the plasma concentrations of the tricyclic antidepressants. Conversely, decreases in plasma levels of the tricyclic antidepressants have been reported upon discontinuation of cimetidine which may result in the loss of the therapeutic efficacy of the tricyclic antidepressant. Other substances, particularly barbiturates and alcohol, induce liver enzyme activity and thereby reduce tricyclic antidepressant plasma levels. Similar effects have been reported with tobacco smoke.

Research on the relationship of plasma level to therapeutic response with the tricyclic antidepressants has produced conflicting results. While some studies report no correlation, many studies cite therapeutic levels for most tricyclics in the range of 50 to 300 nanograms per milliliter. The therapeutic range is different for each tricyclic antidepressant. For desipramine, an optimal range of therapeutic plasma levels has not been established.

INDICATIONS

Norpramin (desipramine hydrochloride) is indicated for relief of symptoms in various depressive syndromes, especially endogenous depression.

CONTRAINDICATIONS

Desipramine hydrochloride should not be given in conjunction with, or within 2 weeks of, treatment with an MAO inhibitor drug; hyperpyretic crises, severe convulsions, and death have occurred in patients taking MAO inhibitors and tricyclic antidepressants. When Norpramin (desipramine hydrochloride) is substituted for an MAO inhibitor, at least 2 weeks should elapse between treatments. Norpramin should then be started cautiously and should be increased gradually.

The drug is contraindicated in the acute recovery period following myocardial infarction. It should not be used in those who have shown prior hypersensitivity to the drug. Cross sensitivity between this and other dibenzazepines is a possibility.

WARNINGS

1. Extreme caution should be used when this drug is given in the following situations:
   a. In patients with cardiovascular disease, because of the possibility of conduction defects, arrhythmias, tachycardias, strokes, and acute myocardial infarction.
   b. In patients with a history of urinary retention or glaucoma, because of the anticholinergic properties of the drug.
   c. In patients with thyroid disease or those taking thyroid medication, because of the possibility of cardiovascular toxicity, including arrhythmias.
   d. In patients with a history of seizure disorder, because this drug has been shown to lower the seizure threshold.
2. This drug is capable of blocking the antihypertensive effect of guanethidine and similarly acting compounds.
3. USE IN PREGNANCY
   Safe use of desipramine hydrochloride during pregnancy and lactation has not been established; therefore, if it is to be given to pregnant patients, nursing mothers, or women of childbearing potential, the possible benefits must be weighed against the possible hazards to mother and child. Animal reproductive studies have been inconclusive.
4. USE IN CHILDREN
   Norpramin (desipramine hydrochloride) is not recommended for use in children since safety and effectiveness in the pediatric age group have not been established. (See ADVERSE REACTIONS, Cardiovascular.)
5. The patient should be cautioned that this drug may impair the mental and/or physical abilities required for the performance of potentially hazardous tasks such as driving a car or operating machinery.
6. In patients who may use alcohol excessively, it should be borne in mind that the potentiation may increase the danger inherent in any suicide attempt or overdosage.

PRECAUTIONS

1. It is important that this drug be dispensed in the least possible quantities to depressed outpatients, since suicide has been accomplished with this class of drug. Ordinary prudence requires that children not have access to this drug or to potent drugs of any kind; if possible, this drug should be dispensed in containers with child-resistant safety closures. Storage of this drug in the home must be supervised responsibly.
2. If serious adverse effects occur, dosage should be reduced or treatment should be altered.
3. Norpramin (desipramine hydrochloride) therapy in patients with manic-depressive illness may induce a hypomanic state after the depressive phase terminates.
4. The drug may cause exacerbation of psychosis in schizophrenic patients.
5. Close supervision and careful adjustment of dosage are required when this drug is given concomitantly with anticholinergic or sympathomimetic drugs.
6. Patients should be warned that while taking this drug their response to alcoholic beverages may be exaggerated.
7. Clinical experience in the concurrent administration of ECT and antidepressant drugs is limited. Thus, if such treatment is essential, the possibility of increased risk relative to benefits should be considered.
8. If Norpramin (desipramine hydrochloride) is to be combined with other psychotropic agents such as tranquilizers or sedative/hypnotics, careful consideration should be given to the pharmacology of the agents employed since the sedative effects of Norpramin and benzodiazepines (e.g., chlordiazepoxide or diazepam) are additive.

Continued on next page

Marion Merrell Dow—Cont.

Both the sedative and anticholinergic effects of the major tranquilizers are also additive to those of Norpramin.

9. Concurrent administration of cimetidine and tricyclic antidepressants can produce clinically significant increases in the plasma levels of the tricyclic antidepressants (see CLINICAL PHARMACOLOGY, *Metabolism*). Conversely, decreases in plasma levels of the tricyclic antidepressants have been reported upon discontinuation of cimetidine which may result in the loss of the therapeutic efficacy of the tricyclic antidepressant.
10. There have been greater than twofold increases of previously stable plasma levels of tricyclic antidepressants when fluoxetine has been administered in combination with these agents.
11. This drug should be discontinued as soon as possible prior to elective surgery because of the possible cardiovascular effects. Hypertensive episodes have been observed during surgery in patients taking desipramine hydrochloride.
12. Both elevation and lowering of blood sugar levels have been reported.
13. Leukocyte and differential counts should be performed in any patient who develops fever and sore throat during therapy; the drug should be discontinued if there is evidence of pathologic neutrophil depression.

ADVERSE REACTIONS

Note: Included in the following listing are a few adverse reactions that have not been reported with this specific drug. However, the pharmacologic similarities among the tricyclic antidepressant drugs require that each of the reactions be considered when Norpramin (desipramine hydrochloride) is given.

Cardiovascular: hypotension, hypertension, palpitations, heart block, myocardial infarction, stroke, arrhythmias, premature ventricular contractions, tachycardia, ventricular tachycardia, ventricular fibrillation, sudden death.

There has been a report of an "acute collapse" and "sudden death" in an eight-year old (18 kg) male, treated for two years for hyperactivity. There have been additional reports of sudden death in children. (See WARNINGS, Use in Children.)

Psychiatric: confusional states (especially in the elderly) with hallucinations, disorientation, delusions; anxiety, restlessness, agitation; insomnia and nightmares; hypomania; exacerbation of psychosis.

Neurologic: numbness, tingling, paresthesias of extremities; incoordination, ataxia, tremors; peripheral neuropathy; extrapyramidal symptoms; seizures; alteration in EEG patterns; tinnitus.

Anticholinergic: dry mouth, and rarely associated sublingual adenitis; blurred vision, disturbance of accommodation, mydriasis, increased intraocular pressure; constipation, paralytic ileus; urinary retention, delayed micturition, dilatation of urinary tract.

Allergic: skin rash, petechiae, urticaria, itching, photosensitization (avoid excessive exposure to sunlight), edema (of face and tongue or general), drug fever, cross sensitivity with other tricyclic drugs.

Hematologic: bone marrow depressions including agranulocytosis, eosinophilia, purpura, thrombocytopenia.

Gastrointestinal: anorexia, nausea and vomiting, epigastric distress, peculiar taste, abdominal cramps, diarrhea, stomatitis, black tongue, hepatitis, jaundice (simulating obstructive), altered liver function, elevated liver function tests, increased pancreatic enzymes.

Endocrine: gynecomastia in the male, breast enlargement and galactorrhea in the female; increased or decreased libido, impotence, painful ejaculation, testicular swelling; elevation or depression of blood sugar levels; syndrome of inappropriate antidiuretic hormone secretion (SIADH).

Other: weight gain or loss; perspiration, flushing; urinary frequency, nocturia; parotid swelling; drowsiness, dizziness, weakness and fatigue, headache; fever; alopecia; elevated alkaline phosphatase.

Withdrawal Symptoms: Though not indicative of addiction, abrupt cessation of treatment after prolonged therapy may produce nausea, headache, and malaise.

DOSAGE AND ADMINISTRATION

Not recommended for use in children.

Lower dosages are recommended for elderly patients and adolescents. Lower dosages are also recommended for outpatients compared to hospitalized patients, who are closely supervised. Dosage should be initiated at a low level and increased according to clinical response and any evidence of intolerance. Following remission, maintenance medication may be required for a period of time and should be at the lowest dose that will maintain remission.

Usual Adult Dose

The usual adult dose is 100 to 200 mg per day. In more severely ill patients, dosage may be further increased gradually to 300 mg/day if necessary. Dosages above 300 mg/day are not recommended.

Dosage should be initiated at a lower level and increased according to tolerance and clinical response.

Treatment of patients requiring as much as 300 mg should generally be initiated in hospitals, where regular visits by the physician, skilled nursing care, and frequent electrocardiograms (ECG's) are available.

The best available evidence of impending toxicity from very high doses of Norpramin is prolongation of the QRS or QT intervals on the ECG. Prolongation of the PR interval is also significant, but less closely correlated with plasma levels. Clinical symptoms of intolerance, especially drowsiness, dizziness, and postural hypotension, should also alert the physician to the need for reduction in dosage. Plasma desipramine measurement would constitute the optimal guide to dosage monitoring.

Initial therapy may be administered in divided doses or a single daily dose.

Maintenance therapy may be given on a once-daily schedule for patient convenience and compliance.

Adolescent and Geriatric Dose

The usual adolescent and geriatric dose is 25 to 100 mg daily. Dosage should be initiated at a lower level and increased according to tolerance and clinical response to a usual maximum of 100 mg daily. In more severely ill patients, dosage may be further increased to 150 mg/day. Doses above 150 mg/day are not recommended in these age groups.

Initial therapy may be administered in divided doses or a single daily dose.

Maintenance therapy may be given on a once-daily schedule for patient convenience and compliance.

OVERDOSAGE

Signs, Symptoms, and Laboratory Findings

Signs and symptoms of toxicity with tricyclic antidepressants most often involve the cardiovascular and central nervous systems. Overdosage with this class of drugs has resulted in death. Within a few hours of ingestion, the patient may become agitated, restless, confused, delirious or stuporous and then comatose. Mydriasis, dry mucous membranes, vomiting, urinary retention, and diminished bowel sounds may occur. Hypotension, shock, respiratory depression, and renal shutdown may ensue. Generalized seizures, both early and later after ingestion, have been reported. Hyperactive reflexes, hyperpyrexia, and muscle rigidity can occur. ECG evidence of impaired conduction and serious disturbances of cardiac rate, rhythm, and output may occur. The duration of the QRS complex on ECG may be a helpful guide to the severity of tricyclic overdose. Physicians should be aware that relapses may occur after apparent recovery.

ORAL LD_{50}

The oral LD_{50} of desipramine is 290 mg/kg in male mice and 320 mg/kg in female rats.

Toxic and Lethal Doses/Plasma Levels

In humans, doses at 10-30 times the usual daily dosage have been considered within the lethal range. The lethal dose for children and geriatric patients would be lower than that for the general adult population. Serious adverse events in general are more frequently associated with plasma levels in excess of 1000 ng/mL.

Dialysis

After overdosage, low plasma desipramine concentrations are found because of the drug's large volume of distribution in the body. Forced diuresis and hemodialysis are, therefore, ineffective in removing tricyclic antidepressants.

Treatment

There is no specific antidote for desipramine overdosage, nor are there specific phenomena of diagnostic value characterizing poisoning by the drug.

Because CNS involvement, respiratory depression, and cardiac arrhythmia can occur suddenly, hospitalization and close observation are generally advisable, even when the amount ingested is thought to be small or the initial degree of intoxication appears slight or moderate. Aggressive supportive therapy of cardiac, neurologic, or acid-base disturbances may be necessary.

The initial phase of therapy in a tricyclic antidepressant overdose should be devoted to protection of the patient's airway, stabilization of the vital signs, establishing an intravenous line, obtaining an ECG, and initiating continuous cardiac monitoring, and maintaining renal output. It should be remembered that rapid deterioration of vital signs, seizures, respiratory failure, and ventricular arrhythmias are common during the first twenty-four hours after ingestion.

Ventricular arrhythmias and intraventricular conduction abnormalities may respond to administration of sodium bicarbonate to correct the metabolic acidosis. During alkalinization, the patient's electrolytes and renal function must be closely monitored with frequent laboratory determinations. Arrhythmias may be treated with standard antiarrhythmic therapy (e.g., lidocaine). Physostigmine may be used with caution to reverse severe cardiovascular abnormalities or coma; too rapid administration may result in seizures.

If the patient is hypotensive, supportive measures (e.g., intravenous fluids) should be used. Vasopressor agents may be used with caution if necessary.

If the patient develops seizures, intravenous diazepam may be used. In addition, longer acting anticonvulsants (e.g., barbiturates) may be necessary for repetitive seizures.

Once the patient is stabilized, gastric lavage with a large bore orogastric tube should be used to evacuate the stomach. The physician must be prepared to protect the airway by endotracheal intubation if seizures or loss of consciousness occur prior to completion of the lavage procedure. Because of the potential for rapid onset of life-threatening events, emesis should not be used to empty the stomach. Activated charcoal (as single or repeated doses) in a water slurry should be given by mouth or instilled through the lavage tube.

Additional information regarding treatment of overdosage may be available from poison control centers.

HOW SUPPLIED

10 mg blue coated tablets imprinted 68-7
  NDC 0068-0007-01: bottles of 100
25 mg yellow coated tablets imprinted NORPRAMIN 25
  NDC 0068-0011-01: bottles of 100
  NDC 0068-0011-61: unit dose dispenser of 100
  NDC 0068-0011-10: bottles of 1000
50 mg green coated tablets imprinted NORPRAMIN 50
  NDC 0068-0015-01: bottles of 100
  NDC 0068-0015-61: unit dose dispenser of 100
  NDC 0068-0015-10: bottles of 1000
75 mg orange coated tablets imprinted NORPRAMIN 75
  NDC 0068-0019-01: bottles of 100
100 mg peach coated tablets imprinted NORPRAMIN 100
  NDC 0068-0020-01: bottles of 100
150 mg white coated tablets imprinted NORPRAMIN 150
  NDC 0068-0021-50: bottles of 50

Norpramin tablets should be stored at room temperature, preferably below 86°F (30°C). Protect from excessive heat.

Product Information as of March, 1991

Shown in Product Identification Section, page 417

NOVAFED® A Capsules ℞

[nō ʹvă-fĕd]

Controlled-Release

Decongestant plus Antihistamine

CAUTION: Federal law prohibits dispensing without prescription.

DESCRIPTION

Each Novafed A capsule for oral use contains 120 mg pseudoephedrine hydrochloride and 8 mg chlorpheniramine maleate. The specially formulated pellets in each capsule are designed to provide continuous therapeutic effect for 12 hours. About one-half of the active ingredients is released soon after administration and the remainder is released slowly over the remaining time period. Each capsule also contains as inactive ingredients: calcium stearate, corn starch, FD&C Blue No. 1, FD&C Red No. 3, FD&C Yellow No. 6, gelatin, pharmaceutical glaze, povidone, sucrose, talc, titanium dioxide, and other ingredients.

Pseudoephedrine hydrochloride is a nasal decongestant. Chemically it is α-[1-(methylamino) ethyl]-[*S*-(*R**, *R**)]-benzenemethanol hydrochloride with the following structure:

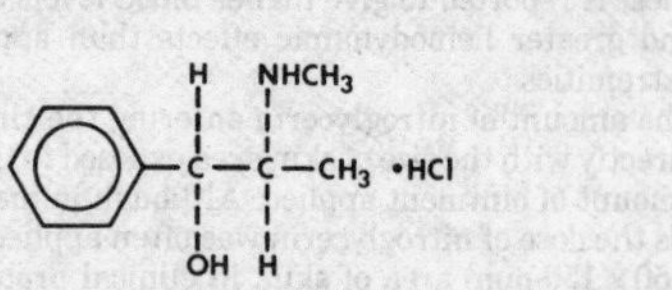

Chlorpheniramine maleate is an antihistamine. Chemically it is γ-(4-chlorophenyl)-N,N-dimethyl-2-pyridinepropanamine with the following structure:

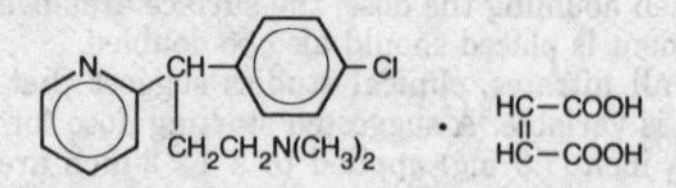

CLINICAL PHARMACOLOGY

Pseudoephedrine is an orally active sympathomimetic amine and exerts a decongestant action on the nasal mucosa. Pseudoephedrine produces peripheral effects similar to those of ephedrine and central effects similar to, but less intense than amphetamines. It has the potential for excitatory side effects. At the recommended oral dosages it has little or no pressor effect in normotensive adults. The serum half-life (T 1/2) of pseudoephedrine is approximately 4 to 6 hours. T 1/2 is decreased with increased excretion of drug at urine pH lower than 6 and may be increased with decreased excretion at urine pH higher than 8.

Chlorpheniramine is an antihistaminic that possesses anticholinergic and sedative effects. It is considered one of the

most effective and least toxic of the histamine antagonists. Chlorpheniramine is an H_1 receptor antagonist. It antagonizes many of the pharmacologic actions of histamine. It prevents released histamine from dilating capillaries and causing edema of the respiratory mucosa. Chlorpheniramine has a duration of action of 4 to 6 hours in clinical studies. Its half-life in serum, however, is 12 to 16 hours.

INDICATIONS AND USAGE

Relief of nasal congestion and eustachian tube congestion associated with the common cold, sinusitus and acute upper respiratory infections. It is also indicated for perennial and seasonal allergic rhinitis, vasomotor rhinitis, allergic conjunctivitis due to inhalant allergens and foods and for mild, uncomplicated allergic skin manifestations of urticaria and angioedema. Decongestants in combination with antihistamines have been used for many years to relieve eustachian tube congestion associated with acute eustachian salpingitis, aerotitis media, acute otitis media and serous otitis media. May be given concomitant with analgesics and antibiotics.

CONTRAINDICATIONS

Patients with severe hypertension, severe coronary artery disease, and in patients on MAO inhibitor therapy. Antihistamines are contraindicated in patients with narrow-angle glaucoma, urinary retention, peptic ulcer, during an asthmatic attack, and in patients receiving MAO inhibitors.
Hypersensitivity: Contraindicated in patients with hypersensitivity or idiosyncrasy to sympathomimetic amines or phenanthrene derivatives.
Nursing Mothers: Contraindicated because of the higher than usual risk for infants from sympathomimetic amines.

WARNINGS

Sympathomimetic amines should be used judiciously and sparingly in patients with hypertension, diabetes mellitus, ischemic heart disease, increased intraocular pressure, hyperthyroidism, or prostatic hypertrophy (see CONTRAINDICATIONS). Sympathomimetics may produce CNS stimulation and convulsions or cardiovascular collapse with accompanying hypotension.
Chlorpheniramine maleate has an atropine-like action and should be used with caution in patients with increased intraocular pressure, cardiovascular disease, hypertension or in patients with a history of bronchial asthma (see CONTRAINDICATIONS). Do not exceed recommended dose.
Use in Elderly: The elderly (60 years and older) are more likely to have adverse reactions to sympathomimetics. Overdosage of sympathomimetics in this age group may cause hallucinations, convulsions, CNS depression and death.

PRECAUTIONS

General: Should be used with caution in patients with diabetes, hypertension, cardiovascular disease and hyperreactivity to ephedrine. The antihistaminic may cause drowsiness and ambulatory patients who operate machinery or motor vehicles should be cautioned accordingly.
Information for Patients: Antihistamines may impair mental and physical abilities required for the performance of potentially hazardous tasks, such as driving a vehicle or operating machinery and mental alertness in children.
Drug Interactions: MAO inhibitors and beta adrenergic blockers increase the effect of sympathomimetics. Sympathomimetics may reduce the antihypertensive effects of methyldopa, mecamylamine, reserpine and veratrum alkaloids. Concomitant use of antihistamines with alcohol, tricyclic antidepressants, barbiturates and other CNS depressants may have an additive effect.
Pregnancy Category C: Animal reproduction studies have not been conducted with Novafed A capsules. It is also not known whether Novafed A capsules can cause fetal harm when administered to a pregnant woman or can affect reproduction capacity. Novafed A capsules may be given to a pregnant woman only if clearly needed.
Nursing Mothers: Pseudoephedrine is contraindicated in nursing mothers because of the higher than usual risk for infants from sympathomimetic amines.

ADVERSE REACTIONS

Hyperreactive individuals may display ephedrine-like reactions such as tachycardia, palpitations, headache, dizziness, or nausea. Patients sensitive to antihistamines may experience mild sedation. Sympathomimetic drugs have been associated with certain untoward reactions including fear, anxiety, tenseness, restlessness, tremor, weakness, pallor, respiratory difficulty, dysuria, insomnia, hallucinations, convulsions, CNS depression, arrhythmias, and cardiovascular collapse with hypotension.
Possible side effects of antihistamines are drowsiness, restlessness, dizziness, weakness, dry mouth, anorexia, nausea, headache, nervousness, blurring of vision, heartburn, dysuria and very rarely dermatitis. Patient idiosyncrasy to adrenergic agents may be manifested by insomnia, dizziness, weakness, tremor or arrhythmias.

OVERDOSAGE

Acute overdosage with Novafed A capsules may produce clinical signs of CNS stimulation and variable cardiovascular effects. Pressor amines should be used with great caution in the presence of pseudoephedrine. Patients with signs of stimulation should be treated conservatively.

DOSAGE AND ADMINISTRATION

One capsule every 12 hours. Do not give to children under 12 years of age.

HOW SUPPLIED

Novafed A is supplied in red and orange-colored hard gelatin capsules monogrammed with the Dow diamond followed by the number 106 or NOVAFED A, in bottles of 100 capsules (NDC 0068-0106-61).

Product Information as of April, 1986

Manufactured by KV Pharmaceutical Company
St. Louis, Mo. 63144

Shown in Product Identification Section, page 417

NOVAFED® Capsules ℞

[*nō ′vă-fĕd*]
(pseudoephedrine hydrochloride)
Controlled-Release Decongestant

DESCRIPTION

Each Novafed capsule contains 120 mg of pseudoephedrine hydrochloride in specially formulated pellets designed to provide continuous therapeutic effect for 12 hours. About one-half of the active ingredient is released soon after administration and the rest slowly over the remaining time period. Each capsule also contains as inactive ingredients: corn starch, FD&C Blue No. 1, FD&C Red No. 3, FD&C Yellow No. 6, gelatin, sucrose, titanium dioxide, and other ingredients.

ACTIONS

Pseudoephedrine (a sympathomimetic) is an orally effective nasal decongestant with peripheral effects similar to epinephrine and central effects similar to, but less intense than, amphetamines. It has the potential for excitatory side effects. At the recommended oral dosage, it has little or no pressor effect in normotensive adults. Patients have not been reported to experience the rebound congestion sometimes experienced with frequent, repeated use of topical decongestants.

INDICATIONS

Relief of nasal congestion or eustachian tube congestion. May be given concomitantly with analgesics, antihistamines, expectorants and antibiotics.

CONTRAINDICATIONS

Patients with severe hypertension, severe coronary artery disease, and patients on MAO inhibitor therapy. Also contraindicated in patients with hypersensitivity or idiosyncrasy to sympathomimetic amines which may be manifested by insomnia, dizziness, weakness, tremor or arrhythmias.
Children under 12: Should not be used by children under 12 years.
Nursing Mothers: Contraindicated because of the higher than usual risk for infants from sympathomimetic amines.

WARNINGS

Use judiciously and sparingly in patients with hypertension, diabetes mellitus, ischemic heart disease, increased intraocular pressure, hyperthyroidism, or prostatic hypertrophy. See, however, Contraindications. Sympathomimetics may produce central nervous stimulation with convulsions or cardiovascular collapse with accompanying hypotension.
Do not exceed recommended dosage.
Use in Pregnancy: Safety in pregnancy has not been established.
Use in Elderly: The elderly (60 years and older) are more likely to have adverse reactions to sympathomimetics. Overdosage of sympathomimetics in the elderly may cause hallucinations, convulsions, CNS depression, and death. Safe use of a short-acting sympathomimetic should be demonstrated in the individual elderly patient before considering the use of a sustained-action formulation.

PRECAUTIONS

Patients with diabetes, hypertension, cardiovascular disease and hyper-reactivity to ephedrine.

ADVERSE REACTIONS

Hyper-reactive individuals may display ephedrine-like reactions such as tachycardia, palpitations, headache, dizziness or nausea. Sympathomimetics have been associated with certain untoward reactions including fear, anxiety, tenseness, restlessness, tremor, weakness, pallor, respiratory difficulty, dysuria, insomnia, hallucinations, convulsions, CNS depression, arrhythmias, and cardiovascular collapse with hypotension.

DRUG INTERACTIONS

MAO inhibitors and beta adrenergic blockers increase the effects of pseudoephedrine. Sympathomimetics may reduce the antihypertensive effects of methyldopa, mecamylamine, reserpine and veratrum alkaloids.

DOSAGE AND ADMINISTRATION

One capsule every 12 hours. Do not give to children under 12 years of age.

HOW SUPPLIED

Brown and orange colored hard gelatin capsules with the identification code DOW or NOVAFED. Bottle of 100 capsules
(NDC 0068-0104-61).

Product Information as of June, 1991

Manufactured by KV Pharmaceutical Company
St. Louis, Mo. 63144 for
Marion Merrell Dow Inc.
Kansas City, MO 64114

Shown in Product Identification Section, page 417

NOVAHISTINE® DH Ⓒ

[*nō″vă-hĭs′tēn*]
Antitussive-Decongestant-Antihistamine

DESCRIPTION

Each 5 ml teaspoonful contains Codeine Phosphate, 10 mg (Warning: may be habit forming), Pseudoephedrine Hydrochloride, 30 mg, Chlorpheniramine Maleate, 2 mg. Also contains: Alcohol, 5%, FD&C Blue No. 1, FD&C Red No. 40, Flavors, Glycerin, Hydrochloric Acid, Invert Sugar, Saccharin Sodium, Sodium Chloride, Sorbitol, and Water.

ACTIONS

Antitussive, decongestant and antihistaminic actions. Codeine, at the recommended dose, causes suppression of the cough reflex by a direct effect on the cough center in the medulla of the brain. Codeine has antitussive, mild analgesic and sedative effects.
Pseudoephedrine hydrochloride, an orally effective nasal decongestant, is a sympathomimetic amine with peripheral effects similar to epinephrine and central effects similar to, but less intense than, amphetamines. Therefore, it has the potential for excitatory side effects. Pseudoephedrine at the recommended oral dosage has little or no pressor effect in normotensive adults. Patients taking pseudoephedrine orally have not been reported to experience the rebound congestion sometimes experienced with frequent, repeated use of topical decongestants. Pseudoephedrine is not known to produce drowsiness.
Chlorpheniramine possesses antihistaminic, mild anticholinergic and sedative effects. It antagonizes many of the pharmacologic actions of histamine. It prevents released histamine from dilating capillaries and causing edema of the respiratory mucosa.

INDICATIONS

For the temporary relief of cough associated with minor throat and bronchial irritation or nasal congestion due to the common cold, sinusitis, and hay fever (allergic rhinitis).
A minimum dosage of codeine is provided for the symptomatic relief of nonproductive cough. Decongestants have been used to relieve eustachian salpingitis, aerotitis, otitis, and serous otitis media. Chlorpheniramine maleate provides temporary relief from runny nose, sneezing, itching of nose or throat, and itchy and watery eyes as may occur in hay fever (allergic rhinitis).
May be used as supportive therapy for acute otitis media and relief of mild otalgia.
May be given concomitantly, when indicated, with analgesics and antibiotics.

CONTRAINDICATIONS

Patients with severe hypertension, severe coronary artery disease, and in patients on MAO inhibitor therapy.
Nursing Mothers: Pseudoephedrine is contraindicated in nursing mothers because of the higher than usual risk for infants from sympathomimetic amines.
Hypersensitivity: This drug is contraindicated in patients with hypersensitivity or idiosyncrasy to its ingredients. Patient idiosyncrasy to adrenergic agents may be manifested by insomnia, dizziness, weakness, tremor or arrhythmias.

WARNINGS

Codeine should be prescribed and administered with the same degree of caution as all oral medications containing a narcotic analgesic. Codeine appears in the milk of nursing mothers.
If sympathomimetic amines are used in patients with hypertension, diabetes mellitus, ischemic heart disease, hyperthyroidism, increased intraocular pressure or prostatic hypertrophy, judicious caution should be exercised. See, however, Contraindications. Sympathomimetics may produce CNS stimulation with convulsions or cardiovascular collapse with accompanying hypotension. Do not exceed recommended dosage.

Continued on next page

Marion Merrell Dow—Cont.

The elderly (60 years and older) are more likely to have adverse reactions to sympathomimetics. Safety for use during pregnancy has not been established.

Antihistamines may cause excitability, especially in children.

PRECAUTIONS

If cough persists for more than one week, tends to recur or is accompanied by fever, rash or headache, discontinue treatment. Other medications containing a narcotic analgesic, phenothiazines, tranquilizers, sedatives, hypnotics and other CNS depressants, including alcohol, may have an additive CNS depressant effect when used concomitantly. The dose should be reduced when such combined therapy is contemplated.

Caution should be exercised if used in patients with high blood pressure, heart disease, asthma, emphysema, diabetes, thyroid disease and hyperreactivity to ephedrine.

The antihistamine may cause drowsiness, and ambulatory patients who operate machinery or motor vehicles should be cautioned accordingly.

ADVERSE REACTIONS

Nausea, vomiting, constipation, dizziness, sedation, palpitations or pruritus may occur. More frequent or higher than recommended dosage may cause respiratory depression, especially in patients with respiratory disease associated with carbon dioxide retention.

Drugs containing sympathomimetic amines have been associated with certain untoward reactions including fear, anxiety, tenseness, restlessness, tremor, weakness, pallor, respiratory difficulty, dysuria, insomnia, hallucinations, convulsions, CNS depression, arrhythmias and cardiovascular collapse with hypotension.

Patients sensitive to antihistamine drugs may experience mild sedation. Other side effects from antihistamines may include dry mouth, dizziness, weakness, anorexia, nausea, vomiting, headache, nervousness, polyuria, heartburn, diplopia, dysuria, and very rarely, dermatitis.

DRUG INTERACTIONS

Codeine may potentiate the effects of other narcotics, general anesthetics, tranquilizers, sedatives and hypnotics, tricyclic antidepressants, MAO inhibitors, alcohol and other CNS depressants.

Beta adrenergic blockers and MAO inhibitors potentiate the sympathomimetic effects of pseudoephedrine. Sympathomimetics may reduce the antihypertensive effects of methyldopa, mecamylamine, reserpine and veratrum alkaloids.

Antihistamines have been shown to enhance one or more of the effects of alcohol, tricyclic antidepressants, barbiturates and other CNS depressants.

DOSAGE

Adults, 2 teaspoonfuls; children 50–90 lbs, ½ to 1 teaspoonful; 25–50 lbs, ¼ to ½ teaspoonful. Repeat every 4 to 6 hours. May be given to children under 2 at the discretion of the physician. *Do not exceed 4 doses in a 24-hour period.*
Product label dosage is as follows: Adults and children 12 years and older, 2 teaspoonfuls every 4 to 6 hours. Children 6 to under 12 years, 1 teaspoonful every 4 to 6 hours. Do not exceed 4 doses in 24 hours. For children under 6 years, give only as directed by a physician.

HOW SUPPLIED

In 4 fluid ounce bottles (NDC 0068-1027-04), and pints (NDC 0068-1027-16).

Product Information as of May, 1986
Shown in Product Identification Section, page 417

NOVAHISTINE® DMX   OTC
[nō"vă-hĭs'tēn]
Antitussive-Decongestant-Expectorant
Liquid

(See PDR For Nonprescription Drugs.)

NOVAHISTINE® ELIXIR   OTC
[nō"vă-hĭs'tēn]
Decongestant—Antihistaminic

(See PDR For Nonprescription Drugs.)

NOVAHISTINE® EXPECTORANT   ℃
[nō"vă-hĭs'tēn]
with Codeine
Antitussive-Decongestant-Expectorant

DESCRIPTION

Each 5 ml teaspoonful contains Codeine Phosphate, 10 mg (Warning: may be habit forming), Pseudoephedrine Hydrochloride, 30 mg, Guaifenesin, 100 mg. Also contains: Alcohol, 7.5%, D&C Yellow No. 10, FD&C Blue No. 1, FD&C Red No. 40, Flavors, Glycerin, Hydrochloric Acid, Invert Sugar, Saccharin Sodium, Sodium Chloride, Sodium Gluconate, Sorbitol, and Water.

ACTIONS

Expectorant, antitussive and decongestant actions. Codeine, at the recommended dose, causes suppression of the cough reflex by a direct effect on the cough center in the medulla of the brain. Codeine has antitussive and mild analgesic and sedative effects.

Pseudoephedrine hydrochloride, an orally effective nasal decongestant, is a sympathomimetic amine with peripheral effects similar to epinephrine and central effects similar to, but less intense than, amphetamines. Therefore, it has the potential for excitatory side effects. Pseudoephedrine at the recommended oral dosage has little or no pressor effect in normotensive adults. Patients taking pseudoephedrine orally have not been reported to experience the rebound congestion sometimes experienced with frequent, repeated use of topical decongestants. Pseudoephedrine is not known to produce drowsiness.

Guaifenesin helps drainage of bronchial tubes by thinning the mucus, and facilitates expectoration by loosening phlegm and bronchial secretions.

INDICATIONS

For loosening tenacious pulmonary secretions associated with cough and respiratory congestion.
A minimum dosage of codeine phosphate is provided for the symptomatic relief of nonproductive cough. Decongestants have been used to relieve eustachian tube congestion associated with acute eustachian salpingitis, aerotitis, otitis and serous otitis media. Guaifenesin helps loosen phlegm (sputum) and bronchial secretions.
May be used as supportive therapy for acute otitis media and relief of mild otalgia.
May be given concomitantly, when indicated, with analgesics and antibiotics.

CONTRAINDICATIONS

Patients with severe hypertension, severe coronary artery disease, and in patients on MAO inhibitor therapy.
Nursing Mothers: Pseudoephedrine is contraindicated in nursing mothers because of the higher than usual risk for infants from sympathomimetic amines.
Hypersensitivity: This drug is contraindicated in patients with hypersensitivity or idiosyncrasy to its ingredients. Patient idiosyncrasy to adrenergic agents may be manifested by insomnia, dizziness, weakness, tremor or arrhythmias.

WARNINGS

Codeine should be prescribed and administered with the same degree of caution as all oral medications containing a narcotic analgesic. Codeine appears in the milk of nursing mothers.

If sympathomimetic amines are used in patients with hypertension, diabetes mellitus, ischemic heart disease, hyperthyroidism, increased intraocular pressure and prostatic hypertrophy, judicious caution should be exercised. See, however, Contraindications. Sympathomimetics may produce CNS stimulation with convulsions or cardiovascular collapse with accompanying hypotension. Do not exceed recommended dosage.

The elderly (60 years and older) are more likely to have adverse reactions to sympathomimetics. Safety for use during pregnancy has not been established.

PRECAUTIONS

If cough persists for more than one week, tends to recur or is accompanied by fever, rash or headache, discontinue treatment.

Other medications containing a narcotic analgesic, phenothiazines, tranquilizers, sedatives, hypnotics, and other CNS depressants, including alcohol, may have an additive CNS depressant effect when used concomitantly. The dose should be reduced when such combined therapy is contemplated. Caution should be exercised if used in patients with high blood pressure, heart disease, asthma, emphysema, diabetes, thyroid disease and hyperreactivity to ephedrine.

ADVERSE REACTIONS

Nausea, vomiting, constipation, dizziness, sedation, palpitations, or pruritus may occur. More frequent or higher than recommended dosage may cause respiratory depression, especially in patients with respiratory disease associated with carbon dioxide retention.

Drugs containing sympathomimetic amines have been associated with certain untoward reactions including fear, anxi-

ety, tenseness, restlessness, tremor, weakness, pallor, respiratory difficulty, dysuria, insomnia, hallucinations, convulsions, CNS depression, arrhythmias and cardiovascular collapse with hypotension.

Note: Guaifenesin interferes with the colorimetric determination of 5-hydroxyindoleacetic acid (5-HIAA) and vanillylmandelic acid (VMA).

DRUG INTERACTIONS

Codeine may potentiate the effects of other narcotics, general anesthetics, tranquilizers, sedatives and hypnotics, tricyclic antidepressants, MAO inhibitors, alcohol and other CNS depressants.

Beta adrenergic blockers and MAO inhibitors potentiate the sympathomimetic effects of pseudoephedrine. Sympathomimetics may reduce the antihypertensive effects of methyldopa, mecamylamine, reserpine and veratrum alkaloids.

DOSAGE

Adults, 2 teaspoonfuls; children 50–90 lbs, ½ to 1 teaspoonful; 25–50 lbs, ¼ to ½ teaspoonful. Repeat every 4 hours. May be given to children under 2 at the discretion of the physician. *Do not exceed 4 doses in a 24-hour period.*
Product label dosage is as follows: Adults and children 12 years and older, 2 teaspoonfuls every 4 hours. Children 6 to under 12 years, 1 teaspoonful every 4 hours. Do not exceed 4 doses in 24 hours. For children under 6 years, give only as directed by a physician.

HOW SUPPLIED

As a liquid in 4 fluid ounce bottles (NDC 0068-1028-04) and pints (NDC 0068-1028-16).

Product Information as of June, 1989
Shown in Product Identification Section, page 417

OS-CAL® 250+D Tablets   OTC
[ahs'kal]
calcium supplement with vitamin D

(See PDR For Nonprescription Drugs.)

OS-CAL® 500 Chewable Tablets   OTC
[ahs'kal]
calcium supplement

(See PDR For Nonprescription Drugs.)

OS-CAL® 500 Tablets   OTC
[ahs'kal]
calcium supplement

(See PDR For Nonprescription Drugs.)

OS-CAL® 500+D Tablets   OTC
[ahs'kal]
calcium supplement with vitamin D

(See PDR For Nonprescription Drugs.)

OS-CAL® FORTIFIED Tablets   OTC
[ahs'kal for'te-fĭd]
multivitamin and minerals supplement
New name—Formerly marketed as Os-Cal Forte

(See PDR For Nonprescription Drugs.)

OS-CAL® PLUS Tablets   OTC
[ahs'kal]
multivitamin and multimineral supplement

(See PDR For Nonprescription Drugs.)

PAVABID® Plateau CAPS®   ℞
[pav'uh-bid]
(papaverine hydrochloride) 150 mg

COMPOSITION

Each capsule contains:
Papaverine hydrochloride .... 150 mg
in a specially prepared base to provide prolonged activity.
Also contains: calcium stearate, starch, stearic acid, sucrose, talc, and other ingredients.

ACTION AND USES

The main actions of papaverine are exerted on cardiac and smooth muscle. Like quinidine, papaverine acts directly on the heart muscle to depress conduction and prolong the re-

fractory period. Papaverine relaxes various smooth muscles. This relaxation may be prominent if spasm exists. The muscle cell is not paralyzed by papaverine, and still responds to drugs and other stimuli causing contraction. The antispasmodic effect is a direct one, and unrelated to muscle innervation. Papaverine is practically devoid of effects on the central nervous system.
Papaverine relaxes the smooth musculature of the larger blood vessels, especially coronary, systemic peripheral, and pulmonary arteries. Perhaps by its direct vasodilating action on cerebral blood vessels, papaverine increases cerebral blood flow and decreases cerebral vascular resistance in normal subjects; oxygen consumption is unaltered. These effects may explain the benefit reported from the drug in cerebral vascular encephalopathy.
The direct actions of papaverine on the heart to depress conduction and irritability and to prolong the refractory period of the myocardium provide the basis for its clinical trial in abrogating atrial and ventricular premature systoles and ominous ventricular arrhythmias. The coronary vasodilator action could be an additional factor of therapeutic value when such rhythms are secondary to insufficiency or occlusion of the coronary arteries.
In patients with acute coronary thrombosis, the occurrence of ventricular rhythms is serious and requires measures designed to decrease myocardial irritability. Papaverine may have advantages over quinidine, used for a similar purpose, in that it may be given in an emergency by the intravenous route, does not depress myocardial contraction or cause cinchonism, and produces coronary vasodilation.

INDICATIONS
For the relief of cerebral and peripheral ischemia associated with arterial spasm and myocardial ischemia complicated by arrhythmias.

PRECAUTIONS
Use with caution in patients with glaucoma. Hepatic hypersensitivity has been reported with gastrointestinal symptoms, jaundice, eosinophilia, and altered liver function tests. Discontinue medication if these occur.

ADVERSE REACTIONS
Although occurring rarely, the reported side effects of papaverine include nausea, abdominal distress, anorexia, constipation, malaise, drowsiness, vertigo, sweating, headache, diarrhea, and skin rash.

DOSAGE AND ADMINISTRATION
One capsule every 12 hours. In difficult cases administration may be increased to one capsule every 8 hours or two capsules every 12 hours.

HOW SUPPLIED
PAVABID® (papaverine hydrochloride) Capsules are available in bottles of 100 (NDC 0088-1555-47). Capsules are imprinted with MARION/1555.

CAUTION
Federal law prohibits dispensing without prescription.

Shown in Product Identification Section, page 417

Issued 2/89

QUINAMM™ 260 mg ℞
[kwĭn 'ăm]
(quinine sulfate tablets)

DESCRIPTION
Quinamm is available as tablets for oral administration. Each tablet contains 260 mg quinine sulfate. Also contains, as inactive ingredients: corn starch, pregelatinized starch, sodium starch glycolate, sucrose, and zinc stearate.
Neuromuscular Agent
Quinine sulfate has the following structural formula:

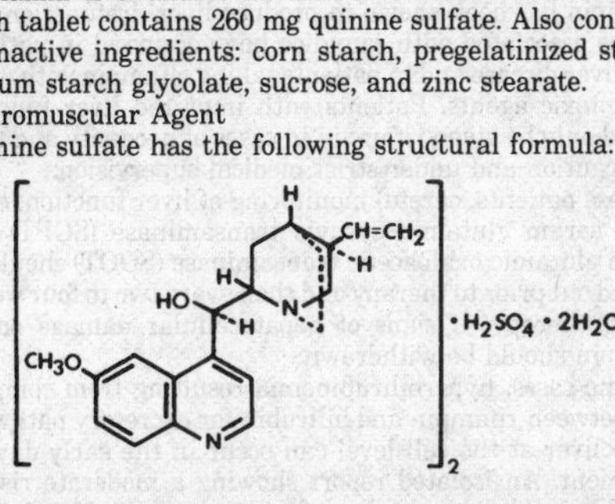

Quinine sulfate occurs as a white, crystalline powder, which darkens on exposure to light. It is odorless and has a persistent, very bitter taste. It is slightly soluble in water, alcohol, chloroform, and ether.

CLINICAL PHARMACOLOGY
Quinine, a cinchona alkaloid, acts on skeletal muscle by three mechanisms: it increases the refractory period by direct action on the muscle fiber, it decreases the excitability of the motor end-plate, an action similar to that of curare, and it affects the distribution of calcium within the muscle fiber. Quinine is readily absorbed when given orally. Absorption occurs mainly from the upper part of the small intestine, and is almost complete even in patients with marked diarrhea. The cinchona alkaloids in large measure are metabolically degraded in the body, especially in the liver; less than 5% of an administered dose is excreted unaltered in the urine. It is reported that there is no accumulation of the drugs in the body upon continued administration. The metabolic degradation products are excreted in the urine, where many of them have been identified as hydroxy derivatives, but small amounts also appear in the feces, gastric juice, bile, and saliva. Renal excretion of quinine is twice as rapid when the urine is acidic as when it is alkaline, due to the greater tubular reabsorption of the alkaloidal base that occurs in an alkaline media. Excretion is also limited by the binding of a large fraction of cinchona alkaloids to plasma proteins.
Peak plasma concentrations of cinchona alkaloids occur within 1 to 3 hours after a single oral dose. The half-life is 4 to 5 hours. After chronic administration of total daily doses of 1 g of drug, the average plasma quinine concentration is approximately 7 μg/ml. After termination of quinine therapy, the plasma level falls rapidly and only a negligible concentration is detectable after 24 hours.
A large fraction (approximately 70%) of the plasma quinine is bound to proteins. This explains in part why the concentration of the alkaloid in cerebrospinal fluid is only 2 to 5% of that in the plasma. However, it can traverse the placental membrane and readily reach fetal tissues.
Tinnitus and impairment of hearing rarely should occur at plasma quinine concentrations of less than 10 μg/ml. While this level would not be anticipated from use of 1 or 2 tablets of Quinamm daily, an occasional patient may have some evidence of cinchonism on this dosage, such as tinnitus. (See WARNINGS section.)

INDICATIONS AND USAGE
For the prevention and treatment of nocturnal recumbency leg muscle cramps.

CONTRAINDICATIONS
Quinamm may cause fetal harm when administered to a pregnant woman. Congenital malformations in the human have been reported with the use of quinine, primarily with large doses (up to 30 g) for attempted abortion. In about half of these reports, the malformation was deafness related to auditory nerve hypoplasia. Among the other abnormalities reported were limb anomalies, visceral defects, and visual changes. In animal tests, teratogenic effects were found in rabbits and guinea pigs and were absent in mice, rats, dogs, and monkeys. Quinamm is contraindicated in women who are or may become pregnant. If this drug is used during pregnancy, or if the patient becomes pregnant while taking this drug, the patient should be apprised of the potential hazard to the fetus.
Because of the quinine content, Quinamm is contraindicated in patients with known quinine hypersensitivity and in patients with glucose-6-phosphate dehydrogenase (G-6-PD) deficiency.
Since thrombocytopenic purpura may follow the administration of quinine in highly sensitive patients, a history of this occurrence associated with previous quinine ingestion contraindicates its further use. Recovery usually occurs following withdrawal of the medication and appropriate therapy.
This drug should not be used in patients with tinnitus or optic neuritis or in patients with a history of blackwater fever.

WARNINGS
Repeated doses or overdosage of quinine in some individuals may precipitate a cluster of symptoms referred to as cinchonism. Such symptoms, in the mildest form, include ringing in the ears, headache, nausea, and slightly disturbed vision; however, when medication is continued or after large single doses, symptoms also involve the gastrointestinal tract, the nervous and cardiovascular systems, and the skin.
Hemolysis (with the potential for hemolytic anemia) has been associated with a G-6-PD deficiency in patients taking quinine. Quinamm should be stopped immediately if evidence of hemolysis appears.
If symptoms occur, drug should be discontinued and supportive measures instituted. In case of overdosage, see OVERDOSAGE section of prescribing information.

PRECAUTIONS
General
Quinamm should be discontinued if there is any evidence of hypersensitivity. (See CONTRAINDICATIONS.) Cutaneous flushing, pruritus, skin rashes, fever, gastric distress, dyspnea, ringing in the ears, and visual impairment are the usual expressions of hypersensitivity, particularly if only small doses of quinine have been taken. Extreme flushing of the skin accompanied by intense, generalized pruritus is the most common form. Hemoglobinuria and asthma from quinine are rare types of idiosyncrasy.
In patients with atrial fibrillation, the administration of quinine requires the same precautions as those for quinidine. (See *Drug Interactions.*)

Drug Interactions
Increased plasma levels of digoxin have been demonstrated in individuals after concomitant quinine administration. Increased plasma levels of digitoxin have been demonstrated in individuals after concomitant quinidine administration. It is therefore recommended that plasma levels of digoxin or digitoxin be determined periodically for those individuals taking either of these glycosides and Quinamm concomitantly.
Concurrent use of aluminum-containing antacids may delay or decrease absorption of quinine.
Cinchona alkaloids, including quinine, have the potential to depress the hepatic enzyme system that synthesizes the vitamin K-dependent factors. The resulting hypoprothrombinemic effect may enhance the action of warfarin and other oral anticoagulants.
The effects of neuromuscular blocking agents (particularly pancuronium, succinylcholine, and tubocurarine) may be potentiated with quinine, and result in respiratory difficulties.
Urinary alkalizers (such as acetazolamide and sodium bicarbonate) may increase quinine blood levels with potential for toxicity.
Drug/Laboratory Interactions
Quinine may produce an elevated value for urinary 17-ketogenic steroids when the Zimmerman method is used.
Carcinogenesis, Mutagenesis, Impairment of Fertility
A study of quinine sulfate administered in drinking water (0.1%) to rats for periods up to 20 months showed no evidence of neoplastic changes.
Mutation studies of quinine (dihydrochloride) in male and female mice gave negative results by the micronucleus test. Intraperitoneal injections (0.5 mM/kg) were given twice, 24 hours apart. Direct *Salmonella typhimurium* tests were negative; when mammalian liver homogenate was added, positive results were found.
Mutation studies of quinine hydrochloride, 100 mg/kg, p.o. in Chinese hamsters showed no genotoxic activity in the sister chromatid exchange (SCE) test, micronucleus test, or chromosome aberration test. In mice given quinine hydrochloride, 100 mg/kg, p.o., the micronucleus test and chromosome aberration test were negative; the SCE test exhibited an increase of SCEs/cell. Tests were repeated in two inbred strains of mice using 55, 75, and 110 mg/kg p.o. The effect was more pronounced in these mice and the increase in SCEs/cell demonstrated a linear dose relationship. One of the inbred strains had positive micronucleus test findings. The chromosome aberration test also revealed an increase of chromatid breaks. The Ames test system results were negative for point mutation.
No information relating to the effect of quinine upon fertility in animal or in man has been found.
Pregnancy
Category X. See CONTRAINDICATIONS.
Nonteratogenic Effects
Because quinine crosses the placenta in humans, the potential for fetal effects is present. Stillbirths in mothers taking quinine have been reported in which no obvious cause for the fetal deaths was shown. Quinine in toxic amounts has been associated with abortion. Whether this action is always due to direct effect on the uterus is questionable.
Nursing Mothers
Caution should be exercised when Quinamm is given to nursing women because quinine is excreted in breast milk (in small amounts).

ADVERSE REACTIONS
The following adverse reactions have been reported with Quinamm in therapeutic or excessive dosage. (Individual or multiple symptoms may represent cinchonism or hypersensitivity.)
Hematologic: acute hemolysis, thrombocytopenic purpura, agranulocytosis, hypoprothrombinemia
CNS: visual disturbances, including blurred vision with scotomata, photophobia, diplopia, diminished visual fields, and disturbed color vision; tinnitus, deafness, and vertigo; headache, nausea, vomiting, fever, apprehension, restlessness, confusion, and syncope
Dermatologic/allergic: cutaneous rashes (urticarial, the most frequent type of allergic reaction, papular, or scarlatinal), pruritus, flushing of the skin, sweating, occasional edema of the face
Respiratory: asthmatic symptoms
Cardiovascular: anginal symptoms
Gastrointestinal: nausea and vomiting (may be CNS-related), epigastric pain, hepatitis

DRUG ABUSE AND DEPENDENCE
Tolerance, abuse, or dependence with Quinamm has not been reported.

OVERDOSAGE
The more common signs and symptoms of overdosage are tinnitus, dizziness, skin rash, and gastrointestinal disturbance (intestinal cramping). With higher doses, cardiovascu-

Continued on next page

Marion Merrell Dow—Cont.

lar and CNS effects may occur, including headache, fever, vomiting, apprehension, confusion, and convulsions. Other effects are listed in the ADVERSE REACTIONS section.

Fatalities with quinine have been reported from single oral doses of 2 to 8 grams; a single fatality reported with a dose of 1.5 grams may reflect an idiosyncratic effect. Several cases of blindness following large overdoses of quinine, with partial recovery of vision in each instance, have been reported. Tinnitus and impaired hearing may occur at plasma quinine concentrations over 10 μg/ml. This level would not be normally attained with the use of 1 or 2 Quinamm tablets daily, but in a hypersensitive patient, as little as 0.3 g of quinine may produce tinnitus.

Treatment

Treatment for overdosage should include initially efforts to remove any residual Quinamm from the stomach by gastric lavage or by emesis induced with syrup of ipecac. The blood pressure should be supported and measures used to maintain renal function. Artificial respiration may be needed. Sedatives, oxygen, and other supportive measures should be used as necessary.

Fluid and electrolyte balance with intravenous fluids should be maintained. Acidification of the urine will promote renal excretion of quinine. In the presence of hemoglobinuria, however, acidification of the urine may augment renal blockade. Quinine should be readily dialyzable by hemodialysis and/or hemoperfusion procedures.

Evidence of angioedema or asthma may require the use of epinephrine, corticosteroids, and antihistamines. In the acute phase of toxic amaurosis caused by quinine, vasodilators administered intravenously may have a salutary effect. Stellate block has also been used effectively for quinine-associated blindness. Residual visual impairment occasionally yields to vasodilators.

DOSAGE AND ADMINISTRATION

1 tablet upon retiring. If needed, 2 tablets may be taken nightly—1 following the evening meal and 1 upon retiring. After several consecutive nights in which recumbency leg cramps do not occur, Quinamm may be discontinued in order to determine whether continued therapy is needed.

HOW SUPPLIED

NDC 0068-0547-15

260 mg tablets in bottles of 100. Tablets are round, white, debossed W one side, Merrell 547 other side.

Store at room temperature, below 86°F (30°C).

Product Information as of May, 1991

Shown in Product Identification Section, page 417

RIFADIN® ℞

[rĭf'ă-dĭn]

(rifampin capsules)

and

RIFADIN® I.V.

(rifampin for injection)

DESCRIPTION

Rifadin (rifampin) capsules for oral administration contain 150 mg or 300 mg rifampin per capsule. The 150 mg capsules also contain, as inactive ingredients: corn starch, edible white ink, FD&C Blue No. 1, FD&C Red No. 3, FD&C Red No. 40, gelatin, magnesium stearate, and titanium dioxide. The 300 mg capsules also contain, as inactive ingredients: corn starch, D&C Red No. 28, FD&C Blue No. 1, FD&C Red No. 40, gelatin, magnesium stearate, and titanium dioxide.

Rifadin I.V. (rifampin for injection) contains rifampin 600 mg, sodium formaldehyde sulfoxylate 10 mg, and sodium hydroxide to adjust pH.

Rifampin is a semisynthetic antibiotic derivative of rifamycin B. The chemical name for rifampin is 3-(4-methyl-1-piperazinyl-iminomethyl)-rifamycin SV. Its chemical structure is:

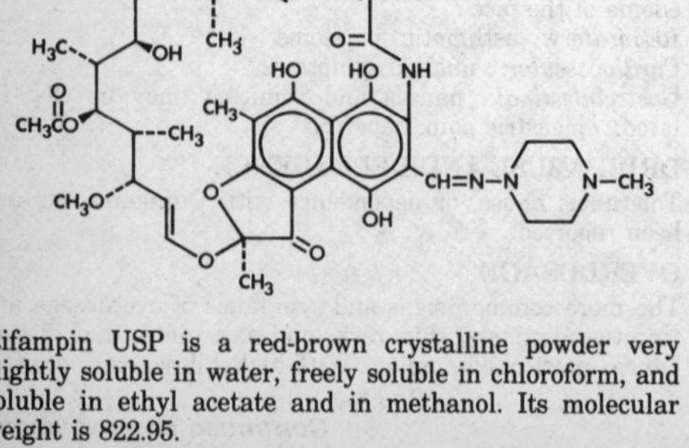

Rifampin USP is a red-brown crystalline powder very slightly soluble in water, freely soluble in chloroform, and soluble in ethyl acetate and in methanol. Its molecular weight is 822.95.

CLINICAL PHARMACOLOGY

Human Pharmacology —Oral

Rifampin is readily absorbed from the gastrointestinal tract. Peak blood levels in normal adults vary widely from individual to individual. The peak level averages 7 μg/mL but may vary from 4 to 32 μg/mL. Absorption of rifampin is reduced when the drug is ingested with food.

In normal subjects, the biological half-life of rifampin in serum averages about 3 hours after a 600 mg oral dose, with increases up to 5.1 hours reported after a 900 mg dose. With repeated administration, the half-life decreases and reaches average values of approximately 2–3 hours. It does not differ in patients with renal failure at doses not exceeding 600 mg daily and, consequently, no dosage adjustment is required. Refer to WARNINGS for information regarding patients with hepatic insufficiency.

After absorption, rifampin is rapidly eliminated in the bile, and an enterohepatic circulation ensues. During this process, rifampin undergoes progressive deacetylation so that nearly all the drug in the bile is in this form in about 6 hours. This metabolite is microbiologically active. Intestinal reabsorption is reduced by deacetylation, and elimination is facilitated. Up to 30% of a dose is excreted in the urine, with about half of this being unchanged drug.

Rifampin is widely distributed throughout the body. It is present in effective concentrations in many organs and body fluids, including cerebrospinal fluid. Rifampin is about 80% protein bound. Most of the unbound fraction is not ionized and therefore diffuses freely into tissues.

Serum Levels in Children

In one recent study, children 6–58 months old were given rifampin suspended in simple syrup or as dry powder mixed with applesauce at a dose of 10 mg/kg body weight. Peak serum levels of 10.7 and 11.5 μg/mL were obtained 1 hour after preprandial ingestion of the drug suspension and the applesauce mixture, respectively. The calculated $t_{1/2}$ for both preparations was 2.9 hrs. It should be noted that in other studies in children, at doses of 10 mg/kg body weight, mean peak serum levels of 3.5 μg/mL to 15 μg/mL have been reported.

Human Pharmacology —I.V.

After intravenous administration of a 300 or 600 mg dose of rifampin infused over 30 minutes to healthy male volunteers (n=11), mean peak plasma concentrations were 9.0 and 17.5 μg/mL, respectively. The average plasma concentrations in these volunteers remained detectable for 8 and 12 hours, respectively (see table).

Rifampin Dosage I.V.	Plasma Concentrations (μg/mL) 30 min.	1 hr	2 hr	4 hr	8 hr	12 hr
300 mg	8.9	4.9	4.0	2.5	<2	<2
600 mg	17.4	11.7	9.4	6.4	3.5	<2

Plasma concentrations after the 600 mg dose, which were disproportionately higher (up to 50% greater than expected) than those found after the 300 mg dose, indicated that the elimination of larger doses was not as rapid.

After repeated once-a-day infusions (3 hr duration) of 600 mg in patients (n=5) for 7 days, concentrations of I.V. rifampin decreased from 5.8 μg/mL 8 hours after the infusion on day 1 to 2.6 μg/mL 8 hours after the infusion on day 7.

The rifampin dose is widely distributed throughout the body. It is present in effective concentrations in many organs and body fluids, including cerebrospinal fluid. Rifampin is about 80% protein bound. Most of the unbound fraction is not ionized and therefore diffuses freely into tissues.

Rifampin is rapidly eliminated in the bile and undergoes progressive enterohepatic circulation and deacetylation to the primary metabolite, 25-desacetyl-rifampin. This metabolite is microbiologically active. Less than 30% of the dose is excreted as rifampin or metabolites. Serum concentrations do not differ in patients with renal failure and, consequently, no dosage adjustment is required.

Serum Concentrations of Rifampin in Children

In patients 0.25 to 12.8 years old (n=12), the mean peak serum concentration of rifampin at the end of a 30 minute infusion of approximately 300 mg/m^2 was 26 μg/mL. In these patients, peak concentrations 1 to 4 days after initiation of therapy ranged from 11.7 to 41.5 μg/mL; peak concentrations 5 to 14 days after initiation of therapy were 13.6 to 37.4 μg/mL. The serum half-life of rifampin decreased significantly from 1.34 to 3.24 hours early in therapy to 1.17 to 3.19 hours 5 to 14 days after therapy was initiated.

Microbiology

Rifampin inhibits DNA-dependent RNA polymerase activity in susceptible cells. Specifically, it interacts with bacterial RNA polymerase but does not inhibit the mammalian enzyme. Rifampin is particularly active against rapidly growing extracellular organisms but has been demonstrated to have intracellular bactericidal activity against susceptible organisms as well.

Cross-resistance to rifampin has been shown only with other rifamycins.

Rifampin has bactericidal activity against slow and intermittently growing *M. tuberculosis*. It also has significant activity against *Neisseria meningitidis* (see INDICATIONS AND USAGE).

In the treatment of both tuberculosis and the meningococcal carrier state (see INDICATIONS AND USAGE), the small number of resistant cells present within large populations of susceptible cells can rapidly become predominant. In addition, resistance to rifampin has been determined to occur as single-step mutations of the DNA-dependent RNA polymerase. Since resistance can emerge rapidly, appropriate susceptibility tests should be performed in the event of persistent positive cultures.

Rifampin has been shown to have initial *in vitro* activity against the following organisms; however, clinical efficacy has not been established (see INDICATIONS AND USAGE): *Mycobacterium leprae, Haemophilus influenzae, Staphylococcus aureus,* and *Staphylococcus epidermidis.* Both penicillinase-producing and non-penicillinase-producing strains, and β-lactam resistant staphylococci (Methicillin Resistant *S. aureus*/MRSA) are initially susceptible to rifampin *in vitro.*

Susceptibility Testing

Use only diagnostic products and methods approved by the Food and Drug Administration for rifampin susceptibility testing of *Mycobacterium tuberculosis* and *Neisseria meningitidis.* Consult the Food and Drug Administration-approved labeling of the diagnostic products for interpretation criteria and quality control parameters.

For the other organisms listed in the microbiology subsection of the labeling, *in vitro* susceptibility testing should be assessed by standardized methods[1,2] developed by the National Committee for Clinical Laboratory Standards.

INDICATIONS AND USAGE

Tuberculosis: Rifampin is indicated in the treatment of all forms of tuberculosis. Rifadin® (rifampin) must always be used in conjunction with at least one other antituberculosis drug. Frequently used regimens are rifampin and isoniazid; rifampin, isoniazid, and pyrazinamide; rifampin, isoniazid, and ethambutol; and rifampin and ethambutol.

Rifadin I.V. is indicated for the initial treatment and retreatment of tuberculosis when the drug cannot be taken by mouth.

Meningococcal Carriers: Rifampin is indicated for the treatment of asymptomatic carriers of *N. meningitidis* to eliminate meningococci from the nasopharynx. *Rifampin is not indicated for the treatment of meningococcal infection because of the possibility of the rapid emergence of resistant organisms.* (See WARNINGS.)

Rifampin should not be used indiscriminately, and therefore diagnostic laboratory procedures, including serotyping and susceptibility testing, should be performed for establishment of the carrier state and the correct treatment. So that the usefulness of rifampin in the treatment of asymptomatic meningococcal carriers is preserved, the drug should be used only when the risk of meningococcal disease is high.

In the treatment of both tuberculosis and the meningococcal carrier state, the small number of resistant cells present within large populations of susceptible cells can rapidly become predominant. Since resistance can emerge rapidly, susceptibility tests should be performed in the event of persistent positive cultures.

CONTRAINDICATIONS

Rifampin is contraindicated in patients with a history of hypersensitivity to any of the rifamycins. (See WARNINGS.)

WARNINGS

Rifampin has been shown to produce liver dysfunction. Fatalities associated with jaundice have occurred in patients with liver disease and in patients taking rifampin with other hepatotoxic agents. Patients with impaired liver function should only be given rifampin in cases of necessity and then with caution and under strict medical supervision.

In these patients, careful monitoring of liver function, especially serum glutamic pyruvic transaminase (SGPT) and serum glutamic oxaloacetic transaminase (SGOT) should be carried out prior to therapy and then every two to four weeks during therapy. If signs of hepatocellular damage occur, rifampin should be withdrawn.

In some cases, hyperbilirubinemia resulting from competition between rifampin and bilirubin for excretory pathways of the liver at the cell level can occur in the early days of treatment. An isolated report showing a moderate rise in bilirubin and/or transaminase level is not in itself an indication for interrupting treatment; rather, the decision should be made after repeating the tests, noting trends in the levels, and considering them in conjunction with the patient's clinical condition.

Rifampin has enzyme-inducing properties, including induction of delta amino levulinic acid synthetase. Isolated reports have associated porphyria exacerbation with rifampin administration.

The possibility of rapid emergence of resistant meningococci restricts the use of Rifadin to short-term treatment of the

asymptomatic carrier state. *Rifadin is not to be used for the treatment of meningococcal disease.*

PRECAUTIONS

General

For the treatment of tuberculosis, rifampin is usually administered on a daily basis. High doses of rifampin (greater than 600 mg) given once or twice weekly have resulted in a high incidence of adverse reactions, including the "flu syndrome" (fever, chills and malaise), hematopoietic reactions (leukopenia, thrombocytopenia, or acute hemolytic anemia), cutaneous, gastrointestinal, and hepatic reactions, shortness of breath, shock and renal failure. Recent studies indicate that regimens using twice-weekly doses of rifampin 600 mg plus isoniazid 15 mg/kg are much better tolerated.

Intermittent therapy may be used if the patient cannot or will not self-administer drugs on a daily basis. Patients on intermittent therapy should be closely monitored for compliance and cautioned against intentional or accidental interruption of prescribed therapy because of the increased risk of serious adverse reactions.

Rifadin I.V.

For intravenous infusion only. Must not be administered by intramuscular or subcutaneous route. Avoid extravasation during injection; local irritation and inflammation due to extravascular infiltration of the infusion have been observed. If these occur, the infusion should be discontinued and restarted at another site.

Information for Patients

The patient should be told that this medication may cause the urine, feces, saliva, sputum, sweat and tears to turn red-orange. Permanent discoloration of soft contact lenses may occur.

The patient should be advised that the reliability of oral contraceptives may be affected; consideration should be given to using alternative contraceptive measures.

Laboratory Tests

A complete blood count (CBC) should be obtained prior to instituting therapy and periodically throughout the course of therapy. Because of a possible transient rise in transaminase and bilirubin values, blood for baseline clinical chemistries should be obtained before rifampin dosing.

Drug Interactions

Rifampin has liver enzyme-inducing properties and may reduce the activity of a number of drugs, including anticoagulants, corticosteroids, cyclosporine, cardiac glycoside preparations, quinidine, oral contraceptives, oral hypoglycemic agents (sulfonylureas), dapsone, narcotics and analgesics. Rifampin also has been reported to diminish the effects of concurrently administered methadone, barbiturates, diazepam, verapamil, beta-adrenergic blockers, clofibrate, progestins, disopyramide, mexiletine, theophylline, chloramphenicol and anticonvulsants. It may be necessary to adjust the dosages of these drugs if they are given concurrently with rifampin.

Patients using oral contraceptives should be advised to change to non-hormonal methods of birth control during rifampin therapy. Also, diabetes may become more difficult to control.

When rifampin is taken with para-aminosalicylic acid (PAS), rifampin levels in the serum may decrease. Therefore, the drugs should be taken at least 8 hours apart.

Probenecid has been reported to increase rifampin blood levels. Halothane, when given concomitantly with rifampin, has been reported to increase the hepatotoxicity of both drugs. Ketoconazole, when given concomitantly with rifampin, has been reported to diminish the serum concentrations of both drugs. Dosage should be adjusted if indicated by the patient's clinical condition. An interaction has also been reported with rifampin-isoniazid and Vitamin D.

Drug/Laboratory Interactions

Therapeutic levels of rifampin have been shown to inhibit standard microbiological assays for serum folate and Vitamin B_{12}. Thus, alternate assay methods should be considered. Transient abnormalities in liver function tests (e.g., elevation in serum bilirubin, abnormal bromsulphalein (BSP) excretion, alkaline phosphatase and serum transaminases), and reduced biliary excretion of contrast media used for visualization of the gallbladder have also been observed. Therefore, these tests should be performed before the morning dose of rifampin.

Carcinogenesis, Mutagenesis, Impairment of Fertility

There are no known human data on long-term potential for carcinogenicity, mutagenicity, or impairment of fertility. A few cases of accelerated growth of lung carcinoma have been reported in man, but a causal relationship with the drug has not been established. An increase in the incidence of hepatomas in female mice (of a strain known to be particularly susceptible to the spontaneous development of hepatomas) was observed when rifampin was administered in doses 2 to 10 times the average daily human dose for 60 weeks followed by an observation period of 46 weeks. No evidence of carcinogencity was found in male mice of the same strain, mice of a different strain, or rats, under similar experimental conditions.

Rifampin has been reported to possess immunosuppressive potential in rabbits, mice, rats, guinea pigs, human lymphocytes *in vitro,* and humans. Antitumor activity *in vitro* has also been shown with rifampin.

There was no evidence of mutagenicity in bacteria, *Drosophila melanogaster,* or mice, nor did rifampin induce chromosome aberrations in human lymphocytes treated *in vitro.* However, an increase in chromatid breaks was noted when whole-blood cell cultures were treated with rifampin.

Pregnancy—Teratogenic Effects

Pregnancy—Category C: Rifampin has been shown to be teratogenic in rodents give oral doses of rifampin 15 to 25 times the human dose. Although rifampin has been reported to cross the placental barrier and appear in cord blood, the effect of Rifadin, alone or in combination with other antituberculosis drugs, on the human fetus is not known. Neonates of rifampin-treated mothers should be carefully observed for any evidence of adverse effects. Isolated cases of fetal malformations have been reported; however, there are no adequate and well-controlled studies in pregnant women. Rifampin should be used during pregnancy only if the potential benefit justifies the potential risk to the fetus. Rifampin in oral doses of 150 to 250 mg/kg produced teratogenic effects in mice and rats. Malformations were primarily cleft palate in the mouse and spina bifida in the rat. The incidence of these anomalies was dose-dependent. When rifampin was given to pregnant rabbits in doses up to 20 times the usual daily human dose, imperfect osteogenesis and embryotoxicity were reported.

When administered during the last few weeks of pregnancy, rifampin can cause postnatal hemorrhages in the mother and infant for which treatment with Vitamin K may be indicated.

Nursing Mothers

Because of the potential for tumorigenicity shown for rifampin in animal studies, a decision should be made whether to discontinue nursing or discontinue the drug, taking into account the importance of the drug to the mother.

Pediatric Use—See CLINICAL PHARMACOLOGY—*Serum Levels in Children;* see also DOSAGE AND ADMINISTRATION

ADVERSE REACTIONS

Gastrointestinal

Heartburn, epigastric distress, anorexia, nausea, vomiting, jaundice, flatulence, cramps and diarrhea have been noted in some patients. Although *C. difficile* has been shown *in vitro* to be sensitive to rifampin, pseudomembranous colitis has been reported with the use of rifampin (and other broad spectrum antibiotics). Therefore, it is important to consider this diagnosis in patients who develop diarrhea in association with antibiotic use. Rarely, hepatitis or a shock-like syndrome with hepatic involvement and abnormal liver function tests has been reported.

Hematologic

Thrombocytopenia has occurred primarily with high dose intermittent therapy, but has also been noted after resumption of interrupted treatment. It rarely occurs during well supervised daily therapy. This effect is reversible if the drug is discontinued as soon as purpura occurs. Cerebral hemorrhage and fatalities have been reported when rifampin administration has been continued or resumed after the appearance of purpura.

Transient leukopenia, hemolytic anemia and decreased hemoglobin have been observed.

Central Nervous System

Headache, fever, drowsiness, fatigue, ataxia, dizziness, inability to concentrate, mental confusion, behavioral changes, muscular weakness, pains in extremities and generalized numbness have been observed.

Rare reports of myopathy have also been observed.

Ocular

Visual disturbances have been observed.

Endocrine

Menstrual disturbances have been observed.

Renal

Elevations in BUN and serum uric acid have been reported. Rarely, hemolysis, hemoglobinuria, hematuria, interstitial nephritis, renal insufficiency and acute renal failure have been noted. These are generally considered to be hypersensitivity reactions. They usually occur during intermittent therapy or when treatment is resumed following intentional or accidental interruption of a daily dosage regimen, and are reversible when rifampin is discontinued and appropriate therapy instituted.

Dermatologic

Cutaneous reactions are mild and self-limiting and do not appear to be hypersensitivity reactions. Typically, they consist of flushing and itching with or without a rash. More serious cutaneous reactions which may be due to hypersensitivity occur but are uncommon.

Hypersensitivity Reactions

Occasionally, pruritus, urticaria, rash, pemphigoid reaction, eosinophilia, sore mouth, sore tongue and conjunctivitis have been observed.

Miscellaneous

Edema of the face and extremities has been reported. Other reactions reported to have occurred with intermittent dosage regimens include "flu" syndrome (such as episodes of fever, chills, headache, dizziness and bone pain), shortness of breath, wheezing, decrease in blood pressure and shock. The "flu" syndrome may also appear if rifampin is taken irregularly by the patient or if daily administration is resumed after a drug free interval.

OVERDOSAGE

Signs and Symptoms

Nausea, vomiting and increasing lethargy will probably occur within a short time after ingestion; unconsciousness may occur when there is severe hepatic disease. Brownish-red or orange discoloration of the skin, urine, sweat, saliva, tears and feces will occur, and its intensity is proportional to the amount ingested.

Liver enlargement, possibly with tenderness, may develop within a few hours after severe overdosage; jaundice may develop rapidly. Hepatic involvement may be more marked in patients with prior impairment of hepatic function. Other physical findings remain essentially normal.

Bilirubin levels may increase rapidly with severe overdosage; hepatic enzyme levels may be affected, especially with prior impairment of hepatic function. A direct effect upon the hematopoietic system, electrolyte levels, or acid-base balance is unlikely.

Acute Toxicity

In animal studies, the LD_{50} of rifampin is approximately 885 mg/kg in the mouse, 1720 mg/kg in the rat, and 2120 mg/kg in the rabbit.

Non-fatal overdoses with as high as 12 g of rifampin have been reported. In one patient who swallowed 12 g of rifampin, vomiting occurred four times within 1 hour of ingestion. Gastric lavage with 20 liters of water was initiated 5 hours after ingestion. Twelve hours after ingestion of rifampin, a plasma concentration of 400 μg of rifampin/mL was measured by microbiological assay. The plasma concentration fell to 64 μg/mL on the following day, and to 0.1 μg/mL on the third day. Urinary rifampin concentration was 313 μg/mL approximately 30 hours after ingestion of the drug, 625 μg/mL after 36 hours, and 78 μg/mL after 40 hours. By the fourth day following the dose, only 0.1 μg/mL rifampin was present in the urine. There was biochemical evidence of mild impairment of liver function. Liver function tests had returned to normal within 5 days, and the patient's recovery was described as uneventful.

One case of fatal overdose is known: a 26-year-old man died after self-administering 60 g of rifampin.

Treatment

Since nausea and vomiting are likely to be present, gastric lavage is probably preferable to induction of emesis. Following evacuation of the gastric contents, the instillation of activated charcoal slurry into the stomach may help absorb any remaining drug from the gastrointestinal tract. Antiemetic medication may be required to control severe nausea and vomiting.

Active diuresis (with measured intake and output) will help promote excretion of the drug. Hemodialysis may be of value in some patients. In patients with previously adequate hepatic function, reversal of liver enlargement and of impaired hepatic excretory function probably will be noted within 72 hours, with a rapid return toward normal thereafter.

DOSAGE AND ADMINISTRATION

Rifampin can be administered by the oral route or by I.V. infusion (see INDICATIONS AND USAGE).

Tuberculosis

Adults: 600 mg in a single daily administration, oral or I.V.

Children: 10–20 mg/kg not to exceed 600 mg/day, oral or I.V.

It is recommended that oral rifampin be administered once daily, either one hour before, or two hours after a meal.

In the treatment of tuberculosis, rifampin should always be administered with at least one other antituberculosis drug.

In general, therapy for tuberculosis should be continued for 6 to 9 months or until at least 6 months have elapsed from conversion of sputum to culture negativity. In patients who cannot be relied on for compliance, intermittent therapy with 600 mg/day two or three times/week under close supervision may be prescribed and substituted for the daily regimen after 1–2 months of an initial daily phase of therapy.

The *9-Month Regimen* ordinarily consists of rifampin and isoniazid, usually supplemented during the initial phase by pyrazinamide, streptomycin or ethambutol.

The *6-Month Regimen* ordinarily consists of an initial *2-month* phase of rifampin, isoniazid and pyrazinamide, and, if clinically indicated, streptomycin or ethambutol; followed by *4 months* of rifampin and isoniazid.

Either of the above regimens is recommended as standard therapy.

The above recommendations apply to patients with drug-susceptible organisms. Patients with drug-resistant organisms may require longer treatment with other drug regimens.

Continued on next page

Marion Merrell Dow—Cont.

Meningococcal Carriers
Adults
For adults, it is recommended that 600 mg rifampin be administered twice daily for two days.
Infants and Children
Children 1 month of age or older: 10 mg/kg every 12 hours for two days.
Children under 1 month of age: 5 mg/kg every 12 hours for two days.
Preparation of Solution for I.V. Infusion
Reconstitute the lyophilized powder by transferring 10 mL of sterile water for injection to a vial containing 600 mg of rifampin for injection. Swirl vial gently to completely dissolve the antibiotic. The reconstituted solution contains 60 mg rifampin per mL and is stable at room temperature for 24 hours. Immediately prior to administration, withdraw from the reconstituted solution a volume equivalent to the amount of rifampin calculated to be administered and add to 500 mL of infusion medium. Mix well and infuse at a rate allowing for complete infusion in 3 hours. In some cases, the amount of rifampin calculated to be administered may be added to 100 mL of infusion medium and infused in 30 minutes. The 500 mL and 100 mL infusion solutions should be prepared and used within a total 4 hour period. Precipitation of rifampin from the infusion solution may occur beyond this time.
CAUTION: Dextrose 5% for injection is the recommended infusion medium. Sterile saline may be used when dextrose is contraindicated, but the stability of rifampin is slightly reduced. Other infusion media are not recommended.
Preparation of Extemporaneous Oral Suspension
For pediatric and adult patients in whom capsule swallowing is difficult or where lower doses are needed, a liquid suspension may be prepared as follows:
Rifadin 1% w/v suspension (10 mg/mL) can be compounded using one of five syrups—Simple Syrup (Syrup NF), Simple Syrup (Humco Laboratories), Simple Syrup (Whiteworth Inc.), Wild Cherry Syrup (Eli Lilly and Company), and Syrpalta® Syrup (Emerson Laboratories).

1. Empty contents of four Rifadin 300 mg capsules or eight Rifadin 150 mg capsules onto a piece of weighing paper.
2. If necessary, gently crush the capsule contents with a spatula to produce a fine powder.
3. Transfer rifampin powder blend to a 4-ounce amber glass prescription bottle.
4. Rinse the paper and spatula with 20 mL of one of the above-mentioned syrups and add the rinse to the bottle. Shake vigorously.
5. Add 100 mL of syrup to the bottle and shake vigorously.

This compounding procedure results in a 1% w/v suspension containing 10 mg rifampin/mL. Stability studies indicate that the suspension is stable when stored at room temperature (25 ± 3°C) or in a refrigerator (2–8°C) for four weeks. This extemporaneously prepared suspension must be shaken well prior to administration.

HOW SUPPLIED

150 mg maroon and scarlet capsules imprinted "RIFADIN 150".
Bottles of 30 (NDC 0068-0510-30)
300 mg maroon and scarlet capsules imprinted "RIFADIN 300".
Bottles of 30 (NDC 0068-0508-30)
Bottles of 60 (NDC 0068-0508-60)
Bottles of 100 (NDC 0068-0508-61)
Storage: Keep tightly closed. Store in a dry place. Avoid excessive heat.
Rifadin I.V. (rifampin for injection) is available in glass vials containing 600 mg rifampin (NDC 0068-0597-01).
Storage: Avoid excessive heat (temperatures above 40°C or 104°F). Protect from light.

1. National Committee for Clinical Laboratory Standards, Approved Standard: Performance Standards for Antimicrobial Disk Susceptibility Tests (M2-T4), December 1988.
2. National Committee for Clinical Laboratory Standards, Approved Standard: Methods for Dilution Antimicrobial Susceptibility Tests for Bacteria that Grow Aerobically (M7-T2), December 1988.

Product Information as of August, 1991
Rifadin 150 mg capsules are manufactured by:
MERRELL DOW PHARMACEUTICALS (CANADA) INC.
Richmond Hill, Ontario, L4C 5H2, CANADA for
Merrell Dow Pharmaceuticals Inc.
Subsidiary of Marion Merrell Dow Inc.
Kansas City, MO 64114
Rifadin I.V. (rifampin for injection) is manufactured by:
GRUPPO LEPETIT S.p.A.
Milan, Italy for
Merrell Dow Pharmaceuticals Inc.
Subsidiary of Marion Merrell Dow Inc.
Kansas City, MO 64114
Shown in Product Identification Section, page 417

RIFAMATE® ℞

[rĭf'ăh-māt]
(rifampin and isoniazid capsules)

> **WARNING**
> Severe and sometimes fatal hepatitis associated with isoniazid therapy may occur and may develop even after many months of treatment. The risk of developing hepatitis is age related. Approximate case rates by age are: 0 per 1,000 for persons under 20 years of age, 3 per 1,000 for persons in the 20–34 year age group, 12 per 1,000 for persons in the 35–49 year age group, 23 per 1,000 for persons in the 50–64 year age group, and 8 per 1,000 for persons over 65 years of age. The risk of hepatitis is increased with daily consumption of alcohol. Precise data to provide a fatality rate for isoniazid-related hepatitis is not available; however, in a U.S. Public Health Service Surveillance Study of 13,838 persons taking isoniazid, there were 8 deaths among 174 cases of hepatitis.
> Therefore, patients given isoniazid should be carefully monitored and interviewed at monthly intervals. Serum transaminase concentration becomes elevated in about 10–20 percent of patients, usually during the first few months of therapy, but it can occur at any time. Usually enzyme levels return to normal despite continuance of drug but in some cases progressive liver dysfunction occurs. Patients should be instructed to report immediately any of the prodromal symptoms of hepatitis, such as fatigue, weakness, malaise, anorexia, nausea, or vomiting. If these symptoms appear or if signs suggestive of hepatic damage are detected, isoniazid should be discontinued promptly, since continued use of the drug in these cases has been reported to cause a more severe form of liver damage.
> Patients with tuberculosis should be given appropriate treatment with alternative drugs. If isoniazid must be reinstituted, it should be reinstituted only after symptoms and laboratory abnormalities have cleared. The drug should be restarted in very small and gradually increasing doses and should be withdrawn immediately if there is any indication of recurrent liver involvement. Treatment should be deferred in persons with acute hepatic diseases.

DESCRIPTION

Rifamate is a combination capsule containing 300 mg rifampin and 150 mg isoniazid. The capsules also contain as inactive ingredients: colloidal silicon dioxide, FD&C Blue No. 1, FD&C Red No. 40, gelatin, magnesium stearate, sodium starch glycolate, and titanium dioxide.
Rifampin is a semisynthetic antibiotic derivative of rifamycin B. The chemical name for rifampin is 3-(4-methyl-1-piperazinyl-iminomethyl) rifamycin SV.
Isoniazid is the hydrazide of isonicotinic acid. It exists as colorless or white crystals or as a white, crystalline powder that is water soluble, odorless, and slowly affected by exposure to air and light.

ACTIONS

Rifampin
Rifampin inhibits DNA-dependent RNA polymerase activity in susceptible cells. Specifically, it interacts with bacterial RNA polymerase but does not inhibit the mammalian enzyme. This is the mechanism of action by which rifampin exerts its therapeutic effect. Rifampin cross resistance has only been shown with other rifamycins.
In a study of 14 normal human adult males, peak blood levels of rifampin occured 1 ½ to 3 hours following oral administration of two Rifamate capsules. The peaks ranged from 6.9 to 14 mcg/ml with an average of 10 mcg/ml.
In normal subjects the $T\frac{1}{2}$ (biological half-life) of rifampin in blood is approximately 3 hours. Elimination occurs mainly through the bile and, to a much lesser extent, the urine.
Isoniazid
Isoniazid acts against actively growing tubercle bacilli.
After oral administration isoniazid produces peak blood levels within 1 to 2 hours which decline to 50% or less within 6 hours. It diffuses readily into all body fluids (cerebrospinal, pleural, and ascitic fluids), tissues, organs and excreta (saliva, sputum, and feces). The drug also passes through the placental barrier and into milk in concentrations comparable to those in the plasma. From 50 to 70% of a dose of isoniazid is excreted in the urine in 24 hours.
Isoniazid is metabolized primarily by acetylation and dehydrazination. The rate of acetylation is genetically determined. Approximately 50% of Blacks and Caucasians are "slow inactivators"; the majority of Eskimos and Orientals are "rapid inactivators."
The rate of acetylation does not significantly alter the effectiveness of isoniazid. However, slow acetylation may lead to higher blood levels of the drug, and thus an increase in toxic reactions.
Pyridoxine deficiency (B_6) is sometimes observed in adults with high doses of isoniazid and is considered probably due to its competition with pyridoxal phosphate for the enzyme apotryptophanase.

INDICATIONS

For pulmonary tuberculosis in which organisms are susceptible, and when the patient has been titrated on the individual components and it has therefore been established that this fixed dosage is therapeutically effective.
This fixed-dosage combination drug is not recommended for initial therapy of tuberculosis or for preventive therapy.
In the treatment of tuberculosis, small numbers of resistant cells, present within large populations of susceptible cells, can rapidly become the predominating type. Since rapid emergence of resistance can occur, culture and susceptibility tests should be performed in the event of persistent positive cultures.
This drug is *not* indicated for the treatment of meningococcal infections or asymptomatic carriers of *N. meningitidis* to eliminate meningococci from the nasopharynx.

CONTRAINDICATIONS

Previous isoniazid-associated hepatic injury; severe adverse reactions to isoniazid, such as drug fever, chills, and arthritis; acute liver disease of any etiology.
A history of previous hypersensitivity reaction to any of the rifamycins or to isoniazid, including drug-induced hepatitis.

WARNINGS

Rifamate (rifampin-isoniazid) is a combination of two drugs, each of which has been associated with liver dysfunction. Liver function tests should be performed prior to therapy with Rifamate and periodically during treatment.
Rifampin
Rifampin has been shown to produce liver dysfunction. There have been fatalities associated with jaundice in patients with liver disease or receiving rifampin concomitantly with other hepatoxic agents. Since an increased risk may exist for individuals with liver disease, benefits must be weighed carefully against the risk of further liver damage.
Several studies of tumorigenicity potential have been done in rodents. In one strain of mice known to be particularly susceptible to the spontaneous development of hepatomas, rifampin given at a level 2–10 times the maximum dosage used clinically, resulted in a significant increase in the occurrence of hepatomas in female mice of this strain after one year of administration. There was no evidence of tumorigenicity in the males of this strain, in males or females of another mouse strain, or in rats.
Isoniazid
See the boxed warning.

PRECAUTIONS

Rifampin
Rifampin is not recommended for intermittent therapy; the patient should be cautioned against intentional or accidental interruption of the daily dosage regimen since rare renal hypersensitivity reactions have been reported when therapy was resumed in such cases.
Rifampin has been observed to increase the requirements for anticoagulant drugs of the coumarin type. The cause of the phenomenon is unknown. In patients receiving anticoagulants and rifampin concurrently, it is recommended that the prothrombin time be performed daily or as frequently as necessary to establish and maintain the required dose of anticoagulant.
Urine, feces, saliva, sputum, sweat and tears may be colored red-orange by rifampin and its metabolites. Soft contact lenses may be permanently stained. Individuals to be treated should be made aware of these possibilities.
It has been reported that the reliability of oral contraceptives may be affected in some patients being treated for tuberculosis with rifampin in combination with at least one other antituberculosis drug. In such cases, alternative contraceptive measures may need to be considered.
It has also been reported that rifampin given in combination with other antituberculosis drugs may decrease the pharmacologic activity of methadone, oral hypoglycemics, digitoxin, quinidine, disopyramide, dapsone and corticosteroids. In these cases, dosage adjustment of the interacting drugs is recommended.
Therapeutic levels of rifampin have been shown to inhibit standard microbiological assays for serum folate and vitamin B_{12}. Alternative methods must be considered when determining folate and vitamin B_{12} concentrations in the presence of rifampin.
Since rifampin has been reported to cross the placental barrier and appear in cord blood and in maternal milk, neonates and newborns of rifampin-treated mothers should be carefully observed for any evidence of untoward effects.

Isoniazid
All drugs should be stopped and an evaluation of the patient should be made at the first sign of a hypersensitivity reaction.
Use of isoniazid should be carefully monitored in the following:
1. Patients who are receiving phenytoin (diphenylhydantoin) concurrently. Isoniazid may decrease the excretion of phenytoin or may enhance its effects. To avoid phenytoin intoxication, appropriate adjustment of the anticonvulsant dose should be made.
2. Daily users of alcohol. Daily ingestion of alcohol may be associated with a higher incidence of isoniazid hepatitis.
3. Patients with current chronic liver disease or severe renal dysfunction.
Periodic ophthalmoscopic examination during isoniazid therapy is recommended when visual symptoms occur.

Usage in Pregnancy and Lactation
Rifampin
Although rifampin has been reported to cross the placental barrier and appear in cord blood, the effect of rifampin, alone or in combination with other antituberculosis drugs, on the human fetus is not known. An increase in congenital malformations, primarily spina bifida and cleft palate, has been reported in the offspring of rodents given oral doses of 150–250 mg/kg/day of rifampin during pregnancy.
The possible teratogenic potential in women capable of bearing children should be carefully weighed against the benefits of therapy.
Isoniazid
It has been reported that in both rats and rabbits, isoniazid may exert an embryocidal effect when administered orally during pregnancy, although no isoniazid-related congenital anomalies have been found in reproduction studies in mammalian species (mice, rats, and rabbits). Isoniazid should be prescribed during pregnancy only when therapeutically necessary. The benefit of preventive therapy should be weighed against a possible risk to the fetus. Preventive treatment generally should be started after delivery because of the increased risk of tuberculosis for new mothers.
Since isoniazid is known to cross the placental barrier and to pass into maternal breast milk, neonates and breast-fed infants of isoniazid treated mothers should be carefully observed for any evidence of adverse effects.
Carcinogenesis:
Isoniazid has been reported to induce pulmonary tumors in a number of strains of mice.

ADVERSE REACTIONS
Rifampin
Nervous system reactions: headache, drowsiness, fatigue, ataxia, dizziness, inability to concentrate, mental confusion, visual disturbances, muscular weakness, pain in extremities and generalized numbness.
Gastrointestinal disturbances: in some patients heartburn, epigastric distress, anorexia, nausea, vomiting, gas, cramps, and diarrhea.
Hepatic reactions: transient abnormalities in liver function tests (e.g., elevations in serum bilirubin, BSP, alkaline phosphatase, serum transaminases) have been observed. Rarely, hepatitis or a shocklike syndrome with hepatic involvement and abnormal liver function tests.
Renal reactions: Elevations in BUN and serum uric acid have been reported. Rarely, hemolysis, hemoglobinuria, hematuria, interstitial nephritis, renal insufficiency and acute renal failure have been noted. These are generally considered to be hypersensitivity reactions. They usually occur during intermittent therapy or when treatment is resumed following intentional or accidental interruption of a daily dosage regimen, and are reversible when rifampin is discontinued and appropriate therapy instituted.
Hematologic reactions: thrombocytopenia, transient leukopenia, hemolytic anemia, eosinophilia and decreased hemoglobin have been observed. Thrombocytopenia has occurred when rifampin and ethambutol were administered concomitantly according to an intermittent dose schedule twice weekly and in high doses.
Allergic and immunological reactions: occasionally pruritus, urticaria, rash, pemphigoid reaction, eosinophilia, sore mouth, sore tongue and exudative conjunctivitis. Rarely, hemolysis, hemoglobinuria, hematuria, renal insufficiency or acute renal failure have been reported which are generally considered to be hypersensitivity reactions. These have usually occurred during intermittent therapy or when treatment was resumed following intentional or accidental interruption of a daily dosage regimen and were reversible when rifampin was discontinued and appropriate therapy instituted.
Although rifampin has been reported to have an immunosuppressive effect in some animal experiments, available human data indicate that this has no clinical significance.
Metabolic reactions: elevations in BUN and serum uric acid have occurred.
Miscellaneous reactions: fever and menstrual disturbances have been noted.

Isoniazid
The most frequent reactions are those affecting the nervous system and the liver.
Nervous system reactions: Peripheral neuropathy is the most common toxic effect. It is dose-related, occurs most often in the malnourished and in those predisposed to neuritis (e.g., alcoholics and diabetics), and is usually preceded by paresthesias of the feet and hands. The incidence is higher in "slow inactivators."
Other neurotoxic effects, which are uncommon with conventional doses, are convulsions, toxic encephalopathy, optic neuritis and atrophy, memory impairment, and toxic psychosis.
Gastrointestinal reactions: Nausea, vomiting, and epigastric distress.
Hepatic reactions: Elevated serum transaminases (SGOT; SGPT), bilirubinemia, bilirubinuria, jaundice, and occasionally severe and sometimes fatal hepatitis. The common prodromal symptoms are anorexia, nausea, vomiting, fatigue, malaise, and weakness. Mild and transient elevation of serum transaminase levels occurs in 10 to 20 percent of persons taking isoniazid. The abnormality usually occurs in the first 4 to 6 months of treatment but can occur at any time during therapy. In most instances, enzyme levels return to normal with no necessity to discontinue medication. In occasional instances, progressive liver damage occurs, with accompanying symptoms. In these cases, the drug should be discontinued immediately. The frequency of progressive liver damage increases with age. It is rare in persons under 20, but occurs in up to 2.3 percent of those over 50 years of age.
Hematologic reactions: agranulocytosis, hemolytic sideroblastic or aplastic anemia, thrombocytopenia and eosinophilia.
Hypersensitivity reactions: fever, skin eruptions (morbilliform, maculopapular, purpuric, or exfoliative), lymphadenopathy and vasculitis.
Metabolic and endocrine reactions: pyridoxine deficiency, pellagra, hyperglycemia, metabolic acidosis, and gynecomastia.
Miscellaneous reactions: rheumatic syndrome and systemic lupus erythematosus-like syndrome.

OVERDOSAGE
Rifampin
Signs and Symptoms
Nausea, vomiting, and increasing lethargy will probably occur within a short time after ingestion; actual unconsciousness may occur with severe hepatic involvement. Brownish-red or orange discoloration of the skin, urine, sweat, saliva, tears, and feces is proportional to amount ingested.
Liver enlargement, possibly with tenderness, can develop within a few hours after severe overdosage and jaundice may develop rapidly. Hepatic involvement may be more marked in patients with prior impairment of hepatic function. Other physical findings remain essentially normal.
Direct and total bilirubin levels may increase rapidly with severe overdosage; hepatic enzyme levels may be affected, especially with prior impairment of hepatic function. A direct effect upon hemopoietic system, electrolyte levels or acid-base balance is unlikely.
Isoniazid
Signs and Symptoms
Isoniazid overdosage produces signs and symptoms within 30 minutes to 3 hours. Nausea, vomiting, dizziness, slurring of speech, blurring of vision, visual hallucinations (including bright colors and strange designs), are among the early manifestations. With marked overdosage, respiratory distress and CNS depression, progressing rapidly from stupor to profound coma, are to be expected, along with severe, intractable seizures. Severe metabolic acidosis, acetonuria, and hyperglycemia are typical laboratory findings.
Rifamate (rifampin and isoniazid capsules)
Treatment
The airway should be secured and adequate respiratory exchange established. Only then should gastric emptying (lavage-aspiration) be attempted; this may be difficult because of seizures. Since nausea and vomiting are likely to be present, gastric lavage is probably preferable to induction of emesis.
Activated charcoal slurry instilled into the stomach following evacuation of gastric contents can help absorb any remaining drug in the GI tract. Antiemetic medication may be required to control severe nausea and vomiting.
Blood samples should be obtained for immediate determination of gases, electrolytes, BUN, glucose, etc. Blood should be typed and crossmatched in preparation for possible hemodialysis.
Rapid control of metabolic acidosis is fundamental to management. Intravenous sodium bicarbonate should be given at once and repeated as needed, adjusting subsequent dosage on the basis of laboratory findings (i.e. serum sodium, pH, etc.). At the same time, anticonvulsants should be given intravenously (i.e., barbiturates, diphenylhydantoin, diazepam) as required, and large doses of intravenous pyridoxine.
Forced osmotic diuresis must be started early and should be continued for some hours after clinical improvement to hasten renal clearance of drug and help prevent relapse. Fluid intake and output should be monitored.
Bile drainage may be indicated in presence of serious impairment of hepatic function lasting more than 24–48 hours. Under these circumstances, and for severe cases extracorporeal hemodialysis may be required; if this is not available, peritoneal dialysis can be used along with forced diuresis.
Along with measures based on initial and repeated determination of blood gases and other laboratory tests as needed, meticulous respiratory and other intensive care should be utilized to protect against hypoxia, hypotension, aspiration, pneumonitis, etc.
In patients with previously adequate hepatic function, reversal of liver enlargement and impaired hepatic excretory function probably will be noted within 72 hours, with rapid return toward normal thereafter.
Untreated or inadequately treated cases of gross isoniazid overdosage can terminate fatally, but good response has been reported in most patients brought under adequate treatment within the first few hours after drug ingestion.

DOSAGE AND ADMINISTRATION
In general, therapy should be continued until bacterial conversion and maximal improvement have occurred.
Adults: Two Rifamate (rifampin-isoniazid) capsules (600 mg rifampin, 300 mg isoniazid) once daily, administered one hour before or two hours after a meal.
Concomitant administration of pyridoxine (B_6) is recommended in the malnourished, in those predisposed to neuropathy (e.g., diabetics) and in adolescents.
Susceptibility Testing
Rifampin
Rifampin susceptibility powders are available for both direct and indirect methods of determining the susceptibility of strains of mycobacteria. The MIC's of susceptible clinical isolates when determined in 7H10 or other non-egg-containing media have ranged from 0.1 to 2 mcg/ml.
Quantitative methods that require measurement of zone diameters give the most precise estimates of antibiotic susceptibility. One such procedure has been recommended for use with discs for testing susceptibility to rifampin. Interpretations correlate zone diameters from the disc test with MIC (minimal inhibitory concentration) values for rifampin.

HOW SUPPLIED
Capsules (opaque red), containing 300 mg rifampin and 150 mg isoniazid; bottles of 60 (NDC 0068-0509-60).

Product Information as of May, 1991
Shown in Product Identification Section, page 417

SELDANE® ℞
[*sĕl 'dān*]
(terfenadine)
60 mg Tablets

CAUTION: Federal law prohibits dispensing without prescription.

DESCRIPTION
Seldane (terfenadine) is available as tablets for oral administration. Each tablet contains 60 mg terfenadine. Tablets also contain, as inactive ingredients: corn starch, gelatin, lactose, magnesium stearate, and sodium bicarbonate.
Terfenadine is a histamine H_1-receptor antagonist with the chemical name α-[4-(1,1-Dimethylethyl) phenyl]-4-(hydroxydiphenylmethyl)-1-piperidinebutanol (±). The molecular weight is 471.68. The molecular formula is $C_{32}H_{41}NO_2$.
It has the following chemical structure:

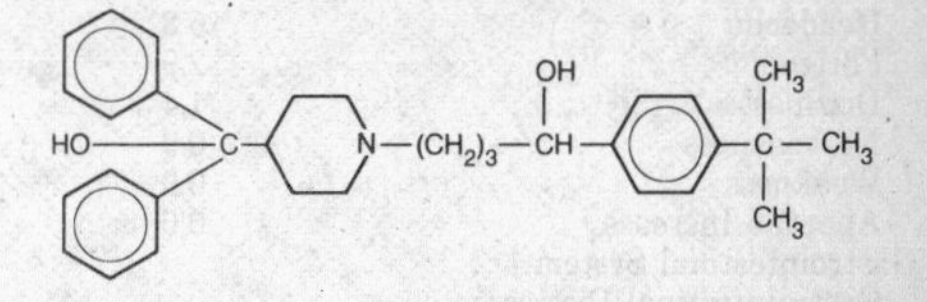

Terfenadine occurs as a white to off-white crystalline powder. It is freely soluble in chloroform, soluble in ethanol, and very slightly soluble in water.

CLINICAL PHARMACOLOGY
Terfenadine is chemically and pharmacologically distinct from other antihistamines.
Histamine skin wheal studies have shown that Seldane in single and repeated doses of 60 mg in 64 subjects has an antihistaminic effect beginning at 1–2 hours, reaching its maximum at 3–4 hours, and lasting in excess of 12 hours.
Clinical trials of Seldane involved about 2,600 patients, most receiving either Seldane, another antihistamine and/or placebo in double-blind, randomized controlled comparisons. The four best controlled and largest trials each lasted 7 days

Continued on next page

Marion Merrell Dow—Cont.

and involved about 1,000 total patients in comparisons of Seldane (60 mg b.i.d.) with an active drug (chlorpheniramine, 4 mg t.i.d.; dexchlorpheniramine, 2 mg t.i.d.; or clemastine 1 mg b.i.d.). In the four trials, about 50–70% of Seldane or other antihistamine recipients had moderate to complete relief of symptoms, compared with 30–50% of placebo recipients, with a significant difference favoring the active drugs in each study. In these studies, Seldane was associated with less frequent drowsiness than the other antihistamines; the frequency of drowsiness with Seldane was similar to the frequency with placebo. None of these studies showed a difference between Seldane and other antihistamines in the frequency of anticholinergic effects. In studies which included 52 subjects in whom EEG assessments were made, no depressant effects have been observed.

Animal studies have demonstrated that terfenadine is a histamine H_1-receptor antagonist. In these animal studies, no sedative or anticholinergic effects were observed at effective antihistaminic doses. Radioactive disposition and autoradiographic studies in rats and radioligand binding studies with guinea pig brain H_1-receptors indicate that, at effective antihistamine doses, neither terfenadine nor its metabolites penetrate the blood brain barrier well.

Relative to a terfenadine suspension, terfenadine tablets are equally bioavailable. On the basis of a mass balance study using ^{14}C labelled terfenadine the oral absorption of terfenadine was estimated to be at least 70%. Terfenadine itself undergoes extensive (99%) first pass metabolism to two primary metabolites, an active acid metabolite and an inactive dealkylated metabolite. Therefore, systemic availability of terfenadine would be low. From information gained in the ^{14}C study it appears that approximately forty percent of the total dose is eliminated renally (40% of this as acid metabolite, 30% dealkyl metabolite, and 30% minor unidentified metabolites). Sixty percent of the dose is eliminated in the feces (50% of it as the acid metabolite, 2% unchanged terfenadine, and the remainder as minor unidentified metabolites). Studies investigating the effect of hepatic and renal insufficiency on the metabolism and excretion of terfenadine are incomplete. Preliminary information indicates that in cases of hepatic impairment, significant concentrations of unchanged terfenadine can be detected with the rate of acid metabolite formation being decreased. In subjects with normal hepatic function unchanged terfenadine plasma concentrations have not been detected.

In vitro studies demonstrate that terfenadine is extensively (97%) bound to human serum protein while the acid metabolite is approximately 70% bound to human serum protein. Based on data gathered from in vitro models of antihistaminic activity, the acid metabolite of terfenadine has approximately 30% of the H_1 blocking activity of terfenadine. The relative contribution of terfenadine and the acid metabolite to the pharmacodynamic effects have not been clearly defined. Since unchanged terfenadine is usually not detected in plasma and active acid metabolite concentrations are relatively high, the acid metabolite may be the entity responsible for the majority of efficacy after oral administration of terfenadine.

In a study involving the administration of a single 60 mg Seldane tablet to 24 subjects, mean peak plasma levels of the acid metabolite were 263 ng/mL (range 133–423 ng/mL) and occurred approximately 2.5 hours after dosing. Plasma concentrations of unchanged terfenadine were not detected. The elimination profile of the acid metabolite was biphasic in nature with an initial mean plasma half-life of 3.5 hours followed by a mean plasma half-life of 6 hours. Ninety percent of the plasma level time curve was associated with these half-lives. Preliminary evidence exists at doses four times of that currently approved, that there may emerge a third phase with a half-life of >14 hours. This third phase was associated with about twenty percent of the plasma level time curve.

After multiple dose administration to steady-state of 60 mg Seldane tablets every 12 hours the observed accumulation of Area Under the Curve during the dosing interval for the active acid metabolite was 1.6[1]. This observed accumulation factor corresponds to an effective pharmacokinetic half-life of 8.5 hours. This 8.5 hour half-life would perdict time to steady-state, steady-state concentrations as well as time for drug elimination after multiple dosing.

[1]Observed Accumulation Factor = ^{AUC}0-12 at steady-state/ ^{AUC}0-12 first dose.

INDICATIONS AND USAGE

Seldane is indicated for the relief of symptoms associated with seasonal allergic rhinitis such as sneezing, rhinorrhea, pruritus, and lacrimation.

CONTRAINDICATIONS

Seldane is contraindicated in patients with a known hypersensitivity to terfenadine or any of its ingredients.

PRECAUTIONS

General

Terfenadine undergoes extensive metabolism in the liver. Patients with impaired hepatic function (alcholic cirrhosis, hepatitis), or on ketoconazole or troleandomycin therapy, or having conditions leading to QT prolongation (e.g., hypokalemia, congenital QT syndrome) may experience QT prolongation and/or ventricular tachycardia at the recommended dose. The effect of terfenadine in patients who are receiving agents which alter the QT interval is not known. These events have also occurred in patients on macrolide antibiotics, including erythromycin, but causality is unclear. The events may be related to altered metabolism of the drug, to electrolyte imbalance, or both.

Information for Patients

Patients taking Seldane should receive the following information and instructions. Antihistamines are prescribed to reduce allergic symptoms. Patients should be questioned about pregnancy or lactation before starting Seldane therapy, since the drug should be used in pregnancy or lactation only if the potential benefit justifies the potential risk to fetus or baby. Patients should be instructed to take Seldane only as needed and not to exceed the prescribed dose. Patients should also be instructed to store this medication in a tightly closed container in a cool, dry place, away from heat or direct sunlight, and away from children.

Drug Interactions

Preliminary evidence exists that concurrent ketoconazole or macrolide administration significantly alters the metabolism of terfenadine. Concurrent use of Seldane with ketoconazole or troleandomycin is not recommended. Concurrent use of other macrolides should be approached with caution.

Carcinogenesis, mutagenesis, impairment of fertility

Oral doses of terfenadine, corresponding to 63 times the recommended human daily dose, in mice for 18 months or in rats for 24 months, revealed no evidence of tumorigenicity. Microbial and micronucleus test assays with terfenadine have revealed no evidence of mutagenesis.

Reproduction and fertility studies in rats showed no effects on male or female fertility at oral doses of up to 21 times the human daily dose. At 63 times the human daily dose there was a small but significant reduction in implants and at 125 times the human daily dose reduced implants and increased post-implantation losses were observed, which were judged to be secondary to maternal toxicity.

Pregnancy Category C

There was no evidence of animal teratogenicity. Reproduction studies have been performed in rats at doses 63 times and 125 times the human daily dose and have revealed decreased pup weight gain and survival when terfenadine was administered throughout pregnancy and lactation. There are no adequate and well-controlled studies in pregnant women. Seldane should be used during pregnancy only if the potential benefit justifies the potential risk to the fetus.

Nonteratogenic effects

Seldane is not recommended for nursing women. The drug has caused decreased pup weight gain and survival in rats given doses 63 times and 125 times the human daily dose throughout pregnancy and lactation. Effects on pups exposed to Seldane only during lactation are not known, and there are no adequate and well-controlled studies in women during lactation.

Pediatric use

Safety and effectiveness of Seldane in children below the age of 12 years have not been established.

ADVERSE REACTIONS

Experience from clinical studies, including both controlled and uncontrolled studies involving more than 2,400 patients who received Seldane, provides information on adverse experience incidence for periods of a few days up to six months. The usual dose in these studies was 60 mg twice daily, but in a small number of patients, the dose was as low as 20 mg twice a day, or a high as 600 mg daily.

In controlled clinical studies using the recommended dose of 60 mg b.i.d., the incidence of reported adverse effects in patients receiving Seldane was similar to that reported in patients receiving placebo. (See Table below.)

ADVERSE EVENTS REPORTED IN CLINICAL TRIALS

Adverse Event	Percent of Patients Reporting				
	Controlled Studies*			All Clinical Studies**	
	Seldane N = 781	Placebo N = 665	Control N = 626***	Seldane N = 2462	Placebo N = 1478
Central Nervous System					
Drowsiness	9.0	8.1	18.1	8.5	8.2
Headache	6.3	7.4	3.8	15.8	11.2
Fatigue	2.9	0.9	5.8	4.5	3.0
Dizziness	1.4	1.1	1.0	1.5	1.2
Nervousness	0.9	0.2	0.6	1.7	1.0
Weakness	0.9	0.6	0.2	0.6	0.5
Appetite Increase	0.6	0.0	0.0	0.5	0.0
Gastrointestinal System					
Gastrointestinal Distress (Abdominal Distress, Nausea, Vomiting, Change in Bowel Habits)	4.6	3.0	2.7	7.6	5.4
Eye, Ear, Nose, and Throat					
Dry Mouth/Nose/Throat	2.3	1.8	3.5	4.8	3.1
Cough	0.9	0.2	0.5	2.5	1.7
Sore Throat	0.5	0.3	0.5	3.2	1.6
Epistaxis	0.0	0.8	0.2	0.7	0.4
Skin					
Eruption (including rash and urticaria) or itching	1.0	1.7	1.4	1.6	2.0

* Duration of treatment in "CONTROLLED STUDIES" was usually 7–14 days.
** Duration of treatment in "ALL CLINICAL STUDIES" was up to 6 months.
*** CONTROL DRUGS: Chlorpheniramine (291 patients), d-Chlorpheniramine (189 patients), Clemastine (146 patients)

Rare reports of severe cardiovascular adverse effects have been received which include arrhythmias (ventricular tachyarrhythmia, torsades de pointes, ventricular fibrillation), hypotension, palpitations, and syncope. In controlled clinical trials in otherwise normal patients with rhinitis, at doses of 60 mg b.i.d. small increases in QTc interval were observed. Changes of this magnitude in a normal population are of doubtful clinical significance. However, in another study (N=20 patients) at 300 mg b.i.d. a mean increase in QTc of 10% (range −4% to +30%) (mean increase of 46 msec) was observed without clinical sign or symptoms.

In addition to the more frequent side effects reported in clinical trials (See Table), adverse effects have been reported at a lower incidence in clinical trials and/or spontaneously during marketing of Seldane that warrant listing as possibly associated with drug administration. These include: alopecia (hair loss or thinning), anaphylaxis, angioedema, bronchospasm, confusion, depression, galactorrhea, insomnia, menstrual disorders (including dysmenorrhea), musculoskeletal symptoms, nightmares, paresthesia, photosensitivity, seizures, sinus tachycardia, sweating, tremor, urinary frequency, and visual disturbances.

In clinical trials, several instances of mild, or in one case, moderate transaminase elevations were seen in patients receiving Seldane. Mild elevations were also seen in placebo treated patients. Marketing experiences include isolated reports of jaundice, cholestatic hepatitis, and hepatitis. In most cases available information is incomplete.

OVERDOSAGE

Generally, signs and symptoms of overdosage are absent or mild (e.g., headache, nausea, confusion). At overdoses of 600 mg/day (300 mg b.i.d.) there may be prolongation of the QT interval. At 900 mg or more there have been rare incidents of ventricular arrhythmia (torsades de pointes or fibrillation). Seizures and syncope have been reported.

Therefore, in cases of overdosage, cardiac monitoring for at least 24 hours is recommended and for as long as QTc is prolonged, along with standard measures to remove any unabsorbed drug. Limited experience with the use of hemoperfu-

sion (N = 1) or hemodialysis (N = 3) was not successful in completely removing the acid metabolite of terfenadine from the blood.

Treatment of the signs and symptoms of overdosage should be symptomatic and supportive after the acute stage.

Oral LD_{50} values for terfenadine were greater than 5000 mg/kg in mature mice and rats. The oral LD_{50} was 438 mg/kg in newborn rats.

DOSAGE AND ADMINISTRATION

One tablet (60 mg) twice daily for adults and children 12 years and older.

HOW SUPPLIED

NDC 0068-0723-61
 60 mg tablets in bottles of 100.
NDC 0068-0723-65
 60 mg tablets in bottles of 500.
 Tablets are round, white, and debossed "SELDANE". Store tablets at controlled room temperature (59°–86°F) (15°–30°C). Protect from exposure to temperatures above 104°F (40°C) and moisture.

Product information as of July, 1990
U.S. Patent 3,878,217
Other patent applications pending.

Shown in Product Identification Section, page 417

SELDANE-D® ℞

(terfenadine and pseudoephedrine hydrochloride)
Extended-Release Tablets

CAUTION: Federal law prohibits dispensing without prescription.

DESCRIPTION

Seldane-D (terfenadine and pseudoephedrine hydrochloride) Extended-Release Tablets are available for oral administration.

Each tablet contains 60 mg terfenadine and 10 mg of pseudoephedrine hydrochloride in an outer press-coat for immediate release and 110 mg of pseudoephedrine hydrochloride in an extended-release core. Tablets also contain, as inactive ingredients: colloidal silicon dioxide, ethylcellulose, glycerin, hydroxypropyl cellulose, hydroxypropyl methylcellulose 2208, hydroxypropyl methylcellulose 2910, lactose, magnesium stearate, microcrystalline cellulose, polysorbate 80, precipitated calcium carbonate, pregelatinized corn starch, sodium lauryl sulfate, sodium starch glycolate, talc, titanium dioxide and zinc stearate.

Terfenadine is a histamine H_1-receptor antagonist with the chemical name α-[4-(1,1-Dimethylethyl)phenyl]-4-(hydroxydiphenylmethyl)-1-piperidinebutanol(+/−). It has the following chemical structure:

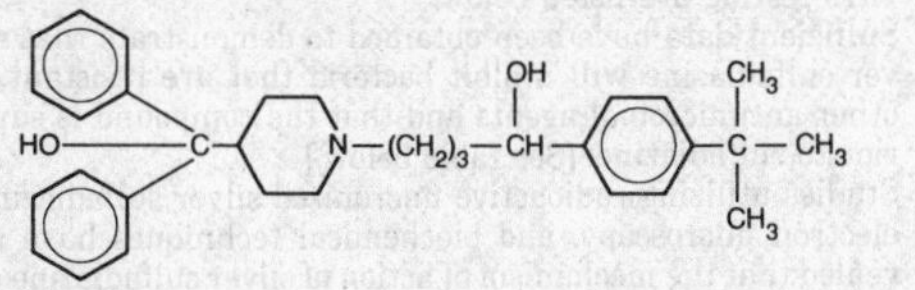

The molecular weight is 471.68. The molecular formula is $C_{32}H_{41}NO_2$.

Terfenadine occurs as a white to off-white crystalline powder. It is freely soluble in chloroform, soluble in ethanol, and very slightly soluble in water.

Pseudoephedrine hydrochloride is an adrenergic (vasoconstrictor) agent with the chemical name [S-(R*,R*)]-α-[1-(methylamino)ethyl]-benzenemethanol hydrochloride. It has the following chemical structure:

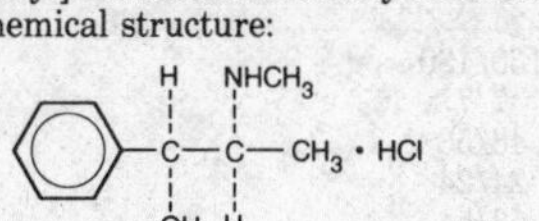

The molecular weight is 201.70. The molecular formula is $C_{10}H_{15}NO \cdot HCl$.

Pseudoephedrine hydrochloride occurs as fine, white to off-white crystals or powder, having a faint characteristic odor. It is very soluble in water; freely soluble in alcohol; and sparingly soluble in chloroform.

CLINICAL PHARMACOLOGY

Terfenadine, a histamine H_1-receptor antagonist, is chemically and pharmacologically distinct from other antihistamines.

Histamine skin wheal studies have shown that terfenadine in single and repeated doses of 60 mg in 64 subjects has an antihistaminic effect beginning at 1–2 hours, reaching its maximum at 3–4 hours, and lasting in excess of 12 hours.

Clinical trials of terfenadine involved more than 2,600 patients, most receiving either terfenadine, another antihistamine and/or placebo in double-blind, randomized controlled comparisons. The four best controlled and largest trials each lasted 7 days and involved about 1,000 total patients in comparisons of terfenadine (60 mg b.i.d.) with active drug (chlorpheniramine, 4 mg t.i.d.; dexchlorpheniramine, 2 mg t.i.d.; or clemastine 1 mg b.i.d.). In the four trials, about 50–70% of terfenadine or other antihistamine recipients had moderate to complete relief of symptoms, compared with 30–50% of placebo recipients, with a significant difference favoring the active drugs in each study. In these studies, terfenadine was associated with less frequent drowsiness than the other antihistamines; the frequency of drowsiness with terfenadine was similar to the frequency with placebo. In studies which included 52 subjects in whom EEG assessments were made, no depressant effects have been observed. Seldane-D has not been studied for effectiveness in relieving the symptoms of the common cold.

Animal studies have demonstrated that terfenadine is a histamine H_1-receptor antagonist. In these animal studies, no sedative or anticholinergic effects were observed at effective antihistaminic doses. Radioactive disposition and autoradiographic studies in rats and radioligand binding studies with guinea pig brain H_1-receptors indicate that, at effective antihistamine doses, neither terfenadine nor its metabolites penetrate the blood brain barrier well.

On the basis of a mass balance study using ^{14}C labeled terfenadine the oral absorption of terfenadine was estimated to be at least 70%. Terfenadine itself undergoes extensive (99%) first pass metabolism to two primary metabolites, an active acid metabolite and an inactive dealkylated metabolite. Therefore, systemic availability of terfenadine would be low. From information gained in the ^{14}C study it appears that approximately forty percent of the total dose is eliminated renally (40% of this as acid metabolite, 30% dealkyl metabolite, and 30% minor unidentified metabolites). Sixty percent of the dose is eliminated in the feces (50% of it as the acid metabolite, 2% unchanged terfenadine, and the remainder as minor unidentified metabolites). Studies investigating the effect of hepatic and renal insufficiency on the metabolism and excretion of terfenadine are incomplete. Preliminary information indicates that in cases of hepatic impairment, significant concentrations of unchanged terfenadine can de detected with the rate of acid metabolite formation being decreased. In subjects with normal hepatic function unchanged terfenadine plasma concentrations have not been detected.

In vitro studies demonstrate that terfenadine is extensively (97%) bound in human serum protein while the acid metabolite is approximately 70% bound to human serum protein. Based on data gathered from in vitro models of antihistaminic activity, the acid metabolite of terfenadine has approximately 30% of the H_1 blocking activity of terfenadine. The relative contribution of terfenadine and the acid metabolite to the pharmacodynamic effects have not been clearly defined. Since unchanged terfenadine is usually not detected in plasma and active metabolite concentrations are relatively high, the acid metabolite may be entirely responsible for the majority of efficacy after oral administration of terfenadine.

In a study involving the administration of a single 60 mg terfenadine tablet to 24 subjects, mean peak plasma levels of the acid metabolite were 263 ng/mL (range 133–423 ng/mL) and occurred approximately 2.5 hours after dosing. Plasma concentrations of unchanged terfenadine were not detected. The elimination profile of the acid metabolite was biphasic in nature with an initial mean plasma half-life of 3.5 hours followed by a mean plasma half-life of 6 hours. Ninety percent of the plasma level time curve was associated with these half-lives. Preliminary evidence exists at doses four times of that currently approved, that there may emerge a third phase with a half-life of >14 hours. This third phase was associated with about twenty percent of the plasma level time curve.

After multiple dose administration to steady-state of 60 mg terfenadine tablets every 12 hours the observed accumulation of Area Under the Curve during the dosing interval for the active acid metabolite was 1.6[(1)]. This observed accumulation factor corresponds to an effective pharmacokinetic half-life of 8.5 hours. This 8.5 hour half-life would predict time to steady-state, steady-state concentrations as well as time for drug elimination after multiple dosing.

Pseudoephedrine is an orally active sympathomimetic amine and exerts a decongestant action on the nasal mucosa. It is recognized as an effective agent for the relief of nasal congestion due to allergic rhinitis. Pseudoephedrine produces peripheral effects similar to those of epinephrine and central effects similar to, but less intense than, amphetamines. It has the potential for excitatory side effects. At the recommended oral dose it has little or no pressor effect in normotensive adults. The serum half-life of pseudoephedrine is approximately 4 to 6 hours. The serum half-life is decreased with increased excretion of drug at urine pH lower than 6 and may be increased with decreased excretion at urine pH higher than 8.

Ingestion of food was found not to affect the absorption of pseudoephedrine from Seldane-D. The effect of food on the absorption of terfenadine from Seldane-D is not known; however, plasma levels of the active metabolite do not appear to be affected by food administered with Seldane-D.

A bioavailability study comparing Seldane-D to immediate-release terfenadine and immediate-release pseudoephedrine, showed that pseudoephedrine is slowly released from Seldane-D to permit twice daily dosage.

[(1)]Observed Accumulation Factor = $AUC_{0\text{-}12 \text{ at steady-state}}/AUC_{0\text{-}12 \text{ at first dose}}$

INDICATIONS AND USAGE

Seldane-D is indicated for the relief of symptoms associated with seasonal allergic rhinitis such as sneezing, rhinorrhea, pruritus, lacrimation, and nasal congestion. It should be administered when both the antihistaminic properties of Seldane (terfenadine) and the nasal decongestant activity of pseudoephedrine hydrochloride are desired (see CLINICAL PHARMACOLOGY).

CONTRAINDICATIONS

Seldane-D is contraindicated in nursing mothers, patients with severe hypertension or severe coronary artery disease, patients receiving monoamine oxidase (MAO) inhibitor therapy, and in patients with a known hypersensitivity to any of its ingredients (see DESCRIPTION section).

WARNINGS

Sympathomimetic amines should be used judiciously and sparingly in patients with hypertension, diabetes mellitus, ischemic heart disease, increased intraocular pressure, hyperthyroidism, or prostatic hypertrophy (see CONTRAINDICATIONS). Sympathomimetic amines may produce CNS stimulation with convulsions or cardiovascular collapse with accompanying hypotension.

Use in Elderly

The elderly are more likely to have adverse reactions to sympathomimetics.

PRECAUTIONS

General

Seldane-D should be used with caution in patients with diabetes, hypertension, cardiovascular disease, and hyperreactivity to ephedrine. Terfenadine undergoes extensive metabolism in the liver. Patients with impaired hepatic function (alcholic cirrhosis, hepatitis), or on ketoconazole or troleandomycin therapy, or having conditions leading to QT prolongation (e.g., hypokalemia, congenital QT syndrome) may experience QT prolongation and/or ventricular tachycardia at the recommended dose. The effect of terfenadine in patients who are receiving agents which alter the QT interval is not known. These events have also occurred in patients on macrolide antibiotics, including erythromycin, but causality is unclear. The events may be related to altered metabolism of the drug, to electrolyte imbalance, or both.

Information for Patients

Patients should be questioned about pregnancy or lactation before starting Seldane-D therapy, since the drug is contraindicated in nursing women and should be used in pregnancy only if the potential benefit justifies the potential risk to fetus. Patients should be instructed to take Seldane-D only as needed and not to exceed the prescribed dose. Patients should be directed to swallow the tablet whole. Patients should also be instructed to store this medication in a tightly closed container in a cool, dry place, away from heat, moisture or direct sunlight, and away from children.

Drug Interactions (see CONTRAINDICATIONS)

Monoamine oxidase (MAO) inhibitors and beta-adrenergic blockers increase the effect of sympathomimetic amines. Sympathomimetic amines may reduce the antihypertensive effects of methyldopa, mecamylamine, and reserpine. MAO inhibitors may prolong and intensify the effects of antihistamines. Preliminary evidence exists that concurrent ketoconazole or macrolide administration significantly alters the metabolism of terfenadine. Concurrent use of Seldane-D with ketoconazole or troleandomycin is not recommended. Concurrent use of other macrolides should be approached with caution.

Carcinogenesis, Mutagenesis, Impairment of Fertility

No studies have been conducted to evaluate the carcinogenic potential of Seldane-D.

Oral doses of terfenadine, corresponding to 63 times the recommended human daily dose, in mice for 18 months or in rats for 24 months, revealed no evidence of tumorigenicity. Microbial and micronucleus test assays with terfenadine have revealed no evidence of mutagenesis.

Reproduction and fertility studies with terfenadine in rats showed no effects on male or female fertility at oral doses of up to 21 times the human daily dose. At 63 times the human daily dose there was a small but significant reduction in implants and at 125 times the human daily dose reduced implants and increased post-implantation losses were observed, which were judged to be secondary to maternal toxicity. Animal reproduction studies have not been carried out with pseudoephedrine.

Continued on next page

Marion Merrell Dow—Cont.

Pregnancy Category C
The combination of terfenadine and pseudoephedrine hydrochloride (in a ratio of 1:2 by weight) has been shown to produce reduced fetal weight in rats and rabbits at 42 times the human dose, and delayed ossification with wavy ribs in a few fetuses when given to rats at a dose of 63 times the human daily dose. There are no adequate and well controlled studies in pregnant women. Seldane-D should be used during pregnancy only if the potential benefit justifies the potential risk to the fetus.

Nursing Mothers (see CONTRAINDICATIONS)
Terfenadine has caused decreased pup weight gain and survival in rats given doses 63 times and 125 times the human daily dose throughout pregnancy and lactation.

Pediatric Use
Safety and effectiveness of Seldane-D in children below the age of 12 years have not been established.

ADVERSE REACTIONS

In double-blind, parallel, controlled studies in over 300 patients in which Seldane-D was compared to extended-release pseudoephedrine, adverse reactions reported for greater than 1% of the patients receiving Seldane-D were not clinically different from those reported for patients receiving pseudoephedrine (see Table at right.)

Pseudoephedrine may cause ephedrine-like reactions such as tachycardia, palpitations, headache, dizziness, or nausea. Sympathomimetic drugs have also been associated with certain untoward reactions including fear, anxiety, tenseness, restlessness, tremor, weakness, pallor, respiratory difficulty, dysuria, insomnia, hallucinations, convulsions, CNS depression, arrhythmias, and cardiovascular collapse with hypotension.

With terfenadine, rare reports of cardiovascular adverse reactions have been received which include arrhythmias (ventricular tachyarrhythmia, torsades de pointes, ventricular fibrillation), hypotension, palpitations, and syncope. In controlled trials in otherwise normal patients with rhinitis, at doses of 60 mg b.i.d. small increases in QTc interval were observed. Changes of this magnitude in a normal population are of doubtful clinical significance. However, in another study ($N = 20$ patients) at 300 b.i.d. a mean increase in QTc of 10% (range -4% to $+30\%$) (mean increase of 46 msec) was observed without clinical signs or symptoms.

In controlled clinical trials with terfenadine, using the recommended daily dose of 60 mg b.i.d., the incidence of adverse events in patients receiving terfenadine was similar to that reported in patients receiving placebo. The effects included: *Central Nervous System* —Drowsiness, headache, fatigue, dizziness, nervousness, weakness, appetite increase; *Gastrointestinal System* —Abdominal distress, nausea, vomiting, change in bowel habits; *Eye, Ear, Nose and Throat* —Dry mouth/nose/throat, cough, sore throat, epistaxis; *Skin* —Eruption (including rash and urticaria) or itching. Also reported spontaneously during the marketing of terfenadine were: alopecia (hair loss or thinning), anaphylaxis, angioedema, bronchospasm, confusion, depression, galactorrhea, insomnia, menstrual disorders (including dysmenorrhea), musculoskeletal symptoms, nightmares, paresthesia, photosensitivity, seizures, sinus tachycardia, sweating, tremor, urinary frequency, and visual disturbances.

Also in clinical trials, several instances of mild, or in one case, moderate transaminase elevations were seen in patients receiving terfenadine. Mild elevations were also seen in placebo treated patients. Marketing experiences include isolated reports of jaundice, cholestatic hepatitis, and hepatitis. In most cases available information is incomplete.

OVERDOSAGE

Acute overdosage with Seldane-D tablets may produce clinical signs of CNS stimulation or depression and various cardiovascular effects, including cardiac collapse and death. Sympathomimetic amines should be used with great caution in the presence of pseudoephedrine. Patients with signs of stimulation should be treated conservatively. At overdoses of 600 mg/day (300 mg b.i.d.) of terfenadine there may be a prolongation of the QT interval. At 900 mg or more there have been rare incidents of ventricular arrhythmias (torsades de pointes or fibrillation). Seizures and syncope have been reported.

Therefore, in cases of overdosage, cardiac monitoring for at least 24 hours is recommended and for as long as QTc is prolonged, along with standard measures to remove any unabsorbed drug. Limited experience with the use of hemoperfusion ($N = 1$) and hemodialysis ($N = 3$) was not successful in completely removing the acid metabolite of terfenadine from the blood.

Oral LD$_{50}$ values for terfenadine were greater than 5000 mg/kg in mature mice and rats. The oral LD$_{50}$ was 438 mg/kg in newborn rats. The LD$_{50}$ of pseudoephedrine hydrochloride alone in male and female rats was 1674 mg/kg, while the LD$_{50}$ of pseudoephedrine hydrochloride administered with terfenadine was 3017 mg/kg.

FREQUENTLY (> 1%) REPORTED ADVERSE EVENTS FOR SELDANE-D IN DOUBLE-BLIND, PARALLEL, CONTROLLED CLINICAL TRIALS*

Adverse Event	Percent of Patients Reporting		
	Seldane-D (N = 374)	Pseudo-Ephedrine (N = 287)	Placebo (N = 193)
Central Nervous System			
Insomnia	25.9	26.8	6.2
Headache	17.4	17.1	22.3
Drowsiness/Sedation	7.2	4.9	11.4
Nervousness	6.7	8.4	1.6
Anorexia	3.7	3.8	0.0
Fatigue	2.1	1.4	2.1
Restlessness	2.1	1.0	0.0
Irritability	1.1	0.0	1.0
Disorientation	1.1	0.0	0.5
Increased Energy	1.1	0.0	0.0
Hyperkinesia	1.1	1.0	0.0
Autonomic			
Dry Mouth/Nose/Throat	21.7	21.3	11.4
Blurring of Vision	1.1	0.3	0.5
Gastrointestinal			
Nausea	4.5	6.6	5.2
Skin			
Rash	1.1	0.0	0.0
Cardiovascular			
Palpitations	2.4	3.8	0.5
Allergy Symptoms			
Sore Throat	1.9	1.7	1.0
Cough	1.6	0.3	1.0
Other			
Infections, Upper Respiratory	1.3	2.4	0.5
Taste Alterations	1.1	1.0	1.0

*Seldane-D B.I.D., pseudoephedrine 120 mg B.I.D.

DOSAGE AND ADMINISTRATION
Adults and children 12 years and older: one tablet swallowed whole, morning and night.

HOW SUPPLIED
Seldane-D Tablets containing 60 mg of terfenadine and 10 mg of pseudoephedrine hydrochloride in an outer press-coat for immediate release and 110 mg of pseudoephedrine hydrochloride in an extended-release core are supplied as follows:
NDC 0068-0722-61: Bottles of 100 tablets.
Tablets are white to off-white, biconvex capsule-shaped; debossed "SELDANE-D". Store at controlled room temperature (59°–86°F) (15°–30°C). Protect from moisture.
Product information as of June, 1991.
Shown in Product Identification Section, page 417

SILVADENE® CREAM 1%   ℞
[*sil'vuh-dēn*]
(silver sulfadiazine)

DESCRIPTION
SILVADENE Cream 1% is a soft, white, water-miscible cream containing the antimicrobial agent silver sulfadiazine in micronized form, which has the following structural formula: [See next column.]

Each gram of SILVADENE Cream 1% contains 10 mg of micronized silver sulfadiazine. The cream vehicle consists of white petrolatum, stearyl alcohol, isopropyl myristate, sorbitan monooleate, polyoxyl 40 stearate, propylene glycol, and water, with methylparaben 0.3% as a preservative.

CLINICAL PHARMACOLOGY
SILVADENE Cream 1% (silver sulfadiazine) spreads easily and can be washed off readily with water.
Silver sulfadiazine has broad antimicrobial activity. It is bactericidal for many gram-negative and gram-positive bacteria as well as being effective against yeast. Results from in vitro testing are listed below.
Sufficient data have been obtained to demonstrate that silver sulfadiazine will inhibit bacteria that are resistant to other antimicrobial agents and that the compound is superior to sulfadiazine. [See table below.]
Studies utilizing radioactive micronized silver sulfadiazine, electron microscopy, and biochemical techniques have revealed that the mechanism of action of silver sulfadiazine on bacteria differs from silver nitrate and sodium sulfadiazine. SILVADENE Cream 1% (silver sulfadiazine) acts only on the cell membrane and cell wall to produce its bactericidal effect.

Genus & Species	Number of Sensitive Strains/Total Strains Tested Concentration of Silver Sulfadiazine	
	50 µg/ml	100 µg/ml
Pseudomonas aeruginosa	130/130	130/130
Pseudomonas maltophilia	7/7	7/7
Enterobacter species	48/50	50/50
Enterobacter cloacae	24/24	24/24
Klebsiella	53/54	54/54
Escherichia coli	63/63	63/63
Serratia	27/28	28/28
Proteus mirabilis	53/53	53/53
Proteus morganii	10/10	10/10
Proteus rettgeri	2/2	2/2
Proteus vulgaris	2/2	2/2
Providencia	1/1	1/1
Citrobacter	10/10	10/10
Herellea	8/9	9/9
Mima	2/2	2/2
Staphylococcus aureus	100/101	101/101
Staphylococcus epidermidis	51/51	51/51
β-Hemolytic *Streptococcus*	4/4	4/4
Enterococcus (group D *Streptococcus*)	52/53	53/53
Corynebacterium diphtheriae	2/2	2/2
Clostridium perfringens	0/2	2/2
Candida albicans	43/50	50/50

INDICATIONS AND USAGE

SILVADENE Cream 1% (silver sulfadiazine) is a topical antimicrobial drug indicated as an adjunct for the prevention and treatment of wound sepsis in patients with second- and third-degree burns.

CONTRAINDICATIONS

Because sulfonamide therapy is known to increase the possibiltiy of kernicterus, SILVADENE Cream 1% should not be used at term pregnancy, on premature infants, or on newborn infants during the first 2 months of life.

WARNINGS

GENERAL. SILVADENE Cream 1% should be administered with great caution to patients with history of hypersensitivity to SILVADENE Cream 1%. There is potential cross-sensitivity between SILVADENE Cream 1% and other sulfonamides. If allergic reactions attributable to treatment with SILVADENE Cream 1% occur, discontinuation of SILVADENE Cream 1% must be considered.

Fungal proliferation in and below the eschar may occur. However, the incidence of clinically reported fungal superinfection is low.

PRECAUTIONS

GENERAL. If hepatic and renal functions become imparied and elimination of drug decreases, accumulation may occur and discontinuation of SILVADENE Cream 1% (silver sulfadiazine) should be weighed against the therapeutic benefit being achieved.

In considering the use of topical proteolytic enzymes in conjunction with SILVADENE Cream 1%, the possibility should be noted that silver may inactivate such enzymes. The use of SILVADENE Cream 1% in some cases of glucose-6-phosphate dehydrogenase-deficient individuals may be hazardous as hemolysis may occur.

LABORATORY TESTS. In the treatment of burn wounds involving extensive areas of the body, the serum sulfa concentrations may approach adult therapeutic levels (8 to 12 mg%). Therefore, in these patients it would be advisable to monitor serum sulfa concentrations. Renal function should be carefully monitored and the urine should be checked for sulfa crystals. Absorption of the propylene glycol vehicle has been reported to affect serum osmolality, which may affect the interpretation of laboratory tests.

CARCINOGENESIS, MUTAGENESIS, IMPAIRMENT OF FERTILITY. Long-term dermal toxicity studies of 24 months' duration in rats and 18 months in mice with concentrations of silver sulfadiazine three to ten times the concentration in SILVADENE Cream 1% revealed no evidence of carcinogenicity.

PREGNANCY CATEGORY B. A reproductive study has been performed in rabbits at concentrations of silver sulfadiazine three to ten times the concentration in SILVADENE Cream 1%. The results of this study showed no harmful effect on the fetus. There are, however, no adequate and well-controlled studies in pregnant women. Because animal reproduction studies are not always predictive of human response, this drug should be used during pregnancy only if clearly needed.

NURSING MOTHERS. It is not known whether SILVADENE Cream 1% is excreted in human milk. However, sulfonamides are known to be excreted in human milk. Since all sulfonamide derivatives are known to increase the possibility of kernicterus, caution should be excercised when SILVADENE Cream 1% is administered to a nursing woman.

ADVERSE REACTIONS

In the original clinical trials, an aggregate of 2,297 patients were treated with SILVADENE Cream 1% and reported 59 drug-related reactions (2.5%). These included burning sensation (2.2%), rash (0.2%), itching (0.1%), and one report of interstitial nephritis.

In postmarketing experience with SILVADENE Cream 1%, there have been additional reports of infrequently occurring events. These include skin necrosis, erythema multiforme, and leukopenia. The propylene glycol vehicle has also been reported to cause hyperosmolality.

Skin discoloration may rarely occur in some patients. The majority of reports to date indicate that this discoloration is transient and subsides upon discontinuation of therapy.

There have also been several cases of transient leukopenia reported in patients receiving silver sulfadiazine therapy. In an uncontrolled study, leukopenia (WBC < 3500) was reported to occur with a frequency of one in 20 patients.[1] However, in a placebo-controlled study in which 69 patients received silver sulfadiazine and 60 received placebo, six (10%) patients in the placebo group and five (7%) patients in the treatment group developed leukopenia[2] (WBC < 5000). The leukopenia associated with silver sulfadiazine is characterized by decreased neutrophil count with maximal white blood cell depression occurring within two to four days of initiation of therapy. Leukocyte levels usually rebound to normal levels within two to three days without discontinuation of therapy.

Absorption of silver sulfadiazine varies depending upon the percent of body surface area and the extent of the tissue damage. Although few have been reported, it is possible that any adverse reaction associated with sulfonamides may occur. Some of the reactions which have been associated with sulfonamides are as follows: blood dyscrasias, including agranulocytosis, aplastic anemia, thrombocytopenia, leukopenia and hemolytic anemia; dermatologic and allergic reactions, including Stevens-Johnson syndrome and exfoliative dermatitis; gastrointestinal reactions; hepatitis and hepatocellular necrosis; CNS reactions; and toxic nephrosis.

DOSAGE AND ADMINISTRATION

Prompt insitution of appropriate regimens for care of the burned patient is of prime importance and includes the control of shock and pain. The burn wounds are then cleansed and debrided and SILVADENE Cream 1% (silver sulfadiazine) is applied with sterile, gloved hand. The burn areas should be covered with SILVADENE Cream 1% at all times. The cream should be applied once to twice daily to a thickness of approximately $\frac{1}{16}$ inch. Whenever necessary, the cream should be reapplied to any areas from which it has been removed by patient activity. Administration may be accomplished in minimal time because dressings are not required. However if individual patient requirements make dressings necessary, they may be used.

When feasible, the patient should be bathed daily. This is an aid in debridement. A whirlpool bath is particularly helpful, but the patient may be bathed in bed or in a shower.

Reduction in bacterial growth after application of topical antibacterial agents has been reported to permit spontaneous healing of deep partial-thickness burns by preventing conversion of the partial thickness to full thickness by sepsis. However, reduction in bacterial colonization has caused delayed separation, in some cases necessitating escharotomy in order to prevent contracture.

Treatment with SILVADENE Cream 1% should be continued until satisfactory healing has occurred or until the burn site is ready for grafting. **The drug should not be withdrawn from the therapeutic regimen while there remains the possibility of infection except if a significant adverse reaction occurs.**

HOW SUPPLIED

SILVADENE Cream 1% (silver sulfadiazine) is available in jars containing 50 grams (NDC 0088-1050-50), 400 grams (NDC 0088-1050-72), and 1,000 grams (NDC 0088-1050-58) and tubes contianing 20 grams (NDC 0088-1050-20) and 85 grams (NDC 0088-1050-85).

BIBLIOGRAPHY

1. Jarret F, Ellerbe S, Demling R: Acute leukopenia during topical burn therapy with silver sulfadiazine. *Amer J Surg* 1978;135:818–819.
2. Kiker RG, Carvajal HF, Micak RP, Larson DL: A controlled study of the effects of silver sulfadiazine on white blood cell counts in burned children. *J Trauma* 1977;17:835–836.

U.S. Patent 3,761,590   Issued 2/88

Shown in Product Identification Section, page 417

SINGLET®   **OTC**
[sĭn ′glĕt]
Long-Acting Tablets
Decongestant-Antihistamine-Analgesic

(See PDR For Nonprescription Drugs.)

TACE®   ℞
(CHLOROTRIANISENE USP)
12 mg and 25 mg
Capsules

WARNINGS

---

1. ESTROGENS HAVE BEEN REPORTED TO INCREASE THE RISK OF ENDOMETRIAL CARCINOMA IN POSTMENOPAUSAL WOMEN.

Close clinical surveillance of all women taking estrogens is important. In all cases of undiagnosed persistent or recurring abnormal vaginal bleeding, adequate diagnostic measures including endometrial sampling when indicated should be undertaken to rule out malignancy. There is currently no evidence that "natural" estrogens are more or less hazardous than "synthetic" estrogens at equiestrogenic doses.

2. ESTROGENS SHOULD NOT BE USED DURING PREGNANCY.

Estrogen therapy during pregnancy is associated with an increased risk of congenital defects in the reproductive organs of the male and female fetus, an increased risk of vaginal adenosis, squamous cell dysplasia of the uterine cervix, and vaginal cancer in the female later in

life. The 1985 Diethylstilbestrol (DES) Task force concluded that women who used DES during their pregnancies may subsequently experience an increased risk of breast cancer. However, a causal relationship is still unproven, and the observed level of risk is similar to that for a number of other breast cancer risk factors. There is no indication for estrogen therapy during pregnancy. Estrogens are ineffective for the prevention or treatment of threatened or habitual abortion.

If TACE (CHLOROTRIANISENE USP) is used during pregnancy, or if the patient becomes pregnant while taking this drug, she should be apprised of the potential risks to the fetus, and the advisability of pregnancy continuation.

DESCRIPTION

TACE (CHLOROTRIANISENE USP) is available in capsule form suitable for oral administration. Each green, soft gelatin capsule contains 12 mg of chlorotrianisene. This capsule also contains inactive ingredients: corn oil (solvent), FD&C Blue No. 1, FD&C Yellow No. 5 (tartrazine, See PRECAUTIONS), gelatin, glycerin, methylparaben, propylparaben, titanium dioxide, and water.

Each two-tone green, hard gelatin capsule contains 25 mg of chlorotrianisene. This capsule also contains inactive ingredients: FD&C Blue No. 1 or FD&C Green No.3, FD&C Blue No. 2, FD&C Red No. 40, FD&C Yellow No. 5 (tartrazine, See PRECAUTIONS), FD&C Yellow No. 6, gelatin, iron oxide, magnesium stearate, titanium dioxide, and tristearin (solvent).

Chlorotrianisene is a long-acting, synthetic estrogen with the chemical name 1,1′,1″-(1-chloro-1-ethenyl-2-ylidene)-tris[4-methoxy]-benzene.

It has the following chemical structure:

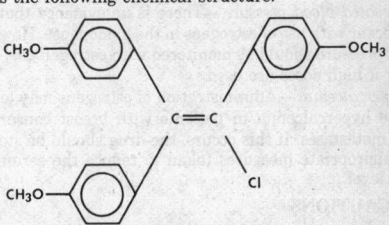

Chlorotrianisene occurs as small, white crystals or as a crystalline powder. It is odorless. It is slightly soluble in alcohol and very slightly soluble in water.

INDICATIONS AND USAGE

TACE is indicated in the treatment of:
1. Advanced androgen-dependent carcinoma of the prostate (for palliation only).
2. Moderate to severe vasomotor symptoms associated with the menopause. There is no adequate evidence that estrogens are effective for nervous symptoms or depression which might occur during menopause and they should not be used to treat these conditions.
3. Atrophic vaginitis.
4. Kraurosis vulvae.
5. Hypoestrogenism due to hypogonadism, castration, or primary ovarian failure.

CONTRAINDICATIONS

TACE is contraindicated in patients with a known hypersensitivity to chlorotrianisene or other ingredients of the formulation.

TACE should not be used in women or men with any of the following conditions:
1. Known or suspected pregnancy. (See Boxed Warning.) Estrogen may cause fetal harm when administered to a pregnant woman.
2. Known or suspected cancer of the breast except in appropriately selected patients being treated for metastatic disease.
3. Known or suspected estrogen-dependent neoplasia.
4. Undiagnosed abnormal genital bleeding.
5. Active thrombophlebitis or thromboembolic disorders— Women on estrogen replacement therapy have not been reported to have an increased risk of thrombophlebitis and/or thromboembolic disease. However, there is insufficient information regarding women who have had previous thromboembolic disease.

WARNINGS

1. *Induction of malignant neoplasms*—Some studies have suggested a possible increased incidence of breast cancer in those women on estrogen therapy taking higher doses for prolonged periods of time. The majority of studies, however, have not shown an association with the usual doses used for estrogen replacement therapy. Women on this therapy should have regular breast examinations and should be instructed in breast self-examination. The reported endome-

Continued on next page

Marion Merrell Dow—Cont.

trial cancer risk among estrogen users was about fourfold or greater than in non-users, and appears dependent on duration of treatment and on estrogen dose. There is no significantly increased risk associated with the use of estrogens for less than one year. The greatest risk appears associated with prolonged use—five years or more. In one study, persistence of risk was demonstrated for 10 years after cessation of estrogen treatment. In another study, a significant decrease in the incidence of endometrial cancer occurred six months after estrogen withdrawal.

Estrogen therapy during pregnancy is associated with an increased risk of fetal congenital reproductive tract disorders. In females, there is an increased risk of vaginal adenosis, squamous cell dysplasia of the cervix, and cancer later in life; in the male, urogenital abnormalities. Although some of these changes are benign, it is not known whether they are precursors of malignancy.

2. *Gallbladder disease*—The risk of surgically confirmed gallbladder disease has been reported to be 2.5 times higher in women receiving postmenopausal estrogens.

3. *Cardiovascular disease*—Large doses of estrogen (5 mg conjugated estrogens per day), comparable to those used to treat cancer of the prostate and breast, have been shown in a large prospective clinical trial in men to increase the risk of non-fatal myocardial infarction, pulmonary embolism, and thrombophlebitis. It cannot necessarily be extrapolated from men to women. However, to avoid the theoretical cardiovascular risk caused by high estrogen doses, the doses for estrogen replacement therapy should not exceed the recommended dose.

4. *Elevated blood pressure*—There is no evidence that this may occur with use of estrogens in the menopause. However, blood pressure should be monitored with estrogen use, especially if high doses are used.

5. *Hypercalcemia*—Administration of estrogens may lead to severe hypercalcemia in patients with breast cancer and bone metastases. If this occurs, the drug should be stopped and appropriate measures taken to reduce the serum calcium level.

PRECAUTIONS

General

1. *Addition of a progestin*—Studies of the addition of a progestin for seven or more days of a cycle of estrogen administration have reported a lowered incidence of endometrial hyperplasia. Morphological and biochemical studies of the endometrium suggest that 10 to 13 days of progestin are needed to provide maximal maturation of the endometrium and to eliminate any hyperplastic changes. Whether this will provide protection from endometrial carcinoma has not been clearly established. There are possible additional risks which may be associated with the inclusion of progestin in estrogen replacement regimens. The potential risks include adverse effects on carbohydrate and lipid metabolism. The choice of progestin and dosage may be important in minimizing these adverse effects.

2. *Physical examination*—A complete medical and family history should be taken prior to the initiation of any estrogen therapy. The pretreatment and periodic physical examinations should include special reference to blood pressure, breasts, abdomen, and pelvic organs, and should include a Papanicolaou smear. As a general rule, estrogen should not be prescribed for longer than 1 year without another physical examination being performed.

3. *Fluid retention*—Because estrogens may cause some degree of fluid retention, conditions which might be influenced by this factor such as asthma, epilepsy, migraine, and cardiac or renal dysfunction, require careful observation.

4. *Uterine bleeding and mastodynia*—Certain patients may develop undesirable manifestations of estrogenic stimulation, such as abnormal uterine bleeding and mastodynia.

5. *Uterine fibroids*—Pre-existing uterine leiomyomata may increase in size during prolonged high-dose estrogen use.

6. *Impaired liver function*—Estrogens may be poorly metabolized in patients with impaired liver function and should be administered with caution.

7. *Hypercalcemia* (and renal insufficiency)—Prolonged use of estrogens can influence the metabolism of calcium and phosphorus. Estrogens should be used with caution in patients with metabolic bone disease or in patients with renal insufficiency.

Information for the Patient

See text of Patient Package Insert which accompanies this drug product.

Laboratory Tests

Clinical response at the smallest dose should generally be the guide to estrogen administration for relief of symptoms for those indications in which symptoms are observable. Tests used to measure adequacy of estrogen replacement therapy include serum estrone and estradiol levels and suppression of serum gonadotropin levels.

Drug/Laboratory Test Interactions

Some of these drug/laboratory test interactions have been observed only with estrogen-progestin combinations (oral contraceptives):

1. Increased prothrombin and factors VII, VIII, IX, and X; decreased antithrombin 3; increased norepinephrine-induced platelet aggregability, decreased fibrinolysis.
2. Increased thyroid-binding globulin (TBG) leading to increased circulating total thyroid hormone, as measured by T_4 levels determined either by column or by radioimmunoassay. Free T_3 resin uptake is decreased, reflecting the elevated TBG; free T_4 concentration is unaltered.
3. Impaired glucose tolerance.
4. Reduced response to metyrapone test.
5. Reduced serum folate concentration.

NOTE: *This product contains FD&C Yellow No. 5 (tartrazine), which may cause allergic-type reactions (including bronchial asthma) in certain susceptible individuals. Although the overall incidence of FD&C Yellow No. 5 (tartrazine) sensitivity in the general population is low, it is frequently seen in patients who also have aspirin hypersensitivity.*

Mutagenesis and Carcinogenesis

Long-term continuous administration of natural and synthetic estrogens in certain animal species increases the frequency of carcinomas of the breast, cervix, vagina, and liver.

Pregnancy Category X

Estrogens should not be used during pregnancy. (See CONTRAINDICATIONS and Boxed Warning.)

Nursing Mothers

As a general principle, the administration of any drug to nursing mothers should be done only when clearly necessary since many drugs are excreted in human milk.

ADVERSE REACTIONS

(See Warnings regarding induction of neoplasia, adverse effects on the fetus, increased incidence of gallbladder disease). The following additional adverse reactions have been reported with estrogen therapy:

1. *Genitourinary system*—Changes in vaginal bleeding pattern and abnormal withdrawal bleeding or flow; breakthrough bleeding, spotting; increase in size of uterine fibromyomata; vaginal candidiasis; change in amount of cervical secretion.
2. *Breasts*—Tenderness, enlargement.
3. *Gastrointestinal*—Nausea, vomiting; abdominal cramps, bloating; cholestatic jaundice.
4. *Skin*—Chloasma or melasma, that may persist when drug is discontinued; erythema multiforme; erythema nodosum; urticaria; hemorrhagic eruption; loss of scalp hair; hirsutism.
5. *Eyes*—Steepening of corneal curvature; intolerance of contact lenses.
6. *CNS*—Headache, migraine, dizziness; mental depression; chorea.
7. *Miscellaneous*—Increase or decrease in weight; reduced carbohydrate tolerance; aggravation of porphyria; edema; changes in libido.

ACUTE OVERDOSAGE

Numerous reports of ingestion of large doses of estrogen-containing oral contraceptives by young children indicate that acute serious ill effects do not occur. Overdoseage of estrogen may cause nausea and vomiting.

DOSAGE AND ADMINISTRATION

1. Advanced androgen-dependent carcinoma of the prostate, for palliation only. The usual dosage is 12 to 25 mg daily (one or two 12 mg capsules or one 25 mg capsule).
2. For treatment of moderate to severe vasomotor symptoms, atrophic vaginitis, or kraurosis vulvae associated with the menopause. The lowest dose that will control symptoms should be chosen and medication should be discontinued as promptly as possible. Administration should be cyclic (e.g., 3 weeks on and 1 week off).
   Attempts to discontinue or taper medication should be made at 3-month to 6-month intervals.
   The usual dosage range for vasomotor symptoms, atrophic vaginitis, or kraurosis vulvae associated with the menopause is 12 to 25 mg daily (one or two 12 mg capsules or one 25 mg capsule) for 30 days; one or more courses may be prescribed.
3. Female hypogonadism; primary ovarian failure.
   The usual dosage is 12 to 25 mg daily (one or two 12 mg capsules or one 25 mg capsule) for 21 days. This course may, if desired, be folowed immediately by the intramuscular injection of 100 mg of progesterone; alternatively, an oral progesterone such as medroxyprogesterone may be given during the last 5 days of TACE (CHLOROTRIANISENE USP) therapy. The next course may begin on the 5th day of the induced uterine bleeding.
   Treated patients with an intact uterus should be monitored closely for signs of endometrial cancer, and appropriate diagnostic measures should be taken to rule out malignancy in the event of persistent or recurrent abnormal vaginal bleeding.

HOW SUPPLIED

TACE 12 mg (CHLOROTRIANISENE CAPSULES USP) green capsules imprinted MERRELL 690
NDC 0068-0690-61: bottles of 100
TACE 25 mg (CHLOROTRIANISENE CAPSULES USP) two-tone green capsules imprinted MERRELL 691
NDC 0068-0691-60: bottles of 60
Patient Information as of June, 1991
TACE 12 mg Capsules
Manufactured By
R.P. Scherer,
North America
Clearwater, Florida 33518
for
Merrell Dow Pharmaceuticals Inc.
Subsidiary of Marion Merrell Dow Inc.
Kansas City, MO 64114

Shown in Product Identification Section, page 417

INFORMATION FOR PATIENTS

TACE (CHLOROTRIANISENE) is a synthetic estrogen supplied in 12 mg and 25 mg capsules.

This leaflet describes when and how to use estrogens and the risks of estrogen treatment.

ESTROGEN DRUGS

Estrogens have several important uses but also some risks. You must decide, with your doctor, whether the risks of estrogens are acceptable in view of their benefits. If you decide to start taking estrogens, check with your doctor to make sure you are using the lowest possible effective dose. The length of treatment with estrogens will depend upon the reason for use. This should also be discussed with your doctor.

USES OF ESTROGEN

1. *To reduce menopausal symptoms*
   Estrogens are hormones produced by the ovaries. The decrease in the amount of estrogen that occurs in all women, usually between ages 45 and 55, causes the menopause. Sometimes the ovaries are removed by an operation, causing "surgical menopause." When the amount of estrogen begins to decrease, some women develop very uncomfortable symptoms, such as feelings of warmth in the face, neck and chest or sudden intense episodes of heat and sweating ("hot flashes"). The use of drugs containing estrogens can help the body adjust to lower estrogen levels.
   Most women have none or only mild menopausal symptoms and do not need estrogens. Other women may need estrogens for a few months while their bodies adjust to lower estrogen levels. The majority of women do not need estrogen replacement for longer than six months for these symptoms.
2. *To treat atrophic vaginitis* (itching, burning, dryness in or around the vagina) and *kraurosis vulvae* (which may cause chronic irritation of the vagina and vulva).
3. *To treat certain cancers*

WHEN ESTROGENS SHOULD NOT BE USED

Estrogens should not be used:

1. *During pregnancy*
   Although the possibility is fairly small, there is a greater risk of having a child born with a birth defect if you take estrogens during pregnancy. A male child may have an increased risk of developing abnormalities of the urinary system and sex organs. A female child may have an increased risk of developing cancer of the vagina or cervix in her teens or twenties. Estrogen is not effective in preventing miscarriage (abortion).
2. *If you have had any heart or circulation problems*
   Estrogen therapy should be used only after consultation with your physician and only in recommended doses. Patients with a tendency for abnormal blood clotting should avoid estrogen use (see below).
3. *If you have had cancer*
   Since estrogens increase the risk of certain cancers, you should not take estrogens if you have ever had cancer of the breast or uterus. In certain situations, your doctor may choose to use estrogen in the treatment of breast cancer or prostate cancer.
4. *When they are ineffective*
   Sometimes women experience nervous symptoms or depression during menopause. There is no evidence that estrogens are effective for such symptoms. You may have heard that taking estrogens for long periods (years) after menopause will keep your skin soft and supple and keep you feeling young. There is no evidence that this is so and such long-term treatment may carry serious risks.

DANGERS OF ESTROGENS

1. *Cancer of the uterus*
   The risk of cancer of the uterus increases the longer estrogens are used and when larger doses are taken. One study showed that when estrogens are discontinued, this increased risk of cancer seems to fall off quickly. In another

study, the persistence of risk was demonstrated for 10 years after stopping estrogen treatment. Because of this risk, *it is important to take the lowest dose of estrogen that will control your symptoms and to take it only as long as you need it.* There is a higher risk of cancer of the uterus if you are overweight, diabetic, or have high blood pressure.
If you have had your uterus removed (total hysterectomy), there is no danger of developing cancer of the uterus.

2. *Cancer of the breast*
The majority of studies have shown no association with the usual doses used for estrogen replacement therapy and breast cancer. Some studies have suggested a possible increased incidence of breast cancer in those women taking estrogens for prolonged periods of time and especially if higher doses are used.
Regular breast examinations by a health professional and self-examination are recommended for women receiving estrogen therapy, as they are for all women.
3. *Gallbladder disease*
Women who use estrogens after menopause are more likely to develop gallbladder disease needing surgery than women who do not use estrogens.
4. *Abnormal blood clotting*
Taking estrogens may increase the risk of blood clots. This can cause a stroke, heart attack or pulmonary embolus, any of which may be fatal.

SIDE EFFECTS

In addition to the risk of estrogens described above, the following side effects have been reported with estrogen use:
1. Nausea and vomiting
2. Breast tenderness or enlargement
3. Enlargement of benign tumors of the uterus
4. Retention of excess fluid This may make some conditions worsen, such as asthma, epilepsy, migraine, heart disease, or kidney disease.
5. A spotty darkening of the skin, particularly on the face.

NOTE: TACE 12 and 25 mg capsules contain a dye (FD&C Yellow No. 5 or tartrazine), which may cause allergic-type reactions (including asthma) in certain suspectible individuals. Although the over-all frequency of tartrazine sensitivity in the general population is low, it is frequently seen in pc 'ients who also have aspirin hypersensitivity.

REDUCING RISK OF ESTROGEN USE

If you decide to take estrogens, you can reduce your risks by carefully monitoring your treatment.
1. *See your doctor regularly*
While you are taking estrogens, it is important that you visit your doctor at least once a year for a physical examination. If members of your family have had breast cancer or if you have ever had breast nodules or an abnormal mammogram (breast x-ray), you may need to have more frequent breast examinations.
2. *Reevaluate your need for estrogens*
You and your doctor should reevaluate your need for estrogens at least every six months.
3. *Be alert for signs of trouble*
Report these or any other unusual side effects to your doctor immediately:
   1. Abnormal bleeding from the vagina
   2. Pains in the calves or chest, a sudden shortness of breath or coughing blood (indicating possible clots in the legs, heart, or lungs)
   3. Severe headache, dizziness, faintness, or changes in vision, indicating possible clots in the brain or eye
   4. Breast lumps
   5. Yellowing of the skin
   6. Pain, swelling, or tenderness in the abdomen.

OTHER INFORMATION

Some physicians may choose to prescribe another hormonal drug to be used in association with estrogen treatment. These drugs, progestins, have been reported to lower the frequency of occurrence of a possible precancerous condition of the uterine lining. Whether this will provide protection from uterine cancer has not been clearly established. There are possible additional risks that may be associated with the inclusion of a progestin in estrogen treatment. The possible risks include unfavorable effects on blood fats and sugars. The choice of progestin and its dosage may be important in minimizing these effects.
Your doctor has prescribed this drug for you and you alone. Do not give the drug to anyone else.
Keep this and all drugs out of the reach of children. In case of overdose, call your doctor, hospital, or poison control center immediately.
This leaflet provides the most important information about estrogens. If you want to read more, ask your doctor or pharmacist to let you read the professional labeling.

HOW SUPPLIED

TACE (CHLOROTRIANISENE CAPSULES USP) is a long-acting synthetic estrogen in capsule form. The capsule is suitable for taking by mouth.
Each green, soft gelatin capsule imprinted MERRELL 690 contains 12 mg of chlorotrianisene. This capsule also contains inactive ingredients: corn oil (solvent), FD&C Blue No. 1, FD&C Yellow No. 5 (tartrazine) as a color additive, gelatin, glycerin, methylparaben, propylparaben, titanium dioxide, and water.
Each two-tone green, hard gelatin capsule imprinted MERRELL 691 contains 25 mg of chlorotrianisene. This capsule also contains inactive ingredients: FD&C Blue No. 1 or FD&C Green No.3, FD&C Blue No. 2, FD&C Red No. 40, FD&C Yellow No. 5 (tartrazine) as a color additive, FD&C Yellow No. 6, gelatin, iron oxide, magnesium stearate, titanium dioxide, and tristearin (solvent).
Patient Information as of June, 1991
TACE 12 mg capsules
Manufactured By
R.P. Scherer,
North America
Clearwater, Florida 33518
for
Marion Merrell Dow
Kansas City, MO 64114

TENUATE® Ⓒ ℞
[*tĕn 'ū-āt*]
(diethylpropion hydrochloride USP)
immediate-release 25 mg tablets
TENUATE DOSPAN® Ⓒ ℞
(diethylpropion hydrochloride USP)
controlled-release
75 mg tablets

DESCRIPTION

Tenuate is available for oral administration in immediate-release tablets containing 25 mg diethylpropion hydrochloride and in controlled-release tablets containing 75 mg diethylpropion hydrochloride. The inactive ingredients in each immediate-release tablet are: corn starch, lactose, magnesium stearate, pregelatinized corn starch, talc, and tartaric acid. The inactive ingredients in each controlled-release tablet are: carbomer 934P, mannitol, povidone, tartaric acid, zinc stearate. Diethylpropion hydrochloride is a sympathomimetic agent. The chemical name for diethylpropion hydrochloride is 1-phenyl-2-diethylamino-1-propanone hydrochloride.
Its chemical structure is:

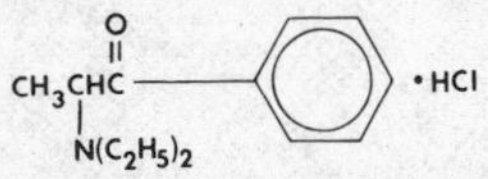

In Tenuate Dospan tablets, diethylpropion hydrochloride is dispersed in a hydrophilic matrix. On exposure to water, the diethylpropion hydrochloride is released at a relatively uniform rate as a result of slow hydration of the matrix. The result is controlled release of the anorectic agent.

CLINICAL PHARMACOLOGY

Diethylpropion hydrochloride is a sympathomimetic amine with some pharmacologic activity similar to that of the prototype drugs of this class used in obesity, the amphetamines. Actions include some central nervous system stimulation and elevation of blood pressure. Tolerance has been demonstrated with all drugs of this class in which these phenomena have been looked for.
Drugs of this class used in obesity are commonly known as "anorectics" or "anorexigenics." It has not been established, however, that the action of such drugs in treating obesity is primarily one of appetite suppression. For example, other central nervous system actions or metabolic effects may be involved.
Adult obese subjects instructed in dietary management and treated with "anorectic" drugs lose more weight on the average than those treated with placebo and diet, as determined in relatively short-term clinical trials.
The magnitude of increased weight loss of drug-treated patients over placebo-treated patients averages some fraction of a pound a week. However, individual weight loss may vary substantially from patient to patient. The rate of weight loss is greatest in the first weeks of therapy for both drug and placebo subjects and tends to decrease in succeeding weeks. The possible origins of the increased weight loss due to the various drug effects are not established. The amount of weight loss associated with the use of an "anorectic" drug varies from trial to trial, and the increased weight loss appears to be related in part to variables other than the drug prescribed, such as the physician/investigator relationship, the population treated, and the diet prescribed. Studies do not permit conclusions as to the relative importance of the drug and non-drug factors on weight loss.
The natural history of obesity is measured in years, whereas most studies cited are restricted to a few weeks duration; thus, the total impact of drug-induced weight loss over that of diet alone is unknown.
Diethylpropion is rapidly absorbed from the GI tract after oral administration and is extensively metabolized through a complex pathway of biotransformation involving N-dealkylation and reduction. Many of these metabolites are biologically active and may participate in the therapeutic action of Tenuate or Tenuate Dospan. Due to the varying lipid solubilities of these metabolites, their circulating levels are affected by urinary pH. Diethylpropion and/or its active metabolites are believed to cross the blood-brain barrier and the placenta.
Diethylpropion and its metabolites are excreted mainly by the kidney. It has been reported that between 75–106% of the dose is recovered in the urine within 48 hours after dosing. Using a phosphorescence assay that is specific for basic compounds containing a benzoyl group, the plasma half-life of the aminoketone metabolites is estimated to be between 4 to 6 hours.
The controlled-release characteristics of Tenuate Dospan have been demonstrated by studies in humans in which plasma levels of diethylpropion-related materials were measured by phosphorescence analysis. Plasma levels obtained with the 75 mg Dospan formulation administered once daily indicated a more gradual release than the immediate-release formulation (three 25 mg tablets given in a single dose).
Tenuate Dospan has not been shown superior in effectiveness to the same dosage of the immediate-release formulation (one 25 mg tablet three times daily). After administration of a single dose of Tenuate Dospan (one 75 mg controlled-release tablet) or diethylpropion hydrochloride solution (75 mg dose) in a crossover study using normal human subjects, the amount of parent compound and its active metabolites recovered in the urine within 48 hours for the two dosage forms were not statistically different.

INDICATIONS AND USAGE

Tenuate and Tenuate Dospan are indicated in the management of exogenous obesity as a short-term adjunct (a few weeks) in a regimen of weight reduction based on caloric restriction. The usefulness of agents of this class (see CLINICAL PHARMACOLOGY) should be measured against possible risk factors inherent in their use such as those described below.

CONTRAINDICATIONS

Advanced arteriosclerosis, hyperthyroidism, known hypersensitivity, or idiosyncrasy to the sympathomimetic amines, glaucoma, severe hypertension. (See PRECAUTIONS.)
Agitated states.
Patients with a history of drug abuse.
During or within 14 days following the administration of monoamine oxidase inhibitors, hypertensive crises may result.

WARNINGS

If tolerance develops, the recommended dose should not be exceeded in an attempt to increase the effect; rather, the drug should be discontinued. Tenuate or Tenuate Dospan may impair the ability of the patient to engage in potentially hazardous activities such as operating machinery or driving a motor vehicle; the patient should therefore be cautioned accordingly.
When central nervous system active agents are used, consideration must always be given to the possibility of adverse interactions with alcohol.

PRECAUTIONS

General
Caution is to be exercised in prescribing Tenuate or Tenuate Dospan for patients with hypertension or with symptomatic cardiovascular disease, including arrhythmias. Tenuate or Tenuate Dospan should not be administered to patients with severe hypertension.
Reports suggest that diethylpropion hydrochloride may increase convulsions in some epileptics. Therefore, epileptics receiving Tenuate of Tenuate Dospan should be carefully monitored. Titration of dose or discontinuance of Tenuate or Tenuate Dospan may be necessary.
The least amount feasible should be prescribed or dispensed at one time in order to minimize the possibility of overdosage.
Information for Patient
The patient should be cautioned about concomitant use of alcohol or other CNS-active drugs and Tenuate or Tenuate Dospan. (See WARNINGS.) The patient should be advised to observe caution when driving or engaging in any potentially hazardous activity.
Laboratory Tests
None
Drug Interactions
Antidiabetic drug requirements (i.e., insulin) may be altered. Concurrent use with general anesthetics may result in arrhythmias. The pressor effects of diethylpropion and those of other drugs may be additive when the drugs are used concomitantly; conversely, diethylpropion may interfere with antihypertensive drugs (i.e., guanethidine, α-methyldopa).

Continued on next page

Marion Merrell Dow—Cont.

Concurrent use of phenothiazines may antagonize the anorectic effect of diethylpropion.

CARCINOGENESIS, MUTAGENESIS, AND IMPAIRMENT OF FERTILITY

No long-term studies have been done to evaluate diethylpropion hydrochloride for carcinogenicity. Mutagenicity studies have not been conducted. Animal reproduction studies revealed no evidence of impairment of fertility (see Pregnancy).

Pregnancy

TERATOGENIC EFFECTS: PREGNANCY CATEGORY B

Reproduction studies have been performed in rats at doses up to 9 times the human dose and have revealed no evidence of impaired fertility or harm to the fetus due to diethylpropion hydrochloride. There are, however, no adequate and well-controlled studies in pregnant women. Because animal reproduction studies are not always predictive of human response, this drug should be used during pregnancy only if clearly needed.

NON-TERATOGENIC EFFECTS

Abuse with diethylpropion hydrochloride during pregnancy may result in withdrawal symptoms in the human neonate.

NURSING MOTHERS

Since diethylpropion hydrochloride and/or its metabolites have been shown to be excreted in human milk, caution should be exercised when Tenuate or Tenuate Dospan is administered to a nursing woman.

PEDIATRIC USE

Since safety and effectiveness in children below the age of 12 have not been established, Tenuate or Tenuate Dospan is *not* recommended for use in children under 12 years of age.

ADVERSE REACTIONS

Cardiovascular: Precordial pain, arrhythmia, ECG changes, tachycardia, elevation of blood pressure, palpitation.
Central Nervous System: In a few epileptics an increase in convulsive episodes has been reported; rarely psychotic episodes at recommended doses; dyskinesia, blurred vision, overstimulation, nervousness, restlessness, dizziness, jitteriness, insomnia, anxiety, euphoria, depression, dysphoria, tremor, mydriasis, drowsiness, malaise, headache.
Gastrointestinal: Vomiting, diarrhea, abdominal discomfort, dryness of the mouth, unpleasant taste, nausea, constipation, other gastrointestinal disturbances.
Allergic: Urticaria, rash, ecchymosis, erythema.
Endocrine: Impotence, changes in libido, gynecomastia, menstrual upset.
Hematopoietic System: Bone marrow depression, agranulocytosis, leukopenia.
Miscellaneous: A variety of miscellaneous adverse reactions has been reported by physicians. These include complaints such as dysuria, dyspnea, hair loss, muscle pain, increased sweating, and polyuria.

DRUG ABUSE AND DEPENDENCE

Tenuate and Tenuate Dospan are schedule IV controlled substances. Diethylpropion hydrochloride has some chemical and pharmacologic similarities to the amphetamines and other related stimulant drugs that have been extensively abused. There have been reports of subjects becoming psychologically dependent on diethylpropion. The possibility of abuse should be kept in mind when evaluating the desirability of including a drug as part of a weight reduction program. Abuse of amphetamines and related drugs may be associated with varying degrees of psychologic dependence and social dysfunction which, in the case of certain drugs, may be severe. There are reports of patients who have increased the dosage to many times that recommended. Abrupt cessation following prolonged high dosage administration results in extreme fatigue and mental depression; changes are also noted on the sleep EEG. Manifestations of chronic intoxication with anorectic drugs include severe dermatoses, marked insomnia, irritability, hyperactivity, and personality changes. The most severe manifestation of chronic intoxication is psychosis, often clinically indistinguishable from schizophrenia.

OVERDOSAGE

Manifestations of acute overdosage include restlessness, tremor, hyperreflexia, rapid respiration, confusion, assaultiveness, hallucinations, panic states.
Fatigue and depression usually follow the central stimulation.
Cardiovascular effects include arrhythmias, hypertension or hypotension and circulatory collapse. Gastrointestinal symptoms include nausea, vomiting, diarrhea, and abdominal cramps. Overdosage of pharmacologically similar compounds has resulted in convulsions, coma and death.
The reported oral LD_{50} for mice is 600 mg/kg, for rats is 250 mg/kg and for dogs is 225 mg/kg.
Management of acute diethylpropion hydrochloride intoxication is largely symptomatic and includes lavage and sedation with a barbiturate. Experience with hemodialysis or peritoneal dialysis is inadequate to permit recommendation

in this regard. Intravenous phentolamine (Regitine®) has been suggested on pharmacologic grounds for possible acute, severe hypertension, if this complicates Tenuate or Tenuate Dospan overdosage.

DOSAGE AND ADMINISTRATION

Tenuate (diethylpropion hydrochloride) immediate-release:
　One immediate-release 25 mg tablet three times daily, one hour before meals, and in midevening if desired to overcome night hunger.
Tenuate Dospan (diethylpropion hydrochloride) controlled-release:
　One controlled-release 75 mg tablet daily, swallowed whole, in midmorning.

HOW SUPPLIED

NDC 0068-0697-61
25 mg immediate-release tablets in bottles of 100
Each white, round tablet is debossed TENUATE 25 or MERRELL 697
Keep tightly closed, store at room temperature, preferably below 86°F.
Protect from excessive heat.
NDC 0068-0698-61
75 mg controlled-release tablets in bottles of 100
NDC 0068-0698-62
75 mg controlled-release tablets in bottles of 250
Each white, capsule-shaped tablet is debossed TENUATE 75 or MERRELL 698
Keep tightly closed. Store at room temperature, below 86°F.
Product Information as of May, 1991
Shown in Product Identification Section, page 417

THROAT DISCS®　　　　　　　　　　　OTC
[thrŏt disks]
Throat Lozenges

(See PDR For Nonprescription Drugs.)

Marlyn Health Care
14851 N. SCOTTSDALE RD.
SCOTTSDALE, AZ 85254

HEP–FORTE®　　　　　　　　　　　　OTC
[hep-for'tay]

DESCRIPTION

Hep Forte is a comprehensive formulation of protein, B factors and other nutritional factors which can be important as a dietary supplement for maintenance and support of normal hepatic function.

COMPOSITION

Each capsule contains:

Vitamin A (Palmitate)	1,200 I.U.
Vitamin E (d-Alpha Tocopherol)	10 I.U.
Vitamin C (Ascorbic Acid)	10 mg.
Folic Acid	0.06 mg.
Vitamin B1 (Thiamine Mononitrate)	1 mg.
Vitamin B2 (Riboflavin)	1 mg.
Niacinamide	10 mg.
Vitamin B6 (Pyridoxine HCl)	0.5 mg.
Vitamin B12 (Cobalamin)	1 mcg.
Biotin	3.3 mcg.
Pantothenic Acid	2 mg.
Choline Bitartrate	21 mg.
Zinc (Zinc Sulfate)	2 mg.
Desiccated Liver	194.4 mg.
Liver Concentrate	64.8 mg.
Liver Fraction Number 2	64.8 mg.
Yeast (Dried)	64.8 mg.
dl-Methionine	10 mg.
Inositol	10 mg.

INDICATIONS

Hep Forte is a balanced formulation of vitamins, minerals, lipotropic factors, and vitamin-protein supplements. It is of value as a nutritional supplement for persons who are receiving professional treatment for alcoholism, hepatic dysfunction due to hepatotoxic drugs and liver poisons, male and female infertility due to hormonal imbalance caused by hepatic dysfunction, and for nutritional supplementation after treatment.

CONTRAINDICATIONS

There are no known contraindications to Hep Forte.

DOSAGE

Three to six capsules daily.

HOW SUPPLIED

Bottles of 100, 300 or 500 capsules.
Literature Available.

MARLYN FORMULA 50®　　　　　　　OTC

PRODUCT OVERVIEW

KEY FACTS

MARLYN FORMULA 50 is a dietary supplement providing a combination of amino acids and B6 in a gelatin capsule which provides protein "building blocks" important to growth and development of all protein containing tissue including nails, hair, and skin.

MAJOR USES

Dermatologists recommend Formula 50 for splitting, peeling nails. Since splitting and peeling nails are often associated with nail fungus, Formula 50 may be recommended in conjunction with drug therapy for nail fungus in order to provide protein necessary to growth and development of nails. OB-Gyn's recommend it for help in controlling excessive hair fall-out after child birth.

SAFETY INFORMATION

There are no known contraindications or adverse reactions.

PRESCRIBING INFORMATION

MARLYN FORMULA 50®

COMPOSITION

Each capsule contains:

Amino Acids	0.3 Gm*
Vitamin B6 (pyridoxine HCl)	1.0 mg.

*Approximate analysis of the amino acids: indispensable amino acids (lysine, tryptophan, phenylalanine, methionine, threonine, leucine, isoleucine, valine), 35.30%; semi-dispensable amino acids (arginine, histidine, tyrosine, cystine, glycine), 19.18%; dispensable amino acids (glutamic acid, alanine, aspartic acid, serine, proline), 45.56%.
Amino acids: Protein "building blocks" important to growth and development of all protein containing tissue including nails, hair, and skin.

DOSAGE AND ADMINISTRATION

The recommended daily dose is 6 capsules daily.

SUPPLY

Bottles of 100, 250 and 500 capsules.

MARLYN FORMULA 50 MEGA FORTE　　OTC

PRODUCT OVERVIEW

KEY FACTS

MARLYN FORMULA 50 MEGA FORTE is a dietary supplement providing a combination of amino acids and B6 in a gelatin capsule which provides protein "building blocks" important to growth and development of all protein containing tissues including nails, hair, and skin.

MAJOR USES

Dermatologists recommend Formula 50 for splitting, peeling nails. Since splitting and peeling nails are often associated with nail fungus, Formula 50 may be recommended in conjunction with drug therapy for nail fungus in order to provide necessary to growth and development of nails. OB-Gyn's recommend it for help in controlling excessive hair fall-out after child birth.

SAFETY INFORMATION

There are no known contraindications or adverse reactions.

PRESCRIBING INFORMATION

MARLYN FORMULA 50 MEGA FORTE

Each 6 capsules contain:

Amino Acids	1980 mg
Vitamin B6	6 mg
Silicon (from Amino Acid Chelate)	90 mg
L-Cysteine HCl (Natural Extract)	120 mg
Mucopolysaccharides (from Bovine cartilage extract)	60 mg

Approximate analysis of amino acids: indispensable amino acids: (lysine, tryptophan, phenylalanine, methionine, threonine, leucine, isoleucine, valine) 35.30%; semi-dispensable amino acids; (arginine, histidine, tyrosine, cystine, glycine, 19.18%; dispensable amino acids (glutamic acids, alanine, aspartic acid, serine, proline), 45.56%.
Amino Acids; Protein "building blocks" important to growth and development of all protein containing tissue including nails, hair, and skin.

DOSAGE AND ADMINISTRATION

The recommended daily dose is 6 capsules daily

SUPPLY

Bottles of 90, 180, 500

PRO-HEPATONE OTC

PRODUCT OVERVIEW

KEY FACTS

PRO-HEPATONE is an all-inclusive formulation of vitamins, hematinic factors, amino acids, lipotropic factors, and other nutritional supplements to help overcome dietary deficiencies of these nutrients.

MAJOR USES

PRO-HEPATONE is specially designed to be of help as a nutritional adjouvant for persons under professional care for the avoidance of liver problems that may result from improper diet or excesses of alcohol or drugs, and to be of assistance in some types of occasional impotence.

SAFETY INFORMATION

There are no known contraindications or adverse reactions.

PRESCRIBING INFORMATION

PRO-HEPATONE

EACH TWO CAPSULES SUPPLY:

Choline Bitartrate	100	mg
Methionine	100	mg
Inositol	100	mg
Lecithin	100	mg
Liver Concentrate	64.8	mg
Desiccated Liver	64.8	mg
Unsaturated Fatty Acid	640	mg
Vitamin E (Alpha Tocopheryl)	20	I.U.
Vitamin C (Ascorbic Acid)	20	mg
Vitamin B_1 (Thiamine)	5	mg
Vitamin B_2 (Riboflavin)	5	mg
Niacinamide (Vitamin P)	20	mg
Vitamin B_6 (Pyridoxine HCl)	5	mg
L-Cysteine HCl	10	mg
Gluthathione	5	mg
Desoxycholic Acid	25	mg
Thiotic Acid	5	mg
d-Calcium Pantothenate	20	mg
Vitamin B_{12} (Cyancobalamin)	64.8	mcg
L-Arginine	5	mg
L-Glutamine	10	mg
L-Aspartic Acid	10	mg
L-Ornithine	5	mg
Ferrous Fumarate	648	mcg
Glycine	100	mg
Fructose	100	mg

DOSAGE AND ADMINISTRATION

The recommended daily dose is 2–3 capsules daily.

SUPPLY

Bottles of 150 capsules

Mason Pharmaceuticals, Inc.

4425 JAMBOREE
NEWPORT BEACH, CA 92660

DAMASON-P Ⓒ℞
[*dă 'mă-sŭn-p*]
(Hydrocodone Bitartrate 5 mg., and Aspirin 500 mg.)

PRODUCT OVERVIEW

KEY FACTS

Damason-P is a narcotic analgesic combining Hydrocodone Bitartrate with aspirin. Hydrocodone exerts its narcotic effects centrally. Aspirin acts both centrally and peripherally in the relief of pain.

MAJOR USES

Damason-P is an analgesic intended for the relief of moderate to moderately severe pain.

SAFETY INFORMATION

Damason-P is contraindicated for patients who have developed a hypersensitivity to aspirin. The benefit/risk potential should be considered before using Damason-P in patients with head injury, head lesions, increased intracranial pressure, or abdominal conditions because of the potential of narcotic induced respiratory depression and the possibility of masking of the diagnosis or clinical course of patients. Damason-P should be avoided in the presence of peptic ulcer and coagulation abnormalities. Use in children and teenagers is also better avoided if flu or chicken pox is suspected.

PRESCRIBING INFORMATION

DAMASON-P Ⓒ℞
[*dă 'mă-sŭn-p*]
(Hydrocodone Bitartrate 5 mg. and Aspirin 500 mg.)

DESCRIPTION

Each pink tablet of DAMASON-P contains:

ACTIVE INGREDIENTS

Hydrocodone Bitartrate	5 mg
(Warning: May be habit forming)	
Aspirin	500 mg

Hydrocodone bitartrate is an opioid analgesic and antitussive and occurs as fine, white crystals or as a crystalline powder. It is affected by light.

Aspirin, Salicylic acid acetate, is a nonopiate, salicylate analgesic, anti-inflammatory and antipyretic which occurs as a white, crystaline tabular or needle like powder and is odorless or has a faint odor.

INACTIVE INGREDIENTS

Pregelatinized Starch
Stearic Acid
D&C Red #7 Lake
Narcotic analgesic tablet for oral administration.

CLINICAL PHARMACOLOGY

Hydrocodone: is a semisynthetic narcotic analgesic and antitussive with multiple actions qualitatively similar to those of codeine. Most of these involve the central nervous system and smooth muscle. The precise mechanism of action of hydrocodone and other opiates is not known, although it is believed to relate to the existence of opiate receptors in the central nervous system. In addition to analgesia, narcotics may produce drowsiness, changes in mood and mental clouding. Radioimmunoassay techniques have recently been developed for the analysis of hydrocodone in human plasma. After a 10 mg oral dose of hydrocodone bitartrate, a mean peak serum drug level of 23.6 ng/ml and an elimination half-life of 3.8 hours were found.

Aspirin: The analgesic, anti-inflammatory and antipyretic effects of aspirin are believed to result from inhibition of the synthesis of certain prostaglandins. Aspirin interferes with clotting mechanisms primarily by diminishing platelet aggregation; at high doses prothrombin synthesis can be inhibited.

Aspirin in solution is rapidly absorbed from the stomach and from the upper small intestine. About 50 percent of an oral dose is absorbed in 30 minutes and peak plasma concentrations are reached in about 40 minutes. Higher than normal stomach pH or the presence of food slightly delays absorption. Once absorbed, aspirin is mainly hydrolyzed to salicylic acid and distributed to all body tissues and fluids, including fetal tissue, breast milk and the central nervous system (CNS). Highest concentrations are found in plasma, liver, renal cortex, heart and lung.

From 50 to 80 percent of salicylic acid and its metabolites in plasma are loosely bound to protein. The plasma half-life of total salicylate is about 3.0 hours, with a 650 mg dose. Higher doses of aspirin cause increases in plasma salicylate half-life. Almost all of the therapeutic dose of aspirin is excreted through the kidneys, either as salicylic acid or its metabolites. Renal clearance of salicylate is greatly augmented by an alkaline urine, as is produced by concurrent administration of sodium bicarbonate or potassium citrate.

Toxic salicylate blood levels are usually above 30 mg/100 ml. The single lethal dose of aspirin in normal adults is approximately 25-30 g., but patients have recovered from much larger doses with appropriate treatment.

INDICATIONS AND USAGE

For the relief of moderate to moderately severe pain.

CONTRAINDICATIONS

Hydrocodone Bitartrate and Aspirin Tablets are contraindicated under the following conditions:

(1) hypersensitivity or intolerance to hydrocodone or aspirin.
(2) severe bleeding, disorders of coagulation or primary hemostasis, including hemophilia, hypoprothrombinemia, von Willebrand's disease, thrombocytopenias, thrombasthenia and other ill-defined hereditary platelet dysfunctions, severe vitamin K deficiency and severe liver damage.
(3) anticoagulant therapy.
(4) peptic ulcer, or other serious gastrointestinal lesions.

WARNINGS

Drugs of this class, salicylates, have been reported to be associated with the development of Reyes Syndrome in children or teenagers with chicken pox, influenza, and influenza-like infections.

Hydrocodone: Respiratory Depressions: At high doses or in sensitive patients, hydrocodone may produce dose-related respiratory depression by acting directly on the brain stem respiratory center. Hydrocodone also affects the center that controls respiratory rhythm, and may produce irregular and periodic breathing.

Head Injury and Increased Intracranial Pressure: The respiratory depressant effects of narcotics and their capacity to elevate cerebrospinal fluid pressure may be markedly exaggerated in the presence of head injury, other intracranial lesions or a pre-existing increase in intracranial pressure. Furthermore, narcotics produce adverse reactions which may obscure the clincial course of patients with head injuries.

Acute Abdominal Conditions: The administration of narcotics may obscure the diagnosis or clinical course of patients with acute abdominal conditions.

Aspirin: Allergic Reactions: Therapeutic doses of aspirin can cause anaphylactic shock and other severe allergic reactions. A history of allergy is often lacking.

Bleeding: Significant bleeding can result from aspirin therapy in patients with peptic ulcer or other gastrointestinal lesions, and in patients with bleeding disorders. Aspirin administered preoperatively may prolong the bleeding time.

PRECAUTIONS:

Special Risk Patients: As with any narcotic analgesic agent, Hydrocodone Bitartrate and Aspirin Tablets should be used with caution in elderly or debilitated patients and those with severe impairment of hepatic or renal function, gallbladder disease or gallstones, respiratory impairment, cardiac arrhythmias, inflammatory disorders of the gastrointestinal tract, hypothyroidism, Addison's disease, prostatic hypertrophy or urethral stricture, coagulation disorders, head injuries or acute abdominal conditions. The usual precautions should be observed and the possibility of respiratory depression should not be overlooked.

Precautions should be taken when administering salicylates to persons with known allergies. Hypersensitivity to aspirin is particularly likely in patients with nasal polyps, and relatively common with asthma.

Information for Patients: Hydrocodone Bitartrate and Aspirin Tablets, like all narcotics, may impair the mental and/or physical abilities required for the performance of potentially hazardous tasks such as driving a car or operating machinery; patients should be cautioned accordingly.

Cough Reflex: Hydrocodone suppresses the cough reflex; as with all narcotics, caution should be exercised when Hydrocodone Bitartrate and Aspirin Tablets are used postoperatively and in patients with pulmonary disease.

Laboratory Tests: Hypersensitivity to aspirin cannot be detected by skin testing or radioimmunoassay procedures.

Drug Interactions:

Hydrocodone: Patients receiving other narcotic analgesics, antipsychotics, antianxiety agents, or other CNS depressants (including alcohol) concomitantly with Hydrocodone Bitartrate and Aspirin Tablets may exhibit additive CNS depression. When combined therapy is contemplated, the dose of one or both agents should be reduced.

The use of MAO inhibitors or tricyclic antidepressants with hydrocodone preparations may increase the effect of either the antidepressant or hydrocodone.

The concurrent use of anticholingergics with hydrocodone, as with all narcotics, may produce paralytic ileus.

Aspirin:

Aspirin may *enhance* the effects of:

(1) oral anticoagulants, causing bleeding by inhibiting prothrombin formation in the liver and displacing anticoagulants from plasma protein binding sites.
(2) oral antidiabetic agents and insulin, causing hypoglycemia by contributing an additive effect, and by displacing the oral antidiabetic agents from secondary binding sites.
(3) 6-mercaptopurine and methotrexate, causing bone marrow toxicity and blood dyscrasias by displacing these drugs from secondary binding sites.
(4) non-sterodial anti-inflammatory agents, increasing the risk of peptic ulceration and bleeding by contributing additive effects.
(5) corticosteroids, potentiating anti-inflammatory effects by displacing steroids from protein binding sites. Aspirin intoxication may occur with corticosteroid withdrawal because steroids promote renal clearance of salicylates.

Aspirin may *diminish* the effects of uricosuric agents, such as probenecid and sulfinpyrazone, in the treatment of gout by competing for protein binding sites.

Drug/Laboratory Test Interactions:

Aspirin: Aspirin may interfere with the following determinations.

In blood: serum amylase, fasting blood glucose, carbon dioxide, cholesterol protein, protein bound iodine, uric acid, prothrombin time, bleeding time, and spectrophotometric detection of barbiturates.

In urine: glucose, 5-hydroxyindoleacetic acid, Gerhardt ketone, vanillylmandelic acid (VMA), protein, uric acid, and diacetic acid.

Teratogenic Effects: Pregnancy Category C.

Hydrocodone: Hydrocodone has been shown to be teratogenic in hamsters when given in doses 700 times the human dose. There are no adequate and well-controlled studies in pregnant women.

Hydrocodone Bitartrate and Aspirin Tablets should be used during pregnancy only if the potential benefit justifies the potential risk to the fetus.

Aspirin: Reproductive studies in rats and mice have shown aspirin to be teratogenic and embryocidal at four to six times

Continued on next page

Mason—Cont.

the human therapeutic dose. Studies in pregnant women, however, have not shown that aspirin increases the risk of abnormalities when administered during the first trimester of pregnancy. In controlled studies involving 41,337 pregnant women and their offspring, there was no evidence that aspirin taken during pregnancy caused stillbirth, neonatal death or reduced birthweight. In controlled studies of 50,282 pregnant women and their offspring, aspirin administration in moderate and heavy doses during the first four months of pregnancy showed no teratogenic effect.

Nonteratogenic Effects:

Hydrocodone: Babies born to mothers who have been taking opioids regularly prior to delivery will be physically dependent. The withdrawal signs include irritability and excessive crying, tremors, hyperactive reflexes, increased respiratory rate, increased stools, sneezing, yawning, vomiting, and fever. The intensity of the syndrome does not always correlate with the duration of maternal opioid use or dose.

There is no consensus on the best method of managing withdrawal. Chlorpromazine 0.7 to 1 mg/kg q6h, and paragoric 2 to 4 drops/kg q4h, have been used to treat withdrawal symptoms in infants. The duration of therapy is 4 to 28 days, with the dosage decreased as tolerated.

Aspirin: Therapeutic doses of aspirin in pregnant women close to term may cause bleeding in the mother, fetus, or neonate. During the last six months of pregnancy, regular use of aspirin in high doses may prolong pregnancy and delivery.

Labor and Delivery: As with all narcotics, administration of Hydrocodone Bitartrate and Aspirin Tablets to the mother shortly before delivery may result in some degree of respiratory depression in the newborn, especially if higher doses are used. Ingestion of aspirin prior to delivery may prolong delivery or lead to bleeding in the mother or neonate.

Nursing Mothers: Aspirin is excreted in human milk in a small amount; the significance of its effect on nursing infants is not known. It is not known whether hydrocodone is excreted in human milk. Because many drugs are excreted in human milk and because of the potential for serious adverse reactions in nursing infants, a decision should be made whether to discontinue nursing or to discontinue the drug, taking into account the importance of the drug to the mother.

Pediatric Use: Safety and effectiveness in children have not been established.

ADVERSE REACTIONS

The most frequently observed adverse reactions include light-headedness, dizziness, sedation, nausea and vomiting. These effects seem to be more prominent in ambulatory than in nonambulatory patients and some of these adverse reactions may be alleviated if the patient lies down.

Other adverse reactions include:

Central Nervous System:

Hydrocodone: Drowsiness, mental clouding, lethargy, impairment of mental and physical performance, anxiety, fear, dysphoria, psychic dependence, mood changes.

Aspirin: Some patients are unable to take aspirin or other salicylates without developing nausea or vomiting. Occasional patients respond to aspirin (usually large doses) with dyspepsia or heartburn, which may be accompanied by occult bleeding. Excessive bruising or bleeding is sometimes seen in patients with mild disorders of primary hemostasis who regularly use low doses of aspirin.

Prolonged use of aspirin can cause painless erosion of gastric mucosa, occult bleeding and, infrequently, iron-deficiency anemia. High doses of aspirin can exacerbate symptoms of peptic ulcer and, occasionally, cause extensive bleeding. Excessive bleeding can follow injury or surgery in patients with or without known bleeding disorders who have taken therapeutic doses of aspirin within the preceding 10 days. Hepatotoxicity has been reported in association with prolonged use of large doses of aspirin in patients with lupus erythematosus, rheumatoid arthritis and rheumatic disease.

Hematologic:

Aspirin: Bone marrow depression, manifested by weakness, fatigue or abnormal bruising or bleeding, has occasionally been reported with aspirin.

In patients with glucose-6-phosphate dehydrogenase deficiency, aspirin can cause a mild degree of hemolytic anemia.

Respiratory:

Hydrocodone: Hydrocodone bitartrate may produce dose-related respiratory depression by acting directly on the brain stem respiratory center. Hydrocodone also affects the center that controls respiratory rhythm, and may produce irregular and periodic breathing. If significant respiratory depression occurs, it may be antagonized by the use of naloxone hydrochloride. Apply other supportive measures when indicated.

Aspirin: Hyperpnea and hyperventilation can occur in response to chronic use of large doses.

Cardiovascular:

Aspirin: Tachycardia can occur in response to chronic use of large doses of aspirin.

Genitourinary:

Hydrocodone: Ureteral spasm, spasm of vesical sphincters and urinary retention have been reported.

Metabolic:

Aspirin: In hyperuricemic persons, low doses of aspirin may reduce the effectiveness of uricosuric therapy or precipitate an attack of gout.

Allergic:

Aspirin: Therapeutic doses of aspirin can induce mild or severe allergic reactions manifested by skin rashes, urticaria, angioedema, rhinorrhea, asthma, abdominal pain, nausea, vomiting, or anaphylactic shock. A history of allergy is often lacking, and allergic reactions may occur even in patients who have previously taken aspirin without any ill effects. Allergic reactions to aspirin are most likely to occur in patients with a history of allergic disease, especially in patients with nasal polyps or asthma.

Other:

Aspirin: Sweating and thirst can occur in response to chronic use of large doses of aspirin.

DRUG ABUSE AND DEPENDENCE

Hydrocodone Bitartrate and Aspirin Tablets are subject to the Federal Controlled Substance Act (Schedule CIII). Psychic dependence, physical dependence, and tolerance may develop upon repeated administration of narcotics; therefore, Hydrocodone Bitartrate and Aspirin Tablets are used for a short time for the treatment of pain.

Physical dependence, the condition in which continued administration of the drug is required to prevent the appearance of a withdrawal syndrome, assumes clinically significant proportions only after several weeks of continued narcotic use, although some mild degree of physical dependence may develop after a few days of narcotic therapy. Tolerance, in which increasingly large doses are required in order to produce the same degree of analgesia, is manifested initially by shortened duration of analgesic effect, and subsequently by decreases in the intensity of analgesia. The rate of development of tolerance varies among patients.

OVERDOSAGE

Hydrocodone:

Signs and Symptoms: Serious overdose with hydrocodone is characterized by respiratory depression (a decrease in respiratory rate and/or tidal volume. Cheyne-Stokes respiration, cyanosis), extreme somnolence progressing to stupor or coma, skeletal muscle flaccidity, cold and clammy skin, and sometimes bradycardia and hypotension. In severe overdosage, apnea, circulatory collapse, cardiac arrest and death may occur.

Treatment: Primary attention should be given to the reestablishment of adequate respiratory exchange through provision of a patent airway and institution of assisted or controlled ventilation. If significant respiratory depression occurs, it may be antagonized by the use of naloxone hydrochloride intravenously (see package insert for dosage and full information). Naloxone promptly reverses the effects of morphine-like opioid antagonists such as hydrocodone. In patients who are physically dependent, small doses of naloxone should therefore be adjusted accordingly in such patients. Since the duration of action of hydrocodone may exceed that of the antagonist, the patient should be kept under continued surveillance and repeated doses of the antagonist should be administered as needed to maintain adequate respiration. A narcotic antagonist should not be administered in the absence of clinically significant respiratory or cardiovascular depression. Oxygen, intravenous fluids, vasopressors and other supportive measures should be employed as indicated. Gastric emptying may be useful in removing unabsorbed drug.

Aspirin:

Signs and Symptoms: The most severe manifestations from aspirin results from cardiovascular and respiratory insufficiency secondary to acid-base and electrolyte disturbances, complicated by hyperthermia and dehydration.

Respiratory alkalosis is characteristic of the early phase of intoxication with aspirin while hyperventilation is occurring, but is quickly followed by metabolic acidosis in most people with severe intoxication.

Concentrations of aspirin in plasma above 30 mg/100 ml are associated with toxicity (See Clinical Pharmacology Section for information on factors influencing aspirin blood levels.) The single lethal dose of aspirin in adults is probably about 25–30 g, but is not known with certainty. Hemodialysis and peritoneal dialysis can be performed to reduce the body aspirin content.

Treatment: Treatment consists primarily of supporting vital functions increasing salicylate elimination, and correcting the acid-base imbalance due primarily to salicylism. Gastric emptying (Syrup of Ipecac) and/or lavage is recommended as soon as possible after ingestion, even if the patient has vomited spontaneously. Administration of activated charcoal as a slurry is beneficial after lavage and/or emesis, if less than three hours have passed since ingestion. Charcoal absorption should NOT be employed prior to emesis or lavage.

Severity of aspirin intoxication is determined by measuring the blood salicylate level. Acid-base status should be closely followed with serial blood gas and serum pH measurements. Fluid and electrolyte balance should also be regularly monitored.

In severe cases, hyperthermia and hypovolemia are the major immediate threats to life. Children should be sponged with tepid water. Replacement fluid should be administered intravenously and augmented with sufficient bicarbonate to correct acidosis, with monitoring of plasma electrolytes and pH, to promote alkaline diuresis of salicylate if renal function is normal. Complete control may also require infusion of glucose to control hypoglycemia.

In patients with renal insufficiency or in cases of life-threatening intoxication, dialysis is usually required. Peritoneal dialysis or exchange transfusion is indicated in infants and young children and hemodialysis in older patients.

DOSAGE AND ADMINISTRATION

Dosage should be adjusted accordingly to the severity of the pain and the response of the patient. However, tolerance to hydrocone can develop with continued use and the incidence of untoward effects is dose related.

The usual adult dosage is one or two tablets every four to six hours as needed for pain. The total 24-hour dose should not exceed eight tablets.

Damason-P Tablets should be taken with food or a full glass of milk or water to lessen gastric irritation.

HOW SUPPLIED

Round, mottled pink tablet containing 5 mg of Hydrocodone Bitartrate (WARNING may be habit forming) and 500 mg of Aspirin. Each tablet is debossed with an "M" on one side and a "D-P" on the other side.

Bottles of 100 tablets ....NDC 12758-057-01
Bottles of 500 tablets ....NDC 12758-057-05
Bottles of 1000 tablets ....NDC 12758-057-10

Storage: Store at controlled room temperature 15–30°C (59–86°F). Protect from moisture.

Dispense in a tight, light-resistant container as defined in the USP/NF with a child-resistant closure.

CAUTION: Federal law prohibits dispensing without prescription. A Schedule CIII Controlled Substance (Narcotic).

Manufactured by:
Central Pharmaceuticals, Inc.
Seymour, IN 47274
Manufactured for:
Mason Pharmaceuticals, Inc.
Newport Beach, CA 92660
7901A Revised July, 1990

Shown in Product Identification Section, page 417

DUOCET™ Ⓒ℞

[du "oset]

Hydrocodone Bitartrate and Acetaminophen Tablets 5 mg/500 mg

DESCRIPTION

Each DuoCet™ tablet (Hydrocodone Bitartrate and Acetaminophen Tablet 5 mg/500 mg) contains:

hydrocodone bitartrate ....5 mg
(**WARNING:** May be habit forming)
acetaminophen ....500 mg

Hydrocodone bitartrate is an opioid analgesic and antitussive and occurs as fine, white crystals or as a crystalline powder. It is affected by light. The chemical name is: 4.5 α-epoxy-3-methoxy-17-methyl-morphinan-6-one tartrate (1:1) hydrate (2.5).

Acetaminophen 4-hydroxyacetamide, is a non-opiate, non-salicylate analgesic and antipyrelic which occurs as a white, odorless, crystalline powder possessing a slightly bitter taste. Inactive ingredients include polacrilin potassium, microcrystalline cellulose, anhydrous lactose, magnesium stearate, corn starch, sodium carboxymethylcellulose, hydrogenated cottonseed oil and silicon dioxide.

HOW SUPPLIED

DuoCet™ tablets [Hydrocodone Bitartrate 5 mg (**WARNING:** May be habit forming) and Acetaminophen 500 mg tablets] are available as white, capsule shaped tablets bisected on one side and debossed with DUOCET on the other side and supplied in:

Bottles of 100, NDC 12758-067-01

Store at controlled room temperature, 15°-30°C (59°-86°F).

Dispense in a tight, light-resistant container with a child-resistant closure.

CAUTION: Federal law prohibits dispensing without prescription.

Manufactured for: Mason Pharmaceuticals, Inc. Newport Beach, CA 92660
By: Watson Laboratories, Inc. Corona, CA 91720

11699
Issued May 1, 1991

Shown in Product Identification Section, page 417

Mayrand Pharmaceuticals, Inc.
P. O. BOX 8869
FOUR DUNDAS CIRCLE
GREENSBORO, NC 27419

ANATUSS® DM SYRUP   OTC

DESCRIPTION
Each 5 ml of ANATUSS DM SYRUP for oral administration contains:

Guaifenesin	100 mg
Pseudoephedrine Hydrochloride	30 mg
Dextromethorphan Hydrochloride	10 mg

In a good tasting cherry flavored vehicle.

HOW SUPPLIED
ANATUSS DM SYRUP is supplied in pints NDC #0259-0383-16.

ANATUSS® DM TABLETS   OTC

DESCRIPTION
Each orange, oval European scored ANATUSS DM TABLET for oral administration contains:

Guaifenesin	400 mg
Pseudoephedrine Hydrochloride	60 mg
Dextromethorphan Hydrochloride	20 mg

HOW SUPPLIED
ANATUSS DM TABLETS are available as orange, oval shaped caplets, deep-scored on one side with an "M" appearing on the left of the score and an "P" appearing on the right of the score and 0382 appearing on the bottom side of the tablet.
In bottles of 100: NDC #0259-0382-01.

ANATUSS® LA TABLETS   ℞

DESCRIPTION
Each off-white European scored Anatuss LA Tablet for oral administration contains:

Guaifenesin	400 mg
Pseudoephedrine Hydrochloride	120 mg

Guaifenesin, 3-(2-methoxyphenoxy)-1,2-Propanediol, a white odorless, crystalline material with a slightly bitter aromatic taste. Pseudoephedrine Hydrochloride, [1-(methylamino) ethyl]benzenemethanol, a white crystalline, almost odorless powder with a bitter taste.
Anatuss LA Tablets also contain the following inactive ingredients: Calcium Phosphate Dibasic; Carnauba wax; and Cellulose Derivative.

CLINICAL PHARMACOLOGY
Guaifenesin has an expectorant action which increases the output of respiratory tract fluid by reducing adhesiveness and surface tension. The increased flow of less viscid secretions promotes ciliary action, lubricating irritated respiratory tract membranes, and facilitates removal of viscous, inspissated mucus. This changes a dry, unproductive cough to a cough that is more productive and less frequent. Pseudoephedrine, a sympathomimetic amine, acts on alpha-adrenergic receptors in the mucosa of the respiratory tract, producing vasoconstriction. The medication shrinks swollen nasal mucous membranes, reduces tissue hyperemia, edema, and nasal congestion, and increases nasal airway patency. Also, drainage of sinus secretions is increased and obstructed eustachian ostia may be opened.

INDICATIONS
Anatuss LA Tablets are indicated for the symptomatic relief of nasal congestion and dry non-productive cough in conditions such as: the common cold, acute bronchitis, allergic asthma, bronchiolitis, croup, emphysema and tracheobronchitis.

CONTRAINDICATIONS
Contraindicated in patients with severe hypertension, severe coronary artery disease and in patients on monoamine oxidase (MAO) inhibitor therapy.

NURSING MOTHERS
Pseudoephedrine is contraindicated in nursing mothers because of the higher than usual risk for infants from sympathomimetic amines.

HYPERSENSITIVITY
This drug is contraindicated in patients with hypersensitivity or idiosyncrasy to its ingredients. Patients with idiosyncrasy to adrenergic agents may be manifested by insomnia, dizziness, weakness, tremor or arrhythmias.

WARNINGS
Anatuss LA Tablets should be used with considerable caution in patients with increased intraocular pressure (narrow

angle glaucoma), symptomatic prostatic, hypertrophy, bladder neck obstruction, hypertension, diabetes mellitus, ischemic heart disease, and hyperthyroidism.

USE IN CHILDREN
As in adults, a sympathomimetic amine can elicit either mild stimulation or mild sedation.

USE IN ELDERLY (Approximately 60 years or older):
The elderly are more likely to exhibit adverse reactions to sympathomimetics. At doses higher than the recommended dose, nervousness, dizziness, or sleeplessness may occur.

PRECAUTIONS
GENERAL:
DO NOT CRUSH OR CHEW ANATUSS LA TABLETS BEFORE INGESTION. As with other sympathomimetic drugs, Anatuss LA Tablets should be used with caution in the presence of hypertension, hyperthyroidism, diabetes, heart disease, glaucoma and prostatic hypertrophy. Tricylic antidepressants may antagonize the effects of pseudoephedrine.
DRUG INTERACTIONS:
Monoamine oxidase (MAO) inhibitors and beta adrenergic blockers may potentiate the affects of sympathomimetic amines. Sympathomimetic amines may reduce the antihypertensive effect of guanethidine, mecamylamine, methyldopa, reserpine and veratrum alkaloids.
DRUG/LABORATORY TEST INTERACTIONS:
Guaifenesin has been shown to produce a color interference with certain clinical laboratory determinations of 5-hydroxy-indoleacetic acid (5-HIAA) and vanillylmandelic acid (VMA).
USAGE IN PREGNANCY: PREGNANCY CATEGORY C:
Reproduction studies have not been performed in animals with Anatuss LA Tablets. There is no adequate information on whether this drug may affect fertility in males and females or has a teratogenic potential or other adverse effect on the fetus.
USAGE IN NURSING MOTHERS:
The components of Anatuss LA Tablets are excreted in breast milk in small amounts but the significance of their effect on nursing infants is not known. Because of the potential for serious adverse reactions in nursing infants from material ingestion of Anatuss LA Tablets a decision should be made whether to discontinue nursing or to discontinue the drug, taking into account the importance of the drug to the mother.

ADVERSE REACTIONS
Possible adverse reactions include nervousness, insomnia, restlessness, tachycardia, headache, nausea, weakness, dizziness, dry mouth or urinary retention in patients with prostatic hypertrophy.

DOSAGE AND ADMINISTRATION
Anatuss LA Tablets: Adults and Children over 12: One (1) tablet every 12 hours; Children (6 to 12): ½ tablet every 12 hours; Children (under 6 years): only as directed by physician. Tablets may be broken in half for ease of administration without affecting release of medication but not crushed or chewed. DO NOT EXCEED RECOMMENDED DOSAGE.

HOW SUPPLIED
Anatuss LA Tablets are available as off-white oval-shaped tablets, deep-scored on one side with an "M" appearing on the left of the score and an "R" appearing on the right of the score and 0379 appearing on the bottom side of the tablet.
In bottles of 100: NDC #0259-0379-01.

STORAGE
Store at controlled room temperature, 15–30 C (59–86 F).
Caution: FEDERAL LAW PROHIBITS DISPENSING WITHOUT PRESCRIPTION.

ANTIOX® CAPSULES   OTC
Antioxidant Nutritional Supplement

DESCRIPTION
Each soft gelatin capsule contains:

Beta Carotene	25 mg
(all-trans-β Carotene)	
Vitamin C	120 mg
(Ascorbic Acid)	
Vitamin E	100 IU
(dl-Alpha-tocopheryl Acetate)	

HOW SUPPLIED
ANTIOX® CAPSULES are available as burnished orange, oval shaped soft gelatin capsules imprinted MP 0384.
In bottles of 60:   NDC 0259-0384-60

ELDERCAPS®   ℞

DESCRIPTION
Each capsule contains: Vitamin A Acetate, 4000 I.U.; Vitamin D₂, 400 I.U.; Vitamin E, 25 I.U.; Ascorbic Acid, 200 mg.;

Thiamine Mononitrate, 10 mg.; Riboflavin, 5 mg.; Pyridoxine HCl, 2 mg.; Niacinamide, 25 mg.; d-Calcium Pantothenate, 10 mg.; Zinc Sulfate, 110 mg.; Magnesium Sulfate, 70 mg.; Manganese Sulfate, 5 mg.; Folic Acid, 1 mg.

HOW SUPPLIED
ELDERCAPS are supplied in bottles of 100: NDC #0259-0337-01.

ELDERTONIC®   OTC

DESCRIPTION
Each 45 ml. contains: Thiamine HCl, 1.5 mg.; Riboflavin, 1.7 mg. (as Riboflavin 5'-Phosphate Sodium); Pyridoxine HCl, 2.0 mg.; Cyanocobalamin, 6.0 mcg.; Dexpanthenol, 10.0 mg.; Niacinamide, 20.0 mg.; Zinc, 15 mg. (as zinc sulfate); Manganese, 2.0 mg. (as manganese sulfate); Magnesium (minimum content as added magnesium), 2.0 mg. (as magnesium sulfate); Alcohol, 13.5%.
In a special sherry wine base.

INDICATIONS
B-complex vitamins with minerals for nutritional supplementation.

DOSAGE
Adults: one tablespoonful three times a day with meals.

WARNING
Do not exceed recommended dosage unless directed by a physician.

USAGE IN PREGNANCY
Safe use of this product in pregnancy has not been established.

CAUTION
Keep out of the reach of children.

HOW SUPPLIED
ELDERTONIC available in 8 oz. bottles: NDC #0259-0351-08, Pint bottles: NDC #0259-0351-16, Quart bottles: NDC #0259-0351-32, Gallons: NDC #0259-0351-28.

MAY–VITA® ELIXIR   ℞

DESCRIPTION
Each 45 ml. contains: Dexpanthenol, 10 mg; Niacinamide, 40 mg.; Pyridoxine HCl (B-6), 4 mg.; Cyanocobalamin (B-12), 12 mcg.; Folic Acid, 1 mg.; Iron, 36 mg. (as polysaccharide iron complex); Zinc, 15 mg. (as zinc sulfate); Manganese, 4 mg. (as manganese sulfate); Alcohol, 13%.

INDICATIONS
For vitamin and mineral replacement therapy in deficiency states and for treatment of iron deficiency anemia and/or nutritional megaloblastic anemias due to inadequate diet.

WARNINGS
Folic acid alone is improper therapy in the treatment of pernicious anemia and other megaloblastic anemias where vitamin B₁₂ is deficient.

PRECAUTIONS
Folic acid, especially in doses above 0.1 mg. daily, may obscure pernicious anemia, in that hematologic remission may occur while neurological manifestations remain progressive.

ADVERSE REACTIONS
Allergic sensitization has been reported following both oral and parenteral administration of folic acid.

USE IN PREGNANCY
Safe use of this product in pregnancy has not been established.

DOSAGE
Usual adult dosage is one tablespoonful three times daily with meals. Do not exceed recommended dosage unless directed by a physician.

HOW SUPPLIED
MAY-VITA ELIXIR is supplied in Pint bottles: NDC #0259-0366-16.

NU-IRON® 150 CAPS   OTC
NU-IRON® Elixir (polysaccharide-iron complex)
Sugar Free

DESCRIPTION
NU-IRON is a highly water soluble complex of iron and a low molecular weight polysaccharide.

Continued on next page

Mayrand—Cont.

Each NU-IRON 150 Capsule contains:
Iron (elemental) .... 150 mg.
  (as Polysaccharide Iron Complex)
Each 5 ml. of NU-IRON Elixir contains:
Iron (elemental) .... 100 mg.
  (as Polysaccharide Iron Complex)
Alcohol 10%

ACTION AND USES
NU-IRON is a non-ionic, easily assimilated, relatively non-toxic form of iron. Full therapeutic doses may be achieved with virtually no gastrointestinal side effects. There is no metallic aftertaste and no staining of teeth.

INDICATIONS
For treatment of uncomplicated iron deficiency anemia.

CONTRAINDICATIONS
Hemochromatosis, hemosiderosis or a known hypersensitivity to any of the ingredients.

DOSAGE
ADULT S:One or two NU-IRON 150 Caps daily, or one or two teaspoonfuls NU-IRON Elixir daily. CHILDREN; 6 to 12 years old; one teaspoonful NU-IRON Elixir daily. For younger children consult physician.

HOW SUPPLIED
NU-IRON 150 CAPSULES in bottles of 100: NDC #0259-0291-01.
NU-IRON ELIXIR in 8 oz bottles: NDC #0259-0292-08.

NU–IRON® PLUS ELIXIR   ℞
(polysaccharide-iron complex)
Sugar Free

DESCRIPTION
Each 5 ml of NU-IRON PLUS ELIXIR contains:
Iron (elemental)   100 mg
Folic Acid   1 mg
Vitamin B12   25 mcg
Alcohol   10%

HOW SUPPLIED
NU-IRON PLUS ELIXIR is supplied in 8 oz bottles: NDC #0259-0342-08.

NU–IRON® V TABLETS   ℞
(polysaccharide-iron complex with vitamins)

DESCRIPTION
Each maroon film-coated tablet contains:
IRON, ELEMENTAL (As a polysaccharide-iron complex) 60 mg; Folic Acid 1 mg; Ascorbic Acid 50 mg. (as sodium ascorbate); Cyanocobalamin (Vitamin B-12) 3 mcg.; Vitamin A 4000 I.U.; Vitamin D-2 400 I.U.; Thiamine Mononitrate 3 mg.; Riboflavin 3 mg.; Pyridoxine Hydrochloride 2 mg.; Niacinamide 10 mg.; Calcium Carbonate 312 mg.

HOW SUPPLIED
NU-IRON V TABLETS are available as maroon film-coated capsule-shaped tablets. In bottles of 100: NDC #0259-0331-01.

SEDAPAP TABLETS   ℞
50 mg/650 mg

DESCRIPTION
Each white, capsule-shaped tablet for oral administration contains:
Butalbital* .... 50 mg
  *(WARNING: May be habit forming.)
Acetaminophen .... 650 mg
Butalbital, 5-allyl-5-isobutylbarbituric acid, a white, odorless, crystalline powder having a slightly bitter taste, is a short- to intermediate-acting barbiturate.
Acetaminophen, 4-hydroxyacetanilide, is a non-opiate, non-salicylate analgesic and antipyretic which occurs as a white, odorless, crystalline powder possessing a slightly bitter taste.

INACTIVE INGREDIENTS
Gelatin, Magnesium Stearate, Microcrystalline Cellulose, Pregelatinized Starch, Sodium Starch Glycolate, Starch.

CLINICAL PHARMACOLOGY
Pharmacologically, SEDAPAP TABLETS combine the analgesic properties of acetaminophen with the anxiolytic and muscle relaxant properties of butalbital.

INDICATIONS AND USAGE
SEDAPAP TABLETS are indicated for the relief of the symptom complex of tension (or muscle contraction) headache.

CONTRAINDICATIONS
Hypersensitivity to acetaminophen or barbiturates. Patients with porphyria.

PRECAUTIONS
General: Barbiturates should be administered with caution, if at all, to patients who are mentally depressed, have suicidal tendencies, or a history of drug abuse.
Elderly or debilitated patients may react to barbiturates with marked excitement, depression, and confusion. In some persons, barbiturates repeatedly produce excitement rather than depression.
Information For Patients: Practitioners should give the following information and instructions to patients receiving barbiturates:
A. The use of barbiturates carries with it an associated risk of psychological and/or physical dependence. The patient should be warned against increasing the dose of the drug without consulting a physician.
B. Barbiturates may impair mental and/or physical abilities required for the performance of potentially hazardous tasks (e.g., driving, operating machinery, etc.).
C. Alcohol should not be consumed while taking barbiturates. Concurrent use of the barbiturates with other CNS depressants (e.g., alcohol, narcotics, tranquilizers, and antihistamines) may result in additional CNS depressant effects.
Drug Interactions: Patients receiving narcotic analgesics, antipsychotics, antianxiety agents, or other CNS depressants (including alcohol) concomitantly with SEDAPAP TABLETS may exhibit additive CNS depressant effects.

DRUGS	EFFECT
Butalbital with coumarin anticoagulants	Decreased effect of anticoagulant because of increased metabolism resulting from enzyme induction
Butalbital with tricyclic antidepressant	Decreased blood levels of the antidepressant

PREGNANCY
Adequate studies have not been performed in animals to determine whether this drug affects fertility in males or females, has teratogenic potential or has other adverse effects on the fetus. Although there is no clearly defined risk, one cannot exclude the possibility of infrequent or subtle damage to the human fetus. SEDAPAP TABLETS should be used in pregnant women only when clearly needed.
Nursing Mothers: The effects of SEDAPAP TABLETS on infants of nursing mothers are not known. Barbiturates are excreted in the breast milk of nursing mothers. The serum levels in infants are believed to be insignificant with therapeutic doses.
Pediatric Use: Safety and effectiveness in children below the age of twelve have not been established.

ADVERSE REACTIONS
The most frequent adverse reactions are drowsiness and dizziness. Less frequent adverse reactions are lightheadedness and gastrointestinal disturbances including nausea, vomiting, and flatulence. Mental confusion or depression can occur due to intolerance or overdosage of butalbital. Several cases of dermatological reactions including toxic epidermal necrolysis and erythema multiforme have been reported.

DRUG ABUSE AND DEPENDENCE
Prolonged use of barbiturates can produce drug dependence, characterized by psychic dependence and tolerance. The abuse liability of SEDAPAP TABLETS is similar to that of other barbiturate-containing drug combinations. Caution should be exercised when prescribing medication for patients with a known propensity for taking excessive quantities of drugs, which is not uncommon in patients with chronic tension headache.

OVERDOSAGE
The toxic effects of acute overdosage of SEDAPAP TABLETS are attributable mainly to its barbiturate component, and, to a lesser extent, acetaminophen.
Barbiturate
SIGNS AND SYMPTOMS: Drowsiness, confusion, coma; respiratory depression; hypotension; shock.
TREATMENT:
1. Maintenance of an adequate airway, with assisted respiration and oxygen administration as necessary.
2. Monitoring of vital signs and fluid balance.
3. If the patient is conscious and has not lost the gag reflex, emesis may be induced with ipecac. Care should be taken to prevent pulmonary aspiration of vomitus. After completion of vomiting, 30 grams of activated charcoal in a glass of water may be administered.

4. If emesis is contraindicated, gastric lavage may be performed with a cuffed endotracheal tube in place with the patient in the facedown position. Activated charcoal may be left in the emptied stomach and a saline cathartic administered.
5. Fluid therapy and other standard treatment for shock, if needed.
6. If renal function is normal, forced diuresis may aid in the elimination of the barbiturate. Alkalinization of the urine increases renal excretion of some barbiturates, especially phenobarbital.
7. Although not recommended as a routine procedure, hemodialysis may be used in severe barbiturate intoxication or if the patient is anuric or in shock.
Acetaminophen
SIGNS AND SYMPTOMS: In acute acetaminophen overdosage, dose-dependent, potentially fatal hepatic necrosis is the most serious adverse effect. Renal tubular necrosis, hypoglycemic coma, and thrombocytopenia may also occur.
In adults, hepatic toxicity has rarely been reported with acute overdoses of less than 10 grams and fatalities with less than 15 grams. Importantly, young children seem to be more resistant than adults to the hepatotoxic effects of an acetaminophen overdose.
Early symptoms following a potentially hepatotoxic overdosage may include: nausea, vomiting, diaphoresis and general malaise. Clinical and laboratory evidence of hepatic toxicity may not be apparent until 48 to 72 hours post-ingestion.
TREATMENT: The stomach should be emptied promptly by lavage or by induction of emesis with syrup of ipecac. Patients' estimates of the quantity of a drug ingested are notoriously unreliable. Therefore, if an acetaminophen overdose is suspected, a serum acetaminophen assay should be obtained as early as possible, but no sooner than four hours following ingestion. Liver function studies should be obtained initially and repeated at 24-hour intervals.
The antidote, N-acetylcysteine, should be administered as early as possible, preferably within 16 hours of the overdose ingestion for optimal results, but in any case, within 24 hours. Following recovery, there are no residual, structural or functional hepatic abnormalities.

DOSAGE AND ADMINISTRATION
One tablet every four hours as needed. Do not exceed 6 tablets per day.

HOW SUPPLIED
SEDAPAP TABLETS [Butalbital 50 mg (WARNING: May be habit forming) and Acetaminophen 650 mg] are available as white, capsule-shaped tablets scored on one side with an "M" appearing on the left side of the score, and an "R" appearing on the right side of the score and "1278" on the other. In bottles of 100, NDC #0259-1278-01.

STERAPRED® UNIPAK   ℞

DESCRIPTION
Each white tablet contains:
Prednisone .... 5 mg

HOW SUPPLIED
STERAPRED UNIPAK Available in 21 tablet tapered dose dispensing pack. NDC #0259-0284-01.

STERAPRED® DS UNIPAK   ℞
STERAPRED® DS 12 DAY UNIPAK

DESCRIPTION
Each white tablet contains:
Prednisone .... 10 mg

HOW SUPPLIED
STERAPRED DS UNIPAK available in 21 tablet tapered dose dispensing pack: NDC #0259-0364-21.
STERAPRED DS 12 DAY UNIPAK available in 48 tablet tapered dose dispensing pack: NDC #0259-0364-48.

Products are cross-indexed by
generic and chemical names
in the
YELLOW SECTION.

McNeil Consumer Products Company

Division of McNeil-PPC, Inc.
FORT WASHINGTON, PA 19034

CHEMET® ℞
SUCCIMER
Capsule 100 mg

DESCRIPTION
CHEMET (succimer) is an orally active, heavy metal chelating agent. The chemical name for succimer is meso 2, 3-dimercaptosuccinic acid (DMSA). Its empirical formula is $C_4H_6O_4S_2$ and molecular weight is 182.2. The meso-structural formula is:

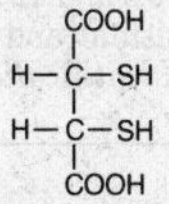

Succimer is a white crystalline powder with an unpleasant, characteristic mercaptan odor and taste.
Each CHEMET opaque white capsule for oral administration contains beads coated with 100 mg of succimer and is imprinted in black with CHEMET 100. Inactive ingredients in medicated beads are: povidone, sodium starch glycolate, starch and sucrose. Inactive ingredients in capsule are: gelatin, iron oxide, titanium dioxide and other ingredients.

CLINICAL PHARMACOLOGY
Succimer is a lead chelator; it forms water soluble chelates and, consequently, increases the urinary excretion of lead.
Preclinical Toxicology: In an ongoing six month chronic oral toxicity study in dogs, thrombocytopenia was observed in animals receiving succimer at 80 or 140 mg/kg/day after three months of dosing. Preliminary gross pathology findings in the affected dogs included ecchymoses in a number of organs. No depressed platelet counts were observed in dogs receiving succimer at 10 mg/kg/day for three months. Platelets were not enumerated in previous oral toxicity studies up to 28 days. In those studies, daily doses of succimer up to 200 mg/kg/day did not produce any significant overt toxicity in rats and dogs. However, six and twenty-eight day oral toxicity studies in dogs have shown that doses of 300 mg/kg/day or higher were toxic and lethal to some dogs. Kidney and gastrointestinal tract were the major target organs for succimer toxicity.
Toxicity was manifested by anorexia, emesis, mucoid and/or bloody diarrhea, increased blood urea nitrogen concentration, increased SGPT, SGOT and alkaline phosphatase levels, renal tubular necrosis, purulent nephritis and severe gastrointestinal bleeding and ulceration. Deaths were due to renal failure.
Pharmacokinetics: In a study performed in healthy adult volunteers, after a single dose of ^{14}C-succimer at 16,32, or 48 mg/kg, absorption was rapid but variable with peak blood radioactivity levels between one and two hours. On average, 49% of the radiolabeled dose was excreted: 39% in the feces, 9% in the urine and 1% as carbon dioxide from the lungs. Since fecal excretion probably represented non-absorbed drug, most of the absorbed drug was excreted by the kidneys. The apparent elimination half-life of the radio-labeled material in the blood was about two days.
In other studies of healthy adult volunteers receiving a single oral dose of 10 mg/kg, the chemical analysis of succimer and its metabolites in the urine showed that succimer was rapidly and extensively metabolized. Approximately 25% of the administered dose was excreted in the urine with the peak blood level and urinary excretion occurring between two and four hours. Of the total amount of drug eliminated in the urine, approximately 90% was eliminated in altered form as mixed succimer-cysteine disulfides; the remaining 10% was eliminated unchanged. The majority of mixed disulfides consisted of succimer in disulfide linkages with two molecules of L-cysteine, the remaining disulfides contained one L-cysteine per succimer molecule.
Pharmacodynamics: Dose ranging studies were performed in 18 men with blood lead levels of 44–96 μg/dL. Three groups of 6 patients received either 10.0, 6.7 or 3.3 mg/kg succimer orally every 8 hours for 5 days. After five days the mean blood levels of the three groups decreased 72.5%, 58.3% and 35.5% respectively. The mean urinary lead excretions in the initial 24 hours were 28.6, 18.6 and 12.3 times the pretreatment 24 hour urinary lead excretion. As the chelatable pool was reduced during therapy, urinary lead output decreased. A mean of 19 mg of lead was excreted during a five-day course of 30 mg/kg/day succimer. Clinical symptoms, such as headache and colic and biochemical indices of lead toxicity also improved. Decrease in urinary excretion of d-aminolevulinic acid (ALA) and coproporphyrin paralleled the improvement in erythrocyte d-aminolevulinic acid dehydratase (ALA-D). Three control patients with lead poisoning of similar severity received $CaNa_2EDTA$ intravenously at a dose of 50 mg/kg/day for five days. The mean blood lead level decreased 47.4% and the mean urinary lead excretion was 21 mg in the control patients.
Effect on Essential Minerals: In the above studies succimer had no significant effect on the urinary elimination of iron, calcium or magnesium. Zinc excretion doubled during treatment. The effect of succimer on the excretion of essential minerals was small compared to that of $CaNa_2EDTA$, which can induce more than a ten-fold increase in urinary excretion of zinc and doubling of copper and iron excretion.
Efficacy: A dose ranging study was performed in 15 children aged 2 to 7 years with blood lead levels of 30–49 μg/dL and positive $CaNa_2EDTA$ lead mobilization tests. Each group of five patients received 350, 233 or 116 mg/m^2 succimer every 8 hours for 5 days. These doses corresponded to 10, 6.7 and 3.3 mg/kg. Six control patients received 1000 mg/m^2/day $CaNa_2EDTA$ intravenously for 5 days. Following therapy, the mean blood lead levels decreased 78, 63 and 42% respectively in the three groups treated with succimer. The response of the 350 mg/m^2 every 8 hours (10 mg/kg q 8 hr) group was significantly better than that of the other succimer treated groups as well as that of the control group, whose mean blood lead level fell 48%. No adverse reactions or changes in essential mineral excretion were reported in the succimer treated groups. In the $CaNa_2EDTA$ treated group, the cumulative amount of urinary lead excreted was slightly but significantly greater than in the succimer group. After $CaNa_2EDTA$, the urinary excretion of copper, zinc, iron and calcium were significantly increased.
As with other chelators, both adults and children experienced a rebound in blood lead levels after discontinuation of CHEMET. In these studies, after treatment with a dose of 350 mg/m^2 (10 mg/kg) every 8 hours for five days, the mean lead level rebounded and plateaued at 60–85% of pretreatment levels two weeks after therapy. The rebound plateau was somewhat higher with lower doses of succimer and with intravenous $CaNa_2EDTA$.
In an attempt to control rebound of blood lead levels, 19 children, ages 1–7 years, with blood lead levels of 42–67 μg/dL, were treated with 350 mg/m^2 succimer every 8 hours for five days and then divided into three groups. One group was followed for two weeks with no further therapy, the second group was treated for two weeks with 350 mg/m^2 daily, and the third with 350 mg/m^2 every 12 hours. After the initial 5 days of therapy, the mean blood lead level in all subjects declined 61%. While the untreated group and the group treated with 350 mg/m^2 daily experienced rebound during the ensuing two weeks, the group who received the 350 mg/m^2 every 12 hours experienced no such rebound during the treatment period and less rebound following cessation of therapy.
In another study, ten children, ages 21 to 72 months, with blood lead levels of 30–57 μg/dL were treated with succimer 350 mg/m^2 every eight hours for five days followed by an additional 19–22 days of therapy at a dose of 350 mg/m^2 every 12 hours. The mean blood lead levels decreased and remained stable at under 15 μg/dL during the extended dosing period.
In addition to the controlled studies, approximately 250 patients with lead poisoning have been treated with succimer either orally or parenterally in open U.S. and foreign studies with similar results reported. Succimer has been used for the treatment of lead poisoning in one patient with sickle cell anemia and in five patients with glucose-6-phosphodehydrogenase (G6PD) deficiency without adverse reactions.
Lead Encephalopathy: Three adults with lead encephalopathy have been reported in the literature to have improved with succimer therapy. However, data are not available regarding the use of succimer for the treatment of this rare and sometimes fatal complication of lead poisoning in children.
Other Heavy Metal Poisoning: No controlled clinical studies have been conducted with succimer in poisoning with other heavy metals. A limited number of patients have received succimer for mercury or arsenic poisoning. These patients showed increased urinary excretion of the heavy metal and varying degrees of symptomatic improvement.

INDICATIONS AND USAGE
CHEMET is indicated for the treatment of lead poisoning in children with blood lead levels above 45 μg/dL. CHEMET is not indicated for prophylaxis of lead poisoning in a lead-containing environment; the use of CHEMET should always be accompanied by identification and removal of the source of the lead exposure.

CONTRAINDICATIONS
CHEMET should not be administered to patients with a history of allergy to the drug.

WARNINGS
Keep out of reach of children. CHEMET is not a substitute for effective abatement of lead exposure.
Mild to moderate neutropenia has been observed in some patients receiving succimer. While a causal relationship to succimer has not been definitely established, neutropenia has been reported with other drugs in the same chemical class. A complete blood count with white blood cell differential and direct platelet counts should be obtained prior to and weekly during treatment with succimer. Therapy should either be withheld or discontinued if the absolute neutrophil count (ANC) is below 1200/μL and the patient followed closely to document recovery of the ANC to above 1500/μL or to the patient's baseline neutrophil count. There is limited experience with reexposure in patients who have developed neutropenia. Therefore, such patients should be rechallenged only if the benefit of succimer therapy clearly outweighs the potential risk of another episode of neutropenia and then only with careful patient monitoring.
Patients treated with succimer should be instructed to promptly report any signs of infection. If infection is suspected, the above laboratory tests should be conducted immediately.

PRECAUTIONS
The extent of clinical experience with CHEMET is limited. Therefore, patients should be carefully observed during treatment.
General: Elevated blood lead levels and associated symptoms may return rapidly after discontinuation of CHEMET because of redistribution of lead from bone stores to soft tissues and blood. After therapy, patients should be monitored for rebound of blood lead levels, by measuring blood lead levels at least once weekly until stable. However, the severity of lead intoxication (as measured by the initial blood lead level and the rate and degree of rebound of blood lead) should be used as a guide for more frequent blood lead monitoring.
All patients undergoing treatment should be adequately hydrated. Caution should be exercised in using CHEMET therapy in patients with compromised renal function. Limited data suggests that CHEMET is dialyzable, but that the lead chelates are not.
Transient mild elevations of serum transaminases have been observed in 6–10% of patients during the course of succimer therapy. Serum transaminases should be monitored before the start of therapy and at least weekly during therapy. Patients with a history of liver disease should be monitored closely. No data are available regarding the metabolism of succimer in patients with liver disease.
Clinical experience with repeated courses is limited. The safety of uninterrupted dosing longer than three weeks has not been established and it is not recommended.
The possibility of allergic or other mucocutaneous reactions to the drug must be borne in mind on readministration (as well as during initial courses). Patients requiring repeated courses of CHEMET should be monitored during each treatment course. One patient experienced recurrent mucocutaneous vesicular eruptions of increasing severity affecting the oral mucosa, the external urethral meatus and the perianal area on the third, fourth and fifth courses of the drug. The reaction resolved between courses and upon discontinuation of therapy.
Information for Patients: Patients should be instructed to maintain adequate fluid intake. If rash occurs, patients should consult their physician. Patients should be instructed to promptly report any indication of infection, which may be a sign of neutropenia (see WARNINGS and ADVERSE REACTIONS).
In young children unable to swallow capsules, the contents of the capsule can be administered in a small amount of food (see DOSAGE AND ADMINISTRATION).
Drug Interaction: CHEMET is not known to interact with other drugs including iron supplements; interactions have not been systematically studied. Concomitant administration of CHEMET with other chelation therapy, such $CaNa_2EDTA$ is not recommended.
Drug/Laboratory Tests Interaction: Succimer may interfere with serum and urinary laboratory tests. *In vitro* studies have shown succimer to cause false positive results for ketones in urine using nitroprusside reagents such as Ketostix® and falsely decreased measurements of serum uric acid and CPK.
Carcinogenesis, Mutagenesis and Impairment of Fertility: CHEMET has not been tested for carcinogenic potential in long-term animal studies. CHEMET has not been tested in animals for its effect on fertility and reproductive performance in males and females. It was not mutagenic in the Ames bacterial assay and in the mammalian cell forward gene mutation assay.
Pregnancy: Teratogenic Effects—Pregnancy Category C. CHEMET has been shown to be teratogenic and fetoxic in pregnant mice when given subcutaneously in a dose range of 410 to 1640 mg/kg/day during the period of organogenesis. There are no adequate and well controlled studies in pregnant women. CHEMET should be used during pregnancy only if the potential benefit justifies the potential risk to the fetus.
Nursing Mothers: It is not known whether this drug is excreted in human milk. Because many drugs and heavy metals are excreted in human milk, nursing mothers requiring

Continued on next page

McNeil Consumer—Cont.

CHEMET therapy should be discouraged from nursing their infants.

Pediatric Use: Refer to the INDICATIONS and DOSAGE AND ADMINISTRATION sections. There is no therapeutic experience with CHEMET in children under one year of age.

ADVERSE REACTIONS

Clinical experience with CHEMET has been limited. Consequently, the full spectrum and incidence of adverse reactions including the possibility of hypersensitivity or idiosyncratic reactions have not been determined. The most common events attributable to succimer, i.e., gastrointestinal symptoms or increases in serum transaminases, have been observed in about 10% of patients (see PRECAUTIONS). Rashes, some necessitating discontinuation of therapy, have been reported in about 4% of patients. If rash occurs, other causes (e.g. measles) should be considered before ascribing the reaction to succimer. Rechallenge with succimer may be considered if lead levels are high enough to warrant retreatment. One allergic mucocutaneous reaction has been reported on repeated administration of the drug (See PRECAUTIONS). Mild to moderate neutropenia has been observed in some patients receiving succimer (see WARNINGS). Table I presents adverse events reported with the administration of succimer for the treatment of lead and other heavy metal intoxication.

TABLE I
INCIDENCE OF ADVERSE EVENTS IN DOMESTIC STUDIES REGARDLESS OF ATTRIBUTION OR SUCCIMER DOSAGE

	Children (191)		Adults (134)	
	%	(n)	%	(n)
Digestive:	12.0	23	20.9	28
Nausea, vomiting, diarrhea, appetite loss, hemorrhoidal symptoms, loose stools, metallic taste in mouth.				
Body as a Whole:	5.2	10	15.7	21
Back pain, abdominal cramps, stomach pains, head pain, rib pain, chills, flank pain, fever, flu-like symptoms, heavy head/tired, head cold, headache, moniliasis.				
Metabolic:	4.2	8	10.4	14
Elevated SGPT, SGOT, alkaline phosphatase, elevated serum cholesterol.				
Nervous:	1.0	2	12.7	17
Drowsiness, dizziness, sensorimotor neuropathy, sleepiness, paresthesia.				
Skin and Appendages:	2.6	5	11.2	15
Papular rash, herpetic rash, rash, mucocutaneous eruptions, pruritus.				
Special Senses:	1.0	2	3.7	5
Cloudy film in eye, ears plugged, otitis media, eyes watery.				
Respiratory:	3.7	7	0.7	1
Throat sore, rhinorrhea, nasal congestion, cough.				
Urogenital:	0.0	—	3.7	5
Decreased urination, voiding difficulty, proteinuria increased.				
Cardiovascular:	0.0	—	1.8	2
Arrhythmia				
Heme/Lymphatic:	0.5*	1	1.5*	2
Mild to moderate neutropenia				
Increased platelet count, intermittent eosinophilia.				
Musculoskeletal:	0.0	—	3.0	4
Kneecap pain, leg pains.				

*Does not include neutropenia - see WARNINGS

OVERDOSAGES

Doses of 2300 mg/kg in the rat and 2400 mg/kg in the mouse produced ataxia, convulsions, labored respiration and frequently death. No case of overdosage has been reported in humans. Limited data indicate that succimer is dialyzable. In case of acute overdosage, induction of vomiting or gastric lavage followed by administration of an activated charcoal slurry and appropriate supportive therapy are recommended.

DOSAGE AND ADMINISTRATION

Start dosage at 10 mg/kg or 350 mg/m^2 every eight hours for five days. Initiation of therapy at higher doses is not recommended. (See Table II for Dosing chart and number of capsules.) Reduce frequency of administration to 10 mg/kg or 350 mg/m^2 every 12 hours (two-thirds of initial daily dosage) for an additional two weeks of therapy. A course of treatment lasts 19 days. Repeated courses may be necessary if indicated by weekly monitoring of blood lead concentration. A minimum of two weeks between courses is recommended unless blood lead levels indicate the need for more prompt treatment.

In young children who cannot swallow capsules, CHEMET can be administered by separating the capsule and sprinkling the medicated beads on a small amount of soft food or putting them in a spoon and following with fruit drink.

Identification of the source of lead in the child's environment and its abatement are critical to a successful therapy outcome. Chelation therapy is not a substitute for preventing further exposure to lead and should not be used to permit continued exposure to lead.

TABLE II
CHEMET (SUCCIMER) PEDIATRIC DOSING CHART

LBS	KG	DOSE (MG)*	Number of CAPSULES*
18–35	8–15	100	1
36–55	16–23	200	2
56–75	24–34	300	3
76–100	35–44	400	4
>100	>45	500	5

*To be administered every 8 hours for 5 days, followed by dosing every 12 hours for 14 days.

Patients who have received $CaNa_2EDTA$ with or without BAL may use CHEMET for subsequent treatment after an interval of four weeks. Data on the concomitant use of CHEMET with $CaNa_2EDTA$ with or without BAL are not available, and such use is not recommended.

HOW SUPPLIED

100 mg capsules in bottle of 100 (NDC 0045-0134-10)

Storage: Store at controlled room temperature (15°–30°C).

CAUTION: Federal Law prohibits dispensing without prescription. Revised November, 1991.

MANUFACTURED FOR:
McNEIL CONSUMER PRODUCTS COMPANY
DIVISION OF McNEIL-PPC, INC.
FORT WASHINGTON, PA 19034 USA 1991
BY:
CENTRAL PHARMACEUTICALS, INC.
SEYMOUR, IN 47274

Shown in Product Identification Section, page 417

IMODIUM® A-D — OTC
(loperamide hydrochloride)

DESCRIPTION

Each 5 ml (teaspoon) of Imodium A-D liquid contains loperamide hydrochloride 1 mg. Imodium A-D liquid is stable, cherry flavored, and clear in color.

Each caplet of Imodium AD contains 2 mg of loperamide and is scored and colored green.

ACTIONS

Imodium A-D contains a clinically proven antidiarrheal medication. Loperamide HCl acts by slowing intestinal motility and by affecting water and electrolyte movement through the bowel.

INDICATION

Imodium A-D is indicated for the control and symptomatic relief of acute nonspecific diarrhea.

USUAL DOSAGE

Adults: Take four teaspoonfuls or two caplets after first loose bowel movement. If needed, take two teaspoonfuls or one caplet after each subsequent loose bowel movement. Do not exceed eight teaspoonfuls or four caplets in any 24 hour period, unless directed by a physician.

9–11 years old (60–95 lbs.): Two teaspoonfuls or one caplet after first loose bowel movement, followed by one teaspoonful or one-half caplet after each subsequent loose bowel movement. Do not exceed six teaspoonfuls or three caplets a day.

6–8 years old (48–59 lbs.): Two teaspoonfuls or one caplet after first loose bowel movement, followed by one teaspoonful or one-half caplet after each subsequent loose bowel movement. Do not exceed four teaspoonfuls or two caplets a day.

Professional Dosage Schedule for children two-five years old (24–47 lbs): one teaspoon after first loose bowel movement, followed by one after each subsequent loose bowel movement. Do not exceed three teaspoonfuls a day.

Warnings: DO NOT USE FOR MORE THAN TWO DAYS UNLESS DIRECTED BY A PHYSICIAN. Do not use if diarrhea is accompanied by high fever (greater than 101°F), or if blood is present in the stool, or if you have had a rash or other allergic reaction to loperamide HCl. If you are taking antibiotics or have a history of liver disease, consult a physician before using this product. As with any drug, if you are pregnant or nursing a baby, seek the advice of a physician before using this product. Keep this and all drugs out of the reach of children. In case of accidental overdose, seek professional assistance or contact a poison control center immediately. Store at room temperature.

OVERDOSAGE

Overdosage of loperamide HCl in man may result in constipation, CNS depression and nausea. A slurry of activated charcoal administered promptly after ingestion of loperamide hydrochloride can reduce the amount of drug which is absorbed. If vomiting occurs spontaneously upon ingestion, a slurry of 100 grams of activated charcoal should be administered orally as soon as fluids can be retained. If vomiting has not occurred, and CNS depression is evident, gastric lavage should be performed followed by administration of 100 gms of the activated charcoal slurry through the gastric tube. In the event of overdosage, patients should be monitored for signs of CNS depression for at least 24 hours. Children may be more sensitive to central nervous system effects than adults. If CNS depression is observed, naloxone may be administered. If responsive to naloxone, vital signs must be monitored carefully for recurrence of symptoms of drug overdose for at least 24 hours after the last dose of naloxone.

INACTIVE INGREDIENTS

Liquid: Alcohol (5.25%), citric acid, flavors, glycerin, methylparaben, propylparaben and purified water.

Caplets: Corn starch, lactose, magnesium stearate, microcrystalline cellulose, FD&C Blue #1 and D&C yellow #10.

HOW SUPPLIED

Cherry flavored liquid (clear) 2 fl. oz., 3 fl. oz., and 4 fl. oz. tamper resistant bottles with child resistant safety caps and special dosage cups.

Green Scored caplets in 6's and 12's and 18's blister packaging which is tamper resistant and child resistant.

Shown in Product Identification Section, page 417

PEDIACARE® Cold-Allergy Chewable Tablets — OTC
PEDIACARE® Cough-Cold Liquid and Chewable Tablets
PEDIACARE® NightRest Cough-Cold Liquid
PEDIACARE® Infants' Oral Decongestant Drops

DESCRIPTION

Each PEDIACARE Cold-Allergy Chewable Tablet contains chlorpheniramine maleate 1 mg and pseudoephedrine hydrochloride 15 mg. Each 5 ml of PEDIACARE Cough-Cold Liquid contains pseudoephedrine hydrochloride 15 mg, chlorpheniramine maleate 1 mg and dextromethorphan hydrobromide 5 mg. Each Pediacare Cough-Cold Formula Chewable Tablet contains pseudoephedrine hydrochloride 15 mg, chlorpheniramine maleate 1 mg and dextromethorphan hydrobromide 5 mg. Each 0.8 ml oral dropper of PEDIACARE Infants' Oral Decongestant Drops contains pseudoephedrine hydrochloride 7.5 mg. PEDIACARE NightRest Cough-Cold liquid contains pseudoephedrine hydrochloride 15 mg, chlorpheniramine maleate 1 mg and dextromethorphan hydrobromide 7.5 mg per 5 ml. PEDIACARE Cough-Cold Liquid and Infants' Drops are stable, cherry flavored and red in color. PEDIACARE Cold-Allergy Chewable Tablets are fruit flavored and pink in color. PEDIACARE Cough-Allergy Chewable Tablets are fruit flavored and pink in color.

ACTIONS

PEDIACARE Products are available in four different formulas, allowing you to select the ideal product to temporarily relieve the patient's symptoms. PEDIACARE Cold-Allergy Chewable Tablets contain an antihistamine and a nasal decongestant to relieve children's cold and allergy symptoms. PEDIACARE Cough-Cold liquid and 6–12 Chewable Tablets contain both of the above ingredients plus a cough suppressant, dextromethorphan hydrobromide, to provide temporary relief of nasal congestion, runny nose, sneezing and coughing due to the common cold, hay fever or other upper respiratory allergies. PEDIACARE NightRest Cough-Cold Liquid contains a decongestant, pseudoephedrine hydrochloride, an antihistamine, chlorpheniramine maleate, and a cough suppressant, dextromethorphan hydrobromide, to provide temporary relief of coughs, nasal congestion, runny nose and sneezing due to the common cold. PEDIACARE NightRest may be used day or night to relieve cough and cold symptoms. PEDIACARE Infants' Oral Decongestant Drops contain a decongestant, pseudoephedrine hydrochloride, to provide temporary relief of nasal congestion due to the common cold, hay fever or other upper respiratory allergies.

Professional Dosage: A calibrated dosage cup is provided for accurate dosing of the PEDIACARE Liquid formulas. A calibrated oral dropper is provided for accurate dosing of PEDIACARE Infants' Drops. All doses of PEDIACARE Cold-Allergy Chewable Tablets, PEDIACARE Cough-Cold Liquid and Chewable Tablets, as well as PEDIACARE Infants' Drops may be repeated every 4–6 hours, not to exceed 4 doses in 24 hours. PEDIACARE NightRest Liquid may be repeated every 6–8 hrs, not to exceed 4 doses in 24 hours.

[See table on next page.]

"**WARNINGS:** Do not use if carton is opened, or if printed plastic bottle wrap or foil inner seal is broken. Keep this and all medication out of the reach of children. In case of accidental overdose, contact a physician or poison control center immediately."

The following information appears on the appropriate package labels:

PEDIACARE Cold-Allergy Chewable Tablets: Do not exceed the recommended dosage because nervousness, dizziness or sleeplessness may occur. Do not give this product to children for more than 7 days. If symptoms do not improve, or are accompanied by fever, consult a physician. May cause excitability especially in children. May cause drowsiness. Do

Age Group	0–3 mos	4–11 mos	12–23 mos	2–3 yrs	4–5 yrs	6–8 yrs	9–10 yrs	11 yrs	Dosage
Weight (lbs)	6–11 lb	12–17 lb	18–23 lb	24–35 lb	36–47 lb	48–59 lb	60–71 lb	72–95 lb	
PEDIACARE Infants' Drops*	½ dropper (0.4 ml)	1 dropper (0.8 ml)	1½ droppers (1.2 ml)	2 droppers (1.6 ml)					q4–6h
PEDIACARE Cold-Allergy Chewable Tablets**				1 tabs	1½ tabs	2 tabs	2½ tabs	3 tabs	q4–6h
PEDIACARE Cough-Cold Liquid**				1 tsp	1½ tsp	2 tsp	2½ tsp	3 tsp	q4–6h
and Chewable Tablets**				1 tabs	1½ tabs	2 tabs	2½ tabs	3 tabs	q4–6h
PEDIACARE NightRest Liquid**				1 tsp	1½ tsp	2 tsp	2½ tsp	3 tsp	q6–8h

* Administer to children under 2 years only on the advice of a physician.
** Administer to children under 6 years only on the advice of a physician.

not give this product to children who have heart disease, high blood pressure, thyroid disease, diabetes, asthma or glaucoma unless directed by a physician.

PEDIACARE Cough-Cold Liquid, NightRest Cough-Cold Liquid and Chewable Tablets: Do not exceed the recommended dosage because nervousness, dizziness or sleeplessness may occur. Do not give this product to children for more than 7 days. If symptoms do not improve, or are accompanied by fever, consult a doctor. A persistent cough may be a sign of a serious condition. If cough persists for more than one week, tends to recur or is accompanied by fever, rash, or persistent headache, consult a doctor. Do not give this product for persistent or chronic cough such as occurs with asthma or if cough is accompanied by excessive phlegm (mucus) unless directed by a doctor. This preparation may cause drowsiness or, in some cases, excitability. Do not give this product to children who have heart disease, high blood pressure, thyroid disease, glaucoma or asthma unless directed by a doctor.

DRUG INTERACTION PRECAUTION: Do not give this product to a child who is taking a prescription drug for high blood pressure or depression, without first consulting the child's doctor.

PEDIACARE Infants' Oral Decongestant Drops: "Do not exceed the recommended dosage because at higher doses nervousness, dizziness or sleeplessness may occur. Do not give this product to children who have heart disease, high blood pressure, thyroid disease or diabetes unless directed by a physician. Do not give this product to children for more than seven days. If symptoms do not improve or are accompanied by fever, consult a physician. Do not give this product to children who are taking a prescription drug for high blood pressure or depression without first consulting a physician. Take by mouth only. Not for nasal use."

PEDIACARE Cold-Allergy Chewable Tablets also contain the warning, "Phenylketonurics: Contains phenylalanine 3 mg per tablet", and the inactive ingredient listing, "Inactive Ingredients: Aspartame, Cellulose, Citric Acid, Corn Starch, Flavors, Mannitol, Colloidal Silicon Dioxide, Stearic Acid, and Red #7."

PEDIACARE Cough-Cold Liquid: Inactive Ingredients: Benzoic acid, citric acid, flavors, glycerin, polyethylene glycol, propylene glycol, sodium benzoate, sorbitol, sucrose, purified water, Red #33, Blue #1 and Red #40.

PEDIACARE NightRest Cough-Cold Liquid: Inactive ingredients: Benzoic acid, citric acid, flavors, glycerin, polyethylene glycol. proplene glycol, sodium benzoate, sorbitol, sucrose, purified water. Red #33, blue #1 and Red #40.

PEDIACARE Cough-Cold Chewable Tablets also contain the warning, "Phenylketonurics: contains phenylalanine 3 mg per tablet", and the inactive ingredient listing, "Inactive Ingredients: Aspartame, cellulose, citric acid, flavors, magnesium stearate, magnesium trisilicate, mannitol, starch and Red #7."

PEDIACARE Infants' Oral Decongestant Drops: "Inactive Ingredients: Benzoic acid, citric acid, flavors, glycerin, polyethylene glycol, propylene glycol, purified water, sodium benzoate, sorbitol, sucrose and Red #40."

OVERDOSAGE

Acute dextromethorphan overdose usually does not result in serious signs and symptoms unless massive amounts have been ingested. Signs and symptoms of a substantial overdose may include nausea and vomiting, visual disturbances, CNS disturbances, and urinary retention. Symptoms from pseudoephedrine overdose consist most often of mild anxiety, tachycardia and/or mild hypertension. Symptoms usually appear within 4 to 8 hours of ingestion and are transient, usually requiring no treatment. Chlorpheniramine toxicity should be treated as you would an antihistamine/anticholinergic overdose and is likely to be present within a few hours after acute ingestion.

HOW SUPPLIED

PEDIACARE Cough-Cold Liquid and NightRest Cough-Cold Liquid (colored red)—bottles of 4 fl. oz. with child-resistant safety cap and calibrated dosage cup. PEDIACARE Cold-Allergy Chewable Tablets (pink, scored)—blister packs of 16. PEDIACARE Cough-Cold Chewable Tablets (pink, scored)—blister packs of 16. PEDIACARE Infants' Drops (colored red)—bottles of ½ fl. oz with calibrated dropper.

Shown in Product Identification Section, page 417

PEDIA-PROFEN® ℞

Ibuprofen Suspension
100 mg/5 ml
SHAKE WELL BEFORE USE

DESCRIPTION

Pedia-Profen (ibuprofen suspension) contains ibuprofen which is (±)-2-(*p*-isobutylphenyl) propionic acid. Ibuprofen is a white powder with a melting point of 74°–77°C and is very slightly soluble in water (< 1 mg/mL) and readily soluble in organic solvents such as ethanol and acetone.

Ibuprofen's structural formula is:

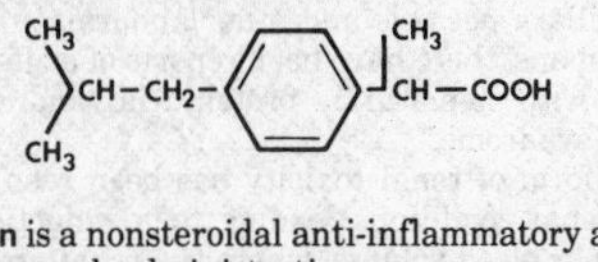

Pedia-Profen is a nonsteroidal anti-inflammatory agent. It is available for oral administration as a sucrose-sweetened, orange colored, berry/vanilla flavored liquid suspension containing 100 mg of ibuprofen per 5 mL. Inactive ingredients include citric acid, flavors, glycerin, polysorbate 80, sodium benzoate, starch, sucrose, purified water, xanthan gum, yellow #10, and red #40.

CLINICAL PHARMACOLOGY

Pedia-Profen is a nonsteroidal anti-inflammatory agent that possesses analgesic and antipyretic activities. Its mode of action, like that of other nonsteroidal anti-inflammatory agents, is not completely understood, but may be related to prostaglandin synthetase inhibition.

In clinical studies in *adult* patients with rheumatoid arthritis and osteoarthritis, ibuprofen has been shown to be comparable to aspirin in controlling pain and inflammation and to be associated with a statistically significant reduction in the milder gastrointestinal side effects (see ADVERSE REACTIONS).

Pedia-Profen may be well tolerated in some patients who have had gastrointestinal side effects with aspirin, but these patients, when treated with **Pedia-Profen,** should be carefully followed for signs and symptoms of gastrointestinal ulceration and bleeding.

Although it is not definitely known whether ibuprofen causes less peptic ulceration than aspirin, in one study involving 885 adult patients with rheumatoid arthritis treated for up to one year, there were no reports of gastric ulceration with ibuprofen whereas frank ulceration was reported in 13 patients in the aspirin group (statistically significant $p < .001$).

Gastroscopic studies at varying doses show an increased tendency toward gastric irritation at higher doses. However, at comparable doses, gastric irritation is approximately half that seen with aspirin. Studies using ^{51}Cr-tagged red cells indicate that fecal blood loss associated with ibuprofen in doses up to 2400 mg daily did not exceed the normal range, and was significantly less than that seen in aspirin-treated patients.

In clinical studies in patients with rheumatoid arthritis, ibuprofen has been shown to be comparable to indomethacin in controlling the signs and symptoms of disease activity and to be associated with a statistically significant reduction of the milder gastrointestinal (see ADVERSE REACTIONS), and CNS side effects.

Pedia-Profen may be used in combination with gold salts and/or corticosteroids.

Controlled studies in adults have demonstrated that ibuprofen is a more effective analgesic than propoxyphene for the relief of episiotomy pain, pain following dental extraction procedures, and for the relief of the symptoms of primary dysmenorrhea.

In patients with primary dysmenorrhea, ibuprofen has been shown to reduce elevated levels of prostaglandin activity in the menstrual fluid and to reduce resting and active intrauterine pressure, as well as the frequency of uterine contractions. The probable mechanism of action is to inhibit prostaglandin synthesis rather than simply to provide analgesia.

Controlled clinical trials comparing doses of 5 and 10 mg/kg ibuprofen and 10–15 mg/kg of acetaminophen have been conducted in children 6 months to 12 years of age with fever primarily due to viral illnesses. In these studies there were no differences between treatments in fever reduction for the first hour and maximum fever reduction occurred between 2 and 4 hours. Response after 1 hour was dependent on both the level of temperature elevation as well as the treatment. In children with baseline temperatures at or below 102.5°F both ibuprofen doses and acetaminophen were equally effective in their maximum effect. In those children with temperatures above 102.5°F, the ibuprofen 10 mg/kg dose was more effective. By 6 hours children treated with ibuprofen 5 mg/kg tended to have recurrence of fever, whereas children treated with ibuprofen 10 mg/ kg still had significant fever reduction at 8 hours. In control groups treated with 10 mg/kg acetaminophen, fever reduction resembled that seen in children treated with 5 mg/kg of ibuprofen, with the exception that temperature elevation tended to return 1–2 hours earlier.

Pharmacokinetics:

Ibuprofen is rapidly absorbed when administered orally. As is true with most tablet and suspension formulations, **Pedia-Profen** is absorbed somewhat faster than the tablet with a time to peak serum level generally within one hour. Peak serum ibuprofen levels are generally attained one to two hours after administration of ibuprofen tablets and within about 1 hour after the suspension. With single, *oral, solid* doses up to 800 mg *in adults,* a linear relationship exists between the amount of drug administered and the integrated area under the serum drug concentration vs. time curve. Above 800 mg, however, the area under the curve increase is less than proportional to the increase in dose. *There is no evidence of age dependent kinetics in patients 2 to 11 years old. With single doses of* **Pedia-Profen** *ranging up to 10 mg/kg, a dose response relationship exists between the amount of drug administered to febrile children and the serum concentration vs. time curve. There is also a correlation between reduction of fever and drug concentration over time, although the peak reduction in fever occurs 2–4 hours after dosing.*

No absorption differences are noticeable when ibuprofen tablets or suspension are given under fasting conditions or immediately before meals. When either product is taken with food, however, the peak levels are somewhat lower (up to 30%) and the time to reach peak levels is slightly prolonged (up to 30 min.) although the extent of absorption is unchanged.

A bioavailability study has shown that there was no interference with the absorption of ibuprofen when given in conjunction with an antacid containing both aluminum hydroxide and magnesium hydroxide.

Ibuprofen is rapidly metabolized and eliminated in the urine. The excretion of ibuprofen is virtually complete 24 hours after the last dose. The serum half-life of ibuprofen is 1.8 to 2.0 hours.

Studies have shown that following ingestion of the drug 45% to 79% of the dose was recovered in the urine within 24 hours as metabolite A(25%), (+)-2-4′-(2-hydroxy-2-methlypropyl)-phenylpropionic acid and metabolite B (37%), (+)-2-4′-(2-carboxypropyl) phenylpropionic acid; the percentages of free and conjugated ibuprofen were approximately 1% and 14%, respectively.

INDICATIONS AND USAGE

Pedia-Profen is indicated for relief of the signs and symptoms of rheumatoid arthritis and osteoarthritis.

Pedia-Profen is indicated for the relief of mild to moderate pain and of primary dysmenorrhea.

Pedia-Profen *is also indicated for the reduction of fever in patients aged 6 months and older.*

Since there have been no controlled trials to demonstrate whether there is any beneficial effect or harmful interaction with the use of ibuprofen in conjunction with aspirin, the combination cannot be recommended (see **Drug Interactions**).

CONTRAINDICATIONS

Pedia-Profen should not be used in patients who have previously exhibited hypersensitivity to ibuprofen, or in individuals with all or part of the syndrome of nasal polyps, angioedema and bronchospastic reactivity to aspirin or other non-

Continued on next page

McNeil Consumer—Cont.

steroidal anti-inflammatory agents. Anaphylactoid reactions have occurred in such patients.

WARNINGS

Risk of GI Ulceration, Bleeding and Perforation with NSAID Therapy. Serious gastrointestinal toxicity such as bleeding, ulceration, and perforation, can occur at any time, with or without warning symptoms, in patients treated chronically with NSAID therapy. Although minor upper gastrointestinal problems, such as dyspepsia, are common, usually developing early in therapy, physicians should remain alert for ulceration and bleeding in patients treated chronically with NSAID even in the absence of previous GI tract symptoms. In patients observed in clinical trials of several months to two years duration, symptomatic upper GI ulcers, gross bleeding or perforation appear to occur in approximately 1% of patients treated for 3–6 months, and in about 2–4% of patients treated for one year. Physicians should inform patients about the signs and/or symptoms of serious GI toxicity and what steps to take if they occur.

Studies to date have not identified any subset of patients not at risk of developing peptic ulceration and bleeding. Except for a prior history of serious GI events and other risk factors known to be associated with peptic ulcer disease, such as alcoholism, smoking, etc., no risk factors (e.g., age, sex) have been associated with increased risk. Elderly or debilitated patients seem to tolerate ulceration or bleeding less well than other individuals and most spontaneous reports of fatal GI events are in this population. Studies to date are inconclusive concerning the relative risk of various NSAIDs in causing such reactions. High doses of any NSAID probably carry a greater risk of these reactions, although controlled clinical trials showing this do not exist in most cases. In considering the use of relatively large doses (within the recommended dosage range), sufficient benefit should be anticipated to offset the potential increased risk of GI toxicity.

PRECAUTIONS

General:
Blurred and/or diminished vision, scotomata, and/or changes in color vision have been reported. If a patient develops such complaints while receiving **Pedia-Profen**, the drug should be discontinued and the patient should have an ophthalmologic examination which includes central visual fields and color vision testing.

Fluid retention and edema have been reported in association with ibuprofen, therefore, the drug should be used with caution in patients with a history of cardiac decompensation or hypertension.

Pedia-Profen, like other nonsteroidal anti-inflammatory agents, can inhibit platelet aggregation, but the effect is quantitatively less and of shorter duration than that seen with aspirin. Ibuprofen has been shown to prolong bleeding time (but within the normal range), in normal subjects. Because this prolonged bleeding effect may be exaggerated in patients with underlying hemostatic defects, **Pedia-Profen** should be used with caution in persons with intrinsic coagulation defects and those on anticoagulant therapy.

Patients on **Pedia-Profen** should report to their physicians signs or symptoms of gastrointestinal ulceration or bleeding, blurred vision or other eye symptoms, skin rash, weight gain, or edema.

In order to avoid exacerbation of disease of adrenal insufficiency, patients who have been on prolonged corticosteroid therapy should have their therapy tapered slowly rather than discontinued abruptly when ibuprofen is added to the treatment program.

The antipyretic and anti-inflammatory activity of **Pedia-Profen** may reduce fever and inflammation, thus diminishing their utility as diagnostic signs in detecting complications of presumed noninfectious, noninflammatory painful conditions.

Liver Effects:
As with other nonsteroidal anti-inflammatory drugs, borderline elevations of one or more liver function tests may occur in up to 15% of patients. These abnormalities may progress, may remain essentially unchanged, or may be transient with continued therapy. The SGPT (ALT) test is probably the most sensitive indicator of liver dysfunction. Meaningful (3 times the upper limit of normal), elevations of SGPT or SGOT (AST) occurred in controlled clinical trials in less than 1% of patients. A patient with symptoms and/or signs suggesting liver dysfunction, or in whom an abnormal liver test has occurred, should be evaluated for evidence of the development of more severe hepatic reactions while on therapy with **Pedia-Profen.** Severe hepatic reactions, including jaundice and cases of fatal hepatitis, have been reported with ibuprofen as with other nonsteroidal anti-inflammatory drugs. Although such reactions are rare, if abnormal liver tests persist or worsen, if clinical signs and symptoms consistent with liver disease develop, or if systemic manifestations occur (e.g. eosinophilia, rash, etc.), **Pedia-Profen** should be discontinued.

Hemoglobin Levels:
In cross-study comparisons with doses ranging from 1200 mg to 3200 mg daily for several weeks, a slight dose-response decrease in hemoglobin/hematocrit was noted. This has been observed with other nonsteroidal anti-inflammatory drugs; the mechanism is unknown. However, even with daily doses of 3200 mg, the total decrease in hemoglobin usually does not exceed 1 gram; if there are no signs of bleeding, it is probably not clinically important.

In two postmarketing clinical studies with ibuprofen the incidence of a decreased hemoglobin level was greater than previously reported. Decrease in hemoglobin of 1 gram or more was observed in 17.1% of 193 patients on 1600 mg ibuprofen daily (osteoarthritis), and in 22.8% of 189 patients taking 2400 mg of ibuprofen daily (rheumatoid arthritis). Positive stool occult blood tests and elevated serum creatinine levels were also observed in these studies.

Aseptic Meningitis:
Aseptic meningitis with fever and coma has been observed on rare occasions in patients on ibuprofen therapy. Although it is probably more likely to occur in patients with systemic lupus erythematosus and related connective tissue diseases, it has been reported in patients who do not have an underlying chronic disease. If signs or symptoms of meningitis develop in a patient on **Pedia-Profen,** the possibility of its being related to ibuprofen should be considered.

Renal Effects:
As with other nonsteroidal anti-inflammatory drugs, long-term administration of ibuprofen to animals has resulted in renal papillary necrosis and other abnormal renal pathology. In humans, there have been reports of acute interstitial nephritis with hematuria, proteinuria, and occasionally nephrotic syndrome.

A second form of renal toxicity has been seen in patients with prerenal conditions leading to a reduction in renal blood flow or blood volume, where the renal prostaglandins have a supportive role in the maintenance of renal perfusion. In these patients administration of a nonsteroidal anti-inflammatory drug may cause a dose dependent reduction in prostaglandin formation and may precipitate overt renal decompensation. Patients at greatest risk of this reaction are those with impaired renal function, heart failure, liver dysfunction, those taking diuretics and the elderly. Discontinuation of nonsteroidal anti-inflammatory drug therapy is typically followed by recovery to the pre-treatment state.

Those patients at high risk who chronically take ibuprofen should have renal function monitored if they have signs or symptoms which may be consistent with mild azotemia, such as malaise, fatigue, loss of appetite, etc. Occasional patients may develop some elevation of serum creatinine and BUN levels without signs or symptoms.

Since ibuprofen is eliminated primarily by the kidneys, patients with significantly impaired renal function should be closely monitored and a reduction in dosage should be anticipated to avoid drug accumulation. Prospective studies on the safety of ibuprofen in patients with chronic renal failure have not be conducted.

Information for Patients:
Pedia-Profen, like other drugs of its class, is not free of side effects. The side effects of these drugs can cause discomfort and, rarely, there are more serious side effects, such as gastrointestinal bleeding, which may result in hospitalization and even fatal outcomes.

NSAIDs (Nonsteroidal Anti-Inflammatory Drugs) are often essential agents in the management of arthritis and have a major role in the treatment of pain, but they also may be commonly employed for conditions which are less serious.

Physicians may wish to discuss with their patients the potential risks (see WARNINGS, PRECAUTIONS, and ADVERSE REACTIONS) and likely benefits of NSAID treatment, particularly when the drugs are used for less serious conditions where treatment without NSAIDs may represent an acceptable alternative to both the patient and physician.

Pedia-Profen Ibuprofen Suspension contains 1.5 grams sucrose and 8 calories per teaspoon which should be taken into consideration when treating patients with impaired glucose tolerance.

LaboratoryTests:
Because serious GI tract ulceration and bleeding can occur without warning symptoms, physicians should follow chronically treated patients for the signs and symptoms of ulceration and bleeding and should inform them of the importance of this follow-up (see WARNINGS).

Drug Interactions:
Coumarin-type anti-coagulants. Several short-term controlled studies failed to show that ibuprofen significantly affected prothrombin times or a variety of other clotting factors administered to individuals on coumarin-type anticoagulants. However, because bleeding has been reported when ibuprofen and other nonsteroidal anti-inflammatory agents have been administered to patients on coumarin-type anti-coagulants, the physician should be cautious when administering **Pedia-Profen** to patients on anti-coagulants.

Aspirin: Animal studies show that aspirin given with nonsteroidal anti-inflammatory agents, including ibuprofen, yields a net decrease in anti-inflammatory activity with lowered blood levels of the non-aspirin drug. Single dose bioavailability studies in normal volunteers have failed to show an effect of aspirin on ibuprofen blood levels. Correlative clinical studies have not been done.

Methotrexate: Ibuprofen, as well as other nonsteroidal anti-inflammatory drugs, has been reported to competitively inhibit methotrexate accumulation in rabbit kidney slices. This may indicate that ibuprofen could enhance the toxicity of methotrexate. Caution should be used if **Pedia-Profen** is administered concomitantly with methotrexate.

H-2 Antagonists: In studies with human volunteers, coadministration of cimetidine or ranitidine with ibuprofen had no substantive effect on ibuprofen serum concentration.

Furosemide: Clinical studies, as well as random observations, have shown that ibuprofen can reduce the natriuretic effect of furosemide and thiazides in some patients. This response has been attributed to inhibition of renal prostaglandin synthesis. During concomitant therapy with **Pedia-Profen,** the patient should be observed closely for signs of renal failure (see PRECAUTIONS, Renal Effects), as well as to assure diuretic efficacy.

Lithium: Ibuprofen produced an elevation of plasma lithium levels and a reduction in renal lithium clearance in a study of eleven normal volunteers. The mean minimum lithium concentration increased 15% and the renal clearance of lithium was decreased by 19% during this period of concomitant drug administration.

This effect has been attributed to inhibition of renal prostaglandin synthesis by ibuprofen. Thus, when **Pedia-Profen** and lithium are administered concurrently, subjects should be observed carefully for signs of lithium toxicity. (Read circulars for lithium preparation before use of such concurrent therapy).

Pregnancy:
Reproductive studies conducted in rats and rabbits at doses somewhat less than the maximal clinical dose did not demonstrate evidence of developmental abnormalities. However, animal reproduction studies are not always predictive of human response. As there are no adequate and well-controlled studies in pregnant women, this drug should be used during pregnancy only if clearly needed. Because of the known effects of nonsteroidal anti-inflammatory drugs on the fetal cardiovascular system (closure of ductus arteriosus), use during late pregnancy should be avoided. As with other drugs known to inhibit prostaglandin synthesis, an increased incidence of dystocia and delayed parturition occurred in rats. Administration of **Pedia-Profen** is not recommended during pregnancy.

Nursing Mothers:
In limited studies, an assay capable of detecting 1 mcg/mL did not demonstrate ibuprofen in the milk of lactating mothers. However, because of the limited nature of the studies and the possible adverse effects of prostaglandin inhibiting drugs on neonates, **Pedia-Profen** is not recommended for use in nursing mothers.

Infants:
Safety and efficacy of **Pedia-Profen** *in children below the age of 6 months has not been established.*

ADVERSE REACTIONS

The most frequent type of adverse reaction occurring with ibuprofen is gastrointestinal. In controlled clinical trials, the percentage of adult patients reporting one or more gastrointestinal complaints ranged from 4% to 16%.

In controlled studies in adults when ibuprofen was compared to aspirin and indomethacin in equally effective doses, the overall incidence of gastrointestinal complaints was about half that seen in either the aspirin- or indomethacin-treated patients.

Adverse reactions observed during controlled clinical trials in adults at an incidence greater than 1% are listed in the chart. Those reactions listed under the heading, Incidence Greater than 1% (but less than 3%) Probable Causal Relationship, encompass observations in approximately 3,000 patients. More than 500 of these patients were treated for periods of at least 54 weeks.

Still other reactions occurring less frequently than 1 in 100 were reported in controlled clinical trials and from marketing experience. These reactions have been divided into two categories: Precise Incidence Unknown (but less than 1%) Probable Causal Relationship, lists reactions with ibuprofen therapy where the probability of causal relationship exists; Precise Incidence Unknown (but less than 1%) Causal Relationship Unknown, lists reactions with ibuprofen therapy where a causal relationship has not been established.

Reported side effects were higher at doses of 3200 mg/day than at doses of 2400 mg or less per day in clinical trials of patients with rheumatoid arthritis. The increases in incidence were slight and still within the ranges reported in the following paragraphs. [See top of next page.]

OVERDOSAGE

Approximately 1½ hours after the reported ingestion of from 7 to 10 ibuprofen tablets (400 mg), a 19-month old child weighing 12 kg was seen in the hospital emergency room,

Incidence Greater than 1%
(but less than 3%)
Probable Causal Relationship

GASTROINTESTINAL: Nausea*, epigastric pain*, heartburn*, diarrhea, abdominal distress, nausea and vomiting, indigestion, constipation, abdominal cramps or pain, fullness of GI tract (bloating and flatulence).
CENTRAL NERVOUS SYSTEM: Dizziness*, headache, nervousness.
DERMATOLOGIC: Rash* (including maculopapular type), pruritus.
SPECIAL SENSES: Tinnitus.
METABOLIC/ENDOCRINE: Decreased appetitie.
CARDIOVASCULAR: Edema, fluid retention (generally responds promptly to drug discontinuation) (see PRECAUTIONS).

Precise Incidence Unknown
(but less than 1%)
Probable Causal Relationship**

GASTROINTESTINAL: Gastric or duodenal ulcer with bleeding and/or perforation, gastrointestinal hemorrhage, pancreatitis, melena, gastritis, hepatitis, jaundice, abnormal liver function tests.
CENTRAL NERVOUS SYSTEM: Depression, insomnia, confusion, emotional lability, somnolence, aseptic meningitis with fever and coma (see PRECAUTIONS).
DERMATOLOGIC: Vesiculobullous eruptions, urticaria, erythema multiforme, Stevens-Johnson syndrome, alopecia.
SPECIAL SENSES: Hearing loss, amblyopia (blurred and/or diminished vision, scotomata and/or changes in color vision) (see PRECAUTIONS).
HEMATOLOGIC: Neutropenia, agranulocytosis, aplastic anemia, hemolytic anemia (sometimes Coombs positive), thrombocytopenia with or without purpura, eosinophilia, decrease in hemoglobin and hematocrit (see PRECAUTIONS).
CARDIOVASCULAR: Congestive heart failure in patients with marginal cardiac function, elevated blood pressure, palpitations.
ALLERGIC: Syndrome of abdominal pain, fever, chills, nausea and vomiting, anaphylaxis, bronchospasm (see CONTRAINDICATIONS).
RENAL: Acute renal failure in patients with pre-existing significantly impaired renal function (see PRECAUTIONS), decreased creatinine clearance, polyuria, azotemia, cystitis, hematuria.
MISCELLANEOUS: Dry eyes and mouth, gingival ulcer, rhinitis.

Precise Incidence Unknown
(but less than 1%)
Causal Relationship Unknown**

CENTRAL NERVOUS SYSTEM: Paresthesias, hallucinations, dream abnormalities, pseudo-tumor cerebri.
DERMATOLOGIC: Toxic epidermal necrolysis, photoallergic skin reactions.
SPECIAL SENSES: Conjunctivitis, diplopia, optic neuritis, cataracts.
HEMATOLOGIC: Bleeding episodes (e.g. epistaxis, menorrhagia).
METABOLIC/ENDOCRINE: Gynecomastia, hypoglycemic reaction, acidosis.
CARDIOVASCULAR: Arrhythmias (sinus tachycardia, sinus bradycardia).
ALLERGIC: Serum sickness, lupus erythematosus syndrome, Henoch-Schönlein vasculitis, angioedema.
RENAL: Renal papillary necrosis.

*Reactions occurring in 3% to 9% of patients treated with ibuprofen. (Those reactions occurring in less than 3% of the patients are unmarked).

**Reactions are classified under "Probable Causal Relationship (PCR)", if there has been one positive rechallenge or if three or more cases occur which might be causally related. Reactions are classified under "Causal Relationship Unknown", if seven or more events have been reported but the criteria for PCR have not been met.

apneic and cyanotic, responding only to painful stimuli. This type of stimulus, however, was sufficient to induce respiration. Oxygen and parenteral fluids were given, a greenish-yellow fluid was aspirated from the stomach with no evidence to indicate the presence of ibuprofen. Two hours after ingestion the child's condition seemed stable, she still responded only to painful stimuli and continued to have periods of apnea lasting from 5 to 10 seconds. She was admitted to intensive care and sodium bicarbonate was administered as well as infusions of dextrose and normal saline. By four hours post-ingestion she could be aroused easily, sit by herself and respond to spoken commands. Blood level of ibuprofen was 102.9 mcg/mL approximately 8½ hours after accidental ingestion. At 12 hours she appeared to be completely recovered.

In two other reported cases where children (each weighing approximately 10 kg) accidentally, acutely ingested approximately 120 mg/kg, there were no signs of acute intoxication or late sequelae. Blood level in one child 90 minutes after ingestion was 700 mcg/mL, about 10 times the peak levels seen in absorption-excretion studies.

A 19-year old male who had taken 8,000 mg of ibuprofen over a period of a few hours complained of dizziness, and nystagmus was noted. After hospitalization, parental hydration and three days bed rest, he recovered with no reported sequelae.

In cases of acute overdosage, the stomach should be emptied by vomiting or lavage, though little drug will likely be recovered if more than an hour has elapsed since ingestion. Because the drug is acidic and is excreted in the urine, it is theoretically beneficial to administer alkali and induce diuresis. In addition to supportive measures, the use of oral activated charcoal may help reduce the absorption and reabsorption of ibuprofen.

DOSAGE AND ADMINISTRATION

Shake well prior to administration.

Do not exceed 3200 mg total daily dose. If gastrointestinal complaints occur, administer ibuprofen with meals or milk.

Rheumatoid arthritis and osteoarthritis, including flare-ups of chronic disease: Suggested *Adult* Dosage; 1200–3200 mg daily (300 mg q.i.d. or 400 mg, 600 mg or 800 mg t.i.d. or q.i.d.). Individual patients may show a better response to 3200 mg daily, as compared with 2400 mg, although in well-controlled clinical trials patients on 3200 mg did not show a better mean response in terms of efficacy. Therefore, when treating patients with 3200 mg/day, the physician should observe sufficient increased clinical benefits to offset potential increased risk.

The dose of **Pedia-Profen** should be tailored to each patient, and may be lowered or raised from the suggested doses depending on the severity of symptoms either at time of initiating drug therapy or as the patient responds or fails to respond.

In general, patients with rheumatoid arthritis seem to require higher doses of ibuprofen than do patients with osteoarthritis.

The smallest dose of **Pedia-Profen** that yield acceptable control should be employed. A linear blood level dose-response relationship exists with single doses up to 800 mg (See CLINICAL PHARAMCOLOGY, Pharmacokinetics for effects of food on rate of absorption).

In chronic conditions, a therapeutic response to ibuprofen therapy is sometimes seen in a few days to a week but most often is observed by two weeks. After a satisfactory response has been achieved, the patient's dose should be reviewed and adjusted as required.

Mild to moderate pain: 400 mg every 4 to 6 hours as necessary for the relief of pain in adults.

In controlled analgesic clinical trials, doses of ibuprofen greater than 400 mg were no more effective than a 400 mg dose.

Dysmenorrhea: For the treatment of dysmenorrhea, beginning with the earliest onset of such pain, **Pedia-Profen** should be given in a dose of 400 mg every 4 hours as necessary for the relief of pain.

FEVER REDUCTION IN CHILDREN 6 months to 12 years of age: Dosage should be adjusted on the basis of the initial temperature level (See CLINICAL PHARMACOLOGY for a description of the controlled clinical trial results). The recommended dose is 5 mg/kg if the baseline temperature is less than 102.5°F or 10 mg/kg if the baseline temperature is greater than 102.5°F. The duration of fever reduction is generally 6–8 hours and is longer with the higher dose. The recommended maximum daily dose is 40 mg/kg.

HOW SUPPLIED

Pedia-Profen Ibuprofen Suspension 100 mg/5 ml (teaspoon)—
orange, berry/vanilla flavored
Bottles of 4 oz (120 ml)NDC 0045-0469-04
Bottles of 16 oz (480 ml)NDC 0045-0469-16
SHAKE WELL BEFORE USING.
Store at room temperature.

Caution: Federal law prohibits dispensing without prescription.

Shown in Product Identification Section, page 417

MAXIMUM STRENGTH SINE-AID® OTC

Sinus Headache Gelcaps, Caplets and Tablets

DESCRIPTION

Each MAXIMUM STRENGTH SINE-AID® Gelcap, Caplet or Tablet contains acetaminophen 500 mg and pseudoephedrine hydrochloride 30 mg.

ACTIONS

MAXIMUM STRENGTH SINE-AID® Gelcaps, Caplets and Tablets contain a clinically proven analgesic-antipyretic and a decongestant. Maximum allowable non-prescription levels of acetaminophen and pseudophedrine provide temporary relief of sinus congestion and pain. Acetaminophen is equal to aspirin in analgesic and antipyretic effectiveness and it is unlikely to produce many of the side effects associated with aspirin and aspirin-containing products. Acetaminophen produces analgesia by elevation of the pain threshold and antipyresis through action on the hypothalamic heat-regulating center. Pseudoephedrine hydrochloride is a sympathomimetic amine that promotes sinus cavity drainage by reducing nasopharyngeal mucosal congestion.

INDICATIONS

MAXIMUM STRENGTH SINE-AID® Gelcaps, Caplets and Tablets provide effective symptomatic relief from sinus headache pain and congestion. SINE-AID® is particularly well-suited in patients with aspirin allergy, hemostatic disturbances (including anticoagulant therapy), and bleeding diatheses (e.g. hemophilia) and upper gastrointestinal disease (e.g. ulcer, gastritis, hiatus hernia).

PRECAUTIONS

If a rare sensitivity occurs, the drug should be discontinued. Although pseudoephedrine is virtually without pressor effect in normotensive patients, it should be used with caution in hypertensives.

USUAL DOSAGE

Adult dosage: Two gelcaps, caplets or tablets every four to six hours. Do not exceed eight gelcaps, caplets or tablets in any 24 hour period. **Warning:** Do not administer to children under 12 or exceed the recommended dosage because at higher doses nervousness, dizziness or sleeplessness may occur. Do not take this product for more than 7 days. If symptoms do not improve or are accompanied by a fever, consult a physician. Do not take this product if you have heart disease, high blood pressure, thyroid disease, diabetes or difficulty in urination due to enlargement of the prostate gland unless directed by a doctor.

Drug Interaction Precaution: Do not take this product if you are presently taking a prescription drug for high blood pressure or depression without first consulting your doctor. **Do not use if carton is open or if blister unit is broken, or if printed neck wrap or printed foil inner seal is broken. Keep this and all medication out of the reach of children. As with any drug, if you are pregnant or nursing a baby, seek the advice of a health professional before using this product. In case of accidental overdosage, contact a physician or poison control center immediately.**

OVERDOSAGE

Acetaminophen in massive overdosage may cause hepatic toxicity in some patients. In adults and adolescents, hepatic toxicity has rarely been reported following ingestion of acute overdoses of less than 10 grams. Fatalities are infrequent (less than 3–4% of untreated cases) and have rarely been reported with overdoses of less than 15 grams. In children, an acute overdosage of less than 150 mg/kg has not been associated with hepatic toxicity.

Early symptoms following a potentially hepatotoxic overdose may include: nausea, vomiting, diaphoresis and general malaise. Clinical and laboratory evidence of hepatic toxicity may not be apparent until 48 to 72 hours postingestion.

In adults and adolescents, regardless of the quantity of acetaminophen reported to have been ingested, administer MUCOMYST® acetylcysteine immediately if 24 hours or less have elapsed from the reported time of ingestion. For full prescribing information, refer to the MUCOMYST package insert. Do not await results of assays for acetaminophen level before initiating treatment with MUCOMYST acetylcysteine. The following additional procedures are recommended: The stomach should be emptied promptly by lavage or by induction of emesis with syrup of ipecac. A serum acetaminophen assay should be obtained as early as possible, but no sooner than four hours following ingestion. Liver function studies should be obtained initially and repeated at 24-hour intervals.

Serious toxicity or fatalities are extremely infrequent in children, possibly due to differences in the way they metabolize acetaminophen. In children, the maximum potential amount ingested can be more easily estimated. If more than 150 mg/kg or an unknown amount was ingested, obtain an acetaminophen plasma level. The acetaminophen plasma level should be obtained as soon as possible, but no sooner than 4 hours following the ingestion. Induce emesis using syrup of ipecac. If the plasma level is obtained and falls above the broken line on the acetaminophen overdose nomogram, the MUCOMYST acetylcysteine therapy should be initiated and continued for a full course of therapy. If acetaminophen plasma assay capability is not available, and the estimated acetaminophen ingestion exceeds 150 mg/kg, MUCOMYST acetylcysteine therapy should be initiated and continued for a full course of therapy.

For additional emergency information, call your regional poison center or call the Rocky Mountain Poison Center toll-free, (1-800-525-6115).

Symptoms from pseudoephedrine overdose consist most often of mild anxiety, tachycardia and/or mild hypertension. Symptoms usually appear within 4 to 8 hours of ingestion and are transient, usually requiring no treatment.

Continued on next page

McNeil Consumer—Cont.

INACTIVE INGREDIENTS

Gelcaps: Benzyl Alcohol, Butylparaben, Castor Oil, Cellulose, Corn Starch, Edetate Calcium Disodium, Gelatin, Hydroxypropyl Methylcellulose, Iron Oxide Black, Magnesium Stearate, Methylparaben, Propylparaben, Sodium Lauryl Sulfate, Sodium Propionate, Sodium Starch Glycolate, Titanium Dioxide, FD&C Red #40.
Caplets: Cellulose, Corn Starch, Hydroxypropyl Methylcellulose, Magnesium Stearate, Polyethylene Glycol, Sodium Starch Glycolate, Titanium Dioxide, Blue #1 and Red #40.
Tablets: Cellulose, Corn Starch, Magnesium Stearate and Sodium Starch Glycolate.

HOW SUPPLIED

Gelcaps (colored red and white imprinted "SINE-AID")—blister package of 20 and tamper resistant bottle of 40.
Caplets (colored white imprinted "Maximum SINE-AID")—blister package of 24 and tamper resistant bottle of 50.
Tablets (colored white embossed "Sine-Aid")—blister package of 24 and tamper resistant bottle of 50.
Shown in Product Identification Section, page 418

CHILDREN'S TYLENOL®   OTC
acetaminophen
Chewable Tablets, Elixir, Drops
Suspension Liquid, Drops

DESCRIPTION

Infants' TYLENOL acetaminophen Drops are stable, alcohol-free, fruit-flavored and orange in color. Infants' TYLENOL Suspension Drops are alcohol-free, grape-flavored and purple in color. Each 0.8 ml (one calibrated dropperful) contains 80 mg acetaminophen. Children's TYLENOL Elixir is stable and alcohol-free, cherry-flavored, and red in color or grape-flavored, and purple in color. Children's TYLENOL Suspension Liquid is alcohol-free, cherry-flavored and red in color. Each 5 ml contains 160 mg acetaminophen. Each Children's TYLENOL Chewable Tablet contains 80 mg acetaminophen in a grape- or fruit-flavored tablet.

ACTIONS

Acetaminophen is a clinically proven analgesic/antipyretic. Acetaminophen produces analgesia by elevation of the pain threshold and antipyresis through action on the hypothalamic heat regulating center. Acetaminophen is equal to aspirin in analgesic and antipyretic effectiveness and it is unlikely to produce many of the side effects associated with aspirin and aspirin containing products.

INDICATIONS

Children's TYLENOL Chewable Tablets, Elixir, Drops, Suspension Liquid and Suspension Drops are designed for treatment of infants and children with conditions requiring temporary relief of fever and discomfort due to colds and "flu," and of simple pain and discomfort due to teething, immunizations and tonsillectomy.

PRECAUTIONS

If a rare sensitivity reaction occurs, the drug should be stopped.

USUAL DOSAGE

All dosages may be repeated every 4 hours, but not more than 5 times daily. Administer to children under 2 years only on the advice of a physician. Children's TYLENOL Chewable Tablets: 2–3 years: two tablets. 4–5 years: three tablets, 6–8 years: four tablets. 9–10 years: five tablets. 11–12 years: six tablets.
Children's TYLENOL Elixir and Suspension Liquid: (special cup for measuring dosage is provided) 4–11 months: one-half teaspoon. 12–23 months: three-quarters teaspoon, 2–3 years: one teaspoon. 4–5 years: one and one-half teaspoons. 6–8 years: 2 teaspoons. 9–10 years: two and one-half teaspoons. 11–12 years: three teaspoons.
Infants' TYLENOL Drops and Suspension Drops: 0–3 months: 0.4 ml. 4–11 months: 0.8 ml. 12–23 months: 1.2 ml. 2–3 years: 1.6 ml. 4–5 years: 2.4 ml.
Warning: Keep this and all medication out of reach of children. In case of accidental overdose, contact a physician or poison control center immediately. Consult your physician if fever persists for more than 3 days or if pain continues for more than 5 days. Store at room temperature.
NOTE: In addition to the above:
Children's TYLENOL Drops and Suspension Drops—Do not use if printed carton overwrap or printed plastic bottle wrap is broken or missing or if carton is opened.
Children's TYLENOL Elixir and Suspension Liquid—Do not use if printed carton overwrap is broken or missing or if carton is opened. Do not use if printed plastic bottle wrap or printed foil inner seal is broken. Not a USP elixir.
Children's TYLENOL Chewables—Do not use if carton is opened or if printed plastic bottle wrap or printed foil inner

seal is broken. Phenylketonurics: contains phenylalanine 3mg per tablet.

OVERDOSAGE

Acetaminophen in massive overdosage may cause hepatic toxicity in some patients. In adults and adolescents, hepatic toxicity has rarely been reported following ingestion of acute overdoses of less than 10 grams. Fatalities are infrequent (less than 3–4% of untreated cases) and have rarely been reported with overdoses of less than 15 grams. In children, an acute overdosage of less than 150 mg/kg has not been associated with hepatic toxicity.
Early symptoms following a potentially hepatotoxic overdose may include: nausea, vomiting, diaphoresis and general malaise. Clinical and laboratory evidence of hepatic toxicity may not be apparent until 48 to 72 hours postingestion.
In adults and adolescents, regardless of the quantity of acetaminophen reported to have been ingested, administer MUCOMYST® acetylcysteine immediately if 24 hours or less have elapsed from the reported time of ingestion. For full prescribing information, refer to the MUCOMYST package insert. Do not await results of assays for acetaminophen level before initiating treatment with MUCOMYST acetylcysteine. The following additional procedures are recommended: The stomach should be emptied promptly by lavage or by induction of emesis with syrup of ipecac. A serum acetaminophen assay should be obtained as early as possible, but no sooner than four hours following ingestion. Liver function studies should be obtained initially and repeated at 24-hour intervals.
Serious toxicity or fatalities are extremely infrequent in children, possibly due to differences in the way they metabolize acetaminophen. In children, the maximum potential amount ingested can be more easily estimated. If more than 150 mg/kg or an unknown amount was ingested, obtain an acetaminophen plasma level. The acetaminophen plasma level should be obtained as soon as possible, but no sooner than 4 hours following the ingestion. Induce emesis using syrup of ipecac. If the plasma level is obtained and falls above the broken line on the acetaminophen overdose nomogram, the MUCOMYST acetylcysteine therapy should be initiated and continued for a full course of therapy. If acetaminophen plasma assay capability is not available, and the estimated acetaminophen ingestion exceeds 150 mg/kg, MUCOMYST acetylcysteine therapy should be initiated and continued for a full course of therapy.
For additional emergency information, call your regional poison center or call the Rocky Mountain Poison Center toll free, (1-800-525-6115).

INACTIVE INGREDIENTS

Children's TYLENOL Chewable Tablets—Aspartame, Cellulose, Citric Acid, Ethylcellulose, Flavors, Hydroxypropyl Methylcellulose, Mannitol, Starch, Magnesium Stearate, Red #7 and Blue #1 (Grape only).
Children's TYLENOL Elixir—Benzoic Acid, Citric Acid, Flavors, Glycerin, Polyethylene Glycol, Propylene Glycol, Sodium Benzoate, Sorbitol, Sucrose, Purified Water, Red #40. In addition to the above ingredients cherry flavored elixir contains Red #33 and grape flavored elixir contains malic acid and Blue #1.
Children's TYLENOL Suspension Liquid—Butylparaben, Cellulose, Citric Acid, Corn Syrup, Flavors, Glycerin, Purified Water, Sodium Benzoate, Sorbitol, Xanthan Gum, FD&C Red #40.
Infant's TYLENOL Drops—Butylparaben, Citric Acid, Glycerin, Polyethylene Glycol, Propylene Glycol, Saccharin, Sodium Citrate, purified water and yellow #6.
Infant's TYLENOL Suspension Drops—Butylparaben, Cellulose, Citric Acid, Corn Syrup, Flavors, Glycerin, Purified Water, Sodium Benzoate, Sorbitol, Xanthan Gum, FD&C Red #33 and FD&C Blue #1.

HOW SUPPLIED

Chewable Tablets (pink colored fruit, purple colored grape, scored, imprinted "TYLENOL")—Bottles of 30 and child resistant blister packs of 48 (fruit only). Elixir (cherry colored red and grape colored purple) Suspension liquid (cherry flavored colored red)—bottles of 2 and 4 fl. oz. Drops (colored orange)— bottles of ½ oz. (15 ml.) and 1 oz. (30 ml.) with calibrated plastic dropper. Suspension drops (grape flavored colored purple)—bottles of ½ oz (15 ml) with calibrated plastic dropper.
All packages listed above have child-resistant safety caps.
Shown in Product Identification Section, page 418

Junior Strength TYLENOL®   OTC
acetaminophen
Coated Caplets and Chewable Tablets

DESCRIPTION

Each Junior Strength Caplet or Chewable tablet contains 160 mg acetaminophen in a small, coated, capsule shaped tablet or grape or fruit chewable tablet.

ACTIONS

Acetaminophen is a clinically proven analgesic/antipyretic. Acetaminophen produces analgesia by elevation of the pain threshold and antipyresis through action on the hypothalamic heat-regulating center. Acetaminophen is equal to aspirin in analgesic and antipyretic effectiveness and it is unlikely to produce many of the side effects associated with aspirin and aspirin-containing products.

INDICATIONS

Junior Strength TYLENOL Caplets are designed for easy swallowability in older children and young adults. Both Junior Strength TYLENOL Caplets and Junior Strength Chewable Tablets provide fast, effective temporary relief of fever and discomfort due to colds and "flu," and pain and discomfort due to simple headaches, minor muscle aches, sprains and overexertion.

PRECAUTIONS

If a rare sensitivity reaction occurs, the drug should be stopped.

USUAL DOSAGE

Caplets should be taken with liquid. Chewable tablets should be well chewed. All dosages may be repeated every 4 hours, but not more than 5 times daily. For ages: 6–8 years: two Caplets or tablets, 9–10 years: two and one-half Caplets or tablets, 11 years: three Caplets or tablets, 12 years: four Caplets or tablets.
Warning: Do not use if carton is opened or if a blister unit is broken. Keep this and all medications out of the reach of children. In case of accidental overdosage, contact a physician or poison control center immediately. Consult your physician if fever persists for more than three days or if pain continues for more than five days. As with any drug, if you are pregnant or nursing a baby, seek the advice of a health professional before using this product. In addition the caplet package states: Not for children who have difficulty swallowing tablets. In addition the chewable tablet package states: Phenylketonurics: contains phenylalanine 5 mg per tablet.

OVERDOSAGE

Acetaminophen in massive overdosage may cause hepatic toxicity in some patients. In adults and adolescents, hepatic toxicity has rarely been reported following ingestion of acute overdosage of less than 10 grams. Fatalities are infrequent (less than 3–4% of untreated cases) and have rarely been reported with overdoses of less than 15 grams. In children, an acute overdosage of less than 150 mg/kg has not been associated with hepatic toxicity.
Early symptoms following a potentially hepatotoxic overdose may include: nausea, vomiting, diaphoresis and general malaise. Clinical and laboratory evidence of hepatic toxicity may not be apparent until 48 to 72 hours postingestion.
In adults and adolescents, regardless of the quantity of acetaminophen reported to have been ingested, administer MUCOMYST® acetylcysteine immediately if 24 hours or less have elapsed from the reported time of ingestion. For full prescribing information, refer to the MUCOMYST package insert. Do not await the results of assays for acetaminophen level before initiating treatment with MUCOMYST acetylcysteine. The following additional procedures are recommended: The stomach should be emptied promptly by lavage or by induction of emesis with syrup of ipecac. A serum acetaminophen assay should be obtained as early as possible, but no sooner than four hours following ingestion. Liver function studies should be obtained initially and repeated at 24-hour intervals.
Serious toxicity or fatalities are extremely infrequent in children, possibly due to differences in the way they metabolize acetaminophen. In children, the maximum potential amount ingested can be more easily estimated. If more than 150 mg/kg or an unknown amount was ingested, obtain an acetaminophen plasma level. The acetaminophen plasma level should be obtained as soon as possible, but no sooner than 4 hours following the ingestion. Induce emesis using syrup of ipecac. If the plasma level is obtained and falls above the broken line on the acetaminophen overdose nomogram, the MUCOMYST acetylcysteine therapy should be initiated and continued for a full course of therapy. If acetaminophen plasma assay capability is not available, and the estimated acetaminophen ingestion exceeds 150 mg/kg, MUCOMYST acetylcysteine therapy should be initiated and continued for a full course of therapy.
For additional emergency information, call your regional poison center or call the Rocky Mountain Poison Center toll-free (1-800-525-6115).

INACTIVE INGREDIENTS

Caplets: Cellulose, Ethylcellulose, Magnesium Stearate, Sodium Lauryl Sulfate, Sodium Starch Glycolate, Starch.
Tablets: Aspartame, Cellulose, Citric Acid, Ethylcellulose, Flavors, Magnesium Stearate, Mannitol, Starch, Blue #1 and Red #7.

HOW SUPPLIED

Coated Caplets, (colored white, coated, scored, imprinted "TYLENOL 160") Package of 30.

Chewable tablets (colored purple or pink, imprinted "TYLENOL 160") Package of 24. All packages are safety sealed and use child resistant blister packaging.

Shown in Product Identification Section, page 418

Regular Strength
TYLENOL® acetaminophen Tablets and Caplets **OTC**

DESCRIPTION
Each Regular Strength TYLENOL Tablet or Caplet contains acetaminophen 325 mg.

ACTIONS
Acetaminophen is a clinically proven analgesic and antipyretic. Acetaminophen produces analgesia by elevation of the pain threshold and antipyresis through action on the hypothalamic heat-regulating center. Acetaminophen is equal to aspirin in analgesic and antipyretic effectiveness and it is unlikely to produce many of the side effects associated with aspirin and aspirin-containing products.

INDICATIONS
Acetaminophen acts safely and quickly to provide temporary relief from: simple headache; minor muscular aches; the minor aches and pains associated with bursitis, neuralgia, sprains, overexertion, menstrual cramps; and from the discomfort of fever due to colds and "flu". Also for temporary relief of minor aches and pains of arthritis and rheumatism.

PRECAUTIONS
If a rare sensitivity reaction occurs, the drug should be discontinued.

USUAL DOSAGE
Adults and Children 12 years of Age and Older: 1 to 2 tablets 3 or 4 times daily. Children (6-12): ½to 1 tablet 3 or 4 times daily. Consult a physician for use by children under 6.

WARNING: DO NOT USE IF PRINTED RED NECK WRAP IS BROKEN OR MISSING. DO NOT TAKE FOR PAIN FOR MORE THAN 10 DAYS OR FOR FEVER FOR MORE THAN 3 DAYS UNLESS DIRECTED BY A PHYSICIAN. SEVERE OR RECURRENT PAIN OR HIGH OR CONTINUED FEVER MAY BE INDICATIVE OF SERIOUS ILLNESS. UNDER THESE CONDITIONS, CONSULT A PHYSICIAN. KEEP THIS AND ALL MEDICATION OUT OF THE REACH OF CHILDREN. AS WITH ANY DRUG, IF YOU ARE PREGNANT OR NURSING A BABY, SEEK THE ADVICE OF A HEALTH PROFESSIONAL BEFORE USING THIS PRODUCT. IN THE CASE OF ACCIDENTAL OVERDOSAGE, CONTACT A PHYSICIAN OR POISON CONTROL CENTER IMMEDIATELY.

OVERDOSAGE
Acetaminophen in massive overdosage may cause hepatic toxicity in some patients. In adults and adolescents, hepatic toxicity has rarely been reported following ingestion of acute overdoses of less than 10 grams. Fatalities are infrequent (less than 3–4% of untreated cases) and have rarely been reported with overdoses of less than 15 grams. In children, an acute overdosage of less than 150 mg/kg has not been associated with hepatic toxicity.

Early symptoms following a potentially hepatotoxic overdose may include: nausea, vomiting, diaphoresis and general malaise. Clinical and laboratory evidence of hepatic toxicity may not be apparent until 48 to 72 hours postingestion.

In adults and adolescents, regardless of the quantity of acetaminophen reported to have been ingested, administer MUCOMYST® acetylcysteine immediately if 24 hours or less have elapsed from the reported time of ingestion. For full prescribing information, refer to the MUCOMYST package insert. Do not await results of assays for acetaminophen level before initiating treatment with MUCOMYST acetylcysteine. The following additional procedures are recommended: The stomach should be emptied promptly by lavage or by induction of emesis with syrup of ipecac. A serum acetaminophen assay should be obtained as early as possible, but no sooner than four hours following ingestion. Liver function studies should be obtained initially and repeated at 24-hour intervals.

Serious toxicity or fatalities are extremely infrequent in children, possibly due to differences in the way they metabolize acetaminophen. In children, the maximum potential amount ingested can be more easily estimated. If more than 150 mg/kg or an unknown amount was ingested, obtain an acetaminophen plasma level. The acetaminophen plasma level should be obtained as soon as possible, but no sooner than 4 hours following the ingestion. Induce emesis using syrup of ipecac. If the plasma level is obtained and falls above the broken line on the acetaminophen overdose nomogram, the MUCOMYST acetylcysteine therapy should be initiated and continued for a full course of therapy. If acetaminophen plasma assay capability is not available, and the estimated acetaminophen ingestion exceeds 150 mg/kg, MUCOMYST acetylcysteine therapy should be initiated and continued for a full course of therapy.

For additional emergency information, call your regional poison center or call the Rocky Mountain Poison Center toll-free (1-800-525-6115).

INACTIVE INGREDIENTS
Tablets—Magnesium Stearate, Cellulose, Sodium Starch Glycolate, and Starch. Caplets—Cellulose, Hydroxpropyl Methylcellulose, Magnesium Stearate, Polyethylene Glycol, Sodium Starch Glycolate, Starch and Red #40 .

HOW SUPPLIED
Tablets (colored white, scored, imprinted "TYLENOL")—tins of 12, and tamper-resistant bottles of 24, 50, 100 and 200. Caplets (colored white, "TYLENOL")—tamper-resistant bottles of 24, 50, 100. For additional pain relief, Extra-Strength TYLENOL® Gelcaps, Caplets and Tablets, 500 mg, and Extra-Strength TYLENOL® Adult Liquid Pain Reliever are available (colored green; 1 fl. oz. = 1000 mg.)

Shown in Product Identification Section, page 418

Extra Strength
TYLENOL® acetaminophen **OTC**
Gelcaps, Caplets, Tablets

DESCRIPTION
Each Extra-Strength TYLENOL Gelcap, Caplet or Tablet contains acetaminophen 500 mg.

ACTIONS
Acetaminophen is a clinically proven analgesic and antipyretic. Acetaminophen produces analgesia by elevation of the pain threshold and antipyresis through action on the hypothalamic heat-regulating center. Acetaminophen is equal to aspirin in analgesic and antipyretic effectiveness and it is unlikely to produce many of the side effects associated with aspirin and aspirin-containing products.

INDICATIONS
For the temporary relief of minor aches, pains, headaches and fever.

PRECAUTIONS
If a rare sensitivity reaction occurs, the drug should be discontinued.

USUAL DOSAGE
Adults and children 12 years of Age and Older: Two Gelcaps, Caplets or Tablets 3 or 4 times daily. No more than a total of 8 Gelcaps, Caplets or Tablets in any 24-hour period.

Warning: Do not take for pain for more than 10 days or for fever for more than 3 days unless directed by a doctor. Severe or recurrent pain or high or continued fever may be indicative of serious illness. Under these conditions, consult a doctor. **Do not use if printed red neck wrap or printed foil inner seal is broken. Keep this and all medication out of the reach of children. As with any drug, if you are pregnant or nursing a baby, seek the advice of a health professional before using this product. In case of accidental overdosage, contact a doctor or poison control center immediately.**

OVERDOSAGE
Acetaminophen in massive overdosage may cause hepatic toxicity in some patients. In adults and adolescents, hepatic toxicity has rarely been reported following ingestion of acute overdosage of less than 10 grams. Fatalities are infrequent (less than 3–4% of untreated cases) and have rarely been reported with overdoses of less than 15 grams. In children, an acute overdosage of less than 150 mg/kg has not been associated with hepatic toxicity.

Early symptoms following a potentially hepatotoxic overdose may include: nausea, vomiting, diaphoresis and general malaise. Clinical and laboratory evidence of hepatic toxicity may not be apparent until 48 to 72 hours postingestion.

In adults and adolescents, regardless of the quantity of acetaminophen reported to have been ingested, administer MUCOMYST® acetylcysteine immediately if 24 hours or less have elapsed from the reported time of ingestion. For full prescribing information, refer to the MUCOMYST package insert. Do not await the results of assays for acetaminophen level before initiating treatment with MUCOMYST acetylcysteine. The following additional procedures are recommended: The stomach should be emptied promptly by lavage or by induction of emesis with syrup of ipecac. A serum acetaminophen assay should be obtained as early as possible, but no sooner than four hours following ingestion. Liver function studies should be obtained initially and repeated at 24-hour intervals.

Serious toxicity or fatalities are extremely infrequent in children, possibly due to differences in the way they metabolize acetaminophen. In children, the maximum potential amount ingested can be more easily estimated. If more than 150 mg/kg or an unknown amount was ingested, obtain an acetaminophen plasma level. The acetaminophen plasma level should be obtained as soon as possible, but no sooner than 4 hours following the ingestion. Induce emesis using syrup of ipecac. If the plasma level is obtained and falls above the broken line on the acetaminophen overdose nomogram, the MUCOMYST acetylcysteine therapy should be initiated and continued for a full course of therapy. If acetaminophen plasma assay capability is not available, and the estimated acetaminophen ingestion exceeds 150 mg/kg, MUCOMYST acetylcysteine therapy should be initiated and continued for a full course of therapy.

For additional emergency information, call your regional poison center or call the Rocky Mountain Poison Center toll-free, (1-800-525-6115).

INACTIVE INGREDIENTS
Tablets—Magnesium Stearate, Cellulose, Sodium Starch Glycolate and Starch. Caplets—Cellulose, Hydroxypropyl Methylcellulose, Magnesium Stearate, Polyethylene Glycol, Sodium Starch Glycolate, Starch and Red #40.

Gelcaps—Benzyl Alcohol, Butylparaben, Castor Oil, Cellulose, Edetate Calcium Disodium, Gelatin, Hydroxypropyl Methylcellulose, Magnesium Stearate, Methylparaben, Propylparaben, Sodium Lauryl Sulfate, Sodium Propionate, Sodium Starch Glycolate, Starch, Titanium Dioxide, Blue #1 and #2, Red #40 and Yellow #10.

HOW SUPPLIED
Tablets (colored white, imprinted "TYLENOL" and "500")—vials of 10 and tamper-resistant bottles of 30, 60, 100, and 200. Caplets (colored white, imprinted "TYLENOL 500 mg")—vials of 10 and tamper-resistant bottles of 24, 50, 100, 175, and 250's.

Gelcaps (colored yellow and red, imprinted "Tylenol 500") tamper-resistant bottles of 24, 50, 100, and 150. For adults who prefer liquids or can't swallow solid medication, Extra-Strength TYLENOL® Adult Liquid Pain Reliever, mint flavored, is also available (colored green; 1 fl. oz. = 1000 mg.).

Shown in Product Identification Section, page 418

EXTRA STRENGTH TYLENOL® **OTC**
Headache Plus
Pain Reliever with Antacid Caplets

DESCRIPTION
Each Extra Strength TYLENOL® Headache Plus Pain Reliever with Antacid caplet contains acetaminophen 500 mg. and calcium carbonate 250 mg.

INDICATIONS
TYLENOL® Headache Plus provides effective temporary relief of minor aches and pains with heartburn or acid indigestion.

ACTIONS
TYLENOL® Headache Plus contains a clinically proven analgesic and antacid. Acetaminophen produces analgesia by elevation of the pain threshold. Acetaminophen is equal to aspirin in analgesic effectiveness, and it is unlikely to produce many of the side effects associated with aspirin and aspirin-containing products. The antacid, calcium carbonate provides fast relief of heartburn, acid indigestion and upset stomach.

USUAL DOSAGE
Adults and children 12 years of age and older: Two caplets every 6 hours. No more than a total of 8 caplets in any 24 hour period or as directed by a physician.

PRECAUTIONS
If a rare sensitivity reaction occurs, the drug should be stopped.

WARNING
Do not give this product to children under 12 years of age. Do not use the maximum dosage of this product for more than 10 days except under the advice and supervision of a physician. Do not take the product for pain for more than 10 days, or for fever for more than 3 days unless directed by a physician. If pain or fever persists or gets worse, if new symptoms occur, or if redness or swelling is present, consult a physician because these could be signs of a serious condition. **Do not use if carton is opened, or if printed neck wrap or printed foil seal is broken. Keep this and all medication out of the reach of children. As with any drug, if you are pregnant or nursing a baby, seek the advice of a health professional before using this product. In the case of accidental overdose, seek professional assistance or contact a poison control center immediately. Prompt medical attention is critical for adults as well as for children even if you do not notice any signs of symptoms.**

OVERDOSAGE
Acetaminophen in massive overdosage may cause hepatic toxicity in some patients. In adults and adolescents, hepatic toxicity has rarely been reported following ingestion of acute overdosage of less than 10 grams. Fatalities are infrequent (less than 3–4% of untreated cases) and have rarely been reported with overdoses of less than 15 grams. In children,

Continued on next page

McNeil Consumer—Cont.

an acute overdosage of less than 150 mg/kg has not been associated with hepatic toxicity.
Early symptoms following a potentially hepatotoxic overdose may include: nausea, vomiting, diaphoresis and general malaise. Clinical and laboratory evidence of hepatic toxicity may not be apparent until 48 to 72 hours postingestion. In adults and adolescents, regardless of the quantity of acetaminophen reported to have been ingested, administer MUCOMYST® acetylcysteine immediately if 24 hours or less have elapsed from the reported time of ingestion. For full prescribing information, refer to the MUCOMYST package insert. Do not await results of assays for acetaminophen level before initiating treatment with MUCOMYST acetylcysteine. The following additional procedures are recommended: The stomach should be emptied promptly by lavage or by induction of emesis with syrup of ipecac. A serum acetaminophen assay should be obtained as early as possible, but no sooner than four hours following ingestion. Liver function studies should be obtained initially and repeated at 24-hour intervals.
Serious toxicity or fatalities are extremely infrequent in children, possibly due to differences in the way they metabolize acetaminophen. In children, the maximum potential amount ingested can be more easily estimated. If more than 150 mg/kg or an unknown amount was ingested, obtain an acetaminophen plasma level. The acetaminophen plasma level should be obtained as soon as possible, but no sooner than 4 hours following the ingestion. Induce emesis using syrup of ipecac. If the plasma level is obtained and falls above the broken line on the acetaminophen overdose nomogram, the MUCOMYST acetylcysteine therapy should be initiated and continued for a full course of therapy. If acetaminophen, plasma assay capability is not available, and the estimated acetaminophen ingestion exceeds 150 mg/kg, MUCOMYST acetylcysteine therapy should be initiated and continued for a full course of therapy.
For additional emergency information, call your regional poison center or call the Rocky Mountain Poison Center toll-free (1-800-525-6115).

INACTIVE INGREDIENTS

Acacia, Cellulose, Corn Starch, Croscarmellose Sodium, Hydroxypropyl Methylcellulose, Magnesium Stearate, Maltodextrin, Propylene Glycol, Sodium Starch Glycolate, Titanium Dioxide, Triacetin, Blue #1 and Blue #2.

HOW SUPPLIED

Caplets (white with royal blue imprinted "TYLENOL Headache Plus"). Tamper resistant bottles of 24, 50 and 100.
Shown in Product Identification Section, page 418

Extra-Strength TYLENOL® acetaminophen Adult Liquid Pain Reliever — OTC

DESCRIPTION

Each 15 ml. (1/2 fl. oz. or one tablespoonful) contains 500 mg. acetaminophen (alcohol 7%).

ACTIONS

TYLENOL acetaminophen is a clinically proven analgesic and antipyretic. Acetaminophen produces analgesia by elevation of the pain threshold and antipyresis through action on the hypothalamic heat-regulating center. Acetaminophen is equal to aspirin in analgesic and antipyretic effectiveness and it is unlikely to produce many of the side effects associated with aspirin and aspirin-containing products.

INDICATIONS

Acetaminophen provides temporary relief of minor aches, pains, headaches and fevers.

PRECAUTIONS

If a rare sensitivity reaction occurs, the drug should be discontinued.

USUAL DOSAGE

Extra-Strength TYLENOL Adult Liquid Pain Reliever is an adult preparation for those adults who prefer liquids or can't swallow solid medication. Not for use in children under 12. Measuring cup is marked for accurate dosage. Extra-Strength Dose—1 fl. oz. (30 ml or 2 tablespoonsful, 1000 mg), which is equivalent to two 500 mg Extra-Strength TYLENOL Tablets, Caplets or Gelcaps. Take every 4–6 hours, no more than 4 doses in any 24-hour period.
"**Warning:** Do not take for pain for more than 10 days or for fever for more than 3 days unless directed by a doctor. Severe or recurrent pain or high or continued fever may be indicative of serious illness. Under these conditions, consult a physician. **Do not use if printed plastic overwrap or printed foil inner seal is broken. Keep this and all medication out of the reach of children. As with any drug, if you are pregnant or nursing a baby, seek the advice of a health professional before using this product. In case of accidental overdosage, contact a doctor or poison control center immediately."**

OVERDOSAGE

Acetaminophen in massive overdosage may cause hepatic toxicity in some patients. In adults and adolescents, hepatic toxicity has rarely been reported following ingestion of acute overdosage of less than 10 grams. Fatalities are infrequent (less than 3–4% of untreated cases) and have rarely been reported with overdoses of less than 15 grams. In children, an acute overdosage of less than 150 mg/kg has not been associated with hepatic toxicity.
Early symptoms following a potentially hepatotoxic overdose may include: nausea, vomiting, diaphoresis and general malaise. Clinical and laboratory evidence of hepatic toxicity may not be apparent until 48 to 72 hours postingestion.
In adults and adolescents, regardless of the quantity of acetaminophen reported to have been ingested, administer MUCOMYST® acetylcysteine immediately if 24 hours or less have elapsed from the reported time of ingestion. For full prescribing information, refer to the MUCOMYST package insert. Do not await the results of assays for acetaminophen level before initiating treatment with MUCOMYST acetylcysteine. The following additional procedures are recommended: The stomach should be emptied promptly by lavage or by induction of emesis with syrup of ipecac. A serum acetaminophen assay should be obtained as early as possible, but no sooner than four hours following ingestion. Liver function studies should be obtained initially and repeated at 24-hour intervals.
Serious toxicity or fatalities are extremely infrequent in children, possibly due to differences in the way they metabolize acetaminophen. In children, the maximum potential amount ingested can be more easily estimated. If more than 150 mg/kg or an unknown amount was ingested, obtain an acetaminophen plasma level. The acetaminophen plasma level should be obtained as soon as possible, but no sooner than 4 hours following the ingestion. Induce emesis using syrup of ipecac. If the plasma level is obtained and falls above the broken line on the acetaminophen overdose nomogram, the MUCOMYST acetylcysteine therapy should be initiated and continued for a full course of therapy. If acetaminophen plasma assay capability is not available, and the estimated acetaminophen ingestion exceeds 150 mg/kg, MUCOMYST acetylcysteine therapy should be initiated and continued for a full course of therapy.
For additional emergency information, call your regional poison center or call the Rocky Mountain Poison Center toll-free, (1-800-525-6115).

INACTIVE INGREDIENTS

Alcohol, Citric Acid, Flavors, Glycerin, Polyethylene Glycol, Purified Water, Sodium Benzoate, Sorbitol, Sucrose, Yellow #6 (Sunset Yellow), Yellow #10 and Blue #1.

HOW SUPPLIED

Mint-flavored liquid (colored green), 8 fl. oz. tamper-resistant bottle with child resistant safety cap and special dosage cup.

EXTRA STRENGTH TYLENOL® PM — OTC
Pain Reliever/Sleep Aid Gelcaps, Caplets and Tablets

DESCRIPTION

Each EXTRA STRENGTH TYLENOL® PM Gelcap, Caplet or Tablet contains acetaminophen 500 mg and diphenhydramine HCl 25 mg.

ACTIONS

EXTRA STRENGTH TYLENOL® PM gelcaps, caplets and tablets contain a clinically proven analgesic-antipyretic and an antihistamine. Maximum allowable non-prescription levels of acetaminophen and diphenhydramine provide temporary relief of occasional headaches and minor aches and pains accompanying sleeplessness. Acetaminophen is equal to aspirin in analgesic and antipyretic effectiveness and it is unlikely to produce many of the side effects associated with aspirin containing products. Acetaminophen produces analgesia by elevation of the pain threshold. Diphenhydramine HCl is an antihistamine with sedative properties.

INDICATIONS

EXTRA STRENGTH TYLENOL® PM gelcaps, caplets and tablets provide effective symptomatic relief from occasional headaches and minor aches and pains with accompanying sleeplessness.

PRECAUTIONS

If a rare sensitivity occurs, the drug should be discontinued.

USUAL DOSAGE

Adults and Children 12 years of Age and Older: Two gelcaps, caplets or tablets at bedtime or as directed by physician. Do not exceed recommended dosage.
"**WARNINGS:** Do not give to children under 12 years of age or use for more than 10 days unless directed by a physician. Consult your physician if symptoms persist or new ones occur, or if fever persists for more than 3 days, or if sleeplessness persists continuously for more than 2 weeks. Insomnia may be a symptom of serious underlying medical illness. Do not take this product if you have asthma, glaucoma, emphysema, chronic pulmonary disease, shortness of breath, difficulty in breathing or difficulty in urination due to enlargement of the prostate gland unless directed by a physician. Avoid alcoholic beverages while taking this product. Do not take if you are taking sedatives or tranquilizers without first consulting your physician. **Do not use if carton is open or if printed neck wrap or printed foil inner seal is broken. Keep this and all medications out of the reach of children. In case of accidental overdose, contact a physician or poison control center immediately. As with any drug, if you are pregnant or nursing a baby, seek the advice of a health professional before using this product.**

CAUTION

This product will cause drowsiness. Do not drive a motor vehicle or operate machinery after use.

OVERDOSAGE

Acetaminophen in massive overdosage may cause hepatic toxicity in some patients. In adults and adolescents, hepatic toxicity has rarely been reported following ingestion of acute overdosage of less than 10 grams. Fatalities are infrequent (less than 3–4% of untreated cases) and have rarely been reported with overdoses of less than 15 grams. In children, an acute overdosage of less than 150 mg/kg has not been associated with hepatic toxicity.
Early symptoms following a potentially hepatotoxic overdose may include: nausea, vomiting, diaphoresis and general malaise. Clinical and laboratory evidence of hepatic toxicity may not be apparent until 48 to 72 hours postingestion.
In adults and adolescents, regardless of the quantity of acetaminophen reported to have been ingested, administer MUCOMYST® acetylcysteine immediately if 24 hours or less have elapsed from the reported time of ingestion. For full prescribing information, refer to the MUCOMYST package insert. Do not await results of assays for acetaminophen level before initiating treatment with MUCOMYST acetylcysteine. The following additional procedures are recommended: The stomach should be emptied promptly by lavage or by induction of emesis with syrup of ipecac. A serum acetaminophen assay should be obtained as early as possible, but no sooner than four hours following ingestion. Liver function studies should be obtained initially and repeated at 24-hour intervals. Serious toxicity or fatalities are extremely infrequent in children, possibly due to differences in the way they metabolize acetaminophen. In children, the maximum potential amount ingested can be more easily estimated. If more than 150 mg/kg or an unknown amount was ingested, obtain an acetaminophen plasma level. The acetaminophen plasma level should be obtained as soon as possible, but no sooner than 4 hours following the ingestion. Induce emesis using syrup of ipecac. If the plasma level is obtained and falls above the broken line on the acetaminophen overdose nomogram, the MUCOMYST acetylcysteine therapy should be initiated and continued for a full course of therapy. If acetaminophen plasma assay capability is not available, and the estimated acetaminophen ingestion exceeds 150 mg/kg, MUCOMYST acetylcysteine therapy should be initiated and continued for a full course of therapy.
For additional emergency information, call your regional poison center or call the Rocky Mountain Poison Center toll-free, (1-800-525-6115).
Diphenhydramine toxicity should be treated as you would an antihistamine/anticholinergic overdose and is likely to be present within a few hours after acute ingestion.

INACTIVE INGREDIENTS

Gelcaps: Benzyl Alcohol, Butylparaben, Castor Oil, Cellulose, Cornstarch, Edetate Calcium Disodium, Gelatin, Hydroxypropyl Methylcellulose, Magnesium Stearate, Propylparaben, Sodium Lauryl Sulfate, Sodium Citrate, Sodium Propionate, Sodium Starch Glycolate, Titanium Dioxide, Blue #1 and Red #28.
Tablets: Cellulose, colloidal silicon dioxide, corn starch, sodium citrate, sodium starch glycolate, stearic acid, and Blue #1. Caplets: Cellulose, colloidal silicon dioxide, corn starch, hydroxypropyl methylcellulose, polyethylene glycol, sodium citrate, sodium starch glycolate, stearic acid, titanium dioxide, Blue #1 and Blue #2.

HOW SUPPLIED

Gelcaps (colored blue and white imprinted "TYLENOL PM") tamper-resistant bottles of 20 and 40.
Caplets (colored light blue imprinted "Tylenol PM") tamper-resistant bottles of 24 and 50. Tablets (colored light blue embossed with "Tylenol" on one side and "PM" on the other) tamper-resistant bottles of 24 and 50.
Shown in Product Identification Section, page 418

CHILDREN'S TYLENOL COLD® OTC
Multi Symptom Chewable Tablets and Liquid

DESCRIPTION
Each Children's Tylenol Cold Chewable Grape-Flavored Tablet contains acetaminophen 80 mg, chlorpheniramine maleate 0.5 mg and pseudoephedrine hydrochloride 7.5 mg. Children's Tylenol Cold Liquid is grape flavored and contains no alcohol. Each teaspoon (5 ml) contains acetaminophen 160 mg, chlorpheniramine maleate 1 mg, and pseudoephedrine hydrochloride 15 mg.

ACTIONS
Children's Tylenol Cold Chewable Tablets and Liquid combine the analgesic-antipyretic acetaminophen with the decongestant pseudoephedrine hydrochloride and the antihistamine chlorpheniramine maleate to help relieve nasal congestion, dry runny noses and prevent sneezing as well as to relieve the fever, aches, pains and general discomfort associated with colds and upper respiratory infections.
Acetaminophen is equal to aspirin in analgesic and antipyretic effectiveness and it is unlikely to produce the side effects often associated with aspirin or aspirin-containing products.

INDICATIONS
Provides fast, effective temporary relief of nasal congestion, runny nose, sneezing, minor aches and pains, headaches and fever due to the common cold, hay fever or other upper respiratory allergies.

USUAL DOSAGE
Administer to children under 6 years only on the advice of a physician. Children's Tylenol Cold Chewable Tablets: 2–5 years—2 tablets, 6–11 years—4 tablets.
Children's Tylenol Cold Liquid Formula: 2–5 years—1 teaspoonful; 6–11 years—2 teaspoonsful. Measuring cup is provided and marked for accurate dosing.
Doses may be repeated every 4-6 hours as needed, not to exceed 4 doses in 24 hours. The Warnings are identical for the two dosage forms except the Liquid Cold Formula does not contain the phenylketonurics statement since the product does not contain aspartame.
Warning: Do not use if carton is opened, or if printed plastic bottle wrap or printed foil inner seal is broken.
Keep this and all medication out of the reach of children. In case of accidental overdosage, contact a physician or poison control center immediately. Phenylketonurics: contains phenylalanine, 4 mg per tablet. Do not exceed the recommended dosage because nervousness, dizziness or sleeplessness may occur. Do not take this product for more than 7 days. If fever persists for more than three days, or if symptoms do not improve or new ones occur within five days or are accompanied by high fever, consult a physician before continuing use. This preparation may cause drowsiness, or in some cases, excitability. Do not give this product to children who have heart disease, high blood pressure, thyroid disease, diabetes, glaucoma or asthma or are taking a prescription drug for high blood pressure or depression, except under the advice and supervision of a physician.

OVERDOSAGE
Acetaminophen in massive overdosage may cause hepatic toxicity in some patients. In adults and adolescents, hepatic toxicity has rarely been reported following ingestion of acute overdosage of less than 10 grams. Fatalities are infrequent (less than 3–4% of untreated cases) and have rarely been reported with overdoses of less than 15 grams. In children, an acute overdosage of less than 150 mg/kg has not been associated with hepatic toxicity.
Early symptoms following a potentially hepatotoxic overdose may include: nausea, vomiting, diaphoresis and general malaise. Clinical and laboratory evidence of hepatic toxicity may not be apparent until 48 to 72 hours postingestion.
In adults and adolescents, regardless of the quantity of acetaminophen reported to have been ingested, administer MUCOMYST® acetylcysteine immediately if 24 hours or less have elapsed from the reported time of ingestion. For full prescribing information, refer to the MUCOMYST package insert. Do not await the results of assays for acetaminophen level before initiating treatment with MUCOMYST acetylcysteine. The following additional procedures are recommended: The stomach should be emptied promptly by lavage or by induction of emesis with syrup of ipecac. A serum acetaminophen assay should be obtained as early as possible, but no sooner than four hours following ingestion. Liver function studies should be obtained initially and repeated at 24-hour intervals.
Serious toxicity or fatalities are extremely infrequent in children, possibly due to differences in the way they metabolize acetaminophen. In children, the maximum potential amount ingested can be more easily estimated. If more than 150 mg/kg or an unknown amount was ingested, obtain an acetaminophen plasma level. The acetaminophen plasma level should be obtained as soon as possible, but no sooner than 4 hours following the ingestion. Induce emesis using syrup of ipecac. If the plasma level is obtained and falls above the broken line on the acetaminophen overdose nomogram, the MUCOMYST acetylcysteine therapy should be initiated and continued for a full course of therapy. If acetaminophen plasma assay capability is not available, and the estimated acetaminophen ingestion exceeds 150 mg/kg, MUCOMYST acetylcysteine therapy should be initiated and continued for a full course of therapy.
For additional emergency information, call your regional poison center or call the Rocky Mountain Poison Center toll-free, (1-800-525-6115).
Chlorpheniramine toxicity should be treated as you would an antihistamine/anticholinergic overdose and is likely to be present within a few hours after acute ingestion.
Symptoms from pseudoephedrine overdose consist most often of mild anxiety, tachycardia and/or mild hypertension. Symptoms usually appear within 4 to 8 hours of ingestion and are transient, usually requiring no treatment.

INACTIVE INGREDIENTS
Chewable Tablets—Aspartame, citric acid, ethylcellulose, flavors, magnesium stearate, mannitol, microcrystalline cellulose, pregelatinized starch, sucrose, Blue #1 and Red #7.
Liquid—Benzoic acid, citric acid, flavors, glycerin, malic acid, polyethylene glycol, propylene glycol, sodium benzoate, sorbitol, sucrose, purified water, Blue #1 and Red #40.

HOW SUPPLIED
Chewable Tablets (colored purple, scored, imprinted "Tylenol Cold") on one side and "TC" on opposite side—bottles of 24. Cold Formula—bottles (colored purple) of 4 fl. oz.
Shown in Product Identification Section, page 418

CHILDREN'S TYLENOL® OTC
COLD PLUS COUGH
Multi Symptom Liquid

DESCRIPTION
Children's Tylenol Cold Plus Cough Liquid is cherry flavored and contains no alcohol. Each teaspoon (5 ml) contains acetaminophen 160 mg, chlorpheniramine maleate 1 mg, dextromethorphan hydrobromide 5 mg and pseudoephedrine hydrochloride 15 mg.

ACTIONS
Children's Tylenol Cold Plus Cough Liquid combine the analgesic-antipyretic acetaminophen with the decongestant pseudoephedrine hydrochloride, the cough suppressant dextromethorphan hydrobromide, and the antihistamine chlorpheniramine maleate to help relieve nasal congestion, coughs, dry runny noses and prevent sneezing as well as to relieve the fever, aches, pains and general discomfort associated with colds and upper respiratory infections.
Acetaminophen is equal to aspirin in analgesic and antipyretic effectiveness and it is unlikely to produce the side effects often associated with aspirin or aspirin-containing products.

INDICATIONS
Provides fast, effective temporary relief of nasal congestion, coughs, runny nose, sneezing, minor aches and pains, headaches and fever due to the common cold, hay fever or other upper respiratory allergies.

USUAL DOSAGE
Administer to children under 6 years only on the advice of a physician.
Children's Tylenol Cold Plus Cough Liquid Formula: 2–5 years—1 teaspoonful; 6–11 years—2 teaspoonsful. Measuring cup is provided and marked for accurate dosing.
Doses may be repeated every 4-6 hours as needed, not to exceed 4 doses in 24 hours.

WARNING
Do not use if carton is opened, or if printed plastic bottle wrap or printed foil inner seal is broken. Keep this and all medication out of the reach of children. In case of accidental overdosage, contact a physician or poison control center immediately. Do not exceed recommended dosage because at higher doses nervousness, dizziness or sleeplessness may occur. Do not give this product to children for more than 7 days. If fever persists for more than 3 days, or if symptoms do not improve or new ones occur within 5 days or are accompanied by fever, consult a physician before continuing use. This preparation may cause drowsiness or in some cases, excitability. Do not give this product to children who have heart disease, high blood pressure, thyroid disease, diabetes, asthma or glaucoma unless directed by a doctor. A persistent cough may be a sign of a serious condition. If cough persists for more than 1 week, tends to recur, or is accompanied by fever, rash or persistent headache, consult a physician. Do not give this product for persistent or chronic cough such as occurs with asthma or if cough is accompanied by excessive phlegm (mucus) unless directed by a physician.

DRUG INTERACTION PRECAUTION
Do not give this product to a child who is taking a prescription drug for high blood pressure or depression without first consulting the child's physician.

OVERDOSAGE
Acetaminophen in massive overdosage may cause hepatic toxicity in some patients. In adults and adolescents, hepatic toxicity has rarely been reported following ingestion of acute overdosage of less than 10 grams. Fatalities are infrequent (less than 3–4% of untreated cases) and have rarely been reported with overdoses of less than 15 grams. In children, an acute overdosage of less than 150 mg/kg has not been associated with hepatic toxicity.
Early symptoms following a potentially hepatotoxic overdose may include: nausea, vomiting, diaphoresis and general malaise. Clinical and laboratory evidence of hepatic toxicity may not be apparent until 48 to 72 hours postingestion.
In adults and adolescents, regardless of the quantity of acetaminophen reported to have been ingested, administer MUCOMYST® acetylcysteine immediately if 24 hours or less have elapsed from the reported time of ingestion. For full prescribing information, refer to the MUCOMYST package insert. Do not await the results of assays for acetaminophen level before initiating treatment with MUCOMYST acetylcysteine. The following additional procedures are recommended: The stomach should be emptied promptly by lavage or by induction of emesis with syrup of ipecac. A serum acetaminophen assay should be obtained as early as possible, but no sooner than four hours following ingestion. Liver function studies should be obtained initially and repeated at 24-hour intervals.
Serious toxicity or fatalities are extremely infrequent in children, possibly due to differences in the way they metabolize acetaminophen. In children, the maximum potential amount ingested can be more easily estimated. If more than 150 mg/kg or an unknown amount was ingested, obtain an acetaminophen plasma level. The acetaminophen plasma level should be obtained as soon as possible, but no sooner than 4 hours following the ingestion. Induce emesis using syrup of ipecac. If the plasma level is obtained and falls above the broken line on the acetaminophen overdose nomogram, the MUCOMYST acetylcysteine therapy should be initiated and continued for a full course of therapy. If acetaminophen plasma assay capability is not available, and the estimated acetaminophen ingestion exceeds 150 mg/kg, MUCOMYST acetylcysteine therapy should be initiated and continued for a full course of therapy.
For additional emergency information, call your regional poison center or call the Rocky Mountain Poison Center toll-free, (1-800-525-6115).
Chlorpheniramine toxicity should be treated as you would an antihistamine/anticholinergic overdose and is likely to be present within a few hours after acute ingestion.
Symptoms from pseudoephedrine overdose consist most often of mild anxiety, tachycardia and/or mild hypertension. Symptoms usually appear within 4 to 8 hours of ingestion and are transient, usually requiring no treatment.

INACTIVE INGREDIENTS
Citric Acid, Corn Syrup, Flavors, Polyethylene Glycol, Propylene Glycol, Sodium Benzoate, Sodium Carboxymethylcellulose, Sorbitol, Purified Water, Red #33 and Red #40.

HOW SUPPLIED
Cold Plus Cough Formula—bottles (red colored) of 4 fl. oz.
Shown in Product Identification Section, page 417

Effervescent Formula OTC
TYLENOL® Cold Medication
Tablets

DESCRIPTION
Each Effervescent TYLENOL Cold Tablet contains acetaminophen 325 mg., chlorpheniramine maleate 2 mg., and phenylpropanolamine hydrochloride 12.5 mg.

ACTIONS
TYLENOL Cold Medication Tablets contain a clinically proven analgesic-antipyretic, decongestant and antihistamine. Acetaminophen produces analgesia by elevation of the pain threshold and antipyresis through action on the hypothalamic heat-regulating center. Acetaminophen is equal to aspirin in analgesic and antipyretic effectiveness and it is unlikely to produce many of the side effects associated with aspirin and aspirin-containing products. Phenylpropanolamine is a sympathomimetic amine which provides temporary relief of nasal congestion. Chlorpheniramine is an antihistamine which helps provide temporary relief of runny nose, sneezing and watery and itchy eyes.

Continued on next page

McNeil Consumer—Cont.

INDICATIONS

TYLENOL Cold Medication provides effective temporary relief of runny nose, sneezing, watery and itchy eyes, nasal congestion, sore throat and aches, pains, and fever due to a cold or "flu."

PRECAUTIONS

If a rare sensitivity reaction occurs, the drug should be stopped. Although phenylpropanolamine is virtually without pressor effect in normotensive patients, it should be used with caution in hypertensives.

USUAL DOSAGE

Effervescent TYLENOL® Cold must be dissolved in water before taking.

ADULTS (12 years and over): 2 tablets every 4 hours, not to exceed 12 tablets in 24 hours.

CHILDREN (6–11): 1 tablet every 4 hours, not to exceed 6 tablets in 24 hours.

"WARNINGS: Do not administer to children under 6. Do not take this product for more than 7 days (Adults) or 5 days (Children) or for fever for more than 3 days unless directed by a doctor. Do not exceed recommended dosage because at higher doses nervousness, dizziness or sleeplessness may occur. May cause excitability, especially in children. May cause drowsiness; alcohol may increase the drowsiness effect. Avoid alcoholic beverages while taking this product. Use caution when driving a motor vehicle or operating machinery. If sore throat is severe, persists for more than 2 days, is accompanied or followed by fever, headache, rash, nausea or vomiting, consult a physician promptly. Do not take this product if you have asthma, glaucoma, emphysema, chronic pulmonary disease, shortness of breath, difficulty in breathing, heart disease, high blood pressure, thyroid disease, diabetes or difficulty in urination due to enlargement of the prostate gland unless directed by a doctor. DO NOT USE IF GLUED CARTON FLAP IS OPENED OR IF FOIL PACK IS TORN OR BROKEN. KEEP THIS AND ALL MEDICATION OUT OF THE REACH OF CHILDREN. AS WITH ANY DRUG, IF YOU ARE PREGNANT OR NURSING A BABY, SEEK THE ADVICE OF A HEALTH PROFESSIONAL BEFORE USING THIS PRODUCT. IN CASE OF ACCIDENTAL OVERDOSAGE, CONTACT A PHYSICIAN OR POISON CONTROL CENTER IMMEDIATELY. DO NOT TAKE THIS PRODUCT IF YOU ARE ON A SODIUM RESTRICTED DIET, EXCEPT UNDER THE ADVICE AND SUPERVISION OF A DOCTOR. EACH TABLET CONTAINS 525 MG. OF SODIUM.

DRUG INTERACTION PRECAUTION: Do not take this product if you are presently taking a prescription drug for high blood pressure or depression without first consulting your doctor."

OVERDOSAGE

Acetaminophen in massive overdosage may cause hepatic toxicity in some patients. In adults and adolescents, hepatic toxicity has rarely been reported following ingestion of acute overdosage of less than 10 grams. Fatalities are infrequent (less than 3–4% of untreated cases) and have rarely been reported with overdoses of less than 15 grams. In children, an acute overdosage of less than 150 mg/kg has not been associated with hepatic toxicity.

Early symptoms following a potentially hepatotoxic overdose may include: nausea, vomiting, diaphoresis and general malaise. Clinical and laboratory evidence of hepatic toxicity may not be apparent until 48 to 72 hours postingestion.

In adults and adolescents, regardless of the quantity of acetaminophen reported to have been ingested, administer MUCOMYST® acetylcysteine immediately if 24 hours or less have elapsed from the reported time of ingestion. For full prescribing information, refer to the MUCOMYST package insert. Do not await results of assays for acetaminophen level before initiating treatment with MUCOMYST acetylcysteine. The following additional procedures are recommended: The stomach should be emptied promptly by lavage or by induction of emesis with syrup of ipecac. A serum acetaminophen assay should be obtained as early as possible, but no sooner than four hours following ingestion. Liver function studies should be obtained initially and repeated at 24-hour intervals.

Serious toxicity or fatalities are extremely infrequent in children, possibly due to differences in the way they metabolize acetaminophen. In children, the maximum potential amount ingested can be more easily estimated. If more than 150 mg/kg or an unknown amount was ingested, obtain an acetaminophen plasma level. The acetaminophen plasma level should be obtained as soon as possible, but no sooner than 4 hours following the ingestion. Induce emesis using syrup of ipecac. If the plasma level is obtained and falls above the broken line on the acetaminophen overdose nomogram, the MUCOMYST acetylcysteine therapy should be initiated and continued for a full course of therapy. If acetaminophen plasma assay capability is not available, and the

estimated acetaminophen ingestion exceeds 150 mg/kg, MUCOMYST acetylcysteine therapy should be initiated and continued for a full course of therapy.

For additional emergency information, call your regional poison center or call the Rocky Mountain Poison Center toll-free, (1-800-525-6115).

Symptoms from phenylpropanolamine overdose consist most often of mild anxiety, tachycardia and/or mild hypertension. Symptoms usually appear within 4 to 8 hours of ingestion and are transient, usually requiring no treatment.

INACTIVE INGREDIENTS: Citric Acid, Flavor, Potassium Benzoate, Povidone, Saccharin, Sodium Bicarbonate, Sodium Carbonate, Sodium Docusate, Sorbitol.

HOW SUPPLIED

Tablets: carton of 20 tablets in 10 foil twin packs; carton of 36 tablets in 18 foil twin packs.

Shown in Product Identification Section, page 418

Hot Medication   OTC
TYLENOL® Cold & Flu Medication
Packets

DESCRIPTION

Each packet of TYLENOL Cold & Flu contains acetaminophen 650 mg., chlorpheniramine maleate 4 mg., pseudoephedrine hydrochloride 60 mg. and dextromethorphan hydrobromide 30 mg.

ACTIONS

TYLENOL Cold and Flu Medication contains a clinically proven analgesic-antipyretic, decongestant, cough suppressant and antihistamine. Acetaminophen produces analgesia by elevation of the pain threshold and antipyresis through action on the hypothalamic heat-regulating center. Acetaminophen is equal to aspirin in analgesic and antipyretic effectiveness and it is unlikely to produce many of the side effects associated with aspirin and aspirin-containing products. Pseudoephedrine hydrochloride is a sympathomimetic amine which provides temporary relief of nasal congestion. Dextromethorphan is a cough suppressant which provides temporary relief of coughs due to minor throat irritations that may occur with the common cold. Chlorpheniramine is an antihistamine which helps provide temporary relief of runny nose, sneezing and watery and itchy eyes.

INDICATIONS

TYLENOL Cold and Flu Medication provides effective temporary relief of runny nose, sneezing, watery and itchy eyes, nasal congestion, sore throat, coughing, and aches, pains, and fever due to a cold or "flu."

PRECAUTIONS

If a rare sensitivity reaction occurs, the drug should be stopped. Although pseudoephedrine is virtually without pressor effect in normotensive patients, it should be used with caution in hypertensives.

USUAL DOSAGE

Adults (12 years and over): Dissolve one packet in 6 oz. cup of hot water. Sip while hot. Sweeten to taste, if desired. May repeat every 6 hours, not to exceed 4 doses in 24 hours.

"WARNINGS: Not recommended for children under 12. Do not take this product for more than 7 days or for fever for more than 3 days unless directed by a doctor. If symptoms do not improve or are accompanied by fever, consult a doctor. A persistent cough may be a sign of a serious condition. If cough persists for more than 1 week, tends to recur or is accompanied by fever, rash or persistent headache, consult a doctor. Do not take this product for persistent or chronic cough such as occurs with smoking, asthma, emphysema, or if cough is accompanied by excessive phlegm (mucus) unless directed by a doctor. Do not exceed recommended dosage because at higher doses nervousness, dizziness, or sleeplessness may occur. May cause excitability, especially in children. If sore throat is severe, persists for more than 2 days, is accompanied or followed by fever, headache, rash, nausea or vomiting, consult a physician promptly. Do not take this product if you have asthma, glaucoma, heart disease, high blood pressure, emphysema, chronic pulmonary disease, shortness of breath, difficulty in breathing, diabetes, thyroid disease or difficulty in urination due to enlargement of the prostate gland unless directed by a doctor. May cause drowsiness, alcohol may increase the drowsiness effect. Avoid alcoholic beverages while taking this product. Use caution when driving a motor vehicle or operating machinery. DO NOT USE IF GLUED CARTON FLAP IS OPENED OR IF FOIL PACKET IS TORN OR BROKEN. KEEP THIS AND ALL MEDICATION OUT OF THE REACH OF CHILDREN. AS WITH ANY DRUG, IF YOU ARE PREGNANT OR NURSING A BABY, SEEK THE ADVICE OF A HEALTH PROFESSIONAL BEFORE USING THIS PRODUCT. IN CASE OF ACCIDENTAL OVERDOSAGE, CONTACT A PHYSICIAN OR POISON CONTROL CENTER IMMEDIATELY. PHENYLKETONURICS: CONTAINS PHENYLALANINE 11 MG PER PACKET.

DRUG INTERACTION PRECAUTION: Do not take this product if you are presently taking a prescription drug for high blood pressure or depression without first consulting your doctor."

OVERDOSAGE

Acetaminophen in massive overdosage may cause hepatic toxicity in some patients. In adults and adolescents, hepatic toxicity has rarely been reported following ingestion of acute overdosage of less than 10 grams. Fatalities are infrequent (less than 3–4% of untreated cases) and have rarely been reported with overdoses of less than 15 grams. In children, an acute overdosage of less than 150 mg/kg has not been associated with hepatic toxicity.

Early symptoms following a potentially hepatotoxic overdose may include: nausea, vomiting, diaphoresis and general malaise. Clinical and laboratory evidence of hepatic toxicity may not be apparent until 48 to 72 hours postingestion.

In adults and adolescents, regardless of the quantity of acetaminophen reported to have been ingested, administer MUCOMYST® acetylcysteine immediately if 24 hours or less have elapsed from the reported time of ingestion. For full prescribing information, refer to the MUCOMYST package insert. Do not await results of assays for acetaminophen level before initiating treatment with MUCOMYST acetylcysteine. The following additional procedures are recommended: The stomach should be emptied promptly by lavage or by induction of emesis with syrup of ipecac. A serum acetaminophen assay should be obtained as early as possible, but no sooner than four hours following ingestion. Liver function studies should be obtained initially and repeated at 24-hour intervals.

Serious toxicity or fatalities are extremely infrequent in children, possibly due to differences in the way they metabolize acetaminophen. In children, the maximum potential amount ingested can be more easily estimated. If more than 150 mg/kg or an unknown amount was ingested, obtain an acetaminophen plasma level. The acetaminophen plasma level should be obtained as soon as possible, but no sooner than 4 hours following the ingestion. Induce emesis using syrup of ipecac. If the plasma level is obtained and falls above the broken line on the acetaminophen overdose nomogram, the MUCOMYST acetylcysteine therapy should be initiated and continued for a full course of therapy. If acetaminophen plasma assay capability is not available, and the estimated acetaminophen ingestion exceeds 150 mg/kg, MUCOMYST acetylcysteine therapy should be initiated and continued for a full course of therapy.

For additional emergency information, call your regional poison center or call the Rocky Mountain Poison Center toll-free, (1-800-525-6115).

Symptoms from pseudoephedrine overdose consist most often of mild anxiety, tachycardia and/or mild hypertension. Symptoms usually appear within 4 to 8 hours of ingestion and are transient, usually requiring no treatment.

Acute dextromethorphan overdose usually does not result in serious signs and symptoms unless massive amounts have been ingested. Signs and symptoms of a substantial overdose may include nausea and vomiting, visual disturbances, CNS disturbances, and urinary retention.

Chlorpheniramine toxicity should be treated as you would an antihistamine/anticholinergic overdose and is likely to be present within a few hours after acute ingestion.

INACTIVE INGREDIENTS

Aspartame, Citric Acid, Flavors, Sodium Citrate, Starch, Sucrose, Tribasic Calcium Phosphate, Red #40 and Yellow #10.

HOW SUPPLIED

Packets of powder (yellow colored) cartons of 6 foil packets and cartons of 12 tamper-resistant foil cartons.

Shown in Product Identification Section, page 418

Multisymptom   OTC
TYLENOL® Cold Medication
Tablets and Caplets

DESCRIPTION

Each TYLENOL Cold Tablet or Caplet contains acetaminophen 325 mg., chlorpheniramine maleate 2 mg., pseudoephedrine hydrochloride 30 mg. and dextromethorphan hydrobromide 15 mg.

ACTIONS

TYLENOL Cold Medication Tablets and Caplets contain a clinically proven analgesic-antipyretic, decongestant, cough suppressant and antihistamine. Acetaminophen produces analgesia by elevation of the pain threshold and antipyresis through action on the hypothalamic heat-regulating center. Acetaminophen is equal to aspirin in analgesic and antipyretic effectiveness and it is unlikely to produce many of the side effects associated with aspirin and aspirin-containing products. Pseudoephedrine hydrochloride is a sympathomimetic amine which provides temporary relief of nasal con-

gestion. Dextromethorphan is a cough suppressant which provides temporary relief of coughs due to minor throat irritations that may occur with the common cold. Chlorpheniramine is an antihistamine which helps provide temporary relief of runny nose, sneezing and watery and itchy eyes.

INDICATIONS

TYLENOL Cold Medication provides effective temporary relief of runny nose, sneezing, watery and itchy eyes, nasal congestion, sore throat, coughing, and aches, pains and fever due to a cold or "flu."

PRECAUTIONS

If a rare sensitivity reaction occurs, the drug should be stopped. Although pseudoephedrine is virtually without pressor effect in normotensive patients, it should be used with caution in hypertensives.

USUAL DOSAGE

Adults: Two tablets or caplets every 6 hours, not to exceed 8 tablets or caplets in 24 hours. Children (6–12 years): One caplet or tablet every 6 hours, not to exceed 4 tablets or caplets in 24 hours for 5 days.

WARNING: Do not administer to children under 6 or exceed the recommended dosage because nervousness, dizziness or sleeplessness may occur. May cause excitability especially in children. Do not take this product for more than 7 days. If fever persists for more than three days, or if symptoms do not improve or are accompanied by high fever, consult a physician. A persistent cough may be a sign of a serious condition. If cough persists for more than 1 week, tends to recur or is accompanied by fever, rash or persistent headache, consult a physician. Do not take this product for persistent or chronic cough such as occurs with smoking, asthma, emphysema or if cough is accompanied by excessive phlegm (mucus) unless directed by a physician. This preparation may cause drowsiness, alcohol may increase the drowsiness effect. Avoid alcoholic beverages while taking this product. Use caution when driving a motor vehicle or operating machinery. If sore throat is severe, persists for more than 2 days, is accompanied or followed by fever, headache, rash, nausea or vomiting, consult a physician promptly. Do not take this product if you have heart disease, high blood pressure, thyroid disease, diabetes, asthma, glaucoma, emphysema, chronic pulmonary disease, shortness of breath, difficulty in breathing or difficulty in urination due to enlargement of the prostate gland unless directed by a physician.

DO NOT USE IF CARTON IS OPENED OR IF A BLISTER UNIT IS BROKEN. KEEP THIS AND ALL MEDICATION OUT OF THE REACH OF CHILDREN. AS WITH ANY DRUG, IF YOU ARE PREGNANT OR NURSING A BABY, SEEK THE ADVICE OF A HEALTH PROFESSIONAL BEFORE USING THIS PRODUCT. IN THE CASE OF ACCIDENTAL OVERDOSAGE CONTACT A PHYSICIAN OR POISON CONTROL CENTER IMMEDIATELY.

DRUG INTERACTION PRECAUTION: Do not take this product if you are presently taking a prescription drug for high blood pressure or depression without first consulting your physician.

OVERDOSAGE

Acetaminophen in massive overdosage may cause hepatic toxicity in some patients. In adults and adolescents, hepatic toxicity has rarely been reported following ingestion of acute overdosage of less than 10 grams. Fatalities are infrequent (less than 3–4% of untreated cases) and have rarely been reported with overdoses of less than 15 grams. In children, an acute overdosage of less than 150 mg/kg has not been associated with hepatic toxicity.

Early symptoms following a potentially hepatotoxic overdose may include: nausea, vomiting, diaphoresis and general malaise. Clinical and laboratory evidence of hepatic toxicity may not be apparent until 48 to 72 hours postingestion.

In adults and adolescents, regardless of the quantity of acetaminophen reported to have been ingested, administer MUCOMYST® acetylcysteine immediately if 24 hours or less have elapsed from the reported time of ingestion. For full prescribing information, refer to the MUCOMYST package insert. Do not await results of assays for acetaminophen level before initiating treatment with MUCOMYST acetylcysteine. The following additional procedures are recommended: The stomach should be emptied promptly by lavage or by induction of emesis with syrup of ipecac. A serum acetaminophen assay should be obtained as early as possible, but no sooner than four hours following ingestion. Liver function studies should be obtained initially and repeated at 24-hour intervals.

Serious toxicity or fatalities are extremely infrequent in children, possibly due to differences in the way they metabolize acetaminophen. In children, the maximum potential amount ingested can be more easily estimated. If more than 150 mg/kg or an unknown amount was ingested, obtain an acetaminophen plasma level. The acetaminophen plasma level should be obtained as soon as possible, but no sooner than 4 hours following the ingestion. Induce emesis using syrup of ipecac. If the plasma level is obtained and falls above the broken line on the acetaminophen overdose nomogram, the MUCOMYST acetylcysteine therapy should be initiated and continued for a full course of therapy. If acetaminophen plasma assay capability is not available, and the estimated acetaminophen ingestion exceeds 150 mg/kg, MUCOMYST acetylcysteine therapy should be initiated and continued for a full course of therapy.

For additional emergency information, call your regional poison center or call the Rocky Mountain Poison Center toll-free, (1-800-525-6115).

Chlorpheniramine toxicity should be treated as you would an antihistamine/anticholinergic overdose and is likely to be present within a few hours after acute ingestion.

Symptoms from pseudoephedrine overdose consist most often of mild anxiety, tachycardia and/or mild hypertension. Symptoms usually appear within 4 to 8 hours of ingestion and are transient, usually requiring no treatment.

Acute dextromethorphan overdose usually does not result in serious signs and symptoms unless massive amounts have been ingested. Signs and symptoms of a substantial overdose may include nausea and vomiting, visual disturbances, CNS disturbances, and urinary retention.

INACTIVE INGREDIENTS

Tablets: Cellulose, Starch, Magnesium Stearate, Yellow #6 and Yellow #10. Caplets: Cellulose, Glyceryl Triacetate, Hydroxypropyl Methylcellulose, Magnesium Stearate, Sodium Starch Glycolate, Corn Starch, Titanium Dioxide, Blue #1 and Yellow #6 & #10.

HOW SUPPLIED

Tablets (colored yellow, imprinted "TYLENOL Cold")—blister packs of 24 and tamper-resistant bottles of 50. Caplets (light yellow, imprinted "TYLENOL Cold")—blister packs of 24 and tamper-resistant bottles of 50.

Shown in Product Identification Section, page 418

TYLENOL® Cold Medication OTC
No Drowsiness Formula
Caplets and Gelcaps

DESCRIPTION

Each TYLENOL Cold Medication No Drowsiness Formula Caplet and Gelcap contains acetaminophen 325 mg., pseudoephedrine hydrochloride 30 mg. and dextromethorphan hydrobromide 15 mg.

ACTIONS

TYLENOL Cold Medication No Drowsiness Formula Caplets and Gelcaps contain a clinically proven analgesic-antipyretic, decongestant and cough suppressant. Acetaminophen produces analgesia by elevation of the pain threshold and antipyresis through action on the hypothalamic heat-regulating center. Acetaminophen is equal to aspirin in analgesic and antipyretic effectiveness and it is unlikely to produce many of the side effects associated with aspirin and aspirin-containing products. Pseudoephedrine hydrochloride is a sympathomimetic amine which provides temporary relief of nasal congestion. Dextromethorphan is a cough suppressant which provides temporary relief of coughs due to minor throat irritations that may occur with the common cold.

INDICATIONS

TYLENOL Cold Medication No Drowsiness Formula provides effective temporary relief of the nasal congestion, sore throat, coughing, and aches, pains and fever due to a cold or "flu."

PRECAUTIONS

If a rare sensitivity reaction occurs, the drug should be stopped. Although pseudoephedrine is virtually without pressor effect in normotensive patients, it should be used with caution in hypertensives.

USUAL DOSAGE

Adults (12 years and older): Two caplets or gelcaps every 6 hours, not to exceed 8 caplets in 24 hours. Children (6–12 years): One caplet or gelcap every 6 hours, not to exceed 4 caplets or gelcaps in 24 hours for 5 days.

WARNING: Do not administer to children under 6 or exceed the recommended dosage because nervousness, dizziness or sleeplessness may occur. Do not take this product for more than 7 days. If fever persists for more than three days, or if symptoms do not improve or are accompanied by high fever, consult a physician. A persistent cough may be a sign of a serious condition. If cough persists for more than 1 week, tends to recur or is accompanied by fever, rash or persistent headache, consult a physician. Do not take this product for persistent or chronic cough such as occurs with smoking, asthma, emphysema or if cough is accompanied by excessive phlegm (mucus) unless directed by a physician. If sore throat is severe, persists for more than 2 days, is accompanied or followed by fever, headache, rash, nausea or vomiting, consult a physician promptly. Do not take this product if you have heart disease, high blood pressure, thyroid disease, diabetes, or difficulty in urination due to enlargement of the prostate gland unless directed by a physician.

DO NOT USE IF CARTON IS OPENED OR IF A BLISTER UNIT IS BROKEN. KEEP THIS AND ALL MEDICATION OUT OF THE REACH OF CHILDREN. AS WITH ANY DRUG, IF YOU ARE PREGNANT OR NURSING A BABY, SEEK THE ADVICE OF HEALTH PROFESSIONAL BEFORE USING THIS PRODUCT. IN THE CASE OF ACCIDENTAL OVERDOSAGE CONTACT A PHYSICIAN OR POISON CONTROL CENTER IMMEDIATELY.

DRUG INTERACTION PRECAUTION: Do not take this product if you are presently taking a prescription drug for high blood pressure or depression without first consulting your physician.

OVERDOSAGE

Acetaminophen in massive overdosage may cause hepatic toxicity in some patients. In adults and adolescents, hepatic toxicity has rarely been reported following ingestion of acute overdosage of less than 10 grams. Fatalities are infrequent (less than 3–4% of untreated cases) and have rarely been reported with overdosage of less than 15 grams. In children, an acute overdosage of less than 150 mg/kg has not been associated with hepatic toxicity.

Early symptoms following a potentially hepatotoxic overdose may include: nausea, vomiting, diaphoresis and general malaise. Clinical and laboratory evidence of hepatic toxicity may not be apparent until 48 to 72 hours postingestion.

In adults and adolescents, regardless of the quantity of acetaminophen reported to have been ingested, administer MUCOMYST® acetylcysteine immediately if 24 hours or less have elapsed from the reported time of ingestion. For full prescribing information, refer to the MUCOMYST package insert. Do not await results of assays for acetaminophen level before initiating treatment with MUCOMYST acetylcysteine. The following additional procedures are recommended: The stomach should be emptied promptly by lavage or by induction of emesis with syrup of ipecac. A serum acetaminophen assay should be obtained as early as possible, but no sooner than four hours following ingestion. Liver function studies should be obtained initially and repeated at 24–hour intervals.

Serious toxicity or fatalities are extremely infrequent in children, possibly due to differences in the way they metabolize acetaminophen. In children, the maximum potential amount ingested can be more easily estimated. If more than 150 mg/kg or an unknown amount was ingested, obtain an acetaminophen plasma level. The acetaminophen plasma level should be obtained as soon as possible, but no sooner than 4 hours following the ingestion. Induce emesis using syrup of ipecac. If the plasma level is obtained and falls above the broken line on the acetaminophen overdose nomogram, the MUCOMYST acetylcysteine therapy should be initiated and continued for a full course of therapy. If acetaminophen plasma assay capability is not available, and the estimated acetaminophen ingestion exceeds 150 mg/kg. MUCOMYST acetylcysteine therapy should be initiated and continued for a full course of therapy.

For additional emergency information, call your regional poison center or call the Rocky Mountain Poison Center toll-free, (1-800-525-6115).

Symptoms from pseudoephedrine overdose consist most often of mild anxiety, tachycardia and/or mild hypertension. Symptoms usually appear within 4 to 8 hours of ingestion and are transient, usually requiring no treatment.

Acute dextromethorphan overdose usually does not result in serious signs and symptoms unless massive amounts have been ingested. Signs and symptoms of a substantial overdose may include nausea and vomiting, visual disturbances, CNS disturbances, and urinary retention.

INACTIVE INGREDIENTS

Caplet: Cellulose, Glyceryl Triacetate, Hydroxypropyl Methylcellulose, Magnesium Stearate, Sodium Starch Glycolate, Starch, Titanium Dioxide, Blue #1 and Yellow #10. Gelcap: Benzyl Alcohol, Butylparaben, Castor Oil, Cellulose, Corn Starch, Edetate Calcium Disodium, Gelatin, Hydroxpropyl Methylcellose, Magnesium Sterate, Methylparaben, Propylparaben, Sodium Propionate, Sodium Lauryl Sulfate, Sodium Starch Glycolate, Titanium Dioxide, Red #40 and Yellow #10.

HOW SUPPLIED

Caplets (colored white, imprinted TYLENOL "cold")—blister packs of 24 and tamper-resistant bottles of 50.

Gelcaps (colored red and tan, imprinted TYLENOL COLD)—blister packs of 20 and tamper-resistant bottles of 40.

Shown in Product Identification Section, page 418

Continued on next page

McNeil Consumer—Cont.

No Drowsiness Formula
TYLENOL® Cold & Flu Hot Medication OTC
Packets

DESCRIPTION

Each packet of No Drowsiness TYLENOL Cold & Flu contains acetaminophen 650 mg., pseudoephedrine hydrochloride 60 mg and dextromethorphan hydrobromide 30 mg.

ACTIONS

No Drowsiness TYLENOL Cold and Flu Hot Medication contains a clinically proven analgesic-antipyretic, decongestant, and cough suppressant. Acetaminophen produces analgesia by elevation of the pain threshold and antipyresis through action on the hypothalamic heat-regulating center. Acetaminophen is equal to aspirin in analgesic and antipyretic effectiveness and it is unlikely to produce many of the side effects associated with aspirin and aspirin-containing products. Pseudoephedrine hydrochloride is a sympathomimetic amine which provides temporary relief of nasal congestion. Dextromethorphan is a cough suppressant which provides temporary relief of coughs due to minor throat irritations that may occur with the common cold.

INDICATIONS

No Drowsiness TYLENOL Cold and Flu Hot Medication provides effective temporary relief of nasal congestion, sore throat, coughing, and aches, pains, and fever due to a cold or "flu."

PRECAUTIONS

If a rare sensitivity reaction occurs, the drug should be stopped. Although pseudoephedrine is virtually without pressor effect in normotensive patients, it should be used with caution in hypertensives.

USUAL DOSAGE

Adults (12 years and over): Dissolve one packet in 6 oz. cup of hot water. Sip while hot. Sweeten to taste, if desired. May repeat every 6 hours, not to exceed 4 doses in 24 hours.

"**WARNING:** Not recommended for children under 12. Do not take this product for more than 7 days or for fever for more than 3 days unless directed by a doctor. If symptoms do not improve or are accompanied by fever, consult a doctor. A persistent cough may be a sign of a serious condition. If cough persists for more than 1 week, tends to recur or is accompanied by fever, rash or persistent headache, consult a doctor. Do not take this product for persistent or chronic cough such as occurs with smoking, asthma, emphysema, or if cough is accompanied by excessive phlegm (mucus) unless directed by a doctor. Do not exceed recommended dosage because at higher doses nervousness, dizziness, or sleeplessness may occur. May cause excitability, especially in children. If sore throat is severe, persists for more than 2 days, is accompanied or followed by fever, headache, rash, nausea or vomiting, consult a physician promptly. Do not take this product if you have asthma, glaucoma, heart disease, high blood pressure, emphysema, chronic pulmonary disease, shortness of breath, difficulty in breathing, diabetes, thyroid disease or difficulty in urination due to enlargement of the prostate gland unless directed by a doctor.

DO NOT USE IF GLUED CARTON FLAP IS OPENED OR IF FOIL PACKET IS TORN OR BROKEN. KEEP THIS AND ALL MEDICATION OUT OF THE REACH OF CHILDREN. AS WITH ANY DRUG, IF YOU ARE PREGNANT OR NURSING A BABY, SEEK THE ADVICE OF A HEALTH PROFESSIONAL BEFORE USING THIS PRODUCT. IN CASE OF ACCIDENTAL OVERDOSAGE, CONTACT A PHYSICIAN OR POISON CONTROL CENTER IMMEDIATELY. PHENYLKETONURICS: CONTAINS PHENYLALANINE 11 MG PER PACKET.

DRUG INTERACTION PRECAUTION: Do not take this product if you are presently taking a prescription drug for high blood pressure or depression without first consulting your doctor."

OVERDOSAGE

Acetaminophen in massive overdosage may cause hepatic toxicity in some patients. In adults and adolescents, hepatic toxicity has rarely been reported following ingestion of acute overdosage of less than 10 grams. Fatalities are infrequent (less than 3–4% of untreated cases) and have rarely been reported with overdoses of less than 15 grams. In children, an acute overdosage of less than 150 mg/kg has not been associated with hepatic toxicity.

Early symptoms following a potentially hepatotoxic overdose may include: nausea, vomiting, diaphoresis and general malaise. Clinical and laboratory evidence of hepatic toxicity may not be apparent until 48 to 72 hours postingestion. In adults and adolescents, regardless of the quantity of acetaminophen reported to have been ingested, administer MUCOMYST® acetylcysteine immediately if 24 hours or less have elapsed from the reported time of ingestion. For full prescribing information, refer to the MUCOMYST package insert. Do not await results of assays for acetaminophen level before initiating treatment with MUCOMYST acetylcysteine. The following additional procedures are recommended. The stomach should be emptied promptly by lavage or by induction of emesis with syrup of ipecac. A serum acetaminophen assay should be obtained as early as possible, but no sooner than four hours following ingestion. Liver function studies should be obtained initially and repeated at 24-hour intervals.

Serious toxicity or fatalities are extremely infrequent in children, possibly due to differences in the way they metabolize acetaminophen. In children, the maximum potential amount ingested can be more easily estimated. If more than 150 mg/kg or an unknown amount was ingested, obtain an acetaminophen plasma level. The acetaminophen plasma level should be obtained as soon as possible, but not sooner than 4 hours following the ingestion. Induce emesis using syrup of ipecac. If the plasma level is obtained and falls above the broken line on the acetaminophen overdose nomogram, the MUCOMYST acetylcysteine therapy should be initiated and continued for a full course of therapy. If acetaminophen plasma assay capability is not available, and the estimated acetaminophen ingestion exceeds 150 mg/kg, MUCOMYST acetylcysteine therapy should be initiated and continued for a full course of therapy.

For additional emergency information, call your regional poison center or call the Rocky Mountain Poison Control toll-free, (1-800-525-6115).

Symptoms from pseudoephedrine overdose consist most often of mild anxiety, tachycardia and/or mild hypertension. Symptoms usually appear within 4 to 8 hours of ingestion and are transient, usually requiring no treatment.

Acute dextromethorphan overdose usually does not result in serious signs and symptoms unless massive amounts have been ingested. Signs and symptoms of a substantial overdose may include nausea and vomiting, visual disturbances. CNS disturbances and urinary retention.

INACTIVE INGREDIENTS

Aspartame, Citric Acid, Flavors, Sodium Citrate, Starch, Sucrose, Tribasic Calcium Phosphate, Red #40 and Yellow #10.

HOW SUPPLIED

Packets of powder (yellow colored) cartons of 6 foil packets and cartons of 12 tamper-resistant foil cartons.

Shown in Product Identification Section, page 418

TYLENOL® Cold Night Time Medication OTC
Liquid

DESCRIPTION

Each 30 ml (1 fl. oz.) contains acetaminophen 650 mg., diphenhydramine hydrochloride 50 mg., pseudoephedrine hydrochloride 60 mg., (alcohol 10%).

ACTIONS

TYLENOL Cold Night Time Medication Liquid contains a clinically proven analgesic-antipyretic, decongestant, cough suppressant and antihistamine. Acetaminophen produces analgesia by elevation of the pain threshold and antipyresis through action on the hypothalamic heat-regulating center. Acetaminophen is equal to aspirin in analgesic and antipyretic effectiveness and it is unlikely to produce many of the side effects associated with aspirin and aspirin-containing products. Pseudoephedrine hydrochloride is a sympathomimetic amine which provides temporary relief of nasal congestion. Diphenhydramine is an antihistamine which helps provide temporary relief of runny nose, sneezing and watery and itchy eyes.

INDICATIONS

TYLENOL Cold Night Time Medication Liquid provides effective temporary relief of runny nose, sneezing, watery and itchy eyes, nasal congestion, and aches, pains, sore throat and fevers due to a cold or "flu."

PRECAUTIONS

If a rare sensitivity reaction occurs, the drug should be stopped. Although pseudoephedrine is virtually without pressor effect in normotensive patients, it should be used with caution in hypertensives.

USUAL DOSAGE

Measuring cup is provided and marked for accurate dosing. Adults (12 years and over): 1 fluid ounce (2 tbsp.) in measuring cup provided every 6 hours, not to exceed 4 doses in 24 hours. Not recommended for children.

WARNINGS: Do not take this product for more than 7 days or for fever for more than 3 days unless directed by a doctor. If symptoms do not improve or are accompanied by fever, consult a doctor. If sore throat is severe, persists for more than 2 days, is accompanied or followed by fever, headache, rash, nausea or vomiting, consult a physician promptly. Do not exceed recommended dosage because at higher doses nervousness, dizziness or sleeplessness may occur. May cause excitability, especially in children. Do not take this product if you have asthma, glaucoma, heart disease, high blood pressure, emphysema, chronic pulmonary disease, shortness of breath, difficulty in breathing, diabetes, thyroid disease or difficulty in urination due to enlargement of the prostate gland, or if you are taking sedatives or tranquilizers, unless directed by a doctor. May cause marked drowsiness; alcohol, sedatives and tranquilizers may increase the drowsiness effect. Avoid alcoholic beverages while taking this product. Use caution when driving a motor vehicle or operating machinery.

DO NOT USE IF CARTON IS OPENED OR IF PRINTED PLASTIC WRAP OR PRINTED FOIL INNER SEAL IS BROKEN. KEEP THIS AND ALL MEDICATION OUT OF THE REACH OF CHILDREN. AS WITH ANY DRUG, IF YOU ARE PREGNANT OR NURSING A BABY, SEEK THE ADVICE OF A HEALTH PROFESSIONAL BEFORE USING THIS PRODUCT. IN CASE OF ACCIDENTAL OVERDOSAGE, CONTACT A PHYSICIAN OR POISON CONTROL CENTER IMMEDIATELY.

DRUG INTERACTION PRECAUTION: Do not take this product if you are presently taking a prescription drug for high blood pressure or depression without first consulting your doctor.

OVERDOSAGE

Acetaminophen in massive overdosage may cause hepatic toxicity in some patients. In adults and adolescents, hepatic toxicity has rarely been reported following ingestion of acute overdosage of less than 10 grams. Fatalities are infrequent (less than 3–4% of untreated cases) and have rarely been reported with overdoses of less than 15 grams. In children, an acute overdosage of less than 150 mg/kg has not been associated with hepatic toxicity.

Early symptoms following a potentially hepatotoxic overdose may include: nausea, vomiting, diaphoresis and general malaise. Clinical and laboratory evidence of hepatic toxicity may not be apparent until 48 to 72 hours postingestion.

In adults and adolescents, regardless of the quantity of acetaminophen reported to have been ingested, administer MUCOMYST® acetylcysteine immediately if 24 hours or less have elapsed from the reported time of ingestion. For full prescribing information, refer to the MUCOMYST package insert. Do not await results of assays for acetaminophen level before initiating treatment with MUCOMYST acetylcysteine. The following additional procedures are recommended: The stomach should be emptied promptly by lavage or by induction of emesis with syrup of ipecac. A serum acetaminophen assay should be obtained as early as possible, but no sooner than four hours following ingestion. Liver function studies should be obtained initially and repeated at 24-hour intervals.

Serious toxicity or fatalities are extremely infrequent in children, possibly due to differences in the way they metabolize acetaminophen. In children, the maximum potential amount ingested can be more easily estimated. If more than 150 mg/kg or an unknown amount was ingested, obtain an acetaminophen plasma level. The acetaminophen plasma level should be obtained as soon as possible, but no sooner than 4 hours following the ingestion. Induce emesis using syrup of ipecac. If the plasma level is obtained and falls above the broken line on the acetaminophen overdose nomogram, the MUCOMYST acetylcysteine therapy should be initiated and continued for a full course of therapy. If acetaminophen plasma assay capability is not available, and the estimated acetaminophen ingestion exceeds 150 mg/kg, MUCOMYST acetylcysteine therapy should be initiated and continued for a full course of therapy.

For additional emergency information, call your regional poison center or call the Rocky Mountain Poison Center toll-free, (1-800-525-6115).

Diphenhydramine toxicity should be treated as you would an antihistamine/anticholinergic overdose and is likely to be present within a few hours after acute ingestion.

Symptoms from pseudoephedrine overdose consist most often of mild anxiety, tachycardia and/or mild hypertension. Symptoms usually appear within 4 to 8 hours of ingestion and are transient, usually requiring no treatment.

INACTIVE INGREDIENTS

Alcohol (10%), Citric Acid, Flavors, Glycerin, Polyethylene Glycol, Purified Water, Sodium Benzoate, Sucrose, Red #40, Red #33 and Blue #1.

HOW SUPPLIED

Cherry flavored (colored red) in 5 oz. bottles with child-resistant safety cap, special dosage cup graded in ounces and tablespoons, and tamper-resistant packaging.

Shown in Product Identification Section, page 418

Maximum-Strength OTC
TYLENOL® Allergy Sinus Medication Caplets, Gelcaps

DESCRIPTION
Each TYLENOL® Allergy Sinus Caplet or Gelcap contains acetaminophen 500 mg, chlorpheniramine maleate 2 mg, and pseudoephedrine hydrochloride 30 mg.

ACTIONS
TYLENOL® Allergy Sinus Caplets or Gelcaps contain a clinically proven analgesic-antipyretic, decongestant, and antihistamine. Acetaminophen produces analgesia by elevation of the pain threshold and antipyresis through action on the hypothalamic heat-regulating center. Acetaminophen is equal to aspirin in analgesic and antipyretic effectiveness, and it is unlikely to produce many of the side effects associated with aspirin and aspirin-containing products. Pseudoephedrine hydrochloride is a sympathomimetic amine which provides temporary relief of nasal congestion. Chlorpheniramine is an antihistamine which helps provide temporary relief of runny nose, sneezing and watery and itchy eyes.

INDICATIONS
TYLENOL® Allergy Sinus provides effective temporary relief of these upper respiratory allergy, hay fever and sinusitis symptoms: sneezing, itchy, watery eyes, runny nose, itching of the nose or throat, nasal and sinus congestion and sinus pain and headaches.

PRECAUTIONS
If a rare sensitivity reaction occurs, the drug should be stopped. Although pseudoephedrine is virtually without pressor effect in normotensive patients, it should be used with caution in hypertensives.

USUAL DOSAGE
Adults: Two caplets or gelcaps every 6 hours, not to exceed 8 caplets or gelcaps in 24 hours.
"WARNING: Do not administer to children under 12 or exceed the recommended dosage because nervousness, dizziness, or sleeplessness may occur. May cause excitability, especially in children. This preparation may cause drowsiness; alcohol may increase the drowsiness effect. Avoid alcoholic beverages when taking this product. Use caution when driving a motor vehicle or operating machinery. Do not take this product if you have heart disease, high blood pressure, thyroid disease, diabetes, asthma, glaucoma, emphysema, chronic pulmonary disease, shortness of breath, difficulty in breathing or difficulty in urination due to enlargement of prostate gland unless directed by a doctor. Do not take this product for more than 7 days. If symptoms do not improve or are accompanied by a high fever, consult a physician." **DO NOT USE IF CARTON IS OPEN OR IF A BLISTER UNIT IS BROKEN. KEEP THIS AND ALL MEDICATION OUT OF THE REACH OF CHILDREN. AS WITH ANY DRUG, IF YOU ARE PREGNANT OR NURSING A BABY, SEEK THE ADVICE OF A HEALTH PROFESSIONAL BEFORE USING THIS PRODUCT. IN THE CASE OF ACCIDENTAL OVERDOSE, CONTACT A PHYSICIAN OR POISON CONTROL CENTER IMMEDIATELY.**
DRUG INTERACTION PRECAUTION: Do not take this product if you are presently taking a prescription drug for high blood pressure or depression without first consulting your doctor.

OVERDOSAGE
Acetaminophen in massive overdosage may cause hepatic toxicity in some patients. In adults and adolescents, hepatic toxicity has rarely been reported following ingestion of acute overdosage of less than 10 grams. Fatalities are infrequent (less than 3–4% of untreated cases) and have rarely been reported with overdoses of less than 15 grams. In children, an acute overdosage of less than 150 mg/kg has not been associated with hepatic toxicity.
Early symptoms following a potentially hepatotoxic overdose may include: nausea, vomiting, diaphoresis and general malaise. Clinical and laboratory evidence of hepatic toxicity may not be apparent until 48 to 72 hours postingestion. In adults and adolescents, regardless of the quantity of acetaminophen reported to have been ingested, administer MUCOMYST® acetylcysteine immediately if 24 hours or less have elapsed from the reported time of ingestion. For full prescribing information, refer to the MUCOMYST package insert. Do not await results of assays for acetaminophen level before initiating treatment with MUCOMYST acetylcysteine. The following additional procedures are recommended: The stomach should be emptied promptly by lavage or by induction of emesis with syrup of ipecac. A serum acetaminophen assay should be obtained as early as possible, but no sooner than four hours following ingestion. Liver function studies should be obtained initially and repeated at 24-hour intervals.
Several toxicity or fatalities are extremely infrequent in children, possibly due to differences in the way they metabolize acetaminophen. In children, the maximum potential amount ingested can be easily estimated. If more than 150 mg/kg or an unknown amount was ingested, obtain an acetaminophen plasma level. The acetaminophen plasma level should be obtained as soon as possible, but no sooner than 4 hours following ingestion. Induce emesis using syrup of ipecac. If the plasma level is obtained and falls above the broken line on the acetaminophen overdose nomogram, the MUCOMYST acetylcysteine therapy should be initiated and continued for a full course of therapy. If acetaminophen plasma assay capability is not available, and the estimated acetaminophen ingestion exceeds 150 mg/kg, MUCOMYST acetylcysteine therapy should be initiated and continued for a full course of therapy.
For additional emergency information, call your regional poison center or call the Rocky Mountain Poison Control Center toll-free, (1-800-525-6115).
Chlorpheniramine toxicity should be treated as you would an antihistamine/anticholinergic overdose and is likely to be present within a few hours after acute ingestion.
Symptoms from pseudoephedrine overdose consist most often of mild anxiety, tachycardia and/or hypertension. Symptoms usually appear within 4 to 8 hours of ingestion and are transient, usually requiring no treatment.

INACTIVE INGREDIENTS
CAPLET: Cellulose, hydroxypropyl cellulose, hydroxypropyl methylcellulose, magnesium stearate, polyethylene glycol, sodium starch glycolate, corn starch, titanium dioxide, blue #1, yellow #6, yellow #10.
GELCAP: Benzyl Alcohol, Butylparaben, Castor oil, Cellulose, Edetate Calcium Disodium, Gelatin, Hydroxypropyl Methylcellulose, Magnesium Stearate, Methylparaben, Propylparaben, Sodium Lauryl Sulfate, Sodium Propionate, Sodium Starch Glycolate, Starch, Titanium Dioxide Blue #1 and #2 and Yellow #10.

HOW SUPPLIED
Caplets: (dark yellow, imprinted "TYLENOL Allergy Sinus")—Blister packs of 24 and tamper-resistant bottles of 50.
Gelcaps: (dark green and dark yellow, imprinted "TYLENOL A/S")—Blister packs of 24 and tamper-resistant bottles of 50.
Shown in Product Identification Section, page 418

MAXIMUM STRENGTH TYLENOL® OTC
COUGH MEDICATION

DESCRIPTION
Each 20 ml (4 tsp.) adult dose contains dextromethorphan HBr 30 mg., and acetaminophen 1,000mg.

ACTIONS
MAXIMUM STRENGTH TYLENOL® COUGH Medication Liquid contains a clinically proven cough suppressant and analgesic-antipyretic. Acetaminophen produces analgesia by elevation of the pain threshold and antipyresis through action on the hypothalamic heat-regulating center. Dextromethorphan is a cough suppressant which provides temporary relief of coughs due to minor throat irritations that may occur with the common cold.

INDICATIONS
MAXIMUM STRENGTH TYLENOL® COUGH Medication provides effective, temporary relief of coughing, and the aches, pains and sore throat that may accompany a cough due to a cold.

USUAL DOSAGE
A specially marked dosage cup is provided for accurate dosing. Adults: (12 years and older) 4 teaspoons or 20ml as marked on dosage cup every 6–8 hours, not to exceed 4 doses in 24 hours. Children: (ages 6–11) 1 1/4 teaspoons or 6.25ml as marked on dosage cup every 4 hours, not to exceed 5 doses in 24 hours. Not recommended for children under 6 years.
"**WARNING:** Do not take this product for more than 10 days or for fever for more than 3 days unless directed by a physician. Severe or recurrent pain or high or continued fever may be indicative of serious illness. Under these conditions, consult a physician. A persistent cough may be a sign of a serious condition. If cough persists for more than 1 week, tends to recur or is accompanied by fever, rash or persistent headache, consult a doctor. Do not take this product for persistent or chronic cough such as occurs with smoking, asthma, emphysema, or if cough is accompanied by excessive phlegm (mucus) unless directed by a doctor. If sore throat is severe, persists for more than 2 days, is accompanied or followed by fever, headache, rash, nausea or vomiting, consult a doctor promptly. Keep this and all medication out of the reach of children. As with any drug, if you are pregnant or nursing a baby, seek the advice of a health professional before using this product. In case of accidental overdosage, contact a doctor or poison control center immediately."

DRUG INTERACTION PRECAUTION
Do not take this product if you are presently taking a prescription drug containing a monoamine oxidase inhibitor (MAOI) without first consulting your doctor.

OVERDOSAGE
Acetaminophen in massive dosage may cause hepatic toxicity in some patients. In adults and adolescents, hepatic toxicity has rarely been reported following ingestion of acute overdosage of less than 10 grams. Fatalities are infrequent (less than 3–4% of untreated cases) and have rarely been reported with overdoses of less than 15 grams. In children, an acute overdosage of less than 150mg/kg has not been associated with hepatic toxicity.
Early symptoms following a potentially hepatotoxic overdose may include: nausea, vomiting, diaphoresis and general malaise. Clinical and laboratory evidence of hepatic toxicity may not be apparent until 48 to 72 hours postingestion. In adults and adolescents, regardless of the quantity of acetaminophen reported to have been ingested, administer MUCOMYST® acetylcysteine immediately if 24 hours or less have elapsed from the reported time of ingestion. For full prescribing information, refer to the MUCOMYST package insert. Do not await results of assays for acetaminophen level before initiating treatment with MUCOMYST acetylcysteine. The following additional procedures are recommended: The stomach should be emptied by lavage or by induction of emesis with syrup of ipecac. A serum acetaminophen assay should be obtained as early as possible, but no sooner than four hours following ingestion. Liver function studies should be obtained initially and repeated at 24-hour intervals.
Serious toxicity or fatalities are extremely infrequent in children, possibly due to differences in the way they metabolize acetaminophen. In children, the maximum potential amount ingested can be more easily estimated. If more than 150mg/kg or an unknown amount was ingested, obtain an acetaminophen plasma level. The acetaminophen plasma level should be obtained as soon as possible, but no sooner than 4 hours following the ingestion. Induce emesis using syrup of ipecac. If the plasma level is obtained and falls above the broken line on the acetaminophen overdose nomogram, the MUCOMYST acetylcysteine therapy should be initiated and continued for a full course of therapy. If acetaminophen plasma assay capability is not available, and the estimated acetaminophen ingestion exceeds 150mg/kg, MUCOMYST acetycysteine therapy should be initiated and continued for a full course of therapy.
For additional emergency information, call your regional poison center or call the Rocky Mountain Poison Center toll free (1-800-526-6115).
Acute dextromethorphan overdose usually does not result in serious signs and symptoms unless massive amounts have been ingested. Signs and symptoms of a substantial overdose may include nausea and vomiting, visual disturbances, CNS disturbances, and urinary retention.

INACTIVE INGREDIENTS
Alcohol (10%), Citric Acid, Flavors, Glycerin, Polyethylene Glycol, Purified Water, Sodium Benzoate, Sodium Carboxymethylcellulose, Sodium Saccharin, Sorbitol, Sucrose, Red #33, and Red #40.

HOW SUPPLIED
MAXIMUM STRENGTH TYLENOL® COUGH is available in a 4 oz. bottle with child-resistant safety cap, special dosing cup marked in ml, and tamper resistant packaging.
Shown in Product Identification Section, page 418

MAXIMUM STRENGTH TYLENOL® OTC
COUGH MEDICATION WITH DECONGESTANT

DESCRIPTION
Each 20 ml (4 tsp.) adult dose contains dextromethorphan HBr 30 mg., and acetaminophen 1,000mg, and pseudoephedrine HCl 60mg.

ACTIONS
MAXIMUM STRENGTH TYLENOL® COUGH Medication Liquid with Decongestant contains a clinically proven cough suppressant, an analgesic-antipyretic, and decongestant. Acetaminophen produces analgesia by elevation of the pain threshold and antipyresis through action on the hypothalamic heat-regulating center. Dextromethorphan is a cough suppressant which provides temporary relief of coughs due to minor throat irritations that may occur with the common cold. Pseudoephedrine hydrochloride is a sympathomimetic amine which provides temporary relief of nasal congestion.

INDICATIONS
MAXIMUM STRENGTH TYLENOL® COUGH Medication provides effective, temporary relief of coughing, and the aches, pains and sore throat that may accompany a cough due to a cold.

USUAL DOSAGE
A specially marked dosage cup is provided for accurate dosing. Adults: (12 years and older) 4 teaspoons or 20ml as marked on dosage cup every 6–8 hours, not to exceed 4 doses

Continued on next page

McNeil Consumer—Cont.

in 24 hours. Children: (ages 6–11) 1 1/4 teaspoons or 6.25ml as marked on dosage cup every 4 hours, not to exceed 5 doses in 24 hours. Not recommended for children under 6 years.

"**WARNING:** Do not take this product for more than 7 days or for fever for more than 3 days unless directed by a doctor. If symptoms do not improve or are accompanied by fever, consult a physician. A persistent cough may be a sign of a serious condition. If cough persists for more than 1 week, tends to recur or is accompanied by fever, rash or persistent headache, consult a doctor. Do not take this product for persistent or chronic cough such as occurs with smoking, asthma, emphysema, or if cough is accompanied by excessive phlegm (mucus) unless directed by a doctor. Do not exceed the recommended dosage because at higher doses nervousness, dizziness or sleeplessness may occur. Do not take this product if you have heart disease, high blood pressure, thyroid disease, diabetes or difficulty in urination due to enlargement of the prostate gland unless directed by a doctor. If sore throat is severe, persists for more than 2 days, is accompanied or followed by fever, headache, rash, nausea or vomiting, consult a doctor promptly. Keep this and all medication out of the reach of children. As with any drug, if you are pregnant or nursing a baby, seek the advice of a health professional before using this product. In case of accidental overdosage, contact a doctor or poison control center immediately."

DRUG INTERACTION PRECAUTION

Do not take this product if you are presently taking a prescription drug containing a monoamine oxidase inhibitor (MAOI) without first consulting your doctor.

OVERDOSAGE

Acetaminophen in massive dosage may cause hepatic toxicity in some patients. In adults and adolescents, hepatic toxicity has rarely been reported following ingestion of acute overdosage of less than 10 grams. Fatalities are infrequent (less than 3–4% of untreated cases) and have rarely been reported with overdoses of less than 15 grams. In children, an acute overdosage of less than 150mg/kg has not been associated with hepatic toxicity.

Early symptoms following a potentially hepatotoxic overdose may include: nausea, vomiting, diaphoresis and general malaise. Clinical and laboratory evidence of hepatic toxicity may not be apparent until 48 to 72 hours postingestion. In adults and adolescents, regardless of the quantity of acetaminophen reported to have been ingested, administer MUCOMYST® acetylcysteine immediately if 24 hours or less have elapsed from the reported time of ingestion. For full prescribing information, refer to the MUCOMYST package insert. Do not await results of assays for acetaminophen level before initiating treatment with MUCOMYST acetylcysteine. The following additional procedures are recommended: The stomach should be emptied by lavage or by induction of emesis with syrup of ipecac. A serum acetaminophen assay should be obtained as early as possible, but no sooner than four hours following ingestion. Liver function studies should be obtained initially and repeated at 24-hour intervals.

Serious toxicity or fatalities are extremely infrequent in children, possibly due to differences in the way they metabolize acetaminophen. In children, the maximum potential amount ingested can be more easily estimated. If more than 150mg/kg or an unknown amount was ingested, obtain an acetaminophen plasma level. The acetaminophen plasma level should be obtained as soon as possible, but no sooner than 4 hours following the ingestion. Induce emesis using syrup of ipecac. If the plasma level is obtained and falls above the broken line on the acetaminophen overdose nomogram, the MUCOMYST acetylcysteine therapy should be initiated and continued for a full course of therapy. If acetaminophen plasma assay capability is not available, and the estimated acetaminophen ingestion exceeds 150mg/kg, MUCOMYST acetycysteine therapy should be initiated and continued for a full course of therapy. For additional emergency information, call your regional poison center or call the Rocky Mountain Poison Center toll free (1-800-526-6115).

Acute dextromethorphan overdose usually does not result in serious signs and symptoms unless massive amounts have been ingested. Signs and symptoms of a substantial overdose may include nausea and vomiting, visual disturbances, CNS disturbances, and urinary retention.

Symptoms from pseudoephedrine overdose consist most often of mild anxiety, tachycardia and/or mild hypertension. Symptoms usually appear witin 4 to 8 hours of ingestion and are transient, usually requiring no treatment.

INACTIVE INGREDIENTS

Alcohol (10%), Citric Acid, Flavors, Glycerin, Polyethylene Glycol, Purified Water, Sodium Benzoate, Sodium Carboxymethylcellulose, Sodium Saccharin, Sorbitol, Sucrose, Red #33, Red #40 and Blue #1.

HOW SUPPLIED

MAXIMUM STRENGTH TYLENOL COUGH with Decongestant is available in a 4 oz. and 8 oz. bottles with child-resistant safety cap, special dosing cup marked in ml, and tamper resistant packaging.

Shown in Product Identification Section, page 418

Maximum-Strength
TYLENOL® Sinus Medication OTC
Gelcaps, Caplets and Tablets

DESCRIPTION

Each Maximum-Strength TYLENOL® Sinus Medication Gelcap, Caplet or Tablet contains acetaminophen 500 mg and pseudoephedrine hydrochloride 30 mg.

ACTIONS

TYLENOL Sinus Medication contains a clinically proven analgesic-antipyretic and a decongestant. Maximum allowable non-prescription levels of acetaminophen and pseudoephedrine provide temporary relief of sinus headache and congestion. Acetaminophen is equal to aspirin in analgesic and antipyretic effectiveness and it is unlikely to produce many of the side effects associated with aspirin and aspirin-containing products.

Acetaminophen produces analgesia by elevation of the pain threshold and antipyresis through action on the hypothalamic heat-regulating center. Pseudoephedrine hydrochloride is a sympathomimetic amine which promotes sinus cavity drainage by reducing nasopharyngeal mucosal congestion.

INDICATIONS

Maximum-Strength TYLENOL Sinus Medication provides effective symptomatic relief from sinus headache pain and congestion. Maximum-Strength TYLENOL Sinus Medication is particularly well-suited in patients with aspirin allergy, hemostatic disturbances (including anticoagulant therapy), and bleeding diatheses (e.g., hemophilia) and upper gastrointestinal disease (e.g., ulcer, gastritis, hiatus hernia).

PRECAUTIONS

If a rare sensitivity occurs, the drug should be discontinued. Although pseudoephedrine is virtually without pressor effect in normotensive patients, it should be used with caution in hypertensives.

USUAL DOSAGE

Adults and Children 12 years of Age and Older: Two Tablets, Caplets or Gelcaps every 4–6 hours. Do not exceed eight Tablets, Caplets or Gelcaps in any 24-hour period. WARNING: Do not administer to children under 12 or exceed the recommended dosage because at higher doses nervousness, dizziness, or sleeplessness may occur. Do not take this product for more than 7 days. If symptoms do not improve or are accompanied by fever, consult a physician. Do not take this product if you have heart disease, high blood pressure, thyroid disease, diabetes, or difficulty in urination due to enlargement of the prostate gland unless directed by a doctor.

DRUG INTERACTION PRECAUTION: Do not take this product if you are presently taking a prescription drug for high blood pressure or depression without first consulting your doctor. **Do not use if carton is opened or if blister unit is broken or if printed green neck wrap or printed foil inner seal is broken. Keep this and all medication out of the reach of children. As with any drug, if you are pregnant or nursing a baby, seek the advice of a health professional before using this product. In case of accidental overdosage, contact a physician or poison control center immediately.**

OVERDOSAGE

Acetaminophen in massive overdosage may cause hepatic toxicity in some patients. In adults and adolescents, hepatic toxicity has rarely been reported following ingestion of acute overdosage of less than 10 grams. Fatalities are infrequent (less than 3–4% of untreated cases) and have rarely been reported with overdoses of less than 15 grams. In children, an acute overdosage of less than 150 mg/kg has not been associated with hepatic toxicity.

Early symptoms following a potentially hepatotoxic overdose may include: nausea, vomiting, diaphoresis and general malaise. Clinical and laboratory evidence of hepatic toxicity may not be apparent until 48 to 72 hours postingestion.

In adults and adolescents, regardless of the quantity of acetaminophen reported to have been ingested, administer MUCOMYST® acetylcysteine immediately if 24 hours or less have elapsed from the reported time of ingestion. For full prescribing information, refer to the MUCOMYST package insert. Do not await the results of assays for acetaminophen level before initiating treatment with MUCOMYST acetylcysteine. The following additional procedures are recommended: The stomach should be emptied promptly by lavage or by induction of emesis with syrup of ipecac. A serum acetaminophen assay should be obtained as early as possible, but no sooner than four hours following ingestion. Liver function studies should be obtained initially and repeated at 24-hour intervals.

Serious toxicity or fatalities are extremely infrequent in children, possibly due to differences in the way they metabolize acetaminophen. In children, the maximum potential amount ingested can be more easily estimated. If more than 150 mg/kg or an unknown amount was ingested, obtain an acetaminophen plasma level. The acetaminophen plasma level should be obtained as soon as possible, but no sooner than 4 hours following the ingestion. Induce emesis using syrup of ipecac. If the plasma level is obtained and falls above the broken line on the acetaminophen overdose nomogram, the MUCOMYST acetylcysteine therapy should be initiated and continued for a full course of therapy. If acetaminophen plasma assay capability is not available, and the estimated acetaminophen ingestion exceeds 150 mg/kg, MUCOMYST acetylcysteine therapy should be initiated and continued for a full course of therapy.

For additional emergency information, call your regional poison center or call the Rocky Mountain Poison Center toll-free, (1-800-525-6115).

Symptoms from pseudoephedrine overdose consist most often of mild anxiety, tachycardia and/or mild hypertension. Symptoms usually appear within 4 to 8 hours of ingestion and are transient, usually requiring no treatment.

INACTIVE INGREDIENTS

Caplets—Cellulose, Hydroxypropyl Methylcellulose, Magnesium Stearate, Polyethylene Glycol, Polysorbate 80, Sodium Starch Glycolate, Starch, Titanium Dioxide, Blue #1, Red #40 and Yellow #10. Tablets—Cellulose, Magnesium Stearate, Sodium Lauryl Sulfate, Starch, Yellow #6, Yellow #10, and Blue #1.

Gelcaps—Benzyl alcohol, butylparaben, castor oil, cellulose, edetate calcium disodium, gelatin, hydroxypropyl methylcellulose, iron oxide black, magnesium stearate, methylparaben, propylparaben, sodium lauryl sulfate, sodium propionate, sodium starch glycolate, starch, titanium dioxide, Blue #1 and Yellow #10.

HOW SUPPLIED

Tablets (colored light green, imprinted "Maximum-Strength TYLENOL Sinus")—tamper-resistant bottles of 24 and 50.

Caplets (light green coating, printed "TYLENOL Sinus" in dark green) tamper-resistant bottles of 24 and 50.

Gelcaps (colored green and white), imprinted "TYLENOL Sinus" in tamper-resistant packages of 20 and 40.

Shown in Product Identification Section, page 418

McNeil Pharmaceutical
SPRING HOUSE, PA 19477-0776

HALDOL® ℞
brand of
haloperidol
[*hal'dawl*]
Tablets/Concentrate/Injection

DESCRIPTION

Haloperidol is the first of the butyrophenone series of major tranquilizers. The chemical designation is 4-[4-(p-chlorophenyl)-4-hydroxy-piperidino]-4'-fluorobutyrophenone and it has the following structural formula:

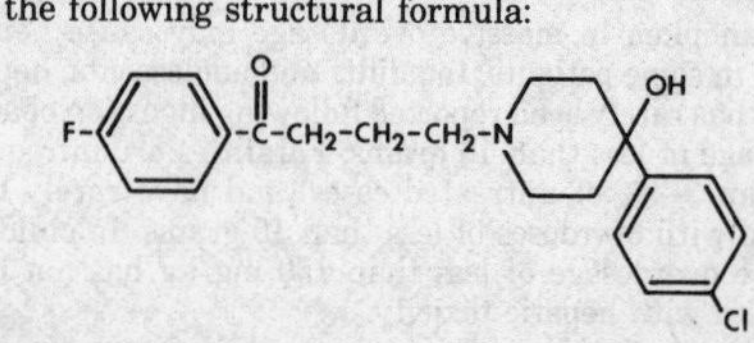

HALDOL haloperidol dosage forms include: tablets (½, 1*, 2, 5*, 10* and 20 mg); a concentrate with 2 mg per mL haloperidol (as the lactate); and a sterile parenteral form for intramuscular injection. The injection provides 5 mg haloperidol (as the lactate) with 1.8 mg methylparaben and 0.2 mg propylparaben per mL, and lactic acid for pH adjustment between 3.0–3.6.

Inactive ingredients: tablets—calcium phosphate, calcium stearate, corn starch, natural flavor—1mg contains FD&C Yellow No. 5*; 2mg contains D&C Red No. 33 and FD&C Blue No. 2; 5mg contains FD&C Blue No. 1 and FD&C Yellow No. 5*; 10 mg contains FD&C Blue No. 1 and FD&C Yellow No. 5*; and 20 mg contains FD&C Red No. 40; concentrate - lactic acid and methylparaben.

ACTIONS

The precise mechanism of action has not been clearly established.

INDICATIONS

HALDOL haloperidol is indicated for use in the management of manifestations of psychotic disorders.

*See Precautions

HALDOL is indicated for the control of tics and vocal utterances of Tourette's Disorder in children and adults.

HALDOL is effective for the treatment of severe behavior problems in children of combative, explosive hyperexcitability (which cannot be accounted for by immediate provocation). HALDOL is also effective in the short-term treatment of hyperactive children who show excessive motor activity with accompanying conduct disorders consisting of some or all of the following symptoms: impulsivity, difficulty sustaining attention, aggressivity, mood lability and poor frustration tolerance.

HALDOL should be reserved for these two groups of children only after failure to respond to psychotherapy or medications other than antipsychotics.

CONTRAINDICATIONS

HALDOL haloperidol is contraindicated in severe toxic central nervous system depression or comatose states from any cause and in individuals who are hypersensitive to this drug or have Parkinson's disease.

WARNINGS

Tardive Dyskinesia

A syndrome consisting of potentially irreversible, involuntary, dyskinetic movements may develop in patients treated with antipsychotic drugs. Although the prevalence of the syndrome appears to be highest among the elderly, especially elderly women, it is impossible to rely upon prevalence estimates to predict, at the inception of antipsychotic treatment, which patients are likely to develop the syndrome. Whether antipsychotic drug products differ in their potential to cause tardive dyskinesia is unknown.

Both the risk of developing tardive dyskinesia and the likelihood that it will become irreversible are believed to increase as the duration of treatment and the total cumulative dose of antipsychotic drugs administered to the patient increase. However, the syndrome can develop, although much less commonly, after relatively brief treatment periods at low doses.

There is no known treatment for established cases of tardive dyskinesia, although the syndrome may remit, partially or completely, if antipsychotic treatment is withdrawn. Antipsychotic treatment, itself, however, may suppress (or partially suppress) the signs and symptoms of the syndrome and thereby may possibly mask the underlying process. The effect that symptomatic suppression has upon the long-term course of the syndrome is unknown.

Given these considerations, antipsychotic drugs should be prescribed in a manner that is most likely to minimize the occurrence of tardive dyskinesia. Chronic antipsychotic treatment should generally be reserved for patients who suffer from a chronic illness that, 1) is known to respond to antipsychotic drugs, and 2) for whom alternative, equally effective, but potentially less harmful treatments are not available or appropriate. In patients who do require chronic treatment, the smallest dose and the shortest duration of treatment producing a satisfactory clinical response should be sought. The need for continued treatment should be reassessed periodically.

If signs and symptoms of tardive dyskinesia appear in a patient on antipsychotics, drug discontinuation should be considered. However, some patients may require treatment despite the presence of the syndrome.

(For further information about the description of tardive dyskinesia and its clinical detection, please refer to ADVERSE REACTIONS.)

Neuroleptic Malignant Syndrome (NMS)

A potentially fatal symptom complex sometimes referred to as Neuroleptic Malignant Syndrome (NMS) has been reported in association with antipsychotic drugs. Clinical manifestations of NMS are hyperpyrexia, muscle rigidity, altered mental status (including catatonic signs) and evidence of autonomic instability (irregular pulse or blood pressure, tachycardia, diaphoresis, and cardiac dysrhythmias). Additional signs may include elevated creatine phosphokinase, myoglobinuria (rhabdomyolysis) and acute renal failure.

The diagnostic evaluation of patients with this syndrome is complicated. In arriving at a diagnosis, it is important to identify cases where the clinical presentation includes both serious medical illness (e.g., pneumonia, systemic infection, etc.) and untreated or inadequately treated extrapyramidal signs and symptoms (EPS). Other important considerations in the differential diagnosis include central anticholinergic toxicity, heat stroke, drug fever and primary central nervous system (CNS) pathology.

The management of NMS should include 1) immediate discontinuation of antipsychotic drugs and other drugs not essential to concurrent therapy, 2) intensive symptomatic treatment and medical monitoring, and 3) treatment of any concomitant serious medical problems for which specific treatments are available. There is no general agreement about specific pharmacological treatment regimens for uncomplicated NMS.

If a patient requires antipsychotic drug treatment after recovery from NMS, the potential reintroduction of drug therapy should be carefully considered. The patient should be carefully monitored, since recurrences of NMS have been reported.

Hyperpyrexia and heat stroke, not associated with the above symptom complex, have also been reported with HALDOL.

Usage in Pregnancy

Rodents given 2 to 20 times the usual maximum human dose of haloperidol by oral or parenteral routes showed an increase in incidence of resorption, reduced fertility, delayed delivery and pup mortality. No teratogenic effect has been reported in rats, rabbits or dogs at dosages within this range, but cleft palate has been observed in mice given 15 times the usual maximum human dose. Cleft palate in mice appears to be a non-specific response to stress or nutritional imbalance as well as to a variety of drugs, and there is no evidence to relate this phenomenon to predictable human risk for most of these agents.

There are no well controlled studies with HALDOL haloperidol in pregnant women. There are reports, however, of cases of limb malformations observed following maternal use of HALDOL along with other drugs which have suspected teratogenic potential during the first trimester of pregnancy. Causal relationships were not established in these cases. Since such experience does not exclude the possibility of fetal damage due to HALDOL, this drug should be used during pregnancy or in women likely to become pregnant only if the benefit clearly justifies a potential risk to the fetus. Infants should not be nursed during drug treatment.

Combined Use of HALDOL and Lithium

An encephalopathic syndrome (characterized by weakness, lethargy, fever, tremulousness and confusion, extrapyramidal symptoms, leukocytosis, elevated serum enzymes, BUN, and FBS) followed by irreversible brain damage has occurred in a few patients treated with lithium plus HALDOL. A causal relationship between these events and the concomitant administration of lithium and HALDOL has not been established; however, patients receiving such combined therapy should be monitored closely for early evidence of neurological toxicity and treatment discontinued promptly if such signs appear.

General

A number of cases of bronchopneumonia, some fatal, have followed the use of antipsychotic drugs, including HALDOL. It has been postulated that lethargy and decreased sensation of thirst due to central inhibition may lead to dehydration, hemoconcentration and reduced pulmonary ventilation. Therefore, if the above signs and symptoms appear, especially in the elderly, the physician should institute remedial therapy promptly.

Although not reported with HALDOL, decreased serum cholesterol and/or cutaneous and ocular changes have been reported in patients receiving chemically-related drugs.

HALDOL may impair the mental and/or physical abilities required for the performance of hazardous tasks such as operating machinery or driving a motor vehicle. The ambulatory patient should be warned accordingly.

The use of alcohol with this drug should be avoided due to possible additive effects and hypotension.

PRECAUTIONS

HALDOL haloperidol should be administered cautiously to patients:

—with severe cardiovascular disorders, because of the possibility of transient hypotension and/or precipitation of anginal pain. Should hypotension occur and a vasopressor be required, epinephrine should not be used since HALDOL may block its vasopressor activity and paradoxical further lowering of the blood pressure may occur. Instead, metaraminol, phenylephrine or norepinephrine should be used.

—receiving anticonvulsant medications, with a history of seizures, or with EEG abnormalities, because HALDOL may lower the convulsive threshold. If indicated, adequate anticonvulsant therapy should be concomitantly maintained.

—with known allergies, or with a history of allergic reactions to drugs.

—receiving anticoagulants, since an isolated instance of interference occurred with the effects of one anticoagulant (phenindione).

If concomitant antiparkinson medication is required, it may have to be continued after HALDOL is discontinued because of the difference in excretion rates. If both are discontinued simultaneously, extrapyramidal symptoms may occur. The physician should keep in mind the possible increase in intraocular pressure when anticholinergic drugs, including antiparkinson agents, are administered concomitantly with HALDOL.

As with other antipsychotic agents, it should be noted that HALDOL may be capable of potentiating CNS depressants such as anesthetics, opiates, and alcohol.

When HALDOL is used to control mania in cyclic disorders, there may be a rapid mood swing to depression.

Severe neurotoxicity (rigidity, inability to walk or talk) may occur in patients with thyrotoxicosis who are also receiving antipsychotic medication, including HALDOL.

No mutagenic potential of haloperidol was found in the Ames Salmonella microsomal activation assay. Negative or inconsistent positive findings have been obtained in in vitro and in vivo studies of effects of haloperidol on chromosome structure and number. The available cytogenetic evidence is considered too inconsistent to be conclusive at this time. Carcinogenicity studies using oral haloperidol were conducted in Wistar rats (dosed at up to 5 mg/kg daily for 24 months) and in Albino Swiss mice (dosed at up to 5 mg/kg daily for 18 months). In the rat study survival was less than optimal in all dose groups, reducing the number of rats at risk for developing tumors. However, although a relatively greater number of rats survived to the end of the study in high dose male and female groups, these animals did not have a greater incidence of tumors than control animals. Therefore, although not optimal, this study does suggest the absence of a haloperidol related increase in the incidence of neoplasia in rats at doses up to 20 times the usual daily human dose for chronic or resistant patients.

In female mice at 5 and 20 times the highest initial daily dose for chronic or resistant patients, there was a statistically significant increase in mammary gland neoplasia and total tumor incidence; at 20 times the same daily dose there was a statistically significant increase in pituitary gland neoplasia. In male mice, no statistically significant differences in incidences of total tumors or specific tumor types were noted.

Antipsychotic drugs elevate prolactin levels; the elevation persists during chronic administration. Tissue culture experiments indicate that approximately one-third of human breast cancers are prolactin dependent in vitro, a factor of potential importance if the prescription of these drugs is contemplated in a patient with a previously detected breast cancer. Although disturbances such as galactorrhea, amenorrhea, gynecomastia, and impotence have been reported, the clinical significance of elevated serum prolactin levels is unknown for most patients. An increase in mammary neoplasms has been found in rodents after chronic administration of antipsychotic drugs. Neither clinical studies nor epidemiologic studies conducted to date, however, have shown an association between chronic administration of these drugs and mammary tumorigenesis; the available evidence is considered too limited to be conclusive at this time.

FD&C Yellow No. 5 (tartrazine) may cause allergic-type reactions (including bronchial asthma) in certain susceptible individuals. Although the overall incidence of FD&C Yellow No. 5 (tartrazine) sensitivity in the general population is low, it is frequently seen in patients who also have aspirin hypersensitivity.

ADVERSE REACTIONS

CNS Effects:

Extrapyramidal Symptoms (EPA) —EPS during the administration of HALDOL (haloperidol) have been reported frequently, often during the first few days of treatment. EPS can be categorized generally as Parkinson-like symptoms, akathisia, or dystonia (including opisthotonos and oculogyric crisis). While all can occur at relatively low doses, they occur more frequently and with greater severity at higher doses. The symptoms may be controlled with dose reductions or administration of antiparkinson drugs such as benztropine mesylate USP or trihexyphenidyl hydrochloride USP. It should be noted that persistent EPS have been reported; the drug may have to be discontinued in such cases.

Withdrawal Emergent Neurological Signs—Generally, patients receiving short term therapy experience no problems with abrupt discontinuation of antipsychotic drugs. However, some patients on maintenance treatment experience transient dyskinetic signs after abrupt withdrawal. In certain of these cases the dyskinetic movements are indistinguishable from the syndrome described below under "Tardive Dyskinesia" except for duration. It is not known whether gradual withdrawal of antipsychotic drugs will reduce the rate of occurrence of withdrawal emergent neurological signs but until further evidence becomes available, it seems reasonable to gradually withdraw use of HALDOL.

Tardive Dyskinesia—As with all antipsychotic agents HALDOL has been associated with persistent dyskinesias. Tardive dyskinesia, a syndrome consisting of potentially irreversible, involuntary, dyskinetic movements, may appear in some patients on long-term therapy or may occur after drug therapy has been discontinued. The risk appears to be greater in elderly patients on high-dose therapy, especially females. The symptoms are persistent and in some patients appear irreversible. The syndrome is characterized by rhythmical involuntary movements of tongue, face, mouth or jaw (e.g., protrusion of tongue, puffing of cheeks, puckering of mouth, chewing movements). Sometimes these may be accompanied by involuntary movements of extremities and the trunk.

Continued on next page

Information on McNeil Pharmaceutical Products is based on labeling in effect in August 1992.

McNeil—Cont.

Psychotic Disorders	0.05 mg/kg/day to 0.15 mg/kg/day
Non-Psychotic Behavior Disorders and Tourette's Disorder	0.05 mg/kg/day to 0.075 mg/kg/day

Severely disturbed psychotic children may require higher doses.

In severely disturbed, non-psychotic children or in hyperactive children with accompanying conduct disorders, who have failed to respond to psychotherapy or medications other than antipsychotics, it should be noted that since these behaviors may be short-lived, short-term administration of HALDOL may suffice. There is no evidence establishing a maximum effective dosage. There is little evidence that behavior improvement is further enhanced in dosages beyond 6 mg per day.

There is no known effective treatment for tardive dyskinesia; antiparkinson agents usually do not alleviate the symptoms of this syndrome. It is suggested that all antipsychotic agents be discontinued if these symptoms appear. Should it be necessary to reinstitute treatment, or increase the dosage of the agent, or switch to a different antipsychotic agent, this syndrome may be masked.

It has been reported that fine vermicular movement of the tongue may be an early sign of tardive dyskinesia and if the medication is stopped at that time the full syndrome may not develop.

Tardive Dystonia —Tardive dystonia, not associated with the above syndrome, has also been reported. Tardive dystonia is characterized by delayed onset of choreic or dystonic movements, is often persistent, and has the potential of becoming irreversible.

Other CNS Effects —Insomnia, restlessness, anxiety, euphoria, agitation, drowsiness, depression, lethargy, headache, confusion, vertigo, grand mal seizures, exacerbation of psychotic symptoms including hallucinations, and catatonic-like behavioral states which may be responsive to drug withdrawal and/or treatment with anticholinergic drugs.

Body as a Whole: Neuroleptic malignant syndrome (NMS), hyperpyrexia and heat stroke have been reported with HALDOL. (See WARNINGS for further information concerning NMS.)

Cardiovascular Effects: Tachycardia, hypotension, hypertension and ECG changes including prolongation of the Q-T interval and ECG pattern changes compatible with the polymorphous configuration of torsades de pointes.

Hematologic Effects: Reports have appeared citing the occurrence of mild and usually transient leukopenia and leukocytosis, minimal decreases in red blood cell counts, anemia, or a tendency toward lymphomonocytosis. Agranulocytosis has rarely been reported to have occurred with the use of HALDOL, and then only in association with other medication.

Liver Effects: Impaired liver function and/or jaundice have been reported.

Dermatologic Reactions: Maculopapular and acneiform skin reactions and isolated cases of photosensitivity and loss of hair.

Endocrine Disorders: Lactation, breast engorgement, mastalgia, menstrual irregularities, gynecomastia, impotence, increased libido, hyperglycemia, hypoglycemia and hyponatremia.

Gastrointestinal Effects: Anorexia, constipation, diarrhea, hypersalivation, dyspepsia, nausea and vomiting.

Autonomic Reactions: Dry mouth, blurred vision, urinary retention, diaphoresis and priapism.

Respiratory Effects: Laryngospasm, bronchospasm and increased depth of respiration.

Special Senses: Cataracts, retinopathy and visual disturbances.

Other: Cases of sudden and unexpected death have been reported in association with the administration of HALDOL. The nature of the evidence makes it impossible to determine definitively what role, if any, HALDOL played in the outcome of the reported cases. The possibility that HALDOL caused death cannot, of course, be excluded, but it is to be kept in mind that sudden and unexpected death may occur in psychotic patients when they go untreated or when they are treated with other antipsychotic drugs.

Postmarketing Events: Hyperammonemia has been reported in a 5½ year old child with citrullinemia, an inherited disorder of ammonia excretion, following treatment with HALDOL.

OVERDOSAGE

Manifestations

In general, the symptoms of overdosage would be an exaggeration of known pharmacologic effects and adverse reactions, the most prominent of which would be: 1) severe extrapyramidal reactions, 2) hypotension, or 3) sedation. The patient would appear comatose with respiratory depression and hypotension which could be severe enough to produce a shock-like state. The extrapyramidal reaction would be manifest by muscular weakness or rigidity and a generalized or localized tremor as demonstrated by the akinetic or agitans types respectively. With accidental overdosage, hypertension rather than hypotension occurred in a two-year old child. The risk of ECG changes associated with torsades de pointes should be considered. (For further information regarding torsades de pointes, please refer to ADVERSE REACTIONS.)

Treatment

Gastric lavage or induction of emesis should be carried out immediately followed by administration of activated charcoal. Since there is no specific antidote, treatment is primarily supportive. A patent airway must be established by use of an oropharyngeal airway or endotracheal tube or, in prolonged cases of coma, by tracheostomy. Respiratory depression may be counteracted by artificial respiration and mechanical respirators. Hypotension and circulatory collapse may be counteracted by use of intravenous fluids, plasma, or concentrated albumin, and vasopressor agents such as metaraminol, phenylephrine and norepinephrine. Epinephrine should not be used. In case of severe extrapyramidal reactions, antiparkinson medication should be administered. ECG and vital signs should be monitored especially for signs of Q-T prolongation or dysrhythmias and monitoring should continue until the ECG is normal. Severe arrhythmias should be treated with appropriate anti-arrhythmic measures.

DOSAGE AND ADMINISTRATION

There is considerable variation from patient to patient in the amount of medication required for treatment. As with all antipsychotic drugs, dosage should be individualized according to the needs and response of each patient. Dosage adjustments, either upward or downward, should be carried out as rapidly as practicable to achieve optimum therapeutic control.

To determine the initial dosage, consideration should be given to the patient's age, severity of illness, previous response to other antipsychotic drugs, and any concomitant medication or disease state. Children, debilitated or geriatric patients, as well as those with a history of adverse reactions to antipsychotic drugs, may require less HALDOL haloperidol. The optimal response in such patients is usually obtained with more gradual dosage adjustments and at lower dosage levels, as recommended below.

Clinical experience suggests the following recommendations:

Oral Administration

Initial Dosage Range

Adults

Moderate Symptomatology	0.5 mg to 2.0 mg b.i.d. or t.i.d.
Severe Symptomatology	3.0 mg to 5.0 mg b.i.d. or t.i.d.

To achieve prompt control, higher doses may be required in some cases.

Geriatric or Debilitated Patients	0.5 mg to 2.0 mg b.i.d. or t.i.d.
Chronic or Resistant Patients	3.0 mg to 5.0 mg b.i.d. or t.i.d.

Patients who remain severely disturbed or inadequately controlled may require dosage adjustment. Daily dosages up to 100 mg may be necessary in some cases to achieve an optimal response. Infrequently, HALDOL has been used in doses above 100 mg for severely resistant patients; however, the limited clinical usage has not demonstrated the safety of prolonged administration of such doses.

	Bottles Containing			Unit Dose Blister Pack	
	100	1000	10×10	31×32	10×32
½mg, white NDC 0045-0240	x	x	x	x	
1mg, yellow NDC 0045-0241	x	x	x	x	
2mg, pink NDC 0045-0242	x	x	x	x	
5mg, green NDC 0045-0245	x	x	x	x	
10mg, aqua NDC 0045-0246	x	x	x	x	
20mg, salmon NDC 0045-0248	x			x	x

Children

The following recommendations apply to children between the ages of 3 and 12 years (weight range 15 to 40 kg). HALDOL is not intended for children under 3 years old. Therapy should begin at the lowest dose possible (0.5 mg per day). If required, the dose should be increased by an increment of 0.5 mg at 5 to 7 day intervals until the desired therapeutic effect is obtained. (See boxed chart top left.)

The total dose may be divided, to be given b.i.d. or t.i.d.

Maintenance Dosage

Upon achieving a satisfactory therapeutic response, dosage should then be gradually reduced to the lowest effective maintenance level.

Intramuscular Administration

Adults

Parenteral medication, administered intramuscularly in doses of 2 to 5 mg, is utilized for prompt control of the acutely agitated patient with moderately severe to very severe symptoms. Depending on the response of the patient, subsequent doses may be given, administered as often as every hour, although 4 to 8 hour intervals may be satisfactory.

Controlled trials to establish the safety and effectiveness of intramuscular administration in children have not been conducted.

Parenteral drug products should be inspected visually for particulate matter and discoloration prior to administration, whenever solution and container permit.

Switchover Procedure

The oral form should supplant the injectable as soon as practicable. In the absence of bioavailability studies establishing bioequivalence between these two dosage forms the following guidelines for dosage are suggested. For an initial approximation of the total daily dose required, the parenteral dose administered in the preceding 24 hours may be used. Since this dose is only an initial estimate, it is recommended that careful monitoring of clinical signs and symptoms, including clinical efficacy, sedation, and adverse effects, be carried out periodically for the first several days following the initiation of switchover. In this way, dosage adjustments, either upward or downward, can be quickly accomplished. Depending on the patient's clinical status, the first oral dose should be given within 12–24 hours following the last parenteral dose.

HOW SUPPLIED

HALDOL® brand of haloperidol Tablets Scored, Imprinted "McNEIL" and "HALDOL":

[See table above.]

HALDOL® brand of haloperidol Concentrate 2 mg per mL (as the lactate) Colorless, Odorless, and Tasteless Solution —NDC 0045-0250, bottles of 15 mL, 120 mL and 240 mL.

HALDOL® brand of haloperidol Injection 5 mg per mL (as the lactate) —NDC 0045-0255, units of 10 × 1 mL ampuls, 10 mL multiple-dose vial and units of 10 × 1 mL disposable Prefilled Syringe.

Dispense HALDOL haloperidol tablets and concentrate in a tight, light-resistant container as defined in the official compendium.

McNeil Pharmaceutical, McNEILAB, INC., Spring House, PA 19477

Revised 12/29/91

Shown in Product Identification Section, page 418

HALDOL® Decanoate 50   R
HALDOL® Decanoate 100   R

[hal 'dawl dek "ah-nō 'ōt]

(haloperidol) Decanoate Injection

NSN 6505-01-241-8602—1 mL Ampul
NSN 6505-01-293-5628—5 mL MDV

PRODUCT OVERVIEW

KEY FACTS

HALDOL Decanoate 50 and HALDOL Decanoate 100 are the long-acting injectable forms of HALDOL. The basic effects of HALDOL Decanoate 50 and HALDOL Decanoate 100 are those of HALDOL, with the exception of duration of action. HALDOL Decanoate 50 and HALDOL Decanoate 100 reach peak plasma concentration about six days after administration, with an apparent half-life of about three weeks. The recommended interval between doses is four weeks.

MAJOR USES

HALDOL Decanoate 50 and HALDOL Decanoate 100 are intended for use in the management of patients requiring prolonged parenteral antipsychotic therapy.

SAFETY INFORMATION

See complete safety information provided below.

PRESCRIBING INFORMATION

HALDOL® Decanoate 50 ℞
HALDOL® Decanoate 100 ℞
[*hal 'dawl dek "ah-nō 'āt*]
(haloperidol) Decanoate Injection

DESCRIPTION

Haloperidol decanoate is the decanoate ester of the butyrophenone, HALDOL haloperidol. It has a markedly extended duration of effect. It is available in sesame oil in sterile form for intramuscular (IM) injection. The structural formula of haloperidol decanoate, 4-(4-chlorophenyl)-1-[4-(4-fluorophenyl)-4-oxobutyl]-4 piperidinyl decanoate, is:

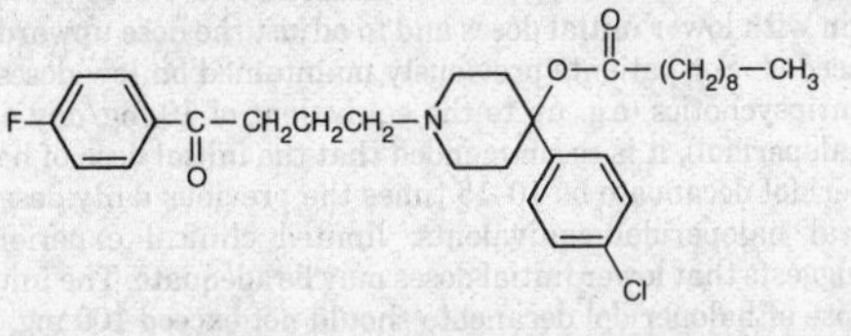

Haloperidol decanoate is almost insoluble in water (0.01 mg/mL), but is soluble in most organic solvents.

Each mL of HALDOL Decanoate 50 for IM injection contains 50 mg haloperidol (present as haloperidol decanoate 70.52 mg) in a sesame oil vehicle, with 1.2% (w/v) benzyl alcohol as a preservative.

Each mL of HALDOL Decanoate 100 for IM injection contains 100 mg haloperidol (present as haloperidol decanoate 141.04 mg) in a sesame oil vehicle, with 1.2% (w/v) benzyl alcohol as a preservative.

CLINICAL PHARMACOLOGY

HALDOL Decanoate 50 and HALDOL Decanoate 100 are the long-acting forms of HALDOL haloperidol. The basic effects of haloperidol decanoate are no different from those of HALDOL with the exception of duration of action. Haloperidol blocks the effects of dopamine and increases its turnover rate; however, the precise mechanism of action is unknown.

Administration of haloperidol decanoate in sesame oil results in slow and sustained release of haloperidol. The plasma concentrations of haloperidol gradually rise, reaching a peak at about 6 days after the injection, and falling thereafter, with an apparent half-life of about 3 weeks. Steady state plasma concentrations are achieved after the third or fourth dose. The relationship between dose of haloperidol decanoate and plasma haloperidol concentration is roughly linear for doses below 450 mg. It should be noted, however, that the pharmacokinetics of haloperidol decanoate following intramuscular injections can be quite variable between subjects.

INDICATIONS AND USAGE

HALDOL Decanoate 50 and HALDOL Decanoate 100 are long-acting parenteral antipsychotic drugs intended for use in the management of patients requiring prolonged parenteral antipsychotic therapy (e.g., patients with chronic schizophrenia).

CONTRAINDICATIONS

Since the pharmacologic and clinical actions of HALDOL Decanoate 50 and HALDOL Decanoate 100 are attributed to HALDOL haloperidol as the active medication, Contraindications, Warnings, and additional information are those of HALDOL, modified only to reflect the prolonged action.

HALDOL is contraindicated in severe toxic central nervous system depression or comatose states from any cause and in individuals who are hypersensitive to this drug or have Parkinson's disease.

WARNINGS

Tardive Dyskinesia

A syndrome consisting of potentially irreversible, involuntary, dyskinetic movements may develop in patients treated with antipsychotic drugs. Although the prevalence of the syndrome appears to be highest among the elderly, especially elderly women, it is impossible to rely upon prevalence estimates to predict, at the inception of antipsychotic treatment, which patients are likely to develop the syndrome. Whether antipsychotic drug products differ in their potential to cause tardive dyskinesia is unknown.

Both the risk of developing tardive dyskinesia and the likelihood that it will become irreversible are believed to increase as the duration of treatment and the total cumulative dose of antipsychotic drugs administered to the patient increase. However, the syndrome can develop, although much less commonly, after relatively brief treatment periods at low doses.

There is no known treatment for established cases of tardive dyskinesia, although the syndrome may remit, partially or completely, if antipsychotic treatment is withdrawn. Antipsychotic treatment, itself, however, may suppress (or partially suppress) the signs and symptoms of the syndrome and thereby may possibly mask the underlying process. The effect that symptomatic suppression has upon the long-term course of the syndrome is unknown.

Given these considerations, antipsychotic drugs should be prescribed in a manner that is most likely to minimize the occurrence of tardive dyskinesia. Chronic antipsychotic treatment should generally be reserved for patients who suffer from a chronic illness that 1) is known to respond to antipsychotic drugs, and 2) for whom alternative, equally effective, but potentially less harmful treatments are **not** available or appropriate. In patients who do require chronic treatment, the smallest dose and the shortest duration of treatment producing a satisfactory clinical response should be sought. The need for continued treatment should be reassessed periodically.

If signs and symptoms of tardive dyskinesia appear in a patient on antipsychotics, drug discontinuation should be considered. However, some patients may require treatment despite the presence of the syndrome. (For further information about the description of tardive dyskinesia and its clinical detection, please refer to ADVERSE REACTIONS.)

Neuroleptic Malignant Syndrome (NMS)

A potentially fatal symptom complex sometimes referred to as Neuroleptic Malignant Syndrome (NMS) has been reported in association with antipsychotic drugs. Clinical manifestations of NMS are hyperpyrexia, muscle rigidity, altered mental status (including catatonic signs) and evidence of autonomic instability (irregular pulse or blood pressure, tachycardia, diaphoresis, and cardiac dysrhythmias). Additional signs may include elevated creatine phosphokinase, myoglobinuria (rhabdomyolysis) and acute renal failure.

The diagnostic evaluation of patients with this syndrome is complicated. In arriving at a diagnosis, it is important to identify cases where the clinical presentation includes both serious medical illness (e.g., pneumonia, systemic infection, etc.) and untreated or inadequately treated extrapyramidal signs and symptoms (EPS). Other important considerations in the differential diagnosis include central anticholinergic toxicity, heat stroke, drug fever and primary central nervous system (CNS) pathology.

The management of NMS should include 1) immediate discontinuation of antipsychotic drugs and other drugs not essential to concurrent therapy, 2) intensive symptomatic treatment and medical monitoring, and 3) treatment of any concomitant serious medical problems for which specific treatments are available. There is no general agreement about specific pharmacological treatment regimens for uncomplicated NMS.

If a patient requires antipsychotic drug treatment after recovery from NMS, the potential reintroduction of drug therapy should be carefully considered. The patient should be carefully monitored, since recurrences of NMS have been reported.

Hyperpyrexia and heat stroke, not associated with the above symptom complex, have also been reported with HALDOL.

General

A number of cases of bronchopneumonia, some fatal, have followed the use of antipsychotic drugs, including HALDOL (haloperidol). It has been postulated that lethargy and decreased sensation of thirst due to central inhibition may lead to dehydration, hemoconcentration and reduced pulmonary ventilation. Therefore, if the above signs and symptoms appear, especially in the elderly, the physician should institute remedial therapy promptly.

Although not reported with HALDOL, decreased serum cholesterol and/or cutaneous and ocular changes have been reported in patients receiving chemically-related drugs.

PRECAUTIONS

HALDOL Decanoate 50 and HALDOL Decanoate 100 should be administered cautiously to patients:

—with severe cardiovascular disorders, because of the possibility of transient hypotension and/or precipitation of anginal pain. Should hypotension occur and a vasopressor be required, epinephrine should not be used since HALDOL haloperidol may block its vasopressor activity, and paradoxical further lowering of the blood pressure may occur. Instead, metaraminol, phenylephrine or norepinephrine should be used.

—receiving anticonvulsant medications, with a history of seizures, or with EEG abnormalities, because HALDOL may lower the convulsive threshold. If indicated, adequate anticonvulsant therapy should be concomitantly maintained.

—with known allergies, or with a history of allergic reactions to drugs.

—receiving anticoagulants, since an isolated instance of interference occurred with the effects of one anticoagulant (phenindione).

If concomitant antiparkinson medication is required, it may have to be continued after HALDOL Decanoate 50 or HALDOL Decanoate 100 is discontinued because of the prolonged action of haloperidol decanoate. If both drugs are discontinued simultaneously, extrapyramidal symptoms may occur. The physician should keep in mind the possible increase in intraocular pressure when anticholinergic drugs, including antiparkinson agents, are administered concomitantly with haloperidol decanoate.

In patients with thyrotoxicosis who are also receiving antipsychotic medication, including haloperidol decanoate, severe neurotoxicity (rigidity, inability to walk or talk) may occur.

When HALDOL is used to control mania in bipolar disorders, there may be a rapid mood swing to depression.

Information for Patients

Haloperidol decanoate may impair the mental and/or physical abilities required for the performance of hazardous tasks such as operating machinery or driving a motor vehicle. The ambulatory patient should be warned accordingly.

The use of alcohol with this drug should be avoided due to possible additive effects and hypotension.

Drug Interactions

An encephalopathic syndrome (characterized by weakness, lethargy, fever, tremulousness and confusion, extrapyramidal symptoms, leukocytosis, elevated serum enzymes, BUN, and FBS) followed by irreversible brain damage has occurred in a few patients treated with lithium plus HALDOL. A causal relationship between these events and the concomitant administration of lithium and HALDOL has not been established; however, patients receiving such combined therapy should be monitored closely for early evidence of neurological toxicity and treatment discontinued promptly if such signs appear.

As with other antipsychotic agents, it should be noted that HALDOL may be capable of potentiating CNS depressants such as anesthetics, opiates, and alcohol.

Carcinogenesis, Mutagenesis, and Impairment of Fertility

No mutagenic potential of haloperidol decanoate was found in the Ames Salmonella microsomal activation assay. Negative or inconsistent positive findings have been obtained in *in vitro* and *in vivo* studies of effects of short-acting haloperidol on chromosome structure and number. The available cytogenetic evidence is considered too inconsistent to be conclusive at this time.

Carcinogenicity studies using oral haloperidol were conducted in Wistar rats (dosed at up to 5 mg/kg daily for 24 months) and in Albino Swiss mice (dosed at up to 5 mg/kg daily for 18 months). In the rat study survival was less than optimal in all dose groups, reducing the number of rats at risk for developing tumors. However, although a relatively greater number of rats survived to the end of the study in high dose male and female groups, these animals did not have a greater incidence of tumors than control animals. Therefore, although not optimal, this study does suggest the absence of a haloperidol related increase in the incidence of neoplasia in rats at doses up to 20 times the usual daily human dose for chronic or resistant patients.

In female mice at 5 and 20 times the highest initial daily dose for chronic or resistant patients, there was a statistically significant increase in mammary gland neoplasia and total tumor incidence; at 20 times the same daily dose there was a statistically significant increase in pituitary gland neoplasia. In male mice, no statistically significant differences in incidences of total tumors or specific tumor types were noted.

Antipsychotic drugs elevate prolactin levels; the elevation persists during chronic administration. Tissue culture experiments indicate that approximately one-third of human breast cancers are prolactin dependent *in vitro*, a factor of potential importance if the prescription of these drugs is contemplated in a patient with a previously detected breast cancer. Although disturbances such as galactorrhea, amenorrhea, gynecomastia, and impotence have been reported, the clinical significance of elevated serum prolactin levels is unknown for most patients.

An increase in mammary neoplasms has been found in rodents after chronic administration of antipsychotic drugs. Neither clinical studies nor epidemiologic studies conducted to date, however, have shown an association between chronic administration of these drugs and mammary tumorigenesis; the available evidence is considered too limited to be conclusive at this time.

Usage in Pregnancy

Pregnancy Category C. Rodents given up to 3 times the usual maximum human dose of haloperidol decanoate showed an increase in incidence of resorption, fetal mortality, and pup mortality. No fetal abnormalities were observed.

Cleft palate has been observed in mice given oral haloperidol at 15 times the usual maximum human dose. Cleft palate in mice appears to be a non-specific response to stress or nutritional imbalance as well as to a variety of drugs, and there is no evidence to relate this phenomenon to predictable human risk for most of these agents.

Continued on next page

Information on McNeil Pharmaceutical Products is based on labeling in effect in August 1992.

McNeil—Cont.

There are no adequate and well-controlled studies in pregnant women. There are reports, however, of cases of limb malformations observed following maternal use of HALDOL along with other drugs which have suspected teratogenic potential during the first trimester of pregnancy. Causal relationships were not established with these cases. Since such experience does not exclude the possibility of fetal damage due to HALDOL, haloperidol decanoate should be used during pregnancy or in women likely to become pregnant only if the benefit clearly justifies a potential risk to the fetus.

Nursing Mothers

Since haloperidol is excreted in human breast milk, infants should not be nursed during drug treatment with haloperidol decanoate.

Pediatric Use

Safety and effectiveness of haloperidol decanoate in children have not been established.

ADVERSE REACTIONS

Adverse reactions following the administration of HALDOL Decanoate 50 or HALDOL Decanoate 100 are those of HALDOL haloperidol. Since vast experience has accumulated with HALDOL, the adverse reactions are reported for that compound as well as for haloperidol decanoate. As with all injectable medications, local tissue reactions have been reported with haloperidol decanoate.

CNS Effects:

Extrapyramidal Symptoms (EPS)—EPS during the administration of HALDOL (haloperidol) have been reported frequently, often during the first few days of treatment. EPS can be categorized generally as Parkinson-like symptoms, akathisia, or dystonia (including opisthotonos and oculogyric crisis). While all can occur at relatively low doses, they occur more frequently and with greater severity at higher doses. The symptoms may be controlled with dose reductions or administration of antiparkinson drugs such as benztropine mesylate USP or trihexyphenidyl hydrochloride USP. It should be noted that persistent EPS have been reported; the drug may have to be discontinued in such cases.

Withdrawal Emergent Neurological Signs—Generally, patients receiving short term therapy experience no problems with abrupt discontinuation of antipsychotic drugs. However, some patients on maintenance treatment experience transient dyskinetic signs after abrupt withdrawal. In certain of these cases the dyskinetic movements are indistinguishable from the syndrome described below under "Tardive Dyskinesia" except for duration. Although the long acting properties of haloperidol decanoate provide gradual withdrawal, it is not known whether gradual withdrawal of antipsychotic drugs will reduce the rate of occurrence of withdrawal emergent neurological signs.

Tardive Dyskinesia—As with all antipsychotic agents HALDOL has been associated with persistent dyskinesias. Tardive dyskinesia, a syndrome consisting of potentially irreversible, involuntary, dyskinetic movements, may appear in some patients on long-term therapy with haloperidol decanoate or may occur after drug therapy has been discontinued. The risk appears to be greater in elderly patients on high-dose therapy, especially females. The symptoms are persistent and in some patients appear irreversible. The syndrome is characterized by rhythmical involuntary movements of tongue, face, mouth, or jaw (e.g., protrusion of tongue, puffing of cheeks, puckering of mouth, chewing movements). Sometimes these may be accompanied by involuntary movements of extremities and the trunk.

There is no known effective treatment for tardive dyskinesia; antiparkinson agents usually do not alleviate the symptoms of this syndrome. It is suggested that all antipsychotic agents be discontinued if these symptoms appear. Should it be necessary to reinstitute treatment, or increase the dosage of the agent, or switch to a different antipsychotic agent, this syndrome may be masked.

It has been reported that fine vermicular movement of the tongue may be an early sign of tardive dyskinesia and if the medication is stopped at that time the full syndrome may not develop.

Tardive Dystonia—Tardive dystonia, not associated with the above syndrome, has also been reported. Tardive dystonia is characterized by delayed onset of choreic or dystonic movements, is often persistent, and has the potential of becoming irreversible.

Other CNS effects—Insomnia, restlessness, anxiety, euphoria, agitation, drowsiness, depression, lethargy, headache, confusion, vertigo, grand mal seizures, exacerbation of psychotic symptoms including hallucinations, and catatonic-like behavioral states which may be responsive to drug withdrawal and/or treatment with anticholinergic drugs.

Body as a Whole: Neuroleptic malignant syndrome (NMS), hyperpyrexia and heat stroke have been reported with HALDOL. (See WARNINGS for further information concerning NMS.)

Cardiovascular Effects: Tachycardia, hypotension, hypertension and ECG changes including prolongation of the Q-T interval and ECG pattern changes compatible with the polymorphous configuration of torsades de pointes.

Hematologic Effects: Reports have appeared citing the occurrence of mild and usually transient leukopenia and leukocytosis, minimal decreases in red blood cell counts, anemia, or a tendency toward lymphomonocytosis. Agranulocytosis has rarely been reported to have occurred with the use of HALDOL, and then only in association with other medication.

Liver Effects: Impaired liver function and/or jaundice have been reported.

Dermatologic Reactions: Maculopapular and acneiform skin reactions and isolated cases of photosensitivity and loss of hair.

Endocrine Disorders: Lactation, breast engorgement, mastalgia, menstrual irregularities, gynecomastia, impotence, increased libido, hyperglycemia, hypoglycemia and hyponatremia.

Gastrointestinal Effects: Anorexia, constipation, diarrhea, hypersalivation, dyspepsia, nausea and vomiting.

Autonomic Reactions: Dry mouth, blurred vision, urinary retention, diaphoresis and priapism.

Respiratory Effects: Laryngospasm, bronchospasm and increased depth of respiration.

Special Senses: Cataracts, retinopathy and visual disturbances.

Other: Cases of sudden and unexpected death have been reported in association with the administration of HALDOL. The nature of the evidence makes it impossible to determine definitively what role, if any, HALDOL played in the outcome of the reported cases. The possibility that HALDOL caused death cannot, of course, be excluded, but it is to be kept in mind that sudden and unexpected death may occur in psychotic patients when they go untreated or when they are treated with other antipsychotic drugs.

Postmarketing Events: Hyperammonemia has been reported in a 5½ year old child with citrullinemia, an inherited disorder of ammonia excretion, following treatment with HALDOL.

OVERDOSAGE

While overdosage is less likely to occur with a parenteral than with an oral medication, information pertaining to HALDOL haloperidol is presented, modified only to reflect the extended duration of action of haloperidol decanoate.

Manifestations—In general, the symptoms of overdosage would be an exaggeration of known pharmacologic effects and adverse reactions, the most prominent of which would be: 1) severe extrapyramidal reactions, 2) hypotension, or 3) sedation. The patient would appear comatose with respiratory depression and hypotension which could be severe enough to produce a shock-like state. The extrapyramidal reactions would be manifested by muscular weakness or rigidity and a generalized or localized tremor, as demonstrated by the akinetic or agitans types, respectively. With accidental overdosage, hypertension rather than hypotension occurred in a two-year old child. The risk of ECG changes associated with torsades de pointes should be considered. (For further information regarding torsades de pointes, please refer to ADVERSE REACTIONS.)

Treatment—Since there is no specific antidote, treatment is primarily supportive. A patent airway must be established by use of an oropharyngeal airway or endotracheal tube or, in prolonged cases of coma, by tracheostomy. Respiratory depression may be counteracted by artificial respiration and mechanical respirators. Hypotension and circulatory collapse may be counteracted by use of intravenous fluids, plasma, or concentrated albumin, and vasopressor agents such as metaraminol, phenylephrine and norepinephrine. Epinephrine should not be used. In case of severe extrapyramidal reactions, antiparkinson medication should be administered, and should be continued for several weeks, and then withdrawn gradually as extrapyramidal symptoms may emerge. ECG and vital signs should be monitored especially for signs of Q-T prolongation or dysrhythmias and monitoring should continue until the ECG is normal. Severe arrhythmias should be treated with appropriate anti-arrhythmic measures.

DOSAGE AND ADMINISTRATION

HALDOL Decanoate 50 and HALDOL Decanoate 100 should be administered by deep intramuscular injection. A 21 gauge needle is recommended. The maximum volume per injection site should not exceed 3 mL. The recommended interval between doses is 4 weeks. DO NOT ADMINISTER INTRAVENOUSLY.

Parenteral drug products should be inspected visually for particulate matter and discoloration prior to administration, whenever solution and container permit.

HALDOL Decanoate 50 and HALDOL Decanoate 100 are intended for use in chronic psychotic patients who require prolonged parenteral antipsychotic therapy. These patients should be previously stabilized on antipsychotic medication before considering a conversion to haloperidol decanoate.

Furthermore, it is recommended that patients being considered for haloperidol decanoate therapy have been treated with, and tolerate well, short-acting HALDOL haloperidol in order to exclude the possibility of an unexpected adverse sensitivity to haloperidol. Close clinical supervision is required during the initial period of dose adjustment in order to minimize the risk of overdosage or reappearance of psychotic symptoms before the next injection. During dose adjustment or episodes of exacerbation of psychotic symptoms, haloperidol decanoate therapy can be supplemented with short-acting forms of haloperidol.

The dose of HALDOL Decanoate 50 and HALDOL Decanoate 100 should be expressed in terms of its haloperidol content. The starting dose of haloperidol decanoate should be based on the patient's clinical history, physical condition, and response to previous antipsychotic therapy. The preferred approach to determining the minimum effective dose is to begin with lower initial doses and to adjust the dose upward as needed. For patients previously maintained on low doses of antipsychotics (e.g. up to the equivalent of 10 mg/day oral haloperidol), it is recommended that the initial dose of haloperidol decanoate be 10–15 times the previous daily dose in oral haloperidol equivalents; limited clinical experience suggests that lower initial doses may be adequate. The initial dose of haloperidol decanoate should not exceed 100 mg, regardless of previous antipsychotic dose requirements. Haloperidol decanoate has been effectively administered at monthly intervals in several clinical studies. However, variation in patient response may dictate a need for adjustment of the dosing interval as well as the dose.

Lower initial doses and more gradual adjustment are recommended for elderly or debilitated patients.

Clinical experience with haloperidol decanoate at doses greater than 300 mg per month has been limited.

HOW SUPPLIED

HALDOL® (haloperidol) Decanoate 50 for IM injection, 50 mg haloperidol as 70.5 mg per mL haloperidol decanoate—NDC 0045-0253, 10 × 1 mL ampuls, 3 × 1 mL ampuls and 5 mL multiple dose vials.

HALDOL®(haloperidol) Decanoate 100 for IM injection, 100 mg haloperidol as 141.04 mg per mL haloperidol decanoate—NDC 0045-0254, 5 × 1 mL ampuls and 5 mL multiple dose vials.

Store at controlled room temperature (15°-30°C, 59°-86°F). Do not refrigerate or freeze.

Protect from light.

McNeil Pharmaceutical, McNEILAB, INC., Spring House, PA 19477

Revised 12/30/91

Shown in Product Identification Section, page 418

PANCREASE®   ℞
[pan 'kre-ace]
(pancrelipase) Capsules
Enteric Coated Microspheres
NSN 6505-01-095-4174—100's
NSN 6505-01-077-2780—250's

DESCRIPTION

PANCREASE pancrelipase capsules are a white, dye-free, orally administered capsule containing enteric coated microspheres of porcine pancreatic enzyme concentrate, predominately steapsin (pancreatic lipase), amylase and protease. Each capsule contains no less than:

Lipase	4,000 U.S.P. Units
Amylase	20,000 U.S.P. Units
Protease	25,000 U.S.P. Units

Inactive ingredients include cellulose acetate phthalate, diethyl phthalate, gelatin, povidone, sodium starch glycollate, corn starch, sugar, talc and titanium dioxide.

CLINICAL PHARMACOLOGY

PANCREASE pancrelipase capsules resist gastric inactivation and deliver predictable, high levels of biologically active enzymes into the duodenum. The enzymes catalyze the hydrolysis of fats into glycerol and fatty acids, protein into proteoses and derived substances, and starch into dextrins and sugars. PANCREASE capsules are effective in controlling steatorrhea and its consequences at low daily dosage levels.

INDICATIONS AND USAGE

PANCREASE pancrelipase capsules are indicated for patients with exocrine pancreatic enzyme deficiency as in but not limited to:

- cystic fibrosis
- chronic pancreatitis
- post-pancreatectomy
- post-gastrointestinal bypass surgery (e.g. Billroth II gastroenterostomy)
- ductal obstruction from neoplasm (e.g. of the pancreas or common bile duct).

CONTRAINDICATIONS

PANCREASE pancrelipase capsules are contraindicated in patients known to be hypersensitive to pork protein.

WARNINGS

Should hypersensitivity occur, discontinue medication and treat symptomatically.

PRECAUTIONS

TO PROTECT ENTERIC COATING, MICROSPHERES SHOULD NOT BE CRUSHED OR CHEWED. Where swallowing of capsules is difficult, they may be opened and the microspheres shaken onto a small quantity of a soft food (e.g. applesauce, gelatin, etc.), which does not require chewing, and swallowed immediately. Contact of the microspheres with foods having a pH greater than 5.5 can dissolve the protective enteric shell.

Pregnancy Category C. Diethyl phthalate, an enteric coating component of PANCREASE pancrelipase capsules has been shown with high intraperitoneal dosing to be tetratogenic in rats. However, when this coating was administered orally to rats up to 100 times the human dose, no teratogenic or embryocidal effects were observed. There were no adequate and well-controlled studies in pregnant women. PANCREASE capsules should be used in pregnancy only if the potential benefit justifies the potential risk to the fetus.

ADVERSE REACTIONS

The most frequently reported adverse reactions to PANCREASE pancrelipase capsules are gastrointestinal in nature. Less frequently, allergic-type reactions have also been observed. Extremely high doses of exogenous pancreatic enzymes have been associated with hyperuricosuria and hyperuricemia.

DOSAGE AND ADMINISTRATION

Usual dosage: One or two capsules during each meal and one capsule with snacks. Occasionally a third capsule with meals may be required depending upon individual requirements for control of steatorrhea.

HOW SUPPLIED

PANCREASE® pancrelipase capsules (white, dye-free, imprinted "McNeil" and "Pancrease") in bottles of:

100	...........NDC 0045-0095-60
250	...........NDC 0045-0095-69

Keep bottle tightly closed. Store at controlled room temperature (15°–30°C, 59°–86°F), in a dry place. Do not refrigerate.

4/18/85

Shown in Product Identification Section, page 418

PANCREASE® MT   ℞
[*pan'kre-ace MT*]
(pancrelipase) Capsules
Enteric Coated Microtablets
    PANCREASE MT 4 (100's)
NSN 6505-01-287-2188
    PANCREASE MT 10 (100's)
NSN 6505-01-287-2187
    PANCREASE MT 16 (100's)
NSN 6505-01-289-2005

PRODUCT OVERVIEW

KEY FACTS

Microtablet formulation allows for higher enzyme concentrations and smaller capsule size than the original PANCREASE capsules—more enzymatic activity per gram of protein. Enteric coating protects against gastric deactivation and allows delivery of predictable, high levels of biologically active enzymes into the duodenum. Available in four convenient capsule strengths for increased dosage flexibility.

MAJOR USES

PANCREASE MT capsules are indicated for patients with exocrine pancreatic enzyme deficiency.

SAFETY INFORMATION

See complete safety information provided below.

PRESCRIBING INFORMATION

PANCREASE® MT   ℞
[*pan'kre-ace MT*]
(pancrelipase) Capsules
Enteric Coated Microtablets

DESCRIPTION

PANCREASE MT pancrelipase capsules are orally administered capsules containing enteric coated microtablets of porcine pancreatic enzyme concentrate, predominately steapsin (pancreatic lipase), amylase and protease.

Each PANCREASE MT 4 capsule contains:

Lipase	4,000 U.S.P. Units
Amylase	12,000 U.S.P. Units
Protease	12,000 U.S.P. Units

Each PANCREASE MT 10 capsule contains:

Lipase	10,000 U.S.P. Units
Amylase	30,000 U.S.P. Units
Protease	30,000 U.S.P. Units

Each PANCREASE MT 16 capsule contains:

Lipase	16,000 U.S.P. Units
Amylase	48,000 U.S.P. Units
Protease	48,000 U.S.P. Units

Each PANCREASE MT 25 capsule contains:

Lipase	25,000 U.S.P. Units
Amylase	75,000 U.S.P. Units
Protease	75,000 U.S.P. Units

Inactive ingredients: benzyl alcohol, cellulose, crospovidone, gelatin, iron oxide, magnesium stearate, methacrylic acid copolymer, methylparaben, polydimethylsiloxane, propylparaben, sodium lauryl sulfate, silicon dioxide, talc, titanium dioxide, triethylcitrate, wax and other trace ingredients.

CLINICAL PHARMACOLOGY

PANCREASE MT pancrelipase capsules resist gastric inactivation and deliver predictable, high levels of biologically active enzymes into the duodenum. The enzymes catalyze the hydrolysis of fats into glycerol and fatty acids, protein into proteoses and derived substances, and starch into dextrins and sugars. PANCREASE MT capsules are effective in controlling steatorrhea and its consequences.

INDICATIONS AND USAGE

PANCREASE MT pancrelipase capsules are indicated for patients with exocrine pancreatic enzyme deficiency such as:

- cystic fibrosis
- chronic pancreatitis
- post-pancreatectomy
- post-gastrointestinal bypass surgery (e.g. Billroth II gastroenterostomy)
- ductal obstruction from neoplasm (e.g. of the pancreas or common bile duct).

CONTRAINDICATIONS

PANCREASE MT pancrelipase capsules are contraindicated in patients known to be hypersensitive to pork protein. PANCREASE MT capsules are contraindicated in patients with acute pancreatitis or with acute exacerbations of chronic pancreatic diseases.

WARNINGS

Should hypersensitivity occur, discontinue medication and treat symptomatically.

PRECAUTIONS

General

TO PROTECT ENTERIC COATING, MICROTABLETS SHOULD NOT BE CRUSHED OR CHEWED. Where swallowing of capsules is difficult, they may be opened and the microtablets shaken onto a small quantity of a soft food (e.g. applesauce, gelatin, etc.), which does not require chewing, and swallowed immediately. Contact of the microtablets with foods having a pH greater than 6.0 can dissolve the protective enteric shell.

Pregnancy Category C. Animal reproduction studies have not been conducted with PANCREASE MT pancrelipase capsules. It is also not known whether PANCREASE MT can cause fetal harm when administered to a pregnant woman or can affect reproduction capacity. PANCREASE MT should be given to a pregnant woman only if clearly needed.

ADVERSE REACTIONS

The most frequently reported adverse reactions to pancrelipase-containing products are gastrointestinal in nature. Less frequently, allergic-type reactions have also been observed. Extremely high doses of exogenous pancreatic enzymes have been associated with hyperuricosuria and hyperuricemia when the preparations given were pancrelipase in powdered or capsule form, or pancreatin in tablet form.

DOSAGE AND ADMINISTRATION

Dosage should be adjusted according to the severity of the exocrine pancreatic enzyme deficiency. The number of capsules or capsule strength given with meals and/or snacks should be estimated by assessing which dose minimizes steatorrhea and maintains good nutritional status.

In some patients with pancreatic enzyme deficiency, satisfactory responses have been achieved with dosages (expressed in U.S.P. units of lipase) similar to the ones stated below. However, dosages should be adjusted according to the response of the patient.

Children 7 to 12 years: 4,000 to 12,000 units (more if necessary) with each meal and with snacks.

Children 1 to 6 years: 4,000 to 8,000 units with each meal and 4,000 units with snacks.

Children under 1 year: Dosage for children under 6 months of age has not been established. Children 6 months to 1 year have responded to 2,000 units of lipase per meal.

The assessment of the end points in children is aided by charting growth curves.

Adults: 4,000 to 25,000 units (more if necessary) with each meal and with snacks.

HOW SUPPLIED

PANCREASE® MT 4 pancrelipase capsules (yellow and clear, printed "McNEIL" and "PANCREASE MT 4") in bottles of 100—NDC 0045-0341-60.

PANCREASE® MT 10 pancrelipase capsules (pink and clear, printed "McNEIL" and "PANCREASE MT 10") in bottles of 100—NDC 0045-0342-60.

PANCREASE® MT 16 pancrelipase capsules (salmon and clear, printed "McNEIL" and "PANCREASE MT 16") in bottles of 100—NDC 0045-0343-60.

PANCREASE® MT 25 pancrelipase capsules (white, printed "McNEIL" and "PANCREASE MT 25") in bottles of 100—NDC 0045-0344-60.

Keep bottle tightly closed. Store at controlled room temperature (15°–30°C, 59°–86°F), in a dry place. Do not refrigerate. Dispense in tight container as defined in the official compendium.

Microtablets manufactured by Nordmark Pharmaceutical, Uetersen, Germany.

McNEIL PHARMACEUTICAL
McNEILAB, INC.
SPRING HOUSE, PA 19477
6834401A   12/12/91

Shown in Product Identification Section, page 418

PARAFLEX® (chlorzoxazone)   ℞
[*par'a-flex*]
Caplets 250 mg
For Painful Musculoskeletal Conditions

DESCRIPTION

Each caplet (capsule-shaped tablet) contains:

chlorzoxazone* .... 250 mg

Inactive ingredients: docusate sodium, FD&C Red No. 40, FD&C Yellow No. 6, hydroxypropyl methylcellulose, lactose (hydrous), magnesium stearate, microcrystalline cellulose, polyethylene glycol, polysorbate 80, pregelatinized corn starch, propylene glycol, sodium benzoate, sodium starch glycolate, titanium dioxide.
*5-chlorobenzoxazolinone

ACTIONS

Chlorzoxazone is a centrally-acting agent for painful musculoskeletal conditions. Data available from animal experiments as well as human study indicate that chlorzoxazone acts primarily at the level of the spinal cord and subcortical areas of the brain where it inhibits multisynaptic reflex arcs involved in producing and maintaining skeletal muscle spasm of varied etiology. The clinical result is a reduction of the skeletal muscle spasm with relief of pain and increased mobility of the involved muscles. Blood levels of chlorzoxazone can be detected in people during the first 30 minutes and peak levels may be reached, in the majority of subjects, in about 1 to 2 hours after oral administration of chlorzoxazone. Chlorzoxazone is rapidly metabolized and is excreted in the urine, primarily in a conjugated form as the glucuronide. Less than one percent of a dose of chlorzoxazone is excreted unchanged in the urine in 24 hours.

INDICATIONS

PARAFLEX chlorzoxazone is indicated as an adjunct to rest, physical therapy, and other measures for the relief of discomfort associated with acute, painful musculoskeletal conditions. The mode of action of this drug has not been clearly identified, but may be related to its sedative properties. Chlorzoxazone does not directly relax tense skeletal muscles in man.

CONTRAINDICATIONS

PARAFLEX chlorzoxazone is contraindicated in patients with known intolerance to the drug.

WARNINGS

The concomitant use of alcohol or other central nervous system depressants may have an additive effect.

Usage in Pregnancy: The safe use of PARAFLEX chlorzoxazone has not been established with respect to the possible adverse effects upon fetal development. Therefore, it should be used in women of childbearing potential only when, in the judgment of the physician, the potential benefits outweigh the possible risks.

PRECAUTIONS

PARAFLEX chlorzoxazone should be used with caution in patients with known allergies or with a history of allergic reac-

Continued on next page

McNeil—Cont.

tions to drugs. If a sensitivity reaction occurs such as urticaria, redness, or itching of the skin, the drug should be stopped.

If any symptoms suggestive of liver dysfunction are observed, the drug should be discontinued.

ADVERSE REACTIONS

After more than twenty-six years of extensive clinical use of chlorzoxazone-containing products in an estimated thirty-two million patients, it is apparent that the drug is well tolerated and seldom produces undesirable side effects. Occasional patients may develop gastrointestinal disturbances. It is possible in rare instances that chlorzoxazone may have been associated with gastrointestinal bleeding. Drowsiness, dizziness, lightheadedness, malaise, or overstimulation may be noted by an occasional patient. Rarely, allergic-type skin rashes, petechiae, or ecchymoses may develop during treatment. Angioneurotic edema or anaphylactic reactions are extremely rare. There is no evidence that the drug will cause renal damage. Rarely, a patient may note discoloration of the urine resulting from a phenolic metabolite of chlorzoxazone. This finding is of no known clinical significance.

Approximately thirty-six patients have been reported in whom the administration of chlorzoxazone-containing products was suspected as being the cause of liver damage. In one case, the jaundice was subsequently considered to be due to a carcinoma of the head of the pancreas rather than to the drug. In a second case, there was no jaundice but an elevated alkaline phosphatase and BSP retention. In this patient there was a malignancy with bony and liver metastases. The role of the drug was difficult to determine. A third and fourth case had cholelithiasis. Diagnosis in a fifth case was submassive hepatic necrosis possibly due to abusive use of the drug for approximately one year. The remaining cases had a clinical picture compatible with either a viral hepatitis or a drug-induced hepatitis. In all these latter cases the drug was stopped, and, with one exception, the patients recovered. It is not possible to state that the hepatitis in these patients was or was not drug-induced.

DOSAGE AND ADMINISTRATION

Usual Adult Dosage: One caplet (250 mg) three or four times daily. Initial dosage for *painful musculoskeletal conditions* should be two caplets (500 mg) three or four times daily. If adequate response is not obtained with this dose, it may be increased to three caplets (750 mg) three or four times daily. As improvement occurs dosage can usually be reduced.

Usual Child's Dosage: One-half to two tablets (125 mg to 500 mg) three or four times daily given according to age and weight. The tablets may be crushed and mixed with food or a suitable vehicle for administration to children.

OVERDOSAGE

Symptoms: Initially, gastrointestinal disturbances such as nausea, vomiting, or diarrhea together with drowsiness, dizziness, lightheadedness or headache may occur. Early in the course there may be malaise or sluggishness followed by marked loss of muscle tone, making voluntary movement impossible. The deep tendon reflexes may be decreased or absent. The sensorium remains intact, and there is no peripheral loss of sensation. Respiratory depression may occur with rapid, irregular respiration and intercostal and substernal retraction. The blood pressure is lowered, but shock has not been observed.

Treatment: Gastric lavage or induction of emesis should be carried out, followed by administration of activated charcoal. Thereafter, treatment is entirely supportive. If respirations are depressed, oxygen and artificial respiration should be employed and a patent airway assured by use of an oropharyngeal airway or endotracheal tube. Hypotension may be counteracted by use of dextran, plasma, concentrated albumin or a vasopressor agent such as norepinephrine. Cholinergic drugs or analeptic drugs are of no value and should not be used.

HOW SUPPLIED

PARAFLEX® (chlorzoxazone) 250 mg caplets (capsule shaped tablet, coated peach, printed "PARAFLEX" "⋏").
NDC 0045-0317, bottles of 100.
Dispense in tight container as defined in the official compendium.
Store at room temperature.

Revised 4/5/90

McNEIL PHARMACEUTICAL
McNEILAB, INC. SPRING HOUSE, PA 19477

PARAFON FORTE™ DSC   ℞
[par'a-fahn for'ta]
(chlorzoxazone) Caplets 500 mg
NSN 6505-01-264-4453—100's
NSN 6505-01-315-5359—500's

DESCRIPTION

Each caplet contains:
Chlorzoxazone* .... 500 mg
Inactive ingredients: FD&C Blue No. 1, microcrystalline cellulose, docusate sodium, lactose (hydrous), magnesium stearate, sodium benzoate, sodium starch glycolate, pregelatinized corn starch, D&C Yellow No. 10.

ACTIONS

Chlorzoxazone is a centrally-acting agent for painful musculoskeletal conditions. Data available from animal experiments as well as human study indicate that chlorzoxazone acts primarily at the level of the spinal cord and subcortical areas of the brain where it inhibits multisynaptic reflex arcs involved in producing and maintaining skeletal muscle spasm of varied etiology. The clinical result is a reduction of the skeletal muscle spasm with relief of pain and increased mobility of the involved muscles. Blood levels of chlorzoxazone can be detected in people during the first 30 minutes and peak levels may be reached, in the majority of the subjects, in about 1 to 2 hours after oral administration of chlorzoxazone. Chlorzoxazone is rapidly metabolized and is excreted in the urine, primarily in a conjugated form as the glucuronide. Less than one percent of a dose of chlorzoxazone is excreted unchanged in the urine in 24 hours.

INDICATIONS

PARAFON FORTE DSC chlorzoxazone is indicated as an adjunct to rest, physical therapy, and other measures for the relief of discomfort associated with acute, painful musculoskeletal conditions. The mode of action of this drug has not been clearly identified, but may be related to its sedative properties. Chlorzoxazone does not directly relax tense skeletal muscles in man.

CONTRAINDICATIONS

PARAFON FORTE DSC chlorzoxazone is contraindicated in patients with known intolerance to the drug.

WARNINGS

The concomitant use of alcohol or other central nervous system depressants may have an additive effect.
Usage in Pregnancy: The safe use of PARAFON FORTE DSC chlorzoxazone has not been established with respect to the possible adverse effects upon fetal development. Therefore, it should be used in women of childbearing potential only when, in the judgment of the physician, the potential benefits outweigh the possible risks.

PRECAUTIONS

PARAFON FORTE DSC chlorzoxazone should be used with caution in patients with known allergies or with a history of allergic reactions to drugs. If a sensitivity reaction occurs such as urticaria, redness, or itching of the skin, the drug should be stopped.
If any signs or symptoms suggestive of liver dysfunction are observed, the drug should be discontinued.

ADVERSE REACTIONS

After more than twenty-six years of extensive clinical use of chlorzoxazone-containing products in an estimated thirty-two million patients, it is apparent that the drug is well tolerated and seldom produces undesirable side effects. Occasional patients may develop gastrointestinal disturbances. It is possible in rare instances that chlorzoxazone may have been associated with gastrointestinal bleeding. Drowsiness, dizziness, lightheadedness, malaise, or overstimulation may be noted by an occasional patient. Rarely, allergic-type skin rashes, petechiae, or ecchymoses may develop during treatment. Angioneurotic edema or anaphylactic reactions are extremely rare. There is no evidence that the drug will cause renal damage. Rarely, a patient may note discoloration of the urine resulting from a phenolic metabolite of chlorzoxazone. This finding is of no known clinical significance.

Approximately thirty-six patients have been reported in whom the administration of chlorzoxazone-containing products was suspected as being the cause of liver damage. In one case, the jaundice was subsequently considered to be due to a carcinoma of the head of the pancreas rather than to the drug. In a second case, there was no jaundice but an elevated alkaline phosphatase and BSP retention. In this patient there was a malignancy with bony and liver metastases. The role of the drug was difficult to determine. A third and fourth case had cholelithiasis. Diagnosis in a fifth case was submassive hepatic necrosis possibly due to abusive use of the drug for approximately one year. The remaining cases had a clinical picture compatible with either a viral hepatitis or a drug-induced hepatitis. In all these latter cases, the drug was stopped, and, with one exception, the patients recovered. It is not possible to state that the hepatitis in these patients was or was not drug-induced.

* 5-chlorobenzoxazolinone

DOSAGE AND ADMINISTRATION

Usual Adult Dosage: One caplet three or four times daily. If adequate reponse is not obtained with this dose, it may be increased to 1½ caplets (750 mg) three or four times daily. As improvement occurs dosage can usually be reduced.

OVERDOSAGE

Symptoms: Initially, gastrointestinal disturbances such as nausea, vomiting, or diarrhea together with drowsiness, dizziness, lightheadedness or headache may occur. Early in the course there may be malaise or sluggishness followed by marked loss of muscle tone, making voluntary movement impossible. The deep tendon reflexes may be decreased or absent. The sensorium remains intact, and there is no peripheral loss of sensation. Respiratory depression may occur with rapid, irregular respiration and intercostal and substernal retraction. The blood pressure is lowered, but shock has not been observed.
Treatment: Gastric lavage or induction of emesis should be carried out, followed by administration of activated charcoal. Thereafter, treatment is entirely supportive. If respirations are depressed, oxygen and artificial respiration should be employed and a patent airway assured by use of an oropharyngeal airway or endotracheal tube. Hypotension may be counteracted by use of dextran, plasma, concentrated albumin or a vasopressor agent such as norepinephrine. Cholinergic drugs or analeptic drugs are of no value and should not be used.

HOW SUPPLIED

PARAFON FORTE™ DSC (chlorzoxazone) 500 mg caplets, (capsule shaped tablet, colored light green, imprinted "PARAFON FORTE DSC" and "McNEIL", scored).
NDC 0045-0325, bottles of 100, 500 and unit dose 100's.
Dispense in a tight container as defined in the official compendium.
Store at room temperature.

Revised 12/20/88

Shown in Product Identification Section, page 418

TOLECTIN® 200 (tolmetin sodium)   ℞
[to-lek 'tin]
  200 mg Tablets
TOLECTIN® DS (tolmetin sodium)   ℞
  400 mg Capsules
TOLECTIN® 600 (tolmetin sodium)   ℞
  600 mg Tablets
For Oral Administration

PRODUCT OVERVIEW

KEY FACTS

TOLECTIN is rapidly and almost completely absorbed with peak plasma levels being reached within 30–60 minutes. A therapeutic response to TOLECTIN can be expected in a few days to a week. TOLECTIN displays a biphasic elimination from the plasma consisting of a rapid phase with a half-life of one to 2 hours followed by a slower phase with a half-life of about 5 hours. Essentially all of the dose is recovered in the urine in 24 hours.

MAJOR USES

TOLECTIN is indicated for the relief of signs and symptoms of rheumatoid arthritis, osteoarthritis and juvenile rheumatoid arthritis.

SAFETY INFORMATION

See complete safety information provided below.

PRESCRIBING INFORMATION

TOLECTIN® 200 (tolmetin sodium)   ℞
[to-lek 'tin]
  200 mg Tablets
  NSN 6505-01-038-7460—100's
TOLECTIN® DS (tolmetin sodium)   ℞
  400 mg Capsules
  NSN 6505-01-091-9624—100's
  NSN 6505-01-091-9624—500's
  NSN 6505-01-091-9624—U/D 100's
TOLECTIN® 600 (tolmetin sodium)   ℞
  600 mg Tablets
  NSN 6505-01-322-8539—100's
  NSN 6505-01-322-8539—500's
For Oral Administration

DESCRIPTION

TOLECTIN 200 (tolmetin sodium) tablets for oral administration contain tolmetin sodium as the dihydrate in an amount equivalent to 200 mg of tolmetin (scored for 100 mg). Each tablet contains 18 mg (0.784 mEq) of sodium and the following inactive ingredients: cellulose, magnesium stearate, silicon dioxide, corn starch and talc.
TOLECTIN DS (tolmetin sodium) capsules for oral administration contain tolmetin sodium as the dihydrate in an amount equivalent to 400 mg of tolmetin. Each capsule contains 36 mg (1.568 mEq) of sodium and the following inactive

ingredients: gelatin, magnesium stearate, corn starch, talc, FD&C Red No. 3, FD&C Yellow No. 6 and titanium dioxide.

TOLECTIN 600 (tolmetin sodium) tablets for oral administration contain tolmetin sodium as the dihydrate in an amount equivalent to 600 mg of tolmetin. Each tablet contains 54 mg (2.35 mEq) of sodium and the following inactive ingredients: cellulose, silicon dioxide, crospovidone, hydroxypropyl methyl cellulose, magnesium stearate, polyethylene glycol, corn starch, titanium dioxide, FD&C Yellow No. 6 and D&C Yellow No. 10.

The pKa of tolmetin is 3.5 and tolmetin sodium is freely soluble in water.

Tolmetin sodium is a nonsteroidal anti-inflammatory agent.

The structural formula is:

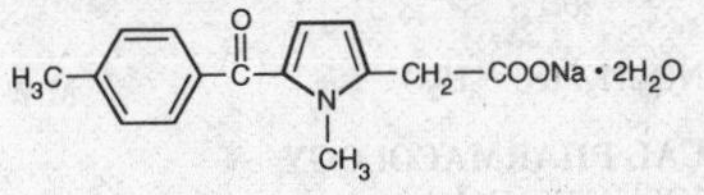

Sodium 1-methyl-5-(4-methylbenzoyl)-1*H*-pyrrole-2-acetate dihydrate.

CLINICAL PHARMACOLOGY

Studies in animals have shown TOLECTIN (tolmetin sodium) to possess anti-inflammatory, analgesic and antipyretic activity. In the rat, TOLECTIN prevents the development of experimentally induced polyarthritis and also decreases established inflammation.

The mode of action of TOLECTIN is not known. However, studies in laboratory animals and man have demonstrated that the anti-inflammatory action of TOLECTIN is *not* due to pituitary-adrenal stimulation. TOLECTIN inhibits prostaglandin synthetase *in vitro* and lowers the plasma level of prostaglandin E in man. This reduction in prostaglandin synthesis may be responsible for the anti-inflammatory action. TOLECTIN does not appear to alter the course of the underlying disease in man.

In patients with rheumatoid arthritis and in normal volunteers, tolmetin sodium is rapidly and almost completely absorbed with peak plasma levels being reached within 30–60 minutes after an oral therapeutic dose. In controlled studies, the time to reach peak tolmetin plasma concentration is approximately 20 minutes longer following administration of a 600 mg tablet, compared to an equivalent dose given as 200 mg tablets. The clinical meaningfulness of this finding, if any, is unknown. Tolmetin displays a biphasic elimination from the plasma consisting of a rapid phase with a half-life of one to 2 hours followed by a slower phase with a half-life of about 5 hours. Peak plasma levels of approximately 40 μg/mL are obtained with a 400 mg oral dose. Essentially all of the administered dose is recovered in the urine in 24 hours either as an inactive oxidative metabolite or as conjugates of tolmetin. An 18-day multiple dose study demonstrated no accumulation of tolmetin when compared with a single dose.

In two fecal blood loss studies of 4 to 6 days duration involving 15 subjects each, TOLECTIN did not induce an increase in blood loss over that observed during a 4-day drug-free control period. In the same studies, aspirin produced a greater blood loss than occurred during the drug-free control period, and a greater blood loss than occurred during the TOLECTIN treatment period. In one of the two studies, indomethacin produced a greater fecal blood loss than occurred during the drug free control period; in the second study, indomethacin did not induce a significant increase in blood loss.

TOLECTIN is effectve in treating both the acute flares and in the long term management of the symptoms of rheumatoid arthritis, osteoarthritis and juvenile rheumatoid arthritis.

In patients with either rheumatoid arthritis or osteoarthritis, TOLECTIN is as effective as aspirin and indomethacin in controlling disease activity, but the frequency of the milder gastrointestinal adverse effects and tinnitus was less than in aspirin-treated patients, and the incidence of central nervous system adverse effects was less than in indomethacin-treated patients.

In patients with juvenile rheumatoid arthritis, TOLECTIN is as effective as aspirin in controlling disease activity, with a similar incidence of adverse reactions. Mean SGOT values, initially elevated in patients on previous aspirin therapy, remained elevated in the aspirin group and decreased in the TOLECTIN group.

TOLECTIN has produced additional therapeutic benefit when added to a regimen of gold salts and, to a lesser extent, with corticosteroids. TOLECTIN should not be used in conjunction with salicylates since greater benefit from the combination is not likely, but the potential for adverse reactions is increased.

INDICATIONS AND USAGE

TOLECTIN (tolmetin sodium) is indicated for the relief of signs and symptoms of rheumatoid arthritis and osteoarthritis. TOLECTIN is indicated in the treatment of acute flares and the long-term management of the chronic disease.

TOLECTIN is also indicated for treatment of juvenile rheumatoid arthritis. The safety and effectiveness of TOLECTIN have not been established in children under 2 years of age (see PRECAUTIONS—Pediatric Use and DOSAGE AND ADMINISTRATION).

CONTRAINDICATIONS

Anaphylactoid reactions have been reported with TOLECTIN as with other nonsteroidal anti-inflammatory drugs. Because of the possibility of cross-sensitivity to other nonsteroidal anti-inflammatory drugs, particularly zomepirac sodium, anaphylactoid reactions may be more likely to occur in patients who have exhibited allergic reactions to these compounds. For this reason, TOLECTIN should not be given to patients in whom aspirin and other nonsteroidal anti-inflammatory drugs induce symptoms of asthma, rhinitis, urticaria and other symptoms of allergic or anaphylactoid reactions. Patients experiencing anaphylactoid reactions on TOLECTIN should be treated with conventional therapy, such as epinephrine, antihistamines and/or steroids.

WARNINGS

Risk of GI Ulceration, Bleeding and Perforation with NSAID Therapy:

Serious gastrointestinal toxicity such as bleeding, ulceration, and perforation, can occur at any time, with or without symptoms, in patients treated chronically with NSAID (Nonsteroidal Anti-Inflammatory Drug) therapy. Although minor upper gastrointestinal problems, such as dyspepsia, are common, usually developng early in therapy, physicians should remain alert for ulceration and bleeding in patients treated chronically with NSAID's even in the absence of previous GI tract symptoms. In patients observed in clinical trials of several months to two years duration, symptomatic upper GI ulcers, gross bleeding or perforation appear to occur in approximately 1% of patients treated for 3–6 months, and in about 2–4% of patients treated for one year. Physicians should inform patients about the signs and/or symptoms of serious GI toxicity and what steps to take if they occur.

Studies to date have not identified any subset of patients not at risk of developing peptic ulceration and bleeding. Except for a prior history of serious GI events and other risk factors known to be associated with peptic ulcer disease, such as alcoholism, smoking, etc., no risk factor (e.g., age, sex) have been associated with increased risk. Elderly or debilitated patients seem to tolerate ulceration or bleeding less well than other individuals and most spontaneous reports of fatal GI events are in this population. Studies to date are inconclusive concerning the relative risk of various NSAID's in causing such reactions. High doses of any NSAID probably carry a greater risk of these reactions, although controlled clinical trials showing this do not exist in most cases. In considering the use of relatively large doses (within the recommended dosage range), sufficient benefit should be anticipated to offset the potential increased risk of GI toxicity.

PRECAUTIONS

General

Because of ocular changes observed in animals and reports of adverse eye findings with nonsteroidal anti-inflammatory agents, it is recommended that patients who develop visual disturbances during treatment with TOLECTIN have ophthalmologic evaluations.

As with other nonsteroidal anti-inflammatory drugs, long-term administration of tolmetin to animals has resulted in renal papillary necrosis and other abnormal renal pathology. In humans, there have been reports of acute interstitial nephritis with hematuria, proteinuria, and occasionally nephrotic syndrome.

A second form of renal toxicity has been seen in patients with prerenal conditions leading to a reduction in renal blood flow or blood volume, where the renal prostaglandins have a supportive role in the maintenance of renal perfusion. In these patients administration of an NSAID may cause a dose dependent reduction in prostaglandin formation and may precipitate overt renal decompensation. Patients at greatest risk of this reaction are those with heart failure, liver dysfunction, those taking diuretics, and the elderly. Discontinuation of NSAID therapy is typically followed by recovery to the pretreatment state.

Since TOLECTIN and its metabolites are eliminated primarily by the kidneys, patients with impaired renal function should be closely monitored, and it should be anticipated that they will require lower doses.

TOLECTIN prolongs bleeding time. Patients who may be adversely affected by prolongation of bleeding time should be carefully observed when TOLECTIN is administered.

In patients receiving concomitant TOLECTIN-steroid therapy, any reduction in steroid dosage should be gradual to avoid the possible complications of sudden steroid withdrawal.

Peripheral edema has been reported in some patients receiving TOLECTIN therapy. Therefore, as with other nonsteroidal anti-inflammatory drugs, TOLECTIN should be used with caution in patients with compromised cardiac function, hypertension, or other conditions predisposing to fluid retention.

The antipyretic and anti-inflammatory activities of the drug may reduce fever and inflammation, thus diminishing their utility as diagnostic signs in detecting complications of presumed non-infectious, non-inflammatory painful conditions.

As with other nonsteroidal anti-inflammatory drugs, borderline elevations of one or more liver tests may occur in up to 15% of patients. These abnormalities may progress, may remain essentially unchanged, or may be transient with continued therapy. The SGPT (ALT) test is probably the most sensitive indicator of liver dysfunction. Meaningful (3 times the upper limit of normal) elevations of SGPT or SGOT (AST) occurred in controlled clinical trials in less than 1% of patients. A patient with symptoms and/or signs suggesting liver dysfunction, or in whom an abnormal liver test has occurred, should be evaluated for evidence of the development of more severe hepatic reaction while on therapy with TOLECTIN. Severe hepatic reactions, including jaundice and fatal hepatitis, have been reported with TOLECTIN as with other nonsteroidal anti-inflammatory drugs. Although such reactions are rare, if abnormal liver tests persist or worsen, if clinical signs and symptoms consistent with liver disease develop, or if systemic manifestations occur (e.g. eosinophilia, rash, etc.), TOLECTIN should be discontinued.

Carcinogenesis, Mutagenesis, Impairment of Fertility

Tolmetin sodium did not possess any carcinogenic liability in the following long-term studies: a 24-month study in rats at doses as high as 75 mg/kg/day, and an 18-month study in mice at doses as high as 50 mg/kg/day.

No mutagenic potential of tolmetin sodium was found in the Ames Salmonella-Microsomal Activation Test.

Reproductive studies revealed no impairment of fertility in animals. Effects on parturition have been shown, however, as with other prostaglandin inhibitors. This information is detailed in the Pregnancy section below.

Pregnancy

Pregnancy Category C. Reproduction studies in rats and rabbits at doses up to 50 mg/kg (1.5 times the maximum clinical dose based on a body weight of 60 kg) revealed no evidence of teratogenesis or impaired fertility due to TOLECTIN. However, TOLECTIN is an inhibitor of prostaglandin synthetase. Drugs in this class have known effects on the fetal cardiovascular system which may cause constriction of the ductus arteriosus *in utero* during the third trimester of pregnancy, which may result in persistent pulmonary hypertension of the newborn.

There are no adequate and well-controlled studies in pregnant women. TOLECTIN should be used during pregnancy only if the potential benefit justifies the potential risk to the fetus.

Non-Teratogenic Effects

Prostaglandin inhibitors have also been shown to increase the incidence of dystocia and delayed parturition in animals.

Nursing Mothers

TOLECTIN has been shown to be secreted in human milk. Because of the possible adverse effects of prostaglandin inhibiting drugs on neonates, use in nursing mothers should be avoided.

Pediatric Use

The safety and effectiveness of TOLECTIN in children under 2 years of age have not been established.

Drug Interactions

The *in vitro* binding of warfarin to human plasma proteins is unaffected by tolmetin, and tolmetin does not alter the prothrombin time of normal volunteers. However, increased prothrombin time and bleeding have been reported in patients on concomitant TOLECTIN and warfarin therapy. Therefore, caution should be exercised when administering TOLECTIN to patients on anticoagulants.

In adult diabetic patients under treatment with either sulfonylureas or insulin there is no change in the clinical effects of either TOLECTIN or the hypoglycemic agents.

Caution should be used if TOLECTIN is administered concomitantly with methotrexate. TOLECTIN and other nonsteroidal anti-inflammatory drugs have been reported to reduce the tubular secretion of methotrexate in an animal model, possibly enhancing the toxicity of methotrexate.

Laboratory Tests

Because serious GI tract ulceration and bleeding can occur without warning symptoms, physicians should follow chronically treated patients for the signs and symptoms of ulceration and bleeding and should inform them of the importance of this follow-up (see WARNINGS—Risk of GI Ulceration, Bleeding and Perforation with NSAID Therapy).

Drug/Laboratory Test Interaction

The metabolites of tolmetin sodium in urine have been found to give positive tests for proteinuria using tests which rely on acid precipitation as their endpoint (e.g. sulfosalicylic acid).

Continued on next page

Information on McNeil Pharmaceutical Products is based on labeling in effect in August 1992.

McNeil—Cont.

No interference is seen in the tests for proteinuria using dye-impregnated commercially available reagent strips (e.g., Albustix®, Uristix®, etc.).

Drug-Food Interaction

In a controlled single dose study, administration of TOLECTIN with milk had no effect on peak plasma tolmetin concentrations, but decreased total tolmetin bioavailability by 16%. When TOLECTIN was taken immediately after a meal, peak plasma tolmetin concentrations were reduced by 50% while total bioavailability was again decreased by 16%.

Information for Patients

TOLECTIN, like other drugs of its class, is not free of side effects. The side effects of these drugs can cause discomfort and, rarely, there are more serious side effects, such as gastrointestinal bleeding, which may result in hospitalization and even fatal outcomes.

NSAID's (Nonsteroidal Anti-Inflammatory Drugs) are often essential agents in the management of arthritis, but they also may be commonly employed for conditions which are less serious.

Physicians may wish to discuss with their patients the potential risks (see WARNINGS, PRECAUTIONS, and ADVERSE REACTIONS sections) and likely benefits of NSAID treatment, particularly when the drugs are used for less serious conditions where treatment without NSAID's may represent an acceptable alternative to both the patient and physician.

ADVERSE REACTIONS

The adverse reactions which have been observed in clinical trials encompass observations in about 4370 patients treated with TOLECTIN (tolmetin sodium), over 800 of whom have undergone at least one year of therapy. These adverse reactions, reported below by body system, are among those typical of nonsteroidal anti-inflammatory drugs and, as expected, gastrointestinal complaints were most frequent. In clinical trials with TOLECTIN, about 10% of patients dropped out because of adverse reactions, mostly gastrointestinal in nature.

Incidence Greater Than 1%

The following adverse reactions which occurred more frequently than 1 in 100 were reported in controlled clinical trials.

Gastrointestinal: Nausea (11%), dyspepsia,* gastrointestinal distress,* abdominal pain,* diarrhea,* flatulence,* vomiting,* constipation, gastritis, and peptic ulcer. Forty percent of the ulcer patients had a prior history of peptic ulcer disease and/or were receiving concomitant anti-inflammatory drugs including corticosteroids, which are known to produce peptic ulceration.

Body as a Whole: Headache,* asthenia,* chest pain

Cardiovascular: Elevated blood pressure,* edema*

Central Nervous System: Dizziness,* drowsiness, depression

Metabolic/Nutritional: Weight gain,* weight loss*

Dermatologic: Skin irritation

Special Senses: Tinnitus, visual disturbance

Hematologic: Small and transient decreases in hemoglobin and hematocrit not associated with gastrointestinal bleeding have occurred. These are similar to changes reported with other nonsteroidal anti-inflammatory drugs.

Urogenital: Elevated BUN, urinary tract infection

*Reactions occurring in 3% to 9% of patients treated with TOLECTIN. Reactions occurring in fewer than 3% of the patients are unmarked.

Incidence Less Than 1%
(Causal Relationship Probable)

The following adverse reactions were reported less frequently than 1 in 100 in controlled clinical trials or were reported since marketing. The probability exists that there is a causal relationship between TOLECTIN and these adverse reactions.

Gastrointestinal: Gastrointestinal bleeding with or without evidence of peptic ulcer, perforation, glossitis, stomatitis, hepatitis, liver function abnormalities

Body as a Whole: Anaphylactoid reactions, fever, lymphadenopathy, serum sickness

Hematologic: Hemolytic anemia, thrombocytopenia, granulocytopenia, agranulocytosis

Cardiovascular: Congestive heart failure in patients with marginal cardiac function

Dermatologic: Urticaria, purpura, erythema multiforme, toxic epidermal necrolysis

Urogenital: Hematuria, proteinuria, dysuria, renal failure

Incidence Less Than 1%
(Causal Relationship Unknown)

Other adverse reactions were reported less frequently than 1 in 100 in controlled clinical trials or were reported since marketing, but a causal relationship between TOLECTIN and the reaction could not be determined. These rarely reported reactions are being listed as alerting information for the physician since the possibility of a causal relationship cannot be excluded.

Body as Whole: Epistaxis

Special Senses: Optic neuropathy, retinal and macular changes

MANAGEMENT OF OVERDOSAGE

In the event of overdosage, the stomach should be emptied by inducing vomiting or by gastric lavage followed by the administration of activated charcoal.

DOSAGE AND ADMINISTRATION

In adults with rheumatoid arthritis or osteoarthritis, the recommended starting dose is 400 mg three times daily (1200 mg daily), preferably including a dose on arising and a dose at bedtime. To achieve optimal therapeutic effect the dose should be adjusted according to the patient's response after one to two weeks. Control is usually achieved at doses of 600–1800 mg daily in divided doses (generally t.i.d.). Doses larger than 1800 mg/kg have not been studied and are not recommended.

The recommended starting dose for children (2 years and older) is 20 mg/kg/day in divided doses (t.i.d. or q.i.d.). When control has been achieved, the usual dose ranges from 15 to 30 mg/kg/day. Doses higher than 30 mg/kg/day have not been studied and, therefore, are not recommended.

A therapeutic response to TOLECTIN (tolmetin sodium) can be expected in a few days to a week. Progressive improvement can be anticipated during succeeding weeks of therapy. If gastrointestinal symptoms occur, TOLECTIN can be administered with antacids other than sodium bicarbonate. TOLECTIN bioavailability and pharmacokinetics are not significantly affected by acute or chronic administration of magnesium and aluminum hydroxides; however, bioavailability is affected by food or milk (see PRECAUTIONS—Drug-Food Interaction).

HOW SUPPLIED

TOLECTIN® 200 (tolmetin sodium) tablets 200 mg (white, scored, imprinted "TOLECTIN," "200" and "McNEIL"), NDC 0045-0412, bottles of 100.

TOLECTIN® DS (tolmetin sodium) capsules 400 mg (colored orange opaque, with contrasting parallel bands, imprinted "TOLECTIN DS" and "McNEIL"), NDC 0045-0414, bottles of 100, 500 and unit dose of 100's.

TOLECTIN® 600 (tolmetin sodium) tablets 600 mg (colored orange, film coated, imprinted "TOLECTIN 600" and "McNEIL"), NDC 0045-0416, bottles of 100 and 500.

Dispense in tight, light-resistant container as defined in the official compendium.

Store at controlled room temperature (15°–30°C, 59°–86°F). Protect from light.

Revised 1/15/91

Shown in Product Identification Section, page 418

TYLENOL® with Codeine ℞

[ti 'len-awl co 'dēn]

(acetaminophen and codeine phosphate tablets and elixir)

Tablets(III) and Elixir(V)

No. 3-NSN 6505-00-400-2054—100's
No. 3-NSN 6505-00-147-8347—500's
No. 3-NSN 6505-01-086-2993—U/D 500's
No. 3-NSN 6505-00-372-3032—1000's
Elixir-NSN 6505-01-035-1963—Pints

DESCRIPTION

Each tablet contains:	
No. 2 Codeine Phosphate*	15 mg
Acetaminophen	300 mg
No. 3 Codeine Phosphate*	30 mg
Acetaminophen	300 mg
No. 4 Codeine Phosphate*	60 mg
Acetaminophen	300 mg
Each 5 mL of elixir contains:	
Codeine Phosphate*	12 mg
Acetaminophen	120 mg
Alcohol 7%	

**Warning*—May be habit forming.

Inactive ingredients: tablets—powdered cellulose, magnesium stearate, sodium metabisulfite†, pregelatinized starch, starch (corn); elixir—alcohol, citric acid, propylene glycol, sodium benzoate, saccharin sodium, sucrose, natural and artificial flavors, FD&C Yellow No.6.

Acetaminophen, 4'-hydroxyacetanilide, is a non-opiate, non-salicylate analgesic and antipyretic which occurs as a white, odorless, crystalline powder, possessing a slightly bitter taste. Its structure is as follows:

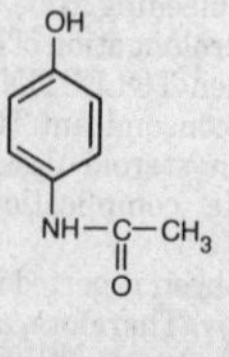

$C_8H_9NO_2$ M.W. 151.16

†See WARNINGS

Codeine is an alkaloid, obtained from opium or prepared from morphine by methylation. Codeine phosphate occurs as fine, white, needle-shaped crystals, or white, crystalline powder. It is affected by light. Its chemical name is: 7,8-didehydro- 4,5α-epoxy-3-methoxy-17- methylmorphinan-6α-ol phosphate (1:1) (salt) hemihydrate. Its structure is as follows:

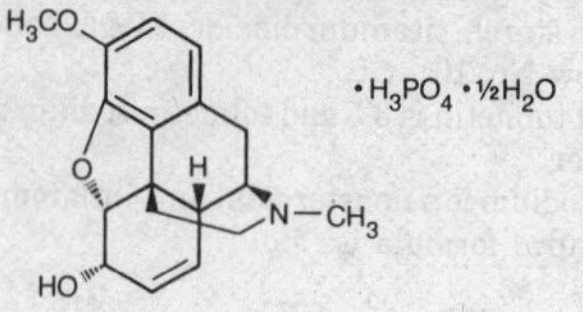

$C_{18}H_{21}NO_3.H_3PO_4. \frac{1}{2}H_2O$ M.W. 406.37

CLINICAL PHARMACOLOGY

TYLENOL with Codeine (acetaminophen and codeine phosphate tablets and elixir) combine the analgesic effects of a centrally acting analgesic, codeine, with a peripherally acting analgesic, acetaminophen. Both ingredients are well absorbed orally. The plasma elimination half-life ranges from 1 to 4 hours for acetaminophen, and from 2.5 to 3 hours for codeine.

Codeine retains at least one-half of its analgesic activity when administered orally. A reduced first-pass metabolism of codeine by the liver accounts for the greater oral efficacy of codeine when compared to most other morphine-like narcotics. Following absorption, codeine is metabolized by the liver and metabolic products are excreted in the urine. Approximately 10 percent of the administered codeine is demethylated to morphine, which may account for its analgesic activity.

Acetaminophen is distributed throughout most fluids of the body, and is metabolized primarily in the liver. Little unchanged drug is excreted in the urine, but most metabolic products appear in the urine within 24 hours.

INDICATIONS AND USAGE

TYLENOL with Codeine tablets (acetaminophen and codeine phosphate tablets) are indicated for the relief of mild to moderately severe pain.

TYLENOL with Codeine elixir (acetaminophen and codeine phosphate elixir) is indicated for the relief of mild to moderate pain.

CONTRAINDICATIONS

TYLENOL with Codeine tablets or elixir (acetaminophen and codeine phosphate tablets and elixir) should not be administered to patients who have previously exhibited hypersensitivity to any component.

WARNINGS

TYLENOL with Codeine tablets (acetaminophen and codeine phosphate tablets) contain sodium metabisulfite, a sulfite that may cause allergic-type reactions including anaphylactic symptoms and life-threatening or less severe asthmatic episodes in certain susceptible people. The overall prevalence of sulfite sensitivity in the general population is unknown and probably low. Sulfite sensitivity is seen more frequently in asthmatic than in nonasthmatic people.

PRECAUTIONS

General

Head Injury and Increased Intracranial Pressure: The respiratory depressant effects of narcotics and their capacity to elevate cerebrospinal fluid pressure may be markedly exaggerated in the presence of head injury, other intracranial lesions or a pre-existing increase in intracranial pressure. Furthermore, narcotics produce adverse reactions which may obscure the clinical course of patients with head injuries.

Acute Abdominal Conditions: The administration of this product or other narcotics may obscure the diagnosis or clinical course of patients with acute abdominal conditions.

Special Risk Patients: This drug should be given with caution to certain patients such as the elderly or debilitated, and those with severe impairment of hepatic or renal function, hypothyroidism, Addison's disease, and prostatic hypertrophy or urethral stricture.

Information for Patients

Codeine may impair the mental and/or physical abilities required for the performance of potentially hazardous tasks such as driving a car or operating machinery. The patient using this drug should be cautioned accordingly.

The patient should understand the single-dose and 24 hour dose limits, and the time interval between doses.

Drug Interactions

Patients receiving other narcotic analgesics, antipsychotics, antianxiety agents, or other CNS depressants (including alcohol) concomitantly with this drug may exhibit an additive CNS depression. When such combined therapy is contemplated, the dose of one or both agents should be reduced.

The concurrent use of anticholinergics with codeine may produce paralytic ileus.

Carcinogenesis, Mutagenesis, Impairment of Fertility

No long-term studies in animals have been performed with acetaminophen or codeine to determine carcinogenic potential or effects on fertility.

Acetaminophen and codeine have been found to have no mutagenic potential using the Ames Salmonella-Microsomal Activation test, the Basc test on Drosophila germ cells, and the Micronucleus test on mouse bone marrow.

Pregnancy

Teratogenic Effects: Pregnancy Category C.

Codeine: A study in rats and rabbits reported no teratogenic effect of codeine administered during the period of organogenesis in doses ranging from 5 to 120 mg/kg. In the rat, doses at the 120 mg/kg level, in the toxic range for the adult animal, were associated with an increase in embryo resorption at the time of implantation. In another study a single 100 mg/kg dose of codeine administered to pregnant mice reportedly resulted in delayed ossification in the offspring.

There are no studies in humans, and the significance of these findings to humans, if any, is not known.

TYLENOL with Codeine (acetaminophen and codeine phosphate tablets and elixir) should be used during pregnancy only if the potential benefit justifies the potential risk to the fetus.

Nonteratogenic Effects:

Dependence has been reported in newborns whose mothers took opiates regularly during pregnancy. Withdrawal signs include irritability, excessive crying, tremors, hyperreflexia, fever, vomiting, and diarrhea. These signs usually appear during the first few days of life.

Labor and Delivery

Narcotic analgesics cross the placental barrier. The closer to delivery and the larger the dose used, the greater the possibility of respiratory depression in the newborn. Narcotic analgesics should be avoided during labor if delivery of a premature infant is anticipated. If the mother has received narcotic analgesics during labor, newborn infants should be observed closely for signs of respiratory depression. Resuscitation may be required (see OVERDOSAGE). The effect of codeine, if any, on the later growth, development, and functional maturation of the child is unknown.

Nursing Mothers

Some studies, but not others, have reported detectable amounts of codeine in breast milk. The levels are probably not clinically significant after usual therapeutic dosage. The possibility of clinically important amounts being excreted in breast milk in individuals abusing codeine should be considered.

Pediatric Use

Safe dosage of TYLENOL with Codeine elixir (acetaminophen and codeine phosphate elixir) has not been established in children below the age of three years.

ADVERSE REACTIONS

The most frequently observed adverse reactions include lightheadedness, dizziness, sedation, shortness of breath, nausea and vomiting. These effects seem to be more prominent in ambulatory than in non-ambulatory patients, and some of these adverse reactions may be alleviated if the patient lies down. Other adverse reactions include allergic reactions, euphoria, dysphoria, constipation, abdominal pain and pruritus.

At higher doses, codeine has most of the disadvantages of morphine including respiratory depression.

DRUG ABUSE AND DEPENDENCE

TYLENOL with Codeine tablets (acetaminophen and codeine phosphate tablets) are a Schedule III controlled substance.

TYLENOL with Codeine elixir (acetaminophen and codeine phosphate elixir) is a Schedule V controlled substance.

Codeine can produce drug dependence of the morphine type and, therefore, has the potential for being abused. Psychic dependence, physical dependence and tolerance may develop upon repeated administration of this drug, and it should be prescribed and administered with the same degree of caution appropriate to the use of other oral narcotic-containing medications.

OVERDOSAGE

Acetaminophen

Signs and Symptoms: In acute acetaminophen overdosage, dose-dependent, potentially fatal hepatic necrosis is the most serious adverse effect. Renal tubular necrosis, hypoglycemic coma and thrombocytopenia may also occur.

In adults, hepatic toxicity has rarely been reported with acute overdoses of less than 10 grams and fatalities with less than 15 grams. Importantly, young children seem to be more resistant than adults to the hepatotoxic effect of an acetaminophen overdose. Despite this, the measures outlined below should be initiated in any adult or child suspected of having ingested an acetaminophen overdose.

Early symptoms following a potentially hepatotoxic overdose may include: nausea, vomiting, diaphoresis and general malaise. Clinical and laboratory evidence of hepatic toxicity may not be apparent until 48 to 72 hours post-ingestion.

Treatment: The stomach should be emptied promptly by lavage or by induction of emesis with syrup of ipecac. Patients' estimates of the quantity of a drug ingested are notoriously unreliable. Therefore, if an acetaminophen overdose is suspected, a serum acetaminophen assay should be obtained as early as possible, but no sooner than four hours following ingestion. Liver function studies should be obtained initially and repeated at 24-hour intervals.

The antidote, N-acetylcysteine, should be administered as early as possible, preferably within 16 hours of the overdose ingestion for optimal results, but in any case, within 24 hours. Following recovery, there are no residual, structural or functional hepatic abnormalities.

Codeine

Signs and Symptoms: Serious overdose with codeine is characterized by respiratory depression (a decrease in respiratory rate and/or tidal volume, Cheyne-Stokes respiration, cyanosis), extreme somnolence progressing to stupor or coma, skeletal muscle flaccidity, cold and clammy skin, and sometimes bradycardia and hypotension. In severe overdosage, apnea, circulatory collapse, cardiac arrest and death may occur.

Treatment: Primary attention should be given to the reestablishment of adequate respiratory exchange through provision of a patent airway and the institution of assisted or controlled ventilation. The narcotic antagonist naloxone is a specific antidote against respiratory depression which may result from overdosage or unusual sensitivity to narcotics, including codeine. Therefore, an appropriate dose of naloxone hydrochloride (see package insert) should be administered, preferably by the intravenous route, and simultaneously with efforts at respiratory resuscitation. Since the duration of action of codeine may exceed that of the antagonist, the patient should be kept under continued surveillance and repeated doses of the antagonist should be administered as needed to maintain adequate respiration.

An antagonist should not be administered in the absence of clinically significant respiratory or cardiovascular depression. Oxygen, intravenous fluids, vasopressors and other supportive measures should be employed as indicated.

Gastric emptying may be useful in removing unabsorbed drug.

DOSAGE AND ADMINISTRATION

Dosage should be adjusted according to severity of pain and response of the patient.

It should be kept in mind, however, that tolerance to codeine can develop with continued use and that the incidence of untoward effects is dose related. Adult doses of codeine higher than 60 mg fail to give commensurate relief of pain but merely prolong analgesia and are associated with an appreciably increased incidence of undesirable side effects. Equivalently high doses in children would have similar effects.

The usual adult dosage for tablets is:

	Single Doses (Range)	Maximum 24 Hour Dose
Codeine Phosphate	15mg–60mg	360mg
Acetaminophen	300mg–1000mg	4000mg

Doses may be repeated up to every 4 hours.

The prescriber must determine the number of tablets per dose, and the maximum number of tablets per 24 hours, based upon the above dosage guidance. This information should be conveyed in the prescription.

For children, the dose of codeine phosphate is 0.5 mg/kg.

TYLENOL with Codeine elixir (acetaminophen and codeine phosphate elixir) contains 120 mg of acetaminophen and 12 mg of codeine phosphate/5 mL and is given orally.

The usual doses are:

Children: *(7 to 12 years):* 10 mL (2 teaspoonfuls) 3 or 4 times daily.
(3 to 6 years): 5 mL (1 teaspoonful) 3 or 4 times daily.
(under 3 years): safe dosage has not been established.

Adults: 15 mL (1 tablespoonful) every 4 hours as needed.

HOW SUPPLIED

TYLENOL with Codeine tablets (acetaminophen and codeine phosphate tablets): (round, white, imprinted "McNEIL", "TYLENOL CODEINE" and either "2", "3", "4"): No.2 - NDC 0045-0511, bottles of 100; No. 3 - NDC 0045-0513, bottles of 100, 500, and 1000; and No. 4 - NDC 0045-0515, bottles of 100 and 500. No. 2, No. 3, and No. 4 also available in unit doses (20 × 25).

TYLENOL with Codeine elixir (acetaminophen and codeine phosphate elixir) contains 120 mg acetaminophen and 12 mg codeine phosphate/5 mL (colored amber, cherry flavored) —NDC 0045-0508, bottles of 1 pint.

Dispense in tight, light-resistant container as defined in the official compendium.

McNeil Pharmaceutical, McNEILAB, INC., Spring House, PA 19477 Revised 7/10/92

Shown in Product Identification Section, page 418

TYLOX® Capsules Ⓒ℞

[ti'lox]

(oxycodone and acetaminophen capsules USP)
NSN 6505-01-210-4450-100's
NSN 6505-01-211-6803-Unit Dose (100's)

DESCRIPTION

Each capsule of TYLOX (oxycodone and acetaminophen capsules USP) contains:

Oxycodone Hydrochloride USP .... 5 mg*
Warning—May be habit forming.
Acetaminophen USP .... 500 mg

Inactive ingredients: docusate sodium, gelatin, magnesium stearate, sodium benzoate, sodium metabisulfite†, corn starch, FD&C Blue No. 1, FD&C Red No. 3, FD&C Red No. 40, and titanium dioxide.

Acetaminophen occurs as a white, odorless crystalline powder, possessing a slightly bitter taste.

The oxycodone component is 14-hydroxydihydrocodeinone, a white, odorless crystalline powder having a saline, bitter taste. It is derived from the opium alkaloid thebaine, and may be represented by the following structural formula:

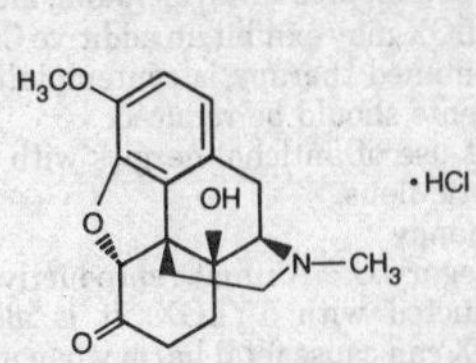

CLINICAL PHARMACOLOGY

The principal ingredient, oxycodone, is a semisynthetic narcotic analgesic with multiple actions qualitatively similar to those of morphine; the most prominent of these involve the central nervous system and organs composed of smooth muscle. The principal actions of therapeutic value of the oxycodone in TYLOX (oxycodone and acetaminophen capsules) are analgesia and sedation.

Oxycodone is similar to codeine and methadone in that it retains at least one-half of its analgesic activity when administered orally.

Acetaminophen is a non-opiate, non-salicylate analgesic and antipyretic.

INDICATIONS AND USAGE

TYLOX (oxycodone and acetaminophen capsules) are indicated for the relief of moderate to moderately severe pain.

CONTRAINDICATIONS

TYLOX (oxycodone and acetaminophen capsules) should not be administered to patients who are hypersensitive to any component.

WARNINGS

Contains sodium metabisulfite, a sulfite that may cause allergic-type reactions including anaphylactic symptoms and life-threatening or less severe asthmatic episodes in certain susceptible people. The overall prevalence of sulfite sensitivity in the general population is unknown and probably low. Sulfite sensitivity is seen more frequently in asthmatic than in nonasthmatic people.

Drug Dependence

Oxycodone can produce drug dependence of the morphine type and, therefore, has the potential for being abused. Psychic dependence, physical dependence and tolerance may develop upon repeated administration of TYLOX (oxycodone and acetaminophen capsules), and it should be prescribed and administered with the same degree of caution appropriate to the use of other oral narcotic-containing medications. Like other narcotic-containing medications, TYLOX is subject to the Federal Control Substances Act (Schedule II).

PRECAUTIONS

General

Head Injury and Increased Intracranial Pressure: The respiratory depressant effects of narcotics and their capacity to elevate cerebrospinal fluid pressure may be markedly exaggerated in the presence of head injury, other intracranial lesions or a pre-existing increase in intracranial pressure. Furthermore, narcotics produce adverse reactions which

*5 mg oxycodone hydrochloride is equivalent to 4.4815 mg oxycodone
†See WARNINGS

Continued on next page

Information on McNeil Pharmaceutical Products is based on labeling in effect in August 1992.

McNeil—Cont.

may obscure the clinical course of patients with head injuries.

Acute Abdominal Conditions: The administration of TYLOX (oxycodone and acetaminophen capsules) or other narcotics may obscure the diagnosis or clinical course in patients with acute abdominal conditions.

Special Risk Patients: TYLOX should be given with caution to certain patients such as the elderly or debilitated, and those with severe impairment of hepatic or renal function, hypothyroidism, Addison's disease, and prostatic hypertrophy or urethral stricture.

Information for Patients

Oxycodone may impair the mental and/or physical abilities required for the performance of potentially hazardous tasks such as driving a car or operating machinery. The patient using TYLOX should be cautioned accordingly.

Drug Interactions

Patients receiving other narcotic analgesics, general anesthetics, phenothiazines, other tranquilizers, sedative-hypnotics or other CNS depressants (including alcohol) concomitantly with TYLOX may exhibit an additive CNS depression. When such combined therapy is contemplated, the dose of one or both agents should be reduced.

The concurrent use of anticholinergics with narcotics may produce paralytic ileus.

Usage in Pregnancy

Pregnancy Category C. Animal reproductive studies have not been conducted with TYLOX. It is also not known whether TYLOX can cause fetal harm when administered to a pregnant woman or can affect reproductive capacity. TYLOX should not be given to a pregnant woman unless in the judgment of the physician, the potential benefits outweigh the possible hazards.

Nonteratogenic Effects: Use of narcotics during pregnancy may produce physical dependence in the neonate.

Labor and Delivery

As with all narcotics, administration of TYLOX to the mother shortly before delivery may result in some degree of respiratory depression in the newborn and the mother, especially if higher doses are used.

Nursing Mothers

It is not known whether the components of TYLOX are excreted in human milk. Because many drugs are excreted in human milk, caution should be exercised when TYLOX is administered to a nursing woman.

Pediatric Use

Safety and effectiveness in children have not been established.

ADVERSE REACTIONS

The most frequently observed adverse reactions include lightheadedness, dizziness, sedation, nausea and vomiting. These effects seem to be more prominent in ambulatory than in non-ambulatory patients, and some of these adverse reactions may be alleviated if the patient lies down.

Other adverse reactions include allergic reactions, euphoria, dysphoria, constipation, skin rash and pruritus. At higher doses, oxycodone has most of the disadvantages of morphine including respiratory depression.

DRUG ABUSE AND DEPENDENCE

TYLOX capsules are a Schedule II controlled substance. Oxycodone can produce drug dependence and has the potential for being abused. (See WARNINGS)

OVERDOSAGE

Acetaminophen

Signs and Symptoms: In acute acetaminophen overdosage, dose-dependent potentially fatal hepatic necrosis is the most serious adverse effect. Renal tubular necrosis, hypoglycemic coma and thrombocytopenia may also occur.

In adults, hepatic toxicity has rarely been reported with acute overdoses of less than 10 grams and fatalities with less than 15 grams. Importantly, young children seem to be more resistant than adults to the hepatotoxic effect of an acetaminophen overdose. Despite this, the measures outlined below should be initiated in any adult or child suspected of having ingested an acetaminophen overdose.

Early symptoms following a potentially hepatotoxic overdose may include: nausea, vomiting, diaphoresis, and general malaise. Clinical and laboratory evidence of hepatic toxicity may not be apparent until 48 to 72 hours post-ingestion.

Treatment: The stomach should be emptied promptly by lavage or by induction of emesis with syrup of ipecac. Patients' estimates of the quantity of a drug ingested are notoriously unreliable. Therefore, if an acetaminophen overdose is suspected, a serum acetaminophen assay should be obtained as early as possible, but no sooner than four hours following ingestion. Liver function studies should be obtained initially and repeated at 24-hour intervals.

The antidote, N-acetylcysteine, should be administered as early as possible, and within 16 hours of the overdose ingestion for optimal results. Following recovery, there are no residual, structural, or functional hepatic abnormalities.

Oxycodone

Signs and symptoms: Serious overdosage with oxycodone is characterized by respiratory depression (a decrease in respiratory rate and/or tidal volume, Cheyne-Stokes respiration, cyanosis), extreme somnolence progressing to stupor or coma, skeletal muscle flaccidity, cold and clammy skin, and sometimes bradycardia and hypotension. In severe overdosage, apnea, circulatory collapse, cardiac arrest, and death may occur.

Treatment: Primary attention should be given to the reestablishment of adequate respiratory exchange through provision of a patent airway and the institution of assisted or controlled ventilation. The narcotic antagonist naloxone hydrochloride is a specific antidote against respiratory depression which may result from overdosage or unusual sensitivity to narcotics, including oxycodone. Therefore, an appropriate dose of naloxone hydrochloride (usual initial adult dose 0.4 mg to 2 mg) should be admininstered preferably by the intravenous route and simultaneously with efforts at respiratory resuscitation (see package insert). Since the duration of action of oxycodone may exceed that of the antagonist, the patient should be kept under continued surveillance and repeated doses of the antagonist should be administered as needed to maintain adequate respiration.

An antagonist should not be administered in the absence of clinically significant respiratory or cardiovascular depression. Oxygen, intravenous fluids, vasopressors and other supportive measures should be employed as indicated.

Gastric emptying may be useful in removing unabsorbed drug.

DOSAGE AND ADMINISTRATION

Dosage should be adjusted according to the severity of the pain and the response of the patient. However, it should be kept in mind that tolerance to oxycodone can develop with continued use and that the incidence of untoward effects is dose related. This product is inappropriate even in high doses for severe or intractable pain.

TYLOX (oxycodone and acetaminophen capsules) are given orally. The usual adult dosage is one TYLOX capsule every 6 hours as needed for pain.

HOW SUPPLIED

TYLOX (oxycodone and acetaminophen capsules USP): (colored red, imprinted "TYLOX" "McNEIL") NDC 0045-0526—bottles of 100 and unit dose 100's.

Dispense in tight, light-resistant container as defined in the official compendium.

Store at controlled room temperature (15°–30° C, 59°–86° F). Protect from moisture.

Revised 4/16/91

Shown in Product Identification Section, page 418

VASCOR® ℞

[vas 'cor]

BEPRIDIL HCl

Tablets

For Oral Administration

DESCRIPTION

VASCOR (bepridil hydrochloride) is an anti-anginal agent that inhibits slow calcium as well as fast sodium channels, interferes with calcium binding to calmodulin and blocks both voltage and receptor operated calcium channels. It is not related chemically to other drugs having similar cardioactivity such as diltiazem hydrochloride, nifedipine and verapamil hydrochloride.

Bepridil hydrochloride monohydrate is a white to off-white, crystalline powder with a bitter taste. It is slightly soluble in water, very soluble in ethanol, methanol and chloroform, and freely soluble in acetone. The molecular weight of bepridil hydrochloride monohydrate is 421.02. Its molecular formula is $C_{24}H_{34}N_2O \cdot HCl \cdot H_2O$. The structural formula is:

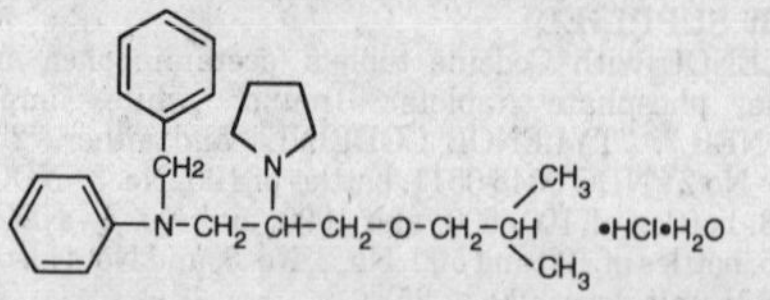

(±)-β-[(2-Methylpropoxy)methyl]-*N*-(phenylmethyl)-1-pyrrolidineethanamine monohydrochloride monohydrate

VASCOR is available as film-coated tablets for oral use containing 200, 300, or 400 mg of bepridil hydrochloride monohydrate. Inactive ingredients: hydroxypropyl methylcellulose, lactose, magnesium stearate, microcrystalline cellulose, polyethylene glycol, silicon dioxide, pregelatinized corn starch, corn starch, titanium dioxide, FD&C Blue #1.

CLINICAL PHARMACOLOGY

VASCOR (bepridil hydrochloride) is a calcium channel blocker anti-anginal agent with Type 1 antiarrhythmic and minimal anti-hypertensive properties. VASCOR has inhibitory effects on both the slow calcium and fast sodium inward currents in myocardial and vascular smooth muscle.

VASCOR inhibits the transmembrane influx of calcium ions into cardiac and vascular smooth muscle. This has been demonstrated in isolated myocardial and vascular smooth muscle preparations in which both the slope of the calcium dose response curve and the maximum calcium-induced inotropic response were significantly reduced by bepridil hydrochloride. In cardiac myocytes *in vitro*, bepridil hydrochloride was shown to be tightly bound to actin. A negative inotropic effect can be seen in the isolated guinea pig atria.

In *in vitro* studies, bepridil hydrochloride has also been demonstrated to inhibit the sodium inward current. Reductions in the maximal upstroke velocity and the amplitude of the action potential, as well as increases in the duration of the normal action potential, have been observed. Additionally, bepridil hydrochloride has been shown to possess local anesthetic activity in isolated myocardial preparations. It effects electrophysiological changes that are observed with several classes of anti-arrhythmic agents.

Clinical Studies

In controlled clinical studies with 200–400 mg of VASCOR, given as a once daily dose, exercise tolerance was improved and angina frequency and daily niitroglycerin use was reduced compared to placebo. Improvement in exercise performance was dose related. In one controlled clinical study, VASCOR was added to propranolol in daily doses of up to 240 mg. The 200–400 mg dose of VASCOR was well tolerated [patients entered were not allowed to be in NYHA Class III or IV heart failure] and there was an added effect of VASCOR on exercise tolerance.

In another controlled clinical study, VASCOR in doses of up to 400 mg/day, significantly improved exercise tolerance compared to diltiazem hydrochloride in patients refractory to diltiazem hydrochloride therapy.

Mechanism of Action: The precise mechanism of action for VASCOR as an anti-anginal agent remains to be fully determined, but is believed to include the following mechanisms: VASCOR regularly reduces heart rate and arterial pressure at rest and at a given level of exercise by dilating peripheral arterioles and reducing total peripheral resistance (afterload) against which the heart works. In exercise tolerance tests in patients with stable angina the heart rate/blood pressure product was reduced with VASCOR for a given work load.

Hemodynamic Effects: VASCOR produces dose dependent slowing of the heart, and reflex tachycardia is not seen. The mean decrease in heart rate in US clinical trials was 3 b.p.m. Orally administered VASCOR also produces modest decreases (less than 5 mm Hg) in systolic and diastolic blood pressure in normotensive patients and somewhat larger decreases in hypertensive patients.

Intravenous administration of VASCOR is associated with a modest reduction in left ventricular contractility (dP/dt), and increased filling pressure, but radionuclide cineangiography studies in angina patients demonstrated improvement in ejection fraction at rest and during exercise following oral VASCOR therapy. Patients with impaired cardiac function [overt heart failure] were not included in these studies.

Electrophysiological Effects: Intravenous administration of VASCOR in man prolongs the effective refractory periods of the atria and ventricles, and the functional refractory period of the AV node. There was a tendency for the AV node effective refractory period and A-H interval to be increased as well. Intravenous and oral administration of VASCOR slow heart rate, prolong the QT and QTc intervals, and alter the morphology of the T-wave (indentation). In clinical trials with angina patients, the mean percent prolongation of the QTc interval was approximately 8%, and of QT about 10%. The prolongation of QT is dose related, varying from about 0.030 sec at doses of 200 mg once a day to 0.055 sec at 400 mg once a day. Upon cessation of therapy, the ECG gradually normalizes. No instances of greater than first-degree heart block have been observed in US controlled or open clinical studies with VASCOR, and first-degree heart block occurred in 0.2% of patients in these studies.

Pulmonary Function: In healthy subjects and asthmatic patients, intravenous VASCOR did not cause bronchoconstriction. VASCOR has been safely used in asthmatic patients and in patients with chronic obstructive lung disease.

Pharmacokinetics and Metabolism: In studies with healthy volunteers, VASCOR is rapidly and completely absorbed after oral administration. The time to peak bepridil plasma concentration is about 2 to 3 hours. Over a ten day period, approximately 70% of a single dose of VASCOR is excreted in the urine and 22% in the feces, as metabolites of bepridil. Excretion of unmetabolized drug is negligible. In healthy male volunteers, the relationship between dose and steady-state blood levels of bepridil was linear over the range of 200 to 400 mg/day. Elimination of bepridil is biphasic, with a distribution half-life of about 2 hours. The terminal

elimination half-life following the cessation of multiple dosing averaged 42 hours (range 26–64 hours). However, during a given dosing interval, decay from the peak concentration occurs relatively rapidly indicating a dosing interval half-life shorter than 24 hours. Following once-daily dosing with therapeutic doses, steady-state was reached in about 8 days in healthy volunteers. The clearance of bepridil decreases after multiple dosing.

Clearance of bepridil in angina patients was lower than that in healthy volunteers, resulting in higher average plasma bepridil concentrations. At steady state, maximum bepridil concentrations averaged 2332 ng/ml (range 1451 to 3609) and mean minimum concentrations were 1174 ng/ml (range 226 to 2639) in angina patients following 300 mg/day doses of VASCOR.

Bepridil is more than 99% bound to plasma proteins. Administration of VASCOR after a meal resulted in a clinically insignificant delay in time to peak concentration, but neither peak bepridil plasma levels nor the extent of absorption was changed.

Bepridil passes through the placental barrier. Bepridil may cause uterine hypotonia.

INDICATIONS AND USAGE

Chronic Stable Angina (Classic Effort-Associated Angina)

VASCOR (bepridil hydrochloride) is indicated for the treatment of chronic stable angina (classic effort-associated angina). Because VASCOR has caused serious ventricular arrhythmias, including torsades de pointes type ventricular tachycardia, and the occurrence of cases of agranulocytosis associated with its use (see WARNINGS), it should be reserved for patients who have failed to respond optimally to, or are intolerant of, other anti-anginal medication.

VASCOR may be used alone or in combination with beta blockers and/or nitrates. Controlled clinical studies have shown an added effect when VASCOR is administered to patients already receiving propranolol.

CONTRAINDICATIONS

VASCOR (bepridil hydrochloride) is contraindicated in patients with a known sensitivity to bepridil hydrochloride.

VASCOR is contraindicated in (1) patients with a history of serious ventricular arrhythmias (see WARNINGS-Induction of New Serious Arrhythmias), (2) patients with sick sinus syndrome or patients with second- or third-degree AV block, except in the presence of a functioning ventricular pacemaker, (3) patients with hypotension (less than 90 mm Hg systolic), (4) patients with uncompensated cardiac insufficiency, (5) patients with congenital QT interval prolongation (see WARNINGS), and (6) patients taking other drugs that prolong QT interval (see PRECAUTIONS-Drug Interactions).

WARNINGS

Induction of New Serious Arrhythmias

VASCOR (bepridil hydrochloride) has Class 1 anti-arrhythmic properties and, like other such drugs, can induce new arrhythmias, including VT/VF. In addition, because of its ability to prolong the QT interval, VASCOR can cause torsades de pointes type ventricular tachycardia. Because of these properties VASCOR should be reserved for patients in whom other anti-anginal agents do not offer a satisfactory effect.

In US clinical trials, the QT and QTc intervals were commonly prolonged by VASCOR in a dose-related fashion. While the mean prolongation of QTc was 8% and of QT was 10%, QTc increases of 25% or more were not uncommon, 5%; 8.7% QT. Increased QT and QTc may be associated with torsades de pointes type VT, which was seen at least briefly, in about 1.0% of patients in US trials; in many cases, however, patients with marked prolongation of QTc were taken off VASCOR therapy. All of the US patients with torsades de pointes had a prolonged QT interval and relatively low serum potassium. French marketing experience has reported over one hundred verified cases of torsades de pointes. While this number, based on total use, represents a rate of only 0.01%, the true rate is undoubtedly much higher, as spontaneous reporting systems all suffer from substantial under reporting.

Torsades de pointes is a polymorphic ventricular tachycardia often but not always associated with a prolonged QT interval, and often drug induced. The relation between the degree of QT prolongation and the development of torsades de pointes is not linear and the likelihood of torsades appears to be increased by hypokalemia, use of potassium wasting diuretics, and the presence of antecedent bradycardia. While the safe upper limit of QT is not defined, it is suggested that the interval not be permitted to exceed 0.52 seconds during treatment. If dose reduction does not eliminate the excessive prolongation, VASCOR should be stopped.

Because most domestic and foreign cases of torsades have developed in patients with hypokalemia, usually

related to diuretic use or significant liver disease, if concomitant diuretics are needed, low doses and addition or primary use of a potassium sparing diuretic should be considered and serum potassium should be monitored.

VASCOR has been associated with the usual range of pro-arrhythmic effects characteristic of Class 1 anti-arrhythmics (increased premature ventricular contraction rates, new sustained VT, and VT/VF that is more difficult than previously to convert to sinus rhythm). Use in patients with severe arrhythmias (who are most susceptible to certain pro-arrhythmic effects) has been limited, so that risk in these patients is not defined.

In the National Heart, Lung and Blood Institute's Cardiac Arrhythmia Suppression Trial (CAST), a long-term, multi-centered, randomized, double-blind study in patients with asymptomatic non-life-threatening ventricular arrhythmias who had myocardial infarctions more than six days but less than two years previously, an excess mortality/non-fatal cardiac arrest rate was seen in patients treated with encainide or flecainide (56/730) compared with that seen in patients assigned to matched placebo-treated groups (22/725). The applicability of these results to other populations (e.g., those without recent myocardial infarction) or to other anti-arrhythmic drugs is uncertain, but at present it is prudent to consider any drug documented to provoke new serious arrhythmias or worsening of pre-existing arrhythmias as having a similar risk and to avoid their use in the post-infarction period.

Agranulocytosis: In US clinical trials of over 800 patients treated with VASCOR for up to five years, two cases of marked leukopenia and neutropenia were reported. Both patients were diabetic and elderly. One died with overwhelming gram-negative sepsis, itself a possible cause of marked leukopenia. The other patient recovered rapidly when VASCOR was stopped.

Congestive Heart Failure: Congestive heart failure has been observed infrequently (about 1%) during US controlled clinical trials, but experience with the use of VASCOR in patients with significantly impaired ventricular function is limited. There is little information on the effect of concomitant administration of VASCOR and digoxin; therefore, caution should be exercised in treating patients with congestive heart failure.

Hepatic Enzyme Elevation: In US clinical studies with VASCOR in about 1000 patients and subjects, clinically significant (at least 2 times the upper limit of normal) transaminase elevations were observed in approximately 1% of the patients. None of these patients became clinically symptomatic or jaundiced and values returned to normal when the drug was stopped.

Hypokalemia: In clinical trials VASCOR has not been reported to reduce serum potassium levels. Because hypokalemia has been associated with ventricular arrhythmias, potassium insufficiency should be corrected before VASCOR therapy is initiated and normal potassium concentrations should be maintained during VASCOR therapy. Serum potassium should be monitored periodically.

PRECAUTIONS

General

Caution should be exercised when using VASCOR (bepridil hydrochloride) in patients with left bundle branch block or sinus bradycardia (less than 50 b.p.m.). Care should also be exercised in patients with serious hepatic or renal disorders because such patients have not been studied and bepridil is highly metabolized, with metabolites excreted primarily in the urine.

Recent Myocardial Infarction

In US clinical trials with VASCOR, patients with myocardial infarctions within three months prior to initiation of drug treatment were excluded. The initiation of VASCOR therapy in such patients, therefore, cannot be recommended.

Information for Patients

Since QT prolongation is not associated with defined symptomatology, patients should be instructed on the importance of maintaining any potassium supplementation or potassium sparing diuretic, and the need for routine electrocardiograms and periodic monitoring of serum potassium.

The following Patient Information is printed on the carton label of each unit of use bottle of 30 tablets:

As with any medication that you take, you should notify your physician of any changes in your overall condition. Insure that you follow your physician's instructions regarding follow-up visits. Please notify any physician who treats you for a medical condition that you are taking VASCOR® (bepridil hydrochloride), as well as any other medications.

Drug Interactions

Nitrates: The concomitant use of VASCOR with long- and short-acting nitrates has been safely tolerated in patients with stable angina pectoris. Sublingual nitroglycerin may be taken if necessary for the control of acute angina attacks during VASCOR therapy.

Beta-blocking Agents: The concomitant use of VASCOR and beta-blocking agents has been well tolerated in patients with stable angina. Available data are not sufficient, however, to predict the effects of concomitant medication on patients with impaired ventricular function or cardiac conduction abnormalities (see CLINICAL PHARMACOLOGY and DOSAGE AND ADMINISTRATION).

Digoxin: In controlled studies in healthy volunteers, bepridil hydrochloride either had no effect (one study) or was associated with modest increases, about 30% (two studies) in steady-state serum digoxin concentrations. Limited clinical data in angina patients receiving concomitant bepridil hydrochloride and digoxin therapy indicate no discernible changes in serum digoxin levels. Available data are neither sufficient to rule out possible increases in serum digoxin with concomitant treatment in some patients, nor other possible interactions, particularly in patients with cardiac conduction abnormalities (Also see WARNINGS-Congestive Heart Failure).

Oral Hypoglycemics: VASCOR has been safely used in diabetic patients without significantly lowering their blood glucose levels or altering their need for insulin or oral hypoglycemic agents.

General Interactions: Certain drugs could increase the likelihood of potentially serious adverse effects with bepridil hydrochloride. In general, these are drugs that have one or more pharmacologic activities similar to bepridil hydrochloride, including anti-arrhythmic agents such as quinidine and procainamide, cardiac glycosides and tricyclic anti-depressants, Anti-arrhythmics and tricyclic anti-depressants could exaggerate the prolongation of the QT interval observed with bepridil hydrochloride. Cardiac glycosides could exaggerate the depression of AV nodal conduction observed with bepridil hydrochloride.

Carcinogenesis, Mutagenesis, Impairment of Fertility

No evidence of carcinogenicity was revealed in one lifetime study in mice at dosages up to 60 times (for a 60 kg subject) the maximum recommended dosage in man. Unilateral follicular adenomas of the thyroid were observed in a study in rats following lifetime administration of high doses of bepridil hydrochloride, i.e., $\geq$ 100 mg/kg/day (20 times the usual recommended dose in man). No mutagenic or other genotoxic potential of bepridil hydrochloride was found in the following standard laboratory tests: the Micronucleus Test for Chromosomal Effects, the Liver Microsome Activated Bacterial Assay for Mutagenicity, the Chinese Hamster Ovary Cell Assay for Mutagenicity, and the Sister Chromatid Exchange Assay. No intrinsic effect on fertility by bepridil hydrochloride was demonstrated in rats.

In monkeys, at 200 mg/kg/day, there was a decrease in testicular weight and spermatogenesis. There were no systematic studies in man related to this point. In rats, at doses up to 300 mg/kg/day, there was no observed alteration of mating behavior nor of reproductive performance.

Usage in Pregnancy

Pregnancy Category C. Reproductive studies (fertility and peri-postnatal) have been conducted in rats. Reduced litter size at birth and decreased pup survival during lactation was observed at maternal dosages 37 times (on a mg/kg basis) the maximum daily recommended therapeutic dosage. In teratology studies, no effects were observed in rats or rabbits at these same dosages. There are no well-controlled studies in pregnant women. Use VASCOR in pregnant or nursing women only if the potential benefit justifies the potential risk.

Nursing Mothers

Bepridil is excreted in human milk. Bepridil concentration in human milk is estimated to reach about one third the concentration in serum. Because of the potential for serious adverse reactions in nursing infants from VASCOR a decision should be made whether to discontinue nursing or to discontinue the drug, taking into account the importance of the drug to the mother.

Pediatric Use

The safety and effectiveness of VASCOR in children have not been established.

ADVERSE REACTIONS

Adverse reactions were assessed in placebo and active-drug controlled trials of 4–12 weeks duration and longer-term uncontrolled studies. The most common side effects occurring more frequently than in control groups were upper gastrointestinal complaints (nausea, dyspepsia or GI distress) in about 22%, diarrhea in about 8%, dizziness in about 15%, asthenia in about 10% and nervousness in about 7%. The adverse reactions seen in at least 2% of bepridil patients in controlled trials are shown in the following table.

[See table on top of next page.]

In one twelve week controlled study, daily doses of 200, 300, and 400 mg were compared to placebo. The following table

Continued on next page

Information on McNeil Pharmaceutical Products is based on labeling in effect in August 1992.

McNeil—Cont.

shows the rates of more common reactions (at least 5% in at least one bepridil group). [See second table at right.]

Although adverse experiences were frequent (at least one being reported in 71% of patients participating in controlled clinical trials), most were well-tolerated. About 15% of patients however, left bepridil treatment because of adverse experiences, in controlled clinical trials, these were principally gastrointestinal (1.0%), dizziness (1.0%) ventricular arrhythmias (1.0%) and syncope (0.6%). The major reasons for discontinuation, with comparison to control agents, are shown below. [See bottom table.]

Across all controlled and uncontrolled trials, VASCOR was evaluated in over 800 patients with chronic angina. In addition to the adverse reactions noted above, the following were observed in 0.5 to 2.0% of the VASCOR patients or are rarer, but potentially important events seen in clinical studies or reported in post marketing experience. In most cases it is not possible to determine whether there is a causal relationship to bepridil treatment.

Body as a Whole: Fever, pain, myalgic asthenia, superinfection, flu syndrome.

Cardiovascular/Respiratory: Sinus tachycardia, sinus bradycardia, hypertension vasodilation, edema, ventricular premature contractions, ventricular tachycardia, prolonged QT interval, rhinitis, cough, pharyngitis.

Gastrointestinal: Flatulence, gastritis, appetite increase, dry mouth, constipation.

Musculoskeletal: Arthritis.

Central Nervous System: Fainting, vertigo, akathisia, drowsiness, insomnia, tremor.

Psychiatric: Depression, anxiousness, adverse behavior effect.

Skin: Rash, sweating, skin irritation.

Special Senses: Blurred vision, tinnitus, taste change.

Urogenital: Loss of libido, impotence.

Abnormal Lab Values: Abnormal liver function test, SGPT increase.

Certain cardiovascular events, such as acute myocardial infarction (about 3% of patients) worsened heart failure (1.9%), worsened angina (4.5%), severe arrhythmia (about 2.4% VT/VF) and sudden death (1.6%) have occurred in patients receiving bepridil, but have not been included as adverse events because they appear to be, and cannot be distinguished from, manifestations of the patient's underlying cardiac disease. Such events as torsades de pointes arrhythmias, prolonged QT/QTc, bradycardia, first degree heart block, which are probably related to bepridil, are included in the tables.

OVERDOSAGE

In the event of overdosage, we recommend close observation in a cardiac care facility for a minimum of 48 hours and use of appropriate supportive measures in addition to gastric lavage. Beta-adrenergic stimulation or parenteral administration of calcium solutions may increase transmembrane calcium ion influx. Clinically significant hypotensive reactions or high-degree AV block should be treated with vasopressor agents or cardiac pacing, respectively. Ventricular tachycardia should be handled by cardioversion and, if persistent, by overdrive pacing.

There has been one experience with overdosage in which a patient inadvertently took a single dose of 1600 mg of VASCOR (bepridil hydrochloride). The patient was observed for 72 hours in intensive care, but no significant adverse experiences were noted.

DOSAGE AND ADMINISTRATION

Therapy with VASCOR (bepridil hydrochloride) should be individualized according to each patient's response and the physician's clinical judgement. The usual starting dose of VASCOR is 200 mg once daily. After 10 days, dosage may be adjusted upward depending upon the patient's response (e.g., ability to perform activities of daily living, QT interval, heart rate, and frequency and severity of angina). This long interval for dosage adjustment is needed because steady-state blood levels are not achieved until 8 days of therapy. In clinical trials, most patients were maintained at a dose of VASCOR of 300 mg once daily. The maximum daily dose of VASCOR is 400 mg and the established minimum effective dose is 200 mg daily.

The starting dose for elderly patients does not differ from that for young patients. After therapeutic response is demonstrated, however, elderly patients may require more frequent monitoring.

Food does not interfere with the absorption of VASCOR. (see CLINICAL PHARMACOLOGY Pharmacokinetics and Metabolism). If nausea is experienced with VASCOR, the drug may be given at meals or at bedtime.

VASCOR has not been studied adequately in patients with impaired hepatic or renal function. It is therefore possible that dosage adjustments may be necessary in these patients.

Adverse Reaction	Bepridil HCl (N = 529)	Nifedipine (N = 50)	Propranolol (N = 88)	Diltiazem (N = 41)	Placebo (N = 190)
Body as a Whole					
Asthenia	9.83	22.00	22.73	12.20	7.37
Headache	11.34	22.00	13.64	7.32	14.21
Flu Syndrome	2.08	8.00	2.27	—α	1.05
Cardiovascular/Respiratory					
Palpitations	2.27	6.00	2.27	0.00	1.58
Dyspnea	3.59	4.00	5.68	4.88	2.11
Respiratory Infection	2.84	4.00	3.41	4.88	3.68
Gastrointestinal					
Dyspepsia	6.81	4.00	5.68	4.88	1.58
G.I. Distress	4.35	10.00	6.82	—α	2.11
Nausea	12.29	14.00	11.36	2.44	3.68
Dry Mouth	3.40	0.00	0.00	2.44	2.63
Anorexia	3.02	0.00	2.27	0.00	1.58
Diarrhea	7.75	2.00	9.09	2.44	2.63
Abdominal Pain	3.02	4.00	1.14	—α	3.16
Constipation	2.84	6.00	1.14	4.88	2.11
Central Nervous System					
Drowsy	3.78	4.00	4.55	—α	3.68
Insomnia	2.65	6.00	3.41	—α	1.05
Dizziness	14.74	30.00	10.23	4.88	9.47
Tremor	4.91	4.00	0.00	—α	1.05
Tremor of Hand	3.02	4.02	0.00	—α	0.53
Paresthesia	2.46	2.00	1.14	4.88	3.16
Psychiatric					
Nervous	7.37	16.00	1.14	2.44	3.68

α No data available.

Adverse Reaction	Bepridil HCl 200 mg (N = 43)	Bepridil HCl 300 mg (N = 46)	Bepridil HCl 400 mg (N = 44)	Placebo (N = 44)
Body as a Whole				
Asthenia	13.95	6.52	11.36	2.27
Headache	6.88	8.70	13.64	15.91
Cardiovascular/Respiratory				
Palpitations	0.00	6.52	4.55	0.00
Dyspnea	2.33	8.70	0.00	2.27
Gastrointestinal				
G.I. Distress	6.98	0.00	4.55	4.55
Nausea	6.98	26.09	18.18	2.27
Anorexia	0.00	2.17	6.82	2.27
Diarrhea	0.00	10.87	6.82	0.00
Central Nervous System				
Drowsy	6.98	6.52	0.00	4.55
Dizziness	11.63	15.22	27.27	6.82
Tremor	6.98	0.00	4.55	0.00
Tremor of Hand	9.30	0.00	4.55	0.00
Psychiatric				
Nervous	11.63	8.70	11.36	0.00
Special Senses				
Tinnitus	0.00	6.52	2.27	2.27

Adverse experiences in long-term open studies were generally similar to those seen in controlled trials.

Most Common Events Resulting in Discontinuation

Adverse Reaction	Bepridil (N = 515) n (%)	Placebo (N = 288) n (%)	Positive Control (N = 119) n (%)
Dizziness	5 (0.97)	0 (0.0)	2 (1.68)
Gastrointestinal Symptoms	5 (0.97)	0 (0.0)	5 (4.20)
Ventricular Arrhythmia	5 (0.97)	0 (0.0)	0 (0.0)
Syncope	3 (0.58)	0 (0.0)	0 (0.0)

Concomitant Use with Other Agents

The concomitant use of VASCOR and beta-blocking agents in patients without heart failure is safely tolerated. Physicians wishing to switch patients from beta-blocker therapy to VASCOR therapy may initiate VASCOR before terminating the beta blocker in the usual gradual fashion (see CLINICAL PHARMACOLOGY and PRECAUTIONS).

HOW SUPPLIED

VASCOR® (bepridil hydrochloride) tablets 200 mg (film coated light blue, scored, printed VASCOR and 200), NDC 0045-0682, bottles of 30 and unit dose of 100s for hospital use.

VASCOR® (bepridil hydrochloride) tablets 300 mg (film coated blue, printed VASCOR and 300), NDC 0045-0683, bottles of 30 and unit dose of 100s for hospital use.

VASCOR® (bepridil hydrochloride) tablets 400 mg (film coated dark blue, printed VASCOR and 400), NDC 0045-0684, bottles of 30 and unit dose of 100s for hospital use.

Store at 15°–25° C (59°–77° F). Protect from light.

Revised 12/27/90

Co-marketed with: **WALLACE LABORATORIES**
Manufactured by: **McNEIL PHARMACEUTICAL**
McNEILAB, Inc. SPRING HOUSE, PA 19477-0776
Shown in product Identification Section, page 418

EDUCATIONAL MATERIAL

Haldol® (haloperidol) Decanoate 50/100 "Feeling Good About Depot Medication" brochure
Available free to physicians and pharmacists through McNeil representatives or directly from McNeil Pharmaceutical (215) 628-5000.

Pancrease® (pancrelipase) and **Pancrease® MT**
"Tree of Life" film and brochure—film available in ½" videotape.

"The Adventures of Mr. Enzyme" Nutritional Video
Target 100%—Growth and Nutrition brochure—for CF patients and families.
Guide to CF for Patients and Families video and workbook.
Mr. Enzyme Activity Books.
Available free to physicians and pharmacists through McNeil representatives or directly from McNeil Pharmaceutical (215) 628-5000.

Parafon Forte™ DSC (chlorzoxazone)
"Remedial Exercises for Low Back Pain" (English and Spanish)
"Remedial Exercises for Cervical Sprain" (English and Spanish)
Both are available free to physicians and pharmacists through McNeil representatives or directly from McNeil Pharmaceutical (215) 628-5000.

Tolectin® (tolmetin sodium)
"Six Steps to Control Your Arthritis Symptoms" (English and Spanish)
Available free to physicians and pharmacists through McNeil representatives or directly from McNeil Pharmaceutical (215) 628-5000.

Vascor® (bepridil hydrochloride) "Patients' Guide" brochure
Available free to physicians and pharmacists through Vascor representatives or directly from McNeil Pharmaceutical (215) 628-5000.

Mead Johnson Laboratories

A Bristol-Myers Squibb Company
P.O. BOX 4500
PRINCETON, NJ 08543-4500

IDENTIFICATION MARKINGS
SOLID ORAL DOSE FORMS

Product	Strengths	Capsules	Tablets One Side
Estrace® (estradiol tablets, USP)	1 mg		MJ755
Estrace® (estradiol tablets, USP)	2 mg		MJ756

[See table above.]

ESTRACE® ℞

[es 'trās]
(estradiol tablets, USP)

Tablets, 1 mg, bottles of 100
NSN 6505-01-281-4829 (M)

WARNING

1. ESTROGENS HAVE BEEN REPORTED TO INCREASE THE RISK OF ENDOMETRIAL CARCINOMA.
Three independent case control studies have shown an increased risk of endometrial cancer in postmenopausal women exposed to exogenous estrogens for prolonged periods.[1-3] This risk was independent of the other known risk factors for endometrial cancer. These studies are further supported by the finding that incidence rates of endometrial cancer have increased sharply since 1969 in eight different areas of the United States with population-based cancer reporting systems, an increase which may be related to the rapidly expanding use of estrogens during the last decade.[4]
The three case control studies reported that the risk of endometrial cancer in estrogen users was about 4.5 to 13.9 times greater than in nonusers. The risk appears to depend on both duration of treatment[1] and on estrogen dose.[3] In view of these findings, when estrogens are used for the treatment of menopausal symptoms, the lowest dose that will control symptoms should be utilized and medication should be discontinued as soon as possible. When prolonged treatment is medically indicated, the patient should be reassessed on at least a semiannual basis to determine the need for continued therapy. Although the evidence must be considered preliminary, one study suggests that cyclic administration of low doses of estrogen may carry less risk than continuous administration[3]; it therefore appears prudent to utilize such a regimen.
Close clinical surveillance of all women taking estrogens is important. In all cases of undiagnosed persistent or recurring abnormal vaginal bleeding, adequate diagnostic measures should be undertaken to rule out malignancy.
There is no evidence at present that "natural" estrogens are more or less hazardous than "synthetic" estrogens at equiestrogenic doses.

2. ESTROGENS SHOULD NOT BE USED DURING PREGNANCY.
The use of female sex hormones, both estrogens and progestogens, during early pregnancy may seriously damage the offspring. It has been shown that females exposed *in utero* to diethylstilbestrol, a nonsteroidal estrogen, have an increased risk of developing in later life a form of vaginal or cervical cancer that is ordinarily extremely rare.[5,6] This risk has been estimated as not greater than 4 per 1,000 exposures.[7] Furthermore, a high percentage of such exposed women (from 30% to 90%) have been found to have vaginal adenosis,[8-12] epithelial changes of the vagina and cervix. Although these changes are histologically benign, it is not known whether they are precursors of malignancy. Although similar data are not available with the use of other estrogens, it cannot be presumed they would not induce similar changes.
Several reports suggest an association between intrauterine exposure to female sex hormones and congenital anomalies, including congenital heart defects and limb reduction defects.[13-16] One case control study[16] estimated a 4.7-fold increased risk of limb reduction defects in infants exposed *in utero* to sex hormones (oral contraceptives, hormone withdrawal tests for pregnancy, or attempted treatment for threatened abortion). Some of these exposures were very short and involved only a few days of treatment. The data suggest that the risk of limb reduction defects in exposed fetuses is somewhat less than 1 per 1,000.
In the past, female sex hormones have been used during pregnancy in an attempt to treat threatened or habitual abortion. There is considerable evidence that estrogens are ineffective for these indications, and there is no evidence from well-controlled studies that progestogens are effective for these uses.
If Estrace is used during pregnancy, or if the patient becomes pregnant while taking this drug, she should be apprised of the potential risks to the fetus and the advisability of pregnancy continuation.

DESCRIPTION

Estrace oral tablets contain 1 or 2 mg of micronized estradiol. Estradiol (17β-estradiol) is a white, crystalline solid, chemically described as estra-1,3,5(10)-triene-3,17β-diol. Estrace oral tablets provide estrogen replacement therapy. The structural formula is:

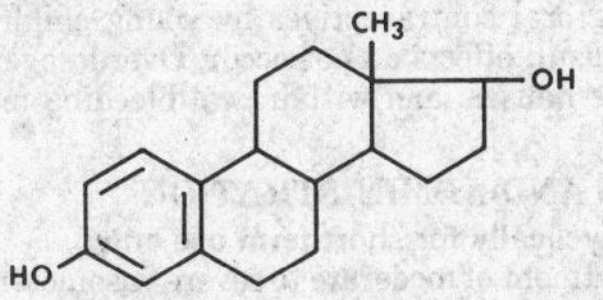

Estrace tablets, 1 mg, contain the following inactive ingredients: acacia, D&C Red No. 27 (aluminum lake), dibasic calcium phosphate, FD&C Blue No. 1 (aluminum lake), lactose, magnesium stearate, colloidal silicon dioxide, starch (corn), and talc.
Estrace tablets, 2 mg, contain the following inactive ingredients: acacia, dibasic calcium phosphate, FD&C Blue No. 1 (aluminum lake), FD&C Yellow No. 5 (tartrazine) (aluminum lake), lactose, magnesium stearate, colloidal silicon dioxide, starch (corn), and talc.

Clinical Pharmacology
17β-Estradiol is the most potent physiologic estrogen and, in fact, is the major estrogenic hormone secreted by the human. Estradiol in Estrace has been micronized and demonstrated to be rapidly and effectively absorbed from the gastrointestinal tract.[17]

INDICATIONS

Estrace affords effective treatment of:
1. Moderate to severe vasomotor symptoms associated with the menopause. (There is no evidence that estrogens are effective for nervous symptoms or depression which might occur during menopause, and they should not be used to treat these conditions.)
2. Atrophic vaginitis.
3. Kraurosis vulvae.
4. Female hypogonadism.
5. Female castration.
6. Primary ovarian failure.
7. Breast cancer (for palliation only) in appropriately selected women and men with metastatic disease.
8. Prostatic carcinoma—palliative therapy of advanced disease.
9. The lowest effective dose appropriate for the specific indication should be utilized. Studies of the addition of a progestogen for seven or more days of a cycle of estrogen administration have reported a lowered incidence of endometrial hyperplasia. Morphological and biochemical studies of endometrium suggest that 10 to 13 days of progestogen are needed to provide maximal maturation of the endometrium and to eliminate any hyperplastic changes. Whether this will provide protection from endometrial carcinoma has not been clearly established. There are possible additional risks which may be associated with the inclusion of progestogen in estrogen replacement regimens. The potential risks include adverse effects on carbohydrate and lipid metabolism. The choice of progestogen and dosage may be important in minimizing these adverse effects.
ESTRACE HAS NOT BEEN SHOWN TO BE EFFECTIVE FOR ANY PURPOSE DURING PREGNANCY AND ITS USE MAY CAUSE SEVERE HARM TO THE FETUS (SEE BOXED WARNING).

CONTRAINDICATIONS

Estrogens should not be used in women (or men) with any of the following conditions:
1. Known or suspected cancer of the breast except in appropriately selected patients being treated for metastatic disease.
2. Known or suspected estrogen-dependent neoplasia.
3. Known or suspected pregnancy (see Boxed Warning).
4. Undiagnosed abnormal genital bleeding.
5. Active thrombophlebitis or thromboembolic disorders.
6. A past history of thrombophlebitis, thrombosis, or thromboembolic disorders associated with previous estrogen use (except when used in treatment of breast or prostatic malignancy).

WARNINGS

1. **Induction of malignant neoplasms.** Long-term continuous administration of natural and synthetic estrogens in certain animal species increases the frequency of carcinomas of the breast, cervix, vagina, and liver. There is now evidence that estrogens increase the risk of carcinoma of the endometrium in humans (see Boxed Warning).
At the present time there is no satisfactory evidence that estrogens given to postmenopausal women increase the risk of cancer of the breast,[18] although a recent long-term follow-up of a single physician's practice has raised this possibility.[19] Because of the animal data there is a need for caution in prescribing estrogens for women with a strong family history of breast cancer or who have breast nodules, fibrocystic disease, or abnormal mammograms.
2. **Gallbladder disease.** A recent study has reported a 2- to 3-fold increase in the risk of surgically confirmed gallbladder disease in women receiving postmenopausal estrogens[18] similar to the 2-fold increase previously noted in users of oral contraceptives.[20,20a] In the case of oral contraceptives, the increased risk appeared after 2 years of use.[34]
3. **Effects similar to those caused by estrogen-progestogen oral contraceptives.** There are several serious adverse effects of oral contraceptives, most of which have not, up to now, been documented as consequences of postmenopausal estrogen therapy. This may reflect the comparatively low doses of estrogen used in postmenopausal women. It would be expected that the larger doses of estrogen used to treat prostatic or breast cancer or postpartum breast engorgement are more likely to result in these adverse effects; in fact, it has been shown that there is an increased risk of thrombosis in men receiving estrogens for prostatic cancer and women for postpartum breast engorgement.[21-24]
a. **Thromboembolic disease.** It is now well established that users of oral contraceptives have an increased risk of various thromboembolic and thrombotic vascular diseases, such as thrombophlebitis, pulmonary embolism, stroke, and myocardial infarction.[25-32] Cases of retinal thrombosis, mesenteric thrombosis, and optic neuritis have been reported in oral contraceptive users. There is evidence that the risk of several of these adverse reactions is related to the dose of the drug.[33,34] An increased risk of postsurgery thromboembolic complications has also been reported in users of oral contraceptives.[35,36] If feasible, estrogen should be discontinued at least 4 weeks before surgery of the type associated with an increased risk of thromboembolism, or during periods of prolonged immobilization.
While an increased rate of thromboembolic and thrombotic disease in postmenopausal users of estrogens has not been found,[19,37] this does not rule out the possibility that such an increase may be present or that subgroups of women who have underlying risk factors or who are receiving relatively large doses of estrogens may have increased risk. Therefore, estrogens should not be used in persons with active thrombophlebitis or thromboembolic disorders, and they should not be used (except in treatment of malignancy) in persons with a history of such disorders in association with estrogen use. They should be used with caution in patients with cerebro-

Continued on next page

Mead Johnson Laboratories—Cont.

vascular or coronary artery disease and only for those in whom estrogens are clearly needed.

Large doses of estrogen (5 mg conjugated estrogens per day), comparable to those used to treat cancer of the prostate and breast, have been shown in a large prospective clinical trial in men[38] to increase the risk of nonfatal myocardial infarction, pulmonary embolism and thrombophlebitis. When estrogen doses of this size are used, any of the thromboembolic and thrombotic adverse effects associated with oral contraceptive use should be considered a clear risk.

b. **Hepatic adenoma.** Hepatic adenomas appear to be associated with the use of oral contraceptives.[39-41] Although rare, these may rupture and may cause death through intraabdominal hemorrhage. Such lesions have not yet been reported in association with other estrogen or progestogen preparations but should be considered in estrogen users having abdominal pain and tenderness, abdominal mass, or hypovolemic shock. Hepatocellular carcinoma has also been reported in women taking estrogen-containing oral contraceptives.[40] The relationship of this malignancy to these drugs is not known at this time.

c. **Elevated blood pressure.** Increased blood pressure is not uncommon in women using oral contraceptives. There is now a report that this may occur with use of estrogens in the menopause[42] and blood pressure should be monitored with estrogen use, especially if high doses are used.

d. **Glucose tolerance.** A worsening of glucose tolerance has been observed in a significant percentage of patients on estrogen-containing oral contraceptives. For this reason, diabetic patients should be carefully observed while receiving estrogen.

4. **Hypercalcemia.** Administration of estrogens may lead to severe hypercalcemia in patients with breast cancer and bone metastases. If this occurs, the drug should be stopped and appropriate measures taken to reduce the serum calcium level.

PRECAUTIONS

A. General Precautions.

1. A complete medical and family history should be taken prior to the initiation of any estrogen therapy. The pretreatment and periodic physical examinations should include special reference to blood pressure, breasts, abdomen, and pelvic organs, and should include a Papanicolaou smear. As a general rule, estrogen should not be prescribed for longer than one year without another physical examination being performed.
2. Fluid retention—Because estrogens may cause some degree of fluid retention, conditions which might be influenced by this factor such as epilepsy, migraine, and cardiac or renal dysfunction, require careful observation.
3. Certain patients may develop undesirable manifestations of excessive estrogenic stimulation, such as abnormal or excessive uterine bleeding, mastodynia, etc.
4. Oral contraceptives appear to be associated with an increased incidence of mental depression. Although it is not clear whether this is due to the estrogenic or progestogenic component of the contraceptive, patients with a history of depression should be carefully observed.
5. Pre-existing uterine leiomyomata may increase in size during estrogen use.
6. The pathologist should be advised of estrogen therapy when relevant specimens are submitted.
7. Patients with a past history of jaundice during pregnancy have an increased risk of recurrence of jaundice while receiving estrogen-containing oral contraceptive therapy. If jaundice develops in any patient receiving estrogen, the medication should be discontinued while the cause is investigated.
8. Estrogens may be poorly metabolized in patients with impaired liver function and they should be administered with caution in such patients.
9. Because estrogens influence the metabolism of calcium and phosphorus, they should be used with caution in patients with metabolic bone diseases that are associated with hypercalcemia or in patients with renal insufficiency.
10. Because of the effects of estrogens on epiphyseal closure, they should be used judiciously in young patients in whom bone growth is not complete.
11. Certain endocrine and liver function tests may be affected by estrogen-containing oral contraceptives. The following similar changes may be expected with larger doses of estrogen:
    a. Increased sulfobromophthalein retention.
    b. Increased prothrombin and factors VII, VIII, IX, and X; decreased antithrombin 3; increased norepinephrine-induced platelet aggregability.
    c. Increased thyroid-binding globulin (TBG) leading to increased circulating total thyroid hormone, as measured by PBI, T4 by volume, or T4 by radioimmunoassay. Free T3 resin uptake is decreased, reflecting the elevated TBG; free T4 concentration is unaltered.
    d. Impaired glucose tolerance.
    e. Decreased pregnanediol excretion.
    f. Reduced response to metyrapone test.
    g. Reduced serum folate concentration.
    h. Increased serum triglyceride and phospholipid concentration.

B. Information for the Patient. See text of Patient Package Insert.

C. Pregnancy Category X. See Contraindications and Boxed Warning.

D. Nursing Mothers. As a general principle, the administration of any drug to nursing mothers should be done only when clearly necessary since many drugs are excreted in human milk.

Estrace 2 mg tablets contain FD&C Yellow No. 5 (tartrazine) which may cause allergic-type reactions (including bronchial asthma) in certain susceptible individuals. Although the overall incidence of FD&C Yellow No. 5 (tartrazine) sensitivity in the general population is low, it is frequently seen in patients who also have aspirin hypersensitivity.

ADVERSE REACTIONS

(See Warnings regarding induction of neoplasia, adverse effects on the fetus, increased incidence of gallbladder disease, and adverse effects similar to those of oral contraceptives, including thromboembolism.) The following additional adverse reactions have been reported with estrogenic therapy, including oral contraceptives:

Genitourinary system. Breakthrough bleeding, spotting, change in menstrual flow. Dysmenorrhea. Premenstrual-like syndrome. Amenorrhea during and after treatment. Increase in size of uterine fibromyomata. Vaginal candidiasis. Change in cervical eversion and in degree of cervical secretion. Cystitis-like syndrome.

Breast. Tenderness, enlargement, secretion.

Gastrointestinal. Nausea, vomiting. Abdominal cramps, bloating. Cholestatic jaundice.

Skin. Chloasma or melasma which may persist when drug is discontinued.

Erythema multiforme. Hemorrhagic eruption. Hirsutism. Erythema nodosum. Loss of scalp hair.

Eyes. Steepening of corneal curvature. Intolerance to contact lenses.

CNS. Headache, migraine, dizziness. Mental depression. Chorea.

Miscellaneous. Increase or decrease in weight. Reduced carbohydrate tolerance. Aggravation of porphyria. Edema. Changes in libido.

OVERDOSAGE

Numerous reports of ingestion of large doses of estrogen-containing oral contraceptives by young children indicate that serious ill effects do not occur. Overdosage of estrogen may cause nausea, and withdrawal bleeding may occur in females.

DOSAGE AND ADMINISTRATION

1. **Given cyclically for short-term use only:**
   For treatment of moderate to severe vasomotor symptoms, atrophic vaginitis, or kraurosis vulvae associated with the menopause. The lowest dose that will control symptoms should be chosen and medication should be discontinued as promptly as possible. Administration should be cyclic (eg, 3 weeks on and 1 week off). Attempts to discontinue or taper medication should be made at 3 to 6 month intervals.
   The usual initial dosage range is 1 or 2 mg daily of micronized estradiol adjusted as necessary to control presenting symptoms. The minimal effective dose for maintenance therapy should be determined by titration.
2. **Given cyclically:**
   Female hypogonadism.
   Female castration.
   Primary ovarian failure.
   Treatment is usually initiated with a dose of 1 or 2 mg daily of micronized estradiol, adjusted as necessary to control presenting symptoms; the minimal effective dose for maintenance therapy should be determined by titration.
3. **Given chronically:**
   Inoperable progressing prostatic cancer—Suggested dosage is 1 to 2 mg three times daily. The effectiveness of therapy can be judged by phosphatase determinations as well as by symptomatic improvement of the patient.
   Inoperable progressing breast cancer in appropriately selected men and postmenopausal women (see INDICATIONS)—Suggested dosage is 10 mg three times daily for a period of at least 3 months.
   Treated patients with an intact uterus should be monitored closely for signs of endometrial cancer and appropriate diagnostic measures should be taken to rule out malignancy in the event of persistent or recurring abnormal vaginal bleeding.

HOW SUPPLIED

Estrace 1 mg; lavender scored tablets

NDC 0087-0755-01	Bottles of 100
NDC 0087-0755-47	Carton of 6 compacts of 25

Estrace 2 mg; turquoise scored tablets

NDC 0087-0756-01	Bottles of 100
NDC 0087-0756-47	Carton of 6 compacts of 25

PATIENT LABELING

WHAT YOU SHOULD KNOW ABOUT ESTROGENS

Estrogens are female hormones produced principally by the ovaries. The ovaries make several different kinds of estrogens. In addition, scientists have been able to make a variety of synthetic estrogens. As far as we know, all these estrogens have the same properties and, therefore, much the same usefulness, side effects, and risks. This leaflet is intended to help you understand what estrogens are used for, the risks involved in their use, and how to use them as safely as possible.

This leaflet includes important information about Estrace and estrogens in general, but not all the information. If you want to know more you can ask your doctor or pharmacist to let you read the professional package insert.

USES OF ESTROGEN

Estrogens are prescribed by doctors for a number of purposes, including:

1. To provide estrogen during a period of adjustment when a woman's ovaries no longer produce it, in order to prevent certain uncomfortable symptoms of estrogen deficiency. (All women normally experience a decrease in the production of estrogens, generally between 45–55; this is called the menopause.)
2. To prevent symptoms of estrogen deficiency when a woman's ovaries have been removed surgically before the natural menopause.
3. To prevent pregnancy. (Some estrogens are given along with a progestogen, another female hormone; these combinations are called oral contraceptives or birth control pills. They will not be discussed in this leaflet.) However, Estrace is not intended for this use.
4. To treat certain cancers in women and men.
5. To prevent painful swelling of the breasts after pregnancy in women who choose not to nurse their babies.

THERE IS NO PROPER USE OF ESTROGENS IN A PREGNANT WOMAN.

ESTROGENS IN THE MENOPAUSE

In the natural course of their lives, all women eventually experience a decrease in estrogen production. This usually occurs between ages 45 and 55 but may occur earlier or later. Sometimes the ovaries may need to be removed before natural menopause by an operation, producing a "surgical menopause."

When the amount of estrogen in the blood begins to decrease, many women may develop typical symptoms: feelings of warmth in the face, neck, and chest or sudden intense episodes of heat and sweating throughout the body (called "hot flashes" or "hot flushes"). These symptoms are sometimes very uncomfortable. A few women eventually develop changes in the vagina (called "atrophic vaginitis") which cause discomfort, especially during and after intercourse.

Estrogens can be prescribed to treat these symptoms of the menopause. It is estimated that considerably more than half of all women undergoing the menopause have only mild symptoms or no symptoms at all and therefore do not need estrogens. Other women may need estrogens for a few months, while their bodies adjust to lower estrogen levels. Sometimes the need will be for periods longer than 6 months. In an attempt to avoid over-stimulation of the uterus (womb), estrogens are usually given cyclically during each month of use, that is, 3 weeks of pills followed by 1 week without pills.

Sometimes women experience nervous symptoms or depression during menopause. There is no evidence that estrogens are effective for such symptoms and they should not be used to treat them, although other treatment may be needed.

You may have heard that taking estrogens for long periods (years) after the menopause will keep your skin soft and supple and keep you feeling young. There is no evidence that this is so, however, and such long-term treatment carries additional risks.

ESTROGENS TO PREVENT SWELLING OF THE BREASTS AFTER PREGNANCY

If you do not breast-feed your baby after delivery, your breasts may fill up with milk and become painful and engorged. This usually begins about 3 to 4 days after delivery and may last for a few days to up to a week or more. Sometimes the discomfort is severe, but usually it is not and can be controlled by pain-relieving drugs such as aspirin and by binding the breasts up tightly. Estrogens can sometimes be used successfully to try to prevent the breasts from filling up. While this treatment is sometimes successful, in many cases the breasts fill up to some degree in spite of treatment. The dose of estrogens needed to prevent pain and swelling of the breasts is much larger than the dose needed to treat symptoms of the menopause and this may increase your chances of developing blood clots in the legs or lungs or other parts of the body (see below, 4. Abnormal Blood Clotting). Therefore, it is important that you discuss the benefits and the risks of estrogen use with your doctor, before using estrogen, if you have decided not to breast-feed your baby.

THE DANGERS OF ESTROGENS

1. Cancer of the uterus. If estrogens are used in the postmenopausal period for more than a year, there is an increased risk of **cancer of the endometrium** (uterine lining). Women taking estrogens have roughly 5 to 15 times as great a chance of getting this cancer as women who take no estrogens. To put this another way, while a postmenopausal woman not taking estrogens has one chance in 1,000 each year of getting cancer of the uterus, a woman taking estrogens has 5 to 15 chances in 1,000 each year. For this reason **it is important to take estrogens only when you really need them.**

The risk of this cancer is greater the longer estrogens are used and also seems to be greater when larger doses are taken. For this reason **it is important to take the lowest dose of estrogen that will control symptoms and to take it only as long as it is needed.** If estrogens are needed for longer periods of time, your doctor will want to reevaluate your need for estrogens at least every 6 months.

Women using estrogens should report any irregular vaginal bleeding to their doctors; such bleeding may be of no importance, but it can be an early warning of cancer of the uterus. If you have undiagnosed vaginal bleeding, you should not use estrogens until a diagnosis is made and you are certain there is no cancer of the uterus.

If you have had your uterus completely removed (total hysterectomy), there is no danger of developing cancer of the uterus.

2. Other possible cancers. Estrogens can cause development of other tumors in animals, such as tumors of the breast, cervix, vagina, or liver, when given for a long time. At present, there is no satisfactory evidence that women using estrogens in the menopause have an increased risk of such tumors, but there is no way yet to be sure they do not; one study raises the possibility that use of estrogens in the menopause may increase the risk of breast cancer many years later. This is a further reason to use estrogens only when clearly needed. While you are taking estrogens, it is important that you go to your doctor at least once a year for a physical examination. Also, if members of your family have had breast cancer or if you have breast nodules or abnormal mammograms (breast x-rays), your doctor may wish to carry out more frequent examinations.

3. Gallbladder disease. Women who use estrogens after menopause are two or three times more likely to develop gallbladder disease needing surgery than women who do not use estrogens. Birth control pills have a similar effect.

4. Abnormal blood clotting. Oral contraceptives increase the risk of blood clotting in various parts of the body. This can occur in different parts of the circulatory system causing thrombophlebitis (clot in the legs or pelvis), retinal thrombosis or optic neuritis (clots affecting vision, including blindness), mesenteric thrombosis (clots in the intestinal blood vessels), stroke (clot in the brain), heart attack (clot in a vessel of the heart) or a pulmonary embolism (clot which eventually lodges in the lungs). These can be fatal.

At this time use of estrogens in the menopause is not known to cause increased blood clotting; this has not been fully studied and there could still prove to be such a risk. It is recommended that if you have had clotting in the legs or lungs or a heart attack or stroke while you were using estrogens or birth control pills, you should not use estrogens (unless they are being used to treat cancer of the breast or prostate). If you have had a stroke or heart attack or if you have angina pectoris, estrogens should be used with great caution and only if clearly needed (for example, if you have severe symptoms of the menopause).

The larger doses of estrogen used to prevent swelling of the breasts after pregnancy have been reported to cause abnormal blood clotting as indicated above.

SPECIAL WARNING ABOUT PREGNANCY

You should not receive estrogen if you are pregnant. If this should occur, there is a greater than usual chance that the developing child will be born with a birth defect, although the possibility remains fairly small. A female child may have an increased risk of developing cancer of the vagina or cervix later in life (in the teens or twenties). Every possible effort should be made to avoid exposure to estrogens during pregnancy. If exposure occurs, see your doctor.

OTHER EFFECTS OF ESTROGENS

In addition to the serious known risks of estrogens described above, estrogens have the following side effects and potential risks which, if occurring, should be discussed promptly with your doctor.

1. Nausea and vomiting. The most common side effect of estrogen therapy is nausea. Vomiting is less common.

2. Effects on breasts. Estrogens may cause breast tenderness or enlargement and may cause the breasts to secrete a liquid.

3. Effects on the uterus. Estrogens may cause benign fibroid tumors of the uterus to get larger. Some women will have menstrual bleeding when estrogens are stopped. But if the bleeding occurs on days you are still taking estrogens, you should report this to your doctor.

4. Effects on liver. Women taking oral contraceptives develop on rare occasions a tumor of the liver which can rupture, bleed into the abdomen, and cause death. So far, these tumors have not been reported in women using estrogens in the menopause, but you should report any swelling or unusual pain or tenderness in the abdomen to your doctor immediately.

Women with a past history of jaundice (yellowing of the skin and white parts of the eyes) may get jaundice again during estrogen use. If this occurs, stop taking estrogens and see your doctor.

5. Other effects. Estrogens may cause excess fluid to be retained in the body. This may make some conditions worse, such as epilepsy, migraine, heart disease, or kidney disease. Mental depression or high blood pressure may occur. A spotty darkening of the skin, particularly of the face, is possible and may persist.

SUMMARY

Estrogens have important uses, and they may have serious risks as well. You must decide, with your doctor, whether the risks are acceptable to you in view of the benefits of treatment. Except where your doctor has prescribed estrogens for use in special cases of cancer of the breast or prostate, you should not use estrogens if you have cancer of the breast or uterus, are pregnant, have undiagnosed abnormal vaginal bleeding, clotting in the legs or lungs or have had a stroke, heart attack or angina, or clotting in the legs or lungs in the past while you were taking estrogens.

You can use estrogens as safely as possible by understanding that your doctor will require regular physical examinations while you are taking them and will try to discontinue the drug as soon as possible and use the smallest dose possible. Be alert for signs of trouble including:
1. Abnormal bleeding from the vagina.
2. Pains in the calves or chest or sudden shortness of breath, or coughing blood (indicating possible clots in the legs, heart, or lungs).
3. Severe headache, dizziness, faintness, or changes in vision (indicating possible developing clots in the brain or eye).
4. Breast lumps (you should ask your doctor how to examine your own breasts).
5. Jaundice (yellowing of the skin).
6. Mental depression.

Based on his or her assessment of your medical needs, your doctor has prescribed this drug for you. Do not give the drug to anyone else.

REFERENCES

1. Ziel HK, Finkel WD: Increased risk of endometrial carcinoma among users of conjugated estrogens. New Eng J Med 293:1167–1170, 1975. **2.** Smith DC, Prentice R, Thompson DJ, Herrmann WL: Association of exogenous estrogen and endometrial carcinoma. New Eng J Med 293:1164–1167, 1975. **3.** Mack TM, Pike MC, Henderson BE, et al: Estrogens and endometrial cancer in a retirement community. New Eng J Med 294:1262–1267, 1976. **4.** Weiss NS, Szekely DR, Austin DF: Increasing incidence of endometrial cancer in the United States. New Eng J Med 294:1259–1262, 1976. **5.** Herbst AL, Ulfelder H, Poskanzer DC: Adenocarcinoma of vagina. New Eng J Med 284:878–881, 1971. **6.** Greenwald P, Barlow J, Nasca P, Burnett W: Vaginal cancer after maternal treatment with synthetic estrogens. New Eng J Med 285:390–392, 1971. **7.** Lanier A, Noller K, Decker D, et al: Cancer and stilbestrol. A follow-up of 1719 persons exposed to estrogens in utero and born 1943–1959. Mayo Clin Proceedings 48:793–799, 1973. **8.** Herbst A, Kurman R, Scully R: Vaginal and cervical abnormalities after exposure to stilbestrol in utero. Obstet Gynec 49:287–298, 1972. **9.** Herbst A, Robboy S, MacDonald G, Scully R: The effects of local progesterone on stilbestrol-associated vaginal adenosis. Am J Obstet Gynec 118:607–615, 1974. **10.** Herbst A, Poskanzer D, Robboy S, et al: Prenatal exposure to stilbestrol, a prospective comparison of exposed female offspring with unexposed controls. New Eng J Med 292:334–339, 1975. **11.** Stafl A, Mattingly R, Foley D, Fetherston W: Clinical diagnosis of vaginal adenosis. Obstet Gynec 43:118–128, 1974. **12.** Sherman AI, Goldrath M, Berlin A, et al: Cervical-vaginal adenosis after in utero exposure to synthetic estrogens. Obstet Gynec 44:531–545, 1974. **13.** Gal I, Kirman B, Stern J: Hormone pregnancy tests and congenital malformation. Nature 216:83, 1967. **14.** Levy EP, Cohen A, Fraser FC: Hormone treatment during pregnancy and congenital heart defects. Lancet 1:611, 1973. **15.** Nora J, Nora A: Birth defects and oral contraceptives. Lancet 1:941–942, 1973. **16.** Janerich DT, Piper JM, Glebatis DM: Oral contraceptives and congenital limb-reduction defects. New Eng J Med 291:697–700, 1974. **17.** Yen SSC, Martin PL, Burnier AM, et al: Circulating estradiol, estrone and gonadotropin levels following the administration of orally active 17β-estradiol in postmenopausal women. J Clin Endocrinol Metab 40:518–521, 1975. **18.** Boston Collaborative Drug Surveillance Program: Surgically confirmed gallbladder disease, venous thromboembolism and breast tumors in relation to post-menopausal estrogen therapy. New Eng J Med 290:15–19, 1974. **19.** Hoover R, Gray LA Sr, Cole P, MacMahon B: Menopausal estrogens and breast cancer. New Eng J Med 295:15–19, 1974. **20.** Boston Collaborative Drug Surveillance Program: Oral contraceptives and venous thromboembolic disease, surgically confirmed gallbladder disease, and breast tumors. Lancet 1:1399–1404, 1973. **20a.** Royal College of General Practitioners: Oral Contraceptives and Health. New York, Pitman Corp, 1974. **21.** Daniel DG, Campbell H, Turnbull AC: Puerperal thromboembolism and suppression of lactation. Lancet 2:287–289, 1967. **22.** The Veterans Administration Cooperative Urological Research Group: Carcinoma of the prostate: treatment comparisons. J Urol 98:516–522, 1967. **23.** Bailar JC: Thromboembolism and oestrogen therapy. Lancet 2:560, 1967. **24.** Blackard C, Doe R, Mellinger G, Byar D: Incidence of cardiovascular disease and death in patients receiving diethylstilbestrol for carcinoma of the prostate. Cancer 26:249–256, 1970. **25.** Royal College of General Practitioners: Oral contraception and thromboembolic disease. J Roy Coll Gen Pract 13:267–279, 1967. **26.** Inman WHW, Vessey MP: Investigation of deaths from pulmonary, coronary, and cerebral thrombosis and embolism in women of child-bearing age. Brit M J 2:193–199, 1968. **27.** Vessey MP, Doll R: Investigation of relation between use of oral contraceptives and thromboembolic disease. A further report. Brit M J 2:651–657, 1969. **28.** Sartwell PE, Masi AT, Arthes FG, et al: Thromboembolism and oral contraceptives: an epidemiological case control study. Am J Epidemiol 90:365–380, 1969. **29.** Collaborative Group for the Study of Stroke in Young Women: Oral contraception and increased risk of cerebral ischemia or thrombosis. New Eng J Med 288:871–878, 1973. **30.** Collaborative Group for the Study of Stroke in Young Women: Oral contraceptives and stroke in young women: Associated risk factors. JAMA 231:718–722, 1975. **31.** Mann JI, Inman WHW: Oral contraceptives and death from myocardial infarction. Brit M J 2:245–248, 1975. **32.** Mann JI, Vessey MP, Thorogood M, Doll R: Myocardial infarction in young women with special reference to oral contraceptive practice. Brit M J 2:241–245, 1975. **33.** Inman WHW, Vessey MP, Westerholm B, Engelund A: Thromboembolic disease and the steroidal content of oral contraceptives. Brit M J 2:203–209, 1970. **34.** Stolley PD, Tonascia JA, Tockman MS, et al: Thrombosis with low-estrogen oral contraceptives. Am J Epidemiol 102:197–208, 1975. **35.** Vessey MP, Doll R, Fairbairn AS, Glober G: Post-operative thromboembolism and the use of the oral contraceptives. Brit M J 3:123–126, 1970. **36.** Greene GR, Sartwell PE: Oral contraceptive use in patients with thromboembolism following surgery, trauma or infection. Am J Pub Health 62:680–685, 1972. **37.** Rosenberg L, Armstrong MB, Jick H: Myocardial infarction and estrogen therapy in postmenopausal women. New Eng J Med 294:1256–1259, 1976. **38.** Coronary Drug Project Research Group: The coronary drug project: initial findings leading to modifications of its research protocol. JAMA 214:1303–1313, 1970. **39.** Baum J, Holtz F, Bookstein JJ, Klein EW: Possible association between benign hepatomas and oral contraceptives. Lancet 2:926–928, 1973. **40.** Mays ET, Christopherson WM, Mahr MM, Williams HC: Hepatic changes in young women ingesting contraceptive steroids, hepatic hemorrhage and primary hepatic tumors. JAMA 235:730–732, 1976. **41.** Edmondson HA, Henderson B, Benton B: Liver cell adenomas associated with the use of oral contraceptives. New Eng J Med 294:470–472, 1976. **42.** Pfeffer RI, Van Den Noort S: Estrogen use and stroke risk in postmenopausal women. Am J Epidemiol 103:445–456, 1976.

Shown in Product Identification Section, page 419

ESTRACE®   ℞
[ĕs′trace]
(Estradiol Vaginal Cream 0.01%)

CAUTION: FEDERAL LAW PROHIBITS DISPENSING WITHOUT PRESCRIPTION

WARNING

1. ESTROGENS HAVE BEEN REPORTED TO INCREASE THE RISK OF ENDOMETRIAL CARCINOMA.

Three independent case control studies have shown an increased risk of endometrial cancer in postmenopausal women exposed to exogenous estrogens for prolonged periods.[1-3] This risk was independent of the other known risk factors for endometrial cancer. These studies are further supported by the finding that incidence rates of endometrial cancer have increased sharply since 1969 in eight different areas of the United States with population based cancer reporting systems, an increase which may be related to the rapidly expanding use of estrogens during the last decade.[4]

The three case control studies reported that the risk of endometrial cancer in estrogen users was about 4.5 to 13.9 times greater than in nonusers. The risk appears to depend on both duration of treatment[1] and on estrogen dose.[3] In view of these findings, when estrogens are used

Continued on next page

Mead Johnson Laboratories—Cont.

for the treatment of menopausal symptoms, the lowest dose that will control symptoms should be utilized and medication should be discontinued as soon as possible. When prolonged treatment is medically indicated, the patient should be reassessed on at least a semiannual basis to determine the need for continued therapy. Although the evidence must be considered preliminary, one study suggests that cyclic administration of low doses of estrogen may carry less risk than continuous administration[3]; it therefore appears prudent to utilize such a regimen.
Close clinical surveillance of all women taking estrogens is important. In all cases of undiagnosed persistent or recurring abnormal vaginal bleeding, adequate diagnostic measures should be undertaken to rule out malignancy.
There is no evidence at present that "natural" estrogens are more or less hazardous than "synthetic" estrogens at equiestrogenic doses.

2. ESTROGENS SHOULD NOT BE USED DURING PREGNANCY.
The use of female sex hormones, both estrogens and progestogens, during early pregnancy may seriously damage the offspring. It has been shown that females exposed *in utero* to diethylstilbestrol, a nonsteroidal estrogen, have an increased risk of developing in later life a form of vaginal or cervical cancer that is ordinarily extremely rare.[5,6] This risk has been estimated as not greater than 4 per 1,000 exposures.[7] Furthermore, a high percentage of such exposed women (from 30% to 90%) have been found to have vaginal adenosis,[8–12] epithelial changes of the vagina and cervix. Although these changes are histologically benign, it is not known whether they are precursors of malignancy. Although similar data are not available with the use of other estrogens, it cannot be presumed they would not induce similar changes.
Several reports suggest an association between intrauterine exposure to female sex hormones and congenital anomalies, including congenital heart defects and limb reduction defects.[13–16] One case control study[16] estimated a 4.7-fold increased risk of limb reduction defects in infants exposed *in utero* to sex hormones (oral contraceptives, hormone withdrawal tests for pregnancy, or attempted treatment for threatened abortion). Some of these exposures were very short and involved only a few days of treatment. The data suggest that the risk of limb reduction defects in exposed fetuses is somewhat less than 1 per 1,000.
In the past, female sex hormones have been used during pregnancy in an attempt to treat threatened or habitual abortion. There is considerable evidence that estrogens are ineffective for these indications, and there is no evidence from well-controlled studies that progestogens are effective for these uses.
If ESTRACE (estradiol vaginal cream) is used during pregnancy, or if the patient becomes pregnant while taking this drug, she should be apprised of the potential risks to the fetus and the advisability of pregnancy continuation.

DESCRIPTION

Each gram of ESTRACE (estradiol vaginal cream) contains 0.1 mg estradiol in a nonliquefying base containing purified water, propylene glycol, stearyl alcohol, white ceresin wax, glyceryl monostearate, hydroxypropyl methylcellulose, 2208 4000 cps, sodium lauryl sulfate, methylparaben, edetate disodium and *tertiary*-butylhydroquinone. Estradiol is chemically described as estra-1,3,5(10)-triene-3, 17β-diol. The structural formula is:

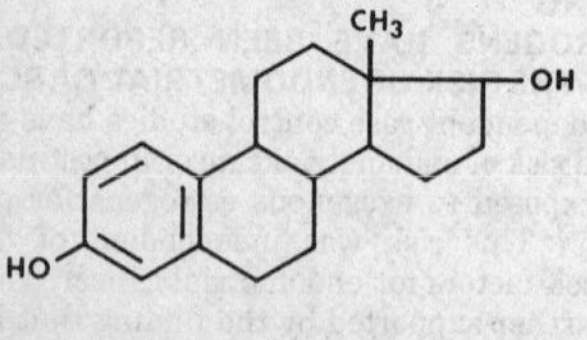

CLINICAL PHARMACOLOGY

Estrogens are important in the development and maintenance of the female reproductive system and secondary sex characteristics. They promote growth and development of the vagina, uterus, and fallopian tubes, and enlargement of the breasts. Indirectly, they contribute to the shaping of the skeleton, maintenance of tone and elasticity or urogenital structures, changes in the epiphyses of the long bones that allow for the pubertal growth spurt and its termination, growth of axillary and pubic hair, and pigmentation of the nipples and genitals. Decline of estrogenic activity at the end of the menstrual cycle can bring on menstruation, although the cessation of progesterone secretion is the most important factor in the mature ovulatory cycle. However, in the preovulatory or nonovulatory cycle, estrogen is the primary determinant in the onset of menstruation. Estrogens also affect the release of pituitary gonadotropins.
Estradiol achieves its pharmacologic effect in estrogen-responsive target tissues via anabolic stimulus at the cellular level. Micronized estradiol in ESTRACE Vaginal Cream is readily absorbed from mucosal surfaces.
In responsive tissues (female genital organs, breasts, hypothalamus, pituitary) estrogens enter the cell and are transported into the nucleus. As a result of estrogen action, specific RNA and protein synthesis occurs.
Metabolism and inactivation occur primarily in the liver. Some estrogens are excreted into the bile; however, they are reabsorbed from the intestine and returned to the liver through the portal venous system.

INDICATIONS AND USAGE

ESTRACE Vaginal Cream is indicated in the treatment of atrophic vaginitis and kraurosis vulvae.
ESTRACE VAGINAL CREAM HAS NOT BEEN SHOWN TO BE EFFECTIVE FOR ANY PURPOSE DURING PREGNANCY AND ITS USE MAY CAUSE SEVERE HARM TO THE FETUS (SEE BOXED WARNING).

CONTRAINDICATIONS

Estrogens should not be used in women (or men) with any of the following conditions:
1. Known or suspected cancer of the breast, except in appropriately selected patients being treated for metastatic disease.
2. Known or suspected estrogen-dependent neoplasia.
3. Known or suspected pregnancy (See Boxed Warning).
4. Undiagnosed abnormal genital bleeding.
5. Active thrombophlebitis or thromboembolic disorders.
6. A past history of thrombophlebitis, thrombosis, or thromboembolic disorders associated with previous estrogen use (except when used in treatment of breast or prostatic malignancy).

WARNINGS

1. **Induction of malignant neoplasms.** Long-term continuous administration of natural and synthetic estrogens in certain animal species increases the frequency of carcinomas of the breast, cervix, vagina, and liver. There is now evidence that estrogens increase the risk of carcinoma of the endometrium in humans. (See Boxed Warning).
At the present time there is no satisfactory evidence that estrogens given to postmenopausal women increase the risk of cancer of the breast,[17] although a recent long-term follow-up of a single physician's practice has raised this possibility.[18] Because of the animal data, there is a need for caution in prescribing estrogens for women with a strong family history of breast cancer or who have breast nodules, fibrocystic disease, or abnormal mammograms.
2. **Gallbladder disease.** A recent study has reported a 2- to 3-fold increase in the risk of surgically confirmed gallbladder disease in women receiving postmenopausal estrogens,[17] similar to the 2-fold increase previously noted in users of oral contraceptives.[19,20] In the case of oral contraceptives, the increased risk appeared after two years of use.[20]
3. **Effects similar to those caused by estrogen-progestogen oral contraceptives.** There are several serious adverse effects of oral contraceptives, most of which have not, up to now, been documented as consequences of postmenopausal estrogen therapy. This may reflect the comparatively low doses of estrogen used in postmenopausal women. It would be expected that the larger doses of estrogen used to treat prostatic or breast cancer or postpartum breast engorgement are more likely to result in these adverse effects; in fact, it has been shown that there is an increased risk of thrombosis in men receiving estrogens for prostatic cancer and women for postpartum breast engorgement.[21–24]

a. **Thromboembolic disease.** It is now well established that users of oral contraceptives have an increased risk of various thromboembolic and thrombotic vascular diseases, such as thrombophlebitis, pulmonary embolism, stroke, and myocardial infarction.[25–32] Cases of retinal thrombosis, mesenteric thrombosis, and optic neuritis have been reported in oral contraceptive users. There is evidence that the risk of several of these adverse reactions is related to the dose of the drug.[33,34] An increased risk of postsurgery thromboembolic complications has also been reported in users of oral contraceptives.[35,36] If feasible, estrogen should be discontinued at least 4 weeks before surgery of the type associated with an increased risk of thromboembolism, or during periods of prolonged immobilization.
While an increased rate of thromboembolic and thrombotic disease in postmenopausal users of estrogens has not been found,[17–37] this does not rule out the possibility that such an increase may be present or that subgroups of women who have underlying risk factors or who are receiving relatively large doses of estrogens may have increased risk. Therefore, estrogens should not be used in persons with active thrombophlebitis or thromboembolic disorders, and they should not be used (except in treatment of malignancy) in persons with a history of such disorders in association with estrogen use. They should be used with caution in patients with cerebrovascular or coronary artery disease and only for those in whom estrogens are clearly needed.
Large doses of estrogen (5 mg conjugated estrogens per day), comparable to those used to treat cancer of the prostate and breast, have been shown in a large prospective clinical trial in men[38] to increase the risk of nonfatal myocardial infarction, pulmonary embolism, and thrombophlebitis. When estrogen doses of this size are used, any of the thromboembolic and thrombotic adverse effects associated with oral contraceptive use should be considered a clear risk.

b. **Hepatic adenoma.** Benign hepatic adenomas appear to be associated with the use of oral contraceptives.[39–41] Although benign and rare, these may rupture and may cause death through intraabdominal hemorrhage. Such lesions have not yet been reported in association with other estrogen or progestogen preparations but should be considered in estrogen users having abdominal pain and tenderness, abdominal mass, or hypovolemic shock. Hepatocellular carcinoma has also been reported in women taking estrogen-containing oral contraceptives.[40] The relationship of this malignancy to these drugs is not known at this time.

c. **Elevated blood pressure.** Increased blood pressure is not uncommon in women using oral contraceptives. There is now a report that this may occur with use of estrogens in the menopause[42] and blood pressure should be monitored with estrogen use, especially if high doses are used.

d. **Glucose tolerance.** A worsening of glucose tolerance has been observed in a significant percentage of patients on estrogen-containing oral contraceptives. For this reason, diabetic patients should be carefully observed while receiving estrogen.

4. **Hypercalcemia.** Administration of estrogens may lead to severe hypercalcemia in patients with breast cancer and bone metastases. If this occurs, the drug should be stopped and appropriate measures taken to reduce the serum calcium level.

PRECAUTIONS

A. General Precautions.

1. A complete medical and family history should be taken prior to the initiation of any estrogen therapy. The pretreatment and periodic physical examinations should include special reference to blood pressure, breasts, abdomen, and pelvic organs, and should include a Papanicolaou smear. As a general rule, estrogen should not be prescribed for longer than one year without another physical examination being performed.
2. Fluid retention — Because estrogens may cause some degree of fluid retention, conditions which might be influenced by this factor such as epilepsy, migraine, and cardiac or renal dysfunction, require careful observation.
3. Certain patients may develop undesirable manifestations of excessive estrogenic stimulation, such as abnormal or excessive uterine bleeding, mastodynia, etc.
4. Oral contraceptives appear to be associated with an increased incidence of mental depression.[20] Although it is not clear whether this is due to the estrogenic or progestogenic component of the contraceptive, patients with a history of depression should be carefully observed.
5. Pre-existing uterine leiomyomata may increase in size during estrogen use.
6. The pathologist should be advised of estrogen therapy when relevant specimens are submitted.
7. Patients with a past history of jaundice during pregnancy have an increased risk of recurrence of jaundice while receiving estrogen-containing oral contraceptive therapy. If jaundice develops in any patient receiving estrogen, the medication should be discontinued while the cause is investigated.
8. Estrogens may be poorly metabolized in patients with impaired liver function and they should be administered with caution in such patients.
9. Because estrogens influence the metabolism of calcium and phosphorus, they should be used with caution in patients with metabolic bone diseases that are associated with hypercalcemia or in patients with renal insufficiency.
10. Because of the effects of estrogens on epiphyseal closure, they should be used judiciously in young patients in whom bone growth is not complete.
11. The lowest effective dose appropriate for the specific indication should be utilized. Studies of the addition of a progestin for seven or more days of a cycle of estrogen administration have reported a lowered incidence of endometrial hyperplasia. Morphological and biochemical studies of endometrium suggest that 10 to 13 days of progestin are needed to provide maximal maturation of the endometrium and to eliminate any hyperplastic changes. Whether this will provide protection from endometrial carcinoma has not been clearly established. There are possible additional risks which may be associated with the inclusion of progestin in estrogen

replacement regimens. The potential risks include adverse effects on carbohydrate and lipid metabolism. The choice of progestin and dosage may be important in minimizing these adverse effects.

B. Information for the Patient. See text which appears after the **REFERENCES** section.

C. Drug/Laboratory Test Interactions: Certain endocrine and liver function tests may be affected by estrogen-containing oral contraceptives. The following similar changes may be expected with larger doses of estrogen.

a. Increased sulfobromophthalein retention.

b. Increased prothrombin and factors VII, VIII, IX, and X; decreased antithrombin 3; increased norepinephrine-induced platelet aggregability.

c. Increased thyroid-binding globulin (TBG) leading to increased circulating total thyroid hormone, as measured by PBI, T4 by volume, or T4 by radioimmunoassay. Free T3 resin uptake is decreased, reflecting the elevated TBG; free T4 concentration is unaltered.

d. Impaired glucose tolerance.

e. Decreased pregnanediol excretion.

f. Reduced response to metyrapone test.

g. Reduced serum folate concentration.

h. Increased serum triglyceride and phospholipid concentration.

D. Pregnancy Category X. See Contraindications and Boxed Warning.

E. Nursing Mothers. As a general principle, the administration of any drug to nursing mothers should be done only when clearly necessary since many drugs are excreted in human milk.

ADVERSE REACTIONS

(See Warnings regarding induction of neoplasia, adverse effects on the fetus, increased incidence of gallbladder disease, and adverse effects similar to those of oral contraceptives, including thromboembolism.) The following additional adverse reactions have been reported with estrogenic therapy, including oral contraceptives:

Genitourinary system. Breakthrough bleeding, spotting, change in menstrual flow. Dysmenorrhea. Premenstrual-like syndrome. Amenorrhea during and after treatment. Increase in size of uterine fibromyomata. Vaginal candidiasis. Change in cervical erosion and in degree of cervical secretion. Cystitis-like syndrome. **Breasts.** Tenderness, enlargement, secretion. **Gastrointestinal.** Nausea, vomiting. Abdominal cramps, bloating. Cholestatic jaundice. **Skin.** Chloasma or melasma which may persist when drug is discontinued. Erythema multiforme. Hemorrhagic eruption. Hirsutism. Erythema nodosum. Loss of scalp hair. **Eyes.** Steepening of corneal curvature. Intolerance to contact lenses. **CNS.** Headache, migraine, dizziness. Mental depression. Chorea. **Miscellaneous.** Increase or decrease in weight. Reduced carbohydrate tolerance. Aggravation of porphyria. Edema. Changes in libido.

OVERDOSAGE

Numerous reports of ingestion of large doses of estrogen-containing oral contraceptives by young children indicate that serious ill effects do not occur. Overdosage of estrogen may cause nausea, and withdrawal bleeding may occur in females.

DOSAGE AND ADMINISTRATION

Given cyclically for short-term use only.

For treatment of atrophic vaginitis or kraurosis vulvae.

The lowest dose that will control symptoms should be chosen and medication should be discontinued as promptly as possible.

Administration should be cyclic (e.g., 3 weeks on and 1 week off).

Attempts to discontinue or taper medication should be made at 3 to 6 month intervals.

Usual Dosage: The usual dosage range is 2 to 4 g (marked on the applicator) daily for one or two weeks, then gradually reduced to one half initial dosage for a similar period. A maintenance dosage of 1 g, one to three times a week, may be used after restoration of the vaginal mucosa has been achieved.

Patients with an intact uterus should be monitored closely for signs of endometrial cancer and appropriate diagnostic measures should be taken to rule out malignancy in the event of persistent or recurring abnormal vaginal bleeding.

HOW SUPPLIED

ESTRACE® (estradiol vaginal cream 0.01%).

NDC 0087-0754-42 42.5 g Tube with a calibrated plastic applicator for delivery of 1, 2, 3, or 4 g.

REFERENCES

1. Ziel HK, Finkel WD: Increased risk of endometrial carcinoma among users of conjugated estrogens. New Eng J Med 293:1167–1170, 1975. **2.** Smith DC, Prentice R, Thompson DJ, Hermann WL: Association of exogenous estrogen and endometrial carcinoma. New Eng J Med 293:1164–1167, 1975. **3.** Mack TM, Pike MC, Henderson BE, *et al:* Estrogens and endometrial cancer in a retirement community. New Eng J Med 294:1262–1267, 1976. **4.** Weiss NS, Szekely DR, Austin DF: Increasing incidence of endometrial cancer in the United States. New Eng J Med 294:1259–1262, 1976. **5.** Herbst AL, Ulfelder H, Poskanzer DC: Adenocarcinoma of vagina. New Eng J Med 284:878–881, 1971. **6.** Greenwald P, Barlow J, Nasca P, Burnett W: Vaginal cancer after maternal treatment with synthetic estrogens. New Eng J Med 285:390–392, 1971. **7.** Lanier A, Noller K, Decker D, *et al:* Cancer and stilbestrol. A follow-up of 1719 persons exposed to estrogens *in utero* and born 1943–1959. Mayo Clin Proceedings 48:793–799, 1973. **8.** Herbst A, Kurman R, Scully R: Vaginal and cervical abnormalities after exposure to stilbestrol *in utero*. Obstet and Gynec 40:287–298, 1972. **9.** Herbst A, Robboy S, MacDonald G, Scully R: The effects of local progesterone on stilbestrol-associated vaginal adenosis. Am J Obstet Gynec 118:607–615, 1974. **10.** Herbst A, Poskanzer D, Robboy S, *et al:* Prenatal exposure to stilbestrol, a prospective comparison of exposed female offspring with unexposed controls. New Eng J Med 292:334–339, 1975. **11.** Stafl A, Mattingly R, Foley D, Fetherston W: Clinical diagnosis of vaginal adenosis. Obstet and Gynec 43:118–128, 1974. **12.** Sherman AI, Goldrath M, Berlin A, *et al:* Cervical-vaginal adenosis after *in utero* exposure to synthetic estrogens. Obstet Gynec 44:531–545, 1974. **13.** Gal I, Kirman B, Stern J: Hormone pregnancy tests and congenital malformation. Nature 216:83, 1967. **14.** Levy EP, Cohen A, Fraser FC: Hormone treatment during pregnancy and congenital heart defects. Lancet 1:611, 1973. **15.** Nora J, Nora A: Birth defects and oral contraceptives. Lancet 1:941–942, 1973. **16.** Janerich DT, Piper JM, Glebatis DM: Oral contraceptives and congenital limb-reduction defects. New Eng J Med 291:697–700, 1974. **17.** Boston Collaborative Drug Surveillance Program: Surgically confirmed gallbladder disease, venous thromboembolism and breast tumors in relation to post-menopausal estrogen therapy. New Eng J Med 290:15–19, 1974. **18.** Hoover R, Gray LA Sr, Cole P, MacMahon B: Menopausal estrogens and breast cancer. New Eng J Med 295:401–405, 1976. **19.** Boston Collaborative Drug Surveillance Program: Oral contraceptives and venous thromboembolic disease, surgically confirmed gallbladder disease, and breast tumors. Lancet 1:1399–1404, 1973. **20.** Royal College of General Practitioners: Oral Contraceptives and Health, New York, Pitman Corp., 1974. **21.** Daniel DG, Campbell H, Turnbull AC: Puerperal thromboembolism and suppression of lactation. Lancet 2:287–289, 1967. **22.** The Veterans Administration Cooperative Urological Research Group: Carcinoma of the prostate; treatment comparisons. J Urol 98:516–522, 1967. **23.** Bailar JC: Thromboembolism and oestrogen therapy. Lancet 2:560, 1967. **24.** Blackard C, Doe R, Mellinger G, Byar D: Incidence of cardiovascular disease and death in patients receiving diethylstilbestrol for carcinoma of the prostate. Cancer 26:249–256, 1970. **25.** Royal College of General Practitioners: Oral contraception and thromboembolic disease. J Roy Coll Gen Pract 13:267–279, 1967. **26.** Inman WHW, Vessey MP: Investigation of deaths from pulmonary, coronary, and cerebral thrombosis and embolism in women of child-bearing age. Brit M J 2:193–199, 1968. **27.** Vessey MP, Doll R: Investigation of relation between use of oral contraceptives and thromboembolic disease. A further report. Brit M J 2:651–657, 1969. **28.** Sartwell PE, Masi AT, Arthes FG, *et al:* Thromboembolism and oral contraceptives: an epidemiological case control study. Am J Epidemiol 90:365–380, 1969. **29.** Collaborative Group for the Study of Stroke in Young Women: Oral contraception and increased risk of cerebral ischemia or thrombosis. New Eng J Med 288:871–878, 1973. **30.** Collaborative Group for the Study of Stroke in Young Women: Oral contraceptives and stroke in young women: Associated risk factors. JAMA 231:718–722, 1975. **31.** Mann JI, Inman WHW: Oral contraceptives and death from myocardial infarction. Brit M J 2:245–248, 1975. **32.** Mann JI, Vessey MP, Thorogood M, Doll R: Myocardial infarction in young women with special reference to oral contraceptive practice. Brit M J 2:241–245, 1975. **33.** Inman WHW, Vessey MP, Westerholm B, Engelund A: Thromboembolic disease and the steroidal content of oral contraceptives. Brit M J 2:203–209, 1970. **34.** Stolley PD, Tonascia JA, Tockman MS, *et al:* Thrombosis with low-estrogen oral contraceptives. Am J Epidemiol 102:197–208, 1975. **35.** Vessey MP, Doll R, Fairbairn AS, Glober G: Post-operative thromboembolism and the use of the oral contraceptives. Brit MJ 3:123–126, 1970. **36.** Greene GR, Sartwell PE: Oral contraceptive use in patients with thromboembolism following surgery, trauma or infection. Am J Pub Health 62:680–685, 1972. **37.** Rosenberg L, Armstrong MB, Jick H: Myocardial infarction and estrogen therapy in post-menopausal women. New Eng J Med 294:1256–1259, 1976. **38.** Coronary Drug Project Research Group: The coronary drug project: initial findings leading to modifications of its research protocol. JAMA 214:1303–1313, 1970. **39.** Baum J, Holtz F, Bookstein JJ, Klein EW: Possible association between benign hepatomas and oral contraceptives. Lancet 2:926–928, 1973. **40.** Mays ET, Christopherson WM, Mahr MM, Williams HC: Hepatic changes in young women ingesting contraceptive steroids, hepatic hemorrhage and primary hepatic tumors. JAMA 235:730–732, 1976. **41.** Edmondson HA, Henderson B, Benton B: Liver cell adenomas associated with the use of oral contraceptives. New Eng J Med 294:470–472, 1976. **42.** Pfeffer RI, Van Den Noort S: Estrogen use and stroke risk in postmenopausal women. Am J Epidemiol 103:445–456, 1976.

INFORMATION FOR THE PATIENT

WHAT YOU SHOULD KNOW ABOUT ESTROGENS

Estrogens are female hormones produced principally by the ovaries. The ovaries make several different kinds of estrogens. In addition, scientists have been able to make a variety of synthetic estrogens. As far as we know, all these estrogens have the same properties and, therefore, much the same usefulness, side effects, and risks. This leaflet is intended to help you understand what estrogens are used for, the risks involved in their use, and how to use them as safely as possible.

This leaflet includes important information about ESTRACE® (estradiol vaginal cream) and estrogens in general, but not all the information. If you want to know more, you can ask your doctor for more information, or you can ask your doctor or pharmacist to let you read the professional package insert.

USES OF ESTROGEN

Estrogens are prescribed by doctors for a number of purposes, including:

1. To provide estrogen during a period of adjustment when a woman's ovaries no longer produce it, in order to prevent certain uncomfortable symptoms of estrogen deficiency. (All women normally stop producing estrogens, generally between 45 and 55; this is called the menopause.)
2. To prevent symptoms of estrogen deficiency when a woman's ovaries have been removed surgically before the natural menopause.
3. To prevent pregnancy. (Some estrogens are given along with a progestogen, another female hormone; these combinations are called oral contraceptives or birth control pills. They will not be discussed in this leaflet.)
4. To treat certain cancers in women and men.
5. To prevent painful swelling of the breasts after pregnancy in women who choose not to nurse their babies.

THERE IS NO PROPER USE OF ESTROGENS IN A PREGNANT WOMAN.

ESTROGENS IN THE MENOPAUSE

In the natural course of their lives, all women eventually experience a decrease in estrogen production. This usually occurs between ages 45 and 55 but may occur earlier or later. Sometimes the ovaries may need to be removed before natural menopause by an operation, producing a "surgical menopause."

When the amount of estrogen in the blood begins to decrease, many women may develop typical symptoms: feelings of warmth in the face, neck, and chest or sudden intense episodes of heat and sweating throughout the body (called "hot flashes" or "hot flushes"). These symptoms are sometimes very uncomfortable. A few women eventually develop changes in the vagina (called "atrophic vaginitis") which cause discomfort, especially during and after intercourse.

Estrogens can be prescribed to treat these symptoms of the menopause. It is estimated that considerably more than half of all women undergoing the menopause have only mild symptoms or no symptoms at all and therefore do not need estrogens. Other women may need estrogens for a few months, while their bodies adjust to lower estrogen levels. Sometimes the need will be for periods longer than six months. In an attempt to avoid over-stimulation of the uterus (womb), estrogens are usually given cyclically during each month of use, that is, three weeks of therapy followed by one week without therapy.

Sometimes women experience nervous symptoms or depression during menopause. There is no evidence that estrogens are effective for such symptoms and they should not be used to treat them, although other treatment may be needed.

You may have heard that taking estrogens for long periods (years) after the menopause will keep your skin soft and supple and keep you feeling young. There is no evidence that this is so, however, and such long-term treatment carries additional risks.

THE DANGERS OF ESTROGENS

1. **Cancer of the uterus.** If estrogens are used in the post-menopausal period for more than a year, there is an increased risk of **endometrial cancer** (cancer of the uterus). Women taking estrogens have roughly 5 to 10 times as great a chance of getting this cancer as women who take no estrogens. To put this another way, while a postmenopausal woman not taking estrogens has one chance in 1,000 each year of getting cancer of the uterus, a woman taking estrogens has 5 to 10 chances in 1,000 each year. For this reason **it is important to take estrogens only when you really need them.**

The risk of this cancer is greater the longer estrogens are used and also seems to be greater when larger doses are taken. For this reason **it is important to take the lowest dose of estrogen that will control symptoms and to take it only as long as it is needed.** If estrogens are needed for longer periods

Continued on next page

Mead Johnson Laboratories—Cont.

of time, your doctor will want to reevaluate your need for estrogens at least every six months.

Women using estrogens should report any irregular vaginal bleeding to their doctors; such bleeding may be of no importance, but it can be an early warning of cancer of the uterus. If you have undiagnosed vaginal bleeding, you should not use estrogens until a diagnosis is made and you are certain there is no cancer of the uterus.

2. **Other possible cancers.** Estrogens can cause development of other tumors in animals, such as tumors of the breast, cervix, vagina, or liver, when given for a long time. At present there is no good evidence that women using estrogens in the menopause have an increased risk of such tumors, but there is no way yet to be sure they do not; and one study raises the possibility that use of estrogens in the menopause may increase the risk of breast cancer many years later. This is a further reason to use estrogens only when clearly needed. While you are taking estrogens, it is important that you go to your doctor at least once a year for a physical examination. Also, if members of your family have had breast cancer or if you have breast nodules or abnormal mammograms (breast x-rays), your doctor may wish to carry out more frequent examinations of your breasts.

3. **Gallbladder disease.** Women who use estrogens after menopause are two or three times more likely to develop gallbladder disease needing surgery than women who do not use estrogens. Birth control pills have a similar effect.

4. **Abnormal blood clotting.** Oral contraceptives increase the risk of blood clotting in various parts of the body. This can result in a stroke (if the clot is in the brain), a heart attack (clot in a vessel of the heart), or a pulmonary embolism (a clot which forms in the legs or pelvis, then breaks off and travels to the lungs). Any of these can be fatal.

At this time, use of estrogens in the menopause is not known to cause such blood clotting, but this has not been fully studied and there could still prove to be such a risk. It is recommended that if you have had clotting in the legs or lungs or a heart attack or stroke while you were using estrogens or birth control pills, you should not use estrogens (unless they are being used to treat cancer of the breast or prostate). If you have had a stroke or heart attack or if you have angina pectoris, estrogens should be used with great caution and only if clearly needed (for example, if you have severe symptoms of the menopause).

SPECIAL WARNING ABOUT PREGNANCY

You should not receive estrogen if you are pregnant. If this should occur, there is a greater than usual chance that the developing child will be born with a birth defect, although the possibility remains fairly small. A female child may have an increased risk of developing cancer of the vagina or cervix later in life (in the teens or twenties). Every possible effort should be made to avoid exposure to estrogens during pregnancy. If exposure occurs, see your doctor.

OTHER EFFECTS OF ESTROGENS

In addition to the serious known risks of estrogens described above, estrogens have the following side effects and potential risks:

1. **Nausea and vomiting.** The most common side effect of estrogen therapy is nausea. Vomiting is less common.

2. **Effects on breasts.** Estrogens may cause breast tenderness or enlargement and may cause the breasts to secrete a liquid. These effects are not dangerous.

3. **Effects on the uterus.** Estrogens may cause benign fibroid tumors of the uterus to get larger.

Some women will have menstrual bleeding when estrogens are stopped. But if the bleeding occurs on days you are still taking estrogens, you should report this to your doctor.

4. **Effects on liver.** Women taking oral contraceptives develop on rare occasions a benign tumor of the liver which can rupture and bleed into the abdomen. So far, these tumors have not been reported in women using estrogens in the menopause, but you should report any swelling or unusual pain or tenderness in the abdomen to your doctor immediately.

Women with a past history of jaundice (yellowing of the skin and white parts of the eyes) may get jaundice again during estrogen use. If this occurs, stop taking estrogens and see your doctor.

5. **Other effects.** Estrogens may cause excess fluid to be retained in the body. This may make some conditions worse, such as epilepsy, migraine, heart disease, or kidney disease.

SUMMARY

Estrogens have important uses, and they may have serious risks as well. You must decide, with your doctor, whether the risks are acceptable to you in view of the benefits of treatment. Except where your doctor has prescribed estrogens for use in special cases of cancer of the breast or prostate, you should not use estrogens if you have cancer of the breast or uterus, are pregnant, have undiagnosed abnormal vaginal bleeding, or have had a stroke, heart attack or angina, or clotting in the legs or lungs in the past while you were taking estrogens.

You can use estrogens as safely as possible by understanding that your doctor will require regular physical examinations while you are taking them and will try to discontinue the drug as soon as possible and use the smallest dose possible. Be alert for signs of trouble including:

1. Abnormal bleeding from the vagina.
2. Pains in the calves or chest or sudden shortness of breath, or coughing blood (indicating possible clots in the legs, heart, or lungs).
3. Severe headache, dizziness, faintness, or changes in vision (indicating possible developing clots in the brain or eye).
4. Breast lumps (you should ask your doctor how to examine your own breasts).
5. Jaundice (yellowing of the skin).
6. Mental depression.

Your doctor has prescribed this drug for you. Do not give this drug to anyone else.

Shown in Product Identification Section, page 419

NATALINS® Tablets   OTC
[nā-tă-lins]
Multivitamin and multimineral supplement with beta-carotene

For pregnant or lactating women
Natural color adopted 1984

COMPOSITION

Each Natalins tablet supplies:
Vitamins

Vitamin A, IU	4,000
Vitamin D, IU	400
Vitamin E, IU	15
Vitamin C (Ascorbic acid), mg	70
Folic acid, mg	0.5
Thiamin (Vitamin B₁), mg	1.5
Riboflavin (Vitamin B₂), mg	1.6
Niacin, mg	17
Vitamin B₆, mg	2.6
Vitamin B₁₂, μg	2.5

Minerals

Calcium, mg	200
Iron, mg	30
Magnesium, mg	100
Copper, mg	1.5
Zinc, mg	15

INGREDIENTS

Calcium carbonate, magnesium hydroxide, ferrous fumarate, sodium ascorbate, povidone, microcrystalline cellulose, dl-alpha-tocopheryl acetate, acacia, zinc oxide, polacrilin potassium, niacinamide, beta-carotene, hydroxypropyl methylcellulose, vitamin A acetate, polyethylene glycol, vitamin D₃, magnesium stearate, pyridoxine hydrochloride, hydroxypropyl cellulose, cupric oxide, riboflavin (color), thiamine mononitrate, silicon dioxide, folic acid, vitamin B₁₂.

INDICATIONS AND USAGE

For supplementing the diet.

DOSAGE AND ADMINISTRATION

One tablet a day or as indicated.
Your physician is the best source of counsel and guidance in vitamin supplementation.

HOW SUPPLIED

Natalins® tablets
0087-0700-01 Bottles of 100
    Shown in Product Identification Section, page 419

NATALINS® RX   ℞
[nā-tă-lins]
Multivitamin and multimineral supplement with beta-carotene
Tablets with 1 mg folic acid and 60 mg Iron
Contains no artificial color or flavor from synthetic sources

Natalins Rx tablets provide twelve vitamins and five minerals to supplement the diet during pregnancy or lactation.

COMPOSITION

Each Natalins Rx tablet supplies:
Vitamins

Vitamin A, IU	4,000
Vitamin D, IU	400
Vitamin E, IU	15
Vitamin C (Ascorbic acid), mg.	80
Folic acid (Folacin), mg.	1
Thiamin (Vitamin B₁), mg.	1.5
Riboflavin (Vitamin B₂), mg.	1.6
Niacin, mg	17
Vitamin B₆, mg	4
Vitamin B₁₂, μg.	2.5
Biotin, mg.	0.03
Pantothenic acid, mg.	7

Minerals

Calcium, mg.	200
Iron, mg.	60
Magnesium, mg.	100
Copper, mg.	3
Zinc, mg.	25

ACTIVE INGREDIENT

Each tablet contains 1 mg folic acid.

OTHER INGREDIENTS

Acacia, biotin, calcium carbonate, calcium pantothenate, beta-carotene, cholecalciferol, colloidal silicon dioxide, cupric oxide, cyanocobalamin, ferrous fumarate, hydroxypropyl cellulose, hydroxypropyl methylcellulose, magnesium hydroxide, magnesium stearate, niacinamide, polacrilin potassium, polyethylene glycol, povidone, pyridoxine hydrochloride, riboflavin, sodium ascorbate, thiamine mononitrate, titanium dioxide, dl-alpha-tocopheryl acetate, vitamin A acetate, zinc oxide.

INDICATIONS AND USAGE

Natalins Rx tablets help assure an adequate intake of the vitamins and minerals listed above. Folic acid helps prevent the development of megaloblastic anemia during pregnancy.

CONTRAINDICATIONS

Supplemental vitamins and minerals should not be prescribed for patients with hemochromatosis or Wilson's disease.

WARNING

Keep Natalins Rx tablets out of the reach of children.

PRECAUTIONS

General—pernicious anemia should be excluded before using this product since folic acid may mask the symptoms of pernicious anemia. The calcium content should be considered before prescribing for patients with kidney stones. Do not exceed the recommended dose.

ADVERSE REACTIONS

No adverse reactions or undesirable side effects have been attributed to the use of Natalins Rx tablets.

DOSAGE AND ADMINISTRATION

One tablet daily, or as prescribed.

HOW SUPPLIED

Natalins® Rx Tablets: (Available on prescription.)
NDC 0087-0702-01 Bottles of 100
NDC 0087-0702-02 Bottles of 1000
    Shown in Product Identification Section, page 419

OVCON® 50   ℞
[ăv'kăn]

21 tablets of norethindrone 1 mg and ethinyl estradiol 0.05 mg. Each green tablet in the 28-day regimen contains inert ingredients.

OVCON® 35   ℞

21 tablets of norethindrone 0.4 mg and ethinyl estradiol 0.035 mg. Each green tablet in the 28-day regimen contains inert ingredients.

Oral contraceptives

DESCRIPTION

28-Day OVCON® 50 and OVCON® 35 tablets (norethindrone and ethinyl estradiol tablets, USP) provide a continuous regimen for oral contraception derived from 21 tablets composed of norethindrone and ethinyl estradiol to be followed by 7 green tablets of inert ingredients.

21-Day OVCON 50 and OVCON 35 tablets provide a regimen for oral contraception derived from 21 tablets composed of norethindrone and ethinyl estradiol. The chemical name for norethindrone is 17-hydroxy-19-nor-17α-pregn-4-en-20-yn-3-one and for ethinyl estradiol the chemical name is 19-nor-17α-pregna-1,3,5 (10)-trien-20-yne-3,17-diol. The structural formulas are:

NORETHINDRONE

[See second chemical structure at top of next column.]

The active OVCON 50 tablets contain 1 mg norethindrone and 0.05 mg ethinyl estradiol. The active OVCON 35 tablets contain 0.4 mg norethindrone and 0.035 mg ethinyl estradiol.

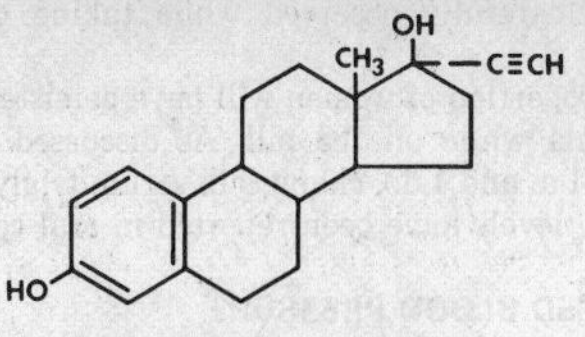

ETHINYL ESTRADIOL

The green tablets contain inert ingredients.

OVCON 50, 21-Day contains the following inactive ingredients: dibasic calcium phosphate, D&C Yellow No. 10 (aluminum lake), FD&C Yellow No. 6 (aluminum lake), lactose, magnesium stearate, povidone, and sodium starch glycolate.

OVCON 50, 28-Day contains the following inactive ingredients: acacia, dibasic calcium phosphate, D&C Yellow No. 10 (aluminum lake), FD&C Blue No. 1 (aluminum lake), FD&C Yellow No. 6 (aluminum lake), lactose, magnesium stearate, povidone, sodium starch glycolate, starch (corn), and talc.

OVCON 35, 21-Day contains the following inactive ingredients: dibasic calcium phosphate, FD&C Yellow No. 6 (aluminum lake), lactose, magnesium stearate, povidone, and sodium starch glycolate.

OVCON 35, 28-Day contains the following inactive ingredients: acacia, dibasic calcium phosphate, D&C Yellow No. 10 (aluminum lake), FD&C Blue No. 1 (aluminum lake), FD&C Yellow No. 6 (aluminum lake), lactose, magnesium stearate, povidone, sodium starch glycolate, starch (corn), and talc.

Clinical Pharmacology

Combination oral contraceptives act by suppression of gonadotropins. Although the primary mechanism of this action is inhibition of ovulation, other alterations include changes in the cervical mucus (which increase the difficulty of sperm entry into the uterus) and the endometrium (which reduce the likelihood of implantation).

INDICATIONS AND USAGE

Oral contraceptives are indicated for the prevention of pregnancy in women who elect to use this product as a method of contraception.

Oral contraceptives are highly effective. Table 1 lists the typical accidental pregnancy rates for users of combination oral contraceptives and other methods of contraception. The efficacy of these contraceptive methods, except sterilization, depends upon the reliability with which they are used. Correct and consistent use of methods can result in lower failure rates. [See Table 1 top of next column.]

CONTRAINDICATIONS

Oral contraceptives should not be used in women who currently have the following conditions:

- Thrombophlebitis or thromboembolic disorders
- A past history of deep vein thrombophlebitis or thromboembolic disorders
- Cerebrovascular or coronary artery disease
- Known or suspected carcinoma of the breast
- Carcinoma of the endometrium or other known or suspected estrogen-dependent neoplasia
- Undiagnosed abnormal genital bleeding
- Cholestatic jaundice of pregnancy or jaundice with prior pill use
- Hepatic adenomas or carcinomas
- Known or suspected pregnancy

WARNINGS

Cigarette smoking increases the risk of serious cardiovascular side effects from oral contraceptive use. This risk increases with age and with heavy smoking (15 or more cigarettes per day) and is quite marked in women over 35 years of age. Women who use oral contraceptives should be strongly advised not to smoke.

The use of oral contraceptives is associated with increased risk of several serious conditions including myocardial infarction, thromboembolism, stroke, hepatic neoplasia, and gallbladder disease, although the risk of serious morbidity or mortality is very small in healthy women without underlying risk factors. The risk of morbidity and mortality increases significantly in the presence of other underlying risk factors such as hypertension, hyperlipidemias, obesity, and diabetes.

Practitioners prescribing oral contraceptives should be familiar with the following information relating to these risks.

The information contained in this package insert is principally based on studies carried out in patients who used oral contraceptives with higher formulations of estrogens and progestogens than those in common use today. The effect of long-term use of the oral contraceptives with lower formulations of both estrogens and progestogens remains to be determined.

Throughout this labeling, epidemiological studies reported are of two types: retrospective or case control studies and prospective or cohort studies. Case control studies provide a measure of the relative risk of a disease, namely, a *ratio* of the incidence of a disease among oral contraceptive users to that among nonusers. The relative risk does not provide information on the actual clinical occurrence of a disease. Cohort studies provide a measure of attributable risk, which is the *difference* in the incidence of disease between oral contraceptive users and nonusers. The attributable risk does provide information about the actual occurrence of a disease in the population.* For further information, the reader is referred to a text on epidemiological methods.

TABLE 1

LOWEST EXPECTED AND TYPICAL FAILURE RATES DURING THE FIRST YEAR OF CONTINUOUS USE OF A METHOD

% of Women Experiencing an Accidental Pregnancy in the First Year of Continuous Use

Method	Lowest Expected*	Typical**
(No contraception)	(89)	(89)
Oral contraceptives		
combined	0.1	N/A***
progestin only	0.5	N/A***
Diaphragm with spermicidal cream or jelly	3	18
Spermicides alone (foam, creams, jellies and vaginal suppositories)	3	21
Vaginal sponge		
nulliparous	5	18
multiparous	>8	>28
IUD (medicated)	1	6#
Condom without spermicides	2	12
Periodic abstinence (all methods)	2–10	20
Female sterilization	0.2	0.4
Male sterilization	0.1	0.15

Reproduced with permission of the Population Council from J. Trussell and K. Kost: Contraceptive failure in the United States: A critical review of the literature. Studies in Family Planning, 18 (5), September–October 1987.

* The authors' best guess of the percentage of women expected to experience an accidental pregnancy among couples who initiate a method (not necessarily for the first time) and who use it consistently and correctly during the first year if they do not stop for any other reason other than pregnancy.

** This term represents "typical" couples who initiate use of a method (not necessarily for the first time), who experience an accidental pregnancy during the first year if they do not stop use for any other reason other than pregnancy.

*** N/A—Data not available

\# Combined typical rate for both medicated and non-medicated IUD. The rate for medicated IUD alone is not available.

1. THROMBOEMBOLIC DISORDERS AND OTHER VASCULAR PROBLEMS

The physician should be alert to the earliest manifestations of thromboembolic thrombotic disorders as discussed below. Should any of these occur or be suspected the drug should be discontinued immediately.

a. **Myocardial Infarction**

An increased risk of myocardial infarction has been associated with oral contraceptive use. This risk is primarily in smokers or women with other underlying risk factors for coronary artery disease such as hypertension, hypercholesterolemia, morbid obesity, and diabetes. The relative risk of heart attack for current oral contraceptive users has been estimated to be two to six. The risk is very low under the age of 30.

Smoking in combination with oral contraceptive use has been shown to contribute substantially to the incidence of myocardial infarctions in women in their mid-thirties or older, with smoking accounting for the majority of excess cases. Mortality rates associated with circulatory disease have been shown to increase substantially in smokers over the age of 35 and nonsmokers over the age of 40 (Figure 1) among women who use oral contraceptives.

[See (Figure 1) at top of next column.]

Oral contraceptives may compound the effects of well-known risk factors, such as hypertension, diabetes, hyperlipidemias, age, and obesity. In particular, some progestogens are known to decrease HDL cholesterol and cause glucose intolerance, while estrogens may create a state of hyperinsulinism. Oral

FIGURE 1

CIRCULATORY DISEASE MORTALITY RATES PER 100,000 WOMAN-YEARS BY AGE, SMOKING STATUS AND ORAL CONTRACEPTIVE USE

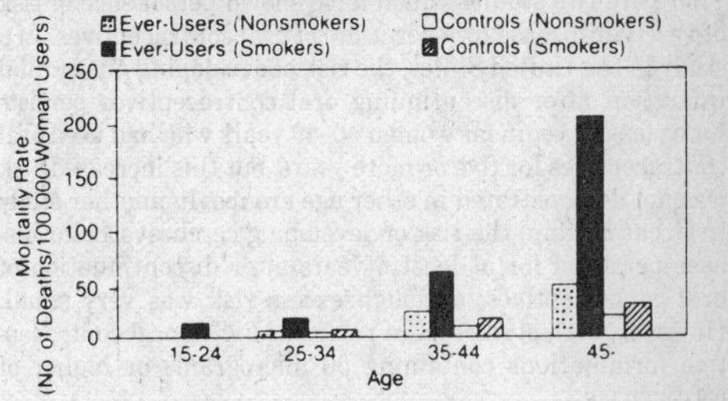

Layde PM, Beral V. Further analyses of mortality in oral contraceptive users: Royal College of General Practitioners' oral contraceptive study. (Table 5) *Lancet* 1981;1:541–546.

contraceptives have been shown to increase blood pressure among users (see section 9 in Warnings). Such increases in risk factors have been associated with an increased risk of heart disease and the risk increases with the number of risk factors present. Oral contraceptives must be used with caution in women with cardiovascular disease risk factors.

b. **Thromboembolism**

An increased risk of thromboembolic and thrombotic disease associated with the use of oral contraceptives is well established. Case control studies have found the relative risk of users compared to nonusers to be 3 for the first episode of superficial venous thrombosis, 4 to 11 for deep vein thrombosis or pulmonary embolism, and 1.5 to 6 for women with predisposing conditions for venous thromboembolic disease. Cohort studies have shown the relative risk to be somewhat lower, about 3 for new cases and about 4.5 for new cases requiring hospitalization. The risk of thromboembolic disease due to oral contraceptives is not related to length of use and disappears after pill use is stopped.

A two- to four-fold increase in relative risk of postoperative thromboembolic complications has been reported with the use of oral contraceptives. The relative risk of venous thrombosis in women who have predisposing conditions is twice that of women without such medical conditions. If feasible, oral contraceptives should be discontinued at least four weeks prior to and for two weeks after elective surgery of a type associated with an increase in risk of thromboembolism and during and following prolonged immobilization. Since the immediate postpartum period is also associated with an increased risk of thromboembolism, oral contraceptives should be started no earlier than four to six weeks after delivery in women who elect not to breastfeed.

c. **Cerebrovascular diseases**

Oral contraceptives have been shown to increase both the relative and attributable risks of cerebrovascular events (thrombotic and hemorrhagic strokes); although, in general, the risk is greatest among older (>35 years), hypertensive women who also smoke. Hypertension was found to be a risk factor for both users and nonusers, for both types of strokes, while smoking interacted to increase the risk for hemorrhagic strokes.

In a large study, the relative risk of thrombotic strokes has been shown to range from 3 for normotensive users to 14 for users with severe hypertension. The relative risk of hemorrhagic stroke is reported to be 1.2 for nonsmokers who used oral contraceptives, 2.6 for smokers who did not use oral contraceptives, 7.6 for smokers who used oral contraceptives, 1.8 for normotensive users and 25.7 for users with severe hypertension. The attributable risk is also greater in older women.

d. **Dose-related risk of vascular disease from oral contraceptives**

A positive association has been observed between the amount of estrogen and progestogen in oral contraceptives and the risk of vascular disease. A decline in serum high density lipoproteins (HDL) has been reported with many progestational agents. A decline in serum high density lipoproteins has been associated with an increased incidence of ischemic heart disease. Because estrogens increase HDL cholesterol, the net effect of an oral contraceptive depends on a balance achieved between doses of estrogen and progestogen and the nature and absolute amount of progestogens used in the contraceptive. The amount of both hormones should be considered in the choice of an oral contraceptive.

Minimizing exposure to estrogen and progestogen is in keeping with good principles of therapeutics. For any particular estrogen/progestogen combination, the dosage regimen prescribed should be one which contains the least amount of estrogen and progestogen that is compatible with a low failure rate and the needs of the individual patient. New acceptors of oral contraceptive agents should be started on preparations containing 0.05 mg or less of estrogen.

*Adapted from Stadel BB: Oral contraceptives and cardiovascular disease. *N Engl J Med.* 1981;305:612–618, 672–677; with author's permission.

Continued on next page

Mead Johnson Laboratories—Cont.

e. Persistence of risk

There are two studies which have shown persistence of risk of vascular disease for ever-users of oral contraceptives. In a study in the United States, the risk of developing myocardial infarction after discontinuing oral contraceptives persists for at least 9 years for women 40–49 years who had used oral contraceptives for five or more years, but this increased risk was not demonstrated in other age groups. In another study in Great Britain, the risk of developing cerebrovascular disease persisted for at least 6 years after discontinuation of oral contraceptives, although excess risk was very small. However, both studies were performed with oral contraceptive formulations containing 50 micrograms or higher of estrogens.

2. ESTIMATES OF MORTALITY FROM CONTRACEPTIVE USE

One study gathered data from a variety of sources which have estimated the mortality rate associated with different methods of contraception at different ages (Table 2).

These estimates include the combined risk of death associated with contraceptive methods plus the risk attributable to pregnancy in the event of method failure. Each method of contraception has its specific benefits and risk. The study concluded that with the exception of oral contraceptive users 35 and older who smoke and 40 and older who do not smoke, mortality associated with all methods of birth control is low and below that associated with childbirth. The observation of a possible increase in risk of mortality with age for oral contraceptive users is based on data gathered in the 1970s—but not reported until 1983. However, current clinical practice involves the use of lower estrogen dose formulations combined with careful restriction of oral contraceptive use to women who do not have the various risk factors listed in this labeling.

Because of these changes in practice and, also, because of some limited new data which suggest that the risk of cardiovascular disease with the use of oral contraceptives may now be less than previously observed (Porter JB, Hunter J, Jick H, et al. Oral contraceptives and nonfatal vascular disease. *Obstet Gynecol* 1985;66:1–4 and Porter JB, Jick H, Walker AM, Mortality among oral contraceptive users. *Obstet Gynecol* 1987;70:29–32), the Fertility and Maternal Health Drugs Advisory Committee was asked to review the topic in 1989. The Committee concluded that although cardiovascular disease risk may be increased with oral contraceptive use after age 40 in healthy nonsmoking women (even with the newer low-dose formulations), there are greater potential health risks associated with pregnancy in older women and with the alternative surgical and medical procedures which may be necessary if such women do not have access to effective and acceptable means of contraception.

Therefore, the Committee recommended that the benefits of oral contraceptive use by healthy nonsmoking women over 40 may outweigh the possible risks. Of course, older women, as all women who take oral contraceptives, should take the lowest possible dose formulation that is effective.

3. CARCINOMA OF THE REPRODUCTIVE ORGANS

Numerous epidemiological studies have been performed on the incidence of breast, endometrial, ovarian, and cervical cancer in women using oral contraceptives. The overwhelming evidence in the literature suggests that use of oral contraceptives is not associated with an increase in the risk of developing breast cancer, regardless of the age and parity of first use or with most of the marketed brands and doses. The Cancer and Steroid Hormone (CASH) study also showed no latent effect on the risk of breast cancer for at least a decade following long-term use. A few studies have shown a slightly increased relative risk of developing breast cancer, although the methodology of these studies, which included differences in examination of users and nonusers and differences in age at start of use, has been questioned.

Some studies suggest that oral contraceptive use has been associated with an increase in the risk of cervical intraepithelial neoplasia in some populations of women.

However, there continues to be controversy about the extent to which such findings may be due to differences in sexual behavior and other factors.

In spite of many studies of the relationship between oral contraceptive use and breast cancer and cervical cancers, a cause-and-effect relationship has not been established.

4. HEPATIC NEOPLASIA

Benign hepatic adenomas are associated with oral contraceptive use, although the occurrence is rare in the United States. Indirect calculations have estimated the attributable risk to be in the range of 3.3 cases/100,000 for users, a risk that increases after four or more years of use. Rupture of hepatic adenomas may cause death through intra-abdominal hemorrhage.

Studies from Britain have shown an increased risk of developing hepatocellular carcinoma in long-term (> 8 years) oral contraceptive users. However, these cancers are extremely rare in the U.S. and the attributable risk (the excess incidence) of liver cancers in oral contraceptive users approaches less than one per million users.

5. OCULAR LESIONS

There have been clincial case reports of retinal thrombosis associated with the use of oral contraceptives. Oral contraceptives should be discontinued if there is unexplained partial or complete loss of vision; onset of proptosis or diplopia; papilledema; or retinal vascular lesions. Appropriate diagnostic and therapeutic measures should be undertaken immediately.

6. ORAL CONTRACEPTIVE USE BEFORE OR DURING EARLY PREGNANCY:

Extensive epidemiological studies have revealed no increased risk of birth defects in women who have used oral contraceptives prior to pregnancy. Studies also do not suggest a teratogenic effect, particularly in so far as cardiac anomalies and limb reduction defects are concerned, when taken inadvertently during early pregnancy.

The administration of oral contraceptives to induce withdrawal bleeding should not be used as a test for pregnancy. Oral contraceptives should not be used during pregnancy to treat threatened or habitual abortion.

It is recommended that for any patient who has missed two consecutive periods, pregnancy should be ruled out before continuing oral contraceptive use. If the patient has not adhered to the prescribed schedule, the possibility of pregnancy should be considered at the time of the first missed period. Oral contraceptive use should be discontinued if pregnancy is confirmed.

7. GALLBLADDER DISEASE

Earlier studies have reported an increased lifetime relative risk of gallbladder surgery in users of oral contraceptives and estrogens. More recent studies, however, have shown that the relative risk of developing gallbladder disease among oral contraceptive users may be minimal.

The recent findings of minimal risk may be related to the use of oral contraceptive formulations containing lower hormonal doses of estrogens and progestogens.

8. CARBOHYDRATE AND LIPID METABOLIC EFFECTS

Oral contraceptives have been shown to cause glucose intolerance in a significant percentage of users. Oral contraceptives containing greater than 75 micrograms of estrogens cause hyperinsulinism, while lower doses of estrogen cause less glucose intolerance. Progestogens increase insulin secretion and create insulin resistance, this effect varying with different progestational agents.

However, in the nondiabetic woman, oral contraceptives appear to have no effect on fasting blood glucose. Because of these demonstrated effects, prediabetic and diabetic women should be carefully observed while taking oral contraceptives.

A small proportion of women will have persistent hypertriglyceridemia while on the pill. As discussed earlier (see Warnings 1.a. and 1.d.), changes in serum triglycerides and lipoprotein levels have been reported in oral contraceptive users.

9. ELEVATED BLOOD PRESSURE

An increase in blood pressure has been reported in women taking oral contraceptives and this increase is more likely in older oral contraceptive users and with continued use. Data from the Royal College of General Practitioners and subsequent randomized trials have shown that the incidence of hypertension increases with increasing concentrations of progestogens.

Women with a history of hypertension or hypertension-related diseases, or renal disease should be encouraged to use another method of contraception. If women elect to use oral contraceptives, they should be monitored closely and if significant elevation of blood pressure occurs, oral contraceptives should be discontinued. For most women, elevated blood pressure will return to normal after stopping oral contraceptives, and there is no difference in the occurrence of hypertension among ever- and never-users.

10. HEADACHE

The onset or exacerbation of migraine or development of headache with a new pattern which is recurrent, persistent, or severe requires discontinuation of oral contraceptives and evaluation of the cause.

11. BLEEDING IRREGULARITIES

Breakthrough bleeding and spotting are sometimes encountered in patients on oral contraceptives, especially during the first three months of use. Nonhormonal causes should be considered and adequate diagnostic measures taken to rule out malignancy or pregnancy in the event of breakthrough bleeding, as in the case of any abnormal vaginal bleeding. If pathology has been excluded, time or a change to another formulation may solve the problem. In the event of amenorrhea, pregnancy should be ruled out.

Women with a history of oligomenorrhea or secondary amenorrhea or young women without regular cycles prior to taking oral contraceptives may again have irregular bleeding or amenorrhea after discontinuation of oral contraceptives.

PRECAUTIONS

1. PHYSICAL EXAMINATION AND FOLLOW-UP

A complete medical history and physical examination should be taken prior to the initiation or reinstitution of oral contraceptives and at least annually during use of oral contraceptives. These physical examinations should include special reference to blood pressure, breasts, abdomen and pelvic organs, including cervical cytology, and relevant laboratory tests. In case of undiagnosed, persistent, or recurrent abnormal vaginal bleeding, appropriate diagnostic measures should be conducted to rule out malignancy. Women with a strong family history of breast cancer or who have breast nodules should be monitored with particular care.

2. LIPID DISORDERS

Women who are being treated for hyperlipidemias should be followed closely if they elect to use oral contraceptives. Some progestogens may elevate LDL levels and may render the control of hyperlipidemias more difficult.

3. LIVER FUNCTION

If jaundice develops in any woman receiving such drugs, the medication should be discontinued. Steroid hormones may be poorly metabolized in patients with impaired liver function.

4. FLUID RETENTION

Oral contraceptives may cause some degree of fluid retention. They should be prescribed with caution, and only with careful monitoring, in patients with conditions which might be aggravated by fluid retention.

5. EMOTIONAL DISORDERS

Women with a history of depression should be carefully observed and the drug discontinued if depression recurs to a serious degree.

Patients becoming significantly depressed while taking oral contraceptives should stop the medication and use an alternate method of contraception in an attempt to determine whether the symptom is drug related.

6. CONTACT LENSES

Contact lens wearers who develop visual changes or changes in lens tolerance should be assessed by an ophthalmologist.

7. DRUG INTERACTIONS

Reduced efficacy and increased incidence of breakthrough bleeding and menstrual irregularities have been associated with concomitant use of rifampin. A similar assocation, though less marked, has been suggested with barbiturates, phenylbutazone, phenytoin sodium, and possibly with griseofulvin, ampicillin, and tetracyclines.

8. INTERACTIONS WITH LABORATORY TESTS

Certain endocrine and liver function tests and blood components may be affected by oral contraceptives:

TABLE 2

ANNUAL NUMBER OF BIRTH-RELATED OR METHOD-RELATED DEATHS ASSOCIATED WITH CONTROL OF FERTILITY PER 100,000 NONSTERILE WOMEN, BY FERTILITY CONTROL METHOD ACCORDING TO AGE

Method of control and outcome	AGE 15–19	20–24	25–29	30–34	35–39	40–44
No fertility control methods*	7.0	7.4	9.1	14.8	25.7	28.2
Oral contraceptives nonsmoker**	0.3	0.5	0.9	1.9	13.8	31.6
Oral contraceptives smoker**	2.2	3.4	6.6	13.5	51.1	117.2
IUD**	0.8	0.8	1.0	1.0	1.4	1.4
Condom*	1.1	1.6	0.7	0.2	0.3	0.4
Diaphragm/spermicide*	1.9	1.2	1.2	1.3	2.2	2.8
Periodic abstinence*	2.5	1.6	1.6	1.7	2.9	3.6

* Deaths are birth related
** Deaths are method related

Ory HW: Mortality associated with fertility and fertility control:1983. *Fam Plann Perspect* 1983;15:50–56.

a. Increased prothrombin and factors VII, VIII, IX, and X; decreased antithrombin 3; increased norepinephrine-induced platelet aggregability.

b. Increased thyroid-binding globulin (TBG) leading to increased circulating total thyroid hormone, as measured by protein-bound iodine (PBI), T4 by column or by radioimmunoassay. Free T3 resin uptake is decreased, reflecting the elevated TBG, free T4 concentration is unaltered.

c. Other binding proteins may be elevated in serum.

d. Sex-binding globulins are increased and result in elevated levels of total circulating sex steroids and corticoids; however, free or biologically active levels remain unchanged.

e. Triglycerides may be increased.

f. Glucose tolerance may be decreased.

g. Serum folate levels may be depressed by oral contraceptive therapy. This may be of clinical significance if a woman becomes pregnant shortly after discontinuing oral contraceptives.

9. CARCINOGENESIS
See **WARNINGS** section.

10. PREGNANCY
Pregnancy Category X. See **CONTRAINDICATIONS** and **WARNINGS** sections.

11. NURSING MOTHERS
Small amounts of oral contraceptive steroids have been identified in the milk of nursing mothers and a few adverse effects on the child have been reported, including jaundice and breast enlargement. In addition, oral contraceptives given in the postpartum period may interfere with lactation by decreasing the quantity and quality of breast milk. If possible, the nursing mother should be advised not to use oral contraceptives but to use other forms of contraception until she has completely weaned her child.

12. SEXUALLY TRANSMITTED DISEASES
Oral contraceptives neither prevent nor are treatment for venereal disease. Also oral contraceptives do not protect against the acquisition of the Auto-Immune Disease Syndrome (AIDS).

13. VOMITING AND/OR DIARRHEA
Although a cause-and-effect relationship has not been clearly established, several cases of oral contraceptive failure have been reported in association with vomiting and/or diarrhea. If significant gastrointestinal disturbance occurs in any woman receiving contraceptive steroids, the use of a back-up method of contraception for the remainder of that cycle is recommended.

INFORMATION FOR THE PATIENT
See Patient Labeling Printed Below.

ADVERSE REACTIONS
An increased risk of the following serious adverse reactions has been associated with the use of oral contraceptives (see Warnings section):
- Thrombophlebitis
- Arterial thromboembolism
- Pulmonary embolism
- Myocardial infarction
- Cerebral hemorrhage
- Cerebral thrombosis
- Hypertension
- Gallbladder disease
- Hepatic adenomas or benign liver tumors

There is evidence of an association between the following conditions and the use of oral contraceptives, although additional confirmatory studies are needed:
- Mesenteric thrombosis
- Retinal thrombosis

The following adverse reactions have been reported in patients receiving oral contraceptives and are believed to be drug related:
- Nausea
- Vomiting
- Gastrointestinal symptoms (such as abdominal cramps and bloating)
- Breakthrough bleeding
- Spotting
- Change in menstrual flow
- Amenorrhea
- Temporary infertility after discontinuation of treatment
- Edema
- Melasma which may persist
- Breast changes: tenderness, enlargement, and secretion
- Change in weight (increase or decrease)
- Change in cervical ectropion and secretion
- Possible diminution in lactation when given immediately postpartum
- Cholestatic jaundice
- Migraine
- Rash (allergic)
- Mental depression
- Reduced tolerance to carbohydrates
- Vaginal candidiasis

- Change in corneal curvature (steepening)
- Intolerance to contact lenses

The following adverse reactions have been reported in users of oral contraceptives, and the association has been neither confirmed nor refuted:
- Premenstrual syndrome
- Cataracts
- Changes in appetite
- Cystitis-like syndrome
- Headache
- Nervousness
- Dizziness
- Hirsutism
- Loss of scalp hair
- Erythema multiforme
- Erythema nodosum
- Hemorrhagic eruption
- Vaginitis
- Porphyria
- Impaired renal function
- Hemolytic uremic syndrome
- Budd-Chiari syndrome
- Acne
- Changes in libido
- Colitis

OVERDOSAGE
Serious ill effects have not been reported following acute ingestion of large doses of oral contraceptives by young children. Overdosage may cause nausea, and withdrawal bleeding may occur in females.

NONCONTRACEPTIVE HEALTH BENEFITS
The following noncontraceptive health benefits related to the use of oral contraceptives are supported by epidemiological studies which largely utilized oral contraceptive formulations containing estrogen doses exceeding 0.035 mg of ethinyl estradiol or 0.05 mg of mestranol.
Effects on menses:
- Increased menstrual cycle regularity
- Decreased blood loss and decreased incidence of iron deficiency anemia
- Decreased incidence of dysmenorrhea
Effects related to inhibition of ovulation:
- Decreased incidence of functional ovarian cysts
- Decreased incidence of ectopic pregnancies
Effects from long-term use:
- Decreased incidence of fibroadenomas and fibrocystic disease of the breast
- Decreased incidence of acute pelvic inflammatory disease
- Decreased incidence of endometrial cancer
- Decreased incidence of ovarian cancer

DOSAGE AND ADMINISTRATION
To achieve maximum contraceptive effectiveness, (OVCON 35 or OVCON 50) must be taken exactly as directed and at intervals not exceeding 24 hours. For the initial cycle of OVCON 35 or OVCON 50 therapy, contraceptive efficacy should not be assumed until after the first seven consecutive days of administration. The possibility of ovulation and conception prior to initiation of medication should be considered.
In subsequent cycles where more than seven days elapse from the first day of menstruation until the first pill containing active contraceptive medication is taken, an additional method of birth control should be used until the oral contraceptive has been taken for seven consecutive days.

28-DAY REGIMEN
Sunday Start
IF THIS IS YOUR FIRST PACKAGE, start taking the yellow or peach tablets on the first Sunday after your period begins, unless your period begins on Sunday. **If your period begins on Sunday, start taking the tablets that very same day.**
Continue to take one tablet each day.
After the last tablet in row 3 has been taken, start taking the green tablets in row 4 the very next day (Sunday).
After the last green tablet in row 4 has been taken, **start your new packet the following day** (Sunday) in the manner described above.
TAKE a tablet every day, without interruption. DO NOT MISS A TABLET. Your period will usually begin while you are taking the green tablets. It may continue during the first few tablets of the next packet.
Should you begin menstrual-like bleeding at another time, or if you do not have a period at all, **continue to take your one tablet daily** and notify your doctor. Your doctor should be informed promptly of any unusual changes in your general health.

Day-Five Start
IF THIS IS YOUR FIRST PACKAGE, count the first day of your menstrual bleeding as Day 1. Take your first yellow or peach tablet on Day 5.
CONTINUE to take one tablet daily. Take the tablets in order—first the yellow or peach, then the green ones.
TAKE a tablet every day, without interruption. DO NOT MISS A TABLET. Your period will usually begin while you are taking the green tablets. It may continue during the first few yellow or peach tablets.

Should you begin menstrual-like bleeding at another time, or if you do not have a period at all, **continue to take your one tablet daily** and notify your doctor. Your doctor should be informed promptly of any unusual changes in your general health.
If you miss a tablet, take it as soon as remembered. Also take the usual tablet for that day. Then resume your tablet-a-day schedule. Each missed tablet increases the possibility that the medication may not work. To reduce this possibility, use an additional method of protection until your next period. Because you are to take a tablet every day, without interruption, always have a new supply of tablets ready to take.

21-DAY REGIMEN
Sunday Start
IF THIS IS YOUR FIRST PACKAGE, start taking the yellow or peach tablets on the first Sunday after your period begins, unless your period begins on Sunday. **If your period begins on Sunday, start taking the tablets that very same day.**
Continue to take one tablet each day.
After the last tablet in row 3 has been taken (on a Saturday), **stop for one week** before starting to take the tablets in your next packet. Start your new packet on Sunday in the manner described above.
TAKE a tablet every day, without interruption. DO NOT MISS A TABLET. Your period will usually begin during your week off therapy. It may continue during the first few tablets of the next packet.
Should you begin menstrual-like bleeding at another time, or if you do not have a period at all, **continue to take your one tablet daily** and notify your doctor. Your doctor should be informed promptly of any unusual changes in your general health.

Day-Five Start
IF THIS IS YOUR FIRST PACKAGE, count the first day of your menstrual bleeding as Day 1. Take your first yellow or peach tablet on Day 5.
CONTINUE to take one tablet daily and take the tablets in order.
AFTER you have taken the last tablet, wait seven days and then begin your next package of tablets. You should begin again on the same day of the week. Thus, three weeks on, one week off therapy.
TAKE a tablet every day, without interruption. DO NOT MISS A TABLET. Your period will usually begin within four days after you have taken your last yellow or peach tablet.
Should you begin menstrual-like bleeding at another time, or if you do not have a period at all, **continue to take your tablets as directed** and notify your doctor. Your doctor should be informed promptly of any unusual changes in your general health.
If you miss a tablet, take it as soon as remembered. Also take the usual tablet for that day. Then resume your tablet-a-day schedule. Each missed tablet increases the possibility that the medication may not work. To reduce this possibility, use an additional method of protection until your next period. Because you are to take a tablet every day for three weeks, without interruption, always have a new supply of tablets ready to take.
Patients should be cautioned to follow the dosage schedule strictly.
If the regimen is interrupted, an additional contraceptive method is recommended for the rest of the cycle. Should spotting or breakthrough bleeding occur, it is recommended that the patient continue medication. If bleeding is persistent or recurrent, the patient should consult her physician.
Use of oral contraceptives in the event of a missed menstrual period:
1. If the patient has not adhered to the prescribed dosage regimen, the possibility of pregnancy should be considered after the first missed period and oral contraceptives should be withheld until pregnancy has been ruled out.
2. If the patient has adhered to the prescribed regimen and misses two consecutive periods, pregnancy should be ruled out before continuing the contraceptive regimen.

HOW SUPPLIED
OVCON® 50 (norethindrone and ethinyl estradiol tablets, USP) is available in 21- and 28-day regimens. Each package contains 21 yellow tablets of 1.0 mg norethindrone and 0.05 mg ethinyl estradiol. Each green tablet in the 28-day regimen contains inert ingredients.
OVCON 50, 21-day
NDC 0087-0584-42   Carton of 6 packages
OVCON 50, 28-Day
NDC 0087-0579-41   Carton of 6 packages
OVCON® 35 (norethindrone and ethinyl estradiol tablets, USP) is available in 21- and 28-day regimens. Each package contains 21 peach tablets of 0.4 mg norethindrone and 0.035 mg ethinyl estradiol. Each green tablet in the 28-day regimen contains inert ingredients.
OVCON 35, 21-Day
NDC 0087-0583-42   Carton of 6 packages

Continued on next page

Mead Johnson Laboratories—Cont.

OVCON 35, 28-Day

NDC 0087-0578-41 Carton of 6 packages
References are available upon request.

PATIENT PACKAGE INSERT
BRIEF SUMMARY

Oral contraceptives, also known as "birth control pills" or "the pill," are taken to prevent pregnancy and when taken correctly, have a failure rate of about 1% per year when used without missing any pills. The typical failure rate of large numbers of pill users is less than 3% per year when women who miss pills are included.

Oral contraceptive use is associated with certain serious diseases that can be life-threatening or may cause temporary or permanent disability. The risks associated with taking oral contraceptives increase significantly if you:

- Smoke
- Have high blood pressure, diabetes, high cholesterol
- Have or have had clotting disorders, heart attack, stroke, angina pectoris, cancer of the breast or sex organs, jaundice or malignant or benign liver tumors.

You should not take the pill if you suspect you are pregnant or have unexplained vaginal bleeding.

Cigarette smoking increases the risk of serious cardiovascular side effects from oral contraceptive use. This risk increases with age and with heavy smoking (15 or more cigarettes per day) and is quite marked in women over 35 years of age. Women who use oral contraceptives are strongly advised not to smoke.

Most side effects of the pill are not serious. The most common such effects are nausea, vomiting, bleeding between menstrual periods, weight gain, breast tenderness, and difficulty wearing contact lenses. These side effects, especially nausea and vomiting, may subside within the first three months of use.

The serious side effects of the pill occur very infrequently, especially if you are in good health and are young. However, you should know that the following medical conditions have been associated with or made worse by the pill:

1. Blood clots in the legs (thrombophlebitis), lungs (pulmonary embolism), stoppage or rupture of a blood vessel in the brain (stroke), blockage of blood vessels in the heart (heart attack or angina pectoris), or other organs of the body. As mentioned above, smoking increases the risk of heart attacks and strokes and subsequent serious medical consequences.
2. Liver tumors, which may rupture and cause severe bleeding. A possible but not definite association has been found with the pill and liver cancer. However, liver cancers are extremely rare. The chance of developing liver cancer from using the pill is thus even rarer.
3. High blood pressure, although blood pressure usually returns to normal when the pill is stopped.

The symptoms associated with these serious side effects are discussed in the detailed leaflet given to you with your supply of pills. Notify your doctor or health-care provider if you notice any unusual physical disturbances while taking the pill. In addition, drugs such as rifampin, as well as some anticonvulsants and some antibiotics may decrease oral contraceptive effectiveness.

Studies to date of women taking the pill have not shown an increase in the incidence of cancer of the breast or cervix. There is, however, insufficient evidence to rule out the possibility that the pill may cause such cancers.

Taking the pill provides some important noncontraceptive effects. These include less painful menstruation, less menstrual blood loss and anemia, fewer pelvic infections, and fewer cancers of the ovary and the lining of the uterus.

Be sure to discuss any medical condition you may have with your health-care provider. Your health-care provider will take a medical and family history before prescribing oral contraceptives and will examine you. You should be reexamined at least once a year while taking oral contraceptives.

The detailed patient information booklet gives you further information which you should read and discuss with your health-care professional.

INSTRUCTIONS TO PATIENTS

See Detailed Package Insert.

PATIENT PACKAGE INSERT

INTRODUCTION

Any woman who considers using oral contraceptives (the birth control pill or the pill) should understand the benefits and risks of using this form of birth control.

Although the oral contraceptives have important advantages over other methods of contraception, they have certain risks that no other method has and some of these risks may continue after you have stopped using the oral contraceptive. This booklet will give you much of the information you will need to make this decision and will also help you determine if you are at risk of developing any of the serious side effects of the pill. It will tell you how to use the pill properly so that it will be as effective as possible. However, this booklet is not a replacement for a careful discussion between you and your health-care professional. You should discuss the information provided in this booklet with him or her, both when you first start taking the pill and during your revisits. You should also follow your health-care professional's advice with regard to regular check-ups while you are on the pill.

EFFECTIVENESS OF ORAL CONTRACEPTIVES

Oral contraceptives or "birth control pills" or "the pill" are used to prevent pregnancy and are more effective than other nonsurgical methods of birth control. The chance of becoming pregnant is less than 1% (1 pregnancy per 100 women per year of use) when the pills are used correctly and no pills are missed. Typical failure rates are actually 3% per year. The chance of becoming pregnant increases with each missed pill during a menstrual cycle.

In comparison, typical accidental pregnancy rates for other nonsurgical methods of birth control during the first year of use are as follows:

IUD: 6%
Diaphragm with spermicides: 18%
Spermicides alone: 21%
Vaginal sponge: 18% to 30%
Condom alone: 12%
Periodic abstinence: 20%
No methods: 89%

WHO SHOULD NOT TAKE ORAL CONTRACEPTIVES

Cigarette smoking increases the risk of serious cardiovascular side effects from oral contraceptive use. This risk increases with age and with heavy smoking (15 or more cigarettes per day) and is quite marked in women over 35 years of age. Women who use oral contraceptives should not smoke.

Some women should not use the pill. For example, you should not take the pill if you are pregnant or think you may be pregnant. You should also not use the pill if you have or have ever had any of the following conditions:

- A history of heart attack or stroke
- Blood clots in the legs (thrombophlebitis), lungs (pulmonary embolism), or eyes
- A history of blood clots in the deep veins of your legs
- Chest pain (angina pectoris)
- Known or suspected breast cancer or cancer of the lining of the uterus
- Unexplained vaginal bleeding (until a diagnosis is reached by your doctor)
- Yellowing of the whites of the eyes or of the skin (jaundice) during pregnancy or during previous use of the pill
- Liver tumor (benign or cancerous)

Tell your health-care professional if you have ever had any of these conditions. Your health-care professional can recommend a safer method of birth control.

OTHER CONSIDERATIONS BEFORE TAKING ORAL CONTRACEPTIVES

Tell your health-care professional if you have:

- Breast nodules, fibrocystic disease of the breast, or an abnormal breast x-ray or mammogram
- Diabetes
- Elevated cholesterol or triglycerides
- High blood pressure
- Migraine or other headaches or epilepsy
- Mental depression
- Gallbladder, heart, or kidney disease
- History of scanty or irregular menstrual periods

Women with any of these conditions should be checked often by their health-care professional if they choose to use oral contraceptives.

Also, be sure to inform your doctor or health-care professional if you smoke or are on any medications.

RISKS OF TAKING ORAL CONTRACEPTIVES

1. Risk of developing blood clots

Blood clots and blockage of blood vessels are the most serious side effects of taking oral contraceptives. In particular, a clot in the legs can cause thrombophlebitis and a clot that travels to the lungs can cause a sudden blocking of the vessel carrying blood to the lungs. Either of these can cause death or disability. Rarely, clots occur in the blood vessels of the eye and may cause blindness, double vision, or impaired vision.

If you take oral contraceptives and need elective surgery, need to stay in bed for a prolonged illness or have recently delivered a baby, you may be at risk of developing blood clots. You should consult your doctor about stopping oral contraceptives three to four weeks before surgery and not taking oral contraceptives for two weeks after surgery or during bed rest. You should also not take oral contraceptives soon after delivery of a baby. It is advisable to wait for at least four weeks after delivery if you are not breastfeeding. If you are breastfeeding see the section on Breastfeeding in General Precautions.

2. Heart attacks and strokes

Oral contraceptives may increase the tendency to develop strokes (stoppage or rupture of blood vessels in the brain) and angina pectoris and heart attacks (blockage of blood vessels in the heart). Any of these conditions can cause death or disability.

Smoking greatly increases the possibility of suffering heart attacks and strokes. Furthermore, smoking and the use of oral contraceptives greatly increase the chances of developing and dying of heart disease.

3. Gallbladder disease

Oral contraceptive users probably have a greater risk than nonusers of having gallbladder disease, although this risk may be related to pills containing high doses of estrogens.

4. Liver tumors

In rare cases, oral contraceptives can cause benign but dangerous liver tumors. These benign liver tumors can rupture and cause fatal internal bleeding. In addition, a possible but not definite, association has been found with the pill and liver cancers in two studies, in which a few women who developed these very rare cancers were found to have used oral contraceptives for long periods. However, liver cancers in general are extremely rare and the chance of developing liver cancer from using the pill is thus even rarer.

5. Cancer of the reproductive organs

There is, at present, no confirmed evidence that oral contraceptives increase the risk of cancer of the reproductive organs and breasts in human studies. Several studies have found no overall increase in the risk of developing breast cancer. However, women who use oral contraceptives and have a strong family history of breast cancer, or who have breast nodules or abnormal mammograms should be closely followed by their doctors.

Some studies have found an increase in the incidence of cancer of the cervix in women who use oral contraceptives. However, this finding may be related to factors other than the use of oral contraceptives.

ESTIMATED RISK OF DEATH FROM A BIRTH CONTROL METHOD OR PREGNANCY

All methods of birth control and pregnancy are associated with a risk of developing certain diseases which may lead to disability or death. An estimate of the number of deaths associated with different methods of birth control and pregnancy has been calculated and is shown in the following table.

[See table at left.]

ANNUAL NUMBER OF BIRTH-RELATED OR METHOD-RELATED DEATHS ASSOCIATED WITH CONTROL OF FERTILITY PER 100,000 NONSTERILE WOMEN, BY FERTILITY CONTROL METHOD ACCORDING TO AGE

Method of control and outcome	AGE 15–19	20–24	25–29	30–34	35–39	40–44
No fertility control methods*	7.0	7.4	9.1	14.8	25.7	28.2
Oral contraceptives nonsmoker**	0.3	0.5	0.9	1.9	13.8	31.6
Oral contraceptives smoker**	2.2	3.4	6.6	13.5	51.1	117.2
IUD**	0.8	0.8	1.0	1.0	1.4	1.4
Condom*	1.1	1.6	0.7	0.2	0.3	0.4
Diaphragm/spermicide*	1.9	1.2	1.2	1.3	2.2	2.8
Periodic abstinence*	2.5	1.6	1.6	1.7	2.9	3.6

* Deaths are birth-related
** Deaths are method-related

It can be seen in the table that for women aged 15 to 39, the risk of death was highest with pregnancy (7–26 deaths per 100,000 women, depending on age). Among pill users who do not smoke, the risk of death was always lower than that associated with pregnancy for any age group, although over the age of 40, the risk increases to 32 deaths per 100,000 women, compared to 28 associated with pregnancy at that age. However, for pill users who smoke and are over the age of 35, the estimated number of deaths exceeds those for other methods of birth control. If a woman is over the age of 40 and smokes, her estimated risk of death is four times higher (117/100,000

women) than the estimated risk associated with pregnancy (28/100,000 women) in that age group.
The suggestion that women over 40 who don't smoke should not take oral contraceptives is based on information from older high-dose pills and on less selective use of pills than is practiced today. An Advisory Committee of the FDA discussed this issue in 1989 and recommended that the benefits of oral contraceptive use by healthy, nonsmoking women over 40 years of age may outweigh the possible risks. However, all women, especially older women, are cautioned to use the lowest dose pill that is effective.
In the above table, the risk of death from any birth control method is less than the risk of childbirth, except for oral contraceptive users over the age of 35 who smoke and pill users over the age of 40 even if they do not smoke.
You should discuss this information with your health-care professional.

WARNING SIGNALS

If any of these adverse conditions occur while you are taking oral contraceptives, call your doctor immediately:

- Sharp chest pain, coughing of blood, or sudden shortness of breath (indicating a possible clot in the lung)
- Pain in the calf (indicating a possible clot in the leg)
- Crushing chest pain or heaviness in the chest (indicating a possible heart attack)
- Sudden severe headache or vomiting, dizziness or fainting, disturbances of vision or speech, weakness, or numbness in an arm or leg (indicating a possible stroke)
- Sudden partial or complete loss of vision (indicating a possible clot in the eye)
- Breast lumps (indicating possible breast cancer or fibrocystic disease of the breast; ask your doctor or health-care professional to show you how to examine your breasts)
- Severe pain or tenderness in the stomach area (indicating a possibly ruptured liver tumor)
- Difficulty in sleeping, weakness, lack of energy, fatigue, or change in mood (possibly indicating severe depression)
- Jaundice or a yellowing of the skin or eyeballs, accompanied frequently by fever, fatigue, loss of appetite, dark-colored urine, or light-colored bowel movements (indicating possible liver problems)
- Abnormal vaginal bleeding (See Side Effects of Oral Contraceptives, 1. Vaginal bleeding, below.)

SIDE EFFECTS OF ORAL CONTRACEPTIVES

In addition to the risks and more serious side effects discussed above (See Risks of Taking Oral Contraceptives, Estimated Risk of Death from a Birth Control Method or Pregnancy and Warning Signals section, above), the following may also occur:

1. Vaginal bleeding
Irregular vaginal bleeding or spotting may occur while you are taking the pills. Irregular bleeding may vary from slight staining between menstrual periods to breakthrough bleeding which is a flow much like a regular period. Irregular bleeding occurs most often during the first few months of oral contraceptive use, but may also occur after you have been taking the pill for some time. Such bleeding may be temporary and usually does not indicate any serious problems. It is important to continue taking your pills on schedule. If the bleeding occurs in more than one cycle or lasts for more than a few days, talk to your doctor or health-care professional.

2. Gastrointestinal effects
The most frequent, unpleasant side effects are nausea and vomiting, stomach cramps, bloating, and a change in appetite.

3. Contact lenses
If you wear contact lenses and notice a change in vision or an inability to wear your lenses, contact your doctor or health-care professional.

4. Fluid retention
Oral contraceptives may cause edema (fluid retention) with swelling of the fingers or ankles and may raise your blood pressure. If you experience fluid retention, contact your doctor or health-care professional.

5. Melasma
A spotty darkening of the skin is possible, particularly of the face.

6. Other side effects
Other side effects may include change in appetite, headache, nervousness, depression, dizziness, loss of scalp hair, rash, and vaginal infections.
If any of these side effects bother you, call your doctor or health-care professional.

GENERAL PRECAUTIONS

1. Missed periods and use of oral contraceptives before or during early pregnancy
There may be times when you may not menstruate regularly after you have completed taking a cycle of pills. If you have taken your pills regularly and miss one menstrual period, continue taking your pills for the next cycle but be sure to inform your health-care professional before doing so. If you have not taken the pills daily as instructed and missed a menstrual period, or if you missed two consecutive menstrual periods, you may be pregnant. Check with your health-care professional immediately to determine whether you are pregnant. Do not continue to take oral contraceptives until you are sure you are not pregnant, but continue to use another method of contraception.
There is no conclusive evidence that oral contraceptive use is associated with an increase in birth defects, when taken inadvertently during early pregnancy. Previously, a few studies had reported that oral contraceptives might be associated with birth defects, but these studies have not been confirmed. Nevertheless, oral contraceptives or any other drugs should not be used during pregnancy unless clearly necessary and prescribed by your doctor. You should check with your doctor about risks to your unborn child of any medication taken during pregnancy.

2. While breastfeeding
If you are breastfeeding, consult your doctor before starting oral contraceptives. Some of the drug will be passed on to the child in the milk. A few adverse effects on the child have been reported, including yellowing of the skin (jaundice) and breast enlargement. In addition, oral contraceptives may decrease the amount and quality of your milk. If possible, do not use oral contraceptives while breastfeeding. You should use another method of contraception since breastfeeding provides only partial protection from becoming pregnant and this partial protection decreases significantly as you breastfeed for longer periods of time. You should consider starting oral contraceptives only after you have weaned your child completely.

3. Laboratory tests
If you are scheduled for any laboratory tests, tell your doctor you are taking birth control pills. Certain blood tests may be affected by birth control pills.

4. Drug interactions
Certain drugs may interact with birth control pills to make them less effective in preventing pregnancy or cause an increase in breakthrough bleeding. Such drugs include rifampin, drugs used for epilepsy such as barbiturates (for example, phenobarbital) and phenytoin (Dilantin is one brand of this drug), phenylbutazone (Butazolidin is one brand) and possibly ampicillin and tetracyclines (several brand names). You may need to use an additional method of contraception when you take drugs which can make oral contraceptives less effective.

HOW TO TAKE ORAL CONTRACEPTIVES

1. General Instructions
You must take your pill every day according to the instructions. Oral contraceptives are most effective if taken no more than 24 hours apart. Take your pill at the same time every day so that you are less likely to forget to take it. You will then maintain an effective dose of the oral contraceptive in your body.

How To Take the Pill So That it Is Most Effective.
To achieve maximum contraceptive effectiveness, OVCON 50 or OVCON 35 must be taken correctly and at intervals not exceeding 24 hours. For the initial cycle of OVCON 35 or OVCON 50 therapy, oral contraceptive efficacy (98% or greater) should not be assumed until after the first seven consecutive days of administration. The possibility of ovulation and conception prior to initiation of medication should be considered.
In subsequent cycles where more than seven days elapse from the first day of menstruation until the first pill containing active contraceptive medication is taken, an additional method of birth control should be used until the oral contraceptive has been taken for seven consecutive days.

28-DAY REGIMEN

Sunday Start
IF THIS IS YOUR FIRST PACKAGE, start taking the yellow or peach tablets on the first Sunday after your period begins, unless your period begins on Sunday. **If your period begins on Sunday, start taking the tablets that very same day.**
CONTINUE to take one tablet each day.
After the last tablet in row 3 has been taken, start taking the green tablets in row 4 the very next day (Sunday).
After the last green tablet in row 4 has been taken, **start your new packet the following day** (Sunday) in the manner described above.
TAKE a tablet every day, without interruption. DO NOT MISS A TABLET. Your period will usually begin while you are taking the green tablets. It may continue during the first few tablets of the next packet.
Should you begin menstrual-like bleeding at another time, or if you do not have a period at all, **continue to take your one tablet daily** and notify your doctor. Your doctor should be informed promptly of any unusual changes in your general health.

Day-Five Start
IF THIS IS YOUR FIRST PACKAGE, count the first day of your menstrual bleeding as Day 1. Take your first yellow or peach tablet on Day 5.
CONTINUE to take one tablet daily. Take the tablets in order—first the yellow or peach, then the green ones.
TAKE a tablet every day, without interruption. DO NOT MISS A TABLET. Your period will usually begin while you are taking the green tablets. It may continue during the first few yellow or peach tablets.
Should you begin menstrual-like bleeding at another time, or if you do not have a period at all, **continue to take your one tablet daily** and notify your doctor. Your doctor should be informed promptly of any unusual changes in your general health.
If you miss a tablet, take it as soon as remembered. Also take the usual tablet for that day. Then resume your tablet-a-day schedule. Each missed tablet increases the possibility that the medication may not work. To reduce this possibility, use an additional method of protection until your next period.
Because you are to take a tablet every day, without interruption, always have a new supply of tablets ready to take.

21-DAY REGIMEN

Sunday Start
IF THIS IS YOUR FIRST PACKAGE, start taking the yellow or peach tablets on the first Sunday after your period begins, unless your period begins on Sunday. **If your period begins on Sunday, start taking the tablets that very same day.**
Continue to take one tablet each day.
After the last tablet in row 3 has been taken (on a Saturday), **stop for one week** before starting to take the tablets in your next packet. Start your new packet on Sunday in the manner described above.
TAKE a tablet every day, without interruption. DO NOT MISS A TABLET. Your period will usually begin your week off therapy. It may continue during the first few tablets of the next packet.
Should you begin menstrual-like bleeding at another time, or if you do not have a period at all, **continue to take your one tablet daily** and notify your doctor. Your doctor should be informed promptly of any unusual changes in your general health.

Day-Five Start
IF THIS IS YOUR FIRST PACKAGE, count the first day of your menstrual bleeding as Day 1. Take your first yellow or peach tablet on Day 5.
CONTINUE to take one tablet daily and take the tablets in order.
TAKE a tablet every day, without interruption. DO NOT MISS A TABLET. Your period will usually begin within four days after you have taken your last yellow or peach tablet.
AFTER you have taken the last tablet, wait seven days and then begin your next package of tablets. You should begin again on the same day of the week. Thus, three weeks on, one week off tablets.
Should you begin menstrual-like bleeding at another time, or if you do not have a period at all, **continue to take your tablets correctly** and notify your doctor. Your doctor will also want you to let him know promptly of any unusual changes in your general health.
If you miss a tablet, take it as soon as remembered. Also take the usual tablet for that day. Then resume your tablet-a-day schedule. Each missed tablet increases the possibility that the medication may not work. To reduce this possibility, use an additional method of protection until your next period.
Because you are to take a tablet every day for three weeks, without interruption, always have a new supply of tablets ready to take.
Patients should be cautioned to follow the dosage schedule strictly. If the regimen is interrupted, an additional contraceptive method is recommended for the rest of the cycle. Should spotting or breakthrough bleeding occur, it is recommended that you continue medication. If bleeding is persistent or recurrent, consult your physician.
Use of oral contraceptives in the event of a missed menstrual period:

a. If you have not adhered to the prescribed dosage regimen, the possibility of pregnancy should be considered after the first missed period (or after 45 days from the last menstrual period if the progestogen-only oral contraceptives are used) and oral contraceptives should be withheld until pregnancy has been ruled out.
b. If you have adhered to the prescribed regimen and miss two consecutive periods, pregnancy should be ruled out before continuing the contraceptive regimen.
c. At times there may be no menstrual period after a cycle of pills. Therefore, if you miss one menstrual period but have taken the pills **exactly as you were supposed to,** continue as usual into the next cycle. If you have not taken the pills correctly and miss a menstrual period, you may be pregnant and should stop taking oral contraceptives until your doctor determines whether or not you are pregnant. Until you can get to your doctor, use another form of contraception. If two consecutive menstrual periods are missed, you should stop taking pills until it is determined whether you are pregnant.

If your doctor has scheduled you for surgery, or you need prolonged bed rest, he or she may suggest that you stop taking the pill four weeks before surgery to avoid an increased risk of blood clots. It is also advisable not to start oral contraceptives sooner than four weeks after delivery of a baby.

Continued on next page

Mead Johnson Laboratories—Cont.

2. **If you forget to take your pill**

If you miss only one pill in a cycle, the change of becoming pregnant is small. Take the missed pill as soon as you realize that you have forgotten it. Since the risk of pregnancy increases with each additional pill you skip, it is very important that you take one pill a day.

At times there may be no menstrual period after a cycle of pills. Therefore, if you miss one menstrual period but have taken the pills **exactly as you were supposed to**, continue as usual into the next cycle. If you have not taken the pills correctly and miss a menstrual period, you may be pregnant and should stop taking oral contraceptives until your doctor determines whether or not you are pregnant. Until you can get to your doctor, use another form of contraception. If two consecutive menstrual periods are missed, you should stop taking pills until it is determined whether you are pregnant.

3. **Pregnancy due to pill failure**

The incidence of pill failure resulting in pregnancy is approximately 1% (ie, one pregnancy per 100 women per year) if taken every day as directed, but more typical failure rates are about 3%. If failure does occur, the risk to the fetus is minimal.

4. **Pregnancy after stopping the pill**

There may be some delay in becoming pregnant after you stop using oral contraceptives, especially if you had irregular menstrual cycles before you used oral contraceptives. It may be advisable to postpone conception until you begin menstruating regularly once you have stopped taking the pill and desire pregnancy.

There does not appear to be any increase in birth defects in newborn babies when pregnancy occurs soon after stopping the pill.

5. **Other**

a. Gastrointestinal upset

If significant vomiting and/or diarrhea occur while you are taking the pill, it is recommended that you use a back-up method of contraception during the remainder of that cycle.

b. Sexually tramsitted diseases

Oral contraceptives are of no value in the treatment or prevention of venereal disease. Neither do oral contraceptives protect against infection with the AIDS virus.

c. Overdosage

Serious ill effects have not been reported following ingestion of large doses of oral contraceptives by young children. Overdosage may cause nausea and withdrawal bleeding in females. In case of overdosage, contact your poison control center, health-care professional, or nearest emergency room. KEEP THIS DRUG AND ALL DRUGS OUT OF THE REACH OF CHILDREN.

d. General medical information.

Your health-care professional will take a medical and family history before prescribing oral contraceptives and will examine you. You should be reexamined at least once a year. Be sure to inform your health-care professional if there is a family history of any of the conditions listed previously in this leaflet. Be sure to keep all appointments with your health-care professional, because this is a time to determine if there are early signs of side effects of oral contraceptive use.

Do not use the drug for any condition other than the one for which it was prescribed. This drug has been prescribed specifically for you; do not give it to others who may want birth control pills.

NONCONTRACEPTIVE EFFECTS OF ORAL CONTRACEPTIVES

In addition to preventing pregnancy, use of oral contraceptives may provide certain benefits. They are:

- Menstrual cycles may become more regular
- Blood flow during menstruation may be lighter and less iron may be lost. Therefore, anemia due to iron deficiency is less likely to occur.
- Pain or other symptoms during menstruation may be encountered less frequently
- Ectopic (tubal) pregnancy may occur less frequently
- Noncancerous cysts or lumps in the breast may occur less frequently
- Acute pelvic inflammatory disease may occur less frequently
- Oral contraceptive use may provide some protection against developing two forms of cancer: cancer of the ovaries and cancer of the lining of the uterus

If you want more information about birth control pills, ask your doctor or pharmacist. They have a more technical leaflet called the Professional Labeling, which you may wish to read.

Shown in Product Identification Section, page 419

STADOL® ℞

[*stā'-dōl*]

(butorphanol tartrate) Injectable

STADOL® NS™ ℞

(butorphanol tartrate)

Nasal Spray

DESCRIPTION

Butorphanol tartrate is a synthetically derived opioid agonist-antagonist analgesic of the phenanthrene series. The chemical name is (-)-17-(cyclobutylmethyl) morphinan-3, 14-diol [S-(R*,R*)] -2,3- dihydroxybutanedioate (1:1) (salt). The molecular formula is $C_{21}H_{29}NO_2.C_4H_6O_6$, which corresponds to a molecular weight of 477.55 and the following structural formula:

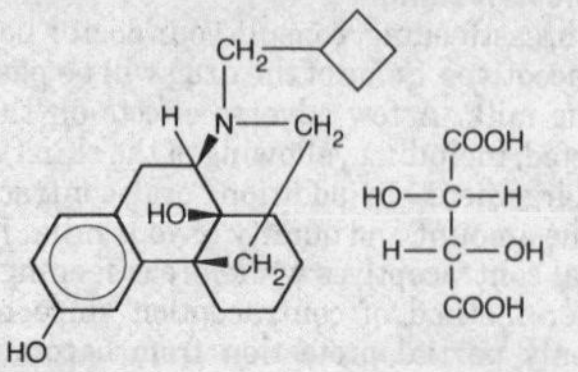

Butorphanol tartrate is a white crystalline substance. The dose is expressed as the tartrate salt. One milligram of the salt is equivalent to 0.68 mg of the free base. The n-octanol/aqueous buffer partition coefficient of butorphanol is 180:1 at pH 7.5.

STADOL® (butorphanol tartrate) Injectable is a sterile, parenteral, aqueous solution of butorphanol tartrate for intravenous or intramuscular administration. In addition to 1 or 2 mg of butorphanol tartrate, each mL of solution contains 3.3 mg of citric acid, 6.4 mg of sodium citrate, and 6.4 mg sodium chloride, and 0.1 mg benzethonium chloride (in multiple dose vial only) as a preservative.

STADOL® NS™ (butorphanol tartrate) Nasal Spray is an aqueous solution of butorphanol tartrate for administration as a metered spray to the nasal mucosa. Each bottle of STADOL NS contains 2.5 mL of a 10 mg/mL solution of butorphanol tartrate with sodium chloride, citric acid, and benzethonium chloride in purified water with sodium hydroxide and/or hydrochloric acid added to adjust the pH to 5.0. The pump reservoir must be fully primed (see PATIENT INSTRUCTIONS) prior to initial use. After initial priming each metered spray delivers an average of 1.0 mg of butorphanol tartrate and the 2.5 mL bottle will deliver an average of 14–15 doses of STADOL NS. If not used for 48 hours or longer, the unit must be re-primed (see PATIENT INSTRUCTIONS). With intermittent use requiring repriming before each dose, the 2.5 mL bottle will deliver an average of 8–10 doses of STADOL NS depending on how much repriming is necessary.

CLINICAL PHARMACOLOGY

General Pharmacology and Mechanism of Action

Butorphanol and its major metabolites are agonists at k-opioid receptors and mixed agonist-antagonists at μ-opioid receptors.

Its interactions with these receptors in the central nervous system apparently mediate most of its pharmacologic effects, including analgesia.

In addition to analgesia, CNS effects include depression of spontaneous respiratory activity and cough, stimulation of the emetic center, miosis and sedation. Effects possibly mediated by non-CNS mechanisms include alteration in cardiovascular resistance and capacitance, bronchomotor tone, gastrointestinal secretory and motor activity and bladder sphincter activity.

In an animal model, the dose of the butorphanol tartrate required to antagonize morphine analgesia by 50% was similar to that for nalorphine, less than that for pentazocine and more than that for naloxone.

The pharmacological activity of butorphanol metabolites has not been studied in humans; in animal studies, butorphanol metabolites have demonstrated some analgesic activity.

In human studies of butorphanol (see CLINICAL TRIALS), sedation is commonly noted at doses of 0.5 mg or more. Narcosis is produced by 10–12 mg doses of butorphanol administered over 10–15 minutes intravenously.

Butorphanol, like other mixed agonist-antagonists with a high affinity for the kappa receptor, may produce unpleasant psychotomimetic effects in some individuals.

Nausea and/or vomiting may be produced by doses of 1 mg or more administered by any route.

In human studies involving individuals without significant respiratory dysfunction, 2 mg of butorphanol IV and 10 mg of morphine sulfate IV depressed respiration to a comparable degree. At higher doses, the magnitude of respiratory depression with butorphanol is not appreciably increased; however, the duration of respiratory depression is longer. Respiratory depression noted after administration of butorphanol to humans by any route is reversed by treatment with naloxone, a specific opioid antagonist (see Treatment in OVERDOSE).

Butorphanol tartrate demonstrates antitussive effects in animals at doses less than those required for analgesia.

Hemodynamic changes noted during cardiac catheterization in patients receiving single 0.025 mg/kg intravenous doses of butorphanol have included increases in pulmonary artery pressure, wedge pressure and vascular resistance, increases in left ventricular end diastolic pressure and in systemic arterial pressure.

Pharmacodynamics

The analgesic effect of butorphanol is influenced by the route of administration. Onset of analgesia is within a few minutes for intravenous administration, within Peak analgesic activity occurs within 30–60 minutes following intravenous and intramuscular administration and within 1–2 hours following the nasal spray administration.

The duration of analgesia varies depending on the pain model as well as the route of administration, but is generally 3–4 hours with IM and IV doses as defined by the time 50% of patients required remedication. In postoperative studies, the duration of analgesia with IV or IM butorphanol was similar to morphine, meperidine and pentazocine when administered in the same fashion at equipotent doses (see CLINICAL TRIALS). Compared to the injectable form and other drugs in this class, STADOL® NS™ (butorphanol tartrate) Nasal Spray has a longer duration of action (4–5 hours) (see CLINICAL TRIALS).

Pharmacokinetics

STADOL Injectable is rapidly absorbed after IM injection and peak plasma levels are reached in 20–40 minutes.

After nasal administration, mean peak blood levels of 0.9–1.04 ng/mL occur at 30–60 minutes after a 1 mg dose (see Table 1). The absolute bioavailability of STADOL NS is 60–70% and is unchanged in patients with allergic rhinitis. In patients using a nasal vasoconstrictor (oxymetazoline) the fraction of the dose absorbed was unchanged, but the rate of absorption was slowed. The peak plasma concentrations were approximately half those achieved in the absence of the vasoconstrictor.

Following its initial absorption/distribution phase, the single dose pharmacokinetics of butorphanol by the intravenous, intramuscular, and nasal routes of administration are similar (see Figure 1).

Figure 1 — Butorphanol Plasma Levels After IV, IM and Nasal Spray Administration of 2 mg Dose

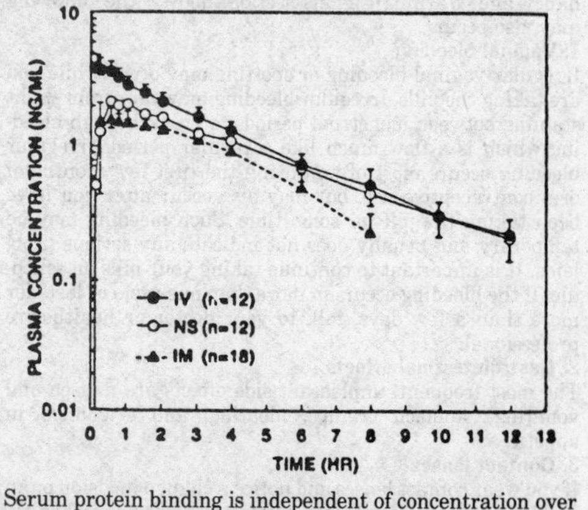

Serum protein binding is independent of concentration over the range achieved in clinical practice (up to 7 ng/mL) with a bound fraction of approximately 80%.

The volume of distribution of butorphanol varies from 305–901 liters and total body clearance from 52–154 liters/hr (see Table 1).

[See table on next page.]

Dose proportionality for STADOL® NS™ (butorphanol tartrate) Nasal Spray has been determined at steady state in doses up to 4 mg at 6 hour intervals. Steady state is achieved within 2 days. The mean peak plasma concentration at steady state was 1.8-fold (maximal 3-fold) following a single dose.

The drug is transported across the blood:brain and placental barriers and into human milk (see Labor and Delivery and Nursing Mothers).

Butorphanol is extensively metabolized in the liver. Metabolism is qualitatively and quantitatively similar following intravenous, intramuscular, or nasal administration. Oral bioavailability is only 5–17% because of extensive first pass metabolism of butorphanol.

The major metabolite of butorphanol is hydroxybutorphanol, while norbutorphanol is produced in small amounts. Both have been detected in plasma following administration of butorphanol. Preliminary evidence suggests the elimination half-life of hydroxybutorphanol may be greater than that of its parent.

Elimination occurs by urine and fecal excretion. When ^3H labelled butorphanol is administered to normal subjects, most (70–80%) of the dose is recovered in the urine, while approximately 15% is recovered in the feces.

About 5% of the dose is recovered in the urine as butorphanol. Forty-nine percent is eliminated in the urine as hydroxybutorphanol. Less than 5% is excreted in the urine as norbutorphanol (see also CLINICAL PHARMACOLOGY above).

Butorphanol pharmacokinetics in the elderly differ from younger patients (see Table 1). The mean absolute bioavailability of STADOL NS in elderly women (48%) was less than that in elderly men (75%), young men (68%) or young women (70%). Elimination of half-life is increased in the elderly (6.6 hours as opposed to 4.7 hours in younger subjects).

In renally impaired patients with creatinine clearances < 30 mL/min the elimination half-life is approximately doubled and the total body clearance is approximately one half (10.5 hours [clearance 150 L/h] as compared to 5.8 hours [clearance 260 L/h] in normals). No effect was observed on Cmax or Tmax after a single dose.

For further recommendations refer to statements on use in Geriatric Patients, Renal Disease, Hepatic Disease, and statement on Drug Interactions in the PRECAUTIONS, and INDIVIDUALIZATION OF DOSAGE sections below.

CLINICAL TRIALS

The effectiveness of opioid analgesics varies in different pain syndromes. Studies with STADOL® (butorphanol tartrate) Injectable have been performed in postoperative (primarily abdominal and orthopedic) pain and pain during labor and delivery, as preoperative and preanesthetic medication, and as a supplement to balanced anesthesia (see CLINICAL TRIALS).

Studies with STADOL NS have been performed in postoperative (general, orthopedic, oral, cesarean section) pain, in post-episiotomy pain, in pain of musculoskeletal origin, and in migraine headache pain (see CLINICAL TRIALS).

USE IN THE MANAGEMENT OF PAIN

Postoperative Analgesia

The analgesic efficacy of STADOL Injectable in postoperative pain was investigated in several double-blind active-controlled studies involving 958 butorphanol-treated patients. The following doses were found to have approximately equivalent analgesic effect: 2 mg butorphanol, 10 mg morphine, 40 mg pentazocine and 80 mg meperidine.

After intravenous administration of STADOL Injectable, onset and peak analgesic effect occurred by the time of first observation (30 minutes). After intramuscular administration, pain relief onset occurred at 30 minutes or less, and peak effect occurred between 30 minutes and one hour. The duration of action of STADOL Injectable was 3–4 hours when defined as the time necessary for pain intensity to return to pretreatment level or the time to retreatment.

The analgesic efficacy of STADOL NS was evaluated (approximately 35 patients per treatment group) in a general and orthopedic surgery trial. Single doses of STADOL NS (1 or 2 mg) and IM meperidine (37.5 or 75 mg) were compared. Analgesia provided by 1 and 2 mg doses of STADOL NS was similar to 37.5 and 75 mg meperidine, respectively, with onset of analgesia within 15 minutes and peak analgesic effect within 1 hour. The median duration of pain relief was 2.5 hours with 1 mg STADOL NS, 3.5 hours with 2 mg STADOL NS and 3.3 hours with either dose of meperidine.

In a postcesarean section trial, STADOL NS administered to 35 patients as two 1 mg doses 60 minutes apart was compared with a single 2 mg dose of STADOL NS or a single 2 mg IV dose of STADOL Injectable (37 patients each). Onset of analgesia was within 15 minutes for all STADOL regimens. Peak analgesic effects of 2 mg intravenous STADOL Injectable and STADOL NS were similar in magnitude. The duration of pain relief provided by both 2 mg STADOL NS regimens was approximately 4.5 hours and was greater than intravenous STADOL Injectable (2.6 h).

Migraine Headache Pain

The analgesic efficacy of two 1 mg doses one hour apart of STADOL NS in migraine headache pain was compared with a single dose of 10 mg IM methadone (31 and 32 patients respectively). Significant onset of analgesia occurred within 15 minutes for both STADOL NS and IM methadone. Peak analgesic effect occurred at 2 hours for STADOL NS and 1.5 hours for methadone. The median duration of pain relief was 6 hours with STADOL NS and 4 hours with methadone as judged by the time when approximately half of the patients remedicated.

In two other trials in patients with migraine headache pain, a 2 mg initial dose of STADOL NS followed by an additional 1 mg dose 1 hr later (76 patients) was compared with either 75 mg IM meperidine (24 patients) or placebo (72 patients). Onset, peak activity and duration were similar with both active treatments; however, the incidence of adverse experiences (nausea, vomiting, dizziness) was higher in these two trials with the 2 mg initial dose of STADOL NS than in the trial with the 1 mg initial dose.

Table 1 — Mean Pharmacokinetic Parameters of Butorphanol in Young and Elderly Subjects[a]

	Intravenous		Nasal	
Parameters	Young	Elderly	Young	Elderly
Tmax[b] (hr)			0.62 (0.32)[e] (0.15–1.50)[g]	1.03 (0.74) (0.25–3.00)
Cmax[c] (ng/mL)			1.04 (0.40) (0.35-1.97)	0.90 (0.57) (0.10–2.68)
AUC (inf)[d] (hr.ng/mL)	7.24 (1.57) (4.40–9.77)	8.71 (2.02) (4.76–13.03)	4.93 (1.24) (2.16–7.27)	5.24 (2.27) (0.30–10.34)
Half-life (hr)	4.56 (1.67) (2.06–8.70)	5.61 (1.36) (3.25–8.79)	4.74 (1.57) (2.89–8.79)	6.56 (1.51) (3.75–9.17)
Absolute Bioavailability (%)			69 (16) (44–113)	61 (25) (3–121)
Volume of Distribution[f] (L)	487 (155) (305–901)	552 (124) (305–737)		
Total body Clearance (L/hr)	99 (23) (70–154)	82 (21) (52–143)		

a) Young subjects (n=24) are from 20 to 40 years old and elderly (n=24) are greater than 65 years of age.
b) Time to peak plasma concentration, median values.
c) Peak plasma concentration normalized to 1 mg dose.
d) Area under the plasma concentration-time curve after a 1 mg dose.
e) Mean (1 S.D.)
f) Derived from IV data.
g) (range of observed values)

Preanesthetic Medication

STADOL® (butorphanol tartrate) Injectable (2 mg and 4 mg) and meperidine (80 mg) were studied for use as preanesthetic medication in hospitalized surgical patients. Patients received a single intramuscular dose of either STADOL Injectable or meperidine approximately 90 minutes prior to anesthesia. The anesthesia regimen included barbiturate induction, followed by nitrous oxide and oxygen with halothane or enflurane, with or without a muscle relaxant.

Anesthetic preparation was rated as satisfactory in all 42 STADOL Injectable patients regardless of the type of surgery.

Balanced Anesthesia

STADOL Injectable administered intravenously (mean dose 2 mg) was compared to intravenous morphine sulfate (mean dose 10 mg) as premedication shortly before thiopental induction, followed by balanced anesthesia in 50 ASA Class 1 and 2 patients. Anesthesia was then maintained by repeated intravenous doses, averaging 4.6 mg STADOL Injectable and 22.8 mg morphine per patient.

Anesthetic induction and maintenance were generally rated as satisfactory with both STADOL Injectable (25 patients) and morphine (25 patients) regardless of the type of surgery performed. Emergence from anesthesia was comparable with both agents.

Labor (see PRECAUTIONS)

The analgesic efficacy of intravenous STADOL Injectable was studied in pain during labor. In a total of 145 patients STADOL Injectable (1 mg and 2 mg) was as effective as 40 mg and 80 mg of meperidine (144 patients) in the relief of pain in labor with no effect on the duration or progress of labor. Both drugs readily crossed the placenta and entered fetal circulation. The condition of the infants in these studies, determined by Apgar scores at 1 and 5 minutes (8 or above) and time to sustained respiration, showed no significant differences between treatment groups.

In these studies neurobehavioral testing in infants exposed to STADOL Injectable at a mean of 18.6 hours after delivery, showed no significant differences between treatment groups.

INDIVIDUALIZATION OF DOSAGE

The usual starting doses of butorphanol are: 1 mg repeated every 3–4 hours IV; 2 mg repeated every 3–4 hours IM; and 1 mg followed by 1 mg in 60–90 minutes nasally repeated every 3–4 hours (see DOSAGE AND ADMINISTRATION).

Use of butorphanol in geriatric patients, patients with renal impairment, patients with hepatic impairment, and during labor requires extra caution (see below and the appropriate sections in PRECAUTIONS).

STADOL Injectable

For pain relief the recommended initial dosage regimen of STADOL Injectable is 1 mg IV or 2 mg IM with repeated doses every three to four hours, as necessary. This dosage regimen is likely to be effective for the majority of patients. Dosage adjustments of STADOL Injectable should be based on observations of its beneficial and adverse effects. The initial dose in the elderly and in patients with renal or hepatic impairment should generally be half the recommended adult dose (0.5 mg IV and 1.0 mg IM). Repeat doses in these patients should be determined by the patient's response rather than at fixed intervals but will generally be no less than 6 hours (see PRECAUTIONS).

The usual preoperative dose is 2 mg IM given 60–90 minutes before surgery or 2 mg IV shortly before induction. This is approximately equivalent in sedative effect to 10 mg morphine or 80 mg of meperidine. The single preoperative dose should be individualized based on age, body weight, physical status, underlying pathological condition, use of other drugs, type of anesthesia to be used and the surgical procedure involved.

During maintenance in balanced anesthesia the usual incremental dose of STADOL Injectable is 0.5 to 1.0 mg IV. The incremental dose may be higher, up to 0.06 mg/kg (4 mg/70 kg), depending on previous sedative, analgesic, and hypnotic drugs administered. The total dose of STADOL Injectable will vary; however, patients seldom require less than 4 mg or more than 12.5 mg (approximately 0.06 to 0.18 mg/kg).

As with other opioids of this class, STADOL Injectable may not provide adequate intraoperative analgesia in every patient or under all conditions. A failure to achieve successful analgesia during balanced anesthesia is commonly reflected by increases in general sympathetic tone. Consequently, if blood pressure or heart rate continue to rise, consideration should be given to adding a potent volatile liquid inhalation anesthetic or another intravenous medication.

In labor, the recommended initial dose of STADOL Injectable is 1 or 2 mg IM or IV in mothers with fetuses of 37 weeks gestation or beyond and without signs of fetal distress. Dosage adjustments of STADOL Injectable in labor should be based on initial response with consideration given to concomitant analgesic or sedative drugs and the expected time of delivery. A dose should not be repeated in less than four hours nor administered less than four hours prior to the anticipated delivery (see PRECAUTIONS).

STADOL® NS™ (butorphanol tartrate) Nasal Spray

Since STADOL NS does not require an injection, it allows the physician to initiate therapy with a low dose and repeat the dose if needed.

The usual recommended dose for initial nasal administration is 1 mg (1 spray in **one** nostril). If adequate pain relief is not achieved within 60–90 minutes, an additional 1 mg dose may be given.

The initial dose sequence outlined above may be repeated in 3–4 hours as required.

For the management of severe pain, an initial dose of 2 mg (1 spray in **each** nostril) may be used in patients who will be able to remain recumbent in the event drowsiness or dizziness occur. In such patients additional doses should not be given for 3–4 hours. The incidence of adverse events is higher with an initial 2 mg dose (see CLINICAL TRIALS).

The initial dose sequence in elderly patients and patients with renal or hepatic impairment should be limited to 1 mg followed by 1 mg in 90–120 minutes. The repeat dose sequence in these patients should be determined by the patients response rather than at fixed times but will generally be no less than at 6 hour intervals (see PRECAUTIONS).

INDICATIONS

STADOL® (butorphanol tartrate) Injectable and STADOL® NS™ (butorphanol tartrate) Nasal Spray are indi-

Continued on next page

Mead Johnson Laboratories—Cont.

cated for the management of pain when the use of an opioid analgesic is appropriate.

STADOL Injectable is also indicated as a preoperative or preanesthetic medication, as a supplement to balanced anesthesia, and for the relief of pain during labor.

CONTRAINDICATIONS

STADOL Injectable and STADOL NS are contraindicated in patients hypersensitive to butorphanol tartrate or the preservative benzethonium chloride in STADOL NS or STADOL Injectable in the multi-dose vial.

WARNINGS

Patients Dependent on Narcotics

Because of its opioid antagonist properties, butorphanol is not recommended for use in patients dependent on narcotics. Such patients should have an adequate period of withdrawal from opioid drugs prior to beginning butorphanol therapy. In patients taking opioid analgesics chronically, butorphanol has precipitated withdrawal symptoms such as anxiety, agitation, mood changes, hallucinations, dysphoria, weakness and diarrhea.

Because of the difficulty in assessing opioid tolerance in patients who have recently received repeated doses of narcotic analgesic medication, caution should be used in the administration of butorphanol to such patients.

PRECAUTIONS

Head Injury and Increased Intracranial Pressure

As with other opioids, the use of butorphanol in patients with head injury may be associated with carbon dioxide retention and secondary elevation of cerebrospinal fluid pressure, drug-induced miosis, and alterations in mental state that would obscure the interpretation of the clinical course of patients with head injuries. In such patients, butorphanol should be used only if the benefits of use outweigh the potential risks.

Disorders of Respiratory Function or Control

Butorphanol may produce respiratory depression, especially in patients receiving other CNS active agents, or patients suffering from CNS diseases or respiratory impairment.

Hepatic and Renal Disease

In patients with severe hepatic or renal disease the initial dosage interval for STADOL Injectable and STADOL NS should be increased to 6–8 hours until the response has been well characterized. Subsequent doses should be determined by patient response rather than being scheduled at fixed intervals (see INDIVIDUALIZATION OF DOSAGE).

Cardiovascular Effects

Because butorphanol may increase the work of the heart, especially the pulmonary circuit (see CLINICAL PHARMACOLOGY), the use of butorphanol in patients with acute myocardial infarction, ventricular dysfunction, or coronary insufficiency should be limited to those situations where the benefits clearly outweigh the risk.

Severe hypertension has been reported rarely during butorphanol therapy. In such cases, butorphanol should be discontinued and the hypertension treated with antihypertensive drugs. In patients who are not opioid dependent, naloxone has also been reported to be effective.

Drug Interactions

Concurrent use of butorphanol with central nervous system depressants (e.g., alcohol, barbiturates, tranquilizers, and antihistamines) may result in increased central nervous system depressant effects. When used concurrently with such drugs, the dose of butorphanol should be the smallest effective dose and the frequency of dosing reduced as much as possible when administered concomitantly with drugs that potentiate the action of opioids.

It is not known if the effects of butorphanol are altered by concomitant medications that affect hepatic metabolism of drugs (cimetidine, erythromycin, theophylline, etc.), but physicians should be alert to the possibility that a smaller initial dose and longer intervals between doses may be needed.

The fraction of STADOL NS absorbed is unaffected by the concomitant administration of a nasal vasoconstrictor (oxymetazoline), but the rate of absorption is decreased. Therefore, a slower onset can be anticipated if STADOL NS is administered concomitantly with, or immediately following, a nasal vasoconstrictor.

No information is available about the use of butorphanol concurrently with MAO inhibitors.

Use in Ambulatory Patients

Drowsiness and dizziness related to the use of butorphanol may impair mental and/or physical abilities required for the performance of potentially hazardous tasks (e.g., driving, operating machinery, etc.). Patients should be told to use caution in such activities until their individual responses to butorphanol have been well characterized.

Alcohol should not be consumed while using butorphanol. Concurrent use of butorphanol with central nervous system depressants (e.g., alcohol, barbiturates, tranquilizers, and antihistamines) may result in increased central nervous system depressant effects.

Patients should be instructed on the proper use of STADOL NS (see PATIENT INSTRUCTIONS).

Carcinogenesis, Mutagenesis, Impairment of Fertility

The carcinogenic potential of butorphanol has not been adequately evaluated.

Butorphanol was not genotoxic in *S. typhimurium* or *E. coli* assays or in unscheduled DNA synthesis and repair assays conducted in cultured human fibroblast cells.

Rats treated orally with 160 mg/kg/day (944 mg/sq.m.) had a reduced pregnancy rate. However, a similar effect was not observed with a 2.5 mg/kg/day (14.75 mg/sq.m.) subcutaneous dose.

Pregnancy

Pregnancy Category C

There are no adequate and well-controlled studies of butorphanol in pregnant women before 37 weeks of gestation (see CLINICAL TRIALS).

Reproduction studies in mice, rats and rabbits during organogenesis did not reveal any teratogenic potential to butorphanol. Pregnant rats treated subcutaneously with butorphanol at 1 mg/kg (5.9 mg/sq.m.) had a higher frequency of stillbirths than controls. Butorphanol at 30 mg/kg/oral (5.1 mg/sq.m.) and 60 mg/kg/oral (10.2 mg/sq.m.) also showed higher incidences of post-implantation loss in rabbits.

Labor and Delivery

Although there have been rare reports of infant respiratory distress/apnea following the administration of STADOL® (butorphanol tartrate) Injectable during labor, this adverse effect was not attributed to STADOL Injectable as used during controlled clinical trials. The reports of respiratory distress/apnea have been associated with administration of a dose two hours or less prior to delivery, use of multiple doses, use with additional analgesic or sedative drugs, or use in preterm pregnancies. In a study of 119 patients, the administration of 1 mg of IV STADOL Injectable during labor was associated with transient (10–90 minutes) sinusoidal fetal heart rate patterns, but was not associated with adverse neonatal outcomes. In the presence of an abnormal fetal heart rate pattern, STADOL Injectable should be used with caution.

STADOL® NS™ (butorphanol tartrate) Nasal Spray is not recommended during labor or delivery because there is no clinical experience with its use in this setting.

Nursing Mothers

Butorphanol has been detected in milk following administration of STADOL Injectable to nursing mothers. The amount an infant would receive is probably clinically insignificant (estimated 4 microgram/liter of milk in a mother receiving 2 mg IM four times a day).

Although there is no clinical experience with the use of STADOL NS in nursing mothers, it should be assumed that butorphanol will appear in the milk in similar amounts following the nasal route of administration.

Pediatric Use

Butorphanol is not recommended for use in patients below 18 years of age because safety and efficacy have not been established in this population.

Geriatric Use

The initial dose of STADOL Injectable recommended for elderly patients is half the usual dose at twice the usual interval. Subsequent doses and intervals should be based on the patient response (see INDIVIDUALIZATION OF DOSAGE).

Initially a 1 mg dose of STADOL NS should generally be used in geriatric patients and 90–120 minutes should elapse before deciding whether a second 1 mg dose is needed (see INDIVIDUALIZATION OF DOSAGE).

Due to changes in clearance, the mean half-life of butorphanol is increased by 25% (to over 6 hours) in patients over the age of 65. Elderly patients may be more sensitive to its side effects. Results from a long-term clinical safety trial suggest that elderly patients may be less tolerant of dizziness due to STADOL NS than younger patients.

Information for Patients

1. Drowsiness and dizziness related to the use of butorphanol may impair mental and/or physical abilities required for the performance of potentially hazardous tasks (e.g., driving, operating machinery, etc.).

2. Alcohol should not be consumed while using butorphanol. Concurrent use of butorphanol with drugs that affect the central nervous system (e.g., alcohol, barbiturates, tranquilizers and antihistamines) may result in increased central nervous system depressant effects such as drowsiness, dizziness and impaired mental function.

3. Patients should be instructed on the proper use of STADOL NS (see PATIENT INSTRUCTIONS).

ADVERSE REACTIONS

A total of 2446 patients were studied in butorphanol clinical trials. Approximately half received STADOL Injectable with the remainder receiving STADOL NS. In nearly all cases the type and incidence of side effects with butorphanol by any route were those commonly observed with opioid analgesics.

The adverse experiences described below are based on data from short- and long-term clinical trials in patients receiving butorphanol by any route and from post-marketing experience with STADOL Injectable. There has been no attempt to correct for placebo effect or to subtract the frequencies reported by placebo treated patients in controlled trials.

REACTIONS

The most frequently reported adverse experiences across all clinical trials with STADOL Injectable and STADOL NS were somnolence (43%), dizziness (19%), nausea and/or vomiting (13%). In long-term trials with STADOL NS only, nasal congestion (13%) and insomnia (11%) were frequently reported.

The following adverse experiences were reported at a frequency of 1% or greater, and were considered to be probably related to the use of butorphanol:

BODY AS A WHOLE: asthenia/lethargy*, headache*, sensation of heat
CARDIOVASCULAR: VASODILATION*, PALPITATIONS
DIGESTIVE: ANOREXIA*, CONSTIPATION*, dry mouth*, nausea and/or vomiting (13%), stomach pain
NERVOUS: anxiety, confusion*, dizziness (19%), euphoria, floating feeling, INSOMNIA (11%), nervousness, paresthesia, somnolence (43%), TREMOR
RESPIRATORY: BRONCHITIS, COUGH, DYSPNEA*, EPISTAXIS*, NASAL CONGESTION (13%), NASAL IRRITATION*, PHARYNGITIS*, RHINITIS*, SINUS CONGESTION*, SINUSITIS, UPPER RESPIRATORY INFECTION*
SKIN AND APPENDAGES: sweating/clammy*, pruritus
SPECIAL SENSES: blurred vision, EAR PAIN, TINNITUS*, UNPLEASANT TASTE* (also seen in short-term trials with STADOL® NS™ [butorphanol tartrate] Nasal Spray).

(Reactions occurring with a frequency of 3–9% are marked with an asterisk.* Reactions reported predominantly from long-term trials with STADOL NS are CAPITALIZED.)

The following adverse experiences were reported with a frequency of less than 1%, in clinical trials or from post-marketing experience, and were considered to be probably related to the use of butorphanol.

CARDIOVASCULAR: hypotension
NERVOUS: abnormal dreams, agitation, *drug dependence*, dysphoria, hallucinations, hostility
SKIN AND APPENDAGES: rash/hives
UROGENITAL: impaired urination

(Reactions reported only from post-marketing experience are *italicized.*)

The following infrequent additional adverse experiences were reported in a frequency of less than 1% of the patients studied in short-term STADOL NS trials and from post-marketing experiences under circumstances where the association between these events and butorphanol administration is unknown. They are being listed as alerting information for the physician.

BODY AS A WHOLE: edema
CARDIOVASCULAR: hypertension
NERVOUS: *convulsion, delusions,* depression
RESPIRATORY: *apnea,* shallow breathing

(Reactions reported only from post-marketing experience are *italicized.*)

DRUG ABUSE AND DEPENDENCE

Although the mixed agonist-antagonist opioid analgesics, as a class, have lower abuse potential than morphine, all such drugs can be and have been reported to be abused.

Chronic use of STADOL® (butorphanol tartrate) Injectable has been reported to result in mild withdrawal syndromes, and reports of overuse and self-reported addiction have been received.

Among 161 patients who used STADOL NS for 2 months or longer approximately 3% had behavioral symptoms suggestive of possible abuse. Approximately 1% of these patients reported significant overuse. Symptoms such as anxiety, agitation, and diarrhea were observed. Symptoms suggestive of opioid withdrawal occurred in 2 patients who stopped the drug abruptly after using 16 mg a day or more for longer than 3 months.

Special care should be exercised in administering butorphanol to emotionally unstable patients and to those with a history of drug misuse. When long-term therapy is necessary, such patients should be closely supervised.

OVERDOSAGE

Clinical Manifestations

The clinical manifestations of overdose are those of opioid drugs, the most serious of which are hypoventilation, cardiovascular insufficiency and/or coma.

Overdose can occur due to accidental or intentional misuse of butorphanol, especially in young children who may gain access to the drug in the home.

Treatment

The management of suspected butorphanol overdosage includes maintenance of adequate ventilation, peripheral perfusion, normal body temperature, and protection of the airway. Patients should be under continuous observation with adequate serial measures of mental state, responsiveness

and vital signs. Oxygen and ventilatory assistance should be available with continual monitoring by pulse oximetry if indicated. In the presence of coma, placement of an artificial airway may be required. An adequate intravenous portal should be maintained to facilitate treatment of hypotension associated with vasodilation.

The use of a specific opioid antagonist such as naloxone should be considered. As the duration of butorphanol action usually exceeds the duration of action of naloxone, repeated dosing with naloxone may be required.

DOSAGE AND ADMINISTRATION

Factors to be considered in determining the dosage are age, body weight, physical status, underlying pathological condition, use of other drugs, type of anesthesia to be used, and surgical procedure involved. Use in the elderly, patients with hepatic or renal disease or in labor requires extra caution (see PRECAUTIONS and INDIVIDUALIZATION OF DOSAGE). The following doses are for patients who do not have impaired hepatic or renal function and who are not on CNS active agents.

Use for Pain

Intravenous: The usual recommended single dose for IV administration is 1 mg repeated every three to four hours as necessary. The effective dosage range, depending on the severity of pain, is 0.5 to 2 mg repeated every three to four hours.

Intramuscular: The usual recommended single dose for IM administration is 2 mg in patients who will be able to remain recumbent, in the event drowsiness or dizziness occurs. This may be repeated every three to four hours, as necessary. The effective dosage range depending on the severity of pain is 1 to 4 mg repeated every three to four hours. There are insufficient clinical data to recommend single doses above 4 mg.

Nasal Spray: The usual recommended dose for initial nasal administration is 1 mg (1 spray in **one** nostril). Adherence to this dose reduces the incidence of drowsiness and dizziness. If adequate pain relief is not achieved within 60–90 minutes, an additional 1 mg dose may be given.

The initial two dose sequence outlined above may be repeated in 3–4 hours as needed.

Depending on the severity of the pain, an initial dose of 2 mg (1 spray in **each** nostril) may be used in patients who will be able to remain recumbent in the event drowsiness or dizziness occur. In such patients single additional 2 mg doses should not be given for 3–4 hours.

Use as Preoperative/Preanesthetic Medication

The preoperative medication dosage of STADOL® (butorphanol tartrate) Injectable should be individualized (see INDIVIDUALIZATION OF DOSAGE). The usual adult dose is 2 mg IM, administered 60–90 minutes before surgery. This is approximately equivalent in sedative effect to 10 mg morphine or 80 mg meperidine.

Use in Balanced Anesthesia

The usual dose of STADOL Injectable is 2 mg IV shortly before induction and/or 0.5 to 1.0 mg IV in increments during anesthesia. The increment may be higher, up to 0.06 mg/kg (4 mg/70 kg), depending on previous sedative, analgesic, and hypnotic drugs administered. The total dose of STADOL Injectable will vary; however, patients seldom require less than 4 mg or more than 12.5 mg (approximately 0.06 to 0.18 mg/kg).

The use of STADOL® NS™ (butorphanol tartrate) Nasal Spray is not recommended, because it has not been studied in induction or maintenance of anesthesia.

Labor

In patients at full term in early labor a 1–2 mg dose of Stadol Injectable IV or IM may be administered and repeated after 4 hours. Alternative analgesia should be used for pain associated with delivery or if delivery is expected to occur within 4 hours.

If concomitant use of STADOL with drugs that may potentiate its effects is deemed necessary (see Drug Interactions in PRECAUTIONS SECTION) the lowest effective dose should be employed.

The use of STADOL NS is not recommended as it has not been studied in labor.

Safety and Handling

STADOL Injectable is supplied in sealed delivery systems that have a low risk of accidental exposure to health care workers. Ordinary care should be taken to avoid aerosol generation while preparing a syringe for use. Following skin contact, rinsing with cool water is recommended.

STADOL NS is an open delivery system with increased risk of exposure to health care workers.

In the priming process, a certain amount of butorphanol may be aerosolized; therefore, the pump sprayer should be aimed away from the patient or other people or animals.

The unit should be disposed of by unscrewing the cap, rinsing the bottle, and placing the parts in a waste container.

HOW SUPPLIED

STADOL Injectable for IM or IV use is available as follows:
NDC 0015-5644-20—2 mg per mL, 2-mL vial
NDC 0015-5645-20—1 mg per mL, 1-mL vial
NDC 0015-5646-20—2 mg per mL, 1-mL vial
NDC 0015-5648-20—2 mg per mL, 10-mL multi-dose vial

STADOL NS is supplied in a child-resistant prescription vial containing a metered-dose spray pump with protective clip and dust cover, a bottle of nasal spray solution, and a patient instruction leaflet. On average, one bottle will deliver 14–15 doses if no repriming is necessary.

NDC 0087-5650-41—10 mg per mL, 2.5-mL bottle.

PHARMACIST ASSEMBLY INSTRUCTIONS FOR STADOL NS NASAL SPRAY

The pharmacist will assemble STADOL NS prior to dispensing to the patient, according to the following instructions:

1. Open the child-resistant prescription vial and remove the spray pump and solution bottle.
2. Assemble STADOL NS by first unscrewing the white cap from the solution bottle and screwing the pump unit tightly onto the bottle. Make sure the clear cover is on the pump unit.
3. Return the STADOL NS bottle to the child-resistant prescription vial for dispensing to the patient.

Storage Conditions

Store below 86°F (30°C). Parenteral drug products should be inspected visually for particulate matter and discoloration prior to administration, whenever solution and container permit.

CAUTION: FEDERAL LAW PROHIBITS DISPENSING WITHOUT PRESCRIPTION

Mead Johnson LABORATORIES
APOTHECON®
A Bristol-Myers Squibb Company
Princeton, New Jersey 08540 USA

Shown in Product Identification Section, page 419

VAGISTAT®-1 ℞

vaginal ointment
(tioconazole 6.5%)

DESCRIPTION

Tioconazole, 1-[2-{(2-chloro-3-thienyl)methoxy}-2(2,4-dichlorophenyl)ethyl]-1H-imidazole, is a topical antifungal agent. Its chemical formula is $C_{16}H_{13}Cl_3N_2OS$ with a molecular weight of 387.7. The structural formula is given below:

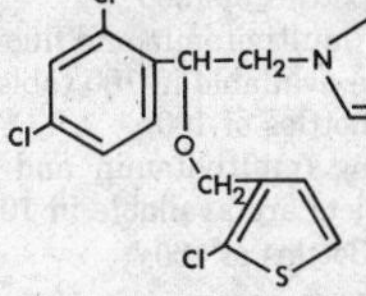

VAGISTAT-1 (tioconazole 6.5%) is formulated in a base of white, soft paraffin and aluminum magnesium silicate with butylated hydroxyanisole (BHA) added as a preservative. Each applicator-full of VAGISTAT-1 provides approximately 4.6 grams of ointment containing 300 mg of tioconazole.

CLINICAL PHARMACOLOGY

Tioconazole is a broad-spectrum antifungal agent that inhibits the growth of human pathogenic yeasts. Tioconazole exhibits fungicidal activity *in vitro* against *Candida albicans*, other species of the genus *Candida*, and against *Torulopsis glabrata*.

Pharmacokinetics: Systemic absorption of tioconazole after a single intravaginal application of VAGISTAT-1 in nonpregnant patients is negligible.

INDICATIONS AND USAGE

VAGISTAT-1 is indicated for the local treatment of vulvovaginal candidiasis (moniliasis). As VAGISTAT-1 has been shown to be effective only for candidal vulvovaginitis, the diagnosis should be confirmed by KOH smears and/or cultures. Other pathogens commonly associated with vulvovaginitis should be ruled out by appropriate methods.

Studies have shown that women taking oral contraceptives have a cure rate similar to those not taking such agents when treated with VAGISTAT-1.

Safety and effectiveness in pregnant and diabetic patients have not been established (see Precautions).

CONTRAINDICATIONS

VAGISTAT-1 is contraindicated in individuals who have been shown to be sensitive to imidazole antifungal agents or to other components of the ointment.

PRECAUTIONS

General: VAGISTAT-1 is intended for intravaginal administration only. Applicators should be opened just prior to administration to prevent contamination. Administration of VAGISTAT-1 just prior to bedtime may be preferred. The VAGISTAT-1 ointment base may interact with rubber or latex products such as condoms or vaginal contraceptive diaphragms; therefore, use of such products within 72 hours following treatment is not recommended.

If clinical symptoms persist, appropriate microbiological tests should be repeated to rule out other pathogens and to confirm the diagnosis.

Information for Patients: The VAGISTAT-1 ointment base may interact with rubber or latex products such as condoms or vaginal contraceptive diaphragms; therefore, use of such products within 72 hours following treatment is not recommended.

Carcinogenesis: No long-term studies in animals have been performed to evaluate the carcinogenic potential of tioconazole.

Mutagenesis: Tioconazole did not demonstrate mutagenic activity at the levels examined in tests at either the chromosomal or subchromosomal level.

Impairment of Fertility: No impairment of fertility was seen in male rats administered tioconazole hydrochloride in oral doses up to 150 mg/kg/day. However, there was evidence of preimplantation loss in female rats at oral dose levels above 35 mg/kg/day.

Pregnancy—Pregnancy Category C: Tioconazole hydrochloride had no adverse effects on fetal viability or growth when administered orally to pregnant rats at doses of 55, 110, and 165 mg/kg/day during the period of organogenesis. A drug-related increase in the incidence of dilated ureters, hydroureters, and hydronephrosis observed in the fetuses of this study was transient and no longer evident in pups raised to 21 days of age. These effects did not occur following intravaginal administration of approximately 10 mg/kg/day in a 2% cream. There was no evidence of major structural anomalies. No embryotoxic or teratogenic effects were observed in rabbits receiving oral dose levels as high as 165 mg/kg/day or daily intravaginal application of approximately 2–3 mg/kg in a 2% tioconazole cream during organogenesis. Tioconazole hydrochloride, like other azole antimycotic agents, causes dystocia in rats when treatment is extended through parturition. Associated effects in rats include prolongation of pregnancy, *in utero* deaths, and impaired pup survival. The "no-effect" level for this phenomenon is 20 mg/kg/day orally and approximately 9 mg/kg/day intravaginally. No effect on parturition occurred in rabbits at 50 mg/kg/day orally.

There are no adequate and well-controlled studies in pregnant women. VAGISTAT-1 (tioconazole 6.5%) should be used during pregnancy only if the potential benefit justifies the potential risk to the fetus.

Nursing Mothers: It is not known whether this drug is excreted in human milk. Because many drugs are excreted in human milk, nursing should be temporarily discontinued while VAGISTAT-1 is administered.

Pediatric Use: Safety and effectiveness in children have not been established.

ADVERSE REACTIONS

The incidence of adverse reactions to VAGISTAT-1 is based on clinical trials involving 1000 patients. Burning and itching were the most frequent side effects occurring in approximately 6% and 5% of the patients, respectively. In most instances these did not interfere with the course of therapy.

There were occasional reports (less than 1%) of other side effects including irritation, discharge, vulvar edema and swelling, vaginal pain, dysuria, nocturia, dyspareunia, dryness of vaginal secretions, desquamation, and burning sensation.

DOSAGE AND ADMINISTRATION

VAGISTAT-1 has been found to be effective as a single-dose treatment for vulvovaginal candidiasis. Using the prefilled applicator, insert one applicator-full intravaginally. Administration of VAGISTAT-1 just prior to bedtime may be preferred.

HOW SUPPLIED

VAGISTAT-1 is supplied in a ready-to-use, prefilled, single-dose vaginal applicator. Each applicator-full will deliver approximately 4.6 grams of VAGISTAT-1 containing 65 mg of tioconazole per gram of ointment. Store at controlled room temperature (59°–86° F).

NDC 0087-0657-40

Manufactured in Canada for Bristol-Myers Squibb Company
Princeton, NJ 08543 by Pfizer Canada, Inc.
Arnprior, Ontario, Canada

Products are
listed alphabetically
in the
PINK SECTION.

Mead Johnson Nutritionals
A Bristol-Myers Squibb Company
2400 W. LLOYD EXPRESSWAY
EVANSVILLE, INDIANA 47721-0001

POLY-VI-FLOR®   ℞
[*pahl-ē-vī'flŏr "*]
- 1.0 mg
- 0.5 mg
- 0.25 mg

Multivitamin and fluoride supplement chewable tablets

DESCRIPTION
[See table at right.]
Active ingredient for caries prophylaxis: Fluoride as sodium fluoride.
Other ingredients: Ascorbic acid, cholecalciferol, colloidal silicon dioxide, cyanocobalamin, dextrates, FD&C Blue No. 2 (aluminum lake), FD&C Red No. 40 (aluminum lake), FD&C Yellow No. 6 (aluminum lake), folic acid, fruit flavors (artificial), lactose, magnesium stearate, niacinamide, pyridoxine hydrochloride, riboflavin, silica gel, sodium ascorbate, sodium chloride, sucrose, thiamine mononitrate, dl-alpha-tocopheryl acetate, vitamin A acetate. The 1.0 mg tablet does not contain lactose.

CLINICAL PHARMACOLOGY
It is well established that fluoridation of the water supply (1 ppm fluoride) during the period of tooth development leads to a significant decrease in the incidence of dental caries. Poly-Vi-Flor chewable tablets provide sodium fluoride, and ten essential vitamins in a chewable tablet. Because the tablets are chewable, they provide a *topical* as well as *systemic* source of fluoride.[1,2]
Hydroxyapatite is the principal crystal for all calcified tissue in the human body. The fluoride ion reacts with the *hydroxyapatite* in the tooth as it is formed to produce the more caries-resistant crystal, *fluorapatite*. The reaction may be expressed by the equation:[3]

$$Ca_{10}(PO_4)_6(OH)_2 + 2F^- \longrightarrow Ca_{10}(PO_4)_6F_2 + 2OH^-$$
(Hydroxyapatite)   (Fluorapatite)

Three stages of fluoride deposition in tooth enamel can be distinguished:[3]
1. Small amounts (reflecting the low levels of fluoride in tissue fluids) are incorporated into the enamel crystals while they are being formed.
2. After enamel has been laid down, fluoride deposition continues in the surface enamel. Diffusion of fluoride from the surface inward is apparently restricted.
3. After eruption, the surface enamel acquires fluoride from water, food, supplementary fluoride and smaller amounts from saliva.

INDICATIONS AND USAGE
Supplementation of the diet with ten essential vitamins. Supplementation of the diet with the fluoride for caries prophylaxis.
Poly-Vi-Flor 1.0 mg chewable tablets provide fluoride in tablet form for children 3 years and above in areas where the water fluoride level is less than 0.3 ppm.[4]
Poly-Vi-Flor 0.5 mg chewable tablets provide fluoride in tablet form for children 2-3 years of age where the drinking water has a fluoride content of less than 0.3 ppm, and for children 3 years of age and above where the drinking water contains 0.3 through 0.7 ppm of fluoride.[4]
Poly-Vi-Flor 0.25 mg chewable tablets provide fluoride in tablet form for children 2–3 years of age where the drinking water contains 0.3 through 0.7 ppm of fluoride.[4]
Poly-Vi-Flor chewable tablets supply significant amounts of vitamins A, D, E, C, thiamine, riboflavin, niacin, pyridoxine, cyanocobalamin and folic acid to supplement the diet, and to help assure that nutritional deficiencies of these vitamins will not develop. Thus, in a single easy-to-use preparation, children obtain ten essential vitamins and the important mineral, fluoride.
The American Academy of Pediatrics recommends that children up to age 16, in areas where drinking water contains less than optimal levels of fluoride, receive daily fluoride supplementation.
Children using Poly-Vi-Flor chewable tablets regularly should receive semiannual dental examinations. The regular brushing of teeth and attention to good oral hygiene practices are also essential.

WARNINGS
As in the case of all medications, keep out of the reach of children.

PRECAUTIONS
The suggested dose *should not be exceeded,* since dental fluorosis may result from continued ingestion of large amounts of fluoride.

	Poly-Vi-Flor chewable tablets			Percentage of U.S. Recommended Daily Allowance	
Each tablet supplies:	1.0 mg	0.5 mg	0.25 mg	Children Age 2–3 Years	Adults & Children Age 4 Years or More
Vitamin A, IU	2500	2500	2500	100	50
Vitamin D, IU	400	400	400	100	100
Vitamin E, IU	15	15	15	150	50
Vitamin C, mg	60	60	60	150	100
Folic acid, mg	0.3	0.3	0.3	150	75
Thiamine, mg	1.05	1.05	1.05	150	70
Riboflavin, mg	1.2	1.2	1.2	150	70
Niacin, mg	13.5	13.5	13.5	150	68
Vitamin B$_6$, mg	1.05	1.05	1.05	150	53
Vitamin B$_{12}$, μg	4.5	4.5	4.5	150	75
Fluoride, mg	1	0.5	0.25	*	*

* U.S. Recommended Daily Allowance has not been established.

Before prescribing Vi-Flor® products:
1. determine the fluoride content of the drinking water.
2. make sure the child is not receiving significant amounts of fluoride from other medications.
3. periodically check to make sure that the child does not develop significant dental fluorosis.

The Council on Dental Therapeutics of the American Dental Association recommends that no more than 264 mg of sodium fluoride should be dispensed at one time.[5] Therefore, no more than 120 Poly-Vi-Flor 1.0 mg chewable tablets (2.2 mg sodium fluoride per tablet) should be dispensed at one time.

ADVERSE REACTIONS
Allergic rash and other idiosyncrasies have been rarely reported.

DOSAGE AND ADMINISTRATION
One tablet daily or as prescribed.

HOW SUPPLIED
Poly-Vi-Flor 1.0 mg (multivitamin and fluoride supplement) chewable tablets are available in 100- and 1000-tablet bottles.
NDC 0087-0474-02 Bottles of 100
NDC 0087-0474-03 Bottles of 1000
Poly-Vi-Flor 0.5 mg (multivitamin and fluoride supplement) chewable tablets are available in 100 tablet bottles.
NDC 0087-0468-41 Bottles of 100
Poly-Vi-Flor 0.25 mg (multivitamin and fluoride supplement) chewable tablets are available in 100-tablet bottles.
NDC 0087-0487-41 Bottles of 100

LITERATURE AVAILABLE
Yes.

REFERENCES
1. Hennon DK, Stookey GK, Muhler JC. The clinical anti-cariogenic effectiveness of supplementary fluoride-vitamin preparations—Results at the end of three years. *J Dentistry for Children.* January 1966;33:3–12.
2. Hennon DK, Stookey GK, Muhler JC. The clinical anti-cariogenic effectiveness of supplementary fluoride-vitamin preparations—Results at the end of four years. *J Dentistry for Children.* November 1967;34:439–443.
3. Brudevold F, McCann HG. Fluoride and caries control—Mechanism of action. In: Nizel AE, ed. *The Science of Nutrition and Its Application in Clinical Dentistry.* Philadelphia: WB Saunders Co; 1966:331–347.
4. American Academy of Pediatrics Committee on Nutrition: Fluoride supplementation. *Pediatrics.*1986;77:758.
5. Council on Dental Therapeutics, Am Dental Assoc. *Accepted Dental Therapeutics.* 1977, 37th ed, p 294.

POLY-VI-FLOR®   ℞
[*pahl-ē-vī'flŏr "*]
- 0.5 mg
- 0.25 mg

Multivitamin and fluoride supplement drops

DESCRIPTION
[See table below.]
See INDICATIONS AND USAGE section below for use by infants and children under two years of age.
Active ingredient for caries prophylaxis: Fluoride as sodium fluoride.
Other ingredients: Ascorbic acid, caramel color, cholecalciferol, cyanocobalamin, ferrous sulfate, fruit flavor (artificial), glycerin, niacinamide, polysorbate 80, pyridoxine hydrochloride, riboflavin-5-phosphate sodium, thiamine hydrochloride, d-alpha-tocopheryl acid succinate, vitamin A palmitate, water, and other ingredients.

CLINICAL PHARMACOLOGY
For information on fluoridation see Poly-Vi-Flor chewable tablets.

INDICATIONS AND USAGE
Supplementation of the diet with nine essential vitamins. Supplementation of the diet with fluoride for caries prophylaxis.
The American Academy of Pediatrics recommends that children up to age 16, in areas where drinking water contains less than optimal levels of fluoride, receive daily fluoride supplementation.
Poly-Vi-Flor 0.5 mg (multivitamin and fluoride supplement) drops provide fluoride in drop form for children ages 2–3 years in areas where the drinking water contains less than 0.3 ppm fluoride; and for children 3 years and above in areas where the drinking water contains 0.3 through 0.7 ppm of fluoride.
Poly-Vi-Flor 0.25 mg (multivitamin and fluoride supplement) drops provide fluoride in drop form for infants and young children from birth to 2 years of age in areas where the drinking water contains less than 0.3 ppm of fluoride and for children ages 2–3 years in areas where the drinking water contains 0.3 through 0.7 ppm of fluoride.
The American Academy of Pediatrics[1] and the American Dental Association[2] currently recommend that infants and children under 2 years of age, in areas where drinking water contains less than 0.3 ppm of fluoride, and children 2-3, in areas where the drinking water contains 0.3 through 0.7 ppm of fluoride, receive 0.25 mg of supplemental fluoride daily which is provided in a full dose (1 mL) of Poly-Vi-Flor® 0.25 mg drops. A half dose (0.5 mL) of Poly-Vi-Flor 0.5 mg drops could also provide a daily fluoride intake of 0.25 mg;

	Poly-Vi-Flor drops		Percentage of U.S. Recommended Daily Allowance	
Each 1.0 mL supplies:	0.5 mg	0.25 mg	Infants	Children Under Age 4 Years
Vitamin A, IU	1500	1500	100	60
Vitamin D, IU	400	400	100	100
Vitamin E, IU	5	5	100	50
Vitamin C, mg	35	35	100	88
Thiamine, mg	0.5	0.5	100	71
Riboflavin, mg	0.6	0.6	100	75
Niacin, mg	8	8	100	89
Vitamin B$_6$, mg	0.4	0.4	100	57
Vitamin B$_{12}$, μg	2	2	100	67
Fluoride, mg	0.5	0.25	*	*

* U.S. Recommended Daily Allowance has not been established.

however, this dosage reduces vitamin supplementation by half.

Poly-Vi-Flor 0.5 mg drops and 0.25 mg drops supply significant amounts of vitamins A, D, E, C, thiamine, riboflavin, niacin, pyridoxine, and cyanocobalamin to supplement the diet, and to help assure that nutritional deficiencies of these vitamins will not develop. Thus in a single easy-to-use preparation, infants and children obtain nine essential vitamins and fluoride.

A comprehensive 5½ year series of studies of the effectiveness of Tri-Vi-Flor® and Poly-Vi-Flor® products in caries protection has been published.[3-6] Children in this continuing study lived in an area where the water supply contained only 0.05 ppm fluoride. The subjects were divided into two groups, one which used only nonfluoridated Vi-Sol® vitamin products and the other Tri-Vi-Flor and Poly-Vi-Flor vitamin-fluoride products.

The three-year interim report showed 63% fewer carious surfaces in primary teeth and 43% fewer carious surfaces in permanent teeth of the children taking Vi-Flor® vitamin-fluoride products.[3]

After four years the studies continued to support the effectiveness of Tri-Vi-Flor and Poly-Vi-Flor, showing a reduction in carious surfaces of 68% in primary teeth and 46% in permanent teeth.[4]

Results at the end of 5½ years further confirmed the previous findings and indicated that significant reductions in dental caries are apparent with the continued use of Vi-Flor vitamin-fluoride products.[5]

WARNINGS
As in the case of all medications, keep out of the reach of children.

PRECAUTIONS
The suggested dose *should not be exceeded* since dental fluorosis may result from continued ingestion of large amounts of fluoride.

When prescribing Vi-Flor products:
1. determine the fluoride content of the drinking water.
2. make sure the child is not receiving significant amounts of fluoride from other medications.
3. periodically check to make sure that the child does not develop significant dental fluorosis.

Poly-Vi-Flor 0.5 mg drops and 0.25 mg drops should be dispensed in the original plastic container, since contact with glass leads to instability and precipitation. (The amount of sodium fluoride in all Poly-Vi-Flor drops is well below the maximum to be dispensed at one time according to recommendations of the American Dental Association.)

ADVERSE REACTIONS
Allergic rash and other idiosyncrasies have been rarely reported.

DOSAGE AND ADMINISTRATION
1.0 mL daily or as prescribed.
Drops may be dropped directly into mouth with 'Safti-Dropper,' or mixed with cereal, fruit juice or other food.

HOW SUPPLIED
Poly-Vi-Flor 0.5 mg (multivitamin and fluoride supplement) drops are available in bottles of 50 mL.
NDC 0087-0472-02 Bottles of 1⅔ fl oz (50 mL)
FSN 6505-080-0967 (50 mL)
Poly-Vi-Flor 0.25 mg (multivitamin and fluoride supplement) drops are available in bottles of 50 mL.
NDC 0087-0451-41 Bottles of 50 mL.

LITERATURE AVAILABLE
Yes.

REFERENCES
1. American Academy of Pediatrics Committee on Nutrition: Fluoride supplementation. *Pediatrics.* 1986;77:758.
2. American Dental Association. *Accepted Dental Therapeutics.* 38th ed. Chicago: 1979:p 321.
3. Hennon DK, Stookey GK, Muhler JC. The clinical anticariogenic effectiveness of supplementary fluoride-vitamin preparations—Results at the end of three years. *J Dentistry for Children.* January 1966;33:3–12.
4. Hennon DK, Stookey GK, Muhler JC. The clinical anticariogenic effectiveness of supplementary fluoride-vitamin preparations—Results at the end of four years. *J Dentistry for Children.* November 1967;34:439–443.
5. Hennon DK, Stookey GK, Muhler JC. The clinical anticariogenic effectiveness of supplementary fluoride-vitamin preparations—Results at the end of five and a half years. *Phar and Ther In Dent.* 1970;1:1.
6. Hennon DK, Stookey GK, Beiswanger BB. Fluoride-vitamin supplements: Effects on dental caries and fluorosis when used in areas with suboptimum fluoride in the water supply. *J Am Dent Assoc.* 1977;95:965.

	Poly-Vi-Flor w/Iron chewable tablets			Percentage of U.S. Recommended Daily Allowance	
Each tablet supplies:	1.0 mg	0.5 mg	0.25 mg	Children Age 2–3 Years	Adults & Children Age 4 Years or More
Vitamin A, IU	2500	2500	2500	100	50
Vitamin D, IU	400	400	400	100	100
Vitamin E, IU	15	15	15	150	50
Vitamin C, mg	60	60	60	150	100
Folic acid, mg	0.3	0.3	0.3	150	75
Thiamine, mg	1.05	1.05	1.05	150	70
Riboflavin, mg	1.2	1.2	1.2	150	70
Niacin, mg	13.5	13.5	13.5	150	68
Vitamin B$_6$, mg	1.05	1.05	1.05	150	53
Vitamin B$_{12}$, µg	4.5	4.5	4.5	150	75
Iron, mg	12	12	12	120	67
Copper, mg	1	1	1	100	50
Zinc, mg	10	10	10	125	67
Fluoride, mg	1	0.5	0.25	*	*

*U.S. Recommended Daily Allowance has not been established.

POLY–VI–FLOR® with Iron   ℞
[pahl-ē-vī'flōr"]
- 1.0 mg
- 0.5 mg
- 0.25 mg
Multivitamin, mineral and fluoride supplement chewable tablets

DESCRIPTION
[See table above.]
Active ingredient for caries prophylaxis: Fluoride as sodium fluoride.
Other ingredients: Ascorbic acid, cholecalciferol, colloidal silicon dioxide, cupric oxide, cyanocobalamin, dextrates, FD&C Red No. 40 (aluminum lake), ferrous fumarate, folic acid, fruit flavors (artificial), lactose, magnesium stearate, niacinamide, pyridoxine hydrochloride, riboflavin, silica gel, sodium ascorbate, sodium chloride, stearic acid, sucrose, thiamine mononitrate, dl-alpha-tocopheryl acetate, vitamin A acetate, zinc oxide. The 1.0 mg tablet does not contain lactose.

CLINICAL PHARMACOLOGY
For information on fluoridation see Poly-Vi-Flor chewable tablets.
Poly-Vi-Flor with Iron chewable tablets provide sodium fluoride, iron, copper, zinc and ten essential vitamins in a chewable tablet. Because the tablets are chewable, they provide a *topical* as well as *systemic* source of fluoride.[1,2]

INDICATIONS AND USAGE
Supplementation of the diet with ten essential vitamins, iron, copper and zinc.
Supplementation of the diet with fluoride, for caries prophylaxis.
The American Academy of Pediatrics recommends that children up to age 16, in areas where drinking water contains less than optimal levels of fluoride, receive daily fluoride supplementation.
Poly-Vi-Flor 1.0 mg with Iron chewable tablets were developed to provide fluoride in tablet form for children 3 years and above in areas where the water fluoride level is less than 0.3 ppm.[3]
Poly-Vi-Flor 0.5 mg with Iron chewable tablets provides fluoride for children 2–3 years of age where the drinking water has fluoride content of less than 0.3 ppm, and for children 3 years of age and above where the drinking water contains 0.3 through 0.7 ppm of fluoride.[3]
Poly-Vi-Flor 0.25 mg with Iron chewable tablets provide fluoride in tablet form for children 2–3 years of age where the drinking water contains 0.3 through 0.7 ppm of fluoride.[3]
Poly-Vi-Flor with Iron chewable tablets supply significant amounts of vitamins A, D, E, C, thiamine, riboflavin, niacin, pyridoxine, cyanocobalamin, and folic acid, and the minerals iron, copper and zinc to supplement the diet, and to help assure that deficiencies of these nutrients will not develop. Thus, in a single easy-to-use preparation, children obtain ten essential vitamins, iron, copper, zinc and fluoride.
Children using Poly-Vi-Flor with Iron chewable tablets regularly should receive semiannual dental examinations. The regular brushing of teeth and attention to good oral hygiene practices are also essential.

WARNINGS
As in the case of all medications, keep out of the reach of children.

PRECAUTIONS
The suggested dose of Poly-Vi-Flor with Iron chewable tablets *should not be exceeded*, since dental fluorosis may result from continued ingestion of large amounts of fluoride.
Before prescribing Vi-Flor® products:
1. determine the fluoride content of the drinking water.
2. make sure the child is not receiving significant amounts of fluoride from other medications.
3. periodically check to make sure that the child does not develop significant dental fluorosis.

ADVERSE REACTIONS
Allergic rash and other idiosyncrasies have been rarely reported.

DOSAGE AND ADMINISTRATION
One tablet daily or as prescribed.

HOW SUPPLIED
Poly-Vi-Flor 1.0 mg with Iron (multivitamin, mineral and fluoride supplement) chewable tablets are available in 100- and 1000-tablet bottles.
NDC 0087-0476-03 Bottles of 100
NDC 0087-0476-04 Bottles of 1000
Poly-Vi-Flor 0.5 mg with Iron (multivitamin, mineral and fluoride supplement) chewable tablets are available only in 100-tablet bottles.
NDC 0087-0482-41 Bottles of 100
Poly-Vi-Flor 0.25 mg with Iron (multivitamin, mineral and fluoride supplement) chewable tablets are available in 100-tablet bottles.
NDC 0087-0488-41 Bottles of 100

LITERATURE AVAILABLE
Yes.

REFERENCES
1. Hennon DK, Stookey GK, Muhler JC. The clinical anticariogenic effectiveness of supplementary fluoride-vitamin preparations— Results at the end of three years. *J Dentistry for Children.* January 1966;33:3–12.
2. Hennon DK, Stookey GK, Muhler JC. The clinical anticariogenic effectiveness of supplementary fluoride-vitamin preparations— Results at the end of four years. *J Dentistry for Children.* November 1967;34:439–443.
3. American Academy of Pediatrics Committee on Nutrition: Fluoride supplementation. *Pediatrics.* 1986;77:758.

POLY–VI–FLOR® with Iron   ℞
[pahl-ē-vī'flōr"]
- 0.5 mg
- 0.25 mg
Multivitamin, iron and fluoride supplement drops

DESCRIPTION
[See table at top of next page.]
See INDICATIONS AND USAGE section below for use by infants and children under two years of age.
Active ingredient for caries prophylaxis: Fluoride as sodium fluoride.
Other ingredients: Ascorbic acid, caramel color, cholecalciferol, ferrous sulfate, fruit flavor (artificial), glycerin, niacinamide, polysorbate 80, pyridoxine hydrochloride, riboflavin 5-phosphate sodium, thiamine hydrochloride, d-alpha-to-

Continued on next page

Mead Johnson Nutritionals—Cont.

copheryl acid succinate, vitamin A palmitate, water, and other ingredients.

CLINICAL PHARMACOLOGY

For information on fluoridation see Poly-Vi-Flor chewable tablets.

INDICATIONS AND USAGE

Supplementation of the diet with eight essential vitamins and iron.

Supplementation of the diet with fluoride for caries prophylaxis.

The American Academy of Pediatrics recommends that children up to age 16, in areas where drinking water contains less than optimal levels of fluoride, receive daily fluoride supplementation.

Poly-Vi-Flor 0.5 mg with Iron (multivitamin, iron, and fluoride supplement) drops provide fluoride in drop form for children ages 2–3 years in areas where the drinking water contains less than 0.3 ppm fluoride; and for children 3 years and above in areas where the drinking water contains 0.3 through 0.7 ppm of fluoride.

Poly-Vi-Flor 0.25 mg with Iron drops provide fluoride in drop form for infants and young children from birth to 2 years of age in areas where the drinking water contains less than 0.3 ppm of fluoride and for children ages 2-3 years in areas where the drinking water contains 0.3 through 0.7 ppm of fluoride.

The American Academy of Pediatrics[1] and the American Dental Association[2] currently recommend that infants and children under 2 years of age, in areas where drinking water contains less than 0.3 ppm of fluoride, and children 2-3, in areas where the drinking water contains 0.3 through 0.7 ppm of fluoride, receive 0.25 mg of supplemental fluoride daily which is provided in a full dose (1 mL) of Poly-Vi-Flor® 0.25 mg with Iron drops. A half dose (0.5 mL) of Poly-Vi-Flor 0.5 mg with Iron drops could also provide a daily fluoride intake of 0.25 mg; however, this dosage reduces vitamin supplementation by half.

Poly-Vi-Flor with Iron drops supply significant amounts of vitamins A, D, E, C, thiamine, riboflavin, niacin, pyridoxine, and ferrous sulfate to supplement the diet, and to help assure that deficiencies of these nutrients will not develop. Thus, in a single easy-to-use preparation, infants and children obtain eight essential vitamins and iron, plus fluoride.

A comprehensive $5\frac{1}{2}$ year series of studies of the effectiveness of Tri-Vi-Flor® and Poly-Vi-Flor® products in caries protection has been published.[3-6] Children in this continuing study lived in an area where the water supply contained only 0.05 ppm fluoride. The subjects were divided into two groups, one which used only nonfluoridated Vi-Sol® vitamin products and the other Tri-Vi-Flor and Poly-Vi-Flor vitamin-fluoride products.

The three-year interim report showed 63% fewer carious surfaces in primary teeth and 43% fewer carious surfaces in permanent teeth of the children taking Vi-Flor® vitamin-fluoride products.[3]

After four years the studies continued to support the effectiveness of Tri-Vi-Flor and Poly-Vi-Flor, showing a reduction in carious surfaces of 68% in primary teeth and 46% in permanent teeth.[4]

Results at the end of $5\frac{1}{2}$ years further confirmed the previous findings and indicated that significant reductions in dental caries are apparent with the continued use of Vi-Flor vitamin-fluoride products.[5]

WARNINGS

As in the case of all medications, keep out of the reach of children.

PRECAUTIONS

The suggested dose *should not be exceeded* since dental fluorosis may result from continued ingestion of large amounts of fluoride.

When prescribing Vi-Flor products:

1. determine the fluoride content of the drinking water.
2. make sure the child is not receiving significant amounts of fluoride from other medications.
3. periodically check to make sure that the child does not develop significant dental fluorosis.

Poly-Vi-Flor with Iron drops should be dispensed in the original plastic container, since contact with glass leads to instability and precipitation. (The amount of sodium fluoride in the 50-mL size is well below the maximum to be dispensed at one time according to recommendations of the American Dental Association.)

ADVERSE REACTIONS

Allergic rash and other idiosyncrasies have been reported rarely.

	Poly-Vi-Flor w/Iron drops		Percentage of U.S. Recommended Daily Allowance	
Each 1.0 mL supplies:	**0.5 mg**	**0.25 mg**	**Infants**	**Children Under Age 4 years**
Vitamin A, IU	1500	1500	100	60
Vitamin D, IU	400	400	100	100
Vitamin E, IU	5	5	100	50
Vitamin C, mg	35	35	100	88
Thiamine, mg	0.5	0.5	100	71
Riboflavin, mg	0.6	0.6	100	75
Niacin, mg	8	8	100	89
Vitamin B₆, mg	0.4	0.4	100	57
Iron, mg	10	10	67	100
Fluoride, mg	0.5	0.25	*	*

*U.S. Recommended Daily Allowance has not been established.

DOSAGE AND ADMINISTRATION

1.0 mL daily or as prescribed.

May be dropped directly into mouth with 'Safti-Dropper,' or mixed with cereal, fruit juice or other foods.

HOW SUPPLIED

Poly-Vi-Flor 0.5 mg with Iron (multivitamin, iron and fluoride supplement) drops are available in bottles of 50 mL.
NDC 0087-0469-41 Bottles of 1⅔ fl oz (50 mL)
Poly-Vi-Flor 0.25 mg with Iron (multivitamin, iron and fluoride supplement) drops are available in bottles of 50 mL.
NDC 0087-0483-41 Bottles of 1⅔ fl oz (50 mL)

LITERATURE AVAILABLE

Yes.

REFERENCES

1. American Academy of Pediatrics Committee on Nutrition: Fluoride supplementation. *Pediatrics.* 1986;77:758.
2. American Dental Association. *Accepted Dental Therapeutics.* 38th ed. Chicago: 1979; p 321.
3. Hennon DK, Stookey GK, Muhler JC. The clinical anticariogenic effectiveness of supplementary fluoride-vitamin preparations—Results at the end of three years. *J Dentistry for Children.* January 1966;33:3–12.
4. Hennon DK, Stookey GK, Muhler JC. The clinical anticariogenic effectiveness of supplementary fluoride-vitamin preparations—Results at the end of four years. *J Dentistry for Children.* November 1967;34:439–443.
5. Hennon DK, Stookey GK, Muhler JC. The clinical anticariogenic effectiveness of supplementary fluoride-vitamin preparations—Results at the end of five and a half years. *Phar and Ther in Dent.* 1970;1:1.
6. Hennon DK, Stookey GK, Beiswanger BB. Fluoride-vitamin supplements: Effects on dental caries and fluorosis when used in areas with suboptimal fluoride in the water supply. *J Am Dent Assoc.* 1977;95:965.

TRI–VI–FLOR® 1.0 mg   ℞

[trī′vī-flōr″]
Vitamins A, D, C and fluoride chewable tablets

DESCRIPTION

[See table below.]

Active ingredient for caries prophylaxis: Fluoride as sodium fluoride.

Other ingredients: Ascorbic acid, cholecalciferol, dextrates, FD&C Blue No. 2 (aluminum lake), FD&C Red No. 40 (aluminum lake), FD&C Yellow No. 6 (aluminum lake), fruit flavors (artificial), magnesium stearate, sodium chloride, sodium ascorbate, stearic acid, sucrose, vitamin A acetate.

CLINICAL PHARMACOLOGY

For information of fluoridation see Poly-Vi-Flor® chewable tablets.

Tri-Vi-Flor tablets provide sodium fluoride (1 mg fluoride) and three basic vitamins in a chewable tablet. Because the tablets are chewable, they provide a *topical* as well as *systemic* source of fluoride.[1,2]

INDICATIONS AND USAGE

Supplementation of the diet with vitamins A, D, and C.

Supplementation of the diet with fluoride for caries prophylaxis.

The American Academy of Pediatrics recommends that children up to age 16, in areas where drinking water contains less than optimal levels of fluoride, receive daily fluoride supplementation.

Tri-Vi-Flor 1.0 mg (vitamins A, D, C and fluoride) chewable tablets provide fluoride in tablet form for children 3 years of age and older where the drinking water contains less than 0.3 ppm of fluoride.[3]

Tri-Vi-Flor 1.0 mg chewable tablets supply vitamins A, D and C to help assure that nutritional deficiencies of these vitamins will not develop.

Tri-Vi-Flor 1.0 mg chewable tablets also provide the important mineral fluoride for caries prophylaxis. Thus in a single easy-to-use preparation, children 3 years of age and above obtain three basic vitamins and the important mineral fluoride.

A study of fluoride tablets given to 121 children revealed the efficacy of sodium fluoride in tablet form. The authors concluded that the caries reduction was comparable to that previously reported for children drinking fluoridated water.[4]

A comprehensive $5\frac{1}{2}$ year series of studies of the effectiveness of Tri-Vi-Flor® and Poly-Vi-Flor® products in caries protection has been published.[1,2,5] Children in this continuing study lived in an area where the water supply contained only 0.05 ppm fluoride. The subjects were divided into two groups, one which used non-fluoridated Vi-Sol® vitamin products and the other Tri-Vi-Flor and Poly-Vi-Flor vitamin-fluoride products.

The three-year interim report showed 63% fewer carious surfaces in primary teeth and 43% fewer carious surfaces in permanent teeth of the children taking Vi-Flor® vitamin-fluoride products.[1]

After four years the studies continued to support the effectiveness of Tri-Vi-Flor and Poly-Vi-Flor, showing a reduction in carious surfaces of 68% in primary teeth and 46% in permanent teeth.[2]

Results at the end of $5\frac{1}{2}$ years further confirmed the previous findings and indicated that significant reductions in dental caries are apparent with the continued use of Vi-Flor vitamin-fluoride products.[5]

Children using Tri-Vi-Flor 1.0 mg chewable tablets regularly should receive semiannual dental examinations. The regular brushing of teeth and attention to good oral hygiene practices are also essential.

WARNINGS

As in the case of all medications, keep out of the reach of children.

PRECAUTIONS

The suggested dose of Tri-Vi-Flor 1.0 mg chewable tablets *should not be exceeded*, since dental fluorosis may result from continued ingestion of large amounts of fluoride.

	Tri-Vi-Flor Chewable Tablets	Percentage of U.S. Recommended Daily Allowance	
Each tablet supplies:	**1.0 mg**	**Children Age 2-3 Years**	**Adults & Children Age 4 Years or More**
Vitamin A, IU	2500	100	50
Vitamin D, IU	400	100	100
Vitamin C, mg	60	150	100
Fluoride, mg	1.0	*	*

*U.S. Recommended Daily Allowance has not been established.

When prescribing Vi-Flor products:
1. determine the fluoride content of the drinking water.
2. make sure the child is not receiving significant amounts of fluoride from other medications.
3. periodically check to make sure that the child does not develop significant dental fluorosis.

The Council on Dental Therapeutics of the American Dental Association recommends that no more than 264 mg of sodium fluoride should be dispensed at one time.[6] Therefore, no more than 120 Tri-Vi-Flor 1.0 mg chewable tablets (2.2 mg sodium fluoride per tablet) should be dispensed at one time.

ADVERSE REACTIONS
Allergic rash and other idiosyncrasies have been rarely reported.

DOSAGE AND ADMINISTRATION
One chewable tablet daily or as prescribed.

HOW SUPPLIED
Tri-Vi-Flor 1.0 mg (vitamins A, D, C and fluoride) chewable tablets are available in 100- and 1000-tablet bottles.
NDC 0087-0477-01 Bottles of 100
NDC 0087-0477-02 Bottles of 1000

LITERATURE AVAILABLE
Yes.

REFERENCES
1. Hennon DK, Stookey GK, Muhler JC. The clinical anticariogenic effectiveness of supplementary fluoride-vitamin preparations—Results at the end of three years. *J Dentistry for Children.* January 1966;33:3–12.
2. Hennon DK, Stookey GK, Muhler JC. The clinical anticariogenic effectiveness of supplementary fluoride-vitamin preparations—Results at the end of four years. *J Dentistry for Children.* November 1967;34:439–443.
3. American Academy of Pediatrics Committee on Nutrition: Fluoride supplementation. *Pediatrics.* 1986;77:758.
4. Arnold FA Jr, McClure FJ, White CL. Sodium fluoride tablets for children. *Dental Progress.* October 1960;1:12–16.
5. Hennon DK, Stookey GK, Muhler JC. The clinical anticariogenic effectiveness of supplementary fluoride-vitamin preparations—Results at the end of five and a half years. *Phar and Ther in Dent.* 1970;1:1.
6. Council on Dental Therapeutics. Am Dental Assoc. *Accepted Dental Therapeutics.* 1977, ed 37, p 294.

TRI-VI-FLOR®   ℞
[*trī'vī-flōr"*]
● 0.5 mg
● 0.25 mg
Vitamins A, D, C and fluoride drops

DESCRIPTION
[See table below.]
See INDICATIONS AND USAGE section below for use by infants and children under two years of age.
Active ingredient for caries prophylaxis: Fluoride as sodium fluoride.
Other ingredients: Ascorbic acid, caramel color, cholecalciferol, fruit flavor (artificial), glycerin, polysorbate 80, sodium hydroxide, vitamin A palmitate, water.

CLINICAL PHARMACOLOGY
For information on fluoridation see Poly-Vi-Flor® chewable tablets.

INDICATIONS AND USAGE
Supplementation of the diet with vitamins A, D and C.
Tri-Vi-Flor drops also provide fluoride for caries prophylaxis.
The American Academy of Pediatrics recommends that children up to age 16, in areas where drinking water contains less than optimal levels of fluoride, receive daily fluoride supplementation.
Tri-Vi-Flor 0.5 mg (vitamins A, D, C and fluoride) drops provide fluoride in drop form for children ages 2-3 years in areas where the drinking water contains less than 0.3 ppm fluoride; and for children 3 years and above in areas where the drinking water contains 0.3 through 0.7 ppm of fluoride.
Tri-Vi-Flor 0.25 mg (vitamins A, D, C and fluoride) drops

provide fluoride in drop form for infants and young children from birth to 2 years of age in areas where the drinking water contains less than 0.3 ppm of fluoride; and for children ages 2-3 years in areas where the drinking water contains 0.3 through 0.7 ppm of fluoride.
The American Academy of Pediatrics[1] and the American Dental Association[6] currently recommend that infants and children under 2 years of age, in areas where drinking water contains less than 0.3 ppm of fluoride, and children 2-3, in areas where the drinking water contains 0.3 through 0.7 ppm of fluoride, receive 0.25 mg of supplemental fluoride daily which is provided in a full dose (1 mL) of Tri-Vi-Flor® 0.25 mg drops. A half dose (0.5 mL) of Tri-Vi-Flor 0.5 mg drops could also provide a daily fluoride intake of 0.25 mg; however, this dosage reduces vitamin supplementation by half.
A comprehensive 5½ year series of studies of the effectiveness of Tri-Vi-Flor® and Poly-Vi-Flor® products in caries protection has been published.[2-5] Children in this continuing study lived in an area where the water supply contained only 0.05 ppm fluoride. The subjects were divided into two groups, one which used only nonfluoridated Vi-Sol® vitamin products and the other Tri-Vi-Flor and Poly-Vi-Flor vitamin-fluoride products.
The three-year interim report showed 63% fewer carious surfaces in primary teeth and 43% fewer carious surfaces in permanent teeth of the children taking Vi-Flor® vitamin-fluoride products.[2]
After four years the studies continued to support the effectiveness of Tri-Vi-Flor and Poly-Vi-Flor, showing a reduction in carious surfaces of 68% in primary teeth and 46% in permanent teeth.[3]
Results at the end of 5½ years further confirmed the previous findings and indicated that significant reductions in dental caries are apparent with the continued use of Vi-Flor vitamin-fluoride products.[4]

WARNINGS
As in the case of all medications, keep out of the reach of children.

PRECAUTIONS
The suggested dose *should not be exceeded* since dental fluorosis may result from continued ingestion of large amounts of fluoride.
When prescribing Vi-Flor products:
1. determine the fluoride content of the drinking water.
2. make sure the child is not receiving significant amounts of fluoride from other medications.
3. periodically check to make sure that the child does not develop significant dental fluorosis.
Tri-Vi-Flor drops should be dispensed in the original plastic container, since contact with glass leads to instability and precipitation. (The amount of sodium fluoride in all Tri-Vi-Flor drops is well below the maximum to be dispensed at one time acccording to recommendations of the American Dental Association.)

ADVERSE REACTIONS
Allergic rash and other idiosyncrasies have been rarely reported.

DOSAGE AND ADMINISTRATION
1.0 mL daily, or as prescribed.
May be dropped directly into mouth with 'Safti-Dropper,' or mixed with cereal, fruit juice or other food.

HOW SUPPLIED
Tri-Vi-Flor 0.5 mg (vitamins A,D,C, and fluoride) drops are available in bottles of 50 mL.
NDC 0087-0473-02 Bottles of 1⅔ fl oz (50 mL)
Tri-Vi-Flor 0.25 mg (vitamins A, D, C and fluoride) drops are available in bottles of 50 mL.
NDC 0087-0452-41 Bottles of 50 mL.

LITERATURE AVAILABLE
Yes.

REFERENCES
1. American Academy of Pediatrics Committee on Nutrition: Fluoride supplementation. *Pediatrics.* 1986; 77:758.
2. Hennon DK, Stookey GK, Muhler JC. The clinical anticariogenic effectiveness of supplementary fluoride-vitamin preparations—Results at the end of three years. *J Dentistry for Children.* January 1966;33:3–12.

3. Hennon DK, Stookey GK, Muhler JC. The clinical anticariogenic effectiveness of supplementary fluoride-vitamin preparations—Results at the end of four years. *J Dentistry for Children.* November 1967;34:439–443.
4. Hennon DK, Stookey GK, Muhler JC. The clinical anticariogenic effectiveness of supplementary fluoride-vitamin preparations—Results at the end of five and a half years. *Phar and Ther in Dent.* 1970;1:1.
5. Hennon DK, Stookey GK, Beiswanger BB. Fluoride-vitamin supplements: Effects on dental caries and fluorosis when used in areas with suboptimum fluoride in the water supply. *J Am Dent Assoc.* 1977;95:965.
6. American Dental Association. *Accepted Dental Therapeutics.* 38th ed. Chicago: 1979;p 321.

TRI-VI-FLOR® 0.25 mg with Iron   ℞
[*trī'vī-flōr"*]
Vitamins A, D, C, iron and fluoride drops

DESCRIPTION

Each 1.0 mL supplies:		Percentage of U.S. Recommended Daily Allowance	
		Infants	Children Under Age 4 Years
Vitamin A, IU	1500	100	60
Vitamin D, IU	400	100	100
Vitamin C, mg	35	100	88
Iron, mg	10	67	100
Fluoride, mg	0.25	*	*

* U.S. Recommended Daily Allowance has not been established.

Active ingredient for caries prophylaxis: Fluoride as sodium fluoride.
Other ingredients: Ascorbic acid, caramel color, cholecalciferol, ferrous sulfate, fruit flavor (artificial), glycerin, polysorbate 80, propylene glycol, sodium hydroxide, vitamin A palmitate, water, and other ingredients.

CLINICAL PHARMACOLOGY
For information on fluoridation see Poly-Vi-Flor® chewable tablets.

INDICATIONS AND USAGE
Supplementation of the diet with vitamins A, D, C and iron.
Supplementation of the diet with fluoride for caries prophylaxis.
The American Academy of Pediatrics[1] recommends that children up to age 16, in areas where drinking water contains less than optimal levels of fluoride, receive daily fluoride supplementation.
Tri-Vi-Flor 0.25 mg with Iron (vitamins A, D, C, iron and fluoride) drops provide fluoride in drop form for infants and young children from birth to 2 years of age in areas where the drinking water contains less than 0.3 ppm of fluoride; and for children ages 2-3 years in areas where the drinking water contains 0.3 through 0.7 ppm of fluoride.

WARNINGS
As in the case of all medications, keep out of the reach of children.

PRECAUTIONS
The suggested dose *should not be exceeded* since dental fluorosis may result from continued ingestion of large amounts of fluoride.
When prescribing Vi-Flor® products:
1. determine the fluoride content of the drinking water.
2. make sure the child is not receiving significant amounts of fluoride from other medications.
3. periodically check to make sure that the child does not develop significant dental fluorosis.
Tri-Vi-Flor 0.25 mg with Iron drops should be dispensed in the original plastic container, since contact with glass leads to instability and precipitation. (The amount of sodium fluoride in the 50-mL size is well below the maximum to be dispensed at one time according to recommendations of the American Dental Association.)

ADVERSE REACTIONS
Allergic rash and other idiosyncrasies have been rarely reported.

DOSAGE AND ADMINISTRATION
1.0 mL daily, or as prescribed. May be dropped directly into mouth with 'Safti-Dropper', or mixed with cereal, fruit juice or other food.
USE FULL DOSAGE.

HOW SUPPLIED
Tri-Vi-Flor 0.25 mg with Iron (vitamins A, D, C, iron and fluoride) drops are available in bottles of 50 mL.

Continued on next page

		Tri-Vi-Flor Drops		Percentage of U.S. Recommended Daily Allowance	
Each 1.0 mL supplies:		0.5 mg	0.25 mg	Infants	Children Under Age 4 Years
Vitamin A, IU		1500	1500	100	60
Vitamin D, IU		400	400	100	100
Vitamin C, mg		35	35	100	88
Fluoride, mg		0.5	0.25	*	*

*U.S. Recommended Daily Allowance has not been established.

Mead Johnson Nutritionals—Cont.

REFERENCES

1. American Academy of Pediatrics Committee on Nutrition: Fluoride supplementation. *Pediatrics.* 1986;77:758.

Mead Johnson Pharmaceuticals
A Bristol-Myers Squibb Company
P.O. Box 4500
PRINCETON, NJ 08543-4500

BUSPAR® ℞
[*būspăr*]
(buspirone HCl)

Tablets, 5 mg, bottles of 100 NSN 6505-01-253-2832 (M)
Tablets, 10 mg, bottles of 100 NSN 6505-01-267-3449 (M)

PRODUCT OVERVIEW

KEY FACTS

BuSpar® (buspirone hydrochloride) is an antianxiety agent that is neither chemically nor pharmacologically related to the benzodiazepines, barbiturates, or other sedative/anxiolytic drugs. BuSpar is less sedating than other anxiolytics. BuSpar has shown no potential for abuse or diversion and there is no evidence that it causes either physical or psychological dependence. BuSpar is not a controlled substance.

MAJOR USES

BuSpar is clinically effective for the management of anxiety disorders or the short-term relief of symptoms of anxiety, even in the presence of coexisting symptoms. The recommended initial dose is 5 mg three times a day, with divided doses of 20 to 30 mg per day commonly employed after titration in 5-mg increments.

SAFETY INFORMATION

BuSpar is contraindicated in patients hypersensitive to buspirone hydrochloride. It is recommended that BuSpar not be used concomitantly with a monoamine oxidase inhibitor. Because BuSpar will not block the withdrawal syndrome often seen with benzodiazepines and other common sedative/hypnotic drugs, it is advisable to withdraw such patients gradually from their prior treatment before starting BuSpar therapy.

PRESCRIBING INFORMATION

BUSPAR® ℞
[*būspăr*]
(buspirone HCl)

DESCRIPTION

BuSpar® (buspirone hydrochloride) is an antianxiety agent that is not chemically or pharmacologically related to the benzodiazepines, barbiturates, or other sedative/anxiolytic drugs.

Buspirone hydrochloride is a white crystalline, water soluble compound with a molecular weight of 422.0. Chemically, buspirone hydrochloride is 8-[4-[4-(2-pyrimidinyl)-1-piperazinyl]butyl]-8-azaspiro[4.5]decane-7,9-dione monohydrochloride. The empirical formula $C_{21}H_{31}N_5O_2 \cdot HCl$ is represented by the following structural formula:

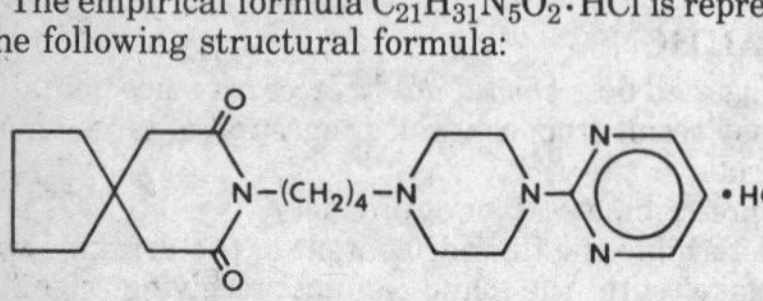

BuSpar is supplied for oral administration in 5 mg and 10 mg white, ovoid-rectangular, scored tablets. BuSpar tablets, 5 mg and 10 mg, contain the following inactive ingredients: colloidal silicon dioxide, lactose, magnesium stearate, microcrystalline cellulose, and sodium starch glycolate.

CLINICAL PHARMACOLOGY

The mechanism of action of buspirone is unknown. Buspirone differs from typical benzodiazepine anxiolytics in that it does not exert anticonvulsant or muscle relaxant effects. It also lacks the prominent sedative effect that is associated with more typical anxiolytics. *In vitro* preclinical studies have shown that buspirone has a high affinity for serotonin ($5\text{-}HT_{1A}$) receptors. Buspirone has no significant affinity for benzodiazepine receptors and does not affect GABA binding *in vitro* or *in vivo* when tested in preclinical models.

Buspirone has moderate affinity for brain D_2-dopamine receptors. Some studies do suggest that buspirone may have indirect effects on other neurotransmitter systems.

BuSpar is rapidly absorbed in man and undergoes extensive first pass metabolism. In a radiolabeled study, unchanged buspirone in the plasma accounted for only about 1% of the radioactivity in the plasma. Following oral administration, plasma concentrations of unchanged buspirone are very low and variable between subjects. Peak plasma levels of 1 to 6 ng/mL have been observed 40 to 90 minutes after single oral doses of 20 mg. The single-dose bioavailability of unchanged buspirone when taken as a tablet is on the average about 90% of an equivalent dose of solution, but there is large variability.

The effects of food upon the bioavailability of BuSpar have been studied in eight subjects. They were given a 20-mg dose with and without food; the area under the plasma concentration-time curve (AUC) and peak plasma concentration (Cmax) of unchanged buspirone increased by 84% and 116% respectively, but the total amount of buspirone immunoreactive material did not change. This suggests that food may decrease the extent of presystemic clearance of buspirone, but the clinical significance of these findings is unknown.

A multiple-dose study conducted in 15 subjects suggests that buspirone has nonlinear pharmacokinetics. Thus, dose increases and repeated dosing may lead to somewhat higher blood levels of unchanged buspirone than would be predicted from results of single-dose studies.

In man, approximately 95% of buspirone is plasma protein bound, but other highly bound drugs, eg, phenytoin, propranolol, and warfarin are not displaced by buspirone from plasma protein *in vitro*. However, *in vitro* binding studies show that buspirone does displace digoxin.

Buspirone is metabolized primarily by oxidation producing several hydroxylated derivatives and a pharmacologically active metabolite, 1-pyrimidinylpiperazine (1-PP). In animal models predictive of anxiolytic potential, 1-PP has about one quarter of the activity of buspirone, but is present in up to 20-fold greater amounts. However, this is probably not important in humans: blood samples from humans chronically exposed to BuSpar do not exhibit high levels of 1-PP; mean values are approximately 3 ng/mL and the highest human blood level recorded among 108 chronically dosed patients was 17 ng/mL, less than 1/200th of 1-PP levels found in animals given large doses of buspirone without signs of toxicity.

In a single-dose study using 14C-labeled buspirone, 29% to 63% of the dose was excreted in the urine within 24 hours, primarily as metabolites; fecal excretion accounted for 18 to 38% of the dose. The average elimination half-life of unchanged buspirone after single doses of 10 to 40 mg is about 2 to 3 hours.

The pharmacokinetics of BuSpar in patients with hepatic or renal dysfunction has not been determined, nor has the effect of age. The effect of BuSpar on drug metabolism or concomitant drug disposition has not been investigated.

INDICATIONS AND USAGE

BuSpar is indicated for the management of anxiety disorders or the short-term relief of the symptoms of anxiety. Anxiety or tension associated with the stress of everyday life usually does not require treatment with an anxiolytic.

The efficacy of BuSpar has been demonstrated in controlled clinical trials of outpatients whose diagnosis roughly corresponds to Generalized Anxiety Disorder (GAD). Many of the patients enrolled in these studies also had coexisting depressive symptoms and BuSpar relieved anxiety in the presence of these coexisting depressive symptoms. The patients evaluated in these studies had experienced symptoms for periods of 1 month to over 1 year prior to the study, with an average symptom duration of 6 months. Generalized Anxiety Disorder (300.02) is described in the American Psychiatric Association's Diagnostic and Statistical Manual, III[1] as follows:

Generalized, persistent anxiety (of at least 1 month continual duration), manifested by symptoms from three of the four following categories.

1. Motor tension: shakiness, jitteriness, jumpiness, trembling, tension, muscle aches, fatigability, inability to relax, eyelid twitch, furrowed brow, strained face, fidgeting, restlessness, easy startle.
2. Autonomic hyperactivity: sweating, heart pounding or racing, cold, clammy hands, dry mouth, dizziness, lightheadedness, paresthesias (tingling in hands or feet), upset stomach, hot or cold spells, frequent urination, diarrhea, discomfort in the pit of the stomach, lump in the throat, flushing, pallor, high resting pulse, and respiration rate.
3. Apprehensive expectation: anxiety, worry, fear, rumination, and anticipation of misfortune to self or others.
4. Vigilance and scanning: hyperattentiveness resulting in distractibility, difficulty in concentrating, insomnia, feeling "on edge," irritability, impatience.

The above symptoms would not be due to another mental disorder, such as a depressive disorder or schizophrenia. However, mild depressive symptoms are common in GAD.

The effectiveness of BuSpar in long-term use, that is, for more than 3 to 4 weeks, has not been demonstrated in controlled trials. There is no body of evidence available that systematically addresses the appropriate duration of treatment for GAD. However, in a study of long-term use, 264 patients were treated with BuSpar for 1 year without ill effect. Therefore, the physician who elects to use BuSpar for extended periods should periodically reassess the usefulness of the drug for the individual patient.

CONTRAINDICATIONS

BuSpar is contraindicated in patients hypersensitive to buspirone hydrochloride.

WARNINGS

The administration of BuSpar to a patient taking a monoamine oxidase inhibitor (MAOI) may pose a hazard. There have been reports of the occurrence of elevated blood pressure when BuSpar has been added to a regimen including an MAOI. Therefore, it is recommended that BuSpar not be used concomitantly with an MAOI.

Because BuSpar has no established antipsychotic activity, it should not be employed in lieu of appropriate antipsychotic treatment.

PRECAUTIONS

General:

Interference with cognitive and motor performance:
Studies indicate that BuSpar is less sedating than other anxiolytics and that it does not produce significant functional impairment. However, its CNS effects in any individual patient may not be predictable. Therefore, patients should be cautioned about operating an automobile or using complex machinery until they are reasonably certain that buspirone treatment does not affect them adversely.

While formal studies of the interaction of BuSpar with alcohol indicate that buspirone does not increase alcohol-induced impairment in motor and mental performance, it is prudent to avoid concomitant use of alcohol and buspirone.

Potential for withdrawal reactions in sedative/hypnotic/anxiolytic drug-dependent patients:
Because BuSpar does not exhibit cross-tolerance with benzodiazepines and other common sedative/hypnotic drugs, it will not block the withdrawal syndrome often seen with cessation of therapy with these drugs. Therefore, before starting therapy with BuSpar, it is advisable to withdraw patients gradually, especially patients who have been using a CNS-depressant drug chronically, from their prior treatment. Rebound or withdrawal symptoms may occur over varying time periods, depending in part on the type of drug, and its effective half-life of elimination.

The syndrome of withdrawal from sedative/hypnotic/anxiolytic drugs can appear as any combination of irritability, anxiety, agitation, insomnia, tremor, abdominal cramps, muscle cramps, vomiting, sweating, flu-like symptoms without fever, and occasionally, even as seizures.

Possible concerns related to buspirone's binding to dopamine receptors:
Because buspirone can bind to central dopamine receptors, a question has been raised about its potential to cause acute and chronic changes in dopamine-mediated neurological function (eg, dystonia, pseudoparkinsonism, akathisia, and tardive dyskinesia). Clinical experience in controlled trials has failed to identify any significant neuroleptic-like activity; however, a syndrome of restlessness, appearing shortly after initiation of treatment, has been reported in some small fraction of buspirone-treated patients. The syndrome may be explained in several ways. For example, buspirone may increase central noradrenergic activity; alternatively, the effect may be attributable to dopaminergic effects (ie, represent akathisia). Obviously, the question cannot be totally resolved at this point in time. Generally, long-term sequelae of any drug's use can be identified only after several years of marketing.

Information for Patients:
To assure safe and effective use of BuSpar, the following information and instructions should be given to patients:

1. Inform your physician about any medications, prescription or nonprescription, alcohol, or drugs that you are now taking or plan to take during your treatment with BuSpar.
2. Inform your physician if you are pregnant, or if you are planning to become pregnant, or if you become pregnant while you are taking BuSpar.
3. Inform your physician if you are breastfeeding an infant.
4. Until you experience how this medication affects you, do not drive a car or operate potentially dangerous machinery.

Laboratory Tests:
There are no specific laboratory tests recommended.

Drug Interactions:
Because the effects of concomitant administration of BuSpar with most other psychotropic drugs have not been studied, the concomitant use of BuSpar with other CNS-active drugs should be approached with caution (see WARNINGS).

There is one report suggesting that the concomitant use of Desyrel® (trazodone hydrochloride) and BuSpar may have caused 3- to 6-fold elevations on SGPT (ALT) in a few patients. In a similar study, attempting to replicate this finding, no interactive effect on hepatic transaminases was identified.

In a study in normal volunteers, concomitant administration of BuSpar and haloperidol resulted in increased serum haloperidol concentrations. The clinical significance of this finding is not clear.

In vitro, buspirone does not displace tightly bound drugs like phenytoin, propranolol, and warfarin from serum proteins.

However, there has been one report of prolonged prothrombin time when buspirone was added to the regimen of a patient treated with warfarin. The patient was also chronically receiving phenytoin, phenobarbital, digoxin, and Synthroid. *In vitro*, buspirone may displace less firmly bound drugs like digoxin. The clinical significance of this property is unknown.

Drug/Laboratory Test Interactions:
Buspirone is not known to interfere with commonly employed clinical laboratory tests.

Carcinogenesis, Mutagenesis, Impairment of Fertility:
No evidence of carcinogenic potential was observed in rats during a 24-month study at approximately 133 times the maximum recommended human oral dose; or in mice, during an 18-month study at approximately 167 times the maximum recommended human oral dose.
With or without metabolic activation, buspirone did not induce point mutations in five strains of *Salmonella typhimurium* (Ames Test) or mouse lymphoma L5178YTK$^+$ cell cultures, nor was DNA damage observed with buspirone in Wi-38 human cells. Chromosomal aberrations or abnormalities did not occur in bone marrow cells of mice given one or five daily doses of buspirone.

Pregnancy: Teratogenic effects:
Pregnancy Category B: No fertility impairment or fetal damage was observed in reproduction studies performed in rats and rabbits at buspirone doses of approximately 30 times the maximum recommended human dose. In humans, however, adequate and well-controlled studies during pregnancy have *not* been performed. Because animal reproduction studies are not always predictive of human response, this drug should be used during pregnancy only if clearly needed.

Labor and Delivery:
The effect of BuSpar on labor and delivery in women is unknown. No adverse effects were noted in reproduction studies in rats.

Nursing Mothers:
The extent of the excretion in human milk of buspirone or its metabolites is not known. In rats, however, buspirone and its metabolites are excreted in milk. BuSpar administration to nursing women should be avoided if clinically possible.

Pediatric Use:
The safety and effectiveness of BuSpar have not been determined in individuals below 18 years of age.

Use in the Elderly:
BuSpar has not been systematically evaluated in older patients; however, several hundred elderly patients have participated in clinical studies with BuSpar and no unusual adverse age-related phenomena have been identified. In 87 elderly patients for whom dosage data were available, the modal total daily dose of BuSpar was 15 mg per day, the same as that in the total sample of patients treated with BuSpar.

Use in Patients with Impaired Hepatic or Renal Function:
Since BuSpar is metabolized by the liver and excreted by the kidneys, its administration to patients with severe hepatic or renal impairment cannot be recommended.

ADVERSE REACTIONS (See also PRECAUTIONS)

Commonly Observed:
The more commonly observed untoward events associated with the use of BuSpar not seen at an equivalent incidence among placebo-treated patients include dizziness, nausea, headache, nervousness, lightheadedness, and excitement.

Associated with Discontinuation of Treatment:
One guide to the relative clinical importance of adverse events associated with BuSpar is provided by the frequency with which they caused drug discontinuation during clinical testing. Approximately 10% of the 2200 anxious patients who participated in the BuSpar premarketing clinical efficacy trials in anxiety disorders lasting 3 to 4 weeks discontinued treatment due to an adverse event. The more common events causing discontinuation included: central nervous system disturbances (3.4%), primarily dizziness, insomnia, nervousness, drowsiness and lightheaded feeling; gastrointestinal disturbances (1.2%), primarily nausea; and miscellaneous disturbances (1.1%), primarily headache and fatigue. In addition, 3.4% of patients had multiple complaints, none of which could be characterized as primary.

Incidence in Controlled Clinical Trials:
The table that follows enumerates adverse events that occurred at a frequency of 1% or more among BuSpar patients who participated in 4-week, controlled trials comparing BuSpar with placebo. The frequencies were obtained from pooled data for 17 trials. The presciber should be aware that these figures cannot be used to predict the incidence of side effects in the course of usual medical practice where patient characteristics and other factors differ from those which prevailed in the clinical trials. Similarly, the cited frequencies cannot be compared with figures obtained from other clinical investigations involving different treatments, uses, and investigators. Comparison of the cited figures, however, does provide the prescribing physician with some basis for estimating the relative contribution of drug and nondrug factors to the side-effect incidence rate in the population studied.

TREATMENT-EMERGENT ADVERSE EXPERIENCE INCIDENCE IN PLACEBO-CONTROLLED CLINICAL TRIALS*
(Percent of Patients Reporting)

Adverse Experience	BuSpar (n=477)	Placebo (n=464)
Cardiovascular		
Tachycardia/Palpitations	1	1
CNS		
Dizziness	12	3
Drowsiness	10	9
Nervousness	5	1
Insomnia	3	3
Lightheadedness	3	—
Decreased Concentration	2	2
Excitement	2	—
Anger/Hostility	2	—
Confusion	2	—
Depression	2	2
EENT		
Blurred Vision	2	—
Gastrointestinal		
Nausea	8	5
Dry Mouth	3	4
Abdominal/Gastric Distress	2	2
Diarrhea	2	—
Constipation	1	2
Vomiting	1	2
Musculoskeletal		
Musculoskeletal Aches/Pains	1	—
Neurological		
Numbness	2	—
Paresthesia	1	—
Incoordination	1	—
Tremor	1	—
Skin		
Skin Rash	1	—
Miscellaneous		
Headache	6	3
Fatigue	4	4
Weakness	2	—
Sweating/Clamminess	1	—

* Events reported by at least 1% of BuSpar patients are included.
—Incidence less than 1%.

Other Events Observed During the Entire Premarketing Evaluation of BuSpar:
During its premarketing assessment, BuSpar was evaluated in over 3500 subjects. This section reports event frequencies for adverse events occurring in approximately 3000 subjects from this group who took multiple doses of BuSpar in the dose range for which BuSpar is being recommended (ie, the modal daily dose of BuSpar fell between 10 and 30 mg for 70% of the patients studied) and for whom safety data were systematically collected. The conditions and duration of exposure to BuSpar varied greatly, involving well-controlled studies as well as experience in open and uncontrolled clinical settings. As part of the total experience gained in clinical studies, various adverse events were reported. In the absence of appropriate controls in some of the studies, a causal relationship to BuSpar treatment cannot be determined. The list includes all undesirable events reasonably associated with the use of the drug.
The following enumeration by organ system describes events in terms of their relative frequency of reporting in this data base. Events of major clinical importance are also described in the PRECAUTIONS section.
The following definitions of frequency are used: Frequent adverse events are defined as those occurring in at least 1/100 patients. Infrequent adverse events are those occurring in 1/100 to 1/1000 patients, while rare events are those occurring in less than 1/1000 patients.

Cardiovascular:
Frequent was nonspecific chest pain; infrequent were syncope, hypotension and hypertension; rare were cerebrovascular accident, congestive heart failure, myocardial infarction, cardiomyopathy and bradycardia.

Central Nervous System:
Frequent were dream disturbances; infrequent were depersonalization, dysphoria, noise intolerance, euphoria, akathisia, fearfulness, loss of interest, dissociative reaction, hallucinations, suicidal ideation and seizures; rare were feelings of claustrophobia, cold intolerance, stupor, and slurred speech and psychosis.

EENT:
Frequent were tinnitus, sore throat, and nasal congestion. Infrequent were redness and itching of the eyes, altered taste, altered smell, and conjunctivitis; rare were inner ear abnormality, eye pain, photophobia, and pressure on eyes.

Endocrine:
Rare were galactorrhea and thyroid abnormality.

Gastrointestinal:
Infrequent were flatulence, anorexia, increased appetite, salivation, irritable colon and rectal bleeding; rare was burning of the tongue.

Genitourinary:
Infrequent were urinary frequency, urinary hesitancy, menstrual irregularity and spotting, and dysuria; rare were amenorrhea, pelvic inflammatory disease, enuresis, and nocturia.

Musculoskeletal:
Infrequent were muscle cramps, muscle spasms, rigid/stiff muscles, and arthralgias.

Neurological:
Infrequent were involuntary movements and slowed reaction time; rare was muscle weakness.

Respiratory:
Infrequent were hyperventilation, shortness of breath, and chest congestion; rare was epistaxis.

Sexual Function:
Infrequent were decreased or increased libido; rare were delayed ejaculation and impotence.

Skin:
Infrequent were edema, pruritus, flushing, easy bruising, hair loss, dry skin, facial edema and blisters; rare were acne and thinning of nails.

Clinical Laboratory:
Infrequent were increases in hepatic aminotransferases (SGOT, SGPT); rare were eosinophilia, leukopenia, and thrombocytopenia.

Miscellaneous:
Infrequent were weight gain, fever, roaring sensation in the head, weight loss, and malaise; rare were alcohol abuse, bleeding disturbance, loss of voice, and hiccoughs.

POSTINTRODUCTION CLINICAL EXPERIENCE

Postmarketing experience has shown an adverse experience profile similar to that given above. Voluntary reports since introduction have included rare occurrences of allergic reactions, cogwheel rigidity, dystonic reactions, ecchymosis, emotional lability, tunnel vision, and urinary retention. Because of the uncontrolled nature of these spontaneous reports, a causal relationship to BuSpar treatment has not been determined.

DRUG ABUSE AND DEPENDENCE

Controlled Substance Class:
BuSpar is not a controlled substance.

Physical and Psychological Dependence:
In human and animal studies, buspirone has shown no potential for abuse or diversion and there is no evidence that it causes tolerance, or either physical or psychological dependence. Human volunteers with a history of recreational drug or alcohol usage were studied in two double-blind clinical investigations. None of the subjects were able to distinguish between BuSpar and placebo. By contrast, subjects showed a statistically significant preference for methaqualone and diazepam. Studies in monkeys, mice, and rats have indicated that buspirone lacks potential for abuse.
Following chronic administration in the rat, abrupt withdrawal of buspirone did not result in the loss of body weight commonly observed with substances that cause physical dependency.
Although there is no direct evidence that BuSpar causes physical dependence or drug-seeking behavior, it is difficult to predict from experiments the extent to which a CNS-active drug will be misused, diverted, and/or abused once marketed. Consequently, physicians should carefully evaluate patients for a history of drug abuse and follow such patients closely, observing them for signs of BuSpar misuse or abuse (eg, development of tolerance, incrementation of dose, drug-seeking behavior).

OVERDOSAGE

Signs and Symptoms:
In clinical pharmacology trials, doses as high as 375 mg/day were administered to healthy male volunteers. As this dose was approached, the following symptoms were observed: nausea, vomiting, dizziness, drowsiness, miosis, and gastric distress. No deaths have been reported in humans either with deliberate or accidental overdosage of BuSpar. Toxicology studies of buspirone yielded the following LD_{50} values: mice, 655 mg/kg; rats, 196 mg/kg; dogs, 586 mg/kg; and monkeys, 356 mg/kg. These dosages are 160–550 times the recommended human daily dose.

Recommended Overdose Treatment:
General symptomatic and supportive measures should be used along with immediate gastric lavage. Respiration, pulse, and blood pressure should be monitored as in all cases of drug overdosage. No specific antidote is known to buspirone, and dialyzability of buspirone has not been determined.

DOSAGE AND ADMINISTRATION

The recommended initial dose is 15 mg daily (5 mg three times a day). To achieve an optimal therapeutic response, at intervals of 2 to 3 days the dosage may be increased 5 mg per day, as needed. The maximum daily dosage should not exceed 60 mg per day. In clinical trials allowing dose titration,

Continued on next page

Mead Johnson—Cont.

divided doses of 20 to 30 mg per day were commonly employed.

HOW SUPPLIED

BuSpar® (buspirone hydrochloride)
Tablets, 5 mg and 10 mg (white, ovoid-rectangular with score, MJ logo, strength, and the name BuSpar embossed) are available in bottles of 100 and 500, and in cartons containing 100 individually packaged tablets.

NDC 0087-0818-41 5 mg tablet	Bottles of 100
NDC 0087-0818-44 5 mg tablet	Bottles of 500
NDC 0087-0818-43 5 mg tablet	Cartons of 100 unit dose
NDC 0087-0819-41 10 mg tablet	Bottles of 100
NDC 0087-0819-44 10 mg tablet	Bottles of 500
NDC 0087-0819-43 10 mg tablet	Cartons of 100 unit dose

U.S. Patent No. 4,182,763
Store at room temperature. Protect from temperatures greater than 86° F (30° C). Dispense in a tight, light-resistant container (USP).

REFERENCE

1. American Psychiatric Association, Ed.: Diagnostic and Statistical Manual of Mental Disorders—III, American Psychiatric Association, May 1980.

Shown in Product Identification Section, page 419

DESYREL® ℞
[des 'ē-rel]
(trazodone HCl)

Tablets, 150 mg, bottles of 100
NSN 6505-01-234-4439 (M&VA)

DESCRIPTION

DESYREL (trazodone hydrochloride) is an antidepressant chemically unrelated to tricyclic, tetracyclic, or other known antidepressant agents. It is a triazolopyridine derivative designated as 2-[3-[4-(3-chlorophenyl)-1-piperazinyl] propyl]-1,2,4-triazolo[4, 3-a]pyridin-3(2H)-one hydrochloride. DESYREL is a white odorless crystalline powder which is freely soluble in water. Its molecular weight is 408.3. The empirical formula is $C_{19}H_{22}ClN_5O \cdot HCl$ and the structural formula is represented as follows:

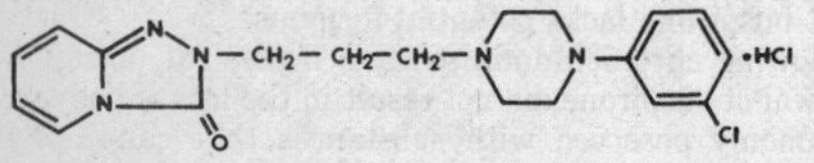

DESYREL is supplied for oral administration in 50 mg, 100 mg, 150 mg and 300 mg tablets.
DESYREL Tablets, 50 mg, contain the following inactive ingredients: dibasic calcium phosphate, castor oil, microcrystalline cellulose, ethylcellulose, FD&C Yellow No. 6 (aluminum lake), lactose, magnesium stearate, povidone, sodium starch glycolate, and starch (corn).
DESYREL Tablets, 100 mg, contain the following inactive ingredients: dibasic calcium phosphate, castor oil, microcrystalline cellulose, ethylcellulose, lactose, magnesium stearate, povidone, sodium starch glycolate, and starch (corn).
DESYREL Tablets, 150 mg, contain the following inactive ingredients: microcrystalline cellulose, FD&C Yellow No. 6 (aluminum lake), magnesium stearate, pregelatinized starch, and stearic acid.
DESYREL Tablets, 300 mg, contain the following inactive ingredients: microcrystalline cellulose, yellow ferric oxide, magnesium stearate, sodium starch glycolate, pregelatinized starch, and stearic acid.

CLINICAL PHARMACOLOGY

The mechanism of DESYREL's antidepressant action in man is not fully understood. In animals, DESYREL selectively inhibits serotonin uptake by brain synaptosomes and potentiates the behavioral changes induced by the serotonin precursor, 5-hydroxytryptophan. Cardiac conduction effects of DESYREL in the anesthetized dog are qualitatively dissimilar and quantitatively less pronounced than those seen with tricyclic antidepressants. DESYREL is not a monoamine oxidase inhibitor and, unlike amphetamine-type drugs, does not stimulate the central nervous system.
In man, DESYREL is well absorbed after oral administration without selective localization in any tissue. When DESYREL is taken shortly after ingestion of food, there may be an increase in the amount of drug absorbed, a decrease in maximum concentration and a lengthening in the time to maximum concentration. Peak plasma levels occur approximately 1 hour after dosing when DESYREL is taken on an empty stomach or 2 hours after dosing when taken with food. Elimination of DESYREL is biphasic, consisting of an initial phase (half-life 3–6 hours) followed by a slower phase (half-life 5–9 hours), and is unaffected by the presence or absence of food. Since the clearance of DESYREL from the body is sufficiently variable, in some patients DESYREL may accumulate in the plasma.
For those patients who responded to DESYREL, one third of the inpatients and one half of the outpatients had a significant therapeutic response by the end of the first week of treatment. Three fourths of all responders demonstrated a significant therapeutic effect by the end of the second week. One fourth of responders required 2–4 weeks for a significant therapeutic response.

INDICATIONS AND USAGE

DESYREL is indicated for the treatment of depression. The efficacy of DESYREL has been demonstrated in both inpatient and outpatient settings and for depressed patients with and without prominent anxiety. The depressive illness of patients studied corresponds to the Major Depressive Episode criteria of the American Psychiatric Association's Diagnostic and Statistical Manual, III.[a]
Major Depressive Episode implies a prominent and relatively persistent (nearly every day for at least 2 weeks) depressed or dysphoric mood that usually interferes with daily functioning, and includes at least four of the following eight symptoms: change in appetite, change in sleep, psychomotor agitation or retardation, loss of interest in usual activities or decrease in sexual drive, increased fatigability, feelings of guilt or worthlessness, slowed thinking or impaired concentration, and suicidal ideation or attempts.

CONTRAINDICATIONS

DESYREL is contraindicated in patients hypersensitive to DESYREL.

WARNINGS

TRAZODONE HAS BEEN ASSOCIATED WITH THE OCCURRENCE OF PRIAPISM. IN APPROXIMATELY ⅓ OF THE CASES REPORTED, SURGICAL INTERVENTION WAS REQUIRED AND, IN A PORTION OF THESE CASES, PERMANENT IMPAIRMENT OF ERECTILE FUNCTION OR IMPOTENCE RESULTED. MALE PATIENTS WITH PROLONGED OR INAPPROPRIATE ERECTIONS SHOULD IMMEDIATELY DISCONTINUE THE DRUG AND CONSULT THEIR PHYSICIAN.
If an erection should persist, promptly contact Bristol-Myers Squibb USPG Medical Services Department (800)321-1335.
The detumescence of priapism and drug-induced penile erections by the intracavernosal injection of alpha-adrenergic stimulants such as epinephrine and metaraminol has been reported.[b-g] For one case of priapism (of some 12-24 hours' duration) in a DESYREL-treated patient in whom the intracavernosal injection of epinephrine was accomplished, prompt detumescence occurred with return of normal erectile activity.
This procedure should be performed under the supervision of a urologist or a physician familiar with the procedure and should not be initiated without urologic consultation if the priapism has persisted for more than 24 hours.
DESYREL is not recommended for use during the initial recovery phase of myocardial infarction.
Caution should be used when administering DESYREL to patients with cardiac disease, and such patients should be closely monitored, since antidepressant drugs (including DESYREL) have been associated with the occurrence of cardiac arrhythmias. Recent clinical studies in patients with pre-existing cardiac disease indicate that DESYREL may be arrhythmogenic in some patients in that population. Arrhythmias identified include isolated PVCs, ventricular couplets, and in two patients short episodes (3–4 beats) of ventricular tachycardia.

PRECAUTIONS

General: The possibility of suicide in seriously depressed patients is inherent in the illness and may persist until significant remission occurs. Therefore, prescriptions should be written for the smallest number of tablets consistent with good patient management.
Hypotension, including orthostatic hypotension and syncope, has been reported to occur in patients receiving DESYREL. Concomitant administration of antihypertensive therapy with DESYREL may require a reduction in the dose of the antihypertensive drug.
Little is known about the interaction between DESYREL and general anesthetics; therefore, prior to elective surgery, DESYREL should be discontinued for as long as clinically feasible.
As with all antidepressants, the use of DESYREL should be based on the consideration of the physician that the expected benefits of therapy outweigh potential risk factors.
Information for Patients: Because priapism has been reported to occur in patients receiving DESYREL, patients with prolonged or inappropriate penile erection should immediately discontinue the drug and consult with the physician (see WARNINGS).
Antidepressants may impair the mental and/or physical ability required for the performance of potentially hazardous tasks, such as operating an automobile or machinery; the patient should be cautioned accordingly.
DESYREL may enhance the response to alcohol, barbiturates, and other CNS depressants.
DESYREL should be given shortly after a meal or light snack. Within any individual patient, total drug absorption may be up to 20% higher when the drug is taken with food rather than on an empty stomach. The risk of dizziness/lightheadedness may increase under fasting conditions.
Laboratory Tests: Occasional low white blood cell and neutrophil counts have been noted in patients receiving DESYREL. These were not considered clinically significant and did not necessitate discontinuation of the drug; however, the drug should be discontinued in any patient whose white blood cell count or absolute neutrophil count falls below normal levels. White blood cell and differential counts are recommended for patients who develop fever and sore throat (or other signs of infection) during therapy.
Drug Interactions: Increased serum digoxin or phenytoin levels have been reported to occur in patients receiving DESYREL concurrently with either of those two drugs.
It is not known whether interactions will occur between monoamine oxidase (MAO) inhibitors and DESYREL. Due to the absence of clinical experience, if MAO inhibitors are discontinued shortly before or are to be given concomitantly with DESYREL, therapy should be initiated cautiously with gradual increase in dosage until optimum response is achieved.
Therapeutic Interactions: Concurrent administration with electroshock therapy should be avoided because of the absence of experience in this area.
There have been reports of increased and decreased prothrombin time occurring in Coumadinized patients who take DESYREL.
Carcinogenesis, Mutagenesis, Impairment of Fertility: No drug- or dose-related occurrence of carcinogenesis was evident in rats receiving DESYREL in daily oral doses up to 300 mg/kg for 18 months.
Pregnancy Category C: DESYREL has been shown to cause increased fetal resorption and other adverse effects on the fetus in two studies using the rat when given at dose levels approximately 30–50 times the proposed maximum human dose. There was also an increase in congenital anomalies in one of three rabbit studies at approximately 15–50 times the maximum human dose. There are no adequate and well-controlled studies in pregnant women. DESYREL should be used during pregnancy only if the potential benefit justifies the potential risk to the fetus.
Nursing Mothers: DESYREL and/or its metabolites have been found in the milk of lactating rats, suggesting that the drug may be secreted in human milk. Caution should be exercised when DESYREL is administered to a nursing woman.
Pediatric Use: Safety and effectiveness in children below the age of 18 have not been established.

ADVERSE REACTIONS

Because the frequency of adverse drug effects is affected by diverse factors (eg, drug dose, method of detection, physician judgment, disease under treatment, etc), a single meaningful estimate of adverse event incidence is difficult to obtain. This problem is illustrated by the variation in adverse event incidence observed and reported from the inpatients and outpatients treated with DESYREL. It is impossible to determine precisely what accounts for the differences observed.
Clinical Trial Reports: The table below is presented solely to indicate the relative frequency of adverse events reported in representative controlled clinical studies conducted to evaluate the safety and efficacy of DESYREL.
The figures cited cannot be used to predict precisely the incidence of untoward events in the course of usual medical practice where patient characteristics and other factors often differ from those which prevailed in the clinical trials. These incidence figures, also, cannot be compared with those obtained from other clinical studies involving related drug products and placebo, as each group of drug trials is conducted under a different set of conditions.
[See table on next page.]
Occasional sinus bradycardia has occurred in long-term studies.
In addition to the relatively common (ie, greater than 1%) untoward events enumerated above, the following adverse events have been reported to occur in association with the use of DESYREL in the controlled clinical studies: akathisia, allergic reaction, anemia, chest pain, delayed urine flow, early menses, flatulence, hallucinations/delusions, hematuria, hypersalivation, hypomania, impaired speech, impotence, increased appetite, increased libido, increased urinary frequency, missed periods, muscle twitches, numbness, and retrograde ejaculation.
Postintroduction Reports:
Although the following adverse reactions have been reported in DESYREL users, the causal association has neither been confirmed nor refuted.

| | Treatment-Emergent Symptom Incidence | | | |
| | Inpts. | | Outpts. | |
	D	P	D	P
Number of Patients	142	95	157	158
% of Patients Reporting				
Allergic				
Skin Condition/Edema	2.8	1.1	7.0	1.3
Autonomic				
Blurred Vision	6.3	4.2	14.7	3.8
Constipation	7.0	4.2	7.6	5.7
Dry Mouth	14.8	8.4	33.8	20.3
Cardiovascular				
Hypertension	2.1	1.1	1.3	*
Hypotension	7.0	1.1	3.8	0.0
Shortness of Breath	*	1.1	1.3	0.0
Syncope	2.8	2.1	4.5	1.3
Tachycardia/Palpitations	0.0	0.0	7.0	7.0
CNS				
Anger/Hostility	3.5	6.3	1.3	2.5
Confusion	4.9	0.0	5.7	7.6
Decreased Concentration	2.8	2.1	1.3	0.0
Disorientation	2.1	0.0	*	0.0
Dizziness/Lightheadedness	19.7	5.3	28.0	15.2
Drowsiness	23.9	6.3	40.8	19.6
Excitement	1.4	1.1	5.1	5.7
Fatigue	11.3	4.2	5.7	2.5
Headache	9.9	5.3	19.8	15.8
Insomnia	9.9	10.5	6.4	12.0
Impaired Memory	1.4	0.0	*	*
Nervousness	14.8	10.5	6.4	8.2
Gastrointestinal				
Abdominal/Gastric Disorder	3.5	4.2	5.7	4.4
Bad Taste in Mouth	1.4	0.0	0.0	0.0
Diarrhea	0.0	1.1	4.5	1.9
Nausea/Vomiting	9.9	1.1	12.7	9.5
Musculoskeletal				
Musculoskeletal Aches/Pains	5.6	3.2	5.1	2.5
Neurological				
Incoordination	4.9	0.0	1.9	0.0
Paresthesia	1.4	0.0	0.0	*
Tremors	2.8	1.1	5.1	3.8
Sexual Function				
Decreased Libido	*	1.1	1.3	*
Other				
Decreased Appetite	3.5	5.3	0.0	*
Eyes Red/Tired/Itching	2.8	0.0	0.0	0.0
Head Full-Heavy	2.8	0.0	0.0	0.0
Malaise	2.8	0.0	0.0	0.0
Nasal/Sinus Congestion	2.8	0.0	5.7	3.2
Nightmares/Vivid Dreams	*	1.1	5.1	5.7
Sweating/Clamminess	1.4	1.1	*	*
Tinnitus	1.4	0.0	0.0	*
Weight Gain	1.4	0.0	4.5	1.9
Weight Loss	*	3.2	5.7	2.5

*Incidence less than 1%.

D = DESYREL   P = Placebo

Voluntary reports received since market introduction include the following: agitation, alopecia, apnea, ataxia, breast enlargement or engorgement, diplopia, edema, extrapyramidal symptoms, grand mal seizures, hallucinations, hemolytic anemia, hyperbilirubinemia, leukonychia, jaundice, lactation, liver enzyme alterations, methemoglobinemia, nausea/vomiting (most frequently), paresthesia, priapism (See WARNINGS and PRECAUTIONS, Information for Patients; some patients have required surgical intervention), pruritus, psychosis, rash, stupor, inappropriate ADH syndrome, tardive dyskinesia, unexplained death, urinary incontinence, urinary retention, urticaria, vasodilation, vertigo, and weakness.

Cardiovascular system effects which have been reported include the following: conduction block, orthostatic hypotension and syncope, palpitations, bradycardia, atrial fibrillation, myocardial infarction, cardiac arrest, arrhythmia, and ventricular ectopic activity, including ventricular tachycardia (see WARNINGS).

OVERDOSE

Animal Oral LD$_{50}$

The oral LD$_{50}$ of the drug is 610 mg/kg in mice, 486 mg/kg in rats, and 560 mg/kg in rabbits.

Signs and Symptoms: Death from overdose has occurred in patients ingesting DESYREL and other drugs concurrently (namely, alcohol; alcohol + chloral hydrate + diazepam; amobarbital; chlordiazepoxide; or meprobamate). The most severe reactions reported to have occurred with overdose of DESYREL alone have been priapism, respiratory arrest, seizures, and EKG changes. The reactions reported most frequently have been drowsiness and vomiting. Over-dosage may cause an increase in incidence or severity of any of the reported adverse reactions (see ADVERSE REACTIONS).

Treatment: There is no specific antidote for DESYREL. Treatment should be symptomatic and supportive in the case of hypotension or excessive sedation. Any patient suspected of having taken an overdose should have the stomach emptied by gastric lavage. Forced diuresis may be useful in facilitating elimination of the drug.

DOSAGE AND ADMINISTRATION

The dosage should be initiated at a low level and increased gradually, noting the clinical response and any evidence of intolerance. Occurrence of drowsiness may require the administration of a major portion of the daily dose at bedtime or a reduction of dosage. DESYREL should be taken shortly after a meal or light snack. Symptomatic relief may be seen during the first week, with optimal antidepressant effects typically evident within 2 weeks. Twenty-five percent of those who respond to DESYREL require more than 2 weeks (up to 4 weeks) of drug administration.

Usual Adult Dosage: An initial dose of 150 mg/day in divided doses is suggested. The dose may be increased by 50 mg/day every 3 to 4 days. The maximum dose for outpatients usually should not exceed 400 mg/day in divided doses. Inpatients (ie, more severely depressed patients) may be given up to but not in excess of 600 mg/day in divided doses.

Maintenance: Dosage during prolonged maintenance therapy should be kept at the lowest effective level. Once an adequate response has been achieved, dosage may be gradually reduced, with subsequent adjustment depending on therapeutic response.

Although there has been no systematic evaluation of the efficacy of DESYREL beyond 6 weeks, it is generally recommended that a course of antidepressant drug treatment should be continued for several months.

HOW SUPPLIED

DESYREL® (trazodone hydrochloride)

Tablets, 50 mg—round, orange/scored, film-sealed (imprinted with DESYREL and MJ 775)

NDC 0087-0775-41	Bottles of 100
NDC 0087-0775-43	Bottles of 1000
NDC 0087-0775-42	Cartons of 100 Unit Doses

Tablets, 100 mg—round, white/scored, film-sealed (imprinted with DESYREL and MJ 776)

NDC 0087-0776-41	Bottles of 100
NDC 0087-0776-43	Bottles of 1000
NDC 0087-0776-42	Cartons of 100 Unit Doses

Tablets, 150 mg—orange, in the Dividose® tablet design (imprinted with MJ and 778 on front; "50," "50," "50" on reverse)

| NDC 0087-0778-43 | Bottles of 100 |
| NDC 0087-0778-44 | Bottles of 500 |

Tablets, 300 mg—yellow, in the Dividose® tablet design (imprinted with MJ and 796 on front; "100," "100," "100" on reverse)

| NDC 0087-0796-41 | Bottles of 100 |

U.S. Patent No. 4,215,104

Store at room temperature. Protect from temperatures above 104°F (40°C).

Dispense in tight, light-resistant container (USP).

REFERENCES

a. Williams JBW, Ed: Diagnostic and Statistical Manual of Mental Disorders-III, American Psychiatric Association, May 1980.

b. Brindley GS: New treatment for priapism, *Lancet* July 28, 1984; ii:220.

c. Goldstein I, et al: Pharmacologic detumescence: The alternative to surgical shunting, *J Urol* April 1986; 135(4:PEII): 308A.

d. Brindley GS: Pilot experiments on the actions of drugs injected into the human corpus cavernosum penis, *Br J Pharmacol* 1986; 87:495-500.

e. Padma-Nathan H, et al: Treatment of prolonged or priapistic erections following intracavernosal papaverine therapy, *Semin Urol* 1986; 4(4):236-238.

f. Lue TF, et al: Priapism: A refined approach to diagnosis and treatment, *J Urol* 1986; 136:104-110.

g. Fabre LF, Feighner JP: Long-term therapy for depression with trazodone, *J Clin Psychiatry* 1983; 44(1):17-21.

Shown in Product Identification Section, page 419

MONOPRIL®   ℞
Fosinopril Sodium Tablets

> ### USE IN PREGNANCY
> **When used in pregnancy during the second and third trimesters, ACE inhibitors can cause injury and even death to the developing fetus.**
> When pregnancy is detected, MONOPRIL should be discontinued as soon as possible. **See WARNINGS: Fetal/Neonatal Morbidity and Mortality.**

DESCRIPTION

MONOPRIL (Fosinopril Sodium) is the sodium salt of fosinopril, the ester prodrug of an angiotensin converting enzyme (ACE) inhibitor, fosinoprilat. It contains a phosphinate group capable of specific binding to the active site of angiotensin converting enzyme. Fosinopril sodium is designated chemically as: L-proline, 4-cyclohexyl-1-[[[2-methyl-1-(1-oxopropoxy) propoxy](4-phenylbutyl) phosphinyl]acetyl]-, sodium salt, *trans*-.

Fosinopril sodium is a white to off-white crystalline powder. It is soluble in water (100 mg/mL), methanol, and ethanol and slightly soluble in hexane.

Its structural formula is:

Its empiric formula is $C_{30}H_{45}NNaO_7P$, and its molecular weight is 585.65.

Continued on next page

Mead Johnson—Cont.

MONOPRIL is available for oral administration as 10 mg and 20 mg tablets. Inactive ingredients include: lactose, microcrystalline cellulose, crospovidone, povidone, and magnesium stearate.

CLINICAL PHARMACOLOGY

Mechanism of Action

In animals and humans, fosinopril sodium is hydrolyzed by esterases to the pharmacologically active form, fosinoprilat, a specific competitive inhibitor of angiotensin converting enzyme (ACE).

ACE is a peptidyl dipeptidase that catalyzes the conversion of angiotensin I to the vasoconstrictor substance, angiotensin II. Angiotensin II also stimulates aldosterone secretion by the adrenal cortex. Inhibition of ACE results in decreased plasma angiotensin II, which leads to decreased vasopressor activity and to decreased aldosterone secretion. The latter decrease may result in a small increase of serum potassium.

In 647 hypertensive patients treated with fosinopril alone for an average of 29 weeks, mean increases in serum potassium of 0.1 mEq/L were observed. Similar increases were observed among all patients treated with fosinopril, including those receiving concomitant diuretic therapy. Removal of angiotensin II negative feedback on renin secretion leads to increased plasma renin activity.

ACE is identical to kininase, an enzyme that degrades bradykinin. Whether increased levels of bradykinin, a potent vasodepressor peptide, play a role in the therapeutic effects of MONOPRIL remains to be elucidated.

While the mechanism through which MONOPRIL lowers blood pressure is believed to be primarily suppression of the renin-angiotensin-aldosterone system, MONOPRIL has an antihypertensive effect even in patients with low-renin hypertension. Although MONOPRIL was antihypertensive in all races studied, black hypertensive patients (usually a low-renin hypertensive population) had a smaller average response to ACE inhibitor monotherapy than non-black patients.

Pharmacokinetics and Metabolism

Following oral administration, fosinopril (the prodrug) is absorbed slowly. The absolute absorption of fosinopril averaged 36% of an oral dose. The primary site of absorption is the proximal small intestine (duodenum/jejunum). While the rate of absorption may be slowed by the presence of food in the gastrointestinal tract, the extent of absorption of fosinopril is essentially unaffected.

Fosinoprilat is highly protein-bound (≥95%), has a relatively small volume of distribution, and has negligible binding to cellular components in blood. After single and multiple oral doses, plasma levels, areas under plasma concentration-time curves (AUCs) and peak concentrations (Cmaxs) are directly proportional to the dose of fosinopril. Times to peak concentrations are independent of dose and are achieved in approximately 3 hours.

After an oral dose of radiolabeled fosinopril, 75% of radioactivity in plasma was present as active fosinoprilat, 20–30% as a glucuronide conjugate of fosinoprilat, and 1–5% as a *p*-hydroxy metabolite of fosinoprilat. Since fosinoprilat is not biotransformed after intravenous administration, fosinopril, not fosinoprilat, appears to be the precursor for the glucuronide and *p*-hydroxy metabolites. In rats, the *p*-hydroxy metabolite of fosinoprilat is as potent an inhibitor of ACE as fosinoprilat; the glucuronide conjugate is devoid of ACE inhibitory activity.

After intravenous administration, fosinoprilat was eliminated approximately equally by the liver and kidney. After oral administration of radiolabeled fosinopril, approximately half of the absorbed dose is excreted in the urine and the remainder is excreted in the feces. In two studies involving healthy subjects, the mean body clearance of intravenous fosinoprilat was between 26 and 39 mL/min.

In healthy subjects, the terminal elimination half-life ($t_{1/2}$) of an intravenous dose of radiolabeled fosinoprilat is approximately 12 hours. In hypertensive patients with normal renal and hepatic function, who received repeated doses of fosinopril, the effective $t_{1/2}$ for accumulation of fosinoprilat averaged 11.5 hours.

In patients with renal insufficiency (creatinine clearance <80 mL/min/1.73m^2), the total body clearance of fosinoprilat is approximately one-half of that in patients with normal renal function, while absorption, bioavailability, and protein-binding are not appreciably altered. The clearance of fosinoprilat does not differ appreciably with degree of renal insufficiency, because the diminished renal elimination is offset by increased hepatobiliary elimination. A modest increase in plasma AUC levels (less than two times that in normals) was observed in patients with various degrees of renal insufficiency, including end-stage renal failure (creatinine clearance <10 mL/min/1.73m^2). (See DOSAGE AND ADMINISTRATION.)

Fosinopril is not well dialyzed. Clearance of fosinoprilat by hemodialysis and peritoneal dialysis averages 2% and 7%, respectively, of urea clearances.

In patients with hepatic insufficiency (alcoholic or biliary cirrhosis), the extent of hydrolysis of fosinopril is not appreciably reduced, although the rate of hydrolysis may be slowed; the apparent total body clearance of fosinoprilat is approximately one-half of that in patients with normal hepatic function.

In elderly (male) subjects (65–74 years old) with clinically normal renal and hepatic function, there appear to be no significant differences in pharmacokinetic parameters for fosinoprilat compared to those of younger subjects (20–35 years old).

Fosinoprilat was found to cross the placenta of pregnant animals.

Studies in animals indicate that fosinopril and fosinoprilat do not cross the blood-brain barrier.

Pharmacodynamics and Clinical Effects

Serum ACE activity was inhibited by ≥90% at 2 to 12 hours after single doses of 10 to 40 mg of fosinopril. At 24 hours, serum ACE activity remained suppressed by 85%, 93%, and 93% in the 10, 20, and 40 mg dose groups, respectively.

Administration of MONOPRIL (Fosinopril Sodium) to patients with mild to moderate hypertension results in a reduction of both supine and standing blood pressure to about the same extent with no compensatory tachycardia. Symptomatic postural hypotension is infrequent, although it can occur in patients who are salt- and/or volume-depleted (see WARNINGS). Use of MONOPRIL in combination with thiazide diuretics gives a blood pressure-lowering effect greater than that seen with either agent alone.

Following oral administration of single doses of 10–40 mg, MONOPRIL lowered blood pressure within one hour, with peak reductions achieved 2–6 hours after dosing. The antihypertensive effect of a single dose persisted for 24 hours. Following four weeks of monotherapy in placebo-controlled trials in patients with mild to moderate hypertension, once daily doses of 20–80 mg lowered supine or seated systolic and diastolic blood pressures 24 hours after dosing by an average of 8–9/6–7 mmHg more than placebo. The trough effect was about 50–60% of the peak diastolic response and about 80% of the peak systolic response.

In most trials, the antihypertensive effect of MONOPRIL (Fosinopril Sodium) increased during the first several weeks of repeated measurements. The antihypertensive effect of MONOPRIL has been shown to continue during long-term therapy for at least 2 years. Abrupt withdrawal of MONOPRIL has not resulted in a rapid increase in blood pressure.

Limited experience in controlled and uncontrolled trials combining fosinopril with a calcium channel blocker or a loop diuretic has indicated no unusual drug-drug interactions. Other ACE inhibitors have had less than additive effects with beta-adrenergic blockers, presumably because both drugs lower blood pressure by inhibiting parts of the renin-angiotensin system.

ACE inhibitors are generally less effective in blacks than in non-blacks. The effectiveness of MONOPRIL was not influenced by age, sex, or weight.

In hemodynamic studies in hypertensive patients, after three months of therapy, responses (changes in BP, heart rate, cardiac index, and PVR) to various stimuli (e.g., isometric exercise, 45° head-up tilt, and mental challenge) were unchanged compared to baseline, suggesting that MONOPRIL does not affect the activity of the sympathetic nervous system. Reduction in systemic blood pressure appears to have been mediated by a decrease in peripheral vascular resistance without reflex cardiac effects. Similarly, renal, splanchnic, cerebral, and skeletal muscle blood flow were unchanged compared to baseline, as was glomerular filtration rate.

INDICATIONS AND USAGE

MONOPRIL is indicated for the treatment of hypertension. It may be used alone or in combination with thiazide diuretics.

In using MONOPRIL, consideration should be given to the fact that another angiotensin converting enzyme inhibitor, captopril, has caused agranulocytosis, particularly in patients with renal impairment or collagen-vascular disease. Available data are insufficient to show that MONOPRIL does not have a similar risk (see WARNINGS).

CONTRAINDICATIONS

MONOPRIL is contraindicated in patients who are hypersensitive to this product or to any other angiotensin converting enzyme inhibitor (e.g., a patient who has experienced angioedema with any other ACE inhibitor therapy).

WARNINGS

Angioedema

Angioedema involving the extremities, face, lips, mucous membranes, tongue, glottis or larynx has been reported in patients treated with ACE inhibitors. If angioedema involves the tongue, glottis or larynx, airway obstruction may occur and be fatal. If laryngeal stridor or angioedema of the face, lips, mucous membranes, tongue, glottis or extremities occurs, treatment with MONOPRIL should be discontinued and appropriate therapy instituted immediately. **Where there is involvement of the tongue, glottis, or larynx, likely to cause airway obstruction, appropriate therapy, e.g., subcutaneous epinephrine solution 1:1000 (0.3 mL to 0.5 mL) should be promptly administered** (see PRECAUTIONS: Information for Patients and ADVERSE REACTIONS).

Hypotension

MONOPRIL can cause symptomatic hypotension. Like other ACE inhibitors, fosinopril has been only rarely associated with hypotension in uncomplicated hypertensive patients. Symptomatic hypotension is most likely to occur in patients who have been volume- and/or salt-depleted as a result of prolonged diuretic therapy, dietary salt restriction, dialysis, diarrhea, or vomiting. Volume and/or salt depletion should be corrected before initiating therapy with MONOPRIL (Fosinopril Sodium).

In patients with congestive heart failure, with or without associated renal insufficiency, ACE inhibitor therapy may cause excessive hypotension, which may be associated with oliguria or azotemia and, rarely, with acute renal failure and death. In such patients, MONOPRIL therapy should be started under close medical supervision; they should be followed closely for the first 2 weeks of treatment and whenever the dose of fosinopril or diuretic is increased.

If hypotension occurs, the patient should be placed in a supine position and, if necessary, treated with intravenous infusion of physiological saline. MONOPRIL treatment usually can be continued following restoration of blood pressure and volume.

Neutropenia/Agranulocytosis

Another angiotensin converting enzyme inhibitor, captopril, has been shown to cause agranulocytosis and bone marrow depression, rarely in uncomplicated patients, but more frequently in patients with renal impairment, especially if they also have a collagen-vascular disease such as systemic lupus erythematosus or scleroderma. Available data from clinical trials of fosinopril are insufficient to show that fosinopril does not cause agranulocytosis at similar rates. Monitoring of white blood cell counts should be considered in patients with collagen-vascular disease, especially if the disease is associated with impaired renal function.

Fetal/Neonatal Morbidity and Mortality

ACE inhibitors can cause fetal and neonatal morbidity and death when administered to pregnant women. Several dozen cases have been reported in the world literature. When pregnancy is detected, ACE inhibitors should be discontinued as soon as possible.

The use of ACE inhibitors during the second and third trimesters of pregnancy has been associated with fetal and neonatal injury, including hypotension, neonatal skull hypoplasia, anuria, reversible or irreversible renal failure, and death. Oligohydramnios has also been reported, presumably resulting from decreased fetal renal function; oligohydramnios in this setting has been associated with fetal limb contractures, craniofacial deformation, and hypoplastic lung development. Prematurity, intrauterine growth retardation, and patent ductus arteriosus have also been reported, although it is not clear whether these occurrences were due to the ACE-inhibitor exposure.

These adverse effects do not appear to have resulted from intrauterine ACE-inhibitor exposure that has been limited to the first trimester. Mothers whose embryos and fetuses are exposed to ACE inhibitors only during the first trimester should be so informed. Nonetheless, when patients become pregnant, physicians should make every effort to discontinue the use of fosinopril as soon as possible.

Rarely (probably less often than once in every thousand pregnancies), no alternative to ACE inhibitors will be found. In these rare cases, the mothers should be apprised of the potential hazards to their fetuses, and serial ultrasound examinations should be performed to assess the intraamniotic environment.

If oligohydramnios is observed, fosinopril should be discontinued unless it is considered life-saving for the mother. Contraction stress testing (CST), a nonstress test (NST), or biophysical profiling (BPP) may be appropriate, depending upon the week of pregnancy. Patients and physicians should be aware, however, that oligohydramnios may not appear until after the fetus has sustained irreversible injury.

Infants with histories of *in utero* exposure to ACE inhibitors should be closely observed for hypotension, oliguria, and hyperkalemia. If oliguria occurs, attention should be directed toward support of blood pressure and renal perfusion. Exchange transfusion or dialysis may be required as a means of reversing hypotension and/or substituting for disordered renal function. Fosinopril is poorly dialyzed from the circulation of adults by hemodialysis and peritoneal dialysis. There is no experience with any procedure for removing fosinopril from the neonatal circulation.

When fosinopril was given to pregnant rats at doses about 80 to 250 times (on a mg/kg basis) the maximum recommended human dose, three similar orofacial malformations and one fetus with *situs inversus* were observed among the offspring. No teratogenic effects of fosinopril were seen in studies in pregnant rabbits at doses up to 25 times (on a mg/kg basis) the maximum recommended human dose.

PRECAUTIONS

General

Impaired Renal Function: As a consequence of inhibiting the renin-angiotensin-aldosterone system, changes in renal function may be anticipated in susceptible individuals. In patients with severe congestive heart failure whose renal function may depend on the activity of the renin-angiotensin-aldosterone system, treatment with angiotensin converting enzyme inhibitors, including MONOPRIL (Fosinopril Sodium), may be associated with oliguria and/or progressive azotemia and (rarely) with acute renal failure and/or death.

In hypertensive patients with renal artery stenosis in a solitary kidney or bilateral renal artery stenosis, increases in blood urea nitrogen and serum creatinine may occur. Experience with another angiotensin converting enzyme inhibitor suggests that these increases are usually reversible upon discontinuation of ACE inhibitor and/or diuretic therapy. In such patients, renal function should be monitored during the first few weeks of therapy. Some hypertensive patients with no apparent pre-existing renal vascular disease have developed increases in blood urea nitrogen and serum creatinine, usually minor and transient, especially when MONOPRIL has been given concomitantly with a diuretic. This is more likely to occur in patients with pre-existing renal impairment. Dosage reduction of MONOPRIL and/or discontinuation of the diuretic may be required.

Evaluation of the hypertensive patient should always include assessment of renal function (see DOSAGE AND ADMINISTRATION).

Impaired renal function decreases total clearance of fosinoprilat and approximately doubles AUC. In general, however, no adjustment of dosing is needed (see CLINICAL PHARMACOLOGY).

Hyperkalemia: In clinical trials, hyperkalemia (serum potassium greater than 10% above the upper limit of normal) has occurred in approximately 2.6% of hypertensive patients receiving MONOPRIL. In most cases, these were isolated values which resolved despite continued therapy. In clinical trials, 0.1% of patients (two patients) were discontinued from therapy due to an elevated serum potassium. Risk factors for the development of hyperkalemia include renal insufficiency, diabetes mellitus, and the concomitant use of potassium-sparing diuretics, potassium supplements, and/or potassium-containing salt substitutes, which should be used cautiously, if at all, with MONOPRIL (Fosinopril Sodium) (see PRECAUTIONS: Drug Interactions).

Cough: Cough has been reported with the use of ACE inhibitors. Characteristically, the cough is nonproductive, persistent, and resolves after discontinuation of therapy. ACE inhibitor-induced cough should be considered as part of the differential diagnosis of cough.

Impaired Liver Function: Since fosinopril is primarily metabolized by hepatic and gut wall esterases to its active moiety, fosinoprilat, patients with impaired liver function could develop elevated plasma levels of unchanged fosinopril. In a study in patients with alcoholic or biliary cirrhosis, the extent of hydrolysis was unaffected, although the rate was slowed. In these patients, the apparent total body clearance of fosinoprilat was decreased and the plasma AUC approximately doubled.

Surgery/Anesthesia: In patients undergoing surgery or during anesthesia with agents that produce hypotension, fosinopril will block the angiotensin II formation that could otherwise occur secondary to compensatory renin release. Hypotension that occurs as a result of this mechanism can be corrected by volume expansion.

Information for Patients

Angioedema: Angioedema, including laryngeal edema, can occur with treatment with ACE inhibitors, especially following the first dose. Patients should be advised to immediately report to their physician any signs or symptoms suggesting angioedema (e.g., swelling of face, eyes, lips, tongue, larynx, mucous membranes, and extremities; difficulty in swallowing or breathing; hoarseness) and to discontinue therapy. (See WARNINGS and ADVERSE REACTIONS.)

Symptomatic Hypotension: Patients should be cautioned that lightheadedness can occur, especially during the first days of therapy, and it should be reported to a physician. Patients should be told that if syncope occurs, MONOPRIL should be discontinued until the physician has been consulted.

All patients should be cautioned that inadequate fluid intake or excessive perspiration, diarrhea, or vomiting can lead to an excessive fall in blood pressure, with the same consequences of lightheadedness and possible syncope.

Hyperkalemia: Patients should be told not to use potassium supplements or salt substitutes containing potassium without consulting the physician.

Neutropenia: Patients should be told to promptly report any indication of infection (e.g., sore throat, fever), which could be a sign of neutropenia.

Pregnancy: Female patients of childbearing age should be told about the consequences of second- and third-trimester exposure to ACE inhibitors, and they should also be told that these consequences do not appear to have resulted from intrauterine ACE-inhibitor exposure that has been limited to the first trimester. These patients should be asked to report pregnancies to their physicians as soon as possible.

Drug Interactions

With diuretics: Patients on diuretics, especially those with intravascular volume depletion, may occasionally experience an excessive reduction of blood pressure after initiation of therapy with MONOPRIL. The possibility of hypotensive effects with MONOPRIL can be minimized by either discontinuing the diuretic or increasing salt intake prior to initiation of treatment with MONOPRIL. If this is not possible, the starting dose should be reduced and the patient should be observed closely for several hours following an initial dose and until blood pressure has stabilized (see DOSAGE AND ADMINISTRATION).

With potassium supplements and potassium-sparing diuretics: MONOPRIL can attenuate potassium loss caused by thiazide diuretics. Potassium-sparing diuretics (spironolactone, amiloride, triamterene, and others) or potassium supplements can increase the risk of hyperkalemia. Therefore, if concomitant use of such agents is indicated, they should be given with caution, and the patient's serum potassium should be monitored frequently.

With lithium: Increased serum lithium levels and symptoms of lithium toxicity have been reported in patients receiving ACE inhibitors during therapy with lithium. These drugs should be coadministered with caution, and frequent monitoring of serum lithium levels is recommended. If a diuretic is also used, the risk of lithium toxicity may be increased.

With antacids: In a clinical pharmacology study, coadministration of an antacid (aluminum hydroxide, magnesium hydroxide, and simethicone) with fosinopril reduced serum levels and urinary excretion of fosinoprilat as compared with fosinopril administrated alone, suggesting that antacids may impair absorption of fosinopril. Therefore, if concomitant administration of these agents is indicated, dosing should be separated by 2 hours.

Other: Neither MONOPRIL nor its metabolites have been found to interact with food. In separate single or multiple dose pharmacokinetic interaction studies with chlorthalidone, nifedipine, propranolol, hydrochlorothiazide, cimetidine, metoclopramide, propantheline, digoxin, and warfarin, the bioavailability of fosinoprilat was not altered by coadministration of fosinopril with any one of these drugs. In a study with concomitant administration of aspirin and MONOPRIL (Fosinopril Sodium), the bioavailability of unbound fosinoprilat was not altered.

In a pharmacokinetic interaction study with warfarin, bioavailability parameters, the degree of protein binding, and the anticoagulant effect (measured by prothrombin time) of warfarin were not significantly changed.

Drug/Laboratory Test Interaction

Fosinopril may cause a false low measurement of serum digoxin levels with the Digi-Tab® RIA Kit for Digoxin. Other kits, such as the Coat-A-Count® RIA Kit, may be used.

Carcinogenesis, Mutagenesis, and Impairment of Fertility

No evidence of a carcinogenic effect was found when fosinopril was given in the diet to mice and rats for up to 24 months at doses up to 400 mg/kg/day. On a body weight basis, the highest dose in mice and rats is about 250 times the maximum human dose of 80 mg, assuming a 50 kg subject. On a body surface area basis, in mice, this dose is 20 times the maximum human dose; in rats, this dose is 40 times the maximum human dose. Male rats given the highest dose level had a slightly higher incidence of mesentery/omentum lipomas.

Neither fosinopril nor the active fosinoprilat was mutagenic in the Ames microbial mutagen test, the mouse lymphoma forward mutation assay, or a mitotic gene conversion assay. Fosinopril was also not genotoxic in a mouse micronucleus test *in vivo* and a mouse bone marrow cytogenetic assay *in vivo*.

In the Chinese hamster ovary cell cytogenetic assay, fosinopril increased the frequency of chromosomal aberrations when tested without metabolic activation at a concentration that was toxic to the cells. However, there was no increase in chromosomal aberrations at lower drug concentrations without metabolic activation or at any concentration with metabolic activation.

There were no adverse reproductive effects in male and female rats treated with 15 or 60 mg/kg daily. On a body weight basis, the high dose of 60 mg/kg is about 38 times the maximum recommended human dose. On a body surface area basis, this dose is 6 times the maximum recommended human dose. There was no effect on pairing time prior to mating in rats until a daily dose of 240 mg/kg, a toxic dose, was given; at this dose, a slight increase in pairing time was observed. On a body weight basis, this dose is 150 times the maximum recommended human dose. On a body surface area basis, this dose is 24 times the maximum recommended human dose.

Pregnancy Categories C (first trimester) and D (second and third trimesters)

See **WARNINGS: Fetal/Neonatal Morbidity and Mortality.**

Nursing Mothers

Ingestion of 20 mg daily for three days resulted in detectable levels of fosinoprilat in breast milk. MONOPRIL (Fosinopril Sodium) should not be administered to nursing mothers.

Geriatric Use

Of the total number of patients who received fosinopril in US clinical studies of MONOPRIL, 13% were 65 and older while 1.3% were 75 and older. No overall differences in effectiveness or safety were observed between these patients and younger patients, and other reported clinical experience has not identified differences in response between the elderly and younger patients, but greater sensitivity of some older individuals cannot be ruled out.

In a pharmacokinetic study comparing elderly (65–74 years old) and non-elderly (20–35 years old) healthy volunteers, there were no differences between the groups in peak fosinoprilat levels or area under the plasma concentration time curve (AUC).

Pediatric Use

Safety and effectiveness in children have not been established.

ADVERSE REACTIONS

MONOPRIL (Fosinopril Sodium) has been evaluated for safety in more than 1500 individuals in hypertension trials, including approximately 450 patients treated for a year or more. Generally adverse events were mild and transient, and their frequency was not prominently related to dose within the recommended daily dosage range.

In placebo-controlled clinical trials (688 fosinopril-treated patients), the usual duration of therapy was two to three months. Discontinuations due to any clinical or laboratory adverse event were 4.1 and 1.1 percent in fosinopril-treated and placebo-treated patients, respectively. The most frequent reasons (0.4 to 0.9%) were headache, elevated transaminases, fatigue, cough (See PRECAUTIONS: General, Cough), diarrhea, and nausea and vomiting.

During clinical trials with any fosinopril regimen, the incidence of adverse events in the elderly (≥ 65 years old) was similar to that seen in younger patients.

Clinical adverse events probably or possibly related or of uncertain relationship to therapy, occurring in at least 1% of patients treated with MONOPRIL (Fosinopril Sodium) alone in placebo-controlled clinical trials are shown in the table below.

Clinical Adverse Events in Placebo-Controlled Trials

	MONOPRIL (N = 688) Incidence (Discontinuation)	Placebo (N = 184) Incidence (Discontinuation)
Headache	3.2 (0.9)	3.3
Cough	2.2 (0.4)	0.0
Dizziness	1.6	0.0
Diarrhea	1.5 (0.4)	1.6
Fatigue	1.5 (0.6)	1.6
Nausea/ Vomiting	1.2 (0.4)	0.5
Sexual Dysfunction	1.0 (0.1)	1.1 (0.5)

Other clinical events probably or possibly related, or of uncertain relationship to therapy occurring in 0.2 to 1.0% of patients (except as noted) treated with MONOPRIL in controlled or uncontrolled clinical trials (N = 1479) and less frequent, clinically significant events include (listed by body system):

General: Chest pain, edema, weakness, excessive sweating.

Cardiovascular: Angina/myocardial infarction, cerebrovascular accident, hypertensive crisis, rhythm disturbances, palpitations, hypotension, syncope, flushing, claudication. Orthostatic hypotension occurred in 1.4% of patients treated with fosinopril monotherapy. Hypotension or orthostatic hypotension was a cause for discontinuation of therapy in 0.1% of patients.

Dermatologic: Urticaria, rash, photosensitivity, pruritus.

Endocrine/Metabolic: Gout, decreased libido.

Gastrointestinal: Pancreatitis, hepatitis, dysphagia, abdominal distention, abdominal pain, flatulence, constipation, heartburn, appetite/weight change, dry mouth.

Hematologic: Lymphadenopathy.

Immunologic: Angioedema.

Musculoskeletal: Arthralgia, musculoskeletal pain, myalgia/muscle cramp.

Nervous/Psychiatric: Memory disturbance, tremor, confusion, mood change, paresthesia, sleep disturbance, drowsiness, vertigo.

Respiratory: Bronchospasm, pharyngitis, sinusitis/rhinitis, laryngitis/hoarseness, epistaxis. A symptom-complex of cough, bronchospasm, and eosinophilia has been observed in two patients treated with fosinopril.

Continued on next page

Mead Johnson—Cont.

Special Senses: Tinnitus, vision disturbance, taste disturbance, eye irritation.
Urogenital: Renal insufficiency, urinary frequency.

Fetal/Neonatal Morbidity and Mortality
See WARNINGS: Fetal/Neonatal Morbidity and Mortality.

Potential Adverse Effects Reported with ACE Inhibitors
Other medically important adverse effects reported with ACE inhibitors include: Cardiac arrest; eosinophilic pneumonitis; neutropenia/agranulocytosis, pancytopenia, anemia (including hemolytic and aplastic), thrombocytopenia; acute renal failure; hepatic failure, jaundice (hepatocellular or cholestatic); symptomatic hyponatremia; bullous pemphigus, exfoliative dermatitis; a syndrome which may include: arthralgia/arthritis, vasculitis, serositis, myalgia, fever, rash or other dermatologic manifestations, a positive ANA, leukocytosis, eosinophilia, or an elevated ESR.

Laboratory Test Abnormalities
Serum Electrolytes: Hyperkalemia, (see PRECAUTIONS); *hyponatremia,* (see PRECAUTIONS: Drug Interactions, With diuretics).
BUN/Serum Creatinine: Elevations, usually transient and minor, of BUN or serum creatinine have been observed. In placebo-controlled clinical trials, there were no significant differences in the number of patients experiencing increases in serum creatinine (outside the normal range or 1.33 times the pre-treatment value) between the fosinopril and placebo treatment groups. Rapid reduction of longstanding or markedly elevated blood pressure by any antihypertensive therapy can result in decreases in the glomerular filtration rate and, in turn, lead to increases in BUN or serum creatinine. (See PRECAUTIONS: General.)
Hematology: In controlled trials, a mean *hemoglobin* decrease of 0.1 g/dL was observed in fosinopril-treated patients. In individual patients decreases in hemoglobin or hematocrit were usually transient, small, and not associated with symptoms. No patient was discontinued from therapy due to the development of anemia. *Other:* Neutropenia (see WARNINGS), leukopenia and eosinophilia.
Liver Function Tests: Elevations of transaminases, LDH, alkaline phosphatase and serum bilirubin have been reported. Fosinopril therapy was discontinued because of serum transaminase elevations in 0.7% of patients. In the majority of cases, the abnormalities were either present at baseline or were associated with other etiologic factors. In those cases which were possibly related to fosinopril therapy, the elevations were generally mild and transient and resolved after discontinuation of therapy.

OVERDOSAGE
The oral LD_{50} of fosinopril in rats is 2600 mg/kg. Human overdoses of fosinopril have not been reported, but the most common manifestation of human fosinopril overdosage is likely to be hypotension.
Laboratory determinations of serum levels of fosinoprilat and its metabolites are not widely available, and such determinations have, in any event, no established role in the management of fosinopril overdose. No data are available to suggest physiological maneuvers (e.g., maneuvers to change the pH of the urine) that might accelerate elimination of fosinopril and its metabolites. Fosinoprilat is poorly removed from the body by both hemodialysis and peritoneal dialysis.
Angiotensin II could presumably serve as a specific antagonist-antidote in the setting of fosinopril overdose, but angiotensin II is essentially unavailable outside of scattered research facilities. Because the hypotensive effect of fosinopril is achieved through vasodilation and effective hypovolemia, it is reasonable to treat fosinopril overdose by infusion of normal saline solution.

DOSAGE AND ADMINISTRATION
The recommended initial dose of MONOPRIL (Fosinopril Sodium) is 10 mg once a day, both as monotherapy and when the drug is added to a diuretic. Dosage should then be adjusted according to blood pressure response at peak (2–6 hours) and trough (about 24 hours after dosing) blood levels. The usual dosage range needed to maintain a response at trough is 20–40 mg but some patients appear to have a further response to 80 mg. In some patients treated with once daily dosing, the antihypertensive effect may diminish toward the end of the dosing interval. If trough response is inadequate, dividing the daily dose should be considered. If blood pressure is not adequately controlled with MONOPRIL alone, a diuretic may be added.
Concomitant administration of MONOPRIL with potassium supplements, potassium salt substitutes, or potassium-sparing diuretics can lead to increases of serum potassium (see PRECAUTIONS).
In patients who are currently being treated with a diuretic, symptomatic hypotension occasionally can occur following the initial dose of MONOPRIL. To reduce the likelihood of hypotension, the diuretic should, if possible, be discontinued two to three days prior to beginning therapy with MONOPRIL (see WARNINGS). Then, if blood pressure is not controlled with MONOPRIL alone, diuretic therapy should be resumed. If diuretic therapy cannot be discontinued, an initial dose of 10 mg of MONOPRIL should be used with careful medical supervision for several hours and until blood pressure has stabilized. (See WARNINGS; PRECAUTIONS: Information for Patients and Drug Interactions.)
Since concomitant administration of MONOPRIL (Fosinopril Sodium) with potassium supplements, or potassium-containing salt substitutes or potassium-sparing diuretics may lead to increases in serum potassium, they should be used with caution.
For Hypertensive Patients With Renal Impairment: In patients with impaired renal function, the total body clearance of fosinoprilat is approximately 50% slower than in patients with normal renal function. Since hepatobiliary elimination partially compensates for diminished renal elimination, the total body clearance of fosinoprilat does not differ appreciably with any degree of renal insufficiency (creatinine clearances < 80 mL/min/1.73m^2), including end-stage renal failure (creatinine clearance < 10 mL/min/1.73m^2). This relative constancy of body clearance of active fosinoprilat, resulting from the dual route of elimination, permits use of the usual dose in patients with any degree of renal impairment.

HOW SUPPLIED
10 mg tablets: White to off-white, biconvex flat-end diamond shaped, compressed tablets with unilog number **158** on one side and **M** on the other. They are supplied in bottles of 100 (NDC 0087-0158-50). Bottles contain a desiccant canister.
20 mg tablets: White to off-white, oval shaped, compressed tablets with unilog number **609** on one side and **M** on the other. They are supplied in bottles of 100 (NDC 0087-0609-50). Bottles contain a desiccant canister.
UNIMATIC® unit-dose packs containing 100 tablets are also available for each potency: **10 mg** (NDC 0087-0158-51) and **20 mg** (NDC 0087-0609-51).

STORAGE
Store between 15°C (59°F) and 30°C (86°F). Avoid prolonged exposure to temperatures above 30°C (86°F). Keep bottles tightly closed (protect from moisture).
Shown in Product Identification Section, page 419

Medicis Dermatologics, Inc.
100 EAST 42nd STREET, 15th FLOOR
NEW YORK, NY 10017

BENZASHAVE™ 5% ℞
Benzoyl Peroxide, USP 5%
Medicated Shave Cream

BENZASHAVE™ 10% ℞
Benzoyl Peroxide, USP 10%
Medicated Shave Cream

DESCRIPTION
BenzaShave 5% and BenzaShave 10% Benzoyl Peroxide, USP (5% and 10%) are topical shave cream preparations for use in the treatment of pseudo folliculitis (*p. barbae;* ingrown hairs, razor bumps) and acne vulgaris associated with shaving. Benzoyl peroxide is an oxidizing agent which possesses antibacterial properties and is classified as a keratolytic agent. Benzoyl peroxide ($C_{14}H_{10}O_4$) is represented by the following chemical structure:

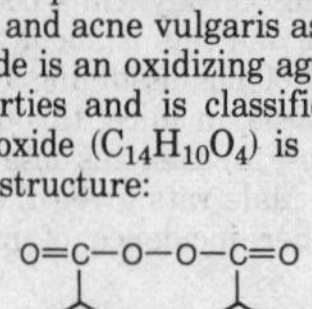

INGREDIENTS
BenzaShave 5% & 10% contain: ACTIVES: Benzoyl Peroxide, USP, 5% or 10%; INACTIVES: Stearic Acid, Mineral Oil, Triethanolamine, Diisopropyl Dimerate, PEG-15 Cocamine, Carbomer 940, Aloe Vera, Purified Water, PRESERVATIVES: Diazolidinyl Urea, Methylparaben and Propylparaben.

CLINICAL PHARMACOLOGY
The mechanism of action of benzoyl peroxide has not been determined but may be related to its antibacterial activity against **Propionibacterium acnes** and its ability to cause drying and peeling. Benzoyl peroxide reduces the concentration of free fatty acids in the sebum. Little is known about the percutaneous penetration, metabolism and excretion of benzoyl peroxide, although it is likely that benzoic acid is a major metabolite. There is no evidence of systemic toxicity caused by benzoyl peroxide in humans.

INDICATIONS AND USAGE
These products are indicated for the topical treatment of acne vulgaris.

CONTRAINDICATIONS
These products are contraindicated in patients with a history of hypersensitivity to any of the components of the preparations.

PRECAUTIONS
General: For external use only. Not for ophthalmic use. If severe irritation develops, discontinue use and institute appropriate therapy. After the reaction clears, treatment may often be resumed with less frequent application. This preparation should not be used in or near the eyes or on mucous membranes.
Information for Patients: Avoid contact with eyes, eyelids, lips and mucous membranes. If accidental contact occurs, rinse with water. May bleach hair and colored fabrics. If excessive irritation develops, discontinue use and consult your physician.
Carcinogensis, Mutagenesis, Impairment of Fertility: Data from several studies using mice known to be highly susceptible to cancer suggest that benzoyl peroxide acts as a tumor promotor. The clinical significance of these findings to humans is unknown.
Pregnancy: Pregnancy Category C: Animal reproduction studies have not been conducted with benzoyl peroxide. It is also *not* known whether benzoyl peroxide can cause fetal harm when administered to a pregnant woman or can affect reproduction capacity. Benzoyl peroxide should be used by a pregnant woman only if clearly needed. There are no data available on the effect of benzoyl peroxide on the growth, development and functional maturation of the unborn child.
Nursing Mothers: It is not known whether this drug is excreted in human milk. Because many drugs are excreted in human milk, caution should be exercised when benzoyl peroxide is administered to a nursing woman.
Pediatric Use: Safety and effectiveness in children have not been established.

ADVERSE REACTIONS
Allergic contact dermatitis has been reported with topical benzoyl peroxide therapy.

DOSAGE AND ADMINISTRATION
Wet area to be shaved. Apply a small amount of BenzaShave with fingertips. Gently rub over entire area and shave.

HOW SUPPLIED
BENZASHAVE™ Benzoyl Peroxide, USP (5%), 4 oz (113.4g) tube, NDC 99207-530-04.
BENZASHAVE™ Benzoyl Peroxide, USP (10%), 4 oz (113.4g) tube, NDC 99207-540-04.
Keep out of reach of children.
Store at Controlled Room Temperature 15°–30°C (59°–86°F).
For external use only. Not for ophthalmic use.
Lot number and expiration date on package.

CAUTION
Federal law prohibit dispensing without prescription.
Mfd. by **Syosset Laboratories Co., Inc.,** Syosset, NY 11791
Dist. by **Medicis Dermatologics, Inc.,** New York, NY 10017

ONYPLEX™ Nail Hardener OTC
Formaldehyde Free

INDICATIONS
Dry Brittle Nails

INGREDIENTS
Ethyl Acetate, Butyl Acetate, Toluene, Nitrocellulose, Polyester Resin, Isopropyl Alcohol, Dibutyl Phthalate, Diisopropyl Dimerate, Acrylates Copolymer, Camphor, Benzophenone-1, Polyvinyl Butyral, Bispyrithione and Magnesium Sulfate, D & C Violet No. 2.

DIRECTIONS
SHAKE WELL BEFORE USING. Apply to clean nail surface. Apply first coat. Let dry, apply second coat. After 3 days remove with nail polish remover and repeat. Use regularly.
For external use only.
Avoid contact with eyes.
Keep away from open flame.
Keep out of reach of children.

HOW SUPPLIED
½ fl. oz. (15 mL) NDC 99207-610-01

PAPLEX™ ℞
Salicylic Acid, USP (17%) in a Solution of Lactic Acid in Flexible Collodion, USP
PAPLEX™ ULTRA ℞
Salicylic Acid, USP (26%) Solution in Flexible Collodion, USP

DESCRIPTION
PAPLEX is a topical preparation containing Salicylic Acid, USP, 17% and Lactic Acid, USP, 17%; in Flexible Collodion, USP. PAPLEX ULTRA is a topical preparation containing

Salicylic Acid, USP, 26% in Flexible Collidion, USP. The pharmacologic activity of PAPLEX and PAPLEX ULTRA is generally attributed to the keratolytic action of Salicylic Acid. The structural formula of Salicylic Acid is:

COOH
OH

CLINICAL PHARMACOLOGY
Although the exact mode of action of Salicylic Acid in the treatment of warts is not known, its activity appears to be associated with its keratolytic action which results in mechanical removal of epidermal cells infected with wart viruses.

INDICATIONS AND USAGE
PAPLEX and PAPLEX ULTRA are indicated in the treatment and removal of common warts and plantar warts.

CONTRAINDICATIONS
PAPLEX and PAPLEX ULTRA should *not* be used on irritated skin, or on any area that is infected or reddened, if you are a diabetic or if you have poor blood circulation. PAPLEX and PAPLEX ULTRA should *not* be used on moles, birthmarks, unusual warts with hair growing from them, or warts on face.

PRECAUTIONS
PAPLEX and PAPLEX ULTRA are for external use only. Do *not* permit PAPLEX and PAPLEX ULTRA to contact eyes or mucous membranes. If contact with eyes or mucous membranes occurs, immediately flush with water for 15 minutes. PAPLEX and PAPLEX ULTRA should *not* be allowed to contact normal skin surrounding wart. Treatment should be discontinued if excessive irritation occurs.
PAPLEX and PAPLEX ULTRA are flammable and should be kept away from fire or flame. Keep bottle tightly capped when not in use.

ADVERSE REACTIONS
A localized irritant reaction may occur if PAPLEX or PAPLEX ULTRA is applied to the normal skin surrounding the wart. Any irritation may normally be controlled by temporarily discontinuing use of PAPLEX and PAPLEX ULTRA and by applying the medication only to the wart site when treatment is resumed.

DOSAGE AND ADMINISTRATION
Prior to application of PAPLEX or PAPLEX ULTRA, soak wart in warm water for five minutes. remove any loosened tissue by gently rubbing with a brush, wash cloth, or emery board. Dry thoroughly. Using the brush applicator supplied, apply twice to affected area, allowing the first application to dry before applying the second. Treatment should be once a day and should continue as directed by physician. Be careful not to apply to surrounding skin.
Clinically visible improvement will normally occur during the first two to four weeks of therapy. Maximum resolution may be expected after six to twelve weeks of drug use.

HOW SUPPLIED
PAPLEX is supplied in a ½ fl oz (15 mL) bottle with brush applicator, NDC 99207-617-01.
PAPLEX ULTRA is supplied in a ½ fl oz (15 mL) bottle with brush applicator, NDC 99207-626-01.
For special handling and storage conditions see PRECAUTIONS section.
Store at Controlled Room Temperature 15°–30°C (59°–86°F). Keep out of reach of children.
For external use only. Not for ophthalmic use.

CAUTION
Federal law prohibits dispensing without prescription.
Mfd. by Syosset Laboratories Co., Inc., Syosset, NY 11791
Dist. by Medicis Dermatologics, Inc. New York, NY 10017

THERAMYCIN™ Z   ℞
ERYTHROMYCIN
TOPICAL SOLUTION 2%

DESCRIPTION
THERAMYCIN Z (Erythromycin Topical Solution 2%) is an antibiotic produced from a strain of *Streptomyces erythraeus*. It is basic and readily forms salts with acids. The active ingredient is represented by the following structure:
[See chemical structure at top of next column.]

CONTENTS
Each mL of THERAMYCIN Z (Erythromycin Topical Solution 2%) Contains: ACTIVE: Erythromycin, USP, 20mg in a clear solution vehicle of; INACTIVES: SD Alcohol 40B 81% (by weight) equivalent to Absolute Alcohol 86% (by volume), Hydroxypropyl Cellulose, Zinc Acetate, Propylene Glycol, Lauramide DEA and Fragrance.

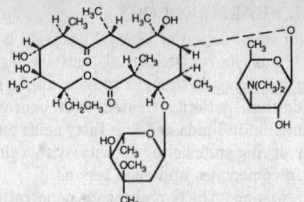

CLINICAL PHARMACOLOGY
Although the mechanism by which Erythromycin Topical Solution 2% acts in reducing inflammatory lesions of acne vulgaris is unknown, it is presumably due to its antibiotic action.

INDICATIONS AND USAGE
Erythromycin Topical Solution 2% is indicated for the topical control of acne vulgaris.

CONTRAINDICATIONS
Erythromycin Topical Solution 2% is contraindicated in persons who have shown hypersensitivity to erythromycin or any of the other listed ingredients.

WARNING
The safe use of Erythromycin Topical Solution 2% during pregnancy or lactation has *not* been established.

PRECAUTIONS
General—The use of antibiotic agents may be associated with the overgrowth of antibiotic-resistant organisms. If this occurs, administration of this drug should be discontinued and appropriate measures taken.
Information for Patients—Erythromycin Topical Solution 2% is for external use only and should be kept away from the eyes, nose, mouth and other mucous membranes. Concomitant topical acne therapy should be used with caution because a cumulative irritant effect may occur, especially with the use of peeling, desquamating, or abrasive agents.
Carcinogenesis, Mutagenesis, Impairment of Fertility—Long-term animal studies to evaluate carcinogenic potential, mutagenicity, or the effect on fertility of erythromycin have *not* been performed.
Pregnancy—Pregnancy Category C. Animal reproduction studies have *not* been conducted with erythromycin. It is also *not* known whether erythromycin can cause fetal harm when administered to a pregnant woman or can affect reproduction capacity. Erythromycin should be given to a pregnant woman only if clearly needed.
Nursing Mothers—Erythromycin is excreted in breast milk. Caution should be exercised when erythromycin is administered to a nursing mother.

ADVERSE REACTIONS
Adverse conditions reported include dryness, pruritus, desquamation, erythema, oiliness, and burning sensation. Irritation of the eyes has also been reported. A case of generalized urticarial reaction, possibly related to the drug, which required the use of systemic steroid therapy has been reported.

DOSAGE AND ADMINISTRATION
The THERAMYCIN Z (Erythromycin Topical Solution 2%) ball type applicator should be rubbed twice a day, once in the morning and once in the evening, to areas usually affected by acne. These areas should be washed with warm water and soap and patted dry before applying the THERAMYCIN Z. Shake well before using and close tightly after each use.

HOW SUPPLIED
THERAMYCIN Z (Erythromycin Topical Solution 2%), 2 fl oz (59.14 mL) in a 60 mL plastic bottle with applicator attached—NDC 99207-550-02.

STORAGE
THERAMYCIN Z (Erythromycin Topical Solution 2%) should be stored at Controlled Room Temperature 15°–30° C (59°–86°F). Preserve in a light-resistant container.

INSTRUCTIONS FOR INSTALLING APPLICATOR
1. Remove and discard temporary shipping cap.
2. Push applicator firmly into bottle using white cap as holder.
3. Screw cap down to seat applicator.

WARNINGS
Contains Alcohol—Do not use near open flame.
For external use only. Not for ophthalmic use.
Keep out of reach of children.

CAUTION
Federal law prohibits dispensing without prescription.
Mfd. by Syosset Laboratories Co., Inc., Syosset, NY 11791
Dist. by Medicis Dermatologics, Inc., New York, NY 10017

THERAPLEX® ClearLotion®   OTC

COMPOSITION
Mineral Oil, Cyclomethicone, Jojoba Oil, Special Petrolatum Fraction.

ACTION AND USES
Theraplex® ClearLotion® is a unique, rapidly penetrating, nongreasy emollient that provides these benefits:
- Special petrolatum fraction and conditioning system relieves dryness and increases moisture retention in the skin.
- The emolliency of Theraplex® ClearLotion® softens, smooths and relieves dryness and scaliness.
- Hypoallergenic, noncomedogenic, preservative and fragrance free.

DIRECTIONS
For best results, use Theraplex® ClearLotion® twice a day (especially after bathing) or as necessary.

HOW SUPPLIED
8 fl oz (240 ml), NDC #99207-102-02, Plastic Bottle

THERAPLEX® Emollient   OTC

COMPOSITION
Special Petrolatum Fraction, Cyclomethicone, Microcrystalline Wax.

ACTIONS AND USES
Theraplex® Emollient is formulated from a highly active emollient fraction of petrolatum and with an Activated Hydrosilicone™ system. Theraplex®:
- Is nongreasy.
- Forms a semipermeable layer that smooths and softens skin against environmental drying.
- Allows the skin to breathe without interfering with normal perspiration and helps moisture from within the skin to hydrate the skin's surface.
- Is nonallergenic, noncomedogenic, free of fragrance and preservatives.

DIRECTIONS
Apply twice daily or as directed by physician.

HOW SUPPLIED
4.3 oz (120 g), NDC # 99207-101-02.

THERAPLEX® HydroLotion®   OTC

COMPOSITION
Water, Dimethicone Copolyol, Cyclomethicone, Special Petrolatum Fraction, SD Alcohol-40, Benzyl Alcohol, Sodium Chloride, Sorbitan Laurate.

ACTION AND USES
Theraplex® HydroLotion® is a unique, greaseless, water in oil emulsion featuring a hydrosilicone moisturizing system. It contains a special petrolatum fraction that provides deep moisturization and rich emolliency to chronically dry skin. Theraplex® HydroLotion® also offers:
- Immediate and sustained relief of dryness, dryness-induced itching and skin tightness.
- Sustained softness.
- Moisture retention within the skin.
- Nonallergenic, noncomedogenic and fragrance free.

DIRECTIONS
Use Theraplex® HydroLotion® twice a day, under makeup, after shaving or as directed by your physician. Keep from freezing.

HOW SUPPLIED
8 fl oz (240 ml), NDC #99207-105-02, Plastic Bottle

THERAPLEX® T Shampoo   OTC

COMPOSITION
Active Ingredient: Coal Tar 1%. Inactive Ingredients: Water, Sodium Laureth Sulfate, Cocamide DEA, Polysorbate 20, Hectorite, Benzyl Alcohol, Hexylene Glycol, Eugenol, Fragrance.

ACTION AND USES
A therapeutic shampoo that relieves the itching, irritation and flaking associated with psoriasis, seborrheic dermatitis and dandruff. Specially formulated in an Activated Delivery System™ with polysorbate 20 to loosen, soften and wash away scales and crusts, and benzyl alcohol to speed delivery

Continued on next page

Medicis—Cont.

of the coal tar through scales and sebum. Contains special conditioners that keep hair lustrous and manageable.

DIRECTIONS

SHAKE WELL BEFORE USING. Wet hair thoroughly. Apply a liberal amount of Theraplex® T Shampoo and massage into a lather. Leave lather on scalp for several minutes. Rinse thoroughly and repeat. Use Theraplex® T Shampoo daily to control problem, then at least twice weekly or as directed by your physician.

PRECAUTIONS

For external use only. Avoid contact with eyes. In case of contact, wash out with water. If irritation occurs, discontinue use and consult physician. In rare instances, discoloration of gray, blond or tinted hair may occur. Keep this and all medications out of the reach of children.

HOW SUPPLIED

8 fl oz (240 ml), NDC # 99207-103-02, Plastic Bottle

THERAPLEX® Z Shampoo   OTC

COMPOSITION

Active Ingredient: Zinc Pyrithione 2%. Inactive Ingredients: Water TEA Lauryl Sulfate Cocamide DEA, Hectorite, Ethylcellulose, Panthenol, Jojoba Oil, Methyl Paraben Fragrance, Tocopherol, Hydrolyzed Animal Protein, Propyl Paraben, FD&C Blue No. 1.

ACTION AND USES

A therapeutic shampoo with special conditioners to relieve the itching, irritation and skin flaking associated with dandruff and seborrheic dermatitis of the scalp. Leaves your hair and scalp clean without overcleaning. The Theraplex® Activated Conditioning System™ conditions and enhances the body, manageability and sheen of your hair while minimizing split ends and premature breakage.

DIRECTION

SHAKE WELL BEFORE USING. Wet hair throughly. Apply a liberal amount of Theraplex® Z Shampoo and massage into a lather. Leave lather on scalp for several minutes. Rinse thoroughly and repeat. Use Theraplex® Z Shampoo daily to control problem, then at least twice weekly or as directed by your physician.

PRECAUTIONS

For external use only. Avoid contact with eyes. In case of contact, wash out with water. If irritation occurs, discontinue use and consult physician. Keep this and all medications out of the reach of children.

HOW SUPPLIED

8 fl oz (240 ml), NDC #99207-104-02, Plastic Bottle

THEROXIDE™ 5%   ℞
(BENZOYL PEROXIDE 5% LOTION)
THEROXIDE™10%   ℞
(BENZOYL PEROXIDE 10% LOTION)
THEROXIDE™ WASH   ℞
(BENZOYL PEROXIDE 10%)

DESCRIPTION

Theroxide 5%, Theroxide 10% Lotions and Theroxide Wash are topical, water-base, benzoyl peroxide containing preparations for use in the treatment of acne vulgaris. Benzoyl peroxide is an oxidizing agent that possesses antibacterial properties and is classified as a keratolytic. Benzoyl peroxide $(C_{14}H_{10}O_4)$ is represented by the following chemical structure:

$$O=C-O-O-C=O$$

Theroxide 5% and Theroxide 10% Lotions contain, respectively, benzoyl peroxide 5% and 10% as the active ingredient in a lotion-based formulation containing purified water, glyceryl stearate, PEG-100 stearate, dried aluminum hydroxide gel, tridecyl stearate, cetyl alcohol, polyethylene glycol (400), glycereth-26, dimethicone copolyol, neopentylglycol dicaprylate/dicaprate, sodium citrate, citric acid, methylparaben, fragrance, menthol, camphor and propylparaben.
Theroxide Wash contains benzoyl peroxide 10% as the active ingredient in a vehicle consisting of purified water, sodium methyl cocoyl taurate, glyceryl stearate SE, cocamidoöropyl betaine, hydroxypropyl methycellulose, C12–C15 alcohols benzoate, citric acid, fragrance and benzoic acid.

CLINICAL PHARMACOLOGY

The mechanism of action of benzoyl peroxide is not totally understood but its antibacterial activity against _Propionibacterium acnes_ is thought to be a major mode of action. In addition, patients treated with benzoyl peroxide show a reduction in lipids and free fatty acids and mild desquamation (drying and peeling activity) with a simultaneous reduction in comedones and acne lesions.
Little is known about the percutaneous penetration, metabolism, and excretion of benzoyl peroxide, although it has been shown that benzoyl peroxide absorbed by the skin is metabolized to benzoic acid and then excreted as benzoate in the urine. There is no evidence of systemic toxicity caused by benzoyl peroxide in humans.

INDICATIONS AND USAGE

Theroxide 5%, Theroxide 10% and Theroxide Wash are indicated for the topical treatment of acne vulgaris.

CONTRAINDICATIONS

These preparations are contraindicated in patients with a history of hypersensitivity to any of their components.

PRECAUTIONS

General: For external use only. If severe irritation develops, discontinue use and institute appropriate therapy. After the reaction clears, treatment may often be resumed with less frequent application. These preparations should not be used in or near the eyes or on mucous membranes.
Information for patients: Avoid contact with eyes, eyelids, lips and mucous membranes. If accidental contact occurs, rinse with water. Contact with any colored material (including hair and fabric) may result in bleaching or discoloration. If excessive irritation develops, discontinue use and consult your physician.
Carcinogenesis, Mutagenesis, Impairment of Fertility: Data from several studies employing a strain of mice that are highly susceptible to developing cancer suggests that benzoyl peroxide acts as a tumor promoter. The clinical significance of these findings to humans is unknown. Benzoyl peroxide has not been found to be mutagenic (Ames Test) and there are no published data indicating it impairs fertility.
Pregnancy: Teratogenic Effects Pregnancy Category C: Animal reproduction studies have not been conducted with benzoyl peroxide. It is not known whether benzoyl peroxide can cause fetal harm when administered to a pregnant woman or can affect reproduction capacity. Benzoyl peroxide should be used by a pregnant woman only if clearly needed. There are no available data on the effect of benzoyl peroxide on the later growth, development and functional maturation of the unborn child.
Nursing Mothers: It is not known whether this drug is excreted in human milk. Because many drugs are excreted in human milk, caution should be exercised when benzoyl peroxide is administered to a nursing woman.
Pediatric Use: Safety and effectiveness in children have not been established.

ADVERSE REACTIONS

Allergic contact dermatitis and dryness have been reported with topical benzoyl peroxide therapy.

OVERDOSAGE

If excessive scaling, erythema or edema occur, the use of this preparation should be discontinued. To hasten resolution of the adverse effects, cool compresses may be used. After symptoms and signs subside, a reduced dosage schedule may be cautiously tried if the reaction is judged to be due to excessive use and not allergenicity.

DOSAGE AND ADMINISTRATION

Theroxide Lotion: Apply once or twice daily to cover affected areas after washing with a mild cleanser and water.
Theroxide Wash: SHAKE WELL BEFORE USE. Wash affected areas once or twice daily, avoid contact with eyes or mucous membranes. Wet skin areas to be treated prior to administration; apply, work to a full lather, rinse thoroughly and pat dry. The amount of drying or peeling may be controlled by modification of dosage frequency.

HOW SUPPLIED

Theroxide 5% Lotion—1.5 oz (42.5 g) tube, NDC 99207-505-15. **Theroxide 10% Lotion**—1.5 oz (42.5 g) tube, NDC 99207-510-15. **Theroxide Wash**—4 oz bottle, NDC 99207-520-04.
Caution: Federal law prohibits dispensing without prescription. Store at controlled room temperature (59°–86°F).
Manufactured for:
Medicis Dermatologics, Inc. New York, NY 10017.
Manufactured by:
Dermatological Products of Texas, Inc., San Antonio, TX 78296.

126564 10/90

Merck & Co., Inc.
WEST POINT, PA 19486

Product Identification Codes

To provide quick and positive identification of Merck products, we have imprinted a code number on tablet and capsule products. In order that you may identify a product by its code number, we have compiled below a numerical list of code numbers with their corresponding product names. We are also listing the code numbers by alphabetical listing of products as a cross reference.
The code number as it appears on tablets and capsules bears the letters MSD plus the numerical code. Decadron® (Dexamethasone) tablets 0.25 mg is identified MSD 20.

Numerical Listing

MSD Code No.	Product	Product No.
14	Vasotec® (Enalapril Maleate) Tablets 2.5 mg	3411
19	Prinivil® (Lisinopril) Tablets 5 mg	3577
20	Decadron® (Dexamethasone) Tablets 0.25 mg	7592
21	Cogentin® (Benztropine Mesylate) Tablets 0.5 mg	3297
25	Indocin® (Indomethacin) Capsules 25 mg	3316
26	Vivactil® (Protriptyline HCl) Tablets 5 mg	3313
41	Decadron® (Dexamethasone) Tablets 0.5 mg	7598
42	HydroDIURIL® (Hydrochlorothiazide) Tablets 25 mg	3263
43	Mephyton® (Phytonadione) Tablets 5 mg	7776
47	Vivactil® (Protriptyline HCl) Tablets 10 mg	3314
49	Daranide® (Dichlorphenamide) Tablets 50 mg	3256
50	Indocin® (Indomethacin) Capsules 50 mg	3317
52	Inversine® (Mecamylamine HCl) Tablets 2.5 mg	3219
53	Hydropres® 25 (Reserpine-Hydrochlorothiazide) Tablets	3265
59	Blocadren® (Timolol Maleate) Tablets 5 mg	3343
60	Cogentin® (Benztropine Mesylate) Tablets 2 mg	3172
62	Periactin® (Cyproheptadine HCl) Tablets 4 mg	3276
63	Decadron® (Dexamethasone) Tablets 0.75 mg	7601
65	Edecrin® (Ethacrynic Acid) Tablets 25 mg	3321
67	Timolide® 10-25 (Timolol Maleate-Hydrochlorothiazide) Tablets	3373
90	Edecrin® (Ethacrynic Acid) Tablets 50 mg	3322
92	Midamor® (Amiloride HCl) Tablets 5 mg	3381
95	Decadron® (Dexamethasone) Tablets 1.5 mg	7638
97	Decadron® (Dexamethasone) Tablets 4 mg	7645
105	HydroDIURIL® (Hydrochlorothiazide) Tablets 50 mg	3264
106	Prinivil® (Lisinopril) Tablets 10 mg	3578
127	Hydropres® 50 (Reserpine-Hydrochlorothiazide) Tablets	3266
135	Aldomet® (Methyldopa) Tablets 125 mg	3341
136	Blocadren® (Timolol Maleate) Tablets 10 mg	3344
140	Prinzide® 12.5 (Lisinopril-Hydrochlorothiazide) Tablets	3594
142	Prinzide® 25 (Lisinopril-Hydrochlorothiazide) Tablets	3595
147	Decadron® (Dexamethasone) Tablets 6 mg	7648
150	Indocin® (Indomethacin) Suppositories 50 mg	3354
207	Prinivil® (Lisinopril) Tablets 20 mg	3579
214	Diuril® (Chlorothiazide) Tablets 250 mg	3244
219	Cortone® (Cortisone Acetate) Tablets 25 mg	7063
230	Diupres-250® (Reserpine-Chlorothiazide) Tablets	3261

Code	Product	Product No.
237	Prinivil® (Lisinopril) Tablets 40 mg	3580
401	Aldomet® (Methyldopa) Tablets 250 mg	3290
403	Urecholine® (Bethanechol Chloride) Tablets 5 mg	7785
405	Diupres-500® (Reserpine-Chlorothiazide) Tablets	3262
410	HydroDIURIL® (Hydrochlorothiazide) Tablets 100 mg	3340
412	Urecholine® (Bethanechol Chloride) Tablets 10 mg	7787
423	Aldoril® 15 (Methyldopa-Hydrochlorothiazide) Tablets	3294
432	Diuril® (Chlorothiazide) Tablets 500 mg	3245
437	Blocadren® (Timolol Maleate) Tablets 20 mg	3371
451	Plendil® (Felodipine) Extended-Release Tablets 5 mg	3585
452	Plendil® (Felodipine) Extended-Release Tablets 10 mg	3586
456	Aldoril® 25 (Methyldopa-Hydrochlorothiazide) Tablets	3295
457	Urecholine® (Bethanechol Chloride) Tablets 25 mg	7788
460	Urecholine® (Bethanechol Chloride) Tablets 50 mg	7790
501	Benemid® (Probenecid) Tablets 0.5 g	3337
516	Aldomet® (Methyldopa) Tablets 500 mg	3292
517	Triavil® 4-50 (Perphenazine-Amitriptyline HCl) Tablets	3364
602	Cuprimine® (Penicillamine) Capsules 250 mg	3299
612	Aldoclor® 150 (Methyldopa-Chlorothiazide) Tablets	3318
614	ColBENEMID® (Probenecid-Colchicine) Tablets	3283
619	Hydrocortone® (Hydrocortisone) Tablets 10 mg	7604
625	Hydrocortone® (Hydrocortisone) Tablets 20 mg	7602
634	Aldoclor® 250 (Methyldopa-Chlorothiazide) Tablets	3319
635	Cogentin® (Benztropine Mesylate) Tablets 1 mg	3334
661	Syprine® (Trientine Hydrochloride) Capsules 250 mg	3408
672	Cuprimine® (Penicillamine) Capsules 125 mg	3350
675	Dolobid® (Diflunisal) Tablets 250 mg	3390
690	Demser® (Metyrosine) Capsules 250 mg	3355
693	Indocin® SR (Indomethacin) Sustained-Release Capsules 75 mg	3370
694	Aldoril® D30 (Methyldopa-Hydrochlorothiazide) Tablets	3362
697	Dolobid® (Diflunisal) Tablets 500 mg	3392
705	Noroxin® (Norfloxacin) Tablets 400 mg	3522
707	Tonocard® (Tocainide HCl) Tablets 400 mg	3409
709	Tonocard® (Tocainide HCl) Tablets 600 mg	3410
712	Vasotec® (Enalapril Maleate) Tablets 5 mg	3412
713	Vasotec® (Enalapril Maleate) Tablets 10 mg	3413
714	Vasotec® (Enalapril Maleate) Tablets 20 mg	3414
720	Vaseretic® 10–25 (Enalapril Maleate-Hydrochlorothiazide) Tablets	3418
726	Zocor® (Simvastatin) Tablets 5 mg	3588
730	Mevacor® (Lovastatin) Tablets 10 mg	3560
731	Mevacor® (Lovastatin) Tablets 20 mg	3561
732	Mevacor® (Lovastatin) Tablets 40 mg	3562
735	Zocor® (Simvastatin) Tablets 10 mg	3589
740	Zocor® (Simvastatin) Tablets 20 mg	3590
742	Prilosec® (Omeprazole) Delayed-Released Capsules 20 mg	3440
749	Zocor® (Simvastatin) Tablets 40 mg	3591
907	Mintezol® (Thiabendazole) Chewable Tablets 500 mg	3332
914	Triavil® 2-10 (Perphenazine-Amitriptyline HCl) Tablets	3328
917	Moduretic® (Amiloride HCl-Hydrochlorothiazide) Tablets	3385
921	Triavil® 2-25 (Perphenazine-Amitriptyline HCl) Tablets	3311
931	Flexeril® (Cyclobenzaprine HCl) Tablets 10 mg	3358
934	Triavil® 4-10 (Perphenazine-Amitriptyline HCl) Tablets	3310
935	Aldoril® D50 (Methyldopa-Hydrochlorothiazide) Tablets	3363
941	Clinoril® (Sulindac) Tablets 150 mg	3360
942	Clinoril® (Sulindac) Tablets 200 mg	3353
946	Triavil® 4-25 (Perphenazine-Amitriptyline HCl) Tablets	3312
963	Pepcid® (Famotidine) Tablets 20 mg	3535
964	Pepcid® (Famotidine) Tablets 40 mg	3536

Alphabetical Listing

MSD Code No.	Product	Product No.
612	Aldoclor® 150 (Methyldopa-Chlorothiazide) Tablets	3318
634	Aldoclor® 250 (Methyldopa-Chlorothiazide) Tablets	3319
135	Aldomet® (Methyldopa) Tablets 125 mg	3341
401	Aldomet® (Methyldopa) Tablets 250 mg	3290
516	Aldomet® (Methyldopa) Tablets 500 mg	3292
423	Aldoril® 15 (Methyldopa-Hydrochlorothiazide) Tablets	3294
456	Aldoril® 25 (Methyldopa-Hydrochlorothiazide) Tablets	3295
694	Aldoril® D30 (Methyldopa-Hydrochlorothiazide) Tablets	3362
935	Aldoril® D50 (Methyldopa-Hydrochlorothiazide) Tablets	3363
501	Benemid® (Probenecid) Tablets 0.5 g	3337
59	Blocadren® (Timolol Maleate) Tablets 5 mg	3343
136	Blocadren® (Timolol Maleate) Tablets 10 mg	3344
437	Blocadren® (Timolol Maleate) Tablets 20 mg	3371
941	Clinoril® (Sulindac) Tablets 150 mg	3360
942	Clinoril® (Sulindac) Tablets 200 mg	3353
21	Cogentin® (Benztropine Mesylate) Tablets 0.5 mg	3297
635	Cogentin® (Benztropine Mesylate) Tablets 1 mg	3334
60	Cogentin® (Benztropine Mesylate) Tablets 2 mg	3172
614	ColBENEMID® (Probenecid-Colchicine) Tablets	3283
219	Cortone® (Cortisone Acetate) Tablets 25 mg	7063
672	Cuprimine® (Penicillamine) Capsules 125 mg	3350
602	Cuprimine® (Penicillamine) Capsules 250 mg	3299
49	Daranide® (Dichlorphenamide) Tablets 50 mg	3256
20	Decadron® (Dexamethasone) Tablets 0.25 mg	7592
41	Decadron® (Dexamethasone) Tablets 0.5 mg	7598
63	Decadron® (Dexamethasone) Tablets 0.75 mg	7601
95	Decadron® (Dexamethasone) Tablets 1.5 mg	7638
97	Decadron® (Dexamethasone) Tablets 4 mg	7645
147	Decadron® (Dexamethasone) Tablets 6 mg	7648
690	Demser® (Metyrosine) Capsules 250 mg	3355
230	Diupres-250® (Reserpine-Chlorothiazide) Tablets	3261
405	Diupres-500® (Reserpine-Chlorothiazide) Tablets	3262
214	Diuril® (Chlorothiazide) Tablets 250 mg	3244
432	Diuril® (Chlorothiazide) Tablets 500 mg	3245
675	Dolobid® (Diflunisal) Tablets 250 mg	3390
697	Dolobid® (Diflunisal) Tablets 500 mg	3392
65	Edecrin® (Ethacrynic Acid) Tablets 25 mg	3321
90	Edecrin® (Ethacrynic Acid) Tablets 50 mg	3322
931	Flexeril® (Cyclobenzaprine HCl) Tablets 10 mg	3358
619	Hydrocortone® (Hydrocortisone) Tablets 10 mg	7604
625	Hydrocortone® (Hydrocortisone) Tablets 20 mg	7602
42	HydroDIURIL® (Hydrochlorothiazide) Tablets 25 mg	3263
105	HydroDIURIL® (Hydrochlorothiazide) Tablets 50 mg	3264
410	HydroDIURIL® (Hydrochlorothiazide) Tablets 100 mg	3340
53	Hydropres® 25 (Reserpine-Hydrochlorothiazide) Tablets	3265
127	Hydropres® 50 (Reserpine-Hydrochlorothiazide) Tablets	3266
25	Indocin® (Indomethacin) Capsules 25 mg	3316
50	Indocin® (Indomethacin) Capsules 50 mg	3317
693	Indocin® SR (Indomethacin) Sustained-Release Capsules 75 mg	3370
150	Indocin® (Indomethacin) Suppositories 50 mg	3354
52	Inversine® (Mecamylamine HCl) Tablets 2.5 mg	3219
43	Mephyton® (Phytonadione) Tablets 5 mg	7776
730	Mevacor® (Lovastatin) Tablets 10 mg	3560
731	Mevacor® (Lovastatin) Tablets 20 mg	3561
732	Mevacor® (Lovastatin) Tablets 40 mg	3562
92	Midamor® (Amiloride HCl) Tablets 5 mg	3381
907	Mintezol® (Thiabendazole) Chewable Tablets 500 mg	3332
917	Moduretic® (Amiloride HCl-Hydrochlorothiazide) Tablets	3385
705	Noroxin® (Norfloxacin) Tablets 400 mg	3522
963	Pepcid® (Famotidine) Tablets 20 mg	3535
964	Pepcid® (Famotidine) Tablets 40 mg	3536
62	Periactin® (Cyproheptadine HCl) Tablets 4 mg	3276
451	Plendil® (Felodipine) Extended-Release Tablets 5 mg	3585
452	Plendil® (Felodipine) Extended-Release Tablets 10 mg	3586
742	Prilosec® (Omeprazole) Delayed-Release Capsules 20 mg	3440
19	Prinivil® (Lisinopril) Tablets 5 mg	3577
106	Prinivil® (Lisinopril) Tablets 10 mg	3578
207	Prinivil® (Lisinopril) Tablets 20 mg	3579
237	Prinivil® (Lisinopril) Tablets 40 mg	3580
140	Prinzide® 12.5 (Lisinopril-Hydrochlorothiazide) Tablets	3594
142	Prinzide® 25 (Lisinopril-Hydrochlorothiazide) Tablets	3595
661	Syprine® (Trientine Hydrochloride) Capsules 250 mg	3408
67	Timolide® 10-25 (Timolol Maleate-Hydrochlorothiazide) Tablets	3373
707	Tonocard® (Tocainide HCl) Tablets 400 mg	3409
709	Tonocard® (Tocainide HCl) Tablets 600 mg	3410
914	Triavil® 2-10 (Perphenazine-Amitriptyline HCl) Tablets	3328
921	Triavil® 2-25 (Perphenazine-Amitriptyline HCl) Tablets	3311
934	Triavil® 4-10 (Perphenazine-Amitriptyline HCl) Tablets	3310
946	Triavil® 4-25 (Perphenazine-Amitriptyline HCl) Tablets	3312

Continued on next page

Information on the Merck & Co. products listed on these pages is the full prescribing information from product circulars in use October 1, 1992.

Merck & Co.—Cont.

ALDOCLOR® Tablets   ℞
(Methyldopa-Chlorothiazide), U.S.P.

WARNING

This fixed combination drug is not indicated for initial therapy of hypertension. Hypertension requires therapy titrated to the individual patient. If the fixed combination represents the dosage so determined, its use may be more convenient in patient management. The treatment of hypertension is not static, but must be re-evaluated as conditions in each patient warrant.

DESCRIPTION

ALDOCLOR* (Methyldopa-Chlorothiazide) combines two antihypertensives: methyldopa and chlorothiazide.
Methyldopa
Methyldopa is an antihypertensive and is the *L*-isomer of alpha-methyldopa. It is levo-3-(3,4-dihydroxyphenyl)-2-methylalanine. Its empirical formula is $C_{10}H_{13}NO_4$, with a molecular weight of 211.22, and its structural formula is:

Methyldopa is a white to yellowish white, odorless fine powder, and is soluble in water.
Chlorothiazide
Chlorothiazide is a diuretic and antihypertensive. It is 6-chloro-2*H*-1, 2, 4-benzothiadiazine-7-sulfonamide 1, 1-dioxide. Its empirical formula is $C_7H_6ClN_3O_4S_2$ and its structural formula is:

It is a white, or practically white crystalline powder with a molecular weight of 295.72, which is very slightly soluble in water, but readily soluble in dilute aqueous sodium hydroxide. It is soluble in urine to the extent of about 150 mg per 100 mL at pH 7.
ALDOCLOR is supplied as tablets in two strengths for oral use:
ALDOCLOR 150, contains 250 mg of methyldopa and 150 mg of chlorothiazide.
ALDOCLOR 250, contains 250 mg of methyldopa and 250 mg of chlorothiazide.

Each tablet contains the following inactive ingredients: calcium disodium edetate, cellulose, citric acid, D&C Yellow 10, ethylcellulose, FD&C Yellow 6, gelatin, glycerin, guar gum, hydroxypropyl methylcellulose, magnesium stearate, starch, talc, and titanium dioxide. ALDOCLOR 150 also contains iron oxides. ALDOCLOR 250 also contains FD&C Blue 2.

*Registered trademark of MERCK & CO., INC.

CLINICAL PHARMACOLOGY

Methyldopa
Methyldopa is an aromatic-amino-acid decarboxylase inhibitor in animals and in man. Although the mechanism of action has yet to be conclusively demonstrated, the antihypertensive effect of methyldopa probably is due to its metabolism to alpha-methylnorepinephrine, which then lowers arterial pressure by stimulation of central inhibitory alpha-adrenergic receptors, false neurotransmission, and/or reduction of plasma renin activity. Methyldopa has been shown to cause a net reduction in the tissue concentration of serotonin, dopamine, norepinephrine, and epinephrine.
Only methyldopa, the *L*-isomer of alpha-methyldopa, has the ability to inhibit dopa decarboxylase and to deplete animal tissues of norepinephrine. In man, the antihypertensive activity appears to be due solely to the *L*-isomer. About twice the dose of the racemate (*DL*-alpha-methyldopa) is required for equal antihypertensive effect.
Methyldopa has no direct effect on cardiac function and usually does not reduce glomerular filtration rate, renal blood flow, or filtration fraction. Cardiac output usually is maintained without cardiac acceleration. In some patients the heart rate is slowed.
Normal or elevated plasma renin activity may decrease in the course of methyldopa therapy.
Methyldopa reduces both supine and standing blood pressure. It usually produces highly effective lowering of the supine pressure with infrequent symptomatic postural hypotension. Exercise hypotension and diurnal blood pressure variations rarely occur.
Chlorothiazide
The mechanism of the antihypertensive effect of thiazides is unknown. Chlorothiazide does not usually affect normal blood pressure.
Chlorothiazide affects the distal renal tubular mechanism of electrolyte reabsorption. At maximal therapeutic dosage all thiazides are approximately equal in their diuretic efficacy. Chlorothiazide increases excretion of sodium and chloride in approximately equivalent amounts. Natriuresis may be accompanied by some loss of potassium and bicarbonate.
After oral use diuresis begins within 2 hours, peaks in about 4 hours and lasts about 6 to 12 hours.
Methyldopa-Chlorothiazide
The concomitant use of methyldopa and chlorothiazide, as provided in ALDOCLOR, frequently produces a more pronounced antihypertensive response than when either compound is the sole therapeutic agent. Particularly in those cases of hypertensive vascular disease where sodium and water retention is a problem, the coadministration of these two drugs in the form of ALDOCLOR will help control the fluid imbalance.
In severe essential hypertension and in malignant hypertension, ALDOCLOR may achieve effective lowering of blood pressure with fewer side effects than occur with other compounds used for this purpose.
ALDOCLOR reduces both supine and standing blood pressure; more effective lowering of the supine pressure with less frequent symptomatic postural hypotension can be obtained with ALDOCLOR than with most other antihypertensive agents. In patients treated with ALDOCLOR, exercise hypotension and diurnal blood pressure variations rarely occur.
Pharmacokinetics and Metabolism
Methyldopa
The maximum decrease in blood pressure occurs four to six hours after oral dosage. Once an effective dosage level is attained, a smooth blood pressure response occurs in most patients in 12 to 24 hours. After withdrawal, blood pressure usually returns to pretreatment levels within 24–48 hours. Methyldopa is extensively metabolized. The known urinary metabolites are: α-methyldopa mono-0-sulfate; 3-0 methyl-α-methyldopa; 3,4,-dihydroxyphenylacetone; α-methyldopamine; 3-0-methyl-α-methyldopamine and their conjugates. Approximately 70 percent of the drug which is absorbed is excreted in the urine as methyldopa and its mono-0-sulfate conjugate. The renal clearance is about 130 mL/min in normal subjects and is diminished in renal insufficiency. The plasma half-life of methyldopa is 105 minutes. After oral doses, excretion is essentially complete in 36 hours. Methyldopa crosses the placental barrier, appears in cord blood, and appears in breast milk.
Chlorothiazide
Chlorothiazide is not metabolized but is eliminated rapidly by the kidney. The plasma half-life is 45–120 minutes. After oral doses, 20–24 percent of the dose is excreted unchanged

in the urine. Chlorothiazide crosses the placental but not the blood-brain barrier and is excreted in breast milk.

INDICATION AND USAGE

Hypertension (see box warning).
Use in Pregnancy. Routine use of diuretics during normal pregnancy is inappropriate and exposes mother and fetus to unnecessary hazard. Diuretics do not prevent development of toxemia of pregnancy and there is no satisfactory evidence that they are useful in the treatment of toxemia.
Edema during pregnancy may arise from pathologic causes or from the physiologic and mechanical consequences of pregnancy. Thiazides are indicated in pregnancy when edema is due to pathologic causes, just as they are in the absence of pregnancy (see PRECAUTIONS, *Pregnancy*). Dependent edema in pregnancy, resulting from restriction of venous return by the gravid uterus, is properly treated through elevation of the lower extremities and use of support stockings. Use of diuretics to lower intravascular volume in this instance is illogical and unnecessary. During normal pregnancy there is hypervolemia which is not harmful to the fetus or the mother in the absence of cardiovascular disease. However, it may be associated with edema, rarely generalized edema. If such edema causes discomfort, increased recumbency will often provide relief. Rarely this edema may cause extreme discomfort which is not relieved by rest. In these instances, a short course of diuretic therapy, may provide relief and be appropriate.

CONTRAINDICATIONS

Active hepatic disease, such as acute hepatitis and active cirrhosis.
If previous methyldopa therapy has been associated with liver disorders (see WARNINGS).
Anuria.
Hypersensitivity to methyldopa, or to chlorothiazide or other sulfonamide-derived drugs.

WARNINGS

Methyldopa
It is important to recognize that a positive Coombs test, hemolytic anemia, and liver disorders may occur with methyldopa therapy. The rare occurrences of hemolytic anemia or liver disorders could lead to potentially fatal complications unless properly recognized and managed. Read this section carefully to understand these reactions.
With prolonged methyldopa therapy, 10 to 20 percent of patients develop a positive direct Coombs test which usually occurs between 6 and 12 months of methyldopa therapy. Lowest incidence is at daily dosage of 1 g or less. This on rare occasions may be associated with hemolytic anemia, which could lead to potentially fatal complications. One cannot predict which patients with a positive direct Coombs test may develop hemolytic anemia.
Prior existence or development of a positive direct Coombs test is not in itself a contraindication to use of methyldopa. If a positive Coombs test develops during methyldopa therapy, the physician should determine whether hemolytic anemia exists and whether the positive Coombs test may be a problem. For example, in addition to a positive direct Coombs test there is less often a positive indirect Coombs test which may interfere with cross matching of blood.
Before treatment is started, it is desirable to do a blood count (hematocrit, hemoglobin, or red cell count) for a baseline or to establish whether there is anemia. Periodic blood counts should be done during therapy to detect hemolytic anemia. It may be useful to do a direct Coombs test before therapy and at 6 and 12 months after the start of therapy.
If Coombs-positive hemolytic anemia occurs, the cause may be methyldopa and the drug should be discontinued. Usually the anemia remits promptly. If not, corticosteroids may be given and other causes of anemia should be considered. If the hemolytic anemia is related to methyldopa, the drug should not be reinstituted.
When methyldopa causes Coombs positivity alone or with hemolytic anemia, the red cell is usually coated with gamma globulin of the IgG (gamma G) class only. The positive Coombs test may not revert to normal until weeks to months after methyldopa is stopped.
Should the need for transfusion arise in a patient receiving methyldopa, both a direct and an indirect Coombs test should be performed. In the absence of hemolytic anemia, usually only the direct Coombs test will be positive. A positive direct Coombs test alone will not interfere with typing or cross matching. If the indirect Coombs test is also positive, problems may arise in the major cross match and the assistance of a hematologist or transfusion expert will be needed. Occasionally, fever has occurred within the first three weeks of methyldopa therapy, associated in some cases with eosinophilia or abnormalities in one or more liver function tests, such as serum alkaline phosphatase, serum transaminases (SGOT, SGPT), bilirubin, and prothrombin time. Jaundice,

with or without fever, may occur with onset usually within the first two to three months of therapy. In some patients the findings are consistent with those of cholestasis. In others the findings are consistent with hepatitis and hepatocellular injury.

Rarely fatal hepatic necrosis has been reported after use of methyldopa. These hepatic changes may represent hypersensitivity reactions. Periodic determination of hepatic function should be done particularly during the first 6 to 12 weeks of therapy or whenever an unexplained fever occurs. If fever, abnormalities in liver function tests, or jaundice appear, stop therapy with methyldopa. If caused by methyldopa, the temperature and abnormalities in liver function characteristically have reverted to normal when the drug was discontinued. Methyldopa should not be reinstituted in such patients.

Rarely, a reversible reduction of the white blood cell count with a primary effect on the granulocytes has been seen. The granulocyte count returned promptly to normal on discontinuance of the drug. Rare cases of granulocytopenia have been reported. In each instance, upon stopping the drug, the white cell count returned to normal. Reversible thrombocytopenia has occurred rarely.

Chlorothiazide

Use with caution in severe renal disease. In patients with renal disease, thiazides may precipitate azotemia. Cumulative effects of the drug may develop in patients with impaired renal function.

Thiazides should be used with caution in patients with impaired hepatic function or progressive liver disease, since minor alterations of fluid and electrolyte balance may precipitate hepatic coma.

Thiazides may add to or potentiate the action of other antihypertensive drugs.

Sensitivity reactions may occur in patients with or without a history of allergy or bronchial asthma.

The possibility of exacerbation or activation of systemic lupus erythematosus has been reported.

Lithium generally should not be given with diuretics (see PRECAUTIONS, *Drug Interactions*).

PRECAUTIONS

General

Methyldopa

Methyldopa should be used with caution in patients with a history of previous liver disease or dysfunction (see WARNINGS).

Some patients taking methyldopa experience clinical edema or weight gain which may be controlled by use of a diuretic. Methyldopa should not be continued if edema progresses or signs of heart failure appear.

Hypertension has recurred occasionally after dialysis in patients given methyldopa because the drug is removed by this procedure.

Rarely involuntary choreoathetotic movements have been observed during therapy with methyldopa in patients with severe bilateral cerebrovascular disease. Should these movements occur, stop therapy.

Chlorothiazide

All patients receiving diuretic therapy should be observed for evidence of fluid or electrolyte imbalance: namely, hyponatremia, hypochloremic alkalosis, and hypokalemia. Serum and urine electrolyte determinations are particularly important when the patient is vomiting excessively or receiving parenteral fluids. Warning signs or symptoms of fluid and electrolyte imbalance, irrespective of cause include dryness of mouth, thirst, weakness, lethargy, drowsiness, restlessness, muscle pains or cramps, muscular fatigue, hypotension, oliguria, tachycardia, and gastrointestinal disturbances such as nausea and vomiting.

Hypokalemia may develop, especially with brisk diuresis, when severe cirrhosis is present, or after prolonged therapy. Interference with adequate oral electrolyte intake will also contribute to hypokalemia. Hypokalemia may cause cardiac arrhythmia and may also sensitize or exaggerate the response of the heart to the toxic effects of digitalis (e.g., increased ventricular irritability). Hypokalemia may be avoided or treated by use of potassium sparing diuretics or potassium supplements such as foods with a high potassium content.

Although any chloride deficit is generally mild and usually does not require specific treatment except under extraordinary circumstances (as in liver disease or renal disease), chloride replacement may be required in the treatment of metabolic alkalosis.

Dilutional hyponatremia may occur in edematous patients in hot weather; appropriate therapy is water restriction, rather than administration of salt, except in rare instances when the hyponatremia is life threatening. In actual salt depletion, appropriate replacement is the therapy of choice. Hyperuricemia may occur or acute gout may be precipitated in certain patients receiving thiazides.

In diabetic patients dosage adjustments of insulin or oral hypoglycemic agents may be required. Hyperglycemia may occur with thiazide diuretics. Thus latent diabetes mellitus may become manifest during thiazide therapy.

The antihypertensive effects of the drug may be enhanced in the postsympathectomy patient.

If progressive renal impairment becomes evident, consider withholding or discontinuing diuretic therapy.

Thiazides have been shown to increase the urinary excretion of magnesium; this may result in hypomagnesemia.

Thiazides may decrease urinary calcium excretion. Thiazides may cause intermittent and slight elevation of serum calcium in the absence of known disorders of calcium metabolism. Marked hypercalcemia may be evidence of hidden hyperparathyroidism. Thiazides should be discontinued before carrying out tests for parathyroid function.

Increases in cholesterol and triglyceride levels may be associated with thiazide diuretic therapy.

Laboratory Tests

Methyldopa

Blood count, Coombs test and liver function tests are recommended before initiating therapy and at periodic intervals (see WARNINGS).

Chlorothiazide

Periodic determination of serum electrolytes to detect possible electrolyte imbalance should be done at appropriate intervals.

Drug Interactions

Methyldopa

When methyldopa is used with other antihypertensive drugs, potentiation of antihypertensive effect may occur. Patients should be followed carefully to detect side reactions or unusual manifestations of drug idiosyncrasy.

Patients may require reduced doses of anesthetics when on methyldopa. If hypotension does occur during anesthesia, it usually can be controlled by vasopressors. The adrenergic receptors remain sensitive during treatment with methyldopa.

Chlorothiazide

When given concurrently the following drugs may interact with thiazide diuretics.

Alcohol, barbiturates, or narcotics—potentiation of orthostatic hypotension may occur.

Antidiabetic drugs (oral agents and insulin)—dosage adjustment of the antidiabetic drug may be required.

Other antihypertensive drugs—additive effect or potentiation.

Corticosteroids, ACTH—intensified electrolyte depletion, particularly hypokalemia.

Pressor amines (e.g., norepinephrine)—possible decreased response to pressor amines but not sufficient to preclude their use.

Skeletal muscle relaxants, nondepolarizing (e.g., tubocurarine)—possible increased responsiveness to the muscle relaxant.

Lithium—generally should not be given with diuretics. Diuretic agents reduce the renal clearance of lithium and add a high risk of lithium toxicity. Refer to the package insert for lithium preparations before use of such preparations with ALDOCLOR.

Non-steroidal Anti-inflammatory Drugs—In some patients, the administration of a non-steroidal anti-inflammatory agent can reduce the diuretic, natriuretic, and antihypertensive effects of loop, potassium-sparing and thiazide diuretics. Therefore, when ALDOCLOR and non-steroidal anti-inflammatory agents are used concomitantly, the patient should be observed closely to determine if the desired effect of the diuretic is obtained.

Drug/Laboratory Test Interactions

Methyldopa

Methyldopa may interfere with measurement of: urinary uric acid by the phosphotungstate method, serum creatinine by the alkaline picrate method, and SGOT by colorimetric methods. Interference with spectrophotometric methods for SGOT analysis has not been reported.

Since methyldopa causes fluorescence in urine samples at the same wave lengths as catecholamines, falsely high levels of urinary catecholamines may be reported. This will interfere with the diagnosis of pheochromocytoma. It is important to recognize this phenomenon before a patient with a possible pheochromocytoma is subjected to surgery. Methyldopa does not interfere with measurement of VMA (vanillylmandelic acid), a test for pheochromocytoma, by those methods which convert VMA to vanillin. Methyldopa is not recommended for the treatment of patients with pheochromocytoma. Rarely, when urine is exposed to air after voiding, it may darken because of breakdown of methyldopa or its metabolites.

Chlorothiazide

Thiazides should be discontinued before carrying out tests for parathyroid function (see PRECAUTIONS, *General*).

Carcinogenesis, Mutagenesis, Impairment of Fertility

Long-term studies in animals have not been performed to evaluate the effects upon fertility, mutagenic or carcinogenic potential of the combination.

Methyldopa

Methyldopa is currently under study in the U.S. Carcinogenesis Testing Program.

Methyldopa did not have mutagenic activity *in vitro* in the Ames microbial mutagen test with or without metabolic activation.

Methyldopa given in a two-litter study in rats at approximately three to six times the usual daily dose did not impair fertility.

Chlorothiazide

Carcinogenic studies have not been done with chlorothiazide.

Chlorothiazide was not mutagenic *in vitro* in the Ames microbial test at a maximum concentration of 5 mg/plate using Strains TA98 and TA100. Chlorothiazide did not produce any significant mutagenicity in the dominant lethal assay in the mouse after 8 oral doses of 50 mg/kg or single intraperitoneal doses of 525 or 644 mg/kg, although early fetal deaths and preimplantation losses were increased beyond control values. In a test using *Aspergillus nidulans*, chlorothiazide was negative and did not induce disjunction.

Chlorothiazide had no effect on fertility in a two-litter study in rats at doses up to 60 mg/kg/day (2 times the maximum recommended human dose).

Pregnancy

Teratogenic Effects—Pregnancy Category B: Reproduction studies in the rat, at doses up to 40 mg/kg/day (3–4 times the maximum recommended human dose), did not impair fertility or cause abnormalities of the fetus due to ALDOCLOR.

There are no adequate and well-controlled studies with ALDOCLOR in pregnant women. Because animal reproduction studies are not always predictive of human response, this drug should be used during pregnancy only if clearly needed. (See INDICATION AND USAGE.)

Chlorothiazide: Thiazides cross the placental barrier and appear in cord blood.

Reproduction studies in the rabbit, the mouse and the rat at doses up to 500 mg/kg/day (25 times the maximum recommended human dose) showed no evidence of external abnormalities of the fetus due to chlorothiazide. Chlorothiazide given in a two-litter study in rats at doses up to 60 mg/kg/day (2 times the maximum recommended human dose) did not impair fertility or produce birth abnormalities in the offspring.

Methyldopa: Reproduction studies have been performed in the rabbit, the mouse, and the rat at doses up to 1000 mg/kg/day (16.6 times the maximum recommended human dose) and have revealed no evidence of impaired fertility or harm to the fetus due to methyldopa. There are, however, no adequate and well-controlled studies in pregnant women in the first trimester of pregnancy. Because animal reproduction studies are not always predictive of human response, methyldopa should be used during pregnancy only if clearly needed.

Published reports of the use of methyldopa during all trimesters indicate that if this drug is used during pregnancy the possibility of fetal harm appears remote. In five studies, three of which were controlled, involving 332 pregnant hypertensive women, treatment with methyldopa was associated with an improved fetal outcome. The majority of these women were in the third trimester when methyldopa therapy was begun.

In one study, women who had begun methyldopa treatment between weeks 16 and 20 of pregnancy gave birth to infants whose average head circumference was reduced by a small amount (34.2 $\pm$ 1.7 cm vs. 34.6 $\pm$ 1.3 cm [mean $\pm$ 1 S.D.]). Long-term follow up of 195 (97.5%) of the children born to methyldopa-treated pregnant women (including those who began treatment between weeks 16 and 20) failed to uncover any significant adverse effect on the children. At four years of age, the developmental delay commonly seen in children born to hypertensive mothers was less evident in those whose mothers were treated with methyldopa during pregnancy than those whose mothers were untreated. The children of the treated group scored consistently higher than the children of the untreated group on five major indices of intellectual and motor development. At age seven and one-half developmental scores and intelligence indices showed no significant differences in children of treated or untreated hypertensive women.

Nonteratogenic Effects: These may include fetal or neonatal jaundice, thrombocytopenia, and possibly other adverse reactions which have occurred in the adult.

Nursing Mothers

Methyldopa and thiazides appear in breast milk. Therefore, because of the potential for serious adverse reactions in nursing infants from chlorothiazide, a decision should be made whether to discontinue nursing or to discontinue the drug, taking into account the importance of the drug to the mother.

Continued on next page

Information on the Merck & Co. products listed on these pages is the full prescribing information from product circulars in use October 1, 1992.

Merck & Co.—Cont.

Pediatric Use
Safety and effectiveness of ALDOCLOR in children has not been established.

ADVERSE REACTIONS

The following adverse reactions have been reported and, within each category, are listed in order of decreasing severity.
Methyldopa
Sedation, usually transient, may occur during the initial period of therapy or whenever the dose is increased. Headache, asthenia, or weakness may be noted as early and transient symptoms. However, significant adverse effects due to methyldopa have been infrequent and this agent usually is well tolerated.
Cardiovascular: Aggravation of angina pectoris, congestive heart failure, prolonged carotid sinus hypersensitivity, orthostatic hypotension (decrease daily dosage), edema or weight gain, bradycardia.
Digestive: Pancreatitis, colitis, vomiting, diarrhea, sialadenitis, sore or "black" tongue, nausea, constipation, distension, flatus, dryness of mouth.
Endocrine: Hyperprolactinemia.
Hematologic: Bone marrow depression, leukopenia, granulocytopenia, thrombocytopenia, hemolytic anemia; positive tests for antinuclear antibody, LE cells, and rheumatoid factor, positive Coombs test.
Hepatic: Liver disorders including hepatitis, jaundice, abnormal liver function tests (see WARNINGS).
Hypersensitivity: Myocarditis, pericarditis, vasculitis, lupus-like syndrome, drug-related fever.
Nervous System/Psychiatric: Parkinsonism, Bell's palsy, decreased mental acuity, involuntary choreoathetotic movements, symptoms of cerebrovascular insufficiency, psychic disturbances including nightmares and reversible mild psychoses or depression, headache, sedation, asthenia or weakness, dizziness, lightheadedness, paresthesias.
Metabolic: Rise in BUN.
Musculoskeletal: Arthralgia, with or without joint swelling; myalgia.
Respiratory: Nasal stuffiness.
Skin: Toxic epidermal necrolysis, rash.
Urogenital: Amenorrhea, breast enlargement, gynecomastia, lactation, impotence, decreased libido.
Chlorothiazide
Body as a Whole: Weakness.
Cardiovascular: Hypotension including orthostatic hypotension (may be aggravated by alcohol, barbiturates, narcotics or antihypertensive drugs).
Digestive: Pancreatitis, jaundice (intrahepatic cholestatic jaundice), diarrhea, vomiting, sialadenitis, cramping, constipation, gastric irritation, nausea, anorexia.
Hematologic: Aplastic anemia, agranulocytosis, leukopenia, hemolytic anemia, thrombocytopenia.
Hypersensitivity: Anaphylactic reactions, necrotizing angiitis (vasculitis and cutaneous vasculitis), respiratory distress including pneumonitis and pulmonary edema, photosensitivity, fever, urticaria, rash, purpura.
Metabolic: Electrolyte imbalance (see PRECAUTIONS), hyperglycemia, glycosuria, hyperuricemia.
Musculoskeletal: Muscle spasm.
Nervous System/Psychiatric: Vertigo, paresthesias, dizziness, headache, restlessness.
Renal: Renal failure, renal dysfunction, interstitial nephritis. (See WARNINGS.)
Special Senses: Transient blurred vision, xanthopsia.
Whenever adverse reactions are moderate or severe, thiazide dosage should be reduced or therapy withdrawn.

OVERDOSAGE

Acute overdosage may produce acute hypotension with other responses attributable to brain and gastrointestinal malfunction (excessive sedation, weakness, bradycardia, dizziness, lightheadedness, constipation, distention, flatus, diarrhea, nausea, vomiting).
In the event of overdosage, symptomatic and supportive measures should be employed. When ingestion is recent, gastric lavage or emesis may reduce absorption. When ingestion has been earlier, infusions may be helpful to promote urinary excretion. Otherwise, management includes special attention to cardiac rate and output, blood volume, electrolyte imbalance, paralytic ileus, urinary function and cerebral activity.
Sympathomimetic drugs [e.g., levarterenol, epinephrine, ARAMINE* (Metaraminol Bitartrate)] may be indicated. Methyldopa is dialyzable.
The oral LD_{50} of methyldopa is greater than 1.5 g/kg in both the mouse and the rat. The oral LD_{50} of chlorothiazide is 8.5 g/kg, greater than 10 g/kg, and greater than 1 g/kg in the mouse, rat, and dog respectively.

*Registered trademark of MERCK & CO., INC.

DOSAGE AND ADMINISTRATION

Dosage: As determined by individual titration (see box warning).
The usual starting dosage is 1 tablet of ALDOCLOR 150 or 1 tablet of ALDOCLOR 250 two or three times a day in the first 48 hours. The daily dosage then may be increased or decreased, preferably at intervals of not less than two days, until an adequate response is achieved. To minimize the sedation associated with methyldopa, start dosage increases in the evening. By adjustment of dosage, morning hypotension may be prevented without sacrificing control of afternoon blood pressure.
When ALDOCLOR is given to patients on other antihypertensives, the dose of these agents may need to be adjusted to effect a smooth transition. When ALDOCLOR is given with antihypertensives other than thiazides, the initial dosage of methyldopa should be limited to 500 mg daily in divided doses.
Although occasional patients have responded to higher doses, the maximum recommended daily dosage is 3 g of methyldopa and 1 to 2 g of chlorothiazide. Once an effective dosage range is attained, a smooth blood pressure response occurs in most patients in 12 to 24 hours. If ALDOCLOR alone does not adequately control blood pressure, additional methyldopa may be given separately to obtain the maximum blood pressure response.
Since both components of ALDOCLOR have a relatively short duration of action, withdrawal is followed by return of hypertension usually within 48 hours. This is not complicated by an overshoot of blood pressure.
Occasionally tolerance may occur, usually between the second and third month of therapy. Increasing the dosage of either methyldopa or chlorothiazide separately or together frequently will restore effective control of blood pressure. Methyldopa is largely excreted by the kidney and patients with impaired renal function may respond to smaller doses of ALDOCLOR. Syncope in older patients may be related to an increased sensitivity and advanced arteriosclerotic vascular disease. This may be avoided by lower doses.

HOW SUPPLIED

No. 3318—Tablets ALDOCLOR 150 are beige, oval, film coated tablets coded MSD 612. Each tablet contains 250 mg of methyldopa and 150 mg of chlorothiazide. They are supplied as follows:
NDC 0006-0612-68 bottles of 100.
   Shown in Product Identification Section, page 419
No. 3319—Tablets ALDOCLOR 250 are green, oval, film coated tablets coded MSD 634. Each tablet contains 250 mg of methyldopa and 250 mg of chlorothiazide. They are supplied as follows:
NDC 0006-0634-68 bottles of 100.
   Shown in Product Identification Section, page 419
Storage
Keep container tightly closed. Protect from light. Store container in carton until contents have been used.
   A.H.F.S. Category: 24:08
   DC 7059834 Issued March 1990
COPYRIGHT © MERCK & CO., INC., 1986
All rights reserved

ALDOMET® Tablets   ℞
(Methyldopa), U.S.P.

ALDOMET® Oral Suspension   ℞
(Methyldopa), U.S.P.

DESCRIPTION

ALDOMET* (Methyldopa) is an antihypertensive drug. Methyldopa, the *L*-isomer of alpha-methyldopa is levo-3-(3,4 - dihydroxyphenyl) -2-methylalanine. Its empirical formula is $C_{10}H_{13}NO_4$, with a molecular weight of 211.22, and its structural formula is:

$$HO-\text{⬡}-CH_2-\underset{NH_2}{\overset{CH_3}{C}}-CO_2H$$

Methyldopa is a white to yellowish white, odorless fine powder, and is soluble in water.
ALDOMET is supplied as tablets, for oral use, in three strengths: 125 mg, 250 mg, or 500 mg of methyldopa per tablet. Inactive ingredients in the tablets are: calcium disodium edetate, cellulose, citric acid, colloidal silicon dioxide, D&C Yellow 10, ethylcellulose, guar gum, hydroxypropyl methylcellulose, iron oxide, magnesium stearate, propylene glycol, talc, and titanium dioxide.

Oral Suspension ALDOMET is supplied as a white to off-white preparation; each 5 mL contains 250 mg of methyldopa and alcohol 1 percent, with benzoic acid 0.1 percent and sodium bisulfite 0.2 percent added as preservatives. Inactive ingredients in the oral suspension are: artificial and natural flavors, cellulose, citric acid, confectioner's sugar, disodium edetate, glycerin, polysorbate, purified water, and sodium carboxymethylcellulose.

*Registered trademark of MERCK & CO., INC.

CLINICAL PHARMACOLOGY

ALDOMET is an aromatic-amino-acid decarboxylase inhibitor in animals and in man. Although the mechanism of action has yet to be conclusively demonstrated, the antihypertensive effect of methyldopa probably is due to its metabolism to alpha-methylnorepinephrine, which then lowers arterial pressure by stimulation of central inhibitory alpha-adrenergic receptors, false neurotransmission, and/or reduction of plasma renin activity. Methyldopa has been shown to cause a net reduction in the tissue concentration of serotonin, dopamine, norepinephrine, and epinephrine.
Only methyldopa, the *L*-isomer of alpha-methyldopa, has the ability to inhibit dopa decarboxylase and to deplete animal tissues of norepinephrine. In man the antihypertensive activity appears to be due solely to the *L*-isomer. About twice the dose of the racemate (*DL*-alpha-methyldopa) is required for equal antihypertensive effect.
Methyldopa has no direct effect on cardiac function and usually does not reduce glomerular filtration rate, renal blood flow, or filtration fraction. Cardiac output usually is maintained without cardiac acceleration. In some patients the heart rate is slowed.
Normal or elevated plasma renin activity may decrease in the course of methyldopa therapy.
ALDOMET reduces both supine and standing blood pressure. Methyldopa usually produces highly effective lowering of the supine pressure with infrequent symptomatic postural hypotension. Exercise hypotension and diurnal blood pressure variations rarely occur.
Pharmacokinetics and Metabolism
The maximum decrease in blood pressure occurs four to six hours after oral dosage. Once an effective dosage level is attained, a smooth blood pressure response occurs in most patients in 12 to 24 hours. After withdrawal, blood pressure usually returns to pretreatment levels within 24–48 hours.
Methyldopa is extensively metabolized. The known urinary metabolites are: α-methyldopa mono-0-sulfate; 3-0-methyl-α-methyldopa; 3,4-dihydroxyphenylacetone; α-methyldopamine; 3-0-methyl-α-methyldopamine and their conjugates. Approximately 70% of the drug which is absorbed is excreted in the urine as methyldopa and its mono-0-sulfate conjugate. The renal clearance is about 130 mL/min in normal subjects and is diminished in renal insufficiency. The plasma half-life of methyldopa is 105 minutes. After oral doses, excretion is essentially complete in 36 hours. Methyldopa crosses the placental barrier, appears in cord blood, and appears in breast milk.

INDICATION AND USAGE

Hypertension.

CONTRAINDICATIONS

Active hepatic disease, such as acute hepatitis and active cirrhosis.
If previous methyldopa therapy has been associated with liver disorders (see WARNINGS).
Hypersensitivity to any component of these products, including sulfites contained in Oral Suspension ALDOMET (see WARNINGS). Tablets ALDOMET do not contain sulfites.

WARNINGS

It is important to recognize that a positive Coombs test, hemolytic anemia, and liver disorders may occur with methyldopa therapy. The rare occurrences of hemolytic anemia or liver disorders could lead to potentially fatal complications unless properly recognized and managed. Read this section carefully to understand these reactions.
With prolonged methyldopa therapy, 10 to 20 percent of patients develop a positive direct Coombs test which usually occurs between 6 and 12 months of methyldopa therapy. Lowest incidence is at daily dosage of 1 g or less. On rare occasions may be associated with hemolytic anemia, which could lead to potentially fatal complications. One cannot predict which patients with a positive direct Coombs test may develop hemolytic anemia.
Prior existence or development of a positive direct Coombs test is not in itself a contraindication to use of methyldopa. If a positive Coombs test develops during methyldopa therapy, the physician should determine whether hemolytic anemia exists and whether the positive Coombs test may be a prob-

lem. For example, in addition to a positive direct Coombs test there is less often a positive indirect Coombs test which may interfere with cross matching of blood.
Before treatment is started, it is desirable to do a blood count (hematocrit, hemoglobin, or red cell count) for a baseline or to establish whether there is anemia. Periodic blood counts should be done during therapy to detect hemolytic anemia. It may be useful to do a direct Coombs test before therapy and at 6 and 12 months after the start of therapy.
If Coombs-positive hemolytic anemia occurs, the cause may be methyldopa and the drug should be discontinued. Usually the anemia remits promptly. If not, corticosteroids may be given and other causes of anemia should be considered. If the hemolytic anemia is related to methyldopa, the drug should not be reinstituted.
When methyldopa causes Coombs positivity alone or with hemolytic anemia, the red cell is usually coated with gamma globulin of the IgG (gamma G) class only. The positive Coombs test may not revert to normal until weeks to months after methyldopa is stopped.
Should the need for transfusion arise in a patient receiving methyldopa, both a direct and an indirect Coombs test should be performed. In the absence of hemolytic anemia, usually only the direct Coombs test will be positive. A positive direct Coombs test alone will not interfere with typing or cross matching. If the indirect Coombs test is also positive, problems may arise in the major cross match and the assistance of a hematologist or transfusion expert will be needed.
Occasionally, fever has occurred within the first 3 weeks of methyldopa therapy, associated in some cases with eosinophilia or abnormalities in one or more liver function tests, such as serum alkaline phosphatase, serum transaminases (SGOT, SGPT), bilirubin, and prothrombin time. Jaundice, with or without fever, may occur with onset usually within the first 2 to 3 months of therapy. In some patients the findings are consistent with those of cholestasis. In others the findings are consistent with hepatitis and hepatocellular injury.
Rarely, fatal hepatic necrosis has been reported after use of methyldopa. These hepatic changes may represent hypersensitivity reactions. Periodic determinations of hepatic function should be done particularly during the first 6 to 12 weeks of therapy or whenever an unexplained fever occurs. If fever, abnormalities in liver function tests, or jaundice appear, stop therapy with methyldopa. If caused by methyldopa, the temperature and abnormalities in liver function characteristically have reverted to normal when the drug was discontinued. Methyldopa should not be reinstituted in such patients.
Rarely, a reversible reduction of the white blood cell count with a primary effect on the granulocytes has been seen. The granulocyte count returned promptly to normal on discontinuance of the drug. Rare cases of granulocytopenia have been reported. In each instance, upon stopping the drug, the white cell count returned to normal. Reversible thrombocytopenia has occurred rarely.
Oral Suspension ALDOMET (but not Tablets ALDOMET) contains sodium bisulfite, a sulfite that may cause allergic-type reactions including anaphylactic symptoms and life-threatening or less severe asthmatic episodes in certain susceptible people. The overall prevalence of sulfite sensitivity in the general population is unknown and probably low. Sulfite sensitivity is seen more frequently in asthmatic than in nonasthmatic people.

PRECAUTIONS

General
Methyldopa should be used with caution in patients with a history of previous liver disease or dysfunction (see WARNINGS).
Some patients taking methyldopa experience clinical edema or weight gain which may be controlled by use of a diuretic. Methyldopa should not be continued if edema progresses or signs of heart failure appear.
Hypertension has recurred occasionally after dialysis in patients given methyldopa because the drug is removed by this procedure.
Rarely involuntary choreoathetotic movements have been observed during therapy with methyldopa in patients with severe bilateral cerebrovascular disease. Should these movements occur, stop therapy.
Laboratory Tests
Blood count, Coombs test, and liver function tests are recommended before initiating therapy and at periodic intervals (see WARNINGS).
Drug Interactions
When methyldopa is used with other antihypertensive drugs, potentiation of antihypertensive effect may occur. Patients should be followed carefully to detect side reactions or unusual manifestations of drug idiosyncrasy.
Patients may require reduced doses of anesthetics when on methyldopa. If hypotension does occur during anesthesia, it usually can be controlled by vasopressors. The adrenergic receptors remain sensitive during treatment with methyldopa.
When methyldopa and lithium are given concomitantly the patient should be carefully monitored for symptoms of lithium toxicity. Read the circular for lithium preparations.
Drug/Laboratory Test Interactions
Methyldopa may interfere with measurement of: urinary uric acid by the phosphotungstate method, serum creatinine by the alkaline picrate method, and SGOT by colorimetric methods. Interference with spectrophotometric methods for SGOT analysis has not been reported.
Since methyldopa causes fluorescence in urine samples at the same wave lengths as catecholamines, falsely high levels of urinary catecholamines may be reported. This will interfere with the diagnosis of pheochromocytoma. It is important to recognize this phenomenon before a patient with a possible pheochromocytoma is subjected to surgery. Methyldopa does not interfere with measurement of VMA (vanillylmandelic acid), a test for pheochromocytoma, by those methods which convert VMA to vanillin. Methyldopa is not recommended for the treatment of patients with pheochromocytoma. Rarely, when urine is exposed to air after voiding, it may darken because of breakdown of methyldopa or its metabolites.
Carcinogenesis, Mutagenesis, Impairment of Fertility
Methyldopa is currently under study in the U.S. Carcinogenesis Testing Program.
Methyldopa did not have mutagenic activity *in vitro* in the Ames microbial mutagen test with or without metabolic activation.
Methyldopa given in a two-litter study in rats at approximately three to six times the usual daily dose did not impair fertility.
Pregnancy
Pregnancy Category B. Reproduction studies have been performed in the rabbit, the mouse, and the rat at doses up to 1000 mg/kg/day (16.6 times the maximum recommended human dose) and have revealed no evidence of impaired fertility or harm to the fetus due to methyldopa. There are, however, no adequate and well-controlled studies in pregnant women in the first trimester of pregnancy. Because animal reproduction studies are not always predictive of human response, ALDOMET should be used during pregnancy only if clearly needed.
Published reports of the use of methyldopa during all trimesters indicate that if this drug is used during pregnancy the possibility of fetal harm appears remote. In five studies, three of which were controlled, involving 332 pregnant hypertensive women, treatment with ALDOMET was associated with an improved fetal outcome. The majority of these women were in the third trimester when methyldopa therapy was begun.
In one study, women who had begun methyldopa treatment between weeks 16 and 20 of pregnancy gave birth to infants whose average head circumference was reduced by a small amount (34.2 ± 1.7 cm vs. 34.6 ± 1.3 cm [mean ± 1 S.D.]). Long-term follow up of 195 (97.5%) of the children born to methyldopa-treated pregnant women (including those who began treatment between weeks 16 and 20) failed to uncover any significant adverse effect on the children. At four years of age, the developmental delay commonly seen in children born to hypertensive mothers was less evident in those whose mothers were treated with methyldopa during pregnancy than those whose mothers were untreated. The children of the treated group scored consistently higher than the children of the untreated group on five major indices of intellectual and motor development. At age seven and one-half developmental scores and intelligence indices showed no significant differences in children of treated or untreated hypertensive women.
Nursing Mothers
Methyldopa appears in breast milk. Therefore, caution should be exercised when methyldopa is given to a nursing woman.

ADVERSE REACTIONS

Sedation, usually transient, may occur during the initial period of therapy or whenever the dose is increased. Headache, asthenia, or weakness may be noted as early and transient symptoms. However, significant adverse effects due to ALDOMET have been infrequent and this agent usually is well tolerated.
The following adverse reactions have been reported and, within each category, are listed in order of decreasing severity.
Cardiovascular: Aggravation of angina pectoris, congestive heart failure, prolonged carotid sinus hypersensitivity, orthostatic hypotension (decrease daily dosage), edema or weight gain, bradycardia.
Digestive: Pancreatitis, colitis, vomiting, diarrhea, sialadenitis, sore or "black" tongue, nausea, constipation, distension, flatus, dryness of mouth.
Endocrine: Hyperprolactinemia.
Hematologic: Bone marrow depression, leukopenia, granulocytopenia, thrombocytopenia, hemolytic anemia; positive tests for antinuclear antibody, LE cells, and rheumatoid factor, positive Coombs test.
Hepatic: Liver disorders including hepatitis, jaundice, abnormal liver function tests (see WARNINGS).
Hypersensitivity: Myocarditis, pericarditis, vasculitis, lupus-like syndrome, drug-related fever.
Nervous System/Psychiatric: Parkinsonism, Bell's palsy, decreased mental acuity, involuntary choreoathetotic movements, symptoms of cerebrovascular insufficiency, psychic disturbances including nightmares and reversible mild psychoses or depression, headache, sedation, asthenia or weakness, dizziness, lightheadedness, paresthesias.
Metabolic: Rise in BUN.
Musculoskeletal: Arthralgia, with or without joint swelling; myalgia.
Respiratory: Nasal stuffiness.
Skin: Toxic epidermal necrolysis, rash.
Urogenital: Amenorrhea, breast enlargement, gynecomastia, lactation, impotence, decreased libido.

OVERDOSAGE

Acute overdosage may produce acute hypotension with other responses attributable to brain and gastrointestinal malfunction (excessive sedation, weakness, bradycardia, dizziness, lightheadedness, constipation, distention, flatus, diarrhea, nausea, vomiting).
In the event of overdosage, symptomatic and supportive measures should be employed. When ingestion is recent, gastric lavage or emesis may reduce absorption. When ingestion has been earlier, infusions may be helpful to promote urinary excretion. Otherwise, management includes special attention to cardiac rate and output, blood volume, electrolyte balance, paralytic ileus, urinary function and cerebral activity.
Sympathomimetic drugs [e.g., levarterenol, epinephrine, ARAMINE* (Metaraminol Bitartrate)] may be indicated. Methyldopa is dialyzable.
The oral LD_{50} of methyldopa is greater than 1.5 g/kg in both the mouse and the rat.

*Registered trademark of MERCK & CO., INC.

DOSAGE AND ADMINISTRATION

ADULTS

Initiation of Therapy
The usual starting dosage of ALDOMET is 250 mg two or three times a day in the first 48 hours. The daily dosage then may be increased or decreased, preferably at intervals of not less than two days, until an adequate response is achieved. To minimize the sedation, start dosage increases in the evening. By adjustment of dosage, morning hypotension may be prevented without sacrificing control of afternoon blood pressure.
When methyldopa is given to patients on other antihypertensives, the dose of these agents may need to be adjusted to effect a smooth transition. When ALDOMET is given with antihypertensives other than thiazides, the initial dosage of ALDOMET should be limited to 500 mg daily in divided doses; when ALDOMET is added to a thiazide, the dosage of thiazide need not be changed.
Maintenance Therapy
The usual daily dosage of ALDOMET is 500 mg to 2 g in two to four doses. Although occasional patients have responded to higher doses, the maximum recommended daily dosage is 3 g. Once an effective dosage range is attained, a smooth blood pressure response occurs in most patients in 12 to 24 hours. Since methyldopa has a relatively short duration of action, withdrawal is followed by return of hypertension usually within 48 hours. This is not complicated by an overshoot of blood pressure.
Occasionally tolerance may occur, usually between the second and third month of therapy. Adding a diuretic or increasing the dosage of methyldopa frequently will restore effective control of blood pressure. A thiazide may be added at any time during methyldopa therapy and is recommended if therapy has not been started with a thiazide or if effective control of blood pressure cannot be maintained on 2 g of methyldopa daily.
Methyldopa is largely excreted by the kidney and patients with impaired renal function may respond to smaller doses. Syncope in older patients may be related to an increased sensitivity and advanced arteriosclerotic vascular disease. This may be avoided by lower doses.

Continued on next page

Information on the Merck & Co. products listed on these pages is the full prescribing information from product circulars in use October 1, 1992.

Merck & Co.—Cont.

CHILDREN

Initial dosage is based on 10 mg/kg of body weight daily in two to four doses. The daily dosage then is increased or decreased until an adequate response is achieved. The maximum dosage is 65 mg/kg or 3 g daily, whichever is less.

HOW SUPPLIED

No. 3341—Tablets ALDOMET, 125 mg, are yellow, film coated, round tablets, coded MSD 135. They are supplied as follows:

NDC 0006-0135-68 bottles of 100.

Shown in Product Identification Section, page 419

No. 3290—Tablets ALDOMET, 250 mg, are yellow, film coated, round tablets, coded MSD 401. They are supplied as follows:

NDC 0006-0401-68 bottles of 100
(6505-00-890-1856, 250 mg 100's)
NDC 0006-0401-28 unit dose packages of 100
(6505-00-149-0090, 250 mg individually sealed 100's)
NDC 0006-0401-78 unit of use bottles of 100
NDC 0006-0401-82 bottles of 1000
(6505-00-931-6646, 250 mg 1000's).

Shown in Product Identification Section, page 419

No. 3292—Tablets ALDOMET, 500 mg, are yellow, film coated, round tablets, coded MSD 516. They are supplied as follows:

NDC 0006-0516-68 bottles of 100
NDC 0006-0516-28 unit dose packages of 100
(6505-01-046-3616, 500 mg individually sealed 100's)
NDC 0006-0516-78 unit of use bottles of 100
NDC 0006-0516-74 bottles of 500
(6505-01-199-8339, 500 mg 500's).

Shown in Product Identification Section, page 419

No. 3382—Oral Suspension ALDOMET, 250 mg per 5 mL, is an off-white, creamy suspension with a citric orange-pineapple flavor. It is supplied as follows:

NDC 0006-3382-74 bottles of 473 mL.

Storage

Store Oral Suspension ALDOMET below 26°C (78°F) in a tight, light-resistant container. Protect from freezing.

A.H.F.S. Category: 24:08
DC 7398625 Issued March 1990

COPYRIGHT © MERCK & CO., INC., 1985
All rights reserved

ALDOMET® Ester HCl Injection (Methyldopate HCl), U.S.P. ℞

DESCRIPTION

Injection ALDOMET* Ester Hydrochloride (Methyldopate HCl) is an antihypertensive agent for intravenous use. Methyldopate hydrochloride [levo-3-(3,4-dihydroxyphenyl)-2-methylalanine, ethyl ester hydrochloride]is the ethyl ester of methyldopa, supplied as the hydrochloride salt with a molecular weight of 275.73. Methyldopate hydrochloride is more soluble and stable in solution than methyldopa and is the preferred form for intravenous use.

The empirical formula for methyldopate hydrochloride is $C_{12}H_{17}NO_4 \cdot HCl$ and its structural formula is:

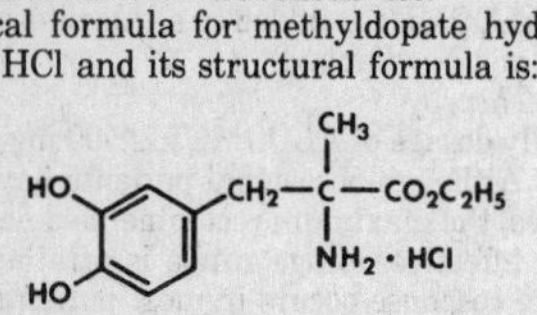

Injection ALDOMET Ester Hydrochloride is supplied as a sterile solution in 5 mL vials each of which contains:

Methyldopate hydrochloride	250.0 mg
Inactive ingredients:	
Citric acid anhydrous	25.0 mg
Disodium edetate	2.5 mg
Monothioglycerol	10.0 mg
Sodium hydroxide to adjust pH	
Water for Injection, q.s. to 5 mL	

Methylparaben 7.5 mg, propylparaben 1 mg, and sodium bisulfite 16 mg added as preservatives.

---

*Registered trademark of MERCK & CO., INC.

CLINICAL PHARMACOLOGY

ALDOMET (Methyldopa), an antihypertensive, is an aromatic-amino-acid decarboxylase inhibitor in animals and in man. Although the mechanism of action has yet to be conclusively demonstrated, the antihypertensive effect of methyldopa probably is due to its metabolism to alpha-methyl-norepinephrine, which then lowers arterial pressure by stimulation of central inhibitory alpha-adrenergic receptors, false neurotransmission, and/or reduction of plasma renin activity. Methyldopa has been shown to cause a net reduction in the tissue concentration of serotonin, dopamine, norepinephrine, and epinephrine.

Only methyldopa, the *L*-isomer of alpha-methyldopa, has the ability to inhibit dopa decarboxylase and to deplete animal tissues of norepinephrine. In man the antihypertensive activity appears to be due solely to the *L*-isomer. About twice the dose of the racemate (*DL*-alpha-methyldopa) is required for equal antihypertensive effect.

Methyldopa has no direct effect on cardiac function and usually does not reduce glomerular filtration rate, renal blood flow, or filtration fraction. Cardiac output usually is maintained without cardiac acceleration. In some patients the heart rate is slowed.

Normal or elevated plasma renin activity may decrease in the course of methyldopa therapy.

Methyldopa reduces both supine and standing blood pressure. It usually produces highly effective lowering of the supine pressure with infrequent symptomatic postural hypotension. Exercise hypotension and diurnal blood pressure variations rarely occur.

Pharmacokinetics and Metabolism

Methyldopate hydrochloride is the ethyl ester of methyldopa hydrochloride and possesses the same pharmacologic attributes.

Methyldopa is extensively metabolized. The known urinary metabolites are: α-methyldopa mono-0-sulfate; 3-0-methyl-α-methyldopa; 3,4-dihydroxyphenylacetone; α-methyldopamine; 3-0-methyl-α-methyldopamine and their conjugates.

Following intravenous administration of methyldopate hydrochloride a decrease in blood pressure may occur in four to six hours and last 10 to 16 hours.

Approximately 49 percent of the dose of methylopate hydrochloride is excreted in the urine as methyldopa and its mono-0-sulfate. The renal clearance of methyldopa following methyldopate hydrochloride is about 156 mL/min in normal subjects and is diminished in renal insufficiency. Following methyldopate hydrochloride injection the plasma half-life of methyldopa is 90–127 mins. Approximately 17 percent of a dose of methyldopate hydrochloride given to normal subjects appears in plasma as free methyldopa.

Methyldopa crosses the placental barrier, appears in cord blood, and appears in breast milk.

INDICATION AND USAGE

Hypertension, when parenteral medication is indicated.

The treatment of hypertensive crises may be initiated with Injection ALDOMET Ester Hydrochloride.

CONTRAINDICATIONS

Active hepatic disease, such as acute hepatitis and active cirrhosis.

If previous methyldopa therapy has been associated with liver disorders (see WARNINGS).

Hypersensitivity to any component of this product, including sulfites (see WARNINGS).

WARNINGS

It is important to recognize that a positive Coombs test, hemolytic anemia, and liver disorders may occur with methyldopa therapy. The rare occurrences of hemolytic anemia or liver disorders could lead to potentially fatal complications unless properly recognized and managed. Read this section carefully to understand these reactions.

With prolonged methyldopa therapy, 10 to 20 percent of patients develop a positive direct Coombs test which usually occurs between 6 and 12 months of methyldopa therapy. Lowest incidence is at daily dosage of 1 g or less. This on rare occasions may be associated with hemolytic anemia, which could lead to potentially fatal complications. One cannot predict which patients with a positive direct Coombs test may develop hemolytic anemia.

Prior existence or development of a positive direct Coombs test is not in itself a contraindication to use of methyldopa. If a positive Coombs test develops during methyldopa therapy, the physician should determine whether hemolytic anemia exists and whether the positive Coombs test may be a problem. For example, in addition to a positive direct Coombs test there is less often a positive indirect Coombs test which may interfere with cross matching of blood.

Before treatment is started, it is desirable to do a blood count (hematocrit, hemoglobin, or red cell count) for a baseline or to establish whether there is anemia. Periodic blood counts should be done during therapy to detect hemolytic anemia. It may be useful to do a direct Coombs test before therapy and at 6 and 12 months after the start of therapy.

If Coombs-positive hemolytic anemia occurs, the cause may be methyldopa and the drug should be discontinued. Usually the anemia remits promptly. If not, corticosteroids may be given and other causes of anemia should be considered. If the hemolytic anemia is related to methyldopa, the drug should not be reinstituted.

When methyldopa causes Coombs positivity alone or with hemolytic anemia, the red cell is usually coated with gamma globulin of the IgG (gamma G) class only. The positive Coombs test may not revert to normal until weeks to months after methyldopa is stopped.

Should the need for transfusion arise in a patient receiving methyldopa, both a direct and an indirect Coombs test should be performed. In the absence of hemolytic anemia, usually only the direct Coombs test will be positive. A positive direct Coombs test alone will not interfere with typing or cross matching. If the indirect Coombs test is also positive, problems may arise in the major cross match and the assistance of a hematologist or transfusion expert will be needed.

Occasionally, fever has occurred within the first three weeks of methyldopa therapy, associated in some cases with eosinophilia or abnormalities in one or more liver function tests, such as serum alkaline phosphatase, serum transaminases (SGOT, SGPT), bilirubin and prothrombin time. Jaundice, with or without fever, may occur with onset usually within the first two to three months of therapy. In some patients the findings are consistent with those of cholestasis. In others the findings are consistent with hepatitis and hepatocellular injury.

Rarely fatal hepatic necrosis has been reported after use of methyldopa. These hepatic changes may represent hypersensitivity reactions. Periodic determination of hepatic function should be done particularly during the first 6 to 12 weeks of therapy or whenever an unexplained fever occurs. If fever, abnormalities in liver function tests, or jaundice appear, stop therapy with methyldopa. If caused by methyldopa, the temperature and abnormalities in liver function characteristically have reverted to normal when the drug was discontinued. Methyldopa should not be reinstituted in such patients.

Rarely, a reversible reduction of the white blood cell count with a primary effect on the granulocytes has been seen. The granulocyte count returned promptly to normal on discontinuance of the drug. Rare cases of granulocytopenia have been reported. In each instance, upon stopping the drug, the white cell count returned to normal. Reversible thrombocytopenia has occurred rarely.

Injection ALDOMET Ester Hydrochloride contains sodium bisulfite, a sulfite that may cause allergic-type reactions including anaphylactic symptoms and life-threatening or less severe asthmatic episodes in certain susceptible people. The overall prevalence of sulfite sensitivity in the general population is unknown and probably low. Sulfite sensitivity is seen more frequently in asthmatic than in nonasthmatic people.

PRECAUTIONS

General

Methyldopa should be used with caution in patients with a history of previous liver disease or dysfunction (see WARNINGS).

Some patients taking methyldopa experience clinical edema or weight gain which may be controlled by use of a diuretic. Methyldopa should not be continued if edema progresses or signs of heart failure appear.

A paradoxical pressor response has been reported with intravenous administration of ALDOMET Ester Hydrochloride.

Hypertension has recurred occasionally after dialysis in patients given methyldopa because the drug is removed by this procedure.

Rarely involuntary choreoathetotic movements have been observed during therapy with methyldopa in patients with severe bilateral cerebrovascular disease. Should these movements occur, stop therapy.

Laboratory Tests

Blood count, Coombs test, and liver function tests are recommended before initiating therapy and at periodic intervals (see WARNINGS).

Drug Interactions

When methyldopa is used with other antihypertensive drugs, potentiation of antihypertensive effect may occur. Patients should be followed carefully to detect side reactions or unusual manifestations of drug idiosyncrasy.

Patients may require reduced doses of anesthetics when on methyldopa. If hypotension does occur during anesthesia, it usually can be controlled by vasopressors. The adrenergic receptors remain sensitive during treatment with methyldopa.

When methyldopa and lithium are given concomitantly the patient should be carefully monitored for symptoms of lithium toxicity. Read the circular for lithium preparations.

Drug/Laboratory Test Interactions

Methyldopa may interfere with measurement of: urinary uric acid by the phosphotungstate method, serum creatinine by the alkaline picrate method, and SGOT by colorimetric methods. Interference with spectrophotometric methods for SGOT analysis has not been reported.

Since methyldopa causes fluorescence in urine samples at the same wave lengths as catecholamines, falsely high levels of urinary catecholamines may be reported. This will interfere with the diagnosis of pheochromocytoma. It is important to recognize this phenomenon before a patient with a possible pheochromocytoma is subjected to surgery. Methyldopa does not interfere with measurement of VMA (vanillylmandelic acid), a test for pheochromocytoma, by those methods which convert VMA to vanillin. Methyldopa is not recommended for the treatment of patients with pheochromocytoma. Rarely, when urine is exposed to air after voiding, it may darken because of breakdown of methyldopa or its metabolites.

Carcinogenesis, Mutagenesis, Impairment of Fertility
Methyldopa is currently under study in the U.S. Carcinogenesis Testing Program.

Methyldopa did not have mutagenic activity *in vitro* in the Ames microbial mutagen test with or without metabolic activation.

Methyldopa given in a two-litter study in rats at approximately three to six times the usual daily human dose did not impair fertility.

Long-term studies in animals have not been performed to evaluate the carcinogenic potential of methyldopate hydrochloride; nor have evaluations of this ester's mutagenic potential or potential to affect fertility been carried out.

Pregnancy
Pregnancy Category C. Animal reproduction studies have not been conducted with ALDOMET Ester Hydrochloride. It is also not known whether ALDOMET Ester Hydrochloride can affect reproduction capacity or can cause fetal harm when given to a pregnant woman. ALDOMET Ester Hydrochloride should be given to a pregnant woman only if clearly needed.

Nursing Mothers
Methyldopa appears in breast milk. Therefore, caution should be exercised when methyldopa is given to a nursing woman.

ADVERSE REACTIONS

Sedation, usually transient, may occur during the initial period of therapy or whenever the dose is increased. Headache, asthenia, or weakness may be noted as early and transient symptoms. However, significant adverse effects due to methyldopa have been infrequent and this agent usually is well tolerated.

The following adverse reactions have been reported and, within each category, are listed in order of decreasing severity.

Cardiovascular: Aggravation of angina pectoris, congestive heart failure, prolonged carotid sinus hypersensitivity, paradoxical pressor response with intravenous use, orthostatic hypotension (decrease daily dosage), edema or weight gain, bradycardia.

Digestive: Pancreatitis, colitis, vomiting, diarrhea, sialadenitis, sore or "black" tongue, nausea, constipation, distension, flatus, dryness of mouth.

Endocrine: Hyperprolactinemia.

Hematologic: Bone marrow depression, leukopenia, granulocytopenia, thrombocytopenia, hemolytic anemia; positive tests for antinuclear antibody, LE cells, and rheumatoid factor, positive Coombs tests.

Hepatic: Liver disorders including hepatitis, jaundice, abnormal liver function tests (see WARNINGS).

Hypersensitivity: Myocarditis, pericarditis, vasculitis, lupus-like syndrome, drug-related fever.

Nervous System/Psychiatric: Parkinsonism, Bell's palsy, decreased mental acuity, involuntary choreoathetotic movements, symptoms of cerebrovascular insufficiency, psychic disturbances including nightmares and reversible mild psychoses or depression, headache, sedation, asthenia or weakness, dizziness, lightheadedness, paresthesias.

Metabolic: Rise in BUN.

Musculoskeletal: Arthralgia, with or without joint swelling; myalgia.

Respiratory: Nasal stuffiness.

Skin: Toxic epidermal necrolysis, rash.

Urogenital: Amenorrhea, breast enlargement, gynecomastia, lactation, impotence, decreased libido.

OVERDOSAGE

Acute overdosage may produce acute hypotension with other responses attributable to brain and gastrointestinal malfunction (excessive sedation, weakness, bradycardia, dizziness, lightheadedness, constipation, distention, flatus, diarrhea, nausea, vomiting).

In the event of overdosage, symptomatic and supportive measures should be employed. Management includes special attention to cardiac rate and output, blood volume, electrolyte balance, paralytic ileus, urinary function and cerebral activity.

Sympathomimetic drugs [e.g. levarterenol, epinephrine, ARAMINE* (Metaraminol Bitartrate)] may be indicated.

The acute intravenous LD_{50} of ALDOMET Ester Hydrochloride in the mouse is 321 mg/kg.

---

*Registered trademark of MERCK & CO., INC.

DOSAGE AND ADMINISTRATION

Injection ALDOMET Ester Hydrochloride, when given intravenously in effective doses, causes a decline in blood pressure that may begin in four to six hours and last 10 to 16 hours after injection.

Add the desired dose of Injection ALDOMET Ester Hydrochloride to 100 mL of 5 percent Dextrose Injection USP. Alternatively the desired dose may be given in 5% dextrose in water in a concentration of 100 mg/10 mL. Give this intravenous infusion slowly over a period of 30 to 60 minutes.

The vial containing Injection ALDOMET Ester Hydrochloride should be inspected visually for particulate matter and discoloration before use whenever solution and container permit.

ADULTS

The usual adult dosage intravenously is 250 to 500 mg at six hour intervals as required. The maximum recommended intravenous dose is 1 g every six hours.

When control has been obtained, oral therapy with Tablets ALDOMET (Methyldopa) may be substituted for intravenous therapy, starting with the same dosage schedule used for the parenteral route. The effectiveness and anticipated responses are described in the circular for Tablets ALDOMET (Methyldopa).

Since methyldopa has a relatively short duration of action, withdrawal is followed by return of hypertension usually within 48 hours. This is not complicated by an overshoot of blood pressure.

Occasionally tolerance may occur, usually between the second and third month of therapy. Adding a diuretic or increasing the dosage of methyldopa frequently will restore effective control of blood pressure. A thiazide may be added at any time during methyldopa therapy and is recommended if therapy has not been started with a thiazide or if effective control of blood pressure cannot be maintained on 2 g of methyldopa daily.

Methyldopa is largely excreted by the kidney and patients with impaired renal function may respond to smaller doses. Syncope in older patients may be related to an increased sensitivity and advanced arteriosclerotic vascular disease. This may be avoided by lower doses.

CHILDREN

The recommended daily dosage is 20 to 40 mg/kg of body weight in divided doses every six hours. The maximum dosage is 65 mg/kg or 3 g daily, whichever is less. When the blood pressure is under control, continue with oral therapy using Tablets ALDOMET (Methyldopa) in the same dosage as for the parenteral route.

HOW SUPPLIED

No. 3293—Injection ALDOMET Ester Hydrochloride, 250 mg per 5 mL, is a clear, colorless solution and is supplied as follows:
NDC 0006-3293-05 in 5 mL vials
(6505-01-096-2735, 5 mL vial).

Storage
Store below 30°C (86°F).
Protect from freezing.

A.H.F.S. Category: 24:08
DC 7347133   Issued March 1990
COPYRIGHT © MERCK & CO., INC., 1989
All rights reserved

ALDORIL® Tablets   ℞
(Methyldopa-Hydrochlorothiazide), U.S.P.

> **WARNING**
> This fixed combination drug is not indicated for initial therapy of hypertension. Hypertension requires therapy titrated to the individual patient. If the fixed combination represents the dosage so determined, its use may be more convenient in patient management. The treatment of hypertension is not static, but must be reevaluated as conditions in each patient warrant.

DESCRIPTION

ALDORIL* (Methyldopa-Hydrochlorothiazide) combines two antihypertensives: methyldopa and hydrochlorothiazide.

Methyldopa
Methyldopa is an antihypertensive and is the *L*-isomer of alphamethyldopa. It is levo-3-(3,4-dihydroxyphenyl)-2-methylalanine. Its empirical formula is $C_{10}H_{13}NO_4$, with a molecular weight of 211.22, and its structural formula is:

Methyldopa is a white to yellowish white, odorless fine powder, and is soluble in water.

Hydrochlorothiazide
Hydrochlorothiazide is a diuretic and antihypertensive. It is the 3,4-dihydro derivative of chlorothiazide. Its chemical name is 6-chloro-3,4-dihydro-2*H*-1,2,4-benzothiadiazine-7-sulfonamide 1,1-dioxide. Its empirical formula is $C_7H_8ClN_3O_4S_2$ and its structural formula is:

Hydrochlorothiazide is a white, or practically white, crystalline powder with a molecular weight of 297.72, which is slightly soluble in water, but freely soluble in sodium hydroxide solution.

ALDORIL is supplied as tablets in four strengths for oral use:
ALDORIL 15, contains 250 mg of methyldopa and 15 mg of hydrochlorothiazide.
ALDORIL 25, contains 250 mg of methyldopa and 25 mg of hydrochlorothiazide.
ALDORIL D30, contains 500 mg of methyldopa and 30 mg of hydrochlorothiazide.
ALDORIL D50, contains 500 mg of methyldopa and 50 mg of hydrochlorothiazide.

Each tablet contains the following inactive ingredients: calcium disodium edetate, calcium phosphate, cellulose, citric acid, colloidal silicon dioxide, ethylcellulose, guar gum, hydroxypropyl methylcellulose, magnesium stearate, propylene glycol, talc, and titanium dioxide. ALDORIL 15 and ALDORIL D30 also contain iron oxide.

---

*Registered trademark of MERCK & CO., INC.

CLINICAL PHARMACOLOGY

Methyldopa
Methyldopa is an aromatic-amino-acid decarboxylase inhibitor in animals and in man. Although the mechanism of action has yet to be conclusively demonstrated, the antihypertensive effect of methyldopa probably is due to its metabolism to alpha-methylnorepinephrine, which then lowers arterial pressure by stimulation of central inhibitory alpha-adrenergic receptors, false neurotransmission, and/or reduction of plasma renin activity. Methyldopa has been shown to cause a net reduction in the tissue concentration of serotonin, dopamine, norepinephrine, and epinephrine.

Only methyldopa, the *L*-isomer of alpha-methyldopa, has the ability to inhibit dopa decarboxylase and to deplete animal tissues of norepinephrine. In man, the antihypertensive activity appears to be due solely to the *L*-isomer. About twice the dose of the racemate (*DL*-alpha-methyldopa) is required for equal antihypertensive effect.

Methyldopa has no direct effect on cardiac function and usually does not reduce glomerular filtration rate, renal blood flow, or filtration fraction. Cardiac output usually is maintained without cardiac acceleration. In some patients the heart rate is slowed.

Normal or elevated plasma renin activity may decrease in the course of methyldopa therapy.

Methyldopa reduces both supine and standing blood pressure. It usually produces highly effective lowering of the supine pressure with infrequent symptomatic postural hypotension. Exercise hypotension and diurnal blood pressure variations rarely occur.

Hydrochlorothiazide
The mechanism of the antihypertensive effect of thiazides is unknown. Hydrochlorothiazide does not usually affect normal blood pressure.

Hydrochlorothiazide affects the distal renal tubular mechanism of electrolyte reabsorption. At maximal therapeutic

Continued on next page

Information on the Merck & Co. products listed on these pages is the full prescribing information from product circulars in use October 1, 1992.

Merck & Co.—Cont.

dosage all thiazides are approximately equal in their diuretic efficacy.

Hydrochlorothiazide increases excretion of sodium and chloride in approximately equivalent amounts. Natriuresis may be accompanied by some loss of potassium and bicarbonate. After oral use diuresis begins within 2 hours, peaks in about 4 hours and lasts about 6 to 12 hours.

Methyldopa-Hydrochlorothiazide

The concomitant use of methyldopa and hydrochlorothiazide, as provided in ALDORIL, frequently produces a more pronounced antihypertensive response than when either compound is the sole therapeutic agent. Particularly in those cases of hypertensive vascular disease where sodium and water retention is a problem, the coadministration of these two drugs in the form of ALDORIL will help control the fluid imbalance.

In severe essential hypertension and in malignant hypertension ALDORIL may achieve effective lowering of blood pressure with fewer side effects than occur with other compounds used for this purpose.

ALDORIL reduces both supine and standing blood pressure; more effective lowering of the supine pressure with less frequent symptomatic postural hypotension can be obtained with ALDORIL than with most other antihypertensive agents. In patients treated with ALDORIL, exercise hypotension and diurnal blood pressure variations rarely occur.

Pharmacokinetics and Metabolism
Methyldopa

The maximum decrease in blood pressure occurs four to six hours after oral dosage. Once an effective dosage level is attained, a smooth blood pressure response occurs in most patients in 12 to 24 hours. After withdrawal, blood pressure usually returns to pretreatment levels within 24–48 hours. Methyldopa is extensively metabolized. The known urinary metabolites are: α-methyldopa mono-0-sulfate; 3-0-methyl-α-methyldopa; 3,4-dihydroxyphenylacetone; α-methyldopamine; 3-0-methyl-α-methyldopamine and their conjugates. Approximately 70 percent of the drug which is absorbed is excreted in the urine as methyldopa and its mono-0-sulfate conjugate. The renal clearance is about 130 mL/min in normal subjects and is diminished in renal insufficiency. The plasma half-life of methyldopa is 105 minutes. After oral doses, excretion is essentially complete in 36 hours. Methyldopa crosses the placental barrier, appears in cord blood, and appears in breast milk.

Hydrochlorothiazide

Hydrochlorothiazide is not metabolized but is eliminated rapidly by the kidney. When plasma levels have been followed for at least 24 hours, the plasma half-life has been observed to vary between 5.6 and 14.8 hours. At least 61 percent of the oral dose is eliminated unchanged within 24 hours. Hydrochlorothiazide crosses the placental but not the blood-brain barrier and is excreted in breast milk.

INDICATION AND USAGE

Hypertension (see box warning).
Use in Pregnancy. Routine use of diuretics during normal pregnancy is inappropriate and exposes mother and fetus to unnecessary hazard. Diuretics do not prevent development of toxemia of pregnancy and there is no satisfactory evidence that they are useful in the treatment of toxemia.

Edema during pregnancy may arise from pathologic causes or from the physiologic and mechanical consequences of pregnancy. Thiazides are indicated in pregnancy when edema is due to pathologic causes, just as they are in the absence of pregnancy (see PRECAUTIONS, *Pregnancy*). Dependent edema in pregnancy, resulting from restriction of venous return by the gravid uterus, is properly treated through elevation of the lower extremities and use of support stockings. Use of diuretics to lower intravascular volume in this instance is illogical and unnecessary. During normal pregnancy there is hypervolemia which is not harmful to the fetus or the mother in the absence of cardiovascular disease. However, it may be associated with edema, rarely generalized edema. If such edema causes discomfort, increased recumbency will often provide relief. Rarely this edema may cause extreme discomfort which is not relieved by rest. In these instances, a short course of diuretic therapy may provide relief and be appropriate.

CONTRAINDICATIONS

Active hepatic disease, such as acute hepatitis and active cirrhosis.
If previous methyldopa therapy has been associated with liver disorders (see WARNINGS).
Anuria.
Hypersensitivity to methyldopa, or to hydrochlorothiazide or other sulfonamide-derived drugs.

WARNINGS

Methyldopa

It is important to recognize that a positive Coombs test, hemolytic anemia, and liver disorders may occur with methyldopa therapy. The rare occurrences of hemolytic anemia or liver disorders could lead to potentially fatal complications unless properly recognized and managed. Read this section carefully to understand these reactions.

With prolonged methyldopa therapy, 10 to 20 percent of patients develop a positive direct Coombs test which usually occurs between 6 and 12 months of methyldopa therapy. Lowest incidence is at daily dosage of 1 g or less. This on rare occasions may be associated with hemolytic anemia, which could lead to potentially fatal complications. One cannot predict which patients with a positive direct Coombs test may develop hemolytic anemia.

Prior existence or development of a positive direct Coombs test is not in itself a contraindication to use of methyldopa. If a positive Coombs test develops during methyldopa therapy, the physician should determine whether hemolytic anemia exists and whether the positive Coombs test may be a problem. For example, in addition to a positive direct Coombs test there is less often a positive indirect Coombs test which may interfere with cross matching of blood.

Before treatment is started it is desirable to do a blood count (hematocrit, hemoglobin, or red cell count) for a baseline or to establish whether there is anemia. Periodic blood counts should be done during therapy to detect hemolytic anemia. It may be useful to do a direct Coombs test before therapy and at 6 and 12 months after the start of therapy.

If Coombs-positive hemolytic anemia occurs, the cause may be methyldopa and the drug should be discontinued. Usually the anemia remits promptly. If not, corticosteroids may be given and other causes of anemia should be considered. If the hemolytic anemia is related to methyldopa, the drug should not be reinstituted.

When methyldopa causes Coombs positivity alone or with hemolytic anemia, the red cell is usually coated with gamma globulin of the IgG (gamma G) class only. The positive Coombs test may not revert to normal until weeks to months after methyldopa is stopped.

Should the need for transfusion arise in a patient receiving methyldopa, both a direct and an indirect Coombs test should be performed. In the absence of hemolytic anemia, usually only the direct Coombs test will be positive. A positive direct Coombs test alone will not interfere with typing or cross matching. If the indirect Coombs test is also positive, problems may arise in the major cross match and the assistance of a hematologist or transfusion expert will be needed.

Occasionally, fever has occurred within the first three weeks of methyldopa therapy, associated in some cases with eosinophilia or abnormalities in one or more liver function tests, such as serum alkaline phosphatase, serum transaminases (SGOT, SGPT), bilirubin, and prothrombin time. Jaundice, with or without fever, may occur with onset usually within the first two to three months of therapy. In some patients the findings are consistent with those of cholestasis. In others the findings are consistent with hepatitis and hepatocellular injury.

Rarely fatal hepatic necrosis has been reported after use of methyldopa. These hepatic changes may represent hypersensitivity reactions. Periodic determination of hepatic function should be done particularly during the first 6 to 12 weeks of therapy or whenever an unexplained fever occurs. If fever, abnormalities in liver function tests, or jaundice appear, stop therapy with methyldopa. If caused by methyldopa, the temperature and abnormalities in liver function characteristically have reverted to normal when the drug was discontinued. Methyldopa should not be reinstituted in such patients.

Rarely, a reversible reduction of the white blood cell count with a primary effect on the granulocytes has been seen. The granulocyte count returned promptly to normal on discontinuance of the drug. Rare cases of granulocytopenia have been reported. In each instance, upon stopping the drug, the white cell count returned to normal. Reversible thrombocytopenia has occurred rarely.

Hydrochlorothiazide

Use with caution in severe renal disease. In patients with renal disease, thiazides may precipitate azotemia. Cumulative effects of the drug may develop in patients with impaired renal function.

Thiazides should be used with caution in patients with impaired hepatic function or progressive liver disease, since minor alterations of fluid and electrolyte balance may precipitate hepatic coma.

Thiazides may add to or potentiate the action of other antihypertensive drugs.

Sensitivity reactions may occur in patients with or without a history of allergy or bronchial asthma.

The possibility of exacerbation or activation of systemic lupus erythematosus has been reported.

Lithium generally should not be given with diuretics (see PRECAUTIONS, *Drug Interactions*).

PRECAUTIONS

General
Methyldopa

Methyldopa should be used with caution in patients with a history of previous liver disease or dysfunction (see WARNINGS).

Some patients taking methyldopa experience clinical edema or weight gain which may be controlled by use of a diuretic. Methyldopa should not be continued if edema progresses or signs of heart failure appear.

Hypertension has recurred occasionally after dialysis in patients given methyldopa because the drug is removed by this procedure.

Rarely involuntary choreoathetotic movements have been observed during therapy with methyldopa in patients with severe bilateral cerebrovascular disease. Should these movements occur, stop therapy.

Hydrochlorothiazide

All patients receiving diuretic therapy should be observed for evidence of fluid or electrolyte imbalance: namely; hyponatremia, hypochloremic alkalosis, and hypokalemia. Serum and urine electrolyte determinations are particularly important when the patient is vomiting excessively or receiving parenteral fluids. Warning signs or symptoms of fluid and electrolyte imbalance, irrespective of cause, include dryness of mouth, thirst, weakness, lethargy, drowsiness, restlessness, muscle pains or cramps, muscular fatigue, hypotension, oliguria, tachycardia, and gastrointestinal disturbances such as nausea and vomiting.

Hypokalemia may develop, especially with brisk diuresis, when severe cirrhosis is present or after prolonged therapy. Interference with adequate oral electrolyte intake will also contribute to hypokalemia. Hypokalemia may cause cardiac arrhythmia and may also sensitize or exaggerate the response of the heart to the toxic effects of digitalis (e.g., increased ventricular irritability). Hypokalemia may be avoided or treated by use of potassium sparing diuretics or potassium supplements such as foods with a high potassium content.

Although any chloride deficit is generally mild and usually does not require specific treatment except under extraordinary circumstances (as in liver disease or renal disease), chloride replacement may be required in the treatment of metabolic alkalosis.

Dilutional hyponatremia may occur in edematous patients in hot weather; appropriate therapy is water restriction, rather than administration of salt, except in rare instances when the hyponatremia is life threatening. In actual salt depletion, appropriate replacement is the therapy of choice. Hyperuricemia may occur or acute gout may be precipitated in certain patients receiving thiazides.

In diabetic patients dosage adjustment of insulin or oral hypoglycemic agents may be required. Hyperglycemia may occur with thiazide diuretics. Thus latent diabetes mellitus may become manifest during thiazide therapy.

The antihypertensive effects of the drug may be enhanced in the postsympathectomy patient.

If progressive renal impairment becomes evident, consider withholding or discontinuing diuretic therapy.

Thiazides have been shown to increase the urinary excretion of magnesium; this may result in hypomagnesemia.

Thiazides may decrease urinary calcium excretion. Thiazides may cause intermittent and slight elevation of serum calcium in the absence of known disorders of calcium metabolism. Marked hypercalcemia may be evidence of hidden hyperparathyroidism. Thiazides should be discontinued before carrying out tests for parathyroid function.

Increases in cholesterol and triglyceride levels may be associated with thiazide diuretic therapy.

Laboratory Tests
Methyldopa

Blood count, Coombs test and liver function test, are recommended before initiating therapy and at periodic intervals (see WARNINGS).

Hydrochlorothiazide

Periodic determination of serum electrolytes to detect possible electrolyte imbalance should be done at appropriate intervals.

Drug Interactions
Methyldopa

When methyldopa is used with other antihypertensive drugs, potentiation of antihypertensive effect may occur. Patients should be followed carefully to detect side reactions or unusual manifestations of drug idiosyncrasy.

Patients may require reduced doses of anesthetics when on methyldopa. If hypotension does occur during anesthesia, it usually can be controlled by vasopressors. The adrenergic receptors remain sensitive during treatment with methyldopa.

Hydrochlorothiazide

When given concurrently the following drugs may interact with thiazide diuretics.

Alcohol, barbiturates, or narcotics—potentiation of orthostatic hypotension may occur.
Antidiabetic drugs (oral agents and insulin)—dosage adjustment of the antidiabetic drug may be required.
Other antihypertensive drugs—additive effect or potentiation.
Corticosteroids, ACTH—intensified electrolyte depletion, particularly hypokalemia.
Pressor amines (e.g., norepinephrine)—possible decreased response to pressor amines but not sufficient to preclude their use.
Skeletal muscle relaxants, nondepolarizing (e.g., tubocurarine)—possible increased responsiveness to the muscle relaxant.
Lithium—generally should not be given with diuretics. Diuretic agents reduce the renal clearance of lithium and add a high risk of lithium toxicity. Refer to the package insert for lithium preparations before use of such preparations with ALDORIL.
Non-steroidal Anti-inflammatory Drugs—In some patients, the administration of a non-steroidal anti-inflammatory agent can reduce the diuretic, natriuretic, and antihypertensive effects of loop, potassium-sparing and thiazide diuretics. Therefore, when ALDORIL and non-steroidal anti-inflammatory agents are used concomitantly, the patient should be observed closely to determine if the desired effect of the diuretic is obtained.
Drug/Laboratory Test Interactions
Methyldopa
Methyldopa may interfere with measurement of: urinary uric acid by the phosphotungstate method, serum creatinine by the alkaline picrate method, and SGOT by colorimetric methods. Interference with spectrophotometric methods for SGOT analysis has not been reported.
Since methyldopa causes fluorescence in urine samples at the same wave lengths as catecholamines, falsely high levels of urinary catecholamines may be reported. This will interfere with the diagnosis of pheochromocytoma. It is important to recognize this phenomenon before a patient with a possible pheochromocytoma is subjected to surgery. Methyldopa does not interfere with measurement of VMA (vanillylmandelic acid), a test for pheochromocytoma, by those methods which convert VMA to vanillin. Methyldopa is not recommended for the treatment of patients with pheochromocytoma. Rarely, when urine is exposed to air after voiding, it may darken because of breakdown of methyldopa or its metabolites.
Hydrochlorothiazide
Thiazides should be discontinued before carrying out tests for parathyroid function (see PRECAUTIONS, *General*).
Carcinogenesis, Mutagenesis,
Impairment of Fertility
Long-term studies in animals have not been performed to evaluate the effects upon fertility, mutagenic or carcinogenic potential of the combination.
Methyldopa
Methyldopa is currently under study in the U.S. Carcinogenesis Testing Program.
Methyldopa did not have mutagenic activity *in vitro* in the Ames microbial mutagen test with or without metabolic activation.
Methyldopa given in a two-litter study in rats at approximately three to six times the usual daily dose did not impair fertility.
Hydrochlorothiazide
Hydrochlorothiazide is currently under study in the U.S. Carcinogenesis Testing Program.
Hydrochlorothiazide was not mutagenic *in vitro*, in the Ames microbial mutagen test at a maximum concentration of 5 mg/plate using Strains TA98 and TA100. Urine samples from patients treated with hydrochlorothiazide did not have mutagenic activity in the Ames test.
The ability of a number of drugs to induce nondisjunction and crossing over was measured using *Aspergillus nidulans*. A large number of drugs, including hydrochlorothiazide, induced nondisjunction.
Hydrochlorothiazide had no effect on fertility in a two-litter study in rats at doses 4–5.6 mg/kg/day (up to 2 times the maximum recommended human dose).
Pregnancy
Teratogenic Effects—Pregnancy Category C: Animal reproduction studies have not been conducted with ALDORIL. It is also not known whether ALDORIL can affect reproduction capacity or can cause fetal harm when given to a pregnant woman. ALDORIL should be given to a pregnant woman only if clearly needed. (See INDICATION AND USAGE.)
Hydrochlorothiazide: Thiazides cross the placental barrier and appear in cord blood.
Reproduction studies in the rabbit, the mouse and the rat at doses up to 100 mg/kg/day (50 times the maximum recommended human dose) showed no evidence of external abnormalities of the fetus due to hydrochlorothiazide. Hydrochlorothiazide given in a two-litter study in rats at doses of 4–5.6 mg/kg/day (approximately 1–2 times the maximum recommended human dose) did not impair fertility or produce birth abnormalities in the offspring.
Methyldopa: Reproduction studies have been performed in the rabbit, the mouse, and the rat at doses up to 1000 mg/kg/day (16.6 times the maximum recommended human dose) and have revealed no evidence of impaired fertility or harm to the fetus due to methyldopa. There are, however, no adequate and well-controlled studies in pregnant women in the first trimester of pregnancy. Because animal reproduction studies are not always predictive of human response, methyldopa should be used during pregnancy only if clearly needed.
Published reports of the use of methyldopa during all trimesters indicate that if this drug is used during pregnancy the possibility of fetal harm appears remote. In five studies, three of which were controlled, involving 332 pregnant hypertensive women, treatment with methyldopa was associated with an improved fetal outcome. The majority of these women were in the third trimester when methyldopa therapy was begun.
In one study, women who had begun methyldopa treatment between weeks 16 and 20 of pregnancy gave birth to infants whose average head circumference was reduced by a small amount (34.2 ± 1.7 cm vs. 34.6 ± 1.3 cm [mean ± 1 S.D.]). Long term follow-up of 195 (97.5%) of the children born to methyldopa-treated pregnant women (including those who began treatment between weeks 16 and 20) failed to uncover any significant adverse effect on the children. At four years of age, the developmental delay commonly seen in children born to hypertensive mothers was less evident in those whose mothers were treated with methyldopa during pregnancy than those whose mothers were untreated. The children of the treated group scored consistently higher than the children of the untreated group on five major indices of intellectual and motor development. At age 7 and one-half developmental scores and intelligence indices showed no significant differences in children of treated or untreated hypertensive women.
Nonteratogenic Effects: These may include fetal or neonatal jaundice, thrombocytopenia, and possibly other adverse reactions which have occurred in the adult.
Nursing Mothers
Methyldopa and thiazides appear in breast milk. Therefore, because of the potential for serious adverse reactions in nursing infants from hydrochlorothiazide, a decision should be made whether to discontinue nursing or to discontinue the drug, taking into account the importance of the drug to the mother.
Pediatric Use
Safety and effectiveness of ALDORIL in children has not been established.

ADVERSE REACTIONS

The following adverse reactions have been reported and, within each category, are listed in order of decreasing severity.
Methyldopa
Sedation, usually transient, may occur during the initial period of therapy or whenever the dose is increased. Headache, asthenia, or weakness may be noted as early and transient symptoms. However, significant adverse effects due to methyldopa have been infrequent and this agent usually is well tolerated.
Cardiovascular: Aggravation of angina pectoris, congestive heart failure, prolonged carotid sinus hypersensitivity, orthostatic hypotension (decrease daily dosage), edema or weight gain, bradycardia.
Digestive: Pancreatitis, colitis, vomiting, diarrhea, sialadenitis, sore or "black" tongue, nausea, constipation, distension, flatus, dryness of mouth.
Endocrine: Hyperprolactinemia.
Hematologic: Bone marrow depression, leukopenia, granulocytopenia, thrombocytopenia, hemolytic anemia; positive tests for antinuclear antibody, LE cells, and rheumatoid factor, positive Coombs test.
Hepatic: Liver disorders including hepatitis, jaundice, abnormal liver function tests (see WARNINGS).
Hypersensitivity: Myocarditis, pericarditis, vasculitis, lupus-like syndrome, drug-related fever.
Nervous System/Psychiatric: Parkinsonism, Bell's palsy, decreased mental acuity, involuntary choreoathetotic movements, symptoms of cerebrovascular insufficiency, psychic disturbances including nightmares and reversible mild psychoses or depression, headache, sedation, asthenia or weakness, dizziness, lightheadedness, paresthesias.
Metabolic: Rise in BUN.
Musculoskeletal: Arthralgia, with or without joint swelling; myalgia.
Respiratory: Nasal stuffiness.
Skin: Toxic epidermal necrolysis, rash.
Urogenital: Amenorrhea, breast enlargement, gynecomastia, lactation, impotence, decreased libido.
Hydrochlorothiazide
Body as a Whole: Weakness.
Cardiovascular: Hypotension including orthostatic hypotension (may be aggravated by alcohol, barbiturates, narcotics or antihypertensive drugs).
Digestive: Pancreatitis, jaundice (intrahepatic cholestatic jaundice), diarrhea, vomiting, sialadenitis, cramping, constipation, gastric irritation, nausea, anorexia.
Hematologic: Aplastic anemia, agranulocytosis, leukopenia, hemolytic anemia, thrombocytopenia.
Hypersensitivity: Anaphylactic reactions, necrotizing angiitis (vasculitis and cutaneous vasculitis), respiratory distress including pneumonitis and pulmonary edema, photosensitivity, fever, urticaria, rash, purpura.
Metabolic: Electrolyte imbalance (see PRECAUTIONS), hyperglycemia, glycosuria, hyperuricemia.
Musculoskeletal: Muscle spasm.
Nervous System/Psychiatric: Vertigo, paresthesias, dizziness, headache, restlessness.
Renal: Renal failure, renal dysfunction, interstitial nephritis. (See WARNINGS.)
Special Senses: Transient blurred vision, xanthopsia.
Whenever adverse reactions are moderate or severe, thiazide dosage should be reduced or therapy withdrawn.

OVERDOSAGE

Acute overdosage may produce acute hypotension with other responses attributable to brain and gastrointestinal malfunction (excessive sedation, weakness, bradycardia, dizziness, lightheadedness, constipation, distention, flatus, diarrhea, nausea, vomiting).
In the event of overdosage, symptomatic and supportive measures should be employed. When ingestion is recent, gastric lavage or emesis may reduce absorption. When ingestion has been earlier, infusions may be helpful to promote urinary excretion. Otherwise, management includes special attention to cardiac rate and output, blood volume, electrolyte balance, paralytic ileus, urinary function and cerebral activity.
Sympathomimetic drugs [e.g., levarterenol, epinephrine, ARAMINE* (Metaraminol Bitartrate)] may be indicated.
Methyldopa is dialyzable.
The oral LD_{50} of methyldopa is greater than 1.5 g/kg in both the mouse and the rat. The oral LD_{50} of hydrochlorothiazide is greater than 10 g/kg in the mouse and rat.

*Registered trademark of MERCK & CO., INC.

DOSAGE AND ADMINISTRATION

Dosage: As determined by individual titration (see box warning).
The usual dosage is 1 tablet of ALDORIL 15, ALDORIL 25, ALDORIL D30, or ALDORIL D50 two or three times a day in the first 48 hours. The daily dosage then may be increased or decreased, preferably at intervals of not less than two days, until an adequate response is achieved. To minimize the sedation associated with methyldopa, start dosage increases in the evening. By adjustment of dosage, morning hypotension may be prevented without sacrificing control of afternoon blood pressure.
When ALDORIL is given to patients on other antihypertensives, the dose of these agents may need to be adjusted to effect a smooth transition. When ALDORIL is given with antihypertensives other than thiazides, the initial dosage of methyldopa should be limited to 500 mg daily in divided doses.
Although occasional patients have responded to higher doses, the maximum recommended daily dosage is 3 g of methyldopa and 100 to 200 mg of hydrochlorothiazide. Once an effective dosage range is attained, a smooth blood pressure response occurs in most patients in 12 to 24 hours. If ALDORIL alone does not adequately control blood pressure, additional methyldopa may be given separately to obtain the maximum blood pressure response.
Since both components of ALDORIL have a relatively short duration of action, withdrawal is followed by return of hypertension usually within 48 hours. This is not complicated by an overshoot of blood pressure.
Occasionally tolerance may occur, usually between the second and third month of therapy. Increasing the dosage of either methyldopa or hydrochlorothiazide separately or together frequently will restore effective control of blood pressure.
Methyldopa is largely excreted by the kidney and patients with impaired renal function may respond to smaller doses of ALDORIL. Syncope in older patients may be related to an

Continued on next page

Information on the Merck & Co. products listed on these pages is the full prescribing information from product circulars in use October 1, 1992.

Merck & Co.—Cont.

increased sensitivity and advanced arteriosclerotic vascular disease. This may be avoided by lower doses.

HOW SUPPLIED

No. 3294—Tablets ALDORIL 15 are salmon, round, film coated tablets, coded MSD 423. Each tablet contains 250 mg of methyldopa and 15 mg of hydrochlorothiazide. They are supplied as follows:
NDC 0006-0423-68 bottles of 100
NDC 0006-0423-82 bottles of 1000.

Shown in Product Identification Section, page 419
No. 3295—Tablets ALDORIL 25 are white, round, film coated tablets, coded MSD 456. Each tablet contains 250 mg of methyldopa and 25 mg of hydrochlorothiazide. They are supplied as follows:
NDC 0006-0456-68 bottles of 100
NDC 0006-0456-28 unit dose packages of 100
NDC 0006-0456-82 bottles of 1000.

Shown in Product Identification Section, page 419
No. 3362—Tablets ALDORIL D30 are salmon, oval, film coated tablets, coded MSD 694. Each tablet contains 500 mg of methyldopa and 30 mg of hydrochlorothiazide. They are supplied as follows:
NDC 0006-0694-68 bottles of 100.

Shown in Product Identification Section, page 419
No. 3363—Tablets ALDORIL D50 are white, oval, film coated tablets, coded MSD 935. Each tablet contains 500 mg of methyldopa and 50 mg of hydrochlorothiazide. They are supplied as follows:
NDC 0006-0935-68 bottles of 100.

Shown in Product Identification Section, page 419
A.H.F.S. Category: 24:08
DC 7059641   Issued March 1990
COPYRIGHT © MERCK & CO., INC., 1986
All rights reserved

AMINOHIPPURATE SODIUM "PAH"   ℞
Injection, U.S.P.

DESCRIPTION

Aminohippurate sodium* is an agent to measure effective renal plasma flow (ERPF). It is the sodium salt of para-aminohippuric acid, commonly abbreviated "PAH." It is water soluble, lipid-insoluble, and has a pKa of 3.83. The empirical formula of the anhydrous salt is $C_9H_9N_2NaO_3$ and its structural formula is:

H₂N————CONHCH₂COONa

It is provided as a sterile, non-preserved 20 percent aqueous solution for injection, with a pH of 6.7 to 7.6. Each 10 mL contains: Aminohippurate sodium 2 g. Inactive ingredients: Sodium hydroxide to adjust pH, water for injection, q.s.

---
* Formerly referred to as Sodium para-Aminohippurate.

CLINICAL PHARMACOLOGY

PAH is filtered by the glomeruli and is actively secreted by the proximal tubules. At low plasma concentrations (1.0 to 2.0 mg/100 mL), an average of 90 percent of PAH is cleared by the kidneys from the renal blood stream in a single circulation. It is ideally suited for measurement of ERPF since it has a high clearance, is essentially nontoxic at the plasma concentrations reached with recommended doses and its analytical determination is relatively simple and accurate. PAH is also used to measure the functional capacity of the renal tubular secretory mechanism or transport maximum (Tm$_{PAH}$). This is accomplished by elevating the plasma concentration to levels (40–60 mg/100 mL) sufficient to saturate the maximal capacity of the tubular cells to secrete PAH. Inulin clearance is generally measured during Tm$_{PAH}$ determinations since glomerular filtration rate (GFR) must be known before calculations of secretory Tm measurements can be done (See *Calculations*).

INDICATIONS AND USAGE

Estimation of effective renal plasma flow.
Measurement of the functional capacity of the renal tubular secretory mechanism.

CONTRAINDICATIONS

Hypersensitivity to this product or to its components.

PRECAUTIONS

General
Intravenous solutions must be given with caution to patients with low cardiac reserve, since a rapid increase in plasma volume can precipitate congestive heart failure.
For measurement of ERPF, small doses of PAH are used. However, in research procedures to measure Tm$_{PAH}$, high plasma levels are required to saturate the capacity of the tubular cells. During these procedures the intravenous administration of PAH solutions should be carried out slowly and with caution. The patient should be continuously observed for any adverse reactions.
Drug Interactions
Renal clearance measurements of PAH cannot be made with any significant accuracy in patients receiving sulfonamides, procaine, or thiazolesulfone. These compounds interfere with chemical color development essential to the analytical procedures.
Probenecid depresses tubular secretion of certain weak acids such as PAH. Therefore, patients receiving probenecid will have erroneously low ERPF and Tm$_{PAH}$ values.
Carcinogenesis, Mutagenesis, Impairment of Fertility
Long-term studies in animals have not been done to evaluate any effects upon fertility or carcinogenic potential of PAH.
Pregnancy
Pregnancy Category C. Animal reproduction studies have not been done with PAH. It is also not known whether PAH can cause fetal harm when given to a pregnant woman or can affect reproduction capacity. PAH should be given to a pregnant woman only if clearly needed.
Nursing Mothers
It is not known whether this drug is excreted in human milk. Because many drugs are excreted in human milk, caution should be exercised when PAH is administered to a nursing woman.
Pediatric Use
Safety and effectiveness in children have not been established.

ADVERSE REACTIONS

Vasomotor disturbances, flushing, tingling, nausea, vomiting, and cramps may occur.
Patients may have a sensation of warmth or the desire to defecate or urinate during or shortly following initiation of infusion.

OVERDOSAGE

The intravenous LD$_{50}$ in female mice is 7.22 g/kg.

DOSAGE AND ADMINISTRATION

For intravenous use only
Clearance measurements using single injection technics are generally inaccurate, particularly in the measurement of ERPF. For this reason, intravenous infusions at fixed rates are used to sustain the plasma PAH concentration at the desired level.
To measure ERPF, the concentration of PAH in the plasma should be maintained at 2 mg per 100 mL, which can be achieved with a priming dose of 6 to 10 mg/kg and an infusion dose of 10 to 24 mg/min.
As a research procedure for the measurement of Tm$_{PAH}$, the plasma level of PAH must be sufficient to saturate the capacity of the tubular secretory cells. Concentrations of from 40 to 60 mg per 100 mL are usually necessary.
Technical details of these tests may be found in Smith[1]; Wesson[2]; Bauer[3]; Pitts[4]; and Schnurr.[5]
Parenteral drug products should be inspected visually for particulate matter and discoloration prior to use, whenever solution and container permit. NOTE: The normal color range for this product is a colorless to yellow/brown solution. The efficacy is not affected by color changes within this range.
Calculations
Effective Renal Plasma Flow (ERPF)
The clearance of PAH, which is extracted almost completely from the plasma during its passage through the renal circulation, constitutes a measure of ERPF. Hence:

$$ERPF = \frac{U_{PAH}V}{P_{PAH}}$$

Where U_{PAH} = concentration of PAH (mg/mL) in the urine
  V = rate of urine excretion (mL/min), and
  P_{PAH} = plasma concentration of PAH (mg/mL).

Example: U_{PAH} = 8.0 mg/mL
  V = 1.5 mL/min
  P_{PAH} = 0.02 mg/mL

$$ERPF = \frac{8.0 \times 1.5}{0.02} = 600 \text{ mL/min.}$$

Based on PAH clearance studies, the normal values for ERPF are:
  men   675 ± 150 mL/min.
  women 595 ± 125 mL/min.
Maximum Tubular Secretory
Mechanism (Tm$_{PAH}$)
The quantity of PAH, secreted by the tubules (Tm$_{PAH}$) is given by the difference between the total rate of excretion ($U_{PAH}V$) and the quantity filtered by the glomeruli (GFR $\times$ P_{PAH}). Hence:
  $Tm_{PAH} = U_{PAH}V - (GFR \times P_{PAH} \times 0.83)$
The factor, 0.83, corrects for that portion of PAH which is bound to plasma protein and hence is unfilterable.
Example: U_{PAH} = 9.55 mg/mL
  V = 16.68 mL/min
  GFR = 120 mL/min
  P_{PAH} = 0.60 mg/mL
Then Tm$_{PAH}$ = 9.55 $\times$ 16.68 − (120 $\times$ 0.60 $\times$ 0.83) = 100 mg/min.
Average normal values of Tm$_{PAH}$ are 80–90 mg/min.
The value of the expression $U_{PAH}V$, used in calculations of ERPF and Tm$_{PAH}$, may be found by determining the amount of PAH in a measured volume of urine excreted within a specific period of time.
These calculations are based on a body surface area of 1.73 m². Corrections for variations in surface area are made by multiplying the values obtained for ERPF and Tm$_{PAH}$ by 1.73/A, where A is the subject surface area.

HOW SUPPLIED

No. 95—Aminohippurate Sodium, 20 percent sterile solution for intravenous injection, is supplied as follows:
NDC 0006-3395-11 in 10 mL vials.
Storage
Avoid storage at temperatures below −20℃ (−4°F) and above 40℃ (104°F).

REFERENCES

1. Smith, H. W.: Lectures on the kidney, University Extension Division, University of Kansas, Lawrence, Kansas, 1943.
2. Wesson, L. G., Jr.: "Physiology of the Human Kidney," New York, Grune & Stratton, 1969, pp. 632–655.
3. Bauer, J. D.; Ackermann, P. G.; Toro, G.: "Brays Clinical Laboratory Methods," ed. 7, St. Louis, Mosby, 1968.
4. Pitts, R. F.: "Physiology of the Kidney and Body Fluids," ed. 2, Chicago, Year Book Medical Publishers, 1968.
5. Schnurr, E., Lahme, W., Kuppers, H.: Measurement of renal clearance of inulin and PAH in the steady state without urine collection; Clinical Nephrology, *13* (1): (26–29), 1980.

A.H.F.S. Category: 36:40
DC 7470618   Issued May 1986
COPYRIGHT © MERCK & CO., INC., 1983
All rights reserved

ANTIVENIN   ℞
(Latrodectus mactans), MSD, U.S.P.
Black Widow Spider Antivenin
Equine Origin

DESCRIPTION

Antivenin (Latrodectus mactans), MSD is a sterile, non-pyrogenic preparation derived by drying a frozen solution of specific venom-neutralizing globulins obtained from the blood serum of healthy horses immunized against venom of black widow spiders (Latrodectus mactans). It is standardized by biological assay on mice, in terms of one dose of antivenin neutralizing the venom in not less than 6000 mouse LD$_{50}$ of Latrodectus mactans. Thimerosal (mercury derivative) 1:10,000 is added as a preservative. When constituted as specified, it is opalescent, ranging in color from light (straw) to very dark (iced tea), and contains not more than 20.0 percent of solids.
Each vial contains not less than 6000 Antivenin units. One unit of Antivenin will neutralize one average mouse lethal dose of black widow spider venom when the Antivenin and the venom are injected simultaneously in mice under suitable conditions.

CLINICAL PHARMACOLOGY

The pharmacological mode of action is unknown and metabolic and pharmacokinetic data in humans are unavailable.

INDICATIONS AND USAGE

Antivenin (Latrodectus mactans), MSD is used to treat patients with symptoms due to bites by the black widow spider (Latrodectus mactans). Early use of the Antivenin is emphasized for prompt relief.

Local muscular cramps begin from 15 minutes to several hours after the bite which usually produces a sharp pain similar to that caused by puncture with a needle. The exact sequence of symptoms depends somewhat on the location of the bite. The venom acts on the myoneural junctions or on the nerve endings, causing an ascending motor paralysis or destruction of the peripheral nerve endings. The groups of muscles most frequently affected at first are those of the thigh, shoulder, and back. After a varying length of time, the pain becomes more severe, spreading to the abdomen, and weakness and tremor usually develop. The abdominal muscles assume a boardlike rigidity, but tenderness is slight. Respiration is thoracic. The patient is restless and anxious. Feeble pulse, cold, clammy skin, labored breathing and speech, light stupor, and delirium may occur. Convulsions also may occur, particularly in small children. The temperature may be normal or slightly elevated. Urinary retention, shock, cyanosis, nausea and vomiting, insomnia, and cold sweats also have been reported. The syndrome following the bite of the black widow spider may be confused easily with any medical or surgical condition with acute abdominal symptoms.

The symptoms of black widow spider bite increase in severity for several hours, perhaps a day, and then very slowly become less severe, gradually passing off in the course of two or three days except in fatal cases. Residual symptoms such as general weakness, tingling, nervousness, and transient muscle spasm may persist for weeks or months after recovery from the acute stage.

If possible, the patient should be hospitalized. Other additional measures giving greatest relief are prolonged warm baths and intravenous injection of 10 mL of 10 percent solution of calcium gluconate repeated as necessary to control muscle pain. Morphine also may be required to control pain. Barbiturates may be used for extreme restlessness. However, as the venom is a neurotoxin, it can cause respiratory paralysis. This must be borne in mind when considering use of morphine or a barbiturate. Adrenocorticosteroids have been used with varying degrees of success. Supportive therapy is indicated by the condition of the patient. Local treatment of the site of the bite is of no value. Nothing is gained by applying a tourniquet or by attempting to remove venom from the site of the bite by incision and suction.

In otherwise healthy individuals between the ages of 16 and 60, the use of Antivenin may be deferred and treatment with muscle relaxants may be considered.

WARNINGS

Prior to treatment with any product prepared from horse serum, a careful review of the patient's history should be taken emphasizing prior exposure to horse serum or any allergies. Serious sickness and even death could result from the use of horse serum in a sensitive patient. A skin or conjunctival test should be performed prior to administration of Antivenin.

Skin test: Inject into (not under) the skin not more than 0.02 mL of the test material (1:10 dilution of normal horse serum in physiologic saline). Evaluate result in 10 minutes. A positive reaction is an urticarial wheal surrounded by a zone of erythema. A control test using Sodium Chloride Injection facilitates interpretation of the results.

Conjunctival test: For adults instill into the conjunctival sac one drop of a 1:10 dilution of horse serum and for children one drop of 1:100 dilution. Itching of the eye and reddening of the conjunctiva indicate a positive reaction, usually within 10 minutes.

Patients should be observed for serum sickness for an average of 8 to 12 days following administration of Antivenin.

Desensitization should be attempted only when the administration of Antivenin is considered necessary to save life. Epinephrine must be available in case of untoward reaction.

Desensitization: If the history is positive or the results of the sensitivity tests are mildly or questionably positive, Antivenin should be administered as follows to reduce the risk of an immediate severe allergic reaction:

1. In separate sterile vials or syringes prepare 1:10 or 1:100 dilutions of Antivenin in Sodium Chloride for Injection.
2. Allow at least 15 but preferably 30 minutes between injections and only proceed with the next dose if no reactions occurred following the previous dose.
3. Using a tuberculin syringe, inject subcutaneously 0.1, 0.2 and 0.5 mL of the 1:100 dilution at 15 or 30 minute intervals; repeat with the 1:10 dilution, and finally the undiluted Antivenin.
4. If there is a reaction after any of the injections, place a tourniquet proximal to the sites of injection and administer epinephrine, 1:1000 (0.3 to 1.0 mL subcutaneously, 0.05 to 0.1 mL intravenously), proximal to the tourniquet or into another extremity. Wait at least 30 minutes before giving another injection of Antivenin, the amount of which should be the same as the last one not evoking a reaction.
5. If no reaction has occurred after 0.5 mL of undiluted Antivenin has been given, it is probably safe to continue the dose at 15 minute intervals until the entire dose has been injected.

PRECAUTIONS

Carcinogenesis, Mutagenesis, Impairment of Fertility

No long term studies in animals have been performed to evaluate the potential for carcinogenesis, mutagenesis, or impairment of fertility.

Pregnancy

Pregnancy Category C. Animal reproduction studies have not been conducted with Black Widow Spider Antivenin. It is also not known whether Black Widow Spider Antivenin can cause fetal harm when administered to a pregnant woman or can affect reproduction capacity. Black Widow Spider Antivenin should be given to a pregnant woman only if clearly needed.

Nursing Mothers

It is not known whether this drug is excreted in human milk. Because many drugs are excreted in human milk, caution should be exercised when Black Widow Spider Antivenin is administered to a nursing woman.

Pediatric Use

Controlled clinical studies for safety and effectiveness in children have not been conducted; however, there have been virtually no adverse effects reported in those children who have received the product.

ADVERSE REACTIONS

Anaphylaxis and serum sickness have been reported following use of Antivenin.

DOSAGE AND ADMINISTRATION

Using a sterile syringe, remove from the accompanying vial 2.5 mL of Sterile Diluent for Antivenin and inject into the vial of Antivenin. With the needle still in the rubber stopper, shake the vial to dissolve the contents completely.

Parenteral drug products should be inspected visually for particulate matter prior to administration, whenever solution and container permit (see DESCRIPTION).

The dose for adults and children is the entire contents of a restored vial (2.5 mL) of Antivenin. It may be given intramuscularly, preferably in the region of the anterolateral thigh so that a tourniquet may be applied in the event of a systemic reaction. Symptoms usually subside in 1 to 3 hours. Although one dose of Antivenin usually is adequate, a second dose may be necessary in some cases.

Antivenin also may be given intravenously in 10 to 50 mL of saline solution over a 15 minute period. It is the preferred route in severe cases, or when the patient is under 12, or in shock. One restored vial usually is enough.

HOW SUPPLIED

No. 4084—Antivenin (Latrodectus mactans), MSD equine origin is a white to grey crystalline powder, each vial containing not less than 6000 Antivenin units. Thimerosal (mercury derivative) 1:10,000 is added as preservative, **NDC** 0006-4084-00. A 2.5 mL vial of Sterile Diluent for Antivenin is included. Also supplied is a 1 mL vial of normal horse serum (1:10 dilution) for sensitivity testing. Thimerosal (mercury derivative) 1:10,000 is added as preservative.

Storage

Antivenin must be stored and shipped at 2–8°C (36–46°F). When reconstituted as directed, the color of Antivenin ranges from light (straw) to very dark (iced tea), but the color has no effect on potency. *Do not freeze.*

A.H.F.S. Category: 80:04

DC 6145213 Issued March 1990

AquaMEPHYTON® Injection ℞
(Phytonadione), U.S.P.
Aqueous Colloidal Solution of Vitamin K_1

> **WARNING—INTRAVENOUS USE**
>
> Severe reactions, including fatalities, have occurred during and immediately after INTRAVENOUS injection of AquaMEPHYTON* (Phytonadione), even when precautions have been taken to dilute the AquaMEPHYTON and to avoid rapid infusion. Typically these severe reactions have resembled hypersensitivity or anaphylaxis, including shock and cardiac and/or respiratory arrest. Some patients have exhibited these severe reactions on receiving AquaMEPHYTON for the first time. Therefore the INTRAVENOUS route should be restricted to those situations where other routes are not feasible and the serious risk involved is considered justified.

*Registered trademark of MERCK & CO., INC.

DESCRIPTION

Phytonadione is a vitamin, which is a clear, yellow to amber, viscous, odorless or nearly odorless liquid. It is insoluble in water, soluble in chloroform and slightly soluble in ethanol. It has a molecular weight of 450.70.

Phytonadione is 2-methyl-3-phytyl-1,4-naphthoquinone. Its empirical formula is $C_{31}H_{46}O_2$ and its structural formula is:

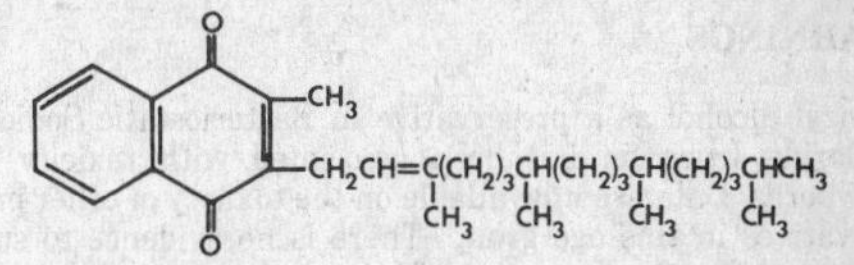

AquaMEPHYTON injection is a yellow, sterile, aqueous colloidal solution of vitamin K_1, with a pH of 5.0 to 7.0, available for injection by the intravenous, intramuscular, and subcutaneous routes. Each milliliter contains:

Phytonadione	2 mg or 10 mg
Inactive ingredients:	
Polyoxyethylated fatty acid derivative	70 mg
Dextrose	37.5 mg
Water for Injection, q.s.	1 mL
Added as preservative:	
Benzyl alcohol	0.9%

CLINICAL PHARMACOLOGY

AquaMEPHYTON aqueous colloidal solution of vitamin K_1 for parenteral injection, possesses the same type and degree of activity as does naturally-occurring vitamin K, which is necessary for the production via the liver of active prothrombin (factor II), proconvertin (factor VII), plasma thromboplastin component (factor IX), and Stuart factor (factor X). The prothrombin test is sensitive to the levels of three of these four factors—II, VII, and X. Vitamin K is an essential cofactor for a microsomal enzyme that catalyzes the post-translational carboxylation of multiple, specific, peptide-bound glutamic acid residues in inactive hepatic precursors of factors II, VII, IX, and X. The resulting gamma-carboxyglutamic acid residues convert the precursors into active coagulation factors that are subsequently secreted by liver cells into the blood.

Phytonadione is readily absorbed following intramuscular administration. After absorption, phytonadione is initially concentrated in the liver, but the concentration declines rapidly. Very little vitamin K accumulates in tissues. Little is known about the metabolic fate of vitamin K. Almost no free unmetabolized vitamin K appears in bile or urine.

In normal animals and humans, phytonadione is virtually devoid of pharmacodynamic activity. However, in animals and humans deficient in vitamin K, the pharmacological action of vitamin K is related to its normal physiological function, that is, to promote the hepatic biosynthesis of vitamin K dependent clotting factors.

The action of the aqueous colloidal solution, when administered intravenously, is generally detectable within an hour or two and hemorrhage is usually controlled within 3 to 6 hours. A normal prothrombin level may often be obtained in 12 to 14 hours.

In the prophylaxis and treatment of hemorrhagic disease of the newborn, phytonadione has demonstrated a greater margin of safety than that of the water-soluble vitamin K analogues.

INDICATIONS AND USAGE

AquaMEPHYTON is indicated in the following coagulation disorders which are due to faulty formation of factors II, VII, IX and X when caused by vitamin K deficiency or interference with vitamin K activity.

AquaMEPHYTON injection is indicated in:

- anticoagulant-induced prothrombin deficiency caused by coumarin or indanedione derivatives;
- prophylaxis and therapy of hemorrhagic disease of the newborn;

Continued on next page

Information on the Merck & Co. products listed on these pages is the full prescribing information from product circulars in use October 1, 1992.

Merck & Co.—Cont.

— hypoprothrombinemia due to antibacterial therapy;
— hypoprothrombinemia secondary to factors limiting absorption or synthesis of vitamin K, e.g., obstructive jaundice, biliary fistula, sprue, ulcerative colitis, celiac disease, intestinal resection, cystic fibrosis of the pancreas, and regional enteritis;
— other drug-induced hypoprothrombinemia where it is definitely shown that the result is due to interference with vitamin K metabolism, e.g., salicylates.

CONTRAINDICATION

Hypersensitivity to any component of this medication.

WARNINGS

Benzyl alcohol as a preservative in Bacteriostatic Sodium Chloride Injection has been associated with toxicity in newborns. Data are unavailable on the toxicity of other preservatives in this age group. There is no evidence to suggest that the small amount of benzyl alcohol contained in AquaMEPHYTON, when used as recommended, is associated with toxicity.
An immediate coagulant effect should not be expected after administration of phytonadione. It takes a minimum of 1 to 2 hours for measurable improvement in the prothrombin time. Whole blood or component therapy may also be necessary if bleeding is severe.
Phytonadione will not counteract the anticoagulant action of heparin.
When vitamin K_1 is used to correct excessive anticoagulant-induced hypoprothrombinemia, anticoagulant therapy still being indicated, the patient is again faced with the clotting hazards existing prior to starting the anticoagulant therapy. Phytonadione is not a clotting agent, but overzealous therapy with vitamin K_1 may restore conditions which originally permitted thromboembolic phenomena. Dosage should be kept as low as possible, and prothrombin time should be checked regularly as clinical conditions indicate.
Repeated large doses of vitamin K are not warranted in liver disease if the response to initial use of the vitamin is unsatisfactory. Failure to respond to vitamin K may indicate that the condition being treated is inherently unresponsive to vitamin K.

PRECAUTIONS

Drug Interactions
Temporary resistance to prothrombin-depressing anticoagulants may result, especially when larger doses of phytonadione are used. If relatively large doses have been employed, it may be necessary when reinstituting anticoagulant therapy to use somewhat larger doses of the prothrombin-depressing anticoagulant, or to use one which acts on a different principle, such as heparin sodium.
Laboratory Tests
Prothrombin time should be checked regularly as clinical conditions indicate.
Carcinogenesis, Mutagenesis, Impairment of Fertility
Studies of carcinogenicity, mutagenesis or impairment of fertility have not been conducted with AquaMEPHYTON.
Pregnancy
Pregnancy Category C: Animal reproduction studies have not been conducted with AquaMEPHYTON. It is also not known whether AquaMEPHYTON can cause fetal harm when administered to a pregnant woman or can affect repro-

duction capacity. AquaMEPHYTON should be given to a pregnant woman only if clearly needed.
Nursing Mothers
It is not known whether this drug is excreted in human milk. Because many drugs are excreted in human milk, caution should be exercised when AquaMEPHYTON is administered to a nursing woman.
Pediatric Use
Hemolysis, jaundice, and hyperbilirubinemia in newborns, particularly in premature infants, may be related to the dose of AquaMEPHYTON. Therefore, the recommended dose should not be exceeded (see ADVERSE REACTIONS and DOSAGE AND ADMINISTRATION).

ADVERSE REACTIONS

Deaths have occurred after intravenous administration. (See Box Warning at beginning of circular.)
Transient "flushing sensations" and "peculiar" sensations of taste have been observed, as well as rare instances of dizziness, rapid and weak pulse, profuse sweating, brief hypotension, dyspnea, and cyanosis.
Pain, swelling, and tenderness at the injection site may occur.
The possibility of allergic sensitivity, including an anaphylactoid reaction, should be kept in mind.
Infrequently, usually after repeated injection, erythematous, indurated, pruritic plaques have occurred; rarely, these have progressed to sclerodermalike lesions that have persisted for long periods. In other cases, these lesions have resembled erythema perstans.
Hyperbilirubinemia has been observed in the newborn following administration of phytonadione. This has occurred rarely and primarily with doses above those recommended. (See PRECAUTIONS, *Pediatric Use.*)

OVERDOSAGE

The intravenous LD_{50} of AquaMEPHYTON in the mouse is 41.5 and 52 mL/kg for the 0.2% and 1% concentrations respectively.

DOSAGE AND ADMINISTRATION

Whenever possible, AquaMEPHYTON should be given by the subcutaneous or intramuscular route. When intravenous administration is considered unavoidable, the drug should be injected very slowly, not exceeding 1 mg per minute.
Protect from light at all times.
Parenteral drug products should be inspected visually for particulate matter and discoloration prior to administration, whenever solution and container permit.
Directions for Dilution
AquaMEPHYTON may be diluted with 0.9% Sodium Chloride Injection, 5% Dextrose Injection, or 5% Dextrose and Sodium Chloride Injection. Benzyl alcohol as a preservative has been associated with toxicity in newborns. *Therefore, all of the above diluents should be preservative-free* (see WARNINGS). *Other diluents should not be used.* When dilutions are indicated, administration should be started immediately after mixture with the diluent, and unused portions of the dilution should be discarded, as well as unused contents of the ampul.
Prophylaxis of Hemorrhagic Disease of the Newborn
The American Academy of Pediatrics recommends that vitamin K_1 be given to the newborn. A single intramuscular dose of AquaMEPHYTON 0.5 to 1 mg within one hour of birth is recommended.

Treatment of Hemorrhagic Disease of the Newborn
Empiric administration of vitamin K_1 should not replace proper laboratory evaluation of the coagulation mechanism. A prompt response (shortening of the prothrombin time in 2 to 4 hours) following administration of vitamin K_1 is usually diagnostic of hemorrhagic disease of the newborn, and failure to respond indicates another diagnosis or coagulation disorder.
AquaMEPHYTON 1 mg should be given either subcutaneously or intramuscularly. Higher doses may be necessary if the mother has been receiving oral anticoagulants.
[See table below.]
Whole blood or component therapy may be indicated if bleeding is excessive. This therapy, however, does not correct the underlying disorder and AquaMEPHYTON should be given concurrently.
Anticoagulant-Induced Prothrombin Deficiency in Adults
To correct excessively prolonged prothrombin time caused by oral anticoagulant therapy—2.5 to 10 mg or up to 25 mg initially is recommended. In rare instances 50 mg may be required. Frequency and amount of subsequent doses should be determined by prothrombin time response or clinical condition (see WARNINGS). If in 6 to 8 hours after parenteral administration the prothrombin time has not been shortened satisfactorily, the dose should be repeated.
In the event of shock or excessive blood loss, the use of whole blood or component therapy is indicated.
Hypoprothrombinemia Due to Other Causes in Adults
A dosage of 2.5 to 25 mg or more (rarely up to 50 mg) is recommended, the amount and route of administration depending upon the severity of the condition and response obtained.
If possible, discontinuation or reduction of the dosage of drugs interfering with coagulation mechanisms (such as salicylates, antibiotics) is suggested as an alternative to administering concurrent AquaMEPHYTON. The severity of the coagulation disorder should determine whether the immediate administration of AquaMEPHYTON is required in addition to discontinuation or reduction of interfering drugs.

HOW SUPPLIED

Injection AquaMEPHYTON is a yellow, sterile, aqueous colloidal solution and is supplied in the following concentrations:
No. 7780—10 mg of vitamin K_1 per mL
NDC 0006-7780-64 boxes of 6 × 1 mL ampuls
(6505-00-854-2499 10 mg 1 mL 6's)
NDC 0006-7780-66 boxes of 25 × 1 mL ampuls.
No. 7782—10 mg of vitamin K_1 per mL
NDC 0006-7782-30 in 2.5 mL multiple dose vials
NDC 0006-7782-03 in 5 mL multiple dose vials.
No. 7784—1 mg of vitamin K_1 per 0.5 mL
NDC 0006-7784-33 boxes of 25 × 0.5 mL ampuls
(6505-00-180-6372 1 mg 0.5 mL 25's).
      A.H.F.S. Category: 88:24
      DC 7498717   Issued March 1991

ARAMINE® Injection   ℞
(Metaraminol Bitartrate), U.S.P.

DESCRIPTION

Metaraminol bitartrate is a potent sympathomimetic amine that increases both systolic and diastolic blood pressure.
Metaraminol bitartrate is $[R-(R^*,S^*)]$-α-(1-aminoethyl)-3-hydroxybenzenemethanol $[R-(R^*,R^*)]$-2,3-dihydroxybutanedioate (1:1) (salt), which is levorotatory. Its empirical formula is $C_9H_{13}NO_2 \cdot C_4H_6O_6$ and its structural formula is:

Metaraminol bitartrate is a white, crystalline powder with a molecular weight of 317.29, is freely soluble in water, slightly soluble in alcohol, and practically insoluble in chloroform and in ether.
Injection ARAMINE* (Metaraminol Bitartrate) is a sterile solution. Each mL contains:

    Metaraminol bitartrate equivalent to
       metaraminol.. 10 mg
    Inactive ingredients:
       Sodium chloride .... 4.4 mg
       Water for Injection q.s. ad................................. 1 mL
       Methylparaben 0.15%, propylparaben 0.02%, and sodium bisulfite 0.2% added as preservatives.

---

*Registered trademark of MERCK & CO., INC.

AquaMEPHYTON
Summary of Dosage Guidelines
(See circular text for details)

Newborns	Dosage
Hemorrhagic Disease of the Newborn	
Prophylaxis	0.5–1 mg IM within 1 hour of birth
Treatment	1 mg SC or IM (Higher doses may be necessary if the mother has been receiving oral anticoagulants)

Adults	Initial Dosage
Anticoagulant-Induced Prothrombin Deficiency (caused by coumarin or indanedione derivatives)	2.5 mg–10 mg or up to 25 mg (rarely 50 mg)
Hypoprothrombinemia due to other causes (Antibiotics; Salicylates or other drugs; Factors limiting absorption or synthesis)	2.5 mg–25 mg or more (rarely up to 50 mg)

CLINICAL PHARMACOLOGY

The pressor effect of ARAMINE begins in 1 to 2 minutes after intravenous infusion, in about 10 minutes after intramuscular injection, and in 5 to 20 minutes after subcutaneous injection. The effect lasts from about 20 minutes to one hour. ARAMINE has a positive inotropic effect on the heart and a peripheral vasoconstrictor action.

Renal, coronary, and cerebral blood flow are a function of perfusion pressure and regional resistance. In patients with insufficient or failing vasoconstriction, there is additional advantage to the peripheral action of ARAMINE, but in most patients with shock, vasoconstriction is adequate and any further increase is unnecessary. Blood flow to vital organs may decrease with ARAMINE if regional resistance increases excessively.

The pressor effect of ARAMINE is decreased but not reversed by alpha-adrenergic blocking agents. Primary or secondary fall in blood pressure and tachyphylactic response to repeated use are uncommon.

INDICATIONS AND USAGE

ARAMINE is indicated for prevention and treatment of the acute hypotensive state occurring with spinal anesthesia. It is also indicated as adjunctive treatment of hypotension due to hemorrhage, reactions to medications, surgical complications, and shock associated with brain damage due to trauma or tumor.

CONTRAINDICATIONS

Use of ARAMINE with cyclopropane or halothane anesthesia should be avoided, unless clinical circumstances demand such use.

Hypersensitivity to any component of this product, including sulfites (see WARNINGS).

WARNINGS

Use of sympathomimetic amines with monoamine oxidase inhibitors or tricyclic antidepressants may result in potentiation of the pressor effect. (See PRECAUTIONS, *Drug Interactions*.)

ARAMINE contains sodium bisulfite, a sulfite that may cause allergic-type reactions including anaphylactic symptoms and life-threatening or less severe asthmatic episodes in certain susceptible people. The overall prevalence of sulfite sensitivity in the general population is unknown and probably low. Sulfite sensitivity is seen more frequently in asthmatic than in nonasthmatic people.

PRECAUTIONS

General

Caution should be used to avoid excessive blood pressure response. Rapidly induced hypertensive responses have been reported to cause acute pulmonary edema, arrhythmias, cerebral hemorrhage, or cardiac arrest.

Patients with cirrhosis should be treated with caution, with adequate restoration of electrolytes if diuresis ensues. Fatal ventricular arrhythmia was reported in one patient with Laennec's cirrhosis while receiving metaraminol bitartrate. In several instances, ventricular extrasystoles that appeared during infusion of this vasopressor subsided promptly when the rate of infusion was reduced.

With the prolonged action of ARAMINE, a cumulative effect is possible. If there is an excessive vasopressor response there may be a prolonged elevation of blood pressure even after discontinuation of therapy.

When vasopressor amines are used for long periods, the resulting vasoconstriction may prevent adequate expansion of circulating volume and may cause perpetuation of shock. There is evidence that plasma volume may be reduced in all types of shock, and that the measurement of central venous pressure is useful in assessing the adequacy of the circulating blood volume. Therefore, blood or plasma volume expanders should be used when the principal reason for hypotension or shock is decreased circulating volume.

Because of its vasoconstrictor effect ARAMINE should be given with caution in heart or thyroid disease, hypertension, or diabetes. Sympathomimetic amines may provoke a relapse in patients with a history of malaria.

Drug Interactions

ARAMINE should be used with caution in digitalized patients, since the combination of digitalis and sympathomimetic amines may cause ectopic arrhythmias.

Monoamine oxidase inhibitors or tricyclic antidepressants may potentiate the action of sympathomimetic amines. Therefore, when initiating pressor therapy in patients receiving these drugs, the initial dose should be small and given with caution. (See WARNINGS.)

Carcinogenesis, Mutagenesis, Impairment of Fertility

Studies in animals have not been performed to evaluate the mutagenic or carcinogenic potential of ARAMINE or its potential to affect fertility.

Pregnancy

Pregnancy Category C. Animal reproduction studies have not been conducted with ARAMINE. It is not known whether ARAMINE can cause fetal harm when given to a pregnant woman or can affect reproduction capacity. ARAMINE should be given to a pregnant woman only if clearly needed.

Nursing Mothers

It is not known whether this drug is secreted in human milk. Because many drugs are secreted in human milk, caution should be exercised when ARAMINE is given to a nursing woman.

Pediatric Use

Safety and effectiveness in children have not been established.

ADVERSE REACTIONS

Sympathomimetic amines, including ARAMINE, may cause sinus or ventricular tachycardia, or other arrhythmias, especially in patients with myocardial infarction. (See PRECAUTIONS.)

In patients with a history of malaria, these compounds may provoke a relapse.

Abscess formation, tissue necrosis, or sloughing rarely may follow the use of ARAMINE. In choosing the site of injection, it is important to avoid those areas recognized as *not* suitable for use of any pressor agent and to discontinue the infusion immediately if infiltration or thrombosis occurs. Although the physician may be forced by the urgent nature of the patient's condition to choose injection sites that are not recognized as suitable, he should, when possible, use the preferred areas of injection. The larger veins of the antecubital fossa or the thigh are preferred to veins in the dorsum of the hand or ankle veins, particularly in patients with peripheral vascular disease, diabetes mellitus, Buerger's disease, or conditions with coexistent hypercoagulability.

OVERDOSAGE

Overdosage may result in severe hypertension accompanied by headache, constricting sensation in the chest, nausea, vomiting, euphoria, diaphoresis, pulmonary edema, tachycardia, bradycardia, sinus arrhythmia, atrial or ventricular arrhythmias, cerebral hemorrhage, myocardial infarction, cardiac arrest or convulsions.

Should an excessive elevation of blood pressure occur, it may be immediately relieved by a sympatholytic agent, e.g. phentolamine. An appropriate antiarrhythmic agent may also be required.

The oral LD_{50} in the rat and mouse is 240 mg/kg and 99 mg/kg, respectively.

DOSAGE AND ADMINISTRATION

ARAMINE may be given intramuscularly, subcutaneously, or intravenously, the route depending on the nature and severity of the indication.

Parenteral drug products should be inspected visually for particulate matter and discoloration prior to use, whenever solution and container permit.

Allow at least 10 minutes to elapse before increasing the dose because the maximum effect is not immediately apparent. When the vasopressor is discontinued, observe the patient carefully as the effect of the drug tapers off, so that therapy can be reinitiated promptly if the blood pressure falls too rapidly. The response to vasopressors may be poor in patients with coexistent shock and acidosis. When indicated, established methods of shock management should be used, such as blood or fluid replacement.

Intramuscular or Subcutaneous Injection (for prevention of hypotension—see INDICATIONS): The recommended dose is 2 to 10 mg (0.2 to 1 mL). As with other agents given subcutaneously, only the preferred sites of injection, as set forth in standard texts, should be used.

Intravenous Infusion (for adjunctive treatment of hypotension—see INDICATIONS): The recommended dose is 15 to 100 mg (1.5 to 10 mL) in 500 mL of Sodium Chloride Injection or 5% Dextrose Injection, adjusting the rate of infusion to maintain the blood pressure at the desired level. Higher concentrations of ARAMINE, 150 to 500 mg per 500 mL of infusion fluid, have been used.

If the patient needs more saline or dextrose solution at a rate of flow that would provide an excessive dose of the vasopressor, the recommended volume of infusion fluid (500 mL) should be increased accordingly. ARAMINE may also be added to *less* than 500 mL of infusion fluid if a smaller volume is desired.

Compatibility Information

In addition to Sodium Chloride Injection and Dextrose Injection 5%, the following infusion solutions were found physically and chemically compatible with Injection ARAMINE when 5 mL of Injection ARAMINE, 10 mg/mL (metaraminol equivalent), was added to 500 mL of infusion solution: Ringer's Injection, Lactated Ringer's Injection, Dextran 6% in Saline†, Normosol®-R pH 7.4†, and Normosol®-M in D5-W†.

When Injection ARAMINE is mixed with an infusion solution, sterile precautions should be observed. Since infusion solutions generally do not contain preservatives, mixtures should be used within 24 hours.

Direct Intravenous Injection: In severe shock, when time is of great importance, this agent should be given by direct intravenous injection. The suggested dose is 0.5 to 5 mg (0.05 to 0.5 mL), followed by an infusion of 15 to 100 mg (1.5 to 10 mL) in 500 mL of infusion fluid as described previously. Vials may be sterilized by autoclaving or by immersion in a sterilizing solution.

†Product of Abbott Laboratories

HOW SUPPLIED

No. 3222X—Injection ARAMINE 1%, containing metaraminol bitartrate equivalent to 10 mg of metaraminol per mL, is a clear, colorless solution and is supplied as follows:
NDC 0006-3222-10 in 10 mL vials
(6505-00-753-9601 10 mL vial).

Storage
Protect from light. Store container in carton until contents have been used.
Avoid storage at temperatures below -20°C (-4°F) and above 40°C (104°F).

A.H.F.S. Category: 12:12
DC 7348522   Issued May 1987
COPYRIGHT © MERCK & CO., INC., 1987
All rights reserved

ATTENUVAX®   ℞
(Measles Virus Vaccine Live, MSD), U.S.P.
(More Attenuated Enders' Strain)

DESCRIPTION

ATTENUVAX* (Measles Virus Vaccine Live, MSD) is a live virus vaccine for immunization against measles (rubeola).

ATTENUVAX is a sterile lyophilized preparation of a more attenuated line of measles virus derived from Enders' attenuated Edmonston strain. The further modification of the virus in ATTENUVAX was achieved in the Merck Institute for Therapeutic Research by multiple passage of Edmonston strain virus in cell cultures of chick embryo at low temperature.

The reconstituted vaccine is for subcutaneous administration. When reconstituted as directed, the dose for injection is 0.5 mL and contains not less than the equivalent of 1,000 $TCID_{50}$ (tissue culture infectious doses) of the U.S. Reference Measles Virus. Each dose also contains approximately 25 mcg of neomycin. The product contains no preservative. Sorbitol and hydrolized gelatin are added as stabilizers.

*Registered trademark of MERCK & CO., INC.

CLINICAL PHARMACOLOGY

ATTENUVAX produces a modified measles infection in susceptible persons. Fever and rash may appear. Extensive clinical trials have demonstrated that ATTENUVAX is highly immunogenic and generally well tolerated. A single injection of the vaccine has been shown to induce measles hemagglutination-inhibiting (HI) antibodies in 97 percent or more of susceptible persons. Vaccine-induced antibody levels have been shown to persist for at least 13 years without substantial decline. Continued surveillance will be necessary to determine further duration of antibody persistence.

INDICATIONS AND USAGE

ATTENUVAX is indicated for immunization against measles (rubeola) in persons 15 months of age or older. A second dose of ATTENUVAX is recommended (see *Revaccination*). Infants who are less than 15 months of age may fail to respond to the vaccine due to presence in the circulation of residual measles antibody of maternal origin; the younger the infant, the lower the likelihood of seroconversion. In geographically isolated or other relatively inaccessible populations for whom immunization programs are logistically difficult, and in population groups in which natural measles

Continued on next page

Merck & Co.—Cont.

infection may occur in a significant proportion of infants before 15 months of age, it may be desirable to give the vaccine to infants at an earlier age. Infants vaccinated under these conditions at less than 12 months of age should be revaccinated after reaching 15 months of age. There is some evidence to suggest that infants immunized at less than one year of age may not develop sustained antibody levels when later reimmunized. The advantage of early protection must be weighed against the chance for failure to respond adequately on reimmunization.

According to ACIP recommendations, most persons born in 1956 or earlier are likely to have been infected naturally and generally need not be considered susceptible. All children, adolescents, and adults born after 1956 are considered susceptible and should be vaccinated, if there are no contraindications. This includes persons who may be immune to measles but who lack adequate documentation of immunity as evidenced by: (1) physician-diagnosed measles, (2) laboratory evidence of measles immunity, or (3) adequate immunization with live measles vaccine on or after the first birthday. ATTENUVAX given immediately after exposure to natural measles may provide some protection. If, however, the vaccine is given a few days before exposure, substantial protection may be provided.

Individuals planning travel outside the United States, if not immune, can acquire measles, mumps or rubella and import these diseases to the United States. Therefore, prior to International travel, individuals known to be susceptible to one or more of these diseases can receive either a single antigen vaccine (measles, mumps or rubella), or a combined antigen vaccine as appropriate. However, M-M-R* II (Measles, Mumps, and Rubella Virus Vaccine Live, MSD) is preferred for persons likely to be susceptible to mumps and rubella; and if single-antigen measles vaccine is not readily available, travelers should receive M-M-R II (Measles, Mumps, and Rubella Virus Vaccine Live, MSD) regardless of their immune status to mumps or rubella.

Revaccination: Children first vaccinated when younger than 12 months of age should be revaccinated at 15 months of age, particularly if vaccine was administered with immune serum globulin or measles immune globulin, a standardized globulin preparation.

The American Academy of Pediatrics (AAP), the Immunization Practices Advisory Committee (ACIP), and some state and local health agencies have recommended guidelines for routine measles revaccination and to help control measles outbreaks.**

Vaccines available for revaccination include monovalent measles vaccine (ATTENUVAX) and polyvalent vaccines containing measles [e.g., M-M-R II (Measles, Mumps, and Rubella Virus Vaccine Live, MSD), M-R-VAX* II (Measles and Rubella Virus Vaccine Live, MSD)]. If the prevention of sporadic measles outbreaks is the sole objective, revaccination with a monovalent measles vaccine should be considered (see appropriate product circular). If concern also exists about immune status regarding mumps or rubella, revaccination with appropriate monovalent or polyvalent vaccines should be considered after consulting the appropriate product circulars. Unnecessary doses of a vaccine are best avoided by ensuring that written documentation of vaccination is preserved and a copy given to each vaccinee's parent or guardian.

Despite the risk of reactions (see ADVERSE REACTIONS), persons born since 1956 who have previously been given inactivated vaccine alone or followed by live vaccine within 3 months should be revaccinated with live vaccine to reduce the risk of the severe atypical form of natural measles that may occur.

Use with other Vaccines

Routine administration of DTP (diphtheria, tetanus, pertussis) and/or OPV (oral poliovirus vaccine) concomitantly with measles, mumps and rubella vaccines is not recommended because there are insufficient data relating to the simultaneous administration of these antigens. However, the American Academy of Pediatrics has noted that in some circumstances, particularly when the patient may not return, some practitioners prefer to administer all these antigens on a single day. If done, separate sites and syringes should be used for DTP and ATTENUVAX.

ATTENUVAX should not be given less than one month before or after administration of other virus vaccines.

---

* Registered trademark of MERCK & CO., INC.
** NOTE: A primary difference among these recommendations is the timing of revaccination: the ACIP recommends routine revaccination at entry into kindergarten or first grade, whereas the AAP recommends routine revaccination at entrance to middle school or junior high school. In addition, some public health jurisdictions mandate the age for revaccination. The complete text of applicable guidelines should be consulted.

CONTRAINDICATIONS

Do not give ATTENUVAX to pregnant females; the possible effects of the vaccine on fetal development are unknown at this time. If vaccination of postpubertal females is undertaken, pregnancy should be avoided for three months following vaccination (see PRECAUTIONS, *Pregnancy*).

Anaphylactic or anaphylactoid reactions to neomycin (each dose of reconstituted vaccine contains approximately 25 mcg of neomycin).

History of anaphylactic or anaphylactoid reactions to eggs (see HYPERSENSITIVITY TO EGGS below).

Any febrile respiratory illness or other active febrile infection.

Active untreated tuberculosis.

Patients receiving immunosuppressive therapy. This contraindication does not apply to patients who are receiving corticosteroids as replacement therapy, e.g., for Addison's disease.

Individuals with blood dyscrasias, leukemia, lymphomas of any type, or other malignant neoplasms affecting the bone marrow or lymphatic systems.

Primary and acquired immunodeficiency states, including patients who are immunosuppressed in association with AIDS or other clinical manifestations of infection with human immunodeficiency viruses; cellular immune deficiencies; and hypogammaglobulinemic and dysgammaglobulinemic states.

Individuals with a family history of congenital or hereditary immunodeficiency, until the immune competence of the potential vaccine recipient is demonstrated.

HYPERSENSITIVITY TO EGGS

Live measles vaccine is produced in chick embryo cell culture. Persons with a history of anaphylactic, anaphylactoid or other immediate reactions (e.g., hives, swelling of the mouth and throat, difficulty breathing, hypotension and shock) subsequent to egg ingestion should not be vaccinated. Evidence indicates that persons are not at increased risk if they have egg allergies that are not anaphylactic or anaphylactoid in nature. Such persons should be vaccinated in the usual manner. There is no evidence to indicate that persons with allergies to chickens or feathers are at increased risk of reaction to the vaccine.

PRECAUTIONS

General

Adequate treatment provisions including epinephrine, should be available for immediate use should an anaphylactic or anaphylactoid reaction occur.

Due caution should be employed in administration of measles vaccine to persons with a history of cerebral injury, individual or family histories of convulsions, or of any other condition in which stress due to fever should be avoided. The physician should be alert to the temperature elevation which may occur following vaccination. (See ADVERSE REACTIONS.)

Children and young adults who are known to be infected with human immunodeficiency viruses but without overt clinical manifestations of immunosuppression may be vaccinated; however, the vaccinees should be monitored closely for vaccine-preventable diseases because immunization may be less effective than for uninfected persons.

Vaccination should be deferred for at least 3 months following blood or plasma transfusions, or administration of human immune serum globulin.

There are no reports of transmission of live attenuated measles virus from vaccinees to susceptible contacts.

It has been reported that attenuated measles virus vaccine, live, may result in a temporary depression of tuberculin skin sensitivity. Therefore, if a tuberculin test is to be done, it should be administered either before or simultaneously with ATTENUVAX.

Children under treatment for tuberculosis have not experienced exacerbation of the disease when immunized with live measles virus vaccine; no studies have been reported to date of the effect of measles virus vaccines on untreated tuberculous children.

As for any vaccine, vaccination with ATTENUVAX may not result in seroconversion in 100% of susceptible persons given the vaccine.

Pregnancy

Pregnancy Category C

Animal reproduction studies have not been conducted with ATTENUVAX. It is also not known whether ATTENUVAX can cause fetal harm when administered to a pregnant woman or can affect reproduction capacity. Therefore, the vaccine should not be administered to pregnant females; furthermore, pregnancy should be avoided for three months following vaccination (see CONTRAINDICATIONS).

Reports have indicated that contracting of natural measles during pregnancy enhances fetal risk. Increased rates of spontaneous abortion, stillbirth, congenital defects and prematurity have been observed subsequent to natural measles

during pregnancy. There are no adequate studies of the attenuated (vaccine) strain of measles virus in pregnancy. However, it would be prudent to assume that the vaccine strain of virus is also capable of inducing adverse fetal effects for up to three months following vaccination.

Vaccine administration to postpubertal females entails a potential for inadvertent immunization during pregnancy. Theoretical risks involved should be weighed against the risks that measles poses to the unimmunized adolescent or adult. Advisory committees reviewing this matter have recommended vaccination of postpubertal females who are presumed to be susceptible to measles and not known to be pregnant. If a measles exposure occurs during pregnancy, one should consider the possibility of providing temporary passive immunity through the administration of immune globulin (human).

Nursing Mothers

It is not known whether measles vaccine virus is secreted in human milk. Therefore, because many drugs are excreted in human milk, caution should be exercised when ATTENUVAX is administered to a nursing woman.

ADVERSE REACTIONS

Burning and/or stinging of short duration at the injection site have been reported.

Anaphylaxis and anaphylactoid reactions have been reported.

Occasional

Moderate fever [101–102.9°F (38.3–39.4°C)] may occur during the month after vaccination. Generally, fever, rash, or both appear between the 5th and the 12th days. Cough and rhinitis have also been reported. Rash, when it occurs, is usually minimal, but rarely may be generalized. Erythema multiforme has also been reported rarely.

Less Common

High fever [over 103°F (39.4°C)].

Mild lymphadenopathy has been reported.

Rare

Reactions at injection site. Allergic reactions such as wheal and flare at the injection site or urticaria have been reported.

Diarrhea has been reported after vaccination with measles-containing vaccines.

Children developing fever may, on rare occasions, exhibit febrile convulsions. Afebrile convulsions or seizures have occurred rarely following vaccination with live attenuated measles vaccine. Syncope, particularly at the time of mass vaccination, has been reported.

Thrombocytopenia and purpura have occurred rarely.

Vasculitis has been reported rarely.

Forms of optic neuritis, including retrobulbar neuritis, papillitis, and retinitis may infrequently follow viral infections, and have been reported to occur 1 to 3 weeks following inoculation with some live virus vaccines.

Experience from more than 80 million doses of all live measles vaccines given in the U.S. through 1975 indicates that significant central nervous system reactions such as encephalitis and encephalopathy, occurring within 30 days after vaccination, have been temporally associated with measles vaccine very rarely. In no case has it been shown that reactions were actually caused by vaccine. The Center for Disease Control has pointed out that "a certain number of cases of encephalitis may be expected to occur in a large childhood population in a defined period of time even when no vaccines are administered". However, the data suggest the possibility that some of these cases may have been caused by measles vaccines. The risk of such serious neurological disorders following live measles virus vaccine administration remains far less than that for encephalitis and encephalopathy with natural measles (one per two thousand reported cases).

There have been rare reports of ocular palsies, Guillain-Barré syndrome, or ataxia occurring after immunization with vaccines containing live attenuated measles virus. The ocular palsies have occurred approximately 3–24 days following vaccination. No definite causal relationship has been established between either of these events and vaccination.

There have been reports of subacute sclerosing panencephalitis (SSPE) in children who did not have a history of natural measles but did receive measles vaccine. Some of these cases may have resulted from unrecognized measles in the first year of life or possibly from the measles vaccination. Based on estimated nationwide measles vaccine distribution, the association of SSPE cases to measles vaccination is about one case per million vaccine doses distributed. This is far less than the association with natural measles, 6–22 cases of SSPE per million cases of measles. The results of a retrospective case-controlled study conducted by the Center for Disease Control suggest that the overall effect of measles vaccine has been to protect against SSPE by preventing measles with its inherent higher risk of SSPE.

Local reactions characterized by marked swelling, redness and vesiculation at the injection site of attenuated live virus measles vaccines, and systemic reactions including atypical measles, have occurred in persons who have previously re-

ceived killed measles vaccine. Rarely, more severe reactions that require hospitalization, including prolonged high fevers, panniculitis, and extensive local reactions, have been reported.

DOSAGE AND ADMINISTRATION

FOR SUBCUTANEOUS ADMINISTRATION
Do not inject intravenously
The dosage of vaccine is the same for all persons. Inject the total volume of the single dose vial (about 0.5 mL) or 0.5 mL of the multiple dose vial of reconstituted vaccine subcutaneously, preferably into the outer aspect of upper arm. *Do not give immune globulin (IG) concurrently with* ATTENUVAX.
During shipment, to insure that there is no loss of potency, the vaccine must be maintained at a temperature of 10°C (50°F) or less.
Before reconstitution, store ATTENUVAX at 2–8°C (36–46°F). *Protect from light.*
CAUTION: A sterile syringe free of preservatives, antiseptics, and detergents should be used for each injection and/or reconstitution of the vaccine because these substances may inactivate the live virus vaccine. A 25 gauge, ⅝" needle is recommended.
To reconstitute, use only the diluent supplied, since it is free of preservatives or other antiviral substances which might inactivate the vaccine.

Single Dose Vial—First withdraw the entire volume of diluent into the syringe to be used for reconstitution. Inject all the diluent in the syringe into the vial of lyophilized vaccine, and agitate to mix thoroughly. Withdraw the entire contents into a syringe and inject the total volume of restored vaccine subcutaneously.
It is important to use a separate sterile syringe and needle for each individual patient to prevent transmission of hepatitis B and other infectious agents from one person to another.

10 Dose Vial (available only to government agencies/institutions)—Withdraw the entire contents (7 mL) of the diluent vial into the sterile syringe to be used for reconstitution, and introduce into the 10 dose vial of lyophilized vaccine. Agitate to ensure thorough mixing. The outer labeling suggests "For Jet Injector or Syringe Use". Use with separate sterile syringes is permitted for containers of 10 doses or less. The vaccine and diluent do not contain preservatives; therefore, the user must recognize the potential contamination hazards and exercise special precautions to protect the sterility and potency of the product. The use of aseptic techniques and proper storage prior to and after restoration of the vaccine and subsequent withdrawal of the individual doses is essential. Use 0.5 mL of the reconstituted vaccine for subcutaneous injection.
It is important to use a separate sterile syringe and needle for each individual patient to prevent transmission of hepatitis B and other infectious agents from one person to another.

50 Dose Vial (available only to government agencies/institutions)—Withdraw the entire contents (30 mL) of diluent vial into the sterile syringe to be used for reconstitution and introduce into the 50 dose vial of lyophilized vaccine. Agitate to ensure thorough mixing. With full aseptic precautions, attach the vial to the sterilized multidose jet injector apparatus. Use 0.5 mL of the reconstituted vaccine for subcutaneous injection.

Each dose of ATTENUVAX contains not less than 1,000 $TCID_{50}$ (tissue culture infectious doses) of measles virus vaccine expressed in terms of the assigned titer of the U.S. Reference Measles Virus.
Parenteral drug products should be inspected visually for particulate matter and discoloration prior to administration. ATTENUVAX, when reconstituted, is clear yellow.

HOW SUPPLIED

No. 4709—ATTENUVAX is supplied as a single-dose vial of lyophilized vaccine, **NDC** 0006-4709-00, and a vial of diluent.
No. 4589X/4309—ATTENUVAX is supplied as follows: (1) a box of 10 single-dose vials of lyophilized vaccine (package A), **NDC** 0006-4589-00; and (2) a box of 10 vials of diluent (package B). To conserve refrigerator space, the diluent may be stored separately at room temperature
(6505-01-038-0794, Ten Pack).
Available only to government agencies/institutions:
No. 4614X—ATTENUVAX is supplied as one 10 dose vial of lyophilized vaccine, **NDC** 0006-4614-00, and one 7 mL vial of diluent.
No. 4591X—ATTENUVAX is supplied as one 50 dose vial of lyophilized vaccine, **NDC** 0006-4591-00, and one 30 mL vial of diluent
(6505-01-222-6467, 50 Dose).
Storage
It is recommended that the vaccine be used as soon as possible after reconstitution. Protect vaccine from light at all times, since such exposure may inactivate the virus. Store reconstituted vaccine in the vaccine vial in a dark place at 2–8°C (36–46°F) and discard if not used within 8 hours.

A.H.F.S. Category: 80:12
DC 7680011 Issued March 1991

BENEMID® Tablets
(Probenecid), U.S.P. ℞

DESCRIPTION

BENEMID* (Probenecid) is a uricosuric and renal tubular transport blocking agent.
Probenecid is the generic name for 4-[(dipropylamino) sulfonyl] benzoic acid (molecular weight 285.36). It has the following structural formula:

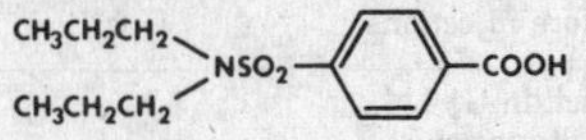

Probenecid is a white or nearly white, fine, crystalline powder. Probenecid is soluble in dilute alkali, in alcohol, in chloroform, and in acetone; it is practically insoluble in water and in dilute acids.
Each tablet contains 0.5 g probenecid and the following inactive ingredients: calcium stearate, D&C Yellow 10, gelatin, hydroxypropyl methylcellulose, iron oxide, magnesium carbonate, polyethylene glycol, starch, talc, and titanium dioxide.

*Registered trademark of MERCK & CO., INC.

ACTIONS

BENEMID is a uricosuric and renal tubular blocking agent. It inhibits the tubular reabsorption of urate, thus increasing the urinary excretion of uric acid and decreasing serum urate levels. Effective uricosuria reduces the miscible urate pool, retards urate deposition, and promotes resorption of urate deposits.
BENEMID inhibits the tubular secretion of penicillin and usually increases penicillin plasma levels by any route the antibiotic is given. A 2-fold to 4-fold elevation has been demonstrated for various penicillins.
BENEMID also has been reported to inhibit the renal transport of many other compounds including aminohippuric acid (PAH), aminosalicylic acid (PAS), indomethacin, sodium iodomethamate and related iodinated organic acids, 17-ketosteroids, pantothenic acid, phenolsulfonphthalein (PSP), sulfonamides, and sulfonylureas. See also DRUG INTERACTIONS.
BENEMID decreases both hepatic and renal excretion of sulfobromophthalein (BSP). The tubular reabsorption of phosphorus is inhibited in hypoparathyroid but not in euparathyroid individuals.
BENEMID does not influence plasma concentrations of salicylates, nor the excretion of streptomycin, chloramphenicol, chlortetracycline, oxytetracycline, or neomycin.

INDICATIONS

For treatment of the hyperuricemia associated with gout and gouty arthritis.
As an adjuvant to therapy with penicillin or with ampicillin, methicillin, oxacillin, cloxacillin, or nafcillin, for elevation and prolongation of plasma levels by whatever route the antibiotic is given.

CONTRAINDICATIONS

Hypersensitivity to this product.
Children under 2 years of age.
Not recommended in persons with known blood dyscrasias or uric acid kidney stones.
Therapy with BENEMID should not be started until an acute gouty attack has subsided.

WARNINGS

Exacerbation of gout following therapy with BENEMID may occur; in such cases colchicine or other appropriate therapy is advisable.
BENEMID increases plasma concentrations of methotrexate in both animals and humans. In animal studies, increased methotrexate toxicity has been reported. If BENEMID is given with methotrexate, the dosage of methotrexate should be reduced and serum levels may need to be monitored.
In patients on BENEMID the use of salicylates in either small or large doses is contraindicated because it antagonizes the uricosuric action of BENEMID. The biphasic action of salicylates in the renal tubules accounts for the so-called "paradoxical effect" of uricosuric agents. In patients on BENEMID who require a mild analgesic agent the use of acetaminophen rather than small doses of salicylates would be preferred.
Rarely, severe allergic reactions and anaphylaxis have been reported with the use of BENEMID. Most of these have been reported to occur within several hours after readministration following prior usage of the drug.
The appearance of hypersensitivity reactions requires cessation of therapy with BENEMID.
Use in Pregnancy: BENEMID crosses the placental barrier and appears in cord blood. The use of any drug in women of childbearing potential requires that the anticipated benefit be weighed against possible hazards.

PRECAUTIONS

General
Hematuria, renal colic, costovertebral pain, and formation of uric acid stones associated with the use of BENEMID in gouty patients may be prevented by alkalization of the urine and a liberal fluid intake (*see* DOSAGE AND ADMINISTRATION). In these cases when alkali is administered, the acid-base balance of the patient should be watched.
Use with caution in patients with a history of peptic ulcer.
BENEMID has been used in patients with some renal impairment but dosage requirements may be increased. BENEMID may not be effective in chronic renal insufficiency particularly when the glomerular filtration rate is 30 mL/minute or less. Because of its mechanism of action, BENEMID is not recommended in conjunction with a penicillin in the presence of *known* renal impairment.
A reducing substance may appear in the urine of patients receiving BENEMID. This disappears with discontinuance of therapy. Suspected glycosuria should be confirmed by using a test specific for glucose.
Drug Interactions
When BENEMID is used to elevate plasma concentrations of penicillin or other beta-lactams, or when such drugs are given to patients taking BENEMID therapeutically, high plasma concentrations of the other drug may increase the incidence of adverse reactions associated with that drug. In the case of penicillin or other beta-lactams, psychic disturbances have been reported.
The use of salicylates antagonizes the uricosuric action of BENEMID (*see* WARNINGS). The uricosuric action of BENEMID is also antagonized by pyrazinamide.
BENEMID produces an insignificant increase in free sulfonamide plasma concentrations but a significant increase in total sulfonamide plasma levels. Since BENEMID decreases the renal excretion of conjugated sulfonamides, plasma concentrations of the latter should be determined from time to time when a sulfonamide and BENEMID are coadministered for prolonged periods. BENEMID may prolong or enhance the action of oral sulfonylureas and thereby increase the risk of hypoglycemia.
It has been reported that patients receiving BENEMID require significantly less thiopental for induction of anesthesia. In addition, ketamine and thiopental anesthesia were significantly prolonged in rats receiving probenecid.
The concomitant administration of probenecid increases the mean plasma elimination half-life of a number of drugs which can lead to increased plasma concentrations. These include agents such as indomethacin, acetaminophen, naproxen, ketoprofen, meclofenamate, lorazepam, and rifampin. Although the clinical significance of this observation has not been established, a lower dosage of the drug may be required to produce a therapeutic effect, and increases in dosage of the drug in question should be made cautiously and in small increments when probenecid is being co-administered. Although specific instances of toxicity due to this potential interaction have not been observed to date physicians should be alert to this possibility.
Probenecid given concomitantly with sulindac had only a slight effect on plasma sulfide levels, while plasma levels of sulindac and sulfone were increased. Sulindac was shown to produce a modest reduction in the uricosuric action of probenecid, which probably is not significant under most circumstances.
In animals and in humans, BENEMID has been reported to increase plasma concentrations of methotrexate (*see* WARNINGS).
Falsely high readings for theophylline have been reported in an *in vitro* study, using the Schack and Waxler technic, when therapeutic concentrations of theophylline and BENEMID were added to human plasma.

ADVERSE REACTIONS

The following adverse reactions have been observed and within each category are listed in order of decreasing severity.

Continued on next page

Information on the Merck & Co. products listed on these pages is the full prescribing information from product circulars in use October 1, 1992.

Merck & Co.—Cont.   BENEMID® (Probenecid)   Penicillin Therapy (Gonorrhea)*

	Recommended Regimens**	Remarks
Uncomplicated gonococcal infection in men and women (urethral, cervical, rectal)	4.8 million units of aqueous procaine penicillin G† I.M., in at least 2 doses injected at different sites at one visit + 1 g of BENEMID (Probenecid) orally just before injections *or* 3.5 g of ampicillin† orally + 1 g of BENEMID orally given simultaneously.	Follow-up: Obtain urethral and other appropriate cultures from men, and cervical, anal, and other appropriate cultures from women, 7 to 14 days after completion of treatment. Treatment of sexual partners: Persons with known recent exposure to gonorrhea should receive same treatment as those known to have gonorrhea. Examination and treatment of male sex partners of persons with gonorrhea are essential because of high prevalence of nonsymptomatic urethral gonococcal infection in such men.
Pharyngeal gonococcal infection in men and women	4.8 million units of aqueous procaine penicillin G† I.M., in at least 2 doses injected at different sites at one visit + 1 g of BENEMID orally just before injections	Pharyngeal gonococcal infections may be more difficult to treat than anogenital gonorrhea. Posttreatment cultures are essential.
Uncomplicated gonorrhea in pregnant patients	4.8 million units of aqueous procaine penicillin G† I.M., in at least 2 doses injected at different sites at one visit *or* 3.5 g of ampicillin† orally + 1 g of BENEMID orally given simultaneously	
Acute gonococcal salpingitis	*Outpatients:* Aqueous procaine penicillin G† or ampicillin† with BENEMID as for gonorrhea in pregnancy, followed by 500 mg of ampicillin 4 times a day for 10 days *Hospitalized patients:* See details in CDC recommendations	Follow-up of patients with acute salpingitis is essential. All patients should receive repeat pelvic examinations and cultures for *Neisseria gonorrhoeae* after treatment. Examination and appropriate treatment of male sex partners are essential because of high prevalence of nonsymptomatic urethral gonorrhea in such men.
Disseminated gonococcal infection (arthritis-dermatitis syndrome)	10 million units of aqueous crystalline penicillin G† I.V. a day for 3 days or till significant clinical improvement occurs. May be followed with 500 mg of ampicillin† 4 times a day orally to complete 7 days of treatment *or* 3.5 g of ampicillin† orally with 1 g of BENEMID, followed by 500 mg of ampicillin† 4 times a day for at least 7 days	
Gonococcal infection in children	For postpubertal children and/or those weighing over 45 kg (100 lb) use the dosage regimens given above for adults Uncomplicated vulvovaginitis and urethritis: aqueous procaine penicillin G† 75,000—100,000 units/kg I.M., with BENEMID 23 mg/kg orally	See CDC recommendations for detailed information about prevention and treatment of neonatal gonococcal infection and gonococcal ophthalmia.

Note: Before treating gonococcal infections in patients with suspected primary or secondary syphilis, perform proper diagnostic procedures including darkfield examinations. If concomitant syphilis is suspected, perform monthly serological tests for at least 4 months.

*   Recommended by Venereal Disease Control Advisory Committee, Center for Disease Control, U.S. Department of Health, Education, and Welfare, Public Health Service (Morbidity and Mortality Weekly Report, Vol. 23: 341, 342, 347, 348, Oct. 11, 1974).

**   See CDC recommendations for definition of regimens of choice, alternative regimens, treatment of hypersensitive patients, and other aspects of therapy.

†   See package circulars of manufacturers for detailed information about contraindications, warnings, precautions, and adverse reactions.

Central Nervous System: headache, dizziness.
Metabolic: precipitation of acute gouty arthritis.
Gastrointestinal: hepatic necrosis, vomiting, nausea, anorexia, sore gums.
Genitourinary: nephrotic syndrome, uric acid stones with or without hematuria, renal colic, costovertebral pain, urinary frequency.
Hypersensitivity: anaphylaxis, fever, urticaria, pruritus.
Hematologic: aplastic anemia, leukopenia, hemolytic anemia which in some patients could be related to genetic deficiency of glucose -6- phosphate dehydrogenase in red blood cells, anemia.
Integumentary: dermatitis, alopecia, flushing.

DOSAGE AND ADMINISTRATION

Gout
Therapy with BENEMID should not be *started* until an acute gouty attack has subsided. However, if an acute attack is precipitated *during* therapy, BENEMID may be continued without changing the dosage, and full therapeutic dosage of colchicine or other appropriate therapy should be given to control the acute attack.

The recommended adult dosage is 0.25 g (½ tablet of BENEMID) twice a day for one week, followed by 0.5 g (1 tablet) twice a day thereafter.

Some degree of renal impairment may be present in patients with gout. A daily dosage of 1 g may be adequate. However, if necessary, the daily dosage may be increased by 0.5 g increments every 4 weeks within tolerance (and usually not above 2 g per day) if symptoms of gouty arthritis are not controlled or the 24 hour uric acid excretion is not above 700 mg. As noted, BENEMID may not be effective in chronic renal insufficiency particularly when the glomerular filtration rate is 30 mL/minute or less.

Gastric intolerance may be indicative of overdosage, and may be corrected by decreasing the dosage.
As uric acid tends to crystallize out of an acid urine, a liberal fluid intake is recommended, as well as sufficient sodium bicarbonate (3 to 7.5 g daily) or potassium citrate (7.5 g daily) to maintain an alkaline urine (see PRECAUTIONS).
Alkalization of the urine is recommended until the serum urate level returns to normal limits and tophaceous deposits disappear, i.e., during the period when urinary excretion of uric acid is at a high level. Thereafter, alkalization of the urine and the usual restriction of purine-producing foods may be somewhat relaxed.
BENEMID should be continued at the dosage that will maintain normal serum urate levels. When acute attacks have been absent for 6 months or more and serum urate levels remain within normal limits, the daily dosage may be decreased by 0.5 g every 6 months. The maintenance dosage should not be reduced to the point where serum urate levels tend to rise.

BENEMID *and Penicillin Therapy (General)*
Adults:
The recommended dosage is 2 g (4 tablets of BENEMID) daily in divided doses. This dosage should be reduced in older patients in whom renal impairment may be present.
Children 2-14 years of age:
Initial dose: 25 mg/kg body weight (*or* 0.7 g/square meter body surface).
Maintenance dose: 40 mg/kg body weight (*or* 1.2 g/square meter body surface) per day, divided into 4 doses.
For children weighing more than 50 kg (110 lb) the adult dosage is recommended.

BENEMID is contraindicated in children under 2 years of age.
The PSP excretion test may be used to determine the effectiveness of BENEMID in retarding penicillin excretion and

maintaining therapeutic levels. The renal clearance of PSP is reduced to about one-fifth the normal rate when dosage of BENEMID is adequate.
Penicillin Therapy (Gonorrhea)
[See table above.]

HOW SUPPLIED

No. 3337—Tablets BENEMID, 0.5 g, are yellow, capsule shaped, scored, film coated tablets, coded MSD 501. They are supplied as follows:
NDC 0006-0501-68 bottles of 100
(6505-00-527-6885 100's)
NDC 0006-0501-28 unit dose packages of 100
NDC 0006-0501-82 bottles of 1000
(6505-00-181-8387 1000's).
    Shown in Product Identification Section, page 419
    A.H.F.S. Category: 40:40
    DC 7399021   Issued August 1988

BIAVAX®II   ℞
(Rubella and Mumps Virus Vaccine Live, MSD), U.S.P.

DESCRIPTION

BIAVAX* II (Rubella and Mumps Virus Vaccine Live, MSD) is a live virus vaccine for immunization against rubella (German measles) and mumps.
BIAVAX II is a sterile lyophilized preparation of the Wistar RA 27/3 strain of live attenuated rubella virus grown in human diploid cell (WI-38) culture; and the Jeryl Lynn (B level) strain of mumps virus grown in cell cultures of chick embryo. The vaccine viruses are the same as those used in the manufacture of MERUVAX* II (Rubella Virus Vaccine Live,

MSD) and MUMPSVAX* (Mumps Virus Vaccine Live, MSD). The two viruses are mixed before being lyophilized. The reconstituted vaccine is for subcutaneous administration. When reconstituted as directed, the dose for injection is 0.5 mL and contains not less than the equivalent of 1,000 $TCID_{50}$ of the U.S. Reference Rubella Virus and 20,000 $TCID_{50}$ of the U.S. Reference Mumps Virus. Each dose contains approximately 25 mcg of neomycin. The product contains no preservative. Sorbitol and hydrolized gelatin are added as stabilizers.

*Registered trademark of MERCK & CO., INC.

CLINICAL PHARMACOLOGY

Clinical studies of 73 double seronegative children 12 months to 2 years of age demonstrated that BIAVAX II is highly immunogenic and generally well tolerated. In these studies, a single injection of the vaccine induced rubella hemagglutination-inhibition (HI) antibodies in 100 percent, and mumps neutralizing antibodies in 97 percent of the susceptible children.

The RA 27/3 rubella strain in BIAVAX II elicits higher immediate post-vaccination HI, complement-fixing and neutralizing antibody levels than other strains of rubella vaccine and has been shown to induce a broader profile of circulating antibodies including anti-theta and anti-iota precipitating antibodies. The RA 27/3 rubella strain immunologically simulates natural infection more closely than other rubella vaccine viruses. The increased levels and broader profile of antibodies produced by RA 27/3 strain rubella virus vaccine appear to correlate with greater resistance to subclinical reinfection with the wild virus, and provide greater confidence for lasting immunity.

Vaccine induced antibody levels following administration of BIAVAX II have been shown to persist for at least two years without substantial decline. Antibody levels after immunization with BIAVAX (Rubella and Mumps Virus Vaccine Live, MSD), containing the HPV-77 strain of rubella, have persisted for 10.5 years without substantial decline. If the present pattern continues, it will provide a basis for the expectation that immunity following vaccination will be permanent. However, continued surveillance will be required to demonstrate this point.

INDICATIONS AND USAGE

BIAVAX II is indicated for simultaneous immunization against rubella and mumps in persons 12 months of age or older. A booster is not needed.

The vaccine is not recommended for infants younger than 12 months because they may retain maternal rubella and mumps neutralizing antibodies which may interfere with the immune response.

Previously unimmunized children of susceptible pregnant women should receive live attenuated rubella vaccine, because an immunized child will be less likely to acquire natural rubella and introduce the virus into the household.

Individuals planning travel outside the United States, if not immune, can acquire measles, mumps or rubella and import these diseases to the United States. Therefore, prior to International travel, individuals known to be susceptible to one or more of these diseases can receive either a single antigen vaccine (measles, mumps, or rubella), or a combined antigen vaccine as appropriate. However, M-M-R* II (Measles, Mumps, and Rubella Virus Vaccine Live, MSD) is preferred for persons likely to be susceptible to mumps and rubella; and if a single-antigen measles vaccine is not readily available, travelers should receive M-M-R II (Measles, Mumps, and Rubella Virus Vaccine Live, MSD) regardless of their immune status to mumps or rubella.

Non-Pregnant Adolescent and Adult Females

Immunization of susceptible non-pregnant adolescent and adult females of childbearing age with live attenuated rubella virus vaccine is indicated if certain precautions are observed (see below and PRECAUTIONS). Vaccinating susceptible postpubertal females confers individual protection against subsequently acquiring rubella infection during pregnancy, which in turn prevents infection of the fetus and consequent congenital rubella injury.

Women of childbearing age should be advised not to become pregnant for three months after vaccination and should be informed of the reasons for this precaution.**

It is recommended that rubella susceptibility be determined by serologic testing prior to immunization.*** If immune, as evidenced by a specific rubella antibody titer of 1:8 or greater (hemagglutination-inhibition test), vaccination is unnecessary. Congenital malformations do occur in up to seven percent of all live births. Their chance appearance after vaccination could lead to misinterpretation of the cause, particularly if the prior rubella-immune status of vaccinees is unknown.

Postpubertal females should be informed of the frequent occurrence of generally self-limited arthralgia and/or arthritis beginning 2 to 4 weeks after vaccination (see ADVERSE REACTIONS).

Postpartum Women

It has been found convenient in many instances to vaccinate rubella-susceptible women in the immediate postpartum period. (See *Nursing Mothers*).

Revaccination: Children vaccinated when younger than 12 months of age should be revaccinated. Based on available evidence, there is no reason to routinely revaccinate persons who were vaccinated originally when 12 months of age or older. However, persons should be revaccinated if there is evidence to suggest that initial immunization was ineffective.

Use with other Vaccines

Routine administration of DTP (diphtheria, tetanus, pertussis) and/or OPV (oral poliovirus vaccine) concomitantly with measles, mumps and rubella vaccines is not recommended because there are insufficient data relating to the simultaneous administration of these antigens. However, the American Academy of Pediatrics has noted that in some circumstances, particularly when the patient may not return, some practitioners prefer to administer all these antigens on a single day. If done, separate sites and syringes should be used for DTP and BIAVAX II.

BIAVAX II should not be given less than one month before or after administration of other virus vaccines.

* Registered trademark of MERCK & CO., INC.

** NOTE: The Immunization Practices Advisory Committee (ACIP) has recommended "In view of the importance of protecting this age group against rubella, reasonable precautions in a rubella immunization program include asking females if they are pregnant, excluding those who say they are, and explaining the theoretical risks to the others."

*** NOTE: The Immunization Practices Advisory Committee (ACIP) has stated "When practical, and when reliable laboratory services are available, potential vaccinees of childbearing age can have serologic tests to determine susceptibility to rubella. . . . However, routinely performing serologic tests for all females of childbearing age to determine susceptibility so that vaccine is given only to proven susceptibles is expensive and has been ineffective in some areas. Accordingly, the ACIP believes that rubella vaccination of a woman who is not known to be pregnant and has no history of vaccination is justifiable without serologic testing."

CONTRAINDICATIONS

Do not give BIAVAX II to pregnant females; the possible effects of the vaccine on fetal development are unknown at this time. If vaccination of postpubertal females is undertaken, pregnancy should be avoided for three months following vaccination. (See PRECAUTIONS, *Pregnancy*).

Anaphylactic or anaphylactoid reactions to neomycin (each dose of reconstituted vaccine contains approximately 25 mcg of neomycin).

History of anaphylactic or anaphylactoid reactions to eggs (see HYPERSENSITIVITY TO EGGS below).

Any febrile respiratory illness or other active febrile infection.

Active untreated tuberculosis.

Patients receiving immunosuppressive therapy. This contraindication does not apply to patients who are receiving corticosteroids as replacement therapy, e.g., for Addison's disease.

Individuals with blood dyscrasias, leukemia, lymphomas of any type, or other malignant neoplasms affecting the bone marrow or lymphatic systems.

Primary and acquired immunodeficiency states, including patients who are immunosuppressed in association with AIDS or other clinical manifestations of infection with human immunodeficiency viruses; cellular immune deficiencies; and hypogammaglobulinemic and dysgammaglobulinemic states.

Individuals with a family history of congenital or hereditary immunodeficiency, until the immune competence of the potential vaccine recipient is demonstrated.

HYPERSENSITIVITY TO EGGS

Live mumps vaccine is produced in chick embryo cell culture. Persons with a history of anaphylactic, anaphylactoid, or other immediate reactions (e.g., hives, swelling of the mouth and throat, difficulty breathing, hypotension, or shock) subsequent to egg ingestion should not be vaccinated. Evidence indicates that persons are not at increased risk if they have egg allergies that are not anaphylactic or anaphylactoid in nature. Such persons may be vaccinated in the usual manner. There is no evidence to indicate that persons with allergies to chickens or feathers are at increased risk of reaction to the vaccine.

PRECAUTIONS

General

Adequate treatment provisions including epinephrine, should be available for immediate use should an anaphylactic or anaphylactoid reaction occur.

Children and young adults who are known to be infected with human immunodeficiency viruses but without overt clinical manifestations of immunosuppression may be vaccinated; however, the vaccinees should be monitored closely for vaccine-preventable diseases because immunization may be less effective than for uninfected persons.

Vaccination should be deferred for at least 3 months following blood or plasma transfusions, or administration of human immune serum globulin.

Excretion of small amounts of the live attenuated rubella virus from the nose and throat has occurred in the majority of susceptible individuals 7–28 days after vaccination. There is no confirmed evidence to indicate that such virus is transmitted to susceptible persons who are in contact with the vaccinated individuals. Consequently, transmission through close personal contact, while accepted as a theoretical possibility, is not regarded as a significant risk. However, transmission of the rubella vaccine virus to infants via breast milk has been documented (see *Nursing Mothers*).

There are no reports of transmission of live attenuated mumps virus from vaccinees to susceptible contacts.

It has been reported that live attenuated rubella and mumps virus vaccines given individually may result in a temporary depression of tuberculin skin sensitivity. Therefore, if a tuberculin test is to be done, it should be administered either before or simultaneously with BIAVAX II.

As for any vaccine, vaccination with BIAVAX II may not result in seroconversion in 100% of susceptible persons given the vaccine.

Pregnancy

Pregnancy Category C

Animal reproduction studies have not been conducted with BIAVAX II. It is also not known whether BIAVAX II can cause fetal harm when administered to a pregnant woman or can affect reproduction capacity. Therefore, the vaccine should not be administered to pregnant females; furthermore, pregnancy should be avoided for three months following vaccination (see CONTRAINDICATIONS).

In counseling women who are inadvertently vaccinated when pregnant or who become pregnant within 3 months of vaccination, the physician should be aware of the following: (1) In a 10 year survey involving over 700 pregnant women who received rubella vaccine within 3 months before or after conception, (of whom 189 received the Wistar RA 27/3 strain) none of the newborns had abnormalities compatible with congenital rubella syndrome; and (2) although mumps virus is capable of infecting the placenta and fetus, there is no good evidence that it causes congenital malformations in humans. Mumps vaccine virus also has been shown to infect the placenta, but the virus has not been isolated from the fetal tissues from susceptible women who were vaccinated and underwent elective abortions.

Nursing Mothers

It is not known whether mumps vaccine virus is secreted in human milk. Recent studies have shown that lactating postpartum women immunized with live attenuated rubella vaccine may secrete the virus in breast milk and transmit it to breast-fed infants. In the infants with serological evidence of rubella infection, none exhibited severe disease; however, one exhibited mild clinical illness typical of acquired rubella. Caution should be exercised when BIAVAX II is administered to a nursing woman.

ADVERSE REACTIONS

Burning and/or stinging of short duration at the injection site have been reported.

The adverse clinical reactions associated with the use of BIAVAX II are those expected to follow administration of the monovalent vaccines given separately. These may include malaise, sore throat, cough, rhinitis, headache, dizziness, fever, rash, nausea, vomiting or diarrhea; mild local reactions such as erythema, induration, tenderness and regional lymphadenopathy; parotitis, orchitis, nerve deafness, thrombocytopenia and purpura; allergic reactions such as wheal and flare at the injection site or urticaria; polyneuritis; and arthralgia and/or arthritis (usually transient and rarely chronic).

Anaphylaxis and anaphylactoid reactions have been reported.

Continued on next page

Information on the Merck & Co. products listed on these pages is the full prescribing information from product circulars in use October 1, 1992.

Merck & Co.—Cont.

Vasculitis has been reported rarely.
Moderate fever [101–102.9°F (38.3–39.4°C)] occurs occasionally, and high fever [above 103°F (39.4°C)] occurs less commonly. On rare occasions, children developing fever may exhibit febrile convulsions. Syncope, particularly at the time of mass vaccination, has been reported. Rash occurs infrequently and is usually minimal, but rarely may be generalized. Erythema multiforme has also been reported rarely.
Forms of optic neuritis, including retrobulbar neuritis and papillitis may infrequently follow viral infections, and have been reported to occur 1 to 3 weeks following inoculation with some live virus vaccines.
Isolated reports of polyneuropathy including Guillain-Barré syndrome have been reported after immunization with rubella-containing vaccines.
Clinical experience with live attenuated rubella and mumps virus vaccines given individually indicates that encephalitis and other nervous system reactions have occurred very rarely. These might occur also with BIAVAX II.
Arthralgia and/or arthritis (usually transient and rarely chronic), and polyneuritis are features of natural rubella and vary in frequency and severity with age and sex, being greatest in adult females and least in prepubertal children. This type of involvement as well as myalgia and paresthesia have also been reported following administration of MERUVAX II (Rubella Virus Vaccine Live, MSD).
Chronic arthritis has been associated with natural rubella infection and has been related to persistent virus and/or viral antigen isolated from body tissues. Only rarely have vaccine recipients developed chronic joint symptoms.
Following vaccination in children, reactions in joints are uncommon and generally of brief duration. In women, incidence rates for arthritis and arthralgia are generally higher than those seen in children (children: 0–3%; women: 12–20%), and the reactions tend to be more marked and of longer duration. Symptoms may persist for a matter of months or on rare occasions for years. In adolescent girls, the reactions appear to be intermediate in incidence between those seen in children and in adult women. Even in older women (35–45 years), these reactions are generally well tolerated and rarely interfere with normal activities.

DOSAGE AND ADMINISTRATION

FOR SUBCUTANEOUS ADMINISTRATION
Do not inject intravenously.
The dosage of vaccine is the same for all persons. Inject the total volume (about 0.5 mL) of reconstituted vaccine subcutaneously, preferably into the outer aspect of upper arm. *Do not give immune globulin (IG) concurrently with* BIAVAX II.
During shipment, to insure that there is no loss of potency, the vaccine must be maintained at a temperature of 10°C (50°F) or less.
Before reconstitution, store BIAVAX II at 2–8°C (36–46°F).
Protect from light.
CAUTION: A sterile syringe free of preservatives, antiseptics, and detergents should be used for each injection of the vaccine because these substances may inactivate the live virus vaccine. A 25 gauge, 5/8" needle is recommended.
To reconstitute, use only the diluent supplied, since it is free of preservatives or other antiviral substances which might inactivate the vaccine. First withdraw the entire volume of diluent into the syringe to be used for reconstitution. Inject all the diluent in the syringe into the vial of lyophilized vaccine, and agitate to mix thoroughly. Withdraw the entire contents into a syringe and inject the total volume of restored vaccine subcutaneously.
It is important to use a separate sterile syringe and needle for each individual patient to prevent transmission of hepatitis B virus and other infectious agents from one person to another.
Each dose of BIAVAX II contains not less than the equivalent of 1,000 $TCID_{50}$ of the U.S. Reference Rubella Virus and 20,000 $TCID_{50}$ of the U.S. Reference Mumps Virus.
Parenteral drug products should be inspected visually for particulate matter and discoloration prior to administration. BIAVAX II, when reconstituted, is clear yellow.

HOW SUPPLIED

No. 4746—BIAVAX II is supplied as a single-dose vial of lyophilized vaccine, **NDC** 0006-4746-00, and a vial of diluent.
No. 4669/4309—BIAVAX II is supplied as follows: (1) a box of 10 single-dose vials of lyophilized vaccine (package A), **NDC** 0006-4669-00; and (2) a box of 10 vials of diluent (package B).
To conserve refrigerator space, the diluent may be stored separately at room temperature.
Storage
It is recommended that the vaccine be used as soon as possible after reconstitution. Protect the vaccine from light at all times, since such exposure may inactivate the virus. Store reconstituted vaccine in the vaccine vial in a dark place at 2–8°C (36–46°F) and discard if not used within eight hours.

A.H.F.S. Category: 80:12
DC 7680114 Issued March 1991
COPYRIGHT © MERCK & CO., INC., 1990
All rights reserved

BLOCADREN® Tablets
(Timolol Maleate), U.S.P. ℞

DESCRIPTION

BLOCADREN* (Timolol Maleate) is a non-selective beta-adrenergic receptor blocking agent. The chemical name for timolol maleate is (S)-1-[(1, 1-dimethylethyl) amino] -3-[[4-(4-morpholinyl)-1, 2, 5-thiadiazol-3-yl]oxy]-2-propanol, (Z)-butenedioate (1:1) salt. It possesses an asymmetric carbon atom in its structure and is provided as the levoisomer. Its empirical formula is $C_{13}H_{24}N_4O_3S \cdot C_4H_4O_4$ and its structural formula is:

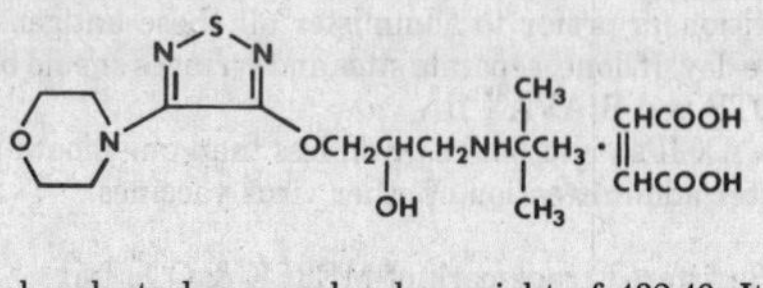

Timolol maleate has a molecular weight of 432.49. It is a white, odorless, crystalline powder which is soluble in water, methanol, and alcohol.
BLOCADREN is supplied as tablets in three strengths containing 5 mg, 10 mg or 20 mg timolol maleate for oral administration. Inactive ingredients are cellulose, FD&C Blue 2, magnesium stearate, and starch.

*Registered trademark of MERCK & CO., INC.

CLINICAL PHARMACOLOGY

BLOCADREN is a $beta_1$ and $beta_2$ (non-selective) adrenergic receptor blocking agent that does not have significant intrinsic sympathomimetic, direct myocardial depressant, or local anesthetic activity.
Pharmacodynamics
Clinical pharmacology studies have confirmed the beta-adrenergic blocking activity as shown by (1) changes in resting heart rate and response of heart rate to changes in posture; (2) inhibition of isoproterenol-induced tachycardia; (3) alteration of the response to the Valsalva maneuver and amyl nitrite administration; and (4) reduction of heart rate and blood pressure changes on exercise.
BLOCADREN decreases the positive chronotropic, positive inotropic, bronchodilator, and vasodilator responses caused by beta-adrenergic receptor agonists. The magnitude of this decreased response is proportional to the existing sympathetic tone and the concentration of BLOCADREN at receptor sites.
In normal volunteers, the reduction in heart rate response to a standard exercise was dose dependent over the test range of 0.5 to 20 mg, with a peak reduction at 2 hours of approximately 30% at higher doses.
Beta-adrenergic receptor blockade reduces cardiac output in both healthy subjects and patients with heart disease. In patients with severe impairment of myocardial function beta-adrenergic receptor blockade may inhibit the stimulatory effect of the sympathetic nervous system necessary to maintain adequate cardiac function.
Beta-adrenergic receptor blockade in the bronchi and bronchioles results in increased airway resistance from unopposed parasympathetic activity. Such an effect in patients with asthma or other bronchospastic conditions is potentially dangerous.
Clinical studies indicate that BLOCADREN at a dosage of 20–60 mg/day reduces blood pressure without causing postural hypotension in most patients with essential hypertension. Administration of BLOCADREN to patients with hypertension results initially in a decrease in cardiac output, little immediate change in blood pressure, and an increase in calculated peripheral resistance. With continued administration of BLOCADREN blood pressure decreases within a few days, cardiac output usually remains reduced, and peripheral resistance falls toward pretreatment levels. Plasma volume may decrease or remain unchanged during therapy with BLOCADREN. In the majority of patients with hypertension BLOCADREN also decreases plasma renin activity. Dosage adjustment to achieve optimal antihypertensive effect may require a few weeks. When therapy with BLOCADREN is discontinued, the blood pressure tends to return to pretreatment levels gradually. In most patients the antihypertensive activity of BLOCADREN is maintained with long-term therapy and is well tolerated.
The mechanism of the antihypertensive effects of beta-adrenergic receptor blocking agents is not established at this time. Possible mechanisms of action include reduction in cardiac output, reduction in plasma renin activity, and a central nervous system sympatholytic action.
A Norwegian multi-center, double-blind study compared the effects of timolol maleate with placebo in 1,884 patients who had survived the acute phase of a myocardial infarction. Patients with systolic blood pressure below 100 mm Hg, sick sinus syndrome and contraindications to beta blockers, including uncontrolled heart failure, second or third degree AV block and bradycardia (<50 beats per minute), were excluded from the multi-center trial. Therapy with BLOCADREN, begun 7 to 28 days following infarction, was shown to reduce overall mortality; this was primarily attributable to a reduction in cardiovascular mortality. BLOCADREN significantly reduced the incidence of sudden deaths (deaths occurring without symptoms or within 24 hours of the onset of symptoms), including those occurring within one hour, and particularly instantaneous deaths (those occurring without preceding symptoms). The protective effect of BLOCADREN was consistent regardless of age, sex or site of infarction. The effect was clearest in patients with a first infarction who were considered at a high risk of dying, defined as those with one or more of the following characteristics during the acute phase: transient left ventricular failure, cardiomegaly, newly appearing atrial fibrillation or flutter, systolic hypotension, or SGOT (ASAT) levels greater than four times the upper limit of normal. Therapy with BLOCADREN also reduced the incidence of non-fatal reinfarction. The mechanism of the protective effect of BLOCADREN is unknown.
BLOCADREN was studied for the prophylactic treatment of migraine headache in placebo-controlled clinical trials involving 400 patients, mostly women between the ages of 18 and 66 years. Common migraine was the most frequent diagnosis. All patients had at least two headaches per month at baseline. Approximately 50 percent of patients who received BLOCADREN had a reduction in the frequency of migraine headache of at least 50 percent, compared to a similar decrease in frequency in 30 percent of patients receiving placebo. The most common cardiovascular adverse effect was bradycardia (5%).
Pharmacokinetics and Metabolism
BLOCADREN is rapidly and nearly completely absorbed (about 90%) following oral ingestion. Detectable plasma levels of timolol occur within one-half hour and peak plasma levels occur in about one to two hours. The drug half-life in plasma is approximately 4 hours and this is essentially unchanged in patients with moderate renal insufficiency. Timolol is partially metabolized by the liver and timolol and its metabolites are excreted by the kidney. Timolol is not extensively bound to plasma proteins; i.e., <10% by equilibrium dialysis and approximately 60% by ultrafiltration. An *in vitro* hemodialysis study, using ^{14}C timolol added to human plasma or whole blood, showed that timolol was readily dialyzed from these fluids; however, a study of patients with renal failure showed that timolol did not dialyze readily. Plasma levels following oral administration are about half those following intravenous administration indicating approximately 50% first pass metabolism. The level of beta sympathetic activity varies widely among individuals, and no simple correlation exists between the dose or plasma level of timolol maleate and its therapeutic activity. Therefore, objective clinical measurements such as reduction of heart rate and/or blood pressure should be used as guides in determining the optimal dosage for each patient.

INDICATIONS AND USAGE

Hypertension
BLOCADREN is indicated for the treatment of hypertension. It may be used alone or in combination with other antihypertensive agents, especially thiazide-type diuretics.
Myocardial Infarction
BLOCADREN is indicated in patients who have survived the acute phase of a myocardial infarction, and are clinically stable, to reduce cardiovascular mortality and the risk of reinfarction.
Migraine
BLOCADREN is indicated for the prophylaxis of migraine headache.

CONTRAINDICATIONS

BLOCADREN is contraindicated in patients with bronchial asthma or with a history of bronchial asthma, or severe chronic obstructive pulmonary disease (see WARNINGS); sinus bradycardia; second and third degree atrioventricular block; overt cardiac failure (see WARNINGS); cardiogenic shock; hypersensitivity to this product.

WARNINGS

Cardiac Failure
Sympathetic stimulation may be essential for support of the circulation in individuals with diminished myocardial contractility, and its inhibition by beta-adrenergic receptor

blockade may precipitate more severe failure. Although beta blockers should be avoided in overt congestive heart failure, they can be used, if necessary, with caution in patients with a history of failure who are well-compensated, usually with digitalis and diuretics. Both digitalis and timolol maleate slow AV conduction. If cardiac failure persists, therapy with BLOCADREN should be withdrawn.

In Patients Without a History of Cardiac Failure continued depression of the myocardium with beta-blocking agents over a period of time can, in some cases, lead to cardiac failure. At the first sign or symptom of cardiac failure, patients receiving BLOCADREN should be digitalized and/or be given a diuretic, and the response observed closely. If cardiac failure continues, despite adequate digitalization and diuretic therapy, BLOCADREN should be withdrawn.

Exacerbation of Ischemic Heart Disease Following Abrupt Withdrawal—Hypersensitivity to catecholamines has been observed in patients withdrawn from beta blocker therapy; exacerbation of angina and, in some cases, myocardial infarction have occurred after *abrupt* discontinuation of such therapy. When discontinuing chronically administered timolol maleate, particularly in patients with ischemic heart disease, the dosage should be gradually reduced over a period of one to two weeks and the patient should be carefully monitored. If angina markedly worsens or acute coronary insufficiency develops, timolol maleate administration should be reinstituted promptly, at least temporarily, and other measures appropriate for the management of unstable angina should be taken. Patients should be warned against interruption or discontinuation of therapy without the physician's advice. Because coronary artery disease is common and may be unrecognized, it may be prudent not to discontinue timolol maleate therapy abruptly even in patients treated only for hypertension.

Obstructive Pulmonary Disease

PATIENTS WITH CHRONIC OBSTRUCTIVE PULMONARY DISEASE (e.g., CHRONIC BRONCHITIS, EMPHYSEMA) OF MILD OR MODERATE SEVERITY, BRONCHOSPASTIC DISEASE OR A HISTORY OF BRONCHOSPASTIC DISEASE (OTHER THAN BRONCHIAL ASTHMA OR A HISTORY OF BRONCHIAL ASTHMA, IN WHICH 'BLOCADREN' IS CONTRAINDICATED, see CONTRAINDICATIONS), SHOULD IN GENERAL NOT RECEIVE BETA BLOCKERS, INCLUDING 'BLOCADREN'. However, if BLOCADREN is necessary in such patients, then the drug should be administered with caution since it may block bronchodilation produced by endogenous and exogenous catecholamine stimulation of $beta_2$ receptors.

Major Surgery

The necessity or desirability of withdrawal of beta-blocking therapy prior to major surgery is controversial. Beta-adrenergic receptor blockade impairs the ability of the heart to respond to beta-adrenergically mediated reflex stimuli. This may augment the risk of general anesthesia in surgical procedures. Some patients receiving beta-adrenergic receptor blocking agents have been subject to protracted severe hypotension during anesthesia. Difficulty in restarting and maintaining the heartbeat has also been reported. For these reasons, in patients undergoing elective surgery, some authorities recommend gradual withdrawal of beta-adrenergic receptor blocking agents.

If necessary during surgery, the effects of beta-adrenergic blocking agents may be reversed by sufficient doses of such agonists as isoproterenol, dopamine, dobutamine or levarterenol (see OVERDOSAGE).

Diabetes Mellitus

BLOCADREN should be administered with caution in patients subject to spontaneous hypoglycemia or to diabetic patients (especially those with labile diabetes) who are receiving insulin or oral hypoglycemic agents. Beta-adrenergic receptor blocking agents may mask the signs and symptoms of acute hypoglycemia.

Thyrotoxicosis

Beta-adrenergic blockade may mask certain clinical signs (e.g., tachycardia) of hyperthyroidism. Patients suspected of developing thyrotoxicosis should be managed carefully to avoid abrupt withdrawal of beta blockade which might precipitate a thyroid storm.

PRECAUTIONS

General

Impaired Hepatic or Renal Function: Since BLOCADREN is partially metabolized in the liver and excreted mainly by the kidneys, dosage reductions may be necessary when hepatic and/or renal insufficiency is present.

Dosing in the Presence of Marked Renal Failure: Although the pharmacokinetics of BLOCADREN are not greatly altered by renal impairment, marked hypotensive responses have been seen in patients with marked renal impairment undergoing dialysis after 20 mg doses. Dosing in such patients should therefore be especially cautious.

Muscle Weakness: Beta-adrenergic blockade has been reported to potentiate muscle weakness consistent with certain myasthenic symptoms (e.g., diplopia, ptosis, and generalized weakness). Timolol has been reported rarely to increase muscle weakness in some patients with myasthenia gravis or myasthenic symptoms.

Cerebrovascular Insufficiency: Because of potential effects of beta-adrenergic blocking agents relative to blood pressure and pulse, these agents should be used with caution in patients with cerebrovascular insufficiency. If signs or symptoms suggesting reduced cerebral blood flow are observed, consideration should be given to discontinuing these agents.

Drug Interactions

Close observation of the patient is recommended when BLOCADREN is administered to patients receiving catecholamine-depleting drugs such as reserpine, because of possible additive effects and the production of hypotension and/or marked bradycardia, which may produce vertigo, syncope, or postural hypotension.

Blunting of the antihypertensive effect of beta-adrenoceptor blocking agents by non-steroidal anti-inflammatory drugs has been reported. When using these agents concomitantly, patients should be observed carefully to confirm that the desired therapeutic effect has been obtained.

Literature reports suggest that oral calcium antagonists may be used in combination with beta-adrenergic blocking agents when heart function is normal, but should be avoided in patients with impaired cardiac function. Hypotension, AV conduction disturbances, and left ventricular failure have been reported in some patients receiving beta-adrenergic blocking agents when an oral calcium antagonist was added to the treatment regimen. Hypotension was more likely to occur if the calcium antagonist were a dihydropyridine derivative, e.g. nifedipine, while left ventricular failure and AV conduction disturbances were more likely to occur with either verapamil or diltiazem.

Intravenous calcium antagonists should be used with caution in patients receiving beta-adrenergic blocking agents.

The concomitant use of beta-adrenergic blocking agents with digitalis and either diltiazem or verapamil may have additive effects in prolonging AV conduction time.

Carcinogenesis, Mutagenesis, Impairment of Fertility

In a two-year study of timolol maleate in rats, there was a statistically significant ($P \leq 0.05$) increase in the incidence of adrenal pheochromocytomas in male rats administered 300 mg/kg/day (250 times* the maximum recommended human dose). Similar differences were not observed in rats administered doses equivalent to approximately 20 or 80 times* the maximum recommended human dose.

In a lifetime study in mice, there were statistically significant ($P \leq 0.05$) increases in the incidence of benign and malignant pulmonary tumors and benign uterine polyps in female mice at 500 mg/kg/day (approximately 400 times* the maximum recommended human dose), but not at 5 or 50 mg/kg/day. In a subsequent supplementary study in female mice at 500 mg/kg/day, a statistically significant increase in the incidence of pulmonary tumors was observed. In the initial study in mice there was also a significant increase in mammary adenocarcinomas at the 500 mg/kg/day dose.

Mammary adenocarcinomas were associated with elevations in serum prolactin which occurred in female mice administered timolol at 500 mg/kg, but not at doses of 5 or 50 mg/kg/day. An increased incidence of mammary adenocarcinomas in rodents has been associated with administration of several other therapeutic agents which elevate serum prolactin, but no correlation between serum prolactin levels and mammary tumors has been established in man. Furthermore, in adult human female subjects who received oral dosages of up to 60 mg of timolol maleate, the maximum recommended human oral dosage, there were no clinically meaningful changes in serum prolactin.

Timolol maleate was devoid of mutagenic potential when evaluated *in vivo* (mouse) in the micronucleus test and cytogenetic assay (doses up to 800 mg/kg) and *in vitro* in a neoplastic cell transformation assay (up to 100 μg/mL). In Ames tests the highest concentrations of timolol employed, 5000 or 10,000 μg/plate, were associated with statistically significant elevations ($P \leq 0.05$) of revertants observed with tester strain TA100 (in seven replicate assays), but not in the remaining three strains. In the assays with tester strain TA100, no consistent dose response relationship was observed, nor did the ratio of test to control revertants reach 2. A ratio of 2 is usually considered the criterion for a positive Ames test.

Reproduction and fertility studies in rats showed no adverse effect on male or female fertility at doses up to 125 times* the maximum recommended human dose.

*Based on patient weight of 50 kg.

Pregnancy

Pregnancy Category C. Teratogenicity studies with timolol in mice and rabbits at doses up to 50 mg/kg/day (50 times the maximum recommended human dose) showed no evidence of fetal malformations. Although delayed fetal ossification was observed at this dose in rats, there were no adverse effects on postnatal development of offspring. Doses of 1000 mg/kg/day (1,000 times the maximum recommended human dose) were maternotoxic in mice and resulted in an increased number of fetal resorptions. Increased fetal resorptions were also seen in rabbits at doses of 100 times the maximum recommended human dose, in this case without apparent maternotoxicity. There are no adequate and well-controlled studies in pregnant women. BLOCADREN should be used during pregnancy only if the potential benefit justifies the potential risk to the fetus.

Nursing Mothers

Because of the potential for serious adverse reactions from timolol in nursing infants, a decision should be made whether to discontinue nursing or to discontinue the drug, taking into account the importance of the drug to the mother.

Pediatric Use

Safety and effectiveness in children have not been established.

ADVERSE REACTIONS

BLOCADREN is usually well tolerated in properly selected patients. Most adverse effects have been mild and transient.

In a multicenter (12-week) clinical trial comparing timolol maleate and placebo in hypertensive patients, the following adverse reactions were reported spontaneously and considered to be causally related to timolol maleate:

	Timolol Maleate (n = 176) %	Placebo (n = 168) %
BODY AS A WHOLE		
fatigue/tiredness	3.4	0.6
headache	1.7	1.8
chest pain	0.6	0
asthenia	0.6	0
CARDIOVASCULAR		
bradycardia	9.1	0
arrhythmia	1.1	0.6
syncope	0.6	0
edema	0.6	1.2
DIGESTIVE		
dyspepsia	0.6	0.6
nausea	0.6	0
SKIN		
pruritus	1.1	0
NERVOUS SYSTEM		
dizziness	2.3	1.2
vertigo	0.6	0
paresthesia	0.6	0
PSYCHIATRIC		
decreased libido	0.6	0
RESPIRATORY		
dyspnea	1.7	0.6
bronchial spasm	0.6	0
rales	0.6	0
SPECIAL SENSES		
eye irritation	1.1	0.6
tinnitus	0.6	0

These data are representative of the incidence of adverse effects that may be observed in properly selected patients treated with BLOCADREN, i.e., excluding patients with bronchospastic disease, congestive heart failure or other contraindications to beta blocker therapy.

In patients with migraine the incidence of bradycardia was 5 percent.

In a coronary artery disease population studied in the Norwegian multi-center trial (see CLINICAL PHARMACOLOGY), the frequency of the principal adverse reactions and the frequency with which these resulted in discontinuation of therapy in the timolol and placebo groups were:

[See table on next page.]

The following additional adverse effects have been reported in clinical experience with the drug: *Body as a Whole:* extremity pain, decreased exercise tolerance, weight loss, fever; *Cardiovascular:* cardiac arrest, cardiac failure, cerebrovascular accident, worsening of angina pectoris, worsening of arterial insufficiency, Raynaud's phenomenon, palpitations, vasodilatation; *Digestive:* gastrointestinal pain, hepatomegaly, vomiting, diarrhea, dyspepsia; *Hematologic:* nonthrombocytopenic purpura; *Endocrine:* hyperglycemia, hypoglycemia; *Skin:* rash, skin irritation, increased pigmentation, sweating, alopecia; *Musculoskeletal:* arthralgia; *Nervous System:* local weakness, increase in signs and symptoms of myasthenia gravis; *Psychiatric:* depression, nightmares,

Continued on next page

Information on the Merck & Co. products listed on these pages is the full prescribing information from product circulars in use October 1, 1992.

Merck & Co.—Cont.

somnolence, insomnia, nervousness, diminished concentration, hallucinations; *Respiratory:* cough; *Special Senses:* visual disturbances, diplopia, ptosis, dry eyes; *Urogenital:* impotence, urination difficulties.

There have been reports of retroperitoneal fibrosis in patients receiving timolol maleate and in patients receiving other beta-adrenergic blocking agents. A causal relationship between this condition and therapy with beta-adrenergic blocking agents has not been established.

Potential Adverse Effects: In addition, a variety of adverse effects not observed in clinical trials with BLOCADREN, but reported with other beta-adrenergic blocking agents, should be considered potential adverse effects of BLOCADREN: *Nervous System:* Reversible mental depression progressing to catatonia; an acute reversible syndrome characterized by disorientation for time and place, short-term memory loss, emotional lability, slightly clouded sensorium, and decreased performance on neuropsychometrics; *Cardiovascular:* Intensification of AV block (see CONTRAINDICATIONS); *Digestive:* Mesenteric arterial thrombosis, ischemic colitis; *Hematologic:* Agranulocytosis, thrombocytopenic purpura; *Allergic:* Erythematous rash, fever combined with aching and sore throat, laryngospasm with respiratory distress; *Miscellaneous:* Peyronie's disease.

There have been reports of a syndrome comprising psoriasiform skin rash, conjunctivitis sicca, otitis, and sclerosing serositis attributed to the beta-adrenergic receptor blocking agent, practolol. This syndrome has not been reported with BLOCADREN.

Clinical Laboratory Test Findings: Clinically important changes in standard laboratory parameters were rarely associated with the administration of BLOCADREN. Slight increases in blood urea nitrogen, serum potassium, uric acid, and triglycerides, and slight decreases in hemoglobin, hematocrit and HDL cholesterol occurred, but were not progressive or associated with clinical manifestations. Increases in liver function tests have been reported.

OVERDOSAGE

No data are available in regard to overdosage in humans. The oral LD_{50} of the drug is 1190 and 900 mg/kg in female mice and female rats, respectively.

An *in vitro* hemodialysis study, using ^{14}C timolol added to human plasma or whole blood, showed that timolol was readily dialyzed from these fluids; however, a study of patients with renal failure showed that timolol did not dialyze readily.

The most common signs and symptoms to be expected with overdosage with a beta-adrenergic receptor blocking agent are symptomatic bradycardia, hypotension, bronchospasm, and acute cardiac failure. Therapy with BLOCADREN should be discontinued and the patient observed closely. The following additional therapeutic measures should be considered:

(1) *Gastric lavage*

(2) *Symptomatic bradycardia:* Use atropine sulfate intravenously in a dosage of 0.25 mg to 2 mg to induce vagal blockade. If bradycardia persists, intravenous isoproterenol hydrochloride should be administered cautiously. In refractory cases the use of a transvenous cardiac pacemaker may be considered.

(3) *Hypotension:* Use sympathomimetic pressor drug therapy, such as dopamine, dobutamine or levarterenol. In refractory cases the use of glucagon hydrochloride has been reported to be useful.

(4) *Bronchospasm:* Use isoproterenol hydrochloride. Additional therapy with aminophylline may be considered.

(5) *Acute cardiac failure:* Conventional therapy with digitalis, diuretics, and oxygen should be instituted immediately. In refractory cases the use of intravenous aminophylline is suggested. This may be followed if necessary by glucagon hydrochloride which has been reported to be useful.

(6) *Heart block (second or third degree):* Use isoproterenol hydrochloride or a transvenous cardiac pacemaker.

DOSAGE AND ADMINISTRATION

Hypertension

The usual initial dosage of BLOCADREN is 10 mg twice a day, whether used alone or added to diuretic therapy. Dosage may be increased or decreased depending on heart rate and blood pressure response. The usual total maintenance dosage is 20–40 mg per day. Increases in dosage to a maximum of 60 mg per day divided into two doses may be necessary. There should be an interval of at least seven days between increases in dosages.

BLOCADREN may be used with a thiazide diuretic or with other antihypertensive agents. Patients should be observed carefully during initiation of such concomitant therapy.

Myocardial Infarction

The recommended dosage for long-term prophylactic use in patients who have survived the acute phase of a myocardial infarction is 10 mg given twice daily (see CLINICAL PHARMACOLOGY).

Migraine

The usual initial dosage of BLOCADREN is 10 mg twice a day. During maintenance therapy the 20 mg daily dosage may be administered as a single dose. Total daily dosage may be increased to a maximum of 30 mg, given in divided doses, or decreased to 10 mg once per day, depending on clinical response and tolerability. If a satisfactory response is not obtained after 6-8 weeks use of the maximum daily dosage, therapy with BLOCADREN should be discontinued.

HOW SUPPLIED

No. 3343—Tablets BLOCADREN, 5 mg, are light blue, round, compressed tablets, with code MSD 59 on one side and BLOCADREN on the other. They are supplied as follows:

NDC 0006-0059-68 bottles of 100.

Shown in Product Identification Section, page 419

No. 3344—Tablets BLOCADREN, 10 mg, are light blue, round, scored, compressed tablets, with code MSD 136 on one side and BLOCADREN on the other. They are supplied as follows:

NDC 0006-0136-68 bottles of 100
(6505-01-132-0651, 10 mg 100's)
NDC 0006-0136-28 unit dose packages of 100.

Shown in Product Identification Section, page 419

No. 3371—Tablets BLOCADREN, 20 mg, are light blue, capsule shaped, scored, compressed tablets, with code MSD 437 on one side and BLOCADREN on the other. They are supplied as follows:

NDC 0006-0437-68 bottles of 100
(6505-01-132-0652, 20 mg 100's)

Shown in Product Identification Section, page 419

Storage

Store in a well-closed container, protected from light.

A.H.F.S. Categories: 24:04, 24:08
DC 7146625 Issued August 1989

COPYRIGHT © MERCK & CO., INC., 1985

CHIBROXIN™ ℞

(Norfloxacin)
Sterile Ophthalmic Solution

DESCRIPTION

CHIBROXIN* (Norfloxacin) Ophthalmic Solution is a synthetic broad-spectrum antibacterial agent supplied as a sterile isotonic solution for topical ophthalmic use. Norfloxacin, a fluoroquinolone, is 1-ethyl-6-fluoro-1,4-dihydro-4-oxo-7-(1-piperazinyl) -3- quinoline-carboxylic acid. Its empirical formula is $C_{16}H_{18}FN_3O_3$ and the structural formula is:

Norfloxacin is a white to pale yellow crystalline powder with a molecular weight of 319.34 and a melting point of about 221°C. It is freely soluble in glacial acetic acid and very slightly soluble in ethanol, methanol and water.

CHIBROXIN Ophthalmic Solution 0.3% is supplied as a sterile isotonic solution. Each mL contains 3 mg norfloxacin. Inactive ingredients: disodium edetate, sodium acetate, sodium chloride, hydrochloric acid (to adjust pH) and water for injection, Benzalkonium chloride 0.0025% is added as preservative. The pH of CHIBROXIN is approximately 5.2 and the osmolarity is approximately 285 mOsmol/liter.

Norfloxacin, a fluoroquinolone, differs from quinolones by having a fluorine atom at the 6 position and a piperazine moiety at the 7 position.

*Trademark of MERCK & CO., INC.

CLINICAL PHARMACOLOGY

Microbiology

Norfloxacin has *in vitro* activity against a broad spectrum of gram-positive and gram-negative aerobic bacteria. The fluorine atom at the 6 position provides increased potency against gram-negative organisms and the piperazine moiety at the 7 position is responsible for anti-pseudomonal activity. Norfloxacin inhibits bacterial deoxyribonucleic acid synthesis and is bactericidal. At the molecular level three specific events are attributed to CHIBROXIN in *E. coli* cells:

1) inhibition of the ATP-dependent DNA supercoiling reaction catalyzed by DNA gyrase;
2) inhibition of the relaxation of supercoiled DNA;
3) promotion of double-stranded DNA breakage.

There is generally no cross-resistance between norfloxacin and other classes of antibacterial agents. Therefore, norfloxacin generally demonstrates activity against indicated organisms resistant to some other antimicrobial agents. When such cross-resistance does occur, it is probably due to decreased entry of the drugs into the bacterial cells. Antagonism has been demonstrated *in vitro* between norfloxacin and nitrofurantoin.

Norfloxacin has been shown to be active against most strains of the following organisms both *in vitro* and clinically in ophthalmic infections (see INDICATIONS AND USAGE):

Gram-positive bacteria including:
Staphylococcus aureus
    (including both penicillinase-producing and methicillin-resistant strains)
Staphylococcus epidermidis
Staphylococcus warneri
Streptococcus pneumoniae
Gram-negative bacteria including:
Acinetobacter calcoaceticus
Aeromonas hydrophila
Haemophilus influenzae
Proteus mirabilis
Serratia marcescens
Norfloxacin has been shown to be active *in vitro* against most strains of the following organisms; however, *the clinical significance of these data in ophthalmic infections is unknown.*
Gram-positive bacteria:
Bacillus cereus
Enterococcus faecalis (formerly *Streptococcus faecalis*)
Staphylococcus saprophyticus
Gram-negative bacteria:
Citrobacter diversus
Citrobacter freundii
Edwardsiella tarda
Enterobacter aerogenes
Enterobacter cloacae
Escherichia coli
Hafnia alvei
Haemophilus aegyptius (Koch-Weeks bacillus)
Klebsiella oxytoca
Klebsiella pneumoniae
Klebsiella rhinoscleromatis

BLOCADREN	Adverse Reaction†		Withdrawal‡	
	Timolol (n = 945) %	Placebo (n = 939) %	Timolol (n = 945) %	Placebo (n = 939) %
Asthenia or Fatigue	5	1	<1	<1
Heart Rate <40 beats/minute	5	<1	4	<1
Cardiac Failure—Nonfatal	8	7	3	2
Hypotension	3	2	3	1
Pulmonary Edema—Nonfatal	2	<1	<1	<1
Claudication	3	3	1	<1
AV Block 2nd or 3rd degree	<1	<1	<1	<1
Sinoatrial Block	<1	<1	<1	<1
Cold Hands and Feet	8	<1	<1	0
Nausea or Digestive Disorders	8	6	1	<1
Dizziness	6	4	1	0
Bronchial Obstruction	2	<1	1	<1

† When an adverse reaction recurred in a patient, it is listed only once.
‡ Only principal reason for withdrawal in each patient is listed.
These adverse reactions can also occur in patients treated for hypertension.

Morganella morganii
Neisseria gonorrhoeae
Proteus vulgaris
Providencia alcalifaciens
Providencia rettgeri
Providencia stuartii
Pseudomonas aeruginosa
Salmonella typhi
Vibrio cholerae
Vibrio parahemolyticus
Yersinia enterocolitica
Other:
Ureaplasma urealyticum
Norfloxacin is not active against obligate anaerobes.

Clinical Studies
Clinical studies were conducted comparing CHIBROXIN Ophthalmic Solution (n=152) with ophthalmic solutions of tobramycin, gentamicin, and chloramphenicol (n=158) in patients with conjunctivitis and positive bacterial cultures. After seven days of therapy with CHIBROXIN Ophthalmic Solution, 72 percent of patients were clinically cured. Of those cured, 85 percent had all their pathogens eradicated. Eradication was also achieved in 62 percent (23/37) of patients whose clinical outcome was not completely cured by day seven. These results were similar among all treatment groups.

Another clinical study compared CHIBROXIN Ophthalmic Solution with placebo in patients with conjunctivitis and positive bacterial cultures. Placebo in this study was the liquid vehicle for CHIBROXIN Ophthalmic Solution and contained the preservative. After five days of therapy, 64 percent (36/56) of patients on CHIBROXIN Ophthalmic Solution were clinically cured compared to 50 percent (23/46) of patients receiving placebo. Of those cured, 78 percent had all their pathogens eradicated. Eradication was also achieved in 50 percent (10/20) of patients whose clinical outcome was not completely cured. The response to CHIBROXIN Ophthalmic Solution was statistically significantly better than the response to placebo.

INDICATIONS AND USAGE

CHIBROXIN Ophthalmic Solution is indicated for the treatment of conjunctivitis when caused by susceptible strains of the following bacteria:
Acinetobacter calcoaceticus*
Aeromonas hydrophila*
Haemophilus influenzae
Proteus mirabilis*
Serratia marcescens*
Staphylococcus aureus
Staphylococcus epidermidis
Staphylococcus warnerii*
Streptococcus pneumoniae
Appropriate monitoring of bacterial response to topical antibiotic therapy should accompany the use of CHIBROXIN Ophthalmic Solution.

---

*Efficacy for this organism was studied in fewer than 10 infections.

CONTRAINDICATIONS

CHIBROXIN Ophthalmic Solution is contraindicated in patients with a history of hypersensitivity to norfloxacin, or the other members of the quinolone group of antibacterial agents or any other component of this medication.

WARNINGS

NOT FOR INJECTION INTO THE EYE.
Serious and occasionally fatal hypersensitivity (anaphylactoid or anaphylactic) reactions, some following the first dose, have been reported in patients receiving systemic quinolone therapy. Some reactions were accompanied by cardiovascular collapse, loss of consciousness, tingling, pharyngeal or facial edema, dyspnea, urticaria, and itching. Only a few patients had a history of hypersensitivity reactions. Serious anaphylactoid or anaphylactic reactions require immediate emergency treatment with epinephrine. Oxygen, intravenous steroids and airway management, including intubation, should be administered as indicated.

PRECAUTIONS

General
As with other antibiotic preparations, prolonged use may result in overgrowth of nonsusceptible organisms, including fungi. If superinfection occurs, appropriate measures should be initiated. Whenever clinical judgment dictates, the patient should be examined with the aid of magnification, such as slit lamp biomicroscopy and, where appropriate, fluorescein staining.

Information For Patients
Patients should be instructed to avoid allowing the tip of the dispensing container to contact the eye or surrounding structures.
Patients should be advised that norfloxacin may be associated with hypersensitivity reactions, even following a single dose, and to discontinue the drug at the first sign of a skin rash or other allergic reaction.

Drug Interactions
Specific drug interaction studies have not been conducted with norfloxacin ophthalmic solution. However, the systemic administration of some quinolones has been shown to elevate plasma concentrations of theophylline, interfere with the metabolism of caffeine, and enhance the effects of the oral anticoagulant warfarin and its derivatives. Elevated serum levels of cyclosporine have been reported with concomitant use of cyclosporine with norfloxacin. Therefore, cyclosporine serum levels should be monitored and appropriate cyclosporine dosage adjustments made when these drugs are used concomitantly.

Carcinogenesis, Mutagenesis, Impairment of Fertility
No increase in neoplastic changes was observed with norfloxacin as compared to controls in a study in rats, lasting up to 96 weeks at doses eight to nine times the usual human oral dose*.
Norfloxacin was tested for mutagenic activity in a number of *in vivo* and *in vitro* tests. Norfloxacin had no mutagenic effect in the dominant lethal test in mice and did not cause chromosomal aberrations in hamsters or rats at doses 30 to 60 times the usual oral dose*. Norfloxacin had no mutagenic activity *in vitro* in the Ames microbial mutagen test, Chinese hamster fibroblasts and V-79 mammalian cell assay. Although norfloxacin was weakly positive in the Rec-assay for DNA repair, all other mutagenic assays were negative including a more sensitive test (V-79).
Norfloxacin did not adversely affect the fertility of male and female mice at oral doses up to 33 times the usual human oral dose*.

Pregnancy
Pregnancy Category C: Norfloxacin has been shown to produce embryonic loss in monkeys when given in doses 10 times the maximum human oral dose* (400 mg b.i.d.), with peak plasma levels that are two to three times those obtained in humans. There has been no evidence of a teratogenic effect in any of the animal species tested (rat, rabbit, mouse, monkey) at 6 to 50 times the human oral dose. There are no adequate and well-controlled studies in pregnant women. CHIBROXIN Ophthalmic Solution should be used during pregnancy only if the potential benefit justifies the potential risk to the fetus.

Nursing Mothers
It is not known whether norfloxacin is excreted in human milk following ocular administration. Because many drugs are excreted in human milk, and because of the potential for serious adverse reactions in nursing infants from norfloxacin, a decision should be made to discontinue nursing or to discontinue the drug, taking into account the importance of the drug to the mother (see ANIMAL PHARMACOLOGY).

Pediatric Use
Safety and effectiveness in infants below the age of one year have not been established.
Although quinolones including norfloxacin have been shown to cause arthropathy in immature animals after oral administration, topical ocular administration of other quinolones to immature animals has not shown any arthropathy and there is no evidence that the ophthalmic dosage form of those quinolones has any effects on the weight-bearing joints.

---

* All factors are based on a standard patient weight of 50 kg. The usual oral dose of norfloxacin is 800 mg daily. One drop of CHIBROXIN Ophthalmic Solution 0.3% contains about 1/6,666 of this dose (0.12 mg).

ADVERSE REACTIONS

In clinical trials, the most frequently reported drug-related adverse reaction was local burning or discomfort. Other drug-related adverse reactions were conjunctival hyperemia, chemosis, photophobia and a bitter taste following instillation.

DOSAGE AND ADMINISTRATION

The recommended dose in adults and pediatric patients (one year and older) is one or two drops of CHIBROXIN Ophthalmic Solution applied topically to the affected eye(s) four times daily for up to seven days. Depending on the severity of the infection, the dosage for the first day of therapy may be one or two drops every two hours during the waking hours.

HOW SUPPLIED

CHIBROXIN Ophthalmic Solution is a clear, colorless to light yellow solution.

No. 3526—CHIBROXIN Ophthalmic Solution 0.3% is supplied in a white, opaque, plastic OCUMETER* ophthalmic dispenser with a controlled drop tip as follows:
NDC 0006-3526-03, 5 mL.
Storage
Store CHIBROXIN Ophthalmic Solution at room temperature, 15°–30°C (59°–86°F). Protect from light.

---

*Registered trademark of MERCK & CO., INC.

ANIMAL PHARMACOLOGY

The oral administration of single doses of norfloxacin, six times the recommended human oral dose**, caused lameness in immature dogs. Histologic examination of the weight-bearing joints of these dogs revealed permanent lesions of the cartilage. Related drugs also produced erosions of the cartilage in weight-bearing joints and other signs of arthropathy in immature animals of various species.

**All factors are based on a standard patient weight of 50 kg. The usual oral dose of norfloxacin is 800 mg daily. One drop of CHIBROXIN Ophthalmic Solution 0.3% contains about 1/6,666 of this dose (0.12 mg).

ADDITIONAL CAUTIONARY INFORMATION

Norfloxacin is available as an oral dosage form in addition to the ophthalmic dosage form. The following adverse effects, while they have not been reported with the ophthalmic dosage form, have been reported with the oral dosage form. However, it should be noted that the usual dosage of oral norfloxacin (800 mg/day) contains 6,666 times the amount in one drop of CHIBROXIN Ophthalmic Solution 0.3% (0.12 mg).
Convulsions have been reported in patients receiving oral norfloxacin. Convulsions, increased intracranial pressure, and toxic psychoses have been reported with other drugs in this class. Orally administered quinolones may also cause central nervous system (CNS) stimulation which may lead to tremors, restlessness, lightheadedness, confusion and hallucinations. If these reactions occur in patients receiving norfloxacin, the drug should be discontinued and appropriate measures instituted.
The effects of norfloxacin on brain function or on the electrical activity of the brain have not been tested. Therefore, as with all quinolones, norfloxacin should be used with caution in patients with known or suspected CNS disorders, such as severe cerebral arteriosclerosis, epilepsy, and other factors which predispose to seizures.
The following adverse effects have been reported with Tablets NOROXIN* (Norfloxacin). *Hypersensitivity Reactions:* Hypersensitivity reactions including anaphylactoid reactions, angioedema, dyspnea, urticaria, arthritis, arthralgia, myalgia; *Gastrointestinal:* Pseudomembranous colitis, hepatitis, pancreatitis; *Hematologic:* Neutropenia, leukopenia, thrombocytopenia; *Nervous System/Psychiatric:* CNS effects characterized as generalized seizures and myoclonus; psychic disturbances including psychotic reactions and confusion, depression; *Skin:* Toxic epidermal necrolysis, Stevens-Johnson syndrome and erythema multiforme, exfoliative dermatitis, rash, photosensitivity; *Special Senses:* Transient hearing loss.
Abnormal laboratory values observed with oral norfloxacin included elevation of ALT (SGPT) and AST (SGOT), alkaline phosphatase, BUN, serum creatinine, and LDH.
Please consult the package circular for Tablets NOROXIN (Norfloxacin) for additional information concerning these and other adverse effects and other cautionary information.

---

*Registered trademark of MERCK & CO., INC.
        A.H.F.S. Category: 52:04
        DC 7679101 Issued June 1991
COPYRIGHT © MERCK & CO., INC., 1991
All rights reserved

CLINORIL® Tablets   ℞
(Sulindac), U.S.P.

DESCRIPTION

Sulindac is a non-steroidal, anti-inflammatory indene derivative designated chemically as (Z)- 5-fluoro-2-methyl - 1 - [[*p*-(methylsulfinyl) phenyl]methylene]-1*H*-indene-3-acetic acid. It is not a salicylate, pyrazolone or propionic acid derivative. Its empirical formula is $C_{20}H_{17}FO_3S$, with a molecular

Continued on next page

Merck & Co.—Cont.

weight of 356.42. Sulindac, a yellow crystalline compound, is a weak organic acid practically insoluble in water below pH 4.5, but very soluble as the sodium salt or in buffers of pH 6 or higher.
CLINORIL* (Sulindac) is available in 150 and 200 mg tablets for oral administration. Each tablet contains the following inactive ingredients: cellulose, magnesium stearate, starch.
Following absorption, sulindac undergoes two major biotransformations—reversible reduction to the sulfide metabolite, and irreversible oxidation to the sulfone metabolite. Available evidence indicates that the biological activity resides with the sulfide metabolite.
The structural formulas of sulindac and its metabolites are:

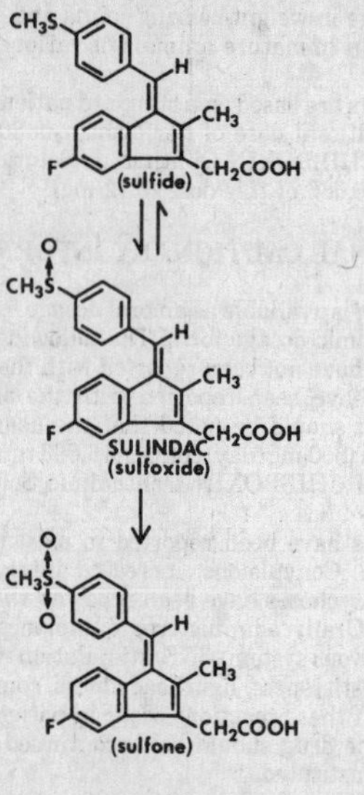

CH_3S
H
CH_3
F
CH_2COOH
(sulfide)
O
CH_3S
H
CH_3
F
CH_2COOH
SULINDAC
(sulfoxide)
O
CH_3S
O
H
CH_3
F
CH_2COOH
(sulfone)

*Registered trademark of MERCK & CO., INC.

CLINICAL PHARMACOLOGY

CLINORIL is a non-steroidal anti-inflammatory drug, also possessing analgesic and antipyretic activities. Its mode of action, like that of other non-steroidal, anti-inflammatory agents, is not known; however, its therapeutic action is not due to pituitary-adrenal stimulation. Inhibition of prostaglandin synthesis by the sulfide metabolite may be involved in the anti-inflammatory action of CLINORIL.
Sulindac is approximately 90% absorbed in man after oral administration. The peak plasma concentrations of the biologically active sulfide metabolite are achieved in about two hours when sulindac is administered in the fasting state, and in about three to four hours when sulindac is administered with food. The mean half-life of sulindac is 7.8 hours while the mean half-life of the sulfide metabolite is 16.4 hours. Sustained plasma levels of the sulfide metabolite are consistent with a prolonged anti-inflammatory action which is the rationale for a twice per day dosage schedule.
Sulindac and its sulfone metabolite undergo extensive enterohepatic circulation relative to the sulfide metabolite in animals. Studies in man have also demonstrated that recirculation of the parent drug, sulindac, and its sulfone metabolite, is more extensive than that of the active sulfide metabolite. The active sulfide metabolite accounts for less than six percent of the total intestinal exposure to sulindac and its metabolites.
The primary route of excretion in man is via the urine as both sulindac and its sulfone metabolite (free and glucuronide conjugates). Approximately 50% of the administered dose is excreted in the urine, with the conjugated sulfone metabolite accounting for the major portion. Less than 1% of the administered dose of sulindac appears in the urine as the sulfide metabolite. Approximately 25% is found in the feces, primarily as the sulfone and sulfide metabolites.
The bioavailability of sulindac, as assessed by urinary excretion, was not changed by concomitant administration of an antacid containing magnesium hydroxide 200 mg and aluminum hydroxide 225 mg per 5 mL.
Because CLINORIL is excreted in the urine primarily as biologically inactive forms, it may possibly affect renal function to a lesser extent than other non-steroidal anti-inflammatory drugs, however, renal adverse experiences have been reported with CLINORIL (see ADVERSE REACTIONS). In a study of patients with chronic glomerular disease treated with therapeutic doses of CLINORIL, no effect was demonstrated on renal blood flow, glomerular filtration rate, or urinary excretion of prostaglandin E_2 and the primary metabolite of prostacyclin, 6-keto-PGF$_{1\alpha}$. However, in other studies in healthy volunteers and patients with liver disease, CLINORIL was found to blunt the renal responses to intravenous furosemide, i.e., the diuresis, natriuresis, increments in plasma renin activity and urinary excretion of prostaglandins. These observations may represent a differentiation of the effects of CLINORIL on renal functions based on differences in pathogenesis of the renal prostaglandin dependence associated with differing dose-response relationships of different NSAIDs to the various renal functions influenced by prostaglandins. These observations need further clarification and in the interim, sulindac should be used with caution in patients whose renal function may be impaired (see PRECAUTIONS).
In healthy men, the average fecal blood loss, measured over a two-week period during administration of 400 mg per day of CLINORIL, was similar to that for placebo, and was statistically significantly less than that resulting from 4800 mg per day of aspirin.
In controlled clinical studies CLINORIL was evaluated in the following five conditions:
1. *Osteoarthritis*
In patients with osteoarthritis of the hip and knee, the anti-inflammatory and analgesic activity of CLINORIL was demonstrated by clinical measurements that included: assessments by both patient and investigator of overall response; decrease in disease activity as assessed by both patient and investigator; improvement in ARA Functional Class; relief of night pain; improvement in overall evaluation of pain, including pain on weight bearing and pain on active and passive motion; improvement in joint mobility, range of motion, and functional activities; decreased swelling and tenderness; and decreased duration of stiffness following prolonged inactivity.
In clinical studies in which dosages were adjusted according to patient needs, CLINORIL 200 to 400 mg daily was shown to be comparable in effectiveness to aspirin 2400 to 4800 mg daily. CLINORIL was generally well tolerated, and patients on it had a lower overall incidence of total adverse effects, of milder gastrointestinal reactions, and of tinnitus than did patients on aspirin. (See ADVERSE REACTIONS.)
2. *Rheumatoid Arthritis*
In patients with rheumatoid arthritis, the anti-inflammatory and analgesic activity of CLINORIL was demonstrated by clinical measurements that included: assessments by both patient and investigator of overall response; decrease in disease activity as assessed by both patient and investigator; reduction in overall joint pain; reduction in duration and severity of morning stiffness; reduction in day and night pain; decrease in time required to walk 50 feet; decrease in general pain as measured on a visual analog scale; improvement in the Ritchie articular index; decrease in proximal interphalangeal joint size; improvement in ARA Functional Class; increase in grip strength; reduction in painful joint count and score; reduction in swollen joint count and score; and increased flexion and extension of the wrist.
In clinical studies in which dosages were adjusted according to patient needs, CLINORIL 300 to 400 mg daily was shown to be comparable in effectiveness to aspirin 3600 to 4800 mg daily. CLINORIL was generally well tolerated, and patients on it had a lower overall incidence of total adverse effects, of milder gastrointestinal reactions, and of tinnitus than did patients on aspirin. (See ADVERSE REACTIONS.)
In patients with rheumatoid arthritis, CLINORIL may be used in combination with gold salts at usual dosage levels. In clinical studies, CLINORIL added to the regimen of gold salts usually resulted in additional symptomatic relief but did not alter the course of the underlying disease.
3. *Ankylosing spondylitis*
In patients with ankylosing spondylitis, the anti-inflammatory and analgesic activity of CLINORIL was demonstrated by clinical measurements that included: assessments by both patient and investigator of overall response; decrease in disease activity as assessed by both patient and investigator; improvement in ARA Functional Class; improvement in patient and investigator evaluation of spinal pain, tenderness and/or spasm; reduction in the duration of morning stiffness; increase in the time to onset of fatigue; relief of night pain; increase in chest expansion; and increase in spinal mobility evaluated by fingers-to-floor distance, occiput to wall distance, the Schober Test, and the Wright Modification of the Schober Test. In a clinical study in which dosages were adjusted according to patient need, CLINORIL 200 to 400 mg daily was as effective as indomethacin 75 to 150 mg daily. In a second study, CLINORIL 300 to 400 mg daily was comparable in effectiveness to phenylbutazone 400 to 600 mg daily. CLINORIL was better tolerated than phenylbutazone. (See ADVERSE REACTIONS.)
4. *Acute painful shoulder (Acute subacromial bursitis/supraspinatus tendinitis)*
In patients with acute painful shoulder (acute subacromial bursitis/supraspinatus tendinitis), the anti-inflammatory and analgesic activity of CLINORIL was demonstrated by clinical measurements that included: assessments by both patient and investigator of overall response; relief of night pain, spontaneous pain, and pain on active motion; decrease in local tenderness; and improvement in range of motion measured by abduction, and internal and external rotation. In clinical studies in acute painful shoulder, CLINORIL 300 to 400 mg daily and oxyphenbutazone 400 to 600 mg daily were shown to be equally effective and well tolerated.
5. *Acute gouty arthritis*
In patients with acute gouty arthritis, the anti-inflammatory and analgesic activity of CLINORIL was demonstrated by clinical measurements that included: assessments by both the patient and investigator of overall response; relief of weight-bearing pain; relief of pain at rest and on active and passive motion; decrease in tenderness; reduction in warmth and swelling; increase in range of motion; and improvement in ability to function. In clinical studies, CLINORIL at 400 mg daily and phenylbutazone at 600 mg daily were shown to be equally effective. In these short-term studies in which reduction of dosage was permitted according to response, both drugs were equally well tolerated.

INDICATIONS AND USAGE

CLINORIL is indicated for acute or long-term use in the relief of signs and symptoms of the following:
1. Osteoarthritis
2. Rheumatoid arthritis*
3. Ankylosing spondylitis
4. Acute painful shoulder (Acute subacromial bursitis/supraspinatus tendinitis)
5. Acute gouty arthritis

*The safety and effectiveness of CLINORIL have not been established in rheumatoid arthritis patients who are designated in the American Rheumatism Association classification as Functional Class IV (incapacitated, largely or wholly bedridden, or confined to wheelchair; little or no self-care).

CONTRAINDICATIONS

CLINORIL should not be used in:
Patients who are hypersensitive to this product.
Patients in whom acute asthmatic attacks, urticaria, or rhinitis are precipitated by aspirin or other non-steroidal anti-inflammatory agents.

WARNINGS

Gastrointestinal Effects
Peptic ulceration and gastrointestinal bleeding have been reported in patients receiving CLINORIL. Fatalities have occurred. Gastrointestinal bleeding is associated with higher morbidity and mortality in patients acutely ill with other conditions, the elderly and patients with hemorrhagic disorders. In patients with active gastrointestinal bleeding or an active peptic ulcer, an appropriate ulcer regimen should be instituted, and the physician must weigh the benefits of therapy with CLINORIL against possible hazards, and carefully monitor the patient's progress. When CLINORIL is given to patients with a history of either upper or lower gastrointestinal tract disease, it should be given under close supervision and only after consulting the ADVERSE REACTIONS section.
Risk of GI Ulcerations, Bleeding and Perforation with NSAID Therapy
Serious gastrointestinal toxicity such as bleeding, ulceration, and perforation, can occur at any time, with or without warning symptoms, in patients treated chronically with NSAID therapy. Although minor upper gastrointestinal problems, such as dyspepsia, are common, usually developing early in therapy, physicians should remain alert for ulceration and bleeding in patients treated chronically with NSAIDs even in the absence of previous GI tract symptoms. In patients observed in clinical trials of several months to two years duration, symptomatic upper GI ulcers, gross bleeding or perforation appear to occur in approximately 1% of patients treated for 3-6 months, and in about 2-4% of patients treated for one year. Physicians should inform patients about the signs and/or symptoms of serious GI toxicity and what steps to take if they occur.
Studies to date have not identified any subset of patients not at risk of developing peptic ulceration and bleeding. Except for a prior history of serious GI events and other risk factors known to be associated with peptic ulcer disease, such as alcoholism, smoking, etc., no risk factors (e.g., age, sex) have been associated with increased risk. Elderly or debilitated patients seem to tolerate ulceration or bleeding less well than other individuals and most spontaneous reports of fatal GI events are in this population. Studies to date are inconclusive concerning the relative risk of various NSAIDs in causing such reactions. High doses of any NSAID probably carry a greater risk of these reactions, although controlled clinical trials showing this do not exist in most cases. In considering the use of relatively large doses (within the recommended dosage range), sufficient benefit should be anticipated to offset the potential increased risk of GI toxicity.

Hypersensitivity
Rarely, fever and other evidence of hypersensitivity (see ADVERSE REACTIONS) including abnormalities in one or more liver function tests and severe skin reactions have occurred during therapy with CLINORIL. Fatalities have occurred in these patients. Hepatitis, jaundice, or both, with or without fever, may occur usually within the first one to three months of therapy. Determinations of liver function should be considered whenever a patient on therapy with CLINORIL develops unexplained fever, rash or other dermatologic reactions or constitutional symptoms. If unexplained fever or other evidence of hypersensitivity occurs, therapy with CLINORIL should be discontinued. The elevated temperature and abnormalities in liver function caused by CLINORIL characteristically have reverted to normal after discontinuation of therapy. Administration of CLINORIL should not be reinstituted in such patients.

Hepatic Effects
In addition to hypersensitivity reactions involving the liver, in some patients the findings are consistent with those of cholestatic hepatitis. As with other non-steroidal anti-inflammatory drugs, borderline elevations of one or more liver tests without any other signs and symptoms may occur in up to 15% of patients. These abnormalities may progress, may remain essentially unchanged, or may be transient with continued therapy. The SGPT (ALT) test is probably the most sensitive indicator of liver dysfunction. Meaningful (3 times the upper limit of normal) elevations of SGPT or SGOT (AST) occurred in controlled clinical trials in less than 1% of patients. A patient with symptoms and/or signs suggesting liver dysfunction, or in whom an abnormal liver test has occurred, should be evaluated for evidence of the development of more severe hepatic reaction while on therapy with CLINORIL. Although such reactions as described above are rare, if abnormal liver tests persist or worsen, if clinical signs and symptoms consistent with liver disease develop, or if systemic manifestations occur (e.g. eosinophilia, rash, etc.), CLINORIL should be discontinued.
In clinical trials with CLINORIL, the use of doses of 600 mg/day has been associated with an increased incidence of mild liver test abnormalities (see DOSAGE AND ADMINISTRATION for maximum dosage recommendation).

PRECAUTIONS

General
Although CLINORIL has less effect on platelet function and bleeding time than aspirin, it is an inhibitor of platelet function; therefore, patients who may be adversely affected should be carefully observed when CLINORIL is administered.
Pancreatitis has been reported in patients receiving CLINORIL (see ADVERSE REACTIONS). Should pancreatitis be suspected, the drug should be discontinued and not restarted, supportive medical therapy instituted, and the patient monitored closely with appropriate laboratory studies (e.g., serum and urine amylase, amylase/creatinine clearance ratio, electrolytes, serum calcium, glucose, lipase, etc.). A search for other causes of pancreatitis as well as those conditions which mimic pancreatitis should be conducted.
Because of reports of adverse eye findings with non-steroidal anti-inflammatory agents, it is recommended that patients who develop eye complaints during treatment with CLINORIL have ophthalmologic studies.
In patients with poor liver function, delayed, elevated and prolonged circulating levels of the sulfide and sulfone metabolites may occur. Such patients should be monitored closely; a reduction of daily dosage may be required.
Edema has been observed in some patients taking CLINORIL. Therefore, as with other non-steroidal anti-inflammatory drugs, CLINORIL should be used with caution in patients with compromised cardiac function, hypertension, or other conditions predisposing to fluid retention.
CLINORIL may allow a reduction in dosage or the elimination of chronic corticosteroid therapy in some patients with rheumatoid arthritis. However, it is generally necessary to reduce corticosteroids gradually over several months in order to avoid an exacerbation of disease or signs and symptoms of adrenal insufficiency. Abrupt withdrawal of chronic corticosteroid treatment is generally not recommended even when patients have had a serious complication of chronic corticosteroid therapy.

Renal Effects
As with other non-steroidal anti-inflammatory drugs, long term administration of sulindac to animals has resulted in renal papillary necrosis and other abnormal renal pathology. In humans, there have been reports of acute interstitial nephritis with hematuria, proteinuria, and occasionally nephrotic syndrome.
A second form of renal toxicity has been seen in patients with prerenal and renal conditions leading to a reduction in renal blood flow or blood volume, where the renal prostaglandins have a supportive role in the maintenance of renal perfusion. In these patients administration of an NSAID may cause a dose dependent reduction in prostaglandin formation and may precipitate overt renal decompensation. CLINORIL may affect renal function less than other NSAIDs in patients with chronic glomerular renal disease (see CLINICAL PHARMACOLOGY). Until these observations are better understood and clarified, however, and because renal adverse experiences have been reported with CLINORIL (see ADVERSE REACTIONS), caution should be exercised when administering the drug to patients with conditions associated with increased risk of the effects of non-steroidal anti-inflammatory drugs on renal function, such as those with renal or hepatic dysfunction, diabetes mellitus, advanced age, extracellular volume depletion from any cause, congestive heart failure, septicemia, pyelonephritis, or concomitant use of any nephrotoxic drug. Discontinuation of NSAID therapy is typically followed by recovery to the pretreatment state.
Since CLINORIL is eliminated primarily by the kidneys, patients with significantly impaired renal function should be closely monitored; a lower daily dosage should be anticipated to avoid excessive drug accumulation.
Sulindac metabolites have been reported rarely as the major or a minor component in renal stones in association with other calculus components. CLINORIL should be used with caution in patients with a history of renal lithiasis, and they should be kept well hydrated while receiving CLINORIL.

Information for Patients
CLINORIL, like other drugs of its class, is not free of side effects. The side effects of these drugs can cause discomfort and, rarely, there are more serious side effects such as gastrointestinal bleeding, which may result in hospitalization and even fatal outcomes.
NSAIDs (Non-steroidal Anti-inflammatory Drugs) are often essential agents in the management of arthritis, but they also may be commonly employed for conditions which are less serious.
Physicians may wish to discuss with their patients the potential risks (see WARNINGS, PRECAUTIONS and ADVERSE REACTIONS) and likely benefits of NSAID treatment, particularly when the drugs are used for less serious conditions where treatment without NSAIDs may represent an acceptable alternative to both the patient and physician.

Laboratory Tests
Because serious GI tract ulceration and bleeding can occur without warning symptoms, physicians should follow chronically treated patients for the signs and symptoms of ulceration and bleeding and should inform them of the importance of this follow-up (see WARNINGS, *Risk of GI Ulcerations, Bleeding and Perforation with NSAID Therapy).*

Use in Pregnancy
CLINORIL is not recommended for use in pregnant women, since safety for use has not been established, and because of the known effect of drugs of this class on the human fetus (closure of the ductus arteriosus, platelet dysfunction with resultant bleeding, renal dysfunction or failure with oligohydramnios, gastrointestinal bleeding or perforation, and myocardial degenerative changes) during the third trimester of pregnancy. In reproduction studies in the rat, a decrease in average fetal weight and an increase in numbers of dead pups were observed on the first day of the postpartum period at dosage levels of 20 and 40 mg/kg/day (2½ and 5 times the usual maximum daily dose in humans), although there was no adverse effect on the survival and growth during the remainder of the postpartum period. CLINORIL prolongs the duration of gestation in rats, as do other compounds of this class which also may cause dystocia and delayed parturition in pregnant animals. Visceral and skeletal malformations observed in low incidence among rabbits in some teratology studies did not occur at the same dosage levels in repeat studies, nor at a higher dosage level in the same species.

Nursing Mothers
Nursing should not be undertaken while a patient is on CLINORIL. It is not known whether sulindac is secreted in human milk; however, it is secreted in the milk of lactating rats.

Use in Children
Safety and effectiveness in children have not been established.

Drug Interactions
DMSO should not be used with sulindac. Concomitant administration has been reported to reduce the plasma levels of the active sulfide metabolite and potentially reduce efficacy. In addition, this combination has been reported to cause peripheral neuropathy.
Although sulindac and its sulfide metabolite are highly bound to protein, studies, in which CLINORIL was given at a dose of 400 mg daily, have shown no clinically significant interaction with oral anticoagulants or oral hypoglycemic agents. However, patients should be monitored carefully until it is certain that no change in their anticoagulant or hypoglycemic dosage is required. Special attention should be paid to patients taking higher doses than those recommended and to patients with renal impairment or other metabolic defects that might increase sulindac blood levels.
The concomitant administration of aspirin with sulindac significantly depressed the plasma levels of the active sulfide metabolite. A double-blind study compared the safety and efficacy of CLINORIL 300 or 400 mg daily given alone or with aspirin 2.4 g/day for the treatment of osteoarthritis. The addition of aspirin did not alter the types of clinical or laboratory adverse experiences for CLINORIL; however, the combination showed an increase in the incidence of gastrointestinal adverse experiences. Since the addition of aspirin did not have a favorable effect on the therapeutic response to CLINORIL, the combination is not recommended.
Caution should be used if CLINORIL is administered concomitantly with methotrexate. Nonsteroidal anti-inflammatory drugs have been reported to decrease the tubular secretion of methotrexate and to potentiate its toxicity.
Administration of non-steroidal anti-inflammatory drugs concomitantly with cyclosporine has been associated with an increase in cyclosporine-induced toxicity, possibly due to decreased synthesis of renal prostacyclin. NSAIDs should be used with caution in patients taking cyclosporine, and renal function should be carefully monitored.
The concomitant administration of CLINORIL and diflunisal in normal volunteers resulted in lowering of the plasma levels of the active sulindac sulfide metabolite by approximately one-third.
Probenecid given concomitantly with sulindac had only a slight effect on plasma sulfide levels, while plasma levels of sulindac and sulfone were increased. Sulindac was shown to produce a modest reduction in the uricosuric action of probenecid, which probably is not significant under most circumstances.
Neither propoxyphene hydrochloride nor acetaminophen had any effect on the plasma levels of sulindac or its sulfide metabolite.

ADVERSE REACTIONS

The following adverse reactions were reported in clinical trials or have been reported since the drug was marketed. The probability exists of a causal relationship between CLINORIL and these adverse reactions. The adverse reactions which have been observed in clinical trials encompass observations in 1,865 patients, including 232 observed for at least 48 weeks.

Incidence Greater Than 1%

Gastrointestinal
The most frequent types of adverse reactions occurring with CLINORIL are gastrointestinal; these include gastrointestinal pain (10%), dyspepsia*, nausea* with or without vomiting, diarrhea*, constipation*, flatulence, anorexia and gastrointestinal cramps.

Dermatologic
Rash*, pruritus.

Central Nervous System
Dizziness*, headache*, nervousness.

Special Senses
Tinnitus.

Miscellaneous
Edema (see PRECAUTIONS).

*Incidence between 3% and 9%. Those reactions occurring in 1 to 3% of patients are not marked with an asterisk.

Incidence Less Than 1 in 100

Gastrointestinal
Gastritis, gastroenteritis or colitis. Peptic ulcer and gastrointestinal bleeding have been reported. GI perforation has been reported rarely.
Liver function abnormalities; jaundice, sometimes with fever; cholestasis; hepatitis; hepatic failure.
Pancreatitis (see PRECAUTIONS).
Ageusia; glossitis.
There have been rare reports of sulindac metabolites in common bile duct "sludge" in patients with symptoms of cholecystitis who underwent a cholecystectomy.

Dermatologic
Stomatitis, sore or dry mucous membranes, alopecia, photosensitivity.
Erythema multiforme, toxic epidermal necrolysis, Stevens-Johnson syndrome, and exfoliative dermatitis have been reported.

Cardiovascular
Congestive heart failure, especially in patients with marginal cardiac function; palpitation; hypertension.

Hematologic
Thrombocytopenia; ecchymosis; purpura; leukopenia; agranulocytosis; neutropenia; bone marrow depression, including aplastic anemia; hemolytic anemia; increased prothrombin time in patients on oral anticoagulants (see PRECAUTIONS).

Continued on next page

Information on the Merck & Co. products listed on these pages is the full prescribing information from product circulars in use October 1, 1992.

Merck & Co.—Cont.

Genitourinary

Urine discoloration; dysuria; vaginal bleeding; hematuria; proteinuria; crystalluria; renal impairment, including renal failure; interstitial nephritis; nephrotic syndrome.

Renal calculi containing sulindac metabolites have been observed rarely.

Metabolic

Hyperkalemia.

Musculoskeletal

Muscle weakness.

Psychiatric

Depression; psychic disturbances including acute psychosis.

Nervous System

Vertigo; insomnia; somnolence; paresthesia; convulsions; syncope; aseptic meningitis.

Special Senses

Blurred vision; visual disturbances; decreased hearing; metallic or bitter taste.

Respiratory

Epistaxis.

Hypersensitivity Reactions

Anaphylaxis; angioneurotic edema; bronchial spasm; dyspnea.

Hypersensitivity vasculitis.

A potentially fatal apparent hypersensitivity syndrome has been reported. This syndrome may include constitutional symptoms (fever, chills, diaphoresis, flushing), cutaneous findings (rash or other dermatologic reactions—see above), conjunctivitis, involvement of major organs (changes in liver function including hepatic failure, jaundice, pancreatitis, pneumonitis with or without pleural effusion, leukopenia, leukocytosis, eosinophilia, disseminated intravascular coagulation, anemia, renal impairment, including renal failure), and other less specific findings (adenitis, arthralgia, arthritis, myalgia, fatigue, malaise, hypotension, chest pain, tachycardia).

Causal Relationship Unknown

Other reactions have been reported in clinical trials or since the drug was marketed, but occurred under circumstances where a causal relationship could not be established. However, in these rarely reported events, that possibility cannot be excluded. Therefore, these observations are listed to serve as alerting information to physicians.

Cardiovascular

Arrhythmia.

Metabolic

Hyperglycemia.

Nervous System

Neuritis.

Special Senses

Disturbances of the retina and its vasculature.

Miscellaneous

Gynecomastia.

MANAGEMENT OF OVERDOSAGE

Cases of overdosage have been reported and rarely, deaths have occurred. The following signs and symptoms may be observed following overdosage: stupor, coma, diminished urine output and hypotension.

In the event of overdosage, the stomach should be emptied by inducing vomiting or by gastric lavage, and the patient carefully observed and given symptomatic and supportive treatment.

Animal studies show that absorption is decreased by the prompt administration of activated charcoal and excretion is enhanced by alkalinization of the urine.

DOSAGE AND ADMINISTRATION

CLINORIL should be administered orally twice a day with food. The maximum dosage is 400 mg per day. Dosages above 400 mg per day are not recommended.

In osteoarthritis, rheumatoid arthritis, and ankylosing spondylitis, the recommended starting dosage is 150 mg twice a day. The dosage may be lowered or raised depending on the response.

A prompt response (within one week) can be expected in about one-half of patients with osteoarthritis, ankylosing spondylitis, and rheumatoid arthritis. Others may require longer to respond.

In acute painful shoulder (acute subacromial bursitis/supraspinatus tendinitis) and acute gouty arthritis, the recommended dosage is 200 mg twice a day. After a satisfactory response has been achieved, the dosage may be reduced according to the response. In acute painful shoulder, therapy for 7–14 days is usually adequate. In acute gouty arthritis, therapy for 7 days is usually adequate.

HOW SUPPLIED

No. 3360—Tablets CLINORIL 150 mg are yellow, hexagon-shaped, compressed tablets, coded MSD 941. They are supplied as follows:

NDC 0006-0941-54 unit of use bottles of 60

NDC 0006-0941-68 in bottles of 100
(6505-01-071-5559 100's)

NDC 0006-0941-78 unit of use bottles of 100

NDC 0006-0941-28 unit dose packages of 100
(6505-01-143-4415, 150 mg individually sealed 100's).

Shown in Product Identification Section, page 419

No. 3353—Tablets CLINORIL 200 mg are yellow, hexagon-shaped, scored, compressed tablets, coded MSD 942. They are supplied as follows:

NDC 0006-0942-54 unit of use bottles of 60

NDC 0006-0942-68 in bottles of 100
(6505-01-072-3426 100's)

NDC 0006-0942-78 unit of use bottles of 100

NDC 0006-0942-28 unit dose packages of 100
(6505-01-143-4416, 200 mg individually sealed 100's)

Shown in Product Identification Section, page 419

A.H.F.S. Category: 28:08.04

DC 7411629   Issued June 1991

COPYRIGHT © MERCK & CO., INC., 1988

All rights reserved

COGENTIN® Tablets
(Benztropine Mesylate), U.S.P.   ℞

COGENTIN® Injection
(Benztropine Mesylate), U.S.P.   ℞

DESCRIPTION

Benztropine mesylate is a synthetic compound containing structural features found in atropine and diphenhydramine. It is designated chemically as 8-azabicyclo[3.2.1] octane, 3-(diphenylmethoxy)-,*endo,* methanesulfonate. Its empirical formula is $C_{21}H_{25}NO \cdot CH_4O_3S$, and its structural formula is:

Benztropine mesylate is a crystalline white powder, very soluble in water, and has a molecular weight of 403.54. COGENTIN* (Benztropine Mesylate) is supplied as tablets in three strengths (0.5 mg, 1 mg, and 2 mg per tablet), and as a sterile injection for intravenous and intramuscular use.

Tablets COGENTIN contain 0.5, 1 or 2 mg of benztropine mesylate. Each tablet contains the following inactive ingredients: calcium phosphate, cellulose, lactose, magnesium stearate and starch.

Each milliliter of the injection contains:

Benztropine mesylate .... 1 mg
Sodium chloride .... 9 mg
Water for Injection q.s. .... 1 mL

*Registered trademark of MERCK & CO., INC.

ACTIONS

COGENTIN possesses both anticholinergic and antihistaminic effects, although only the former have been established as therapeutically significant in the management of parkinsonism.

In the isolated guinea pig ileum, the anticholinergic activity of this drug is about equal to that of atropine; however, when administered orally to unanesthetized cats, it is only about half as active as atropine.

In laboratory animals, its antihistaminic activity and duration of action approach those of pyrilamine maleate.

INDICATIONS

For use as an adjunct in the therapy of all forms of parkinsonism.

Useful also in the control of extrapyramidal disorders (except tardive dyskinesia—see PRECAUTIONS) due to neuroleptic drugs (e.g., phenothiazines).

CONTRAINDICATIONS

Hypersensitivity to COGENTIN tablets or to any component of COGENTIN injection.

Because of its atropine-like side effects, this drug is contraindicated in children under three years of age, and should be used with caution in older children.

WARNINGS

Safe use in pregnancy has not been established.

COGENTIN may impair mental and/or physical abilities required for performance of hazardous tasks, such as operating machinery or driving a motor vehicle.

When COGENTIN is given concomitantly with phenothiazines, haloperidol, or other drugs with anticholinergic or antidopaminergic activity, patients should be advised to report gastrointestinal complaints, fever or heat intolerance promptly. Paralytic ileus, hyperthermia and heat stroke, all of which have sometimes been fatal, have occurred in patients taking anticholinergic-type antiparkinsonism drugs, including COGENTIN, in combination with phenothiazines and/or tricyclic antidepressants.

Since COGENTIN contains structural features of atropine, it may produce anhidrosis. For this reason, it should be administered with caution during hot weather, especially when given concomitantly with other atropine-like drugs to the chronically ill, the alcoholic, those who have central nervous system disease, and those who do manual labor in a hot environment. Anhidrosis may occur more readily when some disturbance of sweating already exists. If there is evidence of anhidrosis, the possibility of hyperthermia should be considered. Dosage should be decreased at the discretion of the physician so that the ability to maintain body heat equilibrium by perspiration is not impaired. Severe anhidrosis and fatal hyperthermia have occurred.

PRECAUTIONS

General

Since COGENTIN has cumulative action, continued supervision is advisable. Patients with a tendency to tachycardia and patients with prostatic hypertrophy should be observed closely during treatment.

Dysuria may occur, but rarely becomes a problem. Urinary retention has been reported with COGENTIN.

The drug may cause complaints of weakness and inability to move particular muscle groups, especially in large doses. For example, if the neck has been rigid and suddenly relaxes, it may feel weak, causing some concern. In this event, dosage adjustment is required.

Mental confusion and excitement may occur with large doses, or in susceptible patients. Visual hallucinations have been reported occasionally. Furthermore, in the treatment of extrapyramidal disorders due to neuroleptic drugs (e.g., phenothiazines), in patients with mental disorders, occasionally there may be intensification of mental symptoms. In such cases, antiparkinsonian drugs can precipitate a toxic psychosis. Patients with mental disorders should be kept under careful observation, especially at the beginning of treatment or if dosage is increased.

Tardive dyskinesia may appear in some patients on long-term therapy with phenothiazines and related agents, or may occur after therapy with these drugs has been discontinued. Antiparkinsonism agents do not alleviate the symptoms of tardive dyskinesia, and in some instances may aggravate them. COGENTIN is not recommended for use in patients with tardive dyskinesia.

The physician should be aware of the possible occurrence of glaucoma. Although the drug does not appear to have any adverse effect on simple glaucoma, it probably should not be used in angle-closure glaucoma.

Drug Interactions

Antipsychotic drugs such as phenothiazines or haloperidol; tricyclic antidepressants (see WARNINGS).

ADVERSE REACTIONS

The adverse reactions below, most of which are anticholinergic in nature, have been reported and within each category are listed in order of decreasing severity.

Cardiovascular

Tachycardia.

Digestive

Paralytic ileus, constipation, vomiting, nausea, dry mouth. If dry mouth is so severe that there is difficulty in swallowing or speaking, or loss of appetite and weight, reduce dosage, or discontinue the drug temporarily.

Slight reduction in dosage may control nausea and still give sufficient relief of symptoms. Vomiting may be controlled by temporary discontinuation, followed by resumption at a lower dosage.

Nervous System

Toxic psychosis, including confusion, disorientation, memory impairment, visual hallucinations; exacerbation of pre-existing psychotic symptoms; nervousness; depression; listlessness; numbness of fingers.

Special Senses

Blurred vision, dilated pupils.

Urogenital

Urinary retention, dysuria.

Metabolic/Immune or Skin
Occasionally, an allergic reaction, e.g., skin rash, develops. If this can not be controlled by dosage reduction, the medication should be discontinued.
Other
Heat stroke, hyperthermia, fever.

DOSAGE AND ADMINISTRATION

COGENTIN tablets should be used when patients are able to take oral medication.
The injection is especially useful for psychotic patients with acute dystonic reactions or other reactions that make oral medication difficult or impossible. It is recommended also when a more rapid response is desired than can be obtained with the tablets.
Since there is no significant difference in onset of effect after intravenous or intramuscular injection, usually there is no need to use the intravenous route. The drug is quickly effective after either route, with improvement sometimes noticeable a few minutes after injection. In emergency situations, when the condition of the patient is alarming, 1 to 2 mL of the injection normally will provide quick relief. If the parkinsonian effect begins to return, the dose can be repeated.
Because of cumulative action, therapy should be initiated with a low dose which is increased gradually at five or six-day intervals to the smallest amount necessary for optimal relief. Increases should be made in increments of 0.5 mg, to a maximum of 6 mg, or until optimal results are obtained without excessive adverse reactions.
Postencephalitic and
Idiopathic Parkinsonism—
The usual daily dose is 1 to 2 mg, with a range of 0.5 to 6 mg orally or parenterally.
As with any agent used in parkinsonism, dosage must be individualized according to age and weight, and the type of parkinsonism being treated. Generally, older patients and thin patients cannot tolerate large doses. Most patients with postencephalitic parkinsonism need fairly large doses and tolerate them well. Patients with a poor mental outlook are usually poor candidates for therapy.
In idiopathic parkinsonism, therapy may be initiated with a single daily dose of 0.5 to 1 mg at bedtime. In some patients, this will be adequate; in others 4 to 6 mg a day may be required.
In postencephalitic parkinsonism, therapy may be initiated in most patients with 2 mg a day in one or more doses. In highly sensitive patients, therapy may be initiated with 0.5 mg at bedtime, and increased as necessary.
Some patients experience greatest relief by taking the entire dose at bedtime; others react more favorably to divided doses, two to four times a day. Frequently, one dose a day is sufficient, and divided doses may be unnecessary or undesirable.
The long duration of action of this drug makes it particularly suitable for bedtime medication when its effects may last throughout the night, enabling patients to turn in bed during the night more easily, and to rise in the morning.
When COGENTIN is started, do not terminate therapy with other antiparkinsonian agents abruptly. If the other agents are to be reduced or discontinued, it must be done gradually. Many patients obtain greatest relief with combination therapy.
COGENTIN may be used concomitantly with SINEMET* (Carbidopa-Levodopa), or with levodopa, in which case periodic dosage adjustment may be required in order to maintain optimum response.
Drug-Induced Extrapyramidal Disorders—In treating extrapyramidal disorders due to neuroleptic drugs (e.g., phenothiazines), the recommended dosage is 1 to 4 mg once or twice a day orally or parenterally. Dosage must be individualized according to the need of the patient. Some patients require more than recommended; others do not need as much.
In acute dystonic reactions, 1 to 2 mL of the injection usually relieves the condition quickly. After that, the tablets, 1 to 2 mg twice a day, usually prevent recurrence.
When extrapyramidal disorders develop soon after initiation of treatment with neuroleptic drugs (e.g., phenothiazines), they are likely to be transient. One to 2 mg of COGENTIN tablets two or three times a day usually provides relief within one or two days. After one or two weeks, the drug should be withdrawn to determine the continued need for it. If such disorders recur, COGENTIN can be reinstituted.
Certain drug-induced extrapyramidal disorders that develop slowly may not respond to COGENTIN.

*Registered trademark of MERCK & CO., INC.

OVERDOSAGE

Manifestations—May be any of those seen in atropine poisoning or antihistamine overdosage: CNS depression, preceded or followed by stimulation; confusion; nervousness; listlessness; intensification of mental symptoms or toxic psychosis in patients with mental illness being treated with neuroleptic drugs (e.g., phenothiazines); hallucinations (especially visual); dizziness; muscle weakness; ataxia; dry mouth; mydriasis; blurred vision; palpitations; tachycardia; elevated blood pressure; nausea; vomiting; dysuria; numbness of fingers; dysphagia; allergic reactions, e.g., skin rash; headache; hot, dry, flushed skin; delirium; coma; shock; convulsions; respiratory arrest; anhidrosis; hyperthermia; glaucoma; constipation.
Treatment—Physostigmine salicylate, 1 to 2 mg, SC or IV, reportedly will reverse symptoms of anticholinergic intoxication.* A second injection may be given after 2 hours if required. Otherwise treatment is symptomatic and supportive. Induce emesis or perform gastric lavage (contraindicated in precomatose, convulsive, or psychotic states). Maintain respiration. A short-acting barbiturate may be used for CNS excitement, but with caution to avoid subsequent depression; supportive care for depression (avoid convulsant stimulants such as picrotoxin, pentylenetetrazol, or bemegride); artificial respiration for severe respiratory depression; a local miotic for mydriasis and cycloplegia; ice bags or other cold applications and alcohol sponges for hyperpyrexia, a vasopressor and fluids for circulatory collapse. Darken room for photophobia.

*Duvoisin, R.C.; Katz, R.J.; Amer. Med. Ass. *206*:1963–1965, Nov. 25, 1968.

HOW SUPPLIED

No. 3297—Tablets COGENTIN, 0.5 mg, are white, round, scored, compressed tablets, coded MSD 21. They are supplied as follows:
NDC 0006-0021-68 in bottles of 100.
Shown in Product Identification Section, page 419
No. 3334—Tablets COGENTIN, 1 mg, are white, oval shaped, scored, compressed tablets, coded MSD 635. They are supplied as follows:
NDC 0006-0635-68 in bottles of 100
NDC 0006-0635-28 unit dose packages of 100.
Shown in Product Identification Section, page 419
No. 3172—Tablets COGENTIN, 2 mg, are white, round, scored, compressed tablets, coded MSD 60. They are supplied as follows:
NDC 0006-0060-68 in bottles of 100
(6505-01-230-8726, 2 mg 100's)
NDC 0006-0060-28 unit dose packages of 100
NDC 0006-0060-82 in bottles of 1000.
Shown in Product Identification Section, page 419
No. 3275—Injection COGENTIN, 1 mg per mL, is a clear, colorless solution and is supplied as follows:
NDC 0006-3275-16 in boxes of 6×2 mL ampuls.
A.H.F.S. Category: 12:08
DC 7398219 Issued November 1991

ColBENEMID® Tablets ℞
(Probenecid-Colchicine), U.S.P.

DESCRIPTION

ColBENEMID* (Probenecid-Colchicine) contains probenecid, which is a uricosuric agent, and colchicine, which has antigout activity, the mechanism of which is unknown.
Probenecid is the generic name for 4-[(dipropylamino) sulfonyl] benzoic acid (molecular weight 285.36). It has the following structural formula:

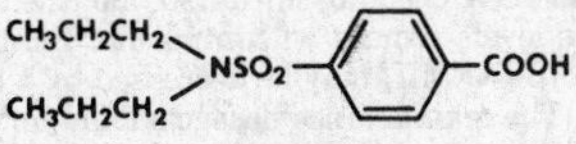
CH3CH2CH2
NSO2
COOH
CH3CH2CH2

Probenecid is a white or nearly white, fine, crystalline powder. It is soluble in dilute alkali, in alcohol, in chloroform, and in acetone; it is practically insoluble in water and in dilute acids.
Colchicine is an alkaloid obtained from various species of Colchicum. The chemical name for colchicine is (*S*)-*N*-(5,6,7,9-tetrahydro-1,2,3,10-tetramethoxy-9-oxobenzo [*a*] heptalen-7-yl) acetamide (molecular weight 399.43). It has the following structural formula:

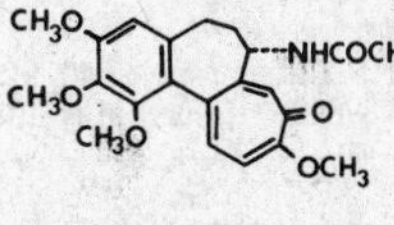
CH3O
CH3O
CH3O
NHCOCH3
O
OCH3

Colchicine consists of pale yellow scales or powder; it darkens on exposure to light. Colchicine is soluble in water, freely soluble in alcohol and in chloroform, and slightly soluble in ether.
Each tablet contains 0.5 g probenecid and 0.5 mg colchicine and the following inactive ingredients: calcium stearate, gelatin, magnesium carbonate, starch.

*Registered trademark of MERCK & CO., INC.

ACTIONS

Probenecid is a uricosuric and renal tubular blocking agent. It inhibits the tubular reabsorption of urate, thus increasing the urinary excretion of uric acid and decreasing serum urate levels. Effective uricosuria reduces the miscible urate pool, retards urate deposition, and promotes resorption of urate deposits.
Probenecid inhibits the tubular secretion of penicillin and usually increases penicillin plasma levels by any route the antibiotic is given. A 2-fold to 4-fold elevation has been demonstrated for various penicillins.
Probenecid also has been reported to inhibit the renal transport of many other compounds including aminohippuric acid (PAH), aminosalicylic acid (PAS), indomethacin, sodium iodomethamate and related iodinated organic acids, 17-ketosteroids, pantothenic acid, phenolsulfonphthalein (PSP), sulfonamides, and sulfonylureas. See also DRUG INTERACTIONS.
Probenecid decreases both hepatic and renal excretion of sulfobromophthalein (BSP). The tubular reabsorption of phosphorus is inhibited in hypoparathyroid but not in euparathyroid individuals.
Probenecid does not influence plasma concentrations of salicylates, nor the excretion of streptomycin, chloramphenicol, chlortetracycline, oxytetracycline, or neomycin.
The mode of action of colchicine in gout is unknown. It is not an analgesic, though it relieves pain in acute attacks of gout. It is not a uricosuric agent and will not prevent progression of gout to chronic gouty arthritis. It does have a prophylactic, suppressive effect that helps to reduce the incidence of acute attacks and to relieve the residual pain and mild discomfort that patients with gout occasionally feel.
In man and certain other animals, colchicine can produce a temporary leukopenia that is followed by leukocytosis.
Colchicine has other pharmacologic actions in animals: It alters neuromuscular function, intensifies gastrointestinal activity by neurogenic stimulation, increases sensitivity to central depressants, heightens response to sympathomimetic compounds, depresses the respiratory center, constricts blood vessels, causes hypertension by central vasomotor stimulation, and lowers body temperature.

INDICATIONS

For the treatment of chronic gouty arthritis when complicated by frequent, recurrent acute attacks of gout.

CONTRAINDICATIONS

Hypersensitivity to this product or to probenecid or colchicine.
Children under 2 years of age.
Not recommended in persons with known blood dyscrasias or uric acid kidney stones.
Therapy with ColBENEMID should not be started until an acute gouty attack has subsided.
Pregnancy: Probenecid crosses the placental barrier and appears in cord blood. Colchicine can arrest cell division in animals and plants. In certain species of animal under certain conditions, colchicine has produced teratogenic effects. The possibility of such effects in humans also has been reported. Because of the colchicine component, ColBENEMID is contraindicated in pregnant patients. The use of any drug in women of childbearing potential requires that the anticipated benefit be weighed against possible hazards.

WARNINGS

Exacerbation of gout following therapy with ColBENEMID may occur; in such cases additional colchicine or other appropriate therapy is advisable.
Probenecid increases plasma concentrations of methotrexate in both animals and humans. In animal studies, increased methotrexate toxicity has been reported. If ColBENEMID is given with methotrexate, the dosage of methotrexate should be reduced and serum levels may need to be monitored.
In patients on ColBENEMID the use of salicylates in either small or large doses is contraindicated because it antagonizes the uricosuric action of probenecid. The biphasic action of salicylates in the renal tubules accounts for the so-called "paradoxical effect" of uricosuric agents. In patients on ColBENEMID who require a mild analgesic agent the use of acetaminophen rather than small doses of salicylates would be preferred.
Rarely, severe allergic reactions and anaphylaxis have been reported with the use of ColBENEMID. Most of these have been reported to occur within several hours after readministration following prior usage of the drug.

Continued on next page

Information on the Merck & Co. products listed on these pages is the full prescribing information from product circulars in use October 1, 1992.

Merck & Co.—Cont.

The appearance of hypersensitivity reactions requires cessation of therapy with ColBENEMID.

Colchicine has been reported to adversely affect spermatogenesis in animals. Reversible azoospermia has been reported in one patient.

PRECAUTIONS

General

Hematuria, renal colic, costovertebral pain, and formation of uric acid stones associated with the use of ColBENEMID in gouty patients may be prevented by alkalization of the urine and a liberal fluid intake (*see* DOSAGE AND ADMINISTRATION). In these cases when alkali is administered, the acid-base balance of the patient should be watched.

Use with caution in patients with a history of peptic ulcer. ColBENEMID has been used in patients with some renal impairment but dosage requirements may be increased. ColBENEMID may not be effective in chronic renal insufficiency particularly when the glomerular filtration rate is 30 mL/minute or less.

A reducing substance may appear in the urine of patients receiving probenecid. This disappears with discontinuance of therapy. Suspected glycosuria should be confirmed by using a test specific for glucose.

Adequate animal studies have not been conducted to determine the carcinogenicity potential of probenecid or this drug combination. Since colchicine is an established mutagen, its ability to act as a carcinogen must be suspected and administration of ColBENEMID should involve a weighing of the benefit-vs-risk when long-term administration is contemplated.

Drug Interactions

When probenecid is used to elevate plasma concentrations of penicillin, or other beta-lactams, or when such drugs are given to patients taking probenecid therapeutically, high plasma concentrations of the other drug may increase the incidence of adverse reactions associated with that drug. In the case of penicillin, or other beta-lactams, psychic disturbances have been reported.

The use of salicylates antagonizes the uricosuric action of probenecid (*see* WARNINGS). The uricosuric action of probenecid is also antagonized by pyrazinamide.

Probenecid produces an insignificant increase in free sulfonamide plasma concentrations but a significant increase in total sulfonamide plasma levels. Since probenecid decreases the renal excretion of conjugated sulfonamides, plasma concentrations of the latter should be determined from time to time when a sulfonamide and ColBENEMID are coadministered for prolonged periods. Probenecid may prolong or enhance the action of oral sulfonylureas and thereby increase the risk of hypoglycemia.

It has been reported that patients receiving probenecid require significantly less thiopental for induction of anesthesia. In addition, ketamine and thiopental anesthesia were significantly prolonged in rats receiving probenecid.

The concomitant administration of probenecid increases the mean plasma elimination half-life of a number of drugs which can lead to increased plasma concentrations. These include agents such as indomethacin, acetaminophen, naproxen, ketoprofen, meclofenamate, lorazepam, and rifampin. Although the clinical significance of this observation has not been established, a lower dosage of the drug may be required to produce a therapeutic effect, and increases in dosage of the drug in question should be made cautiously and in small increments when probenecid is being co-administrated. Although specific instances of toxicity due to this potential interaction have not been observed to date, physicians should be alert to this possibility.

Probenecid given concomitantly with sulindac had only a slight effect on plasma sulfide levels, while plasma levels of sulindac and sulfone were increased. Sulindac was shown to produce a modest reduction in the uricosuric action of probenecid, which probably is not significant under most circumstances.

In animals and in humans, probenecid has been reported to increase plasma concentrations of methotrexate (*see* WARNINGS).

Falsely high readings for theophylline have been reported in an *in vitro* study, using the Schack and Waxler technic, when therapeutic concentrations of theophylline and probenecid were added to human plasma.

ADVERSE REACTIONS

The following adverse reactions have been observed and within each category are listed in order of decreasing severity.

Probenecid

Central Nervous System: headache, dizziness.

Metabolic: precipitation of acute gouty arthritis.

Gastrointestinal: hepatic necrosis, vomiting, nausea, anorexia, sore gums.

Genitourinary: nephrotic syndrome, uric acid stones with or without hematuria, renal colic, costovertebral pain, urinary frequency.

Hypersensitivity: anaphylaxis, fever, urticaria, pruritus.

Hematologic: aplastic anemia, leukopenia, hemolytic anemia which in some patients could be related to genetic deficiency of glucose -6- phosphate dehydrogenase in red blood cells, anemia.

Integumentary: dermatitis, alopecia, flushing.

Colchicine

Side effects due to colchicine appear to be a function of dosage. The possibility of increased colchicine toxicity in the presence of hepatic dysfunction should be considered. The appearance of any of the following symptoms may require reduction of dosage or discontinuance of the drug.

Central Nervous System: peripheral neuritis.

Musculoskeletal: muscular weakness.

Gastrointestinal: nausea, vomiting, abdominal pain, or diarrhea may be particularly troublesome in the presence of peptic ulcer or spastic colon.

Hypersensitivity: urticaria.

Hematologic: aplastic anemia, agranulocytosis.

Integumentary: dermatitis, purpura, alopecia.

At toxic doses, colchicine may cause severe diarrhea, generalized vascular damage, and renal damage with hematuria and oliguria.

DOSAGE AND ADMINISTRATION

Therapy with ColBENEMID should not be *started* until an acute gouty attack has subsided. However, if an acute attack is precipitated *during* therapy, ColBENEMID may be continued without changing the dosage, and additional colchicine or other appropriate therapy should be given to control the acute attack.

The recommended adult dosage is 1 tablet of ColBENEMID daily for one week, followed by 1 tablet twice a day thereafter.

Some degree of renal impairment may be present in patients with gout. A daily dosage of 2 tablets may be adequate. However, if necessary, the daily dosage may be increased by 1 tablet every four weeks within tolerance (and usually not above 4 tablets per day) if symptoms of gouty arthritis are not controlled or the 24 hour uric acid excretion is not above 700 mg. As noted, probenecid may not be effective in chronic renal insufficiency particularly when the glomerular filtration rate is 30 mL/minute or less.

Gastric intolerance may be indicative of overdosage, and may be corrected by decreasing the dosage.

As uric acid tends to crystallize out of an acid urine, a liberal fluid intake is recommended, as well as sufficient sodium bicarbonate (3 to 7.5 g daily) or potassium citrate (7.5 g daily) to maintain an alkaline urine (*see* PRECAUTIONS).

Alkalization of the urine is recommended until the serum urate level returns to normal limits and tophaceous deposits disappear, i.e., during the period when urinary excretion of uric acid is at a high level. Thereafter, alkalization of the urine and the usual restriction of purine-producing foods may be somewhat relaxed.

ColBENEMID (or probenecid) should be continued at the dosage that will maintain normal serum urate levels. When acute attacks have been absent for six months or more and serum urate levels remain within normal limits, the daily dosage of ColBENEMID may be decreased by 1 tablet every six months. The maintenance dosage should not be reduced to the point where serum urate levels tend to rise.

HOW SUPPLIED

No. 3283—Tablets ColBENEMID are white to off-white, capsule-shaped, scored tablets, coded MSD 614. Each tablet contains 0.5 g of probenecid and 0.5 mg of colchicine. They are supplied as follows:

NDC 0006-0614-68 bottles of 100.

Shown in Product Identification Section, page 419

Storage

Protect from light.

        A.H.F.S. Categories: 40:40, 92:00

        DC 7398926 Issued May 1989

CORTONE® Acetate Sterile Suspension   ℞
(Cortisone Acetate), U.S.P.

For intramuscular injection only
NOT FOR INTRAVENOUS USE

DESCRIPTION

Cortisone acetate, a synthetic adrenocortical steroid, is a white or practically white, odorless, crystalline powder. It is

stable in air. It is insoluble in water. The molecular weight is 402.49. It is designated chemically as 21-(acetyloxy)-17-hydroxypregn-4-ene-3,11,20-trione. The empirical formula is $C_{23}H_{30}O_6$ and the structural formula is:

CORTONE* Acetate (Cortisone Acetate) sterile suspension is a sterile suspension containing 50 mg per milliliter of cortisone acetate in an aqueous medium (pH 5.0 to 7.0). Inactive ingredients per mL: sodium chloride, 9 mg; polysorbate 80, 4 mg; sodium carboxymethylcellulose, 5 mg; Water for Injection q.s. 1 mL. Benzyl alcohol, 9 mg, added as preservative. No attempt should be made to alter CORTONE Acetate sterile suspension. Diluting it or mixing it with other substances may affect the state of suspension or change the rate of absorption and reduce its effectiveness.

---

*Registered trademark of MERCK & CO., INC.

ACTIONS

CORTONE Acetate sterile suspension has a slow onset but long duration of action when compared with more soluble preparations. When daily corticosteroid therapy is required and oral therapy is not feasible, the required daily dosage may be given in a single intramuscular injection of this preparation.

Naturally occurring glucocorticoids (hydrocortisone and cortisone), which also have salt-retaining properties, are used as replacement therapy in adrenocortical deficiency states. They are also used for their potent anti-inflammatory effects in disorders of many organ systems.

Glucocorticoids cause profound and varied metabolic effects. In addition, they modify the body's immune responses to diverse stimuli.

INDICATIONS

When oral therapy is not feasible:

1. *Endocrine disorders*

Primary or secondary adrenocortical insufficiency (hydrocortisone or cortisone is the drug of choice; synthetic analogs may be used in conjunction with mineralocorticoids where applicable; in infancy, mineralocorticoid supplementation is of particular importance)

Acute adrenocortical insufficiency (hydrocortisone or cortisone is the drug of choice; mineralocorticoid supplementation may be necessary, particularly when synthetic analogs are used)

Preoperatively, and in the event of serious trauma or illness, in patients with known adrenal insufficiency or when adrenocortical reserve is doubtful

Shock unresponsive to conventional therapy if adrenocortical insufficiency exists or is suspected

    Congenital adrenal hyperplasia

    Nonsuppurative thyroiditis

    Hypercalcemia associated with cancer

2. *Rheumatic disorders*

As adjunctive therapy for short-term administration (to tide the patient over an acute episode or exacerbation) in:

    Post-traumatic osteoarthritis

    Synovitis of osteoarthritis

    Rheumatoid arthritis, including juvenile rheumatoid arthritis (selected cases may require low-dose maintenance therapy)

    Acute and subacute bursitis

    Epicondylitis

    Acute nonspecific tenosynovitis

    Acute gouty arthritis

    Psoriatic arthritis

    Ankylosing spondylitis

3. *Collagen diseases*

During an exacerbation or as maintenance therapy in selected cases of:

    Systemic lupus erythematosus

    Acute rheumatic carditis

    Systemic dermatomyositis (polymyositis)

4. *Dermatologic diseases*

    Pemphigus

    Severe erythema multiforme (Stevens-Johnson syndrome)

    Exfoliative dermatitis

    Bullous dermatitis herpetiformis

    Severe seborrheic dermatitis

    Severe psoriasis

    Mycosis fungoides

5. *Allergic states*

Control of severe or incapacitating allergic conditions intractable to adequate trials of conventional treatment in:

    Bronchial asthma
    Contact dermatitis
    Atopic dermatitis
    Serum sickness
    Seasonal or perennial allergic rhinitis
    Drug hypersensitivity reactions
    Urticarial transfusion reactions
    Acute noninfectious laryngeal edema (epinephrine is the drug of first choice)

6. *Ophthalmic diseases*

Severe acute and chronic allergic and inflammatory processes involving the eye, such as:

    Herpes zoster ophthalmicus
    Iritis, iridocyclitis
    Chorioretinitis
    Diffuse posterior uveitis and choroiditis
    Optic neuritis
    Sympathetic ophthalmia
    Anterior segment inflammation
    Allergic conjunctivitis
    Keratitis
    Allergic corneal marginal ulcers

7. *Gastrointestinal diseases*

To tide the patient over a critical period of the disease in:

    Ulcerative colitis (Systemic therapy)
    Regional enteritis (Systemic therapy)

8. *Respiratory diseases*

    Symptomatic sarcoidosis
    Berylliosis
    Fulminating or disseminated pulmonary tuberculosis when used concurrently with appropriate antituberculous chemotherapy
    Loeffler's syndrome not manageable by other means
    Aspiration pneumonitis

9. *Hematologic disorders*

    Acquired (autoimmune) hemolytic anemia
    Erythroblastopenia (RBC anemia)
    Congenital (erythroid) hypoplastic anemia

10. *Neoplastic diseases*

For palliative management of:

    Leukemias and lymphomas in adults
    Acute leukemia of childhood

11. *Edematous states*

    To induce diuresis or remission of proteinuria in the nephrotic syndrome, without uremia, of the idiopathic type, or that due to lupus erythematosus

12. *Miscellaneous*

    Tuberculous meningitis with subarachnoid block or impending block when used concurrently with appropriate antituberculous chemotherapy
    Trichinosis with neurologic or myocardial involvement.

CONTRAINDICATIONS

Systemic fungal infections
Hypersensitivity to any component of this product

WARNINGS

Because rare instances of anaphylactoid reactions have occurred in patients receiving parenteral corticosteroid therapy, appropriate precautionary measures should be taken prior to administration, especially when the patient has a history of allergy to any drug. Anaphylactoid and hypersensitivity reactions have been reported for Sterile Suspension CORTONE Acetate (see ADVERSE REACTIONS).

In patients on corticosteroid therapy subjected to any unusual stress, increased dosage of rapidly acting corticosteroids before, during, and after the stressful situation is indicated.

Drug-induced secondary adrenocortical insufficiency may result from too rapid withdrawal of corticosteroids and may be minimized by gradual reduction of dosage. This type of relative insufficiency may persist for months after discontinuation of therapy; therefore, in any situation of stress occurring during that period, hormone therapy should be reinstituted. If the patient is receiving steroids already, dosage may have to be increased. Since mineralocorticoid secretion may be impaired, salt and/or a mineralocorticoid should be administered concurrently.

Corticosteroids may mask some signs of infection, and new infections may appear during their use. There may be decreased resistance and inability to localize infection when corticosteroids are used. Moreover, corticosteroids may affect the nitroblue-tetrazolium test for bacterial infection and produce false negative results.

In cerebral malaria, a double-blind trial has shown that the use of corticosteroids is associated with prolongation of coma and a higher incidence of pneumonia and gastrointestinal bleeding.

Corticosteroids may activate latent amebiasis. Therefore, it is recommended that latent or active amebiasis be ruled out before initiating corticosteroid therapy in any patient who has spent time in the tropics or any patient with unexplained diarrhea.

Prolonged use of corticosteroids may produce posterior subcapsular cataracts, glaucoma with possible damage to the optic nerves, and may enhance the establishment of secondary ocular infections due to fungi or viruses.

Usage in pregnancy. Since adequate human reproduction studies have not been done with corticosteroids, use of these drugs in pregnancy or in women of childbearing potential requires that the anticipated benefits be weighed against the possible hazards to the mother and embryo or fetus. Infants born of mothers who have received substantial doses of corticosteroids during pregnancy should be carefully observed for signs of hypoadrenalism.

Corticosteroids appear in breast milk and could suppress growth, interfere with endogenous corticosteroid production, or cause other unwanted effects. Mothers taking pharmacologic doses of corticosteroids should be advised not to nurse.

Average and large doses of cortisone or hydrocortisone can cause elevation of blood pressure, salt and water retention, and increased excretion of potassium. These effects are less likely to occur with the synthetic derivatives except when used in large doses. Dietary salt restriction and potassium supplementation may be necessary. All corticosteroids increase calcium excretion.

Administration of live virus vaccines, including smallpox, is contraindicated in individuals receiving immunosuppressive doses of corticosteroids. If inactivated viral or bacterial vaccines are administered to individuals receiving immunosuppressive doses of corticosteroids, the expected serum antibody response may not be obtained.

The use of CORTONE Acetate sterile suspension in active tuberculosis should be restricted to those cases of fulminating or disseminated tuberculosis in which the corticosteroid is used for the management of the disease in conjunction with an appropriate antituberculous regimen.

If corticosteroids are indicated in patients with latent tuberculosis or tuberculin reactivity, close observation is necessary as reactivation of the disease may occur. During prolonged corticosteroid therapy, these patients should receive chemoprophylaxis.

Literature reports suggest an apparent association between use of corticosteroids and left ventricular free wall rupture after a recent myocardial infarction; therefore, therapy with corticosteroids should be used with great caution in these patients.

PRECAUTIONS

CORTONE Acetate sterile suspension, like many other steroid formulations, is sensitive to heat. Therefore, it should not be autoclaved when it is desirable to sterilize the exterior of the vial.

Following prolonged therapy, withdrawal of corticosteroids may result in symptoms of the corticosteroid withdrawal syndrome including fever, myalgia, arthralgia, and malaise. This may occur in patients even without evidence of adrenal insufficiency.

There is an enhanced effect of corticosteroids in patients with hypothyroidism and in those with cirrhosis.

Corticosteroids should be used cautiously in patients with ocular herpes simplex for fear of corneal perforation.

The lowest possible dose of corticosteroid should be used to control the condition under treatment, and when reduction in dosage is possible, the reduction must be gradual.

Psychic derangements may appear when corticosteroids are used, ranging from euphoria, insomnia, mood swings, personality changes, and severe depression to frank psychotic manifestations. Also, existing emotional instability or psychotic tendencies may be aggravated by corticosteroids.

Aspirin should be used cautiously in conjunction with corticosteroids in hypoprothrombinemia.

Steroids should be used with caution in nonspecific ulcerative colitis, if there is a probability of impending perforation, abscess, or other pyogenic infection, also in diverticulitis, fresh intestinal anastomoses, active or latent peptic ulcer, renal insufficiency, hypertension, osteoporosis, and myasthenia gravis. Signs of peritoneal irritation following gastrointestinal perforation in patients receiving large doses of corticosteroids may be minimal or absent. Fat embolism has been reported as a possible complication of hypercortisonism.

When large doses are given, some authorities advise that antacids be administered between meals to help to prevent peptic ulcer.

Growth and development of infants and children on prolonged corticosteroid therapy should be carefully followed.

Steroids may increase or decrease motility and number of spermatozoa in some patients.

Phenytoin, phenobarbital, ephedrine, and rifampin may enhance the metabolic clearance of corticosteroids, resulting in decreased blood levels and lessened physiologic activity, thus requiring adjustment in corticosteroid dosage.

The prothrombin time should be checked frequently in patients who are receiving corticosteroids and coumarin anticoagulants at the same time because of reports that corticosteroids have altered the response to these anticoagulants. Studies have shown that the usual effect produced by adding corticosteroids is inhibition of response to coumarins, although there have been some conflicting reports of potentiation not substantiated by studies.

When corticosteroids are administered concomitantly with potassium-depleting diuretics, patients should be observed closely for development of hypokalemia.

Injection of a steroid into an infected site is to be avoided.

ADVERSE REACTIONS

Fluid and electrolyte disturbances
    Sodium retention
    Fluid retention
    Congestive heart failure in susceptible patients
    Potassium loss
    Hypokalemic alkalosis
    Hypertension
Musculoskeletal
    Muscle weakness
    Steroid myopathy
    Loss of muscle mass
    Osteoporosis
    Vertebral compression fractures
    Aseptic necrosis of femoral and humeral heads
    Pathologic fracture of long bones
    Tendon rupture
Gastrointestinal
    Peptic ulcer with possible subsequent perforation and hemorrhage
    Perforation of the small and large bowel, particularly in patients with inflammatory bowel disease
    Pancreatitis
    Abdominal distention
    Ulcerative esophagitis
Dermatologic
    Impaired wound healing
    Thin fragile skin
    Petechiae and ecchymoses
    Erythema
    Increased sweating
    May suppress reactions to skin tests
    Other cutaneous reactions, such as allergic dermatitis, urticaria, angioneurotic edema
Neurologic
    Convulsions
    Increased intracranial pressure with papilledema (pseudotumor cerebri) usually after treatment
    Vertigo
    Headache
    Psychic disturbances
Endocrine
    Menstrual irregularities
    Development of cushingoid state
    Suppression of growth in children
    Secondary adrenocortical and pituitary unresponsiveness, particularly in times of stress, as in trauma, surgery, or illness
    Decreased carbohydrate tolerance
    Manifestations of latent diabetes mellitus
    Increased requirements for insulin or oral hypoglycemic agents in diabetics
    Hirsutism
Ophthalmic
    Posterior subcapsular cataracts
    Increased intraocular pressure
    Glaucoma
    Exophthalmos
Metabolic
    Negative nitrogen balance due to protein catabolism
Cardiovascular
    Myocardial rupture following recent myocardial infarction (see WARNINGS).
Other
    Anaphylactoid or hypersensitivity reactions
    Thromboembolism
    Weight gain
    Increased appetite
    Nausea
    Malaise

The following *additional* adverse reactions are related to parenteral corticosteroid therapy:

Continued on next page

Information on Merck & Co. products listed on these pages is the full prescribing information from product circulars in use October 1, 1992.

Merck & Co.—Cont.

Rare instances of blindness associated with intralesional therapy around the face and head
Hyperpigmentation or hypopigmentation
Subcutaneous and cutaneous atrophy
Sterile abscess

OVERDOSAGE

Reports of acute toxicity and/or death following overdosage of glucocorticoids are rare. In the event of overdosage, no specific antidote is available; treatment is supportive and symptomatic.
The intraperitoneal LD_{50} of cortisone acetate in female mice was 1405 mg/kg.

DOSAGE AND ADMINISTRATION

For intramuscular injection only
NOT FOR INTRAVENOUS USE
DOSAGE REQUIREMENTS ARE VARIABLE AND MUST BE INDIVIDUALIZED ON THE BASIS OF THE DISEASE AND THE RESPONSE OF THE PATIENT.
The initial dosage varies from 20 to 300 mg a day depending on the disease being treated. In less severe diseases doses lower than 20 mg may suffice, while in severe diseases doses higher than 300 mg may be required. The initial dosage should be maintained or adjusted until the patient's response is satisfactory. If a satisfactory clinical response does not occur after a reasonable period of time, discontinue COR-TONE Acetate sterile suspension and transfer the patient to other therapy.
After a favorable initial response, the proper maintenance dosage should be determined by decreasing the initial dosage in small amounts to the lowest dosage that maintains an adequate clinical response.
Patients should be observed closely for signs that might require dosage adjustment, including changes in clinical status resulting from remissions or exacerbations of the disease, individual drug responsiveness, and the effect of stress (e.g., surgery, infection, trauma). During stress it may be necessary to increase dosage temporarily.
If the drug is to be stopped after more than a few days of treatment, it usually should be withdrawn gradually.

HOW SUPPLIED

No. 7069—Sterile Suspension CORTONE Acetate is a white, mobile suspension, each mL containing 50 mg cortisone acetate, and is supplied as follows:
Storage
Sensitive to heat. Do not autoclave.
Protect from freezing.
A.H.F.S. Category: 68:04
DC 7411914   Issued March 1988

CORTONE® Acetate Tablets
(Cortisone Acetate), U.S.P.

℞

DESCRIPTION

Glucocorticoids are adrenocortical steroids, both naturally occurring and synthetic, which are readily absorbed from the gastrointestinal tract.
Cortisone acetate is a white or practically white, odorless, crystalline powder. It is stable in air. It is insoluble in water. The molecular weight is 402.49. It is designated chemically as 21-(acetyloxy)-17-hydroxypregn-4-ene-3,11,20-trione. The empirical formula is $C_{23}H_{30}O_6$ and the structural formula is:

CORTONE* Acetate (Cortisone Acetate) tablets contain 25 mg of cortisone acetate in each tablet.
Inactive ingredients are lactose, magnesium stearate, and starch.

*Registered trademark of MERCK & CO., INC.

ACTIONS

Naturally occurring glucocorticoids (hydrocortisone and cortisone), which also have salt-retaining properties, are used as replacement therapy in adrenocortical deficiency states. They are also used for their potent anti-inflammatory effects in disorders of many organ systems.
Glucocorticoids cause profound and varied metabolic effects. In addition, they modify the body's immune responses to diverse stimuli.

INDICATIONS

1. *Endocrine Disorders*
Primary or secondary adrenocortical insufficiency (hydrocortisone or cortisone is the first choice; synthetic analogs may be used in conjunction with mineralocorticoids where applicable; in infancy mineralocorticoid supplementation is of particular importance).
Congenital adrenal hyperplasia
Nonsuppurative thyroiditis
Hypercalcemia associated with cancer
2. *Rheumatic Disorders*
As adjunctive therapy for short-term administration (to tide the patient over an acute episode or exacerbation) in:
Psoriatic arthritis
Rheumatoid arthritis, including juvenile rheumatoid arthritis (selected cases may require low-dose maintenance therapy)
Ankylosing spondylitis
Acute and subacute bursitis
Acute nonspecific tenosynovitis
Acute gouty arthritis
Post-traumatic osteoarthritis
Synovitis of osteoarthritis
Epicondylitis
3. *Collagen Diseases*
During an exacerbation or as maintenance therapy in selected cases of—
Systemic lupus erythematosus
Acute rheumatic carditis
Systemic dermatomyositis (polymyositis)
4. *Dermatologic Diseases*
Pemphigus
Bullous dermatitis herpetiformis
Severe erythema multiforme (Stevens-Johnson syndrome)
Exfoliative dermatitis
Mycosis fungoides
Severe psoriasis
Severe seborrheic dermatitis
5. *Allergic States*
Control of severe or incapacitating allergic conditions intractable to adequate trials of conventional treatment:
Seasonal or perennial allergic rhinitis
Bronchial asthma
Contact dermatitis
Atopic dermatitis
Serum sickness
Drug hypersensitivity reactions
6. *Ophthalmic Diseases*
Severe acute and chronic allergic and inflammatory processes involving the eye and its adnexa, such as—
Allergic conjunctivitis
Keratitis
Allergic corneal marginal ulcers
Herpes zoster ophthalmicus
Iritis and iridocyclitis
Chorioretinitis
Anterior segment inflammation
Diffuse posterior uveitis and choroiditis
Optic neuritis
Sympathetic ophthalmia
7. *Respiratory Diseases*
Symptomatic sarcoidosis
Loeffler's syndrome not manageable by other means
Berylliosis
Fulminating or disseminated pulmonary tuberculosis when used concurrently with appropriate antituberculous chemotherapy
Aspiration pneumonitis
8. *Hematologic Disorders*
Idiopathic thrombocytopenic purpura in adults
Secondary thrombocytopenia in adults
Acquired (autoimmune) hemolytic anemia
Erythroblastopenia (RBC anemia)
Congenital (erythroid) hypoplastic anemia
9. *Neoplastic Diseases*
For palliative management of:
Leukemias and lymphomas in adults
Acute leukemia of childhood
10. *Edematous States*
To induce a diuresis or remission of proteinuria in the nephrotic syndrome, without uremia, of the idiopathic type or that due to lupus erythematosus
11. *Gastrointestinal Diseases*
To tide the patient over a critical period of the disease in:
Ulcerative colitis
Regional enteritis
12. *Miscellaneous*
Tuberculous meningitis with subarachnoid block or impending block when used concurrently with appropriate antituberculous chemotherapy
Trichinosis with neurologic or myocardial involvement

CONTRAINDICATIONS

Systemic fungal infections
Hypersensitivity to this product

WARNINGS

In patients on corticosteroid therapy subjected to unusual stress, increased dosage of rapidly acting corticosteroids before, during, and after the stressful situation is indicated. Drug-induced secondary adrenocortical insufficiency may result from too rapid withdrawal of corticosteroids and may be minimized by gradual reduction of dosage. This type of relative insufficiency may persist for months after discontinuation of therapy; therefore, in any situation of stress occurring during that period, hormone therapy should be reinstituted. If the patient is receiving steroids already, dosage may have to be increased. Since mineralocorticoid secretion may be impaired, salt and/or a mineralocorticoid should be administered concurrently.
Corticosteroids may mask some signs of infection, and new infections may appear during their use. There may be decreased resistance and inability to localize infection when corticosteroids are used. Moreover, corticosteroids may affect the nitroblue-tetrazolium test for bacterial infection and produce false negative results.
In cerebral malaria, a double-blind trial has shown that the use of corticosteroids is associated with prolongation of coma and a higher incidence of pneumonia and gastrointestinal bleeding.
Corticosteroids may activate latent amebiasis. Therefore, it is recommended that latent or active amebiasis be ruled out before initiating corticosteroid therapy in any patient who has spent time in the tropics or any patient with unexplained diarrhea.
Prolonged use of corticosteroids may produce posterior subcapsular cataracts, glaucoma with possible damage to the optic nerves, and may enhance the establishment of secondary ocular infections due to fungi or viruses.
Usage in pregnancy: Since adequate human reproduction studies have not been done with corticosteroids, use of these drugs in pregnancy or in women of childbearing potential requires that the anticipated benefits be weighed against the possible hazards to the mother and embryo or fetus. Infants born of mothers who have received substantial doses of corticosteroids during pregnancy should be carefully observed for signs of hypoadrenalism.
Corticosteroids appear in breast milk and could suppress growth, interefere with endogenous corticosteroid production, or cause other unwanted effects. Mothers taking pharmacologic doses of corticosteroids should be advised not to nurse.
Average and large doses of hydrocortisone or cortisone can cause elevation of blood pressure, salt and water retention, and increased excretion of potassium. These effects are less likely to occur with the synthetic derivatives except when used in large doses. Dietary salt restriction and potassium supplementation may be necessary. All corticosteroids increase calcium excretion.
Administration of live virus vaccines, including smallpox, is contraindicated in individuals receiving immunosuppressive doses of corticosteroids. If inactivated viral or bacterial vaccines are administered to individuals receiving immunosuppressive doses of corticosteroids, the expected serum antibody response may not be obtained. However, immunization procedures may be undertaken in patients who are receiving corticosteroids as replacement therapy, e.g., for Addison's disease.
The use of CORTONE Acetate tablets in active tuberculosis should be restricted to those cases of fulminating or disseminated tuberculosis in which the corticosteroid is used for the management of the disease in conjunction with an appropriate antituberculous regimen.
If corticosteroids are indicated in patients with latent tuberculosis or tuberculin reactivity, close observation is necessary as reactivation of the disease may occur. During prolonged corticosteroid therapy, these patients should receive chemoprophylaxis.
Literature reports suggest an apparent association between use of corticosteroids and left ventricular free wall rupture after a recent myocardial infarction; therefore, therapy with corticosteroids should be used with great caution in these patients.

PRECAUTIONS

Following prolonged therapy, withdrawal of corticosteroids may result in symptoms of the corticosteroid withdrawal

syndrome including fever, myalgia, arthralgia, and malaise. This may occur in patients even without evidence of adrenal insufficiency.

There is an enhanced effect of corticosteroids in patients with hypothyroidism and in those with cirrhosis.

Corticosteroids should be used cautiously in patients with ocular herpes simplex because of possible corneal perforation.

The lowest possible dose of corticosteroid should be used to control the condition under treatment, and when reduction in dosage is possible, the reduction should be gradual.

Psychic derangements may appear when corticosteroids are used, ranging from euphoria, insomnia, mood swings, personality changes, and severe depression, to frank psychotic manifestations. Also, existing emotional instability or psychotic tendencies may be aggravated by corticosteroids.

Aspirin should be used cautiously in conjunction with corticosteroids in hypoprothrombinemia.

Steroids should be used with caution in nonspecific ulcerative colitis, if there is a probability of impending perforation, abscess, or other pyogenic infection, diverticulitis, fresh intestinal anastomoses, active or latent peptic ulcer, renal insufficiency, hypertension, osteoporosis, and myasthenia gravis. Signs of peritoneal irritation following gastrointestinal perforation in patients receiving large doses of corticosteroids may be minimal or absent. Fat embolism has been reported as a possible complication of hypercortisonism.

When large doses are given, some authorities advise that corticosteroids be taken with meals and antacids taken between meals to help to prevent peptic ulcer.

Growth and development of infants and children on prolonged corticosteroid therapy should be carefully observed. Steroids may increase or decrease motility and number of spermatozoa in some patients.

Phenytoin, phenobarbital, ephedrine, and rifampin may enhance the metabolic clearance of corticosteroids, resulting in decreased blood levels and lessened physiologic activity, thus requiring adjustment in corticosteroid dosage.

The prothrombin time should be checked frequently in patients who are receiving corticosteroids and coumarin anticoagulants at the same time because of reports that corticosteroids have altered the response to these anticoagulants. Studies have shown that the usual effect produced by adding corticosteroids is inhibition of response to coumarins, although there have been some conflicting reports of potentiation not substantiated by studies.

When corticosteroids are administered concomitantly with potassium-depleting diuretics, patients should be observed closely for development of hypokalemia.

ADVERSE REACTIONS

Fluid and Electrolyte Disturbances
  Sodium retention
  Fluid retention
  Congestive heart failure in susceptible patients
  Potassium loss
  Hypokalemic alkalosis
  Hypertension

Musculoskeletal
  Muscle weakness
  Steroid myopathy
  Loss of muscle mass
  Osteoporosis
  Vertebral compression fractures
  Aseptic necrosis of femoral and humeral heads
  Pathologic fracture of long bones
  Tendon rupture

Gastrointestinal
  Peptic ulcer with possible perforation and hemorrhage
  Perforation of the small and large bowel, particularly in patients with inflammatory bowel disease
    Pancreatitis
    Abdominal distention
    Ulcerative esophagitis

Dermatologic
  Impaired wound healing
  Thin fragile skin
  Petechiae and ecchymoses
  Erythema
  Increased sweating
  May suppress reactions to skin tests
  Other cutaneous reactions, such as allergic dermatitis, urticaria, angioneurotic edema

Neurologic
  Convulsions
  Increased intracranial pressure with papilledema (pseudotumor cerebri), usually after treatment
    Vertigo
    Headache
    Psychic disturbances

Endocrine
  Menstrual irregularities
  Development of cushingoid state
  Suppression of growth in children
  Secondary adrenocortical and pituitary unresponsiveness, particularly in times of stress, as in trauma, surgery, or illness
  Decreased carbohydrate tolerance
  Manifestations of latent diabetes mellitus
  Increased requirements for insulin or oral hypoglycemic agents in diabetics
  Hirsutism

Ophthalmic
  Posterior subcapsular cataracts
  Increased intraocular pressure
  Glaucoma
  Exophthalmos

Metabolic
  Negative nitrogen balance due to protein catabolism

Cardiovascular
  Myocardial rupture following recent myocardial infarction (see WARNINGS).

Other
  Hypersensitivity
  Thromboembolism
  Weight gain
  Increased appetite
  Nausea
  Malaise
  Psychic disturbances

OVERDOSAGE

Reports of acute toxicity and/or death following overdosage of glucocorticoids are rare. In the event of overdosage, no specific antidote is available; treatment is supportive and symptomatic.

The intraperitoneal LD_{50} of cortisone acetate in female mice was 1405 mg/kg.

DOSAGE AND ADMINISTRATION

For oral administration
DOSAGE REQUIREMENTS ARE VARIABLE AND MUST BE INDIVIDUALIZED ON THE BASIS OF THE DISEASE AND THE RESPONSE OF THE PATIENT.

The initial dosage varies from 25 to 300 mg a day depending on the disease being treated. In less severe diseases doses lower than 25 mg may suffice, while in severe diseases doses higher than 300 mg may be required. The initial dosage should be maintained or adjusted until the patient's response is satisfactory. If satisfactory clinical response does not occur after a reasonable period of time, discontinue CORTONE Acetate tablets and transfer the patient to other therapy.

After a favorable initial response, the proper maintenance dosage should be determined by decreasing the initial dosage in small amounts to the lowest dosage that maintains an adequate clinical response.

Patients should be observed closely for signs that might require dosage adjustment, including changes in clinical status resulting from remissions or exacerbations of the disease, individual drug responsiveness, and the effect of stress (e.g., surgery, infection, trauma). During stress it may be necessary to increase dosage temporarily.

If the drug is to be stopped after more than a few days of treatment, it usually should be withdrawn gradually.

HOW SUPPLIED

No. 7063—Tablets Cortone Acetate, 25 mg each, are white, round, scored, compressed tablets, coded MSD 219. They are supplied as follows:
NDC 0006-0219-68 in bottles of 100.
Shown in Product Identification Section, page 419
A.H.F.S. Category: 68:04
DC 7411828   Issued March 1988

COSMEGEN® Injection   ℞
(Dactinomycin), U.S.P.

+---+
| **WARNING** |
| |
| Dactinomycin is extremely corrosive to soft tissue. |
| If extravasation occurs during intravenous use, |
| severe damage to soft tissues will occur. In at |
| least one instance, this has led to contracture of |
| the arms. |
| |
| **DOSAGE** |
| |
| The dosage of COSMEGEN* (Dactinomycin) is calcu- |
| lated in micrograms (mcg). The usual adult dosage |
| is 500 micrograms (0.5 mg) daily intravenously for |
| a maximum of five days. The dosage for adults or |
| children should not exceed 15 mcg/kg or 400–600 |
| mcg/square |
+---+

meter of body surface daily intravenously for five days. Calculation of the dosage for obese or edematous patients should be on the basis of surface area in an effort to relate dosage to lean body mass.

---

*Registered trademark of MERCK & CO., INC.

DESCRIPTION

Dactinomycin is one of the actinomycins, a group of antibiotics produced by various species of *Streptomyces*. Dactinomycin is the principal component of the mixture of actinomycins produced by *Streptomyces parvullus*. Unlike other species of *Streptomyces*, this organism yields an essentially pure substance that contains only traces of similar compounds differing in the amino acid content of the peptide side chains. The empirical formula is $C_{62}H_{86}N_{12}O_{16}$ and the structural formula is:

COSMEGEN is a sterile, yellow lyophilized powder for injection by the intravenous route or by regional perfusion after reconstitution. Each vial contains 0.5 mg (500 mcg) of dactinomycin and 20.0 mg of mannitol.

CLINICAL PHARMACOLOGY

Action
Generally, the actinomycins exert an inhibitory effect on gram-positive and gram-negative bacteria and on some fungi. However, the toxic properties of the actinomycins (including dactinomycin) in relation to antibacterial activity are such as to preclude their use as antibiotics in the treatment of infectious diseases.

Because the actinomycins are cytotoxic, they have an antineoplastic effect which has been demonstrated in experimental animals with various types of tumor implant. This cytotoxic action is the basis for their use in the palliative treatment of certain types of cancer.

Pharmacokinetics and Metabolism
Results of a study in patients with malignant melanoma indicate that dactinomycin (^3H actinomycin D) is minimally metabolized, is concentrated in nucleated cells, and does not penetrate the blood brain barrier. Approximately 30% of the dose was recovered in urine and feces in one week. The terminal plasma half-life for radioactivity was approximately 36 hours.

INDICATIONS AND USAGE

Wilms' Tumor
The neoplasm responding most frequently to COSMEGEN is Wilms' tumor. With low doses of both dactinomycin and radiotherapy, temporary objective improvement may be as good as and may last longer than with higher doses of each given alone. In the National Wilms' Tumor study, combination therapy with dactinomycin and vincristine together with surgery and radiotherapy, was shown to have significantly improved the prognosis of patients in groups II and III. Dactinomycin and vincristine were given for a total of seven cycles, so that maintenance therapy continued for approximately 15 months.

Postoperative radiotherapy in group I patients and optimal combination chemotherapy for those in group IV are unsettled issues. About 70 percent of lung metastases have disappeared with an appropriate combination of radiation, dactinomycin and vincristine.

Rhabdomyosarcoma
Temporary regression of the tumor and beneficial subjective results have occurred with dactinomycin in rhabdomyosarcoma which, like most soft tissue sarcomas, is comparatively radio-resistant.

Continued on next page

Merck & Co.—Cont.

Several groups have reported successful use of cyclophosphamide, vincristine, dactinomycin and doxorubicin hydrochloride in various combinations. Effective combinations have included vincristine and dactinomycin; vincristine, dactinomycin and cyclophosphamide (VAC therapy) and all four drugs in sequence. At present, the most effective treatment for children with inoperable or metastatic rhabdomyosarcoma has been VAC chemotherapy. Two-thirds of these children were doing well without evidence of disease at a median time of three years after diagnosis.

Carcinoma of Testis and Uterus

The sequential use of dactinomycin and methotrexate, along with meticulous monitoring of human chorionic gonadotropin levels until normal, has resulted in survival in the majority of women with metastatic choriocarcinoma. Sequential therapy is used if there is:

1. Stability in gonadotropin titers following two successive courses of an agent.
2. Rising gonadotropin titers during treatment.
3. Severe toxicity preventing adequate therapy.

In patients with nonmetastatic choriocarcinoma, dactinomycin or methotrexate or both, have been used successfully, with or without surgery.

Dactinomycin has been beneficial as a single agent in the treatment of metastatic nonseminomatour testicular carcinoma when used in cycles of 500 mcg/day for five consecutive days, every 6–8 weeks for periods of four months or longer.

Other Neoplasms

Dactinomycin has been given intravenously or by regional perfusion, either alone or with other antineoplastic compounds or x-ray therapy, in the palliative treatment of Ewing's sarcoma and sarcoma botryoides. For nonmetastatic Ewing's sarcoma, promising results were obtained when dactinomycin (45 mcg/m^2) and cyclophosphamide (1200 mg/m^2) were given sequentially and with radiotherapy, over an 18 month period. Those with metastatic disease remain the subject of continued investigation with a more aggressive chemotherapeutic regimen employed initially.

Temporary objective improvement and relief of pain and discomfort have followed the use of dactinomycin usually in conjunction with radiotherapy for sarcoma botryoides. This palliative effect ranges from transitory inhibition of tumor growth to a considerable but temporary regression in tumor size.

COSMEGEN (Dactinomycin)
and Radiation Therapy

Much evidence suggests that dactinomycin potentiates the effects of x-ray therapy. The converse also appears likely; i.e., dactinomycin may be more effective when radiation therapy also is given.

With combined dactinomycin-radiation therapy, the normal skin, as well as the buccal and pharyngeal mucosa, show early erythema. A smaller than usual x-ray dose when given with dactinomycin causes erythema and vesiculation, which progress more rapidly through the stages of tanning and desquamation. Healing may occur in four to six weeks rather than two to three months. Erythema from previous x-ray therapy may be reactivated by dactinomycin alone, even when irradiation occurred many months earlier, and especially when the interval between the two forms of therapy is brief. This potentiation of radiation effect represents a special problem when the irradiation treatment area includes the mucous membrane. When irradiation is directed toward the nasopharynx, the combination may produce severe oropharyngeal mucositis. *Severe reactions may ensue if high doses of both dactinomycin and radiation therapy are used or if the patient is particularly sensitive to such combined therapy.*

Because of this potentiating effect, dactinomycin may be tried in radio-sensitive tumors not responding to doses of x-ray therapy that can be tolerated. Objective improvement in tumor size and activity may be observed when lower, better tolerated doses of both types of therapy are employed.

COSMEGEN (Dactinomycin)
and Perfusion Technic

Dactinomycin alone or with other antineoplastic agents has also been given by the isolation-perfusion technic, either as palliative treatment or as an adjunct to resection of a tumor. Some tumors considered resistant to chemotherapy and radiation therapy may respond when the drug is given by the perfusion technic. Neoplasms in which dactinomycin has been tried by this technic include various types of sarcoma, carcinoma, and adenocarcinoma.

In some instances tumors regressed, pain was relieved for variable periods, and surgery made possible. On other occasions, however, the outcome has been less favorable. Nevertheless, in selected cases, the drug by perfusion may provide more effective palliation than when given systemically.

Dactinomycin by the isolation-perfusion technic offers certain advantages, provided leakage of the drug through the general circulation into other areas of the body is minimal.

By this technic the drug is in continuous contact with the tumor for the duration of treatment. The dose may be increased well over that used by the systemic route, usually without adding to the danger of toxic effects. If the agent is confined to an isolated part, it should not interfere with the patient's defense mechanism. Systemic absorption of toxic products from neoplastic tissue can be minimized by removing the perfusate when the procedure is finished.

CONTRAINDICATIONS

If dactinomycin is given at or about the time of infection with chicken pox or herpes zoster, a severe generalized disease, which may result in death, may occur.

PRECAUTIONS

General

COSMEGEN should be administered only under the supervision of a physician who is experienced in the use of cancer chemotherapeutic agents.

This drug is highly toxic and both powder and solution must be handled and administered with care. Inhalation of dust or vapors and contact with skin or mucous membranes, especially those of the eyes, must be avoided. Should accidental eye contact occur, copious irrigation with water should be instituted immediately, followed by prompt ophthalmologic consultation. Should accidental skin contact occur, the affected part must be irrigated immediately with copious amounts of water for at least 15 minutes.

As with all antineoplastic agents, dactinomycin is a toxic drug and very careful and frequent observation of the patient for adverse reactions is necessary. These reactions may involve any tissue of the body. The possibility of an anaphylactoid reaction should be borne in mind.

Increased incidence of gastrointestinal toxicity and marrow suppression has been reported when dactinomycin was given with x-ray therapy.

Particular caution is necessary when administering dactinomycin within two months of irradiation for the treatment of right-sided Wilms' tumor, since hepatomegaly and elevated SGOT levels have been noted.

Nausea and vomiting due to dactinomycin make it necessary to give this drug intermittently. It is extremely important to observe the patient daily for toxic side effects when multiple chemotherapy is employed, since a full course of therapy occasionally is not tolerated. If stomatitis, diarrhea, or severe hemopoietic depression appear during therapy, these drugs should be discontinued until the patient has recovered. Recent reports indicate an increased incidence of second primary tumors following treatment with radiation and anti-neoplastic agents, such as dactinomycin. Multi-modal therapy creates the need for careful, long-term observation of cancer survivors.

Laboratory Tests

Many abnormalities of renal, hepatic, and bone marrow function have been reported in patients with neoplastic disease and receiving dactinomycin. It is advisable to check renal, hepatic, and bone marrow functions frequently.

Drug/Laboratory Test Interactions

It has been reported that dactinomycin may interfere with bioassay procedures for the determination of antibacterial drug levels.

Carcinogenesis, Mutagenesis,
Impairment of Fertility

The International Agency on Research on Cancer has judged that dactinomycin is a positive carcinogen in animals. Local sarcomas were produced in mice and rats after repeated subcutaneous or intraperitoneal injection. Mesenchymal tumors occurred in male F344 rats given intraperitoneal injections of 0.05 mg/kg, 2 to 5 times per week for 18 weeks. The first tumor appeared at 23 weeks.

Dactinomycin has been shown to be mutagenic in a number of test systems *in vitro* and *in vivo* including human fibroblasts and leucocytes, and HELA cells. DNA damage and cytogenetic effects have been demonstrated in the mouse and the rat.

Adequate fertility studies have not been reported.

Pregnancy

Pregnancy Category C. COSMEGEN has been shown to cause malformations and embryotoxicity in the rat, rabbit and hamster when given in doses of 50–100 mcg/kg intravenously (3–7 times the maximum recommended human dose). There are no adequate and well-controlled studies in pregnant women. COSMEGEN should be used during pregnancy only if the potential benefit justifies the potential risk to the fetus.

Nursing Mothers

It is not known whether this drug is excreted in human milk. Because many drugs are excreted in human milk and because of the potential for serious adverse reactions in nursing infants from COSMEGEN, a decision should be made whether to discontinue nursing or to discontinue the drug, taking into account the importance of the drug to the mother.

Pediatric Use

The greater frequency of toxic effects of dactinomycin in infants suggest that this drug should be given to infants only over the age of 6 to 12 months.

ADVERSE REACTIONS

Toxic effects (excepting nausea and vomiting) usually do not become apparent until two to four days after a course of therapy is stopped, and may not be maximal before one to two weeks have elapsed. Deaths have been reported. However, adverse reactions are usually reversible on discontinuance of therapy. They include the following:

Miscellaneous: malaise, fatigue, lethargy, fever, myalgia, proctitis, hypocalcemia.

Oral: cheilitis, dysphagia, esophagitis, ulcerative stomatitis, pharyngitis.

Gastrointestinal: anorexia, nausea, vomiting, abdominal pain, diarrhea, gastrointestinal ulceration, liver toxicity including ascites, hepatomegaly, hepatitis, and liver function test abnormalities. Nausea and vomiting, which occur early during the first few hours after administration, may be alleviated by giving antiemetics.

Hematologic: anemia, even to the point of aplastic anemia, agranulocytosis, leukopenia, thrombopenia, pancytopenia, reticulopenia. Platelet and white cell counts should be done *daily* to detect severe hemopoietic depression. If either count markedly decreases, the drug should be withheld to allow marrow recovery. This often takes up to three weeks.

Dermatologic: alopecia, skin eruptions, acne, flare-up of erythema or increased pigmentation of previously irradiated skin.

Soft tissues. Dactinomycin is extremely corrosive. If extravasation occurs during intravenous use, severe damage to soft tissues will occur. In at least one instance, this has led to contracture of the arms.

OVERDOSAGE

The intravenous LD_{50} of COSMEGEN in the rat is 460 mcg/kg.

DOSAGE AND ADMINISTRATION

Toxic reactions due to dactinomycin are frequent and may be severe (see ADVERSE REACTIONS), thus limiting in many instances the amount that may be given. However, the severity of toxicity varies markedly and is only partly dependent on the dose employed. The drug must be given in short courses.

Intravenous Use

The dosage of dactinomycin varies depending on the tolerance of the patient, the size and location of the neoplasm, and the use of other forms of therapy. It may be necessary to decrease the usual dosages suggested below when other chemotherapy or x-ray therapy is used concomitantly or has been used previously.

The dosage for adults or children should not exceed 15 mcg/kg or 400–600 mcg/square meter of body surface daily intravenously for five days. Calculation of the dosage for obese or edematous patients should be on the basis of surface area in an effort to relate dosage to lean body mass.

Adults: The usual adult dosage is 500 mcg (0.5 mg) daily intravenously for a maximum of five days.

Children: In children 15 mcg (0.015 mg) per kilogram of body weight is given intravenously daily for five days. An alternative schedule is a total dosage of 2500 mcg (2.5 mg) per square meter of body surface given intravenously over a one week period.

In both adults and children, a second course may be given after at least three weeks have elapsed, provided all signs of toxicity have disappeared.

Reconstitute COSMEGEN by adding 1.1 ml of **Sterile Water for Injection (without preservative)** using aseptic precautions. The resulting solution of dactinomycin will contain approximately 500 mcg or 0.5 mg per ml.

Parenteral drug products should be inspected visually for particulate matter and discoloration prior to administration, whenever solution and container permit. When reconstituted, COSMEGEN is a clear, gold-colored solution.

Once reconstituted, the solution of dactinomycin can be added to infusion solutions of Dextrose Injection 5 percent or Sodium Chloride Injection either directly or to the tubing of a running intravenous infusion.

Although reconstituted COSMEGEN is chemically stable, the product does not contain a preservative and accidental microbial contamination might result. Any unused portion should be discarded. Use of water containing preservatives (benzyl alcohol or parabens) to reconstitute COSMEGEN for injection, results in the formation of a precipitate.

Partial removal of dactinomycin from intravenous solutions by cellulose ester membrane filters used in some intravenous in-line filters has been reported.

Since dactinomycin is extremely corrosive to soft tissue, precautions for materials of this nature should be observed.

If the drug is given directly into the vein without the use of an infusion, the "two-needle technic" should be used. Reconstitute and withdraw the calculated dose from the vial with one sterile needle. Use another sterile needle for direct injection into the vein.

Discard any unused portion of the dactinomycin solution.

Isolation-Perfusion Technic

The dosage schedules and the technic itself vary from one investigator to another; the published literature, therefore, should be consulted for details. In general, the following doses are suggested:

50 mcg (0.05 mg) per kilogram of body weight for lower extremity or pelvis.

35 mcg (0.035 mg) per kilogram of body weight for upper extremity.

It may be advisable to use lower doses in obese patients, or when previous chemotherapy or radiation therapy has been employed.

Complications of the perfusion technic are related mainly to the amount of drug that escapes into the systemic circulation and may consist of hemopoietic depression, absorption of toxic products from massive destruction of neoplastic tissue, increased susceptibility to infection, impaired wound healing, and superficial ulceration of the gastric mucosa. Other side effects may include edema of the extremity involved, damage to soft tissues of the perfused area, and (potentially) venous thrombosis.

HOW SUPPLIED

No. 3298—Injection COSMEGEN is a lyophilized powder and is supplied as follows: **NDC** 0006-3298-22 in vials containing 0.5 mg (500 micrograms) of dactinomycin and 20.0 mg of mannitol. In the dry form the compound is an amorphous yellow powder. The solution is clear and gold-colored.

Storage

Protect from light.

Special Handling

Due to the drug's toxic and mutagenic properties, appropriate precautions including the use of appropriate safety equipment are recommended for the preparation of COSMEGEN for parenteral administration. The National Institutes of Health presently recommends that the preparation of injectable antineoplastic drugs should be performed in a Class II laminar flow biological safety cabinet and that personnel preparing drugs of this class should wear surgical gloves and a closed front surgical-type gown with knit cuffs.

A.H.F.S. Category: 10:00

DC 7496524 Issued December 1988

COPYRIGHT © MERCK & CO., INC., 1983
All rights reserved

CUPRIMINE® Capsules ℞
(Penicillamine), U.S.P.

> Physicians planning to use penicillamine should thoroughly familiarize themselves with its toxicity, special dosage considerations, and therapeutic benefits. Penicillamine should never be used casually. Each patient should remain constantly under the close supervision of the physician. Patients should be warned to report promptly any symptoms suggesting toxicity.

DESCRIPTION

Penicillamine is a chelating agent used in the treatment of Wilson's disease. It is also used to reduce cystine excretion in cystinuria and to treat patients with severe, active rheumatoid arthritis unresponsive to conventional therapy (see INDICATIONS). It is 3-mercapto-D-valine. It is a white or practically white, crystalline powder, freely soluble in water, slightly soluble in alcohol, and insoluble in ether, acetone, benzene, and carbon tetrachloride. Although its configuration is D, it is levorotatory as usually measured:

$$[\alpha]^{25°}_{D} = -62.5° \pm 2° \text{ (c = 1, 1N NaOH)},$$

calculated on a dried basis.

The empirical formula is $C_5H_{11}NO_2S$, giving it a molecular weight of 149.21. The structural formula is:

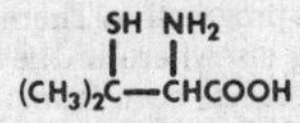

It reacts readily with formaldehyde or acetone to form a thiazolidine-carboxylic acid.

Capsules CUPRIMINE* (Penicillamine) for oral administration contain either 125 mg or 250 mg of penicillamine. Each capsule contains the following inactive ingredients: D & C Yellow 10, gelatin, lactose, magnesium stearate, and titanium dioxide. The 125 mg capsule also contains iron oxide.

*Registered trademark of MERCK & CO., INC.

CLINICAL PHARMACOLOGY

Penicillamine is a chelating agent recommended for the removal of excess copper in patients with Wilson's disease. From *in vitro* studies which indicate that one atom of copper combines with two molecules of penicillamine, it would appear that one gram of penicillamine should be followed by the excretion of about 200 milligrams of copper; however, the actual amount excreted is about one percent of this.

Penicillamine also reduces excess cystine excretion in cystinuria. This is done, at least in part, by disulfide interchange between penicillamine and cystine, resulting in formation of penicillamine-cysteine disulfide, a substance that is much more soluble than cystine and is excreted readily.

Penicillamine interferes with the formation of cross-links between tropocollagen molecules and cleaves them when newly formed.

The mechanism of action of penicillamine in rheumatoid arthritis is unknown although it appears to suppress disease activity. Unlike cytotoxic immunosuppressants, penicillamine markedly lowers IgM rheumatoid factor but produces no significant depression in absolute levels of serum immunoglobulins. Also unlike cytotoxic immunosuppressants which act on both, penicillamine *in vitro* depresses T-cell activity but not B-cell activity.

In vitro, penicillamine dissociates macroglobulins (rheumatoid factor) although the relationship of the activity to its effect in rheumatoid arthritis is not known.

In rheumatoid arthritis, the onset of therapeutic response to CUPRIMINE may not be seen for two or three months. In those patients who respond, however, the first evidence of suppression of symptoms such as pain, tenderness, and swelling is generally apparent within three months. The optimum duration of therapy has not been determined. If remissions occur, they may last from months to years, but usually require continued treatment (see DOSAGE AND ADMINISTRATION).

In all patients receiving penicillamine, it is important that CUPRIMINE be given on an empty stomach, at least one hour before meals or two hours after meals, and at least one hour apart from any other drug, food, or milk. This permits maximum absorption and reduces the likelihood of inactivation by metal binding in the gastrointestinal tract.

Methodology for determining the bioavailability of penicillamine is not available; however, penicillamine is known to be a very soluble substance.

INDICATIONS

CUPRIMINE is indicated in the treatment of Wilson's disease, cystinuria, and in patients with severe, active rheumatoid arthritis who have failed to respond to an adequate trial of conventional therapy. Available evidence suggests that CUPRIMINE is not of value in ankylosing spondylitis.

Wilson's Disease—Wilson's disease (hepatolenticular degeneration) results from the interaction of an inherited defect and an abnormality in copper metabolism. The metabolic defect, which is the consequence of the autosomal inheritance of one abnormal gene from each parent, manifests itself in a greater positive copper balance than normal. As a result, copper is deposited in several organs and appears eventually to produce pathologic effects most prominently seen in the brain, where degeneration is widespread; in the liver, where fatty infiltration, inflammation, and hepatocellular damage progress to postnecrotic cirrhosis; in the kidney, where tubular and glomerular dysfunction results; and in the eye, where characteristic corneal copper deposits are known as Kayser-Fleischer rings.

Two types of patients require treatment for Wilson's disease: (1) the symptomatic, and (2) the asymptomatic in whom it can be assumed the disease will develop in the future if the patient is not treated.

Diagnosis, suspected on the basis of family or individual history, physical examination, or a low serum concentration of ceruloplasmin*, is confirmed by the demonstration of Kayser-Fleischer rings or, particularly in the asymptomatic patient, by the quantitative demonstration in a liver biopsy specimen of a concentration of copper in excess of 250 mcg/g dry weight.

Treatment has two objectives:

(1) to minimize dietary intake and absorption of copper.

(2) to promote excretion of copper deposited in tissues.

The first objective is attained by a daily diet that contains no more than one or two milligrams of copper. Such a diet should exclude, most importantly, chocolate, nuts, shellfish, mushrooms, liver, molasses, broccoli, and cereals enriched with copper, and be composed to as great an extent as possible of foods with a low copper content. Distilled or demineralized water should be used if the patient's drinking water contains more than 0.1 mg of copper per liter.

For the second objective, a copper chelating agent is used. In symptomatic patients this treatment usually produces marked neurologic improvement, fading of Kayser-Fleischer rings, and gradual amelioration of hepatic dysfunction and psychic disturbances.

Clinical experience to date suggests that life is prolonged with the above regimen.

Noticeable improvement may not occur for one to three months. Occasionally, neurologic symptoms become worse during initiation of therapy with CUPRIMINE. Despite this, the drug should not be discontinued permanently, although temporary interruption may result in clinical improvement of the neurological symptoms but it carries an increased risk of developing a sensitivity reaction upon resumption of therapy (see WARNINGS).

Treatment of asymptomatic patients has been carried out for over ten years. Symptoms and signs of the disease appear to be prevented indefinitely if daily treatment with CUPRIMINE can be continued.

Cystinuria—Cystinuria is characterized by excessive urinary excretion of the dibasic amino acids, arginine, lysine, ornithine, and cystine, and the mixed disulfide of cysteine and homocysteine. The metabolic defect that leads to cystinuria is inherited as an autosomal, recessive trait. Metabolism of the affected amino acids is influenced by at least two abnormal factors: (1) defective gastrointestinal absorption and (2) renal tubular dysfunction.

Arginine, lysine, ornithine, and cysteine are soluble substances, readily excreted. There is no apparent pathology connected with their excretion in excessive quantities.

Cystine, however, is so slightly soluble at the usual range of urinary pH that it is not excreted readily, and so crystallizes and forms stones in the urinary tract. Stone formation is the only known pathology in cystinuria.

Normal daily output of cystine is 40 to 80 mg. In cystinuria, output is greatly increased and may exceed 1 g/day. At 500 to 600 mg/day, stone formation is almost certain. When it is more than 300 mg/day, treatment is indicated.

Conventional treatment is directed at keeping urinary cystine diluted enough to prevent stone formation, keeping the urine alkaline enough to dissolve as much cystine as possible, and minimizing cystine production by a diet low in methionine (the major dietary precursor of cystine). Patients must drink enough fluid to keep urine specific gravity below 1.010, take enough alkali to keep urinary pH at 7.5 to 8, and maintain a diet low in methionine. This diet is not recommended in growing children and probably is contraindicated in pregnancy because of its low protein content (see PRECAUTIONS).

When these measures are inadequate to control recurrent stone formation, CUPRIMINE may be used as additional therapy. When patients refuse to adhere to conventional treatment, CUPRIMINE may be a useful substitute. It is capable of keeping cystine excretion to near normal values, thereby hindering stone formation and the serious consequences of pyelonephritis and impaired renal function that develop in some patients.

Bartter and colleagues depict the process by which penicillamine interacts with cystine to form penicillamine-cysteine mixed disulfide as:

$$\text{CSSC} + \text{PS}' \rightleftarrows \text{CS}' + \text{CSSP}$$
$$\text{PSSP} + \text{CS}' \rightleftarrows \text{PS}' + \text{CSSP}$$
$$\text{CSSC} + \text{PSSP} \rightleftarrows 2\ \text{CSSP}$$

CSSC = cystine
CS′ = deprotonated cysteine
PSSP = penicillamine
PS′ = deprotonated penicillamine sulfhydryl
CSSP = penicillamine-cysteine mixed disulfide

In this process, it is assumed that the deprotonated form of penicillamine, PS′, is the active factor in bringing about the disulfide interchange.

Rheumatoid Arthritis—Because CUPRIMINE can cause severe adverse reactions, its use in rheumatoid arthritis should be restricted to patients who have severe, active disease and who have failed to respond to an adequate trial of conventional therapy. Even then, benefit-to-risk ratio should be carefully considered. Other measures, such as rest, physiotherapy, salicylates, and corticosteroids should be used, when indicated, in conjunction with CUPRIMINE (see PRECAUTIONS).

*For quantitative test for serum ceruloplasmin see: Morell, A.G.; Windsor, J.; Sternlieb, I.; Scheinberg, I.H.: Measurement of the concentration of ceruloplasmin in serum by determination of its oxidase activity, in "Laboratory Diagnosis of Liver Disease", F.W. Sunderman; F.W. Sunderman, Jr. (eds.), St. Louis, Warren H. Green, Inc., 1968, pp. 193-195.

Continued on next page

Information on the Merck & Co. products listed on these pages is the full prescribing information from product circulars in use October 1, 1992.

Merck & Co.—Cont.

CONTRAINDICATIONS

Except for the treatment of Wilson's disease or certain cases of cystinuria, use of penicillamine during pregnancy is contraindicated (see WARNINGS).

Although breast milk studies have not been reported in animals or humans, mothers on therapy with penicillamine should not nurse their infants.

Patients with a history of penicillamine-related aplastic anemia or agranulocytosis should not be restarted on penicillamine (see WARNINGS and ADVERSE REACTIONS). Because of its potential for causing renal damage, penicillamine should not be administered to rheumatoid arthritis patients with a history or other evidence of renal insufficiency.

WARNINGS

The use of penicillamine has been associated with fatalities due to certain diseases such as aplastic anemia, agranulocytosis, thrombocytopenia, Goodpasture's syndrome, and myasthenia gravis.

Because of the potential for serious hematological and renal adverse reactions to occur at any time, routine urinalysis, white and differential blood cell count, hemoglobin determination, and direct platelet count must be done every two weeks for at least the first six months of penicillamine therapy and monthly thereafter. Patients should be instructed to report promptly the development of signs and symptoms of granulocytopenia and/or thrombocytopenia such as fever, sore throat, chills, bruising or bleeding. The above laboratory studies should then be promptly repeated.

Leukopenia and thrombocytopenia have been reported to occur in up to five percent of patients during penicillamine therapy. Leukopenia is of the granulocytic series and may or may not be associated with an increase in eosinophils. A confirmed reduction in WBC below $3500/mm^3$ mandates discontinuance of penicillamine therapy. Thrombocytopenia may be on an idiosyncratic basis, with decreased or absent megakaryocytes in the marrow, when it is part of an aplastic anemia. In other cases the thrombocytopenia is presumably on an immune basis since the number of megakaryocytes in the marrow has been reported to be normal or sometimes increased. The development of a platelet count below $100,000/mm^3$, even in the absence of clinical bleeding, requires at least temporary cessation of penicillamine therapy. A progressive fall in either platelet count or WBC in three successive determinations, even though values are still within the normal range, likewise requires at least temporary cessation.

Proteinuria and/or hematuria may develop during therapy and may be warning signs of membranous glomerulopathy which can progress to a nephrotic syndrome. Close observation of these patients is essential. In some patients the proteinuria disappears with continued therapy; in others, penicillamine must be discontinued. When a patient develops proteinuria or hematuria the physician must ascertain whether it is a sign of drug-induced glomerulopathy or is unrelated to penicillamine.

Rheumatoid arthritis patients who develop moderate degrees of proteinuria may be continued cautiously on penicillamine therapy, provided that quantitative 24-hour urinary protein determinations are obtained at intervals of one to two weeks. Penicillamine dosage should not be increased under these circumstances. Proteinuria which exceeds 1 g/24 hours, or proteinuria which is progressively increasing, requires either discontinuance of the drug or a reduction in the dosage. In some patients, proteinuria has been reported to clear following reduction in dosage.

In rheumatoid arthritis patients, penicillamine should be discontinued if unexplained gross hematuria or persistent microscopic hematuria develops.

In patients with Wilson's disease or cystinuria the risks of continued penicillamine therapy in patients manifesting potentially serious urinary abnormalities must be weighed against the expected therapeutic benefits.

When penicillamine is used in cystinuria, an annual x-ray for renal stones is advised. Cystine stones form rapidly, sometimes in six months.

Up to one year or more may be required for any urinary abnormalities to disappear after penicillamine has been discontinued.

Because of rare reports of intrahepatic cholestasis and toxic hepatitis, liver function tests are recommended every six months for the duration of therapy.

Goodpasture's syndrome has occurred rarely. The development of abnormal urinary findings associated with hemoptysis and pulmonary infiltrates on x-ray requires immediate cessation of penicillamine.

Obliterative bronchiolitis has been reported rarely. The patient should be cautioned to report immediately pulmonary symptoms such as exertional dyspnea, unexplained cough or wheezing. Pulmonary function studies should be considered at that time.

Myasthenic syndrome sometimes progressing to myasthenia gravis has been reported. Ptosis and diplopia, with weakness of the extraocular muscles, are often early signs of myasthenia. In the majority of cases, symptoms of myasthenia have receded after withdrawal of penicillamine.

Most of the various forms of pemphigus have occurred during treatment with penicillamine. Pemphigus vulgaris and pemphigus foliaceus are reported most frequently, usually as a late complication of therapy. The seborrhea-like characteristics of pemphigus foliaceus may obscure an early diagnosis. When pemphigus is suspected, CUPRIMINE should be discontinued. Treatment has consisted of high doses of corticosteroids alone or, in some cases, concomitantly with an immunosuppressant. Treatment may be required for only a few weeks or months, but may need to be continued for more than a year.

Once instituted for Wilson's disease or cystinuria, treatment with penicillamine should, as a rule, be continued on a daily basis. Interruptions for even a few days have been followed by sensitivity reactions after reinstitution of therapy.

Use in Pregnancy—Penicillamine has been shown to be teratogenic in rats when given in doses 6 times higher than the highest dose recommended for human use. Skeletal defects, cleft palates and fetal toxicity (resorptions) have been reported.

There are no controlled studies on the use of penicillamine in pregnant women. Although normal outcomes have been reported, characteristic congenital cutis laxa and associated birth defects have been reported in infants born of mothers who received therapy with penicillamine during pregnancy. Penicillamine should be used in women of childbearing potential only when the expected benefits outweigh the possible hazards. Women on therapy with penicillamine who are of childbearing potential should be apprised of this risk, advised to report promptly any missed menstrual periods or other indications of possible pregnancy, and followed closely for early recognition of pregnancy.

Wilson's Disease—Reported experience* shows that continued treatment with penicillamine throughout pregnancy protects the mother against relapse of the Wilson's disease, and that discontinuation of penicillamine has deleterious effects on the mother.

If penicillamine is administered during pregnancy to patients with Wilson's disease, it is recommended that the daily dosage be limited to 1 g. If cesarean section is planned, the daily dosage should be limited to 250 mg during the last six weeks of pregnancy and postoperatively until wound healing is complete.

Cystinuria—If possible, penicillamine should not be given during pregnancy to women with cystinuria (see CONTRA-INDICATIONS). There are reports of women with cystinuria on therapy with penicillamine who gave birth to infants with generalized connective tissue defects who died following abdominal surgery. If stones continue to form in these patients, the benefits of therapy to the mother must be evaluated against the risk to the fetus.

Rheumatoid Arthritis—Penicillamine should not be administered to rheumatoid arthritis patients who are pregnant (see CONTRAINDICATIONS) and should be discontinued promptly in patients in whom pregnancy is suspected or diagnosed.

There is a report that a woman with rheumatoid arthritis treated with less than one gram a day of penicillamine during pregnancy gave birth (cesarean delivery) to an infant with growth retardation, flattened face with broad nasal bridge, low set ears, short neck with loose skin folds, and unusually lax body skin.

---

*Scheinberg, I.H., Sternlieb, I.: N. Engl. J. Med. *293* : 1300-1302, Dec. 18, 1975.

PRECAUTIONS

Some patients may experience drug fever, a marked febrile response to penicillamine, usually in the second to third week following initiation of therapy. Drug fever may sometimes be accompanied by a macular cutaneous eruption.

In the case of drug fever in patients with Wilson's disease or cystinuria, penicillamine should be temporarily discontinued until the reaction subsides. Then penicillamine should be reinstituted with a small dose that is gradually increased until the desired dosage is attained. Systemic steroid therapy may be necessary, and is usually helpful, in such patients in whom toxic reactions develop a second or third time.

In the case of drug fever in rheumatoid arthritis patients, because other treatments are available, penicillamine should be discontinued and another therapeutic alternative tried since experience indicates that the febrile reaction will recur in a very high percentage of patients upon readministration of penicillamine.

The skin and mucous membranes should be observed for allergic reactions. Early and late rashes have occurred.

Early rash occurs during the first few months of treatment and is more common. It is usually a generalized pruritic, erythematous, maculopapular or morbilliform rash and resembles the allergic rash seen with other drugs. Early rash usually disappears within days after stopping penicillamine and seldom recurs when the drug is restarted at a lower dosage. Pruritus and early rash may often be controlled by the concomitant administration of antihistamines. Less commonly, a late rash may be seen, usually after six months or more of treatment, and requires discontinuation of penicillamine. It is usually on the trunk, is accompanied by intense pruritus, and is usually unresponsive to topical corticosteroid therapy. Late rash may take weeks to disappear after penicillamine is stopped and usually recurs if the drug is restarted.

The appearance of a drug eruption accompanied by fever, arthralgia, lymphadenopathy or other allergic manifestations usually requires discontinuation of penicillamine.

Certain patients will develop a positive antinuclear antibody (ANA) test and some of these may show a lupus erythematosus-like syndrome similar to drug-induced lupus associated with other drugs. The lupus erythematosus-like syndrome is not associated with hypocomplementemia and may be present without nephropathy. The development of a positive ANA test does not mandate discontinuance of the drug; however, the physician should be alerted to the possibility that a lupus erythematosus-like syndrome may develop in the future.

Some patients may develop oral ulcerations which in some cases have the appearance of aphthous stomatitis. The stomatitis usually recurs on rechallenge but often clears on a lower dosage. Although rare, cheilosis, glossitis and gingivostomatitis have also been reported. These oral lesions are frequently dose-related and may preclude further increase in penicillamine dosage or require discontinuation of the drug.

Hypogeusia (a blunting or diminution in taste perception) has occurred in some patients. This may last two to three months or more and may develop into a total loss of taste; however, it is usually self-limited despite continued penicillamine treatment. Such taste impairment is rare in patients with Wilson's disease.

Penicillamine should not be used in patients who are receiving concurrently gold therapy, antimalarial or cytotoxic drugs, oxyphenbutazone or phenylbutazone because these drugs are also associated with similar serious hematologic and renal adverse reactions. Patients who have had gold salt therapy discontinued due to a major toxic reaction may be at greater risk of serious adverse reactions with penicillamine but not necessarily of the same type.

Patients who are allergic to penicillin may theoretically have cross-sensitivity to penicillamine. The possibility of reactions from contamination of penicillamine by trace amounts of penicillin has been eliminated now that penicillamine is being produced synthetically rather than as a degradation product of penicillin.

Because of their dietary restrictions, patients with Wilson's disease and cystinuria should be given 25 mg/day of pyridoxine during therapy, since penicillamine increases the requirement for this vitamin. Patients also may receive benefit from a multivitamin preparation, although there is no evidence that deficiency of any vitamin other than pyridoxine is associated with penicillamine. In Wilson's disease, multivitamin preparations must be copper-free.

Rheumatoid arthritis patients whose nutrition is impaired should also be given a daily supplement of pyridoxine. Mineral supplements should not be given, since they may block the response to penicillamine.

Iron deficiency may develop, especially in children and in menstruating women. In Wilson's disease, this may be a result of adding the effects of the low copper diet, which is probably also low in iron, and the penicillamine to the effects of blood loss or growth. In cystinuria, a low methionine diet may contribute to iron deficiency, since it is necessarily low in protein. If necessary, iron may be given in short courses, but a period of two hours should elapse between administration of penicillamine and iron, since orally administered iron has been shown to reduce the effects of penicillamine.

Penicillamine causes an increase in the amount of soluble collagen. In the rat this results in inhibition of normal healing and also a decrease in tensile strength of intact skin. In man this may be the cause of increased skin friability at sites especially subject to pressure or trauma, such as shoulders, elbows, knees, toes, and buttocks. Extravasations of blood may occur and may appear as purpuric areas, with external bleeding if the skin is broken, or as vesicles containing dark blood. Neither type is progressive. There is no apparent association with bleeding elsewhere in the body and no associated coagulation defect has been found. Therapy with penicillamine may be continued in the presence of these lesions. They may not recur if dosage is reduced. Other reported effects probably due to the action of penicillamine on collagen are excessive wrinkling of the skin and development of small, white papules at venipuncture and surgical sites.

The effects of penicillamine on collagen and elastin make it advisable to consider a reduction in dosage to 250 mg/day,

when surgery is contemplated. Reinstitution of full therapy should be delayed until wound healing is complete.

Carcinogenesis—Long-term animal carcinogenicity studies have not been done with penicillamine. There is a report that five of ten autoimmune disease-prone NZB hybrid mice developed lymphocytic leukemia after 6 months' intraperitoneal treatment with a dose of 400 mg/kg penicillamine 5 days per week.

Nursing Mothers —See CONTRAINDICATIONS.

Usage in Children —The efficacy of CUPRIMINE in juvenile rheumatoid arthritis has not been established.

ADVERSE REACTIONS

Penicillamine is a drug with a high incidence of untoward reactions, some of which are potentially fatal. Therefore, it is mandatory that patients receiving penicillamine therapy remain under close medical supervision throughout the period of drug administration (see WARNINGS and PRECAUTIONS).

Reported incidences (%) for the most commonly occurring adverse reactions in rheumatoid arthritis patients are noted, based on 17 representative clinical trials reported in the literature (1270 patients).

Allergic—Generalized pruritus, early and late rashes (5%), pemphigus (see WARNINGS), and drug eruptions which may be accompanied by fever, arthralgia, or lymphadenopathy have occurred (see WARNINGS and PRECAUTIONS). Some patients may show a lupus erythematosus-like syndrome similar to drug-induced lupus produced by other pharmacological agents (see PRECAUTIONS).

Urticaria and exfoliative dermatitis have occurred.

Thyroiditis has been reported; hypoglycemia in association with anti-insulin antibodies has been reported. These reactions are extremely rare.

Some patients may develop a migratory polyarthralgia, often with objective synovitis (see DOSAGE AND ADMINISTRATION).

Gastrointestinal—Anorexia, epigastric pain, nausea, vomiting, or occasional diarrhea may occur (17%).

Isolated cases of reactivated peptic ulcer have occurred, as have hepatic dysfunction and pancreatitis. Intrahepatic cholestasis and toxic hepatitis have been reported rarely. There have been a few reports of increased serum alkaline phosphatase, lactic dehydrogenase, and positive cephalin flocculation and thymol turbidity tests.

Some patients may report a blunting, diminution, or total loss of taste perception (12%); or may develop oral ulcerations. Although rare, cheilosis, glossitis, and gingivostomatitis have been reported (see PRECAUTIONS).

Gastrointestinal side effects are usually reversible following cessation of therapy.

Hematological—Penicillamine can cause bone marrow depression (see WARNINGS). Leukopenia (2%) and thrombocytopenia (4%) have occurred. Fatalities have been reported as a result of thrombocytopenia, agranulocytosis, aplastic anemia, and sideroblastic anemia.

Thrombotic thrombocytopenic purpura, hemolytic anemia, red cell aplasia, monocytosis, leukocytosis, eosinophilia, and thrombocytosis have also been reported.

Renal—Patients on penicillamine therapy may develop proteinuria (6%) and/or hematuria which, in some, may progress to the development of the nephrotic syndrome as a result of an immune complex membranous glomerulopathy (see WARNINGS).

Central Nervous System—Tinnitus, optic neuritis and peripheral sensory and motor neuropathies (including polyradiculoneuropathy, i.e., Guillain-Barre syndrome) have been reported. Muscular weakness may or may not occur with the peripheral neuropathies. Visual and psychic disturbances have been reported.

Neuromuscular—Myasthenia gravis (see WARNINGS).

Other—Adverse reactions that have been reported rarely include thrombophlebitis; hyperpyrexia (see PRECAUTIONS); falling hair or alopecia; lichen planus; polymyositis; dermatomyositis; mammary hyperplasia; elastosis perforans serpiginosa; toxic epidermal necrolysis; anetoderma (cutaneous macular atrophy); and Goodpasture's syndrome, a severe and ultimately fatal glomerulonephritis associated with intra-alveolar hemorrhage (see WARNINGS). Fatal renal vasculitis has also been reported. Allergic alveolitis, obliterative bronchiolitis, interstitial pneumonitis and pulmonary fibrosis have been reported in patients with severe rheumatoid arthritis, some of whom were receiving penicillamine. Bronchial asthma also has been reported.

Increased skin friability, excessive wrinkling of skin, and development of small white papules at venipuncture and surgical sites have been reported (see PRECAUTIONS).

The chelating action of the drug may cause increased excretion of other heavy metals such as zinc, mercury and lead. There have been reports associating penicillamine with leukemia. However, circumstances involved in these reports are such that a cause and effect relationship to the drug has not been established.

DOSAGE AND ADMINISTRATION

In all patients receiving penicillamine, it is important that CUPRIMINE be given on an empty stomach, at least one hour before meals or two hours after meals, and at least one hour apart from any other drug, food, or milk. Because penicillamine increases the requirement for pyridoxine, patients may require a daily supplement of pyridoxine (see PRECAUTIONS).

Wilson's Disease —Optimal dosage can be determined by measurement of urinary copper excretion and the determination of free copper in the serum. The urine must be collected in copper-free glassware, and should be quantitatively analyzed for copper before and soon after initiation of therapy with CUPRIMINE.

Determination of 24-hour urinary copper excretion is of greatest value in the first week of therapy with penicillamine. In the absence of any drug reaction, a dose between 0.75 and 1.5 g that results in an initial 24-hour cupriuresis of over 2 mg should be continued for about three months, by which time the most reliable method of monitoring maintenance treatment is the determination of free copper in the serum. This equals the difference between quantitatively determined total copper and ceruloplasmin-copper. Adequately treated patients will usually have less than 10 mcg free copper/dL of serum. It is seldom necessary to exceed a dosage of 2 g/day. If the patient is intolerant to therapy with CUPRIMINE, alternative treatment is trientine hydrochloride.

In patients who cannot tolerate as much as 1 g/day initially, initiating dosage with 250 mg/day, and increasing gradually to the requisite amount, gives closer control of the effects of the drug and may help to reduce the incidence of adverse reactions.

Cystinuria —It is recommended that CUPRIMINE be used along with conventional therapy. By reducing urinary cystine, it decreases crystalluria and stone formation. In some instances, it has been reported to decrease the size of, and even to dissolve, stones already formed.

The usual dosage of CUPRIMINE in the treatment of cystinuria is 2 g/day for adults, with a range of 1 to 4 g/day. For children, dosage can be based on 30 mg/kg/day. The total daily amount should be divided into four doses. If four equal doses are not feasible, give the larger portion at bedtime. If adverse reactions necessitate a reduction in dosage, it is important to retain the bedtime dose.

Initiating dosage with 250 mg/day, and increasing gradually to the requisite amount, gives closer control of the effects of the drug and may help to reduce the incidence of adverse reactions.

In addition to taking CUPRIMINE, patients should drink copiously. It is especially important to drink about a pint of fluid at bedtime and another pint once during the night when urine is more concentrated and more acid than during the day. The greater the fluid intake, the lower the required dosage of CUPRIMINE.

Dosage must be individualized to an amount that limits cystine excretion to 100–200 mg/day in those with no history of stones, and below 100 mg/day in those who have had stone formation and/or pain. Thus, in determining dosage, the inherent tubular defect, the patient's size, age, and rate of growth, and his diet and water intake all must be taken into consideration.

The standard nitroprusside cyanide test has been reported useful as a qualitative measure of the effective dose*: Add 2 mL of freshly prepared 5 percent sodium cyanide to 5 mL of a 24-hour aliquot of protein-free urine and let stand ten minutes. Add 5 drops of freshly prepared 5 percent sodium nitroprusside and mix. Cystine will turn the mixture magenta. If the result is negative, it can be assumed that cystine excretion is less than 100 mg/g creatinine.

Although penicillamine is rarely excreted unchanged, it also will turn the mixture magenta. If there is any question as to which substance is causing the reaction, a ferric chloride test can be done to eliminate doubt: Add 3 percent ferric chloride dropwise to the urine. Penicillamine will turn the urine an immediate and quickly fading blue. Cystine will not produce any change in appearance.

---

*Lotz, M., Potts, J.T. and Bartter, F.C.: Brit. Med. J. 2 :521, Aug. 28, 1965 (in Medical Memoranda).

Rheumatoid Arthritis —The principal rule of treatment with CUPRIMINE in rheumatoid arthritis is patience. The onset of therapeutic response is typically delayed. Two or three months may be required before the first evidence of a clinical response is noted (see CLINICAL PHARMACOLOGY).

When treatment with CUPRIMINE has been interrupted because of adverse reactions or other reasons, the drug should be reintroduced cautiously by starting with a lower dosage and increasing slowly.

Initial Therapy—The currently recommended dosage regimen in rheumatoid arthritis begins with a single daily dose of 125 mg or 250 mg which is thereafter increased at one to three month intervals, by 125 mg or 250 mg/day, as patient

response and tolerance indicate. If a satisfactory remission of symptoms is achieved, the dose associated with the remission should be continued (see *Maintenance Therapy*). If there is no improvement and there are no signs of potentially serious toxicity after two to three months of treatment with doses of 500–750 mg/day, increases of 250 mg/day at two to three month intervals may be continued until a satisfactory remission occurs (see *Maintenance Therapy*) or signs of toxicity develop (see WARNINGS and PRECAUTIONS). If there is no discernible improvement after three to four months of treatment with 1000 to 1500 mg of penicillamine/day, it may be assumed the patient will not respond and CUPRIMINE should be discontinued.

Maintenance Therapy—The maintenance dosage of CUPRIMINE must be individualized, and may require adjustment during the course of treatment. Many patients respond satisfactorily to a dosage within the 500–750 mg/day range. Some need less.

Changes in maintenance dosage levels may not be reflected clinically or in the erythrocyte sedimentation rate for two to three months after each dosage adjustment.

Some patients will subsequently require an increase in the maintenance dosage to achieve maximal disease suppression. In those patients who do respond, but who evidence incomplete suppression of their disease after the first six to nine months of treatment, the daily dosage of CUPRIMINE may be increased by 125 mg or 250 mg/day at three-month intervals. It is unusual in current practice to employ a dosage in excess of 1 g/day, but up to 1.5 g/day has sometimes been required.

Management of Exacerbations—During the course of treatment some patients may experience an exacerbation of disease activity following an initial good response. These may be self-limited and can subside within twelve weeks. They are usually controlled by the addition of non-steroidal anti-inflammatory drugs, and only if the patient has demonstrated a true "escape" phenomenon (as evidenced by failure of the flare to subside within this time period) should an increase in the maintenance dose ordinarily be considered.

In the rheumatoid patient, migratory polyarthralgia due to penicillamine is extremely difficult to differentiate from an exacerbation of the rheumatoid arthritis. Discontinuance or a substantial reduction in dosage of CUPRIMINE for up to several weeks will usually determine which of these processes is responsible for the arthralgia.

Duration of Therapy—The optimum duration of therapy with CUPRIMINE in rheumatoid arthritis has not been determined. If the patient has been in remission for six months or more, a gradual, stepwise dosage reduction in decrements of 125 mg or 250 mg/day at approximately three month intervals may be attempted.

Concomitant Drug Therapy—CUPRIMINE should not be used in patients who are receiving gold therapy, antimalarial or cytotoxic drugs, oxyphenbutazone, or phenylbutazone (see PRECAUTIONS). Other measures, such as salicylates, other non-steroidal anti-inflammatory drugs, or systemic corticosteroids, may be continued when penicillamine is initiated. After improvement commences, analgesic and anti-inflammatory drugs may be slowly discontinued as symptoms permit. Steroid withdrawal must be done gradually, and many months of treatment with CUPRIMINE may be required before steroids can be completely eliminated.

Dosage Frequency—Based on clinical experience dosages up to 500 mg/day can be given as a single daily dose. Dosages in excess of 500 mg/day should be administered in divided doses.

HOW SUPPLIED

No. 3299—Capsules CUPRIMINE, 250 mg, are ivory-colored capsules containing a white or nearly white powder, and are coded MSD 602. They are supplied as follows:
NDC 0006-0602-68 in bottles of 100
(6505-01-049-9494, 250 mg 100's).
   Shown in Product Identification Section, page 419
No. 3350—Capsules CUPRIMINE, 125 mg, are opaque ivory and gray capsules containing a white or nearly white powder, and are coded MSD 672. They are supplied as follows:
NDC 0006-0672-68 in bottles of 100.
   Shown in Product Identification Section, page 419
Storage
Keep container tightly closed.
     A.H.F.S. Category: 64:00
  DC 7412338   Issued March 1989
COPYRIGHT © MERCK & CO., INC., 1985, 1989
All rights reserved

Continued on next page

Information on the Merck & Co. products listed on these pages is the full prescribing information from product circulars in use October 1, 1992.

Merck & Co.—Cont.

DARANIDE® Tablets
(Dichlorphenamide), U.S.P.   ℞

DESCRIPTION

DARANIDE* (Dichlorphenamide) is an oral carbonic anhydrase inhibitor. Dichlorphenamide, a dichlorinated benzenedisulfonamide, is known chemically as 4,5-dichloro-1,3-benzenedisulfonamide. Its empirical formula is $C_6H_6Cl_2N_2O_4S_2$ and its structural formula is:

Dichlorphenamide is a white or practically white, crystalline compound with a molecular weight of 305.16. It is very slightly soluble in water but soluble in dilute solutions of sodium carbonate and sodium hydroxide. Dilute alkaline solutions of dichlorphenamide are stable at room temperature.

DARANIDE is supplied as tablets, for oral administration, each containing 50 mg dichlorphenamide. Inactive ingredients are D&C Yellow 10, lactose, magnesium stearate, and starch.

*Registered trademark of MERCK & CO., INC.

CLINICAL PHARMACOLOGY

Carbonic anhydrase inhibitors reduce intraocular pressure by partially suppressing the secretion of aqueous humor (inflow), although the mechanism by which they do this is not fully understood. Evidence suggests that HCO_3^- ions are produced in the ciliary body by hydration of carbon dioxide under the influence of carbonic anhydrase and diffuse into the posterior chamber with Na^+ ions. The aqueous fluid contains more Na^+ and HCO_3^- ions than does plasma and consequently is hypertonic. Water is attracted to the posterior chamber by osmosis. Systemic administration of a carbonic anhydrase inhibitor has been shown to inactivate carbonic anhydrase in the ciliary body of the rabbit's eye and to reduce the high concentration of HCO_3^- ions in ocular fluids. As is the case with all carbonic anhydrase inhibitors, DARANIDE in high doses causes some decrease in renal blood flow and glomerular filtration rate.

In man, DARANIDE begins to act within an hour and maximal effect is observed in two to four hours. The lowered intraocular tension may be maintained for approximately 6 to 12 hours.

INDICATIONS AND USAGE

For adjunctive treatment of: chronic simple (open-angle) glaucoma, secondary glaucoma, and preoperatively in acute angle-closure glaucoma where delay of surgery is desired in order to lower intraocular pressure.

CONTRAINDICATIONS

DARANIDE is contraindicated in hepatic insufficiency, renal failure, adrenocortical insufficiency, hyperchloremic acidosis, or in conditions in which serum levels of sodium or potassium are depressed. DARANIDE should not be used in patients with severe pulmonary obstruction who are unable to increase their alveolar ventilation since their acidosis may be increased.

DARANIDE is contraindicated in patients who are hypersensitive to this product.

PRECAUTIONS

General
Potassium excretion is increased by DARANIDE and hypokalemia may develop with brisk diuresis, when severe cirrhosis is present, or during concomitant use of steroids or ACTH.

Interference with adequate oral electrolyte intake will also contribute to hypokalemia. Hypokalemia can sensitize or exaggerate the response of the heart to the toxic effects of digitalis (e.g., increased ventricular irritability). Hypokalemia may be avoided or treated by use of potassium supplements such as foods with a high potassium content. DARANIDE should be used with caution in patients with respiratory acidosis.

Drug Interactions
Caution is advised in patients receiving concomitant high-dose aspirin and carbonic anhydrase inhibitors, as anorexia, tachypnea, lethargy and coma have been rarely reported due to a possible drug interaction.

Carcinogenesis, Mutagenesis, Impairment of Fertility
Long-term studies in animals have not been performed to evaluate the effects upon fertility or carcinogenic potential of DARANIDE.

Pregnancy
Pregnancy Category C. Diclorphenamide has been shown to be teratogenic in the rat (skeletal anomalies) when given in doses 100 times the human dose. There are no adequate and well-controlled studies in pregnant women. DARANIDE should not be used in women of childbearing age or in pregnancy, especially during the first trimester, unless the potential benefits outweigh the potential risks.

Nursing Mothers
It is not known whether diclorphenamide is excreted in human milk. Because many drugs are excreted in human milk, caution should be exercised when diclorphenamide is administered to a nursing woman.

Pediatric Use
Safety and effectiveness in children have not been established.

ADVERSE REACTIONS

Certain side effects characteristic of carbonic anhydrase inhibitors may occur with DARANIDE, particularly with increasing doses. The most common effects include gastrointestinal disturbances (anorexia, nausea, and vomiting), drowsiness and paresthesias.

Included in the listing which follows are some adverse reactions which have not been reported with DARANIDE. However, pharmacological similarities among the carbonic anhydrase inhibitors make it advisable to consider the following reactions when diclorphenamide is administered. *Central Nervous System/Psychiatric:* ataxia, tremor, tinnitus, headache, weakness, nervousness, globus hystericus, lassitude, depression, confusion, disorientation, dizziness; *Gastrointestinal:* constipation, hepatic insufficiency; *Metabolic:* loss of weight, metabolic acidosis, electrolyte imbalance (hypokalemia, hyperchloremia), hyperuricemia; *Hypersensitivity:* skin eruptions, pruritus, fever; *Hematologic:* leukopenia, agranulocytosis, thrombocytopenia; *Genitourinary:* urinary frequency, renal colic, renal calculi, phosphaturia.

OVERDOSAGE

The oral LD_{50} of DARANIDE is 1710 and 2600 mg/kg in the mouse and rat respectively.

Symptoms of overdosage or toxicity may include drowsiness, anorexia, nausea, vomiting, dizziness, paresthesias, ataxia, tremor and tinnitus.

In the event of overdosage, induce emesis or perform gastric lavage. The electrolyte disturbance most likely to be encountered from overdosage is hyperchloremic acidosis that may respond to bicarbonate administration. Potassium supplementation may be required. The patient should be carefully observed and given supportive treatment.

DOSAGE AND ADMINISTRATION

DARANIDE is usually given in conjunction with topical ocular hypotensive agents. In acute angle-closure glaucoma, it may be used together with miotics and osmotic agents in an attempt to reduce intraocular tension rapidly. If this is not quickly relieved, surgery may be mandatory.

Dosage must be adjusted carefully to meet the requirements of the individual patient. A priming dose of 100 to 200 mg of DARANIDE (2 to 4 tablets) is suggested for adults, followed by 100 mg (2 tablets) every 12 hours until the desired response has been obtained. The recommended maintenance dosage for adults is 25 to 50 mg (½ to 1 tablet) once to three times daily.

HOW SUPPLIED

No. 3256—Tablets DARANIDE, 50 mg each, are yellow, round, scored, compressed tablets, coded MSD 49. They are supplied as follows:
NDC 0006-0049-68 bottles of 100.
Shown in Product Identification Section, page 419
A.H.F.S. Category: 52:10
DC 7412517   Issued November 1986
COPYRIGHT © MERCK & CO., INC., 1985
All rights reserved

DECADRON® Elixir   ℞
(Dexamethasone), U.S.P.

DESCRIPTION

Glucocorticoids are adrenocortical steroids, both naturally occurring and synthetic, which are readily absorbed from the gastrointestinal tract.

Dexamethasone, a synthetic adrenocortical steroid, is a white to practically white, odorless, crystalline powder. It is stable in air. It is practically insoluble in water. The molecular weight is 392.47. It is designated chemically as 9-fluoro-11β,17,21-trihydroxy-16α-methylpregna -1, 4- diene-3,20-dione. The empirical formula is $C_{22}H_{29}FO_5$ and the structural formula is:

DECADRON* (Dexamethasone) elixir contains 0.5 mg of dexamethasone in each 5 mL. Benzoic acid, 0.1%, is added as a preservative. It also contains alcohol 5%. Inactive ingredients are FD&C Red 40, flavors, glycerin, purified water, and sodium saccharin.

*Registered trademark of MERCK & CO., INC.

ACTIONS

Naturally occurring glucocorticoids (hydrocortisone and cortisone), which also have salt-retaining properties, are used as replacement therapy in adrenocortical deficiency states. Their synthetic analogs, including dexamethasone, are primarily used for their potent anti-inflammatory effects in disorders of many organ systems.

Glucocorticoids cause profound and varied metabolic effects. In addition, they modify the body's immune responses to diverse stimuli.

At equipotent anti-inflammatory doses, dexamethasone almost completely lacks the sodium-retaining property of hydrocortisone and closely related derivatives of hydrocortisone.

INDICATIONS

1. *Endocrine Disorders*
   Primary or secondary adrenocortical insufficiency (hydrocortisone or cortisone is the first choice; synthetic analogs may be used in conjunction with mineralocorticoids where applicable; in infancy mineralocorticoid supplementation is of particular importance)
      Congenital adrenal hyperplasia
      Nonsuppurative thyroiditis
      Hypercalcemia associated with cancer
2. *Rheumatic Disorders*
   As adjunctive therapy for short-term administration (to tide the patient over an acute episode or exacerbation) in:
      Psoriatic arthritis
      Rheumatoid arthritis, including juvenile rheumatoid arthritis (selected cases may require low-dose maintenance therapy)
      Ankylosing spondylitis
      Acute and subacute bursitis
      Acute nonspecific tenosynovitis
      Acute gouty arthritis
      Post-traumatic osteoarthritis
      Synovitis of osteoarthritis
      Epicondylitis
3. *Collagen Diseases*
   During an exacerbation or as maintenance therapy in selected cases of—
      Systemic lupus erythematosus
      Acute rheumatic carditis
4. *Dermatologic Diseases*
      Pemphigus
      Bullous dermatitis herpetiformis
      Severe erythema multiforme (Stevens-Johnson syndrome)
      Exfoliative dermatitis
      Mycosis fungoides
      Severe psoriasis
      Severe seborrheic dermatitis
5. *Allergic States*
   Control of severe or incapacitating allergic conditions intractable to adequate trials of conventional treatment:
      Seasonal or perennial allergic rhinitis
      Bronchial asthma
      Contact dermatitis
      Atopic dermatitis
      Serum sickness
      Drug hypersensitivity reactions

6. *Ophthalmic Diseases*
Severe acute and chronic allergic and inflammatory processes involving the eye and its adnexa, such as—
    Allergic conjunctivitis
    Keratitis
    Allergic corneal marginal ulcers
    Herpes zoster ophthalmicus
    Iritis and iridocyclitis
    Chorioretinitis
    Anterior segment inflammation
    Diffuse posterior uveitis and choroiditis
    Optic neuritis
    Sympathetic ophthalmia
7. *Respiratory Diseases*
    Symptomatic sarcoidosis
    Loeffler's syndrome not manageable by other means
    Berylliosis
    Fulminating or disseminated pulmonary tuberculosis when used concurrently with appropriate antituberculous chemotherapy
    Aspiration pneumonitis
8. *Hematologic Disorders*
    Idiopathic thrombocytopenic purpura in adults
    Secondary thrombocytopenia in adults
    Acquired (autoimmune) hemolytic anemia
    Erythroblastopenia (RBC anemia)
    Congenital (erythroid) hypoplastic anemia
9. *Neoplastic Diseases*
For palliative management of:
    Leukemias and lymphomas in adults
    Acute leukemia of childhood
10. *Edematous States*
To induce a diuresis or remission of proteinuria in the nephrotic syndrome, without uremia, of the idiopathic type or that due to lupus erythematosus
11. *Gastrointestinal Diseases*
To tide the patient over a critical period of the disease in:
    Ulcerative colitis
    Regional enteritis
12. *Miscellaneous*
Tuberculous meningitis with subarachnoid block or impending block when used concurrently with appropriate antituberculous chemotherapy
Trichinosis with neurologic or myocardial involvement
13. *Diagnostic testing of adrenocortical hyperfunction.*

CONTRAINDICATIONS

Systemic fungal infections
Hypersensitivity to this product

WARNINGS

In patients on corticosteroid therapy subjected to unusual stress, increased dosage of rapidly acting corticosteroids before, during, and after the stressful situation is indicated.
Drug-induced secondary adrenocortical insufficiency may result from too rapid withdrawal of corticosteroids and may be minimized by gradual reduction of dosage. This type of relative insufficiency may persist for months after discontinuation of therapy; therefore, in any situation of stress occurring during that period, hormone therapy should be reinstituted. If the patient is receiving steroids already, dosage may have to be increased. Since mineralocorticoid secretion may be impaired, salt and/or a mineralocorticoid should be administered concurrently.
Corticosteroids may mask some signs of infection, and new infections may appear during their use. There may be decreased resistance and inability to localize infection when corticosteroids are used. Moreover, corticosteroids may affect the nitroblue-tetrazolium test for bacterial infection and produce false negative results.
In cerebral malaria, a double-blind trial has shown that the use of corticosteroids is associated with prolongation of coma and a higher incidence of pneumonia and gastrointestinal bleeding.
Corticosteroids may activate latent amebiasis. Therefore, it is recommended that latent or active amebiasis be ruled out before initiating corticosteroid therapy in any patient who has spent time in the tropics or any patient with unexplained diarrhea.
Prolonged use of corticosteroids may produce posterior subcapsular cataracts, glaucoma with possible damage to the optic nerves, and may enhance the establishment of secondary ocular infections due to fungi or viruses.
Usage in pregnancy: Since adequate human reproduction studies have not been done with corticosteroids, use of these drugs in pregnancy or in women of childbearing potential requires that the anticipated benefits be weighed against the possible hazards to the mother and embryo or fetus. Infants born of mothers who have received substantial doses of corticosteroids during pregnancy should be carefully observed for signs of hypoadrenalism.

Corticosteroids appear in breast milk and could suppress growth, interfere with endogenous corticosteroid production, or cause other unwanted effects. Mothers taking pharmacologic doses of corticosteroids should be advised not to nurse.
Average and large doses of hydrocortisone or cortisone can cause elevation of blood pressure, salt and water retention, and increased excretion of potassium. These effects are less likely to occur with the synthetic derivatives except when used in large doses. Dietary salt restriction and potassium supplementation may be necessary. All corticosteroids increase calcium excretion.
Administration of live virus vaccines, including smallpox, is contraindicated in individuals receiving immunosuppressive doses of corticosteroids. If inactivated viral or bacterial vaccines are administered to individuals receiving immunosuppressive doses of corticosteroids, the expected serum antibody response may not be obtained. However, immunization procedures may be undertaken in patients who are receiving corticosteroids as replacement therapy, e.g., for Addison's disease.
The use of DECADRON elixir in active tuberculosis should be restricted to those cases of fulminating or disseminated tuberculosis in which the corticosteroid is used for the management of the disease in conjunction with an appropriate antituberculous regimen.
If corticosteroids are indicated in patients with latent tuberculosis or tuberculin reactivity, close observation is necessary as reactivation of the disease may occur. During prolonged corticosteroid therapy, these patients should receive chemoprophylaxis.
Literature reports suggest an apparent association between use of corticosteroids and left ventricular free wall rupture after a recent myocardial infarction; therefore, therapy with corticosteroids should be used with great caution in these patients.

PRECAUTIONS

Following prolonged therapy, withdrawal of corticosteroids may result in symptoms of the corticosteroid withdrawal syndrome including fever, myalgia, arthralgia, and malaise. This may occur in patients even without evidence of adrenal insufficiency.
There is an enhanced effect of corticosteroids in patients with hypothyroidism and in those with cirrhosis.
Corticosteroids should be used cautiously in patients with ocular herpes simplex because of possible corneal perforation.
The lowest possible dose of corticosteroid should be used to control the condition under treatment, and when reduction in dosage is possible, the reduction should be gradual.
Psychic derangements may appear when corticosteroids are used, ranging from euphoria, insomnia, mood swings, personality changes, and severe depression, to frank psychotic manifestations. Also, existing emotional instability or psychotic tendencies may be aggravated by corticosteroids.
Aspirin should be used cautiously in conjunction with corticosteroids in hypoprothrombinemia.
Steroids should be used with caution in nonspecific ulcerative colitis, if there is a probability of impending perforation, abscess, or other pyogenic infection, diverticulitis, fresh intestinal anastomoses, active or latent peptic ulcer, renal insufficiency, hypertension, osteoporosis, and myasthenia gravis. Signs of peritoneal irritation following gastrointestinal perforation in patients receiving large doses of corticosteroids may be minimal or absent. Fat embolism has been reported as a possible complication of hypercortisonism.
When large doses are given, some authorities advise that corticosteroids be taken with meals and antacids taken between meals to help to prevent peptic ulcer.
Growth and development of infants and children on prolonged corticosteroid therapy should be carefully observed.
Steroids may increase or decrease motility and number of spermatozoa in some patients.
Phenytoin, phenobarbital, ephedrine, and rifampin may enhance the metabolic clearance of corticosteroids, resulting in decreased blood levels and lessened physiologic activity, thus requiring adjustment in corticosteroid dosage. These interactions may interfere with dexamethasone suppression tests which should be interpreted with caution during administration of these drugs.
False-negative results in the dexamethasone suppression test (DST) in patients being treated with indomethacin have been reported. Thus, results of the DST should be interpreted with caution in these patients.
The prothrombin time should be checked frequently in patients who are receiving corticosteroids and coumarin anticoagulants at the same time because of reports that corticosteroids have altered the response to these anticoagulants. Studies have shown that the usual effect produced by adding corticosteroids is inhibition of response to coumarins, although there have been some conflicting reports of potentiation not substantiated by studies.

When corticosteroids are administered concomitantly with potassium-depleting diuretics, patients should be observed closely for development of hypokalemia.

ADVERSE REACTIONS

Fluid and Electrolyte Disturbances
    Sodium retention
    Fluid retention
    Congestive heart failure in susceptible patients
    Potassium loss
    Hypokalemic alkalosis
    Hypertension
Musculoskeletal
    Muscle weakness
    Steroid myopathy
    Loss of muscle mass
    Osteoporosis
    Vertebral compression fractures
    Aseptic necrosis of femoral and humeral heads
    Pathologic fracture of long bones
    Tendon rupture
Gastrointestinal
    Peptic ulcer with possible perforation and hemorrhage
    Perforation of the small and large bowel, particularly in patients with inflammatory bowel disease
    Pancreatitis
    Abdominal distention
    Ulcerative esophagitis
Dermatologic
    Impaired wound healing
    Thin fragile skin
    Petechiae and ecchymoses
    Erythema
    Increased sweating
    May suppress reactions to skin tests
    Other cutaneous reactions, such as allergic dermatitis, urticaria, angioneurotic edema
Neurologic
    Convulsions
    Increased intracranial pressure with papilledema (pseudotumor cerebri) usually after treatment
    Vertigo
    Headache
    Psychic disturbances
Endocrine
    Menstrual irregularities
    Development of cushingoid state
    Suppression of growth in children
    Secondary adrenocortical and pituitary unresponsiveness, particularly in times of stress, as in trauma, surgery, or illness
    Decreased carbohydrate tolerance
    Manifestations of latent diabetes mellitus
    Increased requirements for insulin or oral hypoglycemic agents in diabetics
    Hirsutism
Ophthalmic
    Posterior subcapsular cataracts
    Increased intraocular pressure
    Glaucoma
    Exophthalmos
Metabolic
    Negative nitrogen balance due to protein catabolism
Cardiovascular
    Myocardial rupture following recent myocardial infarction (see WARNINGS).
Other
    Hypersensitivity
    Thromboembolism
    Weight gain
    Increased appetite
    Nausea
    Malaise
    Hiccups

OVERDOSAGE

Reports of acute toxicity and/or death following overdosage of glucocorticoids are rare. In the event of overdosage, no specific antidote is available; treatment is supportive and symptomatic.
The oral LD_{50} of dexamethasone in female mice was 6.5 g/kg.

Continued on next page

Information on the Merck & Co. products listed on these pages is the full prescribing information from product circulars in use October 1, 1992.

Merck & Co.—Cont.

DOSAGE AND ADMINISTRATION

For oral administration

DOSAGE REQUIREMENTS ARE VARIABLE AND MUST BE INDIVIDUALIZED ON THE BASIS OF THE DISEASE AND THE RESPONSE OF THE PATIENT.

The initial dosage varies from 0.75 to 9 mg a day depending on the disease being treated. In less severe diseases doses lower than 0.75 mg may suffice, while in severe diseases doses higher than 9 mg may be required. The initial dosage should be maintained or adjusted until the patient's response is satisfactory. If satisfactory clinical response does not occur after a reasonable period of time, discontinue DECADRON elixir and transfer the patient to other therapy.

After a favorable initial response, the proper maintenance dosage should be determined by decreasing the initial dosage in small amounts to the lowest dosage that maintains an adequate clinical response.

Patients should be observed closely for signs that might require dosage adjustment, including changes in clinical status resulting from remissions or exacerbations of the disease, individual drug responsiveness, and the effect of stress (e.g., surgery, infection, trauma). During stress it may be necessary to increase dosage temporarily.

If the drug is to be stopped after more than a few days of treatment, it usually should be withdrawn gradually.

The following milligram equivalents facilitate changing to DECADRON from other glucocorticoids:

DECADRON	Methylprednisolone and Triamcinolone	Prednisolone and Prednisone	Hydrocortisone	Cortisone
0.75 mg =	4 mg =	5 mg =	20 mg =	25 mg

Dexamethasone suppression tests

1. Tests for Cushing's syndrome
    Give 1.0 mg of DECADRON orally at 11:00 p.m. Blood is drawn for plasma cortisol determination at 8:00 a.m. the following morning.
    For greater accuracy, give 0.5 mg of DECADRON orally every 6 hours for 48 hours. Twenty-four hour urine collections are made for determination of 17-hydroxycorticosteroid excretion.
2. Test to distinguish Cushing's syndrome due to pituitary ACTH excess from Cushing's syndrome due to other causes
    Give 2.0 mg of DECADRON orally every 6 hours for 48 hours. Twenty-four hour urine collections are made for determination of 17-hydroxycorticosteroid excretion.

HOW SUPPLIED

No. 7622—Elixir DECADRON, 0.5 mg dexamethasone per 5 mL, is a clear, red liquid and is supplied as follows:
NDC 0006-7622-55 bottles of 100 mL with calibrated dropper assembly.
NDC 0006-7622-66 bottles of 237 mL without dropper assembly.
Storage
Store in a container which is kept tightly closed.

A.H.F.S. Category: 68:04
DC 7412726 Issued March 1988

DECADRON® Tablets ℞
(Dexamethasone), U.S.P.

DESCRIPTION

Glucocorticoids are adrenocortical steroids, both naturally occurring and synthetic, which are readily absorbed from the gastrointestinal tract.

Dexamethasone, a synthetic adrenocortical steroid, is a white to practically white, odorless, crystalline powder. It is stable in air. It is practically insoluble in water. The molecular weight is 392.47. It is designated chemically as 9-fluoro-11β, 17, 21-trihydroxy-16α-methylpregna-1, 4-diene-3,20-dione. The empirical formula is $C_{22}H_{29}FO_5$ and the structural formula is: [See top of next column.]

DECADRON* (Dexamethasone) tablets are supplied in six potencies, 0.25 mg, 0.5 mg, 0.75 mg, 1.5 mg, 4 mg, and 6 mg. Inactive ingredients are calcium phosphate, lactose, magnesium stearate, and starch. Tablets DECADRON 0.25 mg also

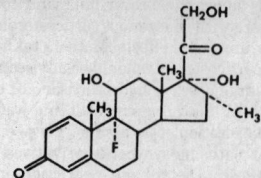

contain FD&C Yellow 6. Tablets DECADRON 0.5 mg also contain D&C Yellow 10 and FD&C Yellow 6. Tablets DECADRON 0.75 mg also contain FD&C Blue 1. Tablets DECADRON 1.5 mg also contain FD&C Red 40. Tablets DECADRON 6 mg also contain FD&C Blue 1 and iron oxide.

*Registered trademark of MERCK & CO., INC.

ACTIONS

Naturally occurring glucocorticoids (hydrocortisone and cortisone), which also have salt-retaining properties, are used as replacement therapy in adrenocortical deficiency states. Their synthetic analogs including dexamethasone are primarily used for their potent anti-inflammatory effects in disorders of many organ systems.

Glucocorticoids cause profound and varied metabolic effects. In addition, they modify the body's immune responses to diverse stimuli.

At equipotent anti-inflammatory doses, dexamethasone almost completely lacks the sodium-retaining property of hydrocortisone and closely related derivatives of hydrocortisone.

INDICATIONS

1. *Endocrine Disorders*
   Primary or secondary adrenocortical insufficiency (hydrocortisone or cortisone is the first choice; synthetic analogs may be used in conjunction with mineralocorticoids where applicable; in infancy mineralocorticoid supplementation is of particular importance)
   Congenital adrenal hyperplasia
   Nonsuppurative thyroiditis
   Hypercalcemia associated with cancer
2. *Rheumatic Disorders*
   As adjunctive therapy for short-term administration (to tide the patient over an acute episode or exacerbation) in:
   Psoriatic arthritis
   Rheumatoid arthritis, including juvenile rheumatoid arthritis (selected cases may require low-dose maintenance therapy)
   Ankylosing spondylitis
   Acute and subacute bursitis
   Acute nonspecific tenosynovitis
   Acute gouty arthritis
   Post-traumatic osteoarthritis
   Synovitis of osteoarthritis
   Epicondylitis
3. *Collagen Diseases*
   During an exacerbation or as maintenance therapy in selected cases of—
   Systemic lupus erythematosus
   Acute rheumatic carditis
4. *Dermatologic Diseases*
   Pemphigus
   Bullous dermatitis herpetiformis
   Severe erythema multiforme (Stevens-Johnson syndrome)
   Exfoliative dermatitis
   Mycosis fungoides
   Severe psoriasis
   Severe seborrheic dermatitis
5. *Allergic States*
   Control of severe or incapacitating allergic conditions intractable to adequate trials of conventional treatment:
   Seasonal or perennial allergic rhinitis
   Bronchial asthma
   Contact dermatitis
   Atopic dermatitis
   Serum sickness
   Drug hypersensitivity reactions
6. *Ophthalmic Diseases*
   Severe acute and chronic allergic and inflammatory processes involving the eye and its adnexa, such as—
   Allergic conjunctivitis
   Keratitis
   Allergic corneal marginal ulcers
   Herpes zoster ophthalmicus
   Iritis and iridocyclitis
   Chorioretinitis
   Anterior segment inflammation
   Diffuse posterior uveitis and choroiditis
   Optic neuritis
   Sympathetic ophthalmia

7. *Respiratory Diseases*
   Symptomatic sarcoidosis
   Loeffler's syndrome not manageable by other means
   Berylliosis
   Fulminating or disseminated pulmonary tuberculosis when used concurrently with appropriate antituberculous chemotherapy
   Aspiration pneumonitis
8. *Hematologic Disorders*
   Idiopathic thrombocytopenic purpura in adults
   Secondary thrombocytopenia in adults
   Acquired (autoimmune) hemolytic anemia
   Erythroblastopenia (RBC anemia)
   Congenital (erythroid) hypoplastic anemia
9. *Neoplastic Diseases*
   For palliative management of:
   Leukemias and lymphomas in adults
   Acute leukemia of childhood
10. *Edematous States*
    To induce a diuresis or remission of proteinuria in the nephrotic syndrome, without uremia, of the idiopathic type or that due to lupus erythematosus
11. *Gastrointestinal Diseases*
    To tide the patient over a critical period of the disease in:
    Ulcerative colitis
    Regional enteritis
12. *Cerebral Edema* associated with primary or metastatic brain tumor, craniotomy, or head injury. Use in cerebral edema is not a substitute for careful neurosurgical evaluation and definitive management such as neurosurgery or other specific therapy.
13. *Miscellaneous*
    Tuberculous meningitis with subarachnoid block or impending block when used concurrently with appropriate antituberculous chemotherapy
    Trichinosis with neurologic or myocardial involvement
14. *Diagnostic testing of adrenocortical hyperfunction.*

CONTRAINDICATIONS

Systemic fungal infections
Hypersensitivity to this drug

WARNINGS

In patients on corticosteroid therapy subjected to unusual stress, increased dosage of rapidly acting corticosteroids before, during, and after the stressful situation is indicated.

Drug-induced secondary adrenocortical insufficiency may result from too rapid withdrawal of corticosteroids and may be minimized by gradual reduction of dosage. This type of relative insufficiency may persist for months after discontinuation of therapy; therefore, in any situation of stress occurring during that period, hormone therapy should be reinstituted. If the patient is receiving steroids already, dosage may have to be increased. Since mineralocorticoid secretion may be impaired, salt and/or a mineralocorticoid should be administered concurrently.

Corticosteroids may mask some signs of infection, and new infections may appear during their use. There may be decreased resistance and inability to localize infection when corticosteroids are used. Moreover, corticosteroids may affect the nitroblue-tetrazolium test for bacterial infection and produce false negative results.

In cerebral malaria, a double-blind trial has shown that the use of corticosteroids is associated with prolongation of coma and a higher incidence of pneumonia and gastrointestinal bleeding.

Corticosteroids may activate latent amebiasis. Therefore, it is recommended that latent or active amebiasis be ruled out before initiating corticosteroid therapy in any patient who has spent time in the tropics or any patient with unexplained diarrhea.

Prolonged use of corticosteroids may produce posterior subcapsular cataracts, glaucoma with possible damage to the optic nerves, and may enhance the establishment of secondary ocular infections due to fungi or viruses.

Usage in pregnancy: Since adequate human reproduction studies have not been done with corticosteroids, use of these drugs in pregnancy or in women of childbearing potential requires that the anticipated benefits be weighed against the possible hazards to the mother and embryo or fetus. Infants born of mothers who have received substantial doses of corticosteroids during pregnancy should be carefully observed for signs of hypoadrenalism.

Corticosteroids appear in breast milk and could suppress growth, interfere with endogenous corticosteroid production, or cause other unwanted effects. Mothers taking pharmacologic doses of corticosteroids should be advised not to nurse.

Average and large doses of hydrocortisone or cortisone can cause elevation of blood pressure, salt and water retention, and increased excretion of potassium. These effects are less likely to occur with the synthetic derivatives except when used in large doses. Dietary salt restriction and potassium supplementation may be necessary. All corticosteroids increase calcium excretion.

Administration of live virus vaccines, including smallpox, is contraindicated in individuals receiving immunosuppressive doses of corticosteroids. If inactivated viral or bacterial vaccines are administered to individuals receiving immunosuppressive doses of corticosteroid the expected serum antibody response may not be obtained. However, immunization procedures may be undertaken in patients who are receiving corticosteroids as replacement therapy, e.g., for Addison's disease.

The use of DECADRON tablets in active tuberculosis should be restricted to those cases of fulminating or disseminated tuberculosis in which the corticosteroid is used for the management of the disease in conjunction with an appropriate antituberculous regimen.

If corticosteroids are indicated in patients with latent tuberculosis or tuberculin reactivity, close observation is necessary as reactivation of the disease may occur. During prolonged corticosteroid therapy, these patients should receive chemoprophylaxis.

Literature reports suggest an apparent association between use of corticosteroids and left ventricular free wall rupture after a recent myocardial infarction; therefore, therapy with corticosteroids should be used with great caution in these patients.

PRECAUTIONS

Following prolonged therapy, withdrawal of the corticosteroid may result in symptoms of the corticosteroid withdrawal syndrome including fever, myalgia, arthralgia, and malaise. This may occur in patients even without evidence of adrenal insufficiency.

There is an enhanced effect of corticosteroids in patients with hypothyroidism and in those with cirrhosis.

Corticosteroids should be used cautiously in patients with ocular herpes simplex because of possible corneal perforation.

The lowest possible dose of corticosteroids should be used to control the condition under treatment, and when reduction in dosage is possible, the reduction should be gradual.

Psychic derangements may appear when corticosteroids are used, ranging from euphoria, insomnia, mood swings, personality changes, and severe depression, to frank psychotic manifestations. Also, existing emotional instability or psychotic tendencies may be aggravated by corticosteroids.

Aspirin should be used cautiously in conjunction with corticosteroids in hypoprothrombinemia.

Steroids should be used with caution in nonspecific ulcerative colitis, if there is a probability of impending perforation, abscess, or other pyogenic infection, diverticulitis, fresh intestinal anastomoses, active or latent peptic ulcer, renal insufficiency, hypertension, osteoporosis, and myasthenia gravis. Signs of peritoneal irritation following gastrointestinal perforation in patients receiving large doses of corticosteroids may be minimal or absent. Fat embolism has been reported as a possible complication of hypercortisonism.

When large doses are given, some authorities advise that corticosteroids be taken with meals and antacids taken between meals to help to prevent peptic ulcer.

Growth and development of infants and children on prolonged corticosteroid therapy should be carefully observed.

Steroids may increase or decrease motility and number of spermatozoa in some patients.

Phenytoin, phenobarbital, ephedrine, and rifampin may enhance the metabolic clearance of corticosteroids, resulting in decreased blood levels and lessened physiologic activity, thus requiring adjustment in corticosteroid dosage. These interactions may interfere with dexamethasone suppression tests which should be interpreted with caution during administration of these drugs.

False-negative results in the dexamethasone suppression test (DST) in patients being treated with indomethacin have been reported. Thus, results of the DST should be interpreted with caution in these patients.

The prothrombin time should be checked frequently in patients who are receiving corticosteroids and coumarin anticoagulants at the same time because of reports that corticosteroids have altered the response to these anticoagulants. Studies have shown that the usual effect produced by adding corticosteroids is inhibition of response to coumarins, although there have been some conflicting reports of potentiation not substantiated by studies.

When corticosteroids are administered concomitantly with potassium-depleting diuretics, patients should be observed closely for development of hypokalemia.

ADVERSE REACTIONS

Fluid and Electrolyte Disturbances
  Sodium retention
  Fluid retention
  Congestive heart failure in susceptible patients
  Potassium loss
  Hypokalemic alkalosis
  Hypertension

Musculoskeletal
  Muscle weakness
  Steroid myopathy
  Loss of muscle mass
  Osteoporosis
  Vertebral compression fractures
  Aseptic necrosis of femoral and humeral heads
  Pathologic fracture of long bones
  Tendon rupture
Gastrointestinal
  Peptic ulcer with possible perforation and hemorrhage
  Perforation of the small and large bowel, particularly in patients with inflammatory bowel disease
  Pancreatitis
  Abdominal distention
  Ulcerative esophagitis
Dermatologic
  Impaired wound healing
  Thin fragile skin
  Petechiae and ecchymoses
  Erythema
  Increased sweating
  May suppress reactions to skin tests
  Other cutaneous reactions, such as allergic dermatitis, urticaria, angioneurotic edema
Neurologic
  Convulsions
  Increased intracranial pressure with papilledema (pseudotumor cerebri) usually after treatment
  Vertigo
  Headache
  Psychic disturbances
Endocrine
  Menstrual irregularities
  Development of cushingoid state
  Suppression of growth in children
  Secondary adrenocortical and pituitary unresponsiveness, particularly in times of stress, as in trauma, surgery, or illness
  Decreased carbohydrate tolerance
  Manifestations of latent diabetes mellitus
  Increased requirements for insulin or oral hypoglycemic agents in diabetics
  Hirsutism
Ophthalmic
  Posterior subcapsular cataracts
  Increased intraocular pressure
  Glaucoma
  Exophthalmos
Metabolic
  Negative nitrogen balance due to protein catabolism
Cardiovascular
  Myocardial rupture following recent myocardial infarction (see WARNINGS).
Other
  Hypersensitivity
  Thromboembolism
  Weight gain
  Increased appetite
  Nausea
  Malaise
  Hiccups

OVERDOSAGE

Reports of acute toxicity and/or death following overdosage of glucocorticoids are rare. In the event of overdosage, no specific antidote is available; treatment is supportive and symptomatic.

The oral LD_{50} of dexamethasone in female mice was 6.5 g/kg.

DOSAGE AND ADMINISTRATION

For oral administration
DOSAGE REQUIREMENTS ARE VARIABLE AND MUST BE INDIVIDUALIZED ON THE BASIS OF THE DISEASE AND THE RESPONSE OF THE PATIENT.
The initial dosage varies from 0.75 to 9 mg a day depending on the disease being treated. In less severe diseases doses lower than 0.75 mg may suffice, while in severe diseases doses higher than 9 mg may be required. The initial dosage should be maintained or adjusted until the patient's response is satisfactory. If satisfactory clinical response does not occur after a reasonable period of time, discontinue DECADRON tablets and transfer the patient to other therapy. After a favorable initial response, the proper maintenance dosage should be determined by decreasing the initial dosage in small amounts to the lowest dosage that maintains an adequate clinical response.

Patients should be observed closely for signs that might require dosage adjustment, including changes in clinical status resulting from remissions or exacerbations of the disease, individual drug responsiveness, and the effect of stress (e.g., surgery, infection, trauma). During stress it may be necessary to increase dosage temporarily.

If the drug is to be stopped after more than a few days of treatment, it usually should be withdrawn gradually.
The following milligram equivalents facilitate changing to DECADRON from other glucocorticoids:

DECADRON	Methylprednisolone and Triamcinolone	Prednisolone and Prednisone	Hydrocortisone	Cortisone
0.75 mg =	4 mg =	5 mg =	20 mg =	25 mg

In *acute, self-limited allergic disorders or acute exacerbations of chronic allergic disorders*, the following dosage schedule combining parenteral and oral therapy is suggested:
DECADRON* Phosphate (Dexamethasone Sodium Phosphate) injection, 4 mg per mL:
First Day
  1 or 2 mL, intramuscularly
DECADRON tablets, 0.75 mg:
Second Day
  4 tablets in two divided doses
Third Day
  4 tablets in two divided doses
Fourth Day
  2 tablets in two divided doses
Fifth Day
  1 tablet
Sixth Day
  1 tablet
Seventh Day
  No treatment
Eighth Day
  Follow-up visit
This schedule is designed to ensure adequate therapy during acute episodes, while minimizing the risk of overdosage in chronic cases.

In *cerebral edema*, DECADRON Phosphate (Dexamethasone Sodium Phosphate) injection is generally administered initially in a dosage of 10 mg intravenously followed by 4 mg every six hours intramuscularly until the symptoms of cerebral edema subside. Response is usually noted within 12 to 24 hours and dosage may be reduced after two to four days and gradually discontinued over a period of five to seven days. For palliative management of patients with recurrent or inoperable brain tumors, maintenance therapy with either DECADRON Phosphate (Dexamethasone Sodium Phosphate) injection or DECADRON tablets in a dosage of two mg two or three times daily may be effective.

Dexamethasone suppression tests
1. Tests for Cushing's syndrome
   Give 1.0 mg of DECADRON orally at 11:00 p.m. Blood is drawn for plasma cortisol determination at 8:00 a.m. the following morning.
   For greater accuracy, give 0.5 mg of DECADRON orally every 6 hours for 48 hours. Twenty-four hour urine collections are made for determination of 17-hydroxycorticosteroid excretion.
2. Test to distinguish Cushing's syndrome due to pituitary ACTH excess from Cushing's syndrome due to other causes
   Give 2.0 mg of DECADRON orally every 6 hours for 48 hours. Twenty-four hour urine collections are made for determination of 17-hydroxycorticosteroid excretion.

*Registered trademark of MERCK & CO., INC.

HOW SUPPLIED

Tablets DECADRON are compressed, pentagonal-shaped tablets, colored to distinguish potency. They are scored and coded on one side and are available as follows:
No. 7648—6 mg, green in color and coded MSD 147.
NDC 0006-0147-50 bottles of 50
NDC 0006-0147-28 single unit packages of 100.
  Shown in Product Identification Section, page 419
No. 7645—4 mg, white in color and coded MSD 97.
NDC 0006-0097-50 bottles of 50
NDC 0006-0097-28 single unit packages of 100.
  Shown in Product Identification Section, page 419

Continued on next page

Merck & Co.—Cont.

No. 7638—1.5 mg, pink in color and coded MSD 95.
NDC 0006-0095-50 bottles of 50
NDC 0006-0095-28 single unit packages of 100.
Shown in Product Identification Section, page 419
No. 7601—0.75 mg, bluish-green in color and coded MSD 63.
NDC 0006-0063-12 5-12 PAK® (package of 12)
NDC 0006-0063-68 bottles of 100
NDC 0006-0063-28 single unit packages of 100.
Shown in Product Identification Section, page 419
No. 7598—0.5 mg, yellow in color and coded MSD 41.
NDC 0006-0041-68 bottles of 100
NDC 0006-0041-28 single unit packages of 100.
Shown in Product Identification Section, page 419
No. 7592—0.25 mg, orange in color and coded MSD 20.
NDC 0006-0020-68 bottles of 100.
Shown in Product Identification Section, page 419
A.H.F.S. Category: 68:04
DC 7420544 Issued March 1988

DECADRON® Phosphate Injection   ℞
(Dexamethasone Sodium Phosphate), U.S.P.

DESCRIPTION

Dexamethasone sodium phosphate, a synthetic adrenocortical steroid, is a white or slightly yellow, crystalline powder. It is freely soluble in water and is exceedingly hygroscopic. The molecular weight is 516.41. It is designated chemically as 9-fluoro-11β, 17-dihydroxy-16α-methyl-21-(phosphonooxy)pregna-1, 4-diene-3, 20-dione disodium salt. The empirical formula is $C_{22}H_{28}FNa_2O_8P$ and the structural formula is:

DECADRON* Phosphate (Dexamethasone Sodium Phosphate) injection is a sterile solution (pH 7.0 to 8.5) of dexamethasone sodium phosphate sealed under nitrogen, and is supplied in two concentrations: 4 mg/mL and 24 mg/mL. The 24 mg/mL concentration offers the advantage of less volume in indications where high doses of corticosteroids by the intravenous route are needed.
Each milliliter of DECADRON Phosphate injection, 4 mg/mL, contains dexamethasone sodium phosphate equivalent to 4 mg dexamethasone phosphate or 3.33 mg dexamethasone. Inactive ingredients per mL: 8 mg creatinine, 10 mg sodium citrate, sodium hydroxide to adjust pH, and Water for Injection q.s., with 1 mg sodium bisulfite, 1.5 mg methylparaben, and 0.2 mg propylparaben added as preservatives.
Each milliliter of DECADRON Phosphate injection, 24 mg/mL, contains dexamethasone sodium phosphate equivalent to 24 mg dexamethasone phosphate or 20 mg dexamethasone. Inactive ingredients per mL: 8 mg creatinine, 10 mg sodium citrate, 0.5 mg disodium edetate, sodium hydroxide to adjust pH, and Water for Injection q.s., with 1 mg sodium bisulfite, 1.5 mg methylparaben, and 0.2 mg propylparaben added as preservatives.

* Registered trademark of MERCK & CO., INC.

ACTIONS

DECADRON Phosphate injection has a rapid onset but short duration of action when compared with less soluble preparations. Because of this, it is suitable for the treatment of acute disorders responsive to adrenocortical steroid therapy.
Naturally occurring glucocorticoids (hydrocortisone and cortisone), which also have salt-retaining properties, are used as replacement therapy in adrenocortical deficiency states. Their synthetic analogs, including dexamethasone, are primarily used for their potent anti-inflammatory effects in disorders of many organ systems.
Glucocorticoids cause profound and varied metabolic effects. In addition, they modify the body's immune responses to diverse stimuli.
At equipotent anti-inflammatory doses, dexamethasone almost completely lacks the sodium-retaining property of hydrocortisone and closely related derivatives of hydrocortisone.

INDICATIONS

A. By intravenous or intramuscular injection when oral therapy is not feasible:

1. *Endocrine disorders*
Primary or secondary adrenocortical insufficiency (hydrocortisone or cortisone is the drug of choice; synthetic analogs may be used in conjunction with mineralocorticoids where applicable; in infancy, mineralocorticoid supplementation is of particular importance)
Acute adrenocortical insufficiency (hydrocortisone or cortisone is the drug of choice; mineralocorticoid supplementation may be necessary, particularly when synthetic analogs are used)
Preoperatively, and in the event of serious trauma or illness, in patients with known adrenal insufficiency or when adrenocortical reserve is doubtful
Shock unresponsive to conventional therapy if adrenocortical insufficiency exists or is suspected
Congenital adrenal hyperplasia
Nonsuppurative thyroiditis
Hypercalcemia associated with cancer
2. *Rheumatic disorders*
As adjunctive therapy for short-term administration (to tide the patient over an acute episode or exacerbation) in:
Post-traumatic osteoarthritis
Synovitis of osteoarthritis
Rheumatoid arthritis, including juvenile rheumatoid arthritis (selected cases may require low-dose maintenance therapy)
Acute and subacute bursitis
Epicondylitis
Acute nonspecific tenosynovitis
Acute gouty arthritis
Psoriatic arthritis
Ankylosing spondylitis
3. *Collagen diseases*
During an exacerbation or as maintenance therapy in selected cases of:
Systemic lupus erythematosus
Acute rheumatic carditis
4. *Dermatologic diseases*
Pemphigus
Severe erythema multiforme (Stevens-Johnson syndrome)
Exfoliative dermatitis
Bullous dermatitis herpetiformis
Severe seborrheic dermatitis
Severe psoriasis
Mycosis fungoides
5. *Allergic states*
Control of severe or incapacitating allergic conditions intractable to adequate trials of conventional treatment in:
Bronchial asthma
Contact dermatitis
Atopic dermatitis
Serum sickness
Seasonal or perennial allergic rhinitis
Drug hypersensitivity reactions
Urticarial transfusion reactions
Acute noninfectious laryngeal edema (epinephrine is the drug of first choice)
6. *Ophthalmic diseases*
Severe acute and chronic allergic and inflammatory processes involving the eye, such as:
Herpes zoster ophthalmicus
Iritis, iridocyclitis
Chorioretinitis
Diffuse posterior uveitis and choroiditis
Optic neuritis
Sympathetic ophthalmia
Anterior segment inflammation
Allergic conjunctivitis
Keratitis
Allergic corneal marginal ulcers
7. *Gastrointestinal diseases*
To tide the patient over a critical period of the disease in:
Ulcerative colitis (Systemic therapy)
Regional enteritis (Systemic therapy)
8. *Respiratory diseases*
Symptomatic sarcoidosis
Berylliosis
Fulminating or disseminated pulmonary tuberculosis when used concurrently with appropriate antituberculous chemotherapy
Loeffler's syndrome not manageable by other means
Aspiration pneumonitis
9. *Hematologic disorders*
Acquired (autoimmune) hemolytic anemia
Idiopathic thrombocytopenic purpura in adults (I.V. only; I.M. administration is contraindicated)
Secondary thrombocytopenia in adults
Erythroblastopenia (RBC anemia)
Congenital (erythroid) hypoplastic anemia
10. *Neoplastic diseases*
For palliative management of:

Leukemias and lymphomas in adults
Acute leukemia of childhood
11. *Edematous states*
To induce diuresis or remission of proteinuria in the nephrotic syndrome, without uremia, of the idiopathic type, or that due to lupus erythematosus
12. *Miscellaneous*
Tuberculous meningitis with subarachnoid block or impending block when used concurrently with appropriate antituberculous chemotherapy
Trichinosis with neurologic or myocardial involvement
13. *Diagnostic testing of adrenocortical hyperfunction*
14. *Cerebral Edema* associated with primary or metastatic brain tumor, craniotomy, or head injury. Use in cerebral edema is not a substitute for careful neurosurgical evaluation and definitive management such as neurosurgery or other specific therapy.
B. By intra-articular or soft tissue injection:
As adjunctive therapy for short-term administration (to tide the patient over an acute episode or exacerbation) in:
Synovitis of osteoarthritis
Rheumatoid arthritis
Acute and subacute bursitis
Acute gouty arthritis
Epicondylitis
Acute nonspecific tenosynovitis
Post-traumatic osteoarthritis.
C. By intralesional injection:
Keloids
Localized hypertrophic, infiltrated, inflammatory lesions of: lichen planus, psoriatic plaques, granuloma annulare, and lichen simplex chronicus (neurodermatitis)
Discoid lupus erythematosus
Necrobiosis lipoidica diabeticorum
Alopecia areata
May also be useful in cystic tumors of an aponeurosis or tendon (ganglia).

CONTRAINDICATIONS

Systemic fungal infections. (See WARNINGS regarding amphotericin B)
Hypersensitivity to any component of this product, including sulfites (see WARNINGS).

WARNINGS

Because rare instances of anaphylactoid reactions have occurred in patients receiving parenteral corticosteroid therapy, appropriate precautionary measures should be taken prior to administration, especially when the patient has a history of allergy to any drug. Anaphylactoid and hypersensitivity reactions have been reported for Injection DECADRON Phosphate (see ADVERSE REACTIONS).
Injection DECADRON Phosphate contains sodium bisulfite, a sulfite that may cause allergic-type reactions including anaphylactic symptoms and life-threatening or less severe asthmatic episodes in certain susceptible people. The overall prevalence of sulfite sensitivity in the general population is unknown and probably low. Sulfite sensitivity is seen more frequently in asthmatic than in nonasthmatic people.
Corticosteroids may exacerbate systemic fungal infections and therefore should not be used in the presence of such infections unless they are needed to control drug reactions due to amphotericin B. Moreover, there have been cases reported in which concomitant use of amphotericin B and hydrocortisone was followed by cardiac enlargement and congestive failure.
In patients on corticosteroid therapy subjected to any unusual stress, increased dosage of rapidly acting corticosteroids before, during, and after the stressful situation is indicated.
Drug-induced secondary adrenocortical insufficiency may result from too rapid withdrawal of corticosteroids and may be minimized by gradual reduction of dosage. This type of relative insufficiency may persist for months after discontinuation of therapy; therefore, in any situation of stress occurring during that period, hormone therapy should be reinstituted. If the patient is receiving steroids already, dosage may have to be increased. Since mineralocorticoid secretion may be impaired, salt and/or a mineralocorticoid should be administered concurrently.
Corticosteroids may mask some signs of infection, and new infections may appear during their use. There may be decreased resistance and inability to localize infection when corticosteroids are used. Moreover, corticosteroids may affect the nitroblue-tetrazolium test for bacterial infection and produce false negative results.
In cerebral malaria, a double-blind trial has shown that the use of corticosteroids is associated with prolongation of coma and a higher incidence of pneumonia and gastrointestinal bleeding.
Corticosteroids may activate latent amebiasis. Therefore, it is recommended that latent or active amebiasis be ruled out before initiating corticosteroid therapy in any patient who

has spent time in the tropics or any patient with unexplained diarrhea.

Prolonged use of corticosteroids may produce posterior subcapsular cataracts, glaucoma with possible damage to the optic nerves, and may enhance the establishment of secondary ocular infections due to fungi or viruses.

Usage in pregnancy. Since adequate human reproduction studies have not been done with corticosteroids, use of these drugs in pregnancy or in women of childbearing potential requires that the anticipated benefits be weighed against the possible hazards to the mother and embryo or fetus. Infants born of mothers who have received substantial doses of corticosteroids during pregnancy should be carefully observed for signs of hypoadrenalism.

Corticosteroids appear in breast milk and could suppress growth, interfere with endogenous corticosteroid production, or cause other unwanted effects. Mothers taking pharmacologic doses of corticosteroids should be advised not to nurse. Average and large doses of cortisone or hydrocortisone can cause elevation of blood pressure, salt and water retention, and increased excretion of potassium. These effects are less likely to occur with the synthetic derivatives except when used in large doses. Dietary salt restriction and potassium supplementation may be necessary. All corticosteroids increase calcium excretion.

Administration of live virus vaccines, including smallpox, is contraindicated in individuals receiving immunosuppressive doses of corticosteroids. If inactivated viral or bacterial vaccines are administered to individuals receiving immunosuppressive doses of corticosteroids, the expected serum antibody response may not be obtained. However, immunization procedures may be undertaken in patients who are receiving corticosteroids as replacement therapy, e.g., for Addison's disease.

The use of DECADRON Phosphate injection in active tuberculosis should be restricted to those cases of fulminating or disseminated tuberculosis in which the corticosteroid is used for the management of the disease in conjunction with an appropriate antituberculous regimen.

If corticosteroids are indicated in patients with latent tuberculosis or tuberculin reactivity, close observation is necessary as reactivation of the disease may occur. During prolonged corticosteroid therapy, these patients should receive chemoprophylaxis.

Literature reports suggest an apparent association between use of corticosteroids and left ventricular free wall rupture after a recent myocardial infarction; therefore, therapy with corticosteroids should be used with great caution in these patients.

PRECAUTIONS

This product, like many other steroid formulations, is sensitive to heat. Therefore, it should not be autoclaved when it is desirable to sterilize the exterior of the vial.

Following prolonged therapy, withdrawal of corticosteroids may result in symptoms of the corticosteroid withdrawal syndrome including fever, myalgia, arthralgia, and malaise. This may occur in patients even without evidence of adrenal insufficiency.

There is an enhanced effect of corticosteroids in patients with hypothyroidism and in those with cirrhosis.

Corticosteroids should be used cautiously in patients with ocular herpes simplex for fear of corneal perforation.

The lowest possible dose of corticosteroid should be used to control the condition under treatment, and when reduction in dosage is possible, the reduction must be gradual.

Psychic derangements may appear when corticosteroids are used, ranging from euphoria, insomnia, mood swings, personality changes, and severe depression to frank psychotic manifestations. Also, existing emotional instability or psychotic tendencies may be aggravated by corticosteroids.

Aspirin should be used cautiously in conjunction with corticosteroids in hypoprothrombinemia.

Steroids should be used with caution in nonspecific ulcerative colitis, if there is a probability of impending perforation, abscess, or other pyogenic infection, also in diverticulitis, fresh intestinal anastomoses, active or latent peptic ulcer, renal insufficiency, hypertension, osteoporosis, and myasthenia gravis. Signs of peritoneal irritation following gastrointestinal perforation in patients receiving large doses of corticosteroids may be minimal or absent. Fat embolism has been reported as a possible complication of hypercortisonism.

When large doses are given, some authorities advise that antacids be administered between meals to help to prevent peptic ulcer.

Growth and development of infants and children on prolonged corticosteroid therapy should be carefully followed.

Steroids may increase or decrease motility and number of spermatozoa in some patients.

Phenytoin, phenobarbital, ephedrine, and rifampin may enhance the metabolic clearance of corticosteroids resulting in decreased blood levels and lessened physiologic activity, thus requiring adjustment in corticosteroid dosage. These

interactions may interfere with dexamethasone suppression tests which should be interpreted with caution during administration of these drugs.

False negative results in the dexamethasone suppression test (DST) in patients being treated with indomethacin have been reported. Thus, results of the DST should be interpreted with caution in these patients.

The prothrombin time should be checked frequently in patients who are receiving corticosteroids and coumarin anticoagulants at the same time because of reports that corticosteroids have altered the response to these anticoagulants. Studies have shown that the usual effect produced by adding corticosteroids is inhibition of response to coumarins, although there have been some conflicting reports of potentiation not substantiated by studies.

When corticosteroids are administered concomitantly with potassium-depleting diuretics, patients should be observed closely for development of hypokalemia.

Intra-articular injection of a corticosteroid may produce systemic as well as local effects.

Appropriate examination of any joint fluid present is necessary to exclude a septic process.

A marked increase in pain accompanied by local swelling, further restriction of joint motion, fever, and malaise is suggestive of septic arthritis. If this complication occurs and the diagnosis of sepsis is confirmed, appropriate antimicrobial therapy should be instituted.

Injection of a steroid into an infected site is to be avoided. Corticosteroids should not be injected into unstable joints. Patients should be impressed strongly with the importance of not overusing joints in which symptomatic benefit has been obtained as long as the inflammatory process remains active.

Frequent intra-articular injection may result in damage to joint tissues.

The slower rate of absorption by intramuscular administration should be recognized.

ADVERSE REACTIONS

Fluid and electrolyte disturbances
Sodium retention
Fluid retention
Congestive heart failure in susceptible patients
Potassium loss
Hypokalemic alkalosis
Hypertension
Musculoskeletal
Muscle weakness
Steroid myopathy
Loss of muscle mass
Osteoporosis
Vertebral compression fractures
Aseptic necrosis of femoral and humeral heads
Pathologic fracture of long bones
Tendon rupture
Gastrointestinal
Peptic ulcer with possible subsequent perforation and hemorrhage
Perforation of the small and large bowel, particularly in patients with inflammatory bowel disease
Pancreatitis
Abdominal distention
Ulcerative esophagitis
Dermatologic
Impaired wound healing
Thin fragile skin
Petechiae and ecchymoses
Erythema
Increased sweating
May suppress reactions to skin tests
Burning or tingling, especially in the perineal area (after I.V. injection)
Other cutaneous reactions, such as allergic dermatitis, urticaria, angioneurotic edema
Neurologic
Convulsions
Increased intracranial pressure with papilledema (pseudotumor cerebri) usually after treatment
Vertigo
Headache
Psychic disturbances
Endocrine
Menstrual irregularities
Development of cushingoid state
Suppression of growth in children
Secondary adrenocortical and pituitary unresponsiveness, particularly in times of stress, as in trauma, surgery, or illness
Decreased carbohydrate tolerance
Manifestations of latent diabetes mellitus
Increased requirements for insulin or oral hypoglycemic agents in diabetics
Hirsutism

Ophthalmic
Posterior subcapsular cataracts
Increased intraocular pressure
Glaucoma
Exophthalmos
Metabolic
Negative nitrogen balance due to protein catabolism
Cardiovascular
Myocardial rupture following recent myocardial infarction (see WARNINGS).
Other
Anaphylactoid or hypersensitivity reactions
Thromboembolism
Weight gain
Increased appetite
Nausea
Malaise
Hiccups

The following *additional* adverse reactions are related to parenteral corticosteroid therapy:

Rare instances of blindness associated with intralesional therapy around the face and head
Hyperpigmentation or hypopigmentation
Subcutaneous and cutaneous atrophy
Sterile abscess
Postinjection flare (following intra-articular use)
Charcot-like arthropathy

OVERDOSAGE

Reports of acute toxicity and/or death following overdosage of glucocorticoids are rare. In the event of overdosage, no specific antidote is available; treatment is supportive and symptomatic.

The oral LD$_{50}$ of dexamethasone in female mice was 6.5 g/kg. The intravenous LD$_{50}$ of dexamethasone sodium phosphate in female mice was 794 mg/kg.

DOSAGE AND ADMINISTRATION

DECADRON Phosphate injection, 4 mg/mL—*For intravenous, intramuscular, intra-articular, intralesional, and soft tissue injection.*
DECADRON Phosphate injection, 24 mg/mL—*For intravenous injection only.*
DECADRON Phosphate injection can be given directly from the vial, or it can be added to Sodium Chloride Injection or Dextrose Injection and administered by intravenous drip. Solutions used for intravenous administration or further dilution of this product should be preservative-free when used in the neonate, especially the premature infant.

When it is mixed with an infusion solution, sterile precautions should be observed. Since infusion solutions generally do not contain preservatives, mixtures should be used within 24 hours.

DOSAGE REQUIREMENTS ARE VARIABLE AND MUST BE INDIVIDUALIZED ON THE BASIS OF THE DISEASE AND THE RESPONSE OF THE PATIENT.

Intravenous and Intramuscular Injection
The initial dosage of DECADRON Phosphate injection varies from 0.5 to 9 mg a day depending on the disease being treated. In less severe diseases doses lower than 0.5 mg may suffice, while in severe diseases doses higher than 9 mg may be required.

The initial dosage should be maintained or adjusted until the patient's response is satisfactory. If a satisfactory clinical response does not occur after a reasonable period of time, discontinue DECADRON Phosphate injection and transfer the patient to other therapy.

After a favorable initial response, the proper maintenance dosage should be determined by decreasing the initial dosage in small amounts to the lowest dosage that maintains an adequate clinical response.

Patients should be observed closely for signs that might require dosage adjustment, including changes in clinical status resulting from remissions or exacerbations of the disease, individual drug responsiveness, and the effect of stress (e.g., surgery, infection, trauma). During stress it may be necessary to increase dosage temporarily.

If the drug is to be stopped after more than a few days of treatment, it usually should be withdrawn gradually.

When the intravenous route of administration is used, dosage usually should be the same as the oral dosage. In certain overwhelming, acute, life-threatening situations, however, administration in dosages exceeding the usual dosages may be justified and may be in multiples of the oral dosages. The

Continued on next page

Merck & Co.—Cont.

slower rate of absorption by intramuscular administration should be recognized.

Shock

There is a tendency in current medical practice to use high (pharmacologic) doses of corticosteroids for the treatment of unresponsive shock. The following dosages of DECADRON phosphate injection have been suggested by various authors:

Author[*]	Dosage
Cavanagh[1]	3 mg/kg of body weight per 24 hours by constant intravenous infusion after an initial intravenous injection of 20 mg
Dietzman[2]	2 to 6 mg/kg of body weight as a single intravenous injection
Frank[3]	40 mg initially followed by repeat intravenous injection every 4 to 6 hours while shock persists
Oaks[4]	40 mg initially followed by repeat intravenous injection every 2 to 6 hours while shock persists
Schumer[5]	1 mg/kg of body weight as a single intravenous injection

Administration of high dose corticosteroid therapy should be continued only until the patient's condition has stabilized and usually not longer than 48 to 72 hours.

Although adverse reactions associated with high dose, short term corticosteroid therapy are uncommon, peptic ulceration may occur.

---

*1. Cavanagh, D.; Singh, K. B.: Endotoxin shock in pregnancy and abortion, in "Corticosteroids in the Treatment of Shock", Schumer, W.; Nyhus, L. M., Editors, Urbana, University of Illinois Press, 1970, pp. 86-96.
2. Dietzman, R. H.; Ersek, R. A.; Bloch, J. M.; Lillehei, R. C.: High-output, low-resistance gram-negative septic shock in man, Angiology *20:* 691-700, Dec. 1969.
3. Frank, E.: Clinical observations in shock and management (In: Shields, T. F., ed.: Symposium on current concepts and management of shock), J. Maine Med. Ass. *59:* 195-200, Oct. 1968.
4. Oaks, W. W.; Cohen, H. E.: Endotoxin shock in the geriatric patient, Geriat. *22:* 120-130, Mar. 1967.
5. Schumer, W.; Nyhus, L. M.: Corticosteroid effect on biochemical parameters of human oligemic shock, Arch. Surg. *100:* 405-408, Apr. 1970.

Cerebral Edema

DECADRON Phosphate injection is generally administered initially in a dosage of 10 mg intravenously followed by 4 mg every six hours intramuscularly until the symptoms of cerebral edema subside. Response is usually noted within 12 to 24 hours and dosage may be reduced after two to four days and gradually discontinued over a period of five to seven days. For palliative management of patients with recurrent or inoperable brain tumors, maintenance therapy with two mg two or three times a day may be effective.

Acute Allergic Disorders

In acute, self-limited allergic disorders or acute exacerbations of chronic allergic disorders, the following dosage schedule combining parenteral and oral therapy is suggested:

DECADRON Phosphate injection, 4 mg/mL: *first day,* 1 or 2 mL (4 or 8 mg), intramuscularly.

DECADRON* (Dexamethasone) tablets, 0.75 mg: *second and third days,* 4 tablets in two divided doses each day; *fourth day,* 2 tablets in two divided doses; *fifth and sixth days,* 1 tablet each day; *seventh day,* no treatment; *eighth day,* follow-up visit.

This schedule is designed to ensure adequate therapy during acute episodes, while minimizing the risk of overdosage in chronic cases.

---

*Registered trademark of MERCK & CO., INC.

Intra-articular, Intralesional, and Soft Tissue Injection

Intra-articular, intralesional, and soft tissue injections are generally employed when the affected joints or areas are limited to one or two sites. Dosage and frequency of injection varies depending on the condition and the site of injection. The usual dose is from 0.2 to 6 mg. The frequency usually ranges from once every three to five days to once every two to three weeks. Frequent intra-articular injection may result in damage to joint tissues.

Some of the usual single doses are: [See table above.]

DECADRON Phosphate injection is particularly recommended for use in conjunction with one of the less soluble, longer-acting steroids for intra-articular and soft tissue injection.

HOW SUPPLIED

No 7628X—Injection DECADRON Phosphate, 4 mg per mL, is a clear, colorless solution, and is available in 1 mL, 5 mL, and 25 mL vials as follows:

Site of Injection	Amount of Dexamethasone Phosphate (mg)
Large Joints (e.g., Knee)	2 to 4
Small Joints (e.g., Interphalangeal, Temporomandibular)	0.8 to 1
Bursae	2 to 3
Tendon Sheaths	0.4 to 1
Soft Tissue Infiltration	2 to 6
Ganglia	1 to 2

NDC 0006-7628-66, boxes of 25 × 1 mL vials
NDC 0006-7628-03, 5 mL vial
(6505-00-963-5355, 5 mL vial)
NDC 0006-7628-25, 25 mL vial.
FOR INTRAVENOUS USE ONLY:
No. 7646—Injection DECADRON Phosphate, 24 mg per mL, is a clear, colorless to light yellow solution and is available in 5 mL and 10 mL vials as follows:
NDC 0006-7646-03, 5 mL vial
NDC 0006-7646-10, 10 mL vial.
Storage
Sensitive to heat. Do not autoclave.
Protect from freezing.
Protect from light. Store container in carton until contents have been used.

A.H.F.S. Category: 68:04
DC 7347225   Issued March 1988

DECADRON® Phosphate with XYLOCAINE® ℞ Injection, Sterile
(Dexamethasone Sodium Phosphate-Lidocaine Hydrochloride)

> **For local injection only**

NOT FOR INTRAVENOUS USE

DESCRIPTION

Dexamethasone sodium phosphate is a white or slightly yellow, crystalline powder. It is freely soluble in water and is exceedingly hygroscopic. The molecular weight is 516.41. It is designated chemically as 9-fluoro-11β,17-dihydroxy-16α-methyl-21-(phosphonooxy)pregna-1,4-diene-3,20-dione disodium salt. The empirical formula is $C_{22}H_{28}FNa_2O_8P$ and the structural formula is:

Lidocaine hydrochloride is a white, crystalline powder that is very soluble in water and alcohol, soluble in chloroform, and insoluble in ether. The molecular weight is 288.82. It is designated chemically as 2-(diethylamino)-*N*-(2,6-dimethylphenyl)acetamide, monohydrochloride, monohydrate. The empirical formula is $C_{14}H_{22}N_2O \cdot HCl \cdot H_2O$ and the structural formula is:

DECADRON* Phosphate with XYLOCAINE** (Dexamethasone Sodium Phosphate-Lidocaine Hydrochloride) injection is provided as a sterile solution (pH 6.5 to 6.9), sealed under nitrogen, for the convenience of physicians who prefer to

treat patients with simultaneous administration of a corticosteroid and a local anesthetic.

Each milliliter contains dexamethasone sodium phosphate equivalent to dexamethasone phosphate, 4 mg; and lidocaine hydrochloride, 10 mg. Inactive ingredients per mL: citric acid anhydrous, 10 mg; creatinine, 8 mg; sodium bisulfite, 0.5 mg; disodium edetate, 0.5 mg; sodium hydroxide to adjust pH; and Water for Injection, q.s., 1 mL.

Methylparaben, 1.5 mg, and propylparaben, 0.2 mg, added as preservatives.

---

*Registered trademark of MERCK & CO., INC.

**Registered trademark of Astra Pharmaceutical Products, Inc.

ACTIONS

DECADRON Phosphate (Dexamethasone Sodium Phosphate) is a synthetic glucocorticoid used primarily for its potent anti-inflammatory effects in disorders of many organ systems. Glucocorticoids cause profound and varied metabolic effects. In addition, they modify the body's immune responses to diverse stimuli.

XYLOCAINE (Lidocaine Hydrochloride) is a local anesthetic with a rapid onset and moderate duration of action.

Local anesthesia appears within a few minutes after injection of DECADRON Phosphate with XYLOCAINE and lasts 45 minutes to one hour. By the time the anesthesia wears off, steroid activity usually has begun. If the anesthesia wears off before full steroid effect appears, there may be some discomfort beginning about an hour after injection and relief of pain may be delayed for a short time.

INDICATIONS

Acute and subacute bursitis
Acute and subacute nonspecific tenosynovitis

CONTRAINDICATIONS

Hypersensitivity to any component of this product, including sulfites (see WARNINGS).
Dexamethasone Sodium Phosphate
  Systemic fungal infections
Lidocaine Hydrochloride
  Patients with known history of hypersensitivity to local anesthetics of the amide type (e.g., mepivacaine, prilocaine)
  Severe shock
  Heart block

WARNINGS

Because rare instances of anaphylactoid reactions have occurred in patients receiving parenteral corticosteroid therapy, appropriate precautionary measures should be taken prior to administration, especially when the patient has a history of allergy to any drug. Anaphylactoid and hypersensitivity reactions have been reported for Injection DECADRON Phosphate with XYLOCAINE (see ADVERSE REACTIONS).

Injection DECADRON Phosphate with XYLOCAINE contains sodium bisulfite, a sulfite that may cause allergic-type reactions including anaphylactic symptoms and life-threatening or less severe asthmatic episodes in certain susceptible people. The overall prevalence of sulfite sensitivity in the general population is unknown and probably low. Sulfite sensitivity is seen more frequently in asthmatic than in nonasthmatic people.

Lidocaine Hydrochloride
RESUSCITATIVE EQUIPMENT AND DRUGS SHOULD BE IMMEDIATELY AVAILABLE WHEN ANY LOCAL ANESTHETIC IS USED.

Usage in pregnancy: The safe use of lidocaine hydrochloride has not been established with respect to adverse effects upon fetal development. Careful consideration should be given to this fact before administering this drug to women of childbearing potential, particularly during early pregnancy.

Dexamethasone Sodium Phosphate
In patients on corticosteroid therapy subjected to unusual stress, increased dosage of rapidly acting corticosteroids before, during, and after the stressful situation is indicated.

Drug-induced secondary adrenocortical insufficiency may result from too rapid withdrawal of corticosteroids and may be minimized by gradual reduction of dosage. This type of relative insufficiency may persist for months after discontinuation of therapy: therefore, in any situation of stress occurring during that period, hormone therapy should be reinstituted. If the patient is receiving steroids already, dosage may have to be increased. Since mineralocorticoid secretion may be impaired, salt and/or a mineralocorticoid should be administered concurrently.

Corticosteroids may mask some signs of infection, and new infections may appear during their use. There may be decreased resistance and inability to localize infection when corticosteroids are used. Moreover, corticosteroids may af-

fect the nitroblue-tetrazolium test for bacterial infection and produce false negative results.

Corticosteroids may activate latent amebiasis. Therefore, it is recommended that latent or active amebiasis be ruled out before initiating corticosteroid therapy in any patient who has spent time in the tropics or any patient with unexplained diarrhea.

Prolonged use of corticosteroids may produce posterior subcapsular cataracts, glaucoma with possible damage to the optic nerves, and may enhance the establishment of secondary ocular infections due to fungi or viruses.

Usage in pregnancy: Since adequate human reproduction studies have not been done with corticosteroids, use of these drugs in pregnancy or in women of childbearing potential requires that the anticipated benefits be weighed against the possible hazards to the mother and embryo or fetus. Infants born of mothers who have received substantial doses of corticosteroids during pregnancy should be carefully observed for signs of hypoadrenalism.

Corticosteroids appear in breast milk and could suppress growth, interfere with endogenous corticosteroid production, or cause other unwanted effects. Mothers taking pharmacologic doses of corticosteroids should be advised not to nurse. Average and large doses of cortisone or hydrocortisone can cause elevation of blood pressure, salt and water retention, and increased excretion of potassium. These effects are less likely to occur with the synthetic derivatives except when used in large doses. Dietary salt restriction and potassium supplementation may be necessary. All corticosteroids increase calcium excretion.

Administration of live virus vaccines, including smallpox, is contraindicated in individuals receiving immunosuppressive doses of corticosteroids. If inactivated viral or bacterial vaccines are administered to individuals receiving immunosuppressive doses of corticosteroids, the expected serum antibody response may not be obtained.

If corticosteroids are indicated in patients with latent tuberculosis or tuberculin reactivity, close observation is necessary as reactivation of the disease may occur. During prolonged corticosteroid therapy, these patients should receive chemoprophylaxis.

Literature reports suggest an apparent association between use of corticosteroids and left ventricular free wall rupture after a recent myocardial infarction; therefore, therapy with corticosteroids should be used with great caution in these patients.

PRECAUTIONS

This product, like many other steroid formulations, is sensitive to heat. Therefore, it should not be autoclaved when it is desirable to sterilize the exterior of the vial.

Therapy with this preparation does not eliminate the need for conventional supportive measures. Although capable of ameliorating symptoms, and even suppressing them completely in some patients, it is not a cure. Neither the hormone nor the anesthetic has any effect on the basic cause of inflammation.

Supportive measures, such as analgesics, pertinent orthopedic procedures, heat or cold, rest, rehabilitation, and physiotherapy must be used as applicable. If physiotherapy is applied immediately following injection, it may cause severe pain.

In some patients, a single injection fully restores mobility. Patients should be strongly impressed with the importance of not overusing the affected part as long as the inflammatory process remains active.

Injection into an infected site is to be avoided.

Dexamethasone Sodium Phosphate
Following prolonged therapy, withdrawal of corticosteroids may result in symptoms of the corticosteroid withdrawal syndrome including fever, myalgia, arthralgia, and malaise. This may occur in patients even without evidence of adrenal insufficiency.

There is an enhanced effect of corticosteroids in patients with hypothyroidism and in those with cirrhosis.

Corticosteroids should be used cautiously in patients with ocular herpes simplex for fear of corneal perforation.

Psychic derangements may appear when corticosteroids are used, ranging from euphoria, insomnia, mood swings, personality changes, and severe depression to frank psychotic manifestations. Also, existing emotional instability or psychotic tendencies may be aggravated by corticosteroids.

Aspirin should be used cautiously in conjunction with corticosteroids in hypoprothrombinemia.

Steroids should be used with caution in non-specific ulcerative colitis, if there is a probability of impending perforation, abscess, or other pyogenic infection, also in diverticulitis, fresh intestinal anastomoses, active or latent peptic ulcer, renal insufficiency, hypertension, osteoporosis, and myasthenia gravis. Signs of peritoneal irritation following gastrointestinal perforation in patients receiving large doses of corticosteroids may be minimal or absent. Fat embolism has been reported as a possible complication of hypercortisonism.

When large doses are given, some authorities advise that antacids be administered between meals to help to prevent peptic ulcer.

Growth and development of infants and children on prolonged corticosteroid therapy should be carefully followed. Steroids may increase or decrease motility and number of spermatozoa in some patients.

Phenytoin, phenobarbital, ephedrine, and rifampin may enhance the metabolic clearance of corticosteroids, resulting in decreased blood levels and lessened physiologic activity, thus requiring adjustment in corticosteroid dosage.

The prothrombin time should be checked frequently in patients who are receiving corticosteroids and coumarin anticoagulants at the same time because of reports that corticosteroids have altered the response to these anticoagulants. Studies have shown that the usual effect produced by adding corticosteroids is inhibition of response to coumarins, although there have been some conflicting reports of potentiation not substantiated by studies.

When corticosteroids are administered concomitantly with potassium-depleting diuretics, patients should be observed closely for development of hypokalemia.

Lidocaine Hydrochloride
The safety and effectiveness of lidocaine hydrochloride depend on proper dosage, correct technique, adequate precautions, and readiness for emergencies.

Injection of repeated doses may cause significant increases in blood levels with each repeated dose due to slow accumulation of the drug or its metabolites. Tolerance varies with the status of the patient. Debilitated, elderly patients, acutely ill patients, and children should be given reduced doses commensurate with their age and physical status. INJECTIONS SHOULD ALWAYS BE MADE SLOWLY AND WITH FREQUENT ASPIRATIONS. Aspiration is advisable since it reduces the possibility of intravascular injection, thereby keeping the incidence of side effects and anesthetic failures to a minimum. Consult standard textbooks for specific techniques and precautions for various local anesthetic procedures.

Lidocaine hydrochloride should be used with caution in persons with known drug sensitivities. Patients allergic to para-aminobenzoic acid derivatives (procaine, tetracaine, benzocaine, etc.) have not shown cross sensitivity to lidocaine hydrochloride.

Local anesthetics react with certain metals and cause the release of their respective ions which, if injected, may cause severe local irritation. Adequate precaution should be taken to avoid this type of interaction.

ADVERSE REACTIONS

Dexamethasone Sodium Phosphate
Fluid and electrolyte disturbances
   Sodium retention
   Fluid retention
   Congestive heart failure in susceptible patients
   Potassium loss
   Hypokalemic alkalosis
   Hypertension

Musculoskeletal
   Muscle weakness
   Steroid myopathy
   Loss of muscle mass
   Osteoporosis
   Vertebral compression fractures
   Aseptic necrosis of femoral and humeral heads
   Pathologic fracture of long bones
   Tendon rupture

Gastrointestinal
   Peptic ulcer with possible subsequent perforation and hemorrhage
   Perforation of the small and large bowel, particularly in patients with inflammatory bowel disease
   Pancreatitis
   Abdominal distention
   Ulcerative esophagitis

Dermatologic
   Impaired wound healing
   Thin fragile skin
   Petechiae and ecchymoses
   Erythema
   Increased sweating
   May suppress reactions to skin tests
   Other cutaneous reactions, such as allergic dermatitis, urticaria, angioneurotic edema

Neurologic
   Convulsions
   Increased intracranial pressure with papilledema (pseudotumor cerebri) usually after treatment
   Vertigo
   Headache
   Psychic disturbances

Endocrine
   Menstrual irregularities
   Development of cushingoid state
   Suppression of growth in children
   Secondary adrenocortical and pituitary unresponsiveness, particularly in times of stress, as in trauma, surgery, or illness
   Decreased carbohydrate tolerance
   Manifestations of latent diabetes mellitus
   Increased requirements for insulin or oral hypoglycemic agents in diabetics

Ophthalmic
   Posterior subcapsular cataracts
   Increased intraocular pressure
   Glaucoma
   Exophthalmos

Metabolic
   Negative nitrogen balance due to protein catabolism

Cardiovascular
   Myocardial rupture following recent myocardial infarction (see WARNINGS).

Other
   Anaphylactoid or hypersensitivity reactions
   Thromboembolism
   Weight gain
   Increased appetite
   Nausea
   Malaise
   Hiccups

The following *additional* adverse reactions are related to parenteral corticosteroid therapy:
   Rare instances of blindness associated with intralesional therapy around the face and head
   Hyperpigmentation or hypopigmentation
   Subcutaneous and cutaneous atrophy
   Sterile abscess
   Charcot-like arthropathy

Lidocaine Hydrochloride
Adverse reactions may result from high plasma levels due to excessive dosage, rapid absorption or inadvertent intravascular injection, or may result from a hypersensitivity, idiosyncrasy or diminished tolerance on the part of the patient. Such reactions are systemic in nature and involve the central nervous system and/or the cardiovascular system.

CNS reactions are excitatory and/or depressant, and may be characterized by nervousness, dizziness, blurred vision, and tremors followed by drowsiness, convulsions, unconsciousness, and possibly respiratory arrest. The excitatory reactions may be very brief or may not occur at all, in which case the first manifestations of toxicity may be drowsiness merging into unconsciousness and respiratory arrest.

Cardiovascular reactions are depressant, and may be characterized by hypotension, myocardial depression, bradycardia and possibly cardiac arrest.

Treatment of a patient with toxic manifestations consists of assuring and maintaining a patent airway and supporting ventilation using oxygen and assisted or controlled respiration as required. This usually will be sufficient in the management of most reactions. Should circulatory depression occur, vasopressors, such as ephedrine or metaraminol, and intravenous fluids may be used. Should a convulsion persist despite oxygen therapy, small increments of an ultra-short acting barbiturate (thiopental or thiamylal) or a short acting barbiturate (pentobarbital or secobarbital) may be given intravenously.

Allergic reactions are characterized by cutaneous lesions, urticaria, edema or anaphylactoid reactions. The detection of sensitivity by skin testing is of doubtful value.

DOSAGE AND ADMINISTRATION

> *For local injection only*

NOT FOR INTRAVENOUS USE
DOSAGE AND FREQUENCY OF INJECTION ARE VARIABLE AND MUST BE INDIVIDUALIZED ON THE BASIS OF THE DISEASE AND THE RESPONSE OF THE PATIENT.

Injections should always be made slowly and with frequent aspiration.

The initial dose ranges from 0.1 to 0.75 mL depending on the disease being treated and the size of the area to be injected. Frequency of injection depends on symptomatic response. In some patients, acute conditions are controlled adequately by a single injection. In others, additional injections are required, usually at intervals of four to seven days. If satisfactory clinical response does not occur after a reasonable pe-

Continued on next page

Information on the Merck & Co. products listed on these pages is the full prescribing information from product circulars in use October 1, 1992.

Merck & Co.—Cont.

riod of time, discontinue DECADRON Phosphate with XY-LOCAINE Injection and transfer the patient to other therapy.

Patients should be observed closely for signs that might require dosage adjustment, including changes in clinical status resulting from remissions or exacerbations of the disease, and individual drug responsiveness.

The usual doses are:

	Acute and Subacute Bursitis	Acute and Subacute Nonspecific Tenosynovitis
Amount of injection (mL)	0.5 to 0.75	0.1 to 0.25
Amount of dexamethasone sodium phosphate (mg)	2 to 3	0.4 to 1
Amount of lidocaine hydrochloride (mg)	5 to 7.5	1 to 2.5

DECADRON Phosphate with XYLOCAINE may be given undiluted directly from the vial, or it may be diluted with Sterile Water for Injection or Sodium Chloride Injection, using up to five parts of diluent to each part of injection. Dilutions should be used within one hour, since there is a possibility of change in pH, and this may adversely affect the stability or activity of the components.

HOW SUPPLIED

No. 7625X—Injection DECADRON Phosphate with XYLO-CAINE, containing 4 mg dexamethasone phosphate equivalent and 10 mg lidocaine hydrochloride per mL, is a clear, colorless solution, and is available as follows:
NDC 0006-7625-03 in 5 mL vials.
Storage
Sensitive to heat. Do not autoclave.
Protect from freezing.
　　　　A.H.F.S. Categories: 68:04-72:00
　　　　DC 7349317　Issued March 1988

DECADRON® Phosphate
(Dexamethasone Sodium Phosphate), U.S.P.
0.05% Dexamethasone Phosphate Equivalent
Sterile Ophthalmic Ointment

℞

DESCRIPTION

Dexamethasone sodium phosphate is 9-fluoro-11β,17-dihydroxy-16α -methyl-21-(phosphonooxy)pregna-1,4-diene-3,20-dione disodium salt. Its empirical formula is $C_{22}H_{28}FNa_2O_8P$ and its structural formula is:

Glucocorticoids are adrenocortical steroids, both naturally occurring and synthetic. Dexamethasone is a synthetic analog of naturally occurring glucocorticoids (hydrocortisone and cortisone). Dexamethasone sodium phosphate is a water soluble, inorganic ester of dexamethasone. Its molecular weight is 516.41.
Sterile Ophthalmic Ointment DECADRON* Phosphate (Dexamethasone Sodium Phosphate) is a topical steroid ointment containing dexamethasone sodium phosphate equivalent to 0.5 mg (0.05%) dexamethasone phosphate in each gram. Inactive ingredients: white petrolatum and mineral oil.
Dexamethasone sodium phosphate is an inorganic ester of dexamethasone.

*Registered trademark of MERCK & CO., INC.

CLINICAL PHARMACOLOGY

Dexamethasone sodium phosphate suppresses the inflammatory response to a variety of agents and it probably delays

or slows healing. No generally accepted explanation of these steroid properties have been advanced.

INDICATIONS AND USAGE

For the treatment of the following conditions:
Steroid responsive inflammatory conditions of the palpebral and bulbar conjunctiva, cornea, and anterior segment of the globe, such as allergic conjunctivitis, acne rosacea, superficial punctate keratitis, herpes zoster keratitis, iritis, cyclitis, selected infective conjunctivitis when the inherent hazard of steroid use is accepted to obtain an advisable diminution in edema and inflammation; corneal injury from chemical or thermal burns, or penetration of foreign bodies.

CONTRAINDICATIONS

Epithelial herpes simplex keratitis (dendritic keratitis).
Acute infectious stages of vaccinia, varicella, and many other viral diseases of the cornea and conjunctiva.
Mycobacterial infection of the eye.
Fungal diseases of ocular structures.
Hypersensitivity to a component of the medication.

WARNINGS

Prolonged use may result in ocular hypertension and/or glaucoma, with damage to the optic nerve, defects in visual acuity and fields of vision, and posterior subcapsular cataract formation. Prolonged use may suppress the host response and thus increase the hazard of secondary ocular infections. In those diseases causing thinning of the cornea or sclera, perforations have been known to occur with the use of topical corticosteroids. In acute purulent conditions of the eye, corticosteroids may mask infection or enhance existing infection. If these products are used for 10 days or longer, intraocular pressure should be routinely monitored even though it may be difficult in children and uncooperative patients.
Employment of corticosteroid medication in the treatment of herpes simplex other than epithelial herpes simplex keratitis, in which it is contraindicated, requires great caution; periodic slit-lamp microscopy is essential.

PRECAUTIONS

General
The possibility of persistent fungal infections of the cornea should be considered after prolonged corticosteroid dosing.
Carcinogenesis, Mutagenesis, Impairment of Fertility
Long-term animal studies have not been performed to evaluate the carcinogenic potential or the effect on fertility of Ophthalmic Ointment DECADRON Phosphate.
Pregnancy
Pregnancy Category C. Dexamethasone has been shown to be teratogenic in mice and rabbits following topical ophthalmic application in multiples of the therapeutic dose.
In the mouse, corticosteroids produce fetal resorptions and a specific abnormality, cleft palate. In the rabbit, corticosteroids have produced fetal resorptions and multiple abnormalities involving the head, ears, limbs, palate, etc.
There are no adequate or well-controlled studies in pregnant women. Ophthalmic Ointment DECADRON Phosphate should be used during pregnancy only if the potential benefit to the mother justifies the potential risk to the embryo or fetus. Infants born of mothers who have received substantial doses of corticosteroids during pregnancy should be observed carefully for signs of hypoadrenalism.
Nursing Mothers
Topically applied steroids are absorbed systemically. Therefore, because of the potential for serious adverse reactions in nursing infants from dexamethasone sodium phosphate, a decision should be made whether to discontinue nursing or discontinue the drug, taking into account the importance of the drug to the mother.
Pediatric Use
Safety and effectiveness in children have not been established.

ADVERSE REACTIONS

Glaucoma with optic nerve damage, visual acuity and field defects, posterior subcapsular cataract formation, secondary ocular infection from pathogens including herpes simplex, perforation of the globe.
Rarely, filtering blebs have been reported when topical steroids have been used following cataract surgery.
Rarely, stinging or burning may occur.

DOSAGE AND ADMINISTRATION

The duration of treatment will vary with the type of lesion and may extend from a few days to several weeks, according to therapeutic response. Relapses, more common in chronic

active lesions than in self-limited conditions, usually respond to retreatment.
Apply a thin coating of ointment three or four times a day. When a favorable response is observed, reduce the number of daily applications to two, and later to one a day as a maintenance dose if this is sufficient to control symptoms.
Ophthalmic Ointment DECADRON Phosphate is particularly convenient when an eye pad is used. It may also be the preparation of choice for patients in whom therapeutic benefit depends on prolonged contact of the active ingredients with ocular tissues.

HOW SUPPLIED

No. 7615—0.05% Sterile Ophthalmic Ointment DECA-DRON Phosphate is a clear unctuous ointment and is supplied as follows:
NDC 0006-7615-04 in 3.5 g tubes
(6505-00-961-5508 0.05% 3.5 g).
　　　　A.H.F.S. Category: 52:08
　　　　DC 6033127　Issued July 1986

DECADRON® Phosphate
(Dexamethasone Sodium Phosphate), U.S.P.
0.1% Dexamethasone Phosphate Equivalent
Sterile Ophthalmic Solution

℞

DESCRIPTION

Dexamethasone sodium phosphate is 9-fluoro-11β,17-dihydroxy-16α -methyl-21-(phosphonooxy)pregna-1,4-diene-3,20-dione disodium salt. Its empirical formula is $C_{22}H_{28}FNa_2O_8P$ and its structural formula is:

Glucocorticoids are adrenocortical steroids, both naturally occurring and synthetic. Dexamethasone is a synthetic analog of naturally occurring glucocorticoids (hydrocortisone and cortisone). Dexamethasone sodium phosphate is a water soluble, inorganic ester of dexamethasone. It is approximately three thousand times more soluble in water at 25℃ than hydrocortisone. Its molecular weight is 516.41.
Ophthalmic Solution DECADRON* Phosphate (Dexamethasone Sodium Phosphate) in the 5 mL OCUMETER* ophthalmic dispenser is a topical steroid solution containing dexamethasone sodium phosphate equivalent to 1 mg (0.1%) dexamethasone phosphate in each milliliter of buffered solution. Inactive ingredients: creatinine, sodium citrate, sodium borate, polysorbate 80, disodium edetate, hydrochloric acid to adjust pH, and water for injection. Sodium bisulfite 0.1%, phenylethanol 0.25% and benzalkonium chloride 0.02% added as preservatives.

*Registered trademark of MERCK & CO., INC.

CLINICAL PHARMACOLOGY

Dexamethasone sodium phosphate suppresses the inflammatory response to a variety of agents and it probably delays or slows healing. No generally accepted explanation of these steroid properties have been advanced.

INDICATIONS AND USAGE

For the treatment of the following conditions:
Ophthalmic:
Steroid responsive inflammatory conditions of the palpebral and bulbar conjunctiva, cornea, and anterior segment of the globe, such as allergic conjunctivitis, acne rosacea, superficial punctate keratitis, herpes zoster keratitis, iritis, cyclitis, selected infective conjunctivitis when the inherent hazard of steroid use is accepted to obtain an advisable diminution in edema and inflammation; corneal injury from chemical or thermal burns, or penetration of foreign bodies.
Otic:
Steroid responsive inflammatory conditions of the external auditory meatus, such as allergic otitis externa, selected purulent and nonpurulent infective otitis externa when the hazard of steroid use is accepted to obtain an advisable diminution in edema and inflammation.

CONTRAINDICATIONS

Epithelial herpes simplex keratitis (dendritic keratitis).
Acute infectious stages of vaccinia, varicella, and many other viral diseases of the cornea and conjunctiva.
Mycobacterial infection of the eye.
Fungal diseases of ocular or auricular structures.
Hypersensitivity to any component of this product, including sulfites (see WARNINGS).
Perforation of a drum membrane.

WARNINGS

Prolonged use may result in ocular hypertension and/or glaucoma, with damage to the optic nerve, defects in visual acuity and fields of vision, and posterior subcapsular cataract formation. Prolonged use may suppress the host response and thus increase the hazard of secondary ocular infections. In those diseases causing thinning of the cornea or sclera, perforations have been known to occur with the use of topical corticosteroids. In acute purulent conditions of the eye or ear, corticosteroids may mask infection or enhance existing infection. If these products are used for 10 days or longer, intraocular pressure should be routinely monitored even though it may be difficult in children and uncooperative patients.
Employment of corticosteroid medication in the treatment of herpes simplex other than epithelial herpes simplex keratitis, in which it is contraindicated, requires great caution; periodic slit-lamp microscopy is essential.
Ophthalmic Solution DECADRON Phosphate contains sodium bisulfite, a sulfite that may cause allergic-type reactions including anaphylactic symptoms and life-threatening or less severe asthmatic episodes in certain susceptible people. The overall prevalence of sulfite sensitivity in the general population is unknown and probably low. Sulfite sensitivity is seen more frequently in asthmatic than in nonasthmatic people.

PRECAUTIONS

General
The possibility of persistent fungal infections of the cornea should be considered after prolonged corticosteroid dosing.
Carcinogenesis, Mutagenesis, Impairment of Fertility
Long-term animal studies have not been performed to evaluate the carcinogenic potential or the effect on fertility of Ophthalmic Solution DECADRON Phosphate.
Pregnancy
Pregnancy Category C. Dexamethasone has been shown to be teratogenic in mice and rabbits following topical ophthalmic application in multiples of the therapeutic dose.
In the mouse, corticosteroids produce fetal resorptions and a specific abnormality, cleft palate. In the rabbit, corticosteroids have produced fetal resorptions and multiple abnormalities involving the head, ears, limbs, palate, etc.
There are no adequate or well-controlled studies in pregnant women. Ophthalmic Solution DECADRON Phosphate should be used during pregnancy only if the potential benefit to the mother justifies the potential risk to the embryo or fetus. Infants born of mothers who have received substantial doses of corticosteroids during pregnancy should be observed carefully for signs of hypoadrenalism.
Nursing Mothers
Topically applied steroids are absorbed systemically. Therefore, because of the potential for serious adverse reactions in nursing infants from dexamethasone sodium phosphate, a decision should be made whether to discontinue nursing or discontinue the drug, taking into account the importance of the drug to the mother.
Pediatric Use
Safety and effectiveness in children have not been established.

ADVERSE REACTIONS

Glaucoma with optic nerve damage, visual acuity and field defects, posterior subcapsular cataract formation, secondary ocular infection from pathogens including herpes simplex, perforation of the globe.
Rarely, filtering blebs have been reported when topical steroids have been used following cataract surgery.
Rarely, stinging or burning may occur.

DOSAGE AND ADMINISTRATION

The duration of treatment will vary with the type of lesion and may extend from a few days to several weeks, according to therapeutic response. Relapses, more common in chronic active lesions than in self-limited conditions, usually respond to retreatment.
Eye—Instill one or two drops of solution into the conjunctival sac every hour during the day and every two hours during the night as initial therapy. When a favorable response is observed, reduce dosage to one drop every four hours. Later, further reduction in dosage to one drop three or four times daily may suffice to control symptoms.
Ear—Clean the aural canal thoroughly and sponge dry. Instill the solution directly into the aural canal. A suggested initial dosage is three or four drops two or three times a day. When a favorable response is obtained, reduce dosage gradually and eventually discontinue.
If preferred, the aural canal may be packed with a gauze wick saturated with solution. Keep the wick moist with the preparation and remove from the ear after 12 to 24 hours. Treatment may be repeated as often as necessary at the discretion of the physician.

HOW SUPPLIED

Sterile Ophthalmic Solution DECADRON Phosphate is a clear, colorless to pale yellow solution.
No. 7643—Ophthalmic Solution DECADRON Phosphate is supplied as follows:
NDC 0006-7643-03 in 5 mL white, opaque, plastic OCUMETER ophthalmic dispenser with a controlled drop tip.
(6505-00-007-4536 0.1% 5 mL).

A.H.F.S. Category: 52:08
DC 7261515 Issued February 1987

DECADRON® Phosphate ℞
RESPIHALER®
(Dexamethasone Sodium Phosphate), U.S.P.

DESCRIPTION

RESPIHALER* DECADRON* Phosphate (Dexamethasone Sodium Phosphate) is an aerosol for oral inhalation which contains dexamethasone sodium phosphate, an inorganic ester of dexamethasone, a synthetic adrenocortical steroid with basic glucocorticoid actions and effects.
Each RESPIHALER DECADRON Phosphate contains an amount sufficient to deliver at least 170 sprays. The metering valve of the aerosol-mechanism of the RESPIHALER dispenses dexamethasone sodium phosphate equivalent to approximately 0.1 mg of dexamethasone phosphate or approximately 0.084 mg of dexamethasone with each activation. On a regimen of 12 inhalations daily, it has been determined that the patient absorbs approximately 0.4-0.6 mg of dexamethasone. The inactive ingredients are fluorochlorohydrocarbons included as propellants. Alcohol 2%.
Dexamethasone sodium phosphate, a synthetic adrenocortical steroid, is a white or slightly yellow, crystalline powder. It is freely soluble in water and is exceedingly hygroscopic. It is prepared by a special process to produce particles in the range of 0.5 to 4 microns in size. The molecular weight is 516.41. It is designated chemically as 9-fluoro-11β,17-dihydroxy-16α-methyl-21-(phosphono-oxy)pregna-1, 4-diene-3, 20-dione disodium salt. The empirical formula is $C_{22}H_{28}FNa_2O_8P$ and the structural formula is:

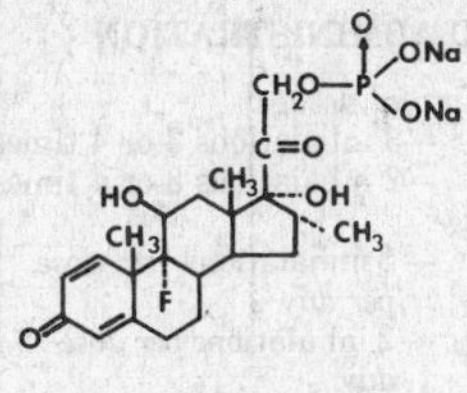

*Registered trademark of MERCK & CO., INC.

ACTIONS

Because of the high water solubility of dexamethasone sodium phosphate, the aerosolized particles dissolve readily in the secretions of the bronchial and bronchiolar mucous membrane.

INDICATIONS

RESPIHALER DECADRON Phosphate is indicated for the treatment of bronchial asthma and related corticosteroid responsive bronchospastic states intractable to adequate trial of conventional therapy.

CONTRAINDICATIONS

Systemic fungal infections.
Hypersensitivity to any component of this medication.
Persistently positive cultures of the sputum for *Candida albicans.*

WARNINGS

Rare instances of laryngeal and pharyngeal fungal infections have been observed in patients using RESPIHALER DECADRON Phosphate. These have usually responded promptly to discontinuation of therapy and institution of antifungal treatment.
In patients on therapy with RESPIHALER DECADRON Phosphate subjected to unusual stress, increased dosage of rapidly acting corticosteroids before, during, and after the stressful situation is indicated.
Drug-induced secondary adrenocortical insufficiency may result from too rapid withdrawal of corticosteroids and may be minimized by gradual reduction of dosage. This type of relative insufficiency may persist for months after discontinuation of therapy; therefore, in any situation of stress occurring during that period, hormone therapy should be reinstituted. If the patient is receiving steroids already, dosage may have to be increased. Since mineralocorticoid secretion may be impaired, salt and/or a mineralocorticoid should be administered concurrently.
Dexamethasone may mask some signs of infection, and new infections may appear during its use. There may be decreased resistance and inability to localize infection when corticosteroids are used. Moreover, dexamethasone may affect the nitroblue-tetrazolium test for bacterial infection and produce false negative results.
Corticosteroids may activate latent amebiasis. Therefore, it is recommended that latent or active amebiasis be ruled out before initiating corticosteroid therapy in any patient who has spent time in the tropics or any patient with unexplained diarrhea.
Prolonged use of RESPIHALER DECADRON Phosphate may produce posterior subcapsular cataracts, glaucoma with possible damage to the optic nerves, and may enhance the establishment of secondary ocular infections due to fungi or viruses.
Usage in pregnancy: Since adequate human reproduction studies have not been done with RESPIHALER DECADRON Phosphate, use of this drug in pregnancy or in women of childbearing potential requires that the anticipated benefits be weighed against the possible hazards to the mother and embryo or fetus. Infants born of mothers who have received substantial doses of dexamethasone during pregnancy, should be carefully observed for signs of hypoadrenalism.
Dexamethasone appears in breast milk and could suppress growth, interfere with endogenous corticosteroid production, or cause other unwanted effects. Mothers taking pharmacologic doses of dexamethasone should be advised not to nurse.
Average and large doses of hydrocortisone or cortisone can cause elevation of blood pressure, salt and water retention, and increased excretion of potassium. These effects are less likely to occur with the synthetic derivatives and with RESPIHALER DECADRON Phosphate, except when used in large doses. Dietary salt restriction and potassium supplementation may be necessary. All corticosteroids increase calcium excretion.
Administration of live virus vaccines, including smallpox, is contraindicated in individuals receiving immunosuppressive doses of corticosteroids. If inactivated viral or bacterial vaccines are administered to individuals receiving immunosuppressive doses of corticosteroids, the expected serum antibody response may not be obtained.
If RESPIHALER DECADRON Phosphate is indicated in patients with latent tuberculosis or tuberculin reactivity, close observation is necessary as reactivation of the disease may occur. During prolonged therapy with RESPIHALER DECADRON Phosphate, these patients should receive chemoprophylaxis.
Literature reports suggest an apparent association between use of corticosteroids and left ventricular free wall rupture after a recent myocardial infarction; therefore, therapy with corticosteroids should be used with great caution in these patients.
Keep out of reach of children.

PRECAUTIONS

RESPIHALER DECADRON Phosphate is *not* indicated for relief of the occasional mild and isolated attack of asthma which is readily responsive to the immediate, though short-lived, action of epinephrine, isoproterenol, aminophylline, etc. Nor should it be employed for the treatment of severe status asthmaticus where intensive measures are required.
RESPIHALER DECADRON Phosphate should be considered only for the following classes of patients: patients not on corticosteroid therapy who have not responded adequately to other treatment; patients already on systemic corticosteroid therapy—in an attempt to reduce or eliminate systemic administration.
Although systemic absorption is low when RESPIHALER DECADRON Phosphate is used in the recommended dosage, adrenal suppression may occur. In addition, other systemic effects of steroid administration must be considered as a possibility.

Continued on next page

Information on the Merck & Co. products listed on these pages is the full prescribing information from product circulars in use October 1, 1992.

Merck & Co.—Cont.

Following prolonged therapy, withdrawal of corticosteroids may result in symptoms of the corticosteroid withdrawal syndrome including fever, myalgia, arthralgia, and malaise. This may occur in patients even without evidence of adrenal insufficiency.

There is an enhanced effect of dexamethasone in patients with hypothyroidism and in those with cirrhosis.

RESPIHALER DECADRON Phosphate should be used cautiously in patients with ocular herpes simplex for fear of corneal perforation.

The lowest possible dose of RESPIHALER DECADRON Phosphate should be used to control the condition under treatment, and when reduction in dosage is possible, the reduction must be gradual.

Psychic derangements may appear when dexamethasone is used, ranging from euphoria, insomnia, mood swings, personality changes, and severe depression, to frank psychotic manifestations. Also, existing emotional instability or psychotic tendencies may be aggravated.

Aspirin should be used cautiously in conjunction with RESPIHALER DECADRON Phosphate in hypoprothrombinemia.

RESPIHALER DECADRON Phosphate should be used with caution in nonspecific ulcerative colitis, if there is a probability of impending perforation, abscess or other pyogenic infection; also in diverticulitis; fresh intestinal anastomoses; active or latent peptic ulcer; renal insufficiency; hypertension; osteoporosis; and myasthenia gravis. Signs of peritoneal irritation following gastrointestinal perforation in patients receiving large doses of corticosteroids may be minimal or absent. Fat embolism has been reported as a possible complication of hypercortisonism.

Growth and development of infants and children on prolonged therapy with RESPIHALER DECADRON Phosphate should be carefully followed.

Dexamethasone may increase or decrease motility and number of spermatozoa in some patients.

Phenytoin, phenobarbital, ephedrine and rifampin may enhance the metabolic clearance of dexamethasone, resulting in decreased blood levels and lessened physiologic activity, thus requiring adjustment in dexamethasone dosage.

The prothrombin time should be checked frequently in patients who are receiving RESPIHALER DECADRON Phosphate and coumarin anticoagulants at the same time because of reports that corticosteroids have altered the response to these anticoagulants. Studies have shown that the usual effect produced by adding corticosteroids is inhibition of response to coumarins, although there have been some conflicting reports of potentiation, not substantiated by studies.

When RESPIHALER DECADRON Phosphate is used concomitantly with potassium-depleting diuretics, patients should be observed closely for development of hypokalemia. Since the contents of RESPIHALER DECADRON Phosphate are under pressure, the container should not be broken, stored in extreme heat, or incinerated. It should be stored at a temperature below 120°F.

ADVERSE REACTIONS

Side effects which may occur in patients treated with RESPIHALER DECADRON Phosphate include throat irritation, hoarseness, coughing, and laryngeal and pharyngeal fungal infections.

Patients should be observed for the hormonal effects described below:

Fluid and Electrolyte Disturbances
  Sodium retention
  Fluid retention
  Congestive heart failure in susceptible patients
  Potassium loss
  Hypokalemic alkalosis
  Hypertension

Musculoskeletal
  Muscle weakness
  Steroid myopathy
  Loss of muscle mass
  Osteoporosis
  Vertebral compression fractures
  Aseptic necrosis of femoral and humeral heads
  Pathologic fracture of long bones
  Tendon rupture

Gastrointestinal
  Peptic ulcer with possible subsequent perforation and hemorrhage
  Perforation of the small and large bowel, particularly in patients with inflammatory bowel disease
  Pancreatitis
  Abdominal distention
  Ulcerative esophagitis

Dermatologic
  Impaired wound healing
  Thin fragile skin
  Petechiae and ecchymoses
  Erythema
  Increased sweating
  May suppress reactions to skin tests
  Other cutaneous reactions, such as allergic dermatitis, urticaria, angioneurotic edema

Neurologic
  Convulsions
  Increased intracranial pressure with papilledema (pseudotumor cerebri) usually after treatment
  Vertigo
  Headache
  Psychic disturbances

Endocrine
  Menstrual irregularities
  Development of cushingoid state
  Suppression of growth in children
  Secondary adrenocortical and pituitary unresponsiveness, particularly in times of stress, as in trauma, surgery, or illness
  Decreased carbohydrate tolerance
  Manifestations of latent diabetes mellitus
  Increased requirements for insulin or oral hypoglycemic agents in diabetics

Ophthalmic
  Posterior subcapsular cataracts
  Increased intraocular pressure
  Glaucoma
  Exophthalmos

Metabolic
  Negative nitrogen balance due to protein catabolism

Cardiovascular
  Myocardial rupture following recent myocardial infarction (see WARNINGS).

Other
  Hypersensitivity
  Thromboembolism
  Weight gain
  Increased appetite
  Nausea
  Malaise
  Hiccups

OVERDOSAGE

Reports of acute toxicity and/or death following overdosage of glucocorticoids are rare. In the event of overdosage, no specific antidote is available; treatment is supportive and symptomatic.

The oral LD_{50} of dexamethasone in female mice was 6.5 g/kg. The intravenous LD_{50} of dexamethasone sodium phosphate in female mice was 794 mg/kg.

DOSAGE AND ADMINISTRATION

Recommended *initial dosage:*
  Adults   —3 inhalations 3 or 4 times per day.
  Children   —2 inhalations 3 or 4 times per day.
Maximum dosage:
  Adults   — 3 inhalations *per dose;* 12 inhalations *per day.*
  Children   — 2 inhalations *per dose;* 8 inhalations *per day.*

When a favorable response is attained, the dose may be gradually reduced. In patients on systemic corticosteroids, it is recommended that systemic therapy be reduced or eliminated before reduction of RESPIHALER dosage is begun. Gradual reduction of systemic corticosteroid therapy must be emphasized to avoid withdrawal symptoms.

HOW SUPPLIED

No. 7626X—RESPIHALER DECADRON Phosphate, aerosol for oral inhalation, is supplied as follows: NDC 0006-7626-13 in a pressurized container, and includes a plastic adapter.

Storage
Store at a temperature below 49°C (120°F).

        A.H.F.S. Category: 68:04
        DC 7413017   Issued August 1989

DECADRON® Phosphate Topical Cream   ℞
(Dexamethasone Sodium Phosphate), U.S.P.
0.1% Dexamethasone Phosphate Equivalent

DESCRIPTION

DECADRON* Phosphate (Dexamethasone Sodium Phosphate) Topical Cream is a topical steroid preparation.

The topical corticosteroids constitute a class of primarily synthetic steroids used as anti-inflammatory and anti-pruritic agents.

Dexamethasone sodium phosphate is 9-fluoro-11β,17-dihydroxy-16α-methyl-21-(phosphonooxy) pregna-1,4-diene-3,20-dione disodium salt. Its empirical formula is $C_{22}H_{28}FNa_2O_8P$ and its structural formula is:

Dexamethasone sodium phosphate has a molecular weight of 516.41.

DECADRON Phosphate Topical Cream contains in each gram: dexamethasone sodium phosphate equivalent to 1 mg (0.1%) dexamethasone phosphate in a greaseless bland base. Inactive ingredients: stearyl alcohol, cetyl alcohol, mineral oil, polyoxyl 40 stearate, sorbitol solution, methyl polysilicone emulsion, creatinine, sodium citrate, disodium edetate, sodium hydroxide to adjust pH, and purified water. Methylparaben, 0.15%, and sorbic acid, 0.1% added as preservatives.

---

*Registered trademark of MERCK & CO., INC.

CLINICAL PHARMACOLOGY

Topical corticosteroids share anti-inflammatory, anti-pruritic and vasoconstrictive actions.

The mechanism of anti-inflammatory activity of the topical corticosteroids is unclear. Various laboratory methods, including vasoconstrictor assays, are used to compare and predict potencies and/or clinical efficacies of the topical corticosteroids. There is some evidence to suggest that a recognizable correlation exists between vasoconstrictor potency and therapeutic efficacy in man.

Pharmacokinetics
The extent of percutaneous absorption of topical corticosteroids is determined by many factors including the vehicle, the integrity of the epidermal barrier, and the use of occlusive dressings.

Topical corticosteroids can be absorbed from normal intact skin. Inflammation and/or other disease processes in the skin increase percutaneous absorption. Occlusive dressings substantially increase the percutaneous absorption of topical corticosteroids. Thus, occlusive dressings may be a valuable therapeutic adjunct for treatment of resistant dermatoses. (See DOSAGE AND ADMINISTRATION)

Once absorbed through the skin, topical corticosteroids are handled through pharmacokinetic pathways similar to systemically administered corticosteroids. Corticosteroids are bound to plasma proteins in varying degrees. Corticosteroids are metabolized primarily in the liver and are then excreted by the kidneys. Some of the topical corticosteroids and their metabolites are also excreted into the bile.

INDICATIONS AND USAGE

DECADRON Phosphate Topical Cream is indicated for relief of the inflammatory and pruritic manifestations of corticosteroid-responsive dermatoses.

CONTRAINDICATIONS

Topical corticosteroids are contraindicated in those patients with a history of hypersensitivity to any of the components of the preparation.

PRECAUTIONS

General
Systemic absorption of topical corticosteroids has produced reversible hypothalamic-pituitary-adrenal (HPA) axis suppression, manifestations of Cushing's syndrome, hyperglycemia, and glycosuria in some patients.

Conditions which augment systemic absorption include the application of the more potent corticosteroids, use over large surface areas, prolonged use, and the addition of occlusive dressings.

Therefore, patients receiving a large dose of a potent topical corticosteroid applied to a large surface area or under an occlusive dressing should be evaluated periodically for evidence of HPA axis suppression by using urinary free cortisol and ACTH stimulation tests. If HPA axis suppression is noted, an attempt should be made to withdraw the drug, to reduce the frequency of application, or to substitute a less potent corticosteroid.

Recovery of HPA axis function is generally prompt and complete upon discontinuation of the drug. Infrequently, signs and symptoms of corticosteroid withdrawal may occur, requiring supplemental systemic corticosteroids.

Children may absorb proportionally larger amounts of topical corticosteroids and thus be more susceptible to systemic toxicity (See PRECAUTIONS, *Pediatric Use*).

If irritation develops, topical corticosteroids should be discontinued and appropriate therapy instituted.

In the presence of dermatological infections, the use of an appropriate antifungal or antibacterial agent should be instituted. If a favorable response does not occur promptly, the corticosteroid should be discontinued until the infection has been adequately controlled.

This product is not for ophthalmic use. However, if applied to the eyelids or skin near the eyes, the drug may enter the eyes. In patients with a history of herpes simplex keratitis, ocular exposure to corticosteroids may lead to a recurrence. Prolonged ocular exposure may cause steroid glaucoma. Generally, occlusive dressings should not be used on weeping or exudative lesions.

If occlusive dressing therapy is used, inspect lesions between dressings for development of infection. If infection develops, the technique should be discontinued and appropriate antimicrobial therapy instituted.

When large areas of the body are covered with an occlusive dressing, thermal homeostasis may be impaired. If elevation of body temperature occurs, use of the occlusive dressing should be discontinued.

Information for the Patient

Patients using topical corticosteroids should receive the following information and instructions:

1. This medication is to be used as directed by the physician. It is for external use only. Avoid contact with the eyes.
2. Patients should be advised not to use this medication for any disorder other than that for which it was prescribed.
3. The treated skin area should not be bandaged or otherwise covered or wrapped so as to be occlusive unless directed by the physician.
4. Patients should report any signs of local adverse reactions, especially under occlusive dressing.
5. Parents of pediatric patients should be advised not to use tight-fitting diapers or plastic pants on a child being treated in the diaper area, as these garments may constitute occlusive dressings.

Laboratory Tests

The following tests may be helpful in evaluating the HPA axis suppression:
● Urinary free cortisol test
● ACTH stimulation test

Carcinogenesis, Mutagenesis, and Impairment of Fertility

Long-term animal studies have not been performed to evaluate the carcinogenic potential or the effect on fertility of topical corticosteroids.

Studies to determine mutagenicity with prednisolone and hydrocortisone have revealed negative results.

Pregnancy

Pregnancy Category C: Corticosteroids are generally teratogenic in laboratory animals when administered systemically at relatively low dosage levels. The more potent corticosteroids have been shown to be teratogenic after dermal application in laboratory animals. There are not adequate and well-controlled studies in pregnant women on teratogenic effects from topically applied corticosteroids. Therefore, topical corticosteroids should be used during pregnancy only if the potential benefit justifies the potential risk to the fetus. Drugs of this class should not be used extensively on pregnant patients, in large amounts, or for prolonged periods of time.

Nursing Mothers

It is not known whether topical administration of corticosteroids could result in sufficient systemic absorption to produce detectable quantities in breast milk. Systemically administered corticosteroids are secreted into breast milk in quantities *not* likely to have a deleterious effect on the infant. Nevertheless, caution should be exercised when topical corticosteroids are administered to a nursing woman.

Pediatric Use

Pediatric patients may demonstrate greater susceptibility to topical corticosteroid-induced HPA axis suppression and Cushing's syndrome than mature patients because of a larger skin surface area to body weight ratio.

Hypothalamic-pituitary-adrenal (HPA) axis suppression, Cushing's syndrome, and intracranial hypertension have been reported in children receiving topical corticosteroids. Manifestations of adrenal suppression in children include linear growth retardation, delayed weight gain, low plasma cortisol levels, and absence of response to ACTH stimulation. Manifestations of intracranial hypertension include bulging fontanelles, headaches, and bilateral papilledema.

Administration of topical corticosteroids to children should be limited to the least amount compatible with an effective therapeutic regimen. Chronic corticosteroid therapy may interfere with the growth and development of children.

ADVERSE REACTIONS

The following adverse reactions are reported infrequently with topical corticosteroids, but may occur more frequently with the use of occlusive dressings. These reactions are listed in an approximate decreasing order of occurrence:

Burning
Itching
Irritation
Dryness
Folliculitis
Hypertrichosis
Acneiform eruptions
Hypopigmentation
Perioral dermatitis
Allergic contact dermatitis
Maceration of the skin
Secondary infection
Skin atrophy
Striae
Miliaria

OVERDOSAGE

Topically applied corticosteroids can be absorbed in sufficient amounts to produce systemic effects (See PRECAUTIONS).

DOSAGE AND ADMINISTRATION

Apply to the affected area as a thin film three or four times daily.

Occlusive dressings may be used for the management of psoriasis or recalcitrant conditions.

Before using this preparation in the *ear*, clean the aural canal thoroughly and sponge dry. Confirm that the eardrum is intact. With a cotton-tipped applicator, apply a thin coating of the cream to the affected canal area three or four times a day.

HOW SUPPLIED

No. 7616X — 0.1% Topical Cream DECADRON Phosphate is a white cream, and is supplied as follows:
NDC 0006-7616-12 in 15 g tubes
NDC 0006-7616-24 in 30 g tubes.
A.H.F.S. Category: 84:06
DC 6005423   Issued April 1983
Copyright © MERCK & CO., INC., 1983
All rights reserved

DECADRON® Phosphate   ℞
TURBINAIRE®
(Dexamethasone Sodium Phosphate), U.S.P.

DESCRIPTION

TURBINAIRE* DECADRON* Phosphate (Dexamethasone Sodium Phosphate) is an aerosol for intranasal application. The inactive ingredients are fluorochlorohydrocarbons as propellants and alcohol 2%. One cartridge delivers an amount sufficient to ensure delivery of 170 metered sprays, each containing dexamethasone sodium phosphate equivalent to approximately 0.1 mg dexamethasone phosphate or to approximately 0.084 mg dexamethasone. Twelve sprays deliver a theoretical maximum of 1.0 mg dexamethasone.

Dexamethasone sodium phosphate, a synthetic adrenocortical steroid, is a white or slightly yellow, crystalline powder. It is freely soluble in water and is exceedingly hygroscopic. The molecular weight is 516.41. It is designated chemically as 9-fluoro-11β, 17-dihydroxy-16α-methyl-21-(phosphonooxy) pregna-1, 4-diene-3, 20-dione disodium salt. The empirical formula is $C_{22}H_{28}FNa_2O_8P$ and the structural formula is:

---

*Registered trademark of MERCK & CO., INC.

ACTION

Inhibition of inflammatory response to inciting agents of mechanical, chemical or immunological nature.

INDICATIONS

Allergic or inflammatory nasal conditions, and nasal polyps (excluding polyps originating within the sinuses).

CONTRAINDICATIONS

Systemic fungal infections.
Hypersensitivity to components.
Tuberculous, viral and fungal nasal conditions, ocular herpes simplex.

WARNINGS

In patients on therapy with TURBINAIRE DECADRON Phosphate subjected to unusual stress, increased dosage of rapidly acting corticosteroids before, during, and after the stressful situation is indicated.

Drug-induced secondary adrenocortical insufficiency may result from too rapid withdrawal of corticosteroids and may be minimized by gradual reduction of dosage. This type of relative insufficiency may persist for months after discontinuation of therapy; therefore, in any situation of stress occurring during that period, hormone therapy should be reinstituted. If the patient is receiving steroids already, dosage may have to be increased. Since mineralocorticoid secretion may be impaired, salt and/or a mineralocorticoid should be administered concurrently.

Dexamethasone may mask some signs of infection, and new infections may appear during its use. There may be decreased resistance and inability to localize infection when corticosteroids are used. Therefore, patients with bacterial infections should also be given appropriate antibiotic therapy if TURBINAIRE DECADRON Phosphate is used. Moreover, dexamethasone may affect the nitroblue-tetrazolium test for bacterial infection and produce false negative results.

Corticosteroids may activate latent amebiasis. Therefore, it is recommended that latent or active amebiasis be ruled out before initiating corticosteroid therapy in any patient who has spent time in the tropics or any patient with unexplained diarrhea.

Prolonged use of TURBINAIRE DECADRON Phosphate may produce posterior subcapsular cataracts, glaucoma with possible damage to the optic nerves, and may enhance the establishment of secondary ocular infections due to fungi or viruses.

Usage in pregnancy: Since adequate human reproduction studies have not been done with TURBINAIRE DECADRON Phosphate, use of this drug in pregnancy or in women of childbearing potential requires that the anticipated benefits be weighed against the possible hazards to the mother and embryo or fetus. Infants born of mothers who have received substantial doses of dexamethasone during pregnancy, should be carefully observed for signs of hypoadrenalism.

Dexamethasone appears in breast milk and could suppress growth, interfere with endogenous corticosteroid production, or cause other unwanted effects. Mothers taking pharmacologic doses of dexamethasone should be advised not to nurse.

Average and large doses of hydrocortisone or cortisone can cause elevation of blood pressure, salt and water retention, and increased excretion of potassium. These effects are less likely to occur with the synthetic derivatives and with TURBINAIRE DECADRON Phosphate, except when used in large doses. Dietary salt restriction and potassium supplementation may be necessary. All corticosteroids increase calcium excretion.

Administration of live virus vaccines, including smallpox, is contraindicated in individuals receiving immunosuppressive doses of corticosteroids. If inactivated viral or bacterial vaccines are administered to individuals receiving immunosuppressive doses of corticosteroids, the expected serum antibody response may not be obtained.

If TURBINAIRE DECADRON Phosphate is indicated in patients with latent tuberculosis or tuberculin reactivity, close observation is necessary as reactivation of the disease may occur. During prolonged therapy with TURBINAIRE DECADRON Phosphate, these patients should receive chemoprophylaxis.

Literature reports suggest an apparent association between use of corticosteroids and left ventricular free wall rupture after a recent myocardial infarction; therefore, therapy with corticosteroids should be used with great caution in these patients.

Keep out of reach of children.

PRECAUTIONS

During local corticosteroid therapy, the possibility of pharyngeal candidiasis should be kept in mind.

Although systemic absorption is low when TURBINAIRE DECADRON Phosphate is used in the recommended dosage, adrenal suppression may occur. In addition, other systemic

Continued on next page

Merck & Co.—Cont.

effects of steroid administration must be considered as a possibility.

Following prolonged therapy, withdrawal of corticosteroids may result in symptoms of the corticosteroid withdrawal syndrome including fever, myalgia, arthralgia, and malaise. This may occur in patients even without evidence of adrenal insufficiency. Replacement of systemic steroid with TURBINAIRE DECADRON Phosphate should be gradual and carefully monitored by the physician.

There is an enhanced effect of dexamethasone in patients with hypothyroidism and in those with cirrhosis.

TURBINAIRE DECADRON Phosphate should be used cautiously in patients with ocular herpes simplex for fear of corneal perforation.

The lowest possible dose of TURBINAIRE DECADRON Phosphate should be used to control the condition under treatment, and when reduction in dosage is possible, the reduction must be gradual. If beneficial effect is not evident within 7 days after initiation of therapy, the patient should be re-evaluated.

Psychic derangements may appear when dexamethasone is used, ranging from euphoria, insomnia, mood swings, personality changes, and severe depression, to frank psychotic manifestations. Also, existing emotional instability or psychotic tendencies may be aggravated.

Aspirin should be used cautiously in conjunction with TURBINAIRE DECADRON Phosphate in hypoprothrombinemia.

TURBINAIRE DECADRON Phosphate should be used with caution in patients with nonspecific ulcerative colitis, if there is a probability of impending perforation, abscess or other pyogenic infection; also in diverticulitis; fresh intestinal anastomoses; active or latent peptic ulcer; renal insufficiency; hypertension; osteoporosis; and myasthenia gravis. Signs of peritoneal irritation following gastrointestinal perforation in patients receiving large doses of corticosteroids may be minimal or absent. Fat embolism has been reported as a possible complication of hypercortisonism.

Because clinical studies have not been done, the use of this product in children under the age of 6 years is not recommended. Growth and development of children 6 years of age or older on prolonged therapy with TURBINAIRE DECADRON Phosphate should be carefully followed.

Dexamethasone may increase or decrease motility and number of spermatozoa in some patients.

Phenytoin, phenobarbital, ephedrine and rifampin may enhance the metabolic clearance of dexamethasone, resulting in decreased blood levels and lessened physiologic activity, thus requiring adjustment in dexamethasone dosage.

The prothrombin time should be checked frequently in patients who are receiving TURBINAIRE DECADRON Phosphate and coumarin anticoagulants at the same time because of reports that corticosteroids have altered the response to these anticoagulants. Studies have shown that the usual effect produced by adding corticosteroids is inhibition of response to coumarins, although there have been some conflicting reports of potentiation, not substantiated by studies.

When TURBINAIRE DECADRON Phosphate is used concomitantly with potassium-depleting diuretics, patients should be observed closely for development of hypokalemia. Since the contents of TURBINAIRE DECADRON Phosphate are under pressure, the container should not be broken, stored in extreme heat, or incinerated. It should be stored at a temperature below 120°F.

ADVERSE REACTIONS

Nasal irritation and dryness are the most common adverse reactions. The following have been reported: headache, lightheadedness, urticaria, nausea, epistaxis, rebound congestion, bronchial asthma, perforation of the nasal septum, and anosmia. Signs of adrenal hypercorticism may occur in some patients, especially with overdosage.

Systemic effects from therapy with TURBINAIRE DECADRON Phosphate are less likely to occur than with oral or parenteral corticosteroid therapy because of a lower total dose administered. Nevertheless, patients should be observed for the hormonal effects described below because of absorption of dexamethasone from the nasal mucosa.

Fluid and Electrolyte Disturbances
  Sodium retention
  Fluid retention
  Congestive heart failure in susceptible patients
  Potassium loss
  Hypokalemic alkalosis
  Hypertension
Musculoskeletal
  Muscle weakness
  Steroid myopathy
  Loss of muscle mass
  Osteoporosis

  Vertebral compression fractures
  Aseptic necrosis of femoral and humeral heads
  Pathologic fracture of long bones
  Tendon rupture
Gastrointestinal
  Peptic ulcer with possible subsequent perforation and hemorrhage
  Perforation of the small and large bowel, particularly in patients with inflammatory bowel disease
  Pancreatitis
  Abdominal distention
  Ulcerative esophagitis
Dermatologic
  Impaired wound healing
  Thin fragile skin
  Petechiae and ecchymoses
  Erythema
  Increased sweating
  May suppress reactions to skin tests
  Other cutaneous reactions, such as allergic dermatitis, urticaria, angioneurotic edema.
Neurologic
  Convulsions
  Increased intracranial pressure with papilledema (pseudotumor cerebri) usually after treatment
  Vertigo
  Headache
  Psychic disturbances
Endocrine
  Menstrual irregularities
  Development of cushingoid state
  Suppression of growth in children
  Secondary adrenocortical and pituitary unresponsiveness, particularly in times of stress, as in trauma, surgery, or illness
  Decreased carbohydrate tolerance
  Manifestations of latent diabetes mellitus
  Increased requirements for insulin or oral hypoglycemic agents in diabetics
Ophthalmic
  Posterior subcapsular cataracts
  Increased intraocular pressure
  Glaucoma
  Exophthalmos
Metabolic
  Negative nitrogen balance due to protein catabolism
Cardiovascular
  Myocardial rupture following recent myocardial infarction (see WARNINGS).
Other
  Hypersensitivity
  Thromboembolism
  Weight gain
  Increased appetite
  Nausea
  Malaise
  Hiccups

OVERDOSAGE

Reports of acute toxicity and/or death following overdosage of glucocorticoids are rare. In the event of overdosage, no specific antidote is available; treatment is supportive and symptomatic.

The oral LD_{50} of dexamethasone in female mice was 6.5 g/kg. The intravenous LD_{50} of dexamethasone sodium phosphate in female mice was 794 mg/kg.

DOSAGE AND ADMINISTRATION

DO NOT EXCEED THE RECOMMENDED DOSAGE.
The usual initial dosage of TURBINAIRE DECADRON Phosphate is:
  Adults—2 sprays in each nostril 2 or 3 times a day.
  Children (6 to 12 years of age)—1 or 2 sprays in each nostril 2 times a day depending on age.
See accompanying instructions on the proper use of TURBINAIRE.
When improvement occurs the dosage should be gradually reduced. Some patients will be symptom-free on one spray in each nostril 2 times a day. The maximum daily dosage for adults is 12 sprays, and for children, 8 sprays. Therapy should be discontinued as soon as feasible. It may be reinstituted if recurrence of symptoms occurs.

HOW SUPPLIED

No. 7634—TURBINAIRE DECADRON Phosphate, aerosol for intranasal application, is supplied as follows: **NDC** 0006-7634-13 in a pressurized container and includes a plastic adapter
(6505-00-885-6302, 12.6 Grams, 170 Metered Doses).

No. 7642—Refill unit for TURBINAIRE DECADRON Phosphate aerosol for intranasal application is supplied as follows: **NDC** 0006-7642-13 in a pressurized container.
Storage
Store at a temperature below 49°C (120°F).
    A.H.F.S. Category: 52:08
    DC 7413123   Issued August 1989

DECADRON-LA® Sterile Suspension   ℞
(Dexamethasone Acetate), U.S.P.

NOT FOR INTRAVENOUS USE

DESCRIPTION

Dexamethasone acetate, a synthetic adrenocortical steroid, is a white to practically white, odorless powder. It is a practically insoluble ester of dexamethasone. The structural formula is:

Dexamethasone acetate is present in DECADRON-LA* (Dexamethasone Acetate) sterile suspension as the monohydrate, with the empirical formula, $C_{24}H_{31}FO_6 \cdot H_2O$, and molecular weight, 452.52. Dexamethasone acetate is designated chemically as 21-(acetyloxy)-9-fluoro-11β,17-dihydroxy-16α-methylpregna-1,4-diene-3,20-dione.

DECADRON-LA sterile suspension is a sterile white suspension (pH 5.0 to 7.5) that settles on standing, but is easily resuspended by mild shaking.

Each milliliter contains dexamethasone acetate equivalent to 8 mg dexamethasone. Inactive ingredients per mL: 6.67 mg sodium chloride; 5 mg creatinine; 0.5 mg disodium edetate; 5 mg sodium carboxymethylcellulose; 0.75 mg polysorbate 80; sodium hydroxide to adjust pH; and Water for Injection, q.s. 1 mL, with 9 mg benzyl alcohol, and 1 mg sodium bisulfite added as preservatives.

*Registered trademark of MERCK & CO., INC.

ACTIONS

DECADRON-LA sterile suspension is a long-acting, repository adrenocorticosteroid preparation with a prompt onset of action. It is suitable for intramuscular or local injection, but not when an immediate effect of short duration is desired. Naturally occurring glucocorticoids (hydrocortisone and cortisone), which also have salt-retaining properties, are used as replacement therapy in adrenocortical deficiency states. Their synthetic analogs, including dexamethasone, are primarily used for their potent anti-inflammatory effects in disorders of many organ systems.

Glucocorticoids cause profound and varied metabolic effects. In addition, they modify the body's immune responses to diverse stimuli.

At equipotent anti-inflammatory doses, dexamethasone almost completely lacks the sodium-retaining property of hydrocortisone.

INDICATIONS

A. By intramuscular injection when oral therapy is not feasible:
1. *Endocrine disorders*
Congenital adrenal hyperplasia
Nonsuppurative thyroiditis
Hypercalcemia associated with cancer
2. *Rheumatic disorders*
As adjunctive therapy for short-term administration (to tide the patient over an acute episode or exacerbation) in:
Post-traumatic osteoarthritis
Synovitis of osteoarthritis
Rheumatoid arthritis, including juvenile rheumatoid arthritis (selected cases may require low-dose maintenance therapy)
Acute and subacute bursitis
Epicondylitis
Acute nonspecific tenosynovitis
Acute gouty arthritis
Psoriatic arthritis
Ankylosing spondylitis
3. *Collagen diseases*
During an exacerbation or as maintenance therapy in selected cases of:

Systemic lupus erythematosus
Acute rheumatic carditis
4. *Dermatologic diseases*
Pemphigus
Severe erythema multiforme (Stevens-Johnson syndrome)
Exfoliative dermatitis
Bullous dermatitis herpetiformis
Severe seborrheic dermatitis
Severe psoriasis
Mycosis fungoides
5. *Allergic states*
Control of severe or incapacitating allergic conditions intractable to adequate trials of conventional treatment in:
Bronchial asthma
Contact dermatitis
Atopic dermatitis
Serum sickness
Seasonal or perennial allergic rhinitis
Drug hypersensitivity reactions
Urticarial transfusion reactions
6. *Ophthalmic diseases*
Severe acute and chronic allergic and inflammatory processes involving the eye, such as:
Herpes zoster ophthalmicus
Iritis, Iridocyclitis
Chorioretinitis
Diffuse posterior uveitis and choroiditis
Optic neuritis
Sympathetic ophthalmia
Anterior segment inflammation
Allergic conjunctivitis
Keratitis
Allergic corneal marginal ulcers
7. *Gastrointestinal diseases*
To tide the patient over a critical period of the disease in:
Ulcerative colitis (Systemic therapy)
Regional enteritis (Systemic therapy)
8. *Respiratory diseases*
Symptomatic sarcoidosis
Berylliosis
Loeffler's syndrome not manageable by other means
Aspiration pneumonitis
9. *Hematologic disorders*
Acquired (autoimmune) hemolytic anemia
Secondary thrombocytopenia in adults
Erythroblastopenia (RBC anemia)
Congenital (erythroid) hypoplastic anemia
10. *Neoplastic diseases*
For palliative management of:
Leukemias and lymphomas in adults
Acute leukemia of childhood
11. *Edematous states*
To induce diuresis or remission of proteinuria in the nephrotic syndrome, without uremia, of the idiopathic type, or that due to lupus erythematosus
12. *Miscellaneous*
Trichinosis with neurologic or myocardial involvement.
B. By intra-articular or soft tissue injection as adjunctive therapy for short-term administration (to tide the patient over an acute episode or exacerbation) in:
Synovitis of osteoarthritis
Rheumatoid arthritis
Acute and subacute bursitis
Acute gouty arthritis
Epicondylitis
Acute nonspecific tenosynovitis
Post-traumatic osteoarthritis.
C. By intralesional injection in:
Keloids
Localized hypertrophic, infiltrated, inflammatory lesions of: lichen planus, psoriatic plaques, granuloma annulare, and lichen simplex chronicus (neurodermatitis)
Discoid lupus erythematosus
Necrobiosis lipoidica diabeticorum
Alopecia areata
May also be useful in cystic tumors of an aponeurosis or tendon (ganglia).

CONTRAINDICATIONS

Systemic fungal infections
Hypersensitivity to any component of this product, including sulfites (see WARNINGS).

WARNINGS

DO NOT INJECT INTRAVENOUSLY
Because rare instances of anaphylactoid reactions have occurred in patients receiving parenteral corticosteroid therapy, appropriate precautionary measures should be taken prior to administration, especially when the patient has a history of allergy to any drug. Anaphylactoid and hypersensitivity reactions have been reported for Sterile Suspension DECADRON-LA (see ADVERSE REACTIONS).

Sterile Suspension DECADRON-LA contains sodium bisulfite, a sulfite that may cause allergic-type reactions including anaphylactic symptoms and life-threatening or less severe asthmatic episodes in certain susceptible people. The overall prevalence of sulfite sensitivity in the general population is unknown and probably low. Sulfite sensitivity is seen more frequently in asthmatic than in nonasthmatic people.
In patients on corticosteroid therapy subjected to any unusual stress, increased dosage of rapidly acting corticosteroids before, during, and after the stressful situation is indicated.
Drug-induced secondary adrenocortical insufficiency may result from too rapid withdrawal of corticosteroids and may be minimized by gradual reduction of dosage. This type of relative insufficiency may persist for months after discontinuation of therapy; therefore, in any situation of stress occurring during that period, hormone therapy should be reinstituted. If the patient is receiving steroids already, dosage may have to be increased. Since mineralocorticoid secretion may be impaired, salt and/or a mineralocorticoid should be administered concurrently.
Corticosteroids may mask some signs of infection, and new infections may appear during their use. There may be decreased resistance and inability to localize infection when corticosteroids are used. Moreover, corticosteroids may affect the nitroblue-tetrazolium test for bacterial infection and produce false negative results.
In cerebral malaria, a double-blind trial has shown that the use of corticosteroids is associated with prolongation of coma and a higher incidence of pneumonia and gastrointestinal bleeding.
Corticosteroids may activate latent amebiasis. Therefore, it is recommended that latent or active amebiasis be ruled out before initiating corticosteroid therapy in any patient who has spent time in the tropics or any patient with unexplained diarrhea.
Prolonged use of corticosteroids may produce posterior subcapsular cataracts, glaucoma with possible damage to the optic nerves, and may enhance the establishment of secondary ocular infections due to fungi or viruses.
Usage in pregnancy. Since adequate human reproduction studies have not been done with corticosteroids, use of these drugs in pregnancy or in women of childbearing potential requires that the anticipated benefits be weighed against the possible hazards to the mother and embryo or fetus. Infants born of mothers who have received substantial doses of corticosteroids during pregnancy should be carefully observed for signs of hypoadrenalism.
Corticosteroids appear in breast milk and could suppress growth, interfere with endogenous corticosteroid production, or cause other unwanted effects. Mothers taking pharmacologic doses of corticosteroids should be advised not to nurse.
Average and large doses of cortisone or hydrocortisone can cause elevation of blood pressure, salt and water retention, and increased excretion of potassium. These effects are less likely to occur with the synthetic derivatives except when used in large doses. Dietary salt restriction and potassium supplementation may be necessary. All corticosteroids increase calcium excretion.
Administration of live virus vaccines, including smallpox, is contraindicated in individuals receiving immunosuppressive doses of corticosteroids. If inactivated viral or bacterial vaccines are administered to individuals receiving immunosuppressive doses of corticosteroids, the expected serum antibody response may not be obtained.
If corticosteroids are indicated in patients with latent tuberculosis or tuberculin reactivity, close observation is necessary as reactivation of the disease may occur. During prolonged corticosteroid therapy, these patients should receive chemoprophylaxis.
Repository adrenocorticosteroid preparations may cause atrophy at the site of injection. To minimize the likelihood and/or severity of atrophy, do not inject subcutaneously, avoid injection into the deltoid muscle, and avoid repeated intramuscular injections into the same site if possible.
Dosage in children under 12 has not been established.
Literature reports suggest an apparent association between use of corticosteroids and left ventricular free wall rupture after a recent myocardial infarction; therefore, therapy with corticosteroids should be used with great caution in these patients.

PRECAUTIONS

DECADRON-LA sterile suspension is not recommended as initial therapy in acute, life-threatening situations.
This product, like many other steroid formulations, is sensitive to heat. Therefore, it should not be autoclaved when it is desirable to sterilize the exterior of the vial.
Following prolonged therapy, withdrawal of corticosteroids may result in symptoms of the corticosteroid withdrawal syndrome including fever, myalgia, arthralgia, and malaise. This may occur in patients even without evidence of adrenal insufficiency.

There is an enhanced effect of corticosteroids in patients with hypothyroidism and in those with cirrhosis.
Corticosteroids should be used cautiously in patients with ocular herpes simplex for fear of corneal perforation.
Psychic derangements may appear when corticosteroids are used, ranging from euphoria, insomnia, mood swings, personality changes, and severe depression to frank psychotic manifestations. Also, existing emotional instability or psychotic tendencies may be aggravated by corticosteroids.
Aspirin should be used cautiously in conjunction with corticosteroids in hypoprothrombinemia.
Steroids should be used with caution in nonspecific ulcerative colitis, if there is a probability of impending perforation, abscess, or other pyogenic infection, also in diverticulitis, fresh intestinal anastomoses, active or latent peptic ulcer, renal insufficiency, hypertension, osteoporosis, and myasthenia gravis. Signs of peritoneal irritation following gastrointestinal perforation in patients receiving large doses of corticosteroids may be minimal or absent. Fat embolism has been reported as a possible complication of hypercortisonism.
When large doses are given, some authorities advise that antacids be administered between meals to help to prevent peptic ulcer.
Growth and development of infants and children on prolonged corticosteroid therapy should be carefully followed.
Steroids may increase or decrease motility and number of spermatozoa in some patients.
Phenytoin, phenobarbital, ephedrine, and rifampin may enhance the metabolic clearance of corticosteroids, resulting in decreased blood levels and lessened physiologic activity, thus requiring adjustment in corticosteroid dosage.
The prothrombin time should be checked frequently in patients who are receiving corticosteroids and coumarin anticoagulants at the same time because of reports that corticosteroids have altered the response to these anticoagulants. Studies have shown that the usual effect produced by adding corticosteroids is inhibition of response to coumarins, although there have been some conflicting reports of potentiation not substantiated by studies.
When corticosteroids are administered concomitantly with potassium-depleting diuretics, patients should be observed closely for development of hypokalemia.
Intra-articular injection of a corticosteroid may produce systemic as well as local effects.
Appropriate examination of any joint fluid present is necessary to exclude a septic process.
A marked increase in pain accompanied by local swelling, further restriction of joint motion, fever, and malaise is suggestive of septic arthritis. If this complication occurs and the diagnosis of sepsis is confirmed, appropriate antimicrobial therapy should be instituted.
Injection of a steroid into an infected site is to be avoided.
Corticosteroids should not be injected into unstable joints.
Patients should be impressed strongly with the importance of not overusing joints in which symptomatic benefit has been obtained as long as the inflammatory process remains active.
Frequent intra-articular injection may result in damage to joint tissues.

ADVERSE REACTIONS

Fluid and electrolyte disturbances
Sodium retention
Fluid retention
Congestive heart failure in susceptible patients
Potassium loss
Hypokalemic alkalosis
Hypertension
Musculoskeletal
Muscle weakness
Steroid myopathy
Loss of muscle mass
Osteoporosis
Vertebral compression fractures
Aseptic necrosis of femoral and humeral heads
Pathologic fracture of long bones
Tendon rupture
Gastrointestinal
Peptic ulcer with possible subsequent perforation and hemorrhage
Perforation of the small and large bowel, particularly in patients with inflammatory bowel disease
Pancreatitis
Abdominal distention
Ulcerative esophagitis

Continued on next page

Merck & Co.—Cont.

Dermatologic
Impaired wound healing
Thin fragile skin
Petechiae and ecchymoses
Erythema
Increased sweating
May suppress reactions to skin tests
Other cutaneous reactions, such as allergic dermatitis, urticaria, angioneurotic edema
Neurologic
Convulsions
Increased intracranial pressure with papilledema (pseudotumor cerebri) usually after treatment
Vertigo
Headache
Psychic disturbances
Endocrine
Menstrual irregularities
Development of cushingoid state
Suppression of growth in children
Secondary adrenocortical and pituitary unresponsiveness, particularly in times of stress, as in trauma, surgery, or illness
Decreased carbohydrate tolerance
Manifestations of latent diabetes mellitus
Increased requirements for insulin or oral hypoglycemic agents in diabetics
Hirsutism
Ophthalmic
Posterior subcapsular cataracts
Increased intraocular pressure
Glaucoma
Exophthalmos
Metabolic
Negative nitrogen balance due to protein catabolism
Cardiovascular
Myocardial rupture following recent myocardial infarction (see WARNINGS).
Other
Anaphylactoid or hypersensitivity reactions
Thromboembolism
Weight gain
Increased appetite
Nausea
Malaise
The following *additional* adverse reactions are related to parenteral corticosteroid therapy:
Rare instances of blindness associated with intralesional therapy around the face and head
Hyperpigmentation or hypopigmentation
Subcutaneous and cutaneous atrophy
Sterile abscess
Postinjection flare (following intra-articular use)
Charcot-like arthropathy
Scarring
Induration
Inflammation
Paresthesia
Delayed pain or soreness
Muscle twitching, ataxia, hiccups, and nystagmus have been reported in low incidence after injection of DECADRON-LA sterile suspension.

OVERDOSAGE

Reports of acute toxicity and/or death following overdosage of glucocorticoids are rare. In the event of overdosage, no specific antidote is available; treatment is supportive and symptomatic.
The intraperitoneal LD_{50} of dexamethasone acetate in female mice was 424 mg/kg.

DOSAGE AND ADMINISTRATION

For intramuscular, intralesional, intra-articular, and soft tissue injection.
Dosage Requirements Are Variable and Must Be Individualized on the Basis of the Disease and the Response of the Patient.
Dosage in children under 12 has not been established.
Intramuscular Injection
Dosage ranges from 1 to 2 mL, equivalent to 8 to 16 mg of dexamethasone. If further treatment is needed, dosage may be repeated at intervals of 1 to 3 weeks.
Intralesional Injection
The usual dose is 0.1 to 0.2 mL, equivalent to 0.8 to 1.6 mg of dexamethasone, per injection site.
Intra-articular and Soft Tissue Injection
The dose varies, depending on the location and the severity of inflammation. The usual dose is 0.5 to 2 mL, equivalent to 4 to 16 mg of dexamethasone. If further treatment is needed,

dosage may be repeated at intervals of 1 to 3 weeks. Frequent intra-articular injection may result in damage to joint tissues.

HOW SUPPLIED

No. 7644—Sterile Suspension DECADRON-LA, 8 mg dexamethasone equivalent per mL, is a sterile white suspension, and is supplied as follows:
NDC 0006-7644-01 in 1 mL vials
NDC 0006-7644-03 in 5 mL vials.
Storage
Sensitive to heat. Do not autoclave.
Protect from freezing.
     A.H.F.S. Category: 68:04
     DC 7350017   Issued March 1988

DECASPRAY® Topical Aerosol   ℞
(Dexamethasone), U.S.P.

DESCRIPTION

Topical Aerosol DECASPRAY* (Dexamethasone) is a topical steroid preparation, each 25 g of which contains 10 mg of dexamethasone. The topical corticosteroids constitute a class of primarily synthetic steroids used as anti-inflammatory and anti-pruritic agents.
Dexamethasone is 9-fluoro-11β,17,21-trihydroxy-16α-methylpregna-1, 4-diene-3, 20 dione. Its empirical formula is $C_{22}H_{29}FO_5$ and its structural formula is:

Dexamethasone has a molecular weight of 392.47.
The inactive ingredients are isopropyl myristate, and isobutane. Each second of spray dispenses approximately 0.075 mg of dexamethasone.

---

*Registered trademark of MERCK & CO., INC.

CLINICAL PHARMACOLOGY

Topical corticosteroids share anti-inflammatory, anti-pruritic, and vasoconstrictive actions.
The mechanism of anti-inflammatory activity of the topical corticosteroids is unclear. Various laboratory methods, including vasoconstrictor assays, are used to compare and predict potencies and/or clinical efficacies of the topical corticosteroids. There is some evidence to suggest that a recognizable correlation exists between vasoconstrictor potency and therapeutic efficacy in man.
Pharmacokinetics
The extent of percutaneous absorption of topical corticosteroids is determined by many factors including the vehicle, the integrity of the epidermal barrier, and the use of occlusive dressings.
Topical corticosteroids can be absorbed from normal intact skin. Inflammation and/or other disease processes in the skin increase percutaneous absorption. Occlusive dressings substantially increase the percutaneous absorption of topical corticosteroids. Thus, occlusive dressings may be a valuable therapeutic adjunct for treatment of resistant dermatoses. (See DOSAGE AND ADMINISTRATION.)
Once absorbed through the skin, topical corticosteroids are handled through pharmacokinetic pathways similar to systemically administered corticosteroids. Corticosteroids are bound to plasma proteins in varying degrees. Corticosteroids are metabolized primarily in the liver and are then excreted by the kidneys. Some of the topical corticosteroids and their metabolites are also excreted into the bile.

INDICATIONS AND USAGE

DECASPRAY Topical Aerosol is indicated for relief of the inflammatory and pruritic manifestations of corticosteroid-responsive dermatoses.

CONTRAINDICATIONS

Topical corticosteroids are contraindicated in those patients with a history of hypersensitivity to any of the components of the preparation.

WARNINGS

Avoid spraying in eyes or nose. Contents under pressure. Do not puncture or burn. Keep out of reach of children. Use only as directed. Intentional misuse by deliberately concentrating and inhaling the contents can be harmful or fatal.

PRECAUTIONS

General
Systemic absorption of topical corticosteroids has produced reversible hypothalamic-pituitary-adrenal (HPA) axis suppression, manifestations of Cushing's syndrome, hyperglycemia, and glycosuria in some patients.
Conditions which augment systemic absorption include the application of the more potent corticosteroids, use over large surface areas, prolonged use, and the addition of occlusive dressings.
Therefore, patients receiving a large dose of a potent topical corticosteroid applied to a large surface area or under an occlusive dressing should be evaluated periodically for evidence of HPA axis suppression by using urinary free cortisol and ACTH stimulation tests. If HPA axis suppression is noted, an attempt should be made to withdraw the drug, to reduce the frequency of application, or to substitute a less potent corticosteroid.
Recovery of HPA axis function is generally prompt and complete upon discontinuation of the drug. Infrequently, signs and symptoms of corticosteroid withdrawal may occur, requiring supplemental systemic corticosteroids.
Children may absorb proportionally larger amounts of topical corticosteroids and thus be more susceptible to systemic toxicity (See PRECAUTIONS, *Pediatric Use*).
If irritation develops, topical corticosteroids should be discontinued and appropriate therapy instituted.
In the presence of dermatological infections, the use of an appropriate antifungal or antibacterial agent should be instituted. If a favorable response does not occur promptly, the corticosteroid should be discontinued until the infection has been adequately controlled.
The product is not for ophthalmic use. However, if applied to the eyelids or skin near the eyes, the drug may enter the eyes. In patients with a history of herpes simplex keratitis ocular exposure to corticosteroids may lead to a recurrence. Prolonged ocular exposure may cause steroid glaucoma.
A few individuals may be sensitive to one or more of the components of this product. If any reaction indicating sensitivity is observed, discontinue use.
Generally, occlusive dressings should not be used on weeping or exudative lesions.
If occlusive dressing therapy is used, inspect lesions between dressings for development of infection. If infection develops, the technique should be discontinued and appropriate antimicrobial therapy instituted.
When large areas of the body are covered with an occlusive dressing, thermal homeostasis may be impaired. If elevation of body temperature occurs, use of the occlusive dressing should be discontinued.
CAUTION: Flammable. Do not use around open flame or while smoking.

Information for the Patient
Patients using topical corticosteroids should receive the following information and instructions:
1. This medication is to be used as directed by the physician. It is for external use only. Avoid contact with the eyes.
2. Patients should be advised not to use this medication for any disorder other than that for which it was prescribed.
3. The treated skin area should not be bandaged or otherwise covered or wrapped so as to be occlusive unless directed by the physician.
4. Patients should report any signs of local adverse reactions, especially under occlusive dressing.
5. Parents of pediatric patients should be advised not to use tight-fitting diapers or plastic pants on a child being treated in the diaper area, as these garments may constitute occlusive dressings.

Laboratory Tests
The following tests may be helpful in evaluating the HPA axis suppression:
• Urinary free cortisol test
• ACTH stimulation test

Carcinogenesis, Mutagenesis, and Impairment of Fertility
Long-term animal studies have not been performed to evaluate the carcinogenic potential or the effect on fertility of topical corticosteroids.
Studies to determine mutagenicity with prednisolone and hydrocortisone have revealed negative results.

Pregnancy
Pregnancy Category C: Corticosteroids are generally teratogenic in laboratory animals when administered systemically at relatively low dosage levels. The more potent corticosteroids have been shown to be teratogenic after dermal appli-

cation in laboratory animals. There are no adequate and well-controlled studies in pregnant women on teratogenic effects from topically applied corticosteroids. Therefore, topical corticosteroids should be used during pregnancy only if the potential benefit justifies the potential risk to the fetus. Drugs of this class should not be used extensively on pregnant patients, in large amounts, or for prolonged periods of time.

Nursing Mothers
It is not known whether topical administration of corticosteroids could result in sufficient systemic absorption to produce detectable quantities in breast milk. Systemically administered corticosteroids are secreted into breast milk in quantities *not* likely to have a deleterious effect on the infant. Nevertheless, caution should be exercised when topical corticosteroids are administered to a nursing woman.

Pediatric Use
Pediatric patients may demonstrate greater susceptibility to topical corticosteroid-induced HPA axis suppression and Cushing's syndrome than mature patients because of a larger skin surface area to body weight ratio.

Hypothalamic-pituitary-adrenal (HPA) axis suppression, Cushing's syndrome, and intracranial hypertension have been reported in children receiving topical corticosteroids. Manifestations of adrenal suppression in children include linear growth retardation, delayed weight gain, low plasma cortisol levels, and absence of response to ACTH stimulation. Manifestations of intracranial hypertension include bulging fontanelles, headaches, and bilateral papilledema. Administration of topical corticosteroids to children should be limited to the least amount compatible with an effective therapeutic regimen. Chronic corticosteroid therapy may interfere with the growth and development of children.

ADVERSE REACTIONS

The following adverse reactions are reported infrequently with topical corticosteroids, but may occur more frequently with the use of occlusive dressings. These reactions are listed in an approximate decreasing order of occurrence:

Burning
Itching
Irritation
Dryness
Folliculitis
Hypertrichosis
Acneiform eruptions
Hypopigmentation
Perioral dermatitis
Allergic contact dermatitis
Maceration of the skin
Secondary infection
Skin atrophy
Striae
Miliaria

OVERDOSAGE

Topically applied corticosteroids can be absorbed in sufficient amounts to produce systemic effects (See PRECAUTIONS).

DOSAGE AND ADMINISTRATION

Patients should be instructed in the correct way to use DECASPRAY. The preparation is readily applied, even on hairy areas. It does not have to be rubbed into the skin. Optimal effects will be obtained with DECASPRAY when these directions are followed:

1. Keep the affected area clean to reduce the possibility of infection.
2. Shake the container *gently* once or twice each time before using. Hold it about six inches from the area to be treated. Effective medication may be obtained with the container held either upright or inverted, since it is fitted with a special valve that dispenses approximately the same dosage in either position.
3. Spray each four inch square of affected area for one or two seconds three or four times a day, depending on the nature of the condition and the response to therapy.
4. When a favorable response is obtained, reduce dosage gradually and eventually discontinue.
5. Occlusive dressings may be used for the management of psoriasis or recalcitrant conditions.

HOW SUPPLIED

No. 7623X—DECASPRAY is supplied as follows:
NDC 0006-7623-25 in a 25 g pressurized container.
A.H.F.S. Category: 84:06
DC 6005318   Issued April 1983
COPYRIGHT © MERCK & CO., INC., 1983
All rights reserved

DEMSER® Capsules   ℞
(Metyrosine), U.S.P.

DESCRIPTION

DEMSER* (Metyrosine) is (−)-α-methyl-*L*-tyrosine or (α-MPT). It has the following structural formula:

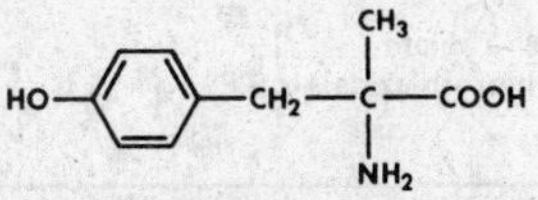

$$HO-\!\!\bigcirc\!\!-CH_2-\underset{\underset{NH_2}{|}}{\overset{\overset{CH_3}{|}}{C}}-COOH$$

Metyrosine is a white, crystalline compound of molecular weight 195. It is very slightly soluble in water, acetone, and methanol, and insoluble in chloroform and benzene. It is soluble in acidic aqueous solutions. It is also soluble in alkaline aqueous solutions, but is subject to oxidative degradation under these conditions.

DEMSER is supplied as capsules, for oral administration. Each capsule contains 250 mg metyrosine. Inactive ingredients are colloidal silicon dioxide, gelatin, hydroxypropyl cellulose, magnesium stearate, and titanium dioxide. The capsules may also contain any combination of D&C Red 33, D&C Yellow 10, FD&C Blue 1, and FD&C Blue 2.

*Registered trademark of MERCK & CO., INC.

CLINICAL PHARMACOLOGY

DEMSER inhibits tyrosine hydroxylase, which catalyzes the first transformation in catecholamine biosynthesis, i.e., the conversion of tyrosine to dihydroxyphenylalanine (DOPA). Because the first step is also the rate-limiting step, blockade of tyrosine hydroxylase activity results in decreased endogenous levels of catecholamines, usually measured as decreased urinary excretion of catecholamines and their metabolites.

In patients with pheochromocytoma, who produce excessive amounts of norepinephrine and epinephrine, administration of one to four grams of DEMSER per day has reduced catecholamine biosynthesis from about 35 to 80 percent as measured by the total excretion of catecholamines and their metabolites (metanephrine and vanillylmandelic acid). The maximum biochemical effect usually occurs within two to three days, and the urinary concentration of catecholamines and their metabolites usually returns to pretreatment levels within three to four days after DEMSER is discontinued. In some patients the total excretion of catecholamines and catecholamine metabolites may be lowered to normal or near normal levels (less than 10 mg/24 hours). In most patients the duration of treatment has been two to eight weeks, but several patients have received DEMSER for periods of one to 10 years.

Most patients with pheochromocytoma treated with DEMSER experience decreased frequency and severity of hypertensive attacks with their associated headache, nausea, sweating, and tachycardia. In patients who respond, blood pressure decreases progressively during the first two days of therapy with DEMSER; after withdrawal, blood pressure usually increases gradually to pretreatment values within two to three days.

Metyrosine is well absorbed from the gastrointestinal tract. From 53 to 88 percent (mean 69 percent) was recovered in the urine as unchanged drug following maintenance oral doses of 600 to 4000 mg/24 hours in patients with pheochromocytoma or essential hypertension. Less than 1% of the dose was recovered as catechol metabolites. These metabolites are probably not present in sufficient amounts to contribute to the biochemical effects of metyrosine. The quantities excreted, however, are sufficient to interfere with accurate determination of urinary catecholamines determined by routine techniques.

Plasma half-life of metyrosine determined over an 8-hour period after single oral doses was 3.4-3.7 hours in three patients.

For further information, refer to: Sjoerdsma, A.; Engelman, K.; Waldman, T. A.; Cooperman, L. H.; Hammond, W. G.: Pheochromocytoma: Current concepts of diagnosis and treatment, Ann. Intern. Med. *65:* 1302–1326, Dec. 1966.

INDICATIONS AND USAGE

DEMSER is indicated in the treatment of patients with pheochromocytoma for:
1. Preoperative preparation of patients for surgery
2. Management of patients when surgery is contraindicated
3. Chronic treatment of patients with malignant pheochromocytoma.
DEMSER is not recommended for the control of essential hypertension.

CONTRAINDICATIONS

DEMSER is contraindicated in persons known to be hypersensitive to this compound.

WARNINGS

Maintain Fluid Volume During and After Surgery
When DEMSER is used preoperatively, alone or especially in combination with alpha-adrenergic blocking drugs, adequate intravascular volume must be maintained intraoperatively (especially after tumor removal) and postoperatively to avoid hypotension and decreased perfusion of vital organs resulting from vasodilatation and expanded volume capacity. Following tumor removal, large volumes of plasma may be needed to maintain blood pressure and central venous pressure within the normal range.

In addition, life-threatening arrhythmias may occur during anesthesia and surgery, and may require treatment with a beta blocker or lidocaine. During surgery, patients should have continuous monitoring of blood pressure and electrocardiogram.

Intraoperative Effects
While the preoperative use of DEMSER in patients with pheochromocytoma is thought to decrease intraoperative problems with blood pressure control, DEMSER does not eliminate the danger of hypertensive crises or arrhythmias during manipulation of the tumor, and the alpha-adrenergic blocking drug, phentolamine, may be needed.

Interaction with Alcohol
DEMSER may add to the sedative effects of alcohol and other CNS depressants, e.g., hypnotics, sedatives, and tranquilizers. (See PRECAUTIONS, *Information for Patients and Drug Interactions.*)

PRECAUTIONS

General
Metyrosine Crystalluria: Crystalluria and urolithiasis have been found in dogs treated with DEMSER (Metyrosine) at doses similar to those used in humans, and crystalluria has also been observed in a few patients. To minimize the risk of crystalluria, patients should be urged to maintain water intake sufficient to achieve a daily urine volume of 2000 mL or more, particularly when doses greater than 2 g per day are given. Routine examination of the urine should be carried out. Metyrosine will crystallize as needles or rods. If metyrosine crystalluria occurs, fluid intake should be increased further. If crystalluria persists, the dosage should be reduced or the drug discontinued.
Relatively Little Data Regarding Long-term Use: The total human experience with the drug is quite limited and few patients have been studied long-term. Chronic animal studies have not been carried out. Therefore, suitable laboratory tests should be carried out periodically in patients requiring prolonged use of DEMSER and caution should be observed in patients with impaired hepatic or renal function.

Information for Patients
When receiving DEMSER, patients should be warned about engaging in activities requiring mental alertness and motor coordination, such as driving a motor vehicle or operating machinery. DEMSER may have additive sedative effects with alcohol and other CNS depressants, e.g., hypnotics, sedatives, and tranquilizers.

Patients should be advised to maintain a liberal fluid intake. (See PRECAUTIONS, *General.*)

Drug Interactions
Caution should be observed in administering DEMSER to patients receiving phenothiazines or haloperidol because the extrapyramidal effects of these drugs can be expected to be potentiated by inhibition of catecholamine synthesis.

Concurrent use of DEMSER with alcohol or other CNS depressants can increase their sedative effects. (See WARNINGS and PRECAUTIONS, *Information for Patients.*)

Laboratory Test Interference
Spurious increases in urinary catecholamines may be observed in patients receiving DEMSER due to the presence of metabolites of the drug.

Carcinogenesis, Mutagenesis, Impairment of Fertility
Long-term carcinogenic studies in animals and studies on mutagenesis and impairment of fertility have not been performed with metyrosine.

Pregnancy
Pregnancy Category C. Animal reproduction studies have not been conducted with DEMSER. It is also not known whether DEMSER can cause fetal harm when administered to a pregnant woman or can affect reproduction capacity. DEMSER should be given to a pregnant woman only if clearly needed.

Nursing Mothers
It is not known whether DEMSER is excreted in human milk. Because many drugs are excreted in human milk, caution should be exercised when DEMSER is administered to a nursing woman.

Continued on next page

Information on the Merck & Co. products listed on these pages is the full prescribing information from product circulars in use October 1, 1992.

Merck & Co.—Cont.

Pediatric Use
Safety and effectiveness in children under 12 years of age have not been established.

ADVERSE REACTIONS

Central Nervous System
Sedation: The most common adverse reaction to DEMSER is moderate to severe sedation, which has been observed in almost all patients. It occurs at both low and high dosages. Sedative effects begin within the first 24 hours of therapy, are maximal after two to three days, and tend to wane during the next few days. Sedation usually is not obvious after one week unless the dosage is increased, but at dosages greater than 2000 mg/day some degree of sedation or fatigue may persist.
In most patients who experience sedation, temporary changes in sleep pattern occur following withdrawal of the drug. Changes consist of insomnia that may last for two or three days and feelings of increased alertness and ambition. Even patients who do not experience sedation while on DEMSER may report symptoms of psychic stimulation when the drug is discontinued.
Extrapyramidal Signs: Extrapyramidal signs such as drooling, speech difficulty, and tremor have been reported in approximately 10 percent of patients. These occasionally have been accompanied by trismus and frank parkinsonism.
Anxiety and Psychic Disturbances: Anxiety and psychic disturbances such as depression, hallucinations, disorientation, and confusion may occur. These effects seem to be dose-dependent and may disappear with reduction of dosage.
Diarrhea
Diarrhea occurs in about 10 percent of patients and may be severe. Anti-diarrheal agents may be required if continuation of DEMSER is necessary.
Miscellaneous
Infrequently, slight swelling of the breast, galactorrhea, nasal stuffiness, decreased salivation, dry mouth, headache, nausea, vomiting, abdominal pain, and impotence or failure of ejaculation may occur. Crystalluria (see PRECAUTIONS) and transient dysuria and hematuria have been observed in a few patients. Hematologic disorders (including eosinophilia, anemia, thrombocytopenia, and thrombocytosis), increased SGOT levels, peripheral edema, and hypersensitivity reactions such as urticaria and pharyngeal edema have been reported rarely.

OVERDOSAGE

Signs of metyrosine overdosage include those central nervous system effects observed in some patients even at low dosages.
At doses exceeding 2000 mg/day, some degree of sedation or feeling of fatigue may persist. Doses of 2000–4000 mg/day can result in anxiety or agitated depression, neuromuscular effects (including fine tremor of the hands, gross tremor of the trunk, tightening of the jaw with trismus), diarrhea, and decreased salivation with dry mouth.
Reduction of drug dose or cessation of treatment results in the disappearance of these symptoms.
The acute toxicity of metyrosine was 442 mg/kg and 752 mg/kg in the female mouse and rat respectively.

DOSAGE AND ADMINISTRATION

The recommended initial dosage of DEMSER for adults and children 12 years of age and older is 250 mg orally four times daily. This may be increased by 250 mg to 500 mg every day to a maximum of 4.0 g/day in divided doses. When used for preoperative preparation, the optimally effective dosage of DEMSER should be given for at least five to seven days.
Optimally effective dosages of DEMSER usually are between 2.0 and 3.0 g/day, and the dose should be titrated by monitoring clinical symptoms and catecholamine excretion. In patients who are hypertensive, dosage should be titrated to achieve normalization of blood pressure and control of clinical symptoms. In patients who are usually normotensive, dosage should be titrated to the amount that will reduce urinary metanephrines and/or vanillylmandelic acid by 50 percent or more.
If patients are not adequately controlled by the use of DEMSER, an alpha-adrenergic blocking agent (phenoxybenzamine) should be added.
Use of DEMSER in children under 12 years of age has been limited and a dosage schedule for this age group cannot be given.

HOW SUPPLIED

No. 3355—Capsules DEMSER, 250 mg, are opaque, two-toned blue capsules coded MSD 690 on one side and DEMSER on the other. They are supplied as follows:

NDC 0006-0690-68 bottles of 100.
Shown in Product Identification Section, page 419
A.H.F.S. Category: 92:00
DC 7111505 Issued September 1985
COPYRIGHT© MERCK & CO., INC., 1985
All rights reserved

DIUPRES® Tablets   ℞
(Reserpine-Chlorothiazide), U.S.P.

> ### WARNING
>
> This fixed combination drug is not indicated for initial therapy of hypertension. Hypertension requires therapy titrated to the individual patient. If the fixed combination represents the dosage so determined, its use may be more convenient in patient management. The treatment of hypertension is not static, but must be re-evaluated as conditions in each patient warrant.

DESCRIPTION

DIUPRES* (Reserpine-Chlorothiazide) combines two antihypertensives: DIURIL* (Chlorothiazide) and reserpine.
Chlorothiazide
Chlorothiazide is a diuretic and antihypertensive. Its chemical name is 6-chloro-2*H*-1,2,4-benzothiadiazine-7-sulfonamide 1,1-dioxide. Its empirical formula is $C_7H_6ClN_3O_4S_2$ and its structural formula is:

Chlorothiazide is a white, or practically white, crystalline powder with a molecular weight of 295.72, which is very slightly soluble in water, but readily soluble in dilute aqueous sodium hydroxide. It is soluble in urine to the extent of about 150 mg per 100 mL at pH 7.
Reserpine
The chemical name of reserpine is 11,17α-dimethoxy-18β-[(3, 4, 5-trimethoxybenzoyl)oxy] -3β,20α-yohimban- 16 β-carboxylic acid methylester. It is a crystalline alkaloid derived from Rauwolfia serpentina. Its empirical formula is $C_{33}H_{40}N_2O_9$ and its structural formula is:

Reserpine is a white or pale buff to slightly yellowish, odorless, crystalline powder with a molecular weight of 608.69, is insoluble in water and freely soluble in glacial acetic acid. DIUPRES is supplied as tablets in two strengths for oral use: DIUPRES-250, contains 250 mg of chlorothiazide and 0.125 mg of reserpine.
DIUPRES-500, contains 500 mg of chlorothiazide and 0.125 mg of reserpine.
Each tablet contains the following inactive ingredients: FD&C Red 3, gelatin, lactose, magnesium stearate, starch and talc.

---

*Registered trademark of MERCK & CO., INC.

CLINICAL PHARMACOLOGY

Chlorothiazide
The mechanism of the antihypertensive effect of thiazides is unknown. Chlorothiazide does not usually affect normal blood pressure.
Chlorothiazide affects the distal renal tubular mechanism of electrolyte reabsorption. At maximal therapeutic dosage all thiazides are approximately equal in their diuretic efficacy. Chlorothiazide increases excretion of sodium and chloride in approximately equivalent amounts. Natriuresis may be accompanied by some loss of potassium and bicarbonate.
After oral use diuresis begins within 2 hours, peaks in about 4 hours and lasts about 6 to 12 hours.
Reserpine
Reserpine has antihypertensive, bradycardic, and tranquilizing properties. It lowers arterial blood pressure by depletion of catecholamines. Reserpine is beneficial in relieving

anxiety, tension, and headache in the hypertensive patient. It acts at the hypothalamic level of the central nervous system to promote relaxation without hypnosis or analgesia. The sleep pattern shown by the electroencephalogram following barbiturates does not occur with this drug. In laboratory animals spontaneous activity and response to external stimuli are decreased, but confusion or difficulty of movement is not evident.
The bradycardic action of reserpine promotes relaxation and may eliminate sinus tachycardia. It is most pronounced in subjects with sinus tachycardia and usually is not prominent in persons with a normal pulse rate.
Miosis, relaxation of the nictitating membrane, ptosis, hypothermia, and increased gastrointestinal activity are noted in animals given reserpine, sometimes in subclinical doses. None of these effects, except increased gastrointestinal activity, has been found to be clinically significant in man with therapeutic doses.
Pharmacokinetics and Metabolism
Chlorothiazide
Chlorothiazide is not metabolized but is eliminated rapidly by the kidney. The plasma half-life of chlorothiazide is 45–120 minutes. After oral doses, 20–24 percent is excreted unchanged in the urine. Chlorothiazide crosses the placental but not the blood-brain barrier and is excreted in breast milk.
Reserpine
Oral reserpine is rapidly absorbed from the gastrointestinal tract. Methylreserpate and trimethoxybenzoic acid are the primary metabolites which result from the hydrolytic cleavage of reserpine. Maximal blood levels are achieved approximately 2 hours after the oral dosage of ^{3}H-reserpine to six normal volunteers; within 96 hours approximately 8 percent was excreted in urine and 62 percent in feces. Reserpine appears in human breast milk. Reserpine crosses the placental barrier in guinea pigs.

INDICATION AND USAGE

Hypertension (see box warning).
Use in Pregnancy. Routine use of diuretics during normal pregnancy is inappropriate and exposes mother and fetus to unnecessary hazard. Diuretics do not prevent development of toxemia of pregnancy and there is no satisfactory evidence that they are useful in the treatment of toxemia.
Edema during pregnancy may arise from pathologic causes or from the physiologic and mechanical consequences of pregnancy. Thiazides are indicated in pregnancy when edema is due to pathologic causes, just as they are in the absence of pregnancy (see PRECAUTIONS, *Pregnancy*). Dependent edema in pregnancy, resulting from restriction of venous return by the gravid uterus, is properly /treated through elevation of the lower extremities and use of support stockings. Use of diuretics to lower intravascular volume in this instance is illogical and unnecessary. During normal pregnancy there is hypervolemia which is not harmful to the fetus or the mother in the absence of cardiovascular disease. However, it may be associated with edema, rarely generalized edema. If such edema causes discomfort, increased recumbency will often provide relief. Rarely this edema may cause extreme discomfort which is not relieved by rest. In these instances, a short course of diuretic therapy may provide relief and be appropriate.

CONTRAINDICATIONS

Chlorothiazide is contraindicated in anuria.
DIUPRES is contraindicated in hypersensitivity to chlorothiazide or other sulfonamide-derived drugs or to reserpine.
Electroshock therapy should not be given to patients while on reserpine, as severe and even fatal reactions have been reported with minimal convulsive electroshock dosage. After discontinuing reserpine, allow at least seven days before starting electroshock therapy.
Active peptic ulcer, ulcerative colitis, and active mental depression, especially suicidal tendencies, are contraindications to reserpine therapy.

WARNINGS

Chlorothiazide
Use with caution in severe renal disease. In patients with renal disease, thiazides may precipitate azotemia. Cumulative effects of the drug may develop in patients with impaired renal function.
Thiazides should be used with caution in patients with impaired hepatic function or progressive liver disease, since minor alterations of fluid and electrolyte balance may precipitate hepatic coma.
Thiazides may add to or potentiate the action of other antihypertensive drugs.
Sensitivity reactions may occur in patients with or without a history of allergy or bronchial asthma.
The possibility of exacerbation or activation of systemic lupus erythematosus has been reported.

Lithium generally should not be given with diuretics (see PRECAUTIONS, *Drug Interactions*).

Reserpine

The occurrence of mental depression due to reserpine in doses of 0.25 mg daily or less is unusual. In any event, DIUPRES should be discontinued at the first sign of depression.

PRECAUTIONS

General

Chlorothiazide

All patients receiving diuretic therapy should be observed for evidence of fluid or electrolyte imbalance: namely, hyponatremia, hypochloremic alkalosis, and hypokalemia. Serum and urine electrolyte determinations are particularly important when the patient is vomiting excessively or receiving parenteral fluids. Warning signs or symptoms of fluid and electrolyte imbalance, irrespective of cause, include dryness of mouth, thirst, weakness, lethargy, drowsiness, restlessness, muscle pains or cramps, muscular fatigue, hypotension, oliguria, tachycardia, and gastrointestinal disturbances such as nausea and vomiting.

Hypokalemia may develop, especially with brisk diuresis, when severe cirrhosis is present or after prolonged therapy. Interference with adequate oral electrolyte intake will contribute to hypokalemia. Hypokalemia may cause cardiac arrhythmia and may also sensitize or exaggerate the response of the heart to the toxic effects of digitalis (e.g., increased ventricular irritability). Hypokalemia may be avoided or treated by use of potassium sparing diuretics or potassium supplements such as foods with a high potassium content.

Although any chloride deficit is generally mild and usually does not require specific treatment except under extraordinary circumstances (as in liver disease or renal disease), chloride replacement may be required in the treatment of metabolic alkalosis.

Dilutional hyponatremia may occur in edematous patients in hot weather. Appropriate therapy is water restriction, rather than administration of salt, except in rare instances when the hyponatremia is life threatening. In actual salt depletion, appropriate replacement is the therapy of choice.

Hyperuricemia may occur or acute gout may be precipitated in certain patients receiving thiazides.

In diabetic patients dosage adjustments of insulin or oral hypoglycemic agents may be required. Hyperglycemia may occur with thiazide diuretics. Thus latent diabetes mellitus may become manifest during thiazide therapy.

The antihypertensive effect of the drug may be enhanced in the postsympathectomy patient.

If progressive renal impairment becomes evident, consider withholding or discontinuing diuretic therapy.

Thiazides have been shown to increase the urinary excretion of magnesium; this may result in hypomagnesemia.

Thiazides may decrease urinary calcium excretion. Thiazides may cause intermittent and slight elevation of serum calcium in the absence of known disorders of calcium metabolism. Marked hypercalcemia may be evidence of hidden hyperparathyroidism. Thiazides should be discontinued before carrying out tests for parathyroid function.

Increases in cholesterol and triglyceride levels may be associated with thiazide diuretic therapy.

Reserpine

Since reserpine may increase gastric secretion and motility, it should be used cautiously in patients with a history of peptic ulcer, ulcerative colitis, or other gastrointestinal disorder. This compound may precipitate biliary colic in patients with gallstones, or bronchial asthma in susceptible persons. Reserpine may cause hypotension including orthostatic hypotension.

Anxiety or depression, as well as psychosis, may develop during reserpine therapy. If depression is present when therapy is begun, it may be aggravated. Mental depression is unusual with reserpine doses of 0.25 mg daily or less. In any case, DIUPRES should be discontinued at the first sign of depression. Extreme caution should be used in treating patients with a history of mental depression, and the possibility of suicide should be kept in mind.

As with most antihypertensive therapy, caution should be exercised when treating hypertensive patients with renal insufficiency, since they adjust poorly to lowered blood pressure.

When two or more antihypertensives are given, the individual dosages may have to be reduced to prevent excessive drop in blood pressure. In hypertensive patients with coronary artery disease, it is important to avoid a precipitous drop in blood pressure.

Laboratory Tests

Periodic determination of serum electrolytes to detect possible electrolyte imbalance should be done at appropriate intervals.

Drug Interactions

Chlorothiazide

When given concurrently the following drugs may interact with thiazide diuretics.

Alcohol, barbiturates, or narcotics —potentiation of orthostatic hypotension may occur.

Antidiabetic drugs (oral agents and insulin)—dosage adjustment of the antidiabetic drug may be required.

Other antihypertensive drugs —additive effect or potentiation.

Corticosteroids, ACTH —intensified electrolyte depletion, particularly hypokalemia.

Pressor amines (e.g., norepinephrine) —possible decreased response to pressor amines but not sufficient to preclude their use.

Skeletal muscle relaxants, nondepolarizing (e.g., tubocurarine) —possible increased responsiveness to the muscle relaxant.

Lithium —generally should not be given with diuretics. Diuretic agents reduce the renal clearance of lithium and add a high risk of lithium toxicity. Refer to the package insert for lithium preparations before use of such preparations with DIUPRES.

Non-steroidal Anti-inflammatory Drugs —In some patients, the administration of a non-steroidal anti-inflammatory agent can reduce the diuretic, natriuretic, and antihypertensive effects of loop, potassium-sparing and thiazide diuretics. Therefore, when DIUPRES and non-steroidal anti-inflammatory agents are used concomitantly, the patient should be observed closely to determine if the desired effect of the diuretic is obtained.

Reserpine

In hypertensive patients on reserpine therapy significant hypotension and bradycardia may develop during surgical anesthesia. The anesthesiologist should be aware that reserpine has been taken, since it may be necessary to give vagal blocking agents parenterally to prevent or reverse hypotension and/or bradycardia.

Use reserpine cautiously with digitalis and quinidine; cardiac arrhythmias have occurred with reserpine preparations.

Barbiturates enhance the central nervous system depressant effects of reserpine.

Drug/Laboratory Test Interactions

Thiazides should be discontinued before carrying out tests for parathyroid function (see PRECAUTIONS, *General*).

Carcinogenesis, Mutagenesis,

Impairment of Fertility

Long-term carcinogenic or mutagenic studies have not been done with DIUPRES.

In a two-litter study in the rat at an oral dose of 50.0/0.25 mg/kg, the combination of chlorothiazide/reserpine did not impair fertility or produce abnormalities in the fetus.

Chlorothiazide

Carcinogenic studies have not been done with chlorothiazide.

Chlorothiazide was not mutagenic *in vitro*, in the Ames microbial mutagen test at a maximum concentration of 5 mg/plate using Strains TA98 and TA100. Chlorothiazide did not produce any significant mutagenicity in the dominant lethal assay in the mouse after 8 oral doses of 50 mg/kg or single intraperitoneal doses of 525 or 644 mg/kg, although early fetal deaths and preimplantation losses were increased beyond control values. In the test using *Aspergillus nidulans*, chlorothiazide was negative and did not induce disjunction. Chlorothiazide had no effect on fertility in a two-litter study in rats at doses up to 60 mg/kg/day (2 times the maximum recommended human dose).

Reserpine

Reserpine at a concentration of 1 to 5000 mcg/plate had no mutagenic activity against four strains of S. typhimurium *in vitro* in the Ames microbial mutagen test with or without metabolic activation. Reserpine did not induce malignant transformation of mouse fibroblasts *in vitro* at concentrations of 0.3 to 10 mcg/mL.

A few chromosomal aberrations were induced by reserpine *in vitro* in cultured mouse mammary carcinoma cells but were considered negative in this study. The drug did not produce chromosomal aberrations in human peripheral leucocyte cultures although an increase in mitotic figures occurred. One study reported chromosomal aberrations and dominant lethal mutations in mice at doses up to 10 mg/kg of reserpine in the form of a pharmaceutical preparation. Another study did not show dominant lethal mutations in mice at IP doses of 0.92 and 4.6 mg/kg of reserpine.

Reserpine did not impair fertility in a two-litter study in the rat at an oral dose of 0.25 mg/kg (35 times the maximum recommended human dose).

Rodent studies have shown that reserpine is an animal tumorigen, causing an increased incidence of mammary fibroadenomas in female mice, malignant tumors of the seminal vesicle in male mice, and malignant adrenal medullary tumors in male rats. These findings arose in two year studies in which the drug was administered in the feed at concentrations of 5 and 10 ppm—about 100 to 300 times the usual human dose. The breast neoplasms are thought to be related to reserpine's prolactin-elevating effect. Several other prolactin-elevating drugs have also been associated with an increased incidence of mammary neoplasia in rodents.

The extent to which these findings indicate a risk to humans is uncertain. Tissue culture experiments show that about one-third of human breast tumors are prolactin-dependent *in vitro*, a factor of considerable importance if the use of the drug is contemplated in a patient with previously detected breast cancer. The possibility of an increased risk of breast cancer in reserpine users has been studied extensively; however, no firm conclusion has emerged. Although a few epidemiologic studies have suggested a slightly increased risk (less than twofold in all studies except one) in women who have used reserpine, other studies of generally similar design have not confirmed this. Epidemiologic studies conducted using other drugs (neuroleptic agents) that, like reserpine, increase prolactin levels and therefore would be considered rodent mammary carcinogens, have not shown an association between chronic administration of the drug and human mammary tumorigenesis. While long-term clinical observation has not suggested such an association, the available evidence is considered too limited to be conclusive at this time. An association of reserpine intake with pheochromocytoma or tumors of the seminal vesicles has not been explored.

Pregnancy

Teratogenic Effects —Pregnancy Category C: There are no adequate and well-controlled studies in pregnant women. DIUPRES may cause fetal harm when given to a pregnant woman. DIUPRES should be used during pregnancy only if the potential benefit justifies the potential risk to the fetus. (See INDICATIONS AND USAGE.)

Reserpine: Reproduction studies in rats have shown that reserpine is teratogenic at doses of 1–2 mg/kg (125–250 times the maximum recommended human dose) IM or IP given early in pregnancy. A variety of abnormalities was produced including anophthalmia, absence of the axial skeleton, hydronephrosis, etc. Pregnancy in rabbits was interrupted when doses as low as 0.04 mg/kg (10 times the maximum recommended human dose) were given early or late in pregnancy.

Chlorothiazide: Thiazides cross the placental barrier and appear in cord blood.

Reproduction studies in the rabbit, the mouse and the rat at doses up to 500 mg/kg/day (25 times the maximum recommended human dose) showed no evidence of external abnormalities of the fetus due to chlorothiazide. Chlorothiazide given in a two-litter study in rats at doses up to 60 mg/kg/day (2 times the maximum recommended human dose) did not impair fertility or produce birth abnormalities in the offspring.

Nonteratogenic Effects

Reserpine: Reserpine has been demonstrated to cross the placental barrier in guinea pigs with depression of adrenal catecholamine stores in the newborn. There is some evidence that side effects such as nasal congestion, lethargy, depressed Moro reflex, and bradycardia may appear in infants born of reserpine-treated mothers.

Chlorothiazide: These may include fetal or neonatal jaundice, thrombocytopenia, and possibly other adverse reactions which have occurred in the adult.

Nursing Mothers

Thiazides and reserpine appear in breast milk. Because of the potential for serious adverse reactions in nursing infants from DIUPRES, a decision should be made whether to discontinue nursing or to discontinue the drug, taking into account the importance of the drug to the mother.

Pediatric Use

Safety and effectiveness of DIUPRES in children has not been established.

ADVERSE REACTIONS

The following adverse reactions have been reported and, within each category, are listed in order of decreasing severity.

Chlorothiazide

Body as a Whole: Weakness.

Cardiovascular: Hypotension including orthostatic hypotension (may be aggravated by alcohol, barbiturates, narcotics or antihypertensive drugs).

Digestive: Pancreatitis, jaundice (intrahepatic cholestatic jaundice), diarrhea, vomiting, sialadenitis, cramping, constipation, gastric irritation, nausea, anorexia.

Hematologic: Aplastic anemia, agranulocytosis, leukopenia, hemolytic anemia, thrombocytopenia.

Hypersensitivity: Anaphylactic reactions, necrotizing angiitis (vasculitis and cutaneous vasculitis), respiratory distress including pneumonitis and pulmonary edema, photosensitivity, fever, urticaria, rash, purpura.

Metabolic: Electrolyte imbalance (see PRECAUTIONS), hyperglycemia, glycosuria, hyperuricemia.

Continued on next page

Information on the Merck & Co. products listed on these pages is the full prescribing information from product circulars in use October 1, 1992.

Merck & Co.—Cont.

Musculoskeletal: Muscle spasm.

Nervous System/Psychiatric: Vertigo, paresthesias, dizziness, headache, restlessness.

Renal: Renal failure, renal dysfunction, interstitial nephritis. (See WARNINGS.)

Special Senses: Transient blurred vision, xanthopsia. Whenever adverse reactions are moderate or severe, thiazide dosage should be reduced or therapy withdrawn.

Reserpine

Cardiovascular: Angina pectoris, arrhythmia, premature ventricular contractions, other direct cardiac effects (e.g., fluid retention, congestive heart failure), bradycardia.

Digestive: Vomiting, diarrhea, nausea, hypersecretion and increased motility, anorexia, dryness of mouth, increased salivation.

Hematologic: Thrombocytopenic purpura, excessive bleeding following prostatic surgery.

Hypersensitivity: Pruritis, rash, flushing of skin.

Metabolic: Weight gain.

Musculoskeletal: Muscular aches.

Nervous System/Psychiatric: Mental depression, dull sensorium, syncope, paradoxical anxiety, excessive sedation, nightmares, headache, dizziness, nervousness, parkinsonism (usually reversible with decreased dosage or discontinuance of therapy).

Respiratory: Dyspnea, epistaxis, nasal congestion, enhanced susceptibility to colds.

Special Senses: Optic atrophy, uveitis, deafness, glaucoma, conjunctival injection, blurred vision.

Urogenital: Dysuria, impotence, decreased libido, non-puerperal lactation.

OVERDOSAGE

Overdosage may lead to excessive sedation, mental depression, severe hypotension, extrapyramidal reactions.

There is no specific antidote. In the event of overdosage, symptomatic and supportive measures should be employed. Emesis should be induced or gastric lavage performed. Correct dehydration, electrolyte imbalance, hepatic coma and hypotension by established procedures. If required, give oxygen or artificial respiration for respiratory impairment. In the event of severe hypotension from the reserpine component, intravenous use of a vasopressor is indicated [e.g., ARAMINE® (Metaraminol Bitartrate, MSD), levarterenol, phenylephrine]. Anticholinergics may be needed to relieve gastrointestinal distress from reserpine. Because the effects of the rauwolfia alkaloids are prolonged, the patient should be closely observed for at least 72 hours.

The oral LD_{50} of chlorothiazide is 8.5 g/kg, greater than 10 g/kg, and greater than 1 g/kg, in the mouse, rat and dog, respectively. The oral LD_{50} of reserpine in the mouse is 390 mg/kg.

DOSAGE AND ADMINISTRATION

The initial dosage of DIUPRES should conform to the dosages of the individual components established during titration (see box warning).

The usual adult dosage of DIUPRES-250* is 1 or 2 tablets once or twice a day; that of DIUPRES-500* is 1 tablet once or twice a day. Dosage may require adjustment according to the blood pressure response of the patient.

*Registered trademark of MERCK & CO., INC.

HOW SUPPLIED

No. 3261—Tablets DIUPRES-250 are pink, round, scored, compressed tablets, coded MSD 230. Each tablet contains 250 mg of chlorothiazide and 0.125 mg of reserpine. They are supplied as follows:

NDC 0006-0230-68 in bottles of 100
NDC 0006-0230-82 in bottles of 1000.

Shown in Product Identification Section, page 419

No. 3262—Tablets DIUPRES-500 are pink, round, scored, compressed tablets, coded MSD 405. Each tablet contains 500 mg of chlorothiazide and 0.125 mg of reserpine. They are supplied as follows:

NDC 0006-0405-68 in bottles of 100
NDC 0006-0405-82 in bottles of 1000.

Shown in Product Identification Section, page 419

Storage

Keep container tightly closed. Protect from light.

A.H.F.S. Category: 24:08

DC 7398838   Issued October 1987

DIURIL® Sodium Intravenous   ℞
(Chlorothiazide Sodium), U.S.P.

DESCRIPTION

Intravenous Sodium DIURIL* (Chlorothiazide Sodium) is a diuretic and antihypertensive. It is 6-chloro-$2H$-1,2,4-benzothiadiazine-7-sulfonamide 1,1-dioxide monosodium salt and its molecular weight is 317.70. Its empirical formula is $C_7H_5ClN_3NaO_4S_2$ and its structural formula is:

Intravenous Sodium DIURIL is a sterile lyophilized white powder and is supplied in a vial containing:

Chlorothiazide sodium equivalent
  to chlorothiazide .... 0.5 g
Inactive ingredients:
  Mannitol .... 0.25 g
Sodium hydroxide to adjust pH, with 0.4 mg thimerosal (mercury derivative) added as preservative.

DIURIL (Chlorothiazide, MSD) is a diuretic and antihypertensive. It is 6-chloro-$2H$-1,2,4-benzothiadiazine-7-sulfonamide 1,1-dioxide. Its empirical formula is $C_7H_6ClN_3O_4S_2$ and its structural formula is:

It is a white, or practically white, crystalline powder with a molecular weight of 295.72, which is very slightly soluble in water, but readily soluble in dilute aqueous sodium hydroxide. It is soluble in urine to the extent of about 150 mg per 100 mL at pH 7.

---

*Registered trademark of MERCK & CO., INC.

CLINICAL PHARMACOLOGY

The mechanism of the antihypertensive effect of thiazides is unknown. DIURIL does not usually affect normal blood pressure.

DIURIL affects the distal renal tubular mechanism of electrolyte reabsorption. At maximal therapeutic dosage all thiazides are approximately equal in their diuretic efficacy. DIURIL increases excretion of sodium and chloride in approximately equivalent amounts. Natriuresis may be accompanied by some loss of potassium and bicarbonate.

After oral use diuresis begins within 2 hours, peaks in about 4 hours and lasts about 6 to 12 hours. Following intravenous use of Sodium DIURIL, onset of the diuretic action occurs in 15 minutes and the maximal action in 30 minutes.

Pharmacokinetics and Metabolism

DIURIL is not metabolized but is eliminated rapidly by the kidney; 96 percent of an intravenous dose is excreted unchanged in the urine within 23 hours. The plasma half-life of chlorothiazide is 45–120 minutes. Chlorothiazide crosses the placental but not the blood-brain barrier and is excreted in breast milk.

INDICATIONS AND USAGE

Intravenous Sodium DIURIL is indicated as adjunctive therapy in edema associated with congestive heart failure, hepatic cirrhosis, and corticosteroid and estrogen therapy.

Intravenous Sodium DIURIL has also been found useful in edema due to various forms of renal dysfunction such as nephrotic syndrome, acute glomerulonephritis, and chronic renal failure.

Use in Pregnancy. Routine use of diuretics during normal pregnancy is inappropriate and exposes mother and fetus to unnecessary hazard. Diuretics do not prevent development of toxemia of pregnancy and there is no satisfactory evidence that they are useful in the treatment of toxemia.

Edema during pregnancy may arise from pathologic causes or from the physiologic and mechanical consequences of pregnancy. Thiazides are indicated in pregnancy when edema is due to pathologic causes, just as they are in the absence of pregnancy (see PRECAUTIONS, *Pregnancy*). Dependent edema in pregnancy, resulting from restriction of venous return by the gravid uterus, is properly treated through elevation of the lower extremities and use of support stockings. Use of diuretics to lower intravascular volume in this instance is illogical and unnecessary. During normal pregnancy there is hypervolemia which is not harmful to the fetus or the mother in the absence of cardiovascular disease. However, it may be associated with edema, rarely generalized edema. If such edema causes discomfort, increased re-

cumbency will often provide relief. Rarely this edema may cause extreme discomfort which is not relieved by rest. In these instances, a short course of diuretic therapy may provide relief and be appropriate.

CONTRAINDICATIONS

Anuria.

Hypersensitivity to any component of this product or to other sulfonamide-derived drugs.

WARNINGS

Intravenous use in infants and children has been limited and is not generally recommended.

Use with caution in severe renal disease. In patients with renal disease, thiazides may precipitate azotemia. Cumulative effects of the drug may develop in patients with impaired renal function.

Thiazides should be used with caution in patients with impaired hepatic function or progressive liver disease, since minor alterations of fluid and electrolyte balance may precipitate hepatic coma.

Thiazides may add to or potentiate the action of other antihypertensive drugs.

Sensitivity reactions may occur in patients with or without a history of allergy or bronchial asthma.

The possibility of exacerbation or activation of systemic lupus erythematosus has been reported.

Lithium generally should not be given with diuretics (see PRECAUTIONS, *Drug Interactions*).

PRECAUTIONS

General

All patients receiving diuretic therapy should be observed for evidence of fluid or electrolyte imbalance: namely, hyponatremia, hypochloremic alkalosis, and hypokalemia. Serum and urine electrolyte determinations are particularly important when the patient is vomiting excessively or receiving parenteral fluids. Warning signs or symptoms of fluid and electrolyte imbalance, irrespective of cause, include dryness of mouth, thirst, weakness, lethargy, drowsiness, restlessness, muscle pains or cramps, muscular fatigue, hypotension, oliguria, tachycardia, and gastrointestinal disturbances such as nausea and vomiting.

Hypokalemia may develop especially with brisk diuresis, when severe cirrhosis is present or after prolonged therapy. Interference with adequate oral electrolyte intake will also contribute to hypokalemia. Hypokalemia may cause cardiac arrhythmias and may also sensitize or exaggerate the response of the heart to the toxic effects of digitalis (e.g., increased ventricular irritability). Hypokalemia may be avoided or treated by use of potassium sparing diuretics or potassium supplements such as foods with a high potassium content.

Although any chloride deficit is generally mild and usually does not require specific treatment except under extraordinary circumstances (as in liver disease or renal disease), chloride replacement may be required in the treatment of metabolic alkalosis.

Dilutional hyponatremia may occur in edematous patients in hot weather; appropriate therapy is water restriction, rather than administration of salt, except in rare instances when the hyponatremia is life threatening. In actual salt depletion, appropriate replacement is the therapy of choice.

Hyperuricemia may occur or acute gout may be precipitated in certain patients receiving thiazides.

In diabetic patients dosage adjustments of insulin or oral hypoglycemic agents may be required. Hyperglycemia may occur with thiazide diuretics. Thus latent diabetes mellitus may become manifest during thiazide therapy.

The antihypertensive effects of the drug may be enhanced in the postsympathectomy patient.

If progressive renal impairment becomes evident, consider withholding or discontinuing diuretic therapy.

Thiazides have been shown to increase the urinary excretion of magnesium; this may result in hypomagnesemia.

Thiazides may decrease urinary calcium excretion. Thiazides may cause intermittent and slight elevation of serum calcium in the absence of known disorders of calcium metabolism. Marked hypercalcemia may be evidence of hidden hyperparathyroidism. Thiazides should be discontinued before carrying out tests for parathyroid function.

Increases in cholesterol and triglyceride levels may be associated with thiazide diuretic therapy.

Laboratory Tests

Periodic determination of serum electrolytes to detect possible electrolyte imbalance should be done at appropriate intervals.

Drug Interactions

When given concurrently the following drugs may interact with thiazide diuretics.

Alcohol, barbiturates, or narcotics —potentiation of orthostatic hypotension may occur.

Antidiabetic drugs —(oral agents and insulin)—dosage adjustment of the antidiabetic drug may be required.
Other antihypertensive drugs —additive effect or potentiation.
Corticosteroids, ACTH —intensified electrolyte depletion, particularly hypokalemia.
Pressor amines (e.g., norepinephrine) —possible decreased response to pressor amines but not sufficient to preclude their use.
Skeletal muscle relaxants, nondepolarizing (e.g., tubocurarine) —possible increased responsiveness to the muscle relaxant.
Lithium —generally should not be given with diuretics. Diuretic agents reduce the renal clearance of lithium and add a high risk of lithium toxicity. Refer to the package insert for lithium preparations before use of such preparations with Sodium DIURIL.
Non-steroidal Anti-inflammatory Drugs —In some patients, the administration of a non-steroidal anti-inflammatory agent can reduce the diuretic, natriuretic, and antihypertensive effects of loop, potassium-sparing and thiazide diuretics. Therefore, when Sodium DIURIL and non-steroidal anti-inflammatory agents are used concomitantly, the patient should be observed closely to determine if the desired effect of the diuretic is obtained.
Drug/Laboratory Test Interactions
Thiazides should be discontinued before carrying out tests for parathyroid function (see PRECAUTIONS, *General*).
Carcinogenesis, Mutagenesis, Impairment of Fertility
Carcinogenic studies have not been done with chlorothiazide.
Chlorothiazide was not mutagenic *in vitro*, in the Ames microbial mutagen test at a maximum concentration of 5 mg/plate using Strains TA98 and TA100. Chlorothiazide did not produce any significant mutagenicity in the dominant lethal assay in the mouse after 8 oral doses of 50 mg/kg or single intraperitoneal doses of 525 or 644 mg/kg, although early fetal deaths and preimplantation losses were increased beyond control values. In a test using *Aspergillus nidulans*, chlorothiazide was negative and did not induce disjunction.
Chlorothiazide had no effect on fertility in a two-litter study in rats at doses up to 60 mg/kg/day (2 times the maximum recommended human dose).
Pregnancy
Teratogenic Effects —Pregnancy Category B: Reproduction studies in the rabbit, the mouse and the rat at doses up to 500 mg/kg/day (25 times the maximum recommended human dose) showed no evidence of external abnormalities of the fetus due to chlorothiazide.
Chlorothiazide given in a two-litter study in rats at doses up to 60 mg/kg/day (2 times the usual daily maximum recommended human dose) did not impair fertility or produce birth abnormalities in the offspring.
There are no adequate and well-controlled studies with Intravenous Sodium DIURIL in pregnant women; however, thiazides cross the placental barrier and appear in cord blood. Since animal reproduction studies are not always predictive of human response, Intravenous Sodium DIURIL should be used during pregnancy only if clearly needed. (See INDICATIONS AND USAGE.)
Nonteratogenic Effects: These may include fetal or neonatal jaundice, thrombocytopenia, and possibly other adverse reactions which have occurred in the adult.
Nursing Mothers
Because of the potential for serious adverse reactions in nursing infants from Intravenous Sodium DIURIL, a decision should be made whether to discontinue nursing or to discontinue the drug, taking into account the importance of the drug to the mother.
Pediatric Use
Safety and effectiveness of Intravenous Sodium DIURIL in children has not been established.

ADVERSE REACTIONS

The following adverse reactions have been reported and, within each category, are listed in order of decreasing severity.
Body as a Whole: Weakness.
Cardiovascular: Hypotension including orthostatic hypotension (may be aggravated by alcohol, barbiturates, narcotics or antihypertensive drugs).
Digestive: Pancreatitis, jaundice (intrahepatic cholestatic jaundice), diarrhea, vomiting, sialadenitis, cramping, constipation, gastric irritation, nausea, anorexia.
Hematologic: Aplastic anemia, agranulocytosis, leukopenia, hemolytic anemia, thrombocytopenia.
Hypersensitivity: Anaphylactic reactions, necrotizing angiitis (vasculitis and cutaneous vasculitis), respiratory distress including pneumonitis and pulmonary edema, photosensitivity, fever, urticaria, rash, purpura.
Metabolic: Electrolyte imbalance (see PRECAUTIONS), hyperglycemia, glycosuria, hyperuricemia.

Musculoskeletal: Muscle spasm.
Nervous System/Psychiatric: Vertigo, paresthesias, dizziness, headache, restlessness.
Special Senses: Transient blurred vision, xanthopsia.
Renal: Renal failure, renal dysfunction, interstitial nephritis (see WARNINGS); hematuria (following intravenous use). Whenever adverse reactions are moderate or severe, thiazide dosage should be reduced or therapy withdrawn.

OVERDOSAGE

The most common signs and symptoms observed are those caused by electrolyte depletion (hypokalemia, hypochloremia, hyponatremia) and dehydration resulting from excessive diuresis. If digitalis has also been administered, hypokalemia may accentuate cardiac arrhythmias.
In the event of overdosage, symptomatic and supportive measures should be employed. Correct dehydration, electrolyte imbalance, hepatic coma and hypotension by established procedures. If required, give oxygen or artificial respiration for respiratory impairment.
The intravenous LD_{50} of chlorothiazide in the mouse is 1.1 g/kg.

DOSAGE AND ADMINISTRATION

Intravenous Sodium DIURIL should be reserved for patients unable to take oral medication or for emergency situations. Therapy should be individualized according to patient response. Use the smallest dosage necessary to achieve the required response.
Intravenous use in infants and children has been limited and is not generally recommended.
When medication can be taken orally, therapy with DIURIL tablets or oral suspension may be substituted for intravenous therapy, using the same dosage schedule as for the parenteral route.
Add 18 mL of Sterile Water for Injection to the vial to form an isotonic solution for intravenous injection. Never add less than 18 mL. Unused solution may be stored at room temperature for 24 hours, after which it must be discarded. Parenteral drug products should be inspected visually for particulate matter and discoloration prior to use whenever solution and container permit. The solution is compatible with dextrose or sodium chloride solutions for intravenous infusion. Avoid simultaneous administration of solutions of chlorothiazide with whole blood or its derivatives.
Extravasation must be rigidly avoided. Do not give subcutaneously or intramuscularly.
The usual adult dosage is 0.5 to 1.0 g once or twice a day. Many patients with edema respond to intermittent therapy, i.e., administration on alternate days or on three to five days each week. With an intermittent schedule, excessive response and the resulting undesirable electrolyte imbalance are less likely to occur.

HOW SUPPLIED

No. 3250—Intravenous Sodium DIURIL is a dry, sterile lyophilized white powder usually in plug form, supplied in vials containing chlorothiazide sodium equivalent to 0.5 g of chlorothiazide.
NDC 0006-3250-32.
Storage
Store reconstituted solution at room temperature and discard unused portion after 24 hours.
A.H.F.S. Category: 40:28
DC 7413527　Issued February 1988

DIURIL® Tablets　　　　　　　　　　　℞
(Chlorothiazide), U.S.P.
DIURIL® Oral Suspension　　　　　　　℞
(Chlorothiazide), U.S.P.

DESCRIPTION

DIURIL* (Chlorothiazide) is a diuretic and antihypertensive. It is 6-chloro-2*H* -1,2,4 -benzothiadiazine-7-sulfonamide 1,1-dioxide. Its empirical formula is $C_7H_6ClN_3O_4S_2$ and its structural formula is:

It is a white, or practically white, crystalline powder with a molecular weight of 295.72, which is very slightly soluble in water, but readily soluble in dilute aqueous sodium hydroxide. It is soluble in urine to the extent of about 150 mg per 100 mL at pH 7.

DIURIL is supplied as 250 mg and 500 mg tablets, for oral use. Each tablet contains the following inactive ingredients: gelatin, magnesium stearate, starch and talc. The 250 mg tablet also contains lactose.
Oral Suspension DIURIL contains 250 mg of chlorothiazide per 5 mL, alcohol 0.5 percent, with methylparaben 0.12 percent, propylparaben 0.02 percent, and benzoic acid 0.1 percent added as preservatives. The inactive ingredients are D&C Yellow 10, flavors, glycerin, purified water, sodium saccharin, sucrose and tragacanth.

*Registered trademark of MERCK & CO., INC.

CLINICAL PHARMACOLOGY

The mechanism of the antihypertensive effect of thiazides is unknown. DIURIL does not usually affect normal blood pressure.
DIURIL affects the distal renal tubular mechanism of electrolyte reabsorption. At maximal therapeutic dosage all thiazides are approximately equal in their diuretic efficacy. DIURIL increases excretion of sodium and chloride in approximately equivalent amounts. Natriuresis may be accompanied by some loss of potassium and bicarbonate.
After oral use diuresis begins within 2 hours, peaks in about 4 hours and lasts about 6 to 12 hours.
Pharmacokinetics and Metabolism
DIURIL is not metabolized but is eliminated rapidly by the kidney. The plasma half-life of chlorothiazide is 45–120 minutes. After oral doses, 20–24 percent of the dose is excreted unchanged in the urine. Chlorothiazide crosses the placental but not the blood-brain barrier and is excreted in breast milk.

INDICATIONS AND USAGE

DIURIL is indicated as adjunctive therapy in edema associated with congestive heart failure, hepatic cirrhosis, and corticosteroid and estrogen therapy.
DIURIL has also been found useful in edema due to various forms of renal dysfunction such as nephrotic syndrome, acute glomerulonephritis, and chronic renal failure.
DIURIL is indicated in the management of hypertension either as the sole therapeutic agent or to enhance the effectiveness of other antihypertensive drugs in the more severe forms of hypertension.
Use in Pregnancy. Routine use of diuretics during normal pregnancy is inappropriate and exposes mother and fetus to unnecessary hazard. Diuretics do not prevent development of toxemia of pregnancy and there is no satisfactory evidence that they are useful in the treatment of toxemia.
Edema during pregnancy may arise from pathologic causes or from the physiologic and mechanical consequences of pregnancy. Thiazides are indicated in pregnancy when edema is due to pathologic causes, just as they are in the absence of pregnancy (see PRECAUTIONS, *Pregnancy*). Dependent edema in pregnancy, resulting from restriction of venous return by the gravid uterus, is properly treated through elevation of the lower extremities and use of support stockings. Use of diuretics to lower intravascular volume in this instance is illogical and unnecessary. During normal pregnancy there is hypervolemia which is not harmful to the fetus or the mother in the absence of cardiovascular disease. However, it may be associated with edema, rarely generalized edema. If such edema causes discomfort, increased recumbency will often provide relief. Rarely this edema may cause extreme discomfort which is not relieved by rest. In these instances, a short course of diuretic therapy may provide relief and be appropriate.

CONTRAINDICATIONS

Anuria.
Hypersensitivity to this product or to other sulfonamide-derived drugs.

WARNINGS

Use with caution in severe renal disease. In patients with renal disease, thiazides may precipitate azotemia. Cumulative effects of the drug may develop in patients with impaired renal function.
Thiazides should be used with caution in patients with impaired hepatic function or progressive liver disease, since minor alterations of fluid and electrolyte balance may precipitate hepatic coma.
Thiazides may add to or potentiate the action of other antihypertensive drugs.

Continued on next page

Merck & Co.—Cont.

Sensitivity reactions may occur in patients with or without a history of allergy or bronchial asthma.
The possibility of exacerbation or activation of systemic lupus erythematosus has been reported.
Lithium generally should not be given with diuretics (see PRECAUTIONS, *Drug Interactions*).

PRECAUTIONS

General
All patients receiving diuretic therapy should be observed for evidence of fluid or electrolyte imbalance: namely, hyponatremia, hypochloremic alkalosis, and hypokalemia. Serum and urine electrolyte determinations are particularly important when the patient is vomiting excessively or receiving parenteral fluids. Warning signs or symptoms of fluid and electrolyte imbalance, irrespective of cause, include dryness of mouth, thirst, weakness, lethargy, drowsiness, restlessness, muscle pains or cramps, muscular fatigue, hypotension, oliguria, tachycardia, and gastrointestinal disturbances such as nausea and vomiting.
Hypokalemia may develop, especially with brisk diuresis, when severe cirrhosis is present or after prolonged therapy. Interference with adequate oral electrolyte intake will also contribute to hypokalemia. Hypokalemia may cause cardiac arrhythmias and may also sensitize or exaggerate the response of the heart to the toxic effects of digitalis (e.g., increased ventricular irritability). Hypokalemia may be avoided or treated by use of potassium sparing diuretics or potassium supplements such as foods with a high potassium content.
Although any chloride deficit is generally mild and usually does not require specific treatment except under extraordinary circumstances (as in liver disease or renal disease), chloride replacement may be required in the treatment of metabolic alkalosis.
Dilutional hyponatremia may occur in edematous patients in hot weather; appropriate therapy is water restriction, rather than administration of salt, except in rare instances when the hyponatremia is life threatening. In actual salt depletion, appropriate replacement is the therapy of choice.
Hyperuricemia may occur or acute gout may be precipitated in certain patients receiving thiazides.
In diabetic patients dosage adjustments of insulin or oral hypoglycemic agents may be required. Hyperglycemia may occur with thiazide diuretics. Thus latent diabetes mellitus may become manifest during thiazide therapy.
The antihypertensive effects of the drug may be enhanced in the post-sympathectomy patient.
If progressive renal impairment becomes evident, consider withholding or discontinuing diuretic therapy.
Thiazides have been shown to increase the urinary excretion of magnesium; this may result in hypomagnesemia.
Thiazides may decrease urinary calcium excretion. Thiazides may cause intermittent and slight elevation of serum calcium in the absence of known disorders of calcium metabolism. Marked hypercalcemia may be evidence of hidden hyperparathyroidism. Thiazides should be discontinued before carrying out tests for parathyroid function.
Increases in cholesterol and triglyceride levels may be associated with thiazide diuretic therapy.

Laboratory Tests
Periodic determination of serum electrolytes to detect possible electrolyte imbalance should be done at appropriate intervals.
Drug Interactions
When given concurrently the following drugs may interact with thiazide diuretics.
Alcohol, barbiturates, or narcotics—potentiation of orthostatic hypotension may occur.
Antidiabetic drugs (oral agents and insulin)—dosage adjustment of the antidiabetic drug may be required.
Other antihypertensive drugs—additive effect or potentiation.
Corticosteroids, ACTH—intensified electrolyte depletion, particularly hypokalemia.
Pressor amines (e.g., norepinephrine)—possible decreased response to pressor amines but not sufficient to preclude their use.
Skeletal muscle relaxants, nondepolarizing (e.g., tubocurarine)—possible increased responsiveness to the muscle relaxant.
Lithium—generally should not be given with diuretics. Diuretic agents reduce the renal clearance of lithium and add a high risk of lithium toxicity. Refer to the package insert for lithium preparations before use of such preparations with DIURIL.
Non-steroidal Anti-inflammatory Drugs—In some patients, the administration of a non-steroidal anti-inflammatory agent can reduce the diuretic, natriuretic, and antihypertensive effects of loop, potassium-sparing and thiazide diuretics. Therefore, when DIURIL and non-steroidal anti-inflammatory agents are used concomitantly, the patient should be observed closely to determine if the desired effect of the diuretic is obtained.
Drug/Laboratory Test Interactions
Thiazides should be discontinued before carrying out tests for parathyroid function (see PRECAUTIONS, *General*).
Carcinogenesis, Mutagenesis,
Impairment of Fertility
Carcinogenic studies have not been done with chlorothiazide.
Chlorothiazide was not mutagenic *in vitro* in the Ames microbial mutagen test at a maximum concentration of 5 mg/plate using Strains TA98 and TA100. Chlorothiazide did not produce any significant mutagenicity in the dominant lethal assay in the mouse after 8 oral doses of 50 mg/kg or single intraperitoneal doses of 525 or 644 mg/kg, although early fetal deaths and preimplantation losses were increased beyond control values. In a test using *Aspergillus nidulans*, chlorothiazide was negative and did not induce disjunction.
Chlorothiazide had no effect on fertility in a two-litter study in rat at doses up to 60 mg/kg/ day (2 times the maximum recommended human dose).

Pregnancy
Teratogenic Effects—Pregnancy Category B: Reproduction studies in the rabbit, the mouse and the rat at doses up to 500 mg/kg/day (25 times the maximum recommended human dose) showed no evidence of external abnormalities of the fetus due to chlorothiazide.
Chlorothiazide given in a two-litter study in rats at doses up to 60 mg/kg/day (2 times the maximum recommended human dose) did not impair fertility.
There are no adequate and well-controlled studies with DIURIL in pregnant women; however, thiazides cross the placental barrier and appear in cord blood. Since animal reproduction studies are not always predictive of human response, DIURIL should be used during pregnancy only if clearly needed. (See INDICATIONS AND USAGE.)
Nonteratogenic Effects: These may include fetal or neonatal jaundice, thrombocytopenia, and possibly other adverse reactions which have occurred in the adult.
Nursing Mothers
Because of the potential for serious adverse reactions in nursing infants from DIURIL, a decision should be made whether to discontinue nursing or to discontinue the drug, taking into account the importance of the drug to the mother.

ADVERSE REACTIONS

The following adverse reactions have been reported and, within each category, are listed in order of decreasing severity.
Body as a Whole: Weakness.
Cardiovascular: Hypotension including orthostatic hypotension (may be aggravated by alcohol, barbiturates, narcotics or antihypertensive drugs).
Digestive: Pancreatitis, jaundice (intrahepatic cholestatic jaundice), diarrhea, vomiting, sialadenitis, cramping, constipation, gastric irritation, nausea, anorexia.
Hematologic: Aplastic anemia, agranulocytosis, leukopenia, hemolytic anemia, thrombocytopenia.
Hypersensitivity: Anaphylactic reactions, necrotizing angiitis (vasculitis and cutaneous vasculitis), respiratory distress including pneumonitis and pulmonary edema, photosensitivity, fever, urticaria, rash, purpura.
Metabolic: Electrolyte imbalance (see PRECAUTIONS), hyperglycemia, glycosuria, hyperuricemia.
Musculoskeletal: Muscle spasm.
Nervous System/Psychiatric: Vertigo, paresthesias, dizziness, headache, restlessness.
Renal: Renal failure, renal dysfunction, interstitial nephritis. (See WARNINGS.)
Special Senses: Transient blurred vision, xanthopsia.
Whenever adverse reactions are moderate or severe, thiazide dosage should be reduced or therapy withdrawn.

OVERDOSAGE

The most common signs and symptoms observed are those caused by electrolyte depletion (hypokalemia, hypochloremia, hyponatremia) and dehydration resulting from excessive diuresis. If digitalis has also been administered, hypokalemia may accentuate cardiac arrhythmias.
In the event of overdosage, symptomatic and supportive measures should be employed. Emesis should be induced or gastric lavage performed. Correct dehydration, electrolyte imbalance, hepatic coma and hypotension by established procedures. If required, give oxygen or artificial respiration for respiratory impairment.
The oral LD_{50} of chlorothiazide is 8.5 g/kg, greater than 10 g/kg, and greater than 1 g/kg, in the mouse, rat and dog respectively.

DOSAGE AND ADMINISTRATION

Therapy should be individualized according to patient response. Use the smallest dosage necessary to achieve the required response.

Adults

For Diuresis
The usual adult dosage is 0.5 to 1.0 g once or twice a day. Many patients with edema respond to intermittent therapy, i.e., administration on alternate days or on three to five days each week. With an intermittent schedule, excessive response and the resulting undesirable electrolyte imbalance are less likely to occur.
For Control of Hypertension
The usual adult starting dosage is 0.5 or 1.0 g a day as a single or divided dose. Dosage is increased or decreased according to blood pressure response. Rarely some patients may require up to 2.0 g a day in divided doses.

Infants and Children

The usual oral pediatric dosage is based on 10 mg of DIURIL per pound of body weight per day in two doses. Infants under 6 months of age may require up to 15 mg per pound per day in two doses.
On this basis, infants up to 2 years of age may be given 125 to 375 mg daily in two doses (2.5 to 7.5 mL, or ½ to 1½ teaspoonfuls of the oral suspension daily). Children from 2 to 12 years of age may be given 375 mg to 1.0 g daily in two doses (7.5 to 20 mL, or 1½ to 4 teaspoonfuls of oral suspension daily). Dosage in both age groups should be based on body weight.

HOW SUPPLIED

No. 3244—Tablets DIURIL, 250 mg, are white, round, scored, compressed tablets, coded MSD 214. They are supplied as follows:
NDC 0006-0214-68 bottles of 100
NDC 0006-0214-82 bottles of 1000.
Shown in Product Identification Section, page 419
No. 3245—Tablets DIURIL, 500 mg, are white, round, scored, compressed tablets, coded MSD 432. They are supplied as follows:
NDC 0006-0432-68 bottles of 100
NDC 0006-0432-28 unit dose packages of 100
NDC 0006-0432-82 bottles of 1000
NDC 0006-0432-86 bottles of 5000.
Shown in Product Identification Section, page 419
No. 3239—Oral Suspension DIURIL, 250 mg of chlorothiazide per 5 mL, is a yellow, creamy suspension, and is supplied as follows:
NDC 0006-3239-66 bottles of 237 mL.
Storage
Oral Suspension DIURIL must be protected from freezing.
A.H.F.S. Category: 40:28
DC 7398750 Issued October 1987
COPYRIGHT © MERCK & CO., INC., 1986
All rights reserved

DOLOBID® Tablets ℞
(Diflunisal), U.S.P.

DESCRIPTION

Diflunisal is 2′, 4′-difluoro-4-hydroxy-3-biphenylcarboxylic acid. Its empirical formula is $C_{13}H_8F_2O_3$ and its structural formula is:

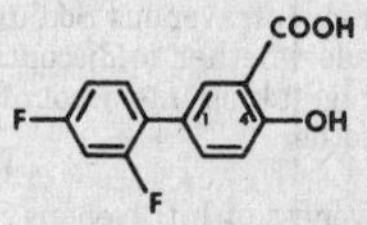

Diflunisal has a molecular weight of 250.20. It is a stable, white, crystalline compound with a melting point of 211–213°C. It is practically insoluble in water at neutral or acidic pH. Because it is an organic acid, it dissolves readily in dilute alkali to give a moderately stable solution at room temperature. It is soluble in most organic solvents including ethanol, methanol, and acetone.
DOLOBID* (Diflunisal) is available in 250 and 500 mg tablets for oral administration. Tablets DOLOBID contain the following inactive ingredients: cellulose, FD&C Yellow 6 hydroxypropyl cellulose, hydroxypropyl methylcellulose, magnesium stearate, starch, talc, and titanium dioxide.

*Registered trademark of MERCK & CO., INC.

CLINICAL PHARMACOLOGY

Action
DOLOBID is a non-steroidal drug with analgesic, anti-inflammatory and antipyretic properties. It is a peripherally-acting non-narcotic analgesic drug. Habituation, tolerance and addiction have not been reported.

Diflunisal is a difluorophenyl derivative of salicylic acid. Chemically, diflunisal differs from aspirin (acetylsalicylic acid) in two respects. The first of these two is the presence of a difluorophenyl substituent at carbon 1. The second difference is the removal of the 0-acetyl group from the carbon 4 position. Diflunisal is not metabolized to salicylic acid, and the fluorine atoms are not displaced from the difluorophenyl ring structure.

The precise mechanism of the analgesic and anti-inflammatory actions of diflunisal is not known. Diflunisal is a prostaglandin synthetase inhibitor. In animals, prostaglandins sensitize afferent nerves and potentiate the action of bradykinin in inducing pain. Since prostaglandins are known to be among the mediators of pain and inflammation, the mode of action of diflunisal may be due to a decrease of prostaglandins in peripheral tissues.

Pharmacokinetics and Metabolism

DOLOBID is rapidly and completely absorbed following oral administration with peak plasma concentrations occurring between 2 to 3 hours. The drug is excreted in the urine as two soluble glucuronide conjugates accounting for about 90% of the administered dose. Little or no diflunisal is excreted in the feces. Diflunisal appears in human milk in concentrations of 2–7% of those in plasma. More than 99% of diflunisal in plasma is bound to proteins.

As is the case with salicylic acid, concentration-dependent pharmacokinetics prevail when DOLOBID is administered; a doubling of dosage produces a greater than doubling of drug accumulation. The effect becomes more apparent with repetitive doses. Following single doses, peak plasma concentrations of 41 ± 11 μg/mL (mean ± S.D.) were observed following 250 mg doses, 87 ± 17 μg/mL were observed following 500 mg and 124 ± 11 μg/mL following single 1000 mg doses. However, following administration of 250 mg b.i.d., a mean peak level of 56 ± 14 μg/mL was observed on day 8, while the mean peak level after 500 mg b.i.d. for 11 days was 190 ± 33 μg/mL. In contrast to salicylic acid which has a plasma half-life of 2½ hours, the plasma half-life of diflunisal is 3 to 4 times longer (8 to 12 hours), because of a difluorophenyl substituent at carbon 1. Because of its long half-life and nonlinear pharmacokinetics, several days are required for diflunisal plasma levels to reach steady state following multiple doses. For this reason, an initial loading dose is necessary to shorten the time to reach steady state levels, and 2 to 3 days of observation are necessary for evaluating changes in treatment regimens if a loading dose is not used.

Studies in baboons to determine passage across the blood-brain barrier have shown that only small quantities of diflunisal, under normal or acidotic conditions are transported into the cerebrospinal fluid (CSF). The ratio of blood/CSF concentrations after intravenous doses of 50 mg/kg or oral doses of 100 mg/kg of diflunisal was 100:1. In contrast, oral doses of 500 mg/kg of aspirin resulted in a blood/CSF ratio of 5:1.

Mild to Moderate Pain

DOLOBID is a peripherally-acting analgesic agent with a long duration of action. DOLOBID produces significant analgesia within 1 hour and maximum analgesia within 2 to 3 hours.

Consistent with its long half-life, clinical effects of DOLOBID mirror its pharmacokinetic behavior, which is the basis for recommending a loading dose when instituting therapy. Patients treated with DOLOBID, on the first dose, tend to have a slower onset of pain relief when compared with drugs achieving comparable peak effects. However, DOLOBID produces longer-lasting responses than the comparative agents.

Comparative single dose clinical studies have established the analgesic efficacy of DOLOBID at various dose levels relative to other analgesics. Analgesic effect measurements were derived from hourly evaluations by patients during eight and twelve-hour postdosing observation periods. The following information may serve as a guide for prescribing DOLOBID.

DOLOBID 500 mg was comparable in analgesic efficacy to aspirin 650 mg, acetaminophen 600 mg or 650 mg, and acetaminophen 650 mg with propoxyphene napsylate 100 mg. Patients treated with DOLOBID had longer lasting responses than the patients treated with the comparative analgesics.

DOLOBID 1000 mg was comparable in analgesic efficacy to acetaminophen 600 mg with codeine 60 mg. Patients treated with DOLOBID had longer lasting responses than the patients who received acetaminophen with codeine.

A loading dose of 1000 mg provides faster onset of pain relief, shorter time to peak analgesic effect, and greater peak analgesic effect than an initial 500 mg dose.

In contrast to the comparative analgesics, a significantly greater proportion of patients treated with DOLOBID did not remedicate and continued to have a good analgesic effect eight to twelve hours after dosing. Seventy-five percent (75%) of patients treated with DOLOBID continued to have a good analgesic response at four hours. When patients having a good analgesic response at four hours were followed, 78% of these patients continued to have a good analgesic response at eight hours and 64% at twelve hours.

Chronic Anti-inflammatory Therapy in Osteoarthritis and Rheumatoid Arthritis

In the controlled, double-blind clinical trials in which DOLOBID (500 mg to 1000 mg a day) was compared with anti-inflammatory doses of aspirin (2–4 grams a day), patients treated with DOLOBID had a significantly lower incidence of tinnitus and of adverse effects involving the gastrointestinal system than patients treated with aspirin. (See also *Effect on Fecal Blood Loss*).

Osteoarthritis

The effectiveness of DOLOBID for the treatment of osteoarthritis was studied in patients with osteoarthritis of the hip and/or knee. The activity of DOLOBID was demonstrated by clinical improvement in the signs and symptoms of disease activity.

In a double-blind multicenter study of 12 weeks' duration in which dosages were adjusted according to patient response, DOLOBID, 500 or 750 mg daily, was shown to be comparable in effectiveness to aspirin, 2000 or 3000 mg daily. In open-label extensions of this study to 24 or 48 weeks, DOLOBID continued to show similar effectiveness and generally was well tolerated.

Rheumatoid Arthritis

In controlled clinical trials, the effectiveness of DOLOBID was established for both acute exacerbations and long-term management of rheumatoid arthritis. The activity of DOLOBID was demonstrated by clinical improvement in the signs and symptoms of disease activity.

In a double-blind multicenter study of 12 weeks' duration in which dosages were adjusted according to patient response, DOLOBID 500 or 750 mg daily was comparable in effectiveness to aspirin 2,600 or 3,900 mg daily. In open-label extensions of this study to 52 weeks, DOLOBID continued to be effective and was generally well tolerated.

DOLOBID 500, 750, or 1000 mg daily was compared with aspirin 2000, 3000, or 4000 mg daily in a multicenter study of 8 weeks' duration in which dosages were adjusted according to patient response. In this study, DOLOBID was comparable in efficacy to aspirin.

In a double-blind multicenter study of 12 weeks' duration in which dosages were adjusted according to patient needs, DOLOBID 500 or 750 mg daily and ibuprofen 1600 or 2400 mg daily were comparable in effectiveness and tolerability.

In a double-blind multicenter study of 12 weeks' duration, DOLOBID 750 mg daily was comparable in efficacy to naproxen 750 mg daily. The incidence of gastrointestinal adverse effects and tinnitus was comparable for both drugs. This study was extended to 48 weeks on an open-label basis. DOLOBID continued to be effective and generally well tolerated.

In patients with rheumatoid arthritis, DOLOBID and gold salts may be used in combination at their usual dosage levels. In clinical studies, DOLOBID added to the regimen of gold salts usually resulted in additional symptomatic relief but did not alter the course of the underlying disease.

Antipyretic Activity

DOLOBID is not recommended for use as an antipyretic agent. In single 250 mg, 500 mg, or 750 mg doses, DOLOBID produced measurable but not clinically useful decreases in temperature in patients with fever; however, the possibility that it may mask fever in some patients, particularly with chronic or high doses, should be considered.

Uricosuric Effect

In normal volunteers, an increase in the renal clearance of uric acid and a decrease in serum uric acid was observed when DOLOBID was administered at 500 mg or 750 mg daily in divided doses. Patients on long-term therapy taking DOLOBID at 500 mg to 1000 mg daily in divided doses showed a prompt and consistent reduction across studies in mean serum uric acid levels, which were lowered as much as 1.4 mg%. It is not known whether DOLOBID interferes with the activity of other uricosuric agents.

Effect on Platelet Function

As an inhibitor of prostaglandin synthetase, DOLOBID has a dose-related effect on platelet function and bleeding time. In normal volunteers, 250 mg b.i.d. for 8 days had no effect on platelet function, and 500 mg b.i.d., the usual recommended dose, had a slight effect. At 1000 mg b.i.d., which exceeds the maximum recommended dosage, however, DOLOBID inhibited platelet function. In contrast to aspirin, these effects of DOLOBID were reversible, because of the absence of the chemically labile and biologically reactive 0-acetyl group at the carbon 4 position. Bleeding time was not altered by a dose of 250 mg b.i.d., and was only slightly increased at 500 mg b.i.d. At 1000 mg b.i.d., a greater increase occurred, but was not statistically significantly different from the change in the placebo group.

Effect on Fecal Blood Loss

When DOLOBID was given to normal volunteers at the usual recommended dose of 500 mg twice daily, fecal blood loss was not significantly different from placebo. Aspirin at 1000 mg four times daily produced the expected increase in fecal blood loss. DOLOBID at 1000 mg twice daily (NOTE: exceeds the recommended dosage) caused a statistically significant increase in fecal blood loss, but this increase was only one-half as large as that associated with aspirin 1300 mg twice daily.

Effect on Blood Glucose

DOLOBID did not affect fasting blood sugar in diabetic patients who were receiving tolbutamide or placebo.

INDICATIONS AND USAGE

DOLOBID is indicated for acute or long-term use for symptomatic treatment of the following:

1. Mild to moderate pain
2. Osteoarthritis
3. Rheumatoid arthritis

CONTRAINDICATIONS

Patients who are hypersensitive to this product.

Patients in whom acute asthmatic attacks, urticaria, or rhinitis are precipitated by aspirin or other non-steroidal anti-inflammatory drugs.

WARNINGS

Peptic ulceration and gastrointestinal bleeding have been reported in patients receiving DOLOBID. Fatalities have occurred rarely. Gastrointestinal bleeding is associated with higher morbidity and mortality in patients acutely ill with other conditions, the elderly and patients with hemorrhagic disorders. In patients with active gastrointestinal bleeding or an active peptic ulcer, the physician must weigh the benefits of therapy with DOLOBID against possible hazards, institute an appropriate ulcer regimen, and carefully monitor the patient's progress. When DOLOBID is given to patients with a history of either upper or lower gastrointestinal tract disease, it should be given only after consulting the ADVERSE REACTIONS section and under close supervision.

Risk of GI Ulcerations, Bleeding and Perforation with NSAID Therapy

Serious gastrointestinal toxicity such as bleeding, ulceration, and perforation, can occur at any time, with or without warning symptoms, in patients treated chronically with NSAID therapy. Although minor upper gastrointestinal problems, such as dyspepsia, are common, usually developing early in therapy, physicians should remain alert for ulceration and bleeding in patients treated chronically with NSAIDs even in the absence of previous GI tract symptoms. In patients observed in clinical trials of several months to two years duration, symptomatic upper GI ulcers, gross bleeding or perforation appear to occur in approximately 1% of patients treated for 3–6 months, and in about 2–4% of patients treated for one year. Physicians should inform patients about the signs and/or symptoms of serious GI toxicity and what steps to take if they occur.

Studies to date have not identified any subset of patients not at risk of developing peptic ulceration and bleeding. Except for a prior history of serious GI events and other risk factors known to be associated with peptic ulcer disease, such as alcoholism, smoking, etc., no risk factors (e.g., age, sex) have been associated with increased risk. Elderly or debilitated patients seem to tolerate ulceration or bleeding less well than other individuals and most spontaneous reports of fatal GI events are in this population. Studies to date are inconclusive concerning the relative risk of various NSAIDs in causing such reactions. High doses of any NSAID probably carry a greater risk of these reactions, although controlled clinical trials showing this do not exist in most cases. In considering the use of relatively large doses (within the recommended dosage range), sufficient benefit should be anticipated to offset the potential increased risk of GI toxicity.

PRECAUTIONS

General

Although DOLOBID has less effect on platelet function and bleeding time than aspirin, at higher doses it is an inhibitor of platelet function; therefore, patients who may be adversely affected should be carefully observed when DOLOBID is administered (see CLINICAL PHARMACOLOGY).

Because of reports of adverse eye findings with agents of this class, it is recommended that patients who develop eye complaints during treatment with DOLOBID have ophthalmologic studies.

Peripheral edema has been observed in some patients taking DOLOBID. Therefore, as with other drugs in this class, DOLOBID should be used with caution in patients with com-

Continued on next page

Information on the Merck & Co. products listed on these pages is the full prescribing information from product circulars in use October 1, 1992.

Merck & Co.—Cont.

promised cardiac function, hypertension, or other conditions predisposing to fluid retention.

Acetylsalicylic acid has been associated with Reye syndrome. Because diflunisal is a derivative of salicylic acid, the possibility of its association with Reye syndrome cannot be excluded.

Hypersensitivity Syndrome

A potentially life-threatening, apparent hypersensitivity syndrome has been reported. This multisystem syndrome includes constitutional symptoms (fever, chills), and cutaneous findings (see ADVERSE REACTIONS, *Dermatologic*). It may also include involvement of major organs (changes in liver function, jaundice, leukopenia, thrombocytopenia, eosinophilia, disseminated intravascular coagulation, renal impairment, including renal failure), and less specific findings (adenitis, arthralgia, myalgia, arthritis, malaise, anorexia, disorientation). If evidence of hypersensitivity occurs, therapy with DOLOBID should be discontinued.

Renal Effects

As with other non-steroidal anti-inflammatory drugs, long term administration of diflunisal to animals has resulted in renal papillary necrosis and other abnormal renal pathology. In humans, there have been reports of acute interstitial nephritis with hematuria and proteinuria and occasionally nephrotic syndrome.

A second form of renal toxicity has been seen in patients with prerenal and renal conditions leading to a reduction in renal blood flow or blood volume, where the renal prostaglandins have a supportive role in the maintenance of renal perfusion. In these patients administration of an NSAID may cause a dose dependent reduction in prostaglandin formation and may precipitate overt renal decompensation. Patients at greatest risk of this reaction are those with conditions such as renal or hepatic dysfunction, diabetes mellitus, advanced age, extracellular volume depletion from any cause, congestive heart failure, septicemia, pyelonephritis, or concomitant use of any nephrotoxic drug. DOLOBID or other NSAIDs should be given with caution and renal function should be monitored in any patient who may have reduced renal reserve. Discontinuation of NSAID therapy is typically followed by recovery to the pretreatment state.

Since DOLOBID is eliminated primarily by the kidneys, patients with significantly impaired renal function should be closely monitored; a lower daily dosage should be anticipated to avoid excessive drug accumulation.

Information for Patients

DOLOBID, like other drugs of its class, is not free of side effects. The side effects of these drugs can cause discomfort and, rarely, there are more serious side effects such as gastrointestinal bleeding, which may result in hospitalization and even fatal outcomes.

NSAIDs (Non-steroidal Anti-inflammatory Drugs) are often essential agents in the management of arthritis and have a major role in the treatment of pain, but they also may be commonly employed for conditions which are less serious.

Physicians may wish to discuss with their patients the potential risks (see WARNINGS, PRECAUTIONS and ADVERSE REACTIONS) and likely benefits of NSAID treatment, particularly when the drugs are used for less serious conditions where treatment without NSAIDs may represent an acceptable alternative to both the patient and physician.

Laboratory Tests

Liver Function Tests: As with other non-steroidal anti-inflammatory drugs, borderline elevations of one or more liver tests may occur in up to 15% of patients. These abnormalities may progress, may remain essentially unchanged, or may be transient with continued therapy. The SGPT (ALT) test is probably the most sensitive indicator of liver dysfunction. Meaningful (3 times the upper limit of normal) elevations of SGPT or SGOT (AST) occurred in controlled clinical trials in less than 1% of patients. A patient with symptoms and/or signs suggesting liver dysfunction, or in whom an abnormal liver test has occurred, should be evaluated for evidence of the development of more severe hepatic reactions while on therapy with DOLOBID. Severe hepatic reactions, including jaundice, have been reported with DOLOBID as well as with other non-steroidal anti-inflammatory drugs. Although such reactions are rare, if abnormal liver tests persist or worsen, if clinical signs and symptoms consistent with liver disease develop, or if systemic manifestations occur (e.g., eosinophilia, rash, etc.), DOLOBID should be discontinued, since liver reactions can be fatal.

Gastrointestinal: Because serious GI tract ulceration and bleeding can occur without warning symptoms, physicians should follow chronically treated patients for the signs and symptoms of ulceration and bleeding and should inform them of the importance of this follow-up (see WARNINGS, *Risk of GI Ulcerations, Bleeding and Perforation with NSAID Therapy*).

Drug Interactions

Oral Anticoagulants: In some normal volunteers, the concomitant administration of DOLOBID and warfarin, acenocoumarol, or phenprocoumon resulted in prolongation of prothrombin time. This may occur because diflunisal competitively displaces coumarins from protein binding sites. Accordingly, when DOLOBID is administered with oral anticoagulants, the prothrombin time should be closely monitored during and for several days after concomitant drug administration. Adjustment of dosage of oral anticoagulants may be required.

Tolbutamide: In diabetic patients receiving DOLOBID and tolbutamide, no significant effects were seen on tolbutamide plasma levels or fasting blood glucose.

Hydrochlorothiazide: In normal volunteers, concomitant administration of DOLOBID and hydrochlorothiazide resulted in significantly increased plasma levels of hydrochlorothiazide. DOLOBID decreased the hyperuricemic effect of hydrochlorothiazide.

Furosemide: In normal volunteers, the concomitant administration of DOLOBID and furosemide had no effect on the diuretic activity of furosemide. DOLOBID decreased the hyperuricemic effect of furosemide.

Antacids: Concomitant administration of antacids may reduce plasma levels of DOLOBID. This effect is small with occasional doses of antacids, but may be clinically significant when antacids are used on a continuous schedule.

Acetaminophen: In normal volunteers, concomitant administration of DOLOBID and acetaminophen resulted in an approximate 50% increase in plasma levels of acetaminophen. Acetaminophen had no effect on plasma levels of DOLOBID. Since acetaminophen in high doses has been associated with hepatotoxicity, concomitant administration of DOLOBID and acetaminophen should be used cautiously, with careful monitoring of patients.

Concomitant administration of DOLOBID and acetaminophen in dogs, but not in rats, at approximately 2 times the recommended maximum human therapeutic dose of each (40-52 mg/kg/day of DOLOBID/acetaminophen), resulted in greater gastrointestinal toxicity than when either drug was administered alone. The clinical significance of these findings has not been established.

Methotrexate: Caution should be used if DOLOBID is administered concomitantly with methotrexate. Non-steroidal anti-inflammatory drugs have been reported to decrease the tubular secretion of methotrexate and to potentiate its toxicity.

Cyclosporine: Administration of non-steroidal anti-inflammatory drugs concomitantly with cyclosporine has been associated with an increase in cyclosporine-induced toxicity, possibly due to decreased synthesis of renal prostacyclin. NSAIDs should be used with caution in patients taking cyclosporine, and renal function should be carefully monitored.

Drug Interactions: Non-steroidal Anti-inflammatory Drugs

The administration of diflunisal to normal volunteers receiving indomethacin decreased the renal clearance and significantly increased the plasma levels of indomethacin. In some patients the combined use of indomethacin and DOLOBID has been associated with fatal gastrointestinal hemorrhage. Therefore, indomethacin and DOLOBID should not be used concomitantly.

Since no further clinical data are available about the safety and effectiveness of DOLOBID when used in combination with other non-steroidal anti-inflammatory drugs, no recommendation for their concomitant use can be made. The following information was obtained from studies in normal volunteers.

Aspirin: In normal volunteers, a small decrease in diflunisal levels was observed when multiple doses of DOLOBID and aspirin were administered concomitantly.

Sulindac: The concomitant administration of DOLOBID and sulindac in normal volunteers resulted in lowering of the plasma levels of the active sulindac sulfide metabolite by approximately one-third.

Naproxen: The concomitant administration of DOLOBID and naproxen in normal volunteers had no effect on the plasma levels of naproxen, but significantly decreased the urinary excretion of naproxen and its glucuronide metabolite. Naproxen had no effect on plasma levels of DOLOBID.

Drug/Laboratory Test Interactions

Serum Salicylate Assays: Caution should be used in interpreting the results of serum salicylate assays when diflunisal is present. Salicylate levels have been found to be falsely elevated with some assay methods.

Carcinogenesis, Mutagenesis, Impairment of Fertility

Diflunisal did not affect the type or incidence of neoplasia in a 105-week study in the rat given doses up to 40 mg/kg/day (equivalent to approximately 1.3 times the maximum recommended human dose), or in long-term carcinogenic studies in mice given diflunisal at doses up to 80 mg/kg/day (equivalent to approximately 2.7 times the maximum recommended human dose). It was concluded that there was no carcinogenic potential for DOLOBID.

Diflunisal passes the placental barrier to a minor degree in the rat. Diflunisal had no mutagenic activity after oral administration in the dominant lethal assay, in the Ames microbial mutagen test or in the V-79 Chinese hamster lung cell assay.

No evidence of impaired fertility was found in reproduction studies in rats at doses up to 50 mg/kg/day.

Pregnancy

Pregnancy Category C. A dose of 60 mg/kg/day of diflunisal (equivalent to two times the maximum human dose) was maternotoxic, embryotoxic, and teratogenic in rabbits. In three of six studies in rabbits, evidence of teratogenicity was observed at doses ranging from 40 to 50 mg/kg/day. Teratology studies in mice, at doses up to 45 mg/kg/day, and in rats at doses up to 100 mg/kg/day, revealed no harm to the fetus due to diflunisal. Aspirin and other salicylates have been shown to be teratogenic in a wide variety of species, including the rat and rabbit, at doses ranging from 50 to 400 mg/kg/day (approximately one to eight times the human dose). There are no adequate and well controlled studies with diflunisal in pregnant women. DOLOBID should be used during the first two trimesters of pregnancy only if the potential benefit justifies the potential risk to the fetus. Because of the known effect of drugs of this class on the human fetus (closure of the ductus arteriosus, platelet dysfunction with resultant bleeding, renal dysfunction or failure with oligohydramnios, gastrointestinal bleeding or perforation, and myocardial degenerative changes), use during the third trimester of pregnancy is not recommended.

In rats at a dose of one and one-half times the maximum human dose, there was an increase in the average length of gestation. Similar increases in the length of gestation have been observed with aspirin, indomethacin, and phenylbutazone, and may be related to inhibition of prostaglandin synthetase. Drugs of this class may cause dystocia and delayed parturition in pregnant animals.

Nursing Mothers

Diflunisal is excreted in human milk in concentrations of 2–7% of those in plasma. Because of the potential for serious adverse reactions in nursing infants from DOLOBID, a decision should be made whether to discontinue nursing or to discontinue the drug, taking into account the importance of the drug to the mother.

Pediatric Use

The adverse effects observed following diflunisal administration to neonatal animals appear to be species, age, and dose-dependent. At dose levels approximately 3 times the usual human therapeutic dose, both aspirin (200 to 400 mg/kg/day) and diflunisal (80 mg/kg/day) resulted in death, leukocytosis, weight loss, and bilateral cataracts in neonatal (4 to 5-day-old) beagle puppies after 2 to 10 doses. Administration of an 80 mg/kg/day dose of diflunisal to 25-day-old puppies resulted in lower mortality, and did not produce cataracts. In newborn rats, a 400 mg/kg/day dose of aspirin resulted in increased mortality and some cataracts, whereas the effects of diflunisal administration at doses up to 140 mg/kg/day were limited to a decrease in average body weight gain.

Safety and effectiveness in infants and children have not been established, and use of the drug in children below the age of 12 years is not recommended.

ADVERSE REACTIONS

The adverse reactions observed in controlled clinical trials encompass observations in 2,427 patients.

Listed below are the adverse reactions reported in the 1,314 of these patients who received treatment in studies of two weeks or longer. Five hundred thirteen patients were treated for at least 24 weeks, 255 patients were treated for at least 48 weeks, and 46 patients were treated for 96 weeks. In general, the adverse reactions listed below were 2 to 14 times less frequent in the 1,113 patients who received short-term treatment for mild to moderate pain.

Incidence Greater Than 1%

Gastrointestinal

The most frequent types of adverse reactions occurring with DOLOBID are gastrointestinal: these include nausea*, vomiting, dyspepsia*, gastrointestinal pain*, diarrhea*, constipation, and flatulence.

Psychiatric

Somnolence, insomnia.

Central Nervous System

Dizziness.

Special Senses

Tinnitus.

Dermatologic

Rash*.

Miscellaneous

Headache*, fatigue/tiredness.

Incidence Less Than 1 in 100

The following adverse reactions, occurring less frequently than 1 in 100, were reported in clinical trials or since the drug was marketed. The probability exists of a causal relationship between DOLOBID and these adverse reactions.

Dermatologic

Erythema multiforme, exfoliative dermatitis, Stevens-Johnson syndrome, toxic epidermal necrolysis, urticaria,

pruritus, sweating, dry mucous membranes, stomatitis, photosensitivity.

Gastrointestinal

Peptic ulcer, gastrointestinal bleeding, anorexia, eructation, gastrointestinal perforation, gastritis.

Liver function abnormalities; jaundice, sometimes with fever; cholestasis; hepatitis.

Hematologic

Thrombocytopenia; agranulocytosis; hemolytic anemia.

Genitourinary

Dysuria; renal impairment, including renal failure; interstitial nephritis; hematuria; proteinuria.

Psychiatric

Nervousness, depression, hallucinations, confusion, disorientation.

Central Nervous System

Vertigo; light-headedness; paresthesias.

Special Senses

Transient visual disturbances including blurred vision.

Hypersensitivity Reactions

Acute anaphylactic reaction with bronchospasm; angioedema.

Hypersensitivity vasculitis.

Hypersensitivity syndrome (see PRECAUTIONS).

Miscellaneous

Asthenia, edema.

Causal Relationship Unknown

Other reactions have been reported in clinical trials or since the drug was marketed, but occurred under circumstances where a causal relationship could not be established. However, in these rarely reported events, that possibility cannot be excluded. Therefore, these observations are listed to serve as alerting information to physicians.

Respiratory

Dyspnea.

Cardiovascular

Palpitation, syncope.

Musculoskeletal

Muscle cramps.

Genitourinary

Nephrotic syndrome.

Miscellaneous

Chest pain.

Potential Adverse Effects

In addition, a variety of adverse effects not observed with DOLOBID in clinical trials or in marketing experience, but reported with other non-steroidal analgesic/anti-inflammatory agents, should be considered potential adverse effects of DOLOBID.

---

*Incidence between 3% and 9%. Those reactions occurring in 1% to 3% are not marked with an asterisk.

OVERDOSAGE

Cases of overdosage have occurred and deaths have been reported. Most patients recovered without evidence of permanent sequelae. The most common signs and symptoms observed with overdosage were drowsiness, vomiting, nausea, diarrhea, hyperventilation, tachycardia, sweating, tinnitus, disorientation, stupor and coma. Diminished urine output and cardiorespiratory arrest have also been reported. The lowest dosage of DOLOBID at which a death has been reported was 15 grams without the presence of other drugs. In a mixed drug overdose, ingestion of 7.5 grams of DOLOBID resulted in death.

In the event of overdosage, the stomach should be emptied by inducing vomiting or by gastric lavage, and the patient carefully observed and given symptomatic and supportive treatment. Because of the high degree of protein binding, hemodialysis may not be effective.

The oral LD$_{50}$ of the drug is 500 mg/kg and 826 mg/kg in female mice and female rats respectively.

DOSAGE AND ADMINISTRATION

Concentration-dependent pharmacokinetics prevail when DOLOBID is administered; a doubling of dosage produces a greater than doubling of drug accumulation. The effect becomes more apparent with repetitive doses.

For mild to moderate pain, an initial dose of 1000 mg followed by 500 mg every 12 hours is recommended for most patients. Following the initial dose, some patients may require 500 mg every 8 hours.

A lower dosage may be appropriate depending on such factors as pain severity, patient response, weight, or advanced age; for example, 500 mg initially, followed by 250 mg every 8–12 hours.

For osteoarthritis and rheumatoid arthritis, the suggested dosage range is 500 mg to 1000 mg daily in two divided doses. The dosage of DOLOBID may be increased or decreased according to patient response.

Maintenance doses higher than 1500 mg a day are not recommended.

DOLOBID may be administered with water, milk or meals. Tablets should be swallowed whole, not crushed or chewed.

HOW SUPPLIED

Tablets DOLOBID are capsule-shaped, film-coated tablets supplied as follows:

No. 3390—250 mg peach colored, coded MSD 675
NDC 0006-0675-28 unit dose package of 100
NDC 0006-0675-61 unit of use bottles of 60
(6505-01-164-0581, 250 mg 60's)

Shown in Product Identification Section, page 419

No. 3392—500 mg orange colored, coded MSD 697
NDC 0006-0697-28 unit dose package of 100
NDC 0006-0697-61 unit of use bottles of 60
(6505-01-144-9724, 500 mg 60's)

Shown in Product Identification Section, page 419

A.H.F.S. Category: 28:08
DC 7327726   Issued March 1990
COPYRIGHT © MERCK & CO., INC., 1988
All rights reserved

EDECRIN® Tablets   ℞
(Ethacrynic Acid), U.S.P.
Intravenous
SODIUM EDECRIN®   ℞
(Ethacrynate Sodium), U.S.P.

EDECRIN* (Ethacrynic Acid) is a potent diuretic which, if given in excessive amounts, may lead to profound diuresis with water and electrolyte depletion. Therefore, careful medical supervision is required, and dose and dose schedule must be adjusted to the individual patient's needs (see DOSAGE AND ADMINISTRATION).

DESCRIPTION

Ethacrynic acid is an unsaturated ketone derivative of an aryloxyacetic acid. It is designated chemically as [2,3-dichloro-4-(2-methylene-1-oxobutyl)phenoxy] acetic acid, and has a molecular weight of 303.14. Ethacrynic acid is a white, or practically white, crystalline powder, very slightly soluble in water, but soluble in most organic solvents such as alcohols, chloroform, and benzene. Its empirical formula is $C_{13}H_{12}Cl_2O_4$ and its structural formula is:

Ethacrynate sodium, the sodium salt of ethacrynic acid, is soluble in water at 25°C to the extent of about 7 percent. Solutions of the sodium salt are relatively stable at about pH 7 at room temperature for short periods, but as the pH or temperature increases the solutions are less stable. The molecular weight of ethacrynate sodium is 325.12. Its empirical formula is $C_{13}H_{11}Cl_2NaO_4$ and its structural formula is:

EDECRIN is supplied as 25 mg and 50 mg tablets for oral use. Each tablet contains the following inactive ingredients: colloidal silicon dioxide, lactose, magnesium stearate, starch and talc. The 50 mg tablet also contains D&C Yellow 10, FD&C Blue 1 and FD&C Yellow 6. Intravenous SODIUM EDECRIN* (Ethacrynate Sodium) is a sterile freeze-dried powder and is supplied in a vial containing:

Ethacrynate sodium equivalent to ethacrynic
acid .... 50.0 mg
Inactive ingredients:
Mannitol .... 62.5 mg
with 0.1 mg thimerosal (mercury derivative) added as preservative.

---

*Registered trademark of MERCK & CO., INC.

CLINICAL PHARMACOLOGY

Pharmacokinetics and Metabolism

EDECRIN acts on the ascending limb of the loop of Henle and on the proximal and distal tubules. Urinary output is usually dose dependent and related to the magnitude of fluid accumulation. Water and electrolyte excretion may be increased several times over that observed with thiazide diuretics, since EDECRIN inhibits reabsorption of a much greater proportion of filtered sodium than most other diuretic agents. Therefore, EDECRIN is effective in many patients who have significant degrees of renal insufficiency (see WARNINGS concerning deafness). EDECRIN has little or no effect on glomerular filtration or on renal blood flow, except following pronounced reductions in plasma volume when associated with rapid diuresis.

The electrolyte excretion pattern of ethacrynic acid varies from that of the thiazides and mercurial diuretics. Initial sodium and chloride excretion is usually substantial and chloride loss exceeds that of sodium. With prolonged administration, chloride excretion declines, and potassium and hydrogen ion excretion may increase. EDECRIN is effective whether or not there is clinical acidosis or alkalosis.

Although EDECRIN, in carefully controlled studies in animals and experimental subjects, produces a more favorable sodium/potassium excretion ratio than the thiazides, in patients with increased diuresis excessive amounts of potassium may be excreted.

Onset of action is rapid, usually within 30 minutes after an oral dose of EDECRIN or within 5 minutes after an intravenous injection of SODIUM EDECRIN. After oral use, diuresis peaks in about 2 hours and lasts about 6 to 8 hours.

The sulfhydryl binding propensity of ethacrynic acid differs somewhat from that of the organomercurials. Its mode of action is not by carbonic anhydrase inhibition.

Ethacrynic acid does not cross the blood-brain barrier.

INDICATIONS AND USAGE

EDECRIN is indicated for treatment of edema when an agent with greater diuretic potential than those commonly employed is required.

1. Treatment of the edema associated with congestive heart failure, cirrhosis of the liver, and renal disease, including the nephrotic syndrome.
2. Short-term management of ascites due to malignancy, idiopathic edema, and lymphedema.
3. Short-term management of hospitalized pediatric patients, other than infants, with congenital heart disease or the nephrotic syndrome.
4. Intravenous SODIUM EDECRIN is indicated when a rapid onset of diuresis is desired, e.g., in acute pulmonary edema, or when gastrointestinal absorption is impaired or oral medication is not practicable.

CONTRAINDICATIONS

All diuretics, including ethacrynic acid, are contraindicated in anuria. If increasing electrolyte imbalance, azotemia, and/or oliguria occur during treatment of severe, progressive renal disease, the diuretic should be discontinued.

In a few patients this diuretic has produced severe, watery diarrhea. If this occurs, it should be discontinued and not used again.

Until further experience in infants is accumulated, therapy with oral and parenteral EDECRIN is contraindicated.

Hypersensitivity to any component of this product.

WARNINGS

The effects of EDECRIN on electrolytes are related to its renal pharmacologic activity and are dose dependent. The possibility of profound electrolyte and water loss may be avoided by weighing the patient throughout the treatment period, by careful adjustment of dosage, by initiating treatment with small doses, and by using the drug on an intermittent schedule when possible. When excessive diuresis occurs, the drug should be withdrawn until homeostasis is restored. When excessive electrolyte loss occurs, the dosage should be reduced or the drug temporarily withdrawn.

Initiation of diuretic therapy with EDECRIN in the cirrhotic patient with ascites is best carried out in the hospital. When maintenance therapy has been established, the individual can be satisfactorily followed as an outpatient.

EDECRIN should be given with caution to patients with advanced cirrhosis of the liver, particularly those with a history of previous episodes of electrolyte imbalance or hepatic encephalopathy. Like other diuretics it may precipitate hepatic coma and death.

Continued on next page

Merck & Co.—Cont.

Too vigorous a diuresis, as evidenced by rapid and excessive weight loss, may induce an acute hypotensive episode. In elderly cardiac patients, rapid contraction of plasma volume and the resultant hemoconcentration should be avoided to prevent the development of thromboembolic episodes, such as cerebral vascular thromboses and pulmonary emboli which may be fatal. Excessive loss of potassium in patients receiving digitalis glycosides may precipitate digitalis toxicity. Care should also be exercised in patients receiving potassium-depleting steroids.

A number of possibly drug-related deaths have occurred in critically ill patients refractory to other diuretics. These generally have fallen into two categories: (1) patients with severe myocardial disease who have been receiving digitalis and presumably developed acute hypokalemia with fatal arrhythmia; (2) patients with severely decompensated hepatic cirrhosis with ascites, with or without accompanying encephalopathy, who were in electrolyte imbalance and died because of intensification of the electrolyte defect.

Deafness, tinnitus, and vertigo with a sense of fullness in the ears have occurred, most frequently in patients with severe impairment of renal function. These symptoms have been associated most often with intravenous administration and with doses in excess of those recommended. The deafness has usually been reversible and of short duration (one to 24 hours). However, in some patients the hearing loss has been permanent. A number of these patients were also receiving drugs known to be ototoxic. EDECRIN may increase the ototoxic potential of other drugs (see PRECAUTIONS, subsection *Drug Interactions*).

Lithium generally should not be given with diuretics (see PRECAUTIONS, subsection *Drug Interactions*).

PRECAUTIONS

General

Weakness, muscle cramps, paresthesias, thirst, anorexia, and signs of hyponatremia, hypokalemia, and/or hypochloremic alkalosis may occur following vigorous or excessive diuresis and these may be accentuated by rigid salt restriction. Rarely tetany has been reported following vigorous diuresis. *During therapy with ethacrynic acid, liberalization of salt intake and supplementary potassium chloride are often necessary.*

When a metabolic alkalosis may be anticipated, e.g., in cirrhosis with ascites, the use of potassium chloride or a potassium-sparing agent before and during therapy with EDECRIN may mitigate or prevent the hypokalemia.

Loop diuretics have been shown to increase the urinary excretion of magnesium; this may result in hypomagnesemia.

The safety and efficacy of ethacrynic acid in hypertension have not been established. However, the dosage of coadministered antihypertensive agents may require adjustment.

Orthostatic hypotension may occur in patients receiving other antihypertensive agents when given ethacrynic acid.

EDECRIN has little or no effect on glomerular filtration or on renal blood flow, except following pronounced reductions in plasma volume when associated with rapid diuresis. A transient increase in serum urea nitrogen may occur. Usually, this is readily reversible when the drug is discontinued.

As with other diuretics used in the treatment of renal edema, hypoproteinemia may reduce responsiveness to ethacrynic acid and the use of salt-poor albumin should be considered.

A number of drugs, including ethacrynic acid, have been shown to displace warfarin from plasma protein; a reduction in the usual anticoagulant dosage may be required in patients receiving both drugs.

EDECRIN may increase the risk of gastric hemorrhage associated with corticosteroid treatment.

Laboratory Tests

Frequent serum electrolyte, CO_2 and BUN determinations should be performed early in therapy and periodically thereafter during active diuresis. Any electrolyte abnormalities should be corrected or the drug temporarily withdrawn.

Increases in blood glucose and alterations in glucose tolerance tests have been observed in patients receiving EDECRIN.

Drug Interactions

Lithium generally should not be given with diuretics because they reduce its renal clearance and add a high risk of lithium toxicity. Read circulars for lithium preparations before use of such concomitant therapy.

EDECRIN may increase the ototoxic potential of other drugs such as aminoglycoside and some cephalosporin antibiotics. Their concurrent use should be avoided.

A number of drugs, including ethacrynic acid, have been shown to displace warfarin from plasma protein; a reduction in the usual anticoagulant dosage may be required in patients receiving both drugs.

In some patients, the administration of a non-steroidal anti-inflammatory agent can reduce the diuretic, natriuretic, and antihypertensive effects of loop, potassium-sparing and thiazide diuretics. Therefore, when EDECRIN and non-steroidal anti-inflammatory agents are used concomitantly, the patient should be observed closely to determine if the desired effect of the diuretic is obtained.

Carcinogenesis, Mutagenesis, Impairment of Fertility

There was no evidence of a tumorigenic effect in a 79-week oral chronic toxicity study in rats at doses up to 45 times the human dose.

Ethacrynic acid had no effect on fertility in a two-litter study in rats or a two-generation study in mice at 10 times the human dose.

Pregnancy

Pregnancy Category B: Reproduction studies in the mouse and rabbit at doses up to 50 times the human dose showed no evidence of external abnormalities of the fetus due to EDECRIN.

In a two-litter study in the dog and rat, oral doses of 5 or 20 mg/kg/day (2½ or 10 times the human dose), respectively, did not interfere with pregnancy or with growth and development of the pups. Although there was reduction in the mean body weights of the fetuses in a teratogenic study in the rat at a dose level of 100 mg/kg (50 times the human dose), there was no effect on mortality or postnatal development. Functional and morphologic abnormalities were not observed.

There are, however, no adequate and well-controlled studies in pregnant women. Since animal reproduction studies are not always predictive of human response, EDECRIN should be used during pregnancy only if clearly needed.

Nursing Mothers

It is not known whether this drug is excreted in human milk. Because many drugs are excreted in human milk and because of the potential for serious adverse reactions in nursing infants from EDECRIN, a decision should be made whether to discontinue nursing or to discontinue the drug, taking into account the importance of the drug to the mother.

Pediatric Use

For information on oral use in pediatrics, other than infants, see INDICATIONS AND USAGE and DOSAGE AND ADMINISTRATION.

Safety and effectiveness in infants have not been established (see CONTRAINDICATIONS).

Safety and effectiveness of intravenous use in children have not been established (see DOSAGE AND ADMINISTRATION, *Intravenous Use*).

ADVERSE REACTIONS

Gastrointestinal

Anorexia, malaise, abdominal discomfort or pain, dysphagia, nausea, vomiting, and diarrhea have occurred. These are more frequent with large doses or after one to three months of continuous therapy. A few patients have had sudden onset of profuse, watery diarrhea. Discontinue EDECRIN if diarrhea is severe and do not give it again. Gastrointestinal bleeding has occurred in some patients. Rarely, acute pancreatitis has been reported.

Metabolic

Reversible hyperuricemia and acute gout have been reported. Acute symptomatic hypoglycemia with convulsions occurred in two uremic patients who received doses above those recommended. Hyperglycemia has been reported. Rarely, jaundice and abnormal liver function tests have been reported in seriously ill patients receiving multiple drug therapy, including EDECRIN.

Hematologic

Agranulocytosis or severe neutropenia has been reported in a few critically ill patients also receiving agents known to produce this effect. Thrombocytopenia has been reported rarely. Henoch-Schönlein purpura has been reported rarely in patients with rheumatic heart disease receiving multiple drug therapy, including EDECRIN.

Special Senses (See WARNINGS)

Deafness, tinnitus and vertigo with a sense of fullness in the ears, and blurred vision have occurred.

Central Nervous System

Headache, fatigue, apprehension, confusion.

Miscellaneous

Skin rash, fever, chills, hematuria.

SODIUM EDECRIN occasionally has caused local irritation and pain after intravenous use.

OVERDOSAGE

Overdosage may lead to excessive diuresis with electrolyte depletion and dehydration.

In the event of overdosage, symptomatic and supportive measures should be employed. Emesis should be induced or gastric lavage performed. Correct dehydration, electrolyte imbalance, hepatic coma, and hypotension by established procedures. If required, give oxygen or artificial respiration for respiratory impairment.

In the mouse, the oral LD_{50} of ethracrynic acid is 627 mg/kg and the intravenous LD_{50} of ethacrynate sodium is 175 mg/kg.

DOSAGE AND ADMINISTRATION

Dosage must be regulated carefully to prevent a more rapid or substantial loss of fluid or electrolyte than is indicated or necessary. The magnitude of diuresis and natriuresis is largely dependent on the degree of fluid accumulation present in the patient. Similarly, the extent of potassium excretion is determined in large measure by the presence and magnitude of aldosteronism.

Oral Use

EDECRIN is available for oral use as 25 mg and 50 mg tablets.

Dosage: To Initiate Diuresis

In Adults: The smallest dose required to produce gradual weight loss (about 1 to 2 pounds per day) is recommended. Onset of diuresis usually occurs at 50 to 100 mg for adults. After diuresis has been achieved, the minimally effective dose (usually from 50 to 200 mg daily) may be given on a continuous or intermittent dosage schedule. Dosage adjustments are usually in 25 to 50 mg increments to avoid derangement of water and electrolyte excretion.

The patient should be weighed under standard conditions before and during the institution of diuretic therapy with this compound. Small alterations in dose should effectively prevent a massive diuretic response. The following schedule may be helpful in determining the smallest effective dose.

Day 1—50 mg (single dose) after a meal
Day 2—50 mg twice daily after meals, if necessary
Day 3—100 mg in the morning and 50 to 100 mg following the afternoon or evening meal, depending upon response to the morning dose

A few patients may require initial and maintenance doses as high as 200 mg twice daily. These higher doses, which should be achieved gradually, are most often required in patients with severe, refractory edema.

In children (excluding infants, see CONTRAINDICATIONS): The initial dose should be 25 mg. Careful stepwise increments in dosage of 25 mg should be made to achieve effective maintenance.

Maintenance Therapy

It is usually possible to reduce the dosage and frequency of administration once dry weight has been achieved.

EDECRIN (Ethacrynic Acid) may be given intermittently after an effective diuresis is obtained with the regimen outlined above. Dosage may be on an alternate daily schedule or more prolonged periods of diuretic therapy may be interspersed with rest periods. Such an intermittent dosage schedule allows time for correction of any electrolyte imbalance and may provide a more efficient diuretic response.

The chloruretic effect of this agent may give rise to retention of bicarbonate and a metabolic alkalosis. This may be corrected by giving chloride (ammonium chloride or arginine chloride). Ammonium chloride should not be given to cirrhotic patients.

EDECRIN has additive effects when used with other diuretics. For example, a patient who is on maintenance dosage of an oral diuretic may require additional intermittent diuretic therapy, such as an organomercurial, for the maintenance of basal weight. The intermittent use of EDECRIN orally may eliminate the need for injections of organomercurials. Small doses of EDECRIN may be added to existing diuretic regimens to maintain basal weight. This drug may potentiate the action of carbonic anhydrase inhibitors, with augmentation of natriuresis and kaliuresis. Therefore, when adding EDECRIN the initial dose and changes of dose should be in 25 mg increments, to avoid electrolyte depletion. Rarely, patients who failed to respond to ethacrynic acid have responded to older established agents.

While many patients do not require supplemental potassium, the use of potassium chloride or potassium-sparing agents, or both, during treatment with EDECRIN is advisable, especially in cirrhotic or nephrotic patients and in patients receiving digitalis.

Salt liberalization usually prevents the development of hyponatremia and hypochloremia. During treatment with EDECRIN, salt may be liberalized to a greater extent than with other diuretics. Cirrhotic patients, however, usually require at least moderate salt restriction concomitant with diuretic therapy.

Intravenous Use

Intravenous SODIUM EDECRIN is for intravenous use when oral intake is impractical or in urgent conditions, such as acute pulmonary edema.

The usual intravenous dose for the average sized adult is 50 mg, or 0.5 to 1.0 mg per kg of body weight. Usually only one dose has been necessary; occasionally a second dose at a new injection site, to avoid possible thrombophlebitis, may be required. A single intravenous dose not exceeding 100 mg has been used in critical situations.

Insufficient pediatric experience precludes recommendation for this age group.

To reconstitute the dry material, add 50 mL of 5 percent Dextrose Injection, or Sodium Chloride Injection to the vial. Occasionally, some 5 percent Dextrose Injection solutions may have a low pH (below 5). The resulting solution with

such a diluent may be hazy or opalescent. Intravenous use of such a solution is not recommended. Inspect the vial containing Intravenous SODIUM EDECRIN for particulate matter and discoloration before use.
The solution may be given slowly through the tubing of a running infusion or by direct intravenous injection over a period of several minutes. Do not mix this solution with whole blood or its derivatives. Discard unused reconstituted solution after 24 hours.
SODIUM EDECRIN should not be given subcutaneously or intramuscularly because of local pain and irritation.

HOW SUPPLIED

No. 3321—Tablets EDECRIN, 25 mg, are white, capsule shaped, scored tablets, coded MSD 65. They are supplied as follows:
NDC 0006-0065-68 in bottles of 100.
Shown in Product Identification Section, page 419
No. 3322—Tablets EDECRIN, 50 mg, are green, capsule shaped, scored tablets, coded MSD 90. They are supplied as follows:
NDC 0006-0090-68 in bottles of 100.
Shown in Product Identification Section, page 419
No. 3330—Intravenous SODIUM EDECRIN is a dry white material either in a plug form or as a powder. It is supplied in vials containing ethacrynate sodium equivalent to 50 mg of ethacrynic acid, **NDC** 0006-3330-50.
A.H.F.S. Category: 40:28
DC 7413624 Issued October 1985
COPYRIGHT © MERCK & CO., INC., 1984
All rights reserved

ELAVIL* Tablets ℞
(Amitriptyline HCl), U.S.P.
ELAVIL* Injection ℞
(Amitriptyline HCl), U.S.P.

This product is marketed by Stuart Pharmaceuticals. Please refer to Stuart for prescribing information.

*Registered trademark of ICI Americas Inc.

ELSPAR® ℞
(Asparaginase, MSD)

WARNING

IT IS RECOMMENDED THAT ASPARAGINASE BE ADMINISTERED TO PATIENTS ONLY IN A HOSPITAL SETTING UNDER THE SUPERVISION OF A PHYSICIAN WHO IS QUALIFIED BY TRAINING AND EXPERIENCE TO ADMINISTER CANCER CHEMOTHERAPEUTIC AGENTS, BECAUSE OF THE POSSIBILITY OF SEVERE REACTIONS, INCLUDING ANAPHYLAXIS AND SUDDEN DEATH. THE PHYSICIAN MUST BE PREPARED TO TREAT ANAPHYLAXIS AT EACH ADMINISTRATION OF THE DRUG.
IN THE TREATMENT OF EACH PATIENT THE PHYSICIAN MUST WEIGH CAREFULLY THE POSSIBILITY OF ACHIEVING THERAPEUTIC BENEFIT VERSUS THE RISK OF TOXICITY. THE FOLLOWING DATA SHOULD BE THOROUGHLY REVIEWED BEFORE ADMINISTERING THE COMPOUND.

DESCRIPTION

ELSPAR* (Asparaginase, MSD) contains the enzyme L-asparagine amidohydrolase, type EC-2, derived from *Escherichia coli.* It is a white crystalline powder that is freely soluble in water and practically insoluble in methanol, acetone and chloroform. Its activity is expressed in terms of International Units (I.U.) according to the recommendation of the International Union of Biochemistry. The specific activity of ELSPAR is at least 225 I.U. per milligram of protein and each vial contains 10,000 I.U. of asparaginase and 80 mg of mannitol, an inactive ingredient, as a sterile, white lyophilized plug or powder for intravenous or intramuscular injection after reconstitution.

*Registered trademark of MERCK & CO., INC.

CLINICAL PHARMACOLOGY

Action
In a significant number of patients with acute leukemia, particularly lymphocytic, the malignant cells are dependent on an exogenous source of asparagine for survival. Normal cells, however, are able to synthesize asparagine and thus are affected less by the rapid depletion produced by treatment with the enzyme asparaginase. This is a unique approach to therapy based on a metabolic defect in asparagine synthesis of some malignant cells. ELSPAR, derived from *Escherichia coli,* is effective in inducing remissions in some patients with acute lymphocytic leukemia.

Asparagine Dependence Test
An asparagine dependence test has been utilized during the investigational studies. In this test leukemic cells obtained from some marrow cultures could be shown to require asparagine in *vitro,* suggesting sensitivity to asparaginase therapy in *vivo.* However, present data indicate that the correlation between asparagine dependence in such tests and the final response to therapy is sufficiently poor that the test is not recommended as a basis for selection of patients for treatment.
Pharmacokinetics and Metabolism
In a study in patients with metastatic cancer and leukemia, initial plasma levels of L-asparaginase following intravenous administration were correlated to dose. Daily administration resulted in a cumulative increase in plasma levels. Plasma half-life varied from 8 to 30 hours; it did not appear to be influenced by dosage, either single or repetitive, and could not be correlated with age, sex, surface area, renal or hepatic function, diagnosis or extent of disease. Apparent volume of distribution was approximately 70–80% of estimated plasma volume. There was some slow movement of asparaginase from vascular to extravascular, extracellular space. L-asparaginase was detected in the lymph. Cerebrospinal fluid levels were less than 1% of concurrent plasma levels. Only trace amounts appeared in the urine.
In a study in which patients with leukemia and metastatic cancer received intramuscular L-asparaginase, peak plasma levels of asparaginase were reached 14 to 24 hours after dosing. Plasma half-life was 39 to 49 hours. No asparaginase was detected in the urine.

INDICATIONS AND USAGE

ELSPAR is indicated in the therapy of patients with acute lymphocytic leukemia. This agent is useful primarily in combination with other chemotherapeutic agents in the induction of remissions of the disease in children. ELSPAR should not be used as the sole induction agent unless combination therapy is deemed inappropriate. ELSPAR is not recommended for maintenance therapy.

CONTRAINDICATIONS

ELSPAR is contraindicated in patients with pancreatitis or a history of pancreatitis. Acute hemorrhagic pancreatitis, in some instances fatal, has been reported following asparaginase administration. Asparaginase is also contraindicated in patients who have had previous anaphylactic reactions to it.

WARNINGS

Allergic reactions to asparaginase are frequent and may occur during the primary course of therapy. They are not completely predictable on the basis of the intradermal skin test. Anaphylaxis and death have occurred even in a hospital setting with experienced observers.
Once a patient has received ELSPAR as part of a treatment regimen, retreatment with this agent at a later time is associated with increased risk of hypersensitivity reactions. In patients found by skin testing to be hypersensitive to asparaginase, and in any patient who has received a previous course of therapy with asparaginase, therapy with this agent should be instituted or reinstituted only after successful desensitization, and then only if in the judgement of the physician the possible benefit is greater than the increased risk. Desensitization itself may be hazardous. (See DOSAGE AND ADMINISTRATION, *Intradermal Skin Test.*)
In view of the unpredictability of the adverse reactions to asparaginase, it is recommended that this product be used in a hospital setting. Asparaginase has an adverse effect on liver function in the majority of patients. Therapy with asparaginase may increase pre-existing liver impairment caused by prior therapy or the underlying disease. Because of this there is a possibility that asparaginase may increase the toxicity of other medications.
The administration of ELSPAR *intravenously concurrently with or immediately before* a course of vincristine and prednisone may be associated with increased toxicity. (See DOSAGE AND ADMINISTRATION, *Recommended Induction Regimens.*)

PRECAUTIONS

General
This drug may be a contact irritant and both powder and solution must be handled and administered with care. Inhalation of dust or vapors and contact with skin or mucous membranes, especially those of the eyes, must be avoided. In case of contact, wash with copious amounts of water for at least 15 minutes.
Asparaginase has been reported to have immunosuppressive activity in animal experiments. Accordingly, the possibility that use of the drug in man may predispose to infection should be considered.
Asparaginase toxicity is reported to be greater in adults than in children.
Laboratory Tests
The fall in circulating lymphoblasts often is quite marked; normal or below normal leukocyte counts are noted frequently within the first several days after initiating therapy. This may be accompanied by a marked rise in serum uric acid. The possible development of uric acid nephropathy should be borne in mind. Appropriate preventive measures should be taken, e.g., allopurinol, increased fluid intake, alkalization of urine. As a guide to the effects of therapy, the patient's peripheral blood count and bone marrow should be monitored frequently.
Frequent serum amylase determinations should be obtained to detect early evidence of pancreatitis. If pancreatitis occurs, therapy should be stopped and not reinstituted.
Blood sugar should be monitored during therapy with ELSPAR because hyperglycemia may occur.
Drug Interactions
Tissue culture and animal studies indicate that ELSPAR can diminish or abolish the effect of methotrexate on malignant cells. This effect on methotrexate activity persists as long as plasma asparagine levels are suppressed. These results would seem to dictate against the clinical use of methotrexate with ELSPAR, or during the period following ELSPAR therapy when plasma asparagine levels are below normal.
Drug/Laboratory Test Interactions
L-asparaginase has been reported to interfere with the interpretation of thyroid function tests by producing a rapid and marked reduction in serum concentrations of thyroxine-binding globulin within two days after the first dose. Serum concentrations of thyroxine-binding globulin returned to pretreatment values within four weeks of the last dose of L-asparaginase.
Animal Toxicology
A one-month intravenous toxicity study of ELSPAR in dogs at doses of 250, 1000, and 2000 I.U./kg/day revealed reduced serum total protein and albumin with loss of body weight at the highest dose level and anorexia, emesis, and diarrhea at all dosage levels. A similar study in monkeys at doses of 100, 300, and 1000 I.U./kg/day also revealed reduction of serum total protein and albumin and body weight loss at all dosage levels. Bromsulfalein retention and fatty changes in the liver were noted in monkeys that were given 300 and 1000 I.U./kg/day. The rabbit was unusually sensitive to ELSPAR since a single intravenous dose of 1000 I.U./kg caused hypocalcemia associated with necrosis of the parathyroid cells, convulsions, and death in about one third of the animals. Some rabbits that died showed small thymic and lymph node hemorrhages and necrosis of the germinal centers in the lymph nodes and spleen. The intravenous administration of calcium gluconate alleviated or prevented the adverse effects.
Changes in the pancreatic islets (not pancreatitis) ranging from edema to necrosis were observed in the rabbits in the acute intravenous toxicity studies (doses of 12,500 to 50,000 I.U./kg) but not in rabbits that received 1000 I.U./kg. The anatomical changes and the hypocalcemia found in the rabbits were not observed in the subacute intravenous studies in the dogs and monkeys.
Carcinogenesis, Mutagenesis, Impairment of Fertility
The intraperitoneal injection of 2500 I.U./kg/ day for 4 days in newborn Swiss mice resulted in a small increase in pulmonary adenomas; lymphatic leukemia was not increased.
L-asparaginase at concentrations of 152-909 I.U./plate was not mutagenic in the Ames microbial mutagen test with or without metabolic activation.
There are no adequate studies on the effects of asparaginase on fertility.
Pregnancy
Pregnancy Category C. In mice and rats ELSPAR has been shown to retard the weight gain of mothers and fetuses when given in doses of more than 1000 I.U./kg (the recommended human dose). Resorptions, gross abnormalities and skeletal abnormalities were observed. The intravenous administration of 50 or 100 I.U./kg (one-twentieth or one-tenth of the human dose) to pregnant rabbits on Day 8 and 9 of gestation resulted in dose dependent embryotoxicity and gross abnormalities. There are no adequate and well-controlled studies in pregnant women. ELSPAR should be used during pregnancy only if the potential benefit justifies the potential risk to the fetus.

Continued on next page

Information on the Merck & Co. products listed on these pages is the full prescribing information from product circulars in use October 1, 1992.

Merck & Co.—Cont.

Nursing Mothers
It is not known whether this drug is secreted in human milk. Because many drugs are secreted in human milk and because of the potential for serious adverse reactions in nursing infants from ELSPAR, a decision should be made whether to discontinue nursing or to discontinue the drug, taking into account the importance of the drug to the mother.

ADVERSE REACTIONS

Allergic reactions, including skin rashes, urticaria, arthralgia, respiratory distress, and acute anaphylaxis have been reported. (See WARNINGS.) Acute reactions have occurred in the absence of a positive skin test and during continued maintenance of therapeutic serum levels of ELSPAR.
In children with advanced leukemia, a lower incidence of anaphylaxis has been reported with intramuscular administration, although there was a higher incidence of milder hypersensitivity reactions than with intravenous administration.
Fatal hyperthermia has been reported.
Pancreatitis, sometimes fulminant and fatal, has occurred during or following therapy with ELSPAR.
Hyperglycemia with glucosuria and polyuria has been reported in low incidence. Serum and urine acetone usually have been absent or negligible in these patients; this syndrome thus resembles hyperosmolar, nonketotic, hyperglycemia induced by a variety of other agents. This complication usually responds to discontinuance of ELSPAR, judicious use of intravenous fluid, and insulin, but may be fatal on occasion.
In addition to hypofibrinogenemia, depression of various other clotting factors has been reported. Most marked has been a decrease in plasma levels of factors V and VIII with a variable decrease in factors VII and IX. A decrease in circulating platelets has occurred in low incidence which, together with the increased levels of fibrin degradation products in the serum, may indicate development of a consumption coagulopathy. Bleeding has been a problem in only a minority of patients with demonstrable coagulopathy. However, intracranial hemorrhage and fatal bleeding associated with low fibrinogen levels have been reported. Increased fibrinolytic activity, apparently compensatory in nature, also has occurred.
Some patients have shown central nervous system effects consisting of depression, somnolence, fatigue, coma, confusion, agitation, and hallucinations varying from mild to severe. Rarely, a Parkinson-like syndrome has occurred, with tremor and a progressive increase in muscular tone. These side effects usually have reversed spontaneously after treatment was stopped. Therapy with ELSPAR is associated with an increase in blood ammonia during the conversion of asparagine to asparatic acid by the enzyme. No clear correlation exists between the degree of elevation of blood ammonia levels and the appearance of CNS changes. Chills, fever, nausea, vomiting, anorexia, abdominal cramps, weight loss, headache, and irritability may occur and usually are mild.
Azotemia, usually pre-renal, occurs frequently. Acute renal shut down and fatal renal insufficiency have been reported during treatment. Proteinuria has occurred infrequently.
A variety of liver function abnormalities have been reported, including elevations of SGOT, SGPT, alkaline phosphatase, bilirubin (direct and indirect), and depression of serum albumin, cholesterol (total and esters), and plasma fibrinogen. Increases and decreases of total lipids have occurred. Marked hypoalbuminemia associated with peripheral edema has been reported. However, these abnormalities usually are reversible on discontinuance of therapy and some reversal may occur during the course of therapy. Fatty changes in the liver have been documented by biopsy. Malabsorption syndrome has been reported.
Rarely, transient bone marrow depression has been observed, as evidenced by a delay in return of hemoglobin or hematocrit levels to normal in patients undergoing hematologic remission of leukemia. Marked leukopenia has been reported.

OVERDOSAGE

The acute intravenous LD_{50} of ELSPAR for mice was about 500,000 I.U./kg and for rabbits about 22,000 I.U./kg.

DOSAGE AND ADMINISTRATION

As a component of selected multiple agent induction regimens, ELSPAR may be administered by either the intravenous or the intramuscular route. When administered intravenously this enzyme should be given over a period of not less than thirty minutes through the side arm of an already running infusion of Sodium Chloride Injection or Dextrose Injection 5% (D_5W). ELSPAR has little tendency to cause phlebitis when given intravenously. Anaphylactic reactions require the immediate use of epinephrine, oxygen, and intravenous steroids.
When administering ELSPAR intramuscularly, the volume at a single injection site should be limited to 2 ml. If a volume greater than 2 ml is to be administered, two injection sites should be used.
Unfavorable interactions of ELSPAR with some antitumor agents have been demonstrated. It is recommended therefore, that ELSPAR be used in combination regimens only by physicians familiar with the benefits and risks of a given regimen. During the period of its inhibition of protein synthesis and cell replication ELSPAR may interfere with the action of drugs such as methotrexate which require cell replication for their lethal effect. ELSPAR may interfere with the enzymatic detoxification of other drugs, particularly in the liver.
Recommended Induction Regimens:
When using chemotherapeutic agents in combination for the induction of remissions in patients with acute lymphocytic leukemia, regimens are sought which provide maximum chance of success while avoiding excessive cumulative toxicity or negative drug interactions.
One of the following combination regimens incorporating ELSPAR is recommended for acute lymphocytic leukemia in children:
In the regimens below, Day 1 is considered to be the first day of therapy.
Regimen I
Prednisone 40 mg/square meter of body surface area per day orally in three divided doses for 15 days, followed by tapering of the dosage as follows:
20 mg/square meter for 2 days, 10 mg/square meter for 2 days, 5 mg/square meter for 2 days, 2.5 mg/square meter for 2 days and then discontinue.
Vincristine sulfate 2 mg/square meter of body surface area intravenously once weekly on Days 1, 8, and 15 of the treatment period. The maximum single dose should not exceed 2.0 mg.
Asparaginase 1,000 I.U./kg/day intravenously for ten successive days beginning on Day 22 of the treatment period.
Regimen II
Prednisone 40 mg/square meter of body surface area per day orally in three divided doses for 28 days (the total daily dose should be to the nearest 2.5 mg), following which the dosage of prednisone should be discontinued gradually over a 14 day period.
Vincristine sulfate 1.5 mg/square meter of body surface area intravenously weekly for four doses, on Days 1, 8, 15, and 22 of the treatment period. The maximum single dose should not exceed 2.0 mg.
Asparaginase 6,000 I.U./square meter of body surface area intramuscularly on Days 4, 7, 10, 13, 16, 19, 22, 25, and 28 of the treatment period. When a remission is obtained with either of the above regimens, appropriate maintenance therapy must be instituted. ELSPAR should not be used as part of a maintenance regimen. The above regimens do not preclude a need for special therapy directed toward the prevention of central nervous system leukemia.
It should be noted that ELSPAR has been used in combination regimens other than those recommended above. It is important to keep in mind that ELSPAR administered intravenously concurrently with or immediately before a course of vincristine and prednisone may be associated with increased toxicity. Physicians using a given regimen should be thoroughly familiar with its benefits and risks. Clinical data are insufficient for a recommendation concerning the use of combination regimens in adults. Asparaginase toxicity is reported to be greater in adults than in children.
Use of ELSPAR as the sole induction agent should be undertaken only in an unusual situation when a combined regimen is inappropriate because of toxicity or other specific patient-related factors, or in cases refractory to other therapy. When ELSPAR is to be used as the sole induction agent for children or adults the recommended dosage regimen is 200 I.U./kg/ day intravenously for 28 days. When complete remissions were obtained with this regimen, they were of short duration, 1 to 3 months. ELSPAR has been used as the sole induction agent in other regimens. Physicians using a given regimen should be thoroughly familiar with its benefits and risks.
Patients undergoing induction therapy must be carefully monitored and the therapeutic regimen adjusted according to response and toxicity.
Such adjustments should always involve decreasing dosages of one or more agents or discontinuation depending on the degree of toxicity. Patients who have received a course of ELSPAR, if retreated, have an increased risk of hypersensitivity reactions. Therefore, retreatment should be undertaken only when the benefit of such therapy is weighed against the increased risk.
Intradermal Skin Test:
Because of the occurrence of allergic reactions, an intradermal skin test should be performed prior to the initial administration of ELSPAR and when ELSPAR is given after an interval of a week or more has elapsed between doses. The skin test solution may be prepared as follows: Reconstitute the contents of a 10,000 I.U. vial with 5.0 ml of diluent. From this solution (2,000 I.U./ml) withdraw 0.1 ml and inject it into another vial containing 9.9 ml of diluent, yielding a skin test solution of approximately 20.0 I.U./ml. Use 0.1 ml of this solution (about 2.0 I.U.) for the intradermal skin test. The skin test site should be observed for at least one hour for the appearance of a wheal or erythema either of which indicates a positive reaction. An allergic reaction even to the skin test dose in certain sensitized individuals may rarely occur. A negative skin test reaction does not preclude the possibility of the development of an allergic reaction.

Desensitization:
Desensitization should be performed before administering the first dose of ELSPAR on initiation of therapy in positive reactors, and on retreatment of any patient in whom such therapy is deemed necessary after carefully weighing the increased risk of hypersensitivity reactions. Rapid desensitization of the patient may be attempted with progressively increasing amounts of intravenously administered ELSPAR provided adequate precautions are taken to treat an acute allergic reaction should it occur. One reported schedule begins with a total of 1 I.U. given intravenously and doubles the dose every 10 minutes, provided no reaction has occurred, until the accumulated total amount given equals the planned doses for that day.
For convenience the following table is included to calculate the number of doses necessary to reach the patient's total dose for that day:

Injection Number	ELSPAR Dose in I.U.	Accumulated Total Dose
1	1	1
2	2	3
3	4	7
4	8	15
5	16	31
6	32	63
7	64	127
8	128	255
9	256	511
10	512	1023
11	1024	2047
12	2048	4095
13	4096	8191
14	8192	16383
15	16384	32767
16	32768	65535
17	65536	131071
18	131072	262143

For example: A patient weighing 20 kg who is to receive 200 I.U./kg (total dose 4000 I.U.) would receive injections 1 through 12 during desensitization.

DIRECTIONS FOR RECONSTITUTION

Parenteral drug products should be inspected visually for particulate matter and discoloration prior to administration whenever solution and container permit. When reconstituted, ELSPAR should be a clear, colorless solution. If the solution becomes cloudy, discard.
For Intravenous Use
Reconstitute with Sterile Water for Injection or with Sodium Chloride Injection. The volume recommended for reconstitution is 5 ml for the 10,000 unit vials. Ordinary shaking during reconstitution does not inactivate the enzyme. This solution may be used for direct intravenous administration within an eight hour period following restoration. For administration by infusion, solutions should be diluted with the isotonic solutions, Sodium Chloride Injection or Dextrose Injection 5%. These solutions should be infused within eight hours and only if clear.
Occasionally, a very small number of gelatinous fiber-like particles may develop on standing. Filtration through a 5.0 micron filter during administration will remove the particles with no resultant loss in potency. Some loss of potency has been observed with the use of a 0.2 micron filter.
For Intramuscular Use
When ELSPAR is administered intramuscularly according to the schedule cited in the induction regimen, reconstitution is carried out by adding 2 ml Sodium Chloride Injection to the 10,000 unit vial. The resulting solution should be used within eight hours and only if clear.

HOW SUPPLIED

No. 4612 — ELSPAR is a white lyophilized plug or powder supplied as follows:
NDC 0006-4612-00 in a sterile 10 ml vial containing 10,000 I.U. of asparaginase and 80 mg mannitol, an inactive ingredient.

Personnel preparing ELSPAR should avoid drug contact with skin, mucous membranes, or eyes and avoid inhaling the dust or vapor.

Store at 2–8°C (36–46°F). ELSPAR does not contain a preservative. Unused, reconstituted solution should be stored at 2 to 8°C (36 to 46°F) and discarded after eight hours, or sooner if it becomes cloudy.

A.H.F.S. Category: 44:00
DC 7407109 Issued September 1983
COPYRIGHT © MERCK & CO., INC., 1983
All rights reserved

FLEXERIL® Tablets   ℞
(Cyclobenzaprine HCl), U.S.P.

DESCRIPTION

Cyclobenzaprine hydrochloride is a white, crystalline tricyclic amine salt with the empirical formula $C_{20}H_{21}N \cdot HCl$ and a molecular weight of 311.9. It has a melting point of 217°C, and a pK_a of 8.47 at 25°C. It is freely soluble in water and alcohol, sparingly soluble in isopropanol, and insoluble in hydrocarbon solvents. If aqueous solutions are made alkaline, the free base separates. Cyclobenzaprine HCl is designated chemically as 3-(5H -dibenzo[a,d]cyclohepten-5-ylidene)-N, N -dimethyl-1-propanamine hydrochloride, and has the following structural formula:

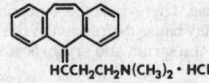

HCCH₂CH₂N(CH₃)₂ · HCl

FLEXERIL* (Cyclobenzaprine HCl) is supplied as 10 mg tablets for oral administration.

Tablets FLEXERIL contain the following inactive ingredients: hydroxypropyl cellulose, hydroxypropyl methylcellulose, iron oxide, lactose, magnesium stearate, starch, and titanium dioxide.

*Registered trademark of MERCK & CO., INC.

CLINICAL PHARMACOLOGY

Cyclobenzaprine HCl relieves skeletal muscle spasm of local origin without interfering with muscle function. It is ineffective in muscle spasm due to central nervous system disease. Cyclobenzaprine reduced or abolished skeletal muscle hyperactivity in several animal models. Animal studies indicate that cyclobenzaprine does not act at the neuromuscular junction or directly on skeletal muscle. Such studies show that cyclobenzaprine acts primarily within the central nervous system at brain stem as opposed to spinal cord levels, although its action on the latter may contribute to its overall skeletal muscle relaxant activity. Evidence suggests that the net effect of cyclobenzaprine is a reduction of tonic somatic motor activity, influencing both gamma (γ) and alpha (α) motor systems.

Pharmacological studies in animals showed a similarity between the effects of cyclobenzaprine and the structurally related tricyclic antidepressants, including reserpine antagonism, norepinephrine potentiation, potent peripheral and central anticholinergic effects, and sedation. Cyclobenzaprine caused slight to moderate increase in heart rate in animals.

Cyclobenzaprine is well absorbed after oral administration, but there is a large intersubject variation in plasma levels. Cyclobenzaprine is eliminated quite slowly with a half-life as long as one to three days. It is highly bound to plasma proteins, is extensively metabolized primarily to glucuronidelike conjugates, and is excreted primarily via the kidneys. No significant effect on plasma levels or bioavailability of FLEXERIL or aspirin was noted when single or multiple doses of the two drugs were administered concomitantly. Concomitant administration of FLEXERIL and aspirin is usually well tolerated and no unexpected or serious clinical or laboratory adverse effects have been observed. No studies have been performed to indicate whether FLEXERIL enhances the clinical effect of aspirin or other analgesics, or whether analgesics enhance the clinical effect of FLEXERIL in acute musculoskeletal conditions.

Clinical Studies
Controlled clinical studies show that FLEXERIL significantly improves the signs and symptoms of skeletal muscle spasm as compared with placebo. The clinical responses include improvement in muscle spasm as determined by palpation, reduction in local pain and tenderness, increased range of motion, and less restriction in activities of daily living. When daily observations were made, clinical improvement was observed as early as the first day of therapy.

Eight double-blind controlled clinical studies were performed in 642 patients comparing FLEXERIL, diazepam*, and placebo. Muscle spasm, local pain and tenderness, limitation of motion, and restriction in activities of daily living

were evaluated. In three of these studies there was a significantly greater improvement with FLEXERIL than with diazepam, while in the other studies the improvement following both treatments was comparable.

Although the frequency and severity of adverse reactions observed in patients treated with FLEXERIL were comparable to those observed in patients treated with diazepam, dry mouth was observed more frequently in patients treated with FLEXERIL and dizziness more frequently in those treated with diazepam. The incidence of drowsiness, the most frequent adverse reaction, was similar with both drugs. Analysis of the data from controlled studies shows that FLEXERIL produces clinical improvement whether or not sedation occurs.

*VALIUM® (diazepam, Roche)

Surveillance Program
A post-marketing surveillance program was carried out in 7607 patients with acute musculoskeletal disorders, and included 297 patients treated for 30 days or longer. The overall effectiveness of FLEXERIL was similar to that observed in the double-blind controlled studies; the overall incidence of adverse effects was less (see ADVERSE REACTIONS).

INDICATIONS AND USAGE

FLEXERIL is indicated as an adjunct to rest and physical therapy for relief of muscle spasm associated with acute, painful musculoskeletal conditions.

Improvement is manifested by relief of muscle spasm and its associated signs and symptoms, namely, pain, tenderness, limitation of motion, and restriction in activities of daily living.

FLEXERIL (Cyclobenzaprine HCl) should be used only for short periods (up to two or three weeks) because adequate evidence of effectiveness for more prolonged use is not available and because muscle spasm associated with acute, painful musculoskeletal conditions is generally of short duration and specific therapy for longer periods is seldom warranted.

FLEXERIL has not been found effective in the treatment of spasticity associated with cerebral or spinal cord disease, or in children with cerebral palsy.

CONTRAINDICATIONS

Hypersensitivity to the drug.

Concomitant use of monoamine oxidase inhibitors or within 14 days after their discontinuation.

Acute recovery phase of myocardial infarction, and patients with arrhythmias, heart block or conduction disturbances, or congestive heart failure.

Hyperthyroidism.

WARNINGS

Cyclobenzaprine is closely related to the tricyclic antidepressants, e.g., amitriptyline and imipramine. In short term studies for indications other than muscle spasm associated with acute musculoskeletal conditions, and usually at doses somewhat greater than those recommended for skeletal muscle spasm, some of the more serious central nervous system reactions noted with the tricyclic antidepressants have occurred (see WARNINGS, below, and ADVERSE REACTIONS).

FLEXERIL may interact with monoamine oxidase (MAO) inhibitors. Hyperpyretic crisis, severe convulsions, and deaths have occurred in patients receiving tricyclic antidepressants and MAO inhibitor drugs.

Tricyclic antidepressants have been reported to produce arrhythmias, sinus tachycardia, prolongation of the conduction time leading to myocardial infarction and stroke.

FLEXERIL may enhance the effects of alcohol, barbiturates, and other CNS depressants.

PRECAUTIONS

General
Because of its atropine-like action, FLEXERIL should be used with caution in patients with a history of urinary retention, angle-closure glaucoma, increased intraocular pressure, and in patients taking anticholinergic medication.

Information for Patients
FLEXERIL may impair mental and/or physical abilities required for performance of hazardous tasks, such as operating machinery or driving a motor vehicle.

Drug Interactions
FLEXERIL may enhance the effects of alcohol, barbiturates, and other CNS depressants.

Tricyclic antidepressants may block the antihypertensive action of guanethidine and similarly acting compounds.

Carcinogenesis, Mutagenesis, Impairment of Fertility
In rats treated with FLEXERIL for up to 67 weeks at doses of approximately 5 to 40 times the maximum recommended human dose, pale, sometimes enlarged, livers were noted and there was a dose-related hepatocyte vacuolation with lipido-

sis. In the higher dose groups this microscopic change was seen after 26 weeks and even earlier in rats which died prior to 26 weeks; at lower doses, the change was not seen until after 26 weeks.

Cyclobenzaprine did not affect the onset, incidence or distribution of neoplasia in an 81-week study in the mouse or in a 105-week study in the rat.

At oral doses of up to 10 times the human dose, cyclobenzaprine did not adversely affect the reproductive performance or fertility of male or female rats. Cyclobenzaprine did not demonstrate mutagenic activity in the male mouse at dose levels of up to 20 times the human dose.

Pregnancy
Pregnancy Category B: Reproduction studies have been performed in rats, mice and rabbits at doses up to 20 times the human dose, and have revealed no evidence of impaired fertility or harm to the fetus due to FLEXERIL. There are, however, no adequate and well-controlled studies in pregnant women. Because animal reproduction studies are not always predictive of human response, this drug should be used during pregnancy only if clearly needed.

Nursing Mothers
It is not known whether this drug is excreted in human milk. Because cyclobenzaprine is closely related to the tricyclic antidepressants, some of which are known to be excreted in human milk, caution should be exercised when FLEXERIL is administered to a nursing woman.

Pediatric Use
Safety and effectiveness of FLEXERIL in children below the age of 15 have not been established.

ADVERSE REACTIONS

The following list of adverse reactions is based on the experience in 473 patients treated with FLEXERIL in controlled clinical studies, 7607 patients in the post-marketing surveillance program, and reports received since the drug was marketed. The overall incidence of adverse reactions among patients in the surveillance program was less than the incidence in the controlled clinical studies.

The adverse reactions reported most frequently with FLEXERIL were drowsiness, dry mouth and dizziness. The incidence of these common adverse reactions was lower in the surveillance program than in the controlled clinical studies:

	Clinical Studies	Surveillance Program
drowsiness	39%	16%
dry mouth	27%	7%
dizziness	11%	3%

Among the less frequent adverse reactions, there was no appreciable difference in incidence in controlled clinical studies or in the surveillance program. Adverse reactions which were reported in 1% to 3% of the patients were: fatigue/tiredness, asthenia, nausea, constipation, dyspepsia, unpleasant taste, blurred vision, headache, nervousness, and confusion.

Incidence Less Than 1 in 100
The following adverse reactions have been reported at an incidence of less than 1 in 100:

Body as a Whole: Syncope; malaise.

Cardiovascular: Tachycardia; arrhythmia; vasodilatation; palpitation; hypotension.

Digestive: Vomiting; anorexia; diarrhea; gastrointestinal pain; gastritis; thirst; flatulence; edema of the tongue; abnormal liver function and rare reports of hepatitis, jaundice and cholestasis.

Hypersensitivity: Anaphylaxis; angioedema; pruritus; facial edema; urticaria; rash.

Musculoskeletal: Local weakness.

Nervous System and Psychiatric: Ataxia; vertigo; dysarthria; tremors; hypertonia; convulsions; muscle twitching; disorientation; insomnia; depressed mood; abnormal sensations; anxiety; agitation; abnormal thinking and dreaming; hallucinations; excitement; paresthesia; diplopia.

Skin: Sweating.

Special Senses: Ageusia; tinnitus.

Urogenital: Urinary frequency and/or retention.

Causal Relationship Unknown
Other reactions, reported rarely for FLEXERIL under circumstances where a causal relationship could not be established or reported for other tricyclic drugs, are listed to serve as alerting information to physicians:

Body as a Whole: Chest pain; edema.

Cardiovascular: Hypertension; myocardial infarction; heart block; stroke.

Digestive: Paralytic ileus; tongue discoloration; stomatitis; parotid swelling.

Continued on next page

Information on the Merck & Co. products listed on these pages is the full prescribing information from product circulars in use October 1, 1992.

Merck & Co.—Cont.

Endocrine: Inappropriate ADH syndrome.
Hematic and Lymphatic: Purpura; bone marrow depression; leukopenia; eosinophilia; thrombocytopenia.
Metabolic, Nutritional and Immune: Elevation and lowering of blood sugar levels; weight gain or loss.
Musculoskeletal: Myalgia.
Nervous System and Psychiatric: Decreased or increased libido; abnormal gait; delusions; peripheral neuropathy; Bell's palsy; alteration in EEG patterns; extrapyramidal symptoms.
Respiratory: Dyspnea.
Skin: Photosensitization; alopecia.
Urogenital: Impaired urination; dilatation of urinary tract; impotence; testicular swelling; gynecomastia; breast enlargement; galactorrhea.

DRUG ABUSE AND DEPENDENCE

Pharmacologic similarities among the tricyclic drugs require that certain withdrawal symptoms be considered when FLEXERIL is administered, even though they have not been reported to occur with this drug. Abrupt cessation of treatment after prolonged administration may produce nausea, headache, and malaise. These are not indicative of addiction.

OVERDOSAGE

Manifestations: High doses may cause temporary confusion, disturbed concentration, transient visual hallucinations, agitation, hyperactive reflexes, muscle rigidity, vomiting, or hyperpyrexia, in addition to anything listed under ADVERSE REACTIONS. Based on the known pharmacologic actions of the drug, overdosage may cause drowsiness, hypothermia, tachycardia and other cardiac rhythm abnormalities such as bundle branch block, ECG evidence of impaired conduction, and congestive heart failure. Other manifestations may be dilated pupils, convulsions, severe hypotension, stupor, and coma.
The acute oral LD_{50} of FLEXERIL is approximately 338 and 425 mg/kg in mice and rats, respectively.
Treatment: Treatment is symptomatic and supportive. Empty the stomach as quickly as possible by emesis, followed by gastric lavage. After gastric lavage, activated charcoal may be administered. Twenty to 30 g of activated charcoal may be given every four to six hours during the first 24 to 48 hours after ingestion. An ECG should be taken and close monitoring of cardiac function must be instituted if there is any evidence of dysrhythmia. Maintenance of an open airway, adequate fluid intake, and regulation of body temperature are necessary.
The intravenous administration of 1-3 mg of physostigmine salicylate is reported to reverse symptoms of poisoning by atropine and other drugs with anticholinergic activity. Physostigmine may be helpful in the treatment of cyclobenzaprine overdose. Because physostigmine is rapidly metabolized, the dosage of physostigmine should be repeated as required, particularly if life-threatening signs such as arrhythmias, convulsions, and deep coma recur or persist after the initial dosage of physostigmine. Because physostigmine itself may be toxic, it is not recommended for routine use. Standard medical measures should be used to manage circulatory shock and metabolic acidosis. Cardiac arrhythmias may be treated with neostigmine, pyridostigmine, or propranolol. When signs of cardiac failure occur, the use of a short-acting digitalis preparation should be considered. Close monitoring of cardiac function for not less than five days is advisable.
Anticonvulsants may be given to control seizures.
Dialysis is probably of no value because of low plasma concentrations of the drug.
Since overdosage is often deliberate, patients may attempt suicide by other means during the recovery phase. Deaths by deliberate or accidental overdosage have occurred with this class of drugs.

DOSAGE AND ADMINISTRATION

The usual dosage of FLEXERIL is 10 mg three times a day, with a range of 20 to 40 mg a day in divided doses. Dosage should not exceed 60 mg a day. Use of FLEXERIL for periods longer than two or three weeks is not recommended. (See INDICATIONS AND USAGE.)

HOW SUPPLIED

No. 3358—Tablets FLEXERIL, 10 mg, are butterscotch yellow, D-shaped, film coated tablets, coded MSD 931. They are supplied as follows:
NDC 0006-0931-68 in bottles of 100
(6505-01-062-8010, 10 mg 100's)
NDC 0006-0931-28 unit dose packages of 100.

Shown in Product Identification Section, page 419
A.H.F.S. Category: 12:20
DC 7399212 Issued August 1990
COPYRIGHT © MERCK & CO., INC., 1985
All rights reserved

FLOROPRYL® Sterile Ophthalmic Ointment   ℞
(Isoflurophate), U.S.P.
For Topical Application into the
Conjunctival Sac Only

DESCRIPTION

FLOROPRYL* (Isoflurophate) is available as 0.025% sterile ophthalmic ointment in polyethylene mineral oil gel. Isoflurophate has a molecular weight of 184.15 and is known chemically as bis (1-methylethyl) phosphorofluoridate. Its empirical formula is $C_6H_{14}FO_3P$ and its structural formula is:

$$(CH_3)_2CH-O-\overset{\overset{\displaystyle F}{|}}{\underset{\underset{\displaystyle O}{\|}}{P}}-O-CH(CH_3)_2$$

*Registered trademark of MERCK & CO., INC.

CLINICAL PHARMACOLOGY

FLOROPRYL is a cholinesterase inhibitor with sustained activity. Application to the eye produces intense miosis and ciliary muscle contraction due to inhibition of cholinesterase, allowing acetylcholine to accumulate at sites of cholinergic transmission.
FLOROPRYL *irreversibly* inactivates cholinesterase. Thus, following use of FLOROPRYL in the eye, cholinesterase must be either regenerated or supplied from depots elsewhere in the body before ophthalmic action dependent on cholinesterase returns.
If given systemically in sufficient amounts, FLOROPRYL reduces plasma cholinesterase to zero. However, when applied locally to the eye, plasma cholinesterase is usually reduced only slightly.

INDICATIONS AND USAGE

Open-angle glaucoma (FLOROPRYL should be used in glaucoma only when shorter-acting miotics have proven inadequate.)
Conditions obstructing aqueous outflow, such as synechial formation, that are amenable to miotic therapy
Following iridectomy
Accommodative esotropia (accommodative convergent strabismus)

CONTRAINDICATIONS

Hypersensitivity to any component of this product.
Because of the toxicity of cholinesterase inhibitors in general, FLOROPRYL is contraindicated in women who are or who may become pregnant. If this drug is used during pregnancy, or if the patient becomes pregnant while taking this drug, the patient should be apprised of the potential hazard to the fetus.
Because miotics may aggravate inflammation, FLOROPRYL should not be used in active uveal inflammation and/or glaucoma associated with iridocyclitis.

WARNINGS

In patients receiving cholinesterase inhibitors such as FLOROPRYL, succinylcholine should be administered with extreme caution before and during general anesthesia because of possible respiratory and cardiovascular collapse.
Because of possible adverse additive effects, FLOROPRYL should be administered only with extreme caution to patients with myasthenia gravis who are receiving systemic anticholinesterase therapy; conversely, extreme caution should be exercised in the use of an anticholinesterase drug for the treatment of myasthenia gravis patients who are already undergoing topical therapy with cholinesterase inhibitors.

PRECAUTIONS

General
FLOROPRYL should be used with caution in patients with chronic angle-closure (narrow-angle) glaucoma or in patients with narrow angles, because of the possibility of producing pupillary block and increasing angle blockage.
Gonioscopy is recommended prior to medication with FLOROPRYL.

When an intraocular inflammatory process is present, the intensity and persistence of miosis and ciliary muscle contraction that result from anticholinesterase therapy require abstention from, or cautious use of, FLOROPRYL.
Systemic effects are infrequent when FLOROPRYL is applied carefully. The hands should be washed immediately following application.
Discontinue FLOROPRYL if salivation, urinary incontinence, diarrhea, profuse sweating, muscle weakness, respiratory difficulties, shock, or cardiac irregularities occur.
Persons receiving cholinesterase inhibitors who are exposed to organophosphate-type insecticides and pesticides (gardeners, organophosphate plant or warehouse workers, farmers, residents of communities which are undergoing insecticide spraying or dusting, etc.) should be warned of the added systemic effects possible from absorption through the respiratory tract or skin. Wearing of respiratory masks, frequent washing, and clothing changes may be advisable.
Anticholinesterase drugs should be used with extreme caution, if at all, in patients with marked vagotonia, bronchial asthma, spastic gastrointestinal disturbances, peptic ulcer, pronounced bradycardia and hypotension, recent myocardial infarction, epilepsy, parkinsonism, and other disorders that may respond adversely to vagotonic effects.
After long-term use of FLOROPRYL, dilation of blood vessels and resulting greater permeability increase the possibility of hyphema during ophthalmic surgery. Therefore, this drug should be discontinued before surgery.
Despite observance of all precautions and the use of only the recommended dose, there is some evidence that repeated administration may cause depression of the concentration of cholinesterase in the serum and erythrocytes, with resultant systemic effects.
Drug Interactions
See WARNINGS regarding possible drug interactions of FLOROPRYL with succinylcholine or with other anticholinesterase agents.
Carcinogenesis, Mutagenesis, Impairment of Fertility
Long-term studies in animals have not been performed to evaluate the effects of FLOROPRYL on fertility or carcinogenic potential.
Pregnancy
Pregnancy Category X: See CONTRAINDICATIONS.
Nursing Mothers
It is not known whether this drug is excreted in human milk. Because of the potential for serious adverse reactions in nursing infants from FLOROPRYL, a decision should be made whether to discontinue nursing or to discontinue the drug, taking into account the importance of the drug to the mother.
Pediatric Use
The occurrence of iris cysts is more frequent in children. (See ADVERSE REACTIONS and DOSAGE AND ADMINISTRATION.)
Extreme caution should be exercised in children receiving FLOROPRYL who may require general anesthesia (see WARNINGS).
Since FLOROPRYL is a potent cholinesterase inhibitor it should be kept out of the reach of children.

ADVERSE REACTIONS

Stinging, burning, lacrimation, lid muscle twitching, conjunctival and ciliary redness, brow ache, headache, and induced myopia with visual blurring may occur.
As with all miotic therapy, retinal detachment has been reported occasionally.
Activation of latent iritis or uveitis may occur.
Iris cysts may form, enlarge, and obscure vision. Occurrence is more frequent in children. The iris cyst usually shrinks upon discontinuance of the miotic. Rarely, the cyst may rupture or break free into the aqueous. Frequent examination for this occurrence is advised.
Prolonged use may cause conjunctival thickening and obstruction of nasolacrimal canals.
Systemic effects, which occur rarely, are suggestive of increased cholinergic activity. Such effects may include nausea, vomiting, abdominal cramps, diarrhea, urinary incontinence, salivation, sweating, difficulty in breathing, bradycardia, or cardiac irregularities. Medical management of systemic effects may be indicated (see TREATMENT OF ADVERSE EFFECTS).
Lens opacities have been reported in patients on miotic therapy. Routine slit-lamp examinations, including the lens, should accompany prolonged use.
Paradoxical increase in intraocular pressure may follow anticholinesterase application. This may be alleviated by pupil-dilating medication.

TREATMENT OF ADVERSE EFFECTS

If FLOROPRYL is taken systemically by accident, or if systemic effects occur after topical application in the eye or from accidental skin contact, atropine sulfate in a dose (for adults) of 0.4 to 0.6 mg or more should be given parenterally

(intravenously if necessary). The recommended dosage of atropine in infants and children up to 12 years of age is 0.01 mg/kg repeated every two hours as needed until the desired effect is obtained, or adverse effects of atropine preclude further usage. The maximum single dose should not exceed 0.4 mg.
The use of much larger doses of atropine in treating anticholinesterase intoxication in adults has been reported in the literature. Initially 2 to 6 mg may be given followed by 2 mg every hour or more often, as long as muscarinic effects continue. The greater possibility of atropinization with large doses, particularly in sensitive individuals, should be borne in mind.
Pralidoxime* chloride has been reported to be useful in treatment of systemic effects due to cholinesterase inhibitors. However, its use is recommended in addition to and not as a substitute for atropine.
A short-acting barbiturate is indicated if convulsions occur that are not entirely relieved by atropine. Barbiturate dosage should be carefully adjusted to avoid central respiratory depression. Marked weakness or paralysis of muscles of respiration should be treated promptly by artificial respiration and maintenance of a clear airway.
The oral LD_{50} of FLOROPRYL is 37 mg/kg in the mouse, 5–10 mg/kg in the rat, and 4–10 mg/kg in the rabbit.

*PROTOPAM® Chloride (Pralidoxime Chloride). Ayerst Laboratories.

DOSAGE AND ADMINISTRATION

FLOROPRYL *is intended solely for topical use in the conjunctival sac.*
Isoflurophate hydrolyzes in the presence of water to form hydrofluoric acid. To prevent absorption of moisture and loss of potency, the ointment tube should be kept tightly closed; the tip of the tube should not be washed or allowed to touch the eyelid or other moist surface.
Whenever possible, FLOROPRYL should be applied at night before retiring to lessen blurring of vision. As it is an extremely potent drug, it should be used with great care and only by those familiar with its use and thoroughly indoctrinated in the technic of application.
The required dose is applied in the conjunctival sac, with the patient supine, care being taken not to touch the cornea with the tip of the tube. *Wash the hands immediately after administration.*
FLOROPRYL *should not be used more often than directed. Caution is necessary to avoid overdosage.*
Keep frequency of use to a minimum in all patients, but especially in children, to reduce the chance of iris cyst development (see ADVERSE REACTIONS). If tolerance develops, another miotic should be used. FLOROPRYL may be resumed later.

Glaucoma
For initial therapy 1/4 inch strip of ophthalmic ointment FLOROPRYL 0.025 per cent is placed in the glaucomatous eye every 8 to 72 hours. A decrease in intraocular pressure should occur within a few hours. During this period, keep the patient under supervision and make tonometric examinations at least hourly for 3 or 4 hours to be sure that no immediate rise in pressure occurs (see ADVERSE REACTIONS).

Strabismus
Essentially equal visual acuity of both eyes is a prerequisite to successful treatment. For initial evaluation FLOROPRYL may be used as a diagnostic aid to determine if an accomodative factor exists. This is especially useful preoperatively in young children and in patients with normal hypermetropic refractive errors. Not more than 1/4 inch strip of ointment is administered every night for 2 weeks. If the eyes become straighter, an accommodative factor is demonstrated. This technic may supplement or complement standard testing with atropine and trial with glasses for the accommodative factor.
In esotropia uncomplicated by amblyopia or anisometropia, ophthalmic ointment FLOROPRYL may be used in both eyes, not more than 1/4 inch strip at a time every night for 2 weeks, as too severe a degree of miosis may interfere with vision. The dosage is then reduced to from 1/4 inch strip every other day to 1/4 inch strip once a week for 2 months, after which the patient's status should be re-evaluated.
If benefit can not be maintained with a dosage interval of at least 48 hours, therapy with FLOROPRYL should be stopped. Frequency of administration and duration of maintenance therapy depend on how long the eyes remain straight without medication. Intervals between administration should be gradually increased to the greatest length compatible with good results. Therapy may need to be continued for many years in some patients; in others, it has been possible to discontinue therapy after several months.

HOW SUPPLIED

No. 7742—Sterile Ophthalmic Ointment FLOROPRYL 0.025 per cent is an opaque white, smooth, unctuous ointment and is supplied as follows:
NDC 0006-7742-04 in a 3.5 g tube.

Storage
Protect from moisture, freezing and excessive heat.
A.H.F.S. Category: 52:20
DC 7413720 Issued October 1987
COPYRIGHT © MERCK & CO., INC., 1987
All rights reserved

HEP-B-GAMMAGEE® ℞
(Hepatitis B Immune Globulin [Human], MSD), U.S.P.

DESCRIPTION

HEP-B-GAMMAGEE* [Hepatitis B Immune Globulin (Human), MSD] is a sterile solution of human immunoglobulin (10–18% protein) intended for intramuscular injection. The high levels of antibody to hepatitis B surface antigen (anti-HBs) found in the product are derived from a small group of well-monitored individuals who were hyperimmunized with hepatitis B vaccine. The potency is adjusted by the addition of IgG obtained from large pools of normal plasma. The pooled plasma is processed by MSD and/or Armour Pharmaceutical Company using Cohn cold ethanol fractionation procedures. The product is dissolved in 0.3 molar glycine and contains thimerosal (mercury derivative) 1:10,000 added as a preservative. The solution has a pH of 6.8 ± 0.4 adjusted with hydrochloric acid or sodium hydroxide. Each vial of HEP-B-GAMMAGEE contains anti-HBs equivalent to or exceeding the potency of anti-HBs in a U.S. reference Hepatitis B Immune Globulin (Office of Biologics Research and Review FDA).
There is no evidence to suggest that the causative virus of AIDS (HIV) has been transmitted by HEP-B-GAMMAGEE prepared by the Cohn cold ethanol process.

*Registered trademark of MERCK & CO., INC.

CLINICAL PHARMACOLOGY

Hepatitis B Immune Globulin (Human) provides passive immunization for individuals exposed to the hepatitis B virus (HBV) as evidenced by a reduction in the attack rate of hepatitis B following its use. The administration of the usual recommended dose of HEP-B-GAMMAGEE generally results in a detectable level of circulating antibody to hepatitis B surface antigen (anti-HBs) which persists for approximately 2 months or longer. Peak serum levels of anti-HBs are seen at 3–7 days after intramuscular administration of hepatitis B immunoglobulin. The half-life of this antibody ranges from 17.5–25 days. The possibility of hepatitis B transmission is remote, as it is with other immune globulins prepared by the cold ethanol process.

INDICATIONS AND USAGE

HEP-B-GAMMAGEE is indicated for post-exposure prophylaxis following either parenteral exposure, direct mucous membrane contact, sexual exposure or oral ingestion involving HBsAg-positive materials such as blood, plasma or serum. Such exposures might occur by accidental "needlestick", accidental splash, or a pipetting accident. HEP-B-GAMMAGEE is also indicated for post-exposure prophylaxis in infants born to hepatitis B-positive (HBsAg-positive) mothers.

CONTRAINDICATIONS

Hypersensitivity to any component of the product.

WARNINGS

Persons with isolated immunoglobulin A deficiency have the potential for developing antibodies to immunoglobulin A and could have anaphylactic reactions to subsequent administration of blood products that contain immunoglobulin A. Therefore, as with any immunoglobulin preparation, Hepatitis B Immune Globulin (Human) should be given to such persons only if the expected benefits outweigh the potential risks.
In patients who have severe thrombocytopenia or any coagulation disorder that would contraindicate intramuscular injections, Hepatitis B Immune Globulin (Human) should be given only if the expected benefits outweigh the potential risks.

PRECAUTIONS

General
HEP-B-GAMMAGEE should be given with caution to patients with a history of prior systemic allergic reactions following the administration of human immune globulin preparations. Hypersensitivity reactions to injections of immunoglobulin occur rarely. The incidence of these reactions may be increased in patients receiving large intramuscular doses or in patients receiving repeated injections of immunoglobulin.
HEP-B-GAMMAGEE *must not be administered intravenously* because of the potential for serious reactions. Injections should be made intramuscularly. Care should be taken to draw back on the plunger of the syringe before injection in order to be certain that the needle is not in a blood vessel.
Epinephrine should be available for treatment of acute allergic symptoms.
There is no evidence that the causative virus of AIDS (HIV-1) is transmitted by HEP-B-GAMMAGEE which is prepared by the Cohn cold ethanol process.
Some investigational intravenous immunoglobulin products have been linked to transmission of non-A, non-B hepatitis; however, there have been no reports of this in association with HEP-B-GAMMAGEE.

Drug Interactions
Antibodies present in immunoglobulin preparations may interfere with the immune response to live virus vaccines such as measles, mumps, and rubella. Therefore, vaccination with live virus vaccines should be deferred until approximately three months after administration of Hepatitis B Immune Globulin (Human). It may be necessary to revaccinate persons who received Hepatitis B Immune Globulin (Human) shortly after live virus vaccination.

Pregnancy
Pregnancy Category C. Animal reproduction studies have not been conducted with HEP-B-GAMMAGEE. It is also not known whether HEP-B-GAMMAGEE can cause fetal harm when administered to a pregnant woman or can affect reproduction capacity. HEP-B-GAMMAGEE should be given to a pregnant woman only if clearly needed.

Nursing Mothers
It is not known whether this drug is excreted in human milk. Because many drugs are excreted in human milk, caution should be exercised when HEP-B-GAMMAGEE is administered to a nursing woman.

ADVERSE REACTIONS

Local pain and tenderness at the injection site, urticaria and angioedema may occur. Anaphylactic reactions, although rare, have been reported following the injection of human immunoglobulin preparations. Anaphylaxis is more likely to occur if Hepatitis B Immune Globulin (Human) is given intravenously; therefore, Hepatitis B Immune Globulin (Human) must be administered *only* intramuscularly. In highly allergic individuals, repeated injections may lead to anaphylactic shock.

OVERDOSAGE

Although no data are available, clinical experience with other immunoglobulin preparations suggests that the only manifestations would be pain and tenderness at the injection site.

DOSAGE AND ADMINISTRATION

Parenteral drug products should be inspected visually for particulate matter and discoloration prior to administration, whenever solution and container permit. HEP-B-GAMMAGEE is a clear, very slightly amber, moderately viscous liquid.
HEP-B-GAMMAGEE is administered *intramuscularly. It must not be injected intravenously.*
It is important to use a separate sterile syringe and needle for each individual patient to prevent transmission of hepatitis B and other infectious agents from one person to another.

Known or Presumed Exposure to HBsAg
There are no prospective studies directly testing the efficacy of a combination of Hepatitis B Immune Globulin (Human) and hepatitis B vaccine (HEPTAVAX-B† (Hepatitis B Vaccine, MSD) or RECOMBIVAX HB† [Hepatitis B Vaccine (Recombinant), MSD]) in preventing clinical hepatitis B following percutaneous, ocular or mucous membrane exposure to hepatitis B virus. However, since most persons with such exposures (e.g., health-care workers) are candidates for the hepatitis B vaccine and since combined Hepatitis B Immune Globulin (Human) plus vaccine is more efficacious than Hepatitis B Immune Globulin (Human) alone in perinatal exposures, the following guidelines are recommended for persons who have been exposed to hepatitis B virus such as through (1) percutaneous (needlestick), ocular, mucous membrane exposure to blood known or presumed to contain HBsAg, (2) human bites by known or presumed HBsAg carri-

Continued on next page

Information on the Merck & Co. products listed on these pages is the full prescribing information from product circulars in use October 1, 1992.

Merck & Co.—Cont.

ers, that penetrate the skin, or (3) following intimate sexual contact with known or presumed HBsAg carriers:

Recommendations for adults who have not been previously vaccinated against hepatitis B:

Hepatitis B Immune Globulin (Human) (0.06 mL/kg) should be given intramuscularly as soon as possible after exposure and within 24 hours if possible. Hepatitis B vaccine (see HEPTAVAX-B (Hepatitis B Vaccine, MSD) or RECOM-BIVAX HB [Hepatitis B Vaccine (Recombinant), MSD] circular for appropriate dosage recommendations) should be given intramuscularly within 7 days of exposure and second and third doses given one and six months, respectively, after the first dose.

Recommendations for adults who have been previously vaccinated against hepatitis B:

Prior recipients of a recommended course of hepatitis B vaccine should have their anti-HBs titer checked promptly. For those with known adequate antibody (10 MIU/mL anti-HBs, approximately equal to 10 SRU) nothing is required. Those with inadequate or unknown titers should receive a dose of Hepatitis B Immune Globulin (Human) and a dose of hepatitis B vaccine simultaneously at two different sites as soon as possible.

Dosage for Infants Born of HBsAg Positive Mothers:

Infants born to HBsAg positive mothers are at high risk of becoming chronic carriers of hepatitis B virus and of developing the chronic sequelae of hepatitis B virus infection. Well-controlled studies have shown that administration of three 0.5 mL doses of Hepatitis B Immune Globulin (Human) starting at birth is 75% effective in preventing establishment of the chronic carrier state in these infants during the first year of life. Protection can be transient, whereupon the effectiveness of the Hepatitis B Immune Globulin (Human) would decline thereafter. Results from clinical studies indicate that administration of one 0.5 mL dose of Hepatitis B Immune Globulin (Human) at birth and the recommended three doses of HEPTAVAX-B (Hepatitis B Vaccine, MSD) or RECOM-BIVAX HB [Hepatitis B Vaccine (Recombinant), MSD] (see Table below), were effective in preventing establishment of the chronic carrier state in infants born to HBsAg and HBeAg positive mothers.

Testing for HBsAg and anti-HBs is recommended at 12–15 months of age. If HBsAg is not detectable, and anti-HBs is present, the child has been protected.

The recommended dosage for infants born to HBsAg positive mothers is as follows:

	Birth	Within 7 days	1 month	6 months
Hepatitis B vaccine**		0.5 mL*	0.5 mL	0.5 mL
Hepatitis B Immune Globulin (Human)	0.5 mL	—	—	—

* The first dose of hepatitis B vaccine may be given at birth at the same time as Hepatitis B Immune Globulin (Human); but should be administered in the opposite anterolateral thigh.

** See DOSAGE AND ADMINISTRATION section of RECOMBIVAX HB [Hepatitis B Vaccine (Recombinant), MSD] circular.

† Registered trademark of MERCK & CO., INC.

HOW SUPPLIED

No. 4692—HEP-B-GAMMAGEE is supplied as follows:
NDC 0006-4692-00 in 5 mL vials.
Store at 2–8°C (36–46°F). Do not freeze. Do not use after expiration date.

A.H.F.S. Category: 80:04
DC 7413910   Issued April 1992
COPYRIGHT © MERCK & CO., INC., 1988
All rights reserved

HUMORSOL® Sterile Ophthalmic Solution   ℞
(Demecarium Bromide), U.S.P.
For Topical Application into the
Conjunctival Sac Only

DESCRIPTION

Ophthalmic Solution HUMORSOL* (Demecarium Bromide) is a sterile solution supplied in two dosage strengths: 0.125 percent and 0.25 percent. The inactive ingredients are sodium chloride and water for injection; benzalkonium chloride 1:5000 is added as preservative. Demecarium bromide is a quaternary ammonium compound with a molecular weight of 716.60. Its chemical name is 3,3′-[1,10-decanediylbis [(methylimino)carbonyloxy]] bis [*N,N,N*-trimethylbenzenaminium] dibromide. Its empirical formula is $C_{32}H_{52}Br_2N_4O_4$ and its structural formula is:

*Registered trademark of MERCK & CO., INC.

CLINICAL PHARMACOLOGY

HUMORSOL is a cholinesterase inhibitor with sustained activity. It acts mainly on true (erythrocyte) cholinesterase. Application of HUMORSOL to the eye produces intense miosis and ciliary muscle contraction due to inhibition of cholinesterase, allowing acetylcholine to accumulate at sites of cholinergic transmission. These effects are accompanied by increased capillary permeability of the ciliary body and iris, increased permeability of the blood-aqueous barrier, and vasodilation. Myopia may be induced or, if present, may be augmented by the increased refractive power of the lens that results from the accommodative effect of the drug. HUMORSOL indirectly produces some of the muscarinic and nicotinic effects of acetylcholine as quantities of the latter accumulate.

INDICATIONS AND USAGE

Open-angle glaucoma (HUMORSOL should be used in glaucoma only when shorter-acting miotics have proved inadequate.)
Conditions obstructing aqueous outflow, such as synechial formation, that are amenable to miotic therapy
Following iridectomy
Accommodative esotropia (accommodative convergent strabismus)

CONTRAINDICATIONS

Hypersensitivity to any component of this product.
Because of the toxicity of cholinesterase inhibitors in general, HUMORSOL is contraindicated in women who are or who may become pregnant. If this drug is used during pregnancy, or if the patient becomes pregnant while taking this drug, the patient should be apprised of the potential hazard to the fetus.
Because miotics may aggravate inflammation, HUMORSOL should not be used in active uveal inflammation and/or glaucoma associated with iridocyclitis.

WARNINGS

In patients receiving cholinesterase inhibitors such as HUMORSOL, succinylcholine should be administered with extreme caution before and during general anesthesia.
Because of possible adverse additive effects, HUMORSOL should be administered only with extreme caution to patients with myasthenia gravis who are receiving systemic anticholinesterase therapy; conversely, extreme caution should be exercised in the use of an anticholinesterase drug for the treatment of myasthenia gravis patients who are already undergoing topical therapy with cholinesterase inhibitors.

PRECAUTIONS

General
Gonioscopy is recommended prior to medication with HUMORSOL.
HUMORSOL should be used with caution in patients with chronic angle-closure (narrow-angle) glaucoma or in patients with narrow angles, because of the possibility of producing pupillary block and increasing angle blockage.
When an intraocular inflammatory process is present, the intensity and persistence of miosis and ciliary muscle contraction that result from anticholinesterase therapy require abstention from, or cautious use of, HUMORSOL.
Systemic effects are infrequent when HUMORSOL is instilled carefully. Compression of the lacrimal duct for several seconds immediately following instillation minimizes drainage into the nasal chamber with its extensive absorption surface. Wash the hands immediately after instillation. Discontinue HUMORSOL if salivation, urinary incontinence, diarrhea, profuse sweating, muscle weakness, respiratory difficulties, shock, or cardiac irregularities occur.
Persons receiving cholinesterase inhibitors who are exposed to organophosphate-type insecticides and pesticides (gardeners, organophosphate plant or warehouse workers, farmers,

residents of communities which are undergoing insecticide spraying or dusting, etc.) should be warned of the added systemic effects possible from absorption through the respiratory tract or skin. Wearing of respiratory masks, frequent washing, and clothing changes may be advisable.
Anticholinesterase drugs should be used with extreme caution, if at all, in patients with marked vagotonia, bronchial asthma, spastic gastrointesinal disturbances, peptic ulcer, pronounced bradycardia and hypotension, recent myocardial infarction, epilepsy, parkinsonism, and other disorders that may respond adversely to vagotonic effects.
After long-term use of HUMORSOL, dilation of blood vessels and resulting greater permeability increase the possibility of hyphema during ophthalmic surgery. Therefore, this drug should be discontinued before surgery.
Despite observance of all precautions and the use of only the recommended dose, there is some evidence that repeated administration may cause depression of the concentration of cholinesterase in the serum and erythrocytes, with resultant systemic effects.

Drug Interactions
See WARNINGS regarding possible drug interactions of HUMORSOL with succinylcholine or with other anticholinesterase agents.

Carcinogenesis, Mutagenesis, Impairment of Fertility
Long-term studies in animals have not been performed to evaluate the effects of HUMORSOL on fertility or carcinogenic potential.

Pregnancy
Pregnancy Category X: See CONTRAINDICATIONS.

Nursing Mothers
It is not known whether this drug is excreted in human milk. Because of the potential for serious adverse reactions in nursing infants from HUMORSOL, a decision should be made whether to discontinue nursing or to discontinue the drug, taking into account the importance of the drug to the mother.

Pediatric Use
The occurrence of iris cysts is more frequent in children. (See ADVERSE REACTIONS and DOSAGE AND ADMINISTRATION.)
Extreme caution should be exercised in children receiving HUMORSOL who may require general anesthesia (see WARNINGS).
Since HUMORSOL is a potent cholinesterase inhibitor it should be kept out of the reach of children.

ADVERSE REACTIONS

Stinging, burning, lacrimation, lid muscle twitching, conjunctival and ciliary redness, brow ache, headache, and induced myopia with visual blurring may occur.
Activation of latent iritis or uveitis may occur.
As with all miotic therapy, retinal detachment has been reported occasionally.
Iris cysts may form, enlarge, and obscure vision. Occurrence is more frequent in children. The iris cyst usually shrinks upon discontinuance of the miotic. Rarely, the cyst may rupture or break free into the aqueous. Frequent examination for this occurrence is advised.
Lens opacities have been reported in patients on miotic therapy. Routine slit-lamp examinations, including the lens, should accompany prolonged use.
Paradoxical increase in intraocular pressure may follow anticholinesterase instillation. This may be alleviated by pupil-dilating medication.
Prolonged use may cause conjunctival thickening and obstruction of nasolacrimal canals.
Systemic effects, which occur rarely, are suggestive of increased cholinergic activity. Such effects may include nausea, vomiting, abdominal cramps, diarrhea, urinary incontinence, salivation, sweating, difficulty in breathing, bradycardia, or cardiac irregularities. Medical management of systemic effects may be indicated (see TREATMENT OF ADVERSE EFFECTS).

TREATMENT OF ADVERSE EFFECTS

If HUMORSOL is taken systemically by accident, or if systemic effects occur after topical application in the eye or from accidental skin contact, administer atropine sulfate parenterally (intravenously if necessary) in a dose (for adults) of 0.4 to 0.6 mg or more. The recommended dosage of atropine in infants and children up to 12 years of age is 0.01 mg/kg repeated every two hours as needed until the desired effect is obtained, or adverse effects of atropine preclude further usage. The maximum single dose should not exceed 0.4 mg.
The use of much larger doses of atropine in treating anticholinesterase intoxication in adults has been reported in the literature. Initially 2 to 6 mg may be given followed by 2 mg every hour or more often, as long as muscarinic effects continue. The greater possibility of atropinization with large doses, particularly in sensitive individuals, should be borne in mind.

Pralidoxime* chloride has been reported to be useful in treating systemic effects due to cholinesterase inhibitors. However, its use is recommended in addition to and not as substitute for atropine.

A short-acting barbiturate is indicated if convulsions occur that are not entirely relieved by atropine. Barbiturate dosage should be carefully adjusted to avoid central respiratory depression. Marked weakness or paralysis of muscles of respiration should be treated promptly by artificial respiration and maintenance of a clear airway.

The oral LD_{50} of HUMORSOL is 2.96 mg/kg in the mouse.

---

*PROTOPAM® Chloride (Pralidoxime Chloride). Ayerst Laboratories

DOSAGE AND ADMINISTRATION

HUMORSOL *is intended solely for topical use in the conjunctival sac.*

As HUMORSOL is an extremely potent drug, the physician should thoroughly familiarize himself with its use and the technic of instillation.

The required dose is applied in the conjunctival sac, with the patient supine, care being taken not to touch the cornea with the tip of the OCUMETER** ophthalmic dispenser. *The patient or person administering the medication should apply continuous gentle pressure on the lacrimal duct with the index finger for several seconds immediately following instillation of the drops. This is to prevent drainage overflow of solution into the nasal and pharyngeal spaces, which might cause systemic absorption. Wash the hands immediately after administration.*

HUMORSOL *should not be used more often than directed. Caution is necessary to avoid overdosage.*

Initial titration and dosage adjustments with HUMORSOL must be individualized to obtain maximal therapeutic effect. The patient must be closely observed during the initial period. If the response is not adequate within the first 24 hours, other measures should be considered.

Keep frequency of use to a minimum in all patients, but especially in children, to reduce the chance of iris cyst development (see ADVERSE REACTIONS).

Glaucoma

For initial therapy with HUMORSOL (0.125 percent or 0.25 percent) place 1 drop (children) or 1 or 2 drops (adults) in the glaucomatous eye. A decrease in intraocular pressure should occur within a few hours. During this period, keep the patient under supervision and make tonometric examinations at least hourly for 3 or 4 hours to be sure that no immediate rise in pressure occurs (see ADVERSE REACTIONS).

Duration of effect varies with the individual. The usual dosage can vary from as much as 1 or 2 drops twice a day to as little as 1 or 2 drops twice a week. The 0.125 percent strength used twice a day usually results in smooth control of the physiologic diurnal variation in intraocular pressure. This is probably the preferred dosage for most wide (open) angle glaucoma patients.

Strabismus

Essentially equal visual acuity of both eyes is a prerequisite to the successful treatment of esotropia with HUMORSOL. For initial evaluation it may be used as a diagnostic aid to determine if an accommodative factor exists. This is especially useful preoperatively in young children and in patients with normal hypermetropic refractive errors. One drop is given daily for 2 weeks, then 1 drop every 2 days for 2 to 3 weeks. If the eyes become straighter, an accommodative factor is demonstrated. This technic may supplement or complement standard testing with atropine and trial with glasses for the accommodative factor.

In esotropia uncomplicated by amblyopia or anisometropia, HUMORSOL may be instilled in both eyes, *not more than 1 drop at a time every day for 2 to 3 weeks,* as too severe a degree of miosis may interfere with vision. Then reduce the dosage to 1 drop every other day for 3 to 4 weeks and reevaluate the patient's status.

HUMORSOL may be continued in a dosage of 1 drop every 2 days to 1 drop twice a week. (The latter dosage may be maintained for several months.) Evaluate the patient's condition every 4 to 12 weeks. If improvement continues, change the schedule to 1 drop once a week and eventually to a trial without medication. However, if after 4 months, control of the condition still requires 1 drop every 2 days, therapy with HUMORSOL should be stopped.

**Registered trademark of MERCK & CO., INC.

HOW SUPPLIED

Sterile Ophthalmic Solution HUMORSOL is a clear, colorless, aqueous solution and is supplied in a 5 mL white, opaque, plastic OCUMETER ophthalmic dispenser with a controlled-drop tip:

No. 3255—0.125 percent solution.
  NDC 0006-3255-03.
No. 3267—0.25 percent solution.
  NDC 0006-3267-03.

Storage

Protect from freezing and excessive heat.
  A.H.F.S. Category: 52:20
  DC 7414311 Issued October 1987

HYDELTRASOL® Injection, Sterile ℞
(Prednisolone Sodium Phosphate), U.S.P.

DESCRIPTION

Prednisolone sodium phosphate, a synthetic adrenocortical steroid, is a white or slightly yellow powder that is slightly hygroscopic and is freely soluble in water. The molecular weight is 484.39. It is designated chemically as $11\beta,17$-dihydroxy-21-(phosphonooxy)pregna-1,4-diene-3,20-dione disodium salt. The empirical formula is $C_{21}H_{27}Na_2O_8P$ and the structural formula is:

HYDELTRASOL* (Prednisolone Sodium Phosphate) injection is a sterile solution (pH 7.0 to 8.0) sealed under nitrogen, for intravenous, intramuscular, intra-articular, intralesional, and soft tissue administration.

Each milliliter contains prednisolone sodium phosphate equivalent to 20 mg prednisolone phosphate. Inactive ingredients per mL: niacinamide, 25 mg; sodium hydroxide to adjust pH; disodium edetate, 0.5 mg; Water for Injection, q.s. 1 mL. Sodium bisulfite, 1 mg, and phenol, 5 mg, added as preservatives.

* Registered trademark of MERCK & CO., INC.

ACTIONS

HYDELTRASOL injection has a rapid onset but short duration of action when compared with less soluble preparations. Because of this, it is suitable for the treatment of acute disorders responsive to adrenocortical steroid therapy.

Naturally occurring glucocorticoids (hydrocortisone and cortisone), which also have salt-retaining properties, are used as replacement therapy in adrenocortical deficiency states. Their synthetic analogs, including prednisolone, are primarily used for their potent anti-inflammatory effects in disorders of many organ systems.

Glucocorticoids cause profound and varied metabolic effects. In addition, they modify the body's immune responses to diverse stimuli.

At equipotent anti-inflammatory doses, prednisolone has less tendency to cause salt and water retention than either hydrocortisone or cortisone.

INDICATIONS

A. By intravenous or intramuscular injection when oral therapy is not feasible:
1. *Endocrine disorders*
  Primary or secondary adrenocortical insufficiency (hydrocortisone or cortisone is the drug of choice; synthetic analogs may be used in conjunction with mineralocorticoids where applicable; in infancy, mineralocorticoid supplementation is of particular importance)
  Acute adrenocortical insufficiency (hydrocortisone or cortisone is the drug of choice; mineralocorticoid supplementation may be necessary, particularly when synthetic analogs are used)
  Preoperatively, and in the event of serious trauma or illness, in patients with known adrenal insufficiency or when adrenocortical reserve is doubtful
    Congenital adrenal hyperplasia
    Nonsuppurative thyroiditis
    Hypercalcemia associated with cancer
2. *Rheumatic disorders*
  As adjunctive therapy for short-term administration (to tide the patient over an acute episode or exacerbation) in:
    Post-traumatic osteoarthritis
    Synovitis of osteoarthritis
    Rheumatoid arthritis, including juvenile rheumatoid arthritis (selected cases may require low-dose maintenance therapy)

    Acute and subacute bursitis
    Epicondylitis
    Acute nonspecific tenosynovitis
    Acute gouty arthritis
    Psoriatic arthritis
    Ankylosing spondylitis
3. *Collagen diseases*
  During an exacerbation or as maintenance therapy in selected cases of:
    Systemic lupus erythematosus
    Acute rheumatic carditis
    Systemic dermatomyositis (polymyositis)
4. *Dermatologic diseases*
    Pemphigus
    Severe erythema multiforme (Stevens-Johnson syndrome)
    Exfoliative dermatitis
    Bullous dermatitis herpetiformis
    Severe seborrheic dermatitis
    Severe psoriasis
    Mycosis fungoides
5. *Allergic states*
  Control of severe or incapacitating allergic conditions intractable to adequate trials of conventional treatment in:
    Bronchial asthma
    Contact dermatitis
    Atopic dermatitis
    Serum sickness
    Seasonal or perennial allergic rhinitis
    Drug hypersensitivity reactions
    Urticarial transfusion reactions
    Acute noninfectious laryngeal edema (epinephrine is the drug of first choice)
6. *Ophthalmic diseases*
  Severe acute and chronic allergic and inflammatory processes involving the eye, such as:
    Herpes zoster ophthalmicus
    Iritis, iridocyclitis
    Chorioretinitis
    Diffuse posterior uveitis and choroiditis
    Optic neuritis
    Sympathetic ophthalmia
    Anterior segment inflammation
    Allergic conjunctivitis
    Keratitis
    Allergic corneal marginal ulcers
7. *Gastrointestinal diseases*
  To tide the patient over a critical period of the disease in:
    Ulcerative colitis (Systemic therapy)
    Regional enteritis (Systemic therapy)
8. *Respiratory diseases*
    Symptomatic sarcoidosis
    Berylliosis
  Fulminating or disseminated pulmonary tuberculosis when used concurrently with appropriate antituberculous chemotherapy
    Loeffler's syndrome not manageable by other means
    Aspiration pneumonitis
9. *Hematologic disorders*
    Acquired (autoimmune) hemolytic anemia
    Idiopathic thrombocytopenic purpura in adults (I.V. only; I.M. administration is contraindicated)
    Secondary thrombocytopenia in adults
    Erythroblastopenia (RBC anemia)
    Congenital (erythroid) hypoplastic anemia
10. *Neoplastic diseases*
  For palliative management of:
    Leukemias and lymphomas in adults
    Acute leukemia of childhood
11. *Edematous states*
  To induce diuresis or remission of proteinuria in the nephrotic syndrome, without uremia, of the idiopathic type, or that due to lupus erythematosus
12. *Miscellaneous*
    Tuberculous meningitis with subarachnoid block or impending block when used concurrently with appropriate antituberculous chemotherapy
    Trichinosis with neurologic or myocardial involvement.
B. By intra-articular or soft tissue injection:
  As adjunctive therapy for short-term administration (to tide the patient over an acute episode or exacerbation) in:
    Synovitis of osteoarthritis
    Rheumatoid arthritis
    Acute and subacute bursitis
    Acute gouty arthritis
    Epicondylitis
    Acute nonspecific tenosynovitis
    Post-traumatic osteoarthritis.

Continued on next page

Information on the Merck & Co. products listed on these pages is the full prescribing information from product circulars in use October 1, 1992.

Merck & Co.—Cont.

C. By intralesional injection:
Keloids
Localized hypertrophic, infiltrated, inflammatory lesions of: lichen planus, psoriatic plaques, granuloma annulare, and lichen simplex chronicus (neurodermatitis)
Discoid lupus erythematosus
Necrobiosis lipoidica diabeticorum
Alopecia areata
May also be useful in cystic tumors of an aponeurosis or tendon (ganglia).

CONTRAINDICATIONS

Systemic fungal infections (see WARNINGS regarding amphotericin B)
Hypersensitivity to any component of this product, including sulfites (see WARNINGS).

WARNINGS

Because rare instances of anaphylactoid reactions have occurred in patients receiving parenteral corticosteroid therapy, appropriate precautionary measures should be taken prior to administration, especially when the patient has a history of allergy to any drug. Anaphylactoid and hypersensitivity reactions have been reported for Injection HYDELTRASOL (see ADVERSE REACTIONS).
Injection HYDELTRASOL contains sodium bisulfite, a sulfite that may cause allergic-type reactions including anaphylactic symptoms and life-threatening or less severe asthmatic episodes in certain susceptible people. The overall prevalence of sulfite sensitivity in the general population is unknown and probably low. Sulfite sensitivity is seen more frequently in asthmatic than in nonasthmatic people.
Corticosteroids may exacerbate systemic fungal infections and therefore should not be used in the presence of such infections unless they are needed to control drug reactions due to amphotericin B. Moreover, there have been cases reported in which concomitant use of amphotericin B and hydrocortisone was followed by cardiac enlargement and congestive failure.
In patients on corticosteroid therapy subjected to any unusual stress, increased dosage of rapidly acting corticosteroids before, during, and after the stressful situation is indicated.
Drug-induced secondary adrenocortical insufficiency may result from too rapid withdrawal of corticosteroids and may be minimized by gradual reduction of dosage. This type of relative insufficiency may persist for months after discontinuation of therapy; therefore, in any situation of stress occurring during that period, hormone therapy should be reinstituted. If the patient is receiving steroids already, dosage may have to be increased. Since mineralocorticoid secretion may be impaired, salt and/or a mineralocorticoid should be administered concurrently.
Corticosteroids may mask some signs of infection, and new infections may appear during their use. There may be decreased resistance and inability to localize infection when corticosteroids are used. Moreover, corticosteroids may affect the nitroblue-tetrazolium test for bacterial infection and produce false negative results.
In cerebral malaria, a double-blind trial has shown that the use of corticosteroids is associated with prolongation of coma and a higher incidence of pneumonia and gastrointestinal bleeding.
Corticosteroids may activate latent amebiasis. Therefore, it is recommended that latent or active amebiasis be ruled out before initiating corticosteroid therapy in any patient who has spent time in the tropics or any patient with unexplained diarrhea.
Prolonged use of corticosteroids may produce posterior subcapsular cataracts, glaucoma with possible damage to the optic nerves, and may enhance the establishment of secondary ocular infections due to fungi or viruses.
Usage in pregnancy. Since adequate human reproduction studies have not been done with corticosteroids, use of these drugs in pregnancy or in women of childbearing potential requires that the anticipated benefits be weighed against the possible hazards to the mother and embryo or fetus. Infants born of mothers who have received substantial doses of corticosteroids during pregnancy should be carefully observed for signs of hypoadrenalism.
Corticosteroids appear in breast milk and could suppress growth, interfere with endogenous corticosteroid production, or cause other unwanted effects. Mothers taking pharmacologic doses of corticosteroids should be advised not to nurse.
Average and large doses of cortisone or hydrocortisone can cause elevation of blood pressure, salt and water retention, and increased excretion of potassium. These effects are less likely to occur with the synthetic derivatives except when used in large doses. Dietary salt restriction and potassium supplementation may be necessary. All corticosteroids increase calcium excretion.
Administration of live virus vaccines, including smallpox, is contraindicated in individuals receiving immunosuppressive doses of corticosteroids. If inactivated viral or bacterial vaccines are administered to individuals receiving immunosuppressive doses of corticosteroids, the expected serum antibody response may not be obtained. However, immunization procedures may be undertaken in patients who are receiving corticosteroids as replacement therapy, e.g., for Addison's disease.
The use of HYDELTRASOL injection in active tuberculosis should be restricted to those cases of fulminating or disseminated tuberculosis in which the corticosteroid is used for the management of the disease in conjunction with appropriate antituberculous regimen.
If corticosteroids are indicated in patients with latent tuberculosis or tuberculin reactivity, close observation is necessary as reactivation of the disease may occur. During prolonged corticosteroid therapy, these patients should receive chemoprophylaxis.
Literature reports suggest an apparent association between use of corticosteroids and left ventricular free wall rupture after a recent myocardial infarction; therefore, therapy with corticosteroids should be used with great caution in these patients.

PRECAUTIONS

This product, like many other steroid formulations, is sensitive to heat. Therefore, it should not be autoclaved when it is desirable to sterilize the exterior of the vial.
Following prolonged therapy, withdrawal of corticosteroids may result in symptoms of the corticosteroid withdrawal syndrome including fever, myalgia, arthralgia, and malaise. This may occur in patients even without evidence of adrenal insufficiency.
There is an enhanced effect of corticosteroids in patients with hypothyroidism and in those with cirrhosis.
Corticosteroids should be used cautiously in patients with ocular herpes simplex for fear of corneal perforation.
The lowest possible dose of corticosteroid should be used to control the condition under treatment, and when reduction in dosage is possible, the reduction must be gradual.
Psychic derangements may appear when corticosteroids are used, ranging from euphoria, insomnia, mood swings, personality changes, and severe depression to frank psychotic manifestations. Also, existing emotional instability or psychotic tendencies may be aggravated by corticosteroids.
Aspirin should be used cautiously in conjunction with corticosteroids in hypoprothrombinemia.
Steroids should be used with caution in nonspecific ulcerative colitis, if there is a probability of impending perforation, abscess, or other pyogenic infection, also in diverticulitis, fresh intestinal anastomoses, active or latent peptic ulcer, renal insufficiency, hypertension, osteoporosis, and myasthenia gravis. Signs of peritoneal irritation following gastrointestinal perforation in patients receiving large doses of corticosteroids may be minimal or absent. Fat embolism has been reported as a possible complication of hypercortisonism.
When large doses are given, some authorities advise that antacids be administered between meals to help to prevent peptic ulcer.
Growth and development of infants and children on prolonged corticosteroid therapy should be carefully followed.
Steroids may increase or decrease motility and number of spermatozoa in some patients.
Phenytoin, phenobarbital, ephedrine, and rifampin may enhance the metabolic clearance of corticosteroids, resulting in decreased blood levels and lessened physiologic activity, thus requiring adjustment in corticosteroid dosage.
The prothrombin time should be checked frequently in patients who are receiving corticosteroids and coumarin anticoagulants at the same time because of reports that corticosteroids have altered the response to these anticoagulants. Studies have shown that the usual effect produced by adding corticosteroids is inhibition of response to coumarins, although there have been some conflicting reports of potentiation not substantiated by studies.
When corticosteroids are administered concomitantly with potassium-depleting diuretics, patients should be observed closely for development of hypokalemia.
Intra-articular injection of a corticosteroid may produce systemic as well as local effects.
Appropriate examination of any joint fluid present is necessary to exclude a septic process.
A marked increase in pain accompanied by local swelling, further restriction of joint motion, fever, and malaise is suggestive of septic arthritis. If this complication occurs and the diagnosis of sepsis is confirmed, appropriate antimicrobial therapy should be instituted.
Injection of a steroid into an infected site is to be avoided.
Corticosteroids should not be injected into unstable joints.
Patients should be impressed strongly with the importance of not overusing joints in which symptomatic benefit has been obtained as long as the inflammatory process remains active.
Frequent intra-articular injection may result in damage to joint tissues.
The slower rate of absorption by intramuscular administration should be recognized.

ADVERSE REACTIONS

Fluid and electrolyte disturbances
Sodium retention
Fluid retention
Congestive heart failure in susceptible patients
Potassium loss
Hypokalemic alkalosis
Hypertension
Musculoskeletal
Muscle weakness
Steroid myopathy
Loss of muscle mass
Osteoporosis
Vertebral compression fractures
Aseptic necrosis of femoral and humeral heads
Pathologic fracture of long bones
Tendon rupture
Gastrointestinal
Peptic ulcer with possible subsequent perforation and hemorrhage
Perforation of the small and large bowel, particularly in patients with inflammatory bowel disease
Pancreatitis
Abdominal distention
Ulcerative esophagitis
Dermatologic
Impaired wound healing
Thin fragile skin
Petechiae and ecchymoses
Erythema
Increased sweating
May suppress reactions to skin tests
Burning or tingling, especially in the perineal area (after I.V. injection)
Other cutaneous reactions, such as allergic dermatitis, urticaria, angioneurotic edema
Neurologic
Convulsions
Increased intracranial pressure with papilledema (pseudotumor cerebri) usually after treatment
Vertigo
Headache
Psychic disturbances
Endocrine
Menstrual irregularities
Development of cushingoid state
Suppression of growth in children
Secondary adrenocortical and pituitary unresponsiveness, particularly in times of stress, as in trauma, surgery, or illness
Decreased carbohydrate tolerance
Manifestations of latent diabetes mellitus
Increased requirements for insulin or oral hypoglycemic agents in diabetics
Hirsutism
Ophthalmic
Posterior subcapsular cataracts
Increased intraocular pressure
Glaucoma
Exophthalmos
Metabolic
Negative nitrogen balance due to protein catabolism
Cardiovascular
Myocardial rupture following recent myocardial infarction (see WARNINGS).
Other
Anaphylactoid or hypersensitivity reactions
Thromboembolism
Weight gain
Increased appetite
Nausea
Malaise
The following *additional* adverse reactions are related to parenteral corticosteroid therapy:
Rare instances of blindness associated with intralesional therapy around the face and head
Hyperpigmentation or hypopigmentation
Subcutaneous and cutaneous atrophy
Sterile abscess
Postinjection flare (following intra-articular use)
Charcot-like arthropathy.

Site of Injection	Amount of Injection (mL)	Amount of Prednisolone Phosphate (mg)
	Doses	
Large Joints (e.g., Knee)	0.5 to 1	10 to 20
Small Joints (e.g., Interphalangeal, Temporomandibular)	0.2 to 0.25	4 to 5
Bursae	0.5 to 0.75	10 to 15
Tendon Sheaths	0.1 to 0.25	2 to 5
Soft Tissue Infiltration	0.5 to 1.5	10 to 30
Ganglia	0.25 to 0.5	5 to 10

OVERDOSAGE

Reports of acute toxicity and/or death following overdosage of glucocorticoids are rare. In the event of overdosage, no specific antidote is available; treatment is supportive and symptomatic.
The intraperitoneal LD_{50} of prednisolone phosphate disodium in female mice was 1190 mg/kg.

DOSAGE AND ADMINISTRATION

For intravenous, intramuscular, intra-articular, intralesional, and soft tissue injection.
DOSAGE REQUIREMENTS ARE VARIABLE AND MUST BE INDIVIDUALIZED ON THE BASIS OF THE DISEASE AND THE RESPONSE OF THE PATIENT.

Intravenous and Intramuscular Injection

HYDELTRASOL injection can be given directly from the vial, or it can be added to Sodium Chloride Injection or Dextrose Injection and given by intravenous drip.
Benzyl alcohol as a preservative has been associated with toxicity in premature infants. Solutions used for intravenous administration or further dilution of this product should be preservative-free when used in the neonate, especially the premature infant.
When it is mixed with an infusion solution, sterile precautions should be observed. Since infusion solutions generally do not contain preservatives, mixtures should be used within 24 hours.
The initial dosage varies from 4 to 60 mg a day depending on the disease being treated. In less severe diseases doses lower than 4 mg may suffice, while in severe diseases doses higher than 60 mg may be required. Usually the daily parenteral dose of HYDELTRASOL injection is the same as the daily oral dose of prednisolone and the dosage interval is every 4 to 8 hours.
The initial dosage should be maintained or adjusted until the patient's response is satisfactory. If a satisfactory clinical response does not occur after a reasonable period of time, discontinue HYDELTRASOL injection and transfer the patient to other therapy.
After a favorable initial response, the proper maintenance dosage should be determined by decreasing the initial dosage in small amounts to the lowest dosage that maintains an adequate clinical response.
Patients should be observed closely for signs that might require dosage adjustment, including changes in clinical status resulting from remissions or exacerbations of the disease, individual drug responsiveness, and the effect of stress (e.g., surgery, infection, trauma). During stress it may be necessary to increase dosage temporarily.
If the drug is to be stopped after more than a few days of treatment, it usually should be withdrawn gradually.

Intra-articular, Intralesional, and Soft Tissue Injection

Intra-articular, intralesional, and soft tissue injections are generally employed when the affected joints or areas are limited to one or two sites. Dosage and frequency of injection vary depending on the condition being treated and the site of injection. The usual dose is from 2 to 30 mg. The frequency usually ranges from once every three to five days to once every two to three weeks. Frequent intra-articular injection may result in damage to joint tissues.
Some of the usual single doses are:
[See table above.]
HYDELTRASOL injection is particularly recommended for use in conjunction with one of the less soluble, longer-acting steroids, such as HYDELTRA-T.B.A.® (Prednisolone Tebutate, MSD) suspension or HYDROCORTONE® Acetate (Hydrocortisone Acetate, MSD) sterile suspension, available for intra-articular and soft tissue injection.

HOW SUPPLIED

No. 7577X—Injection HYDELTRASOL, 20 mg prednisolone phosphate equivalent per mL, is a clear, colorless to slightly yellow solution, and is supplied as follows:
NDC 0006-7577-02 in 2 mL vials
NDC 0006-7577-03 in 5 mL vials
(6505-00-890-1496 20 mg/mL 5 mL vial).
Storage
Sensitive to heat. Do not autoclave.
Protect from light. Store container in carton until contents have been used.

A.H.F.S. Category: 68:04
DC 7407226 Issued March 1988

HYDELTRA-T.B.A.® Sterile Suspension (Prednisolone Tebutate), U.S.P. ℞

For intra-articular, intralesional, and soft tissue injection only.

NOT FOR INTRAVENOUS USE

DESCRIPTION

Prednisolone tebutate, a synthetic adrenocortical steroid, is a white to slightly yellow powder sparingly soluble in alcohol, freely soluble in chloroform, and very slightly soluble in water. The molecular weight is 476.61 (monohydrate). It is designated chemically as 11β,17-dihydroxy-21-[(3,3-dimethyl-1-oxobutyl)oxy]pregna-1,4-diene-3,20-dione. The empirical formula is $C_{27}H_{38}O_6$ and the structural formula is:

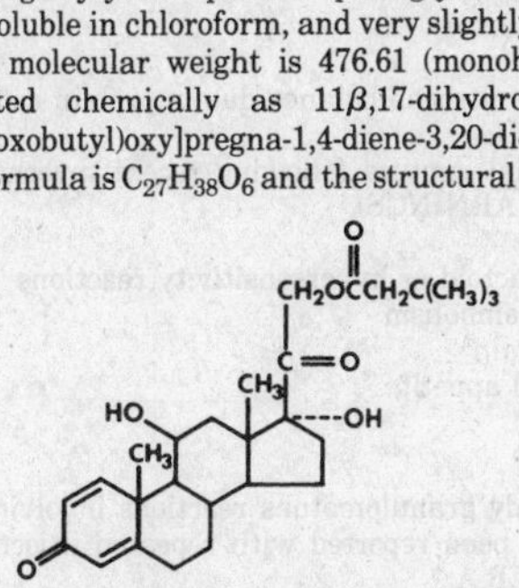

HYDELTRA-T.B.A.* (Prednisolone Tebutate) sterile suspension is a white to slightly yellow suspension (pH 6.0 to 8.0) that settles upon standing. Each mL contains prednisolone tebutate, 20 mg. Inactive ingredients per mL: sodium citrate, 1 mg; polysorbate 80, 1 mg; sorbitol solution, 0.5 mL (equal to 450 mg d-sorbitol); Water for Injection, q.s., 1 mL. Benzyl alcohol, 9 mg, added as preservative.

*Registered trademark of MERCK & CO., INC.

ACTIONS

HYDELTRA-T.B.A. has a slow onset but long duration of action when compared with more soluble preparations. Because of its slight solubility, it is suitable for intra-articular, intralesional, and soft tissue injection where its anti-inflammatory effects are confined mainly to the area in which it has been injected, although it is capable of producing systemic hormonal effects.
Naturally occurring glucocorticoids (hydrocortisone and cortisone), which also have salt-retaining properties, are used as replacement therapy in adrenocortical deficiency states. Their synthetic analogs, including prednisolone, are primarily used for their potent anti-inflammatory effects in disorders of many organ systems.
Glucocorticoids cause profound and varied metabolic effects. In addition, they modify the body's immune responses to diverse stimuli.

INDICATIONS

A. By intra-articular or soft tissue injection:
As adjunctive therapy for short-term administration (to tide the patient over an acute episode or exacerbation) in:
- Synovitis of osteoarthritis
- Rheumatoid arthritis
- Acute and subacute bursitis
- Acute gouty arthritis
- Epicondylitis
- Acute nonspecific tenosynovitis
- Post-traumatic osteoarthritis

B. By intralesional injection:
May be useful in cystic tumors of an aponeurosis or tendon (ganglia).

CONTRAINDICATIONS

Systemic fungal infections
Hypersensitivity to any component of this product

WARNINGS

Because rare instances of anaphylactoid reactions have occurred in patients receiving parenteral corticosteroid therapy, appropriate precautionary measures should be taken prior to administration, especially when the patient has a history of allergy to any drug. Anaphylactoid and hypersensitivity reactions have been reported for Sterile Suspension HYDELTRA-T.B.A. (see ADVERSE REACTIONS).
In patients on corticosteroid therapy subjected to any unusual stress, increased dosage of rapidly acting corticosteroids before, during, and after the stressful situation is indicated.
Drug-induced secondary adrenocortical insufficiency may result from too rapid withdrawal of corticosteroids and may be minimized by gradual reduction of dosage. This type of relative insufficiency may persist for months after discontinuation of therapy; therefore, in any situation of stress occurring during that period, hormone therapy should be reinstituted. If the patient is receiving steroids already, dosage may have to be increased. Since mineralocorticoid secretion may be impaired, salt and/or a mineralocorticoid should be administered concurrently.
Corticosteroids may mask some signs of infection, and new infections may appear during their use. There may be decreased resistance and inability to localize infection when corticosteroids are used. Moreover, corticosteroids may affect the nitroblue-tetrazolium test for bacterial infection and produce false negative results.
In cerebral malaria, a double-blind trial has shown that the use of corticosteroids is associated with prolongation of coma and a higher incidence of pneumonia and gastrointestinal bleeding.
Corticosteroids may activate latent amebiasis. Therefore, it is recommended that latent or active amebiasis be ruled out before initiating corticosteroid therapy in any patient who has spent time in the tropics or any patient with unexplained diarrhea.
Prolonged use of corticosteroids may produce posterior subcapsular cataracts, glaucoma with possible damage to the optic nerves, and may enhance the establishment of secondary ocular infections due to fungi or viruses.
Usage in pregnancy. Since adequate human reproduction studies have not been done with corticosteroids, use of these drugs in pregnancy or in women of childbearing potential requires that the anticipated benefits be weighed against the possible hazards to the mother and embryo or fetus. Infants born of mothers who have received substantial doses of corticosteroids during pregnancy should be carefully observed for signs of hypoadrenalism.
Corticosteroids appear in breast milk and could suppress growth, interfere with endogenous corticosteroid production, or cause other unwanted effects. Mothers taking pharmacologic doses of corticosteroids should be advised not to nurse.
Average and large doses of cortisone or hydrocortisone can cause elevation of blood pressure, salt and water retention, and increased excretion of potassium. These effects are less

Continued on next page

Information on the Merck & Co. products listed on these pages is the full prescribing information from product circulars in use October 1, 1992.

Merck & Co.—Cont.

likely to occur with the synthetic derivatives except when used in large doses. Dietary salt restriction and potassium supplementation may be necessary. All corticosteroids increase calcium excretion.

Administration of live virus vaccines, including smallpox, is contraindicated in individuals receiving immunosuppressive doses of corticosteroids. If inactivated viral or bacterial vaccines are administered to individuals receiving immunosuppressive doses of corticosteroids, the expected serum antibody response may not be obtained.

If corticosteroids are indicated in patients with latent tuberculosis or tuberculin reactivity, close observation is necessary as reactivation of the disease may occur. During prolonged corticosteroid therapy, these patients should receive chemoprophylaxis.

Literature reports suggest an apparent association between use of corticosteroids and left ventricular free wall rupture after a recent myocardial infarction; therefore, therapy with corticosteroids should be used with great caution in these patients.

PRECAUTIONS

This product, like many other steroid formulations, is sensitive to heat. Therefore, it should not be autoclaved when it is desirable to sterilize the exterior of the vial.

Following prolonged therapy, withdrawal of corticosteroids may result in symptoms of the corticosteroid withdrawal syndrome including fever, myalgia, arthralgia, and malaise. This may occur in patients even without evidence of adrenal insufficiency.

There is an enhanced effect of corticosteroids in patients with hypothyroidism and in those with cirrhosis.

Corticosteroids should be used cautiously in patients with ocular herpes simplex for fear of corneal perforation.

Psychic derangements may appear when corticosteroids are used, ranging from euphoria, insomnia, mood swings, personality changes, and severe depression to frank psychotic manifestations. Also, existing emotional instability or psychotic tendencies may be aggravated by corticosteroids.

Aspirin should be used cautiously in conjunction with corticosteroids in hypoprothrombinemia.

Steroids should be used with caution in nonspecific ulcerative colitis, if there is a probability of impending perforation, abscess, or other pyogenic infection, also in diverticulitis, fresh intestinal anastomoses, active or latent peptic ulcer, renal insufficiency, hypertension, osteoporosis, and myasthenia gravis. Signs of peritoneal irritation following gastrointestinal perforation in patients receiving large doses of corticosteroids may be minimal or absent. Fat embolism has been reported as a possible complication of hypercortisonism.

When large doses are given, some authorities advise that antacids be administered between meals to help to prevent peptic ulcer.

Growth and development of infants and children on prolonged corticosteroid therapy should be carefully followed. Steroids may increase or decrease motility and number of spermatozoa in some patients.

Phenytoin, phenobarbital, ephedrine, and rifampin may enhance the metabolic clearance of corticosteroids, resulting in decreased blood levels and lessened physiologic activity, thus requiring adjustment in corticosteroid dosage.

The prothrombin time should be checked frequently in patients who are receiving corticosteroids and coumarin anticoagulants at the same time because of reports that corticosteroids have altered the response to these anticoagulants. Studies have shown that the usual effect produced by adding corticosteroids is inhibition of response to coumarins, although there have been some conflicting reports of potentiation not substantiated by studies.

When corticosteroids are administered concomitantly with potassium-depleting diuretics, patients should be observed closely for development of hypokalemia.

Intra-articular injection of a corticosteroid may produce systemic as well as local effects.

Appropriate examination of any joint fluid present is necessary to exclude a septic process.

A marked increase in pain accompanied by local swelling, further restriction of joint motion, fever, and malaise is suggestive of septic arthritis. If this complication occurs and the diagnosis of sepsis is confirmed, appropriate antimicrobial therapy should be instituted.

Injection of a steroid into an infected site is to be avoided.

Corticosteroids should not be injected into unstable joints.

Patients should be impressed strongly with the importance of not overusing joints in which symptomatic benefit has been obtained as long as the inflammatory process remains active.

Frequent intra-articular injection may result in damage to joint tissues.

ADVERSE REACTIONS

Fluid and electrolyte disturbances
  Sodium retention
  Fluid retention
  Congestive heart failure in susceptible patients
  Potassium loss
  Hypokalemic alkalosis
  Hypertension
Musculoskeletal
  Muscle weakness
  Steroid myopathy
  Loss of muscle mass
  Osteoporosis
  Vertebral compression fractures
  Aseptic necrosis of femoral and humeral heads
  Pathologic fracture of long bones
  Tendon rupture
Gastrointestinal
  Peptic ulcer with possible subsequent perforation and hemorrhage
  Perforation of the small and large bowel, particularly in patients with inflammatory bowel disease
  Pancreatitis
  Abdominal distention
  Ulcerative esophagitis
Dermatologic
  Impaired wound healing
  Thin fragile skin
  Petechiae and ecchymoses
  Erythema
  Increased sweating
  May suppress reactions to skin tests
  Other cutaneous reactions, such as allergic dermatitis, urticaria, angioneurotic edema
Neurologic
  Convulsions
  Increased intracranial pressure with papilledema (pseudotumor cerebri) usually after treatment
  Vertigo
  Headache
  Psychic disturbances
Endocrine
  Menstrual irregularities
  Development of cushingoid state
  Suppression of growth in children
  Secondary adrenocortical and pituitary unresponsiveness, particularly in times of stress, as in trauma, surgery, or illness
  Decreased carbohydrate tolerance
  Manifestations of latent diabetes mellitus
  Increased requirements for insulin or oral hypoglycemic agents in diabetics
  Hirsutism
Ophthalmic
  Posterior subcapsular cataracts
  Increased intraocular pressure
  Glaucoma
  Exophthalmos
Metabolic
  Negative nitrogen balance due to protein catabolism
Cardiovascular
  Myocardial rupture following recent myocardial infarction (see WARNINGS).
Other
  Anaphylactoid or hypersensitivity reactions
  Thromboembolism
  Weight gain
  Increased appetite
  Nausea
  Malaise

Foreign body granulomatous reactions involving the synovium have been reported with repeated injections of HYDELTRA-T.B.A.

Localized pain and swelling, sometimes distal to the site of injection and persisting for several days, have been reported. The following *additional* adverse reactions are related to injection of corticosteroids:

  Rare instances of blindness associated with intralesional therapy around the face and head
  Hyperpigmentation or hypopigmentation
  Subcutaneous and cutaneous atrophy
  Sterile abscess
  Postinjection flare (following intra-articular use)
  Charcot-like arthropathy

DOSAGE AND ADMINISTRATION

> *For intra-articular, intralesional, and soft tissue injection only.*

NOT FOR INTRAVENOUS USE

DOSAGE AND FREQUENCY OF INJECTION ARE VARIABLE AND MUST BE INDIVIDUALIZED ON THE BASIS OF THE DISEASE AND THE RESPONSE OF THE PATIENT.

The initial dose varies from 4 to 40 mg depending on the disease being treated and the size of the area to be injected. Frequency of injection depends on symptomatic response, and usually is once every two or three weeks. Severe conditions may require injection once a week. Frequent intra-articular injection may result in damage to joint tissues. If satisfactory clinical response does not occur after a reasonable period of time, discontinue HYDELTRA-T.B.A. sterile suspension and transfer the patient to other therapy.

Patients should be observed closely for signs that might require dosage adjustment, including changes in clinical status resulting from remissions or exacerbations of the disease, and individual drug responsiveness.

For rapid onset of action, a soluble adrenocortical hormone preparation, such as DECADRON* Phosphate (Dexamethasone Sodium Phosphate) injection or HYDELTRASOL* (Prednisolone Sodium Phosphate) injection, may be given with HYDELTRA-T.B.A.

If desired, a local anesthetic may be used, and may be injected before HYDELTRA-T.B.A., or mixed in a syringe with HYDELTRA-T.B.A. and given simultaneously.

If used prior to intra-articular injection of the steroid, inject most of the anesthetic into the soft tissues of the surrounding area and instill a small amount into the joint.

If given together, mixing should be done in the injection syringe by drawing the steroid in *first*, then the anesthetic. In this way, the anesthetic will not be introduced inadvertently into the vial of steroid. *The mixture must be used immediately and any unused portion discarded.*

Some of the usual single doses are:

Large Joints (e.g., Knee)	20 mg (1 mL), occasionally 30 mg (1.5 mL). Doses over 40 mg (2 mL) not recommended.
Small Joints (e.g., Interphalangeal, Temporomandibular)	8 to 10 mg (0.4 to 0.5 mL).
Bursae	20 to 30 mg (1 to 1.5 mL).
Tendon Sheaths	4 to 10 mg (0.2 to 0.5 mL).
Ganglia	10 to 20 mg (0.5 to 1 mL).

*Registered trademark of MERCK & CO., Inc.

HOW SUPPLIED

No. 7572—Sterile Suspension HYDELTRA-T.B.A., 20 mg per mL, is a white, milky suspension, and is supplied as follows:
NDC 0006-7572-01 in 1 mL vials
(6505-00-225-7499 1 mL vial)
NDC 0006-7572-03 in 5 mL vials
(6505-00-890-1353 5 mL vial).
Storage
Sensitive to heat. Do not autoclave.
Protect from freezing.
Protect from light. Store container in carton until contents have been used.

A.H.F.S. Category: 68:04
DC 7349125   Issued March 1988

HYDROCORTONE®   R
Acetate Sterile Suspension
(Hydrocortisone Acetate), U.S.P.

For intra-articular, intralesional, and soft tissue injection only.

NOT FOR INTRAVENOUS USE

DESCRIPTION

Hydrocortisone acetate, a synthetic adrenocortical steroid, is a white to practically white, odorless, crystalline powder. It is insoluble in water and slightly soluble in alcohol and chloroform. The molecular weight is 404.50. It is designated chemically as 21-(acetyloxy)-11β,17-dihydroxypregn-4-ene-3,20-dione. The empirical formula is $C_{23}H_{32}O_6$ and the structural formula is:
[See chemical structure at top of next column.]

HYDROCORTONE* Acetate (Hydrocortisone Acetate) sterile suspension is a sterile suspension of hydrocortisone acetate (pH 5.0 to 7.0) in a suitable aqueous medium. It is supplied in two strengths, one containing 25 mg hydrocortisone acetate per milliliter, the other containing 50 mg per milliliter. Inactive ingredients per mL: sodium chloride, 9 mg; polysorbate 80, 4 mg; sodium carboxymethylcellulose, 5 mg; and Water for Injection, q.s., 1 mL. Benzyl alcohol, 9 mg, added as preservative.

---

*Registered trademark of MERCK & CO., INC.

ACTIONS

HYDROCORTONE Acetate sterile suspension has a slow onset but long duration of action when compared with more soluble preparations. Because of its insolubility, it is suitable for intra-articular, intralesional, and soft tissue injection where its anti-inflammatory effects are confined mainly to the area in which it has been injected, although it is capable of producing systemic hormonal effects.

Naturally occurring glucocorticoids (hydrocortisone and cortisone), which also have salt-retaining properties, are used as replacement therapy in adrenocortical deficiency states. They are also used for their potent anti-inflammatory effect in disorders of many organ systems.

Glucocorticoids cause profound and varied metabolic effects. In addition, they modify the body's immune responses to diverse stimuli.

INDICATIONS

A. By intra-articular or soft tissue injection:
   As adjunctive therapy for short-term administration (to tide the patient over an acute episode or exacerbation) in:
   Synovitis of osteoarthritis
   Rheumatoid arthritis
   Acute and subacute bursitis
   Acute gouty arthritis
   Epicondylitis
   Acute nonspecific tenosynovitis
   Post-traumatic osteoarthritis
B. By intralesional injection:
   Keloids
   Localized hypertrophic, infiltrated, inflammatory lesions of: lichen planus, psoriatic plaques, granuloma annulare, and lichen simplex chronicus (neurodermatitis)
   Discoid lupus erythematosus
   Necrobiosis lipoidica diabeticorum
   Alopecia areata
   May also be useful in cystic tumors of an aponeurosis or tendon (ganglia).

CONTRAINDICATIONS

Systemic fungal infections
Hypersensitivity to any component of this product

WARNINGS

Because rare instances of anaphylactoid reactions have occurred in patients receiving parenteral corticosteroid therapy, appropriate precautionary measures should be taken prior to administration, especially when the patient has a history of allergy to any drug.

In patients on corticosteroid therapy subjected to any unusual stress, increased dosage of rapidly acting corticosteroids before, during, and after the stressful situation is indicated.

Drug-induced secondary adrenocortical insufficiency may result from too rapid withdrawal of corticosteroids and may be minimized by gradual reduction of dosage. This type of relative insufficiency may persist for months after discontinuation of therapy; therefore, in any situation of stress occurring during that period, hormone therapy should be reinstituted. If the patient is receiving steroids already, dosage may have to be increased. Since mineralocorticoid secretion may be impaired, salt and/or a mineralocorticoid should be administered concurrently.

Corticosteroids may mask some signs of infection, and new infections may appear during their use. There may be decreased resistance and inability to localize infection when corticosteroids are used. Moreover, corticosteroids may affect the nitroblue-tetrazolium test for bacterial infection and produce false negative results.

In cerebral malaria, a double-blind trial has shown that the use of corticosteroids is associated with prolongation of coma and a higher incidence of pneumonia and gastrointestinal bleeding.

Corticosteroids may activate latent amebiasis. Therefore, it is recommended that latent or active amebiasis be ruled out before initiating corticosteroid therapy in any patient who has spent time in the tropics or any patient with unexplained diarrhea.

Prolonged use of corticosteroids may produce posterior subcapsular cataracts, glaucoma with possible damage to the optic nerves, and may enhance the establishment of secondary ocular infections due to fungi or viruses.

Usage in pregnancy: Since adequate human reproduction studies have not been done with corticosteroids, use of these drugs in pregnancy or in women of childbearing potential requires that the anticipated benefits be weighed against the possible hazards to the mother and embryo or fetus. Infants born of mothers who have received substantial doses of corticosteroids during pregnancy should be carefully observed for signs of hypoadrenalism.

Corticosteroids appear in breast milk and could suppress growth, interfere with endogenous corticosteroid production, or cause other unwanted effects. Mothers taking pharmacologic doses of corticosteroids should be advised not to nurse.

Average and large doses of cortisone or hydrocortisone can cause elevation of blood pressure, salt and water retention, and increased excretion of potassium. These effects are less likely to occur with the synthetic derivatives except when used in large doses. Dietary salt restriction and potassium supplementation may be necessary. All corticosteroids increase calcium excretion.

Administration of live virus vaccines, including smallpox, is contraindicated in individuals receiving immunosuppressive doses of corticosteroids. If inactivated viral or bacterial vaccines are administered to individuals receiving immunosuppressive doses of corticosteroids, the expected serum antibody response may not be obtained.

If corticosteroids are indicated in patients with latent tuberculosis or tuberculin reactivity, close observation is necessary as reactivation of the disease may occur. During prolonged corticosteroid therapy, these patients should receive chemoprophylaxis.

Literature reports suggest an apparent association between use of corticosteroids and left ventricular free wall rupture after a recent myocardial infarction; therefore, therapy with corticosteroids should be used with great caution in these patients.

PRECAUTIONS

This product, like many other steroid formulations, is sensitive to heat. Therefore, it should not be autoclaved when it is desirable to sterilize the exterior of the vial.

Following prolonged therapy, withdrawal of corticosteroids may result in symptoms of the corticosteroid withdrawal syndrome including fever, myalgia, arthralgia, and malaise. This may occur in patients even without evidence of adrenal insufficiency.

There is an enhanced effect of corticosteroids in patients with hypothyroidism and in those with cirrhosis.

Corticosteroids should be used cautiously in patients with ocular herpes simplex for fear of corneal perforation.

Psychic derangements may appear when corticosteroids are used, ranging from euphoria, insomnia, mood swings, personality changes, and severe depression to frank psychotic manifestations. Also, existing emotional instability or psychotic tendencies may be aggravated by corticosteroids.

Aspirin should be used cautiously in conjunction with corticosteroids in hypoprothrombinemia.

Steroids should be used with caution in nonspecific ulcerative colitis, if there is a probability of impending perforation, abscess, or other pyogenic infection, also in diverticulitis, fresh intestinal anastomoses, active or latent peptic ulcer, renal insufficiency, hypertension, osteoporosis, and myasthenia gravis. Signs of peritoneal irritation following gastrointestinal perforation in patients receiving large doses of corticosteroids may be minimal or absent. Fat embolism has been reported as a possible complication of hypercortisonism.

When large doses are given, some authorities advise that antacids be administered between meals to help to prevent peptic ulcer.

Growth and development of infants and children on prolonged corticosteroid therapy should be carefully followed. Steroids may increase or decrease motility and number of spermatozoa in some patients.

Phenytoin, phenobarbital, ephedrine, and rifampin may enhance the metabolic clearance of corticosteroids resulting in decreased blood levels and lessened physiologic activity, thus requiring adjustment in corticosteroid dosage.

The prothrombin time should be checked frequently in patients who are receiving corticosteroids and coumarin anticoagulants at the same time because of reports that corticosteroids have altered the response to these anticoagulants. Studies have shown that the usual effect produced by adding corticosteroids is inhibition of response to coumarins, although there have been some conflicting reports of potentiation not substantiated by studies.

When corticosteroids are administered concomitantly with potassium-depleting diuretics, patients should be observed closely for development of hypokalemia.

Intra-articular injection of a corticosteroid may produce systemic as well as local effects.

Appropriate examination of any joint fluid present is necessary to exclude a septic process.

A marked increase in pain accompanied by local swelling, further restriction of joint motion, fever, and malaise is suggestive of septic arthritis. If this complication occurs and the diagnosis of sepsis is confirmed, appropriate antimicrobial therapy should be instituted.

Injection of a steroid into an infected site is to be avoided. Corticosteroids should not be injected into unstable joints. Patients should be impressed strongly with the importance of not overusing joints in which symptomatic benefit has been obtained as long as the inflammatory process remains active.

Frequent intra-articular injection may result in damage to joint tissues.

ADVERSE REACTIONS

Fluid and electrolyte disturbances
   Sodium retention
   Fluid retention
   Congestive heart failure in susceptible patients
   Potassium loss
   Hypokalemic alkalosis
   Hypertension
Musculoskeletal
   Muscle weakness
   Steroid myopathy
   Loss of muscle mass
   Osteoporosis
   Vertebral compression fractures
   Aseptic necrosis of femoral and humeral heads
   Pathologic fracture of long bones
   Tendon rupture
Gastrointestinal
   Peptic ulcer with possible subsequent perforation and hemorrhage
   Perforation of the small and large bowel, particularly in patients with inflammatory bowel disease
   Pancreatitis
   Abdominal distention
   Ulcerative esophagitis
Dermatologic
   Impaired wound healing
   Thin fragile skin
   Petechiae and ecchymoses
   Erythema
   Increased sweating
   May suppress reactions to skin tests
   Other cutaneous reactions, such as allergic dermatitis, urticaria, angioneurotic edema
Neurologic
   Convulsions
   Increased intracranial pressure with papilledema (pseudotumor cerebri) usually after treatment
   Vertigo
   Headache
   Psychic disturbances
Endocrine
   Menstrual irregularities
   Development of cushingoid state
   Suppression of growth in children
   Secondary adrenocortical and pituitary unresponsiveness, particularly in times of stress, as in trauma, surgery, or illness
   Decreased carbohydrate tolerance
   Manifestations of latent diabetes mellitus
   Increased requirements for insulin or oral hypoglycemic agents in diabetics
   Hirsutism
Ophthalmic
   Posterior subcapsular cataracts
   Increased intraocular pressure
   Glaucoma
   Exophthalmos

Continued on next page

Merck & Co.—Cont.

Metabolic
Negative nitrogen balance due to protein catabolism
Cardiovascular
Myocardial rupture following recent myocardial infarction (see WARNINGS).
Other
Anaphylactoid or hypersensitivity reactions
Thromboembolism
Weight gain
Increased appetite
Nausea
Malaise
The following *additional* adverse reactions are related to injection of corticosteroids:
Rare instances of blindness associated with intralesional therapy around the face and head
Hyperpigmentation or hypopigmentation
Subcutaneous and cutaneous atrophy
Sterile abscess
Postinjection flare (following intra-articular use)
Charcot-like arthropathy.

OVERDOSAGE

Reports of acute toxicity and/or death following overdosage of glucocorticoids are rare. In the event of overdosage, no specific antidote is available; treatment is supportive and symptomatic.

DOSAGE AND ADMINISTRATION

For intra-articular, intralesional, and soft tissue injection only

NOT FOR INTRAVENOUS USE

DOSAGE AND FREQUENCY OF INJECTION ARE VARIABLE AND MUST BE INDIVIDUALIZED ON THE BASIS OF THE DISEASE AND THE RESPONSE OF THE PATIENT.
The initial dose varies from 5 to 75 mg depending on the disease being treated and the size of the area to be injected. Frequency of injection depends on symptomatic response, and usually is once every two or three weeks. Severe conditions may require injection once a week. Frequent intra-articular injection may result in damage to joint tissues. If satisfactory clinical response does not occur after a reasonable period of time, discontinue HYDROCORTONE Acetate sterile suspension and transfer the patient to other therapy.
Patients should be observed closely for signs that might require dosage adjustment, including changes in clinical status resulting from remissions or exacerbations of the disease, and individual drug responsiveness.
Some of the usual single doses are:

Large Joints (e.g., Knee)	25 mg, occasionally 37.5 mg. Doses over 50 mg not recommended
Small Joints (e.g, Interphalangeal, Temporomandibular	10 to 25 mg
Bursae	25 to 37.5 mg
Tendon Sheaths	5 to 12.5 mg
Soft Tissue Infiltration	25 to 50 mg, occasionally 75 mg
Ganglia	12.5 to 25 mg

For rapid onset of action, a soluble adrenocortical hormone preparation, such as DECADRON* Phosphate (Dexamethasone Sodium Phosphate) injection or HYDELTRASOL* (Prednisolone Sodium Phosphate) injection, may be given with HYDROCORTONE Acetate sterile suspension.
If desired, a local anesthetic may be used, and may be injected before HYDROCORTONE Acetate sterile suspension or mixed in a syringe with HYDROCORTONE Acetate sterile suspension and given simultaneously.
If used prior to intra-articular injection of the steroid, inject most of the anesthetic into the soft tissues of the surrounding area and instill a small amount into the joint.
If given together, mixing should be done in the injection syringe by drawing the steroid in *first* , then the anesthetic. In this way, the anesthetic will not be introduced inadvertently into the vial of steroid. *The mixture must be used immediately and any unused portion discarded.*

---

* Registered trademark of MERCK & CO., INC.

HOW SUPPLIED

No. 7501—Sterile suspension HYDROCORTONE Acetate is a white, mobile suspension, containing 25 mg hydrocortisone acetate in each mL, and is supplied as follows:
NDC 0006-7501-03 in 5 mL vials.
No. 7519—Sterile suspension HYDROCORTONE Acetate is a white, mobile suspension, containing 50 mg hydrocortisone acetate in each mL, and is supplied as follows:
NDC 0006-7519-03 in 5 mL vials.
Storage
Sensitive to heat. Do not autoclave.
Protect from freezing.
A.H.F.S. Category: 68:04
DC 7348726 Issued March 1988

HYDROCORTONE® Phosphate Injection, Sterile   ℞
(Hydrocortisone Sodium Phosphate), U.S.P.

DESCRIPTION

Hydrocortisone sodium phosphate, a synthetic adrenocortical steroid, is a white to light yellow, odorless or practically odorless powder. It is freely soluble in water and is exceedingly hygroscopic. The molecular weight is 486.41. It is designated chemically as 11β,17-dihydroxy-21-(phosphonooxy)-pregn-4-ene-3,20-dione disodium salt. The empirical formula is $C_{21}H_{29}Na_2O_8P$ and the structural formula is:

HYDROCORTONE* Phosphate (Hydrocortisone Sodium Phosphate) injection is a sterile solution (pH 7.5 to 8.5), sealed under nitrogen, for intravenous, intramuscular, and subcutaneous administration.
Each milliliter contains hydrocortisone sodium phosphate equivalent to 50 mg hydrocortisone. Inactive ingredients per mL: 8 mg creatinine, 10 mg sodium citrate, sodium hydroxide to adjust pH, and Water for Injection, q.s. 1 mL, with 3.2 mg sodium bisulfite, 1.5 mg methylparaben, and 0.2 mg propylparaben added as preservatives.

---

* Registered trademark of MERCK & CO., INC.

ACTIONS

HYDROCORTONE Phosphate injection has a rapid onset but short duration of action when compared with less soluble preparations. Because of this, it is suitable for the treatment of acute disorders responsive to adrenocortical steroid therapy.
Naturally occurring glucocorticoids (hydrocortisone and cortisone), which also have salt-retaining properties, are used as replacement therapy in adrenocortical deficiency states. They are also used for their potent anti-inflammatory effects in disorders of many organ systems.
Glucocorticoids cause profound and varied metabolic effects. In addition, they modify the body's immune responses to diverse stimuli.

INDICATIONS

When oral therapy is not feasible:
1. *Endocrine disorders*
Primary or secondary adrenocortical insufficiency (hydrocortisone or cortisone is the drug of choice; synthetic analogs may be used in conjunction with mineralocorticoids where applicable; in infancy, mineralocorticoid supplementation is of particular importance)
Acute adrenocortical insufficiency (hydrocortisone or cortisone is the drug of choice; mineralocorticoid supplementation may be necessary, particularly when synthetic analogs are used)
Preoperatively, and in the event of serious trauma or illness, in patients with known adrenal insufficiency or when adrenocortical reserve is doubtful
Shock unresponsive to conventional therapy if adrenocortical insufficiency exists or is suspected
Congenital adrenal hyperplasia
Nonsuppurative thyroiditis
Hypercalcemia associated with cancer
2. *Rheumatic disorders*
As adjunctive therapy for short-term administration (to tide the patient over an acute episode or exacerbation) in:

Post-traumatic osteoarthritis
Synovitis of osteoarthritis
Rheumatoid arthritis, including juvenile rheumatoid arthritis (selected cases may require low-dose maintenance therapy)
Acute and subacute bursitis
Epicondylitis
Acute nonspecific tenosynovitis
Acute gouty arthritis
Psoriatic arthritis
Ankylosing spondylitis
3. *Collagen diseases*
During an exacerbation or as maintenance therapy in selected cases of:
Systemic lupus erythematosus
Acute rheumatic carditis
Systemic dermatomyositis (polymyositis)
4. *Dermatologic diseases*
Pemphigus
Severe erythema multiforme (Stevens-Johnson syndrome)
Exfoliative dermatitis
Bullous dermatitis herpetiformis
Severe seborrheic dermatitis
Severe psoriasis
Mycosis fungoides
5. *Allergic states*
Control of severe or incapacitating allergic conditions intractable to adequate trials of conventional treatment in:
Bronchial asthma
Contact dermatitis
Atopic dermatitis
Serum sickness
Seasonal or perennial allergic rhinitis
Drug hypersensitivity reactions
Urticarial transfusion reactions
Acute noninfectious laryngeal edema (epinephrine is the drug of first choice)
6. *Ophthalmic diseases*
Severe acute and chronic allergic and inflammatory processes involving the eye, such as:
Herpes zoster ophthalmicus
Iritis, iridocyclitis
Chorioretinitis
Diffuse posterior uveitis and choroiditis
Optic neuritis
Sympathetic ophthalmia
Anterior segment inflammation
Allergic conjunctivitis
Keratitis
Allergic corneal marginal ulcers
7. *Gastrointestinal diseases*
To tide the patient over a critical period of the disease in:
Ulcerative colitis (Systemic therapy)
Regional enteritis (Systemic therapy)
8. *Respiratory diseases*
Symptomatic sarcoidosis
Berylliosis
Fulminating or disseminated pulmonary tuberculosis when used concurrently with appropriate antituberculous chemotherapy
Loeffler's syndrome not manageable by other means
Aspiration pneumonitis
9. *Hematologic disorders*
Acquired (autoimmune) hemolytic anemia
Idiopathic thrombocytopenic purpura in adults (I.V. only; I.M. administration is contraindicated)
Secondary thrombocytopenia in adults
Erythroblastopenia (RBC anemia)
Congenital (erythroid) hypoplastic anemia
10. *Neoplastic diseases*
For palliative management of:
Leukemias and lymphomas in adults
Acute leukemia of childhood
11. *Edematous states*
To induce diuresis or remission of proteinuria in the nephrotic syndrome, without uremia, of the idiopathic type, or that due to lupus erythematosus
12. *Miscellaneous*
Tuberculous meningitis with subarachnoid block or impending block when used concurrently with appropriate antituberculous chemotherapy
Trichinosis with neurologic or myocardial involvement

CONTRAINDICATIONS

Systemic fungal infections (see WARNINGS regarding amphotericin B)
Hypersensitivity to any component of this product, including sulfites (see WARNINGS).

WARNINGS

Because rare instances of anaphylactoid reactions have occurred in patients receiving parenteral corticosteroid therapy, appropriate precautionary measures should be taken

prior to administration, especially when the patient has a history of allergy to any drug. Anaphylactoid and hypersensitivity reactions have been reported for Injection HYDROCORTONE Phosphate (see ADVERSE REACTIONS).

Injection HYDROCORTONE Phosphate contains sodium bisulfite, a sulfite that may cause allergic-type reactions including anaphylactic symptoms and life-threatening or less severe asthmatic episodes in certain susceptible people. The overall prevalence of sulfite sensitivity in the general population is unknown and probably low. Sulfite sensitivity is seen more frequently in asthmatic than in nonasthmatic people.

Corticosteroids may exacerbate systemic fungal infections and therefore should not be used in the presence of such infections unless they are needed to control drug reactions due to amphotericin B. Moreover, there have been cases reported in which concomitant use of amphotericin B and hydrocortisone was followed by cardiac enlargement and congestive failure.

In patients on corticosteroid therapy subjected to any unusual stress, increased dosage of rapidly acting corticosteroids before, during, and after the stressful situation is indicated.

Drug-induced secondary adrenocortical insufficiency may result from too rapid withdrawal of corticosteroids and may be minimized by gradual reduction of dosage. This type of relative insufficiency may persist for months after discontinuation of therapy; therefore, in any situation of stress occurring during that period, hormone therapy should be reinstituted. If the patient is receiving steroids already, dosage may have to be increased. Since mineralocorticoid secretion may be impaired, salt and/or a mineralocorticoid should be administered concurrently.

Corticosteroids may mask some signs of infection, and new infections may appear during their use. There may be decreased resistance and inability to localize infection when corticosteroids are used. Moreover, corticosteroids may affect the nitroblue-tetrazolium test for bacterial infection and produce false negative results.

In cerebral malaria, a double-blind trial has shown that the use of corticosteroids is associated with prolongation of coma and a higher incidence of pneumonia and gastrointestinal bleeding.

Corticosteroids may activate latent amebiasis. Therefore, it is recommended that latent or active amebiasis be ruled out before initiating corticosteroid therapy in any patient who has spent time in the tropics or any patient with unexplained diarrhea.

Prolonged use of corticosteroids may produce posterior subcapsular cataracts, glaucoma with possible damage to the optic nerves, and may enhance the establishment of secondary ocular infections due to fungi or viruses.

Usage in pregnancy. Since adequate human reproduction studies have not been done with corticosteroids, use of these drugs in pregnancy or in women of childbearing potential requires that the anticipated benefits be weighed against the possible hazards to the mother and embryo or fetus. Infants born of mothers who have received substantial doses of corticosteroids during pregnancy should be carefully observed for signs of hypoadrenalism.

Corticosteroids appear in breast milk and could suppress growth, interfere with endogenous corticosteroid production, or cause other unwanted effects. Mothers taking pharmacologic doses of corticosteroids should be advised not to nurse.

Average and large doses of cortisone or hydrocortisone can cause elevation of blood pressure, salt and water retention, and increased excretion of potassium. These effects are less likely to occur with the synthetic derivatives except when used in large doses. Dietary salt restriction and potassium supplementation may be necessary. All corticosteroids increase calcium excretion.

Administration of live virus vaccines, including smallpox, is contraindicated in individuals receiving immunosuppressive doses of corticosteroids. If inactivated viral or bacterial vaccines are administered to individuals receiving immunosuppressive doses of corticosteroids, the expected serum antibody response may not be obtained. However, immunization procedures may be undertaken in patients who are receiving corticosteroids as replacement therapy, e.g., for Addison's disease.

The use of HYDROCORTONE Phosphate injection in active tuberculosis should be restricted to those cases of fulminating or disseminated tuberculosis in which the corticosteroid is used for the management of the disease in conjunction with an appropriate antituberculous regimen.

If corticosteroids are indicated in patients with latent tuberculosis or tuberculin reactivity, close observation is necessary as reactivation of the disease may occur. During prolonged corticosteroid therapy, these patients should receive chemoprophylaxis.

Literature reports suggest an apparent association between use of corticosteroids and left ventricular free wall rupture after a recent myocardial infarction; therefore, therapy with corticosteroids should be used with great caution in these patients.

PRECAUTIONS

This product, like many other steroid formulations, is sensitive to heat. Therefore, it should not be autoclaved when it is desirable to sterilize the exterior of the vial.

Following prolonged therapy, withdrawal of corticosteroids may result in symptoms of the corticosteroid withdrawal syndrome including fever, myalgia, arthralgia, and malaise. This may occur in patients even without evidence of adrenal insufficiency.

There is an enhanced effect of corticosteroids in patients with hypothyroidism and in those with cirrhosis.

Corticosteroids should be used cautiously in patients with ocular herpes simplex for fear of corneal perforation.

The lowest possible dose of corticosteroid should be used to control the condition under treatment, and when reduction in dosage is possible, the reduction must be gradual.

Psychic derangements may appear when corticosteroids are used, ranging from euphoria, insomnia, mood swings, personality changes, and severe depression to frank psychotic manifestations. Also, existing emotional instability or psychotic tendencies may be aggravated by corticosteroids.

Aspirin should be used cautiously in conjunction with corticosteroids in hypoprothrombinemia.

Steroids should be used with caution in nonspecific ulcerative colitis, if there is a probability of impending perforation, abscess, or other pyogenic infection, also in diverticulitis, fresh intestinal anastomoses, active or latent peptic ulcer, renal insufficiency, hypertension, osteoporosis, and myasthenia gravis. Signs of peritoneal irritation following gastrointestinal perforation in patients receiving large doses of corticosteroids may be minimal or absent. Fat embolism has been reported as a possible complication of hypercortisonism.

When large doses are given, some authorities advise that antacids be administered between meals to help to prevent peptic ulcer.

Growth and development of infants and children on prolonged corticosteroid therapy should be carefully followed.

Steroids may increase or decrease motility and number of spermatozoa in some patients.

Phenytoin, phenobarbital, ephedrine, and rifampin may enhance the metabolic clearance of corticosteroids, resulting in decreased blood levels and lessened physiologic activity, thus requiring adjustment in corticosteroid dosage.

The prothrombin time should be checked frequently in patients who are receiving corticosteroids and coumarin anticoagulants at the same time because of reports that corticosteroids have altered the response to these anticoagulants. Studies have shown that the usual effect produced by adding corticosteroids is inhibition of response to coumarins, although there have been some conflicting reports of potentiation not substantiated by studies.

When corticosteroids are administered concomitantly with potassium-depleting diuretics, patients should be observed closely for development of hypokalemia.

Injection of a steroid into an infected site is to be avoided.

The slower rate of absorption by intramuscular administration should be recognized.

ADVERSE REACTIONS

Fluid and electrolyte disturbances
- Sodium retention
- Fluid retention
- Congestive heart failure in susceptible patients
- Potassium loss
- Hypokalemic alkalosis
- Hypertension

Musculoskeletal
- Muscle weakness
- Steroid myopathy
- Loss of muscle mass
- Osteoporosis
- Vertebral compression fractures
- Aseptic necrosis of femoral and humeral heads
- Pathologic fracture of long bones
- Tendon rupture

Gastrointestinal
- Peptic ulcer with possible subsequent perforation and hemorrhage
- Perforation of the small and large bowel, particularly in patients with inflammatory bowel disease
- Pancreatitis
- Abdominal distention
- Ulcerative esophagitis

Dermatologic
- Impaired wound healing
- Thin fragile skin
- Petechiae and ecchymoses
- Erythema
- Increased sweating
- May suppress reactions to skin tests
- Burning or tingling, especially in the perineal area (after I.V. injection)
- Other cutaneous reactions, such as allergic dermatitis, urticaria, angioneurotic edema

Neurologic
- Convulsions
- Increased intracranial pressure with papilledema (pseudotumor cerebri) usually after treatment
- Vertigo
- Headache
- Psychic disturbances

Endocrine
- Menstrual irregularities
- Development of cushingoid state
- Suppression of growth in children
- Secondary adrenocortical and pituitary unresponsiveness, particularly in times of stress, as in trauma, surgery, or illness
- Decreased carbohydrate tolerance
- Manifestations of latent diabetes mellitus
- Increased requirements for insulin or oral hypoglycemic agents in diabetics
- Hirsutism

Ophthalmic
- Posterior subcapsular cataracts
- Increased intraocular pressure
- Glaucoma
- Exophthalmos

Metabolic
- Negative nitrogen balance due to protein catabolism

Cardiovascular
- Myocardial rupture following recent myocardial infarction (see WARNINGS).

Other
- Anaphylactoid or hypersensitivity reactions
- Thromboembolism
- Weight gain
- Increased appetite
- Nausea
- Malaise

The following *additional* adverse reactions are related to parenteral corticosteroid therapy:
- Rare instances of blindness associated with intralesional therapy around the face and head
- Hyperpigmentation or hypopigmentation
- Subcutaneous and cutaneous atrophy
- Sterile abscess

OVERDOSAGE

Reports of acute toxicity and/or death following overdosage of glucocorticoids are rare. In the event of overdosage, no specific antidote is available; treatment is supportive and symptomatic.

The intraperitoneal LD_{50} of hydrocortisone in female mice was 1740 mg/kg.

DOSAGE AND ADMINISTRATION

For intravenous, intramuscular, and subcutaneous injection.
HYDROCORTONE Phosphate injection can be given directly from the vial, or it can be added to Sodium Chloride Injection or Dextrose Injection and administered by intravenous drip.

Benzyl alcohol as a preservative has been associated with toxicity in premature infants. Solutions used for intravenous administration or further dilution of this product should be preservative-free when used in the neonate, especially the premature infant.

When it is mixed with an infusion solution, sterile precautions should be observed. Since infusion solutions generally do not contain preservatives, mixtures should be used within 24 hours.

DOSAGE REQUIREMENTS ARE VARIABLE AND MUST BE INDIVIDUALIZED ON THE BASIS OF THE DISEASE AND THE RESPONSE OF THE PATIENT.

The initial dosage varies from 15 to 240 mg a day depending on the disease being treated. In less severe diseases doses lower than 15 mg may suffice, while in severe diseases doses higher than 240 mg may be required. Usually the parenteral dosage ranges are one-third to one-half the oral dose given every 12 hours. However, in certain overwhelming, acute, life-threatening situations, administration in dosages exceeding the usual dosages may be justified and may be in multiples of the oral dosages.

The initial dosage should be maintained or adjusted until the patient's response is satisfactory. If a satisfactory clinical response does not occur after a reasonable period of time, discontinue HYDROCORTONE Phosphate injection and transfer the patient to other therapy.

Continued on next page

Information on the Merck & Co. products listed on these pages is the full prescribing information from product circulars in use October 1, 1992.

Merck & Co.—Cont.

After a favorable initial response, the proper maintenance dosage should be determined by decreasing the initial dosage in small amounts to the lowest dosage that maintains an adequate clinical response.

Patients should be observed closely for signs that might require dosage adjustment, including changes in clinical status resulting from remissions or exacerbations of the disease, individual drug responsiveness, and the effect of stress (e.g., surgery, infection, trauma). During stress it may be necessary to increase dosage temporarily.

If the drug is to be stopped after more than a few days of treatment, it usually should be withdrawn gradually.

HOW SUPPLIED

No. 7633—Injection HYDROCORTONE Phosphate, 50 mg hydrocortisone equivalent per mL, is a clear, light yellow solution, and is supplied as follows:

NDC 0006-7633-04 in 2 mL multiple dose vials
NDC 0006-7633-10 in 10 mL multiple dose vials.
Storage
Sensitive to heat. Do not autoclave.

A.H.F.S. Category: 68:04
DC 7349525 Issued March 1988

HYDROCORTONE® Tablets   Ɓ
(Hydrocortisone), U.S.P.

DESCRIPTION

Glucocorticoids are adrenocortical steroids, both naturally occurring and synthetic, which are readily absorbed from the gastrointestinal tract.

Hydrocortisone is a white to practically white, odorless, crystalline powder, very slightly soluble in water. The molecular weight is 362.47. It is designated chemically as 11β,17,21-trihydroxypregn-4-ene-3,20-dione. The empirical formula is $C_{21}H_{30}O_5$ and the structural formula is:

Hydrocortisone is believed to be the principal hormone secreted by the adrenal cortex.
HYDROCORTONE* (Hydrocortisone) tablets are supplied in two potencies, 10 mg and 20 mg.
Inactive ingredients are lactose, magnesium stearate, and starch.

* Registered trademark of MERCK & CO., INC.

ACTIONS

Naturally occurring glucocorticoids (hydrocortisone and cortisone), which also have salt-retaining properties, are used as replacement therapy in adrenocortical deficiency states. They are also used for their potent anti-inflammatory effects in disorders of many organ systems.
Glucocorticoids cause profound and varied metabolic effects. In addition, they modify the body's immune responses to diverse stimuli.

INDICATIONS

1. *Endocrine Disorders*
   Primary or secondary adrenocortical insufficiency (hydrocortisone or cortisone is the first choice; synthetic analogs may be used in conjunction with mineralocorticoids where applicable; in infancy mineralocorticoid supplementation is of particular importance)
   Congenital adrenal hyperplasia
   Nonsuppurative thyroiditis
   Hypercalcemia associated with cancer
2. *Rheumatic Disorders*
   As adjunctive therapy for short-term administration (to tide the patient over an acute episode or exacerbation) in:
   Psoriatic arthritis
   Rheumatoid arthritis, including juvenile rheumatoid arthritis (selected cases may require low-dose maintenance therapy)
   Ankylosing spondylitis
   Acute and subacute bursitis
   Acute nonspecific tenosynovitis
   Acute gouty arthritis

Post-traumatic osteoarthritis
Synovitis of osteoarthritis
Epicondylitis
3. *Collagen Diseases*
   During an exacerbation or as maintenance therapy in selected cases of—
   Systemic lupus erythematosus
   Acute rheumatic carditis
   Systemic dermatomyositis (polymyositis)
4. *Dermatologic Diseases*
   Pemphigus
   Bullous dermatitis herpetiformis
   Severe erythema multiforme (Stevens-Johnson syndrome)
   Exfoliative dermatitis
   Mycosis fungoides
   Severe psoriasis
   Severe seborrheic dermatitis
5. *Allergic States*
   Control of severe or incapacitating allergic conditions intractable to adequate trials of conventional treatment:
   Seasonal or perennial allergic rhinitis
   Bronchial asthma
   Contact dermatitis
   Atopic dermatitis
   Serum sickness
   Drug hypersensitivity reactions
6. *Ophthalmic Diseases*
   Severe acute and chronic allergic and inflammatory processes involving the eye and its adnexa, such as—
   Allergic conjunctivitis
   Keratitis
   Allergic corneal marginal ulcers
   Herpes zoster ophthalmicus
   Iritis and iridocyclitis
   Chorioretinitis
   Anterior segment inflammation
   Diffuse posterior uveitis and choroiditis
   Optic neuritis
   Sympathetic ophthalmia
7. *Respiratory Diseases*
   Symptomatic sarcoidosis
   Loeffler's syndrome not manageable by other means
   Berylliosis
   Fulminating or disseminated pulmonary tuberculosis when used concurrently with appropriate antituberculous chemotherapy
   Aspiration pneumonitis
8. *Hematologic Disorders*
   Idiopathic thrombocytopenic purpura in adults
   Secondary thrombocytopenia in adults
   Acquired (autoimmune) hemolytic anemia
   Erythroblastopenia (RBC anemia)
   Congenital (erythroid) hypoplastic anemia
9. *Neoplastic Diseases*
   For palliative management of:
   Leukemias and lymphomas in adults
   Acute leukemia of childhood
10. *Edematous States*
    To induce a diuresis or remission of proteinuria in the nephrotic syndrome, without uremia, of the idiopathic type or that due to lupus erythematosus
11. *Gastrointestinal Diseases*
    To tide the patient over a critical period of the disease in:
    Ulcerative colitis
    Regional enteritis
12. *Miscellaneous*
    Tuberculous meningitis with subarachnoid block or impending block when used concurrently with appropriate antituberculous chemotherapy
    Trichinosis with neurologic or myocardial involvement

CONTRAINDICATIONS

Systemic fungal infections
Hypersensitivity to this product

WARNINGS

In patients on corticosteroid therapy subjected to unusual stress, increased dosage of rapidly acting corticosteroids before, during, and after the stressful situation is indicated.
Drug-induced secondary adrenocortical insufficiency may result from too rapid wthdrawal of corticosteroids and may be minimized by gradual reduction of dosage. This type of relative insufficiency may persist for months after discontinuation of therapy; therefore, in any situation of stress occurring during that period, hormone therapy should be reinstituted. If the patient is receiving steroids already, dosage may have to be increased. Since mineralocorticoid secretion may be impaired, salt and/or a mineralocorticoid should be administered concurrently.
Corticosteroids may mask some signs of infection, and new infections may appear during their use. There may be decreased resistance and inability to localize infection when corticosteroids are used. Moreover, corticosteroids may af-

fect the nitroblue-tetrazolium test for bacterial infection and produce false negative results.
In cerebral malaria, a double-blind trial has shown that the use of corticosteroids is associated with prolongation of coma and a higher incidence of pneumonia and gastrointestinal bleeding.
Corticosteroids may activate latent amebiasis. Therefore, it is recommended that latent or active amebiasis be ruled out before initiating corticosteroid therapy in any patient who has spent time in the tropics or any patient with unexplained diarrhea.
Prolonged use of corticosteroids may produce posterior subcapsular cataracts, glaucoma with possible damage to the optic nerves, and may enhance the establishment of secondary ocular infections due to fungi or viruses.
Usage in pregnancy: Since adequate human reproduction studies have not been done with corticosteroids, use of these drugs in pregnancy or in women of childbearing potential requires that the anticipated benefits be weighed against the possible hazards to the mother and embryo or fetus. Infants born of mothers who have received substantial doses of corticosteroids during pregnancy should be carefully observed for signs of hypoadrenalism.
Corticosteroids appear in breast milk and could suppress growth, interfere with endogenous corticosteroid production, or cause other unwanted effects. Mothers taking pharmacologic doses of corticosteroids should be advised not to nurse.
Average and large doses of hydrocortisone or cortisone can cause elevation of blood pressure, salt and water retention, and increased excretion of potassium. These effects are less likely to occur with the synthetic derivatives except when used in large doses. Dietary salt restriction and potassium supplementation may be necessary. All corticosteroids increase calcium excretion.
Administration of live virus vaccines, including smallpox, is contraindicated in individuals receiving immunosuppressive doses of corticosteroids. If inactivated viral or bacterial vaccines are administered to individuals receiving immunosuppressive doses of corticosteroids, the expected serum antibody response may not be obtained. However, immunization procedures may be undertaken in patients who are receiving corticosteroids as replacement therapy, e.g., for Addison's disease.
The use of HYDROCORTONE tablets in active tuberculosis should be restricted to those cases of fulminating or disseminated tuberculosis in which the corticosteroid is used for the management of the disease in conjunction with an appropriate antituberculous regimen.
If corticosteroids are indicated in patients with latent tuberculosis or tuberculin reactivity, close observation is necessary as reactivation of the disease may occur. During prolonged corticosteroid therapy, these patients should receive chemoprophylaxis.
Literature reports suggest an apparent association between use of corticosteroids and left ventricular free wall rupture after a recent myocardial infarction; therefore, therapy with corticosteroids should be used with great caution in these patients.

PRECAUTIONS

Following prolonged therapy, withdrawal of corticosteroids may result in symptoms of the corticosteroid withdrawal syndrome including fever, myalgia, arthralgia, and malaise. This may occur in patients even without evidence of adrenal insufficiency.
There is an enhanced effect of corticosteroids in patients with hypothyroidism and in those with cirrhosis.
Corticosteroids should be used cautiously in patients with ocular herpes simplex because of possible corneal perforation.
The lowest possible dose of corticosteroid should be used to control the condition under treatment, and when reduction in dosage is possible, the reduction should be gradual.
Psychic derangements may appear when corticosteroids are used, ranging from euphoria, insomnia, mood swings, personality changes, and severe depression, to frank psychotic manifestations. Also, existing emotional instability or psychotic tendencies may be aggravated by corticosteroids.
Aspirin should be used cautiously in conjunction with corticosteroids in hypoprothrombinemia.
Steroids should be used with caution in nonspecific ulcerative colitis, if there is a probability of impending perforation, abscess, or other pyogenic infection, diverticulitis, fresh intestinal anastomoses, active or latent peptic ulcer, renal insufficiency, hypertension, osteoporosis, and myasthenia gravis. Signs of peritoneal irritation following gastrointestinal perforation in patients receiving large doses of corticosteroids may be minimal or absent. Fat embolism has been reported as a possible complication of hypercortisonism.
When large doses are given, some authorities advise that corticosteroids be taken with meals and antacids taken between meals to help to prevent peptic ulcer.
Growth and development of infants and children on prolonged corticosteroid therapy should be carefully observed.

Steroids may increase or decrease motility and number of spermatozoa in some patients.

Phenytoin, phenobarbital, ephedrine, and rifampin may enhance the metabolic clearance of corticosteroids, resulting in decreased blood levels and lessened physiologic activity, thus requiring adjustment in corticosteroid dosage.

The prothrombin time should be checked frequently in patients who are receiving corticosteroids and coumarin anticoagulants at the same time because of reports that corticosteroids have altered the response to these anticoagulants. Studies have shown that the usual effect produced by adding corticosteroids is inhibition of response to coumarins, although there have been some conflicting reports of potentiation not substantiated by studies.

When corticosteroids are administered concomitantly with potassium-depleting diuretics, patients should be observed closely for development of hypokalemia.

ADVERSE REACTIONS

Fluid and Electrolyte Disturbances
Sodium retention
Fluid retention
Congestive heart failure in susceptible patients
Potassium loss
Hypokalemic alkalosis
Hypertension
Musculoskeletal
Muscle weakness
Steroid myopathy
Loss of muscle mass
Osteoporosis
Vertebral compression fractures
Aseptic necrosis of femoral and humeral heads
Pathologic fracture of long bones
Tendon rupture
Gastrointestinal
Peptic ulcer with possible perforation and hemorrhage
Perforation of the small and large bowel, particularly in patients with inflammatory bowel disease
Pancreatitis
Abdominal distention
Ulcerative esophagitis
Dermatologic
Impaired wound healing
Thin fragile skin
Petechiae and ecchymoses
Erythema
Increased sweating
May suppress reactions to skin tests
Other cutaneous reactions, such as allergic dermatitis, urticaria, angioneurotic edema
Neurologic
Convulsions
Increased intracranial pressure with papilledema (pseudotumor cerebri) usually after treatment
Vertigo
Headache
Psychic disturbances
Endocrine
Menstrual irregularities
Development of cushingoid state
Suppression of growth in children
Secondary adrenocortical and pituitary unresponsiveness, particularly in times of stress, as in trauma, surgery, or illness
Decreased carbohydrate tolerance
Manifestations of latent diabetes mellitus
Increased requirements for insulin or oral hypoglycemic agents in diabetics
Hirsutism
Ophthalmic
Posterior subcapsular cataracts
Increased intraocular pressure
Glaucoma
Exophthalmos
Metabolic
Negative nitrogen balance due to protein catabolism
Cardiovascular
Myocardial rupture following recent myocardial infarction (see WARNINGS).
Other
Hypersensitivity
Thromboembolism
Weight gain
Increased appetite
Nausea
Malaise

OVERDOSAGE

Reports of acute toxicity and/or death following overdosage of glucocorticoids are rare. In the event of overdosage, no specific antidote is available; treatment is supportive and symptomatic.

The intraperitoneal LD_{50} of hydrocortisone in female mice was 1740 mg/kg.

DOSAGE AND ADMINISTRATION

For oral administration
DOSAGE REQUIREMENTS ARE VARIABLE AND MUST BE INDIVIDUALIZED ON THE BASIS OF THE DISEASE AND THE RESPONSE OF THE PATIENT.
The initial dosage varies from 20 to 240 mg a day depending on the disease being treated. In less severe diseases doses lower than 20 mg may suffice, while in severe diseases doses higher than 240 mg may be required. The initial dosage should be maintained or adjusted until the patient's response is satisfactory. If satisfactory clinical response does not occur after a reasonable period of time, discontinue HYDROCORTONE tablets and transfer the patient to other therapy.

After a favorable initial response, the proper maintenance dosage should be determined by decreasing the initial dosage in small amounts to the lowest dosage that maintains an adequate clinical response.

Patients should be observed closely for signs that might require dosage adjustment, including changes in clinical status resulting from remissions or exacerbations of the disease, individual drug responsiveness, and the effect of stress (e.g, surgery, infection, trauma). During stress it may be necessary to increase dosage temporarily.

If the drug is to be stopped after more than a few days of treatment, it usually should be withdrawn gradually.

HOW SUPPLIED

No. 7604—Tablets HYDROCORTONE, 10 mg each, are white, oval shaped compressed tablets, scored on one side, coded MSD 619, and are supplied as follows:
NDC 0006-0619-68 in bottles of 100.
Shown in Product Identification Section, page 419
No. 7602—Tablets HYDROCORTONE, 20 mg each, are white, oval shaped compressed tablets, scored on one side, coded MSD 625, and are supplied as follows:
NDC 0006-0625-68 in bottles of 100.
Shown in Product Identification Section, page 419
A.H.F.S. Category: 68:04
DC 7414424 Issued March 1988

HydroDIURIL® Tablets   ℞
(Hydrochlorothiazide), U.S.P.

DESCRIPTION

HydroDIURIL* (Hydrochlorothiazide) is a diuretic and antihypertensive. It is the 3,4-dihydro derivative of chlorothiazide. Its chemical name is 6-chloro-3,4-dihydro-2H-1,2,4-benzothiadiazine-7-sulfonamide 1,1-dioxide. Its empirical formula is $C_7H_8ClN_3O_4S_2$ and its structural formula is:

It is a white, or practically white, crystalline powder with a molecular weight of 297.72, which is slightly soluble in water, but freely soluble in sodium hydroxide solution.
HydroDIURIL is supplied as 25 mg, 50 mg and 100 mg tablets for oral use. Each tablet contains the following inactive ingredients: calcium phosphate, FD&C Yellow 6, gelatin, lactose, magnesium stearate, starch and talc.

*Registered trademark of MERCK & CO., INC.

CLINICAL PHARMACOLOGY

The mechanism of the antihypertensive effect of thiazides is unknown. HydroDIURIL does not usually affect normal blood pressure.
HydroDIURIL affects the distal renal tubular mechanism of electrolyte reabsorption. At maximal therapeutic dosage all thiazides are approximately equal in their diuretic efficacy. HydroDIURIL increases excretion of sodium and chloride in approximately equivalent amounts. Natriuresis may be accompanied by some loss of potassium and bicarbonate.
After oral use diuresis begins within 2 hours, peaks in about 4 hours and lasts about 6 to 12 hours.
Pharmacokinetics and Metabolism
HydroDIURIL is not metabolized but is eliminated rapidly by the kidney. When plasma levels have been followed for at least 24 hours, the plasma half-life has been observed to vary between 5.6 and 14.8 hours. At least 61 percent of the oral dose is eliminated unchanged within 24 hours. Hydrochloro-

thiazide crosses the placental but not the blood-brain barrier and is excreted in breast milk.

INDICATIONS AND USAGE

HydroDIURIL is indicated as adjunctive therapy in edema associated with congestive heart failure, hepatic cirrhosis, and corticosteroid and estrogen therapy.
HydroDIURIL has also been found useful in edema due to various forms of renal dysfunction such as nephrotic syndrome, acute glomerulonephritis, and chronic renal failure.
HydroDIURIL is indicated in the management of hypertension either as the sole therapeutic agent or to enhance the effectiveness of other antihypertensive drugs in the more severe forms of hypertension.
Use in Pregnancy. Routine use of diuretics during normal pregnancy is inappropriate and exposes mother and fetus to unnecessary hazard. Diuretics do not prevent development of toxemia of pregnancy and there is no satisfactory evidence that they are useful in the treatment of toxemia. Edema during pregnancy may arise from pathologic causes or from the physiologic and mechanical consequences of pregnancy. Thiazides are indicated in pregnancy when edema is due to pathologic causes, just as they are in the absence of pregnancy (see PRECAUTIONS, *Pregnancy*). Dependent edema in pregnancy, resulting from restriction of venous return by the gravid uterus, is properly treated through elevation of the lower extremities and use of support stockings. Use of diuretics to lower intravascular volume in this instance is illogical and unnecessary. During normal pregnancy there is hypervolemia which is not harmful to the fetus or the mother in the absence of cardiovascular disease. However, it may be associated with edema, rarely generalized edema. If such edema causes discomfort, increased recumbency will often provide relief. Rarely this edema may cause extreme discomfort which is not relieved by rest. In these instances, a short course of diuretic therapy may provide relief and be appropriate.

CONTRAINDICATIONS

Anuria.
Hypersensitivity to this product or to other sulfonamide-derived drugs.

WARNINGS

Use with caution in severe renal disease. In patients with renal disease, thiazides may precipitate azotemia. Cumulative effects of the drug may develop in patients with impaired renal function.
Thiazides should be used with caution in patients with impaired hepatic function or progressive liver disease, since minor alterations of fluid and electrolyte balance may precipitate hepatic coma.
Thiazides may add to or potentiate the action of other antihypertensive drugs.
Sensitivity reactions may occur in patients with or without a history of allergy or bronchial asthma.
The possibility of exacerbation or activation of systemic lupus erythematosus has been reported.
Lithium generally should not be given with diuretics (see PRECAUTIONS, *Drug Interactions*).

PRECAUTIONS

General
All patients receiving diuretic therapy should be observed for evidence of fluid or electrolyte imbalance: namely, hyponatremia, hypochloremic alkalosis, and hypokalemia. Serum and urine electrolyte determinations are particularly important when the patient is vomiting excessively or receiving parenteral fluids. Warning signs or symptoms of fluid and electrolyte imbalance, irrespective of cause, include dryness of mouth, thirst, weakness, lethargy, drowsiness, restlessness, muscle pains or cramps, muscular fatigue, hypotension, oliguria, tachycardia, and gastrointestinal disturbances such as nausea and vomiting.
Hypokalemia may develop, especially with brisk diuresis, when severe cirrhosis is present or after prolonged therapy. Interference with adequate oral electrolyte intake will also contribute to hypokalemia. Hypokalemia may cause cardiac arrhythmia and may also sensitize or exaggerate the response of the heart to the toxic effects of digitalis (e.g., increased ventricular irritability). Hypokalemia may be avoided or treated by use of potassium sparing diuretics or potassium supplements such as foods with a high potassium content.

Continued on next page

Information on the Merck & Co. products listed on these pages is the full prescribing information from product circulars in use October 1, 1992.

Merck & Co.—Cont.

Although any chloride deficit is generally mild and usually does not require specific treatment except under extraordinary circumstances (as in liver disease or renal disease), chloride replacement may be required in the treatment of metabolic alkalosis.

Dilutional hyponatremia may occur in edematous patients in hot weather; appropriate therapy is water restriction, rather than administration of salt, except in rare instances when the hyponatremia is life threatening. In actual salt depletion, appropriate replacement is the therapy of choice.

Hyperuricemia may occur or acute gout may be precipitated in certain patients receiving thiazides.

In diabetic patients dosage adjustments of insulin or oral hypoglycemic agents may be required. Hyperglycemia may occur with thiazide diuretics. Thus latent diabetes mellitus may become manifest during thiazide therapy.

The antihypertensive effects of the drug may be enhanced in the post-sympathectomy patient.

If progressive renal impairment becomes evident, consider withholding or discontinuing diuretic therapy.

Thiazides have been shown to increase the urinary excretion of magnesium; this may result in hypomagnesemia.

Thiazides may decrease urinary calcium excretion. Thiazides may cause intermittent and slight elevation of serum calcium in the absence of known disorders of calcium metabolism. Marked hypercalcemia may be evidence of hidden hyperparathyroidism. Thiazides should be discontinued before carrying out tests for parathyroid function.

Increases in cholesterol and triglyceride levels may be associated with thiazide diuretic therapy.

Laboratory Tests

Periodic determination of serum electrolytes to detect possible electrolyte imbalance should be done at appropriate intervals.

Drug Interactions

When given concurrently the following drugs may interact with thiazide diuretics.

Alcohol, barbiturates, or narcotics —potentiation of orthostatic hypotension may occur.

Antidiabetic drugs —(oral agents and insulin)—dosage adjustment of the antidiabetic drug may be required.

Other antihypertensive drugs —additive effect or potentiation.

Corticosteroids, ACTH —intensified electrolyte depletion, particularly hypokalemia.

Pressor amines (e.g., norepinephrine) —possible decreased response to pressor amines but not sufficient to preclude their use.

Skeletal muscle relaxants, nondepolarizing (e.g., tubocurarine) —possible increased responsiveness to the muscle relaxant.

Lithium —generally should not be given with diuretics. Diuretic agents reduce the renal clearance of lithium and add a high risk of lithium toxicity. Refer to the package insert for lithium preparations before use of such preparations with HydroDIURIL.

Non-steroidal Anti-inflammatory Drugs —In some patients, the administration of a non-steroidal anti-inflammatory agent can reduce the diuretic, natriuretic, and antihypertensive effects of loop, potassium-sparing and thiazide diuretics. Therefore, when HydroDIURIL and non-steroidal anti-inflammatory agents are used concomitantly, the patient should be observed closely to determine if the desired effect of the diuretic is obtained.

Drug/Laboratory Test Interactions

Thiazides should be discontinued before carrying out tests for parathyroid function (see PRECAUTIONS, *General*).

Carcinogenesis, Mutagenesis, Impairment of Fertility

Hydrochlorothiazide is currently under study in the U.S. Carcinogenesis Testing Program.

Hydrochlorothiazide was not mutagenic *in vitro*, in the Ames microbial mutagen test at a maximum concentration of 5 mg/plate using Strains TA98 and TA100. Urine samples of patients treated with hydrochlorothiazide did not have mutagenic activity in the Ames test.

The ability of a number of drugs to induce nondisjunction and crossing-over was measured using *Aspergillus nidulans*. A large number of drugs, including hydrochlorothiazide, induced nondisjunction.

Hydrochlorothiazide had no effect on fertility in a two-litter study in rats at doses of 4-5.6 mg/kg/day (up to 2 times the maximum recommended human dose).

Pregnancy

Teratogenic Effects —Pregnancy Category B: Reproduction studies in the rabbit, the mouse and the rat at doses up to 100 mg/kg/day (50 times the maximum human dose) showed no evidence of external abnormalities of the fetus due to hydrochlorothiazide. Hydrochlorothiazide given in a two-litter study in rats at doses of 4-5.6 mg/kg/day (approximately 1–2 times the maximum recommended human dose) did not impair fertility or produce birth abnormalities in the offspring.

There are no adequate and well-controlled studies with HydroDIURIL in pregnant women; however, thiazides cross the placental barrier and appear in cord blood. Since animal reproduction studies are not always predictive of human response, HydroDIURIL should be used during pregnancy only if clearly needed. (See INDICATIONS AND USAGE.)

Nonteratogenic effects: These may include fetal or neonatal jaundice, thrombocytopenia, and possibly other adverse reactions which have occurred in the adult.

Nursing Mothers

Because of the potential for serious adverse reactions in nursing infants from HydroDIURIL, a decision should be made whether to discontinue nursing or to discontinue the drug, taking into account the importance of the drug to the mother.

ADVERSE REACTIONS

The following adverse reactions have been reported and, within each category, are listed in order of decreasing severity.

Body as a Whole: Weakness.

Cardiovascular: Hypotension including orthostatic hypotension (may be aggravated by alcohol, barbiturates, narcotics or antihypertensive drugs).

Digestive: Pancreatitis, jaundice (intrahepatic cholestatic jaundice), diarrhea, vomiting, sialadenitis, cramping, constipation, gastric irritation, nausea, anorexia.

Hematologic: Aplastic anemia, agranulocytosis, leukopenia, hemolytic anemia, thrombocytopenia.

Hypersensitivity: Anaphylactic reactions, necrotizing angiitis (vasculitis and cutaneous vasculitis), respiratory distress including pneumonitis and pulmonary edema, photosensitivity, fever, urticaria, rash, purpura.

Metabolic: Electrolyte imbalance (see PRECAUTIONS), hyperglycemia, glycosuria, hyperuricemia.

Musculoskeletal: Muscle spasm.

Nervous System/Psychiatric: Vertigo, paresthesias, dizziness, headache, restlessness.

Renal: Renal failure, renal dysfunction, interstitial nephritis. (See WARNINGS.)

Special Senses: Transient blurred vision, xanthopsia.

Whenever adverse reactions are moderate or severe, thiazide dosage should be reduced or therapy withdrawn.

OVERDOSAGE

The oral LD_{50} of hydrochlorothiazide is greater than 10 g/kg in the mouse and rat.

The most common signs and symptoms observed are those caused by electrolyte depletion (hypokalemia, hypochloremia, hyponatremia) and dehydration resulting from excessive diuresis. If digitalis has also been administered, hypokalemia may accentuate cardiac arrhythmias.

In the event of overdosage, symptomatic and supportive measures should be employed. Emesis should be induced or gastric lavage performed. Correct dehydration, electrolyte imbalance, hepatic coma and hypotension by established procedures. If required, give oxygen or artificial respiration for respiratory impairment.

DOSAGE AND ADMINISTRATION

Therapy should be individualized according to patient response. Use the smallest dosage necessary to achieve the required response.

Adults

For Diuresis

The usual adult dosage is 50 to 100 mg once or twice a day. Many patients with edema respond to intermittent therapy, i.e., administration on alternate days or on three to five days each week. With an intermittent schedule, excessive response and the resulting undesirable electrolyte imbalance are less likely to occur.

For Control of Hypertension

The usual adult starting dosage is 50 or 100 mg a day as a single or divided dose. Dosage is increased or decreased according to blood pressure response. Rarely some patients may require up to 200 mg a day in divided doses.

Patients usually do not require doses in excess of 50 mg of hydrochlorothiazide daily when used concomitantly with other antihypertensive agents.

Infants and Children

The usual pediatric dosage is based on 1.0 mg of HydroDIURIL per pound of body weight per day in two doses. Infants under 6 months of age may require up to 1.5 mg per pound per day in two doses.

On this basis, infants up to 2 years of age may be given 12.5 to 37.5 mg daily in two doses. Children from 2 to 12 years of age may be given 37.5 to 100 mg daily in two doses. Dosage in both age groups should be based on body weight.

HOW SUPPLIED

No. 3263—Tablets HydroDIURIL, 25 mg, are peach-colored, round, scored, compressed tablets, coded MSD 42. They are supplied as follows:

NDC 0006-0042-68 bottles of 100

NDC 0006-0042-28 unit dose packages of 100

NDC 0006-0042-82 bottles of 1000.

Shown in Product Identification Section, page 419

No. 3264—Tablets HydroDIURIL, 50 mg, are peach-colored, round, scored, compressed tablets, coded MSD 105. They are supplied as follows:

NDC 0006-0105-68 bottles of 100

NDC 0006-0105-28 unit dose packages of 100

NDC 0006-0105-82 bottles of 1000

NDC 0006-0105-86 bottles of 5000.

Shown in Product Identification Section, page 419

No. 3340—Tablets HydroDIURIL, 100 mg, are peach-colored, round, scored, compressed tablets, coded MSD 410. They are supplied as follows:

NDC 0006-0410-68 bottles of 100.

Shown in Product Identification Section, page 419

A.H.F.S. Category: 40:28

DC 7398042 Issued October 1987

COPYRIGHT © MERCK & CO., INC., 1986

HYDROPRES® Tablets ℞
(Reserpine-Hydrochlorothiazide), U.S.P.

WARNING

This fixed combination drug is not indicated for initial therapy of hypertension. Hypertension requires therapy titrated to the individual patient. If the fixed combination represents the dosage so determined, its use may be more convenient in patient management. The treatment of hypertension is not static, but must be re-evaluated as conditions in each patient warrant.

DESCRIPTION

HYDROPRES* (Reserpine-Hydrochlorothiazide) combines two antihypertensives: HydroDIURIL* (Hydrochlorothiazide) and reserpine.

Hydrochlorothiazide

Hydrochlorothiazide is a diuretic and antihypertensive. It is the 3,4-dihydro derivative of chlorothiazide. Its chemical name is 6-chloro-3,4-dihydro-2H -1,2,4-benzothiadiazine-7-sulfonamide 1,1-dioxide. Its empirical formula is $C_7H_8ClN_3O_4S_2$ and its structural formula is:

Hydrochlorothiazide is a white, or practically white, crystalline powder with a molecular weight of 297.72, which is slightly soluble in water, but freely soluble in sodium hydroxide solution.

Reserpine

The chemical name for reserpine is (11, 17α-dimethoxy -18β-[(3,4,5-trimethoxybenzoyl) oxy]-3β, 20α-yohimban-16β-carboxylic acid methyl ester). It is a crystalline alkaloid derived from Rauwolfia serpentina. Its empirical formula is $C_{33}H_{40}N_2O_9$ and its structural formula is:

Reserpine is a white or pale buff to slightly yellowish, odorless, crystalline powder with a molecular weight of 608.69, is insoluble in water, and freely soluble in glacial acetic acid.

HYDROPRES is supplied as tablets in two strengths for oral use:

HYDROPRES 25, contains 25 mg of hydrochlorothiazide and 0.125 mg of reserpine.

HYDROPRES 50, contains 50 mg of hydrochlorothiazide and 0.125 mg of reserpine.
Each tablet contains the following inactive ingredients: calcium phosphate, D&C Yellow 10, FD&C Blue 1, FD&C Yellow 6, lactose, magnesium stearate, starch and talc.

*Registered trademark of MERCK & CO., INC.

CLINICAL PHARMACOLOGY

Hydrochlorothiazide
The mechanism of the antihypertensive effect of thiazides is unknown. Hydrochlorothiazide does not usually affect normal blood pressure.
Hydrochlorothiazide affects the distal renal tubular mechanism of electrolyte reabsorption. At maximal therapeutic dosage all thiazides are approximately equal in their diuretic efficacy.
Hydrochlorothiazide increases excretion of sodium and chloride in approximately equivalent amounts. Natriuresis may be accompanied by some loss of potassium and bicarbonate.
After oral use, diuresis begins within 2 hours, peaks in about 4 hours and lasts about 6 to 12 hours.
Reserpine
Reserpine has antihypertensive, bradycardic, and tranquilizing properties. It lowers arterial blood pressure by depletion of catecholamines. Reserpine is beneficial in relieving anxiety, tension, and headache in the hypertensive patient. It acts at the hypothalamic level of the central nervous system to promote relaxation without hypnosis or analgesia. The sleep pattern shown by the electroencephalogram following barbiturates does not occur with this drug. In laboratory animals spontaneous activity and response to external stimuli are decreased, but confusion or difficulty of movement is not evident.
The bradycardic action of reserpine promotes relaxation and may eliminate sinus tachycardia. It is most pronounced in subjects with sinus tachycardia and usually is not prominent in persons with a normal pulse rate.
Miosis, relaxation of the nictitating membrane, ptosis, hypothermia, and increased gastrointestinal activity are noted in animals given reserpine, sometimes in subclinical doses. None of these effects, except increased gastrointestinal activity, has been found to be clinically significant in man with therapeutic doses.
Pharmacokinetics and Metabolism
Hydrochlorothiazide
Hydrochlorothiazide is not metabolized but is eliminated rapidly by the kidney. When plasma levels have been followed for at least 24 hours, the plasma half-life has been observed to vary between 5.6 and 14.8 hours. At least 61 percent of the oral dose is eliminated unchanged within 24 hours. Hydrochlorothiazide crosses the placental but not the blood-brain barrier and is excreted in breast milk.
Reserpine
Oral reserpine is rapidly absorbed from the gastrointestinal tract. Methylreserpate and trimethoxybenzoic acid are the primary metabolites which result from the hydrolytic cleavage of reserpine. Maximal blood levels were achieved approximately 2 hours after the oral dosage of ^{3}H-reserpine to six normal volunteers; within 96 hours approximately 8 percent was excreted in urine and 62 percent in feces. Reserpine appears in human breast milk. Reserpine crosses the placental barrier in guinea pigs.

INDICATION AND USAGE

Hypertension (see box warning).
Use in Pregnancy. Routine use of diuretics during normal pregnancy is inappropriate and exposes mother and fetus to unnecessary hazard. Diuretics do not prevent development of toxemia of pregnancy and there is no satisfactory evidence that they are useful in the treatment of toxemia.
Edema during pregnancy may arise from pathologic causes or from the physiologic and mechanical consequences of pregnancy. Thiazides are indicated in pregnancy when edema is due to pathologic causes, just as they are in the absence of pregnancy (see PRECAUTIONS, *Pregnancy*).
Dependent edema in pregnancy, resulting from restriction of venous return by the gravid uterus, is properly treated through elevation of the lower extremities and use of support stockings. Use of diuretics to lower intravascular volume in this instance is illogical and unnecessary. During normal pregnancy there is hypervolemia which is not harmful to the fetus or the mother in the absence of cardiovascular disease. However, it may be associated with edema, rarely generalized edema. If such edema causes discomfort, increased recumbency will often provide relief. Rarely this edema may cause extreme discomfort which is not relieved by rest. In these instances, a short course of diuretic therapy may provide relief and be appropriate.

CONTRAINDICATIONS

Hydrochlorothiazide is contraindicated in anuria.
HYDROPRES is contraindicated in hypersensitivity to hydrochlorothiazide or other sulfonamide-derived drugs or to reserpine.
Electroshock therapy should not be given to patients while on reserpine, as severe and even fatal reactions have been reported with minimal convulsive electroshock dosage. After discontinuing reserpine, allow at least seven days before starting electroshock therapy.
Active peptic ulcer, ulcerative colitis, and active mental depression, especially suicidal tendencies, are contraindications to reserpine therapy.

WARNINGS

Hydrochlorothiazide
Use with caution in severe renal disease. In patients with renal disease, thiazides may precipitate azotemia. Cumulative effects of the drug may develop in patients with impaired renal function.
Thiazides should be used with caution in patients with impaired hepatic function or progressive liver disease, since minor alterations of fluid and electrolyte balance may precipitate hepatic coma.
Thiazides may add to or potentiate the action of other antihypertensive drugs.
Sensitivity reactions may occur in patients with or without a history of allergy or bronchial asthma.
The possibility of exacerbation or activation of systemic lupus erythematosus has been reported.
Lithium generally should not be given with diuretics (see PRECAUTIONS, *Drug Interactions*).
Reserpine
The occurrence of mental depression due to reserpine in doses of 0.25 mg daily or less is unusual. In any event, HYDROPRES should be discontinued at the first sign of depression.

PRECAUTIONS

General
Hydrochlorothiazide
All patients receiving diuretic therapy should be observed for evidence of fluid or electrolyte imbalance: namely, hyponatremia, hypochloremic alkalosis, and hypokalemia. Serum and urine electrolyte determinations are particularly important when the patient is vomiting excessively or receiving parenteral fluids. Warning signs or symptoms of fluid and electrolyte imbalance irrespective of cause, include dryness of mouth, thirst, weakness, lethargy, drowsiness, restlessness, muscle pains or cramps, muscular fatigue, hypotension, oliguria, tachycardia, and gastrointestinal disturbances such as nausea and vomiting.
Hypokalemia may develop, especially with brisk diuresis, when severe cirrhosis is present or after prolonged therapy. Interference with adequate oral electrolyte intake will contribute to hypokalemia. Hypokalemia may cause cardiac arrhythmia and may also sensitize or exaggerate the response of the heart to the toxic effects of digitalis (e.g., increased ventricular irritability). Hypokalemia may be avoided or treated by use of potassium sparing diuretic or potassium supplements such as foods with a high potassium content.
Although any chloride deficit is generally mild and usually does not require specific treatment except under extraordinary circumstances (as in liver disease or renal disease), chloride replacement may be required in the treatment of metabolic alkalosis.
Dilutional hyponatremia may occur in edematous patients in hot weather. Appropriate therapy is water restriction, rather than administration of salt, except in rare instances when the hyponatremia is life threatening. In actual salt depletion, appropriate replacement is the therapy of choice.
Hyperuricemia may occur or acute gout may be precipitated in certain patients receiving thiazides.
In diabetic patients dosage adjustment of insulin or oral hypoglycemic agents may be required. Hyperglycemia may occur with thiazide diuretics. Thus latent diabetes mellitus may become manifest during thiazide therapy.
The antihypertensive effect of the drug may be enhanced in the postsympathectomy patient.
If progressive renal impairment becomes evident, consider withholding or discontinuing diuretic therapy.
Thiazides have been shown to increase the urinary excretion of magnesium; this may result in hypomagnesemia.
Thiazides may decrease urinary calcium excretion. Thiazides may cause intermittent and slight elevation of serum calcium in the absence of known disorders of calcium metabolism. Marked hypercalcemia may be evidence of hidden hyperparathyroidism. Thiazides should be discontinued before carrying out tests for parathyroid function.
Increases in cholesterol and triglyceride levels may be associated with thiazide diuretic therapy.
Reserpine
Since reserpine may increase gastric secretion and motility, it should be used cautiously in patients with a history of peptic ulcer, ulcerative colitis, or other gastrointestinal disorder. This compound may precipitate biliary colic in patients with gallstones, or bronchial asthma in susceptible persons.
Reserpine may cause hypotension including orthostatic hypotension.
Anxiety or depression, as well as psychosis, may develop during reserpine therapy. If depression is present when therapy is begun, it may be aggravated. Mental depression is unusual with reserpine doses of 0.25 mg daily or less. In any case, HYDROPRES should be discontinued at the first sign of depression. Extreme caution should be used in treating patients with a history of mental depression, and the possibility of suicide should be kept in mind.
As with most antihypertensive therapy, caution should be exercised when treating hypertensive patients with renal insufficiency, since they adjust poorly to lowered blood pressure.
When two or more antihypertensives are given, the individual dosages may have to be reduced to prevent excessive drop in blood pressure. In hypertensive patients with coronary artery disease, it is important to avoid a precipitous drop in blood pressure.
Laboratory Tests
Periodic determination of serum electrolytes to detect possible electrolyte imbalance should be done at appropriate intervals.
Drug Interactions
Hydrochlorothiazide
When given concurrently the following drugs may interact with thiazide diuretics.
Alcohol, barbiturates, or narcotics—potentiation of orthostatic hypotension may occur.
Antidiabetic drugs (oral agents and insulin)—dosage adjustment of the antidiabetic drug may be required.
Other antihypertensive drugs—additive effect or potentiation.
Corticosteroids, ACTH—intensified electrolyte depletion, particularly hypokalemia.
Pressor amines (e.g., norepinephrine)—possible decreased response to pressor amines but not sufficient to preclude their use.
Skeletal muscle relaxants, nondepolarizing (e.g., tubocurarine)—possible increased responsiveness to the muscle relaxant.
Lithium—generally should not be given with diuretics. Diuretic agents reduce the renal clearance of lithium and add a high risk of lithium toxicity. Refer to the package insert for lithium preparations before use of such preparations with HYDROPRES.
Non-steroidal Anti-inflammatory Drugs—In some patients, the administration of a non-steroidal anti-inflammatory agent can reduce the diuretic, natriuretic, and antihypertensive effects of loop, potassium-sparing and thiazide diuretics. Therefore, when HYDROPRES and non-steroidal anti-inflammatory agents are used concomitantly, the patient should be observed closely to determine if the desired effect of the diuretic is obtained.
Reserpine
In hypertensive patients on reserpine therapy significant hypotension and bradycardia may develop during surgical anesthesia. The anesthesiologist should be aware that reserpine has been taken, since it may be necessary to give vagal blocking agents parenterally to prevent or reverse hypotension and/or bradycardia.
Use reserpine cautiously with digitalis and quinidine; cardiac arrhythmias have occurred with reserpine preparations.
Barbiturates enhance the central nervous system depressant effects of reserpine.
Drug/Laboratory Test Interactions
Thiazides should be discontinued before carrying out tests for parathyroid function (see PRECAUTIONS, *General*).
Carcinogenesis, Mutagenesis, Impairment of Fertility
Long-term carcinogenic or mutagenic studies have not been done with HYDROPRES.
In a two-litter study in the rat at an oral dose of 5.0/0.25 mg/kg, the combination of hydrochlorothiazide/reserpine did not impair fertility or produce abnormalities in the fetus.
Hydrochlorothiazide
Hydrochlorothiazide is currently under study in the U.S. Carcinogenesis Testing Program.
Hydrochlorothiazide was not mutagenic *in vitro*, in the Ames microbial mutagen test at a maximum concentration of 5 mg/plate using Strains TA98 and TA100. Urine samples

Continued on next page

Information on the Merck & Co. products listed on these pages is the full prescribing information from product circulars in use October 1, 1992.

Merck & Co.—Cont.

from patients treated with hydrochlorothiazide did not have mutagenic activity in the Ames test.

The ability of a number of drugs to induce nondisjunction and crossing-over was measured with *Aspergillus nidulans.* A large number of drugs, including hydrochlorothiazide, induced nondisjunction.

Hydrochlorothiazide had no effect on fertility in a two-litter study in rats at doses of 4–5.6 mg/kg/day (up to 2 times the maximum recommended human dose).

Reserpine

Reserpine at a concentration of 1 to 5000 mcg/plate had no mutagenic activity against four strains of S. typhimurium *in vitro* in the Ames microbial mutagen test with or without metabolic activation. Reserpine did not induce malignant transformation of mouse fibroblasts *in vitro* at concentrations of 0.3 to 10 mcg/mL.

A few chromosomal aberrations were induced by reserpine *in vitro* in cultured mouse mammary carcinoma cells but were considered negative in this study. The drug did not produce chromosomal aberrations in human peripheral leucocyte cultures although an increase in mitotic figures occurred. One study reported chromosomal aberrations and dominant lethal mutations in mice at doses up to 10 mg/kg of reserpine in the form of a pharmaceutical preparation. Another study did not show dominant lethal mutations in mice at IP doses of 0.92 and 4.6 mg/kg of reserpine. Reserpine did not impair fertility in a two-litter study in the rat at an oral dose of 0.25 mg/kg (35 times the maximum recommended human dose).

Rodent studies have shown that reserpine is an animal tumorigen, causing an increased incidence of mammary fibroadenomas in female mice, malignant tumors of the seminal vesicles in male mice, and malignant adrenal medullary tumors in male rats. These findings arose in 2 year studies in which the drug was administered in the feed at concentrations of 5 and 10 ppm—about 100 to 300 times the usual human dose. The breast neoplasms are thought to be related to reserpine's prolactin-elevating effect. Several other prolactin-elevating drugs have also been associated with an increased incidence of mammary neoplasia in rodents.

The extent to which these findings indicate a risk to humans is uncertain. Tissue culture experiments show that about one-third of human breast tumors are prolactin-dependent *in vitro,* a factor of considerable importance if the use of the drug is contemplated in a patient with previously detected breast cancer. The possibility of an increased risk of breast cancer in reserpine users has been studied extensively; however, no firm conclusion has emerged. Although a few epidemiologic studies have suggested a slightly increased risk (less than twofold in all studies except one) in women who have used reserpine, other studies of generally similar design have not confirmed this. Epidemiologic studies conducted using other drugs (neuroleptic agents) that, like reserpine, increase prolactin levels and therefore would be considered rodent mammary carcinogens, have not shown an association between chronic administration of the drug and human mammary tumorigenesis. While long-term clinical observation has not suggested such an association, the available evidence is considered too limited to be conclusive at this time. An association of reserpine intake with pheochromocytoma or tumors of the seminal vesicles has not been explored.

Pregnancy

Teratogenic Effects —Pregnancy Category C: HYDROPRES may cause fetal harm when given to a pregnant woman. There are no adequate and well-controlled studies in pregnant women. HYDROPRES should be used during pregnancy only if the potential benefit justifies the potential risk to the fetus. (See INDICATIONS AND USAGE.)

Reserpine: Reproduction studies in rats have shown that reserpine is teratogenic at doses of 1–2 mg/kg (125 to 250 times the maximum recommended human dose) IM or IP given early in pregnancy. A variety of abnormalities was produced including anophthalmia, absence of the axial skeleton, hydronephrosis, etc. Pregnancy in rabbits was interrupted when doses as low as 0.04 mg/kg (10 times the maximum recommended human dose) were given early or late in pregnancy.

Hydrochlorothiazide: Thiazides cross the placental barrier and appear in cord blood.

Reproduction studies in the rabbit, the mouse and the rat at doses up to 100 mg/kg/day (50 times the maximum recommended human dose) showed no evidence of external abnormalities of the fetus due to hydrochlorothiazide. Hydrochlorothiazide given in a two-litter study in rats at doses of 4–5.6 mg/kg/day (approximately 1–2 times the maximum recommended human dose) did not impair fertility or produce abnormalities in the offspring.

Nonteratogenic Effects

Reserpine: Reserpine has been demonstrated to cross the placental barrier in guinea pigs with depression of adrenal catecholamine stores in the newborn. There is some evidence that side effects such as nasal congestion, lethargy, de-

pressed Moro reflex, and bradycardia may appear in infants born of reserpine-treated mothers.

Hydrochlorothiazide: These may include fetal or neonatal jaundice, thrombocytopenia, and possibly other adverse reactions which have occurred in the adult.

Nursing Mothers

Thiazides and reserpine appear in breast milk. Because of the potential for serious adverse reactions in nursing infants from HYDROPRES, a decision should be made whether to discontinue nursing or to discontinue the drug, taking into account the importance of the drug to the mother.

Pediatric Use

Safety and effectiveness of HYDROPRES in children has not been established.

ADVERSE REACTIONS

The following adverse reactions have been reported and, within each category, are listed in order of decreasing severity.

Hydrochlorothiazide

Body as a Whole: Weakness.

Cardiovascular: Hypotension including orthostatic hypotension (may be aggravated by alcohol, barbiturates, narcotics or antihypertensive drugs).

Digestive: Pancreatitis, jaundice (intrahepatic cholestatic jaundice), diarrhea, vomiting, sialadenitis, cramping, constipation, gastric irritation, nausea, anorexia.

Hematologic: Aplastic anemia, agranulocytosis, leukopenia, hemolytic anemia, thrombocytopenia.

Hypersensitivity: Anaphylactic reactions, necrotizing angiitis (vasculitis and cutaneous vasculitis), respiratory distress including pneumonitis and pulmonary edema, photosensitivity, fever, urticaria, rash, purpura.

Metabolic: Electrolyte imbalance (see PRECAUTIONS), hyperglycemia, glycosuria, hyperuricemia.

Musculoskeletal: Muscle spasm.

Nervous System/Psychiatric: Vertigo, paresthesias, dizziness, headache, restlessness.

Renal: Renal failure, renal dysfunction, interstitial nephritis. (See WARNINGS.)

Special Senses: Transient blurred vision, xanthopsia.

Whenever adverse reactions are moderate or severe, thiazide dosage should be reduced or therapy withdrawn.

Reserpine

Cardiovascular: Angina pectoris, arrhythmia, premature ventricular contractions, other direct cardiac effects (e.g., fluid retention, congestive heart failure), bradycardia.

Digestive: Vomiting, diarrhea, nausea, hypersecretion and increased motility, anorexia, dryness of mouth, increased salivation.

Hematologic: Thrombocytopenic purpura, excessive bleeding following prostatic surgery.

Hypersensitivity: Pruritus, rash, flushing of skin.

Metabolic: Weight gain.

Musculoskeletal: Muscular aches.

Nervous System/Psychiatric: Mental depression, dull sensorium, syncope, paradoxical anxiety, excessive sedation, nightmares, headache, dizziness, nervousness, parkinsonism (usually reversible with decreased dosage or discontinuance of therapy).

Respiratory: Dyspnea, epistaxis, nasal congestion, enhanced susceptibility to colds.

Special Senses: Optic atrophy, uveitis, deafness, glaucoma, conjunctival injection, blurred vision.

Urogenital: Dysuria, impotence, decreased libido, nonpuerperal lactation.

OVERDOSAGE

Overdosage may lead to excessive sedation, mental depression, severe hypotension, extrapyramidal reactions.

There is no specific antidote. In the event of overdosage, symptomatic and supportive measures should be employed. Emesis should be induced or gastric lavage performed. Correct dehydration, electrolyte imbalance, hepatic coma and hypotension by established procedures. If required, give oxygen or artificial respiration for respiratory impairment. In the event of severe hypotension from the reserpine component, intravenous use of a vasopressor is indicated [e.g., ARAMINE® (Metaraminol Bitartrate, MSD), levarterenol, phenylephrine]. Anticholinergics may be needed to relieve gastrointestinal distress from reserpine. Because the effects of the rauwolfia alkaloids are prolonged, the patient should be closely observed for at least 72 hours.

The oral LD_{50} of hydrochlorothiazide is greater than 10 g/kg in the mouse and rat. The oral LD_{50} of reserpine in the mouse is 390 mg/kg.

DOSAGE AND ADMINISTRATION

The initial dosage of HYDROPRES should conform to the dosages of the individual components established during titration (see box warning).

The usual adult dosage of HYDROPRES 25 is 1 or 2 tablets once a day; that of HYDROPRES 50 is 1 tablet once a day. Patients usually do not require doses in excess of 50 mg of hydrochlorothiazide daily when combined with other antihypertensive agents. Dosage may require adjustment according to the blood pressure response of the patient.

HOW SUPPLIED

No. 3265—Tablets HYDROPRES 25 are green, round, scored, compressed tablets, coded MSD 53. Each tablet contains 25 mg of hydrochlorothiazide and 0.125 mg of reserpine. They are supplied as follows:
NDC 0006-0053-68 in bottles of 100
NDC 0006-0053-82 in bottles of 1000.
Shown in Product Identification Section, page 419
No. 3266—Tablets HYDROPRES 50 are green, round, scored, compressed tablets, coded MSD 127. Each tablet contains 50 mg of hydrochlorothiazide and 0.125 mg of reserpine. They are supplied as follows:
NDC 0006-0127-68 in bottles of 100
NDC 0006-0127-82 in bottles of 1000.
Shown in Product Identification Section, page 419
Storage
Keep container tightly closed. Protect from light.
    A.H.F.S. Category: 24:08
    DC 7414638   Issued October 1987
COPYRIGHT © MERCK & CO., INC., 1986
All rights reserved

INDOCIN® Capsules, Oral Suspension and   ℞
Suppositories
(Indomethacin), U.S.P.
INDOCIN® SR Capsules   ℞
(Indomethacin), U.S.P.

DESCRIPTION

INDOCIN* (Indomethacin) cannot be considered a simple analgesic and should not be used in conditions other than those recommended under INDICATIONS.

INDOCIN is supplied in four dosage forms. Capsules INDOCIN for oral administration contain either 25 mg or 50 mg of indomethacin and the following inactive ingredients: colloidal silicon dioxide, FD & C Blue 1, FD & C Red 3, gelatin, lactose, lecithin, magnesium stearate, and titanium dioxide. Capsules INDOCIN SR for sustained release oral administration contain 75 mg of indomethacin and the following inactive ingredients: cellulose, confectioner's sugar, FD & C Blue 1, FD & C Blue 2, FD & C Red 3, gelatin, hydroxypropyl methylcellulose, magnesium stearate, polyvinyl acetate-crotonic acid copolymer, starch, and titanium dioxide. Capsules INDOCIN SR conform to the requirements of the USP Drug Release Test 1 for Indomethacin Extended-release Capsules. Suspension INDOCIN for oral use contains 25 mg of indomethacin per 5 mL, alcohol 1%, and sorbic acid 0.1% added as a preservative and the following inactive ingredients: antifoam AF emulsion, flavors, purified water, sodium hydroxide or hydrochloric acid to adjust pH, sorbitol solution, tragacanth. Suppositories INDOCIN for rectal use contain 50 mg of indomethacin and the following inactive ingredients: butylated hydroxyanisole, butylated hydroxytoluene, edetic acid, glycerin, polyethylene glycol 3350, polyethylene glycol 8000 and sodium chloride. Indomethacin is a non-steroidal anti-inflammatory indole derivative designated chemically as 1-(4-chlorobenzoyl)-5-methoxy-2-methyl-1*H*-indole-3-acetic acid. Indomethacin is practically insoluble in water and sparingly soluble in alcohol. It has a pKa of 4.5 and is stable in neutral or slightly acidic media and decomposes in strong alkali. The suspension has a pH of 4.0–5.0. The structural formula is:

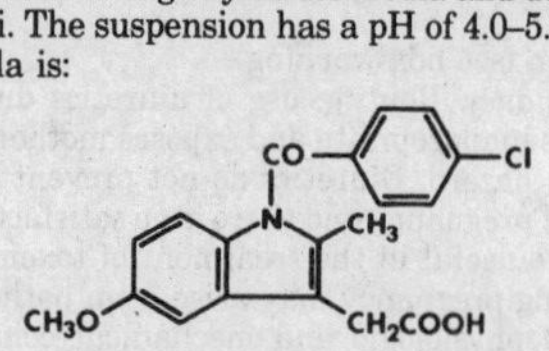

*Registered trademark of MERCK & CO., INC.

CLINICAL PHARMACOLOGY

INDOCIN is a non-steroidal drug with anti-inflammatory, antipyretic and analgesic properties. Its mode of action, like that of other anti-inflammatory drugs, is not known. However, its therapeutic action is not due to pituitary-adrenal stimulation.

INDOCIN is a potent inhibitor of prostaglandin synthesis *in vitro.* Concentrations are reached during therapy which have been demonstrated to have an effect *in vivo* as well. Prostaglandins sensitize afferent nerves and potentiate the action of bradykinin in inducing pain in animal models.

Moreover, prostaglandins are known to be among the mediators of inflammation. Since indomethacin is an inhibitor of prostaglandin synthesis, its mode of action may be due to a decrease of prostaglandins in peripheral tissues.

INDOCIN has been shown to be an effective anti-inflammatory agent, appropriate for long-term use in rheumatoid arthritis, ankylosing spondylitis, and osteoarthritis.

INDOCIN affords relief of symptoms; it does not alter the progressive course of the underlying disease.

INDOCIN suppresses inflammation in rheumatoid arthritis as demonstrated by relief of pain, and reduction of fever, swelling and tenderness. Improvement in patients treated with INDOCIN for rheumatoid arthritis has been demonstrated by a reduction in joint swelling, average number of joints involved, and morning stiffness; by increased mobility as demonstrated by a decrease in walking time; and by improved functional capability as demonstrated by an increase in grip strength.

Indomethacin has been reported to diminish basal and CO_2 stimulated cerebral blood flow in healthy volunteers following acute oral and intravenous administration. In one study after one week of treatment with orally administered indomethacin, this effect on basal cerebral blood flow had disappeared. The clinical significance of this effect has not been established.

Capsules INDOCIN have been found effective in relieving the pain, reducing the fever, swelling, redness, and tenderness of acute gouty arthritis. Capsules INDOCIN rather than Capsules INDOCIN SR are recommended for treatment of acute gouty arthritis—see INDICATIONS.

Following single oral doses of Capsules INDOCIN 25 mg or 50 mg, indomethacin is readily absorbed, attaining peak plasma concentrations of about 1 and 2 mcg/mL, respectively, at about 2 hours. Orally administered Capsules INDOCIN are virtually 100% bioavailable, with 90% of the dose absorbed within 4 hours. A single 50 mg dose of Oral Suspension INDOCIN was found to be bioequivalent to a 50 mg INDOCIN capsule when each was administered with food.

Capsules INDOCIN SR 75 mg are designed to release 25 mg of the drug initially and the remaining 50 mg over approximately 12 hours (90% of dose absorbed by 12 hours). When measured over a 24-hour period, the cumulative amount and time-course of indomethacin absorption from a single Capsule INDOCIN SR are comparable to those of 3 doses of 25 mg Capsules INDOCIN given at 4–6 hour intervals.

Plasma concentrations of indomethacin fluctuate less and are more sustained following administration of Capsules INDOCIN SR than following administration of 25 mg Capsules INDOCIN given at 4–6 hour intervals. In multiple-dose comparisons, the mean daily steady-state plasma level of indomethacin attained with daily administration of Capsules INDOCIN SR 75 mg was indistinguishable from that following Capsules INDOCIN 25 mg given at 0, 6 and 12 hours daily. However, there was a significant difference in indomethacin plasma levels between the two dosage regimens especially after 12 hours.

Controlled clinical studies of safety and efficacy in patients with osteoarthritis have shown that one Capsule INDOCIN SR was clinically comparable to one 25 mg Capsule INDOCIN t.i.d.; and in controlled clinical studies in patients with rheumatoid arthritis, one Capsule INDOCIN SR taken in the morning and one in the evening were clinically indistinguishable from one 50 mg Capsule INDOCIN t.i.d.

Indomethacin is eliminated via renal excretion, metabolism, and biliary excretion. Indomethacin undergoes appreciable enterohepatic circulation. The mean half-life of indomethacin is estimated to be about 4.5 hours. With a typical therapeutic regimen of 25 or 50 mg t.i.d., the steady-state plasma concentrations of indomethacin are an average 1.4 times those following the first dose.

The rate of absorption is more rapid from the rectal suppository than from Capsules INDOCIN. Ordinarily, therefore, the total amount absorbed from the suppository would be expected to be at least equivalent to the capsule. In controlled clinical trials, however, the amount of indomethacin absorbed was found to be somewhat less (80–90%) than that absorbed from Capsules INDOCIN. This is probably because some subjects did not retain the material from the suppository for the one hour necessary to assure complete absorption. Since the suppository dissolves rather quickly rather than melting slowly, it is seldom recovered in recognizable form if the patient retains the suppository for more than a few minutes.

Indomethacin exists in the plasma as the parent drug and its desmethyl, desbenzoyl, and desmethyl-desbenzoyl metabolites, all in the unconjugated form. About 60 percent of an oral dosage is recovered in urine as drug and metabolites (26 percent as indomethacin and its glucuronide), and 33 percent is recovered in feces (1.5 percent as indomethacin).

About 99% of indomethacin is bound to protein in plasma over the expected range of therapeutic plasma concentrations.

In a gastroscopic study in 45 healthy subjects, the number of gastric mucosal abnormalities was significantly higher in the group receiving Capsules INDOCIN than in the group taking Suppositories INDOCIN or placebo.

In a double-blind comparative clinical study involving 175 patients with rheumatoid arthritis, however, the incidence of upper gastrointestinal adverse effects with Suppositories or Capsules INDOCIN was comparable. The incidence of lower gastrointestinal adverse effects was greater in the suppository group.

INDICATIONS

Indomethacin has been found effective in active stages of the following:
1. Moderate to severe rheumatoid arthritis including acute flares of chronic disease.
2. Moderate to severe ankylosing spondylitis.
3. Moderate to severe osteoarthritis.
4. Acute painful shoulder (bursitis and/or tendinitis).
5. Acute gouty arthritis.

Capsules INDOCIN SR are recommended for all of the indications for Capsules INDOCIN except acute gouty arthritis.

INDOCIN may enable the reduction of steroid dosage in patients receiving steroids for the more severe forms of rheumatoid arthritis. In such instances the steroid dosage should be reduced slowly and the patients followed very closely for any possible adverse effects.

The use of INDOCIN in conjunction with aspirin or other salicylates is not recommended. Controlled clinical studies have shown that the combined use of INDOCIN and aspirin does not produce any greater therapeutic effect than the use of INDOCIN alone. Furthermore, in one of these clinical studies, the incidence of gastrointestinal side effects was significantly increased with combined therapy (see DRUG INTERACTIONS).

CONTRAINDICATIONS

INDOCIN should not be used in:
Patients who are hypersensitive to this product.
Patients in whom acute asthmatic attacks, urticaria, or rhinitis are precipitated by aspirin or other non-steroidal anti-inflammatory agents.
Suppositories INDOCIN are contraindicated in patients with a history of proctitis or recent rectal bleeding.

WARNINGS

General:
Because of the variability of the potential of INDOCIN to cause adverse reactions in the individual patient, the following are strongly recommended:
1. The lowest possible effective dose for the individual patient should be prescribed. Increased dosage tends to increase adverse effects, particularly in doses over 150–200 mg/day, without corresponding increase in clinical benefits.
2. Careful instructions to, and observations of, the individual patient are essential to the prevention of serious adverse reactions. As advancing years appear to increase the possibility of adverse reactions, INDOCIN should be used with greater care in the aged.
3. Effectiveness of INDOCIN in children has not been established. INDOCIN should not be prescribed for children 14 years of age and younger unless toxicity or lack of efficacy associated with other drugs warrants the risk.
   In experience with more than 900 children reported in the literature or to Merck Sharp and Dohme who were treated with Capsules INDOCIN, side effects in children were comparable to those reported in adults. Experience in children has been confined to the use of Capsules INDOCIN. If a decision is made to use indomethacin for children two years of age or older, such patients should be monitored closely and periodic assessment of liver function is recommended. There have been cases of hepatotoxicity reported in children with juvenile rheumatoid arthritis, including fatalities.
   If indomethacin treatment is instituted, a suggested starting dose is 2 mg/kg/day given in divided doses. Maximum daily dosage should not exceed 4 mg/kg/day or 150–200 mg/day, whichever is less. As symptoms subside, the total daily dosage should be reduced to the lowest level required to control symptoms, or the drug should be discontinued.
4. If Capsules INDOCIN SR are used for initial therapy or during dosage adjustment, observe the patient closely (see DOSAGE AND ADMINISTRATION).

Gastrointestinal Effects:
Single or multiple ulcerations, including perforation and hemorrhage of the esophagus, stomach, duodenum or small and large intestine, have been reported to occur with INDOCIN. Fatalities have been reported in some instances. Rarely, intestinal ulceration has been associated with stenosis and obstruction.
Gastrointestinal bleeding without obvious ulcer formation and perforation of pre-existing sigmoid lesions (diverticulum, carcinoma, etc.) have occurred. Increased abdominal pain in ulcerative colitis patients or the development of ulcerative colitis and regional ileitis have been reported to occur rarely.

Because of the occurrence, and at times severity, of gastrointestinal reactions to INDOCIN, the prescribing physician must be continuously alert for any sign or symptom signaling a possible gastrointestinal reaction. The risks of continuing therapy with INDOCIN in the face of such symptoms must be weighed against the possible benefits to the individual patient.

INDOCIN should not be given to patients with active gastrointestinal lesions or with a history of recurrent gastrointestinal lesions except under circumstances which warrant the very high risk and where patients can be monitored very closely.

The gastrointestinal effects may be reduced by giving Capsules INDOCIN or Capsules INDOCIN SR immediately after meals, with food, or with antacids.

Risk of GI Ulcerations, Bleeding and Perforation with NSAID Therapy
Serious gastrointestinal toxicity such as bleeding, ulceration, and perforation, can occur at any time, with or without warning symptoms, in patients treated chronically with NSAID therapy. Although minor upper gastrointestinal problems, such as dyspepsia, are common, usually developing early in therapy, physicians should remain alert for ulceration and bleeding in patients treated chronically with NSAIDs even in the absence of previous GI tract symptoms. In patients observed in clinical trials of several months to two years duration, symptomatic upper GI ulcers, gross bleeding or perforation appear to occur in approximately 1% of patients treated for 3–6 months, and in about 2–4% of patients treated for one year. Physicians should inform patients about the signs and/or symptoms of serious GI toxicity and what steps to take if they occur.

Studies to date have not identified any subset of patients not at risk of developing peptic ulceration and bleeding. Except for a prior history of serious GI events and other risk factors known to be associated with peptic ulcer disease, such as alcoholism, smoking, etc., no risk factors (e.g., age, sex) have been associated with increased risk. Elderly or debilitated patients seem to tolerate ulceration or bleeding less well than other individuals and most spontaneous reports of fatal GI events are in this population. Studies to date are inconclusive concerning the relative risk of various NSAIDs in causing such reactions. High doses of any NSAID probably carry a greater risk of these reactions, although controlled clinical trials showing this do not exist in most cases. In considering the use of relatively large doses (within the recommended dosage range), sufficient benefit should be anticipated to offset the potential increased risk of GI toxicity.

Renal Effects:
As with other non-steroidal anti-inflammatory drugs, long term administration of indomethacin to animals has resulted in renal papillary necrosis and other abnormal renal pathology. In humans, there have been reports of acute interstitial nephritis with hematuria, proteinuria, and occasionally nephrotic syndrome.

A second form of renal toxicity has been seen in patients with prerenal and renal conditions leading to a reduction in renal blood flow or blood volume, where the renal prostaglandins have a supportive role in the maintenance of renal perfusion. In these patients administration of an NSAID may cause a dose dependent reduction in prostaglandin formation and may precipitate overt renal decompensation. Patients at greatest risk of this reaction are those with conditions such as renal or hepatic dysfunction, diabetes mellitus, advanced age, extracellular volume depletion from any cause, congestive heart failure, septicemia, pyelonephritis, or concomitant use of any nephrotoxic drug. INDOCIN or other NSAIDs should be given with caution and renal function should be monitored in any patient who may have reduced renal reserve. Discontinuation of NSAID therapy is typically followed by recovery to the pretreatment state.

Increases in serum potassium concentration, including hyperkalemia, have been reported, even in some patients without renal impairment. In patients with normal renal function, these effects have been attributed to a hyporeninemichypoaldosteronism state (see PRECAUTIONS, *Drug Interactions*).

Since INDOCIN is eliminated primarily by the kidneys, patients with significantly impaired renal function should be closely monitored; a lower daily dosage should be anticipated to avoid excessive drug accumulation.

Ocular Effects:
Corneal deposits and retinal disturbances, including those of the macula, have been observed in some patients who had received prolonged therapy with INDOCIN. The prescribing

Continued on next page

Information on the Merck & Co. products listed on these pages is the full prescribing information from product circulars in use October 1, 1992.

Merck & Co.—Cont.

physician should be alert to the possible association between the changes noted and INDOCIN. It is advisable to discontinue therapy if such changes are observed. Blurred vision may be a significant symptom and warrants a thorough ophthalmological examination. Since these changes may be asymptomatic, ophthalmologic examination at periodic intervals is desirable in patients where therapy is prolonged.

Central Nervous System Effects:
INDOCIN may aggravate depression or other psychiatric disturbances, epilepsy, and parkinsonism, and should be used with considerable caution in patients with these conditions. If severe CNS adverse reactions develop, INDOCIN should be discontinued.

INDOCIN may cause drowsiness; therefore, patients should be cautioned about engaging in activities requiring mental alertness and motor coordination, such as driving a car. INDOCIN may also cause headache. Headache which persists despite dosage reduction requires cessation of therapy with INDOCIN.

Use in Pregnancy and the Neonatal Period
INDOCIN is not recommended for use in pregnant women, since safety for use has not been established, and because of the known effect of drugs of this class on the human fetus (closure of the ductus arteriosus, platelet dysfunction with resultant bleeding, renal dysfunction or failure with oligohydramnios, gastrointestinal bleeding or perforation, and myocardial degenerative changes) during the third trimester of pregnancy.

Teratogenic studies were conducted in mice and rats at dosages of 0.5, 1.0, 2.0, and 4.0 mg/kg/day. Except for retarded fetal ossification at 4 mg/kg/day considered secondary to the decreased average fetal weights, no increase in fetal malformations was observed as compared with control groups. Other studies in mice reported in the literature using higher doses (5 to 15 mg/kg/day) have described maternal toxicity and death, increased fetal resorptions, and fetal malformations. Comparable studies in rodents using high doses of aspirin have shown similar maternal and fetal effects.

As with other non-steroidal anti-inflammatory agents which inhibit prostaglandin synthesis, indomethacin has been found to delay parturition in rats.

In rats and mice, 4.0 mg/kg/day given during the last three days of gestation caused a decrease in maternal weight gain and some maternal and fetal deaths. An increased incidence of neuronal necrosis in the diencephalon in the live-born fetuses was observed. At 2.0 mg/kg/day, no increase in neuronal necrosis was observed as compared to the control groups. Administration of 0.5 or 4.0 mg/kg/day during the first three days of life did not cause an increase in neuronal necrosis at either dose level.

Use in Nursing Mothers
INDOCIN is excreted in the milk of lactating mothers. INDOCIN is not recommended for use in nursing mothers.

PRECAUTIONS

INDOCIN may mask the usual signs and symptoms of infection. Therefore, the physician must be continually on the alert for this and should use the drug with extra care in the presence of existing controlled infection.

Fluid retention and peripheral edema have been observed in some patients taking INDOCIN. Therefore, as with other non-steroidal anti-inflammatory drugs, INDOCIN should be used with caution in patients with cardiac dysfunction, hypertension, or other conditions predisposing to fluid retention.

In a study of patients with severe heart failure and hyponatremia, INDOCIN was associated with significant deterioration of circulatory hemodynamics, presumably due to inhibition of prostaglandin dependent compensatory mechanisms.

INDOCIN, like other non-steroidal anti-inflammatory agents, can inhibit platelet aggregation. This effect is of shorter duration than that seen with aspirin and usually disappears within 24 hours after discontinuation of INDOCIN. INDOCIN has been shown to prolong bleeding time (but within the normal range) in normal subjects. Because this effect may be exaggerated in patients with underlying hemostatic defects, INDOCIN should be used with caution in persons with coagulation defects.

As with other non-steroidal anti-inflammatory drugs, borderline elevations of one or more liver tests may occur in up to 15% of patients. These abnormalities may progress, may remain essentially unchanged, or may be transient with continued therapy. The SGPT (ALT) test is probably the most sensitive indicator of liver dysfunction. Meaningful (3 times the upper limit of normal) elevations of SGPT or SGOT (AST) occurred in controlled clinical trials in less than 1% of patients. A patient with symptoms and/or signs suggesting liver dysfunction, or in whom an abnormal liver test has occurred, should be evaluated for evidence of the development of more severe hepatic reaction while on therapy with INDOCIN. Severe hepatic reactions, including jaundice and

cases of fatal hepatitis, have been reported with INDOCIN as with other non-steroidal anti-inflammatory drugs. Although such reactions are rare, if abnormal liver tests persist or worsen, if clinical signs and symptoms consistent with liver disease develop, or if systemic manifestations occur (e.g., eosinophilia, rash, etc.), INDOCIN should be discontinued.

Information for Patients
INDOCIN, like other drugs of its class, is not free of side effects. The side effects of these drugs can cause discomfort and, rarely, there are more serious side effects such as gastrointestinal bleeding, which may result in hospitalization and even fatal outcomes.

NSAIDs (Non-steroidal Anti-inflammatory Drugs) are often essential agents in the management of arthritis; but they also may be commonly employed for conditions which are less serious.

Physicians may wish to discuss with their patients the potential risks (see WARNINGS, PRECAUTIONS and ADVERSE REACTIONS) and likely benefits of NSAID treatment, particularly when the drugs are used for less serious conditions where treatment without NSAIDs may represent an acceptable alternative to both the patient and physician.

Laboratory Tests
Because serious GI tract ulceration and bleeding can occur without warning symptoms, physicians should follow chronically treated patients for the signs and symptoms of ulceration and bleeding and should inform them of the importance of this follow-up (see WARNINGS, *Risk of GI Ulcerations, Bleeding and Perforation with NSAID Therapy*).

Carcinogenesis, Mutagenesis, Impairment of Fertility
In an 81-week chronic oral toxicity study in the rat at doses up to 1 mg/kg/day, indomethacin had no tumorigenic effect.

Incidence greater than 1%	*Incidence less than 1%*	
GASTROINTESTINAL		
nausea* with or without vomiting	anorexia	gastrointestinal bleeding without obvious ulcer formation and perforation of pre-existing sigmoid lesions (diverticulum, carcinoma, etc.) development of ulcerative colitis and regional ileitis ulcerative stomatitis toxic hepatitis and jaundice (some fatal cases have been reported)
dyspepsia* (including indigestion, heartburn and epigastric pain)	bloating (includes distention)	
diarrhea	flatulence	
abdominal distress or pain	peptic ulcer	
constipation	gastroenteritis	
	rectal bleeding	
	proctitis	
	single or multiple ulcerations, including perforation and hemorrhage of the esophagus, stomach, duodenum or small and large intestines	
	intestinal ulceration associated with stenosis and obstruction	
CENTRAL NERVOUS SYSTEM		
headache (11.7%)	anxiety (includes nervousness)	light-headedness
dizziness*	muscle weakness	syncope
vertigo	involuntary muscle movements	paresthesia
somnolence	insomnia	aggravation of epilepsy and parkinsonism
depression and fatigue (including malaise and listlessness)	muzziness	depersonalization
	psychic disturbances including psychotic episodes	coma
	mental confusion	peripheral neuropathy
	drowsiness	convulsions
		dysarthria
SPECIAL SENSES		
tinnitus	ocular—corneal deposits and retinal disturbances, including those of the macula, have been reported in some patients on prolonged therapy with INDOCIN	blurred vision diplopia hearing disturbances, deafness
CARDIOVASCULAR		
none	hypertension	congestive heart failure
	hypotension	arrhythmia; palpitations
	tachycardia	
	chest pain	
METABOLIC		
none	edema	hyperglycemia
	weight gain	glycosuria
	fluid retention	hyperkalemia
	flushing or sweating	
INTEGUMENTARY		
none	pruritus	exfoliative dermatitis
	rash; urticaria	erythema nodosum
	petechiae or ecchymosis	loss of hair
		Stevens-Johnson syndrome
		erythema multiforme
		toxic epidermal necrolysis
HEMATOLOGIC		
none	leukopenia	aplastic anemia
	bone marrow depression	hemolytic anemia
	anemia secondary to obvious or occult gastrointestinal bleeding	agranulocytosis
		thrombocytopenic purpura
		disseminated intravascular coagulation

Continued

Incidence greater than 1%	*Incidence less than 1%*	
HYPERSENSITIVITY		
none	acute anaphylaxis acute respiratory distress rapid fall in blood pressure resembling a shock-like state angioedema	dyspnea asthma purpura angiitis pulmonary edema fever
GENITOURINARY		
none	hematuria vaginal bleeding proteinuria nephrotic syndrome interstitial nephritis	BUN elevation renal insufficiency, including renal failure
MISCELLANEOUS		
none	epistaxis breast changes, including enlargement and tenderness, or gynecomastia	

*Reactions occurring in 3% to 9% of patients treated with INDOCIN. (Those reactions occurring in less than 3% of the patients are unmarked.)

Indomethacin produced no neoplastic or hyperplastic changes related to treatment in carcinogenic studies in the rat (dosing period 73–110 weeks) and the mouse (dosing period 62–88 weeks) at doses up to 1.5 mg/kg/day.

Indomethacin did not have any mutagenic effect in *in vitro* bacterial tests (Ames test and *E. coli* with or without metabolic activation) and a series of *in vivo* tests including the host-mediated assay, sex-linked recessive lethals in *Drosophila,* and the micronucleus test in mice.

Indomethacin at dosage levels up to 0.5 mg/kg/day had no effect on fertility in mice in a two generation reproduction study or a two litter reproduction study in rats.

Drug Interactions

In normal volunteers receiving indomethacin, the administration of diflunisal decreased the renal clearance and significantly increased the plasma levels of indomethacin. In some patients, combined use of INDOCIN and diflunisal has been associated with fatal gastrointestinal hemorrhage. Therefore, diflunisal and INDOCIN should not be used concomitantly.

In a study in normal volunteers, it was found that chronic concurrent administration of 3.6 g of aspirin per day decreases indomethacin blood levels approximately 20%.

Clinical studies have shown that INDOCIN does not influence the hypoprothrombinemia produced by anticoagulants. However, when any additional drug, including INDOCIN, is added to the treatment of patients on anticoagulant therapy, the patients should be observed for alterations of the prothrombin time.

When INDOCIN is given to patients receiving probenecid, the plasma levels of indomethacin are likely to be increased. Therefore, a lower total daily dosage of INDOCIN may produce a satisfactory therapeutic effect. When increases in the dose of INDOCIN are made, they should be made carefully and in small increments.

Caution should be used if INDOCIN is administered simultaneously with methotrexate. INDOCIN has been reported to decrease the tubular secretion of methotrexate and to potentiate its toxicity.

Administration of non-steroidal anti-inflammatory drugs concomitantly with cyclosporine has been associated with an increase in cyclosporine-induced toxicity, possibly due to decreased synthesis of renal prostacyclin. NSAIDs should be used with caution in patients taking cyclosporine, and renal function should be monitored.

Capsules INDOCIN 50 mg t.i.d. produced a clinically relevant elevation of plasma lithium and reduction in renal lithium clearance in psychiatric patients and normal subjects with steady state plasma lithium concentrations. This effect has been attributed to inhibition of prostaglandin synthesis. As a consequence, when INDOCIN and lithium are given concomitantly, the patient should be carefully observed for signs of lithium toxicity. (Read circulars for lithium preparations before use of such concomitant therapy.) In addition, the frequency of monitoring serum lithium concentration should be increased at the outset of such combination drug treatment.

INDOCIN given concomitantly with digoxin has been reported to increase the serum concentration and prolong the half-life of digoxin. Therefore, when INDOCIN and digoxin are used concomitantly, serum digoxin levels should be closely monitored.

In some patients, the administration of INDOCIN can reduce the diuretic, natriuretic, and, antihypertensive effects of loop, potassium-sparing, and thiazide diuretics. Therefore, when INDOCIN and diuretics are used concomitantly, the patient should be observed closely to determine if the desired effect of the diuretic is obtained.

INDOCIN reduces basal plasma renin activity (PRA), as well as those elevations of PRA induced by furosemide administration, or salt or volume depletion. These facts should be considered when evaluating plasma renin activity in hypertensive patients.

It has been reported that the addition of triamterene to a maintenance schedule of INDOCIN resulted in reversible acute renal failure in two of four healthy volunteers. INDOCIN and triamterene should not be administered together.

INDOCIN and potassium-sparing diuretics each may be associated with increased serum potassium levels. The potential effects of INDOCIN and potassium-sparing diuretics on potassium kinetics and renal function should be considered when these agents are administered concurrently.

Most of the above effects concerning diuretics have been attributed, at least in part, to mechanisms involving inhibition of prostaglandin synthesis by INDOCIN.

Blunting of the antihypertensive effect of beta-adrenoceptor blocking agents by non-steroidal anti-inflammatory drugs including INDOCIN has been reported. Therefore, when using these blocking agents to treat hypertension, patients should be observed carefully in order to confirm that the desired therapeutic effect has been obtained. There are reports that INDOCIN can reduce the antihypertensive effect of captopril in some patients.

False-negative results in the dexamethasone suppression test (DST) in patients being treated with INDOCIN have been reported. Thus, results of the DST should be interpreted with caution in these patients.

Pediatric Use

Effectiveness in children 14 years of age and younger has not been established (see WARNINGS).

ADVERSE REACTIONS

The adverse reactions for Capsules INDOCIN listed in the following table have been arranged into two groups: (1) incidence greater than 1%; and (2) incidence less than 1%. The incidence for group (1) was obtained from 33 double-blind controlled clinical trials reported in the literature (1,092 patients). The incidence for group (2) was based on reports in clinical trials, in the literature, and on voluntary reports since marketing. The probability of a causal relationship exists between INDOCIN and these adverse reactions, some of which have been reported only rarely.

In controlled clinical trials, the incidence of adverse reactions to Capsules INDOCIN SR and equal 24-hour doses of Capsules INDOCIN were similar.

The adverse reactions reported with Capsules INDOCIN may occur with use of the suppositories. In addition, rectal irritation and tenesmus have been reported in patients who have received the suppositories.

The adverse reactions reported with Capsules INDOCIN may also occur with use of the suspension.

[See table.]

Causal relationship unknown: Other reactions have been reported but occurred under circumstances where a causal relationship could not be established. However, in these rarely reported events, the possibility cannot be excluded. Therefore, these observations are being listed to serve as alerting information to physicians:

Cardiovascular: Thrombophlebitis

Hematologic: Although there have been several reports of leukemia, the supporting information is weak.

Genitourinary: Urinary frequency.

OVERDOSAGE

The following symptoms may be observed following overdosage: nausea, vomiting, intense headache, dizziness, mental confusion, disorientation, or lethargy. There have been reports of paresthesias, numbness, and convulsions.

Treatment is symptomatic and supportive. The stomach should be emptied as quickly as possible if the ingestion is recent. If vomiting has not occurred spontaneously, the patient should be induced to vomit with syrup of ipecac. If the patient is unable to vomit, gastric lavage should be performed. Once the stomach has been emptied, 25 or 50 g of activated charcoal may be given. Depending on the condition of the patient, close medical observation and nursing care may be required. The patient should be followed for several days because gastrointestinal ulceration and hemorrhage have been reported as adverse reactions of indomethacin. Use of antacids may be helpful.

The oral LD_{50} of indomethacin in mice and rats (based on 14 day mortality response) was 50 and 12 mg/kg, respectively.

DOSAGE AND ADMINISTRATION

INDOCIN is available as 25 and 50 mg Capsules INDOCIN, 75 mg Capsules INDOCIN SR for oral use, Oral Suspension INDOCIN, containing 25 mg of indomethacin per 5 mL, and 50 mg Suppositories INDOCIN for rectal use. Capsules INDOCIN SR 75 mg once a day can be substituted for Capsules INDOCIN 25 mg t.i.d. However, there will be significant differences between the two dosage regimens in indomethacin blood levels, especially after 12 hours (see CLINICAL PHARMACOLOGY). In addition, Capsules INDOCIN SR 75 mg b.i.d. can be substituted for Capsules INDOCIN 50 mg t.i.d. Capsules INDOCIN SR may be substituted for all the indications for Capsules INDOCIN except acute gouty arthritis.

Adverse reactions appear to correlate with the size of the dose of INDOCIN in most patients but not all. Therefore, every effort should be made to determine the smallest effective dosage for the individual patient.

Always give Capsules INDOCIN, Capsules INDOCIN SR, or Oral Suspension INDOCIN with food, immediately after meals, or with antacids to reduce gastric irritation.

Pediatric Use

INDOCIN ordinarily should not be prescribed for children 14 years of age and under (see WARNINGS).

Adult Use

Dosage Recommendations for Active Stages of the Following:

1. Moderate to severe rheumatoid arthritis including acute flares of chronic disease; moderate to severe ankylosing spondylitis; and moderate to severe osteoarthritis.

   Suggested Dosage:

   Capsules INDOCIN 25 mg b.i.d. or t.i.d. If this is well tolerated, increase the daily dosage by 25 or by 50 mg, if required by continuing symptoms, at weekly intervals until a satisfactory response is obtained or until a total daily dose of 150–200 mg is reached. DOSES ABOVE THIS AMOUNT GENERALLY DO NOT INCREASE THE EFFECTIVENESS OF THE DRUG.

In patients who have persistent night pain and/or morning stiffness, the giving of a large portion, up to a maximum of 100 mg, of the total daily dose at bedtime, either orally or by rectal suppositories, may be helpful in affording relief. The total daily dose should not exceed 200 mg. In acute flares of chronic rheumatoid arthritis, it may be necessary to increase the dosage by 25 mg or, if required, by 50 mg daily.

If Capsules INDOCIN SR 75 mg are used for initiating indomethacin treatment, one capsule daily should be the usual starting dose in order to observe patient tolerance since 75 mg per day is the maximum recommended starting dose for indomethacin (see above). If Capsules INDOCIN SR are used to increase the daily dose, patients should be observed for possible signs and symptoms of intolerance since the daily increment will exceed the daily increment recommended for the other dosage forms. For patients who require 150 mg of INDOCIN per day and have demonstrated acceptable tolerance, INDOCIN SR may be prescribed as one capsule twice daily.

If minor adverse effects develop as the dosage is increased, reduce the dosage rapidly to a tolerated dose and OBSERVE THE PATIENT CLOSELY.

If severe adverse reactions occur, STOP THE DRUG. After the acute phase of the disease is under control, an attempt to reduce the daily dose should be made repeatedly until the patient is receiving the smallest effective dose or the drug is discontinued.

Careful instructions to, and observations of, the individual patient are essential to the prevention of serious, irreversible, including fatal, adverse reactions.

Continued on next page

Information on the Merck & Co. products listed on these pages is the full prescribing information from product circulars in use October 1, 1992.

Merck & Co.—Cont.

As advancing years appear to increase the possibility of adverse reactions, INDOCIN should be used with greater care in the aged.

2. Acute painful shoulder (bursitis and/or tendinitis).
   Initial Dose:
   75–150 mg daily in 3 or 4 divided doses.
   The drug should be discontinued after the signs and symptoms of inflammation have been controlled for several days. The usual course of therapy is 7–14 days.
3. Acute gouty arthritis.
   Suggested Dosage:
   Capsules INDOCIN 50 mg t.i.d. until pain is tolerable. The dose should then be rapidly reduced to complete cessation of the drug. Definite relief of pain has been reported within 2 to 4 hours. Tenderness and heat usually subside in 24 to 36 hours, and swelling gradually disappears in 3 to 5 days.

HOW SUPPLIED

No. 3316—Capsules INDOCIN, 25 mg are opaque blue and white capsules, coded MSD 25. They are supplied as follows:
NDC 0006-0025-68 bottles of 100
(6505-00-926-2154, 25 mg 100's)
NDC 0006-0025-78 unit of use bottles of 100
NDC 0006-0025-28 unit dose packages of 100
(6505-00-118-2776, 25 mg individually sealed 100's)
NDC 0006-0025-82 bottles of 1000
(6505-00-931-0680, 25 mg 1000's).

Shown in Product Identification Section, page 419

No. 3317—Capsules INDOCIN, 50 mg are opaque blue and white capsules, coded MSD 50. They are supplied as follows:
NDC 0006-0050-68 bottles of 100
NDC 0006-0050-28 unit dose packages of 100
(6505-01-049-6811, 50 mg individually sealed 100's).

Shown in Product Identification Section, page 419

No. 3376—Oral Suspension INDOCIN, 25 mg per 5 mL, is an off-white suspension with a pineapple coconut mint flavor. It is supplied as follows:
NDC 0006-3376-66 in bottles of 237 mL.

No. 3370—Capsules INDOCIN SR, 75 mg each, are capsules with an opaque blue cap and clear body containing a mixture of blue and white pellets, coded MSD 693. They are supplied as follows:
NDC 0006-0693-31 unit of use bottles of 30
(6505-01-135-7391, 75 mg 30's)
NDC 0006-0693-61 unit of use bottles of 60
(6505-01-137-4629, 75 mg 60's).

Shown in Product Identification Section, page 419

No. 3354—Suppositories INDOCIN, 50 mg each, are white, opaque, rectal suppositories and are supplied as follows:
NDC 0006-0150-30, boxes of 30.

Shown in Product Identification Section, page 419

Storage
Store Oral Suspension INDOCIN below 30°C (86°F). Avoid temperatures above 50°C (122°F). Protect from freezing.
Store Suppositories INDOCIN below 30°C (86°F). Avoid transient temperatures above 40°C (104°F).

Suppositories INDOCIN are distributed by:
MERCK SHARP & DOHME, Division of Merck & Co., INC.
West Point, Pa. 19486
Manufactured by:
MERCK SHARP & DOHME
(Italia) S.p.A.
27100—Pavia, Italy
Capsules and Oral Suspension INDOCIN® and Capsules INDOCIN® SR are distributed and manufactured by:
MERCK SHARP & DOHME, Division of Merck & Co., INC.
West Point, Pa. 19486
A.H.F.S. Category: 28:08.04
DC 7342920 Issued May 1991
COPYRIGHT © MERCK & CO., INC., 1988
All rights reserved

INDOCIN® I.V. ℞
(Indomethacin Sodium Trihydrate)

DESCRIPTION

Sterile INDOCIN* I.V. (Indomethacin Sodium Trihydrate) for intravenous administration is lyophilized indomethacin sodium trihydrate. Each vial contains indomethacin sodium trihydrate equivalent to 1 mg indomethacin as a white to yellow lyophilized powder or plug. Variations in the size of the lyophilized plug and the intensity of color have no relationship to the quality or amount of indomethacin present in the vial.
Indomethacin sodium trihydrate is designated chemically as 1-(4-chlorobenzoyl) -5- methoxy-2-methyl-1*H* -indole-3-acetic acid, sodium salt, trihydrate. Its molecular weight is 433.82. Its empirical formula is $C_{19}H_{15}ClNNaO_4 \cdot 3H_2O$ and its structural formula is:

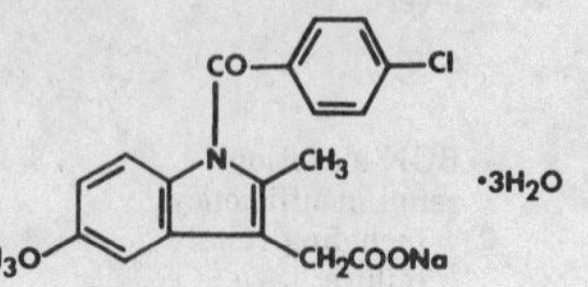

*Registered trademark of MERCK & CO., INC.

CLINICAL PHARMACOLOGY

Although the exact mechanism of action through which indomethacin causes closure of a patent ductus arteriosus is not known, it is believed to be through inhibition of prostaglandin synthesis. Indomethacin has been shown to be a potent inhibitor of prostaglandin synthesis, both *in vitro* and *in vivo*. In human newborns with certain congenital heart malformations, PGE 1 dilates the ductus arteriosus. In fetal and newborn lambs, E type prostaglandins have also been shown to maintain the patency of the ductus, and as in human newborns, indomethacin causes its constriction.
Studies in healthy young animals and in premature infants with patent ductus arteriosus indicated that, after the first dose of intravenous indomethacin, there was a transient reduction in cerebral blood flow velocity and cerebral blood flow. The clinical significance of this effect has not been established.
In double-blind placebo-controlled studies of INDOCIN I.V. in 460 small pre-term infants, weighing 1750 g or less, the infants treated with placebo had a ductus closure rate after 48 hours of 25 to 30 percent, whereas those treated with INDOCIN I.V. had a 75 to 80 percent closure rate. In one of these studies, a multicenter study, involving 405 pre-term infants, later re-opening of the ductus arteriosus occurred in 26 percent of infants treated with INDOCIN I.V., however, 70 percent of these closed subsequently without the need for surgery or additional indomethacin.
Pharmacokinetics and Metabolism
The disposition of indomethacin following intravenous administration (0.2 mg/kg) in pre-term neonates with patent ductus arteriosus has not been extensively evaluated. Even though the plasma half-life of indomethacin was variable among premature infants, it was shown to vary inversely with postnatal age and weight. In one study, of 28 infants who could be evaluated, the plasma half-life in those infants less than 7 days old averaged 20 hours (range: 3–60 hours, n = 18). In infants older than 7 days, the mean plasma half-life of indomethacin was 12 hours (range: 4–38 hours, n = 10). Grouping the infants by weight, mean plasma half-life in those weighing less than 1000 g was 21 hours (range: 9–60 hours, n = 10); in those infants weighing more than 1000 g, the mean plasma half-life was 15 hours (range: 3–52 hours, n = 18).
Following intravenous administration in adults, indomethacin is eliminated via renal excretion, metabolism, and biliary excretion. Indomethacin undergoes appreciable enterohepatic circulation. The mean plasma half-life of indomethacin is 4.5 hours. In the absence of enterohepatic circulation, it is 90 minutes.
In adults, about 99 percent of indomethacin is bound to protein in plasma over the expected range of therapeutic plasma concentrations. The percent bound in neonates has not been studied. In controlled trials in premature infants, however, no evidence of bilirubin displacement has been observed as evidenced by increased incidence of bilirubin encephalopathy (kernicterus).

INDICATIONS AND USAGE

INDOCIN I.V. is indicated to close a hemodynamically significant patent ductus arteriosus in premature infants weighing between 500 and 1750 g when after 48 hours usual medical management (e.g., fluid restriction, diuretics, digitalis, respiratory support, etc.) is ineffective. Clear-cut clinical evidence of a hemodynamically significant patent ductus arteriosus should be present, such as respiratory distress, a continuous murmur, a hyperactive precordium, cardiomegaly and pulmonary plethora on chest x-ray.

CONTRAINDICATIONS

INDOCIN I.V. is contraindicated in: infants with proven or suspected infection that is untreated; infants who are bleeding, especially those with active intracranial hemorrhage or gastrointestinal bleeding; infants with thrombocytopenia; infants with coagulation defects; infants with or who are suspected of having necrotizing enterocolitis; infants with significant impairment of renal function; infants with congenital heart disease in whom patency of the ductus arteriosus is necessary for satisfactory pulmonary or systemic blood flow (e.g., pulmonary atresia, severe tetralogy of Fallot, severe coarctation of the aorta).

WARNINGS

Gastrointestinal Effects:
In the collaborative study, major gastrointestinal bleeding was no more common in those infants receiving indomethacin than in those infants on placebo. However, minor gastrointestinal bleeding (i.e., chemical detection of blood in the stool) was more commonly noted in those infants treated with indomethacin. Severe gastrointestinal effects have been reported in adults with various arthritic disorders treated chronically with oral indomethacin. [For further information, see package circular for Capsules INDOCIN* (Indomethacin)].
Central Nervous System Effects:
Prematurity per se, is associated with an increased incidence of spontaneous intraventricular hemorrhage. Because indomethacin may inhibit platelet aggregation, the potential for intraventricular bleeding may be increased. However, in the large multi-center study of INDOCIN I.V. (see CLINICAL PHARMACOLOGY), the incidence of intraventricular hemorrhage in babies treated with INDOCIN I.V. was not significantly higher than in the control infants.
Renal Effects:
INDOCIN I.V. may cause significant reduction in urine output (50 percent or more) with concomitant elevations of blood urea nitrogen and creatinine, and reductions in glomerular filtration rate and creatinine clearance. These effects in most infants are transient, disappearing with cessation of therapy with INDOCIN I.V. However, because adequate renal function can depend upon renal prostaglandin synthesis, INDOCIN I.V. may precipitate renal insufficiency, including acute renal failure, especially in infants with other conditions that may adversely affect renal function (e.g., extracellular volume depletion from any cause, congestive heart failure, sepsis, concomitant use of any nephrotoxic drug, hepatic dysfunction). When significant suppression of urine volume occurs after a dose of INDOCIN I.V., no additional dose should be given until the urine output returns to normal levels.
INDOCIN I.V. in pre-term infants may suppress water excretion to a greater extent than sodium excretion. When this occurs, a significant reduction in serum sodium values (i.e., hyponatremia) may result. Infants should have serum electrolyte determinations done during therapy with INDOCIN I.V. Renal function and serum electrolytes should be monitored (see PRECAUTIONS, *Drug Interactions* and DOSAGE AND ADMINISTRATION).

* Registered trademark of MERCK & CO., INC.

PRECAUTIONS

General
INDOCIN (Indomethacin) may mask the usual signs and symptoms of infection. Therefore, the physician must be continually on the alert for this and should use the drug with extra care in the presence of existing controlled infection.
Severe hepatic reactions have been reported in adults treated chronically with oral indomethacin for arthritic disorders. [For further information, see package circular for Capsules INDOCIN (Indomethacin)]. If clinical signs and symptoms consistent with liver disease develop in the neonate, or if systemic manifestations occur, INDOCIN I.V. should be discontinued.
INDOCIN I.V. may inhibit platelet aggregation. In one small study, platelet aggregation was grossly abnormal after indomethacin therapy (given orally to premature infants to close the ductus arteriosus). Platelet aggregation returned to normal by the tenth day. Premature infants should be observed for signs of bleeding.
The drug should be administered carefully to avoid extravascular injection or leakage as the solution may be irritating to tissue.
Drug Interactions
Since renal function may be reduced by INDOCIN I.V., consideration should be given to reduction in dosage of those medications that rely on adequate renal function for their elimination. Because the half-life of digitalis (given frequently to pre-term infants with patent ductus arteriosus and associated cardiac failure) may be prolonged when given concomitantly with indomethacin, the infant should be observed closely; frequent ECGs and serum digitalis levels may be required to prevent or detect digitalis toxicity early. Furthermore, in one study of premature infants treated with INDOCIN I.V. and also receiving either gentamicin or amikacin, both peak and trough levels of these aminoglycosides were significantly elevated.

Therapy with indomethacin may blunt the natriuretic effect of furosemide. This response has been attributed to inhibition of prostaglandin synthesis by non-steroidal anti-inflammatory drugs. In a study of 19 premature infants with patent ductus arteriosus treated with either INDOCIN I.V. alone or a combination of INDOCIN I.V. and furosemide, results showed that infants receiving both INDOCIN I.V. and furosemide had significantly higher urinary output, higher levels of sodium and chloride excretion, and higher glomerular filtration rates than did those infants receiving INDOCIN I.V. alone. In this study, the data suggested that therapy with furosemide helped to maintain renal function in the premature infant when INDOCIN I.V. was added to the treatment of patent ductus arteriosus.

Neonatal Effects
In rats and mice, oral indomethacin 4.0 mg/kg/day given during the last three days of gestation caused a decrease in maternal weight gain and some maternal and fetal deaths. An increased incidence of neuronal necrosis in the diencephalon in the live-born fetuses was observed. At 2.0 mg/kg/day, no increase in neuronal necrosis was observed as compared to the control groups. Administration of 0.5 or 4.0 mg/kg/day during the first three days of life did not cause an increase in neuronal necrosis at either dose level.
Pregnant rats, given 2.0 mg/kg/day and 4.0 mg/kg/day during the last trimester of gestation, delivered offspring whose pulmonary blood vessels were both reduced in number and excessively muscularized. These findings are similar to those observed in the syndrome of persistent pulmonary hypertension of the newborn.

ADVERSE REACTIONS

In a double-blind placebo-controlled trial of 405 premature infants weighing less than or equal to 1750 g with evidence of large ductal shunting, in those infants treated with indomethacin (n = 206), there was a statistically significantly greater incidence of bleeding problems, including gross or microscopic bleeding into the gastrointestinal tract, oozing from the skin after needle stick, pulmonary hemorrhage, and disseminated intravascular coagulation. There was no statistically significant difference between treatment groups with reference to intracranial hemorrhage.
The infants treated with indomethacin sodium trihydrate also had a significantly higher incidence of transient oliguria and elevations of serum creatinine (greater than or equal to 1.8 mg/dL) than did the infants treated with placebo.
The incidences of retrolental fibroplasia (grades III and IV) and pneumothorax in infants treated with INDOCIN I.V. were no greater than in placebo controls and were statistically significantly lower than in surgically-treated infants.
The following additional adverse reactions in infants have been reported from the collaborative study, anecdotal case reports, and from other studies using rectal, oral, or intravenous indomethacin for treatment of patent ductus arteriosus. The rates are based on the experience of 849 indomethacin-treated infants reported in the medical literature, regardless of the route of administration. One year follow-up is available on 175 infants and shows no long-term sequelae which could be attributed to indomethacin. In controlled clinical studies, only electrolyte imbalance and renal dysfunction (of the reactions listed below) occurred statistically significantly more frequently after INDOCIN I.V. than after placebo.
Renal: renal dysfunction in 41 percent of infants, including one or more of the following: reduced urinary output; reduced urine sodium, chloride, or potassium, urine osmolality, free water clearance, or glomerular filtration rate; elevated serum creatinine or BUN; uremia.
Cardiovascular: intracranial bleeding**, pulmonary hypertension.
Gastrointestinal: gastrointestinal bleeding*, vomiting, abdominal distention, transient ileus, localized perforation(s) of the small and/or large intestine.
Metabolic: hyponatremia*, elevated serum potassium*, reduction in blood sugar, including hypoglycemia, increased weight gain (fluid retention).
Coagulation: decreased platelet aggregation (see PRECAUTIONS).
The following adverse reactions have also been reported in infants treated with indomethacin, however, a causal relationship to therapy with INDOCIN I.V. has not been established:
Cardiovascular: bradycardia.
Respiratory: apnea, exacerbation of pre-existing pulmonary infection.
Metabolic: acidosis/alkalosis.
Hematologic: disseminated intravascular coagulation.
Gastrointestinal: necrotizing enterocolitis.
Ophthalmic: retrolental fibroplasia.**
A variety of additional adverse experiences have been reported in adults treated with oral indomethacin for moderate to severe rheumatoid arthritis, osteoarthritis, ankylosing spondylitis, acute painful shoulder and acute gouty arthritis (see section ADDITIONAL ADVERSE REACTIONS—

ADULTS). Their relevance to the pre-term neonate receiving indomethacin for patent ductus arteriosus is unknown, however, the possibility exists that these experiences may be associated with the use of INDOCIN I.V. in pre-term neonates.

*Incidence 3–9 percent. Those reactions which are unmarked occurred in 1–3 percent of patients.
**Incidence in both indomethacin and placebo-treated infants 3–9 percent. Those reactions which are unmarked occurred in less than 3 percent.

DOSAGE AND ADMINISTRATION

FOR INTRAVENOUS ADMINISTRATION ONLY.
Dosage recommendations for closure of the ductus arteriosus depends on the age of the infant at the time of therapy. A course of therapy is defined as three intravenous doses of INDOCIN I.V. given at 12–24 hour intervals, with careful attention to urinary output. If anuria or marked oliguria (urinary output < 0.6 mL/kg/hr) is evident at the scheduled time of the second or third dose of INDOCIN I.V., no additional doses should be given until laboratory studies indicate that renal function has returned to normal (see WARNINGS, *Renal Effects*).
Dosage according to age is as follows:

AGE at 1st dose	DOSAGE (mg/kg)		
	1st	2nd	3rd
Less than 48 hours	0.2	0.1	0.1
2–7 days	0.2	0.2	0.2
over 7 days	0.2	0.25	0.25

If the ductus arteriosus closes or is significantly reduced in size after an interval of 48 hours or more from completion of the first course of INDOCIN I.V., no further doses are necessary. If the ductus arteriosus re-opens, a second course of 1–3 doses may be given, each dose separated by a 12–24 hour interval as described above.
If the infant remains unresponsive to therapy with INDOCIN I.V. after 2 courses, surgery may be necessary for closure of the ductus arteriosus. If severe adverse reactions occur, STOP THE DRUG.
Directions for Use
Parenteral drug products should be inspected visually for particulate matter and discoloration prior to administration whenever solution and container permit.
The solution should be prepared only with 1 to 2 mL of preservative-free sterile Sodium Chloride Injection, 0.9 percent or preservative-free Sterile Water for Injection. Benzyl alcohol as a preservative has been associated with toxicity in newborns. Therefore, all diluents should be preservative-free. If 1 mL of diluent is used, the concentration of indomethacin in the solution will equal approximately 0.1 mg/0.1 mL; if 2 mL of diluent are used, the concentration of the solution will equal approximately 0.05 mg/0.1 mL. Any unused portion of the solution should be discarded because there is no preservative contained in the vial. A fresh solution should be prepared just prior to each administration. Once reconstituted, the indomethacin solution may be injected intravenously over 5–10 seconds.
Further dilution with intravenous infusion solutions is not recommended. INDOCIN I.V. is not buffered, and reconstitution with solutions at pH values below 6.0 may result in precipitation of the insoluble indomethacin free acid moiety.

HOW SUPPLIED

No. 3406—Sterile INDOCIN I.V. is a lyophilized white to yellow powder or plug supplied as single dose vials containing indomethacin sodium trihydrate, equivalent to 1 mg indomethacin.
NDC 0006-3406-17.
Storage
Store below 30°C (86°F). *Protect from light.* Store container in carton until contents have been used.

ADDITIONAL ADVERSE REACTIONS—ADULTS

The following adverse reactions have been reported in adults treated with oral indomethacin for moderate to severe rheumatoid arthritis, osteoarthritis, ankylosing spondylitis, acute painful shoulder and acute gouty arthritis. Complaints not of relevance in the treatment of the premature infant, such as anorexia, psychic disturbances, and blurred vision, are not listed. [See table next column.]
See package circular for Capsules INDOCIN (Indomethacin) for additional information concerning adverse reactions and other cautionary statements.
A.H.F.S. Category: 28:08.04
DC 7414812   Issued November 1991

Incidence 1% to 3%	Incidence less than 1%	
GASTROINTESTINAL		
diarrhea	bloating (includes	gastrointestinal
constipation	distention)	bleeding without
	flatulence	obvious ulcer
	peptic ulcer	formation and
	gastroenteritis	perforation of
	rectal bleeding	pre-existing sigmoid
	proctitis	lesions
	single or multiple	development of
	ulcerations, includ-	ulcerative stomatitis
	ing perforation and	toxic hepatitis and
	hemorrhage of the	jaundice (some fatal
	esophagus, stomach,	cases have been
	duodenum or small	reported)
	and large intestines	
	intestinal ulceration	
	associated with	
	stenosis and	
	obstruction	
CENTRAL NERVOUS SYSTEM		
none	involuntary muscle	aggravation of epilepsy
	movements	coma
		peripheral neuropathy
		convulsions
SPECIAL SENSES		
none	hearing disturbances,	
	deafness	
CARDIOVASCULAR		
none	hypertension	arrhythmia
	hypotension	congestive heart
	tachycardia	failure
		thrombophlebitis
METABOLIC		
none	edema	hyperglycemia
	weight gain	glycosuria
	flushing	hyperkalemia
INTEGUMENTARY		
none	rash; urticaria	exfoliative dermatitis
	petechiae or	erythema nodosum
	ecchymosis	loss of hair
		Stevens-Johnson
		syndrome
		erythema multiforme
		toxic epidermal
		necrolysis
HEMATOLOGIC		
none	leukopenia	aplastic anemia
	bone marrow	hemolytic anemia
	depression	agranulocytosis
	anemia secondary to	thrombocytopenic
	obvious or occult	purpura
	gastrointestinal	
	bleeding	
HYPERSENSITIVITY		
none	acute anaphylaxis	dyspnea
	acute respiratory	asthma
	distress	purpura
	rapid fall in blood	angiitis
	pressure resembling	pulmonary edema
	a shock-like state	
GENITOURINARY		
none	hematuria	renal insufficiency,
	vaginal bleeding	including renal
		failure
MISCELLANEOUS		
none	epistaxis	
	breast changes,	
	including en-	
	largement and	
	tenderness, or	
	gynecomastia	

INVERSINE® Tablets   ℞
(Mecamylamine HCl), U.S.P.

DESCRIPTION

INVERSINE* (Mecamylamine HCl) is a potent, oral antihypertensive agent and ganglion blocker, and is a secondary amine. It is *N*,2,3,3-tetramethylbicyclo[2.2.1] heptan-2-amine hydrochloride. Its empirical formula is $C_{11}H_{21}N \cdot HCl$ and its structural formula is:
[See chemical structure at top of next column.]

Continued on next page

Merck & Co.—Cont.

It is a white, odorless, or practically odorless, crystalline powder, is highly stable, soluble in water and has a molecular weight of 203.75.

INVERSINE is supplied as tablets for oral use, each containing 2.5 mg mecamylamine HCl. Inactive ingredients are acacia, calcium phosphate, D&C Yellow 10, FD&C Yellow 6, lactose, magnesium stearate, starch, and talc.

---

*Registered trademark of MERCK & CO., INC.

CLINICAL PHARMACOLOGY

Mecamylamine reduces blood pressure in both normotensive and hypertensive individuals. It has a gradual onset of action ($\frac{1}{2}$ to 2 hours) and a long-lasting effect (usually 6 to 12 hours or more). A small oral dosage often produces a smooth and predictable reduction of blood pressure. Although this antihypertensive effect is predominantly orthostatic, the supine blood pressure is also significantly reduced.

Pharmacokinetics and Metabolism

Mecamylamine is almost completely absorbed from the gastrointestinal tract, resulting in consistent lowering of blood pressure in most patients with hypertensive cardiovascular disease. Mecamylamine is excreted slowly in the urine in the unchanged form. The rate of its renal elimination is influenced markedly by urinary pH. Alkalinization of the urine reduces, and acidification promotes, renal excretion of mecamylamine.

Mecamylamine crosses the blood-brain and placental barriers.

INDICATIONS AND USAGE

For the management of moderately severe to severe essential hypertension and in uncomplicated cases of malignant hypertension.

CONTRAINDICATIONS

INVERSINE should not be used in mild, moderate, labile hypertension and may prove unsuitable in uncooperative patients. It is contraindicated in coronary insufficiency or recent myocardial infarction.

INVERSINE should be given with great discretion, if at all, when renal insufficiency is manifested by a rising or elevated BUN. The drug is contraindicated in uremia. Patients receiving antibiotics and sulfonamides should generally not be treated with ganglion blockers. Other contraindications are glaucoma, organic pyloric stenosis or hypersensitivity to the product.

WARNINGS

Mecamylamine, a secondary amine, readily penetrates into the brain and thus may produce central nervous sytem effects. Tremor, choreiform movements, mental aberrations, and convulsions may occur rarely. These have occurred most often when large doses of INVERSINE were used, especially in patients with cerebral or renal insufficiency.

When ganglion blockers or other potent antihypertensive drugs are discontinued suddenly, hypertensive levels return. In patients with malignant hypertension and others, this may occur abruptly and may cause fatal cerebral vascular accidents or acute congestive heart failure. When INVERSINE is withdrawn, this should be done gradually and other antihypertensive therapy usually must be substituted. On the other hand, the effects of INVERSINE sometimes may last from hours to days after therapy is discontinued.

PRECAUTIONS

General

The patient's condition should be evaluated carefully, particularly as to renal and cardiovascular function. When renal, cerebral, or coronary blood flow is deficient, any additional impairment, which might result from added hypotension, must be avoided. The use of INVERSINE in patients with marked cerebral and coronary arteriosclerosis or after a recent cerebral accident requires caution.

The action of INVERSINE may be potentiated by excessive heat, fever, infection, hemorrhage, pregnancy, anesthesia, surgery, vigorous exercise, other antihypertensive drugs, alcohol, and salt depletion as a result of diminished intake or increased excretion due to diarrhea, vomiting, excessive sweating, or diuretics.

During therapy with INVERSINE, sodium intake should not be restricted but, if necessary, the dosage of the ganglion blocker must be adjusted.

Since urinary retention may occur in patients on ganglion blockers, caution is required in patients with prostatic hypertrophy, bladder neck obstruction, and urethral stricture. Frequent loose bowel movements with abdominal distention and decreased borborygmi may be the first signs of paralytic ileus. If these are present, INVERSINE should be discontinued immediately and remedial steps taken.

Information for Patients

INVERSINE may cause dizziness, lightheadedness, or fainting, especially when rising from a lying or sitting position. This effect may be increased by alcoholic beverages, exercise, or during hot weather. Getting up slowly may help alleviate such a reaction.

Drug Interactions

Patients receiving antibiotics and sulfonamides generally should not be treated with ganglion blockers.

The action of INVERSINE may be potentiated by anesthesia, other antihypertensive drugs and alcohol.

Carcinogenesis, Mutagenesis, Impairment of Fertility

Long-term studies in animals have not been performed to evaluate the effects upon fertility, mutagenic or carcinogenic potential of INVERSINE.

Pregnancy

Pregnancy Category C. Animal reproduction studies have not been conducted with INVERSINE. It is not known whether INVERSINE can cause fetal harm when given to a pregnant woman or can affect reproductive capacity. INVERSINE should be given to a pregnant woman only if clearly needed.

Nursing Mothers

Because of the potential for serious adverse reactions in nursing infants from INVERSINE, a decision should be made whether to discontinue nursing or to discontinue the drug, taking into account the importance of the drug to the mother.

ADVERSE REACTIONS

The following adverse reactions have been reported and within each category are listed in order of decreasing severity.

Gastrointestinal: Ileus, constipation (sometimes preceded by small, frequent liquid stools), vomiting, nausea, anorexia, glossitis and dryness of mouth.

Cardiovascular: Orthostatic dizziness and syncope, postural hypotension.

Nervous System/Psychiatric: Convulsions, choreiform movements, mental aberrations, tremor, and paresthesias (see WARNINGS).

Respiratory: Interstitial pulmonary edema and fibrosis.

Urogenital: Urinary retention, impotence, decreased libido.

Special Senses: Blurred vision, dilated pupils.

Miscellaneous: Weakness, fatigue, sedation.

OVERDOSAGE

Signs of overdosage include: hypotension (which may progress to peripheral vascular collapse), postural hypotension, nausea, vomiting, diarrhea, constipation, paralytic ileus, urinary retention, dizziness, anxiety, dry mouth, mydriasis, blurred vision, or palpitations. A rise in intraocular pressure may occur.

Pressor amines may be used to counteract excessive hypotension. Since patients being treated with ganglion blockers are more than normally reactive to pressor amines, small doses of the latter are recommended to avoid excessive response. The oral LD_{50} of mecamylamine in the mouse is 92 mg/kg.

DOSAGE AND ADMINISTRATION

Therapy is usually started with one 2.5 mg tablet of INVERSINE twice a day. This initial dosage should be modified by increments of one 2.5 mg tablet at intervals of not less than 2 days until the desired blood pressure response occurs (the criterion being a dosage just under that which causes signs of mild postural hypotension).

The average total daily dosage of INVERSINE is 25 mg, usually in three divided doses. However, as little as 2.5 mg daily may be sufficient to control hypertension in some patients. A range of two to four or even more doses may be required in severe cases when smooth control is difficult to obtain. In severe or urgent cases, larger increments at smaller intervals may be needed. Partial tolerance may develop in certain patients, requiring an increase in the daily dosage of INVERSINE.

Administration of INVERSINE after meals may cause a more gradual absorption and smoother control of excessively high blood pressure. The timing of doses in relation to meals should be consistent. Since the blood pressure response to antihypertensive drugs is increased in the early morning, the larger dose should be given at noontime and perhaps in the evening. The morning dose, as a rule, should be relatively small and in some instances may even be omitted.

The *initial regulation of dosage* should be determined by blood pressure readings in the erect position at the time of maximal effect of the drug, as well as by other signs and symptoms of orthostatic hypertension.

The *effective maintenance dosage* should be regulated by blood pressure readings in the erect position and by limitation of dosage to that which causes slight faintness or dizziness in this position. If the patient or a relative can use a sphygmomanometer, instructions may be given to reduce or omit a dose if readings fall below a designated level or if faintness or lightheadedness occurs. *However, no change should be instituted without the knowledge of the physician.* Close supervision and education of the patient, as well as critical adjustment of dosage, are essential to successful therapy.

Other Antihypertensive Agents

When INVERSINE is given with other antihypertensive drugs, the dosage of these other agents, as well as that of INVERSINE, should be reduced to avoid excessive hypotension. However, thiazides should be continued in their usual dosage, while that of INVERSINE is decreased by at least 50 percent.

HOW SUPPLIED

No. 3219—Tablets INVERSINE, 2.5 mg, are yellow, round, scored, compressed tablets, coded MSD 52. They are supplied as follows:

NDC 0006-0052-68 in bottles of 100.
    Shown in Product Identification Section, page 419
    A.H.F.S. Category: 24:08
    DC 6041721   Issued September 1985
COPYRIGHT © MERCK & CO., INC., 1985
All rights reserved

LACRISERT® Sterile Ophthalmic Insert   ℞
(Hydroxypropyl Cellulose), U.S.P.

DESCRIPTION

LACRISERT* (Hydroxypropyl Cellulose) is a sterile, translucent, rod-shaped, water soluble, ophthalmic insert made of hydroxypropyl cellulose, for administration into the inferior cul-de-sac of the eye.

The chemical name for hydroxypropyl cellulose is cellulose, 2-hydroxypropyl ether. It is an ether of cellulose in which hydroxypropyl groups (-CH$_2$CHOHCH$_3$) are attached to the hydroxyls present in the anhydroglucose rings of cellulose by ether linkages. A representative structure of the monomer is:

$$R = CH_2CHCH_3$$
$$OH$$

The molecular weight is typically 1×10^6.

Hydroxypropyl cellulose is an off-white, odorless, tasteless powder. It is soluble in water below 38°C, and in many polar organic solvents such as ethanol, propylene glycol, dioxane, methanol, isopropyl alcohol (95%), dimethyl sulfoxide, and dimethyl formamide.

Each LACRISERT is 5 mg of hydroxypropyl cellulose. LACRISERT contains no preservatives or other ingredients. It is about 1.27 mm in diameter by about 3.5 mm long.

LACRISERT is supplied in packages of 60 units, together with illustrated instructions and a special applicator for removing LACRISERT from the unit dose blister and inserting it into the eye. A spare applicator is included in each package.

---

*Registered trademark of MERCK & CO., INC.

CLINICAL PHARMACOLOGY

Pharmacodynamics

LACRISERT acts to stabilize and thicken the precorneal tear film and prolong the tear film breakup time which is usually accelerated in patients with dry eye states. LACRISERT also acts to lubricate and protect the eye.

LACRISERT usually reduces the signs and symptoms resulting from moderate to severe dry eye syndromes, such as conjunctival hyperemia, corneal and conjunctival staining with rose bengal, exudation, itching, burning, foreign body sensation, smarting, photophobia, dryness and blurred or cloudy vision. Progressive visual deterioration which occurs in some patients may be retarded, halted, or sometimes reversed.

In a multicenter crossover study the 5 mg LACRISERT administered once a day during the waking hours was compared to artificial tears used four or more times daily. There was a prolongation of tear film breakup time and a decrease in foreign body sensation associated with dry eye syndrome in patients during treatment with inserts as compared to artificial tears; these findings were statistically significantly different between the treatment groups. Improvement, as measured by amelioration of symptoms, by slit-lamp examination and by rose bengal staining of the cornea and conjunctiva, was greater in most patients with moderate to severe symptoms during treatment with LACRISERT. Patient comfort was usually better with LACRISERT than with artificial tears solution, and most patients preferred LACRISERT.

In most patients treated with LACRISERT for over one year, improvement was observed as evidenced by amelioration of symptoms generally associated with keratoconjunctivitis sicca such as burning, tearing, foreign body sensation, itching, photophobia and blurred or cloudy vision.

During studies in healthy volunteers, a thickened precorneal tear film was usually observed through the slit-lamp while LACRISERT was present in the conjunctival sac.

Pharmacokinetics and Metabolism

Hydroxypropyl cellulose is a physiologically inert substance. In a study of rats fed hydroxypropyl cellulose or unmodified cellulose at levels up to 5% of their diet, it was found that the two were biologically equivalent in that neither was metabolized.

Studies conducted in rats fed ^{14}C-labeled hydroxypropyl cellulose demonstrated that when orally administered, hydroxypropyl cellulose is not absorbed from the gastrointestinal tract and is quantitatively excreted in the feces.

Dissolution studies in rabbits showed that hydroxypropyl cellulose inserts became softer within 1 hour after they were placed in the conjunctival sac. Most of the inserts dissolved completely in 14 to 18 hours; with a single exception, all had disappeared by 24 hours after insertion. Similar dissolution of the inserts was observed during prolonged administration (up to 54 weeks).

INDICATIONS AND USAGE

LACRISERT is indicated in patients with moderate to severe dry eye syndromes, including keratoconjunctivitis sicca. LACRISERT is indicated especially in patients who remain symptomatic after an adequate trial of therapy with artificial tear solutions.

LACRISERT is also indicated for patients with:

- Exposure keratitis
- Decreased corneal sensitivity
- Recurrent corneal erosions

CONTRAINDICATIONS

LACRISERT is contraindicated in patients who are hypersensitive to hydroxypropyl cellulose.

WARNINGS

Instructions for inserting and removing LACRISERT should be carefully followed.

PRECAUTIONS

General

If improperly placed, LACRISERT may result in corneal abrasion (see DOSAGE AND ADMINISTRATION).

Information for Patients

Patients should be advised to follow the instructions for using LACRISERT which accompany the package.

Because this product may produce transient blurring of vision, patients should be instructed to exercise caution when operating hazardous machinery or driving a motor vehicle.

Drug Interactions

Application of hydroxypropyl cellulose inserts to the eyes of unanesthetized rabbits immediately prior to or two hours before instilling pilocarpine, proparacaine HCl (0.5%), or phenylephrine (5%) did not markedly alter the magnitude and/or duration of the miotic, local corneal anesthetic, or mydriatic activity, respectively, of these agents.

Under various treatment schedules, the anti-inflammatory effect of ocularly instilled dexamethasone (0.1%) in unanesthetized rabbits with primary uveitis was not affected by the presence of hydroxypropyl cellulose inserts.

Carcinogenesis, Mutagenesis, Impairment of Fertility

Feeding of hydroxypropyl cellulose to rats at levels up to 5% of their diet produced no gross or histopathologic changes or other deleterious effects.

ADVERSE REACTIONS

The following adverse reactions have been reported in patients treated with LACRISERT, but were in most instances mild and transient:

- Transient blurring of vision (See PRECAUTIONS)
- Ocular discomfort or irritation
- Matting or stickiness of eyelashes
- Photophobia
- Hypersensitivity
- Edema of the eyelids
- Hyperemia

DOSAGE AND ADMINISTRATION

One LACRISERT ophthalmic insert in each eye once daily is usually sufficient to relieve the symptoms associated with moderate to severe dry eye syndromes. Individual patients may require more flexibility in the use of LACRISERT; some patients may require twice daily use for optimal results.

Clinical experience with LACRISERT indicates that in some patients several weeks may be required before satisfactory improvement of symptoms is achieved.

LACRISERT is inserted into the inferior cul-de-sac of the eye beneath the base of the tarsus, not in apposition to the cornea, nor beneath the eyelid at the level of the tarsal plate. If not properly positioned, it will be expelled into the interpalpebral fissure, and may cause symptoms of a foreign body. Illustrated instructions are included in each package. While in the licensed practitioner's office, the patient should read the instructions, then practice insertion and removal of LACRISERT until proficiency is achieved.

NOTE: Occasionally LACRISERT is inadvertently expelled from the eye, especially in patients with shallow conjunctival fornices. The patient should be cautioned against rubbing the eye(s) containing LACRISERT, especially upon awakening, so as not to dislodge or expel the insert. If required, another LACRISERT ophthalmic insert may be inserted. If experience indicates that transient blurred vision develops in an individual patient, the patient may want to remove LACRISERT a few hours after insertion to avoid this. Another LACRISERT ophthalmic insert may be inserted if needed.

If LACRISERT causes worsening of symptoms, the patient should be instructed to inspect the conjunctival sac to make certain LACRISERT is in the proper location, deep in the inferior cul-de-sac of the eye beneath the base of the tarsus. If these symptoms persist, LACRISERT should be removed and the patient should contact the practitioner.

HOW SUPPLIED

No. 3380—LACRISERT, a sterile, translucent, rod-shaped, water soluble, ophthalmic insert made of hydroxypropyl cellulose, 5 mg, is supplied as follows:

NDC 0006-3380-60 in packages containing 60 unit doses, two reusable applicators and a storage container.

(6505-01-153-4360, 5 mg 60's).

Storage

Store below 30°C (86°F).

DC 7415108 Issued August 1989

COPYRIGHT © MERCK & CO., INC., 1988
All rights reserved

M-M-R® II ℞

(Measles, Mumps, and Rubella Virus Vaccine Live, MSD), U.S.P.

DESCRIPTION

M-M-R* II (Measles, Mumps, and Rubella Virus Vaccine Live, MSD) is a live virus vaccine for immunization against measles (rubeola), mumps and rubella (German measles).

M-M-R II is a sterile lyophilized preparation of (1) ATTENUVAX* (Measles Virus Vaccine Live, MSD), a more attenuated line of measles virus, derived from Enders' attenuated Edmonston strain and grown in cell cultures of chick embryo; (2) MUMPSVAX* (Mumps Virus Vaccine Live, MSD), the Jeryl Lynn (B level) strain of mumps virus grown in cell cultures of chick embryo; and (3) MERUVAX* II (Rubella Virus Vaccine Live, MSD), the Wistar RA 27/3 strain of live attenuated rubella virus grown in human diploid cell (WI-38) culture. The vaccine viruses are the same as those used in the manufacture of ATTENUVAX (Measles Virus Vaccine Live, MSD), MUMPSVAX (Mumps Virus Vaccine Live, MSD) and MERUVAX II (Rubella Virus Vaccine Live, MSD). The three viruses are mixed before being lyophilized. The product contains no preservative.

The reconstituted vaccine is for subcutaneous administration. When reconstituted as directed, the dose for injection is 0.5 mL and contains not less than the equivalent of 1,000 $TCID_{50}$ (tissue culture infectious doses) of the U.S. Reference Measles Virus; 20,000 $TCID_{50}$ of the U.S. Reference Mumps Virus; and 1,000 $TCID_{50}$ of the U.S. Reference Rubella Virus. Each dose contains approximately 25 mcg of neomycin. The product contains no preservative. Sorbitol and hydrolyzed gelatin are added as stabilizers.

---

*Registered trademark of MERCK & CO., INC.

CLINICAL PHARMACOLOGY

Clinical studies of 279 triple seronegative children, 11 months to 7 years of age, demonstrated that M-M-R II is highly immunogenic and generally well tolerated. In these studies, a single injection of the vaccine induced measles hemagglutination-inhibition (HI) antibodies in 95 percent, mumps neutralizing antibodies in 96 percent, and rubella HI antibodies in 99 percent of susceptible persons.

The RA 27/3 rubella strain in M-M-R II elicits higher immediate post-vaccination HI, complement-fixing and neutralizing antibody levels than other strains of rubella vaccine and has been shown to induce a broader profile of circulating antibodies including anti-theta and anti-iota precipitating antibodies. The RA 27/3 rubella strain immunologically simulates natural infection more closely than other rubella vaccine viruses. The increased levels and broader profile of antibodies produced by RA 27/3 strain rubella virus vaccine appear to correlate with greater resistance to subclinical reinfection with the wild virus, and provide greater confidence for lasting immunity.

Vaccine induced antibody levels following administration of M-M-R II have been shown to persist up to 11 years without substantial decline. Continued surveillance will be necessary to determine further duration of antibody persistence.

INDICATIONS AND USAGE

M-M-R II is indicated for simultaneous immunization against measles, mumps, and rubella in persons 15 months of age or older. A second dose of M-M-R II or monovalent measles vaccine is recommended (see *Revaccination*).

Infants who are less than 15 months of age may fail to respond to the measles component of the vaccine due to presence in the circulation of residual measles antibody of maternal origin, the younger the infant, the lower the likelihood of seroconversion. In geographically isolated or other relatively inaccessible populations for whom immunization programs are logistically difficult, and in population groups in which natural measles infection may occur in a significant proportion of infants before 15 months of age, it may be desirable to give the vaccine to infants at an earlier age. Infants vaccinated under these conditions at less than 12 months of age should be revaccinated after reaching 15 months of age. There is some evidence to suggest that infants immunized at less than one year of age may not develop sustained antibody levels when later reimmunized. The advantage of early protection must be weighed against the chance for failure to respond adequately on reimmunization.

Previously unimmunized children of susceptible pregnant women should receive live attenuated rubella vaccine, because an immunized child will be less likely to acquire natural rubella and introduce the virus into the household.

Individuals planning travel outside the United States, if not immune, can acquire measles, mumps or rubella and import these diseases to the United States. Therefore, prior to International travel, individuals known to be susceptible to one or more of these diseases can receive either a single antigen vaccine (measles, mumps or rubella), or a combined antigen vaccine as appropriate. However, M-M-R II is preferred for persons likely to be susceptible to mumps and rubella; and if single-antigen measles vaccine is not readily available, travelers should receive M-M-R II regardless of their immune status to mumps or rubella.

Non-Pregnant Adolescent and Adult Females

Immunization of susceptible non-pregnant adolescent and adult females of childbearing age with live attenuated rubella virus vaccine is indicated if certain precautions are observed (see below and PRECAUTIONS). Vaccinating susceptible postpubertal females confers individual protection against subsequently acquiring rubella infection during pregnancy, which in turn prevents infection of the fetus and consequent congenital rubella injury.

Women of childbearing age should be advised not to become pregnant for three months after vaccination and should be informed of the reasons for this precaution.*

It is recommended that rubella susceptibility be determined by serologic testing prior to immunization.** If immune, as evidenced by a specific rubella antibody titer of 1:8 or greater (hemagglutination-inhibition test), vaccination is unnecessary. Congenital malformations do occur in up to seven percent of all live births. Their chance appearance after vaccination could lead to misinterpretation of the cause, particu-

Continued on next page

Information on the Merck & Co. products listed on these pages is the full prescribing information from product circulars in use October 1, 1992.

Merck & Co.—Cont.

larly if the prior rubella-immune status of vaccinees is unknown.

Postpubertal females should be informed of the frequent occurrence of generally self-limited arthralgia and/or arthritis beginning 2 to 4 weeks after vaccination (see ADVERSE REACTIONS).

Postpartum Women

It has been found convenient in many instances to vaccinate rubella-susceptible women in the immediate postpartum period. (See *Nursing Mothers*).

Revaccination: Children first vaccinated when younger than 12 months of age should be revaccinated at 15 months of age.

The American Academy of Pediatrics (AAP), the Immunization Practices Advisory Committee (ACIP), and some state and local health agencies have recommended guidelines for routine measles revaccination and to help control measles outbreaks.†

Vaccines available for revaccination include monovalent measles vaccine [ATTENUVAX (Measles Virus Vaccine Live, MSD)] and polyvalent vaccines containing measles [e.g., M-M-R II, M-R-VAX‡ II (Measles and Rubella Virus Vaccine Live, MSD)]. If the prevention of sporadic measles outbreaks is the sole objective, revaccination with a monovalent measles vaccine should be considered (see appropriate product circular). If concern also exists about immune status regarding mumps or rubella, revaccination with appropriate monovalent or polyvalent vaccine should be considered after consulting the appropriate product circulars. Unnecessary doses of a vaccine are best avoided by ensuring that written documentation of vaccination is preserved and a copy given to each vaccinee's parent or guardian.

Use with other Vaccines

Routine administration of DTP (diphtheria, tetanus, pertussis) and/or OPV (oral poliovirus vaccine) concomitantly with measles, mumps, and rubella vaccines is not recommended because there are limited data relating to the simultaneous administration of these antigens. M-M-R II should be given one month before or after administration of other vaccines. However, other schedules have been used. For example, the American Academy of Pediatrics has noted that when the patient may not return, some practitioners prefer to administer DTP, OPV, and M-M-R II on a single day. If done, separate sites and syringes should be used for DTP and M-M-R II. The Immunization Practices Advisory Committee (ACIP) recommends routine simultaneous administration of M-M-R II, DTP and OPV or inactivated polio vaccine (IPV) to all children ≥ 15 months who are eligible to receive these vaccines on the basis that there are equivalent antibody responses and no clinically significant increases in the frequency of adverse events when DTP, M-M-R II and OPV or IPV are administered either simultaneously at different sites or separately.†† Administration of M-M-R II at 15 months followed by DTP and OPV (or IPV) at 18 months remains an acceptable alternative, especially for children with caregivers known to be generally compliant with other health-care recommendations.

---

*NOTE: The Immunization Practices Advisory Committee (ACIP) has recommended "In view of the importance of protecting this age group against rubella, reasonable precautions in a rubella immunization program include asking females if they are pregnant, excluding those who say they are, and explaining the theoretical risks to the others."

**NOTE: The Immunization Practices Advisory Committee (ACIP) has stated "When practical, and when reliable laboratory services are available, potential vaccinees of childbearing age can have serologic tests to determine susceptibility to rubella. . . . However, routinely performing serologic tests for all females of childbearing age to determine susceptibility so that vaccine is given only to proven susceptibles is expensive and has been ineffective in some areas. Accordingly, the ACIP believes that rubella vaccination of a woman who is not known to be pregnant and has no history of vaccination is justifiable without serologic testing."

†NOTE: A primary difference among these recommendations is the timing of revaccination: the ACIP recommends routine revaccination at entry into kindergarten or first grade, whereas the AAP recommends routine revaccination at entrance to middle school or junior high school. In addition, some public health jurisdictions mandate the age for revaccination. The complete text of applicable guidelines should be consulted.

††NOTE: The Immunization Practices Advisory Committee (ACIP) recommends administering M-M-R II concomitantly with the fourth dose of DTP and the third dose of OPV to children 15 months of age or older providing that 6 months have elapsed since DTP-3; or, if fewer than three DTPs have been received, at least 6 weeks have elapsed since the last dose of DTP and OPV.

‡Registered trademark of MERCK & CO., INC.

CONTRAINDICATIONS

Do not give M-M-R II to pregnant females; the possible effects of the vaccine on fetal development are unknown at this time. If vaccination of postpubertal females is undertaken, pregnancy should be avoided for three months following vaccination. (See PRECAUTIONS, *Pregnancy*).

Anaphylactic or anaphylactoid reactions to neomycin (each dose of reconstituted vaccine contains approximately 25 mcg of neomycin).

History of anaphylactic or anaphylactoid reactions to eggs (see HYPERSENSITIVITY TO EGGS below).

Any febrile respiratory illness or other active febrile infection.

Active untreated tuberculosis.

Patients receiving immunosuppressive therapy. This contraindication does not apply to patients who are receiving corticosteroids as replacement therapy, e.g., for Addison's disease.

Individuals with blood dyscrasias, leukemia, lymphomas of any type, or other malignant neoplasms affecting the bone marrow or lymphatic systems.

Primary and acquired immunodeficiency states, including patients who are immunosuppressed in association with AIDS or other clinical manifestations of infection with human immunodeficiency viruses; cellular immune deficiencies; and hypogammaglobulinemic and dysgammaglobulinemic states.

Individuals with a family history of congenital or hereditary immunodeficiency, until the immune competence of the potential vaccine recipient is demonstrated.

HYPERSENSITIVITY TO EGGS

Live measles vaccine and live mumps vaccine are produced in chick embryo cell culture. Persons with a history of anaphylactic, anaphylactoid, or other immediate reactions (e.g., hives, swelling of the mouth and throat, difficulty breathing, hypotension, or shock) subsequent to egg ingestion should not be vaccinated. Evidence indicates that persons are not at increased risk if they have egg allergies that are not anaphylactic or anaphylactoid in nature. Such persons may be vaccinated in the usual manner. There is no evidence to indicate that persons with allergies to chickens or feathers are at increased risk of reaction to the vaccine.

PRECAUTIONS

General

Adequate treatment provisions including epinephrine, should be available for immediate use should an anaphylactic or anaphylactoid reaction occur.

Due caution should be employed in administration of M-M-R II to persons with a history of cerebral injury, individual or family histories of convulsions, or any other condition in which stress due to fever should be avoided. The physician should be alert to the temperature elevation which may occur following vaccination. (See ADVERSE REACTIONS).

Children and young adults who are known to be infected with human immunodeficiency viruses but without overt clinical manifestations of immunosuppression may be vaccinated; however, the vaccinees should be monitored closely for vaccine-preventable diseases because immunization may be less effective than for uninfected persons.

Vaccination should be deferred for at least 3 months following blood or plasma transfusions, or administration of human immune serum globulin.

Excretion of small amounts of the live attenuated rubella virus from the nose or throat has occurred in the majority of susceptible individuals 7–28 days after vaccination. There is no confirmed evidence to indicate that such virus is transmitted to susceptible persons who are in contact with the vaccinated individuals. Consequently, transmission through close personal contact, while accepted as a theoretical possibility, is not regarded as a significant risk. However, transmission of the rubella vaccine virus to infants via breast milk has been documented (see *Nursing Mothers*).

There are no reports of transmission of live attenuated measles or mumps viruses from vaccinees to susceptible contacts. It has been reported that live attenuated measles, mumps and rubella virus vaccines given individually may result in a temporary depression of tuberculin skin sensitivity. Therefore, if a tuberculin test is to be done, it should be administered either before or simultaneously with M-M-R II.

Children under treatment for tuberculosis have not experienced exacerbation of the disease when immunized with live measles virus vaccine; no studies have been reported to date of the effect of measles virus vaccines on untreated tuberculous children.

As for any vaccine, vaccination with M-M-R II may not result in seroconversion in 100% of susceptible persons given the vaccine.

Pregnancy
Pregnancy Category C

Animal reproduction studies have not been conducted with M-M-R II. It is also not known whether M-M-R II can cause fetal harm when administered to a pregnant woman or can affect reproduction capacity. Therefore, the vaccine should not be administered to pregnant females; furthermore, pregnancy should be avoided for three months following vaccination (see CONTRAINDICATIONS).

In counseling women who are inadvertently vaccinated when pregnant or who become pregnant within 3 months of vaccination, the physician should be aware of the following: (1) In a 10 year survey involving over 700 pregnant women who received rubella vaccine within 3 months before or after conception (of whom 189 received the Wistar RA 27/3 strain), none of the newborns had abnormalities compatible with congenital rubella syndrome; (2) Although mumps virus is capable of infecting the placenta and fetus, there is no good evidence that it causes congenital malformations in humans. Mumps vaccine virus also has been shown to infect the placenta, but the virus has not been isolated from the fetal tissues from susceptible women who were vaccinated and underwent elective abortions; and (3) Reports have indicated that contracting of natural measles during pregnancy enhances fetal risk. Increased rates of spontaneous abortion, stillbirth, congenital defects and prematurity have been observed subsequent to natural measles during pregnancy. There are no adequate studies of the attenuated (vaccine) strain of measles virus in pregnancy. However, it would be prudent to assume that the vaccine strain of virus is also capable of inducing adverse fetal effects.

Nursing Mothers

It is not known whether measles or mumps vaccine virus is secreted in human milk. Recent studies have shown that lactating postpartum women immunized with live attenuated rubella vaccine may secrete the virus in breast milk and transmit it to breast-fed infants. In the infants with serological evidence of rubella infection, none exhibited severe disease; however, one exhibited mild clinical illness typical of acquired rubella. Caution should be exercised when M-M-R II is administered to a nursing woman.

ADVERSE REACTIONS

Burning and/or stinging of short duration at the injection site have been reported.

The adverse clinical reactions associated with the use of M-M-R II are those expected to follow administration of the monovalent vaccines given separately. These may include malaise, sore throat, cough, rhinitis, headache, dizziness, fever, rash, nausea, vomiting or diarrhea; mild local reactions such as erythema, induration, tenderness and regional lymphadenopathy; parotitis, orchitis, nerve deafness, thrombocytopenia and purpura; allergic reactions such as wheal and flare at the injection site or urticaria; polyneuritis; and arthralgia and/or arthritis (usually transient and rarely chronic).

Anaphylaxis and anaphylactoid reactions have been reported.

Vasculitis has been reported rarely.

Otitis media and conjunctivitis have been reported.

Moderate fever [101-102.9°F (38.3-39.4°C)] occurs occasionally, and high fever [above 103°F (39.4°C)] occurs less commonly. On rare occasions, children developing fever may exhibit febrile convulsions. Afebrile convulsions or seizures have occurred rarely following vaccination with live attenuated measles vaccine. Syncope, particularly at the time of mass vaccination, has been reported. Rash occurs infrequently and is usually minimal, but rarely may be generalized. Erythema multiforme has also been reported rarely. Forms of optic neuritis, including retrobulbar neuritis, papillitis, and retinitis may infrequently follow viral infections, and have been reported to occur 1 to 3 weeks following inoculation with some live virus vaccines.

Clinical experience with live attenuated measles, mumps and rubella virus vaccines given individually indicates that encephalitis and other nervous system reactions have occurred very rarely. These might occur also with M-M-R II. Experience from more than 80 million doses of all live measles vaccines given in the U.S. through 1975 indicates that significant central nervous system reactions such as encephalitis and encephalopathy, occurring within 30 days after vaccination, have been temporally associated with measles vaccine very rarely. In no case has it been shown that reactions were actually caused by vaccine. The Center for Disease Control has pointed out that "a certain number of cases of encephalitis may be expected to occur in a large childhood population in a defined period of time even when no vaccines are administered". However, the data suggest the possibility that some of these cases may have been caused by measles vaccines. The risk of such serious neurological disorders following live measles virus vaccine administration remains far less than that for encephalitis and encephalopathy with natural measles (one per two thousand reported cases).

There have been rare reports of ocular palsies, Guillain-Barré syndrome, or ataxia occurring after immunization with vaccines containing live attenuated measles virus. The ocular palsies have occurred approximately 3–24 days following vaccination. No definite causal relationship has been established between these events and vaccination. Isolated reports of polyneuropathy including Guillain-Barré syndrome have also been reported after immunization with rubella-containing vaccines.

There have been reports of subacute sclerosing panencephalitis (SSPE) in children who did not have a history of natural measles but did receive measles vaccine. Some of these cases may have resulted from unrecognized measles in the first year of life or possibly from the measles vaccination. Based on estimated nationwide measles vaccine distribution, the association of SSPE cases to measles vaccination is about one case per million vaccine doses distributed. This is far less than the association with natural measles, 6–22 cases of SSPE per million cases of measles. The results of a retrospective case-controlled study conducted by the Center for Disease Control suggest that the overall effect of measles vaccine has been to protect against SSPE by preventing measles with its inherent higher risk of SSPE.

Local reactions characterized by marked swelling, redness and vesiculation at the injection site of attenuated live measles virus vaccines, and systemic reactions including atypical measles, have occurred in persons who received killed measles vaccine previously. M-M-R II was not given under this condition in clinical trials. Rarely, more severe reactions that require hospitalization, including prolonged high fevers and extensive local reactions, have been reported. Panniculitis has been reported rarely following administration of measles vaccine.

Arthralgia and/or arthritis (usually transient and rarely chronic), and polyneuritis are features of natural rubella and vary in frequency and severity with age and sex, being greatest in adult females and least in prepubertal children. This type of involvement as well as myalgia and paresthesia, have also been reported following administration of MERUVAX II (Rubella Virus Vaccine Live, MSD).

Chronic arthritis has been associated with natural rubella infection and has been related to persistent virus and/or viral antigen isolated from body tissues. Only rarely have vaccine recipients developed chronic joint symptoms.

Following vaccination in children, reactions in joints are uncommon and generally of brief duration. In women, incidence rates for arthritis and arthralgia are generally higher than those seen in children (children: 0–3%; women: 12–20%), and the reactions tend to be more marked and of longer duration. Symptoms may persist for a matter of months or on rare occasions for years. In adolescent girls, the reactions appear to be intermediate in incidence between those seen in children and in adult women. Even in older women (35–45 years), these reactions are generally well tolerated and rarely interfere with normal activities.

DOSAGE AND ADMINISTRATION

FOR SUBCUTANEOUS ADMINISTRATION

Do not inject intravenously.

The dosage of vaccine is the same for all persons. Inject the total volume of the single dose vial (about 0.5 mL) or 0.5 mL of the 10 dose vial of reconstituted vaccine subcutaneously, preferably into the outer aspect of upper arm. *Do not give immune globulin (IG) concurrently with* M-M-R II.

During shipment, to insure that there is no loss of potency, the vaccine must be maintained at a temperature of 10°C (50°F) or less.

Before reconstitution, store M-M-R II at 2–8°C (36–46°F). *Protect from light.*

CAUTION: A sterile syringe free of preservatives, antiseptics, and detergents should be used for each injection and/or reconstitution of the vaccine because these substances may inactivate the live virus vaccine. A 25 gauge, 5/8" needle is recommended.

To reconstitute, use only the diluent supplied, since it is free of preservatives or other antiviral substances which might inactivate the vaccine.

Single Dose Vial—First withdraw the entire volume of diluent into the syringe to be used for reconstitution. Inject all the diluent in the syringe into the vial of lyophilized vaccine, and agitate to mix thoroughly. Withdraw the entire contents into a syringe and inject the total volume of restored vaccine subcutaneously.

It is important to use a separate sterile syringe and needle for each individual patient to prevent transmission of hepatitis B and other infectious agents from one person to another.

10 Dose Vial (available only to government agencies/institutions)

Withdraw the entire contents (7 mL) of the diluent vial into the sterile syringe to be used for reconstitution, and introduce into the 10 dose vial of lyophilized vaccine. Agitate to ensure thorough mixing. The outer labeling suggests "For Jet Injector or Syringe Use". Use with separate sterile syringes is permitted for containers of 10 doses or less. The vaccine and diluent do not contain preservatives; therefore, the user must recognize the potential contamination hazards and exercise special precautions to protect the sterility and potency of the product. The use of aseptic techniques and proper storage prior to and after restoration of the vaccine and subsequent withdrawal of the individual doses is essential. Use 0.5 mL of the reconstituted vaccine for subcutaneous injection.

It is important to use a separate sterile syringe and needle for each individual patient to prevent transmission of hepatitis B and other infectious agents from one person to another.

Each dose contains not less than the equivalent of 1,000 $TCID_{50}$ of the U.S. Reference Measles Virus, 20,000 $TCID_{50}$ of the U.S. Reference Mumps Virus and 1,000 $TCID_{50}$ of the U.S. Reference Rubella Virus.

Parenteral drug products should be inspected visually for particulate matter and discoloration prior to administration. M-M-R II, when reconstituted, is clear yellow.

HOW SUPPLIED

No. 4749—M-M-R II is supplied as a single-dose vial of lyophilized vaccine, **NDC** 0006-4749-00, and a vial of diluent.

No. 4681/4309—M-M-R II is supplied as follows: (1) a box of 10 single-dose vials of lyophilized vaccine (package A), **NDC** 0006-4681-00; and (2) a box of 10 vials of diluent (package B). To conserve refrigerator space, the diluent may be stored separately at room temperature (6505-00-165-6519, Ten Pack).

Available only to government agencies/institutions

No. 4682X—M-M-R II is supplied as one 10 dose vial of lyophilized vaccine, **NDC** 0006-4682-00, and one 7 mL vial of diluent.

Storage

It is recommended that the vaccine be used as soon as possible after reconstitution. Protect vaccine from light at all times, since such exposure may inactivate the virus. Store reconstituted vaccine in the vaccine vial in a dark place at 2–8°C (36–46°F) and discard if not used within 8 hours.

A.H.F.S. Category: 80:12

DC 7678913 Issued March 1991

Copyright © MERCK & CO., INC., 1990
All rights reserved

M-R-VAX®II ℞

(Measles and Rubella Virus Vaccine Live, MSD), U.S.P.

DESCRIPTION

M-R-VAX* II (Measles and Rubella Virus Vaccine Live, MSD) is a live virus vaccine for immunization against measles (rubeola) and rubella (German measles).

M-R-VAX II is a sterile lyophilized preparation of (1) ATTENUVAX* (Measles Virus Vaccine Live, MSD), a more attenuated line of measles virus, derived from Enders' attenuated Edmonston strain and grown in cell cultures of chick embryo; and (2) MERUVAX* II (Rubella Virus Vaccine Live, MSD), the Wistar RA 27/3 strain of live attenuated rubella virus grown in human diploid cell (WI-38) culture. The vaccine viruses are the same as those used in the manufacture of ATTENUVAX (Measles Virus Vaccine Live, MSD) and MERUVAX II (Rubella Virus Vaccine Live, MSD). The two viruses are mixed before being lyophilized. The product contains no preservative.

The reconstituted vaccine is for subcutaneous administration. When reconstituted as directed, the dose for injection is 0.5 mL and contains not less than the equivalent of 1,000 $TCID_{50}$ (tissue culture infectious doses) of the U.S. Reference Measles Virus; and 1,000 $TCID_{50}$ of the U.S. Reference Rubella Virus. Each dose contains approximately 25 mcg of neomycin. The product contains no preservative. Sorbitol and hydrolized gelatin are added as stabilizers.

*Registered trademark of MERCK & CO., INC.

CLINICAL PHARMACOLOGY

Clinical studies of 237 double seronegative children, 10 months to 10 years of age, demonstrated that M-R-VAX II is highly immunogenic and generally well tolerated. In these studies, a single injection of the vaccine induced measles hemagglutination-inhibition (HI) antibodies in 95 percent and rubella HI antibodies in 99 percent of susceptible persons.

The RA 27/3 rubella strain in M-R-VAX II elicits higher immediate post-vaccination HI, complement-fixing and neutralizing antibody levels than other strains of rubella vaccine and has been shown to induce a broader profile of circulating antibodies including anti-theta and anti-iota precipitating antibodies. The RA 27/3 rubella strain immunologically simulates natural infection more closely than other rubella vaccine viruses. The increased levels and broader profile of antibodies produced by RA 27/3 strain rubella virus vaccine appear to correlate with greater resistance to subclinical reinfection with the wild virus, and provide greater confidence for lasting immunity.

Vaccine induced antibody levels following administration of M-R-VAX II have been shown to persist up to 11 years without substantial decline. Continued surveillance will be necessary to determine further duration of antibody persistence.

INDICATIONS AND USAGE

M-R-VAX II is indicated for simultaneous immunization against measles and rubella in persons 15 months of age or older. A second dose of M-R-VAX II or monovalent measles vaccine is recommended (see *Revaccination*).

Infants who are less than 15 months of age may fail to respond to the measles component of the vaccine due to presence in the circulation of residual measles antibody of maternal origin; the younger the infant, the lower the likelihood of seroconversion. In geographically isolated or other relatively inaccessible populations for whom immunization programs are logistically difficult, and in population groups in which natural measles infection may occur in a significant proportion of infants before 15 months of age, it may be desirable to give the vaccine to infants at an earlier age. Infants vaccinated under these conditions at less than 12 months of age should be revaccinated after reaching 15 months of age. There is some evidence to suggest that infants immunized at less than one year of age may not develop sustained antibody levels when later reimmunized. The advantage of early protection must be weighed against the chance for failure to respond adequately on reimmunization.

Previously unimmunized children of susceptible pregnant women should receive live attenuated rubella vaccine, because an immunized child will be less likely to acquire natural rubella and introduce the virus into the household.

Individuals planning travel outside the United States, if not immune, can acquire measles, mumps or rubella and import these diseases to the United States. Therefore, prior to International travel, individuals known to be susceptible to one or more of these diseases can receive either a single antigen vaccine (measles, mumps, or rubella), or a combined antigen vaccine as appropriate. However, M-M-R† II (Measles, Mumps, and Rubella Virus Vaccine Live, MSD) is preferred for persons likely to be susceptible to mumps and rubella; and if a single-antigen measles vaccine is not readily available, travelers should receive M-M-R II (Measles, Mumps, and Rubella Virus Vaccine Live, MSD) regardless of their immune status to mumps or rubella.

Non-Pregnant Adolescent and Adult Females

Immunization of susceptible non-pregnant adolescent and adult females of childbearing age with live attenuated rubella virus vaccine is indicated if certain precautions are observed (see below and PRECAUTIONS). Vaccinating susceptible postpubertal females confers individual protection against subsequently acquiring rubella infection during pregnancy, which in turn prevents infection of the fetus and consequent congenital rubella injury.

Women of childbearing age should be advised not to become pregnant for three months after vaccination and should be informed of the reason for this precaution.*

It is recommended that rubella susceptibility be determined by serologic testing prior to immunization.** If immune, as evidenced by a specific rubella antibody titer of 1:8 or greater (hemagglutination-inhibition test), vaccination is unnecessary. Congenital malformations do occur in up to seven percent of all live births. Their chance appearance after vaccination could lead to misinterpretation of the cause, particularly if the prior rubella-immune status of vaccinees is unknown.

Postpubertal females should be informed of the frequent occurrence of generally self-limited arthralgia and/or arthritis beginning 2 to 4 weeks after vaccination (see ADVERSE REACTIONS).

Postpartum Women

It has been found convenient in many instances to vaccinate rubella-susceptible women in the immediate postpartum period. (See *Nursing Mothers*).

Revaccination: Children first vaccinated when younger than 12 months of age should be revaccinated at 15 months of age.

The American Academy of Pediatrics (AAP), the Immunization Practices Advisory Committee (ACIP), and some state and local health agencies have recommended guidelines for routine measles revaccination and to help control measles outbreaks.***

Continued on next page

Information on the Merck & Co. products listed on these pages is the full prescribing information from product circulars in use October 1, 1992.

Merck & Co.—Cont.

Vaccines available for revaccination include monovalent measles vaccine [ATTENUVAX (Measles Virus Vaccine Live, MSD)] and polyvalent vaccines containing measles [e.g., M-M-R II (Measles, Mumps, and Rubella Virus Vaccine Live, MSD), M-R-VAX II]. If the prevention of sporadic measles outbreaks is the sole objective, revaccination with a monovalent measles vaccine should be considered (see appropriate product circular). If concern also exists about immune status regarding mumps or rubella, revaccination with appropriate monovalent or polyvalent vaccines should be considered after consulting the appropriate product circulars. Unnecessary doses of a vaccine are best avoided by ensuring that written documentation of vaccination is preserved and a copy given to each vaccinee's parent or guardian.

Use with other Vaccines

Routine administration of DTP (diphtheria, tetanus, pertussis) and/or OPV (oral poliovirus vaccine) concomitantly with measles, mumps and rubella vaccines is not recommended because there are insufficient data relating to the simultaneous administration of these antigens. However, the American Academy of Pediatrics has noted that in some circumstances, particularly when the patient may not return, some practitioners prefer to administer all these antigens on a single day. If done, separate sites and syringes should be used for DTP and M-R-VAX II.

M-R-VAX II should not be given less than one month before or after administration of other virus vaccines.

---

† Registered trademark of MERCK & CO., INC.

* NOTE: The Immunization Practices Advisory Committee (ACIP) has recommended "In view of the importance of protecting this age group against rubella, reasonable precautions in a rubella immunization program include asking females if they are pregnant, excluding those who say they are, and explaining the theoretical risks to the others."

** NOTE: The Immunization Practices Advisory Committee (ACIP) has stated "When practical, and when reliable laboratory services are available, potential vaccinees of childbearing age can have serologic tests to determine susceptibility to rubella.... However, routinely performing serologic tests for all females of childbearing age to determine susceptibility so that vaccine is given only to proven susceptibles is expensive and has been ineffective in some areas. Accordingly, the ACIP believes that rubella vaccination of a woman who is not known to be pregnant and has no history of vaccination is justifiable without serologic testing."

*** NOTE: A primary difference among these recommendations is the timing of revaccination: the ACIP recommends routine revaccination at entry into Kindergarten or first grade, whereas the AAP recommends routine revaccination at entrance to middle school or junior high school. In addition, some public health jurisdictions mandate the age for revaccination. The complete text of applicable guidelines should be consulted.

CONTRAINDICATIONS

Do not give M-R-VAX II to pregnant females; the possible effects of the vaccine on fetal development are unknown at this time. If vaccination of postpubertal females is undertaken, pregnancy should be avoided for three months following vaccination. (See PRECAUTIONS, *Pregnancy*).

Anaphylactic or anaphylactoid reactions to neomycin (each dose of reconstituted vaccine contains approximately 25 mcg of neomycin).

History of anaphylactic or anaphylactoid reactions to eggs (see HYPERSENSITIVITY TO EGGS below).

Any febrile respiratory illness or other active febrile infection.

Active untreated tuberculosis.

Patients receiving immunosuppressive therapy. This contraindication does not apply to patients who are receiving corticosteroids as replacement therapy, e.g., for Addison's disease.

Individuals with blood dyscrasias, leukemia, lymphomas of any type, or other malignant neoplasms affecting the bone marrow or lymphatic systems.

Primary and acquired immunodeficiency states, including patients who are immunosuppressed in association with AIDS or other clinical manifestations of infection with human immunodeficiency viruses; cellular immune deficiencies; and hypogammaglobulinemic and dysgammaglobulinemic states.

Individuals with a family history of congenital or hereditary immunodeficiency, until the immune competence of the potential vaccine recipient is demonstrated.

HYPERSENSITIVITY TO EGGS

Live measles vaccine is produced in chick embryo cell culture. Persons with a history of anaphylactic, anaphylactoid, or other immediate reactions (e.g., hives, swelling of the mouth and throat, difficulty breathing, hypotension, or shock) subsequent to egg ingestion should not be vaccinated. Evidence indicates that persons are not at increased risk if they have egg allergies that are not anaphylactic or anaphylactoid in nature. Such persons may be vaccinated in the usual manner. There is no evidence to indicate that persons with allergies to chickens or feathers are at increased risk of reaction to the vaccine.

PRECAUTIONS

General

Adequate treatment provisions including epinephrine, should be available for immediate use should an anaphylactic or anaphylactoid reaction occur.

Due caution should be employed in administration of M-R-VAX II to persons with a history of cerebral injury, individual or family histories of convulsions, or any other condition in which stress due to fever should be avoided. The physician should be alert to the temperature elevation which may occur following vaccination. (See ADVERSE REACTIONS.)

Children and young adults who are known to be infected with human immunodeficiency viruses but without overt clinical manifestations of immunosuppression may be vaccinated; however, the vaccinees should be monitored closely for vaccine-preventable diseases because immunization may be less effective than for uninfected persons.

Vaccination should be deferred for at least 3 months following blood or plasma transfusions, or administration of human immune serum globulin.

Excretion of small amounts of the live attenuated rubella virus from the nose or throat has occurred in the majority of susceptible individuals 7–28 days after vaccination. There is no confirmed evidence to indicate that such virus is transmitted to susceptible persons who are in contact with the vaccinated individuals. Consequently, transmission through close personal contact, while accepted as a theoretical possibility, is not regarded as a significant risk. However, transmission of the rubella vaccine virus to infants via breast milk has been documented (see *Nursing Mothers*).

There are no reports of transmission of live attenuated measles virus from vaccinees to susceptible contacts.

It has been reported that live attenuated measles and rubella virus vaccines given individually may result in a temporary depression of tuberculin skin sensitivity. Therefore, if a tuberculin test is to be done, it should be administered either before or simultaneously with M-R-VAX II.

Children under treatment for tuberculosis have not experienced exacerbation of the disease when immunized with live measles virus vaccine; no studies have been reported to date of the effect of measles virus vaccines on untreated tuberculous children.

As for any vaccine, vaccination with M-R-VAX II may not result in seroconversion in 100% of susceptible persons given the vaccine.

Pregnancy

Pregnancy Category C

Animal reproduction studies have not been conducted with M-R-VAX II. It is also not known whether M-R-VAX II can cause fetal harm when administered to a pregnant woman or can affect reproduction capacity. Therefore, the vaccine should not be administered to pregnant females; futhermore, pregnancy should be avoided for three months following vaccination (see CONTRAINDICATIONS).

In counseling women who are inadvertently vaccinated when pregnant or who become pregnant within 3 months of vaccination, the physician should be aware of the following: (1) In a 10 year survey involving over 700 pregnant women who received rubella vaccine within 3 months before or after conception, (of whom 189 received the Wistar RA 27/3 strain), none of the newborns had abnormalities compatible with congenital rubella syndrome; (2) Reports have indicated that contracting of natural measles during pregnancy enhances fetal risk. Increased rates of spontaneous abortion, stillbirth, congenital defects and prematurity have been observed subsequent to natural measles during pregnancy. There are no adequate studies of the attenuated (vaccine) strain of measles virus in pregnancy. However, it would be prudent to assume that the vaccine strain of virus is also capable of inducing adverse fetal effects.

Nursing Mothers

It is not known whether measles vaccine virus is secreted in human milk. Recent studies have shown that lactating postpartum women immunized with live attenuated rubella vaccine may secrete the virus in breast milk and transmit it to breast-fed infants. In the infants with serological evidence of rubella infection, none exhibited severe disease; however, one exhibited mild clinical illness typical of acquired rubella. Caution should be exercised when M-R-VAX II is administered to a nursing woman.

ADVERSE REACTIONS

Burning and/or stinging of short duration at the injection site have been reported.

The adverse clinical reactions associated with the use of M-R-VAX II are those expected to follow administration of the monovalent vaccines given separately. These may include malaise, sore throat, cough, rhinitis, headache, dizziness, fever, rash, nausea, vomiting or diarrhea; mild local reactions such as erythema, induration, tenderness and regional lymphadenopathy; thrombocytopenia and purpura; allergic reactions such as wheal and flare at the injection site or urticaria; polyneuritis, and arthralgia and/or arthritis (usually transient and rarely chronic).

Anaphylaxis and anaphylactoid reactions have been reported.

Vasculitis has been reported rarely.

Moderate fever [101–102.9°F (38.3–39.4°C)] occurs occasionally, and high fever [above 103°F (39.4°C)] occurs less commonly. On rare occasions, children developing fever may exhibit febrile convulsions. Afebrile convulsions or seizures have occurred rarely following vaccination with live attenuated measles vaccine. Syncope, particularly at the time of mass vaccination, has been reported. Rash occurs infrequently and is usually minimal, but rarely may be generalized. Erythema multiforme has also been reported rarely. Forms of optic neuritis, including retrobulbar neuritis, papillitis, and retinitis may infrequently follow viral infections, and have been reported to occur 1 to 3 weeks following inoculation with some live virus vaccines.

Clinical experience with live attenuated measles and rubella virus vaccines given individually indicates that encephalitis and other nervous system reactions have occurred very rarely. These might occur also with M-R-VAX II.

Experience from more than 80 million doses of all live measles vaccines given in the U.S. through 1975 indicates that significant central nervous system reactions such as encephalitis and encephalopathy, occurring within 30 days after vaccination, have been temporally associated with measles vaccine very rarely. In no case has it been shown that reactions were actually caused by vaccine. The Center for Disease Control has pointed out that "a certain number of cases of encephalitis may be expected to occur in a large childhood population in a defined period of time even when no vaccines are administered". However, the data suggest the possibility that some of these cases may have been caused by measles vaccines. The risk of such serious neurological disorders following live measles virus vaccine administration remains far less than that for encephalitis and encephalopathy with natural measles (one per two thousand reported cases).

There have been rare reports of ocular palsies, Guillain-Barré syndrome, or ataxia occurring after immunization with vaccines containing live attenuated measles virus. The ocular palsies have occurred approximately 3–24 days following vaccination. No definite causal relationship has been established between these events and vaccination. Isolated reports of polyneuropathy including Guillain-Barré syndrome have also been reported after immunization with rubella-containing vaccines.

There have been reports of subacute sclerosing panencephalitis (SSPE) in children who did not have a history of natural measles but did receive measles vaccine. Some of these cases may have resulted from unrecognized measles in the first year of life or possibly from the measles vaccination. Based on estimated nationwide measles vaccine distribution, the association of SSPE cases to measles vaccination is about one case per million vaccine doses distributed. This is far less than the association with natural measles, 6–22 cases of SSPE per million cases of measles. The results of a retrospective case-controlled study conducted by the Center for Disease Control suggest that the overall effect of measles vaccine has been to protect against SSPE by preventing measles with its inherent higher risk of SSPE.

Local reactions characterized by marked swelling, redness and vesiculation at the injection site of attenuated live measles virus vaccines, and systemic reactions including atypical measles, have occurred in persons who received killed measles vaccine previously. M-R-VAX II was not given under this condition in clinical trials. Rarely, more severe reactions that require hospitalization, including prolonged high fevers and extensive local reactions, have been reported. Panniculitis has been reported rarely following administration of measles vaccine.

Arthralgia and/or arthritis (usually transient and rarely chronic), and polyneuritis are features of natural rubella and vary in frequency and severity with age and sex, being greatest in adult females and least in prepubertal children. This type of involvement as well as myalgia and paresthesia have also been reported following administration of MERUVAX II (Rubella Virus Vaccine Live, MSD).

Chronic arthritis has been associated with natural rubella infection and has been related to persistent virus and/or viral antigen isolated from body tissues. Only rarely have vaccine recipients developed chronic joint symptoms.

Following vaccination in children, reactions in joints are uncommon and generally of brief duration. In women, incidence rates for arthritis and arthralgia are generally higher than those seen in children (children: 0–3%; women: 12–20%), and the reactions tend to be more marked and of longer duration. Symptoms may persist for a matter of months or on rare occasions for years. In adolescent girls, the reactions appear to be intermediate in incidence between those seen in children and in adult women. Even in older women (35–45 years), these reactions are generally well tolerated and rarely interfere with normal activities.

DOSAGE AND ADMINISTRATION

FOR SUBCUTANEOUS ADMINISTRATION
Do not inject intravenously
The dosage of vaccine is the same for all persons. Inject the total volume of the single dose vial (about 0.5 mL) or 0.5 mL of the multiple dose vial of reconstituted vaccine subcutaneously, preferably into the outer aspect of upper arm. *Do not give immune globulin (IG) concurrently with* M-R-VAX II.
During shipment, to insure that there is no loss of potency, the vaccine must be maintained at a temperature of 10°C (50°F) or less.
Before reconstitution, store M-R-VAX II at 2–8°C (36–46°F). *Protect from light.*
CAUTION: A sterile syringe free of preservatives, antiseptics, and detergents should be used for each injection and/or reconstitution of the vaccine because these substances may inactivate the live virus vaccine. A 25 gauge, 5/8" needle is recommended.
To reconstitute, use only the diluent supplied, since it is free of preservatives or other antiviral substances which might inactivate the vaccine.

Single Dose Vial—First withdraw the entire volume of diluent into the syringe to be used for reconstitution. Inject all the diluent in the syringe into the vial of lyophilized vaccine, and agitate to mix thoroughly. Withdraw the entire contents into a syringe and inject the total volume of restored vaccine subcutaneously.
It is important to use a separate sterile syringe and needle for each individual patient to prevent transmission of hepatitis B and other infectious agents from one person to another.

10 Dose Vial (available only to government agencies/institutions)—Withdraw the entire contents (7 mL) of the diluent vial into the sterile syringe to be used for reconstitution, and introduce into the 10 dose vial of lyophilized vaccine. Agitate to ensure thorough mixing. The outer labeling suggests "For Jet Injector or Syringe Use". Use with separate sterile syringes is permitted for containers of 10 doses or less. The vaccine and diluent do not contain preservatives; therefore, the user must recognize the potential contamination hazards and exercise special precautions to protect the sterility and potency of the product. The use of aseptic techniques and proper storage prior to and after restoration of the vaccine and subsequent withdrawal of the individual doses is essential. Use 0.5 mL of the reconstituted vaccine for subcutaneous injection.
It is important to use a separate sterile syringe and needle for each individual patient to prevent transmission of hepatitis B and other infectious agents from one person to another.

50 Dose Vial (available only to government agencies/institutions)—Withdraw the entire contents (30 mL) of diluent vial into the sterile syringe to be used for reconstitution and introduce into the 50 dose vial of lyophilized vaccine. Agitate to ensure thorough mixing. With full aseptic precautions, attach the vial to the sterilized multidose jet injector apparatus. Use 0.5 mL of the reconstituted vaccine for subcutaneous injection.

Each dose contains not less than the equivalent of 1,000 $TCID_{50}$ of the U.S. Reference Measles Virus and 1,000 $TCID_{50}$ of the U.S. Reference Rubella Virus.
Parenteral drug products should be inspected visually for particulate matter and discoloration prior to administration. M-R-VAX II, when reconstituted, is clear yellow.

HOW SUPPLIED

No. 4751—M-R-VAX II is supplied as a single-dose vial of lyophilized vaccine, **NDC** 0006-4751-00, and a vial of diluent.
No. 4677/4309—M-R-VAX II is supplied as follows: (1) a box of 10 single-dose vials of lyophilized vaccine (package A), **NDC** 0006-4677-00; and (2) a box of 10 vials of diluent (package B). To conserve refrigerator space, the diluent may be stored separately at room temperature (6505-01-098-8004, Ten Pack).
Available only to government agencies/institutions:
No. 4678—M-R-VAX II is supplied as one 10 dose vial of lyophilized vaccine, **NDC** 0006-4678-00, and one 7 mL vial of diluent.
No. 4679—M-R-VAX II is supplied as one 50 dose vial of lyophilized vaccine, **NDC** 0006-4679-00, and one 30 mL vial of diluent (6505-01-098-8005, 50 dose).

Storage
It is recommended that the vaccine be used as soon as possible after reconstitution. Protect vaccine from light at all times, since such exposure may inactivate the virus. Store reconstituted vaccine in the vaccine vial in a dark place at 2–8°C (36–46°F) and discard if not used within 8 hours.

A.H.F.S. Category: 80:12
DC 7680215 Issued March 1991

COPYRIGHT © MERCK & CO., INC., 1990
All rights reserved

MEFOXIN® ℞
(Cefoxitin Sodium), U.S.P.

DESCRIPTION

MEFOXIN* (Sterile Cefoxitin Sodium) is a semi-synthetic, broad-spectrum cepha antibiotic sealed under nitrogen for parenteral administration. It is derived from cephamycin C, which is produced by *Streptomyces lactamdurans.* It is the sodium salt of 3-(hydroxymethyl)-7α-methoxy-8-oxo-7-[2-(2-thienyl) acetamido]-5-thia-1-azabicyclo [4.2.0] oct-2-ene-2-carboxylate carbamate (ester). The empirical formula is $C_{16}H_{16}N_3NaO_7S_2$, and the structural formula is:

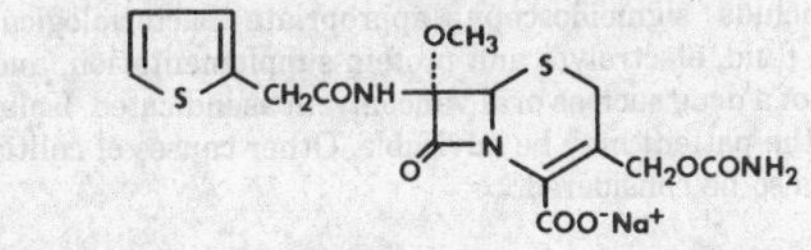

MEFOXIN contains approximately 53.8 mg (2.3 milliequivalents) of sodium per gram of cefoxitin activity. Solutions of MEFOXIN range from colorless to light amber in color. The pH of freshly constituted solutions usually ranges from 4.2 to 7.0.

*Registered trademark of MERCK & CO., INC.

CLINICAL PHARMACOLOGY

Clinical Pharmacology
After intramuscular administration of a 1 gram dose of MEFOXIN to normal volunteers, the mean peak serum concentration was 24 mcg/mL. The peak occurred at 20 to 30 minutes. Following an intravenous dose of 1 gram, serum concentrations were 110 mcg/mL at 5 minutes, declining to less than 1 mcg/mL at 4 hours. The half-life after an intravenous dose is 41 to 59 minutes; after intramuscular administration, the half-life is 64.8 minutes. Approximately 85 percent of cefoxitin is excreted unchanged by the kidneys over a 6-hour period, resulting in high urinary concentrations. Following an intramuscular dose of 1 gram, urinary concentrations greater than 3000 mcg/mL were observed. Probenecid slows tubular excretion and produces higher serum levels and increases the duration of measurable serum concentrations.
Cefoxitin passes into pleural and joint fluids and is detectable in antibacterial concentrations in bile.
Clinical experience has demonstrated that MEFOXIN can be administered to patients who are also receiving carbenicillin, kanamycin, gentamicin, tobramycin, or amikacin (see PRECAUTIONS and ADMINISTRATION).

Microbiology
The bactericidal action of cefoxitin results from inhibition of cell wall synthesis. Cefoxitin has *in vitro* activity against a wide range of gram-positive and gram-negative organisms. The methoxy group in the 7α position provides MEFOXIN with a high degree of stability in the presence of beta-lactamases, both penicillinases and cephalosporinases, of gram-negative bacteria. Cefoxitin is usually active against the following organisms *in vitro* and in clinical infections:

Gram-positive
- *Staphylococcus aureus,* including penicillinase and non-penicillinase producing strains.
- *Staphylococcus epidermidis*
- Beta-hemolytic and other streptococci (most strains of enterococci, e.g., *Streptococcus faecalis,* are resistant)
- *Streptococcus pneumoniae*

Gram-negative
- *Escherichia coli*
- *Klebsiella* species (including *K. pneumoniae*)
- *Hemophilus influenzae*
- *Neisseria gonorrhoeae,* including penicillinase and non-penicillinase producing strains
- *Proteus mirabilis*
- *Morganella morganii*
- *Proteus vulgaris*
- *Providencia* species, including *Providencia rettgeri*

Anaerobic organisms
- *Peptococcus* species
- *Peptostreptococcus* species
- *Clostridium* species
- *Bacteroides* species, including the *B. fragilis* group (includes *B. fragilis, B. distasonis, B. ovatus, B. thetaiotaomicron, B. vulgatus*)

MEFOXIN is inactive *in vitro* against most strains of *Pseudomonas aeruginosa* and enterococci and many strains of *Enterobacter cloacae.*
Methicillin-resistant staphylococci are almost uniformly resistant to MEFOXIN.

Susceptibility Tests
For fast-growing aerobic organisms, quantitative methods that require measurements of zone diameters give the most precise estimates of antibiotic susceptibility. One such procedure* has been recommended for use with discs to test susceptibility to cefoxitin. Interpretation involves correlation of the diameters obtained in the disc test with minimal inhibitory concentration (MIC) values for cefoxitin.
Reports from the laboratory giving results of the standardized single disc susceptibility test* using a 30 mcg cefoxitin disc should be interpreted according to the following criteria: Organisms producing zones of 18 mm or greater are considered susceptible, indicating that the tested organism is likely to respond to therapy.
Organisms of intermediate susceptibility produce zones of 15 to 17 mm, indicating that the tested organism would be susceptible if high dosage is used or if the infection is confined to tissues and fluids (e.g., urine) in which high antibiotic levels are attained.
Resistant organisms produce zones of 14 mm or less, indicating that other therapy should be selected.
The cefoxitin disc should be used for testing cefoxitin susceptibility.
Cefoxitin has been shown by *in vitro* tests to have activity against certain strains of *Enterobacteriaceae* found resistant when tested with the cephalosporin class disc. For this reason, the cefoxitin disc should not be used for testing susceptibility to cephalosporins, and cephalosporin discs should not be used for testing susceptibility to cefoxitin.
Dilution methods, preferably the agar plate dilution procedure, are most accurate for susceptibility testing of obligate anaerobes.
A bacterial isolate may be considered susceptible if the MIC value for cefoxitin† is not more than 16 mcg/mL. Organisms are considered resistant if the MIC is greater than 32 mcg/mL.

* Bauer, A. W.; Kirby, W. M. M.; Sherris, J. C.; Turck, M.: Antibiotic susceptibility testing by a standardized single disc method, Amer. J. Clin. Path. *45*: 493–496, Apr. 1966. Standardized disc susceptibility test, Federal Register *37*: 20527–20529, 1972. National Committee for Clinical Laboratory Standards: Approved Standard: ASM-2, Performance Standards for Antimicrobial Disc Susceptibility Tests, July 1975.

† Determined by the ICS agar dilution method (Ericsson and Sherris, Acta Path. Microbiol. Scand. (B) Suppl. No. 217, 1971) or any other method that has been shown to give equivalent results.

INDICATIONS AND USAGE

Treatment
MEFOXIN is indicated for the treatment of serious infections caused by susceptible strains of the designated microorganisms in the diseases listed below.
(1) Lower respiratory tract infections, including pneumonia and lung abscess, caused by *Streptococcus pneumoniae,* other streptococci (excluding enterococci, e.g., *Streptococcus faecalis*), *Staphylococcus aureus* (penicillinase and non-penicillinase producing), *Escherichia coli, Klebsiella* species, *Hemophilus influenzae,* and *Bacteroides* species.
(2) Genitourinary infections. Urinary tract infections caused by *Escherichia coli, Klebsiella* species, *Proteus mirabilis,* indole-positive Proteus (which include the organisms now called *Morganella morganii* and *Proteus vulgaris),* and *Providencia* species (including *Providencia rettgeri).* Uncomplicated gonorrhea due to *Neisseria gonorrhoeae* (penicillinase and non-penicillinase producing).
(3) Intra-abdominal infections, including peritonitis and intra-abdominal abscess, caused by *Escherichia coli, Klebsiella* species, *Bacteroides* species including the *Bacteroides fragilis* group**, and *Clostridium* species.
(4) Gynecological infections, including endometritis, pelvic cellulitis, and pelvic inflammatory disease caused by *Escherichia coli, Neisseria gonorrhoeae* (penicillinase and non-peni-

Continued on next page

Information on the Merck & Co. products listed on these pages is the full prescribing information from product circulars in use October 1, 1992.

Merck & Co.—Cont.

cillinase producing), *Bacteroides* species including the *Bacteroides fragilis* group**, *Clostridium* species, *Peptococcus* species, *Peptostreptococcus* species, and Group B streptococci.

(5) Septicemia caused by *Streptococcus pneumoniae, Staphylococcus aureus* (penicillinase and non-penicillinase producing), *Escherichia coli, Klebsiella* species, and *Bacteroides* species including the *Bacteroides fragilis* group.**

(6) Bone and joint infections caused by *Staphylococcus aureus* (penicillinase and non-penicillinase producing).

(7) Skin and skin structure infections caused by *Staphylococcus aureus* (penicillinase and non-penicillinase producing), *Staphylococcus epidermidis,* streptococci (excluding enterococci, e.g., *Streptococcus faecalis*), *Escherichia coli, Proteus mirabilis, Klebsiella* species, *Bacteroides* species including the *Bacteroides fragilis* group**, *Clostridium* species, *Peptococcus* species, and *Peptostreptococcus* species.

Appropriate culture and susceptibility studies should be performed to determine the susceptibility of the causative organisms to MEFOXIN. Therapy may be started while awaiting the results of these studies.

In randomized comparative studies, MEFOXIN and cephalothin were comparably safe and effective in the management of infections caused by gram-positive cocci and gram-negative rods susceptible to the cephalosporins. MEFOXIN has a high degree of stability in the presence of bacterial beta-lactamases, both penicillinases and cephalosporinases.

Many infections caused by aerobic and anaerobic gram-negative bacteria resistant to some cephalosporins respond to MEFOXIN. Similarly, many infections caused by aerobic and anaerobic bacteria resistant to some penicillin antibiotics (ampicillin, carbenicillin, penicillin G) respond to treatment with MEFOXIN. Many infections caused by mixtures of susceptible aerobic and anaerobic bacteria respond to treatment with MEFOXIN.

Prevention

When compared to placebo in randomized controlled studies in patients undergoing gastrointestinal surgery, vaginal hysterectomy, abdominal hysterectomy and cesarean section, the prophylactic use of MEFOXIN resulted in a significant reduction in the number of postoperative infections.

The prophylactic administration of MEFOXIN may reduce the incidence of certain postoperative infections in patients undergoing surgical procedures (e.g., hysterectomy, gastrointestinal surgery and transurethral prostatectomy) that are classified as contaminated or potentially contaminated.

The perioperative use of MEFOXIN may be effective in surgical patients in whom subsequent infection at the operative site would present a serious risk, e.g., prosthetic arthroplasty.

Effective prophylactic use depends on the time of administration. MEFOXIN usually should be given one-half to one hour before the operation, which is sufficient time to achieve effective levels in the wound during the procedure. Prophylactic administration should usually be stopped within 24 hours since continuing administration of any antibiotic increases the possibility of adverse reactions but, in the majority of surgical procedures, does not reduce the incidence of subsequent infection. However, in patients undergoing prosthetic arthroplasty, it is recommended that MEFOXIN be continued for 72 hours after the surgical procedure.

If there are signs of infection, specimens for culture should be obtained for identification of the causative organism so that appropriate treatment may be instituted.

**B. fragilis, B. distasonis, B. ovatus, B. thetaiotaomicron, B. vulgatus.*

CONTRAINDICATIONS

MEFOXIN is contraindicated in patients who have shown hypersensitivity to cefoxitin and the cephalosporin group of antibiotics.

WARNINGS

BEFORE THERAPY WITH 'MEFOXIN' IS INSTITUTED, CAREFUL INQUIRY SHOULD BE MADE TO DETERMINE WHETHER THE PATIENT HAS HAD PREVIOUS HYPERSENSITIVITY REACTIONS TO CEFOXITIN, CEPHALOSPORINS, PENICILLINS, OR OTHER DRUGS. THIS PRODUCT SHOULD BE GIVEN WITH CAUTION TO PENICILLIN-SENSITIVE PATIENTS. ANTIBIOTICS SHOULD BE ADMINISTERED WITH CAUTION TO ANY PATIENT WHO HAS DEMONSTRATED SOME FORM OF ALLERGY, PARTICULARLY TO DRUGS. IF AN ALLERGIC REACTION TO 'MEFOXIN' OCCURS, DISCONTINUE THE DRUG. SERIOUS HYPERSENSITIVITY REACTIONS MAY REQUIRE EPINEPHRINE AND OTHER EMERGENCY MEASURES.

Pseudomembranous colitis has been reported with virtually all antibiotics (including cephalosporins); therefore, it is important to consider its diagnosis in patients who develop diarrhea in association with antibiotic use. This colitis may range from mild to life threatening in severity.

Treatment with broad-spectrum antibiotics alters normal flora of the colon and may permit overgrowth of clostridia. Studies indicate a toxin produced by *Clostridium difficile* is one primary cause of antibiotic-associated colitis.

Mild cases of pseudomembranous colitis may respond to drug discontinuance alone. In more severe cases, management may include sigmoidoscopy, appropriate bacteriological studies, fluid, electrolyte and protein supplementation, and the use of a drug such as oral vancomycin as indicated. Isolation of the patient may be advisable. Other causes of colitis should also be considered.

PRECAUTIONS

General

The total daily dose should be reduced when MEFOXIN is administered to patients with transient or persistent reduction of urinary output due to renal insufficiency (see DOSAGE), because high and prolonged serum antibiotic concentrations can occur in such individuals from usual doses.

Antibiotics (including cephalosporins) should be prescribed with caution in individuals with a history of gastrointestinal disease, particularly colitis.

As with other antibiotics, prolonged use of MEFOXIN may result in overgrowth of nonsusceptible organisms. Repeated evaluation of the patient's condition is essential. If superinfection occurs during therapy, appropriate measures should be taken.

Drug Interactions

Increased nephrotoxicity has been reported following concomitant administration of cephalosporins and aminoglycoside antibiotics.

Drug/Laboratory Test Interactions

As with cephalothin, high concentrations of cefoxitin (>100 micrograms/mL) may interfere with measurement of serum and urine creatinine levels by the Jaffé reaction, and produce false increases of modest degree in the levels of creatinine reported. Serum samples from patients treated with cefoxitin should not be analyzed for creatinine if withdrawn within 2 hours of drug administration.

High concentrations of cefoxitin in the urine may interfere with measurement of urinary 17-hydroxy-corticosteroids by the Porter-Silber reaction, and produce false increases of modest degree in the levels reported.

A false-positive reaction for glucose in the urine may occur. This has been observed with CLINITEST* reagent tablets.

Carcinogenesis, Mutagenesis, Impairment of Fertility

Long-term studies in animals have not been performed with cefoxitin to evaluate carcinogenic or mutagenic potential. Studies in rats treated intravenously with 400 mg/kg of cefoxitin (approximately three times the maximum recommended human dose) revealed no effects on fertility or mating ability.

Pregnancy

Pregnancy Category B. Reproduction studies performed in rats and mice at parenteral doses of approximately one to seven and one-half times the maximum recommended human dose did not reveal teratogenic or fetal toxic effects, although a slight decrease in fetal weight was observed. There are, however, no adequate and well-controlled studies in pregnant women. Because animal reproduction studies are not always predictive of human response, this drug should be used during pregnancy only if clearly needed.

In the rabbit, cefoxitin was associated with a high incidence of abortion and maternal death. This was not considered to be a teratogenic effect but an expected consequence of the rabbit's unusual sensitivity to antibiotic-induced changes in the population of the microflora of the intestine.

Nursing Mothers

MEFOXIN is excreted in human milk in low concentrations. Caution should be exercised when MEFOXIN is administered to a nursing woman.

Pediatric Use

Safety and efficacy in infants from birth to three months of age have not yet been established. In children three months of age and older, higher doses of MEFOXIN have been associated with an increased incidence of eosinophilia and elevated SGOT.

---

* Registered trademark of Ames Company, Division of Miles Laboratories, Inc.

ADVERSE REACTIONS

MEFOXIN is generally well tolerated. The most common adverse reactions have been local reactions following intravenous or intramuscular injection. Other adverse reactions have been encountered infrequently.

Local Reactions

Thrombophlebitis has occurred with intravenous administration. Pain, induration, and tenderness after intramuscular injections have been reported.

Allergic Reactions

Rash (including exfoliative dermatitis), pruritus, eosinophilia, fever, dyspnea, and other allergic reactions including anaphylaxis have been noted.

Cardiovascular

Hypotension

Gastrointestinal

Diarrhea, including documented pseudomembranous colitis which can appear during or after antibiotic treatment. Nausea and vomiting have been reported rarely.

Blood

Eosinophilia, leukopenia, including granulocytopenia, neutropenia, anemia, including hemolytic anemia, thrombocytopenia, and bone marrow depression. A positive direct Coombs test may develop in some individuals, especially those with azotemia.

Liver Function

Transient elevations in SGOT, SGPT, serum LDH, serum alkaline phosphatase; and jaundice have been reported.

Renal Function

Elevations in serum creatinine and/or blood urea nitrogen levels have been observed. As with the cephalosporins, acute renal failure has been reported rarely. The role of MEFOXIN in changes in renal function tests is difficult to assess, since factors predisposing to prerenal azotemia or to impaired renal function usually have been present.

OVERDOSAGE

The acute intravenous LD_{50} in the adult female mouse and rabbit was about 8.0 g/kg and greater than 1.0 g/kg respectively. The acute intraperitoneal LD_{50} in the adult rat was greater than 10.0 g/kg.

DOSAGE

TREATMENT

Adults

The usual adult dosage range is 1 gram to 2 grams every six to eight hours. Dosage and route of administration should be determined by susceptibility of the causative organisms, severity of infection, and the condition of the patient (see Table 1 for dosage guidelines).

MEFOXIN may be used in patients with reduced renal function with the following dosage adjustments:

In adults with renal insufficiency, an initial loading dose of 1 gram to 2 grams may be given. After a loading dose, the recommendations for *maintenance dosage* (Table 2) may be used as a guide.

[See Table 2 on next page.]

When only the serum creatinine level is available, the following formula (based on sex, weight, and age of the patient) may be used to convert this value into creatinine clearance. The serum creatinine should represent a steady state of renal function.

Table 1—Guidelines for Dosage of MEFOXIN

Type of Infection	Daily Dosage	Frequency and Route
Uncomplicated forms* of infections such as pneumonia, urinary tract infection, cutaneous infection	3–4 grams	1 gram every 6–8 hours IV or IM
Moderately severe or severe infections	6–8 grams	1 gram every 4 hours *or* 2 grams every 6–8 hours IV
Infections commonly needing antibiotics in higher dosage (e.g., gas gangrene)	12 grams	2 grams every 4 hours *or* 3 grams every 6 hours IV

*Including patients in whom bacteremia is absent or unlikely

Males:

$$\frac{\text{Weight (kg)} \times (140 - \text{age})}{72 \times \text{serum creatinine (mg/100 mL)}}$$

Females:　0.85 × above value

In patients undergoing hemodialysis, the loading dose of 1 to 2 grams should be given after each hemodialysis, and the maintenance dose should be given as indicated in Table 2. Antibiotic therapy for group A beta-hemolytic streptococcal infections should be maintained for at least 10 days to guard against the risk of rheumatic fever or glomerulonephritis. In staphylococcal and other infections involving a collection of pus, surgical drainage should be carried out where indicated. The recommended dosage of MEFOXIN **for uncomplicated gonorrhea** is 2 grams intramuscularly, with 1 gram of BENE-MID* (Probenecid) given by mouth at the same time or up to ½ hour before MEFOXIN.

Infants and Children
The recommended dosage in children three months of age and older is 80 to 160 mg/kg of body weight per day divided into four to six equal doses. The higher dosages should be used for more severe or serious infections. The total daily dosage should not exceed 12 grams.
At this time no recommendation is made for children from birth to three months of age (See PRECAUTIONS).
In children with renal insufficiency the dosage and frequency of dosage should be modified consistent with the recommendations for adults (see Table 2).

PREVENTION
General
For prophylactic use in surgery, the following doses are recommended:
　Adults:
　1) 2 grams administered intravenously or intramuscularly just prior to surgery (approximately one-half to one hour before the initial incision).
　2) 2 grams every 6 hours after the first dose for no more than 24 hours (continued for 72 hours after prosthetic arthroplasty).
　Children (3 months and older):
　30 to 40 mg/kg doses may be given at the times designated above.

Obstetric-Gynecologic
For prophylactic use in vaginal hysterectomy, a single 2.0 gram dose administered intramuscularly one-half to one hour prior to surgery is recommended.
For patients undergoing cesarean section, a single 2.0 gram dose should be administered intravenously as soon as the umbilical cord is clamped. A 3-dose regimen may be more effective than a single dose regimen in preventing postoperative infection (esp. endometritis) following cesarean section. Such a regimen would consist of 2.0 grams given intravenously as soon as the umbilical cord is clamped, followed by 2.0 grams 4 and 8 hours after the initial dose.

Transurethral prostatectomy patients:
One gram administered just prior to surgery; 1 gram every 8 hours for up to five days.

* Registered trademark of MERCK & CO., INC.

PREPARATION OF SOLUTION

Table 3 is provided for convenience in constituting MEFOXIN for both intravenous and intramuscular administration.
For intravenous use, 1 gram should be constituted with at least 10 mL of Sterile Water for Injection, and 2 grams, with 10 or 20 mL. The 10 gram bulk package should be constituted with 43 or 93 mL of Sterile Water for Injection or any of the solutions listed under the *Intravenous* portion of the COMPATIBILITY AND STABILITY section. CAUTION: THE 10 GRAM BULK STOCK SOLUTION IS NOT FOR DIRECT INFUSION. One or 2 grams of MEFOXIN for infusion may be constituted with 50 or 100 mL of 0.9 percent Sodium Chloride Injection, 5 percent or 10 percent Dextrose Injection, or any of the solutions listed under the *Intravenous* portion of the COMPATIBILITY AND STABILITY section.

Benzyl alcohol as a preservative has been associated with toxicity in neonates. While toxicity has not been demonstrated in infants greater than three months of age, in whom use of MEFOXIN may be indicated, small infants in this age range may also be at risk for benzyl alcohol toxicity. Therefore, diluent containing benzyl alcohol should not be used

Table 3—Preparation of Solution

MEFOXIN

Strength	Amount of Diluent to be Added (mL)*	Approximate Withdrawable Volume (mL)	Approximate Average Concentration (mg/mL)
1 gram Vial	2 (Intramuscular)	2.5	400
2 gram Vial	4 (Intramuscular)	5	400
1 gram Vial	10 (IV)	10.5	95
2 gram Vial	10 or 20 (IV)	11.1 or 21.0	180 or 95
1 gram Infusion Bottle	50 or 100 (IV)	50 or 100	20 or 10
2 gram Infusion Bottle	50 or 100 (IV)	50 or 100	40 or 20
10 gram Bulk	43 or 93 (IV)	49 or 98.5	200 or 100

*Shake to dissolve and let stand until clear.

when MEFOXIN is constituted for administration to infants.
For ADD-Vantage®† vials, see separate INSTRUCTIONS FOR USE OF MEFOXIN IN ADD-Vantage® VIALS. MEFOXIN in ADD-Vantage® vials should be constituted with ADD-Vantage® diluent containers containing 50 mL or 100 mL of either 0.9 percent Sodium Chloride Injection or 5 percent Dextrose Injection. MEFOXIN in ADD-Vantage® vials is for IV use only.
For intramuscular use, each gram of MEFOXIN may be constituted with 2 mL of Sterile Water for Injection, or—
For intramuscular use ONLY: each gram of MEFOXIN may be constituted with 2 mL of 0.5 percent lidocaine hydrochloride solution** (without epinephrine) to minimize the discomfort of intramuscular injection.

†Registered trademark of Abbott Laboratories.
**See package circular of manufacturer for detailed information concerning contraindications, warnings, precautions, and adverse reactions.

ADMINISTRATION

MEFOXIN may be administered intravenously or intramuscularly after constitution.
Parenteral drug products should be inspected visually for particulate matter and discoloration prior to administration whenever solution and container permit.

Intravenous Administration
The intravenous route is preferable for patients with bacteremia, bacterial septicemia, or other severe or life-threatening infections, or for patients who may be poor risks because of lowered resistance resulting from such debilitating conditions as malnutrition, trauma, surgery, diabetes, heart failure, or malignancy, particularly if shock is present or impending.
For intermittent intravenous administration, a solution containing 1 gram or 2 grams in 10 mL of Sterile Water for Injection can be injected over a period of three to five minutes. Using an infusion system, it may also be given over a longer period of time through the tubing system by which the patient may be receiving other intravenous solutions. However, during infusion of the solution containing MEFOXIN, it is advisable to temporarily discontinue administration of any other solutions at the same site.
For the administration of higher doses by continuous intravenous infusion, a solution of MEFOXIN may be added to an intravenous bottle containing 5 percent Dextrose Injection, 0.9 percent Sodium Chloride Injection, 5 percent Dextrose and 0.9 percent Sodium Chloride Injection, or 5 percent Dextrose Injection with 0.02 percent sodium bicarbonate solution. BUTTERFLY† or scalp vein-type needles are preferred for this type of infusion.
Solutions of MEFOXIN, like those of most beta-lactam antibiotics, should not be added to aminoglycoside solutions (e.g., gentamicin sulfate, tobramycin sulfate, amikacin sulfate) because of potential interaction. However, MEFOXIN and aminoglycosides may be administered separately to the same patient.

Intramuscular Administration
As with all intramuscular preparations, MEFOXIN should be injected well within the body of a relatively large muscle such as the upper outer quadrant of the buttock (i.e., gluteus maximus); aspiration is necessary to avoid inadvertent injection into a blood vessel.

† Registered trademark of Abbott Laboratories.

COMPATIBILITY AND STABILITY

Intravenous
MEFOXIN, as supplied in vials or the bulk package and constituted to 1 gram/10 mL with Sterile Water for Injection, Bacteriostatic Water for Injection (see PREPARATION OF SOLUTION), 0.9 percent Sodium Chloride Injection, or 5 percent Dextrose Injection, maintains satisfactory potency for 24 hours at room temperature, for one week under refrigeration (below 5℃), and for at least 30 weeks in the frozen state.
These primary solutions may be further diluted in 50 to 1000 mL of the following solutions and maintain potency for 24 hours at room temperature and at least 48 hours under refrigeration:
Sterile Water for Injection‡
0.9 percent Sodium Chloride Injection
5 percent or 10 percent Dextrose Injection‡
5 percent Dextrose and 0.9 percent Sodium Chloride Injection
5 percent Dextrose Injection with 0.02 percent sodium bicarbonate solution
5 percent Dextrose Injection with 0.2 percent or 0.45 percent saline solution
Ringer's Injection
Lactated Ringer's Injection‡
5 percent dextrose in Lactated Ringer's Injection‡
5 percent or 10 percent invert sugar in water
10 percent invert sugar in saline solution
5 percent Sodium Bicarbonate Injection
Neut (sodium bicarbonate)*‡
M/6 sodium lactate solution
NORMOSOL-M in D5-W*‡
IONOSOL B w/Dextrose 5 percent*‡
POLYONIC M 56 in 5 percent Dextrose**
Mannitol 5% and 2.5%
Mannitol 10%‡
ISOLYTE*** E
ISOLYTE*** E with 5% dextrose
MEFOXIN, as supplied in infusion bottles and constituted with 50 to 100 mL of 0.9 percent Sodium Chloride Injection, or 5 percent or 10 percent Dextrose Injection, maintains satisfactory potency for 24 hours at room temperature or for 1 week under refrigeration (below 5℃).
MEFOXIN is supplied in single dose ADD-Vantage® vials and should be prepared as directed in the accompanying INSTRUCTIONS FOR USE OF MEFOXIN IN ADD-Vantage® VIALS using ADD-Vantage® diluent containers containing 50 mL or 100 mL of either 0.9 percent Sodium Chloride Injection or 5 percent Dextrose Injection. When prepared with either of these diluents, MEFOXIN maintains satisfactory potency for 24 hours at room temperature.
Limited studies with solutions of MEFOXIN in 0.9 percent Sodium Chloride Injection, Lactated Ringer's Injection, and 5 percent Dextrose Injection in VIAFLEX† intravenous bags show stability for 24 hours at room temperature, 48 hours under refrigeration or 26 weeks in the frozen state and 24 hours at room temperature thereafter. Also, solutions of MEFOXIN in 0.9 percent Sodium Chloride Injection show similar stability in plastic tubing, drip chambers, and volume control devices of common intravenous infusion sets.
After constitution with Sterile Water for Injection and subsequent storage in disposable plastic syringes, MEFOXIN is stable for 24 hours at room temperature and 48 hours under refrigeration.
After the periods mentioned above, any unused solutions or frozen material should be discarded. Do not refreeze.
Intramuscular
MEFOXIN, as constituted with Sterile Water for Injection, Bacteriostatic Water for Injection, or 0.5 percent or 1 percent lidocaine hydrochloride solution (without epinephrine),

Continued on next page

Information on the Merck & Co. products listed on these pages is the full prescribing information from product circulars in use October 1, 1992.

Table 2—Maintenance Dosage of MEFOXIN in Adults with Reduced Renal Function

Renal Function	Creatinine Clearance (mL/min)	Dose (grams)	Frequency
Mild impairment	50–30	1–2	every 8–12 hours
Moderate impairment	29–10	1–2	every 12–24 hours
Severe impairment	9–5	0.5–1	every 12–24 hours
Essentially no function	<5	0.5–1	every 24–48 hours

Merck & Co.—Cont.

maintains satisfactory potency for 24 hours at room temperature, for one week under refrigeration (below 5°C), and for at least 30 weeks in the frozen state.
After the periods mentioned above, any unused solutions or frozen material should be discarded. Do not refreeze.
MEFOXIN has also been found compatible when admixed in intravenous infusions with the following:
Heparin 0.1 units/mL at room temperature—8 hours
Heparin 100 units/mL at room temperature—24 hours
M.V.I.†† concentrate at room temperature 24 hours; under refrigeration 48 hours
BEROCCA††† C-500 at room temperature 24 hours; under refrigeration 48 hours
Insulin in Normal Saline at room temperature 24 hours; under refrigeration 48 hours
Insulin in 10% invert sugar at room temperature 24 hours; under refrigeration 48 hours

- * Registered trademark of Abbott Laboratories.
- ** Registered trademark of Cutter Laboratories, Inc.
- *** Registered trademark of American Hospital Supply Corporation.
- ‡ In these solutions, MEFOXIN has been found to be stable for a period of one week under refrigeration.
- † Registered trademark of Baxter International, Ltd.
- †† Registered trademark of USV Pharmaceutical Corp.
- ††† Registered trademark of Roche Laboratories.

HOW SUPPLIED

Sterile MEFOXIN is a dry white to off-white powder supplied in vials and infusion bottles containing cefoxitin sodium as follows:
No. 3356—1 gram cefoxitin equivalent
NDC 0006-3356-45 in trays of 25 vials
(6505-01-119-6005, 1 g 25's).
No. 3368—1 gram cefoxitin equivalent
NDC 0006-3368-71 in trays of 10 infusion bottles
(6505-01-195-0649, 1 g infusion bottle 10's).
No. 3357—2 gram cefoxitin equivalent
NDC 0006-3357-53 in trays of 25 vials
(6505-01-104-6393, 2 g 25's).
No. 3369—2 gram cefoxitin equivalent
NDC 0006-3369-73 in trays of 10 infusion bottles
(6505-01-185-2624, 2 g infusion bottle 10's).
No. 3388—10 gram cefoxitin equivalent
NDC 0006-3388-67 in trays of 6 bulk bottles
(6505-01-263-0730, 10 g 6's).
No. 3548—1 gram cefoxitin equivalent
NDC 0006-3548-45 in trays of 25 ADD-Vantage® vials.
(6505-01-262-9509, 1 g ADD-Vantage® 25's).
No. 3549—2 gram cefoxitin equivalent
NDC 0006-3549-53 in trays of 25 ADD-Vantage® vials.
(6505-01-263-4531, 2 g ADD-Vantage® 25's).
Special storage instructions
MEFOXIN in the dry state should be stored below 30°C. Avoid exposure to temperatures above 50°C. The dry material as well as solutions tend to darken, depending on storage conditions; product potency, however, is not adversely affected.

A.H.F.S. Category: 8:12.07
DC 7057130 Issued January 1992
COPYRIGHT © MERCK & CO., INC., 1985
All rights reserved

MEFOXIN® Premixed Intravenous Solution (Cefoxitin Sodium Injection), U.S.P. ℞

DESCRIPTION

Cefoxitin sodium is a semi-synthetic, broad-spectrum cepha antibiotic for parenteral administration. It is derived from cephamycin C, which is produced by *Streptomyces lactamdurans*. It is the sodium salt of 3-(hydroxymethyl) -7α- methoxy-8-oxo -7- [2- (2-thienyl) acetamido]-5-thia-1-azabicyclo [4.2.0] oct-2-ene-2-carboxylate carbamate (ester). The empirical formula is $C_{16}H_{16}N_3NaO_7S_2$, and the structural formula is:

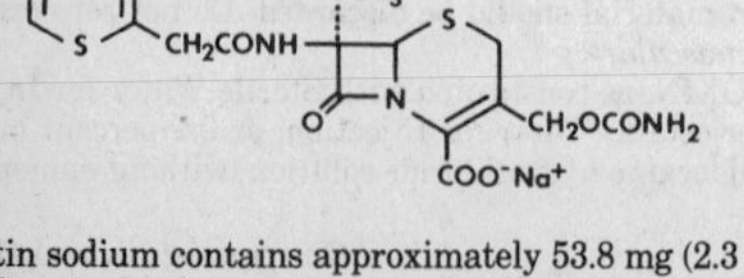

Cefoxitin sodium contains approximately 53.8 mg (2.3 milliequivalents) of sodium per gram of cefoxitin activity.
Premixed Intravenous Solution MEFOXIN* (Cefoxitin Sodium Injection) is supplied as a sterile, nonpyrogenic, frozen solution of cefoxitin sodium in an iso-osmotic diluent in plastic containers. Each 50 mL contains cefoxitin sodium equivalent to either 1 gram or 2 grams of cefoxitin in 5% Dextrose (2.5 g dextrose hydrous USP, Water for Injection q.s. to 50 mL). The pH is adjusted with sodium bicarbonate and may be adjusted with hydrochloric acid. The pH is approximately 6.5. After thawing, the solution is intended for intravenous use only. Solutions of MEFOXIN range from colorless to light amber.
The plastic container is fabricated from specially formulated polyvinyl chloride. Solutions in contact with the plastic container can leach out certain of the container's chemical components, e.g., di-2-ethylhexyl phthalate (DEHP), in very small amounts (up to 5 parts per million) within the expiration period. The safety of the plastic has been demonstrated by animal tests according to the USP biological tests for plastic containers, as well as by tissue culture toxicity studies.
MEFOXIN is also available in dry powder form in vials and infusion bottles containing sterile cefoxitin sodium equivalent to either 1 gram or 2 grams of cefoxitin, and in vials for pharmacy bulk use containing sterile cefoxitin sodium equivalent to 10 grams of cefoxitin, for constitution and either intravenous or intramuscular administration (see appropriate product circular).

*Registered trademark of MERCK & CO., INC.

CLINICAL PHARMACOLOGY

Clinical Pharmacology
Following an intravenous dose of 1 gram of cefoxitin, serum concentrations were 110 mcg/mL at 5 minutes, declining to less than 1 mcg/mL at 4 hours. The half-life after an intravenous dose is 41 to 59 minutes. Approximately 85 percent of cefoxitin is excreted unchanged by the kidneys over a 6-hour period, resulting in high urinary concentrations. Probenecid slows tubular excretion and produces higher serum levels and increases the duration of measurable serum concentrations.
Cefoxitin passes into pleural and joint fluids and is detectable in antibacterial concentrations in bile.
Clinical experience has demonstrated that cefoxitin can be administered to patients who are also receiving carbenicillin, kanamycin, gentamicin, tobramycin, or amikacin (see PRECAUTIONS and ADMINISTRATION).
Microbiology
The bactericidal action of cefoxitin results from inhibition of cell wall synthesis. Cefoxitin has *in vitro* activity against a wide range of gram-positive and gram-negative organisms. The methoxy group in the 7α position provides MEFOXIN with a high degree of stability in the presence of beta-lactamases, both penicillinases and cephalosporinases, of gram-negative bacteria. Cefoxitin is usually active against the following organisms *in vitro* and in clinical infections:
Gram-positive
Staphylococcus aureus, including penicillinase and non-penicillinase producing strains
Staphylococcus epidermidis
Beta-hemolytic and other streptococci (most strains of enterococci, e.g., *Streptococcus faecalis,* are resistant)
Streptococcus pneumoniae
Gram-negative
Escherichia coli
Klebsiella species (including *K. pneumoniae*)
Hemophilus influenzae
Neisseria gonorrhoeae, including penicillinase and non-penicillinase producing strains
Proteus mirabilis
Morganella morganii
Proteus vulgaris
Providencia species, including *Providencia rettgeri*
Anaerobic organisms
Peptococcus species
Peptostreptococcus species
Clostridium species
Bacteroides species, including the *B. fragilis* group (includes *B. fragilis, B. distasonis, B. ovatus, B. thetaiotaomicron, B. vulgatus*)
MEFOXIN is inactive *in vitro* against most strains of *Pseudomonas aeruginosa* and enterococci and many strains of *Enterobacter cloacae.*
Methicillin-resistant staphylococci are almost uniformly resistant to MEFOXIN.
Susceptibility Tests
For fast-growing aerobic organisms, quantitative methods that require measurements of zone diameters give the most precise estimates of antibiotic susceptibility. One such procedure* has been recommended for use with discs to test susceptibility to cefoxitin. Interpretation involves correlation of the diameters obtained in the disc test with minimal inhibitory concentration (MIC) values for cefoxitin.
Reports from the laboratory giving results of the standardized single disc susceptibility test* using a 30 mcg cefoxitin disc should be interpreted according to the following criteria:
Organisms producing zones of 18 mm or greater are considered susceptible, indicating that the tested organism is likely to respond to therapy.
Organisms of intermediate susceptibility produce zones of 15 to 17 mm, indicating that the tested organism would be susceptible if high dosage is used or if the infection is confined to tissues and fluids (e.g., urine) in which high antibiotic levels are attained.
Resistant organisms produce zones of 14 mm or less, indicating that other therapy should be selected.
The cefoxitin disc should be used for testing cefoxitin susceptibility.
Cefoxitin has been shown by *in vitro* tests to have activity against certain strains of *Enterobacteriaceae* found resistant when tested with the cephalosporin class disc. For this reason, the cefoxitin disc should not be used for testing susceptibility to cephalosporins, and cephalosporin discs should not be used for testing susceptibility to cefoxitin.
Dilution methods, preferably the agar plate dilution procedure, are most accurate for susceptibility testing of obligate anaerobes.
A bacterial isolate may be considered susceptible if the MIC value for cefoxitin** is not more than 16 mcg/mL. Organisms are considered resistant if the MIC is greater than 32 mcg/mL.

* Bauer, A. W.; Kirby, W. M. M.; Sherris, J. C.; Turck, M.: Antibiotic susceptibility testing by a standardized single disc method, Amer. J. Clin. Path. *45*: 493–496, Apr. 1966. Standardized disc susceptibility test, Federal Register *37*: 20527–20529, 1972. National Committee for Clinical Laboratory Standards: Approved Standard: M2-A3, Performance Standards for Antimicrobial Disk Susceptibility Tests, 1984.
** Determined by the ICS agar dilution method (Ericsson and Sherris, Acta Path. Microbiol. Scand. [B] Suppl. No. 217, 1971) or any other method that has been shown to give equivalent results.

INDICATIONS AND USAGE

MEFOXIN, supplied as a premixed solution in plastic containers, is intended for intravenous use only. For indications specifically concerning the intramuscular use of cefoxitin (e.g., gonococcal urethritis) or for adverse reactions associated only with intramuscular administration, please refer to the product circular for MEFOXIN (Sterile Cefoxitin Sodium) supplied as dry powder.
Treatment
MEFOXIN is indicated for the treatment of serious infections caused by susceptible strains of the designated microorganisms in the diseases listed below.
(1) **Lower respiratory tract infections,** including pneumonia and lung abscess, caused by *Streptococcus pneumoniae,* other streptococci (excluding enterococci, e.g., *Streptococcus faecalis*), *Staphylococcus aureus* (penicillinase and non-penicillinase producing), *Escherichia coli, Klebsiella* species, *Hemophilus influenzae,* and *Bacteroides* species.
(2) **Genitourinary infections.** Urinary tract infections caused by *Escherichia coli, Klebsiella* species, *Proteus mirabilis,* indole-positive Proteus , (which include *Morganella morganii* and *Proteus vulgaris*), and *Providencia* species (including *Providencia rettgeri*). Uncomplicated gonorrhea due to *Neisseria gonorrhoeae* (penicillinase and non-penicillinase producing).
(3) **Intra-abdominal infections,** including peritonitis and intra-abdominal abscess, caused by *Escherichia coli, Klebsiella* species, *Bacteroides* species including the *Bacteroides fragilis* group***, and *Clostridium* species.
(4) **Gynecological infections,** including endometritis, pelvic cellulitis, and pelvic inflammatory disease caused by *Escherichia coli, Neisseria gonorrhoeae* (penicillinase and non-penicillinase producing), *Bacteroides* species including the *Bacteroides fragilis* group***, *Clostridium* species, *Peptococcus* species, *Peptostreptococcus* species, and Group B streptococci.
(5) **Septicemia** caused by *Streptococcus pneumoniae, Staphylococcus aureus* (penicillinase and non-penicillinase producing), *Escherichia coli, Klebsiella* species, and *Bacteroides* species including the *Bacteroides fragilis* group.***
(6) **Bone and joint infections** caused by *Staphylococcus aureus* (penicillinase and non-penicillinase producing).
(7) **Skin and skin structure infections** caused by *Staphylococcus aureus* (penicillinase and non-penicillinase producing), *Staphylococcus epidermidis,* streptococci (excluding enterococci, e.g., *Streptococcus faecalis*), *Escherichia coli, Proteus mirabilis, Klebsiella* species, *Bacteroides* species including the *Bacteroides fragilis* group***, *Clostridium* species, *Peptococcus* species, and *Peptostreptococcus* species.
Appropriate culture and susceptibility studies should be performed to determine the susceptibility of the causative organisms to MEFOXIN. Therapy may be started while awaiting the results of these studies.
In randomized comparative studies, cefoxitin and cephalothin were comparably safe and effective in the management of infections caused by gram-positive cocci and gram-negative rods susceptible to the cephalosporins. MEFOXIN has a high degree of stability in the presence of bacterial beta-lactamases, both penicillinases and cephalosporinases.

Many infections caused by aerobic and anaerobic gram-negative bacteria resistant to some cephalosporins respond to MEFOXIN. Similarly, many infections caused by aerobic and anaerobic bacteria resistant to some penicillin antibiotics (ampicillin, carbenicillin, penicillin G) respond to treatment with MEFOXIN. Many infections caused by mixtures of susceptible aerobic and anaerobic bacteria respond to treatment with MEFOXIN.

Prevention
When compared to placebo in randomized controlled studies in patients undergoing gastrointestinal surgery, vaginal hysterectomy, abdominal hysterectomy and cesarean section, the prophylactic use of cefoxitin resulted in a significant reduction in the number of postoperative infections.
The prophylactic administration of MEFOXIN may reduce the incidence of certain postoperative infections in patients undergoing surgical procedures (e.g., hysterectomy, gastrointestinal surgery and transurethral prostatectomy) that are classified as contaminated or potentially contaminated.
The perioperative use of MEFOXIN may be effective in surgical patients in whom infection at the operative site would present a serious risk, e.g., prosthetic arthroplasty.
Effective prophylactic use depends on the time of administration. MEFOXIN usually should be given one-half to one hour before the operation, which is sufficient time to achieve effective levels in the wound during the procedure. Prophylactic administration should usually be stopped within 24 hours since continuing administration of any antibiotic increases the possibility of adverse reactions but, in the majority of surgical procedures, does not reduce the incidence of subsequent infection. However, in patients undergoing prosthetic arthroplasty, it is recommended that MEFOXIN be continued for 72 hours after the surgical procedure.
If there are signs of infection, specimens for culture should be obtained for identification of the causative organism so that appropriate treatment may be instituted.

*** *B. fragilis, B. distasonis, B. ovatus, B. thetaiotaomicron, B. vulgatus.*

CONTRAINDICATIONS

MEFOXIN is contraindicated in patients who have shown hypersensitivity to cefoxitin and the cephalosporin group of antibiotics.

WARNINGS

BEFORE THERAPY WITH 'MEFOXIN' IS INSTITUTED, CAREFUL INQUIRY SHOULD BE MADE TO DETERMINE WHETHER THE PATIENT HAS HAD PREVIOUS HYPERSENSITIVITY REACTIONS TO CEFOXITIN, CEPHALOSPORINS, PENICILLINS, OR OTHER DRUGS. THIS PRODUCT SHOULD BE GIVEN WITH CAUTION TO PENICILLIN-SENSITIVE PATIENTS. ANTIBIOTICS SHOULD BE ADMINISTERED WITH CAUTION TO ANY PATIENT WHO HAS DEMONSTRATED SOME FORM OF ALLERGY, PARTICULARLY TO DRUGS. IF AN ALLERGIC REACTION TO 'MEFOXIN' OCCURS, DISCONTINUE THE DRUG. SERIOUS HYPERSENSITIVITY REACTIONS MAY REQUIRE EPINEPHRINE AND OTHER EMERGENCY MEASURES.

Pseudomembranous colitis has been reported with virtually all antibiotics (including cephalosporins); therefore, it is important to consider its diagnosis in patients who develop diarrhea in association with antibiotic use. This colitis may range from mild to life threatening in severity.

Treatment with broad-spectrum antibiotics alters normal flora of the colon and may permit overgrowth of clostridia. Studies indicate a toxin produced by *Clostridium difficile* is one primary cause of antibiotic-associated colitis.

Mild cases of pseudomembranous colitis may respond to drug discontinuance alone. In more severe cases, management may include sigmoidoscopy, appropriate bacteriological studies, fluid, electrolyte and protein supplementation, and the use of a drug such as oral vancomycin as indicated. Isolation of the patient may be advisable. Other causes of colitis should also be considered.

PRECAUTIONS

General
The total daily dose should be reduced when MEFOXIN is administered to patients with transient or persistent reduction of urinary output due to renal insufficiency (see DOSAGE), because high and prolonged serum antibiotic concentrations can occur in such individuals from usual doses.
Antibiotics (including cephalosporins) should be prescribed with caution in individuals with a history of gastrointestinal disease, particularly colitis.
As with other antibiotics, prolonged use of MEFOXIN may result in overgrowth of nonsusceptible organisms. Repeated evaluation of the patient's condition is essential. If superinfection occurs during therapy, appropriate measures should be taken.

Table 1—Guidelines for Dosage of MEFOXIN

Type of Infection	Daily Dosage	Frequency and Route
Uncomplicated forms* of infections such as pneumonia, urinary tract infection, cutaneous infection	3–4 grams	1 gram every 6–8 hours IV
Moderately severe or severe infections	6–8 grams	1 gram every 4 hours *or* 2 grams every 6–8 hours IV
Infections commonly needing antibiotics in higher dosage (e.g., gas gangrene)	12 grams	2 grams every 4 hours *or* 3 grams every 6 hours IV

*Including patients in whom bacteremia is absent or unlikely.

Do not use unless solution is clear and seal is intact.
Drug Interactions
Increased nephrotoxicity has been reported following concomitant administration of cephalosporins and aminoglycoside antibiotics.
Drug/Laboratory Test Interactions
As with cephalothin, high concentrations of cefoxitin (> 100 micrograms/mL) may interfere with measurement of serum and urine creatinine levels by the Jaffé reaction, and produce false increases of modest degree in the levels of creatinine reported. Serum samples from patients treated with cefoxitin should not be analyzed for creatinine if withdrawn within 2 hours of drug administration.
High concentrations of cefoxitin in the urine may interfere with measurement of urinary 17-hydroxy-corticosteroids by the Porter-Silber reaction, and produce false increases of modest degree in the levels reported.
A false-positive reaction for glucose in the urine may occur. This has been observed with CLINITEST* reagent tablets.

---
* Registered trademark of Ames Company, Division of Miles Laboratories, Inc.

Carcinogenesis, Mutagenesis, Impairment of Fertility
Long term studies in animals have not been performed with cefoxitin to evaluate carcinogenic or mutagenic potential. Studies in rats treated intravenously with 400 mg/kg of cefoxitin (approximately three times the maximum recommended human dose) revealed no effects on fertility or mating ability.
Pregnancy
Pregnancy Category B. Reproduction studies performed in rats and mice at parenteral doses of approximately one to seven and one-half times the maximum recommended human dose did not reveal teratogenic or fetal toxic effects, although a slight decrease in fetal weight was observed.
There are, however, no adequate and well-controlled studies in pregnant women. Because animal reproduction studies are not always predictive of human response, this drug should be used during pregnancy only if clearly needed.
In the rabbit, cefoxitin was associated with a high incidence of abortion and maternal death. This was not considered to be a teratogenic effect but an expected consequence of the rabbit's unusual sensitivity to antibiotic-induced changes in the population of the microflora of the intestine.
Nursing Mothers
Cefoxitin is excreted in human milk in low concentrations. Caution should be exercised when MEFOXIN is administered to a nursing woman.
Pediatric Use
Safety and efficacy in infants from birth to three months of age have not yet been established. In children three months of age and older, higher doses of cefoxitin have been associated with an increased incidence of eosinophilia and elevated SGOT.

ADVERSE REACTIONS

Cefoxitin is generally well tolerated. The most common adverse reactions have been local reactions following intravenous injection. Other adverse reactions have been encountered infrequently.
Local Reactions
Thrombophlebitis has occurred with intravenous administration.
Allergic Reactions
Rash (including exfoliative dermatitis), pruritus, eosinophilia, fever, dyspnea, and other allergic reactions including anaphylaxis and angioedema have been noted.
Cardiovascular
Hypotension
Gastrointestinal
Diarrhea, including documented pseudomembranous colitis which can appear during or after antibiotic treatment. Nausea and vomiting have been reported rarely.

Blood
Eosinophilia, leukopenia including granulocytopenia, neutropenia, anemia, including hemolytic anemia, thrombocytopenia, and bone marrow depression. A positive direct Coombs test may develop in some individuals, especially those with azotemia.
Liver Function
Transient elevations in SGOT, SGPT, serum LDH, and serum alkaline phosphatase; and jaundice have been reported.
Renal Function
Elevations in serum creatinine and/or blood urea nitrogen levels have been observed. As with the cephalosporins, acute renal failure has been reported rarely. The role of MEFOXIN in changes in renal function tests is difficult to assess, since factors predisposing to prerenal azotemia or to impaired renal function usually have been present.

OVERDOSAGE

The acute intravenous LD$_{50}$ in the adult female mouse and rabbit was about 8.0 g/kg and greater than 1.0 g/kg respectively. The acute intraperitoneal LD$_{50}$ in the adult rat was greater than 10.0 g/kg.

DOSAGE

TREATMENT
Adults
The usual adult dosage range is 1 gram to 2 grams every six to eight hours. Dosage and route of administration should be determined by susceptibility of the causative organisms, severity of infection, and the condition of the patient (see Table 1 for dosage guidelines).
MEFOXIN may be used in patients with reduced renal function with the following dosage adjustments:
In adults with renal insufficiency, an initial loading dose of 1 gram to 2 grams may be given. After a loading dose, the recommendations for *maintenance dosage* (Table 2) may be used as a guide.
When only the serum creatinine level is available, the following formula (based on sex, weight, and age of the patient) may be used to convert this value into creatinine clearance. The serum creatinine should represent a steady state of renal function.

Males: $$\frac{\text{Weight (kg)} \times (140 - \text{age})}{72 \times \text{serum creatinine (mg/100 mL)}}$$

Females: 0.85 × above value

In patients undergoing hemodialysis, the loading dose of 1 to 2 grams should be given after each hemodialysis, and the maintenance dose should be given as indicated in Table 2.
Antibiotic therapy for group A beta-hemolytic streptococcal infections should be maintained for at least 10 days to guard against the risk of rheumatic fever or glomerulonephritis. In staphylococcal and other infections involving a collection of pus, surgical drainage should be carried out where indicated.
Infants and Children
The recommended dosage in children three months of age and older is 80 to 160 mg/kg of body weight per day divided into four to six equal doses. The higher dosages should be used for more severe or serious infections. The total daily dosage should not exceed 12 grams.
At this time no recommendation is made for children from birth to three months of age (see PRECAUTIONS).
In children with renal insufficiency the dosage and frequency of dosage should be modified consistent with the recommendations for adults (see Table 2). [See next page.]

Continued on next page

Merck & Co.—Cont.

Table 2—Maintenance Dosage of MEFOXIN in Adults with Reduced Renal Function

Renal Function	Creatinine Clearance (mL/min)	Dose (grams)	Frequency
Mild impairment	50–30	1–2	every 8–12 hours
Moderate impairment	29–10	1–2	every 12–24 hours
Severe impairment	9–5	0.5–1	every 12–24 hours
Essentially no function	<5	0.5–1	every 24–48 hours

PREVENTION
General
For prophylactic use in surgery, the following doses are recommended:
Adults:
(1) 2 grams administered intravenously just prior to surgery (approximately one-half to one hour before the initial incision).
(2) 2 grams every 6 hours after the first dose for no more than 24 hours (continued for 72 hours after prosthetic arthroplasty).
Children (3 months and older):
30 to 40 mg/kg doses may be given at the times designated above.
Cesarean section patients:
A single 2 gram dose should be administered intravenously as soon as the umbilical cord is clamped. A 3-dose regimen may be more effective than a single dose regimen in preventing postoperative infection (esp. endometritis) following cesarean section. Such a regimen would consist of 2 grams given intravenously as soon as the umbilical cord is clamped, followed by 2 grams 4 and 8 hours after the initial dose.
Transurethral prostatectomy patients:
One gram administered just prior to surgery; 1 gram every 8 hours for up to five days.

ADMINISTRATION

This premixed solution is for intravenous use only. Thaw the container at room temperature. After thawing, check for minute leaks by squeezing the bag firmly. If leaks are found or if the seal is not intact, discard the solution since sterility may be compromised. Additives should not be introduced into this solution.
Parenteral drug products should be inspected visually for particulate matter and discoloration prior to administration, whenever solution and container permit. Do not use if the solution is cloudy or a precipitate has formed. Solutions of MEFOXIN tend to darken, depending on storage conditions; product potency, however, is not adversely affected.
The intravenous route is preferred for patients with bacteremia, bacterial septicemia, or other severe or life-threatening infections, or for patients who may be poor risks because of lowered resistance resulting from such debilitating conditions as malnutrition, trauma, surgery, diabetes, heart failure, or malignancy, particularly if shock is present or impending.
Premixed Intravenous Solution MEFOXIN supplied as a sterile, nonpyrogenic, frozen solution in plastic containers is to be administered as a continuous or intermittent intravenous infusion. Scalp vein type needles are preferred for this type of infusion.
Use sterile equipment. It is recommended that the intravenous administration apparatus be replaced at least once every 48 hours.
CAUTION: Do not use plastic containers in series connections. Such use would result in air embolism due to residual air being drawn from the primary container before administration of the fluid from the secondary container is complete.
Preparation for administration:
1. Suspend container from eyelet support.
2. Remove plastic protector from outlet port at bottom of container.
3. Attach administration set. Refer to complete directions accompanying set.
MEFOXIN may be administered through the tubing system by which the patient may be receiving other intravenous solutions. However, during infusion of the solution containing MEFOXIN, it is advisable to temporarily discontinue administration of any other solutions at the same site.
Solutions of MEFOXIN, like those of most beta-lactam antibiotics, should not be added to aminoglycoside solutions (e.g., gentamicin sulfate, tobramycin sulfate, amikacin sulfate) because of potential interaction. However, MEFOXIN and aminoglycosides may be administered separately to the same patient.

STABILITY

MEFOXIN, as supplied premixed in 5% Dextrose in plastic containers, maintains satisfactory potency after thawing for 24 hours at room temperature and 5 days if stored under refrigeration [2 to 8°C (36 to 46°F)]. After these periods, any unused thawed solutions should be discarded.
DO NOT REFREEZE.

HOW SUPPLIED

Premixed Intravenous Solution MEFOXIN is supplied in single dose plastic containers containing cefoxitin sodium as follows:
No. 2B3506—1 gram cefoxitin equivalent in 50 mL 5% Dextrose
NDC 0006-3506-24 in boxes of 24.
No. 2B3507—2 gram cefoxitin equivalent in 50 mL 5% Dextrose
NDC 0006-3507-25 in boxes of 24.
Special storage instructions
Do not store above −20°C (−4°F). After thawing, do not refreeze.
Manufactured for:
MERCK SHARP & DOHME
Div. of MERCK & CO, INC., WEST POINT, PA 19486, USA
By:
BAXTER HEALTHCARE CORPORATION
Deerfield, Illinois 60015, USA
A.H.F.S. Category 8:12.07
DC 7407413   Issued January 1992
COPYRIGHT © MERCK & CO., INC., 1985
All rights reserved

MEPHYTON® Tablets   ℞
(Phytonadione), U.S.P.
Vitamin K₁

DESCRIPTION

Phytonadione is a vitamin which is a clear, yellow to amber, viscous, and nearly odorless liquid. It is insoluble in water, soluble in chloroform and slightly soluble in ethanol. It has a molecular weight of 450.70.
Phytonadione is 2-methyl-3-phytyl-1, 4-naphthoquinone. Its empirical formula is $C_{31}H_{46}O_2$ and its structural formula is:

MEPHYTON* (Phytonadione) tablets containing 5 mg of phytonadione are yellow, compressed tablets, scored on one side. Inactive ingredients are acacia, calcium phosphate, colloidal silicon dioxide, lactose, magnesium stearate, starch, and talc.

* Registered trademark of MERCK & CO., INC.

CLINICAL PHARMACOLOGY

MEPHYTON tablets possess the same type and degree of activity as does naturally-occurring vitamin K, which is necessary for the production via the liver of active prothrombin (factor II), proconvertin (factor VII), plasma thromboplastin component (factor IX), and Stuart factor (factor X). The prothrombin test is sensitive to the levels of three of these four factors—II, VII, and X. Vitamin K is an essential cofactor for a microsomal enzyme that catalyzes the post-translational carboxylation of multiple, specific, peptide-bound glutamic acid residues in inactive hepatic precursors of factors II, VII, IX, and X. The resulting gamma-carboxyglutamic acid residues convert the precursors into active coagulation factors that are subsequently secreted by liver cells into the blood. Oral phytonadione is adequately absorbed from the gastrointestinal tract only if bile salts are present. After absorption, phytonadione is initially concentrated in the liver, but the concentration declines rapidly. Very little vitamin K accumulates in tissues. Little is known about the metabolic fate of vitamin K. Almost no free unmetabolized vitamin K appears in bile or urine.
In normal animals and humans, phytonadione is virtually devoid of pharmacodynamic activity. However, in animals and humans deficient in vitamin K, the pharmacological action of vitamin K is related to its normal physiological function; that is, to promote the hepatic biosynthesis of vitamin K-dependent clotting factors.
MEPHYTON tablets generally exert their effect within 6 to 10 hours.

INDICATIONS AND USAGE

MEPHYTON is indicated in the following coagulation disorders which are due to faulty formation of factors II, VII, IX and X when caused by vitamin K deficiency or interference with vitamin K activity.
MEPHYTON tablets are indicated in:
—anticoagulant-induced prothrombin deficiency caused by coumarin or indanedione derivatives;
—hypoprothrombinemia secondary to antibacterial therapy;
—hypoprothrombinemia secondary to administration of salicylates;
—hypoprothrombinemia secondary to obstructive jaundice or biliary fistulas but only if bile salts are administered concurrently, since otherwise the oral vitamin K will not be absorbed.

CONTRAINDICATION

Hypersensitivity to any component of this medication.

WARNINGS

An immediate coagulant effect should not be expected after administration of phytonadione.
Phytonadione will not counteract the anticoagulant action of heparin.
When vitamin K₁ is used to correct excessive anticoagulant-induced hypoprothrombinemia, anticoagulant therapy still being indicated, the patient is again faced with the clotting hazards existing prior to starting the anticoagulant therapy. Phytonadione is not a clotting agent, but overzealous therapy with vitamin K₁ may restore conditions which originally permitted thromboembolic phenomena. Dosage should be kept as low as possible, and prothrombin time should be checked regularly as clinical conditions indicate.
Repeated large doses of vitamin K are not warranted in liver disease if the response to initial use of the vitamin is unsatisfactory. Failure to respond to vitamin K may indicate a congenital coagulation defect or that the condition being treated is unresponsive to vitamin K.

PRECAUTIONS

General
Temporary resistance to prothrombin-depressing anticoagulants may result, especially when larger doses of phytonadione are used. If relatively large doses have been employed, it may be necessary when reinstituting anticoagulant therapy to use somewhat larger doses of the prothrombin-depressing anticoagulant, or to use one which acts on a different principle, such as heparin sodium.
Laboratory Tests
Prothrombin time should be checked regularly as clinical conditions indicate.
Carcinogenesis, Mutagenesis, Impairment of Fertility
Studies of carcinogenicity or impairment of fertility have not been performed with MEPHYTON. MEPHYTON at concentrations up to 2000 mcg/plate with or without metabolic activation, was negative in the Ames microbial mutagen test.
Pregnancy
Pregnancy Category C: Animal reproduction studies have not been conducted with MEPHYTON. It is also not known whether MEPHYTON can cause fetal harm when administered to a pregnant woman or can affect reproduction capacity. MEPHYTON should be given to a pregnant woman only if clearly needed.
Pediatric Use
Safety and effectiveness in children have not been established with MEPHYTON. Hemolysis, jaundice, and hyperbilirubinemia in newborns, particularly in premature infants, have been reported with vitamin K.
Nursing Mothers
It is not known whether this drug is excreted in human milk. Because many drugs are excreted in human milk, caution should be exercised when MEPHYTON is administered to a nursing woman.

ADVERSE REACTIONS

Transient "flushing sensations" and "peculiar" sensations of taste have been observed with parenteral phytonadione, as well as rare instances of dizziness, rapid and weak pulse, profuse sweating, brief hypotension, dyspnea, and cyanosis. Hyperbilirubinemia has been observed in the newborn following administration of parenteral phytonadione. This has

occurred rarely and primarily with doses above those recommended.

OVERDOSAGE

The intravenous and oral LD_{50}s in the mouse are approximately 1.17 g/kg and greater than 24.18 g/kg, respectively.

DOSAGE AND ADMINISTRATION

MEPHYTON
Summary of Dosage Guidelines
(See circular text for details)

Adults	Initial Dosage
Anticoagulant-Induced Prothrombin Deficiency (caused by coumarin or indanedione derivatives)	2.5 mg–10 mg or up to 25 mg (rarely 50 mg)
Hypoprothrombinemia due to other causes (Antibiotics; Salicylates or other drugs; Factors limiting absorption or synthesis)	2.5 mg–25 mg or more (rarely up to 50 mg)

Anticoagulant-Induced Prothrombin Deficiency in Adults
To correct excessively prolonged prothrombin times caused by oral anticoagulant therapy—2.5 to 10 mg or up to 25 mg initially is recommended. In rare instances 50 mg may be required. Frequency and amount of subsequent doses should be determined by prothrombin time response or clinical condition. (See WARNINGS.) If, in 12 to 48 hours after oral administration, the prothrombin time has not been shortened satisfactorily, the dose should be repeated.
Hypoprothrombinemia Due to Other Causes in Adults
If possible, discontinuation or reduction of the dosage of drugs interfering with coagulation mechanisms (such as salicylates, antibiotics) is suggested as an alternative to administering concurrent MEPHYTON. The severity of the coagulation disorder should determine whether the immediate administration of MEPHYTON is required in addition to discontinuation or reduction of interfering drugs.
A dosage of 2.5 to 25 mg or more (rarely up to 50 mg) is recommended, the amount and route of administration depending upon the severity of the condition and response obtained.
The oral route should be avoided when the clinical disorder would prevent proper absorption. Bile salts must be given with the tablets when the endogenous supply of bile to the gastrointestinal tract is deficient.

HOW SUPPLIED

No. 7776—Tablets MEPHYTON, 5 mg vitamin K_1, are yellow, round, scored, compressed tablets, coded MSD 43. They are supplied as follows:
NDC 0006-0043-68 bottles of 100
(6505-00-560-0460, 5 mg 100's).
Shown in Product Identification Section, page 419
Storage:
Protect from light.
A.H.F.S. Category: 88:24
DC 7469513 Issued March 1991
COPYRIGHT © MERCK & CO., INC., 1986, 1991
All rights reserved

MERUVAX®$_{II}$ ℞
(Rubella Virus Vaccine Live, MSD), U.S.P.
(Wistar RA 27/3 Strain)

DESCRIPTION

MERUVAX* II (Rubella Virus Vaccine Live, MSD) is a live virus vaccine for immunization against rubella (German measles).
MERUVAX II is a sterile lyophilized preparation of the Wistar Institute RA 27/3 strain of live attenuated rubella virus. The virus was adapted to and propagated in human diploid cell (WI-38) culture.
The reconstituted vaccine is for subcutaneous administration. When reconstituted as directed, the dose for injection is 0.5 mL and contains not less than the equivalent of 1,000 $TCID_{50}$ (tissue culture infectious doses) of the U.S. Reference Rubella Virus. Each dose also contains approximately 25 mcg of neomycin. The product contains no preservative. Sorbitol and hydrolized gelatin are added as stabilizers.

*Registered trademark of MERCK & CO., INC.

CLINICAL PHARMACOLOGY

MERUVAX II produces a modified, non-communicable rubella infection in susceptible persons.
Extensive clinical trials of rubella virus vaccines, prepared using RA 27/3 strain rubella virus, have been carried out in more than 28,000 human subjects (approximately 11,000 with MERUVAX II) in the U.S.A. and more than 20 additional countries. A single injection of the vaccine has been shown to induce rubella hemagglutination-inhibiting (HI) antibodies in 97% or more of susceptible persons. The RA 27/3 rubella strain elicits higher immediate post-vaccination HI, complement-fixing and neutralizing antibody levels than other strains of rubella vaccine and has been shown to induce a broader profile of circulating antibodies including anti-theta and anti-iota precipitating antibodies. The RA 27/3 rubella strain immunologically simulates natural infection more closely than other rubella vaccine viruses. The increased levels and broader profile of antibodies produced by RA 27/3 strain rubella virus vaccine appear to correlate with greater resistance to subclinical reinfection with the wild virus, and provide greater confidence for lasting immunity.
Vaccine-induced antibody levels have been shown to persist for at least 10 years without substantial decline. If the present pattern continues, it will provide a basis for the expectation that immunity following vaccination will be permanent. However, continued surveillance will be required to demonstrate this point.

INDICATIONS AND USAGE†

1. *Children Between 12 Months of Age and Puberty*
MERUVAX II is indicated for immunization against rubella (German measles) in persons from 12 months of age to puberty. A booster is not needed. It is not recommended for infants younger than 12 months because they may retain maternal rubella neutralizing antibodies that may interfere with the immune response. Children in kindergarten and the first grades of elementary school deserve priority for vaccination because often they are epidemiologically the major source of virus dissemination in the community. A history of rubella illness is usually not reliable enough to exclude children from immunization.
Previously unimmunized children of susceptible pregnant women should receive live attenuated rubella vaccine, because an immunized child will be less likely to acquire natural rubella and introduce the virus into the household.
2. *Adolescent and Adult Males*
Vaccination of adolescent or adult males may be a useful procedure in preventing or controlling outbreaks of rubella in circumscribed population groups (e.g., military bases and schools).
3. *Non-Pregnant Adolescent and Adult Females*
Immunization of susceptible non-pregnant adolescent and adult females of childbearing age with live attenuated rubella virus vaccine is indicated if certain precautions are observed (see below and PRECAUTIONS). Vaccinating susceptible postpubertal females confers individual protection against subsequently acquiring rubella infection during pregnancy, which in turn prevents infection of the fetus and consequent congenital rubella injury.
Women of childbearing age should be advised not to become pregnant for three months after vaccination and should be informed of the reason for this precaution.*
It is recommended that rubella susceptibility be determined by serologic testing prior to immunization.** If immune, as evidenced by a specific rubella antibody titer of 1:8 or greater (hemagglutination-inhibition test), vaccination is unnecessary. Congenital malformations do occur in up to seven percent of all live births. Their chance appearance after vaccination could lead to misinterpretation of the cause, particularly if the prior rubella-immune status of vaccinees is unknown.
Postpubertal females should be informed of the frequent occurrence of generally self-limited arthralgia and/or arthritis beginning 2 to 4 weeks after vaccination (see ADVERSE REACTIONS).
4. *Postpartum Women*
It has been found convenient in many instances to vaccinate rubella-susceptible women in the immediate postpartum period (see *Nursing Mothers*).
5. *International Travelers*
Individuals planning travel outside the United States, if not immune, can acquire measles, mumps or rubella and import these diseases to the United States. Therefore, prior to International travel, individuals known to be susceptible to one or more of these diseases can receive either a single antigen vaccine (measles, mumps or rubella), or a combined antigen vaccine as appropriate. However, M-M-R‡ II (Measles, Mumps, and Rubella Virus Vaccine Live, MSD) is preferred for persons likely to be susceptible to mumps and rubella; and if single-antigen measles vaccine is not readily available, travelers should receive M-M-R II (Measles, Mumps, and Rubella Virus Vaccine Live, MSD) regardless of their immune status to mumps or rubella.
Revaccination:
Children vaccinated when younger than 12 months of age should be revaccinated. Based on available evidence, there is no reason to routinely revaccinate persons who were vaccinated originally when 12 months of age or older. However, persons should be revaccinated if there is evidence to suggest that initial immunization was ineffective.
Use with Other Vaccines
Routine administration of DTP (diphtheria, tetanus, pertussis) and/or OPV (oral poliovirus vaccine) concomitantly with measles, mumps and rubella vaccines is not recommended because there are insufficient data relating to the simultaneous administration of these antigens. However, the American Academy of Pediatrics has noted that in some circumstances, particularly when the patient may not return, some practitioners prefer to administer all these antigens on a single day. If done, separate sites and syringes should be used for DTP and MERUVAX II.
MERUVAX II should not be given less than one month before or after administration of other virus vaccines.

†Based in part on the recommendation for rubella vaccine use of the Immunization Practices Advisory Committee (ACIP), Morbidity and Mortality Weekly Report: *33* (22): 301–310, 315–318, June 8, 1984.
*NOTE: The Immunization Practices Advisory Committee (ACIP) has recommended "In view of the importance of protecting this age group against rubella, reasonable precautions in a rubella immunization program include asking females if they are pregnant, excluding those who say they are, and explaining the theoretical risks to the others."
**NOTE: The Immunization Practices Advisory Committee (ACIP) has stated "When practical, and when reliable laboratory services are available, potential vaccinees of childbearing age can have serologic tests to determine susceptibility to rubella. . . . However, routinely performing serologic tests for all females of childbearing age to determine susceptibility so that vaccine is given only to proven susceptibles is expensive and has been ineffective in some areas. Accordingly, the ACIP believes that rubella vaccination of a woman who is not known to be pregnant and has no history of vaccination is justifiable without serologic testing."
‡Registered trademark of MERCK & CO., INC.

CONTRAINDICATIONS

Do not give MERUVAX II to pregnant females; the possible effects of the vaccine on fetal development are unknown at this time. If vaccination of postpubertal females is undertaken, pregnancy should be avoided for three months following vaccination. (See PRECAUTIONS, *Pregnancy*).
Anaphylactic or anaphylactoid reactions to neomycin (each dose of reconstituted vaccine contains approximately 25 mcg of neomycin).
Any febrile respiratory illness or other active febrile infection.
Active untreated tuberculosis.
Patients receiving immunosuppressive therapy. This contraindication does not apply to patients who are receiving corticosteroids as replacement therapy, e.g., for Addison's disease.
Individuals with blood dyscrasias, leukemia, lymphomas of any type, or other malignant neoplasms affecting the bone marrow or lymphatic systems.
Primary and acquired immunodeficiency states, including patients who are immunosuppressed in association with AIDS or other clinical manifestations of infection with human immunodeficiency viruses; cellular immune deficiencies; and hypogammaglobulinemic and dysgammaglobulinemic states.
Individuals with a family history of congenital or hereditary immunodeficiency, until the immune competence of the potential vaccine recipient is demonstrated.

PRECAUTIONS

General
Adequate treatment provisions including epinephrine, should be available for immediate use should an anaphylactic or anaphylactoid reaction occur.
Excretion of small amounts of the live attenuated rubella virus from the nose or throat has occurred in the majority of susceptible individuals 7–28 days after vaccination. There is no confirmed evidence to indicate that such virus is transmitted to susceptible persons who are in contact with the vaccinated individuals. Consequently, transmission through close personal contact, while accepted as a theoretical possibility, is not regarded as a significant risk. However, trans-

Continued on next page

Information on the Merck & Co. products listed on these pages is the full prescribing information from product circulars in use October 1, 1992.

Merck & Co.—Cont.

mission of the vaccine virus to infants via breast milk has been documented (see *Nursing Mothers*).
There is no evidence that live rubella virus vaccine given after exposure to natural rubella virus will prevent illness. There is, however, no contraindication to vaccinating children already exposed to natural rubella.
Children and young adults who are known to be infected with human immunodeficiency viruses but without overt clinical manifestations of immunosuppression may be vaccinated; however, the vaccinees should be monitored closely for vaccine-preventable diseases because immunization may be less effective than for uninfected persons.
Vaccination should be deferred for at least three months following blood or plasma transfusions, or administration of human immune serum globulin. However, susceptible postpartum patients who received blood products may receive MERUVAX II prior to discharge provided that a repeat HI titer is drawn 6–8 weeks after vaccination to insure seroconversion. Similarly, although studies with other live rubella virus vaccines suggest that MERUVAX II may be given in the immediate postpartum period to those non-immune women who have received anti-Rho (D) globulin (human) without interfering with vaccine effectiveness, a follow-up post-vaccination HI titer should also be determined.
It has been reported that attenuated rubella virus vaccine, live, may result in a temporary depression of tuberculin skin sensitivity. Therefore, if a tuberculin test is to be done, it should be administered either before or simultaneously with MERUVAX II.
As for any vaccine, vaccination with MERUVAX II may not result in seroconversion in 100% of susceptible persons given the vaccine.
Pregnancy
Pregnancy Category C
Animal reproduction studies have not been conducted with MERUVAX II. It is also not known whether MERUVAX II can cause fetal harm when administered to a pregnant woman or can affect reproduction capacity. There is evidence suggesting transmission of rubella vaccine viruses to products of conception. Therefore, rubella vaccine should not be administered to pregnant females (see CONTRAINDICATIONS).
In counseling women who are inadvertently vaccinated when pregnant or who become pregnant within 3 months of vaccination, the physician should be aware of the following: In a 10 year survey involving over 700 pregnant women who received rubella vaccine within 3 months before or after conception, (of whom 189 received the Wistar RA 27/3 strain) none of the newborns had abnormalities compatible with congenital rubella syndrome.
Nursing Mothers
Recent studies have shown that lactating postpartum women immunized with live attenuated rubella vaccine may secrete the virus in breast milk and transmit it to breast-fed infants. In the infants with serological evidence of rubella infection, none exhibited severe disease; however, one exhibited mild clinical illness typical of acquired rubella. Caution should be exercised when MERUVAX II is administered to a nursing woman.

ADVERSE REACTIONS

Burning and/or stinging of short duration at the injection site have been reported.
Symptoms of the same kind as those seen following natural rubella may occur after vaccination. These include mild regional lymphadenopathy, urticaria, rash, malaise, sore throat, fever, headache, dizziness, nausea, vomiting, diarrhea, polyneuritis, and arthralgia and/or arthritis (usually transient and rarely chronic). Local pain, wheal and flare, induration, and erythema may occur at the site of injection. Reactions are usually mild and transient. Erythema multiforme has also been reported rarely.
Cough and rhinitis have also been reported.
Vasculitis has been reported rarely.
Anaphylaxis and anaphylactoid reactions have been reported.
Moderate fever [101–102.9°F (38.3–39.4°C)] occurs occasionally, and high fever [over 103°F (39.4°C)] occurs less commonly.
Syncope, particularly at the time of mass vaccination, has been reported.
Chronic arthritis has been associated with natural rubella infection and has been related to persistent virus and/or viral antigen isolated from body tissues. Only rarely have vaccine recipients developed chronic joint symptoms.
Following vaccination in children, reactions in joints are uncommon and generally of brief duration. In women, incidence rates for arthritis and arthralgia are generally higher than those seen in children (children: 0–3%; women: 12–20%) and the reactions tend to be more marked and of longer duration. Symptoms may persist for a matter of months or on rare occasions for years. In adolescent girls, the reactions appear to be intermediate in incidence between those seen in children and in adult women. Even in older women (35–45 years), these reactions are generally well tolerated and rarely interfere with normal activities. Myalgia and paresthesia have been reported rarely after administration of MERUVAX II.
Forms of optic neuritis, including retrobulbar neuritis and papillitis may infrequently follow viral infections, and have been reported to occur 1 to 3 weeks following inoculation with some live virus vaccines.
Isolated reports of polyneuropathy including Guillain-Barré syndrome have been reported after immunization with rubella-containing vaccines.
Clinical experience with live rubella vaccines thus far indicates that encephalitis and other nervous system reactions have occurred very rarely in subjects who were given the vaccines, but a cause and effect relationship has not been established.
Thrombocytopenia with or without purpura has been reported.

DOSAGE AND ADMINISTRATION

FOR SUBCUTANEOUS ADMINISTRATION
Do not inject intravenously
The dosage of vaccine is the same for all persons. Inject the total volume of the single dose vial (about 0.5 mL) or 0.5 mL of the multiple dose vial of reconstituted vaccine subcutaneously, preferably into the outer aspect of upper arm. *Do not give immune globulin (IG) concurrently with* MERUVAX II.
To insure that there is no loss of potency during shipment, the vaccine must be maintained at a temperature of 10°C (50°F) or less.
Before reconstitution, store MERUVAX II at 2–8°C (36–46°F). *Protect from light.*
CAUTION: A sterile syringe free of preservatives, antiseptics, and detergents should be used for each injection and/or reconstitution of the vaccine because these substances may inactivate the live virus vaccine. A 25 gauge, ⅝" needle is recommended.
To reconstitute, use only the diluent supplied, since it is free of preservatives or other antiviral substances which might inactivate the vaccine.
Single Dose Vial—First withdraw the entire volume of diluent into the syringe to be used for reconstitution. Inject all the diluent in the syringe into the vial of lyophilized vaccine, and agitate to mix thoroughly. Withdraw the entire contents into a syringe and inject the total volume of restored vaccine subcutaneously.
It is important to use a separate sterile syringe and needle for each individual patient to prevent transmission of hepatitis B and other infectious agents from one person to another.
10 Dose Vial (available only to government agencies/institutions)—Withdraw the entire contents (7 mL) of the diluent vial into the sterile syringe to be used for reconstitution, and introduce into the 10 dose vial of lyophilized vaccine. Agitate to ensure thorough mixing. The outer labeling suggests "For Jet Injector or Syringe Use". Use with separate sterile syringes is permitted for containers of 10 doses or less. The vaccine and diluent do not contain preservatives; therefore, the user must recognize the potential contamination hazards and exercise special precautions to protect the sterility and potency of the product. The use of aseptic techniques and proper storage prior to and after restoration of the vaccine and subsequent withdrawal of the individual doses is essential. Use 0.5 mL of the reconstituted vaccine for subcutaneous injection.
It is important to use a separate sterile syringe and needle for each individual patient to prevent transmission of hepatitis B and other infectious agents from one person to another.
50 Dose Vial (available only to government agencies/institutions)—Withdraw the entire contents (30 mL) of diluent vial into the sterile syringe to be used for reconstitution and introduce into the 50 dose vial of lyophilized vaccine. Agitate to ensure thorough mixing. With full aseptic precautions, attach the vial to the sterilized multidose jet injector apparatus. Use 0.5 mL of the reconstituted vaccine for subcutaneous injection.
Each dose contains not less than the equivalent of 1,000 $TCID_{50}$ of the U.S. Reference Rubella Virus.
Parenteral drug products should be inspected visually for particulate matter and discoloration prior to administration. MERUVAX II, when reconstituted, is clear yellow.

HOW SUPPLIED

No. 4747—MERUVAX II is supplied as a single-dose vial of lyophilized vaccine,
NDC 0006-4747-00, and a vial of diluent.
No. 4673/4309—MERUVAX II is supplied as follows: (1) a box of 10 single-dose vials of lyophilized vaccine (package A), **NDC** 0006-4673-00; and (2) a box of 10 vials of diluent (package B). To conserve refrigerator space, the diluent may be stored separately at room temperature.
(6505-00-145-0180, Ten Pack).
Available only to government agencies/institutions:
No. 4674—MERUVAX II is supplied as one 10 dose vial of lyophilized vaccine,
NDC 0006-4674-00, and one 7 mL vial of diluent.
No. 4675—MERUVAX II is supplied as one 50 dose vial of lyophilized vaccine,
NDC 0006-4675-00, and one 30 mL vial of diluent.
(6505-01-222-6468, 50 Dose).
Storage
It is recommended that the vaccine be used as soon as possible after reconstitution. Protect vaccine from light at all times, since such exposure may inactivate the virus. Store reconstituted vaccine in the vaccine vial in a dark place at 2–8°C (36–46°F) and discard if not used within 8 hours.

A.H.F.S. Category: 80:12
DC 7680315 Issued March 1991

COPYRIGHT © MERCK & CO., INC., 1990
All rights reserved

MEVACOR® Tablets ℞
(Lovastatin)

DESCRIPTION

MEVACOR* (Lovastatin), is a cholesterol lowering agent isolated from a strain of *Aspergillus terreus.* After oral ingestion, lovastatin, which is an inactive lactone, is hydrolyzed to the corresponding β-hydroxyacid form. This is a principal metabolite and an inhibitor of 3-hydroxy-3-methylglutaryl-coenzyme A (HMG-CoA) reductase. This enzyme catalyzes the conversion of HMG-CoA to mevalonate, which is an early and rate limiting step in the biosynthesis of cholesterol.
Lovastatin is [1*S*-[1α(*R* *),3α,7β,8β(2*S* *,4*S* *),8aβ]]-1,2,3,7,8,8a-hexahydro-3,7-dimethyl-8-[2-(tetrahydro-4-hydroxy-6-oxo-2*H*-pyran-2-yl)ethyl]-1-naphthalenyl 2-methylbutanoate. The empirical formula of lovastatin is $C_{24}H_{36}O_5$ and its molecular weight is 404.55. Its structural formula is:

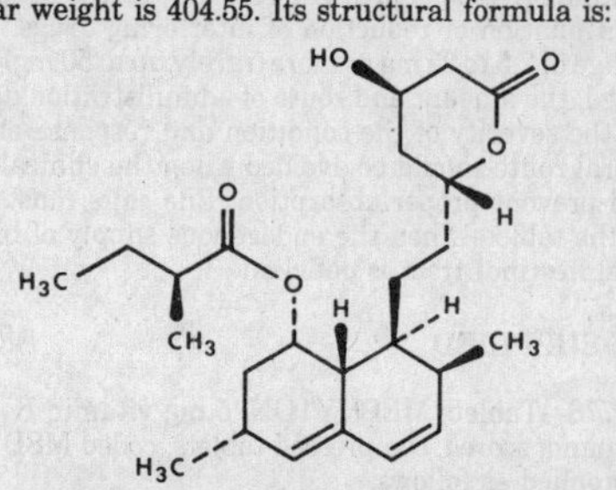

Lovastatin is a white, nonhygroscopic crystalline powder that is insoluble in water and sparingly soluble in ethanol, methanol, and acetonitrile.
Tablets MEVACOR are supplied as 10 mg, 20 mg and 40 mg tablets for oral administration. In addition to the active ingredient lovastatin, each tablet contains the following inactive ingredients: cellulose, lactose, magnesium stearate, and starch. Butylated hydroxyanisole (BHA) is added as a preservative. Tablets MEVACOR 10 mg also contain red ferric oxide and yellow ferric oxide. Tablets MEVACOR 20 mg also contain FD&C Blue 2. Tablets MEVACOR 40 mg also contain D&C Yellow 10 and FD&C Blue 2.

*Registered trademark of MERCK & CO., INC.

CLINICAL PHARMACOLOGY

The involvement of low-density lipoprotein (LDL) cholesterol in atherogenesis has been well-documented in clinical and pathological studies, as well as in many animal experiments. Epidemiological studies have established that high LDL (low-density lipoprotein) cholesterol and low HDL (high-density lipoprotein) cholesterol are both risk factors for coronary heart disease. The Lipid Research Clinics Coronary Primary Prevention Trial (LRC-CPPT), coordinated by the National Institutes of Health (NIH) studied men aged 35–59 with total cholesterol levels 265 mg/dL (6.8 mmol/L) or greater, LDL cholesterol values 175 mg/dL (4.5 mmol/L) or greater and triglyceride levels not more than 300 mg/dL (3.4 mmol/L). This seven-year, double-blind, placebo-controlled study demonstrated that lowering LDL cholesterol with diet and cholestyramine decreased the combined rate of coronary heart disease death plus non-fatal myocardial infarction.
MEVACOR has been shown to reduce both normal and elevated LDL cholesterol concentrations. The effect of lovastatin-induced changes in lipoprotein levels, including reduction of serum cholesterol, on cardiovascular morbidity or mortality has not been established.

TABLE I
FAMILIAL HYPERCHOLESTEROLEMIA STUDY
DOSE RESPONSE OF MEVACOR
(Percent Change from Baseline After 6 Weeks)

DOSAGE	N	TOTAL-C (mean)	LDL-C (mean)	HDL-C (mean)	LDL-C/ HDL-C (mean)	TOTAL-C/ HDL-C (mean)	TRIG. (median)
Placebo	21	−1	−2	+1	−1	0	+3
MEVACOR							
20 mg q.p.m.	20	−18	−19	+10	−26	−24	−7
40 mg q.p.m.	21	−24	−27	+10	−32	−29	−22
10 mg b.i.d.	19	−22	−25	+6	−28	−25	−11
20 mg b.i.d.	20	−27	−31	+12	−38	−34	−18
40 mg b.i.d.	20	−34	−39	+8	−43	−38	−12

LDL is formed from VLDL and is catabolized predominantly by the high affinity LDL receptor. The mechanism of the LDL-lowering effect of MEVACOR may involve both reduction of VLDL cholesterol concentration, and induction of the LDL receptor, leading to reduced production and/or increased catabolism of LDL cholesterol. Apolipoprotein B also falls substantially during treatment with MEVACOR. Since each LDL particle contains one molecule of apolipoprotein B, and since little apolipoprotein B is found in other lipoproteins, this strongly suggests that MEVACOR does not merely cause cholesterol to be lost from LDL, but also reduces the concentration of circulating LDL particles. In addition, MEVACOR can produce increases of variable magnitude in HDL cholesterol, and modestly reduces VLDL cholesterol and plasma triglycerides (see Tables I–IV under *Clinical Studies*). The effects of MEVACOR on Lp(a), fibrinogen, and certain other indpendent biochemical risk markers for coronary heart disease are unknown.

MEVACOR is a specific inhibitor of HMG-CoA reductase, the enzyme which catalyzes the conversion of HMG-CoA to mevalonate. The conversion of HMG-CoA to mevalonate is an early step in the biosynthetic pathway for cholesterol.

Pharmacokinetics
Lovastatin is a lactone which is readily hydrolyzed *in vivo* to the corresponding β-hydroxyacid, a potent inhibitor of HMG-CoA reductase. Inhibition of HMG-CoA reductase is the basis for an assay in pharmacokinetic studies of the β-hydroxyacid metabolites (active inhibitors) and, following base hydrolysis, active plus latent inhibitors (total inhibitors) in plasma following administration of lovastatin.
Following an oral dose of ^{14}C-labeled lovastatin in man, 10% of the dose was excreted in urine and 83% in feces. The latter represents absorbed drug equivalents excreted in bile, as well as any unabsorbed drug. Plasma concentrations of total radioactivity (lovastatin plus ^{14}C-metabolites) peaked at 2 hours and declined rapidly to about 10% of peak by 24 hours postdose. Absorption of lovastatin, estimated relative to an intravenous reference dose, in each of four animal species tested, averaged about 30% of an oral dose. In animal studies, after oral dosing, lovastatin had high selectivity for the liver, where it achieved substantially higher concentrations than in non-target tissues. Lovastatin undergoes extensive first-pass extraction in the liver, its primary site of action, with subsequent excretion of drug equivalents in the bile. As a consequence of extensive hepatic extraction of lovastatin, the availability of drug to the general circulation is low and variable. In a single dose study in four hypercholesterolemic patients, it was estimated that less than 5% of an oral dose of lovastatin reaches the general circulation as active inhibitors. Following administration of lovastatin tablets the coefficient of variation, based on between-subject variability, was approximately 40% for the area under the curve (AUC) of total inhibitory activity in the general circulation.

Both lovastatin and its β-hydroxyacid metabolite are highly bound (>95%) to human plasma proteins. Animal studies demonstrated that lovastatin crosses the blood-brain and placental barriers.

The major active metabolites present in human plasma are the β-hydroxyacid of lovastatin, its 6'-hydroxy derivative, and two additional metabolites. Peak plasma concentrations of both active and total inhibitors were attained within 2 to 4 hours of dose administration. While the recommended therapeutic dose range is 20 to 80 mg/day, linearity of inhibitory activity in the general circulation was established by a single dose study employing lovastatin tablet dosages from 60 to as high as 120 mg. With a once-a-day dosing regimen, plasma concentrations of total inhibitors over a dosing interval achieved a steady state between the second and third days of therapy and were about 1.5 times those following a single dose. When lovastatin was given under fasting conditions, plasma concentrations of total inhibitors were on average about two-thirds those found when lovastatin was administered immediately after a standard test meal.

In a study of patients with severe renal insufficiency (creatinine clearance 10–30 mL/min), the plasma concentrations of total inhibitors after a single dose of lovastatin were approximately two-fold higher than those in healthy volunteers.

Clinical Studies
MEVACOR has been shown to be highly effective in reducing total and LDL cholesterol in heterozygous familial and non-familial forms of primary hypercholesterolemia and in mixed hyperlipidemia. A marked response was seen within 2 weeks, and the maximum therapeutic response occurred within 4–6 weeks. The response was maintained during continuation of therapy. Single daily doses given in the evening were more effective than the same dose given in the morning, perhaps because cholesterol is synthesized mainly at night.

In multicenter, double-blind studies in patients with familial or non-familial hypercholesterolemia, MEVACOR, administered in doses ranging from 20 mg q.p.m. to 40 mg b.i.d., was compared to placebo. MEVACOR consistently and significantly decreased total plasma cholesterol (TOTAL-C), LDL cholesterol (LDL-C), total cholesterol/HDL cholesterol (TOTAL-C/HDL-C) ratio and LDL cholesterol/HDL cholesterol (LDL-C/HDL-C) ratio. In addition, MEVACOR produced increases of variable magnitude in HDL cholesterol (HDL-C), and modestly decreased VLDL cholesterol (VLDL-C) and plasma triglycerides (TRIG.) (see Tables I and IV for dose response results).

MEVACOR was compared to cholestyramine in a randomized open parallel study and to probucol in a double-blind, parallel study. Both studies were performed with patients with hypercholesterolemia who were at high risk of myocardial infarction. Summary results of these two comparative studies are presented in Tables II & III.

Expanded Clinical Evaluation of Lovastatin (EXCEL) Study
MEVACOR was compared to placebo in 8,245 patients with hypercholesterolemia (total cholesterol 240–300 mg/dL [6.2 mmol/L–7.6 mmol/L], LDL cholesterol >160 mg/dL [4.1 mmol/L]) in the randomized, double-blind, parallel, 48-week EXCEL study. All changes in the lipid measurements (Table IV) in MEVACOR treated patients were dose-related and significantly different from placebo (p ≤ 0.001). These results were sustained throughout the study.

Eye
There was a high prevalence of baseline lenticular opacities in the patient population included in the early clinical trials with lovastatin. During these trials the appearance of new opacities was noted in both the lovastatin and placebo groups. There was no clinically significant change in visual acuity in the patients who had new opacities reported nor was any patient, including those with opacities noted at baseline, discontinued from therapy because of a decrease in visual acuity.

An interim analysis was performed at 2 years in 192 hypercholesterolemic patients who participated in a placebo-controlled, parallel, double-blind study to assess the effect of lovastatin on the human lens. There were no clinically significant differences between the lovastatin and placebo groups in the incidence, type, or progression of lenticular opacities.

INDICATIONS AND USAGE

Therapy with lipid-altering agents should be a component of multiple risk factor intervention in those individuals at significantly increased risk for artherosclerotic vascular disease due to hypercholesterolemia. MEVACOR is indicated as an adjunct to diet for the reduction of elevated total and LDL cholesterol levels in patients with primary hypercholesterolemia (Types IIa and IIb[1]), when the response to diet restricted in saturated fat and cholesterol and to other nonpharmacological measures alone has been inadequate.

Prior to initiating therapy with lovastatin, secondary causes for hypercholesterolemia (e.g., poorly controlled diabetes mellitus, hypothyroidism, nephrotic syndrome, dysproteinemias, obstructive liver disease, other drug therapy, alcoholism) should be excluded, and a lipid profile performed to measure TOTAL-C, HDL-C, and triglycerides (TG). For patients with TG less than 400 mg/dL (<4.5 mmol/L), LDL-C can be estimated using the following equation:

$$LDL\text{-}C = Total\ cholesterol - [0.2 \times (triglycerides) + HDL\text{-}C]$$

For TG levels >400 mg/dL (>4.5 mmol/L), this equation is less accurate and LDL-C concentrations should be determined by ultracentrifugation. In hypertriglyceridemic patients, LDL-C may be low or normal despite elevated TOTAL-C. In such cases, MEVACOR is not indicated.

The effect of lovastatin-induced changes in lipoprotein levels, including reduction of serum cholesterol, on cardiovascular morbidity or mortality has not been established.

The National Cholesterol Education Program (NCEP) Treatment Guidelines[§] are summarized below:

[See table on next page.]

TABLE II
MEVACOR vs. Cholestyramine
(Percent Change from Baseline After 12 Weeks)

TREATMENT	N	TOTAL-C (mean)	LDL-C (mean)	HDL-C (mean)	LDL-C/ HDL-C (mean)	TOTAL-C/ HDL-C (mean)	VLDL-C (median)	TRIG. (median)
MEVACOR								
20 mg b.i.d.	85	−27	−32	+9	−36	−31	−34	−21
40 mg b.i.d.	88	−34	−42	+8	−44	−37	−31	−27
Cholestyramine								
12 g b.i.d.	88	−17	−23	+8	−27	−21	+2	+11

TABLE III
MEVACOR vs. Probucol
(Percent Change from Baseline After 14 Weeks)

TREATMENT	N	TOTAL-C (mean)	LDL-C (mean)	HDL-C (mean)	LDL-C/ HDL-C (mean)	TOTAL-C/ HDL-C (mean)	VLDL-C (median)	TRIG. (median)
MEVACOR								
40 mg q.p.m.	47	−25	−32	+9	−38	−31	−37	−18
80 mg q.p.m.	49	−30	−37	+11	−42	−36	−27	−17
40 mg b.i.d.	47	−33	−40	+12	−45	−39	−40	−25
Probucol								
500 mg b.i.d.	97	−10	−8	−23	+26	+23	−13	+1

TABLE IV
MEVACOR vs. Placebo
(Percent Change from Baseline—
Average Values Between Weeks 12 and 48)

DOSAGE	N*	TOTAL-C (mean)	LDL-C (mean)	HDL-C (mean)	LDL-C/ HDL-C (mean)	TOTAL-C/ HDL-C (mean)	TRIG. (median)
Placebo	1663	+0.7	+0.4	+2.0	+0.2	+0.6	+4
MEVACOR							
20 mg q.p.m.	1642	−17	−24	+6.6	−27	−21	−10
40 mg q.p.m.	1645	−22	−30	+7.2	−34	−26	−14
20 mg b.i.d.	1646	−24	−34	+8.6	−38	−29	−16
40 mg b.i.d.	1649	−29	−40	+9.5	−44	−34	−19

*Patients enrolled

Continued on next page

Information on the Merck & Co. products listed on these pages is the full prescribing information from product circulars in use October 1, 1992.

Merck & Co.—Cont.

	LDL Cholesterol mg/dL (mmol/L) Initiation Level	LDL Cholesterol mg/dL (mmol/L) Minimum Goal	Total Cholesterol mg/dL (mmol/L) Minimum Goal
Without Definite CHD or Two Other Risk Factors*	≥190 (≥4.9)	<160 (<4.1)	<240 (<6.2)
With Definite CHD or Two Other Risk Factors*	≥160 (≥4.1)	<130 (<3.4)	<200 (<5.2)

* Other risk factors for coronary heart disease (CHD) include: male sex, family history of premature CHD, cigarette smoking, hypertension, confirmed HDL-C <35 mg/dL (<0.91 mmol/L), diabetes mellitus, definite cerebrovascular or peripheral vascular disease, or severe obesity.

§ For adult diabetics, a modification of these guidelines is recommended—see: American Diabetes Association Consensus Statement: Role of cardiovascular risk factors in prevention and treatment of macrovascular disease in diabetes, Diabetes Care 12(8): 573–79, 1989.

Since the goal of treatment is to lower LDL-C, the NCEP recommends that LDL-C levels be used to initiate and assess treatment response. Only if LDL-C levels are not available, should the TOTAL-C be used to monitor therapy.

Although MEVACOR may be useful to reduce elevated LDL cholesterol levels in patients with combined hypercholesterolemia and hypertriglyceridemia where hypercholesterolemia is the major abnormality (Type IIb hyperlipoproteinemia), it has not been studied in conditions where the major abnormality is elevation of chylomicrons, VLDL or IDL (i.e., hyperlipoproteinemia types I, III, IV, or V).[1]

[1] Classification of Hyperlipoproteinemias

Type	Lipoproteins elevated	Lipid Elevations major	Lipid Elevations minor
I (rare)	chylomicrons	TG	↑→C
IIa	LDL	C	—
IIb	LDL, VLDL	C	TG
III (rare)	IDL	C/TG	—
IV	VLDL	TG	↑→C
V (rare)	chylomicrons, VLDL	TG	↑→C

C = cholesterol, TG = triglycerides,
LDL = low-density lipoprotein,
VLDL = very low-density lipoprotein,
IDL = intermediate-density lipoprotein.

CONTRAINDICATIONS

Hypersensitivity to any component of this medication.

Active liver disease or unexplained persistent elevations of serum transaminases (see WARNINGS).

Pregnancy and lactation.

Atherosclerosis is a chronic process and the discontinuation of lipid-lowering drugs during pregnancy should have little impact on the outcome of long-term therapy of primary hypercholesterolemia. Moreoever, cholesterol and other products of the cholesterol biosynthesis pathway are essential components for fetal development, including synthesis of steroids and cell membranes. Because of the ability of inhibitors of HMG-CoA reductase such as MEVACOR to decrease the synthesis of cholesterol and possibly other products of the cholesterol biosynthesis pathway, MEVACOR may cause fetal harm when administered to a pregnant woman. Therefore, lovastatin is contraindicated during pregnancy. Lovastatin should be administered to women of childbearing age only when such patients are highly unlikely to conceive. If the patient becomes pregnant while taking this drug, lovastatin should be discontinued and the patient should be apprised of the potential hazard to the fetus.

WARNINGS

Liver Dysfunction

Marked persistent increases (to more than 3 times the upper limit of normal) in serum transaminases occurred in 1.9% of adult patients who received lovastatin for at least one year in early clinical trials (see ADVERSE REACTIONS). When the drug was interrupted or discontinued in these patients, the transaminase levels usually fell slowly to pretreatment levels. The increases usually appeared 3 to 12 months after the start of therapy with lovastatin, and were not associated with jaundice or other clinical signs or symptoms. There was no evidence of hypersensitivity. In the EXCEL study (see CLINICAL PHARMACOLOGY, *Clinical Studies*), the incidence of marked persistent increases in serum transaminases over 48 weeks was 0.1% for placebo, 0.1% at 20 mg/day, 0.9% at 40 mg/day, and 1.5% at 80 mg/day in patients on lovastatin. However, in post-marketing experience with MEVACOR, symptomatic liver disease has been reported rarely at all dosages (see ADVERSE REACTIONS).

It is recommended that liver function tests be performed during therapy with lovastatin. Serum transaminases, including ALT (SGPT), should be monitored before treatment begins, every 6 weeks during the first 3 months, every 8 weeks during the remainder of the first year, and periodically thereafter (e.g., at approximately 6 month intervals). Special attention should be paid to patients who develop elevated serum transaminase levels, and in these patients, measurements should be repeated promptly and then performed more frequently. If the transaminase levels show evidence of progression, particularly if they rise to three times the upper limit of normal and are persistent, the drug should be discontinued. Liver biopsy should be considered if elevations are persistent beyond the discontinuation of the drug.

The drug should be used with caution in patients who consume substantial quantities of alcohol and/or have a past history of liver disease. Active liver disease or unexplained transaminase elevations are contraindications to the use of lovastatin.

As with other lipid-lowering agents, moderate (less than three times the upper limit of normal) elevations of serum transaminases have been reported following therapy with MEVACOR (see ADVERSE REACTIONS). These changes appeared soon after initiation of therapy with MEVACOR, were often transient, were not accompanied by any symptoms and interruption of treatment was not required.

Skeletal Muscle

Rhabdomyolysis has been associated with lovastatin therapy alone, when combined with immunosuppressive therapy including cyclosporine in cardiac transplant patients, and when combined in non-transplant patients with either gemfibrozil or lipid-lowering doses (≥ 1 g/day) of nicotinic acid. Some of the affected patients had pre-existing renal insufficiency, usually as a consequence of long-standing diabetes. Acute renal failure from rhabdomyolysis has been seen more commonly with the lovastatin-gemfibrozil combination, and has also been reported in transplant patients receiving lovastatin plus cyclosporine.

Rhabdomyolysis with or without renal impairment has been reported in seriously ill patients receiving erythromycin concomitantly with lovastatin. Therefore, patients receiving concomitant lovastatin and erythromycin should be carefully monitored.

Fulminant rhabdomyolysis has been seen as early as three weeks after initiation of combined therapy with gemfibrozil and lovastatin, but may be seen after several months. For these reasons, it is felt that, in most subjects who have had an unsatisfactory lipid response to either drug alone, the possible benefits of combined therapy with lovastatin and gemfibrozil do not outweigh the risks of severe myopathy, rhabdomyolysis, and acute renal failure. While it is not known whether this interaction occurs with fibrates other than gemfibrozil, myopathy and rhabdomyolysis have occasionally been associated with the use of other fibrates alone, including clofibrate. Therefore, the combined use of lovastatin with other fibrates should generally be avoided.

Physicians contemplating combined therapy with lovastatin and lipid-lowering doses of nicotinic acid or with immunosuppressive drugs should carefully weigh the potential benefits and risks and should carefully monitor patients for any signs and symptoms of muscle pain, tenderness, or weakness, particularly during the initial months of therapy and during any periods of upward dosage titration of either drug. Periodic CPK determinations may be considered in such situations, but there is no assurance that such monitoring will prevent the occurrence of severe myopathy. The monitoring of lovastatin drug and metabolite levels may be considered in transplant patients who are treated with immunosuppressives and lovastatin.

Lovastatin therapy should be temporarily withheld or discontinued in any patient with an acute, serious condition suggestive of a myopathy or having a risk factor predisposing to the development of renal failure secondary to rhabdomyolysis, including: severe acute infection, hypotension, major surgery, trauma, severe metabolic, endocrine and electrolyte disorders, and uncontrolled seizures.

Myalgia has been associated with lovastatin therapy. Transient, mildly elevated creatine phosphokinase levels are commonly seen in lovastatin-treated patients. However, in early clinical trials, approximately 0.5% of patients developed a myopathy, i.e., myalgia or muscle weakness associated with markedly elevated CPK levels. In the EXCEL study (see CLINICAL PHARMACOLOGY, *Clinical Studies*), five (0.1%) patients taking lovastatin alone (one at 40 mg q.p.m., and four at 40 mg b.i.d.) developed myopathy (muscle symptoms and CPK levels >10 times the upper limit of normal). Myopathy should be considered in any patient with diffuse myalgias, muscle tenderness or weakness, and/or marked elevation of CPK. Patients should be advised to report promptly unexplained muscle pain, tenderness or weakness, particularly if accompanied by malaise or fever. Lovastatin therapy should be discontinued if markedly elevated CPK levels occur or myopathy is diagnosed or suspected.

Most of the patients who have developed myopathy (including rhabdomyolysis) while taking lovastatin were receiving concomitant therapy with immunosuppressive drugs, gemfibrozil or lipid-lowering doses of nicotinic acid. In clinical trials, about 30 percent of patients on concomitant immunosuppressive therapy including cyclosporine developed myopathy; the corresponding percentages for gemfibrozil and niacin were approximately 5 percent and 2 percent respectively.

In six patients with cardiac transplants taking immunosuppressive therapy including cyclosporine concomitantly with lovastatin 20 mg/day, the average plasma level of active metabolites derived from lovastatin was elevated to approximately four times the expected levels. Because of an apparent relationship between increased plasma levels of active metabolites derived from lovastatin and myopathy, the daily dosage in patients taking immunosuppressants should not exceed 20 mg/day (see DOSAGE AND ADMINISTRATION). Even at this dosage, the benefits and risks of using lovastatin in patients taking immunosuppressants should be carefully considered.

PRECAUTIONS

General

Before instituting therapy with MEVACOR, an attempt should be made to control hypercholesterolemia with appropriate diet, exercise, weight reduction in obese patients, and to treat other underlying medical problems (see INDICATIONS AND USAGE).

Lovastatin may elevate creatine phosphokinase and transaminase levels (see WARNINGS and ADVERSE REACTIONS). This should be considered in the differential diagnosis of chest pain in a patient on therapy with lovastatin.

Homozygous Familial Hypercholesterolemia

MEVACOR is less effective in patients with the rare homozygous familial hypercholesterolemia, possibly because these patients have no functional LDL receptors. MEVACOR appears to be more likely to raise serum transaminases (see ADVERSE REACTIONS) in these homozygous patients.

Information for Patients

Patients should be advised to report promptly unexplained muscle pain, tenderness or weakness, particularly if accompanied by malaise or fever.

Drug Interactions

Immunosuppressive Drugs, Gemfibrozil, Niacin (Nicotinic Acid), Erythromycin: See WARNINGS, *Skeletal Muscle.*

Coumarin Anticoagulants: In a small clinical trial in which lovastatin was administered to warfarin treated patients, no effect on prothrombin time was detected. However, another HMG-CoA reductase inhibitor has been found to produce a less than two seconds increase in prothrombin time in healthy volunteers receiving low doses of warfarin. Also, bleeding and/or increased prothrombin time have been reported in a few patients taking coumarin anticoagulants concomitantly with lovastatin. It is recommended that in patients taking anticoagulants, prothrombin time be determined before starting lovastatin and frequently enough during early therapy to insure that no significant alteration of prothrombin time occurs. Once a stable prothrombin time has been documented, prothrombin times can be monitored at the intervals usually recommended for patients on coumarin anticoagulants. If the dose of lovastatin is changed, the same procedure should be repeated. Lovastatin therapy has not been associated with bleeding or with changes in prothrombin time in patients not taking anticoagulants.

Antipyrine: Because lovastatin had no effect on the pharmacokinetics of antipyrine or its metabolites, interactions of other drugs metabolized via the same cytochrome isozymes are not expected.

Propranolol: In normal volunteers, there was no clinically significant pharmacokinetic or pharmacodynamic interaction with concomitant administration of single doses of lovastatin and propranolol.

Digoxin: In patients with hypercholesterolemia, concomitant administration of lovastatin and digoxin resulted in no effect on digoxin plasma concentrations.

Other Concomitant Therapy: Although specific interaction studies were not performed, in clinical studies, lovastatin was used concomitantly with beta blockers, calcium channel blockers, diuretics and nonsteroidal anti-inflammatory drugs (NSAIDs) without evidence of clinically significant adverse interactions.

Endocrine Function

HMG-CoA reductase inhibitors interfere with cholesterol synthesis and as such might theoretically blunt adrenal and/or gonadal steroid production. Results of clinical trials with drugs in this class have been inconsistent with regard to drug effects on basal and reserve steroid levels. However, clinical studies have shown that lovastatin does not reduce basal plasma cortisol concentration or impair adrenal reserve, and does not reduce basal plasma testosterone concentration. Another HMG-CoA reductase inhibitor has been

	MEVACOR (N=613) %	Placebo (N=82) %	Cholestyramine (N=88) %	Probucol (N=97) %
Gastrointestinal				
Constipation	4.9	—	34.1	2.1
Diarrhea	5.5	4.9	8.0	10.3
Dyspepsia	3.9	—	13.6	3.1
Flatus	6.4	2.4	21.6	2.1
Abdominal pain/cramps	5.7	2.4	5.7	5.2
Heartburn	1.6	—	8.0	—
Nausea	4.7	3.7	9.1	6.2
Musculoskeletal				
Muscle cramps	1.1	—	1.1	—
Myalgia	2.4	1.2	—	—
Nervous System/Psychiatric				
Dizziness	2.0	1.2	—	1.0
Headache	9.3	4.9	4.5	8.2
Skin				
Rash/pruritus	5.2	—	4.5	—
Special Senses				
Blurred vision	1.5	—	1.1	3.1
Dysgeusia	0.8	—	1.1	—

shown to reduce the plasma testosterone response to HCG. In the same study, the mean testosterone response to HCG was slightly but not significantly reduced after treatment with lovastatin 40 mg daily for 16 weeks in 21 men. The effects of HMG-CoA reductase inhibitors on male fertility have not been studied in adequate numbers of male patients. The effects, if any, on the pituitary-gonadal axis in premenopausal women are unknown. Patients treated with lovastatin who develop clinical evidence of endocrine dysfunction should be evaluated appropriately. Caution should also be exercised if an HMG-CoA reductase inhibitor or other agent used to lower cholesterol levels is administered to patients also receiving other drugs (e.g., ketoconazole, spironolactone, cimetidine) that may decrease the levels or activity of endogenous steroid hormones.

CNS Toxicity
Lovastatin produced optic nerve degeneration (Wallerian degeneration of retinogeniculate fibers) in clinically normal dogs in a dose-dependent fashion starting at 60 mg/kg/day, a dose that produced mean plasma drug levels about 30 times higher than the mean drug level in humans taking the highest recommended dose (as measured by total enzyme inhibitory activity). Vestibulocochlear Wallerian-like degeneration and retinal ganglion cell chromatolysis were also seen in dogs treated for 14 weeks at 180 mg/kg/day, a dose which resulted in a mean plasma drug level (C_{max}) similar to that seen with the 60 mg/kg/day dose.
CNS vascular lesions, characterized by perivascular hemorrhage and edema, mononuclear cell infiltration of perivascular spaces, perivascular fibrin deposits and necrosis of small vessels, were seen in dogs treated with lovastatin at a dose of 180 mg/kg/day, a dose which produced plasma drug levels (C_{max}) which were about 30 times higher than the mean values in humans taking 80 mg/day.
Similar optic nerve and CNS vascular lesions have been observed with other drugs of this class.

Carcinogenesis, Mutagenesis, Impairment of Fertility
In a 21-month carcinogenic study in mice, there was a statistically significant increase in the incidence of hepatocellular carcinomas and adenomas in both males and females at 500 mg/kg/day. This dose produced a total plasma drug exposure 3 to 4 times that of humans given the highest recommended dose of lovastatin (drug exposure was measured as total HMG-CoA reductase inhibitory activity in extracted plasma). Tumor increases were not seen at 20 and 100 mg/kg/day, doses that produced drug exposures of 0.3 to 2 times that of humans at the 80 mg/day dose. A statistically signifi-

cant increase in pulmonary adenomas was seen in female mice at approximately 4 times the human drug exposure. (Although mice were given 300 times the human dose [HD] on a mg/kg body weight basis, plasma levels of total inhibitory activity were only 4 times higher in mice than in humans given 80 mg of MEVACOR.)
There was an increase in incidence of papilloma in the nonglandular mucosa of the stomach of mice beginning at exposures of 1 to 2 times that of humans. The glandular mucosa was not affected. The human stomach contains only glandular mucosa.
In a 24-month carcinogenicity study in rats, there was a positive dose response relationship for hepatocellular carcinogenicity in males at drug exposures between 2–7 times that of human exposure at 80 mg/day (doses in rats were 5, 30 and 180 mg/kg/day).
A chemically similar drug in this class was administered to mice for 72 weeks at 25, 100, and 400 mg/kg body weight, which resulted in mean serum drug levels approximately 3, 15, and 33 times higher than the mean human serum drug concentration (as total inhibitory activity) after a 40 mg oral dose. Liver carcinomas were significantly increased in high dose females and mid- and high dose males, with a maximum incidence of 90 percent in males. The incidence of adenomas of the liver was significantly increased in mid- and high dose females. Drug treatment also significantly increased the incidence of lung adenomas in mid- and high dose males and females. Adenomas of the Harderian gland (a gland of the eye of rodents) were significantly higher in high dose mice than in controls.
No evidence of mutagenicity was observed in a microbial mutagen test using mutant strains of *Salmonella typhimurium* with or without rat or mouse liver metabolic activation. In addition, no evidence of damage to genetic material was noted in an *in vitro* alkaline elution assay using rat or mouse hepatocytes, a V-79 mammalian cell forward mutation study, an *in vitro* chromosome aberration study in CHO cells, or an *in vivo* chromosomal aberration assay in mouse bone marrow.
Drug-related testicular atrophy, decreased spermatogenesis, spermatocytic degeneration and giant cell formation were seen in dogs starting at 20 mg/kg/day. Similar findings were seen with another drug in this class. No drug-related effects on fertility were found in studies with lovastatin in rats. However, in studies with a similar drug in this class, there was decreased fertility in male rats treated for 34 weeks at 25 mg/kg body weight, although this effect was not observed

in a subsequent fertility study when this same dose was administered for 11 weeks (the entire cycle of spermatogenesis, including epididymal maturation). In rats treated with this same reductase inhibitor at 180 mg/kg/day, seminiferous tubule degeneration (necrosis and loss of spermatogenic epithelium) was observed. No microscopic changes were observed in the testes from rats of either study. The clinical significance of these findings is unclear.

Pregnancy
Pregnancy Category X
See CONTRAINDICATIONS.
Safety in pregnant women has not been established. Lovastatin has been shown to produce skeletal malformations at plasma levels 40 times the human exposure (for mouse fetus) and 80 times the human exposure (for rat fetus) based on mg/m² surface area (doses were 800 mg/kg/day). No drug-induced changes were seen in either species at multiples of 8 times (rat) or 4 times (mouse) based on surface area. No evidence of malformations was noted in rabbits at exposures up to 3 times the human exposure (dose of 15 mg/kg/day, highest tolerated dose). MEVACOR should be administered to women of child-bearing potential only when such patients are highly unlikely to conceive and have been informed of the potential hazards. If the woman becomes pregnant while taking MEVACOR, it should be discontinued and the patient advised again as to the potential hazards to the fetus.

Nursing Mothers
It is not known whether lovastatin is excreted in human milk. Because a small amount of another drug in this class is excreted in human breast milk and because of the potential for serious adverse reactions in nursing infants, women taking MEVACOR should not nurse their infants (see CONTRAINDICATIONS).

Pediatric Use
Safety and effectiveness in children and adolescents have not been established. Because children and adolescents are not likely to benefit from cholesterol lowering for at least a decade and because experience with this drug is limited (no studies in subjects below the age of 20 years), treatment of children with lovastatin is not recommended at this time.

ADVERSE REACTIONS

MEVACOR is generally well tolerated; adverse reactions usually have been mild and transient. Less than 1% of patients were discontinued from controlled clinical studies of up to 14 weeks due to adverse experiences attributable to MEVACOR. About 3% of patients were discontinued from extensions of these studies due to adverse experiences attributable to MEVACOR; about half of these patients were discontinued due to increases in serum transaminases. The median duration of therapy in these extensions was 5.2 years.
In the EXCEL study (see CLINICAL PHARMACOLOGY, *Clinical Studies*), 4.6% of the patients treated up to 48 weeks were discontinued due to clinical or laboratory adverse experiences which were rated by the investigator as possibly, probably or definitely related to therapy with MEVACOR. The value for the placebo group was 2.5%.

Clinical Adverse Experiences
Adverse experiences reported in patients treated with MEVACOR in controlled clinical studies are shown in the table below:

Laboratory Tests
Marked persistent increases of serum transaminases have been noted (see WARNINGS).
About 11% of patients had elevations of creatine phosphokinase (CPK) levels of at least twice the normal value on one or more occasions. The corresponding values for the control agents were cholestyramine, 9 percent and probucol, 2 percent. This was attributable to the noncardiac fraction of CPK. Large increases in CPK have sometimes been reported (see WARNINGS, *Skeletal Muscle*).

Expanded Clinical Evaluation of Lovastatin (EXCEL) Study
Clinical Adverse Experiences
MEVACOR was compared to placebo in 8,245 patients with hypercholesterolemia (total cholesterol 240–300 mg/dL [6.2–7.8 mmol/L]) in the randomized, double-blind, parallel, 48-week EXCEL study. Clinical adverse experiences reported as possibly, probably or definitely drug-related in ≥1% in any treatment group are shown in the second table. For no event was the incidence on drug and placebo statistically different.
[See table at left.]
Other clinical adverse experiences reported as possibly, probably or definitely drug-related in 0.5 to 1.0 percent of patients in any drug-related group are listed next. In all

	Placebo (N=1663) %	MEVACOR 20 mg q.p.m. (N=1642) %	MEVACOR 40 mg q.p.m. (N=1645) %	MEVACOR 20 mg b.i.d. (N=1646) %	MEVACOR 40 mg b.i.d. (N=1649) %
Body As a Whole					
Asthenia	1.4	1.7	1.4	1.5	1.2
Gastrointestinal					
Abdominal pain	1.6	2.0	2.0	2.2	2.5
Constipation	1.9	2.0	3.2	3.2	3.5
Diarrhea	2.3	2.6	2.4	2.2	2.6
Dyspepsia	1.9	1.3	1.3	1.0	1.6
Flatulence	4.2	3.7	4.3	3.9	4.5
Nausea	2.5	1.9	2.5	2.2	2.2
Musculoskeletal					
Muscle cramps	0.5	0.6	0.8	1.1	1.0
Myalgia	1.7	2.6	1.8	2.2	3.0
Nervous System/Psychiatric					
Dizziness	0.7	0.7	1.2	0.5	0.5
Headache	2.7	2.6	2.8	2.1	3.2
Skin					
Rash	0.7	0.8	1.0	1.2	1.3
Special Senses					
Blurred vision	0.8	1.1	0.9	0.9	1.2

Continued on next page

Information on the Merck & Co. products listed on these pages is the full prescribing information from product circulars in use October 1, 1992.

Merck & Co.—Cont.

these cases the incidence on drug and placebo was not statistically different.

Body as a Whole: chest pain; *Gastrointestinal:* acid regurgitation, dry mouth, vomiting; *Musculoskeletal:* leg pain, shoulder pain, arthralgia; *Nervous System/Psychiatric:* insomnia, paresthesia; *Skin:* alopecia, pruritus; *Special Senses:* eye irritation.

Concomitant Therapy

In controlled clinical studies in which lovastatin was administered concomitantly with cholestyramine, no adverse reactions peculiar to this concomitant treatment were observed. The adverse reactions that occurred were limited to those reported previously with lovastatin or cholestyramine. Other lipid-lowering agents were not administered concomitantly with lovastatin during controlled clinical studies. Preliminary data suggests that the addition of either probucol or gemfibrozil to therapy with lovastatin is not associated with greater reduction in LDL cholesterol than that achieved with lovastatin alone. In uncontrolled clinical studies, most of the patients who have developed myopathy were receiving concomitant therapy with immunosuppressive drugs, gemfibrozil or niacin (nicotinic acid) (see WARNINGS, *Skeletal Muscle*).

The following effects have been reported with drugs in this class:

Skeletal: myopathy, rhabdomyolysis, arthralgias.

Neurological: dysfunction of certain cranial nerves (including alteration of taste, impairment of extra-ocular movement, facial paresis), tremor, vertigo, memory loss, paresthesia, peripheral neuropathy, peripheral nerve palsy, anxiety, insomnia, depression.

Hypersensitivity Reactions: An apparent hypersensitivity syndrome has been reported rarely which has included one or more of the following features: anaphylaxis, angioedema, lupus erythematous-like syndrome, polymyalgia rheumatica, vasculitis, purpura, thrombocytopenia, leukopenia, hemolytic anemia, positive ANA, ESR increase, arthritis, arthralgia, urticaria, asthenia, photosensitivity, fever, chills, flushing, malaise, dyspnea, toxic epidermal necrolysis, erythema multiforme, including Stevens-Johnson syndrome.

Gastrointestinal: pancreatitis, hepatitis, including chronic active hepatitis, cholestatic jaundice, fatty change in liver; and rarely, cirrhosis, fulminant hepatic necrosis, and hepatoma; anorexia, vomiting.

Skin: alopecia.

Reproductive: gynecomastia, loss of libido, erectile dysfunction.

Eye: progression of cataracts (lens opacities), ophthalmoplegia.

Laboratory Abnormalities: elevated transaminases, alkaline phosphatase, and bilirubin; thyroid function abnormalities.

OVERDOSAGE

After oral administration of MEVACOR to mice the median lethal dose observed was >15 g/m^2.

Five healthy human volunteers have received up to 200 mg of lovastatin as a single dose without clinically significant adverse experiences. A few cases of accidental overdosage have been reported; no patients had any specific symptoms, and all patients recovered without sequelae. The maximum dose taken was 5–6 g.

Until further experience is obtained, no specific treatment of overdosage with MEVACOR can be recommended.

The dialyzability of lovastatin and its metabolites in man is not known at present.

DOSAGE AND ADMINISTRATION

The patient should be placed on a standard cholesterol-lowering diet before receiving MEVACOR and should continue on this diet during treatment with MEVACOR. MEVACOR should be given with meals.

The recommended starting dose is 20 mg once a day given with the evening meal. The recommended dosing range is 20–80 mg/day in single or divided doses; the maximum recommended dose is 80 mg/day. Adjustments of dosage should be made at intervals of 4 weeks or more. Doses should be individualized according to the patient's response (see Tables I to IV under CLINICAL PHARMACOLOGY, *Clinical Studies* for dose response results).

In patients taking immunosuppressive drugs concomitantly with lovastatin (see WARNINGS, *Skeletal Muscle*), therapy should begin with 10 mg of MEVACOR and should not exceed 20 mg/day.

Cholesterol levels should be monitored periodically and consideration should be given to reducing the dosage of MEVACOR if cholesterol levels fall below the targeted range.

Concomitant Therapy

Preliminary evidence suggests that the cholesterol-lowering effects of lovastatin and the bile acid sequestrant, cholestyramine, are additive.

Dosage in Patients with Renal Insufficiency

In patients with severe renal insufficiency (creatinine clearance <30 mL/min), dosage increases above 20 mg/day should be carefully considered and, if deemed necessary, implemented cautiously (see CLINICAL PHARMACOLOGY and WARNINGS, *Skeletal Muscle*).

HOW SUPPLIED

No. 3560—Tablets MEVACOR 10 mg are peach, octagonal tablets, coded MSD 730. They are supplied as follows:

NDC 0006-0730-61 unit of use bottles of 60.

No. 3561—Tablets MEVACOR 20 mg are light blue, octagonal tablets, coded MSD 731. They are supplied as follows:

NDC 0006-0731-37 unit of use bottles of 30

NDC 0006-0731-61 unit of use bottles of 60 (6505-01-267-2497, 20 mg 60's)

NDC 0006-0731-94 unit of use bottles of 90

NDC 0006-0731-28 unit dose packages of 100

NDC 0006-0731-78 unit of use bottles of 100

NDC 0006-0731-98 unit of use bottles of 180.

No. 3562—Tablets MEVACOR 40 mg are green, octagonal tablets, coded MSD 732. They are supplied as follows:

NDC 0006-0732-61 unit of use bottles of 60 (6505-01-310-0615, 40 mg 60's)

NDC 0006-0732-94 unit of use bottles of 90.

Storage

Store between 5–30°C (41–86°F). Tablets MEVACOR must be protected from light and stored in a well-closed, light-resistant container.

Distributed by:
MERCK SHARP & DOHME
DIV OF MERCK & CO., INC.,
WEST POINT, PA 19486, USA

Manufactured by:
MERCK SHARP & DOHME QUIMICA
DE PUERTO RICO, INC.
Caguas, Puerto Rico 00626

Certain manufacturing operations have been performed by other firms.

A.H.F.S. Category: 24:06

DC 7526520 Issued December 1991

COPYRIGHT © MERCK & CO., INC., 1987, 1989, 1991
All rights reserved

Shown in Product Identification Section, page 420

MIDAMOR® Tablets ℞
(Amiloride HCl), U.S.P.

DESCRIPTION

Amiloride HCl, an antikaliuretic-diuretic agent, is a pyrazine-carbonyl-guanidine that is unrelated chemically to other known antikaliuretic or diuretic agents. It is the salt of a moderately strong base (pKa 8.7). It is designated chemically as 3,5-diamino-6-chloro-*N*-(diaminomethylene) pyrazinecarboxamide monohydrochloride, dihydrate and has a molecular weight of 302.14. Its empirical formula is $C_6H_8ClN_7O \cdot HCl \cdot 2H_2O$ and its structural formula is:

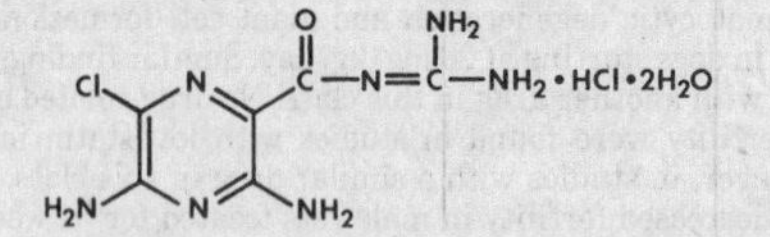

MIDAMOR* (Amiloride HCl) is available for oral use as tablets containing 5 mg of anhydrous amiloride HCl. Each tablet contains the following inactive ingredients: calcium phosphate, D&C Yellow 10, iron oxide, lactose, magnesium stearate and starch.

*Registered trademark of MERCK & CO., INC.

CLINICAL PHARMACOLOGY

MIDAMOR is a potassium-conserving (antikaliuretic) drug that possesses weak (compared with thiazide diuretics) natriuretic, diuretic, and antihypertensive activity. These effects have been partially additive to the effects of thiazide diuretics in some clinical studies. When administered with a thiazide or loop diuretic, MIDAMOR has been shown to decrease the enhanced urinary excretion of magnesium which occurs when a thiazide or loop diuretic is used alone. MIDAMOR has potassium-conserving activity in patients receiving kaliuretic-diuretic agents.

MIDAMOR is not an aldosterone antagonist and its effects are seen even in the absence of aldosterone.

MIDAMOR exerts its potassium sparing effect through the inhibition of sodium reabsorption at the distal convoluted tubule, cortical collecting tubule and collecting duct; this decreases the net negative potential of the tubular lumen and reduces both potassium and hydrogen secretion and their subsequent excretion. This mechanism accounts in large part for the potassium sparing action of amiloride.

MIDAMOR usually begins to act within 2 hours after an oral dose. Its effect on electrolyte excretion reaches a peak between 6 and 10 hours and lasts about 24 hours. Peak plasma levels are obtained in 3 to 4 hours and the plasma half-life varies from 6 to 9 hours. Effects on electrolytes increase with single doses of amiloride HCl up to approximately 15 mg.

Amiloride HCl is not metabolized by the liver but is excreted unchanged by the kidneys. About 50 percent of a 20 mg dose of MIDAMOR is excreted in the urine and 40 percent in the stool within 72 hours. MIDAMOR has little effect on glomerular filtration rate or renal blood flow. Because amiloride HCl is not metabolized by the liver, drug accumulation is not anticipated in patients with hepatic dysfunction, but accumulation can occur if the hepatorenal syndrome develops.

INDICATIONS AND USAGE

MIDAMOR is indicated as adjunctive treatment with thiazide diuretics or other kaliuretic-diuretic agents in congestive heart failure or hypertension to:

a. help restore normal serum potassium levels in patients who develop hypokalemia on the kaliuretic diuretic
b. prevent development of hypokalemia in patients who would be exposed to particular risk if hypokalemia were to develop, e.g., digitalized patients or patients with significant cardiac arrhythmias.

The use of potassium-conserving agents is often unnecessary in patients receiving diuretics for uncomplicated essential hypertension when such patients have a normal diet.

MIDAMOR has little additive diuretic or antihypertensive effect when added to a thiazide diuretic.

MIDAMOR should rarely be used alone. It has weak (compared with thiazides) diuretic and antihypertensive effects. Used as single agents, potassium sparing diuretics, including MIDAMOR, result in an increased risk of hyperkalemia (approximately 10% with amiloride). MIDAMOR should be used alone only when persistent hypokalemia has been documented and only with careful titration of the dose and close monitoring of serum electrolytes.

CONTRAINDICATIONS

Hyperkalemia

MIDAMOR should not be used in the presence of elevated serum potassium levels (greater than 5.5 mEq per liter).

Antikaliuretic Therapy or Potassium Supplementation

MIDAMOR should not be given to patients receiving other potassium-conserving agents, such as spironolactone or triamterene. Potassium supplementation in the form of medication, potassium-containing salt substitutes or a potassium-rich diet should not be used with MIDAMOR except in severe and/or refractory cases of hypokalemia. Such concomitant therapy can be associated with rapid increases in serum potassium levels. If potassium supplementation is used, careful monitoring of the serum potassium level is necessary.

Impaired Renal Function

Anuria, acute or chronic renal insufficiency, and evidence of diabetic nephropathy are contraindications to the use of MIDAMOR. Patients with evidence of renal functional impairment (blood urea nitrogen [BUN] levels over 30 mg per 100 mL or serum creatinine levels over 1.5 mg per 100 mL) or diabetes mellitus should not receive the drug without careful, frequent and continuing monitoring of serum electrolytes, creatinine, and BUN levels. Potassium retention associated with the use of an antikaliuretic agent is accentuated in the presence of renal impairment and may result in the rapid development of hyperkalemia.

Hypersensitivity

MIDAMOR is contraindicated in patients who are hypersensitive to this product.

WARNINGS

Hyperkalemia

Like other potassium-conserving agents, amiloride may cause hyperkalemia (serum potassium levels greater than 5.5 mEq per liter) which, if uncorrected, is potentially fatal. Hyperkalemia occurs commonly (about 10%) when amiloride is used without a kaliuretic diuretic. This incidence is greater in patients with renal impairment, diabetes mellitus (with or without recognized renal insufficiency), and in the elderly. When MIDAMOR is used concomitantly with a thiazide diuretic in patients without these complications, the risk of hyperkalemia is reduced to about 1–2 percent. It is thus essential to monitor serum potassium levels carefully in any patient receiving amiloride, particularly when it is first introduced, at the time of diuretic dosage adjustments, and during any illness that could affect renal function.

The risk of hyperkalemia may be increased when potassium-conserving agents, including MIDAMOR, are administered concomitantly with an angiotensin-converting enzyme inhibitor. (See PRECAUTIONS, *Drug Interactions.*) Warning signs or symptoms of hyperkalemia include paresthesias, muscular weakness, fatigue, flaccid paralysis of the extremities, bradycardia, shock, and ECG abnormalities. Monitoring of the serum potassium level is essential because mild hyperkalemia is not usually associated with an abnormal ECG. When abnormal, the ECG in hyperkalemia is characterized primarily by tall, peaked T waves or elevations from previous tracings. There may also be lowering of the R wave and increased depth of the S wave, widening and even disappearance of the P wave, progressive widening of the QRS complex, prolongation of the PR interval, and ST depression.

Treatment of hyperkalemia: If hyperkalemia occurs in patients taking MIDAMOR, the drug should be discontinued immediately. If the serum potassium level exceeds 6.5 mEq per liter, active measures should be taken to reduce it. Such measures include the intravenous administration of sodium bicarbonate solution or oral or parenteral glucose with a rapid-acting insulin preparation. If needed, a cation exchange resin such as sodium polystyrene sulfonate may be given orally or by enema. Patients with persistent hyperkalemia may require dialysis.

Diabetes Mellitus
In diabetic patients, hyperkalemia has been reported with the use of all potassium-conserving diuretics, including MIDAMOR, even in patients without evidence of diabetic nephropathy. Therefore, MIDAMOR should be avoided, if possible, in diabetic patients and, if it is used, serum electrolytes and renal function must be monitored frequently. MIDAMOR should be discontinued at least three days before glucose tolerance testing.

Metabolic or Respiratory Acidosis
Antikaliuretic therapy should be instituted only with caution in severely ill patients in whom respiratory or metabolic acidosis may occur, such as patients with cardiopulmonary disease or poorly controlled diabetes. If MIDAMOR is given to these patients, frequent monitoring of acid-base balance is necessary. Shifts in acid-base balance alter the ratio of extracellular/intracellular potassium, and the development of acidosis may be associated with rapid increases in serum potassium levels.

PRECAUTIONS

General
Electrolyte Imbalance and BUN Increases
Hyponatremia and hypochloremia may occur when MIDAMOR is used with other diuretics and increases in BUN levels have been reported. These increases usually have accompanied vigorous fluid elimination, especially when diuretic therapy was used in seriously ill patients, such as those who had hepatic cirrhosis with ascites and metabolic alkalosis, or those with resistant edema. Therefore, when MIDAMOR is given with other diuretics to such patients, careful monitoring of serum electrolytes and BUN levels is important. In patients with pre-existing severe liver disease, hepatic encephalopathy, manifested by tremors, confusion, and coma, and increased jaundice, have been reported in association with diuretics, including amiloride HCl.

Drug Interactions
When amiloride HCl is administered concomitantly with an angiotensin-converting enzyme inhibitor, the risk of hyperkalemia may be increased. Therefore, if concomitant use of these agents is indicated because of demonstrated hypokalemia, they should be used with caution and with frequent monitoring of serum potassium. (See WARNINGS.)
Lithium generally should not be given with diuretics because they reduce its renal clearance and add a high risk of lithium toxicity. Read circulars for lithium preparations before use of such concomitant therapy.
In some patients, the administration of a non-steroidal anti-inflammatory agent can reduce the diuretic, natriuretic, and antihypertensive effects of loop, potassium-sparing and thiazide diuretics. Therefore, when MIDAMOR and non-steroidal anti-inflammatory agents are used concomitantly, the patient should be observed closely to determine if the desired effect of the diuretic is obtained. Since indomethacin and potassium-sparing diuretics, including MIDAMOR, each may be associated with increased serum potassium levels, the potential effects on potassium kinetics and renal function should be considered when these agents are administered concurrently.

Carcinogenicity, Mutagenicity, Impairment of Fertility
There was no evidence of a tumorigenic effect when amiloride HCl was administered for 92 weeks to mice at doses up to 10 mg/kg/day (25 times the maximum daily human dose). Amiloride HCl has also been administered for 104 weeks to male and female rats at doses up to 6 and 8 mg/kg/day (15 and 20 times the maximum daily dose for humans, respectively) and showed no evidence of carcinogenicity.

Amiloride HCl was devoid of mutagenic activity in various strains of *Salmonella typhimurium* with or without a mammalian liver microsomal activation system (Ames test).
Pregnancy
Pregnancy Category B. Teratogenicity studies with amiloride HCl in rabbits and mice given 20 and 25 times the maximum human dose, respectively, revealed no evidence of harm to the fetus, although studies showed that the drug crossed the placenta in modest amounts. Reproduction studies in rats at 20 times the expected maximum daily dose for humans showed no evidence of impaired fertility. At approximately 5 or more times the expected maximum daily dose for humans, some toxicity was seen in adult rats and rabbits and a decrease in rat pup growth and survival occurred. There are, however, no adequate and well-controlled studies in pregnant women. Because animal reproduction studies are not always predictive of human response, this drug should be used during pregnancy only if clearly needed.
Nursing Mothers
Studies in rats have shown that amiloride is excreted in milk in concentrations higher than that found in blood, but it is not known whether MIDAMOR is excreted in human milk. Because many drugs are excreted in human milk and because of the potential for serious adverse reactions in nursing infants from MIDAMOR, a decision should be made whether to discontinue nursing or to discontinue the drug, taking into account the importance of the drug to the mother.
Pediatric Use
Safety and effectiveness in children have not been established.

ADVERSE REACTIONS

MIDAMOR is usually well tolerated and, except for hyperkalemia (serum potassium levels greater than 5.5 mEq per liter—see WARNINGS), significant adverse effects have been reported infrequently. Minor adverse reactions were reported relatively frequently (about 20%) but the relationship of many of the reports to amiloride HCl is uncertain and the overall frequency was similar in hydrochlorothiazide treated groups. Nausea/anorexia, abdominal pain, flatulence, and mild skin rash have been reported and probably are related to amiloride. Other adverse experiences that have been reported with amiloride are generally those known to be associated with diuresis, or with the underlying disease being treated.
The adverse reactions for MIDAMOR listed in the following table have been arranged into two groups: (1) incidence greater than one percent; and (2) incidence one percent or less. The incidence for group (1) was determined from clinical studies conducted in the United States (837 patients treated with MIDAMOR). The adverse effects listed in group (2) include reports from the same clinical studies and voluntary reports since marketing. The probability of a causal relationship exists between MIDAMOR and these adverse reactions, some of which have been reported only rarely.
[See table above.]

Causal Relationship Unknown
Other reactions have been reported but occurred under circumstances where a causal relationship could not be established. However, in these rarely reported events, that possibility cannot be excluded. Therefore, these observations are listed to serve as alerting information to physicians.

    Activation of probable pre-existing peptic ulcer
    Aplastic anemia
    Neutropenia
    Abnormal liver function

OVERDOSAGE

No data are available in regard to overdosage in humans. The oral LD_{50} of amiloride hydrochloride (calculated as the base) is 56 mg/kg in mice and 36 to 85 mg/kg in rats, depending on the strain.
It is not known whether the drug is dialyzable.
The most likely signs and symptoms to be expected with overdosage are dehydration and electrolyte imbalance. These can be treated by established procedures. Therapy with MIDAMOR should be discontinued and the patient observed closely. There is no specific antidote. Emesis should be induced or gastric lavage performed. Treatment is symptomatic and supportive. If hyperkalemia occurs, active measures should be taken to reduce the serum potassium levels.

DOSAGE AND ADMINISTRATION

MIDAMOR should be administered with food.
MIDAMOR, one 5 mg tablet daily, should be added to the usual antihypertensive or diuretic dosage of a kaliuretic diuretic. The dosage may be increased to 10 mg per day, if necessary. More than two 5 mg tablets of MIDAMOR daily usually are not needed, and there is little controlled experience with such doses. If persistent hypokalemia is documented with 10 mg, the dose can be increased to 15 mg, then 20 mg, with careful monitoring of electrolytes.

	Incidence > 1%	Incidence ≤ 1%
Body as a Whole		
	Headache*	Back pain
	Weakness	Chest pain
	Fatigability	Neck/shoulder ache
		Pain, extremities
Cardiovascular		
	None	Angina pectoris
		Orthostatic hypotension
		Arrhythmia
		Palpitation
Digestive		
	Nausea/anorexia*	Jaundice
	Diarrhea*	GI bleeding
	Vomiting*	Abdominal fullness
	Abdominal pain	GI disturbance
	Gas pain	Thirst
	Appetite changes	Heartburn
	Constipation	Flatulence
		Dyspepsia
Metabolic		
	Elevated serum potassium levels (> 5.5 mEq per liter)†	None
Integumentary		
	None	Skin rash
		Itching
		Dryness of mouth
		Pruritus
		Alopecia
Musculoskeletal		
	Muscle cramps	Joint pain
		Leg ache
Nervous		
	Dizziness	Paresthesia
	Encephalopathy	Tremors
		Vertigo
Psychiatric		
	None	Nervousness
		Mental confusion
		Insomnia
		Decreased libido
		Depression
		Somnolence
Respiratory		
	Cough	Shortness of breath
	Dyspnea	
Special Senses		
	None	Visual disturbances
		Nasal congestion
		Tinnitus
		Increased intraocular pressure
Urogenital		
	Impotence	Polyuria
		Dysuria
		Urinary frequency
		Bladder spasms

* Reactions occurring in 3% to 8% of patients treated with MIDAMOR. (Those reactions occurring in less than 3% of the patients are unmarked.)
† See WARNINGS.

In treating patients with congestive heart failure after an initial diuresis has been achieved, potassium loss may also decrease and the need for MIDAMOR should be reevaluated. Dosage adjustment may be necessary. Maintenance therapy may be on an intermittent basis.
If it is necessary to use MIDAMOR alone (see INDICATIONS), the starting dosage should be one 5 mg tablet daily. This dosage may be increased to 10 mg per day, if necessary. More than two 5 mg tablets usually are not needed, and there is little controlled experience with such doses. If persistent hypokalemia is documented with 10 mg, the dose can be increased to 15 mg, then 20 mg, with careful monitoring of electrolytes.

HOW SUPPLIED

No. 3381—Tablets MIDAMOR, 5 mg, are yellow, diamond-shaped, compressed tablets, coded MSD 92. They are supplied as follows:
NDC 0006-0092-68 bottles of 100.
    Shown in Product Identification Section, page 420

Continued on next page

Information on the Merck & Co. products listed on these pages is the full prescribing information from product circulars in use October 1, 1992.

Merck & Co.—Cont.

Storage
Protect from moisture, freezing and excessive heat.
A.H.F.S. Category: 40:28
DC 7212513 Issued May 1988
COPYRIGHT © MERCK & CO., INC., 1985
All rights reserved

MINTEZOL® Chewable Tablets   ℞
(Thiabendazole), U.S.P.
MINTEZOL® Suspension   ℞
(Thiabendazole), U.S.P.

DESCRIPTION

MINTEZOL* (Thiabendazole) is an anthelmintic provided as 500 mg chewable tablets, and as a suspension, containing 500 mg thiabendazole per 5 mL. The suspension also contains sorbic acid 0.1% added as a preservative. Inactive ingredients in the tablets are acacia, calcium phosphate, flavors, lactose, magnesium stearate, mannitol, methylcellulose, and sodium saccharin. Inactive ingredients in the suspension are an antifoam agent, flavors, polysorbate, purified water, sorbitol solution, and tragacanth.
Thiabendazole is a white to off-white odorless powder with a molecular weight of 201.26, which is practically insoluble in water but readily soluble in dilute acid and alkali. Its chemical name is 2-(4-thiazolyl)-1H-benzimidazole. The empirical formula is $C_{10}H_7N_3S$ and the structural formula is:

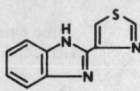

*Registered trademark of MERCK & CO., INC.

CLINICAL PHARMACOLOGY

In man, thiabendazole is rapidly absorbed and peak plasma concentration is reached within 1 to 2 hours after the oral administration of a suspension. It is metabolized almost completely to the 5-hydroxy form which appears in the urine as glucuronide or sulfate conjugates. In 48 hours, about 5% of the administered dose is recovered from the feces and about 90% from the urine. Most is excreted in the first 24 hours.
Mechanism of Action
The precise mode of action of thiabendazole on the parasite is unknown, but it may inhibit the helminth-specific enzyme fumarate reductase.
Thiabendazole is vermicidal and/or vermifugal against *Ascaris lumbricoides* ("common roundworm"), *Strongyloides stercoralis* (threadworm), *Necator americanus*, and *Ancylostoma duodenale* (hookworm), *Trichuris trichiura* (whipworm), *Ancylostoma braziliense* (dog and cat hookworm), *Toxocara canis* and *Toxocara cati* (ascarids), and *Enterobius vermicularis* (pinworm).
Its effect on larvae of *Trichinella spiralis* that have migrated to muscle is questionable.
Thiabendazole also suppresses egg and/or larval production and may inhibit the subsequent development of those eggs or larvae which are passed in the feces.

INDICATIONS AND USAGE

MINTEZOL is indicated for the treatment of:
   Strongyloidiasis (threadworm)
   Cutaneous larva migrans (creeping eruption)
   Visceral larva migrans
   Trichinosis: Relief of symptoms and fever and a reduction of eosinophilia have followed the use of MINTEZOL during the invasion stage of the disease.
Although not indicated as primary therapy, when enterobiasis (pinworm) occurs with any of the conditions listed above, additional therapy is not required for most patients. MINTEZOL should be used only in the following infestations when more specific therapy is not available or cannot be used or when further therapy with a second agent is desirable: Uncinariasis (hookworm: *Necator americanus* and *Ancylostoma duodenale*); Trichuriasis (whipworm); Ascariasis (large roundworm).

CONTRAINDICATION

Hypersensitivity to this product.

WARNINGS

If hypersensitivity reactions occur, the drug should be discontinued immediately and not be resumed. Erythema multiforme has been associated with thiabendazole therapy; in severe cases (Stevens-Johnson syndrome), fatalities have occurred.
Because CNS side effects may occur quite frequently, activities requiring mental alertness should be avoided.

PRECAUTIONS

General
MINTEZOL is not suitable for the treatment of mixed infections with ascaris because it may cause these worms to migrate.
Ideally, supportive therapy is indicated for anemic, dehydrated or malnourished patients prior to initiation of the anthelmintic therapy.
In the presence of hepatic or renal dysfunction, patients should be carefully monitored.
MINTEZOL should be used only in patients in whom susceptible worm infestation has been diagnosed and should not be used prophylactically.
Information for Patients
Because CNS side effects may occur quite frequently, activities requiring mental alertness should be avoided.
Laboratory Tests
Rarely, a transient rise in cephalin flocculation and SGOT has occurred in patients receiving MINTEZOL.
Drug Interactions
Thiabendazole may compete with other drugs, such as theophylline, for sites of metabolism in the liver, thus elevating the serum levels of such compounds to potentially toxic levels. Therefore, when concomitant use of thiabendazole and xanthine derivatives is anticipated, it may be necessary to monitor blood levels and/or reduce the dosage of such compounds. Such concomitant use should be administered under careful medical supervision.
Carcinogenesis, Mutagenesis,
Impairment of Fertility
Thiabendazole has been used in numerous short- and long-term studies in animals at doses up to 15 times the usual human dose and was without carcinogenic effects. It did not adversely affect fertility in the mouse at 2½ times the usual human dose or in the rat at a dose equivalent to the usual human dose. Thiabendazole had no mutagenic activity in *in vitro* microbial mutagen test, the micronucleus test and the host mediated assay *in vivo*.
Pregnancy
Pregnancy Category C: Reproduction and teratogenic studies done in the rabbit at a dose up to 15 times the usual human dose, in the rat at a dose equivalent to the human dose, and in the mouse at a dose up to 2½ times the usual human dose, revealed no evidence of harm to the fetus. In an additional study in the mouse, no defects were observed when thiabendazole was given in an aqueous suspension, at a dose 10 times the usual human dose; however, cleft palate and axial skeletal defects were observed when thiabendazole was suspended in olive oil and given at the same dose. There are no adequate and well controlled studies in pregnant women. MINTEZOL should be used during pregnancy only if the potential benefit justifies the potential risk to the fetus.
Nursing Mothers
It is not known whether this drug is excreted in human milk. Because of the potential for serious adverse reactions in nursing infants from MINTEZOL, a decision should be made whether to discontinue nursing or to discontinue the drug, taking into account the importance of the drug to the mother.

Pediatric Use
The safety and effectiveness of thiabendazole for the treatment of Strongyloidiasis, Ascariasis, Uncinariasis, Trichuriasis and Trichinosis in children weighing less than 30 lbs has been limited.

ADVERSE REACTIONS

Gastrointestinal: anorexia, nausea, vomiting, diarrhea, epigastric distress, jaundice, cholestasis and parenchymal liver damage.
Central Nervous System: dizziness, weariness, drowsiness, giddiness, headache, numbness, hyperirritability, convulsions, collapse, psychic disturbances.
Special Senses: tinnitus, abnormal sensation in eyes, xanthopsia, blurring of vision, drying of mucous membranes (mouth, eyes, etc.).
Cardiovascular: hypotension.
Metabolic: hyperglycemia.
Hematologic: transient leukopenia.
Genitourinary: hematuria, enuresis, malodor of the urine, crystalluria.
Hypersensitivity: pruritus, fever, facial flush, chills, conjunctival injection, angioedema, anaphylaxis, skin rashes (including perianal), erythema multiforme (including Stevens-Johnson syndrome), and lymphadenopathy.
Miscellaneous: appearance of live Ascaris in the mouth and nose.

OVERDOSAGE

Overdosage may be associated with transient disturbances of vision and psychic alterations.
There is no specific antidote in the event of overdosage. Therefore, symptomatic and supportive measures should be employed. Emesis should be induced or gastric lavage performed carefully.
The oral LD_{50} of MINTEZOL is 3.6 g/kg, 3.1 g/kg and 3.8 g/kg in the mouse, rat, and rabbit respectively.

DOSAGE AND ADMINISTRATION

The recommended maximum daily dose of MINTEZOL is 3 grams.
MINTEZOL should be given after meals if possible. Tablets MINTEZOL should be chewed before swallowing. Dietary restriction, complementary medications and cleansing enemas are not needed.
The usual dosage schedule for all conditions is two doses per day. The dosage is determined by the patient's weight. A weight-dose chart follows:

Weight	Each Dose	
	g	mL
30 lb	0.25	2.5
	(½ tablet)	(½ teaspoon)
50 lb	0.5	5.0
	(1 tablet)	(1 teaspoon)
75 lb	0.75	7.5
	(1½ tablets)	(1½ teaspoons)
100 lb	1.0	10.0
	(2 tablets)	(2 teaspoons)
125 lb	1.25	12.5
	(2½ tablets)	(2½ teaspoons)
150 lb	1.5	15.0
& over	(3 tablets)	(3 teaspoons)

The regimen for each indication follows: [See table below.]

Therapeutic Regimens

Indication	Regimen	Comments
*STRONGYLOIDIASIS	2 doses per day for 2 successive days.	A single dose of 20 mg/lb or 50 mg/kg may be employed as an alternative schedule, but a higher incidence of side effects should be expected.
CUTANEOUS LARVA MIGRANS (Creeping Eruption)	2 doses per day for 2 successive days.	If active lesions are still present 2 days after completion of therapy, a second course is recommended.
VISCERAL LARVA MIGRANS	2 doses per day for 7 successive days.	Safety and efficacy data on the seven-day treatment course are limited.
*TRICHINOSIS	2 doses per day for 2–4 successive days according to the response of the patient.	The optimal dosage for the treatment of trichinosis has not been established.
Other Indications		
* Intestinal roundworms (including Ascariasis, Uncinariasis and Trichuriasis)	2 doses per day for 2 successive days.	A single dose of 20 mg/lb or 50 mg/kg may be employed as an alternative schedule, but a higher incidence of side effects should be expected.

* Clinical experience with thiabendazole for treatment of each of these conditions in children weighing less than 30 lbs has been limited.

HOW SUPPLIED

No. 3331 — MINTEZOL Suspension, 500 mg per 5 mL, is white to off-white and is supplied as follows:
NDC 0006-3331-60 in bottles of 120 mL
(6505-00-935-5835, 0.5 g/5 mL, 120 mL).
No. 3332 — MINTEZOL Chewable Tablets, 500 mg, are white to off-white, orange-flavored, round, scored, compressed tablets, coded MSD 907. They are supplied as follows:
NDC 0006-0907-36 in boxes of 36 strip packaged, individually foil-wrapped tablets
(6505-01-226-9909, 500 mg chewable, 36's).
Shown in Product Identification Section, page 420
A.H.F.S. Category: 8:08
DC 7528210 Issued June 1985
COPYRIGHT © MERCK & CO., INC., 1983
All rights reserved

MODURETIC® Tablets ℞
(Amiloride HCl-Hydrochlorothiazide), U.S.P.

DESCRIPTION

MODURETIC* (Amiloride HCl-Hydrochlorothiazide) combines the potassium-conserving action of amiloride HCl with the natriuretic action of hydrochlorothiazide.
Amiloride HCl is designated chemically as 3,5-diamino-6- chloro -*N*- (diaminomethylene) pyrazinecarboxamide monohydrochloride, dihydrate and has a molecular weight of 302.14. Its empirical formula is $C_6H_8ClN_7O \cdot HCl \cdot 2H_2O$ and its structural formula is:

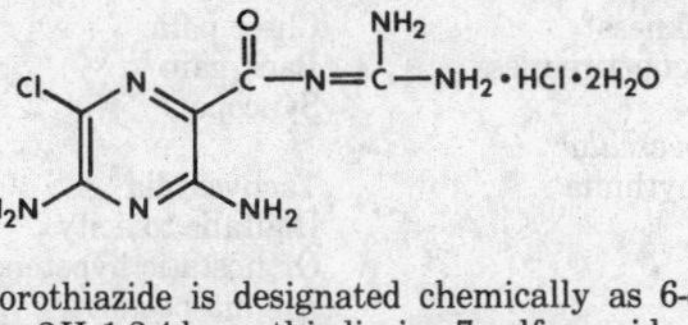

Hydrochlorothiazide is designated chemically as 6-chloro-3,4-dihydro-2*H*-1,2,4-benzothiadiazine-7-sulfonamide 1,1-dioxide. Its empirical formula is $C_7H_8ClN_3O_4S_2$ and its structural formula is:

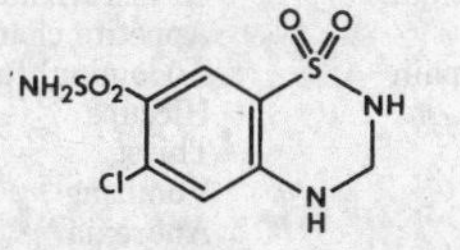

It is a white, or practically white, crystalline powder with a molecular weight of 297.72, which is slightly soluble in water, but freely soluble in sodium hydroxide solution.

MODURETIC is available for oral use as tablets containing 5 mg of anhydrous amiloride HCl and 50 mg of hydrochlorothiazide. Each tablet contains the following inactive ingredients: calcium phosphate, FD&C Yellow 6, guar gum, lactose, magnesium stearate and starch.

*Registered trademark of MERCK & CO., INC.

CLINICAL PHARMACOLOGY

MODURETIC provides diuretic and antihypertensive activity (principally due to the hydrochlorothiazide component), while acting through the amiloride component to prevent the excessive potassium loss that may occur in patients receiving a thiazide diuretic. Due to its amiloride component, the urinary excretion of magnesium is less with MODURETIC than with a thiazide or loop diuretic used alone (see PRECAUTIONS). The onset of the diuretic action of MODURETIC is within 1 to 2 hours and this action appears to be sustained for approximately 24 hours.

Amiloride HCl
Amiloride HCl is a potassium-conserving (antikaliuretic) drug that possesses weak (compared with thiazide diuretics) natriuretic, diuretic, and antihypertensive activity. These effects have been partially additive to the effects of thiazide diuretics in some clinical studies. Amiloride HCl has potassium-conserving activity in patients receiving kaliuretic-diuretic agents.

Amiloride HCl is not an aldosterone antagonist and its effects are seen even in the absence of aldosterone.
Amiloride HCl exerts its postassium sparing effect through the inhibition of sodium reabsorption at the distal convoluted tubule, cortical collecting tubule and collecting duct; this decreases the net negative potential of the tubular lumen and reduces both potassium and hydrogen secretion and their subsequent excretion. This mechanism accounts in large part for the potassium sparing action of amiloride.
Amiloride HCl usually begins to act within 2 hours after an oral dose. Its effect on electrolyte excretion reaches a peak between 6 and 10 hours and lasts about 24 hours. Peak plasma levels are obtained in 3 to 4 hours and the plasma half-life varies from 6 to 9 hours. Effects on electrolytes increase with single doses of amiloride HCl up to approximately 15 mg.

Amiloride HCl is not metabolized by the liver but is excreted unchanged by the kidneys. About 50 percent of a 20 mg dose of amiloride HCl is excreted in the urine and 40 percent in the stool within 72 hours. Amiloride HCl has little effect on glomerular filtration rate or renal blood flow. Because amiloride HCl is not metabolized by the liver, drug accumulation is not anticipated in patients with hepatic dysfunction, but accumulation can occur if the hepatorenal syndrome develops.

Hydrochlorothiazide
The mechanism of the antihypertensive effect of thiazides is unknown. Thiazides do not usually affect normal blood pressure.

Hydrochlorothiazide is a diuretic and antihypertensive. It affects the distal renal tubular mechanism of electrolyte reabsorption. Hydrochlorothiazide increases excretion of sodium and chloride in approximately equivalent amounts. Natriuresis may be accompanied by some loss of potassium and bicarbonate.

After oral use diuresis begins within two hours, peaks in about four hours and lasts about 6 to 12 hours.
Hydrochlorothiazide is not metabolized but is eliminated rapidly by the kidney. When plasma levels have been followed for at least 24 hours, the plasma half-life has been observed to vary between 5.6 and 14.8 hours. At least 61 percent of the oral dose is eliminated unchanged within 24 hours. Hydrochlorothiazide crosses the placental but not the blood-brain barrier and is excreted in breast milk.

INDICATIONS AND USAGE

MODURETIC is indicated in those patients with hypertension or with congestive heart failure who develop hypokalemia when thiazides or other kaliuretic diuretics are used alone, or in whom maintenance of normal serum potassium levels is considered to be clinically important, e.g., digitalized patients, or patients with significant cardiac arrhythmias.

The use of potassium-conserving agents is often unnecessary in patients receiving diuretics for uncomplicated essential hypertension when such patients have a normal diet.

MODURETIC may be used alone or as an adjunct to other antihypertensive drugs, such as methyldopa or beta blockers. Since MODURETIC enhances the action of these agents, dosage adjustments may be necessary to avoid an excessive fall in blood pressure and other unwanted side effects.

This fixed combination drug is not indicated for the initial therapy of edema or hypertension except in individuals in whom the development of hypokalemia cannot be risked.

CONTRAINDICATIONS

Hyperkalemia
MODURETIC should not be used in the presence of elevated serum potassium levels (greater than 5.5 mEq per liter).
Antikaliuretic Therapy or Potassium Supplementation
MODURETIC should not be given to patients receiving other potassium-conserving agents, such as spironolactone or triamterene. Potassium supplementation in the form of medication, potassium-containing salt substitutes or a potassium-rich diet should not be used with MODURETIC except in severe and/or refractory cases of hypokalemia. Such concomitant therapy can be associated with rapid increases in serum potassium levels. If potassium supplementation is used, careful monitoring of the serum potassium level is necessary.
Impaired Renal Function
Anuria, acute or chronic renal insufficiency, and evidence of diabetic nephropathy are contraindications to the use of MODURETIC. Patients with evidence of renal functional impairment (blood urea nitrogen [BUN] levels over 30 mg per 100 mL or serum creatinine levels over 1.5 mg per 100 mL) or diabetes mellitus should not receive the drug without careful, frequent and continuing monitoring of serum electrolytes, creatinine, and BUN levels. Potassium retention associated with the use of an antikaliuretic agent is accentuated in the presence of renal impairment and may result in the rapid development of hyperkalemia.
Hypersensitivity
MODURETIC is contraindicated in patients who are hypersensitive to this product, or to other sulfonamide-derived drugs.

WARNINGS

Hyperkalemia

> Like other potassium-conserving diuretic combinations, MODURETIC may cause hyperkalemia (serum potassium levels greater than 5.5 mEq per liter). In patients without renal impairment or diabetes mellitus, the risk of hyperkalemia with MODURETIC is about 1-2 percent. This risk is higher in patients with renal impairment or diabetes mellitus (even without recognized diabetic nephropathy). Since hyperkalemia, if uncorrected, is potentially fatal, it is essential to monitor serum potassium levels carefully in any patient receiving MODURETIC, particularly when it is first introduced, at the time of dosage adjustments, and during any illness that could affect renal function.

The risk of hyperkalemia may be increased when potassium-conserving agents, including MODURETIC, are administered concomitantly with an angiotensin-converting enzyme inhibitor. (See PRECAUTIONS, *Drug Interactions.*) Warning signs or symptoms of hyperkalemia include paresthesias, muscular weakness, fatigue, flaccid paralysis of the extremities, bradycardia, shock, and ECG abnormalities. Monitoring of the serum potassium level is essential because mild hyperkalemia is not usually associated with an abnormal ECG.
When abnormal, the ECG in hyperkalemia is characterized primarily by tall, peaked T waves or elevations from previous tracings. There may also be lowering of the R wave and increased depth of the S wave, widening and even disappearance of the P wave, progressive widening of the QRS complex, prolongation of the PR interval, and ST depression.
Treatment of hyperkalemia: If hyperkalemia occurs in patients taking MODURETIC, the drug should be discontinued immediately. If the serum potassium level exceeds 6.5 mEq per liter, active measures should be taken to reduce it. Such measures include the intravenous administration of sodium bicarbonate solution or oral or parenteral glucose with a rapid-acting insulin preparation. If needed, a cation exchange resin such as sodium polystyrene sulfonate may be given orally or by enema. Patients with persistent hyperkalemia may require dialysis.
Diabetes Mellitus
In diabetic patients, hyperkalemia has been reported with the use of all potassium-conserving diuretics, including amiloride HCl, even in patients without evidence of diabetic nephropathy. Therefore, MODURETIC should be avoided, if possible, in diabetic patients and, if it is used, serum electrolytes and renal function must be monitored frequently.
MODURETIC should be discontinued at least three days before glucose tolerance testing.
Metabolic or Respiratory Acidosis
Antikaliuretic therapy should be instituted only with caution in severely ill patients in whom respiratory or metabolic acidosis may occur, such as patients with cardiopulmonary disease or poorly controlled diabetes. If MODURETIC is given to these patients, frequent monitoring of acid-base balance is necessary. Shifts in acid-base balance alter the ratio of extracellular/intracellular potassium, and the development of acidosis may be associated with rapid increases in serum potassium levels.

PRECAUTIONS

General
Electrolyte Imbalance and BUN Increases
Determination of serum electrolytes to detect possible electrolyte imbalance should be performed at appropriate intervals.
Patients should be observed for clinical signs of fluid or electrolyte imbalance: i.e., hyponatremia, hypochloremic alkalosis, and hypokalemia. Serum and urine electrolyte determinations are particularly important when the patient is vomiting excessively or receiving parenteral fluids. Warning signs or symptoms of fluid and electrolyte imbalance, irrespective of cause, include dryness of mouth, thirst, weakness, lethargy, drowsiness, restlessness, seizures, muscle pains or cramps, muscular fatigue, hypotension, oliguria, tachycardia, and gastrointestinal disturbances such as nausea and vomiting.
Hyponatremia and hypochloremia may occur during the use of thiazides and other diuretics. Any chloride deficit during thiazide therapy is generally mild and may be lessened by the amiloride HCl component of MODURETIC. Hypochloremia usually does not require specific treatment except under extraordinary circumstances (as in liver disease or renal disease). Dilutional hyponatremia may occur in edematous patients in hot weather; appropriate therapy is water restric-

Continued on next page

Information on the Merck & Co. products listed on these pages is the full prescribing information from product circulars in use October 1, 1992.

Merck & Co.—Cont.

tion, rather than administration of salt, except in rare instances when the hyponatremia is life threatening. In actual salt depletion, appropriate replacement is the therapy of choice.

Hypokalemia may develop during thiazide therapy, especially with brisk diuresis, when severe cirrhosis is present, during concomitant use of corticosteroids or ACTH, or after prolonged therapy. However, this usually is prevented by the amiloride HCl component of MODURETIC.

Interference with adequate oral electrolyte intake will also contribute to hypokalemia. Hypokalemia may cause cardiac arrhythmia and may also sensitize or exaggerate the response of the heart to the toxic effects of digitalis (e.g., increased ventricular irritability).

Thiazides have been shown to increase the urinary excretion of magnesium; this may result in hypomagnesemia. Amiloride HCl, a component of MODURETIC, has been shown to decrease the enhanced urinary excretion of magnesium which occurs when a thiazide or loop diuretic is used alone.

Increases in BUN levels have been reported with amiloride HCl and with hydrochlorothiazide. These increases usually have accompanied vigorous fluid elimination, especially when diuretic therapy was used in seriously ill patients, such as those who had hepatic cirrhosis with ascites and metabolic alkalosis, or those with resistant edema. Therefore, when MODURETIC is given to such patients, careful monitoring of serum electrolyte and BUN levels is important. In patients with pre-existing severe liver disease, hepatic encephalopathy, manifested by tremors, confusion, and coma, and increased jaundice, have been reported in association with diuretic therapy including amiloride HCl and hydrochlorothiazide.

In patients with renal disease, diuretics may precipitate azotemia. Cumulative effects of the components of MODURETIC may develop in patients with impaired renal function. If renal impairment becomes evident, MODURETIC should be discontinued (see CONTRAINDICATIONS and WARNINGS).

Drug Interactions

In some patients, the administration of a non-steroidal anti-inflammatory agent can reduce the diuretic, natriuretic, and antihypertensive effects of loop, potassium-sparing and thiazide diuretics. Therefore, when MODURETIC and non-steroidal anti-inflammatory agents are used concomitantly, the patient should be observed closely to determine if the desired effect of the diuretic is obtained. Since indomethacin and potassium-sparing diuretics, including MODURETIC, each may be associated with increased serum potassium levels, the potential effects on potassium kinetics and renal function should be considered when these agents are administered concurrently.

Amiloride HCl

When amiloride HCl is administered concomitantly with an angiotensin-converting enzyme inhibitor, the risk of hyperkalemia may be increased. Therefore, if concomitant use of these agents in indicated because of demonstrated hypokalemia, they should be used with caution and with frequent monitoring of serum potassium. (See WARNINGS.)

Hydrochlorothiazide

When given concurrently the following drugs may interact with thiazide diuretics.

Alcohol, barbiturates, or narcotics—potentiation of orthostatic hypotension may occur.

Antidiabetic drugs (oral agents and insulin)—dosage adjustment of the antidiabetic drug may be required.

Other antihypertensive drugs—additive effect or potentiation.

Corticosteroids, ACTH—intensified electrolyte depletion, particularly hypokalemia.

Pressor amines (e.g., norepinephrine)—possible decreased response to pressor amines but not sufficient to preclude their use.

Skeletal muscle relaxants, nondepolarizing (e.g., tubocurarine)—possible increased responsiveness to the muscle relaxant.

Lithium—generally should not be given with diuretics. Diuretic agents reduce the renal clearance of lithium and add a high risk of lithium toxicity. Refer to the package insert for lithium preparations before use of such preparations with MODURETIC.

Metabolic and Endocrine Effects

In diabetic patients, insulin requirements may be increased, decreased, or unchanged due to the hydrochlorothiazide component. Diabetes mellitus that has been latent may become manifest during administration of thiazide diuretics.

Because calcium excretion is decreased by thiazides, MODURETIC should be discontinued before carrying out tests for parathyroid function. Pathologic changes in the parathyroid glands, with hypercalcemia and hypophosphatemia have been observed in a few patients on prolonged thiazide therapy; however, the common complications of hyperparathyroidism such as renal lithiasis, bone resorption, and peptic ulceration have not been seen.

Hyperuricemia may occur or acute gout may be precipitated in certain patients receiving thiazide therapy.

Other Precautions

In patients receiving thiazides, sensitivity reactions may occur with or without a history of allergy or bronchial asthma. The possibility of exacerbation or activation of systemic lupus erythematosus has been reported with the use of thiazides.

Increases in cholesterol and triglyceride levels may be associated with thiazide diuretic therapy.

Carcinogenicity, Mutagenicity, Impairment of Fertility

Long-term studies in animals have not been performed to evaluate the effects upon fertility, mutagenicity or carcinogenic potential of MODURETIC.

Amiloride HCl

There was no evidence of a tumorigenic effect when amiloride HCl was administered for 92 weeks to mice at doses up to 10 mg/kg/day (25 times the maximum daily human dose). Amiloride HCl has also been administered for 104 weeks to male and female rats at doses up to 6 and 8 mg/kg/day (15 and 20 times the maximum daily dose for humans, respectively) and showed no evidence of carcinogenicity.

Amiloride HCl was devoid of mutagenic activity in various strains of *Salmonella typhimurium* with or without a mammalian liver microsomal activation system (Ames test).

Hydrochlorothiazide

Hydrochlorothiazide is currently under study in the U.S. Carcinogenesis Testing Program.

Hydrochlorothiazide was not mutagenic *in vitro*, in the Ames microbial mutagen test at a maximum concentration of 5 mg/plate using Strains TA98 and TA100. Urine samples of patients treated with hydrochlorothiazide did not have mutagenic activity in the Ames test.

The ability of a number of drugs to induce nondisjunction and crossing-over was measured using *Aspergillus nidulans*. A large number of drugs, including hydrochlorothiazide, induced nondisjunction.

Hydrochlorothiazide had no effect on fertility in a two-litter study in rats at doses of 4–5.6 mg/kg/day (up to 2 times the maximum recommended human dose).

Pregnancy

Pregnancy Category B. Teratogenicity studies have been performed with combinations of amiloride HCl and hydrochlorothiazide in rabbits and mice at doses up to 25 times the expected maximum daily dose for humans and have revealed no evidence of harm to the fetus. No evidence of impaired fertility in rats was apparent at dosage levels up to 25 times the expected maximum human daily dose. A perinatal and postnatal study in rats showed a reduction in maternal body weight gain during and after gestation at a daily dose of 25 times the expected maximum daily dose for humans. The body weights of alive pups at birth and at weaning were also reduced at this dose level. There are no adequate and well controlled studies in pregnant women. Because animal reproduction studies are not always predictive of human responses, and because of the data listed below with the individual components, this drug should be used during pregnancy only if clearly needed.

Amiloride HCl

Teratogenicity studies with amiloride HCl in rabbits and mice given 20 and 25 times the maximum human dose, respectively, revealed no evidence of harm to the fetus, although studies showed that the drug crossed the placenta in modest amounts. Reproduction studies in rats at 20 times the expected maximum daily dose for humans showed no evidence of impaired fertility. At approximately 5 or more times the expected maximum daily dose for humans, some toxicity was seen in adult rats and rabbits and a decrease in rat pup growth and survival occurred.

Hydrochlorothiazide

Teratogenic Effects: Reproduction studies in the rabbit, the mouse and the rat at doses up to 100 mg/kg/day (50 times the maximum human dose) showed no evidence of external abnormalities of the fetus due to hydrochlorothiazide. Hydrochlorothiazide given in a two-litter study in rats at doses of 4–5.6 mg/kg/day (approximately 1–2 times the maximum recommended human dose) did not impair fertility or produce birth abnormalities in the offspring.

Thiazides cross the placental barrier and appear in the cord blood.

Nonteratogenic Effects: These may include fetal or neonatal jaundice, thrombocytopenia, and possibly other adverse reactions which have occurred in the adult.

Nursing Mothers

Studies in rats have shown that amiloride is excreted in milk in concentrations higher than that found in blood, but it is not known whether amiloride HCl is excreted in human milk. However, thiazides appear in breast milk. Because of the potential for serious adverse reactions in nursing infants, a decision should be made whether to discontinue nursing or to discontinue the drug, taking into account the importance of the drug to the mother.

Pediatric Use

Safety and effectiveness in children have not been established.

ADVERSE REACTIONS

MODURETIC is usually well tolerated and significant clinical adverse effects have been reported infrequently. The risk of hyperkalemia (serum potassium levels greater than 5.5 mEq per liter) with MODURETIC is about 1–2 percent in patients without renal impairment or diabetes mellitus (see WARNINGS). Minor adverse reactions to amiloride HCl have been reported relatively frequently (about 20%) but the relationship of many of the reports to amiloride HCl is uncertain and the overall frequency was similar in hydrochlorothiazide treated groups. Nausea/anorexia, abdominal pain, flatulence, and mild skin rash have been reported and probably are related to amiloride. Other adverse experiences that have been reported with MODURETIC are generally those known to be associated with diuresis, thiazide therapy, or with the underlying disease being treated. Clinical trials have not demonstrated that combining amiloride and hydrochlorothiazide increases the risk of adverse reactions over those seen with the individual components.

The adverse reactions for MODURETIC listed in the following table have been arranged into two groups: (1) incidence greater than one percent; and (2) incidence one percent or less. The incidence for group (1) was determined from clinical studies conducted in the United States (607 patients treated with MODURETIC). The adverse effects listed in group (2) include reports from the same clinical studies and voluntary reports since marketing. The probability of a causal relationship exists between MODURETIC and these adverse reactions, some of which have been reported only rarely.

Incidence > 1%	*Incidence ≤ 1%*
Body as a Whole	
Headache*	Malaise
Weakness*	Chest pain
Fatigue/tiredness	Back pain
	Syncope
Cardiovascular	
Arrhythmia	Tachycardia
	Digitalis toxicity
	Orthostatic hypotension
	Angina pectoris
Digestive	
Nausea/anorexia*	Constipation
Diarrhea	GI bleeding
Gastrointestinal pain	GI disturbance
	Appetite changes
Abdominal pain	Abdominal fullness
	Hiccups
	Thirst
	Vomiting
	Anorexia
	Flatulence
Metabolic	
Elevated serum potassium levels (> 5.5 mEq per liter)†	Gout
	Dehydration
	Symptomatic hyponatremia**
Integumentary	
Rash*	Flushing
Pruritus	Diaphoresis
Musculoskeletal	
Leg ache	Muscle cramps/spasm
	Joint pain
Nervous	
Dizziness*	Paresthesia/numbness
	Stupor
	Vertigo
Psychiatric	
None	Insomnia
	Nervousness
	Depression
	Sleepiness
	Mental confusion
Respiratory	
Dyspnea	None
Special Senses	
None	Bad taste
	Visual disturbance
	Nasal congestion
Urogenital	
None	Impotence
	Nocturia
	Dysuria
	Incontinence
	Renal dysfunction including renal failure

* Reactions occurring in 3% to 8% of patients treated with MODURETIC. (Those reactions occurring in less than 3% of the patients are unmarked.)

† See WARNINGS.

** See PRECAUTIONS.

Other adverse reactions that have been reported with the individual components and within each category are listed in order of decreasing severity:

Amiloride—Body as a Whole: Painful extremities, neck/shoulder ache, fatigability; *Cardiovascular:* Palpitation; *Digestive:* Activation of probable pre-existing peptic ulcer, abnormal liver function, jaundice, dyspepsia, heartburn; *Hematologic:* Aplastic anemia, neutropenia; *Integumentary:* Alopecia, itching, dry mouth; *Nervous System/Psychiatric:* Encephalopathy, tremors, decreased libido; *Respiratory:* Shortness of breath, cough; *Special Senses:* Increased intraocular pressure, tinnitus; *Urogenital:* Bladder spasms, polyuria, urinary frequency.

Hydrochlorothiazide—Digestive: Pancreatitis, jaundice (intrahepatic cholestatic jaundice), sialadenitis, cramping, gastric irritation; *Hematologic:* Aplastic anemia, agranulocytosis, leukopenia, hemolytic anemia, thrombocytopenia; *Hypersensitivity:* Anaphylactic reactions, necrotizing angiitis (vasculitis, cutaneous vasculitis), respiratory distress including pneumonitis and pulmonary edema, photosensitivity, fever, urticaria, purpura; *Metabolic:* Electrolyte imbalance (see PRECAUTIONS), hyperglycemia, glycosuria, hyperuricemia; *Nervous System/Psychiatric:* Restlessness; *Special Senses:* Transient blurred vision, xanthopsia; *Urogenital:* Interstitial nephritis (see WARNINGS).

OVERDOSAGE

No data are available in regard to overdosage in humans. The oral LD_{50} of the combination drug is 189 and 422 mg/kg for female mice and female rats, respectively.

It is not known whether the drug is dialyzable.

No specific information is available on the treatment of overdosage with MODURETIC, and no specific antidote is available. Treatment is symptomatic and supportive. Therapy with MODURETIC should be discontinued and the patient observed closely. Suggested measures include induction of emesis and/or gastric lavage.

Amiloride HCl: No data are available in regard to overdosage in humans.

The oral LD_{50} of amiloride HCl (calculated as the base) is 56 mg/kg in mice and 36 to 85 mg/kg in rats, depending on the strain.

The most common signs and symptoms to be expected with overdosage are dehydration and electrolyte imbalance. If hyperkalemia occurs, active measures should be taken to reduce the serum potassium levels.

Hydrochlorothiazide: The oral LD_{50} of hydrochlorothiazide is greater than 10.0 g/kg in both mice and rats.

The most common signs and symptoms observed are those caused by electrolyte depletion (hypokalemia, hypochloremia, hyponatremia) and dehydration resulting from excessive diuresis. If digitalis has also been administered, hypokalemia may accentuate cardiac arrhythmias.

DOSAGE AND ADMINISTRATION

MODURETIC should be administered with food.

The usual starting dosage is 1 tablet a day. The dosage may be increased to 2 tablets a day, if necessary. More than 2 tablets of MODURETIC daily usually are not needed and there is no controlled experience with such doses. The daily dose is usually given as a single dose but may be given in divided doses. Once an initial diuresis has been achieved, dosage adjustment may be necessary. Maintenance therapy may be on an intermittent basis.

HOW SUPPLIED

No. 3385—Tablets MODURETIC are peach-colored, diamond-shaped, scored, compressed tablets, coded MSD 917. Each tablet contains 5 mg of anhydrous amiloride HCl and 50 mg of hydrochlorothiazide. They are supplied as follows:
NDC 0006-0917-68 in bottles of 100
(6505-01-139-1498 100's)
NDC 0006-0917-28 unit dose packages of 100.

Shown in Product Identification Section, page 420

Storage
Protect from moisture, freezing and excessive heat.

A.H.F.S. Category: 40:28
DC 7168018 Issued May 1988
COPYRIGHT © MERCK & CO., INC., 1988
All rights reserved

MUMPSVAX®   ℞
(Mumps Virus Vaccine Live, MSD), U.S.P.
Jeryl Lynn Strain

DESCRIPTION

MUMPSVAX* (Mumps Virus Vaccine Live, MSD) is a live virus vaccine for immunization against mumps.
MUMPSVAX is a sterile lyophilized preparation of the Jeryl Lynn (B level) strain of mumps virus. The virus was adapted to and propagated in cell cultures of chick embryo free of avian leukosis virus and other adventitious agents.

The reconstituted vaccine is for subcutaneous administration. When reconstituted as directed, the dose for injection is 0.5 mL and contains not less than the equivalent of 20,000 $TCID_{50}$ (tissue culture infectious doses) of the U.S. Reference Mumps Virus. Each dose contains approximately 25 mcg of neomycin. The product contains no preservative. Sorbitol and hydrolized gelatin are added as stabilizers.

---

* Registered trademark of MERCK & CO., INC.

CLINICAL PHARMACOLOGY

MUMPSVAX produces a modified, non-communicable mumps infection in susceptible persons. Extensive clinical trials have demonstrated that MUMPSVAX is highly immunogenic and well tolerated. A single injection of the vaccine has been shown to induce mumps neutralizing antibodies in approximately 97 percent of susceptible children and approximately 93 percent of susceptible adults. The pattern of antibody response closely resembles that observed for natural mumps. Although the antibody level is significantly lower than that following natural infection, it is protective and long lasting. Vaccine-induced antibody levels have been shown to persist for at least 15 years with a rate of decline comparable to that seen in natural infection. If the present pattern continues, it will provide a basis for the expectation that immunity following vaccination will be permanent. However, continued surveillance will be required to demonstrate this point.

INDICATIONS AND USAGE

MUMPSVAX is indicated for immunization against mumps in persons 12 months of age or older. Most adults are likely to have been infected naturally and generally may be considered immune, even if they did not have clinically recognizable disease. A booster is not needed. It is not recommended for infants younger than 12 months because they may retain maternal mumps neutralizing antibodies which may interfere with the immune response.

Evidence indicates that the vaccine will not offer protection when given after exposure to natural mumps. Passively acquired antibody can interfere with the response to live, attenuated-virus vaccines. Therefore, administration of mumps virus vaccine should be deferred until approximately three months after passive immunization.

Individuals planning travel outside the United States, if not immune, can acquire measles, mumps or rubella and import these diseases to the United States. Therefore, prior to International travel, individuals known to be susceptible to one or more of these diseases can receive either a single antigen vaccine (measles, mumps or rubella), or a combined antigen vaccine as appropriate. However, M-M-R* II (Measles, Mumps, and Rubella Virus Vaccine Live, MSD) is preferred for persons likely to be susceptible to mumps and rubella; and if single-antigen measles vaccine is not readily available, travelers should receive M-M-R II (Measles, Mumps, and Rubella Virus Vaccine Live, MSD) regardless of their immune status to mumps or rubella.

Revaccination: Children vaccinated when younger than 12 months of age should be revaccinated. Based on available evidence, there is no reason to routinely revaccinate persons who were vaccinated originally when 12 months of age or older. However, persons should be revaccinated if there is evidence to suggest that initial immunization was ineffective.

Use with other Vaccines
Routine administration of DTP (diphtheria, tetanus, pertussis) and/or OPV (oral poliovirus vaccine) concomitantly with measles, mumps and rubella vaccines is not recommended because there are insufficient data relating to the simultaneous administration of these antigens. However, the American Academy of Pediatrics has noted that in some circumstances, particularly when the patient may not return, some practitioners prefer to administer all these antigens on a single day. If done, separate sites and syringes should be used for DTP and MUMPSVAX.

MUMPSVAX should not be given less than one month before or after administration of other virus vaccines.

---

* Registered trademark of MERCK & CO., INC.

CONTRAINDICATIONS

Do not give MUMPSVAX to pregnant females; the possible effects of the vaccine on fetal development are unknown at this time. If vaccination of postpubertal females is undertaken, pregnancy should be avoided for three months following vaccination (see PRECAUTIONS, *Pregnancy*).

Anaphylactic or anaphylactoid reactions to neomycin (each dose of reconstituted vaccine contains approximately 25 mcg of neomycin).

History of anaphylactic or anaphylactoid reactions to eggs (see HYPERSENSITIVITY TO EGGS below).

Any febrile respiratory illness or other active febrile infection.

Active untreated tuberculosis.

Patients receiving immunosuppressive therapy. This contraindication does not apply to patients who are receiving corticosteroids as replacement therapy, e.g., for Addison's disease.

Individuals with blood dyscrasias, leukemia, lymphomas of any type, or other malignant neoplasms affecting the bone marrow or lymphatic systems.

Primary and acquired immunodeficiency states, including patients who are immunosuppressed in association with AIDS or other clinical manifestations of infection with human immunodeficiency viruses; cellular immune deficiencies; and hypogammaglobulinemic and dysgammaglobulinemic states.

Individuals with a family history of congenital or hereditary immunodeficiency, until the immune competence of the potential vaccine recipient is demonstrated.

HYPERSENSITIVITY TO EGGS

Live mumps vaccine is produced in chick embryo cell culture. Persons with a history of anaphylactic, anaphylactoid, or other immediate reactions (e.g., hives, swelling of the mouth and throat, difficulty breathing, hypotension, or shock) subsequent to egg ingestion should be vaccinated only with extreme caution. Evidence indicates that persons are not at increased risk if they have egg allergies that are not anaphylactic or anaphylactoid in nature. Such persons may be vaccinated in the usual manner. There is no evidence to indicate that persons with allergies to chickens or feathers are at increased risk of reaction to the vaccine.

PRECAUTIONS

General
Adequate treatment provisions including epinephrine, should be available for immediate use should an anaphylactic or anaphylactoid reaction occur.

Children and young adults who are known to be infected with human immunodeficiency viruses but without overt clinical manifestations of immunosuppression may be vaccinated; however, the vaccinees should be monitored closely for vaccine-preventable diseases because immunization may be less effective than for uninfected persons.

Vaccination should be deferred for at least 3 months following blood or plasma transfusions, or administration of human immune serum globulin.

There are no reports of transmission of live mumps virus from vaccinees to susceptible contacts.

It has been reported that mumps virus vaccine, live, may result in a temporary depression of tuberculin skin sensitivity. Therefore, if a tuberculin test is to be done, it should be administered either before or simultaneously with MUMPSVAX.

As for any vaccine, vaccination with MUMPSVAX may not result in seroconversion in 100% of susceptible persons given the vaccine.

Pregnancy
Pregnancy Category C
Animal reproduction studies have not been conducted with MUMPSVAX. It is also not known whether MUMPSVAX can cause fetal harm when administered to a pregnant woman or can affect reproduction capacity. Therefore, mumps virus vaccine should not be given to persons known to be pregnant; furthermore, pregnancy should be avoided for three months following vaccination. Although mumps virus is capable of infecting the placenta and fetus, there is no good evidence that it causes congenital malformations in humans. Mumps vaccine virus also has been shown to infect the placenta, but the virus has not been isolated from the fetal tissues from susceptible women who were vaccinated and underwent elective abortions.

Nursing Mothers
It is not known whether mumps vaccine virus is secreted in human milk. Therefore, because many drugs are excreted in human milk, caution should be exercised when MUMPSVAX is administered to a nursing woman.

ADVERSE REACTIONS

Burning and/or stinging of short duration at the injection site have been reported.

Continued on next page

Information on the Merck & Co. products listed on these pages is the full prescribing information from product circulars in use October 1, 1992.

Merck & Co.—Cont.

Anaphylaxis and anaphylactoid reactions have been reported.

Mild fever occurs occasionally. Fever above 103°F (39.4°C) is uncommon.

Mild lymphadenopathy has been reported.

Cough and rhinitis have been reported after vaccination with other mumps-containing vaccines.

Diarrhea has been reported after vaccination with mumps-containing vaccines.

Vasculitis has been reported rarely after vaccination with other mumps-containing vaccines.

Parotitis has been reported to occur in very low incidence, and orchitis rarely, in persons who were vaccinated. In most instances investigated, prior exposure to natural mumps was established. In other instances, whether or not this was due to vaccine or to prior natural mumps exposure or to other causes has not been established. Erythema multiforme has also been reported rarely.

Reports of purpura and allergic reactions such as wheal and flare at the injection site or urticaria have been extremely rare.

Forms of optic neuritis, including retrobulbar neuritis and papillitis may infrequently follow viral infections, and have been reported to occur 1 to 3 weeks following inoculation with some live virus vaccines.

Syncope, particularly at the time of mass vaccination, has been reported.

Very rarely encephalitis, febrile seizures, nerve deafness and other nervous system reactions have occurred in vaccinees. A cause-effect relationship has not been established.

DOSAGE AND ADMINISTRATION

FOR SUBCUTANEOUS ADMINISTRATION
Do not inject intravenously
The dosage of vaccine is the same for all persons. Inject the total volume (about 0.5 mL) of reconstituted vaccine subcutaneously, preferably into the outer aspect of upper arm. *Do not give immune serum globulin (ISG) concurrently with* MUMPSVAX.

During shipment, to insure that there is no loss of potency, the vaccine must be maintained at a temperature of 10°C (50°F) or less.

Before reconstitution, store MUMPSVAX at 2–8°C (36–46°F). *Protect from light.*

CAUTION: A sterile syringe free of preservatives, antiseptics, and detergents should be used for each injection and/or reconstitution of the vaccine because these substances may inactivate the live virus vaccine. A 25 gauge, ⅝″ needle is recommended.

To reconstitute, use only the diluent supplied, since it is free of preservatives or other antiviral substances which might inactivate the vaccine.

Single Dose Vial —First withdraw the entire volume of diluent into the syringe to be used for reconstitution. Inject all the diluent in the syringe into the vial of lyophilized vaccine, and agitate to mix thoroughly. Withdraw the entire contents into a syringe and inject the total volume of restored vaccine subcutaneously.

It is important to use a separate sterile syringe and needle for each individual patient to prevent transmission of hepatitis B and other infectious agents from one person to another.

10 Dose Vial (available only to government agencies/institutions) —Withdraw the entire contents (7 mL) of the diluent vial into the sterile syringe to be used for reconstitution, and introduce into the 10 dose vial of lyophilized vaccine. Agitate to ensure thorough mixing. The outer labeling suggests "For Jet Injector or Syringe Use". Use with separate sterile syringes is permitted for containers of 10 doses or less. The vaccine and diluent do not contain preservatives; therefore, the user must recognize the potential contamination hazards and exercise special precautions to protect the sterility and potency of the product. The use of aseptic techniques and proper storage prior to and after restoration of the vaccine and subsequent withdrawal of the individual doses is essential. Use 0.5 mL of the reconstituted vaccine for subcutaneous injection.

It is important to use a separate sterile syringe and needle for each individual patient to prevent transmission of hepatitis B and other infectious agents from one person to another.

50 Dose Vial (available only to government agencies/institutions) —Withdraw the entire contents (30 mL) of the diluent vial into the sterile syringe to be used for reconstitution and introduce into the 50 dose vial of lyophilized vaccine. Agitate to ensure thorough mixing. With full aseptic precautions, attach the vial to the sterilized multidose jet injector apparatus. Use 0.5 mL of the reconstituted vaccine for subcutaneous injection.

Each dose of MUMPSVAX contains not less than the equivalent of 20,000 $TCID_{50}$ of the U.S. Reference Mumps Virus. Parenteral drug products should be inspected visually for particulate matter and discoloration prior to administration. MUMPSVAX, when reconstituted, is clear yellow.

HOW SUPPLIED

No. 4753—MUMPSVAX is supplied as a single-dose vial of lyophilized vaccine, **NDC** 0006-4753-00, and a vial of diluent.
No. 4584X/4309—MUMPSVAX is supplied as follows: (1) a box of 10 single-dose vials of lyophilized vaccine (package A), **NDC** 0006-4584-00; and (2) a box of 10 vials of diluent (package B). To conserve refrigerator space, the diluent may be stored separately at room temperature (6505-01-037-6792, Ten Pack).
Available only to government agencies/institutions:
No. 4664X—MUMPSVAX is supplied as one 10 dose vial of lyophilized vaccine, **NDC** 0006-4664-00, and one 7 mL vial of diluent.
No. 4593X—MUMPSVAX is supplied as one 50 dose vial of lyophilized vaccine, **NDC** 0006-4593-00, and one 30 mL vial of diluent.
Storage
It is recommended that the vaccine be used as soon as possible after reconstitution. Protect vaccine from light at all times, since such exposure may inactivate the virus. Store reconstituted vaccine in the vaccine vial in a dark place at 2–8°C (36–46°F) and discard if not used within 8 hours.
A.H.F.S. Category: 80:12
DC 7680410   Issued March 1991
COPYRIGHT © MERCK & CO., INC., 1990
All rights reserved

MUSTARGEN®, Trituration of ℞
(Mechlorethamine HCl for Injection), U.S.P.

DESCRIPTION

MUSTARGEN* (Mechlorethamine HCl), an antineoplastic nitrogen mustard also known as HN2 hydrochloride, is a nitrogen analog of sulfur mustard. It is a white, crystalline, hygroscopic powder that is very soluble in water and also soluble in alcohol.
Mechlorethamine hydrochloride is designated chemically as 2-chloro-N-(2-chloroethyl)-N-methylethanamine hydrochloride. The molecular weight is 192.52 and the melting point is 108–111°C. The empirical formula is $C_5H_{11}Cl_2N \cdot HCl$, and the structural formula is:

$$CH_3N(CH_2CH_2Cl)_2 \cdot HCl$$

Trituration of MUSTARGEN is a sterile, white crystalline powder for injection by the intravenous or intracavitary routes after dissolution. Each vial of MUSTARGEN contains 10 mg of mechlorethamine hydrochloride triturated with sodium chloride q.s. 100 mg. When dissolved with 10 mL Sterile Water for Injection or 0.9% Sodium Chloride Injection, the resulting solution has a pH of 3–5 at a concentration of 1 mg mechlorethamine HCl per mL.

*Registered trademark of MERCK & CO., INC.

CLINICAL PHARMACOLOGY

Mechlorethamine, a biologic alkylating agent, has a cytotoxic action which inhibits rapidly proliferating cells.
Pharmacokinetics and Metabolism
In water or body fluids, mechlorethamine undergoes rapid chemical transformation and combines with water or reactive compounds of cells, so that the drug is no longer present in active form a few minutes after administration.

INDICATIONS AND USAGE

Before using MUSTARGEN see CONTRAINDICATIONS, WARNINGS, PRECAUTIONS, ADVERSE REACTIONS, DOSAGE AND ADMINISTRATION, and HOW SUPPLIED, Special Handling.
MUSTARGEN, administered intravenously, is indicated for the palliative treatment of Hodgkin's disease (Stages III and IV), lymphosarcoma, chronic myelocytic or chronic lymphocytic leukemia, polycythemia vera, mycosis fungoides, and bronchogenic carcinoma.
MUSTARGEN, administered intrapleurally, intraperitoneally, or intrapericardially, is indicated for the palliative treatment of metastatic carcinoma resulting in effusion.

CONTRAINDICATIONS

The use of MUSTARGEN is contraindicated in the presence of known infectious diseases and in patients who have had previous anaphylactic reactions to MUSTARGEN.

WARNINGS

Extravasation of the drug into subcutaneous tissues results in a painful inflammation. The area usually becomes indurated and sloughing may occur. If leakage of drug is obvious, prompt infiltration of the area with sterile isotonic sodium thiosulfate (⅙ molar) and application of an ice compress for 6 to 12 hours may minimize the local reaction. For a ⅙ molar solution of sodium thiosulfate, use 4.14 g of sodium thiosulfate per 100 mL of Sterile Water for Injection or 2.64 g of anhydrous sodium thiosulfate per 100 mL or dilute 4 mL of Sodium Thiosulfate Injection (10%) with 6 mL of Sterile Water for Injection.

Before using MUSTARGEN, an accurate histologic diagnosis of the disease, a knowledge of its natural course, and an adequate clinical history are important. The hematologic status of the patient must first be determined. It is essential to understand the hazards and therapeutic effects to be expected. Careful clinical judgment must be exercised in selecting patients. If the indication for its use is not clear, the drug should not be used.
As nitrogen mustard therapy may contribute to extensive and rapid development of amyloidosis, it should be used only if foci of acute and chronic suppurative inflammation are absent.
Usage in Pregnancy
Mechlorethamine hydrochloride can cause fetal harm when administered to a pregnant woman. MUSTARGEN has been shown to produce fetal malformations in the rat and ferret when given as single subcutaneous injections of 1 mg/kg (2–3 times the maximum recommended human dose). There are no adequate and well controlled studies in pregnant women. If this drug is used during pregnancy, or if the patient becomes pregnant while taking this drug, the patient should be apprised of the potential hazard to the fetus. Women of childbearing potential should be advised to avoid becoming pregnant.

PRECAUTIONS

General
This drug is highly toxic and both powder and solution must be handled and administered with care. Since MUSTARGEN is a powerful vesicant, it is intended primarily for intravenous use, and in most instances is given by this route. Inhalation of dust or vapors and contact with skin or mucous membranes, especially those of the eyes, must be avoided. Rubber gloves should be worn when handling MUSTARGEN. (See DOSAGE AND ADMINISTRATION and HOW SUPPLIED, *Special Handling.*)
Because of the toxicity of MUSTARGEN, and the unpleasant side effects following its use, the potential risk and discomfort from the use of this drug in patients with inoperable neoplasms or in the terminal stage of the disease must be balanced against the limited gain obtainable. These gains will vary with the nature and the status of the disease under treatment. The routine use of MUSTARGEN in all cases of widely disseminated neoplasms is to be discouraged.
The use of MUSTARGEN in patients with leukopenia, thrombocytopenia, and anemia, due to invasion of the bone marrow by tumor carries a greater risk. In such patients a good response to treatment with disappearance of the tumor from the bone marrow may be associated with improvement of bone marrow function. However, in the absence of a good response or in patients who have been previously treated with chemotherapeutic agents, hematopoiesis may be further compromised, and leukopenia, thrombocytopenia and anemia may become more severe and lead to the demise of the patient.
Tumors of bone and nervous tissue have responded poorly to therapy. Results are unpredictable in disseminated and malignant tumors of different types.
Precautions must be observed with the use of MUSTARGEN and x-ray therapy or other chemotherapy in alternating courses. Hematopoietic function is characteristically depressed by either form of therapy, and neither MUSTARGEN following x-ray therapy nor x-ray therapy subsequent to the drug should be given until bone marrow function has recovered. In particular, irradiation of such areas as sternum, ribs, and vertebrae shortly after a course of nitrogen mustard may lead to hematologic complications.
MUSTARGEN has been reported to have immunosuppressive activity. Therefore, it should be borne in mind that use of the drug may predispose the patient to bacterial, viral, or fungal infection.
Hyperuricemia may develop during therapy with MUSTARGEN. The problem of urate precipitation should be anticipated, particularly in the treatment of the lymphomas, and adequate methods for control of hyperuricemia should be instituted and careful attention directed toward adequate fluid intake before treatment.

Since drug toxicity, especially sensitivity to bone marrow failure, seems to be more common in chronic lymphatic leukemia than in other conditions, the drug should be given in this condition with great caution, if at all.

Extreme caution must be used in exceeding the average recommended dose. (See OVERDOSAGE.)

Laboratory Tests

Many abnormalities of renal, hepatic, and bone marrow function have been reported in patients with neoplastic disease and receiving mechlorethamine. It is advisable to check renal, hepatic, and bone marrow functions frequently.

Carcinogenesis, Mutagenesis, Impairment of Fertility

Therapy with alkylating agents such as MUSTARGEN may be associated with an increased incidence of a second malignant tumor, especially when such therapy is combined with other antineoplastic agents or radiation therapy.

Young-adult female RF mice were injected intravenously with four doses of 2.4 mg/kg of mechlorethamine (0.1% solution) at 2-week intervals with observations for up to 2 years. An increased incidence of thymic lymphomas and pulmonary adenomas was observed. Painting mechlorethamine on the skin of mice for periods up to 33 weeks resulted in squamous cell tumors in 9 of 33 mice.

Mechlorethamine induced mutations in the Ames test, in *E. coli*, and *Neurospora crassa*. Mechlorethamine caused chromosome aberrations in a variety of plant and mammalian cells. Dominant lethal mutations were produced in ICR/Ha Swiss mice.

Mechlorethamine impaired fertility in the rat at a daily dose of 500 mg/kg intravenously for two weeks.

Pregnancy

Pregnancy Category D. See WARNINGS.

Nursing Mothers

It is not known whether this drug is excreted in human milk. Because many drugs are excreted in human milk and because of the potential for serious adverse reactions in nursing infants from MUSTARGEN, a decision should be made whether to discontinue nursing or to discontinue the drug, taking into account the importance of the drug to the mother.

Pediatric Use

Safety and effectiveness in children have not been established by well-controlled studies. Use of MUSTARGEN in children has been quite limited. MUSTARGEN has been used in Hodgkin's disease, stages III and IV, in combination with other oncolytic agents (MOPP schedule). The MOPP chemotherapy combination includes mechlorethamine, vincristine, procarbazine, and prednisone or prednisolone.

ADVERSE REACTIONS

Clinical use of MUSTARGEN *usually is accompanied by toxic manifestations.*

Local Toxicity

Thrombosis and thrombophlebitis may result from direct contact of the drug with the intima of the injected vein. Avoid high concentration and prolonged contact with the drug, especially in cases of elevated pressure in the antebrachial vein (e.g., in mediastinal tumor compression from severe vena cava syndrome).

Systemic Toxicity

General: Hypersensitivity reactions, including anaphylaxis, have been reported. Nausea, vomiting and depression of formed elements in the circulating blood are dose-limiting side effects and usually occur with the use of full doses of MUSTARGEN. Jaundice, alopecia, vertigo, tinnitus and diminished hearing may occur infrequently. Rarely, hemolytic anemia associated with such diseases as the lymphomas and chronic lymphocytic leukemia may be precipitated by treatment with alkylating agents including MUSTARGEN. Also, various chromosomal abnormalities have been reported in association with nitrogen mustard therapy.

MUSTARGEN is given preferably at night in case sedation for side effects is required. Nausea and vomiting usually occur 1 to 3 hours after use of the drug. Emesis may disappear in the first 8 hours, but nausea may persist for 24 hours. Nausea and vomiting may be so severe as to precipitate vascular accidents in patients with a hemorrhagic tendency. Premedication with antiemetics, in addition to sedatives, may help control severe nausea and vomiting. Anorexia, weakness and diarrhea may also occur.

Hematologic: The usual course of MUSTARGEN (total dose of 0.4 mg/kg either given as a single intravenous dose or divided into two or four daily doses of 0.2 or 0.1 mg/kg respectively) generally produces a lymphocytopenia within 24 hours after the first injection; significant granulocytopenia occurs within 6 to 8 days and lasts for 10 days to 3 weeks. Agranulocytosis appears to be relatively infrequent and recovery from leukopenia in most cases is complete within two weeks of the maximum reduction. Thrombocytopenia is variable but the time course of the appearance and recovery from reduced platelet counts generally parallels the sequence of granulocyte levels. In some cases severe thrombocytopenia may lead to bleeding from the gums and gastrointestinal tract, petechiae, and small subcutaneous hemor-

rhages; these symptoms appear to be transient and in most cases disappear with return to a normal platelet count. However, a severe and even uncontrollable depression of the hematopoietic system occasionally may follow the usual dose of MUSTARGEN, particularly in patients with widespread disease and debility and in patients previously treated with other antineoplastic agents or x-ray. Persistent pancytopenia has been reported. In rare instances, hemorrhagic complications may be due to hyperheparinemia. Erythrocyte and hemoglobin levels may decline during the first 2 weeks after therapy but rarely significantly. Depression of the hematopoietic system may be found up to 50 days or more after starting therapy.

Integumentary: Occasionally, a maculopapular skin eruption occurs, but this may be idiosyncratic and does not necessarily recur with subsequent courses of the drug. Erythema multiforme has been observed. Herpes zoster, a common complicating infection in patients with lymphomas, may first appear after therapy is instituted and on occasion may be precipitated by treatment. Further treatment should be discontinued during the acute phase of this illness to avoid progression to generalized herpes zoster.

Reproductive: Since the gonads are susceptible to MUSTARGEN, treatment may be followed by delayed catamenia, oligomenorrhea, or temporary or permanent amenorrhea. Impaired spermatogenesis, azoospermia, and total germinal aplasia have been reported in male patients treated with alkylating agents, especially in combination with other drugs. In some instances spermatogenesis may return in patients in remission, but this may occur only several years after intensive chemotherapy has been discontinued. Patients should be warned of the potential risk to their reproductive capacity.

OVERDOSAGE

With total doses exceeding 0.4 mg/kg of body weight for a single course, severe leukopenia, anemia, thrombocytopenia and a hemorrhagic diathesis with subsequent delayed bleeding may develop. Death may follow. The only treatment in instances of excessive dosage appears to be repeated blood product transfusions, antibiotic treatment of complicating infections and general supportive measures.

The intravenous LD$_{50}$ of MUSTARGEN is 2 mg/kg and 1.6 mg/kg in the mouse and rat, respectively.

DOSAGE AND ADMINISTRATION

Intravenous Administration

The dosage of MUSTARGEN varies with the clinical situation, the therapeutic response and the magnitude of hematologic depression. A total dose of 0.4 mg/kg of body weight for each course usually is given either as a single dose or in divided doses of 0.1 to 0.2 mg/kg per day. Dosage should be based on ideal dry body weight. The presence of edema or ascites must be considered so that dosage will be based on actual weight unaugmented by these conditions.

The margin of safety in therapy with MUSTARGEN *is narrow and considerable care must be exercised in the matter of dosage.* Repeated examinations of blood are *mandatory* as a guide to subsequent therapy. (See OVERDOSAGE.)

Within a few minutes after intravenous injection, MUSTARGEN undergoes chemical transformation, combines with reactive compounds, and is no longer present in its active form in the blood stream. Subsequent courses should not be given until the patient has recovered hematologically from the previous course; this is best determined by repeated studies of the peripheral blood elements awaiting their return to normal levels. It is often possible to give repeated courses of MUSTARGEN as early as three weeks after treatment.

Preparation of Solution for Intravenous Administration

This drug is highly toxic and both powder and solution must be handled and administered with care. Since MUSTARGEN is a powerful vesicant, it is intended primarily for intravenous use, and in most instances is given by this route. Inhalation of dust or vapors and contact with skin or mucous membranes, especially those of the eyes, must be avoided. Rubber gloves should be worn when handling MUSTARGEN. Should accidental eye contact occur, copious irrigation with water, normal saline or a balanced salt ophthalmic irrigating solution should be instituted immediately, followed by prompt ophthalmologic consultation. Should accidental skin contact occur, the affected part must be irrigated immediately with copious amounts of water, for at least 15 minutes, followed by 2 percent sodium thiosulfate solution. (See also box warning and *Special Handling*.)

Each vial of MUSTARGEN contains 10 mg of mechlorethamine hydrochloride triturated with sodium chloride q.s. 100 mg. In neutral or alkaline aqueous solution it undergoes rapid chemical transformation and is highly unstable. Although solutions prepared according to instructions are acidic and do not decompose as rapidly, they should be prepared immediately before each injection since they will decompose on standing. When reconstituted, MUSTARGEN is a clear colorless solution. *Do not use if the solution is discol-*

ored or if droplets of water are visible within the vial prior to reconstitution.

Using a sterile 10 mL syringe, inject 10 mL of Sterile Water for Injection or 10 mL Sodium Chloride Injection into a vial of MUSTARGEN. With the needle (syringe attached) still in the rubber stopper, shake the vial several times to dissolve the drug completely. The resultant solution contains 1 mg of mechlorethamine hydrochloride per mL.

Parenteral drug products should be inspected visually for particulate matter and discoloration prior to administration whenever solution and container permit.

Special Handling

Due to the drug's toxic and mutagenic properties, appropriate precautions including the use of appropriate safety equipment are recommended for the preparation of MUSTARGEN for parenteral administration. The National Institutes of Health presently recommends that the preparation of injectable anti-neoplastic drugs should be performed in a Class II laminar flow biological safety cabinet and that personnel preparing drugs of this class should wear surgical gloves and a closed front surgical-type gown with knit cuffs. Several other guidelines for proper handling and disposal of anti-cancer drugs have been published and should be considered. There is no general agreement that all of the procedures recommended in the guidelines are necessary or appropriate.

Accidental contact: Should accidental eye contact occur, copious irrigation with water, normal saline or a balanced salt ophthalmic irrigating solution should be instituted immediately, followed by prompt ophthalmologic consultation. Should accidental skin contact occur, the affected part must be irrigated immediately with copious amounts of water, for at least 15 minutes, followed by 2 percent sodium thiosulfate solution. (See also box warning.)

Technique for Intravenous Administration

Withdraw into the syringe the calculated volume of solution required for a single injection. *Dispose of any remaining solution after neutralization* (see below). Although the drug may be injected directly into any suitable vein, it is injected preferably into the rubber or plastic tubing of a flowing intravenous infusion set. This reduces the possibility of severe local reactions due to extravasation or high concentration of the drug. Injecting the drug into the tubing rather than adding it to the entire volume of the infusion fluid minimizes a chemical reaction between the drug and the solution. The rate of injection apparently is not critical provided it is completed within a few minutes.

Intracavitary Administration

Nitrogen mustard has been used by intracavitary administration with varying success in certain malignant conditions for the control of pleural, peritoneal, and pericardial effusions caused by malignant cells.

The technic and the dose used by any of these routes varies. Therefore, if MUSTARGEN is given by the intracavitary route, the published articles concerning such use should be consulted. *Because of the inherent risks involved, the physician should be experienced in the appropriate injection technics, and be thoroughly aware of the indications, dosages, hazards, and precautions as set forth in the published literature. When using* MUSTARGEN *by the intracavitary route, the general precautions concerning this agent should be borne in mind.*

As a general guide, reference is made especially to the technics of Weisberger et al. Intracavitary use is indicated in the presence of pleural, peritoneal, or pericardial effusion due to metastatic tumors. Local therapy with nitrogen mustard is used only when malignant cells are demonstrated in the effusion. Intracavitary injection is not recommended when the accumulated fluid is chylous in nature, since results are likely to be poor.

Paracentesis is first performed with most of the fluid being removed from the pleural or peritoneal cavity. The intracavitary use of MUSTARGEN may exert at least some of its effect through production of a chemical poudrage. Therefore, the removal of excess fluid allows the drug to more easily contact the peritoneal and pleural linings. For intrapleural or intrapericardial injection nitrogen mustard is introduced directly through the thoracentesis needle. For intraperitoneal injection it is given through a rubber catheter inserted into the trocar used for paracentesis or through a No. 18 gauge needle inserted at another site. This drug should be injected slowly, with frequent aspiration to ensure that a free flow of fluid is present. If fluid cannot be aspirated, pain and necrosis due to injection of solution outside the cavity may occur. Free flow of fluid also is necessary to prevent injection into a loculated pocket and to ensure adequate dissemination of nitrogen mustard.

Continued on next page

Information on the Merck & Co. products listed on these pages is the full prescribing information from product circulars in use October 1, 1992.

Merck & Co.—Cont.

The usual dose of nitrogen mustard for intracavitary injection is 0.4 mg/kg of body weight, though 0.2 mg/kg (or 10 to 20 mg) has been used by the intrapericardial route. The solution is prepared, as previously described for intravenous injection, by adding 10 mL of Sterile Water for Injection or 10 mL of Sodium Chloride Injection to the vial containing 10 mg of mechlorethamine hydrochloride. (Amounts of diluent of 50 to 100 mL of normal saline have also been used.) The position of the patient should be changed every 5 to 10 minutes for an hour after injection to obtain more uniform distribution of the drug throughout the serous cavity. The remaining fluid may be removed from the pleural or peritoneal cavity by paracentesis 24 to 36 hours later. The patient should be followed carefully by clinical and x-ray examination to detect reaccumulation of fluid.

Pain occurs rarely with intrapleural use; it is common with intraperitoneal injection and is often associated with nausea, vomiting, and diarrhea of 2 to 3 days duration. Transient cardiac irregularities may occur with intrapericardial injection. Death, possibly accelerated by nitrogen mustard, has been reported following the use of this agent by the intracavitary route. Although absorption of MUSTARGEN when given by the intracavitary route is probably not complete because of its rapid deactivation by body fluids, the systemic effect is unpredictable. The acute side effects such as nausea and vomiting are usually mild. Bone marrow depression is generally milder than when the drug is given intravenously. Care should be taken to avoid use by the intracavitary route when other agents which may suppress bone marrow function are being used systemically.

Neutralization of Equipment and Unused Solution

To clean rubber gloves, tubing, glassware, etc., after giving MUSTARGEN, soak them in an aqueous solution containing equal volumes of sodium thiosulfate (5%) and sodium bicarbonate (5%) for 45 minutes. Excess reagents and reaction products are washed away easily with water. Any unused injection solution should be neutralized by mixing with an equal volume of sodium thiosulfate/sodium bicarbonate solution. Allow the mixture to stand for 45 minutes. Vials that have contained MUSTARGEN should be treated in the same way with thiosulfate/bicarbonate solution before disposal.

HOW SUPPLIED

No. 7753—Trituration of MUSTARGEN is a white crystalline powder, each vial containing 10 mg mechlorethamine hydrochloride with sodium chloride q.s. 100 mg, and is supplied as follows:

NDC 0006-7753-31 in treatment sets of 4 vials.

Storage

Store at room temperature. Solutions of mechlorethamine HCl decompose on standing; therefore, solutions of the drug should be prepared immediately before use.

A.H.F.S. Category: 10:00

DC 7417928 Issued July 1987

COPYRIGHT © MERCK & CO., INC., 1985
All rights reserved

MYOCHRYSINE® Injection (Gold Sodium Thiomalate), U.S.P. ℞

Physicians planning to use MYOCHRYSINE* *(Gold Sodium Thiomalate) should thoroughly familiarize themselves with its toxicity and its benefits. The possibility of toxic reactions should always be explained to the patient before starting therapy. Patients should be warned to report promptly any symptoms suggesting toxicity. Before each injection of* MYOCHRYSINE, *the physician should review the results of laboratory work, and see the patient to determine the presence or absence of adverse reactions since some of these can be severe or even fatal.*

*Registered trademark of MERCK & CO., INC.

DESCRIPTION

MYOCHRYSINE is a sterile aqueous solution of gold sodium thiomalate. It contains 0.5 percent benzyl alcohol added as a preservative. The pH of the product is 5.8–6.5.

Gold sodium thiomalate is a mixture of the mono- and disodium salts of gold thiomalic acid. The structural formula is:

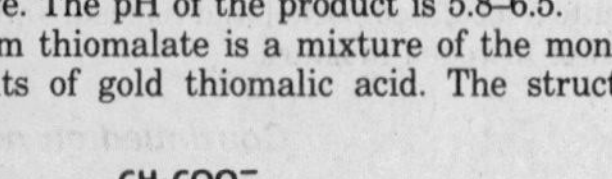

mercaptobutanedioic acid, monogold (1+) sodium salt

The molecular weight for $C_4H_3AuNa_2O_4S$ (the disodium salt) is 390.07 and for $C_4H_4AuNaO_4S$ (the monosodium salt) is 368.09.

MYOCHRYSINE is supplied as a solution for intramuscular injection containing 25 mg or 50 mg of gold sodium thiomalate per mL.

CLINICAL PHARMACOLOGY

The mode of action of gold sodium thiomalate is unknown. The predominant action appears to be a suppressive effect on the synovitis of active rheumatoid disease.

INDICATIONS AND USAGE

MYOCHRYSINE is indicated in the treatment of selected cases of active rheumatoid arthritis— both adult and juvenile type. The greatest benefit occurs in the early active stage. In late stages of the illness when cartilage and bone damage have occurred, gold can only check the progression of rheumatoid arthritis and prevent further structural damage to joints. It cannot repair damage caused by previously active disease.

MYOCHRYSINE should be used only as *one part* of a complete program of therapy; alone it is not a complete treatment.

CONTRAINDICATIONS

Hypersensitivity to any component of this product.

Severe toxicity resulting from previous exposure to gold or other heavy metals.

Severe debilitation.

Systemic lupus erythematosus.

WARNINGS

Before treatment is started, the patient's hemoglobin, erythrocyte, white blood cell, differential and platelet counts should be determined, and urinalysis should be done to serve as basic reference. Urine should be analyzed for protein and sediment changes prior to each injection. Complete blood counts including platelet estimation should be made before every second injection throughout treatment. The occurrence of purpura or ecchymoses at any time always requires a platelet count.

Danger signals of possible gold toxicity include: rapid reduction of hemoglobin, leukopenia below 4000 WBC/mm^3, eosinophilia above 5 percent, platelet decrease below 100,000/mm^3, albuminuria, hematuria, pruritus, skin eruption, stomatitis, or persistent diarrhea. No additional injections of MYOCHRYSINE should be given unless further studies show these abnormalities to be caused by conditions other than gold toxicity.

PRECAUTIONS

General

Gold salts should not be used concomitantly with penicillamine.

The safety of coadministration with cytotoxic drugs has not been established.

Caution is indicated in the use of MYOCHRYSINE in patients with the following:

1. a history of blood dyscrasias such as granulocytopenia or anemia caused by drug sensitivity,
2. allergy or hypersensitivity to medications,
3. skin rash,
4. previous kidney or liver disease,
5. marked hypertension,
6. compromised cerebral or cardiovascular circulation.

Diabetes mellitus or congestive heart failure should be under control before gold therapy is instituted.

Carcinogenicity

Renal adenomas have been reported in long-term toxicity studies of rats receiving MYOCHRYSINE at high dose levels (2 mg/kg weekly for 45 weeks, followed by 6 mg/kg daily for 47 weeks), approximately 2 to 42 times the usual human dose. These adenomas are histologically similar to those produced in rats by chronic administration of experimental gold compounds and other heavy metals, such as lead. No reports have been received of renal adenomas in man in association with the use of MYOCHRYSINE.

Pregnancy

Pregnancy Category C.

MYOCHRYSINE has been shown to be teratogenic during the organogenetic period in rats and rabbits when given in doses, respectively, of 140 and 175 times the usual human dose. Hydrocephaly and microphthalmia were the malformations observed in rats when MYOCHRYSINE was administered subcutaneously at a dose of 25 mg/kg/day from day 6 through day 15 of gestation. In rabbits, limb malformations and gastroschisis were the malformations observed when MYOCHRYSINE was administered subcutaneously at doses of 20–45 mg/kg/day from day 6 through day 18 of gestation.

There are no adequate and well-controlled studies in pregnant women. MYOCHRYSINE should be used during pregnancy only if the potential benefit to the mother justifies the potential risk to the fetus.

Nursing Mothers

The presence of gold has been demonstrated in the milk of lactating mothers. In addition, gold has been found in the serum and red blood cells of a nursing infant. In view of the above findings and because of the potential for serious adverse reactions in nursing infants from MYOCHRYSINE, a decision should be made whether to discontinue nursing or to discontinue the drug, taking into account the importance of the drug to the mother. The slow excretion and persistence of gold in the mother, even after therapy is discontinued, must also be kept in mind.

ADVERSE REACTIONS

A variety of adverse reactions may develop during the initial phase (weekly injections) of therapy or during maintenance treatment. Adverse reactions are observed most frequently when the cumulative dose of MYOCHRYSINE administered is between 400 and 800 mg. Very uncommonly, complications occur days to months after cessation of treatment.

Cutaneous reactions: Dermatitis is the most common reaction. *Any eruption, especially if pruritic, that develops during treatment with* MYOCHRYSINE *should be considered a reaction to gold until proven otherwise.* Pruritus often exists before dermatitis becomes apparent, and therefore should be considered a warning signal of impending cutaneous reaction. The most serious form of cutaneous reaction is generalized exfoliative dermatitis which may lead to alopecia and shedding of nails. Gold dermatitis may be aggravated by exposure to sunlight or an actinic rash may develop.

Mucous membrane reactions: Stomatitis is the second most common adverse reaction. Shallow ulcers on the buccal membranes, on the borders of the tongue, and on the palate or in the pharynx may occur as the only adverse reaction, or along with dermatitis. Sometimes diffuse glossitis or gingivitis develops. A metallic taste may precede these oral mucous membrane reactions and should be considered a warning signal.

Conjunctivitis is a rare reaction.

Renal reactions: Gold may be toxic to the kidney and produce a nephrotic syndrome or glomerulitis with hematuria. These renal reactions are usually relatively mild and subside completely if recognized early and treatment is discontinued. They may become severe and chronic if treatment is continued after onset of the reaction. Therefore, it is important to perform a *urinalysis before every injection,* and to discontinue treatment promptly if proteinuria or hematuria develops.

Hematologic reactions: Blood dyscrasia due to gold toxicity is rare, but because of the potential serious consequences it must be constantly watched for and recognized early by frequent blood examinations done throughout treatment. Granulocytopenia; thrombocytopenia, with or without purpura; hypoplastic and aplastic anemia; and eosinophilia have all been reported. These hematologic disorders may occur separately or in combinations.

Nitritoid and allergic reactions: Reactions of the "nitritoid type" which may resemble anaphylactoid effects have been reported. Flushing, fainting, dizziness and sweating are most frequently reported. Other symptoms that may occur include: nausea, vomiting, malaise, headache, and weakness. More severe, but less common effects include: anaphylactic shock, syncope, bradycardia, thickening of the tongue, difficulty in swallowing and breathing, and angioneurotic edema. These effects may occur almost immediately after injection or as late as 10 minutes following injection. They may occur at any time during the course of therapy and if observed, treatment with MYOCHRYSINE should be discontinued.

Miscellaneous reactions: Gastrointestinal reactions have been reported, including nausea, vomiting, anorexia, abdominal cramps and diarrhea. Ulcerative enterocolitis, which can be severe or even fatal, has been reported rarely.

There have been rare reports of reactions involving the eye such as iritis, corneal ulcers, and gold deposits in ocular tissues. Peripheral and central nervous system complications have been reported rarely. Peripheral neuropathy, with or without fasciculations, sensorimotor effects (including Guillain-Barré syndrome) and elevated spinal fluid protein have been reported. Central nervous system complications have included confusion, hallucinations and seizures. Usually these signs and symptoms cleared upon discontinuation of gold therapy.

Hepatitis, jaundice, with or without cholestasis, gold bronchitis, pulmonary injury manifested by interstitial pneumonitis and fibrosis, partial or complete hair loss and fever have also been reported.

Sometimes arthralgia occurs for a day or two after an injection of MYOCHRYSINE; this reaction usually subsides after the first few injections.

MANAGEMENT OF ADVERSE REACTIONS

Treatment with MYOCHRYSINE should be discontinued immediately when toxic reactions occur. Minor complications such as localized dermatitis, mild stomatitis, or slight proteinuria generally require no other therapy and resolve spontaneously with suspension of MYOCHRYSINE. Moderately severe skin and mucous membrane reactions often benefit from topical corticosteroids, oral antihistaminics, and soothing or anesthetic lotions.

If stomatitis or dermatitis becomes severe or more generalized, systemic corticosteroids (generally, prednisone 10 to 40 mg daily in divided doses) may provide symptomatic relief.

For serious renal, hematologic, pulmonary, and enterocolitic complications, high doses of systemic corticosteroids (prednisone 40 to 100 mg daily in divided doses) are recommended. The optimum duration of corticosteroid treatment varies with the response of the individual patient. Therapy may be required for many months when adverse effects are unusually severe or progressive.

In patients whose complications do not improve with high-dose corticosteroid treatment, or who develop significant steroid-related adverse reactions, a chelating agent may be given to enhance gold excretion. Dimercaprol (BAL) has been used successfully, but patients must be monitored carefully as numerous untoward reactions may attend its use. Corticosteroids and a chelating agent may be used concomitantly.

MYOCHRYSINE *should not be reinstituted after severe or idiosyncratic reactions.*

MYOCHRYSINE may be readministered following resolution of mild reactions, using a reduced dosage schedule. If an initial test dose of 5 mg MYOCHRYSINE is well-tolerated, progressively larger doses (5 to 10 mg increments) may be given at weekly to monthly intervals until a dose of 25 to 50 mg is reached.

DOSAGE AND ADMINISTRATION

MYOCHRYSINE should be administered only by intramuscular injection, preferably intragluteally. It should be given with the patient lying down. He should remain recumbent for approximately 10 minutes after the injection.

Therapeutic effects from MYOCHRYSINE occur slowly. Early improvement, often limited to a reduction in morning stiffness, may begin after six to eight weeks of treatment, but beneficial effects may not be observed until after months of therapy.

Parenteral drug products should be inspected visually for particulate matter and discoloration prior to administration. Do not use if material has darkened. Color should not exceed pale yellow.

For the adult of average size the following dosage schedule is suggested:

Weekly Injections

1st injection ....10 mg
2nd injection ....25 mg
3rd and subsequent injections, 25 to 50 mg
until there is toxicity or major clinical improvement, or, in the absence of either of these, the cumulative dose of MYOCHRYSINE reaches one gram.

MYOCHRYSINE is continued until the cumulative dose reaches one gram unless toxicity or major clinical improvement occurs. If significant clinical improvement occurs before a cumulative dose of one gram has been administered, the dose may be decreased or the interval between injections increased as with maintenance therapy. Maintenance doses of 25 to 50 mg every other week for two to 20 weeks are recommended. If the clinical course remains stable, injections of 25 to 50 mg may be given every third and subsequently every fourth week indefinitely. Some patients may require maintenance treatment at intervals of one to three weeks. Should the arthritis exacerbate during maintenance therapy, weekly injections may be resumed temporarily until disease activity is suppressed.

Should a patient fail to improve during initial therapy (cumulative dose of one gram), several options are available:

1— the patient may be considered to be unresponsive and MYOCHRYSINE is discontinued
2— the same dose (25 to 50 mg) of MYOCHRYSINE may be continued for approximately ten additional weeks
3— the dose of MYOCHRYSINE may be increased by increments of 10 mg every one to four weeks, not to exceed 100 mg in a single injection.

If significant clinical improvement occurs using option 2 or 3, the maintenance schedule described above should be initiated. If there is no significant improvement or if toxicity occurs, therapy with MYOCHRYSINE should be stopped. The higher the individual dose of MYOCHRYSINE, the greater the risk of gold toxicity. Selection of one of these options for chrysotherapy should be based upon a number of factors, including the physician's experience with gold salt therapy, the course of the patient's condition, the choice of alternative treatments, and the availability of the patient for the close supervision required.

Juvenile Rheumatoid Arthritis

The pediatric dose of MYOCHRYSINE is proportional to the adult dose on a weight basis. After the initial test dose of 10 mg, the recommended dose for children is one mg per kilogram body weight, not to exceed 50 mg for a single injection. Otherwise, the guidelines given above for administration to adults also apply to children.

Concomitant Drug Therapy—Gold salts should not be used concomitantly with penicillamine.

The safety of coadministration with cytotoxic drugs has not been established. Other measures, such as salicylates, other non-steroidal anti-inflammatory drugs, or systemic corticosteroids, may be continued when MYOCHRYSINE is initiated. After improvement commences, analgesic and anti-inflammatory drugs may be discontinued slowly as symptoms permit.

HOW SUPPLIED

Injection MYOCHRYSINE is a light yellow to yellow solution, depending on potency, which must be protected from light. It is supplied as follows:

No. 7764—25 mg of gold sodium thiomalate per mL as
NDC 0006-7764-64 in boxes of 6 x 1 mL ampuls.
No. 7762—50 mg of gold sodium thiomalate per mL as
NDC 0006-7762-64 in boxes of 6 x 1 mL ampuls
NDC 0006-7762-10 in 10 mL vials
(6505-00-973-8579, 10 mL vial).

Storage

Protect from light.
Store container in carton until contents have been used.

A.H.F.S. Category: 60:00
DC 7594527 Revised July 1989

COPYRIGHT © MERCK & CO., INC., 1985
All rights reserved

NEODECADRON® Sterile Ophthalmic Ointment ℞
(Neomycin Sulfate-Dexamethasone Sodium Phosphate), U.S.P.

DESCRIPTION

Sterile ophthalmic ointment NEODECADRON* (Neomycin Sulfate-Dexamethasone Sodium Phosphate) is a topical corticosteroid-antibiotic ointment for use in certain disorders of the anterior segment of the eye.

Ophthalmic ointment NEODECADRON contains in each gram: dexamethasone sodium phosphate equivalent to 0.5 mg (0.05%) dexamethasone phosphate and neomycin sulfate equivalent to 3.5 mg neomycin base. Inactive ingredients: white petrolatum and mineral oil.

Dexamethasone sodium phosphate is an inorganic ester of dexamethasone. Its empirical formula is $C_{22}H_{28}FNa_2O_8P$.

Neomycin sulfate is the sulfate salt of neomycin, an antibacterial substance produced by the growth of *Streptomyces fradiae* Waksman (Fam. Streptomycetaceae).

*Registered trademark of MERCK & CO., INC.

CLINICAL PHARMACOLOGY

Dexamethasone sodium phosphate, a corticosteroid, suppresses the inflammatory response to a variety of agents, and it probably delays or slows healing. Since corticosteroids may inhibit the body's defense mechanism against infection, a concomitant antimicrobial drug may be used when this inhibition is considered to be clinically significant in a particular case.

Neomycin sulfate, the anti-infective component in the combination, is included to provide action against specific organisms susceptible to it. Neomycin sulfate is considered active mainly against gram-negative organisms, except *Bacteroides* spp. and *Pseudomonas aeruginosa,* which are resistant. Gram-positive organisms except for *Staphylococcus aureus* are usually resistant.

When a decision to administer both a corticosteroid and an antimicrobial is made, the administration of such drugs in combination has the advantage of greater patient compliance and convenience, with the added assurance that the appropriate dosage of both drugs is administered, plus assured compatibility of ingredient when both types of drug are in the same formulation and, particularly, that the correct volume of drug is delivered and retained.

The relative potency of corticosteroids depends on the molecular structure, concentration, and release from the vehicle.

INDICATIONS AND USAGE

For steroid-responsive inflammatory ocular conditions for which a corticosteroid is indicated and where bacterial infection or a risk of bacterial ocular infection exists.

Ocular steroids are indicated in inflammatory conditions of the palpebral and bulbar conjunctiva, cornea, and anterior segment of the globe where the inherent risk of steroid use in certain infective conjunctivitides is accepted to obtain a diminution in edema and inflammation. They are also indicated in chronic anterior uveitis and corneal injury from chemical, radiation, or thermal burns, or penetration of foreign bodies.

The use of a combination drug with an anti-infective component is indicated where the risk of infection is high or where there is an expectation that potentially dangerous numbers of bacteria will be present in the eye.

The particular anti-infective drug in this product is active against the following common bacterial eye pathogens:

Staphylococcus aureus
Escherichia coli
Haemophilus influenzae
Klebsiella/Enterobacter species
Neisseria species

The product does not provide adequate coverage against:

Pseudomonas aeruginosa
Serratia marcescens
Streptococci, including *Streptococcus pneumoniae*

CONTRAINDICATIONS

Epithelial herpes simplex keratitis (dendritic keratitis), acute infectious stages of vaccinia, varicella, and many other viral diseases of the cornea and conjunctiva. Mycobacterial infection of the eye. Fungal diseases of ocular structures. Hypersensitivity to a component of the medication (hypersensitivity to the antibiotic component occurs at a higher rate than for other components).

The use of these combinations is always contraindicated after uncomplicated removal of a corneal foreign body.

WARNINGS

Prolonged use may result in glaucoma, with damage to the optic nerve, defects in visual acuity and fields of vision, and posterior subcapsular cataract formation. Prolonged use may suppress the host response and thus increase the hazard of secondary ocular infections. In those diseases causing thinning of the cornea or sclera, perforations have been known to occur with the use of topical corticosteroids. In acute purulent conditions of the eye, corticosteroids may mask infection or enhance existing infection. If these products are used for 10 days or longer, intraocular pressure should be routinely monitored even though it may be difficult in children and uncooperative patients.

Employment of corticosteroid medication in the treatment of herpes simplex requires great caution: periodic slit-lamp microscopy is recommended.

Any substance (e.g. neomycin sulfate) may occasionally cause cutaneous sensitization. If any reaction indicating such sensitivity is observed, discontinue use.

PRECAUTIONS

The initial prescriptions and renewal of the medication order beyond 8 grams should be made by a physician only after examination of the patient with the aid of magnification, such as slit-lamp biomicroscopy and, where appropriate, fluorescein staining.

The possibility of persistent fungal infections of the cornea should be considered after prolonged corticosteroid dosing.

Usage in Pregnancy

Safety of intensive or protracted use of topical corticosteroids during pregnancy has not been substantiated.

ADVERSE REACTIONS

Adverse reactions have occurred with corticosteroid/anti-infective combination drugs which can be attributed to the corticosteroid component, the anti-infective component, or the combination. Exact incidence figures are not available since no denominator of treated patients is available.

Reactions occurring most often from the presence of the anti-infective ingredient are allergic sensitizations. The reactions due to the corticosteroid component in decreasing order of frequency are: elevation of intraocular pressure (IOP) with possible development of glaucoma, and infrequent optic nerve damage; posterior subcapsular cataract formation; and delayed wound healing.

Secondary Infection: The development of secondary infection has occurred after use of combinations containing corticosteroids and antimicrobials. Fungal infections of the cornea are particularly prone to develop coincidentally with long-term applications of corticosteroid. The possibility of

Continued on next page

Information on the Merck & Co. products listed on these pages is the full prescribing information from product circulars in use October 1, 1992.

Merck & Co.—Cont.

fungal invasion must be considered in any persistent corneal ulceration where corticosteroid treatment has been used. Secondary bacterial ocular infection following suppression of host responses also occurs.

DOSAGE AND ADMINISTRATION

The duration of treatment will vary with the type of lesion and may extend from a few days to several weeks, according to therapeutic response. Relapses, more common in chronic active lesions than in self-limited conditions, usually respond to retreatment.
Apply a thin coating of ophthalmic ointment NEODECADRON three or four times a day. When a favorable response is observed, reduce the number of daily applications to two, and later to one a day as maintenance dose if this is sufficient to control symptoms.
Not more than 8 grams should be prescribed initially and the prescription should not be refilled without further evaluation as outlined in PRECAUTIONS above.
Ophthalmic ointment NEODECADRON is particularly convenient when an eye pad is used. It may also be the preparation of choice for patients in whom therapeutic benefit depends on prolonged contact of the active ingredients with ocular tissues.

HOW SUPPLIED

No. 7617—Sterile Ophthalmic Ointment NEODECADRON is a clear, unctuous ointment, and is supplied as follows:
NDC 0006-7617-04 in 3.5 g tubes
(6505-00-823-7956 0.05% 3.5 g)
A.H.F.S. Category: 52:08
DC 6167722 Issued June 1982

NEODECADRON® Sterile Ophthalmic Solution ℞
(Neomycin Sulfate-Dexamethasone Sodium Phosphate), U.S.P.

DESCRIPTION

Ophthalmic solution NEODECADRON* (Neomycin Sulfate-Dexamethasone Sodium Phosphate) is a topical corticosteroid-antibiotic solution for use in certain disorders of the anterior segment of the eye.
Each milliliter of buffered ophthalmic solution NEODECADRON in the OCUMETER* ophthalmic dispenser contains: dexamethasone sodium phosphate equivalent to 1 mg (0.1%) dexamethasone phosphate, and neomycin sulfate equivalent to 3.5 mg neomycin base. Inactive ingredients: creatinine, sodium citrate, sodium borate, polysorbate 80, disodium edetate, hydrochloric acid to adjust pH to 6.6–7.2, and water for injection. Benzalkonium chloride 0.02% and sodium bisulfite 0.1% added as preservatives.
Dexamethasone sodium phosphate is a water soluble, inorganic ester of dexamethasone. Its empirical formula is $C_{22}H_{28}FNa_2O_8P$. It is approximately three thousand times more soluble in water at 25°C than hydrocortisone.
Neomycin sulfate is the sulfate salt of neomycin, an antibacterial substance produced by the growth of *Streptomyces fradiae* Waksman (Fam. Streptomycetaceae).

*Registered trademark of MERCK & CO., INC.

CLINICAL PHARMACOLOGY

Dexamethasone sodium phosphate, a corticosteroid, suppresses the inflammatory response to a variety of agents, and it probably delays or slows healing. Since corticosteroids may inhibit the body's defense mechanism against infection, a concomitant antimicrobial drug may be used when this inhibition is considered to be clinically significant in a particular case. Neomycin sulfate, the anti-infective component in the combination, is included to provide action against specific organisms susceptible to it. Neomycin sulfate is considered active mainly against gram-negative organisms, except *Bacteroides* spp. and *Pseudomonas aeruginosa*, which are resistant. Gram-positive organisms except for *Staphylococcus aureus* are usually resistant.
When a decision to administer both a corticosteroid and an antimicrobial is made, the administration of such drugs in combination has the advantage of greater patient compliance and convenience, with the added assurance that the appropriate dosage of both drugs is administered, plus assured compatibility of ingredients when both types of drug are in the same formulation and, particularly, that the correct volume of drug is delivered and retained.
The relative potency of corticosteroids depends on the molecular structure, concentration, and release from the vehicle.

INDICATIONS AND USAGE

For steroid-responsive inflammatory ocular conditions for which a corticosteroid is indicated and where bacterial infection or a risk of bacterial ocular infection exists.
Ocular steroids are indicated in inflammatory conditions of the palpebral and bulbar conjunctiva, cornea, and anterior segment of the globe where the inherent risk of steroid use in certain infective conjunctivitides is accepted to obtain a diminution in edema and inflammation. They are also indicated in chronic anterior uveitis and corneal injury from chemical, radiation, or thermal burns, or penetration of foreign bodies.
The use of a combination drug with an anti-infective component is indicated where the risk of infection is high or where there is an expectation that potentially dangerous numbers of bacteria will be present in the eye.
The particular anti-infective drug in this product is active against the following common bacterial eye pathogens:
Staphylococcus aureus
Escherichia coli
Haemophilus influenzae
Klebsiella/Enterobacter species
Neisseria species
The product does not provide adequate coverage against:
Pseudomonas aeruginosa
Serratia marcescens
Streptococci, including *Streptococcus pneumoniae*

CONTRAINDICATIONS

Epithelial herpes simplex keratitis (dendritic keratitis), acute infectious stages of vaccinia, varicella, and many other viral diseases of the cornea and conjunctiva. Mycobacterial infection of the eye. Fungal diseases of ocular structures. Hypersensitivity to any component of this product, including sulfites (see WARNINGS). (Hypersensitivity to the antibiotic component occurs at a higher rate than for other components.)
The use of these combinations is always contraindicated after uncomplicated removal of a corneal foreign body.

WARNINGS

Prolonged use may result in glaucoma, with damage to the optic nerve, defects in visual acuity and fields of vision, and posterior subcapsular cataract formation. Prolonged use may suppress the host response and thus increase the hazard of secondary ocular infections. In those diseases causing thinning of the cornea or sclera, perforations have been known to occur with the use of topical corticosteroids. In acute purulent conditions of the eye, corticosteroids may mask infection or enhance existing infection. If these products are used for 10 days or longer, intraocular pressure should be routinely monitored even though it may be difficult in children and uncooperative patients.
Employment of corticosteroid medication in the treatment of herpes simplex requires great caution: periodic slit-lamp microscopy is recommended.
Any substance (e.g., neomycin sulfate) may occasionally cause cutaneous sensitization. If any reaction indicating such sensitivity is observed, discontinue use.
Ophthalmic Solution NEODECADRON contains sodium bisulfite, a sulfite that may cause allergic-type reactions including anaphylactic symptoms and life-threatening or less severe asthmatic episodes in certain susceptible people. The overall prevalence of sulfite sensitivity in the general population is unknown and probably low. Sulfite sensitivity is seen more frequently in asthmatic than in nonasthmatic people.

PRECAUTIONS

The initial prescription and renewal of the medication order beyond 20 milliliters should be made by a physician only after examination of the patient with the aid of magnification, such as slit-lamp biomicroscopy and, where appropriate, fluorescein staining.
The possibility of persistent fungal infections of the cornea should be considered after prolonged corticosteroid dosing.
Usage in Pregnancy
Safety of intensive or protracted use of topical corticosteroids during pregnancy has not been substantiated.

ADVERSE REACTIONS

Adverse reactions have occurred with corticosteroid/anti-infective combination drugs which can be attributed to the corticosteroid component, the anti-infective component, the combination, or any other component of the product. Exact incidence figures are not available since no denominator of treated patients is available.
Reactions occurring most often from the presence of the anti-infective ingredient are allergic sensitizations. The reactions due to the corticosteroid component in decreasing order of frequency are: elevation of intraocular pressure (IOP) with possible development of glaucoma, and infrequent optic nerve damage; posterior subcapsular cataract formation; and delayed wound healing.
Secondary Infection: The development of secondary infection has occurred after use of combinations containing corticosteroids and antimicrobials. Fungal infections of the cornea are particularly prone to develop coincidentally with long-term applications of corticosteroid. The possibility of fungal invasion must be considered in any persistent corneal ulceration where corticosteroid treatment has been used. Secondary bacterial ocular infection following suppression of host responses also occurs.

DOSAGE AND ADMINISTRATION

The duration of treatment will vary with the type of lesion and may extend from a few days to several weeks, according to therapeutic response. Relapses, more common in chronic active lesions than in self-limited conditions, usually respond to retreatment.
Instill one or two drops of ophthalmic solution NEODECADRON into the conjunctival sac every hour during the day and every two hours during the night as initial therapy. When a favorable response is observed, reduce dosage to one drop every four hours. Later, further reduction in dosage to one drop three or four times daily may suffice to control symptoms.
Not more than 20 milliliters should be prescribed initially and the prescription should not be refilled without further evaluation as outlined in PRECAUTIONS above.

HOW SUPPLIED

Sterile ophthalmic solution NEODECADRON is a clear, colorless to pale yellow solution.
No. 7639—Ophthalmic solution NEODECADRON is supplied as follows:
NDC 0006-7639-03 in 5 mL white opaque, plastic OCUMETER ophthalmic dispenser with a controlled drop tip.
(6505-01-039-4352 0.1% 5 mL).
A.H.F.S. Category: 52:08
DC 7261319 Issued February 1987

NEODECADRON® Topical Cream ℞
(Neomycin Sulfate-Dexamethasone Sodium Phosphate), U.S.P.

DESCRIPTION

NEODECADRON* (Neomycin Sulfate-Dexamethasone Sodium Phosphate) Topical Cream is a topical steroid-antibiotic preparation.
NEODECADRON Topical Cream contains in each gram: dexamethasone sodium phosphate equivalent to 1 mg (0.1%) dexamethasone phosphate, and neomycin sulfate equivalent to 3.5 mg neomycin base, in a greaseless bland base. Inactive ingredients: stearyl alcohol, cetyl alcohol, mineral oil, polyoxyl 40 stearate, sorbitol solution, methyl polysilicone emulsion, creatinine, disodium edetate, sodium citrate, sodium hydroxide to adjust pH, and purified water. Methylparaben 0.15%, sodium bisulfite 0.18%, and sorbic acid 0.1% added as preservatives.
Dexamethasone sodium phosphate is 9-fluoro-11β,17-dihydroxy-16α-methyl-21-(phosphonooxy)pregna-1,4-diene-3,20-dione disodium salt. Its empirical formula is $C_{22}H_{28}FNa_2O_8P$ and its structural formula is:

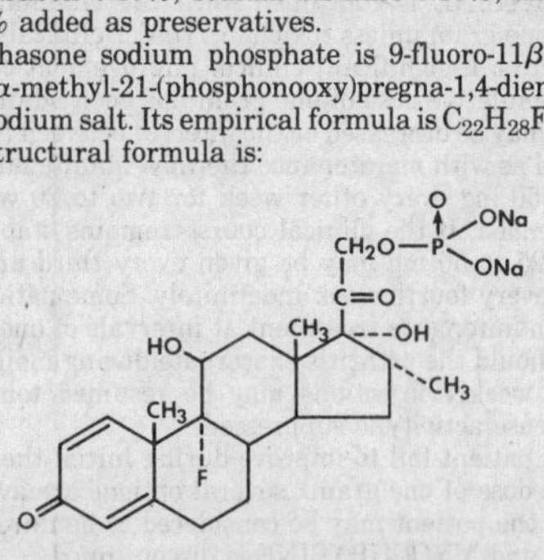

Dexamethasone sodium phosphate has a molecular weight of 516.41.
Glucocorticoids are adrenocortical steroids, both naturally occurring and synthetic. Dexamethasone is a synthetic analog of naturally occurring glucocorticoids (hydrocortisone and cortisone).
Neomycin sulfate is a mixture of the sulfate salts of neomycin, an antibacterial substance produced by the growth of *Streptomyces fradiae* Waksman (Fam. Streptomycetaceae).
Neomycin is a complex typically containing 8–13% neomycin C, less than 0.2% neomycin A and the rest, neomycin B. The empirical formulas and molecular weights for the three components are: neomycin B, $C_{23}H_{46}N_6O_{13}$, molecular weight 614.65; neomycin C, $C_{23}H_{46}N_6O_{13}$, molecular weight 614.65; neomycin A, (also referred to as neamine),

$C_{12}H_{26}N_4O_6$, molecular weight 322.36. The structural formula for neomycin B sulfate is:

neamine

Neomycin B

*Registered trademark of MERCK & CO., INC.

CLINICAL PHARMACOLOGY

Topical corticosteroids share anti-inflammatory, anti-pruritic, and vasoconstrictive actions.

The mechanism of anti-inflammatory activity of the topical corticosteroids is unclear. Various laboratory methods, including vasoconstrictor assays, are used to compare and predict potencies and/or clinical efficacies of the topical corticosteroids. There is some evidence to suggest that a recognizable correlation exists between vasoconstrictor potency and therapeutic efficacy in man.

Pharmacokinetics

The extent of percutaneous absorption of topical corticosteroids is determined by many factors including the vehicle, the integrity of the epidermal barrier, and the use of occlusive dressings.

Topical corticosteroids can be absorbed from normal intact skin. Inflammation and/or other disease processes in the skin increase percutaneous absorption. Occlusive dressings substantially increase the percutaneous absorption of topical corticosteroids. Thus, occlusive dressings may be a valuable therapeutic adjunct for treatment of resistant dermatoses. (See DOSAGE AND ADMINISTRATION.)

Once absorbed through the skin, topical corticosteroids are handled through pharmacokinetic pathways similar to systemically administered corticosteroids. Corticosteroids are bound to plasma proteins in varying degrees. Corticosteroids are metabolized primarily in the liver and are then excreted by the kidneys. Some of the topical corticosteroids and their metabolites are also excreted into the bile.

The antibiotic component, neomycin, is bactericidal to many gram-positive and gram-negative bacteria.

INDICATIONS AND USAGE

For the treatment of corticosteroid-responsive dermatoses with secondary infection. It has not been demonstrated that this steroid-antibiotic combination provides greater benefit than the steroid component alone after 7 days of treatment (see WARNINGS).

CONTRAINDICATIONS

Hypersensitivity to any component of this product, including sulfites (see WARNINGS).

WARNINGS

Topical Cream NEODECADRON contains sodium bisulfite, a sulfite that may cause allergic-type reactions including anaphylactic symptoms and life-threatening or less severe asthmatic episodes in certain susceptible people. The overall prevalence of sulfite sensitivity in the general population is unknown and probably low. Sulfite sensitivity is seen more frequently in asthmatic than in nonasthmatic people.

Because of the concern of nephrotoxicity and ototoxicity associated with neomycin, this combination product should not be used over a wide area or for extended periods of time.

PRECAUTIONS

General

Systemic absorption of topical corticosteroids has produced reversible hypothalamic-pituitary-adrenal (HPA) axis suppression, manifestations of Cushing's syndrome, hyperglycemia, and glycosuria in some patients.

Conditions which augment systemic absorption include the application of the more potent corticosteroids, use over large surface areas, prolonged use, and the addition of occlusive dressings.

Therefore, patients receiving a large dose of a potent topical corticosteroid applied to a large surface area or under an occlusive dressing should be evaluated periodically for evidence of HPA axis suppression by using urinary free cortisol

and ACTH stimulation tests. If HPA axis suppression is noted, an attempt should be made to withdraw the drug, to reduce the frequency of application, or to substitute a less potent corticosteroid.

Recovery of HPA axis function is generally prompt and complete upon discontinuation of the drug. Infrequently, signs and symptoms of corticosteroid withdrawal may occur, requiring supplemental systemic corticosteroids.

Children may absorb proportionally larger amounts of topical corticosteroids and thus be more susceptible to systemic toxicity (see PRECAUTIONS, *Pediatric Use*).

Corticosteroids may mask some signs of infection, and new infections may appear during their use. There may be decreased resistance and inability to localize infection when corticosteroids are used. Therefore, patients with bacterial infections should also be given appropriate antibiotic therapy if Topical Cream NEODECADRON is used. Moreover, corticosteroids may affect the nitroblue-tetrazolium test for bacterial infection and produce false-negative results.

Corticosteroid therapy exerts its major immunosuppressive effects by impairing the normal function of the T-lymphocyte population and macrophages. When T-cell and/or macrophage function is impaired, latent disease may be activated or there may be an exacerbation of intercurrent infections due to pathogens, including those caused by Candida, Mycobacterium, Ameba, Toxoplasma, Strongyloides, Pneumocystis, Cryptococcus, Nocardia, etc. Products containing steroids should be used with caution in patients with impaired T-cell function or in patients receiving other immunosuppressive therapy.

In the presence of dermatological infections, the use of an appropriate antifungal or antibacterial agent should be instituted. If a favorable response does not occur promptly, the corticosteroid should be discontinued until the infection has been adequately controlled.

If irritation develops, topical corticosteroids should be discontinued and appropriate therapy instituted.

This product is not for ophthalmic use. However, if applied to the eyelids or skin near the eyes, the drug may enter the eyes. In patients with a history of herpes simplex keratitis, ocular exposure to corticosteroids may lead to a recurrence. Prolonged ocular exposure may cause steroid glaucoma.

A few individuals may be sensitive to one or more of the components of this product. Sensitivity to neomycin may occasionally develop, especially when it is applied to abraded skin. If any reaction indicating sensitivity is observed, discontinue use. There are reports in the current medical literature that indicate an increase in the prevalence of persons sensitive to neomycin.

Generally, occlusive dressings should not be used on weeping or exudative lesions.

If the occlusive dressing technique is employed, caution should be exercised with regard to the use of plastic films which are often inflammable and may pose a suffocation hazard for children.

When large areas of the body are covered with an occlusive dressing, thermal homeostasis may be impaired. If elevation of body temperature occurs, use of the occlusive dressing should be discontinued.

Information for the Patient

Patients using topical corticosteroids should receive the following information and instructions:

1. This medication is to be used as directed by the physician. It is for external use only. Avoid contact with the eyes.
2. Patients should be advised not to use this medication for any disorder other than that for which it was prescribed.
3. The treated skin area should not be bandaged or otherwise covered or wrapped so as to be occlusive unless directed by the physician.
4. Patients should report any signs of local adverse reactions, especially under occlusive dressings.
5. Parents of pediatric patients should be advised not to use tight-fitting diapers or plastic pants on a child being treated in the diaper area, as these garments may constitute occlusive dressings.

Laboratory Tests

The following tests may be helpful in evaluating the HPA axis suppression:

- Urinary free cortisol test
- ACTH stimulation test

Carcinogenesis, Mutagenesis and Impairment of Fertility

Long-term animal studies have not been performed to evaluate the carcinogenic potential or the effect on fertility of Topical Cream NEODECADRON.

Studies to determine mutagenicity with prednisolone and hydrocortisone have revealed negative results.

Pregnancy

Pregnancy Category C: Corticosteroids are generally teratogenic in laboratory animals when administered systemically at relatively low dosage levels. The more potent corticosteroids have been shown to be teratogenic after dermal application in laboratory animals. There are no adequate and well controlled studies in pregnant women on teratogenic effects from topically applied corticosteroids. Therefore, topical corticosteroids should be used during pregnancy only if the potential benefit justifies the potential risk to the fetus.

Drugs of this class should not be used extensively on pregnant patients, in large amounts, or for prolonged periods of time.

Nursing Mothers

It is not known whether topical administration of corticosteroids could result in sufficient systemic absorption to produce detectable quantities in breast milk. Systemically administered corticosteroids are secreted into breast milk in quantities *not* likely to have a deleterious effect on the infant. Nevertheless, caution should be exercised when topical corticosteroids are administered to a nursing woman.

Pediatric Use

Pediatric patients may demonstrate greater susceptibility to topical corticosteroid-induced HPA axis suppression and Cushing's syndrome than mature patients bcause of a larger skin surface area to body weight ratio.

Hypothalamic-pituitary-adrenal (HPA) axis suppression, Cushing's syndrome, and intracranial hypertension have been reported in children receiving topical corticosteroids. Manifestations of adrenal suppression in children include linear growth retardation, delayed weight gain, low plasma cortisol levels, and absence of response to ACTH stimulation. Manifestations of intracranial hypertension include bulging fontanelles, headaches, and bilateral papilledema.

Administration of topical corticosteroids to children should be limited to the least amount compatible with an effective therapeutic regimen. Chronic corticosteroid therapy may interfere with the growth and development of children.

ADVERSE REACTIONS

The following adverse reactions are reported infrequently with topical corticosteroids, but may occur more frequently with the use of occlusive dressings. These reactions are listed in an approximate decreasing order of occurrence:

Burning
Itching
Irritation
Dryness
Folliculitis
Hypertrichosis
Acneiform eruptions
Hypopigmentation
Perioral dermatitis
Allergic contact dermatitis
Maceration of the skin
Secondary infection
Skin atrophy
Striae
Miliaria

Prevalence of neomycin hypersensitivity is increasing. Ototoxicity and nephrotoxicity have been reported with prolonged use or use of large amounts of topical neomycin preparations.

OVERDOSAGE

Topically applied corticosteroids can be absorbed in sufficient amounts to produce systemic effects (see PRECAUTIONS).

DOSAGE AND ADMINISTRATION

Apply to the affected area as a thin film three or four times daily.

Before using NEODECADRON Topical Cream in the *ear*, clean the aural canal thoroughly and sponge dry. Confirm that the eardrum is intact. With a cotton-tipped applicator, apply a thin coating of the cream to the affected canal area two or three times a day. When a favorable response is obtained, reduce the number of daily applications to one or two, and eventually discontinue.

HOW SUPPLIED

No. 7607—Topical Cream NEODECADRON is a white cream, and is supplied as follows:
NDC 0006-7607-12 in 15 g tubes
NDC 0006-7607-24 in 30 g tubes
A.H.F.S. Category: 84:06
DC 7612427 Issued October 1989
COPYRIGHT © MERCK & CO. INC., 1985
All rights reserved

Continued on next page

Merck & Co.—Cont.

NOROXIN® Tablets ℞
(Norfloxacin), U.S.P.

DESCRIPTION

NOROXIN* (Norfloxacin) is a synthetic, broad-spectrum antibacterial agent for oral administration. Norfloxacin, a fluoroquinolone, is 1-ethyl-6-fluoro-1,4-dihydro-4-oxo-7-(1-piperazinyl)-3-quinolinecarboxylic acid. Its empirical formula is $C_{16}H_{18}FN_3O_3$ and the structural formula is:

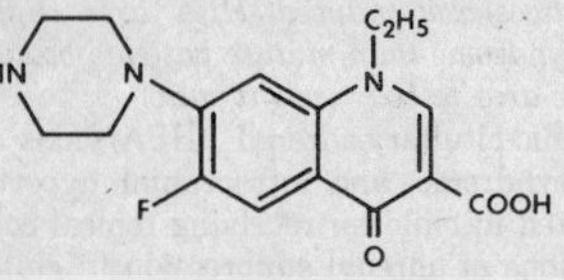

Norfloxacin is a white to pale yellow crystalline powder with a molecular weight of 319.34 and a melting point of about 221°C. It is freely soluble in glacial acetic acid, and very slightly soluble in ethanol, methanol and water.
NOROXIN is available in 400-mg tablets. Each tablet contains the following inactive ingredients: cellulose, croscarmellose sodium, hydroxypropyl cellulose, hydroxypropyl methylcellulose, iron oxide, magnesium stearate, and titanium dioxide.
Norfloxacin, a fluoroquinolone, differs from non-fluorinated quinolones by having a fluorine atom at the 6 position and a piperazine moiety at the 7 position.

*Registered trademark of MERCK & CO., INC.

CLINICAL PHARMACOLOGY

In fasting healthy volunteers, at least 30–40% of an oral dose of NOROXIN is absorbed. Absorption is rapid following single doses of 200 mg, 400 mg and 800 mg. At the respective doses, mean peak serum and plasma concentrations of 0.8, 1.5 and 2.4 mcg/mL are attained approximately one hour after dosing. The presence of food may decrease absorption. The effective half-life of norfloxacin in serum and plasma is 3–4 hours. Steady-state concentrations of norfloxacin will be attained within two days of dosing.
In healthy elderly volunteers (65–75 years of age with normal renal function for their age), norfloxacin is eliminated more slowly because of their slightly decreased renal function. Drug absorption appears unaffected. However, the effective half-life of norfloxacin in these elderly subjects is 4 hours.
The disposition of norfloxacin in patients with creatinine clearance rates greater than 30 mL/min/1.73m^2 is similar to that in healthy volunteers. In patients with creatinine clearance rates equal to or less than 30 mL/min/1.73m^2, the renal elimination of norfloxacin decreases so that the effective serum half-life is 6.5 hours. In these patients, alteration of dosage is necessary (see DOSAGE AND ADMINISTRATION). Drug absorption appears unaffected by decreasing renal function.
Norfloxacin is eliminated through metabolism, biliary excretion, and renal excretion. After a single 400-mg dose of NOROXIN, mean antimicrobial activities equivalent to 278, 773, and 82 mcg of norfloxacin/g of feces were obtained at 12, 24, and 48 hours, respectively. Renal excretion occurs by both glomerular filtration and tubular secretion as evidenced by the high rate of renal clearance (approximately 275 mL/min). Within 24 hours of drug administration, 26 to 32% of the administered dose is recovered in the urine as norfloxacin with an additional 5–8% being recovered in the urine as six active metabolites of lesser antimicrobial potency. Only a small percentage (less than 1%) of the dose is recovered thereafter. Fecal recovery accounts for another 30% of the administered dose.
Two to three hours after a single 400-mg dose, urinary concentrations of 200 mcg/mL or more are attained in the urine. In healthy volunteers, mean urinary concentrations of norfloxacin remain above 30 mcg/mL for at least 12 hours following a 400-mg dose. The urinary pH may affect the solubility of norfloxacin. Norfloxacin is least soluble at urinary pH of 7.5 with greater solubility occurring at pHs above and below this value. The serum protein binding of norfloxacin is between 10 and 15%.
The following are mean concentrations of norfloxacin in various fluids and tissues measured 1 to 4 hours post-dose after two 400-mg doses, unless otherwise indicated:

Renal Parenchyma	7.3 μg/g
Prostate	2.5 μg/g
Seminal Fluid	2.7 μg/mL
Testicle	1.6 μg/g
Uterus/Cervix	3.0 μg/g
Vagina	4.3 μg/g
Fallopian Tube	1.9 μg/g
Bile	6.9 μg/mL (after two 200-mg doses)

Microbiology
Norfloxacin has *in vitro* activity against a broad range of gram-positive and gram-negative aerobic bacteria. The fluorine atom at the 6 position provides increased potency against gram-negative organisms, and the piperazine moiety at the 7 position is responsible for anti-pseudomonal activity.
Norfloxacin inhibits bacterial deoxyribonucleic acid synthesis and is bactericidal. At the molecular level, three specific events are attributed to norfloxacin in *E. coli* cells:
1) inhibition of the ATP-dependent DNA supercoiling reaction catalyzed by DNA gyrase,
2) inhibition of the relaxation of supercoiled DNA,
3) promotion of double-stranded DNA breakage.
Resistance to norfloxacin due to spontaneous mutation *in vitro* is a rare occurrence (range: 10^{-9} to 10^{-12} cells). Resistant organisms have emerged during therapy with norfloxacin in less than 1% of patients treated. Organisms in which development of resistance is greatest are the following:
Pseudomonas aeruginosa
Klebsiella pneumoniae
Acinetobacter species
Enterococcus species
For this reason, when there is a lack of satisfactory clinical response, repeat culture and susceptibility testing should be done. Nalidixic acid-resistant organisms are generally susceptible to norfloxacin *in vitro;* however, these organisms may have higher MICs to norfloxacin than nalidixic acid-susceptible strains. There is generally no cross-resistance between norfloxacin and other classes of antibacterial agents. Therefore, norfloxacin may demonstrate activity against indicated organisms resistant to some other antimicrobial agents including the aminoglycosides, penicillins, cephalosporins, tetracyclines, macrolides, and sulfonamides, including combinations of sulfamethoxazole and trimethoprim. Antagonism has been demonstrated *in vitro* between norfloxacin and nitrofurantoin.
Norfloxacin has been shown to be active against most strains of the following organisms both *in vitro* and in clinical infections (see INDICATIONS AND USAGE):
Gram-positive aerobes:
Enterococcus faecalis
Staphylococcus aureus
Staphylococcus epidermidis
Staphylococcus saprophyticus
Streptococcus agalactiae
Gram-negative aerobes:
Citrobacter freundii
Enterobacter aerogenes
Enterobacter cloacae
Escherichia coli
Klebsiella pneumoniae
Neisseria gonorrhoeae
Proteus mirabilis
Proteus vulgaris
Pseudomonas aeruginosa
Serratia marcescens
Norfloxacin has been shown to be active *in vitro* against most strains of the following organisms; however, the clinical significance of these data is unknown.
Gram-positive aerobes:
Bacillus cereus
Gram-negative aerobes:
Acinetobacter calcoaceticus
Aeromonas species
Alcaligenes species
Campylobacter species
Citrobacter diversus
Edwardsiella tarda
Flavobacterium species
Hafnia alvei
Klebsiella oxytoca
Klebsiella rhinoscleromatis
Morganella morganii
Providencia alcalifaciens
Providencia rettgeri
Providencia stuartii
Salmonella species
Shigella species
Vibrio cholerae
Vibrio parahemolyticus
Yersinia enterocolitica
Other:
Ureaplasma urealyticum
NOROXIN is not generally active against obligate anaerobes.
Norfloxacin has not been shown to be active against *Treponema pallidum*. (See WARNINGS.)
Susceptibility Tests
Diffusion Techniques: Quantitative methods that require measurement of zone diameters give the most precise estimate of the susceptibility of bacteria to antimicrobial agents. One such procedure is the National Committee for Clinical Laboratory Standards (NCCLS) approved procedure (M2-A4–Performance Standards for Antimicrobial Disk Susceptibility Tests 1990). This method has been recommended for use with the 10-mcg norfloxacin disk to test susceptibility to norfloxacin. Interpretation involves correlation of the diameters obtained in the disk test with minimum inhibitory concentration (MIC) for norfloxacin. Reports from the laboratory giving results of the standard single-disk susceptibility test with a 10-mcg norfloxacin disk should be interpreted according to the following criteria **(these criteria only apply to isolates from urinary tract infections):**

Zone diameter (mm)	Interpretation
≥17	(S) Susceptible
13–16	(I) Intermediate
≤12	(R) Resistant

A report of "Susceptible" indicates that the pathogen is likely to be inhibited by generally achievable urine levels. A report of "Intermediate" indicates that the test results be considered equivocal or indeterminate. A report of "Resistant" indicates that achievable concentrations of the antibiotic are unlikely to be inhibitory and other therapy should be selected.
Standardized procedures require the use of laboratory control organisms. The 10-mcg norfloxacin disk should give the following zone diameter:

Organism	Zone diameter (mm)
E. coli ATCC 25922	28–35
P. aeruginosa ATCC 27853	22–29
S. aureus ATCC 25923	17–28

Other quinolone antibacterial disks should not be substituted when performing susceptibility tests for norfloxacin because of spectrum differences with norfloxacin. The 10-mcg norfloxacin disk should be used for all *in vitro* testing of isolates using diffusion techniques.
Dilution Techniques: Broth and agar dilution methods, such as those recommended by the NCCLS (M7-A2—Methods for Dilution Antimicrobial Susceptibility Tests for Bacteria that Grow Aerobically 1990), may be used to determine the minimum inhibitory concentration (MIC) of norfloxacin. MIC test results should be interpreted according to the following criteria **(these criteria only apply to isolates from urinary tract infections):**

MIC (mcg/mL)	Interpretation
≤4	(S) Susceptible
8	(I) Intermediate
≥16	(R) Resistant

As with standard diffusion methods, dilution procedures require the use of laboratory control organisms. Standard norfloxacin powder should give the following MIC values:

Organism	MIC range (mcg/mL)
E. coli ATCC 25922	0.03–0.12
E. faecalis ATCC 29212	2.0–8.0
P. aeruginosa ATCC 27853	1.0–4.0
S. aureus ATCC 29213	0.05–2.0

INDICATIONS AND USAGE

NOROXIN is indicated for the treatment of adults with the following infections caused by susceptible strains of the designated microorganisms:
Urinary tract infections:
Uncomplicated urinary tract infections (including cystitis) due to *Enterococcus faecalis, Escherichia coli, Klebsiella pneumoniae, Proteus mirabilis, Pseudomonas aeruginosa, Staphylococcus epidermidis, Staphylococcus saprophyticus, Citrobacter freundii**, *Enterobacter aerogenes**, *Enterobacter cloacae**, *Proteus vulgaris**, *Staphylococcus aureus**, or *Streptococcus agalactiae**.
Complicated urinary tract infections due to *Enterococcus faecalis, Escherichia coli, Klebsiella pneumoniae, Proteus mirabilis, Pseudomonas aeruginosa,* or *Serratia marcescens**.
Sexually transmitted diseases (See WARNINGS.):
Uncomplicated urethral and cervical gonorrhea due to *Neisseria gonorrhoeae.*
(See DOSAGE AND ADMINISTRATION for appropriate dosing instructions.)
Penicillinase production should have no effect on norfloxacin activity.
Appropriate culture and susceptibility tests should be performed before treatment in order to isolate and identify organisms causing the infection and to determine their susceptibility to norfloxacin. Therapy with norfloxacin may be initiated before results of these tests are known; once results become available, appropriate therapy should be given. Repeat culture and susceptibility testing performed periodically during therapy will provide information not only on the therapeutic effect of the antimicrobial agents but also on the possible emergence of bacterial resistance.

*Efficacy for this organism in this organ system was studied in fewer than 10 infections.

CONTRAINDICATIONS

NOROXIN is contraindicated in patients with a history of hypersensitivity to norfloxacin or the other members of the quinolone group of antibacterial agents.

WARNINGS

THE SAFETY AND EFFICACY OF ORAL NORFLOXACIN IN CHILDREN, ADOLESCENTS (UNDER THE AGE OF 18), PREGNANT WOMEN, AND NURSING MOTHERS HAVE NOT BEEN ESTABLISHED. (See PRECAUTIONS—*Pregnancy, Nursing Mothers* and *Pediatric Use.*) The oral administration of single doses of norfloxacin, 6 times† the recommended human clinical dose (on a mg/kg basis), caused lameness in immature dogs. Histologic examination of the weight-bearing joints of these dogs revealed permanent lesions of the cartilage. Other quinolones also produced erosions of the cartilage in weight-bearing joints and other signs of arthropathy in immature animals of various species. (See ANIMAL PHARMACOLOGY.)

Norfloxacin has not been shown to be effective in the treatment of syphilis. Antimicrobial agents used in high doses for short periods of time to treat gonorrhea may mask or delay the symptoms of incubating syphilis. All patients with gonorrhea should have a serologic test for syphilis at the time of diagnosis. Patients treated with norfloxacin should have a follow-up serologic test for syphilis after three months.

Serious and occasionally fatal hypersensitivity (anaphylactoid or anaphylactic) reactions, some following the first dose, have been reported in patients receiving quinolone therapy. Some reactions were accompanied by cardiovascular collapse, loss of consciousness, tingling, pharyngeal or facial edema, dyspnea, urticaria and itching. Only a few patients had a history of hypersensitivity reactions. If an allergic reaction to norfloxacin occurs, discontinue the drug. Serious acute hypersensitivity reactions may require immediate emergency treatment with epinephrine. Oxygen, intravenous fluids, antihistamines, corticosteroids, pressor amines, and airway management, including intubation, should be administered as indicated.

Convulsions have been reported in patients receiving norfloxacin. Convulsions, increased intracranial pressure, and toxic psychoses have been reported in patients receiving drugs in this class. Quinolones may also cause central nervous system (CNS) stimulation which may lead to tremors, restlessness, lightheadedness, confusion, and hallucinations. If these reactions occur in patients receiving norfloxacin, the drug should be discontinued and appropriate measures instituted.

The effects of norfloxacin on brain function or on the electrical activity of the brain have not been tested. Therefore, until more information becomes available, norfloxacin, like all other quinolones, should be used with caution in patients with known or suspected CNS disorders, such as severe cerebral arteriosclerosis, epilepsy, and other factors which predispose to seizures. (See ADVERSE REACTIONS.)

†Based on a patient weight of 50 kg.

PRECAUTIONS

General:

Needle-shaped crystals were found in the urine of some volunteers who received either placebo, 800 mg norfloxacin, or 1600 mg norfloxacin (at or twice the recommended daily dose, respectively) while participating in a double-blind, crossover study comparing single doses of norfloxacin with placebo. While crystalluria is not expected to occur under usual conditions with a dosage regimen of 400 mg b.i.d., as a precaution, the daily recommended dosage should not be exceeded and the patient should drink sufficient fluids to ensure a proper state of hydration and adequate urinary output.

Alteration in dosage regimen is necessary for patients with impaired renal function (see DOSAGE AND ADMINISTRATION).

Moderate to severe phototoxicity reactions have been observed in patients who are exposed to excessive sunlight while receiving some members of this drug class. Excessive sunlight should be avoided. Therapy should be discontinued if phototoxicity occurs.

Information for Patients

Patients should be advised:

—to drink fluids liberally.

—that norfloxacin should be taken at least one hour before or at least two hours after a meal.

—that multivitamins or other products containing iron or zinc, or antacids should not be taken within the two-hour period before or within the two-hour period after taking norfloxacin. (See *Drug Interactions.*)

—that norfloxacin can cause dizziness and lightheadedness and, therefore, patients should know how they react to norfloxacin before they operate an automobile or machinery or engage in activities requiring mental alertness and coordination.

—that norfloxacin may be associated with hypersensitivity reactions, even following the first dose, and to discontinue the drug at the first sign of a skin rash or other allergic reaction.

—to avoid undue exposure to excessive sunlight while receiving norfloxacin and to discontinue therapy if phototoxicity occurs.

—that some quinolones may increase the effects of theophylline and/or caffeine. (See *Drug Interactions.*)

Drug Interactions

Elevated plasma levels of theophylline have been reported with concomitant quinolone use. There have been reports of theophylline-related side effects in patients on concomitant therapy with norfloxacin and theophylline. Therefore, monitoring of theophylline plasma levels should be considered and dosage of theophylline adjusted as required.

Elevated serum levels of cyclosporine have been reported with concomitant use of cyclosporine with norfloxacin. Therefore cyclosporine serum levels should be monitored and appropriate cyclosporine dosage adjustments made when these drugs are used concomitantly.

Quinolones, including norfloxacin, may enhance the effects of the oral anticoagulant warfarin or its derivatives. When these products are administered concomitantly, prothrombin time or other suitable coagulation tests should be closely monitored.

Diminished urinary excretion of norfloxacin has been reported during the concomitant administration of probenecid and norfloxacin.

The concomitant use of nitrofurantoin is not recommended since nitrofurantoin may antagonize the antibacterial effect of NOROXIN in the urinary tract.

Multivitamins, or other products containing iron or zinc, antacids or sucralfate should not be administered concomitantly with, or within 2 hours of, the administration of norfloxacin, because they may interfere with absorption resulting in lower serum and urine levels of norfloxacin.

Some quinolones have also been shown to interfere with the metabolism of caffeine. This may lead to reduced clearance of caffeine and a prolongation of its plasma half-life.

Carcinogenesis, Mutagenesis, Impairment of Fertility

No increase in neoplastic changes was observed with norfloxacin as compared to controls in a study in rats, lasting up to 96 weeks at doses 8–9 times† the usual human dose (on a mg/kg basis).

Norfloxacin was tested for mutagenic activity in a number of *in vivo* and *in vitro* tests. Norfloxacin had no mutagenic effect in the dominant lethal test in mice and did not cause chromosomal aberrations in hamsters or rats at doses 30–60 times† the usual human dose (on a mg/kg basis). Norfloxacin had no mutagenic activity *in vitro* in the Ames microbial mutagen test, Chinese hamster fibroblasts and V-79 mammalian cell assay. Although norfloxacin was weakly positive in the Rec-assay for DNA repair, all other mutagenic assays were negative including a more sensitive test (V-79).

Norfloxacin did not adversely affect the fertility of male and female mice at oral doses up to 30 times† the usual human dose (on a mg/kg basis).

Pregnancy

Teratogenic Effects. Pregnancy Category C. Norfloxacin has been shown to produce embryonic loss in monkeys when given in doses 10 times† the maximum daily total human dose (on a mg/kg basis). At this dose, peak plasma levels obtained in monkeys were approximately 2 times those obtained in humans. There has been no evidence of a teratogenic effect in any of the animal species tested (rat, rabbit, mouse, monkey) at 6–50 times† the maximum daily human dose (on a mg/kg basis). There are, however, no adequate and well controlled studies in pregnant women. Norfloxacin should be used during pregnancy only if the potential benefit justifies the potential risk to the fetus.

Nursing Mothers

It is not known whether norfloxacin is excreted in human milk.

When a 200-mg dose of NOROXIN was administered to nursing mothers, norfloxacin was not detected in human milk. However, because the dose studied was low, because other drugs in this class are secreted in human milk, and because of the potential for serious adverse reactions from norfloxacin in nursing infants, a decision should be made to discontinue nursing or to discontinue the drug, taking into account the importance of the drug to the mother.

Pediatric Use

The safety and effectiveness of oral norfloxacin in children and adolescents below the age of 18 years have not been established. Norfloxacin causes arthropathy in juvenile animals of several animal species. (See WARNINGS and ANIMAL PHARMACOLOGY.)

†Based on a patient weight of 50 kg.

ADVERSE REACTIONS

Urinary Tract Infections

In clinical trials involving 1869 patients/subjects, 3.5% reported drug-related adverse experiences. However, the incidence figures below were calculated without reference to drug relationship.

The most common adverse experiences (>1%) were: nausea (4.3%), headache (2.9%), dizziness (1.8%), and fatigue (1.1%).

Additional reactions (0.3%–1%) were: rash, abdominal pain, dyspepsia, somnolence, depression, insomnia, constipation, flatulence, heartburn, dry mouth, diarrhea, fever, vomiting, pruritus, loose stools, back pain and hyperhidrosis.

Less frequent reactions included: erythema, anorexia, bitter taste, and asthenia.

Abnormal laboratory values observed in these patient/subjects were: elevation of ALT (SGPT) (1.6%), decreased WBC and neutrophil count (1.6%), elevation of AST (SGOT) (1.4%), eosinophilia (1.4%), and increased alkaline phosphatase (1.2%). Those occurring less frequently included increased BUN, serum creatinine, and LDH, and decreased hematocrit.

Gonorrhea

In clinical trials involving 228 patients who received a single 800-mg dose, 7.0% of patients reported drug-related adverse experiences. However, the following incidence figures were calculated without reference to drug relationship.

The most common adverse experiences (1%–3.5%) were: dizziness (3.5%), nausea (2.2%), abdominal cramping (1.8%), diarrhea (1.3%), anorexia (1.3%), headache (1.3%), and hyperhidrosis (1.3%).

Additional reactions (0.3%–1%) were: vomiting, constipation, dyspepsia, and tingling of the fingers.

Laboratory adverse changes considered drug-related were reported in 2.2% of patients who received a single 800-mg dose of norfloxacin. These laboratory changes were: decreased hemoglobin and hematocrit (0.9%), decreased platelet count (0.9%), and increased AST (0.4%).

Post Marketing

The most frequently reported adverse reaction in post-marketing experience is rash.

CNS effects characterized as generalized seizures and myoclonus have been reported with NOROXIN. A causal relationship to NOROXIN has not been established (see WARNINGS). Visual disturbances have been reported with drugs in this class.

The following additional adverse reactions have been reported since the drug was marketed:

Hypersensitivity Reactions

Hypersensitivity reactions have been reported including anaphylactoid reactions, angioedema, dyspnea, vasculitis, urticaria, arthritis, arthralgia and myalgia (see WARNINGS).

Skin

Toxic epidermal necrolysis, Stevens-Johnson syndrome and erythema multiforme, exfoliative dermatitis, pruritus, photosensitivity

Gastrointestinal

Pseudomembranous colitis, hepatitis, jaundice, including cholestatic jaundice, pancreatitis (rare), stomatitis, anorexia

Renal

Interstitial nephritis, renal failure

Nervous System/Psychiatric

Neurologic changes such as ataxia, diplopia and weakness, possible exacerbation of myasthenia gravis, psychic disturbances including psychotic reactions and confusion, paresthesia

Hematologic

Neutropenia, leukopenia, thrombocytopenia

Special Senses

Transient hearing loss (rare), tinnitus

Other adverse events reported with quinolones include: agranulocytosis, albuminuria, candiduria, crystalluria, cylindruria, dysphagia, elevation of blood glucose, elevation of serum cholesterol, elevation of serum potassium, elevation of serum triglycerides, hematuria, hepatic necrosis, nystagmus, postural hypotension, prolongation of prothrombin time, and vaginal candidiasis.

OVERDOSAGE

No significant lethality was observed in male and female mice and rats at single oral doses up to 4 g/kg.

In the event of acute overdosage, the stomach should be emptied by inducing vomiting or by gastric lavage, and the patient carefully observed and given symptomatic and supportive treatment. Adequate hydration must be maintained.

DOSAGE AND ADMINISTRATION

Tablets NOROXIN should be taken at least one hour before or at least two hours after a meal with a glass of water. Patients receiving NOROXIN should be well hydrated (see PRECAUTIONS).

Continued on next page

Information on the Merck & Co. products listed on these pages is the full prescribing information from product circulars in use October 1, 1992.

Merck & Co.—Cont.

Normal Renal Function

The recommended daily dose of NOROXIN is as described in the following chart:

[See table at right.]

Renal Impairment

NOROXIN may be used for the treatment of urinary tract infections in patients with renal insufficiency. In patients with a creatinine clearance rate of 30 mL/min/1.73m² or less, the recommended dosage is one 400-mg tablet once daily for the duration given above. At this dosage, the urinary concentration exceeds the MICs for most urinary pathogens susceptible to norfloxacin, even when the creatinine clearance is less than 10 mL/min/1.73m².

When only the serum creatinine level is available, the following formula (based on sex, weight, and age of the patient) may be used to convert this value into creatinine clearance. The serum creatinine should represent a steady state of renal function.

Males: $= \dfrac{\text{(weight in kg)} \times (140 - \text{age})}{(72) \times \text{serum creatinine (mg/100 mL)}}$

Females: $= (0.85) \times \text{(above value)}$

Elderly

Elderly patients being treated for urinary tract infections who have a creatinine clearance of greater than 30 mL/min/1.73m² should receive the dosages recommended under *Normal Renal Function.*

Elderly patients being treated for urinary tract infections who have a creatinine clearance of 30 mL/min/1.73m² or less should receive 400 mg once daily as recommended under *Renal Impairment.*

HOW SUPPLIED

No. 3522—Tablets NOROXIN 400 mg are dark pink, oval shaped, film-coated tablets, coded MSD 705 on one side and NOROXIN on the other. They are supplied as follows:

NDC 0006-0705-68 bottles of 100
(6505-01-258-9542 100's)
NDC 0006-0705-20 unit of use bottles of 20
NDC 0006-0705-28 unit dose packages of 100.

Storage

Tablets NOROXIN should be stored in a tightly-closed container. Avoid storage at temperatures above 40°C (104°F).

ANIMAL PHARMACOLOGY

Norfloxacin and related drugs have been shown to cause arthropathy in immature animals of most species tested (see WARNINGS).

Crystalluria has occurred in laboratory animals tested with norfloxacin. In dogs, needle-shaped drug crystals were seen in the urine at doses of 50 mg/kg/day. In rats, crystals were reported following doses of 200 mg/kg/day.

Embryo lethality and slight maternotoxicity (vomiting and anorexia) were observed in cynomolgus monkeys at doses of 150 mg/kg/day or higher.

Ocular toxicity, seen with some related drugs, was not observed in any norfloxacin-treated animals.

A.H.F.S. Category: 8:22
DC 7455415   Issued May 1992
COPYRIGHT © MERCK & CO., INC., 1986, 1989
All rights reserved

Shown in Product Identification Section, page 420

PedvaxHIB®   ℞
[Haemophilus b Conjugate Vaccine
(Meningococcal Protein Conjugate), MSD]

DESCRIPTION

PedvaxHIB* [Haemophilus b Conjugate Vaccine (Meningococcal Protein Conjugate), MSD] is a highly purified capsular polysaccharide (polyribosylribitol phosphate or PRP) of *Haemophilus influenzae* type b (Haemophilus b, Ross strain) that is covalently bound to an outer membrane protein complex (OMPC) of the B11 strain of *Neisseria meningitidis* serogroup B. The covalent bonding of the PRP to the OMPC which is necessary for enhanced immunogenicity of the PRP is confirmed by analysis of the conjugate's components by chemical treatment which yields a unique amino acid. This PRP-OMPC conjugate vaccine is a lyophilized preparation containing lactose as a stabilizer.

PedvaxHIB, when reconstituted as directed, is a sterile suspension for intramuscular use formulated to contain: 15 mcg of Haemophilus b PRP, 250 mcg of *Neisseria meningitidis* OMPC, 225 mcg of aluminum as aluminum hydroxide, thimerosal (a mercury derivative) at 1:20,000 as a preservative, and 2.0 mg of lactose, in 0.9% sodium chloride.

* Registered trademark of MERCK & CO., INC.

CLINICAL PHARMACOLOGY

Haemophilus influenzae type b (Haemophilus b) is the most frequent cause of bacterial meningitis and a leading cause of serious, systemic bacterial disease in young children worldwide.

Haemophilus b disease occurs primarily in children under 5 years of age and in the United States prior to the initiation of a vaccine program was estimated to account for nearly 20,000 cases of invasive infections annually, approximately 12,000 of which are meningitis. The mortality rate from Haemophilus b meningitis is about 5%. In addition, up to 35% of survivors develop neurologic sequelae including seizures, deafness, and mental retardation. Other invasive diseases caused by this bacterium include cellulitis, epiglottitis, sepsis, pneumonia, septic arthritis, osteomyelitis and pericarditis.

It has been estimated that 17% of all cases of Haemophilus b disease occur in infants less than 6 months of age. The peak incidence of Haemophilus b meningitis occurs between 6 to 11 months of age. Forty-seven percent of all cases occur by one year of age with the remaining 53% of cases occurring over the next four years.

Among children under 5 years of age, the risk of invasive Haemophilus b disease is further increased in certain populations including the following:

• Daycare attendees
• Lower socio-economic groups
• Blacks (especially those who lack the Km(1) immunoglobulin allotype)
• Caucasians who lack the G2m(n or 23) immunoglobulin allotype
• Native Americans
• Household contacts of cases
• Individuals with asplenia, sickle cell disease, or antibody deficiency syndromes

An important virulence factor of the Haemophilus b bacterium is its polysaccharide capsule (PRP). Antibody to PRP (anti-PRP) has been shown to correlate with protection against Haemophilus b disease. While the anti-PRP level associated with protection using conjugated vaccines has not yet been determined, the level of anti-PRP associated with protection in studies using bacterial polysaccharide immune globulin or nonconjugated PRP vaccines ranged from ≥ 0.15 to ≥ 1.0 mcg/mL.

Nonconjugated PRP vaccines are capable of stimulating B-lymphocytes to produce antibody without the help of T-lymphocytes (T-independent). The responses to many other antigens are augmented by helper T-lymphocytes (T-dependent). PedvaxHIB is a PRP-conjugate vaccine in which the PRP is covalently bound to the OMPC carrier producing an antigen which is postulated to convert the T-independent antigen (PRP alone) into a T-dependent antigen resulting in both an enhanced antibody response and immunologic memory.

Clinical Evaluation of PedvaxHIB

The protective efficacy, safety, and antibody responses to PedvaxHIB were evaluated in 3,486 Native American (Navajo) infants who completed the primary two-dose regimen in a randomized, double-blind, placebo-controlled study (The Protective Efficacy Study). This population has a much higher incidence of Haemophilus b disease than the United States population as a whole and also has a lower antibody response to Haemophilus b conjugate vaccines, including PedvaxHIB.

Each infant in this study received two doses of either placebo or PedvaxHIB with the first dose administered at a mean of 8 weeks of age and the second administered approximately two months later; DTP and OPV were administered concomitantly. Antibody levels were measured in a subset of each group (Table 1). [See table below.]

In this study, 22 cases of invasive Haemophilus b disease occurred in the placebo group (8 cases after the first dose and 14 cases after the second dose) and only 1 case in the vaccine group (none after the first dose and 1 after the second dose). Following the recommended two-dose regimen, the protective efficacy of PedvaxHIB was calculated to be 93% with a 95% confidence interval of 57%–98% (p = 0.001, two-tailed). In the two months between the first and second doses, the difference in number of cases of disease between placebo and vaccine recipients (8 vs 0 cases, respectively) was statistically significant (p = 0.008, two-tailed); however, a primary two-dose regimen is required for infants 2–14 months of age. A subset of 1,368 infants from this study was followed to 15 months of age with no additional cases of invasive Haemophilus b disease occurring after the primary two-dose regimen of PedvaxHIB (see DOSAGE AND ADMINISTRATION, including *Booster Dose*).

Since protective efficacy with PedvaxHIB was demonstrated in such a high risk population, it would be expected to be predictive of efficacy in other populations.

The safety and immunogenicity of PedvaxHIB were evaluated in infants and children in other clinical studies that were conducted in various locations throughout the United States. PedvaxHIB was highly immunogenic in all age groups studied.

Antibody responses from these clinical studies (excluding Native Americans) are shown in Table 2. These data were derived by evaluating the sera in one laboratory using a radioimmunoassay which correlated with both the Finnish National Public Health Institute assay and that recommended by the Center for Biologics Evaluation and Research of the FDA (Table 1, Table 2). [See table 2 next page.]

Since the magnitude of initial antibody response is lower among younger infants, a booster dose is required in infants

Infection	Description	Unit Dose	Frequency	Duration	Daily Dose
Urinary Tract	Uncomplicated UTI's (cystitis) due to *E. coli,* *K. pneumoniae,* or *P. mirabilis*	400 mg	q12h	3 days	800 mg
	Uncomplicated UTI's due to other indicated organisms	400 mg	q12h	7–10 days	800 mg
	Complicated UTI's	400 mg	q12h	10–21 days	800 mg
Sexually Transmitted Diseases	Uncomplicated Gonorrhea	800 mg	single dose	1 day	800 mg

TABLE 1
Antibody Responses in Navajo Infants

Vaccine	No. of Subjects	Time	% Subjects with > 0.15 mcg/mL	% Subjects with > 1.0 mcg/mL	Anti-PRP GMT (mcg/mL)
PedvaxHIB*	416†	Pre-Vaccination	44	10	0.16
	416	Dose 1	88	52	0.95
	416	Dose 2	91	60	1.43
Placebo*	461†	Pre-Vaccination	44	9	0.16
	461	Dose 1	21	2	0.09
	461	Dose 2	14	1	0.08
PedvaxHIB	27**	Prebooster	70	33	0.51
	27	Postbooster***	100	89	8.39

  * Post vaccination values obtained approximately 1–3 months after each dose.
  † The Protective Efficacy Study.
  ** Immunogenicity Trial.
*** Booster given at 12 months of age; post vaccination values obtained 1 month after administration of booster dose.

TABLE 2
Antibody Responses* to PedvaxHIB in Other Clinical Studies

Age (Months)	Time	No. of Subjects	% Subjects Responding with > 0.15 mcg/mL	% Subjects Responding with > 1.0 mcg/mL	Post-Vaccination Anti-PRP GMT (mcg/mL)
2–3	Dose 1**	113	97	81	2.48
	Dose 2***	113	98	88	4.60
4–14	Dose 1**	252	98	75	2.53
	Dose 2***	252	100	92	6.04
15–17	Single Dose***	59	100	83	3.11
18–23	Single Dose***	59	98	97	7.43
24–71	Dose ***	52	98	92	10.55

* Only subjects with prevaccination anti-PRP ≤ 0.15 mcg/mL are included in this table (excluding native Americans).
** Two months post vaccination.
*** One month post vaccination.

TABLE 3
Antibody Responses* After Two Doses of PedvaxHIB Among
Infants Initially Vaccinated at 2–3 Months of Age
By Racial/Ethnic Group

Racial/Ethnic Groups	No. of Subjects	% With Anti-PRP > 0.15 mcg/mL	% With Anti-PRP > 1.0 mcg/mL	GMT (mcg/mL)
Native American†	44	95	68	2.24
Caucasian	155	99	85	4.00
Hispanic	16	100	94	4.60
Black	18	100	94	8.57

† Apache and Navajo
* One month after the second dose

TABLE 4
Fever or Local Reactions in Subjects 2 to 71 Months of Age
Vaccinated with PedvaxHIB Alone
Other Clinical Studies

Age (Months)	Reaction	No. of Subjects Evaluated	Dose 1 6 hr	Dose 1 24	Dose 1 48	No. of Subjects Evaluated	Dose 2 6 hr	Dose 2 24	Dose 2 48
					Percentage				
2–14*	Fever > 38.3°C (101°F) Rectal	532	2.4	3.8	1.9	329	3.0	4.3	3.6
	Erythema > 2.5 cm diameter	1026	0.2	1.0	0.4	585	0.9	1.2	0.7
	Swelling/ Induration > 2.5 cm diameter	1026	0.6	1.5	1.6	585	0.9	2.8	3.7
15–71**	Fever > 38.3°C (101°F) Rectal	149	4.0	4.0	6.7				
	Erythema > 2.5 cm diameter	572	0.0	0.3	0.2				
	Swelling/ Induration > 2.5 cm diameter	572	0.9	2.1	1.4				

*Additional complaints reported following vaccination with the first and second dose of PedvaxHIB, respectively, in the indicated number of subjects were: nausea, vomiting and/or diarrhea (101, 41), crying for more than one-half hour (43, 15), rash (16, 17), and unusual high-pitched crying (4, 4).
**Additional complaints reported following vaccination with 1 dose of PedvaxHIB in the indicated number of subjects were: nausea, vomiting and/or diarrhea (44), crying for more than one-half hour (19), rash (12), and unusual high-pitched crying (0).

who complete the primary two-dose regimen before 12 months of age (see Table 1 and DOSAGE AND ADMINIS-TRATION).

Antibodies to the OMPC of *N. meningitidis* (see DESCRIPTION) have been demonstrated in vaccinee sera but the clinical relevance of these antibodies has not been established. In a multicenter study of immunogenicity and safety in different subpopulations in the United States, antibody responses to PedvaxHIB were evaluated in infants initially vaccinated between the ages of 2 and 3 months (Table 3).

PedvaxHIB induced antibody levels greater than 1.0 mcg/mL in children who were poor responders to nonconjugated PRP vaccines. In a study involving such a subpopulation 34 children ranging in age from 27 to 61 months who developed invasive Haemophilus b disease despite previous vaccination with nonconjugated PRP vaccines were randomly assigned to 2 groups. One group (n = 14) was immunized with PedvaxHIB and the other group (n = 20) with a nonconjugated PRP vaccine at a mean interval of approximately 12 months after recovery from disease. All 14 children immunized with PedvaxHIB but only 6 of 20 children re-immunized with a nonconjugated PRP vaccine achieved an antibody level of > 1.0 mcg/mL. The 14 children who had not responded to revaccination with the nonconjugated PRP vaccine were then immunized with a single dose of PedvaxHIB; following this vaccination, all achieved antibody levels of > 1.0 mcg/mL. In addition, PedvaxHIB has been studied in children at high risk of Haemophilus b disease because of genetically-related

deficiencies [Blacks who were Km(1) allotype negative and Caucasians who were G2m(23) allotype negative] and are considered hyporesponsive to nonconjugated PRP vaccines on this basis. The hyporesponsive children had anti-PRP responses comparable to those of allotype positive children of similar age range when vaccinated with PedvaxHIB. All children achieved anti-PRP levels of > 1.0 mcg/mL.

INDICATIONS AND USAGE

PedvaxHIB is indicated for routine immunization against invasive disease caused by *Haemophilus influenzae* type b in infants and children 2 to 71 months of age.

PedvaxHIB will not protect against disease caused by *Haemophilus influenzae* other than type b or against other microorganisms that cause invasive disease such as meningitis or sepsis.

Revaccination
Infants completing the primary two-dose regimen before 12 months of age should receive a booster dose (see DOSAGE AND ADMINISTRATION).

Use with Other Vaccines
Studies have been conducted in which PedvaxHIB has been administered concomitantly with the primary vaccination series of DTP and OPV, or concomitantly with M-M-R* II (Measles, Mumps, and Rubella Virus Vaccine Live, MSD) (using separate sites and syringes) or with a booster dose of OPV plus DTP (using separate sites and syringes for PedvaxHIB and DTP). No impairment of immune response to individual tested vaccine antigens was demonstrated. The type, frequency and severity of adverse experiences observed in these studies with PedvaxHIB were similar to those seen when the other vaccines were given alone.

PedvaxHIB IS NOT RECOMMENDED FOR USE IN INFANTS YOUNGER THAN 2 MONTHS OF AGE.

*Registered trademark of MERCK & CO., INC.

CONTRAINDICATIONS

Hypersensitivity to any component of the vaccine or the diluent.

WARNINGS

USE ONLY THE ALUMINUM HYDROXIDE DILUENT SUPPLIED.

If PedvaxHIB is used in persons with malignancies or those receiving immunosuppressive therapy or who are otherwise immunocompromised, the expected immune response may not be obtained.

PRECAUTIONS

General
As for any vaccine, adequate treatment provisions, including epinephrine, should be available for immediate use should an anaphylactoid reaction occur.

As with other vaccines, PedvaxHIB may not induce protective antibody levels immediately following vaccination.

As with any vaccine, vaccination with PedvaxHIB may not result in a protective antibody response in all individuals given the vaccine.

As reported with Haemophilus b Polysaccharide Vaccine and another Haemophilus b Conjugate Vaccine, cases of Haemophilus b disease may occur in the week after vaccination, prior to the onset of the protective effects of the vaccines.

There is insufficient evidence that PedvaxHIB given immediately after exposure to natural *Haemophilus influenzae* type b will prevent illness.

Any acute infection or febrile illness is reason for delaying use of PedvaxHIB except when in the opinion of the physician, withholding the vaccine entails a greater risk.

Laboratory Test Interactions
Sensitive tests (e.g., Latex Agglutination Kits) may detect PRP derived from the vaccine in urine of some vaccinees for up to seven days following vaccination with PedvaxHIB; in clinical studies with PedvaxHIB, such children demonstrated normal immune response to the vaccine.

Carcinogenesis, Mutagenesis, and Impairment of Fertility
PedvaxHIB has not been evaluated for its carcinogenic or mutagenic potential, or its potential to impair fertility.

Pregnancy
Pregnancy Category C: Animal reproduction studies have not been conducted with PedvaxHIB. It is also not known whether PedvaxHIB can cause fetal harm when adminis-

Continued on next page

Information on the Merck & Co. products listed on these pages is the full prescribing information from product circulars in use October 1, 1992.

Merck & Co.—Cont.

tered to a pregnant woman or can affect reproductive capacity. PedvaxHIB is not recommended for use in a pregnant woman.

ADVERSE REACTIONS

In early clinical studies involving the administration of 8,086 doses of PedvaxHIB alone to 5,027 healthy infants and children 2 months to 71 months of age, PedvaxHIB was generally well tolerated. No serious adverse reactions were reported.

During a two-day period following vaccination with PedvaxHIB in a subset of these infants and children, the most frequently reported adverse reactions, excluding those shown in Table 4, in decreasing order of frequency included irritability, sleepiness, respiratory infection/symptoms and ear infection/otitis media. Urticaria was reported in two children. Thrombocytopenia was seen in one child. A cause and effect relationship between these side effects and the vaccination has not been established.

Selected objective observations reported by parents over a 48-hour period in infants and children 2 to 71 months of age following primary vaccination with PedvaxHIB alone are summarized in Table 4.

In The Protective Efficacy Study (see CLINICAL PHARMACOLOGY), 4,459 healthy Navajo infants 6 to 12 weeks of age received PedvaxHIB or placebo. Most of these infants received DTP/OPV concomitantly. No differences were seen in the type and frequency of serious health problems expected in this Navajo population or in serious adverse experiences reported among those who received PedvaxHIB and those who received placebo, and none was reported to be related to PedvaxHIB. Only one serious reaction (tracheitis) was reported as possibly related to PedvaxHIB and only one (diarrhea) as possibly related to placebo. Seizures occurred infrequently in both groups (9 occurred in vaccine recipients, 8 of whom also received DTP; 8 occurred in placebo recipients, 7 of whom also received DTP) and were not reported to be related to PedvaxHIB. The frequencies of fever and local reactions occurring in a subset of these infants during a 48-hour period following each dose were similar to those seen in early clinical studies (Table 4).

[See Table 4 on preceding page.]

As with any vaccine, there is the possibility that broad use of PedvaxHIB could reveal adverse reactions not observed in clinical trials.

Potential Adverse Reactions

The use of Haemophilus b Polysaccharide Vaccines and another Haemophilus b Conjugate Vaccine has been associated with the following additional adverse effects: early onset Haemophilus b disease and Guillain-Barré syndrome. A cause and effect relationship between these side effects and the vaccination was not established.

DOSAGE AND ADMINISTRATION

FOR INTRAMUSCULAR ADMINISTRATION
DO NOT INJECT INTRAVENOUSLY

2 to 14 Months of Age

Infants 2 to 14 months of age should receive a 0.5 mL dose of vaccine ideally beginning at 2 months of age followed by a 0.5 mL dose 2 months later (or as soon as possible thereafter). When the primary two-dose regimen is completed before 12 months of age, a booster dose is required (see below and Table 5).

15 Months of Age and Older

Children 15 months of age and older previously unvaccinated against Haemophilus b disease should receive a single 0.5 mL dose of vaccine.

Booster Dose

In infants completing the primary two-dose regimen before 12 months of age, a booster dose (0.5 mL) should be administered at 12 to 15 months of age but not earlier than 2 months after the second dose.

DATA ARE NOT AVAILABLE REGARDING THE INTERCHANGEABILITY OF OTHER HAEMOPHILUS b CONJUGATE VACCINES AND PedvaxHIB.

Vaccination regimens by age group are outlined in Table 5.

TABLE 5
(see circular text above for details)

Age (Months) at First Dose	Primary	Age (Months) at Booster Dose
2–10	2 doses, 2 mo. apart	12–15
11–14	2 doses, 2 mo. apart	—
15–71	1 dose	—

TO RECONSTITUTE, USE ONLY THE ALUMINUM HYDROXIDE DILUENT SUPPLIED.

First, agitate the diluent vial, then, using sterile technique, withdraw the entire volume of aluminum hydroxide diluent into the syringe to be used for reconstitution. Inject all the aluminum hydroxide diluent in the syringe into the vial of lyophilized vaccine, and agitate to mix thoroughly.

Withdraw the entire contents into the syringe and inject the total volume of reconstituted vaccine (0.5 mL) intramuscularly, preferably into the anterolateral thigh or the outer aspect of the upper arm.

It is recommended that the vaccine be used as soon as possible after reconstitution. Store reconstituted vaccine in the vaccine vial at 2–8°C (36–46°F) and discard if not used with 24 hours. Agitate prior to injection.

Parenteral drug products should be inspected visually for extraneous particulate matter and discoloration prior to administration whenever solution and container permit. Aluminum hydroxide diluent and PedvaxHIB when reconstituted are slightly opaque white suspensions.

Special care should be taken to ensure that the injection does not enter a blood vessel.

It is important to use a separate sterile syringe and needle for each patient to prevent transmission of hepatitis B or other infectious agents from one person to another.

HOW SUPPLIED

No. 4792—PedvaxHIB is supplied as a single-dose vial of lyophilized vaccine, **NDC** 0006-4792-00, and a vial of aluminum hydroxide diluent.

No. 4797—PedvaxHIB is supplied as follows: a box of 5 single-dose vials of lyophilized vaccine, **NDC** 0006-4797-00, and 5 vials of aluminum hydroxide diluent.

Storage

Before reconstitution, store PedvaxHIB at 2–8°C (36–46°F). Store reconstituted vaccine in the vaccine vial at 2–8°C (36–46°F) and discard if not used within 24 hours.

DO NOT FREEZE the aluminum hydroxide diluent or the reconstituted vaccine.

A.H.F.S. Category: 80:12
DC 7611803 Issued October 1991

COPYRIGHT © MERCK & CO., INC., 1990
All rights reserved

PEPCID® Tablets ℞
(Famotidine), U.S.P.
PEPCID® Oral Suspension ℞
(Famotidine for Oral Suspension)
PEPCID® I.V. ℞
(Famotidine)

DESCRIPTION

The active ingredient in PEPCID* (Famotidine), is a histamine H_2-receptor antagonist. Famotidine is N'-(aminosulfonyl) -3- [[[2-[(diaminomethylene)amino] -4- thiazolyl]methyl]thio]propanimidamide. The empirical formula of famotidine is $C_8H_{15}N_7O_2S_3$ and its molecular weight is 337.43. Its structural formula is:

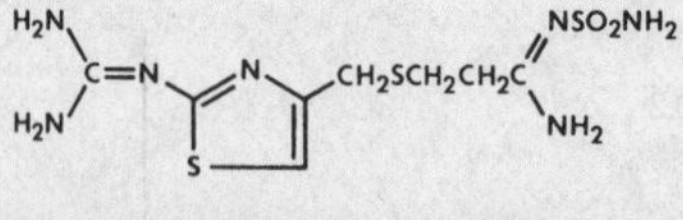

Famotidine is a white to pale yellow crystalline compound that is freely soluble in glacial acetic acid, slightly soluble in methanol, very slightly soluble in water, and practically insoluble in ethanol.

Famotidine is supplied in three dosage forms: PEPCID Tablets, PEPCID Oral Suspension, and PEPCID I.V.

Each tablet for oral administration contains either 20 mg or 40 mg of famotidine and the following inactive ingredients: hydroxypropyl cellulose, hydroxypropyl methylcellulose, iron oxides, magnesium stearate, microcrystalline cellulose, starch, talc, titanium dioxide.

Each 5 mL of the oral suspension when prepared as directed contains 40 mg of famotidine and the following inactive ingredients: citric acid, flavors, microcrystalline cellulose and carboxymethylcellulose sodium, sucrose and xanthan gum. Added as preservatives are sodium benzoate 0.1%, sodium methylparaben 0.1%, and sodium propylparaben 0.02%.

Each mL of the solution for intravenous injection contains 10 mg of famotidine and the following inactive ingredients: L-aspartic acid 4 mg, mannitol 20 mg, and Water for Injection q.s. 1 mL. The multidose injection also contains benzyl alcohol 0.9% added as preservative.

*Registered trademark of MERCK & CO., INC.

CLINICAL PHARMACOLOGY

GI Effects

PEPCID is a competitive inhibitor of histamine H_2-receptors. The primary clinically important pharmacologic activity of PEPCID is inhibition of gastric secretion. Both the acid concentration and volume of gastric secretion are suppressed by PEPCID, while changes in pepsin secretion are proportional to volume output.

In normal volunteers and hypersecretors, PEPCID inhibited basal and nocturnal gastric secretion, as well as secretion stimulated by food and pentagastrin. After oral administration, the onset of the antisecretory effect occurred within one hour; the maximum effect was dose-dependent, occurring within one to three hours. Duration of inhibition of secretion by doses of 20 and 40 mg was 10 to 12 hours.

After intravenous administration, the maximum effect was achieved within 30 minutes. Single intravenous doses of 10 and 20 mg inhibited nocturnal secretion for a period of 10 to 12 hours. The 20 mg dose was associated with the longest duration of action in most subjects.

Single evening oral doses of 20 and 40 mg inhibited basal and nocturnal acid secretion in all subjects; mean nocturnal gastric acid secretion was inhibited by 86% and 94%, respectively, for a period of at least 10 hours. The same doses given in the morning suppressed food-stimulated acid secretion in all subjects. The mean suppression was 76% and 84% respectively 3 to 5 hours after administration, and 25% and 30% respectively 8 to 10 hours after administration. In some subjects who received the 20 mg dose, however, the antisecretory effect was dissipated within 6–8 hours. There was no cumulative effect with repeated doses. The nocturnal intragastric pH was raised by evening doses of 20 and 40 mg of PEPCID to mean values of 5.0 and 6.4, respectively. When PEPCID was given after breakfast, the basal daytime interdigestive pH at 3 and 8 hours after 20 or 40 mg of PEPCID was raised to about 5.

PEPCID had little or no effect on fasting or postprandial serum gastrin levels. Gastric emptying and exocrine pancreatic function were not affected by PEPCID.

Other Effects

Systemic effects of PEPCID in the CNS, cardiovascular, respiratory or endocrine systems were not noted in clinical pharmacology studies. Also, no antiandrogenic effects were noted. (See ADVERSE REACTIONS.) Serum hormone levels, including prolactin, cortisol, thyroxine (T_4), and testosterone, were not altered after treatment with PEPCID.

Pharmacokinetics

PEPCID is incompletely absorbed. The bioavailability of oral doses is 40–45%. PEPCID Tablets and PEPCID Oral Suspension are bioequivalent. Bioavailability may be slightly increased by food, or slightly decreased by antacids; however, these effects are of no clinical consequence. PEPCID undergoes minimal first-pass metabolism. After oral doses, peak plasma levels occur in 1–3 hours. Plasma levels after multiple doses are similar to those after single doses. Fifteen to 20% of PEPCID in plasma is protein bound. PEPCID has an elimination half-life of 2.5–3.5 hours. PEPCID is eliminated by renal (65–70%) and metabolic (30–35%) routes. Renal clearance is 250–450 mL/min, indicating some tubular excretion. Twenty-five to 30% of an oral dose and 65–70% of an intravenous dose are recovered in the urine as unchanged compound. The only metabolite identified in man is the S-oxide.

There is a close relationship between creatinine clearance values and the elimination half-life of PEPCID. In patients with severe renal insufficiency, i.e., creatinine clearance less than 10 mL/min, PEPCID elimination half-life may exceed 20 hours and adjustment of dose or dosing intervals may be necessary (see PRECAUTIONS, DOSAGE AND ADMINISTRATION).

In elderly patients, there are no clinically significant age-related changes in the pharmacokinetics of PEPCID.

Clinical Studies

Duodenal Ulcer

In a U.S. multicenter, double-blind study in outpatients with endoscopically confirmed duodenal ulcer, orally administered PEPCID was compared to placebo. As shown in Table 1, 70% of patients treated with PEPCID 40 mg h.s. were healed by week 4.

Table 1
Outpatients with Endoscopically
Confirmed Healed Duodenal Ulcers

	PEPCID 40 mg h.s. (N=89)	PEPCID 20 mg b.i.d. (N=84)	Placebo h.s. (N=97)
Week 2	*32%	*38%	17%
Week 4	*70%	*67%	31%

*Statistically significantly different than placebo ($p < 0.001$)

Patients not healed by week 4 were continued in the study. By week 8, 83% of patients treated with PEPCID had healed versus 45% of patients treated with placebo. The incidence of

ulcer healing with PEPCID was significantly higher than with placebo at each time point based on proportion of endoscopically confirmed healed ulcers.

In this study, time to relief of daytime and nocturnal pain was significantly shorter for patients receiving PEPCID than for patients receiving placebo; patients receiving PEPCID also took less antacid than the patients receiving placebo.

Long-Term Maintenance

Treatment of Duodenal Ulcers

PEPCID, 20 mg p.o. h.s. was compared to placebo h.s. as maintenance therapy in two double-blind, multicenter studies of patients with endoscopically confirmed healed duodenal ulcers. In the U.S. study the observed ulcer incidence within 12 months in patients treated with placebo was 2.4 times greater than in the patients treated with PEPCID. The 89 patients treated with PEPCID had a cumulative observed ulcer incidence of 23.4% compared to an observed ulcer incidence of 56.6% in the 89 patients receiving placebo ($p < 0.01$). These results were confirmed in an international study where the cumulative observed ulcer incidence within 12 months in the 307 patients treated with PEPCID was 35.7%, compared to an incidence of 75.5% in the 325 patients treated with placebo ($p < 0.01$).

Gastric Ulcer

In both a U.S. and an international multicenter, double-blind study in patients with endoscopically confirmed active benign gastric ulcer, orally administered PEPCID, 40 mg h.s., was compared to placebo h.s. Antacids were permitted during the studies, but consumption was not significantly different between the PEPCID and placebo groups. As shown in Table 2, the incidence of ulcer healing (dropouts counted as unhealed) with PEPCID was statistically significantly better than placebo at weeks 6 and 8 in the U.S. study, and at weeks 4, 6 and 8 in the international study, based on the number of ulcers that healed, confirmed by endoscopy.

Table 2

Patients with Endoscopically
Confirmed Healed Gastric Ulcers

	U.S. Study		International Study	
	PEPCID 40 mg h.s. (N=74)	Placebo h.s. (N=75)	PEPCID 40 mg h.s. (N=149)	Placebo h.s. (N=145)
Week 4	45%	39%	**47%	31%
Week 6	**66%	44%	**65%	46%
Week 8	*78%	64%	**80%	54%

*,** Statistically significantly better than placebo ($p \le 0.05$, $p \le 0.01$ respectively)

Time to complete relief of daytime and nighttime pain was statistically significantly shorter for patients receiving PEPCID than for patients receiving placebo; however, in neither study was there a statistically significant difference in the proportion of patients whose pain was relieved by the end of the study (week 8).

Gastroesophageal Reflux Disease (GERD)

PEPCID was compared to placebo in a U.S. study that enrolled patients with symptoms of GERD and without endoscopic evidence of erosion or ulceration of the esophagus. PEPCID 20 mg b.i.d. was statistically significantly superior to 40 mg h.s. and to placebo in providing a successful symptomatic outcome, defined as moderate or excellent improvement of symptoms (Table 3).

Table 3

% Successful Symptomatic Outcome

	PEPCID 20 mg b.i.d. (N=154)	PEPCID 40 mg h.s. (N=149)	Placebo (N=73)
Week 6	82**	69	62

**$p \le 0.01$) vs Placebo

By two weeks of treatment, symptomatic success was observed in a greater percentage of patients taking PEPCID 20 mg b.i.d. compared to placebo ($p \le 0.01$).

Symptomatic improvement and healing of endoscopically verified erosion and ulceration were studied in two additional trials. Healing was defined as complete resolution of all erosions or ulcerations visible with endoscopy. The U.S. study comparing PEPCID 40 mg b.i.d. to placebo and PEPCID 20 mg b.i.d., showed a significantly greater percentage of healing for PEPCID 40 mg b.i.d. at weeks 6 and 12 (Table 4).

Table 4

% Endoscopic Healing—U.S. Study

	PEPCID 40 mg b.i.d. (N=127)	PEPCID 20 mg b.i.d. (N=125)	Placebo (N=66)
Week 6	48**,++	32	18
Week 12	69**,+	54**	29

** $p \le 0.01$ vs Placebo
+ $p \le 0.05$ vs PEPCID 20 mg b.i.d.
++ $p \le 0.01$ vs PEPCID 20 mg b.i.d.

As compared to placebo, patients who received PEPCID had faster relief of daytime and nighttime heartburn and a greater percentage of patients experienced complete relief of nighttime heartburn. These differences were statistically significant.

In the international study, when PEPCID 40 mg b.i.d., was compared to ranitidine 150 mg b.i.d., a statistically signifi-

cantly greater percentage of healing was observed with PEPCID 40 mg b.i.d. at week 12 (Table 5). There was, however, no significant difference among treatments in symptom relief.

Table 5

% Endoscopic Healing—International Study

	PEPCID 40 mg b.i.d. (N=175)	PEPCID 20 mg b.i.d. (N=93)	Ranitidine 150 mg b.i.d. (N=172)
Week 6	48	52	42
Week 12	71*	68	60

* $p \le 0.05$ vs Ranitidine 150 mg b.i.d.

Pathological Hypersecretory Conditions (e.g., Zollinger-Ellison Syndrome, Multiple Endocrine Adenomas)

In studies of patients with pathological hypersecretory conditions such as Zollinger-Ellison Syndrome with or without multiple endocrine adenomas, PEPCID significantly inhibited gastric acid secretion and controlled associated symptoms. Doses from 20 to 160 mg q 6 h maintained basal acid secretion below 10 mEq/hr; initial doses were titrated to the individual patient need and subsequent adjustments were necessary with time in some patients. PEPCID was well tolerated at these high dose levels for prolonged periods (greater than 12 months) in eight patients, and there were no cases reported of gynecomastia, increased prolactin levels, or impotence which were considered to be due to the drug.

INDICATIONS AND USAGE

PEPCID is indicated in:

1. *Short term treatment of active duodenal ulcer.* Most patients heal within 4 weeks; there is rarely reason to use PEPCID at full dosage for longer than 6 to 8 weeks. Studies have not assessed the safety of famotidine in uncomplicated active duodenal ulcer for periods of more than eight weeks.

2. *Maintenance therapy for duodenal ulcer patients at reduced dosage after healing of an active ulcer.* Controlled studies have not extended beyond one year.

3. *Short term treatment of active benign gastric ulcer.* Most patients heal within 6 weeks. Studies have not assessed the safety or efficacy of famotidine in uncomplicated active benign gastric ulcer for periods of more than 8 weeks.

4. *Short term treatment of gastroesophageal reflux disease (GERD).* PEPCID is indicated for short term treatment of patients with symptoms of GERD (see CLINICAL PHARMACOLOGY, *Clinical Studies*).
PEPCID is also indicated for the short term treatment of esophagitis due to GERD including erosive or ulcerative disease diagnosed by endoscopy (see CLINICAL PHARMACOLOGY, *Clinical Studies*).

5. *Treatment of pathological hypersecretory conditions (e.g., Zollinger-Ellison Syndrome, multiple endocrine adenomas).*
PEPCID I.V. is indicated in some hospitalized patients with pathological hypersecretory conditions or intractable ulcers, or as an alternative to the oral dosage forms for short-term use in patients who are unable to take oral medication.

CONTRAINDICATIONS

Hypersensitivity to any component of these products.

PRECAUTIONS

General

Symptomatic response to therapy with PEPCID does not preclude the presence of gastric malignancy.

Patients with Severe Renal Insufficiency

Longer intervals between doses or lower doses may need to be used in patients with severe renal insufficiency (creatinine clearance < 10 mL/min) to adjust for the longer elimination half-life of famotidine. (See CLINICAL PHARMACOLOGY and DOSAGE AND ADMINISTRATION.) However, currently, no drug-related toxicity has been found with high plasma concentrations of famotidine.

Information for Patients

The patient should be instructed to shake the oral suspension vigorously for 5–10 seconds prior to each use. Unused constituted oral suspension should be discarded after 30 days.

Drug Interactions

No drug interactions have been identified. Studies with famotidine in man, in animal models, and *in vitro* have shown no significant interference with the disposition of compounds metabolized by the hepatic microsomal enzymes, e.g., cytochrome P450 system. Compounds tested in man include warfarin, theophylline, phenytoin, diazepam, aminopyrine and antipyrine. Indocyanine green as an index of hepatic drug extraction has been tested and no significant effects have been found.

Carcinogenesis, Mutagenesis, Impairment of Fertility

In a 106 week study in rats and a 92 week study in mice given oral doses of up to 2000 mg/kg/day (approximately 2500 times the recommended human dose for active duodenal ulcer), there was no evidence of carcinogenic potential for PEPCID.

Famotidine was negative in the microbial mutagen test (Ames test) using *Salmonella typhimurium* and *Escherichia coli* with or without rat liver enzyme activation at concentrations up to 10,000 mcg/plate. In *in vivo* studies in mice, with a micronucleus test and a chromosomal aberration test, no evidence of a mutagenic effect was observed.

In studies with rats given oral doses of up to 2000 mg/kg/day or intravenous doses of up to 200 mg/kg/day fertility and reproductive performance were not affected.

Pregnancy

Pregnancy Category B

Reproductive studies have been performed in rats and rabbits at oral doses of up to 2000 and 500 mg/kg/day respectively and in both species at I.V. doses of up to 200 mg/kg/day, and have revealed no significant evidence of impaired fertility or harm to the fetus due to PEPCID. While no direct fetotoxic effects have been observed, sporadic abortions occurring only in mothers displaying marked decreased food intake were seen in some rabbits at oral doses of 200 mg/kg/day (250 times the usual human dose) or higher. There are, however, no adequate or well-controlled studies in pregnant women. Because animal reproductive studies are not always predictive of human response, this drug should be used during pregnancy only if clearly needed.

Nursing Mothers

Studies performed in lactating rats have shown that famotidine is secreted into breast milk. Transient growth depression was observed in young rats suckling from mothers treated with maternotoxic doses of at least 600 times the usual human dose. It is not known whether this drug is secreted into human milk. Because many drugs are secreted into human milk and because of the potential for serious adverse reactions in nursing infants from PEPCID, a decision should be made whether to discontinue nursing or discontinue the drug, taking into account the importance of the drug to the mother.

Pediatric Use

Safety and effectiveness in children have not been established.

Use in Elderly Patients

No dosage adjustment is required based on age (see CLINICAL PHARMACOLOGY, *Pharmacokinetics).* Dosage adjustment in the case of severe renal impairment may be necessary.

ADVERSE REACTIONS

The adverse reactions listed below have been reported during domestic and international clinical trials in approximately 2500 patients. In those controlled clinical trials in which PEPCID Tablets were compared to placebo, the incidence of adverse experiences in the group which received PEPCID Tablets, 40 mg at bedtime, was similar to that in the placebo group.

The following adverse reactions have been reported to occur in more than 1% of patients on therapy with PEPCID in controlled clinical trials, and may be causally related to the drug: headache (4.7%), dizziness (1.3%), constipation (1.2%) and diarrhea (1.7%).

The following other adverse reactions have been reported infrequently in clinical trials or since the drug was marketed. The relationship to therapy with PEPCID has been unclear in many cases. Within each category the adverse reactions are listed in order of decreasing severity:

Body as a Whole: fever, asthenia, fatigue
Cardiovascular: arrhythmia, AV block, palpitation
Gastrointestinal: cholestatic jaundice, liver enzyme abnormalities, vomiting, nausea, abdominal discomfort, anorexia, dry mouth
Hematologic: rare cases of agranulocytosis, pancytopenia, leukopenia, thrombocytopenia
Hypersensitivity: anaphylaxis, angioedema, orbital or facial edema, urticaria, rash, conjunctival injection
Musculoskeletal: musculoskeletal pain, arthralgia
Nervous System/Psychiatric: grand mal seizure; psychic disturbances, which were reversible in cases for which follow-up was obtained, including hallucinations, confusion, agitation, depression, anxiety, decreased libido; paresthesia; insomnia; somnolence
Respiratory: bronchospasm
Skin: alopecia, acne, pruritus, dry skin, flushing
Special Senses: tinnitus, taste disorder
Other: rare cases of impotence have been reported; however, in controlled clinical trials, the incidence was not greater than that seen with placebo.

The adverse reactions reported for PEPCID Tablets may also occur with PEPCID Oral Suspension or PEPCID I.V. In addi-

Continued on next page

Information on the Merck & Co. products listed on these pages is the full prescribing information from product circulars in use October 1, 1992.

Merck & Co.—Cont.

tion, transient irritation at the injection site has been observed with PEPCID I.V.

OVERDOSAGE

There is no experience to date with deliberate overdosage. Doses of up to 640 mg/day have been given to patients with pathological hypersecretory conditions with no serious adverse effects. In the event of overdosage, treatment should be symptomatic and supportive. Unabsorbed material should be removed from the gastrointestinal tract, the patient should be monitored, and supportive therapy should be employed.

The oral LD_{50} of famotidine in male and female rats and mice was greater than 3000 mg/kg and the minimum lethal acute oral dose in dogs exceeded 2000 mg/kg. Famotidine did not produce overt effects at high oral doses in mice, rats, cats and dogs, but induced significant anorexia and growth depression in rabbits starting with 200 mg/kg/day orally. The intravenous LD_{50} of famotidine for mice and rats ranged from 254–563 mg/kg and the minimum lethal single I.V. dose in dogs was approximately 300 mg/kg. Signs of acute intoxication in I.V. treated dogs were emesis, restlessness, pallor of mucous membranes or redness of mouth and ears, hypotension, tachycardia and collapse.

DOSAGE AND ADMINISTRATION

Duodenal Ulcer
Acute Therapy: The recommended adult oral dosage for active duodenal ulcer is 40 mg once a day at bedtime. Most patients heal within 4 weeks; there is rarely reason to use PEPCID at full dosage for longer than 6 to 8 weeks. A regimen of 20 mg b.i.d. is also effective.
Maintenance Therapy: The recommended oral dose is 20 mg once a day at bedtime.
Benign Gastric Ulcer
Acute Therapy: The recommended adult oral dosage for active benign gastric ulcer is 40 mg once a day at bedtime.
Gastroesophageal Reflux Disease (GERD)
The recommended oral dosage for treatment of patients with symptoms of GERD is 20 mg b.i.d. for up to 6 weeks. The recommended oral dosage for the treatment of patients with esophagitis including erosions and ulcerations and accompanying symptoms due to GERD is 20 or 40 mg b.i.d. for up to 12 weeks (see CLINICAL PHARMACOLOGY, *Clinical Studies*).
Pathological Hypersecretory Conditions (e.g., Zollinger-Ellison Syndrome, Multiple Endocrine Adenomas)
The dosage of PEPCID in patients with pathological hypersecretory conditions varies with the individual patient. The recommended adult oral starting dose for pathological hypersecretory conditions is 20 mg q 6 h. In some patients, a higher starting dose may be required. Doses should be adjusted to individual patient needs and should continue as long as clinically indicated. Doses up to 160 mg q 6 h have been administered to some patients with severe Zollinger-Ellison Syndrome.
Oral Suspension
PEPCID Oral Suspension may be substituted for PEPCID Tablets in any of the above indications. Each five mL contains 40 mg of famotidine after constitution of the powder with 46 mL of Purified Water as directed.
Directions for Preparing PEPCID Oral Suspension
Prepare suspension at time of dispensing. Slowly add 46 mL of Purified Water. Shake vigorously for 5–10 seconds immediately after adding the water and immediately before use.
Stability of PEPCID Oral Suspension
Unused constituted oral suspension should be discarded after 30 days.
Intravenous Administration
In some hospitalized patients with pathological hypersecretory conditions or intractable ulcers, or in patients who are unable to take oral medication, PEPCID I.V. may be administered. The recommended dosage is 20 mg q 12 h.
The doses and regimen for parenteral administration in patients with GERD have not been established.
Preparation of PEPCID Intravenous Solutions
Dilute 2 mL of PEPCID I.V. (solution containing 10 mg/mL) with 0.9% Sodium Chloride Injection or other compatible intravenous solution to a total volume of either 5 mL or 10 mL and inject over a period of not less than 2 minutes.
Preparation of PEPCID Intravenous Infusion Solutions
PEPCID I.V. may also be administered as an infusion, 2 mL diluted with 100 mL of 5% dextrose or other compatible solution, and infused over a 15–30 minute period.
Stability of PEPCID I.V.
PEPCID I.V. is stable for 48 hours at room temperature when added to or diluted with most commonly used intravenous solutions, e.g., Water for Injection, 0.9% Sodium Chloride Injection, 5% and 10% Dextrose Injection, Lactated Ringer's Injection, or Sodium Bicarbonate Injection, 5%.

Parenteral drug products should be inspected visually for particulate matter and discoloration prior to administration whenever solution and container permit.
Concomitant Use of Antacids
Antacids may be given concomitantly if needed.
Dosage Adjustment for Patients with Severe Renal Insufficiency
In patients with severe renal insufficiency, i.e., with a creatinine clearance less than 10 mL/min, the elimination half-life of PEPCID may exceed 20 hours, reaching approximately 24 hours in anuric patients. Although no relationship of adverse effects to high plasma levels has been established, to avoid excess accumulation of the drug, the dose of PEPCID may be reduced to 20 mg h.s. or the dosing interval may be prolonged to 36–48 hours as indicated by the patient's clinical response.

HOW SUPPLIED

No. 3535—Tablets PEPCID, 20 mg, are beige colored, U-shaped, film-coated tablets coded MSD 963. They are supplied as follows:
NDC 0006-0963-31 unit of use bottles of 30
(6505-01-260-0902, 20 mg 30's)
NDC 0006-0963-94 unit of use bottles of 90
NDC 0006-0963-58 unit of use bottles of 100
NDC 0006-0963-28 unit dose package of 100
NDC 0006-0963-98 unit of use bottles of 180.
    Shown in Product Identification Section, page 420
No. 3536—Tablets PEPCID, 40 mg, are light brownish-orange, U-shaped, film-coated tablets coded MSD 964. They are supplied as follows:
NDC 0006-0964-31 unit of use bottles of 30
(6505-01-257-3164, 40 mg 30's)
NDC 0006-0964-94 unit of use bottles of 90
NDC 0006-0964-58 unit of use bottles of 100
NDC 0006-0964-28 unit dose package of 100
(6505-01-318-0464, 40 mg individually sealed 100's).
    Shown in Product Identification Section, page 420
No. 3538—Oral Suspension PEPCID is a white to off-white powder containing 400 mg of famotidine for constitution. When constituted as directed, PEPCID Oral Suspension is a smooth, mobile, off-white, homogeneous suspension with a cherry-banana-mint flavor, containing 40 mg of famotidine per 5 mL.
NDC 0006-3538-92, bottles containing 400 mg famotidine.
FOR INTRAVENOUS USE ONLY
No. 3539—Injection PEPCID I.V. 10 mg per 1 mL, is a non-preserved, clear, colorless solution and is supplied as follows:
NDC 0006-3539-04, 10 × 2 mL single dose vials
(6505-01-281-1249, 10 mg per mL, 2 mL 10's).
No. 3541—Injection PEPCID I.V. 10 mg per 1 mL, is a clear, colorless solution and is supplied as follows:
NDC 0006-3541-14, 4 mL vials
(6505-01-282-1180, 10 mg per mL, 4 mL).
Storage
Avoid storage of PEPCID Tablets at temperatures above 40°C (104°F).
Avoid storage of the powder for oral suspension at temperatures above 40°C (104°F). After constitution store the suspension below 30°C (86°F). Do not freeze. Discard unused suspension after 30 days.
Store PEPCID I.V. at 2–8°C (36–46°F). If solution freezes, bring to room temperature; allow sufficient time to solubilize all the components.
When diluted as recommended (see DOSAGE AND ADMINISTRATION) PEPCID I.V. is stable for 48 hours at room temperature.

A.H.F.S. Category: 56:40
DC 7545318   Issued December 1991
COPYRIGHT © MERCK & CO., INC., 1986, 1988, 1991
All rights reserved

PERIACTIN® Tablets   ℞
(Cyproheptadine HCl), U.S.P.
PERIACTIN® Syrup   ℞
(Cyproheptadine HCl), U.S.P.

DESCRIPTION

PERIACTIN* (Cyproheptadine HCl) is an antihistaminic and antiserotonergic agent.
Cyproheptadine hydrochloride is a white to slightly yellowish, crystalline solid, with a molecular weight of 350.89, which is soluble in water, freely soluble in methanol, sparingly soluble in ethanol, soluble in chloroform, and practically insoluble in ether. It is the sesquihydrate of 4-(5*H*-dibenzo[*a,d*]cyclohepten-5-ylidene)-1-methylpiperidine hydrochloride. The empirical formula of the anhydrous salt is $C_{21}H_{21}N\cdot HCl$ and the structural formula of the anhydrous salt is:
[See chemical structure at top of next column.]
PERIACTIN is available in tablets, containing 4 mg of cyproheptadine hydrochloride, and as a syrup in which 5 mL con-

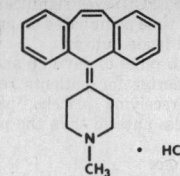

tains 2 mg of cyproheptadine hydrochloride, with a pH range of 3.5 to 4.5.
The tablets also contain the following inactive ingredients: calcium phosphate, lactose, magnesium stearate, and starch. The syrup contains the following inactive ingredients: alcohol 5%, D & C Yellow 10, artificial flavors, glycerin, purified water, sodium saccharin, and sucrose, with sorbic acid 0.1% added as preservative.

---

*Registered trademark of MERCK & CO., INC.

CLINICAL PHARMACOLOGY

PERIACTIN is a serotonin and histamine antagonist with anticholinergic and sedative effects. Antiserotonin and antihistamine drugs appear to compete with serotonin and histamine, respectively, for receptor sites.
Pharmacokinetics and Metabolism
After a single 4 mg oral dose of ^{14}C-labelled cyproheptadine HCl in normal subjects, given as tablets or syrup, 2-20% of the radioactivity was excreted in the stools. Only about 34% of the stool radioactivity was unchanged drug, corresponding to less than 5.7% of the dose. At least 40% of the administered radioactivity was excreted in the urine. No significant difference in the mean urinary excretion exists between the tablet and syrup formulations. No detectable amounts of unchanged drug were present in the urine of patients on chronic 12-20 mg daily doses of PERIACTIN Syrup. The principle metabolite found in human urine has been identified as a quaternary ammonium glucuronide conjugate of cyproheptadine. Elimination is diminished in renal insufficiency.

INDICATIONS AND USAGE

Perennial and seasonal allergic rhinitis
Vasomotor rhinitis
Allergic conjunctivitis due to inhalant allergens and foods
Mild, uncomplicated allergic skin manifestations of urticaria and angioedema
Amelioration of allergic reactions to blood or plasma
Cold urticaria
Dermatographism
As therapy for anaphylactic reactions *adjunctive* to epinephrine and other standard measures after the acute manifestations have been controlled.

CONTRAINDICATIONS

Newborn or Premature Infants
This drug should *not* be used in newborn or premature infants.
Nursing Mothers
Because of the higher risk of antihistamines for infants generally and for newborns and prematures in particular, antihistamine therapy is contraindicated in nursing mothers.
Other Conditions
Hypersensitivity to cyproheptadine and other drugs of similar chemical structure:
    Monoamine oxidase inhibitor therapy
        (see DRUG INTERACTIONS)
    Angle-closure glaucoma
    Stenosing peptic ulcer
    Symptomatic prostatic hypertrophy
    Bladder neck obstruction
    Pyloroduodenal obstruction
    Elderly, debilitated patients

WARNINGS

Children
Overdosage of antihistamines, particularly in infants and children, may produce hallucinations, central nervous system depression, convulsions, and death.
Antihistamines may diminish mental alertness; conversely, particularly, in the young child, they may occasionally produce excitation.
CNS Depressants
Antihistamines may have additive effects with alcohol and other CNS depressants, e.g., hypnotics, sedatives, tranquilizers, antianxiety agents.
Activities Requiring Mental Alertness
Patients should be warned about engaging in activities requiring mental alertness and motor coordination, such as driving a car or operating machinery.

Antihistamines are more likely to cause dizziness, sedation, and hypotension in elderly patients.

PRECAUTIONS

General

Cyproheptadine has an atropine-like action and, therefore, should be used with caution in patients with:

- History of bronchial asthma
- Increased intraocular pressure
- Hyperthyroidism
- Cardiovascular disease
- Hypertension

Information for Patients

Antihistamines may diminish mental alertness; conversely, particularly, in the young child, they may occasionally produce excitation.

Patients should be warned about engaging in activities requiring mental alertness and motor coordination, such as driving a car or operating machinery.

Drug Interactions

MAO inhibitors prolong and intensify the anticholinergic effects of antihistamines.

Antihistamines may have additive effects with alcohol and other CNS depressants, e.g., hypnotics, sedatives, tranquilizers, antianxiety agents.

Carcinogenesis, Mutagenesis, Impairment of Fertility

Long-term carcinogenic studies have not been done with cyproheptadine.

Cyproheptadine had no effect on fertility in a two-litter study in rats or a two generation study in mice at about 10 times the human dose.

Cyproheptadine did not produce chromosome damage in human lymphocytes or fibroblasts *in vitro;* high doses (10^{-4} M) were cytotoxic. Cyproheptadine did not have any mutagenic effect in the Ames microbial mutagen test; concentrations of above 500 mcg/plate inhibited bacterial growth.

Pregnancy

Pregnancy Category B: Reproduction studies have been performed in rabbits, mice, and rats at oral or subcutaneous doses up to 32 times the maximum recommended human oral dose and have revealed no evidence of impaired fertility or harm to the fetus due to cyproheptadine. Cyproheptadine has been shown to be fetotoxic in rats when given by intraperitoneal injection in doses four times the maximum recommended human oral dose. Two studies in pregnant women, however, have not shown that cyproheptadine increases the risk of abnormalities when administered during the first, second and third trimesters of pregnancy. No teratogenic effects were observed in any of the newborns. Nevertheless, because the studies in humans cannot rule out the possibility of harm, cyproheptadine should be used during pregnancy only if clearly needed.

Nursing Mothers

It is not known whether this drug is excreted in human milk. Because many drugs are excreted in human milk, and because of the potential for serious adverse reactions in nursing infants from PERIACTIN, a decision should be made whether to discontinue nursing or to discontinue the drug, taking into account the importance of the drug to the mother (see CONTRAINDICATIONS).

Pediatric Use

Safety and effectiveness in children below the age of two have not been established. See CONTRAINDICATIONS, *Newborn Premature Infants,* and WARNINGS, *Children.*

ADVERSE REACTIONS

Adverse reactions which have been reported with the use of antihistamines are as follows:

Central Nervous System: Sedation and sleepiness (often transient), dizziness, disturbed coordination, confusion, restlessness, excitation, nervousness, tremor, irritability, insomnia, paresthesias, neuritis, convulsions, euphoria, hallucinations, hysteria, faintness.

Integumentary: Allergic manifestation of rash and edema, excessive perspiration, urticaria, photosensitivity.

Special Senses: Acute labyrinthitis, blurred vision, diplopia, vertigo, tinnitus.

Cardiovascular: Hypotension, palpitation, tachycardia, extrasystoles, anaphylactic shock.

Hematologic: Hemolytic anemia, leukopenia, agranulocytosis, thrombocytopenia.

Digestive System: Dryness of mouth, epigastric distress, anorexia, nausea, vomiting, diarrhea, constipation, jaundice.

Genitourinary: Urinary frequency, difficult urination, urinary retention, early menses.

Respiratory: Dryness of nose and throat, thickening of bronchial secretions, tightness of chest and wheezing, nasal stuffiness.

Miscellaneous: Fatigue, chills, headache.

OVERDOSAGE

Antihistamine overdosage reactions may vary from central nervous system depression to stimulation especially in children. Also, atropine-like signs and symptoms (dry mouth; fixed, dilated pupils; flushing, etc.) as well as gastrointestinal symptoms may occur.

If vomiting has not occurred spontaneously the patient should be induced to vomit with syrup of ipecac.

If the patient is unable to vomit, perform gastric lavage followed by activated charcoal. Isotonic or ½ isotonic saline is the lavage of choice. Precautions against aspiration must be taken especially in infants and children.

When life threatening CNS signs and symptoms are present, intravenous physostigmine salicylate may be considered. Dosage and frequency of administration are dependent on age, clinical response, and recurrence after response. (See package circulars for physostigmine products.)

Saline cathartics, as milk of magnesia, by osmosis draw water into the bowel and, therefore, are valuable for their action in rapid dilution of bowel content.

Stimulants should *not* be used.

Vasopressors may be used to treat hypotension.

The oral LD_{50} of cyproheptadine is 123 mg/kg, and 295 mg/kg in the mouse and rat, respectively.

DOSAGE AND ADMINISTRATION

DOSAGE SHOULD BE INDIVIDUALIZED ACCORDING TO THE NEEDS AND THE RESPONSE OF THE PATIENT.

Each PERIACTIN tablet contains 4 mg of cyproheptadine hydrochloride. Each 5 mL of PERIACTIN syrup contains 2 mg of cyproheptadine hydrochloride.

Although intended primarily for administration to children, the syrup is also useful for administration to adults who cannot swallow tablets.

Children

The total daily dosage for children may be calculated on the basis of body weight or body area using approximately 0.25 mg/kg/day (0.11 mg/lb/day) or 8 mg per square meter of body surface (8 mg/M^2). In small children for whom the calculation of dosage based upon body size is most important, it may be necessary to use PERIACTIN syrup to permit accurate dosage.

Age 2 to 6 years

The usual dose is 2 mg (½ tablet or 1 teaspoon) two or three times a day, adjusted as necessary to the size and response of the patient. The dose is not to exceed 12 mg a day.

Age 7 to 14 years

The usual dose is 4 mg (1 tablet or 2 teaspoons) two or three times a day, adjusted as necessary to the size and response of the patient. The dose is not to exceed 16 mg a day.

Adults

The total daily dose for adults should not exceed 0.5 mg/kg/day (0.23 mg/lb/day).

The therapeutic range is 4 to 20 mg a day, with the majority of patients requiring 12 to 16 mg a day. An occasional patient may require as much as 32 mg a day for adequate relief. It is suggested that dosage be initiated with 4 mg (1 tablet or 2 teaspoons) three times a day and adjusted according to the size and response of the patient.

HOW SUPPLIED

No. 3276—Tablets PERIACTIN, containing 4 mg of cyproheptadine hydrochloride each, are white, round, scored, compressed tablets, coded MSD 62. They are supplied as follows:

NDC 0006-0062-68 bottles of 100

(6505-00-890-1884 4 mg 100's).

Shown in Product Identification Section, page 420

No. 3289X—Syrup PERIACTIN, 2 mg per 5 mL is a clear, yellow, syrupy liquid and is supplied as follows:

NDC 0006-3289-74 bottles of 473 mL.

Storage

Store Tablets PERIACTIN in a well-closed container. Avoid storage at temperatures above 40°C (104°F).

Store Syrup PERIACTIN in a container which is kept tightly closed. Avoid storage at temperatures below −20°C (−4°F) and above 40°C (104°F).

A.H.F.S. Category: 4:00

DC 7398318 Issued January 1992

COPYRIGHT © MERCK & CO., INC., 1985
All rights reserved

PLENDIL® ℞
(Felodipine)
Extended-Release Tablets

DESCRIPTION

PLENDIL* (Felodipine) is a calcium antagonist (calcium channel blocker). Felodipine is a dihydropyridine derivative that is chemically described as ± ethyl methyl 4-(2,3-dichlorophenyl)-1, 4-dihydro-2,6-dimethyl-3,5-pyridine-dicarboxylate. Its empirical formula is $C_{18}H_{19}Cl_2NO_4$ and its structural formula is:

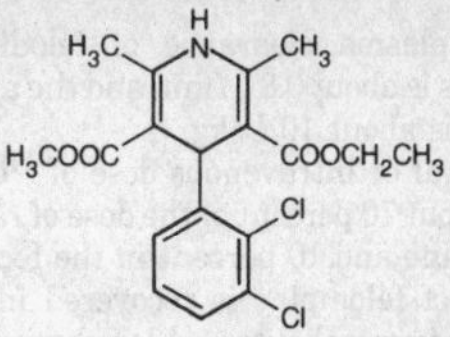

Felodipine is a slightly yellowish, crystalline powder with a molecular weight of 384.26. It is insoluble in water and is freely soluble in dichloromethane and ethanol. Felodipine is a racemic mixture.

Tablets PLENDIL provide extended release of felodipine. They are available as tablets containing 5 mg or 10 mg of felodipine for oral administration. In addition to the active ingredient felodipine, each tablet contains the following inactive ingredients: cellulose, iron oxides, lactose, polyethylene glycol, sodium stearyl fumarate, titanium dioxide and other ingredients.

*Registered trademark of AB Astra

CLINICAL PHARMACOLOGY

Mechanism of Action

Felodipine is a member of the dihydropyridine class of calcium channel antagonists (calcium channel blockers). It reversibly competes with nitrendipine and/or other calcium channel blockers for dihydropyridine binding sites, blocks voltage-dependent Ca^{++} currents in vascular smooth muscle and cultured rabbit atrial cells and blocks potassium-induced contracture of the rat portal vein.

In vitro studies show that the effects of felodipine on contractile processes are selective, with greater effects on vascular smooth muscle than cardiac muscle. Negative inotropic effects can be detected *in vitro,* but such effects have not been seen in intact animals.

The effect of felodipine on blood pressure is principally a consequence of a dose-related decrease of peripheral vascular resistance in man, with a modest reflex increase in heart rate (see *Cardiovascular Effects*). With the exception of a mild diuretic effect seen in several animal species and man, the effects of felodipine are accounted for by its effects on peripheral vascular resistance.

Pharmacokinetics and Metabolism

Following oral administration, felodipine is almost completely absorbed and undergoes extensive first-pass metabolism. The systemic bioavailability of PLENDIL is approximately 20 percent. Mean peak concentrations following the administration of PLENDIL are reached in 2.5 to 5 hours. Both peak plasma concentration and the area under the plasma concentration time curve (AUC) increase linearly with doses up to 20 mg. Felodipine is greater than 99 percent bound to plasma proteins.

Following intravenous administration, the plasma concentration of felodipine declined triexponentially with mean disposition half-lives of 4.8 minutes, 1.5 hours and 9.1 hours. The mean contributions of the three individual phases to the overall AUC were 15, 40 and 45 percent, respectively, in the order of increasing $t_{1/2}$.

Following oral administration of the immediate-release formulation, the plasma level of felodipine also declined polyexponentially with a mean terminal $t_{1/2}$ of 11 to 16 hours. The mean peak and trough steady-state plasma concentrations achieved after 10 mg of the immediate-release formulation given once a day to normal volunteers, were 20 and 0.5 nmol/L, respectively. The trough plasma concentration of felodipine in most individuals was substantially below the concentration needed to effect a half-maximal decline in blood pressure (EC_{50}) [4–6 nmol/L for felodipine], thus precluding once a day dosing with the immediate-release formulation.

Following administration of a 10-mg dose of PLENDIL, the extended-release formulation, to young, healthy volunteers, mean peak and trough steady-state plasma concentrations of felodipine were 7 and 2 nmol/L, respectively. Corresponding values in hypertensive patients (mean age 64) after a 20-mg dose of PLENDIL were 23 and 7 nmol/L. Since the EC_{50} for felodipine is 4 to 6 nmol/L, a 5 to 10-mg dose of PLENDIL in some patients, and a 20-mg dose in others, would be expected to provide an antihypertensive effect that persists for 24 hours (see *Cardiovascular Effects* below and DOSAGE AND ADMINISTRATION).

Continued on next page

Information on the Merck & Co. products listed on these pages is the full prescribing information from product circulars in use October 1, 1992.

Merck & Co.—Cont.

The systemic plasma clearance of felodipine in young healthy subjects is about 0.8 L/min and the apparent volume of distribution is about 10 L/kg.
Following an oral or intravenous dose of ^{14}C-labeled felodipine in man, about 70 percent of the dose of radioactivity was recovered in urine and 10 percent in the feces. A negligible amount of intact felodipine is recovered in the urine and feces (<0.5%). Six metabolites, which account for 23 percent of the oral dose, have been identified; none has significant vasodilating activity.
Following administration of PLENDIL to hypertensive patients, mean peak plasma concentrations at steady state are about 20 percent higher than after a single dose. Blood pressure response is correlated with plasma concentrations of felodipine.
The bioavailability of PLENDIL is not influenced by the presence of food in the gastrointestinal tract. In a study of six patients, the bioavailability of felodipine was increased more than two-fold when taken with doubly concentrated grapefruit juice, compared to when taken with water or orange juice. A similar finding has been seen with some other dihydropyridine calcium antagonists, but to a lesser extent than that seen with felodipine.
Age Effects: Plasma concentrations of felodipine, after a single dose and at steady state, increase with age. Mean clearance of felodipine in elderly hypertensives (mean age 74) was only 45 percent of that of young volunteers (mean age 26). At steady state mean AUC for young patients was 39 percent of that for the elderly. Data for intermediate age ranges suggest that the AUC's fall between the extremes of the young and the elderly.
Hepatic Dysfunction: In patients with hepatic disease, the clearance of felodipine was reduced to about 60 percent of that seen in normal young volunteers.

Renal impairment does not alter the plasma concentration profile of felodipine; although higher concentrations of the metabolites are present in the plasma due to decreased urinary excretion, these are inactive.
Animal studies have demonstrated that felodipine crosses the blood-brain barrier and the placenta.
Cardiovascular Effects
Following administration of PLENDIL, a reduction in blood pressure generally occurs within two to five hours. During chronic administration, substantial blood pressure control lasts for 24 hours, with trough reductions in diastolic blood pressure approximately 40–50 percent of peak reductions. The antihypertensive effect is dose-dependent and correlates with the plasma concentration of felodipine.
A reflex increase in heart rate frequently occurs during the first week of therapy; this increase attenuates over time. Heart rate increases of 5–10 beats per minute may be seen during chronic dosing. The increase is inhibited by beta-blocking agents.
The P-R interval of the ECG is not affected by felodipine when administered alone or in combination with a beta-blocking agent. Felodipine alone or in combination with a beta-blocking agent has been shown, in clinical and electrophysiologic studies, to have no significant effect on cardiac conduction (P-R, P-Q and H-V intervals).
In clinical trials in hypertensive patients without clinical evidence of left ventricular dysfunction, no symptoms suggestive of a negative inotropic effect were noted; however none would be expected in this population (see PRECAUTIONS).
Renal/Endocrine Effects
Renal vascular resistance is decreased by felodipine while glomerular filtration rate remains unchanged. Mild diuresis, natriuresis and kaliuresis have been observed during the first week of therapy. No significant effects on serum electrolytes were observed during short- and long-term therapy.
In clinical trials increases in plasma noradrenaline levels have been observed.
Clinical Studies
Felodipine produces dose-related decreases in systolic and diastolic blood pressure as demonstrated in six placebo-controlled, dose response studies using either immediate-release or extended-release dosage forms. These studies enrolled over 800 patients on active treatment, at total daily doses ranging from 2.5 to 20 mg. In those studies felodipine was administered either as monotherapy or was added to beta blockers. The results of the two studies with PLENDIL given once daily as monotherapy are shown in the table above:
[See table top of next column.]

MEAN REDUCTIONS IN BLOOD PRESSURE (mmHg)*
Systolic/Diastolic

Dose	N	Mean Peak Response	Mean Trough Response	Trough/Peak Ratios (%s)
Study 1 (8 weeks)				
2.5 mg	68	9.4/4.7	2.7/2.5	29/53
5 mg	69	9.5/6.3	2.4/3.7	25/59
10 mg	67	18.0/10.8	10.0/6.0	56/56
Study 2 (4 weeks)				
10 mg	50	5.3/7.2	1.5/3.2	33/40**
20 mg	50	11.3/10.2	4.5/3.2	43/34**

* Placebo response subtracted
** Different number of patients available for peak and trough measurements

INDICATIONS AND USAGE

PLENDIL is indicated for the treatment of hypertension. PLENDIL may be used alone or concomitantly with other antihypertensive agents.

CONTRAINDICATIONS

PLENDIL is contraindicated in patients who are hypersensitive to this product.

PRECAUTIONS

General
Hypotension: Felodipine, like other calcium antagonists, may occasionally precipitate significant hypotension and rarely syncope. It may lead to reflex tachycardia which in susceptible individuals may precipitate angina pectoris. (See ADVERSE REACTIONS.)
Heart Failure: Although acute hemodynamic studies in a small number of patients with NYHA Class II or III heart failure treated with felodipine have not demonstrated negative inotropic effects, safety in patients with heart failure has not been established. Caution therefore should be exercised when using PLENDIL in patients with heart failure or compromised ventricular function, particularly in combination with a beta blocker.
Elderly Patients or Patients with Impaired Liver Function: Patients over 65 years of age or patients with impaired liver function may have elevated plasma concentrations of felodipine and may therefore respond to lower doses of PLENDIL. These patients should have their blood pressure monitored closely during dosage adjustment of PLENDIL and should rarely require doses above 10 mg. (See CLINICAL PHARMACOLOGY and DOSAGE AND ADMINISTRATION.)
Peripheral Edema: Peripheral edema, generally mild and not associated with generalized fluid retention, was the most common adverse event in the clinical trials. The incidence of peripheral edema was both dose- and age-dependent. Frequency of peripheral edema ranged from about 10 percent in patients under 50 years of age taking 5 mg daily to about 30 percent in those over 60 years of age taking 20 mg daily. This adverse effect generally occurs within 2–3 weeks of the initiation of treatment.
Information for Patients
Patients should be instructed to take PLENDIL whole and not to crush or chew the tablets. They should be told that mild gingival hyperplasia (gum swelling) has been reported. Good dental hygiene decreases its incidence and severity.
NOTE: As with many other drugs, certain advice to patients being treated with PLENDIL is warranted. This information is intended to aid in the safe and effective use of this medication. It is not a disclosure of all possible adverse or intended effects.
Drug Interactions
Beta-Blocking Agents: A pharmacokinetic study of felodipine in conjunction with metoprolol demonstrated no significant effects on the pharmacokinetics of felodipine. The AUC and C_{max} of metoprolol, however, were increased approximately 31 and 38 percent, respectively. In controlled clinical trials, however, beta blockers including metoprolol were concurrently administered with felodipine and were well tolerated.
Cimetidine: In healthy subjects pharmacokinetic studies showed an approximately 50 percent increase in the area under the plasma concentration time curve (AUC) as well as the C_{max} of felodipine when given concomitantly with cimetidine. It is anticipated that a clinically significant interaction may occur in some hypertensive patients. Therefore, it is recommended that low doses of PLENDIL be used when given concomitantly with cimetidine.
Digoxin: When given concomitantly with felodipine the peak plasma concentration of digoxin was significantly increased. There was, however, no significant change in the AUC of digoxin.
Other Concomitant Therapy: In healthy subjects there were no clinically significant interactions when felodipine was given concomitantly with indomethacin or spironolactone.
Interaction with Food: See CLINICAL PHARMACOLOGY, *Pharmacokinetics and Metabolism.*
Carcinogenesis, Mutagenesis, Impairment of Fertility
In a two-year carcinogenicity study in the rats fed felodipine at doses of 7.7, 23.1 or 69.3 mg/kg/day (up to 28 times* the maximum recommended human dose on a mg/m^2 basis), a dose-related increase in the incidence of benign interstitial cell tumors of the testes (Leydig cell tumors) was observed in treated male rats. These tumors were not observed in a similar study in mice at doses up to 138.6 mg/kg/day (28 times* the maximum recommended human dose on a mg/m^2 basis). Felodipine, at the doses employed in the two-year rat study, has been shown to lower testicular testosterone and to produce a corresponding increase in serum luteinizing hormone in rats. The Leydig cell tumor development is possibly secondary to these hormonal effects which have not been observed in man.
In this same rate study a dose-related increase in the incidence of focal squamous cell hyperplasia compared to control was observed in the esophageal groove of male and female rats in all dose groups. No other drug-related esophageal or gastric pathology was observed in the rats or with chronic administration in mice and dogs. The latter species, like man, has no anatomical structure comparable to the esophageal groove.
Felodipine was not carcinogenic when fed to mice at doses of up to 138.6 mg/kg/day (28 times* the maximum recommended human dose on a mg/m^2 basis) for periods of up to 80 weeks in males and 99 weeks in females.
Felodipine did not display any mutagenic activity *in vitro* in the Ames microbial mutagenicity test or in the mouse lymphoma forward mutation assay. No clastogenic potential was seen *in vivo* in the mouse micronucleus test at oral doses up to 2500 mg/kg (506 times* the maximum recommended human dose on a mg/m^2 basis) or *in vitro* in a human lymphocyte chromosome aberration assay.
A fertility study in which male and female rats were administered doses of 3.8, 9.6 or 26.9 mg/kg/day showed no significant effect of felodipine on reproductive performance.

*Based on patient weight of 50 kg

Pregnancy
Pregnancy Category C
Teratogenic Effects: Studies in pregnant rabbits administered doses of 0.46, 1.2, 2.3 and 4.6 mg/kg/day (from 0.4 to 4 times* the maximum recommended human dose on a mg/m^2 basis) showed digital anomalies consisting of reduction in size and degree of ossification of the terminal phalanges in the fetuses. The frequency and severity of the changes appeared dose-related and were noted even at the lowest dose. These changes have been shown to occur with other members of the dihydropyridine class and are possibly a result of compromised uterine blood flow. Similar fetal anomalies were not observed in rats given felodipine.
In a teratology study in cynomolgus monkeys no reduction in the size of the terminal phalanges was observed but an abnormal position of the distal phalanges was noted in about 40 percent of the fetuses.

*Based on patient weight of 50 kg

Nonteratogenic Effects: A prolongation of parturition with difficult labor and an increased frequency of fetal and early postnatal deaths were observed in rats administered doses of 9.6 mg/kg/day (4 times* the maximum human dose on a mg/m^2 basis) and above.
Significant enlargement of the mammary glands in excess of the normal enlargement for pregnant rabbits was found with doses greater than or equal to 1.2 mg/kg/day (equal to the maximum human dose on a mg/m^2 basis). This effect occurred only in pregnant rabbits and regressed during lactation. Similar changes in the mammary glands were not observed in rats or monkeys.
There are no adequate and well-controlled studies in pregnant woman. If felodipine is used during pregnancy, or if the patient becomes pregnant while taking this drug, she should be apprised of the potential hazard to the fetus, possible digital anomalies of the infant, and the potential effects of felodipine on labor and delivery, and on the mammary glands of pregnant females.

*Based on patient weight of 50 kg

Nursing Mothers
It is not known whether this drug is secreted in human milk and because of the potential for serious adverse reactions from felodipine in the infant, a decision should be made whether to discontinue nursing or to discontinue the drug, taking into account the importance of the drug to the mother.
Pediatric Use
Safety and effectiveness in children have not been established.

ADVERSE REACTIONS

In controlled studies in the United States and overseas approximately 3000 patients were treated with felodipine as either the extended-release or the immediate-release formulation.
The most common clinical adverse experiences reported with PLENDIL administered as monotherapy in all settings and with all dosage forms of felodipine were peripheral edema and headache. Peripheral edema was generally mild,

but it was age- and dose-related and resulted in discontinuation of therapy in about 4 percent of the enrolled patients. Discontinuation of therapy due to any clinical adverse experience occurred in about 9 percent of the patients receiving PLENDIL, principally for peripheral edema, headache, or flushing.

Adverse experiences that occurred with an incidence of 1.5 percent or greater during monotheraphy with PLENDIL without regard to causality are compared to placebo in the table below.

Percent of Patients with Adverse Effects in Controlled Trials of PLENDIL as Monotherapy (Incidence of discontinuations shown in parentheses)

Adverse Effect	PLENDIL % N=730		Placebo % N=283
Peripheral Edema	22.3	(4.2)	3.5
Headache	18.6	(2.1)	10.6
Flushing	6.4	(1.0)	1.1
Dizziness	5.8	(0.8)	3.2
Upper Respiratory Infection	5.5	(0.1)	1.1
Asthenia	4.7	(0.1)	2.8
Cough	2.9	(0.0)	0.4
Paresthesia	2.5	(0.1)	1.8
Dyspepsia	2.3	(0.0)	1.4
Chest Pain	2.1	(0.1)	1.4
Nausea	1.9	(0.8)	1.1
Muscle Cramps	1.9	(0.0)	1.1
Palpitation	1.8	(0.5)	2.5
Abdominal Pain	1.8	(0.3	1.1
Constipation	1.6	(0.1)	1.1
Diarrhea	1.6	(0.1)	1.1
Pharyngitis	1.6	(0.0)	0.4
Rhinorrhea	1.6	(0.0)	0.0
Back Pain	1.6	(0.0)	1.1
Rash	1.5	(0.1)	1.1

In the two dose response studies using PLENDIL as monotherapy, the following table describes the incidence (percent) of adverse experiences that were dose-related:

Adverse Effect	Placebo N=121	2.5 mg N=71	5.0 mg N=72	10.0 mg N=123	20 mg N=50
Peripheral Edema	2.5	1.4	13.9	19.5	36.0
Palpitation	0.8	1.4	0.0	2.4	12.0
Headache	12.4	11.3	11.1	18.7	28.0
Flushing	0.0	4.2	2.8	8.1	20.0

In addition, adverse experiences that occurred in 0.5 up to 1.5 percent of patients who received PLENDIL in all controlled clinical studies (listed in order of decreasing severity within each category) and serious adverse events that occurred at a lower rate or were found during marketing experience (those lower rate events are in italics) were: *Body as a Whole:* Facial edema, warm sensation; *Cardiovascular:* Tachycardia, *myocardial infarction, hypotension, syncope, angina pectoris,* arrhythmia; *Digestive:* Vomiting, dry mouth, flatulence; *Hematologic: Anemia; Musculoskeletal:* Athralgia, arm pain, knee pain, leg pain, foot pain, hip pain, myalgia; *Nervous/Psychiatric:* Depression, anxiety disorders, insomnia, irritability, nervousness, somnolence; *Respiratory:* Bronchitis, influenza, sinusitis, dyspnea, epistaxis, respiratory infection, sneezing; *Skin:* Contusion, erythema, urticaria; *Urogenital:* Decreased libido, impotence, urinary frequency, urinary urgency, dysuria.

Felodipine, as an immediate release formulation, has also been studied as monotherapy in 680 patients with hypertension in U.S. and overseas controlled clinical studies. Other adverse experiences not listed above and with an incidence of 0.5 percent or greater include: *Body as a Whole:* Fatigue; *Digestive:* Gastrointestinal pain; *Musculoskeletal:* Arthritis, local weakness, neck pain, shoulder pain, ankle pain; *Nervous/Psychiatric:* Tremor; *Respiratory:* Rhinitis; *Skin:* Hyperhidrosis, pruritus; *Special Senses:* Blurred vision, tinnitus; *Urogenital:* Nocturia.

Gingival Hyperplasia: Gingival hyperplasia, usually mild, occurred in <0.5 percent of patients in controlled studies. This condition may be avoided or may regress with improved dental hygiene. (See PRECAUTIONS, *Information for Patients.*)

Clinical Laboratory Test Findings

Serum Electrolytes: No significant effects on serum electrolytes were observed during short- and long-term therapy (see CLINICAL PHARMACOLOGY, *Renal/Endocrine Effects*).

Serum Glucose: No significant effects on fasting serum glucose were observed in patients treated with PLENDIL in the U.S. controlled study.

Liver Enzymes: One of two episodes of elevated serum transaminases decreased once drug was discontinued in clinical studies; no follow-up was available for the other patient.

OVERDOSAGE

Oral doses of 240 mg/kg and 264 mg/kg in male and female mice, respectively and 2390 mg/kg and 2250 mg/kg in male and female rats, respectively, caused significant lethality.

In a suicide attempt, one patient took 150 mg felodipine together with 15 tablets each of atenolol and spironolactone and 20 tablets of nitrazepam. The patient's blood pressure and heart rate were normal on admission to hospital; he subsequently recovered without significant sequelae.

Overdosage might be expected to cause excessive peripheral vasodilation with marked hypotension and possibly bradycardia.

If severe hypotension occurs, symptomatic treatment should be instituted. The patient should be placed supine with the legs elevated. The admistration of intravenous fluids may be useful to treat hypotension due to overdosage with calcium antagonists. In case of accompanying bradycardia, atropine (0.5–1 mg) should be administered intravenously. Sympathomimetic drugs may also be given if the physician feels they are warranted.

It has not been established whether felodipine can be removed from the circulation by hemodialysis.

DOSAGE AND ADMINISTRATION

The recommended initial dose is 5 mg once a day. Therapy should be adjusted individually according to patient response, generally at intervals of not less than two weeks. The usual dosage range is 5–10 mg once daily. The maximum recommended daily dose is 20 mg once a day. That dose in clinical trials showed an increased blood pressure response but a large increase in the rate of peripheral edema and other vasodilatory adverse events (see ADVERSE REACTIONS). Modification of the recommended dosage is usually not required in patients with renal impairment.

PLENDIL should be swallowed whole and not crushed or chewed.

Use in the Elderly or Patients with Impaired Liver Function: Patients over 65 years of age or patients with impaired liver function, because they may develop higher plasma concentrations of felodipine, should have their blood pressure monitored closely during dosage adjustment (see PRECAUTIONS). In general, doses above 10 mg should not be considered in these patients.

HOW SUPPLIED

No. 3585—Tablets PLENDIL, 5 mg, are light red-brown, round convex tablets, with code MSD 451 on one side and PLENDIL on the other. They are supplied as follows:

NDC 0006-0451-28 unit dose packages of 100
NDC 0006-0451-58 unit of use bottles of 100
NDC 0006-0451-31 unit of use bottles of 30.

Shown in Product Identification Section, page 420

No. 3586—Tablets PLENDIL, 10 mg, are red-brown, round convex tablets, with code MSD 452 on one side and PLENDIL on the other. They are supplied as follows:

NDC 0006-0452-28 unit dose packages of 100
NDC 0006-0452-58 unit of use bottles of 100
NDC 0006-0452-31 unit of use bottles of 30.

Shown in Product Identification Section, page 420

Storage

Store below 30°C (86°F). Keep container tightly closed. Protect from light.

A.H.F.S. Category: 24:04
DC 7650202 Issued July 1991

COPYRIGHT © MERCK & CO., INC., 1991
All rights reserved

PNEUMOVAX® 23 ℞
(Pneumococcal Vaccine Polyvalent, MSD)

DESCRIPTION

PNEUMOVAX* 23 (Pneumococcal Vaccine Polyvalent, MSD), is a sterile, liquid vaccine for intramuscular or subcutaneous injection. It consists of a mixture of highly purified capsular polysaccharides from the 23 most prevalent or invasive pneumococcal types accounting for at least 90% of pneumococcal blood isolates and at least 85% of all pneumococcal isolates from sites which are generally sterile as determined by ongoing surveillance of U.S. data.

PNEUMOVAX 23 is manufactured according to methods developed by the MERCK SHARP & DOHME Research Laboratories. Each 0.5 mL dose of vaccine contains 25 μg of each polysaccharide type dissolved in isotonic saline solution containing 0.25% phenol as preservative.

Type 6B pneumococcal polysaccharide exhibits somewhat greater stability in purified form than does Type 6A. A high degree of cross-reactivity between the two types has been demonstrated in adult volunteers. Therefore, Type 6B has replaced Type 6A, which had been used in the 14-valent vaccine. Although contained in the 14-valent vaccine, Type 25 is not included in PNEUMOVAX 23 because it has recently become a rare isolate in many parts of the world including the United States, Canada and Europe.

[See first table at bottom of next page.]

*Registered trademark of MERCK & CO., INC.

CLINICAL PHARMACOLOGY

Pneumococcal infection is a leading cause of death throughout the world and a major cause of pneumonia, meningitis, and otitis media. The emergence of strains of pneumococci with increased resistance to one or more of the common antibiotics and recent isolations of pneumococci with multiple antibiotic resistance emphasize the importance of vaccine prophylaxis against pneumococcal disease. Based on projection from limited observations in the United States, it has been estimated that 400,000 to 500,000 cases of pneumococcal pneumonia may occur annually. The overall case fatality rate ranges from 5–10%. Populations at high risk are the elderly; individuals with immune deficiencies; patients with asplenia or splenic deficiencies, including sickle cell anemia and other severe hemoglobinopathies; alcoholics; and patients with the following diseases: Hodgkin's disease, multiple myeloma and nephrotic syndrome. About 25% of all persons with pneumococcal pneumonia develop bacteremia. Death occurs in about 28% of these bacteremic patients over 50 years of age. Of all patients with pneumococcal bacteremia who died despite treatment with penicillin or tetracycline, as many as 60% died within five days of onset of the illness.

The annual incidence of pneumococcal meningitis is approximately 1.5 to 2.5 per 100,000 population. One-half of the cases occur in children, in whom the fatality rate is about 40%. Children with sickle cell disease have been estimated to have a risk of pneumococcal meningitis nearly 600 times greater than normal children. Other illnesses caused by pneumococci include acute exacerbations of chronic bronchitis, sinusitis, arthritis and conjunctivitis.

Invasive pneumococcal disease causes high morbidity and mortality in spite of effective antimicrobial control by antibiotics. These effects of pneumococcal disease appear due to irreversible physiologic damage caused by the bacteria during the first 5 days following onset of illness, and occur irrespective of antimicrobial therapy. Vaccination offers an effective means of further reducing the mortality and morbidity of this disease.

At present, there are 83 known pneumococcal capsular types. However, the preponderance of pneumococcal diseases is caused by only some capsular types. For example, a 10-year (1952–1962) surveillance at a New York medical center, showed that 56% of all deaths due to pneumococcal pneumonia were caused by 6 capsular types and that approximately 78% of all pneumococcal pneumonias were caused by 12 capsular types. Such unequal distribution of pneumococcal capsular types causing disease has been shown throughout the world. It is on the basis of this information that the pneumococcal vaccine is composed of 23 capsular types, designed to provide coverage of approximately 90% of the most frequently reported types.

It has been established that the purified pneumococcal capsular polysaccharides induce antibody production and that such antibody is effective in preventing pneumococcal disease. Studies in humans have demonstrated the immunogenicity (antibody-stimulating capability) of each of the 23 capsular types when tested in polyvalent vaccines. Adults of all ages responded immunologically to the vaccines. Earlier studies with 12- and 14-valent pneumococcal vaccines in children two years of age and older and in adults showed immunogenic responses. Protective capsular type-specific antibody levels develop by the third week following vaccination.

The protective efficacy of pneumococcal vaccines containing 6 and 12 capsular polysaccharides was investigated in controlled studies of gold miners in South Africa, in whom there is a high attack rate for pneumococcal pneumonia. Capsular type-specific attack rates for pneumococcal pneumonia were observed for the period from 2 weeks through about 1 year after vaccination. The rates for pneumonia caused by the same capsular types represented in the vaccines are given in the table. Protective efficacy was 76% and 92%, respectively, in the two studies for the capsular types represented.

[See second table at bottom of next page.]

In similar studies carried out by Dr. R. Austrian and associates using similar pneumococcal vaccines prepared for the National Institute of Allergy and Infectious Diseases, the reduction in pneumonias caused by the capsular types contained in the vaccines was 79%. Reduction in type-specific pneumococcal bacteremia was 82%. A preliminary report suggests that in patients with sickle cell anemia and/or anatomical or functional asplenia, the vaccine was highly effective in persons over two years of age in preventing severe pneumococcal disease and bacteremia.

The duration of protective effect of PNEUMOVAX 23 is presently unknown, but it has been shown in previous stud-

Continued on next page

Information on the Merck & Co. products listed on these pages is the full prescribing information from product circulars in use October 1, 1992.

Merck & Co.—Cont.

ies with other pneumococcal vaccines that antibody induced by the vaccine may persist for as long as 5 years. Type-specific antibody levels induced by PNEUMOVAX (Pneumococcal Vaccine, Polyvalent, MSD) (14-valent) have been observed to decline over a 42-month period of observation, but remain significantly above prevaccination levels in almost all recipients who manifest an initial response.

INDICATIONS AND USAGE

PNEUMOVAX 23 is indicated for immunization against pneumococcal disease caused by those pneumococcal types included in the vaccine. Effectiveness of the vaccine in the prevention of pneumococcal pneumonia and pneumococcal bacteremia has been demonstrated in controlled trials. PNEUMOVAX 23 *will not immunize against capsular types of pneumococcus other than those contained in the vaccine. Use in selected individuals over 2 years of age as follows:* (1) patients who have anatomical asplenia or who have splenic dysfunction due to sickle cell disease or other causes; (2) persons with chronic illnesses in which there is an increased risk of pneumococcal disease, such as functional impairment of cardiorespiratory, hepatic and renal systems; (3) persons 50 years of age or older; (4) patients with other chronic illnesses who may be at greater risk of developing pneumococcal infection or experiencing more severe pneumococcal illness as a result of alcohol abuse or coexisting diseases including diabetes mellitus, chronic cerebrospinal fluid leakage, or conditions associated with immunosuppression; (5) patients with Hodgkin's disease if immunization can be given at least 10 days prior to treatment. For maximal antibody response immunization should be given at least 14 days prior to the start of treatment with radiation or chemotherapy. Immunization of patients less than 10 days prior to or during treatment is not recommended. (see CONTRAINDICATIONS.) *Use in communities.* Persons over 2 years of age as follows: (1) closed groups such as those in residential schools, nursing homes and other institutions. (To decrease the likelihood of acute outbreaks of pneumococcal disease in closed institutional populations where there is increased risk that the disease may be severe, vaccination of the entire closed population should be considered where there are no other contraindications.); (2) groups epidemiologically at risk in the community when there is a generalized outbreak in the population due to a single pneumococcal type included in the vaccine; (3) patients at high risk of influenza complications, particularly pneumonia.
PNEUMOVAX 23 may not be effective in preventing infection resulting from basilar skull fracture or from external communication with cerebrospinal fluid.
Simultaneous administration of pneumococcal polysaccharide vaccine and whole-virus influenza vaccine gives satisfactory antibody response without increasing the occurrence of adverse reactions. Simultaneous administration of the pneumococcal vaccine and split-virus influenza vaccine may also be expected to yield satisfactory results.
Revaccination
Routine revaccination of adults previously vaccinated with PNEUMOVAX 23 is not recommended because an increased incidence and severity of adverse reactions have been reported among healthy adults revaccinated with pneumococcal vaccines at intervals under three years. This was probably due to sustained high antibody levels.
Based on a clinical study, revaccination with PNEUMOVAX 23 is recommended for adults at highest risk of fatal pneumococcal infection who were initially vaccinated with PNEUMOVAX* (Pneumococcal Vaccine Polyvalent, MSD) (14-valent) without serious or severe reaction four or more years previously.**
Children at highest risk for pneumococcal infection (e.g., children with asplenia, sickle cell disease or nephrotic syndrome) may have lower peak antibody levels and/or more

rapid antibody decline than do healthy adults. There is evidence that some of these high-risk children, (e.g., asplenic children) benefit from revaccination with vaccine containing antigen types 7F, 8, 19F. The Immunization Practices Advisory Committee (ACIP) recommends that revaccination after three to five years should be considered for children at highest risk for pneumococcal infection (e.g., children with asplenia, sickle cell disease or nephrotic syndrome) who would be ten years old or younger at revaccination.

* Registered trademark of MERCK & CO., INC.
** NOTE: The Immunization Practices Advisory Committee (ACIP) has stated that, without more information: persons who received the 14-valent pneumococcal vaccine should not be routinely revaccinated with the 23-valent vaccine, as increased coverage is modest and duration of protection is not well defined. However, revaccination with the 23-valent vaccine should be strongly considered for persons who received the 14-valent vaccine if they are at highest risk of fatal pneumococcal infection (e.g., asplenic patients). Revaccination should also be considered for adults at highest risk who received the 23-valent vaccine ≥ 6 years before and for those shown to have rapid decline in pneumococcal antibody levels (e.g., patients with nephrotic syndrome, renal failure, or transplant recipients).

CONTRAINDICATIONS

Hypersensitivity to any component of the vaccine. Epinephrine injection (1:1000) must be immediately available should an acute anaphylactoid reaction occur due to any component of the vaccine.
Revaccination of adults with PNEUMOVAX 23 is contraindicated except as described under INDICATIONS AND USAGE.
Patients with Hodgkin's disease immunized less than 7 to 10 days prior to immunosuppressive therapy have in some instances been found to have post-immunization antibody levels below their pre-immunization levels. Because of these results, immunization less than 10 days prior to or during treatment is contraindicated.
Patients with Hodgkin's disease who have received extensive chemotherapy and/or nodal irradiation have been shown to have an impaired antibody response to a 12-valent pneumococcal vaccine. Because, in some intensively treated patients, administration of that vaccine depressed pre-existing levels of antibody to some pneumococcal types, PNEUMOVAX 23 is not recommended at this time for patients who have received these forms of therapy for Hodgkin's disease.

WARNINGS

If the vaccine is used in persons receiving immunosuppressive therapy, the expected serum antibody response may not be obtained.
Intradermal administration may cause severe local reactions.

PRECAUTIONS

General
Caution and appropriate care should be exercised in administering PNEUMOVAX 23 to individuals with severely compromised cardiac and/or pulmonary function in whom a systemic reaction would pose a significant risk.
Any febrile respiratory illness or other active infection is reason for delaying use of PNEUMOVAX 23, except when, in the opinion of the physician, withholding the agent entails even greater risk.
In patients who require penicillin (or other antibiotic) prophylaxis against pneumococcal infection, such prophylaxis should not be discontinued after vaccination with PNEUMOVAX 23.
Pregnancy
Pregnancy Category C: Animal reproduction studies have not been conducted with PNEUMOVAX 23. It is also not

known whether PNEUMOVAX 23 can cause fetal harm when administered to a pregnant woman or can affect reproduction capacity. PNEUMOVAX 23 should be given to a pregnant woman only if clearly needed.
Nursing Mothers
It is not known whether this drug is excreted in human milk. Because many drugs are excreted in human milk, caution should be exercised when PNEUMOVAX 23 is administered to a nursing woman.
Pediatric Use
Children less than 2 years of age do not respond satisfactorily to the capsular types of PNEUMOVAX 23 that are most often the cause of pneumococcal disease in this age group. Safety and effectiveness in children below the age of 2 years have not been established. Accordingly, PNEUMOVAX 23 is not recommended in this age group.

ADVERSE REACTIONS

Local reactions including local injection site soreness, erythema and swelling, usually of less than 48 hours duration, occurs commonly; local induration occurs less commonly. In a study of PNEUMOVAX 22 (containing 22 capsular types) in 29 adults, 21 (71%) showed local reaction characterized principally by local soreness and/or induration at the injection site within 2 days after vaccination.
Rash, urticaria, arthritis, arthralgia, serum sickness, and adenitis have been reported rarely.
Low grade fever (less than 100.9°F) occurs occasionally and is usually confined to the 24-hour period following vaccination. Although rare, fever over 102°F has been reported. Malaise, myalgia, headache, and asthenia also have been reported. Patients with otherwise stabilized idiopathic thrombocytopenic purpura have, on rare occasions, experienced a relapse in their thrombocytopenia, occurring 2 to 14 days after vaccination, and lasting up to 2 weeks.
Reactions of greater severity, duration, or extent are unusual. Neurological disorders such as paresthesias and acute radiculoneuropathy including Guillain-Barré syndrome have been rarely reported in temporal association with administration of pneumococcal vaccine. No cause and effect relationship has been established. Rarely, anaphylactoid reactions have been reported.

DOSAGE AND ADMINISTRATION

Do not inject intravenously. Intradermal administration should be avoided.
Parenteral drug products should be inspected visually for particulate matter and discoloration prior to administration, whenever solution and container permit. PNEUMOVAX 23 is a clear, colorless solution.
Administer a single 0.5 mL dose of PNEUMOVAX 23 subcutaneously or intramuscularly (preferably in the deltoid muscle or lateral mid-thigh), with appropriate precautions to avoid intravascular administration.
Single-Dose and 5-Dose Vials
For Syringe Use Only: Withdraw 0.5 mL from the vial using a sterile needle and syringe free of preservatives, antiseptics and detergents.
It is important to use a separate sterile syringe and needle for each individual patient to prevent transmission of hepatitis B and other infectious agents from one person to another. Store unopened and opened vials at 2–8°C (36–46°F). The vaccine is used directly as supplied. No dilution or reconstitution is necessary. Phenol 0.25% added as preservative. All vaccine must be discarded after the expiration date.

HOW SUPPLIED

No. 4739—PNEUMOVAX 23 contains one 5-dose vial of liquid vaccine, **NDC** 0006-4739-00. For use with syringe only (6505-01-092-0391).
No. 4741—PNEUMOVAX 23 is supplied as follows: **NDC** 0006-4741-00. A box of 5 individual cartons, each containing a single-dose vial of vaccine.
A.H.F.S. Category: 80:12
DC 7497407   Issued July 1990

---

23 Pneumococcal Capsular Types Included in PNEUMOVAX 23

Nomenclature	Pneumococcal Types																						
Danish	1	2	3	4	5	6B	7F	8	9N	9V	10A	11A	12F	14	15B	17F	18C	19F	19A	20	22F	23F	33F
U.S.	1	2	3	4	5	26	51	8	9	68	34	43	12	14	54	17	56	19	57	20	22	23	70

PNEUMOVAX 23

Number of Capsular Types in Pneumococcal Vaccine	Rate/1000 for Pneumonia Caused by Homologous Capsular Types		Protective Efficacy
	Vaccinated Group	Control Group	
6	9.2	38.3	76%
12	1.8	22.0	92%

PRILOSEC® Delayed-Release Capsules   ℞
(Omeprazole)

DESCRIPTION

The active ingredient in PRILOSEC* (Omeprazole) Delayed-Release Capsules is a substituted benzimidazole, 5-methoxy-2-[[(4-methoxy-3,5-dimethyl-2-pyridinyl)methyl] sulfinyl]-1*H*-benzimidazole, a compound that inhibits gastric acid secretion. Its empirical formula is $C_{17}H_{19}N_3O_3S$, with a molecular weight of 345.42. The structural formula is:
[See chemical structure at top of next page.]

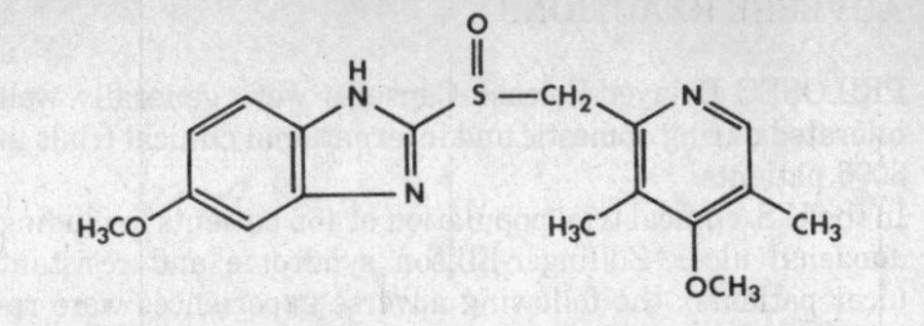

Omeprazole is a white to off-white crystalline powder which melts with decomposition at about 155°C. It is a weak base, freely soluble in ethanol and methanol, and slightly soluble in acetone and isopropanol and very slightly soluble in water. The stability of omeprazole is a function of pH; it is rapidly degraded in acid media, but has acceptable stability under alkaline conditions.
PRILOSEC is supplied as delayed-release capsules for oral administration. Each delayed-release capsule contains 20 mg of omeprazole in the form of enteric-coated granules with the following inactive ingredients: cellulose, disodium hydrogen phosphate, hydroxpropyl cellulose, hydroxpropyl methycellulose, lactose, mannitol, sodium lauryl sulfate and other ingredients. The capsule shell has the following inactive ingredients: gelatin, FD&C Blue #1, FD&C Red #40, titanium dioxide, synthetic black iron oxide, isopropanol, butyl alcohol, FD&C Blue #2, and D&C Red #7 Calcium Lake.

* Registered trademark of AB Astra

CLINICAL PHARMACOLOGY

Pharmacokinetics and Metabolism
PRILOSEC Delayed-Release Capsules contain an enteric-coated granule formulation of omeprazole (because omeprazole is acid-labile), so that absorption of omeprazole begins only after the granules leave the stomach. Absorption is rapid, with peak plasma levels of omeprazole occurring within 0.5 to 3.5 hours. Peak plasma concentrations of omeprazole and AUC are approximately proportional to doses up to 40 mg, but because of a saturable first-pass effect, a greater than linear response in peak plasma concentration and AUC occurs with doses greater than 40 mg. Absolute bioavailability (compared to intravenous administration) is about 30–40% at doses of 20–40 mg, due in large part to presystemic metabolism. In healthy subjects the plasma half-life is 0.5 to 1 hour, and the total body clearance is 500–600 mL/min. Protein binding is approximately 95%.
The bioavailability of omeprazole increases slightly upon repeated administration of PRILOSEC Delayed-Release Capsules.
Following single dose oral administration of a buffered solution of omeprazole, little if any unchanged drug was excreted in urine. The majority of the dose (about 77%) was eliminated in urine as at least six metabolites. Two were identified as hydroxyomeprazole and the corresponding carboxylic acid. The remainder of the dose was recoverable in feces. This implies a significant biliary excretion of the metabolites of omeprazole. Three metabolites have been identified in plasma—the sulfide and sulfone derivatives of omeprazole, and hydroxyomeprazole. These metabolites have very little or no antisecretory activity.
In patients with chronic hepatic disease, the bioavailability increased to approximately 100% compared to an I.V. dose, reflecting decreased first-pass effect, and the plasma half-life of the drug increased to nearly 3 hours compared to the half-life in normals of 0.5–1 hour. Plasma clearance averaged 70 mL/min, compared to a value of 500–600 mL/min in normal subjects.
In patients with chronic renal impairment, whose creatinine clearance ranged between 10 and 62 mL/min/1.73 m^2, the disposition of omeprazole was very similar to that in healthy volunteers, although there was a slight increase in bioavailability. Because urinary excretion is a primary route of excretion of omeprazole metabolites, their elimination slowed in proportion to the decreased creatinine clearance.
The elimination rate of omeprazole was somewhat decreased in the elderly, and bioavailability was increased. Omeprazole was 76% bioavailable when a single 40 mg oral dose of omeprazole (buffered solution) was administered to healthy elderly volunteers, versus 58% in young volunteers given the same dose. Nearly 70% of the dose was recovered in urine as metabolites of omeprazole and no unchanged drug was detected. The plasma clearance of omeprazole was 250 mL/min (about half that of young volunteers) and its plasma half-life averaged one hour, about twice that of young healthy volunteers.
Pharmacodynamics
Mechanism of Action
Omeprazole belongs to a new class of antisecretory compounds, the substituted benzimidazoles, that do not exhibit anticholinergic or H_2 histamine antagonistic properties, but that suppress gastric acid secretion by specific inhibition of the H^+/K^+ ATPase enzyme system at the secretory surface of the gastric parietal cell. Because this enzyme system is regarded as the acid (proton) pump within the gastric mucosa, omeprazole has been characterized as a gastric acid-pump inhibitor, in that it blocks the final step of acid production. This effect is dose-related and leads to inhibition of both basal and stimulated acid secretion irrespective of the stimulus. Animal studies indicate that after rapid disappearance from plasma, omeprazole can be found within the gastric mucosa for a day or more.
Antisecretory Activity
After oral administration, the onset of the antisecretory effect of omeprazole occurs within one hour, with the maximum effect occurring within two hours. Inhibition of secretion is about 50% of maximum at 24 hours and the duration of inhibition lasts up to 72 hours. The antisecretory effect thus lasts far longer than would be expected from the very short (less than one hour) plasma half-life, apparently due to prolonged binding to the parietal H^+/K^+ ATPase enzyme. When the drug is discontinued, secretory activity returns gradually, over 3 to 5 days. The inhibitory effect of omeprazole on acid secretion increases with repeated once-daily dosing, reaching a plateau after four days.
Results from numerous studies of the antisecretory effect of multiple doses of 20 mg and 40 mg of omeprazole in normal volunteers and patients are shown below. The "max" value represents determinations at a time of maximum effect (2–6 hours after dosing), while "min" values are those 24 hours after the last dose of omeprazole.

Range of Mean Values from Multiple Studies of the Mean Antisecretory Effects of Omeprazole After Multiple Daily Dosing

Parameter	Omeprazole 20 mg Max	Omeprazole 20 mg Min	Omeprazole 40 mg Max	Omeprazole 40 mg Min
% Decrease in Basal Acid Output	78*	58–80	94*	80–93
% Decrease in Peak Acid Output	79*	50–59	88*	62–68
% Decrease in 24-hr. Intragastric Acidity		80–97		92–94

* Single Studies

Single daily oral doses of omeprazole ranging from a dose of 10 mg to 40 mg have produced 100% inhibition of 24-hour intragastric acidity in some patients.
Enterochromaffin-like (ECL) Cell Effects
In 24-month carcinogenicity studies in rats, a dose-related significant increase in gastric carcinoid tumors and ECL cell hyperplasia was observed in both male and female animals (see PRECAUTIONS, *Carcinogenesis, Mutagenesis, Impairment of Fertility*). Hypergastrinemia secondary to prolonged and sustained hypochlorhydria has been postulated to be the mechanism by which ECL cell hyperplasia and gastric carcinoid tumors develop. Omeprazole may also affect other cells in the gastrointestinal tract (e.g., G cells), either directly or by inducing sustained hypochlorhydria, but this possibility has not been extensively studied.
Human gastric biopsy specimens from about 200 patients treated continuously with omeprazole for an average of over 12 months have not detected ECL cell effects of omeprazole similar to those seen in rats. Longer term data are needed to rule out the possibility of an increased risk for the development of gastric tumors in patients receiving long-term therapy with omeprazole.
Serum Gastrin Effects
In studies involving more than 200 patients, serum gastrin levels increased during the first 1 to 2 weeks of once-daily administration of therapeutic doses of omeprazole in parallel with inhibition of acid secretion. No further increase in serum gastrin occurred with continued treatment. In comparison with histamine H_2-receptor antagonists, the median increases produced by 20 mg doses of omeprazole were higher (1.3 to 3.6 fold vs. 1.1 to 1.8 fold increase). Gastrin values returned to pretreatment levels, usually within 1 to 2 weeks after discontinuation of therapy.
Other Effects
Systemic effects of omeprazole in the CNS, cardiovascular and respiratory systems have not been found to date. Omeprazole, given in oral doses of 30 or 40 mg for 2 to 4 weeks, had no effect on thyroid function, carbohydrate metabolism, or circulating levels of parathyroid hormone, cortisol, estradiol, testosterone, prolactin, cholecystokinin or secretin.
No effect on gastric emptying of the solid and liquid components of a test meal was demonstrated after a single dose of omeprazole 90 mg. In healthy subjects, a single I.V. dose of omeprazole (0.35 mg/kg) had no effect on intrinsic factor secretion. No systematic dose-dependent effect has been observed on basal or stimulated pepsin output in humans. However, when intragastric pH is maintained at 4.0 or above, basal pepsin output is low, and pepsin activity is decreased.
As do other agents that elevate intragastric pH, omeprazole administered for 14 days in healthy subjects produced a significant increase in the intragastric concentrations of viable bacteria. The pattern of the bacterial species was unchanged from that commonly found in saliva. All changes resolved within three days of stopping treatment.
Clinical Studies
Duodenal Ulcer Disease
Active Duodenal Ulcer: In a multicenter, double-blind, placebo-controlled study of 147 patients with endoscopically documented duodenal ulcer, the percentage of patients healed (per protocol) at 2 and 4 weeks was significantly higher with PRILOSEC 20 mg once a day than with placebo ($p \leq 0.01$).

Treatment of Active Duodenal Ulcer
% of Patients Healed

	PRILOSEC 20 mg a.m. (n=99)	Placebo a.m. (n=48)
Week 2	*41	13
Week 4	*75	27

*($p \leq 0.01$)

Complete daytime and nighttime pain relief occurred significantly faster ($p \leq 0.01$) in patients treated with PRILOSEC 20 mg than in patients treated with placebo. At the end of the study, significantly more patients who had received PRILOSEC had complete relief of daytime pain ($p \leq 0.05$) and nighttime pain ($p \leq 0.01$).
In a multicenter, double-blind study of 293 patients with endoscopically documented duodenal ulcer, the percentage of patients healed (per protocol) at 4 weeks was significantly higher with PRILOSEC 20 mg once a day than with ranitidine 150 mg b.i.d. ($p < 0.01$).

Treatment of Active Duodenal Ulcer
% of Patients Healed

	PRILOSEC 20 mg a.m. (n=145)	Ranitidine 150 mg b.i.d. (n=148)
Week 2	42	34
Week 4	*82	63

*($p < 0.01$)

Healing occurred significantly faster in patients treated with PRILOSEC than in those treated with ranitidine 150 mg b.i.d. ($p < 0.01$).
In a foreign multinational randomized, double-blind study of 105 patients with endoscopically documented duodenal ulcer, 20 mg and 40 mg of PRILOSEC were compared to 150 mg b.i.d. of ranitidine at 2, 4 and 8 weeks. At 2 and 4 weeks both doses of PRILOSEC were statistically superior (per protocol) to ranitidine, but 40 mg was not superior to 20 mg of PRILOSEC, and at 8 weeks there was no significant difference between any of the active drugs.

Treatment of Active Duodenal Ulcer
% of Patients Healed

	PRILOSEC 20 mg (n=34)	PRILOSEC 40 mg (n=36)	Ranitidine 150 mg b.i.d. (n=35)
Week 2	*83	*83	53
Week 4	*97	*100	82
Week 8	100	100	94

*($p \leq 0.01$)

Gastroesophageal Reflux Disease (GERD)
In a U.S. multicenter double-blind placebo controlled study of 20 mg or 40 mg of PRILOSEC Delayed-Release Capsules in patients with symptomatic esophagitis and endoscopically diagnosed erosive esophagitis of grade 2 or above, the percentage healing rates (per protocol) were as follows:

Week	20 mg PRILOSEC (n=83)	40 mg PRILOSEC (n=87)	Placebo (n=43)
4	39**	45**	7
8	74**	75**	14

**($p < 0.01$) PRILOSEC versus placebo.

In this study, the 40 mg dose was not superior to the 20 mg dose of PRILOSEC in the percentage healing rate. Other controlled clinical trials have also shown that PRILOSEC is effective in severe GERD. In comparisons with histamine H_2-receptor antagonists in patients with erosive esophagitis, grade 2 or above, PRILOSEC in a dose of 20 mg was significantly more effective than the active controls. Complete daytime and nighttime heartburn relief occurred significantly faster ($p < 0.01$) in patients treated with PRILOSEC than in those taking placebo or histamine H_2-receptor antagonists.
Pathological Hypersecretory Conditions
In open studies of 136 patients with pathological hypersecretory conditions, such as Zollinger-Ellison (ZE) syndrome with or without multiple endocrine adenomas, PRILOSEC Delayed-Release Capsules significantly inhibited gastric acid

Continued on next page

Information on the Merck & Co. products listed on these pages is the full prescribing information from product circulars in use October 1, 1992.

Merck & Co.—Cont.

secretion and controlled associated symptoms of diarrhea, anorexia, and pain. Doses ranging from 20 mg every other day to 360 mg per day maintained basal acid secretion below 10 mEq/hr in patients without prior gastric surgery, and below 5 mEq/hr in patients with prior gastric surgery.
Initial doses were titrated to the individual patient need, and adjustments were necessary with time in some patients (see DOSAGE AND ADMINISTRATION). PRILOSEC was well tolerated at these high dose levels for prolonged periods (> 5 years in some patients). In most ZE patients, serum gastrin levels were not modified by PRILOSEC. However, in some patients serum gastrin increased to levels greater than those present prior to initiation of omeprazole therapy. At least 2 patients with ZE syndrome on long-term treatment with PRILOSEC developed gastric carcinoids. This finding was believed to be a manifestation of the underlying condition, which is known to be associated with such tumors, rather than the result of the administration of PRILOSEC.

INDICATIONS AND USAGE

Short-Term Treatment of Active Duodenal Ulcer
PRILOSEC Delayed-Release Capsules are indicated for short-term treatment of active duodenal ulcer. Most patients heal within four weeks. Some patients may require an additional four weeks of therapy.
PRILOSEC SHOULD NOT BE USED AS MAINTENANCE THERAPY FOR TREATMENT OF PATIENTS WITH DUODENAL ULCER DISEASE. (See boxed WARNING.)
Gastroesophageal Reflux Disease (GERD)
Severe Erosive Esophagitis
PRILOSEC Delayed-Release Capsules are indicated for the short-term treatment (4–8 weeks) of severe erosive esophagitis (grade 2 or above) which has been diagnosed by endoscopy (see CLINICAL PHARMACOLOGY, *Clinical Studies*).
Poorly Responsive Symptomatic GERD
PRILOSEC Delayed-Release Capsules are also indicated for the short-term treatment (4–8 weeks) of symptomatic gastroesophageal reflux disease (esophagitis) poorly responsive to customary medical treatment, usually including an adequate course of a histamine H₂-receptor antagonist.
The efficacy of PRILOSEC used for longer than 8 weeks in these patients has not been established. In the rare instance of a patient not responding to 8 weeks of treatment, it may be helpful to give up to an additional 4 weeks of treatment. If there is recurrence of severe or symptomatic GERD poorly responsive to customary medical treatment, additional 4–8 week courses of omeprazole may be considered. THE DRUG SHOULD NOT BE USED AS MAINTENANCE THERAPY. (See boxed WARNING.)
Pathological Hypersecretory Conditions
PRILOSEC Delayed-Release Capsules are indicated for the long-term treatment of pathological hypersecretory conditions (e.g., Zollinger-Ellison syndrome, multiple endocrine adenomas and systemic mastocytosis).

CONTRAINDICATIONS

PRILOSEC Delayed-Release Capsules are contraindicated in patients with known hypersensitivity to any component of the formulation.

> **WARNING**
>
> In long-term (2 year) studies in rats, omeprazole produced a dose-related increase in gastric carcinoid tumors (see PRECAUTIONS, *Carcinogenesis, Mutagenesis, Impairment of Fertility*). While available endoscopic evaluations and histologic examinations of biopsy specimens from human stomachs have not detected a risk from short-term exposure to PRILOSEC, further human data on the effect of sustained hypochlorhydria and hypergastrinemia are needed to rule out the possibility of an increased risk for the development of tumors in humans receiving long-term therapy with PRILOSEC. PRILOSEC should be prescribed only for the conditions, dosage and duration described (see INDICATIONS AND USAGE and DOSAGE AND ADMINISTRATION).

PRECAUTIONS

General
Symptomatic response to therapy with omeprazole does not preclude the presence of gastric malignancy.
Information for Patients
PRILOSEC Delayed-Release Capsules should be taken before eating. Patients should be cautioned that the PRILOSEC Delayed-Release Capsule should not be opened, chewed or crushed, and should be swallowed whole.

Drug Interactions
Omeprazole can prolong the elimination of diazepam, warfarin and phenytoin, drugs that are metabolized by oxidation in the liver. Although in normal subjects no interaction with theophylline or propranolol was found, there have been reports of interaction with other drugs metabolized via the cytochrome P-450 system (e.g., cyclosporine, disulfiram). Patients should be monitored to determine if it is necessary to adjust the dosage of these drugs when taken concomitantly with PRILOSEC.
Because of its profound and long lasting inhibition of gastric acid secretion, it is theoretically possible that omeprazole may interfere with absorption of drugs where gastric pH is an important determinant of their bioavailability (e.g., ketoconazole, ampicillin esters, and iron salts). In the clinical trials, antacids were used concomitantly with the administration of PRILOSEC.

Carcinogenesis, Mutagenesis, Impairment of Fertility
In two 24-month carcinogenicity studies in rats, omeprazole at daily doses of 1.7, 3.4, 13.8, 44.0 and 140.8 mg/kg/day (approximately 4 to 352 times the human dose, based on a patient weight of 50 kg and a human dose of 20 mg) produced gastric ECL cell carcinoids in a dose-related manner in both male and female rats; the incidence of this effect was markedly higher in female rats, which had higher blood levels of omeprazole. Gastric carcinoids seldom occur in the untreated rat. In addition, ECL cell hyperplasia was present in all treated groups of both sexes. In one of these studies, female rats were treated with 13.8 mg omeprazole/kg/day (approximately 35 times the human dose) for one year, then followed for an additional year without the drug. No carcinoids were seen in these rats. An increased incidence of treatment-related ECL cell hyperplasia was observed at the end of one year (94% treated vs 10% controls). By the second year the difference between treated and control rats was much smaller (46% vs 26%) but still showed more hyperplasia in the treated group. An unusual primary malignant tumor in the stomach was seen in one rat (2%). No similar tumor was seen in male or female rats treated for two years. For this strain of rat no similar tumor has been noted historically, but a finding involving only one tumor is difficult to interpret. A 78-week mouse carcinogenicity study of omeprazole did not show increased tumor occurrence, but the study was not conclusive.
Omeprazole was not mutagenic in an *in vitro* Ames *Salmonella typhimurium* assay, an *in vitro* mouse lymphoma cell assay and an *in vivo* rat liver DNA damage assay. A mouse micronucleus test at 625 and 6250 times the human dose gave a borderline result, as did an *in vivo* bone marrow chromosome aberration test. A second mouse micronucleus study at 2000 times the human dose, but with different (suboptimal) sampling times, was negative.
In a rat fertility and general reproductive performance test, omeprazole in a dose range of 13.8 to 138.0 mg/kg/day (approximately 35 to 345 times the human dose) was not toxic or deleterious to the reproductive performance of parental animals.

Pregnancy
Pregnancy Category C
Teratology studies conducted in pregnant rats at doses up to 138 mg/kg/day (approximately 345 times the human dose) and in pregnant rabbits at doses up to 69 mg/kg/day (approximately 172 times the human dose) did not disclose any evidence for a teratogenic potential of omeprazole.
In rabbits, omeprazole in a dose range of 6.9 to 69.1 mg/kg/day (approximately 17 to 172 times the human dose) produced dose-related increases in embryo-lethality, fetal resorptions and pregnancy disruptions. In rats, dose-related embryo/fetal toxicity and postnatal developmental toxicity were observed in offspring resulting from parents treated with omeprazole 13.8 to 138.0 mg/kg/day (approximately 35 to 345 times the human dose). There are no adequate or well-controlled studies in pregnant women. Omeprazole should be used during pregnancy only if the potential benefit justifies the potential risk to the fetus.

Nursing Mothers
It is not known whether omeprazole is excreted in human milk. In rats, omeprazole administration during late gestation and lactation at doses of 13.8 to 138 mg/kg/day (35 to 345 times the human dose) resulted in decreased weight gain in pups. Because many drugs are excreted in human milk, because of the potential for serious adverse reactions in nursing infants from omeprazole, and because of the potential for tumorigenicity shown for omeprazole in rat carcinogenicity studies, a decision should be made whether to discontinue nursing or to discontinue the drug, taking into account the importance of the drug to the mother.

Pediatric Use
Safety and effectiveness in children have not been established.

ADVERSE REACTIONS

PRILOSEC Delayed-Release Capsules were generally well tolerated during domestic and international clinical trials in 3096 patients.
In the U.S. clinical trial population of 465 patients (including duodenal ulcer, Zollinger-Ellison syndrome and resistant ulcer patients), the following adverse experiences were reported to occur in 1% or more of patients on therapy with PRILOSEC. Numbers in parentheses indicate percentages of the adverse experiences considered by investigators as possibly, probably or definitely related to the drug:

	Omeprazole (n = 465)	Placebo (n = 64)	Ranitidine (n = 195)
Headache	6.9 (2.4)	6.3	7.7 (2.6)
Diarrhea	3.0 (1.9)	3.1 (1.6)	2.1 (0.5)
Abdominal Pain	2.4 (0.4)	3.1	2.1
Nausea	2.2 (0.9)	3.1	4.1 (0.5)
URI	1.9	1.6	2.6
Dizziness	1.5 (0.6)	0.0	2.6 (1.0)
Vomiting	1.5 (0.4)	4.7	1.5 (0.5)
Rash	1.5 (1.1)	0.0	0.0
Constipation	1.1 (0.9)	0.0	0.0
Cough	1.1	0.0	1.5
Asthenia	1.1 (0.2)	1.6 (1.6)	1.5 (1.0)
Back Pain	1.1	0.0	0.5

The following adverse reactions which occurred in 1% or more of omeprazole-treated patients have been reported in international double-blind, and open-label, clinical trials in which 2,631 patients and subjects received omeprazole.

	Incidence of Adverse Experiences ≥ 1% Causal Relationship not Assessed	
	Omeprazole (n = 2631)	Placebo (n = 120)
Body as a Whole, site unspecified		
Abdominal pain	5.2	3.3
Asthenia	1.3	0.8
Digestive System		
Constipation	1.5	0.8
Diarrhea	3.7	2.5
Flatulence	2.7	5.8
Nausea	4.0	6.7
Vomiting	3.2	10.0
Acid regurgitation	1.9	3.3
Nervous System/Psychiatric		
Headache	2.9	2.5

Additional adverse experiences occurring in <1% of patients or subjects in domestic and/or international trials, or occurring since the drug was marketed, are shown below within each body system. In many instances, the relationship to PRILOSEC was unclear.
Body As a Whole: Fever, pain, fatigue, malaise, abdominal swelling
Cardiovascular: Chest pain or angina, tachycardia, bradycardia, palpitation, elevated blood pressure, peripheral edema
Digestive: Hepatitis including hepatic failure (rarely), elevated ALT (SGPT), elevated AST (SGOT), elevated γ-glutamyl transpeptidase, elevated alkaline phosphatase, elevated bilirubin (jaundice), anorexia, irritable colon, flatulence, fecal discoloration, esophageal candidiasis, mucosal atrophy of the tongue, dry mouth
Metabolic/Nutritional: Hypoglycemia, weight gain
Musculoskeletal: Muscle cramps, myalgia, joint pain, leg pain
Nervous System/Psychiatric: Psychic disturbances including depression, aggression, hallucinations, confusion, insomnia, nervousness, tremors, apathy, somnolence, anxiety, dream abnormalities; vertigo; paresthesia; hemifacial dysesthesia
Respiratory: Epistaxis, pharyngeal pain
Skin: Rash, skin inflammation, urticaria, angioedema, pruritus, alopecia, dry skin, hyperhidrosis
Special Senses: Tinnitus, taste perversion
Urogenital: Urinary tract infection, microscopic pyuria, urinary frequency, elevated serum creatinine, proteinuria, hematuria, glycosuria, testicular pain, gynecomastia
Hematologic: Agranulocytosis has been reported in a 65 year old diabetic male on several drugs in addition to omeprazole; the relationship of the agranulocytosis to omeprazole is uncertain. Pancytopenia, thrombocytopenia, neutropenia, anemia, leucocytosis, hemolytic anemia.
The incidence of clinical adverse experiences in patients greater than 65 years of age was similar to that in patients 65 years of age or less.

OVERDOSAGE

There is no experience to date with deliberate overdosage. Dosages of up to 360 mg/day have been well tolerated. No

specific antidote is known. Omeprazole is extensively protein bound and is, therefore, not readily dialyzable. In the event of overdosage, treatment should be symptomatic and supportive.

Lethal doses of omeprazole after single oral administration are about 1500 mg/kg in mice and greater than 4000 mg/kg in rats, and about 100 mg/kg in mice and greater than 40 mg/kg in rats given single intravenous injections. Animals given these doses showed sedation, ptosis, convulsions, and decreased activity, body temperature, and respiratory rate and increased depth of respiration.

DOSAGE AND ADMINISTRATION

Short-Term Treatment of Active Duodenal Ulcer
The recommended adult oral dose is 20 mg once daily. Most patients heal within four weeks. Some patients may require an additional four weeks of therapy. (See INDICATIONS AND USAGE.)
Severe Erosive Esophagitis or Poorly Responsive Gastroesophageal Reflux Disease (GERD)
The recommended adult oral dose is 20 mg daily for 4 to 8 weeks (see INDICATIONS AND USAGE).
Pathological Hypersecretory Conditions
The dosage of PRILOSEC in patients with pathological hypersecretory conditions varies with the individual patient. The recommended adult oral starting dose is 60 mg once a day. Doses should be adjusted to individual patient needs and should continue for as long as clinically indicated. Doses up to 120 mg t.i.d. have been administered. Daily dosages of greater than 80 mg should be administered in divided doses. Some patients with Zollinger-Ellison syndrome have been treated continuously with PRILOSEC for more than 5 years. No dosage adjustment is necessary for patients with renal impairment, hepatic dysfunction or for the elderly.
PRILOSEC Delayed-Release Capsules should be taken before eating. In the clinical trials, antacids were used concomitantly with PRILOSEC.
Patients should be cautioned that the PRILOSEC Delayed-Release Capsule should not be opened, chewed or crushed, and should be swallowed whole.

HOW SUPPLIED

No. 3440—PRILOSEC Delayed-Release Capsules, 20 mg, are opaque, hard gelatin, amethyst colored capsules, coded MSD 742. They are supplied as follows:
NDC 0006-0742-31 unit of use bottles of 30 (6505-01-314-2716, 20 mg 30's)
NDC 0006-0742-28 unit dose package of 100 (6505-01-314-2717, 20 mg individually sealed 100's).
Shown in Product Identification Section, page 420
Storage
Store PRILOSEC Delayed-Release Capsules in a tight container protected from light and moisture. Store between 59°F and 86°F (15°C and 30°C).
Jointly manufactured by:
MERCK SHARP & DOHME, Division of Merck & Co., INC.
West Point, Pa. 19486
and
AB ASTRA
Södertälje, Sweden
    A.H.F.S. Category: 56:40
    DC 7685405   Issued January 1992
Copyright © MERCK & CO., INC., 1987, 1990, 1991
All rights reserved

PRIMAXIN® I.M.   ℞
(Imipenem-Cilastatin Sodium for Suspension)

For Intramuscular Injection Only

DESCRIPTION

Sterile PRIMAXIN† I.M. (Imipenem-Cilastatin Sodium for Suspension) is a formulation of imipenem (a thienamycin antibiotic) and cilastatin sodium (the inhibitor of the renal dipeptidase, dehydropeptidase I). PRIMAXIN I.M. is a potent broad spectrum antibacterial agent for intramuscular administration.
Imipenem (N-formimidoylthienamycin monohydrate) is a crystalline derivative of thienamycin, which is produced by *Streptomyces cattleya*. Its chemical name is [5R-[5α, 6α (R*)]]-6-(1-hydroxyethyl)-3-[[2-[(iminomethyl)amino] ethyl] thio]-7-oxo-1-azabicyclo [3.2.0] hept-2-ene-2-carboxylic acid monohydrate. It is an off-white, nonhygroscopic crystalline compound with a molecular weight of 317.37. It is sparingly soluble in water, and slightly soluble in methanol. Its empirical formula is $C_{12}H_{17}N_3O_4S \cdot H_2O$, and its structural formula is:
[See chemical structure at top of next column.]
Cilastatin sodium is the sodium salt of a derivatized heptenoic acid. Its chemical name is [R-[R*,S*-(Z)]]-7-[(2-amino-2-carboxyethyl)thio]-2-[[(2, 2-dimethylcyclopropyl)

carbonyl]amino]-2-heptenoic acid, monosodium salt. It is an off-white to yellowish-white, hygroscopic, amorphous compound with a molecular weight of 380.43. It is very soluble in water and in methanol. Its empirical formula is $C_{16}H_{25}N_2O_5SNa$, and its structural formula is:

PRIMAXIN I.M. 500 contains 32 mg of sodium (1.4 mEq) and PRIMAXIN I.M. 750 contains 48 mg of sodium (2.1 mEq). Prepared PRIMAXIN I.M. suspensions are white to light tan in color. Variations of color within this range do not affect the potency of the product.

---

† Registered trademark of MERCK & CO., INC.

CLINICAL PHARMACOLOGY

Following intramuscular administrations of 500 or 750 mg doses of imipenem-cilastatin sodium in a 1:1 ratio with 1% lidocaine, peak plasma levels of imipenem antimicrobial activity occur within 2 hours and average 10 and 12 mcg/mL, respectively. For cilastatin, peak plasma levels average 24 and 33 mcg/mL, respectively, and occur within 1 hour. When compared to intravenous administration of imipenem-cilastatin sodium, imipenem is approximately 75% bioavailable following intramuscular administration while cilastatin is approximately 95% bioavailable. The absorption of imipenem from the IM injection site continues for 6 to 8 hours while that for cilastatin is essentially complete within 4 hours. This prolonged absorption of imipenem following the administration of the intramuscular formulation of imipenem-cilastatin sodium results in an effective plasma half-life of imipenem of approximately 2 to 3 hours and plasma levels of the antibiotic which remain above 2 mcg/mL for at least 6 or 8 hours, following a 500 mg or 750 mg dose, respectively. This plasma profile for imipenem permits IM administration of the intramuscular formulation of imipenem-cilastatin sodium every 12 hours with no accumulation of cilastatin and only slight accumulation of imipenem.
A comparison of plasma levels of imipenem after a single dose of 500 mg or 750 mg of imipenem-cilastatin sodium (intravenous formulation) administered intravenously or of imipenem-cilastatin sodium (intramuscular formulation) diluted with 1% lidocaine and administered intramuscularly is as follows:

PLASMA CONCENTRATIONS OF IMIPENEM
(mcg/mL)

TIME	500 MG I.V.	500 MG I.M.	750 MG I.V.	750 MG I.M.
25 min	45.1	6.0	57.0	6.7
1 hr	21.6	9.4	28.1	10.0
2 hr	10.0	9.9	12.0	11.4
4 hr	2.6	5.6	3.4	7.3
6 hr	0.6	2.5	1.1	3.8
12 hr	ND†	0.5	ND†	0.8

† ND: Not Detectable (<0.3 mcg/mL)

Imipenem urine levels remain above 10 mcg/mL for the 12 hour dosing interval following the administration of 500 mg or 750 mg doses of the intramuscular formulation of imipenem-cilastatin sodium. Total urinary excretion of imipenem averages 50% while that for cilastatin averages 75% following either dose of the intramuscular formulation of imipenem-cilastatin sodium.
Imipenem, when administered alone, is metabolized in the kidneys by dehydropeptidase I resulting in relatively low levels in urine. Cilastatin sodium, an inhibitor of this enzyme, effectively prevents renal metabolism of imipenem so that when imipenem and cilastatin sodium are given concomitantly increased levels of imipenem are achieved in the urine. The binding of imipenem to human serum proteins is approximately 20% and that of cilastatin is approximately 40%.
In a clinical study in which a 500 mg dose of the intramuscular formulation of imipenem-cilastatin sodium was administered to healthy subjects, the average peak level of imipenem in interstitial fluid (skin blister fluid) was approximately 5.0 mcg/mL within 3.5 hours after administration.

Imipenem-cilastatin sodium is hemodialyzable. However, usefulness of this procedure in the overdosage setting is questionable (see OVERDOSAGE).
Microbiology
The bactericidal activity of imipenem results from the inhibition of cell wall synthesis. Its greatest affinity is for penicillin-binding proteins (PBPs) 1A, 1B, 2, 4, 5 and 6 of *Escherichia coli*, and 1A, 1B, 2, 4 and 5 of *Pseudomonas aeruginosa*. The lethal effect is related to binding to PBP 2 and PBP 1B. Imipenem has a high degree of stability in the presence of beta-lactamases, including penicillinases and cephalosporinases produced by gram-negative and gram-positive bacteria. It is a potent inhibitor of beta-lactamases from certain gram-negative bacteria which are inherently resistant to many beta-lactam antibiotics, e.g., *Pseudomonas aeruginosa*, *Serratia* spp. and *Enterobacter* spp.
Imipenem has *in vitro* activity against a wide range of gram-positive and gram-negative organisms. Imipenem is active against most strains of the following microorganisms *in vitro* and in clinical infections treated with the intramuscular formulation of imipenem-cilastatin sodium (see INDICATIONS AND USAGE).
Gram-positive aerobes:
  Staphylococcus aureus including penicillinase-producing strains
    (NOTE: Methicillin-resistant staphylococci should be reported as resistant to imipenem.)
  Group D streptococcus including *Enterococcus faecalis* (formerly *S. faecalis*)
    (NOTE: Imipenem is inactive *in vitro* against *Enterococcus faecium* [formerly *S. faecium*].)
  Streptococcus pneumoniae
  Streptococcus pyogenes (Group A streptococcus)
  Streptococcus viridans group
Gram-negative aerobes:
  Acinetobacter spp., including *A. calcoaceticus*
  Citrobacter spp.
  Enterobacter cloacae
  Escherichia coli
  Haemophilus influenzae
  Klebsiella pneumoniae
  Pseudomonas aeruginosa
    (NOTE: Imipenem is inactive *in vitro* against *Xanthomonas (Pseudomonas) maltophilia* and *P. cepacia*.)
Gram-positive anaerobes:
  Peptostreptococcus spp.
Gram-negative anaerobes:
  Bacteroides spp., including
    Bacteroides distasonis
    Bacteroides intermedius (formerly *B. melaninogenicus intermedius*)
    Bacteroides fragilis
    Bacteroides thetaiotaomicron
  Fusobacterium spp.
Imipenem has been shown to be active *in vitro* against the following microorganisms; however, the clinical significance of these data is unknown.
Gram-positive aerobes:
  Listeria monocytogenes
  Nocardia spp.
  Staphylococcus epidermidis including penicillinase-producing strains.
    (NOTE: Methicillin-resistant staphylococci should be reported as resistant to imipenem.)
  Streptococcus agalactiae (Group B streptococcus)
  Group C streptococcus
  Group G streptococcus
Gram-negative aerobes:
  Achromobacter spp.
  Aeromonas hydrophila
  Alcaligenes spp.
  Bordetella bronchiseptica
  Campylobacter spp.
  Enterobacter spp.
  Gardnerella vaginalis
  Haemophilus parainfluenzae
  Hafnia spp., including *H. alvei*
  Klebsiella spp., including *K. oxytoca*
  Moraxella spp.
  Morganella morganii
  Neisseria gonorrhoeae including penicillinase-producing strains
  Pasteurella multocida
  Plesiomonas shigelloides
  Proteus mirabilis
  Proteus vulgaris
  Providencia rettgeri

Continued on next page

Information on the Merck & Co. products listed on these pages is the full prescribing information from product circulars in use October 1, 1992.

Merck & Co.—Cont.

Providencia stuartii
Salmonella spp.
Serratia spp., including *S. marcescens* and *S. proteamaculans* (formerly *S. liquefaciens*)
Shigella spp.
Yersinia spp., including *Y. enterocolitica* and *Y. pseudotuberculosis*
Gram-positive anaerobes:
Actinomyces spp.
Clostridium spp., including *C. perfringens*
Eubacterium spp.
Peptococcus niger
Propionibacterium spp., including *P. acnes*
Gram-negative anaerobes:
Bacteroides bivius
Bacteroides disiens
Bacteroides ovatus
Bacteroides vulgatus
Porphyromonas asaccharolytica (formerly *Bacteroides asaccharolyticus*)
Veillonella spp.
In vitro tests show imipenem to act synergistically with aminoglycoside antibiotics against some isolates of *Pseudomonas aeruginosa*.
Susceptibility Tests:
Diffusion techniques:
Quantitative methods that require measurement of zone diameters give the most precise estimate of antibiotic susceptibility. One such standard procedure[1], which has been recommended for use with disks to test susceptibility of organisms to imipenem, uses the 10-mcg imipenem disk. Interpretation involves the correlation of the diameters obtained in the disk test with the minimum inhibitory concentration (MIC) for imipenem.
Reports from the laboratory giving results of the standard single-disk susceptibility test with a 10-mcg imipenem disk should be interpreted according to the following criteria:

Zone Diameter (mm)	Interpretation
≥ 16	Susceptible
14–15	Moderately Susceptible
≤ 13	Resistant

A report of "susceptible" indicates that the pathogen is likely to be inhibited by generally achievable blood levels. A report of "moderately susceptible" suggests that the organism would be susceptible if high dosage is used or if the infection is confined to tissues and fluids in which high antibiotic levels are attained. A report of "resistant" indicates that achievable concentrations are unlikely to be inhibitory and other therapy should be selected.
Standardized procedures require the use of laboratory control organisms. The 10-mcg imipenem disk should give the following zone diameters:

Organism	Zone Diameter (mm)
E. coli ATCC 25922	26–32
P. aeruginosa ATCC 27853	20–28

Dilution techniques:
Use a standardized dilution method[2] (broth, agar, microdilution) or equivalent with imipenem powder. The MIC values obtained should be interpreted according to the following criteria:

MIC (mcg/mL)	Interpretation
≤ 4	Susceptible
8	Moderately Susceptible
≥ 16	Resistant

As with standard diffusion techniques, dilution methods require the use of laboratory control organisms. Standard imipenem powder should provide the following MIC values:

Organism	MIC (mcg/mL)
E. coli ATCC 25922	0.06–0.25
S. aureus ATCC 29213	0.015–0.06
E. faecalis ATCC 29212	0.5–2.0
P. aeruginosa ATCC 27853	1.0–4.0

For anaerobic bacteria, the MIC of imipenem can be determined by agar or broth dilution (including microdilution) techniques.[3]

INDICATIONS AND USAGE

PRIMAXIN I.M. is indicated for the treatment of serious infections (listed below) of mild to moderate severity for which intramuscular therapy is appropriate. **PRIMAXIN I.M. is not intended for the therapy of severe or life-threatening infections, including bacterial sepsis or endocarditis, or in instances of major physiological impairments such as shock.**
PRIMAXIN I.M. is indicated for the treatment of infections caused by susceptible strains of the designated microorganisms in the conditions listed below:
(1) **Lower respiratory tract infections,** including pneumonia and bronchitis as an exacerbation of COPD, caused by *Streptococcus pneumoniae* and *Haemophilus influenzae*.

(2) **Intra-abdominal infections,** including acute gangrenous or perforated appendicitis and appendicitis with peritonitis, caused by Group D streptococcus including *Enterococcus faecalis**; *Streptococcus viridans* group*; *Escherichia coli; Klebsiella pneumoniae**; *Pseudomonas aeruginosa**; *Bacteroides* species including *B. fragilis, B. distasonis*, B. intermedius** and *B. thetaiotaomicron**; *Fusobacterium* species and *Peptostreptococcus** species.
(3) **Skin and skin structure infections,** including abscesses, cellulitis, infected skin ulcers and wound infections caused by *Staphylococcus aureus* including penicillinase-producing strains; *Streptococcus pyogenes**; Group D streptococcus including *Enterococcus faecalis*; *Acinetobacter* species* including *A. calcoaceticus**; *Citrobacter* species*; *Escherichia coli; Enterobacter cloacae; Klebsiella pneumoniae**; *Pseudomonas aeruginosa** and *Bacteroides* species* including *B. fragilis**.
(4) **Gynecologic infections,** including postpartum endomyometritis, caused by Group D streptococcus including *Enterococcus faecalis**; *Escherichia coli; Klebsiella pneumoniae**; *Bacteroides intermedius**; and *Peptostreptococcus* species*.
As with other beta-lactam antibiotics, some strains of *Pseudomonas aeruginosa* may develop resistance fairly rapidly during treatment with PRIMAXIN I.M. During therapy of *Pseudomonas aeruginosa* infections, periodic susceptibility testing should be done when clinically appropriate.

---

*Efficacy for this organism in this organ system was studied in fewer than 10 infections.

CONTRAINDICATIONS

PRIMAXIN I.M. is contraindicated in patients who have shown hypersensitivity to any component of this product. Due to the use of lidocaine hydrochloride diluent, this product is contraindicated in patients with a known hypersensitivity to local anesthetics of the amide type and in patients with severe shock or heart block. (Refer to the package circular for lidocaine hydrochloride.)

WARNINGS

SERIOUS AND OCCASIONALLY FATAL HYPERSENSITIVITY (anaphylactic) REACTIONS HAVE BEEN REPORTED IN PATIENTS RECEIVING THERAPY WITH BETA-LACTAMS. THESE REACTIONS ARE MORE LIKELY TO OCCUR IN INDIVIDUALS WITH A HISTORY OF SENSITIVITY TO MULTIPLE ALLERGENS. THERE HAVE BEEN REPORTS OF INDIVIDUALS WITH A HISTORY OF PENICILLIN HYPERSENSITIVITY WHO HAVE EXPERIENCED SEVERE REACTIONS WHEN TREATED WITH ANOTHER BETA-LACTAM. BEFORE INITIATING THERAPY WITH PRIMAXIN® I.M., CAREFUL INQUIRY SHOULD BE MADE CONCERNING PREVIOUS HYPERSENSITIVITY REACTIONS TO PENICILLINS, CEPHALOSPORINS, OTHER BETA-LACTAMS, AND OTHER ALLERGENS. IF AN ALLERGIC REACTION OCCURS, PRIMAXIN® SHOULD BE DISCONTINUED. SERIOUS ANAPHYLACTIC REACTIONS REQUIRE IMMEDIATE EMERGENCY TREATMENT WITH EPINEPHRINE. OXYGEN, INTRAVENOUS STEROIDS, AND AIRWAY MANAGEMENT, INCLUDING INTUBATION, MAY ALSO BE ADMINISTERED AS INDICATED.
Pseudomembranous colitis has been reported with nearly all antibacterial agents, including PRIMAXIN, and may range in severity from mild to life-threatening. Therefore, it is important to consider this diagnosis in patients who present with diarrhea subsequent to the administration of antibacterial agents.
Treatment with antibacterial agents alters the normal flora of the colon and may permit overgrowth of clostridia. Studies indicate that a toxin produced by *Clostridium difficile* is one primary cause of "antibiotic-associated colitis".
After the diagnosis of pseudomembranous colitis has been established, therapeutic measures should be initiated. Mild cases of pseudomembranous colitis usually respond to drug discontinuation alone. In moderate to severe cases, consideration should be given to management with fluids and electrolytes, protein supplementation and treatment with an antibacterial drug effective against *C. difficile*.
Lidocaine HCl —Refer to the package circular for lidocaine HCl.

PRECAUTIONS

General
CNS adverse experiences such as myoclonic activity, confusional states, or seizures have been reported with PRIMAXIN I.V. (Imipenem-Cilastatin Sodium for Injection). These experiences have occurred most commonly in patients with CNS disorders (e.g., brain lesions or history of seizures) who also have compromised renal function. However, there were reports in which there was no recognized or documented underlying CNS disorder. These adverse CNS effects

have not been seen with PRIMAXIN I.M.; however, should they occur during treatment, PRIMAXIN I.M. should be discontinued. Anticonvulsant therapy should be continued in patients with a known seizure disorder.
As with other antibiotics, prolonged use of PRIMAXIN I.M. may result in overgrowth of nonsusceptible organisms. Repeated evaluation of the patient's condition is essential. If superinfection occurs during therapy, appropriate measures should be taken.
Caution should be taken to avoid inadvertent injection into a blood vessel (see DOSAGE AND ADMINISTRATION). For additional precautions, refer to the package circular for lidocaine HCl.
Drug Interactions
Since concomitant administration of PRIMAXIN (Imipenem-Cilastatin Sodium) and probenecid results in only minimal increases in plasma levels of imipenem and plasma half-life, it is not recommended that probenecid be given with PRIMAXIN I.M.
PRIMAXIN I.M. should not be mixed with or physically added to other antibiotics. However, PRIMAXIN I.M. may be administered concomitantly with other antibiotics, such as aminoglycosides.
Carcinogenesis, Mutagenesis, Impairment of Fertility
Long term studies in animals have not been performed to evaluate carcinogenic potential of imipenem-cilastatin. Genetic toxicity studies were performed in a variety of bacterial and mammalian tests in vivo and in vitro. The tests used were: V79 mammalian cell mutagenesis assay (imipenem-cilastatin sodium alone and imipenem alone), Ames test (cilastatin sodium alone and imipenem alone), unscheduled DNA synthesis assay (imipenem-cilastatin sodium) and in vivo mouse cytogenetics test (imipenem-cilastatin sodium). None of these tests showed any evidence of genetic alterations.
Reproductive tests in male and female rats were performed with imipenem-cilastatin sodium at dosage levels up to 11 times† the maximum daily recommended human dose of the intramuscular formulation (on a mg/kg basis). Slight decreases in live fetal body weight were restricted to the highest dosage level. No other adverse effects were observed on fertility, reproductive performance, fetal viability, growth or postnatal development of pups. Similarly, no adverse effects on the fetus or on lactation were observed when imipenem-cilastatin sodium was administered to rats late in gestation.
Pregnancy: Teratogenic Effects
Pregnancy Category C: Teratology studies with cilastatin sodium in rabbits and rats at 10 and 33 times† the maximum recommended daily human dose of the intramuscular formulation (30 mg/kg/day) of PRIMAXIN, respectively, showed no evidence of adverse effects on the fetus. No evidence of teratogenicity was observed in rabbits and rats given imipenem at doses up to 2 and 30 times† the maximum recommended daily human dose of the intramuscular formulation of PRIMAXIN, respectively.
Teratology studies with imipenem-cilastatin sodium at doses up to 11 times† the maximum recommended human dose in pregnant mice and rats during the period of major organogenesis revealed no evidence of teratogenicity.
Imipenem-cilastatin sodium, when administered to pregnant rabbits at dosages above the usual human dose of the intramuscular formulation (1000–1500 mg/day), caused body weight loss, diarrhea, and maternal deaths. When comparable doses of imipenem-cilastatin sodium were given to nonpregnant rabbits, body weight loss, diarrhea, and deaths were also observed. This intolerance is not unlike that seen with other beta-lactam antibiotics in this species and is probably due to alteration of gut flora.
A teratology study in pregnant cynomolgus monkeys given imipenem-cilastatin sodium at doses of 40 mg/kg/day (bolus intravenous injection) or 160 mg/kg/day (subcutaneous injection) resulted in maternal toxicity including emesis, inappetence, body weight loss, diarrhea, abortion and death in some cases. In contrast, no significant toxicity was observed when nonpregnant cynomolgus monkeys were given doses of imipenem-cilastatin sodium up to 180 mg/kg/day (subcutaneous injection). When doses of imipenem-cilastatin sodium (approximately 100 mg/kg/day or approximately 3 times† the maximum daily recommended human dose of the intramuscular formulation) were administered to pregnant cynomolgus monkeys at an intraveous infusion rate which mimics human clinical use, there was minimal maternal intolerance (occasional emesis), no maternal deaths, no evidence of teratogenicity, but an increase in embryonic loss relative to the control groups.
There are, however, no adequate and well-controlled studies in pregnant women. PRIMAXIN I.M. should be used during pregnancy only if the potential benefit justifies the potential risk to the mother and fetus.
Nursing Mothers
It is not known whether imipenem-cilastatin sodium or lidocaine HCl (diluent) is excreted in human milk. Because many drugs are excreted in human milk, caution should be exercised when PRIMAXIN I.M. is administered to a nursing woman.

Pediatric Use
Safety and effectiveness in children below the age of 12 years have not been established.

---

† Based on patient weight of 50 kg.

ADVERSE REACTIONS

PRIMAXIN I.M.
In 686 patients in multiple dose clinical trials of PRIMAXIN I.M., the following adverse reactions were reported:
Local Adverse Reactions
The most frequent adverse local clinical reaction that was reported as possibly, probably or definitely related to therapy with PRIMAXIN I.M. was pain at the injection site (1.2%).
Systemic Adverse Reactions
The most frequently reported systemic adverse clinical reactions that were reported as possibly, probably or definitely related to PRIMAXIN I.M. were nausea (0.6%), diarrhea (0.6%), vomiting (0.3%) and rash (0.4%).
Adverse Laboratory Changes
Adverse laboratory changes without regard to drug relationship that were reported during clinical trials were:
Hemic: decreased hemoglobin and hematocrit, eosinophilia, increased and decreased WBC, increased and decreased platelets, decreased erythrocytes, and increased prothrombin time.
Hepatic: increased AST, ALT, alkaline phosphatase, and bilirubin.
Renal: increased BUN and creatinine.
Urinalysis: presence of red blood cells, white blood cells, casts, and bacteria in the urine.
Potential ADVERSE EFFECTS:
In addition, a variety of adverse effects, not observed in clinical trials with PRIMAXIN I.M., have been reported with intravenous administration of PRIMAXIN I.V. (Imipenem-Cilastatin Sodium for Injection). Those listed below are to serve as alerting information to physicians.
Systemic Adverse Reactions
The most frequently reported systemic adverse clinical reactions that were reported as possibly, probably or definitely related to PRIMAXIN I.V. (Imipenem-Cilastatin Sodium for Injection) were fever, hypotension, seizures (see PRECAUTIONS), dizziness, pruritus, urticaria, and somnolence.
Additional adverse systemic clinical reactions reported possibly, probably or definitely drug related or reported since the drug was marketed are listed within each body system in order of decreasing severity: *Gastrointestinal:* pseudomembranous colitis (the onset of pseudomembranous colitis symptoms may occur during or after antibiotic treatment, see WARNINGS), hemorrhagic colitis, hepatitis, jaundice, gastroenteritis, abdominal pain, glossitis, tongue papillar hypertrophy, staining of the teeth, heartburn, pharyngeal pain, increased salivation; *Hematologic:* thrombocytopenia, neutropenia, leukopenia; *CNS:* encephalopathy, tremor, confusion, myoclonus, paresthesia, vertigo, headache, psychic disturbances; *Special Senses:* hearing loss, tinnitus, taste perversion; *Respiratory:* chest discomfort, dyspnea, hyperventilation, thoracic spine pain; *Cardiovascular:* palpitations, tachycardia; *Renal:* acute renal failure, oliguria/anuria, polyuria, urine discoloration; *Skin:* toxic epidermal necrolysis, erythema multiforme, angioneurotic edema, flushing, cyanosis, hyperhidrosis, skin texture changes, candidiasis, pruritus vulvae; *Body as a whole:* polyarthralgia, asthenia/weakness.
Adverse Laboratory Changes
Adverse laboratory changes without regard to drug relationship that were reported during clinical trials or reported since the drug was marketed were:
Hepatic: increased LDH; *Hemic:* positive Coombs test, decreased neutrophils, agranulocytosis, increased monocytes, abnormal prothrombin time, increased lymphocytes, increased basophils; *Electrolytes:* decreased serum sodium, increased potassium, increased chloride; *Urinalysis:* presence of urine protein, urine bilirubin, and urine urobilinogen.
Lidocaine HCl —Refer to the package circular for lidocaine HCl.

OVERDOSAGE

The acute intravenous toxicity of imipenem-cilastatin sodium in a ratio of 1:1 was studied in mice at doses of 751 to 1359 mg/kg. Following drug administration, ataxia was rapidly produced and clonic convulsions were noted in about 45 minutes. Deaths occurred within 4–56 minutes at all doses. The acute intravenous toxicity of imipenem-cilastatin sodium was produced within 5–10 minutes in rats at doses of 771 to 1583 mg/kg. In all dosage groups, females had decreased activity, bradypnea and ptosis with clonic convulsions preceding death; in males, ptosis was seen at all dose levels while tremors and clonic convulsions were seen at all but the lowest dose (771 mg/kg). In another rat study, female rats showed ataxia, bradypnea and decreased activity in all

DOSAGE GUIDELINES

Type†/Location of Infection	Severity	Dosage Regimen
Lower respiratory tract Skin and skin structure Gynecologic	Mild/Moderate	500 or 750 mg q 12 h depending on the severity of infection
Intra-abdominal	Mild/Moderate	750 mg q 12 h

†See INDICATIONS AND USAGE section.

but the lowest dose (550 mg/kg); deaths were preceded by clonic convulsions. Male rats showed tremors at all doses and clonic convulsions and ptosis were seen at the two highest doses (1130 and 1734 mg/kg). Deaths occurred between 6 and 88 minutes with doses of 771 to 1734 mg/kg.
In the case of overdosage, discontinue PRIMAXIN I.M., treat symptomatically, and institute supportive measures as required. Imipenem-cilastatin sodium is hemodialyzable. However, usefulness of this procedure in the overdosage setting is questionable.

DOSAGE AND ADMINISTRATION

PRIMAXIN I.M. is for intramuscular use only.
The dosage recommendations for PRIMAXIN I.M. represent the quantity of imipenem to be administered. An equivalent amount of cilastatin is also present.
Patients with lower respiratory tract infections, skin and skin structure infections, and gynecologic infections of mild to moderate severity may be treated with 500 mg or 750 mg administered every 12 hours depending on the severity of the infection.
Intra-abdominal infection may be treated with 750 mg every 12 hours.
[See table above.]

Total daily IM dosages greater than 1500 mg per day are not recommended.
The dosage for any particular patient should be based on the location of and severity of the infection, the susceptibility of the infecting pathogen(s), and renal function.
The duration of therapy depends upon the type and severity of the infection. Generally, PRIMAXIN I.M. should be continued for at least two days after the signs and symptoms of infection have resolved. Safety and efficacy of treatment beyond fourteen days have not been established.
PRIMAXIN I.M. should be administered by deep intramuscular injection into a large muscle mass (such as the gluteal muscles or lateral part of the thigh) with a 21 gauge 2" needle. Aspiration is necessary to avoid inadvertent injection into a blood vessel.

ADULTS WITH IMPAIRED RENAL FUNCTION
The safety and efficacy of PRIMAXIN I.M. have not been studied in patients with creatinine clearance of less than 20 mL/ min/1.73m². Serum creatinine alone may not be a sufficiently accurate measure of renal function. Creatinine clearance (T_{cc}) may be estimated from the following equation:

$$T_{cc} \text{ (Males)} = \frac{(\text{wt. in kg}) \, (140 - \text{age})}{(72) \, (\text{creatinine in mg/dL})}$$

$$T_{cc} \text{ (Females)} = 0.85 \times \text{above value}$$

PREPARATION FOR ADMINISTRATION

PRIMAXIN I.M. should be prepared for use with 1.0% lidocaine HCl solution† (without epinephrine). PRIMAXIN I.M. 500 should be prepared with 2 mL and PRIMAXIN I.M. 750 with 3 mL of lidocaine HCl. Agitate to form a suspension then withdraw and inject the entire contents of vial intramuscularly. The suspension of PRIMAXIN I.M. in lidocaine HCl should be used within one hour after preparation. **Note: The IM formulation is not for IV use.**

---

† Refer to the package circular for lidocaine HCl for detailed information concerning CONTRAINDICATIONS, WARNINGS, PRECAUTIONS, and ADVERSE REACTIONS.

COMPATIBILITY AND STABILITY

Before reconstitution:
The dry powder should be stored at a temperature below 30°C (86°F).
Suspensions for IM Administration
Suspensions of PRIMAXIN I.M. are white to light tan in color. Variations of color within this range do not affect the potency of the product.
The suspension of PRIMAXIN I.M. in lidocaine HCl should be used within one hour after preparation.
PRIMAXIN I.M. should not be mixed with or physically added to other antibiotics. However, PRIMAXIN I.M. may be administered concomitantly but at separate sites with other antibiotics, such as aminoglycosides.

HOW SUPPLIED

PRIMAXIN I.M. is supplied as a sterile powder mixture in vials for IM administration as follows:
No. 3582—500 mg imipenem equivalent and 500 mg cilastatin equivalent
NDC 0006-3582-75 in trays of 10 vials
(6505-01-337-3131 500 mg, 10's).
No. 3583—750 mg imipenem equivalent and 750 mg cilastatin equivalent
NDC 0006-3583-76 in trays of 10 vials
(6505-01-337-3130 750 mg, 10's).

REFERENCES

1. National Committee for Clinical Laboratory Standards, Performance Standards for Antimicrobial Disk Susceptibility Tests—Fourth Edition. Approved Standard NCCLS Document M2-A4, Vol. 10, No. 7 NCCLS, Villanova, PA, 1990.
2. National Committee for Clinical Laboratory Standards, Methods for Dilution Antimicrobial Susceptibility Tests for Bacteria that Grow Aerobically—Second Edition. Approved Standard NCCLS Document M7-A2, Vol. 10, No. 8 NCCLS, Villanova, PA, 1990.
3. National Committee for Clinical Laboratory Standards, Methods for Antimicrobial Susceptibility Testing of Anaerobic Bacteria—Second Edition. Tentative Standard NCCLS Document M11-T2, Villanova, PA, 1988.
    A.H.F.S. Category: 8:12.07
    DC 7632904   Issued May 1992
COPYRIGHT© MERCK & CO., INC., 1985, 1990

PRIMAXIN® I.V.   ℞
(Imipenem-Cilastatin Sodium for Injection)

DESCRIPTION

PRIMAXIN† I.V. (Imipenem-Cilastatin Sodium for Injection) is a sterile formulation of imipenem, a thienamycin antibiotic, and cilastatin sodium, the inhibitor of the renal dipeptidase, dehydropeptidase I, with sodium bicarbonate added as a buffer. PRIMAXIN I.V. is a potent broad spectrum antibacterial agent for intravenous administration. Imipenem (N-formimidoylthienamycin monohydrate) is a crystalline derivative of thienamycin, which is produced by *Streptomyces cattleya*. Its chemical name is [5R-[5α, 6α (R*)]]-6-(1-hydroxyethyl)-3-[[2-[(iminomethyl)amino] ethyl] thio]-7-oxo-1-azabicyclo [3.2.0] hept-2-ene-2-carboxylic acid monohydrate. It is an off-white, nonhygroscopic crystalline compound with a molecular weight of 317.37. It is sparingly soluble in water, and slightly soluble in methanol. Its empirical formula is $C_{12}H_{17}N_3O_4S \cdot H_2O$, and its structural formula is:

Cilastatin sodium is the sodium salt of a derivatized heptenoic acid. Its chemical name is [R-[R*,S*-(Z)]]-7-[(2-amino-2-carboxyethyl)thio]-2-[[(2, 2-dimethylcyclopropyl) carbonyl]amino]-2-heptenoic acid, monosodium salt. It is an off-white to yellowish-white, hygroscopic, amorphous compound with a molecular weight of 380.43. It is very soluble in water and in methanol. Its empirical formula is $C_{16}H_{25}N_2O_5S$ Na, and its structural formula is:
[See chemical structure at top of next page.]
PRIMAXIN I.V. is buffered to provide solutions in the pH range of 6.5 to 7.5. There is no significant change in pH when

Continued on next page

Merck & Co.—Cont.

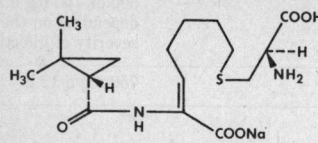

solutions are prepared and used as directed. (See COMPATI-BILITY AND STABILITY.) PRIMAXIN I.V. 250 contains 18.8 mg of sodium (0.8 mEq) and PRIMAXIN I.V. 500 contains 37.5 mg of sodium (1.6 mEq). Solutions of PRIMAXIN I.V. range from colorless to yellow. Variations of color within this range do not affect the potency of the product.

---

†Registered trademark of MERCK & CO., INC.

CLINICAL PHARMACOLOGY

Intravenous Administration
Intravenous infusion of PRIMAXIN I.V. over 20 minutes results in peak plasma levels of imipenem antimicrobial activity that range from 14 to 24 mcg/mL for the 250 mg dose, from 21 to 58 mcg/mL for the 500 mg dose and from 41 to 83 mcg/mL for the 1000 mg dose. At these doses, plasma levels of imipenem antimicrobial activity decline to below 1 mcg/mL or less in 4 to 6 hours. Peak plasma levels of cilastatin following a 20-minute intravenous infusion of PRIMAXIN I.V., range from 15 to 25 mcg/mL for the 250 mg dose, from 31 to 49 mcg/mL for the 500 mg dose and from 56 to 88 mcg/mL for the 1000 mg dose.

General
The plasma half-life of each component is approximately 1 hour. The binding of imipenem to human serum proteins is approximately 20% and that of cilastatin is approximately 40%. Approximately 70% of the administered imipenem is recovered in the urine within 10 hours after which no further urinary excretion is detectable. Urine concentrations of imipenem in excess of 10 mcg/mL can be maintained for up to 8 hours with PRIMAXIN I.V. at the 500 mg dose. Approximately 70% of the cilastatin sodium dose is recovered in the urine within 10 hours of administration of PRIMAXIN I.V. No accumulation of PRIMAXIN I.V. in plasma or urine is observed with regimens administered as frequently as every 6 hours in patients with normal renal function.
Imipenem, when administered alone, is metabolized in the kidneys by dehydropeptidase I resulting in relatively low levels in urine. Cilastatin sodium, an inhibitor of this enzyme, effectively prevents renal metabolism of imipenem so that when imipenem and cilastatin sodium are given concomitantly fully adequate antibacterial levels of imipenem are achieved in the urine.
After a 1 gram dose of PRIMAXIN I.V., the following average levels of imipenem were measured (usually at 1 hour post-dose except where indicated) in the tissues and fluids listed:
[See table below.]

Microbiology
The bactericidal activity of imipenem results from the inhibition of cell wall synthesis. Its greatest affinity is for penicillin binding proteins (PBP) 1A, 1B, 2, 4, 5, and 6 of *Escherichia coli*, and 1A, 1B, 2, 4 and 5 of *Pseudomonas aeruginosa*. The lethal effect is related to binding to PBP 2 and PBP 1B.
Imipenem has *in vitro* activity against a wide range of gram-positive and gram-negative organisms.
Imipenem has a high degree of stability in the presence of beta-lactamases, both penicillinases and cephalosporinases produced by gram-negative and gram-positive bacteria. It is a potent inhibitor of beta-lactamases from certain gram-negative bacteria which are inherently resistant to most beta-lactam antibiotics, e.g., *Pseudomonas aeruginosa*, *Serratia* spp., and *Enterobacter* spp.

In vitro, imipenem is active against most strains of clinical isolates of the following microorganisms:

Gram-positive:
Group D streptococci (including enterococci e.g., *Streptococcus faecalis*)
   NOTE: Imipenem is inactive against *Streptococcus faecium*.
Streptococcus pyogenes (Group A streptococci)
Streptococcus agalactiae (Group B streptococci)
Group C streptococci
Group G streptococci
Viridans streptococci
Streptococcus pneumoniae (formerly *Diplococcus pneumoniae*)
Staphylococcus aureus including penicillinase producing strains
Staphylococcus epidermidis including penicillinase producing strains
   NOTE: Many strains of methicillin-resistant staphylococci are resistant to imipenem.

Gram-negative:
Escherichia coli
Proteus mirabilis
Proteus vulgaris
Morganella morganii
Providencia rettgeri
Providencia stuartii
Citrobacter spp.
Klebsiella spp. including *K. pneumoniae* and *K. oxytoca*
Enterobacter spp.
Hafnia spp. including *H. alvei*
Serratia marcescens
Serratia spp. including *S. liquefaciens*
Haemophilus parainfluenzae
H. influenzae
Gardnerella vaginalis
Acinetobacter spp.
Pseudomonas aeruginosa
   NOTE: Imipenem is inactive against *P. maltophilia* and some strains of *P. cepacia*.

Anaerobes:
Bacteroides spp. including *Bacteroides bivius*, *Bacteroides fragilis*, *Bacteroides melaninogenicus*
Clostridium spp. including *C. perfringens*
Eubacterium spp.
Fusobacterium spp.
Peptococcus spp.
Peptostreptococcus spp.
Propionibacterium spp. including *P. acnes*
Actinomyces spp.
Veillonella spp.
Imipenem has been shown to be active *in vitro* against the following microorganisms; however, clinical efficacy has not yet been established:

Gram-positive:
Listeria monocytogenes
Nocardia spp.

Gram-negative:
Salmonella spp.
Shigella spp.
Yersinia spp. including *Yersinia enterocolitica*, *Yersinia pseudotuberculosis*
Bordetella bronchiseptica
Campylobacter spp.
Achromobacter spp.
Alcaligenes spp.
Moraxella spp.
Pasteurella multocida
Aeromonas hydrophila
Plesiomonas shigelloides
Neisseria gonorrhoeae (including penicillinase-producing strains)

Anaerobes:
Bacteroides asaccharolyticus
Bacteroides disiens

Bacteroides distasonis
Bacteroides ovatus
Bacteroides thetaiotaomicron
Bacteroides vulgatus
In vitro tests show imipenem to act synergistically with aminoglycoside antibiotics against some isolates of *Pseudomonas aeruginosa*.

Susceptibility Testing
Quantitative methods that require measurement of zone diameters give the most precise estimate of antibiotic susceptibility. One such procedure has been recommended for use with discs to test susceptibility to imipenem.
Reports from the laboratory giving results of the standard single-disc susceptibility test with a 10 mcg imipenem disc should be interpreted according to the following criteria.
Fully susceptible organisms produce zones of 16 mm or greater, indicating that the test organism is likely to respond to doses of 2 g per day or less (see DOSAGE AND ADMINISTRATION.)
Moderately susceptible organisms produce zones of 14 to 15 mm and are expected to be susceptible if the maximum recommended dosage is used or if infection is confined to tissues and fluids in which high antibiotic levels are attained.
Resistant organisms produce zones of 13 mm or less, indicating that other therapy should be selected.
A bacterial isolate may be considered fully susceptible if the MIC value for imipenem is equal to or less than 4 mcg/mL. Organisms are considered moderately susceptible if the MIC value is 8 mcg/mL. Organisms are considered resistant if the MIC is equal to or greater than 16 mcg/mL.
The standardized quality control procedure requires use of control organisms. The 10 mcg imipenem disc should give the zone diameters listed below for the quality control strains.

Organism	ATCC	Zone Size Range
E. coli	25922	26–32 mm
Ps. aeruginosa	27853	20–28 mm

Dilution susceptibility tests should give MICs between the ranges listed below for the quality control strains.

Organism	ATCC	MIC (mcg/mL)
E. coli	25922	0.06–0.25
S. aureus	29213	0.015–0.06
S. faecalis	29212	0.5–2.0
Ps. aeruginosa	27853	1.0–4.0

Based on blood levels of imipenem achieved in man, breakpoint criteria have been adopted for imipenem.

Category	Zone Diameter (mm)	Recommended MIC Breakpoint (mcg/mL)
Fully Susceptible	≥ 16	≤ 4
Moderately Susceptible	14–15	8
Resistant	≤ 13	≥ 16

INDICATIONS AND USAGE

PRIMAXIN I.V. is indicated for the treatment of serious infections caused by susceptible strains of the designated microorganisms in the diseases listed below:
(1) **Lower respiratory tract infections.** *Staphylococcus aureus* (penicillinase producing strains), *Escherichia coli*, *Klebsiella* species, *Enterobacter* species, *Haemophilus influenzae*, *Haemophilus parainfluenzae**, *Acinetobacter* species, *Serratia marcescens*.
(2) **Urinary tract infections** (Complicated and uncomplicated). *Staphylococcus aureus* (penicillinase producing strains)*, Group D streptococci (enterococci), *Escherichia coli*, *Klebsiella* species, *Enterobacter* species, *Proteus vulgaris**, *Providencia rettgeri**, *Morganella morganii**, *Pseudomonas aeruginosa*.
(3) **Intra-abdominal infections.** *Staphylococcus aureus* (penicillinase producing strains)*, *Staphylococcus epidermidis*, Group D streptococci (enterococci), *Escherichia coli*, *Klebsiella* species, *Enterobacter* species, *Proteus* species (indole positive and indole negative), *Morganella morganii**, *Pseudomonas aeruginosa*, *Citrobacter* species, *Clostridium* species, Gram-positive anaerobes, including *Peptococcus* species, *Peptostreptococcus* species, *Eubacterium* species, *Propionibacterium* species*, *Bifidobacterium* species, *Bacteroides* species, including *B. fragilis*, *Fusobacterium* species.
(4) **Gynecologic infections.** *Staphylococcus aureus* (penicillinase producing strains)*, *Staphylococcus epidermidis*, Group B streptococci, Group D streptococci (enterococci), *Escherichia coli*, *Klebsiella* species*, *Proteus* species (indole positive and indole negative), *Enterobacter* species*,

Tissue or Fluid	n	Imipenem Level mcg/mL or mcg/g	Range
Vitreous Humor	3	3.4 (3.5 hours post dose)	2.88–3.6
Aqueous Humor	5	2.99 (2 hours post dose)	2.4–3.9
Lung Tissue	8	5.6 (median)	3.5–15.5
Sputum	1	2.1	—
Pleural	1	22.0	—
Peritoneal	12	23.9 S.D. ±5.3 (2 hours post dose)	—
Bile	2	5.3 (2.25 hours post dose)	4.6 to 6.0
CSF (uninflamed)	5	1.0 (4 hours post dose)	0.26–2.0
CSF (inflamed)	7	2.6 (2 hours post dose)	0.5–5.5
Fallopian Tubes	1	13.6	—
Endometrium	1	11.1	—
Myometrium	1	5.0	—
Bone	10	2.6	0.4–5.4
Interstitial Fluid	12	16.4	10.0–22.6
Skin	12	4.4	NA
Fascia	12	4.4	NA

Gram-positive anaerobes, including *Peptococcus* species*, *Peptostreptococcus* species, *Propionibacterium* species*, *Bifidobacterium* species*, *Bacteroides* species, *B. fragilis**, *Gardnerella vaginalis*.

(5) **Bacterial septicemia.** *Staphylococcus aureus* (penicillinase producing strains), Group D streptococci (enterococci), *Escherichia coli*, *Klebsiella* species, *Pseudomonas aeruginosa*, *Serratia* species*, *Enterobacter* species, *Bacteroides* species, *B. fragilis**.

(6) **Bone and joint infections.** *Staphylococcus aureus* (penicillinase producing strains), *Staphylococcus epidermidis*, Group D streptococci (enterococci), *Enterobacter* species, *Pseudomonas aeruginosa*.

(7) **Skin and skin structure infections.** *Staphylococcus aureus* (penicillinase producing strains), *Staphylococcus epidermidis*, Group D streptococci (enterococci), *Escherichia coli*, *Klebsiella* species, *Enterobacter* species, *Proteus vulgaris*, *Providencia rettgeri**, *Morganella morganii*, *Pseudomonas aeruginosa*, *Serratia* species, *Citrobacter* species, *Acinetobacter* species, Gram-positive anaerobes, including *Peptococcus* species and *Peptostreptococcus* species, *Bacteroides* species, including *B. fragilis*, *Fusobacterium* species*.

(8) **Endocarditis.** *Staphylococcus aureus* (penicillinase producing strains).

(9) **Polymicrobic infections.** PRIMAXIN I.V. is indicated for polymicrobic infections including those in which *S. pneumoniae* (pneumonia, septicemia), Group A beta-hemolytic streptococcus (skin and skin structure), or nonpenicillinase-producing *S. aureus* is one of the causative organisms. However, monobacterial infections due to these organisms are usually treated with narrower spectrum antibiotics, such as penicillin G.

PRIMAXIN I.V. is not indicated in patients with meningitis because safety and efficacy have not been established.

Because of its broad spectrum of bactericidal activity against gram-positive and gram-negative aerobic and anaerobic bacteria, PRIMAXIN I.V. is useful for the treatment of mixed infections and as presumptive therapy prior to the identification of the causative organisms.

Although clinical improvement has been observed in patients with cystic fibrosis, chronic pulmonary disease, and lower respiratory tract infections caused by *Pseudomonas aeruginosa*, bacterial eradication may not necessarily be achieved.

As with other beta-lactam antibiotics, some strains of *Pseudomonas aeruginosa* may develop resistance fairly rapidly on treatment with PRIMAXIN I.V. When clinically appropriate during therapy of *Pseudomonas aeruginosa* infections, periodic susceptibility testing should be done.

Infections resistant to other antibiotics, for example, cephalosporins, penicillin, and aminoglycosides, have been shown to respond to treatment with PRIMAXIN I.V.

*Efficacy for this organism in this organ system was studied in fewer than 10 infections.

CONTRAINDICATIONS

PRIMAXIN I.V. is contraindicated in patients who have shown hypersensitivity to any component of this product.

WARNINGS

SERIOUS AND OCCASIONALLY FATAL HYPERSENSITIVITY (anaphylactic) REACTIONS HAVE BEEN REPORTED IN PATIENTS RECEIVING THERAPY WITH BETA-LACTAMS. THESE REACTIONS ARE MORE APT TO OCCUR IN PERSONS WITH A HISTORY OF SENSITIVITY TO MULTIPLE ALLERGENS.

THERE HAVE BEEN REPORTS OF PATIENTS WITH A HISTORY OF PENICILLIN HYPERSENSITIVITY WHO HAVE EXPERIENCED SEVERE HYPERSENSITIVITY REACTIONS WHEN TREATED WITH ANOTHER BETA-LACTAM. BEFORE INITIATING THERAPY WITH 'PRIMAXIN I.V.', CAREFUL INQUIRY SHOULD BE MADE CONCERNING PREVIOUS HYPERSENSITIVITY REACTIONS TO PENICILLINS, CEPHALOSPORINS, OTHER BETA-LACTAMS, AND OTHER ALLERGENS. IF AN ALLERGIC REACTION TO 'PRIMAXIN I.V.' OCCURS, DISCONTINUE THE DRUG. SERIOUS HYPERSENSITIVITY REACTIONS MAY REQUIRE EPINEPHRINE AND OTHER EMERGENCY MEASURES.

Pseudomembranous colitis has been reported with virtually all antibiotics, including PRIMAXIN I.V.; therefore it is important to consider its diagnosis in patients who develop diarrhea in association with antibiotic use. This colitis may range in severity from mild to life threatening.

Mild cases of pseudomembranous colitis may respond to drug discontinuance alone. In more severe cases, management may include sigmoidoscopy, appropriate bacteriological studies, fluid, electrolyte and protein supplementation, and the use of a drug such as oral vancomycin, as indicated. Isolation of the patient may be advisable. Other causes of colitis should also be considered.

PRECAUTIONS

General

CNS adverse experiences such as confusional states, myoclonic activity, and seizures have been reported during treatment with PRIMAXIN I.V., especially when recommended dosages were exceeded. These experiences have occurred most commonly in patients with CNS disorders (e.g., brain lesions or history of seizures) and/or compromised renal function. However, there have been reports of CNS adverse experiences in patients who had no recognized or documented underlying CNS disorder or compromised renal function.

Patients with severe or marked impairment of renal function, whether or not undergoing hemodialysis, had a higher risk of seizure activity when receiving maximum recommended doses than those with no impairment of renal function; therefore, maximum recommended doses should be used only where clearly indicated (see DOSAGE AND ADMINISTRATION).

Patients with creatinine clearances of ≤ 5 mL/min/1.73 m^2 should not receive PRIMAXIN I.V. unless hemodialysis is instituted within 48 hours.

For patients on hemodialysis, PRIMAXIN I.V. is recommended only when the benefit outweighs the potential risk of seizures.

Close adherence to the recommended dosage and dosage schedules is urged, especially in patients with known factors that predispose to convulsive activity. Anticonvulsant therapy should be continued in patients with known seizure disorders. If focal tremors, myoclonus, or seizures occur, patients should be evaluated neurologically, placed on anticonvulsant therapy if not already instituted, and the dosage of PRIMAXIN I.V. re-examined to determine whether it should be decreased or the antibiotic discontinued.

As with other antibiotics, prolonged use of PRIMAXIN I.V. may result in overgrowth of nonsusceptible organisms. Repeated evaluation of the patient's condition is essential. If superinfection occurs during therapy, appropriate measures should be taken.

While PRIMAXIN I.V. possesses the characteristic low toxicity of the beta-lactam group of antibiotics, periodic assessment of organ system function during prolonged therapy is advisable.

Drug Interactions

Generalized seizures have been reported in patients who received ganciclovir and PRIMAXIN I.V. These drugs should not be used concomitantly unless the potential benefits outweigh the risks.

Since concomitant administration of PRIMAXIN I.V. and probenecid results in only minimal increases in plasma levels of imipenem and plasma half-life, it is not recommended that probenecid be given with PRIMAXIN I.V.

PRIMAXIN I.V. should not be mixed with or physically added to other antibiotics. However, PRIMAXIN I.V. may be administered concomitantly with other antibiotics, such as aminoglycosides.

Carcinogenesis, Mutagenesis, Impairment of Fertility

Gene toxicity studies were performed in a variety of bacterial and mammalian tests *in vivo* and *in vitro*. The tests were: V79 mammalian cell mutation assay (PRIMAXIN I.V. alone and imipenem alone), Ames test (cilastatin sodium alone), unscheduled DNA synthesis assay (PRIMAXIN I.V.) and *in vivo* mouse cytogenicity test (PRIMAXIN I.V.). None of these tests showed any evidence of genetic damage.

Reproduction tests in male and female rats were performed with PRIMAXIN I.V. at dosage levels up to 8 times the usual human dose. Slight decreases in live fetal body weight were restricted to the highest dosage level. No other adverse effects were observed on fertility, reproductive performance, fetal viability, growth or postnatal development of pups. Similarly, no adverse effects on the fetus or on lactation were observed when PRIMAXIN I.V. was administered to rats late in gestation.

Pregnancy

Pregnancy Category C. Teratogenicity studies with cilastatin sodium in rabbits and rats at 10 and 33 times the usual human dose, respectively, showed no evidence of adverse effect on the fetus. No evidence of teratogenicity or adverse effect on postnatal growth or behavior was observed in rats given imipenem at dosage levels up to 30 times the usual human dose. Similarly, no evidence of adverse effect on the fetus was observed in teratology studies in rabbits with imipenem at dosage levels at the usual human dose.

Teratology studies with PRIMAXIN I.V. at doses up to 11 times the usual human dose in pregnant mice and rats during the period of major organogenesis revealed no evidence of teratogenicity.

Data from preliminary studies suggests an apparent intolerance to PRIMAXIN I.V. (including emesis, inappetence, body weight loss, diarrhea and death) at doses equivalent to the average human dose in pregnant rabbits and cynomolgus monkeys that is not seen in non-pregnant animals in these or other species. In other studies, PRIMAXIN I.V. was well tolerated in equivalent or higher doses (up to 11 times the average human dose) in pregnant rats and mice. Further studies are underway to evaluate these findings.

There are, however, no adequate and well-controlled studies in pregnant women. PRIMAXIN I.V. should be used during pregnancy only if the potential benefit justifies the potential risk to the fetus.

Nursing Mothers

It is not known whether this drug is excreted in human milk. Because many drugs are excreted in human milk, caution should be exercised when PRIMAXIN I.V. is administered to a nursing woman.

Pediatric Use

Safety and effectiveness in infants and children below 12 years of age have not yet been established.

ADVERSE REACTIONS

PRIMAXIN I.V. is generally well tolerated. Many of the 1,723 patients treated in clinical trials were severely ill and had multiple background diseases and physiological impairments, making it difficult to determine causal relationship of adverse experiences to therapy with PRIMAXIN I.V.

Local Adverse Reactions

Adverse local clinical reactions that were reported as possibly, probably or definitely related to therapy with PRIMAXIN I.V. were:

Phlebitis/thrombophlebitis—3.1%
Pain at the injection site—0.7%
Erythema at the injection site—0.4%
Vein induration—0.2%
Infused vein infection—0.1%

Systemic Adverse Reactions

The most frequently reported systemic adverse clinical reactions that were reported as possibly, probably, or definitely related to PRIMAXIN I.V. were nausea (2.0%) (see *Granulocytopenic Patients* below), diarrhea (1.8%), vomiting (1.5%), rash (0.9%), fever (0.5%), hypotension (0.4%), seizures (0.4%) (see PRECAUTIONS), dizziness (0.3%), pruritus (0.3%), urticaria (0.2%), somnolence (0.2%).

Additional adverse systemic clinical reactions reported as possibly, probably or definitely drug related occurring in less than 0.2% of the patients or reported since the drug was marketed are listed within each body system in order of decreasing severity: *Gastrointestinal*—pseudomembranous colitis (see WARNINGS), hemorrhagic colitis, hepatitis (rarely), jaundice, gastroenteritis, abdominal pain, glossitis, tongue papillar hypertrophy, staining of the teeth, heartburn, pharyngeal pain, increased salivation; *Hematologic*—agranulocytosis, thrombocytopenia, neutropenia, leukopenia; *CNS*—encephalopathy, tremor, confusion, myoclonus, paresthesia, vertigo, headache, psychic disturbances; *Special Senses*—hearing loss, tinnitus, taste perversion; *Respiratory*—chest discomfort, dyspnea, hyperventilation, thoracic spine pain; *Cardiovascular*—palpitations, tachycardia; *Skin*—toxic epidermal necrolysis (rarely), erythema multiforme, angioneurotic edema, flushing, cyanosis, hyperhidrosis, skin texture changes, candidiasis, pruritus vulvae; *Body as a whole*—polyarthralgia, asthenia/weakness; *Renal*—acute renal failure (rarely), oliguria/anuria, polyuria, urine discoloration. The role of PRIMAXIN I.V. in changes in renal function is difficult to assess, since factors predisposing to pre-renal azotemia or to impaired renal function usually have been present.

Granulocytopenic Patients

Drug-related nausea and/or vomiting appear to occur more frequently in granulocytopenic patients than in non-granulocytopenic patients treated with PRIMAXIN I.V.

Adverse Laboratory Changes

Adverse laboratory changes without regard to drug relationship that were reported during clinical trials or reported since the drug was marketed were:

Hepatic: Increased SGPT, SGOT, alkaline phosphatase, bilirubin and LDH.

Hemic: Increased eosinophils, positive Coombs test, increased WBC, increased platelets, decreased hemoglobin and hematocrit, increased monocytes, abnormal prothrombin time, increased lymphocytes, increased basophils.

Electrolytes: Decreased serum sodium, increased potassium, increased chloride.

Renal: Increased BUN, creatinine.

Urinalysis: Presence of urine protein, urine red blood cells, urine white blood cells, urine casts, urine bilirubin, and urine urobilinogen.

Continued on next page

Information on the Merck & Co. products listed on these pages is the full prescribing information from product circulars in use October 1, 1992.

Merck & Co.—Cont.

OVERDOSAGE

The intravenous LD_{50} of imipenem is greater than 2000 mg/kg in the rat and approximately 1500 mg/kg in the mouse. The intravenous LD_{50} of cilastatin sodium is approximately 5000 mg/kg in the rat and approximately 8700 mg/kg in the mouse. The intravenous LD_{50} of PRIMAXIN I.V. is approximately 1000 mg/kg in the rat and approximately 1100 mg/kg in the mouse.
Information on overdosage in humans is not available.

DOSAGE AND ADMINISTRATION

The dosage recommendations for PRIMAXIN I.V. represent the quantity of imipenem to be administered. An equivalent amount of cilastatin is also present in the solution. Each 250 mg or 500 mg dose should be given by intravenous administration over 20 to 30 minutes. Each 1000 mg dose should be infused over 40 to 60 minutes. In patients who develop nausea during the infusion, the rate of infusion may be slowed. The total daily dosage for PRIMAXIN I.V. should be based on the type or severity of infection and given in equally divided doses based on consideration of degree of susceptibility of the pathogen(s), renal function and body weight. Patients with impaired renal function, as judged by creatinine clearance ≤ 70 mL/min/1.73 m^2, require adjustment of dosage as described in the succeeding section of these guidelines.
Dosage regimens in column A in the Table for Adults with Normal Renal Function are recommended for infections caused by fully susceptible organisms which represent the majority of pathogenic species. Dosage regimens in column B of this Table are recommended for infections caused by organisms with moderate susceptibility to imipenem, primarily some strains of *Ps. aeruginosa*.
Doses cited in the Table below are based on a body weight of 70 kg. A further proportionate reduction in dose administered must be made for patients with a body weight less than 70 kg by multiplying the selected dose by the patient's weight in kg divided by 70.

INTRAVENOUS DOSAGE SCHEDULE FOR ADULTS WITH NORMAL RENAL FUNCTION

Type or Severity of Infection	A Fully susceptible organisms including gram-positive and gram-negative aerobes and anaerobes	B Moderately susceptible organisms, primarily some strains of *Ps. aeruginosa*
Mild	250 mg q6h	500 mg q6h
Moderate	500 mg q8h 500 mg q6h	500 mg q6h 1 g q8h
Severe, life threatening	500 mg q6h	1 g q8h 1 g q6h
Uncomplicated urinary tract infection	250 mg q6h	250 mg q6h
Complicated urinary tract infection	500 mg q6h	500 mg q6h

Maximum Recommended Intravenous Dosage of PRIMAXIN I.V. in Adults With Impaired Renal Function

Creatinine Clearance (mL/min/1.73 m^2)	Renal Function	A Fully susceptible organisms including gram-positive and gram-negative aerobes and anaerobes	B Moderately susceptible organisms, primarily some strains of *Ps. aeruginosa*
31–70	Mild Impairment	500 mg q8h	500 mg q6h
21–30	Moderate Impairment	500 mg q12h	500 mg q8h
6–20	Severe to Marked Impairment	250 mg q12h See Text Below	500 mg q12h See Text Below
0–5	None, but on Hemodialysis		

Due to the high antimicrobial activity of PRIMAXIN I.V., it is recommended that the maximum total daily dosage not exceed 50 mg/kg/day or 4.0 g/day, whichever is lower. There is no evidence that higher doses provide greater efficacy. However, patients over twelve years of age with cystic fibrosis and normal renal function have been treated with PRIMAXIN I.V. at doses up to 90 mg/kg/day in divided doses, not exceeding 4.0 g/day.

INTRAVENOUS DOSAGE SCHEDULE FOR ADULTS WITH IMPAIRED RENAL FUNCTION

Patients with creatinine clearance of ≤ 70 mL/min/1.73 m^2 require adjustment of the dosage of PRIMAXIN I.V. as indicated in the Table below. Creatinine clearance may be calculated from serum creatinine concentration by the following equation:

$$T_{cc} \text{ (Males)} = \frac{(\text{wt. in kg}) (140 - \text{age})}{(72) (\text{creatinine in mg/dL})}$$

$$T_{cc} \text{ (Females)} = 0.85 \times \text{above value}$$

Column A of the following Table shows maximum dosages recommended in each category of impaired renal function for infections caused by fully susceptible organisms which represent the majority of pathogenic species. The maximum dosages in column B are recommended only for infections caused by organisms with moderate susceptibility to imipenem, primarily some strains of *Ps. aeruginosa*. Doses cited are based on a body weight of 70 kg. A further proportionate reduction in dose administered must be made for patients with a body weight less than 70 kg by multiplying the selected dose by the patient's weight in kg divided by 70.
Patients with creatinine clearance ≤ 5 mL/min/1.73 m^2 should not receive PRIMAXIN I.V. unless hemodialysis is instituted within 48 hours. There is inadequate information to recommend usage of PRIMAXIN I.V. for patients undergoing peritoneal dialysis.
[See table below.]
Patients with creatinine clearances of 6 to 20 mL/min/1.73 m^2 should be treated with 250 mg (or 3.5 mg/kg whichever is lower) every 12 hours for most pathogens. When the 500 mg dose is used in these patients, there may be an increased risk of seizures.
Similar dosage and safety considerations apply in the treatment of patients with creatinine clearances of ≤ 5 mL/min/1.73 m^2 who are undergoing hemodialysis. Both imipenem and cilastatin are cleared from the circulation during hemodialysis. The patient should receive PRIMAXIN I.V. after hemodialysis and at 12 hour intervals timed from the end of that hemodialysis session. Dialysis patients, especially those with background CNS disease, should be carefully monitored; for patients on hemodialysis, PRIMAXIN I.V. is recommended only when the benefit outweighs the potential risk of seizures (see PRECAUTIONS).

PREPARATION OF SOLUTION

Infusion Bottles
Contents of the infusion bottles of PRIMAXIN I.V. Powder should be restored with 100 mL of diluent (see list of diluents under COMPATIBILITY AND STABILITY) and shaken until a clear solution is obtained.
Vials
Contents of the vials must be suspended and transferred to 100 mL of an appropriate infusion solution.
A suggested procedure is to add approximately 10 mL from the appropriate infusion solution (see list of diluents under COMPATIBILITY AND STABILITY) to the vial. Shake well and transfer the resulting suspension to the infusion solution container.

CAUTION: THE SUSPENSION IS NOT FOR DIRECT INFUSION.
Repeat with an additional 10 mL of infusion solution to ensure complete transfer of vial contents to the infusion solution. **The resulting mixture should be agitated until clear.**
ADD-Vantage ®† Vials
See separate INSTRUCTIONS FOR USE OF 'PRIMAXIN I.V.' IN ADD-Vantage® VIALS.
PRIMAXIN I.V. in ADD-Vantage® vials should be reconstituted with ADD-Vantage® diluent containers containing 100 mL of either 0.9 percent Sodium Chloride Injection or 100 mL 5% Dextrose Injection.

COMPATIBILITY AND STABILITY

Before reconstitution:
The dry powder should be stored at a temperature below 30°C.
Reconstituted solutions:
Solutions of PRIMAXIN I.V. range from colorless to yellow. Variations of color within this range do not affect the potency of the product.
PRIMAXIN I.V., as supplied in infusion bottles and vials and reconstituted as above with the following diluents, maintains satisfactory potency for four hours at room temperature or for 24 hours under refrigeration (5°C) (note exception below). Solutions of PRIMAXIN I.V. should not be frozen.
0.9% Sodium Chloride Injection*
5% or 10% Dextrose Injection
5% Dextrose Injection with 0.02% sodium bicarbonate solution
5% Dextrose and 0.9% Sodium Chloride Injection
5% Dextrose Injection with 0.225% or 0.45% saline solution
NORMOSOL†–M in D5-W
5% Dextrose Injection with 0.15% potassium chloride solution
Mannitol 2.5%, 5% and 10%
PRIMAXIN I.V. is supplied in single dose ADD-Vantage® vials and should be prepared as directed in the accompanying INSTRUCTIONS FOR USE OF 'PRIMAXIN I.V.' IN ADD-Vantage® VIALS using ADD-Vantage® diluent containers containing 100 mL of either 0.9% Sodium Chloride Injection or 5% Dextrose Injection. When prepared with either of these diluents, PRIMAXIN I.V. maintains satisfactory potency for 8 hours at room temperature.
PRIMAXIN I.V. should not be mixed with or physically added to other antibiotics. However, PRIMAXIN I.V. may be administered concomitantly with other antibiotics, such as aminoglycosides.

* PRIMAXIN I.V. has been found to be stable in 0.9% Sodium Chloride Injection for 10 hours at room temperature or 48 hours under refrigeration.
† Registered trademark of Abbott Laboratories, Inc.

HOW SUPPLIED

PRIMAXIN I.V. is supplied as a sterile powder mixture in vials and infusion bottles containing imipenem (anhydrous equivalent) and cilastatin sodium as follows:
No. 3514—250 mg imipenem equivalent and 250 mg cilastatin equivalent and 10 mg sodium bicarbonate as a buffer
NDC 0006-3514-58 in trays of 25 vials (6505-01-332-4793 250 mg, 25's).
No. 3516—500 mg imipenem equivalent and 500 mg cilastatin equivalent and 20 mg sodium bicarbonate as a buffer
NDC 0006-3516-59 in trays of 25 vials (6505-01-332-4794 500 mg, 25's).
No. 3515—250 mg imipenem equivalent and 250 mg cilastatin equivalent and 10 mg sodium bicarbonate as a buffer
NDC 0006-3515-74 in trays of 10 infusion bottles (6505-01-246-4126 infusion bottle, 10's).
No. 3517—500 mg imipenem equivalent and 500 mg cilastatin equivalent and 20 mg sodium bicarbonate as a buffer
NDC 0006-3517-75 in trays of 10 infusion bottles (6505-01-234-0240 infusion bottle, 10's).
No. 3551—250 mg imipenem equivalent and 250 mg cilastatin equivalent and 10 mg sodium bicarbonate as a buffer
NDC 0006-3551-58 in trays of 25 ADD-Vantage® vials.
No. 3552—500 mg imipenem equivalent and 500 mg cilastatin equivalent and 20 mg sodium bicarbonate as a buffer
NDC 0006-3552-59 in trays of 25 ADD-Vantage® vials (6505-01-279-9627 500 mg ADD-Vantage®, 25's).
A.H.F.S. Category: 8:12.28
DC 7362417 Issued August 1992
COPYRIGHT© MERCK & CO., INC., 1987

PRINIVIL® Tablets ℞
(Lisinopril)

USE IN PREGNANCY
When used in pregnancy during the second and third trimesters, ACE inhibitors can cause injury and even death to the developing fetus. When pregnancy is detected, PRINIVIL should be discontinued as soon as possible. See WARNINGS, *Fetal/Neonatal Morbidity and Mortality.*

DESCRIPTION

PRINIVIL* (Lisinopril), a synthetic peptide derivative, is an oral long-acting angiotensin converting enzyme inhibitor. Lisinopril is chemically described as (*S*)-1-[N^2-(1-carboxy-3-phenylpropyl)-L-lysyl]-L-proline dihydrate. Its empirical formula is $C_{21}H_{31}N_3O_5 \cdot 2H_2O$ and its structural formula is:

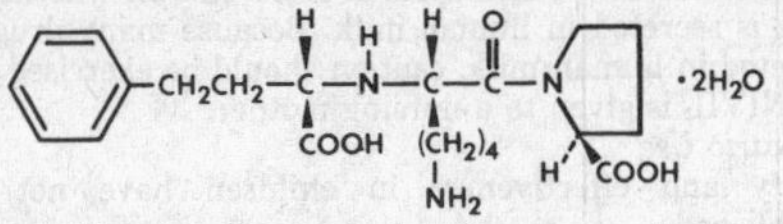

Lisinopril is a white to off-white, crystalline powder, with a molecular weight of 441.52. It is soluble in water and sparingly soluble in methanol and practically insoluble in ethanol.
PRINIVIL is supplied as 5 mg, 10 mg, 20 mg and 40 mg tablets for oral administration. In addition to the active ingredient lisinopril, each tablet contains the following inactive ingredients: calcium phosphate, mannitol, magnesium stearate, and starch. The 10 mg, 20 mg and 40 mg tablets also contain iron oxide.

*Registered trademark of MERCK & CO., INC.

CLINICAL PHARMACOLOGY

Mechanism of Action
Lisinopril inhibits angiotensin-converting enzyme (ACE) in human subjects and animals. ACE is a peptidyl dipeptidase that catalyzes the conversion of angiotensin I to the vasoconstrictor substance, angiotensin II. Angiotensin II also stimulates aldosterone secretion by the adrenal cortex. Inhibition of ACE results in decreased plasma angiotensin II which leads to decreased vasopressor activity and to decreased aldosterone secretion. The latter decrease may result in a small increase of serum potassium. In hypertensive patients with normal renal function treated with PRINIVIL alone for up to 24 weeks, the mean increase in serum potassium was approximately 0.1 mEq/L; however, approximately 15 percent of patients had increases greater than 0.5 mEq/L and approximately six percent had a decrease greater than 0.5 mEq/L. In the same study, patients treated with PRINIVIL and hydrochlorothiazide for up to 24 weeks had a mean decrease in serum potassium of 0.1 mEq/L; approximately 4 percent of patients had increases greater than 0.5 mEq/L and approximately 12 percent had a decrease greater than 0.5 mEq/L. (See PRECAUTIONS.) Removal of angiotensin II negative feedback on renin secretion leads to increased plasma renin activity.
ACE is identical to kininase, an enzyme that degrades bradykinin. Whether increased levels of bradykinin, a potent vasodepressor peptide, play a role in the therapeutic effects of PRINIVIL remains to be elucidated.
While the mechanism through which PRINIVIL lowers blood pressure is believed to be primarily suppression of the renin-angiotensin-aldosterone system, PRINIVIL is antihypertensive even in patients with low-renin hypertension. Although PRINIVIL was antihypertensive in all races studied, black hypertensive patients (usually a low-renin hypertensive population) had a smaller average response to monotherapy than non-black patients.
Concomitant administration of PRINIVIL and hydrochlorothiazide further reduced blood pressure in black and non-black patients and any racial difference in blood pressure response was no longer evident.
Pharmacokinetics and Metabolism
Following oral administration of PRINIVIL, peak serum concentrations of lisinopril occur within about 7 hours. Declining serum concentrations exhibit a prolonged terminal phase which does not contribute to drug accumulation. This terminal phase probably represents saturable binding to ACE and is not proportional to dose. Lisinopril does not appear to be bound to other serum proteins.
Lisinopril does not undergo metabolism and is excreted unchanged entirely in the urine. Based on urinary recovery, the mean extent of absorption of lisinopril is approximately 25 percent, with large intersubject variability (6–60 percent) at all doses tested (5–80 mg). Lisinopril absorption is not influenced by the presence of food in the gastrointestinal tract.
Upon multiple dosing, lisinopril exhibits an effective half-life of accumulation of 12 hours.
Impaired renal function decreases elimination of lisinopril, which is excreted principally through the kidneys, but this decrease becomes clinically important only when the glomerular filtration rate is below 30 mL/min. Above this glomerular filtration rate, the elimination half-life is little changed. With greater impairment, however, peak and trough lisinopril levels increase, time to peak concentration increases and time to attain steady state is prolonged. Older patients, on average, have (approximately doubled) higher blood levels and area under the plasma concentration time curve (AUC) than younger patients. (See DOSAGE AND ADMINISTRATION.) Lisinopril can be removed by hemodialysis.
Studies in rats indicate that lisinopril crosses the blood-brain barrier poorly. Multiple doses of lisinopril in rats do not result in accumulation in any tissues. Milk of lactating rats contains radioactivity following administration of ^{14}C lisinopril. By whole body autoradiography, radioactivity was found in the placenta following administration of labeled drug to pregnant rats, but none was found in the fetuses.
Pharmacodynamics
Administration of PRINIVIL to patients with hypertension results in a reduction of supine and standing blood pressure to about the same extent with no compensatory tachycardia. Symptomatic postural hypotension is usually not observed although it can occur and should be anticipated in volume and/or salt-depleted patients. (See WARNINGS.) When given together with thiazide-type diuretics, the blood pressure lowering effects of the two drugs are approximately additive.
In most patients studied, onset of antihypertensive activity was seen at one hour after oral administration of an individual dose of PRINIVIL, with peak reduction of blood pressure achieved by six hours. Although an antihypertensive effect was observed 24 hours after dosing with recommended single daily doses, the effect was more consistent and the mean effect was considerably larger in some studies with doses of 20 mg or more than with lower doses. However, at all doses studied, the mean antihypertensive effect was substantially smaller 24 hours after dosing than it was six hours after dosing.
In some patients achievement of optimal blood pressure reduction may require two to four weeks of therapy.
The antihypertensive effects of PRINIVIL are maintained during long-term therapy. Abrupt withdrawal of PRINIVIL has not been associated with a rapid increase in blood pressure or a significant increase in blood pressure compared to pretreatment levels.
Two dose-response studies utilizing a once daily regimen were conducted in 438 mild to moderate hypertensive patients not on a diuretic. Blood pressure was measured 24 hours after dosing. An antihypertensive effect of PRINIVIL was seen with 5 mg in some patients. However, in both studies blood pressure reduction occurred sooner and was greater in patients treated with 10, 20, or 80 mg of PRINIVIL. In controlled clinical studies, PRINIVIL 20–80 mg has been compared in patients with mild to moderate hypertension to hydrochlorothiazide 12.5–50 mg and with atenolol 50–200 mg; and in patients with moderate to severe hypertension to metoprolol 100–200 mg. It was superior to hydrochlorothiazide in effects on systolic and diastolic blood pressure in a population that was ¾ Caucasian. PRINIVIL was approximately equivalent to atenolol and metoprolol in effects on diastolic blood pressure and had somewhat greater effects on systolic blood pressure.
PRINIVIL had similar effectiveness and adverse effects in younger and older (>65 years) patients. It was less effective in blacks than in Caucasians.
In hemodynamic studies in patients with essential hypertension, blood pressure reduction was accompanied by a reduction in peripheral arterial resistance with little or no change in cardiac output and in heart rate. In a study in nine hypertensive patients, following administration of PRINIVIL, there was an increase in mean renal blood flow that was not significant. Data from several small studies are inconsistent with respect to the effect of PRINIVIL on glomerular filtration rate in hypertensive patients with normal renal function, but suggest that changes, if any, are not large.
In patients with renovascular hypertension PRINIVIL has been shown to be well tolerated and effective in controlling blood pressure (see PRECAUTIONS).

INDICATIONS AND USAGE

PRINIVIL is indicated for the treatment of hypertension. It may be used alone as initial therapy or concomitantly with other classes of antihypertensive agents.
In using PRINIVIL, consideration should be given to the fact that another angiotensin converting enzyme inhibitor, captopril, has caused agranulocytosis, particularly in patients with renal impairment or collagen vascular disease, and that available data are insufficient to show that PRINIVIL does not have a similar risk. (See WARNINGS.)

CONTRAINDICATIONS

PRINIVIL is contraindicated in patients who are hypersensitive to this product and in patients with a history of angioedema related to previous treatment with an angiotensin converting enzyme inhibitor.

WARNINGS

Angioedema
Angioedema of the face, extremities, lips, tongue, glottis and/or larynx has been reported in patients treated with angiotensin converting enzyme inhibitors, including PRINIVIL. In such cases PRINIVIL should be promptly discontinued and appropriate therapy and monitoring should be provided until complete and sustained resolution of signs and symptoms has occurred. In instances where swelling has been confined to the face and lips the condition has generally resolved without treatment, although antihistamines have been useful in relieving symptoms. Angioedema associated with laryngeal edema may be fatal. **Where there is involvement of the tongue, glottis or larynx, likely to cause airway obstruction, appropriate therapy, e.g., subcutaneous epinephrine solution 1:1000 (0.3 mL to 0.5 mL) and/or measures necessary to ensure a patent airway, should be promptly provided.** (See ADVERSE REACTIONS.)
Patients with a history of angioedema unrelated to ACE inhibitor therapy may be at increased risk of angioedema while receiving an ACE inhibitor (see also CONTRAINDICATIONS).
Hypotension
Excessive hypotension was rarely seen in uncomplicated hypertensive patients but is a possible consequence of the use of PRINIVIL in salt/volume-depleted persons, such as those treated vigorously with diuretics or patients on dialysis. (See PRECAUTIONS, *Drug Interactions* and ADVERSE REACTIONS.) In patients with severe congestive heart failure, with or without associated renal insufficiency, excessive hypotension has been observed and may be associated with oliguria and/or progressive azotemia, and rarely with acute renal failure and/or death. Because of the potential fall in blood pressure in these patients, therapy should be started under very close medical supervision. Such patients should be followed closely for the first two weeks of treatment and whenever the dose of PRINIVIL and/or diuretic is increased. Similar considerations apply to patients with ischemic heart or cerebrovascular disease in whom an excessive fall in blood pressure could result in a myocardial infarction or cerebrovascular accident.
If hypotension occurs, the patient should be placed in supine position and, if necessary, receive an intravenous infusion of normal saline. A transient hypotensive response is not a contraindication to further doses which usually can be given without difficulty once the blood pressure has increased after volume expansion.
Neutropenia/Agranulocytosis
Another angiotensin converting enzyme inhibitor, captopril, has been shown to cause agranulocytosis and bone marrow depression, rarely in uncomplicated patients but more frequently in patients with renal impairment especially if they also have a collagen vascular disease. Available data from clinical trials of PRINIVIL are insufficient to show that PRINIVIL does not cause agranulocytosis at similar rates. Marketing experience has revealed rare cases of neutropenia and bone marrow depression in which a causal relationship to lisinopril cannot be excluded. Periodic monitoring of white blood cell counts in patients with collagen vascular disease and renal disease should be considered.
Fetal/Neonatal Morbidity and Mortality
ACE inhibitors can cause fetal and neonatal morbidity and death when administered to pregnant women. Several dozen cases have been reported in the world literature. When pregnancy is detected, ACE inhibitors should be discontinued as soon as possible.
The use of ACE inhibitors during the second and third trimesters of pregnancy has been associated with fetal and neonatal injury, including hypotension, neonatal skull hypoplasia, anuria, reversible or irreversible renal failure, and death. Oligohydramnios has also been reported, presumably resulting from decreased fetal renal function; oligohydramnios in this setting has been associated with fetal limb contractures, craniofacial deformation, and hypoplastic lung development. Prematurity, intrauterine growth retardation, and patent ductus arteriosus have also been reported, although it is not clear whether these occurrences were due to the ACE-inhibitor exposure.
These adverse effects do not appear to have resulted from intrauterine ACE-inhibitor exposure that has been limited

Continued on next page

Information on the Merck & Co. products listed on these pages is the full prescribing information from product circulars in use October 1, 1992.

Merck & Co.—Cont.

to the first trimester. Mothers whose embryos and fetuses are exposed to ACE inhibitors only during the first trimester should be so informed. Nonetheless, when patients become pregnant, physicians should make every effort to discontinue the use of PRINIVIL as soon as possible.

Rarely (probably less often than once in every thousand pregnancies), no alternative to ACE inhibitors will be found. In these rare cases, the mothers should be apprised of the potential hazards to their fetuses, and serial ultrasound examinations should be performed to assess the intraamniotic environment.

If oligohydramnios is observed, PRINIVIL should be discontinued unless it is considered lifesaving for the mother. Contraction stress testing (CST), a non-stress test (NST), or biophysical profiling (BPP) may be appropriate, depending upon the week of pregnancy. Patients and physicians should be aware, however, that oligohydramnios may not appear until after the fetus has sustained irreversible injury.

Infants with histories of *in utero* exposure to ACE inhibitors should be closely observed for hypotension, oliguria, and hyperkalemia. If oliguria occurs, attention should be directed toward support of blood pressure and renal perfusion. Exchange transfusion or dialysis may be required as means of reversing hypotension and/or substituting for disordered renal function. Lisinopril, which crosses the placenta, has been removed from neonatal circulation by peritoneal dialysis with some clinical benefit, and theoretically may be removed by exchange transfusion, although there is no experience with the latter procedure.

No teratogenic effects of lisinopril were seen in studies of pregnant rats, mice, and rabbits. On a mg/kg basis, the doses used were up to 625 times (in mice), 188 times (in rats), and 0.6 times (in rabbits) the maximum recommended human dose.

PRECAUTIONS

General

Impaired Renal Function: As a consequence of inhibiting the renin-angiotensin-aldosterone system, changes in renal function may be anticipated in susceptible individuals. In patients with severe congestive heart failure whose renal function may depend on the activity of the renin-angiotensin-aldosterone system, treatment with angiotensin converting enzyme inhibitors, including PRINIVIL, may be associated with oliguria and/or progressive azotemia and rarely with acute renal failure and/or death.

In hypertensive patients with unilateral or bilateral renal artery stenosis, increases in blood urea nitrogen and serum creatinine may occur. Experience with another angiotensin converting enzyme inhibitor suggests that these increases are usually reversible upon discontinuation of PRINIVIL and/or diuretic therapy. In such patients renal function should be monitored during the first few weeks of therapy. Some hypertensive patients with no apparent pre-existing renal vascular disease have developed increases in blood urea nitrogen and serum creatinine, usually minor and transient, especially when PRINIVIL has been given concomitantly with a diuretic. This is more likely to occur in patients with pre-existing renal impairment. Dosage reduction of PRINIVIL and/or discontinuation of the diuretic may be required.

Evaluation of the hypertensive patient should always include assessment of renal function. (See DOSAGE AND ADMINISTRATION.)

Hemodialysis Patients: Anaphylactoid reactions have been reported in patients dialyzed with high-flux membranes (e.g., AN 69*) and treated concomitantly with an ACE inhibitor. In these patients consideration should be given to using a different type of dialysis membrane or a different class of antihypertensive agent.

Hyperkalemia: In clinical trials hyperkalemia (serum potassium greater than 5.7 mEq/L) occurred in approximately 2.2 percent of hypertensive patients and 4.0 percent of patients with congestive heart failure. In most cases these were isolated values which resolved despite continued therapy. Hyperkalemia was a cause of discontinuation of therapy in approximately 0.1 percent of hypertensive patients. Risk factors for the development of hyperkalemia include renal insufficiency, diabetes mellitus, and the concomitant use of potassium-sparing diuretics, potassium supplements and/or potassium-containing salt substitutes, which should be used cautiously, if at all, with PRINIVIL. (See *Drug Interactions*.)

Cough: Cough has been reported with the use of ACE inhibitors. Characteristically, the cough is nonproductive, persistent and resolves after discontinuation of therapy. ACE inhibitor-induced cough should be considered as part of the differential diagnosis of cough.

Surgery/Anesthesia: In patients undergoing major surgery or during anesthesia with agents that produce hypotension, PRINIVIL may block angiotensin II formation secondary to compensatory renin release. If hypotension occurs and is

---

considered to be due to this mechanism, it can be corrected by volume expansion.

---

* Registered trademark of Hospal Ltd.

Information for Patients

Angioedema: Angioedema, including laryngeal edema, may occur especially following the first dose of PRINIVIL. Patients should be so advised and told to report immediately any signs or symptoms suggesting angioedema (swelling of face, extremities, eyes, lips, tongue, difficulty in swallowing or breathing) and to take no more drug until they have consulted with the prescribing physician.

Symptomatic Hypotension: Patients should be cautioned to report lightheadedness especially during the first few days of therapy. If actual syncope occurs, the patients should be told to discontinue the drug until they have consulted with the prescribing physician.

All patients should be cautioned that excessive perspiration and dehydration may lead to an excessive fall in blood pressure because of reduction in fluid volume. Other causes of volume depletion such as vomiting or diarrhea may also lead to a fall in blood pressure; patients should be advised to consult with their physician.

Hyperkalemia: Patients should be told not to use salt substitutes containing potassium without consulting their physician.

Neutropenia: Patients should be told to report promptly any indication of infection (e.g., sore throat, fever) which may be a sign of neutropenia.

Pregnancy: Female patients of childbearing age should be told about the consequences of second- and third-trimester exposure to ACE inhibitors, and they should also be told that these consequences do not appear to have resulted from intrauterine ACE-inhibitor exposure that has been limited to the first trimester. These patients should be asked to report pregnancies to their physicians as soon as possible.

NOTE: As with many other drugs, certain advice to patients being treated with PRINIVIL is warranted. This information is intended to aid in the safe and effective use of this medication. It is not a disclosure of all possible adverse or intended effects.

Drug Interactions

Hypotension—Patients on Diuretic Therapy: Patients on diuretics, and especially those in whom diuretic therapy was recently instituted, may occasionally experience an excessive reduction of blood pressure after initiation of therapy with PRINIVIL. The possibility of hypotensive effects with PRINIVIL can be minimized by either discontinuing the diuretic or increasing the salt intake prior to initiation of treatment with PRINIVIL. If it is necessary to continue the diuretic, initiate therapy with PRINIVIL at a dose of 5 mg daily, and provide close medical supervision after the initial dose for at least two hours and until blood pressure has stabilized for at least an additional hour. (See WARNINGS, and DOSAGE AND ADMINISTRATION.) When a diuretic is added to the therapy of a patient receiving PRINIVIL, an additional antihypertensive effect is usually observed. Studies with ACE inhibitors in combination with diuretics indicate that the dose of the ACE inhibitor can be reduced when it is given with a diuretic. (See DOSAGE AND ADMINISTRATION.)

Indomethacin: In a study in 36 patients with mild to moderate hypertension where the antihypertensive effects of PRINIVIL alone were compared to PRINIVIL given concomitantly with indomethacin, the use of indomethacin was associated with a reduced effect, although the difference between the two regimens was not significant.

Other Agents: PRINIVIL has been used concomitantly with nitrates and/or digoxin without evidence of clinically significant adverse interactions. No clinically important pharmacokinetic interactions occurred when PRINIVIL was used concomitantly with propranolol or hydrochlorothiazide. The presence of food in the stomach does not alter the bioavailability of PRINIVIL.

Agents Increasing Serum Potassium: PRINIVIL attenuates potassium loss caused by thiazide-type diuretics. Use of PRINIVIL with potassium-sparing diuretics (e.g., spironolactone, triamterene, or amiloride), potassium supplements, or potassium-containing salt substitutes may lead to significant increases in serum potassium. Therefore, if concomitant use of these agents is indicated because of demonstrated hypokalemia, they should be used with caution and with frequent monitoring of serum potassium.

Lithium: Lithium toxicity has been reported in patients receiving lithium concomitantly with drugs which cause elimination of sodium, including ACE inhibitors. Lithium toxicity was usually reversible upon discontinuation of lithium and the ACE inhibitor. It is recommended that serum lithium levels be monitored frequently if PRINIVIL is administered concomitantly with lithium.

Carcinogenesis, Mutagenesis, Impairment of Fertility

There was no evidence of a tumorigenic effect when lisinopril was administered for 105 weeks to male and female rats at doses up to 90 mg/kg/day (about 56 times* the maximum recommended daily human dose) or when lisinopril was ad-

---

ministered for 92 weeks to (male and female) mice at doses up to 135 mg/kg/day (about 84 times* the maximum recommended daily human dose).

Lisinopril was not mutagenic in the Ames microbial mutagen test with or without metabolic activation. It was also negative in a forward mutation assay using Chinese hamster lung cells. Lisinopril did not produce single strand DNA breaks in an *in vitro* alkaline elution rat hepatocyte assay. In addition, lisinopril did not produce increases in chromosomal aberrations in an *in vitro* test in Chinese hamster ovary cells or in an *in vivo* study in mouse bone marrow. There were no adverse effects on reproductive performance in male and female rats treated with up to 300 mg/kg/day of lisinopril.

Pregnancy

Pregnancy Categories C (first trimester) *and D* (second and third trimesters). See WARNINGS, *Fetal/Neonatal Morbidity and Mortality.*

Nursing Mothers

Milk of lactating rats contains radioactivity following administration of ^{14}C lisinopril. It is not known whether this drug is secreted in human milk. Because many drugs are secreted in human milk, caution should be exercised when PRINIVIL is given to a nursing mother.

Pediatric Use

Safety and effectiveness in children have not been established.

---

* Based on patient weight of 50 kg

ADVERSE REACTIONS

PRINIVIL has been found to be generally well tolerated in controlled clinical trials involving 2003 patients and subjects.

The most frequent clinical adverse experiences in controlled trials with PRINIVIL were: dizziness (6.3 percent), headache (5.3 percent), fatigue (3.3 percent), diarrhea (3.2 percent), upper respiratory symptoms (3.0 percent) and cough (2.9 percent), all of which were more frequent than in placebo-treated patients. For the most part, adverse experiences were mild and transient in nature. Discontinuation of therapy was required in 6.0 percent of patients. In clinical trials, the overall frequency of adverse experiences could not be related to total daily dosage within the recommended therapeutic dosage range.

For adverse experiences which occurred in more than one percent of patients and subjects treated with PRINIVIL or PRINIVIL plus hydrochlorothiazide in controlled clinical trials, comparative incidence data are listed in the table below.

[See table on next page.]

Clinical adverse experiences occurring in 0.3 to 1.0 percent of patients treated with PRINIVIL monotherapy in the controlled trials and rarer, serious, possibly drug-related events reported in uncontrolled studies or marketing experience are listed below and, within each category, are in order of decreasing severity.

Body as a Whole: Anaphylactoid reactions (see PRECAUTIONS, *Hemodialysis Patients*), chest discomfort, fever, flushing, malaise.

Cardiovascular: Myocardial infarction or cerebrovascular accident, possibly secondary to excessive hypotension in high risk patients (see WARNINGS, *Hypotension*); angina pectoris, orthostatic hypotension, rhythm disturbances, tachycardia, peripheral edema, vasculitis, palpitation.

Digestive: Pancreatitis, hepatitis (hepatocellular or cholestatic jaundice), abdominal pain, anorexia, constipation, flatulence, dry mouth.

Metabolism: Gout.

Musculoskeletal: Joint pain, shoulder pain.

Nervous System/Psychiatric: Depression, somnolence, insomnia, stroke, nervousness, confusion.

Respiratory System: Bronchitis, sinusitis, pharyngeal pain.

Skin: Urticaria, pruritus, diaphoresis.

Special Senses: Blurred vision.

Urogenital: Oliguria, progressive azotemia, acute renal failure, urinary tract infection.

A symptom complex has been reported which may include a positive ANA, an elevated erythrocyte sedimentation rate, arthralgia/arthritis, myalgia and fever.

Angioedema: Angioedema has been reported in patients receiving PRINIVIL (0.1 percent). Angioedema associated with laryngeal edema may be fatal. If angioedema of the face, extremities, lips, tongue, glottis and/or larynx occurs, treatment with PRINIVIL should be discontinued and appropriate therapy instituted immediately. (See WARNINGS.)

Hypotension: In hypertensive patients, hypotension occurred in 1.2 percent and syncope occurred in 0.1 percent of patients. Hypotension or syncope was a cause for discontinuation of therapy in 0.5 percent of hypertensive patients. (See WARNINGS.)

In patients with congestive heart failure, hypotension occurred in 5.0 percent and syncope occurred in 1.0 percent of

	PRINIVIL (n=2003*) Incidence (discontinuation)	Percent of Patients in Controlled Studies PRINIVIL/ Hydrochlorothiazide (n=644) Incidence (discontinuation)	Placebo (n=207) Incidence
Dizziness	6.3 (0.6)	9.0 (0.9)	1.9
Headache	5.3 (0.2)	4.3 (0.5)	1.9
Fatigue	3.3 (0.2)	3.9 (0.5)	1.0
Diarrhea	3.2 (0.3)	2.6 (0.3)	2.4
Upper Respiratory Symptoms	3.0 (0.0)	4.5 (0.0)	0.0
Cough	2.9 (0.4)	4.5 (0.8)	1.0
Nausea	2.3 (0.3)	2.5 (0.2)	2.4
Hypotension	1.8 (0.8)	1.6 (0.5)	0.5
Rash	1.5 (0.4)	1.6 (0.2)	0.5
Orthostatic Effects	1.4 (0.0)	3.4 (0.2)	1.0
Asthenia	1.3 (0.4)	2.0 (0.1)	1.0
Chest Pain	1.3 (0.1)	1.2 (0.0)	1.4
Vomiting	1.3 (0.2)	1.4 (0.0)	0.5
Dyspnea	1.1 (0.0)	0.5 (0.0)	1.4
Dyspepsia	1.0 (0.0)	1.9 (0.0)	0.0
Paresthesia	0.8 (0.0)	2.0 (0.2)	0.0
Impotence	0.7 (0.2)	1.6 (0.3)	0.0
Muscle Cramps	0.6 (0.0)	2.8 (0.6)	0.5
Back Pain	0.5 (0.0)	1.1 (0.0)	1.4
Nasal Congestion	0.3 (0.0)	1.2 (0.0)	0.0
Decreased Libido	0.2 (0.1)	1.2 (0.0)	0.0
Vertigo	0.1 (0.0)	1.1 (0.2)	0.0

*Includes 420 patients treated for congestive heart failure who were receiving concomitant digitalis and/or diuretic therapy.

patients. These adverse experiences were causes for discontinuation of therapy in 1.3 percent of these patients.

Fetal/Neonatal Morbidity and Mortality: See WARNINGS, *Fetal/Neonatal Morbidity and Mortality.*

Cough: See PRECAUTIONS, *Cough.*

Clinical Laboratory Test Findings

Serum Electrolytes: Hyperkalemia (see PRECAUTIONS).

Creatinine, Blood Urea Nitrogen: Minor increases in blood urea nitrogen and serum creatinine, reversible upon discontinuation of therapy, were observed in about 2.0 percent of patients with essential hypertension treated with PRINIVIL alone. Increases were more common in patients receiving concomitant diuretics and in patients with renal artery stenosis. (See PRECAUTIONS.) Reversible minor increases in blood urea nitrogen and serum creatinine were observed in approximately 9.1 percent of patients with congestive heart failure on concomitant diuretic therapy. Frequently, these abnormalities resolved when the dosage of the diuretic was decreased.

Hemoglobin and Hematocrit: Small decreases in hemoglobin and hematocrit (mean decreases of approximately 0.4 g percent and 1.3 vol percent, respectively) occurred frequently in patients treated with PRINIVIL but were rarely of clinical importance in patients without some other cause of anemia. In clinical trials, less than 0.1 percent of patients discontinued therapy due to anemia.

Other (Causal Relationship Unknown): Rarely, elevations of liver enzymes and/or serum bilirubin have occurred. In marketing experience, rare cases of neutropenia and bone marrow depression have been reported.

Overall, 2.0 percent of patients discontinued therapy due to laboratory adverse experiences, principally elevations in blood urea nitrogen (0.6 percent), serum creatinine (0.5 percent) and serum potassium (0.4 percent).

OVERDOSAGE

The oral LD_{50} of lisinopril is greater than 20 g/kg in mice and rats. The most likely manifestation of overdosage would be hypotension, for which the usual treatment would be intravenous infusion of normal saline solution.

Lisinopril can be removed by hemodialysis.

DOSAGE AND ADMINISTRATION

Initial Therapy: In patients with uncomplicated essential hypertension not on diuretic therapy, the recommended initial dose is 10 mg once a day. Dosage should be adjusted according to blood pressure response. The usual dosage range is 20 to 40 mg per day administered in a single daily dose. The antihypertensive effect may diminish toward the end of the dosing interval regardless of the administered dose, but most commonly with a dose of 10 mg daily. This can be evaluated by measuring blood pressure just prior to dosing to determine whether satisfactory control is being maintained for 24 hours. If it is not, an increase in dose should be considered. Doses up to 80 mg have been used but do not appear to give a greater effect. If blood pressure is not controlled with PRINIVIL alone, a low dose of a diuretic may be added. Hydrochlorothiazide 12.5 mg has been shown to pro-

vide an additive effect. After the addition of a diuretic, it may be possible to reduce the dose of PRINIVIL.

Diuretic Treated Patients: In hypertensive patients who are currently being treated with a diuretic, symptomatic hypotension may occur occasionally following the initial dose of PRINIVIL. The diuretic should be discontinued, if possible, for two to three days before beginning therapy with PRINIVIL to reduce the likelihood of hypotension. (See WARNINGS.) The dosage of PRINIVIL should be adjusted according to blood pressure response. If the patient's blood pressure is not controlled with PRINIVIL alone, diuretic therapy may be resumed as described above.

If the diuretic cannot be discontinued, an initial dose of 5 mg should be used under medical supervision for at least two hours and until blood pressure has stabilized for at least an additional hour. (See WARNINGS and PRECAUTIONS, *Drug Interactions.*)

Concomitant administration of PRINIVIL with potassium supplements, potassium salt substitutes, or potassium-sparing diuretics may lead to increases of serum potassium (see PRECAUTIONS).

Use in Elderly: In general, blood pressure response and adverse experiences were similar in younger and older patients given similar doses of PRINIVIL. Pharmacokinetic studies, however, indicate that maximum blood levels and area under the plasma concentration time curve (AUC) are doubled in older patients so that dosage adjustments should be made with particular caution.

Dosage Adjustment in Renal Impairment: The usual dose of PRINIVIL (10 mg) is recommended for patients with a creatinine clearance > 30 mL/min (serum creatinine of up to approximately 3 mg/dL). For patients with creatinine clearance ≥ 10 mL/min ≤ 30 mL/min (serum creatinine ≥ 3 mg/dL), the first dose is 5 mg once daily. For patients with creatinine clearance < 10 mL/min (usually on hemodialysis) the recommended initial dose is 2.5 mg. The dosage may be titrated upward until blood pressure is controlled or to a maximum of 40 mg daily.

Renal Status	Creatinine-Clearance mL/min	Initial Dose mg/day
Normal Renal Function to Mild Impairment	> 30 mL/min	10 mg
Moderate to Severe Impairment	≥ 10 ≤ 30 mL/min	5 mg
Dialysis Patients*	< 10 mL/min	2.5 mg**

* See PRECAUTIONS, *Hemodialysis Patients*

** Dosage or dosing interval should be adjusted depending on the blood pressure response.

HOW SUPPLIED

No. 3577—Tablets PRINIVIL, 5 mg, are white, shield shaped, scored, compressed tablets, with code MSD 19 on

one side and PRINIVIL on the other. They are supplied as follows:

NDC 0006-0019-28 unit dose packages of 100

NDC 0006-0019-58 unit of use bottles of 100.

(6505-01-281-2771, 5 mg 100's)

NDC 0006-0019-94 unit of use bottles of 90.

Shown in Product Identification Section, page 420

No. 3578—Tablets PRINIVIL, 10 mg, are light yellow, shield shaped, compressed tablets, with code MSD 106 on one side and PRINIVIL on the other. They are supplied as follows:

NDC 0006-0106-28 unit dose packages of 100

NDC 0006-0106-31 unit of use bottles of 30

NDC 0006-0106-58 unit of use bottles of 100.

(6505-01-275-0061, 10 mg 100's)

NDC 0006-0106-94 unit of use bottles of 90.

Shown in Product Identification Section, page 420

No. 3579—Tablets PRINIVIL, 20 mg, are peach, shield shaped, compressed tablets, with code MSD 207 on one side and PRINIVIL on the other. They are supplied as follows:

NDC 0006-0207-28 unit dose packages of 100

NDC 0006-0207-31 unit of use bottles of 30

NDC 0006-0207-58 unit of use bottles of 100.

(6505-01-282-6327, 20 mg 100's)

NDC 0006-0207-94 unit of use bottles of 90.

Shown in Product Identification Section, page 420

No. 3580—Tablets PRINIVIL, 40 mg, are rose red, shield shaped, compressed tablets, with code MSD 237 on one side and PRINIVIL on the other. They are supplied as follows:

NDC 0006-0237-58 unit of use bottles of 100.

Shown in Product Identification Section, page 420

Storage

Protect from moisture, freezing and excessive heat.

Dispense in a tight container, if product package is subdivided.

A.H.F.S. Category: 24:08

DC 7507520   Issued May 1992

COPYRIGHT © MERCK & CO., INC., 1988, 1989, 1992

All rights reserved

PRINZIDE® Tablets   ℞
(Lisinopril-Hydrochlorothiazide)

> ### USE IN PREGNANCY
> When used in pregnancy during the second and third trimesters, ACE inhibitors can cause injury and even death to the developing fetus. When pregnancy is detected, PRINZIDE should be discontinued as soon as possible. See WARNINGS, *Pregnancy, Lisinopril, Fetal/Neonatal Morbidity and Mortality.*

DESCRIPTION

PRINZIDE* (Lisinopril-Hydrochlorothiazide) combines an angiotensin converting enzyme inhibitor, lisinopril, and a diuretic, hydrochlorothiazide.

Lisinopril, a synthetic peptide derivative, is an oral long-acting angiotensin converting enzyme inhibitor. It is chemically described as (S)-1-[N^2-(1-carboxy-3-phenylpropyl)-L-lysyl]-L-proline dihydrate. Its empirical formula is $C_{21}H_{31}N_3O_5 \cdot 2H_2O$ and its structural formula is:

Lisinopril is a white to off-white, crystalline powder, with a molecular weight of 441.52. It is soluble in water, sparingly soluble in methanol, and practically insoluble in ethanol. Hydrochlorothiazide is 6-chloro-3,4-dihydro-2H-1,2,4-benzothiadiazine-7-sulfonamide 1,1-dioxide. Its empirical formula is $C_7H_8ClN_3O_4S_2$ and its structural formula is:

Hydrochlorothiazide is a white, or practically white, crystalline powder with a molecular weight of 297.72, which is slightly soluble in water, but freely soluble in sodium hydroxide solution.

Continued on next page

Merck & Co.—Cont.

PRINZIDE is available for oral use in two tablet combinations of lisinopril with hydrochlorothiazide: PRINZIDE 12.5, containing 20 mg lisinopril and 12.5 mg hydrochlorothiazide and PRINZIDE 25, containing 20 mg lisinopril and 25 mg hydrochlorothiazide.

Inactive ingredients are calcium phosphate, iron oxide, magnesium stearate, mannitol, and starch.

* Registered trademark of MERCK & CO., INC.

CLINICAL PHARMACOLOGY

Lisinopril-Hydrochlorothiazide

As a result of its diuretic effects, hydrochlorothiazide increases plasma renin activity, increases aldosterone secretion, and decreases serum potassium. Administration of lisinopril blocks the renin-angiotensin-aldosterone axis and tends to reverse the potassium loss associated with the diuretic.

In clinical studies, the extent of blood pressure reduction seen with the combination of lisinopril and hydrochlorothiazide was approximately additive. The combination appeared somewhat less effective in black patients, but relatively few black patients were studied. In most patients, the antihypertensive effect of PRINZIDE was sustained for at least 24 hours.

In a randomized, controlled comparison, the mean antihypertensive effects of PRINZIDE 12.5 and PRINZIDE 25 were similar, suggesting that many patients who respond adequately to the latter combination may be controlled with PRINZIDE 12.5. (See DOSAGE AND ADMINISTRATION.)

Concomitant administration of lisinopril and hydrochlorothiazide has little or no effect on the bioavailability of either drug. The combination tablet is bioequivalent to concomitant administration of the separate entities.

Lisinopril

Mechanism of Action

Lisinopril inhibits angiotensin-converting enzyme (ACE) in human subjects and animals. ACE is a peptidyl dipeptidase that catalyzes the conversion of angiotensin I to the vasoconstrictor substance, angiotensin II. Angiotensin II also stimulates aldosterone secretion by the adrenal cortex. Inhibition of ACE results in decreased plasma angiotensin II which leads to decreased vasopressor activity and to decreased aldosterone secretion. The latter decrease may result in a small increase of serum potassium. Removal of angiotensin II negative feedback on renin secretion leads to increased plasma renin activity. In hypertensive patients with normal renal function treated with lisinopril alone for up to 24 weeks, the mean increase in serum potassium was less than 0.1 mEq/L; however, approximately 15 percent of patients had increases greater than 0.5 mEq/L and approximately six percent had a decrease greater than 0.5 mEq/L. In the same study, patients treated with lisinopril plus a thiazide diuretic showed essentially no change in serum potassium. (See PRECAUTIONS.)

ACE is identical to kininase, an enzyme that degrades bradykinin. Whether increased levels of bradykinin, a potent vasodepressor peptide, play a role in the therapeutic effects of lisinopril remains to be elucidated.

While the mechanism through which lisinopril lowers blood pressure is believed to be primarily suppression of the renin-angiotensin-aldosterone system, lisinopril is antihypertensive even in patients with low-renin hypertension. Although lisinopril was antihypertensive in all races studied, black hypertensive patients (usually a low-renin hypertensive population) had a smaller average response to lisinopril monotherapy than non-black patients.

Pharmacokinetics and Metabolism

Following oral administration of lisinopril, peak serum concentrations occur within about 7 hours. Declining serum concentrations exhibit a prolonged terminal phase which does not contribute to drug accumulation. This terminal phase probably represents saturable binding to ACE and is not proportional to dose. Lisinopril does not appear to be bound to other serum proteins.

Lisinopril does not undergo metabolism and is excreted unchanged entirely in the urine. Based on urinary recovery, the mean extent of absorption of lisinopril is approximately 25 percent, with large intersubject variability (6–60 percent) at all doses tested (5–80 mg). Lisinopril absorption is not influenced by the presence of food in the gastrointestinal tract.

Upon multiple dosing, lisinopril exhibits an effective half-life of accumulation of 12 hours.

Impaired renal function decreases elimination of lisinopril, which is excreted principally through the kidneys, but this decrease becomes clinically important only when the glomerular filtration rate is below 30 mL/min. Above this glomerular filtration rate, the elimination half-life is little changed. With greater impairment, however, peak and trough lisinopril levels increase, time to peak concentration increases and time to attain steady state is prolonged. Older

patients, on average, have (approximately doubled) higher blood levels and area under the plasma concentration time curve (AUC) than younger patients. (See DOSAGE AND ADMINISTRATION.) Lisinopril can be removed by hemodialysis.

Studies in rats indicate that lisinopril crosses the blood-brain barrier poorly. Multiple doses of lisinopril in rats do not result in accumulation in any tissues. However, milk of lactating rats contains radioactivity following administration of ^{14}C lisinopril. By whole body autoradiography, radioactivity was found in the placenta following administration of labeled drug to pregnant rats, but none was found in the fetuses.

Pharmacodynamics

Administration of lisinopril to patients with hypertension results in a reduction of supine and standing blood pressure to about the same extent with no compensatory tachycardia. Symptomatic postural hypotension is usually not observed although it can occur and should be anticipated in volume and/or salt-depleted patients. (See WARNINGS.)

In most patients studied, onset of antihypertensive activity was seen at one hour after oral administration of an individual dose of lisinopril, with peak reduction of blood pressure achieved by six hours.

In some patients achievement of optimal blood pressure reduction may require two to four weeks of therapy.

At recommended single daily doses, antihypertensive effects have been maintained for at least 24 hours after dosing, although the effect at 24 hours was substantially smaller than the effect six hours after dosing.

The antihypertensive effects of lisinopril have continued during long-term therapy. Abrupt withdrawal of lisinopril has not been associated with a rapid increase in blood pressure; nor with a significant overshoot of pretreatment blood pressure.

In hemodynamic studies in patients with essential hypertension, blood pressure reduction was accompanied by a reduction in peripheral arterial resistance with little or no change in cardiac output and in heart rate. In a study in nine hypertensive patients, following administration of lisinopril, there was an increase in mean renal blood flow that was not significant. Data from several small studies are inconsistent with respect to the effect of lisinopril on glomerular filtration rate in hypertensive patients with normal renal function, but suggest that changes, if any, are not large.

In patients with renovascular hypertension lisinopril has been shown to be well tolerated and effective in controlling blood pressure (see PRECAUTIONS).

Hydrochlorothiazide

The mechanism of the antihypertensive effect of thiazides is unknown. Thiazides do not usually affect normal blood pressure.

Hydrochlorothiazide is a diuretic and antihypertensive. It affects the distal renal tubular mechanism of electrolyte reabsorption. Hydrochlorothiazide increases excretion of sodium and chloride in approximately equivalent amounts. Natriuresis may be accompanied by some loss of potassium and bicarbonate.

After oral use diuresis begins within two hours, peaks in about four hours and lasts about 6 to 12 hours.

Hydrochlorothiazide is not metabolized but is eliminated rapidly by the kidney. When plasma levels have been followed for at least 24 hours, the plasma half-life has been observed to vary between 5.6 and 14.8 hours. At least 61 percent of the oral dose is eliminated unchanged within 24 hours. Hydrochlorothiazide crosses the placental but not the blood-brain barrier.

INDICATIONS AND USAGE

PRINZIDE is indicated for the treatment of hypertension in patients for whom combination therapy is appropriate.

This fixed dose combination is not indicated for initial therapy. Patients already receiving a diuretic when lisinopril is initiated, or given a diuretic and lisinopril simultaneously, can develop symptomatic hypotension. In the initial titration of the individual entities, it is important, if possible, to stop the diuretic for several days before starting lisinopril or, if this is not possible, begin lisinopril at a low initial dose. (See DOSAGE AND ADMINISTRATION.)

In using PRINZIDE, consideration should be given to the fact that an angiotensin converting enzyme inhibitor, captopril, has caused agranulocytosis, particularly in patients with renal impairment or collagen vascular disease, and that available data are insufficient to show that lisinopril does not have a similar risk. (See WARNINGS.)

CONTRAINDICATIONS

PRINZIDE is contraindicated in patients who are hypersensitive to any component of this product and in patients with a history of angioedema related to previous treatment with an angiotensin converting enzyme inhibitor. Because of the hydrochlorothiazide component, this product is contraindi-

cated in patients with anuria or hypersensitivity to other sulfonamide-derived drugs.

WARNINGS

General

Lisinopril

Angioedema: Angioedema of the face, extremities, lips, tongue, glottis and/or larynx has been reported rarely in patients treated with angiotensin converting enzyme inhibitors, including lisinopril. In such cases PRINZIDE should be promptly discontinued and appropriate therapy and monitoring should be provided until complete and sustained resolution of signs and symptoms has occurred. In instances where swelling has been confined to the face and lips the condition has generally resolved without treatment, although antihistamines have been useful in relieving symptoms. Angioedema associated with laryngeal edema may be fatal. **Where there is involvement of the tongue, glottis or larynx, likely to cause airway obstruction, subcutaneous epinephrine solution 1:1000 (0.3 mL to 0.5 mL) and/or measures necessary to ensure a patent airway, should be promptly provided. (See ADVERSE REACTIONS.)**

Patients with a history of angioedema unrelated to ACE inhibitor therapy may be at increased risk of angioedema while receiving an ACE inhibitor (see also CONTRAINDICATIONS).

Hypotension and Related Effects: Excessive hypotension was rarely seen in uncomplicated hypertensive patients but is a possible consequence of lisinopril use in salt/volume-depleted persons, such as those treated vigorously with diuretics or patients on dialysis. (See PRECAUTIONS, *Drug Interactions* and ADVERSE REACTIONS.)

Syncope has been reported in 0.8 percent of patients receiving PRINZIDE. In patients with hypertension receiving lisinopril alone, the incidence of syncope was 0.1 percent. The overall incidence of syncope may be reduced by proper titration of the individual components. (See PRECAUTIONS, *Drug Interactions*, ADVERSE REACTIONS and DOSAGE AND ADMINISTRATION.)

In patients with severe congestive heart failure, with or without associated renal insufficiency, excessive hypotension has been observed and may be associated with oliguria and/or progressive azotemia, and rarely with acute renal failure and/or death. Because of the potential fall in blood pressure in these patients, therapy should be started under very close medical supervision. Such patients should be followed closely for the first two weeks of treatment and whenever the dose of lisinopril and/or diuretic is increased. Similar considerations apply to patients with ischemic heart or cerebrovascular disease in whom an excessive fall in blood pressure could result in a myocardial infarction or cerebrovascular accident.

If hypotension occurs, the patient should be placed in supine position and, if necessary, receive an intravenous infusion of normal saline. A transient hypotensive response is not a contraindication to further doses which usually can be given without difficulty once the blood pressure has increased after volume expansion.

Neutropenia/Agranulocytosis: Another angiotensin converting enzyme inhibitor, captopril, has been shown to cause agranulocytosis and bone marrow depression, rarely in uncomplicated patients but more frequently in patients with renal impairment, especially if they also have a collagen vascular disease. Available data from clinical trials of lisinopril are insufficient to show that lisinopril does not cause agranulocytosis at similar rates. Marketing experience has revealed rare cases of neutropenia and bone marrow depression in which a causal relationship to lisinopril cannot be excluded. Periodic monitoring of white blood cell counts in patients with collagen vascular disease and renal disease should be considered.

Hydrochlorothiazide

Thiazides should be used with caution in severe renal disease. In patients with renal disease, thiazides may precipitate azotemia. Cumulative effects of the drug may develop in patients with impaired renal function.

Thiazides should be used with caution in patients with impaired hepatic function or progressive liver disease, since minor alterations of fluid and electrolyte balance may precipitate hepatic coma.

Sensitivity reactions may occur in patients with or without a history of allergy or bronchial asthma.

The possibility of exacerbation or activation of systemic lupus erythematosus has been reported.

Lithium generally should not be given with thiazides (see PRECAUTIONS, *Drug Interactions, Lisinopril* and *Hydrochlorothiazide*).

Pregnancy

Lisinopril-Hydrochlorothiazide

Teratogenicity studies were conducted in mice and rats with up to 90 mg/kg/day of lisinopril (56 times the maximum recommended human dose) in combination with 10 mg/kg/day of hydrochlorothiazide (2.5 times the maximum recommended human dose). Maternal or fetotoxic effects were not

seen in mice with the combination. In rats decreased maternal weight gain and decreased fetal weight occurred down to 3/10 mg/kg/day (the lowest dose tested). Associated with the decreased fetal weight was a delay in fetal ossification. The decreased fetal weight and delay in fetal ossification were not seen in saline-supplemented animals given 90/10 mg/kg/day.

If PRINZIDE is used during pregnancy or if the patient becomes pregnant while taking PRINZIDE, the patient should be apprised of the potential hazards to the fetus. (See *Lisinopril, Fetal/Neonatal Morbidity and Mortality,* below.)

Lisinopril

Fetal/Neonatal Morbidity and Mortality:

ACE inhibitors can cause fetal and neonatal morbidity and death when administered to pregnant women. Several dozen cases have been reported in the world literature. When pregnancy is detected, ACE inhibitors should be discontinued as soon as possible.

The use of ACE inhibitors during the second and third trimesters of pregnancy has been associated with fetal and neonatal injury, including hypotension, neonatal skull hypoplasia, anuria, reversible or irreversible renal failure, and death. Oligohydramnios has also been reported, presumably resulting from decreased fetal renal function; oligohydramnios in this setting has been associated with fetal limb contractures, craniofacial deformation, and hypoplastic lung development. Prematurity, intrauterine growth retardation, and patent ductus arteriosus have also been reported, although it is not clear whether these occurrences were due to the ACE-inhibitor exposure.

These adverse effects do not appear to have resulted from intrauterine ACE-inhibitor exposure that has been limited to the first trimester. Mothers whose embryos and fetuses are exposed to ACE inhibitors only during the first trimester should be so informed. Nonetheless, when patients become pregnant, physicians should make every effort to discontinue the use of PRINZIDE as soon as possible.

Rarely (probably less often than once in every thousand pregnancies), no alternative to ACE inhibitors will be found. In these rare cases, the mothers should be apprised of the potential hazards to their fetuses, and serial ultrasound examinations should be performed to assess the intraamniotic environment.

If oligohydramnios is observed, PRINZIDE should be discontinued unless it is considered lifesaving for the mother. Contraction stress testing (CST), a non-stress test (NST), or biophysical profiling (BPP) may be appropriate, depending upon the week of pregnancy. Patients and physicians should be aware, however, that oligohydramnios may not appear until after the fetus has sustained irreversible injury.

Infants with histories of *in utero* exposure to ACE inhibitors should be closely observed for hypotension, oliguria, and hyperkalemia. If oliguria occurs, attention should be directed toward support of blood pressure and renal perfusion. Exchange transfusion or dialysis may be required as means of reversing hypotension and/or substituting for disordered renal function. Lisinopril, which crosses the placenta, has been removed from neonatal circulation by peritoneal dialysis with some clinical benefit, and theoretically may be removed by exchange transfusion, although there is no experience with the latter procedure.

No teratogenic effects of lisinopril were seen in studies of pregnant rats, mice, and rabbits. On a mg/kg basis, the doses used were up to 625 times (in mice), 188 times (in rats), 0.6 times (in rabbits) the maximum recommended human dose.

Hydrochlorothiazide

Teratogenic Effects: Reproduction studies in the rabbit, the mouse and the rat at doses up to 100 mg/kg/day (50 times the human dose) showed no evidence of external abnormalities of the fetus due to hydrochlorothiazide. Hydrochlorothiazide given in a two-litter study in rats at doses of 4 - 5.6 mg/kg/day (approximately 1 - 2 times the usual daily human dose) did not impair fertility or produce birth abnormalities in the offspring. Thiazides cross the placental barrier and appear in cord blood.

Nonteratogenic Effects: These may include fetal or neonatal jaundice, thrombocytopenia, and possibly other adverse reactions which have occurred in the adult.

PRECAUTIONS

General

Lisinopril

Impaired Renal Function: As a consequence of inhibiting the renin-angiotensin-aldosterone system, changes in renal function may be anticipated in susceptible individuals. In patients with severe congestive heart failure whose renal function may depend on the activity of the renin-angiotensin-aldosterone system, treatment with angiotensin converting enzyme inhibitors, including lisinopril, may be associated with oliguria and/or progressive azotemia and rarely with acute renal failure and/or death.

In hypertensive patients with unilateral or bilateral renal artery stenosis, increases in blood urea nitrogen and serum creatinine may occur. Experience with another angiotensin converting enzyme inhibitor suggests that these increases are usually reversible upon discontinuation of lisinopril and/ or diuretic therapy. In such patients renal function should be monitored during the first few weeks of therapy.

Some hypertensive patients with no apparent pre-existing renal vascular disease have developed increases in blood urea and serum creatinine, usually minor and transient, especially when lisinopril has been given concomitantly with a diuretic. This is more likely to occur in patients with pre-existing renal impairment. Dosage reduction of lisinopril and/or discontinuation of the diuretic may be required.

Evaluation of the hypertensive patient should always include assessment of renal function. (See DOSAGE AND ADMINISTRATION.)

Hemodialysis Patients: Anaphylactoid reactions have been reported in patients dialyzed with high-flux membranes (e.g., AN 69*) and treated concomitantly with an ACE inhibitor. In these patients consideration should be given to using a different type of dialysis membrane or a different class of antihypertensive agent.

Hyperkalemia: In clinical trials hyperkalemia (serum potassium greater than 5.7 mEq/L) occurred in approximately 1.4 percent of hypertensive patients treated with lisinopril plus hydrochlorothiazide. In most cases these were isolated values which resolved despite continued therapy. Hyperkalemia was not a cause of discontinuation of therapy. Risk factors for the development of hyperkalemia include renal insufficiency, diabetes mellitus, and the concomitant use of potassium-sparing diuretics, potassium supplements and/or potassium-containing salt substitutes, which should be used cautiously if at all with PRINZIDE. (See *Drug Interactions.*)

Cough: Cough has been reported with the use of ACE inhibitors. Characteristically, the cough is nonproductive, persistent and resolves after discontinuation of therapy. ACE inhibitor-induced cough should be considered as part of the differential diagnosis of cough.

Surgery/Anesthesia: In patients undergoing major surgery or during anesthesia with agents that produce hypotension, lisinopril may block angiotensin II formation secondary to compensatory renin release. If hypotension occurs and is considered to be due to this mechanism, it can be corrected by volume expansion.

* Registered trademark of Hospal Ltd.

Hydrochlorothiazide

Periodic determination of serum electrolytes to detect possible electrolyte imbalance should be performed at appropriate intervals.

All patients receiving thiazide therapy should be observed for clinical signs of fluid or electrolyte imbalance: namely, hyponatremia, hypochloremic alkalosis, and hypokalemia. Serum and urine electrolyte determinations are particularly important when the patient is vomiting excessively or receiving parenteral fluids. Warning signs or symptoms of fluid and electrolyte imbalance, irrespective of cause, include dryness of mouth, thirst, weakness, lethargy, drowsiness, restlessness, confusion, seizures, muscle pains or cramps, muscular fatigue, hypotension, oliguria, tachycardia, and gastrointestinal disturbances such as nausea and vomiting.

Hypokalemia may develop, especially with brisk diuresis, when severe cirrhosis is present, or after prolonged therapy. Interference with adequate oral electrolyte intake will also contribute to hypokalemia. Hypokalemia may cause cardiac arrhythmia and may also sensitize or exaggerate the response of the heart to the toxic effects of digitalis (e.g., increased ventricular irritability). Because lisinopril reduces the production of aldosterone, concomitant therapy with lisinopril attenuates the diuretic-induced potassium loss (see *Drug Interactions, Agents Increasing Serum Potassium*).

Although any chloride deficit is generally mild and usually does not require specific treatment, except under extraordinary circumstances (as in liver disease or renal disease), chloride replacement may be required in the treatment of metabolic alkalosis.

Dilutional hyponatremia may occur in edematous patients in hot weather; appropriate therapy is water restriction, rather than administration of salt except in rare instances when the hyponatremia is life-threatening. In actual salt depletion, appropriate replacement is the therapy of choice.

Hyperuricemia may occur or frank gout may be precipitated in certain patients receiving thiazide therapy.

In diabetic patients dosage adjustments of insulin or oral hypoglycemic agents may be required. Hyperglycemia may occur with thiazide diuretics. Thus latent diabetes mellitus may become manifest during thiazide therapy.

The antihypertensive effects of the drug may be enhanced in the postsympathectomy patient.

If progressive renal impairment becomes evident consider withholding or discontinuing diuretic therapy.

Thiazides have been shown to increase the urinary excretion of magnesium; this may result in hypomagnesemia.

Thiazides may decrease urinary calcium excretion. Thiazides may cause intermittent and slight elevation of serum calcium in the absence of known disorders of calcium metabolism. Marked hypercalcemia may be evidence of hidden hyperparathyroidism. Thiazides should be discontinued before carrying out tests for parathyroid function.

Increases in cholesterol and triglyceride levels may be associated with thiazide diuretic therapy.

Information for Patients

Angioedema: Angioedema, including laryngeal edema, may occur especially following the first dose of lisinopril. Patients should be so advised and told to report immediately any signs or symptoms suggesting angioedema (swelling of face, extremities, eyes, lips, tongue, difficulty in swallowing or breathing) and to take no more drug until they have consulted with the prescribing physician.

Symptomatic Hypotension: Patients should be cautioned to report lightheadedness especially during the first few days of therapy. If actual syncope occurs, the patients should be told to discontinue the drug until they have consulted with the prescribing physician.

All patients should be cautioned that excessive perspiration and dehydration may lead to an excessive fall in blood pressure because of reduction in fluid volume. Other causes of volume depletion such as vomiting or diarrhea may also lead to a fall in blood pressure; patients should be advised to consult with their physician.

Hyperkalemia: Patients should be told not to use salt substitutes containing potassium without consulting their physician.

Neutropenia: Patients should be told to report promptly any indication of infection (e.g., sore throat, fever) which may be a sign of neutropenia.

Pregnancy: Female patients of childbearing age should be told about the consequences of second- and third-trimester exposure to ACE inhibitors, and they should also be told that these consequences do not appear to have resulted from intrauterine ACE-inhibitor exposure that has been limited to the first trimester. These patients should be asked to report pregnancies to their physicians as soon as possible.

NOTE: As with many other drugs, certain advice to patients being treated with PRINZIDE is warranted. This information is intended to aid in the safe and effective use of this medication. It is not a disclosure of all possible adverse or intended effects.

Drug Interactions

Lisinopril

Hypotension —Patients on Diuretic Therapy: Patients on diuretics, and especially those in whom diuretic therapy was recently instituted, may occasionally experience an excessive reduction of blood pressure after initiation of therapy with lisinopril. The possibility of hypotensive effects with lisinopril can be minimized by either discontinuing the diuretic or increasing the salt intake prior to initiation of treatment with lisinopril. If it is necessary to continue the diuretic, initiate therapy with lisinopril at a dose of 5 mg daily, and provide close medical supervision after the initial dose for at least two hours and until blood pressure has stabilized for at least an additional hour. (See WARNINGS and DOSAGE AND ADMINISTRATION.)

When a diuretic is added to the therapy of a patient receiving lisinopril, an additional antihypertensive effect is usually observed. (See DOSAGE AND ADMINISTRATION.)

Indomethacin: In a study in 36 patients with mild to moderate hypertension where the antihypertensive effects of lisinopril alone were compared to lisinopril given concomitantly with indomethacin, the use of indomethacin was associated with a reduced effect, although the difference between the two regimens was not significant.

Other Agents: Lisinopril has been used concomitantly with nitrates and/or digoxin without evidence of clinically significant adverse interactions. No meaningful clinically important pharmacokinetic interactions occurred when lisinopril was used concomitantly with propranolol, digoxin, or hydrochlorothiazide. The presence of food in the stomach does not alter the bioavailability of lisinopril.

Agents Increasing Serum Potassium: Lisinopril attenuates potassium loss caused by thiazide-type diuretics. Use of lisinopril with potassium-sparing diuretics (e.g., spironolactone, triamterene, or amiloride), potassium supplements, or potassium-containing salt substitutes may lead to significant increases in serum potassium. Therefore, if concomitant use of these agents is indicated, because of demonstrated hypokalemia, they should be used with caution and with frequent monitoring of serum potassium.

Lithium: Lithium toxicity has been reported in patients receiving lithium concomitantly with drugs which cause elimination of sodium, including ACE inhibitors. Lithium toxicity was usually reversible upon discontinuation of lithium and the ACE inhibitor. It is recommended that serum

Continued on next page

Information on the Merck & Co. products listed on these pages is the full prescribing information from product circulars in use October 1, 1992.

Merck & Co.—Cont.

lithium levels be monitored frequently if lisinopril is administered concomitantly with lithium.

Hydrochlorothiazide

When administered concurrently the following drugs may interact with thiazide diuretics.

Alcohol, barbiturates, or narcotics—potentiation of orthostatic hypotension may occur.

Antidiabetic drugs (oral agents and insulin)—dosage adjustment of the antidiabetic drug may be required.

Other antihypertensive drugs—additive effect or potentiation.

Cholestyramine and colestipol resins—Cholestyramine and colestipol resins bind the hydrochlorothiazide and reduce its absorption from the gastrointestinal tract by up to 85 and 43 percent, respectively. Thiazides may be administered two to four hours before the resin when the two drugs are used concomitantly.

Corticosteroids, ACTH—intensified electrolyte depletion, particularly hypokalemia.

Pressor amines (e.g., norepinephrine)—possible decreased response to pressor amines but not sufficient to preclude their use.

Skeletal muscle relaxants, nondepolarizing (e.g., tubocurarine)—possible increased responsiveness to the muscle relaxant.

Lithium—should not generally be given with diuretics. Diuretic agents reduce the renal clearance of lithium and add a high risk of lithium toxicity. Refer to the package insert for lithium preparations before use of such preparations with PRINZIDE.

Non-steroidal Anti-inflammatory Drugs—In some patients, the administration of a non-steroidal anti-inflammatory agent can reduce the diuretic, natriuretic, and antihypertensive effects of loop, potassium-sparing and thiazide diuretics. Therefore, when PRINZIDE and non-steroidal anti-inflammatory agents are used concomitantly, the patient should be observed closely to determine if the desired effect of PRINZIDE is obtained.

Carcinogenesis, Mutagenesis, Impairment of Fertility

Lisinopril-Hydrochlorothiazide

Lisinopril in combination with hydrochlorothiazide was not mutagenic in a microbial mutagen test using *Salmonella typhimurium* (Ames test) or *Escherichia coli* with or without metabolic activation or in a forward mutation assay using Chinese hamster lung cells. Lisinopril-hydrochlorothiazide did not produce DNA single strand breaks in an *in vitro* alkaline elution rat hepatocyte assay. In addition, it did not produce increases in chromosomal aberrations in an *in vitro* test in Chinese hamster ovary cells or in an *in vivo* study in mouse bone marrow.

Lisinopril

There was no evidence of a tumorigenic effect when lisinopril was administered for 105 weeks to male and female rats at doses up to 90 mg/kg/day (about 56 times* the maximum recommended daily human dose). Lisinopril has also been administered for 92 weeks to (male and female) mice at doses up to 135 mg/kg/day (about 84 times* the maximum recommended daily human dose) and showed no evidence of carcinogenicity.

Lisinopril was not mutagenic in the Ames microbial mutagen test with or without metabolic activation. It was also negative in a forward mutation assay using Chinese hamster lung cells. Lisinopril did not produce single strand DNA breaks in an *in vitro* alkaline elution rat hepatocyte assay. In addition, lisinopril did not produce increases in chromosomal aberrations in an *in vitro* test in Chinese hamster ovary cells or in an *in vivo* study in mouse bone marrow.

There were no adverse effects on reproductive performance in male and female rats treated with up to 300 mg/kg/day of lisinopril.

*Based on patient weight of 50 kg

Hydrochlorothiazide

Two-year feeding studies in mice and rats conducted under the auspices of the National Toxicology Program (NTP) uncovered no evidence of a carcinogenic potential of hydrochlorothiazide in female mice (at doses of up to approximately 600 mg/kg/day) or in male and female rats (at doses of up to approximately 100 mg/kg/day). The NTP, however, found equivocal evidence for hepatocarcinogenicity in male mice.

Hydrochlorothiazide was not genotoxic *in vitro* in the Ames mutagenicity assay of *Salmonella typhimurium* strains TA 98, TA 100, TA 1535, TA 1537, and TA 1538 and in the Chinese Hamster Ovary (CHO) test for chromosomal aberrations, or *in vivo* in assays using mouse germinal cell chromosomes, Chinese hamster bone marrow chromosomes, and the *Drosophila* sex-linked recessive lethal trait gene. Positive test results were obtained only in the *in vitro* CHO Sister Chromatid Exchange (clastogenicity) and in the Mouse Lymphoma Cell (mutagenicity) assays, using concentrations of hydrochlorothiazide from 43 to 1300 μg/mL, and in the *Aspergillus nidulans* non-disjunction assay at an unspecified concentration.

Hydrochlorothiazide had no adverse effects on the fertility of mice and rats of either sex in studies wherein these species were exposed, via their diet, to doses of up to 100 and 4 mg/kg, respectively, prior to conception and throughout gestation.

Pregnancy

Pregnancy Categories C (first trimester) *and D* (second and third trimesters). See WARNINGS, *Pregnancy, Lisinopril, Fetal/Neonatal Morbidity and Mortality.*

Nursing Mothers

It is not known whether lisinopril is secreted in human milk. However, milk of lactating rats contains radioactivity following administration of ^{14}C lisinopril. In another study, lisinopril was present in rat milk at levels similar to plasma levels in the dams. Thiazides do appear in human milk. Because of the potential for serious reactions in nursing infants from hydrochlorothiazide and the unknown effects of lisinopril in infants, a decision should be made whether to discontinue nursing or to discontinue PRINZIDE, taking into account the importance of the drug to the mother.

Pediatric Use

Safety and effectiveness in children have not been established.

ADVERSE REACTIONS

PRINZIDE has been evaluated for safety in 930 patients, including 100 patients treated for 50 weeks or more.

In clinical trials with PRINZIDE no adverse experiences peculiar to this combination drug have been observed. Adverse experiences that have occurred have been limited to those that have been previously reported with lisinopril or hydrochlorothiazide.

The most frequent clinical adverse experiences in controlled trials (including open label extensions) with any combination of lisinopril and hydrochlorothiazide were: dizziness (7.5 percent), headache (5.2 percent), cough (3.9 percent), fatigue (3.7 percent) and orthostatic effects (3.2 percent), all of which were more common than in placebo-treated patients. Generally, adverse experiences were mild and transient in nature; but see WARNINGS regarding angioedema and excessive hypotension or syncope. Discontinuation of therapy due to adverse effects was required in 4.4 percent of patients, principally because of dizziness, cough, fatigue and muscle cramps.

Adverse experiences occurring in greater than one percent of patients treated with lisinopril plus hydrochlorothiazide in controlled clinical trials are shown below.

[See table below.]

	Percent of Patients in Controlled Studies: Lisinopril-Hydrochlorothiazide (n=930) Incidence (discontinuation)	Placebo (n=207) Incidence
Dizziness	7.5 (0.8)	1.9
Headache	5.2 (0.3)	1.9
Cough	3.9 (0.6)	1.0
Fatigue	3.7 (0.4)	1.0
Orthostatic Effects	3.2 (0.1)	1.0
Diarrhea	2.5 (0.2)	2.4
Nausea	2.2 (0.1)	2.4
Upper Respiratory Infection	2.2 (0.0)	0.0
Muscle Cramps	2.0 (0.4)	0.5
Asthenia	1.8 (0.2)	1.0
Paresthesia	1.5 (0.1)	0.0
Hypotension	1.4 (0.3)	0.5
Vomiting	1.4 (0.1)	0.5
Dyspepsia	1.3 (0.0)	0.0
Rash	1.2 (0.1)	0.5
Impotence	1.2 (0.3)	0.0

Clinical adverse experiences occurring in 0.3 to 1.0 percent of patients in controlled trials included: *Body as a Whole:* Chest pain, abdominal pain, syncope, chest discomfort, fever, trauma, virus infection. *Cardiovascular:* Palpitation, orthostatic hypotension. *Digestive:* Gastrointestinal cramps, dry mouth, constipation, heartburn. *Musculoskeletal:* Back pain, shoulder pain, knee pain, back strain, myalgia, foot pain. *Nervous/Psychiatric:* Decreased libido, vertigo, depression, somnolence. *Respiratory:* Common cold, nasal congestion, influenza, bronchitis, pharyngeal pain, dyspnea, pulmonary congestion, chronic sinusitis, allergic rhinitis, pharyngeal discomfort. *Skin:* Flushing, pruritus, skin inflammation, diaphoresis. *Special Senses:* Blurred vision, tinnitus, otalgia. *Urogenital:* Urinary tract infection.

Angioedema: Angioedema of the face, extremities, lips, tongue, glottis and/or larynx has been reported rarely. (See WARNINGS.)

Hypotension: In clinical trials, adverse effects relating to hypotension occurred as follows: hypotension (1.4), orthostatic hypotension (0.5), other orthostatic effects (3.2). In addition syncope occurred in 0.8 percent of patients. (See WARNINGS.)

Cough: See PRECAUTIONS, *Cough.*

Clinical Laboratory Test Findings

Serum Electrolytes: See PRECAUTIONS.

Creatinine, Blood Urea Nitrogen: Minor reversible increases in blood urea nitrogen and serum creatinine were observed in patients with essential hypertension treated with PRINZIDE. More marked increases have also been reported and were more likely to occur in patients with renal artery stenosis. (See PRECAUTIONS.)

Serum Uric Acid, Glucose, Magnesium, Cholesterol, Triglycerides and Calcium: See PRECAUTIONS.

Hemoglobin and Hematocrit: Small decreases in hemoglobin and hematocrit (mean decreases of approximately 0.5 g percent and 1.5 vol percent, respectively) occurred frequently in hypertensive patients treated with PRINZIDE but were rarely of clinical importance unless another cause of anemia coexisted. In clinical trials, 0.4 percent of patients discontinued therapy due to anemia.

Other (Causal Relationship Unknown): Rarely, elevations of liver enzymes and/or serum bilirubin have occurred.

Other adverse reactions that have been reported with the individual components are listed below:

Lisinopril—Lisinopril has been evaluated for safety in 2003 patients. In clinical trials adverse reactions which occurred with lisinopril were also seen with PRINZIDE. In addition, and since lisinopril has been marketed, the following adverse reactions have been reported. *Body as a Whole:* Anaphylactoid reactions (see PRECAUTIONS, *Hemodialysis Patients*), malaise; *Cardiovascular:* Myocardial infarction or cerebrovascular accident, possibly secondary to excessive hypotension in high risk patients (see WARNINGS, *Hypotension*); angina pectoris, rhythm disturbances, tachycardia, peripheral edema, vasculitis; *Digestive:* Pancreatitis, hepatitis (hepatocellular or cholestatic jaundice), anorexia, flatulence; *Hematologic:* Rare cases of neutropenia and bone marrow depression have been reported in which a causal relationship to lisinopril cannot be excluded; *Metabolic:* Gout; *Musculoskeletal:* Joint pain; *Nervous System/Psychiatric:* Insomnia, stroke, nervousness, confusion; *Skin:* Urticaria; *Urogenital:* Oliguria, progressive azotemia, acute renal failure.

A symptom complex has been reported which may include a positive ANA, an elevated erythrocyte sedimentation rate, arthralgia/arthritis, myalgia and fever.

Fetal/Neonatal Morbidity and Mortality: See WARNINGS, *Pregnancy, Lisinopril, Fetal/Neonatal Morbidity and Mortality.*

Hydrochlorothiazide—*Body as a Whole:* Weakness; *Digestive:* Anorexia, gastric irritation, cramping, jaundice (intrahepatic cholestatic jaundice), pancreatitis, sialadenitis, constipation; *Hematologic:* Leukopenia, agranulocytosis, thrombocytopenia, aplastic anemia, hemolytic anemia; *Musculoskeletal:* Muscle spasm; *Nervous System/Psychiatric:* Restlessness; *Renal:* Renal failure, renal dysfunction, interstitial nephritis (see WARNINGS); *Skin:* Erythema multiforme including Stevens-Johnson syndrome, exfoliative dermatitis including toxic epidermal necrolysis, alopecia; *Special Senses:* Xanthopsia; *Hypersensitivity:* Purpura, photosensitivity, urticaria, necrotizing angiitis (vasculitis and cutaneous vasculitis), respiratory distress including pneumonitis and pulmonary edema, anaphylactic reactions.

OVERDOSAGE

No specific information is available on the treatment of overdosage with PRINZIDE. Treatment is symptomatic and supportive. Therapy with PRINZIDE should be discontinued and the patient observed closely. Suggested measures in-

clude induction of emesis and/or gastric lavage, and correction of dehydration, electrolyte imbalance and hypotension by established procedures.

Lisinopril

The oral LD_{50} of lisinopril is greater than 20 g/kg in mice and rats. The most likely manifestation of overdosage would be hypotension, for which the usual treatment would be intravenous infusion of normal saline solution.

Lisinopril can be removed by hemodialysis.

Hydrochlorothiazide

The oral LD_{50} of hydrochlorothiazide is greater than 10.0 g/kg in both mice and rats. The most common signs and symptoms observed are those caused by electrolyte depletion (hypokalemia, hypochloremia, hyponatremia) and dehydration resulting from excessive diuresis. If digitalis has also been administered, hypokalemia may accentuate cardiac arrhythmias.

DOSAGE AND ADMINISTRATION

DOSAGE MUST BE INDIVIDUALIZED. THE FIXED COMBINATION IS NOT FOR INITIAL THERAPY. IT MAY BE SUBSTITUTED FOR THE TITRATED INDIVIDUAL COMPONENTS. ALTERNATIVELY, PATIENTS WHO HAVE RECEIVED LISINOPRIL MONOTHERAPY 20 OR 40 MG MAY BE GIVEN 'PRINZIDE' 12.5, THEN 'PRINZIDE' 25, THUS TITRATING THE HYDROCHLOROTHIAZIDE COMPONENT USING THE COMBINATION.

The usual dose is one or two tablets of PRINZIDE 12.5 or PRINZIDE 25 once daily. (See INDICATIONS AND USAGE and WARNINGS.) However, because data from a clinical trial suggest that the mean group antihypertensive response is similar when lisinopril 20 mg is combined with hydrochlorothiazide 12.5 mg or 25 mg, patients whose blood pressure is controlled with lisinopril 20 mg plus hydrochlorothiazide 25 mg ordinarily should be given a trial of PRINZIDE 12.5 before PRINZIDE 25 is used. (See CLINICAL PHARMACOLOGY, *Lisinopril-Hydrochlorothiazide.*)

Patients usually do not require doses in excess of 50 mg of hydrochlorothiazide daily, particularly when it is combined with other antihypertensive agents.

For lisinopril monotherapy the recommended initial dose in patients not on diuretics is 10 mg of lisinopril once a day. Dosage should be adjusted according to blood pressure response. The usual dosage range of lisinopril is 20 to 40 mg administered in a single daily dose; the maximum recommended dose is 80 mg in a single daily dose. Blood pressure should be measured at the interdosing interval to ensure that there is an adequate antihypertensive response at that time. If blood pressure is not controlled with lisinopril alone, a diuretic may be added. Hydrochlorothiazide 12.5 mg has been shown to provide an additive effect. After addition of the diuretic it may be possible to reduce the dose of lisinopril.

In patients who are currently being treated with a diuretic, symptomatic hypotension occasionally may occur following the initial dose of lisinopril. The diuretic should, if possible, be discontinued for two to three days before beginning therapy with lisinopril to reduce the likelihood of hypotension. (See WARNINGS.) If the patient's blood pressure is not controlled with lisinopril alone, diuretic therapy may be resumed.

If the diuretic cannot be discontinued an initial dose of 5 mg of lisinopril should be used under medical supervision for at least two hours and until blood pressure has stabilized for at least an additional hour. (See WARNINGS and PRECAUTIONS, *Drug Interactions.*)

Concomitant administration of PRINZIDE with potassium supplements, potassium salt substitutes, or potassium sparing diuretics may lead to increases of serum potassium (see PRECAUTIONS).

Dosage Adjustment in Renal Impairment

The usual dose of PRINZIDE is recommended for patients with a creatinine clearance > 30 mL/min (serum creatinine of up to approximately 3 mg/dL).

When concomitant diuretic therapy is required in patients with severe renal impairment, a loop diuretic rather than a thiazide diuretic is preferred for use with lisinopril; therefore, for patients with severe renal dysfunction the lisinopril-hydrochlorothiazide combination tablet is not recommended.

HOW SUPPLIED

No. 3594—Tablets PRINZIDE 12.5, are yellow, round, fluted-edge tablets, coded MSD 140 on one side and PRINZIDE on the other. Each tablet contains 20 mg of lisinopril and 12.5 mg of hydrochlorothiazide. They are supplied as follows:

NDC 0006-0140-31 unit of use bottles of 30

NDC 0006-0140-58 unit of use bottles of 100.

Shown in Product Indentification Section, page 420

No. 3595—Tablets PRINZIDE 25, are peach, round, fluted-edge tablets, coded MSD 142 on one side and PRINZIDE on the other. Each tablet contains 20 mg of lisinopril and 25 mg of hydrochlorothiazide. They are supplied as follows:

NDC 0006-0142-31 unit of use bottles of 30

NDC 0006-0142-58 unit of use bottles of 100.

Shown in Product Identification Section, page 420

Storage

Avoid storage at temperatures above 40°C (104°F).

Dispense in a well-closed container, if product package is subdivided.

A.H.F.S. Category: 24:08, 40:28

DC 7615012 Issued May 1992

COPYRIGHT © MERCK & CO., INC., 1989, 1992
All rights reserved

PROSCAR® Tablets ℞
(Finasteride)

DESCRIPTION

PROSCAR* (finasteride), a synthetic 4-azasteroid compound, is a specific inhibitor of steroid 5α-reductase, an intracellular enzyme that converts testosterone into the potent androgen 5α-dihydrotestosterone (DHT).

Finasteride is 4-azaandrost-1-ene-17-carboxamide, *N*-(1,1-dimethylethyl)-3-oxo-,(5α, 17β)-. The empirical formula of finasteride is $C_{23}H_{36}N_2O_2$ and its molecular weight is 372.55. Its structural formula is:

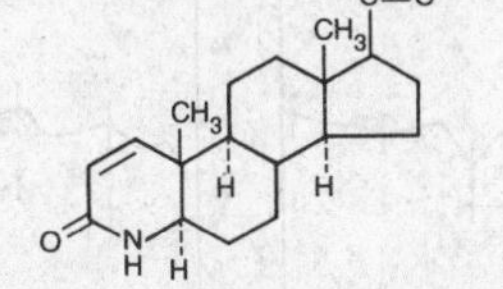

Finasteride is a white crystalline powder with a melting point near 250°C. It is freely soluble in chloroform and in lower alcohol solvents, but is practically insoluble in water.

PROSCAR (finasteride) tablets for oral administration are film-coated tablets that contain 5 mg of finasteride and the following inactive ingredients: docusate sodium, FD&C Blue 2 aluminum lake, hydrous lactose, hydroxypropyl cellulose LF, hydroxypropylmethyl cellulose, magnesium stearate, microcrystalline cellulose, pregelatinized starch, purified water, sodium starch glycolate, talc, titanium dioxide and yellow iron oxide.

*Registered trademark of MERCK & CO., INC.

CLINICAL PHARMACOLOGY

Progressive enlargement of the prostate gland is often associated with urinary symptoms and a decrease in urine flow, although a precise correlation between increased gland size and symptoms has not been demonstrated. Benign prostatic hyperplasia (BPH) produces symptoms in the majority of men over the age of 50 and its prevalence increases with age.

The development of the prostate gland is dependent on the potent androgen, 5α-dihydrotestosterone (DHT). The enzyme 5α-reductase metabolizes testosterone to DHT in the prostate gland, liver and skin. DHT induces androgenic effects by binding to androgen receptors in the cell nuclei of these organs.

Finasteride is a competitive and specific inhibitor of 5α-reductase. This has been demonstrated both *in vivo* and *in vitro*. Finasteride has no affinity for the androgen receptor. In man, the 5α-reduced steroid metabolites in blood and urine are decreased after administration of finasteride.

In man, a single 5-mg oral dose of PROSCAR produces a rapid reduction in serum DHT concentration, with the maximum effect observed 8 hours after the first dose. The suppression of DHT is maintained throughout the 24-hour dosing interval and with continued treatment. Daily dosing of PROSCAR at 5 mg/day for up to 24 months has been shown to reduce the serum DHT concentration by approximately 70%. The median circulating level of testosterone increased by 10% but remained within the physiologic range.

Adult males with genetically inherited 5α-reductase deficiency also have decreased levels of DHT. Except for the associated urogenital defects present at birth, no other clinical abnormalities related to 5α-reductase deficiency have been observed in these individuals. These individuals have a small prostate gland throughout life and do not develop BPH.

In patients with BPH treated with finasteride (1–100 mg/day) for 7–10 days prior to prostatectomy, an approximate 80% lower DHT content was measured in prostatic tissue removed at surgery, compared to placebo; testosterone tissue concentration was increased up to 10 times over pretreatment levels, relative to placebo. Intraprostatic content of prostate-specific antigen (PSA) was also decreased.

In healthy male volunteers treated with PROSCAR for 14 days, discontinuation of therapy resulted in a return of DHT levels to pretreatment levels in approximately 2 weeks.

In patients with BPH, PROSCAR had no effect on circulating levels of cortisol, estradiol, prolactin, thyroid-stimulating hormone, or thyroxine. Nor did it affect the plasma lipid profile (i.e. total cholesterol, low density lipoproteins, high density lipoproteins and triglycerides) of 56 patients receiving PROSCAR for 12 weeks. The effects of long-term administration of PROSCAR on the plasma lipid profile are unknown. Increases of about 10% were observed in luteinizing hormone (LH), follicle-stimulating hormone (FSH) and testosterone levels in patients receiving PROSCAR, but levels remained within the normal range. In healthy volunteers, treatment with PROSCAR did not alter the response of LH and FSH to gonadotropin-releasing hormone, indicating that the hypothalamic-pituitary-testicular axis was not affected.

Pharmacokinetics

Following an oral dose of ^{14}C-finasteride in man, a mean of 39% (range, 32–46%) of the dose was excreted in the urine in the form of metabolites; 57% (range, 51–64%) was excreted in the feces. The major compound isolated from urine was the monocarboxylic acid metabolite; virtually no unchanged drug was recovered. The t-butyl side chain monohydroxylated metabolite has been isolated from plasma. These metabolites possess no more than 20% of the 5α-reductase inhibitory activity of finasteride.

In a study in 15 healthy male subjects, the mean bioavailability of a 5-mg PROSCAR tablet was 63% (range, 34–108%), based on the ratio of AUC relative to a 5-mg intravenous dose infused over 60 minutes. Maximum finasteride plasma concentration averaged 37 ng/mL (range, 27–49 ng/mL) and was reached 1 to 2 hours postdose. The mean plasma half-life of elimination was 6 hours (range, 3–16 hours). Following the intravenous infusion, mean plasma clearance was 165 mL/min (range, 70–279 mL/min) and mean steady-state volume of distribution was 76 liters (range, 44–96 liters). In a separate study, the bioavailability of finasteride was not affected by food.

Approximately 90% of circulating finasteride is bound to plasma proteins. Finasteride has been found to cross the blood-brain barrier.

There is a slow accumulation phase for finasteride after multiple dosing. After dosing with 5 mg/day of finasteride for 17 days, plasma concentrations of finasteride were 47% and 54% higher than after the first dose in men 45–60 years old (n=12) and ≥70 years old (n=12), respectively. Mean trough concentrations after 17 days of dosing were 6.2 ng/mL (range, 2.4–9.8 ng/mL) and 8.1 ng/mL (range, 1.8–19.7 ng/mL), respectively in the two age groups. Although steady state was not reached in this study, mean trough plasma concentration in another study in patients with BPH (mean age, 65 years) receiving 5 mg/day was 9.4 ng/mL (range, 7.1–13.3 ng/mL; n=22) after over a year of dosing.

The elimination rate of finasteride is decreased in the elderly, but no dosage adjustment is necessary. The mean terminal half-life of finasteride in subjects ≥70 years of age was approximately 8 hours (range, 6–15 hours) compared to 6 hours (range, 4–12 hours) in subjects 45–60 years of age. As a result, mean AUC (0–24 hr) after 17 days of dosing was 15% higher in subjects ≥70 years of age (p=0.02).

No dosage adjustment is necessary in patients with renal insufficiency. In patients with chronic renal impairment, with creatinine clearances ranging from 9.0 to 55 mL/min, area under the curve, maximum plasma concentration, half-life, and protein binding after a single dose of ^{14}C-finasteride were similar to values obtained in healthy volunteers. Urinary excretion of metabolites was decreased in patients with renal impairment. This decrease was associated with an increase in fecal excretion of metabolites. Plasma concentrations of metabolites were significantly higher in patients with renal impairment (based on a 60% increase in total radioactivity AUC). However, finasteride has been well tolerated in BPH patients with normal renal function receiving up to 80 mg/day for 12 weeks where exposure of these patients to metabolites would presumably be much greater.

In 16 subjects receiving PROSCAR 5 mg/day, finasteride concentrations in semen ranged from undetectable (<1 ng/mL) to 21 ng/mL. Based on a 5 mL ejaculate volume, the amount of finasteride in ejaculate was estimated to be less than 1/50 of the dose of finasteride (5 micrograms) that had no effect on circulating DHT levels in adults.

Clinical Studies

Twelve-Month Controlled Clinical Trials

In a North American and in an international multicenter, double-blind, placebo-controlled, 12-month study in patients with BPH treated with PROSCAR 5 mg/day, statistically significant regression of the enlarged prostate gland was noted at the first evaluation at 3 months and was maintained during the studies (Table 1). In both studies, the maximum urinary flow rates showed statistically significant increases

Continued on next page

Information on the Merck & Co. products listed on these pages is the full prescribing information from product circulars in use October 1, 1992.

Merck & Co.—Cont.

from baseline in patients treated with PROSCAR from week 2 throughout the 12-month studies. Compared to placebo, statistically significant increases in maximum urinary flow rates were maintained in the North American study from month 4 through 12 in patients treated with PROSCAR. The maximum urinary flow rates in the international study were statistically significantly greater than placebo at months 7, 8, 11 and 12 (Figures 1–3 and Table 2).

TABLE 1
Median % Change in Prostate Volume†
from Baseline

	North American Study		International Study	
	PROSCAR 5 mg (n=297)[a]	Placebo (n=300)[a]	PROSCAR 5 mg (n=246)[a]	Placebo (n=255)[a]
Baseline volume (cc)	52.1	50.0	45.5	41.5
	%	%	%	%
Month 3	−12.1***	−2.4	−19.1***	−6.0
Month 6	−17.4***	−2.8	−21.9***	−5.5
Month 12	−19.2***	−3.0	−24.0***	−6.1

† Prostate volume was measured by magnetic resonance imaging (N. Am.) and ultrasound (Int'l). (Prostate volume was not measured at month 9.)
[a] Enrolled at baseline
*** $p < 0.001$ vs placebo

FIGURE 1
Maximum Urinary Flow Rate†

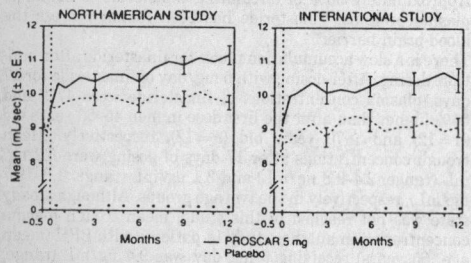

* $p < 0.05$ vs Placebo
† Maximum urinary flow rates (voided volumes ≥ 150 mL) were measured with a non-invasive urinary flow meter.
NOTE: Area of the graph to the left of time 0 is a two-week placebo run-in period.

TABLE 2
Mean Increase in Maximum Urinary Flow Rate
(mL/sec)† from Baseline

	North American Study		International Study	
	PROSCAR 5 mg (n=297)	Placebo (n=300)	PROSCAR 5 mg (n=246)	Placebo (n=255)
Baseline flow rate (mL/sec)	9.6	9.6	9.2	8.6
Week 2	0.5*	−0.2	0.6	0.2
Month 1	0.5	0.2	0.7	0.3
Month 2	0.9*	0.3	1.1	0.6
Month 3	0.8	0.3	0.8	0.2
Month 4	1.0*	0.4	1.0	0.6
Month 5	1.0**	0.2	0.9	0.8
Month 6	0.8*	0.1	1.1	0.7
Month 7	1.2**	0.4	1.3*	0.4
Month 8	1.4***	0.3	1.3*	0.5
Month 9	1.3**	0.3	1.2	0.4
Month 10	1.5***	0.5	1.3	0.7
Month 11	1.4***	0.3	1.5**	0.4
Month 12	1.6***	0.2	1.3*	0.4

† Maximum urinary flow rates (voided volumes ≥ 150 mL) were measured with a non-invasive urinary flow meter.
*,**,*** $p < 0.05$, $p < 0.01$, $p < 0.001$ vs placebo, respectively

Symptomatic improvement was also evaluated in these multicenter studies. Obstructive and total symptom scores were calculated based on patient responses to a validated questionnaire. The obstructive symptoms evaluated were hesitancy, feeling of incomplete bladder emptying, interruption of urinary stream, impairment of size and force of urinary stream and terminal urinary dribbling. The total symptom score also included straining to start urinary flow, dysuria, frequency of clothes wetting and urgency to urinate. On a

FIGURE 2
Mean Increase in Maximum Urinary Flow Rate (mL/sec)†
(Pooled Data)

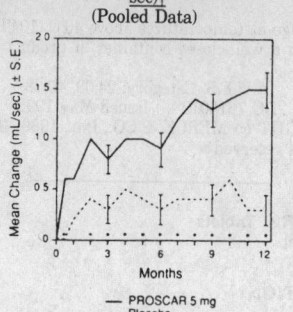

* $p < 0.05$ vs Placebo
† Maximum urinary flow rates (voided volumes ≥ 150 mL) were measured with a non-invasive urinary flow meter.

FIGURE 3
Percent of Patients with a Maximum Urinary Flow Rate Increase ≥ 3 mL/sec

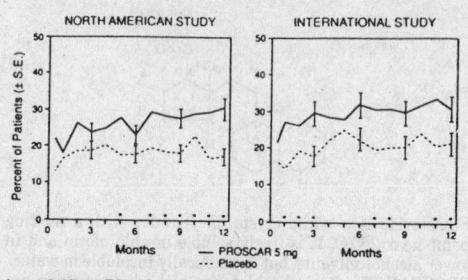

* $p < 0.05$ vs Placebo

scale of 0 (absence of all symptoms) to 36 (worst response for all symptoms), the mean baseline total symptom scores for the North American and international studies were 10.1 and 10.6, respectively.
The mean total symptom scores of patients in the North American and international studies decreased from baseline starting at week 2 of treatment with either PROSCAR or placebo; from week 2 the scores of the patients treated with PROSCAR were numerically lower than those of placebo and remained so throughout the 12-month study. These scores became statistically significantly lower than placebo ($p < 0.05$) starting at month 7 in the international study and at month 10 in the North American study (Figure 4). Similar results were observed with the obstructive symptom scores.

FIGURE 4
Mean Change in Total Symptom Scores
from Baseline

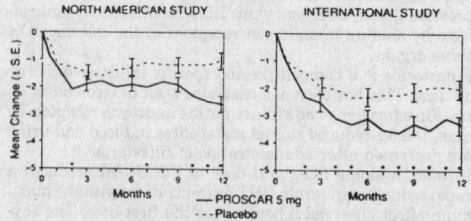

* $p < 0.05$ vs Placebo

Blinded global assessments of overall urinary function and symptoms were performed. Greater improvement in patients treated with PROSCAR as compared to placebo was demonstrated by both the investigator's assessment (N. Am. and Int'l, $p \leq 0.01$) and the patient's own assessment (N. Am., $p \leq 0.01$; Int'l, $p \leq 0.1$).
In both of these 12-month studies, patients treated with PROSCAR 5 mg had progressively decreasing prostate volumes, increasing maximum urinary flow rates and improvement of symptoms associated with BPH, suggesting an arrest in the disease process. Controlled clinical data beyond 12 months are not available.

Long-Term Open Extensions
In long-term uncontrolled extensions of these studies in approximately 300 patients receiving PROSCAR 5 mg/day for 24 months, prostate volume was reduced by a median of 25.5% (baseline, 52.2 cc), maximum flow rate increased by a mean of 2.2 mL/sec (baseline, 11.3 mL/sec) and the total symptom score improved by a mean of 3.4 points (baseline, 9.6 points).

In addition, regression of the enlarged prostate gland and a decrease in PSA levels were maintained in approximately 50 patients who were treated with PROSCAR for 36 months.

INDICATIONS AND USAGE

PROSCAR is indicated for the treatment of symptomatic benign prostatic hyperplasia (BPH). Although there is a rapid regression of the enlarged prostate gland in most treated patients, less than 50% of patients experience an increase in urinary flow and improvement in symptoms of BPH when treated with PROSCAR for 12 months. (See CLINICAL PHARMACOLOGY.)
The long-term effects of PROSCAR on the incidence of surgery, acute urinary obstruction or other complications of BPH are yet to be determined.
A minimum of 6 months treatment may be necessary to determine whether an individual will respond to PROSCAR. It is not possible to identify prospectively those patients who will respond.
Prior to initiating therapy with PROSCAR, appropriate evaluation should be performed to identify other conditions, such as infection, prostate cancer, stricture disease, hypotonic bladder or other neurogenic disorders, that might mimic BPH.

CONTRAINDICATIONS

PROSCAR is contraindicated in the following:
Hypersensitivity to any component of this medication.
Pregnancy. Finasteride is contraindicated in women who are or may become pregnant. Because of the ability of 5α-reductase inhibitors to inhibit the conversion of testosterone to DHT, finasteride may cause abnormalities of the external genitalia of a male fetus of a pregnant woman who receives finasteride. If this drug is used during pregnancy, or if pregnancy occurs while taking this drug, the pregnant woman should be apprised of the potential hazard to the male fetus. (See also WARNINGS, *Exposure of Women—Risk to Male Fetus* and PRECAUTIONS, *Information for Patients* and *Pregnancy.*) In female rats, low doses of finasteride administered during pregnancy have produced abnormalities of the external genitalia in male offspring.

WARNINGS

PROSCAR is not indicated for use in children (see PRECAUTIONS, *Pediatric Use*) or women (see also CLINICAL PHARMACOLOGY, *Pharmacokinetics;* WARNINGS, *Exposure of Women—Risk to Male Fetus;* PRECAUTIONS, *Information for Patients* and *Pregnancy;* and HOW SUPPLIED).
Exposure of Women—Risk to Male Fetus
It is not known whether the amount of finasteride that could potentially be absorbed by a pregnant woman through either direct contact with crushed PROSCAR tablets or from the semen of a patient taking PROSCAR can adversely affect a developing male fetus (see CLINICAL PHARMACOLOGY, *Pharmacokinetics;* CONTRAINDICATIONS; PRECAUTIONS, *Information for Patients* and *Pregnancy;* and HOW SUPPLIED). Therefore, because of the potential risk to a male fetus, a woman who is pregnant or who may become pregnant should not handle crushed PROSCAR tablets; in addition, when the patient's sexual partner is or may become pregnant, the patient should either avoid exposure of his partner to semen or he should discontinue PROSCAR.

PRECAUTIONS

General
Digital rectal examinations, as well as other evaluations for prostate cancer, should be performed on patients with BPH prior to initiating therapy with PROSCAR and periodically thereafter. Although currently not indicated for this purpose, serum PSA is being increasingly used as one of the components of the screening process to detect prostate cancer.[1] Generally, a baseline PSA > 10 ng/mL (Hybritech) prompts further evaluation and consideration of biopsy; for PSA levels between 4 and 10 ng/mL, further evaluation is generally considered advisable. The physician should be aware that a baseline PSA < 4 ng/mL does not exclude the diagnosis of prostate cancer.
PROSCAR causes a decrease in serum PSA levels in patients with BPH even in the presence of prostate cancer (see *Drug/Laboratory Test Interactions*). This reduction of PSA levels should be considered when evaluating PSA laboratory data and does not suggest a beneficial effect of PROSCAR on prostate cancer. In controlled clinical trials PROSCAR did not appear to alter the rate of prostate cancer detection.
Any sustained increases in PSA levels while on PROSCAR should be carefully evaluated, including consideration of non-compliance to therapy with PROSCAR (see *Drug/Laboratory Test Interactions*).
Since not all patients demonstrate a response to PROSCAR, patients with a large residual urinary volume and/or severely diminished urinary flow should be carefully moni-

tored for obstructive uropathy. These patients may not be candidates for this therapy.
Caution should be used in the administration of PROSCAR in those patients with liver function abnormalities, as finasteride is metabolized extensively in the liver.

[1] Catalona, W.J.; Smith, D.S.; Ratliff, T.I.; Dodds, K.M.; Coplen, M.D.; Yuan, J.J.J.; Petros, J.A.; Andriole, G.L.: Measurement of prostate-specific antigen in serum as a screening test for prostate cancer, N.Eng.J.Med. *324*(17): 1156–1161, April 25, 1991.

Information for Patients
Crushed PROSCAR tablets should not be handled by a woman who is pregnant or who may become pregnant because of the potential for absorption of finasteride and the subsequent potential risk to the male fetus. Similarly, when the patient's sexual partner is or may become pregnant, the patient should either avoid exposure of his partner to semen or he should discontinue PROSCAR (see CLINICAL PHARMACOLOGY, *Pharmacokinetics;* CONTRAINDICATIONS; WARNINGS, *Exposure of Women—Risk to Male Fetus;* PRECAUTIONS, *Pregnancy;* and HOW SUPPLIED).
Physicians should inform patients that the volume of ejaculate may be decreased in some patients during treatment with PROSCAR. This decrease does not appear to interfere with normal sexual function. However, impotence and decreased libido may occur in patients treated with PROSCAR (see ADVERSE REACTIONS, *Twelve-Month Controlled Clinical Trials).*
Drug/Laboratory Test Interactions
When PSA laboratory determinations are evaluated, consideration should be given to the fact that PSA levels are decreased in patients treated with PROSCAR. In controlled clinical trials in patients with BPH treated with PROSCAR, PSA levels decreased from baseline by a median of 41% (95% confidence interval of the median: 38–45%) at month 6 and by a median of 48% (95% confidence interval of the median: 45–52%) at month 12.
Drug Interactions
Antipyrine: Antipyrine is used as a model for drugs that are metabolized by the same isoenzymatic cytochrome P450 system. In 12 subjects receiving PROSCAR 10 mg/day for 28 days, PROSCAR had no effect on the pharmacokinetic parameters of antipyrine or its metabolites.
Propranolol: In 19 normal volunteers receiving PROSCAR 5 mg/day for 10 days, PROSCAR did not affect the beta-adrenergic blocking activity or plasma concentrations of propranolol enantiomers after a single dose of propranolol.
Digoxin: In 17 normal volunteers receiving PROSCAR 5 mg/day for 10 days, concomitant administration of multiple doses of PROSCAR and a single dose of digoxin resulted in no effect on plasma concentrations of digoxin and its immunoreactive metabolites.
Theophylline: In 12 normal volunteers receiving PROSCAR 5 mg/day for 8 days, PROSCAR significantly increased theophylline clearance by 7% and decreased its half-life by 10% after intravenous administration of aminophylline. These changes were not clinically significant.
Warfarin: In 12 patients chronically treated with warfarin, the prothrombin times and plasma concentrations of warfarin enantiomers were not altered after treatment with PROSCAR 5 mg/day for 14 days.
Other Concomitant Therapy: Although specific interaction studies were not performed, PROSCAR was concomitantly used in clinical studies with α-blockers, angiotensin-converting enzyme (ACE) inhibitors, analgesics, anti-convulsants, beta-adrenergic blocking agents, diuretics, calcium channel blockers, cardiac nitrates, HMG-CoA reductase inhibitors, nonsteroidal anti-inflammatory drugs (NSAIDs), benzodiazepines, H_2 antagonists and quinolone antiinfectives without evidence of clinically significant adverse interactions.
Carcinogenesis, Mutagenesis, Impairment of Fertility
No evidence of a tumorigenic effect was observed in a 24-month study in Sprague-Dawley rats receiving doses of finasteride up to 160 mg/kg/day in males and 320 mg/kg/day in females. These doses produced respective systemic exposure in rats of 111 and 274 times those observed in man receiving the recommended human dose of 5 mg/day. All exposure calculations were based on calculated AUC(0–24hr) for animals and mean AUC(0–24hr) for man (0.4 μg·hr/mL).
In a 19-month carcinogenicity study in CD-1 mice, a statistically significant ($p \leq 0.05$) increase in the incidence of testicular Leydig cell adenomas was observed at a dose of 250 mg/kg/day (228 times the human exposure). In mice at a dose of 25 mg/kg/day (23 times the human exposure, estimated) and in rats at a dose of ≥40 mg/kg/day (39 times the human exposure) an increase in the incidence of Leydig cell hyperplasia was observed. A positive correlation between the proliferative changes in the Leydig cells and an increase in serum LH levels (2–3 fold above control) has been demonstrated in both rodent species treated with high doses of finasteride. No drug-related Leydig cell changes were seen in either rats or dogs treated with finasteride for 1 year at doses of 20 mg/kg/day and 45 mg/kg/day (30 and 350 times, respectively, the human exposure) or in mice treated for 19 months at a dose of 2.5 mg/kg/day (2.3 times the human exposure, estimated).
No evidence of mutagenicity was observed in an *in vitro* bacterial mutagenesis assay, a mammalian cell mutagenesis assay, or in an *in vitro* alkaline elution assay. In an *in vitro* chromosome aberration assay, when Chinese hamster ovary cells were treated with high concentrations (450–550 μmol) of finasteride, there was a slight increase in chromosome aberrations. These concentrations correspond to 4000–5000 times the peak plasma levels in man given a total dose of 5 mg. Further, the concentrations (450–550 μmol) used in *in vitro* studies are not achievable in a biological system. In an *in vivo* chromosome aberration assay in mice, no treatment-related increase in chromosome aberration was observed with finasteride at the maximum tolerated dose of 250 mg/kg/day (228 times the human exposure) as determined in the carcinogenicity studies.
In sexually mature male rabbits treated with finasteride at 80 mg/kg/day (543 times the human exposure) for up to 12 weeks, no effect on fertility, sperm count, or ejaculate volume was seen. In sexually mature male rats treated with 80 mg/kg/day of finasteride (61 times the human exposure), there were no significant effects on fertility after 6 or 12 weeks of treatment; however, when treatment was continued for up to 24 or 30 weeks, there was an apparent decrease in fertility, fecundity and an associated significant decrease in the weights of the seminal vesicles and prostate. All these effects were reversible within 6 weeks of discontinuation of treatment. No drug-related effect on testes or on mating performance has been seen in rats or rabbits. This decrease in fertility in finasteride-treated rats is secondary to its effect on accessory sex organs (prostate and seminal vesicles) resulting in failure to form a seminal plug. The seminal plug is essential for normal fertility in rats and is not relevant in man.
Pregnancy
Pregnancy Category X
See CONTRAINDICATIONS.
PROSCAR is not indicated for use in women.
Administration of finasteride to pregnant rats at doses ranging from 100 μg/kg/day to 100 mg/kg/day (1–1000 times the recommended human dose) resulted in dose-dependent development of hypospadias in 3.6 to 100% of male offspring. Pregnant rats produced male offspring with decreased prostatic and seminal vesicular weights, delayed preputial separation and transient nipple development when given finasteride at ≥30 μg/kg/day (≥3/10 of the recommended human dose) and decreased anogenital distance when given finasteride at ≥3 μg/kg/day (≥3/100 of the recommended human dose). The critical period during which these effects can be induced in male rats has been defined to be days 16–17 of gestation. The changes described above are expected pharmacological effects of drugs belonging to the class of 5α-reductase inhibitors and are similar to those reported in male infants with a genetic deficiency of 5α-reductase. No abnormalities were observed in female offspring exposed to any dose of finasteride *in utero.*
No developmental abnormalities have been observed in first filial generation (F_1) male or female offspring resulting from mating finasteride-treated male rats (80 mg/kg/day; 61 times the human exposure) with untreated females. Administration of finasteride at 3 mg/kg/day (30 times the recommended human dose) during the late gestation and lactation period resulted in slightly decreased fertility in F_1 male offspring. No effects were seen in female offspring. No evidence of malformations has been observed in rabbit fetuses exposed to finasteride *in utero* from days 6–18 of gestation at doses up to 100 mg/kg/day (1000 times the recommended human dose). However, effects on male genitalia would not be expected since the rabbits were not exposed during the critical period of genital system development.
Nursing Mothers
PROSCAR is not indicated for use in women.
It is not known whether finasteride is excreted in human milk.
Pediatric Use
PROSCAR is not indicated for use in children.
Safety and effectiveness in children have not been established.

ADVERSE REACTIONS

PROSCAR is generally well tolerated; adverse reactions usually have been mild and transient.
Twelve-Month Controlled Clinical Trials
In North American and international clinical trials, 543 patients were treated with 5 mg of PROSCAR for 12 months. Seven of these patients (1.3%) were discontinued due to adverse experiences that were considered to be possibly, probably or definitely drug-related; only 1 of these patients (0.2%) discontinued therapy with PROSCAR because of a sexual adverse experience.
The following clinical adverse reactions were reported as possibly, probably or definitely drug-related in ≥1% of patients treated for 12 months with 5 mg/day of PROSCAR or placebo, respectively: impotence (3.7%, 1.1%), decreased libido (3.3%, 1.6%), decreased volume of ejaculate (2.8%, 0.9%).
The adverse experience profile for an additional 547 patients treated with 1 mg/day of PROSCAR for 12 months was similar to that observed in patients treated for 12 months with 5 mg/day of PROSCAR.
Long-Term Open Extensions
The adverse experience profile for approximately 300 patients who were maintained on PROSCAR 5 mg/day for 24 months was similar to that observed in the controlled studies. In addition, a similar safety profile was observed in 50 patients treated with PROSCAR 5 mg/day for 36 months.

OVERDOSAGE

Patients have received single doses of PROSCAR up to 400 mg and multiple doses of PROSCAR up to 80 mg/day for three months without adverse effects. Until further experience is obtained, no specific treatment for an overdose with PROSCAR can be recommended.
Significant lethality was observed in male and female mice at single oral doses of 1500 mg/m^2 (500 mg/kg) and in female and male rats at single oral doses of 2360 mg/m^2 (400 mg/kg) and 5900 mg/m^2 (1000 mg/kg), respectively.

DOSAGE AND ADMINISTRATION

The recommended dose is 5 mg once a day.
Although early improvement may be seen, at least 6–12 months of therapy with PROSCAR may be necessary in some patients to assess whether a beneficial response has been achieved. Periodic follow-up evaluations should be performed to determine whether a clinical response has occurred.
PROSCAR may be administered with or without meals.
No dosage adjustment is necessary for patients with renal impairment or for the elderly (see CLINICAL PHARMACOLOGY, *Pharmacokinetics*).

HOW SUPPLIED

No. 3094—PROSCAR tablets 5 mg are blue, modified apple-shaped, film-coated tablets, with the code MSD 72 on one side and PROSCAR on the other. They are supplied as follows:
NDC 0006-0072-31 unit of use bottles of 30
NDC 0006-0072-58 unit of use bottles of 100
NDC 0006-0072-28 unit dose packages of 100.
Shown in Product Identification Section, page 420
Storage and Handling
Store at room temperatures below 30°C (86°F). Protect from light and keep container tightly closed.
If the film coating of PROSCAR tablets has been broken (e.g., crushed), the tablets should not be handled by a woman who is pregnant or who may become pregnant because of the potential for absorption of finasteride and the subsequent potential risk to a male fetus (see CLINICAL PHARMACOLOGY, *Pharmacokinetics;* WARNINGS, *Exposure of Women—Risk to Male Fetus;* and PRECAUTIONS, *Information for Patients* and *Pregnancy*).
Distributed by:
MERCK SHARP & DOHME
DIV OF MERCK & CO., INC.,
WEST POINT, PA 19486, USA
Manufactured by:
MERCK SHARP & DOHME Ltd.
Hoddesdon, Herts, U.K.
EN11 9BU
DC 7735800 Issued May 1992
COPYRIGHT © MERCK & CO., INC., 1992
All rights reserved.

RECOMBIVAX HB® ℞

[Hepatitis B Vaccine (Recombinant), MSD]

DESCRIPTION

RECOMBIVAX HB* [Hepatitis B Vaccine (Recombinant), MSD] is a non-infectious subunit viral vaccine derived from Hepatitis B surface antigen (HBsAg) produced in yeast cells. A portion of the hepatitis B virus gene, coding for HBsAg, is cloned into yeast, and the vaccine for hepatitis B is produced from cultures of this recombinant yeast strain according to methods developed in the Merck Sharp & Dohme Research Laboratories.

Continued on next page

Information on the Merck & Co. products listed on these pages is the full prescribing information from product circulars in use October 1, 1992.

Merck & Co.—Cont.

The antigen is harvested and purified from fermentation cultures of a recombinant strain of the yeast *Saccharomyces cerevisiae* containing the gene for the *adw* subtype of HBsAg. The HBsAg protein is released from the yeast cells by cell disruption and purified by a series of physical and chemical methods. The vaccine contains no detectable yeast DNA but may contain not more than 1% yeast protein. The vaccine produced by the Merck method has been shown to be comparable to the plasma-derived vaccine in terms of animal potency (mouse, monkey, and chimpanzee) and protective efficacy (chimpanzee and human).

The vaccine against hepatitis B, prepared from recombinant yeast cultures, is free of association with human blood or blood products.

Each lot of hepatitis B vaccine is tested for safety, in mice and guinea pigs, and for sterility.

RECOMBIVAX HB is a sterile suspension for intramuscular injection. However, for persons at risk of hemorrhage following intramuscular injection, the vaccine may be administered subcutaneously. (See DOSAGE AND ADMINISTRATION).

Hepatitis B Vaccine (Recombinant), MSD, is supplied in two dosage strengths.

RECOMBIVAX HB [Hepatitis B Vaccine (Recombinant), MSD] contains 10 mcg of HBsAg/mL. Each 1 mL dose of RECOMBIVAX HB contains 10 mcg of hepatitis B surface antigen adsorbed onto approximately 0.5 mg of aluminum provided as aluminum hydroxide; each 0.5 mL dose contains 5 mcg of hepatitis B surface antigen adsorbed onto approximately 0.25 mg of aluminum provided as aluminum hydroxide; and each 0.25 mL dose contains 2.5 mcg of hepatitis B surface antigen adsorbed onto approximately 0.125 mg of aluminum provided as aluminum hydroxide.

RECOMBIVAX HB [Hepatitis B Vaccine (Recombinant), MSD] Dialysis Formulation is a sterile suspension for intramuscular injection. RECOMBIVAX HB Dialysis Formulation contains 40 mcg of HBsAg/mL. Each 1 mL dose of RECOMBIVAX HB Dialysis Formulation contains 40 mcg of hepatitis B surface antigen adsorbed onto approximately 0.5 mg of aluminum provided as aluminum hydroxide.

Both dosage strengths contain thimerosal (mercury derivative) 1:20,000 added as a preservative and have been treated with formaldehyde prior to adsorption onto aluminum hydroxide. The vaccine is of the *adw* subtype. RECOMBIVAX HB is indicated for vaccination of persons at risk of infection from hepatitis B virus including all known subtypes. RECOMBIVAX HB Dialysis Formulation is indicated for vaccination of adult predialysis and dialysis patients against infection caused by all known subtypes of hepatitis B virus.

---

*Registered trademark of MERCK & CO., INC.

CLINICAL PHARMACOLOGY

Hepatitis B virus is one of at least three hepatitis viruses that cause a systemic infection, with a major pathology in the liver. The others are hepatitis A virus, and non-A, non-B hepatitis viruses.

Hepatitis B virus is an important cause of viral hepatitis. There is no specific treatment for this disease. The incubation period for hepatitis B is relatively long; six weeks to six months may elapse between exposure and the onset of clinical symptoms. The prognosis following infection with hepatitis B virus is variable and dependent on at least three factors: (1) Age—Infants and younger children usually experience milder initial disease than older persons; (2) Dose of virus—The higher the dose, the more likely acute icteric hepatitis B will result; and, (3) Severity of associated underlying disease—underlying malignancy or pre-existing hepatic disease predisposes to increased mortality and morbidity.

Persistence of viral infection (the chronic hepatitis B virus carrier state) occurs in 5–10% of persons following acute hepatitis B, and occurs more frequently after initial anicteric hepatitis B than after initial icteric disease. Consequently, carriers of hepatitis B surface antigen (HBsAg) frequently give no history of having had recognized acute hepatitis. It has been estimated that more than 170 million people in the world today are persistently infected with hepatitis B virus. The Centers for Disease Control (CDC) estimates that there are approximately 0.75 to 1 million chronic carriers of hepatitis B virus in the USA. Chronic carriers represent the largest human reservoir of hepatitis B virus.

The serious complications and sequelae of hepatitis B virus infection include massive hepatic necrosis, cirrhosis of the liver, chronic active hepatitis, and hepatocellular carcinoma. Chronic carriers of HBsAg appear to be at increased risk of developing hepatocellular carcinoma. Although a number of etiologic factors are associated with development of hepatocellular carcinoma, the single most important etiologic factor appears to be active infection with the hepatitis B virus.

There is also evidence that several diseases other than hepatitis have been associated with hepatitis B virus infection through an immunologic mechanism involving antigen-antibody complexes. Such diseases include a syndrome with rash, urticaria, and arthralgia resembling serum sickness; periarteritis nodosa; membranous glomerulonephritis; and infantile papular acrodermatitis.

Although the vehicles for transmission of the virus are often blood and blood products, viral antigen has also been found in tears, saliva, breast milk, urine, semen and vaginal secretions. Hepatitis B virus is capable of surviving for days on environmental surfaces exposed to body fluids containing hepatitis B virus. Infection may occur when hepatitis B virus, transmitted by infected body fluids, is implanted via mucous surfaces or percutaneously introduced through accidental or deliberate breaks in the skin.

Transmission of hepatitis B virus infection is often associated with close interpersonal contact with an infected individual and with crowded living conditions. In such circumstances, transmission by inoculation via routes other than overt percutaneous ones may be quite common. Perinatal transmission of hepatitis B infection from infected mother to child, at or shortly after birth, can occur if the mother is a hepatitis B surface antigen (HBsAg) carrier or if the mother has an acute hepatitis B infection in the third trimester. Infection in infancy by the hepatitis B virus usually leads to the chronic carrier state. Among infants born to women whose sera are positive for both the hepatitis B surface antigen and the e antigen, 85–90% are infected and become chronic carriers. Well-controlled studies have shown that administration of three 0.5 mL doses of Hepatitis B Immune Globulin (Human) starting at birth is 75% effective in preventing establishment of the chronic carrier state in these infants during the first year of life. However, the protective effect of Hepatitis B Immune Globulin (Human) is transient.

Hepatitis B is endemic throughout the world and is a serious medical problem in population groups at increased risk. (Refer to INDICATIONS AND USAGE.)

Numerous epidemiological studies have shown that persons who develop anti-HBs following active infection with the hepatitis B virus are protected against the disease on reexposure to the virus.

Clinical studies have established that RECOMBIVAX HB when injected into the deltoid muscle induced protective levels of antibody in 96% of 1213 healthy adults who received the recommended 3-dose regimen. Antibody responses varied with age; a protective level of antibody was induced in 98% of 787 young adults 20–29 years of age, 94% of 249 adults 30–39 years of age and in 89% of 177 adults ≥ 40 years of age. Studies with hepatitis B vaccine derived from plasma have shown that a lower response rate (81%) to vaccine may be obtained if the vaccine is administered as a buttock injection. Seroconversion rates and geometric mean antibody titers were measured 1 to 2 months after the 3rd dose. A protective antibody (anti-HBs) level has been defined as 1) 10 or more sample ratio units (SRU) as determined by radioimmunoassay or 2) a positive result as determined by enzyme immunoassay. Note: 10 SRU is comparable to 10 mIU/mL of antibody.

RECOMBIVAX HB is highly immunogenic in younger individuals. In clinical studies, 99% of 94 infants under 1 year of age born of non-carrier mothers, 96% of 48 children 1–10 years of age, and 99% of 112 children and adolescents 11–19 years of age developed a protective level of antibody following the recommended 3-dose regimen of vaccine (see DOSAGE AND ADMINISTRATION).

The protective efficacy of three 5 mcg doses of RECOMBIVAX HB has been demonstrated in neonates born of mothers positive for both HBsAg and HBeAg (a core-associated antigenic complex which correlates with high infectivity). In a clinical study of infants who received one dose of Hepatitis B Immune Globulin at birth followed by the recommended three dose regimen of RECOMBIVAX HB, chronic infection had not occurred in 96% of 130 infants after nine months of follow-up. The estimated efficacy in prevention of chronic hepatitis B infection was 95% as compared to the infection rate in untreated historical controls. Significantly fewer neonates became chronically infected when given one dose of Hepatitis B Immune Globulin at birth followed by the recommended three dose regimen of RECOMBIVAX HB when compared to historical controls who received only a single dose of Hepatitis B Immune Globulin. Testing for HBsAg and anti-HBs is recommended at 12–15 months of age. If HBsAg is not detectable, and anti-HBs is present, the child has been protected.

As demonstrated in the above study, Hepatitis B Immune Globulin, when administered simultaneously with RECOMBIVAX HB at separate body sites, did not interfere with the induction of protective antibodies against hepatitis B virus elicited by the vaccine.

Predialysis and Dialysis Patients

Predialysis and dialysis adult patients respond less well to hepatitis B vaccines than do healthy individuals. In addition, the responses to these vaccines may be lower if the vaccine is administered as a buttock injection. When 40 mcg of Hepatitis B Vaccine (Recombinant), MSD, was administered in the deltoid muscle, 89% of 28 participants developed anti-HBs with 86% achieving levels ≥ 10 mIU/mL. However, when the same dosage of this vaccine was administered inappropriately either in the buttock or a combination of buttock and deltoid, 62% of 47 participants developed anti-HBs with 55% achieving levels of ≥ 10 mIU/mL.

The duration of protective effect of RECOMBIVAX HB is unknown at present, and the need for booster doses is not yet defined. However, a booster dose or revaccination with RECOMBIVAX HB Dialysis Formulation may be considered in predialysis/dialysis patients if the anti-HBs level is less than 10 mIU/mL 1 to 2 months after the 3rd dose.

Reports in the literature describe a more virulent form of hepatitis B associated with superinfections or coinfections by delta virus, an imcomplete RNA virus. Delta virus can only infect and cause illness in persons infected with hepatitis B virus since the delta agent requires a coat of HBsAg in order to become infectious. Therefore, persons immune to hepatitis B virus infection should also be immune to delta virus infection.

Interchangeability of Plasma-Derived and Recombinant Hepatitis B Vaccines

Recombinant-derived vaccine is produced in yeast by the hepatitis B virus gene which codes for the hepatitis B surface antigen (HBsAg). Like plasma-derived vaccine, recombinant-derived vaccine is a protein aggregate or particle visible by electron microscopy containing important vaccine antigen epitopes as determined by monoclonal antibody analyses.

Recombinant-derived vaccine has been shown by *in vitro* analyses to induce antibodies (anti-HBs) which are biochemically and immunologically comparable by extent of binding, and both avidity and affinity of binding to virus-derived antigen, to antibodies induced by plasma-derived vaccine. In cross absorption studies, the spectra of antibodies induced in man to plasma-derived or to recombinant hepatitis B vaccines were indistinguishable.

The recommended doses of HEPTAVAX-B* (Hepatitis B Vaccine, MSD) and RECOMBIVAX HB have resulted in similar seroconversion rates in healthy persons; the geometric mean titers (GMTs) following RECOMBIVAX HB have been lower in some studies and equivalent in others but were many times greater than the minimum level associated with protection (≥ 10 mIU/mL). A single injection of the recommended dose of RECOMBIVAX HB induced significant anamnestic antibody responses in 97% of 31 healthy adults vaccinated 5 to 7 years previously with HEPTAVAX-B (Hepatitis B Vaccine, MSD).

There have been no clinical studies in which a three-dose vaccine series was initiated with HEPTAVAX-B (Hepatitis B Vaccine, MSD) and completed with RECOMBIVAX HB, or vice versa. However, based on the comparability of the plasma-derived and recombinant-derived vaccines in extensive *in vitro* and *in vivo* studies as described above, it is possible to interchange the use of these two vaccines (but see CONTRAINDICATIONS).

---

*Registered trademark of MERCK & CO., INC.

INDICATIONS AND USAGE

RECOMBIVAX HB is indicated for vaccination against infection caused by all known subtypes of hepatitis B virus. **RECOMBIVAX HB Dialysis Formulation** is indicated for vaccination of adult predialysis and dialysis patients against infection caused by all known subtypes of hepatitis B virus.

Vaccination with RECOMBIVAX HB is recommended in persons of all ages, who are or will be at increased risk of infection with hepatitis B virus. In areas with high prevalence of infection, most of the population are at risk of acquiring hepatitis B infection at a young age. Therefore, vaccination should be targeted to prevent such transmission. In areas of low prevalence, vaccination should be limited to those who are in groups identified as being at increased risk of infection, for example:

- *Health Care Personnel*
  - Dentists and oral surgeons.
  - Physicians and surgeons.
  - Nurses.
  - Paramedical personnel and custodial staff who may be exposed to the virus via blood or other patient specimens.
  - Dental hygienists and dental nurses.
  - Laboratory personnel handling blood, blood products, and other patient specimens.
  - Dental, medical and nursing students.
- *Selected Patients and Patient Contacts*
  - Staff in hemodialysis units and hematology/oncology units.
  - Patients requiring frequent and/or large volume blood tranfusions or clotting factor concentrates (e.g., persons with hemophilia, thalassemia).
  - Clients (residents) and staff of institutions for the mentally handicapped.

Classroom contacts of deinstitutionalized mentally handicapped persons who have persistent hepatitis B surface antigenemia and who show aggressive behavior.

Household and other intimate contacts of persons with persistent hepatitis B surface antigenemia.

- *Infants Born to HBsAg Positive Mothers whether HBeAg positive or negative (See DOSAGE AND ADMINISTRATION)*
- *Sub-populations with a known high incidence of the disease,* such as:
  Alaskan Eskimos.
  Indochinese refugees.
  Haitian refugees.
- *Military Personnel identified as being at increased risk*
- *Morticians and Embalmers*
- *Blood bank and plasma fractionation workers*
- *Persons at Increased Risk of the Disease Due to Their Sexual Practices,* such as:
  Persons who have heterosexual activity with multiple partners.
  Persons who repeatedly contract sexually transmitted diseases.
  Homosexually active males.
  Female prostitutes.
- *Prisoners*
- *Users of illicit injectable drugs*

Neither dosage strength will prevent hepatitis caused by other agents, such as hepatitis A virus, non-A, non-B hepatitis viruses, or other viruses known to infect the liver.
Revaccination
See CLINICAL PHARMACOLOGY

CONTRAINDICATIONS

Hypersensitivity to yeast or any component of the vaccine.

WARNINGS

Patients who develop symptoms suggestive of hypersensitivity after an injection should not receive further injections of the vaccine (see CONTRAINDICATIONS).

Because of the long incubation period for hepatitis B, it is possible for unrecognized infection to be present at the time the vaccine is given. The vaccine may not prevent hepatitis B in such patients.

PRECAUTIONS

General
As with any percutaneous vaccine, epinephrine should be available for immediate use should an anaphylactoid reaction occur.

Any serious active infection is reason for delaying use of the vaccine except when in the opinion of the physician, withholding the vaccine entails a greater risk.

Caution and appropriate care should be exercised in administering the vaccine to individuals with severely compromised cardiopulmonary status or to others in whom a febrile or systemic reaction could pose a significant risk.

Pregnancy
Pregnancy Category C: Animal reproduction studies have not been conducted with the vaccine. It is also not known whether the vaccine can cause fetal harm when administered to a pregnant woman or can affect reproduction capacity. The vaccine should be given to a pregnant woman only if clearly needed.

Nursing Mothers
It is not known whether the vaccine is excreted in human milk. Because many drugs are excreted in human milk, cautions should be exercised when the vaccine is administered to a nursing woman.

Pediatric Use
RECOMBIVAX HB has been shown to be usually well-tolerated and highly immunogenic in infants and children of all ages. Newborns also respond well; maternally transferred antibodies do not interfere with the active immune response to the vaccine. See DOSAGE AND ADMINISTRATION for recommended pediatric dosage and for recommended dosage for infants born to HBsAg positive mothers.

The safety and effectiveness of RECOMBIVAX HB Dialysis Formulation in children have not been established.

ADVERSE REACTIONS

RECOMBIVAX HB and RECOMBIVAX HB Dialysis Formulation are generally well-tolerated. No serious adverse reactions attributable to the vaccine have been reported during the course of clinical trials. No adverse experiences were reported during clinical trials which could be related to changes in the titers of antibodies to yeast. As with any vaccine, there is the possibility that broad use of the vaccine could reveal adverse reactions not observed in clinical trials. In a group of studies, 3258 doses of RECOMBIVAX HB were administered to 1252 healthy adults who were monitored for 5 days after each dose. Injection site and systemic complaints were reported following 17% and 15% of the injections, respectively. The following adverse reactions were reported:

*Incidence Equal to or
Greater Than 1% of Injections*
LOCAL REACTION (INJECTION SITE)
Injection site reactions consisting principally of soreness, and including pain, tenderness, pruritus, erythema, ecchymosis, swelling, warmth, and nodule formation.
BODY AS A WHOLE
The most frequent systemic complaints include fatigue/weakness; headache; fever (≥ 100°F); and malaise.
DIGESTIVE SYSTEM
Nausea; and diarrhea
RESPIRATORY SYSTEM
Pharyngitis; and upper respiratory infection
Incidence Less than 1% of Injections
BODY AS A WHOLE
Sweating; achiness; sensation of warmth; lightheadedness; chills; and flushing
DIGESTIVE SYSTEM
Vomiting; abdominal pains/cramps; dyspepsia; and diminished appetite
RESPIRATORY SYSTEM
Rhinitis; influenza; and cough
NERVOUS SYSTEM
Vertigo/dizziness; and paresthesia
INTEGUMENTARY SYSTEM
Pruritus; rash (non-specified); angioedema; and urticaria
MUSCULOSKELETAL SYSTEM
Arthralgia including monoarticular; myalgia; back pain; neck pain; shoulder pain; and neck stiffness
HEMIC/LYMPHATIC SYSTEM
Lymphadenopathy
PSYCHIATRIC/BEHAVIORAL
Insomnia/Disturbed sleep
SPECIAL SENSES
Earache
UROGENITAL SYSTEM
Dysuria
CARDIOVASCULAR SYSTEM
Hypotension
The following additional adverse reactions have been reported with use of the marketed vaccine. In many instances, the relationship to the vaccine was unclear.
Hypersensitivity
Anaphylaxis and symptoms of immediate hypersensitivity reactions including rash, pruritus, urticaria, edema, angioedema, dyspnea, chest discomfort, bronchial spasm, palpitation, or symptoms consistent with a hypotensive episode have been reported within the first few hours after vaccination. An apparent hypersensitivity syndrome (serum-sickness-like) of delayed onset has been reported days to weeks after vaccination, including: arthralgia/arthritis (usually transient), fever, and dermatologic reactions such as urticaria, erythema multiforme, ecchymoses and erythema nodosum (See WARNINGS and PRECAUTIONS).
Digestive System
Elevation of liver enzymes; constipation.
Nervous System
Peripheral neuropathy including Bell's Palsy; muscle weakness; Guillain-Barré syndrome; radiculopathy; herpes zoster; hypesthesia; migraine.
Integumentary System
Stevens-Johnson Syndrome; petechiae.
Hematologic
Increased erythrocyte sedimentation rate.
Psychiatric/Behavioral
Irritability; agitation; somnolence.
Special Senses
Optic neuritis; tinnitus; conjunctivitis.
Cardiovascular System
Syncope; tachycardia.
Potential ADVERSE EFFECTS:
In addition, a variety of adverse effects, not observed in clinical trials with RECOMBIVAX HB or RECOMBIVAX HB Dialysis Formulation have been reported with HEPTAVAX-B (plasma-derived hepatitis B vaccine). Those listed below are to serve as alerting information to physicians:
Nervous System: Neurological disorders such as myelitis including transverse myelitis.
Hematologic
Thrombocytopenia
Special Senses
Visual disturbances
The following adverse reaction has been reported with another Heaptitis B Vaccine (Recombinant) but not with RECOMBIVAX HB: keratitis.

DOSAGE AND ADMINISTRATION

Do not inject intravenously or intradermally.
RECOMBIVAX HB [Hepatitis B Vaccine (Recombinant), MSD] DIALYSIS FORMULATION (40 mcg/mL) IS IN-TENDED ONLY FOR ADULT PREDIALYSIS/DIALYSIS PATIENTS
RECOMBIVAX HB [Hepatitis B Vaccine (Recombinant), MSD] (10 mcg/mL) IS NOT INTENDED FOR USE IN PREDIALYSIS/DIALYSIS PATIENTS
RECOMBIVAX HB and RECOMBIVAX HB Dialysis Formulation are for intramuscular injection. The *deltoid muscle* is the preferred site for intramuscular injection in adults. Data suggests that injections given in the buttocks frequently are given into fatty tissue instead of into muscle. Such injections have resulted in a lower seroconversion rate than was expected. The *anterolateral thigh* is the recommended site for intramuscular injection in infants and young children.
For persons at risk of hemorrhage following intramuscular injection, RECOMBIVAX HB may be administered subcutaneously. However, when other aluminum-adsorbed vaccines have been administered subcutaneously, an increased incidence of local reactions including subcutaneous nodules has been observed. Therefore, subcutaneous administration should be used only in persons (e.g., hemophiliacs) who are at risk of hemorrhage following intramuscular injections.
The vaccine should be used as supplied; no dilution or reconstitution is necessary. The full recommended dose of the vaccine should be used.
It is important to use a separate sterile syringe and needle for each individual patient to prevent transmission of hepatitis and other infectious agents from one person to another.
Shake well before withdrawal and use. Thorough agitation at the time of administration is necessary to maintain suspension of the vaccine.
Parenteral drug products should be inspected visually for particulate matter and discoloration prior to administration. After thorough agitation, the vaccine is a slightly opaque, white suspension.
RECOMBIVAX HB
The vaccination regimen consists of 3 doses of vaccine given according to the following schedule:
1st dose: at elected date
2nd dose: 1 month later
3rd dose: 6 months after the first dose
The volume of vaccine to be given on each occasion is as follows:

Age Group	Initial	1 month	6 months
Birth* through 10 years of age	0.25 mL (2.5 mcg)	0.25 mL (2.5 mcg)	0.25 mL (2.5 mcg)
11–19 years of age	0.5 mL (5 mcg)	0.5 mL (5 mcg)	0.5 mL (5 mcg)
≥ 20 years	1 mL (10 mcg)	1 mL (10 mcg)	1 mL (10 mcg)

*Infants born of HBsAg negative mothers.

For Syringe Use Only: Withdraw the recommended dose from the vial using a sterile needle and syringe free of preservatives, antiseptics, and detergents.
Use of a 1 mL hubless syringe, one in which the needle is permanently attached to the syringe, will permit accurate withdrawal of 0.25 mL doses for pediatric use. However, injection must be accomplished with a needle long enough to ensure intramuscular deposition of the vaccine.
Revaccination
Whenever revaccination or administration of a booster dose is appropriate, RECOMBIVAX HB may be used (see CLINICAL PHARMACOLOGY).
*Dosage For Infants Born
of HBsAg Positive Mothers*
The recommended regimen for infants born of HBsAg positive mothers is as follows:

	Birth	Within 7 days	1 month	6 months
RECOMBIVAX HB	0.5 mL** (5 mcg)	0.5 mL (5 mcg)		0.5 mL (5 mcg)
HEPATITIS B IMMUNE GLOBULIN	0.5 mL	—	—	—

** The first 0.5 mL dose of RECOMBIVAX HB may be given at birth at the same time as Hepatitis B Immune Globulin, but should be administered in the opposite anterolateral thigh.

Known or Presumed Exposure to HBsAg
There are no prospective studies directly testing the efficacy of a combination of Hepatitis B Immune Globulin (Human)

Continued on next page

Merck & Co.—Cont.

and RECOMBIVAX HB in preventing clinical hepatitis B following percutaneous, ocular or mucous membrane exposure to hepatitis B virus. However, since most persons with such exposures (e.g., health-care workers) are candidates for RECOMBIVAX HB and since combined Hepatitis B Immune Globulin (Human) plus vaccine is more efficacious than Hepatitis B Immune Globulin (Human) alone in perinatal exposures, the following guidelines are recommended for persons who have been exposed to hepatitis B virus such as through (1) percutaneous (needlestick), ocular, mucous membrane exposure to blood known or presumed to contain HBsAg, (2) human bites by known or presumed HBsAg carriers, that penetrate the skin, or (3) following intimate sexual contact with known or presumed HBsAg carriers:

Hepatitis B Immune Globulin (Human) (0.06 mL/kg) should be given intramuscularly as soon as possible after exposure and within 24 hours if possible. RECOMBIVAX HB (see dosage recommendation) should be given intramuscularly at a separate site within 7 days of exposure and second and third doses given one and six months, respectively, after the first dose.

RECOMBIVAX HB Dialysis Formulation

The recommended vaccination regimen for predialysis/dialysis patients is as follows:

Group	Formulation	Initial	1 month	6 months
Predialysis and Dialysis Patients	Dialysis 40 mcg/mL	1 mL	1 mL	1 mL

For Syringe Use Only: Withdraw the recommended dose from the vial using a sterile needle and syringe free of preservatives, antiseptics, and detergents.

Revaccination

A booster dose or revaccination with RECOMBIVAX HB Dialysis Formulation may be considered in predialysis/dialysis patients if the anti-HBs level is less than 10 mIU/mL 1 to 2 months after the 3rd dose.

HOW SUPPLIED

No. 4773—RECOMBIVAX HB is supplied as 10 mcg/mL of HBsAg in a 3 mL vial, **NDC** 0006-4773-00.
(6505-01-266-3780 10 mcg/mL, 3 mL).

No. 4775—RECOMBIVAX HB is supplied as 10 mcg/mL of HBsAg in a 1 mL vial, **NDC** 0006-4775-00.

No. 4776—RECOMBIVAX HB Dialysis Formulation is supplied as a single dose vial of vaccine, 40 mcg/mL of HBsAg in a 1 mL vial, **NDC** 0006-4776-00
(6505-01-317-1132 40 mcg/mL, 1 mL).

Storage

Store vials at 2–8°C (36°–46°F). Storage above or below the recommended temperature may reduce potency.
Do not freeze since freezing destroys potency.

A.H.F.S. Category: 80:12

DC 7462208 Issued September 1991

COPYRIGHT © MERCK & CO., INC., 1986, 1989
All rights reserved

SINEMET® Tablets ℞
(Carbidopa-Levodopa), U.S.P.

This product is marketed by Du Pont Pharmaceuticals. Please refer to Du Pont for prescribing information.

Shown in Product Identification Section, page 409

SYPRINE® Capsules ℞
(Trientine Hydrochloride), U.S.P.
(Formerly 'CUPRID®')

DESCRIPTION

Trientine hydrochloride is *N,N'*-bis (2-aminoethyl)-1,2-ethanediamine dihydrochloride. It is a white to pale yellow crystalline hygroscopic powder. It is freely soluble in water, soluble in methanol, slightly soluble in ethanol, and insoluble in chloroform and ether.

The empirical formula is $C_6H_{18}N_4 \cdot 2HCl$ with a molecular weight of 219.2. The structural formula is:

$$NH_2(CH_2)_2NH(CH_2)_2NH(CH_2)_2NH_2 \cdot 2HCl$$

Trientine hydrochloride is a chelating compound for removal of excess copper from the body. SYPRINE* (Trientine Hydrochloride) is available as 250 mg capsules for oral administration. Capsules SYPRINE contain gelatin, iron oxides, stearic acid, and titanium dioxide as inactive ingredients.

*Registered trademark of MERCK & CO., INC.

CLINICAL PHARMACOLOGY

Introduction

Wilson's disease (hepatolenticular degeneration) is an autosomal inherited metabolic defect resulting in an inability to maintain a near-zero balance of copper. Excess copper accumulates possibly because the liver lacks the mechanism to excrete free copper into the bile. Hepatocytes store excess copper but when their capacity is exceeded copper is released into the blood and is taken up into extrahepatic sites. This condition is treated with a low copper diet and the use of chelating agents that bind copper to facilitate its excretion from the body.

Clinical Summary

Forty-one patients (18 male and 23 female) between the ages of 6 and 54 with a diagnosis of Wilson's disease and who were intolerant of d-penicillamine were treated in two separate studies with trientine hydrochloride. The dosage varied from 450 to 2400 mg per day. The average dosage required to achieve an optimal clinical response varied between 1000 mg and 2000 mg per day. The mean duration of trientine hydrochloride therapy was 48.7 months (range 2–164 months). Thirty-four of the 41 patients improved, 4 had no change in clinical global response, 2 were lost to follow-up and one showed deterioration in clinical condition. One of the patients who improved while on therapy with trientine hydrochloride experienced a recurrence of the symptoms of systemic lupus erythematosus which had appeared originally during therapy with penicillamine. Therapy with trientine hydrochloride was discontinued. No other adverse reactions, except iron deficiency, were noted among any of these 41 patients.

One investigator treated 13 patients with trientine hydrochloride following their development of intolerance to d-penicillamine. Retrospectively, he compared these patients to an additional group of 12 patients with Wilson's disease who were both tolerant of and controlled with d-penicillamine therapy, but who failed to continue any copper chelation therapy. The mean age at onset of disease of the latter group was 12 years as compared to 21 years for the former group. The trientine hydrochloride group received d-penicillamine for an average of 4 years as compared to an average of 10 years for the non-treated group.

Various laboratory parameters showed changes in favor of the patients treated with trientine hydrochloride. Free and total serum copper, SGOT, and serum bilirubin all showed mean increases over baseline in the untreated group which were significantly larger than with the patients treated with trientine hydrochloride. In the 13 patients treated with trientine hydrochloride, previous symptoms and signs relating to d-penicillamine intolerance disappeared in 8 patients, improved in 4 patients, and remained unchanged in one patient. The neurological status in the trientine hydrochloride group was unchanged or improved over baseline, whereas in the untreated group, 6 patients remained unchanged and 6 worsened. Kayser-Fleischer rings improved significantly during trientine hydrochloride treatment.

The clinical outcome of the two groups also differed markedly. Of the 13 patients on therapy with trientine hydrochloride (mean duration of therapy 4.1 years; range 1 to 13 years), all were alive at the data cutoff date, and in the non-treated group (mean years with no therapy 2.7 years; range 3 months to 9 years), 9 of the 12 died of hepatic disease.

Chelating Properties

Preclinical Studies

Studies in animals have shown that trientine hydrochloride has cupriuretic activities in both normal and copper-loaded rats. In general, the effects of trientine hydrochloride on urinary copper excretion are similar to those of equimolar doses of penicillamine, although in one study they were significantly smaller.

Human Studies

Renal clearance studies were carried out with penicillamine and trientine hydrochloride on separate occasions in selected patients treated with penicillamine for at least one year. Six-hour excretion rates of copper were determined off treatment and after a single dose of 500 mg of penicillamine or 1.2 g of trientine hydrochloride. The mean urinary excretion rates of copper were as follows:

No. of Patients	Single Dose Treatment	Basal Excretion Rate ($\mu g\ Cu^{++}/6hr$)	Test-dose Excretion Rate ($\mu g\ Cu^{++}/6hr$)
6	Trientine, 1.2 g	19	234
4	Penicillamine, 500 mg	17	320

In patients *not* previously treated with chelating agents, a similar comparison was made:

No. of Patients	Single Dose Treatment	Basal Excretion Rate ($\mu g\ Cu^{++}/6hr$)	Test-dose Excretion Rate ($\mu g\ Cu^{++}/6hr$)
8	Trientine, 1.2 g	71	1326
7	Penicillamine, 500 mg	68	1074

These results demonstrate that SYPRINE is effective as a cupriuretic agent in patients with Wilson's disease although on a molar basis it appears to be less potent or less effective than penicillamine. Evidence from a radio-labelled copper study indicates that the different cupriuretic effect between these two drugs could be due to a difference in selectivity of the drugs for different copper pools within the body.

Pharmacokinetics

Data on the pharmacokinetics of trientine hydrochloride are not available. Dosage adjustment recommendations are based upon clinical use of the drug (see DOSAGE AND ADMINISTRATION).

INDICATIONS AND USAGE

SYPRINE is indicated in the treatment of patients with Wilson's disease who are intolerant of penicillamine. Clinical experience with SYPRINE is limited and alternate dosing regimens have not been well-characterized; all endpoints in determining an individual patient's dose have not been well defined. SYPRINE and penicillamine cannot be considered interchangeable. SYPRINE should be used when continued treatment with penicillamine is no longer possible because of intolerable or life endangering side effects.

Unlike penicillamine, SYPRINE is not recommended in cystinuria or rheumatoid arthritis. The absence of a sulfhydryl moiety renders it incapable of binding cystine and, therefore, it is of no use in cystinuria. In 15 patients with rheumatoid arthritis, SYPRINE was reported not to be effective in improving any clinical or biochemical parameter after 12 weeks of treatment.

SYPRINE is not indicated for treatment of biliary cirrhosis.

CONTRAINDICATIONS

Hypersensitivity to this product.

WARNINGS

Patient experience with trientine hydrochloride is limited (see CLINICAL PHARMACOLOGY). Patients receiving SYPRINE should remain under regular medical supervision throughout the period of drug administration. Patients (especially women) should be closely monitored for evidence of iron deficiency anemia.

PRECAUTIONS

General

There are no reports of hypersensitivity in patients who have been administered trientine hydrochloride for Wilson's disease. However, there have been reports of asthma, bronchitis and dermatitis occurring after prolonged environmental exposure in workers who use trientine hydrochloride as a hardener of epoxy resins. Patients should be observed closely for signs of possible hypersensitivity.

Information for Patients

Patients should be directed to take SYPRINE on an empty stomach, at least one hour before meals or two hours after meals and at least one hour apart from any other drug, food, or milk. The capsules should be swallowed whole with water and should not be opened or chewed. Because of the potential for contact dermatitis, any site of exposure to the capsule contents should be washed with water promptly. For the first month of treatment, the patient should have his temperature taken nightly, and he should be asked to report any symptom such as fever or skin eruption.

Laboratory Tests

The most reliable index for monitoring treatment is the determination of free copper in the serum, which equals the difference between quantitatively determined total copper and ceruloplasmin-copper. Adequately treated patients will usually have less than 10 mcg free copper/dL of serum.

Therapy may be monitored with a 24 hour urinary copper analysis periodically (i.e., every 6–12 months). Urine must be collected in copper-free glassware. Since a low copper diet should keep copper absorption down to less than one milligram a day, the patient probably will be in the desired state of negative copper balance if 0.5 to 1.0 milligram of copper is present in a 24-hour collection of urine.

Drug Interactions

In general, mineral supplements should not be given since they may block the absorption of SYPRINE. However, iron deficiency may develop, especially in children and menstruating or pregnant women, or as a result of the low copper diet recommended for Wilson's disease. If necessary, iron may be given in short courses, but since iron and SYPRINE each

inhibit absorption of the other, two hours should elapse between administration of SYPRINE and iron.
It is important that SYPRINE be taken on an empty stomach, at least one hour before meals or two hours after meals and at least one hour apart from any other drug, food, or milk. This permits maximum absorption and reduces the likelihood of inactivation of the drug by metal binding in the gastrointestinal tract.
Carcinogenesis, Mutagenesis, Impairment of Fertility
Data on carcinogenesis, mutagenesis, and impairment of fertility are not available.
Pregnancy
Pregnancy Category C. Trientine hydrochloride was teratogenic in rats at doses similar to the human dose. The frequencies of both resorptions and fetal abnormalities, including hemorrhage and edema, increased while fetal copper levels decreased when trientine hydrochloride was given in the maternal diets of rats. There are no adequate and well-controlled studies in pregnant women. SYPRINE should be used during pregnancy only if the potential benefit justifies the potential risk to the fetus.
Nursing Mothers
It is not known whether this drug is excreted in human milk. Because many drugs are excreted in human milk, caution should be exercised when SYPRINE is administered to a nursing mother.
Pediatric Use
Controlled studies of the safety and effectiveness of SYPRINE in children have not been conducted. It has been used clinically in children as young as 6 years with no reported adverse experiences.

ADVERSE REACTIONS

Clinical experience with SYPRINE has been limited. The following adverse reactions have been reported in patients with Wilson's disease who were on therapy with trientine hydrochloride: iron deficiency, systemic lupus erythematosus (see CLINICAL PHARMACOLOGY).
SYPRINE is not indicated for treatment of biliary cirrhosis, but in one study of 4 patients treated with trientine hydrochloride for primary biliary cirrhosis, the following adverse reactions were reported: heartburn; epigastric pain and tenderness; thickening, fissuring and flaking of the skin; hypochromic microcytic anemia; acute gastritis; aphthoid ulcers; abdominal pain; melena; anorexia; malaise; cramps; muscle pain; weakness; rhabdomyolysis. A causal relationship of these reactions to drug therapy could not be rejected or established.

OVERDOSAGE

There is a report of an adult woman who ingested 30 grams of trientine hydrochloride without apparent ill effects. No other data on overdosage are available.

DOSAGE AND ADMINISTRATION

Systemic evaluation of dose and/or interval between dose has not been done. However, on limited clinical experience, the recommended initial dose of SYPRINE is 500–750 mg/day for children and 750–1250 mg/day for adults given in divided doses two, three or four times daily. This may be increased to a maximum of 2000 mg/day for adults or 1500 mg/day for children age 12 or under. The daily dose of SYPRINE should be increased only when the clinical response is not adequate or the concentration of free serum copper is persistently above 20 mcg/dL. Optimal long-term maintenance dosage should be determined at 6–12 month intervals (see PRECAUTIONS, *Laboratory Tests*).
It is important that SYPRINE be given on an empty stomach, at least one hour before meals or two hours after meals and at least one hour apart from any other drug, food, or milk. The capsules should be swallowed whole with water and should not be opened or chewed.

HOW SUPPLIED

No. 3408—Capsules SYPRINE, 250 mg, are light brown opaque capsules and are coded MSD 661. They are supplied as follows:
NDC 0006-0661-68 in bottles of 100.
Shown in Product Identification Section, page 420
Storage
Keep container tightly closed.
Store at 2°–8°C (36°–46°F).
A.H.F.S. Category: 64:00
DC 7664600 Issued March 1989

TIMOLIDE® Tablets ℞
(Timolol Maleate-Hydrochlorothiazide), U.S.P.

DESCRIPTION

TIMOLIDE* (Timolol Maleate-Hydrochlorothiazide) is for the treatment of hypertension. It combines the antihypertensive activity of two agents: a non-selective beta-adrenergic receptor blocking agent (timolol maleate) and a diuretic (hydrochlorothiazide).
Timolol maleate is (S)-1-[(1, 1-dimethylethyl) amino]-3-[[4- (4-morpholinyl)-1, 2, 5-thiadiazol -3- yl] oxy]-2-propanol, (Z)-butenedioate (1:1) salt. Its empirical formula is $C_{13}H_{24}N_4O_3S \cdot C_4H_4O_4$ and its structural formula is:

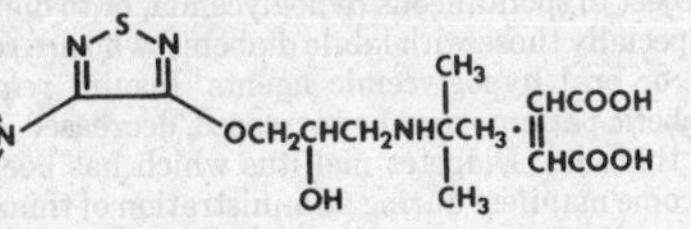

Timolol maleate has a molecular weight of 432.49. It is a white, odorless, crystalline powder which is soluble in water, methanol, and alcohol.
Hydrochlorothiazide is 6-chloro-3,4-dihydro-2*H*-1,2,4-benzothiadiazine-7-sulfonamide 1, 1- dioxide. Its empirical formula is $C_7H_8ClN_3O_4S_2$ and its structural formula is:

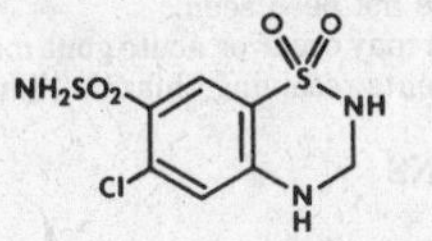

Hydrochlorothiazide has a molecular weight of 297.72. It is a white, or practically white, crystalline powder which is slightly soluble in water, but freely soluble in sodium hydroxide solution.
TIMOLIDE is supplied as tablets containing 10 mg of timolol maleate and 25 mg of hydrochlorothiazide for oral administration. Inactive ingredients are cellulose, FD&C Blue 2, magnesium stearate, and starch.

*Registered trademark of MERCK & CO., INC.

CLINICAL PHARMACOLOGY

TIMOLIDE
Timolol maleate and hydrochlorothiazide have been used singly and concomitantly for the treatment of hypertension. The antihypertensive effects of these agents are additive. The two components of TIMOLIDE have similar dosage schedules, and studies have shown that there is no interference with bioavailability when these agents are given together in the single combination tablet. Therefore, this combination provides a convenient formulation for the concomitant administration of these two entities.
In controlled clinical trials with TIMOLIDE in selected patients with mild to moderate essential hypertension, about 90 percent had a good to excellent response. In patients with more severe hypertension, TIMOLIDE may be administered with other antihypertensives such as ALDOMET* (Methyldopa) or a vasodilator.
Although the mechanisms of action of timolol maleate and hydrochlorothiazide in the treatment of hypertension have not been established, they are thought to be different; for example, hydrochlorothiazide increases plasma renin activity while timolol maleate reduces plasma renin activity.
Timolol Maleate
Timolol maleate is a $beta_1$ and $beta_2$ (non-selective) adrenergic receptor blocking agent that does not have significant intrinsic sympathomimetic, direct myocardial depressant, or local anesthetic activity.
Pharmacodynamics
Clinical pharmacology studies have confirmed the beta-adrenergic blocking activity as shown by (1) changes in resting heart rate and response of heart rate to changes in posture; (2) inhibition of isoproterenol-induced tachycardia; (3) alteration of the response to the Valsalva maneuver and amyl nitrite administration; and (4) reduction of heart rate and blood pressure changes on exercise.
Timolol maleate decreases the positive chronotropic, positive inotropic, bronchodilator, and vasodilator responses caused by beta-adrenergic receptor agonists. The magnitude of this decreased response is proportional to the existing sympathetic tone and the concentration of timolol maleate at receptor sites.
In normal volunteers, the reduction in heart rate response to a standard exercise was dose dependent over the test range of 0.5 to 20 mg, with a peak reduction at 2 hours of approximately 30% at higher doses.
Beta-adrenergic receptor blockade reduces cardiac output in both healthy subjects and patients with heart disease. In patients with severe impairment of myocardial function beta-adrenergic receptor blockade may inhibit the stimulatory effect of the sympathetic nervous system necessary to maintain adequate cardiac function.
Beta-adrenergic receptor blockade in the bronchi and bronchioles results in increased airway resistance from unopposed parasympathetic activity. Such an effect in patients with asthma or other bronchospastic conditions is potentially dangerous.
Clinical studies indicate that timolol maleate at a dosage of 20–60 mg/day reduces blood pressure without causing postural hypotension in most patients with essential hypertension. Administration of timolol maleate to patients with hypertension results initially in a decrease in cardiac output, little immediate change in blood pressure, and an increase in calculated peripheral resistance. With continued administration of timolol maleate blood pressure decreases within a few days, cardiac output usually remains reduced, and peripheral resistance falls toward pretreatment levels. Plasma volume may decrease or remain unchanged during therapy with timolol maleate. In the majority of patients with hypertension timolol maleate also decreases plasma renin activity. Dosage adjustment to achieve optimal antihypertensive effect may require a few weeks. When therapy with timolol maleate is discontinued, the blood pressure tends to return to pretreatment levels gradually. In most patients the antihypertensive activity of timolol maleate is maintained with long-term therapy and is well tolerated.
The mechanism of the antihypertensive effects of beta-adrenergic receptor blocking agents is not established at this time. Possible mechanisms of action include reduction in cardiac output, reduction in plasma renin activity, and a central nervous system sympatholytic action.
Pharmacokinetics and Metabolism
Timolol maleate is rapidly and nearly completely absorbed (about 90%) following oral ingestion. Detectable plasma levels of timolol occur within one-half hour and peak plasma levels occur in about one to two hours. The drug half-life in plasma is approximately 4 hours and this is essentially unchanged in patients with moderate renal insufficiency. Timolol is partially metabolized by the liver and timolol and its metabolites are excreted by the kidney. Timolol is not extensively bound to plasma proteins; i.e., $<10\%$ by equilibrium dialysis and approximately 60% by ultrafiltration. An *in vitro* hemodialysis study, using ^{14}C timolol added to human plasma or whole blood, showed that timolol was readily dialyzed from these fluids; however, a study of patients with renal failure showed that timolol did not dialyze readily. Plasma levels following oral administration are about half those following intravenous administration indicating approximately 50% first pass metabolism. The level of beta sympathetic activity varies widely among individuals, and no simple correlation exists between the dose or plasma level of timolol maleate and its therapeutic activity. Therefore, objective clinical measurements such as reduction of heart rate and/or blood pressure should be used as guides in determining the optimal dosage for each patient.
Hydrochlorothiazide
Hydrochlorothiazide is a diuretic and antihypertensive agent. It affects the renal tubular mechanism of electrolyte reabsorption. Hydrochlorothiazide increases excretion of sodium and chloride in approximately equivalent amounts. Natriuresis may be accompanied by some loss of potassium and bicarbonate. The mechanism of the antihypertensive effect of thiazides may be related to the excretion and redistribution of body sodium. Hydrochlorothiazide usually does not cause clinically important changes in normal blood pressure.

*Registered trademark of MERCK & CO., INC.

INDICATIONS AND USAGE

TIMOLIDE is indicated for the treatment of hypertension.
This fixed combination drug is not indicated for initial therapy of hypertension. If the fixed combination represents the dose titrated to an individual patient's needs, it may be more convenient than the separate components.

CONTRAINDICATIONS

TIMOLIDE is contraindicated in patients with bronchial asthma or with a history of bronchial asthma, or severe chronic obstructive pulmonary disease (see WARNINGS); sinus bradycardia; second and third degree atrioventricular block; overt cardiac failure (see WARNINGS); cardiogenic shock; anuria; hypersensitivity to this product or to sulfonamide-derived drugs.

Continued on next page

Information on the Merck & Co. products listed on these pages is the full prescribing information from product circulars in use October 1, 1992.

Merck & Co.—Cont.

WARNINGS

Cardiac Failure
Sympathetic stimulation may be essential for support of the circulation in individuals with diminished myocardial contractility, and its inhibition by beta-adrenergic receptor blockade may precipitate more severe failure. Although beta blockers should be avoided in overt congestive heart failure, they can be used, if necessary, with caution in patients with a history of failure who are well-compensated, usually with digitalis and diuretics. Both digitalis and timolol maleate slow AV conduction. If cardiac failure persists, therapy with TIMOLIDE should be withdrawn.
In Patients Without a History of Cardiac Failure continued depression of the myocardium with beta-blocking agents over a period of time can, in some cases, lead to cardiac failure. At the first sign or symptom of cardiac failure, patients receiving TIMOLIDE should be digitalized and/or be given additional diuretic therapy. Observe the patient closely. If cardiac failure continues, despite adequate digitalization and diuretic therapy, TIMOLIDE should be withdrawn.
Renal and Hepatic Disease and Electrolyte Disturbances
Since timolol maleate is partially metabolized in the liver and excreted mainly by the kidneys, dosage reductions may be necessary when hepatic and/or renal insufficiency is present.
Although the pharmacokinetics of timolol maleate are not greatly altered by renal impairment, marked hypotensive responses have been seen in patients with marked renal impairment undergoing dialysis after 20 mg doses. Dosing in such patients should therefore be especially cautious.
In patients with renal disease, thiazides may precipitate azotemia, and cumulative effects may develop in the presence of impaired renal function. If progressive renal impairment becomes evident, TIMOLIDE should be discontinued.
In patients with impaired hepatic function or progressive liver disease, even minor alterations in fluid and electrolyte balance may precipitate hepatic coma. Hepatic encephalopathy, manifested by tremors, confusion, and coma, has been reported in association with diuretic therapy including hydrochlorothiazide.

Exacerbation of Ischemic Heart Disease Following Abrupt Withdrawal—Hypersensitivity to catecholamines has been observed in patients withdrawn from beta blocker therapy; exacerbation of angina and, in some cases, myocardial infarction have occurred after *abrupt* discontinuation of such therapy. When discontinuing chronically administered timolol maleate, particularly in patients with ischemic heart disease, the dosage should be gradually reduced over a period of one to two weeks and the patient should be carefully monitored. If angina markedly worsens or acute coronary insufficiency develops, timolol maleate administration should be reinstituted promptly, at least temporarily, and other measures appropriate for the management of unstable angina should be taken. Patients should be warned against interruption or discontinuation of therapy without the physician's advice. Because coronary artery disease is common and may be unrecognized, it may be prudent not to discontinue timolol maleate therapy abruptly even in patients treated only for hypertension.

Obstructive Pulmonary Disease
PATIENTS WITH CHRONIC OBSTRUCTIVE PULMONARY DISEASE (e.g., CHRONIC BRONCHITIS, EMPHYSEMA) OF MILD OR MODERATE SEVERITY, BRONCHOSPASTIC DISEASE OR A HISTORY OF BRONCHOSPASTIC DISEASE (OTHER THAN BRONCHIAL ASTHMA OR A HISTORY OF BRONCHIAL ASTHMA, IN WHICH 'TIMOLIDE' IS CONTRAINDICATED, see CONTRAINDICATIONS), SHOULD IN GENERAL NOT RECEIVE BETA BLOCKERS, INCLUDING 'TIMOLIDE'. However, if TIMOLIDE is necessary in such patients, then the drug should be administered with caution since it may block bronchodilation produced by endogenous and exogenous catecholamine stimulation of $beta_2$ receptors.
Major Surgery
The necessity or desirability of withdrawal of beta-blocking therapy prior to major surgery is controversial. Beta-adrenergic receptor blockade impairs the ability of the heart to respond to beta-adrenergically mediated reflex stimuli. This may augment the risk of general anesthesia in surgical procedures. Some patients receiving beta-adrenergic receptor blocking agents have been subject to protracted severe hypotension during anesthesia. Difficulty in restarting and maintaining the heartbeat has also been reported. For these reasons, in patients undergoing elective surgery, some authorities recommend gradual withdrawal of beta-adrenergic receptor blocking agents.
If necessary during surgery, the effects of beta-adrenergic blocking agents may be reversed by sufficient doses of such agonists as isoproterenol, dopamine, dobutamine or levarterenol (see OVERDOSAGE).
Metabolic and Endocrine Effects
Beta-adrenergic blockade may mask certain clinical signs (e.g., tachycardia) of hyperthyroidism. Patients suspected of developing thyrotoxicosis should be managed carefully to avoid abrupt withdrawal of beta blockade which might precipitate a thyroid storm. Thiazides may decrease serum PBI levels without signs of thyroid disturbance.
Beta-adrenergic receptor blocking agents may mask the signs and symptoms of acute hypoglycemia. Therefore, TIMOLIDE should be administered with caution to patients subject to spontaneous hypoglycemia, or to diabetic patients (especially those with labile diabetes) who are receiving insulin or oral hypoglycemic agents. Insulin requirements in diabetic patients may be increased, decreased, or unchanged by thiazides. Diabetes mellitus which has been latent may become manifest during administration of thiazide diuretics.
Because calcium excretion is decreased by thiazides, TIMOLIDE should be discontinued before carrying out tests for parathyroid function. Pathologic changes in the parathyroid glands, with hypercalcemia and hypophosphatemia, have been observed in a few patients on prolonged thiazide therapy; however, the common complications of hyperparathyroidism such as renal lithiasis, bone resorption, and peptic ulceration have not been seen.
Hyperuricemia may occur or acute gout may be precipitated in certain patients receiving thiazide therapy.

PRECAUTIONS

General
Electrolyte and Fluid Balance Status: Periodic determination of serum electrolytes to detect possible electrolyte imbalance should be performed at appropriate intervals.
Patients should be observed for clinical signs of fluid or electrolyte imbalance, i.e., hyponatremia, hypochloremic alkalosis, and hypokalemia. Serum and urine electrolyte determinations are particularly important when the patient is vomiting excessively or receiving parenteral fluids. Warning signs or symptoms of fluid and electrolyte imbalance include dryness of the mouth, thirst, weakness, lethargy, drowsiness, restlessness, muscle pains or cramps, muscular fatigue, hypotension, oliguria, tachycardia, and gastrointestinal disturbances such as nausea and vomiting.
Hypokalemia may develop, especially with brisk diuresis, when severe cirrhosis is present, or during concomitant use of corticosteroids or ACTH.
Interference with adequate oral electrolyte intake will also contribute to hypokalemia. Hypokalemia can sensitize or exaggerate the response of the heart to the toxic effects of digitalis (e.g., increased ventricular irritability). Hypokalemia may be avoided or treated by use of potassium supplements or foods with a high potassium content.
Any chloride deficit during thiazide therapy is generally mild and usually does not require specific treatment except under extraordinary circumstances (as in liver disease or renal disease). Dilutional hyponatremia may occur in edematous patients in hot weather; appropriate therapy is water restriction rather than administration of salt except in rare instances when the hyponatremia is life threatening. In actual salt depletion, appropriate replacement is the therapy of choice.
Thiazides have been shown to increase urinary excretion of magnesium, which may result in hypomagnesemia.
Muscle Weakness: Beta-adrenergic blockade has been reported to potentiate muscle weakness consistent with certain myasthenic symptoms (e.g., diplopia, ptosis, and generalized weakness). Timolol has been reported rarely to increase muscle weakness in some patients with myasthenia gravis or myasthenic symptoms.
Cerebrovascular Insufficiency: Because of potential effects of beta-adrenergic blocking agents relative to blood pressure and pulse, these agents should be used with caution in patients with cerebrovascular insufficiency. If signs or symptoms suggesting reduced cerebral blood flow are observed, consideration should be given to discontinuing these agents.
Drug Interactions
TIMOLIDE may potentiate the action of other antihypertensive agents used concomitantly. Close observation of the patient is recommended when TIMOLIDE is administered to patients receiving catecholamine-depleting drugs such as reserpine, because of possible additive effects and the production of hypotension and/or marked bradycardia, which may produce vertigo, syncope, or postural hypotension.
Blunting of the antihypertensive effect of beta-adrenoceptor blocking agents by non-steroidal anti-inflammatory drugs has been reported. In some patients, the administration of a non-steroidal anti-inflammatory agent can reduce the diuretic, natriuretic, and antihypertensive effects of loop, potassium-sparing and thiazide diuretics. Therefore, when TIMOLIDE and non-steroidal anti-inflammatory agents are used concomitantly, the patient should be observed closely to determine if the desired therapeutic effect has been obtained.
Literature reports suggest that oral calcium antagonists may be used in combination with beta-adrenergic blocking agents when heart function is normal, but should be avoided in patients with impaired cardiac function. Hypotension, AV conduction disturbances, and left ventricular failure have been reported in some patients receiving beta-adrenergic blocking agents when an oral calcium antagonist was added to the treatment regimen. Hypotension was more likely to occur if the calcium antagonist were a dihydropyridine derivative, e.g., nifedipine, while left ventricular failure and AV conduction disturbances were more likely to occur with either verapamil or diltiazem.
Intravenous calcium antagonists should be used with caution in patients receiving beta-adrenergic blocking agents.
The concomitant use of beta-adrenergic blocking agents with digitalis and either diltiazem or verapamil may have additive effects in prolonging AV conduction time.
Thiazides may decrease arterial responsiveness to norepinephrine. This diminution is not sufficient to preclude the therapeutic effectiveness of norepinephrine. Thiazides may increase the responsiveness to tubocurarine.
Lithium generally should not be given with diuretics because they reduce its renal clearance and add a high risk of lithium toxicity. Read circulars for lithium preparations before use of such preparations with TIMOLIDE.
Other Precautions
In patients receiving thiazides, sensitivity reactions may occur with or without a history of allergy or bronchial asthma. The possible exacerbation or activation of systemic lupus erythematosus has been reported. The antihypertensive effects of thiazides may be enhanced in the post-sympathectomy patient.
Increases in cholesterol and triglyceride levels may be associated with thiazide diuretic therapy.
Carcinogenesis, Mutagenesis, Impairment of Fertility
In a two-year study of timolol maleate in rats, there was a statistically significant ($P \leq 0.05$) increase in the incidence of adrenal pheochromocytomas in male rats administered 300 times the maximum recommended human dose (1 mg/kg/day). Similar differences were not observed in rats administered doses equivalent to 25 or 100 times the maximum recommended human dose. In a lifetime study in mice, there were statistically significant ($P \leq 0.05$) increases in the incidence of benign and malignant pulmonary tumors and benign uterine polyps in female mice at 500 mg/kg/day, but not at 5 or 50 mg/kg/day. There was also a significant increase in mammary adenocarcinomas at the 500 mg/kg/day dose. This was associated with elevations in serum prolactin which occurred in female mice administered timolol at 500 mg/kg, but not at doses of 5 or 50 mg/kg/day. An increased incidence of mammary adenocarcinomas in rodents has been associated with administration of several other therapeutic agents which elevate serum prolactin, but no correlation between serum prolactin levels and mammary tumors has been established in man. Furthermore, in adult human female subjects who received oral dosages of up to 60 mg of timolol maleate, the maximum recommended human oral dosage, there were no clinically meaningful changes in serum prolactin.
There was a statistically significant increase ($P \leq 0.05$) in the overall incidence of neoplasms in female mice at the 500 mg/kg/day dosage level.
Timolol maleate was devoid of mutagenic potential when evaluated *in vivo* (mouse) in the micronucleus test and cytogenetic assay (doses up to 800 mg/kg) and *in vitro* in a neoplastic cell transformation assay (up to 100 μg/mL). In Ames tests the highest concentrations of timolol employed, 5000 or 10,000 μg/plate, were associated with statistically significant elevations ($P \leq 0.05$) of revertants observed with tester strain TA100 (in seven replicate assays), but not in the remaining three strains. In the assays with tester strain TA100, no consistent dose response relationship was observed, nor did the ratio of test to control revertants reach 2. A ratio of 2 is usually considered the criterion for a positive Ames test.
Reproduction and fertility studies in rats showed no adverse effect on male or female fertility at doses up to 150 times the maximum recommended human dose.
Pregnancy
Pregnancy Category C. Combinations of timolol maleate and hydrochlorothiazide were studied for teratogenic potential in the mouse and rabbit. The timolol maleate/hydrochlorothiazide combinations were administered orally to pregnant mice and pregnant rabbits at dosage levels of 1/2.5, 4/10, or 8/10 mg/kg/day. No teratogenic, embryotoxic, fetotoxic, or maternotoxic effects attributable to treatment were observed in either species. There are no adequate and well-controlled studies in pregnant women with TIMOLIDE. Because of the data listed below with the individual components, TIMOLIDE should be used during pregnancy only if the potential benefit justifies the potential risk to the fetus.
Timolol Maleate: Teratogenicity studies with timolol maleate in mice and rabbits at doses up to 50 mg/kg/day (50 times the maximum recommended human dose) showed no evi-

dence of fetal malformations. Although delayed fetal ossification was observed at this dose in rats, there were no adverse effects on postnatal development of offspring. Doses of 1000 mg/kg/day (1,000 times the maximum recommended human dose) were maternotoxic in mice and resulted in an increased number of fetal resorptions. Increased fetal resorptions were also seen in rabbits at doses of 100 times the maximum recommended human dose, in this case without apparent maternotoxicity.

Hydrochlorothiazide: TIMOLIDE contains hydrochlorothiazide. Thiazides cross the placental barrier and appear in cord blood. The possible hazards to the fetus include fetal or neonatal jaundice, thrombocytopenia, and possibly other adverse reactions which have occurred in the adult.

Nursing Mothers
Because of the potential for serious adverse reactions from timolol and hydrochlorothiazide in nursing infants, a decision should be made whether to discontinue nursing or to discontinue the drug, taking into account the importance of the drug to the mother.

Pediatric Use
Safety and effectiveness in children have not been established.

ADVERSE REACTIONS

TIMOLIDE is usually well tolerated in properly selected patients. Most adverse effects have been mild and transient. The adverse reactions listed in the following table were spontaneously reported and have been arranged into two groups: (1) incidence greater than 1%; and (2) incidence less than 1%. The incidence was obtained from clinical studies conducted in the United States (257 patients treated with TIMOLIDE).

Incidence Greater Than 1%	Incidence Less Than 1%
BODY AS A WHOLE	
fatigue/tiredness (1.9%)	chest pain
asthenia (1.9%)	headache
CARDIOVASCULAR	
hypotension (1.6%)	arrhythmia
bradycardia (1.2%)	syncope
	cardiac failure
DIGESTIVE SYSTEM	
none	diarrhea
	dyspepsia
	nausea
	gastrointestinal pain
	constipation
INTEGUMENTARY	
none	rash
	increased pigmentation
	dry mucous membranes
MUSCULOSKELETAL	
none	myalgia
NERVOUS SYSTEM	
dizziness (1.2%)	none
PSYCHIATRIC	
none	insomnia
	decreased libido
	nervousness
	confusion
	trouble concentrating
	somnolence
RESPIRATORY	
bronchial spasm (1.6%)	rales
dyspnea (1.2%)	
UROGENITAL	
none	renal colic

The following additional adverse effects have been reported in clinical experience with the drug: cerebral ischemia, cerebral vascular accident, gout, muscle cramps, oculogyric crisis, worsening of chronic obstructive pulmonary disease, earache, and impotence.

Other adverse reactions that have been reported with the individual components are listed below:

Timolol Maleate—Body as a Whole: extremity pain, decreased exercise tolerance, weight loss, fever; *Cardiovascular:* cardiac arrest, cerebral vascular accident, worsening of angina pectoris, sinoatrial block, AV block, worsening of arterial insufficiency, Raynaud's phenomenon, claudication, palpitations, vasodilatation, cold hands and feet, edema; *Digestive:* hepatomegaly, elevated liver function tests, vomiting; *Hematologic:* nonthrombocytopenic purpura; *Endocrine:* hyperglycemia, hypoglycemia; *Skin:* skin irritation, pruritus, sweating, alopecia; *Musculoskeletal:* arthralgia; *Nervous System:* local weakness, vertigo, paresthesia, increase in signs and symptoms of myasthenia gravis; *Psychiatric:* depression, nightmares, hallucinations; *Respiratory:* cough; *Special Senses:* visual disturbances, diplopia, ptosis, eye irritation, dry eyes, tinnitus; *Urogenital:* urination difficulties.

There have been reports of retroperitoneal fibrosis in patients receiving timolol maleate and in patients receiving other beta-adrenergic blocking agents. A causal relationship between this condition and therapy with beta-adrenergic blocking agents has not been established.

Hydrochlorothiazide —Body as a Whole: weakness; *Digestive:* anorexia, gastric irritation, vomiting, cramping, jaundice (intrahepatic cholestatic jaundice), pancreatitis, sialadenitis; *Nervous System/Psychiatric:* vertigo, paresthesias, restlessness; *Hematologic:* Leukopenia, agranulocytosis, thrombocytopenia, aplastic anemia, hemolytic anemia; *Cardiovascular:* orthostatic hypotension (may be aggravated by alcohol, barbiturates, or narcotics); *Hypersensitivity:* purpura, photosensitivity, urticaria, necrotizing angiitis (vasculitis, cutaneous vasculitis), fever, respiratory distress including pneumonitis and pulmonary edema, anaphylactic reactions; *Metabolic:* hyperglycemia, glycosuria, hyperuricemia, electrolyte imbalance (see PRECAUTIONS); *Musculoskeletal:* muscle spasm; *Special Senses:* transient blurred vision, xanthopsia.

Potential Adverse Effects: In addition, a variety of adverse effects not observed in clinical trials with timolol maleate, but reported with other beta-adrenergic blocking agents, should be considered potential adverse effects of timolol maleate: *Nervous System:* Reversible mental depression progressing to catatonia; an acute reversible syndrome characterized by disorientation for time and place, short-term memory loss, emotional lability, slightly clouded sensorium, and decreased performance on neuropsychometrics; *Cardiovascular:* Intensification of AV block (see CONTRAINDICATIONS); *Digestive:* Mesenteric arterial thrombosis, ischemic colitis; *Hematologic:* Agranulocytosis, thrombocytopenic purpura; *Allergic:* Erythematous rash, fever combined with aching and sore throat, laryngospasm with respiratory distress; *Miscellaneous:* Peyronie's disease.

There have been reports of a syndrome comprising psoriasiform skin rash, conjunctivitis sicca, otitis, and sclerosing serositis attributed to the beta-adrenergic receptor blocking agent, practolol. This syndrome has not been reported with TIMOLIDE or BLOCADREN* (Timolol Maleate).

Clinical Laboratory Test Findings: Clinically important changes in standard laboratory parameters were rarely associated with the administration of TIMOLIDE. The changes in laboratory parameters were not progressive and usually were not associated with clinical manifestations. The most common changes were increases in serum triglycerides and uric acid and decreases in serum potassium and chloride. Decreases in HDL cholesterol have been reported.

---

*Registered trademark of MERCK & CO., INC.

OVERDOSAGE

No data are available in regard to overdosage in humans. Pretreatment of mice with hydrochlorothiazide (5 mg/kg) did not alter the LD_{50} of timolol (1320 mg/kg compared to 1300 mg/kg without pretreatment).

No specific information is available on the treatment of overdosage with TIMOLIDE, and no specific antidote is available. Treatment is symptomatic and supportive. Therapy with TIMOLIDE should be discontinued and the patient observed closely. Suggested measures include induction of emesis and/or gastric lavage, and correction of dehydration, electrolyte imbalance, and hypotension by established procedures.

Timolol Maleate
No data are available in regard to overdosage in humans. The oral LD_{50} of the drug is 1190 and 900 mg/kg in female mice and female rats, respectively.

An *in vitro* hemodialysis study, using ¹⁴C timolol added to human plasma or whole blood, showed that timolol was readily dialyzed from these fluids; however, a study of patients with renal failure showed that timolol did not dialyze readily.

The most common signs and symptoms to be expected with overdosage with a beta-adrenergic receptor blocking agent are symptomatic bradycardia, hypotension, bronchospasm, and acute cardiac failure. If overdosage occurs the following therapeutic measures should be considered:

(1) *Gastric lavage.*
(2) *Symptomatic bradycardia:* Use atropine sulfate intravenously in a dosage of 0.25 mg to 2 mg to induce vagal blockade. If bradycardia persists, intravenous isoproterenol hydrochloride should be administered cautiously. In refractory cases the use of a transvenous cardiac pacemaker may be considered.
(3) *Hypotension:* Use sympathomimetic pressor drug therapy, such as dopamine, dobutamine or levarterenol. In refractory cases the use of glucagon hydrochloride has been reported to be useful.
(4) *Bronchospasm:* Use isoproterenol hydrochloride. Additional therapy with aminophylline may be considered.
(5) *Acute cardiac failure:* Conventional therapy with digitalis, diuretics, and oxygen should be instituted immediately. In refractory cases the use of intravenous aminophyl-

line is suggested. This may be followed, if necessary, by glucagon hydrochloride which has been reported to be useful.
(6) *Heart block (second or third degree):* Use isoproterenol hydrochloride or a transvenous cardiac pacemaker.

Hydrochlorothiazide
The most common signs and symptoms observed with hydrochlorothiazide overdosage are those caused by electrolyte depletion (hypokalemia, hypochloremia, hyponatremia) and dehydration resulting from excessive diuresis. If digitalis has also been administered, hypokalemia may accentuate cardiac arrhythmias.

DOSAGE AND ADMINISTRATION

The recommended starting and maintenance dosage is 1 tablet twice a day or 2 tablets once a day. If the antihypertensive response is not satisfactory, another antihypertensive agent may be added.

HOW SUPPLIED

No. 3373—Tablets TIMOLIDE 10-25 are light blue, flat, hexagonal-shaped, compressed tablets, with MSD 67 code on one side and TIMOLIDE on the other. Each tablet contains 10 mg of timolol maleate and 25 mg of hydrochlorothiazide. They are supplied as follows:
NDC 0006-0067-68 bottles of 100.
Shown in Product Identification Section, page 420
Storage
Store in a well-closed container, protected from light.
A.H.F.S. Category: 24:08
DC 7244226 Issued August 1987
COPYRIGHT © MERCK & CO., INC., 1985
All rights reserved

TIMOPTIC® Sterile Ophthalmic Solution ℞
(Timolol Maleate), U.S.P.

DESCRIPTION

TIMOPTIC* (Timolol Maleate) Ophthalmic Solution is a non-selective beta-adrenergic receptor blocking agent. Its chemical name is (S)- 1- [(1, 1-dimethylethyl)amino] -3- [[4- (4-morpholinyl) -1, 2, 5-thiadiazol-3-yl]oxy] -2- propanol, (Z)-butenedioate (1:1) salt. Timolol maleate possesses an asymmetric carbon atom in its structure and is provided as the levo isomer. The nominal optical rotation of timolol maleate is:
$$[\alpha]^{25°}_{405\,nm} \text{ in } 0.1N \text{ HCl } (C = 5\%) = -12.2°.$$

Its empirical formula is $C_{13}H_{24}N_4O_3S \cdot C_4H_4O_4$ and its structural formula is:

Timolol maleate has a molecular weight of 432.49. It is a white, odorless, crystalline powder which is soluble in water, methanol, and alcohol. TIMOPTIC is stable at room temperature.

TIMOPTIC Ophthalmic Solution is supplied as a sterile, isotonic, buffered, aqueous solution of timolol maleate in two dosage strengths: Each mL of TIMOPTIC 0.25% contains 2.5 mg of timolol (3.4 mg of timolol maleate). Each mL of TIMOPTIC 0.5% contains 5.0 mg of timolol (6.8 mg of timolol maleate). Inactive ingredients: monobasic and dibasic sodium phosphate, sodium hydroxide to adjust pH, and water for injection. Benzalkonium chloride 0.01% is added as preservative.

---

*Registered trademark of MERCK & CO., INC.

CLINICAL PHARMACOLOGY

Timolol maleate is a $beta_1$ and $beta_2$ (non-selective) adrenergic receptor blocking agent that does not have significant intrinsic sympathomimetic, direct myocardial depressant, or local anesthetic (membrane-stabilizing) activity.

Beta-adrenergic receptor blockade reduces cardiac output in both healthy subjects and patients with heart disease. In patients with severe impairment of myocardial function beta-adrenergic receptor blockade may inhibit the stimula-

Continued on next page

Merck & Co.—Cont.

tory effect of the sympathetic nervous system necessary to maintain adequate cardiac function.

Beta-adrenergic receptor blockade in the bronchi and bronchioles results in increased airway resistance from unopposed para-sympathetic activity. Such an effect in patients with asthma or other bronchospastic conditions is potentially dangerous.

TIMOPTIC Ophthalmic Solution, when applied topically in the eye, has the action of reducing elevated as well as normal intraocular pressure, whether or not accompanied by glaucoma. Elevated intraocular pressure is a major risk factor in the pathogenesis of glaucomatous visual field loss. The higher the level of intraocular pressure, the greater the likelihood of glaucomatous visual field loss and optic nerve damage.

The onset of reduction in intraocular pressure following administration of TIMOPTIC can usually be detected within one-half hour after a single dose. The maximum effect usually occurs in one to two hours and significant lowering of intraocular pressure can be maintained for periods as long as 24 hours with a single dose. Repeated observations over a period of one year indicate that the intraocular pressure-lowering effect of TIMOPTIC is well maintained.

The precise mechanism of the ocular hypotensive action of TIMOPTIC is not clearly established at this time. Tonography and fluorophotometry studies in man suggest that its predominant action may be related to reduced aqueous formation. However, in some studies a slight increase in outflow facility was also observed. Unlike miotics, TIMOPTIC reduces intraocular pressure with little or no effect on accommodation or pupil size. Thus, changes in visual acuity due to increased accommodation are uncommon, and dim or blurred vision and night blindness produced by miotics are not evident. In addition, in patients with cataracts the inability to see around lenticular opacities when the pupil is constricted is avoided.

In the clinical studies which are reported below, ocular pressure reductions to less than 22 mmHg were used as a reasonable reference point to allow comparisons between treatments. Reduction of ocular pressure to just below 22 mmHg may not be optimal for all patients; therapy should be individualized.

In controlled multiclinic studies in patients with untreated intraocular pressures of 22 mmHg or greater, TIMOPTIC 0.25 percent or 0.5 percent administered twice a day produced a greater reduction in intraocular pressure than 1, 2, 3, or 4 percent pilocarpine solution administered four times a day or 0.5, 1, or 2 percent epinephrine hydrochloride solution administered twice a day.

In the multiclinic studies comparing TIMOPTIC with pilocarpine, 61 percent of patients treated with TIMOPTIC had intraocular pressure reduced to less than 22 mmHg compared to 32 percent of patients treated with pilocarpine. For patients completing these studies, the mean reduction in pressure at the end of the study from pretreatment was 30.7 percent for patients treated with TIMOPTIC and 21.7 percent for patients treated with pilocarpine.

In the multiclinic studies comparing TIMOPTIC with epinephrine, 69 percent of patients treated with TIMOPTIC had intraocular pressure reduced to less than 22 mmHg compared to 42 percent of patients treated with epinephrine. For patients completing these studies, the mean reduction in pressure at the end of the study from pretreatment was 33.2 percent for patients treated with TIMOPTIC and 28.1 percent for patients treated with epinephrine.

In these studies, TIMOPTIC was generally well tolerated and produced fewer and less severe side effects than either pilocarpine or epinephrine. A slight reduction of resting heart rate in some patients receiving TIMOPTIC (mean reduction 2.9 beats/minute standard deviation 10.2) was observed.

TIMOPTIC has also been used in patients with glaucoma wearing conventional (PMMA) hard contact lenses, and has generally been well tolerated. TIMOPTIC has not been studied in patients wearing lenses made with materials other than PMMA.

INDICATIONS AND USAGE

TIMOPTIC Ophthalmic Solution has been shown to be effective in lowering intraocular pressure and may be used in:
Patients with chronic open-angle glaucoma
Patients with aphakic glaucoma
Some patients with secondary glaucoma
Other patients with elevated intraocular pressure who are at sufficient risk to require lowering of the ocular pressure.
Clinical trials have also shown that in patients who respond inadequately to multiple antiglaucoma drug therapy the addition of TIMOPTIC may produce a further reduction of intraocular pressure.

CONTRAINDICATIONS

TIMOPTIC is contraindicated in patients with bronchial asthma or with a history of bronchial asthma, or severe chronic obstructive pulmonary disease (see WARNINGS); sinus bradycardia; second and third degree atrioventricular block; overt cardiac failure (see WARNINGS); cardiogenic shock; hypersensitivity to any component of this product.

WARNINGS

As with other topically applied ophthalmic drugs, this drug may be absorbed systemically.

The same adverse reactions found with systemic administration of beta-adrenergic blocking agents may occur with topical administration. For example, severe respiratory reactions and cardiac reactions, including death due to bronchospasm in patients with asthma, and rarely death in association with cardiac failure, have been reported following administration of TIMOPTIC (Timolol Maleate) (see CONTRAINDICATIONS).

Cardiac Failure
Sympathetic stimulation may be essential for support of the circulation in individuals with diminished myocardial contractility, and its inhibition by beta-adrenergic receptor blockade may precipitate more severe failure.

In Patients Without a History of Cardiac Failure continued depression of the myocardium with beta-blocking agents over a period of time can, in some cases, lead to cardiac failure. At the first sign or symptom of cardiac failure TIMOPTIC should be discontinued.

Obstructive Pulmonary Disease
PATIENTS WITH CHRONIC OBSTRUCTIVE PULMONARY DISEASE (e.g., CHRONIC BRONCHITIS, EMPHYSEMA) OF MILD OR MODERATE SEVERITY, BRONCHOSPASTIC DISEASE OR A HISTORY OF BRONCHOSPASTIC DISEASE (OTHER THAN BRONCHIAL ASTHMA OR A HISTORY OF BRONCHIAL ASTHMA, IN WHICH 'TIMOPTIC' IS CONTRAINDICATED, see CONTRAINDICATIONS), SHOULD IN GENERAL NOT RECEIVE BETA BLOCKERS, INCLUDING 'TIMOPTIC'. However, if TIMOPTIC is necessary in such patients, then the drug should be administered with caution since it may block bronchodilation produced by endogenous and exogenous catecholamine stimulation of beta₂ receptors.

Major Surgery
The necessity or desirability of withdrawal of beta-adrenergic blocking agents prior to major surgery is controversial. Beta-adrenergic receptor blockade impairs the ability of the heart to respond to beta-adrenergically mediated reflex stimuli. This may augment the risk of general anesthesia in surgical procedures. Some patients receiving beta-adrenergic receptor blocking agents have been subject to protracted severe hypotension during anesthesia. Difficulty in restarting and maintaining the heartbeat has also been reported. For these reasons, in patients undergoing elective surgery, some authorities recommend gradual withdrawal of beta-adrenergic receptor blocking agents.

If necessary during surgery, the effects of beta-adrenergic blocking agents may be reversed by sufficient doses of such agonists as isoproterenol, dopamine, dobutamine or levarterenol (see OVERDOSAGE).

Diabetes Mellitus
Beta-adrenergic blocking agents should be administered with caution in patients subject to spontaneous hypoglycemia or to diabetic patients (especially those with labile diabetes) who are receiving insulin or oral hypoglycemic agents. Beta-adrenergic receptor blocking agents may mask the signs and symptoms of acute hypoglycemia.

Thyrotoxicosis
Beta-adrenergic blocking agents may mask certain clinical signs (e.g., tachycardia) of hyperthyroidism. Patients suspected of developing thyrotoxicosis should be managed carefully to avoid abrupt withdrawal of beta-adrenergic blocking agents which might precipitate a thyroid storm.

PRECAUTIONS

General
Patients who are receiving a beta-adrenergic blocking agent orally and TIMOPTIC should be observed for a potential additive effect either on the intraocular pressure or on the known systemic effects of beta blockade.
Patients should not receive two topical ophthalmic beta-adrenergic blocking agents concurrently (see DOSAGE AND ADMINISTRATION).
Because of potential effects of beta-adrenergic blocking agents relative to blood pressure and pulse, these agents should be used with caution in patients with cerebrovascular insufficiency. If signs or symptoms suggesting reduced cerebral blood flow develop following initiation of therapy with TIMOPTIC, alternative therapy should be considered.
Muscle Weakness: Beta-adrenergic blockade has been reported to potentiate muscle weakness consistent with certain myasthenic symptoms (e.g., diplopia, ptosis, and gener-

alized weakness). Timolol has been reported rarely to increase muscle weakness in some patients with myasthenia gravis or myasthenic symptoms.

In patients with angle-closure glaucoma, the immediate objective of treatment is to reopen the angle. This requires constricting the pupil with a miotic. TIMOPTIC has little or no effect on the pupil. When TIMOPTIC is used to reduce elevated intraocular pressure in angle-closure glaucoma, it should be used with a miotic and not alone.

As with the use of other antiglaucoma drugs, diminished responsiveness to TIMOPTIC after prolonged therapy has been reported in some patients. However, in one long-term study in which 96 patients have been followed for at least 3 years, no significant difference in mean intraocular pressure has been observed after initial stabilization.

Drug Interactions
Although TIMOPTIC used alone has little or no effect on pupil size, mydriasis resulting from concomitant therapy with TIMOPTIC and epinephrine has been reported occasionally.

Close observation of the patient is recommended when a beta blocker is administered to patients receiving catecholamine-depleting drugs such as reserpine, because of possible additive effects and the production of hypotension and/or marked bradycardia, which may produce vertigo, syncope, or postural hypotension.

Caution should be used in the coadministration of beta-adrenergic blocking agents, such as TIMOPTIC, and oral or intravenous calcium antagonists, because of possible atrioventricular conduction disturbances, left ventricular failure, and hypotension. In patients with impaired cardiac function, coadministration should be avoided.

The concomitant use of beta-adrenergic blocking agents with digitalis and calcium antagonists may have additive effects in prolonging atrioventricular conduction time.

Animal Studies
No adverse ocular effects were observed in rabbits and dogs administered TIMOPTIC topically in studies lasting one and two years respectively.

Carcinogenesis, Mutagenesis, Impairment of Fertility
In a two-year oral study of timolol maleate in rats, there was a statistically significant (P ≤ 0.05) increase in the incidence of adrenal pheochromocytomas in male rats administered 300 times the maximum recommended human oral dose* (1 mg/kg/day). Similar differences were not observed in rats administered oral doses equivalent to 25 or 100 times the maximum recommended human oral dose. In a lifetime oral study in mice, there were statistically significant (P ≤ 0.05) increases in the incidence of benign and malignant pulmonary tumors and benign uterine polyps in female mice at 500 mg/kg/day, but not at 5 or 50 mg/kg/day. There was also a significant increase in mammary adenocarcinomas at the 500 mg/kg/day dose. This was associated with elevations in serum prolactin which occurred in female mice administered timolol at 500 mg/kg, but not at doses of 5 or 50 mg/kg/day. An increased incidence of mammary adenocarcinomas in rodents has been associated with administration of several other therapeutic agents which elevate serum prolactin, but no correlation between serum prolactin levels and mammary tumors has been established in man. Furthermore, in adult human female subjects who received oral dosages of up to 60 mg of timolol maleate, the maximum recommended human oral dosage, there were no clinically meaningful changes in serum prolactin.

There was a statistically significant increase (P ≤ 0.05) in the overall incidence of neoplasms in female mice at the 500 mg/kg/day dosage level.

Timolol maleate was devoid of mutagenic potential when evaluated *in vivo* (mouse) in the micronucleus test and cytogenetic assay (doses up to 800 mg/kg) and *in vitro* in a neoplastic cell transformation assay (up to 100 μg/mL). In Ames tests the highest concentrations of timolol employed, 5000 or 10,000 μg/plate, were associated with statistically significant elevations (P ≤ 0.05) of revertants observed with tester strain TA100 (in seven replicate assays), but not in the remaining three strains. In the assays with tester strain TA100, no consistent dose response relationship was observed, nor did the ratio of test to control revertants reach 2. A ratio of 2 is usually considered the criterion for a positive Ames test.

Reproduction and fertility studies in rats showed no adverse effect on male or female fertility at doses up to 150 times the maximum recommended human oral dose.

*The maximum recommended single oral dose is 30 mg of timolol. One drop of TIMOPTIC 0.5% contains about 1/150 of this dose which is about 0.2 mg.

Pregnancy
Pregnancy Category C. Teratogenicity studies with timolol in mice and rabbits at doses up to 50 mg/kg/day (50 times the maximum recommended human oral dose) showed no evidence of fetal malformations. Although delayed fetal ossification was observed at this dose in rats, there were no adverse effects on postnatal development of offspring. Doses of 1000 mg/kg/day (1,000 times the maximum recommended human oral dose) were maternotoxic in mice and resulted in

an increased number of fetal resorptions. Increased fetal resorptions were also seen in rabbits at doses of 100 times the maximum recommended human oral dose, in this case without apparent maternotoxicity. There are no adequate and well-controlled studies in pregnant women. TIMOPTIC should be used during pregnancy only if the potential benefit justifies the potential risk to the fetus.

Nursing Mothers

Because of the potential for serious adverse reactions from timolol in nursing infants, a decision should be made whether to discontinue nursing or to discontinue the drug, taking into account the importance of the drug to the mother.

Pediatric Use

Safety and effectiveness in children have not been established by adequate and well-controlled studies.

ADVERSE REACTIONS

TIMOPTIC Ophthalmic Solution is usually well tolerated. The following adverse reactions have been reported either in clinical trials of up to 3 years duration prior to release in 1978 or since the drug has been marketed.

BODY AS A WHOLE
Headache, asthenia, chest pain.

CARDIOVASCULAR
Bradycardia, arrhythmia, hypotension, syncope, heart block, cerebral vascular accident, cerebral ischemia, cardiac failure, palpitation, cardiac arrest.

DIGESTIVE
Nausea, diarrhea.

NERVOUS SYSTEM/PSYCHIATRIC
Dizziness, depression, increase in signs and symptoms of myasthenia gravis, paresthesia.

SKIN
Hypersensitivity, including localized and generalized rash; urticaria, alopecia.

RESPIRATORY
Bronchospasm (predominantly in patients with pre-existing bronchospastic disease), respiratory failure, dyspnea, nasal congestion, cough.

ENDOCRINE
Masked symptoms of hypoglycemia in insulin-dependent diabetics (See WARNINGS).

SPECIAL SENSES
Signs and symptoms of ocular irritation, including conjunctivitis, blepharitis, keratitis, blepharoptosis, decreased corneal sensitivity, visual disturbances including refractive changes (due to withdrawal of miotic therapy in some cases), diplopia, ptosis.

Causal Relationship Unknown: The following adverse effects have been reported, and a causal relationship to therapy with TIMOPTIC has not been established: *Body as a Whole:* Fatigue; *Cardiovascular:* Hypertension, pulmonary edema, worsening of angina pectoris; *Digestive:* Dyspepsia, anorexia, dry mouth; *Nervous System/Psychiatric:* Behavioral changes including confusion, hallucinations, anxiety, disorientation, nervousness, somnolence, and other psychic disturbances; *Special Senses:* Aphakic cystoid macular edema; *Urogenital:* Retroperitoneal fibrosis, impotence.

The following additional adverse effects have been reported in clinical experience with oral timolol maleate, and may be considered potential effects of ophthalmic timolol maleate: *Body as a Whole:* Extremity pain, decreased exercise tolerance, weight loss; *Cardiovascular:* Edema, worsening of arterial insufficiency, Raynaud's phenomenon, vasodilatation; *Digestive:* Gastrointestinal pain, hepatomegaly, vomiting; *Hematologic:* Nonthrombocytopenic purpura; *Endocrine:* Hyperglycemia, hypoglycemia; *Skin:* Pruritus, skin irritation, increased pigmentation, sweating, cold hands and feet; *Musculoskeletal:* Arthralgia, claudication; *Nervous System/Psychiatric:* Vertigo, local weakness, decreased libido, nightmares, insomnia, diminished concentration; *Respiratory:* Rales, bronchial obstruction; *Special Senses:* Tinnitus, dry eyes; *Urogenital:* Urination difficulties.

Potential Adverse Effects: In addition, a variety of adverse effects have been reported with other beta-adrenergic blocking agents and may be considered potential effects of ophthalmic timolol maleate: *Digestive:* Mesenteric arterial thrombosis, ischemic colitis; *Hematologic:* Agranulocytosis, thrombocytopenic purpura; *Nervous System:* Reversible mental depression progressing to catatonia; an acute reversible syndrome characterized by disorientation for time and place, short-term memory loss, emotional lability, slightly clouded sensorium, and decreased performance on neuropsychometrics; *Allergic:* Erythematous rash, fever combined with aching and sore throat, laryngospasm with respiratory distress; *Urogenital:* Peyronie's disease.

There have been reports of a syndrome comprising psoriasiform skin rash, conjunctivitis sicca, otitis and sclerosing serositis attributed to the beta- adrenergic receptor blocking agent, practolol. This syndrome has not been reported with timolol maleate.

OVERDOSAGE

No data are available in regard to overdosage in humans. The oral LD_{50} of the drug is 1190 and 900 mg/kg in female mice and female rats, respectively.

An *in vitro* hemodialysis study, using ^{14}C timolol added to human plasma or whole blood, showed that timolol was readily dialyzed from these fluids; however, a study of patients with renal failure showed that timolol did not dialyze readily.

The most common signs and symptoms to be expected with overdosage with administration of a systemic beta-adrenergic receptor blocking agent are symptomatic bradycardia, hypotension, bronchospasm, and acute cardiac failure. The following therapeutic measures should be considered:

(1) *Gastric lavage:* If ingested.
(2) *Symptomatic bradycardia:* Use atropine sulfate intravenously in a dosage of 0.25 mg to 2 mg to induce vagal blockade. If bradycardia persists, intravenous isoproterenol hydrochloride should be administered cautiously. In refractory cases the use of a transvenous cardiac pacemaker may be considered.
(3) *Hypotension:* Use sympathomimetic pressor drug therapy, such as dopamine, dobutamine or levarterenol. In refractory cases the use of glucagon hydrochloride has been reported to be useful.
(4) *Bronchospasm:* Use isoproterenol hydrochloride. Additional therapy with aminophylline may be considered.
(5) *Acute cardiac failure:* Conventional therapy with digitalis, diuretics, and oxygen should be instituted immediately. In refractory cases the use of intravenous aminophylline is suggested. This may be followed if necessary by glucagon hydrochloride which has been reported to be useful.
(6) *Heart block (second or third degree):* Use isoproterenol hydrochloride or a transvenous cardiac pacemaker.

DOSAGE AND ADMINISTRATION

TIMOPTIC Ophthalmic Solution is available in concentrations of 0.25 and 0.5 percent. The usual starting dose is one drop of 0.25 percent TIMOPTIC in the affected eye(s) twice a day. If the clinical response is not adequate, the dosage may be changed to one drop of 0.5 percent solution in the affected eye(s) twice a day.

Since in some patients the pressure-lowering response to TIMOPTIC may require a few weeks to stabilize, evaluation should include a determination of intraocular pressure after approximately 4 weeks of treatment with TIMOPTIC.

If the intraocular pressure is maintained at satisfactory levels, the dosage schedule may be changed to one drop once a day in the affected eye(s). Because of diurnal variations in intraocular pressure, satisfactory response to the once-a-day dose is best determined by measuring the intraocular pressure at different times during the day.

Dosages above one drop of 0.5 percent TIMOPTIC twice a day generally have not been shown to produce further reduction in intraocular pressure. If the patient's intraocular pressure is still not at a satisfactory level on this regimen, concomitant therapy with pilocarpine and other miotics, and/or epinephrine, and/or systemically administered carbonic anhydrase inhibitors, such as acetazolamide, can be instituted.

When a patient is transferred from another topical ophthalmic beta-adrenergic blocking agent, that agent should be discontinued after proper dosing on one day and treatment with TIMOPTIC started on the following day with 1 drop of 0.25 percent TIMOPTIC in the affected eye(s) twice a day. The dose may be increased to one drop of 0.5 percent TIMOPTIC twice a day if the clinical response is not adequate.

When a patient is transferred from a single antiglaucoma agent, other than a topical ophthalmic beta-adrenergic blocking agent, continue the agent already being used and add one drop of 0.25 percent TIMOPTIC in the affected eye(s) twice a day. On the following day, discontinue the previously used antiglaucoma agent completely and continue with TIMOPTIC. If a higher dosage of TIMOPTIC is required, substitute one drop of 0.5 percent solution in the affected eye(s) twice a day.

When a patient is transferred from several concomitantly administered antiglaucoma agents, individualization is required. If any of the agents is an ophthalmic beta-adrenergic blocker, it should be discontinued before starting TIMOPTIC. Additional adjustments should involve one agent at a time and usually should be made at intervals of not less than one week. A recommended approach is to continue the agents being used and to add one drop of 0.25 percent TIMOPTIC in the affected eye(s) twice a day. On the following day, discontinue one of the other antiglaucoma agents. The remaining antiglaucoma agents may be decreased or discontinued according to the patient's response to treatment. If a higher dosage of TIMOPTIC is required, substitute

one drop of 0.5 percent solution in the affected eye(s) twice a day. The physician may be able to discontinue some or all of the other antiglaucoma agents.

HOW SUPPLIED

Sterile Ophthalmic Solution TIMOPTIC is a clear, colorless to light yellow solution.

No. 3366—TIMOPTIC Ophthalmic Solution, 0.25% timolol equivalent, is supplied in a white, opaque, plastic OCUMETER* ophthalmic dispenser with a controlled drop tip as follows:

NDC 0006-3366-32, 2.5 mL
NDC 0006-3366-03, 5 mL
(6505-01-069-6518, 0.25% 5 mL)
NDC 0006-3366-10, 10 mL
(6505-01-093-5458, 0.25% 10 mL)
NDC 0006-3366-12, 15 mL.

No. 3367—TIMOPTIC Ophthalmic Solution, 0.5% timolol equivalent, is supplied in a white, opaque, plastic OCUMETER ophthalmic dispenser with a controlled drop tip as follows:

NDC 0006-3367-32, 2.5 mL
NDC 0006-3367-03, 5 mL
(6505-01-069-6519, 0.5% 5 mL)
NDC 0006-3367-10, 10 mL
(6505-01-092-0422, 0.5% 10 mL)
NDC 0006-3367-12, 15 mL.

* Registered trademark of MERCK & CO., INC.
Storage
Protect from light. Store at room temperature.
A.H.F.S. Category: 52:36
DC 7115427   Issued August 1990
COPYRIGHT © MERCK & CO., INC., 1985
All rights reserved

TIMOPTIC®   ℞
(Timolol Maleate)
in OCUDOSE® (Dispenser), U.S.P.
Preservative-Free Sterile Ophthalmic Solution
in a Sterile Ophthalmic Unit Dose Dispenser

DESCRIPTION

Timolol maleate is a non-selective beta-adrenergic receptor blocking agent. Its chemical name is (S)-1- [(1, 1-dimethyl-ethyl)amino]-3-[[4- (4- morpholinyl) -1, 2, 5-thiadiazol-3-yl]-oxy] -2-propanol, (Z)-butenedioate (1:1) salt. Timolol maleate possesses an asymmetric carbon atom in its structure and is provided as the levo isomer. The nominal optical rotation of timolol maleate is

$[\alpha]_{405\ nm}^{25°}$ in 0.1N HCl (C = 5%) = $-12.2°$.

Its empirical formula is $C_{13}H_{24}N_4O_3S \cdot C_4H_4O_4$ and its structural formula is:

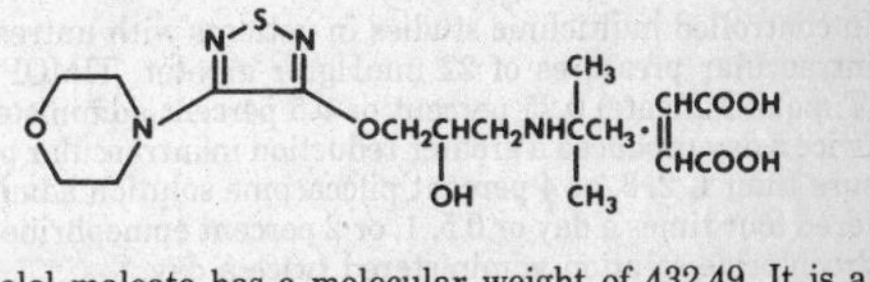

Timolol maleate has a molecular weight of 432.49. It is a white, odorless, crystalline powder which is soluble in water, methanol, and alcohol. Timolol maleate is stable at room temperature.

Timolol maleate ophthalmic solution is supplied in two formulations: Ophthalmic Solution TIMOPTIC* (Timolol Maleate), which contains the preservative, benzalkonium chloride; and Ophthalmic Solution TIMOPTIC* (Timolol Maleate), the preservative-free formulation.

Preservative-free Ophthalmic Solution TIMOPTIC is supplied in OCUDOSE*, a unit dose container as a sterile, isotonic, buffered, aqueous solution of timolol maleate in two dosage strengths: Each mL of Preservative-free TIMOPTIC in OCUDOSE 0.25% contains 2.5 mg of timolol (3.4 mg of timolol maleate). Each mL of Preservative-free TIMOPTIC in OCUDOSE 0.5% contains 5.0 mg of timolol (6.8 mg of timolol maleate). Inactive ingredients: monobasic and dibasic sodium phosphate, sodium hydroxide to adjust pH, and water for injection.

---

* Registered trademark of MERCK & CO., INC.

Continued on next page

Merck & Co.—Cont.

CLINICAL PHARMACOLOGY

Timolol maleate is a beta$_1$ and beta$_2$ (non-selective) adrenergic receptor blocking agent that does not have significant intrinsic sympathomimetic, direct myocardial depressant, or local anesthetic (membrane-stabilizing) activity.

Beta-adrenergic receptor blockade reduces cardiac output in both healthy subjects and patients with heart disease. In patients with severe impairment of myocardial function beta-adrenergic receptor blockade may inhibit the stimulatory effect of the sympathetic nervous system necessary to maintain adequate cardiac function.

Beta-adrenergic receptor blockade in the bronchi and bronchioles results in increased airway resistance from unopposed parasympathetic activity. Such an effect in patients with asthma or other bronchospastic conditions is potentially dangerous.

TIMOPTIC (Timolol Maleate), when applied topically in the eye, has the action of reducing elevated as well as normal intraocular pressure, whether or not accompanied by glaucoma. Elevated intraocular pressure is a major risk factor in the pathogenesis of glaucomatous visual field loss. The higher the level of intraocular pressure, the greater the likelihood of glaucomatous visual field loss and optic nerve damage.

The onset of reduction in intraocular pressure following administration of TIMOPTIC (Timolol Maleate) can usually be detected within one-half hour after a single dose. The maximum effect usually occurs in one to two hours and significant lowering of intraocular pressure can be maintained for periods as long as 24 hours with a single dose. Repeated observations over a period of one year indicate that the intraocular pressure-lowering effect of TIMOPTIC (Timolol Maleate) is well maintained.

The precise mechanism of the ocular hypotensive action of TIMOPTIC (Timolol Maleate) is not clearly established at this time. Tonography and fluorophotometry studies in man suggest that its predominant action may be related to reduced aqueous formation. However, in some studies a slight increase in outflow facility was also observed. Unlike miotics, TIMOPTIC (Timolol Maleate) reduces intraocular pressure with little or no effect on accommodation or pupil size. Thus, changes in visual acuity due to increased accommodation are uncommon, and dim or blurred vision and night blindness produced by miotics are not evident. In addition, in patients with cataracts the inability to see around lenticular opacities when the pupil is constricted is avoided.

Clinical studies have shown that the mean percent reductions in intraocular pressure with Preservative-free TIMOPTIC and TIMOPTIC (Timolol Maleate) were similar. Preservative-free TIMOPTIC was generally well tolerated.

In the clinical studies which are reported below, ocular pressure reductions to less than 22 mmHg were used as a reasonable reference point to allow comparisons between treatments. Reduction of ocular pressure to just below 22 mmHg may not be optimal for all patients; therapy should be individualized.

In controlled multiclinic studies in patients with untreated intraocular pressures of 22 mmHg or greater, TIMOPTIC (Timolol Maleate) 0.25 percent or 0.5 percent administered twice a day produced a greater reduction in intraocular pressure than 1, 2, 3, or 4 percent pilocarpine solution administered four times a day or 0.5, 1, or 2 percent epinephrine hydrochloride solution administered twice a day.

In the multiclinic studies comparing TIMOPTIC (Timolol Maleate) with pilocarpine, 61 percent of patients treated with TIMOPTIC (Timolol Maleate) had intraocular pressure reduced to less than 22 mmHg compared to 32 percent of patients treated with pilocarpine. For patients completing these studies, the mean reduction in pressure at the end of the study from pretreatment was 30.7 percent for patients treated with TIMOPTIC (Timolol Maleate) and 21.7 percent for patients treated with pilocarpine.

In the multiclinic studies comparing TIMOPTIC (Timolol Maleate) with epinephrine, 69 percent of patients treated with TIMOPTIC (Timolol Maleate) had intraocular pressure reduced to less than 22 mmHg compared to 42 percent of patients treated with epinephrine. For patients completing these studies, the mean reduction in pressure at the end of the study from pretreatment was 33.2 percent for patients treated with TIMOPTIC (Timolol Maleate) and 28.1 percent for patients treated with epinephrine.

In these studies, TIMOPTIC (Timolol Maleate) was generally well tolerated and produced fewer and less severe side effects than either pilocarpine or epinephrine. A slight reduction of resting heart rate in some patients receiving TIMOPTIC (Timolol Maleate) (mean reduction 2.9 beats/minute standard deviation 10.2) was observed.

TIMOPTIC (Timolol Maleate) has also been used in patients with glaucoma wearing conventional (PMMA) hard contact lenses, and has generally been well tolerated. TIMOPTIC (Timolol Maleate) has not been studied in patients wearing lenses made with materials other than PMMA.

INDICATIONS AND USAGE

TIMOPTIC (Timolol Maleate) has been shown to be effective in lowering intraocular pressure. Clinical studies have shown that the mean percent reductions in intraocular pressure with Preservative-free TIMOPTIC and TIMOPTIC (Timolol Maleate) are similar. When a patient is sensitive to the preservative, benzalkonium chloride, or when use of a preservative-free topical medication is advisable, Preservative-free TIMOPTIC may be used in:

   Patients with chronic open-angle glaucoma
   Patients with aphakic glaucoma
   Some patients with secondary glaucoma
   Other patients with elevated intraocular pressure who are at sufficient risk to require lowering of the ocular pressure. Clinical trials have also shown that in patients who respond inadequately to multiple antiglaucoma drug therapy the addition of TIMOPTIC (Timolol Maleate) may produce a further reduction of intraocular pressure.

CONTRAINDICATIONS

Preservative-free TIMOPTIC in OCUDOSE is contraindicated in patients with bronchial asthma or with a history of bronchial asthma, or severe chronic obstructive pulmonary disease (see WARNINGS); sinus bradycardia; second and third degree atrioventricular block; overt cardiac failure (see WARNINGS); cardiogenic shock; hypersensitivity to any component of this product.

WARNINGS

As with other topically applied ophthalmic drugs, this drug may be absorbed systemically.
The same adverse reactions found with systemic administration of beta-adrenergic blocking agents may occur with topical administration. For example, severe respiratory reactions and cardiac reactions, including death due to bronchospasm in patients with asthma, and rarely death in association with cardiac failure, have been reported following administration of TIMOPTIC (Timolol Maleate) (see CONTRAINDICATIONS).
Cardiac Failure
Sympathetic stimulation may be essential for support of the circulation in individuals with diminished myocardial contractility, and its inhibition by beta-adrenergic receptor blockade may precipitate more severe failure.
In Patients Without a History of Cardiac Failure continued depression of the myocardium with beta-blocking agents over a period of time can, in some cases, lead to cardiac failure. At the first sign or symptom of cardiac failure Preservative-free TIMOPTIC in OCUDOSE should be discontinued.
Obstructive Pulmonary Disease
PATIENTS WITH CHRONIC OBSTRUCTIVE PULMONARY DISEASE (e.g., CHRONIC BRONCHITIS, EMPHYSEMA) OF MILD OR MODERATE SEVERITY, BRONCHOSPASTIC DISEASE OR A HISTORY OF BRONCHOSPASTIC DISEASE (OTHER THAN BRONCHIAL ASTHMA OR A HISTORY OF BRONCHIAL ASTHMA, IN WHICH 'Preservative-free TIMOPTIC in OCUDOSE' IS CONTRAINDICATED, see CONTRAINDICATIONS), SHOULD IN GENERAL NOT RECEIVE BETA BLOCKERS, INCLUDING 'Preservative-free TIMOPTIC in OCUDOSE'. However, if Preservative-free TIMOPTIC in OCUDOSE is necessary in such patients, then the drug should be administered with caution since it may block bronchodilation produced by endogenous and exogenous catecholamine stimulation of beta$_2$ receptors.
Major Surgery
The necessity or desirability of withdrawal of beta-adrenergic blocking agents prior to major surgery is controversial. Beta-adrenergic receptor blockade impairs the ability of the heart to respond to beta-adrenergically mediated reflex stimuli. This may augment the risk of general anesthesia in surgical procedures. Some patients receiving beta-adrenergic receptor blocking agents have been subject to protracted severe hypotension during anesthesia. Difficulty in restarting and maintaining the heartbeat has also been reported. For these reasons, in patients undergoing elective surgery, some authorities recommend gradual withdrawal of beta-adrenergic receptor blocking agents.
If necessary during surgery, the effects of beta-adrenergic blocking agents may be reversed by sufficient doses of such agonists as isoproterenol, dopamine, dobutamine or levarterenol (see OVERDOSAGE).
Diabetes Mellitus
Beta-adrenergic blocking agents should be administered with caution in patients subject to spontaneous hypoglycemia or to diabetic patients (especially those with labile diabetes) who are receiving insulin or oral hypoglycemic agents. Beta-adrenergic receptor blocking agents may mask the signs and symptoms of acute hypoglycemia.
Thyrotoxicosis
Beta-adrenergic blocking agents may mask certain clinical signs (e.g., tachycardia) of hyperthyroidism. Patients sus-

pected of developing thyrotoxicosis should be managed carefully to avoid abrupt withdrawal of beta-adrenergic blocking agents which might precipitate a thyroid storm.

PRECAUTIONS

General
Patients who are receiving a beta-adrenergic blocking agent orally and Preservative-free TIMOPTIC in OCUDOSE should be observed for a potential additive effect either on the intraocular pressure or on the known systemic effects of beta blockade.
Patients should not receive two topical ophthalmic beta-adrenergic blocking agents concurrently (see DOSAGE AND ADMINISTRATION).
Because of potential effects of beta-adrenergic blocking agents relative to blood pressure and pulse, these agents should be used with caution in patients with cerebrovascular insufficiency. If signs or symptoms suggesting reduced cerebral blood flow develop following initiation of therapy with Preservative-free TIMOPTIC in OCUDOSE, alternative therapy should be considered.
Muscle Weakness: Beta-adrenergic blockade has been reported to potentiate muscle weakness consistent with certain myasthenic symptoms (e.g., diplopia, ptosis, and generalized weakness). Timolol has been reported rarely to increase muscle weakness in some patients with myasthenia gravis or myasthenic symptoms.
In patients with angle-closure glaucoma, the immediate objective of treatment is to reopen the angle. This requires constricting the pupil with a miotic. TIMOPTIC (Timolol Maleate) has little or no effect on the pupil. When Preservative-free TIMOPTIC in OCUDOSE is used to reduce elevated intraocular pressure in angle-closure glaucoma, it should be used with a miotic and not alone.
As with the use of other antiglaucoma drugs, diminished responsiveness to TIMOPTIC (Timolol Maleate) after prolonged therapy has been reported in some patients. However, in one long-term study in which 96 patients have been followed for at least 3 years, no significant difference in mean intraocular pressure has been observed after initial stabilization.
Information for Patients
Patients should be instructed about the use of Preservative-free TIMOPTIC in OCUDOSE.
Since sterility cannot be maintained after the individual unit is opened, patients should be instructed to use the product immediately after opening, and to discard the individual unit and any remaining contents immediately after use.
Drug Interactions
Although TIMOPTIC (Timolol Maleate) used alone has little or no effect on pupil size, mydriasis resulting from concomitant therapy with TIMOPTIC (Timolol Maleate) and epinephrine has been reported occasionally.
Close observation of the patient is recommended when a beta blocker is administered to patients receiving catecholamine-depleting drugs such as reserpine, because of possible additive effects and the production of hypotension and/or marked bradycardia, which may produce vertigo, syncope, or postural hypotension.
Caution should be used in the coadministration of beta-adrenergic blocking agents, such as Preservative-free TIMOPTIC in OCUDOSE, and oral or intravenous calcium antagonists, because of possible atrioventricular conduction disturbances, left ventricular failure, and hypotension. In patients with impaired cardiac function, coadministration should be avoided.
The concomitant use of beta-adrenergic blocking agents with digitalis and calcium antagonists may have additive effects in prolonging atrioventricular conduction time.
Animal Studies
No adverse ocular effects were observed in rabbits and dogs administered TIMOPTIC (Timolol Maleate) topically in studies lasting one and two years respectively.
Carcinogenesis, Mutagenesis, Impairment of Fertility
In a two-year oral study of timolol maleate in rats, there was a statistically significant (P ≤ 0.05) increase in the incidence of adrenal pheochromocytomas in male rats administered 300 times the maximum recommended human oral dose* (1 mg/kg/day). Similar differences were not observed in rats administered oral doses equivalent to 25 or 100 times the maximum recommended human oral dose. In a lifetime oral study in mice, there were statistically significant (P ≤ 0.05) increases in the incidence of benign and malignant pulmonary tumors and benign uterine polyps in female mice at 500 mg/kg/day, but not at 5 or 50 mg/kg/day. There was also a significant increase in mammary adenocarcinomas at the 500 mg/kg/day dose. This was associated with elevations in serum prolactin which occurred in female mice administered timolol at 500 mg/kg, but not at doses of 5 or 50 mg/kg/day. An increased incidence of mammary adenocarcinomas in rodents has been associated with administration of several other therapeutic agents which elevate serum prolactin, but no correlation between serum prolactin levels and mammary tumors has been established in man. Furthermore, in

adult human female subjects who received oral dosages of up to 60 mg of timolol maleate, the maximum recommended human oral dosage, there were no clinically meaningful changes in serum prolactin.

There was a statistically significant increase (P ≤ 0.05) in the overall incidence of neoplasms in female mice at the 500 mg/kg/day dosage level.

Timolol maleate was devoid of mutagenic potential when evaluated *in vivo* (mouse) in the micronucleus test and cyto-genetic assay (doses up to 800 mg/kg) and *in vitro* in a neo-plastic cell transformation assay (up to 100 μg/mL). In Ames tests the highest concentrations of timolol employed, 5000 or 10,000 μg/plate, were associated with statistically signifi-cant elevations (P ≤ 0.05) of revertants observed with tester strain TA 100 (in seven replicate assays), but not in the re-maining three strains. In the assays with tester strain TA 100, no consistent dose response relationship was observed, nor did the ratio of test to control revertants reach 2. A ratio of 2 is usually considered the criterion for a positive Ames test.

Reproduction and fertility studies in rats showed no adverse effect on male or female fertility at doses up to 150 times the maximum recommended human oral dose.

---

* The maximum recommended single oral dose is 30 mg of timolol. One drop of Preservative-free TIMOPTIC in OCU-DOSE 0.5% contains about $1/150$ of this dose which is about 0.2 mg.

Pregnancy
Pregnancy Category C. Teratogenicity studies with timolol in mice and rabbits at doses up to 50 mg/kg/day (50 times the maximum recommended human oral dose) showed no evi-dence of fetal malformations. Although delayed fetal ossifi-cation was observed at this dose in rats, there were no ad-verse effects on postnatal development of offspring. Doses of 1000 mg/kg/day (1,000 times the maximum recommended human oral dose) were maternotoxic in mice and resulted in an increased number of fetal resorptions. Increased fetal resorptions were also seen in rabbits at doses of 100 times the maximum recommended human oral dose, in this case with-out apparent maternotoxicity. There are no adequate and well-controlled studies in pregnant women. Preservative-free TIMOPTIC in OCUDOSE should be used during preg-nancy only if the potential benefit justifies the potential risk to the fetus.
Nursing Mothers
Because of the potential for serious adverse reactions from timolol in nursing infants, a decision should be made whether to discontinue nursing or to discontinue the drug, taking into account the importance of the drug to the mother.
Pediatric Use
Safety and effectiveness in children have not been estab-lished by adequate and well-controlled studies.

ADVERSE REACTIONS

Preservative-free TIMOPTIC in OCUDOSE Ophthalmic Solution is usually well tolerated. The following adverse reactions have been reported with TIMOPTIC (Timolol Mal-eate), either in clinical trials of up to 3 years duration prior to release in 1978 or since the drug has been marketed, and may be expected to occur with Preservative-free TIMOPTIC.
BODY AS A WHOLE
Headache, asthenia, chest pain.
CARDIOVASCULAR
Bradycardia, arrhythmia, hypotension, syncope, heart block, cerebral vascular accident, cerebral ischemia, cardiac fail-ure, palpitation, cardiac arrest.
DIGESTIVE
Nausea, diarrhea.
NERVOUS SYSTEM/PSYCHIATRIC
Dizziness, depression, increase in signs and symptoms of myasthenia gravis, paresthesia.
SKIN
Hypersensitivity, including localized and generalized rash; urticaria, alopecia.
RESPIRATORY
Bronchospasm (predominantly in patients with pre-existing bronchospastic disease), respiratory failure, dyspnea, nasal congestion, cough.
ENDOCRINE
Masked symptoms of hypoglycemia in insulin-dependent diabetics (See WARNINGS).
SPECIAL SENSES
Signs and symptoms of ocular irritation, including conjunc-tivitis, blepharitis, keratitis, blepharoptosis, decreased cor-neal sensitivity, visual disturbances including refractive changes (due to withdrawal of miotic therapy in some cases), diplopia, ptosis.
Causal Relationship Unknown: The following adverse ef-fects have been reported, and a causal relationship to ther-apy with ophthalmic timolol maleate has not been estab-lished: *Body as a Whole:* Fatigue; *Cardiovascular:* Hyperten-

sion, pulmonary edema, worsening of angina pectoris; *Diges-tive:* Dyspepsia, anorexia, dry mouth; *Nervous System/Psy-chiatric:* Behavioral changes including confusion, hallucina-tions, anxiety, disorientation, nervousness, somnolence, and other psychic disturbances; *Special Senses:* Aphakic cystoid macular edema; *Urogenital:* Retroperitoneal fibrosis, impotence.
The following additional adverse effects have been reported in clinical experience with oral timolol maleate, and may be considered potential effects of ophthalmic timolol maleate: *Body as a Whole:* Extremity pain, decreased exercise toler-ance, weight loss; *Cardiovascular:* Edema, worsening of arte-rial insufficiency, Raynaud's phenomenon, vasodilatation; *Digestive:* Gastrointestinal pain, hepatomegaly, vomiting; *Hematologic:* Nonthrombocytopenic purpura; *Endocrine:* Hyperglycemia, hypoglycemia; *Skin:* Pruritus, skin irrita-tion, increased pigmentation, sweating, cold hands and feet; *Musculoskeletal:* Arthralgia, claudication; *Nervous System/ Psychiatric:* Vertigo, local weakness, decreased libido, night-mares, insomnia, diminished concentration; *Respiratory:* Rales, bronchial obstruction; *Special Senses:* Tinnitus, dry eyes; *Urogenital:* Urination difficulties.
Potential Adverse Effects: In addition, a variety of adverse effects have been reported with other beta-adrenergic block-ing agents and may be considered potential effects of oph-thalmic timolol maleate: *Digestive:* Mesenteric arterial thrombosis, ischemic colitis; *Hematologic:* Agranulocytosis, thrombocytopenic purpura; *Nervous System:* Reversible men-tal depression progressing to catatonia; an acute reversible syndrome characterized by disorientation for time and place, short-term memory loss, emotional lability, slightly clouded sensorium, and decreased performance on neuropsychomet-rics; *Allergic:* Erythematous rash, fever combined with ach-ing and sore throat, laryngospasm with respiratory distress; *Urogenital:* Peyronie's disease.
There have been reports of a syndrome comprising psoriasi-form skin rash, conjunctivitis sicca, otitis and sclerosing serositis attributed to the beta-adrenergic receptor blocking agent, practolol. This syndrome has not been reported with timolol maleate.

OVERDOSAGE

No data are available in regard to overdosage in humans. The oral LD_{50} of timolol maleate is 1190 and 900 mg/kg in female mice and female rats, respectively.
An *in vitro* hemodialysis study, using ^{14}C timolol added to human plasma or whole blood, showed that timolol was readily dialyzed from these fluids; however, a study of pa-tients with renal failure showed that timolol did not dialyze readily.
The most common signs and symptoms to be expected with overdosage with administration of a systemic beta-adrener-gic receptor blocking agent are symptomatic bradycardia, hypotension, bronchospasm, and acute cardiac failure. The following additional therapeutic measures should be considered:
(1) *Gastric lavage:* If ingested.
(2) *Symptomatic bradycardia:* Use atropine sulfate intrave-nously in a dosage of 0.25 mg to 2 mg to induce vagal block-ade. If bradycardia persists, intravenous isoproterenol hy-drochloride should be administered cautiously. In refractory cases the use of a transvenous cardiac pacemaker may be considered.
(3) *Hypotension:* Use sympathomimetic pressor drug therapy, such as dopamine, dobutamine or levarterenol. In refractory cases the use of glucagon hydrochloride has been reported to be useful.
(4) *Bronchospasm:* Use isoproterenol hydrochloride. Addi-tional therapy with aminophylline may be considered.
(5) *Acute cardiac failure:* Conventional therapy with digitalis, diuretics, and oxygen should be instituted immediately. In refractory cases the use of intravenous aminophylline is suggested. This may be followed if necessary by glucagon hydrochloride which has been reported to be useful.
(6) *Heart block (second or third degree):* Use isoproterenol hydrochloride or a transvenous cardiac pacemaker.

DOSAGE AND ADMINISTRATION

Preservative-free TIMOPTIC in OCUDOSE is a sterile solu-tion that does not contain a preservative. The solution from one individual unit is to be used immediately after opening for administration to one or both eyes. Since sterility cannot be guaranteed after the individual unit is opened, the re-maining contents should be discarded immediately after administration.
Preservative-free TIMOPTIC in OCUDOSE is available in concentrations of 0.25 and 0.5 percent. The usual starting dose is one drop of 0.25 percent Preservative-free TIMOPTIC in OCUDOSE in the affected eye(s) administered twice a day. Apply enough gentle pressure on the individual container to obtain a single drop of solution. If the clinical response is not adequate, the dosage may be changed to one drop of 0.5 per-cent solution in the affected eye(s) administered twice a day.

Since in some patients the pressure-lowering response to Preservative-free TIMOPTIC in OCUDOSE may require a few weeks to stabilize, evaluation should include a determi-nation of intraocular pressure after approximately 4 weeks of treatment with Preservative-free TIMOPTIC in OCU-DOSE.
If the intraocular pressure is maintained at satisfactory lev-els, the dosage schedule may be changed to one drop once a day in the affected eye(s). Because of diurnal variations in intraocular pressure, satisfactory response to the once-a-day dose is best determined by measuring the intraocular pres-sure at different times during the day.
Dosages above one drop of 0.5 percent TIMOPTIC (Timolol Maleate) twice a day generally have not been shown to pro-duce further reduction in intraocular pressure. If the pa-tient's intraocular pressure is not at a satisfactory level dur-ing treatment with Preservative-free TIMOPTIC in OCU-DOSE 0.5 percent, concomitant therapy with pilocarpine and other miotics, and/or epinephrine, and/or systemically administered carbonic anhydrase inhibitors, such as aceta-zolamide, can be instituted taking into consideration that the preparation(s) used concomitantly may contain one or more preservatives.
When a patient is transferred from another topical ophthal-mic beta-adrenergic blocking agent, that agent should be discontinued after proper dosing on one day and treatment with Preservative-free TIMOPTIC in OCUDOSE started on the following day with one drop of 0.25 percent Preservative-free TIMOPTIC in OCUDOSE in the affected eye(s) twice a day. The dose may be increased to one drop of 0.5 percent Preservative-free TIMOPTIC in OCUDOSE twice a day if the clinical response is not adequate.
When a patient is transferred from a single antiglaucoma agent, other than a topical ophthalmic beta-adrenergic blocking agent, continue the agent already being used and add one drop of 0.25 percent Preservative-free TIMOPTIC in OCUDOSE in the affected eye(s) twice a day. On the follow-ing day, discontinue the previously used antiglaucoma agent completely and continue with Preservative-free TIMOPTIC in OCUDOSE. If a higher dosage of Preservative-free TIMOPTIC in OCUDOSE is required, substitute one drop of 0.5 percent solution in the affected eye(s) twice a day.
When a patient is transferred from several concomitantly administered antiglaucoma agents, individualization is re-quired. If any of the agents is an ophthalmic beta-adrenergic blocker, it should be discontinued before starting Preserva-tive-free TIMOPTIC in OCUDOSE. Additional adjustments should involve one agent at a time and usually should be made at intervals of not less than one week. A recommended approach is to continue the agents being used and to add one drop of 0.25 percent Preservative-free TIMOPTIC in OCU-DOSE in the affected eye(s) twice a day. On the following day, discontinue one of the other antiglaucoma agents. The re-maining antiglaucoma agents may be decreased or discontin-ued according to the patient's response to treatment. If a higher dosage of Preservative-free TIMOPTIC in OCUDOSE is required, substitute one drop of 0.5 percent solution in the affected eye(s) twice a day. The physician may be able to dis-continue some or all of the other antiglaucoma agents.

HOW SUPPLIED

Preservative-free Sterile Ophthalmic Solution TIMOPTIC in OCUDOSE is a clear, colorless to light yellow solution.
No. 3542—Preservative-free TIMOPTIC, 0.25% timolol equivalent, is supplied in OCUDOSE, a clear polyethylene unit dose container. Each individual unit contains 0.45 mL of solution, and is available in a foil laminate overwrapped pouch as follows:
NDC 0006-3542-60; 60 Individual Unit Doses
(6505-01-316-8791, 0.25% 60 Individual Unit Doses).
No. 3543—Preservative-free TIMOPTIC, 0.5% timolol equiv-alent, is supplied in OCUDOSE, a clear polyethylene unit dose container. Each individual unit contains 0.45 mL of solution, and is available in a foil laminate overwrapped pouch as follows:
NDC 0006-3543-60; 60 Individual Unit Doses
(6505-01-284-5154, 0.5% 60 Individual Unit Doses).
Storage
Store Preservative-free TIMOPTIC in OCUDOSE at room temperature.
Because evaporation can occur through the unprotected polyethylene unit dose container and prolonged exposure to direct light can modify the product, the unit dose container should be kept in the protective foil overwrap and used within one month after the foil package has been opened.

Continued on next page

Information on the Merck & Co. products listed on these pages is the full prescribing information from product circulars in use October 1, 1992.

Merck & Co.—Cont.

Manufactured by:
MERCK SHARP & DOHME, Division of Merck & Co., INC.
West Point, Pa. 19486
Filled by:
PACO
Lakewood, NJ 08701

A.H.F.S. Category: 52:36
DC 7475304 Issued August 1990

COPYRIGHT © MERCK & CO., INC., 1986
All rights reserved

TONOCARD® Tablets ℞
(Tocainide HCl), U.S.P.

WARNINGS

Blood Dyscrasias: Agranulocytosis, bone marrow depression, leukopenia, neutropenia, aplastic/hypoplastic anemia, thrombocytopenia and sequelae such as septicemia and septic shock have been reported in patients receiving TONOCARD. Most of these patients received TONOCARD within the recommended dosage range. Fatalities have occurred (with approximately 25 percent mortality in reported agranulocytosis cases). Since most of these events have been noted during the first 12 weeks of therapy, it is recommended that complete blood counts, including white cell, differential and platelet counts be performed, optimally, at weekly intervals for the first three months of therapy; and frequently thereafter. Complete blood counts should be performed promptly if the patient develops any signs of infection (such as fever, chills, sore throat, or stomatitis), bruising, or bleeding. If any of these hematologic disorders is identified, TONOCARD should be discontinued and appropriate treatment should be instituted if necessary. Blood counts usually return to normal within one month of discontinuation. Caution should be used in patients with pre-existing marrow failure or cytopenia of any type. (See ADVERSE REACTIONS.)

Pulmonary Fibrosis: Pulmonary fibrosis, interstitial pneumonitis, fibrosing alveolitis, pulmonary edema, and pneumonia have been reported in patients receiving TONOCARD. Many of these events occurred in patients who were seriously ill. Fatalities have been reported. The experiences are usually characterized by bilateral infiltrates on x-ray and are frequently associated with dyspnea and cough. Fever may or may not be present. Patients should be instructed to promptly report the development of any pulmonary symptoms such as exertional dyspnea, cough or wheezing. Chest x-rays are advisable at that time. If these pulmonary disorders develop, TONOCARD should be discontinued. (See ADVERSE REACTIONS.)

DESCRIPTION

TONOCARD* (Tocainide HCl) is a primary amine analog of lidocaine with antiarrhythmic properties useful in the treatment of ventricular arrhythmias. The chemical name for tocainide hydrochloride is 2-amino-*N*-(2,6-dimethylphenyl) propanamide hydrochloride. Its empirical formula is $C_{11}H_{16}N_2O \cdot HCl$, with a molecular weight of 228.72. The structural formula is:

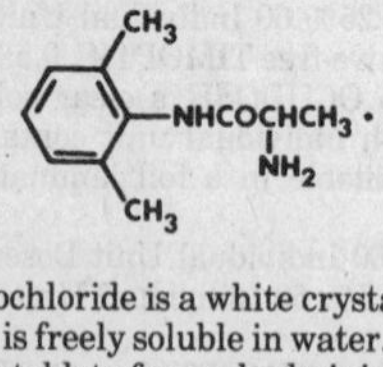

Tocainide hydrochloride is a white crystalline powder with a bitter taste and is freely soluble in water. It is supplied as 400 mg and 600 mg tablets for oral administration. Each tablet contains the following inactive ingredients: hydroxypropyl methylcellulose, iron oxide, magnesium stearate, methylcellulose, polyethylene glycol, and titanium dioxide.

* Registered trademark of Astra Pharmaceutical Products, Inc.

CLINICAL PHARMACOLOGY

Action

Tocainide, like lidocaine, produces dose dependent decreases in sodium and potassium conductance, thereby decreasing the excitability of myocardial cells. In experimental animal models, the dose-related depression of sodium current is more pronounced in ischemic tissue than in normal tissue.

Electrophysiology

Tocainide is a Class I antiarrhythmic compound with electrophysiologic properties in man similar to those of lidocaine, but dissimilar from quinidine, procainamide, and disopyramide.

In studies of isolated dog Purkinje fibers, tocainide in concentrations of 1–50 mcg/mL had no significant effect on resting membrane potential, but reduced the amplitude and rate of depolarization (dv/dt) of the action potential. Tocainide decreased the effective refractory period (ERP) to a lesser extent than the action potential duration (APD) resulting in an increase in the ERP/APD ratio.

In patients with cardiac disease, TONOCARD produced no clinically significant changes in sinus nodal function, effective refractory periods, or intracardiac conduction times when studied under electrophysiologic testing procedures.

Tocainide, like lidocaine, characteristically does not prolong ventricular depolarization (QRS duration) or repolarization (QT intervals) as measured by electrocardiography. Theoretically, therefore, TONOCARD may be useful in the treatment of ventricular arrhythmias associated with a prolonged QT interval.

Patients who respond to lidocaine also respond to TONOCARD in a majority of cases. Failure to respond to lidocaine usually predicts failure to respond to TONOCARD, but there are exceptions to this.

In a controlled comparison with quinidine, 600 mg b.i.d. of TONOCARD produced a mean reduction of 42 percent in PVC count, compared to a 54 percent reduction by quinidine 300 mg every 6 hours. Among all patients entered into the study, about one-fifth of tocainide recipients and one-third of quinidine recipients had 75 percent or greater reductions in PVC count or had elimination of ventricular tachycardia.

Pharmacokinetics

Following oral administration of tocainide, peak plasma concentrations occur within 0.5 to 2 hours. The average plasma half-life in patients is approximately 15 hours. Although the effective plasma concentration may vary from patient to patient, the usual therapeutic plasma range (as defined by 50–80 percent PVC suppression) is 4–10 mcg/mL (18–45 micromole/L), expressed as tocainide hydrochloride. Tocainide is approximately 10 percent bound to plasma protein.

In contrast to lidocaine, tocainide undergoes negligible first pass hepatic degradation. Following oral administration, the bioavailability of TONOCARD approaches 100 percent. The extent of its bioavailability is unaffected by food. Tocainide has no cardioactive metabolites. Approximately 40 percent of the administered dose of tocainide is excreted unchanged in the urine. Acidification of the urine has not been shown to significantly alter tocainide excretion in the urine, but alkalinization of the urine results in a significant decrease in the percent of tocainide excreted unchanged in the urine. Animal data indicate that tocainide crosses the blood-brain barrier; however, it has less lipid solubility than lidocaine.

Hemodynamics

Cardiac catheterization studies in man utilizing intravenous tocainide infusions (0.5–0.75 mg/kg/min over 15 min) have shown that tocainide usually produces a small degree of depression of parameters of left ventricular function, such as left ventricular dP/dt, and left ventricular end diastolic pressure. There were usually no changes in cardiac output or clinical evidence of increasing congestive heart failure in the well-compensated patients studied. Small but statistically significant increases in aortic and pulmonary arterial pressures have been consistently observed and are probably related to small increases in vascular resistance. When used concomitantly with a beta-blocking drug, tocainide further reduced cardiac index and left ventricular dP/dt and further increased pulmonary wedge pressure.

No clinically significant changes in heart rate, blood pressure, or signs of myocardial depression were observed in a study of 72 post-myocardial infarction patients receiving long-term therapy with oral TONOCARD at usual doses (400 mg q8h). When tocainide was administered orally at a dose of 120 mg/kg to anesthetized dogs (14 times the initial maximum dose recommended for humans), a negative inotropic effect was observed: the rate of change of left ventricular pressure decreased by up to 29 percent of control at 3 hours after administration. This effect was not observed at lower doses (60 mg/kg). Tocainide has been used safely in patients with acute myocardial infarction and various degrees of congestive heart failure. It has, however, a small negative inotropic effect and can increase peripheral resistance slightly. It therefore should be used cautiously in patients with known heart failure, particularly if a beta blocker is given as well. (See PRECAUTIONS).

INDICATIONS AND USAGE

TONOCARD is indicated for the treatment of life-threatening ventricular arrhythmias. However, because TONOCARD has the potential to produce serious and sometimes fatal hematologic disorders (0.18 percent in clinical trials) particularly leukopenia, agranulocytosis or aplastic/hypoplastic anemia as well as pulmonary fibrosis (sometimes fatal), the risk/benefit decision is most difficult (see Box WARNINGS). The use of TONOCARD should be reserved for patients in whom, in the opinion of the physician, the benefits of treatment outweigh the risks, keeping in mind the possible alternative therapies for the patient.

Like all other antiarrhythmics, tocainide has not been shown to prevent sudden death in patients with serious ventricular ectopic activity, and also, like all other antiarrhythmics, it has potentially serious adverse effects, including the ability to worsen arrhythmias. It is therefore essential that each patient given tocainide be evaluated electrocardiographically and clinically prior to, and during, tocainide therapy to determine whether the response to tocainide supports continued treatment.

CONTRAINDICATIONS

Patients who are hypersensitive to this product or to local anesthetics of the amide type.

Patients with second or third degree atrioventricular block in the absence of an artificial ventricular pacemaker.

WARNINGS

Acceleration of Ventricular Rate: Acceleration of ventricular rate occurs infrequently when antiarrhythmics are administered to patients with atrial flutter or fibrillation (see ADVERSE REACTIONS).

PRECAUTIONS

General

In patients with known heart failure or minimal cardiac reserve, TONOCARD should be used with caution because of the potential for aggravating the degree of heart failure.

Caution should be used in the institution or continuation of antiarrhythmic therapy in the presence of signs of increasing depression of cardiac conductivity.

In patients with severe liver or kidney disease, the rate of drug elimination may be significantly decreased (see DOSAGE AND ADMINISTRATION).

Since antiarrhythmic drugs may be ineffective in patients with hypokalemia, the possibility of a potassium deficit should be explored and, if present, the deficit should be corrected.

Like all other oral antiarrhythmics, TONOCARD has been reported to increase arrhythmias in some patients (see ADVERSE REACTIONS).

Information for Patients

Patients should be instructed to promptly report the development of bruising or bleeding; any signs of infections such as fever, chills, sore throat, or soreness and ulcers in the mouth; or any pulmonary symptoms, such as exertional dyspnea, cough, or wheezing; rash.

Laboratory Tests

As with other antiarrhythmics, abnormal liver function tests, particularly in the early stages of therapy, have been reported. Periodic monitoring of liver function should be considered. Hepatitis and jaundice have been reported in some patients.

Drug Interactions

Tocainide and lidocaine are pharmacodynamically similar. The concomitant use of these two agents may cause an increased incidence of adverse reactions, including central nervous system adverse reactions such as seizure.

Specific interaction studies with cimetidine, digoxin, metoprolol and warfarin have been conducted, no clinically significant interaction was seen with cimetidine, digoxin or warfarin; but tocainide and metoprolol had additive effects on wedge pressure and cardiac index. TONOCARD has also been used in open studies with digitalis, beta-blocking agents, other antiarrhythmic agents, anticoagulants, and diuretics, without evidence of clinically significant interactions. Nevertheless, caution should be exercised in the use of multiple drug therapy.

TONOCARD is equally effective in digitalized and non-digitalized patients. In 17 patients with refractory ventricular arrhythmias on concomitant therapy, serum digoxin levels (1.1 ± 0.4 ng/mL) remained in the expected normal range (0.5–2.5 ng/mL) during tocainide administration.

Carcinogenesis, Mutagenesis, Impairment of Fertility

The carcinogenic potential of tocainide was studied in mice using oral doses up to 300 mg/kg/day (about 6 times the maximum recommended human dose) for up to 94 weeks in males and 102 weeks in females and in rats at doses up to 200 mg/kg/day for 24 months. Tocainide did not affect the type or incidence of neoplasia in the two studies.

Tocainide did not show any mutagenic potential when evaluated *in vivo* in the micronucleus test using mice at oral doses up to 187.5 mg/kg/day (about 7 times the usual human dose). Also, no mutagenic activity was seen *in vitro* in the Ames

microbial mutagen test or in the mouse lymphoma forward mutation assay.

Reproduction and fertility studies in rats showed no adverse effects on male or female fertility at oral doses up to 200 mg/kg/day (about 8 times the usual human dose).

Pregnancy

Pregnancy Category C. In a teratogenicity study in rabbits, tocainide was administered orally at doses of 25, 50, and 100 mg/kg/day (about 1 to 4 times the usual human dose). No evidence of a drug-related teratogenic effect was noted; however, these doses were maternotoxic and produced a dose-related increase in abortions and stillbirths. In a teratogenicity study in rats, an oral dose of 300 mg/kg/day (about 12 times the usual human dose) showed no evidence of treatment-related fetal malformations, but maternotoxicity and an increase in fetal resorptions were noted. An oral dose of 30 mg/kg/day (about twice the usual human dose) did not produce any adverse effects.

In reproduction studies in rats at maternotoxic oral doses of 200 and 300 mg/kg/day (about 8 and 12 times the usual human dose, respectively), dystocia, and delayed parturition occurred which was accompanied by an increase in stillbirths and decreased survival in offspring during the first week postpartum. Growth and viability of surviving offspring were not affected for the remainder of the lactation period.

There are no adequate and well-controlled studies in pregnant women. TONOCARD should be used during pregnancy only if the potential benefit justifies the potential risk to the fetus.

Nursing Mothers

It is not known whether tocainide is secreted in human milk. Because many drugs are secreted in human milk and because of the potential for serious adverse reactions in nursing infants from TONOCARD, a decision should be made whether to discontinue nursing or to discontinue the drug, taking into account the importance of the drug to the mother.

Pediatric Use

Safety and effectiveness in children have not been established.

ADVERSE REACTIONS

TONOCARD commonly produces minor, transient, nervous system and gastrointestinal adverse reactions, but is otherwise generally well tolerated. TONOCARD has been evaluated in both short-term (n = 1,358) and long-term (n = 262) controlled studies as well as a compassionate use program. Dosages were lower in most of the controlled studies (1200 mg/day) and higher in the compassionate use program (1800 mg and more). In long-term (2–6 months) controlled studies, the most frequent adverse reactions were dizziness/vertigo (15.3 percent), nausea (14.5 percent), paresthesia (9.2 percent), and tremor (8.4 percent). These reactions are generally mild, transient, dose-related and reversible with a reduction in dosage, by taking the drug with food, or by therapy discontinuation. Tremor, when present, may be useful as a clinical indicator that the maximum dose is being approached. Adverse reactions leading to therapy discontinuation occurred in 21 percent of patients in long-term controlled trials and were usually related to the nervous system or digestive system.

Adverse reactions occurring in greater than one percent of patients from the short-term and long-term controlled studies appear in the following table: [See table at top of next column.]

An additional group of about 2,000 patients has been treated in a program allowing for the use of TONOCARD under compassionate use circumstances. These patients were seriously ill with the large majority on multiple drug therapy, and comparatively high doses of TONOCARD were used. Fifty-four percent of the patients continued in the program for one year or longer, and 12 percent were treated for longer than three years, with the longest duration of therapy being nine years. Adverse reactions leading to therapy discontinuation occurred in 12 percent of patients (usually central nervous system effects or rash). A tabulation of adverse reactions occurring in one percent or more of patients follows: [See second table at right.]

Adverse reactions occurring in less than one percent of patients in either the controlled studies or the compassionate use program or since the drug was marketed are as follows:

Body as a Whole: Septicemia; septic shock; syncope; vasovagal episodes; edema; fever; chills; cinchonism; asthenia; malaise.

Cardiovascular: Ventricular fibrillation; extension of acute myocardial infarction; cardiogenic shock; pulmonary embolism; angina; AV block; hypertension; claudication; increased QRS duration; pleurisy/pericarditis; prolonged QT interval; right bundle branch block; cardiomegaly; sinus arrest; vasculitis; orthostatic hypotension; cold extremities.

Digestive: Hepatitis, jaundice (see PRECAUTIONS), abnormal liver function tests; pancreatitis; abdominal pain/discomfort; constipation; dysphagia; gastrointestinal symptoms (including dyspepsia); stomatitis; dry mouth; thirst.

	Percent of Patients Controlled Studies	
	Short-term (n = 1,358)	Long-term (n = 262)
BODY AS A WHOLE		
Tiredness/drowsiness/fatigue/ lethargy/lassitude/ sleepiness	1.6	0.8
Hot/cold feelings	0.5	1.5
CARDIOVASCULAR		
Hypotension	3.4	2.7
Bradycardia	1.8	0.4
Palpitations	1.8	0.4
Chest pain	1.6	0.4
Conduction disorders	1.5	0.0
Left ventricular failure	1.4	0.0
DIGESTIVE		
Nausea	15.2	14.5
Vomiting	8.3	4.6
Anorexia	1.2	1.9
Diarrhea/loose stools	0.0	3.8
NERVOUS SYSTEM/PSYCHIATRIC		
Dizziness/vertigo	8.0	15.3
Paresthesia	3.5	9.2
Tremor	2.9	8.4
Confusion/disorientation/ hallucinations	2.1	2.7
Headache	2.1	4.6
Nervousness	1.5	0.4
Altered mood/awareness	1.5	3.4
Incoordination/unsteadiness/ walking disturbances	1.2	0.0
Anxiety	1.1	1.5
Ataxia	0.2	3.0
SKIN		
Diaphoresis	5.1	2.3
Rash/skin lesion	0.4	8.4
SPECIAL SENSES		
Blurred vision/visual disturbances	1.3	1.5
Tinnitus/hearing loss	0.4	1.5
Nystagmus	0.0	1.1

Hematologic: Agranulocytosis; bone marrow depression; aplastic/hypoplastic anemia; hemolytic anemia; anemia; leukopenia; neutropenia; thrombocytopenia; eosinophilia.

Metabolic and Immune: Hypersensitivity Reaction (including some of the following symptoms or signs: rash, fever, joint pains, abnormal liver function tests, eosinophilia); increased ANA.

Musculoskeletal: Muscle cramps; muscle twitching/spasm; neck pain; pain radiating from neck; pressure on shoulder.

Nervous System/Psychiatric: Coma; convulsions/seizures; myasthenia gravis; depression; psychosis; psychic disturbances; agitation; decreased mental acuity; dysarthria; impaired memory; increased stuttering/slurred speech; insomnia/sleeping disturbances; local anesthesia; dream abnormalities.

Respiratory: Respiratory arrest; pulmonary edema; pulmonary fibrosis; fibrosing alveolitis; pneumonia; interstitial pneumonitis; dyspnea; hiccough; yawning.

Skin: Stevens-Johnson syndrome; exfoliative dermatitis; erythema multiforme; urticaria; alopecia; pruritus; pallor/flushed face.

Special Senses: Diplopia; earache; taste perversion/smell perversion.

Urogenital: Urinary retention; polyuria/increased diuresis.

Agranulocytosis, bone marrow depression, leukopenia, neutropenia, aplastic/hypoplastic anemia, and thrombocytopenia have been reported (0.18 percent) in patients receiving TONOCARD in controlled trials and the compassionate use program. Most of these events have been noted during the first 12 weeks of therapy. (See Box WARNINGS.)

Pulmonary fibrosis, interstitial pneumonitis, fibrosing alveolitis, pulmonary edema, and pneumonia, possibly drug related, have been reported in patients receiving TONOCARD. The incidence of pulmonary fibrosis (including interstitial pneumonitis and fibrosing alveolitis) was 0.11 percent in controlled trials and the compassionate use program. These events usually occurred in seriously ill patients. Symptoms of these pulmonary disorders and/or x-ray changes usually occurred following 3–18 weeks of therapy. Fatalities have been reported. (See Box WARNINGS.)

A number of disorders, in which a causal relationship with TONOCARD has not been established, have been reported in seriously ill patients. These include: renal failure, renal dysfunction, myocardial infarction, cerebrovascular accidents and transient ischemic attacks. These disorders may be related to the patients underlying condition.

	Percent of Patients Compassionate Use (n = 1,927)
CARDIOVASCULAR	
Increased ventricular arrhythmias/PVCs	10.9
CHF/progression of CHF	4.0
Tachycardia	3.2
Hypotension	1.8
Conduction disorders	1.3
Bradycardia	1.0
DIGESTIVE	
Nausea	24.6
Anorexia	11.3
Vomiting	9.0
Diarrhea/loose stools	6.8
MUSCULOSKELETAL	
Arthritis/arthralgia	4.7
Myalgia	1.7
NERVOUS SYSTEM/PSYCHIATRIC	
Dizziness/vertigo	25.3
Tremor	21.6
Nervousness	11.5
Confusion/disorientation/ hallucinations	11.2
Altered mood/awareness	11.0
Ataxia	10.8
Paresthesia	9.2
SKIN	
Rash/skin lesion	12.2
Diaphoresis	8.3
Lupus	1.6
SPECIAL SENSES	
Blurred vision/vision disturbances	10.0
Nystagmus	1.1

DRUG ABUSE AND DEPENDENCE

Drug withdrawal after chronic treatment has not shown any indication of psychological or physical dependence.

OVERDOSAGE

The initial and most important signs and symptoms of overdosage would be expected to be related to the central nervous system. Other adverse reactions, such as gastrointestinal disturbances, may follow. (See ADVERSE REACTIONS). Should convulsions or cardiopulmonary depression or arrest develop, the patency of the airway and adequacy of ventilation must be assured immediately. Should convulsions persist despite ventilatory therapy with oxygen, small increments of anticonvulsive agents may be given intravenously. Examples of such agents include a benzodiazepine (e.g., diazepam), an ultra-short-acting barbiturate (e.g., thiopental or thiamylal), or a short-acting barbiturate (e.g., pentobarbital or secobarbital).

The oral LD_{50} of tocainide was calculated to be about 800 mg/kg in mice, 1000 mg/kg in rats, and 230 mg/kg in guinea pigs; deaths were usually preceded by convulsions.

Studies in normal individuals to date indicate that tocainide has a hemodialysis clearance approximately equivalent to its renal clearance.

DOSAGE AND ADMINISTRATION

The dosage of TONOCARD must be individualized on the basis of antiarrhythmic response and tolerance, both of which are dose related. Clinical and electrocardiographic evaluation (including Holter monitoring if necessary for evaluation) are needed to determine whether the desired antiarrhythmic response has been obtained and to guide titration and dose adjustment. Adverse effects appearing shortly after dosing, for example, suggest a need for dividing the dose further with a shorter dose-interval. Loss of arrhythmia control prior to the next dose suggests use of a shorter dose interval and/or a dose increase. Absence of a clear response suggests reconsideration of therapy.

The recommended initial dosage is 400 mg every 8 hours. The usual adult dosage is between 1200 and 1800 mg/day in a three dose daily divided regimen. Doses beyond 2400 mg per day have been administered infrequently. Patients who tolerate the t.i.d. regimen may be tried on a twice daily regimen with careful monitoring.

Some patients, particularly those with renal or hepatic impairment, may be adequately treated with less than 1200 mg/day.

Continued on next page

Merck & Co.—Cont.

HOW SUPPLIED

No. 3409—Tablets TONOCARD, 400 mg, are oval, yellow, scored, film-coated tablets, coded MSD 707. They are supplied as follows:
NDC 0006-0707-68 bottles of 100
(6505-01-203-6240 100's)
NDC 0006-0707-28 unit dose packages of 100.
Shown in Product Identification Section, page 420
No. 3410—Tablets TONOCARD, 600 mg, are oblong, yellow, scored, film-coated tablets, coded MSD 709. They are supplied as follows:
NDC 0006-0709-68 bottles of 100
(6505-01-206-0273 100's)
NDC 0006-0709-28 unit dose packages of 100.
Shown in Product Identification Section, page 420
A.H.F.S. Category: 24:04
DC 7369908 Issued June 1989
COPYRIGHT © MERCK & CO., INC., 1987, 1989
All rights reserved

TRIAVIL® Tablets ℞
(Perphenazine-Amitriptyline HCl), U.S.P.

DESCRIPTION

TRIAVIL* (Perphenazine-Amitriptyline HCl), a broad-spectrum psychotherapeutic agent for the management of outpatients and hospitalized patients with psychoses or neuroses characterized by mixtures of anxiety or agitation with symptoms of depression, is a combination of perphenazine and amitriptyline HCl. Since such mixed syndromes can occur in patients with various degrees of intensity of mental illness, TRIAVIL tablets are provided in multiple combinations to afford dosage flexibility for optimum management.
TRIAVIL is a combination of perphenazine, a piperazine phenothiazine, and amitriptyline HCl, a dibenzocycloheptadiene.
Perphenazine
Perphenazine is 4-[3-(2-chloro-10*H*-phenothiazin-10-yl)-propyl]-1-piperazineethanol. Its empirical formula is $C_{21}H_{26}ClN_3OS$ and its structural formula is:

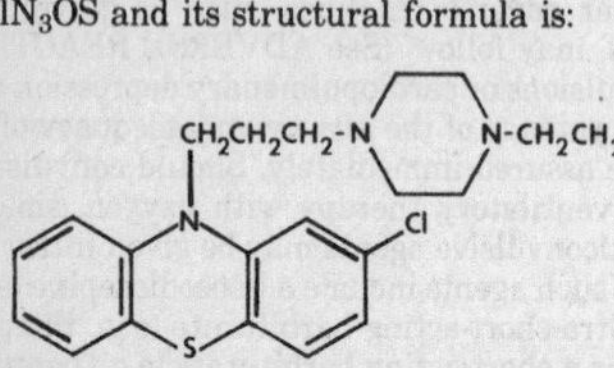

Perphenazine has a molecular weight of 403.97. It is a white, odorless, bitter-tasting powder that is insoluble in water.
Amitriptyline HCl
Amitriptyline hydrochloride is 3-(10,11-dihydro-5*H*-dibenzo[*a,d*]cyclohepten-5-ylidene)-*N,N*-dimethyl-1-propanamine hydrochloride. Its empirical formula is $C_{20}H_{23}N \cdot HCl$ and its structural formula is:

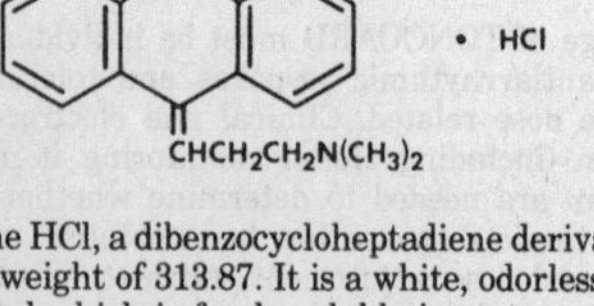

Amitriptyline HCl, a dibenzocycloheptadiene derivative, has a molecular weight of 313.87. It is a white, odorless, crystalline compound which is freely soluble in water.
Tablets TRIAVIL are supplied in 5 potencies:
TRIAVIL 2-10, containing 2 mg of perphenazine and 10 mg of amitriptyline HCl.
TRIAVIL 2-25, containing 2 mg of perphenazine and 25 mg of amitriptyline HCl.
TRIAVIL 4-10, containing 4 mg of perphenazine and 10 mg of amitriptyline HCl.
TRIAVIL 4-25, containing 4 mg of perphenazine and 25 mg of amitriptyline HCl.
TRIAVIL 4-50, containing 4 mg of perphenazine and 50 mg of amitriptyline HCl.
Inactive ingredients are calcium phosphate, cellulose, hydroxypropyl cellulose, hydroxypropyl methylcellulose, lactose, magnesium stearate, starch, talc, and titanium dioxide. TRIAVIL 2-10 also contains FD&C Blue 1. TRIAVIL 2-25 and 4-50 also contain FD&C Yellow 6. TRIAVIL 4-10 also contains iron oxide. TRIAVIL 4-25 also contains D&C Yellow 10 and FD&C Yellow 6.

*Registered trademark of MERCK & CO., INC.

ACTIONS

Perphenazine—In common with all members of the piperazine group of phenothiazine derivatives, perphenazine has greater behavioral potency than phenothiazine derivatives of other groups without a corresponding increase in autonomic, hematologic, or hepatic side effects.
Extrapyramidal effects, however, may occur more frequently. These effects are interpreted as neuropharmacologic. They usually regress after discontinuation of the drug.
Perphenazine is a potent tranquilizer and also a potent antiemetic. Orally, its milligram potency is about five or six times that of chlorpromazine with respect to behavorial effects. It is capable of alleviating symptoms of anxiety, tension, psychomotor excitement, and other manifestations of emotional stress without apparent dulling of mental acuity.
Amitriptyline HCl is an antidepressant with sedative effects. Its mechanism of action in man is not known. It is not a monoamine oxidase inhibitor and it does not act primarily by stimulation of the central nervous system.

INDICATIONS

TRIAVIL is recommended for treatment of (1) patients with *moderate to severe anxiety and/or agitation and depressed mood,* (2) patients with *depression in whom anxiety and/or agitation are severe,* and (3) patients with *depression and anxiety in association with chronic physical disease.* In many of these patients anxiety masks the depressive state so that, although therapy with a tranquilizer appears to be indicated, the administration of a tranquilizer alone will not be adequate.
Schizophrenic patients who have associated depressive symptoms should be considered for therapy with TRIAVIL.
Many patients presenting symptoms such as agitation, anxiety, insomnia, psychomotor retardation, functional somatic complaints, a feeling of tiredness, loss of interest, and anorexia have responded well to therapy with TRIAVIL.

CONTRAINDICATIONS

TRIAVIL is contraindicated in depression of the central nervous system from drugs (barbiturates, alcohol, narcotics, analgesics, antihistamines); in the presence of evidence of bone marrow depression; and in patients known to be hypersensitive to phenothiazines or amitriptyline.
It should not be given concomitantly with monoamine oxidase inhibitors. Hyperpyretic crises, severe convulsions, and deaths have occurred in patients receiving tricyclic antidepressants and monoamine oxidase inhibitors simultaneously. When it is desired to replace a monoamine oxidase inhibitor with TRIAVIL, a minimum of 14 days should be allowed to elapse after the former is discontinued. TRIAVIL should then be initiated cautiously with gradual increase in dosage until optimum response is achieved.
Amitriptyline HCl is not recommended for use during the acute recovery phase following myocardial infarction.

WARNINGS

Tardive dyskinesia
Tardive dyskinesia, a syndrome consisting of potentially irreversible, involuntary dyskinetic movements may develop in patients treated with neuroleptic (antipsychotic) drugs. Although the prevalence of the syndrome appears to be highest among the elderly, especially elderly women, it is impossible to rely upon prevalence estimates to predict, at the inception of neuroleptic treatment, which patients are likely to develop the syndrome. Whether neuroleptic drug products differ in their potential to cause tardive dyskinesia is unknown.
Both the risk of developing the syndrome and the likelihood that it will become irreversible are believed to increase as the duration of treatment and the total cumulative dose of neuroleptic drugs administered to the patient increase. However, the syndrome can develop, although much less commonly, after relatively brief treatment periods at low doses.
There is no known treatment for established cases of tardive dyskinesia, although the syndome may remit, partially or completely, if neuroleptic treatment is withdrawn. Neuroleptic treatment, itself, however, may suppress (or partially suppress) the signs and symptoms of the syndrome and thereby may possibly mask the underlying disease process. The effect that symptomatic suppression has upon the long-term course of the syndrome is unknown.
Given these considerations, neuroleptics should be prescribed in a manner that is most likely to minimize the occurrence of tardive dyskinesia. Chronic neuroleptic treatment should generally be reserved for patients who suffer from a chronic mental illness that, 1) is known to respond to neuroleptic drugs, and, 2) for whom alternative, equally effective, but potentially less harmful treatments are *not* available or appropriate. In patients who do require chronic treatment, the smallest dose and the shortest duration of treatment producing a satisfactory clinical response should be sought. The need for continued treatment should be reassessed periodically.
If signs and symptoms of tardive dyskinesia appear in a patient on neuroleptics, drug discontinuation should be considered. However, some patients may require treatment despite the presence of the syndrome.
(For further information about the description of tardive dyskinesia and its clinical detection, please refer to the section on ADVERSE REACTIONS).
Neuroleptic Malignant Syndrome (NMS)
A potentially fatal symptom complex sometimes referred to as Neuroleptic Malignant Syndrome (NMS) has been reported in association with antipsychotic drugs. Clinical manifestations of NMS are hyperpyrexia, muscle rigidity, altered mental status and evidence of autonomic instability (irregular pulse or blood pressure, tachycardia, diaphoresis, and cardiac dysrhythmias).
The diagnostic evaluation of patients with this syndrome is complicated. In arriving at a diagnosis, it is important to identify cases where the clinical presentation includes both serious medical illness (e.g., pneumonia, systemic infection, etc.) and untreated or inadequately treated extrapyramidal signs and symptoms (EPS). Other important considerations in the differential diagnosis include central anticholinergic toxicity, heat stroke, drug fever and primary central nervous system (CNS) pathology.
The management of NMS should include 1) immediate discontinuation of antipsychotic drugs and other drugs not essential to concurrent therapy, 2) intensive symptomatic treatment and medical monitoring, and 3) treatment of any concomitant serious medical problems for which specific treatments are available. There is no general agreement about specific pharmacological treatment regimens for uncomplicated NMS.
If a patient requires antipsychotic drug treatment after recovery from NMS, the potential reintroduction of drug therapy should be carefully considered. The patient should be carefully monitored, since recurrences of NMS have been reported.
General
TRIAVIL should not be given concomitantly with guanethidine or similarly acting compounds, since amitriptyline, like other tricyclic antidepressants, may block the antihypertensive effect of these compounds.
Because of the atropine-like activity of amitriptyline, TRIAVIL should be used with caution in patients with a history of urinary retention, or with angle-closure glaucoma or increased intraocular pressure. In patients with angle-closure glaucoma, even average doses may precipitate an attack.
It should be used with caution also in patients with convulsive disorders. Dosage of anticonvulsive agents may have to be increased.
Patients with cardiovascular disorders should be watched closely. Tricyclic antidepressants, including amitriptyline HCl, particularly when given in high doses, have been reported to produce arrhythmias, sinus tachycardia, and prolongation of the conduction time. Myocardial infarction and stroke have been reported with drugs of this class.
Close supervision is required when amitriptyline HCl is given to hyperthyroid patients or those receiving thyroid medication.
TRIAVIL may enhance the response to alcohol and the effects of barbiturates and other CNS depressants. In patients who may use alcohol excessively, it should be borne in mind that the potentiation may increase the danger inherent in any suicide attempt or overdosage. Delirium has been reported with concurrent administration of amitriptyline and disulfiram.
Usage in Pregnancy—TRIAVIL is not recommended for use in pregnant patients or in nursing mothers at this time. Reproduction studies in rats have shown no fetal abnormalities; however, clinical experience and follow-up in pregnancy have been limited, and the possibility of adverse effects on fetal development must be considered.
Usage in Children—Since dosage for children has not been established, TRIAVIL is not recommended for use in children.

PRECAUTIONS

General
The possibility of suicide in depressed patients remains during treatment and until significant remission occurs. Such patients should not have access to large quantities of this drug.

Perphenazine
As with all phenothiazine compounds, perphenazine should not be used indiscriminately. Caution should be observed in giving it to patients who have previously exhibited severe adverse reactions to other phenothiazines.
Some of the untoward actions of perphenazine tend to appear more frequently when high doses are used. However, as with other phenothiazine compounds, patients receiving perphenazine in any dosage should be kept under close supervision.

The antiemetic effect of perphenazine may obscure signs of toxicity due to overdosage of other drugs, or render more difficult the diagnosis of disorders such as brain tumors or intestinal obstruction.
A significant, not otherwise explained, rise in body temperature may suggest individual intolerance to perphenazine, in which case TRIAVIL should be discontinued.
Neuroleptic drugs elevate prolactin levels; the elevation persists during chronic administration. Tissue culture experiments indicate that approximately one third of human breast cancers are prolactin dependent *in vitro*, a factor of potential importance if the prescription of these drugs is contemplated in a patient with a previously detected breast cancer. Although disturbances such as galactorrhea, amenorrhea, gynecomastia, and impotence have been reported, the clinical significance of elevated serum prolactin levels is unknown for most patients. An increase in mammary neoplasms has been found in rodents after chronic administration of neuroleptic drugs. Neither clinical studies nor epidemiologic studies conducted to date, however, have shown an association between chronic administration of these drugs and mammary tumorigenesis; the available evidence is considered too limited to be conclusive at this time.

Amitriptyline HCl
Depressed patients, particularly those with known manic depressive illness, may experience a shift to mania or hypomania. Patients with paranoid symptomatology may have an exaggeration of such symptoms. The tranquilizing effect of TRIAVIL seems to reduce the likelihood of these effects.
Concurrent administration of amitriptyline HCl and electroshock therapy may increase the hazards associated with such therapy. Such treatment should be limited to patients for whom it is essential.
Discontinue the drug several days before elective surgery if possible.
Both elevation and lowering of blood sugar levels have been reported.
Amitriptyline HCl should be used with caution in patients with impaired liver function.
Information for Patients
While on therapy with TRIAVIL, patients should be advised as to the possible impairment of mental and/or physical abilities required for performance of hazardous tasks, such as operating machinery or driving a motor vehicle.
Drug Interactions
Perphenazine
If hypotension develops, epinephrine should not be employed, as its action is blocked and partially reversed by perphenazine.
Phenothiazines may potentiate the action of central nervous system depressants (opiates, analgesics, antihistamines, barbiturates, alcohol) and atropine. In concurrent therapy with any of these, TRIAVIL should be given in reduced dosage. Phenothiazines also may potentiate the action of heat and phosphorous insecticides.
Amitriptyline HCl
When amitriptyline HCl is given with anticholinergic agents or sympathomimetic drugs, including epinephrine combined with local anesthetics, close supervision and careful adjustment of dosages are required.
Hyperpyrexia has been reported when amitriptyline HCl is administered with anticholinergic agents or with neuroleptic drugs, particularly during hot weather.
Paralytic ileus may occur in patients taking tricyclic antidepressants in combination with anticholinergic-type drugs.
Cimetidine is reported to reduce hepatic metabolism of certain tricyclic antidepressants, thereby delaying elimination and increasing steady-state concentrations of these drugs. Clinically significant effects have been reported with the tricyclic antidepressants when used concomitantly with cimetidine. Increases in plasma levels of tricyclic antidepressants, and in the frequency and severity of side effects, particularly anticholinergic, have been reported when cimetidine was added to the drug regimen. Discontinuation of cimetidine in well-controlled patients receiving tricyclic antidepressants and cimetidine may decrease the plasma levels and efficacy of the antidepressants.
Caution is advised if patients receive large doses of ethchlorvynol concurrently. Transient delirium has been reported in patients who were treated with 1 g of ethchlorvynol and 75-150 mg of amitriptyline HCl.

ADVERSE REACTIONS

To date, clinical evaluation of TRIAVIL has not revealed any adverse reactions peculiar to the combination. The adverse reactions that occurred were limited to those that have been reported previously for perphenazine and amitriptyline.
Treatment with TRIAVIL is commonly associated with sedation, hypotension, neurological impairments, and dry mouth.
Perphenazine
The common acute neurological effects of neuroleptic drugs, including perphenazine, consist of dystonia, akathisia or motor restlessness, and pseudoparkinsonism.
More chronic use of neuroleptics may be associated with the development of tardive dyskinesia. The salient features of this syndrome are described in the WARNINGS section and below.
The following adverse reactions have been reported and, within each category, are listed in order of decreasing severity.
Neurological:
Tardive dyskinesia:
The syndrome is characterized by involuntary choreoathetoid movements which variously involve the tongue, face, mouth, lips, or jaw (e.g., protrusion of the tongue, puffing of cheeks, puckering of the mouth, chewing movements), trunk and extremities. The severity of the syndrome and the degree of impairment produced vary widely.
The syndrome may become clinically recognizable either during treatment, upon dosage reduction, or upon withdrawal of treatment. Movements may decrease in intensity and may disappear altogether if further treatment with neuroleptics is withheld. It is generally believed that reversibility is more likely after short rather than long term neuroleptic exposure. Consequently, early detection of tardive dyskinesia is important. To increase the likelihood of detecting the syndrome at the earliest possible time, the dosage of neuroleptic drug should be reduced periodically (if clinically possible) and the patient observed for signs of the disorder. It has been suggested that fine vermicular movements of the tongue may be an early sign of the syndrome, and that the full-blown syndrome may not develop if medication is stopped when lingual vermiculation appears.
1. Dystonia
This may present as acute, reversible torticollis, opisthotonos, carpopedal spasm, trismus, dysphagia, respiratory difficulty, oculogyric crisis, and protrusion of the tongue. Treatment consists of the parenteral administration of either an anticholinergic antiparkinsonian agent or diphenhydramine.
2. Akathisia
Akathisia presents as constant motor restlessness. The patient with akathisia often complains, *when asked*, about his/her inability to stop moving. Akathisia should *not* be treated with an increased dose of neuroleptic; rather, the dose of antipsychotic may be lowered until the motor restlessness has subsided. The efficacy of anticholinergic treatment of this side effect is unestablished.
3. Pseudoparkinsonism
Pseudoparkinsonism refers to a drug-induced state similar to the classic syndrome. Generally, anticholinergic antiparkinsonian agents (i.e., benztropine, biperiden, procyclidine, or trihexphenidyl) and amantadine are helpful in alleviating symptoms that cannot be managed by neuroleptic dose reduction. The value of prophylactic antiparkinsonian drug therapy has not been established. The need for continued use of antiparkinsonian medication should be re-evaluated periodically.
Cardiovascular: Hypotension, hypertension, tachycardia, peripheral edema, occasional change in pulse rate, ECG abnormalities (quinidine-like effect), reversed epinephrine effect.
CNS and Neuromuscular: Neuroleptic malignant syndrome (see WARNINGS); extrapyramidal symptoms, including acute dyskinesia (see *Neurological*); reactivation of psychoses and production of catatonic-like states; paradoxical excitement; ataxia; muscle weakness; hypnotic effects; mild insomnia; lassitude; headache; hyperflexia; altered cerebrospinal fluid proteins.
Autonomic: Urinary frequency or incontinence, dry mouth or salivation, nasal congestion.
Allergic: Anaphylactoid reactions, laryngeal edema, asthma, angioneurotic edema.
Hematologic: Blood dyscrasias including pancytopenia, agranulocytosis, leukopenia, thrombocytopenic purpura, eosinophilia.
Gastrointestinal: Liver damage (jaundice, biliary stasis), obstipation, vomiting, nausea, constipation, anorexia.
Dermatologic: Eczema up to exfoliative dermatitis, urticaria, erythema, itching, photosensitivity.
Ophthalmic: Pigmentation of the cornea and lens, blurred vision.
Endocrine: Lactation, galactorrhea, hyperglycemia, gynecomastia, disturbances in menstrual cycle.
Other: False-positive pregnancy tests, including immunologic.
Other adverse reactions that should be considered because they have been reported with various phenothiazine compounds, but not with perphenazine, include:
CNS and Neuromuscular: Grand mal convulsions, cerebral edema.
Gastrointestinal: Polyphagia.
Dermatologic: Photophobia, pigmentation.
Ophthalmic: Pigmentary retinopathy.
Endocrine: Failure of ejaculation.
Amitriptyline HCl
Within each category the following adverse reactions are listed in order of decreasing severity. Included in the listing are a few adverse reactions which have not been reported with this specific drug. However, pharmacological similarities among the tricyclic antidepressant drugs require that each of the reactions be considered when amitriptyline is administered.
Cardiovascular: Myocardial infarction; stroke; heart block; arrhythmias; hypotension, particularly orthostatic hypotension; hypertension; tachycardia; palpitation.
CNS and Neuromuscular: Coma; seizures; hallucinations; delusions; confusional states; disorientation; incoordination; ataxia; tremors; peripheral neuropathy; numbness, tingling, and paresthesias of the extremities; extrapyramidal symptoms; dysarthria; disturbed concentration; excitement; anxiety; insomnia; restlessness; nightmares; drowsiness; dizziness; weakness; fatigue; headache; syndrome of inappropriate ADH (antidiuretic hormone) secretion; tinnitus; alteration in EEG patterns.
Anticholinergic: Paralytic ileus; hyperpyrexia; urinary retention, dilatation of the urinary tract; constipation; blurred vision, disturbance of accommodation, increased intraocular pressure, mydriasis; dry mouth.
Allergic: Skin rash; urticaria; photosensitization; edema of face and tongue.
Hematologic: Bone marrow depression including agranulocytosis, leukopenia, thrombocytopenia; purpura; eosinophilia.
Gastrointestinal: Rarely hepatitis (including altered liver function and jaundice); nausea; epigastric distress; vomiting; anorexia; stomatitis; peculiar taste; diarrhea; parotid swelling; black tongue.
Endocrine: Testicular swelling and gynecomastia in the male; breast enlargement and galactorrhea in the female; increased or decreased libido; elevation and lowering of blood sugar levels.
Other: Alopecia; edema; weight gain or loss; urinary frequency; increased perspiration.
Withdrawal Symptoms: After prolonged administration, abrupt cessation of treatment may produce nausea, headache, and malaise. Gradual dosage reduction has been reported to produce within two weeks, transient symptoms including irritability, restlessness, and dream and sleep disturbance. These symptoms are not indicative of addiction. Rare instances have been reported of mania or hypomania occurring within 2-7 days following cessation of chronic therapy wih tricyclic antidepressants.

DOSAGE AND ADMINISTRATION

Since dosage for children has not been established, TRIAVIL is not recommended for use in children.
The total daily dose of TRIAVIL should not exceed four tablets of the 4-50 or eight tablets of any other dosage strength.

Initial Dosage
In psychoneurotic patients when anxiety and depression are of such a degree as to warrant combined therapy, one tablet of TRIAVIL 2-25 or TRIAVIL 4-25 three or four times a day or one tablet of TRIAVIL 4-50 twice a day is recommended.
In more severely ill patients with schizophrenia, TRIAVIL 4-25 is recommended in an initial dose of two tablets three times a day. If necessary, a fourth dose may be given at bedtime.
In elderly patients and adolescents, and some other patients in whom anxiety tends to predominate, TRIAVIL 4-10 may be administered three or four times a day initially, then adjusted as required for subsequent adequate therapy.

Maintenance Dosage
Depending on the condition being treated, therapeutic response may take from a few days to a few weeks or even longer. After a satisfactory response is noted, dosage should be reduced to the smallest amount necessary to obtain relief from the symptoms for which TRIAVIL is being administered. A useful maintenance dosage is one tablet of TRIAVIL 2-25 or 4-25 two to four times a day or one tablet of TRIAVIL 4-50 twice a day. TRIAVIL 2-10 and 4-10 can be used to increase flexibility in adjusting maintenance dosage to the lowest amount consistent with relief of symptoms. In some patients, maintenance dosage is required for many months.

OVERDOSAGE

Manifestations—High doses may cause temporary confusion, disturbed concentration, or transient visual hallucinations. Overdosage may cause drowsiness; hypothermia; tachycardia and other arrhythmic abnormalities, such as bundle branch block; ECG evidence of impaired conduction; congestive heart failure; dilated pupils; disorders of ocular motility; convulsions; severe hypotension; stupor; and coma. Other symptoms may be agitation, hyperactive reflexes, muscle

Continued on next page

Information on the Merck & Co. products listed on these pages is the full prescribing information from product circulars in use October 1, 1992.

Merck & Co.—Cont.

rigidity, vomiting, hyperpyrexia, or any of the adverse reactions listed for perphenazine or amitriptyline.
Levarterenol (norepinephrine) may be used to treat hypotension, but not epinephrine.
All patients suspected of having taken an overdosage should be admitted to a hospital as soon as possible. *Treatment* is symptomatic and supportive. Empty the stomach as quickly as possible by emesis followed by gastric lavage upon arrival at the hospital. Saline emetics should not be used as the antiemetic effect of perphenazine may cause retention of the saline load and subsequent hypernatremia. Following gastric lavage, activated charcoal may be administered. Twenty to 30 g of activated charcoal may be given every four to six hours during the first 24 to 48 hours after ingestion. An ECG should be taken and close monitoring of cardiac function instituted if there is any sign of abnormality. Maintain an open airway and adequate fluid intake; regulate body temperature.
The intravenous administration of 1–3 mg of physostigmine salicylate is reported to reverse the symptoms of tricyclic antidepressant poisoning. Because physostigmine is rapidly metabolized, the dosage of physostigmine should be repeated as required particularly if life threatening signs such as arrhythmias, convulsions, and deep coma recur or persist after the initial dosage of physostigmine. On this basis, in severe overdosage with perphenazine-amitriptyline combinations, symptomatic treatment of central anticholinergic effects with physostigmine salicylate should be considered. Because physostigmine itself may be toxic, it is not recommended for routine use.
Standard measures should be used to manage circulatory shock and metabolic acidosis. Cardiac arrhythmias may be treated with neostigmine, pyridostigmine, or propranolol. Should cardiac failure occur, the use of digitalis should be considered. Close monitoring of cardiac function for not less than five days is advisable.
Anticonvulsants may be given to control convulsions. Amitriptyline and perphenazine increase the CNS depressant action but not the anticonvulsant action of barbiturates; therefore, an inhalation anesthetic, diazepam, or paraldehyde is recommended for control of convulsions. The management of acute symptoms of parkinsonism resulting from perphenazine intoxication may be treated with appropriate doses of COGENTIN* (Benztropine Mesylate) or diphenhydramine hydrochloride.**
Dialysis is of no value because of low plasma concentrations of the drug.
Since overdosage is often deliberate, patients may attempt suicide by other means during the recovery phase.
Deaths by deliberate or accidental overdosage have occurred with this class of drugs.

* Registered trademark of MERCK & CO., INC.
** BENADRYL® (Diphenhydramine Hydrochloride), Parke, Davis & Co.

HOW SUPPLIED

No. 3328—Tablets TRIAVIL 2–10 are blue, triangular, film coated tablets, coded MSD 914. They are supplied as follows:
NDC 0006-0914-68 bottles of 100
NDC 0006-0914-28 unit dose package of 100
NDC 0006-0914-74 bottles of 500.
Shown in Product Identification Section, page 420
No. 3311—Tablets TRIAVIL 2–25 are orange, triangular, film coated tablets, coded MSD 921. They are supplied as follows:
NDC 0006-0921-68 bottles of 100
NDC 0006-0921-28 unit dose package of 100
NDC 0006-0921-74 bottles of 500.
(6505-01-210-4467 500's)
Shown in Product Identification Section, page 420
No. 3310—Tablets TRIAVIL 4–10 are salmon, triangular, film coated tablets, coded MSD 934. They are supplied as follows:
NDC 0006-0934-68 bottles of 100
NDC 0006-0934-74 bottles of 500.
Shown in Product Identification Section, page 420
No. 3312—Tablets TRIAVIL 4–25 are yellow, triangular, film coated tablets, coded MSD 946. They are supplied as follows:
NDC 0006-0946-68 bottles of 100
(6505-01-210-4468 100's)
NDC 0006-0946-28 unit dose package of 100
NDC 0006-0946-74 bottles of 500.
Shown in Product Identification Section, page 420
No. 3364—Tablets TRIAVIL 4-50 are orange, diamond shaped, film coated tablets, coded MSD 517. They are supplied as follows:
NDC 0006-0517-60 bottles of 60
NDC 0006-0517-68 bottles of 100.
Shown in Product Identification Section, page 420
Storage
Store Tablets TRIAVIL in a well-closed container. Avoid storage at temperatures above 40°C (104°F). In addition, Tablets TRIAVIL 2–10 must be protected from light and stored in a well-closed, light-resistant container.
A.H.F.S. Categories: 28:16:04, 28:16:08
DC 7398431 Issued September 1990
COPYRIGHT © MERCK & CO., INC., 1985
All rights reserved

TURBINAIRE®—see under DECADRON® Phosphate, TURBINAIRE® (Dexamethasone Sodium Phosphate)

URECHOLINE® Tablets ℞
(Bethanechol Chloride), U.S.P.
URECHOLINE® Injection ℞
(Bethanechol Chloride), U.S.P.

DESCRIPTION

URECHOLINE* (Bethanechol Chloride), a cholinergic agent, is a synthetic ester which is structurally and pharmacologically related to acetylcholine.
It is designated chemically as 2-[(aminocarbonyl)oxy]-*N, N, N*-trimethyl-1-propanaminium chloride. Its empirical formula is $C_7H_{17}ClN_2O_2$ and its structural formula is:

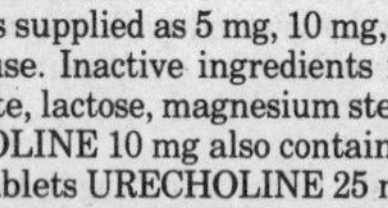

It is a white, hygroscopic crystalline compound having a slight amine-like odor, freely soluble in water, and has a molecular weight of 196.68.
URECHOLINE is supplied as 5 mg, 10 mg, 25 mg, and 50 mg tablets for oral use. Inactive ingredients in the tablets are calcium phosphate, lactose, magnesium stearate, and starch. Tablets URECHOLINE 10 mg also contain FD&C Red 3 and FD&C Red 40. Tablets URECHOLINE 25 mg and 50 mg also contain D&C Yellow 10 and FD&C Yellow 6.
URECHOLINE is also supplied as a sterile solution **for subcutaneous use only.** The sterile solution is essentially neutral. Each milliliter contains bethanechol chloride, 5 mg, and Water for Injection, q.s., 1 mL. It may be autoclaved at 120° C for 20 minutes without discoloration or loss of potency.

*Registered trademark of MERCK & CO., INC.

CLINICAL PHARMACOLOGY

Bethanechol chloride acts principally by producing the effects of stimulation of the parasympathetic nervous system. It increases the tone of the detrusor urinae muscle, usually producing a contraction sufficiently strong to initiate micturition and empty the bladder. It stimulates gastric motility, increases gastric tone, and often restores impaired rhythmic peristalsis.
Stimulation of the parasympathetic nervous system releases acetylcholine at the nerve endings. When spontaneous stimulation is reduced and therapeutic intervention is required, acetylcholine can be given, but it is rapidly hydrolyzed by cholinesterase, and its effects are transient. Bethanechol chloride is not destroyed by cholinesterase and its effects are more prolonged than those of acetylcholine.
Effects on the GI and urinary tracts sometimes appear within 30 minutes after oral administration of bethanechol chloride, but more often 60–90 minutes are required to reach maximum effectiveness. Following oral administration, the usual duration of action of bethanechol is one hour, although large doses (300–400 mg) have been reported to produce effects for up to six hours. Subcutaneous injection produces a more intense action on bladder muscle than does oral administration of the drug.
Because of the selective action of bethanechol, nicotinic symptoms of cholinergic stimulation are usually absent or minimal when orally or subcutaneously administered in therapeutic doses, while muscarinic effects are prominent. Muscarinic effects usually occur within 5–15 minutes after subcutaneous injection, reach a maximum in 15–30 minutes, and disappear within two hours. Doses that stimulate micturition and defecation and increase peristalsis do not ordinarily stimulate ganglia or voluntary muscles. Therapeutic test doses in normal human subjects have little effect on heart rate, blood pressure, or peripheral circulation.
Bethanechol chloride does not cross the blood-brain barrier because of its charged quaternary amine moiety. The metabolic fate and mode of excretion of the drug have not been elucidated.
A clinical study* was conducted on the relative effectiveness of oral and subcutaneous doses of bethanechol chloride on the stretch response of bladder muscle in patients with urinary retention. Results showed that 5 mg of the drug given subcutaneously stimulated a response that was more rapid in onset and of larger magnitude than an oral dose of 50 mg, 100 mg, or 200 mg. All the oral doses, however, had a longer duration of effect than the subcutaneous dose. Although the 50 mg oral dose caused little change in intravesical pressure in this study, this dose has been found in other studies to be clinically effective in the rehabilitation of patients with decompensated bladders.

*Diokno, A. C.; Lapides, J., Urol. *10:* 23–24, July 1977.

INDICATIONS AND USAGE

For the treatment of acute postoperative and postpartum nonobstructive (functional) urinary retention and for neurogenic atony of the urinary bladder with retention.

CONTRAINDICATIONS

Hypersensitivity to URECHOLINE tablets or to any component of URECHOLINE injection, hyperthyroidism, peptic ulcer, latent or active bronchial asthma, pronounced bradycardia or hypotension, vasomotor instability, coronary artery disease, epilepsy, and parkinsonism.
URECHOLINE should not be employed when the strength or integrity of the gastrointestinal or bladder wall is in question, or in the presence of mechanical obstruction; when increased muscular activity of the gastrointestinal tract or urinary bladder might prove harmful, as following recent urinary bladder surgery, gastrointestinal resection and anastomosis, or when there is possible gastrointestinal obstruction; in bladder neck obstruction, spastic gastrointestinal disturbances, acute inflammatory lesions of the gastrointestinal tract, or peritonitis; or in marked vagotonia.

WARNING

The sterile solution is for subcutaneous use only. It should never be given intramuscularly or intravenously. Violent symptoms of cholinergic over-stimulation, such as circulatory collapse, fall in blood pressure, abdominal cramps, bloody diarrhea, shock, or sudden cardiac arrest are likely to occur if the drug is given by either of these routes. Although rare, these same symptoms have occurred after subcutaneous injection, and may occur in cases of hypersensitivity or overdosage.

PRECAUTIONS

General
In urinary retention, if the sphincter fails to relax as URECHOLINE contracts the bladder, urine may be forced up the ureter into the kidney pelvis. If there is bacteriuria, this may cause reflux infection.
Information for Patients
URECHOLINE tablets should preferably be taken one hour before or two hours after meals to avoid nausea or vomiting. Dizziness, lightheadedness or fainting may occur, especially when getting up from a lying or sitting position.
Drug Interactions
Special care is required if this drug is given to patients receiving ganglion blocking compounds because a critical fall in blood pressure may occur. Usually, severe abdominal symptoms appear before there is such a fall in the blood pressure.
Carcinogenesis, Mutagenesis, Impairment of Fertility
Long-term studies in animals have not been performed to evaluate the effects upon fertility, mutagenic or carcinogenic potential of URECHOLINE.
Pregnancy
Pregnancy Category C. Animal reproduction studies have not been conducted with URECHOLINE. It is also not known whether URECHOLINE can cause fetal harm when administered to a pregnant woman or can affect reproduction capacity. URECHOLINE should be given to a pregnant woman only if clearly needed.
Nursing Mothers
It is not known whether this drug is secreted in human milk. Because many drugs are secreted in human milk and because of the potential for serious adverse reactions from URECHOLINE in nursing infants, a decision should be made whether to discontinue nursing or to discontinue the drug, taking into account the importance of the drug to the mother.
Pediatric Use
Safety and effectiveness in children have not been established.

ADVERSE REACTIONS

Adverse reactions are rare following oral administration of bethanechol, but are more common following subcutaneous

injection. Adverse reactions are more likely to occur when dosage is increased.
The following adverse reactions have been observed: *Body as a Whole:* malaise; *Digestive:* abdominal cramps or discomfort, colicky pain, nausea and belching, diarrhea, borborygmi, salivation; *Renal:* urinary urgency; *Nervous System:* headache; *Cardiovascular:* a fall in blood pressure with reflex tachycardia, vasomotor response; *Skin:* flushing producing a feeling of warmth, sensation of heat about the face, sweating; *Respiratory:* bronchial constriction, asthmatic attacks; *Special Senses:* lacrimation, miosis.

OVERDOSAGE

Early signs of overdosage are abdominal discomfort, salivation, flushing of the skin ("hot feeling"), sweating, nausea and vomiting.
Atropine is a specific antidote. The recommended dose for adults is 0.6 mg (1/100 grain). Repeat doses can be given every two hours, according to clinical response. The recommended dosage in infants and children up to 12 years of age is 0.01 mg/kg (to a maximum single dose of 0.4 mg) repeated every two hours as needed until the desired effect is obtained, or adverse effects of atropine preclude further usage. Subcutaneous injection of atropine is preferred except in emergencies when the intravenous route may be employed.
When URECHOLINE is administered subcutaneously, a syringe containing a dose of atropine sulfate should always be available to treat symptoms of toxicity.
The oral LD_{50} of bethanechol chloride is 1510 mg/kg in the mouse.

DOSAGE AND ADMINISTRATION

Dosage and route of administration must be individualized, depending on the type and severity of the condition to be treated.
Preferably give the drug when the stomach is empty. If taken soon after eating, nausea and vomiting may occur.
Oral—The usual adult dosage is 10 to 50 mg three or four times a day. The minimum effective dose is determined by giving 5 or 10 mg initially and repeating the same amount at hourly intervals until satisfactory response occurs or until a maximum of 50 mg has been given. The effects of the drug sometimes appear within 30 minutes and usually within 60 to 90 minutes. They persist for about an hour.
Subcutaneous—The usual dose is 1 mL (5 mg), although some patients respond satisfactorily to as little as 0.5 mL (2.5 mg). The minimum effective dose is determined by injecting 0.5 mL (2.5 mg) initially and repeating the same amount at 15 to 30 minute intervals to a maximum of four doses until satisfactory response is obtained, unless disturbing reactions appear. The minimum effective dose may be repeated thereafter three or four times a day as required.
Rarely, single doses up to 2 mL (10 mg) may be required. Such large doses may cause severe reactions and should be used only after adequate trial of single doses of 0.5 to 1 mL (2.5 to 5 mg) has established that smaller doses are not sufficient.
URECHOLINE is usually effective in 5 to 15 minutes after subcutaneous injection.
If necessary, the effects of the drug can be abolished promptly by atropine (see OVERDOSAGE).
Parenteral drug products should be inspected visually for particulate matter and discoloration prior to administration, whenever solution and container permit.

HOW SUPPLIED

Tablets URECHOLINE are round, compressed tablets, scored on one side. They are supplied as follows:
No. 7785—5 mg, white in color, coded MSD 403.
NDC 0006-0403-68 in bottles of 100
NDC 0006-0403-28 unit dose packages of 100.
Shown in Product Identification Section, page 420
No. 7787—10 mg, pink in color, coded MSD 412.
NDC 0006-0412-68 in bottles of 100
(6505-00-616-7856 10 mg 100's)
NDC 0006-0412-28 unit dose packages of 100.
(6505-01-153-3547, 10 mg individually sealed 100's).
Shown in Product Identification Section, page 420
No. 7788—25 mg, yellow in color, coded MSD 457.
NDC 0006-0457-68 in bottles of 100
NDC 0006-0457-28 unit dose packages of 100.
Shown in Product Identification Section, page 420
No. 7790 — 50 mg, yellow in color, coded MSD 460.
NDC 0006-0460-68 in bottles of 100
NDC 0006-0460-28 in unit dose packages of 100.
Shown in Product Identification Section, page 420
No. 7786—Injection URECHOLINE, 5 mg per mL, is a clear, colorless solution, and is supplied as follows:
NDC 0006-7786-29 in box of 6 × 1 mL vials
(6505-00-616-8947 in box of 6 × 1 mL vials).
Storage
Store Tablets URECHOLINE in a tightly-closed container. Avoid storage at temperatures above 40°C (104°F).
Avoid storage of Injection URECHOLINE at temperatures below −20°C (−4°F) and above 40°C (104°F).
A.H.F.S. Category: 12:04
DC 6208430 Issued May 1986
COPYRIGHT © MERCK & CO., INC., 1984
All rights reserved

VASERETIC® Tablets ℞
(Enalapril Maleate-Hydrochlorothiazide)

USE IN PREGNANCY
When used in pregnancy during the second and third trimesters, ACE inhibitors can cause injury and even death to the developing fetus. When pregnancy is detected, VASERETIC should be discontinued as soon as possible. See WARNINGS, *Pregnancy, Enalapril Maleate, Fetal/Neonatal Morbidity and Mortality.*

DESCRIPTION

VASERETIC* (Enalapril Maleate-Hydrochlorothiazide) combines an angiotensin converting enzyme inhibitor, enalapril maleate, and a diuretic, hydrochlorothiazide.
Enalapril maleate is the maleate salt of enalapril, the ethyl ester of a long-acting angiotensin converting enzyme inhibitor, enalaprilat. Enalapril maleate is chemically described as (*S*)-1-[*N*-[1-(ethoxycarbonyl)-3-phenylpropyl]-L-alanyl]-L-proline, (*Z*)-2-butenedioate salt (1:1). Its empirical formula is $C_{20}H_{28}N_2O_5 \cdot C_4H_4O_4$, and its structural formula is:

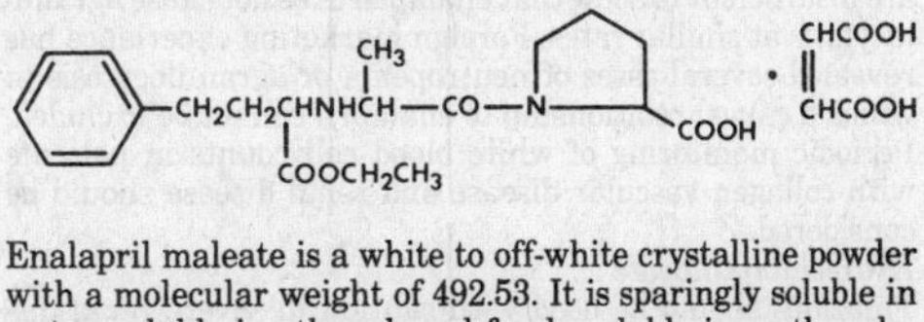

Enalapril maleate is a white to off-white crystalline powder with a molecular weight of 492.53. It is sparingly soluble in water, soluble in ethanol, and freely soluble in methanol.
Enalapril is a pro-drug; following oral administration, it is bioactivated by hydrolysis of the ethyl ester to enalaprilat, which is the active angiotensin converting enzyme inhibitor.
Hydrochlorothiazide is 6-chloro-3,4-dihydro-2*H*-1,2,4-benzothiadiazine-7-sulfonamide 1,1-dioxide. Its empirical formula is $C_7H_8ClN_3O_4S_2$ and its structural formula is:

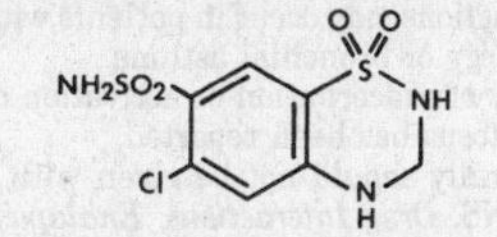

It is a white, or practically white, crystalline powder with a molecular weight of 297.72, which is slightly soluble in water, but freely soluble in sodium hydroxide solution.
VASERETIC is available for oral use as tablets containing 10 mg of enalapril maleate, 25 mg of hydrochlorothiazide and the following inactive ingredients: iron oxides, lactose, magnesium stearate, starch and other ingredients.

*Registered trademark of MERCK & CO., INC.

CLINICAL PHARMACOLOGY

As a result of its diuretic effects, hydrochlorothiazide increases plasma renin activity, increases aldosterone secretion, and decreases serum potassium. Administration of enalapril maleate blocks the renin-angiotensin-aldosterone axis and tends to reverse the potassium loss associated with the diuretic.
In clinical studies, the extent of blood pressure reduction seen with the combination of enalapril maleate and hydrochlorothiazide was approximately additive. The antihypertensive effect of VASERETIC was usually sustained for at least 24 hours.
Concomitant administration of enalapril maleate and hydrochlorothiazide has little, or no effect on the bioavailability of either drug. The combination tablet is bioequivalent to concomitant administration of the separate entities.
Enalapril Maleate
Mechanism of Action: Enalapril, after hydrolysis to enalaprilat, inhibits angiotensin-converting enzyme (ACE) in human subjects and animals. ACE is a peptidyl dipeptidase that catalyzes the conversion of angiotensin I to the vasoconstrictor substance, angiotensin II. Angiotensin II also stimulates aldosterone secretion by the adrenal cortex. Inhibition of ACE results in decreased plasma angiotensin II, which leads to decreased vasopressor activity and to decreased aldosterone secretion. Although the latter decrease is small, it results in small increases of serum potassium. In hypertensive patients treated with enalapril maleate alone for up to 48 weeks, mean increases in serum potassium of approximately 0.2 mEq/L were observed. In patients treated with enalapril maleate plus a thiazide diuretic, there was essentially no change in serum potassium. (See PRECAUTIONS.)
Removal of angiotensin II negative feedback on renin secretion leads to increased plasma renin activity.
ACE is identical to kininase, an enzyme that degrades bradykinin. Whether increased levels of bradykinin, a potent vasodepressor peptide, play a role in the therapeutic effects of enalapril remains to be elucidated.
While the mechanism through which enalapril lowers blood pressure is believed to be primarily suppression of the renin-angiotensin-aldosterone system, enalapril is antihypertensive even in patients with low-renin hypertension. Although enalapril was antihypertensive in all races studied, black hypertensive patients (usually a low-renin hypertensive population) had a smaller average response to enalapril maleate monotherapy than non-black patients. In contrast, hydrochlorothiazide was more effective in black patients than enalapril. Concomitant administration of enalapril maleate and hydrochlorothiazide was equally effective in black and non-black patients.
Pharmacokinetics and Metabolism: Following oral administration of enalapril maleate, peak serum concentrations of enalapril occur within about one hour. Based on urinary recovery, the extent of absorption of enalapril is approximately 60 percent. Enalapril absorption is not influenced by the presence of food in the gastrointestinal tract. Following absorption, enalapril is hydrolyzed to enalaprilat, which is a more potent angiotensin converting enzyme inhibitor than enalapril; enalaprilat is poorly absorbed when administered orally. Peak serum concentrations of enalaprilat occur three to four hours after an oral dose of enalapril maleate. Excretion of enalaprilat and enalapril is primarily renal. Approximately 94 percent of the dose is recovered in the urine and feces as enalaprilat or enalapril. The principal components in urine are enalaprilat, accounting for about 40 percent of the dose, and intact enalapril. There is no evidence of metabolites of enalapril, other than enalaprilat.
The serum concentration profile of enalaprilat exhibits a prolonged terminal phase, apparently representing a small fraction of the administered dose that has been bound to ACE. The amount bound does not increase with dose, indicating a saturable site of binding. The effective half-life for accumulation of enalaprilat following multiple doses of enalapril maleate is 11 hours.
The disposition of enalapril and enalaprilat in patients with renal insufficiency is similar to that in patients with normal renal function until the glomerular filtration rate is 30 mL/min or less. With glomerular filtration rate ≤30 mL/min, peak and trough enalaprilat levels increase, time to peak concentration increases and time to steady state may be delayed. The effective half-life of enalaprilat following multiple doses of enalapril maleate is prolonged at this level of renal insufficiency. Enalaprilat is dialyzable at the rate of 62 mL/min.
Studies in dogs indicate that enalapril crosses the blood-brain barrier poorly, if at all; enalaprilat does not enter the brain. Multiple doses of enalapril maleate in rats do not result in accumulation in any tissues. Milk of lactating rats contains radioactivity following administration of ^{14}C enalapril maleate. Radioactivity was found to cross the placenta following administration of labeled drug to pregnant hamsters.
Pharmacodynamics: Administration of enalapril maleate to patients with hypertension of severity ranging from mild to severe results in a reduction of both supine and standing blood pressure usually with no orthostatic component. Symptomatic postural hypotension is infrequent with enalapril alone but it can be anticipated in volume-depleted patients, such as patients treated with diuretics. In clinical trials with enalapril and hydrochlorothiazide administered concurrently, syncope occurred in 1.3 percent of patients. (See WARNINGS and DOSAGE AND ADMINISTRATION.)
In most patients studied, after oral administration of a single dose of enalapril maleate, onset of antihypertensive activity was seen at one hour with peak reduction of blood pressure achieved by four to six hours.
At recommended doses, antihypertensive effects of enalapril maleate monotherapy have been maintained for at least 24 hours. In some patients the effects may diminish toward the end of the dosing interval; this was less frequently observed with concomitant administration of enalapril maleate and hydrochlorothiazide.

Continued on next page

Information on the Merck & Co. products listed on these pages is the full prescribing information from product circulars in use October 1, 1992.

Merck & Co.—Cont.

Achievement of optimal blood pressure reduction may require several weeks of enalapril therapy in some patients. The antihypertensive effects of enalapril have continued during long term therapy. Abrupt withdrawal of enalapril has not been associated with a rapid increase in blood pressure.

In hemodynamic studies in patients with essential hypertension, blood pressure reduction produced by enalapril was accompanied by a reduction in peripheral arterial resistance with an increase in cardiac output and little or no change in heart rate. Following administration of enalapril maleate, there is an increase in renal blood flow; glomerular filtration rate is usually unchanged. The effects appear to be similar in patients with renovascular hypertension.

In a clinical pharmacology study, indomethacin or sulindac was administered to hypertensive patients receiving enalapril maleate. In this study there was no evidence of a blunting of the antihypertensive action of enalapril maleate.

Hydrochlorothiazide

The mechanism of the antihypertensive effect of thiazides is unknown. Thiazides do not usually affect normal blood pressure. Hydrochlorothiazide is a diuretic and antihypertensive. It affects the distal renal tubular mechanism of electrolyte reabsorption. Hydrochlorothiazide increases excretion of sodium and chloride in approximately equivalent amounts. Natriuresis may be accompanied by some loss of potassium and bicarbonate. After oral use diuresis begins within two hours, peaks in about four hours and lasts about 6 to 12 hours. Hydrochlorothiazide is not metabolized but is eliminated rapidly by the kidney. When plasma levels have been followed for at least 24 hours, the plasma half-life has been observed to vary between 5.6 and 14.8 hours. At least 61 percent of the oral dose is eliminated unchanged within 24 hours. Hydrochlorothiazide crosses the placental but not the blood-brain barrier.

INDICATIONS AND USAGE

VASERETIC is indicated for the treatment of hypertension in patients for whom combination therapy is appropriate. **This fixed dose combination is not indicated for initial therapy. Patients already receiving a diuretic when enalapril is initiated, or given a diuretic and enalapril simultaneously, can develop symptomatic hypotension. In the initial titration of the individual entities, it is important, if possible, to stop the diuretic for several days before starting enalapril or, if this is not possible, begin enalapril at a low initial dose (see DOSAGE AND ADMINISTRATION). This fixed dose combination is not suitable for titration but may be substituted for the individual components if the titrated doses are the same as those in the combination.**

In using VASERETIC, consideration should be given to the fact that another angiotensin converting enzyme inhibitor, captopril, has caused agranulocytosis, particularly in patients with renal impairment or collagen vascular disease, and that available data are insufficient to show that enalapril does not have a similar risk. (See WARNINGS.)

CONTRAINDICATIONS

VASERETIC is contraindicated in patients who are hypersensitive to any component of this product and in patients with a history of angioedema related to previous treatment with an angiotensin converting enzyme inhibitor. Because of the hydrochlorothiazide component, this product is contraindicated in patients with anuria or hypersensitivity to other sulfonamide-derived drugs.

WARNINGS

General
Enalapril Maleate
Hypotension: Excessive hypotension was rarely seen in uncomplicated hypertensive patients but is a possible consequence of enalapril use in severely salt/volume depleted persons such as those treated vigorously with diuretics or patients on dialysis.

Syncope has been reported in 1.3 percent of patients receiving VASERETIC. In patients receiving enalapril alone, the incidence of syncope is 0.5 percent. The overall incidence of syncope may be reduced by proper titration of the individual components. (See PRECAUTIONS, *Drug Interactions,* ADVERSE REACTIONS and DOSAGE AND ADMINISTRATION.)

In patients with severe congestive heart failure, with or without associated renal insufficiency, excessive hypotension has been observed and may be associated with oliguria and/or progressive azotemia, and rarely with acute renal failure and/or death. Because of the potential fall in blood pressure in these patients, therapy should be started under very close medical supervision. Such patients should be followed closely for the first two weeks of treatment and when-

ever the dose of enalapril and/or diuretic is increased. Similar considerations may apply to patients with ischemic heart or cerebrovascular disease, in whom an excessive fall in blood pressure could result in a myocardial infarction or cerebrovascular accident.

If hypotension occurs, the patient should be placed in the supine position and, if necessary, receive an intravenous infusion of normal saline. A transient hypotensive response is not a contraindication to further doses, which usually can be given without difficulty once the blood pressure has increased after volume expansion.

Angioedema: Angioedema of the face, extremities, lips, tongue, glottis and/or larynx has been reported in patients treated with angiotensin converting enzyme inhibitors, including enalapril. In such cases VASERETIC should be promptly discontinued and appropriate therapy and monitoring should be provided until complete and sustained resolution of signs and symptoms has occurred. In instances where swelling has been confined to the face and lips the condition has generally resolved without treatment, although antihistamines have been useful in relieving symptoms. Angioedema associated with laryngeal edema may be fatal. **Where there is involvement of the tongue, glottis or larynx, likely to cause airway obstruction, appropriate therapy, e.g., subcutaneous epinephrine solution 1:1000 (0.3 mL to 0.5 mL) and/or measures necessary to ensure a patent airway, should be promptly provided.** (See ADVERSE REACTIONS.)

Patients with a history of angioedema unrelated to ACE inhibitor therapy may be at increased risk of angioedema while receiving an ACE inhibitor (see also CONTRAINDICATIONS).

Neutropenia/Agranulocytosis: Another angiotensin converting enzyme inhibitor, captopril, has been shown to cause agranulocytosis and bone marrow depression, rarely in uncomplicated patients but more frequently in patients with renal impairment especially if they also have a collagen vascular disease. Available data from clinical trials of enalapril are insufficient to show that enalapril does not cause agranulocytosis at similar rates. Foreign marketing experience has revealed several cases of neutropenia or agranulocytosis in which a causal relationship to enalapril cannot be excluded. Periodic monitoring of white blood cell counts in patients with collagen vascular disease and renal disease should be considered.

Hydrochlorothiazide
Thiazides should be used with caution in severe renal disease. In patients with renal disease, thiazides may precipitate azotemia. Cumulative effects of the drug may develop in patients with impaired renal function.

Thiazides should be used with caution in patients with impaired hepatic function or progressive liver disease, since minor alterations of fluid and electrolyte balance may precipitate hepatic coma.

Sensitivity reactions may occur in patients with or without a history of allergy or bronchial asthma.

The possibility of exacerbation or activation of systemic lupus erythematosus has been reported.

Lithium generally should not be given with thiazides (see PRECAUTIONS, *Drug Interactions, Enalapril Maleate* and *Hydrochlorothiazide*).

Pregnancy
Enalapril-Hydrochlorothiazide
There was no teratogenicity in rats given up to 90 mg/kg/day of enalapril (150 times the maximum human dose) in combination with 10 mg/kg/day of hydrochlorothiazide ($2\frac{1}{2}$ times the maximum human dose) or in mice given up to 30 mg/kg/day of enalapril (50 times the maximum human dose) in combination with 10 mg/kg/day of hydrochlorothiazide ($2\frac{1}{2}$ times the maximum human dose). At these doses, fetotoxicity expressed as a decrease in average fetal weight occurred in both species. No fetotoxicity occurred at lower doses; 30/10 mg/kg/day of enalapril-hydrochlorothiazide in rats and 10/10 mg/kg/day of enalapril-hydrochlorothiazide in mice.

If VASERETIC is used during pregnancy or if the patient becomes pregnant while taking VASERETIC, the patient should be apprised of the potential hazards to the fetus. (See *Enalapril Maleate, Fetal/Neonatal Morbidity and Mortality,* below.)

Enalapril Maleate
Fetal/Neonatal Morbidity and Mortality: ACE inhibitors can cause fetal and neonatal morbidity and death when administered to pregnant women. Several dozen cases have been reported in the world literature. When pregnancy is detected, ACE inhibitors should be discontinued as soon as possible.

The use of ACE inhibitors during the second and third trimesters of pregnancy has been associated with fetal and neonatal injury, including hypotension, neonatal skull hypoplasia, anuria, reversible or irreversible renal failure, and death. Oligohydramnios has also been reported, presumably resulting from decreased fetal renal function; oligohydramnios in this setting has been associated with fetal limb contractures, craniofacial deformation, and hypoplastic lung development. Prematurity, intrauterine growth retardation,

and patent ductus arteriosus have also been reported, although it is not clear whether these occurrences were due to the ACE-inhibitor exposure.

These adverse effects do not appear to have resulted from intrauterine ACE-inhibitor exposure that has been limited to the first trimester. Mothers whose embryos and fetuses are exposed to ACE inhibitors only during the first trimester should be so informed. Nonetheless, when patients become pregnant, physicians should make every effort to discontinue the use of VASERETIC as soon as possible.

Rarely (probably less often than once in every thousand pregnancies), no alternative to ACE inhibitors will be found. In these rare cases, the mothers should be apprised of the potential hazards to their fetuses, and serial ultrasound examinations should be performed to assess the intraamniotic environment.

If oligohydramnios is observed, VASERETIC should be discontinued unless it is considered lifesaving for the mother. Contraction stress testing (CST), a non-stress test (NST), or biophysical profiling (BPP) may be appropriate, depending upon the week of pregnancy. Patients and physicians should be aware, however, that oligohydramnios may not appear until after the fetus has sustained irreversible injury.

Infants with histories of *in utero* exposure to ACE inhibitors should be closely observed for hypotension, oliguria, and hyperkalemia. If oliguria occurs, attention should be directed toward support of blood pressure and renal perfusion. Exchange transfusion or dialysis may be required as means of reversing hypotension and/or substituting for disordered renal functon. Enalapril, which crosses the placenta, has been removed from neonatal circulation by peritoneal dialysis with some clinical benefit, and theoretically may be removed by exchange transfusion, although there is no experience with the latter procedure.

No teratogenic effects of enalapril were seen in studies of pregnant rats, and rabbits. On a mg/kg basis, the doses used were up to 333 times (in rats), and 50 times (in rabbits) the maximum recommended human dose.

Hydrochlorothiazide
Teratogenic Effects: Reproduction studies in the rabbit, the mouse and the rat at doses up to 100 mg/kg/day (50 times the human dose) showed no evidence of external abnormalities of the fetus due to hydrochlorothiazide. Hydrochlorothiazide given in a two-litter study in rats at doses of 4–5.6 mg/kg/day (approximately 1–2 times the usual daily human dose) did not impair fertility or produce birth abnormalities in the offspring. Thiazides cross the placental barrier and appear in cord blood.

Nonteratogenic Effects: These may include fetal or neonatal jaundice, thrombocytopenia, and possibly other adverse reactions which have occurred in the adult.

PRECAUTIONS

General
Enalapril Maleate
Impaired Renal Function: As a consequence of inhibiting the renin-angiotensin-aldosterone system, changes in renal function may be anticipated in susceptible individuals. In patients with severe congestive heart failure whose renal function may depend on the activity of the renin-angiotensin-aldosterone system, treatment with angiotensin converting enzyme inhibitors, including enalapril, may be associated with oliguria and/or progressive azotemia and rarely with acute renal failure and/or death.

In clinical studies in hypertensive patients with unilateral or bilateral renal artery stenosis, increases in blood urea nitrogen and serum creatinine were observed in 20 percent of patients. These increases were almost always reversible upon discontinuation of enalapril and/or diuretic therapy. In such patients renal function should be monitored during the first few weeks of therapy.

Some patients with hypertension or heart failure with no apparent pre-existing renal vascular disease have developed increases in blood urea and serum creatinine, usually minor and transient, especially when enalapril has been given concomitantly with a diuretic. This is more likely to occur in patients with pre-existing renal impairment. Dosage reduction of enalapril and/or discontinuation of the diuretic may be required.

Evaluation of the hypertensive patient should always include assessment of renal function.

Hemodialysis Patients: Anaphylactoid reactions have been reported in patients dialyzed with high-flux membranes (e.g., AN 69*) and treated concomitantly with an ACE inhibitor. In these patients consideration should be given to using a different type of dialysis membrane or a different class of antihypertensive agent.

Hyperkalemia: Elevated serum potassium (greater than 5.7 mEq/L) was observed in approximately one percent of hypertensive patients in clinical trials treated with enalapril alone. In most cases these were isolated values which resolved despite continued therapy, although hyperkalemia was a cause of discontinuation of therapy in 0.28 percent of hypertensive patients. Hyperkalemia was less frequent (ap-

proximately 0.1 percent) in patients treated with enalapril plus hydrochlorothiazide. Risk factors for the development of hyperkalemia include renal insufficiency, diabetes mellitus, and the concomitant use of potassium-sparing diuretics, potassium supplements and/or potassium-containing salt substitutes, which should be used cautiously, if at all, with enalapril. (See *Drug Interactions.*)

Cough: Cough has been reported with the use of ACE inhibitors. Characteristically, the cough is nonproductive, persistent and resolves after discontinuation of therapy. ACE inhibitor-induced cough should be considered as part of the differential diagnosis of cough.

Surgery/Anesthesia: In patients undergoing major surgery or during anesthesia with agents that produce hypotension, enalapril may block angiotensin II formation secondary to compensatory renin release. If hypotension occurs and is considered to be due to this mechanism, it can be corrected by volume expansion.

---

* Registered trademark of Hospal Ltd.

Hydrochlorothiazide

Periodic determination of serum electrolytes to detect possible electrolyte imbalance should be performed at appropriate intervals. All patients receiving thiazide therapy should be observed for clinical signs of fluid or electrolyte imbalance: namely hyponatremia, hypochloremic alkalosis, and hypokalemia. Serum and urine electrolyte determinations are particularly important when the patient is vomiting excessively or receiving parenteral fluids. Warning signs or symptoms of fluid and electrolyte imbalance, irrespective of cause, include dryness of mouth, thirst, weakness, lethargy, drowsiness, restlessness, confusion, seizures, muscle pains or cramps, muscular fatigue, hypotension, oliguria, tachycardia, and gastrointestinal disturbances such as nausea and vomiting.

Hypokalemia may develop, especially with brisk diuresis, when severe cirrhosis is present, or after prolonged therapy. Interference with adequate oral electrolyte intake will also contribute to hypokalemia. Hypokalemia may cause cardiac arrhythmia and may also sensitize or exaggerate the response of the heart to the toxic effects of digitalis (e.g., increased ventricular irritability). Because enalapril reduces the production of aldosterone, concomitant therapy with enalapril attenuates the diuretic-induced potassium loss (see *Drug Interactions, Agents Increasing Serum Potassium*).

Although any chloride deficit is generally mild and usually does not require specific treatment except under extraordinary circumstances (as in liver disease or renal disease), chloride replacement may be required in the treatment of metabolic alkalosis.

Dilutional hyponatremia may occur in edematous patients in hot weather; appropriate therapy is water restriction, rather than administration of salt except in rare instances when the hyponatremia is life-threatening. In actual salt depletion, appropriate replacement is the therapy of choice.

Hyperuricemia may occur or frank gout may be precipitated in certain patients receiving thiazide therapy.

In diabetic patients dosage adjustments of insulin or oral hypoglycemic agents may be required. Hyperglycemia may occur with thiazide diuretics. Thus latent diabetes mellitus may become manifest during thiazide therapy.

The antihypertensive effects of the drug may be enhanced in the postsympathectomy patient.

If progressive renal impairment becomes evident consider withholding or discontinuing diuretic therapy.

Thiazides have been shown to increase the urinary excretion of magnesium; this may result in hypomagnesemia.

Thiazides may decrease urinary calcium excretion. Thiazides may cause intermittent and slight elevation of serum calcium in the absence of known disorders of calcium metabolism. Marked hypercalcemia may be evidence of hidden hyperparathyroidism. Thiazides should be discontinued before carrying out tests for parathyroid function.

Increases in cholesterol and triglyceride levels may be associated with thiazide diuretic therapy.

Information for Patients

Angioedema: Angioedema, including laryngeal edema, may occur especially following the first dose of enalapril. Patients should be so advised and told to report immediately any signs or symptoms suggesting angioedema (swelling of face, extremities, eyes, lips, tongue, difficulty in swallowing or breathing) and to take no more drug until they have consulted with the prescribing physician.

Hypotension: Patients should be cautioned to report lightheadedness especially during the first few days of therapy. If actual syncope occurs, the patients should be told to discontinue the drug until they have consulted with the prescribing physician.

All patients should be cautioned that excessive perspiration and dehydration may lead to an excessive fall in blood pressure because of reduction in fluid volume. Other causes of volume depletion such as vomiting or diarrhea may also lead to a fall in blood pressure; patients should be advised to consult with the physician.

Hyperkalemia: Patients should be told not to use salt substitutes containing potassium without consulting their physician.

Neutropenia: Patients should be told to report promptly any indication of infection (e.g., sore throat, fever) which may be a sign of neutropenia.

Pregnancy: Female patients of childbearing age should be told about the consequences of second- and third-trimester exposure to ACE inhibitors, and they should also be told that these consequences do not appear to have resulted from intrauterine ACE-inhibitor exposure that has been limited to the first trimester. These patients should be asked to report pregnancies to their physicians as soon as possible.

NOTE: As with many other drugs, certain advice to patients being treated with VASERETIC is warranted. This information is intended to aid in the safe and effective use of this medication. It is not a disclosure of all possible adverse or intended effects.

Drug Interactions

Enalapril Maleate

Hypotension—Patients on Diuretic Therapy: Patients on diuretics and especially those in whom diuretic therapy was recently instituted, may occasionally experience an excessive reduction of blood pressure after initiation of therapy with enalapril. The possibility of hypotensive effects with enalapril can be minimized by either discontinuing the diuretic or increasing the salt intake prior to initiation of treatment with enalapril. If it is necessary to continue the diuretic, provide medical supervision for at least two hours and until blood pressure has stabilized for at least an additional hour. (See WARNINGS, and DOSAGE AND ADMINISTRATION.)

Agents Causing Renin Release: The antihypertensive effect of enalapril is augmented by antihypertensive agents that cause renin release (e.g., diuretics).

Other Cardiovascular Agents: Enalapril has been used concomitantly with beta adrenergic-blocking agents, methyldopa, nitrates, calcium-blocking agents, hydralazine and prazosin without evidence of clinically significant adverse interactions.

Agents Increasing Serum Potassium: Enalapril attenuates diuretic-induced potassium loss. Potassium-sparing diuretics (e.g., spironolactone, triamterene, or amiloride), potassium supplements, or potassium-containing salt substitutes may lead to significant increases in serum potassium. Therefore, if concomitant use of these agents is indicated because of demonstrated hypokalemia they should be used with caution and with frequent monitoring of serum potassium.

Lithium: Lithium toxicity has been reported in patients receiving lithium concomitantly with drugs which cause elimination of sodium, including ACE inhibitors. A few cases of lithium toxicity have been reported in patients receiving concomitant enalapril and lithium and were reversible upon discontinuation of both drugs. It is recommended that serum lithium levels be monitored frequently if enalapril is administered concomitantly with lithium.

Hydrochlorothiazide

When administered concurrently the following drugs may interact with thiazide diuretics:

Alcohol, barbiturates, or narcotics—potentiation of orthostatic hypotension may occur.

Antidiabetic drugs (oral agents and insulin)—dosage adjustment of the antidiabetic drug may be required.

Other antihypertensive drugs—additive effect or potentiation.

Cholestyramine and colestipol resins—Cholestyramine and colestipol resins bind the hydrochlorothiazide and reduce its absorption from the gastrointestinal tract by up to 85 and 43 percent, respectively. Thiazides may be administered two to four hours before the resin when the two drugs are used concomitantly.

Corticosteroids, ACTH—intensified electrolyte depletion, particularly hypokalemia.

Pressor amines (e.g., norepinephrine)—possible decreased response to pressor amines but not sufficient to preclude their use.

Skeletal muscle relaxants, nondepolarizing (e.g., tubocurarine)—possible increased responsiveness to the muscle relaxant.

Lithium—should not generally be given with diuretics. Diuretic agents reduce the renal clearance of lithium and add a high risk of lithium toxicity. Refer to the package insert for lithium preparations before use of such preparations with VASERETIC.

Non-steroidal Anti-inflammatory Drugs—In some patients, the administration of a non-steroidal anti-inflammatory agent can reduce the diuretic, natriuretic, and antihypertensive effects of loop, potassium-sparing and thiazide diuretics. Therefore, when VASERETIC and non-steroidal anti-inflammatory agents are used concomitantly, the patient should be observed closely to determine if the desired effect of the diuretic is obtained.

Carcinogenesis, Mutagenesis, Impairment of Fertility

Enalapril in combination with hydrochlorothiazide was not mutagenic in the Ames microbial mutagen test with or without metabolic activation. Enalapril-hydrochlorothiazide did not produce DNA single strand breaks in an *in vitro* alkaline elution assay in rat hepatocytes or chromosomal aberrations in an *in vivo* mouse bone marrow assay.

Enalapril Maleate

There was no evidence of a tumorigenic effect when enalapril was administered for 106 weeks to rats at doses up to 90 mg/kg/day (150 times* the maximum daily human dose). Enalapril has also been administered for 94 weeks to male and female mice at doses up to 90 and 180 mg/kg/day, respectively, (150 and 300 times* the maximum daily dose for humans) and showed no evidence of carcinogenicity.

Neither enalapril maleate nor the active diacid was mutagenic in the Ames microbial mutagen test with or without metabolic activation. Enalapril was also negative in the following genotoxicity studies: rec-assay, reverse mutation assay with *E. coli*, sister chromatid exchange with cultured mammalian cells, and the micronucleus test with mice, as well as in an *in vivo* cytogenic study using mouse bone marrow.

There were no adverse effects on reproductive performance in male and female rats treated with 10 to 90 mg/kg/day of enalapril.

---

* Based on patient weight of 50 kg

Hydrochlorothiazide

Two-year feeding studies in mice and rats conducted under the auspices of the National Toxicology Program (NTP) uncovered no evidence of a carcinogenic potential of hydrochlorothiazide in female mice (at doses of up to approximately 600 mg/kg/day) or in male and female rats (at doses of up to approximately 100 mg/kg/day). The NTP, however, found equivocal evidence for hepatocarcinogenicity in male mice.

Hydrochlorothiazide was not genotoxic *in vitro* in the Ames mutagenicity assay of *Salmonella typhimurium* strains TA 98, TA 100, TA 1535, TA 1537, and TA 1538 and in the Chinese Hamster Ovary (CHO) test for chromosomal aberrations, or *in vivo* in assays using mouse germinal cell chromosomes, Chinese hamster bone marrow chromosomes, and the *Drosophila* sex-linked recessive lethal trait gene. Positive test results were obtained only in the *in vitro* CHO Sister Chromatid Exchange (clastogenicity) and in the Mouse Lymphoma Cell (mutagenicity) assays, using concentrations of hydrochlorothiazide from 43 to 1300 μg/mL, and in the *Aspergillus nidulans* non-disjunction assay at an unspecified concentration.

Hydrochlorothiazide had no adverse effects on the fertility of mice and rats of either sex in studies wherein these species were exposed, via their diet, to doses of up to 100 and 4 mg/kg, respectively, prior to conception and throughout gestation.

Pregnancy

Pregnancy Categories C (first trimester) *and D* (second and third trimesters). See WARNINGS, *Pregnancy, Enalapril Maleate, Fetal/Neonatal Morbidity and Mortality.*

Nursing Mothers

Enalapril and enalaprilat are detected in human milk in trace amounts. Thiazides do appear in human milk. Because of the potential for serious reactions in nursing infants from hydrochlorothiazide, a decision should be made whether to discontinue nursing or to discontinue VASERETIC, taking into account the importance of the drug to the mother.

Pediatric Use

Safety and effectiveness in children have not been established.

ADVERSE REACTIONS

VASERETIC has been evaluated for safety in more than 1500 patients, including over 300 patients treated for one year or more. In clinical trials with VASERETIC no adverse experiences peculiar to this combination drug have been observed. Adverse experiences that have occurred, have been limited to those that have been previously reported with enalapril or hydrochlorothiazide.

The most frequent clinical adverse experiences in controlled trials were: dizziness (8.6 percent), headache (5.5 percent), fatigue (3.9 percent) and cough (3.5 percent). Generally, adverse experiences were mild and transient in nature. Adverse experiences occurring in greater than two percent of patients treated with VASERETIC in controlled clinical trials are shown . [See table at top of next page.]

Continued on next page

Information on the Merck & Co. products listed on these pages is the full prescribing information from product circulars in use October 1, 1992.

Merck & Co.—Cont.

	Percent of Patients in Controlled Studies VASERETIC (n=1580) Incidence (discontinuation)		Placebo (n=230) Incidence
Dizziness	8.6	(0.7)	4.3
Headache	5.5	(0.4)	9.1
Fatigue	3.9	(0.8)	2.6
Cough	3.5	(0.4)	0.9
Muscle Cramps	2.7	(0.2)	0.9
Nausea	2.5	(0.4)	1.7
Asthenia	2.4	(0.3)	0.9
Orthostatic Effects	2.3	(<0.1)	0.0
Impotence	2.2	(0.5)	0.5
Diarrhea	2.1	(<0.1)	1.7

Clinical adverse experiences occurring in 0.5 to 2.0 percent of patients in controlled trials included: *Body As A Whole:* Syncope, chest pain, abdominal pain; *Cardiovascular:* Orthostatic hypotension, palpitation, tachycardia; *Digestive:* Vomiting, dyspepsia, constipation, flatulence, dry mouth; *Nervous/Psychiatric:* Insomnia, nervousness, paresthesia, somnolence, vertigo; *Skin:* Pruritus, rash; *Other:* Dyspnea, gout, back pain, arthralgia, diaphoresis, decreased libido, tinnitus, urinary tract infection.

Angioedema: Angioedema has been reported in patients receiving VASERETIC (0.6 percent). Angioedema associated with laryngeal edema may be fatal. If angioedema of the face, extremities, lips, tongue, glottis and/or larynx occurs, treatment with VASERETIC should be discontinued and appropriate therapy instituted immediately. (See WARNINGS.)

Hypotension: In clinical trials, adverse effects relating to hypotension occurred as follows: hypotension (0.9 percent), orthostatic hypotension (1.5 percent), other orthostatic effects (2.3 percent). In addition syncope occurred in 1.3 percent of patients. (See WARNINGS.)

Cough: See PRECAUTIONS, *Cough.*

Clinical Laboratory Test Findings

Serum Electrolytes: See PRECAUTIONS.

Creatinine, Blood Urea Nitrogen: In controlled clinical trials minor increases in blood urea nitrogen and serum creatinine, reversible upon discontinuation of therapy, were observed in about 0.6 percent of patients with essential hypertension treated with VASERETIC. More marked increases have been reported in other enalapril experience. Increases are more likely to occur in patients with renal artery stenosis. (See PRECAUTIONS.)

Serum Uric Acid, Glucose, Magnesium, and Calcium: See PRECAUTIONS.

Hemoglobin and Hematocrit: Small decreases in hemoglobin and hematocrit (mean decreases of approximately 0.3 g percent and 1.0 vol percent, respectively) occur frequently in hypertensive patients treated with VASERETIC but are rarely of clinical importance unless another cause of anemia coexists. In clinical trials, less than 0.1 percent of patients discontinued therapy due to anemia.

Other (Causal Relationship Unknown): Rarely, elevations of liver enzymes and/or serum bilirubin have occurred.

Other adverse reactions that have been reported with the individual components are listed below and, within each category, are in order of decreasing severity.

Enalapril Maleate—Enalapril has been evaluated for safety in more than 10,000 patients. In clinical trials adverse reactions which occurred with enalapril were also seen with VASERETIC. However, since enalapril has been marketed, the following adverse reactions have been reported: *Body As A Whole:* Anaphylactoid reactions (see PRECAUTIONS, *Hemodialysis Patients*); *Cardiovascular:* Cardiac arrest; myocardial infarction or cerebrovascular accident, possibly secondary to excessive hypotension in high risk patients (see WARNINGS, *Hypotension*); pulmonary embolism and infarction; pulmonary edema; rhythm disturbances including atrial tachycardia and bradycardia, atrial fibrillation; hypotension; angina pectoris; *Digestive:* Ileus, pancreatitis, hepatic failure, hepatitis (hepatocellular [proven on rechallenge] or cholestatic jaundice), melena, anorexia, glossitis, stomatitis, dry mouth; *Hematologic:* Rare cases of neutropenia, thrombocytopenia and bone marrow depression as well as a few cases of hemolysis in patients with G6PD deficiency have been reported; in which a causal relationship to enalapril cannot be excluded; *Nervous System/Psychiatric:* Depression, confusion, ataxia; *Urogenital:* Renal failure, oliguria, renal dysfunction, (see PRECAUTIONS and DOSAGE AND ADMINISTRATION), flank pain, gynecomastia; *Respiratory:* Bronchospasm, pneumonia, bronchitis, rhinorrhea, sore throat and hoarseness, asthma, upper respiratory infection; *Skin:* Exfoliative dermatitis, toxic epidermal necrolysis, Stevens-Johnson syndrome, herpes zoster, erythema multiforme, urticaria, alopecia, flushing; *Special Senses:* Blurred vision, taste alteration, anosmia, conjunctivitis, dry eyes, tearing.

A symptom complex has been reported which may include a positive ANA, an elevated erythrocyte sedimentation rate, arthralgia/arthritis, myalgia, fever, serositis, vasculitis, leukocytosis, eosinophilia, photosensitivity, rash and other dermatologic manifestations.

Fetal/Neonatal Morbidity and Mortality: See WARNINGS, *Pregnancy, Enalapril Maleate, Fetal/Neonatal Morbidity and Mortality.*

Hydrochlorothiazide—Body as a Whole: Weakness; *Digestive:* Pancreatitis, jaundice (intrahepatic cholestatic jaundice), sialadenitis, cramping, gastric irritation, anorexia; *Hematologic:* Aplastic anemia, agranulocytosis, leukopenia, hemolytic anemia, thrombocytopenia; *Hypersensitivity:* Purpura, photosensitivity, urticaria, necrotizing angiitis (vasculitis and cutaneous vasculitis), fever, respiratory distress including pneumonitis and pulmonary edema, anaphylactic reactions; *Musculoskeletal:* Muscle spasm; *Nervous system/Psychiatric:* Restlessness; *Renal:* Renal failure, renal dysfunction, interstitial nephritis (see WARNINGS); *Skin:* Erythema multiforme including Stevens-Johnson syndrome, exfoliative dermatitis including toxic epidermal necrolysis, alopecia; *Special Senses:* Transient blurred vision, xanthopsia.

OVERDOSAGE

No specific information is available on the treatment of overdosage with VASERETIC. Treatment is symptomatic and supportive. Therapy with VASERETIC should be discontinued and the patient observed closely. Suggested measures include induction of emesis and/or gastric lavage, and correction of dehydration, electrolyte imbalance and hypotension by established procedures.

Enalapril Maleate—The oral LD_{50} of enalapril is 2000 mg/kg in mice and rats. The most likely manifestation of overdosage would be hypotension, for which the usual treatment would be intravenous infusion of normal saline solution. Enalaprilat may be removed from general circulation by hemodialysis and has been removed from neonatal circulation by peritoneal dialysis.

Hydrochlorothiazide—The oral LD_{50} of hydrochlorothiazide is greater than 10.0 g/kg in both mice and rats. The most common signs and symptoms observed are those caused by electrolyte depletion (hypokalemia, hypochloremia, hyponatremia) and dehydration resulting from excessive diuresis. If digitalis has also been administered, hypokalemia may accentuate cardiac arrhythmias.

DOSAGE AND ADMINISTRATION

DOSAGE MUST BE INDIVIDUALIZED. THE FIXED COMBINATION IS NOT FOR INITIAL THERAPY. THE DOSE OF 'VASERETIC' SHOULD BE DETERMINED BY THE TITRATION OF THE INDIVIDUAL COMPONENTS.

Once the patient has been successfully titrated with the individual components as described below, VASERETIC (one or two 10-25 tablets once daily) may be substituted if the titrated doses are the same as those in the fixed combination. (See INDICATIONS AND USAGE and WARNINGS.)

Patients usually do not require doses in excess of 50 mg of hydrochlorothiazide daily when combined with other antihypertensive agents. Therefore, since each tablet of VASERETIC includes 25 mg of hydrochlorothiazide, the daily dosage of VASERETIC should not exceed two tablets. If further blood pressure control is indicated, additional doses of enalapril or other nondiuretic antihypertensive agents should be considered.

For enalapril monotherapy the recommended initial dose in patients not on diuretics is 5 mg of enalapril once a day. Dosage should be adjusted according to blood pressure response. The usual dosage range of enalapril is 10 to 40 mg per day administered in a single dose or two divided doses. In some patients treated once daily, the antihypertensive effects may diminish toward the end of the dosing interval. In such patients, an increase in dosage or twice daily administration should be considered. If blood pressure is not controlled with enalapril alone, a diuretic may be added.

In patients who are currently being treated with a diuretic, symptomatic hypotension occasionally may occur following the initial dose of enalapril. The diuretic should, if possible, be discontinued for two to three days before beginning therapy with enalapril to reduce the likelihood of hypotension. (See WARNINGS.) If the patient's blood pressure is not controlled with enalapril alone, diuretic therapy may be resumed.

If the diuretic cannot be discontinued an initial dose of 2.5 mg of enalapril should be used under medical supervision for at least two hours and until blood pressure has stabilized for at least an additional hour. (See WARNINGS and PRECAUTIONS, *Drug Interactions.*)

Concomitant administration of VASERETIC with potassium supplements, potassium salt substitutes, or potassium sparing agents may lead to increases of serum potassium. (See PRECAUTIONS.)

Dosage Adjustment in Renal Impairment: The usual dose of VASERETIC is recommended for patients with a creatinine clearance >30 mL/min (serum creatinine of up to approximately 3 mg/dL).

When concomitant diuretic therapy is required in patients with severe renal impairment, a loop diuretic, rather than a thiazide diuretic is preferred for use with enalapril; therefore, for patients with severe renal dysfunction the enalapril maleate-hydrochlorothiazide combination tablet is not recommended.

HOW SUPPLIED

No. 3418—Tablets VASERETIC 10-25, are rust, squared capsule-shaped, compressed tablets, coded MSD 720 on one side and VASERETIC on the other. Each tablet contains 10 mg of enalapril maleate and 25 mg of hydrochlorothiazide. They are supplied as follows:

NDC 0006-0720-68 bottles of 100 (with desiccant).

Shown in Product Identification Section, page 420

Storage

Store below 30°C (86°F) and avoid transient temperatures above 50°C (122°F). Keep container tightly closed. Protect from moisture.

Dispense in a tight container, if product package is subdivided.

A.H.F.S. Category: 24:08, 40:28

DC 7432316 Issued May 1992

COPYRIGHT © MERCK & CO., INC., 1989, 1992
All rights reserved

VASOTEC® I.V. Injection ℞
(Enalaprilat)

USE IN PREGNANCY
When used in pregnancy during the second and third timesters, ACE inhibitors can cause injury and even death to the developing fetus. When pregnancy is detected, VASOTEC I.V. should be discontinued as soon as possible. See WARNINGS. *Fetal/Neonatal Morbidity and Mortality.*

DESCRIPTION

VASOTEC* I.V. (Enalaprilat) is a sterile aqueous solution for intravenous administration. Enalaprilat is an angiotensin converting enzyme inhibitor. It is chemically described as (*S*)-1-[*N*-(1-carboxy-3-phenylpropyl)-L-alanyl]-L-proline dihydrate. Its empirical formula is $C_{18}H_{24}N_2O_5 \cdot 2H_2O$ and its structural formula is:

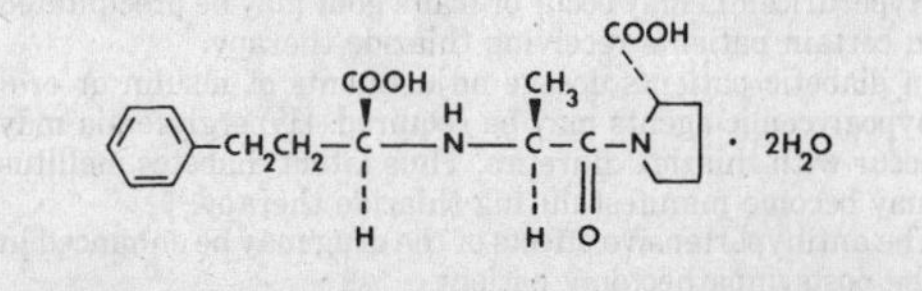

Enalaprilat is a white to off-white, crystalline powder with a molecular weight of 384.43. It is sparingly soluble in methanol and slightly soluble in water.

Each milliliter of VASOTEC I.V. contains 1.25 mg enalaprilat (anhydrous equivalent); sodium chloride to adjust tonicity; sodium hydroxide to adjust pH; water for injection, q.s.; with benzyl alcohol, 9 mg, added as a preservative.

*Registered trademark of MERCK & CO., INC.

CLINICAL PHARMACOLOGY

Enalaprilat, an angiotensin-converting enzyme (ACE) inhibitor when administered intravenously, is the active metabolite of the orally administered pro-drug, enalapril maleate. Enalaprilat is poorly absorbed orally.

Mechanism of Action

Intravenous enalaprilat, or oral enalapril, after hydrolysis to enalaprilat, inhibits ACE in human subjects and animals. ACE is a peptidyl dipeptidase that catalyzes the conversion of angiotensin I to the vasoconstrictor substance, angiotensin II. Angiotensin II also stimulates aldosterone secretion by the adrenal cortex. Inhibition of ACE results in decreased plasma angiotensin II, which leads to decreased vasopressor activity and to decreased aldosterone secretion. Although the latter decrease is small, it results in small increases of serum potassium. In hypertensive patients treated with enalapril alone for up to 48 weeks, mean increases in serum potassium of approximately 0.2 mEq/L were observed. In patients treated with enalapril plus a thiazide diuretic, there was essentially no change in serum potassium. (See PRE-

CAUTIONS.) Removal of angiotensin II negative feedback on renin secretion leads to increased plasma renin activity.

ACE is identical to kininase, an enzyme that degrades bradykinin. Whether increased levels of bradykinin, a potent vasodepressor peptide, play a role in the therapeutic effects of enalaprilat remains to be elucidated.

While the mechanism through which enalaprilat lowers blood pressure is believed to be primarily suppression of the renin-angiotensin-aldosterone system, enalaprilat has antihypertensive activity even in patients with low-renin hypertension. In clinical studies, black hypertensive patients (usually a low-renin hypertensive population) had a smaller average response to enalaprilat monotherapy than non-black patients.

Pharmacokinetics and Metabolism

Following intravenous administration of a single dose, the serum concentration profile of enalaprilat is polyexponential with a prolonged terminal phase, apparently representing a small fraction of the administered dose that has been bound to ACE. The amount bound does not increase with dose, indicating a saturable site of binding. The effective half-life for accumulation of enalaprilat, as determined from oral administration of multiple doses of enalapril maleate, is approximately 11 hours. Excretion of enalaprilat is primarily renal with more than 90 percent of an administered dose recovered in the urine as unchanged drug within 24 hours. Enalaprilat is poorly absorbed following oral administration. The disposition of enalaprilat in patients with renal insufficiency is similar to that in patients with normal renal function until the glomerular filtration rate is 30 mL/min or less. With glomerular filtration rate ≤30 mL/min, peak and trough enalaprilat levels increase, time to peak concentration increases and time to steady state may be delayed. The effective half-life of enalaprilat is prolonged at this level of renal insufficiency. (See DOSAGE AND ADMINISTRATION.) Enalaprilat is dialyzable at the rate of 62 mL/min.

Studies in dogs indicate that enalaprilat does not enter the brain, and that enalapril crosses the blood-brain barrier poorly, if at all. Multiple doses of enalapril maleate in rats do not result in accumulation in any tissues. Milk in lactating rats contains radioactivity following administration of ^{14}C enalapril maleate. Radioactivity was found to cross the placenta following administration of labeled drug to pregnant hamsters.

Pharmacodynamics

VASOTEC I.V. results in the reduction of both supine and standing systolic and diastolic blood pressure, usually with no orthostatic component. Symptomatic postural hypotension is therefore infrequent, although it might be anticipated in volume-depleted patients (see WARNINGS). The onset of action usually occurs within fifteen minutes of administration with the maximum effect occurring within one to four hours. The abrupt withdrawal of enalaprilat has not been associated with a rapid increase in blood pressure.

The duration of hemodynamic effects appears to be dose-related. However, for the recommended dose, the duration of action in most patients is approximately six hours.

Following administration of enalapril, there is an increase in renal blood flow; glomerular filtration rate is usually unchanged. The effects appear to be similar in patients with renovascular hypertension.

INDICATIONS AND USAGE

VASOTEC I.V. is indicated for the treatment of hypertension when oral therapy is not practical.

VASOTEC I.V. has been studied with only one other antihypertensive agent, furosemide, which showed approximately additive effects on blood pressure. Enalapril, the pro-drug of enalaprilat, has been used extensively with a variety of other antihypertensive agents, without apparent difficulty except for occasional hypotension.

In using VASOTEC I.V., consideration should be given to the fact that another angiotensin converting enzyme inhibitor, captopril, has caused agranulocytosis, particularly in patients with renal impairment or collagen vascular disease, and that available data are insufficient to show that VASOTEC I.V. does not have a similar risk. (See WARNINGS.)

CONTRAINDICATIONS

VASOTEC I.V. is contraindicated in patients who are hypersensitive to any component of this product and in patients with a history of angioedema related to previous treatment with an angiotensin converting enzyme inhibitor.

WARNINGS

Hypotension

Excessive hypotension is rare in uncomplicated hypertensive patients but is a possible consequence of the use of enalaprilat especially in severely salt/volume depleted persons such as those treated vigorously with diuretics or patients on dialysis. Patients at risk for excessive hypotension, sometimes associated with oliguria and/or progressive azotemia, and rarely with acute renal failure and/or death, include those with the following conditions or characteristics: heart failure, hyponatremia, high dose diuretic therapy, recent intensive diuresis or increase in diuretic dose, renal dialysis, or severe volume and/or salt depletion of any etiology. It may be advisable to eliminate the diuretic, reduce the diuretic dose or increase salt intake cautiously before initiating therapy with VASOTEC I.V. in patients at risk for excessive hypotension who are able to tolerate such adjustment. (See PRECAUTIONS, *Drug Interactions,* ADVERSE REACTIONS, and DOSAGE AND ADMINISTRATION.) In patients with heart failure, with or without associated renal insufficiency, excessive hypotension has been observed and may be associated with oliguria and/or progressive azotemia, and rarely with acute renal failure and/or death. Because of the potential for an excessive fall in blood pressure especially in these patients, therapy should be followed closely whenever the dose of enalaprilat is adjusted and/or diuretic is increased. Similar consideration may apply to patients with ischemic heart or cerebrovascular disease, in whom an excessive fall in blood pressure could result in a myocardial infarction or cerebrovascular accident.

If hypotension occurs, the patient should be placed in the supine position and, if necessary, receive an intravenous infusion of normal saline. A transient hypotensive response is not a contraindication to further doses, which usually can be given without difficulty once the blood pressure has increased after volume expansion.

Angioedema

Angioedema of the face, extremities, lips, tongue, glottis and/or larynx has been reported in patients treated with angiotensin converting enzyme inhibitors, including enalaprilat. In such cases VASOTEC I.V. should be promptly discontinued and appropriate therapy and monitoring should be provided until complete and sustained resolution of signs and symptoms has occurred. In instances where swelling has been confined to the face and lips the condition has generally resolved without treatment, although antihistamines have been useful in relieving symptoms. Angioedema associated with laryngeal edema may be fatal. **Where there is involvement of the tongue, glottis or larynx, likely to cause airway obstruction, appropriate therapy, e.g., subcutaneous epinephrine solution 1:1000 (0.3 mL to 0.5 mL) and/or measures necessary to ensure a patent airway, should be promptly provided.** (See ADVERSE REACTIONS.)

Patients with a history of angioedema unrelated to ACE inhibitor therapy may be at increased risk of angioedema while receiving an ACE inhibitor (see also CONTRAINDICATIONS).

Neutropenia/Agranulocytosis

Another angiotensin converting enzyme inhibitor, captopril, has been shown to cause agranulocytosis and bone marrow depression, rarely in uncomplicated patients but more frequently in patients with renal impairment especially if they also have a collagen vascular disease. Available data from clinical trials of enalapril are insufficient to show that enalapril does not cause agranulocytosis in similar rates. Foreign marketing experience has revealed several cases of neutropenia, or agranulocytosis in which a causal relationship to enalapril cannot be excluded. Periodic monitoring of white blood cell counts in patients with collagen vascular disease and renal disease should be considered.

Fetal/Neonatal Morbidity and Mortality

ACE inhibitors can cause fetal and neonatal morbidity and death when administered to pregnant women. Several dozen caes have been reported in the world literature. When pregnancy is detected, ACE inhibitors should be discontinued as soon as possible.

The use of ACE inhibitors during the second and third trimesters of pregnancy has been associated with fetal and neonatal injury, including hypotension, neonatal skull hypoplasia, anuria, reversible or irreversible renal failure, and death. Oligohydramnios has also bee reported, presumably resulting from decreased fetal renal function: oligohydramnois in this setting has been associated with fetal limb contractures, craniofacial deformation, and hypoplastic lung development. Prematurity, intrauterine growth retardation, and patent ductus arteriosus have also been reported, although it is not clear whether these occurrences were due to the ACE-inhibitor exposure.

These adverse effects do not appear to have resulted from intrauterine ACE-inhibitor exposure that has been limited to the first trimester. Mothers whose embryos and fetuses are exposed to ACE inhibitors only during the first trimester should be so informed. Nonetheless, when patients become pregnant, physicians should make every effort to discontinue the use of VASOTEC I.V. as soon as possible.

Rarely (probably less often than once in every thousand pregnancies), no alternative to ACE inhibitors will be found. In these rare cases, the mothers should be apprised of the potential hazards to their fetuses, and serial ultrasound examinations should be performed to assess the intraamniotic environment.

If oligohydramnois is observed, VASOTEC I.V. should be discontinued unless it is considered lifesaving for the mother. Contraction stress testing (CST, a non-stress test (NST), or biophysical profiling (BPP) may be appropriate, depending upon the week of pregnancy. Patients and physicians should be aware, however, that oligohydramnois may not appear until after the fetus has sustained irreversible injury.

Infants with histories of *in utero* exposure to ACE inhibitors should be closely observed for hypotension, oliguria, and hyperkalemia. If oliguria occurs, attention should be directed toward support of blood pressure and renal perfusion. Exchange transfusion or dialysis may be required as means of reversing hypotension and/or substituting for disordered renal function. Enalapril, which crosses the placenta, has been removed from neonatal circulation by peritoneal dialysis with some clinical benefit, and theoretically may be removed by exchange transfusion, although there is no experience with the latter procedure.

No teratogenic effects of oral enalapril were seen in studies of pregnant rats and rabbits. On a mg/kg basis, the doses used were up to 333 times (in rats) and 50 times (in rabbits) the maximum recommended human dose.

PRECAUTIONS

General

Impaired Renal Function: As a consequence of inhibiting the renin-angiotensin-aldosterone system, changes in renal function may be anticipated in susceptible individuals. In patients with severe heart failure whose renal function may depend on the activity of the renin-angiotensin-aldosterone system, treatment with angiotensin converting enzyme inhibitors, including enalapril or enalaprilat, may be associated with oliguria and/or progressive azotemia and rarely with acute renal failure and/or death.

In clinical studies in hypertensive patients with unilateral or bilateral renal artery stenosis, increases in blood urea nitrogen and serum creatinine were observed in 20 percent of patients receiving enalapril. These increases were almost always reversible upon discontinuation of enalapril or enalaprilat and/or diuretic therapy. In such patients renal function should be monitored during the first few weeks of therapy.

Some hypertensive patients with no apparent pre-existing renal vascular disease have developed increases in blood urea and serum creatinine, usually minor and transient, especially when enalaprilat has been given concomitantly with a diuretic. This is more likely to occur in patients with pre-existing renal impairment. Dosage reduction of enalaprilat and/or discontinuation of the diuretic may be required.

Evaluation of the hypertensive patient should always include assessment of renal function. (See DOSAGE AND ADMINISTRATION.)

Hemodialysis Patients: Anaphylactoid reactions have been reported in patients dialyzed with high-flux membranes (e.g., AN 69*) and treated concomitantly with an ACE inhibitor. In these patients consideration should be given to using a different type of dialysis membrane or a different class of antihypertensive agent.

Hyperkalemia: Elevated serum potassium (greater than 5.7 mEq/L) was observed in approximately one percent of hypertensive patients in clinical trials receiving enalapril. In most cases these were isolated values which resolved despite continued therapy. Hyperkalemia was a cause of discontinuation of therapy in 0.28 percent of hypertensive patients. Risk factors for the development of hyperkalemia include renal insufficiency, diabetes mellitus, and the concomitant use of potassium-sparing agents or potassium supplements, which should be used cautiously, if at all, with VASOTEC I.V. (See *Drug Interactions.*)

Cough: Cough has been reported with the use of ACE inhibitors. Characteristically, the cough is nonproductive, persistent and resolves after discontinuation of therapy. ACE inhibitor-induced cough should be considered as part of the differential diagnosis of cough.

Surgery/Anesthesia: In patients undergoing major surgery or during anesthesia with agents that produce hypotension, enalapril may block angiotensin II formation secondary to compensatory renin release. If hypotension occurs and is considered to be due to this mechanism, it can be corrected by volume expansion.

*Registered trademark of Hospal Ltd.

Drug Interactions

Hypotension—Patients on Diuretic Therapy: Patients on diuretics and especially those in whom diuretic therapy was recently instituted, may occasionally experience an excessive reduction of blood pressure after initiation of therapy with enalaprilat. The possibility of hypotensive effects with

Continued on next page

Information on the Merck & Co. products listed on these pages is the full prescribing information from product circulars in use October 1, 1992.

Merck & Co.—Cont.

enalaprilat can be minimized by administration of an intravenous infusion of normal saline, discontinuing the diuretic or increasing the salt intake prior to initiation of treatment with enalaprilat. If it is necessary to continue the diuretic, provide close medical supervision for at least one hour after the initial dose of enalaprilat. (See WARNINGS.)

Agents Causing Renin Release: The antihypertensive effect of VASOTEC I.V. appears to be augmented by antihypertensive agents that cause renin release (e.g., diuretics.)

Other Cardiovascular Agents: VASOTEC I.V. has been used concomitantly with digitalis, beta adrenergic-blocking agents, methyldopa, nitrates, calcium-blocking agents, hydralazine and prazosin without evidence of clinically significant adverse interactions.

Agents Increasing Serum Potassium: VASOTEC I.V. attenuates potassium loss caused by thiazide-type diuretics. Potassium-sparing diuretics (e.g., spironolactone, triamterene, or amiloride), potassium supplements, or potassium-containing salt substitutes may lead to significant increases in serum potassium. Therefore, if concomitant use of these agents is indicated because of demonstrated hypokalemia, they should be used with caution and with frequent monitoring of serum potassium.

Lithium: Lithium toxicity has been reported in patients receiving lithium concomitantly with drugs which cause elimination of sodium, including ACE inhibitors. A few cases of lithium toxicity have been reported in patients receiving concomitant enalapril and lithium and were reversible upon discontinuation of both drugs. It is recommended that serum lithium levels be monitored frequently if enalapril is administered concomitantly with lithium.

Carcinogenesis, Mutagenesis, Impairment of Fertility
Carcinogenicity studies have not been done with VASOTEC I.V.

VASOTEC I.V. is the bioactive form of its ethyl ester, enalapril maleate. There was no evidence of a tumorigenic effect when enalapril was administered orally for 106 weeks to rats at doses up to 90 mg/kg/day (150 times* the maximum daily human dose). Enalapril has also been administered for 94 weeks to male and female mice at oral doses up to 90 and 180 mg/kg/day, respectively (150 and 300 times* the maximum oral daily dose for humans), and showed no evidence of carcinogenicity.

VASOTEC I.V. was not mutagenic in the Ames microbial mutagen test with or without metabolic activation. Enalapril showed no drug-related changes in the following genotoxicity studies: rec-assay, reverse mutation assay with *E. coli*, sister chromatid exchange with cultured mammalian cells, the micronucleus test with mice, and in an *in vivo* cytogenic study using mouse bone marrow. There were no adverse effects on reproductive performance in male and female rats treated with 10 to 90 mg enalapril/kg/day.

* Based on patient weight of 50 kg

Pregnancy
Pregnancy Categories C (first trimester) and *D* (second and third trimesters). See WARNINGS, *Fetal/Neonatal Morbidity and Mortality.*

Nursing Mothers
Enalapril and enalaprilat are detected in human milk in trace amounts. Caution should be exercised when VASOTEC I.V. is given to a nursing mother.

Pediatric Use
Safety and effectiveness in children have not been established.

ADVERSE REACTIONS

VASOTEC I.V. has been found to be generally well tolerated in controlled clinical trials involving 349 patients (168 with hypertension, 153 with congestive heart failure and 28 with coronary artery disease). The most frequent clinically significant adverse experience was hypotension (3.4 percent), occurring in eight patients (5.2 percent) with congestive heart failure, three (1.8 percent) with hypertension and one with coronary artery disease. Other adverse experiences occurring in greater than one percent of patients were: headache (2.9 percent) and nausea (1.1 percent).

Adverse experiences occurring in 0.5 to 1.0 percent of patients in controlled clinical trials included: myocardial infarction, fatigue, dizziness, fever, rash and constipation.

Angioedema: Angioedema has been reported in patients receiving enalaprilat. Angioedema associated with laryngeal edema may be fatal. If angioedema of the face, extremities, lips, tongue, glottis and/or larynx occurs, treatment with enalaprilat should be discontinued and appropriate therapy instituted immediately. (See WARNINGS.)

Cough: See PRECAUTIONS, *Cough.*

Enalapril Maleate
Since enalapril is converted to enalaprilat, those adverse experiences associated with enalapril might also be expected to occur with VASOTEC I.V.

The following adverse experiences have been reported with enalapril and, within each category, are listed in order of decreasing severity.

Body As A Whole: Syncope, orthostatic effects, anaphylactoid reactions (see PRECAUTIONS, *Hemodialysis Patients*), chest pain, abdominal pain, asthenia.

Cardiovascular: Cardiac arrest; myocardial infarction or cerebrovascular accident, possibly secondary to excessive hypotension in high risk patients (see WARNINGS, *Hypotension*); pulmonary embolism and infarction; pulmonary edema; rhythm disturbances including atrial tachycardia and bradycardia; atrial fibrillation; orthostatic hypotension; angina pectoris; palpitation.

Digestive: Ileus, pancreatitis, hepatic failure, hepatitis (hepatocellular [proven on rechallenge] or cholestatic jaundice), melena, diarrhea, vomiting, dyspepsia, anorexia, glossitis, stomatitis, dry mouth.

Musculoskeletal: Muscle cramps.

Nervous/Psychiatric: Depression, vertigo, confusion, ataxia, somnolence, insomnia, nervousness, paresthesia.

Respiratory: Bronchospasm, dyspnea, pneumonia, bronchitis, cough, rhinorrhea, sore throat and hoarseness, asthma, upper respiratory infection.

Skin: Exfoliative dermatitis, toxic epidermal necrolysis, Stevens-Johnson syndrome, herpes zoster, erythema multiforme, urticaria, pruritus, alopecia, flushing, diaphoresis.

Special Senses: Blurred vision, taste alteration, anosmia, tinnitus, conjunctivitis, dry eyes, tearing.

Urogenital: Renal failure, oliguria, renal dysfunction (see PRECAUTIONS and DOSAGE AND ADMINISTRATION), urinary tract infection, flank pain, gynecomastia, impotence.

A symptom complex has been reported which may include a positive ANA, an elevated erythrocyte sedimentation rate, arthralgia/arthritis, myalgia, fever, serositis, vasculitis, leukocytosis, eosinophilia, photosensitivity, rash and other dermatologic manifestations.

Angioedema: Angioedema has been reported in patients receiving enalapril (0.2 percent). Angioedema associated with laryngeal edema may be fatal. If angioedema of the face, extremities, lips, tongue, glottis and/or larynx occurs, treatment with enalapril should be discontinued and appropriate therapy instituted immediately. (See WARNINGS.)

Hypotension: Combining the results of clinical trials in patients with hypertension or congestive heart failure, hypotension (including postural hypotension, and other orthostatic effects) was reported in 2.3 percent of patients following the initial dose of enalapril or during extended therapy. In the hypertensive patients, hypotension occurred in 0.9 percent and syncope occurred in 0.5 percent of patients. Hypotension or syncope was a cause for discontinuation of therapy in 0.1 percent of hypertensive patients. (See WARNINGS.)

Fetal/Neonatal Morbidity and Mortality: See WARNINGS, *Fetal/Neonatal Morbidity and Mortality.*

Clinical Laboratory Test Findings
Serum Electrolytes: Hyperkalemia (see PRECAUTIONS), hyponatremia.

Creatinine, Blood Urea Nitrogen: In controlled clinical trials minor increases in blood urea nitrogen and serum creatinine, reversible upon discontinuation of therapy, were observed in about 0.2 percent of patients with essential hypertension treated with enalapril alone. Increases are more likely to occur in patients receiving concomitant diuretics or in patients with renal artery stenosis. (See PRECAUTIONS.)

Hemoglobin and Hematocrit: Small decreases in hemoglobin and hematocrit (mean decreases of approximately 0.3 g percent and 1.0 vol percent, respectively) occur frequently in hypertensive patients treated with enalapril but are rarely of clinical importance unless another cause of anemia coexists. In clinical trials, less than 0.1 percent of patients discontinued therapy due to anemia.

Other (Causal Relationship Unknown): In marketing experience, rare cases of neutropenia, thrombocytopenia and bone marrow depression have been reported. A few cases of hemolysis have been reported in patients with G6PD deficiency.

Liver Function Tests: Elevations of liver enzymes and/or serum bilirubin have occurred.

OVERDOSAGE

In clinical studies, some hypertensive patients received a maximum dose of 80 mg of enalaprilat intravenously over a fifteen minute period. At this high dose, no adverse effects beyond those as associated with the recommended dosages were observed.

The intravenous LD_{50} of enalaprilat is 3740–5890 mg/kg in female mice.

The most likely manifestation of overdosage would be hypotension, for which the usual treatment would be intravenous infusion of normal saline solution.

Enalaprilat may be removed from general circulation by hemodialysis and has been removed from neonatal circulation by peritoneal dialysis.

DOSAGE AND ADMINISTRATION

FOR INTRAVENOUS ADMINISTRATION ONLY

The dose in hypertension is 1.25 mg every six hours administered intravenously over a five minute period. A clinical response is usually seen within 15 minutes. Peak effects after the first dose may not occur for up to four hours after dosing. The peak effects of the second and subsequent doses may exceed those of the first.

No dosage regimen for VASOTEC I.V. has been clearly demonstrated to be more effective in treating hypertension than 1.25 mg every six hours. However, in controlled clinical studies in hypertension, doses as high as 5 mg every six hours were well tolerated for up to 36 hours. There has been inadequate experience with doses greater than 20 mg per day. In studies of patients with hypertension, VASOTEC I.V. has not been administered for periods longer than 48 hours. In other studies, patients have received VASOTEC I.V. for as long as seven days.

The dose for patients being converted to VASOTEC I.V. from oral therapy for hypertension with enalapril maleate is 1.25 mg every six hours. For conversion from intravenous to oral therapy, the recommended initial dose of Tablets VASOTEC (Enalapril Maleate) is 5 mg once a day with subsequent dosage adjustments as necessary.

Patients on Diuretic Therapy
For patients on diuretic therapy the recommended starting dose for hypertension is 0.625 mg administered intravenously over a five minute period. A clinical response is usually seen within 15 minutes. Peak effects after the first dose may not occur for up to four hours after dosing, although most of the effect is usually apparent within the first hour. If after one hour there is an inadequate clinical response, the 0.625 mg dose may be repeated. Additional doses of 1.25 mg may be administered at six hour intervals.

For conversion from intravenous to oral therapy, the recommended initial dose of Tablets VASOTEC (Enalapril Maleate) for patients who have responded to 0.625 mg of enalaprilat every six hours is 2.5 mg once a day with subsequent dosage adjustment as necessary.

Dosage Adjustment in Renal Impairment
The usual dose of 1.25 mg of enalaprilat every six hours is recommended for patients with a creatinine clearance > 30 mL/min (serum creatinine of up to approximately 3 mg/dL). For patients with creatinine clearance ≤ 30 mL/min (serum creatinine ≥ 3 mg/dL), the initial dose is 0.625 mg. (See WARNINGS.)

If after one hour there is an inadequate clinical response, the 0.625 mg dose may be repeated. Additional doses of 1.25 mg may be administered at six hour intervals.

For dialysis patients, the initial dose should be 0.625 mg q.6.h.

For conversion from intravenous to oral therapy, the recommended initial dose of Tablets VASOTEC (Enalapril Maleate) is 5 mg once a day for patients with creatinine clearance > 30 mL/min and 2.5 mg once daily for patients with creatinine clearance ≤ 30 mL/min. Dosage should then be adjusted according to blood pressure response.

Administration
VASOTEC I.V. should be administered as a slow intravenous infusion, as indicated above, over at least five minutes. It may be administered as provided or diluted with up to 50 mL of a compatible diluent.

Parenteral drug products should be inspected visually for particulate matter and discoloration prior to use whenever solution and container permit.

Compatibility and Stability
VASOTEC I.V. as supplied and mixed with the following intravenous diluents has been found to maintain full activity for 24 hours at room temperature:

5 percent Dextrose Injection
0.9 percent Sodium Chloride Injection
0.9 percent Sodium Chloride Injection in 5 percent Dextrose
5 percent Dextrose in Lactated Ringer's Injection
McGaw ISOLYTE* E.

* Registered trademark of American Hospital Supply Corporation.

HOW SUPPLIED

No. 3508—VASOTEC I.V., 1.25 mg per mL, is a clear, colorless solution and is supplied in vials containing 1 mL and 2 mL.

NDC 0006-3508-01, 1 mL vials.
NDC 0006-3508-04, 2 mL vials.

Storage
Store below 30°C (86°F).

A.H.F.S. Category: 24:08

DC 7494617   Issued May 1992

VASOTEC® Tablets ℞
(Enalapril Maleate), U.S.P.

> **USE IN PREGNANCY**
> **When used in pregnancy during the second and third trimesters, ACE inhibitors can cause injury and even death to the developing fetus.** When pregnancy is detected, VASOTEC should be discontinued as soon as possible. See WARNINGS. *Fetal/Neonatal Morbidity and Mortality.*

DESCRIPTION

VASOTEC* (Enalapril Maleate) is the maleate salt of enalapril, the ethyl ester of a long-acting angiotensin converting enzyme inhibitor, enalaprilat. Enalapril maleate is chemically described as (*S*)-1-[*N*-[1-(ethoxycarbonyl)-3-phenylpropyl]-L-alanyl]-L-proline, (*Z*)-2-butenedioate salt (1:1). Its empirical formula is $C_{20}H_{28}N_2O_5 \cdot C_4H_4O_4$, and its structural formula is:

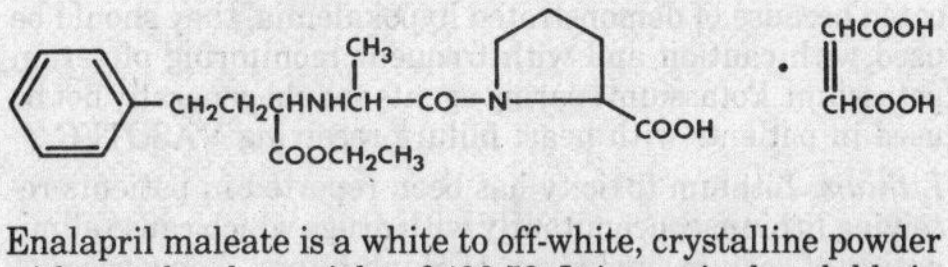

Enalapril maleate is a white to off-white, crystalline powder with a molecular weight of 492.53. It is sparingly soluble in water, soluble in ethanol, and freely soluble in methanol.
Enalapril is a pro-drug; following oral administration, it is bioactivated by hydrolysis of the ethyl ester to enalaprilat, which is the active angiotensin converting enzyme inhibitor.
Enalapril maleate is supplied as 2.5 mg, 5 mg, 10 mg, and 20 mg tablets for oral administration. In addition to the active ingredient enalapril maleate, each tablet contains the following inactive ingredients: lactose, magnesium stearate, starch, and other ingredients. The 2.5 mg, 10 mg and 20 mg tablets also contain iron oxides.

*Registered trademark of MERCK & CO., INC.

CLINICAL PHARMACOLOGY

Mechanism of Action
Enalapril, after hydrolysis to enalaprilat, inhibits angiotensin-converting enzyme (ACE) in human subjects and animals. ACE is a peptidyl dipeptidase that catalyzes the conversion of angiotensin I to the vasoconstrictor substance, angiotensin II. Angiotensin II also stimulates aldosterone secretion by the adrenal cortex. The beneficial effects of enalapril in hypertension and heart failure appear to result primarily from suppression of the renin-angiotensin-aldosterone system. Inhibition of ACE results in decreased plasma angiotensin II, which leads to decreased vasopressor activity and to decreased aldosterone secretion. Although the latter decrease is small, it results in small increases of serum potassium. In hypertensive patients treated with VASOTEC alone for up to 48 weeks, mean increases in serum potassium of approximately 0.2 mEq/L were observed. In patients treated with VASOTEC plus a thiazide diuretic, there was essentially no change in serum potassium. (See PRECAUTIONS.)
Removal of angiotensin II negative feedback on renin secretion leads to increased plasma renin activity.
ACE is identical to kininase, an enzyme that degrades bradykinin. Whether increased levels of bradykinin, a potent vasodepressor peptide, play a role in the therapeutic effects of VASOTEC remains to be elucidated.
While the mechanism through which VASOTEC lowers blood pressure is believed to be primarily suppression of the renin-angiotensin-aldosterone system, VASOTEC is antihypertensive even in patients with low-renin hypertension. Although VASOTEC was antihypertensive in all races studied, black hypertensive patients (usually a low-renin hypertensive population) had a smaller average response to enalapril monotherapy than non-black patients.
Pharmacokinetics and Metabolism
Following oral administration of VASOTEC, peak serum concentrations of enalapril occur within about one hour. Based on urinary recovery, the extent of absorption of enalapril is approximately 60 percent. Enalapril absorption is not influenced by the presence of food in the gastrointestinal tract. Following absorption, enalapril is hydrolyzed to enalaprilat, which is a more potent angiotensin converting enzyme inhibitor than enalapril; enalaprilat is poorly absorbed when administered orally. Peak serum concentrations of enalaprilat occur three to four hours after an oral dose of enalapril maleate. Excretion of VASOTEC is primarily renal. Approximately 94 percent of the dose is recovered in the urine and feces as enalaprilat or enalapril. The principal components in urine are enalaprilat, accounting for about 40 percent of the dose, and intact enalapril. There is no evidence of metabolites of enalapril, other than enalaprilat.
The serum concentration profile of enalaprilat exhibits a prolonged terminal phase, apparently representing a small fraction of the administered dose that has been bound to ACE. The amount bound does not increase with dose, indicating a saturable site of binding. The effective half-life for accumulation of enalaprilat following multiple doses of enalapril maleate is 11 hours.
The disposition of enalapril and enalaprilat in patients with renal insufficiency is similar to that in patients with normal renal function until the glomerular filtration rate is 30 mL/min or less. With glomerular filtration rate ≤30 mL/min, peak and trough enalaprilat levels increase, time to peak concentration increases and time to steady state may be delayed. The effective half-life of enalaprilat following multiple doses of enalapril maleate is prolonged at this level of renal insufficiency. (See DOSAGE AND ADMINISTRATION.) Enalaprilat is dialyzable at the rate of 62 mL/min.
Studies in dogs indicate that enalapril crosses the blood-brain barrier poorly, if at all; enalaprilat does not enter the brain. Multiple doses of enalapril maleate in rats do not result in accumulation in any tissues. Milk of lactating rats contains radioactivity following administration of ^{14}C enalapril maleate. Radioactivity was found to cross the placenta following administration of labeled drug to pregnant hamsters.
Pharmacodynamics and Clinical Effects
Hypertension: Administration of VASOTEC to patients with hypertension of severity ranging from mild to severe results in a reduction of both supine and standing blood pressure usually with no orthostatic component. Symptomatic postural hypotension is therefore infrequent, although it might be anticipated in volume-depleted patients. (See WARNINGS.)
In most patients studied, after oral administration of a single dose of enalapril, onset of antihypertensive activity was seen at one hour with peak reduction of blood pressure achieved by four to six hours.
At recommended doses, antihypertensive effects have been maintained for at least 24 hours. In some patients the effects may diminish toward the end of the dosing interval (see DOSAGE AND ADMINISTRATION).
In some patients achievement of optimal blood pressure reduction may require several weeks of therapy.
The antihypertensive effects of VASOTEC have continued during long term therapy. Abrupt withdrawal of VASOTEC has not been associated with a rapid increase in blood pressure.
In hemodynamic studies in patients with essential hypertension, blood pressure reduction was accompanied by a reduction in peripheral arterial resistance with an increase in cardiac output and little or no change in heart rate. Following administration of VASOTEC, there is an increase in renal blood flow; glomerular filtration rate is usually unchanged. The effects appear to be similar in patients with renovascular hypertension.
When given together with thiazide-type diuretics, the blood pressure lowering effects of VASOTEC are approximately additive.
In a clinical pharmacology study, indomethacin or sulindac was administered to hypertensive patients receiving VASOTEC. In this study there was no evidence of a blunting of the antihypertensive action of VASOTEC.
Heart Failure: In trials in patients treated with digitalis and diuretics, treatment with enalapril resulted in decreased systemic vascular resistance, blood pressure, pulmonary capillary wedge pressure and heart size, and increased cardiac output and exercise tolerance. Heart rate was unchanged or slightly reduced, and mean ejection fraction was unchanged or increased. There was a beneficial effect on severity of heart failure as measured by the New York Heart Association (NYHA) classification and on symptoms of dyspnea and fatigue. Hemodynamic effects were observed after the first dose, and appeared to be maintained in uncontrolled studies lasting as long as four months. Effects on exercise tolerance, heart size, and severity and symptoms of heart failure were observed in placebo-controlled studies lasting from eight weeks to over one year. From the results of one trial involving an ACE inhibitor other than enalapril, it appears that the symptomatic benefit associated with that ACE inhibitor's use does not depend upon digitalis being present.
Heart Failure, Mortality Trials: In a multicenter, placebo-controlled clinical trial (SOLVD), from more than 39,000 patients screened, 2569 patients with all degrees of symptomatic heart failure and ejection fraction ≤35 percent were randomized to placebo or enalapril and followed for up to 55 months. Use of enalapril was associated with an 11 percent reduction in all-cause mortality and a 30 percent reduction in hospitalization for heart failure. Diseases that excluded patients from enrollment in the study included severe stable angina (>2 attacks/day), hemodynamically significant valvular or outflow tract obstruction, renal failure (creatinine >2.5 mg/dL), cerebral vascular disease (e.g., significant carotid artery disease), advanced pulmonary disease, malignancies, active myocarditis and constrictive pericarditis.
In another multicenter, placebo-controlled trial (CONSENSUS) limited to patients with NYHA Class IV congestive heart failure and radiographic evidence of cardiomegaly, use of enalapril was associated with improved survival. The results are shown in the following table.

	SURVIVAL (%) Six Months	One Year
VASOTEC (n = 127)	74	64
Placebo (n = 126)	56	48

In both trials, patients were also usually receiving digitalis, diuretics or both.

INDICATIONS AND USAGE

Hypertension
VASOTEC is indicated for the treatment of hypertension.
VASOTEC is effective alone or in combination with other antihypertensive agents, especially thiazide-type diuretics. The blood pressure lowering effects of VASOTEC and thiazides are approximately additive.
Heart Failure
VASOTEC is indicated for the treatment of symptomatic congestive heart failure, usually in combination with diuretics and digitalis. In these patients VASOTEC improves symptoms, increases survival, and decreases the frequency of hospitalization (see CLINICAL PHARMACOLOGY, *Heart Failure, Mortality Trials* for details and limitations of survival trials).
In using VASOTEC consideration should be given to the fact that another angiotensin converting enzyme inhibitor, captopril, has caused agranulocytosis, particularly in patients with renal impairment or collagen vascular disease, and that available data are insufficient to show that VASOTEC does not have a similar risk. (See WARNINGS.)

CONTRAINDICATIONS

VASOTEC is contraindicated in patients who are hypersensitive to this product and in patients with a history of angioedema related to previous treatment with an angiotensin converting enzyme inhibitor.

WARNINGS

Angioedema
Angioedema of the face, extremities, lips, tongue, glottis and/or larynx has been reported in patients treated with angiotensin converting enzyme inhibitors, including VASOTEC. In such cases VASOTEC should be promptly discontinued and appropriate therapy and monitoring should be provided until complete and sustained resolution of signs and symptoms has occurred. In instances where swelling has been confined to the face and lips the condition has generally resolved without treatment, although antihistamines have been useful in relieving symptoms. Angioedema associated with laryngeal edema may be fatal. **Where there is involvement of the tongue, glottis or larynx, likely to cause airway obstruction, appropriate therapy, e.g., subcutaneous epinephrine solution 1:1000 (0.3 mL to 0.5 mL) and/or measures necessary to ensure a patent airway, should be promptly provided.** (See ADVERSE REACTIONS).
Patients with a history of angioedema unrelated to ACE inhibitor therapy may be at increased risk of angioedema while receiving an ACE inhibitor (see also CONTRAINDICATIONS).
Hypotension
Excessive hypotension is rare in uncomplicated hypertensive patients treated with VASOTEC alone. Patients with heart failure given VASOTEC commonly have some reduction in blood pressure, especially with the first dose, but discontinuation of therapy for continuing symptomatic hypotension usually is not necessary when dosing instructions are followed; caution should be observed when initiating therapy. (See DOSAGE AND ADMINISTRATION.) Patients at risk for excessive hypotension, sometimes associated with oliguria and/or progressive azotemia, and rarely with acute renal failure and/or death, include those with the following conditions or characteristics: heart failure, hyponatremia, high dose diuretic therapy, recent intensive diuresis or increase in diuretic dose, renal dialysis, or severe volume and/or salt depletion of any etiology. It may be advisable to eliminate the diuretic (except in patients with heart failure), reduce the diuretic dose or increase salt intake cautiously before initiating therapy with VASOTEC in patients at risk for excessive hypotension who are able to tolerate such adjustments. (See PRECAUTIONS, *Drug Interactions* and ADVERSE REACTIONS.) In patients at risk for excessive hypo-

Continued on next page

Information on the Merck & Co. products listed on these pages is the full prescribing information from product circulars in use October 1, 1992.

Merck & Co.—Cont.

tension, therapy should be started under very close medical supervision and such patients should be followed closely for the first two weeks of treatment and whenever the dose of enalapril and/or diuretic is increased. Similar considerations may apply to patients with ischemic heart or cerebrovascular disease, in whom an excessive fall in blood pressure could result in a myocardial infarction or cerebrovascular accident.

If excessive hypotension occurs, the patient should be placed in the supine position and, if necessary, receive an intravenous infusion of normal saline. A transient hypotensive response is not a contraindication to further doses of VASOTEC, which usually can be given without difficulty once the blood pressure has stabilized. If symptomatic hypotension develops, a dose reduction or discontinuation of VASOTEC or concomitant diuretic may be necessary.

Neutropenia/Agranulocytosis

Another angiotensin converting enzyme inhibitor, captopril, has been shown to cause agranulocytosis and bone marrow depression, rarely in uncomplicated patients but more frequently in patients with renal impairment especially if they also have a collagen vascular disease. Available data from clinical trials of enalapril are insufficient to show that enalapril does not cause agranulocytosis at similar rates. Foreign marketing experience has revealed several cases of neutropenia or agranulocytosis in which a causal relationship to enalapril cannot be excluded. Periodic monitoring of white blood cell counts in patients with collagen vascular disease and renal disease should be considered.

Fetal/Neonatal Morbidity and Mortality

ACE inhibitors can cause fetal and neonatal morbidity and death when administered to pregnant women. Several dozen cases have been reported in the world literature. When pregnancy is detected, ACE inhibitors should be discontinued as soon as possible.

The use of ACE inhibitors during the second and third trimesters of pregnancy has been associated with fetal and neonatal injury, including hypotension, neonatal skull hypoplasia, anuria, reversible or irreversible renal failure, and death. Oligohydramnios has also been reported, presumably resulting from decreased fetal renal function: oligohydramnois in this setting has been associated with fetal limb contractures, craniofacial deformation, and hypoplastic lung development. Prematurity, intrauterine growth retardation, and patent ductus arteriosus have also been reported, although it is not clear whether these occurrences were due to the ACE-inhibitor exposure.

These adverse effects do not appear to have resulted from intrauterine ACE-inhibitor exposure that has been limited to the first trimester. Mothers whose embryos and fetuses are exposed to ACE inhibitors only during the first trimester should be so informed. Nonetheless, when patients become pregnant, physicians should make every effort to discontinue the use of VASOTEC as soon as possible.

Rarely (probably less often than once in every thousand pregnancies), no alternative to ACE inhibitors will be found. In these rare cases, the mothers should be apprised of the potential hazards to their fetuses, and serial ultrasound examinations should be performed to assess the intraamniotic environment.

If oligohydramnois is observed, VASOTEC should be discontinued unless it is considered lifesaving for the mother. Contraction stress testing (CST, a non-stress test (NST), or biophysical profiling (BPP) may be appropriate, depending upon the week of pregnancy. Patients and physicians should be aware, however, that oligohydramnois may not appear until after the fetus has sustained irreversible injury.

Infants with histories of *in utero* exposure to ACE inhibitors should be closely observed for hypotension, oliguria, and hyperkalemia. If oliguria occurs, attention should be directed toward support of blood pressure and renal perfusion. Exchange transfusion or dialysis may be required as means of reversing hypotension and/or substituting for disordered renal function. Enalapril, which crosses the placenta, has been removed from neonatal circulation by peritoneal dialysis with some clinical benefit, and theoretically may be removed by exchange transfusion, although there is no experience with the latter procedure.

No teratogenic effects of oral enalapril were seen in studies of pregnant rats and rabbits. On a mg/kg basis, the doses used were up to 333 times (in rats), and 50 times (in rabbits) the maximum recommended human dose.

PRECAUTIONS

General

Impaired Renal Function: As a consequence of inhibiting the renin-angiotensin-aldosterone system, changes in renal function may be anticipated in susceptible individuals. In patients with severe heart failure whose renal function may depend on the activity of the renin-angiotensin-aldosterone system, treatment with angiotensin converting enzyme inhibitors, including VASOTEC, may be associated with oliguria and/or progressive azotemia and rarely with acute renal failure and/or death.

In clinical studies in hypertensive patients with unilateral or bilateral renal artery stenosis, increases in blood urea nitrogen and serum creatinine were observed in 20 percent of patients. These increases were almost always reversible upon discontinuation of enalapril and/or diuretic therapy. In such patients renal function should be monitored during the first few weeks of therapy.

Some patients with hypertension or heart failure with no apparent pre-existing renal vascular disease have developed increases in blood urea and serum creatinine, usually minor and transient, especially when VASOTEC has been given concomitantly with a diuretic. This is more likely to occur in patients with pre-existing renal impairment. Dosage reduction and/or discontinuation of the diuretic and/or VASOTEC may be required.

Evaluation of patients with hypertension or heart failure should always include assessment of renal function. (See DOSAGE AND ADMINISTRATION.)

Hemodialysis Patients: Anaphylactoid reactions have been reported in patients dialyzed with high-flux membranes (e.g., AN 69*) and treated concomitantly with an ACE inhibitor. In these patients consideration should be given to using a different type of dialysis membrane or a different class of antihypertensive agent.

Hyperkalemia: Elevated serum potassium (greater than 5.7 mEq/L) was observed in approximately one percent of hypertensive patients in clinical trials. In most cases these were isolated values which resolved despite continued therapy. Hyperkalemia was a cause of discontinuation of therapy in 0.28 percent of hypertensive patients. In clinical trials in heart failure, hyperkalemia was observed in 3.8 percent of patients but was not a cause for discontinuation.

Risk factors for the development of hyperkalemia include renal insufficiency, diabetes mellitus, and the concomitant use of potassium-sparing diuretics, potassium supplements and/or potassium-containing salt substitutes, which should be used cautiously, if at all, with VASOTEC. (See *Drug Interactions.*)

Cough: Cough has been reported with the use of ACE inhibitors. Characteristically, the cough is nonproductive, persistent and resolves after discontinuation of therapy. ACE inhibitor-induced cough should be considered as part of the differential diagnosis of cough.

Surgery/Anesthesia: In patients undergoing major surgery or during anesthesia with agents that produce hypotension, enalapril may block angiotensin II formation secondary to compensatory renin release. If hypotension occurs and is considered to be due to this mechanism, it can be corrected by volume expansion.

*Registered trademark of Hospal Ltd.

Information for Patients

Angioedema: Angioedema, including laryngeal edema, may occur especially following the first dose of enalapril. Patients should be so advised and told to report immediately any signs or symptoms suggesting angioedema (swelling of face, extremities, eyes, lips, tongue, difficulty in swallowing or breathing) and to take no more drug until they have consulted with the prescribing physician.

Hypotension: Patients should be cautioned to report lightheadedness, especially during the first few days of therapy. If actual syncope occurs, the patients should be told to discontinue the drug until they have consulted with the prescribing physician.

All patients should be cautioned that excessive perspiration and dehydration may lead to an excessive fall in blood pressure because of reduction in fluid volume. Other causes of volume depletion such as vomiting or diarrhea may also lead to a fall in blood pressure; patients should be advised to consult with the physician.

Hyperkalemia: Patients should be told not to use salt substitutes containing potassium without consulting their physician.

Neutropenia: Patients should be told to report promptly any indication of infection (e.g., sore throat, fever) which may be a sign of neutropenia.

Pregnancy: Female patients of childbearing age should be told about the consequences of second- and third-trimester exposure to ACE inhibitors, and they should also be told that these consequences do not appear to have resulted from intrauterine ACE-inhibitor exposure that has been limited to the first trimester. These patients should be asked to report pregnancies to their physicians as soon as possible.

NOTE: As with many other drugs, certain advice to patients being treated with enalapril is warranted. This information is intended to aid in the safe and effective use of this medication. It is not a disclosure of all possible adverse or intended effects.

Drug Interactions

Hypotension—Patients on Diuretic Therapy: Patients on diuretics and especially those in whom diuretic therapy was recently instituted, may occasionally experience an excessive reduction of blood pressure after initiation of therapy with enalapril. The possibility of hypotensive effects with enalapril can be minimized by either discontinuing the diuretic or increasing the salt intake prior to initiation of treatment with enalapril. If it is necessary to continue the diuretic, provide close medical supervision after the initial dose for at least two hours and until blood pressure has stabilized for at least an additional hour. (See WARNINGS and DOSAGE AND ADMINISTRATION.)

Agents Causing Renin Release: The antihypertensive effect of VASOTEC is augmented by antihypertensive agents that cause renin release (e.g., diuretics).

Other Cardiovascular Agents: VASOTEC has been used concomitantly with beta adrenergic-blocking agents, methyldopa, nitrates, calcium-blocking agents, hydralazine, prazosin and digoxin without evidence of clinically significant adverse interactions.

Agents Increasing Serum Potassium: VASOTEC attenuates potassium loss caused by thiazide-type diuretics. Potassium-sparing diuretics (e.g., spironolactone, triamterene, or amiloride), potassium supplements, or potassium-containing salt substitutes may lead to significant increases in serum potassium. Therefore, if concomitant use of these agents is indicated because of demonstrated hypokalemia, they should be used with caution and with frequent monitoring of serum potassium. Potassium sparing agents should generally not be used in patients with heart failure receiving VASOTEC.

Lithium: Lithium toxicity has been reported in patients receiving lithium concomitantly with drugs which cause elimination of sodium, including ACE inhibitors. A few cases of lithium toxicity have been reported in patients receiving concomitant VASOTEC and lithium and were reversible upon discontinuation of both drugs. It is recommended that serum lithium levels be monitored frequently if enalapril is administered concomitantly with lithium.

Carcinogenesis, Mutagenesis, Impairment of Fertility

There was no evidence of a tumorigenic effect when enalapril was administered for 106 weeks to rats at doses up to 90 mg/kg/day (150 times* the maximum daily human dose). Enalapril has also been administered for 94 weeks to male and female mice at doses up to 90 and 180 mg/kg/day, respectively, (150 and 300 times* the maximum daily dose for humans) and showed no evidence of carcinogenicity.

Neither enalapril maleate nor the active diacid was mutagenic in the Ames microbial mutagen test with or without metabolic activation. Enalapril was also negative in the following genotoxicity studies: rec-assay, reverse mutation assay with *E. coli,* sister chromatid exchange with cultured mammalian cells, and the micronucleus test with mice, as well as in an *in vivo* cytogenic study using mouse bone marrow.

There were no adverse effects on reproductive performance in male and female rats treated with 10 to 90 mg/kg/day of enalapril.

*Based on patient weight of 50 kg

Pregnancy

Pregnancy Categories C (first trimester) and *D* (second and third trimesters). See WARNINGS, *Fetal/Neonatal Morbidity and Mortality.*

Nursing Mothers

Enalapril and enalaprilat are detected in human milk in trace amounts. Caution should be exercised when VASOTEC is given to a nursing mother.

Pediatric Use

Safety and effectiveness in children have not been established.

ADVERSE REACTIONS

VASOTEC has been evaluated for safety in more than 10,000 patients, including over 1000 patients treated for one year or more. VASOTEC has been found to be generally well tolerated in controlled clinical trials involving 2987 patients.

For the most part, adverse experiences were mild and transient in nature. In clinical trials, discontinuation of therapy due to clinical adverse experiences was required in 3.3 percent of patients with hypertension and in 5.7 percent of patients with heart failure. The frequency of adverse experiences was not related to total daily dosage within the usual dosage ranges. In patients with hypertension the overall percentage of patients treated with VASOTEC reporting adverse experiences was comparable to placebo.

HYPERTENSION

Adverse experiences occurring in greater than one percent of patients with hypertension treated with VASOTEC in controlled clinical trials are shown below. In patients treated with VASOTEC, the maximum duration of therapy was three years; in placebo treated patients the maximum duration of therapy was 12 weeks.

[See table top left next page.]

	VASOTEC (n = 2314) Incidence (discontinuation)	Placebo (n = 230) Incidence
Body As A Whole		
Fatigue	3.0 (<0.1)	2.6
Orthostatic Effects	1.2 (<0.1)	0.0
Asthenia	1.1 (0.1)	0.9
Digestive		
Diarrhea	1.4 (<0.1)	1.7
Nausea	1.4 (0.2)	1.7
Nervous/Psychiatric		
Headache	5.2 (0.3)	9.1
Dizziness	4.3 (0.4)	4.3
Respiratory		
Cough	1.3 (0.1)	0.9
Skin		
Rash	1.4 (0.4)	0.4

HEART FAILURE

Adverse experiences occurring in greater than one percent of patients with heart failure treated with VASOTEC are shown below. The incidences represent the experiences from both controlled and uncontrolled clinical trials (maximum duration of therapy was approximately one year). In the placebo treated patients, the incidences reported are from the controlled trials (maximum duration of therapy is 12 weeks). The percentage of patients with severe heart failure (NYHA Class IV) was 29 percent and 43 percent for patients treated with VASOTEC and placebo, respectively.

	VASOTEC (n = 673) Incidence (discontinuation)	Placebo (n = 339) Incidence
Body As A Whole		
Orthostatic Effects	2.2 (0.1)	0.3
Syncope	2.2 (0.1)	0.9
Chest Pain	2.1 (0.0)	2.1
Fatigue	1.8 (0.0)	1.8
Abdominal Pain	1.6 (0.4)	2.1
Asthenia	1.6 (0.1)	0.3
Cardiovascular		
Hypotension	6.7 (1.9)	0.6
Orthostatic Hypotension	1.6 (0.1)	0.3
Angina Pectoris	1.5 (0.1)	1.8
Myocardial Infarction	1.2 (0.3)	1.8
Digestive		
Diarrhea	2.1 (0.1)	1.2
Nausea	1.3 (0.1)	0.6
Vomiting	1.3 (0.0)	0.9
Nervous/Psychiatric		
Dizziness	7.9 (0.6)	0.6
Headache	1.8 (0.1)	0.9
Vertigo	1.6 (0.1)	1.2
Respiratory		
Cough	2.2 (0.0)	0.6
Bronchitis	1.3 (0.0)	0.9
Dyspnea	1.3 (0.1)	0.4
Pneumonia	1.0 (0.0)	2.4
Skin		
Rash	1.3 (0.0)	2.4
Urogenital		
Urinary Tract Infection	1.3 (0.0)	2.4

Other serious clinical adverse experiences occurring since the drug was marketed or adverse experiences occurring in 0.5 to 1.0 percent of patients with hypertension or heart failure in clinical trials are listed below and, within each category, are in order of decreasing severity.

Body As A Whole: Anaphylactoid reactions (see PRECAUTIONS, *Hemodialysis Patients*).

Cardiovascular: Cardiac arrest; myocardial infarction or cerebrovascular accident, possibly secondary to excessive hypotension in high risk patients (see WARNINGS, *Hypotension*); pulmonary embolism and infarction; pulmonary edema; rhythm disturbances including atrial tachycardia and bradycardia; atrial fibrillation; palpitation.

Digestive: Ileus, pancreatitis, hepatic failure, hepatitis (hepatocellular [proven on rechallenge] or cholestatic jaundice), melena, anorexia, dyspepsia, constipation, glossitis, stomatitis, dry mouth.

Musculoskeletal: Muscle cramps.

Nervous/Psychiatric: Depression, confusion, ataxia, somnolence, insomnia, nervousness, paresthesia.

Respiratory: Bronchospasm, rhinorrhea, sore throat and hoarseness, asthma, upper respiratory infection.

Skin: Exfoliative dermatitis, toxic epidermal necrolysis, Stevens-Johnson syndrome, herpes zoster, erythema multiforme, urticaria, pruritus, alopecia, flushing, diaphoresis.

Special Senses: Blurred vision, taste alteration, anosmia, tinnitus, conjunctivitis, dry eyes, tearing.

Urogenital: Renal failure, oliguria, renal dysfunction (see PRECAUTIONS and DOSAGE AND ADMINISTRATION), flank pain, gynecomastia, impotence.

A symptom complex has been reported which may include a positive ANA, an elevated erythrocyte sedimentation rate, arthralgia/arthritis, myalgia, fever, serositis, vasculitis, leukocytosis, eosinophilia, photosensitivity, rash and other dermatologic manifestations.

Angioedema: Angioedema has been reported in patients receiving VASOTEC (0.2 percent). Angioedema associated with laryngeal edema may be fatal. If angioedema of the face, extremities, lips, tongue, glottis and/or larynx occurs, treatment with VASOTEC should be discontinued and appropriate therapy instituted immediately. (See WARNINGS.)

Hypotension: In the hypertensive patients, hypotension occurred in 0.9 percent and syncope occurred in 0.5 percent of patients following the initial dose or during extended therapy. Hypotension or syncope was a cause for discontinuation of therapy in 0.1 percent of hypertensive patients. In heart failure patients, hypotension occurred in 6.7 percent and syncope occurred in 2.2 percent of patients. Hypotension or syncope was a cause for discontinuation of therapy in 1.9 percent of patients with heart failure. (See WARNINGS.)

Fetal/Neonatal Morbidity and Mortality: See WARNINGS, Fetal/Neonatal Morbidity and Mortality.

Cough: See PRECAUTIONS, Cough.

Clinical Laboratory Test Findings

Serum Electrolytes: Hyperkalemia (see PRECAUTIONS), hyponatremia.

Creatinine, Blood Urea Nitrogen: In controlled clinical trials minor increases in blood urea nitrogen and serum creatinine, reversible upon discontinuation of therapy, were observed in about 0.2 percent of patients with essential hypertension treated with VASOTEC alone. Increases are more likely to occur in patients receiving concomitant diuretics or in patients with renal artery stenosis. (See PRECAUTIONS.) In patients with heart failure who were also receiving diuretics with or without digitalis increases in blood urea nitrogen or serum creatinine, usually reversible upon discontinuation of VASOTEC and/or other concomitant diuretic therapy, were observed in about 11 percent of patients. Increases in blood urea nitrogen or creatinine were a cause for discontinuation in 1.2 percent of patients.

Hemoglobin and Hematocrit: Small decreases in hemoglobin and hematocrit (mean decreases of approximately 0.3 g percent and 1.0 vol percent, respectively) occur frequently in either hypertension or congestive heart failure patients treated with VASOTEC but are rarely of clinical importance unless another cause of anemia coexists. In clinical trials, less than 0.1 percent of patients discontinued therapy due to anemia.

Other (Causal Relationship Unknown): In marketing experience, rare cases of neutropenia, thrombocytopenia, and bone marrow depression have been reported. A few cases of hemolysis have been reported in patients with G6PD deficiency.

Liver Function Tests: Elevations of liver enzymes and/or serum bilirubin have occurred.

OVERDOSAGE

Limited data are available in regard to overdosage in humans.

The oral LD_{50} of enalapril is 2000 mg/kg in mice and rats. The most likely manifestation of overdosage would be hypotension, for which the usual treatment would be intravenous infusion of normal saline solution.

Enalaprilat may be removed from general circulation by hemodialysis and has been removed from neonatal circulation by peritoneal dialysis.

DOSAGE AND ADMINISTRATION

Hypertension

In patients who are currently being treated with a diuretic, symptomatic hypotension occasionally may occur following the initial dose of VASOTEC. The diuretic should, if possible, be discontinued for two to three days before beginning therapy with VASOTEC to reduce the likelihood of hypotension. (See WARNINGS.) If the patient's blood pressure is not controlled with VASOTEC alone, diuretic therapy may be resumed.

If the diuretic cannot be discontinued an initial dose of 2.5 mg should be used under medical supervision for at least two hours and until blood pressure has stabilized for at least an additional hour. (See WARNINGS and PRECAUTIONS, Drug Interactions.)

The recommended initial dose in patients not on diuretics is 5 mg once a day. Dosage should be adjusted according to blood pressure response. The usual dosage range is 10 to 40 mg per day administered in a single dose or two divided doses. In some patients treated once daily, the antihypertensive effect may diminish toward the end of the dosing interval. In such patients, an increase in dosage or twice daily administration should be considered. If blood pressure is not controlled with VASOTEC alone, a diuretic may be added. Concomitant administration of VASOTEC with potassium supplements, potassium salt substitutes, or potassium-spar-

ing diuretics may lead to increases of serum potassium (see PRECAUTIONS).

Dosage Adjustment in Hypertensive Patients with Renal Impairment

The usual dose of enalapril is recommended for patients with a creatinine clearance > 30 mL/min (serum creatinine of up to approximately 3 mg/dL). For patients with creatinine clearance ≤ 30 mL/min (serum creatinine ≥ 3 mg/dL), the first dose is 2.5 mg once daily. The dosage may be titrated upward until blood pressure is controlled or to a maximum of 40 mg daily.

Renal Status	Creatinine-Clearance mL/min	Initial Dose mg/day
Normal Renal Function	> 80 mL/min	5 mg
Mild Impairment	≤ 80 > 30 mL/min	5 mg
Moderate to Severe Impairment	≤ 30 mL/min	2.5 mg
Dialysis Patients*	—	2.5 mg on dialysis days**

*See PRECAUTIONS, *Hemodialysis Patients*

**Dosage on nondialysis days should be adjusted depending on the blood pressure response.

Heart Failure

VASOTEC is indicated for the treatment of symptomatic congestive heart failure, usually in combination with diuretics and digitalis.

The recommended starting dose is 2.5 mg administered once or twice daily. The usual therapeutic dosing range is 5 to 20 mg daily, given as a single dose or two divided doses; the majority of patient experience in clinical studies has been with twice daily dosing. Dosage may be adjusted depending upon clinical response (see WARNINGS). In the placebo-controlled studies which demonstrated improved survival, the dose of VASOTEC was titrated upward as tolerated by the patient. The maximum daily dose administered in clinical trials was 40 mg.

After the initial dose of VASOTEC, the patient should be observed under medical supervision for at least two hours and until blood pressure has stabilized for at least an additional hour. (See WARNINGS and PRECAUTIONS, *Drug Interactions.*) If possible, the dose of any concomitant diuretic should be reduced which may diminish the likelihood of hypotension. The appearance of hypotension after the initial dose of VASOTEC does not preclude subsequent careful dose titration with the drug, following effective management of the hypotension.

Dosage Adjustment in Patients with Heart Failure and Renal Impairment or Hyponatremia

In patients with heart failure who have hyponatremia (serum sodium less than 130 mEq/L) or with serum creatinine greater than 1.6 mg/dL, therapy should be initiated at 2.5 mg daily under close medical supervision. (See DOSAGE AND ADMINISTRATION, Heart Failure, WARNINGS and PRECAUTIONS, Drug Interactions.) The dose may be increased to 2.5 mg b.i.d., then 5 mg b.i.d. and higher as needed, usually at intervals of four days or more if at the time of dosage adjustment there is not excessive hypotension or significant deterioration of renal function. The maximum daily dose is 40 mg.

HOW SUPPLIED

No. 3411—Tablets VASOTEC, 2.5 mg, are yellow, biconvex barrel shaped, scored, compressed tablets with code MSD 14 on one side and VASOTEC on the other. They are supplied as follows:

NDC 0006-0014-94 unit of use bottles of 90 (with desiccant)
NDC 0006-0014-68 bottles of 100 (with desiccant)
NDC 0006-0014-28 unit dose packages of 100
NDC 0006-0014-98 unit of use bottles of 180 (with desiccant).

Shown in Product Identification Section, page 420

No. 3412—Tablets VASOTEC, 5 mg. are white, barrel shaped, scored, compressed tablets, with code MSD 712 on one side and VASOTEC on the other. They are supplied as follows:

NDC 0006-0712-94 unit of use bottles of 90 (with desiccant)
NDC 0006-0712-68 bottles of 100 (with desiccant)
(6505-01-236-8880, 5 mg 100's)
NDC 0006-0712-28 unit dose packages of 100
NDC 0006-0712-98 unit of use bottles of 180) with desiccant).

Shown in Product Identification Section, page 420

Continued on next page

Information on the Merck & Co. products listed on these pages is the full prescribing information from product circulars in use October 1, 1992.

Merck & Co.—Cont.

No. 3413—Tablets VASOTEC, 10 mg, are salmon, barrel shaped, compressed tablets, with code MSD 713 on one side and VASOTEC on the other. They are supplied as follows:
NDC 0006-0713-94 unit of use bottles of 90 (with desiccant)
NDC 0006-0713-68 bottles of 100 (with desiccant)
(6505-01-236-8881, 10 mg 100's)
NDC 0006-0713-28 unit dose packages of 100
NDC 0006-0713-98 unit of use bottles of 180 (with desiccant)
Shown in Product Identification Section, page 420
No. 3414—Tablets VASOTEC, 20 mg, are peach, barrel shaped, compressed tablets, with code MSD 714 on one side and VASOTEC on the other. They are supplied as follows:
NDC 0006-0714-94 unit of use bottles of 90 (with desiccant)
NDC 0006-0714-68 bottles of 100 (with desiccant)
(6505-01-237-0545, 20 mg 100's)
NDC 0006-0714-28 unit dose packages of 100.
Shown in Product Identification Section, page 420
Storage
Store below 30°C (86°F) and avoid transient temperatures above 50°C (122°F). Keep container tightly closed. Protect from moisture.
Dispense in a tight container, if product package is subdivided.

A.H.F.S. Category: 24:04
DC 7576634   Issued May 1992
COPYRIGHT © MERCK & CO., INC., 1988, 1989, 1992
All rights reserved

VIVACTIL® Tablets   ℞
(Protriptyline HCl), U.S.P.

DESCRIPTION

Protriptyline HCl is *N*-methyl-5*H*-dibenzo[*a,d*]-cyclohep-tene-5-propanamine hydrochloride. Its empirical formula is $C_{19}H_{21}N \cdot HCl$ and its structural formula is:

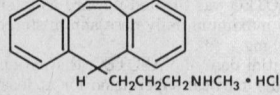

Protriptyline HCl, a dibenzocycloheptene derivative, has a molecular weight of 299.84. It is a white to yellowish powder that is freely soluble in water and soluble in dilute HCl.
VIVACTIL* (Protriptyline HCl) is supplied as 5 mg and 10 mg film coated tablets. Inactive ingredients are calcium phosphate, cellulose, guar gum, hydroxypropyl cellulose, hydroxypropyl methylcellulose, lactose, magnesium stearate, starch, talc, and titanium dioxide. Tablets VIVACTIL 5 mg and 10 mg also contain FD&C Yellow 6. Tablets VIVACTIL 10 mg also contain D&C Yellow 10.

---

*Registered trademark of MERCK & CO., INC.

ACTIONS

VIVACTIL is an antidepressant agent. The mechanism of its antidepressant action in man is not known. It is not a monoamine oxidase inhibitor, and it does not act primarily by stimulation of the central nervous system.
VIVACTIL has been found in some studies to have a more rapid onset of action than imipramine or amitriptyline. The initial clinical effect may occur within one week. Sedative and tranquilizing properties are lacking. The rate of excretion is slow.

INDICATIONS

VIVACTIL is indicated for the treatment of symptoms of mental depression in patients who are under close medical supervision. Its activating properties make it particularly suitable for withdrawn and anergic patients.

CONTRAINDICATIONS

VIVACTIL is contraindicated in patients who have shown prior hypersensitivity to it.
It should not be given concomitantly with a monoamine oxidase inhibiting compound. Hyperpyretic crises, severe convulsions, and deaths have occurred in patients receiving tricyclic antidepressant and monoamine oxidase inhibiting drugs simultaneously. When it is desired to substitute VIVACTIL for a monoamine oxidase inhibitor, a minimum of 14 days should be allowed to elapse after the latter is discontinued. VIVACTIL should then be initiated cautiously with gradual increase in dosage until optimum response is achieved.
This drug should not be used during the acute recovery phase following myocardial infarction.

WARNINGS

VIVACTIL may block the antihypertensive effect of guanethidine or similarly acting compounds.
VIVACTIL should be used with caution in patients with a history of seizures, and, because of its autonomic activity, in patients with a tendency to urinary retention, or increased intraocular tension.
Tachycardia and postural hypotension may occur more frequently with VIVACTIL than with other antidepressant drugs. VIVACTIL should be used with caution in elderly patients and patients with cardiovascular disorders; such patients should be observed closely because of the tendency of the drug to produce tachycardia, hypotension, arrhythmias, and prolongation of the conduction time. Myocardial infarction and stroke have occurred with drugs of this class.
On rare occasions, hyperthyroid patients or those receiving thyroid medication may develop arrhythmias when this drug is given.
In patients who may use alcohol excessively, it should be borne in mind that the potentiation may increase the danger inherent in any suicide attempt or overdosage.
Usage in Children
This drug is not recommended for use in children because safety and effectiveness in the pediatric age group have not been established.
Usage in Pregnancy
Safe use in pregnancy and lactation has not been established; therefore, use in pregnant women, nursing mothers or women who may become pregnant requires that possible benefits be weighed against possible hazards to mother and child.
In mice, rats, and rabbits, doses about ten times greater than the recommended human doses had no apparent adverse effects on reproduction.

PRECAUTIONS

When protriptyline HCl is used to treat the depressive component of schizophrenia, psychotic symptoms may be aggravated. Likewise, in manic-depressive psychosis, depressed patients may experience a shift toward the manic phase if they are treated with an antidepressant drug. Paranoid delusions, with or without associated hostility, may be exaggerated. In any of these circumstances, it may be advisable to reduce the dose of VIVACTIL or to use a major tranquilizing drug concurrently.
Symptoms, such as anxiety or agitation, may be aggravated in overactive or agitated patients.
When VIVACTIL is given with anticholinergic agents or sympathomimetic drugs, including epinephrine combined with local anesthetics, close supervision and careful adjustment of dosages are required.
Hyperpyrexia has been reported when tricyclic antidepressants are administered with anticholinergic agents or with neuroleptic drugs, particularly during hot weather.
Cimetidine is reported to reduce hepatic metabolism of certain tricyclic antidepressants, thereby delaying elimination and increasing steady-state concentrations of these drugs. Clinically significant effects have been reported with the tricyclic antidepressants when used concomitantly with cimetidine. Increases in plasma levels of tricyclic antidepressants, and in the frequency and severity of side effects, particularly anticholinergic, have been reported when cimetidine was added to the drug regimen. Discontinuation of cimetidine in well-controlled patients receiving tricyclic antidepressants and cimetidine may decrease the plasma levels and efficacy of the antidepressants.
It may enhance the response to alcohol and the effects of barbiturates and other CNS depressants.
The possibility of suicide in depressed patients remains during treatment and until significant remission occurs. This type of patient should not have access to large quantities of the drug.
Concurrent administration of VIVACTIL and electroshock therapy may increase the hazards of therapy. Such treatment should be limited to patients for whom it is essential. Discontinue the drug several days before elective surgery, if possible.
Both elevation and lowering of blood sugar levels have been reported.
Information for Patients
While on therapy with VIVACTIL, patients should be advised as to the possible impairment of mental and/or physical abilities required for performance of hazardous tasks, such as operating machinery or driving a motor vehicle.

ADVERSE REACTIONS

Within each category the following adverse reactions are listed in order of decreasing severity. Included in the listing are a few adverse reactions which have not been reported with this specific drug. However, the pharmacological similarities among the tricyclic antidepressant drugs require

that each of the reactions be considered when protriptyline is administered. VIVACTIL is more likely to aggravate agitation and anxiety and produce cardiovascular reactions such as tachycardia and hypotension.
Cardiovascular: Myocardial infarction; stroke; heart block; arrhythmias; hypotension, particularly orthostatic hypotension; hypertension; tachycardia; palpitation.
Psychiatric: Confusional states (especially in the elderly) with hallucinations, disorientation, delusions, anxiety, restlessness, agitation; hypomania; exacerbation of psychosis; insomnia, panic, and nightmares.
Neurological: Seizures; incoordination; ataxia; tremors; peripheral neuropathy; numbness, tingling, and paresthesias of extremities; extrapyramidal symptoms; drowsiness; dizziness; weakness and fatigue; headache; syndrome of inappropriate ADH (antidiuretic hormone) secretion; tinnitus; alteration in EEG patterns.
Anticholinergic: Paralytic ileus; hyperpyrexia; urinary retention, delayed micturition, dilatation of the urinary tract; constipation; blurred vision, disturbance of accommodation, increased intraocular pressure, mydriasis; dry mouth and rarely associated sublingual adenitis.
Allergic: Drug fever; petechiae, skin rash, urticaria, itching, photosensitization (avoid excessive exposure to sunlight); edema (general, or of face and tongue).
Hematologic: Agranulocytosis; bone marrow depression; leukopenia; thrombocytopenia; purpura; eosinophilia.
Gastrointestinal: Nausea and vomiting; anorexia; epigastric distress; diarrhea; peculiar taste; stomatitis; abdominal cramps; black tongue.
Endocrine: Impotence, increased or decreased libido; gynecomastia in the male; breast enlargement and galactorrhea in the female; testicular swelling; elevation or depression of blood sugar levels.
Other: Jaundice (simulating obstructive); altered liver function; parotid swelling; alopecia; flushing; weight gain or loss, urinary frequency, nocturia; perspiration.
Withdrawal Symptoms: Though not indicative of addiction, abrupt cessation of treatment after prolonged therapy may produce nausea, headache, and malaise.

DOSAGE AND ADMINISTRATION

Dosage should be initiated at a low level and increased gradually, noting carefully the clinical response and any evidence of intolerance.
Usual Adult Dosage—Fifteen to 40 mg a day divided into 3 or 4 doses. If necessary, dosage may be increased to 60 mg a day. Dosages above this amount are not recommended. Increases should be made in the morning dose.
Adolescent and Elderly Patients—In general, lower dosages are recommended for these patients. Five mg 3 times a day may be given initially, and increased gradually if necessary. In elderly patients, the cardiovascular system must be monitored closely if the daily dose exceeds 20 mg.
When satisfactory improvement has been reached, dosage should be reduced to the smallest amount that will maintain relief of symptoms.
Minor adverse reactions require reduction in dosage. Major adverse reactions or evidence of hypersensitivity require prompt discontinuation of the drug.
Usage in Children—This drug is not recommended for use in children because safety and effectiveness in the pediatric age group have not been established.

OVERDOSAGE

Manifestations—High doses may cause temporary confusion, disturbed concentration, or transient visual hallucinations. Overdosage may cause drowsiness; hypothermia; tachycardia and other arrhythmic abnormalities, for example, bundle branch block; ECG evidence of impaired conduction; congestive heart failure; dilated pupils; convulsions; severe hypotension; stupor; and coma. Other symptoms may be agitation, hyperactive reflexes, muscle rigidity, vomiting, hyperpyrexia, or any of those listed under ADVERSE REACTIONS.
Experience in the management of overdosage with protriptyline is limited. The following recommendations are based on the management of overdosage with other tricyclic antidepressants.
All patients suspected of having taken an overdosage should be admitted to a hospital as soon as possible. *Treatment* is symptomatic and supportive. Empty the stomach as quickly as possible by emesis followed by gastric lavage upon arrival at the hospital. Following gastric lavage, activated charcoal may be administered. Twenty to 30 g of activated charcoal may be given every four to six hours during the first 24 to 48 hours after ingestion. An ECG should be taken and close monitoring of cardiac function instituted if there is any sign of abnormality. Maintain an open airway and adequate fluid intake; regulate body temperature.
The intravenous administration of 1-3 mg of physostigmine salicylate is reported to reverse the symptoms of other tricyclic antidepressant poisoning in humans. Because physostig-

mine is rapidly metabolized, the dosage of physostigmine should be repeated as required particularly if life threatening signs such as arrhythmias, convulsions, and deep coma recur or persist after the initial dosage of physostigmine. Because physostigmine itself may be toxic, it is not recommended for routine use.
Standard measures should be used to manage circulatory shock and metabolic acidosis. Cardiac arrhythmias may be treated with neostigmine, pyridostigmine, or propranolol. Should cardiac failure occur, the use of digitalis should be considered. Close monitoring of cardiac function for not less than five days is advisable.
Anticonvulsants may be given to control convulsions.
Dialysis is of no value because of low plasma concentrations of the drug.
Since overdosage is often deliberate, patients may attempt suicide by other means during the recovery phase.
Deaths by deliberate or accidental overdosage have occurred with this class of drugs.

HOW SUPPLIED

No. 3313—Tablets VIVACTIL, 5 mg, are orange, oval, film coated tablets, coded MSD 26. They are supplied as follows:
NDC 0006-0026-68 bottles of 100.
Shown in Product Identification Section, page 420
No. 3314—Tablets VIVACTIL, 10 mg, are yellow, oval, film coated tablets, coded MSD 47. They are supplied as follows:
NDC 0006-0047-68 bottles of 100
(6505-00-462-7353, 10 mg 100's)
NDC 0006-0047-28 unit dose packages of 100.
Shown in Product Identification Section, page 420
Storage
Store Tablets VIVACTIL in a tightly closed container. Avoid storage at temperatures above 40°C (104°F).

METABOLISM

Metabolic studies indicate that protriptyline is well absorbed from the gastrointestinal tract and is rapidly sequestered in tissues. Relatively low plasma levels are found after administration, and only a small amount of unchanged drug is excreted in the urine of dogs and rabbits. Preliminary studies indicate that demethylation of the secondary amine moiety occurs to a significant extent, and that metabolic transformation probably takes place in the liver. It penetrates the brain rapidly in mice and rats, and moreover that which is present in the brain is almost all unchanged drug.
Studies on the disposition of radioactive protriptyline in human test subjects showed significant plasma levels within 2 hours, peaking at 8 to 12 hours, then declining gradually. Urinary excretion studies in the same subjects showed significant amounts of radioactivity in 2 hours. The rate of excretion was slow. Cumulative urinary excretion during 16 days accounted for approximately 50% of the drug. The fecal route of excretion did not seem to be important.

A.H.F.S. Category: 28:16:04
DC 7398519 Issued July 1986

ZOCOR® Tablets ℞
(Simvastatin)

DESCRIPTION

ZOCOR* (Simvastatin) is a cholesterol lowering agent that is derived synthetically from a fermentation product of *Aspergillus terreus*. After oral ingestion, simvastatin, which is an inactive lactone, is hydrolyzed to the corresponding β-hydroxyacid form. This is an inhibitor of 3-hydroxy-3-methylglutaryl-coenzyme A (HMG-CoA) reductase. This enzyme catalyzes the conversion of HMG-CoA to mevalonate, which is an early and rate-limiting step in the biosynthesis of cholesterol.
Simvastatin is butanoic acid, 2,2-dimethyl-, 1,2,3,7,8,8a-hexahydro-3,7-dimethyl-8-[2-(tetrahydro-4-hydroxy-6-oxo-2*H*-pyran-2-yl) ethyl]-1-napthalenyl ester, [1*S*-[1α,3α,7β, 8β(2*S**, 4*S**),-8aβ]]. The empirical formula of simvastatin is $C_{25}H_{38}O_5$ and its molecular weight is 418.57. Its structural formula is:

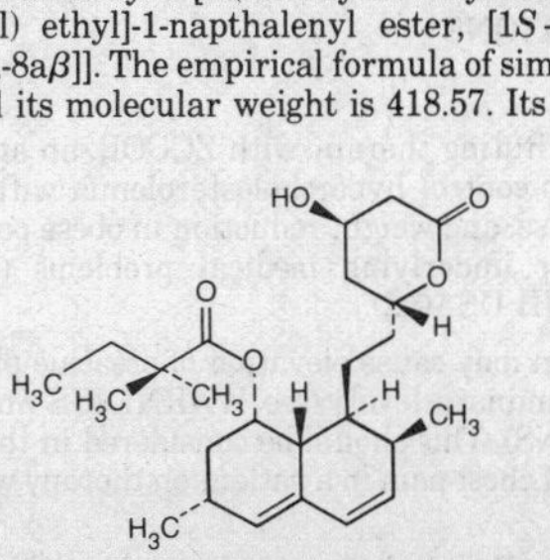

Simvastatin is a white to off-white, nonhygroscopic, crystalline powder that is practically insoluble in water, and freely soluble in chloroform, methanol and ethanol.

TABLE I
Dose Response in Patients with Primary Hypercholesterolemia
(Mean Percent Change from Baseline After 8 Weeks)

TREATMENT	N	TOTAL-C	LDL-C	HDL-C	LDL-C/ HDL-C	TOTAL-C/ HDL-C	TRIG.
Placebo	28	−3	−4	+2	−4	−3	+7
ZOCOR							
5 mg q.p.m.	28	−17	−24	+7	−27	−22	−10
10 mg q.p.m.	27	−24	−33	+9	−37	−29	−10
20 mg q.p.m.	26	−25	−33	+11	−36	−30	−19
40 mg q.p.m.	29	−28	−40	+12	−46	−36	−19

Tablets ZOCOR for oral administration contain either 5 mg, 10 mg, 20 mg or 40 mg of simvastatin and the following inactive ingredients: cellulose, hydroxypropyl cellulose, hydroxypropyl methylcellulose, iron oxides, lactose, magnesium stearate, starch, talc, titanium dioxide and other ingredients. Butylated hydroxyanisole is added as a preservative.

*Registered trademark of MERCK & CO., INC.

CLINICAL PHARMACOLOGY

The involvement of low-density lipoprotein (LDL) cholesterol in atherogenesis has been well-documented in clinical and pathological studies, as well as in many animal experiments. Epidemiological studies have established that high LDL (low-density lipoprotein) cholesterol and low HDL (high-density lipoprotein) cholesterol are both risk factors for coronary heart disease. The Lipid Research Clinics Coronary Primary Prevention Trial (LRC-CPPT), coordinated by the National Institutes of Health (NIH), studied men aged 35–59 with total cholesterol levels of 265 mg/dL (6.8 mmol/L) or greater, LDL cholesterol values 175 mg/dL (4.5 mmol/L) or greater, and triglyceride levels not more than 300 mg/dL (3.4 mmol/L). This seven-year, double-blind, placebo-controlled study demonstrated that lowering LDL cholesterol with diet and cholestyramine decreased the combined rate of coronary heart disease death plus non-fatal myocardial infarction.
ZOCOR has been shown to reduce both normal and elevated LDL cholesterol concentrations. The effect of simvastatin-induced changes in lipoprotein levels, including reduction of serum cholesterol, on cardiovascular morbidity or mortality has not been established.
LDL is formed from very-low-density lipoprotein (VLDL) and is catabolized predominantly by the high affinity LDL receptor. The mechanism of the LDL-lowering effect of ZOCOR may involve both reduction of VLDL cholesterol concentration, and induction of the LDL receptor, leading to reduced production and/or increased catabolism of LDL cholesterol. Apolipoprotein B also falls substantially during treatment with ZOCOR. Since each LDL particle contains one molecule of apolipoprotein B, and since little apolipoprotein B is found in other lipoproteins, this strongly suggests that ZOCOR does not merely cause cholesterol to be lost from LDL, but also reduces the concentration of circulating LDL particles. In addition, ZOCOR modestly reduces VLDL cholesterol and plasma triglycerides and can produce increases of variable magnitude in HDL cholesterol. The effects of ZOCOR on Lp(a), fibrinogen, and certain other independent biochemical risk markers for coronary heart disease are unknown.
ZOCOR is a specific inhibitor of HMG-CoA reductase, the enzyme that catalyzes the conversion of HMG-CoA to mevalonate. The conversion of HMG-CoA to mevalonate is an early step in the biosynthetic pathway for cholesterol.
Pharmacokinetics
Simvastatin is a lactone that is readily hydrolyzed *in vivo* to the corresponding β-hydroxyacid, a potent inhibitor of HMG-CoA reductase. Inhibition of HMG-CoA reductase is the basis for an assay in pharmacokinetic studies of the β-hydroxyacid metabolites (active inhibitors) and, following base hydrolysis, active plus latent inhibitors (total inhibitors) in plasma following administration of simvastatin.
Following an oral dose of ^{14}C-labeled simvastatin in man, 13% of the dose was excreted in urine and 60% in feces. The latter represents absorbed drug equivalents excreted in bile, as well as any unabsorbed drug. Plasma concentrations of total radioactivity (simvastatin plus ^{14}C-metabolites) peaked at 4 hours and declined rapidly to about 10% of peak by 12 hours postdose. Absorption of simvastatin, estimated relative to an intravenous reference dose, in each of two animal species tested, averaged about 85% of an oral dose. In animal studies, after oral dosing, simvastatin achieved substantially higher concentrations in the liver than in nontarget tissues. Simvastatin undergoes extensive first-pass extraction in the liver, its primary site of action, with subsequent excretion of drug equivalents in the bile. As a consequence of extensive hepatic extraction of simvastatin (estimated to be > 60% in man), the availability of drug to the general circulation is low. In a single-dose study in nine healthy subjects, it was estimated that less than 5% of an oral dose of simvastatin reaches the general circulation as active inhibitors. Following administration of simvastatin tablets, the coefficient of variation, based on between-subject variability, was approximately 48% for the area under the concentration-time curve (AUC) for total inhibitory activity in the general circulation.
Both simvastatin and its β-hydroxyacid metabolite are highly bound (approximately 95%) to human plasma proteins. Animal studies have not been performed to determine whether simvastatin crosses the blood-brain and placental barriers. However, when radiolabeled simvastatin was administered to rats, simvastatin-derived radioactivity crossed the blood-brain barrier.
The major active metabolites of simvastatin present in human plasma are the β-hydroxyacid of simvastatin and its 6′-hydroxy, 6′-hydroxy methyl, and 6′-exomethylene derivatives. Peak plasma concentrations of both active and total inhibitors were attained within 1.3 to 2.4 hours postdose. While the recommended therapeutic dose range is 5 to 40 mg/day, there was no substantial deviation from linearity of AUC of inhibitors in the general circulation with an increase in dose to as high as 120 mg. Relative to the fasting state, the plasma profile of inhibitors was not affected when simvastatin was administered immediately before an A.H.A. recommended low-fat meal.
Kinetic studies with another reductase inhibitor, having a similar principal route of elimination, have suggested that for a given dose level higher systemic exposure may be achieved in patients with severe renal insufficiency (as measured by creatinine clearance).
Clinical Studies
ZOCOR has been shown to be highly effective in reducing total and LDL cholesterol in heterozygous familial and non-familial forms of hypercholesterolemia and in mixed hyperlipidemia. A marked response was seen within 2 weeks, and the maximum therapeutic response occurred within 4–6 weeks. The response was maintained during chronic therapy.
In a multicenter, double-blind, placebo-controlled, dose-response study in patients with familial or non-familial hypercholesterolemia, ZOCOR given as a single-dose in the evening (the recommended dosing) was similarly effective as when given on a twice-daily basis. ZOCOR consistently and significantly decreased total plasma cholesterol (TOTAL-C), LDL cholesterol (LDL-C), total cholesterol/HDL cholesterol (TOTAL-C/HDL-C) ratio, and LDL cholesterol/HDL cholesterol (LDL-C/HDL-C) ratio. ZOCOR also modestly decreased triglycerides (TRIG) and produced increases of variable magnitude in HDL cholesterol (HDL-C).
The results of a dose response study in patients with primary hypercholesterolemia are presented in Table I.
ZOCOR was compared to cholestyramine, probucol, or gemfibrozil, respectively, in double-blind parallel studies involving 1102 patients. All studies were performed in patients who were at moderate to high risk of coronary events based on serum cholesterol levels. At all dosage levels tested, ZOCOR produced a significantly greater reduction of total plasma cholesterol, LDL cholesterol, VLDL cholesterol, triglycerides, and total cholesterol/HDL cholesterol ratio when compared to cholestyramine or probucol. The increase in HDL seen with ZOCOR was not significantly greater than the increase seen with cholestyramine but was significantly different from the decrease seen with probucol (see Tables II and III).
[See tables on next page.]
In a study designed to evaluate the possible effects of simvastatin on reproductive hormones and sperm characteristics in men with familial hypercholesterolemia, there was a small decrease in the mean percentage of vital sperm and a small increase in the mean percentage of abnormal forms, with these changes achieving statistical significance at week 14. However, there was no effect on numbers or concentration of motile sperm. Simvastatin had no effect on basal reproductive hormone levels (prolactin, luteinizing hormone, follicle-stimulating hormone, and plasma testosterone). Provocative testing (HCG stimulation) was not done. Treatment with another HMG-CoA reductase inhibitor resulted in a statistically significant decrease in plasma testosterone response to HCG.

Continued on next page

Information on the Merck & Co. products listed on these pages is the full prescribing information from product circulars in use October 1, 1992.

Merck & Co.—Cont.

TABLE II
ZOCOR vs. Cholestyramine
(Percent Change from Baseline After 12 Weeks)

TREATMENT	N	TOTAL-C (mean)	LDL-C (mean)	HDL-C (mean)	LDL-C/ HDL-C (mean)	TOTAL-C/ HDL-C (mean)	VLDL-C (median)	TRIG. (mean)
ZOCOR								
20 mg q.p.m.	84	−27	−32	+10	−36	−31	−8	−13
40 mg q.p.m.	82	−33	−41	+10	−45	−38	−28	−21
Cholestyramine								
4–24 g/day*	85	−15	−21	+8	−25	−19	+7	+15

*maximum tolerated dose (mean dose taken, 18 g/day)

TABLE III
ZOCOR vs. Probucol
(Percent Change from Baseline After 12 Weeks)

TREATMENT	N	TOTAL-C (mean)	LDL-C (mean)	HDL-C (mean)	LDL-C/ HDL-C (mean)	TOTAL-C/ HDL-C (mean)	VLDL-C (median)	TRIG. (mean)
ZOCOR								
20 mg q.p.m.	82	−27	−34	+10	−39	−34	−18	−17
40 mg q.p.m.	86	−30	−40	+13	−45	−37	−14	−19
Probucol								
500 mg b.i.d.	81	−13	−8	−27	+31	+25	+11	−0.4

In a study to evaluate the effect of simvastatin on adrenocortical function in patients with Type II hypercholesterolemia, simvastatin had no effect on basal adrenocortical function as assessed by determination of morning plasma cortisol levels, urine free cortisol, and urinary excretion of 17-hydroxy steroids. Simvastatin also had no effect on adrenocortical reserve as evaluated by the plasma cortisol response to ACTH stimulation and insulin-induced hypoglycemia.

INDICATIONS AND USAGE

Therapy with lipid-altering agents should be a component of multiple risk factor intervention in those individuals at significantly increased risk for atherosclerotic vascular disease due to hypercholesterolemia. ZOCOR is indicated as an adjunct to diet for the reduction of elevated total and LDL cholesterol levels in patients with primary hypercholesterolemia (Types IIa and IIb[1]), when the response to a diet restricted in saturated fat and cholesterol and other nonpharmacological measures alone has been inadequate.

Prior to initiating therapy with simvastatin, secondary causes for hypercholesterolemia (e.g., poorly controlled diabetes mellitus, hypothyroidism, nephrotic syndrome, dysproteinemias, obstructive liver disease, other drug therapy, alcoholism) should be excluded, and a lipid profile performed to measure TOTAL-C, HDL-C, and triglycerides (TG). For patients with TG less than 400 mg/dL (<4.5 mmol/L), LDL-C can be estimated using the following equation:

LDL-C = Total cholesterol − [0.20 × (triglycerides) + HDL-C]

For TG levels >400 mg/dL (>4.5 mmol/L), this equation is less accurate and LDL-C concentrations should be determined by ultracentrifugation. In many hypertriglyceridemic patients, LDL-C may be low or normal despite elevated TOTAL-C. In such cases, ZOCOR is not indicated.

Lipid determinations should be performed at intervals of no less than four weeks and dosage adjusted according to the patient's response to therapy.

The National Cholesterol Education Program (NCEP) Treatment Guidelines† are summarized below:

	LDL Cholesterol mg/dL (mmol/L) Initiation Level	Minimum Goal	Total Cholesterol mg/dL (mmol/L) Minimum Goal
Without Definite CHD or Two Other Risk Factors*	≥190 (≥4.9)	<160 (<4.1)	<240 (<6.2)
With Definite CHD or Two Other Risk Factors*	≥160 (≥4.1)	<130 (<3.4)	<200 (<5.2)

*Other risk factors for coronary heart disease (CHD) include: male sex, family history of premature CHD, cigarette smoking, hypertension, confirmed HDL-C <35 mg/dL (<0.91 mmol/L), diabetes mellitus, definite cerebrovascular or peripheral vascular disease, or severe obesity.

Since the goal of treatment is to lower LDL-C, the NCEP recommends that LDL-C levels be used to initiate and assess treatment response. Only if LDL-C levels are not available, should the TOTAL-C be used to monitor therapy.

Although ZOCOR may be useful to reduce elevated LDL cholesterol levels in patients with combined hypercholesterolemia and hypertriglyceridemia where hypercholesterolemia is the major abnormality (Type IIb hyperlipoproteinemia), it has not been studied in conditions where the major abnormality is elevation of chylomicrons, VLDL or IDL (i.e., hyperlipoproteinemia types I, III, IV, or V).[1]

The effect of simvastatin-induced changes in lipoprotein levels, including reduction of serum cholesterol, on cardiovascular morbidity or mortality has not been established.

[1]Classification of Hyperlipoproteinemias

Type	Lipoproteins elevated	Lipid Elevations major	minor
I (rare)	chylomicrons	TG	↑→C
IIa	LDL	C	—
IIb	LDL, VLDL	C	TG
III (rare)	IDL	C/TG	—
IV	VLDL	TG	↑→C
V (rare)	chylomicrons, VLDL	TG	↑→C

C = cholesterol, TG = triglycerides,
LDL = low-density lipoprotein,
VLDL = very-low-density lipoprotein,
IDL = intermediate-density lipoprotein.

†For adult diabetics, a modification of these guidelines is recommended—see: American Diabetes Association Consensus Statement: Role of cardiovascular risk factors in prevention and treatment of macrovascular disease in diabetes, Diabetes Care *12* (8): 573–79, 1989.

CONTRAINDICATIONS

Hypersensitivity to any component of this medication.

Active liver disease or unexplained persistent elevations of serum transaminases (see WARNINGS).

Pregnancy and lactation. Atherosclerosis is a chronic process and the discontinuation of lipid-lowering drugs during pregnancy should have little impact on the outcome of long-term therapy of primary hypercholesterolemia. Moreoever, cholesterol and other products of the cholesterol biosynthesis pathway are essential components for fetal development, including synthesis of steroids and cell membranes. Because of the ability of inhibitors of HMG-CoA reductase such as ZOCOR to decrease the synthesis of cholesterol and possibly other products of the cholesterol biosynthesis pathway, ZOCOR may cause fetal harm when administered to a pregnant woman. Therefore, simvastatin is contraindicated during pregnancy and in nursing mothers. **Simvastatin should be administered to women of childbearing age only when such patients are highly unlikely to conceive.** If the patient becomes pregnant while taking this drug, simvastatin should be discontinued and the patient should be apprised of the potential hazard to the fetus.

WARNINGS

Liver Dysfunction

Persistent increases (to more than 3 times the upper limit of normal) in serum transaminases have occurred in 1% of patients who received simvastatin in clinical trials. When drug treatment was interrupted or discontinued in these patients, the transaminase levels usually fell slowly to pretreatment levels. The increases were not associated with jaundice or other clinical signs or symptoms. There was no evidence of hypersensitivity.

It is recommended that liver function tests be performed during therapy with simvastatin. Serum transaminase levels, including ALT (SGPT), should be monitored before treatment begins, every six weeks for the first three months, every eight weeks during the remainder of the first year, and periodically thereafter (e.g., at approximately 6 month intervals). Special attention should be paid to patients who develop elevated serum transaminase levels, and in these patients, measurements should be repeated promptly and then performed more frequently. If the transaminase levels show evidence of progression, particularly if they rise to three times the upper limit of normal and are persistent, the drug should be discontinued. Liver biopsy should be considered if elevations persist beyond discontinuation of drug.

The drug should be used with caution in patients who consume substantial quantities of alcohol and/or have a past history of liver disease. Active liver diseases or unexplained transaminase elevations are contraindications to the use of simvastatin.

As with other lipid-lowering agents, moderate (less than three times the upper limit of normal) elevations of serum transaminases have been reported following therapy with simvastatin. These changes appeared soon after initiation of therapy with simvastatin, were often transient, were not accompanied by any symptoms and did not require interruption of treatment.

Skeletal Muscle

Rare cases of rhabdomyolysis with acute renal failure secondary to myoglobinuria have been associated with simvastatin therapy. Rhabdomyolysis has also been associated with other HMG-CoA reductase inhibitors when they were administered alone or concomitantly with 1) immunosuppressive therapy, including cyclosporine in cardiac transplant patients; 2) gemfibrozil or lipid-lowering doses (≥ 1 g/day) of nicotinic acid in non-transplant patients, or 3) erythromycin in seriously ill patients. Some of the patients who had rhabdomyolysis in association with the reductase inhibitors had preexisting renal insufficiency, usually as a consequence of long-standing diabetes. In most subjects who have had an unsatisfactory lipid response to either simvastatin or gemfibrozil alone, the possible benefits of combined therapy with these drugs are not considered to outweigh the risk of severe myopathy, rhabdomyolysis, and acute renal failure. While it is not known whether this interaction occurs with fibrates other than gemfibrozil, myopathy and rhabdomyolysis have occasionally been associated with the use of other fibrates alone, including clofibrate. Therefore, the combined use of simvastatin with other fibrates should generally be avoided.

Physicians contemplating combined therapy with simvastatin and lipid-lowering doses of nicotinic acid, or with immunosuppressive drugs should carefully weigh the potential benefits and risks and should carefully monitor patients for any signs and symptoms of muscle pain, tenderness, or weakness, particularly during the initial months of therapy and during any periods of upward dosage titration of either drug. Periodic creatine phosphokinase (CPK) determinations may be considered in such situations, but there is no assurance that such monitoring will prevent the occurrence of severe myopathy.

Because of an apparent relationship between increased plasma levels of active metabolites derived from other HMG-CoA reductase inhibitors and myopathy, in patients taking cyclosporine, the daily dosage should not exceed 10 mg/day (see DOSAGE AND ADMINISTRATION).

Simvastatin therapy should be temporarily withheld or discontinued in any patient with an acute, serious condition suggestive of a myopathy or having a risk factor predisposing to the development of renal failure secondary to rhabdomyolysis, (e.g., severe acute infection, hypotension, major surgery, trauma, severe metabolic, endocrine and electrolyte disorders, and uncontrolled seizures).

Myopathy should be considered in any patient with diffuse myalgias, muscle tenderness or weakness, and/or marked elevation of CPK. Patients should be advised to report promptly unexplained muscle pain, tenderness or weakness, particularly if accompanied by malaise or fever. Simvastatin therapy should be discontinued if markedly elevated CPK levels occur or myopathy is diagnosed or suspected.

PRECAUTIONS

General

Before instituting therapy with ZOCOR, an attempt should be made to control hypercholesterolemia with appropriate diet, exercise, and weight reduction in obese patients, and to treat other underlying medical problems (see INDICATIONS AND USAGE).

Simvastatin may cause elevation of creatine phosphokinase and transaminase levels (see WARNINGS and ADVERSE REACTIONS). This should be considered in the differential diagnosis of chest pain in a patient on therapy with simvastatin.

Homozygous Familial Hypercholesterolemia

ZOCOR is less effective in patients with the rare homozygous familial hypercholesterolemia, possibly because these patients have few functional LDL receptors.

Information for Patients
Patients should be advised to report promptly unexplained muscle pain, tenderness, or weakness, particularly if accompanied by malaise or fever.
Drug Interactions
Immunosuppressive Drugs, Gemfibrozil, Niacin (Nicotinic Acid), Erythromycin: See WARNINGS, *Skeletal Muscle.*
Antipyrine: Because simvastatin had no effect on the pharmacokinetics of antipyrine, interactions with other drugs metabolized via the same cytochrome isozymes are not expected.
Propranolol: In healthy male volunteers there was a significant decrease in mean C_{max}, but no change in AUC, for simvastatin total and active inhibitors with concomitant administration of single doses of ZOCOR and propranolol. The clinical relevance of this finding is unclear. The pharmacokinetics of the enantiomers of propranolol were not affected.
Digoxin: Concomitant administration of a single dose of digoxin in healthy male volunteers receiving simvastatin resulted in a slight elevation (less than 0.3 ng/mL) in digoxin concentrations in plasma (as measured by a radioimmunoassay) compared to concomitant administration of placebo and digoxin. Patients taking digoxin should be monitored appropriately when simvastatin is initiated.
Warfarin: Simvastatin therapy appeared to enhance slightly the anticoagulant effect of warfarin (mean changes in prothrombin time less than two seconds) in normal volunteers maintained in a state of low therapeutic anticoagulation. With other reductase inhibitors, clinically evident bleeding and/or increased prothrombin time has been reported in a few patients taking coumarin anticoagulants concomitantly. In such patients, prothrombin time should be determined before starting simvastatin and frequently enough during early therapy to insure that no significant alteration of prothrombin time occurs. Once a stable prothrombin time has been documented, prothrombin times can be monitored at the intervals usually recommended for patients on coumarin anticoagulants. If the dose of simvastatin is changed, the same procedure should be repeated. Simvastatin therapy has not been associated with bleeding or with changes in prothrombin time in patients not taking anticoagulants.
Other Concomitant Therapy: Although specific interaction studies were not performed, in clinical studies, simvastatin was used concomitantly with angiotensin-converting enzyme (ACE) inhibitors, beta blockers, calcium-channel blockers, diuretics and nonsteroidal anti-inflammatory drugs (NSAIDs) without evidence of clinically significant adverse interactions. The effect of cholestyramine on the absorption and kinetics of simvastatin has not been determined.
Endocrine Function
HMG-CoA reductase inhibitors interfere with cholesterol synthesis and as such might theoretically blunt adrenal and/or gonadal steroid production. However, clinical studies have shown that simvastatin does not reduce basal plasma cortisol concentration or impair adrenal reserve, and does not reduce basal plasma testosterone concentration (see CLINICAL PHARMACOLOGY, *Clinical Studies*). Another HMG-CoA reductase inhibitor has been shown to reduce the plasma testosterone response to HCG; the effect of simvastatin on HCG-stimulated testosterone secretion has not been studied.
Results of clinical trials with drugs in this class have been inconsistent with regard to drug effects on basal and reserve steroid levels. The effects of HMG-CoA reductase inhibitors on male fertility have not been studied in adequate numbers of male patients. The effects, if any, on the pituitary-gonadal axis in pre-menopausal women are unknown. Patients treated with simvastatin who develop clinical evidence of endocrine dysfunction should be evaluated appropriately. Caution should also be exercised if an HMG-CoA reductase inhibitor or other agent used to lower cholesterol levels is administered to patients also receiving other drugs (e.g., ketoconazole, spironolactone, cimetidine) that may decrease the levels or activity of endogenous steroid hormones.
CNS Toxicity
Optic nerve degeneration was seen in clinically normal dogs treated with simvastatin for 14 weeks at 180 mg/kg/day, a dose that produced mean plasma drug levels about 44 times higher than the mean drug level in humans taking 40 mg/day.
CNS vascular lesions, characterized by perivascular hemorrhage and edema, mononuclear cell infiltration of perivascular spaces, perivascular fibrin deposits and necrosis of small vessels were seen in dogs treated with simvastatin at a dose of 360 mg/kg/day, a dose that produced plasma drug levels that were about 50 times higher than the mean drug levels in humans taking 40 mg/day. Similar CNS vascular lesions have been observed with several other drugs of this class.
A chemically similar drug in this class also produced optic nerve degeneration (Wallerian degeneration of retinogeniculate fibers) in clinically normal dogs in a dose-dependent fashion starting at 60 mg/kg/day, a dose that produced mean plasma drug levels about 30 times higher than the mean drug level in humans taking the highest recommended dose (as measured by total enzyme inhibitory activity). This same drug also produced vestibulocochlear Wallerian-like degeneration and retinal ganglion cell chromatolysis in dogs treated for 14 weeks at 180 mg/kg/day, a dose that resulted in a mean plasma drug level similar to that seen with the 60 mg/kg/day dose.

	ZOCOR (N=1583) %	Placebo (N=157) %	Cholestyramine (N=179) %	Probucol (N=81) %
Body as a Whole				
Abdominal pain	3.2	3.2	8.9	2.5
Asthenia	1.6	2.5	1.1	1.2
Gastrointestinal				
Constipation	2.3	1.3	29.1	1.2
Diarrhea	1.9	2.5	7.8	3.7
Dyspepsia	1.1	—	4.5	3.7
Flatulence	1.9	1.3	14.5	6.2
Nausea	1.3	1.9	10.1	2.5
Nervous System/Psychiatric				
Headache	3.5	5.1	4.5	3.7
Respiratory				
Upper respiratory infection	2.1	1.9	3.4	6.2

Carcinogenesis, Mutagenesis, Impairment of Fertility
In a 72-week carcinogenicity study, mice were administered daily doses of simvastatin of 25, 100, and 400 mg/kg body weight, which resulted in mean plasma drug levels approximately 3, 15, and 33 times higher than the mean human plasma drug concentration (as total inhibitory activity) after a 40 mg oral dose. Liver carcinomas were significantly increased in high-dose females and mid- and high-dose males with a maximum incidence of 90 percent in males. The incidence of adenomas of the liver was significantly increased in mid- and high-dose females. Drug treatment also significantly increased the incidence of lung adenomas in mid- and high-dose males and females. Adenomas of the Harderian gland (a gland of the eye of rodents) were significantly higher in high-dose mice than in controls. No evidence of a tumorigenic effect was observed at 25 mg/kg/day. Although mice were given up to 500 times the human dose (HD) on a mg/kg/body weight basis, blood levels of HMG-CoA reductase inhibitory activity were only 3–33 times higher in mice than in humans given 40 mg of ZOCOR.
In a separate 92-week carcinogenicity study in mice at doses up to 25 mg/kg/day, no evidence of a tumorigenic effect was observed. Although mice were given up to 31 times the human dose on a mg/kg basis, plasma drug levels were only 2–4 times higher than humans given 40 mg simvastatin as measured by AUC.
In a two-year study in rats, there was a statistically significant increase in the incidence of thyroid follicular adenomas in female rats exposed to approximately 45 times higher levels of simvastatin than humans given 40 mg simvastatin (as measured by AUC). Preliminary results from a second two-year rat study indicate an increase in the incidence of thyroid and liver tumors in male and female rats at doses that produce exposure levels ≥ 29 times (based on AUC) that achieved in humans at a dosage of 40 mg/day. Liver tumors are found in rodents with all the chemically similar drugs of this class. No increased incidence of tumors was observed at doses that produce exposure levels 15 times (based on AUC) those seen in man.
No evidence of mutagenicity was observed in a microbial mutagen test using mutant strains of *Salmonella typhimurium* with or without rat or mouse liver metabolic activation. In addition, no evidence of damage to genetic material was noted in an *in vitro* alkaline elution assay using rat hepatocytes, a V-79 mammalian cell forward mutation study, an *in vitro* chromosome aberration study in CHO cells, or an *in vivo* chromosomal aberration assay in mouse bone marrow.
There was decreased fertility in male rats treated with simvastatin for 34 weeks at 25 mg/kg body weight (15 times the maximum human exposure level, based on AUC, in patients receiving 40 mg/day); however, this effect was not observed during a subsequent fertility study in which simvastatin was administered at this same dose level to male rats for 11 weeks (the entire cycle of spermatogenesis including epididymal maturation). No microscopic changes were observed in the testes of rats from either study. At 180 mg/kg/day, (which produces exposure levels 44 times higher than those in humans taking 40 mg/day), seminiferous tubule degeneration (necrosis and loss of spermatogenic epithelium) was observed. In dogs, there was drug-related testicular atrophy, decreased spermatogenesis, spermatocytic degeneration and giant cell formation at 10 mg/kg/day (approximately 7 times the human exposure level, based on AUC, at 40 mg/day). The clinical significance of these findings is unclear.
Pregnancy
Pregnancy Category X
See CONTRAINDICATIONS.
Safety in pregnant women has not been established. Simvastatin was not teratogenic in rats at doses of 25 mg/kg/day or in rabbits at doses up to 10 mg/kg daily. These doses resulted in 6 times (rat) or 4 times (rabbit) the human exposure based on mg/m^2 surface area. However, in studies with another structurally-related HMG-CoA reductase inhibitor, skeletal malformations were observed in rats and mice. Simvastatin should be administered to women of child-bearing potential only when such patients are highly unlikely to conceive and have been informed of the potential hazards. If the woman becomes pregnant while taking simvastatin, it should be discontinued and the patient advised again as to the potential hazards to the fetus.
Nursing Mothers
It is not known whether simvastatin is excreted in human milk. Because a small amount of another drug in this class is excreted in human milk and because of the potential for serious adverse reactions in nursing infants, women taking simvastatin should not nurse their infants (see CONTRAINDICATIONS).
Pediatric Use
Safety and effectiveness in children and adolescents have not been established. Because children and adolescents are not likely to benefit from cholesterol lowering for at least a decade and because experience with this drug is limited (no studies in subjects below the age of 20 years), treatment of children or adolescents with simvastatin is not recommended at this time.

ADVERSE REACTIONS

In the controlled clinical studies and their open extensions (2423 patients with mean duration of follow-up of approximately 18 months), 1.4% of patients were discontinued due to adverse experiences attributable to ZOCOR. Adverse reactions have usually been mild and transient. ZOCOR has been evaluated for serious adverse reactions in more than 21,000 patients and is generally well-tolerated.
Clinical Adverse Experiences
Adverse experiences occurring at an incidence of 1 percent or greater in patients treated with ZOCOR, regardless of causality, in controlled clinical studies are shown in the table above.
The following effects have been reported with drugs in this class:
Skeletal: myopathy, rhabdomyolysis, arthralgias.
Neurological: dysfunction of certain cranial nerves (including alteration of taste, impairment of extra-ocular movement, facial paresis), tremor, vertigo, memory loss, paresthesia, peripheral neuropathy, peripheral nerve palsy, anxiety, insomnia, depression.
Hypersensitivity Reactions: An apparent hypersensitivity syndrome has been reported rarely which has included one or more of the following features: anaphylaxis, angioedema, lupus erythematous-like syndrome, polymyalgia rheumatica, vasculitis, purpura, thrombocytopenia, leukopenia, hemolytic anemia, positive ANA, ESR increase, arthritis, arthralgia, urticaria, asthenia, photosensitivity, fever, chills, flushing, malaise, dyspnea, toxic epidermal necrolysis, erythema multiforme, including Stevens-Johnson syndrome.
Gastrointestinal: pancreatitis, hepatitis, including chronic active hepatitis, cholestatic jaundice, fatty change in liver, and, rarely, cirrhosis, fulminant hepatic necrosis, and hepatoma; anorexia, vomiting.
Skin: alopecia.
Reproductive: gynecomastia, loss of libido, erectile dysfunction.
Eye: progression of cataracts (lens opacities), ophthalmoplegia.
Laboratory Abnormalities: elevated transaminases, alkaline phosphatase, and bilirubin; thyroid function abnormalities.
Laboratory Tests
Marked persistent increases of serum transaminases have been noted (see WARNINGS, *Liver Dysfunction*). About 5%

Continued on next page

Information on the Merck & Co. products listed on these pages is the full prescribing information from product circulars in use October 1, 1992.

Merck & Co.—Cont.

of patients had elevations of creatine phosphokinase (CPK) levels of 3 or more times the normal value on one or more occasions. This was attributable to the noncardiac fraction of CPK. Muscle pain or dysfunction usually was not reported (see WARNINGS, *Skeletal Muscle*).

Concomitant Therapy

In controlled clinical studies in which simvastatin was administered concomitantly with cholestyramine, no adverse reactions peculiar to this concomitant treatment were observed. The adverse reactions that occurred were limited to those reported previously with simvastatin or cholestyramine. The combined use of simvastatin with fibrates should generally be avoided (see WARNINGS, *Skeletal Muscle*).

OVERDOSAGE

Significant lethality was observed in mice after a single oral dose of 9 g/m^2. No evidence of lethality was observed in rats or dogs treated with doses of 30 and 100 g/m^2, respectively. No specific diagnostic signs were observed in rodents. At these doses the only signs seen in dogs were emesis and mucoid stools.

There have been no cases of clinically significant overdosage with ZOCOR in humans. Until further experience is obtained, no specific treatment of overdosage with ZOCOR can be recommended.

DOSAGE AND ADMINISTRATION

Prior to initiating ZOCOR, the patient should be placed on a standard cholesterol-lowering diet (A.H.A. Phase I or N.C.E.P. Step I) for a minimum of three to six months, depending upon the severity of the lipid alteration. Dietary therapy should continue during treatment with ZOCOR.

The recommended starting dose is 5–10 mg once a day in the evening. The recommended dosing range is 5–40 mg/day as a single dose in the evening; the maximum recommended dose is 40 mg/day. Doses should be individualized according to baseline LDL-C levels, the recommended goal of therapy (see NCEP Guidelines) and the patient's response. A starting dose of 5 mg/day should be considered for patients with LDL-C (on diet) of ≤190 mg/dL (4.9 mmol/L) and for the elderly. Patients with LDL-C levels >190 mg/dL (4.9 mmol/L) should be started on 10 mg/day. Adjustments of dosage should be made at intervals of 4 weeks or more.

In the elderly, maximum reductions in LDL cholesterol may be achieved with daily doses of 20 mg or less.

Cholesterol levels should be monitored periodically and consideration should be given to reducing the dosage of ZOCOR if cholesterol falls below the targeted range.

Concomitant Therapy

ZOCOR is effective alone or when used concomitantly with bile-acid sequestrants. Use of ZOCOR with fibrate-type drugs such as gemfibrozil or clofibrate should generally be avoided (see WARNINGS, *Skeletal Muscle*).

In patients taking immunosuppressive drugs concomitantly with simvastatin (see WARNINGS, *Skeletal Muscle*), therapy should begin with 5 mg of ZOCOR and should not exceed 10 mg/day.

Dosage in Patients with Renal Insufficiency

Because ZOCOR does not undergo significant renal excretion, modification of dosage should not be necessary in patients with mild to moderate renal insufficiency. However, caution should be exercised when ZOCOR is administered to patients with severe renal insufficiency; such patients should be started at 5 mg/day and be closely monitored (see CLINICAL PHARMACOLOGY, *Pharmacokinetics*).

HOW SUPPLIED

No. 3588—Tablets ZOCOR 5 mg are buff, shield-shaped, film-coated tablets, coded MSD 726. They are supplied as follows:

NDC 0006-0726-61 unit of use bottles of 60

NDC 0006-0726-54 unit of use bottles of 90

NDC 0006-0726-28 unit dose packages of 100.

Shown in Product Identification Section, page 420

No. 3589—Tablets ZOCOR 10 mg are peach, shield-shaped, film-coated tablets, coded MSD 735. They are supplied as follows:

NDC 0006-0735-61 unit of use bottles of 60

NDC 0006-0735-54 unit of use bottles of 90

NDC 0006-0735-28 unit dose packages of 100.

Shown in Product Identification Section, page 420

No. 3590—Tablets ZOCOR 20 mg are tan, shield-shaped, film-coated tablets, coded MSD 740. They are supplied as follows:

NDC 0006-0740-61 unit of use bottles of 60.

Shown in Product Identification Section, page 420

No. 3591—Tablets ZOCOR 40 mg are brick-red, shield-shaped, film-coated tablets, coded MSD 749. They are supplied as follows:

NDC 0006-0749-61 unit of use bottles of 60.

Shown in Product Identification Section, page 420

Storage

Store between 5–30°C (41–86°F).

A.H.F.S. Category: 24:06

DC 7713902 Issued December 1991

COPYRIGHT © MERCK & CO., INC., 1991
All rights reserved

Information on the Merck Sharp & Dohme products listed on these pages is the full prescribing information from product circulars in use October 1, 1991.

Miles Inc.

Consumer Healthcare Products
P.O. BOX 340
ELKHART, IN 46515

ALKA-MINTS® OTC
Chewable Antacid Rich in Calcium

(See PDR For Nonprescription Drugs.)

ALKA-SELTZER® OTC
Effervescent Antacid & Pain Reliever
With Specially Buffered Aspirin
[*al-kuh-selt-sir*]

ACTIVE INGREDIENTS

Each tablet contains: aspirin 325 mg., heat treated sodium bicarbonate 1916 mg., citric acid 1000 mg. ALKA-SELTZER® in water contains principally the antacid sodium citrate and the analgesic sodium acetylsalicylate. Buffered pH is between 6 and 7.

INACTIVE INGREDIENTS

None.

INDICATIONS

ALKA-SELTZER® Effervescent Antacid & Pain Reliever is an analgesic and an antacid and is indicated for relief of sour stomach, acid indigestion or heartburn with headache or body aches and pains. Also for fast relief of upset stomach with headache from overindulgence in food and drink—especially recommended for taking before bed and again on arising. Effective for pain relief alone: headache or body and muscular aches and pains.

ACTIONS

When the ALKA-SELTZER® Effervescent Antacid & Pain Reliever tablet is dissolved in water, the acetylsalicylate ion differs from acetylsalicylic acid chemically, physically and pharmacologically. Being fat insoluble, it is not absorbed by the gastric mucosal cells. Studies and observations in animals and man including radiochrome determinations of fecal blood loss, measurement of ion fluxes and direct visualization with gastrocamera, have shown that, as contrasted with acetylsalicylic acid, the acetylsalicylate ion delivered in the solution does not alter gastric mucosal permeability to permit back-diffusion of hydrogen ion, and gastric damage and acute gastric mucosal lesions are therefore not seen after administration of the product.

ALKA-SELTZER® Effervescent Antacid & Pain Reliever has the capacity to neutralize gastric hydrochloric acid quickly and effectively. In-vitro, 154 ml. of 0.1 N hydrochloric acid are required to decrease the pH of one tablet of ALKA-SELTZER® Effervescent Antacid & Pain Reliever in solution to 4.0. Measured against the in vitro standard established by the Food and Drug Administration one tablet neutralizes 17.2 mEq of acid. In vivo, the antacid activity of two ALKA-SELTZER® Antacid & Pain Reliever tablets is comparable to that of 10 ml. of milk of magnesia. ALKA-SELTZER® Effervescent Antacid & Pain Reliever is able to resist pH changes caused by the continuing secretion of acid in the normal individual and to maintain an elevated pH until emptying occurs.

ALKA-SELTZER® Effervescent Antacid & Pain Reliever provides highly water soluble acetylsalicylate ions which are fat insoluble. Acetylsalicylate ions are not absorbed from the stomach. They empty from the stomach and thereby become available for absorption from the duodenum. Thus, fast drug absorption and high plasma acetylsalicylate levels are achieved. Plasma levels of salicylate following the administration of ALKA-SELTZER® Effervescent Antacid & Pain Reliever solution (acetylsalicylate ion equivalent to 648 mg. acetylsalicylic acid) can reach 29 mg./liter in 10 minutes and rise to peak levels as high as 55 mg./liter within 30 minutes.

WARNINGS

Children and teenagers should not use this medicine for chicken pox or flu symptoms before a doctor is consulted about Reye syndrome, a rare but serious illness reported to be associated with aspirin. As with any drug, if you are pregnant or nursing a baby, seek the advice of a health professional before using this product. **IT IS ESPECIALLY IMPORTANT NOT TO USE ASPIRIN DURING THE LAST 3 MONTHS OF PREGNANCY UNLESS SPECIFICALLY DIRECTED TO DO SO BY A DOCTOR BECAUSE IT MAY CAUSE PROBLEMS IN THE UNBORN CHILD OR COMPLICATIONS DURING DELIVERY.** Except under the advice and supervision of a physician, do not take more than, Adults: 8 tablets in a 24 hour period. (60 years of age or older: 4 tablets in a 24 hour period), or use the daily maximum dosage for more than 10 days. Do not use if you are allergic to aspirin or have asthma, if you have a coagulation (bleeding) disease, or if you are on a sodium restricted diet. Each tablet contains 567 mg. of sodium.

Keep this and all drugs out of the reach of children.

DOSAGE AND ADMINISTRATION

ALKA-SELTZER® Effervescent Antacid & Pain Reliever is taken in solution, approximately three ounces of water per tablet is sufficient.

Adults: 2 tablets every 4 hours. CAUTION: If symptoms persist or recur frequently, or if you are under treatment for ulcer, consult your physician.

PROFESSIONAL LABELING

ASPIRIN FOR MYOCARDIAL INFARCTION

INDICATION

The Aspirin contained in ALKA-SELTZER is indicated to reduce the risk of death and/or non-fatal myocardial infarction in patients with a previous infarction or unstable angina pectoris.

CLINICAL TRIALS

The indication is supported by the results of six, large, randomized multicenter, placebo-controlled studies[1–7] involving 10,816 predominantly male, post-myocardial infarction (MI) patients and one randomized placebo-controlled study of 1,266 men with unstable angina. Therapy with aspirin was begun at intervals after the onset of acute MI varying from less than 3 days to more than 5 years and continued for periods of from less than one year to four years. In the unstable angina study, treatment was started within 1 month after the onset of unstable angina and continued for 12 weeks and complicating conditions such as congestive heart failure were not included in the study.

Aspirin therapy in MI patients was associated with about a 20 percent reduction in the risk of subsequent death and/or non-fatal reinfarction, a median absolute decrease of 3 percent from the 12 to 22 percent event rates in the placebo groups. In aspirin-treated unstable angina patients the reduction in risk was about 50 percent, a reduction in event rate of 5 percent from the 10 percent rate in the placebo group over the 12 weeks of the study.

Daily dosage of aspirin in the post-myocardial infarction studies was 300 mg in one study and 900 to 1500 mg in five studies. A dose of 325 mg was used in the study of unstable angina.

ADVERSE REACTIONS

Gastrointestinal Reactions: Symptoms and signs of gastrointestinal irritation were not significantly increased in subjects treated for unstable angina with buffered aspirin in solution. (ALKA-SELTZER®.) Doses of 1000 mg per day of aspirin tablets caused gastrointestinal symptoms and bleeding that in some cases were clinically significant. In the largest post-infarction study (the Aspirin Myocardial Infarction Study (AMIS) with 4,500 people), the percentage incidences of gastrointestinal symptoms for the aspirin (1000 mg of a standard, solid-tablet formulation) and placebo-treated subjects, respectively, were: stomach pain (14.5%; 4.4%); heartburn (11.9%; 4.8%); nausea and/or vomiting (7.6%; 2.1%); hospitalization for gastrointestinal disorder (4.9%; 3.5%). In the AMIS and other trials, aspirin treated patients had increased rates of gross gastrointestinal bleeding. As with all aspirin products ALKA-SELTZER is contraindicated in patients with aspirin sensitivity, with asthma, or with coagulation disease.

CARDIOVASCULAR AND BIOCHEMICAL

In the AMIS trial, the dosage of 1000 mg per day of aspirin was associated with small increases in systolic blood pressure (BP) (average 1.5 to 2.1 mm) and diastolic BP (0.5 to 0.6 mm), depending upon whether maximal or last available readings were used. Blood urea nitrogen and uric acid levels were also increased, but by less than 1.0 mg%. Subjects with marked hypertension or renal insufficiency had been excluded from the trial so that the clinical importance of these observations for such subjects or for any subjects treated over more prolonged periods is not known. It is recommended that patients placed on long-term aspirin treatment, even at doses of 300 mg per day, be seen at regular intervals to assess changes in these measurements.

SODIUM IN BUFFERED ASPIRIN FOR SOLUTION FORMULATIONS

One tablet daily of buffered aspirin in solution adds 567 mg of sodium to that in the diet and may not be tolerated by pa-

tients with active sodium-retaining states such as congestive heart or renal failure. This amount of sodium adds about 30 percent to the 70 to 90 meq intake suggested as appropriate for dietary treatment of essential hypertension in the 1984 Report of the Joint National Committee on Detection, Evaluation, and Treatment of High Blood Pressure[8].

DOSAGE AND ADMINISTRATION

Although most of the studies used dosages exceeding 300 mg, daily, two trials used only 300 mg and pharmacologic data indicate that this dose inhibits platelet function fully. Therefore, 300 mg or a conventional 325 mg aspirin dose daily is a reasonable, routine dose that would minimize gastrointestinal adverse reactions. This use of aspirin applies to both solid, oral dosage forms (buffered and plain aspirin) and buffered aspirin in solution.

REFERENCES

(1) Elwood, P. C., et al., "A Randomized Controlled Trial of Acetysalicylic Acid in the Secondary Prevention of Mortality from Myocardial Infarction," *British Medical Journal* 1:436–440, 1974.
(2) The Coronary Drug Project Research Group, "Aspirin in Coronary Heart Disease," *Journal of Chronic Diseases*, 29:625–642, 1976.
(3) Breddin, K., et al., "Secondary Prevention of Myocardial Infarction: A Comparison of Acetylsalicylic Acid, Phenprocoumon or Placebo," *International Congress Series* 470:263–268, 1979.
(4) Aspirin Myocardial Infarction Study Research Group, "A Randomized, Controlled Trial of Aspirin in Persons Recovered from Myocardial Infarction," *Journal American Medical Association* 245:661–669, 1980.
(5) Elwood, P. C., and P. M. Sweetnam, "Aspirin and Secondary Mortality after Myocardial Infarction." *Lancet* pp. 1313–1315, December 22–29, 1979.
(6) The Persantine-Aspirin Reinfarction Study Research Group, "Persantine and Aspirin in Coronary Heart Disease," *Circulation*, 62: 449–460, 1980.
(7) Lewis, H. D., et al., "Protective Effects of Aspirin Against Acute Myocardial Infarction and Death in Men with Unstable Angina, Results of a Veterans Administration Cooperative Study," *New England Journal of Medicine* 309:396–403, 1983.
(8) "1984 Report of the Joint National Committee on Detection, Evaluation, Treatment of High Blood Pressure," U.S. Department of Health and Human Services and United States Public Health Service, National Institutes of Health.

HOW SUPPLIED

Tablets: foil sealed; box of 12, 24, 36 and 72 in twin packs; carton of 100 in twin packs.

Flavored ALKA-SELTZER® — OTC

Effervescent Antacid & Pain Reliever
[al-kuh-selt-sir]

ACTIVE INGREDIENTS

Each tablet contains: Aspirin 325 mg, heat treated sodium bicarbonate 1710 mg, citric acid 1220 mg. Alka-Seltzer in water contains principally the antacid sodium citrate and the analgesic sodium acetylsalicylate.

INACTIVE INGREDIENTS

Flavors, Saccharin Sodium.

INDICATIONS

SPARKLING FRESH TASTE!
Flavored Alka-Seltzer®
For speedy relief of ACID INDIGESTION, SOUR STOMACH or HEARTBURN with HEADACHE, or BODY ACHES AND PAINS. Also for fast relief of UPSET STOMACH with HEADACHE from overindulgence in food and drink—especially recommended for taking before bed and again on arising. EFFECTIVE FOR PAIN RELIEF ALONE: HEADACHE or BODY and MUSCULAR ACHES and PAINS.

WARNINGS

Children and teenagers should not use this medicine for chicken pox and flu symptoms before a doctor is consulted about Reye syndrome, a rare but serious illness reported to be associated with aspirin.
As with any drug, if you are pregnant or nursing a baby, seek the advice of a health professional before using this product. **IT IS ESPECIALLY IMPORTANT NOT TO USE ASPIRIN DURING THE LAST 3 MONTHS OF PREGNANCY UNLESS SPECIFICALLY DIRECTED TO DO SO BY A DOCTOR BECAUSE IT MAY CAUSE PROBLEMS IN THE UNBORN CHILD OR COMPLICATIONS DURING DELIVERY.**
Except under the advice and supervision of a physician: Do not take more than, ADULTS: 6 tablets in a 24-hour period, (60 years of age or older: 4 tablets in a 24-hour period), or use the daily maximum dosage for more than 10 days. Do not use if you are allergic to aspirin or have asthma, if you have a coagulation (bleeding) disease, or if you are on a sodium restricted diet. Each tablet contains 506 mg of sodium.
KEEP this and all drugs out of the reach of children.

DIRECTIONS

Alka-Seltzer must be dissolved in water before taking. ADULTS: 2 tablets every 4 hours. CAUTION: If symptoms persist or recur frequently or if you are under treatment for ulcer, consult your physician.

PROFESSIONAL LABELING

ASPIRIN FOR MYOCARDIAL INFARCTION

INDICATION

The Aspirin contained in Alka-Seltzer is indicated to reduce the risk of death and/or non-fatal myocardial infarction in patients with a previous infarction or unstable angina pectoris.

CLINICAL TRIALS

The indication is supported by the results of six, large, randomized multicenter, placebo-controlled studies[1–7] involving 10,816, predominantly male, post-myocardial infarction (MI) patients and one randomized placebo-controlled study of 1,266 men with unstable angina. Therapy with aspirin was begun at intervals after the onset of acute MI varying from less than 3 days to more than 5 years and continued for periods of from less than one year to four years. In the unstable angina study, treatment was started within 1 month after the onset of unstable angina and continued for 12 weeks and complicating conditions such as congestive heart failure were not included in the study.
Aspirin therapy in MI patients was associated with about a 20 percent reduction in the risk of subsequent death and/or non-fatal reinfarction, a median absolute decrease of 3 percent from the 12 to 22 percent event rates in the placebo groups. In aspirin-treated unstable angina patients the reduction in risk was about 50 percent, a reduction in event rate of 5 percent from the 10 percent rate in the placebo group over the 12 week of the study.
Daily dosage of aspirin in the post-myocardial infarction studies was 300 mg in one study and 900 to 1500 mg in five studies. A dose of 325 mg was used in the study of unstable angina.

ADVERSE REACTIONS

Gastrointestinal Reactions: Symptoms and signs of gastrointestinal irritation were not significantly increased in subjects treated for unstable angina with buffered aspirin in solution (ALKA-SELTZER®). Doses of 1000 mg per day of aspirin tablets caused gastrointestinal symptoms and bleeding that in some cases were clinically significant. In the largest post-infarction study (the Aspirin Myocardial Infarction Study (AMIS) with 4,500 people), the percentage incidences of gastrointestinal symptoms for the aspirin (1000 mg of a standard, solid-tablet formulation) and placebo-treated subjects, respectively, were: stomach pain (14.5%; 4.4%); heartburn (11.9%; 4.8%); nausea and/or vomiting (7.6%; 2.1%); hospitalization for gastrointestinal disorder (4.9%; 3.5%). In the AMIS and other trials, aspirin treated patients had increased rates of gross gastrointestinal bleeding. As with all aspirin products Alka-Seltzer is contraindicated in patients with aspirin sensitivity, with asthma, or with coagulation disease.
Cardiovascular and Biochemical: In the AMIS trial, the dosage of 1000 mg per day of aspirin was associated with small increases in systolic blood pressure (BP) (average 1.5 to 2.1 mm) and diastolic BP (0.5 to 0.6 mm), depending upon whether maximal or last available readings were used. Blood urea nitrogen and uric acid levels were also increased, but by less than 1.0 mg%. Subjects with marked hypertension or renal insufficiency had been excluded from the trial so that the clinical importance of these observations for such subjects or for any subjects treated over more prolonged periods is not known. It is recommended that patients placed on long-term aspirin treatment, even at doses of 300 mg per day, be seen at regular intervals to assess changes in these measurements.
Sodium in Buffered Aspirin for Solution Formulations: One tablet daily of flavored buffered aspirin in solution adds 506 mg of sodium to that in the diet and may not be tolerated by patients with active sodium-retaining states such as congestive heart or renal failure. This amount of sodium adds about 30 percent to the 70 to 90 meq intake suggested as appropriate for dietary treatment of essential hypertension in the 1984 Report of the Joint National Committee on Detection, Evaluation, and Treatment of High Blood Pressure[8].

DOSAGE AND ADMINISTRATION

Although most of the studies used dosages exceeding 300 mg, daily, two trials used only 300 mg and pharmacologic data indicate that this dose inhibits platelet function fully. Therefore, 300 mg or a conventional 325 mg aspirin dose daily is a reasonable, routine dose that would minimize gastrointestinal adverse reactions. This use of aspirin applies to both solid, oral dosage forms (buffered and plain aspirin) and buffered aspirin in solution.

REFERENCES

(1) Elwood, P. C., et al., A Randomized Controlled Trial of Acetysalicylic Acid in the Secondary Prevention of Mortality from Myocardial Infarction," *British Medical Journal* 1:436–440, 1974.
(2) The Coronary Drug Project Research Group, "Aspirin in Coronary Heart Disease," *Journal of Chronic Diseases*, 29:625–642, 1976.
(3) Breddin K., et al., "Secondary Prevention of Myocardial Infarction: A Comparison of Acetylsalicylic Acid, Phenprocoumon or Placebo," *Int. Congr. Series* 470:263–268, 1979.
(4) Aspirin Myocardial Infarction Study Research Group, "A Randomized, Controlled Trial of Aspirin in Persons Recovered from Myocardial Infarction," *Journal American Medical Association* 245:661–669, 1980.
(5) Elwood, P. C., and P. M. Sweetnam, "Aspirin and Secondary Mortality after Myocardial Infarction," *Lancet* pp. 1313–1315, December 22–29, 1979.
(6) The Persantine-Aspirin Reinfarction Study Research Group, "Persantine and Aspirin in Coronary Heart Disease," *Circulation*, 62: 449–460, 1980.
(7) Lewis, H. D., et al., "Protective Effects of Aspirin Against Acute Myocardial Infarction and Death in Men with Unstable Angina, Results of a Veterans Administration Cooperative Study," *New England Journal of Medicine* 309:396–403, 1983.
(8) "1984 Report of the Joint National Committee on Detection, Evaluation, Treatment of High Blood Pressure," U.S. Department of Health and Human Services and United States Public Health Service, National Institutes of Health.

HOW SUPPLIED

Tablets: foil sealed; box of 12, 24, and 36 in twin packs.

ALKA-SELTZER® Extra Strength — OTC

Antacid & Pain Reliever

ACTIVE INGREDIENTS

Each tablet contains: Aspirin 500mg, heat treated sodium bicarbonate 1985mg, citric acid 1000mg. Alka-Seltzer in water contains principally the antacid sodium citrate and the analgesic sodium acetylsalicylate.

INACTIVE INGREDIENTS

Flavors.

INDICATIONS

For speedy relief of acid indigestion, sour stomach or heartburn with headache or body aches and pains. Also, for fast relief of upset stomach with headache from overindulgence in food and drink—especially recommended for taking before bed and again on arising. Effective for pain relief alone: Headache or body and muscular aches and pains.

WARNINGS

Children and teenagers should not use this medicine for chicken pox or flu symptoms before a doctor is consulted about Reye syndrome, a rare but serious illness reported to be associated with aspirin. As with any drug, if you are pregnant or nursing a baby, seek the advice of a health professional before using this product. **IT IS ESPECIALLY IMPORTANT NOT TO USE ASPIRIN DURING THE LAST 3 MONTHS OF PREGNANCY UNLESS SPECIFICALLY DIRECTED TO DO SO BY A DOCTOR BECAUSE IT MAY CAUSE PROBLEMS IN THE UNBORN CHILD OR COMPLICATIONS DURING DELIVERY.** Except under the advice and supervision of a physician: Do not take more than, Adults: 7 tablets in a 24-hour period (60 years of age or older, 4 tablets in a 24-hour period), or use the daily maximum dosage for more than 10 days. Do not use if you are allergic to aspirin or have asthma, if you have a coagulation (bleeding) disease, or if you are on a sodium restricted diet. Each tablet contains 588mg of sodium. Keep this and all drugs out of the reach of children.

DOSAGE AND ADMINISTRATION

Extra Strength Alka-Seltzer must be dissolved in water before taking. Adults: 2 tablets every 4 hours. Caution: If symptoms persist, or recur frequently, or if you are under treatment for ulcer, consult your physician.

HOW SUPPLIED

Tablets: foil sealed; Boxes of 12 and 24 in twin packs.

Continued on next page

Miles Consumer—Cont.

ALKA-SELTZER®   OTC
Effervescent Antacid
[al-kuh-selt-sir]

ACTIVE INGREDIENTS
Each tablet contains heat treated sodium bicarbonate 958 mg., citric acid 832 mg., potassium bicarbonate 312 mg. ALKA-SELTZER® Effervescent Antacid in water contains principally the antacids sodium citrate and potassium citrate.

INACTIVE INGREDIENTS
A tableting aid.

INDICATIONS
ALKA-SELTZER® Effervescent Antacid is indicated for relief of acid indigestion, sour stomach or heartburn.

ACTIONS
The ALKA-SELTZER® Effervescent Antacid solution provides quick and effective neutralization of gastric acid. Measured by the in vitro standard established by the Food and Drug Administration one tablet will neutralize 10.6 mEq of acid.

WARNINGS
Except under the advice and supervision of a physician, do not take more than: Adults: 8 tablets in a 24 hour period (60 years of age or older: 7 tablets in a 24 hour period), Children 4 tablets in a 24 hour period; or use the maximum dosage of this product for more than 2 weeks.
Do not use this product if you are on a sodium restricted diet. Each tablet contains 311 mg. of sodium.
Keep this and all drugs out of the reach of children. As with any drug, if you are pregnant or nursing a baby, seek the advice of a health professional before using this product.

DOSAGE AND ADMINISTRATION
ALKA-SELTZER® Effervescent Antacid is taken in solution; approximately 3 oz. of water per tablet is sufficient. Adults: one or two tablets every 4 hours as needed. Children: ½ the adult dosage.

HOW SUPPLIED
Tablets: foil sealed; box of 20 and 36 in twin packs.

ALKA-SELTZER PLUS®   OTC
Cold Medicine

(See PDR For Nonprescription Drugs.)

ALKA-SELTZER PLUS® MAXIMUM STRENGTH   OTC
Sinus Allergy Medicine

(See PDR For Nonprescription Drugs.)

ALKA-SELTZER PLUS® NIGHT-TIME   OTC
Cold Medicine

(See PDR For Nonprescription Drugs.)

BACTINE® Antiseptic · Anesthetic   OTC
First Aid Spray
[bak-tēn]

(See PDR For Nonprescription Drugs.)

BACTINE® First Aid Antibiotic Ointment   OTC

(See PDR For Nonprescription Drugs.)

BACTINE® Hydrocortisone (0.5%)   OTC
Skin Care Cream
[bak-tēn]

(See PDR For Nonprescription Drugs.)

Maximum Strength
BACTINE® Anti-Itch Cream   OTC
[bac-tēn]
1.0% Hydrocortisone
Previously Available only by Prescription

INDICATIONS
For the temporary relief of itching associated with minor skin irritations, inflammation and rashes due to:
Eczema
Poison Sumac
Soaps
Jewelry
Insect Bites
Poison Oak
Detergents
Seborrheic Dermatitis
Psoriasis
Poison Ivy
Cosmetics
Other uses of this product should be only under the advice and supervision of a physician.

DIRECTIONS
For Adults and Children 2 years of age and older. Apply to affected area not more than 3 or 4 times daily. Children under 2 years of age: Do not use, consult a physician.

WARNINGS
For external use only. Avoid contact with the eyes. If condition worsens or if symptoms persist for more than seven days or clear up and occur again within a few days, stop use of this product and do not begin use of any other hydrocortisone product unless you have consulted a physician. Do not use for the treatment of diaper rash. Consult a physician.
Keep this and all drugs out of the reach of children. In case of accidental ingestion, seek professional assistance or contact a Poison Control Center immediately.

ACTIVE INGREDIENTS
Hydrocortisone 1.0%.

INACTIVE INGREDIENTS
Aluminum Sulfate, Beeswax, Calcium Acetate, Cetearyl Alcohol, Dextrin, Glycerin, Hydrocortisone Alcohol, Light Mineral Oil, Methylparaben, Purified Water, Sodium Lauryl Sulfate, White Petrolatum.
Miles Inc.
Elkhart, IN 46515, USA

BUGS BUNNY® Children's   OTC
Chewable Vitamins (Sugar Free)

(See PDR For Nonprescription Drugs.)

BUGS BUNNY® Complete Children's   OTC
Chewable Vitamins + Minerals
With Iron and Calcium (Sugar Free)

(See PDR For Nonprescription Drugs.)

BUGS BUNNY® Plus Iron Children's   OTC
Chewable Vitamins
(Sugar Free)

(See PDR For Nonprescription Drugs.)

BUGS BUNNY® With Extra C   OTC
Children's Chewable Vitamins
(Sugar Free)
Multivitamin Supplement

(See PDR For Nonprescription Drugs.)

DOMEBORO® ASTRINGENT SOLUTION   OTC

(See PDR For Nonprescription Drugs.)

FLINTSTONES® Children's   OTC
Chewable Vitamins

(See PDR For Nonprescription Drugs.)

FLINTSTONES® Plus Iron Children's   OTC
Chewable Vitamins

(See PDR For Nonprescription Drugs.)

FLINTSTONES® COMPLETE   OTC
With Iron, Calcium & Minerals
Children's Chewable Vitamins

(See PDR For Nonprescription Drugs.)

FLINTSTONES® With Extra C   OTC
Children's Chewable Vitamins
Multivitamin Supplement

(See PDR For Nonprescription Drugs.)

MILES® NERVINE   OTC
NIGHTTIME SLEEP-AID

(See PDR For Nonprescription Drugs.)

MYCELEX® OTC ANTIFUNGAL   OTC
(CREAM OR SOLUTION)

ACTIVE INGREDIENT
Clotrimazole 1%

INACTIVE INGREDIENTS
Benzyl alcohol (1%) as a preservative, cetostearyl alcohol, cetyl esters wax, octyldodecanol, polysorbate 60, purified water, sorbitan monostearate.
Store between 2°–30°C (36°–86°F).

INDICATIONS
Cures athlete's foot (tinea pedis), jock itch (tinea cruris) and ringworm (tinea corporis). For effective relief of the itching, cracking, burning and discomfort which can accompany these conditions.

WARNINGS
For external use only. Do not use on children under 2 years of age except under the advice and supervision of a doctor. If irritation occurs or if there is no improvement within 4 weeks (for athlete's foot or ringworm) or within 2 weeks (for jock itch) discontinue use and consult a doctor or pharmacist. Keep this and all drugs out of the reach of children. In case of accidental ingestion seek professional assistance or contact a Poison Control Center immediately. Use only as directed.

DOSAGE AND ADMINISTRATION
Cleanse skin with soap and water and dry thoroughly. Apply a thin layer and gently massage over affected area morning and evening or as directed by a doctor. For athlete's foot, pay special attention to the spaces between the toes. It is also helpful to wear well-fitting, ventilated shoes and to change shoes and socks at least once daily. Best results in athlete's foot and ringworm are usually obtained with 4 weeks' use of this product and in jock itch with 2 weeks' use. If satisfactory results have not occurred within these times, consult a doctor or pharmacist. Children under 12 years of age should be supervised in the use of this product. This product is not effective on the scalp or nails.

HOW SUPPLIED
CREAM (Tube 15g) and SOLUTION (Bottle 10mL)

MYCELEX®-7   OTC
Clotrimazole Vaginal Cream 1%
Clotrimazole Vaginal Inserts (100 mg)

DESCRIPTION
MYCELEX®-7 Antifungal Vaginal Cream and Vaginal Inserts can kill the yeast that may cause vaginal infection. It does not stain clothes. The cream is greaseless.
Active Ingredient: Cream—clotrimazole 1%.
Insert—100 mg clotrimazole.
Inactive Ingredients: Cream—Benzyl alcohol, cetostearyl alcohol, cetyl esters wax, octyldodecanol, polysorbate 60, purified water, sorbitan monostearate.
Inserts—Corn starch, lactose, magnesium stearate, povidone.

INDICATIONS
For treatment of vaginal yeast (Candida) infection.
IF THIS IS THE FIRST TIME YOU HAVE HAD VAGINAL ITCH AND DISCOMFORT, CONSULT YOUR DOCTOR. IF YOU HAVE HAD A DOCTOR DIAGNOSE A VAGINAL YEAST INFECTION BEFORE AND HAVE THE SAME

SYMPTOMS NOW, USE CREAM OR INSERTS AS DIRECTED FOR 7 CONSECUTIVE DAYS.
WARNING: DO NOT USE IF YOU HAVE ABDOMINAL PAIN, FEVER, OR FOUL-SMELLING DISCHARGE. CONTACT YOUR DOCTOR IMMEDIATELY.
Before using, read the enclosed phamplet.

DIRECTIONS

Cream: Fill the applicator and insert one applicatorful of cream into the vagina, preferably at bedtime. Repeat this procedure daily for 7 consecutive days.

Inserts: Unwrap one insert, place it in the applicator, and use the applicator to place the insert into the vagina, preferably at bedtime. Repeat this procedure daily for 7 consecutive days.

WARNING: IF YOU DO NOT IMPROVE IN 3 DAYS OR IF YOU DO NOT GET WELL IN 7 DAYS, YOU MAY HAVE A CONDITION OTHER THAN A YEAST INFECTION. CONSULT YOUR DOCTOR. Do not use during pregnancy except under the advice and supervision of a doctor. Do not use tampons while using this medication. If symptoms return within a two-month period, contact your doctor. Keep this and all drugs out of reach of children. In case of accidental ingestion, seek professional assistance or contact a Poison Control Center immediately. NOT FOR USE IN CHILDREN LESS THAN 12 YEARS OF AGE.

If you have any questions about MYCELEX®-7 or vaginal yeast infection, contact your physician.

Store at room temperature between 2° and 30°C (36° and 86°F). See end panel of carton and tube crimp or foil wrappers for lot number and expiration date.

Miles Inc.
Elkhart, IN 46515, USA

ONE–A–DAY® Essential Vitamins　　OTC
with Beta Carotene

(See PDR For Nonprescription Drugs.)

ONE–A–DAY® Maximum Formula　　OTC
Vitamins and Minerals with Beta Carotene

(See PDR For Nonprescription Drugs.)

ONE–A–DAY® Plus Extra C　　OTC
Vitamins with Beta Carotene

(See PDR For Nonprescription Drugs.)

ONE–A–DAY STRESSGARD®　　OTC
Stress Formula Vitamins with Beta Carotene

(See PDR For Nonprescription Drugs.)

ONE–A–DAY WITHIN®　　OTC
Multivitamin for Women with Calcium, Extra Iron, Zinc and Beta Carotene

(See PDR For Nonprescription Drugs.)

Miles Inc.
Pharmaceutical Division
400 MORGAN LANE
WEST HAVEN, CT 06516

PRODUCT IDENTIFICATION CODES

To provide an accurate identification of Miles Inc. Pharmaceutical Division products, each solid dosage form is coded with the name Miles and a 3 digit product identification number.

PRODUCT	PRODUCT IDENTIFICATION CODE NUMBER
ORAL DOSAGE FORMS	
Adalat Capsules 10 mg (nifedipine/Miles)	811
Adalat Capsules 20 mg (nifedipine/Miles)	821
Biltricide Tablets 600 mg (praziquantel)	521
Cipro Tablets 250 mg (ciprofloxacin HCl/Miles)	512
Cipro Tablets 500 mg (ciprofloxacin HCl/Miles)	513
Cipro Tablets 750 mg (ciprofloxacin HCl/Miles)	514
Lithane® Tablets 300 mg (lithium carbonate)	951
Mycelex® Troche 10 mg (clotrimazole)	095
Niclocide® Chewable Tablets 500 mg (niclosamide)	721
Nimotop® Capsules 30 mg (nimodipine/Miles)	855
Stilphostrol® Tablets 50 mg (diethylstilbestrol diphosphate)	132

NON-ORAL DOSAGE FORMS

Mycelex®-G 500 mg Vaginal Tablets (clotrimazole)	097

ADALAT®　　℞
Capsules
(nifedipine/Miles)
For Oral Use

DESCRIPTION

ADALAT® (nifedipine) is an antianginal drug belonging to a class of pharmacological agents, the calcium channel blockers. Nifedipine is 3,5-pyridinedicarboxylic acid, 1,4-dihydro-2,6-dimethyl-4-(2-nitrophenyl)-, dimethyl ester, $C_{17}H_{18}N_2O_6$, and has the structural formula:

Nifedipine is a yellow crystalline substance, practically insoluble in water but soluble in ethanol. It has a molecular weight of 346.3. ADALAT® CAPSULES are formulated as soft gelatin capsules for oral administration each containing 10 mg or 20 mg of nifedipine.

Inert ingredients in the formulations are: glycerin; peppermint oil; polyethylene glycol 400; soft gelatin capsules (which contain FD&C Yellow No. 6, Red Ferric Oxide and other inert ingredients), and water. The 10 mg capsules also contain saccharin sodium.

CLINICAL PHARMACOLOGY

ADALAT® is a calcium ion influx inhibitor (slow channel blocker or calcium ion antagonist) and inhibits the transmembrane influx of calcium ions into cardiac muscle and smooth muscle. The contractile processes of cardiac muscle and vascular smooth muscle are dependent upon the movement of extracellular calcium ions into these cells through specific ion channels. ADALAT® selectively inhibits calcium ion influx across the cell membrane of cardiac muscle and vascular smooth muscle without changing serum calcium concentrations.

Mechanism of Action
The precise means by which this inhibition relieves angina has not been fully determined, but includes at least the following two mechanisms:

1) Relaxation and Prevention of Coronary Artery Spasm
ADALAT® dilates the main coronary arteries and coronary arterioles, both in normal and ischemic regions, and is a potent inhibitor of coronary artery spasm, whether spontaneous or ergonovine-induced. This property increases myocardial oxygen delivery in patients with coronary artery spasm, and is responsible for the effectiveness of ADALAT® in vasospastic (Prinzmetal's or variant) angina. Whether this effect plays any role in classical angina is not clear, but studies of exercise tolerance have not shown an increase in the maximum exercise rate-pressure product, a widely accepted measure of oxygen utilization. This suggests that, in general, relief of spasm or dilation of coronary arteries is not an important factor in classical angina.

2) Reduction of Oxygen Utilization
ADALAT® regularly reduces arterial pressure at rest and at a given level of exercise by dilating peripheral arterioles and reducing the total peripheral resistance (afterload) against which the heart works. This unloading of the heart reduces myocardial energy consumption and oxygen requirements and probably accounts for the effectiveness of ADALAT® in chronic stable angina.

Pharmacokinetics and Metabolism
ADALAT® is rapidly and fully absorbed after oral administration. The drug is detectable in serum 10 minutes after oral administration, and peak blood levels occur in approximately 30 minutes. Bioavailability is proportional to dose from 10 to 30 mg; half-life does not change significantly with dose. There is little difference in relative bioavailability

when ADALAT® capsules are given orally and swallowed whole, bitten and swallowed, or bitten and held sublingually. However, biting through the capsule prior to swallowing does result in slightly earlier plasma concentrations (27 ng/mL 10 minutes after 10 mg) than if capsules are swallowed intact. It is highly bound by serum proteins. ADALAT® is extensively converted to inactive metabolites and approximately 80 percent of ADALAT® and metabolites are eliminated via the kidneys. The half-life of nifedipine in plasma is approximately two hours. Since hepatic biotransformation is the predominant route for the disposition of nifedipine, the pharmacokinetics may be altered in patients with chronic liver disease. Patients with hepatic impairment (liver cirrhosis) have a longer disposition half-life and higher bioavailability of nifedipine than healthy volunteers. The degree of serum protein binding of nifedipine is high (92–98%). Protein binding may be greatly reduced in patients with renal or hepatic impairment.

Hemodynamics
Like other slow channel blockers, ADALAT® exerts a negative inotropic effect on isolated myocardial tissue. This is rarely, if ever, seen in intact animals or man, probably because of reflex responses to its vasodilating effects. In man, ADALAT® causes decreased peripheral vascular resistance and a fall in systolic and diastolic pressure, usually modest (5–10mm Hg systolic), but sometimes larger. There is usually a small increase in heart rate, a reflex response to vasodilation. Measurements of cardiac function in patients with normal ventricular function have generally found a small increase in cardiac index without major effects on ejection fraction, left ventricular end diastolic pressure (LVEDP) or volume (LVEDV). In patients with impaired ventricular function, most acute studies have shown some increase in ejection fraction and reduction in left ventricular filling pressure.

Electrophysiologic Effects
Although like other members of its class, ADALAT® decreases sinoatrial node function and atrioventricular conduction in isolated myocardial preparations, such effects have not been seen in studies in intact animals or in man. In formal electrophysiologic studies, predominantly in patients with normal conduction system, ADALAT® has had no tendency to prolong atrioventricular conduction, prolong sinus node recovery time, or slow sinus rate.

INDICATIONS AND USAGE

I. Vasospastic Angina
ADALAT® (nifedipine) is indicated for the management of vasospastic angina confirmed by any of the following criteria: 1) classical pattern of angina at rest accompanied by ST segment elevation, 2) angina or coronary artery spasm provoked by ergonovine, or 3) angiographically demonstrated coronary artery spasm. In those patients who have had angiography, the presence of significant fixed obstructive disease is not incompatible with the diagnosis of vasospastic angina, provided that the above criteria are satisfied. ADALAT® may also be used where the clinical presentation suggests a possible vasospastic component but where vasospasm has not been confirmed, e.g., where pain has a variable threshold on exertion or in unstable angina where electrocardiographic findings are compatible with intermittent vasospasm, or when angina is refractory to nitrates and/or adequate doses of beta blockers.

II. Chronic Stable Angina
(Classical Effort-Associated Angina)
ADALAT® is indicated for the management of chronic stable angina (effort-associated angina) without evidence of vasospasm in patients who remain symptomatic despite adequate dose of beta blockers and/or organic nitrates or who cannot tolerate those agents.

In chronic stable angina (effort-associated angina) ADALAT® has been effective in controlled trials of up to eight weeks duration in reducing angina frequency and increasing exercise tolerance, but confirmation of sustained effectiveness and evaluation of long term safety in these patients are incomplete.

Controlled studies in small numbers of patients suggest concomitant use of ADALAT® and beta blocking agents may be beneficial in patients with chronic stable angina, but available information is not sufficient to predict with confidence the effects of concurrent treatment, especially in patients with compromised left ventricular function or cardiac conduction abnormalities. When introducing such concomitant therapy, care must be taken to monitor blood pressure closely since severe hypotension can occur from the combined effects of the drugs (See WARNINGS).

CONTRAINDICATIONS

Known hypersensitivity reaction to ADALAT®.

WARNINGS

Excessive Hypotension
Although in most patients, the hypotensive effect of ADALAT® is modest and well tolerated, occasional patients have had excessive and poorly tolerated hypotension. These re-

Continued on next page

Miles—Cont.

sponses have usually occurred during initial titration or at the time of subsequent upward dosage adjustment, and may be more likely in patients on concomitant beta blockers. Severe hypotension and/or increased fluid volume requirements have been reported in patients receiving ADALAT® together with a beta blocking agent who underwent coronary artery bypass surgery using high dose fentanyl anesthesia. The interaction with high dose fentanyl appears to be due to the combination of ADALAT® and a beta blocker, but the possibility that it may occur with ADALAT® alone, with low doses of fentanyl, in other surgical procedures, or with other narcotic analgesics cannot be ruled out. In ADALAT® treated patients where surgery using high dose fentanyl anesthesia is contemplated, the physician should be aware of these potential problems and, if the patient's condition permits, sufficient time (at least 36 hours) should be allowed for ADALAT® to be washed out of the body prior to surgery.

Increased Angina and/or Myocardial Infarction

Rarely, patients, particularly those who have severe obstructive coronary artery disease, have developed well documented increased frequency, duration and/or severity of angina or acute myocardial infarction on starting ADALAT® or at the time of dosage increase. The mechanism of this effect is not established.

Beta Blocker Withdrawal

Patients recently withdrawn from beta blockers may develop a withdrawal syndrome with increased angina, probably related to increased sensitivity to catecholamines. Initiation of ADALAT® treatment will not prevent this occurrence and might be expected to exacerbate it by provoking reflex catecholamine release. There have been occasional reports of increased angina in a setting of beta blocker withdrawal and ADALAT® initiation. It is important to taper beta blockers if possible, rather than stopping them abruptly before beginning ADALAT®.

Congestive Heart Failure

Rarely, patients (usually those receiving a beta blocker) have developed heart failure after beginning ADALAT®. Patients with tight aortic stenosis may be at greater risk for such an event since the unloading effect of ADALAT® would be expected to be of less benefit to these patients, owing to the fixed impedance to flow across the aortic valve.

PRECAUTIONS

General: Hypotension: Because ADALAT® decreases peripheral vascular resistance, careful monitoring of blood pressure during the initial administration and titration of ADALAT® is suggested. Close observation is especially recommended for patients already taking medications that are known to lower blood pressure (See WARNINGS).

Peripheral Edema: Mild to moderate peripheral edema, typically associated with arterial vasodilation and not due to left ventricular dysfunction, occurs in about one in ten patients treated with ADALAT® (nifedipine). This edema occurs primarily in the lower extremities and usually responds to diuretic therapy. With patients whose angina is complicated by congestive heart failure, care should be taken to differentiate this peripheral edema from the effects of increasing left ventricular dysfunction.

Laboratory Tests: Rare, usually transient, but occasionally significant elevations of enzymes such as alkaline phosphatase, CPK, LDH, SGOT and SGPT have been noted. The relationship to ADALAT® therapy is uncertain in most cases, but probable in some. These laboratory abnormalities have rarely been associated with clinical symptoms, however, cholestasis with or without jaundice has been reported. Rare instances of allergic hepatitis have been reported.

ADALAT®, like other calcium channel blockers, decreases platelet aggregation *in vitro*. Limited clinical studies have demonstrated a moderate but statistically significant decrease in platelet aggregation and increase in bleeding time in some ADALAT® patients. This is thought to be a function of inhibition of calcium transport across the platelet membrane. No clinical significance for these findings has been demonstrated.

Positive direct Coombs test with/without hemolytic anemia has been reported.

Although ADALAT® has been used safely in patients with renal dysfunction and has been reported to exert a beneficial effect in certain cases, rare, reversible elevations in BUN and serum creatinine have been reported in patients with pre-existing chronic renal insufficiency. The relationship to ADALAT® therapy is uncertain in most cases, but probable in some.

Drug Interactions: *Beta-adrenergic blocking agents:* (See INDICATIONS and WARNINGS). Experience in over 1400 patients in a non-comparative clinical trial has shown that concomitant administration of ADALAT® and beta blocking agents is usually well tolerated, but there have been occasional literature reports suggesting that the combination may increase the likelihood of congestive heart failure, severe hypotension or exacerbation of angina.

Long acting nitrates: ADALAT® may be safely co-administered with nitrates, but there have been no controlled studies to evaluate the antianginal effectiveness of this combination.

Digitalis: Since there have been isolated reports of patients with elevated digoxin levels, and there is a possible interaction between digoxin and nifedipine, it is recommended that digoxin levels be monitored when initiating, adjusting and discontinuing nifedipine to avoid possible over- or under-digitalization.

Coumarin anticoagulants: There have been rare reports of increased prothrombin time in patients taking coumarin anticoagulants to whom ADALAT® was administered. However, the relationship to ADALAT® therapy is uncertain.

Cimetidine: A study in six healthy volunteers has shown a significant increase in peak nifedipine plasma levels (80%) and area-under-the-curve (74%) after a one week course of cimetidine at 1000 mg per day and nifedipine at 40 mg per day. Ranitidine produced smaller, non-significant increases. The effect may be mediated by the known inhibition of cimetidine on hepatic cytochrome P-450, the enzyme system probably responsible for the first-pass metabolism of nifedipine. If nifedipine therapy is initiated in a patient currently receiving cimetidine, cautious titration is advised.

Quinidine: There have been rare reports of an interaction between quinidine and nifedipine (with a decreased plasma level of quinidine).

Carcinogenesis, Mutagenesis, Impairment of Fertility: Nifedipine was administered orally to rats for two years and was not shown to be carcinogenic. When given to rats prior to mating, nifedipine caused reduced fertility at a dose approximately 30 times the maximum recommended human dose. *In vivo* mutagenicity studies were negative.

Pregnancy: Pregnancy Category C. Nifedipine has been shown to be teratogenic in rats when given in doses 30 times the maximum recommended human dose. Nifedipine was embryotoxic (increased fetal resorptions, decreased fetal weight, increased stunted forms, increased fetal deaths, decreased neonatal survival) in rats, mice and rabbits at doses of from 3 to 10 times the maximum recommended human dose. In pregnant monkeys, doses ⅔ and twice the maximum recommended human dose resulted in small placentas and underdeveloped chorionic villi. In rats doses three times maximum human dose and higher caused prolongation of pregnancy. There are no adequate and well controlled studies in pregnant women. ADALAT® should be used during pregnancy only if the potential benefit justifies the potential risk to the fetus.

Nursing Mothers: Nifedipine is excreted in human milk. Therefore, a decision should be made to discontinue nursing or to discontinue the drug, taking into account the importance of the drug to the mother.

ADVERSE REACTION

In multiple-dose U.S. and foreign controlled studies in which adverse reactions were reported spontaneously, adverse effects were frequent but generally not serious and rarely required discontinuation of therapy or dosage adjustment. Most were expected consequences of the vasodilator effects of ADALAT®.

Adverse Effect	ADALAT® (%) (N=226)	Placebo (%) (N=235)
Dizziness, lightheaded-ness, giddiness	27	15
Flushing, heat sensation	25	8
Headache	23	20
Weakness	12	10
Nausea, heartburn	11	8
Muscle cramps, tremor	8	3
Peripheral edema	7	1
Nervousness, mood changes	7	4
Palpitation	7	5
Dyspnea, cough, wheezing	6	3
Nasal congestion, sore throat	6	8

There is also a large uncontrolled experience in over 2100 patients in the United States. Most of the patients had vasospastic or resistant angina pectoris, and about half had concomitant treatment with beta-adrenergic blocking agents. The most common adverse events were:

Incidence Approximately 10%

Cardiovascular: peripheral edema
Central Nervous System: dizziness or lightheadedness
Gastrointestinal: nausea
Systemic: headache and flushing, weakness.

Incidence Approximately 5%

Cardiovascular: transient hypotension.

Incidence 2% or Less

Cardiovascular: palpitation
Respiratory: nasal and chest congestion, shortness of breath
Gastrointestinal: diarrhea, constipation, cramps, flatulence
Musculoskeletal: inflammation, joint stiffness, muscle cramps
Central Nervous System: shakiness, nervousness, jitteriness, sleep disturbances, blurred vision, difficulties in balance
Other: dermatitis, pruritus, urticaria, fever, sweating, chills, sexual difficulties.

Incidence Approximately 0.5%

Cardiovascular: syncope. Syncopal episodes did not recur with reduction in the dose of ADALAT® or concomitant antianginal medication.

Incidence Less Than 0.5%

Hematologic: thrombocytopenia, anemia, leukopenia, purpura
Gastrointestinal: allergic hepatitis
Oral: gingival hyperplasia
CNS: depression, paranoid syndrome
Musculosketal: myalgia
Special Senses: transient blindness at the peak of plasma level
Urogenital: nocturia, polyuria
Other: erythromelalgia, arthritis with ANA (+), gynecomastia, exfoliative dermatitis.

Several of these side effects appear to be dose related. Peripheral edema occurred in about one in 25 patients at doses less than 60 mg per day and in about one patient in eight at 120 mg per day or more. Transient hypotension, generally mild to moderate severity and seldom requiring discontinuation of therapy, occurred in one of 50 patients at less than 60 mg per day and in one of 20 patients at 120 mg per day or more. Very rarely, introduction of ADALAT® therapy was associated with an increase in anginal pain, possibly due to associated hypotension.

In addition, more serious adverse events were observed, not readily distinguishable from the natural history of the disease in these patients. It remains possible, however, that some or many of these events were drug related. Myocardial infarction occurred in about 4% of patients and congestive heart failure or pulmonary edema in about 2%. Ventricular arrhythmias or conduction disturbances each occurred in fewer than 0.5% of patients.

In a subgroup of over 1000 patients receiving ADALAT® with concomitant beta blocker therapy, the pattern and incidence of adverse experiences were not different from that of the entire group of ADALAT® (nifedipine) treated patients (See PRECAUTIONS).

In a subgroup of approximately 250 patients with a diagnosis of congestive heart failure as well as angina, dizziness or lightheadedness, peripheral edema, headache or flushing each occurred in one in eight patients. Hypotension occurred in about one in 20 patients. Syncope occurred in approximately one patient in 250. Myocardial infarction or symptoms of congestive heart failure each occurred in about one patient in 15. Atrial or ventricular dysrhythmias each occurred in about one patient in 150.

OVERDOSAGE

Experience with nifedipine overdosage is limited. Generally, overdosage with nifedipine leading to pronounced hypotension calls for active cardiovascular support including monitoring of cardiovascular and respiratory function, elevation of extremities, judicious use of calcium infusion, pressor agents and fluids. Clearance of nifedipine would be expected to be prolonged in patients with impaired liver function. Since nifedipine is highly protein bound, dialysis is not likely to be of any benefit; however, plasmapheresis may be beneficial.

DOSAGE AND ADMINISTRATION

The dosage of ADALAT® needed to suppress angina and that can be tolerated by the patient must be established by titration. Excessive doses can result in hypotension.

Therapy should be initiated with the 10 mg capsule. The starting dose is one 10 mg capsule, swallowed whole, 3 times/day. The usual effective dose range is 10–20 mg three times daily. Some patients, especially those with evidence of coronary artery spasm, respond only to higher doses, more frequent administration, or both. In such patients, doses of 20–30 mg three or four times daily may be effective. Doses above 120 mg daily are rarely necessary. More than 180 mg per day is not recommended.

In most cases, ADALAT® titration should proceed over a 7–14 day period so that the physician can assess the response to each dose level and monitor the blood pressure before proceeding to higher doses.

If symptoms so warrant, titration may proceed more rapidly provided that the patient is assessed frequently. Based on the patient's physical activity level, attack frequency, and sublingual nitroglycerin consumption, the dose of ADALAT® may be increased from 10 mg t.i.d. to 20 mg t.i.d. and then to 30 mg t.i.d. over a three-day period.

In hospitalized patients under close observation, the dose may be increased in 10 mg increments over four to six-hour periods as required to control pain and arrhythmias due to ischemia. A single dose should rarely exceed 30 mg.

No "rebound effect" has been observed upon discontinuation of ADALAT®. However, if discontinuation of ADALAT® is necessary, sound clinical practice suggests that the dosage should be decreased gradually with close physician supervision.

Co-Administration with Other Antianginal Drugs

Sublingual nitroglycerin may be taken as required for the control of acute manifestations of angina, particularly during ADALAT® titration. See **PRECAUTIONS, Drug Interactions,** for information on co-administration of ADALAT® with beta blockers or long acting nitrates.

HOW SUPPLIED

ADALAT® soft gelatin capsules are supplied in:

Bottles of 100:   10 mg (NDC 0026-8811-51) orange
    20 mg (NDC 0026-8821-51)
    orange and light brown

Bottles of 300:   10 mg (NDC 0026-8811-18) orange
    20 mg (NDC 0026-8821-18)
    orange and light brown

Unit dose
packages of 100:   10 mg (NDC 0026-8811-48) orange
    20 mg (NDC 0026-8821-48) orange and
    light brown

The capsules are identified as follows: 10 mg (Miles 811), 20 mg (Miles 821).

The capsules should be protected from light and moisture and stored at controlled room temperature 59° to 77°F (15° to 25°C). Dispense in tight, light resistant containers (USP).

Miles Inc.
Pharmacuetical Division
400 Morgan Lane
West Haven, CT 06516

Encapsulated by
R.P. Scherer N.A., Clearwater, FL 33518

Caution: Federal (USA) law prohibits dispensing without prescription.

PD100727   04/91   BAY a 1040 1477
© 1991 Miles Inc.
Shown in Product Identification Section, page 420

BILTRICIDE® Tablets   ℞
(praziquantel)

DESCRIPTION

BILTRICIDE® (praziquantel) is a trematodicide provided in tablet form for the oral treatment of schistosome infections and infections due to liver fluke.

BILTRICIDE® (praziquantel) is 2-(cyclohexylcarbonyl)-1,2,3,6,7, 11b-hexahydro-4H-pyrazino [2, 1-a] isoquinolin-4-one with the molecular formula; $C_{19}H_{24}N_2O_2$. The structural formula is as follows:

Praziquantel is a white to nearly white crystalline powder of bitter taste. The compound is stable under normal conditions and melts at 136–140°C with decomposition. The active substance is hygroscopic. Praziquantel is easily soluble in chloroform and dimethylsulfoxide, soluble in ethanol and very slightly soluble in water.

BILTRICIDE® tablets contain 600 mg of praziquantel. Inactive ingredients: corn starch, magnesium stearate, microcrystalline cellulose, povidone, sodium lauryl sulfate, polyethylene glycol, titanium dioxide and HPM cellulose.

CLINICAL PHARMACOLOGY

BILTRICIDE® induces a rapid contraction of schistosomes by a specific effect on the permeability of the cell membrane. The drug further causes vacuolization and disintegration of the schistosome tegument.

After oral administration BILTRICIDE® is rapidly absorbed (80%), subjected to a first pass effect, metabolized and eliminated by the kidneys. Maximal serum concentration is achieved 1–3 hours after dosing. The half-life of praziquantel in serum is 0.8–1.5 hours.

INDICATIONS AND USAGE

BILTRICIDE® is indicated for the treatment of infections due to: all species of schistosoma (eg. *Schistosoma mekongi, Schistosoma japonicum, Schistosoma mansoni* and *Schistosoma hematobium)*, and infections due to the liver flukes, *Clonorchis sinensis/Opisthorchis viverrini* (approval of this indication was based on studies in which the two species were not differentiated).

CONTRAINDICATIONS

BILTRICIDE® should not be given to patients who previously have shown hypersensitivity to the drug. Since parasite destruction within the eye may cause irreparable lesions, ocular cysticercosis should not be treated with this compound.

PRECAUTIONS

Information for the patient: Patients should be warned not to drive a car and not to operate machinery on the day of BILTRICIDE® treatment and the following day.

Minimal increases in liver enzymes have been reported in some patients.

When schistosomiasis or fluke infection is found to be associated with cerebral cysticercosis it is advised to hospitalize the patient for the duration of treatment.

Drug Interactions: No data are available regarding interaction of BILTRICIDE® with other drugs.

Mutagenesis, Carcinogenesis: Mutagenic effects in Salmonella tests found by one laboratory have not been confirmed in the same tested strain by other laboratories. Long term carcinogenicity studies in rats and golden hamsters did not reveal any carcinogenic effect.

Pregnancy Category B: Reproduction studies have been performed in rats and rabbits at doses up to 40 times the human dose and have revealed no evidence of impaired fertility or harm to the fetus due to BILTRICIDE® . There are, however, no adequate and well-controlled studies in pregnant women. An increase of the abortion rate was found in rats at three times the single human therapeutic dose. While animal reproduction studies are not always predictive of human response, this drug should be used during pregnancy only if clearly needed.

Nursing mothers: BILTRICIDE® appeared in the milk of nursing women at a concentration of about ¼ that of maternal serum. Women should not nurse on the day of BILTRICIDE® treatment and during the subsequent 72 hours.

Pediatric use: Safety in children under 4 years of age has not been established.

ADVERSE EFFECTS

In general BILTRICIDE® is very well tolerated. Side effects are usually mild and transient and do not require treatment. The following side effects were observed generally in order of severity: malaise, headache, dizziness, abdominal discomfort with or without nausea, rise in temperature and, rarely, urticaria. Such symptoms can, however, also result from the infection itself. Such side effects may be more frequent and/or serious in patients with a heavy worm burden. In patients with liver impairment caused by the infection, no adverse effects of BILTRICIDE® have occurred which would necessitate restriction in use.

OVERDOSAGE

In rats and mice the acute LD_{50} was about 2,500 mg/kg. No data are available in humans. In the event of overdose a fast-acting laxative should be given.

DOSAGE AND ADMINISTRATION

The dosage recommended for the treatment of schistosomiasis is: 3×20 mg/kg bodyweight as a one day treatment. The recommended dose for clonorchiasis and opisthorchiasis is: 3×25 mg/kg as a one day treatment. The tablets should be washed down unchewed with some liquid during meals. Keeping the tablets or segments thereof in the mouth can reveal a bitter taste which can promote gagging or vomiting. The interval between the individual doses should not be less than 4 and not more than 6 hours.

HOW SUPPLIED

BILTRICIDE® is supplied as a 600 mg white to orange tinged, filmcoated, oblong tablets with three scores. When broken each of the four segments contain 150 mg of active ingredient so that the dosage can be easily adjusted to the patient's bodyweight.

Segments are broken off by pressing the score (notch) with thumbnails. If ¼ of a tablet is required, this is best achieved by breaking the segment from the outer end.

BILTRICIDE® is available in bottles of 6 tablets.

Strength	NDC	Tablet ID
Bottles of 6: 600 mg	0026-2521-06	521

Store below 86°F (30°C).
Miles Inc.
Pharmaceutical Division
400 Morgan Lane
West Haven, CT 06516 USA
Made in Germany

Caution: Federal (USA) law prohibits dispensing without prescription.

PD100722   7/91   EMBAY 8440   1568
© 1991 Miles Inc
Shown in Product Identification Section, page 420

CIPRO®   ℞
(ciprofloxacin hydrochloride)
TABLETS

DESCRIPTION

Cipro® (ciprofloxacin hydrochloride) is a synthetic broad spectrum antibacterial agent for oral administration. Ciprofloxacin, a fluoroquinolone, is available as the monohydrochloride monohydrate salt of 1-cyclopropyl-6-fluoro-1, 4-dihydro-4-oxo-7-(1-piperazinyl)-3-quinolinecarboxylic acid. It is a faintly yellowish to light yellow crystalline substance with a molecular weight of 385.8. Its empirical formula is $C_{17}H_{18}FN_3O_3 \cdot HCl \cdot H_2O$ and its chemical structure is as follows:

Cipro® is available in 250-mg, 500-mg and 750-mg (ciprofloxacin equivalent) film-coated tablets. The inactive ingredients are starch, microcrystalline cellulose, silicon dioxide, crospovidone, magnesium stearate, hydroxypropyl methylcellulose, titanium dioxide, polyethylene glycol and water. Ciprofloxacin differs from other quinolones in that it has a fluorine atom at the 6-position, a piperazine moiety at the 7-position, and a cyclopropyl ring at the 1-position. Examples of other antibacterial drugs in the quinolone class are nalidixic acid, cinoxacin, and norfloxacin.

CLINICAL PHARMACOLOGY

Cipro® tablets are rapidly and well absorbed from the gastrointestinal tract after oral administration. The absolute bioavailability is approximately 70% with no substantial loss by first pass metabolism. Serum concentrations increase proportionally with the dose as shown:

Dose (mg)	Maximum Serum Concentration (mcg/mL)	Area Under Curve (AUC) (mcg·hr/mL)
250	1.2	4.8
500	2.4	11.6
750	4.3	20.2
1000	5.4	30.8

Maximum serum concentrations are attained 1 to 2 hours after oral dosing. Mean concentrations 12 hours after dosing with 250, 500, or 750 mg are 0.1, 0.2, and 0.4 mcg/mL, respectively. The serum elimination half-life in subjects with normal renal function is approximately 4 hours.

Approximately 40 to 50% of an orally administered dose is excreted in the urine as unchanged drug. After a 250-mg oral dose, urine concentrations of ciprofloxacin usually exceed 200 mcg/mL during the first two hours and are approximately 30 mcg/mL at 8 to 12 hours after dosing. The urinary excretion of ciprofloxacin is virtually complete within 24 hours after dosing. The renal clearance of ciprofloxacin, which is approximately 300 mL/minute, exceeds the normal glomerular filtration rate of 120 mL/minute. Thus, active tubular secretion would seem to play a significant role in its elimination. Co-administration of probenecid with ciprofloxacin results in about a 50% reduction in the ciprofloxacin renal clearance and a 50% increase in its concentration in the systemic circulation. Although bile concentrations of ciprofloxacin are several fold higher than serum concentrations after oral dosing, only a small amount of the dose administered is recovered from the bile as unchanged drug. An additional 1–2% of the dose is recovered from the bile in the form of metabolites. Approximately 20 to 35% of an oral dose is recovered from the feces within 5 days after dosing. This may arise from either biliary clearance or transintestinal elimination. Four metabolites have been identified in human urine which together account for approximately 15% of an oral dose. The metabolites have antimicrobial activity, but are less active than unchanged ciprofloxacin.

When Cipro® is given concomitantly with food, there is a delay in the absorption of the drug, resulting in peak concentrations that are closer to 2 hours after dosing rather than 1 hour. The overall absorption, however, is not substantially affected. Concurrent administration of antacids containing magnesium hydroxide or aluminum hydroxide may reduce the bioavailability of ciprofloxacin by as much as 90% (See Precautions).

Concomitant administration of ciprofloxacin with theophylline decreases the clearance of theophylline resulting in elevated serum theophylline levels, and increased risk of a patient developing CNS or other adverse reactions (See Precautions).

In patients with reduced renal function, the half-life of ciprofloxacin is slightly prolonged. Dosage adjustments may be required (See Dosage and Administration).

In preliminary studies in patients with stable chronic liver cirrhosis, no significant changes in ciprofloxacin pharmaco-

Continued on next page

Miles—Cont.

kinetics have been observed. The kinetics of ciprofloxacin in patients with acute hepatic insufficiency, however, have not been fully elucidated.

The binding of ciprofloxacin to serum proteins is 20 to 40% which is not likely to be high enough to cause significant protein binding interactions with other drugs.

After oral administration ciprofloxacin is widely distributed throughout the body. Tissue concentrations often exceed serum concentrations in both men and women, particularly in genital tissue including the prostate. Ciprofloxacin is present in active form in the saliva, nasal and bronchial secretions, sputum, skin blister fluid, lymph, peritoneal fluid, bile and prostatic secretions. Ciprofloxacin has also been detected in lung, skin, fat, muscle, cartilage, and bone. The drug diffuses into the cerebrospinal fluid (CSF); however, CSF concentrations are generally less than 10% of peak serum concentrations. Low levels of the drug have been detected in the aqueous and vitreous humors of the eye.

Microbiology: Ciprofloxacin has *in vitro* activity against a wide range of gram-negative and gram-positive organisms. The bactericidal action of ciprofloxacin results from interference with the enzyme DNA gyrase which is needed for the synthesis of bacterial DNA.

While *in vitro* studies have demonstrated the susceptibility of most strains of the following microorganisms, clinical efficacy for infections other than those included in the Indications and Usage Section has not been documented:

Gram-Negative: *Escherichia coli; Klebsiella pneumoniae; Klebsiella oxytoca; Enterobacter aerogenes; Enterobacter cloacae; Citrobacter diversus; Citrobacter freundii; Edwardsiella tarda; Salmonella enteritidis; Salmonella typhi; Shigella sonnei; Shigella flexneri; Proteus mirabilis; Proteus vulgaris; Providencia stuartii; Providencia rettgeri; Morganella morganii; Serratia marcescens; Yersinia enterocolitica; Pseudomonas aeruginosa; Acinetobacter calcoaceticus subsp. Iwoffi; Acinetobacter calcoaceticus subsp. anitratus; Haemophilus influenzae; Haemophilus parainfluenzae; Haemophilus ducreyi; Neisseria gonorrhoeae; Neisseria meningitidis; Moraxella (Branhamella) catarrhalis; Campylobacter jejuni; Campylobacter coli; Aeromonas hydrophila; Aeromonas caviae; Vibrio cholerae; Vibrio parahaemolyticus; Vibrio vulnificus; Brucella melitensis; Pasteurella multocida; Legionella pneumophila.*

Gram-Positive: *Staphylococcus aureus* (including methicillin-susceptible and methicillin-resistant strains); *Staphylococcus epidermidis; Staphylococcus haemolyticus; Staphylococcus hominis; Staphylococcus saprophyticus; Streptococcus pyogenes; Streptococcus pneumoniae.*

Most strains of streptococci including *Streptococcus faecalis* are only moderately susceptible to ciprofloxacin as are *Mycobacterium tuberculosis* and *Chlamydia trachomatis.*

Most strains of *Pseudomonas cepacia* and some strains of *Pseudomonas maltophilia* are resistant to ciprofloxacin as are most anaerobic bacteria, including *Bacteroides fragilis* and *Clostridium difficile.*

Ciprofloxacin is slightly less active when tested at acidic pH. The inoculum size has little effect when tested *in vitro.* The minimum bactericidal concentration (MBC) generally does not exceed the minimum inhibitory concentration (MIC) by more than a factor of 2. Resistance to ciprofloxacin *in vitro* develops slowly (multiple-step mutation). Rapid one-step development of resistance has not been observed.

Ciprofloxacin does not cross-react with other antimicrobial agents such as beta-lactams or aminoglycosides; therefore, organisms resistant to these drugs may be susceptible to ciprofloxacin.

In vitro studies have shown that additive activity often results when ciprofloxacin is combined with other antimicrobial agents such as beta-lactams, aminoglycosides, clindamycin, or metronidazole; antagonism is observed only rarely.

Susceptibility Tests

Diffusion Techniques: Quantitative methods that require measurement of zone diameters give the most precise estimates of antibiotic susceptibility. One such procedure recommended for use with the 5-mcg ciprofloxacin disk is the National Committee for Clinical Laboratory Standards (NCCLS) approved procedure. Only a 5-mcg ciprofloxacin disk should be used, and it should not be used for testing susceptibility to less active quinolones; there are no suitable surrogate disks.

Results of laboratory tests using 5-mcg ciprofloxacin disks should be interpreted using the following criteria:

Zone Diameter (mm)	Interpretation
≥ 21	(S) Susceptible
16–20	(I) Intermediate (Moderately Susceptible)
≤ 15	(R) Resistant

Dilution Techniques: Broth and agar dilution methods, such as those recommended by the NCCLS, may be used to determine the minimum inhibitory concentration (MIC) of ciprofloxacin. MIC test results should be interpreted according to the following criteria:

MIC (mcg/mL)	Interpretation
≤ 1	(S) Susceptible
> 1–≤ 2	(I) Intermediate (Moderately Susceptible)
> 2	(R) Resistant

For any susceptibility test, a report of "susceptible" indicates that the pathogen is likely to respond to ciprofloxacin therapy. A report of "resistant" indicates that the pathogen is not likely to respond. A report of "intermediate" (moderately susceptible) indicates that the pathogen is expected to be susceptible to ciprofloxacin if high doses are used, or if the infection is confined to tissues and fluids in which high ciprofloxacin levels are obtained.

The Quality Control strains should have the following assigned daily ranges for ciprofloxacin.

QC Strains	Disk Zone Diameter (mm)	MIC (mcg/mL)
S. aureus (ATCC 25923)	22–30	—
S. aureus (ATCC 29213)	—	0.25–1.0
E. coli (ATCC 25922)	30–40	0.008–0.03
P. aeruginosa (ATCC 27853)	25–33	0.25–1.0

INDICATIONS AND USAGE

Cipro® is indicated for the treatment of infections caused by susceptible strains of the designated microorganisms in the conditions listed below:

Lower Respiratory Infections caused by *Escherichia coli, Klebsiella pneumoniae, Enterobacter cloacae, Proteus mirabilis, Pseudomonas aeruginosa, Haemophilus influenzae, Haemophilus parainfluenzae,* and *Streptococcus pneumoniae.*

Skin and Skin Structure Infections caused by *Escherichia coli, Klebsiella pneumoniae, Enterobacter cloacae, Proteus mirabilis, Proteus vulgaris, Providencia stuartii, Morganella morganii, Citrobacter freundii, Pseudomonas aeruginosa, Staphylococcus aureus, Staphylococcus epidermidis,* and *Streptococcus pyogenes.*

Bone and Joint Infections caused by *Enterobacter cloacae, Serratia marcescens,* and *Pseudomonas aeruginosa.*

Urinary Tract Infections caused by *Escherichia coli, Klebsiella pneumoniae, Enterobacter cloacae, Serratia marcescens, Proteus mirabilis, Providencia rettgeri, Morganella morganii, Citrobacter diversus, Citrobacter freundii, Pseudomonas aeruginosa, Staphylococcus epidermidis,* and *Streptococcus faecalis.*

Infectious Diarrhea caused by *Escherichia coli* (enterotoxigenic strains), *Campylobacter jejuni, Shigella flexneri** and *Shigella sonnei** when antibacterial therapy is indicated.

Appropriate culture and susceptibility tests should be performed before treatment in order to isolate and identify organisms causing infection and to determine their susceptibility to ciprofloxacin. Therapy with Cipro® may be initiated before results of these tests are known; once results become available appropriate therapy should be continued. As with other drugs, some strains of *Pseudomonas aeruginosa* may develop resistance fairly rapidly during treatment with ciprofloxacin. Culture and susceptibility testing performed periodically during therapy will provide information not only on the therapeutic effect of the antimicrobial agent but also on the possible emergence of bacterial resistance.

CONTRAINDICATIONS

A history of hypersensitivity to ciprofloxacin is a contraindication to its use. A history of hypersensitivity to other quinolones may also contraindicate the use of ciprofloxacin.

WARNINGS

THE SAFETY AND EFFECTIVENESS OF CIPROFLOXACIN IN CHILDREN, ADOLESCENTS (LESS THAN 18 YEARS OF AGE), PREGNANT WOMEN, AND LACTATING WOMEN HAVE NOT BEEN ESTABLISHED. (SEE PRECAUTIONS-PEDIATRIC USE, PREGNANCY AND NURSING MOTHERS SUBSECTIONS.) Ciprofloxacin causes lameness in immature dogs. Histopathological examination of the weight-bearing joints of these dogs revealed permanent lesions of the cartilage. Related quinolone-class drugs also produce erosions of cartilage of weight-bearing joints and other signs of arthropathy in immature animals of various species. (See ANIMAL PHARMACOLOGY.)

Convulsions have been reported in patients receiving ciprofloxacin. Convulsions, increased intracranial pressure, and toxic psychosis have been reported in patients receiving ciprofloxacin and other drugs of this class. Quinolones may also cause central nervous system (CNS) stimulation which may lead to tremors, restlessness, lightheadedness, confusion and hallucinations. If these reactions occur in patients receiving ciprofloxacin, the drug should be discontinued and appropriate measures instituted. As with all quinolones, ciprofloxacin should be used with caution in patients with known or suspected CNS disorders, such as severe cerebral arteriosclerosis, epilepsy, and other factors that predispose to seizures. (See ADVERSE REACTIONS.)

*Efficacy for this organism in this organ system was studied in fewer than 10 infections.

SERIOUS AND FATAL REACTIONS HAVE BEEN REPORTED IN PATIENTS RECEIVING CONCURRENT ADMINISTRATION OF CIPROFLOXACIN AND THEOPHYLLINE. These reactions have included cardiac arrest, seizure, status epilepticus and respiratory failure. Although similar serious adverse events have been reported in patients receiving theophylline alone, the possibility that these reactions may be potentiated by ciprofloxacin cannot be eliminated. If concomitant use cannot be avoided, serum levels of theophylline should be monitored and dosage adjustments made as appropriate.

Serious and occasionally fatal hypersensitivity (anaphylactic) reactions, some following the first dose, have been reported in patients receiving quinolone therapy. Some reactions were accompanied by cardiovascular collapse, loss of consciousness, tingling, pharyngeal or facial edema, dyspnea, urticaria, and itching. Only a few patients had a history of hypersensitivity reactions. Serious anaphylactic reactions require immediate emergency treatment with epinephrine and other resuscitation measures, including oxygen, intravenous antihistamines, corticosteroids, pressor amines and airway management, as clinically indicated.

Severe hypersensitivity reactions characterized by rash, fever, eosinophilia, jaundice, and hepatic necrosis with fatal outcome have also been reported extremely rarely in patients receiving ciprofloxacin along with other drugs. The possibility that these reactions were related to ciprofloxacin cannot be excluded. Ciprofloxacin should be discontinued at the first appearance of a skin rash or any other sign of hypersensitivity.

Pseudomembranous colitis has been reported with nearly all antibacterial agents, including ciprofloxacin, and may range in severity from mild to life-threatening. Therefore, it is important to consider this diagnosis in patients who present with diarrhea subsequent to the administration of antibacterial agents.

Treatment with antibacterial agents alters the normal flora of the colon and may permit overgrowth of clostridia. Studies indicate that a toxin produced by *Clostridium difficile* is one primary cause of "antibiotic-associated colitis".

After the diagnosis of pseudomembranous colitis has been established, therapeutic measures should be initiated. Mild cases of pseudomembranous colitis usually respond to drug discontinuation alone. In moderate to severe cases, consideration should be given to management with fluids and electrolytes, protein supplementation and treatment with an antibacterial drug effective against *C. difficile.*

PRECAUTIONS

General: Crystals of ciprofloxacin have been observed rarely in the urine of human subjects but more frequently in the urine of laboratory animals, which is usually alkaline. (See ANIMAL PHARMACOLOGY.) Crystalluria related to ciprofloxacin has been reported only rarely in humans because human urine is usually acidic. Alkalinity of the urine should be avoided in patients receiving ciprofloxacin. Patients should be well hydrated to prevent the formation of highly concentrated urine.

Alteration of the dosage regimen is necessary for patients with impairment of renal function. (See DOSAGE AND ADMINISTRATION.)

Moderate to severe phototoxicity manifested by an exaggerated sunburn reaction has been observed in some patients who were exposed to direct sunlight while receiving some members of the quinolone class of drugs. Excessive sunlight should be avoided.

As with any potent drug, periodic assessment of organ system functions, including renal, hepatic, and hematopoietic, is advisable during prolonged therapy.

Information for Patients: Patients should be advised that ciprofloxacin may be taken with or without meals. The preferred time of dosing is two hours after a meal. Patients should also be advised to drink fluids liberally and not take antacids containing magnesium, aluminum, or calcium, products containing iron, or multivitamins containing zinc. However, usual dietary intake of calcium has not been shown to alter the absorption of ciprofloxacin.

Patients should be advised that ciprofloxacin may be associated with hypersensitivity reactions, even following a single dose, and to discontinue the drug at the first sign of a skin rash or other allergic reaction.

Ciprofloxacin may cause dizziness and lightheadedness; therefore patients should know how they react to this drug before they operate an automobile or machinery or engage in activities requiring mental alertness or coordination.

Patients should be advised that ciprofloxacin may increase the effects of theophylline and caffeine. There is a possibility of caffeine accumulation when products containing caffeine are consumed while taking quinolones.

Drug Interactions: As with other quinolones, concurrent administration of ciprofloxacin with theophylline may lead to elevated serum concentrations of theophylline and prolongation of its elimination half-life. This may result in increased risk of theophylline-related adverse reactions. (See WARNINGS.) If concomitant use cannot be avoided, serum

levels of theophylline should be monitored and dosage adjustments made as appropriate.
Some quinolones, including ciprofloxacin, have also been shown to interfere with the metabolism of caffeine. This may lead to reduced clearance of caffeine and a prolongation of its serum half-life.
Concurrent administration of ciprofloxacin with antacids containing magnesium, aluminum, or calcium; with sucralfate or divalent and trivalent cations such as iron may substantially interfere with the absorption of ciprofloxacin, resulting in serum and urine levels considerably lower than desired. To a lesser extent this effect is demonstrated with zinc-containing multivitamins. (See DOSAGE AND ADMINISTRATION for concurrent administration of these agents with ciprofloxacin.)
Some quinolones, including ciprofloxacin, have been associated with transient elevations in serum creatinine in patients receiving cyclosporine concomitantly.
Quinolones have been reported to enhance the effects of the oral anticoagulant warfarin or its derivatives. When these products are administered concomitantly, prothrombin time or other suitable coagulation tests should be closely monitored.
Probenecid interferes with renal tubular secretion of ciprofloxacin and produces an increase in the level of ciprofloxacin in the serum. This should be considered if patients are receiving both drugs concomitantly.
As with other broad spectrum antimicrobial agents, prolonged use of ciprofloxacin may result in overgrowth of nonsusceptible organisms. Repeated evaluation of the patient's condition and microbial susceptibility testing is essential. If superinfection occurs during therapy, appropriate measures should be taken.

Carcinogenesis, Mutagenesis, Impairment of Fertility: Eight *in vitro* mutagenicity tests have been conducted with ciprofloxacin and the test results are listed below:

- Salmonella/Microsome Test (Negative)
- *E. coli* DNA Repair Assay (Negative)
- Mouse Lymphoma Cell Forward Mutation Assay (Positive)
- Chinese Hamster V_{79} Cell HGPRT Test (Negative)
- Syrian Hamster Embryo Cell Transformation Assay (Negative)
- *Saccharomyces cerevisiae* Point Mutation Assay (Negative)
- *Saccharomyces cerevisiae* Mitotic Crossover and Gene Conversion Assay (Negative)
- Rat Hepatocyte DNA Repair Assay (Positive)

Thus 2 of the 8 tests were positive but results of the following 3 *in vivo* test systems gave negative results:

- Rat Hepatocyte DNA Repair Assay
- Micronucleus Test (Mice)
- Dominant Lethal Test (Mice)

Long term carcinogenicity studies in mice and rats have been completed. After daily oral dosing for up to 2 years, there is no evidence that ciprofloxacin had any carcinogenic or tumorigenic effects in these species.

Pregnancy: Teratogenic Effects. Pregnancy Category C: Reproduction studies have been performed in rats and mice at doses up to 6 times the usual daily human dose and have revealed no evidence of impaired fertility or harm to the fetus due to ciprofloxacin. In rabbits, ciprofloxacin (30 and 100 mg/kg orally) produced gastrointestinal disturbances resulting in maternal weight loss and an increased incidence of abortion. No teratogenicity was observed at either dose. After intravenous administration of doses up to 20 mg/kg, no maternal toxicity was produced, and no embryotoxicity or teratogenicity was observed. There are, however, no adequate and well-controlled studies in pregnant women. Ciprofloxacin should be used during pregnancy only if the potential benefit justifies the potential risk to the fetus. (See WARNINGS.)

Nursing Mothers: Ciprofloxacin is excreted in human milk. Because of the potential for serious adverse reactions in infants nursing from mothers taking ciprofloxacin, a decision should be made either to discontinue nursing or to discontinue the drug, taking into account the importance of the drug to the mother.

Pediatric Use: Safety and effectiveness in children and adolescents less than 18 years of age have not been established. Ciprofloxacin causes arthropathy in juvenile animals. (See WARNINGS.)

ADVERSE REACTIONS

During clinical investigation, 2,799 patients received 2,868 courses of the drug. Adverse events that were considered likely to be drug related occurred in 7.3% of courses, possibly related in 9.2%, (total of 16.5% thought to be possibly or probably related to drug therapy), and remotely related in 3.0%. Ciprofloxacin was discontinued because of an adverse event in 3.5% of courses, primarily involving the gastrointestinal system (1.5%), skin (0.6%), and central nervous system (0.4%). Those events typical of quinolones are italicized.
The most frequently reported events, drug related or not, were *nausea* (5.2%), *diarrhea* (2.3%), *vomiting* (2.0%), *abdominal pain/discomfort* (1.7%), *headache* (1.2%), *restlessness* (1.1%), and *rash* (1.1%).

DOSAGE GUIDELINES

Location of Infection	Type or Severity	Unit Dose	Frequency	Daily Dose
Urinary Tract	Mild/Moderate	250 mg	q 12 h	500 mg
	Severe/Complicated	500 mg	q 12 h	1000 mg
Lower Respiratory Tract; Bone and Joint; Skin & Skin Structure	Mild/Moderate	500 mg	q 12 h	1000 mg
	Severe/Complicated	750 mg	q 12 h	1500 mg
Infectious Diarrhea	Mild/Moderate/Severe	500 mg	q 12 h	1000 mg

Additional events that occurred in less than 1% of ciprofloxacin courses are listed below.
GASTROINTESTINAL: *(See above),* painful oral mucosa, oral candidiasis, dysphagia, intestinal perforation, gastrointestinal bleeding.
CENTRAL NERVOUS SYSTEM: *(See above), dizziness, lightheadedness, insomnia, nightmares, hallucinations, manic reaction, irritability, tremor, ataxia, convulsive seizures, lethargy, drowsiness, weakness, malaise, anorexia, phobia, depersonalization, depression, paresthesia, toxic psychosis.*
SKIN/HYPERSENSITIVITY: *(See above), pruritus, urticaria, photosensitivity, flushing, fever, chills, angioedema, edema of the face, neck, lips, conjunctivae or hands;* cutaneous candidiasis, hyperpigmentation, erythema nodosum. Allergic reactions ranging from urticaria to anaphylactic reactions have been reported (See WARNINGS).
SPECIAL SENSES: *blurred vision, disturbed vision (change in color perception, overbrightness of lights), decreased visual acuity, diplopia, eye pain, tinnitus, hearing loss, bad taste.*
MUSCULOSKELETAL: *joint or back pain, joint stiffness,* achiness, neck or chest pain, flare up of gout.
RENAL/UROGENITAL: *interstitial nephritis, nephritis, renal failure,* polyuria, urinary retention, urethral bleeding, vaginitis, acidosis.
CARDIOVASCULAR: palpitation, atrial flutter, ventricular ectopy, syncope, hypertension, angina pectoris, myocardial infarction, cardiopulmonary arrest, cerebral thrombosis.
RESPIRATORY: epistaxis, laryngeal or pulmonary edema, hiccough, hemoptysis, dyspnea, bronchospasm, pulmonary embolism.
Most of the adverse events reported were described as only mild or moderate in severity, abated soon after the drug was discontinued, and required no treatment.
In several instances nausea, vomiting, tremor, irritability or palpitation were judged by investigators to be related to elevated plasma levels of theophylline possibly as a result of drug interaction with ciprofloxacin.
Other adverse events reported in the postmarketing phase include anaphylactic reactions, erythema multiforme/Stevens-Johnson syndrome, exfoliative dermatitis, toxic epidermal necrolysis, vasculitis, jaundice, hepatic necrosis, postural hypotension, possible exacerbation of myasthenia gravis, anosmia, confusion, dysphasia, nystagmus, pseudomembranous colitis, pancreatitis, dyspepsia, flatulence, and constipation. Also reported were hemolytic anemia; agranulocytosis; elevation of serum triglycerides, serum cholesterol, blood glucose, serum potassium; prolongation of prothrombin time; albuminuria; candiduria, vaginal candidiasis; renal calculi, and change in serum phenytoin (See PRECAUTIONS).

Adverse Laboratory Changes: Changes in laboratory parameters listed as adverse events without regard to drug relationship:
Hepatic—Elevations of: ALT (SGPT) (1.9%), AST (SGOT) (1.7%), Alkaline Phosphatase (0.8%), LDH (0.4%), serum bilirubin (0.3%).
Cholestatic jaundice has been reported
Hematologic—Eosinophilia (0.6%), leukopenia (0.4%), decreased blood platelets (0.1%), elevated blood platelets (0.1%), pancytopenia (0.1%).
Renal—Elevations of: Serum creatinine (1.1%), BUN (0.9%).
CRYSTALLURIA, CYLINDRURIA AND HEMATURIA HAVE BEEN REPORTED.
Other changes occurring in less than 0.1% of courses were: Elevation of serum gammaglutamyl transferase, elevation of serum amylase, reduction in blood glucose, elevated uric acid, decrease in hemoglobin, anemia, bleeding diathesis, increase in blood monocytes, leukocytosis.

OVERDOSAGE

In the event of acute overdosage the stomach should be emptied by inducing vomiting or by gastric lavage. The patient should be carefully observed and given supportive treatment. Adequate hydration must be maintained. Only a small amount of ciprofloxacin (< 10%) is removed from the body after hemodialysis or peritoneal dialysis.

DOSAGE AND ADMINISTRATION

The usual adult dosage for patients with urinary tract infections is 250 mg every 12 hours. For patients with complicated infections caused by organisms not highly susceptible, 500 mg may be administered every 12 hours.
Lower respiratory tract infections, skin and skin structure infections, and bone and joint infections may be treated with 500 mg every 12 hours. For more severe or complicated infections, a dosage of 750 mg may be given every 12 hours.
The recommended dosage for Infectious Diarrhea is 500 mg every 12 hours.
[See table above.]
The determination of dosage for any particular patient must take into consideration the severity and nature of the infection, the susceptibility of the causative organism, the integrity of the patient's host-defense mechanisms, and the status of renal function.
The duration of treatment depends upon the severity of infection. Generally ciprofloxacin should be continued for at least 2 days after the signs and symptoms of infection have disappeared. The usual duration is 7 to 14 days; however, for severe and complicated infections more prolonged therapy may be required. Bone and joint infections may require treatment for 4 to 6 weeks or longer. Infectious Diarrhea may be treated for 5–7 days.

Impaired Renal Function: Ciprofloxacin is eliminated primarily by renal excretion; however, the drug is also metabolized and partially cleared through the biliary system of the liver and through the intestine. These alternate pathways of drug elimination appear to compensate for the reduced renal excretion in patients with renal impairment. Nonetheless, some modification of dosage is recommended, particularly for patients with severe renal dysfunction. The following table provides dosage guidelines for use in patients with renal impairment; however, monitoring of serum drug levels provides the most reliable basis for dosage adjustment:

RECOMMENDED STARTING AND MAINTENANCE DOSES FOR PATIENTS WITH IMPAIRED RENAL FUNCTION

Creatinine Clearance (mL/min)	Dose
> 50	See Usual Dosage
30–50	250–500 mg q 12 h
5–29	250–500 mg q 18 h
Patients on hemodialysis or Peritoneal dialysis	250–500 mg q 24 h (after dialysis)

When only the serum creatinine concentration is known, the following formula may be used to estimate creatinine clearance.
Men: Creatinine clearance

$$(\text{mL/min}) = \frac{\text{Weight (kg)} \times (140 - \text{age})}{72 \times \text{serum creatinine (mg/dL)}}$$

Women: 0.85 × the value calculated for men.
The serum creatinine should represent a steady state of renal function.
In patients with severe infections and severe renal impairment, a unit dose of 750 mg may be administered at the intervals noted above; however, patients should be carefully monitored and the serum ciprofloxacin concentration should be measured periodically. Peak concentrations (1–2 hours after dosing) should generally range from 2 to 4 mcg/mL.
For patients with changing renal function or for patients with renal impairment and hepatic insufficiency, measurement of serum concentrations of ciprofloxacin will provide additional guidance for adjusting dosage.

HOW SUPPLIED

Cipro® (ciprofloxacin hydrochloride) is available as round, slightly yellowish film-coated tablets containing 250 mg ciprofloxacin. The 250-mg tablet is coded with the word "Miles" on one side and "512" on the reverse side. Cipro® is also available as capsule shaped, slightly yellowish film-coated tablets containing 500 mg or 750 mg ciprofloxacin. The 500-mg tablet is coded with the word "Miles" on one side and "513" on the reverse side; the 750-mg tablet is coded with the word "Miles" on one side and "514" on the reverse side.

Continued on next page

Miles—Cont.

	Strength	NDC Code	Tablet Identification
Bottles of 50:	750 mg	NDC 0026-8514-50	Miles 514
Bottles of 100:	250 mg	NDC 0026-8512-51	Miles 512
	500 mg	NDC 0026-8513-51	Miles 513
Unit Dose	250 mg	NDC 0026-8512-48	Miles 512
Package of 100:	500 mg	NDC 0026-8513-48	Miles 513
	750 mg	NDC 0026-8514-48	Miles 514

Available in bottles of 50's, 100's and in Unit Dose packages of 100. [See table above.]

Store below 86°F (30°C).

ANIMAL PHARMACOLOGY

Ciprofloxacin and related drugs have been shown to cause arthropathy in immature animals of most species tested (See WARNINGS). Damage of weight bearing joints was observed in juvenile dogs and rats. In young beagles 100 mg/kg ciprofloxacin given daily for 4 weeks, caused degenerative articular changes of the knee joint. At 30 mg/kg the effect on the joint was minimal. In a subsequent study in beagles removal of weight bearing from the joint reduced the lesions but did not totally prevent them.

Crystalluria, sometimes associated with secondary nephropathy, occurs in laboratory animals dosed with ciprofloxacin. This is primarily related to the reduced solubility of ciprofloxacin under alkaline conditions, which predominate in the urine of test animals; in man, crystalluria is rare since human urine is typically acidic. In rhesus monkeys, crystalluria without nephropathy has been noted after single oral doses as low as 5 mg/kg. After 6 months of intravenous dosing at 10 mg/kg/day, no nephropathological changes were noted; however, nephropathy was observed after dosing at 20 mg/kg/day for the same duration.

In dogs, ciprofloxacin at 3 and 10 mg/kg by rapid IV injection (15 sec.) produces pronounced hypotensive effects. These effects are considered to be related to histamine release since they are partially antagonized by pyrilamine, an antihistamine. In rhesus monkeys, rapid IV injection also produces hypotension but the effect in this species is inconsistent and less pronounced.

In mice, concomitant administration of nonsteroidal anti-inflammatory drugs such as fenbufen, phenylbutazone and indomethacin, with quinolones has been reported to enhance the CNS stimulatory effect of quinolones.

Ocular toxicity seen with some related drugs has not been observed in ciprofloxacin-treated animals.

Miles Inc.
Pharmaceutical Division
400 Morgan Lane
West Haven, CT 06516 USA

Caution: Federal (USA) Law prohibits dispensing without a prescription.

PZ100735   8/91   Bay o 9867   5202-2-A-U.S.-3
©1991 Miles Inc.   1577
Shown in Product Identification Section, page 420

CIPRO® I.V.   ℞
(ciprofloxacin)
For Intravenous Infusion

DESCRIPTION

Cipro® I.V. (ciprofloxacin) is a synthetic broad-spectrum antimicrobial agent for intravenous (iv) administration. Ciprofloxacin, a fluoroquinolone, is 1-cyclopropyl-6-fluoro-1, 4-dihydro-4-oxo-7-(1-piperazinyl)-3-quinolinecarboxylic acid. Its empirical formula is $C_{17}H_{18}FN_3O_3$ and its chemical structure is:

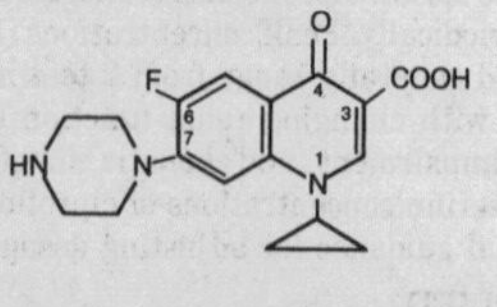

Ciprofloxacin is a faint to light yellow crystalline powder with a molecular weight of 331.4. It is soluble in dilute (0.1N) hydrochloric acid and is practically insoluble in water and ethanol. Ciprofloxacin differs from other quinolones in that it has a fluorine atom at the 6-position, a piperazine moiety at the 7-position, and a cyclopropyl ring at the 1-position. Cipro® I.V. solutions are available as 1.0% aqueous concentrates, which are intended for dilution prior to administration, and as a 0.2% ready-for-use infusion solution in 5% Dextrose Injection. All formulas contain lactic acid as a solubilizing agent and hydrochloric acid for pH adjustment. The pH range for the 1.0% aqueous concentrates in vials is 3.3 to 3.9. The pH range for the 0.2% ready-for-use infusion solutions is 3.5 to 4.6.

The plastic container is fabricated from a specially formulated polyvinyl chloride. Solutions in contact with the plastic container can leach out certain of its chemical components in very small amounts within the expiration period, e.g., di(2-ethylhexyl) phthalate (DEHP), up to 5 parts per million. The suitability of the plastic has been confirmed in tests in animals according to USP biological tests for plastic containers as well as by tissue culture toxicity studies.

CLINICAL PHARMACOLOGY

Following 60-minute intravenous infusions of 200 mg and 400 mg ciprofloxacin to normal volunteers, the mean maximum serum concentrations achieved were 2.1 and 4.6 $\mu g/mL$, respectively; the concentrations at 12 hours were 0.1 and 0.2 $\mu g/mL$, respectively.

Steady-state Ciprofloxacin Serum Concentrations ($\mu g/mL$) After 60-minute IV Infusions q 12 h.

	Time after starting the infusion					
Dose	30 min.	1 hr	3 hr	6 hr	8 hr	12 hr
200 mg	1.7	2.1	0.6	0.3	0.2	0.1
400 mg	3.7	4.6	1.3	0.7	0.5	0.2

The pharmacokinetics of ciprofloxacin are linear over the dose range of 200 to 400 mg administered intravenously. The serum elimination half-life is approximately 5–6 hours and the total clearance is around 35 L/hr. Comparison of the pharmacokinetic parameters following the 1st and 5th iv dose on a q 12 h regimen indicates no evidence of drug accumulation.

The absolute bioavailability of oral ciprofloxacin is within a range of 70-80% with no substantial loss by first pass metabolism. An intravenous infusion of 400 mg ciprofloxacin given over 60 minutes every 12 hours has been shown to produce an area under the serum concentration time curve (AUC) equivalent to that produced by a 500 mg oral dose given every 12 hours. A 400 mg iv dose administered over 60 minutes every 12 hours results in a C_{max} similar to that observed with a 750 mg oral dose. An infusion of 200 mg ciprofloxacin given every 12 hours produces an AUC equivalent to that produced by a 250 mg oral dose given every 12 hours.

After intravenous administration, approximately 50% to 70% of the dose is excreted in the urine as unchanged drug. Following a 200 mg iv dose, concentrations in the urine usually exceed 200 $\mu g/mL$ 0–2 hours after dosing and are generally greater than 15 $\mu g/mL$ 8–12 hours after dosing. Following a 400 mg iv dose, urine concentrations generally exceed 400 $\mu g/mL$ 0–2 hours after dosing and are usually greater than 30 $\mu g/mL$ 8–12 hours after dosing. The renal clearance is approximately 22 L/hr. The urinary excretion of ciprofloxacin is virtually complete by 24 hours after dosing.

Co-administration of probenecid with ciprofloxacin results in about a 50% reduction in the ciprofloxacin renal clearance and a 50% increase in its concentration in the systemic circulation. Although bile concentrations of ciprofloxacin are severalfold higher than serum concentrations after intravenous dosing, only a small amount of the administered dose (<1%) is recovered from the bile as unchanged drug. Approximately 15% of an iv dose is recovered from the feces within 5 days after dosing.

After iv administration, three metabolites of ciprofloxacin have been identified in human urine which together account for approximately 10% of the intravenous dose.

In patients with reduced renal function, the half-life of ciprofloxacin is slightly prolonged and dosage adjustments may be required. (See DOSAGE AND ADMINISTRATION.)

In preliminary studies in patients with stable chronic liver cirrhosis, no significant changes in ciprofloxacin pharmacokinetics have been observed. However, the kinetics of ciprofloxacin in patients with acute hepatic insufficiency have not been fully elucidated.

The binding of ciprofloxacin to serum proteins is 20 to 40%. After intravenous administration, ciprofloxacin is present in saliva, nasal and bronchial secretions, sputum, skin blister fluid, lymph, peritoneal fluid, bile and prostatic secretions. It has also been detected in the lung, skin, fat, muscle, cartilage and bone. Although the drug diffuses into cerebrospinal fluid (CSF), CSF concentrations are generally less than 10% of peak serum concentrations. Levels of the drug in the aqueous and vitreous chambers of the eye are lower than in serum.

Microbiology: Ciprofloxacin has *in vitro* activity against a wide range of gram-negative and gram-positive organisms.

The bactericidal action of ciprofloxacin results from interference with the enzyme DNA gyrase which is needed for the synthesis of bacterial DNA.

Ciprofloxacin has been shown to be active against most strains of the following organisms both *in vitro* and in clinical infections. (See INDICATIONS AND USAGE section.)

Gram-positive bacteria
Enterococcus faecalis (Many strains are only moderately susceptible)
Staphylococcus aureus
Staphylococcus epidermidis
Streptococcus pneumoniae
Streptococcus pyogenes

Gram-negative bacteria
Citrobacter diversus
Citrobacter freundii
Enterobacter cloacae
Escherichia coli
Haemophilus influenzae
Haemophilus parainfluenzae
Klebsiella pneumoniae
Morganella morganii
Proteus mirabilis
Proteus vulgaris
Providencia rettgeri
Providencia stuartii
Pseudomonas aeruginosa
Serratia marcescens

Ciprofloxacin has been shown to be active *in vitro* against most strains of the following organisms; however, *the clinical significance of these data is unknown.*

Gram-positive bacteria
Staphylococcus haemolyticus
Staphylococcus hominis
Staphylococcus saprophyticus

Gram-negative bacteria
Acinetobacter calcoaceticus
Aeromonas caviae
Aeromonas hydrophila
Brucella melitensis
Campylobacter coli
Campylobacter jejuni
Edwardsiella tarda
Enterobacter aerogenes
Haemophilus ducreyi
Klebsiella oxytoca
Legionella pneumophila
Moraxella (Branhamella) catarrhalis
Neisseria gonorrhoeae
Neisseria meningitidis
Pasteurella multocida
Salmonella enteritidis
Salmonella typhi
Shigella flexneri
Shigella sonnei
Vibrio cholerae
Vibrio parahaemolyticus
Vibrio vulnificus
Yersinia enterocolitica

Other organisms
Chlamydia trachomatis (only moderately susceptible)
Mycobacterium tuberculosis (only moderately susceptible)
Most strains of *Pseudomonas cepacia* and some strains of *Pseudomonas maltophilia* are resistant to ciprofloxacin as are most anaerobic bacteria, including *Bacteroides fragilis* and *Clostridium difficile.*

Ciprofloxacin is slightly less active when tested at acidic pH. The inoculum size has little effect when tested *in vitro*. The minimum bactericidal concentration (MBC) generally does not exceed the minimum inhibitory concentration (MIC) by more than a factor of 2. Resistance to ciprofloxacin *in vitro* usually develops slowly (multiple-step mutation).

Ciprofloxacin does not cross-react with other antimicrobial agents such as beta-lactams or aminoglycosides; therefore, organisms resistant to these drugs may be susceptible to ciprofloxacin.

In vitro studies have shown that additive activity often results when ciprofloxacin is combined with other anti-microbial agents such as beta-lactams, aminoglycosides, clindamycin, or metronidazole. Synergy has been reported particularly with the combination of ciprofloxacin and a beta-lactam; antagonism is observed only rarely.

Susceptibility Tests

Diffusion Techniques: Quantitative methods that require measurement of zone diameters give the most precise estimates of antibiotic susceptibility. One such procedure recommended for use with the 5-μg ciprofloxacin disk is the National Committee for Clinical Laboratory Standards (NCCLS) approved procedure (M2-A4—Performance Standards for Antimicrobial Disc Susceptibility Tests 1990). Only a 5-μg ciprofloxacin disk should be used, and it should not be used for testing susceptibility to less active quinolones; there are no suitable surrogate disks.

Results of laboratory tests using 5-μg ciprofloxacin disks should be interpreted using the following criteria:

Zone Diameter (mm)	Interpretation
≥ 21	(S) Susceptible
16 — 20	(MS) Moderately Susceptible
≤ 15	(R) Resistant

Dilution Techniques: Broth and agar dilution methods, such as those recommended by the NCCLS (M7-A2—Methods for Dilution Antimicrobial Susceptibility Tests for Bacteria that Grow Aerobically 1990), may be used to determine the minimum inhibitory concentration (MIC) of ciprofloxacin. MIC test results should be interpreted according to the following criteria:

MIC (µg/mL)	Interpretation
≤ 1	(S) Susceptible
2	(MS) Moderately Susceptible
≥ 4	(R) Resistant

For any susceptibility test, a report of "susceptible" indicates that the pathogen is likely to be inhibited by generally achievable blood levels. A report of "resistant" indicates that the pathogen is not likely to respond. A report of "moderately susceptible" indicates that the pathogen is expected to be susceptible to ciprofloxacin if high doses are used, or if the infection is confined to tissues and fluids in which high ciprofloxacin levels are attained.

The Quality Control (QC) strains should have the following assigned daily ranges for ciprofloxacin.

QC Strains	Disk Zone Diameter (mm)	MIC (µg/mL)
S. aureus (ATCC 25923)	22–30	—
S. aureus (ATCC 29213)	—	0.12–0.5
E. coli (ATCC 25922)	30–40	0.004–0.015
P. aeruginosa (ATCC 27853)	25–33	0.25–1.0
E. faecalis (ATCC 29212)	—	0.25–2.0

INDICATIONS AND USAGE

Cipro® I.V. is indicated for the treatment of infections caused by susceptible strains of the designated microorganisms in the conditions listed below when the intravenous administration offers a route of administration advantageous to the patient:

Urinary Tract Infections—mild, moderate, severe and complicated infections caused by *Escherichia coli*, (including cases with secondary bacteremia), *Klebsiella pneumoniae* subspecies *pneumoniae*, *Enterobacter cloacae*, *Serratia marcescens*, *Proteus mirabilis*, *Providencia rettgeri*, *Morganella morganii*, *Citrobacter diversus*, *Citrobacter freundii*, *Pseudomonas aeruginosa*, *Staphylococcus epidermidis*, and *Enterococcus faecalis*.

Cipro® I.V. is also indicated for the treatment of mild to moderate lower respiratory tract infections, skin and skin structure infections and bone and joint infections due to the organisms listed in each section below. In severe and complicated lower respiratory tract infections, skin and skin structure infections and bone and joint infections, safety and effectiveness of the iv formulation have not been established.

Lower Respiratory Infections—mild to moderate infections caused by *Escherichia coli*, *Klebsiella pneumoniae* subspecies *pneumoniae*, *Enterobacter cloacae*, *Proteus mirabilis*, *Pseudomonas aeruginosa*, *Haemophilus influenzae*, *Haemophilus parainfluenzae*, and *Streptococcus pneumoniae*.

Skin and Skin Structure Infections—mild to moderate infections caused by *Escherichia coli*, *Klebsiella pneumoniae* subspecies *pneumoniae*, *Enterobacter cloacae*, *Proteus mirabilis*, *Proteus vulgaris*, *Providencia stuartii*, *Morganella morganii*, *Citrobacter freundii*, *Pseudomonas aeruginosa*, *Staphylococcus aureus*, *Staphylococcus epidermidis*, and *Streptococcus pyogenes*.

Bone and Joint Infections—mild to moderate infections caused by *Enterobacter cloacae*, *Serratia marcescens*, and *Pseudomonas aeruginosa*.

If anaerobic organisms are suspected of contributing to the infection, appropriate therapy should be administered.

Appropriate culture and susceptibility tests should be performed before treatment in order to isolate and identify organisms causing infection and to determine their susceptibility to ciprofloxacin. Therapy with Cipro® I.V. may be initiated before results of these tests are known; once results become available, appropriate therapy should be continued. As with other drugs, some strains of *Pseudomonas aeruginosa* may develop resistance fairly rapidly during treatment with ciprofloxacin. Culture and susceptibility testing performed periodically during therapy will provide information not only on the therapeutic effect of the antimicrobial agent but also on the possible emergence of bacterial resistance.

CONTRAINDICATIONS

Cipro® I.V. (ciprofloxacin) is contraindicated in persons with a history of hypersensitivity to ciprofloxacin or any member of the quinolone class of antimicrobial agents.

WARNINGS

THE SAFETY AND EFFECTIVENESS OF CIPROFLOXACIN IN CHILDREN, ADOLESCENTS (LESS THAN 18 YEARS OF AGE), PREGNANT WOMEN, AND LACTATING WOMEN HAVE NOT BEEN ESTABLISHED. (SEE PRECAUTIONS—PEDIATRIC USE, PREGNANCY AND NURSING MOTHERS SUBSECTIONS.) Ciprofloxacin causes lameness in imma-

ture dogs. Histopathological examination of the weight-bearing joints of these dogs revealed permanent lesions of the cartilage. Related quinolone-class drugs also produce erosions of cartilage of weight-bearing joints and other signs of arthropathy in immature animals of various species. (See ANIMAL PHARMACOLOGY.)

Convulsions have been reported in patients receiving ciprofloxacin. Convulsions, increased intracranial pressure, and toxic psychosis have been reported in patients receiving ciprofloxacin and other drugs of this class. Quinolones may also cause central nervous system (CNS) stimulation which may lead to tremors, restlessness, lightheadedness, confusion and hallucinations. If these reactions occur in patients receiving ciprofloxacin, the drug should be discontinued and appropriate measures instituted. As with all quinolones, ciprofloxacin should be used with caution in patients with known or suspected CNS disorders, such as severe cerebral arteriosclerosis, epilepsy, and other factors that predispose to seizures. (See ADVERSE REACTIONS.)

SERIOUS AND FATAL REACTIONS HAVE BEEN REPORTED IN PATIENTS RECEIVING CONCURRENT ADMINISTRATION OF INTRAVENOUS CIPROFLOXACIN AND THEOPHYLLINE. These reactions have included cardiac arrest, seizure, status epilepticus and respiratory failure. Although similar serious adverse events have been reported in patients receiving theophylline alone, the possibility that these reactions may be potentiated by ciprofloxacin cannot be eliminated. If concomitant use cannot be avoided, serum levels of theophylline should be monitored and dosage adjustments made as appropriate.

Serious and occasionally fatal hypersensitivity (anaphylactic) reactions, some following the first dose, have been reported in patients receiving quinolone therapy. Some reactions were accompanied by cardiovascular collapse, loss of consciousness, tingling, pharyngeal or facial edema, dyspnea, urticaria, and itching. Only a few patients had a history of hypersensitivity reactions. Serious anaphylactic reactions require immediate emergency treatment with epinephrine and other resuscitation measures, including oxygen, intravenous fluids, intravenous antihistamines, corticosteroids, pressor amines and airway management, as clinically indicated.

Severe hypersensitivity reactions characterized by rash, fever, eosinophilia, jaundice, and hepatic necrosis with fatal outcome have also been reported extremely rarely in patients receiving ciprofloxacin along with other drugs. The possibility that these reactions were related to ciprofloxacin cannot be excluded. Ciprofloxacin should be discontinued at the first appearance of a skin rash or any other sign of hypersensitivity.

Pseudomembranous colitis has been reported with nearly all antibacterial agents, including ciprofloxacin, and may range in severity from mild to life-threatening. Therefore, it is important to consider this diagnosis in patients who present with diarrhea subsequent to the administration of antibacterial agents.

Treatment with antibacterial agents alters the normal flora of the colon and may permit overgrowth of clostridia. Studies indicate that a toxin produced by *Clostridium difficile* is one primary cause of "antibiotic-associated colitis".

After the diagnosis of pseudomembranous colitis has been established, therapeutic measures should be initiated. Mild cases of pseudomembranous colitis usually respond to drug discontinuation alone. In moderate to severe cases, consideration should be given to management with fluids and electrolytes, protein supplementation and treatment with an antibacterial drug effective against *C. difficile*.

PRECAUTIONS

General: INTRAVENOUS CIPROFLOXACIN SHOULD BE ADMINISTERED BY SLOW INFUSION OVER A PERIOD OF 60 MINUTES. Local iv site reactions have been reported with the intravenous administration of ciprofloxacin. These reactions are more frequent if infusion time is 30 minutes or less or if small veins of the hand are used. (See ADVERSE REACTIONS.)

Crystals of ciprofloxacin have been observed rarely in the urine of human subjects but more frequently in the urine of laboratory animals, which is usually alkaline. (See ANIMAL PHARMACOLOGY.) Crystalluria related to ciprofloxacin has been reported only rarely in humans because human urine is usually acidic. Alkalinity of the urine should be avoided in patients receiving ciprofloxacin. Patients should be well hydrated to prevent the formation of highly concentrated urine.

Alteration of the dosage regimen is necessary for patients with impairment of renal function. (See DOSAGE AND ADMINISTRATION.)

Moderate to severe phototoxicity manifested by an exaggerated sunburn reaction has been observed in some patients who were exposed to direct sunlight while receiving some members of the quinolone class of drugs. Excessive sunlight should be avoided.

As with any potent drug, periodic assessment of organ system functions, including renal, hepatic, and hematopoietic, is advisable during prolonged therapy.

Information for Patients: Patients should be advised that ciprofloxacin may be associated with hypersensitivity reactions, even following a single dose, and to discontinue the drug at the first sign of a skin rash or other allergic reaction. Ciprofloxacin may cause dizziness and lightheadedness; therefore, patients should know how they react to this drug before they operate an automobile or machinery or engage in activities requiring mental alertness or coordination.

Patients should be advised that ciprofloxacin may increase the effects of theophylline and caffeine. There is a possibility of caffeine accumulation when products containing caffeine are consumed while taking quinolones.

Drug Interactions: As with other quinolones, concurrent administration of ciprofloxacin with theophylline may lead to elevated serum concentrations of theophylline and prolongation of its elimination half-life. This may result in increased risk of theophylline-related adverse reactions. (See WARNINGS.) If concomitant use cannot be avoided, serum levels of theophylline should be monitored and dosage adjustments made as appropriate.

Some quinolones, including ciprofloxacin, have also been shown to interfere with the metabolism of caffeine. This may lead to reduced clearance of caffeine and a prolongation of its serum half-life.

Some quinolones, including ciprofloxacin, have been associated with transient elevations in serum creatinine in patients receiving cyclosporine concomitantly.

Quinolones have been reported to enhance the effects of the oral anticoagulant warfarin or its derivatives. When these products are administered concomitantly, prothrombin time or other suitable coagulation tests should be closely monitored.

Probenecid interferes with renal tubular secretion of ciprofloxacin and produces an increase in the level of ciprofloxacin in the serum. This should be considered if patients are receiving both drugs concomitantly.

As with other broad-spectrum antimicrobial agents, prolonged use of ciprofloxacin may result in overgrowth of nonsusceptible organisms. Repeated evaluation of the patient's condition and microbial susceptibility testing are essential. If superinfection occurs during therapy, appropriate measures should be taken.

Carcinogenesis, Mutagenesis, Impairment of Fertility: Eight *in vitro* mutagenicity tests have been conducted with ciprofloxacin. Test results are listed below:

Salmonella/Microsome Test (Negative)
E. coli DNA Repair Assay (Negative)
Mouse Lymphoma Cell Forward Mutation Assay (Positive)
Chinese Hamster V_{79} Cell HGPRT Test (Negative)
Syrian Hamster Embryo Cell Transformation Assay (Negative)
Saccharomyces cerevisiae Point Mutation Assay (Negative)
Saccharomyces cerevisiae Mitotic Crossover and Gene Conversion Assay (Negative)
Rat Hepatocyte DNA Repair Assay (Positive)

Thus, two of the eight tests were positive, but results of the following three *in vivo* test systems gave negative results:

Rat Hepatocyte DNA Repair Assay
Micronucleus Test (Mice)
Dominant Lethal Test (Mice)

Long-term carcinogenicity studies in mice and rats have been completed. After daily oral dosing for up to 2 years, there is no evidence that ciprofloxacin has any carcinogenic or tumorigenic effects in these species.

Pregnancy: Teratogenic Effects. Pregnancy Category C: Reproduction studies have been performed in rats and mice at doses up to 6 times the usual daily human dose and have revealed no evidence of impaired fertility or harm to the fetus due to ciprofloxacin. In rabbits, ciprofloxacin (30 and 100 mg/kg orally) produced gastrointestinal disturbances resulting in maternal weight loss and an increased incidence of abortion. No teratogenicity was observed at either dose. After intravenous administration of doses up to 20 mg/kg, no maternal toxicity was produced, and no embryotoxicity or teratogenicity was observed. There are, however, no adequate and well-controlled studies in pregnant women. Ciprofloxacin should be used during pregnancy only if the potential benefit justifies the potential risk to the fetus. (See WARNINGS.)

Nursing Mothers: Ciprofloxacin is excreted in human milk. Because of the potential for serious adverse reactions in infants nursing from mothers taking ciprofloxacin, a decision should be made either to discontinue nursing or to discontinue the drug, taking into account the importance of the drug to the mother.

Pediatric Use: Safety and effectiveness in children and adolescents less than 18 years of age have not been established. Ciprofloxacin causes arthropathy in juvenile animals. (See WARNINGS.)

ADVERSE REACTIONS

The most frequently reported events, without regard to drug relationship, among patients treated with intravenous ciprofloxacin were nausea, diarrhea, central nervous system dis-

Continued on next page

Miles—Cont.

turbance, local iv site reactions, abnormalities of liver associated enzymes (hepatic enzymes) and eosinophilia. Headache, restlessness and rash were also noted in greater than 1% of patients treated with the most common doses of ciprofloxacin.

Local iv site reactions have been reported with the intravenous administration of ciprofloxacin. These reactions are more frequent if the infusion time is 30 minutes or less. These may appear as local skin reactions which resolve rapidly upon completion of the infusion. Subsequent intravenous administration is not contraindicated unless the reactions recur or worsen.

Additional events, without regard to drug relationship or route of administration, that occurred in 1% or less of ciprofloxacin courses are listed below:

GASTROINTESTINAL: ileus; jaundice; gastrointestinal bleeding; *C. difficile* associated diarrhea; pseudomembranous colitis; pancreatitis; hepatic necrosis; intestinal perforation; dyspepsia; epigastric or abdominal pain; vomiting; constipation; oral ulceration; oral candidiasis; mouth dryness; anorexia; dysphagia; flatulence.

CENTRAL NERVOUS SYSTEM: convulsive seizures, paranoia, toxic psychosis, depression, dysphasia, phobia, depersonalization, manic reaction, unresponsiveness, ataxia, confusion, hallucinations, dizziness, lightheadedness, paresthesia, anxiety, tremor, insomnia, nightmares, weakness, drowsiness, irritability, malaise, lethargy.

SKIN/HYPERSENSITIVITY: anaphylactic reactions; erythema multiforme/Stevens-Johnson syndrome; exfoliative dermatitis; toxic epidermal necrolysis; vasculitis; angioedema; edema of the lips, face, neck, conjunctivae, hands or lower extremities; purpura; fever; chills; flushing; pruritus; urticaria; cutaneous candidiasis; vesicles; increased perspiration; hyperpigmentation; erythema nodosum; photosensitivity.

Allergic reactions ranging from urticaria to anaphylactic reactions have been reported. (See WARNINGS.)

SPECIAL SENSES: decreased visual acuity, blurred vision, disturbed vision (flashing lights, change in color perception, overbrightness of lights, diplopia), eye pain, anosmia, hearing loss, tinnitus, nystagmus, a bad taste.

MUSCULOSKELETAL: joint pain; jaw, arm or back pain; joint stiffness; neck and chest pain; achiness; flare up of gout.

RENAL/UROGENITAL: renal failure, interstitial nephritis, hemorrhagic cystitis, renal calculi, frequent urination, acidosis, urethral bleeding, polyuria, urinary retention, gynecomastia, candiduria, vaginitis. Crystalluria, cylindruria, hematuria, and albuminuria have also been reported.

CARDIOVASCULAR: cardiovascular collapse, cardiopulmonary arrest, myocardial infarction, arrhythmia, tachycardia, palpitation, cerebral thrombosis, syncope, cardiac murmur, hypertension, hypotension, angina pectoris.

RESPIRATORY: respiratory arrest, pulmonary embolism, dyspnea, pulmonary edema, respiratory distress, pleural effusion, hemoptysis, epistaxis, hiccough.

IV INFUSION SITE: thrombophlebitis, burning, pain, pruritus, paresthesia, erythema, swelling.

Also reported were agranulocytosis, prolongation of prothrombin time and possible exacerbation of myasthenia gravis.

Many of these events were described as only mild or moderate in severity, abated soon after the drug was discontinued and required no treatment.

In several instances, nausea, vomiting, tremor, irritability or palpitation were judged by investigators to be related to elevated serum levels of theophylline possibly as a result of drug interaction with ciprofloxacin.

Adverse Laboratory Changes: The most frequently reported changes in laboratory parameters with intravenous ciprofloxacin therapy, without regard to drug relationship, were:

Hepatic—Elevations of AST (SGOT), ALT (SGPT), alkaline phosphatase, LDH and serum bilirubin.

Hematologic—Elevated eosinophil and platelet counts, decreased platelet counts, hemoglobin and/or hematocrit.

Renal—Elevations of serum creatinine, BUN, uric acid.

Other—Elevations of serum creatine phosphokinase, serum theophylline (in patients receiving theophylline concomitantly), blood glucose, and triglycerides.

Other changes occurring infrequently were: decreased leukocyte count, elevated atypical lymphocyte count, immature WBCs, elevated serum calcium, elevation of serum gamma-glutamyl transpeptidase (γ GT), decreased BUN, decreased uric acid, decreased total serum protein, decreased serum albumin, decreased serum potassium, elevated serum potassium, elevated serum cholesterol.

Other changes occurring rarely during administration of ciprofloxacin were: elevation of serum amylase, decrease of blood glucose, pancytopenia, leukocytosis, elevated sedimentation rate, change in serum phenytoin, decreased prothrombin time, hemolytic anemia, and bleeding diathesis.

OVERDOSAGE

In the event of acute overdosage, the patient should be carefully observed and given supportive treatment. Adequate hydration must be maintained. Only a small amount of ciprofloxacin (< 10%) is removed from the body after hemodialysis or peritoneal dialysis.

DOSAGE AND ADMINISTRATION

The recommended adult dosage for urinary tract infections of mild to moderate severity is 200 mg every 12 hours. For severe or complicated urinary tract infections the recommended dosage is 400 mg every 12 hours.

The recommended adult dosage for lower respiratory tract infections, skin and skin structure infections and bone and joint infections of mild to moderate severity is 400 mg every 12 hours.

The determination of dosage for any particular patient must take into consideration the severity and nature of the infection, the susceptibility of the causative organism, the integrity of the patient's host-defense mechanisms and the status of renal and hepatic function.

[See table below.]

Cipro® I.V. should be administered by intravenous infusion over a period of 60 minutes.

The duration of treatment depends upon the severity of infection. Generally, ciprofloxacin should be continued for at least 2 days after the signs and symptoms of infection have disappeared. The usual duration is 7 to 14 days. Bone and joint infections may require treatment for 4 to 6 weeks or longer.

Ciprofloxacin hydrochloride tablets (Cipro®) for oral administration are available. Parenteral therapy may be changed to oral Cipro® tablets when the condition warrants, at the discretion of the physician. For complete dosage and administration information, see Cipro® tablet package insert.

Impaired Renal Function: The following table provides dosage guidelines for use in patients with renal impairment; however, monitoring of serum drug levels provides the most reliable basis for dosage adjustment.

RECOMMENDED STARTING AND MAINTENANCE DOSES FOR PATIENTS WITH IMPAIRED RENAL FUNCTION

Creatinine Clearance (mL/min)	Dosage
≥ 30	See usual dosage
5–29	200–400 mg q 18–24 hr

When only the serum creatinine concentration is known, the following formula may be used to estimate creatinine clearance.

Men: Creatinine clearance

$$(\text{mL/min}) = \frac{\text{Weight (kg)} \times (140 - \text{age})}{72 \times \text{serum creatinine (mg/dL)}}$$

Women: 0.85 × the value calculated for men.

The serum creatinine should represent a steady state of renal function.

For patients with changing renal function or for patients with renal impairment and hepatic insufficiency, measurement of serum concentrations of ciprofloxacin will provide additional guidance for adjusting dosage.

DOSAGE GUIDELINES

Location of Infection	Type or Severity	Intravenous Unit Dose	Frequency	Daily Dose
Urinary tract	Mild/Moderate	200 mg	q 12 h	400 mg
	Severe/Complicated	400 mg	q 12 h	800 mg
Lower Respiratory tract; Skin and Skin Structure; Bone and Joint	Mild/Moderate	400 mg	q 12 h	800 mg

INTRAVENOUS ADMINISTRATION

Cipro® I.V. should be administered by intravenous infusion over a period of 60 minutes. Slow infusion of a dilute solution into a large vein will minimize patient discomfort and reduce the risk of venous irritation.

Vials (Injection Concentrate): THIS PREPARATION MUST BE DILUTED BEFORE USE. The intravenous dose should be prepared by aseptically withdrawing the appropriate volume of concentrate from the vials of Cipro® I.V. This should be diluted with a suitable intravenous solution to a final concentration of 1–2 mg/mL. (See COMPATIBILITY AND STABILITY.) The resulting solution should be infused over a period of 60 minutes by direct infusion or through a Y-type intravenous infusion set which may already be in place.

If this method or the "piggyback" method of administration is used, it is advisable to discontinue temporarily the administration of any other solutions during the infusion of Cipro® I.V.

Flexible Containers: Cipro® I.V. is also available as a 0.2% premixed solution in 5% dextrose in flexible containers of 100 mL or 200 mL. The solutions in flexible containers may be infused as described above.

COMPATIBILITY AND STABILITY

Ciprofloxacin injection 1% (10 mg/mL), when diluted with the following intravenous solutions to concentrations of 0.5 to 2.0 mg/mL, is stable for up to 14 days at refrigerated or room temperature storage.

0.9% Sodium Chloride Injection, USP

5% Dextrose Injection, USP

If Cipro® I.V. is to be given concomitantly with another drug, each drug should be given separately in accordance with the recommended dosage and route of administration for each drug.

HOW SUPPLIED

Cipro® I.V. (ciprofloxacin) is available as a clear, colorless to slightly yellowish solution. Cipro® I.V. is available in 200 mg and 400 mg strengths. The concentrate is supplied in vials while the premixed solution is supplied in flexible containers as follows:

CONTAINER	SIZE	STRENGTH	NDC NUMBER
Vial:	20 mL	200 mg, 1%	0026-8562-20
	40 mL	400 mg, 1%	0026-8564-64
Flexible Container:	100 mL 5% dextrose	200 mg, 0.2%	0026-8552-26
	200 mL 5% dextrose	400 mg, 0.2%	0026-8554-63

STORAGE

Vials: Store between 41–77°F (5–25°C).

Flexible Container: Store between 41–77°F (5–25°C).

Protect from light, avoid excessive heat, protect from freezing.

Ciprofloxacin is also available as Cipro® (ciprofloxacin HCl) Tablets 250, 500 and 750 mg.

ANIMAL PHARMACOLOGY

Ciprofloxacin and other quinolones have been shown to cause arthropathy in immature animals of most species tested. (See WARNINGS.) Damage of weight-bearing joints was observed in juvenile dogs and rats. In young beagles, 100 mg/kg ciprofloxacin given daily for 4 weeks caused degenerative articular changes of the knee joint. At 30 mg/kg, the effect on the joint was minimal. In a subsequent study in beagles, removal of weight-bearing from the joint reduced the lesions but did not totally prevent them.

Crystalluria, sometimes associated with secondary nephropathy, occurs in laboratory animals dosed with ciprofloxacin. This is primarily related to the reduced solubility of ciprofloxacin under alkaline conditions, which predominate in the urine of test animals; in man, crystalluria is rare since human urine is typically acidic. In rhesus monkeys, crystalluria without nephropathy has been noted after intravenous doses as low as 5 mg/kg. After 6 months of intravenous dosing at 10 mg/kg/day, no nephropathological changes were noted; however, nephropathy was observed after dosing at 20 mg/kg/day for the same duration.

In dogs, ciprofloxacin administered at 3 and 10 mg/kg by rapid intravenous injection (15 sec.) produces pronounced hypotensive effects. These effects are considered to be related to histamine release because they are partially antagonized by pyrilamine, an antihistamine. In rhesus monkeys, rapid intravenous injection also produces hypotension, but the effect in this species is inconsistent and less pronounced.

In mice, concomitant administration of nonsteroidal anti-inflammatory drugs, such as fenbufen, phenylbutazone and indomethacin, with quinolones has been reported to enhance the CNS stimulatory effect of quinolones.

Ocular toxicity, seen with some related drugs, has not been observed in ciprofloxacin-treated animals.

Miles Inc.
Pharmaceutical Division
400 Morgan Lane
West Haven, CT 06516 USA

Caution: Federal (USA) Law prohibits dispensing without a prescription.

PZ100736 9/91 BAY q 3939
5202-4-A-U.S.-1

© 1991 Miles Inc. 1628
06-4745

CIPRO® I.V. ℞
(ciprofloxacin)
For Intravenous Infusion

PHARMACY BULK PACKAGE—NOT FOR DIRECT INFUSION

DESCRIPTION

The pharmacy bulk package is a single-entry container of a sterile preparation for parenteral use that contains many single doses. It contains ciprofloxacin as a 1% aqueous solution concentrate. The contents are intended for use in a pharmacy admixture program and are restricted to the preparation of admixtures for intravenous infusion.
Cipro® I.V. (ciprofloxacin) is a synthetic broad-spectrum antimicrobial agent for intravenous (iv) administration. Ciprofloxacin, a fluoroquinolone, is 1-cyclopropyl-6-fluoro-1, 4-dihydro-4-oxo-7-(1-piperazinyl)-3-quinolinecarboxylic acid. Its empirical formula is $C_{17}H_{18}FN_3O_3$ and its chemical structure is:

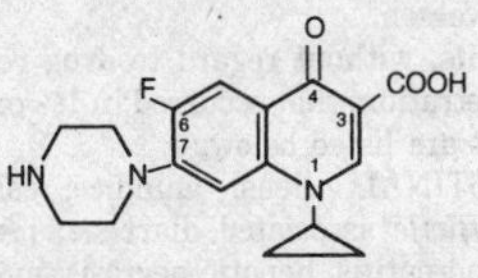

Ciprofloxacin is a faint to light yellow crystalline powder with a molecular weight of 331.4. It is soluble in dilute (0.1N) hydrochloric acid and is practically insoluble in water and ethanol. Ciprofloxacin differs from other quinolones in that it has a fluorine atom at the 6-position, a piperazine moiety at the 7-position, and cyclopropyl ring at the 1-position. Cipro® I.V. solution is available as 1.0% aqueous concentrate, which is intended for dilution prior to administration. Ciprofloxacin solution contains lactic acid as a solubilizing agent and hydrochloric acid for pH adjustment. The pH range for the 1.0% aqueous concentrate is 3.3 to 3.9.

CLINICAL PHARMACOLOGY

Following 60-minute intravenous infusions of 200 mg and 400 mg ciprofloxacin to normal volunteers, the mean maximum serum concentrations achieved were 2.1 and 4.6 μg/mL, respectively; the concentrations at 12 hours were 0.1 and 0.2 μg/mL, respectively.

Steady-state Ciprofloxacin
Serum Concentrations (μg/mL)
After 60-minute IV Infusions q 12 h.

	Time after starting the infusion					
Dose	**30 min.**	**1 hr**	**3 hr**	**6 hr**	**8 hr**	**12 hr**
200 mg	1.7	2.1	0.6	0.3	0.2	0.1
400 mg	3.7	4.6	1.3	0.7	0.5	0.2

The pharmacokinetics of ciprofloxacin are linear over the dose range of 200 to 400 mg administered intravenously. The serum elimination half-life is approximately 5–6 hours and the total clearance is around 35 L/hr. Comparison of the pharmacokinetic parameters following the 1st and 5th iv dose on a q 12 h regimen indicates no evidence of drug accumulation.
The absolute bioavailability of oral ciprofloxacin is within a range of 70–80% with no substantial loss by first pass metabolism. An intravenous infusion of 400 mg ciprofloxacin given over 60 minutes every 12 hours has been shown to produce an area under the serum concentration time curve (AUC) equivalent to that produced by a 500 mg oral dose given every 12 hours. A 400 mg iv dose administered over 60 minutes every 12 hours results in a C_{max} similar to that observed with a 750 mg oral dose. An infusion of 200 mg ciprofloxacin given every 12 hours produces an AUC equivalent to that produced by a 250 mg oral dose given every 12 hours.
After intravenous administration, approximately 50% to 70% of the dose is excreted in the urine as unchanged drug. Following a 200 mg iv dose, concentrations in the urine usually exceed 200 μg/mL 0–2 hours after dosing and are generally greater than 15 μg/mL 8–12 hours after dosing. Following a 400 mg iv dose, urine concentrations generally exceed 400 μg/mL 0–2 hours after dosing and are usually greater than 30 μg/mL 8–12 hours after dosing. The renal clearance is approximately 22 L/hr. The urinary excretion of ciprofloxacin is virtually complete by 24 hours after dosing.
Co-administration of probenecid with ciprofloxacin results in about a 50% reduction in the ciprofloxacin renal clearance and a 50% increase in its concentration in the systemic circulation. Although bile concentrations of ciprofloxacin are severalfold higher than serum concentrations after intravenous dosing, only a small amount of the administered dose (<1%) is recovered from the bile as unchanged drug. Approximately 15% of an iv dose is recovered from the feces within 5 days after dosing.
After iv administration, three metabolites of ciprofloxacin have been identified in human urine which together account for approximately 10% of the intravenous dose.
In patients with reduced renal function, the half-life of ciprofloxacin is slightly prolonged and dosage adjustments may be required. (See DOSAGE AND ADMINISTRATION.)
In preliminary studies in patients with stable chronic liver cirrhosis, no significant changes in ciprofloxacin pharmacokinetics have been observed. However, the kinetics of ciprofloxacin in patients with acute hepatic insufficiency have not been fully elucidated.
The binding of ciprofloxacin to serum proteins is 20 to 40%.
After intravenous administration, ciprofloxacin is present in saliva, nasal and bronchial secretions, sputum, skin blister fluid, lymph, peritoneal fluid, bile and prostatic secretions. It has also been detected in the lung, skin, fat, muscle, cartilage and bone. Although the drug diffuses into cerebrospinal fluid (CSF), CSF concentrations are generally less than 10% of peak serum concentrations. Levels of the drug in the aqueous and vitreous chambers of the eye are lower than in serum.
Microbiology: Ciprofloxacin has *in vitro* activity against a wide range of gram-negative and gram-positive organisms. The bactericidal action of ciprofloxacin results from interference with the enzyme DNA gyrase which is needed for the synthesis of bacterial DNA.
Ciprofloxacin has been shown to be active against most strains of the following organisms both *in vitro* and in clinical infections. (See INDICATIONS AND USAGE section.)

Gram-positive bacteria
Enterococcus faecalis (Many strains are only moderately susceptible)
Staphylococcus aureus
Staphylococcus epidermidis
Streptococcus pneumoniae
Streptococcus pyogenes

Gram-negative bacteria

Citrobacter diversus	*Morganella morganii*
Citrobacter freundii	*Proteus mirabilis*
Enterobacter cloacae	*Proteus vulgaris*
Escherichia coli	*Providencia rettgeri*
Haemophilus influenzae	*Providencia stuartii*
Haemophilus parainfluenzae	*Pseudomonas aeruginosa*
Klebsiella pneumoniae	*Serratia marcescens*

Ciprofloxacin has been shown to be active *in vitro* against most strains of the following organisms; however, *the clinical significance of these data is unknown.*

Gram-positive bacteria
Staphylococcus haemolyticus
Staphylococcus hominis
Staphylococcus saprophyticus

Gram-negative bacteria

Acinetobacter calcoaceticus	*Neisseria gonorrhoeae*
Aeromonas caviae	*Neisseria meningitidis*
Aeromonas hydrophila	*Pasteurella multocida*
Brucella melitensis	*Salmonella enteritidis*
Campylobacter coli	*Salmonella typhi*
Campylobacter jejuni	*Shigella flexneri*
Edwardsiella tarda	*Shigella sonnei*
Enterobacter aerogenes	*Vibrio cholerae*
Haemophilus ducreyi	*Vibrio parahaemolyticus*
Klebsiella oxytoca	*Vibrio vulunificus*
Legionella pneumophila	*Yersinia enterocolitica*
Moraxella (Branhamella) catarrhalis	

Other organisms
Chlamydia trachomatis (only moderately susceptible)
Mycobacterium tuberculosis (only moderately susceptible)

Most strains of *Pseudomonas cepacia* and some strains of *Pseudomonas maltophilia* are resistant to ciprofloxacin as are most anaerobic bacteria, including *Bacteroides fragilis* and *Clostridium difficile.*
Ciprofloxacin is slightly less active when tested at acidic pH. The inoculum size has little effect when tested *in vitro.* The minimum bactericidal concentration (MBC) generally does not exceed the minimum inhibitory concentration (MIC) by more than a factor of 2. Resistance to ciprofloxacin *in vitro* usually develops slowly (multiple-step mutation).
Ciprofloxacin does not cross-react with other antimicrobial agents such as beta-lactams or aminoglycosides; therefore, organisms resistant to these drugs may be susceptible to ciprofloxacin.
In vitro studies have shown that additive activity often results when ciprofloxacin is combined with other antimicrobial agents such as beta-lactams, aminoglycosides, clindamycin, or metronidazole. Synergy has been reported particularly with the combination of ciprofloxacin and a beta-lactam; antagonism is observed only rarely.

Susceptibility Tests
Diffusion Techniques: Quantitative methods that require measurement of zone diameters give the most precise estimates of antibiotic susceptibility. One such procedure recommended for use with the 5-μg ciprofloxacin disk is the National Committee for Clinical Laboratory Standards (NCCLS) approved procedure M2-A4—Performance Standards for Antimicrobial Disc Susceptibility Tests 1990). Only a 5-μg ciprofloxacin disk should be used, and it should not be used for testing susceptibility to less active quinolones; there are no suitable surrogate disks.
Results of laboratory tests using 5μg ciprofloxacin disks should be interpreted using the following criteria:

Zone Diameter (mm)	**Interpretation**
≥21	(S) Susceptible
16-20	(MS) Moderately Susceptible
≤15	(R) Resistant

Dilution Techniques: Broth and agar dilution methods, such as those recommended by the NCCLS (M7-A2—Methods for Dilution Antimicrobial Susceptibility Tests for Bacteria that Grow Aerobically 1990), may be used to determine the minimum inhibitory concentration (MIC) of ciprofloxacin. MIC test results should be interpreted according to the following criteria:

MIC (μg/mL	**Interpretation**
≤1	(S) Susceptible
2	(MS) Moderately Susceptible
≥4	(R) Resistant

For any susceptibility test, a report of "susceptible" indicates that the pathogen is likely to be inhibited by generally achievable blood levels. A report of "resistant" indicates that the pathogen is not likely to respond. A report of "moderately susceptible" indicates that the pathogen is expected to be susceptible to ciprofloxacin if high doses are used, or if the infection is confined to tissues and fluids in which high ciprofloxacin levels are attained.
The Quality Control (QC) strains should have the following assigned daily ranges for ciprofloxacin.

QC Strains	**Disk Zone Diameter (mm)**	**MIC (μg/mL)**
S. aureus (ATCC 25923)	22-30	—
S. aureus (ATCC 29213)	—	0.12–0.5
E. coli (ATCC 25922)	30-40	0.004–0.015
P. aeruginosa (ATCC 27853)	25-33	0.25–1.0
E. faecalis (ATCC 29212)	—	0.25–2.0

INDICATIONS AND USAGE

Cipro® I.V. is indicated for the treatment of infections caused by susceptible strains of the designated microorganisms in the conditions listed below when the intravenous administration offers a route of administration advantageous to the patient:
Urinary Tract Infections—mild, moderate, severe and complicated infections caused by *Escherichia coli,* (including cases with secondary bacteremia), *Klebsiella pneumoniae* subspecies *pneumoniae, Enterobacter cloacae, Serratia marcescens, Proteus mirabilis, Providencia rettgeri, Morganella morganii, Citrobacter diversus, Citrobacter freundii, Pseudomonas aeruginosa, Staphylococcus epidermidis,* and *Enterococcus faecalis.*
Cipro® I.V. is also indicated for the treatment of mild to moderate lower respiratory tract infections, skin and skin structure infections and bone and joint infections due to the organisms listed in each section below. In severe and complicated lower respiratory tract infections, skin and skin structure infections and bone and joint infections, safety and effectiveness of the iv formulation have not been established.
Lower Respiratory Infections—mild to moderate infections caused by *Escherichia coli, Klebsiella pneumoniae* subspecies *pneumoniae, Enterobacter cloacae, Proteus mirabilis, Pseudomonas aeruginosa, Haemophilus influenzae, Haemophilus parainfluenzae,* and *Streptococcus pneumoniae.*
Skin and Skin Structure Infections—mild to moderate infections caused by *Escherichia coli, Klebsiella pneumoniae* subspecies *pneumoniae, Enterobacter cloacae, Proteus mirabilis, Proteus vulgaris, Providencia stuartii, Morganella morganii, Citrobacter freundii, Pseudomonas aeruginosa, Staphylococcus aureus, Staphylococcus epidermidis,* and *Streptococcus pyogenes.*
Bone and Joint Infections—mild to moderate infections caused by *Enterobacter cloacae, Serratia marcescens, and Pseudomonas aeruginosa.*
If anaerobic organisms are suspected of contributing to the infection, appropriate therapy should be administered.
Appropriate culture and susceptibility tests should be performed before treatment in order to isolate and identify organisms causing infection and to determine their susceptibility to ciprofloxacin. Therapy with Cipro® I.V. may be initiated before results of these tests are known; once results become available, appropriate therapy should be continued.

Continued on next page

Miles—Cont.

As with other drugs, some strains of *Pseudomonas aeruginosa* may develop resistance fairly rapidly during treatment with ciprofloxacin. Culture and susceptibility testing performed periodically during therapy will provide information not only on the therapeutic effect of the antimicrobial agent but also on the possible emergence of bacterial resistance.

CONTRAINDICATIONS

Cipro® I.V. (ciprofloxacin) is contraindicated in persons with a history of hypersensitivity to ciprofloxacin or any member of the quinolone class of antimicrobial agents.

WARNINGS

THE SAFETY AND EFFECTIVENESS OF CIPROFLOXACIN IN CHILDREN, ADOLESCENTS (LESS THAN 18 YEARS OF AGE), PREGNANT WOMEN, AND LACTATING WOMEN HAVE NOT BEEN ESTABLISHED. (SEE PRECAUTIONS—PEDIATRIC USE, PREGNANCY AND NURSING MOTHERS SUBSECTIONS.) Ciprofloxacin causes lameness in immature dogs. Histopathological examination of the weight-bearing joints of these dogs revealed permanent lesions of the cartilage. Related quinolone-class drugs also produce erosions of cartilage of weight-bearing joints and other signs of arthropathy in immature animals of various species. (See ANIMAL PHARMACOLOGY.)

Convulsions have been reported in patients receiving ciprofloxacin. Convulsions, increased intracranial pressure, and toxic psychosis have been reported in patients receiving ciprofloxacin and other drugs of this class. Quinolones may also cause central nervous system (CNS) stimulation which may lead to tremors, restlessness, lightheadedness, confusion and hallucinations. If these reactions occur in patients receiving ciprofloxacin, the drug should be discontinued and appropriate measures instituted. As with all quinolones, ciprofloxacin should be used with caution in patients with known or suspected CNS disorders, such as severe cerebral arteriosclerosis, epilepsy, and other factors that predispose to seizures. (See ADVERSE REACTIONS.)

SERIOUS AND FATAL REACTIONS HAVE BEEN REPORTED IN PATIENTS RECEIVING CONCURRENT ADMINISTRATION OF INTRAVENOUS CIPROFLOXACIN AND THEOPHYLLINE. These reactions have included cardiac arrest, seizure, status epilepticus and respiratory failure. Although similar serious adverse events have been reported in patients receiving theophylline alone, the possibility that these reactions may be potentiated by ciprofloxacin cannot be eliminated. If concomitant use cannot be avoided, serum levels of theophylline should be monitored and dosage adjustments made as appropriate.

Serious and occasionally fatal hypersensitivity (anaphylactic) reactions, some following the first dose, have been reported in patients receiving quinolone therapy. Some reactions were accompanied by cardiovascular collapse, loss of consciousness, tingling, pharyngeal or facial edema, dyspnea, urticaria, and itching. Only a few patients had a history of hypersensitivity reactions. Serious anaphylactic reactions require immediate emergency treatment with epinephrine and other resuscitation measures, including oxygen, intravenous fluids, intravenous antihistamines, corticosteroids, pressor amines and airway management, as clinically indicated.

Severe hypersensitivity reactions characterized by rash, fever, eosinophilia, jaundice, and hepatic necrosis with fatal outcome have also been reported extremely rarely in patients receiving ciprofloxacin along with other drugs. The possibility that these reactions were related to ciprofloxacin cannot be excluded. Ciprofloxacin should be discontinued at the first appearance of a skin rash or any other sign of hypersensitivity.

Pseudomembranous colitis has been reported with nearly all antibacterial agents, including ciprofloxacin, and may range in severity from mild to life-threatening. Therefore, it is important to consider this diagnosis in patients who present with diarrhea subsequent to the administration of antibacterial agents.

Treatment with antibacterial agents alters the normal flora of the colon and may permit overgrowth of clostridia. Studies indicate that a toxin produced by *Clostridium difficile* is one primary cause of "antibiotic-associated colitis."

After the diagnosis of pseudomembranous colitis has been established, therapeutic measures should be initiated. Mild cases of pseudomembranous colitis usually respond to drug discontinuation alone. In moderate to severe cases, consideration should be given to management with fluids and electrolytes, protein supplementation and treatment with an antibacterial drug effective against *C. difficile.*

PRECAUTIONS

General: INTRAVENOUS CIPROFLOXACIN SHOULD BE ADMINISTERED BY SLOW INFUSION OVER A PERIOD OF 60 MINUTES. Local iv site reactions have been reported with the intravenous administration of ciprofloxacin. These reactions are more frequent if infusion time is 30 minutes or less or if small veins of the hand are used. (See ADVERSE REACTIONS.)

Crystals of ciprofloxacin have been observed rarely in the urine of human subjects but more frequently in the urine of laboratory animals, which is usually alkaline. (See ANIMAL PHARMACOLOGY.) Crystalluria related to ciprofloxacin has been reported only rarely in humans because human urine is usually acidic. Alkalinity of the urine should be avoided in patients receiving ciprofloxacin. Patients should be well hydrated to prevent the formation of highly concentrated urine.

Alteration of the dosage regimen is necessary for patients with impairment of renal function. (See DOSAGE AND ADMINISTRATION.)

Moderate to severe phototoxicity manifested by an exaggerated sunburn reaction has been observed in some patients who were exposed to direct sunlight while receiving some members of the quinolone class of drugs. Excessive sunlight should be avoided.

As with any potent drug, periodic assessment of organ system functions, including renal, hepatic, and hematopoietic, is advisable during prolonged therapy.

Information for Patients: Patients should be advised that ciprofloxacin may be associated with hypersensitivity reactions, even following a single dose, and to discontinue the drug at the first sign of a skin rash or other allergic reaction.

Ciprofloxacin may cause dizziness and lightheadedness; therefore, patients should know how they react to this drug before they operate an automobile or machinery or engage in activities requiring mental alertness or coordination.

Patients should be advised that ciprofloxacin may increase the effects of theophylline and caffeine. There is a possibility of caffeine accumulation when products containing caffeine are consumed while taking quinolones.

Drug Interactions: As with other quinolones, concurrent administration of ciprofloxacin with theophylline may lead to elevated serum concentrations of theophylline and prolongation of its elimination half-life. This may result in increased risk of theophylline-related adverse reactions. (See WARNINGS.) If concomitant use cannot be avoided, serum levels of theophylline should be monitored and dosage adjustments made as appropriate.

Some quinolones, including ciprofloxacin, have also been shown to interfere with the metabolism of caffeine. This may lead to reduced clearance of caffeine and a prolongation of its serum half-life.

Some quinolones, including ciprofloxacin, have been associated with transient elevations in serum creatinine in patients receiving cyclosporine concomitantly.

Quinolones have been reported to enhance the effects of the oral anticoagulant warfarin or its derivatives. When these products are administered concomitantly, prothrombin time or other suitable coagulation tests should be closely monitored.

Probenecid interferes with renal tubular secretion of ciprofloxacin and produces an increase in the level of ciprofloxacin in the serum. This should be considered if patients are receiving both drugs concomitantly.

As with other broad-spectrum antimicrobial agents, prolonged use of ciprofloxacin may result in overgrowth of nonsusceptible organisms. Repeated evaluation of the patient's condition and microbial susceptibility testing are essential. If superinfection occurs during therapy, appropriate measures should be taken.

Carcinogenesis, Mutagenesis, Impairment of Fertility: Eight *in vitro* mutagenicity tests have been conducted with ciprofloxacin. Test results are listed below:

Salmonella/Microsome Test (Negative)
E. coli DNA Repair Assay (Negative)
Mouse Lymphoma Cell Forward Mutation Assay (Positive)
Chinese Hamster V_{79} Cell HGPRT Test (Negative)
Syrian Hamster Embryo Cell Transformation Assay (Negative)
Saccharomyces cerevisiae Point Mutation Assay (Negative)
Saccharomyces cerevisiae Mitotic Crossover and Gene Conversion Assay (Negative)
Rat Hepatocyte DNA Repair Assay (Positive)

Thus, two of the eight tests were positive, but results of the following three *in vivo* test systems gave negative results:

Rat Hepatocyte DNA Repair Assay
Micronucleus Test (Mice)
Dominant Lethal Test (Mice)

Long-term carcinogenicity studies in mice and rats have been completed. After daily oral dosing for up to 2 years, there is no evidence that ciprofloxacin has any carcinogenic or tumorigenic effects in these species.

Pregnancy: Teratogenic Effects. Pregnancy Category C: Reproduction studies have been performed in rats and mice at doses up to 6 times the usual daily human dose and have revealed no evidence of impaired fertility or harm to the fetus due to ciprofloxacin. In rabbits, ciprofloxacin (30 and 100 mg/kg orally) produced gastrointestinal disturbances resulting in maternal weight loss and an increased incidence of abortion. No teratogenicity was observed at either dose. After intravenous administration of doses up to 20 mg/kg, no maternal toxicity was produced, and no embryotoxicity or teratogenicity was observed. There are, however, no adequate and well-controlled studies in pregnant women. Ciprofloxacin should be used during pregnancy only if the potential benefit justifies the potential risk to the fetus. (See WARNINGS.)

Nursing Mothers: Ciprofloxacin is excreted in human milk. Because of the potential for serious adverse reactions in infants nursing from mothers taking ciprofloxacin, a decision should be made either to discontinue nursing or to discontinue the drug, taking into account the importance of the drug to the mother.

Pediatric Use: Safety and effectiveness in children and adolescents less than 18 years of age have not been established. Ciprofloxacin causes arthropathy in juvenile animals. (See WARNINGS.)

ADVERSE REACTIONS

The most frequently reported events, without regard to drug relationship, among patients treated with intravenous ciprofloxacin were nausea, diarrhea, central nervous system disturbance, local iv site reactions, abnormalities of liver associated enzymes (hepatic enzymes) and eosinophilia. Headache, restlessness and rash were also noted in greater than 1% of patients treated with the most common doses of ciprofloxacin.

Local iv site reactions have been reported with the intravenous administration of ciprofloxacin. These reactions are more frequent if the infusion time is 30 minutes or less. These may appear as local skin reactions which resolve rapidly upon completion of the infusion. Subsequent intravenous administration is not contraindicated unless the reactions recur or worsen.

Additional events, without regard to drug relationship or route of administration, that occurred in 1% or less of ciprofloxacin courses are listed below:

GASTROINTESTINAL: ileus; jaundice; gastrointestinal bleeding; *C. difficile* associated diarrhea; pseudomembranous colitis; pancreatitis; hepatic necrosis; intestinal perforation; dyspepsia; epigastric or abdominal pain; vomiting; constipation; oral ulceration; oral candidiasis; mouth dryness; anorexia; dysphagia; flatulence.

CENTRAL NERVOUS SYSTEM: convulsive seizures, paranoia, toxic psychosis, depression, dysphasia, phobia, depersonalization, manic reaction, unresponsiveness, ataxia, confusion, hallucinations, dizziness, lightheadedness, paresthesia, anxiety, tremor, insomnia, nightmares, weakness, drowsiness, irritability, malaise, lethargy.

SKIN/HYPERSENSITIVITY: anaphylactic reactions; erythema multiforme/Stevens-Johnson syndrome; exfoliative dermatitis; toxic epidermal necrolysis; vasculitis; angioedema; edema of the lips, face, neck, conjunctivae, hands or lower extremities; purpura; fever; chills; flushing; pruritus; urticaria; cutaneous candidiasis; vesicles; increased perspiration; hyperpigmentation; erythema nodosum; photosensitivity.

Allergic reactions ranging from urticaria to anaphylactic reactions have been reported. (See WARNINGS.)

SPECIAL SENSES: decreased visual acuity, blurred vision, disturbed vision (flashing lights, change in color perception, overbrightness of lights, diplopia), eye pain, anosmia, hearing loss, tinnitus, nystagmus, a bad taste.

MUSCULOSKELETAL: joint pain; jaw, arm or back pain; joint stiffness; neck and chest pain; achiness; flare up of gout.

RENAL/UROGENITAL: renal failure, interstitial nephritis, hemorrhagic cystitis, renal calculi, frequent urination, acidosis, urethral bleeding, polyuria, urinary retention, gynecomastia, candiduria, vaginitis. Crystalluria, cylindruria, hematuria, and albuminuria have also been reported.

CARDIOVASCULAR: cardiovascular collapse, cardiopulmonary arrest, myocardial infarction, arrhythmia, tachycardia, palpitation, cerebral thrombosis, syncope, cardiac murmur, hypertension, hypotension, angina pectoris.

RESPIRATORY: respiratory arrest, pulmonary embolism, dyspnea, pulmonary edema, respiratory distress, pleural effusion hemoptysis, epistaxis, hiccough.

IV INFUSION SITE: thrombophlebitis, burning, pain, pruritus, paresthesia, erythema, swelling.

Also reported were agranulocytosis, prolongation of prothrombin time and possible exacerbation of myasthenia gravis.

Many of these events were described as only mild or moderate in severity, abated soon after the drug was discontinued and required no treatment.

In several instances, nausea, vomiting, tremor, irritability or palpitation were judged by investigators to be related to elevated serum levels of theophylline possibly as a result of drug interaction with ciprofloxacin.

Adverse Laboratory Changes: The most frequently reported changes in laboratory parameters with intravenous ciprofloxacin therapy, without regard to drug relationship, were:

Hepatic	—	Elevations of AST (SGOT), ALT (SGPT), alkaline phosphatase, LDH and serum billirubin.
Hematologic	—	Elevated eosinophil and platelet counts, decreased platelet counts, hemoglobin and/or hematocrit.
Renal	—	Elevations of serum creatinine, BUN, uric acid.
Other	—	Elevations of serum creatine phosphokinase, serum theophylline (in patients receiving theophylline concomitantly), blood glucose, and triglycerides.

Other changes occurring infrequently were: decreased leukocyte count, elevated atypical lymphocyte count, immature WBCs, elevated serum calcium, elevation of serum gamma-glutamyl transpeptidase (γ GT), decreased BUN, decreased uric acid, decreased total serum protein, decreased serum albumin, decreased serum potassium, elevated serum potassium, elevated serum cholesterol.

Other changes occurring rarely during administration of ciprofloxacin were: elevation of serum amylase, decrease of blood glucose, pancytopenia, leukocytosis, elevated sedimentation rate, change in serum phenytoin, decreased prothrombin time, hemolytic anemia, and bleeding diathesis.

OVERDOSAGE

In the event of acute overdosage, the patient should be carefully observed and given supportive treatment. Adequate hydration must be maintained. Only a small amount of ciprofloxacin (< 10%) is removed from the body after hemodialysis or peritoneal dialysis.

DOSAGE AND ADMINISTRATION

The recommended adult dosage for urinary tract infections of mild to moderate severity is 200 mg every 12 hours. For severe or complicated urinary tract infections the recommended dosage is 400 mg every 12 hours.

The recommended adult dosage for lower respiratory tract infections, skin and skin structure infections and bone and joint infections of mild to moderate severity is 400 mg every 12 hours.

The determination of dosage for any particular patient must take into consideration the severity and nature of the infection, the susceptibility of the causative organism, the integrity of the patient's host-defense mechanisms and the status of renal and hepatic function. [See table above.]

After dilution Cipro® I.V. should be administered by intravenous infusion over a period of 60 minutes.

The duration of treatment depends upon the severity of infection. Generally, ciprofloxacin should be continued for at least 2 days after the signs and symptoms of infection have disappeared. The usual duration is 7 to 14 days. Bone and joint infections may require treatment for 4 to 6 weeks or longer.

Cipro® (ciprofloxacin hydrochloride) Tablets for oral administration are available. Parenteral therapy may be changed to oral Cipro® tablets when the condition warrants, at the discretion of the physician. For complete dosage and administration information, see Cipro® tablet package insert.

Impaired Renal Function: The following table provides dosage guidelines for use in patients with renal impairment; however, monitoring of serum drug levels provides the most reliable basis for dosage adjustment.

RECOMMENDED STARTING AND MAINTENANCE DOSES FOR PATIENTS WITH IMPAIRED RENAL FUNCTION

Creatinine Clearance (mL/min)	Dosage
≥ 30	See usual dosage
5–29	200–400 mg q 18–24 hr

When only the serum creatinine concentration is known, the following formula may be used to estimate creatinine clearance.

$$\text{Men: Creatinine clearance (mL/min)} = \frac{\text{Weight (kg)} \times (140 - \text{age})}{72 \times \text{serum creatinine (mg/dL)}}$$

Women: 0.85 × the value calculated for men.

The serum creatinine should represent a steady state of renal function.

For patients with changing renal function or for patients with renal impairment and hepatic insufficiency, measurement of serum concentrations of ciprofloxacin will provide additional guidance for adjusting dosage.

INTRAVENOUS ADMINISTRATION

After dilution Cipro® I.V. should be administered by intravenous infusion over a period of 60 minutes. Slow infusion of a dilute solution into a large vein will minimize patient discomfort and reduce the risk of venous irritation.

PHARMACY BULK PACKAGE: The pharmacy bulk package is a single-entry container of a sterile preparation for parenteral use that contains many single doses. It contains ciprofloxacin as a 1% aqueous solution concentrate. The

contents are intended for use in a pharmacy admixture program and are restricted to the preparation of admixtures for intravenous infusion. **THE CLOSURE SHALL BE PENETRATED ONLY ONE TIME** with a suitable sterile transfer set or dispensing device which allows measured dispensing of the contents.

The pharmacy bulk package is to be used only in a suitable work area such as laminar flow hood or an equivalent clean air or compounding area. **THIS PREPARATION MUST BE DILUTED BEFORE USE.** The intravenous dose should be prepared by aseptically withdrawing the Cipro® I.V. concentrate from the pharmacy bulk package and diluting the appropriate volume with a suitable intravenous solution to a final concentration of 0.5–2 mg/mL (See COMPATIBILITY AND STABILITY). The resulting solution should be infused over a period of 60 minutes by direct infusion or through a Y-type intravenous set which may already be in place. If this method or the "piggyback" method of administration is used, it is advisable to discontinue the administration of any other intravenous solutions during the infusion of Cipro® I.V.

COMPATIBILITY AND STABILITY

Ciprofloxacin injection 1% (10 mg/mL), when diluted with the following intravenous solutions to concentrations of 0.5 to 2.0 mg/mL, is stable for up to 14 days at refrigerated or room temperature storage.

  0.9% Sodium Chloride Injection, USP

  5% Dextrose Injection, USP

If Cipro® I.V. is to be given with another drug, each drug should be given separately in accordance with the recommended dosage and route of administration for each drug.

HOW SUPPLIED

Cipro® I.V. (ciprofloxacin) is a clear, colorless to slightly yellowish solution supplied in the pharmacy bulk package as follows:

CONTAINER	SIZE	STRENGTH	NDC NUMBER
Pharmacy Bulk Package	120 mL	1200 mg, 1%	0026-8566-65

STORAGE

Store between 41–86°F (5–30°C).

Protect from light, avoid excessive heat, protect from freezing.

Cipro® I.V. (ciprofloxacin) is also available as follows:

CONTAINER	SIZE	STRENGTH	NDC NUMBER
Vial	20 mL	200 mg, 1%	0026-8562-20
	40 mL	400 mg, 1%	0026-8564-64
Flexible Container	100 mL 5% dextrose	200 mg, 0.2%	0026-8552-36
	200 mL 5% dextrose	400 mg, 0.2%	0026-8554-63

Ciprofloxacin is also available as Cipro® (ciprofloxacin HCl) Tablets 250, 500 and 750 mg.

ANIMAL PHARMACOLOGY

Ciprofloxacin and other quinolones have been shown to cause arthropathy in immature animals of most species tested. (See WARNINGS.) Damage of weight-bearing joints was observed in juvenile dogs and rats. In young beagles, 100 mg/kg ciprofloxacin given daily for 4 weeks caused degenerative articular changes of the knee joint. At 30 mg/kg, the effect on the joint was minimal. In a subsequent study in beagles, removal of weight-bearing on the joint reduced the lesions but did not totally prevent them.

Crystalluria, sometimes associated with secondary nephropathy, occurs in laboratory animals dosed with ciprofloxacin. This is primarily related to the reduced solubility of ciprofloxacin under alkaline conditions, which predominate in the urine of test animals; in man, crystalluria is rare since human urine is typically acidic. In rhesus monkeys, crystalluria without nephropathy has been noted after intravenous doses as low as 5 mg/kg. After 6 months of intravenous dosing at 10 mg/kg/day, no nephropathological changes were noted; however, nephropathy was observed after dosing at 20 mg/kg/day for the same duration.

In dogs, ciprofloxacin administered at 3 and 10 mg/kg by rapid intravenous injection (15 sec.) produces pronounced hypotensive effects. These effects are considered to be related to histamine release because they are partially antago-

nized by pyrilamine, an antihistamine. In rhesus monkeys, rapid intravenous injection also produces hypotension, but the effect in this species is inconsistent and less pronounced. In mice, concomitant administration of nonsteroidal anti-inflammatory drugs, such as fenbufen, phenylbutazone and indomethacin, with quinolones has been reported to enhance the CNS stimulatory effect of quinolones.

Ocular toxicity, seen with some related drugs, has not been observed in ciprofloxacin-treated animals.

  Miles Inc.
  Pharmaceutical Division
  400 Morgan Lane
  West Haven, CT 06516 USA

Caution: Federal (USA) Law prohibits dispensing without a prescription.

| PD100742 | 7/92 | BAY q 3939 |
| 5202-4-A-U.S.-1 | © 1992 Miles Inc. | 2084 |

DTIC–Dome®   ℞
(dacarbazine)
Sterile

WARNING

It is recommended that DTIC-Dome (dacarbazine) be administered under the supervision of a qualified physician experienced in the use of cancer chemotherapeutic agents.

1. Hemopoietic depression is the most common toxicity with DTIC-Dome (See Warnings).
2. Hepatic necrosis has been reported (See Warnings).
3. Studies have demonstrated this agent to have a carcinogenic and teratogenic effect when used in animals.
4. In treatment of each patient, the physician must weigh carefully the possibility of achieving therapeutic benefit against the risk of toxicity.

DESCRIPTION

DTIC-Dome Sterile (dacarbazine) is a colorless to an ivory colored solid which is light sensitive. Each vial contains 100 mg of dacarbazine, or 200 mg of dacarbazine (the active ingredient), anhydrous citric acid and mannitol. DTIC-Dome is reconstituted and administered intravenously (pH 3–4). DTIC-Dome is an anticancer agent. Chemically, DTIC-Dome is 5-(3,3-dimethyl-1-triazeno)-imidazole-4-carboxamide (DTIC) with the following structural formula:

$$(CH_3)_2N-N-N \qquad\qquad$$

$C_6H_{10}N_6O$

CLINICAL PHARMACOLOGY

After intravenous administration of DTIC-Dome, the volume of distribution exceeds total body water content suggesting localization in some body tissue, probably the liver. Its disappearance from the plasma is biphasic with initial half-life of 19 minutes and a terminal half-life of 5 hours.[1] In a patient with renal and hepatic dysfunctions, the half-lives were lengthened to 55 minutes and 7.2 hours.[1] The average cumulative excretion of unchanged DTIC in the urine is 40% of the injected dose in 6 hours.[1] DTIC is subject to renal tubular secretion rather than glomerular filtration. At therapeutic concentrations DTIC is not appreciably bound to human plasma protein.

In man, DTIC is extensively degraded. Besides unchanged DTIC, 5-aminoimidazole -4 carboxamide (AIC) is a major metabolite of DTIC excreted in the urine. AIC is not derived endogenously but from the injected DTIC, because the administration of radioactive DTIC labeled with ^{14}C in the imidazole portion of the molecule (DTIC-2-^{14}C) gives rise to AIC-2-^{14}C.[1]

Although the exact mechanism of action of DTIC-Dome is not known, three hypotheses have been offered:

Continued on next page

Miles—Cont.

1. inhibition of DNA synthesis by acting as a purine analog
2. action as an alkylating agent
3. interaction with SH groups

INDICATIONS AND USAGE

DTIC-Dome is indicated in the treatment of metastatic malignant melanoma. In addition, DTIC-Dome is also indicated for Hodgkin's disease as a secondary-line therapy when used in combination with other effective agents.

CONTRAINDICATIONS

DTIC-Dome is contraindicated in patients who have demonstrated a hypersensitivity to it in the past.

WARNINGS

Hemopoietic depression is the most common toxicity with DTIC-Dome and involves primarily the leukocytes and platelets, although, anemia may sometimes occur. Leukopenia and thrombocypenia may be severe enough to cause death. The possible bone marrow depression requires careful monitoring of white blood cells, red blood cells, and platelet levels. Hemopioetic toxicity may warrant temporary suspension or cessation of therapy with DTIC-Dome.

Hepatic toxicity accompanied by hepatic vein thrombosis and hepatocellular necrosis resulting in death, has been reported. The incidence of such reactions has been low; approximately 0.01% of patients treated. This toxicity has been observed mostly when DTIC-Dome has been administered concomitantly with other anti-neoplastic drugs; however, it has also been reported in some patients treated with DTIC-Dome alone.

Anaphylaxis can occur following the administration of DTIC-Dome.

PRECAUTIONS

Hospitalization is not always necessary but adequate laboratory study capability must be available. Extravasation of the drug subcutaneously during intravenous administration may result in tissue damage and severe pain. Local pain, burning sensation, and irritation at the site of injection may be relieved by locally applied hot packs.

Carcinogenicity of DTIC was studied in rats and mice. Proliferative endocardial lesions, including fibrosarcomas and sarcomas were induced by DTIC in rats. In mice, administration of DTIC resulted in the induction of angiosarcomas of the spleen.

Pregnancy Category C. DTIC-Dome has been shown to be teratogenic in rats when given in doses 20 times the human daily dose on day 12 of gestation. DTIC when administered in 10 times the human daily dose to male rats (twice weekly for 9 weeks) did not affect the male libido, although female rats mated to male rats had higher incidence of resorptions than controls. In rabbits, DTIC daily dose 7 times the human daily dose given on Days 6–15 of gestation resulted in fetal skeletal anomalies. There are no adequate and well controlled studies in pregnant women. DTIC-Dome should be used during pregnancy only if the potential benefit justifies the potential risk to the fetus.

It is not known whether this drug is excreted in human milk. Because many drugs are excreted in human milk and because of the potential for tumorigenicity shown for DTIC-Dome in animal studies, a decision should be made whether to discontinue nursing or to discontinue the drug, taking into account the importance of the drug to the mother.

ADVERSE REACTIONS

Symptoms of anorexia, nausea, and vomiting are the most frequently noted of all toxic reactions. Over 90% of patients are affected with the initial few doses. The vomiting lasts 1–12 hours and is incompletely and unpredictably palliated with phenobarbital and/or prochlorperazine. Rarely, intractable nausea and vomiting have necessitated discontinuance of therapy with DTIC-Dome. Rarely, DTIC-Dome has caused diarrhea. Some helpful suggestions include restricting the patient's oral intake of food for 4–6 hours prior to treatment. The rapid toleration of these symptoms suggests that a central nervous system mechanism may be involved, and usually these symptoms subside after the first 1 or 2 days.

There are a number of minor toxicities that are infrequently noted. Patients have experienced an influenza-like syndrome of fever to 39°C, myalgias and malaise. These symptoms occur usually after large single doses, may last for several days, and they may occur with successive treatments.

Alopecia has been noted as has facial flushing and facial paresthesia. There have been few reports of significant liver or renal function test abnormalities in man. However, these abnormalities have been observed more frequently in animal studies.

Erythematous and urticarial rashes have been observed infrequently after administration of DTIC-Dome. Rarely, photosensitivity reactions may occur.

OVERDOSAGE

Give supportive treatment and monitor blood cell counts.

DOSAGE AND ADMINISTRATION

Malignant Melanoma: The recommended dosage is 2 to 4.5mg/kg/day for 10 days. Treatment may be repeated at 4 week intervals.[2]

An alternate recommended dosage is 250mg/square meter body surface/day I.V. for 5 days. Treatment may be repeated every 3 weeks.[3,4]

Hodgkin's Disease: The recommended dosage of DTIC-Dome in the treatment of Hodgkin's Disease is 150mg/square meter body surface/day for 5 days, in combination with other effective drugs. Treatment may be repeated every 4 weeks.[5] An alternative recommended dosage is 375mg/square meter body surface on day 1, in combination with other effective drugs, to be repeated every 15 days.[6]

DTIC-Dome (dacarbazine) 100mg/vial and 200mg/vial are reconstituted with 9.9 mL and 19.7 mL, respectively, of Sterile Water for Injection, U.S.P. The resulting solution contains 10mg/mL of dacarbazine having a pH of 3.0 to 4.0. The calculated dose of the resulting solution is drawn into a syringe and administered *only* intravenously.

The reconstituted solution may be further diluted with 5% dextrose injection, U.S.P. or sodium chloride injection, U.S.P. and administered as an intravenous infusion.

After reconstitution and prior to use, the solution in the vial may be stored at 4°C for up to 72 hours or at normal room conditions (temperature and light) for up to 8 hours. If the reconstituted solution is further diluted in 5% dextrose, injection, U.S.P. or sodium chloride injection, U.S.P., the resulting solution may be stored at 4°C for up to 24 hours or at normal room conditions for up to 8 hours.

Procedures for proper handling and disposal of anticancer drugs should be considered. Several guidelines on this subject have been published.[7–12] There is no general agreement that all of the procedures recommended in the guidelines are necessary or appropriate.

HOW SUPPLIED

10 mL vials containing 100 mg or 20 mL vials containing 200 mg of DTIC-Dome as sterile dacarbazine in boxes of 12. Store in a refrigerator 2°C to 8°C (36°F to 46°F).

REFERENCES

1. Loo, T.J., *et al.:* Mechanism of action and pharmacology studies with DTIC (NSC-45388). Cancer Treatment Reports 60: 149–152, 1976.
2. Nathanson, L., *et al.:* Characteristics of prognosis and response to an imidazole carboxamide in malignant melanoma. Clinical Pharmacology and Therapeutics 12: 955–962, 1971.
3. Costanza, M.E., *et al.:* Therapy of malignant melanoma with an imidazole carboxamide and bischloroethyl nitrosourea. Cancer 30: 1457–1461, 1972.
4. Luce, J.K., *et al.:* Clinical trials with the antitumor agent 5-(3, 3-dimethyl-l-triazeno) imidazole-4-carboxamide (NSC-45388). Cancer Chemotherapy Reports 54: 119–124, 1970.
5. Bonadonna, G., *et al.:* Combined Chemotherapy (MOPP or ABVD)—radiotherapy approach in advanced Hodgkin's disease. Cancer Treatment Reports 61: 769–777, 1977.
6. Santoro, A., and Bonadonna, G.: Prolonged disease-free survival in MOPP-resistant Hodgkin's disease after treatment with adriamycin, bleomycin, vinblastine and decarbazine (ABVD). Cancer Chemotherapy Pharmacol. 2: 101–105, 1979.
7. Recommendations for the Safe Handling of Parenteral Antineoplastic Drugs. NIH Publication No. 83-2621. For sale by the Superintendent of Documents, U.S. Government Printing Office, Washington, D.C. 20402.
8. AMA Council Report. Guidelines for Handling Parenteral Antineoplastics. JAMA, March 15, 1985.
9. National Study Commission on Cytotoxic Exposure—Recommendations for Handling Cytotoxic Agents. Available from Louis P. Jeffrey, Sc. D., Director of Pharmacy Services, Rhode Island Hospital, 593 Eddy Street, Providence, Rhode Island 02902.
10. Clinical Oncological Society of Australia: Guidelines and recommendations for safe handling of antineoplastic agents. Med. J. Australia 1: 426–428, 1983.
11. Jones, R.B., *et al.:* Safe handling of chemotherapeutic agents: A report from the Mount Sinai Medical Center. Ca-A Cancer Journal for Clinicians Sept./Oct. 258–263, 1983.
12. American Society of Hospital Pharmacists technical assistance bulletin on handling cytotoxic drugs in hospitals. Am. J. Hosp. Pharm. 42: 131–137, 1985.

Manufactured by:
Ben Venue Laboratories
Bedford, Ohio 44146

Distributed by:
Miles Inc.
Pharmaceutical Division
400 Morgan Lane
West Haven, CT 06516 USA
PD100688-0561 ©1988 Miles Inc. 6/88
Made in USA

LITHANE® ℞

(lithium carbonate)
TABLETS
For Control of Manic Episodes in Manic-Depressive Psychosis

Warning

> Lithium toxicity is closely related to serum lithium levels, and can occur at doses close to therapeutic levels. Facilities for prompt and accurate serum lithium determinations should be available before initiating therapy.

DESCRIPTION

Lithium carbonate is a white, light, alkaline powder with molecular formula Li_2CO_3 and molecular weight 73.89. Lithium is an element of the alkali-metal group with atomic number 3, atomic weight 6.94, and an emission line at 671 nm on the flame photometer.

Inert ingredients are: Blue 1 Lake; dibasic calcium phosphate; magnesium stearate; polyethylene glycol; sodium lauryl sulfate; starch; Yellow 5 Lake.

ACTIONS

Preclinical studies have shown that lithium alters sodium transport in nerve and muscle cells and effects a shift toward intraneuronal metabolism of catecholamines, but the specific biochemical mechanism of lithium action in mania is unknown.

INDICATIONS

Lithium carbonate is indicated in the treatment of manic episodes of manic-depressive illness. Maintenance therapy prevents or diminishes the intensity of subsequent episodes in those manic-depressive patients with a history of mania.

Typical symptoms of mania include pressure of speech, motor hyperactivity, reduced need for sleep, flight of ideas, grandiosity, elation, poor judgment, aggressiveness, and possibly hostility. When given to a patient experiencing a manic episode, lithium may produce a normalization of symptomatology within 1 to 3 weeks.

WARNINGS

Lithium should generally not be given to patients with significant renal or cardiovascular disease, severe debilitation or dehydration, or sodium depletion, and to patients receiving diuretics, since the risk of lithium toxicity is very high in such patients. If the psychiatric indication is life-threatening, and if such a patient fails to respond to other measures, lithium treatment may be undertaken with extreme caution, including daily serum lithium determinations and adjustment to the usually low doses ordinarily tolerated by these individuals. In such instances, hospitalization is a necessity.

Chronic lithium therapy may be associated with diminution of renal concentrating ability, occasionally presenting as nephrogenic diabetes insipidus, with polyuria and polydipsia. Such patients should be carefully managed to avoid dehydration with resulting lithium retention and toxicity. This condition is usually reversible when lithium is discontinued.

Morphologic changes with glomerular and interstitial fibrosis and nephron atrophy have been reported in patients on chronic lithium therapy. Morphologic changes have also been seen in manic-depressive patients never exposed to lithium. The relationship between renal functional and morphologic changes and their association with lithium therapy have not been established.

When kidney function is assessed, for baseline data prior to starting lithium therapy or thereafter, routine urinalysis and other tests may be used to evaluate tubular function (e.g. urine specific gravity or osmolality following a period of water deprivation, or 24 hour urine volume) and glomerular function (e.g. serum creatinine or creatinine clearance). During lithium therapy, progressive or sudden changes in renal function, even within the normal range, indicate the need for reevaluation of treatment.

Lithium therapy has been reported in some cases to be associated with morphologic changes in the kidneys. The relationship between such changes and renal function has not been established.

An encephalopathic syndrome (characterized by weakness, lethargy, fever, tremulousness and confusion, extrapyramidal symptoms, leukocytosis, elevated serum enzymes, BUN and FBS) followed by irreversible brain damage has occurred in a few patients treated with lithium plus haloperidol. A causal relationship between these events and the concomitant administration of lithium and haloperidol has not been

established; however, patients receiving such combined therapy should be monitored closely for early evidence of neurologic toxicity and treatment discontinued promptly if such signs appear. The possibility of similar adverse interactions with other antipsychotic medication exists.

Lithium toxicity is closely related to serum lithium levels, and can occur at doses close to therapeutic levels (see DOSAGE AND ADMINISTRATION).

Outpatients and their families should be warned that the patient must discontinue lithium carbonate therapy and contact his physician if such clinical signs of lithium toxicity as diarrhea, vomiting, tremor, mild ataxia, drowsiness, or muscular weakness occur.

Lithium carbonate may impair mental and/or physical abilities. Caution patients about activities requiring alertness (e.g., operating vehicles or machinery).

Lithium may prolong the effects of neuromuscular blocking agents. Therefore, neuromuscular blocking agents should be given with caution to patients receiving lithium.

Usage in Pregnancy: Adverse effects on nidation in rats, embryo viability in mice, and metabolism *in vitro* of rat testis and human spermatozoa have been attributed to lithium, as have teratogenicity in submammalian species and cleft palates in mice. Studies in rats, rabbits, and monkeys have shown no evidence of lithium-induced teratology.

In humans, lithium carbonate may cause fetal harm when administered to a pregnant woman. Data from lithium birth registries suggest an increase in cardiac and other anomalies, especially Ebstein' anomaly. If this drug is used during pregnancy, or if a patient becomes pregnant while taking this drug, the patient should be apprised of the potential hazard to the fetus.

There are lithium birth registries in the United States and elsewhere; however there is at the present time insufficient data to determine the effects of lithium carbonate on human fetuses. Therefore, at this point, lithium should not be used in pregnancy, especially the first trimester, unless in the opinion of the physician, the potential benefits outweigh the possible hazards.

Usage in Nursing Mothers: Lithium is excreted in human milk. Nursing should not be undertaken during lithium therapy except in rare and unusual circumstances where, in the view of the physician, the potential benefits to the mother outweigh possible hazards to the child.

Usage in Children: Since information regarding the safety and effectiveness of lithium carbonate in children under 12 years of age is not available, its use in such patients is not recommended at this time. There has been a report of a transient syndrome of acute dystonia and hyperreflexia occurring in a 15 kg child who ingested 300 mg of lithium carbonate.

PRECAUTIONS

The ability to tolerate lithium is greater during the acute manic phase and decreases when manic symptoms subside (see DOSAGE AND ADMINISTRATION).

Drug Interactions: Caution should be used when lithium and diuretics or angiotensin converting enzyme (ACE) inhibitors are used concomitantly because sodium loss may reduce the renal clearance of lithium and increase serum lithium levels with risk of lithium toxicity. When such combinations are used, the lithium dosage may need to be decreased, and more frequent monitoring of lithium plasma levels is recommended.

The distribution space of lithium approximates that of total body water. Lithium is primarily excreted in urine with insignificant excretion in feces. Renal excretion of lithium is proportional to its plasma concentration. The half-life of elimination of lithium is approximately 24 hours. Lithium decreases sodium reabsorption by the renal tubules which could lead to sodium depletion. Therefore, it is essential for the patient to maintain a normal diet, including salt, and an adequate fluid intake (2500–3000 ml) at least during the initial stabilization period. Decreased tolerance to lithium has been reported to ensue from protracted sweating or diarrhea and, if such occur, supplemental fluid and salt should be administered.

In addition to sweating and diarrhea, concomitant infection with elevated temperatures may also necessitate a temporary reduction or cessation of medication.

Previously existing underlying thyroid disorders do not necessarily constitute a contraindication to lithium treatment; where hypothyroidism exists, careful monitoring of thyroid function during lithium stabilization and maintenance allows for correction of changing thyroid parameters, if any; where hypothroidism occurs during lithium stabilization and maintenance, supplemental thyroid treatment may be used.

This product contains FD&C Yellow No. 5 (tartrazine) which may cause allergic-type reactions (including bronchial asthma) in certain susceptible individuals. Although the over-all incidence of FD&C Yellow No. 5 (tartrazine) sensitivity in the general population is low, it is frequently seen in patients who also have aspirin hypersensitivity.

Indomethacin and piroxican has been reported to increase significantly, steady state plasma lithium levels. In some cases lithium toxicity has resulted from such interactions. There is also some evidence that other nonsteroidal, anti-inflammatory agents may have a similar effect. When such combinations are used, increased plasma lithium level monitoring is recommended.

ADVERSE REACTIONS

Adverse reactions are seldom encountered at serum lithium levels below 1.5 mEq./l., except in the occasional patient sensitive to lithium. Mild to moderate toxic reactions may occur at levels from 1.5–2.5 mEq./l., and moderate to severe reactions may be seen at levels from 2.0–2.5 mEq./l., depending upon individual response to the drug.

Fine hand tremor, polyuria, and mild thirst may occur during initial therapy for the acute manic phase, and may persist throughout treatment. Transient and mild nausea and general discomfort may also appear during the first few days of lithium administration.

These side effects are an inconvenience rather than a disabling condition, and usually subside with continued treatment or a temporary reduction or cessation of dosage. If persistent, a cessation of dosage is indicated.

Diarrhea, vomiting, drowsiness, muscular weakness, and lack of coordination may be early signs of lithium intoxication, and can occur at lithium levels below 2.0 mEq./l. At higher lcvels, giddiness, ataxia, blurred vision, tinnitus, and a large output of dilute urine may be seen. Serum lithium levels above 3.0 mEq./l. may produce a complex clinical picture involving multiple organs and organ systems. Serum lithium levels should not be permitted to exceed 2.0 mEq./l, during the acute treatment phase.

The following reactions have been reported and appear to be related to serum lithium levels, including levels within the therapeutic range:

Neurological: Cases of pseudotumor cerebri (increased intracranial pressure and papilledema) have been reported with lithium use. If undetected, this condition may result in enlargement of the blind spot, constriction of visual fields and eventual blindness due to optic atrophy. Lithium should be discontinued, if clinically possible, if this syndrome occurs.

Neuromuscular: tremor, muscle hyperirritability (fasciculations, twitching, clonic movements of whole limbs), ataxia, choreo-athetotic movements, hyperactive deep tendon reflexes.

Central Nervous System: blackout spells, epileptiform seizures, slurred speech, dizziness, vertigo, incontinence of urine or feces, somnolence, psychomotor retardation, restlessness, confusion stupor, coma, acute dystonia, and downbeat nystagmus.

Cardiovascular: cardiac arrhythmia, hypotension, peripheral circulatory collapse.

Gastrointestinal: anorexia, nausea, vomiting, diarrhea.

Genitourinary: albuminuria, oliguria, polyuria, glycosuria.

Dermatologic: drying and thinning of hair, anesthesia of skin, chronic folliculitis, xerosis cutis, alopecia, and exacerbation of psoriasis.

Autonomic Nervous System: blurred vision, dry mouth.

Thyroid Abnormalities: Euthyroid goiter and/or hypothyroidism (including myxedema) accompanied by lower T_3 and T_4. I^{131} iodine uptake may be elevated. (See **Precautions.**) Paradoxically, rare cases of hyperthyroidism have been reported.

EEG. Changes: diffuse slowing, widening of frequency spectrum, potentiation and disorganization of background rhythm.

EKG. Changes: reversible flattening, isoelectricity or inversion of T-waves.

Miscellaneous: fatigue, lethargy, tendency to sleep, dehydration, weight loss, transient scotomata.

Miscellaneous reactions unrelated to dosage are: transient electroencephalographic and electrocardiographic changes, leucocytosis, headache, diffuse non-toxic goiter with or without hypothyroidism, transient hyperglycemia, generalized pruritus with or without rash, cutaneous ulcers, albuminuria, worsening of organic brain syndromes, excessive weight gain, edematous swelling of ankles or wrists, and thirst or polyuria, sometimes resembling diabetes insipidus, and metallic taste. A single report has been received of the development of painful discoloration of fingers and toes and coldness of the extremities within one day of the starting of treatment of lithium. The mechanism through which these symptoms (resembling Raynaud's Syndrome) developed is not known. Recovery followed discontinuance.

DOSAGE AND ADMINISTRATION

Acute Mania: Optimal patient response to lithium carbonate usually can be established and maintained with 600 mg t.i.d. Such doses will normally produce an effective serum lithium level ranging between 1.0 and 1.5 mEq./l. Dosage must be individualized according to serum levels and clinical response. Regular monitoring of the patient's clinical state and of serum lithium levels is necessary. Serum levels should be determined twice per week during the acute phase, and until the serum level and clinical condition of the patient have been stabilized.

Long term Control: The desirable lithium levels are 0.6 to 1.2 mEq./l. Dosage will vary from one individual to another, but usually 300 mg t.i.d. or q.i.d. will maintain this level. Serum lithium levels in uncomplicated cases receiving maintenance therapy during remission should be monitored at least every two months.

Patients abnormally sensitive to lithium may exhibit toxic signs at serum levels of 1.0 to 1.5 mEq./l. Elderly patients often respond to reduced dosage, and may exhibit signs of toxicity at serum levels ordinarily tolerated by other patients.

N.B.: Blood samples for serum lithium determinations should be drawn immediately prior to the next dose when lithium concentrations are relatively stable (i.e., 8–12 hours after the previous dose). Total reliance must not be placed on serum levels alone. Accurate patient evaluation requires both clinical and laboratory analysis.

OVERDOSAGE

The toxic levels for lithium are close to the therapeutic levels. It is therefore important that patients and their families be cautioned to watch for early toxic symptoms and to discontinue the drug and inform the physician should they occur. Toxic symptoms are listed in detail under ADVERSE REACTIONS.

Treatment: No specific antidote for lithium poisoning is known. Early symptoms of lithium toxicity can usually be treated by reduction or cessation of dosage of the drug and resumption of the treatment at a lower dose after 24 to 48 hours. In severe cases of lithium poisoning, the first and foremost goal of treatment consists of elimination of this ion from the organism.

Treatment is essentially the same as that used in barbiturate poisoning: 1) lavage, 2) correction of fluid and electrolyte imbalance, and 3) regulation of kidney functioning. Urea, mannitol, and aminophylline all produce significant increases in lithium excretion. Hemodialysis is an effective and rapid means of removing the ion from the severely toxic patient. Infection prophylaxis, regular chest X-rays, and preservation of adequate respiration are essential.

HOW SUPPLIED

Lithane (lithium carbonate) is available as scored tablets containing 300 mg of lithium carbonate in bottles of 100 (NDC 0026-2951-51), and 1000 (NDC 0026-2951-54).

Manufactured for
Miles Pharmaceuticals
Divison of Miles Laboratories, Inc.
West Haven, Connecticut 06516 USA
by Pfizer, Inc., New York, N.Y. 10017
PD 100733 Revised July 1991

Shown in Product Identification Section, page 420

MEZLIN® ℞

Sterile mezlocillin sodium
for intravenous or intramuscular use.
BAYPEN®

DESCRIPTION

MEZLIN® (sterile mezlocillin sodium) is a semisynthetic broad spectrum penicillin antibiotic for parenteral administration. It is the monohydrate sodium salt of 6-{D-2 [3-(methyl-sulfonyl) -2- OXO-imidazolidine -1- carboxamido] - 2-phenyl acetamido} penicillanic acid.

Structural Formula:

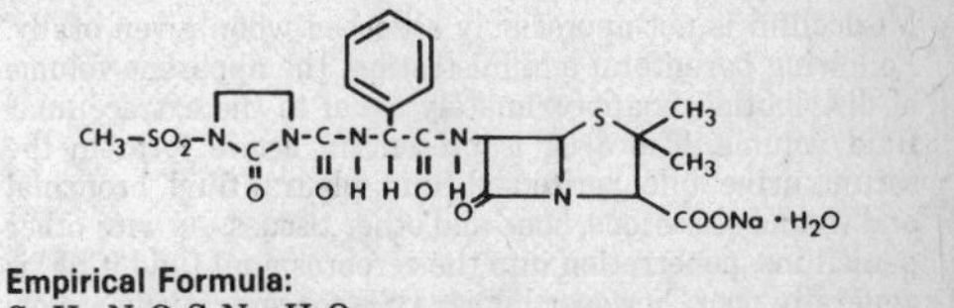

Empirical Formula:
$C_{21}H_{24}N_5O_8S_2Na \cdot H_2O$

MEZLIN® has a molecular weight of 579.6 and contains 42.6 mg (1.85 mEq) of sodium per one gram of mezlocillin activity. The dosage form is supplied as a sterile white to pale yellow crystalline powder, which is freely soluble in water. When reconstituted, solutions of MEZLIN® are clear and range from colorless to pale yellow with a pH of 4.5 to 8.0.

CLINICAL PHARMACOLOGY

Intravenous Administration. In healthy adult volunteers, mean serum levels of mezlocillin 5 minutes after a 5-minute intravenous injection of 1g, 2g, or 5g are 100, 253, or 411 mcg/mL, respectively. Serum levels, as noted below, lack dose proportionality: [See table at top of next page.]

Continued on next page

Miles—Cont.

MEZLOCILLIN SERUM LEVELS IN ADULTS (mcg/mL) 5 MIN. IV INJECTION

DOSE	0	5 min.	10 min.	20 min.	30 min.	1 hr.	2 hr.	3 hr.	4 hr.	6 hr.	8 hr.
1g	149 (132–185)	100 (64–143)	66 (47–87)	50 (31–87)	40 (22–83)	18 (8–31)	5.3 (3.3–7.7)	2.5 (1.7–3.7)	1.7 (0.7–2.8)	0.5 (0–1.2)	0.1 (0–0.2)
2g	314 (207–362)	253 (161–364)	161 (113–214)	117 (76–174)	82 (55–112)	56 (23–88)	20 (7.5–32)	11 (3.8–16)	4.4 (1.6–8.7)	1.5 (0.5–2.6)	0.6 (0.1–1.4)
5g	547 (268–854)	411 (199–597)	357 (246–456)	250 (203–353)	226 (190–333)	131 (104–193)	76 (59–104)	31 (20–40)	13 (6.4–17)	4.6 (2.1–9.4)	1.9 (1.1–3.6)

MEZLOCILLIN SERUM LEVELS IN ADULTS (mcg/mL) 2–5 MIN. IV INJECTION

DOSE	0	15 min.	30 min.	45 min.	1 hr.	2 hr.	3 hr.	4 hr.	6 hr.
4g	—	254 (155–400)	163 (99–260)	122 (78–215)	93 (67–133)	47 (22–96)	20 (8–45)	9.1 (6–13)	8.4 (5–17)

Fifteen minutes after a 4g intravenous injection (2-5 min.), the concentration in serum is 254 mcg/mL; 1 hour and 4 hours later levels are 93 mcg/mL and 9.1 mcg/mL, respectively: [See second table above.]

After an intravenous infusion (15 min.) of 3g, mean levels 15 minutes after dosing are 269 mcg/mL (170-280).

A 30-minute intravenous infusion of 3g produces mean peak concentrations of 263 mcg/mL; 1 hour and 4 hours later the concentrations are 57 mcg/mL and 4.4 mcg/mL, respectively: [See table below.]

Following intravenous infusion (2 hr.) of a 3g dose of mezlocillin every 4 hours for 7 days, mean peak serum concentrations are higher than 100 mcg/mL, and levels above 50 mcg/mL are maintained throughout dosing.

Intramuscular Administration. MEZLIN® is rapidly absorbed after intramuscular injection. In healthy volunteers, the mean peak serum concentration occurs approximately 45 minutes after a single dose of 1g and is about 15 mcg/mL. The oral administration of 1g probenecid before injection produces an increase in mezlocillin serum levels of about 50%. After repetitive intramuscular doses of 1g mezlocillin every 6 hours, peak levels in the serum generally range between 35 and 45 mcg/mL. The relationship between the pharmacokinetics of intramuscular and intravenous dosing has not yet been clearly established.

General. As with other penicillins, mezlocillin is excreted primarily by glomerular filtration and tubular secretion. The rate of elimination is dose dependent and related to the degree of renal functional impairment. In patients with normal renal function, approximately 55% of the administered dose is recovered from the urine within the first 6 hours after dosing. Two hours after an intravenous injection of 2g, concentrations of active drug in urine generally exceed 4000 mcg/mL. By 4-6 hours after injection, concentrations usually decline to a range of about 50 to 200 mcg/mL. The serum elimination half-life of mezlocillin after intravenous dosing is approximately 55 minutes.

In patients with reduced renal function, the half-life is only slightly prolonged. Dosage adjustments are usually not necessary except in patients with severe renal impairment. (See Dosage and Administration.) As with other penicillins, mezlocillin is metabolized only slightly; less than 10% of the drug excreted in the urine is in the form of the penicilloate or penilloate. The drug is readily removed from the serum by hemodialysis and, to a lesser extent, by peritoneal dialysis. Up to 26% of a dose of mezlocillin is recovered from the bile of patients with normal liver function. Following intravenous doses of 2g to 5g, concentrations of active drug in bile generally range from 500 to 2500 mcg/mL. The biliary excretion of mezlocillin is reduced in patients with common bile duct obstruction.

Mezlocillin is not appreciably absorbed when given orally. Following parenteral administration, the apparent volume of distribution is approximately equal to the extracellular fluid volume. The drug is present in active form in the serum, urine, bile, peritoneal fluid, pleural fluid, bronchial and wound secretions, bone and other tissues. As with other penicillins, penetration into the cerebrospinal fluid (CSF) is generally poor, however higher CSF concentrations are obtained in the presence of meningeal inflammation.

Protein binding studies indicate that the degree of mezlocillin binding is low (16-42%) and depends upon testing methods and concentrations of drug studied.

Microbiology

Mezlocillin is a bactericidal antibiotic which acts by interfering with synthesis of cell wall components. It is active against a variety of gram-negative and gram-positive bacteria, including aerobic and anaerobic strains. Mezlocillin is usually active *in vitro* against most strains of the following organisms:

Gram-negative bacteria

Escherichia coli

Proteus mirabilis

Proteus vulgaris

Morganella morganii (formerly *P. morganii*)

Providencia rettgeri (formerly *Proteus rettgeri*)

Providencia stuartii

Citrobacter species*

Klebsiella species (including *K. pneumoniae*)

Enterobacter species

Shigella species*

Pseudomonas aeruginosa (and other species)

Haemophilus influenzae

Haemophilus parainfluenzae

Neisseria species

Many strains of *Serratia*, *Salmonella**, and *Acinetobacter** are also susceptible.

Gram-positive bacteria

Staphylococcus aureus (non-penicillinase producing strains)

Beta-hemolytic *streptococci* (Groups A and B)

Streptococcus pneumoniae (formerly *Diplococcus Pneumoniae*)

Streptococcus faecalis (enterococcus)

Anaerobic Organisms

Peptococcus species

Peptostreptococcus species

Clostridium species*

Bacteroides species (including *B. fragilis* group)

Fusobacterium species*

Veillonella species*

Eubacterium species*

*Mezlocillin has been shown to be active *in vitro* against these organisms, however clinical efficacy has not yet been established.

Noteworthy is mezlocillin's broadened spectrum of *in vitro* activity against important pathogenic aerobic gram-negative bacteria, including strains of *Pseudomonas*, *Klebsiella*, *Enterobacter*, *Serratia*, *Proteus*, *Escherichia* and *Haemophilus*, as well as *Bacteroides* and other anaerobes; and its excellent inhibitory effect against gram-positive organisms including *Streptococcus faecalis* (enterococcus). It is inactive against penicillinase-producing strains of *Staphylococcus aureus*.

In vitro studies have shown that mezlocillin combined with an aminoglycoside (e.g., gentamicin, tobramycin, amikacin, sisomicin) acts synergistically against strains of *Streptococcus faecalis* and *Pseudomonas aeruginosa*. In some instances, this combination also acts synergistically *in vitro* against other gram-negative bacteria such as *Serratia*, *Klebsiella* and *Acinetobacter* species.

Mezlocillin is slightly more active when tested at alkaline pH and, as with other penicillins, has reduced activity when tested *in vitro* with increasing inoculum. The minimum bactericidal concentration (MBC) generally exceeds the minimum inhibitory concentration (MIC) by a factor of 2 or 3. Resistance to mezlocillin *in vitro* develops slowly (multiple step mutation). Some strains of *Pseudomonas aeruginosa* have developed resistance fairly rapidly. Mezlocillin is not stable in the presence of penicillinase and strains of *Staphylococcus aureus* resistant to penicillin are also resistant to mezlocillin.

Susceptibility Tests

Quantitative methods that require measurement of zone diameters give good estimates of bacterial susceptibility. One such procedure* has been recommended for use with discs to test susceptibility to antimicrobials. When the causative organism is tested by the Kirby-Bauer method of disc susceptibility, a 75 mcg mezlocillin disc should give a zone of 18 mm or greater to indicate susceptibility. Zone sizes of 14 mm or less indicate resistance. Zone sizes of 15 to 17 mm indicate intermediate susceptibility. Susceptibile strains of *Haemophilus* and *Neisseria* species give zones of ≥ 29 mm, resistant strains ≤ 28 mm. With this procedure, a report from the laboratory of "Susceptibile" indicates that the infecting organism is likely to respond to therapy. A report of "Resistant" indicates that the infecting organism is not likely to respond to therapy; other therapy should be selected. A report of "Intermediate Susceptibility" suggests that the organism may be susceptible if the infection is confined to tissues and fluids (e.g., urine), in which high antibiotic levels are attained. The mezlocillin disc should be used for testing susceptibility to mezlocillin. In certain conditions, it may be desirable to do additional susceptibility testing by broth or agar dilution techniques. Dilution methods, preferably the agar plate dilution procedure, are most accurate for susceptibility testing of obligate anaerobes. *Enterobacteriaceae*, *Pseudomonas* species and *Acinetobacter* species are considered susceptible if the MIC of mezlocillin is no greater than 64 mcg/mL and are considered resistant if the MIC is greater than 128 mcg/mL. *Haemophilus* species and *Neisseria* species are considered susceptible if the MIC of mezlocillin is less than or equal to 1 mcg/mL. Mezlocillin standard is available for broth or agar dilution studies.

*Bauer, A.W., Kirby, W.M., Sherris, J.C., and Turck, M.: Antibiotic Testing by a Standardized Single Disc Method, Am. J. Clin. Pathol., 45:493, 1966; Standardized Disc Susceptibility Test, FEDERAL REGISTER, 39:19182–19184, 1974.

INDICATIONS AND USAGE

MEZLIN® is indicated for the treatment of serious infections caused by susceptible strains of the designated microorganisms in the conditions listed below:

LOWER RESPIRATORY TRACT INFECTIONS including pneumonia and lung abscess caused by *Haemophilus influenzae*, *Klebsiella* species including *K. pneumoniae*, *Proteus mirabilis*, *Pseudomonas* species including *P. aeruginosa*, *E. coli*, and *Bacteroides* species including *B. fragilis*.

INTRA-ABDOMINAL INFECTIONS including acute cholecystitis, cholangitis, peritonitis, hepatic abscess and intra-abdominal abscess caused by susceptible *E. coli*, *Proteus mirabilis*, *Klebsiella* species, *Pseudomonas* species, *S. faecalis* (enterococcus), *Bacteroides* species, *Peptococcus* species, and *Peptostreptococcus* species.

URINARY TRACT INFECTIONS caused by susceptible *E. coli*, *Proteus mirabilis*, the indole positive *Proteus* species, *Morganella morganii*; *Klebsiella* species, *Enterobacter* species, *Serratia* species, *Pseudomonas* species, *S. faecalis* (enterococcus).

Uncomplicated gonorrhea due to susceptible *Neisseria* gonorrhoeae.

GYNECOLOGICAL INFECTIONS including endometritis, pelvic cellulitis, and pelvic inflammatory disease associated with susceptible *Neisseria gonorrhoeae*, *Peptococcus* species, *Peptostreptococcus* species, *Bacteroides* species, *E. coli*, *Proteus mirabilis*, *Klebsiella* species, and *Enterobacter* species.

SKIN AND SKIN STRUCTURE INFECTIONS caused by susceptible *S. faecalis* (enterococcus), *E. coli*, *Proteus mirabilis*, the indole positive *Proteus* species, *Proteus vulgaris*, and *Providencia rettgeri*; *Klebsiella* species, *Enterobacter* species, *Pseudomonas* species, *Peptococcus* species, and *Bacteroides* species.

SEPTICEMIA including bacteremia caused by susceptible *E. coli*, *Klebsiella* species, *Enterobacter* species, *Pseudomonas* species, *Bacteroides* species, and *Peptococcus* species.

Mezlocillin has also been shown to be effective for the treatment of infections caused by *Streptococcus* species including Group A Beta-hemolytic *Streptococcus* and *Streptococcus pneumoniae* (formerly *Diplococcus pneumoniae*) however, infections caused by these organisms are ordinarily treated with more narrow spectrum penicillins.

Appropriate culture and susceptibility tests should be performed before treatment in order to isolate and identify organisms causing infection and to determine their susceptibility to mezlocillin. Therapy with MEZLIN® may be initiated before results of these tests are known; once results become available, appropriate therapy should be continued.

MEZLOCILLIN SERUM LEVELS IN ADULTS (mcg/mL) 30 MIN. IV INFUSION

DOSE	0	5 min.	15 min.	30 min.	45 min.	1 hr.	2 hr.	3 hr.	4 hr.	6 hr.	8 hr.
3g	263 (87–489)	170 (63–371)	141 (75–301)	109 (56–288)	79 (41–135)	57 (28–100)	26 (14–55)	12 (5.8–26)	4.4 (2.2–6.5)	1.6 (1.0–3.4)	<1

MEZLIN® DOSAGE GUIDE (ADULTS)

Condition	Daily Dosage Range	Usual Daily Dosage	Frequency and Route of Administration
Urinary tract infection (uncomplicated)	100–125 mg/kg	6-8g	1.5–2g every 6 hours IV or IM
Urinary tract infection (complicated)	150–200 mg/kg	12g	3g every 6 hours IV
Lower respiratory tract infection Intra-abdominal infection Gynecological infection Skin & skin structure infection Septicemia	225–300 mg/kg	16–18g	4g every 6 hours or 3g every 4 hours IV

Mezlocillin's broad spectrum of activity makes it particularly useful for treating mixed infections caused by susceptible strains of both gram-negative and gram-positive aerobic or anaerobic bacteria. It is not effective, however, against infections caused by penicillinase-producing *Staphylococcus aureus*.

In certain severe infections, when the causative organisms are unknown, MEZLIN® may be administered in conjunction with an aminoglycoside or a cephalosporin antibiotic as initial therapy. As soon as results of culture and susceptibility tests become available, antimicrobial therapy should be adjusted if indicated. Culture and sensitivity testing, performed periodically during therapy, will provide information on the therapeutic effect of the antimicrobial and will monitor for the possible emergence of bacterial resistance.

MEZLIN® has been used effectively in combination with an aminoglycoside antibiotic for the treatment of life-threatening infections caused by *Pseudomonas aeruginosa*. For the treatment of febrile episodes in immunosuppressed patients with granulocytopenia, MEZLIN® should be combined with an aminoglycoside or a cephalosporin antibiotic.

Prevention: The administration of MEZLIN® perioperatively (preoperatively, intraoperatively, and postoperatively) may reduce the incidence of infections in patients undergoing surgical procedures (e.g. vaginal hysterectomy and colorectal surgery) that may be classified as contaminated or potentially contaminated. Effective perioperative use for surgery depends on the time of administration. To achieve effective tissue levels, MEZLIN® should be given ½ hour to 1½ hours before surgery.

In patients undergoing Caesarean section, intraoperative (after clamping the umbilical cord) and postoperative use of MEZLIN® may reduce the incidence of certain postoperative infections. (See DOSAGE AND ADMINISTRATION section.)

For patients undergoing colorectal surgery, preoperative bowel preparation by mechanical cleansing as well as with a non-absorbable antibiotic (e.g. neomycin) is recommended.

If there are signs of infection, specimens for culture should be obtained for identification of the causative organism so that appropriate therapy may be instituted.

CONTRAINDICATIONS

MEZLIN® is contraindicated in patients with a history of hypersensitivity reactions to any of the penicillins.

WARNINGS

Serious and occasionally fatal hypersensitivity (anaphylactic) reactions have occurred in patients receiving a penicillin. These reactions are more apt to occur in individuals with a history of sensitivity to multiple allergens. There have been reports of individuals with a history of penicillin hypersensitivity reactions who have experienced severe hypersensitivity reactions when treated with cephalosporin. Before therapy with mezlocillin is instituted, careful inquiry should be made to determine whether the patient has had previous hypersensitivity reactions to penicillins, cephalosporins or other drugs. Antibiotics should be used with caution in any patient who has demonstrated some form of allergy, particularly to drugs.

If an allergic reaction occurs during therapy with mezlocillin, the drug should be discontinued. SERIOUS ANAPHYLACTOID REACTIONS REQUIRE IMMEDIATE EMERGENCY TREATMENT. EPINEPHRINE, OXYGEN, INTRAVENOUS STEROIDS, AND AIRWAY MANAGEMENT, INCLUDING INTUBATION, SHOULD BE PROVIDED AS INDICATED.

PRECAUTIONS

General

Although MEZLIN® shares with other penicillins the low potential for toxicity, as with any potent drug, periodic assessment of organ system functions, including renal, hepatic and hematopoietic, is advisable during prolonged therapy.

MEZLIN® has been reported rarely to cause acute interstitial nephritis.

Bleeding manifestations have occurred in some patients receiving beta-lactam antibiotics. These reactions have been associated with abnormalities of coagulation tests, such as clotting time, platelet aggregation and prothrombin time and are more likely to occur in patients with renal impairment. Although MEZLIN® has rarely been associated with clinical bleeding, the possibility of this occurring should be kept in mind, particularly in patients with severe renal impairment receiving maximum doses of the drug.

MEZLIN® has only rarely been reported to cause hypokalemia; however, the possibility of this occurring should also be kept in mind, particularly when treating patients with fluid and electrolyte imbalance. Periodic monitoring of serum potassium may be advisable in patients receiving prolonged therapy.

MEZLIN® is a monosodium salt containing only 42.6 mg (1.85 mEq) of sodium per gram of mezlocillin. This should be considered when treating patients requiring restricted salt intake.

As with any penicillin, an allergic reaction, including anaphylaxis, may occur during MEZLIN® administration, particularly in a hypersensitive individual.

As with other antibiotics, prolonged use of MEZLIN® may result in overgrowth of non-susceptible organisms. If this occurs, appropriate measures should be taken.

MEZLIN®, along with other ureidopenicillins, has been reported in one study to prolong neuromuscular blockage of vecuronium. Caution is indicated when mezlocillin is used perioperatively.

Antimicrobials used in high doses for short periods to treat gonorrhea may mask or delay the symptoms of incubating syphilis. Therefore, prior to treatment, patients with gonorrhea should also be evaluated for syphilis. Specimens for dark field examination should be obtained from any suspected primary lesion and serologic tests should be performed. Patients treated with MEZLIN® should undergo follow-up serologic tests three months after therapy.

Interactions with Drugs and Laboratory Tests

As with other penicillins, the mixing of mezlocillin with an aminoglycoside in solutions for parenteral administration can result in substantial inactivation of the aminoglycoside.

Probenecid interferes with the renal tubular secretion of mezlocillin, thereby increasing serum concentrations and prolonging serum half-life of the antibiotic.

High urine concentrations of mezlocillin may produce false positive protein reactions (pseudoproteinuria) with the following methods: sulfosalicylic acid and boiling test, acetic acid test, biuret reaction, and nitric acid test. The bromphenol blue (Multi-stix®) reagent strip test has been reported to be reliable.

Pregnancy Category B

Reproduction studies have been performed in rats and mice at doses up to 2 times the human dose, and have revealed no evidence of impaired fertility or harm to the fetus, due to MEZLIN®. There are however no adequate and well-controlled studies in pregnant women. Because animal reproductive studies are not always predictive of human response, this drug should be used during pregnancy only if clearly needed. Mezlocillin crosses the placenta and is found in low concentrations in cord blood and amniotic fluid.

Nursing Mothers

Mezlocillin is detected in low concentrations in the milk of nursing mothers, therefore caution should be exercised when MEZLIN® is administered to a nursing woman.

ADVERSE REACTIONS

As with other penicillins, the following adverse reactions may occur:

Hypersensitivity reactions: skin rash, pruritus, urticaria, drug fever, acute interstitial nephritis and anaphylactic reactions.

Gastrointestinal disturbances: abnormal taste sensation, nausea, vomiting and diarrhea. If diarrhea persists, pseudomembranous colitis should be considered.

Hemic and Lymphatic Systems: thrombocytopenia, leukopenia, neutropenia, eosinophilia, reduction of hemoglobin or hematocrit, and positive Coombs' test.

Abnormalities of hepatic and renal function tests: elevation of serum aspartate aminotransferase (SGOT), serum alanine aminotransferase (SGPT), serum alkaline phosphatase, serum bilirubin. Elevation of serum creatinine and/or BUN. Reduction in serum potassium.

Central nervous system: convulsive seizures or neuromuscular hyperirritability.

Local reactions: thrombophlebitis with intravenous administration, pain with intramuscular injection.

OVERDOSAGE

As with other penicillins, MEZLIN® in overdosage has the potential to cause neuromuscular hyperirritability or convulsive seizures. Hemodialysis, if necessary, will aid in the removal of drug from the blood.

DOSAGE AND ADMINISTRATION

MEZLIN® (sterile mezlocillin sodium) may be administered intravenously or intramuscularly. For serious infections, the intravenous route of administration should be used. Intramuscular doses should not exceed 2g per injection.

The recommended adult dosage for serious infections is 200-300 mg/kg per day given in 4 to 6 divided doses. The usual dose is 3g given every 4 hours (18g/day) or 4g given every 6 hours (16g/day). For life-threatening infections, up to 350 mg/kg per day may be administered, but the total daily dosage should ordinarily not exceed 24g.

[See table above.]

For patients with life-threatening infections, 4g may be administered every 4 hours (24g/day).

Dosage for any individual patient must take into consideration the site and severity of infection, the susceptibility of the organisms causing infection, and the status of the patient's host defense mechanism.

The duration of therapy depends upon the severity of infection. Generally, MEZLIN® should be discontinued for at least 2 days after the signs and symptoms of infection have disappeared. The usual duration is 7 to 10 days; however, in difficult and complicated infections, more prolonged therapy may be required. Antibiotic therapy for Group A Beta-hemolytic streptococcal infections should be maintained for at least 10 days to reduce the risk of rheumatic fever or glomerulonephritis.

In certain deep-seated infections, involving abscess formation, appropriate surgical drainage should be performed in conjunction with antimicrobial therapy.

For acute, uncomplicated gonococcal urethritis, the usual dose is 1-2g given once intravenously or by intramuscular injection. Probenecid 1g may be given orally at the time of dosing or up to ½ -hour before. (For full prescribing information, refer to probenecid package insert.)

Prevention

To prevent postoperative infection in contaminated or potentially contaminated surgery, the following doses are recommended:

4g IV given ½ hour to 1½ hours prior to the start of surgery.

4g IV given 6 hours and 12 hours later.

Caesarean Section Patients.

The first dose of 4g is given intravenously as soon as the umbilical cord is clamped. The second and third doses of 4g should be given intravenously 4 and 8 hours, respectively, after the first dose.

Patients with Impaired Renal Function

The rate of elimination of mezlocillin is dose dependent and related to the degree of renal function impairment. After an intravenous dose of 3g, the serum half-life is approximately 1 hour in patients with creatinine clearances above 60 mL/min., 1.3 hr. in those with clearances of 30–59 mL/min., 1.6 hr. in those with clearances of 10–29 mL/min. and approximately 3.6 hr. in patients with clearances of less than 10 mL/min. Dosage adjustments of MEZLIN® are not required in patients with mild impairment of renal function. For patients with a creatinine clearance of ≤ 30 mL/min. (serum creatinine of approximately 3.0 mg% or greater), the following dosage guide may be used:

[See first table on next page.]

For life-threatening infections, 3g may be given every 6 hours to patients with creatinine clearances between 10–30 mL/min. and 2g every 6 hours to those with clearances less than 10 mL/min.

For patients with serious systemic infection undergoing hemodialysis for renal failure, 3–4g may be administered after each dialysis and then every 12 hours. Patients undergoing peritoneal dialysis may receive 3g every 12 hours.

For patients with renal failure and hepatic insufficiency, measurement of serum levels of mezlocillin will provide additional guidance for adjusting dosage.

Intravenous Administration

MEZLIN® may be administered intravenously by intermittent infusion or by direct intravenous injection.

Infusion. Each gram of mezlocillin should be reconstituted by vigorous shaking with at least 9–10 mL of Sterile Water for Injection, 5% Dextrose Injection or 0.9% Sodium Chloride Injection. The dissolved drug should be further diluted to desired volume (50–100 mL) with an appropriate intravenous solution. (See Compatibility and Stability section.) The

Continued on next page

Miles—Cont.

solution of reconstituted drug may then be administered over a period of 30 minutes by direct infusion, or through a Y-type intravenous infusion set which may already be in place. If this method or the "piggyback" method of administration is used, it is advisable to discontinue temporarily the administration of any other solutions during the infusion of MEZLIN®.

Injection. The reconstituted solution of MEZLIN® may also be injected directly into a vein or into intravenous tubing; when administered this way, the injection should be given slowly over a period of 3–5 minutes. To minimize venous irritation, the concentration of drug should not exceed 10%. When MEZLIN® is given in combination with another antimicrobial, such as an aminoglycoside, each drug should be given separately in accordance with the recommended dosage and routes of administration for each drug.

Intramuscular Administration

Each gram of mezlocillin may be reconstituted by vigorous shaking with 3–4 mL of sterile water for injection or with 3–4 mL of 0.5 or 1.0% lidocaine hydrochloride solution (without epinephrine). (For full prescribing information, refer to lidocaine package insert.) Intramuscular doses of MEZLIN® should not exceed 2g per injection.

As with all intramuscular preparations, MEZLIN® should be injected well within the body of a relatively large muscle, such as the upper outer quadrant of the buttock (i.e., gluteus maximus); aspiration will help avoid unintentional injection into a blood vessel. Slow injection (12–15 sec.) will minimize the discomfort associated with intramuscular administration.

Infants and Children

Only limited data are available on the safety and effectiveness of MEZLIN® in the treatment of infants and children with documented serious infection. In the event a child has an infection for which MEZLIN® may be judged particularly appropriate, the following dosage guide may be used:
[See second table below.]

For infants beyond one month of age and children up to the age of 12 years, 50 mg/kg may be administered every 4 hours (300 mg/kg/day).

The drug may be infused intravenously over 30-minutes or be given by intramuscular injection.

COMPATIBILITY AND STABILITY

MEZLIN® at concentrations of 10 mg/mL and 100 mg/mL is stable (loss of potency less than 10%) in the following intravenous solutions for the time periods stated.

[See table at bottom of page.]
MEZLIN® at concentrations up to 250 mg/mL is stable for 24 hours at room temperature in the following diluents:
Sterile Water for Injection, USP
0.9% Sodium Chloride Injection, USP
0.5% and 1.0% Lidocaine Hydrochloride solution (without epinephrine)
MEZLIN® is stable for up to 28 days when frozen at −12℃ at concentrations up to 100 mg/mL in the following diluents:
Sterile Water for Injection, USP
0.9% Sodium Chloride Injection, USP or 5% Dextrose Injection, USP

HOW SUPPLIED

MEZLIN® (sterile mezlocillin sodium) is a white to pale yellow crystalline powder supplied as listed below:
MEZLIN® is available in vials, infusion bottles, pharmacy bulk packages and ADD-Vantage® vials containing mezlocillin sodium equivalent to mezlocillin, as specified:

	NDC Number
1g Vial	0026-8211-10
2g Vial	0026-8212-30
2g Infusion Bottle	0026-8212-36
3g Vial	0026-8213-35
3g Infusion Bottle	0026-8213-36
3g ADD-Vantage® Vial	0026-8213-19
4g Vial	0026-8214-35
4g Infusion Bottle	0026-8214-36
4g ADD-Vantage® Vial	0026-8214-19
20g Pharmacy Bulk Package	0026-8220-31

Unreconstituted MEZLIN® should be stored at temperatures not exceeding 86℉ (30℃). The powder as well as the reconstituted solution of drug may darken slightly, depending upon storage conditions, but potency is not affected.
Miles Inc.
Pharmaceutical Division
400 Morgan Lane
West Haven, CT 06516 USA
Made in Germany

PD100724 3/91 BAY f 1353 5202/4/A/US/MILES
© 1991 Miles Inc. 1426

MEZLIN®   ℞
Sterile mezlocillin sodium
BAYPEN®

DESCRIPTION

A pharmacy bulk package is a container of a sterile preparation for parenteral use that contains many single doses. The contents are intended for use in a pharmacy admixture program and are restricted to the preparation of admixtures for intravenous infusion, or the filling of empty sterile syringes for intravenous injection for patients with individualized dosing requirements (see Dosage and Administration section).

MEZLIN® (sterile mezlocillin sodium) is a semisynthetic broad spectrum penicillin antibiotic for parenteral administration. It is the monohydrate sodium salt of 6-{D-2 [3-(methyl-sulfonyl) -2-OXO -imidazolidine -1- carboxamido] -2-phenyl acetamido} penicillanic acid.

Structural Formula:

Empirical Formula: $C_{21}H_{24}N_5O_8S_2Na \cdot H_2O$
MEZLIN® has a molecular weight of 579.6 and contains 42.6 mg (1.85 mEq) of sodium per one gram of mezlocillin activity. The dosage form is supplied as a sterile white to pale yellow crystalline powder, which is freely soluble in water. When reconstituted, solutions of MEZLIN® are clear and range from colorless to pale yellow with a pH of 4.5 to 8.0.

CLINICAL PHARMACOLOGY

Intravenous Administration. In healthy adult volunteers, mean serum levels of mezlocillin 5 minutes after a 5-minute intravenous injection of 1g, 2g, or 5g are 100, 253, or 411 mcg/mL, respectively. Serum levels, as noted below, lack dose proportionality:
[See first table on next page.]
Fifteen minutes after a 4g intravenous injection (2-5 min.), the concentration in serum is 254 mcg/mL; 1 hour and 4 hours later levels are 93 mcg/mL and 9.1 mcg/mL, respectively:
[See second table on next page.]
After an intravenous infusion (15 min.) of 3g, mean levels 15 minutes after dosing are 269 mcg/mL (170-280).
A 30-minute intravenous infusion of 3g produces mean peak concentrations of 263 mcg/mL; 1 hour and 4 hours later the concentrations are 57 mcg/mL and 4.4 mcg/mL, respectively:
[See third table on next page.]
Following intravenous infusion (2 hr.) of a 3g dose of mezlocillin every 4 hours for 7 days, mean peak serum concentrations are higher than 100 mcg/mL, and levels above 50 mcg/mL are maintained throughout dosing.
Intramuscular Administration. MEZLIN® is rapidly absorbed after intramuscular injection. In healthy volunteers, the mean peak serum concentration occurs approximately 45 minutes after a single dose of 1g and is about 15 mcg/mL. The oral administration of 1g probenecid before injection produces an increase in mezlocillin serum levels of about 50%. After repetitive intramuscular doses of 1g mezlocillin every 6 hours, peak levels in the serum generally range between 35 and 45 mcg/mL. The relationship between the pharmacokinetics of intramuscular and intravenous dosing has not yet been clearly established.
General. As with other penicillins, mezlocillin is excreted primarily by glomerular filtration and tubular secretion. The rate of elimination is dose dependent and related to the degree of renal functional impairment. In patients with normal renal function, approximately 55% of the administered dose is recovered from the urine within the first 6 hours after dosing. Two hours after an intravenous injection of 2g, concentrations of active drug in urine generally exceed 4000 mcg/mL. By 4-6 hours after injection, concentrations usually decline to a range of about 50 to 200 mcg/mL. The serum elimination half-life of mezlocillin after intravenous dosing is approximately 55 minutes.
In patients with reduced renal function, the half-life is only slightly prolonged. Dosage adjustments are usually not necessary except in patients with severe renal impairment. (See Dosage and Administration.) As with other penicillins, mezlocillin is metabolized only slightly; less than 10% of the drug excreted in the urine is in the form of the penicilloate or penilloate. The drug is readily removed from the serum by hemodialysis and, to a lesser extent, by peritoneal dialysis. Up to 26% of a dose of mezlocillin is recovered from the bile of patients with normal liver function. Following intravenous doses of 2 to 5g, concentrations of active drug in bile generally range from 500 to 2500 mcg/mL. The biliary excretion of mezlocillin is reduced in patients with common bile duct obstruction.
Mezlocillin is not appreciably absorbed when given orally. Following parenteral administration, the apparent volume of distribution is approximately equal to the extracellular fluid volume. The drug is present in active form in the serum, urine, bile, peritoneal fluid, pleural fluid, bronchial and wound secretions, bone and other tissues. As with other penicillins, penetration into the cerebrospinal fluid (CSF) is generally poor, however higher CSF concentrations are obtained in the presence of meningeal inflammation.

MEZLIN® DOSAGE GUIDE FOR PATIENTS WITH IMPAIRED RENAL FUNCTION

Creatinine Clearance mL/min.	Urinary Tract Infection (Uncomplicated)	Urinary Tract Infection (Complicated)	Serious Systemic Infection
> 30	Usual Recommended Dosage		
10–30	1.5g every 8 hours	1.5g every 6 hours	3g every 8 hours
< 10	1.5g every 8 hours	1.5g every 8 hours	2g every 8 hours

MEZLIN® DOSAGE GUIDE (NEWBORNS)

BODY WEIGHT (gm)	AGE ≤7 DAYS	>7 DAYS
≤2000	75 mg/kg every 12 hours (150 mg/kg/day)	75 mg/kg every 8 hours (225 mg/kg/day)
>2000	75 mg/kg every 12 hours (150 mg/kg/day)	75 mg/kg every 6 hours (300 mg/kg/day)

STABILITY

INTRAVENOUS SOLUTION	Controlled Room Temperature	Refrigeration
Sterile Water for Injection, USP	48 hours	7 days
0.9% Sodium Chloride Injection, USP	48 hours	7 days
5% Dextrose Injection, USP	48 hours	7 days
5% Dextrose in 0.225% Sodium Chloride Injection, USP	72 hours	7 days
Lactated Ringer's Injection, USP	24 hours	7 days
5% Dextrose in Electrolyte #75 Injection	72 hours	7 days
5% Dextrose in 0.45% Sodium Chloride Injection, USP*	48 hours	48 hours
Ringer's Injection	24 hours	24 hours
10% Dextrose Injection	24 hours	24 hours
5% Fructose Injection	24 hours	24 hours

If precipitation should occur under refrigeration, the product should be warmed to 37℃ for 20 minutes in a water bath and shaken well.
*This solution is stable from 10 mg/mL to 50 mg/mL under refrigeration.

MEZLOCILLIN SERUM LEVELS IN ADULTS (mcg/mL) 5 MIN. IV INJECTION

DOSE	0	5 min	10 min	20 min	30 min	1 hr	2 hr	3 hr	4 hr	6 hr	8 hr
1g	**149** (132–185)	**100** (64–143)	**66** (47–87)	**50** (31–87)	**40** (22–83)	**18** (8–31)	**5.3** (3.3–7.7)	**2.5** (1.7–3.7)	**1.7** (0.7–2.8)	**0.5** (0–1.2)	**0.1** (0–0.2)
2g	**314** (207–362)	**253** (161–364)	**161** (113–214)	**117** (76–174)	**82** (55–112)	**56** (23–88)	**20** (7.5–32)	**11** (3.8–16)	**4.4** (1.6–8.7)	**1.5** (0.5–2.6)	**0.6** (0.1–1.4)
5g	**547** (268–854)	**411** (199–597)	**357** (246–456)	**250** (203–353)	**226** (190–333)	**131** (104–193)	**76** (59–104)	**31** (20–40)	**13** (6.4–17)	**4.6** (2.1–9.4)	**1.9** (1.1–3.6)

MEZLOCILLIN SERUM LEVELS IN ADULTS (mcg/mL) 2–5 MIN. IV INJECTION

DOSE	0	15 min	30 min	45 min	1 hr	2 hr	3 hr	4 hr	6 hr
4g	—	**254** (155–400)	**163** (99–260)	**122** (78–215)	**93** (67–133)	**47** (22–96)	**20** (8–45)	**9.1** (6–13)	**8.4** (5–17)

Protein binding studies indicate that the degree of mezlocillin binding is low (16-42%) and depends upon testing methods and concentrations of drug studied.

Microbiology

Mezlocillin is a bactericidal antibiotic which acts by interfering with synthesis of cell wall components. It is active against a variety of gram-negative and gram-positive bacteria, including aerobic and anaerobic strains. Mezlocillin is usually active *in vitro* against most strains of the following organisms:

Gram-negative bacteria

Escherichia coli
Proteus mirabilis
Proteus vulgaris
Morganella morganii (formerly *P. morganii*)
Providencia rettgeri (formerly *Proteus rettgeri*)
Providencia stuartii
Citrobacter species*
Klebsiella species (including *K. pneumoniae*)
Enterobacter species
Shigella species*
Pseudomonas aeruginosa (and other species)
Haemophilus influenzae
Haemophilus parainfluenzae
Neisseria species

Many strains of *Serratia, Salmonella**, and *Acinetobacter** are also susceptible.

Gram-positive bacteria

Staphylococcus aureus (non-penicillinase producing strains)
Beta-hemolytic *streptococci* (Groups A and B)
Streptococcus pneumoniae (formerly *Diplococcus pneumoniae*)
Streptococcus faecalis (enterococcus)

Anaerobic Organisms

Peptococcus species
Peptostreptococcus species
Clostridium species*
Bacteroides species (including *B. fragilis* group)
Fusobacterium species*
Veillonella species*
Eubacterium species*

*Mezlocillin has been shown to be active *in vitro* against these organisms, however clinical efficacy has not yet been established.

Noteworthy is mezlocillin's broadened spectrum of *in vitro* activity against important pathogenic aerobic gram-negative bacteria, including strains of *Pseudomonas, Klebsiella, Enterobacter, Serratia, Proteus, Escherichia* and *Haemophilus*, as well as *Bacteroides* and other anaerobes; and its excellent inhibitory effect against gram-positive organisms including *Streptococcus faecalis* (enterococcus). It is inactive against penicillinase-producing strains of *Staphylococcus aureus*.

In vitro studies have shown that mezlocillin combined with an aminoglycoside (e.g., gentamicin, tobramycin, amikacin, sisomicin) acts synergistically against strains of *Streptococcus faecalis* and *Pseudomonas aeruginosa*. In some instances, this combination also acts synergistically *in vitro* against other gram-negative bacteria such as *Serratia, Klebsiella* and *Acinetobacter species.*

Mezlocillin is slightly more active when tested at alkaline pH and, as with other penicillins, has reduced activity when tested *in vitro* with increasing inoculum. The minimum bactericidal concentration (MBC) generally exceeds the minimum inhibitory concentration (MIC) by a factor of 2 or 3. Resistance to mezlocillin in vitro develops slowly (multiple step mutation). Some strains of *Pseudomonas aeruginosa* have developed resistance fairly rapidly. Mezlocillin is not stable in the presence of penicillinase and strains of *Staphylococcus aureus* resistant to penicillin are also resistant to mezlocillin.

Susceptibility Tests

Quantitative methods that require measurement of zone diameters give good estimates of bacterial susceptibility. One such procedure* has been recommended for use with discs to test susceptibility to antimicrobials. When the causative organism is tested by the Kirby-Bauer method of disc susceptibility, a 75 mcg mezlocillin disc should give a zone of 18 mm or greater to indicate susceptibility. Zone sizes of 14 mm or less indicate resistance. Zone sizes of 15 to 17 mm indicate intermediate susceptibility. Susceptibile strains of *Haemophilus* and *Neisseria* species give zones of ≥29 mm, resistant strains ≤28 mm. With this procedure, a report from the laboratory of "Susceptibile" indicates that the infecting organism is likely to respond to therapy. A report of "Resistant" indicates that the infecting organism is not likely to respond to therapy; other therapy should be selected. A report of "Intermediate Susceptibility" suggests that the organism may be susceptible if the infection is confined to tissues and fluids (e.g., urine), in which high antibiotic levels are attained. The mezlocillin disc should be used for testing susceptibility to mezlocillin. In certain conditions, it may be desirable to do additional susceptibility testing by broth or agar dilution techniques. Dilution methods, preferably the agar plate dilution procedure, are most accurate for susceptibility testing of obligate anaerobes. *Enterobacteriaceae, Pseudomonas* species and *Acinetobacter* species are considered susceptible if the MIC of mezlocillin is no greater than 64 mcg/mL and are considered resistant if the MIC is greater than 128 mcg/mL. *Haemophilus* species and *Neisseria* species are considered susceptible if the MIC of mezlocillin is less than or equal to 1 mcg/mL. Mezlocillin standard is available for broth or agar dilution studies.

*Bauer, A.W., Kirby, W.M., Sherris, J.C., and Turck, M.: Antibiotic Testing by a Standardized Single Disc Method, Am. J. Clin. Pathol., 45:493, 1966; Standardized Disc Susceptibility Test, FEDERAL REGISTER, 39: 19182-19184, 1974.

INDICATIONS AND USAGE

MEZLIN® is indicated for the treatment of serious infections caused by susceptible strains of the designated microorganisms in the conditions listed below:

LOWER RESPIRATORY TRACT INFECTIONS including pneumonia and lung abscess caused by *Haemophilus influenzae, Klebsiella* species including *K. pneumoniae, Proteus mirabilis, Pseudomonas* species including *P. aeruginosa, E. coli,* and *Bacteroides* species including *B. fragilis.*

INTRA-ABDOMINAL INFECTIONS including acute cholecystitis, cholangitis, peritonitis, hepatic abscess and intra-abdominal abscess caused by susceptible *E. coli, Proteus mirabilis, Klebsiella* species, *Pseudomonas* species, *S. faecalis* (enterococcus), *Bacteroides* species, *Peptococcus* species, and *Peptostreptococcus* species.

URINARY TRACT INFECTIONS caused by susceptible *E. coli, Proteus mirabilis,* the indole positive *Proteus* species, *Morganella morganii; Klebsiella* species, *Enterobacter* species, *Serratia* species, *Pseudomonas* species, *S. faecalis* (enterococcus).

Uncomplicated gonorrhea due to susceptible *Neisseria gonorrhoeae.*

GYNECOLOGICAL INFECTIONS including endometritis, pelvic cellulitis, and pelvic inflammatory disease associated with susceptible *Neisseria gonorrhoeae, Peptococcus* species, *Peptostreptococcus* species, *Bacteroides species, E. coli, Proteus mirabilis, Klebsiella* species, and *Enterobacter* species.

SKIN AND SKIN STRUCTURE INFECTIONS caused by susceptible *S. faecalis* (enterococcus), *E. coli, Proteus mirabilis,* the indole positive *Proteus* species, *Proteus vulgaris,* and *Providencia rettgeri; Klebsiella* species, *Enterobacter* species, *Pseudomonas* species, *Peptococcus* species, and *Bacteroides* species.

SEPTICEMIA including bacteremia caused by susceptible *E. coli, Klebsiella* species, *Enterobacter* species, *Pseudomonas* species, *Bacteroides* species, and *Peptococcus* species.

Mezlocillin has also been shown to be effective for the treatment of infections caused by *Streptococcus* species including Group A Beta-hemolytic *Streptococcus* and *Streptococcus pneumoniae* (formerly *Diplococcus pneumoniae*) however, infections caused by these organisms are ordinarily treated with more narrow spectrum penicillins.

Appropriate culture and susceptibility tests should be performed before treatment in order to isolate and identify organisms causing infection and to determine their susceptibility to mezlocillin. Therapy with MEZLIN® may be initiated before results of these tests are known; once results become available, appropriate therapy should be continued.

Mezlocillin's broad spectrum of activity makes it particularly useful for treating mixed infections caused by susceptible strains of both gram-negative and gram-positive aerobic or anaerobic bacteria. It is not effective, however, against infections caused by penicillinase-producing *Staphylococcus aureus.*

In certain severe infections, when the causative organisms are unknown, MEZLIN® may be administered in conjunction with an aminoglycoside or a cephalosporin antibiotic as initial therapy. As soon as results of culture and susceptibility tests become available, antimicrobial therapy should be adjusted if indicated. Culture and sensitivity testing, performed periodically during therapy, will provide information on the therapeutic effect of the antimicrobial and will monitor for the possible emergence of bacterial resistance.

MEZLIN® has been used effectively in combination with an aminoglycoside antibiotic for the treatment of life-threatening infections caused by *Pseudomonas aeruginosa.* For the treatment of febrile episodes in immunosuppressed patients with granulocytopenia, MEZLIN® should be combined with an aminoglycoside or a cephalosporin antibiotic.

Prevention: The administration of MEZLIN® perioperatively (preoperatively, intraoperatively, and postoperatively) may reduce the incidence of infections in patients undergoing surgical procedures (e.g. vaginal hysterectomy and colorectal surgery) that may be classified as contaminated or potentially contaminated. Effective perioperative use for surgery depends on the time of administration. To achieve effective tissue levels, MEZLIN® should be given ½ hour to 1½ hours before surgery.

In patients undergoing Caesarean section, intraoperative (after clamping the umbilical cord) and postoperative use of MEZLIN® may reduce the incidence of certain postoperative infections. (See DOSAGE AND ADMINISTRATION section.)

For patients undergoing colorectal surgery, preoperative bowel preparation by mechanical cleansing as well as with a non-absorbable antibiotic (e.g. neomycin) is recommended.

If there are signs of infection, specimens for culture should be obtained for identification of the causative organism so that appropriate therapy may be instituted.

CONTRAINDICATIONS

MEZLIN® is contraindicated in patients with a history of hypersensitivity reactions to any of the penicillins.

WARNINGS

Serious and occasionally fatal hypersensitivity (anaphylactic) reactions have occurred in patients receiving a penicillin. These reactions are more apt to occur in individuals with a history of sensitivity to multiple allergens. There have been reports of individuals with a history of penicillin hypersensitivity reactions who have experienced severe hypersensitivity reactions when treated with cephalosporin. Before therapy with mezlocillin is instituted, careful inquiry should be

MEZLOCILLIN SERUM LEVELS IN ADULTS (mcg/mL) 30 MIN. IV INFUSION

DOSE	0	5 min	15 min	30 min	45 min	1 hr	2 hr	3 hr	4 hr	6 hr	8 hr
3g	**263** (87–489)	**170** (63–371)	**141** (75–301)	**109** (56–288)	**79** (41–135)	**57** (28–100)	**26** (14–55)	**12** (5.8–26)	**4.4** (2.2–6.5)	**1.6** (1.0–3.4)	<1

Miles—Cont.

made to determine whether the patient has had previous hypersensitivity reactions to penicillins, cephalosporins or other drugs. Antibiotics should be used with caution in any patient who has demonstrated some form of allergy, particularly to drugs.

If an allergic reaction occurs during therapy with mezlocillin, the drug should be discontinued. SERIOUS ANAPHYLACTOID REACTIONS REQUIRE IMMEDIATE EMERGENCY TREATMENT. EPINEPHRINE, OXYGEN, INTRAVENOUS STEROIDS, AND AIRWAY MANAGEMENT, INCLUDING INTUBATION, SHOULD BE PROVIDED AS INDICATED.

PRECAUTIONS
General
Although MEZLIN® shares with other penicillins the low potential for toxicity, as with any other potent drug, periodic assessment of organ system functions, including renal, hepatic and hematopoietic, is advisable during prolonged therapy. MEZLIN® has been reported rarely to cause acute interstitial nephritis.

Bleeding manifestations have occurred in some patients receiving beta-lactam antibiotics. These reactions have been associated with abnormalities of coagulation tests, such as clotting time, platelet aggregation and prothrombin time and are more likely to occur in patients with renal impairment. Although MEZLIN® has rarely been associated with clinical bleeding, the possibility of this occurring should be kept in mind, particularly in patients with severe renal impairment receiving maximum doses of the drug.

MEZLIN® has only rarely been reported to cause hypokalemia; however, the possibility of this occurring should also be kept in mind, particularly when treating patients with fluid and electrolyte imbalance. Periodic monitoring of serum potassium may be advisable in patients receiving prolonged therapy.

MEZLIN® is a monosodium salt containing only 42.6 mg (1.85 mEq) of sodium per gram of mezlocillin. This should be considered when treating patients requiring restricted salt intake.

As with any penicillin, an allergic reaction, including anaphylaxis, may occur during MEZLIN® administration, particularly in a hypersensitive individual.

As with other antibiotics, prolonged use of MEZLIN® may result in overgrowth of non-susceptible organisms. If this occurs, appropriate measures should be taken.

MEZLIN®, along with other ureidopenicillins, has been reported in one study to prolong neuromuscular blockage of vecuronium. Caution is indicated when mezlocillin is used perioperatively.

Antimicrobials used in high doses for short periods to treat gonorrhea may mask or delay the symptoms of incubating syphilis. Therefore, prior to treatment, patients with gonorrhea should also be evaluated for syphilis. Specimens for dark field examination should be obtained from any suspected primary lesion and serologic tests should be performed. Patients treated with MEZLIN® should undergo follow-up serologic tests three months after therapy.

Interactions with Drugs and Laboratory Tests
As with other penicillins, the mixing of mezlocillin with an aminoglycoside in solutions for parenteral administration can result in substantial inactivation of the aminoglycoside.

Probenecid interferes with the renal tubular secretion of mezlocillin, thereby increasing serum concentrations and prolonging serum half-life of the antibiotic.

High urine concentrations of mezlocillin may produce false positive protein reactions (pseudoproteinuria) with the following methods: sulfosalicylic acid and boiling test, acetic acid test, biuret reaction, and nitric acid test. The bromphenol blue (Multi-stix®) reagent strip test has been reported to be reliable.

Pregnancy Category B
Reproduction studies have been performed in rats and mice at doses up to 2 times the human dose, and have revealed no evidence of impaired fertility or harm to the fetus, due to MEZLIN®. There are however no adequate and well-controlled studies in pregnant women. Because animal reproductive studies are not always predictive of human response, this drug should be used during pregnancy only if clearly needed. Mezlocillin crosses the placenta and is found in low concentrations in cord blood and amniotic fluid.

Nursing Mothers
Mezlocillin is detected in low concentrations in the milk of nursing mothers. Therefore caution should be exercised when MEZLIN® is administered to a nursing woman.

ADVERSE REACTIONS
As with other penicillins, the following adverse reactions may occur:

MEZLIN® DOSAGE GUIDE (ADULTS)

Condition	Daily Dosage Range	Usual Daily Dosage	Frequency and Route of Administration
Urinary tract infection (uncomplicated)	100–125 mg/kg	6-8g	1.5–2g every 6 hours IV or IM
Urinary tract infection (complicated)	150–200 mg/kg	12g	3g every 6 hours IV
Lower respiratory tract infection			
Intra-abdominal infection			
Gynecological infection	225–300 mg/kg	16–18g	4g every 6 hours or 3g every 4 hours IV
Skin & skin structure infection			
Septicemia			

MEZLIN® DOSAGE GUIDE FOR PATIENTS WITH IMPAIRED RENAL FUNCTION

Creatinine Clearance mL/min	Urinary Tract Infection (Uncomplicated)	Urinary Tract Infection (Complicated)	Serious Systemic Infection
>30	Usual Recommended Dosage		
10–30	1.5g every 8 hours	1.5g every 6 hours	3g every 8 hours
<10	1.5g every 8 hours	1.5g every 8 hours	2g every 8 hours

Hypersensitivity reactions: skin rash, pruritus, urticaria, drug fever, acute interstitial nephritis and anaphylactic reactions.

Gastrointestinal disturbances: abnormal taste sensation, nausea, vomiting and diarrhea. If diarrhea persists, pseudomembranous colitis should be considered.

Hematologic and Lymphatic Systems: thrombocytopenia, leukopenia, neutropenia, eosinophilia, reduction of hemoglobin or hematocrit, and positive Coombs' test.

Abnormalities of hepatic and renal function tests: elevation of serum aspartate aminotransferase (SGOT), serum alanine aminotransferase (SGPT), serum alkaline phosphatase, serum bilirubin. Elevation of serum creatinine and/or BUN. Reduction in serum potassium.

Central nervous system: convulsive seizures or neuromuscular hyperirritability.

Local reactions: thrombophlebitis with intravenous administration, pain with intramuscular injection.

OVERDOSAGE
As with other penicillins, MEZLIN® in overdosage has the potential to cause neuromuscular hyperirritability or convulsive seizures. Hemodialysis, if necessary, will aid in the removal of drug from the blood.

DOSAGE AND ADMINISTRATION
MEZLIN® (sterile mezlocillin sodium) may be administered intravenously or intramuscularly. For serious infections, the intravenous route of administration should be used. Intramuscular doses should not exceed 2g per injection.

The 20g pharmacy bulk package is intended for the preparation of solutions for intravenous use. When intramuscular administration is required, the MEZLIN® vial should be used.

The recommended adult dosage for serious infections is 200-300 mg/kg per day given in 4 to 6 divided doses. The usual dose is 3g given every 4 hours (18g/day) or 4g given every 6 hours (16g/day). For life-threatening infections, up to 350 mg/kg per day may be administered, but the total daily dosage should ordinarily not exceed 24g.
[See table above.]

For patients with life-threatening infections, 4g may be administered every 4 hours (24g/day).

Dosage for any individual patient must take into consideration the site and severity of infection, the susceptibility of the organisms causing infection, and the status of the patient's host defense mechanism.

The duration of therapy depends upon the severity of infection. Generally, MEZLIN® should be discontinued for at least 2 days after the signs and symptoms of infection have disappeared. The usual duration is 7 to 10 days; however, in difficult and complicated infections, more prolonged therapy may be required. Antibiotic therapy for Group A Beta-hemolytic streptococcal infections should be maintained for at least 10 days to reduce the risk of rheumatic fever or glomerulonephritis.

In certain deep-seated infections, involving abscess formation, appropriate surgical drainage should be performed in conjunction with antimicrobial therapy.

For acute, uncomplicated gonococcal urethritis, the usual dose is 1-2g given once intravenously or by intramuscular injection. Probenecid 1g may be given orally at the time of dosing or up to ½-hour before. (For full prescribing information, refer to probenecid package insert.)

Prevention
To prevent postoperative infection in contaminated or potentially contaminated surgery, the following doses are recommended:

4g IV given ½ hour to 1½ hours prior to the start of surgery.

4g IV given 6 hours and 12 hours later.

Caesarean Section Patients.

The first dose of 4g is given intravenously as soon as the umbilical cord is clamped. The second and third doses of 4g should be given intravenously 4 and 8 hours, respectively, after the first dose.

Patients with Impaired Renal Function
The rate of elimination of mezlocillin is dose dependent and related to the degree of renal function impairment. After an intravenous dose of 3g, the serum half-life is approximately 1 hour in patients with creatinine clearances above 60 mL/min., 1.3 hr. in those with clearances of 30-59 mL/min., 1.6 hr. in those with clearances of 10-29 mL/min. and approximately 3.6 hr. in patients with clearances of less than 10 mL/min. Dosage adjustments of MEZLIN® are not required in patients with mild impairment of renal function. For patients with a creatinine clearance of ≤30 mL/min. (serum creatinine of approximately 3.0 mg% or greater), the following dosage guide may be used: [See second table .]

For life-threatening infections, 3g may be given every 6 mL/min. to patients with creatinine clearances between 10-30 mL/min. and 2g every 6 hours to those with clearances less than 10 mL/min.

For patients with serious systemic infection undergoing hemodialysis for renal failure, 3-4g may be administered after each dialysis and then every 12 hours. Patients undergoing peritoneal dialysis may receive 3g every 12 hours.

For patients with renal failure and hepatic insufficiency, measurement of serum levels of mezlocillin will provide additional guidance for adjusting dosage.

Directions for Proper Use of 20 gram Pharmacy Bulk Package
A pharmacy bulk package is a container of a sterile preparation for parenteral use that contains many single doses. The contents are intended for use in a pharmacy admixture program and are restricted to the preparation of admixtures for intravenous infusion, or the filling of empty sterile syringes for intravenous injection for patients with individualized dosing requirements.

THE CLOSURE SHALL BE PENETRATED ONLY ONE TIME AFTER RECONSTITUTION with a suitable sterile transfer set or dispensing device which allows measured dispensing of the contents. The pharmacy bulk package is to be used only in a suitable work area such as a laminar flow hood or an equivalent clean air compounding area.

Reconstitute by vigorous shaking with 186 mL of Sterile Water for Injection, 5% Dextrose Injection or 0.9% Sodium Chloride Injection resulting in a solution containing approximately 100 mg/mL which should be stored at controlled room temperature or under refrigeration. Within 8 hours of reconstitution, the desired dosages should be withdrawn and may be further diluted with an appropriate intravenous solution (see Compatability & Stability section).

Intravenous Administration
MEZLIN® may be administered by intermittent infusion or by direct intravenous injection.

INTRAVENOUS SOLUTION

Sterile Water for Injection, USP
0.9% Sodium Chloride Injection, USP
5% Dextrose Injection, USP
5% Dextrose in 0.225% Sodium Chloride Injection, USP
Lactated Ringer's Injection, USP
5% Dextrose in Electrolyte #75 Injection
5% Dextrose in 0.45% Sodium Chloride Injection, USP*
Ringer's Injection
10% Dextrose Injection
5% Fructose Injection

STABILITY

Controlled Room Temperature	Refrigeration
48 hours	7 days
48 hours	7 days
48 hours	7 days
72 hours	7 days
72 hours	7 days
72 hours	7 days
48 hours	48 hours
24 hours	24 hours
24 hours	24 hours
24 hours	24 hours

If precipitation should occur under refrigeration, the product should be warmed to 37°C for 20 minutes in a water bath and shaken well.

*This solution is stable from 10 mg/mL to 50 mg/mL under refrigeration.

Infusion. The dissolved drug should be further diluted to desired volume (50-100 mL) with an appropriate intravenous solution. (See Compatibility and Stability section.) The solution of reconstituted drug may then be administered over a period of 30 minutes by direct infusion, or through a Y-type intravenous infusion set which may already be in place. If this method or the"piggyback" method of administration is used, it is advisable to discontinue temporarily the administration of any other solutions during the infusion of MEZLIN®.

Injection. The reconstituted solution of MEZLIN® may also be injected directly into a vein or into intravenous tubing; when administered this way, the injection should be given slowly over a period of 3-5 minutes. To minimize venous irritation, the concentration of drug should not exceed 10%. When MEZLIN® is given in combination with another antimicrobial, such as an aminoglycoside, each drug should be given separately in accordance with the recommended dosage and routes of administration for each drug.

Intramuscular Administration
For intramuscular administration, please refer to the Dosage and Administration section of the MEZLIN® vial package insert.

Infants and Children
Only limited data are available on the safety and effectiveness of MEZLIN® in the treatment of infants and children with documented serious infection. In the event a child has an infection for which MEZLIN® may be judged particularly appropriate, the following dosage guide may be used:

MEZLIN DOSAGE GUIDE (NEWBORNS)

BODY WEIGHT	AGE	
(gm)	≤7 DAYS	>7 DAYS
≤2000	75 mg/kg every 12 hours (150 mg/kg/day)	75 mg/kg every 8 hours (225 mg/kg/day)
>2000	75 mg/kg every 12 hours (150 mg/kg/day)	75 mg/kg every 6 hours (300 mg/kg/day)

For infants beyond one month of age and children up to the age of 12 years, 60 mg/kg may be administered every 4 hours (300 mg/kg/day).
The drug may be infused intravenously over 30-minutes or be given by intramuscular injection.

COMPATIBILITY AND STABILITY

MEZLIN® at concentrations of 10 mg/mL and 100 mg/mL is stable (loss of potency less than 10%) in the following intravenous solutions for the time periods stated (includes time retained in pharmacy bulk package after reconstitution): [See table at top of page.]
MEZLIN® is stable for up to 28 days when frozen at −12°C at concentrations up to 100 mg/mL in the following diluents:
Sterile Water for Injection, USP
0.9% Sodium Chloride Injection, USP or 5% Dextrose Injection, USP

HOW SUPPLIED

MEZLIN® (sterile mezlocillin sodium) is a white to pale yellow crystalline powder supplied as listed below:
MEZLIN® is available in vials, infusion bottles, pharmacy bulk packages and ADD-Vantage® vials containing mezlocillin sodium equivalent to mezlocillin, as specified:

	NDC Number
1g Vial	0026-8211-10
2g Vial	0026-8212-30
2g Infusion Bottle	0026-8212-36
3g Vial	0026-8213-35
3g Infusion Bottle	0026-8213-36
3g ADD-Vantage® Vial	0026-8213-19
4g Vial	0026-8214-35
4g Infusion Bottle	0026-8214-36
4g ADD-Vantage® Vial	0026-8214-19
20g Pharmacy Bulk Package	0026-8220-31

Unreconstituted MEZLIN® should be stored at temperatures not exceeding 86°F (30°C). The powder as well as the reconstituted solution of drug may darken slightly, depending upon storage conditions, but potency is not affected.

Miles Inc.
Pharmaceutical Division
400 Morgan Lane
West Haven, CT 06516 USA
PD100668 9/88 BAY f 1353   5202/4/A/US/MILES
© 1988 Miles Inc.   0626

MITHRACIN®   ℞
(plicamycin)
FOR INTRAVENOUS USE

WARNING

IT IS RECOMMENDED THAT MITHRACIN (plicamycin) BE ADMINISTERED ONLY TO HOSPITALIZED PATIENTS BY OR UNDER THE SUPERVISION OF A QUALIFIED PHYSICIAN WHO IS EXPERIENCED IN THE USE OF CANCER CHEMOTHERAPEUTIC AGENTS, BECAUSE OF THE POSSIBILITY OF SEVERE REACTIONS. FACILITIES FOR THE DETERMINATION OF NECESSARY LABORATORY STUDIES MUST BE AVAILABLE.
SEVERE THROMBOCYTOPENIA, A HEMORRHAGIC TENDENCY AND EVEN DEATH MAY RESULT FROM THE USE OF MITHRACIN. ALTHOUGH SEVERE TOXICITY IS MORE APT TO OCCUR IN PATIENTS WHO HAVE FAR-ADVANCED DISEASE OR ARE OTHERWISE CONSIDERED POOR RISKS FOR THERAPY, SERIOUS TOXICITY MAY ALSO OCCASIONALLY OCCUR EVEN IN PATIENTS WHO ARE IN RELATIVELY GOOD CONDITION.
IN THE TREATMENT OF EACH PATIENT, THE PHYSICIAN MUST WEIGH CAREFULLY THE POSSIBILITY OF ACHIEVING THERAPEUTIC BENEFIT VERSUS THE RISK OF TOXICITY WHICH MAY OCCUR WITH MITHRACIN THERAPY, THE FOLLOWING DATA CONCERNING THE USE OF MITHRACIN IN THE TREATMENT OF TESTICULAR TUMORS, HYPERCALCEMIC AND/OR HYPERCALCIURIC CONDITIONS ASSOCIATED WITH VARIOUS ADVANCED MALIGNANCIES, SHOULD BE THOROUGHLY REVIEWED BEFORE ADMINISTERING THIS COMPOUND.

DESCRIPTION

Mithracin is a yellow crystalline compound which is produced by a microorganism, *Streptomyces plicatus.* Mithracin is available in vials as a freeze-dried, sterile preparation for intravenous administration. Each vial contains 2500 mcg (2.5 mg) of Mithracin with 100 mg of mannitol and sufficient disodium phosphate to adjust to pH 7. After reconstitution with sterile water for injection, the solution has a pH of 7. The drug is unstable in acid solutions with a pH below 4. Mithracin is an antineoplastic agent. It has an empirical formula of $C_{52}H_{76}O_{24}$. The following structural formula has been proposed for this compound.

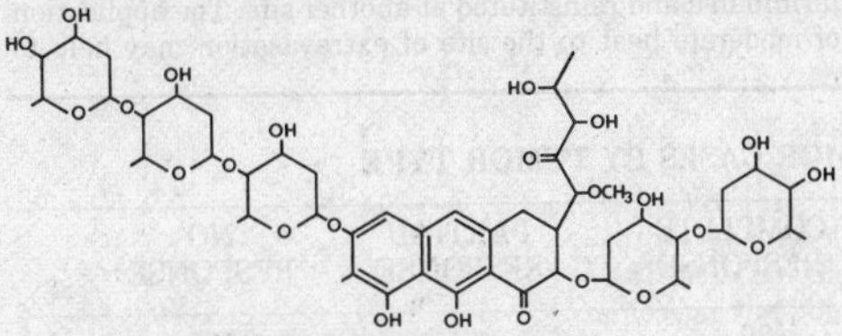

CLINICAL PHARMACOLOGY

Although the exact mechanism by which Mithracin causes tumor inhibition is not yet known, studies have indicated that this compound forms a complex with deoxyribonucleic acid (DNA) and inhibits cellular ribonucleic acid (RNA) and enzymic RNA synthesis. The binding of Mithracin to DNA in the presence of Mg^{++} (or other divalent cations) is responsible for the inhibition of DNA-dependent or DNA-directed RNA synthesis. This action presumably accounts for the biological properties of Mithracin.
Mithracin shows potent cytotoxicity against malignant cells of human origin (Hela cells) growing in tissue culture. Mithracin is lethal to Hela cells in 48 hours at concentrations as low as 0.5 micrograms per milliliter of tissue culture medium. Mithracin has shown significant anti-tumor activity against experimental leukemia in mice when administered intraperitoneally.
Plicamycin may lower serum calcium levels; the exact mechanism (or mechanisms) by which the drug exerts this effect is unknown. It appears that plicamycin may block the hypercalcemic action of pharmacologic doses of vitamin D. It has also been suggested that plicamycin may lower calcium serum levels by inhibiting the effect of parathyroid hormone upon osteoclasts. Plicamycin's inhibition of DNA-dependent RNA synthesis appears to render osteoclasts unable to fully respond to parathyroid hormone with the biosynthesis necessary for osteolysis. Decreases in serum phosphate levels and urinary calcium excretion accompany the lowering of serum calcium concentrations.
Radioautography studies[1] with ³H-labeled plicamycin in C3H mice slow that the greatest concentrations of the isotope are in the Kupffer cells of the liver and cells of the renal tubules. Plicamycin is rapidly cleared from the blood within the first 2 hours and excretion is also rapid. Sixty-seven percent of measured excretion occurs within 4 hours, 75% within 8 hours, and 90% is recovered in the first 24 hours after injection. There is no evidence of protein binding, nor is there any evidence of metabolism of the carbohydrate moiety of the drug to carbon dioxide and water with loss through respiration. Plicamycin crosses the blood-brain barrier; the concentration found in brain tissue is low but it persists longer than in other tissues. The experimental results in animals correlate closely with results achieved in man.[2]

INDICATIONS

Mithracin is a potent antineoplastic agent which has been shown to be useful in the treatment of carefully selected hospitalized patients with malignant tumors of the testis in whom successful treatment by surgery and/or radiation is impossible. Also, on the basis of limited clinical experience to date, it may be considered in the treatment of certain symptomatic patients with hypercalcemia and hypercalciuria associated with a variety of advanced neoplasms.
The use of Mithracin in other types of neoplastic disease is not recommended at the present time.

CONTRAINDICATIONS

Mithracin (plicamycin) is contraindicated in patients with thrombocytopenia, thrombocytopathy, coagulation disorder or an increased susceptibility to bleeding due to other causes. Mithracin should not be administered to any patient with impairment of bone marrow function.
Mithracin may cause fetal harm when administered to a pregnant woman. Mithracin is contraindicated in women who are or may become pregnant. If this drug is used during pregnancy or if the patient becomes pregnant while taking this drug, the patient should be apprised of the potential hazard to the fetus.

PRECAUTIONS

General: Mithracin should be administered only to patients who are hospitalized and who can be observed carefully and frequently during and after therapy.
Severe thrombocytopenia, a hemorrhagic tendency and even death may result from the use of Mithracin. Although severe toxicity is more apt to occur in patients who have far-advanced disease or are otherwise considered poor risks for therapy, serious toxicity may also occasionally occur even in patients who are in relatively good condition.
Electrolyte imbalance, especially hypocalcemia, hypokalemia, and hypophosphatemia, should be corrected with appropriate electrolyte therapy prior to treatment with Mithracin.
Mithracin should be used with extreme caution in patients with significant impairment of renal or hepatic function.
Mithracin should not normally be administered to patients who are pregnant or to mothers who are breast feeding.
In the treatment of each patient, the physician must weigh carefully the possibility of achieving therapeutic benefit versus the risk of toxicity which may occur with Mithracin therapy.
Laboratory Tests: The following laboratory studies should be obtained frequently during therapy and for several days following the last dose: platelet count, prothrombin time, bleeding time. The occurrence of thrombocytopenia or a significant prolongation of prothrombin time or bleeding time is an indication for the termination of therapy.
Carcinogenesis, mutagenesis, impairment of fertility: No long-term studies in animals have been performed to evaluate the carcinogenic potential of Mithracin. Histologic evidence of inhibition of spermatogenesis was observed in a substantial number of male rats receiving doses of 0.6 mg/kg/day and above.
Pregnancy Category X: See "Contraindications" section.
Nursing Mothers: It is not known whether this drug is excreted in human milk. Because many drugs are excreted in human milk and because of the potential for serious adverse reactions in nursing infants from Mithracin, a decision should be made whether to discontinue nursing or to discon-

Miles—Cont.

tinue the drug, taking into account the importance of the drug to the mother.

ADVERSE REACTIONS

THE MOST IMPORTANT FORM OF TOXICITY ASSOCIATED WITH THE USE OF MITHRACIN CONSISTS OF A BLEEDING SYNDROME WHICH USUALLY BEGINS WITH AN EPISODE OF EPISTAXIS. This bleeding tendency may only consist of a single or several episodes of epistaxis and progress no further. However, in some cases, this hemorrhagic syndrome can start with an episode of hematemesis which may progress to more wide-spread hemorrhage in the gastrointestinal tract or to a more generalized bleeding tendency. This hemorrhagic diathesis is most likely due to abnormalities in multiple clotting factors.

A detailed analysis of the clinical data in 1,160 patients treated with Mithracin indicates that the hemorrhagic syndrome is dose related. With doses of 30 mcg/kg/day or less for 10 or fewer doses, the incidence of bleeding episodes has been 5.4% with an associated drug-related mortality rate of 1.6%. With doses greater than 30 mcg/kg/day and/or for more than 10 doses, a significantly larger number of bleeding episodes occurred (11.9%) and the associated drug-related mortality rate was also significantly higher (5.7%).

The most common side effects reported with the use of Mithracin consist of gastrointestinal symptoms: anorexia, nausea, vomiting, diarhea, and stomatitis. Other less frequently reported side effects include fever, drowsiness, weakness, lethargy, malaise, headache, depression, phlebitis, facial flushing, and skin rash.

The following laboratory abnormalities have been reported during therapy with Mithracin (plicamycin) and in most instances were reversible following cessation of treatment:

Hematologic Abnormalities: Depression of platelet count, white count, hemoglobin and prothrombin content; elevation of clotting time and bleeding time; abnormal clot retraction. Thrombocytopenia may be rapid in onset and may occur at any time during therapy or within several days following the last dose. With the occurrence of severe thrombocytopenia, the infusion of platelet concentrates of platelet-rich plasma may be helpful in elevating the platelet count.

The occurrence of leukopenia with the use of Mithracin is relatively uncommon, occurring only in approximately 6% of patients.

It has been uncommon for abnormalities in clotting time or clot retraction to be demonstrated prior to the onset of an overt bleeding episode noted in some patients treated with Mithracin. Nevertheless, the performance of these tests periodically is recommended because in a few instances, an abnormality in one of these studies may have served as a warning to terminate therapy because of impeding serious toxicity.

Abnormal Liver Function Tests: Increased levels of serum glutamic oxalacetic transaminase, serum glutamic pyruvic transaminase, lactic dehydrogenase, alkaline phosphatase, serum bilirubin, ornithine carbamyl transferase, isocitric dehydrogenase, and increased retention of bromsulphalein.

Abnormal Renal Function Tests: Increased blood urea nitrogen and serum creatinine; proteinuria.

Abnormalities in Electrolyte Concentrations: Depression of serum calcium, phosphorus, and potassium.

OVERDOSAGE

Generally, adverse effects following the use of Mithracin, especially the hemorrhagic syndrome, are dose related. Therefore, following administration of an overdose, patients can be expected to experience an exaggeration of the usual adverse effects. Close monitoring of the hematologic picture, including factors involved in the clotting mechanism, hepatic and renal functions, and serum electrolytes, is necessary. No specific antidote for Mithracin is known. Management of overdosage would include general supportive measures to sustain the patient through the period of toxicity.

DOSAGE

The daily dose of Mithracin is based on the patient's body weight. If a patient has abnormal fluid retention such as edema, hydrothorax or ascites, the patient's ideal weight rather than actual body weight should be used to calculate the dose.

Treatment of Testicular Tumors: In the treatment of patients with testicular tumors the recommended daily dose of Mithracin (plicamycin) is 25 to 30 mcg (0.025–0.030 mg) per kilogram of body weight. Therapy should be continued for a period of 8 to 10 days unless significant side effects or toxicity occur during therapy. A course of therapy consisting of more than 10 daily doses is not recommended. Individual daily doses should not exceed 30 mcg (0.030 mg) per kilogram of body weight.

In those patients with responsive tumors, some degree of tumor regression is usually evident within 3 or 4 weeks following the initial course of therapy. If tumor masses remain unchanged following an initial course of therapy, additional courses of therapy at monthly intervals are warranted.

When a significant tumor regression is obtained, it is suggested that additional courses of therapy be given at monthly intervals until a complete regression of tumor masses is achieved or until definite tumor progression or new tumor masses occur in spite of continued courses of therapy.

Treatment of Hypercalcemia and Hypercalciuria: Reversal of hypercalcemia and hypercalciuria can usually be achieved with Mithracin at doses considerably lower than those recommended for use in the treatment of testicular tumors.

In hypercalcemia and hypercalciuria associated with advanced malignancy the recommended course of treatment with Mithracin is 25 mcg (0.025 mg) per kilogram of body weight per day for 3 or 4 days.

If the desired degree of reversal of hypercalcemia or hypercalciuria is not achieved with the initial course of therapy, additional courses of therapy may then be administered at intervals of one week or more to achieve the desired result or to maintain serum calcium and urinary calcium excretion at normal levels. It may be possible to maintain normal calcium balance with single, weekly doses or with a schedule of 2 or 3 doses per week.

NOTE: BECAUSE OF THE DRUG'S TOXICITY AND THE LIMITED CLINICAL EXPERIENCE TO DATE IN THESE INDICATIONS, THE FOLLOWING RECOMMENDATIONS SHOULD BE KEPT IN MIND BY THE PHYSICIAN.

1. **CONSIDER CASES OF HYPERCALCEMIA AND HYPERCALCIURIA NOT RESPONSIVE TO CONVENTIONAL TREATMENT.**
2. **APPLY SAME CONTRAINDICATIONS AND PRECAUTIONARY MEASURES AS IN ANTITUMOR TREATMENT.**
3. **RENAL FUNCTION SHOULD BE CAREFULLY MONITORED BEFORE, DURING, AND AFTER TREATMENT.**
4. **BENEFITS OF USE DURING PREGNANCY OR IN WOMEN OF CHILD-BEARING AGE SHOULD BE WEIGHED AGAINST POTENTIAL TOXICITY TO EMBRYO OR FETUS.**

ADMINISTRATION

By IV administration only. The appropriate daily dose of Mithracin should be diluted in one liter of 5% Dextrose Injection, USP or Sodium Chloride Injection, USP and administered by slow intravenous infusion over a period of 4 to 6 hours. Rapid direct intravenous injection of Mithracin should be avoided as it may be associated with a higher incidence and greater severity of gastrointestinal side effects. Extravasation of solutions of Mithracin may cause local irritation and cellulitis at injection sites. Should thrombophlebitis or perivascular cellulitis occur, the infusion should be terminated and reinstituted at another site. The application of moderate heat to the site of extravasation may help to disperse the compound and minimize discomfort and local tissue irritation. The use of antiemetic compounds prior to and during treatment with Mithracin may be helpful in relieving nausea and vomiting.

Procedures for proper handling and disposal of anti-cancer drugs should be considered. Several guidelines on this subject have been published.[3–8] There is no general agreement that all of the procedures recommended in the guidelines are necessary or appropriate.

HOW SUPPLIED

Mithracin is available in vials as a freeze-dried preparation for intravenous administration. Each vial contains 2500 mcg (2.5 mg) of Mithracin with 100 mg of mannitol and sufficient disodium phosphate to adjust to pH 7. These vials should be stored at refrigerator temperatures between 2°C. to 8°C. (36°F. to 46°F.).

To reconstitute, add aseptically 4.9 ml of Sterile Water for Injection to the contents of the vial and shake to dissolve. Each ml of the resulting solution will then contain 500 mcg (0.5 mg) of Mithracin. NOTE: 1 mg (milligram)=1000 mcg (micrograms). AFTER REMOVAL OF THE APPROPRIATE DOSE, THE REMAINING UNUSED SOLUTION MUST BE DISCARDED, FRESH SOLUTIONS MUST BE PREPARED IN THE ABOVE MANNER EACH DAY OF THERAPY.

ANIMAL PHARMACOLOGY AND TOXICOLOGY

In mice the average intravenous LD_{50} of Mithracin is 2,000 mcg/kg of body weight. When administered orally, it is not toxic to mice even at doses 100 times greater than the intravenous LD_{50}. In rats the average intravenous LD_{50} of Mithracin is 1,700 mcg/kg of body weight. It is not toxic to rats when administered orally at doses 17 times greater than the intravenous LD_{50}. In dogs and monkeys Mithracin is essentially non-toxic when administered intravenously for 24 days at daily doses as high as 50 and 24 mcg/kg of body weight, respectively. However, at higher doses of 100 mcg/kg/day intravenously it is lethal to dogs and monkeys. Signs of toxicity in dogs and monkeys included anorexia, vomiting, listlessness, nelena, anemia, lymphopenia, elevated alkaline phosphatase, serum glutamic oxalacetic transaminase, serum glutamic pyruvic transaminase values, hypochloremia, and azotemia. Dogs also showed marked thrombocytopenia, hyponatremia, hypokalemia, hypocalcemia, and decreased prothrombin consumption. Necropsy findings consisted of necrosis of lymphoid tissue and multiple generalized hemorrhages. Mithracin (plicamycin) was only mildly irritating when injected intramuscularly in rabbits and subcutaneously in guinea pigs. Histologic evidence of inhibition of spermatogenesis was observed in a substantial number of male rats receiving doses of 0.6 mg/kg/day and above. This preclinical finding of selective drug effect constituted the scientific rationale for clinical trials in testicular tumors.

Clinical Reports:

Treatment of Patients with Inoperable Testicular Tumors: In a combined series of 305 patients with inoperable testicular tumors treated with Mithracin, 33 patients (10.8%) showed a complete disappearance of tumor masses and an additional 80 patients (26.2%) responded with significant partial regression of tumor masses. The longest duration of a continuing complete response is now over 8½ years. The therapeutic responses in this series of patients have been summarized by type of testicular tumor in the accompanying table.

[See table below.]

Mithracin may be useful in the treatment of patients with testicular tumors which are resistant to other chemotherapeutic agents. Prior radiation therapy or prior chemotherapy did not alter the response rate with Mithracin. This suggests that there is no significant cross resistance between Mithracin (plicamycin) and other chemotherapeutic agents.

Treatment of Patients with Hypercalcemia and Hypercalciuria: A limited number of patients with hypercalcemia (range: 12.0–25.8 mg%) and patients with hypercalciuria (range 215–492 mg/day) associated with malignant disease were treated with Mithracin. Hypercalcemia and hypercalciuria were promptly reversed in all patients. In some patients, the primary malignancy was of non-testicular origin.

MITHRACIN

RESULTS IN 305 TESTICULAR TUMOR CASES BY TUMOR TYPE

TYPE OF TESTICULAR TUMOR	TOTAL	COMPLETE RESPONSE	PARTIAL RESPONSE	NO RESPONSE
EMBRYONAL CELL	173	26	42	105
TERATOMA	5	0	1	4
TERATOCARCINOMA	23	0	5	18
SEMINOMA	18	0	7	11
CHORIOCARCINOMA	13	1	6	6
MIXED TUMOR	73	6	19	48
TOTALS	305	33	80	192

REFERENCES

1. Kennedy, B.D., et al: Cancer Res. *27*:1534, 1967.
2. Ransohoff, J., et al: Cancer Chemother. Rep. *49*:51, 1965.
3. Recommendations for the Safe Handling of Parenteral Antieoplastic Drugs. NIH Publication No. 83-2621. For sale by the Superintendent of Documents, U.S. Government Printing Office, Washington, D.C. 20402.
4. AMA Council Report. Guidelines for Handling Parenteral Antineoplastics. JAMA, March 15, 1985.
5. National Study Commission on Cytotoxic Exposure—Recommendations for Handling Cytotoxic Agents. Available from Louis P. Jeffrey, Sc.D., Director of Pharmacy Services, Rhode Island Hospital, 593 Eddy Street, Providence, Rhode Island 02902.
6. Clinical Oncological Society of Australia: Guidelines and recommendations for safe handling of antineoplastic agents. Med J Australia *1*:426–428, 1983.
7. Jones, R.B., et al: Safe handling of chemotherapeutic agents: A report from the Mount Sinai Medical Center.

Ca—A Cancer Journal for Clinicians, Sept/Oct. 258–263, 1983.

8. American Society of Hospital Pharmacists technical assistance bulletin on handling cytotoxic drugs in hospitals. Am J Hosp Pharm 42:131–137, 1985.

Manufactured for
Miles Inc.
Pharmaceutical Division
400 Morgan Lane
West Haven, CT 06516
by Ben Venue Laboratories
Bedford, Ohio 44146
PD100654—60-4178-81-4   Revised September, 1987

MYCELEX®   ℞
(clotrimazole) TROCHE
FOR TOPICAL ORAL ADMINISTRATION

PRODUCT OVERVIEW

KEY FACTS

MYCELEX® Troche is a slow-dissolving tablet (lozenge) containing 10 mg of clotrimazole, a synthetic antifungal agent for topical use in the mouth. Clotrimazole is a broad-spectrum antifungal which exhibits fungicidal activity *in vitro* against *Candida albicans* and other species of the genus *Candida*. No single-step or multiple-step resistance to clotrimazole has developed during successive passages of *Candida albicans* in the laboratory.

MAJOR USES

MYCELEX® Troche has been proven effective in the treatment of oropharyngeal candidiasis (oral thrush) in patients over 3 years of age.

SAFETY INFORMATION

MYCELEX® Troches are contra-indicated in patients who are hypersensitive to any of its components. MYCELEX Troches are not indicated for the treatment of systemic mycoses. Since elevated SGOT levels have been reported, periodic assessment of hepatic function is advisable, particularly, in patients with pre-existing hepatic impairment.

PRESCRIBING INFORMATION

MYCELEX®   ℞
(clotrimazole) TROCHE
FOR TOPICAL ORAL ADMINISTRATION

DESCRIPTION

Each Mycelex® Troche contains 10 mg clotrimazole [1-(o-chloro-α,α-diphenylbenzyl) imidazole], a synthetic antifungal agent, for topical use in the mouth.
Structural Formula:

Chemical Formula:
$C_{22}H_{17}ClN_2$

The troche dosage form is a large, slowly dissolving tablet (lozenge) containing 10 mg of clotrimazole dispersed in dextrose, microcrystalline cellulose, povidone, and magnesium stearate.

CLINICAL PHARMACOLOGY

Clotrimazole is a broad-spectrum antifungal agent that inhibits the growth of pathogenic yeasts by altering the permeability of cell membranes. The action of clotrimazole is fungistatic at concentrations of drug up to 20 mcg/mL and may be fungicidal *in vitro* against *Candida albicans* and other species of the genus *Candida* at higher concentrations. No single-step or multiple-step resistance to clotrimazole has developed during successive passages of *Candida albicans* in the laboratory; however, individual organism tolerance has been observed during successive passages in the laboratory. Such *in vitro* tolerance has resolved once the organism has been removed from the antifungal environment.
After oral administration of a 10 mg clotrimazole troche to healthy volunteers, concentrations sufficient to inhibit most species of *Candida* persist in saliva for up to three hours following the approximately 30 minutes needed for a troche to dissolve. The long term persistence of drug in saliva appears to be related to the slow release of clotrimazole from the oral mucosa to which the drug is apparently bound. Repetitive dosing at three hour intervals maintains salivary levels above the minimum inhibitory concentrations of most strains of *Candida*; however, the relationship between *in*

vitro susceptibility of pathogenic fungi to clotrimazole and prophylaxis or cure of infections in humans has not been established.
In another study, the mean serum concentrations were 4.98 ± 3.7 and 3.23 ± 1.4 nanograms/mL of clotrimazole at 30 and 60 minutes, respectively, after administration as a troche.

INDICATIONS AND USAGE

Mycelex® Troches are indicated for the local treatment of oropharyngeal candidiasis. The diagnosis should be confirmed by a KOH smear and/or culture prior to treatment. Mycelex Troches are also indicated prophylactically to reduce the incidence of oropharyngeal candidiasis in patients immunocompromised by conditions that include chemotherapy, radiotherapy, or steroid therapy utilized in the treatment of leukemia, solid tumors, or renal transplantation. There are no data from adequate and well-controlled trials to establish the safety and efficacy of this product for prophylactic use in patients immunocompromised by etiologies other than those listed in the previous sentence. (See DOSAGE AND ADMINISTRATION.)

CONTRAINDICATIONS

Mycelex® Troches are contraindicated in patients who are hypersensitive to any of its components.

WARNING

Mycelex® Troches are not indicated for the treatment of systemic mycoses including systemic candidiasis.

PRECAUTIONS

Abnormal liver function tests have been reported in patients treated with clotrimazole troches; elevated SGOT levels were reported in about 15% of patients in the clinical trials. In most cases the elevations were minimal and it was often impossible to distinguish effects of clotrimazole from those of other therapy and the underlying disease (malignancy in most cases). Periodic assessment of hepatic function is advisable particularly in patients with pre-existing hepatic impairment.
Since patients must be instructed to allow each troche to dissolve slowly in the mouth in order to achieve maximum effect of the medication, they must be of such an age and physical and/or mental condition to comprehend such instructions.
Carcinogenesis: An 18 month dosing study with clotrimazole in rats has not revealed any carcinogenic effect.
Usage in Pregnancy: Pregnancy Category C: Clotrimazole has been shown to be embryotoxic in rats and mice when given in doses 100 times the adult human dose (in mg/kg), possibly secondary to maternal toxicity. The drug was not teratogenic in mice, rabbits, and rats when given in doses up to 200, 180, and 100 times the human dose.
Clotrimazole given orally to mice from nine weeks before mating through weaning at a dose 120 times the human dose was associated with impairment of mating, decreased number of viable young, and decreased survival to weaning. No effects were observed at 60 times the human dose. When the drug was given to rats during a similar time period at 50 times the human dose, there was a slight decrease in the number of pups per litter and decreased pup viability. There are no adequate and well controlled studies in pregnant women. Clotrimazole troches should be used during pregnancy only if the potential benefit justifies the potential risk to the fetus.

PEDIATRIC USE

Safety and effectiveness of clotrimazole in children below the age of 3 years have not been established; therefore, its use in such patients is not recommended.
The safety and efficacy of the prophylactic use of clotrimazole troches in children have not been established.

ADVERSE REACTIONS

Abnormal liver function tests have been reported in patients treated with clotrimazole troches; elevated SGOT levels were reported in about 15% of patients in the clinical trials (See Precautions section).
Nausea, vomiting, unpleasant mouth sensations and pruritus have also been reported with the use of the troche.

OVERDOSAGE

No data available.

DRUG ABUSE AND DEPENDENCE

No data available.

DOSAGE AND ADMINISTRATION

Mycelex® Troches are administered only as a lozenge that must be slowly dissolved in the mouth. The recommended dose is one troche five times a day for fourteen consecutive days. Only limited data are available on the safety and effectiveness of the clotrimazole troche after prolonged administration; therefore, therapy should be limited to short term use, if possible.
For prophylaxis to reduce the incidence of oropharyngeal candidiasis in patients immunocompromised by conditions that include chemotherapy, radio-therapy, or steroid therapy utilized in the treatment of leukemia, solid tumors, or

renal transplantation, the recommended dose is one troche three times daily for the duration of chemotherapy or until steroids are reduced to maintenance levels.

HOW SUPPLIED

Mycelex® Troches, white discoid, uncoated tablets are supplied in bottles of 70 and 140. Mycelex Troches are also available for institutional use in foil packages of 70 tablets. Each tablet will be identified with the following: Miles 095.
Store below 86°F (30°C).
Avoid freezing.

Miles Inc.
Pharmaceutical Division
400 Morgan Lane
West Haven, CT 06516 USA
PD100717   BAY 5097   2147
© 1992 Miles Inc   8/92
Shown in Product Identification Section, page 420

MYCELEX®-G 1%   ℞
(clotrimazole) Vaginal Cream

PRODUCT OVERVIEW

KEY FACTS

Mycelex®-G-1% Vaginal Cream is an effective vaginal antifungal cream. Each applicatorful of Mycelex-G-1% Vaginal Cream contains approximately 50 mg of clotrimazole. Clotrimazole is a broad spectrum antifungal which exhibits fungicidal activity *in vitro* against *Candida albicans* and other species of the genus *Candida*. No single-step or multiple-step resistance to clotrimazole has developed during successive passages of *Candida albicans*.

MAJOR USES

Mycelex®-G-1% Vaginal Cream has been proven clinically effective for the local treatment of patients with vulvovaginal candidiasis.

SAFETY INFORMATION

Mycelex®-G-1% Vaginal Cream is contraindicated in women who have shown hypersensitivity to any of the components. If there is a lack of response to treatment with Mycelex®-G-1% Vaginal Cream, appropriate microbiological studies should be repeated to confirm the diagnosis and rule out other pathogens before instituting another course of antimycotic therapy. No adequate and well-controlled studies in pregnany women during the first trimester of pregnancy.

PRESCRIBING INFORMATION

MYCELEX®-G 1%   ℞
(clotrimazole) Vaginal Cream

DESCRIPTION

Mycelex-G is clotrimazole [1-(o-Chloro-α, α-diphenylbenzyl) imidazole], a synthetic antifungal agent having the chemical formula, $C_{22}H_{17}ClN_2$, and following chemical structure:

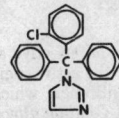

Each applicatorful of Mycelex-G Vaginal Cream contains approximately 50 mg clotrimazole dispersed in sorbitan monostearate, polysorbate 60, cetyl esters wax, cetostearyl alcohol, 2-octyldodecanol, purified water, and as a preservative, benzyl alcohol (1%).

ACTIONS

Clotrimazole is a broad spectrum antifungal agent that inhibits the growth of pathogenic yeasts. Clotrimazole exhibits fungicidal activity *in vitro* against *Candida albicans* and other species of the genus *Candida*.
No single-step or multiple-step resistance to clotrimazole has developed during successive passages of *Candida albicans*.

INDICATIONS

Mycelex®-G Vaginal Cream is indicated for the local treatment of patients with vulvovaginal candidiasis (moniliasis). As Mycelex-G Vaginal Cream has been shown to be effective only for candidal vulvovaginitis, the diagnosis should be confirmed by KOH smears and/or cultures. Other pathogens commonly associated with vulvovaginitis (*Trichomonas* and *Hemophilus vaginalis*) should be ruled out by appropriate laboratory methods.
Studies have shown that women taking oral contraceptives had a cure rate similar to those not taking oral contraceptives.

Continued on next page

Miles—Cont.

CONTRAINDICATIONS

Mycelex®-G Vaginal Cream is contraindicated in women who have shown hypersensitivity to any of the components of the preparation.

PRECAUTIONS

Laboratory Tests: If there is a lack of response to Mycelex-G Vaginal Cream, appropriate microbiological studies should be repeated to confirm the diagnosis and rule out other pathogens before instituting another course of antimycotic therapy.

Usage in Pregnancy: While Mycelex-G Vaginal Cream has not been studied in the first trimester of pregnancy, use in the second and third trimesters has not been associated with ill effects.

Application of ^{14}C-labeled clotrimazole has shown negligible absorption (peak serum level of 0.01 mcg/mL 24 hours after insertion of vaginal cream containing 50 mg of active drug) from both normal and inflamed human vaginal mucosa.

ADVERSE REACTIONS

Three (0.5%) of the 653 patients treated with Mycelex-G Vaginal Cream reported complaints during therapy that were possibly drug related. Vaginal burning occurred in one patient; erythema, irritation and burning in another; intercurrent cystitis was reported in the third.

DOSAGE AND ADMINISTRATION

Mycelex-G Vaginal Cream has been found to be effective when used from seven to fourteen days; studies have shown that patients treated for fourteen days had a significantly higher cure rate. The recommended dose is one applicatorful a day for seven to fourteen consecutive days; using the applicator supplied, insert one applicatorful of cream (approximately 5 grams) intravaginally preferably at bedtime.

HOW SUPPLIED

Mycelex-G Vaginal Cream 1% is supplied in 45 and 90 gram tubes with a measured-dose applicator, for seven-day and for fourteen-day treatments.

	NDC Numbers
45g	0026-3094-45
90g	0026-3094-46

Caution: Federal (USA) law prohibits dispensing without prescription.

Store below 86°F (30°C).
Miles Inc.
Pharmaceutical Division
400 Morgan Lane
West Haven, CT 06516 USA
PD100679-0290   2/88   BAY 5097
© 1989 Miles Inc.

MYCELEX®-G 500 mg ℞
brand of clotrimazole
Vaginal Tablets

PRODUCT OVERVIEW

KEY FACTS

Mycelex®-G 500 mg is an effective antifungal containing 500 mg of clotrimazole (the active ingredient). Clotrimazole is a broad spectrum antifungal which exhibits fungicidal activity *in vitro* against *Candida albicans* and other species of the genus *Candida*. No single-step or multiple-step resistance to clotrimazole has developed during successive passages of *Candida albicans*.

MAJOR USES

Mycelex®-G 500 mg has proved to be clinically effective for local treatment of vulvovaginal candidiasis when one day therapy is felt warranted. In the case of severe vulvovaginal candidiasis longer antimycotic therapy such as Mycelex®-G 100 mg tablets or Mycelex®-G Cream is recommended.

SAFETY INFORMATION

Mycelex®-G 500 Vaginal Tablets are contraindicated in women who have shown hypersensitivity to any components of the compound. If there is a lack of response to treatment with Mycelex®-G 500 mg, appropriate microbiological studies should be repeated to confirm the diagnosis and rule out other pathogens before instituting another course of antimycotic therapy. No adequate and well-controlled studies in pregnant women during the first trimester of pregnancy.

PRESCRIBING INFORMATION

MYCELEX®-G 500mg ℞
brand of clotrimazole
Vaginal Tablets

DESCRIPTION

Each Mycelex®-G 500 mg Vaginal Tablet contains 500 mg clotrimazole (the active ingredient) dispersed in lactose, microcrystalline cellulose, lactic acid, corn starch, crospovi-

done, calcium lactate, magnesium stearate, silicon dioxide and hydroxypropyl methylcellulose. Chemically, clotrimazole is [1-(o-Chloro-α, α-diphenylbenzyl) imidazole], a synthetic antifungal agent having the chemical formula $C_{22}H_{17}ClN_2$; a molecular weight of 344.84; and the following chemical structure:

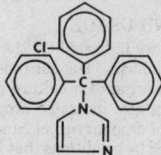

Clotrimazole is an odorless, white crystalline substance, practically insoluble in water, sparingly soluble in ether, soluble in carbon tetrachloride, and very soluble in ethanol and chloroform.

CLINICAL PHARMACOLOGY

Serum levels and levels in vaginal secretions of clotrimazole were measured in six healthy volunteers who had one 500 mg vaginal tablet inserted. Although serum levels of clotrimazole were higher than those in other volunteers given 100 mg and 200 mg vaginal tablets these levels did not exceed 10 nanograms/mL. It has been estimated that three to ten percent of a vaginal dose of clotrimazole may be absorbed, but the drug rapidly and efficiently degrades to microbiologically inactive metabolites. The clotrimazole concentrations remaining in vaginal secretions were still in the mg/mL range for 48 hours and in two of the six subjects at 72 hours.

The findings of high clotrimazole concentrations in vaginal secretions for up to 72 hours and low concentrations in the serum suggest that nearly all the clotrimazole given in the 500 mg vaginal tablet remains in the vagina for 48 hours, and in some cases 72 hours, in fungicidal concentrations.

Clotrimazole is a broad-spectrum antifungal agent. It has been postulated that the compound affects the permeability characteristics of the membrane allowing the leakage of essential intracellular components with a consequent inhibition of the synthesis of such macromolecules as protein, lipid, DNA, and polysaccharides.

At concentrations as low as 2–5 µg/mL, clotrimazole exhibits fungicidal activity *in vitro* against *Candida albicans* and other species of the genus *Candida*.

No single-step or multiple-step resistance to clotrimazole has developed during successive passages of *Candida albicans*.

INDICATIONS

Mycelex-G 500 mg Vaginal Tablets are indicated for the local treatment of vulvovaginal candidiasis when one day therapy is felt warranted. In the case of severe vulvovaginitis due to candidiasis, longer antimycotic therapy is recommended. The diagnosis should be confirmed by KOH smears and/or cultures. Other pathogens commonly associated with vulvovaginitis, *Trichomonas* and *Gardnerella (Haemophilus) vaginalis*, should be ruled out by appropriate laboratory methods.

CONTRAINDICATIONS

Mycelex-G 500 mg Vaginal Tablets are contraindicated in women who have shown hypersensitivity to any components of the preparation.

WARNINGS

None.

PRECAUTIONS

If there is a lack of response to Mycelex-G 500 mg Vaginal Tablets, appropriate microbiological studies should be repeated to confirm the diagnosis and rule out other pathogens before instituting another course of antimycotic therapy.

CARCINOGENESIS

No long term studies in animals have been performed to evaluate the carcinogenic potential of Mycelex-G 500 mg Vaginal Tablets intravaginally. A long term study in rats (Wistar strains) where clotrimazole was administered orally provided no indication of carcinogenicity.

USAGE IN PREGNANCY

Category B: The disposition of ^{14}C-clotrimazole has been studied in humans and animals. Clotrimazole is poorly absorbed following intravaginal administration to humans, whereas it is rather well absorbed after oral administration. In clinical trials, use of vaginally applied clotrimazole in pregnant women in their second and third trimesters has not been associated with ill effects. There are, however, no adequate and well-controlled studies in pregnant women during the first trimester of pregnancy.

Studies in pregnant rats given repeated intravaginal doses up to 100 mg/kg/day have revealed no evidence of harm to the fetus due to clotrimazole.

Repeated high oral doses of clotrimazole in rats and mice ranging from 50 to 120 mg/kg resulted in embryotoxicity (possibly secondary to maternal toxicity), impairment of mating, decreased litter size and number of viable young and

decreased pup survival to weaning. However, clotrimazole was not teratogenic in mice, rabbits and rats at oral doses up to 200, 180 and 100 mg/kg, respectively. Oral absorption in the rat amounts to approximately 90% of the administered dose.

Because animal reproduction studies are not always predictive of human response, this drug should be used only if clearly indicated during the first trimester of pregnancy.

ADVERSE REACTIONS

Of 297 patients in double-blind studies with the 500 mg vaginal tablet, 3 of 149 patients treated with active drug and 3 of 148 patients treated with placebo reported complaints during therapy that were possibly drug related. In the active drug group, vomiting occurred in one patient, vaginal soreness with coitus in another, and complaints of vaginal irritation, itching, burning and dyspareunia in the third patient. In the placebo group, clitoral irritation occurred in one patient and dysuria, described as remotely related to drug, in the other. A third patient in the placebo group developed bacterial vaginitis which the investigator classed as possibly related to drug.

Eighteen (1.6%) of the 1116 patients treated with Mycelex-G in other formulations in double-blind studies reported complaints during therapy that were possibly drug-related. Mild burning occurred in six patients while other complaints such as skin rash, itching, vulval irritation, lower abdominal cramps and bloating, slight cramping, slight urinary frequency, and burning or irritation in the sexual partner, occurred rarely.

OVERDOSAGE

No data available.

DRUG ABUSE AND DEPENDENCE

Drug abuse and dependence with Mycelex-G 500 mg Vaginal Tablets has not been reported.

DOSAGE AND ADMINISTRATION

The recommended dose is one tablet inserted intravaginally one time only, preferably at bedtime. In the event of treatment failure, that is, persistence of signs and symptoms of vaginitis after five days, other pathogens commonly responsible for vaginitis should be ruled out before instituting another course of antimycotic therapy.

HOW SUPPLIED

Mycelex-G 500 mg Vaginal Tablets are white, bullet shaped, uncoated tablets, coded with Miles on one side and 097 on the other, supplied as a single 500 mg tablet with plastic applicator and patient instructions, or in twin pack with Mycelex 1% cream 7g tube.

Store Below 86°F (30°C).
U.S. Patent Numbers 3,660,577; 3,705,172; 3,839,573; 4,457,938.
Manufactured by
Miles Inc.
Pharmaceutical Division
400 Morgan Lane
West Haven, CT 06516
PD100689-0563   6/88   BAY 5097
© 1989 Miles Inc.
Shown in Product Identification Section, page 420

NICLOCIDE® ℞
(niclosamide)
Chewable Tablets

DESCRIPTION

NICLOCIDE (niclosamide) is an anthelmintic provided in chewable tablet form at a strength of 500 mg per tablet. Niclosamide is 2', 5-Dichloro-4'-nitrosalicylanilide. Inactive ingredients: corn starch, magnesium stearate, povidone, sodium lauryl sulfate, sodium saccharin, talc and vanillin. The empirical formula is $C_{13}H_8Cl_2N_2O_4$ with the following structural formula:

CLINICAL PHARMACOLOGY

NICLOCIDE inhibits oxidative phosphorylation in the mitochondria of cestodes. Both *in vitro* and *in vivo*, the scolex and proximal segments are killed on contact with the drug. The scolex of the tapeworm, loosened from the gut wall, may be digested in the intestine, and thus may not be identified in the feces even after extensive purging.

The use of NICLOCIDE has not been associated with the development of anemia, leukopenia or thrombocytopenia nor have there been any effects on normal renal and hepatic functions.

INDICATIONS AND USAGE

NICLOCIDE (niclosamide) is indicated for the treatment of tapeworm infections by *Taenia saginata* (beef tapeworm), *Diphyllobothrium latum* (fish tapeworm) and *Hymenolepis nana* (dwarf tapeworm).

CONTRAINDICATIONS

NICLOCIDE™ Tablets are contraindicated in individuals who have shown hypersensitivity to any of its components.

PRECAUTIONS

NICLOCIDE affects the cestodes of the intestine only. It is without effect in cysticercosis.

Drug Interactions: No data are available regarding interaction of niclosamide with other drugs.

Carcinogenesis, mutagenesis, impairment of fertility:

Carcinogenicity Potential: Although carcinogenicity studies on niclosamide *per se* have not been done, long-term feeding studies on its ethanolamine salt in rats and mice did not show carcinogenicity. Mutagenicity tests have not been performed.

Pregnancy: Pregnancy Category B: Reproduction studies in rabbits and rats at doses of 25 times the human therapeutic dose and in mice at 12 times the human therapeutic dose, have revealed no evidence of impaired fertility or harm to the fetus due to niclosamide. There are, however, no adequate and well-controlled studies in pregnant women. Because animal studies are not always predictive of human response, the drug should be used during pregnancy only if clearly needed.

Nursing Mothers: No studies are available.

Pediatric Use: In children under 2 years of age, the safety of the drug has not been established.

ADVERSE REACTIONS

The incidence of side effects has been reported as follows: nausea/vomiting 4.1%, abdominal discomfort including loss of appetite 3.4%, diarrhea 1.6%, drowsiness, dizziness, and or headache 1.4%, and skin rash including pruritus ani 0.3%. Other side effects listed in decreasing order of frequency were: oral irritation, fever, rectal bleeding, weakness, bad taste in mouth, sweating, palpitations, constipation, alopecia, edema of an arm, backache and irritability. There was also one instance of a transient rise in SGOT in an i.v. narcotic addict. Two cases of urticaria reported may be related to the breakdown products of the tapeworm. All side effects were mild or moderate and transitory and did not necessitate discontinuation of the treatment.

OVERDOSAGE

Insufficient data are available. In the event of overdose a fast-acting laxative and enema should be given. Vomiting should not be induced.

DOSAGE AND ADMINISTRATION

1. *Taenia saginata* and *Diphyllobothrium latum*
   a. Adults: 4 tablets (2.0 g) chewed thoroughly in a single dose.
   b. Children weighing more than 34 kg (75 lbs): 3 tablets (1.5 g) chewed thoroughly in a single dose.
   c. Children weighing between 11 and 34 kg (25 to 75 lbs): 2 tablets (1.0 g) chewed thoroughly in a single dose.
2. *Hymenolepis nana*
   a. Adults: 4 tablets (2.0 g) chewed thoroughly as a single daily dose for 7 days.
   b. Children weighing more than 34 kg (75 lbs): 3 tablets (1.5g) chewed thoroughly on the first day, then 2 tablets (1.0 g) daily for next 6 days.
   c. Children weighing between 11 and 34 kg (25 to 75 lbs): 2 tablets (1.0 g) to be chewed thoroughly on the first day, then one tablet (0.5 g) daily for next 6 days.

   T. saginata and *D. latum* infections are usually due to a single adult worm and require an intermediate host in their life cycle. With *Hymenolepis nana* multiple infections are the rule. No intermediate host is required; both larval and adult stages of the worm may be found in the human intestine where the complete life cycle occurs. Since the drug is more effective against the mature than the larval stage, therapy must be extended over several days to cover all stages of maturation.

   Patients with *H. nana* must be instructed to observe strict personal and environmental hygiene to avoid autoinfection with this parasite.
3. NICLOCIDE™ must be thoroughly chewed and then swallowed with a little water. No special dietary restrictions are necessary before or after treatment. The best time to take the drug is after a light meal (e.g., breakfast). A mild laxative may be desirable in constipated patients to achieve a normal bowel movement. Young children should have the tablets crushed to a fine powder and mixed with a small amount of water to form a paste.

   NICLOCIDE has a vanilla taste which is not unpleasant to most persons.

   NICLOCIDE is suitable for administration on an ambulatory or outpatient basis.
4. Follow-up:

   As the vermicidal action of NICLOCIDE renders the tapeworm, especially the scolex and proximal segments, vulnerable to destruction during their passage through the gut, it is not always possible to identify the scolex in stools. The sooner the tapeworm is passed and examined after treatment, the better the chance of identification of the scolex. Segments and/or ova of beef or fish tapeworm may be present in the stool for up to 3 days after therapy. Persistent *T. saginata* or *D. latum* segments and/or ova on the seventh day post therapy indicate failure. A second identical course of treatment may be given at that time.

   No patient should be considered cured unless the stool has been negative for a minimum of three months.

HOW SUPPLIED

NICLOCIDE is available as round, light yellow chewable tablets, scored on one side, coded with the word Miles and number 721, each containing 500 mg of niclosamide, and is supplied in boxes of 4 tablets.

Storage Conditions: Store below 86°F (30°C), avoid freezing.

Miles Inc.
Pharmaceutical Division
400 Morgan Lane
West Haven, CT 06516
PD100697-0617 BAY 2353 June 1985

Shown in Product Identification Section, page 420

NIMOTOP® ℞
(nimodipine)
CAPSULES
For Oral Use

DESCRIPTION

Nimotop® (nimodipine) belongs to the class of pharmacological agents known as calcium channel blockers. Nimodipine is isopropyl (2 - methoxyethyl) 1, 4 - dihydro - 2, 6 - dimethyl - 4 - (3 - nitrophenyl) - 3, 5 - pyridine - dicarboxylate. It has a molecular weight of 418.5 and a molecular formula of $C_{21}H_{26}N_2O_7$. The structural formula is:

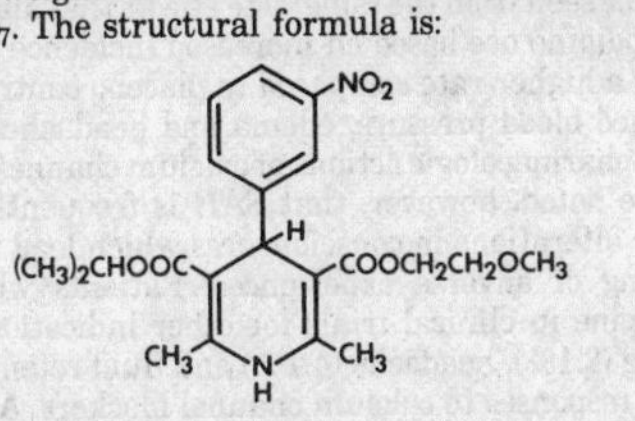

Nimodipine is a yellow crystalline substance, practically insoluble in water.

NIMOTOP® capsules are formulated as soft gelatin capsules for oral administration. Each liquid filled capsule contains 30 mg of nimodipine in a vehicle of glycerin, peppermint oil, purified water and polyethylene glycol 400. The soft gelatin capsule shell contains gelatin, glycerin, purified water and titanium dioxide.

CLINICAL PHARMACOLOGY

Mechanism of Action: Nimodipine is a calcium channel blocker. The contractile processes of smooth muscle cells are dependent upon calcium ions, which enter these cells during depolarization as slow ionic transmembrane currents. Nimodipine inhibits calcium ion transfer into these cells and thus inhibits contractions of vascular smooth muscle. In animal experiments, nimodipine had a greater effect on cerebral arteries than on arteries elsewhere in the body perhaps because it is highly lipophilic, allowing it to cross the blood-brain barrier; concentrations of nimodipine as high as 12.5 ng/mL have been detected in the cerebrospinal fluid of nimodipine treated subarachnoid hemorrhage (SAH) patients.

Based on animal experiments, it was hoped that nimodipine would prevent cerebral arterial spasm in SAH patients. While the clinical studies described below demonstrate a favorable effect by nimodipine on the severity of neurological deficits caused by cerebral vasospasm following SAH, there is no arteriographic evidence that the drug either prevents or relieves the spasm of these arteries. The actual mechanism of action in humans is, therefore, unknown.

Pharmacokinetics and Metabolism: In man, nimodipine is rapidly absorbed after oral administration, and peak concentrations are generally attained within one hour. The terminal elimination half-life is approximately 8 to 9 hours but earlier elimination rates are much more rapid, equivalent to a half-life of 1–2 hours; a consequence is the need for frequent (every 4 hours) dosing. There were no signs of accumulation when nimodipine was given three times a day for seven days. Nimodipine is over 95% bound to plasma proteins. The binding was concentration independent over the range of 10 ng/mL to 10 μg/mL. Nimodipine is eliminated almost exclusively in the form of metabolites and less than 1% is recovered in the urine as unchanged drug. Numerous metabolites, all of which are either inactive or considerably less active than the parent compound, have been identified. Because of a high first-pass metabolism, the bioavailability of nimodipine averages 13% after oral administration. The bioavailability is significantly increased in patients with hepatic cirrhosis, with C_{max} approximately double that in normals which necessitates lowering the dose in this group of patients (see Dosage and Administration). The influence of food on the pharmacokinetics of nimodipine capsules has not been studied.

Clinical Trials: Nimodipine has been shown, in 4 randomized, placebo-controlled trials, to reduce the severity of neurological deficits resulting from vasospasm in patients who have had a recent subarachnoid hemorrhage (SAH). The trials used doses ranging from 20–30 mg to 90 mg every 4 hours, with drug given for 21 days in 3 studies, and for at least 18 days in the other. Three of the four trials followed patients for 3–6 months. Three of the trials studied relatively well patients, with all or most patients in Hunt and Hess Grades I–II (essentially free of focal deficits after the initial bleed); the fourth studied much sicker patients, Hunt and Hess Grades III–V. Two studies, one domestic, one French, were similar in design, with relatively unimpaired SAH patients randomized to nimodipine or placebo. In each, a judgment was made as to whether any late-developing deficit was due to spasm or other causes, and the deficits were graded. Both studies showed significantly fewer severe deficits due to spasm in the nimodipine group; the second (French) study showed fewer spasm-related deficits of all severities. No effect was seen on deficits not related to spasm.

[See table below.]

A Canadian study entered much sicker patients, who had a high rate of death and disability, and used a dose of 90 mg every 4 hours, but was otherwise similar to the first two studies. Analysis of delayed ischemic deficits, many of which result from spasm, showed a significant reduction in spasm-related deficits. Among analyzed patients (72 nimodipine, 82 placebo), there were the following outcomes.

[See table at top of next page.]

A fourth, large, study was performed in the United Kingdom in SAH patients with all grades of severity (but about 90% were in Grades I–III). Outcomes were not defined as spasm related or not but there was a significant reduction in the overall rate of infarction and severely disabling neurological outcome at 3 months:

	Nimodipine	Placebo
Total patients	278	276
Good recovery	199*	169
Moderate disability	24	16
Severe disability	12**	31
Death	43***	60

* $p = 0.0444$—good and moderate vs severe and dead
** $p = 0.001$—severe disability
*** $p = 0.056$—death

A dose-ranging study comparing 30, 60 and 90 mg doses found a generally low rate of spasm-related neurological deficits but no significant relation of response to dose.

The effect of nimodipine on mortality is not yet clear. The large United Kingdom study showed near-significantly improved survival. The two smaller studies (domestic, French) had too few deaths to contribute to this question. The Canadian study, despite showing markedly decreased spasm-related deficits, showed overall (all patients randomized) greater 90 day mortality, 49/91 (54%) on nimodipine vs 38/97 (39%) on placebo, a significant difference. Most of the

Study	Dose	Grade*	Number Analyzed	Patients: Any Deficit Due to Spasm	Patients: Numbers With Severe Deficit
1.	20–30 mg	I–III	Nimodipine 56	13	1
			Placebo 60	16	8**
2.	60 mg	I–III	Nimodipine 31	4	2
			Placebo 39	11	10**

*Hunt and Hess Grade
**p = 0.03

Continued on next page

Miles—Cont.

deaths appeared, in this very severely ill group (Hunt and Hess Grades III–V), to be consequences of SAH, but a drug effect cannot be ruled out. In this study 90 mg every 4 hours was the dose used, perhaps too high for the very ill population studied. The 90 mg dose is not recommended nor is treatment of Hunt and Hess Grades IV–V patients.

INDICATIONS AND USAGE

Nimotop® (nimodipine) is indicated for the improvement of neurological outcome by reducing the incidence and severity of ischemic deficits in patients with subarachnoid hemorrhage from ruptured congenital aneurysms who are in good neurological condition post-ictus (e.g., Hunt and Hess Grades I–III).

CONTRAINDICATIONS

None known.

PRECAUTIONS

General: Blood Pressure: Nimodipine has the hemodynamic effects expected of a calcium channel blocker, although they are generally not marked. In patients with subarachnoid hemorrhage given Nimotop® in clinical studies, about 5% were reported to have had lowering of the blood pressure and about 1% left the study because of this (not all could be attributed to nimodipine). Nevertheless, blood pressure should be carefully monitored during treatment with Nimotop® based on its known pharmacology and the known effects of calcium channel blockers.

Hepatic Disease: The metabolism of Nimotop® is decreased in patients with impaired hepatic function. Such patients should have their blood pressure and pulse rate monitored closely and should be given a lower dose (see Dosage and Administration).

Intestinal pseudo-obstruction and ileus have been reported rarely in patients treated with nimodipine. A causal relationship has not been established. The condition has responded to conservative management.

Laboratory Test Interactions: None known.

Drug Interaction: It is possible that the cardiovascular action of other calcium channel blockers could be enhanced by the addition of Nimotop®.

In Europe, Nimotop® was observed to occasionally intensify the effect of antihypertensive compounds taken concomitantly by patients suffering from hypertension; this phenomenon was not observed in North American clinical trials.

A study in eight healthy volunteers has shown a 50% increase in mean peak nimodipine plasma concentrations and a 90% increase in mean area under the curve, after a one-week course of cimetidine at 1,000 mg/day and nimodipine at 90 mg/day. This effect may be mediated by the known inhibition of hepatic cytochrome P-450 by cimetidine, which could decrease first-pass metabolism of nimodipine.

Carcinogenesis, Mutagenesis, Impairment of Fertility: In a two-year study, higher incidences of adenocarcinoma of the uterus and Leydig-cell adenoma of the testes were observed in rats given a diet containing 1800 ppm nimodipine (equivalent to 91 to 121 mg/kg/day nimodipine) than in placebo controls. The differences were not statistically significant, however, and the higher rates were well within historical control range for these tumors in the Wistar strain. Nimodipine was found not to be carcinogenic in a 91-week mouse study but the high dose of 1800 ppm nimodipine-in-feed (546 to 774 mg/kg/day) shortened the life expectancy of the animals. Mutagenicity studies, including the Ames, micronucleus and dominant lethal tests were negative.

Nimodipine did not impair the fertility and general reproductive performance of male and female Wistar rats following oral doses of up to 30 mg/kg/day when administered daily for more than 10 weeks in the males and 3 weeks in the females prior to mating and continued to day 7 of pregnancy. This dose in a rat is about 4 times the equivalent clinical dose of 60 mg q4h in a 50 kg patient.

Pregnancy: Pregnancy Category C. Nimodipine has been shown to have a teratogenic effect in Himalayan rabbits. Incidences of malformations and stunted fetuses were increased at oral doses of 1 and 10 mg/kg/day administered (by gavage) from day 6 through day 18 of pregnancy but not at 3.0 mg/kg/day in one of two identical rabbit studies. In the second study an increased incidence of stunted fetuses was seen at 1.0 mg/kg/day but not at higher doses. Nimodipine was embryotoxic, causing resorption and stunted growth of fetuses, in Long Evans rats at 100 mg/kg/day administered by gavage from day 6 through day 15 of pregnancy. In two other rat studies, doses of 30 mg/kg/day nimodipine administered by gavage from day 16 of gestation and continued until sacrifice (day 20 of pregnancy or day 21 post partum) were associated with higher incidences of skeletal variation, stunted fetuses and stillbirths but no malformations. There are no adequate and well controlled studies in pregnant women to directly assess the effect on human fetuses. Nimodipine should be used during pregnancy only if the potential benefit justifies the potential risk to the fetus.

	Delayed Ischemic Deficits (DID)		Permanent Deficits	
	Nimodipine n (%)	Placebo n (%)	Nimodipine n (%)	Placebo n (%)
DID Spasm alone	8 (11)*	25 (31)	5 (7)*	22 (27)
DID Spasm Contributing	18 (25)	21 (26)	16 (22)	17 (21)
DID Without Spasm	7 (10)	8 (10)	6 (8)	7 (9)
No DID	39 (54)	28 (34)	45 (63)	36 (44)

*P = 0.001, nimodipine vs placebo

Nursing Mothers: Nimodipine and/or its metabolites have been shown to appear in rat milk at concentrations much higher than in maternal plasma. It is not known whether the drug is excreted in human milk. Because many drugs are excreted in human milk, nursing mothers are advised not to breast feed their babies when taking the drug.

Pediatric Use: Safety and effectiveness in children have not been established.

ADVERSE REACTIONS

Adverse experiences were reported by 92 of 823 patients with subarachnoid hemorrhage (11.2%) who were given nimodipine. The most frequently reported adverse experience was decreased blood pressure in 4.4% of these patients. Twenty-nine of 479 (6.1%) placebo treated patients also reported adverse experiences. The events reported with a frequency greater than 1% are displayed below by dose. [See table below.]

There were no other adverse experiences reported by the patients who were given 0.35 mg/kg q4h, 30 mg q4h or 120 mg q4h. Adverse experiences with an incidence rate of less than 1% in the 60 mg q4h dose group were: hepatitis; itching; gastrointestinal hemorrhage; thrombocytopenia; anemia; palpitations; vomiting; flushing; diaphoresis; wheezing; phenytoin toxicity; lightheadedness; dizziness; rebound vasospasm; jaundice; hypertension; hematoma.

Adverse experiences with an incidence rate less than 1% in the 90 mg q4h dose group were: itching, gastrointestinal hemorrhage; thrombocytopenia; neurological deterioration; vomiting; diaphoresis; congestive heart failure; hyponatremia; decreasing platelet count; disseminated intravascular coagulation; deep vein thrombosis.

As can be seen from the table, side effects that appear related to nimodipine use based on increased incidence with higher dose or a higher rate compared to placebo control, included decreased blood pressure, edema and headaches which are known pharmacologic actions of calcium channel blockers. It must be noted, however, that SAH is frequently accompanied by alterations in consciousness which lead to an under reporting of adverse experiences. Patients who received nimodipine in clinical trials for other indications reported flushing (2.1%), headache (4.1%) and fluid retention (0.3%), typical responses to calcium channel blockers. As a calcium channel blocker, nimodipine may have the potential to exacerbate heart failure in susceptible patients or to interfere with A-V conduction, but these events were not observed. No clinically significant effects on hematologic factors, renal or hepatic function or carbohydrate metabolism have been causally associated with oral nimodipine. Isolated cases of non-fasting elevated serum glucose levels (0.8%), elevated LDH levels (0.4%), decreased platelet counts (0.3%), elevated alkaline phosphatase levels (0.2%) and elevated SGPT levels (0.2%) have been reported rarely.

DRUG ABUSE AND DEPENDENCE

There have been no reported instances of drug abuse or dependence with Nimotop®.

OVERDOSAGE

There have been no reports of overdosage from the oral administration of Nimotop®. Symptoms of overdosage would be expected to be related to cardiovascular effects such as excessive peripheral vasodilation with marked systemic hypotension. Clinically significant hypotension due to Nimotop® overdosage may require active cardiovascular support. Norepinephrine or dopamine may be helpful in restoring blood pressure. Since Nimotop® is highly protein-bound, dialysis is not likely to be of benefit.

DOSAGE AND ADMINISTRATION

Nimotop is given orally in the form of ivory colored, soft gelatin 30 mg capsules for subarachnoid hemorrhage. The oral dose is 60 mg (two 30 mg capsules) every 4 hours for 21 consecutive days. Oral Nimotop® therapy should commence within 96 hours of the subarachnoid hemorrhage.

If the capsule cannot be swallowed, e.g., at the time of surgery, or if the patient is unconscious, a hole should be made in both ends of the capsule with an 18 gauge needle, and the contents of the capsule extracted into a syringe. The contents should then be emptied into the patient's *in situ* naso-gastric tube and washed down the tube with 30 mL of normal saline (0.9%).

Patients with hepatic cirrhosis have substantially reduced clearance and approximately doubled C_{max}. Dosage should be reduced to 30 mg every 4 hours, with close monitoring of blood pressure and heart rate.

HOW SUPPLIED

Each ivory colored, soft gelatin NIMOTOP® capsule is imprinted with the word Miles and the number 855 and contains 30 mg of nimodipine. The 30 mg capsules are packaged in unit dose foil pouches and supplied in cartons containing 100 capsules. The capsules should be stored in the manufacturer's original foil package at a controlled room temperature of 59°F to 86°F (15°C to 30°C).

Capsules should be protected from light and freezing.

Unit Dose	Strength	NDC Code	Capsule Identification
Package of 100:	30 mg	0026-2855-48	Miles 855

Manufactured by: Miles Inc.
Pharmaceutical Division
400 Morgan Lane
West Haven, CT 06516
Encapsulated by: R.P. Scherer North America
Division of R.P. Scherer Corp.
Clearwater, FL 33518
Caution: Federal (USA) law prohibits dispensing without prescription.

PD100729   5/91   BAY e 9736   5202-7-A-U.S.-2
© 1991 Miles Inc.   1494
Shown in Product Identification Section, page 420

DOSE q4h
Number of Patients (%)

Sign/Symptom	Nimodipine					Placebo
	0.35 mg/kg (n = 82)	30 mg (n = 71)	60 mg (n = 494)	90 mg (n = 172)	120 mg (n = 4)	(n = 479)
Decreased Blood Pressure	1 (1.2)	0	19 (3.8)	14 (8.1)	2 (50.0)	6 (1.2)
Abnormal Liver Function Test	1 (1.2)	0	2 (0.4)	1 (0.6)	0	7 (1.5)
Edema	0	0	2 (0.4)	2 (1.2)	0	3 (0.6)
Diarrhea	0	3 (4.2)	0	3 (1.7)	0	3 (0.6)
Rash	2 (2.4)	0	3 (0.6)	2 (1.2)	0	3 (0.6)
Headache	0	1 (1.4)	6 (1.2)	0	0	1 (0.2)
Gastrointestinal Symptoms	2 (2.4)	0	0	2 (1.2)	0	0
Nausea	1 (1.2)	1 (1.4)	6 (1.2)	1 (0.6)	0	0
Dyspnea	1 (1.2)	0	0	0	0	0
EKG Abnormalities	0	1 (1.4)	0	1 (0.6)	0	0
Tachycardia	0	1 (1.4)	0	0	0	0
Bradycardia	0	0	5 (1.0)	1 (0.6)	0	0
Muscle Pain/Cramp	0	1 (1.4)	1 (0.2)	1 (0.6)	0	0
Acne	0	1 (1.4)	0	0	0	0
Depression	0	1 (1.4)	0	0	0	0

Otic DOMEBORO®
Solution Acid pH

℞

DESCRIPTION

Otic Domeboro® Solution contains 2% acetic acid as the active ingredient, in modified Burow's solution (water, aluminum acetate, and sodium acetate) with boric acid as a stabilizer. Otic Domeboro® Solution is instilled in the external auditory canal. Acetic acid is an astringent and antimicrobial agent. The pH range is from 4.5 to 6.0.
Chemically, acetic acid is $C_2H_4O_2$ and has the following structural formula:

$$H-\overset{\overset{\textstyle H}{|}}{\underset{\underset{\textstyle H}{|}}{C}}-\overset{\overset{\textstyle }{}}{\underset{\underset{\textstyle O}{\|}}{C}}-OH$$

CLINICAL PHARMACOLOGY

Acetic acid is antibacterial and antifungal; and is effective against microorganisms (bacteria and fungi) that infect the ears of patients with acute diffuse external otitis. In *in vitro* tests, minimum lethal-time was less than 0.25 minutes when bacteria and fungi isolated from patients with otitis externa were exposed to 2% acetic acid. Quantitative absorption of acetic acid 2% from external auditory canal is not known.

INDICATIONS AND USAGE

Otic Domeboro® Solution is indicated for the treatment of superficial infections of the external auditory canal caused by organisms susceptible to the action of the antimicrobial.

CONTRAINDICATIONS

Hypersensitivity to acetic acid or any of the ingredients of this product. Perforated tympanic membrane is considered a contraindication to the use of any medication in the external ear canal.

WARNINGS

Avoid use or use with caution in patients with perforated tympanic membrane (see CONTRAINDICATIONS).

PRECAUTIONS

General
Care should be taken to assure that the Otic Domeboro® Solution gets into the ear canal and stays in contact with the affected area long enough for the drug to act.
Discontinue promptly if sensitization or irritation occurs.
Carcinogenesis, Mutagenesis, Impairment of Fertility: No long term studies in animals have been performed to evaluate the carcinogenic potential of Otic Domeboro® Solution.

ADVERSE REACTIONS

Irritation may occur.

OVERDOSAGE

No toxic effect has been reported with overdosage of Otic Domeboro® Solution.

DOSAGE AND ADMINISTRATION

Patient should lie on his side with affected ear uppermost. Instill 4 to 6 drops into the external auditory canal and maintain this position for five minutes. Repeat the procedure every 2 to 3 hours.
Store below 86°F (30°C), avoid freezing.
Otic Domeboro® Solution is a clear colorless liquid.

HOW SUPPLIED

Otic Domeboro® solution is supplied in 2 oz. dropper bottle.

	NDC
2 oz.	0026-4312-02

Miles Inc.
Pharmaceutical Division
400 Morgan Lane
West Haven, CT 06516 USA
CAUTION: Federal (USA) law prohibits dispensing without prescription.
PY100666 7/88   ©1988 Miles Inc.   0591

STILPHOSTROL®
(diethylstilbestrol diphosphate)

℞

DESCRIPTION

STILPHOSTROL (diethylstilbestrol diphosphate) is available as tablets containing 50 mg diethylstilbestrol diphosphate, colored white to off-white with grey to tan mottling. Inactive ingredients: corn starch, lactose, magnesium stearate and talc. STILPHOSTROL is also available for intravenous administration as a sterile solution in 5 mL ampules containing 0.25 gram diethylstilbestrol diphosphatase its sodium salt. The solution is clear, colorless to light straw-colored, with a pH of 9.0 to 10.5, and may darken with age and exposure to heat and light.
STILPHOSTROL is a phosphoryiated, nonsteroidal estrogen with the chemical name: Diethylstilbestrol 4,4'-Diphosphoric ester, an empirical formula of $C_{18}H_{22}O_8P_2$, and the following structural formula:

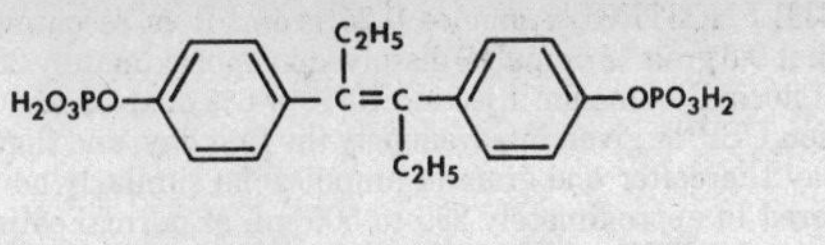

$$H_2O_3PO-\!\!\!-\!\!\!\overset{\displaystyle C_2H_5}{\underset{\displaystyle C_2H_5}{C}}\!\!=\!\!C-\!\!\!-\!\!\!OPO_3H_2$$

CLINICAL PHARMACOLOGY

Putative receptor proteins for estrogens have been detected in estrogen-responsive tissues. Estrogens are first bound to a cytoplasmic receptor protein. Following modification, the estrogen-protein complex is translocated to the nucleus where ultimate binding of the estrogen containing complex occurs. As a result of such binding characteristic metabolic alterations ensue.
In the male patient with androgenic hormone dependent conditions such as metastatic carcinoma of the prostate gland, estrogens counter the androgenic influence by competing for the receptor sites. As a result of treatment with estrogens, metastatic lesions in the bone may also show improvement.
It has been demonstrated in animal studies that diethylstilbestrol diphosphate is rapidly hydrolysed to diethylstilbestrol through phosphatase activity in the blood and tissues.[1] When diethylstilbestrol diphosphate (92 mg/kg body wt.) was injected intravenously into rabbits over a period of 2 to 3 minutes, free diethylstilbestrol appeared in the blood stream as early as 5 minutes after termination of injection, and within 15 minutes had reached a concentration of 16.3 ug/mL of plasma. This was followed by a rapid decline in concentration, only 1.2 ug/mL remaining after 2 hours.[1] It is, therefore, expected that the high concentration of serum acid phosphatase in patients with prostatic carcinoma will hydrolyse diethylstilbestrol diphosphate to free, active diethylstilbestrol.
Diethylstilbestrol is metabolized by the body in much the same manner as the endogenous hormones. Inactivation of estrogen is carried out mainly in the liver. A certain proportion of the estrogen reaching that organ is excreted into the bile, only to be reabsorbed from the intestine. During this enterohepatic circulation, degradation of estrogen occurs through conversion to less active products, through oxidation to nonestrogenic substances, and through conjugation with sulfuric and glucuronic acids. These water-soluble conjugates are strong acids and are thus fully ionized in the body fluids; penetration into cells is therefore limited, and excretion by the kidney is favored because little tubular reabsorption is possible.

INDICATION AND USAGE

STILPHOSTROL (diethylstilbestrol diphosphate) is indicated in the treatment of prostatic carcinoma—palliative therapy of advanced disease.

CONTRAINDICATIONS

Estrogens should not be used in men with any of the following conditions:
1. Known or suspected cancer of the breast except in appropriately selected patients being treated for metastatic disease.
2. Known or suspected estrogen-dependent neoplasia.
3. Active thrombophlebitis or thromboembolic disorders.
STILPHOSTROL IS NOT INDICATED IN THE TREATMENT OF ANY DISORDER IN WOMEN.

WARNINGS

1. Induction of malignant neoplasms: Long-term continuous administration of natural and synthetic estrogens in certain animal species increases the frequency of carcinomas of the breast, cervix, vagina, and liver.
2. Gallbladder disease: A study has reported a 2- to 3-fold increase in the risk of surgically confirmed gallbladder disease in women receiving postmenopausal estrogens,[2] similar to a 2-fold increase previously noted in users of oral contraceptives.[3,9]
3. Effects similar to those caused by estrogen-progestogen oral contraceptives: There are several serious adverse effects of oral contraceptives. It has been shown that there is an increased risk of thrombosis in men receiving estrogens for prostatic cancer and women for postpartum breast engorgement.[4-7]
   a. Thromboembolic disease: It is now well established that users of oral contraceptives have an increased risk of various thromboembolic and thrombotic vascular diseases, such as thrombophlebitis, pulmonary embolism, stroke, and myocardial infarction.[8-16] Cases of retinal thrombosis, mesenteric thrombosis, and optic neuritis have been reported in oral contraceptive users. There is evidence that the risk of several of these adverse reactions is related to the dose of the drug.[17,18] An increased risk of postsurgery thromboembolic complications has also been reported in users of oral contraceptives.[19,20] If feasible, estrogen should be discontinued at least 4 weeks before surgery of the type associated with an increased risk of thromboembolism or during periods of prolonged immobilization.
   Estrogens should not be used in persons with active thrombophlebitis or thromboembolic disorders. They

should be used with caution in patients with cerebral vascular or coronary artery disease and only for those in whom estrogens are clearly indicated.
   Large doses of estrogen (5 mg conjugated estrogens per day), comparable to those used to treat cancer of the prostate, have been shown in a large prospective clinical trial in men[21] to increase the risk of nonfatal myocardial infarction, pulmonary embolism and thrombophlebitis. When estrogen doses of this size are used, any of the thromboembolic and thrombotic adverse effects associated with oral contraceptive use should be considered a clear risk.
   b. Hepatic adenoma: Benign hepatic adenomas appear to be associated with the use of oral contraceptives.[22-24] Although benign, and rare, these may rupture and may cause death through intra-abdominal hemorrhage. Such lesions have not yet been reported in association with other estrogen or progestogen preparations but should be considered in estrogen users having abdominal pain and tenderness, abdominal mass, or hypovolemic shock. Hepatocellular carcinoma has also been reported in women taking estrogen-containing oral contraceptives.[23] The relationship of this malignancy to these drugs is not known at this time.
   c. Elevated blood pressure: Women using oral contraceptives sometimes experience increased blood pressure which, in most cases, returns to normal on discontinuing the drug. There is now a report that this may occur with use of estrogens in the menopause[25] and blood pressure should be monitored with estrogen use, especially if high doses are used.
   d. Glucose tolerance: A worsening of glucose tolerance has been observed in a significant percentage of patients on estrogen-containing oral contraceptives. For this reason, diabetic patients should be carefully observed while receiving estrogen.
4. Hypercalcemia: Administration of estrogens may lead to severe hypercalcemia in patients with breast cancer and bone metastases. If this occurs, the drug should be stopped and appropriate measures taken to reduce the serum calcium level.

PRECAUTIONS

General:
1. A complete medical and family history should be taken prior to the initiation of any estrogen therapy. The pretreatment and periodic physical examinations should include special reference to blood pressure, breasts, abdomen and pelvic organs. As a general rule, estrogen should not be prescribed for longer than one year without another physical examination being performed.
2. Fluid retention—Because estrogens may cause some degree of fluid retention, conditions which might be influenced by this factor such as asthma, epilepsy, migraine, and cardiac or renal dysfunction, require careful observation.
3. Certain patients may develop undesirable manifestations of excessive estrogenic stimulation, such as gynecomastia.
4. Oral contraceptives appear to be associated with an increased incidence of mental depression. Although it is not clear whether this is due to the estrogenic or progestogenic component of the contraceptive, patients with a history of depression should be carefully observed.
5. If jaundice develops in any patient receiving estrogen, the medication should be discontinued while the cause is investigated.
6. Estrogens may be poorly metabolized in patients with impaired liver function and they should be administered with caution in such patients.
7. Because estrogens influence the metabolism of calcium and phosphorus, they should be used with caution in patients with metabolic bone diseases that are associated with hypercalcemia or in patients with renal insufficiency.
Information for Patients:
1. Stilphostrol should not be used by women.
2. The following side effects have been reported in patients being treated with Stilphostrol. If they occur they should be reported promptly to your physician:
   ● Mood changes, depression
   ● Nervousness, dizziness
   ● Loss of appetite, nausea, vomiting, abdominal cramps, bloating
   ● Skin rash
   ● Chest pain and shortness of breath
   ● Numbness or tingling about the nose or mouth
   ● Fluid accumulation
   ● Swelling or tenderness of breasts
   ● Disturbances of vision
   ● Frequent or uncomfortable urination
   ● Painful swelling of extremities
3. The patient should consult a physician regularly for evaluation of blood pressure and heart rate.

Continued on next page

Miles—Cont.

4. Diabetic patients should monitor urines very carefully. Test of blood sugar may be necessary as well.
5. The following clinical problems are associated with the use of Stilphostrol:
   - Hepatic cutaneous prophyria
   - Erythema nodosum
   - Erythema multiforme

   A significant association has been shown between the use of estrogen containing drugs and the following serious reactions:
   1. Thrombophlebitis
   2. Pulmonary embolism
   3. Cerebral thrombosis
   4. There is suggestive evidence that there may be a relationship with coronary thrombosis.

The following adverse reactions are known to have occurred in patients receiving estrogens:
- Change in body weight
- Headache
- Loss of sex drive
- Post injection flare
- Aggravation of migraine headaches
- Loss of scalp hair
- Hemorrhagic eruption
- Fatigue
- Backache

Drug/Laboratory Test Interactions:
1. The pathologist should be advised of estrogen therapy when relevant specimens are submitted.
2. Certain endocrine and liver function tests may be affected by estrogen-containing oral contraceptives.

The following similar changes may be expected with larger doses of estrogen.
a. Increased sulfobromophthalein retention.
b. Increased prothrombin and factors VII, VIII, IX, and X; decreased antithrombin 3; increased norepinephrine-induced platelet aggregability.
c. Increased thyroid binding globulin (TBG) leading to increased circulating total thyroid hormone, as measured by PBI, T4 by column, or T4 by radioimmunoassay. Free T3 resin uptake is decreased, reflecting the elevated TBG; free T4 concentration is unaltered.
d. Impaired glucose tolerance.
e. Reduced response to metyrapone test.
f. Reduced serum folate concentration.
g. Increased serum triglyceride and phospholipid concentration.

Carcinogenesis, mutagenesis, impairment of fertility: (See Warnings regarding induction of neoplasia.)
Pregnancy: Pregnancy Category X. STILPHOSTROL IS NOT INDICATED IN THE TREATMENT OF ANY DISORDER IN WOMEN.
Pediatric Use: Because of the effects of estrogens on epiphyseal closure, they should be used judiciously in young patients in whom bone growth is not complete.

ADVERSE REACTIONS

(See Warnings regarding induction of neoplasia, increased incidence of gallbladder disease, and adverse effects similar to those of oral contraceptives, including thromboembolism.)
The following additional adverse reactions have been reported with estrogenic therapy, including oral contraceptives:
1. Breasts: Tenderness, enlargement, secretion.
2. Gastrointestinal: Nausea, vomiting; abdominal cramps, bloating; cholestatic jaundice.
3. Skin: Chloasma or melasma which may persist when drug is discontinued; erythema multiforme, erythema nodosum; hemorrhagic eruption; loss of scalp hair; hirsutism.
4. Eyes: Steepening of corneal curvature; intolerance to contact lenses.
5. CNS: Headache, migraine, dizziness, mental depression; chorea.
6. Miscellaneous: Increase or decrease in weight; reduced carbohydrate tolerance; aggravation of porphyria; edema; changes in libido; transient itching and burning sensation in the perineal region.

OVERDOSAGE

Numerous reports of ingestion of large doses of estrogen-containing oral contraceptives by young children indicate that acute serious ill effects do not occur. Overdosage of estrogen may cause nausea.

DOSAGE AND ADMINISTRATION

Inoperable, progressing prostatic cancer.
STILPHOSTROL Tablets 50 mg: Start with one tablet three times a day and increase this dose level to four or more tablets three times a day, depending on the tolerance of the patient. Maximum daily dose not to exceed one gram.
Alternatively, if relief is not obtained with high oral dosages, STILPHOSTROL may be administered intravenously. STILPHOSTROL solution must be diluted before intravenous infusion.
STILPHOSTROL Ampules 0.25 gram: It is recommended that 0.5 gram (2 ampules) dissolved in approximately 250 mL of normal saline for injection USP, or 5% dextrose for injection USP, be given intravenously the first day, and that each day thereafter one gram (4 ampules) be similarly administered in approximately 250 to 500 mL of normal saline for injection USP, or 5% dextrose for injection USP.
The infusion should be administered slowly (20–30 drops per minute) during the first 10–15 minutes and then the rate of flow adjusted so that the entire amount is given in a period of about one hour. This procedure should be followed for five days or more depending on the response of the patient. Following the first intensive course of therapy, 0.25–0.5 gram (1 or 2 ampules) may be administered in a similar manner once or twice weekly or maintenance obtained with STILPHOSTROL Tablets.
Stability of Solution: After reconstitution, if storage is desired, the solution should be kept at room temperature and away from direct light. Under these conditions the solution is stable for about 5 days, so long as cloudiness or evidence of a precipitate has not occurred.

HOW SUPPLIED

STILPHOSTROL Tablets–Bottles of 50 tablets.
Each scored tablet, white to off-white with grey to tan mottling, contains diethylstilbestrol diphosphate 50 mg. Each tablet is identified with: Miles 132.
STORAGE: Store at controlled room temperature (59°–86°F), protect from light.
STILPHOSTROL Ampules—Boxes of 20 ampules.
Each 5 mL ampule contains diethylstilbestrol diphosphate 0.25 gram as a solution of its sodium salt.
STORAGE: Store at controlled room temperature (59°–86°F), protect from light.

REFERENCES

1. Johnson, W., et al: Proc. Soc. Exp. Biol. Med. 106:327–330, 1961.
2. Boston Collaborative Drug Surveillance Program: N. Eng. J. Med. 290:15–19, 1974.
3. Boston Collaborative Drug Surveillance Program: Lancet 1:1399–1404, 1973.
4. Daniel, D.G., et al: Lancet 2:287–289, 1967.
5. The Veterans Administration Cooperative Urological Research Group: J. Urol. 98:516–522, 1967.
6. Bailar, J.C.: Lancet 2-560, 1967.
7. Blackard, C., et al: Cancer 26:249–256, 1970.
8. Royal College of General Practitioners: R. Coll. Gen. Pract. 13:267–279, 1967.
9. Royal College of General Practitioners: Oral Contraceptives and Health, New York, Pitman Corp., 1974.
10. Inman, W.H.W., et al: Br. Med. J. 2:193–199, 1968.
11. Vessey, M.P., et al: Br. Med. J. 2:651–657, 1969.
12. Sartwell, P.E., et al: Am.J. Epidemiol. 90:365–380, 1969.
13. Collaborative Group for the Study of Stroke in Young Women: N. Eng. J. Med. 288:871–878, 1973.
14. Collaborative Group for the Study of Stroke in Young Women: J.A.M.A. 231:718–722, 1975.
15. Mann, J.I., et al: Br. Med. J. 2:245–248, 1975.
16. Mann, J.I., et al: Br. Med. J. 2:241–245, 1975.
17. Inman, W.H.W., et al: Br. Med. J. 2:203–209, 1970.
18. Stolley, P.D., et al: Am. J. Epidemiol. 102:197–208, 1975.
19. Vessey, M.P., et al: Br. Med. J. 3:123–126, 1970.
20. Greene, G.R., et al: Am. J. Public Health 62:680–685, 1972.
21. Coronary Drug Project Research Group: J.A.M.A. 214:1303–1313, 1970.
22. Baum, J., et al: Lancet 2:926–928, 1973.
23. Mays, E.T., et al: J.A.M.A. 235:730–732, 1976.
24. Edmondson, H.A., et al: N. Eng. J. Med. 294:470–472, 1976.
25. Pfeffer, R.I., et al: Am. J. Epidemiol. 103:445–456, 1976.

Ampules manufactured by:
Ben Venue Laboratories, Inc.
Bedford, OH 44146
Distributed by
Miles Inc.
Pharmaceutical Division
400 Morgan Lane
West Haven, CT 06516
PD 100708-0760 3/89
Shown in Product Identification Section, page 420

TRIDESILON® 0.05% ℞
(desonide)
cream

DESCRIPTION

Tridesilon® Cream contains microdispersed desonide (the active ingredient) in a compatible vehicle buffered to the pH range of normal skin. Each gram of Tridesilon® Cream contains 0.5 milligrams of desonide. Tridesilon® Cream is applied topically.
Tridesilon® (desonide) is a non-fluorinated corticosteroid. Chemically, desonide is Pregna-1,4-diene-3,20-dione,11,21-dihydroxy-16,17-[(1-methylethylidene)bis(oxy)]-,(11β,16α)-with the following structural formula:

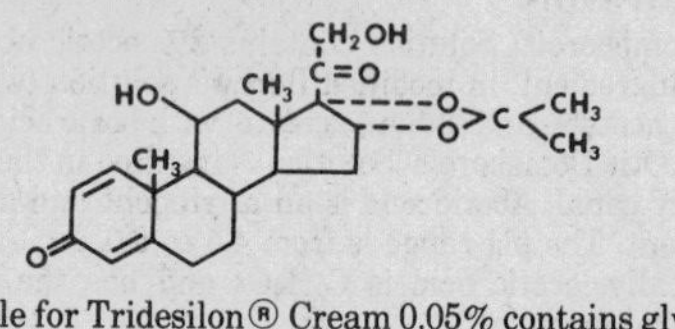

The vehicle for Tridesilon® Cream 0.05% contains glycerin, sodium lauryl sulfate, aluminum sulfate, calcium acetate, dextrin, purified water, cetyl stearyl alcohol, synthetic beeswax, (B-wax), white petrolatum, and light mineral oil. Preserved with methylparaben.

EMPIRICAL FORMULA	MOLECULAR WEIGHT	CAS REGISTRY NUMBER
$C_{24}H_{32}O_6$	416.51	638-94-8

CLINICAL PHARMACOLOGY

Topical corticosteroids share anti-inflammatory, anti-pruritic and vasoconstrictive actions.
The mechanism of anti-inflammatory activity of the topical corticosteroids is unclear. Various laboratory methods, including vasoconstrictor assays, are used to compare and predict potencies and/or clinical efficacies of the topical corticosteroids. There is some evidence to suggest that a recognizable correlation exists between vasoconstrictor potency and therapeutic efficacy in man.

Pharmacokinetics
The extent of percutaneous absorption of topical corticosteroids is determined by many factors including the vehicle, the integrity of the epidermal barrier, and the use of occlusive dressings.
Topical corticosteroids can be absorbed from normal intact skin. Inflammation and/or other disease processes in the skin increase percutaneous absorption. Occlusive dressings substantially increase the percutaneous absorption of topical corticosteroids. Thus, occlusive dressings may be a valuable therapeutic adjunct for treatment of resistant dermatoses. (See DOSAGE AND ADMINISTRATION).
Once absorbed through the skin, topical corticosteroids are handled through pharmacokinetic pathways similar to systemically administered corticosteroids. Corticosteroids are bound to plasma proteins in varying degrees. Corticosteroids are metabolized primarily in the liver and are then excreted by the kidneys. Some of the topical corticosteroids and their metabolites are also excreted into the bile.

INDICATIONS AND USAGE

Topical corticosteroids are indicated for the relief of the inflammatory and pruritic manifestations of corticosteroid-responsive dermatoses.

CONTRAINDICATIONS

Topical corticosteroids are contraindicated in those patients with a history of hypersensitivity to any of the components of the preparation.

PRECAUTIONS

General
Systemic absorption of topical corticosteroids has produced reversible hypothalmic-pituitary-adrenal (HPA) axis suppression, manifestations of Cushing's syndrome, hyperglycemia, and glycosuria in some patients.
Conditions which augment systemic absorption include the application of the more potent steroids, use over large surface areas, prolonged use, and the addition of occlusive dressings.
Therefore, patients receiving a large dose of a potent topical steroid applied to a large surface area or under an occlusive dressing should be evaluated periodically for evidence of HPA axis suppression by using the urinary free cortisol and ACTH stimulation tests. If HPA axis suppression is noted, an attempt should be made to withdraw the drug, to reduce the frequency of application, or to substitute a less potent steroid.
Recovery of HPA axis function is generally prompt and complete upon discontinuation of the drug. Infrequently, signs and symptoms of steroid withdrawal may occur, requiring supplemental systemic corticosteroids.
Children may absorb proportionally larger amounts of topical corticosteroids and thus be more susceptible to systemic toxicity. (See PRECAUTIONS—Pediatric Use).
If irritation develops, topical corticosteroids should be discontinued and appropriate therapy instituted.
In the presence of dermatological infections, the use of an appropriate antifungal or antibacterial agent should be instituted. If a favorable response does not occur promptly, the corticosteroid should be discontinued until the infection has been adequately controlled.

Information for the Patient
Patients using topical corticosteroids should receive the following information and instructions:
1. This medication is to be used as directed by the physician. It is for external use only. Avoid contact with eyes.

2. Patients should be advised not to use this medication for any disorder other than for which it was prescribed.
3. The treated skin area should not be bandaged or otherwise covered or wrapped as to be occlusive unless directed by the physician.
4. Patients should report any signs of local adverse reactions especially under occlusive dressing.
5. Parents of pediatric patients should be advised not to use tightfitting diapers or plastic pants on a child being treated in the diaper area, as these garments may constitute occlusive dressings.

Laboratory Tests
The following tests may be helpful in evaluating the HPA axis suppression:
Urinary free cortisol test
ACTH stimulation test

Carcinogenesis, Mutagenesis, and Impairment of Fertility
Long-term animal studies have not been performed to evaluate the carcinogenic potential or the effect on fertility of topical corticosteroids.
Studies to determine mutagenicity with prednisolone and hydrocortisone have revealed negative results.

Pregnancy Category C
Corticosteroids are generally teratogenic in laboratory animals when administered systemically at relatively low dosage levels. The more potent corticosteroids have been shown to be teratogenic after dermal application in laboratory animals. There are no adequate and well-controlled studies in pregnant women on teratogenic effects from topically applied corticosteroids. Therefore, topical corticosteroids should be used during pregnancy only if the potential benefit justifies the potential risk to the fetus. Drugs of this class should not be used extensively on pregnant patients, in large amounts, or for prolonged periods of time.

Nursing Mothers
It is not known whether topical administration of corticosteroids could result in sufficient systemic absorption to produce detectable quantities in breast milk. Systemically administered corticosteroids are secreted into breast milk in quantities *not* likely to have a deleterious effect on the infant. Nevertheless, caution should be exercised when topical corticosteroids are administered to a nursing woman.

Pediatric Use
Pediatric patients may demonstrate greater susceptibility to topical corticosteroid-induced HPA axis suppression and Cushing's syndrome than mature patients because of a larger skin surface area to body weight ratio.
Hypothalamic-pituitary-adrenal (HPA) axis suppression. Cushing's syndrome, and intracranial hypertension have been reported in children receiving topical corticosteroids. Manifestations of adrenal supression in children include linear growth retardation, delayed weight gain, low plasma cortisol levels, and absence of response to ACTH stimulation. Manifestations of intracranial hypertension include bulging fontanelles, headaches, and bilateral papilledema.
Administration of topical corticosteroids to children should be limited to the least amount compatible with an effective therapeutic regimen. Chronic corticosteroid therapy may interfere with the growth and development of children.

ADVERSE REACTIONS
The following local adverse reactions are reported infrequently with topical corticosteroids, but may occur more frequently with the use of occlusive dressings. These reactions are listed in an approximate decreasing order of occurrence:
Burning
Itching
Irritation
Dryness
Folliculitis
Hypertrichosis
Acneiform eruptions
Hypopigmentation
Perioral dermatitis
Allergic contact dermatitis
Maceration of the skin
Secondary infection
Skin atrophy
Striae
Miliaria

OVERDOSAGE
Topically applied corticosteroids can be absorbed in sufficient amounts to produce systemic effects. (See PRECAUTIONS).

DOSAGE AND ADMINISTRATION
Topical corticosteroids are generally applied to the affected area as a thin film from two to four times daily depending on the severity of the condition.
Occlusive dressings may be used for management of psoriasis or recalcitrant conditions.
If an infection develops, the use of occlusive dressings should be discontinued and appropriate antimicrobial therapy instituted.

HOW SUPPLIED
Tridesilon® (desonide) Cream 0.05% is supplied in 15 and 60 gram tubes and in 5 pound jars. It is a white semi-solid.
Store below 86°F (30°C), avoid freezing.

	NDC Number
15g	0026-5561-61
60g	0026-5561-62
5lb	0026-5561-92

Miles Inc.
Pharmaceutical Division
400 Morgan Lane
West Haven, CT 06516 USA

CAUTION
Federal (USA) law prohibits dispensing without a prescription.
 PD100672 0229

TRIDESILON® 0.05% ℞
(desonide)
ointment

DESCRIPTION
Tridesilon® Ointment contains microdispersed desonide (the active ingredient) in white petrolatum. Each gram of Tridesilon® Ointment contains 0.5 miligrams of desonide. Tridesilon® Ointment is applied topically.
Tridesilon® (desonide) is a non-fluorinated corticosteroid. Chemically, desonide is Pregna-1,4-diene-3,20-dione,11,21-dihydroxy-16,17-[(1-methylethylidene)bis(oxy)]-,11β,16α)- with the following structural formula:

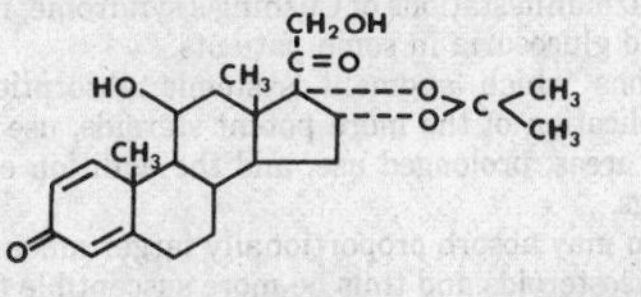

EMPIRICAL FORMULA	MOLECULAR WEIGHT	CAS REGISTRY NUMBER
$C_{24}H_{32}O_6$	416.51	638-94-8

CLINICAL PHARMACOLOGY
Topical corticosteroids share anti-inflammatory, anti-puritic and vasoconstrictive actions.
The mechanism of anti-inflammatory activity of the topical corticosteroids is unclear. Various laboratory methods, including vasoconstrictor assays, are used to compare and predict potencies and/or clinical efficacies of the topical corticosteroids. There is some evidence to suggest that a recognizable correlation exists between vasoconstrictor potency and therapeutic efficacy in man.

Pharmacokinetics
The extent of percutaneous absorption of topical corticosteroids is determined by many factors including the vehicle, the integrity of the epidermal barrier, and the use of occlusive dressings.
Topical corticosteroids can be absorbed from normal intact skin. Inflammation and/or other disease processes in the skin increase percutaneous absorption. Occlusive dressings substantially increase the percutaneous absorption of topical corticosteroids. Thus, occlusive dressings may be a valuable therapeutic adjunct for treatment of resistant dermatoses. (See DOSAGE AND ADMINISTRATION).
Once absorbed through the skin, topical corticosteroids are handled through pharmacokinetic pathways similar to systemically administered corticosteroids. Corticosteroids are bound to plasma proteins in varying degrees. Corticosteroids are metabolized primarily in the liver and are then excreted by the kidneys. Some of the topical corticosteroids and their metabolites are also excreted into the bile.

INDICATIONS AND USAGE
Topical corticosteroids are indicated for the relief of the inflammatory and pruritic manifestations of corticosteroid-responsive dermatoses.

CONTRAINDICATIONS
Topical corticosteroids are contraindicated in those patients with a history of hypersensitivity to any of the components of the preparation.

PRECAUTIONS
General
Systemic absorption of topical corticosteroids has produced reversible hypothalamic-pituitary-adrenal (HPA) axis suppression, manifestations of Cushing's syndrome, hyperglycemia, and glycosuria in some patients.
Conditions which augment systemic absorption include the application of the more potent steroids, use over large surface areas, prolonged use, and the addition of occlusive dressings.
Therefore, patients receiving a large dose of a potent topical steroid applied to a large surface area or under an occlusive dressing should be evaluated periodically for evidence of HPA axis suppression by using the urinary free cortisol and ACTH stimulation tests. If HPA axis suppression is noted, an attempt should be made to withdraw the drug, to reduce the frequency of application, or to substitute a less potent steroid.
Recovery of HPA axis functions is generally prompt and complete upon discontinuation of the drug. Infrequently, signs and symptoms of steroid withdrawal may occur, requiring supplemental systemic corticosteroids.
Children may absorb proportionally larger amounts of topical corticosteroids and thus be more susceptible to systemic toxicity. (See PRECAUTIONS—Pediatric Use).
If irritation develops, topical corticosteroids should be discontinued and appropriate therapy instituted.
In the presence of dermatological infections, the use of an appropriate antifungal or antibacterial agent should be instituted. If a favorable response does not occur promptly, the corticosteroid should be discontinued until the infection has been adequately controlled.

Information for the Patient
Patients using topical corticosteroids should receive the following information and instructions:
1. This medication is to be used as directed by the physician. It is for external use only. Avoid contact with the eyes.
2. Patients should be advised not to use this medication for any disorder other than for which it was prescribed.
3. The treated skin area should not be bandaged or otherwise covered or wrapped so as to be occlusive unless directed by the physician.
4. Patients should report any signs of local adverse reactions especially under occlusive dressing.
5. Parents of pediatric patients should be advised not to use tight-fitting diapers or plastic pants on a child being treated in the diaper area, as these garments may constitute occlusive dressings.

Laboratory Tests
The following tests may be helpful in evaluating the HPA axis suppression.
Urinary free cortisol test
ACTH stimulation test

Carcinogenesis, Mutagenesis, and Impairment of Fertility
Long-term animal studies have not been performed to evaluate the carcinogenic potential or the effect on fertility of topical corticosteroids.
Studies to determine mutagenicity with prednisolone and hydrocortisone have revealed negative results.

Pregnancy Category C
Corticosteroids are generally teratogenic in laboratory animals when administered systemically at relatively low dosage levels. The more potent corticosteroids have been shown to be teratogenic after dermal application in laboratory animals. There are no adequate and well-controlled studies in pregnant women on teratogenic effects from topically applied corticosteroids. Therefore, topical corticosteroids should be used during pregnancy only if the potential benefit justifies the potential risk to the fetus. Drugs of this class should not be used extensively on pregnant patients, in large amounts, or for prolonged periods of time.

Nursing Mothers
It is not known whether topical administration of corticosteroids could result in sufficient systemic absorption to produce detectable quantities in breast milk. Systemically administered corticosteroids are secreted into breast milk in quantities *not* likely to have a deleterious effect on the infant. Nevertheless, caution should be exercised when topical corticosteroids are administered to a nursing woman.

Pediatric Use
Pediatric patients may demonstrate greater susceptibility to topical corticosteroid-induced HPA axis and Cushing's syndrome than mature patients because of a larger skin surface area to body weight ratio.
Hypothalamic-pituitary-adrenal (HPA) axis suppression, Cushing's syndrome, and intracranial hypertension have been reported in children receiving topical corticosteroids. Manifestations of adrenal suppression in children include linear growth retardation, delayed weight gain, low plasma cortisol levels, and absence of response to ACTH stimulation. Manifestations of intracranial hypertension include bulging fontanelles, headaches, and bilateral papilledema.
Administration of topical corticosteroids to children should be limited to the least amount compatible with an effective therapeutic regimen. Chronic corticosteroid therapy may interfere with the growth and development of children.

ADVERSE REACTIONS
The following local adverse reactions are reported infrequently with topical corticosteroids, but may occur more frequently with the use of occlusive dressings. These reactions are listed in an approximate decreasing order of occurrence:
Burning
Itching
Irritation

Continued on next page

Miles—Cont.

Dryness
Folliculitis
Hypertrichosis
Acneiform eruptions
Hypopigmentation
Perioral dermatitis
Allergic contact dermatitis
Maceration of the skin
Secondary infection
Skin atrophy
Striae
Miliaria

OVERDOSAGE
Topically applied corticosteroids can be absorbed in sufficient amounts to produce systemic effects. (See PRECAUTIONS).

DOSAGE AND ADMINISTRATION
Topical corticosteroids are generally applied to the affected area as a thin film from two to four times daily depending on the severity of the condition.
Occlusive dressings may be used for the management of psoriasis or recalcitrant conditions.
If an infection develops, the use of occlusive dressings should be discontinued and appropriate antimicrobial therapy instituted.

HOW SUPPLIED
Tridesilon® (desonide) Ointment 0.05% is supplied in 15 and 60 gram tubes. It is white or faintly yellowish, transparent semisolid.
Store below 86°F (30°C). Avoid freezing.

	NDC Number
15g	0026-5591-61
60g	0026-5591-62

Miles Inc.
Pharmaceutical Division
400 Morgan Lane
West Haven, CT 06516 USA
CAUTION: Federal (USA) law prohibits dispensing without a prescription.

PD100671 0227
© 1988 Miles Inc.

OTIC TRIDESILON® 0.05%   ℞
(desonide 0.05%–acetic acid 2%)
solution

DESCRIPTION
Otic Tridesilon® Solution contains desonide 0.05% and acetic acid 2% (the active ingredients) in a compatible vehicle buffered to the pH range of the normal ear. Otic Tridesilon® Solution is instilled into the external auditory canal. Tridesilon® (desonide) is a non-fluorinated corticosteroid. Chemically, desonide is Pregna-1,4-diene-3,20-dione,11,21-dihydroxy-16,17-[(1-methylethylidene)bis(oxy)] -,(11β,16α)- with the following structural formula:

EMPIRICAL FORMULA	MOLECULAR WEIGHT	CAS REGISTRY NUMBER
$C_{24}H_{32}O_6$	416.51	638-94-8

Acetic acid is an astringent and antimicrobial agent. Chemically, it is $C_2H_4O_2$ with the following structural formula:

The base is composed of purified water, propylene glycol, sodium acetate, and citric acid.

CLINICAL PHARMACOLOGY
Topical corticosteroids share anti-inflammatory, anti-pruritic and vasoconstrictive actions.
The mechanism of anti-inflammatory activity of the topical corticosteroids is unclear. Various laboratory methods, including vasoconstrictor assays, are used to compare and predict potencies and/or clinical efficacies of the topical corticosteroids. There is some evidence to suggest that a recognizable correlation exists between vasoconstrictor potency and therapeutic efficacy in man.

Pharmacokinetics
The extent of percutaneous absorption of topical corticosteroids is determined by many factors including the vehicle, the integrity of the epidermal barrier, and the use of occlusive dressings.
Topical corticosteroids can be absorbed from normal intact skin. Inflammation and/or other disease processes in the skin increase percutaneous absorption. Occlusive dressings substantially increase the percutaneous absorption of topical corticosteroids.
Once absorbed through the skin, topical corticosteroids are handled through pharmacokinetic pathways similar to systemically administered corticosteroids. Corticosteroids are bound to plasma proteins in varying degrees. Corticosteroids are metabolized primarily in the liver and are then excreted by the kidneys. Some of the topical corticosteroids and their metabolites are also excreted into the bile.

INDICATIONS AND USAGE
Otic Tridesilon® Solution is indicated for the treatment of superficial infections of the external auditory canal caused by organisms susceptible to the action of the antimicrobial and accompanied by inflammation.

CONTRAINDICATIONS
Otic Tridesilon® Solution (desonide 0.05%–acetic acid 2%) is contraindicated in those patients who have shown hypersensitivity to any of the components of the preparation. Perforated tympanic membranes are frequently considered a contraindication to the use of external ear canal medication.

PRECAUTIONS
General
Systemic absorption of topical corticosteroids has produced reversible hypothalamic-pituitary-adrenal (HPA) axis suppression, manifestations of Cushing's syndrome, hyperglycemia, and glucosuria in some patients.
Conditions which augment systemic absorption include the application of the more potent steroids, use over large surface areas, prolonged use, and the addition of occlusive dressings.
Children may absorb proportionally larger amounts of topical corticosteroids and thus be more susceptible to systemic toxicity (See PRECAUTIONS—Pediatric Use).
If irritation develops, the product should be discontinued and appropriate therapy instituted.
If infection persists or new infection appears, appropriate therapy should be instituted. If a favorable response does not occur promptly, the corticosteroid should be discontinued until the infection has been adequately controlled.

Information for the Patient
Patients using topical corticosteroids should receive the following information and instructions:
1. This medication is to be used as directed by the physician. It is for external use only. Avoid contact with the eyes.
2. Patients should be advised not to use this medication for any disorder other than for which it was prescribed.

Laboratory Tests
The following tests may be helpful in evaluating the HPA axis suppression:
Urinary free cortisol test
ACTH stimulation test

Carcinogenesis, Mutagenesis, and Impairment of Fertility
Long-term animal studies have not been preformed to evaluate the carcinogenic potential or the effect on fertility of topical corticosteroids.
Studies to determine mutagenicity with prednisolone and hydrocortisone have revealed negative results.

Pregnancy Category C
Corticosteroids are generally teratogenic in laboratory animals when administered systemically at relatively low dosage levels. The more potent corticosteroids have been shown to be teratogenic after dermal application in laboratory animals. There are no adequate and well-controlled studies in pregnant women on teratogenic effects from topically applied corticosteroids. Therefore, topical corticosteroids should be used during pregnancy only if the potential benefit justifies the potential risk to the fetus. Drugs of this class should not be used extensively on pregnant patients, in large amounts, or for prolonged periods of time.

Nursing Mothers
It is not known whether topical administration of corticosteroids could result in sufficient systemic absorption to produce detectable quantities in breast milk. Systemically administered corticosteroids are secreted into breast milk in quantities *not* likely to have a deleterious effect on the infant. Nevertheless, caution should be exercised when topical corticosteroids are administered to a nursing woman.

Pediatric Use
Pediatric patients may demonstrate greater susceptibility to topical corticosteroid-induced HPA axis suppression and Cushing's syndrome than mature patients because of a larger skin surface area to body weight ratio.
Hypothalamic-pituitary-adrenal (HPA) axis suppression. Cushing's syndrome, and intracranial hypertension have been reported in children receiving topical corticosteroids.
Manifestations of adrenal suppression in children include

linear growth retardation, delayed weight gain, low plasma cortisol levels, and absence of response to ACTH stimulation. Manifestations of intracranial hypertension include bulging fontanelles, headaches, and bilateral papilledema.
Administration of topical corticosteroids to children should be limited to the least amount compatible with an effective therapeutic regimen. Chronic corticosteroid therapy may interfere with the growth and development of children.

ADVERSE REACTIONS
The following local adverse reactions may occur infrequently with otic use of topical corticosteroids. These reactions are listed in an approximate decreasing order of occurrence.

Burning	Hypopigmentation
Itching	Allergic contact dermatitis
Irritation	Maceration of the skin
Dryness	Secondary infection
Folliculitis	Skin atrophy
Hypertrichosis	

OVERDOSAGE
Topically applied corticosteroids can be absorbed in sufficient amounts to produce systemic effects (See PRECAUTIONS).

DOSAGE AND ADMINISTRATION
All ceruminous material and debris should be carefully removed to permit Otic Tridesilon® Solution (desonide 0.05%–acetic acid 2%) to contact the infected surfaces. Instill 3 to 4 drops into the ear 3 to 4 times daily. If preferred, a gauze or cotton wick saturated with the solution may be inserted in the ear canal and allowed to remain in situ. It should be kept moist by further addition of the solution, as required.

HOW SUPPLIED
Otic Tridesilon® Solution (desonide 0.05%–acetic acid 2%) is supplied in 10cc bottles with dropper.
Otic Tridesilon® is a clear colorless solution.

	NDC Number
10 mL	0026-7210-10

Store below 86°F (30°C), avoid freezing.

Miles Inc.
Pharmaceutical Division
400 Morgan Lane
West Haven, CT 06516 USA
CAUTION: Federal (USA) law prohibits dispensing without a prescription. For external use only.

PD100698 0627   10/88   © 1988 Miles Inc.

Miles Inc.
Pharmaceutical Division
Allergy Products
400 MORGAN LANE
WEST HAVEN, CT 06516

ANA-KIT®   ℞
ANAPHYLAXIS EMERGENCY TREATMENT KIT

DESCRIPTION
Epinephrine Injection, USP, (1:1000), contained in a sterile, 1 mL syringe, designed to deliver 2 doses of 0.3 mL each. Product is intended for subcutaneous or intramuscular use. Each mL of Epinephrine Injection, USP, (1:1000) contains 1 mg *l*-epinephrine as the hydrochloride, 8.5 mg sodium chloride, not more than 5 mg chlorobutanol (chloral derivative) and 1.5 mg sodium bisulfite.
Epinephrine is a sympathomimetic catecholamine. Its naturally occurring levo isomer, which is twenty times as active as the *d* isomer, is now obtained in pure form by separation from the synthetically produced racemate.
Chemically, epinephrine is α-(3,4-dihydroxyphenyl)-β-(methylamino)ethanol with the following structure:

Chlo-Amine® Chlorpheniramine Maleate Tablets: 4 chewable tablets, each containing 2 mg chlorpheniramine maleate, USP, for oral administration. Contains FD&C Yellow No. 6 (Sunset Yellow) as a color additive. Chlorpheniramine maleate is an antihistamine having the chemical name γ-(4-chlorophenyl)-N,N-dimethyl-2-pyridinepropanamine, (Z)-2-butenedioate(1:1) with the following structure:
[See chemical structure at top of next page.]
DEVICES: 2 sterile pads containing isopropyl alcohol 70% by volume. One tourniquet.

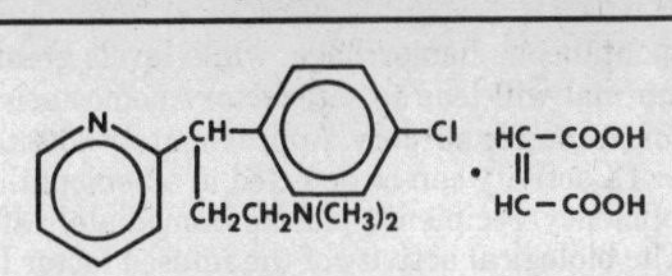

CLINICAL PHARMACOLOGY

EPINEPHRINE: The most valuable drug for the emergency treatment of severe allergic reactions is epinephrine. The vasoconstrictor effect of epinephrine on the capillary directly antagonizes the generalized vasodilation produced by histamine. Epinephrine reverses the increased permeability of dilated capillaries to plasma. The shock of severe allergic reactions is due to the loss of circulating blood volume by pooling in the dilated capillary beds and loss of plasma into the tissues. Epinephrine quickly restores circulating blood volume and blood pressure by constricting the capillary bed. The itching during episodes of hives or angioedema is promptly relieved by epinephrine. Epinephrine is a powerful relaxer of the smooth muscle of the bronchioles, stomach, intestine, pregnant uterus and urinary bladder wall. The bronchospasm, wheezing and dyspnea of the acute allergic reactions are relieved. Where abdominal cramping, defecation or involuntary urination have occurred during severe allergic attacks, epinephrine rapidly produces relief. Subcutaneously or intramuscularly administered epinephrine has a rapid onset and short duration of action. Subcutaneous administration during asthmatic attacks may produce bronchodilation within 5 to 10 minutes, and maximal effects may occur within 20 minutes.

CHLO-AMINE: Chlo-Amine is an effective agent in nullifying the characteristic effects of histamine and is especially valuable in the prophylaxis and relief of many allergic symptoms. It is readily absorbed from the intestinal tract and released into the tissues from the bloodstream. This action is both prompt and sustained. Elimination of the drug is such that there is a low incidence of side effects.

INDICATIONS AND USAGE

HOLLISTER-STIER Anaphylaxis Emergency Treatment Kit (Ana-Kit®) is indicated for use by adult and pediatric patients under the following situations:

1. Allergic reactions including anaphylactic shock due to stinging insects (primarily of the Hymenoptera order, which includes bees, wasps, hornets, yellow jackets, bumble bees, and fire ants.
2. Severe allergic or anaphylactoid reactions due to allergy injections, exposures to pollens, dusts, molds, foods, drugs, and exercise or unknown substances (so-called idiopathic anaphylaxis).
3. Severe, life-threatening asthma attacks characterized by wheezing, dyspnea and inability to breathe.

In the sensitive patient, severe allergic reactions and anaphylactic shock may occur within minutes of the insect sting or exposure to an allergenic substance.

Symptoms may include bronchoconstriction, wheezing, sneezing, hoarseness, urticaria, angioedema, erythema, pruritis, tachycardia, thready pulse, falling blood pressure, sense of oppression or impending doom, disorientation, cramping abdominal pain, incontinance, faintness, loss of consciousness.

The Ana-Kit is compactly designed to be carried and used by patients when severe symptoms arise, and the patient is out of reach of immediate attention by a doctor or hospital.

CONTRAINDICATIONS

EPINEPHRINE: Epinephrine must not be given intra-arterially as marked vasoconstriction may result in gangrene. **This unit is not intended for intravenous use.** Further dilution would be necessary and is not practical with this emergency syringe.

Epinephrine Injection, USP, (1:1000) must not be used if there is hypersensitivity to any of the components.

Epinephrine is contraindicated in narrow-angle glaucoma; cardiogenic, traumatic, or hemorrhagic shock; cardiac dilation; cerebral arteriosclerosis; and organic brain damage.

Epinephrine should not be used to counteract circulatory collapse or hypotension due to phenothiazines, since such agents may reverse the pressor effect of epinephrine, leading to a further lowering of blood pressure.

Epinephrine should not be administered concomitantly with other sympathomimetic agents, since the effects are additive and may be detrimental to the patient.

CHLO-AMINE: No known contraindications.

WARNINGS

EPINEPHRINE: Overdosage or accidental intravenous administration of conventional subcutaneous doses may induce severe or fatal hypertension, or cerebrovascular hemorrhage. Fatalities may also occur from pulmonary edema resulting from peripheral constriction and cardiac stimulation. The marked pressor effects may be counteracted by use of rapidly acting vasodilators, such as the nitrites and alpha-adrenergic blockers.

Deaths have been reported in asthmatics treated with epinephrine following the use of isoproterenol or orciprenaline. Epinephrine is the preferred treatment for serious allergic or other emergency situations even though this product contains sodium bisulfite, a sulfite that may in other products cause allergic-type reactions including anaphylactic symptoms or life-threatening or less severe asthmatic episodes in certain susceptible persons. The alternatives to using epinephrine in a life-threatening situation may not be satisfactory. The presence of a sulfite(s) in this product should not deter administration of the drug for treatment of serious allergic or other emergency situations.

Epinephrine must be administered with great caution, if at all, in patients with cardiac arrhythmias, coronary artery or organic heart disease, and hypertension. In patients with coronary insufficiency or ischemic heart disease, epinephrine may precipitate or aggravate angina pectoris as well as produce potentially fatal ventricular arrhythmias. Epinephrine should be administered only with great caution to elderly patients, those with diabetes mellitus, hyperthyroidism or psychoneurotic disorders; also to those with long-standing bronchial asthma or emphysema if such individuals may also have degenerative heart disease, and to pregnant women (see "Pregnancy").

CHLO-AMINE®: Chlorpheniramine maleate should be used with extreme caution in patients with stenosing peptic ulcer, pyloroduodenal obstruction, prostatic hypertrophy, or bladder neck obstruction. These compounds have an atropine-like action and therefore should be used with caution in patients with a history of increased intraocular pressure, cardiovascular disease, or hypertension. The asthmatic patient should take the chlorpheniramine maleate tablets with caution.

PRECAUTIONS

GENERAL: Hollister-Stier Ana-Kit® is not intended to be a substitute for medical attention or hospital care. The kit is designed to be compact and easy to carry, and to provide emergency treatment when medical care is not immediately available. Highly sensitive individuals should have the kit readily available at all times. Because of its small size it can be carried by outdoor sportsmen, golfers, gardeners, or any sensitive individual who may be exposed to stinging insects (wasps, hornets, yellow jackets, fire ants or bees) or other potentially life-threatening allergens. The drugs in the Ana-Kit®, when used as directed immediately following exposure to an allergen, may prove life-saving. Certain changes in the emergency instructions and in the kit itself may be made by the doctor according to the needs of the patient. IN ALL CASES THE PHYSICIAN SHOULD INSTRUCT THE PATIENT, AND/OR ANY OTHER PERSON WHO MIGHT BE IN A POSITION TO ADMINISTER THE EPINEPHRINE, IN THE PROPER USE OF THE SYRINGE AND THE OTHER COMPONENTS OF THIS KIT.

The effects of epinephrine may be potentiated by **tricyclic antidepressants**, sodium levothyroxine, and certain antihistamines, notably chlorpheniramine, tripeiennamine, and diphenhydramine.

Carcinogenesis, Mutagenesis, Impairment of Fertility: There are no data from either animal or human studies regarding the carcinogenicity or mutagenicity of epinephrine or Chlo-Amine, and no studies have been conducted to determine their potential for the impairment of fertility.

Pregnancy: Teratogenic Effects. Pregnancy Category C—Epinephrine has been shown to be teratogenic in rats and hamsters at dose levels hundreds of times as high as the maximal human dose. Although there are no adequate or well-controlled studies in pregnant women, epinephrine crosses the placenta and its use during pregnancy may cause anoxia in the fetus. Epinephrine should be used in pregnancy only if the potential benefit justifies the potential risk to the fetus.

Pediatric Use: Administer Epinephrine or Chlo-Amine with caution to infants and children (see "Dosage and Administration"). Syncope has occurred following the administration of epinephrine to asthmatic children.

INFORMATION FOR PATIENTS: Complete patient information, including dosage, directions for proper administration, and precautions, can be found at the end of this package insert, as well as inside each Ana-Kit® kit.

ADVERSE REACTIONS

EPINEPHRINE: Adverse reactions include transient, moderate anxiety, apprehensiveness, restlessness, tremor, weakness, dizziness, sweating, palpitations, pallor, nausea and vomiting, headache, and respiratory difficulties. These symptoms occur in some persons receiving therapeutic doses of epinephrine, but are more likely to occur, or to occur in exaggerated form, in those with hypertension or hyperthyroidism. Excessive doses cause acute hypertension and cardiac arrhythmias.

CHLO-AMINE: Drowsiness, dizziness, blurred vision, dry mouth and gastrointestinal upsets may occur. Patients should not drive or operate machinery after taking the drug. Large doses produce central nervous system depression and occasionally tremors or convulsions. Reports of hematological disorders are rare.

OVERDOSAGE

EPINEPHRINE: Epinephrine is rapidly inactivated in the body, and treatment is primarily supportive. If necessary, pressor effects may be counteracted by rapidly acting vasodilators or alpha-adrenergic blocking drugs. If prolonged hypotension follows such measures, it may be necessary to administer another pressor drug, such as levarterenol.

If an epinephrine overdose induces pulmonary edema that interferes with respiration, treatment consists of a rapidly acting alpha-adrenergic blocking drug such as phentolamine and/or intermittent positive-pressure respiration.

Epinephrine overdosage can also cause transient bradycardia followed by tachycardia, and these may be accompanied by potentially fatal cardiac arrhythmias. Ventricular premature contractions may appear within one minute after injection and may be followed by multilocal ventricular tachycardia (prefibrillation rhythm). Subsidence of the ventricular effects may be followed by atrial tachycardia and occasionally by atrioventricular block. Treatment of arrhythmias consists of administration of beta-adrenergic blocking drug such as propranolol.

Overdosage sometimes also results in extreme pallor and coldness of the skin, metabolic acidosis, and kidney failure. Suitable corrective measures must be taken.

CHLO-AMINE: Overdose symptoms may be sedation, apnea, cardiovascular collapse to stimulation, insomnia, hallucinations, tremors or convulsions. Also there may be dizziness, tinnitus, ataxia, blurred vision, hypotension, dry mouth, flushing, and abdominal symptoms.

Treatment—The patient should be induced to vomit, preferably with ipecac syrup—and large amounts of water. Prevent aspiration of vomitus. Gastric lavage may be necessary using activated charcoal and saline. Hyperosmotic cathartics such as Milk of Magnesia may hasten elimination of residual cling. Vasopressors can be used to correct hypotension. Diazepan may be used to control seizures. Hyperpyrexia can be treated with cool sponges or a hypothermic blanket.

DOSAGE AND ADMINISTRATION

The physician who prescribes the Ana-Kit® should review the package insert in detail with the patient. This review should include the proper use of the 2-dose epinephrine syringe to insure that subcutaneous or intramuscular injections are given into the deltoid region of the arm or the anteriolateral aspect of the thigh. See also the PATIENT DIRECTIONS FOR USE.

EPINEPHRINE: For subcutaneous or intramuscular injection only.

Adults and children over 12 years: 0.3 mL; 6–12 years: 0.2 mL; 2–6 years: 0.15 mL; Infants to 2 years: 0.05 to 0.1 mL.

When syringe is properly set up, as directed in the Patient Instruction Sheet, a 0.3 mL dose is administered when plunger is pushed until it stops. Syringe barrel has 0.1 mL graduations so that smaller doses can be measured. (Operation of syringe is explained in the Patient Directions For Use section at the end of this package insert.)

If after 10 minutes from the first injection symptoms are not noticeably improved, administer a second dose of epinephrine from the syringe.

CHLO-AMINE: Tablets are chewable antihistamines. Adults and children over 12 years: 4 tablets; children 6–12 years: 2 tablets; children under 6 years: 1 tablet.

HOW SUPPLIED

HOLLISTER-STIER ANAPHYLAXIS EMERGENCY TREATMENT KIT (ANA-KIT®) CONTAINS:

SYRINGE: One sterile syringe containing 1 mL Epinephrine Injection, USP, (1:1000). Syringe delivers two 0.3 mL doses.

TABLETS: Four 2 mg chewable Chlo-Amine® tablets, Chlorpheniramine Maleate Tablets.

DEVICES: Two sterile pads containing 70% isopropyl alcohol (by volume) and 1 tourniquet.

PROTECT FROM LIGHT. KEEP AT ROOM TEMPERATURE, APPROX. 25°C (77°F), PROTECT FROM FREEZING.

CAUTION: U.S. Federal Law Prohibits Dispensing Without Prescription.

Epinephrine Mfg. by: Wyeth Laboratories, Inc.,
Philadelphia, PA 19101

Pkgd. and Dist. by:
Hollister-Stier
Miles Inc.
Pharmaceutical Division
Spokane, WA 99207 USA

PATIENT DIRECTIONS FOR USE

ANA-KIT® Anaphylaxis Emergency Treatment Kit

(Please read entire direction sheet before an emergency arises.)

The Ana-Kit® **IS TO BE USED ONLY WHEN PRESCRIBED BY A PHYSICIAN**, for patients who are highly allergic to pollens, foods, dusts, insect stings, and drugs which may produce a life-threatening anaphylactic reaction, or have severe asthma attacks.

Continued on next page

Miles Allergy—Cont.

IN THE EVENT OF A LIFE-
THREATENING SITUATION,
FOLLOW THESE STEPS IM-
MEDIATELY TO ADMINISTER
THE EPINEPHRINE.

1. Remove red rubber needle cover.
Hold syringe upright and push
plunger to expel air and excess
epinephrine (plunger will stop).

Expel

2. Rotate rectangular plunger $\frac{1}{4}$
turn to the right. Plunger will
align with slot in barrel of syringe
Wipe injection site with alcohol
swab.

Rotate Plunger

3. Insert needle straight into arm or
thigh as illustrated.

4. Push plunger until it stops.
Syringe will inject a 0.3 mL dose
for adults and children over 12
years.

Insert and Inject

Children: Syringe barrel has 0.1
mL graduations so that smaller
doses can be measured. Administer to infants to 2 years:
0.05 to 0.1 mL; 2–6 years: 0.15 mL;
and 6–12 years: 0.2 mL.

ONCE THE INITIAL EPINEPHRINE
INJECTION HAS BEEN ADMINIS-
TERED, FOLLOW THESE ADDI-
TIONAL STEPS.

1. CONTACT PHYSICIAN, IF
POSSIBLE.

2. REMOVE STINGER if stung
by insect. (Use fingernails. DO
NOT push, pinch or squeeze, or
further imbed the stinger into
the skin as this may cause
further venom to be injected.)

Remove Stinger

3. APPLY TOURNIQUET. If
exposure to life-threatening
agent was by injection (allergic
extract, drug) or insect sting on an
arm or leg, place tourniquet
between injection or sting site
and body. (If exposure is elsewhere—neck, face, or body—
proceed immediately to Step 5.)

Apply Tourniquet

4. TIGHTEN TOURNIQUET. To tight-
en, pull on the end of ONE STRING.
Then, at least every ten minutes,
loosen the tourniquet by pulling on
the small metal ring.

5. CHEW AND SWALLOW CHLO-
AMINE TABLETS. For adults and
children over 12 years, take 4 tablets;
children 6–12 years take 2 tablets;
children under 6 years take 1 tablet.
These tablets are chewable antihistamine which is generally tolerated.

Chew Chlo-Amine

6. PREPARE SYRINGE FOR A POS-
SIBLE SECOND INJECTION. Turn
the rectangular plunger $\frac{1}{4}$ turn to
the right to line up with rectangular
slot in the syringe. (A slight wig-
gling may aid the turning and alignment of the plunger.)

Rotate Plunger

7. THE SECOND INJECTION. If after
10 minutes from the first injection
symptoms are not noticeably improved, a second injection is required.
Cleanse skin area with alcohol swab
and make second injection as in
STEPS 3 and 4 for the first epinephrine injection. (A small amount of
epinephrine will remain in syringe
after the second dose and cannot be
expelled.) Note: Dispose of
syringe and remaining contents if
second injection is not required.

8. APPLY ICE PACKS IF AVAILABLE,
AT THE SITE OF THE DRUG
OR ALLERGY INJECTION, OR
INSECT STING (if applicable).

9. KEEP PATIENT WARM AND
AVOID EXERTION.

PRECAUTIONS

EPINEPHRINE: For subcutaneous or intramuscular injection only. Not intended for intravenous use.

Epinephrine Injection, USP, contains sodium bisulfite. Patients with a suspected sulfite sensitivity should consult
their physician well in advance before the need to use this
product becomes critical.
Epinephrine is light sensitive and should be stored in box
provided. KEEP AT ROOM TEMPERATURE, approximately 25°C (77°F). Protect from freezing. Any epinephrine
solution in contact with the needle may cause rusting of the
metal. Do not try to force air out of the syringe until you are
ready to use the epinephrine. This may rupture the seal and
allow the epinephrine solution to contact the metal promoting deterioration. Never remove rubber protector over needle
until ready to use syringe as this may cause needle and contents to become contaminated.
Periodically check contents of the syringe. If discoloration or
precipitate is present, DO NOT USE. Obtain replacement
syringe from physician. Periodically check expiration date
on syringe. If expiration date is near, re-order new syringe
and discard outdated syringe after new syringe has been
received.

CHLO-AMINE: As with any drug, if you are pregnant or
nursing a baby, seek the advice of a health professional before using this product.
Patients should not drive or operate machinery after taking
Chlo-Amine. Drowsiness, dizziness, blurred vision, dry
mouth and gastrointestinal upsets may occur. Keep out of
reach of children.
The asthmatic patient should take the chlorpheniramine
maleate tablets with caution.

LIMITED WARRANTY: A number of factors beyond our
control could reduce the efficacy of this product or even result in an ill effect following its use. These include storage
and handling of the product after it leaves our hands, diagnosis, dosage, method of administration and biological differences in individual patients. Because of these factors, it is
important that this product be stored properly and that the
directions be followed carefully during use.
The foregoing statement is made in lieu of any other warranty, express or implied, including any warranty of merchantability or fitness. Representatives of the Company are
not authorized to vary the terms of this warranty or the contents of any printed labeling for this product except by
printed notice from the Company's Spokane, WA office. The
prescriber and user of this product must accept the terms
hereof.

Epinephrine Mfg. by: Wyeth Laboratories, Inc.,
Philadelphia, PA 19101
Pkgd. and Dist. by:
Miles Inc.
Hollister-   Pharmaceutical Division
Stier   Spokane, WA 99207 USA
Phys: 471103 M03 3/91   © 1988 Miles Inc.
Cr. Ref. 471104

Miles Inc.

**Pharmaceutical Division
Biological Products
400 MORGAN LANE
WEST HAVEN, CT 06516**

Factor IX Complex   ℞
KONȲNE® 80
Heat-Treated at 80°C

DESCRIPTION

Factor IX Complex, Konȳne® 80, heat-treated at 80°C for 72
hours, is a sterile, dried, plasma fraction comprising coagulation factors II, IX, X and low levels of factor VII.

Factor:	Nomenclature Synonyms:
II	prothrombin
VII	proconvertin
IX	plasma thromboplastin com-ponent, PTC, Christmas factor
X	Stuart-Prower factor

Konȳne 80 is standardized in terms of factor IX content and
each vial of Konȳne 80 is labeled for factor IX. One international unit (IU) of factor IX as defined by the World Health
Organization standard for blood coagulation factor IX is approximately equal to the level of factor IX found in 1.0 mL of
fresh, normal plasma.
The factor IX content is approximately 50 times purified
over whole plasma, and when reconstituted as directed,
Konȳne 80 contains 25 times as much factor IX as an equal
volume of fresh plasma. Konȳne 80, containing approximately 1000 IU of factor IX administered in 40 mL, contains
the factor IX content of 1 liter of fresh plasma. Konȳne 80
must be administered intravenously.

CLINICAL PHARMACOLOGY

Factor IX Complex raises the plasma level of factor IX and
restores hemostasis in patients with factor IX deficiency. In
general, a level of factor IX less than 5% of normal will give

---

rise to spontaneous hemorrhage, while levels greater than
20% of normal will lead to satisfactory hemostasis even in
the face of trauma or surgery. Approximately 30% to 50% of
the factor IX activity can be detected in a hemophilia B (factor IX deficiency) recipient's plasma immediately after infusion.[1,2] The biological activity of the infused factor IX disappears from the plasma with a half-life of approximately 24
hours.[2] Pharmacokinetic studies in six patients treated with
Konȳne 80 have shown a mean half-life of 11.98 ± 1.46 hours
(mean $\pm$ SD), with a mean recovery of $43.42\% \pm 16\%$. It
must be noted that administration of Factor IX Complex
causes an increase in blood levels of factors II, VII, IX and X.
Factors II, VII, IX and X are the vitamin K dependent coagulation factors and are synthesized in the liver. Congenital
deficiencies of each of the four factors do occur and may result in a bleeding tendency. Naturally low levels of the vitamin K dependent factors may also be found in vitamin K
deficiency and in severe liver disease.
This product has been heated at 80°C for 72 hours and there
is no evidence of adverse effects upon the product. In a study[3]
designed to assess the effectiveness of heat treatment at 68°C
for 72 hours, hepatitis naive chimpanzees were inoculated
with heated Antihemophilic Factor (Human) and Factor IX
Complex preparations to which had been previously added
non-A, non-B hepatitis Hutchinson Strain[4] to a total level of
2500 chimpanzee infectious doses (CID). The chimpanzees
receiving heated preparations failed to exhibit any symptoms of non-A, non-B hepatitis. In contrast, one chimpanzee
receiving Antihemophilic Factor (Human) concentrate
which was not heated after the non-A, non-B inoculum was
added, developed abnormally elevated alanine aminotransferase (ALT) levels beginning 10 weeks postinoculation and
liver histopathology at 6 weeks. From these results, it was
concluded that the heat treatment employed inactivated a
known quantity of non-A, non-B hepatitis: at least 2500 CID.
Additional in vitro studies[5] on the effect of heating Factor IX
Complex, Konȳne® 80, in a dried state at 80°C for 72 hours,
on virus inactivation were carried out with a number of
viruses, including human immunodeficiency virus (HIV),
added to Factor IX Complex prior to heating. The following
table shows the amount of each model virus inactivated by
the process:

Virus	Starting Amount Logs*	Logs Inactivated
Vesicular Stomatitis Virus	8.0	≥ 7.5
Vaccinia Virus	5.75	1.0
Sindbis Virus	7.25	≥ 6.75
Bovine Parvovirus	4.5	3.5
Human Immunodeficiency Virus (HIV), HIV-1	4.8	≥ 4.3

*$\log_{10}$ TCID$_{50}$/mL (for HIV-1, $\log_{10}$ TCID$_{50}$)

INDICATIONS AND USAGE

Factor IX Complex, Konȳne® 80 is indicated for the preven-
tion and control of bleeding caused by Factor IX deficiency
due to hemophilia B.
Konȳne 80 is not indicated for use in the treatment of factor
VII deficiency.
Konȳne 80 is appropriate for use in:

1. Hemophilia B (Christmas disease); demonstrated factor IX
deficiency in children or adults with real or impending
bleeding episodes. Spontaneous bleeding can occur even in
the absence of any trauma.

2. Reversal of coumarin anticoagulant induced hemorrhage;
in situations where prompt reversal is required (e.g., preceding emergency surgery, trauma, etc.), administration
of fresh-frozen plasma should be initially considered as
treatment; however, Konȳne 80 may be considered as a
secondary approach if the risk of transmitting hepatitis is
considered justifiable in the face of a life-threatening situation.[6–8]

3. Treatment of bleeding episodes in patients with hemophilia A (factor VIII deficiency) who have inhibitors to
factor VIII.[9]
In addition to coumarin anticoagulant induced deficiencies, low levels of factors II, VII, IX and X may be found in
vitamin K deficiency, in patients with gut sterilization due
to oral antibiotics, in patients with liver disease, and in
those with nephrotic syndrome. However, Factor IX Complex, Konȳne 80® is not indicated in these situations and
treatment should be aimed at correcting the primary condition.

Note: For publications on the clinical use of Konȳne®,
please refer to references 1,2, 6–18.

CONTRAINDICATIONS

None known.

WARNINGS

1. Hepatitis and Viral Diseases
This product is prepared from pooled human plasma
which may contain the causative agents of hepatitis
and other viral diseases. Prescribed manufacturing
procedures utilized at the plasma collection centers,

plasma testing laboratories, and the fractionation facilities are designed to reduce the risk of transmitting viral infection. However, the risk of viral infectivity from this product cannot be totally eliminated.

Individuals who receive infusions of blood or plasma products may develop signs and/or symptoms of some viral infections, particularly non-A, non-B hepatitis.[19] It is emphasized that hepatitis B vaccination is essential for patients with hemophilia and it is recommended that this be done at birth or diagnosis.[20]

Konȳne 80 is a plasma fraction obtained from many paid donors. The presence of hepatitis viruses should be assumed and the hazard of administering Konȳne 80 should be weighed against the medical consequences of withholding it, particularly in persons with few previous transfusions of blood or blood products.

2. Thrombosis

Cases of patients developing postoperative thrombosis after treatment with Factor IX Complex have been described. Although thrombosis is a well-known risk of the postoperative period, it is found to be greater in these patients.[13-15] No other data are presently available. Until further surveys and more conclusive studies are available, Konȳne 80 is only advised for patients undergoing elective surgery where the expected beneficial effects of its use outweigh the increased risk of the possibility of thrombosis. This applies especially to those who may be predisposed to thrombosis. Do not use in cases of known liver disease where there is any suspicion of intravascular coagulation or fibrinolysis.

PRECAUTIONS

General

1. Reconstitute only with Sterile Water for Injection, USP.
2. Administer within 3 hours after reconstitution. Do not refrigerate after reconstitution.
3. Administer only by the intravenous route.
4. The administration equipment and any reconstituted Factor IX Complex, Konȳne® 80 not immediately used should be discarded.
5. ε -aminocaproic acid should not be administered with Factor IX Complex as this may increase the risk of thrombosis.
6. Patients who receive Konȳne 80 either postoperatively or with known liver disease should be kept under close observation for signs and symptoms of intravascular coagulation or thrombosis. Any suspicious findings of this nature indicate the dosage should be markedly decreased if the patient's conditions are such that the treatment cannot be discontinued entirely. In the event of thrombohemorrhagic disorders occurring, reduction in dosage should be considered, and treatment with heparin may be warranted. Although this preparation does not contain heparin, it has been suggested that reconstitution with heparin in a concentration of 2–5 IU per mL may reduce the risk of development of thrombosis.[18] However, thrombosis can occur even in the presence of heparin.
7. Patients receiving Konȳne 80 for prolonged periods should be continually monitored at least for levels of factors II, IX and X. The same comments as in No. 6 above are indicated.

Pregnancy Category C

Animal reproduction studies have not been conducted with Konȳne 80. It is also not known whether Konȳne 80 can cause fetal harm when administered to a pregnant woman or can affect reproduction capacity. Konȳne 80 should be given to a pregnant woman only if clearly needed.

ADVERSE REACTIONS

In some patients the rapid administration of Konȳne 80 can cause transient fever, chills, headache, flushing or tingling.

DOSAGE AND ADMINISTRATION

Each bottle of Konȳne 80 has the factor IX activity, in IU, stated on the bottle label. One IU is defined as the activity present in 1 mL of fresh, normal plasma. The potency is standardized in terms of factor IX content.

The amount of Konȳne 80 required for normalizing hemostasis will depend upon the patient and upon the circumstances. Sufficient Konȳne 80 should be administered to achieve and maintain a plasma level of at least 20% until hemostasis is achieved.

The dosage guidelines may be derived from the table below. The following formulas may be used as guidelines to calculate an appropriate dose or to estimate the expected percentage increase obtained from a given dose.:

$$\text{Expected factor IX increase (in \% of normal)} = \frac{\text{IU administered} \times 1.0}{\text{body weight (in kg)}}$$

IU required = body weight (kg) × desired factor IX increase (% normal) × 1.0

Thus, in order to bring a 70 kg patient from 0% to 50% of normal, the patient would require 70 × 50 × 1.0 = 3500 IU or 50 IU/kg body weight.

Prophylaxis

The ideal treatment for proven congenital deficiency of the procoagulants is prophylactic administration. A dosage of 10–20 IU per kg body weight once or twice per week may be

sufficient to prevent spontaneous bleeding in patients with hemophilia B (congenital factor IX deficiency). Maintenance dosage should be adapted to the individual patient's needs. Additional Factor IX Complex, Konȳne ® 80 should be administered when a patient on prophylaxis is exposed to trauma or surgery.

Maintenance Dose

Maintenance dosage should be administered according to the clinical response and the factor IX level achieved. Such dosage is usually about 10–20 IU per kg body weight per day.

Inhibitor Patients

For treatment of bleeding episodes in patients with hemophilia A (factor VIII deficiency) who have inhibitors to factor VIII, the recommended dose should be 75 IU/kg. A second dose may be administered after 12 hours if necessary.[9] [See table above.]

Reconstitution

Vacuum Transfer

1. Warm the unopened diluent and concentrate to room temperature (NMT 37°C, 99°F).
2. After removing the plastic flip-top caps (Fig. A) aseptically cleanse the rubber stoppers of both bottles.
3. Remove the protective cover from the plastic transfer-needle cartridge with tamper-proof seal and penetrate the stopper of the diluent bottle (Fig. B).
4. Remove the remaining portion of the plastic cartridge. Invert the diluent bottle and penetrate the rubber seal on the concentrate bottle (Fig. C) with the needle at an angle. Alternate method of transferring sterile water: With a sterile needle and syringe, withdraw the appropriate volume of diluent and transfer to the bottle of lyophilized concentrate.
5. Hold the diluent bottle at an angle to the concentrate bottle in order to direct the jet of diluent against the wall of the concentrate bottle. The vacuum will draw the diluent into the concentrate bottle. Avoid excessive foaming. Do not shake the concentrate bottle.
6. After removing the diluent bottle and transfer-needle (Fig. D), optimal reconstitution time is achieved by swirling continuously until completely dissolved (Fig. E). Reconstitution can also be achieved by very gently agitating until dissolved.

Parenteral drug products should be inspected visually for particulate matter and discoloration prior to administration, whenever solution and container permit.

7. After the concentrate powder is completely dissolved, withdraw the Factor IX Complex, Konȳne® 80 solution into the syringe through the filter needle which is supplied in the package (Fig. F). Replace the filter needle with an appropriate sterile injection needle, e.g., 21 gauge × 1 inch, and inject intravenously.
8. If the same patient is to receive more than one bottle of Konȳne 80, the contents of two bottles may be drawn into the same syringe through filter needles before attaching the vein needle.

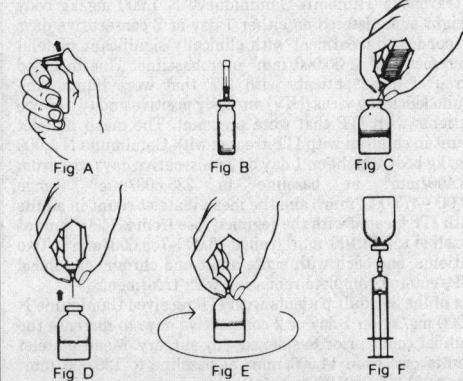

Fig A   Fig B   Fig C

Fig D   Fig E   Fig F

Rate of Administration

The rate of administration should be adapted to the response of the individual patient, but is generally well-tolerated at a rate of approximately 100 IU per minute.

The Pharmacology of Factor IX
(adapted from[1])

Factor	Minor spontaneous hemorrhage, % of normal	Major trauma or surgery, % of normal	Dosage/kg Body Weight*		Metabolic half-life (hours)	% increase in plasma level/dose of 1 U/kg body wt.
			Initial (Loading)	Daily Maintenance		
IX	10–15	20–25	40–60 IU	5–10 IU b.i.d.	10.5–13.5	about 1.0

*In general, 25% is considered the minimal hemostatic level for most patients while undergoing surgery or severe accidental trauma.

The range of values in normal clinical practice is likely to be much wider than those shown above. This is due to differences between patients, their clinical condition and the type of assay employed.

HOW SUPPLIED

Factor IX Complex, Konȳne® 80 is supplied in single dose bottles with the total IU of factor IX activity stated on the label of each bottle. A suitable volume of Sterile Water for Injection, USP, a sterile double-ended transfer needle, and a sterile filter needle are provided.

Product Code	Approximate Factor IX Activity	Diluent
626–20	500 IU	20 mL
626–50	1000 IU	40 mL

STORAGE

Konȳne 80 should be stored under refrigeration (2°–8°C; 35°–46°F). Freezing should be avoided as breakage of the diluent bottle might occur.

Konȳne 80 concentrate may be stored for a period of up to 1 month at temperatures not to exceed 25°C (77°F) during travel.

CAUTION

U.S. federal law prohibits dispensing without prescription.

LIMITED WARRANTY

A number of factors beyond our control could reduce the efficacy of this product or even result in an ill effect following its use. These include improper storage and handling of the product after it leaves our hands, diagnosis, dosage, method of administration, and biological differences in individual patients. Because of these factors it is important that this product be stored properly, that the directions be followed carefully during use, and that the risk of transmitting viruses be carefully weighed before the product is prescribed. No warranty, express or implied, including any warranty of merchantability or fitness is made. Representatives of the Company are not authorized to vary the terms or contents of the printed labeling, including the package insert, for this product except by printed notice from the Company's headquarters. The prescriber and user of this product must accept the terms hereof.

REFERENCES

1. Johnson AJ, Aronson DL, Williams WJ: Preparation and clinical use of plasma and plasma fractions. In: Williams WJ (ed): *Hematology*, 2d ed, New York, McGraw-Hill, 1977, ch 169, pp 1561–83.
2. Zauber NP, Levin J: Factor IX levels in patients with hemophilia B (Christmas disease) following transfusion with concentrates of factor IX or fresh frozen plasma (FFP). *Medicine* (Baltimore) 56(3): 213–24, 1977.
3. Mozen MM, Louie RE, Mitra G: Heat inactivation of viruses in antihemophilic factor concentrates. Abstracts, XVIth International Congress of the World Federation of Hemophilia, Rio de Janeiro, Aug. 24–28, 1984. Number 240.
4. Feinstone SM, Alter HJ, Dienes HP, et al: Non-A, non-B hepatitis in chimpanzees and marmosets. *J Infect Dis* 144(6):588–98, 1981.
5. Unpublished data in files of Miles Inc., Cutter Biological.
6. Taberner DA, Thompson JM, Poller L: Comparison of prothrombin complex concentrate and vitamin K_1 in oral anticoagulant reversal. *Br Med J* 2(6027):83–5, 1976.
7. Menache D, Roberts HR: Summary report and recommendations of the task force members and consultants. *Thromb Diath Haemorrh* 33:645–7, 1975.
8. Aronson DL: Factor IX Complex. *Semin Thromb Hemostas* 6(1):28–43, 1979.
9. Lusher JM, Shapiro SS, Palascak JE, et al: Efficacy of prothrombin-complex concentrates in hemophiliacs with antibodies to factor VIII: a multicenter therapeutic trial. *N Engl J Med* 303(8):421–5, 1980.
10. Hoag MS, Johnson FF, Robinson AJ, et al: Treatment of hemophilia B with a new clotting-factor concentrate. *N Engl J Med* 280(11):581–6, 1969.
11. Hoag MS, Johnson FF, Robinson AJ, et al: Use of plasma concentrate in congenital factor VII and IX deficiencies. *Clin Res* 17:152, 1969.

Continued on next page

Miles Biological—Cont.

12. Breen FA Jr, Tullis JL: Prothrombin concentrates in treatment of Christmas disease and allied disorders. *JAMA* 208(10):1848–52, 1969.
13. Kasper CK: Postoperative thrombosis in hemophilia. *N Engl J Med* 289(3):160, 1973.
14. Kasper CK: Surgical operation in hemophilia B. Use of factor IX concentrate. *Calif Med* 113(1):4–8, 1970.
15. George JN, Breckenridge RT: The use of factor VIII and factor IX concentrates during surgery. *JAMA* 214(9):1673–6, 1970.
16. Gunay U, Choi HS, Maurer HS, et al: Commercial preparations of prothrombin complex. A clinical comparison. *Am J Dis Child* 126(6):775–7, 1973.
17. O'Leary DS, Ruymann FB, Conrad ME: Therapeutic approaches to factor X deficiency with emphasis on the use of a new clotting-factor concentrate (Konyne®). *J Lab Clin Med* 77(1):23–32, 1971.
18. White GC 2d, Lundblad RL, Kingdon HS: Prothrombin complex concentrates: preparation, properties, and clinical uses. *Curr Top Hematol* 2:203–44, 1979.
19. Colombo M, Mannucci PM, Carnelli V, et al: Transmission of non-A, non-B hepatitis by heat-treated factor VIII concentrate. *Lancet* 2(8445):1–4, 1985.
20. National Hemophilia Foundation Medical and Scientific Advisory Council. Hemophilia Information Exchange—AIDS Update: Recommendations concerning AIDS and the treatment of hemophilia. HIV infection, Section I.G. (Rev. Jan., 1988).

U.S. License No. 8
Miles Inc.
Cutter Biological
Elkhart, IN 46515 USA
14-7626-000 (Rev. April 1991)

IMMUNE GLOBULIN INTRAVENOUS (HUMAN) ℞
GAMIMUNE® N

DESCRIPTION

Immune Globulin Intravenous (Human)—Gamimune® N is a sterile 4.5%–5.5% solution of human protein in 9%–11% maltose; it contains no preservative. Each milliliter (mL) contains approximately 50 mg of protein, not less than 98% of which has the electrophoretic mobility of gamma globulin. Not less than 90% of the gamma globulin is monomer. Also present are traces of IgA and of IgM. The distribution of IgG subclasses is similar to that found in normal serum. Gamimune N has a buffer capacity of 16.5 mEq/L of solution (~ 0.3 mEq/g of protein). The calculated osmolality is 309 milliosmoles per kilogram of solvent (water) and the calculated osmolarity is 278 milliosmoles per liter of solution.

The product is made by cold ethanol fractionation of large pools of human plasma. Part of the fractionation may be performed by another licensed manufacturer. The immunoglobulin is isolated from Cohn Effluent III by diafiltration and ultrafiltration. The protein has not been chemically modified other than in the adjustment of the pH of the solution to 4.0–4.5.[1] Isotonicity is achieved by the addition of maltose. The product is intended for intravenous administration.

CLINICAL PHARMACOLOGY

Gamimune N supplies a broad spectrum of opsonic and neutralizing IgG antibodies for the prevention or attenuation of a wide variety of infectious diseases. As Gamimune N is administered intravenously, essentially 100% of the infused IgG antibodies are immediately available in the recipient's circulation.[2] A relatively rapid fall in serum IgG level in the first week postinfusion is to be expected; this decrease averages 40% of the peak level achieved immediately postinfusion and is mainly due to the equilibration of IgG between the plasma and the extravascular space.[2,10,11,14] The in vivo half-life of Gamimune N equals or exceeds the 3-week half-life reported for IgG in the literature, but individual patient variation in half-life has been observed.[2] Thus, this variable as well as the amount of immune globulin administered per dose is important in determining the frequency of administration of the drug for each individual patient.

While Gamimune N has been shown to be effective in some cases of idiopathic thrombocytopenic purpura (ITP) (see INDICATIONS AND USAGE), the mechanism of action has not been fully elucidated.

The intravenous administration of solutions of maltose has been studied by several investigators.[4–8] Healthy subjects tolerated the infusions well, and no adverse effects were observed at a rate of 0.25 g maltose/kg body weight per hour.[5] In safety studies conducted by Cutter Biological, infusions of 10% maltose administered at 0.27–0.62 g maltose/kg per hour[8] to normal subjects produced either mild side effects (e.g., headache) or no adverse reaction.[2] Following intravenous administrations of maltose, maltose was detected in the peripheral blood; there was a dose-dependent excretion of maltose and glucose in the urine and a mild diuretic effect.[2] These alterations were well-tolerated without significant adverse effects.[2] The highest recommended infusion rate, 0.08 mL/kg body weight per minute (see DOSAGE AND ADMINISTRATION), is equivalent to 0.48 g maltose/kg body weight per hour.

The buffer capacity of Immune Globulin Intravenous (Human)—Gamimune® N is 16.5 mEq/L (~ 0.3 mEq/g protein); a dose of 150–400 mg/kg (3–8 mL/kg) body weight therefore represents an acid load of 0.0495–0.1320 mEq/kg body weight. The total buffering capacity of whole blood in a normal individual is 45–50 mEq/L of blood, or 3.6 mEq/kg body weight.[9] Thus, the acid load delivered in the largest dose of Gamimune N would be neutralized by the buffering capacity of whole blood alone, even if the dose were infused instantaneously. (An infusion usually lasts several hours.)

In Phase I human studies, no change in arterial blood pH measurements was detected following the intravenous administration of Gamimune N at a dose of 150 mg/kg body weight;[2] following a dose of 400 mg/kg body weight in 37 patients, there were no clinically important differences in mean venous pH or bicarbonate measurements in patients who received Gamimune N compared with those who received a chemically modified intravenous immunoglobulin preparation with a pH of 6.8.[2]

In patients with limited or compromised acid-base compensatory mechanisms, consideration should be given to the effect of the additional acid load Gamimune N might present.

INDICATIONS AND USAGE

Primary Humoral Immunodeficiency

Gamimune N is efficacious in the treatment of primary immunodeficiency states in which severe impairment of antibody forming capacity has been shown, such as: congenital agammaglobulinemias, common variable immunodeficiency, Wiskott-Aldrich syndrome, x-linked immunodeficiency with hyper IgM, and severe combined immunodeficiencies.[3,12–15] Gamimune N is especially useful when high levels or rapid elevation of circulating antibodies are desired or when intramuscular injections are contraindicated.

Idiopathic Thrombocytopenic Purpura (ITP)

In clinical situations in which a rapid rise in platelet count is needed to control bleeding or to allow a patient with ITP to undergo surgery, administration of Gamimune N should be considered; in patients in whom a response is achieved, the rise of platelets is generally rapid (within 1–5 days), transient (most often lasting from several days to several weeks) and should not be considered curative. It is presently not possible to predict which patients with ITP will respond to therapy, although the increase in platelet counts in children seems to be better than that in adults.

Two different dosing regimens of Gamimune N have been studied in clinical investigations: a regimen consisting of 400 mg/kg body weight daily for 5 consecutive days, and a high dose treatment regimen consisting of 1,000 mg/kg body weight administered on either 1 day or 2 consecutive days.

In clinical studies of Gamimune N, five of six (83.3%) children and 12 of 16 (75%) adults with acute or chronic ITP treated with 400 mg/kg body weight for 5 consecutive days demonstrated clinically significant platelet increments of $\geq$30,000/mm^3 over baseline. The mean platelet count in children with ITP rose from 27,800/mm^3 at baseline to 297,000/mm^3 (range 50,000–455,000/mm^3) and the mean platelet count in adults with ITP rose from 27,900/mm^3 at baseline to 124,900/mm^3 (range 11,000–341,000/mm^3). Two of three children with acute ITP rapidly went into complete remission. However, childhood ITP may respond spontaneously without treatment.

Thirteen of 14 children (92.9%) and 26 of 29 adults (89.7%) with acute or chronic ITP treated with Immune Globulin Intravenous (Human)—Gamimune® N 1,000 mg/kg body weight administered on either 1 day or 2 consecutive days responded to treatment with clinically significant platelet increments of $\geq$30,000/mm^3 over baseline. This included three of three patients with ITP that were human immunodeficiency virus (HIV) antibody positive and two of two patients with ITP that were pregnant. The mean platelet count in children with ITP treated with Gamimune N 1,000 mg/kg body weight on 1 day or 2 consecutive days rose from 44,400/mm^3 at baseline to 285,600/mm^3 (range 89,000–473,000/mm^3) and the mean platelet count in adults with ITP treated with the regimen rose from 23,400/mm^3 at baseline to 173,100/mm^3 (range 28,000–709,000/mm^3). Two patients, one each with acute adult and chronic childhood ITP, entered complete remission with treatment.

Six of the 29 adult patients with ITP received Gamimune N 1,000 mg/kg on 1 day or 2 consecutive days to increase the platelet count prior to splenectomy surgery. Mean platelet counts rose from 14,500/mm^3 at baseline to 129,300/mm^3 (range 51,000–242,000/mm^3) prior to surgery.

The duration of the platelet rise following treatment of ITP with either treatment regimen of Gamimune N was variable, ranging from several days to 12 months or more. Some ITP patients have demonstrated continuing responsiveness over many months to intermittent infusions of Gamimune N 400–1,000 mg/kg body weight, administered as a single maintenance dose, at intervals as indicated by the platelet count.

CONTRAINDICATIONS

Gamimune N is contraindicated in individuals who are known to have had an anaphylactic or severe systemic response to Immune Globulin (Human). Individuals with selective IgA deficiencies who have known antibody against IgA (anti-IgA antibody) should not receive Gamimune N since these patients may experience severe reactions to the IgA which may be present.[13]

WARNINGS

Gamimune N should be administered only intravenously as the intramuscular and subcutaneous routes have not been evaluated.

Gamimune N may, on rare occasions, cause a precipitous fall in blood pressure and a clinical picture of anaphylaxis, even when the patient is not known to be sensitive to immune globulin preparations. These reactions may be related to the rate of infusion. Accordingly, the infusion rate given under DOSAGE AND ADMINISTRATION should be closely followed, at least until the physician has had sufficient experience with a given patient. The patient's vital signs should be monitored continuously and careful observation made for any symptoms throughout the entire infusion. Epinephrine should be available for the treatment of an acute anaphylactic reaction.

PRECAUTIONS

General

Any vial that has been entered should be used promptly. Partially used vials should be discarded. Do not use if turbid. Solution which has been frozen should not be used.

Drug Interactions

If dilution is required, Immune Globulin Intravenous (Human)—Gamimune® N may be diluted with 5% dextrose in water (D5/W). No other drug interactions or compatibilities have been evaluated. It is recommended that infusion of Gamimune N be given by a separate line, by itself, without mixing with other intravenous fluids or medications the patient might be receiving.

Pregnancy Category C

Animal reproduction studies have not been conducted with Gamimune N. It is not known whether Gamimune N can cause fetal harm when administered to a pregnant woman or can affect reproduction capacity. Gamimune N should be given to a pregnant woman only if clearly needed.

ADVERSE REACTIONS

In a study of 37 patients with immunodeficiency syndromes receiving Gamimune N at a monthly dose of 400 mg/kg body weight, reactions were seen in 5.2% of the infusions of Gamimune N. Symptoms reported with Gamimune N included malaise, a feeling of faintness, fever, chills, headache, nausea, vomiting, chest tightness, dyspnea and chest, back or hip pain. In addition, mild erythema following infiltration of Gamimune N at the infusion site was reported in some cases.

In studies of Gamimune N administered at a dose of 400 mg/kg body weight in the treatment of adult and pediatric patients with ITP, systemic reactions were noted in only 4 of 154 (2.6%) infusions, and all but one occurred at rates of infusion greater than 0.04 mL/kg body weight per minute. The symptoms reported included chest tightness, a sense of tachycardia (pulse was 84 beats per minute), and a burning sensation in the head; these symptoms were all mild and transient.

In studies of Gamimune N administered at a dose of 1,000 mg/kg body weight either as a single dose or as two doses on consecutive days in the treatment of adult and pediatric patients with ITP, adverse reactions were noted in only 25 of 251 (10%) infusions. Symptoms reported included headache, nausea, fever, chills, back pain, chest tightness, and shortness of breath. In children, the high dose regimen has been well-tolerated at the highest rates of infusion. In adults, however, the frequency of adverse reactions tended to increase with infusion rates in excess of 0.06 mL/kg/min. In general, reactions reported with infusion of Gamimune N in these studies were reported as mild or moderate, and responded to slowing of the infusion rate.

In the studies undertaken to date, other types of reactions have not been reported with Gamimune N. It may be, however, that adverse effects will be similar to those previously reported with intravenous and intramuscular immunoglobulin administration. Potential reactions therefore, may also include anxiety, flushing, wheezing, abdominal cramps, myalgias, arthralgia, and dizziness; rash has been reported only rarely. Reactions to intravenous immunoglobulin tend to be related to the rate of infusion.

True anaphylactic reactions to Immune Globulin Intravenous (Human)—Gamimune® N may occur in recipients with documented prior histories of severe allergic reactions to intramuscular immunoglobulin, but some patients may tolerate cautiously administered intravenous immunoglobulin without adverse effects.[2,16] Very rarely an anaphylactoid reaction may occur in patients with no prior history of severe

allergic reactions to either intramuscular or intravenous immunoglobulin.[2]

DOSAGE AND ADMINISTRATION

Primary Humoral Immunodeficiency

The usual dosage of Gamimune N for prophylaxis in primary immunodeficiency syndromes is 100–200 mg/kg (2–4 mL/kg) of body weight administered approximately once a month by intravenous infusion. The dosage may be given more frequently or increased as high as 400 mg/kg (8 mL/kg) body weight, if the clinical response is inadequate, or the level of IgG achieved in the circulation is felt to be insufficient. The minimum level of IgG required for protection has not been determined.

Idiopathic Thrombocytopenic Purpura (ITP)

Induction: An increase in platelet count has been observed in children and some adults with acute or chronic ITP receiving Gamimune N 400 mg/kg body weight daily for 5 days, or alternatively, 1,000 mg/kg body weight daily for 1 day or 2 consecutive days. In the latter treatment regimen, if an adequate increase in the platelet count is observed at 24 hours, the second dose of 1,000 mg/kg body weight may be withheld. The high dose regimen (1,000 mg/kg $\times$ 1–2 days) is not recommended for individuals with expanded fluid volumes or where fluid volume may be a concern. With both treatment regimens, a response usually occurs within several days and is maintained for a variable period of time. In general, a response is seen less often in adults than in children. **Maintenance:** In adults and children with ITP, if after induction therapy the platelet count falls to less than 30,000/mm[3] and/or the patient manifests clinically significant bleeding, Gamimune N 400 mg/kg body weight may be given as a single infusion. If an adequate response does not result, the dose can be increased to 800–1,000 mg/kg of body weight given as a single infusion. Maintenance infusions may be administered intermittently as clinically indicated to maintain a platelet count greater than 30,000/mm[3].

Investigations indicate that Gamimune N is well-tolerated and less likely to produce side effects when infused at the indicated rate. It is recommended that Gamimune N be infused by itself at a rate of 0.01 to 0.02 mL/kg body weight per minute for 30 minutes; if well-tolerated, the rate may be **gradually** increased to a maximum of 0.08 mL/kg body weight per minute. If side effects occur, the rate may be reduced, or the infusion interrupted until symptoms subside. The infusion may then be resumed at the rate which is comfortable for the patient.

Parenteral drug products should be inspected visually for particulate matter and discoloration prior to administration, whenever solution and container permit.

HOW SUPPLIED

Gamimune® N is supplied in the following sizes:

Size	Grams Protein
10 mL	0.5
50 mL	2.5
100 mL	5.0
250 mL	12.5

STORAGE

Store at 2°–8°C (35°–46°F). Do not freeze. Do not use after expiration date.

CAUTION

U.S. federal law prohibits dispensing without prescription.

LIMITED WARRANTY

A number of factors beyond our control could reduce the efficacy of this product or even result in an ill effect following its use. These include improper storage and handling of the product after it leaves our hands, diagnosis, dosage, method of administration, and biological differences in individual patients. Because of these factors, it is important that this product be stored properly and that the directions be followed carefully during use.

The foregoing statement is made in lieu of any other warranty, express or implied, including any warranty of merchantability or fitness. Representatives of the Company are not authorized to vary the terms of this warranty or the contents of any printed labeling for this product except by printed notice from the Company's headquarters. The prescriber and user of this product must accept the terms hereof.

REFERENCES

1. Tenold RA, inventor; Cutter Laboratories, assignee. Intravenously injectable immune serum globulin. U.S. Patent 4,396,608 August 2, 1983.
2. Data on file at Miles Inc., Cutter Biological.
3. Ochs HD, Buckley RH, Pirofsky B, et al: Safety and patient acceptability of intravenous immune globulin in 10% maltose. *Lancet* 2(8205):1158–9, 1980.
4. Berg G, Matzkies F: Wirkung von Maltose nach intravenöser Dauerinfusion auf den Stoffwechsel. *Z Ernährungswiss* 15:255–62, 1976.
5. Förster H, Hoos I, Boecker S: Versuche mit Probanden zur parenteralen Verwertung von Maltose. *Z Ernährungswiss* 15(3):284–93, 1976.
6. Finke C, Reinauer H: Utilization of maltose and oligosaccharides after intravenous infusion in man. *Nutr Metab* 21(Suppl 1):115–7, 1977.
7. Young EA, Drummond A, Cioletti L, et al: Metabolism of continuously infused intravenous maltose. [abstract] *Clin Res* 925(3):543A, 1977.
8. Soroff HS, Hansen LM, Sasvary D, et al: Clinical pharmacology and metabolism of maltose in normal human volunteers. *Clin Res* [abstract] 26(3):286A, 1978.
9. Guyton AC: *Textbook of Medical Physiology.* 5th ed. Philadelphia, W.B. Saunders Company, 1976, pp 499–500.
10. Pirofsky B, Campbell SM, Montanaro A: Individual patient variations in the kinetics of intravenous immunoglobulin administration. *J Clin Immunol* 2 (2):7S–14S, 1982.
11. Pirofsky B: Intravenous immune globulin therapy in hypogammaglobulinemia. *Amer J Med* 76(3A): 53–60, 1984.
12. Nolte MT, Pirofsky B, Gerritz GA, et al: Intravenous immunoglobulin therapy for antibody deficiency. *Clin Exp Immunol* 36:237–43, 1979.
13. Buckley RH: Immunoglobulin replacement therapy: indications and contraindications for use and variable IgG levels achieved. In: Alving BM (ed.): *Immunoglobulins: characteristics and uses of intravenous preparations.* Washington, D.C., U.S. Government Printing Office (1980), pp 3–8.
14. Pirofsky B, Anderson CJ, Bardana EJ Jr.: Therapeutic and detrimental effects of intravenous immunoglobulin therapy. In: Alving BM (ed.): *Immunoglobulins: characteristics and uses of intravenous preparations.* Washington, D.C., U.S. Government Printing Office (1980), pp 15–22.
15. Ochs HD: Intravenous immunoglobulin therapy of patients with primary immunodeficiency syndromes: efficacy and safety of a new modified immune globulin preparation. In: Alving BM (ed.): *Immunoglobulins: characteristics and uses of intravenous preparations.* Washington, D.C., U.S. Government Printing Office (1980), pp 9–14.
16. Peerless AG, Stiehm ER: Intravenous gammaglobulin for reaction to intramuscular preparation. [letter] *Lancet* 2(8347):461, 1983.

Shown in Product Identification Section, page 420

HYPERAB®   ℞
[hī'per-ab″]
Rabies Immune Globulin (Human), USP

DESCRIPTION

Rabies Immune Globulin (Human), USP—Hyperab® is a sterile solution of antirabies immunoglobulin for intramuscular administration. This product is prepared from human plasma. It is prepared by cold alcohol fractionation from the plasma of donors hyperimmunized with rabies vaccine. Hyperab is a 15%–18% solution of human protein stabilized in 0.21–0.32 M glycine. The pH of the solution has been adjusted to 6.4–7.2 with sodium carbonate. Hyperab contains the mercurial preservative sodium ethylmercurithiosalicylate (thimerosal), 80–120 μg/mL as measured by mercury assay. The product is standardized against the U.S. Standard Rabies Immune Globulin to contain an average potency value of 150 IU/mL. The U.S. unit of potency is equivalent to the International Unit (IU) for rabies antibody.

CLINICAL PHARMACOLOGY

The usefulness of prophylactic rabies antibody in preventing rabies in man when administered immediately after exposure was dramatically demonstrated in a group of persons bitten by a rabid wolf in Iran.[1,2] Similarly, beneficial results were later reported from the U.S.S.R.[3] Studies coordinated by WHO helped determine the optimal conditions under which antirabies serum of equine origin and rabies vaccine can be used in man.[4-7] These studies showed that serum can interfere to a variable extent with the active immunity induced by the vaccine, but could be minimized by booster doses of vaccine after the end of the usual dosage series. Preparation of rabies immune globulin of human origin with adequate potency was reported by Cabasso et al.[8] In carefully controlled clinical studies, this globulin was used in conjunction with rabies vaccine of duck-embryo origin (DEV).[8,9] These studies determined that a human globulin dose of 20 IU/kg of rabies antibody, given simultaneously with the first DEV dose, resulted in amply detectable levels of passive rabies antibody 24 hours after injection in all recipients. The injections produced minimal, if any, interference with the subject's endogenous antibody response to DEV.

More recently, human diploid cell rabies vaccines (HDCV) prepared from tissue culture fluids containing rabies virus have received substantial clinical evaluation in Europe and the United States.[10-16] In a study in adult volunteers, the administration of Rabies Immune Globulin (Human) did not interfere with antibody formation induced by HDCV when given in a dose of 20 IU per kilogram body weight simultaneously with the first dose of vaccine.[15]

INDICATIONS AND USAGE

Rabies vaccine and Rabies Immune Globulin (Human), USP—Hyperab® should be given to all persons suspected of exposure to rabies with one exception: persons who have been previously immunized with rabies vaccine and have a confirmed adequate rabies antibody titer should receive only vaccine. Hyperab should be administered as promptly as possible after exposure, but can be administered up to the eighth day after the first dose of vaccine is given.

Recommendations for use of passive and active immunization after exposure to an animal suspected of having rabies have been detailed by the U.S. Public Health Service Advisory Committee on Immunization Practices (ACIP).[17]

Every exposure to possible rabies infection must be individually evaluated. The following factors should be considered before specific antirabies treatment is initiated:

1. **Species of Biting Animal**

Carnivorous wild animals (especially skunks, foxes, coyotes, raccoons, and bobcats) and bats are the animals most commonly infected with rabies and have caused most of the indigenous cases of human rabies in the United States since 1960.[18] Unless the animal is tested and shown not to be rabid, postexposure prophylaxis should be initiated upon bite or nonbite exposure to these animals (see item 3 below). If treatment has been initiated and subsequent testing in a competent laboratory shows the exposing animal is not rabid, treatment can be discontinued.

In the United States, the likelihood that a domestic dog or cat is infected with rabies varies from region to region; hence, the need for postexposure prophylaxis also varies. However, in most of Asia and all of Africa and Latin America, the dog remains the major source of human exposure; exposures to dogs in such countries represent a special threat. Travelers to those countries should be aware that >50% of the rabies cases among humans in the United States result from exposure to dogs outside the United States.

Rodents (such as squirrels, hamsters, guinea pigs, gerbils, chipmunks, rats, and mice) and lagomorphs (including rabbits and hares) are rarely found to be infected with rabies and have not been known to cause human rabies in the United States. However, from 1971 through 1988, woodchucks accounted for 70% of the 179 cases of rabies among rodents reported to CDC.[19] In these cases, the state or local health department should be consulted before a decision is made to initiate postexposure antirabies prophylaxis.

2. **Circumstances of Biting Incident**

An unprovoked attack is more likely to mean that the animal is rabid. (Bites during attempts to feed or handle an apparently healthy animal may generally be regarded as provoked.)

3. **Type of Exposure**

Rabies is transmitted only when the virus is introduced into open cuts or wounds in skin or mucous membranes. If there has been no exposure (as described in this section), postexposure treatment is not necessary. Thus, the likelihood that rabies infection will result from exposure to a rabid animal varies with the nature and extent of the exposure. Two categories of exposure should be considered:
Bite: any penetration of the skin by teeth. Bites to the face and hands carry the highest risk, but the site of the bite should not influence the decision to begin treatment.[20]
Nonbite: scratches, abrasions, open wounds or mucous membranes contaminated with saliva or any potentially infectious material, such as brain tissue, from a rabid animal constitute nonbite exposures. If the material containing the virus is dry, the virus can be considered noninfectious. Casual contact, such as petting a rabid animal and contact with the blood, urine, or feces (e.g., guano) of a rabid animal, does not constitute an exposure and is not an indication for prophylaxis. Instances of airborne rabies have been reported rarely. Adherence to respiratory precautions will minimize the risk of airborne exposure.[21]
The only documented cases of rabies from human-to-human transmission have occurred in patients who received corneas transplanted from persons who died of rabies undiagnosed at the time of death. Stringent guidelines for acceptance of donor corneas have reduced this risk.
Bite and nonbite exposures from humans with rabies theoretically could transmit rabies, although no cases of rabies acquired this way have been documented.

4. **Vaccination Status of Biting Animal**

A properly immunized animal has only a minimal chance of developing rabies and transmitting the virus.

5. **Presence of Rabies in Region**

If adequate laboratory and field records indicate that there is no rabies infection in a domestic species within a given region, local health officials are justified in considering this in making recommendations on antirabies treat-

Continued on next page

Miles Biological—Cont.

ment following a bite by that particular species. Such officials should be consulted for current interpretations.

Rabies Postexposure Prophylaxis

The following recommendations are only a guide. In applying them, take into account the animal species involved, the circumstances of the bite or other exposure, the vaccination status of the animal, and presence of rabies in the region. Local or state public health officials should be consulted if questions arise about the need for rabies prophylaxis.

Local Treatment of Wounds: Immediate and thorough washing of all bite wounds and scratches with soap and water is perhaps the most effective measure for preventing rabies. In experimental animals, simple local wound cleansing has been shown to reduce markedly the likelihood of rabies.

Tetanus prophylaxis and measures to control bacterial infection should be given as indicated.

Active Immunization: Active immunization should be initiated as soon as possible after exposure. Many dosage schedules have been evaluated for the currently available rabies vaccines and their respective manufacturers' literature should be consulted.

Passive Immunization: A combination of active and passive immunization (vaccine and immune globulin) is considered the acceptable postexposure prophylaxis except for those persons who have been previously immunized with rabies vaccine and who have documented adequate rabies antibody titer. These individuals should receive vaccine only. For passive immunization, Rabies Immune Globulin (Human) is preferred over antirabies serum, equine.[16,17] It is recommended both for treatment of all bites by animals suspected of having rabies and for non-bite exposure inflicted by animals suspected of being rabid. Rabies Immune Globulin (Human) should be used in conjunction with rabies vaccine and can be administered through the seventh day after the first dose of vaccine is given. Beyond the seventh day, Rabies Immune Globulin (Human) is not indicated since an antibody response to cell culture vaccine is presumed to have occurred.

[See table below.]

CONTRAINDICATONS

None known.

WARNINGS

Rabies Immune Globulin (Human), USP—Hyperab® should be given with caution to patients with a history of prior systemic allergic reactions following the administration of human immunoglobulin preparations or in patients who are known to have had an allergic response to thimerosal.

The attending physician who wishes to administer Hyperab to persons with isolated immunoglobulin A (IgA) deficiency must weigh the benefits of immunization against the potential risks of hypersensitivity reactions. Such persons have increased potential for developing antibodies to IgA and could have anaphylactic reactions to subsequent administration of blood products that contain IgA.[22]

As with all preparations administered by the intramuscular route, bleeding complications may be encountered in patients with thrombocytopenia or other bleeding disorders.

PRECAUTIONS

General

Hyperab should **not** be administered intravenously because of the potential for serious reactions. Although systemic reactions to immunoglobulin preparations are rare, epinephrine should be available for treatment of acute anaphylactoid symptoms.

Drug Interactions

Repeated doses of Rabies Immune Globulin (Human), USP—Hyperab® should not be administered once vaccine treatment has been initiated as this could prevent the full expression of active immunity expected from the rabies vaccine. Other antibodies in the Hyperab preparation may interfere with the response to live vaccines such as measles, mumps, polio or rubella. Therefore, immunization with live vaccines should not be given within 3 months after Hyperab administration.

Pregnancy Category C

Animal reproduction studies have not been conducted with Hyperab. It is also not known whether Hyperab can cause fetal harm when administered to a pregnant woman or can affect reproduction capacity. Hyperab should be given to a pregnant woman only if clearly needed.

ADVERSE REACTIONS

Soreness at the site of injection and mild temperature elevations may be observed at times. Sensitization to repeated injections has occurred occasionally in immunoglobulin-deficient patients. Angioneurotic edema, skin rash, nephrotic syndrome, and anaphylactic shock have rarely been reported after intramuscular injection, so that a causal relationship between immunoglobulin and these reactions is not clear.

DOSAGE AND ADMINISTRATION

The recommended dose for Hyperab is 20 IU/kg (0.133 mL/kg) of body weight given preferably at the time of the first vaccine dose.[8,9] It may also be given through the seventh day after the first dose of vaccine is given. If anatomically feasible, up to one-half the dose of Hyperab should be thoroughly infiltrated in the area around the wound and the rest should be administered intramuscularly in the gluteal area. Because of risk of injury to the sciatic nerve, the central region of the gluteal area MUST be avoided; only the upper, outer quadrant should be used.[23] Rabies Immune Globulin (Human), USP—Hyperab® should never be administered in the same syringe or into the same anatomical site as vaccine. Parenteral drug products should be inspected visually for particulate matter and discoloration prior to administration, whenever solution and container permit.

HOW SUPPLIED

Hyperab is packaged in 2 mL and 10 mL vials with an average potency value of 150 International Units per mL (IU/mL). The 2 mL vial contains a total of 300 IU which is sufficient for a child weighing 15 kg. The 10 mL vial contains a total of 1500 IU which is sufficient for an adult weighing 75 kg.

STORAGE

Hyperab should be stored under refrigeration (2°–8°C, 35°–46°F). Solution that has been frozen should not be used.

CAUTION

U.S. federal law prohibits dispensing without prescription.

LIMITED WARRANTY

A number of factors beyond our control could reduce the efficacy of this product or even result in an ill effect following its use. These include improper storage and handling of the product after it leaves our hands, diagnosis, dosage, method of administration, and biological differences in individual patients. Because of these factors, it is important that this product be stored properly and that the directions be followed carefully during use.

No warranty, express or implied, including any warranty of merchantability or fitness is made. Representatives of the Company are not authorized to vary the terms or the contents of the printed labeling, including the package insert for this product, except by printed notice from the Company's headquarters. The prescriber and user of this product must accept the terms hereof.

REFERENCES

1. Baltazard M, Bahmanyar M, Ghodssi M, et al: Essai pratique du sérum antirabique chez les mordus par loups enragés. *Bull WHO* 13:747–72, 1955.
2. Habel K, Koprowski H: Laboratory data supporting the clinical trial of antirabies serum in persons bitten by a rabid wolf. *Bull WHO* 13:773–9, 1955.
3. Selimov M, Boltucij L, Semenova E, et al: [The use of antirabies gamma globulin in subjects severely bitten by rabid wolves or other animals.] *J Hyg Epidemiol Microbiol Immunol (Praha)* 3:168–80, 1959.
4. Atanasiu P, Bahmanyar M, Baltazard M, et al: Rabies neutralizing antibody response to different schedules of serum and vaccine inoculations in non-exposed persons. *Bull WHO* 14:593–611, 1956.
5. Atanasiu P, Bahmanyar M, Baltazard M, et al: Rabies neutralizing antibody response to different schedules of serum and vaccine inoculations in non-exposed persons: Part II. *Bull WHO* 17:911–32, 1957.
6. Atanasiu P, Cannon DA, Dean DJ, et al: Rabies neutralizing antibody response to different schedules of serum and vaccine inoculations in non-exposed persons: Part 3. *Bull WHO* 25:103–14, 1961.
7. Atanasiu P, Dean DJ, Habel K, et al: Rabies neutralizing antibody response to different schedules of serum and vaccine inoculations in non-exposed persons: Part 4. *Bull WHO* 36:361–5, 1967.
8. Cabasso VJ, Loofbourow JC, Roby RE, et al: Rabies immune globulin of human origin: preparation and dosage determination in non-exposed volunteer subjects. *Bull WHO* 45:303–15, 1971.
9. Loofbourow JC, Cabasso VJ, Roby RE, et al: Rabies immune globulin (human): clinical trials and dose determination. *JAMA* 217(13): 1825–31, 1971.
10. Plotkin SA: New rabies vaccine halts disease — without severe reactions. *Mod Med* 45(20):45–8, 1977.
11. Plotkin SA, Wiktor TJ, Koprowski H, et al: Immunization schedules for the new human diploid cell vaccine against rabies. *Am J Epidemiol* 103(1):75–80, 1976.
12. Hafkin B, Hattwick MA, Smith JS, et al: A comparison of a WI-38 vaccine and duck embryo vaccine for preexposure rabies prophylaxis. *Am J Epidemiol* 107(5):439–43, 1978.
13. Kuwert EK, Marcus I, Höher PG; Neutralizing and complement-fixing antibody responses in pre- and post-exposure vaccinees to a rabies vaccine produced in human diploid cells. *J Biol Stand* 4(4):249–62, 1976.
14. Grandien M: Evaluation of tests for rabies antibody and analysis of serum responses after administration of three different types of rabies vaccines. *J Clin Microbiol* 5(3):263–7, 1977.
15. Kuwert EK, Marcus I, Werner J, et al: Postexpositionelle Schutzimpfung des Menschen gegen Tollwut mit einer neuentwickelten Gewebekulturvakzine (HDCS-Impfstoff). *Zentralbl Bakteriol [A]* 239(4):437–58, 1977.
16. Bahmanyar M, Fayaz A, Nour-Salehi S, et al: Successful protection of humans exposed to rabies infection: postexposure treatment with the new human diploid cell rabies vaccine and antirabies serum. *JAMA* 236(24):2751–4, 1976.
17. Recommendations of the Immunization Practices Advisory Committee (ACIP): Rabies prevention—United States, 1991. *MMWR* 40(RR–3):1–19, 1991.
18. Reid-Sanden FL, Dobbins JG, Smith JS, et al: Rabies surveillance in the United States during 1989. *J Am Vet Med Assoc* 197(12):1571–83, 1990.
19. Fishbein DB, Belotto AJ, Pacer RE, et al: Rabies in rodents and lagomorphs in the United States, 1971–1984: increased cases in the woodchuck (*Marmota monax*) in mid-Atlantic states. *J Wildl Dis* 22(2):151–5, 1986.
20. Hattwick MAW: Human rabies. *Public Health Rev* 3(3):229–74, 1974.
21. Garner JS, Simmons BP: Guideline for isolation precautions in hospitals. *Infect Control*.
22. Fudenberg HH: Sensitization to immunoglobulins and hazards of gamma globulin therapy. In: Merler E (ed.):

Rabies Postexposure Prophylaxis Guide[17]

Animal species	Condition of animal at time of attack	Treatment of exposed person [1]
Dog and cat	Healthy and available for 10 days of observation	None, unless animal develops rabies [2]
	Rabid or suspected rabid	RIGH [3] and HDCV
	Unknown (escaped)	Consult public health officials
Skunk, bat, fox, coyote raccoon, bobcat, and other carnivores; woodchuck	Regard as rabid unless geographic area is known to be free of rabies or proven negative by laboratory tests [4]	RIGH [3] and HDCV
Livestock, rodents, and lagomorphs (rabbits and hares)	Consider individually. Local and state public health officials should be consulted on questions about the need for rabies prophylaxis. In most geographical areas bites of squirrels, hamsters, guinea pigs, gerbils, chipmunks, rats, mice, other rodents, rabbits, and hares almost never call for antirabies prophylaxis.	

[1] ALL BITES AND WOUNDS SHOULD IMMEDIATELY BE THOROUGHLY CLEANSED WITH SOAP AND WATER. If antirabies treatment is indicated, both Rabies Immune Globulin (Human) [RIGH] and human diploid cell rabies vaccine (HDCV) should be given as soon as possible, REGARDLESS of the interval from exposure.

[2] During the usual holding period of 10 days, begin treatment with RIGH and vaccine (HDCV) at first sign of rabies in a dog or cat that has bitten someone. The symptomatic animal should be killed immediately and tested.

[3] If RIGH is not available, use antirabies serum, equine (ARS). Do not use more than the recommended dosage.

[4] The animal should be killed and tested as soon as possible. Holding for observation is not recommended. Discontinue vaccine if immunofluorescence test results of the animal are negative.

Immunoglobulins: biologic aspects and clinical uses. Washington, DC, Nat Acad Sci, 1970, pp 211–20.
23. Recommendations of the Immunization Practices Advisory Committee (ACIP): General recommendations on immunization. *MMWR* 38(13):205–14; 219–27, 1989.

HYPERHEP®   ℞

[hī'per-hep"]
Hepatitis B Immune Globulin (Human)

DESCRIPTION

Hepatitis B Immune Globulin (Human)—HyperHep® is a sterile solution of immunoglobulin (15%-18% protein) which is prepared by cold alcohol fractionation from pooled plasma of individuals with high titers of antibody to the hepatitis B surface antigen (anti-HBs). The product is stabilized with 0.21-0.32 M glycine and is preserved with 80-120 μg/mL thimerosal (a mercury derivative), by mercury assay. The solution has a pH of 6.4-7.2 adjusted with sodium carbonate. Each vial contains anti-HBs antibody equivalent to or exceeding the potency of anti-HBs in a U.S. reference hepatitis B immune globulin (Center for Biologics Evaluation and Research, FDA). The U.S. reference has been tested against the World Health Organization standard Hepatitis B Immune Globulin and found to be equal to 217 international units (IU) per mL. HyperHep must be administered intramuscularly.

CLINICAL PHARMACOLOGY

Hepatitis B Immune Globulin (Human) provides passive immunization for individuals exposed to the hepatitis B virus (HBV) as evidenced by a reduction in the attack rate of hepatitis B following its use.[1-6] The administration of the usual recommended dose of this immune globulin generally results in a detectable level of circulating anti-HBs which persists for approximately 2 months or longer. The highest antibody (IgG) serum levels were seen in the following distribution of subjects studied:[7]

DAY	% OF SUBJECTS
3	38.9%
7	41.7%
14	11.1%
21	8.3%

Mean values for half-life were between 17.5 and 25 days, with the shortest being 5.9 days and the longest 35 days.[7] Cases of type B hepatitis are rarely seen following exposure to HBV in persons with pre-existing anti-HBs. No confirmed instance of transmission of hepatitis B has been associated with this product.

INDICATIONS AND USAGE

Hepatitis B Immune Globulin (Human)—HyperHep® is indicated for postexposure prophylaxis following either parenteral exposure, e.g., by accidental "needle-stick," or direct mucous membrane contact (accidental splash), or oral ingestion (pipetting accident) involving HBsAg-positive materials such as blood, plasma or serum.

HyperHep is also indicated for prophylaxis of infants born to HBsAg-positive mothers. Such infants are at risk of being infected with hepatitis B virus and becoming chronic carriers.[5,8-10] The risk is especially great if the mother is HBeAg-positive.[11,12] For perinatal exposure to an HBsAg-positive, HBeAg-positive mother, a regimen combining one dose of Hepatitis B Immune Globulin (Human) at birth with the Hepatitis B Vaccine series started soon after birth is 94% effective in preventing development of the HB carrier state.[13] Regimens involving either multiple doses of Hepatitis B Immune Globulin (Human) alone, or Hepatitis B Vaccine series alone, have a 70%-75% efficacy, while a single dose of Hepatitis B Immune Globulin (Human) alone has only 50% efficacy.[14]

Administration of Hepatitis B Immune Globulin (Human) either preceding or concomitant with the commencement of active immunization with Hepatitis B Vaccine provides for more rapid achievement of protective levels of hepatitis B antibody, than when the vaccine alone is administered.[15] Rapid achievement of protective levels of antibody to hepatitis B virus may be desirable in certain clinical situations, as in cases of accidental inoculations with contaminated medical instruments.[15] Administration of Hepatitis B Immune Globulin (Human) either 1 month preceding or at the time of commencement of a program of active vaccination with Hepatitis B Vaccine has been shown not to interfere with the active immune response to the vaccine.[15]

CONTRAINDICATIONS

None known.

WARNINGS

HyperHep should be given with caution to patients with a history of prior systemic allergic reactions following the administration of human immune globulin preparations or in patients who are known to have had an allergic response to thimerosal. Epinephrine should be available.

In patients who have severe thrombocytopenia or any coagulation disorder that would contraindicate intramuscular injections, Hepatitis B Immune Globulin (Human) should be given only if the expected benefits outweigh the risks.

PRECAUTIONS

General
Hepatitis B Immune Globulin (Human)—HyperHep® should **not** be administered intravenously because of the potential for serious reactions. Injections should be made intramuscularly, and care should be taken to draw back on the plunger of the syringe before injection in order to be certain that the needle is not in a blood vessel.

Intramuscular injections are preferably administered in the anterolateral aspects of the upper thigh and the deltoid muscle of the upper arm. The gluteal region should not be used routinely as an injection site because of the risk of injury to the sciatic nerve. An individual decision as to which muscle is injected must be made for each patient based on the volume of material to be administered. If the gluteal region is used when very large volumes are to be injected or multiple doses are necessary, the central region MUST be avoided; only the upper, outer quadrant should be used.[16]

Laboratory Tests
None required.

Drug Interactions
Although administration of Hepatitis B Immune Globulin (Human) did not interfere with measles vaccination,[17] it is not known whether Hepatitis B Immune Globulin (Human) may interfere with other live virus vaccines. Therefore, use of such vaccines should be deferred until approximately three months after Hepatitis B Immune Globulin (Human) administration. Hepatitis B Vaccine may be administered at the same time, but at a different injection site, without interfering with the immune response.[15] No interactions with other products are known.

Pregnancy Category C
Animal reproduction studies have not been conducted with HyperHep. It is also not known whether HyperHep can cause fetal harm when administered to a pregnant woman or can affect reproduction capacity. HyperHep should be given to a pregnant woman only if clearly needed.

ADVERSE REACTIONS

Local pain and tenderness at the injection site, urticaria and angioedema may occur; anaphylactic reactions, although rare, have been reported following the injection of human immune globulin preparations.[18]

OVERDOSAGE

Although no data are available, clinical experience with other immunoglobulin preparations suggests that the only manifestations would be pain and tenderness at the injection site.

DOSAGE AND ADMINISTRATION

Acute Exposure to Blood Containing HBsAg[14]
The following table summarizes prophylaxis for percutaneous (needlestick or bite), ocular, or mucous-membrane exposure to blood according to the source of exposure and vaccination status of the exposed person. For greatest effectiveness, passive prophylaxis with Hepatitis B Immune Globulin (Human) should be given as soon as possible after exposure (its value beyond 7 days of exposure is unclear). If Hepatitis B Immune Globulin (Human) is indicated (see table below), an injection of 0.06 mL/kg of body weight should be administered intramuscularly (See PRECAUTIONS). Consult Hepatitis B Vaccine package insert for dosage information regarding that product. [See table above.]

For persons who refuse Hepatitis B Vaccine, a second dose of Hepatitis B Immune Globulin (Human)—HyperHep® should be given 1 month after the first dose.

Prophylaxis of Infants Born to HBsAg and HBeAg Positive Mothers
Efficacy of prophylactic Hepatitis B Immune Globulin (Human) in infants at risk depends on administering Hepatitis B Immune Globulin (Human) on the day of birth. It is therefore vital that HBsAg-positive mothers be identified before delivery.

Hepatitis B Immune Globulin (Human) (0.5 mL) should be administered intramuscularly (IM) to the newborn infant after physiologic stabilization of the infant and preferably within 12 hours of birth. Hepatitis B Immune Globulin (Human) efficacy decreases markedly if treatment is delayed beyond 48 hours. Hepatitis B Vaccine should be administered IM in three doses of 0.5 mL of vaccine (10 μg) each. The first dose should be given within 7 days of birth and may be given concurrently with Hepatitis B Immune Globulin (Human) but at a separate site. The second and third doses of vaccine should be given 1 month and 6 months, respectively, after the first. If administration of the first dose of Hepatitis B Vaccine is delayed for as long as 3 months, then a 0.5 mL dose of Hepatitis B Immune Globulin (Human)—HyperHep® should be repeated at 3 months. If Hepatitis B Vaccine is refused, the 0.5 mL dose of Hepatitis B Immune Globulin (Human) should be repeated at 3 and 6 months. Hepatitis B Immune Globulin (Human) administered at birth should not interfere with oral polio and diphtheria-tetanus-pertussis vaccines administered at 2 months of age.[14]

Hepatitis B Immune Globulin (Human) may be administered at the same time (but at a different site), or up to 1 month preceding Hepatitis B Vaccination without impairing the active immune response from Hepatitis B Vaccination.[15] Parenteral drug products should be inspected visually for particulate matter and discoloration prior to administration, whenever solution and container permit.

Administer intramuscularly. Do not inject intravenously.

HOW SUPPLIED

HyperHep is supplied in a 0.5 mL neonatal single dose syringe, a 1 mL and a 5 mL multiple dose vial.

STORAGE

Store at 2°-8°C (35°-46°F). Do not freeze. Do not use after expiration date.

CAUTION

U.S. federal law prohibits dispensing without prescription.

LIMITED WARRANTY

A number of factors beyond our control could reduce the efficacy of this product or even result in an ill effect following its use. These include improper storage and handling of the product after it leaves our hands, diagnosis, dosage, method of administration and biological differences in individual patients. Because of these factors, it is important that this product be stored properly and that the directions be followed carefully during use.

The foregoing statement is made in lieu of any other warranty, express or implied, including any warranty of merchantability or fitness. Representatives of the Company are

Continued on next page

Recommendations for Hepatitis B Prophylaxis Following Percutaneous Exposure

	Exposed Person	
Source	**Unvaccinated**	**Vaccinated**
HBsAg-Positive	1. Hepatitis B Immune Globulin (Human)×1 immediately* 2. Initiate HB Vaccine series†	1. Test exposed person for anti-HBs. 2. If inadequate antibody,‡ Hepatitis B Immune Globulin (Human) (×1) immediately plus HB Vaccine booster dose.
Known Source (High Risk)	1. Initiate HB Vaccine series 2. Test source for HBsAg. If positive, Hepatitis B Immune Globulin (Human)×1	1. Test Source for HBsAg only if exposed is vaccine nonresponder; if source is HBsAg-positive, give Hepatitis B Immune Globulin (Human)×1 immediately plus HB Vaccine booster dose.
Low Risk HBsAg-Positive	Initiate HB Vaccine series.	Nothing required.
Unknown Source	Initiate HB Vaccine series.	Nothing required.

* Hepatitis B Immune Globulin (Human), dose 0.06 mL/kg IM.
† HB Vaccine dose 20 μg IM for adults; 10 μg IM for infants or children under 10 years of age. First dose within 1 week; second and third doses, 1 and 6 months later.
‡ Less than 10 sample ratio units (SRU) by radioimmunoassay (RIA), negative by enzyme immunoassay (EIA).

Miles Biological—Cont.

not authorized to vary the terms of this warranty or the contents of any printed labeling for this product except by printed notice from the Company's headquarters. The prescriber and user of this product must accept the terms hereof.

REFERENCES

1. Grady GF, Lee VA: Hepatitis B immune globulin—prevention of hepatitis from accidental exposure among medical personnel. *N Engl J Med* 293(21): 1067-70, 1975.
2. Seeff LB, Zimmerman HJ, Wright EC, et al: Efficacy of hepatitis B immune serum globulin after accidental exposure. *Lancet* 2(7942):939-41, 1975.
3. Krugman S, Giles JP: Viral hepatitis, type B (MS-2-strain). Further observations on natural history and prevention. *N Engl J Med* 288(15):755-60, 1973.
4. Current trends: Health status of Indochinese refugees: malaria and hepatitis B. *MMWR* 28(39):463-4; 469-70, 1979.
5. Jhaveri R, Rosenfeld W, Salazar JD, et al: High titer multiple dose therapy with HBIG in newborn infants of HBsAg positive mothers. *J Pediatr* 97(2):305-8, 1980.
6. Hoofnagle JH, Seeff LB, Bales ZB, et al: Passive-active immunity from hepatitis B immune globulin. *Ann Intern Med* 91(6):813-8, 1979.
7. Scheiermann N, Kuwert EK: Uptake and elimination of hepatitis B immunoglobulins after intramuscular application in man. *Dev Biol Stand* 54:347-55, 1983.
8. Stevens CE, Beasley RP, Tsui J, et al: Vertical transmission of hepatitis B antigen in Taiwan. *N Engl J Med* 292(15):771-4, 1975.
9. Shiraki K, Yoshihara N, Kawana T, et al: Hepatitis B surface antigen and chronic hepatitis in infants born to asymptomatic carrier mothers. *Am J Dis Child* 131(6):644-7, 1977.
10. Recommendation of the Immunization Practices Advisory Committee (ACIP): Immune globulins for protection against viral hepatitis. *MMWR* 30(34):423-8; 433-5, 1981.
11. Okada K, Kamiyama I, Inomata M, et al: e antigen and anti-e in the serum of asymptomatic carrier mothers as indicators of positive and negative transmission of hepatitis B virus to their infants. *N Engl J Med* 294(14):746-9, 1976.
12. Beasley RP, Trepo C, Stevens CE, et al: The e antigen and vertical transmission of hepatitis B surface antigen. *Am J Epidemiol* 105(2):94-8, 1977.
13. Beasley RP, Hwang LY, Lee GCY, et al: Prevention of perinatally transmitted hepatitis B virus infections with hepatitis B immune globulin and hepatitis B vaccine. *Lancet* 2(8359):1099-102, 1983.
14. Recommendation of the Immunization Practices Advisory Committee (ACIP): Recommendations for protection against viral hepatitis. *MMWR* 34(22):313-35, 1985.
15. Szmuness W, Stevens CE, Olesko WR, et al: Passive-active immunisation against hepatitis B: Immunogenicity studies in adult Americans. *Lancet* 1:575-77, 1981.
16. Recommendations of the Immunization Practices Advisory Committee (ACIP): General recommendations on immunization. *MMWR* 38(13):205-14; 219-27, 1989.
17. Beasley RP, Hwang LY: Measles vaccination not interfered with by hepatitis B immune globulin. *Lancet* 1:161, 1982.
18. Ellis EF, Henney CS: Adverse reactions following administration of human gamma globulin. *J Allerg* 43(1):45-54, 1969.

HYPER-TET® ℞

[*hī'per-tet"*]

Tetanus Immune Globulin (Human), USP
250 Units

DESCRIPTION

Tetanus Immune Globulin (Human), USP—Hyper-Tet® is a sterile solution of tetanus hyperimmune immunoglobulin, primarily immunoglobulin G (IgG), containing 15%–18% protein, of which not less than 90% is gamma globulin. This product has been prepared from large pools of plasma obtained from individuals immunized with tetanus toxoid. Hyper-Tet is stabilized with 0.21–0.32 M glycine and contains the mercurial preservative sodium ethylmercurithiosalicylate (thimerosal), 80–120 μg per mL as measured by mercury assay. The pH is adjusted to 6.4–7.2 with sodium carbonate or acetic acid as required. The product is standardized against the U.S. Standard Antitoxin and the U.S. Control Tetanus Toxin and contains not less than 250 tetanus antitoxin units per container. Hyper-Tet must be administered intramuscularly.

CLINICAL PHARMACOLOGY

Hyper-Tet supplies passive immunity to those individuals who have low or no immunity to the toxin produced by the tetanus organism, *Clostridium tetani*. The antibodies act to neutralize the free form of the powerful exotoxin produced by this bacterium. Historically, such passive protection was provided by antitoxin derived from equine or bovine serum; however, the foreign protein in these heterologous products often produced severe allergic manifestations, even in individuals who demonstrated negative skin and/or conjunctival tests prior to administration. Estimates of the frequency of these foreign protein reactions following antitoxin of equine origin varied from 5%–30%.[1–4]

Several studies suggest the value of human tetanus antitoxin in the treatment of active tetanus.[5,6] In 1961 and 1962, Nation et al,[5] using Hyper-Tet treated 20 patients with tetanus using single doses of 3,000 to 6,000 antitoxin units in combination with other accepted clinical and nursing procedures. Six patients, all over 45 years of age, died of causes other than tetanus. The authors felt that the mortalilty rate (30%) compared favorably with their previous experience using equine antitoxin in larger doses and that the results were much better than the 60% national death rate for tetanus reported from 1951 to 1954.[7] Blake et al,[8] however, found in a data analysis of 545 cases of tetanus reported to the Centers for Disease Control from 1965 to 1971 that survival was no better with 8,000 units of human tetanus immune globulin (TIG) than with 500 units; however, an optimal dose could not be determined.

Passive immunization with Hyper-Tet may be undertaken concomitantly with active immunization using tetanus toxoid in those persons who must receive an immediate injection of tetanus antitoxin and in whom it is desirable to begin the process of active immunization. Based on the work of Rubbo,[9] McComb and Dwyer,[10] and Levine at al, [11] the physician may thus supply immediate passive protection against tetanus, and at the same time begin formation of active immunization in the injured individual which upon completion of a **full toxoid series** will preclude future need for antitoxin.

Peak blood levels of IgG are obtained approximately 2 days after intramuscular injection. The half-life of IgG in the circulation of individuals with normal IgG levels is approximately 23 days.[12]

INDICATIONS AND USAGE

Tetanus Immune Globulin (Human), USP—Hyper-Tet® is indicated for prophylaxis against tetanus following injury in patients whose immunization is incomplete or uncertain (see below). It is also indicated, although evidence of effectiveness is limited, in the regimen of treatment of active cases of tetanus.[5,6,13]

The following table is a summary guide to tetanus prophylaxis in wound management: [See table below.]

CONTRAINDICATIONS

None known.

WARNINGS

Hyper-Tet should be given with caution to patients with a history of prior systemic allergic reactions following the administration of human immunoglobulin preparations, or in patients who are known to have had an allergic response to thimerosal.

In patients who have severe thrombocytopenia or any coagulation disorder that would contraindicate intramuscular injections, Hyper-Tet should be given only if the expected benefits outweigh the risks.

PRECAUTIONS

General

Hyper-Tet should not be given intravenously. Intravenous injection of immunoglobulin intended for intramuscular use can, on occasion, cause a precipitous fall in blood pressure, and a picture not unlike anaphylaxis. Injections should only be made **intramuscularly** and care should be taken to draw back on the plunger of the syringe before injection in order to be certain that the needle is not in a blood vessel. Intramuscular injections are preferably administered in the anterolateral aspects of the upper thigh and the deltoid muscle of the upper arm. The gluteal region should not be used routinely as an injection site because of the risk of injury to the sciatic nerve. If the gluteal region is used, the central region MUST be avoided; only the upper, outer quadrant should be used.[15]

Skin tests should not be done. The intradermal injection of concentrated IgG solutions often causes a localized area of inflammation which can be misinterpreted as a positive allergic reaction. In actuality, this does not represent an allergy; rather, it is localized tissue irritation. Misinterpretation of the results of such tests can lead the physician to withhold needed human antitoxin from a patient who is not actually allergic to this material. True allergic responses to human IgG given in the prescribed intramuscular manner are rare.

Although systemic reactions to human immunoglobulin preparations are rare, epinephrine should be available for treatment of acute anaphylactic reactions.

Drug Interactions

Antibodies in immunoglobulin preparations may interfere with the response to live viral vaccines such as measles, mumps, polio, and rubella. Therefore, use of such vaccines should be deferred until approximately 3 months after Tetanus Immune Globulin (Human), USP—Hyper-Tet® administration.

No interactions with other products are known.

Pregnancy Category C

Animal reproduction studies have not been conducted with Hyper-Tet. It is also not known whether Hyper-Tet can cause fetal harm when administered to a pregnant woman or can affect reproduction capacity. Hyper-Tet should be given to a pregnant woman only if clearly needed.

ADVERSE REACTIONS

Slight soreness at the site of injection and slight temperature elevation may be noted at times. Sensitization to repeated injections of human immunoglobulin is extremely rare.

In the course of routine injections of large numbers of persons with immunoglobulin there have been a few isolated occurrences of angioneurotic edema, nephrotic syndrome, and anaphylactic shock after injection.

OVERDOSAGE

Although no data are available, clinical experience with other immunoglobulin preparations suggests that the only manifestations would be pain and tenderness at the injection site.

DOSAGE AND ADMINISTRATION

Routine prophylactic dosage schedule:

Adults and children 7 years and older: Hyper-Tet, 250 units should be given by deep intramuscular injection (see PRECAUTIONS). At the same time, but in a different extremity and with a separate syringe, Tetanus and Diphtheria Toxoids Adsorbed (For Adult Use) (Td) should be administered according to the manufacturer's package insert.

Children less than 7 years old: In small children the routine prophylactic dose of Hyper-Tet may be calculated by the body weight (4.0 units/kg). However, it may be advisable to administer the entire contents of the vial or syringe of Hyper-Tet (250 units) regardless of the child's size, since theoretically the same amount of toxin will be produced in the child's body by the infecting tetanus organism as it will in an adult's body. At the same time but in a different extremity and with a different syringe, Diphtheria and Tetanus Toxoids and Pertussis Vaccine Adsorbed (DTP) or Diphtheria and Tetanus Toxoids Adsorbed (For Pediatric

Guide to Tetanus Prophylaxis in Wound Management[14]

History of Tetanus Immunization	Clean, Minor Wounds		All Other Wounds	
(Doses)	Td*	TIG§	Td	TIG
Uncertain or less than 3	Yes	No	Yes	Yes
3 or more†	No‡	No	No£	No

* Adult type tetanus and diphtheria toxoids. If the patient is less than 7 years old, DT or DTP is given (see Dosage and Administration).

§ Tetanus Immune Globulin (Human)

† If only three doses of fluid tetanus toxoid have been received, a fourth dose of toxoid, preferably an adsorbed toxoid, should be given.

‡ Yes if more than 10 years since the last dose.

£ Yes if more than 5 years since the last dose.

Use)(DT), if pertussis vaccine is contraindicated, should be administered per the manufacturer's package insert. Note: The single injection of tetanus toxoid only initiates the series for producing active immunity in the recipient. The physician must impress upon the patient the need for further toxoid injections in 1 month and 1 year. Without such, the active immunization series is incomplete. Current recommendations for wound management of patients definitely known to have completed a full tetanus toxoid series indicate tetanus toxoid booster only if more than 5 to 10 years have elapsed since the last dose of toxoid.[14] The prophylactic dosage schedule for these patients and for those with incomplete or uncertain immunity is shown on the table in INDICATIONS AND USAGE. Since tetanus is actually a local infection, proper initial wound care is of paramount importance. The use of antitoxin is adjunctive to this procedure. However, in approximately 10% of recent tetanus cases, no wound or other breach in skin or mucous membrane could be implicated.[16]

Treatment of active cases of tetanus:
Standard therapy for the treatment of active tetanus including the use of Hyper-Tet must be implemented immediately. The dosage should be adjusted according to the severity of the infection.[5,6]

Parenteral drug products should be inspected visually for particulate matter and discoloration prior to administration, whenever solution and container permit. They should not be used if particulate matter and/or discoloration are present.

HOW SUPPLIED

Tetanus Immune Globulin (Human), USP—Hyper-Tet® is supplied in 250 unit prefilled disposable syringes and 250 unit vials.

STORAGE

Store at 2°–8°C (35°–46°F). Solution that has been frozen should not be used.

CAUTION

U.S. federal law prohibits dispensing without prescription.

LIMITED WARRANTY

A number of factors beyond our control could reduce the efficacy of this product or even result in an ill effect following its use. These include improper storage and handling of the product after it leaves our hands, diagnosis, dosage, method of administration, and biological differences in individual patients. Because of these factors it is important that this product be stored properly and that the directions be followed carefully during use.

The foregoing statement is made in lieu of any other warranty, express or implied, including any warranty of merchantability or fitness. Representatives of the Company are not authorized to vary the terms or the contents of the printed labeling for this product except by printed notice from the Company's headquarters. The prescriber and user of this product must accept the terms hereof.

REFERENCES

1. Moynihan NH: Tetanus prophylaxis and serum sensitivity tests. *Br Med J* 1:260–4, 1956.
2. Scheibel I: The uses and results of active tetanus immunization. *Bull WHO* 13:381–94, 1955.
3. Edsall G: Specific prophylaxis of tetanus. *JAMA* 171(4):417–27, 1959.
4. Bardenwerper HW: Serum neuritis from tetanus antitoxin. *JAMA* 179(10):763–6, 1962.
5. Nation NS, Pierce NF, Adler SJ, et al: Tetanus: the use of human hyperimmune globulin in treatment. *Calif Med* 98(6):305–6, 1963.
6. Ellis M: Human antitetanus serum in the treatment of tetanus. *Br Med J* 1(5338):1123–6, 1963.
7. Axnick NW, Alexander ER: Tetanus in the United States: A review of the problem. *Am J Public Health* 47(12):1493–1501, 1957.
8. Blake PA, Feldman RA, Buchanan TM, et al: Serologic therapy of tetanus in the United States, 1965–1971. *JAMA* 235(1):42–4, 1976.
9. Rubbo SD: New approaches to tetanus prophylaxis. *Lancet* 2(7461):449–53, 1966.
10. McComb JA, Dwyer RC: Passive-active immunization with tetanus immune globulin (human). *N Engl J Med* 268(16):857–62, 1963.
11. Levine L, McComb JA, Dwyer RC, et al: Active-passive tetanus immunization; choice of toxoid, dose of tetanus immune globulin and timing of injections. *N Engl J Med* 274(4):186–90, 1966.
12. Waldmann TA, Strober W, Blaese RM: Variations in the metabolism of immunoglobulins measured by turnover rates. In Merler E (ed.): Immunoglobulins: biologic aspects and clinical uses. Washington, DC, Nat Acad Sci, 1970, p 33–51.
13. McCracken GH Jr., Dowell DL, Marshall FN: Double-blind trial of equine antitoxin and human immune globulin in tetanus neonatorum. *Lancet* 1(7710):1146–9, 1971.
14. American Academy of Pediatrics, Committee on Infectious Diseases: Report ed. 20. Evanston, 1986, p. 355–9.
15. Recommendations of the Immunization Practices Advisory Committee (ACIP): General recommendations on immunization. *MMWR* 38(13): 205–14; 219–27, 1989.
16. Tetanus-Rates by year, United States, 1955–1984. Annual Summary 1984. *MMWR* 33 (54):61, 1986.

HypRho®-D Mini-Dose   ℞
[hī"prō-d']
Rho(D) Immune Globulin (Human)

DESCRIPTION

Rho(D) Immune Globulin (Human)—HypRho®-D Mini-Dose—is a sterile solution of immune globulin containing antibodies to Rho(D) which is for intramuscular injection only. It is prepared from human plasma collected from carefully screened donors. It contains 15%–18% protein stabilized with 0.21–0.32 M glycine and preserved with 80–120 μg/mL thimerosal (a mercury derivative, as measured by mercury assay. The pH is adjusted with sodium carbonate. One dose of HypRho-D Mini-Dose contains not less than one-sixth the quantity of Rho(D) antibody contained in one standard dose of Rho(D) Immune Globulin (Human), USP and it will suppress the immunizing potential of 2.5 mL of Rho(D) positive packed red blood cells or the equivalent of whole blood (5 mL). The quantity of Rho(D) antibody in HypRho-D Mini-Dose is not less than one-sixth of that contained in 1 mL of the U.S. Food and Drug Administration Reference Rho(D) Immune Globulin (Human).

CLINICAL PHARMACOLOGY

Rh sensitization may occur in nonsensitized Rho(D) negative women following transplacental hemorrhage resulting from spontaneous or induced abortions.[1–2] The risk of sensitization is higher in women undergoing induced abortions than in those aborting spontaneously.[1–3]

HypRho-D Mini-Dose is used to prevent the formation of anti-Rho(D) antibody in Rho(D) negative women who are exposed to the Rho(D) antigen at the time of spontaneous or induced abortion (up to 12 weeks' gestation).[3–5] HypRho-D Mini-Dose suppresses the stimulation of active immunity by Rho(D) positive fetal erythrocytes that may enter the maternal circulation at the time of termination of the pregnancy. The amount of anti-Rho(D) in HypRho-D Mini-Dose has been shown to effectively prevent maternal isosensitization to the Rho(D) antigens following spontaneous or induced abortion occurring up to the 12th week of gestation.[6–8] After the 12th week of gestation, a standard dose of Rho(D) Immune Globulin (Human), USP—HypRho®-D is indicated.

INDICATIONS AND USAGE

Rho(D) Immune Globulin (Human)—HypRho®-D Mini-Dose is recommended to prevent the isoimmunization of Rho(D) negative women at the time of spontaneous or induced abortion of up to 12 weeks' gestation provided the following criteria are met:
1. The mother must be Rho(D) negative and must not already be sensitized to the Rho(D) antigen.
2. The father is not known to be Rho(D) negative.
3. Gestation is not more than 12 weeks at termination.

Note: Rho(D) Immune Globulin (Human) prophylaxis is not indicated if the fetus or father can be determined to be Rh negative. If the Rh status of the fetus is unknown, the fetus must be assumed to be Rho(D) positive, and HypRho-D Mini-Dose should be administered to the mother.

FOR ABORTIONS OR MISCARRIAGES OCCURRING AFTER 12 WEEKS' GESTATION, A STANDARD DOSE OF Rho(D) IMMUNE GLOBULIN (HUMAN), USP IS INDICATED.

HypRho-D Mini-Dose should be administered within 3 hours or as soon as possible after spontaneous passage or surgical removal of the products of conception. However, if HypRho-D Mini-Dose is not given within this time period, consideration should still be given to its administration since clinical studies in male volunteers have demonstrated the effectiveness of Rho(D) Immune Globulin (Human), USP in preventing isoimmunization as long as 72 hours after infusion of Rho(D) positive red cells.[9]

CONTRAINDICATIONS

None known.

WARNINGS

NEVER ADMINISTER HYPRHO-D MINI-DOSE INTRAVENOUSLY. INJECT ONLY INTRAMUSCULARLY. ADMINISTER ONLY TO WOMEN POST-ABORTION OR POST-MISCARRIAGE OF UP TO 12 WEEKS' GESTATION.
HypRho-D Mini-Dose should be given with caution to patients with a history of prior systemic allergic reactions following the administration of human immune globulin preparations or in patients who are known to have had an allergic response to thimerosal.
The attending physician who wishes to administer HypRho-D Mini-Dose to persons with isolated immunoglobulin A (IgA) deficiency must weigh the benefits of immunization against the potential risks of hypersensitivity reactions. Such persons have increased potential for developing antibodies to IgA and could have anaphylactic reactions to subsequent administration of blood products that contain IgA. As with all preparations administered by the intramuscular route, bleeding complications may be encountered in patients with thrombocytopenia or other bleeding disorders.

PRECAUTIONS

General
Although systemic reactions to immunoglobulin preparations are rare, epinephrine should be available for treatment of acute anaphylactic symptoms.

Drug Interactions
Other antibodies in the Rho(D) Immune Globulin (Human) —HypRho®-D Mini-Dose preparation may interfere with the response to live vaccines such as measles, mumps, polio or rubella. Therefore, immunization with live vaccines should not be given within 3 months after HypRho-D Mini-Dose administration.

Pregnancy Category C
Animal reproduction studies have not been conducted with HypRho-D Mini-Dose. It is also not known whether HypRho-D Mini-Dose can cause fetal harm when administered to a pregnant woman or can affect reproduction capacity. It should be again noted, however, that HypRho-D Mini-Dose is **not** indicated for use during pregnancy and it should be administered only post-abortion or post-miscarriage.

ADVERSE REACTIONS

Reactions to HypRho-D Mini-Dose are infrequent in Rho (D) negative individuals and consist primarily of slight soreness at the site of injection and slight temperature elevation. While sensitization to repeated injections of human globulin is extremely rare, it has occurred.

DOSAGE AND ADMINISTRATION

One syringe of HypRho-D Mini-Dose provides sufficient antibody to prevent Rh sensitization to 2.5 mL Rho(D) positive packed red cells or the equivalent (5 mL) of whole blood. This dose is sufficient to provide protection against maternal Rh sensitization for women undergoing spontaneous or induced abortion of up to 12 weeks' gestation.

HypRho-D Mini-Dose should be administered within 3 hours or as soon as possible following spontaneous or induced abortion. If prompt administration is not possible, HypRho-D Mini-Dose should be given within 72 hours following termination of the pregnancy.

HypRho-D Mini-Dose is administered **intramuscularly,** preferably in the anterolateral aspects of the upper thigh and the deltoid muscle of the upper arm. The gluteal region should not be used routinely as an injection site because of the risk of injury to the sciatic nerve. If the gluteal region is used, the central region must be avoided; only the upper, outer quadrant should be used.[10]

Parenteral drug products should be inspected visually for particulate matter and discoloration prior to administration, whenever solution and container permit.

HOW SUPPLIED

Each HypRho-D Mini-Dose package contains ten single dose syringes.

STORAGE

Store at 2°–8°C (35°–46°F). Do not freeze.

CAUTION

U.S. federal law prohibits dispensing without prescription.

LIMITED WARRANTY

A number of factors beyond our control could reduce the efficacy of this product or even result in an ill effect following its use. These include improper storage and handling of the product after it leaves our hands, diagnosis, dosage, method of administration, and biological differences in individual patients. Because of these factors, it is important that this product be stored properly and that the directions be followed carefully during use.

No warranty, express or implied, including any warranty of merchantability or fitness is made. Representatives of the Company are not authorized to vary the terms or the contents of the printed labeling, including the package insert for this product, except by printed notice from the Company's headquarters. The prescriber and user of this product must accept the terms hereof.

REFERENCES

1. Queenan JT, Shah S, Kubarych SF, *et al*: Role of induced abortion in rhesus immunisation. *Lancet* 1(7704): 815–7, 1971.
2. Goldman JA, Eckerling B: Prevention of Rh immunization after abortion with anti-Rho(D)-immunoglobulin. *Obstet Gynecol* 40(3):366–70, 1972.
3. The selective use of Rho(D) immune globulin (RhIG). *ACOG Tech Bull* 61, 1981.

Continued on next page

Miles Biological—Cont.

4. Prevention of Rh sensitization. *WHO Tech Rep Ser* 468, 1971.
5. Recommendation of the Public Health Service Advisory Committee on Immunization Practices: Rh immune globulin. *MMWR* 21(15):126–7, 1972.
6. Stewart FH, Burnhill MS, Bozorgi N: Reduced dose of Rh immunoglobulin following first trimester pregnancy termination. *Obstet Gynecol* 51(3):318–22, 1978.
7. McMaster conference on prevention of Rh immunization, 28-30 September, 1977. *Vox Sang* 36(1):50–64, 1979.
8. Simonovits I: Efficiency of anti-D IgG prevention after induced abortion. *Vox Sang* 26(4):361–7, 1974.
9. Freda VJ, Gorman JG, Pollack W: Prevention of Rh-hemolytic disease with Rh-immune globulin. *Am J Obstet Gynecol* 128(4):456–60, 1977.
10. Recommendations of the Immunization Practices Advisory Committee (ACIP): General recommendations on immunization. *MMWR* 38(13):205–14; 219–27, 1989.

14-7621-055
(Rev Sept 1990)

HypRho®-D Full Dose ℞
[*hī″prō-d′*]
Rh_o(D) Immune
Globulin (Human), USP

DESCRIPTION

Rh_o(D) Immune Globulin (Human), USP—HypRho®-D is a sterile solution of immune globulin containing antibodies to Rh_o(D) which is intended for intramuscular injection. This product has been prepared from large pools of human plasma. It contains 15%–18% protein stabilized with 0.21–0.32 M glycine and is preserved with 80–120 μg/mL thimerosal (a mercury derivative), as measured by mercury assay. The pH is adjusted with sodium carbonate. The potency is equal to or greater than that of the U.S. Food and Drug Administration Reference Rh_o(D) Immune Globulin. Each single dose vial or syringe contains sufficient anti-Rh_o(D) (approximately 300 μg*) to effectively suppress the immunizing potential of 15 mL of Rh_o(D) positive red blood cells.[2–4]

CLINICAL PHARMACOLOGY

HypRho-D is used to prevent isoimmunization in the Rh_o(D) negative individual exposed to Rh_o(D) positive blood as a result of a fetomaternal hemorrhage occurring during a delivery of an Rh_o(D) positive infant, abortion (either spontaneous or induced), or following amniocentesis or abdominal trauma. Similarly, immunization resulting in the production of anti-Rh_o(D) following transfusion of Rh positive red cells to an Rh_o(D) negative recipient may be prevented by administering Rh_o(D) Immune Globulin (Human), USP.[5,6]

Rh hemolytic disease of the newborn is the result of the active immunization of an Rh_o(D) negative mother by Rh_o(D) positive red cells entering the maternal circulation during a previous delivery, abortion, amniocentesis, abdominal trauma, or as a result of red cell transfusion.[7,8] HypRho-D acts by suppressing the immune response of Rh_o(D) negative individuals to Rh_o(D) positive red blood cells. The mechanism of action of HypRho-D is not fully understood.

The administration of Rh_o(D) Immune Globulin (Human), USP within 72 hours of a full-term delivery of an Rh_o(D) positive infant by an Rh_o(D) negative mother reduces the incidence of Rh isoimmunization from 12%–13% to 1%–2%.[9] The 1%–2% treatment failures are probably due to isoimmunization occurring during the latter part of pregnancy or following delivery.[10] Bowman and Pollock[11] have reported that the incidence of isoimmunization can be further reduced from approximately 1.6% to less than 0.1% by administering Rh_o(D) Immune Globulin (Human), USP in two doses, one antenatal at 28 weeks' gestation and another following delivery.

INDICATIONS AND USAGE

Pregnancy and Other Obstetric Conditions

Rh_o(D) Immune Globulin (Human), USP—HypRho®-D is recommended for the prevention of Rh hemolytic disease of the newborn by its administration to the Rh_o(D) negative mother within 72 hours after birth of an Rh_o(D) positive infant,[12] providing the following criteria are met:

1. The mother must be Rh_o(D) negative, and must not already be sensitized to the Rh_o(D) factor.
2. Her child must be Rh_o(D) positive, and should have a negative direct antiglobulin test (see PRECAUTIONS).

If HypRho-D is administered antepartum, it is essential that the mother receive another dose of HypRho-D after delivery of an Rh_o(D) positive infant.

If the father can be determined to be Rh_o(D) negative, HypRho-D need not be given.

HypRho-D should be administered within 72 hours to all nonimmunized Rh_o(D) negative women who have undergone spontaneous or induced abortion, following ruptured tubal pregnancy, amniocentesis or abdominal trauma unless the blood group of the fetus or the father is known to be Rh_o(D) negative.[7,8] If the fetal blood group cannot be determined, one must assume that it is Rh_o(D) positive,[2] and HypRho-D should be administered to the mother.

Transfusion

HypRho-D may be used to prevent isoimmunization in Rh_o(D) negative individuals who have been transfused with Rh_o(D) positive red blood cells or blood components containing red blood cells.[5,13]

CONTRAINDICATIONS

None known.

WARNINGS

NEVER ADMINISTER HYPRHO-D INTRAVENOUSLY. INJECT ONLY INTRAMUSCULARLY. NEVER ADMINISTER TO THE NEONATE.

Rh_o(D) Immune Globulin (Human), USP should be given with caution to patients with a history of prior systemic allergic reactions following the administration of human immunoglobulin preparations or to patients who are known to have had an allergic respose to thimerosal.

The attending physician who wishes to administer Rh_o(D) Immune Globulin (Human), USP to persons with isolated immunoglobulin A (IgA) deficiency must weigh the benefits of immunization against the potential risks of hypersensitivity reactions. Such persons have increased potential for developing antibodies to IgA and could have anaphylactic reactions to subsequent administration of blood products that contain IgA.

As with all preparations administered by the intramuscular route, bleeding complications may be encountered in patients with thrombocytopenia or other bleeding disorders.

PRECAUTIONS

General

A large fetomaternal hemorrhage late in pregnancy or following delivery may cause a weak mixed field positive D^u test result. If there is any doubt about the mother's Rh type, she should be given Rh_o(D) Immune Globulin (Human), USP.

A screening test to detect fetal red blood cells may be helpful in such cases.

If more than 15 mL of D-positive fetal red blood cells are present in the mother's circulation, more than a single dose of Rh_o(D) Immune Globulin (Human), USP—HypRho®-D is required. Failure to recognize this may result in the administration of an inadequate dose.

Although systemic reactions to human immunoglobulin preparations are rare, epinephrine should be available for treatment of acute anaphylactic reactions.

Drug Interactions

Other antibodies in the Rh_o(D) Immune Globulin (Human), USP preparation may interfere with the response to live vaccines such as measles, mumps, polio or rubella. Therefore, immunization with live vaccines should not be given within 3 months after Rh_o(D) Immune Globulin (Human), USP administration.

Drug/Laboratory Interactions

Babies born of women given Rh_o(D) Immune Globulin (Human), USP antepartum may have a weakly positive direct antiglobulin test at birth.

Passively acquired anti-Rh_o(D) may be detected in maternal serum if antibody screening tests are performed subsequent to antepartum or postpartum administration of Rh_o(D) Immune Globulin (Human), USP.

Pregnancy Category C

Animal reproduction studies have not been conducted with HypRho-D. It is also not known whether HypRho-D can cause fetal harm when administered to a pregnant woman or can affect reproduction capacity. HypRho-D should be given to a pregnant woman only if clearly needed.

ADVERSE REACTIONS

Reactions to Rh_o(D) Immune Globulin (Human), USP are infrequent in Rh_o(D) negative individuals and consist primarily of slight soreness at the site of injection and slight temperature elevation. While sensitization to repeated injections of human immune globulin is extremely rare, it has occurred. Elevated bilirubin levels have been reported in some individuals receiving multiple doses of Rh_o(D) Immune Globulin (Human), USP following mismatched tranfusions. This is believed to be due to a relatively rapid rate of foreign red cell destruction.

DOSAGE AND ADMINISTRATION

Pregnancy and Other Obstetric Conditions

1. For postpartum prophylaxis, administer one vial or syringe of HypRho-D (300 μg*), preferably within 72 hours of delivery. Although a lesser degree of protection is afforded if Rh antibody is administered beyond the 72-hour period, HypRho-D may still be given.[7,14] Full-term deliveries can vary in their dosage requirements depending on the magnitude of the fetomaternal hemorrhage. One 300 μg* vial or syringe of HypRho-D provides sufficient antibody to prevent Rh sensitization if the volume of red blood cells that has entered the circulation is 15 mL or less.[2–4] In instances where a large (greater than 30 mL of whole blood or 15 mL red blood cells) fetomaternal hemorrhage is suspected, a fetal red cell count by an approved laboratory technique (e.g., modified Kleihauer-Betke acid elution stain technique) should be performed to determine the dosage of immune globulin required.[8,15] The red blood cell volume of the calculated fetomaternal hemorrhage is divided by 15 mL to obtain the number of vials or syringes of Rh_o(D) Immune Globulin (Human), USP—HypRho®-D for administration.[3,8,13] If more than 15 mL of red cells is suspected or if the dose calculation results in a fraction, administer the next higher whole number of vials or syringes (e.g., if 1.4, give 2 vials or syringes).
2. For antenatal prophylaxis, one 300 μg* vial or syringe of HypRho(D) is administered at approximately 28 weeks' gestation. This **must** be followed by another 300 μg* dose, preferably within 72 hours following delivery, if the infant is Rh positive.
3. Following threatened abortion at any stage of gestation with continuation of pregnancy, it is recommended that 300 μg* of HypRho-D be given. If more than 15 mL of red cells is suspected due to fetomaternal hemorrhage, the same dose modification in No. 1 above applies.
4. Following miscarriage, abortion, or termination of ectopic pregnancy at or beyond 13 weeks' gestation, it is recommended that 300 μg* of HypRho-D be given. If more than 15 mL of red blood cells is suspected due to fetomaternal hemorrhage, the same dose modification in No. 1 above applies. If pregnancy is terminated prior to 13 weeks' gestation, a single dose of HypRho®-D Mini-Dose (approximately 50 μg*) may be used instead of HypRho-D.
5. Following amniocentesis at either 15 to 18 weeks' gestation or during the third trimester, or following abdominal trauma in the second or third trimester, it is recommended that 300 μg* of HypRho-D be administered. If there is a fetomaternal hemorrhage in excess of 15 mL of red cells, the same dose modification in No. 1 applies.

If abdominal trauma, amniocentesis, or other adverse event requires the administration of HypRho-D at 13 to 18 weeks' gestation, another 300 μg* dose should be given at 26 to 28 weeks. To maintain protection throughout pregnancy, the level of passively acquired anti-Rh_o(D) should not be allowed to fall below the level required to prevent an immune response to Rh positive red cells. The half-life of IgG is 23 to 26 days. In any case, a dose of HypRho-D should be given within 72 hours after delivery if the baby is Rh positive. If delivery occurs within 3 weeks after the last dose, the postpartum dose may be withheld unless there is a fetomaternal hemorrhage in excess of 15 mL of red blood cells.[16]

Transfusion

In the case of a transfusion of Rh_o(D) positive red cells to an Rh_o(D) negative recipient, the volume of Rh positive whole blood administered is multiplied by the hematocrit of the donor unit giving the volume of red blood cells transfused. The volume of red blood cells is divided by 15 mL which provides the number of vials or syringes of HypRho-D to be administered.

If the dose calculated results in a fraction, the next higher whole number of vials or syringes should be administered (e.g., if 1.4, give 2 vials or 2 syringes). HypRho-D should be administered within 72 hours after an incompatible transfusion, but preferably as soon as possible.

Injection Procedure

DO NOT INJECT INTRAVENOUSLY. DO NOT INJECT NEONATE. Rh_o(D) Immune Globulin (Human), USP—HypRho®-D is administered **intramuscularly**, preferably in the anterolateral aspects of the upper thigh and the deltoid muscle of the upper arm. The gluteal region should not be used routinely as an injection site because of the risk of injury to the sciatic nerve. If the gluteal region is used, the central region MUST be avoided; only the upper, outer quadrant should be used.[17]

A. Single Vial or Syringe Dose
INJECT ENTIRE CONTENTS OF THE VIAL OR SYRINGE INTO THE INDIVIDUAL INTRAMUSCULARLY.

B. Multiple Vial or Syringe Dose
1. Calculate the number of vials or syringes of HypRho-D to be given (See Dosage section above).

*See footnote under DESCRIPTION.

*A full dose of Rh_o(D) Immune Globulin (Human), USP has traditionally been referred to as a "300 μg" dose and this usage is employed here for convenience in terminology. **It should not be construed as the actual anti-D content.** Each full dose of Rh_o(D) Immune Globulin (Human), USP must contain at least as much anti-D as 1 mL of the U.S. Reference Rh_o(D) Immune Globulin. Studies performed at the FDA have shown that the U.S. Reference contains 820 international units (IU) of anti-D per mL. When the conversion factor determined for the International (WHO) Reference Preparation[1] is used, 820 IU per mL is equivalent to 164 μg per mL of anti-D.

2. The total volume of HypRho-D can be given in divided doses at different sites at one time or the total dose may be divided and injected at intervals, provided the total dosage is given within 72 hours of the fetomaternal hemorrhage or transfusion. USING STERILE TECHNIQUE, INJECT THE ENTIRE CONTENTS OF THE CALCULATED NUMBER OF VIALS OR SYRINGES INTRAMUSCULARLY INTO THE PATIENT.

Parenteral drug products should be inspected visually for particulate matter and discoloration prior to administration, whenever solution and container permit.

HOW SUPPLIED

HypRho-D is available in individual and multiple-pack single dose syringes and vials.

STORAGE

Store at 2°-8°C (35°-46°F). Do not freeze.

CAUTION

U.S. federal law prohibits dispensing without prescription.

LIMITED WARRANTY

A number of factors beyond our control could reduce the efficacy of this product or even result in an ill effect following its use. These include improper storage and handling of the product after it leaves our hands, diagnosis, dosage, method of administration, and biological differences in individual patients. Because of these factors, it is important that this product be stored properly and that the directions be followed carefully during use.

The foregoing statement is made in lieu of any other warranty, express or implied, including any warranty of merchantability or fitness. Representatives of the Company are not authorized to vary the terms of this warranty or the contents of any printed labeling for this product except by printed notice from the Company's headquarters. The prescriber and user of this product must accept the terms hereof.

REFERENCES

1. Gunson HH, Bowell PJ, Kirkwood TBL: Collaborative study to recalibrate the International Reference Preparation of Anti-D Immunoglobulin. *J Clin Pathol* 33:249–53, 1980.
2. Rh_o(D) immune globulin (human). *Med Lett Drugs Ther* 16(1):3–4, 1974.
3. Pollack W, Ascari WQ, Kochesky RJ, et al: Studies on Rh prophylaxis I. Relationship between doses of anti-Rh and size of antigenic stimulus. *Transfusion* 11(6):333–9, 1971.
4. Unpublished data in files of Miles Inc., Cutter Biological.
5. Pollack W, Asceri WQ, Crispen JF, et al: Studies on Rh prophylaxis. II. Rh immune prophylaxis after transfusion with Rh-positive blood. *Transfusion* 11 (6):340–4, 1971.
6. Keith LG, Houser GH: Anti-Rh immune globulin after a massive transfusion accident. *Transfusion* 11(3):176, 1971.
7. The selective use of Rh_o(D) Immune Globulin (RhIG). *ACOG Tech Bull* 61, 1981.
8. Current uses of Rh_o immune globulin and detection of antibodies. *ACOG Tech Bull* 35, 1976.
9. Pollack W: Rh hemolytic disease of the newborn; its cause and prevention. *Prog Clin Biol Res* 70:185–203, 1981.
10. Bowman JM, Chown B, Lewis M, et al: Rh isoimmunization during pregnancy: antenatal prophylaxis. *Can Med Assoc J* 118(6):623–7, 1978.
11. Bowman JM, Pollock JM: Antenatal prophylaxis of Rh isommunization: 28-weeks'-gestation service program. *Can Med Assoc J* 118(6):627–30, 1978.
12. Ascari WQ, Allen AE, Baker WJ, et al: Rh_o(D) immune globulin (human): evaluation in women at risk of Rh immunization. *JAMA* 205(1): 1–4, 1968.
13. Prevention of Rh sensitization, *WHO Tech Rep Ser* 468:25, 1971.
14. Samson D, Mollison PL: Effect on primary Rh immunization of delayed administration of anti-Rh. *Immunology* 28:349–57, 175.
15. Finn R, Harper DT, Stallings, SA, et al: Transplacental hemorrhage. *Transfusion* 3(2):114–24, 1963.
16. Garraty G (ed): Hemolytic disease of the newborn. Arlington, VA, American Association of Blood Banks, 1984, p 78.
17. Recommendations of the Immunization Practices Advisory Committee (ACIP): General recommendations on immunization. *MMWR* 38(13):205–14; 219–27, 1989.

KOĀTE®-HP ℞

[kō'ate]

Antihemophilic Factor (Human)
(Factor VIII, AHF, AHG)

DESCRIPTION

Antihemophilic Factor (Human), Koāte®-HP, is a sterile, stable, purified, dried concentrate of human Antihemophilic Factor (AHF, factor VIII, AHG) which has been treated with tri-n-butyl phosphate (TNBP) and polysorbate 80 and is intended for use in therapy of classical hemophilia (hemophilia A).

Koāte-HP is purified from the cold insoluble fraction of pooled fresh-frozen plasma by modification and refinements of the methods first described by Hershgold, Pool, and Pappenhagen.[1] Koāte-HP contains purified and concentrated factor VIII. The factor VIII is 300-1000 times purified over whole plasma. When reconstituted as directed, Koāte-HP contains approximately 50-150 times as much factor VIII as an equal volume of fresh plasma. The specific activity, after addition of Albumin (Human), is in the range of 9-22 IU/mg protein. Koāte-HP must be administered by the intravenous route.

Each bottle of Koāte-HP contains the labeled amount of antihemophilic factor activity in International Units (IU). One IU, as defined by the World Health Organization Standard for Blood Coagulation factor VIII, human, is approximately equal to the level of AHF found in 1.0 mL of fresh pooled human plasma. The final product when reconstituted as directed contains not more than (NMT) 5 units heparin/mL, NMT 1500 ppm polyethylene glycol (PEG), NMT 0.05 M glycine, NMT 25 ppm polysorbate 80, NMT 5 ppm tri-n-butyl phosphate (TNBP), NMT 3 mM calcium chloride, NMT 1 ppm aluminum, NMT 0.06 M histidine, and NMT 10 mg/mL Albumin (Human).

CLINICAL PHARMACOLOGY

Hemophilia A is a hereditary bleeding disorder characterized by deficient coagulant activity of the specific plasma protein clotting factor, factor VIII. In afflicted individuals, hemorrhages may occur spontaneously or after only minor trauma. Surgery on such individuals is not feasible without first correcting the clotting abnormality. The administration of Koāte-HP provides an increase in plasma levels of factor VIII and can temporarily correct the coagulation defect in these patients.

After infusion of Koāte-HP, there is usually an instantaneous rise in the coagulant level followed by an initial rapid decrease in activity, and then a subsequent much slower rate of decrease in activity.[2–4] The early rapid phase may represent the time of equilibration with the extravascular compartment, and the second or slow phase of the survival curve presumably is the result of degradation and reflects the true biologic half-life of the infused Antihemophilic Factor (Human).[3] Studies with Koāte-HP in hemophilic patients have demonstrated a biologic half-life of approximately 9 to 14 hours.[2]

In 1984, Prince, et al,[5] described the susceptibility of hepatitis B virus (HBV) and the Hutchinson strain of non-A, non-B hepatitis virus to inactivation by ether and polysorbate 80. This method is known to disrupt lipid-containing enveloped viruses. Subsequently, others[6,7] using tri-n-butyl phosphate as an alternative organic solvent to the hazardous ethyl ether in combination with a number of different detergents including polysorbate 80, sodium deoxycholate, sodium cholate, or Triton x-100, showed these forms of chemical treatment to be rapidly effective in inactivating certain lipid-enveloped viruses. These viruses included vesicular stomatitis virus (VSV), sindbis virus, and sendai virus[6] as well as, in a later study,[7] human immunodeficiency virus (HIV), HBV and non-A, non-B virus. Similar studies undertaken at Miles Inc., Cutter Biological using TNBP and polysorbate 80 treatment of factor VIII concentrate immediately prior to a gel permeation chromatography purifying/concentrating procedure have confirmed the inactivation of VSV, visna, and sindbis viruses.

Antihemophilic Factor (Human), Koāte®-HP is purified by virtue of a gel permeation chromatography step serving the dual purpose of removing the TNBP and polysorbate 80 as well as increasing the purity of the Factor VIII. Recently, concerns have been expressed concerning alterations to immune function occurring in asymptomatic hemophiliacs,[8–15] with some of the abnormalities being independent of HIV exposure. It has been suggested that the underlying mechanisms might include repeated exposure to viral agents, repeated allostimulation and/or possible contaminants in factor VIII preparations (e.g., IgG aggregates). More highly purified preparations which have minimized risks of viral transmission may therefore be desirable.[6]

INDICATIONS AND USAGE

Koāte-HP is indicated for the treatment of classical hemophilia (hemophilia A) in which there is a demonstrated deficiency of activity of the plasma clotting factor, factor VIII. Koāte-HP provides a means of temporarily replacing the missing clotting factor in order to correct or prevent bleeding episodes, or in order to perform emergency and elective surgery on hemophiliacs.

Koāte-HP has not been investigated for efficacy in the treatment of von Willebrand's disease, and hence is not approved for such usage.

CONTRAINDICATIONS

None known.

WARNINGS

This product is prepared from pooled human plasma which may contain the causative agents of hepatitis and other viral diseases. Prescribed manufacturing procedures utilized at the plasma collection centers, plasma testing laboratories, and the fractionation facilities are designed to reduce the risk of transmitting viral infection. However, the risk of viral infectivity from this product cannot be totally eliminated. The presence of hepatitis viruses should be assumed.

Individuals who receive infusions of blood or plasma products may develop signs and/or symptoms of some viral infections, particularly non-A, non-B hepatitis. It is emphasized that hepatitis B vaccination is essential for patients with hemophilia and it is recommended that this be done at birth or diagnosis.[16,17]

Fletcher et al,[18] have concluded that those who have had little exposure to blood products have a higher risk of developing hepatitis after introduction of clotting factor concentrates. For such patients, especially those with mild hemophilia, Kasper and Kipnis[19] recommend single donor products. For patients with moderate or severe hemophilia who have received numerous infusions of blood or blood products, they feel that the risk of hepatitis is small. They believe that the clotting factor concentrates have so greatly improved the management of severe hemophilia that these products should not be denied to appropriate patients. The physician and patient should consider that factor VIII concentrates may be associated with the trasmission of hepatitis and weigh the benefits of therapy accordingly.

PRECAUTIONS

General

1. Antihemophilic Factor (Human), Koāte-HP is intended for treatment of bleeding disorders arising from a deficiency in factor VIII. This deficiency should be proven prior to administering Koāte-HP.
2. Administer within 3 hours after reconstitution. Do not refrigerate after reconstitution.
3. Administer only by the intravenous route.
4. Filter needle should be used prior to administering.
5. Koāte-HP contains levels of blood group isoagglutinins which are not clinically significant when controlling relatively minor bleeding episodes. When large or frequently repeated doses are required, patients of blood groups A, B, or AB should be monitored by means of hematocrit for signs of progressive anemia, as well as by direct Coombs' tests.
6. Administration equipment and any reconstituted Koāte-HP not used should be appropriately discarded.

Pregnancy Category C

Animal reproduction studies have not been conducted with Koāte-HP. It is also not known whether Koāte-HP can cause fetal harm when administered to a pregnant woman or can affect reproduction capacity. Koāte-HP should be given to a pregnant woman only if clearly needed.

ADVERSE REACTIONS

Allergic-type reactions may result from the administration of Antihemophilic Factor (Human) preparations.[20,21]

DOSAGE AND ADMINISTRATION

Each bottle of Koāte-HP has the Antihemophilic Factor (Human) content in International Units per bottle stated on the label of the bottle. The reconstituted product must be administered intravenously by either direct syringe injection or drip infusion.

Shanbrom et al,[22] based upon studies in hemophiliacs, have suggested a linear dose-response relation with an approximate rise of 2.5% in Factor VIII activity for each unit of Antihemophilic Factor (Human) transfused per kg of body weight. Abildgaard et al,[23] in work with hemophilic children 8 months to 14 years of age, reported a response factor of 0.5 units/kg. Clinical experience with Koāte-HP has demonstrated a similar dose-response relationship.[2] The following formulas can provide a guide for dosage calculations:

Expected factor VIII increase (% of normal) =

$$\frac{\text{IU administered}}{\text{body weight (kg)} \times 0.4\ \text{IU/kg}}$$

Example: $\frac{840\ \text{IU}}{70\ \text{kg} \times 0.4\ \text{IU/kg}} = 30\%$

or

IU required = body weight (kg) × desired factor VIII increase (% normal) × 0.4 IU/kg

Example: 70 kg × 0.4 IU/kg × 30% = 840 IU

All efforts should be made to follow the course of therapy with factor VIII level assays. It may be dangerous to assume

Continued on next page

Miles Biological—Cont.

any certain level has been reached unless direct evidence is obtained.

Prophylaxis of Spontaneous Hemorrhage

The level of factor VIII required to prevent spontaneous hemorrhage is approximately 5% of normal, while a level of 30% of normal is the minimum required for hemostasis following trauma and surgery.[24–26] Mild superficial or early hemorrhages may respond to a single dose of 10 IU per kg,[4,27] leading to an in vivo rise of approximately 20% in the factor VIII level. In patients with early hemarthrosis (mild pain, minimal or no swelling, erythema, warmth, and minimal or no joint limitation), if treated promptly, even smaller doses may be adequate.[27–29]

Mild Hemorrhage

In cases of mild hemorrhage, therapy need not be repeated unless there is evidence of further bleeding.

Moderate Hemorrhage and Minor Surgery

For more serious hemorrhages and for minor surgical procedures, the patient's plasma factor VIII level should be raised to 30%–50% of normal for optimum hemostasis.[27,30] This usually requires an initial dose of 15–25 IU per kg; and if further therapy is required, a maintenance dose of 10–15 IU per kg every 8–12 hours.

Severe Hemorrhage

In patients with life-threatening bleeding, or hemorrhage involving vital structures (central nervous system, retropharyngeal and retroperitoneal spaces, iliopsoas sheath), it may be desirable to raise the factor VIII level to 80%–100% of normal in order to achieve hemostasis.[27,30–32] This may be achieved with an initial Koāte-HP dose of 40–50 IU per kg and a maintenance dose of 20–25 IU per kg every 8–12 hours.

Major Surgery

For major surgical procedures, Kasper[30] recommends that a dose of Antihemophilic Factor (Human) sufficient to achieve a level of 80%–100% of normal be given an hour before the procedure. It is recommended that the factor VIII level be checked prior to going to surgery to assure the expected level is achieved. A second dose, half the size of the priming dose, should be given about 5 hours after the first dose. The factor VIII level should be maintained at a daily minimum of at least 30% for a healing period of 10–14 days, depending on the nature of the operative procedure.

The above discussion is presented as a reference and a guideline. It should be emphasized that the dosage of Antihemophilic Factor (Human), Koāte®-HP required for normalizing hemostasis must be individualized according to the needs of the patient. Factors to be considered include the weight of the patient, the severity of the deficiency, the severity of the hemorrhage, the presence of inhibitors, and the factor VIII level desired. All efforts should be made to follow the course of therapy with factor VIII level assays.

The clinical effect of Koāte-HP is the most important element in evaluating the effectiveness of treatment. It may be necessary to administer more Koāte-HP than would be estimated in order to attain satisfactory clinical results. If the calculated dose fails to attain the expected factor VIII levels, or if bleeding is not controlled after adequate calculated dosage, the presence of a factor VIII inhibitor should be suspected. Its presence should be substantiated and the inhibitor level quantitated by appropriate laboratory procedure. When an inhibitor is present, the dosage requirement for Koāte-HP is extremely variable and the dosage can be determined only by the clinical response.

Parenteral drug products should be inspected visually for particulate matter and discoloration prior to administration, whenever solution and container permit.

Reconstitution

Vacuum Transfer

1. Warm the unopened diluent and the concentrate to room temperature (NMT 37°C, 99°F).
2. After removing the plastic flip-top caps (Fig. A), aseptically cleanse the rubber stoppers of both bottles.
3. Remove the protective cover from the plastic transfer-needle cartridge with tamper-proof seal and penetrate the stopper of the diluent bottle (Fig. B).
4. Remove the remaining portion of the plastic cartridge, invert the diluent bottle and penetrate the rubber seal on the concentrate bottle (Fig. C) with the needle at an angle. Alternate method of transferring sterile water: With a sterile needle and syringe, withdraw the appropriate volume of diluent and transfer to the bottle of lyophilized concentrate.
5. The vacuum will draw the diluent into the concentrate bottle. Hold the diluent bottle at an angle to the concentrate bottle in order to direct the jet of diluent against the wall of the concentrate bottle (Fig. C). Avoid excessive foaming.
6. After removing the diluent bottle and transfer needle (Fig. D), swirl continuously until completely dissolved (Fig. E).
7. After the concentrate powder is completely dissolved, withdraw solution into the syringe through the filter nee-

dle which is supplied in the package (Fig. F). Replace the filter needle with the administration set provided and inject intravenously.

8. If the same patient is to receive more than one bottle, the contents of two bottles may be drawn into the same syringe through a separate unused filter needle before attaching the vein needle.

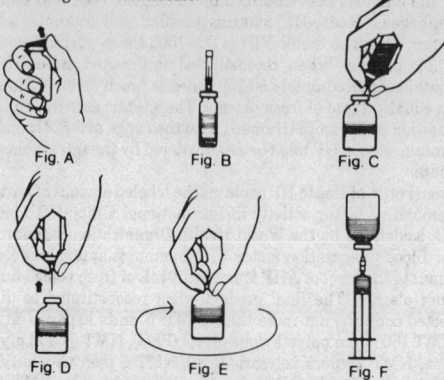

Fig. A   Fig. B   Fig. C

Fig. D   Fig. E   Fig. F

Rate of Administration

The rate of administration should be adapted to the response of the individual patient, but administration of the entire dose in 5 to 10 minutes is generally well-tolerated.

HOW SUPPLIED

Antihemophilic Factor (Human), Koāte®-HP is supplied in the following single dose bottles with the total units of factor VIII activity stated on the label of each bottle. A suitable volume of Sterile Water for Injection, USP, a sterile double-ended transfer needle, a sterile filter needle, and a sterile administration set are provided.

Approximate Factor VIII

Product Code	Activity	Diluent
664-20	250 IU	5 mL
664-30	500 IU	5 mL
664-50	1000 IU	10 mL
664-60	1500 IU	10 mL

STORAGE

Koāte-HP should be stored under refrigeration (2°–8°C; 35°–46°F). Storage of lyophilized powder at room temperature (up to 25°C or 77°F) for 6 months, such as in home treatment situations, may be done without loss of factor VIII activity. Freezing should be avoided as breakage of the diluent bottle might occur.

CAUTION

U.S. federal law prohibits dispensing without prescription.

LIMITED WARRANTY

A number of factors beyond our control could reduce the efficacy of this product or even result in an ill effect following its use. These include improper storage and handling of the product after it leaves our hands, diagnosis, dosage, method of administration, and biological differences in individual patients. Because of these factors, it is important that this product be stored properly, that the directions be followed carefully during use, and that the risk of transmitting viruses be carefully weighed before the product is prescribed. No warranty, express or implied, including any warranty of merchantability or fitness is made. Representatives of the Company are not authorized to vary the terms or the contents of the printed labeling, including the package insert for this product, except by printed notice from the Company's headquarters. The prescriber and user of this product must accept the terms hereof.

REFERENCES

1. Hershgold EJ, Pool JG, Pappenhagen AR: The potent antihemophilic globulin concentrate derived from a cold insoluble fraction of human plasma: characterization and further data on preparation and clinical trial. *J Lab Clin Med* 67(1):23–32, 1966.
2. Unpublished data in files of Miles Inc., Cutter Biological.
3. Aronson DL: Factor VIII (antihemophilic globulin). *Semin Thromb Hemostas* 6(1):12–27, 1979.
4. Britton M, Harrison J, Abildgaard CF: Early treatment of hemophilic hemarthroses with minimal dose of new factor VIII concentrate. *J Pediatr* 85(2):245–7, 1974.
5. Prince AM, Horowitz B, Brotman B, et al: Inactivation of hepatitis B and Hutchinson strain non-A, non-B hepatitis viruses by exposure to Tween 80 and ether. *Vox Sang* 46:36–43, 1984.
6. Horowitz B, Wiebe ME, Lippin A, et al: Inactivation of viruses in labile blood derivatives. I. Distruption of lipid-enveloped viruses by tri(n-butyl) phosphate detergent combinations. *Transfusion* 25(6):516–22, 1985.
7. Piet MPJ, Chin S, Prince AM, et al: Inactivtion of viruses in plasma on treatment with tri(n-butyl) phosphate (TNBP) detergent mixtures. [abstract] *Thromb Haemost* 58(1):370, 1987.

8. Lederman MM, Ratnoff OD, Scillian JJ, et al: Impaired cell-mediated immunity in patients with classic hemophilia. *N Engl J Med* 308(2):79–83, 1983.
9. Weintrub PS, Koerper MA, Addiego JE Jr, et al: Immunologic abnormalities in patients with hemophilia A. *J Pediatr* 103(5):692–5, 1983.
10. Goldsmith JC, Moseley PL, Monick M, et al: T-lymphocyte subpopulation abnormalities in apparently healthy patients with hemophilia. *Ann Intern Med* 98:294–6, 1983.
11. Saidi P, Kim HC, Raska K Jr: T-cell subsets in hemophilia. [letter] *N Engl J Med* 308(21):1291–3, 1983.
12. Landay A, Poon MC, Abo T, et al: Immunologic studies in asymptomatic hemophilia patients: relationship to acquired immune deficiency syndrome (AIDS). *J Clin Invest* 71(5):1500–4, 1983.
13. Jones P, Proctor S, Dickinson A, et al: Altered immunology in haemophilia. [letter] *Lancet* 1:120–1, 1983.
14. Mannhalter JW, Zlabinger GJ, Ahmad R, et al: A functional defect in the early phase of the immune response observed in patients with hemophilia A. *Clin Immunol Immunopathol* 38:390–7, 1986.
15. Frydecka I, Kowalewska B, Lesiecki A, et al: Immunologic studies in asymptomatic hemophiliac patients. *Folia Haematol* 113(5):708–15, 1986.
16. Fletcher ML, Trowell JM, Craske J, et al: Non-A, non-B hepatitis after transfusion of factor VIII in infrequently treated patients. *Br Med J* 287(6407):1754–7, 1983.
17. National Hemophilia Foundation Medical and Scientific Advisory Council. Hemophilia Information Exchange —AIDS Update: Recommendations concerning HIV infection, AIDS and the treatment of hemophilia. Section I.G. (Rev. Jan., 1988).
18. Safety of therapeutic products used for hemophilia patients. *MMWR* 37(29):441–4, 449–50,1988.
19. Kasper CK, Kipnis SA: Hepatitis and clotting-factor concentrates. *JAMA* 221(5):510, 1972.
20. Eyster ME, Bowman HS, Haverstick JN: Adverse reactions to factor VIII infusions. [letter] *Ann Intern Med* 87(2):248, 1977.
21. Prager D, Djerassi I, Eyster ME, et al: Pennsylvania state-wide hemophilia program: summary of immediate reactions with the use of factor VIII and factor IX concentrate. *Blood* 53(5):1012–3, 1979.
22. Shanbrom E, Thelin GM: Experimental prophylaxis of severe hemophilia with a factor VIII concentrate. *JAMA* 208(10):1853–6, 1969.
23. Abildgaard CF, Simone JV, Corrigan JJ, et al: Treatment of hemophilia with glycine-precipitated factor VIII. *N Engl J Med* 275(9):471–5, 1966.
24. Biggs R, MacFarlane RG: Haemophilia and related conditions: a survey of 187 cases. *Br J Haematol* 4(1):1–27, 1958.
25. Langdell RD, Wagner RH, Brinkhous KM: Antihemophilic factor (AHF) levels following transfusions of blood, plasma and plasma fractions. *Proc Soc Exp Biol Med* 88(2):212–5, 1955.
26. Shulman NR, Cowan DH, Libre EP, et al: The physiologic basis for therapy of classic hemophilia (factor VIII deficiency) and related disorders. *Ann Intern Med* 67(4):856–82, 1967.
27. Abildgaard CF: Current concepts in the management of hemophilia. *Semin Hematol* 12(3):223–32, 1975.
28. Penner JA, Kelly PE: Low doses of factor VIII for hemophilia. [letter] *N Engl J Med* 297(7):401, 1977.
29. Ashenhurst JB, Langehennig PL, Seller RA: Early treatment of bleeding episodes with 10 U/kg of factor VIII. [letter] *Blood* 50(1):181–2, 1977.
30. Kasper CK: Hematologic care. In: Boone DC (ed.): Comprehensive management of hemophilia. Philadelphia, Davis, 1976, pp 3–17.
31. Edson JR: Hemophilia and related conditions. In: Conn HF (ed): Current therapy. Philadelphia, Saunders, 1980, pp 264–9.
32. Hilgartner MW; Management of hemophilia: the routine and the crises. *Drug Ther* 8(2):141–54, 1978.

PLAGUE VACCINE, USP   ℞

DESCRIPTION

Plague Vaccine is a sterile, liquid vaccine for intramuscular injection. It contains at the time of manufacture $1.8-2.2 \times 10^9$ per mL of formaldehyde-killed plague bacilli (*Yersinia pestis*) in Sodium Chloride Injection, USP. The product may also contain trace amounts of: beef heart extract, yeast extract, the peptones and peptides of soya and casein, agar and not more than 0.019% formaldehyde. It is preserved with 0.5% phenol.

CLINICAL PHARMACOLOGY

Plague Vaccine is used to promote active immunity to plague in individuals considered at high risk of infection. Inactivated bacilli present in plague vaccine promote the production of plague antibody; plague antibody neutralizes the ba-

cilli so that the incidence and severity of infection are reduced.

Plague is caused by the bacterium, *Yersinia pestis*, an organism which occurs naturally in rodents and their ectoparasites. Plague may develop in humans following exposure to or handling of infected wild rodents or their fleas and, less commonly, following exposure to or handling of other infected wild animals (e.g., bobcats, coyotes, rabbits) or domestic animals (e.g., cats, dogs). In the U.S., plague has been found in ground squirrels, prairie dogs, jack rabbits, and pack rats. Worldwide, camels, goats, sheep, coyotes, deer, dogs, and cats may be exposed to plague infection either by feeding on infected carcasses or by becoming infested with infected fleas.

Transmission of plague from rodent to rodent or rodent to human is generally mediated by the bite(s) of an infected flea(s). Human infection from an infected flea bite(s) most frequently results in bubonic plague with an incubation period of 2-8 days. Bubonic plague may rarely progress to pneumonic plague by hematogenous (septicemic) transport of *Y. pestis* to the lungs. Virulent encapsulated droplets of *Y. pestis* can then be transmitted from individual to individual by the respiratory route without insect vectors. The incubation period for pneumonic plague is 2-5 days.

Y. pestis contains at least 19 different antigenic components. Five components (i.e., Fraction 1 capsular antigen, the V and W antigens, exotoxin and endotoxin) correlate with immunogenic activity and virulence, whereas the remaining components have not been demonstrated to correlate with plague immunity or infection. Fraction 1 capsular antigen is the principal antigen involved with both virulence and immunity. Antibody to Fraction 1 capsular antigen, determined by passive hemagglutination (PHA) test, correlates with protection against *Y. pestis* infection in experimental animals; a comparable correlation between the titer for antibody to Fraction 1 capsular antigen (determined by PHA) and immunity appears to exist in humans. Although some experts consider a titer of antibody to Fraction 1 capsular antigen (determined by PHA) of at least 1:32 to be indicative of protection, the U.S. Public Health Service Immunization Practices Advisory Committee (ACIP) states that the minimum titer of antibody to Fraction 1 capsular antigen (determined by PHA) indicative of adequate protection against plague infection is 1:128 in animals.

The presumptive protective titer of antibody to Fraction 1 capsular antigen (1:128) is generally reached following IM administration of an initial 1 mL dose of Plague Vaccine followed by a second dose of 0.2 mL. The titer increases following administration of a third dose of 0.2 mL of the vaccine and persists for about 6-12 months. In one study in 29 adult male volunteers,[1] following IM administration of Plague Vaccine in doses of 1, 0.2, and 0.2 mL on days 0, 90, and 270, respectively, the mean titer of antibody to Fraction 1 capsular antigen determined by passive hemagglutination (PHA) test, was 1:25, 1:140, and 1:576 at 15, 105 and 285 days, respectively. However, in this study, 7% of the individuals failed to produce detectable antibodies even after the second booster dose. Thus individual variation in the response to the vaccine does exist.

It is generally believed that the use of plague vaccine greatly increases the chances of recovery in those vaccinated individuals who may develop the insect-borne (bubonic) form of the infection.[2] The degree of protection afforded against the pneumonic form is unknown and vaccinated persons exposed to pneumonic form should be given daily, adequate doses of a suitable antibiotic over a 7-10 day period.

The duration of protection against infection following administration of the primary series of these injections of Plague Vaccine is brief (i.e., 6-12 months) and booster doses in approximate 6-month intervals are required for continued protection.

INDICATIONS AND USAGE

Immunization with this vaccine is recommended for those persons at particularly high risk of exposure to plague. High risk areas include rural mountains or upland areas of South America, Asia and Africa. Routine vaccination is not necessary for persons residing in plague-enzootic areas (such as those in the western United States) nor for travelers in countries where cases have been reported particularly if travel is limited to urban areas.[3] Use of the vaccine is recommended in the following situations:[3]

1. Following natural disaster and/or at times when regular sanitary practices are interrupted;
2. All laboratory and field personnel who are working with *Y. pestis* organisms resistant to antimicrobics;
3. Persons engaged in aerosol experiments with *Y. pestis*;
4. Persons engaged in field operations in plague-enzootic areas where prevention of exposure is not possible (such as some disaster areas).

Selective plague vaccination might be considered for:

1. Laboratory personnel regularly working with *Y. pestis* or plague-infected rodents;
2. Workers (for example, Peace Corps volunteers and agricultural advisors) who reside in plague-enzootic or plague-epidemic rural areas where avoidance of rodents and fleas is impossible;
3. Persons whose vocation brings them into regular contact with wild rodents or rabbits in plague-enzootic areas.

Table 1
Recommended doses, by volume (mL), for immunization against plague:

Dose number	Age (Years) <1	1-4	5-10	>10
1	0.2 mL	0.4 mL	0.6 mL	1.0 mL
2 & 3	0.04 mL	0.08 mL	0.12 mL	0.2 mL
Boosters	0.02-0.04 mL	0.04-0.08 mL	0.06-0.12 mL	0.1-0.2 mL

CONTRAINDICATIONS

Plague Vaccine should not be administered to anyone with a known hypersensitivity to any of the product constituents, such as beef protein, soya, casein, phenol, and formaldehyde. Patients who have had severe local or systemic reactions to Plague Vaccine injections should not be revaccinated.

Plague Vaccine should not be administered to patients who have severe thrombocytopenia or any coagulation disorder that would contraindicate intramuscular injections.

WARNINGS

Immunization of individuals with severe febrile illness should generally be deferred until they have recovered to avoid superimposing adverse effects of the vaccine on the underlying illness or to avoid mistakenly concluding that a manifestation of the underlying illness resulted from vaccination. Public health officials should be consulted regarding the need for prophylaxis in these individuals. Administration of plague vaccine to individuals with minor illnesses (e.g., mild upper respiratory infections) should not be postponed.

PRECAUTIONS

General

Epinephrine should be available for immediate treatment of an anaphylactic reaction if it occurs.

Drug Interactions

When practical, Plague Vaccine should not be given on the same occasion as typhoid or cholera vaccines to avoid the possibility of accentuated side effects.[4]

Pregnancy Category C

Animal reproduction studies have not been conducted with Plague Vaccine. It is also not known whether Plague Vaccine can cause fetal harm when administered to a pregnant woman or can affect reproduction capacity. Plague Vaccine should be given to a pregnant woman only if clearly needed.

Pediatric Use

Although clinical studies have not been conducted in children, the Immunization Practices Advisory Committee (ACIP) recommends immunization of children who are at risk.[3]

ADVERSE REACTIONS

Adverse reactions are usually mild following primary immunization with Plague Vaccine. Adverse reactions may occur more frequently and with more severity following repeated doses of the vaccine. The increased frequency and severity of adverse reactions following repeated doses appear to depend on the number of doses received, the method by which the doses are administered, and the reactivity of the individual.

Local Effects

Erythema and induration at the site of injection occur in about 10% of patients receiving Plague Vaccine but may occur more frequently following repeated injections. Other adverse local reactions to the vaccine include tenderness and edema. Most adverse local reactions to the vaccine subside within 2 days. Sterile abscesses occur rarely.

Systemic Effects

Malaise, headache, lymphadenopathy, and fever occur in about 10% of patients receiving Plague Vaccine but may occur more frequently following repeated doses. Other adverse systemic reactions to the vaccine include arthralgia, myalgia, leukocytosis, nausea, and vomiting. Adverse systemic effects of the vaccine usually persist for only a few days.

Sensitivity reactions, manifested by anaphylactic shock, tachycardia, urticaria, asthma and/or hypotension, have occurred rarely following administration of Plague Vaccine.

DOSAGE AND ADMINISTRATION

Plague Vaccine is administered by intramuscular injection preferably into the deltoid muscle. It may be used with the jet injector gun. The product should be well shaken before use.

Adults and Children Over 10 Years Old:

Primary immunization consists of series of two to three injections. The first injection consists of 1.0 mL of Plague Vaccine followed after 1 to 3 months by a second injection of 0.2 mL.[5] This series of two injections will produce adequate protection in the vast majority of human beings who have never received this vaccine..[1] Generally, plague antibody titers are increased by a third injection. Some individuals not responding to the first two injections may produce an adequate response following the third injection. A third injection of 0.2 mL 3 to 6 months after the second injection is strongly recommended.

Booster injections of 0.1 to 0.2 mL should be administered at 6-month intervals to individuals remaining in a known plague area. The smaller dose should be approached as the total number of such injections increases. It should be noted, however, that booster doses at intervals of greater than 6 months, e.g., 1-2 years, may be appropriate for persons who have received three or more booster doses at 6-month intervals. In persons who have an unusually high risk of infection or who have a history of serious reactions to the vaccine, passive hemagglutination titers (PHA) should be determined in order to govern the frequency of booster doses.[3]

Children Less Than 10 Years Old:

The same technique and time schedule holds true for primary and booster injections in children; however, in both primary and booster injections the following dosage formula should be used:

Under 1 year	1/5 adult primary or booster dose
1-4 years	2/5 adult primary or booster dose
5-10 years	3/5 adult primary or booster dose
11 years and over	adult primary or booster dose

Table 1 summarizes the recommended doses for primary and booster vaccinations.

Parenteral drug products should be inspected visually for particulate matter and discoloration prior to administration, whenever solution and container permit.

HOW SUPPLIED

Plague Vaccine is supplied in a 20 mL vial.

STORAGE

Store at 2°-8°C (35°-46°F). Do not freeze. Do not use after expiration date.

CAUTION

U.S. federal law prohibits dispensing without prescription.

LIMITED WARRANTY

A number of factors beyond our control could reduce the efficacy of this product or even result in an ill effect following its use. These include improper storage and handling of the product after it leaves our hands, diagnosis, dosage, method of administration, and biological differences in individual patients. Because of these factors, it is important that this product be stored properly and that the directions be followed carefully during use.

The foregoing statement is made in lieu of any other warranty, express or implied, including any warranty of merchantability or fitness. Representatives of the Company are not authorized to vary the terms of this warranty or the contents of any printed labeling for this product except by printed notice from the Company's headquarters. The prescriber and user of this product must accept the terms hereof.

REFERENCES

1. Bartelloni PJ, Marshall JD Jr, Cavanaugh DC: Clinical and serological responses to plague vaccine USP. *Milit Med* 138:720-2, 1973.
2. Cavanaugh DC, Elisberg BL, Llewellyn CH, et al: Plague immunization. V. Indirect evidence for the efficacy of plague vaccine. *J Infect Dis* 129:S37-S40, 1974.
3. Plague vaccine. *Morbidity Mortality Weekly Report* 31(22):301-4, 1982.
4. General recommendations on immunization. *Morbidity Mortality Weekly Report* 32(1):1-18, 1983.
5. Meyer KF: Effectiveness of live or killed plague vaccines in man. *Bull WHO* 42:653-66, 1970.

Continued on next page

Miles Biological—Cont.

ALPHA$_1$-PROTEINASE INHIBITOR (HUMAN) ℞
PROLASTIN®
[pro-las 'tin]

DESCRIPTION

Alpha$_1$-Proteinase Inhibitor (Human), Prolastin®, is a sterile, stable, lyophilized preparation of purified human Alpha$_1$-Proteinase Inhibitor (alpha$_1$-PI) also known as alpha$_1$-antitrypsin. Alpha$_1$-Proteinase Inhibitor (Human) is intended for use in therapy of congenital alpha$_1$-antitrypsin deficiency.

Alpha$_1$-Proteinase Inhibitor (Human) is prepared from pooled human plasma of normal donors by modification and refinements of the cold ethanol method of Cohn.[1] In order to reduce the potential risk of transmission of infectious agents, Alpha$_1$-Proteinase Inhibitor (Human) has been heat-treated in solution at 60±0.5°C for not less than 10 hours. However, no procedure has been found to be totally effective in removing viral infectivity from plasma fractionation products.

The specific activity of Alpha$_1$-Proteinase Inhibitor (Human) is ≥0.35 mg functional alpha$_1$-PI/mg protein and when reconstituted as directed, the concentration of alpha$_1$-PI is ≥20 mg/mL. When reconstituted, Alpha$_1$-Proteinase Inhibitor (Human) has a pH of 6.6–7.4, a sodium content of 100–210 mEq/L, a chloride content of 60–180 mEq/L, a sodium phosphate content of 0.015–0.025 M, a polyethylene glycol content of not more than (NMT) 5 ppm, NMT 0.1% sucrose. Alpha$_1$-Proteinase Inhibitor (Human) contains small amounts of other plasma proteins including alpha$_2$-plasmin inhibitor, alpha$_1$-antichymotrypsin, C_1-esterase inhibitor, haptoglobin, antithrombin III, alpha$_1$-lipoprotein, albumin, and IgA.[1]

Each vial of Prolastin contains the labeled amount of functionally active alpha$_1$-PI in milligrams per vial (mg/vial), as determined by capacity to neutralize porcine pancreatic elastase.[1] Alpha$_1$-Proteinase Inhibitor (Human) contains no preservative and must be administered by the intravenous route.

CLINICAL PHARMACOLOGY

Alpha$_1$-antitrypsin deficiency is a chronic hereditary, usually fatal, autosomal recessive disorder in which a low concentration of alpha$_1$-PI (alpha$_1$-antitrypsin) is associated with slowly progressive, severe, panacinar emphysema that most often manifests itself in the third to fourth decades of life.[2–9] [Although the terms "Alpha$_1$-Proteinase Inhibitor" and "alpha$_1$-antitrypsin" are used interchangeably in the scientific literature, the hereditary disorder associated with a reduction in the serum level of alpha$_1$-PI is conventionally referred to as "alpha$_1$-antitrypsin deficiency" while the deficient protein is referred to as "Alpha$_1$-Proteinase Inhibitor"[10]]. The emphysema is typically worse in the lower lung zones.[4,8,9] The pathogenesis of development of emphysema in alpha$_1$-antitrypsin deficiency is not well understood at this time. It is believed, however, to be due to a chronic biochemical imbalance between elastase (an enzyme capable of degrading elastin tissues, released by inflammatory cells, primarily neutrophils, in the lower respiratory tract) and alpha$_1$-PI (the principal inhibitor of neutrophil elastase) which is deficient in alpha$_1$-antitrypsin disease.[11–15] As a result, it is believed that alveolar structures are unprotected from chronic exposure to elastase released from a chronic, low level burden of neutrophils in the lower respiratory tract, resulting in progressive degradation of elastin tissues.[11–15] The eventual outcome is the development of emphysema. Neonatal hepatitis with cholestatic jaundice appears in approximately 10% of newborns with alpha$_1$-antitrypsin deficiency.[15] In some adults, alpha$_1$-antitrypsin deficiency is complicated by cirrhosis.[15]

A large number of phenotypic variants of alpha$_1$-antitrypsin deficiency exists.[15] The most severely affected individuals are those with the PiZZ variant, typically characterized by alpha$_1$-PI serum levels <35% normal.[15] Epidemiologic studies of individuals with various phenotypes of alpha$_1$-antitrypsin deficiency have demonstrated that individuals with endogenous serum levels of alpha$_1$-PI ≤50 mg/dL (based on commercial standards) have a risk of >80% of developing emphysema over a lifetime.[3–6,8,9,16] However, individuals with endogenous alpha$_1$-PI levels >80 mg/dL, in general, do not manifest an increased risk for development of emphysema above the general population background risk.[5,15] From these observations, it is believed that the "threshold" level of alpha$_1$-PI in the serum required to provide adequate anti-elastase activity in the lung of individuals with alpha$_1$-antitrypsin deficiency is about 80 mg/dL (based on commercial standards for immunologic assay of alpha$_1$-PI).[12,15,17]

In clinical studies of Alpha$_1$-Proteinase Inhibitor (Human), Prolastin®, 23 subjects with the PiZZ variant of congenital deficiency of alpha$_1$-antitrypsin deficiency and documented destructive lung disease participated in a study of acute and/or chronic replacement therapy with Alpha$_1$-Proteinase Inhibitor (Human).[18] The mean in vivo recovery of alpha$_1$-PI was 4.2 mg (immunologic) dL per mg (functional)/kg body weight administered.[18,19] The half-life of alpha$_1$-PI in vivo was approximately 4.5 days.[18,19] Based on these observations, a program of chronic replacement therapy was developed. Nineteen of the subjects in these studies received Alpha$_1$-Proteinase Inhibitor (Human) replacement therapy, 60 mg/kg body weight, once weekly for up to 26 weeks (average 24 weeks of therapy). With this schedule of replacement therapy, blood levels of alpha$_1$-PI were maintained above 80 mg/dL (based on the commercial standards for alpha$_1$-PI immunologic assay).[18–20]. Within a few weeks of commencing this program, bronchoalveolar lavage studies demonstrated significantly increased levels of alpha$_1$-PI and functional antineutrophil elastase capacity in the epithelial lining fluid of the lower respiratory tract of the lung, as compared to levels prior to commencing the program of chronic replacement therapy with Alpha$_1$-Proteinase Inhibitor (Human).[18–20].

All 23 individuals who participated in the investigations were immunized with Hepatitis B Vaccine and received a single dose of Hepatitis B Immune Globulin (Human) on entry into the investigation. Although no other steps were taken to prevent hepatitis, neither hepatitis B nor non-A, non-B hepatitis occurred in any of the subjects.[18,19] All subjects remained seronegative for HIV antibody. None of the subjects developed any detectable antibody to alpha$_1$-PI or other serum protein.

Long-term controlled clinical trials to evaluate the effect of chronic replacement therapy with Alpha$_1$-Proteinase Inhibitor (Human), Prolastin®, on the development of or progression of emphysema in patients with congenital alpha$_1$-antitrypsin deficiency have not been performed. Estimates of the sample size required of this rare disorder and the slow progressive nature of the clinical course have been considered impediments in the ability to conduct such a trial.[21] Studies to monitor the long-term effects will continue as part of the postapproval process.

INDICATIONS AND USAGE

Congenital Alpha$_1$-Antitrypsin Deficiency

Alpha$_1$-Proteinase Inhibitor (Human) is indicated for chronic replacement therapy of individuals having congenital deficiency of alpha$_1$-PI (alpha$_1$-antitrypsin deficiency) with clinically demonstrable panacinar emphysema. Clinical and biochemical studies have demonstrated that with such therapy, it is possible to increase plasma levels of alpha$_1$-PI, and that levels of functionally active alpha$_1$-PI in the lung epithelial lining fluid are increased proportionately.[18–20] As some individuals with alpha$_1$-antitrypsin deficiency will not go on to develop panacinar emphysema, only those with early evidence of such disease should be considered for chronic replacement therapy with Alpha$_1$-Proteinase Inhibitor (Human).[22] Subjects with the PiMZ or PiMS phenotypes of alpha$_1$-antitrypsin deficiency should not be considered for such treatment as they appear to be at small risk for panacinar emphysema.[22] Clinical data are not available as to the long-term effects derived from chronic replacement therapy of individuals with alpha$_1$-antitrypsin deficiency with Alpha$_1$-Proteinase Inhibitor (Human). Only adult subjects have received Alpha$_1$-Proteinase Inhibitor (Human) to date.

Alpha$_1$-Proteinase Inhibitor (Human) is not indicated for use in patients other than those with PiZZ, PiZ(null), or Pi(null) (null) phenotypes.

CONTRAINDICATIONS

Individuals with selective IgA deficiencies who have known antibody against IgA (anti-IgA antibody) should not receive Alpha$_1$-Proteinase Inhibitor (Human), since these patients may experience severe reactions, including anaphylaxis, to IgA which may be present.

WARNINGS

This product is prepared from pooled human plasma which may contain the causative agents of hepatitis and other viral diseases. Prescribed manufacturing procedures utilized at the plasma collection centers, plasma testing laboratories, and the fractionation facilities are designed to reduce the risk of transmitting viral infection. However, the risk of viral infectivity from this product cannot be totally eliminated.

Individuals who receive infusions of blood or plasma products may develop signs and/or symptoms of some viral infections, particularly non-A, non-B hepatitis.

Alpha$_1$-Proteinase Inhibitor (Human) has been heat-treated in solution at 60°C for 10 hours in order to reduce the potential for transmission of infectious agents.[1] No cases of hepatitis, either hepatitis B or non-A, non-B hepatitis have been recorded to date in individuals receiving Alpha$_1$-Proteinase Inhibitor (Human).[18] However, as all individuals received prophylaxis against hepatitis B, no conclusion can be drawn at this time regarding potential transmission of hepatitis B virus.

PRECAUTIONS

General

1. Administer within 3 hours after reconstitution. Do not refrigerate after reconstitution.
2. Administer only by the intravenous route.
3. As with any colloid solution there will be an increase in plasma volume following intravenous administration of Alpha$_1$-Proteinase Inhibitor (Human).[23] Caution should therefore be used in patients at risk for circulatory overload.
4. It is recommended that in preparation for receiving Alpha$_1$-Proteinase Inhibitor (Human), recipients be immunized against hepatitis B using a licensed Hepatitis B Vaccine according to the manufacturer's recommendations. Should it become necessary to treat an individual with Alpha$_1$-Proteinase Inhibitor (Human), and time is insufficient for adequate antibody response to vaccination, individuals should receive a single dose of Hepatitis B Immune Globulin (Human), 0.06 mL/kg body weight, intramuscularly, at the time of administration of the initial dose of Hepatitis B Vaccine.
5. Alpha$_1$-Proteinase Inhibitor (Human) should be given alone, without mixing with other agents or diluting solutions.
6. Administration equipment and any reconstituted Alpha$_1$-Proteinase Inhibitor (Human) not used should be appropriately discarded.

Carcinogenesis, Mutagenesis, Impairment of Fertility

Long-term studies in animals to evaluate carcinogenesis, mutagenesis or impairment of fertility have not been conducted.

Pregnancy Category C

Animal reproduction studies have not been conducted with Prolastin. It is also not known whether Prolastin can cause fetal harm when administered to a pregnant woman or can affect reproduction capacity. Prolastin should be given to a pregnant woman only if clearly needed.

Nursing Mothers

It is not known whether Prolastin is excreted in human milk. Because many drugs are excreted in human milk, caution should be exercised when Prolastin is administered to a nursing woman.

Pediatric Use

Safety and effectiveness in children have not been established.

ADVERSE REACTIONS

Therapeutic administration of Alpha$_1$-Proteinase Inhibitor (Human), 60 mg/kg weekly, has been demonstrated to be well-tolerated. In clinical studies, six reactions were observed with 517 infusions of Alpha$_1$-Proteinase Inhibitor (Human), or 1.16%. None of the reactions was severe.[18] The adverse reactions reported included delayed fever (maximum temperature rise was 38.9°C, resolving spontaneously over 24 hours) occurring up to 12 hours following treatment (0.77%), light-headedness (0.19%), and dizziness (0.19%).[18] Mild transient leukocytosis and dilutional anemia several hours after infusion have also been noted.[18] Since market entry, occasional reports of other flu-like symptoms, allergic-like reactions, chills, dyspnea, rash, tachycardia, and, rarely, hypotension have also been received.

DOSAGE AND ADMINISTRATION

Each bottle of Alpha$_1$-Proteinase Inhibitor (Human) has the functional activity, as determined by inhibition of porcine pancreatic elastase,[1] stated on the label of the bottle.

The "threshold" level of alpha$_1$-PI in the serum believed to provide adequate anti-elastase activity in the lung of individuals with alpha$_1$-antitrypsin deficiency is 80 mg/dL (based on commercial standards for alpha$_1$-PI immunologic assay).[12,15,17] However, assays of alpha$_1$-PI based on commercial standards measure antigenic activity of alpha$_1$-PI whereas the labeled potency value of alpha$_1$-PI is expressed as actual functional activity, i.e., actual capacity to neutralize porcine pancreatic elastase. As functional activity may be less than antigenic activity, serum levels of alpha$_1$-PI determined using commercial immunologic assays may not accurately reflect actual functional alpha$_1$-PI levels. Therefore, although it may be helpful to monitor serum levels of alpha$_1$-PI in individuals receiving Alpha$_1$-Proteinase Inhibitor (Human), Prolastin®, using currently available commercial assays of antigenic activity, results of these assays should not be used to determine the required therapeutic dosage.

The recommended dosage of Alpha$_1$-Proteinase Inhibitor (Human) is 60 mg/kg body weight administered once weekly. This dose is intended to increase and maintain a level of functional alpha$_1$-PI in the epithelial lining of the lower respiratory tract providing adequate anti-elastase activity in the lung of individuals with alpha$_1$-antitrypsin deficiency.

Alpha$_1$-Proteinase Inhibitor (Human) may be given at a rate of 0.08 mL/kg/min or greater and must be administered intravenously. The recommended dosage of 60 mg/kg takes approximately 30 minutes to infuse.

Parenteral drug products should be inspected visually for particulate matter and discoloration prior to administration, whenever solution and container permit.

Reconstitution

1. Warm the unopened diluent and concentrate to room temperature (NMT 37°C, 99°F).
2. After removing the plastic flip-top caps (Fig. A), aseptically cleanse rubber stoppers of both bottles.
3. Remove the protective cover from the plastic transfer needle cartridge with tamper-proof seal and penetrate the stopper of the diluent bottle (Fig. B).
4. Remove the remaining portion of the plastic cartridge. Invert the diluent bottle and penetrate the rubber seal on the concentrate bottle (Fig. C) with the needle at an angle.
5. The vacuum will draw the diluent into the concentrate bottle. For best results, and to avoid foaming, hold the diluent bottle at an angle to the concentrate bottle in order to direct the jet of diluent against the wall of the concentrate bottle (Fig. C).
6. After removing the diluent bottle and transfer needle (Fig. D), gently swirl the concentrate bottle until the powder is completely dissolved (Fig. E).
7. Swab top of reconstituted bottle of Alpha$_1$-Proteinase Inhibitor (Human), Prolastin® again.
8. Attach the sterile filter needle provided to syringe. With filter needle in place, insert syringe into reconstituted bottle of Prolastin and withdraw Prolastin solution into syringe (Fig. F).
9. To administer Prolastin, replace filter needle with appropriate injection needle and follow procedure for I.V. administration.
10. The contents of more than one bottle of Prolastin may be drawn into the same syringe before administration. If more than one bottle of Prolastin is used, withdraw contents from bottles using aseptic technique. Place contents into an administration container (plastic minibag or glass bottle) using a syringe.* Avoid pushing an I.V. administration set spike into the product container stopper as this has been known to force the stopper into the vial, with a resulting loss of sterility.

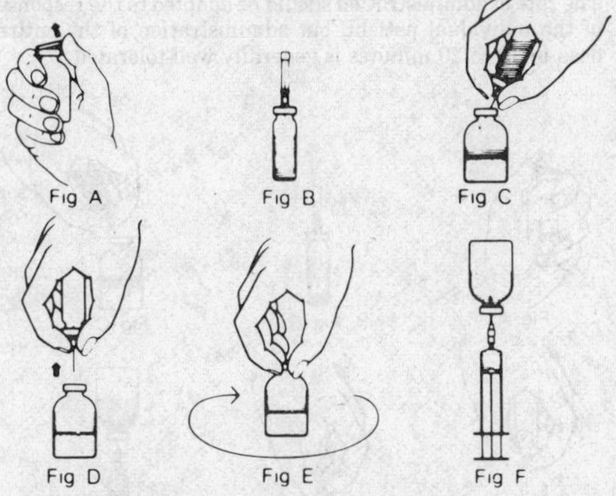
Fig A
Fig B
Fig C
Fig D
Fig E
Fig F

HOW SUPPLIED

Alpha$_1$-Proteinase Inhibitor (Human), Prolastin®, is supplied in the following single dose vials with the total alpha$_1$-PI functional activity, in milligrams, stated on the label of each vial. A suitable volume of Sterile Water for Injection, USP is provided.

Product Code	Approximate Alpha$_1$-PI Functional Activity	Diluent
601-30	500 mg	20 mL
601-35	1000 mg	40 mL

STORAGE

Alpha$_1$-Proteinase Inhibitor (Human) should be stored under refrigeration (2°-8°C; 35°-46°F). Freezing should be avoided as breakage of the diluent bottle might occur.

CAUTION

U.S. federal law prohibits dispensing without prescription.

LIMITED WARRANTY

A number of factors beyond our control could reduce the efficacy of this product or even result in an ill effect following its use. These include improper storage and handling of the product after it leaves our hands, diagnosis, dosage, method of administration, and biological differences in individual patients. Because of these factors, it is important that this product be stored properly, that the directions be followed carefully during use, and that the risk of transmitting viruses be carefully weighed before the product is prescribed. No warranty, express or implied, including any warranty of merchantability or fitness is made. Representatives of the Company are not authorized to vary the terms or the contents of the printed labeling, including the package insert for this product, except by printed notice from the Company's headquarters. The prescriber and user of this product must accept the terms hereof.

*For a patient of average weight (about 70 kg), the volume needed will exceed the limit of one syringe.

REFERENCES

1. Coan MH, Brockway WJ, Eguizabal H, et al: Preparation and properties of alpha$_1$-proteinase inhibitor concentrate from human plasma. *Vox Sang* 48(6):333–42, 1985.
2. Laurell CB, Eriksson S: The electrophoretic alpha$_1$-globulin pattern of serum in alpha$_1$-antitrypsin deficiency. *Scand J Clin Lab Invest* 15:132–40, 1963.
3. Eriksson S: Pulmonary emphysema and alpha$_1$-antitrypsin deficiency. *Acta Med Scand* 175(2):197–205, 1964.
4. Eriksson S: Studies in alpha$_1$-antitrypsin deficiency. *Acta Med Scand* Suppl 432:1–85, 1965.
5. Kueppers F, Black LF: Alpha$_1$-antitrypsin and its deficiency. *Am Rev Respir Dis* 110(2):176–94, 1974.
6. Morse JO: Alpha$_1$-antitrypsin deficiency. *N Engl J Med* 299:1045–8; 1099–105, 1978.
7. Black LF, Kueppers F: Alpha$_1$-antitrypsin deficiency in nonsmokers. *Am Rev Respir Dis* 117(3):421–8, 1978.
8. Tobin JM, Cook PJ, Hutchison DC: Alpha$_1$-antitrypsin deficiency: the clinical and physiological features of pulmonary emphysema in subjects homozygous for Pi type Z. A survey by the British Thoracic Association. *Br J Dis Chest* 77(1):14–27, 1983.
9. Larsson C. Natural history and life expectancy in severe alpha$_1$-antitrypsin deficiency, Pi Z. *Acta Med Scand* 204(5):345–51, 1978.
10. Pannell R, Johnson D, Travis J: Isolation and properties of human plasma alpha$_1$-proteinase inhibitor. *Biochemistry* 13(26):5439–45, 1974.
11. Lieberman J: Elastase, collagenase, emphysema, and alpha$_1$-antitrypsin deficiency. *Chest* 70(1):62–7, 1976.
12. Gadek JE, Fells GA, Zimmerman RL, et al: Antielastases of the human alveolar structures: implications for the protease-antiprotease theory of emphysema. *J Clin Invest* 68(4):889–98, 1981.
13. Beatty K, Bieth J, Travis J: Kinetics of association of serine proteinases with native and oxidized alpha-1-proteinase inhibitor and alpha-1-antichymotrypsin. *J Biol Chem* 255(9):3931–4, 1980.
14. Janoff A, White R, Carp H, et al: Lung injury induced by leukocytic proteases. *Am J Pathol* 97(1):111–36, 1979.
15. Gadek JE, Crystal RG: Alpha$_1$-antitrypsin deficiency. In: Stanbury JB, Wyngaarden JB, Frederickson DS, et al, eds.: *The Metabolic Basis of Inherited Disease* 5th ed. New York, McGraw-Hill, 1983, p. 1450–67.
16. Larsson C, Dirksen H, Sundstrom G, et al: Lung function studies in asymptomatic individuals with moderately (Pi SZ) and severely (Pi Z) reduced levels of alpha$_1$-antitrypsin. *Scand J Respir Dis* 57(6):267–80, 1976.
17. Gadek JE, Klein HG, Holland PV, et al: Replacement therapy of alpha$_1$-antitrypsin deficiency: reversal of protease-antiprotease imbalance within the alveolar structures of PiZ subjects. *J Clin Invest* 68(5):1158–65, 1981.
18. Data on file, Miles Inc., Cutter Biological.
19. Wewers MD, Casolaro MA, Sellers SE, et al: Replacement therapy for alpha$_1$-antitrypsin deficiency associated with emphysema. *N Engl J Med* 316(17):1055–62, 1987.
20. Wewers MD, Casolaro MA, Crystal RG: Comparison of alpha-1-antitrypsin levels and antineutrophil elastase capacity of blood and lung in a patient with the alpha-1-antitrypsin phenotype null-null before and during alpha-1-antitrypsin augmentation therapy. *Am Rev Respir Dis* 135(3):539-43, 1987.
21. Burrows B: A clinical trial of efficacy of antiproteolytic therapy: can it be done? *Am Rev Respir Dis* 127(2:2):S42–3, 1983.
22. Cohen AB: Unraveling the mysteries of alpha$_1$-antitrypsin deficiency. *N Engl J Med* 314(12):778–9, 1986.
23. Finlayson JS: Albumin products. *Semin Thromb Hemost* 6(2);85-120, 1980.

ANTITHROMBIN III (HUMAN) ℞
THROMBATE III™ AT-III

DESCRIPTION

Antithrombin III (Human), THROMBATE III™, is a sterile, stable, lyophilized preparation of purified human antithrombin III.

THROMBATE III is prepared from pooled units of human plasma from normal donors by modifications and refinements of the cold ethanol method of Cohn.[1] When reconstituted, THROMBATE III has a pH of 6.0–7.5, a sodium content of 110–210 mEq/L, a chloride content of 110–210 mEq/L, an alanine content of 0.075–0.125 M and a heparin content of not more than 0.004 unit/IU AT-III. THROMBATE III contains no preservative and must be administered by the intravenous route. In addition, THROMBATE III has been heat-treated in solution at 60°C ± 0.5°C for not less than 10 hours.

Each vial of THROMBATE III contains the labeled amount of antithrombin III in international units (IU) per vial. The potency assignment has been determined with a standard calibrated against a World Health Organization (WHO) antithrombin III reference preparation.

CLINICAL PHARMACOLOGY

Antithrombin III (AT-III), an alpha$_2$-glycoprotein of molecular weight 58,000, is normally present in human plasma at a concentration of approximately 12.5 mg/dL[2,3] and is the major plasma inhibitor of thrombin.[4] Inactivation of thrombin by AT-III occurs by formation of a covalent bond resulting in an inactive 1:1 stoichiometric complex between the two, involving an interaction of the active serine of thrombin and an arginine reactive site on AT-III.[4] AT-III is also capable of inactivating other components of the coagulation cascade including factors IXa, Xa, XIa, and XIIa, as well as plasmin.[4]

The neutralization rate of serine proteases by AT-III proceeds slowly in the absence of heparin, but is greatly accelerated in the presence of heparin.[4] As the therapeutic antithrombotic effect in vivo of heparin is mediated by AT-III, heparin is ineffective in the absence or near absence of AT-III.[4–8]

The prevalence of the hereditary deficiency of AT-III is estimated to be one per 2000 to 5000 in the general population.[4,7] The pattern of inheritance is autosomal dominant. In affected individuals, spontaneous episodes of thrombosis and pulmonary embolism may be associated with AT-III levels of 40%–60% of normal.[7] These episodes usually appear after the age of 20, the risk increasing with age and in association with surgery, pregnancy and delivery. The frequency of thromboembolic events in hereditary antithrombin III (AT-III) deficiency during pregnancy has been reported to be 70%, and several studies of the beneficial use of Antithrombin III (Human) concentrates during pregnancy in women with hereditary deficiency have been reported.[9–11] In many cases, however, no precipitating factor can be identified for venous thrombosis or pulmonary embolism.[7] Greater than 85% of individuals with hereditary AT-III deficiency have had at least one thrombotic episode by the age of 50 years.[7] In about 60% of patients thrombosis is recurrent. Clinical signs of pulmonary embolism occur in 40% of affected individuals.[7] In some individuals, treatment with oral anticoagulants leads to an increase of the endogenous levels of AT-III, and treatment with oral anticoagulants may be effective in the prevention of thrombosis in such individuals.[6,7]

In clinical studies of Antithrombin III (Human), THROMBATE III™ conducted in 10 asymptomatic subjects with hereditary deficiency of AT-III, the mean in vivo recovery of AT-III was 1.6% per unit per kg administered based on immunologic AT-III assays, and 1.4% per unit per kg administered based on functional AT-III assays.[12] The mean 50% disappearance time (the time to fall to 50% of the peak plasma level following an initial administration) was approximately 22 hours and the biologic half-life was 2.5 days based on immunologic assays and 3.8 days based on functional assays of AT-III.[12] These values are similar to the half-life for radiolabeled Antithrombin III (Human) reported in the literature of 2.8–4.8 days.[13–15]

In clinical studies of THROMBATE III, none of the 13 patients with hereditary AT-III deficiency and histories of thromboembolism treated prophylactically on 16 separate occasions with THROMBATE III for high thrombotic risk situations (11 surgical procedures, 5 deliveries) developed a thrombotic complication. Heparin was also administered in 3 of the 11 surgical procedures and all 5 deliveries. Eight patients with hereditary AT-III deficiency were treated therapeutically with THROMBATE III as well as heparin for major thrombotic or thromboembolic complications, with seven patients recovering. Treatment with THROMBATE III reversed heparin resistance in two patients with hereditary AT-III deficiency being treated for thrombosis or thromboembolism.

During clinical investigation of THROMBATE III, none of the 12 subjects monitored for a median of 8 months (range 2–19 months) after receiving THROMBATE III, became antibody positive to human immunodeficiency virus (HIV-1). None of 14 subjects monitored for ≥ 3 months demonstrated any evidence of hepatitis, either non-A, non-B hepatitis or hepatitis B.

INDICATIONS AND USAGE

THROMBATE III is indicated for the treatment of patients with hereditary antithrombin III deficiency in connection with surgical or obstetrical procedures or when they suffer from thromboembolism.

Subjects with AT-III deficiency should be informed about the risk of thrombosis in connection with pregnancy and surgery and about the inheritance of the disease.

The diagnosis of hereditary antithrombin III (AT-III) deficiency should be based on a clear family history of venous

Continued on next page

Miles Biological—Cont.

thrombosis as well as decreased plasma AT-III levels, and the exclusion of acquired deficiency.

AT-III in plasma may be measured by amidolytic assays using synthetic chromogenic substrates, by clotting assays, or by immunoassays. The latter does not detect all hereditary AT-III deficiencies.[16]

The AT-III level in neonates of parents with hereditary AT-III deficiency should be measured immediately after birth. (Fatal neonatal thromboembolism, such as aortic thrombi in children of women with hereditary antithrombin III deficiency, has been reported.)[17]

Plasma levels of AT-III are lower in neonates than adults, averaging approximately 60% in normal term infants.[18,19] AT-III levels in premature infants may be much lower.[18,19] Low plasma AT-III levels, especially in a premature infant, therefore, do not necessarily indicate hereditary deficiency. It is recommended that testing and treatment with Antithrombin III (Human), THROMBATE III™ of neonates be discussed with an expert on coagulation.[11]

CONTRAINDICATIONS

None known.

WARNINGS

This product is prepared from pooled human plasma which may contain the causative agents of hepatitis and other viral diseases. Prescribed manufacturing procedures utilized at the plasma collection centers, plasma testing laboratories, and the fractionation facilities are designed to reduce the risk of transmitting viral infection. However, the risk of viral infectivity from this product cannot be totally eliminated.

Individuals who receive multiple infusions of blood or plasma products may develop signs and/or symptoms of some viral infections, particularly non-A, non-B hepatitis.

The anticoagulant effect of heparin is enhanced by concurrent treatment with THROMBATE III in patients with hereditary AT-III deficiency. Thus, in order to avoid bleeding, reduced dosage of heparin is recommended during treatment with THROMBATE III.

PRECAUTIONS

General

1. Administer within 3 hours after reconstitution. Do not refrigerate after reconstitution.
2. Administer only by the intravenous route.
3. THROMBATE III should be given alone, without mixing with other agents or diluting solutions.
4. Administration equipment and any reconstituted THROMBATE III not used should be appropriately discarded.

The diagnosis of hereditary antithrombin III (AT-III) deficiency should be based on a clear family history of venous thrombosis as well as decreased plasma AT-III levels, and the exclusion of acquired deficiency.

Laboratory Tests

It is recommended that AT-III plasma levels be monitored during the treatment period. Functional levels of AT-III in plasma may be measured by amidolytic assays using chromogenic substrates or by clotting assays.

Drug Interactions

The anticoagulant effect of heparin is enhanced by concurrent treatment with Antithrombin III (Human), THROMBATE III™ in patients with hereditary AT-III deficiency. Thus, in order to avoid bleeding, reduced dosage of heparin is recommended during treatment with THROMBATE III.

Pregnancy Category C

Animal reproduction studies have not been conducted with THROMBATE III. It is also not known whether THROMBATE III can cause fetal harm when administered to a pregnant woman or can affect reproduction capacity. THROMBATE III should be given to a pregnant woman only if clearly needed.

Pediatric Use

Safety and effectiveness in children have not been established. The AT-III level in neonates of parents with hereditary AT-III deficiency should be measured immediately after birth. (Fatal neonatal thromboembolism, such as aortic thrombi in children of women with hereditary antithrombin III deficiency, has been reported.)[17]

Plasma levels of AT-III are lower in neonates than adults, averaging approximately 60% in normal term infants.[18,19] AT-III levels in premature infants may be much lower.[18,19] Low plasma AT-III levels, especially in a premature infant, therefore, do not necessarily indicate hereditary deficiency. It is recommended that testing and treatment with THROMBATE III of neonates be discussed with an expert on coagulation.[11]

ADVERSE REACTIONS

In clinical studies involving THROMBATE III, adverse reactions were reported in association with 17 of the 340 infusions during the clinical studies. Included were dizziness (7), chest tightness (3), nausea (3), foul taste in mouth (3), chills (2), cramps (2), shortness of breath (1), chest pain (1), film over eye (1), light-headedness (1), bowel fullness (1), hives (1), fever (1), and oozing and hematoma formation (1). If adverse reactions are experienced, the infusion rate should be decreased, or if indicated, the infusion should be interrupted until symptoms abate.

DOSAGE AND ADMINISTRATION

Each bottle of THROMBATE III has the functional activity, in international units (IU), stated on the label of the bottle. The potency assignment has been determined with a standard calibrated against a World Health Organization antithrombin III reference preparation.

Dosage should be determined on an individual basis based on the pre-therapy plasma antithrombin III (AT-III) level, in order to increase plasma AT-III levels to the level found in normal human plasma (100%). Dosage of THROMBATE III can be calculated from the following formula:

$$\text{units required (IU)} = \frac{[\text{desired - baseline AT-III level}^*] \times \text{weight (kg)}}{1.4}$$

*expressed as % normal level based on functional AT-III assay

The above formula is based on an expected incremental in vivo recovery above baseline levels for Antithrombin III (Human). THROMBATE III™ of 1.4% per IU per kg administered.[12] Thus, if a 70 kg individual has a baseline AT-III level of 57%, in order to increase plasma AT-III to 120%, the initial THROMBATE III dose would be $[(120-57) \times 70]/1.4 =$ 3150 IU total.

However, recovery may vary, and initially levels should be drawn at baseline and 20 minutes postinfusion. Subsequent doses can be calculated based on the recovery of the first dose. These recommendations are intended only as a guide for therapy. The exact loading dose and maintenance intervals should be individualized for each patient.

It is recommended that following an initial dose of THROMBATE III, plasma levels of AT-III be initially monitored at least every 12 hours and before the next infusion of THROMBATE III to maintain plasma AT-III levels greater than 80%. In some situations, e.g., following surgery,[20] hemorrhage or acute thrombosis, and during intravenous heparin administration,[13,21–23] the half-life of Antithrombin III (Human) has been reported to be shortened. In such conditions, plasma AT-III levels should be monitored more frequently, and THROMBATE III administered as necessary.

When an infusion of THROMBATE III is indicated for a patient with hereditary deficiency to control an acute thrombotic episode or prevent thrombosis following surgical or obstetrical procedures, it is desirable to raise the AT-III level to normal and maintain this level for 2 to 8 days, depending on the indication for treatment, type and extent of surgery, patient's medical condition, past history and physician's judgment. Concomitant administration of heparin in each of these situations should be based on the medical judgment of the physician.

As a general recommendation, the following therapeutic program may be utilized as a starting program for treatment, modifying the program based on the actual plasma AT-III levels achieved:

a) An initial loading dose of THROMBATE III calculated to elevate the plasma AT-III level to 120%, assuming an expected rise over the baseline plasma AT-III level of 1.4% (functional activity) per IU per kg of THROMBATE III administered. Thus, if an individual has a baseline AT-III level of 57%, the initial THROMBATE III dose would be $(120-57)/1.4 = 45$ IU/kg.

b) Measure preinfusion and 20 minutes postinfusion (peak) plasma antithrombin III levels following the initial dose, plasma antithrombin III level after 12 hours, then preceding the next infusion (trough level). Subsequently measure antithrombin III levels preceding and 20 minutes after each infusion until predictable peak and trough levels have been achieved, generally between 80%–120%. Plasma levels between 80%–120% may be maintained by administration of maintenance doses of 60% of the initial loading dose, administered every 24 hours. Adjustments in the maintenance dose and/or interval between doses should be made based on actual plasma AT-III levels achieved.

The above recommendations for dosing are provided as a general guideline for therapy only. The exact loading and maintenance dosages and dosing intervals should be individualized for each subject, based on the individual clinical conditions, response to therapy, and actual plasma AT-III levels achieved. In some situations, e.g., following surgery,[20] with hemorrhage or acute thrombosis and during intravenous heparin administration,[13,21–23] in vivo survival of infused Antithrombin III (Human), THROMBATE III™ has been reported to be shortened, resulting in the need to administer THROMBATE III more frequently.

THROMBATE III should be reconstituted with Sterile Water for Injection, USP and brought to room temperature prior to administration. THROMBATE III should be filtered through a sterile filter needle as supplied in the package prior to use, and should be administered within 3 hours following reconstitution. THROMBATE III may be infused over 10–20 minutes. THROMBATE III must be administered intravenously.

Parenteral drug products should be inspected visually for particulate matter and discoloration prior to administration, whenever solution and container permit.

Reconstitution

Vacuum Transfer

1. Warm the unopened diluent and the concentrate to room temperature (NMT 37°C, 99°F).
2. After removing the plastic flip-top caps (Fig. A), aseptically cleanse the rubber stoppers of both bottles.
3. Remove the protective cover from the plastic transfer needle cartridge with tamper-proof seal and penetrate the stopper of the diluent bottle (Fig. B).
4. Remove the remaining portion of the plastic cartridge, invert the diluent bottle and penetrate the rubber seal on the concentrate bottle (Fig. C) with the needle at an angle. Alternate method of transferring sterile water: With a sterile needle and syringe, withdraw the appropriate volume of diluent and transfer to the bottle of lyophilized concentrate.
5. The vacuum will draw the diluent into the concentrate bottle. Hold the diluent bottle at an angle to the concentrate bottle in order to direct the jet of diluent against the wall of the concentrate bottle (Fig. C). Avoid excessive foaming.
6. After removing the diluent bottle and transfer needle (Fig. D), swirl continuously until completely dissolved (Fig. E).
7. After the concentrate powder is completely dissolved, withdraw solution into the syringe through the filter needle which is supplied in the package (Fig. F). Replace the filter needle with an administration set (not provided) and inject intravenously.
8. If the same patient is to receive more than one bottle, the contents of two bottles may be drawn into the same syringe through a separate unused filter needle before attaching the vein needle.

Rate of Administration

The rate of administration should be adapted to the response of the individual patient, but administration of the entire dose in 10 to 20 minutes is generally well-tolerated.

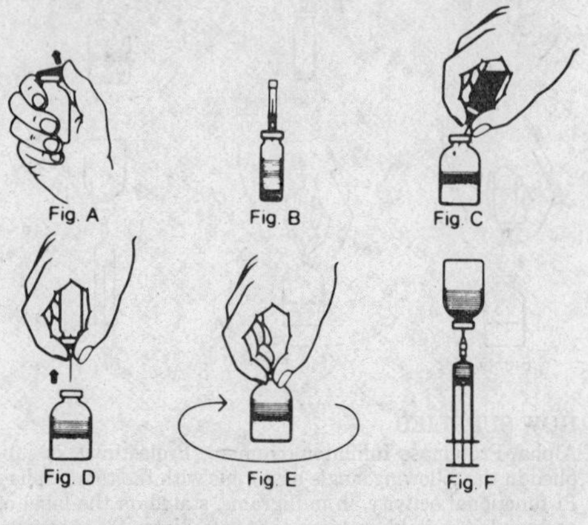
Fig. A
Fig. B
Fig. C
Fig. D
Fig. E
Fig. F

HOW SUPPLIED

Antithrombin III (Human), THROMBATE III™ is supplied in the following single dose vials with the potency in international units stated on the label of each vial. A suitable volume of Sterile Water for Injection, USP, a sterile double-ended transfer needle, and a sterile filter needle are provided.

NDC No.	Approximate Antithrombin III Potency	Diluent
0161-0603-20	500 IU	10 mL
0161-0603-30	1000 IU	20 mL

STORAGE

THROMBATE III should be stored under refrigeration (2°–8°C; 35°–46°F). Freezing should be avoided as breakage of the diluent bottle might occur.

CAUTION

U.S. federal law prohibits dispensing without prescription.

LIMITED WARRANTY

A number of factors beyond our control could reduce the efficacy of this product or even result in an ill effect following its use. These include improper storage and handling of the product after it leaves our hands, diagnosis, dosage, method of administration, and biological differences in individual patients. Because of these factors, it is important that this product be stored properly, that the directions be followed carefully during use, and that the risk of transmitting viruses be carefully weighed before the product is prescribed. No warranty, express or implied, including any warranty of

merchantability or fitness is made. Representatives of the Company are not authorized to vary the terms or the contents of the printed labeling, including the package insert for this product, except by printed notice from the Company's headquarters. The prescriber and user of this product must accept the terms hereof.

REFERENCES

1. Cohn EJ, Strong LE, Hughes WL Jr, et al: Preparation and properties of serum and plasma proteins. IV. A system for the separation into fractions of the protein and lipoprotein components of biological tissues and fluids. *J Am Chem Soc* 68(3):459–75, 1946.
2. Rosenberg RD, Bauer KA, Marcum JA: Antithrombin III "the heparin-antithrombin system." *Rev Hematol* 2:351–416, 1986.
3. Murano G, Williams L, Miller-Andersson M: Some properties of antithrombin-III and its concentration in human plasma. *Thromb Res* 18(1–2):259–62, 1980.
4. Rosenberg RD: Action and interactions of antithrombin and heparin. *N Engl J Med* 292(3):146–51, 1975.
5. Winter JH, Fenech A, Ridley W, et al: Familial antithrombin III deficiency. *Q J Med* 51(204):373–95, 1982.
6. Marciniak E, Farley CH, DeSimone PA: Familial thrombosis due to antithrombin III deficiency. *Blood* 43(2):219–31, 1974.
7. Thaler E, Lechner K: Antithrombin III deficiency and thromboembolism. *Clin Haematol* 10(2):369–90, 1981.
8. Blauhut B, Necek S, Kramar H, et al: Activity of antithrombin III and effect of heparin on coagulation in shock. *Thromb Res* 19(6):775–82, 1980.
9. Samson D, Stirling Y, Woolf L, et al: Management of planned pregnancy in a patient with congenital antithrombin III deficiency. *Br J Haematol* 56(2):243–9, 1984.
10. Brandt P: Observations during the treatment of antithrombin-III deficient women with heparin and antithrombin concentrate during pregnancy, parturition, and abortion. *Thromb Res* 22(1–2):15–24, 1981.
11. Hellgren M, Tengborn L, Abildgaard U: Pregnancy in women with congenital antithrombin III deficiency; experience of treatment with heparin and antithrombin. *Gynecol Obstet Invest* 14(2):127–41, 1982.
12. Schwartz RS, Bauer KA, Rosenberg RD, et al: Clinical experience with antithrombin III concentrate in treatment of congenital and acquired deficiency of antithrombin. *Am J Med* 87 (Suppl 3B): 53S–60S, 1989.
13. Collen D, Schetz J, de Cock F, et al: Metabolism of antithrombin III (heparin cofactor) in man; effects of venous thrombosis and of heparin administration. *Eur J Clin Invest* 7(1):27–35, 1977.
14. Knot EAR, de Jong E, ten Cate JW, et al: Purified radiolabeled antithrombin III metabolism in three families with hereditary AT III deficiency: application of a three-compartment model. *Blood* 67(1):93–8, 1986.
15. Tengborn L, Frohm B, Nilsson LE, et al: Antithrombin III concentrate; its catabolism in health and in antithrombin III deficiency. *Scand J Clin Lab Invest* 41(5):469–77, 1981.
16. Sas G, Blasko G, Banhegyi D, et al: Abnormal antithrombin III (antithrombin III "Budapest") as a cause of familial thrombophilia. *Thromb Diath Haemorrh* 32(1):105–15, 1974.
17. Bjarke B, Herin P, Blomback M: Neonatal aortic thrombosis. A possible clinical manifestation of congenital antithrombin III deficiency. *Acta Paediatr Scand* 63:297–301, 1974.
18. Hathaway WE, Bonnar J: Perinatal coagulation, New York, Grune & Stratton, 1978, p.68.
19. Peters M, Jansen E, ten Cate JW, et al: Neonatal antithrombin III. *Br J Haematol* 58(4):579–87, 1984.
20. Mannucci PM, Boyer C, Wolf M, et al: Treatment of congenital antithrombin III deficiency with concentrates. *Br J Haematol* 50(3):531–5, 1982.
21. Marciniak E, Gockerman JP: Heparin-induced decrease in circulating antithrombin-III. *Lancet* 2(8038):581–4, 1977.
22. O'Brien JR, Etherington MD: Effect of heparin and warfarin on antithrombin III. *Lancet* 2(8050):1232, 1977.
23. Kakkar VV, Bentley PG, Scully MF, et al: Antithrombin III and heparin. *Lancet* 1(8159):103–4, 1980.

U.S. License No. 8
Miles Inc,
Cutter Biological
Elkart, IN 46515 USA

Milex Products, Inc.
**5915 NORTHWEST HIGHWAY
CHICAGO, IL 60631**

AMINO-CERV™   ℞
[ah-me 'no-serv]
pH 5.5 Cervical Creme

ACTIVE INGREDIENTS
Urea 8.34%, Sodium Propionate 0.50%, Methionine 0.83%, Cystine 0.35%, Inositol 0.83%, Benzalkonium Chloride 0.000004%. Buffered to pH of 5.5 in a water-miscible creme base.

DESCRIPTION
An AMINO-ACID and UREA creme specifically formulated for cervical treatment: Cervicitis (mild), postpartum cervicitis, postpartum cervical tears, post cauterization, post cryo-surgery and post conization.

ADVANTAGES
METHIONINE and CYSTINE are amino-acids necessary for wound healing and forming of epithelial tissue. INOSITOL acts as an essential growth factor and promotes epithelialization.
UREA aids in debridement, dissolves the coagulum and promotes epithelialization. Its solvent action on fibroblasts prevents the formation of excessive tissue—thus preventing stenosis when used as directed.
BENZALKONIUM CHLORIDE serves to lower surface tension and thus aids in spreading the medication. Along with SODIUM PROPIONATE it also exerts a bacteriostatic effect.
AMINO-CERV is geared to the higher pH of the healthy cervix in contrast with pH 4 vaginal preparations. With its pH factor of 5.5 Amino-Cerv promotes faster healing of the cervix, yet will not adversely affect a healthy vagina.

DIRECTIONS
When immediate postpartum bleeding has subsided (usually from 24 to 48 hours after delivery), one Milex-Jector full of AMINO-CERV creme should be applied nightly for four weeks. In mild CERVICITIS (not requiring cautery or cryo-surgery) one applicatorful of AMINO-CERV should be injected in the vagina nightly upon retiring for 2 weeks.
A small amount of AMINO-CERV should be applied immediately after HOT CAUTERIZATION, HOT CONIZATION and CRYOSURGERY. One applicatorful should be injected nightly upon retiring for 2 to 4 weeks (the duration of treatment depends on extent of cauterization or hot conization or cryosurgery). During the weekly office visit for (2 to 4 visits) the physician should again apply a small amount of AMINO-CERV with a probe or applicator. The canal is to be completely probed on the last visit.
After COLD CONING, one applicatorful should be injected upon retiring about 24 hours after surgery and nightly thereafter for four weeks. During the four weekly office visits following cold coning, a small amount of AMINO-CERV should be applied with a probe or applicator into the canal by the physician. The canal is to be completely probed on the last visit.
Reasons For Variation of Directions:
(1) After hot conization, cauterization and cryosurgery immediate use of AMINO-CERV is indicated to aid in dissolving dead or burned tissue.
(2) After cold coning, there is no dead tissue to slough off. Therefore, a wait of 24 hours or longer is desirable for normal healing to take place and for some fibroblasts to be laid down before applying the AMINO-CERV (which has a solvent action on both the fibroblasts and the absorbable sutures). When NONABSORBABLE sutures are used, AMINO-CERV can be used immediately.

CONTRAINDICATIONS
Deleterious side effects have not been a problem at the doses recommended. The usual precautions against allergic reactions should be observed.

STORAGE
Store at room temperature.

PACKAGING
2¾ oz. tube with Milex-Jector (2 weeks supply, 14 applications).
Available only on hospital direct orders: 5½ oz. tube with MILEX-JECTOR (4 weeks supply, 28 applications).

PRO-CEPTION   OTC
[pro-sep 'shun]

DESCRIPTION
PRO-CEPTION is a precoital douche to help promote conception. It provides in a convenient form supplementary nutrient immediately available to the sperm for metabolism and movement. Also effective for removal of a thick tenacious mucous plug of the cervix.

DIRECTIONS
The screw cap is used as a measuring device and filled level with the powder which is then dissolved in eight ounces of lukewarm water. The woman is told to douche while in a recumbent position and to retain the solution (10 to 15 minutes). Following coitus the patient should remain recumbent for two hours or more. May be used as a companion with Milex Oligospermia Cups.

CONTRAINDICATIONS
None.

PACKAGING
Available in 12 douche container.

Mission Pharmacal Company
**1325 E. DURANGO ST.
SAN ANTONIO, TX 78210**

CALCET®   OTC
[kăl 'cet]
Calcium Supplement
NDC-0178-0251-01

HOW SUPPLIED
CALCET® tablets are supplied as yellow, oval shaped, coated tablets in bottles of 100 tablets.

CALCET PLUS™   OTC
[kăl 'cet]
Calcium-Iron-Zinc-Multivitamin
NDC 0178-0252-60

HOW SUPPLIED
CALCET PLUS tablets are supplied as white, oval shaped, coated tablets in bottles of 60's.

CITRACAL®   OTC
[sit 'ra-cal]
Ultradense Calcium Citrate 950 mg

HOW SUPPLIED
CITRACAL® NDC 0178-0800-01 is supplied as white, bolus shaped, sugar coated tablets in bottles of 100 tablets each. For product information call: 1-800-531-3333
                                  In Texas: 1-800-292-7364

CITRACAL® Caplets +D   OTC
Ultradense Calcium Citrate 1500 mg

HOW SUPPLIED
CITRACAL® CAPLETS NDC 0178-0815-60 is supplied as white capsule shaped, sugar coated tablets in bottles of 60 tablets each. For product information call: 1-800-531-3333
                                  In Texas: 1-800-292-7364

CITRACAL® LIQUITAB   OTC
[sit 'ra-cal lĭc 'wĭ-tab]
**Presolubilized Calcium Citrate
Effervescent Citrus Flavored Tablets**

HOW SUPPLIED
CITRACAL® LIQUITAB NDC 0178-0811-30 is supplied as white wafers in bottles of 30 tablets each. For product information call: 1-800-531-3333
                                  In Texas: 1-800-292-7364

COMPETE®   OTC
[kŏm 'pēt]
Multivitamins with Iron and Zinc
NDC-0178-0221-01

HOW SUPPLIED
COMPETE® is supplied as orange, football-shaped, sugar coated tablets in bottles of 100.

Continued on next page

Mission Pharamcal—Cont.

FERRALET®   OTC
[fer "a-lét]
Ferrous Gluconate
NDC-0178-0082-01

HOW SUPPLIED
FERRALET® is packaged in bottles of 100 tablets.

FOSFREE®   OTC
[fos 'frē]
Calcium—Vitamins—Iron
NDC-0178-0031-01

HOW SUPPLIED
FOSFREE® is supplied as yellow capsule shaped coated tablets in bottles of 100 tablets.

IROMIN-G®   OTC
[i 'rŏ-min]
Hematinic Supplement
NDC-0178-0081-01

HOW SUPPLIED
IROMIN-G® is supplied as red football shaped coated tablets in bottles of 100 tablets.

MEDILAX™   OTC
[měd 'i-laks]
Phenolphthalein tablets, U.S.P.
NDC 0178-0095-24

HOW SUPPLIED
MEDILAX™ is supplied in yellow scored tablets in film strip package of 24 tablets.

MISSION PHARMACAL UROLOGICALS

CALCIBIND®   ℞
[kal 'sē-bĭnd]
Cellulose Sodium Phosphate
Oral Powder

DESCRIPTION
Cellulose Sodium Phosphate (CSP), the active ingredient in CALCIBIND®, is a synthetic compound made by phosphorylation of cellulose and has the following structural formula:

Where n indicates the degree of polymerization and has an average value of approximately 3000. The molecular weight of CSP monomer is 286.1 and the average molecular weight of the polymer is 858,000.
It has an inorganic bound phosphate of 31–36%, free phosphate of 3.5%, sodium content of approximately 11% and a calcium binding capacity of 1.8 mmol of Ca per gram of the oral powder. It has excellent ion exchange properties, the sodium ion exchanging for calcium. When taken orally, CSP binds calcium, the complex of calcium and cellulose phosphate being excreted in feces. The dosage of CALCIBIND® is powder for oral administration.

HOW SUPPLIED
CALCIBIND® NDC 0178-0255-30 is available for oral administration in bottles of 300 grams of CSP bulk powder.

LITHOSTAT®   ℞
[lith 'o-stat]
Acetohydroxamic Acid (AHA)

DESCRIPTION
Acetohydroxamic acid (AHA) is a stable, synthetic compound derived from hydroxylamine and ethyl acetate. Its molecular structure is similar to urea:

ACETOHYDROXAMIC ACID (AHA)
AHA is weakly acidic, highly soluble in water, and chelates metals - notably iron. The molecular weight is 75.068. AHA has a PKA of 9.32 and a melting point of 89–91°C. Available as 250 mg tablets.

HOW SUPPLIED
LITHOSTAT®, NDC 0178-0500-01, is available for oral administration as 250 mg scored tablets, in unit of use packages of 100 tablets.

THIOLA™   ℞
[thi-ŏl-a]
Tiopronin Tablets

DESCRIPTION
THIOLA™ (Tiopronin) is a reducing and complexing thiol compound. Tiopronin is N-(2-Mercaptopropionyl) glycine and has the following structure:

$$CH_3\text{-}CH\text{-}CONHCH_2\text{-}COOH$$
$$SH$$

Tiopronin has the empirical formula $C_5H_9NO_3S$ and a molecular weight of 163.20. It has one asymmetric center and therefore exists as dl (racemic) mixture.
Tiopronin is a white crystalline powder which is freely soluble in water.
THIOLA™ tablets are white sugar coated tablets, each containing 100 mg. of Tiopronin and are taken orally.

HOW SUPPLIED
THIOLA™ (NDC 0178-0900-01), is available for oral administration as 100 mg. round, white, sugar coated tablets in bottles of 100 tablets each.
For product information call: 1-800-531-3333
In Texas call: 1-800-292-7364

UROCIT®-K   ℞
[yu 'ro-cĭt kay]
Potassium Citrate
WAX MATRIX TABLETS

DESCRIPTION
Urocit®-K is a citrate salt of potassium. Its empirical formula is $K_3C_6H_5O_7 \cdot H_2O$, and its structural formula is:

$$CH_2\text{---}COOK$$
$$HO\text{---}C\text{---}COOK \cdot H_2O$$
$$CH_2\text{---}COOK$$

Potassium citrate is a white granular powder that is soluble in water at 154g/100 ml, almost insoluble in alcohol, and insoluble in organic solvents.
Urocit®-K is supplied as wax matrix tablets, containing 5 meq (540 mg) potassium citrate each, for oral administration.

HOW SUPPLIED
Urocit®-K (NDC 0178-0600-01) is available for oral administration in tablet form (5 meq potassium citrate/tablet), in bottles each containing 100 tablets.

MISSION PRENATAL SERIES

MISSION PRENATAL®   OTC
Vitamins—Iron—Calcium—.4 mg. Folic Acid
NDC 0178-132-01

MISSION PRENATAL® F.A.   OTC
Vitamins—Iron—Calcium—.8 mg. Folic Acid and Zinc
NDC 0178-0153-01

MISSION PRENATAL® H.P.   OTC
Vitamins—Iron—Calcium—0.8 mg. Folic Acid
NDC 0178-0161-01

HOW SUPPLIED
MISSION® PRENATAL is supplied as pink, football-shaped, sugar-coated tablets in bottles of 100.
MISSION® PRENATAL F.A. is supplied as blue, football-shaped, sugar coated tablets in bottles of 100.
MISSION® PRENATAL H.P. is supplied as green, football-shaped, sugar-coated tablets in bottles of 100.

MISSION PRENATAL™ Rx   ℞
Prenatal Supplement with
Vitamins and Minerals
NDC 0178-0007-01

HOW SUPPLIED
MISSION PRENATAL Rx is supplied as pink, football shape, film-coated tablets in bottles of 100.

MISSION® SURGICAL SUPPLEMENT   OTC
A dietary supplement for pre-surgical and
post-surgical patients. NDC 0178-0168-01

HOW SUPPLIED
MISSION® PRE-SURGICAL is supplied as a light green, bolus-shaped, sugar coated tablet in bottles of 100.

PRULET®   OTC
[prŭ-let']
Phenolphthalein Tablets U.S.P.
NDC 0178-0090-01

HOW SUPPLIED
PRULET® is supplied in green scored tablets in film strip packages of 12 and 40 tables.

SUPAC®   OTC
[sŭ 'pac]
Analgesic Compound
NDC-0178-0100-01

HOW SUPPLIED
SUPAC® is supplied as white scored tablets in bottles of 100 and 1000 tablets.

THERABID®   OTC
[thĕr 'a-bid]
Therapeutic Multivitamin
NDC 0178-0171-01

HOW SUPPLIED
THERABID® is supplied as green capsule shaped sugar coated tablets in bottles of 100 tablets.

THERA-GESIC®   OTC
[ther 'a-jē-zik]
Analgesic Creme Balm
Methyl Salicylate and Menthol

DESCRIPTION
THERA-GESIC® contains Methyl Salicylate and Menthol in a rapidly absorbed greaseless base.

ACTIONS
Topical analgesic, counterirritant.

INDICATIONS
For the temporary relief of pain associated with musculo-skeletal soreness and discomfort; additionally, as a topical adjunct in arthritis, rheumatism, and bursitis.

CONTRAINDICATIONS
Do not use in patients with Aspirin or Salicylate idiosyncrasy.

WARNINGS
Use only as directed. Keep away from children to avoid accidental poisoning. Keep away from eyes, mucous membranes, broken or irritated skin. If skin irritation develops, or if pain lasts 10 days or more, or if redness is present, discontinue use and consult a physician. DO NOT SWALLOW. If swallowed, induce vomiting, call a physician.

PRECAUTIONS
Do not use excessive amounts of THERA-GESIC® or occlude a fresh application of THERA-GESIC®. Do not heat pack THERA-GESIC® covered skin. For use by adults only.

ADVERSE REACTIONS
Adverse reactions related to the Salicylate and Menthol components are possible. These include excessive irritation, tinnitus, nausea or vomiting if excessive or extreme dosage is employed.

DOSAGE AND ADMINISTRATION
Gently massage THERA-GESIC® in thin applications into the sore or painful area as well as into the area immediately surrounding the painful area. The number of thin applications applied controls the intensity of the action of THERA-GESIC®. One application provides a mild effect, two provide a strong effect and three applications provide a very strong effect. Once THERA-GESIC® has penetrated the skin, the area may be washed, leaving the area dry, clean and free from the typical wintergreen odor without decreasing the effectiveness of the product. If you intend to bandage or wrap the area, the area should be washed first to avoid excessive irritation.

HOW SUPPLIED
NDC-0178-0320-03 Tubes–3 oz.
NDC-0178-0320-05 Tubes–5 oz.

Muro Pharmaceutical, Inc.
890 EAST STREET
TEWKSBURY, MA 01876-9987

BROMFED® CAPSULES ℞
[brōm 'fĕd]

A light green and clear capsule containing white beads. Timed-Release.
Each capsule contains:
Brompheniramine maleate .... 12 mg
Pseudoephedrine hydrochloride .... 120 mg
in a specially prepared base to provide prolonged action.

BROMFED-PD® CAPSULES ℞
A dark green and clear capsule containing white beads. Timed-Release.
Each capsule contains:
Brompheniramine maleate .... 6 mg
Pseudoephedrine hydrochloride .... 60 mg
in a specially prepared base to provide prolonged action.

BROMFED® and BROMFED-PD® CAPSULES also contain inactive ingredients: benzyl alcohol, butyl paraben, carboxymethylcellulose sodium, D & C yellow #10, edetate calcium disodium, FD&C blue #1, FD&C yellow #6, gelatin, methyl paraben, pharmaceutical glaze, propyl paraben, sodium lauryl sulfate, sodium propionate, starch, sucrose and other ingredients.

BROMFED® TABLETS ℞
A white scored tablet.
Each tablet contains:
Brompheniramine maleate .... 4 mg
Pseudoephedrine hydrochloride .... 60 mg
Also contains as inactive ingredients colloidal silicon dioxide, lactose, magnesium stearate, microcrystalline cellulose and sodium starch glycolate.

BROMFED® contains ingredients of the following therapeutic classes: antihistamine and decongestant.

CLINICAL PHARMACOLOGY
Brompheniramine maleate is an alkylamine type antihistamine. This group of antihistamines are among the most active histamine antagonists and are generally effective in relatively low doses. The drugs are not so prone to produce drowsiness and are among the most suitable agents for day time use; but again, a significant proportion of patients do experience this effect. Pseudoephedrine hydrochloride is a sympathomimetic which acts predominantly on alpha receptors and has little action on beta receptors. It therefore functions as an oral nasal decongestant with minimal CNS stimulation.

INDICATIONS
For the temporary relief of symptoms of seasonal and perennial allergic rhinitis, and vasomotor rhinitis, including nasal obstruction (congestion).

CONTRAINDICATIONS
Hypersensitivity to any of the ingredients. Also contraindicated in patients with severe hypertension, severe coronary artery disease, patients on MAO inhibitor therapy, patients with narrow-angle glaucoma, urinary retention, peptic ulcer and during an asthmatic attack.

WARNINGS
Considerable caution should be exercised in patients with hypertension, diabetes mellitus, ischemic heart disease, hyperthyroidism, increased intraocular pressure and prostatic hypertrophy. The elderly (60 years or older) are more likely to exhibit adverse reactions. Antihistamines may cause excitability, especially in children. At dosages higher than the recommended dose, nervousness, dizziness or sleeplessness may occur.

PRECAUTIONS
General: Caution should be exercised in patients with high blood pressure, heart disease, diabetes or thyroid disease. The antihistamine in this product may exhibit additive effects with other CNS depressants, including alcohol.
Information for Patients: Antihistamine may cause drowsiness and ambulatory patients who operate machinery or motor vehicles should be cautioned accordingly.
Drug Interactions: MAO inhibitors and beta adrenergic blockers increase the effects of sympathomimetics. Sympathomimetics may reduce the antihypertensive effects of methyldopa, mecamylamine, reserpine and veratrum alkaloids. Concomitant use of antihistamines with alcohol and other CNS depressants may have an additive effect.
Pregnancy: The safety of use of this product in pregnancy has not been established.

ADVERSE REACTIONS
Adverse reactions include drowsiness, lassitude, nausea, giddiness, dryness of mouth, blurred vision, cardiac palpitations, flushing, increased irritability or excitement (especially in children).

DOSAGE AND ADMINISTRATION
BROMFED® CAPSULES Adults and children over 12 years of age—1 capsule every 12 hours.
BROMFED-PD® CAPSULES Adults and children over 12 years of age—1 or 2 capsules every 12 hours. Children 6 to 12 years of age—1 capsule every 12 hours.
BROMFED® TABLETS Adults and children 12 and over: One tablet every 4 hours not to exceed 6 doses in 24 hours. Children 6 to 12 years: One-half tablet every 4 hours not to exceed 6 doses in 24 hours. Do not give to children under 6 years except under the advice and supervision of a physician.

HOW SUPPLIED
BROMFED® CAPSULES. Bottle of 100 (NDC 0451-4000-50) and 500 (NDC 0451-4000-60). Each capsule is coded "BROMFED" "MURO 12-120".
BROMFED-PD® CAPSULES. Bottle of 100 (NDC 0451-4001-50) and 500 (NDC 0451-4001-60). Each capsule is coded "BROMFED-PD" "MURO 6-60".
BROMFED® TABLETS. Bottle of 100 (NDC 0451-4060-50). Each tablet is coded "MURO 4060" on one side and scored on the reverse side.
Dispense in tight child-resistant containers as defined in USP. Store between 15°–30°C (59°–86°F).
CAUTION: FEDERAL (U.S.A.) LAW PROHIBITS DISPENSING WITHOUT A PRESCRIPTION.

BROMFED® SYRUP OTC
[brōm 'fĕd]

(See PDR For Nonprescription Drugs.)

BROMFED-DM® COUGH SYRUP ℞
[brōm 'fĕd]

Each teaspoonful contains:
Brompheniramine maleate .... 2 mg
Pseudoephedrine hydrochloride .... 30 mg
Dextromethorphan hydrobromide .... 10 mg

HOW SUPPLIED
NDC #0451-4101-16—16 fl. oz.

GUAIFED® CAPSULES ℞
[gwī 'ah-fed]

A white opaque and clear capsule containing white beads.
Each capsule contains:
Pseudoephedrine hydrochloride .... 120 mg
in a specially prepared base to provide prolonged action.
Guaifenesin .... 250 mg
designed for immediate release to provide rapid action.

GUAIFED–PD® CAPSULE ℞
A blue and clear capsule containing white beads.
Each capsule contains:
Pseudoephedrine hydrochloride .... 60 mg
in a specially prepared base to provide prolonged action.
Guaifenesin .... 300 mg
designed for immediate release to provide rapid action.

GUAIFED® and GUAIFED-PD® CAPSULES also contain as inactive ingredients: Benzyl Alcohol, Butyl Paraben, Edetate Calcium Disodium, Gelatin, Methyl Paraben, Pharmaceutical Glaze, Propyl Paraben, Sodium Lauryl Sulfate, Sodium Propionate, Starch, Sucrose, Titanium Dioxide, FD&C Blue #1 (GUAIFED-PD only) and other ingredients.

GUAIFED® and **GUAIFED-PD®** contains ingredients of the following therapeutic classes: nasal decongestant and expectorant.

CLINICAL PHARMACOLOGY
Pseudoephedrine hydrochloride is a sympathomimetic which acts predominantly on alpha adrenergic receptors in the mucosa of the respiratory tract, producing vasoconstriction and has little action on beta receptors. It therefore functions as an oral nasal decongestant with minimal CNS stimulation. Pseudoephedrine hydrochloride also increases sinus drainage and secretions. Guaifenesin is an expectorant which increases the output of phlegm (sputum) and bronchial secretions by reducing adhesiveness and surface tension. The increased flow of less viscid secretions promotes ciliary action and changes a dry, unproductive cough to one that is more productive and less frequent.

INDICATIONS
For temporary relief of nasal congestion and dry non-productive cough associated with the common cold and other respiratory allergies. Helps drainage of the bronchial tubes by thinning the mucus.

CONTRAINDICATIONS
This product is contraindicated in patients with a known hypersensitivity to any of its ingredients. Also contraindicated in patients with severe hypertension, severe coronary artery disease and patients on MAO inhibitor therapy. Should not be used during pregnancy or in nursing mothers. Considerable caution should be exercised in patients with hypertension, diabetes mellitus, ischemic heart disease, hyperthyroidism, increased intraocular pressure and prostatic hypertrophy. The elderly (60 years or older) are more likely to exhibit adverse reactions. At dosages higher than the recommended dose, nervousness, dizziness or sleeplessness may occur.

PRECAUTIONS
General: Caution should be exercised in patients with high blood pressure, heart disease, diabetes or thyroid disease and in patients who exhibit difficulty in urination due to enlargement of the prostate gland. Check with a physician if symptoms do not improve within 7 days or if accompanied by high fever, rash or persistent headache.
Drug Interactions: Do not take this product if you are presently taking a prescription drug for high blood pressure or depression, without first consulting a physician. MAO inhibitors and beta adrenergic blockers may increase the effect of sympathomimetics. Sympathomimetics may reduce the antihypertensive effects of methyldopa, mecamylamine, reserpine and veratrum alkaloids. Pseudoephedrine hydrochloride may increase the possibility of cardiac arrhythmias in patients presently taking digitalis glycosides.
Pregnancy: Pregnancy Catagory B. It has been shown that pseudoephedrine hydrochloride can cause reduced average weight, length, and rate of skeletal ossification in the animal fetus.
Nursing Mothers: Pseudoephedrine is excreted in breast milk; use by nursing mother is not recommended because of the higher than usual risk of side effects from sympathomimetic amines for infants, especially newborn and premature infants.
Geriatrics: Pseudoephedrine should be used with caution in the elderly because they may be more sensitive to the effects of the sympathomimetics.

WARNINGS
Do not take this product for persistent or chronic cough such as occurs with smoking, asthma, or emphysema, or where cough is accompanied by excessive secretions except under the advice and supervision of a physician. This medication should be taken a few hours prior to bedtime to minimize the possibility of sleeplessness. Take this medication with a glass of water after each dose, to help loosen mucus in the lungs.

ADVERSE REACTIONS
Adverse reactions include nausea, cardiac palpitations, increased irritability or excitement, headache, dizziness, tachycardia, diarrhea, drowsiness, stomach pain, seizures, slowed heart rate, shortness of breath and/or troubled breathing.

OVERDOSAGE
KEEP THIS AND ALL DRUGS OUT OF THE REACH OF CHILDREN. IN CASE OF SUSPECTED OVERDOSE, IMMEDIATELY CALL YOUR REGIONAL POISON CONTROL CENTER and/or SEEK PROFESSIONAL ASSISTANCE.
Symptoms of overdosage may be caused by pseudoephedrine. Symptoms of overdosage with pseudoephedrine include anxiety, tenseness, respiratory difficulty, headache and awareness of the slow forceful heartbeat.

TREATMENT OF OVERDOSE
The stomach should be emptied promptly by emetics and/or gastric lavage. The installation of activated charcoal also

Continued on next page

Muro—Cont.

should be considered. Cardiac function and serum electrolytes should be monitored and treatment instigated if indicated. If convulsions or marked CNS excitement occurs, diazepam may be used.

DOSAGE AND ADMINISTRATION
GUAIFED® CAPSULES Adults and children over 12 years of age: 1 capsule every 12 hours.
GUAIFED-PD® CAPSULES Adults and children over 12 years of age: 1 or 2 capsules every 12 hours. Children 6 to 12 years of age—1 capsule every 12 hours.

HOW SUPPLIED
GUAIFED® CAPSULES Bottle of 100 (NDC 0451-4002-50) and 500 (NDC 0451-4002-60). Each capsule is coded "GUAIFED" "MURO 120-250".
GUAIFED-PD® CAPSULES Bottle of 100 (NDC 0451-4003-50) and 500 (NDC 0451-4003-60). Each capsule is coded "GUAIFED-PD" "MURO 60-300".
Dispense in tight containers as defined in USP. Store at controlled room temperature, between 15°–30°C (59°–86°F).
Dispense in child resistant container.
Keep this and all drugs out of reach of children.
CAUTION: FEDERAL (U.S.A.) LAW PROHIBITS DISPENSING WITHOUT A PRESCRIPTION.

GUAIFED® SYRUP   OTC

(See PDR For Nonprescription Drugs.)

GUAITAB™ TABLETS   OTC

(See PDR For Nonprescription Drugs.)

IOTUSS® LIQUID   Ⓒ ℞
[ī'ō-tŭs]

Each teaspoonful contains:
Iodinated glycerol, 30 mg (15 mg organically bound iodine), codeine phosphate, (Warning: may be habit forming), 10 mg.

HOW SUPPLIED
NDC 0451-6500-16—16 fl. oz.

IOTUSS–DM® LIQUID   ℞
[ī'ō-tŭs]

Each teaspoonful contains:
Iodinated glycerol, 30 mg (15 mg organically bound iodine), dextromethorphan hydrobromide, 10 mg.

HOW SUPPLIED
NDC 0451-8200-16—16 fl. oz.

LIQUID PRED® SYRUP   ℞

Each teaspoonful contains:
Prednisone 5mg/5mL

HOW SUPPLIED
NDC-0451-1201-04–4 fl. oz. (120 mL)
NDC-0451-1201-08–8 fl. oz. (240 mL)

PRELONE® SYRUP   ℞
(Prednisolone 15 mg per 5 mL)

Each 5 mL of *PRELONE ® Syrup* contains **15 mg** of prednisolone for oral administration. Benzoic acid 0.1% is added as a preservative. It also contains: alcohol 5%, citric acid, edetate disodium, FD&C Blue #1 and Red #40, glycerin, propylene glycol, purified water, sodium saccharin, sucrose, artificial flavor.

HOW SUPPLIED
PRELONE ® Syrup containing **15 mg** of Prednisolone in each 5 mL (teaspoonful) is a red, cherry flavored clear liquid and is supplied in 240 mL bottles. NDC #0451-1500-08.

SALINEX® NASAL MIST AND DROPS   OTC
[sal'i-nĕx]
(Buffered isotonic sodium chloride solution)

(See PDR For Nonprescription Drugs.)

Mylan Pharmaceuticals Inc.
781 CHESTNUT RIDGE ROAD
P.O. BOX 4310
MORGANTOWN, WV 26505-4310

The following list of Mylan products is provided to facilitate identification. It includes the color(s) and identification codes for all tablets and capsules.

PRODUCT GENERIC NAME Description Color(s)	IDENTIFICATION CODE (Front/Back*)
ALBUTEROL SULFATE Tablets, 2 mg. ℞ White	M255/Blank
ALBUTEROL SULFATE Tablets, 4 mg. ℞ White	M572/Blank
ALLOPURINOL Tablets, USP, 100 mg. ℞ White	M31/Blank
ALLOPURINOL Tablets, USP, 300 mg. ℞ White	M71/Blank
AMILORIDE HYDROCHLORIDE and HYDROCHLOROTHIAZIDE Tablets, USP, 5 mg./50 mg. ℞ Lt. Orange	M577/Blank
AMITRIPTYLINE HYDROCHLORIDE Tablets, USP, 10 mg. ℞ White	M77/Blank
AMITRIPTYLINE HYDROCHLORIDE Tablets, USP, 25 mg. ℞ Lt. Green	M51/Blank
AMITRIPTYLINE HYDROCHLORIDE Tablets, USP, 50 mg. ℞ Brown	M36/Blank
AMITRIPTYLINE HYDROCHLORIDE Tablets, USP, 75 mg. ℞ Blue	M37/Blank
AMITRIPTYLINE HYDROCHLORIDE Tablets, USP, 100 mg. ℞ Orange	M38/Blank
AMITRIPTYLINE HYDROCHLORIDE Tablets, USP, 150 mg. ℞ Flesh	M39/Blank
AMOXICILLIN TRIHYDRATE Capsules, USP, 250 mg. ℞ Caramel & Buff	MYLAN 204
AMOXICILLIN TRIHYDRATE Capsules, USP, 500 mg. ℞ Buff & Buff	MYLAN 205
AMOXICILLIN TRIHYDRATE for Oral Suspension, USP, 125 mg./5 ml. ℞	—
AMOXICILLIN TRIHYDRATE for Oral Suspension, USP, 250 mg./5 ml. ℞	—
AMPICILLIN TRIHYDRATE Capsules, USP, 250 mg. ℞ Scarlet & Lt. Gray	MYLAN 115
AMPICILLIN TRIHYDRATE Capsules, USP, 500 mg. ℞ Scarlet & Lt. Gray	MYLAN 116
AMPICILLIN TRIHYDRATE for Oral Suspension, USP, 125 mg./5 ml. ℞	—
AMPICILLIN TRIHYDRATE for Oral Suspension, USP, 250 mg./5 ml. ℞	—
ATENOLOL Tablets, 50 mg. ℞ White	M/231
ATENOLOL Tablets, 100 mg. ℞ White	M/757
CHLORDIAZEPOXIDE and AMITRIPTYLINE HYDROCHLORIDE Tablets, USP, 5 mg./12.5 mg. Ⓒ/℞ Green	MYLAN/211
CHLORDIAZEPOXIDE and AMITRIPTYLINE HYDROCHLORIDE Tablets, USP, 10 mg./25 mg. Ⓒ/℞ White	MYLAN/277
CHLOROTHIAZIDE Tablets, USP, 250 mg. ℞ White	M50
CHLOROTHIAZIDE Tablets, USP, 500 mg. ℞ White	MYLAN 162/Blank
CHLORPROPAMIDE Tablets, USP, 100 mg. ℞ Green	MYLAN 197/100
CHLORPROPAMIDE Tablets, USP, 250 mg. ℞ Green	MYLAN 210/250

PRODUCT	IDENTIFICATION CODE
CHLORTHALIDONE Tablets, USP, 25 mg. ℞ Lt. Yellow	M35/Blank
CHLORTHALIDONE Tablets, USP, 50 mg. ℞ Lt. Green	M75/Blank
CLONIDINE HYDROCHLORIDE Tablets, USP, 0.1 mg. ℞ White	MYLAN 152/Blank
CLONIDINE HYDROCHLORIDE Tablets, USP, 0.2 mg. ℞ White	MYLAN 186/Blank
CLONIDINE HYDROCHLORIDE Tablets, USP, 0.3 mg. ℞ White	MYLAN 199/Blank
CLONIDINE HYDROCHLORIDE and CHLORTHALIDONE Tablets, USP, 0.1 mg./15 mg. ℞ Yellow	M1/Blank
CLONIDINE HYDROCHLORIDE and CHLORTHALIDONE Tablets, USP, 0.2 mg./15 mg. ℞ Yellow	M27/Blank
CLONIDINE HYDROCHLORIDE and CHLORTHALIDONE Tablets, USP, 0.3 mg./15 mg. ℞ Yellow	M72/Blank
CLORAZEPATE DIPOTASSIUM Tablets, 3.75 mg. Ⓒ/℞ Blue	M30/Blank
CLORAZEPATE DIPOTASSIUM Tablets, 7.5 mg. Ⓒ/℞ Peach	M40/Blank
CLORAZEPATE DIPOTASSIUM Tablets, 15 mg. Ⓒ/℞ White	M70/Blank
CYCLOBENZAPRINE HYDROCHLORIDE Tablets, USP, 10 mg. ℞ Butterscotch-Yellow	M/751
CYPROHEPTADINE HYDROCHLORIDE Tablets, USP, 4 mg. ℞ White	M44/Blank
DIAZEPAM Tablets, USP, 2 mg. Ⓒ/℞ White	MYLAN 271/Scored
DIAZEPAM Tablets, USP, 5 mg. Ⓒ/℞ Orange	MYLAN 345/Scored
DIAZEPAM Tablets, USP, 10 mg. Ⓒ/℞ Green	MYLAN 477/Scored
DILTIAZEM HYDROCHLORIDE Tablets, USP, 30 mg. ℞ White	M23/Blank
DILTIAZEM HYDROCHLORIDE Tablets, USP, 60 mg. ℞ White	M45/Blank
DILTIAZEM HYDROCHLORIDE Tablets, USP, 90 mg. ℞ White	M135/Blank
DILTIAZEM HYDROCHLORIDE Tablets, USP, 120 mg. ℞ White	M525/Blank
DIPHENOXYLATE HYDROCHLORIDE and ATROPINE SULFATE Tablets, USP, 2.5 mg./0.025 mg. Ⓒ/℞ White	M15/Blank
DOXEPIN HYDROCHLORIDE Capsules, USP, 10 mg. ℞ Buff & Buff	MYLAN 1049
DOXEPIN HYDROCHLORIDE Capsules, USP, 25 mg. ℞ Ivory & White	MYLAN 3125
DOXEPIN HYDROCHLORIDE Capsules, USP, 50 mg. ℞ Ivory & Ivory	MYLAN 4250
DOXEPIN HYDROCHLORIDE Capsules, USP, 75 mg. ℞ Lt. Green & Lt. Green	MYLAN 5375
DOXEPIN HYDROCHLORIDE Capsules, USP, 100 mg. ℞ Lt. Green & White	MYLAN 6410
DOXYCYCLINE HYCLATE Capsules, USP, 50 mg. ℞ Aqua Blue & White	MYLAN 145
DOXYCYCLINE HYCLATE Capsules, USP, 100 mg. ℞ Aqua Blue & Aqua Blue	MYLAN 148
DOXYCYCLINE HYCLATE Tablets, USP, 100 mg. ℞ Beige	MYLAN 167/100
ERYTHROMYCIN ETHYLSUCCINATE Tablets, USP, 400 mg. ℞ Beige	M400/Blank

Drug	Code
ERYTHROMYCIN STEARATE Tablets, USP, 250 mg. ℞ *Yellow*	MYLAN 106/250
ERYTHROMYCIN STEARATE Tablets, USP, 500 mg. ℞ *Yellow*	MYLAN 107/500
FENOPROFEN CALCIUM Tablets, USP, 600 mg. ℞ *Lt. Orange*	M471/Scored
FLUPHENAZINE HYDROCHLORIDE Tablets, USP, 1 mg. ℞ *White*	M/4
FLUPHENAZINE HYDROCHLORIDE Tablets, USP, 2.5 mg. ℞ *Yellow*	M/9
FLUPHENAZINE HYDROCHLORIDE Tablets, USP, 5 mg. ℞ *Green*	M/74
FLUPHENAZINE HYDROCHLORIDE Tablets, USP, 10 mg. ℞ *Orange*	M/97
FLURAZEPAM HYDROCHLORIDE Capsules, USP, 15 mg. ℂ/℞ *White & Powder Blue*	MYLAN 4415
FLURAZEPAM HYDROCHLORIDE Capsules, USP, 30 mg. ℂ/℞ *Powder Blue & Powder Blue*	MYLAN 4430
FUROSEMIDE Tablets, USP, 20 mg. ℞ *White*	M2/Blank
FUROSEMIDE Tablets, USP, 40 mg. ℞ *White*	MYLAN 216/40
FUROSEMIDE Tablets, USP, 80 mg. ℞ *White*	MYLAN 232/80
HALOPERIDOL Tablets, USP, 0.5 mg. ℞ *Orange*	MYLAN 351/Scored
HALOPERIDOL Tablets, USP, 1 mg. ℞ *Orange*	MYLAN 257/Scored
HALOPERIDOL Tablets, USP, 2 mg. ℞ *Orange*	MYLAN 214/Scored
HALOPERIDOL Tablets, USP, 5 mg. ℞ *Orange*	MYLAN 327/Scored
IBUPROFEN Tablets, USP, 400 mg. ℞ *White*	MYLAN/401
IBUPROFEN Tablets, USP, 600 mg. ℞ *White*	MYLAN/601
IBUPROFEN Tablets, USP, 800 mg. ℞ *White*	MYLAN/801
INDOMETHACIN Capsules, USP, 25 mg. ℞ *Lt. Green & Lt. Green*	MYLAN 143
INDOMETHACIN Capsules, USP, 50 mg. ℞ *Lt. Green & Lt. Green*	MYLAN 147
LOPERAMIDE HYDROCHLORIDE Capsules, USP, 2 mg. ℞ *Lt. Brown & Lt. Brown*	MYLAN 2100
LORAZEPAM Tablets, USP, 0.5 mg. ℂ/℞ *White*	M/321
LORAZEPAM Tablets, USP, 1 mg. ℂ/℞ *White*	MYLAN 457/Blank
LORAZEPAM Tablets, USP, 2 mg ℂ/℞ *White*	MYLAN 777/Blank
MAPROTILINE HYDROCHLORIDE Tablets, USP, 25 mg. ℞ *White*	M/60
MAPROTILINE HYDROCHLORIDE Tablets, USP, 50 mg. ℞ *Blue*	M/87
MAPROTILINE HYDROCHLORIDE Tablets, USP, 75 mg. ℞ *White*	M/92
MECLOFENAMATE SODIUM Capsules, USP, 50 mg. ℞ *Coral & Coral*	MYLAN 2150
MECLOFENAMATE SODIUM Capsules, USP, 100 mg. ℞ *Coral & White*	MYLAN 3000
METHOTREXATE Tablets, USP, 2.5 mg. ℞ *Orange*	M14/Blank
METHYCLOTHIAZIDE Tablets, USP, 5 mg. ℞ *Blue*	M29/Blank
METHYLDOPA Tablets, USP, 250 mg. ℞ *Beige*	MYLAN/611
METHYLDOPA Tablets, USP, 500 mg. ℞ *Beige*	MYLAN/421
METHYLDOPA and HYDROCHLOROTHIAZIDE Tablets, USP, 250 mg./15 mg. ℞ *Green*	MYLAN/507
METHYLDOPA and HYDROCHLOROTHIAZIDE Tablets, USP, 250 mg./25 mg. ℞ *White*	MYLAN/711
NITROGLYCERIN TRANSDERMAL SYSTEM Patches, 0.2 mg./hr. ℞	Nitroglycerin 0.2 mg/hr
NITROGLYCERIN TRANSDERMAL SYSTEM Patches, 0.4 mg./hr. ℞	Nitroglycerin 0.4 mg/hr
NITROGLYCERIN TRANSDERMAL SYSTEM Patches, 0.6 mg./hr. ℞	Nitroglycerin 0.6 mg/hr
PENICILLIN V POTASSIUM Tablets (Oval), USP, 250 mg. ℞ *White*	M11/Blank
PENICILLIN V POTASSIUM Tablets (Round), USP, 250 mg. ℞ *White*	M95/Blank
PENICILLIN V POTASSIUM Tablets (Oval), USP, 500 mg. ℞ *White*	M98/Blank
PENICILLIN V POTASSIUM Tablets (Round), USP, 500 mg. ℞ *White*	M12/Blank
PERPHENAZINE and AMITRIPTYLINE HYDROCHLORIDE Tablets, USP, 2 mg./10 mg. ℞ *White*	MYLAN/330
PERPHENAZINE and AMITRIPTYLINE HYDROCHLORIDE Tablets, USP, 2 mg./25 mg. ℞ *Purple*	MYLAN/442
PERPHENAZINE and AMITRIPTYLINE HYDROCHLORIDE Tablets, USP, 4 mg./10 mg. ℞ *Blue*	MYLAN/727
PERPHENAZINE and AMITRIPTYLINE HYDROCHLORIDE Tablets, USP, 4 mg./25 mg. ℞ *Orange*	MYLAN/574
PERPHENAZINE and AMITRIPTYLINE HYDROCHLORIDE Tablets, USP, 4 mg./50 mg. ℞ *Purple*	MYLAN/73
PIROXICAM Capsules, USP, 10 mg. ℞ *Maroon & Blue*	MYLAN 1010
PIROXICAM Capsules, USP, 20 mg. ℞ *Maroon & Maroon*	MYLAN 2020
PRAZOSIN HYDROCHLORIDE Capsules, USP, 1 mg. ℞ *Dk. Green & Brown*	MYLAN 1101
PRAZOSIN HYDROCHLORIDE Capsules, USP, 2 mg. ℞ *Brown & Brown*	MYLAN 2302
PRAZOSIN HYDROCHLORIDE Capsules, USP, 5 mg. ℞ *Lt. Blue & Brown*	MYLAN 3205
PROBENECID Tablets, USP. 500 mg. ℞ *Yellow*	MYLAN 156/500
PROPOXYPHENE HYDROCHLORIDE and ACETAMINOPHEN Tablets, USP, 65 mg./ 650 mg. ℂ/℞ *Orange*	MYLAN/130
PROPOXYPHENE NAPSYLATE and ACETAMINOPHEN Tablets, USP, 100 mg./650 mg. ℂ/℞ *Pink*	MYLAN/155
PROPOXYPHENE NAPSYLATE and ACETAMINOPHEN Tablets, USP, 100 mg./650 mg. ℂ/℞ *White*	MYLAN/521
PROPRANOLOL HYDROCHLORIDE Tablets, USP, 10 mg. ℞ *Orange*	MYLAN 182/10
PROPRANOLOL HYDROCHLORIDE Tablets, USP, 20 mg. ℞ *Blue*	MYLAN 183/20
PROPRANOLOL HYDROCHLORIDE Tablets, USP, 40 mg. ℞ *Green*	MYLAN 184/40
PROPRANOLOL HYDROCHLORIDE Tablets, USP, 80 mg. ℞ *Yellow*	MYLAN 185/80
PROPRANOLOL HYDROCHLO- RIDE and HYDROCHLOROTHIAZIDE Tablets, 40 mg./25 mg. ℞ *White*	MYLAN 731/Scored
PROPRANOLOL HYDROCHLO- RIDE and HYDROCHLOROTHIAZIDE Tablets, 80 mg./25 mg. ℞ *White*	MYLAN 347/Scored
RESERPINE and CHLOROTHIAZIDE Tablets, USP, 0.125 mg./250 mg. ℞ *Lt. Orange*	M33/Blank
RESERPINE and CHLOROTHIAZIDE Tablets, USP, 0.125 mg./500 mg. ℞ *Lt. Orange*	M43/Blank
SPIRONOLACTONE Tablets, USP, 25 mg. ℞ *White*	MYLAN 146/25
SPIRONOLACTONE and HYDROCHLOROTHIAZIDE Tablets, 25 mg./25 mg. ℞ *Ivory*	M41/Blank
TEMAZEPAM Capsules, 15 mg. ℂ/℞ *Peach & Peach*	MYLAN 4010
TEMAZEPAM Capsules, 30 mg. ℂ/℞ *Yellow & Yellow*	MYLAN 5050
TETRACYCLINE HYDROCHLORIDE Capsules, USP, 250 mg. ℞ *Orange & Yellow*	MYLAN 101
TETRACYCLINE HYDROCHLORIDE Capsules, USP, 500 mg. ℞ *Black & Yellow*	MYLAN 102
THIORIDAZINE HYDROCHLORIDE Tablets, USP, 10 mg. ℞ *Orange*	M54/10
THIORIDAZINE HYDROCHLORIDE Tablets, USP, 25 mg. ℞ *Orange*	M58/25
THIORIDAZINE HYDROCHLORIDE Tablets, USP, 50 mg. ℞ *Orange*	M59/50
THIORIDAZINE HYDROCHLORIDE Tablets, USP, 100 mg. ℞ *Orange*	M61/100
THIOTHIXENE Capsules, USP, 1 mg. ℞ *Caramel & Powder Blue*	MYLAN 1001
THIOTHIXENE Capsules, USP, 2 mg. ℞ *Caramel & Yellow*	MYLAN 2002
THIOTHIXENE Capsules, USP, 5 mg. ℞ *Caramel & White*	MYLAN 3005
THIOTHIXENE Capsules, USP, 10 mg. ℞ *Caramel & Peach*	MYLAN 5010
TIMOLOL MALEATE Tablets, USP, 5 mg. ℞ *Green*	M55/Blank
TIMOLOL MALEATE Tablets, USP, 10 mg. ℞ *Green*	M221/Blank
TIMOLOL MALEATE Tablets, USP, 20 mg. ℞ *Green*	M715/Blank
TOLAZAMIDE Tablets, USP, 250 mg. ℞ *White*	MYLAN 217/250
TOLAZAMIDE Tablets, USP, 500 mg. ℞ *White*	MYLAN 551/Blank
TOLBUTAMIDE Tablets, USP, 500 mg. ℞ *White*	M13/Blank
VERAPAMIL Tablets, 80 mg. ℞ *White*	MYLAN 512/Blank
VERAPAMIL Tablets, 120 mg. ℞ *White*	MYLAN 772/Blank

*Front/Back Side for Tablets
or Left and Right Side
for Capsules.

Products are cross-indexed by
generic and chemical names in the
YELLOW SECTION.

Nature's Bounty, Inc.
90 ORVILLE DRIVE
BOHEMIA, NY 11716

ENER–B®   OTC
Intra-nasal Vitamin B-12 Gel
Dietary Supplement

DESCRIPTION
ENER-B® is the first intra-nasal application for Vitamin B-12. Each delivery supplies 400 mcg. of Vitamin B-12. This method of delivery provides the highest Vitamin B-12 blood levels that can be obtained without a prescription. Clinical tests show that ENER-B produced 8.4 to 10 times more Vitamin B-12 in the blood than tablets.

Measured Vitamin B-12 Increase in Blood Levels

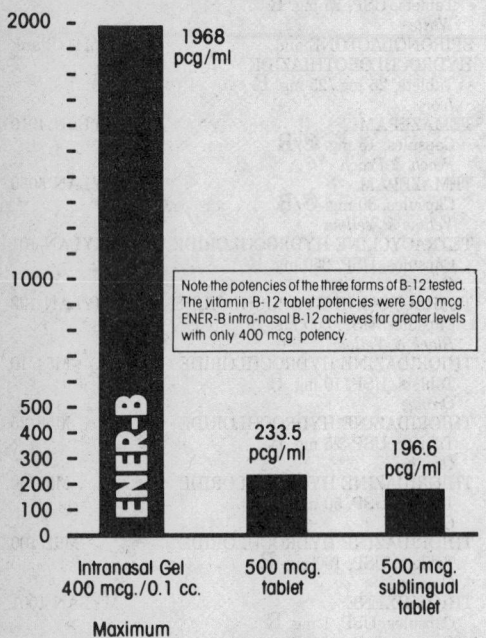

Note the potencies of the three forms of B-12 tested. The vitamin B-12 tablet potencies were 500 mcg. ENER-B intra-nasal B-12 achieves far greater levels with only 400 mcg. potency.

	Intranasal Gel 400 mcg./0.1 cc.	500 mcg. tablet	500 mcg. sublingual tablet
	1968 pcg/ml	233.5 pcg/ml	196.6 pcg/ml
	Maximum blood levels achieved in 1.6 hours	Maximum B-12 blood levels in 25.6 hours	Maximum B-12 blood levels in 5.7 hours

Clinical Test results are available by writing Nature's Bounty.

POTENCY AND ADMINISTRATION
Each nasal applicator delivers $\frac{1}{10}$ cc of gel into the nose which adheres to the mucous membranes providing 400 mcg. of Vitamin B-12. Odorless and non-irritating to the nose.

DIRECTIONS
As a dietary supplement, one unit every two to three days.

HOW SUPPLIED
Packages of 12 unit doses. Supplies 400 mcg. of B-12 each.
Shown in Product Identification Section, page 420

Neutrogena Dermatologics
5760 WEST 96th STREET
LOS ANGELES, CA 90045

MELANEX®   ℞
Topical Solution
(3% Hydroquinone)
FOR EXTERNAL USE ONLY

CAUTION: Federal law prohibits dispensing without prescription.

DESCRIPTION
Each package includes a cap with a plastic rod applicator (for small, more precise application) and an Appliderm® Applicator for larger areas of skin involvement. If neither applicator is specified on prescription, install the Appliderm® Applicator (sponge top) unit.
[See chemical structure at top of next column.]

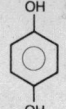

$C_6H_6O_2$ 110.11
1,4 DIHYDROXYBENZENE
Hydroquinone

Melanex® Topical Solution (3% Hydroquinone) contains:
Active Ingredient: 3% Hydroquinone. Each ml contains 30 mg of Hydroquinone.
Other ingredients: Purified Water, SD Alcohol 40 (45%), Laureth-4, Isopropyl Alcohol (4%), Propylene Glycol, Ascorbic Acid.
Pharmacological class: Depigmenting agent.

CLINICAL PHARMACOLOGY
It has been suggested the primary action of hydroquinone is directed at tyrosinase.[1] The selective inhibition of the enzyme affects melanogenesis in the melanocytes resulting in cessation of melanin formation and subsequent reduction in pigmentation. Additional studies indicate hydroquinone acts on the essential subcellular metabolic processes of melanocytes with resultant cytolysis, i.e., nonenzymediated depigmentation.[2]

INDICATIONS AND USAGE
Melanex® is indicated in the temporary bleaching of hyperpigmented skin conditions such as chloasma, melasma, freckles, senile lentigines, and other forms of melanin hyperpigmentation.

DOSAGE AND ADMINISTRATION
Apply to affected areas twice daily, in the morning and before bedtime. During the day, an effective broad spectrum sunscreen like Neutrogena® Sunblock SPF 15 or SPF 30 should be used and unnecessary solar exposure avoided, or protective clothing should be worn to cover bleached skin in order to prevent repigmentation from occurring.

CONTRAINDICATIONS
Melanex® is contraindicated in persons who have shown hypersensitivity to hydroquinone or any of the other ingredients. The safety of topical treatment with hydroquinone during pregnancy has not been established.

PRECAUTIONS
Concurrent use of Melanex® with peroxide products may result in transient dark staining of skin areas so treated. This is due to the oxidation of hydroquinone by the peroxide. This transient staining can be removed by discontinuing concurrent usage and normal soap cleansing.

FOR EXTERNAL USE ONLY
Hydroquinone preparations may produce skin irritation in susceptible individuals and have a slight potential to produce allergic response. Therefore, the physician should use appropriate caution. If rash or irritation develops, discontinue use and consult physician. Do not use on children under 12 years.
If no improvement is seen after two months of treatment, use of product should be discontinued. Avoid contact with eyes. In case of accidental contact, patient should rinse eyes thoroughly with water and contact physician. A bitter taste and anesthetic effect may occur if applied to lips. Keep out of reach of children. Use of Melanex® in paranasal and infraorbital areas increases the chance of irritation (see **ADVERSE REACTIONS**).
A Patient Instruction Sheet for using Melanex® is available to the physician and may be given to the patient at the discretion of the doctor.

ADVERSE REACTIONS
The following have been reported: dryness and fissuring of the paranasal and infraorbital areas, erythema, and stinging. Hydroquinone has been known to produce irritation and sensitization in susceptible individuals.

INSTRUCTIONS TO PHARMACIST
HOW SUPPLIED: 1 fl. oz. (30 ML) bottle with plastic rod and Appliderm® Applicator unit.
NOTE: Slight darkening of the Melanex® solution is normal and will not affect potency. See expiration date on bottle.
[See Instructions above.]
INSTRUCTIONS FOR INSTALLING APPLIDERM® FILTER/APPLICATOR:

(1) JIMBOW K., OBATHA H., PATHAK M., FITZPATRICK T.B. Mechanism and Depigmentation of Hydroquinone, Journal of Investigative Dermatology 1974, 62:436–449.
(2) op. cit.

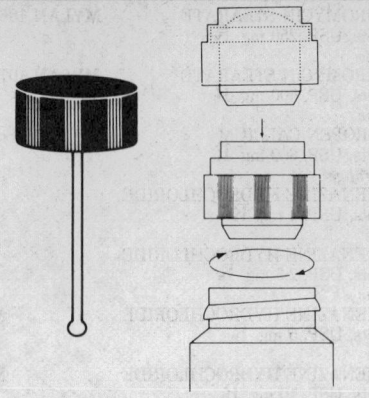

1. Remove black cap with plastic rod.
2. Push applicator firmly into bottle using brown cap as holder.
3. Important: Screw cap all the way down to seat the applicator.
Cap should be kept tightly closed to avoid leakage.

Store at room temperature or below. Avoid excessive heat.
For additional information please call:
Neutrogena Technical Department toll-free (800) 421-6857; in California call collect (310) 642-1150.
NDC #10812-9300-1
Distributed by
Neutrogena Dermatologics
5760 W. 96th St.
Los Angeles, CA 90045
Manufactured by
Packaging Corporation of America
Los Angeles, CA 90058
Shown in Product Identification Section, page 420

Niché Pharmaceuticals, Inc.
300 TROPHY CLUB DRIVE #400
ROANOKE, TX 76262

MAGTAB® SR
[*măg-tăb*]
(Magnesium L-lactate dihydrate)
Sustained release Magnesium Supplement

DESCRIPTION
MagTab® SR is a sustained release oral magnesium supplement. Each pale yellow caplet contains 7mEq (84 Mg) magnesium as magnesium lactate in a wax matrix.

INGREDIENTS
Each caplet contains 7mEq (84 Mg) elemental magnesium as magnesium L.Lactate dihydrate (835 Mg) in a sustained release wax matrix formulation. Inactive ingredients: polyethylene glycol, microcrystalline cellulose, carnauba wax, stearic acid, calcium stearate, and D & C yellow No. 10 aluminum lake.

INDICATIONS/USES
As a dietary supplement, MagTab® SR is indicated for patients with, or at risk for, magnesium deficiency. Hypomagnesemia and/or magnesium deficiency can result from inadequate nutritional intake or absorption, magnesium depleting drugs such as diuretics, or alcoholism.

WARNINGS
Patients with renal disease should not take magnesium supplements without the advice and direct supervision of a physician.

SIDE EFFECTS
Excessive dosage of magnesium can cause loose stools or diarrhea.

DOSAGE
As a dietary supplement, take 1 or 2 caplets b.i.d. or as directed by a physician. Four caplets of MagTab® SR will meet the USRDA range for average adult males and females (300–350 mg) where magnesium depleting drugs are being used, supplementation with higher dosages may be required and should be considered.

HOW SUPPLIED
MagTab® SR is available for oral administration as uncoated yellow caplets, coded Niche/420. Caplets are supplied as follows:
59016-42016	Bottles of 60
59016-42017	Bottles of 100
Store at 15°–30°C (59°–86°F)
U.S. Patent Number: 5,002,774

Nordisk-USA
(See Novo Nordisk Pharmaceuticals Inc.)

Northampton Medical, Inc.
3039 AMWILER RD
SUITE 122
ATLANTA, GA 30360

FEMCET®   ℞
(Butalbital, Acetaminophen, and Caffeine)

DESCRIPTION
Each FEMCET® capsule for oral administration contains:
Butalbital* .... 50 mg
*WARNING: May be habit forming.
Acetaminophen .... 325 mg
Caffeine .... 40 mg

HOW SUPPLIED
Bottles of 100.

FERROCON™   OTC
Extended Release Iron Caplets

DESCRIPTION
Each caplet contains 160 mg dried ferrous sulfate USP, equivalent to 50 mg elemental iron. Also contains corn starch, glyceryl monostearate, maltodextrin, hydroxypropyl methylcellulose, polyethylene glycol, titanium dioxide.

HOW SUPPLIED
Bottles of 100.

NUTRAVESCENT   OTC
Calcium With Biostatic Effervescence

DESCRIPTION
Each dosepack contains two 500 mg tablets and offers:

		Adult % US RDA
Elemental Calcium (from Calcium Citrate)	1000 mg	100%
Vitamin D (from Cholecalciferol)	400 IU	100%
Vitamin A (from Beta-Carotene)	1000 IU	20%

Contains less than 2% of the U.S. RDA of Protein, Vitamin C, Thiamine, Riboflavin, Niacin and Iron.

HOW SUPPLIED
52 orange-flavored tablets in 26 foil dosepacks.

PDRx .25   ℞
for the removal of warts
(including condylomas)

DESCRIPTION
25% Podophyllin (Podophyllum Rhizome Resin USP) in Tincture of Benzoin, USP, Disposable Applicator.

HOW SUPPLIED
10 × 0.5 mL Disposable applicator units/box NDC 38245-668-22.

PRECARE Caplets   ℞
Vitamin and Mineral Supplements
for Pre- and Postnatal Periods

DESCRIPTION
Each peach film-coated caplet contains:
Vitamin D (cholecalciferol) .... 6 mcg
Vitamin E (dl-α-tocopherol
   acetate) .... 3.5 mg
Vitamin C (ascorbic acid) .... 50 mg
Folic Acid (folate) .... 1 mg
Vitamin B$_6$ (pyridoxine
   hydrochloride) .... 2 mg
Calcium (as calcium
   carbonate) .... 250 mg
Magnesium (as magnesium
   oxide) .... 50 mg
Iron (as ferrous fumarate) .... 40 mg
Zinc (as zinc sulfate) .... 15 mg
Copper (as cupric sulfate) .... 2 mg

HOW SUPPLIED
Bottles of 100.

Norwich Eaton
Pharmaceuticals, Inc.
NORWICH, NY 13815-1799

See Procter & Gamble Pharmaceuticals, Inc.

Novo Nordisk Pharmaceuticals Inc.
SUITE 200
100 OVERLOOK CENTER
PRINCETON, NJ 08540-7810

STANDARD INSULIN
REGULAR INSULIN
Insulin Injection
USP (Pork) 100 units/ml

DESCRIPTION
Regular Insulin, Insulin Injection USP, 100 units of insulin per milliliter, is a clear, colorless solution which has a short duration of action. The effect of Regular Insulin begins approximately ½ hour after injection. The effect is maximal between 2½ and 5 hours and ends approximately 8 hours after injection. The time course of action of any insulin may vary considerably in different individuals, or at different times in the same individual. Because of this variation, the time periods listed here should be considered as general guidelines only.

STORAGE
Insulin should be stored in a cold place, preferably in a refrigerator, but not in the freezing compartment. Do not let it freeze. Keep the insulin vial in its carton so that it will stay clean and protected from light. If refrigeration is not possible, the bottle of insulin which you are currently using can be kept unrefrigerated as long as it is kept as cool as possible and away from heat and sunlight.
Never use Regular Insulin if it becomes viscous (thickened) or cloudy; use it only if it is clear and colorless.
Never use insulin after the expiration date which is printed on the vial label and carton.

SEMILENTE® INSULIN
Prompt Insulin Zinc Suspension
USP (Beef) 100 units/ml

DESCRIPTION
Semilente® Insulin, Prompt Insulin Zinc Suspension USP, 100 units of insulin per milliliter, is a cloudy or milky suspension of amorphous beef insulin. The insulin substance (the cloudy material) settles at the bottom of the vial, therefore, the vial must be gently agitated or rotated so that the contents are uniformly mixed before a dose is withdrawn. The effect of Semilente® Insulin begins approximately 1½ hours after injection. The effect is maximal between 5 and 10 hours and ends approximately 16 hours after injection. The time course of action of any insulin may vary considerably in different individuals, or at different times in the same individual. Because of this variation, the time periods listed here should be considered as general guidelines only.

STORAGE
Insulin should be stored in a cold place, preferably in a refrigerator, but not in the freezing compartment. Do not let it freeze. Keep the insulin vial in its carton so that it will stay clean and protected from light. If refrigeration is not possible, the bottle of insulin which you are currently using can be kept unrefrigerated as long as it is kept as cool as possible and away from heat and sunlight.
Never use Semilente® Insulin if the precipitate (the white deposit at the bottom of the vial) has become lumpy or granular in appearance or has formed a deposit of solid particles on the wall of the vial. This insulin should not be used if the liquid in the vial remains clear after the vial has been gently agitated.
Never use insulin after the expiration date which is printed on the vial label and carton.

LENTE® INSULIN
Insulin Zinc Suspension
USP (Beef) 100 units/ml

DESCRIPTION
LENTE® Insulin, Insulin Zinc Suspension USP, 100 units of insulin per milliliter, is a cloudy or milky suspension of 70% crystalline and 30% amorphous beef insulin. The insulin substance (the cloudy material) settles at the bottom of the vial, therefore, the vial must be gently agitated or rotated so that the contents are uniformly mixed before a dose is withdrawn. Lente® Insulin has an intermediate duration of action. The effect of Lente® Insulin begins approximately 2½ hours after injection. The effect is maximal between 7 and 15 hours and ends approximately 24 hours after injection. The time course of action of any insulin may vary considerably in different individuals, or at different times in the same individual. Because of this variation, the time periods listed here should be considered as general guidelines only.

STORAGE
Insulin should be stored in a cold place, preferably in a refrigerator, but not in the freezing compartment. Do not let it freeze. Keep the insulin vial in its carton so that it will stay clean and protected from light. If refrigeration is not possible, the bottle of insulin which you are currently using can be kept unrefrigerated as long as it is kept as cool as possible and away from heat and sunlight.
Never use Lente® Insulin if the precipitate (the white deposit at the bottom of the vial) has become lumpy or granular in appearance or has formed a deposit of solid particles on the wall of the vial. This insulin should not be used if the liquid in the vial remains clear after the vial has been gently agitated.
Never use insulin after the expiration date which is printed on the vial label and carton.

NPH INSULIN
Isophane Insulin Suspension USP (Beef) 100 units/ml

DESCRIPTION
NPH Insulin, Isophane Insulin Suspension USP, 100 units of insulin per milliliter, is a cloudy or milky suspension of beef insulin with protamine and zinc. The insulin substance (the cloudy material) settles at the bottom of the vial, therefore, the vial must be gently agitated or rotated so that the contents are uniformly mixed before a dose is withdrawn. NPH Insulin has an intermediate duration of action. The effect of NPH Insulin begins approximately 1½ hours after injection. The effect is maximal between 4 and 12 hours and ends approximately 24 hours after injection. The time course of action of any insulin may vary considerably in different individuals, or at different times in the same individual. Because of this variation, the time periods listed here should be considered as general guidelines only.

STORAGE
Insulin should be stored in a cold place, preferably in a refrigerator, but not in the freezing compartment. Do not let it freeze. Keep the insulin vial in its carton so that it will stay clean and protected from light. If refrigeration is not possible, the bottle of insulin which you are currently using can be kept unrefrigerated as long as it is kept as cool as possible and away from heat and sunlight.
Never use NPH Insulin if the precipitate (the white deposit at the bottom of the vial) has become lumpy or granular in appearance or has formed a deposit of solid particles on the wall of the vial. This insulin should not be used if the liquid in the vial remains clear after the vial has been gently agitated.
Never use insulin after the expiration date which is printed on the vial label and carton.

ULTRALENTE® INSULIN
Extended Insulin Zinc
Suspension USP (Beef) 100 units/ml

DESCRIPTION
Ultralente® Insulin, Extended Insulin Zinc Suspension USP, 100 units of insulin per milliliter, is a cloudy or milky suspension of crystalline beef insulin. The insulin substance (the cloudy material) settles at the bottom of the vial, therefore, the vial must be gently agitated or rotated so that the contents are uniformly mixed before a dose is withdrawn. The effect of Ultralente® Insulin begins approximately 4 hours after injection. The effect is maximal between 10 and 30 hours and ends approximately 36 hours after injection. The time course of action of any insulin may vary considerably in different individuals, or at different times in the same individual. Because of this variation, the time periods listed here should be considered as general guidelines only.

STORAGE
Insulin should be stored in a cold place, preferably in a refrigerator, but not in the freezing compartment. Do not let it freeze. Keep the insulin vial in its carton so that it will stay clean and protected from light. If refrigeration is not possible, the bottle of insulin which you are currently using can be

Continued on next page

Novo Nordisk—Cont.

kept unrefrigerated as long as it is kept as cool as possible and away from heat and sunlight.
Never use **Ultralente® Insulin** if the precipitate (the white deposit at the bottom of the vial) has become lumpy or granular in appearance or has formed a deposit of solid particles on the wall of the vial. This insulin should not be used if the liquid in the vial remains clear after the vial has been gently agitated.
Never use insulin after the expiration date which is printed on the vial label and carton.

PURIFIED INSULIN

REGULAR PURIFIED PORK INSULIN INJECTION USP 100 units/ml

DESCRIPTION

Regular Purified Pork Insulin Injection, USP, 100 units of insulin per milliliter, is a clear, colorless solution which has a short duration of action. The effect of **Regular Purified Insulin** begins approximately 1/2 hour after injection. The effect is maximal between 2 1/2 and 5 hours and ends approximately 8 hours after injection. The time course of action of any insulin may vary considerably in different individuals, or at different times in the same individual. Because of this variation, the time periods listed here should be considered as general guidelines only.
The word "purified" on the label indicates that this insulin differs from standard insulin in that it has undergone additional purification steps (i.e., molecular sieve and ion-exchange chromatography).

STORAGE

Insulin should be stored in a cold place, preferably in a refrigerator, but not in the freezing compartment. **Do not let it freeze.** Keep the insulin vial in its carton so that it will stay clean and protected from light. If refrigeration is not possible, the bottle of insulin which you are currently using can be kept unrefrigerated as long as it is kept as cool as possible and away from heat and sunlight.
Never use Regular Purified Insulin if it becomes viscous (thickened) or cloudy; use it only if it is clear and colorless.
Never use insulin after the expiration date which is printed on the vial label and carton.

LENTE® PURIFIED PORK INSULIN ZINC SUSPENSION USP 100 units/ml

DESCRIPTION

Lente® Purified Pork Insulin Zinc Suspension, USP, 100 units of insulin per milliliter, is a cloudy or milky suspension of 70% crystalline and 30% amorphous purified pork insulin. The insulin substance (the cloudy material) settles at the bottom of the vial, therefore, the vial must be gently agitated or rotated so that the contents are uniformly mixed before a dose is withdrawn. **Lente® Purified Insulin** has an intermediate duration of action. The effect of **Lente® Purified Insulin** begins approximately 2 1/2 hours after injection. The effect is maximal between 7 and 15 hours and ends approximately 22 hours after injection. The time course of action of any insulin may vary considerably in different individuals, or at different times in the same individual. Because of this variation, the time periods listed here should be considered as general guidelines only.
The word "purified" on the label indicates that this insulin differs from standard insulin in that it has undergone additional purification steps (i.e., molecular sieve and ion-exchange chromatography).

STORAGE

Insulin should be stored in a cold place, preferably in a refrigerator, but not in the freezing compartment. **Do not let it freeze.** Keep the insulin vial in its carton so that it will stay clean and protected from light. If refrigeration is not possible, the bottle of insulin which you are currently using can be kept unrefrigerated as long as it is kept as cool as possible and away from heat and sunlight.
Never use **Lente® Purified Insulin** if the precipitate (the white deposit at the bottom of the vial) has become lumpy or granular in appearance or has formed a deposit of solid particles on the wall of the vial. This insulin should not be used if the liquid in the vial remains clear after the vial has been gently agitated.
Never use insulin after the expiration date which is printed on the vial label and carton.

NPH PURIFIED PORK ISOPHANE INSULIN SUPSENSION USP 100 units/ml

DESCRIPTION

NPH Purified Pork Isophane Insulin Suspension, USP, 100 units of insulin per milliliter, is a cloudy or milky suspension of purified pork insulin with protamine and zinc. The insulin substance (the cloudy material) settles at the bottom of the vial, therefore, the vial must be gently agitated or rotated so that the contents are uniformly mixed before a dose is withdrawn. **NPH Purified Insulin** has an intermediate duration of action. The effect of **NPH Purified Insulin** begins approximately 1 1/2 hours after injection. The effect is maximal between 4 and 12 hours and ends approximately 24 hours after injection. The time course of action of any insulin may vary considerably in different individuals, or at different times in the same individual. Because of this variation, the time periods listed here should be considered as general guidelines only.
The word "purified" on the label indicates that this insulin differs from standard insulin in that it has undergone additional purification steps (i.e., molecular sieve and ion-exchange chromatography).

STORAGE

Insulin should be stored in a cold place, preferably in a refrigerator, but not in the freezing compartment. **Do not let it freeze.** Keep the insulin vial in its carton so that it will stay clean and protected from light. If refrigeration is not possible, the bottle of insulin which you are currently using can be kept unrefrigerated as long as it is kept as cool as possible and away from heat and sunlight.
Never use **NPH Purified Insulin** if the precipitate (the white deposit at the bottom of the vial) has become lumpy or granular in appearance or has formed a deposit of solid particles on the wall of the vial. This insulin should not be used if the liquid in the vial remains clear after the vial has been gently agitated.
Never use insulin after the expiration date which is printed on the vial label and carton.

INSULATARD® NPH

Purified Pork Isophane Insulin Suspension 100 units/ml

DESCRIPTION

Insulatard® NPH is a suspension of protamine insulin crystals obtained from pork pancreas only. It has a slower onset of action than Velosulin® (Regular) insulin. The effect on the blood sugar begins approximately 1 1/2 hours after the injection and lasts up to approximately 24 hours, having its maximum effect between the 4th and 12th hour.
The time course of action of any insulin may vary considerably in different individuals, or at different times in the same individual. Because of this variation, the time periods listed here should be considered as general guidelines only.
Rotate the vial carefully to obtain a uniformly cloudy suspension of the crystals. Avoid heavy foaming. Do not use a vial if the insulin remains clear after it has been rotated. Also do not use it if you see lumps that float or stick to the sides of the vial.

STORAGE

Insulin should be stored in a cold place, preferably in a refrigerator, but not in the freezing compartment. **Do not let it freeze.** Keep the insulin vial in its carton so that it will stay clean and protected from light. If refrigeration is not possible, the bottle of insulin which you are currently using can be kept unrefrigerated as long as it is kept as cool as possible and away from heat and sunlight.

Never use insulin after the expiration date which is printed on the vial label and carton.

See NOVOLIN® 70/30 for package insert information on syringes; important statement; preparing the injection; usage in pregnancy; insulin reaction and shock; diabetic ketoacidosis and coma; adverse reactions; and important notes.

MIXTARD® 70/30

70% Purified Pork Isophane Insulin Suspension and 30% Purified Pork Insulin Injection 100 units/ml

DESCRIPTION

Mixtard® 70/30 is a standard mixture of 30% Velosulin® (corresponding to Regular insulin) and 70% Insulatard® NPH obtained from pork pancreas only. The content of Velosulin® gives the preparation a rapid onset of effect on the blood sugar, approximately 1/2 hour after the injection. The content of Insulatard® NPH gives it a duration of up to 24 hours, depending on the size of the dose. The maximal effect is between the 4th and the 8th hour after injection.
The time course of action of any insulin may vary considerably in different individuals, or at different times in the same individual. Because of this variation, the time periods listed here should be considered as general guidelines only.
Rotate the vial carefully to obtain a uniformly cloudy suspension of the crystals. Avoid heavy foaming. Do not use a vial if the insulin remains clear after it has been rotated. Also, do not use it if you see lumps that float or stick to the sides of the vial.

STORAGE

Insulin should be stored in a cold place, preferably in a refrigerator, but not in the freezing compartment. **Do not let it freeze.** Keep the insulin vial in its carton so that it will stay clean and protected from light. If refrigeration is not possible, the bottle of insulin which you are currently using can be kept unrefrigerated as long as it is kept as cool as possible and away from heat and sunlight.

Never use insulin after the expiration date which is printed on the vial label and carton.

See NOVOLIN® 70/30 for package insert information on syringes; important statement; preparing the injection; usage in pregnancy; insulin reaction and shock; diabetic ketoacidosis and coma; adverse reactions; and important notes.

VELOSULIN®

Regular Purified Pork Insulin Injection 100 units/ml

DESCRIPTION

Velosulin® is a clear solution of insulin obtained from pork pancreas only. It has a rapid onset of action, approximately 1/2 hour after the injection. The effect lasts up to approximately 8 hours with a maximal effect between the 1st and 3rd hour.
The time course of action of any insulin may vary considerably in different individuals, or at different times in the same individual. Because of this variation, the time periods listed here should be considered as general guidelines only.
Do not use the preparation if the color has become other than water clear or if the liquid has become viscous.

STORAGE

Insulin should be stored in a cold place, preferably in a refrigerator, but not in the freezing compartment. **Do not let it freeze.** Keep the insulin vial in its carton so that it will stay clean and protected from light. If refrigeration is not possible, the bottle of insulin which you are currently using can be kept unrefrigerated as long as it is kept as cool as possible and away from heat and sunlight.

Never use insulin after the expiration date which is printed on the vial label and carton.

MIXING TWO TYPES OF INSULIN

Different insulins should be mixed only under instruction from a physician. Hypodermic syringes may vary in the amount of space between the bottom line and the needle ("dead space"), so if you are mixing two types of insulin be sure to discuss any change in the model and brand of syringe you are using with your physician or pharmacist. When you are mixing two types of insulin, always draw the Regular (clear) insulin into the syringe first.

Velosulin® should not be mixed with Lente®-type insulins, because the buffering agent in Velosulin® could interact with the other insulin and change its activity. This could lead to an unpredictable effect on blood sugar.

See NOVOLIN® 70/30 for package insert information on syringes; important statement; preparing the injection; usage in pregnancy; insulin reaction and shock; diabetic ketoacidosis and coma; adverse reactions; and important notes.

NOVOLIN® 70/30

70% NPH, Human Insulin Isophane Suspension and 30% Regular, Human Insulin Injection (recombinant DNA origin) 100 units/ml

WARNING

ANY CHANGE OF INSULIN SHOULD BE MADE CAUTIOUSLY AND ONLY UNDER MEDICAL SUPERVISION. CHANGES IN REFINEMENT, PURITY, STRENGTH, BRAND (MANUFACTURER), TYPE (REGULAR, NPH, LENTE®, ETC.), SPECIES (BEEF, PORK, BEEF-PORK, HUMAN) AND/OR METHOD OF MANUFACTURE (RECOMBINANT DNA VERSUS ANIMAL-SOURCE INSULIN) MAY RESULT IN THE NEED FOR A CHANGE IN DOSAGE.
SPECIAL CARE SHOULD BE TAKEN WHEN THE TRANSFER IS FROM A STANDARD BEEF OR MIXED SPECIES INSULIN TO A PURIFIED PORK OR HUMAN INSULIN. IF A DOSAGE ADJUSTMENT IS NEEDED, IT WILL USUALLY

BECOME APPARENT EITHER IN THE FIRST FEW DAYS OR OVER A PERIOD OF SEVERAL WEEKS. ANY CHANGE IN TREATMENT SHOULD BE CAREFULLY MONITORED. PLEASE READ THE SECTIONS "INSULIN REACTION AND SHOCK" AND "DIABETIC KETOACIDOSIS AND COMA" FOR SYMPTOMS OF HYPOGLYCEMIA (LOW BLOOD GLUCOSE) AND HYPERGLYCEMIA (HIGH BLOOD GLUCOSE).

INSULIN USE IN DIABETES

Your physician has explained that you have diabetes and that your treatment involves injections of insulin. Insulin is normally produced by the pancreas, a gland that lies behind the stomach. Without insulin, glucose (a simple sugar made from digested food) is trapped in the bloodstream and cannot enter the cells of the body. Some patients who don't make enough of their own insulin, or who cannot use the insulin they do make properly, must take insulin by injection in order to control their blood glucose levels.

Each case of diabetes is different and requires direct and continued medical supervision. Your physician has told you the type, strength and amount of insulin you should use and the time(s) at which you should inject it, and has also discussed with you a diet and exercise schedule. You should contact your physician if you experience any difficulties or if you have questions.

TYPES OF INSULINS

Standard and purified animal insulins as well as human insulins are available. Standard and purified insulins differ in their degree of purification and content of noninsulin material. Standard and purified insulins also vary in species source: they may be of beef, pork, or mixed beef and pork origin. Human insulin is identical in structure to the insulin produced by the human pancreas, and thus differs from animal insulins. Insulins vary in time of action and in strength; see PRODUCT DESCRIPTION and SYRINGES for additional information.

Your physician has prescribed the insulin that is right for you; be sure you have purchased the correct insulin and check it carefully before you use it.

PRODUCT DESCRIPTION

This vial contains **Novolin® 70/30** which is a mixture of 70% NPH, Human Insulin Isophane Suspension (recombinant DNA origin) and 30% Regular, Human Insulin Injection (recombinant DNA origin) USP. The concentration of this product is 100 units of insulin per milliliter. It is a cloudy or milky suspension of human insulin with protamine and zinc. The insulin substance (the cloudy material) settles at the bottom of the vial, therefore, the vial must be gently agitated or rotated so that the contents are uniformly mixed before a dose is withdrawn. **Novolin® 70/30** has an intermediate duration of action. The effect of **Novolin® 70/30** begins approximately ½ hour after injection. The effect is maximal between 2 and approximately 12 hours. The full duration of action may last up to 24 hours after injection.

The time course of action of any insulin may vary considerably in different individuals, or at different times in the same individual. Because of this variation, the time periods listed here should be considered as general guidelines only.

This human insulin (recombinant DNA origin) is structurally identical to the insulin produced by the human pancreas. This human insulin is produced by recombinant DNA technology utilziing Saccharomyces cerevisiae (bakers' yeast) as the production organism.

STORAGE

Insulin should be stored in a cold place, preferebly in a refrigerator, but not in the freezing compartment. **Do not let it freeze.** Keep the insulin vial in its carton so that it will stay clean and protected from light. If refrigeration is not possible, the bottle of insulin which you are currently using can be kept unrefrigerated as long as it is kept as cool as possible and away from heat and sunlight.

Never use **Novolin® 70/30** if the precipitate (the white deposit at the bottom of the vial) has become lumpy or granular in appearance or has formed a deposit of solid particles on the wall of the vial. This insulin should not be used if the liquid in the vial remains clear after the vial has been gently agitated.

Never use insulin after the expiration date which is printed on the vial label and carton.

SYRINGES

Use the Correct Syringe

Doses of insulin are measured in units. Some insulins are available in two strengths: U-100 and U-40. One milliliter (ml) of U-100 contains 100 units of insulin. One milliliter (ml) of U-40 contains 40 units of insulin. Be sure to use the proper syringe for the strength of the insulin prescribed for you. Syringes are clearly marked "**For use with U-100 insulin**" or "**For use with U-40 insulin**". Low dose U-100 syringes are also available. Failure to use the proper syringe can lead to mistakes in dosage.

Disposable Syringes

Disposable syringes and needles require no sterilization provided the package is intact. They should be used only once and discarded.

Reusable Syringes

Reusable syringes and needles must be sterilized before each use.

1. Boil the syringe parts and needles in a pan of water for at least five minutes. Keep a special pan for this purpose. Heavily chlorinated water should not be used; distilled water is preferable.
   If boiling is not possible, the syringe parts and needles may be sterilized by immersion in 70% ethyl alcohol or 91% isopropyl alcohol for at least five minutes. **Do not use bathing, rubbing or medicated alcohol for sterilization.**
2. Assemble the syringe and fit the needle on the tip of the syringe being careful not to touch the surface of the plunger or needle.
3. Push the plunger in and out several times until the water (or alcohol) has been completely expelled. (The syringe should be thoroughly dried before its use.)

IMPORTANT

Failure to comply with the above and the following antiseptic measures may lead to infections at the injection site.

PREPARING THE INJECTION

1. Clean your hands and the injection site with soap and water or with alcohol. Wipe the rubber stopper with an alcohol swab. (Note: remove the tamper-resistant cap at first use. If the cap has already been removed, do not use this product, return it to your pharmacy.)
2. For insulin suspensions, roll the vial of insulin gently in your hands to mix it. Vigorous shaking immediately before the dose is drawn into the syringe may result in the formation of bubbles or froth which could cause dosage errors.
3. Pull back the plunger until the black tip reaches the marking for the number of units you will inject.
4. Push the needle through the rubber stopper into the vial.
5. Push the plunger all the way in. This inserts air into the bottle.
6. Turn the vial and syringe upside down and slowly pull the plunger back to a few units beyond the correct dose.
7. If there are air bubbles, flick the syringe firmly with your finger to raise the air bubbles to the needle, then slowly push the plunger to the correct unit marking.
8. Lift the vial off the syringe.

GIVING THE INJECTION

1. The following areas are suitable for subcutaneous insulin injection: thighs, upper arms, buttocks, abdomen. Do not change areas without consulting your physician. The actual point of injection should be changed each time; injection sites should be about an inch apart.
2. The injection site should be clean and dry. Pinch up skin area to be injected and hold it firmly.
3. Hold the syringe like a pencil and push the needle quickly and firmly into the pinched-up area. If you go straight in it will probably sting less. Pull back the plunger slightly. If blood comes into the syringe, the needle has entered a blood vessel. Remove the needle and make the injection in another spot.
4. If blood does not appear in the syringe, release skin and push plunger all the way in to inject insulin beneath the skin. Do not inject into a muscle unless your physician has advised it. You should never inject insulin into a vein.
5. Remove needle. If slight bleeding occurs, press lightly with a dry cotton swab for a few seconds—**do not rub.**

Note:

The dose should be injected over 2–4 seconds. Preparations of insulin suspensions which are injected slowly may clog the tip of the needle, resulting in an inability to complete the injection. Syringe plugging does not occur when the drug is injected more rapidly.

MIXING INSULIN

Novolin® 70/30 is a premixed insulin containing 70% NPH, Human Insulin Isophane Suspension, recombinant DNA origin (**Novolin® N**) and 30% Regular, Human Insulin Injection, recombinant DNA origin (**Novolin® R**). You should not attempt to change the ratio of this product by adding additional NPH or Regular insulin to this vial. If your physician has prescribed insulin mixed in a proportion other than 70% NPH and 30% Regular, you should use the separate insulin formulations (**Novolin® N** and **Novolin® R**) in the amounts recommended by your physician.

USAGE IN PREGNANCY

It is particularly important to maintain good control of your diabetes during pregnancy and special attention must be paid to your diet, exercise and insulin regimens. If you are pregnant or nursing a baby, consult your physician or nurse educator.

INSULIN REACTION AND SHOCK

Insulin reaction ("hypoglycemia") occurs when the blood glucose falls very low. This can happen if you take too much insulin, miss or delay a meal, exercise more than usual or work too hard without eating, or become ill (especially with vomiting or fever). The first symptoms of an insulin reaction usually come on suddenly. They may include a cold sweat, fatigue, nervousness or shakiness, rapid heartbeat, or nausea. Personality change or confusion may also occur. If you drink or eat something right away (a glass of milk or orange juice, or several sugar candies), you can often stop the progression of symptoms. If symptoms persist, call your physician — an insulin reaction can lead to unconsciousness. If a reaction results in loss of consciousness, emergency medical care should be obtained immediately. If you have had repeated reactions or if an insulin reaction has led to a loss of consciousness, contact your physician.

In certain cases, the nature and intensity of the warning symptoms of hypoglycemia may change. A few patients have reported that after being transferred to human insulin, the early warning symptoms of hypoglycemia were less pronounced than they had been with animal-source insulin.

DIABETIC KETOACIDOSIS AND COMA

Diabetic ketoacidosis may develop if your body has too little insulin. The most common causes are acute illness or infection or failure to take enough insulin by injection. If you are ill you should check your urine for ketones. The symptoms of diabetic ketoacidosis usually come on gradually, over a period of hours or days, and include a drowsy feeling, flushed face, thirst and loss of appetite. Notify your physician right away if the urine test is positive for ketones (acetone) or if you have any of these symptoms. Fast, heavy breathing and rapid pulse are more severe symptoms and you should have medical attention right away as diabetic coma can result.

ADVERSE REACTIONS

A few people with diabetes develop red, swollen and itchy skin where the insulin has been injected. This is called a "local reaction" and it may occur if the injection is not properly made, if the skin is sensitive to the cleansing solution, or if you are allergic to the insulin being used. If you have a local reaction, tell your physician.

Generalized insulin allergy occurs rarely, but when it does it may cause a serious reaction, including skin rash over the body, shortness of breath, fast pulse, sweating, and a drop in blood pressure. If any of these symptoms develop, you should seek emergency medical care.

If severe allergic reactions to insulin have occurred (i.e., generalized rash, swelling or breathing difficulties) you should be skin-tested with **each** new insulin preparation before it is used.

IMPORTANT NOTES

1. A change in the type, strength, species or purity of insulin could require a dosage adjustment. Any change in insulin should be made under medical supervision.
2. You may have learned how to test your urine or your blood for glucose. It is important to do these tests regularly and to record the results for review with your physician or nurse educator.
3. If you have an acute illness, especially with vomiting or fever, continue taking your insulin. If possible, stay on your regular diet. If you have trouble eating, drink fruit juices, regular soft drinks, or clear soups; if you can, eat small amounts of bland foods. Test your urine for glucose and ketones and, if possible, test your blood glucose. Note the results and contact your physician for possible insulin dose adjustment. If you have severe and prolonged vomiting, seek emergency medical care.
4. You should always carry identification which states that you have diabetes.

Always consult your physician if you have any questions about your condition or the use of insulin.

Helpful information for people with diabetes is published by American Diabetes Association, 1660 Duke Street, Alexandria, VA 22314.

For information contact: Novo Nordisk Pharmaceuticals Inc., Princeton, NJ 08540

Manufactured by Novo Nordisk A/S, DK-2880 Bagsvaerd, Denmark

NOVOLIN® L

Lente® Human Insulin Zinc Suspension (recombinant DNA origin)

100 units/ml

DESCRIPTION

Novolin® L is generically known as Lente® Human Insulin Zinc Suspension (recombinant DNA origin). The concentration of this product is 100 units of insulin per milliliter. It is a cloudy or milky suspension of 70% crystalline and 30% amorphous human insulin. The insulin substance (the cloudy material) settles at the bottom of the vial, therefore, the vial must be gently agitated or rotated so that the con-

Continued on next page

Novo Nordisk—Cont.

tents are uniformly mixed before a dose is withdrawn. **Novolin® L** has an intermediate duration of action. The effect of **Novolin® L** begins approximately 2½ hours after injection. The effect is maximal between 7 and 15 hours and ends approximately 22 hours after injection. The time course of action for any insulin may vary considerably in different individuals or at different times in the same individual. Because of this variation, the periods listed here should be considered as general guidelines only.
This human insulin (recombinant DNA origin) is structurally identical to the insulin produced by the human pancreas. This human insulin is produced by recombinant DNA technology utilizing *Saccharomyces cerevisiae* (bakers' yeast) as the production organism.

STORAGE

Insulin should be stored in a cold place, preferably in a refrigerator, but not in the freezing compartment. **Do not let it freeze.** Keep the insulin vial in its carton so that it will stay clean and protected from light. If refrigeration is not possible, the bottle of insulin which you are currently using can be kept unrefrigerated as long as it is kept as cool as possible and away from heat and sunlight.
Never use **Novolin® L** if the precipitate (the white deposit at the bottom of the vial) has become lumpy or granular in appearance or has formed a deposit of solid particles on the wall of the vial. This insulin should not be used if the liquid in the vial remains clear after the vial has been gently agitated.

Never use insulin after the expiration date which is printed on the vial label and carton.

MIXING TWO TYPES OF INSULIN

Different insulins should be mixed only under instruction from a physician. Hypodermic syringes may vary in the amount of space between the bottom line and the needle ("dead space"), so if you are mixing two types of insulin be sure to discuss any change in the model and brand of syringe you are using with your physician or pharmacist. When you are mixing two types of insulin, always draw the Regular (clear) insulin into the syringe first.

SEE NOVOLIN® 70/30 for complete package insert information on syringes; important statement; preparing the injection; usage in pregnancy, insulin reaction and shock; diabetic ketoacidosis and coma; adverse reactions; and important notes.

NOVOLIN® N

NPH, Human Insulin Isophane Suspension (recombinant DNA origin)
100 units/ml

DESCRIPTION

Novolin® N is generically known as NPH, Human Insulin Isophane Suspension (recombinant DNA origin). The concentration of this product is 100 units of insulin per milliliter. It is a cloudy or milky suspension of human insulin with protamine and zinc. The insulin substance (the cloudy material) settles at the bottom of the vial, therefore, the vial must be gently agitated or rotated so that the contents are uniformly mixed before a dose is withdrawn. **Novolin® N** has an intermediate duration of action. The effect of **Novolin® N** begins approximately 1½ hours after injection. The effect is maximal between 4 and 12 hours. The full duration of action may last up to 24 hours after injection. The time course of action for any insulin may vary considerably in different individuals, or at different times in the same individual. Because of this variation, the periods listed here should be considered as general guidelines only.
This human insulin (recombinant DNA origin) is structurally identical to the insulin produced by the human pancreas. This human insulin is produced by recombinant DNA technology utilizing *Saccharomyces cerevisiae* (bakers' yeast) as the production organism.

STORAGE

Insulin should be stored in a cold place, preferably in a refrigerator, but not in the freezing compartment. **Do not let it freeze.** Keep the insulin vial in its carton so that it will stay clean and protected from light. If refrigeration is not possible, the bottle of insulin which you are currently using can be kept unrefrigerated as long as it is kept as cool as possible and away from heat and sunlight.
Never use **Novolin® N** if the precipitate (the white deposit at the bottom of the vial) has become lumpy or granular in appearance or has formed a deposit of solid particles on the wall of the vial. This insulin should not be used if the liquid in the vial remains clear after the vial has been gently agitated.

Never use insulin after the expiration date which is printed on the vial label and carton.

MIXING TWO TYPES IF INSULIN

Different insulins should be mixed only under instruction from a physician. Hypodermic syringes may vary in the amount of space between the bottom line and the needle ("dead space"), so if you are mixing two types of insulin be sure to discuss any change in the model and brand of syringe you are using with your physician or pharmacist. When you are mixing two types of insulin, always draw the Regular (clear) insulin into the syringe first.
SEE NOVOLIN® 70/30 for complete package insert information on syringes; important statement; preparing the injection; usage in pregnancy, insulin reaction and shock; diabetic ketoacidosis and coma; adverse reactions; and important notes.

HUMAN INSULIN

NOVOLIN® R

Regular, Human Insulin Injection (recombinant DNA origin) USP
100 units/ml

DESCRIPTION

Novolin® R is generically known as Regular, Human Insulin Injection (recombinant DNA origin) USP. The concentration of this product is 100 units of insulin per milliliter. It is a clear, colorless solution which has a short duration of action. The effect of **Novolin® R** begins approximately ½ hour after injection. The effect is maximal between 2½ and 5 hours and ends approximately 8 hours after injection. The time course of action of any insulin may vary considerably in different individuals or at different times in the same individual. Because of this variation, the time periods listed here should be considered as general guidelines only.
This human insulin (recombinant DNA origin) is structurally identical to the insulin produced by the human pancreas. This human insulin is produced by recombinant DNA technology utilizing *Saccharomyces cerevisiae* (bakers' yeast) as the production organism.

STORAGE

Insulin should be stored in a cold place, preferably in a refrigerator, but not in the freezing compartment. **Do not let it freeze.** Keep the insulin vial in its carton so that it will stay clean and protected from light. If refrigeration is not possible, the bottle of insulin which you are currently using can be kept unrefrigerated as long as it is kept as cool as possible and away from heat and sunlight.
Never use **Novolin® R** if it becomes viscous (thickened) or cloudy; use it only if it is clear and colorless.

Never use insulin after the expiration date which is printed on the vial label and carton.

MIXING TWO TYPES OF INSULIN—SEE NOVOLIN® N.

IMPORTANT NOTES

1. Due to risk of precipitation in some pump catheters, Novolin® R is not recommended for use in insulin pumps.
2. A change in the type, strength, species or purity of insulin could require a dosage adjustment. Any change in insulin should be made under medical supervision.
3. You may have learned how to test your urine or your blood for glucose. It is important to do these tests regularly and to record the results for review with your physician or nurse educator.
4. If you have an acute illness, especially with vomiting or fever, continue taking your insulin. If possible, stay on your regular diet. If you have trouble eating, drink fruit juices, regular soft drinks, or clear soups; if you can, eat small amounts of bland foods. Test your urine for glucose and ketones and, if possible, test your blood glucose. Note the results and contact your physician for possible insulin dose adjustment. If you have severe and prolonged vomiting, seek emergency medical care.
5. You should always carry identification which states that you have diabetes.

See Novolin® 70/30 for complete package insert information on syringes; important statement; preparing the injection; usage in pregnancy, insulin reaction and shock; diabetic ketoacidosis and coma; adverse reactions; and important notes.

INSULATARD® NPH, HUMAN

Human Insulin Isophane Suspension (semi-synthetic)
100 units/ml

DESCRIPTION

Insulatard® NPH, Human is a suspension of protamine insulin crystals. It has a slower onset of action than Velosulin® Human (Regular) insulin. The effect on the blood sugar begins approximately 1½ hours after the injection and lasts up to approximately 24 hours, having its maximum effect between the 4th and 12th hour.
The time course of action of any insulin may vary considerably in different individuals, or at different times in the same individual. Because of this variation, the time periods listed here should be considered as general guidelines only.
Rotate the vial carefully to obtain a uniformly cloudy suspension of the crystals. Avoid heavy foaming. Do not use a vial if the insulin remains clear after it has been rotated. Also, do not use it if you see lumps that float or stick to the sides of the vial.
This human insulin is structurally identical to the insulin produced by the pancreas in the human body. This structural identity is obtained by enzymatic conversion of the purified pork insulin.

STORAGE

Insulin should be stored in a cold place, preferably in a refrigerator, but not in the freezing compartment. **Do not let it freeze.** Keep the insulin vial in its carton so that it will stay clean and protected from light. If refrigeration is not possible, the bottle of insulin which you are currently using can be kept unrefrigerated as long as it is kept as cool as possible and away from heat and sunlight.

Never use insulin after the expiration date which is printed on the vial label and carton.

See NOVOLIN® 70/30 for package insert information on syringes; important statement; preparing the injection; usage in pregnancy; insulin reaction and shock; diabetic ketoacidosis and coma; adverse reactions; and important notes.

MIXTARD® HUMAN 70/30

70% Human Insulin Isophane Suspension and
30% Human Insulin Injection (semi-synthetic)
100 units/ml

DESCRIPTION

Mixtard® Human 70/30 is a standard mixture of 30% Velosulin® Human (corresponding to Regular insulin) and 70% Insulatard® NPH Human. The content of Velosulin® Human gives the preparation a rapid onset of effect on the blood sugar, approximately ½ hour after the injection. The content of Insulatard® NPH Human gives it a duration of up to 24 hours, depending on the size of the dose. The maximal effect lies between the 4th and the 8th hour after injection.
The time course of action of any insulin may vary considerably in different individuals, or at different times in the same individual. Because of this variation, the time periods listed here should be considered as general guidelines only.
Rotate the vial carefully to obtain a uniformly cloudy suspension of the crystals. Avoid heavy foaming. Do not use a vial if the insulin remains clear after it has been rotated. Also, do not use it if you see lumps that float or stick to the sides of the vial.
This human insulin is structurally identical to the insulin produced by the pancreas in the human body. This structural identity is obtained by enzymatic conversion of purified pork insulin.

STORAGE

Insulin should be stored in a cold place, preferably in a refrigerator, but not in the freezing compartment. **Do not let it freeze.** Keep the insulin vial in its carton so that it will stay clean and protected from light. If refrigeration is not possible, the bottle of insulin which you are currently using can be kept unrefrigerated as long as it is kept as cool as possible and away from heat and sunlight.

Never use insulin after the expiration date which is printed on the vial label and carton.

See NOVOLIN® 70/30 for package insert information on syringes; important statement; preparing the injection; usage in pregnancy; insulin reaction and shock; diabetic ketoacidosis and coma; adverse reactions; and important notes.

VELOSULIN® HUMAN

Regular Human Insulin Injection (semi-synthetic)
100 units/ml

DESCRIPTION

Velosulin® Human is a clear solution of insulin. It has a rapid onset of action, approximately ½ hour after the injection. The effect lasts up to approximately 8 hours with a maximal effect between the 1st and 3rd hour.
The time course of action of any insulin may vary considerably in different individuals, or at different times in the same individual. Because of this variation, the time periods listed here should be considered as general guidelines only.
Do not use the preparation if the color has become other than water clear or if the liquid has become viscous.
This human insulin is structurally identical to the insulin produced by the pancreas in the human body. This structural

identity is obtained by enzymatic conversion of purified pork insulin.

STORAGE

Insulin should be stored in a cold place, preferably in a refrigerator, but not in the freezing compartment. **Do not let it freeze.** Keep the insulin vial in its carton so that it will stay clean and protected from light. If refrigeration is not possible, the bottle of insulin which you are currently using can be kept unrefrigerated as long as it is kept as cool as possible and away from heat and sunlight.

Never use insulin after the expiration date which is printed on the vial label and carton.

MIXING TWO TYPES OF INSULIN

Different insulins should be mixed only under instruction from a physician. Hypodermic syringes may vary in the amount of space between the bottom line and the needle ("dead space"), so if you are mixing two types of insulin be sure to discuss any change in the model and brand of syringe you are using with your physician or pharmacist. When you are mixing two types of insulin, always draw the Regular (clear) insulin into the syringe first.

Velosulin® Human should not be mixed with Lente®-type insulins, because the buffering agent in Velosulin® Human could interact with the other insulin and change its activity. This could lead to an unpredictable effect on blood sugar.

See NOVOLIN® 70/30 for package insert information on syringes; important statement; preparing the injection; usage in pregnancy; insulin reaction and shock; diabetic ketoacidosis and coma; adverse reactions; and important notes.

HUMAN INSULIN DELIVERY SYSTEM

NOVOLIN® R PenFill®
Regular, Human Insulin Injection (recombinant DNA origin)
100 units/ml
5 x 1.5 ml cartridges
PenFill® cartridge is for single person use only.

DESCRIPTION

Novolin® R PenFill® cartridges contain **Novolin® R**, generically known as Regular, Human Insulin Injection (recombinant DNA origin). The concentration of this product is 100 units of insulin per milliliter. It is a clear, colorless solution which has a short duration of action. The effect of **Novolin® R** begins approximately ½ hour after injection. The effect is maximal between 2½ and 5 hours and ends approximately 8 hours after injection. The time course of action of any insulin may vary considerably in different individuals, or at different times in the same individual. Because of this variation, the time periods listed here should be considered as general guidelines only.
This human insulin (recombinant DNA origin) is structurally identical to the insulin produced by the human pancreas. This human insulin is produced by recombinant DNA technology utilizing *Saccharomyces cerevisiae* (bakers' yeast) as the production organism.
Novolin® PenFill® cartridges are designed for specific use with **NovoPen®** and/or **NovolinPen®** Insulin Delivery Systems.

STORAGE

Insulin should be stored in a cold place, preferably in a refrigerator, but not in the freezing compartment. **Do not let it freeze.** Keep **Novolin® R PenFill®** cartridges in the carton so that they will stay clean and protected from light. **Novolin® R PenFill®** cartridges can be kept unrefrigerated for one (1) month. Unrefrigerated cartridges must be used within this time period or discarded. Be sure to protect cartridges from sunlight and extreme heat or cold.
Never use any **Novolin® PenFill®** if it becomes viscous (thickened) or cloudy; use it only if it is clear and colorless.

Never use insulin after the expiration date which is printed on the cartridge label and carton.

See NOVOLIN® 70/30 for package insert information on syringes; important statement; preparing the injection; usage in pregnancy; insulin reaction and shock; diabetic ketoacidosis and coma; adverse reactions; and important notes.

NOVOLIN® N PenFill®
NPH, Human Insulin Isophane Suspension (recombinant DNA origin)
100 units/ml
5 × 1.5 ml cartridges
PenFill® cartridge is for single person use only.

DESCRIPTION

Novolin® N PenFill® cartridges contain **Novolin® N**, generically known as NPH, Human Insulin Isophane Suspension (recombinant DNA origin). The concentration of this product is 100 units of insulin per milliliter. It is a cloudy or milky suspension of human insulin with protamine and zinc. The insulin substance (the cloudy material) settles at the

bottom of the cartridge; therefore, the cartridge must be turned up and down at least 10 times or until the liquid appears uniformly white and cloudy (a glass ball inside the cartridge facilitates mixing).
Novolin® N has an intermediate duration of action. The effect of **Novolin® N** begins approximately 1½ hours after injection. The effect is maximal between 4 and 12 hours. The full duration of action may last up to 24 hours after injection. The time course of action for any insulin may vary considerably in different individuals, or at different times in the same individual. Because of this variation, the time periods listed here should be considered as general guidelines only.
This human insulin (recombinant DNA origin) is structurally identical to the insulin produced by the human pancreas. This human insulin is produced by recombinant DNA technology utilizing *Saccharomyces cerevisiae* (bakers' yeast) as the production organism.
Novolin® PenFill® cartridges are designed for specific use with **NovoPen®** and/or **NovolinPen®** Insulin Delivery Systems.

STORAGE

Insulin should be stored in a cold place, preferably in a refrigerator, but not in the freezing compartment. **Do not let it freeze.** Keep the **Novolin® N PenFill®** cartridges in the carton so that they will stay clean and protected from light. **Novolin® N PenFill®** cartridges can be kept unrefrigerated for one (1) week. Unrefrigerated cartridges must be used within this time period or discarded. Be sure to protect cartridges from sunlight and extreme heat or cold.
Never use **Novolin® N PenFill®** cartridge if the precipitate (the white deposit) has become lumpy or granular in appearance or has formed a deposit of solid particles on the wall of the cartridge. This insulin should not be used if the liquid in the cartridge remains clear after it has been mixed.

Never use insulin after the expiration date which is printed on the cartridge label and carton.

See NOVOLIN® 70/30 for package insert information on syringes; important statement; preparing the injection; usage in pregnancy; insulin reaction and shock; diabetic ketoacidosis and coma; adverse reactions; and important notes.

NOVOLIN® 70/30 PenFill®
70% NPH, Human Insulin Isophane Suspension and
30% Regular, Human Insulin Injection
(recombinant DNA origin)
100 units/ml
5 × 1.5 ml cartridges
PenFill® cartridge is for single person use only.

DESCRIPTION

Novolin® 70/30 PenFill® cartridges contain **Novolin® 70/30**, a mixture of 70% NPH, Human Insulin Isophane Suspension and 30% Regular, Human Insulin Injection (recombinant DNA origin) USP. The concentration of this product is 100 units of insulin per milliliter. It is a cloudy or milky suspension of human insulin with protamine and zinc. The insulin substance (the cloudy material) settles at the bottom of the cartridge; therefore, the cartridge must be turned up and down at least 10 times or until the liquid appears uniformly white and cloudy (a glass ball inside the cartridge facilitates mixing).
Novolin® 70/30 has an intermediate duration of action. The effect of **Novolin® 70/30** begins approximately ½ hour after injection. The effect is maximal between 2 and approximately 12 hours. The full duration of action may last up to 24 hours after injection. The time course of action for any insulin may vary considerably in different individuals, or at different times in the same individual. Because of this variation, the time periods listed here should be considered as general guidelines only.
This human insulin (recombinant DNA origin) is structurally identical to the insulin produced by the human pancreas. This human insulin is produced by recombinant DNA technology utilizing *Saccharomyces cerevisiae* (bakers' yeast) as the production organism.
Novolin® PenFill® cartridges are designed for specific use with **NovoPen®** and/or **NovolinPen®** Insulin Delivery Systems.

STORAGE

Insulin should be stored in a cold place, preferably in a refrigerator, but not in the freezing compartment. **Do not let it freeze.** Keep **Novolin® 70/30 PenFill®** cartridges in the carton so that they will stay clean and protected from light. **Novolin® 70/30 PenFill®** cartridges can be kept unrefrigerated for one (1) week. Unrefrigerated cartridges must be used within this time period or discarded. Be sure to protect cartridges from sunlight and extreme heat or cold.
Never use any **Novolin® 70/30 PenFill®** cartridge if the precipitate (the white deposit) has become lumpy or granular in appearance or has formed a deposit of solid particles on the wall of the cartridge. This insulin should not be used if

the liquid in the cartridge remains clear after it has been mixed.

Never use insulin after the expiration date which is printed on the cartridge label and carton.

See NOVOLIN® 70/30 for package insert information on syringes; important statement; preparing the injection; usage in pregnancy; insulin reaction and shock; diabetic ketoacidosis and coma; adverse reactions; and important notes.

NOVOLIN PREFILLED™
PREFILLED INSULIN SYRINGES

NOVOLIN 70/30 PREFILLED™
70% NPH, Human Insulin Isophane Suspension and
30% Regular, Human Insulin Injection
(recombinant DNA origin)
in a 1.5 ml Prefilled Syringe
100 units/ml
This prefilled syringe is specifically designed for use with PenNeedle® Disposable Needle.

Insulin Information For The Patient
Novolin 70/30 Prefilled™ syringe is for single person use only. See important notes section.

WARNING

ANY CHANGE OF INSULIN SHOULD BE MADE CAUTIOUSLY AND ONLY UNDER MEDICAL SUPERVISION. CHANGES IN PURITY, STRENGTH, BRAND (MANUFACTURER), TYPE (REGULAR, NPH, LENTE®, ETC.), SPECIES (BEEF, PORK, BEEF-PORK, HUMAN), AND/OR METHOD OF MANUFACTURE (RECOMBINANT DNA VERSUS ANIMAL-SOURCE INSULIN) MAY RESULT IN THE NEED FOR A CHANGE IN DOSAGE.
SPECIAL CARE SHOULD BE TAKEN WHEN THE TRANSFER IS FROM A STANDARD BEEF OR MIXED SPECIES INSULIN TO A PURIFIED PORK OR HUMAN INSULIN. IF A DOSAGE ADJUSTMENT IS NEEDED, IT WILL USUALLY BECOME APPARENT EITHER IN THE FIRST FEW DAYS OR OVER A PERIOD OF SEVERAL WEEKS. ANY CHANGE IN TREATMENT SHOULD BE CAREFULLY MONITORED.

PRODUCT DESCRIPTION

The package contains five (5) **Novolin 70/30 Prefilled™** insulin syringes. **Novolin® 70/30** is a mixture of 70% NPH, Human Insulin Isophane Suspension (recombinant DNA origin) and 30% Regular, Human Insulin Injection (recombinant DNA origin) USP. The concentration of this product is 100 units of insulin per milliliter. It is a cloudy or milky suspension of human insulin with protamine and zinc. The insulin substance (the cloudy material) settles at the bottom of the insulin reservoir, therefore, the syringe must be rotated up and down so that the contents are uniformly mixed before the dose is given.
Novolin® 70/30 has an intermediate duration of action. The effect of **Novolin® 70/30** begins approximately ½ hour after injection. The effect is maximal between 2 and approximately 12 hours. The full duration of action may last up to 24 hours after injection.
The time course of action of any insulin may vary considerably in different individuals, or at different times in the same individual. Because of the variation, the time periods listed here should be considered as general guidelines only.
This human insulin (recombinant DNA origin) is structurally identical to the insulin produced by the human pancreas. This human insulin is produced by recombinant DNA technology utilizing Saccharomyces cerevisiae (bakers' yeast) as the production organism.

STORAGE

Novolin 70/30 Prefilled™ should be stored in a cold place, preferably in a refrigerator, but not in the freezing compartment. **Do not let it freeze.** Keep **Novolin 70/30 Prefilled™** insulin syringes in the carton so that they will stay clean and protected from light. **Novolin 70/30 Prefilled™** can be kept unrefrigerated for one (1) week. Unrefrigerated syringes must be used within this time period or discarded. Be sure to protect syringes from sunlight and extreme heat or cold. Never use any **Novolin 70/30 Prefilled™** syringe if the precipitate (the white deposit) has become lumpy or granular in appearance or has formed a deposit of solid particles on the wall of the insulin reservoir. This insulin should not be used if the liquid in the insulin reservoir remains clear after it has been mixed.

Never use insulin after the expiration date which is printed on the label and carton.

IMPORTANT

Failure to comply with the following antiseptic measures may lead to infections at the injection site.

Continued on next page

Novo Nordisk—Cont.

—PenNeedle® disposable needles are for single use; they should be used only once and discarded properly.
—Clean your hands and the injection site with soap and water or with alcohol.
—Wipe the rubber stopper with an alcohol swab.

PREPARING THE INJECTION

Never place a PenNeedle® single-use needle on your insulin delivery device until you are ready to give an injection. If the needle is not removed, some liquid may be expelled from the syringe causing a change in the insulin concentration (strength). The cloudy material in an insulin suspension will settle to the bottom of the insulin reservoir, so the syringes contain a glass ball to aid mixing. Rotate the syringe up and down so that the contents are uniformly mixed before the dose is given.

GIVING THE INJECTION

1. The following areas are suitable for subcutaneous insulin injection: Thighs, upper arms, buttocks, abdomen. Do not change areas without consulting your physician. The actual point of injection should be changed each time; injection sites should be about an inch apart.
2. The injection site should be clean and dry. Pinch up skin area to be injected and hold it firmly.
3. Hold the device like a pencil and push the needle quickly and firmly into the pinched-up area. If you go straight in it will probably sting less.
4. Do not inject into a muscle unless your physician has advised it. You should never inject insulin into a vein.
5. Remove needle. If slight bleeding occurs, press lightly with a dry cotton swab for a few seconds—do not rub.

IMPORTANT NOTES

1. A change in the type, strength, species or purity of insulin could require a dosage adjustment. Any change in insulin should be made under medical supervision.
2. To avoid possible transmission of disease, Novolin 70/30 Prefilled™ syringe is for single person use only.
3. You may have learned how to test your urine or your blood for glucose. It is important to do these tests regularly and to record the results for review with your physician or nurse educator.
4. If you have an acute illness, especially with vomiting or fever, continue taking your insulin. If possible, stay on your regular diet. If you have trouble eating, drink fruit juices, regular soft drinks, or clear soups; if you can, eat small amounts of bland foods. Test your urine for glucose and ketones and, if possible, test your blood glucose. Note the results and contact your physician for possible insulin dose adjustment. If you have severe and prolonged vomiting, seek emergency medical care.
5. You should always carry identification which states that you have diabetes.
Always consult your physician if you have any questions about your condition or the use of insulin.
See full package insert enclosed with the Novolin 70/30 Prefilled™ syringe for instructions on using the prefilled syringe.

NOVOPEN®
Insulin Delivery Device

DESCRIPTION

NovoPen® Insulin Delivery Device is made of nickel and chromium-plated brass, is 6 inches in length and 7 ounces in weight, designed to utilize a replaceable 1.5 ml cartridge of Novolin® human insulin (PenFill®) and a single-use disposable needle (PenNeedle®) to deliver 2 or more units of insulin by a push-button mechanism. Dosage accuracy was evaluated over a wide range of units and resulted in a standard deviation of 0.12 units for a dose from the test cartridges. NovoPen® should not be stored in the refrigerator or exposed to extremely hot temperatures. NovoPen® can be cleaned by wiping it with a moistened clean cloth. NovoPen® should only be used with Novolin® PenFill® cartridges and PenNeedle® disposable needles.

PenNeedle®
Disposable Needle

DESCRIPTION

The self-contained disposable needle consists of a protective plastic outer cap, a smooth plastic needle cap and a protective tab. (The needle should not be used if the protective tab is missing or damaged.)
Each PenNeedle® is beveled and siliconized throughout its length to ensure minimal friction with the skin. Each PenNeedle® is 27 gauge, one-half (½) inch (12.5mm) in length and is intended for single use only. The product is sold

in boxes containing 100 single-use PenNeedle® disposable needles.
This disposable needle is specifically designed to be used with NOVOPEN®, NOVOLINPEN®, and NOVOLIN PRE-FILLED™ Products.

EDUCATIONAL MATERIAL

PATIENT EDUCATION MATERIALS
NOVO DIABETES CARE™
SERVICE PROGRAMS THAT
EDUCATE AND SUPPORT
Novo Diabetes Care™ is a comprehensive service program encompassing patient education materials, professional education programs and a wide variety of services to support health care professionals and their patients with diabetes. Some of the items available from Novo Diabetes Care™ are:
Professional Education
● CME & CPE Programs
● Speakers
● ProFile informative newsletter
Patient Education
● Self-management materials
● Modules for individualized treatment
   —for children with diabetes and their parents
   —for patients with type II diabetes
   —for patients with complications
For additional information call 1-800-727-6500.

Novopharm, Inc.
165 EAST COMMERCE DRIVE, SUITES 100-101-200
SCHAUMBURG, IL 60173-5326

The following list of Novopharm, Inc. products is provided to facilitate identification. It includes the color(s) and identification codes for all tablets and capsules. NDC Numbers are also provided for each product.

PRODUCT GENERIC NAME Description Color(s)	IDENTIFICATION CODE (Front/Back-Tablets) (Left/Right-Capsules) NDC NUMBER
AMOXICILLIN Capsules USP, 250MG Rx Caramel/Buff	N 724/250 NDC: 55953-724
AMOXICILLIN Capsules USP, 500mg Rx Buff/Buff	N 716/500 NDC: 55953-716
AMOXICILLIN For Oral Suspension USP, 125MG/5ML, Rx	— NDC: 55953-149
AMOXICILLIN For Oral Suspension USP, 250MG/5ML, Rx	— NDC: 55953-130
CEPHALEXIN Capsules USP, 250mg Rx Gray/Swedish Orange	N 084/250 NDC: 55953-084
CEPHALEXIN Capsules USP, 500mg Rx Swedish Orange/Swedish Orange	N 114/500 NDC: 55953-114
CEPHALEXIN For Oral Suspension USP 125MG/5ML Rx	— NDC: 55953-106
CEPHALEXIN For Oral Suspension USP 250MG/5ML Rx	— NDC: 55953-092
CLOFIBRATE Capsules, USP, 500MG Rx Yellow	L/N 382 NDC: 55953-382
INDOMETHACIN Capsules, 25MG Rx Light Green/Light Green	N 420/25 NDC: 55953-420
INDOMETHACIN Capsules, 50MG Rx Light Green/Light Green	N 439/50 NDC: 55953-439
LOPERAMIDE HYDROCHLORIDE Capsules USP, 2MG Rx White Opaque/White Opaque	N 020/2 NDC: 55953-020
METHYLDOPA Tablets USP, 125MG Rx White	N/463 NDC: 55953-463
METHYLDOPA Tablets USP, 250MG Rx White	N/471 NDC: 55953-471
METHYLDOPA Tablets USP, 500MG Rx White	N/498 NDC: 55953-498
METHYLDOPA AND **HYDROCHLOROTHIAZIDE** Tablets USP, 250MG/15MG Rx Light Green	N/634 NDC: 55953-634
METHYLDOPA AND **HYDROCHLOROTHIAZIDE** Tablets USP, 250MG/25MG Rx White	N/642 NDC: 55953-642
METHYLDOPA AND **HYDROCHLOROTHIAZIDE** Tablets USP, 500MG/30MG Rx Dark Green	N/635 NDC: 55953-635
METHYLDOPA AND **HYDROCHLOROTHIAZIDE** Tablets USP, 500MG/50MG Rx White	N/643 NDC: 55953-643
NIFEDIPINE Capsules USP, 10MG Rx Brown	N 040/10 NDC: 55953-040
NIFEDIPINE Capsules USP, 10MG Rx Yellow	497/Blank NDC: 55953-040
NIFEDIPINE Capsules USP, 20MG Rx Reddish Brown	530/Blank NDC: 55953-045
TOLMETIN SODIUM Capsules USP, 400MG Rx Opaque Red/Opaque Red	N 815/400 NDC: 55953-815

Nutripharm Laboratories, Inc.
8 BARTLES CORNER ROAD, SUITE 101
FLEMINGTON, NJ 08822

ISOCOM®   ℞

CAUTION
Federal law prohibits dispensing without prescription.

DESCRIPTION
Each capsule contains Isometheptene Mucate 65 mg., Dichloralphenazone 100 mg., and Acetaminophen 325 mg. Isometheptene Mucate is a white crystalline powder having a characteristic aromatic odor and bitter taste. It is an unsaturated aliphatic amine with sympathomimetic properties. Dichloralphenazone is a white microcrystalline powder, with slight odor and tastes saline at first, becoming acrid. It is a mild sedative.
Acetaminophen, a non-salicylate, occurs as a white, odorless, crystalline powder possessing a slightly bitter taste.

ACTIONS
Isometheptene Mucate, a sympathomimetic amine, acts by constricting dilated cranial and cerebral arterioles, thus reducing the stimuli that lead to vascular headaches. Dichloralphenazone, a mild sedative, reduces the patient's emotional reaction to the pain of both vascular and tension headaches. Acetaminophen raises the threshold to painful stimuli, thus exerting an analgesic effect against all types of headaches.

INDICATIONS
For relief of vascular and tension headaches.

Based on a review for this drug (isometheptene mucate), The National Academy of Sciences—National Research Council and/or other information, FDA has classified the other indication as "possibly" effective in the treatment of migraine headache.
Final classification of the less-than-effective indication requires further investigation.

CONTRAINDICATIONS
Isocom is contraindicated in Glaucoma and/or severe cases of renal disease, hypertension, organic heart disease, hepatic disease and in those patients who are on monoamineoxidase (MAO) inhibitor therapy.

PRECAUTIONS
Caution should be observed in hypertension, peripheral vascular disease and after recent cardiovascular attacks.

ADVERSE REACTIONS
Transient dizziness and skin rash may appear in hypersensitive patients. This can usually be eliminated by reducing the dose.

DOSAGE AND ADMINISTRATION

FOR RELIEF OF MIGRAINE HEADACHE: The usual adult dose is two capsules at once, followed by one capsule every hour until relieved, up to 5 capsules within a twelve hour period.

FOR RELIEF OF TENSION HEADACHE: The usual adult dose is one or two capsules every four hours up to 8 capsules a day.

HOW SUPPLIED

Bottles of 50 capsules, NDC 51081-424-05, bottles of 100 capsules, NDC 51081-424-10, bottles of 250 capsules, NDC 51081-424-25.

NUTRIPHARM LABORATORIES, INC.
Flemington, N.J. 08822

Oclassen Pharmaceuticals, Inc.
100 PELICAN WAY
SAN RAFAEL, CA 94901

CONDYLOX®   ℞
[con 'de-lox]
(podofilox)
0.5% topical solution

DESCRIPTION

Condylox® is the brand name of podofilox, an antimitotic drug which can be chemically synthesized or purified from the plant families *Coniferae* and *Berberidaceae* (e.g. species of *Juniperus* and *Podophyllum*). Condylox® 0.5% solution is formulated for topical administration. Each milliliter of solution contains 5 mg of podofilox, in a vehicle containing lactic acid and sodium lactate in alcohol 95%, USP.

Podofilox has a molecular weight of 414.4 daltons, and is soluble in alcohol and sparingly soluble in water. Its chemical name is 5,8,8a,9-Tetrahydro-9-hydroxy-5-(3,4,5-trimethoxylphenyl)furo [3',4':6,7] naphtho [2,3,d] -1,3-dioxol-6(5aH)-one. Podofilox has the following structural formula:

CLINICAL PHARMACOLOGY
Mechanism of Action
Treatment of genital warts with podofilox results in necrosis of visible wart tissue. The exact mechanism of action is unknown.

Pharmacokinetics
In systemic absorption studies in 52 patients, topical applications of 0.05 mL of 0.5% podofilox solution to external genitalia did not result in detectable serum levels. Applications of 0.1 to 1.5 mL resulted in peak serum levels of 1 to 17 ng/mL one to two hours after application. The elimination half-life ranged from 1.0 to 4.5 hours. The drug was not found to accumulate after multiple treatments.

CLINICAL STUDIES
In clinical studies with Condylox® Solution, the test product and its vehicle were applied in a double-blind fashion to comparable patient groups. Patients were treated for two to four weeks, and reevaluated at a two-week follow-up examination. Although the number of patients and warts evaluated at each time period varied, the results among investigators were relatively consistent.

The following table represents the responses noted in terms of frequency of response by lesions treated and the overall response by patients. Data are presented for the 2-week follow-up only for those patients evaluated at that time point.

Responses in Treated Patients

	Initially Cleared*	Recurred after Clearing*	Cleared at 2-Week Follow-Up*
% Warts (n=524)	79% (412/524)	35% (146/412)	60% (269/449)
% Patients (n=70)	50% (35/70)	60% (21/35)	25% (14/57)

*Cleared and clearing mean no visible wart tissue remained at the treated sites

INDICATIONS AND USAGE
Condylox® 0.5% solution is indicated for the topical treatment of external genital warts (Condyloma acuminatum). This product is *not* indicated in the treatment of perianal or mucous membrane warts (see PRECAUTIONS).

Diagnosis
Although genital warts have a characteristic appearance, histopathologic confirmation should be obtained if there is any doubt of the diagnosis. Differentiating warts from squamous cell carcinoma (so-called "Bowenoid papulosis") is of particular concern. Squamous cell carcinoma may also be associated with human papillomavirus but should not be treated with Condylox® 0.5% solution.

CONTRAINDICATIONS
Condylox® 0.5% solution is contraindicated for patients who develop hypersensitivity or intolerance to any component of the formulation.

WARNINGS
Correct diagnosis of the lesions to be treated is essential. See the "Diagnosis" subsection of the INDICATIONS AND USAGE statement.

Condylox® 0.5% solution is intended for cutaneous use only. **Avoid contact with the eye. If eye contact occurs, patients should immediately flush the eye with copious quantities of water and seek medical advice.**

PRECAUTIONS
General
Data are not available on the safe and effective use of this product for treatment of warts occurring in the perianal area or mucous membranes of the genital area (including the urethra, rectum and vagina). The recommended method of application, frequency of application, and duration of usage should not be exceeded (see DOSAGE AND ADMINISTRATION).

Information for Patients
The patient should be provided with a Patient Information leaflet when a Condylox® prescription is filled.

Carcinogenesis, Mutagenesis and Impairment of Fertility
Reports of lifetime carcinogenicity studies in mice are not available. Published animal studies, in general, have not shown the drug substance, podofilox, to be carcinogenic.[1,2,3,4,5] There are published reports that, in mouse studies, crude podophyllin resin (containing podofilox) applied topically to the cervix produced changes resembling carcimona *in situ*.[6] These changes were reversible at five weeks after cessation of treatment. In one reported experiment, epidermal carcinoma of the vagina and cervix was found in 1 out of 18 mice after 120 applications of podophyllin[7] (the drug was applied twice weekly over a 15-month period). Podofilox was not mutagenic in the Ames plate reverse mutation assay at concentrations up to 5 mg/plate, with and without metabolic activation. No cell transformation related to potential oncogenicity was observed in BALB/3T3 cells after exposure to podofilox at concentrations up to 0.008 μg/mL without metabolic activation and 12 μg/mL podofilox with metabolic activation. Results from the mouse micronucleus *in vivo* assay using podofilox 0.5% solution in concentrations up to 25 mg/kg, indicate that podofilox should be considered a potential clastogen (a chemical that induces disruption and breakage of chromosomes).

Daily topical applications of Condylox® 0.5% Solution at doses up to the equivalent of 0.2 mg/kg (5 times the recommended maximum human dose) to rats throughout gametogenesis, mating, gestation, parturition and lactation for two generations demonstrated no impairment of fertility.

Pregnancy
Pregnancy Category C: Podofilox was not teratogenic in the rabbit following topical application of up to 0.21 mg/kg (5 times the maximum human dose) once daily for 13 days. The scientific literature contains references that podofilox is embryotoxic in rats when administered systemically in a dose approximately 250 times the recommended maximum human dose.[8,9] Teratogenicity and embryotoxicity have not been studied with intravaginal application. Many antimitotic drug products are known to be embryotoxic. There are no adequate and well-controlled studies in pregnant women. Podofilox should be used in pregnancy only if the potential benefit justifies the potential risk to the fetus.

Nursing Mothers
It is not known whether this drug is excreted in human milk. Because of the potential for serious adverse reactions in nursing infants from podofilox, a decision should be made whether to discontinue nursing or to discontinue the drug, taking into account the importance of the drug to the mother.

Pediatric Use
Safety and effectiveness in children have not been established.

ADVERSE REACTIONS
In clinical trials, the following local adverse reactions were reported at some point during treatment.

Adverse Experience	Males	Females
Burning	64%	78%
Pain	50%	72%
Inflammation	71%	63%
Erosion	67%	67%
Itching	50%	65%

Reports of burning and pain were more frequent and of greater severity in women than in men.

Adverse effects reported in less than 5% of the patients included pain with intercourse, insomnia, tingling, bleeding, tenderness, chafing, malodor, dizziness, scarring, vesicle formation, crusting, edema, dryness/peeling, foreskin irretraction, hematuria, vomiting and ulceration.

OVERDOSAGE
Topically applied podofilox may be absorbed systemically (see CLINICAL PHARMACOLOGY section). Toxicity reported following systemic administration of podofilox in investigational use for cancer treatment included: nausea, vomiting, fever, diarrhea, bone marrow depression, and oral ulcers. Following 5 to 10 daily intravenous doses of 0.5 to 1 mg/kg/day, significant hematological toxicity occurred but was reversible. Other toxicities occurred at lower doses. Toxicity reported following systemic administration of podophyllum resin included: nausea, vomiting, fever, diarrhea, peripheral neuropathy, altered mental status, lethargy, coma, tachypnea, respiratory failure, leukocytosis, pancytosis, hematuria, renal failure, and seizures. Treatment of topical overdosage should include washing the skin free of any remaining drug and symptomatic and supportive therapy.

DOSAGE AND ADMINISTRATION
In order to ensure that the patient is fully aware of the correct method of therapy and to identify which specific warts should be treated, the technique for initial application of the medication should be demonstrated by the prescriber.

Apply twice daily morning and evening (every 12 hours), for 3 consecutive days, then withhold use for 4 consecutive days. This one week cycle of treatment may be repeated up to four times until there is no visible wart tissue. **If there is incomplete response after four treatment weeks, alternative treatment should be considered. Safety and effectiveness of more than four treatment weeks have not been established.**

Condylox® 0.5% solution is applied to the warts with a cotton-tipped applicator supplied with the drug. The drug-dampened applicator should be touched to the wart to be treated, applying the minimum amount of solution necessary to cover the lesion. **Treatment should be limited to less than 10 cm² of wart tissue and to no more than 0.5 mL of the solution per day.** There is no evidence to suggest that more frequent application will increase efficacy, but additional applications would be expected to increase the rate of local adverse reactions and systemic absorption.

Care should be taken to allow the solution to dry before allowing the return of opposing skin surfaces to their normal positions. After each treatment, the used applicator should be carefully disposed of and the patient should wash his or her hands.

HOW SUPPLIED
3.5 mL of Condylox® 0.5% solution is supplied as a clear liquid in amber glass bottles with child-resistant screw caps. NDC #55515-101-01. Store at controlled room temperature between 15° and 30°C (59° and 86°F). **Avoid excessive heat. Do not freeze.**

Caution—Federal law prohibits dispensing without prescription.

REFERENCES
1. Berenblum, 1951. J. Natl. Cancer Inst. *11:* 839–841
2. H.A. Kaminetsky and M. Swerdlow, 1965. Am. J. Obst. Gyn. *93:* 486–490
3. E.A. McGrew and H.A. Kaminetsky. 1961. Am J. Clin. Pathol. *35:* 538–545
4. F.J.C. Roe and M.H. Salaman, 1955. Brit. J. Cancer. *9:* 177–203
5. H.S. Taper, 1977. Z. Kerbsforsch, *90:* 197–210
6. H.A. Kaminetsky and E.A. McGrew, and R.L. Phillips, 1959. Am. J. Obst. Gyn. *14:* 1–3
7. H.A. Kaminetsky and E.A. McGrew, 1963. Arch. Path. *73:* 481–485
8. K. Didcock, D. Jackson, and J.M. Robson, 1956. Brit. J. Pharmacol. *11:* 437–441
9. J. Thiersch, 1963. Soc. Exptl. Biol. Med. Proc. *113:* 124–127
Revised: Dec., 1990
Mfd. for
OCLASSEN
Pharmaceuticals, Inc.
San Rafael, CA 94901
By Abbott Laboratories
N. Chicago, IL 60064

01-2428-R1

Shown in Product Identification Section, page 420

Continued on next page

Oclassen—Cont.

MONODOX® ℞

DOXYCYCLINE MONOHYDRATE CAPSULES
[mon′o-dox]

DESCRIPTION

Doxycycline is a broad-spectrum antibiotic synthetically derived from oxytetracycline. Monodox® 100 mg & 50 mg capsules contain doxycycline monohydrate equivalent to 100 mg or 50 mg of doxycycline for oral administration. The chemical designation of the light-yellow crystalline powder is alpha-6-deoxy-5-oxytetracycline.

Structural formula:

$C_{22}H_{24}N_2O_8 \cdot H_2O$ M.W. = 462.46

Doxycycline has a high degree of lipid solubility and a low affinity for calcium binding. It is highly stable in normal human serum.

Doxycycline will not degrade into an epianhydro form.

Inert ingredients: colloidal silicon dioxide; hard gelatin capsule; magnesium stearate; microcrystalline cellulose; and sodium starch glycolate.

CLINICAL PHARMACOLOGY

Tetracyclines are readily absorbed and are bound to plasma proteins in varying degrees. They are concentrated by the liver in the bile and excreted in the urine and feces at high concentrations in a biologically active form. Doxycycline is virtually completely absorbed after oral administration.

Following a 200 mg dose of doxycycline monohydrate, 24 normal adult volunteers averaged the following serum concentration values:

Time (hr):	0.5	1.0	1.5	2.0	3.0	4.0
Conc. (mcg/mL)	1.02	2.26	2.67	3.01	3.16	3.03

Time (hr):	8.0	12.0	24.0	48.0	72.0
Conc. (mcg/mL)	2.03	1.62	0.95	0.37	0.15

Average Observed Values	
Maximum Concentration	3.61 mcg/mL (± 0.9 sd)
Time of Maximum Concentration	2.60 hr (± 1.10 sd)
Elimination Rate Constant	0.049 per hr (± 0.030 sd)
Half-Life	16.33 hr (± 4.53 sd)

Excretion of doxycycline by the kidney is about 40%/72 hours in individuals with normal function (creatinine clearance about 75 mL/min). This percentage excretion may fall as low as 1-5%/72 hours in individuals with severe renal insufficiency (creatinine clearance below 10 mL/min). Studies have shown no significant difference in serum half-life of doxycycline (range 18-22 hours) in individuals with normal and severely impaired renal function.

Hemodialysis does not alter serum half-life.

Microbiology: The tetracyclines are primarily bacteriostatic and are thought to exert their antimicrobial effect by the inhibition of protein synthesis. The tetracyclines, including doxycycline, have a similar antimicrobial spectrum of activity against a wide range of gram-positive and gram-negative organisms. Cross-resistance of these organisms to tetracyclines is common.

While in vitro studies have demonstrated the susceptibility of most strains of the following microorganisms, clinical efficacy for infections other than those included in the INDICATIONS AND USAGE section has not been documented.

GRAM-NEGATIVE BACTERIA:

Neisseria gonorrhoeae
Haemophilus ducreyi
Haemophilus influenzae
Yersinia pestis (formerly *Pasteurella pestis*)
Francisella tularensis (formerly *Pasteurella tularensis*)
Vibrio cholerae (formerly *Vibrio comma*)
Bartonella bacilliformis
Brucella species

Because many strains of the following groups of gram-negative microorganisms have been shown to be resistant to tetracyclines, culture and susceptibility testing are recommended:

Escherichia coli
Klebsiella species
Enterobacter aerogenes
Shigella species
Acinetobacter species (formerly *Mima* species and *Herellea* species)
Bacteroides species

GRAM-POSITIVE BACTERIA:

Because many strains of the following groups of gram-positive microorganisms have been shown to be resistant to tetracyclines, culture and susceptibility testing are recommended.

Up to 44 percent of strains of *Streptococcus pyogenes* and 74 percent of *Streptococcus faecalis* have been found to be resistant to tetracycline drugs. Therefore, tetracyclines should not be used to treat streptococcal infections unless the organism has been demonstrated to be susceptible.

Streptococcus pyogenes
Streptococcus pneumoniae
Enterococcus group (*Streptococcus faecalis* and *Streptococcus faecium*)
Alpha-hemolytic streptococci (*viridans* group)

OTHER MICROORGANISMS:

Chlamydia psittaci
Chlamydia trachomatis
Ureaplasma urealyticum
Borrelia recurrentis
Treponema pallidum
Treponema pertenue
Clostridium species
Fusobacterium fusiforme
Actinomyces species
Bacillus anthracis
Propionibacterium acnes
Entamoeba species
Balantidium coli

Susceptibility tests: Diffusion Techniques: Quantitative methods that require measurement of zone diameters give the most precise estimate of the susceptibility of bacteria to antimicrobial agents.

One such standard procedure which has been recommended for use with disks to test susceptibility of organisms to doxycycline uses the 30-mcg tetracycline-class disk or the 30-mcg doxycycline disk. Interpretation involves the correlation of the diameter obtained in the disk test with the minimum inhibitory concentration (MIC) for tetracycline or doxycycline, respectively.

Reports from the laboratory giving results of the standard single-disk susceptibility test with a 30-mcg tetracycline-class disk or the 30-mcg doxycycline disk should be interpreted according to the following criteria.

Zone Diameter (mm)		Interpretation
tetracycline	doxycycline	
≥ 19	≥ 16	Susceptible
15–18	13–15	Intermediate
≤ 14	≤ 12	Resistant

A report of "susceptible" indicates that the pathogen is likely to be inhibited by generally achievable blood levels. A report "intermediate" suggests that the organism would be susceptible if a high dosage is used or if the infection is confined to tissues and fluids in which high antimicrobial levels are attained. A report of "resistant" indicates that achievable concentrations are unlikely to be inhibitory, and other therapy should be selected.

Standardized procedures require the use of laboratory control organisms. The 30-mcg tetracycline-class disk or the 30-mcg doxycycline disk should give the following zone diameters:

Organism	Zone Diameter	
	tetracycline	doxycycline
E. coli ATCC 25922	18–25	18–24
S. aureus ATCC 25923	19–28	23–29

Dilution Techniques:

Use a standard dilution method[2] (broth, agar, microdilution) or equivalent with tetracycline powder. The MIC values obtained should be interpreted according to the following criteria:

MIC (mcg/mL)	Interpretation
≤ 4	Susceptible
8	Intermediate
≥ 16	Resistant

As with standard diffusion techniques, dilution methods require the use of laboratory control organisms. Standard tetracycline powder should provide the following MIC values:

Organism	MIC (mcg/mL)
S. aureus ATCC 29213	0.25–1
E. faecalis ATCC 29212	8–32
E. coli ATCC 25922	1–4
P. aeruginosa ATCC 27853	8–32

INDICATIONS AND USAGE

Doxycycline is indicated for the treatment of the following infections:

Rocky mountain spotted fever, typhus fever and the typhus group, Q fever, rickettsialpox, and tick fevers caused by Rickettsiae.

Respiratory tract infections caused by *Mycoplasma pneumoniae*.

Lymphogranuloma venereum caused by *Chlamydia trachomatis*.

Psittacosis (ornithosis) caused by *Chlamydia psittaci*.

Trachoma caused by *Chlamydia trachomatis*, although the infectious agent is not always eliminated as judged by immunofluorescence.

Inclusion conjunctivitis caused by *Chlamydia trachomatis*.

Uncomplicated urethral, endocervical or rectal infections in adults caused by *Chlamydia trachomatis*.

Nongonococcal urethritis caused by *Ureaplasma urealyticum*.

Relapsing fever due to *Borrelia recurrentis*.

Doxycycline is also indicated for the treatment of infections caused by the following gram-negative microorganisms:

Chancroid caused by *Haemophilus ducreyi*.

Plague due to *Yersinia pestis* (formerly *Pasteurella pestis*).

Tularemia due to *Francisella tularensis* (formerly *Pasteurella tularensis*).

Cholera caused by *Vibrio cholerae* (formerly *Vibrio comma*).

Campylobacter fetus infections caused by *Campylobacter fetus* (formerly *Vibrio fetus*).

Brucellosis due to *Brucella* species (in conjunction with streptomycin).

Bartonellosis due to *Bartonella bacilliformis*.

Granuloma inguinale caused by *Calymmatobacterium granulomatis*.

Because many strains of the following groups of microorganisms have been shown to be resistant to doxycycline, culture and susceptibility testing are recommended.

Doxycycline is indicated for treatment of infections caused by the following gram-negative microorganisms, when bacteriologic testing indicates appropriate susceptibility to the drug:

Escherichia coli
Enterobacter aerogenes (formerly *Aerobacter aerogenes*)
Shigella species
Acinetobacter species (formerly *Mima* species and *Herellea* species)
Respiratory tract infections caused by *Haemophilus influenzae*.
Respiratory tract and urinary tract infections caused by *Klebsiella species*.

Doxycycline is indicated for treatment of infections caused by the following gram-positive microorganisms when bacteriologic testing indicates appropriate susceptibility to the drug:

Upper respiratory infections caused by *Streptococcus pneumoniae* (formerly *Diplococcus pneumoniae*).

Skin and skin structure infections caused by *Staphylococcus aureus*. Doxycycline is not the drug of choice in the treatment of any type of staphylococcal infections.

When penicillin is contraindicated, doxycycline is an alternative drug in the treatment of the following infections:

Uncomplicated gonorrhea caused by *Neisseria gonorrhoeae*.

Syphillis caused by *Treponema pallidum*.

Yaws caused by *Treponema pertenue*.

Listeriosis due to *Listeria monocytogenes*.

Anthrax due to *Bacillus anthracis*.

Vincent's infection caused by *Fusobacterium fusiforme*.

Actinomycosis caused by *Actinomyces israelli*.

Infections caused by *Clostridium* species .

In acute intestinal amebiasis, doxycycline may be a useful adjunct to amebicides.

In severe acne, doxycycline may be useful adjunctive therapy.

CONTRAINDICATIONS

This drug is contraindicated in persons who have shown hypersensitivity to any of the tetracyclines.

WARNINGS

THE USE OF DRUGS OF THE TETRACYCLINE CLASS DURING TOOTH DEVELOPMENT (LAST HALF OF PREGNANCY, INFANCY, AND CHILDHOOD TO THE AGE OF 8 YEARS) MAY CAUSE PERMANENT DISCOLORATION OF THE TEETH (YELLOW-GRAY-BROWN).

This adverse reaction is more common during long term use of the drugs but has been observed following repeated short-term courses. Enamel hypoplasia has also been reported. TETRACYCLINE DRUGS, THEREFORE, SHOULD NOT BE USED IN THIS AGE GROUP UNLESS OTHER DRUGS ARE NOT LIKELY TO BE EFFECTIVE OR ARE CONTRAINDICATED.

All tetracyclines form a stable calcium complex in any bone-forming tissue. A decrease in the fibula growth rate has been observed in prematures given oral tetracycline in doses of 25 mg/kg every six hours. This reaction was shown to be reversible when the drug was discontinued.

Results of animal studies indicate that tetracyclines cross the placenta, are found in fetal tissues, and can have toxic effects on the developing fetus (often related to retardation of skeletal development). Evidence of embryo toxicity has been noted in animals treated early in pregnancy. If any tetracycline is used during pregnancy or if the patient becomes pregnant while taking these drugs, the patient should be apprised of the potential hazard to the fetus.

The antianabolic action of the tetracyclines may cause an increase in BUN. Studies to date indicate that this does not

occur with the use of doxycycline in patients with impaired renal function.

Photosensitivity manifested by an exaggerated sunburn reaction has been observed in some individuals taking tetracyclines. Patients apt to be exposed to direct sunlight or ultraviolet light should be advised that this reaction can occur with tetracycline drugs, and treatment should be discontinued at the first evidence of skin erythema.

PRECAUTIONS

General: As with other antibiotic preparations, use of this drug may result in overgrowth of non-susceptible organisms, including fungi. If superinfection occurs, the antibiotic should be discontinued and appropriate therapy instituted.

Bulging fontanels in infants and benign intracranial hypertension in adults have been reported in individuals receiving tetracyclines. These conditions disappeared when the drug was discontinued.

Incision and drainage or other surgical procedures should be performed in conjunction with antibiotic therapy when indicated.

Laboratory tests: In venereal disease when coexistent syphillis is suspected, a dark-field examination should be done before treatment is started and the blood serology repeated monthly for at least four months.

In long-term therapy, periodic laboratory evaluations of organ systems, including hematopoietic, renal, and hepatic studies should be performed.

Drug interactions: Because tetracyclines have been shown to depress plasma prothrombin activity, patients who are on anticoagulant therapy may require downward adjustment of their anticoagulant dosage.

Since bacteriostatic drugs may interfere with the bactericidal action of penicillin, it is advisable to avoid giving tetracyclines in conjunction with penicillin.

Absorption of tetracyclines is impaired by antacids containing aluminum, calcium, or magnesium, and iron-containing preparations.

Barbiturates, carbamazepine, and phenytoin decrease the half-life of doxycycline.

The concurrent use of tetracycline and methoxyflurane has been reported to result in fatal renal toxicity.

Concurrent use of tetracycline may render oral contraceptives less effective.

Drug/laboratory test interactions: False elevations of urinary catecholamine levels may occur due to interference with the fluorescence test.

Carcinogenesis, mutagenesis, impairment of fertility: Long-term studies in animals to evaluate the carcinogenic potential of doxycycline have not been conducted. However, there has been evidence of oncogenic activity in rats in studies with related antibiotics, oxytetracycline (adrenal and pituitary tumors) and minocycline (thyroid tumors). Likewise, although mutagenicity studies of doxycycline have not been conducted, positive results in *in vitro* mammalian cell assays have been reported for related antibiotics (tetracycline, oxytetracycline). Doxycycline administered orally at dosage levels as high as 250 mg/kg/day had no apparent effect on the fertility of female rats. Effect on male fertility has not been studied.

Pregnancy: Pregnancy Category D. (See WARNINGS).

Labor and Delivery: The effect of tetracyclines on labor and delivery is unknown.

Nursing mothers: Tetracyclines are present in the milk of lactating women who are taking a drug in this class. Because of the potential for serious adverse reactions in nursing infants from the tetracyclines, a decision should be made whether to discontinue nursing or discontinue the drug, taking into account the importance of the drug to the mother. (See WARNINGS).

Pediatric Use: See Warnings and Dosage and Administration sections.

ADVERSE REACTIONS

Due to oral doxycycline's virtually complete absorption, side effects to the lower bowel, particularly diarrhea, have been infrequent. The following adverse reactions have been observed in patients receiving tetracyclines.

Gastrointestinal: Anorexia, nausea, vomiting, diarrhea, glossitis, dysphagia, enterocolitis, and inflammatory lesions (with monilial overgrowth) in the anogenital region. These reactions have been caused by both the oral and parenteral administration of tetracyclines. Rare instances of esophagitis and esophageal ulcerations have been reported in patients receiving capsule and tablet forms of drugs in the tetracycline class. Most of these patients took medications immediately before going to bed. (See DOSAGE AND ADMINISTRATION).

Skin: Maculopapular and erythematous rashes. Exfoliative dermatitis has been reported but is uncommon. Photosensitivity is discussed above. (See WARNINGS).

Renal toxicity: Rise in BUN has been reported and is apparently dose related. (See WARNINGS).

Hypersensitivity reactions: urticaria, angioneurotic edema, anaphylaxis, anaphylactoid purpura, pericarditis, and exacerbation of systemic lupus erythematosus.

Blood: Hemolytic anemia, thrombocytopenia, neutropenia, and eosinophilia have been reported with tetracyclines.

Other: Bulging fontanels in infants and intracranial hypertension in adults. (See PRECAUTIONS—General).

When given over prolonged periods, tetracyclines have been reported to produce brown-black microscopic discoloration of the thyroid gland. No abnormalities of thyroid function are known to occur.

OVERDOSAGE

In case of overdosage, discontinue medication, treat symptomatically and institute supportive measures. Dialysis does not alter serum half-life, and it would not be of benefit in treating cases of overdosage.

DOSAGE AND ADMINISTRATION

THE USUAL DOSAGE AND FREQUENCY OF ADMINISTRATION OF DOXYCYCLINE DIFFERS FROM THAT OF THE OTHER TETRACYCLINES. EXCEEDING THE RECOMMENDED DOSAGE MAY RESULT IN AN INCREASED INCIDENCE OF SIDE EFFECTS.

Adults: The usual dose of oral doxycycline is 200 mg on the first day of treatment (administered 100 mg every 12 hours or 50 mg every 6 hours) followed by a maintenance dose of 100 mg/day. The maintenance dose may be administered as a single dose or as 50 mg every 12 hours. In the management of more severe infections (particularly chronic infections of the urinary tract), 100 mg every 12 hours is recommended.

For children above eight years of age: The recommended dosage schedule for children weighing 100 pounds or less is 2 mg/lb of body weight divided into two doses on the first day of treatment, followed by 1 mg/lb of body weight given as a single daily dose or divided into two doses, on subsequent days. For more severe infections, up to 2 mg/lb of body weight may be used. For children over 100 lbs the usual adult dose should be used.

Uncomplicated gonococcal infections in adults (except anorectal infections in men): 100 mg by mouth, twice a day for 7 days. As an alternate single visit dose, administer 300 mg stat followed in one hour by a second 300 mg dose.

Acute epididymo-orchitis caused by *N. gonorrhoeae*: 100 mg by mouth, twice a day for at least 10 days.

Primary and secondary syphilis: 300 mg a day in divided doses for at least 10 days.

Uncomplicated urethral, endocervical, or rectal infection in adults caused by *Chlamydia trachomatis*: 100 mg. by mouth, twice a day for at least 7 days.

Nongonococcal urethritis caused by *C. trachomatis* and *U. urealyticum*: 100 mg. by mouth, twice a day for at least 7 days.

Acute epididymo-orchitis caused by *C. trachomatis*: 100 mg. by mouth, twice a day for at least 10 days.

When used in streptococcal infections, therapy should be continued for 10 days.

Administration of adequate amounts of fluid along with capsule and tablet forms of drugs in the tetracycline class is recommended to wash down the drugs and reduce the risk of esophageal irritation and ulceration. (See ADVERSE REACTIONS). If gastric irritation occurs, doxycycline may be given with food. Ingestion of a high fat meal has been shown to delay the time to peak plasma concentrations by an average of one hour and 20 minutes. However, in the same study, food enhanced the average peak concentration by 7.5% and the area under the curve by 5.7%.

HOW SUPPLIED

MONODOX® 50 mg Capsules have a white opaque body with a yellow opaque cap. The capsule bears the inscription "MONODOX 50" in white and "M 260" in brown. Each capsule contains doxycycline monohydrate equivalent to 50 mg doxycycline.

MONODOX® 50 mg is available in:
Bottles of 100 capsules ....NDC 55515-260-06

MONODOX® 100 mg Capsules have a yellow opaque body with a brown opaque cap. The capsule bears the inscription "MONODOX 100" in white and "M 259" in brown. Each capsule contains doxycycline monohydrate equivalent to 100 mg of doxycycline.

MONODOX® 100 mg is available in:
Bottles of 50 capsules ....NDC 55515-259-04
Bottles of 250 capsules ....NDC 55515-259-07

STORE AT CONTROLLED ROOM TEMPERATURE 15°-30°C (59°-86°F). PROTECT FROM LIGHT.

ANIMAL PHARMACOLOGY AND ANIMAL TOXICOLOGY

Hyperpigmentation of the thyroid has been produced by members of the tetracycline class in the following species: in rats by oxytetracycline, doxycycline, tetracycline PO$_4$, and methacycline; in minipigs by doxycycline, minocycline, tetracycline PO$_4$, and methacycline; in dogs by doxycycline and minocycline; in monkeys by minocycline.

Minocycline, tetracycline PO$_4$, methacycline, doxycycline, tetracycline base, oxytetracycline HCl and tetracycline HCl were goitrogenic in rats fed a low iodine diet. This goitrogenic effect was accompanied by high radioactive iodine uptake. Administration of minocycline also produced a large

goiter with high radioiodine uptake in rats fed a relatively high iodine diet.

Treatment of various animal species with this class of drugs has also resulted in the induction of thyroid hyperplasia in the following: in rats and dogs (minocycline), in chickens (chlortetracycline) and in rats and mice (oxytetracycline). Adrenal gland hyperplasia has been observed in goats and rats treated with oxytetracycline.

References:

1. National Committee for Clinical Laboratory Standards, *Performance Standards for Antimicrobial Disk Susceptibility Tests,* Fourth Edition. Approved Standard NCCLS Document M2-A4, Vol. 10, No. 7 NCCLS, Villanova, PA, April 1990.
2. National Committee for Clinical Laboratory Standards, *Methods for Dilution Antimicrobial Susceptibility Tests for Bacteria That Grow Aerobically,* Second Edition. Approved Standard NCCLS Document M7-A2, Vol. 10, No. 8 NCCLS, Villanova, PA, April 1990.

Caution—Federal law prohibits dispensing without prescription.

Manufactured for
OCLASSEN
Pharmaceuticals, Inc.
San Rafael, CA 94901
by Medicopharma, Inc.
Charlotte, N.C.
revised March 1992   02-6534/R1
Shown in Product Identification Section, page 420

Organon Inc.
375 MT. PLEASANT AVE.
WEST ORANGE, NJ 07052

Currently available products are listed below. For complete product line information and price lists, direct inquiries to Organon Inc. Customer Service. For specific product information, contact Organon Inc. Professional Services Department.

ARDUAN®   ℞
(pipecuronium bromide) for injection

HOW SUPPLIED
10 mL vials/10 mg—boxes of 6 vials—NDC-0052-0446-36

BCG VACCINE U.S.P.   ℞
(FOR INTRAVESICAL OR PERCUTANEOUS USE)
TICE® BCG

DESCRIPTION
TICE® BCG, a BCG Vaccine for intravesical or percutaneous use, is an attenuated, live culture preparation of the Bacillus of Calmette and Guerin (BCG) strain *Mycobacterium bovis.*[1] The TICE strain was developed at the University of Illinois from a strain originated at the Pasteur Institute. The medium in which the BCG organism is grown for preparation of the freeze-dried cake is composed of the following ingredients: glycerin, asparagine, citric acid, potassium phosphate, magnesium sulfate, and iron ammonium citrate. The final preparation prior to freeze-drying also contains lactose. The freeze-dried BCG preparation is delivered in glass-sealed ampules, each containing 1 to 8 × 10^8 colony forming units (CFU) of TICE BCG which is equivalent to approximately 50 mg wet weight.
No preservatives have been added.

CLINICAL PHARMACOLOGY
Intravesical Use for Carcinoma In Situ of the Bladder. TICE BCG induces a granulomatous reaction at the local site of administration.[2] Intravesical TICE BCG has been used as a therapy for and prophylaxis against recurrent tumors in patients with carcinoma in situ (CIS) of the bladder. The precise mechanism of action is unknown. A variety of different treatment regimens have been used with the TICE[3-6] and other BCG substrains.[7-12]
An evaluation of intravesical administration of TICE BCG in patients with carcinoma in situ of the urinary bladder was recently completed. Bladder cancer patients were identified who had been treated with TICE BCG under six different Investigational New Drug (IND) applications in which the most important shared aspect was the use of an induction plus maintenance schedule. Comparison of demographic data between the six INDs revealed uniformity. Among these six studies were 119 evaluable patients who received intravesical treatment of CIS of the bladder. Patients with

Continued on next page

Organon—Cont.

biopsy-proven CIS received TICE BCG (50 mg; 1–8 × 10^8 CFU) intravesically, once weekly for at least 6 weeks and once monthly thereafter for up to 12 months. A longer maintenance was given in some cases. Follow-up cystoscopies were performed at 3 month intervals, as were urine cytologies for most patients (71 of 119). Urine cytology was obtained at the time of the 1989 follow-up for all patients who responded to TICE BCG treatment, (CR and CRNC, see below). The median time post treatment for these follow-up cytologies was 47 months.
The study population consisted of 153 patients; 132 males, 19 females and 2 unidentified as to gender. Thirty patients lacking baseline documentation of CIS and 4 patients lost to follow-up were not evaluable for treatment response. Therefore, 119 patients with biopsy or cystoscopy proven CIS prior to TICE BCG administration were available for efficacy evaluation. Some of these patients had undergone transurethral resection (TUR) one or more weeks prior to BCG, primarily for the treatment of papillomatous disease. The mean age for the CIS population was 68.8 ± 9.7 years s.d. (range: 38–97 years). Sixty-three evaluable patients had received intravesical chemotherapy treatment for their bladder malignancy prior to TICE BCG treatment and had been diagnosed as treatment failures. The treatment had been as follows: thiotepa (30), mitomycin C (10), doxorubicin (1), mitomycin C and thiotepa (14), doxorubicin and thiotepa (1), doxorubicin and mitomycin C (1), thiotepa, mitomycin C and doxorubicin (2), interferon (1), interferon and thiotepa (1), cyclophosphamide IV (1), and cisplatin and thiotepa (1).
For the 119 patients with biopsy or cystoscopy proven CIS, the TICE BCG induction dosage consisted of a mean of 6.6 instillations (± 1.5 standard error of the mean). These patients also received a mean of 10.0 maintenance instillations after completing the induction phase. Twenty patients (16.8%) required TICE BCG reinduction at some point in the study. Nine patients in one of the six studies received a percutaneous dose along with intravesical instillation. Data from a recent study show that a percutaneous dose with CIS is unnecessary.[13]
Clinical response criteria were defined as follows:
Complete Histological Response (CR): Complete resolution of carcinoma in situ documented by biopsy or, if a biopsy was not obtained, then by negative cystoscopy. All patients in this category were required to have urine cytology tests that were negative upon examination.
Complete Clinical Response Without Cytology (CRNC): Patients in this category had an apparent complete disappearance of tumor that was not confirmed by urine cytology tests. Complete resolution of carcinoma in situ documented by a biopsy or, if a biopsy was not obtained, then by negative cystoscopy.
Failure/Progression: Patients in this category had urine cytology tests that were found to be positive, although biopsy or cystoscopy was negative. This category also includes patients who continued to have evidence of malignant lesions, or a progression to a higher stage or grade; the appearance of new lesions; reappearance of old lesions.
A 75.6 percent response rate was reported for 119 evaluable patients (Table 1).

TABLE 1: RESPONSE OF PATIENTS TO TICE BCG IN CIS BLADDER CANCER

	Entered	Evaluable	CR	CRNC	Overall Response
No. of Patients	153	119	54	36	90
% Response		—	45.4%	30.2%	75.6%

The median duration of follow-up for the 1989 update, presented in Table 2, is 47 months. Of the 54 patients classified as CR in 1987, 30 remained without evidence of disease (CR) in 1989, whereas 6 patients died of unrelated disease and 18 relapsed. The 15 of 36 patients classified as CRNC in 1987 who remained without evidence of disease in 1989 were all found to meet the criteria of CR status on the basis of negative cytologies. In the interim, 4 CRNC patients died of unrelated diseases, 2 died of unknown causes, and 15 relapsed. Therefore, of the 90 overall responders (75.6%), 36.7 percent of patients relapsed, 13.3 percent died of other diseases, and 50 percent remained in CR. In addition, two patients who relapsed were reinduced in complete response by a second course of TICE BCG. [See Table 2 above.]
Among the 119 evaluable patients there was no significant difference in response rates between patients with or without prior intravesical chemotherapy: 45 of 63 (71%) versus 45 of 56 (80%), p >.05. Similarly, for the patients remaining in CR at the time of the 1989 evaluation, there was no significant difference between those with or without prior chemotherapy.
The median duration of response, calculated from the Kaplan-Meier curve as median time to recurrence, is estimated at 4 years or greater. The median duration of follow-up was

TABLE 2: THERAPEUTIC EFFICACY OF TICE BCG IN CIS BLADDER CANCER 1989 STATUS OF 90 RESPONDERS (CR OR CRNC)

Response	1987/CR n = 54	1987/CRNC n = 36	1987 Response n = 90	Percent
CR	30	15	45	50.0
CRNC	0	0	0	0.0
Unrelated Deaths	6	6	12	13.3
Failure	18	15	33	36.7

47 months. Of the total 90 responders, 45 patients (50%) remained without evidence of disease.
At a median follow-up of 47 months, 85 (71.4%) of the 119 evaluable patients remain alive. Thirteen patients (10.9%) died from causes unrelated to bladder cancer: cardiovascular disease (6 patients), second primary cancer (3 patients), and other (4 patients). Three patients died from unknown causes and bladder cancer cannot be ruled out. The bladder cancer related deaths were 18 (15%) of the 119. Historical data prior to the use of BCG, in a series of CIS patients treated usually with electrofulguration, indicate 82% of the patients recurred, 60% of the patients developed invasive cancer, and 34% of the patients died of their disease within 5 years.[14]
The incidence of cystectomy for 90 patients who achieved a complete response (CR or CRNC) with TICE BCG was 11%. For 29 patients who did not achieve CR or CRNC, the incidence of cystectomy was 55%, which is consistent with cystectomy rates reported in the literature for CIS patients who were not treated with intravesical therapies.[15]
The median time to cystectomy in patients who achieved a complete response (CR or CRNC) exceeded 74 months, whereas the median time to cystectomy for non-responders was 31 months.
Percutaneous Use for Immunization Against Tuberculosis. Immunization with BCG vaccine lowers the risk of serious complications of primary tuberculosis in children.[16–19] Estimates of efficacy from observational studies in areas where vaccination is performed at birth show that the incidence of tuberculous meningitis and miliary tuberculosis is 50%–100% lower and that the incidence of pulmonary tuberculosis 2%–80% lower in vaccinated children less than 15 years of age than in unvaccinated controls.[16–21] However, estimates of vaccine efficacy may be distorted because of the following: vaccination was not allocated randomly in observational studies; there were differences in BCG strains, methods, and routes of administration; and there were differences in the characteristics of the populations and environments in which the vaccines have been studied.[22]

INDICATIONS AND USAGE

Intravesical Use for Carcinoma In Situ of the Bladder. Intravesical instillation of TICE BCG is indicated for the treatment of carcinoma in situ of the bladder in the following situations: (1) primary treatment in the absence of an associated invasive cancer without papillary tumors or with papillary tumors after TUR, (2) secondary treatment in the absence of an associated invasive cancer, in patients failing to respond or relapsing after intravesical chemotherapy with other agents, (3) primary or secondary treatment in the absence of invasive cancer for patients with medical contraindications to radical surgery. TICE BCG is not indicated for the treatment of papillary tumors occurring alone.
Percutaneous Use for Immunization Against Tuberculosis.
Exposed tuberculin skin test-negative infants and children: BCG vaccination is recommended for infants and children with negative tuberculin skin test who are (1) at high risk to intimate and prolonged exposure to persistently untreated or ineffectively treated patients with infectious pulmonary tuberculosis and who cannot be removed from the source of exposure and cannot be placed on long-term preventive therapy, or (2) continuously exposed to persons with tuberculosis who have bacilli resistant to isoniazid and rifampin.[22]
Groups with an excessive rate of new infections: BCG vaccination is also recommended for tuberculin-negative infants and children in groups in which the rate of new infections exceeds 1% per year and for whom the usual surveillance and treatment programs have been attempted but are not operationally feasible. These groups include persons without regular access to health care, those for whom usual health care is culturally or socially unacceptable, or groups who have demonstrated an inability to effectively use existing accessible care.
The US Immunization Practices Advisory Committee (ACIP) no longer recommends the use of BCG vaccination of health care workers at risk of repeated exposure to tuberculosis but recommends that these individuals be under tuberculin skin testing surveillance and receive isoniazid prophylaxis in case of tuberculin skin test conversion.[22]
For international travelers, the Centers for Disease Control (CDC) recommends that BCG vaccination be considered only for travelers with insignificant reaction to tuberculin skin test who will be in a high-risk environment for prolonged periods of time without access to tuberculin skin test surveillance.[22]

CONTRAINDICATIONS

Intravesical Use for Carcinoma In Situ of the Bladder. TICE BCG should not be used in immunosuppressed patients or persons with congenital or acquired immune deficiencies, whether due to concurrent disease (e.g., AIDS, leukemia, lymphoma) or cancer therapy (e.g., cytotoxic drugs, radiation). TICE BCG should be avoided in asymptomatic carriers with a positive HIV serology and in patients receiving steroids at immunosuppressive doses or other immunosuppressive therapies because of the possibility of the vaccine establishing a systemic infection.
Treatment should be postponed until resolution of a concurrent febrile illness, urinary tract infection, or gross hematuria. Seven to fourteen days should elapse before BCG is administered following biopsy, TUR, or traumatic catheterization.
A positive Mantoux test is a contraindication only if there is evidence of an active tuberculosis infection.
In the absence of safety data, intravesical TICE BCG should not be given to pregnant or lactating women.
Percutaneous Use for Immunization Against Tuberculosis. TICE BCG Vaccine for the prevention of tuberculosis should not be given to persons with impaired immune responses, whether they be congenital, disease produced, drug or therapy induced (i.e., cytotoxic drugs and radiation used in cancer therapy). The concurrent use of steroids requires caution because of the possibility of the vaccine establishing a systemic infection. If necessary, the infection can be treated with anti-tuberculous drugs.

WARNINGS

Intravesical Use for Carcinoma In Situ of the Bladder. **TICE BCG is not a vaccine for the prevention of cancer.**
There are currently no data on the effectiveness of intravesical installation of TICE BCG in the treatment of invasive bladder cancer.
The use of TICE BCG may cause tuberculin sensitivity. Since this is a valuable aid in the diagnosis of tuberculosis, it may therefore be useful to determine the tuberculin reactivity by PPD skin testing before treatment.
Intravesical instillations should be postponed in the presence of fever, suspected infection, or during treatment with antibiotics, since antimicrobial therapy may interfere with the effectiveness of TICE BCG.
Instillation of TICE BCG onto a bleeding mucosa may promote systemic BCG infection.[23] Death has been reported as a result of systemic BCG infection and sepsis. Patients should be monitored for the presence of symptoms and signs of toxicity after each intravesical treatment. Febrile episodes with flu-like symptoms lasting more than 48 hours, fever ≥ 103°F, systemic manifestations increasing in intensity with repeated instillations, or persistent abnormalities of liver function tests suggest systemic BCG infection and require antituberculous therapy (see **ADVERSE REACTIONS** section).
Small bladder capacity has been associated with increased risk of severe local reactions and should be considered in deciding to use TICE BCG therapy.
Percutaneous Use for Immunization Against Tuberculosis. Administration should be percutaneous with the multiple puncture disc as described below. DO NOT INJECT INTRAVENOUSLY, SUBCUTANEOUSLY, OR INTRADERMALLY. TICE BCG Vaccine should not be used in infants, children, or adults with severe immune deficiency syndromes. Children with family history of immune deficiency disease should not be vaccinated. If they are, an infectious disease specialist should be consulted and anti-tuberculous therapy[24] administered if clinically indicated.

PRECAUTIONS

General: TICE BCG contains live bacteria and should be used with aseptic technique. All equipment, supplies, and receptacles in contact with TICE BCG should be handled and disposed of as biohazardous.
The possibility of allergic reactions should be assessed. TICE BCG administration should not be attempted in individuals with severe immune deficiency disease. TICE BCG Vaccine should be administered with caution to persons in groups at high risk for HIV infection.
Intravesical Use for Carcinoma In Situ of the Bladder.
General: Care should be taken not to traumatize the urinary tract or to introduce contaminants into the urinary system. Seven to fourteen days should elapse before BCG is administered following TUR, biopsy, or traumatic catheterization.
Information For Patients: TICE BCG is retained in the bladder 2 hours and then voided. Patients should void while seated for safety reasons following instillation of suspension. Within 6 hours after treatment, urine voided should be disinfected for 15 minutes with an equal volume of household bleach before flushing. Patients should be instructed to increase fluid intake to "flush" the bladder in the hours following BCG treatment. Patients may experience burning with the first void after treatment. Patients should be attentive to side effects, such as fever, chills, malaise, flu-like symptoms,

or increased fatigue. If patient experiences severe urinary side effects, such as burning or pain on urination, urgency, frequency of urination, blood in urine, joint pain, cough, or skin rash, the physician should be notified.

Drug Interaction: Drug combinations containing immunosuppressants and/or bone marrow depressants and/or radiation interfere with the development of the immune response and should not be used in combination with TICE BCG. Antimicrobial therapy for other infections may interfere with the effectiveness of TICE BCG therapy.

Pregnancy Category C: Animal reproduction studies have not been conducted with TICE BCG. It is also not known whether TICE BCG can cause fetal harm when administered to a pregnant woman or can affect reproductive capacity. TICE BCG should be given to a pregnant woman only if clearly needed. Women should be advised not to become pregnant while on therapy.

Nursing Mothers: It is not known whether TICE BCG is excreted in human milk. Because many drugs are excreted in human milk and because of the potential for serious adverse reactions from TICE BCG in nursing infants, a decision should be made whether to discontinue nursing or to discontinue the drug, taking into account the importance of the drug to the mother.

Pediatric Use: Safety and effectiveness of carcinoma in situ of the urinary bladder in children have not been established.

Percutaneous Use for Immunization Against Tuberculosis.

Normal Reaction: The intensity and duration of the local reaction depends on the depth of penetration of the multiple-puncture disc and individual variations in patients' tissue reactions. The initial skin lesions usually appear within 10–14 days and consist of small red papules at the site. The papules reach maximum diameter (about 3 mm) after 4 to 6 weeks, after which they may scale and then slowly subside. Six months afterward there is usually no visible sign of the vaccination, but on occasion a faintly discernible pattern of the disc points may be visible. On people whose skin tends to keloid formation, there may be slightly more visible evidence of the vaccination.

Vaccination is recommended only for those who are tuberculin negative to a recent skin test with 5 tuberculin units (5TU). Otherwise, vaccination of persons highly sensitive to mycobacterial antigens can result in hypersensitivity reactions including fever, anorexia, myalgia, and neuralgia, which last a few days.

After TICE BCG vaccination, it is usually not possible to clearly distinguish between a tuberculin reaction caused by persistent postvaccination sensitivity and one caused by a virulent suprainfection. Caution is advised in attributing a positive skin test to TICE BCG vaccination. A sharp rise in the tuberculin reaction since the latest test should be further investigated (except in the immediate postvaccination period).

Information For Patients: Keep the vaccination site clean until the local reaction has disappeared.

Drug Interaction: Antimicrobial or immunosuppressive agents may interfere with the development of the immune response and should be used only under medical supervision.

Pregnancy Category C: Animal reproduction studies have not been conducted with TICE BCG. It is also not known whether TICE BCG can cause fetal harm when administered to a pregnant woman or can affect reproduction capacity. TICE BCG should be given to a pregnant woman only if clearly needed.

Nursing Mothers: It is not known whether TICE BCG is excreted in human milk. Because many drugs are excreted in human milk and because of the potential for serious adverse reactions in nursing infants from TICE BCG, a decision should be made whether to discontinue nursing or not to vaccinate, taking into account the importance of tuberculosis vaccination to the mother.

Pediatric Use: See **Treatment and Schedule** under **DOSAGE AND ADMINISTRATION** section. Precautions should be taken with respect to infants vaccinated with BCG and exposed to persons with active tuberculosis.[25]

ADVERSE REACTIONS

Intravesical Use for Carcinoma In Situ of the Bladder. Adverse reactions are often localized to the bladder but may be accompanied by systemic manifestations. Symptoms of bladder irritability, related to the inflammatory response induced by intravesical TICE BCG, are reported in 60 percent of cases. They begin 3–4 hours after instillation and last 24–72 hours. The urinary side effects are usually seen after the third treatment and tend to increase in severity after each administration. There were, however, no long-term urinary complications in this group of patients.

A summary of adverse reactions seen with 674 patients with superficial bladder cancer, including 153 CIS patients treated intravesically with TICE BCG is shown in Table 3.[26] Irritative bladder adverse effects associated with BCG administration can be managed symptomatically with pyridium, propantheline bromide or oxybutynin chloride, and acetaminophen or ibuprofen.[27] Systemic adverse effects such as malaise, fever, and chills may reflect hypersensitivity reactions and can be treated with antihistamines.[27] The "flu-like" syndrome of 1–2 days' duration that frequently accompanies intravesical BCG administration should be managed by standard symptomatic treatment. Symptoms persisting longer than 2 days suggest continued infection, and consideration should be given to therapy with isoniazid. Localized (e.g., prostatitis, epididymitis) as well as systemic infection can occur with intravesical BCG administration. For systemic infection, an infectious diseases specialist should be consulted and the patient promptly treated with anti-tuberculous therapy as advised.[28] At least two deaths have been reported as a result of systemic BCG infection and sepsis.[27] There have been two cases of nephrogenic adenoma, a benign lesion of bladder epithelium, associated with intravesical BCG therapy.[29] In general, the adverse effects of BCG therapy in bladder carcinoma have been of short duration and moderate morbidity.

TABLE 3: SUMMARY OF ADVERSE EFFECTS SEEN IN 674 PATIENTS WITH SUPERFICIAL BLADDER CANCER, INCLUDING 153 WITH CARCINOMA IN SITU

Local Adverse Effects	Number of Patients	Percent (%)	Toxicity by Grade (%)* Mild	Moderate	Severe	Not Stated
Dysuria	401	59.5	28.2	18.1	10.7	2.5
Urinary Frequency	272	40.4	17.2	15.7	7.4	—
Hematuria	175	26.0	8.2	9.6	7.4	0.8
Cystitis	40	5.9	1.6	2.4	1.9	—
Urgency	39	5.8	1.2	1.8	1.3	1.5
Nocturia	30	4.5	1.3	1.8	0.6	0.7
Cramps/Pain	27	4.0	0.9	1.3	0.9	0.9
Urinary Incontinence	16	2.4	0.4	0.9	—	1.2
Urinary Debris	15	2.2	0.2	1.0	0.4	0.6
Genital Inflammation/ Abscess	12	1.8	0.3	0.4	0.4	0.6
Urinary Tract Infection	10	1.5	0.2	0.3	0.9	0.2
Urethritis	8	1.2	0.3	0.6	—	0.3
Pyuria	5	0.7	0.2	0.1	0.1	0.3
Epididymitis/Prostatitis	2	0.3	—	—	—	0.3
Urinary Obstruction	2	0.3	—	—	—	0.3
Contracted Bladder	1	0.2	—	—	—	0.2
Orchitis	1	0.2	—	—	—	0.2
Systemic Adverse Effects	**Number of Patients**	**Percent (%)**	**Toxicity by Grade (%) Mild**	**Moderate**	**Severe**	**Not Stated**
Flu-like Syndrome**	224	33.2	9.3	10.9	9.0	4.0
Fever	134	19.9	6.1	5.3	7.6	0.9
Malaise/Fatigue	50	7.4	2.7	3.1	—	1.6
Shaking Chills	22	3.3	0.2	1.5	1.0	0.6
Nausea/Vomiting	20	3.0	1.0	1.6	0.3	—
Arthritis/Myalgia	18	2.7	0.3	1.0	0.4	0.9
Headache/Dizziness	16	2.4	0.3	0.9	—	1.2
Anorexia/Weight Loss	15	2.2	0.4	1.3	0.1	0.5
Allergic	14	2.1	0.6	0.7	0.4	0.3
Cardiac	13	1.9	—	0.3	1.3	0.3
Respiratory (Unclassified)	11	1.6	0.4	0.4	0.2	0.6
Abdominal Pain	10	1.5	—	0.6	0.6	0.3
Anemia	9	1.3	0.2	0.6	0.4	0.1
Diarrhea	8	1.2	0.2	0.6	0.1	0.3
Pneumonitis	8	1.2	0.2	—	0.6	0.4
Gastrointestinal (Unclassified)	7	1.0	0.2	0.1	—	0.7
Neurologic	6	0.9	0.1	—	0.3	0.4
Rash	4	0.6	—	0.4	0.2	—
BCG Sepsis	3	0.4	—	—	0.4	—
Coagulopathy	2	0.3	—	—	0.3	—
Leukopenia	2	0.3	0.2	0.1	—	—
Thrombocytopenia	2	0.3	0.2	0.1	—	—
Hepatic Granuloma	1	0.2	—	—	0.2	—
Hepatitis	1	0.2	—	—	0.2	—

*Grade was determined using ECOG scale of toxicity criteria, Mild = Grade 1, Moderate = Grade 2, Severe = Grade 3 or 4.
**Flu-like syndrome includes fever, shaking chills, malaise and myalgia.

Percutaneous Use for Immunization Against Tuberculosis. Occasionally, lymphadenopathy of the regional lymph node, which spontaneously resolves itself, is seen in young children. Only rarely does the node create a fistula followed by a short period of drainage. The usual treatment is to maintain cleanliness of the site of drainage and allow the lesion to heal spontaneously without medical intervention.

Other rare events are osteomyelitis, lupoid reactions, disseminated BCG infection, and death. Osteomyelitis has been reported to occur at a rate of about 1 per 1,000,000 vaccinees.[22] Disseminated BCG infection and death are very rare (about 1 per 5,000,000 vaccinees)[30] and occur almost exclusive in children with impaired immune responses. [See table above.]

OVERDOSAGE

Intravesical Use for Carcinoma In Situ of the Bladder. Overdosage occurs if more than one ampule of TICE BCG is administered per instillation. The patient should be closely monitored for signs of systemic BCG infection and treated with anti-tuberculous medication (see **ADVERSE REACTIONS** section).

Percutaneous Use of Immunization Against Tuberculosis. Accidental overdosages if treated immediately with anti-tuberculous drugs have not led to complications.[31] If the vaccination response is allowed to progress it can still be treated successfully with anti-tuberculous drugs but complications can include regional adenitis, lupus vulgaris, subcutaneous cold abscesses, ocular lesions, and others.[32]

DOSAGE AND ADMINISTRATION

Intravesical Use for Carcinoma In Situ of the Bladder. The intravesical dose consists of one ampule of TICE BCG suspended in 50 mL preservative-free saline. **Preparation of Agent:** The preparation of the TICE BCG suspension should be done using sterile technique. The pharmacist or individual responsible for mixing the agent should wear gloves, mask, and gown to avoid inadvertent exposure of open sores or inhalation of BCG organisms. Draw 1 mL of sterile, preservative-free saline (0.9% Sodium Chloride Injection USP) at 4°–25°C, into a small (e.g., 3 mL) syringe and add to one ampule of TICE BCG to resuspend. Draw the mixture into the syringe and gently expel back into the ampule three times to ensure thorough mixing. This mixing minimizes the clumping of the mycobacteria. Dispense the cloudy BCG suspension into the top end of a catheter-tip syringe which contains 49 mL saline diluent bringing the total volume to 50 mL. Gently rotate the syringe. The suspended TICE BCG should be used immediately after preparation. Discard after 2 hours.

Note: DO NOT filter the contents of the TICE BCG ampule. Precautions should be taken to avoid exposing the TICE BCG to light. Bacteriostatic solutions must be avoided. In addition, use only sterile preservative-free saline, 0.9% Sodium Chloride Injection USP, as diluent and perform all mixing operations in sterile glass or thermosetting plastic containers and syringes.

Treatment and Schedule: Allow 7–14 days to elapse after bladder biopsy or TUR before TICE BCG is administered. Patients should not drink fluids for 4 hours before treatment and should empty their bladder prior to TICE BCG administration. The reconstituted TICE BCG is instilled into the bladder by gravity flow via the catheter. DO NOT depress plunger and force the flow of the TICE BCG. The TICE BCG

Continued on next page

Organon—Cont.

is retained in the bladder 2 hours and then voided. Patients unable to retain the suspension for 2 hours should be allowed to void sooner, if necessary. While the TICE BCG is retained in the bladder, the patient may be repositioned from left side to right side and also may alternately lie upon the back and the abdomen, changing these positions every 15 minutes to maximize bladder surface exposure to the agent.

A standard treatment schedule consists of one intravesical instillation per week for 6 weeks. This schedule may be repeated once if tumor remission has not been achieved and if the clinical circumstances warrant. Thereafter, intravesical TICE BCG administration should continue at approximately monthly intervals for at least 6–12 months.

Percutaneous Use for Immunization Against Tuberculosis.

Preparation of Agent: Using sterile methods, 1 mL of sterile water for injection, USP at 4°–25°C, is added to one ampule of vaccine (see **Pediatric Dose** below for pediatric use). Draw the mixture into a syringe and expel it back into the ampule three times to ensure thorough mixing.

Parenteral drug products should be inspected visually for particulate matter and discoloration prior to administration, whenever solution and container permit. Reconstitution should result in a uniform suspension of the bacilli.

Treatment and Schedule: The vaccine is to be administered after fully explaining the risks and benefits to the vacinee, parent, or guardian. After the vaccine is prepared, the immunizing dose of 0.2–0.3 mL is dropped on the cleansed surface of the skin, and the vaccine is administered percutaneously utilizing a sterile multiple-puncture disc. The multiple-puncture disc is a thin wafer-like stainless steel plate $\frac{7}{8}'' \times 1\frac{1}{8}''$, from which 36 points protrude. The disc is held by a magnet type holder. In this method a drop of vaccine is placed on the arm and spread with the wide edge of disc. The disc is placed gently over the vaccine and the magnet is centered. The arm is grasped firmly from underneath, tensing the skin appreciably. Downward pressure is applied on the magnet so the points of the disc are well buried in skin. With pressure still exerted, the disc is rocked forward and backward and from side to side several times. Pressure underneath the arm is then released and the magnetic is slid off the disc. In a successful procedure, the points remain in the skin. If the points are on top of the skin, the procedure must be repeated. Remove the disc after successful puncture and spread vaccine evenly over the puncture area with the wide edge of the disc. Discs should only be used once and discarded after autoclaving. Between individual vaccinations the magnet should be sterilized (see instructions for use provided with the device). Discs may be purchased separately from Organon Teknika Corporation, 115 South Sangamon Street, Chicago, Illinois 60607; telephone number (800) 662-6842.

After vaccination the vaccine should flow into the wounds and dry. No dressing is required; however, it is recommended that the site be kept dry for 24 hours. The patient should be advised that the vaccine contains live organisms. Although the vaccine will not survive in a dry state, infection of others is possible.

Reconstituted vaccine should be kept refrigerated, protected from exposure to light, and used within 2 hours. Vaccination should be repeated for those who remain tuberculin negative to 5TU of tuberculin after 2–3 months.

Pediatric Dose: In infants less than 1 month old the dosage of vaccine should be reduced by one half, by using 2 mL of sterile water when reconstituting. If a vaccinated infant remains tuberculin negative to 5TU on skin testing, and if indications for vaccination persist, the infant should receive a full dose after 1 year of age.

HOW SUPPLIED

TICE BCG vaccine is supplied in a box of one 2 mL ampule of TICE BCG. Each ampule contains 1 to 8×10^8 CFU, which is equivalent to approximately 50 mg (wet weight), as lyophilized (freeze-dried) powder, NDC 0052-0601-01.

STORAGE

Storage of the intact ampules of TICE BCG should be at refrigerated temperatures of 2–8°C (36–46°F). This agent contains live bacteria and should be protected from light. The product should not be used after the expiration date printed on the label.

REFERENCES

1. Guerin C: The history of BCG. In: Rosenthal SR (ed); BCG Vaccine: Tuberculosis-Cancer. Littleton, MA, PSG Publishing Co., Inc. 1980, pp. 35–43.
2. Kelley DR, Haaff E, Becich M, et al.: Prognostic value of purified protein derivative skin test and granuloma formation in patients treated with intravesical bacillus Calmette-Guerin. J Urol 1986; 135:268–271.
3. Brosman SA: The use of bacillus Calmette-Guerin in the therapy of bladder carcinoma in situ. J Urol 1985; 134:36–39.
4. DeKernion JB, Huang M. Linder A, et al.: The management of superficial bladder tumors and carcinoma in situ with intravesical bacillus Calmette-Guerin. J Urol 1985; 133:598–601.
5. Guinan P, Batenhorst R: BCG in the treatment of superficial bladder cancer (Abstract). J Urol 1987; 137:180A.
6. Soloway M, Perry A: Bacillus Calmette-Guerin for treatment of superficial transitional cell carcinoma of the bladder in patients who have failed thiotepa and/or mitomycin C. J Urol 1987; 137:871–873.
7. Morales A: Long-term results and complications of intracavitary bacillus Calmette-Guerin therapy for bladder cancer. J Urol 1984; 132:457–459.
8. Haaff E, Dresner SM, Ratliff TL, Catalona WJ: Two courses of intravesical bacillus Calmette-Guerin for transitional cell carcinoma of the bladder. J Urol 1986; 136:820–824.
9. Herr HW, Pinsky CM, Whitmore WF, et al.: Effect of intravesical bacillus Calmette-Guerin (BCG) on carcinoma in situ. Cancer 1983; 51:1323–1326.
10. Kelley DR, Ratliff T, Catalona WJ, et al.: Intravesical bacillus Calmette-Guerin therapy for superficial bladder cancer. Effect of bacillus Calmette-Guerin viability on treatment results. J Urol 1985; 134:48–53.
11. Schellhammer PF, Ladaga LE, Fillion MB: Bacillus Calmette-Guerin for therapy of superficial transitional cell carcinoma of the bladder. J Urol 1986; 135:261–264.
12. Lamm DL: BCG immunotherapy in bladder cancer. In: Urology Annual 1987. Vol. 1, Appleton & Lange, Norwalk, CT, 1987; pp. 67–86.
13. Lamm DL, Sarosdy MS, DeHaven JI: Percutaneous, oral, or intravesical BCG administration: What is the optimal route? EORTC Genitourinary Group Monograph 6: BCG in Superficial Bladder Cancer. Alan R. Liss, Inc., New York, NY, 1989; pp. 301–310.
14. Utz DC, Hanash KA, Farrow GM: The plight of the patient with carcinoma in situ of the bladder. J Urol 1970; 103: 160–164.
15. Herr HW, Pinsky CM, Whitmore WF Jr., et al.: Long-term effect of intravesical bacillus Calmette-Guerin on flat carcinoma in situ of the bladder. J Urol 1986; 135:265–267.
16. Romanus V: Tuberculosis in bacillus Calmette-Guerin immunized and unimmunized children in Sweden: a ten-year evaluation following the cessation of general bacillus Calmette-Guerin immunization of the newborn in 1975. Pediatr Infect Dis 1987; 6:272–280.
17. Smith PG: Case-control studies of the efficacy of BCG against tuberculosis. In: International Union Against Tuberculosis, Proceedings of the XXXVIth IUAT World Conference on Tuberculosis and Respiratory Diseases, Singapore. Professional Postgraduate Services, International, Japan, 1987; 73–79.
18. Padungchan S, Konjanart S, Kasiratta S, et al.: The effectiveness of BCG vaccination of the newborn against childhood tuberculosis in Bangkok. Bull WHO 1986; 64:247–258.
19. Tidjani O, Amedone A, ten Dam HG: The protective effect of BCG vaccination of the newborn against childhood tuberculosis in an African community. Tubercle 1986; 67:269–281.
20. Young TK, Hershfield ES: A case-control study to evaluate the effectiveness of mass neonatal BCG vaccination among Canadian Indians. Am J Public Health 1986; 76:783–786.
21. Shapiro C, Cook N, Evans D, et al.: A case-control study of BCG and childhood tuberculosis in Cali, Columbia. Int H Epidemiol 1985; 14:441–446.
22. Morbidity and Mortality Weekly Report 37, No. 43 1988; pp. 663–675.
23. Rawls WH, Lamm DL, Eyolfson MF: Septic complications in the use of bacillus Calmette-Guerin (BCG) for noninvasive transitional cell carcinoma. Presented at: 1988 Annual Meeting, American Urological Association, Boston, MA.
24. Lorin MI, Hsu KHK, Jacob SC: Treatment of tuberculosis in children. In: Symposium on anti-infective therapy. Pediatric Clinics of North America, 1983; 30:333–348.
25. Report of the Committee on the Control of Infectious Diseases. American Academy of Pediatrics 1988; 21st Edition.
26. Data on file. Organon Teknika Corporation/Biotechnology Research Institute, Rockville, MD.
27. Lamm DL, Steg A, Boccon-Gibod L, et al.: Complications of bacillus Calmette-Guerin immunotherapy: Review of 2602 patients and comparison of chemotherapy complications. EORTC Genitourinary Group Monograph 6: BCG in Superficial Bladder Cancer. Alan R. Liss, Inc., New York, NY, 1989; pp. 335–355.
28. Standard Therapy for Tuberculosis, 1985. Presented at: National Consensus Conference on Tuberculosis. Chest, 1985; 87 (Suppl):117S–124S.
29. Oates R, Siroky M: Nephrogenic adenoma of urinary bladder due to intravesical BCG therapy. J Urol 1986; 135:186.
30. Mande R: BCG Vaccination. Dawsons, London, 1968.
31. Griffith AH: Ten cases of BCG overdose treated with isoniazid. Tubercle 1963; 44:247–250.
32. Watkins SM: Unusual complications of BCG vaccination. Brit Med J 1971; 1:442.

Manufactured by: Organon Teknika Corporation
100 Akzo Avenue
Durham, NC 27704
Manufactured at: Chicago, IL 60607
Distributed by: Organon Inc.
West Orange, NJ 07052
U.S. License No. 956 Issue Date: August, 1990
TICE® is a trademark licensed from the University of Illinois.

CALDEROL® ℞

[kal-dah 'rol]

(calcifediol capsules, USP)

HOW SUPPLIED

20 μg (white, soft elastic capsules) bottle of 60
50 μg (orange, soft elastic capsules) bottle of 60

Shown in Product Identification Section, page 420

CORTROSYN® ℞

Cosyntropin is α 1–24 corticotropin, a synthetic subunit of ACTH.

HOW SUPPLIED

Box containing: 10 Vials of Cortrosyn® (cosyntropin) for injection 0.25 mg
10 ampuls of solvent (sodium chloride for injection, USP)

COTAZYM® ℞

[kōt 'a zīm]

(pancrelipase capsules, USP)

DESCRIPTION

Cotazym (Pancrelipase, USP) is a powder containing enzymes obtained from the pancreas of the hog. These include amylase and protease but principally lipase. Each capsule contains:

Lipase—8,000 USP Units
Protease—30,000 USP Units
Amylase—30,000 USP Units
Precipitated calcium carbonate 25 mg.

Each capsule also contains the inactive ingredients: cornstarch, gelatin, magnesium stearate, talc, FD&C green #3, FD&C yellow #10 as coloring and titanium dixoide.

INDICATIONS AND USAGE

It is indicated in conditions where pancreatic enzymes are either absent or deficient with resultant inadequate fat digestion. Such conditions include but are not limited to chronic pancreatitis, pancreatectomy, cystic fibrosis and steatorrhea of diverse etiologies.

CONTRAINDICATIONS

Known hypersensitivity to pork protein.

PRECAUTIONS

In the event that capsules are opened for any reason care should be taken so that powder is not inhaled or spilled on hands since it may prove irritating to the skin or mucous membranes.

ADVERSE REACTIONS

No adverse reactions have been reported. It should be noted, however, that extremely high doses of exogenous pancreatic enzymes have been associated with hyperuricosuria and hyperuricemia.

DOSAGE AND ADMINISTRATION

One to three capsules just prior to each meal or snack. Individual cases may require higher dosage and dietery adjustment.

STORAGE

Not to exceed 25°C (77°F). Store in dry place when opened.

DISPENSE

In tight container as defined in the USP.

SUPPLIED

Cotazym capsules (regular) bottles of 100 and 500.
NDC # 0052-0381-91, NDC # 0052-0381-95.

Shown in Product Identification Section, page 420

COTAZYM®-S   ℞
[kōt'a zīm-s]
(pancrelipase, USP)
Enteric coated spheres

Each capsule contains
5,000	USP Units of Lipase
20,000	USP Units of Protease
20,000	USP Units of Amylase

HOW SUPPLIED
Bottles of 100 capsules
Bottles of 500 capsules
Shown in Product Identification Section, page 420

DECA–DURABOLIN®   ⒸⅡⅠ ℞
(nandrolone decanoate injection, USP)

HOW SUPPLIED
100 mg/mL—2 mL vials, 1 mL prefilled syringe.
200 mg/mL—1 mL vials, 1 mL prefilled syringe.

DURABOLIN®   ⒸⅡⅠ ℞
(nandrolone phenpropionate injection, USP)

HOW SUPPLIED
25 mg/mL—5 mL vials.
50 mg/mL—2 mL vials.

HEXADROL® Elixir   ℞
(dexamethasone elixir, USP)

Each 5 mL contains: 0.5 mg dexamethasone with 5% alcohol.

HOW SUPPLIED
Elixir (0.5 mg/5 mL)—Bottle of 120 mL

HEXADROL®   ℞
(dexamethasone tablets, USP)

HOW SUPPLIED
Tablets (4 mg green, scored)—bottle of 100
Tablets (4 mg green, scored)—box of 100
    (10 strips—10 per strip)
Shown in Product Identification Section, page 420

HEXADROL®   ℞
Phosphate Injection
(dexamethasone sodium phosphate injection, USP)

HOW SUPPLIED
Available in two potencies:
4 mg/mL—5 mL vials, 1 mL prefilled syringe.
10 mg/mL—10 mL vials, 1 mL prefilled syringe.

HYDROCORTISONE, USP   ℞
Micronized Powder
Non-Sterile: For Prescription Compounding Only

HOW SUPPLIED
Available in 25 and 100 gram containers.

JENEST™-28 Tablets   ℞
(norethindrone/ethinyl estradiol)

COMBINATION ORAL CONTRACEPTIVES
JENEST™-28 Tablets are a combination oral contraceptive containing the progestational compound norethindrone and the estrogenic compound ethinyl estradiol. Each white tablet contains 0.5 mg of norethindrone and 0.035 mg of ethinyl estradiol. Inactive ingredients include lactose, magnesium stearate and pregelatinized starch. Each peach tablet contains 1 mg norethindrone and 0.035 mg ethinyl estradiol. Inactive ingredients include FD&C Yellow No. 6, lactose, magnesium stearate and pregelatinized starch. Each green tablet contains only inert ingredients, as follows: D&C Yellow No. 10 Aluminum Lake, FD&C Blue No. 2 Aluminum Lake, lactose, magnesium stearate, microcrystalline cellulose and pregelatinized starch.
The chemical name for norethindrone is 17-hydroxy-19-nor-17α-pregn-4-en-20-yn-3-one, for ethinyl estradiol is 19-nor-17α-pregna-1,3,5(10)-trien-20-yne-3,17-diol. Their structural formulas are as follows:

norethindrone   ethinyl estradiol

CLINICAL PHARMACOLOGY
COMBINATION ORAL CONTRACEPTIVES
Combination oral contraceptives act by suppression of gonadotropins. Although the primary mechanism of this action is inhibition of ovulation, other alterations include changes in the cervical mucus (which increase the difficulty of sperm entry into the uterus) and the endometrium (which reduce the likelihood of implantation).

INDICATIONS AND USAGE
JENEST™-28 is indicated for the prevention of pregnancy in women who elect to use this product as a method of contraception.
Oral contraceptives are highly effective. Table I lists the typical accidental pregnancy rates for users of combination oral contraceptives and other methods of contraception. The efficacy of these contraceptive methods, except sterilization, depends upon the reliability with which they are used. Correct and consistent use of methods can result in lower failure rates.

TABLE I: LOWEST EXPECTED AND TYPICAL FAILURE RATES DURING THE FIRST YEAR OF CONTINUOUS USE OF A METHOD
% of Women Experiencing an Accidental Pregnancy in the First Year of Continuous Use

Method	Lowest Expected*	Typical**
(No contraception)	(89)	(89)
Oral contraceptives		3
combined	0.1	N/A***
progestin only	0.5	N/A***
Diaphragm with spermicidal cream or jelly	3	18
Spermicides alone (foam, creams, jellies and vaginal suppositories)	3	21
Vaginal sponge		
nulliparous	5	18
multiparous	>8	>28
IUD (medicated)	1	6#
Condom without spermicides	2	12
Periodic abstinence (all methods)	2–10	20
Female sterilization	0.2	0.4
Male sterilization	0.1	0.15

Adapted from J. Trussell and K. Kost, Table II, ref. #1.
   * The authors' best guess of the percentage of women expected to experience an accidental pregnancy among couples who initiate a method (not necessarily for the first time) and who use it consistently and correctly during the first year if they do not stop for any other reason.
  ** This term represents "typical" couples who initiate use of a method (not necessarily for the first time), who experience an accidental pregnancy during the first year if they do not stop use for any other reason.
*** N/A—Data not available.
  # Combined typical rate for both medicated and non-medicated IUD. The rate for medicated IUD alone is not available.

CONTRAINDICATIONS
Oral contraceptives should not be used in women who currently have the following conditions:
- Thrombophlebitis or thromboembolic disorders
- A past history of deep vein thrombophlebitis or thromboembolic disorders
- Cerebral vascular or coronary artery disease
- Known or suspected carcinoma of the breast
- Carcinoma of the endometrium or other known or suspected estrogen-dependent neoplasia
- Undiagnosed abnormal genital bleeding
- Cholestatic jaundice of pregnancy or jaundice with prior pill use
- Hepatic adenomas or carcinomas
- Known or suspected pregnancy

WARNINGS

> Cigarette smoking increases the risk of serious cardiovascular side effects from oral contraceptive use. This risk increases with age and with heavy smoking (15 or more cigarettes per day) and is quite marked in women over 35 years of age. Women who use oral contraceptives should be strongly advised not to smoke.

The use of oral contraceptives is associated with increased risks of several serious conditions including myocardial infarction, thromboembolism, stroke, hepatic neoplasia, and gallbladder disease, although the risk of serious morbidity or mortality is very small in healthy women without underlying risk factors. The risk of morbidity and mortality increases significantly in the presence of other underlying risk factors such as hypertension, hyperlipidemias, obesity and diabetes.
Practitioners prescribing oral contraceptives should be familiar with the following information relating to these risks. The information contained in this package insert is principally based on studies carried out in patients who used oral contraceptives with higher formulations of estrogens and progestogens than those in common use today. The effect of long term use of the oral contraceptives with lower formulations of both estrogens and progestogens remains to be determined.
Throughout this labeling, epidemiological studies reported are of two types: retrospective or case control studies and prospective or cohort studies. Case control studies provide a measure of the relative risk of a disease, namely, a *ratio* of the incidence of a disease among oral contraceptive users to that among nonusers. The relative risk does not provide information on the actual clinical occurrence of a disease. Cohort studies provide a measure of attributable risk, which is the *difference* in the incidence of disease between oral contraceptive users and nonusers. The attributable risk does provide information about the actual occurrence of a disease in the population (adapted from refs. 2 and 3 with the authors' permission). For further information, the reader is referred to a text on epidemiological methods.
1. THROMBOEMBOLIC DISORDERS AND OTHER VASCULAR PROBLEMS
a. Myocardial Infarction
An increased risk of myocardial infarction has been associated with oral contraceptive use. This risk is primarily in smokers or women with other underlying risk factors for coronary artery disease such as hypertension, hypercholesterolemia, morbid obesity, and diabetes. The relative risk of heart attack for current oral contraceptive users has been estimated to be two to six[4–10]. The risk is very low under the age of 30.
Smoking in combination with oral contraceptive use has been shown to contribute substantially to the incidence of myocardial infarctions in women in their mid-thirties or older with smoking accounting for the majority of excess cases[11]. Mortality rates associated with circulatory disease have been shown to increase substantially in smokers, especially in those 35 years of age and older among women who use oral contraceptives.

CIRCULATORY DISEASE MORTALITY RATES PER 100,000 WOMAN-YEARS BY AGE, SMOKING STATUS AND ORAL CONTRACEPTIVE USE

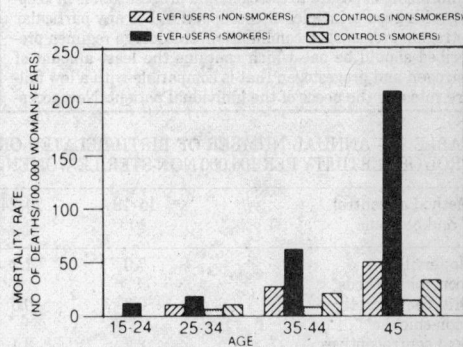

TABLE II. (Adapted from P.M. Layde and V. Beral, ref. #12.)

Oral contraceptives may compound the effects of well-known risk factors, such as hypertension, diabetes, hyperlipidemias, age and obesity[13]. In particular, some progestogens are known to decrease HDL cholesterol and cause glucose intolerance, while estrogens may create a state of hyperinsulinism[14–18]. Oral contraceptives have been shown to increase blood pressure among users (see section 9 in WARNINGS).

Continued on next page

Organon—Cont.

Similar effects on risk factors have been associated with an increased risk of heart disease. Oral contraceptives must be used with caution in women with cardiovascular disease risk factors.

b. Thromboembolism

An increased risk of thromboembolic and thrombotic disease associated with the use of oral contraceptives is well established. Case control studies have found the relative risk of users compared to non-users to be 3 for the first episode of superficial venous thrombosis, 4 to 11 for deep vein thrombosis or pulmonary embolism, and 1.5 to 6 for women with predisposing conditions for venous thromboembolic disease[2,3,19–24]. Cohort studies have shown the relative risk to be somewhat lower, about 3 for new cases and about 4.5 for new cases requiring hospitalization[25]. The risk of thromboembolic disease associated with oral contraceptives is not related to length of use and disappears after pill use is stopped[2].

A two- to four-fold increase in relative risk of post-operative thromboembolic complications has been reported with the use of oral contraceptives[9]. The relative risk of venous thrombosis in women who have predisposing conditions is twice that of women without such medical conditions[26]. If feasible, oral contraceptives should be discontinued at least four weeks prior to and for two weeks after elective surgery of a type associated with an increase in risk of thromboembolism and during and following prolonged immobilization. Since the immediate postpartum period is also associated with an increased risk of thromboembolism, oral contraceptives should be started no earlier than four weeks after delivery in women who elect not to breast feed.

c. Cerebrovascular diseases

Oral contraceptives have been shown to increase both the relative and attributable risks of cerebrovascular events (thrombotic and hemorrhagic strokes), although, in general, the risk is greatest among older (> 35 years), hypertensive women who also smoke. Hypertension was found to be a risk factor for both users and non-users, for both types of strokes, and smoking interacted to increase the risk of stroke[27–29].

In a large study, the relative risk of thrombotic strokes has been shown to range from 3 for normotensive users to 14 for users with severe hypertension[30]. The relative risk of hemorrhagic stroke is reported to be 1.2 for non-smokers who used oral contraceptives, 2.6 for smokers who did not use oral contraceptives, 7.6 for smokers who used oral contraceptives, 1.8 for normotensive users and 25.7 for users with severe hypertension[30]. The attributable risk is also greater in older women[3].

d. Dose-related risk of vascular disease from oral contraceptives

A positive association has been observed between the amount of estrogen and progestogen in oral contraceptives and the risk of vascular disease[31–33]. A decline in serum high density lipoproteins (HDL) has been reported with many progestational agents[14–16]. A decline in serum high density lipoproteins has been associated with an increased incidence of ischemic heart disease. Because estrogens increase HDL cholesterol, the net effect of an oral contraceptive depends on a balance achieved between doses of estrogen and progestogen and the activity of the progestogen used in the contraceptive. The activity and amount of both hormones should be considered in the choice of an oral contraceptive.

Minimizing exposure to estrogen and progestogen is in keeping with good principles of therapeutics. For any particular estrogen/progestogen combination, the dosage regimen prescribed should be one which contains the least amount of estrogen and progestogen that is compatible with a low failure rate and the needs of the individual patient. New acceptors of oral contraceptive agents should be started on preparations containing 0.035 mg or less of estrogen.

e. Persistence of risk of vascular disease

There are two studies which have shown persistence of risk of vascular disease for ever-users of oral contraceptives. In a study in the United States, the risk of developing myocardial infarction after discontinuing oral contraceptives persists for at least 9 years for women 40–49 years who had used oral contraceptives for five or more years, but this increased risk was not demonstrated in other age groups[8]. In another study in Great Britain, the risk of developing cerebrovascular disease persisted for at least 6 years after discontinuation of oral contraceptives, although excess risk was very small[34]. However, both studies were performed with oral contraceptive formulations containing 50 micrograms or higher of estrogens.

2. ESTIMATES OF MORTALITY FROM CONTRACEPTIVE USE

One study gathered data from a variety of sources which have estimated the mortality rate associated with different methods of contraception at different ages (Table III). These estimates include the combined risk of death associated with contraceptive methods plus the risk attributable to pregnancy in the event of method failure. Each method of contraception has its specific benefits and risks. The study concluded that with the exception of oral contraceptive users 35 and older who smoke and 40 and older who do not smoke, mortality associated with all methods of birth control is low and below that associated with childbirth. However, smokers 35 and older and non-smokers 40 and older who use oral contraceptives have a significant increase in mortality higher than those using other methods of birth control. These facts must be weighed in conjunction with failure rates for other methods and the risk associated with subsequent pregnancy. (See Table I.)

[See also Table III below.]

3. CARCINOMA OF THE REPRODUCTIVE ORGANS

Numerous epidemiological studies have been performed on the incidence of breast, endometrial, ovarian and cervical cancer in women using oral contraceptives. While there are conflicting reports, most studies suggest that use of oral contraceptives is not associated with an overall increase in the risk of developing breast cancer. Some studies have reported an increased relative risk of developing breast cancer, particularly at a younger age. This increased relative risk appears to be related to duration of use[36–44,79–89].

Some studies suggest that oral contraceptive use has been associated with an increase in the risk of cervical intraepithelial neoplasia in some populations of women[45–48]. However, there continues to be controversy about the extent to which such findings may be due to differences in sexual behavior and other factors.

4. HEPATIC NEOPLASIA

Benign hepatic adenomas are associated with oral contraceptives use, although the incidence of benign tumors is rare in the United States. Indirect calculations have estimated the attributable risk to be in the range of 3.3 cases/100,000 for users, a risk that increases after four or more years of use especially with oral contraceptives of higher dose[49]. Rupture of benign, hepatic adenomas may cause death through intra-abdominal hemorrhage[50,51].

Studies from Britain have shown an increased risk of developing hepatocellular carcinoma[52–54] in long-term (> 8 years) oral contraceptive users. However, these cancers are rare in the U.S. and the attributable risk (the excess incidence) of liver cancers in oral contraceptive users approaches less than one per million users.

5. OCULAR LESIONS

There have been clinical case reports of retinal thrombosis associated with the use of oral contraceptives. Oral contraceptives should be discontinued if there is unexplained partial or complete loss of vision; onset of proptosis or diplopia; papilledema; or retinal vascular lesions. Appropriate diagnostic and therapeutic measures should be undertaken immediately.

6. ORAL CONTRACEPTIVE USE BEFORE OR DURING EARLY PREGNANCY

Extensive epidemiological studies have revealed no increased risk of birth defects in women who have used oral contraceptives prior to pregnancy[56,57]. The majority of recent studies also do not indicate a teratogenic effect, particularly in so far as cardiac anomalies and limb reduction defects are concerned[55,56,58,59], when taken inadvertently during early pregnancy.

The administration of oral contraceptives to induce withdrawal bleeding should not be used as a test for pregnancy. Oral contraceptives should not be used during pregnancy to treat threatened or habitual abortion.

It is recommended that for any patient who has missed two consecutive periods, pregnancy should be ruled out before continuing oral contraceptive use. If the patient has not adhered to the prescribed schedule, the possibility of pregnancy should be considered at the time of the first missed period. Oral contraceptive use should be discontinued until pregnancy is ruled out.

7. GALLBLADDER DISEASE

Earlier studies have reported an increased lifetime relative risk of gallbladder surgery in users of oral contraceptives and estrogens[60,61]. More recent studies, however, have shown that the relative risk of developing gallbladder disease among oral contraceptive users may be minimal[62–64]. The recent findings of minimal risk may be related to the use of oral contraceptive formulations containing lower hormonal doses of estrogens and progestogens.

8. CARBOHYDRATE AND LIPID METABOLIC EFFECTS

Oral contraceptives have been shown to cause a decrease in glucose tolerance in a significant percentage of users[17]. This effect has been shown to be directly related to estrogen dose[65]. Progestogens increase insulin secretion and create insulin resistance, this effect varying with different progestational agents[17,66]. However, in the non-diabetic woman, oral contraceptives appear to have no effect on fasting blood glucose[67]. Because of these demonstrated effects, prediabetic and diabetic women in particular should be carefully monitored while taking oral contraceptives.

A small proportion of women will have persistent hypertriglyceridemia while on the pill. As discussed earlier (see WARNINGS 1a and 1d), changes in serum triglycerides and lipoprotein levels have been reported in oral contraceptive users.

9. ELEVATED BLOOD PRESSURE

An increase in blood pressure has been reported in women taking oral contraceptives[68] and this increase is more likely in older oral contraceptive users[69] and with extended duration of use[61]. Data from the Royal College of General Practitioners[12] and subsequent randomized trials have shown that the incidence of hypertension increases with increasing progestational activity.

Women with a history of hypertension or hypertension-related diseases, or renal disease[70] should be encouraged to use another method of contraception. If women elect to use oral contraceptives, they should be monitored closely and if significant elevation of blood pressure occurs, oral contraceptives should be discontinued. For most women, elevated blood pressure will return to normal after stopping oral contraceptives, and there is no difference in the occurrence of hypertension between former and never users[68–71].

10. HEADACHE

The onset or exacerbation of migraine or development of headache with a new pattern which is recurrent, persistent or severe requires discontinuation of oral contraceptives and evaluation of the cause.

11. BLEEDING IRREGULARITIES

Breakthrough bleeding and spotting are sometimes encountered in patients on oral contraceptives, especially during the first three months of use. Non-hormonal causes should be considered and adequate diagnostic measures taken to rule out malignancy or pregnancy in the event of breakthrough bleeding, as in the case of any abnormal vaginal bleeding. If pathology has been excluded, time or a change to another formulation may solve the problem. In the event of amenorrhea, pregnancy should be ruled out.

Some women may encounter post-pill amenorrhea or oligomenorrhea, especially when such a condition was preexistent.

PRECAUTIONS

1. PHYSICAL EXAMINATION AND FOLLOW UP

A complete medical history and physical examination should be taken prior to the initiation or reinstitution of oral contraceptives and at least annually during use of oral contraceptives. These physical examinations should include special reference to blood pressure, breasts, abdomen and pelvic organs, including cervical cytology, and relevant laboratory tests. In case of undiagnosed, persistent or recurrent abnormal vaginal bleeding, appropriate diagnostic measures

TABLE III—ANNUAL NUMBER OF BIRTH-RELATED OR METHOD-RELATED DEATHS ASSOCIATED WITH CONTROL OF FERTILITY PER 100,000 NON-STERILE WOMEN, BY FERTILITY CONTROL METHOD ACCORDING TO AGE

Method of control and outcome	15–19	20–24	25–29	30–34	35–39	40–44
No fertility control methods*	7.0	7.4	9.1	14.8	25.7	28.2
Oral contraceptives non-smoker**	0.3	0.5	0.9	1.9	13.8	31.6
Oral contraceptives smoker**	2.2	3.4	6.6	13.5	51.1	117.2
IUD**	0.8	0.8	1.0	1.0	1.4	1.4
Condom*	1.1	1.6	0.7	0.2	0.3	0.4
Diaphragm/ spermicide*	1.9	1.2	1.2	1.3	2.2	2.8
Periodic abstinence*	2.5	1.6	1.6	1.7	2.9	3.6

*Deaths are birth-related

**Deaths are method-related

Adapted from H.W. Ory, ref. #35.

should be conducted to rule out malignancy. Women with a strong family history of breast cancer or who have breast nodules should be monitored with particular care.

2. LIPID DISORDERS

Women who are being treated for hyperlipidemias should be followed closely if they elect to use oral contraceptives. Some progestogens may elevate LDL levels and may render the control of hyperlipidemias more difficult.

3. LIVER FUNCTION

If jaundice develops in any woman receiving such drugs, the medication should be discontinued. Steroid hormones may be poorly metabolized in patients with impaired liver function.

4. FLUID RETENTION

Oral contraceptives may cause some degree of fluid retention. They should be prescribed with caution, and only with careful monitoring, in patients with conditions which might be aggravated by fluid retention.

5. EMOTIONAL DISORDERS

Women with a history of depression should be carefully observed and the drug discontinued if depression recurs to a serious degree.

6. CONTACT LENSES

Contact lens wearers who develop visual changes or changes in lens tolerance should be assessed by an ophthalmologist.

7. DRUG INTERACTIONS

Reduced efficacy and increased incidence of breakthrough bleeding and menstrual irregularities have been associated with concomitant use of rifampin. A similar association, though less marked, has been suggested with barbiturates, phenylbutazone, phenytoin sodium, and possibly with griseofulvin, ampicillin and tetracyclines[72].

8. INTERACTIONS WITH LABORATORY TESTS

Certain endocrine and liver function tests and blood components may be affected by oral contraceptives:

a. Increased prothrombin and factors VII, VIII, IX, and X; decreased antithrombin 3; increased norepinephrine-induced platelet aggregability.

b. Increased thyroid binding globulin (TBG) leading to increased circulating total thyroid hormone, as measured by protein-bound iodine (PBI), T4 by column or by radio-immunoassay. Free T3 resin uptake is decreased, reflecting the elevated TBG, free T4 concentration is unaltered.

c. Other binding proteins may be elevated in serum.

d. Sex-binding globulins are increased and result in elevated levels of total circulating sex steroids and corticoids; however, free or biologically active levels remain unchanged.

e. Triglycerides may be increased.

f. Glucose tolerance may be decreased.

g. Serum folate levels may be depressed by oral contraceptive therapy. This may be of clinical significance if a woman becomes pregnant shortly after discontinuing oral contraceptives.

9. CARCINOGENESIS

See WARNINGS section.

10. PREGNANCY

Pregnancy Category X. See CONTRAINDICATIONS and WARNINGS sections.

11. NURSING MOTHERS

Small amounts of oral contraceptive steroids have been identified in the milk of nursing mothers and a few adverse effects on the child have been reported, including jaundice and breast enlargement. In addition, oral contraceptives given in the postpartum period may interfere with lactation by decreasing the quantity and quality of breast milk. If possible, the nursing mother should be advised not to use oral contraceptives but to use other forms of contraception until she has completely weaned her child.

INFORMATION FOR THE PATIENT

See Patient Labeling Printed Below

ADVERSE REACTIONS

An increased risk of the following serious adverse reactions has been associated with the use of oral contraceptives (see WARNINGS section).

- Thrombophlebitis and venous thrombosis with or without embolism
- Arterial thromboembolism
- Pulmonary embolism
- Myocardial infarction
- Cerebral hemorrhage
- Cerebral thrombosis
- Hypertension
- Gallbladder disease
- Hepatic adenomas or benign liver tumors

The following adverse reactions have been reported in patients receiving oral contraceptives and are believed to be drug-related:

- Nausea
- Vomiting
- Gastrointestinal symptoms (such as abdominal cramps and bloating)
- Breakthrough bleeding
- Spotting
- Change in menstrual flow
- Amenorrhea
- Temporary infertility after discontinuation of treatment
- Edema
- Melasma which may persist
- Breast changes: tenderness, enlargement, secretion
- Change in weight (increase or decrease)
- Change in cervical erosion and secretion
- Diminution in lactation when given immediately postpartum
- Cholestatic jaundice
- Migraine
- Rash (allergic)
- Mental depression
- Reduced tolerance to carbohydrates
- Vaginal candidiasis
- Change in corneal curvature (steepening)
- Intolerance to contact lenses

The following adverse reactions have been reported in users of oral contraceptives and the association has been neither confirmed nor refuted:

- Pre-menstrual syndrome
- Cataracts
- Changes in appetite
- Cystitis-like syndrome
- Headache
- Nervousness
- Dizziness
- Hirsutism
- Loss of scalp hair
- Erythema multiforme
- Erythema nodosum
- Hemorrhagic eruption
- Vaginitis
- Porphyria
- Impaired renal function
- Hemolytic uremic syndrome
- Acne
- Changes in libido
- Colitis

OVERDOSAGE

Serious ill effects have not been reported following acute ingestion of large doses of oral contraceptives by young children. Overdosage may cause nausea, and withdrawal bleeding may occur in females.

NON-CONTRACEPTIVE HEALTH BENEFITS

The following non-contraceptive health benefits related to the use of combination oral contraceptives are supported by epidemiological studies which largely utilized oral contraceptive formulations containing estrogen doses exceeding 0.035 mg of estrogen[73–78].

Effects on menses:

- increased menstrual cycle regularity
- decreased blood loss and decreased incidence of iron deficiency anemia
- decreased incidence of dysmenorrhea

Effects related to inhibition of ovulation:

- decreased incidence of functional ovarian cysts
- decreased incidence of ectopic pregnancies

Other effects:

- decreased incidence of fibroadenomas and fibrocystic disease of the breast
- decreased incidence of acute pelvic inflammatory disease
- decreased incidence of endometrial cancer
- decreased incidence of ovarian cancer

DOSAGE AND ADMINISTRATION

To achieve maximum contraceptive effectiveness, JENEST™-28 Tablets must be taken exactly as directed and at intervals not exceeding 24 hours.

28-Day Regimen (Sunday Start)

When taking JENEST™-28, the first white tablet should be taken on the first Sunday after menstruation begins. If period begins on Sunday, the first white tablet is taken on that day. If switching directly from another oral contraceptive, the first white tablet should be taken on the first Sunday after the last ACTIVE tablet of the previous product. Tablets are taken without interruption as follows: one white tablet daily for 7 days, one peach tablet daily for 14 days, then one green tablet daily for 7 days. After 28 tablets have been taken, a white tablet is then taken the next day (Sunday), etc.

The use of JENEST™-28 for contraception may be initiated postpartum. When the tablets are administered during the postpartum period, the increased risk of thromboembolic disease associated with the postpartum period must be considered. (See CONTRAINDICATIONS and WARNINGS concerning thromboembolic disease.) The possibility of ovulation and conception prior to initiation of medication should be considered. If the patient misses more than one tablet, the patient should begin taking tablets again as soon as remembered and another method of contraception used for the balance of that tablet cycle.

All Oral Contraceptives

Breakthrough bleeding, spotting, and amenorrhea are frequent reasons for patients discontinuing oral contraceptives. In breakthrough bleeding, as in all cases of irregular bleeding from the vagina, nonfunctional causes should be borne in mind. In undiagnosed persistent or recurrent abnormal bleeding from the vagina, adequate diagnostic measures are indicated to rule out pregnancy or malignancy. If pathology has been excluded, time or a change to another formulation may solve the problem. Changing to an oral contraceptive with a higher estrogen content, while potentially useful in minimizing menstrual irregularity, should be done only if necessary since this may increase the risk of thromboembolic disease.

Use of oral contraceptives in the event of a missed menstrual period:

1. If the patient has not adhered to the prescribed schedule, the possibility of pregnancy should be considered at the time of the first missed period and oral contraceptive use should be discontinued until pregnancy is ruled out.
2. If the patient has adhered to the prescribed regimen and misses two consecutive periods, pregnancy should be ruled out before continuing oral contraceptive use.

HOW SUPPLIED

JENEST™-28 Tablets are available in boxes of 6 Cyclic Tablet Dispensers (NDC 0052-0269-06). Each Cyclic Tablet Dispenser contains 28 tablets, as follows: 7 white tablets (0.5 mg norethindrone and 0.035 mg ethinyl estradiol), 14 peach tablets (1 mg norethindrone and 0.035 mg ethinyl estradiol) and 7 green tablets containing inert ingredients. The white tablets are unscored with "ORG" and "07" debossed on each side; the peach tablets are unscored with "ORG" and "14" debossed on each side; the green tablets are unscored with "ORG" debossed on each side.

REFERENCES

1. Reproduced with permission of the Population Council from J. Trussell and K. Kost: Contraceptive failure in the United States: A critical review of the literature. Studies in Family Planning, 18 (5), September–October 1987. **2.** Stadel BV. Oral contraceptives and cardiovascular disease. (Pt. 1). N Engl J Med 1981; *305*:612–618. **3.** Stadel BV. Oral contraceptives and cardiovascular disease. (Pt. 2). N Engl J Med 1981; *305*:672–677. **4.** Adam SA, Thorogood M. Oral contraception and myocardial infarction revisited: the effects of new preparations and prescribing patterns. Br J Obstet Gynaecol 1981; *88*:838–845. **5.** Mann JI, Inman WH. Oral contraceptives and death from myocardial infarction. Br Med J 1975; *2(5965)*:245–248. **6.** Mann JI, Vessey MP, Thorogood M, Doll R. Myocardial infarction in young women with special reference to oral contraceptive practice. Br Med J 1975; *2(5956)*:241–245. **7.** Royal College of General Practitioners' Oral Contraception Study: Further analyses of mortality in oral contraceptive users. Lancet 1981; *1*:541–546. **8.** Slone D, Shapiro S, Kaufman DW, Rosenberg L, Miettinen OS, Stolley PD. Risk of myocardial infarction in relation to current and discontinued use of oral contraceptives. N Engl J Med 1981; *305*:420–424. **9.** Vessey MP. Female hormones and vascular disease—an epidemiological overview. Br J Fam Plann 1980; *6(Supplement)*:1–12. **10.** Russell-Briefel RG, Ezzati TM, Fulwood R, Perlman JA, Murphy RS. Cardiovascular risk status and oral contraceptive use, United States, 1976–80. Prevent Med 1986; *15*:352–362. **11.** Goldbaum GM, Kendrick JS, Hogelin GC, Gentry EM. The relative impact of smoking and oral contraceptive use on women in the United States. JAMA 1987; *258*:1339–1342. **12.** Layde PM, Beral V. Further analyses of mortality in oral contraceptive users: Royal College of General Practitioners' Oral Contraception Study. (Table 5) Lancet 1981; *1*:541–546. **13.** Knopp RH. Arteriosclerosis risk: the roles of oral contraceptives and postmenopausal estrogens. J Reprod Med 1986; *31(9) (Supplement)*:913–921. **14.** Krauss RM, Roy S, Mishell DR, Casagrande J, Pike MC. Effects of two low-dose oral contraceptives on serum lipids and lipoproteins: Differential changes in high-density lipoproteins subclasses. Am J Obstet 1983; *145*:446–452. **15.** Wahl P, Walden C, Knopp R, Hoover J, Wallace R, Heiss G, Rifkind B. Effect of estrogen/progestin potency on lipid/lipoprotein cholesterol. N Engl J Med 1983; *308*:862–867. **16.** Wynn V, Niththyananthan R. The effect of progestin in combined oral contraceptives on serum lipids with special reference to high density lipoproteins. Am J Obstet Gynecol 1982; *142*:766–771. **17.** Wynn V, Godsland I. Effects of oral contraceptives on carbohydrate metabolism. J Reprod Med 1986; *31(9)(Supplement)*:892–897. **18.** La Rosa JC. Atherosclerotic risk factors in cardiovascular disease. J Reprod Med 1986; *31(9)(Supplement)*:906–912. **19.** Inman WH, Vessey MP. Investigation of death from pulmonary, coronary, and cerebral thrombosis and embolism in women of child-bearing age. Br Med J 1968; *2(5599)*:193–199. **20.** Maguire MG, Tonascia J, Sartwell PE, Stolley PD, Tockman MS. Increased risk of thrombosis due to oral contraceptives: a further report. Am J Epidemiol 1979; *110(2)*:188–195. **21.** Petitti DB, Wingerd J, Pellegrin F, Ramacharan S. Risk of

Continued on next page

Organon—Cont.

vascular disease in women: smoking, oral contraceptives, noncontraceptive estrogens, and other factors. JAMA 1979; 242:1150–1154. **22.** Vessey MP, Doll R. Investigation of relation between use of oral contraceptives and thromboembolic disease. Br Med J 1968; 2(5599):199–205. **23.** Vessey MP, Doll R. Investigation of relation between use of oral contraceptives and thromboembolic disease. A further report. Br Med J 1969; 2(5658):651–657. **24.** Porter JB, Hunter JR, Danielson DA, Jick H, Stergachis A. Oral contraceptives and non-fatal vascular disease—recent experience. Obstet Gynecol 1982; 59(3):299–302. **25.** Vessey M, Doll R, Peto R, Johnson B, Wiggins P. A long-term follow-up study of women using different methods of contraception: an interim report. J Biosocial Sci 1976; 8:375–427. **26.** Royal College of General Practitioners: Oral Contraceptives, venous thrombosis, and varicose veins. J Royal Coll Gen Pract 1978; 28:393–399. **27.** Collaborative Group for the Study of Stroke in Young Women: Oral contraception and increased risk of cerebral ischemia or thrombosis. N Engl J Med 1973; 288:871–878. **28.** Petitti DB, Wingerd J. Use of oral contraceptives, cigarette smoking, and risk of subarachnoid hemorrhage. Lancet **1978;** 2:234–236. **29.** Inman WH. Oral contraceptives and fatal subarachnoid hemorrhage. Br Med J 1979; 2(6203):1468–1470. **30.** Collaborative Group for the Study of Stroke in Young Women: Oral Contraceptives and stroke in young women:associated risk factors. JAMA 1975; 231:718–722. **31.** Inman WH, Vessey MP, Westerholm B, Engelund A. Thromboembolic disease and the steroidal content of oral contraceptives. A report to the Committee on Safety of Drugs. Br Med J 1970; 2:203–209. **32.** Meade TW, Greenberg G, Thompson SG. Progestogens and cardiovascular reactions associated with oral contraceptives and a comparison of the safety of 50- and 35-mcg oestrogen preparations. Br Med J 1980; 280(6224):1157–1161. **33.** Kay CR. Progestogens and arterial disease—evidence from the Royal College of General Practitioners' Study. Am J Obstet Gynecol 1982; 142:762–765. **34.** Royal College of General Practitioners: Incidence of arterial disease among oral contraceptive users. J Royal Coll Gen Pract 1983; 33:75–82. **35.** Ory HW. Mortality associated with fertility and fertility control: 1983. Family Planning Perspectives 1983; 15:50–56. **36.** The Cancer and Steroid Hormone Study of the Centers for Disease Control and the National Institute of Child Health and Human Development: Oral contraceptive use and the risk of breast cancer. N Engl J Med 1986; 315:405–411. **37.** Pike MC, Henderson BE, Krailo MD, Duke A, Roy S. Breast cancer in young women and use of oral contraceptives: possible modifying effect of formulation and age at use. Lancet 1983; 2:926–929. **38.** Paul C, Skegg DG, Spears GFS, Kaldor JM. Oral contraceptives and breast cancer: A national study. Br Med J 1986; 293:723–725. **39.** Miller DR, Rosenberg L, Kaufman DW, Schottenfeld D, Stolley PD, Shapiro S. Breast cancer risk in relation to early oral contraceptive use. Obstet Gynecol 1986; 68:863–868. **40.** Olson H, Olson KL, Moller TR, Ranstam J, Holm P. Oral contraceptive use and breast cancer in young women in Sweden (letter). Lancet 1985; 2:748–749. **41.** McPherson K, Vessey M, Neil A, Doll R, Jones L, Roberts M. Early contraceptive use and breast cancer: Results of another case-control study. Br J Cancer 1987; 56:653–660. **42.** Huggins GR, Zucker PF. Oral contraceptives and neoplasia: 1987 update. Fertil Steril 1987; 47:733–761. **43.** McPherson K, Drife JO. The pill and breast cancer: why the uncertainty? Br Med J 1986; 293:709–710. **44.** Shapiro S. Oral contraceptives-time to take stock. N Engl J Med 1987; 315:450–451. **45.** Ory H, Naib Z, Conger SB, Hatcher RA, Tyler CW, Contraceptive choice and prevalence of cervical dysplasia and carcinoma in situ. Am J Obstet Gynecol 1976; 124:573–577. **46.** Vessey MP, Lawless M, McPherson K, Yeates D. Neoplasia of the cervix uteri and contraception: a possible adverse effect of the pill. Lancet 1983; 2:930. **47.** Brinton LA, Huggins GR, Lehman HF, Malli K, Savitz DA, Trapido E, Rosenthal J, Hoover R. Long term use of oral contraceptives and risk of invasive cervical cancer. Int J Cancer 1986; 38:339–344. **48.** WHO Collaborative Study of Neoplasia and Steroid Contraceptives: Invasive cervical cancer and combined oral contraceptives. Br Med J 1985; 290:961–965. **49.** Rooks JB, Ory HW, Ishak KG, Strauss LT, Greenspan JR, Hill AP, Tyler CW. Epidemiology of hepatocellular adenoma: the role of oral contraceptive use. JAMA 1979; 242:644–648. **50.** Bein NN, Goldsmith HS. Recurrent massive hemorrhage from benign hepatic tumors secondary to oral contraceptives. Br J Surg 1977; 64:433–435. **51.** Klatskin G. Hepatic tumors: possible relation to use of oral contraceptives. Gastroenterology 1977; 73:386–394. **52.** Henderson BE, Preston-Martin S, Edmondson HA, Peters RL, Pike MC. Hepatocellular carcinoma and oral contraceptives. Br J Cancer 1983; 48:437–440. **53.** Neuberger J, Forman D, Doll R, Williams R. Oral contraceptives and hepatocellular carcinoma. Br Med J 1986; 292:1355–1357. **54.** Forman D, Vincent TJ, Doll R. Cancer of the liver and oral contraceptives. Br Med J 1986; 292:1357–1361. **55.** Harlap S, Eldor J. Births following oral contraceptive failures. Obstet Gynecol 1980; 55:447–452. **56.** Savolainen E, Saksela E, Saxen L. Teratogenic hazards of oral contraceptives analyzed in a national malformation register. Am J Obstet Gynecol 1981; 140:521–524. **57.** Janerich DT, Piper JM, Glebatis DM. Oral contraceptives and birth defects. Am J Epidemiol 1980; 112:73–79. **58.** Ferencz C, Matanoski GM, Wilson PD, Rubin JD, Neill CA, Gutberlet R. Maternal hormone therapy andcongenital heart disease. Teratology 1980; 21:225–239. **59.** Rothman KJ, Fyler DC, Goldblatt A, Kreidberg MB. Exogenous hormones and other drug exposures of children with congenital heart disease. Am J Epidemiol 1979; 109:433–439. **60.** Boston Collaborative Drug Surveillance Program: Oral contraceptives and venous thromboembolic disease, surgically confirmed gallbladder disease, and breast tumors. Lancet 1973; 1:1399–1404. **61.** Royal College of General Practitioners: Oral contraceptives and health. New York, Pittman 1974. **62.** Layde PM, Vessey MP, Yeates D. Risk of gallbladder disease: a cohort study of young women attending family planning clinics. J Epidemiol Community Health 1982; 36:274–278. **63.** Rome Group for Epidemiology and Prevention of Cholelithiasis (GREPCO): Prevalence of gallstone disease in an Italian adult female population. Am J Epidemiol 1984; 119:796–805. **64.** Storm BL, Tamragouri RT, Morse ML, Lazar EL, West SL, Stolley PD, Jones JK. Oral contraceptives and other risk factors for gallbladder disease. Clin Pharmacol Ther 1986; 39:335–341. **65.** Wynn V, Adams PW, Godsland IF, Melrose J, Niththyananthan R, Oakley NW, Seedj A. Comparison of effects of different combined oral contraceptive formulations on carbohydrate and lipid metabolism. Lancet 1979; 1:1045–1049. **66.** Wynn V. Effect of progesterone and progestins on carbohydrate metabolism. In: Progesterone and Progestin. Bardin CW, Milgrom E, Mauvis-Jarvis P. eds. New York, Raven Pres 1983; pp. 395–410. **67.** Perlman JA, Roussell-Briefel RG, Ezzati TM, Lieberknecht G. Oral glucose tolerance and the potency of oral contraceptive progestogens. J Chronic Dis 1985; 38:857–864. **68.** Royal College of General Practitioners' Oral Contraception Study: Effect on hypertension and benign breast disease of progestogen component in combined oral contraceptives. Lancet 1977; 1:624. **69.** Fisch IR, Frank J. Oral contraceptives and blood pressure. JAMA 1977; 237:2499–2503. **70.** Laragh AJ. Oral contraceptive induced hypertension—nine years later. Am J Obstet Gynecol 1976; 126:141–147. **71.** Ramcharan S, Peritz E, Pellegrin FA, Williams WT. Incidence of hypertension in the Walnut Creek Contraceptive Drug Study cohort: In: Pharmacology of steroid contraceptive drugs. Garattini S, Berendes HW. Eds. New York, Raven Press, 1977; pp. 277–288, (Monographs of the Mario Negri Institute for Pharmacological Research Milan.) **72.** Stockley I. Interactions with oral contraceptives. J Pharm 1976; 216:140–143. **73.** The Cancer and Steroid Hormone Study of the Centers for Disease Control and the National Institute of Child Health and Human Development: Oral contraceptive use and the risk of ovarian cancer. JAMA 1983; 249:1596–1599. **74.** The Cancer and Steroid Hormone Study of the Centers for Disease Control and the National Institute of Child Health and Human Development: Combination oral contraceptive use and the risk of endometrial cancer. JAMA 1987; 257:796–800. **75.** Ory HW. Functional ovarian cysts and oral contraceptives: negative association confirmed surgically. JAMA 1974; 228:68–69. **76.** Ory HW, Cole P, MacMahon B, Hoover R. Oral contraceptives and reduced risk of benign breast disease. N Engl J Med 1976; 294:419–422. **77.** Ory HW. The noncontraceptive health benefits from oral contraceptive use. Fam Plann Perspect 1982; 14:182–184. **78.** Ory HW, Forrest JD, Lincoln R. Making choices: Evaluating the health risks and benefits of birth control methods. New York, The Alan Guttmacher Institute, 1983; p. 1. **79.** Schlesselman J, Stadel BV, Murray P. Lai S. Breast cancer in relation to early use of oral contraceptives. JAMA 1988; 259:1828–1833. **80.** Hennekens CH, Speizer FE, Lipnick RJ, Rosner B, Bain C, Belanger C, Stampfer MJ, Willett W, Peto R. A case-control study of oral contraceptive use and breast cancer. JNCI 1984; 72:39–42. **81.** LaVecchia C, Decarli A, Fasoli M, Franceschi S, Gentile A, Negri E, Parazzini F, Tognoni G. Oral contraceptives and cancers of the breast and of the female genital tract. Interim results from a case-control study. Br J Cancer 1986; 54:311–317. **82.** Meirik O, Lund E, Adami H, Bergstrom R, Christoffersen T, Bergsjo P. Oral contraceptive use and breast cancer in young women. A Joint National Case-control study in Sweden and Norway. Lancet 1986; II:650–654. **83.** Kay CR, Hannaford PC. Breast cancer and the pill—A further report from the Royal College of General Practitioners' oral contraception study. Br J Cancer 1988; 58:675–680. **84.** Stadel BV, Lai S, Schlesselman JJ, Murray P. Oral contraceptives and premenopausal breast cancer in nulliparous women. Contraception 1988; 38:287–299. **85.** Miller DR, Rosenberg L, Kaufman DW, Stolley P, Warshauer ME, Shapiro S. Breast cancer before age 45 and oral contraceptive use: New Findings. Am J Epidemiol 1989; 129:269–280. **86.** The UK National Case-Control Study Group, Oral contraceptive use and breast cancer risk in young women. Lancet 1989; 1:973–982. **87.** Schlesselman JJ. Cancer of the breast and reproductive tract in relation to use of oral contraceptives. Contraception 1989; 40:1–38. **88.** Vessey MP, McPherson K, Villard-Mackintosh L, Yeates D. Oral contraceptives and breast cancer: latest findings in a large cohort study. Br J Cancer 1989; 59:613–617. **89.** Jick SS, Walker AM, Stergachis A, Jick H. Oral contraceptives and breast cancer. Br J Cancer 1989; 59:618–621.

BRIEF SUMMARY PATIENT PACKAGE INSERT

Oral contraceptives, also known as "birth control pills" or "the pill", are taken to prevent pregnancy and when taken correctly, have a failure rate of less than 1% per year when used without missing any pills. The typical failure rate of large numbers of pill users is less than 3% per year when women who miss pills are included. For most women oral contraceptives are also free of serious or unpleasant side effects. However, forgetting to take pills considerably increases the chances of pregnancy.

For the majority of women, oral contraceptives can be taken safely. But there are some women who are at high risk of developing certain serious diseases that can be fatal or may cause temporary or permanent disability. The risks associated with taking oral contraceptives increase significantly if you:

- smoke
- are over the age 40
- have high blood pressure, diabetes, high cholesterol
- have or have had clotting disorders, heart attack, stroke, angina pectoris, cancer of the breast or sex organs, jaundice or malignant or benign liver tumors.

You should not take the pill if you suspect you are pregnant or have unexplained vaginal bleeding.

Cigarette smoking increases the risk of serious cardiovascular side effects from oral contraceptive use. This risk increases with age and with heavy smoking (15 or more cigarettes per day) and is quite marked in women over 35 years of age. Women who use oral contraceptives are strongly advised not to smoke.

Most side effects of the pill are not serious. The most common such effects are nausea, vomiting, bleeding between menstrual periods, weight gain, breast tenderness, and difficulty wearing contact lenses. These side effects, especially nausea and vomiting, may subside within the first three months of use.

The serious side effects of the pill occur very infrequently, especially if you are in good health and are young. However, you should know that the following medical conditions have been associated with or made worse by the pill:

1. Blood clots in the legs (thrombophlebitis), lungs (pulmonary embolism), stoppage or rupture of a blood vessel in the brain (stroke), blockage of blood vessels in the heart (heart attack or angina pectoris) or other organs of the body. As mentioned above, smoking increases the risk of heart attacks and strokes and subsequent serious medical consequences.
2. Liver tumors, which may rupture and cause severe bleeding. A possible but not definite association has been found with the pill and liver cancer. However, liver cancers are extremely rare. The chance of developing liver cancer from using the pill is thus even rarer.
3. High blood pressure, although blood pressure usually returns to normal when the pill is stopped.

The symptoms associated with these serious side effects are discussed in the detailed leaflet given to you with your supply of pills. Notify your doctor or health care provider if you notice any unusual physical disturbances while taking the pill. In addition, drugs such as rifampin, as well as some anticovulsants and some antibiotics may decrease oral contraceptive effectiveness.

There is conflict among studies regarding breast cancer and oral contraceptive use. Some studies have reported an increase in the risk of developing breast cancer, particularly at a younger age. This increased risk appears to be related to duration of use. The majority of studies have found no overall increase in the risk of developing breast cancer. Some studies have found an increase in the incidence of cancer of the cervix in women who use oral contraceptives. However, this finding may be related to factors other than the use of oral contraceptives. There is insufficient evidence to rule out the possibility pills may cause such cancers.

Taking the combination pill provides some important noncontraceptive benefits. These include less painful menstruation, less menstrual blood loss and anemia, fewer pelvic infections, and fewer cancers of the ovary and the lining of the uterus.

Be sure to discuss any medical condition you may have with your health care provider. Your health care provider will take a medical and family history before prescribing oral contraceptives and will examine you. You should be reexamined at least once a year while taking oral contraceptives. Your pharmacist should have given you the detailed patient information labeling which gives you further information which you should read and discuss with your health care provider.

DETAILED PATIENT LABELING

PLEASE NOTE: This labeling is revised from time to time as important new medical information becomes available. Therefore, please review this labeling carefully.

The following oral contraceptive product contains a combination of an estrogen and progestogen, the two kinds of female hormones.

JENEST™-28   28 Day Regimen

Each white tablet contains 0.5 mg norethindrone and 0.035 mg ethinyl estradiol. Each peach tablet contains 1 mg norethindrone and 0.035 mg ethinyl estradiol. Each green tablet contains inert ingredients.

INTRODUCTION

Any woman who considers using oral contraceptives (the birth control pill or the pill) should understand the benefits and risks of using this form of birth control. This patient labeling will give you much of the information you will need to make this decision and will also help you determine if you are at risk of developing any of the serious side effects of the pill. It will tell you how to use the pill properly so that it will be as effective as possible. However, this labeling is not a replacement for a careful discussion between you and your health care provider. You should discuss the information provided in this labeling with him or her, both when you first start taking the pill and during your revisits. You should also follow your health care provider's advice with regard to regular check-ups while you are on the pill.

EFFECTIVENESS OF ORAL CONTRACEPTIVES

Oral contraceptives or "birth control pills" or "the pill" are used to prevent pregnancy and are more effective than other non-surgical methods of birth control. When they are taken correctly, the chance of becoming pregnant is less than 1% (1 pregnancy per 100 women per year of use) when used perfectly, without missing any pills. Typical failure rates are actually 3% per year. The chance of becoming pregnant increases with each missed pill during a menstrual cycle.

In comparison, typical failure rates for other non-surgical methods of birth control during the first year of use are as follows:

IUD: 6%
Diaphragm with spermicides: 18%
Spermicides alone: 21%
Vaginal sponge: 18% to 30%
Condom alone: 12%
Periodic abstinence: 20%
No methods: 89%

WHO SHOULD NOT TAKE ORAL CONTRACEPTIVES

> Cigarette smoking increases the risk of serious cardiovascular side effects from oral contraceptive use. This risk increases with age and with heavy smoking (15 or more cigarettes per day) and is quite marked in women over 35 years of age. Women who use oral contraceptives are strongly advised not to smoke.

Some women should not use the pill. For example, you should not take the pill if you are pregnant or think you may be pregnant. You should also not use the pill if you have any of the following conditions:
- A history of heart attack or stroke
- Blood clots in the legs (thrombophlebitis), lungs (pulmonary embolism), or eyes
- A history of blood clots in the deep veins of your legs
- Chest pain (angina pectoris)
- Known or suspected breast cancer or cancer of the lining of the uterus, cervix or vagina
- Unexplained vaginal bleeding (until a diagnosis is reached by your doctor)
- Yellowing of the whites of the eyes or of the skin (jaundice) during pregnancy or during previous use of the pill
- Liver tumor (benign or cancerous)
- Known or suspected pregnancy

Tell your health care provider if you have ever had any of these conditions. Your health care provider can recommend a safer method of birth control.

OTHER CONSIDERATIONS BEFORE TAKING ORAL CONTRACEPTIVES

Tell your health care provider if you have or have had:
- Breast nodules, fibrocystic disease of the breast, an abnormal breast x-ray or mammogram
- Diabetes
- Elevated cholesterol or triglycerides
- High blood pressure
- Migraine or other headaches or epilepsy
- Mental depression
- Gallbladder, heart or kidney disease
- History of scanty or irregular menstrual periods

Women with any of these conditions should be checked often by their health care provider if they choose to use oral contraceptives.

Also, be sure to inform your doctor or health care provider if you smoke or are on any medications.

ANNUAL NUMBER OF BIRTH-RELATED OR METHOD-RELATED DEATHS ASSOCIATED WITH CONTROL OF FERTILITY PER 100,000 NONSTERILE WOMEN, BY FERTILITY CONTROL METHOD ACCORDING TO AGE

Method of control and outcome	15–19	20–24	25–29	30–34	35–39	40–44
No fertility control methods*	7.0	7.4	9.1	14.8	25.7	28.2
Oral contraceptives non-smoker**	0.3	0.5	0.9	1.9	13.8	31.6
Oral contraceptives smoker**	2.2	3.4	6.6	13.5	51.1	117.2
IUD**	0.8	0.8	1.0	1.0	1.4	1.4
Condom*	1.1	1.6	0.7	0.2	0.3	0.4
Diaphragm/ spermicide*	1.9	1.2	1.2	1.3	2.2	2.8
Periodic abstinence*	2.5	1.6	1.6	1.7	2.9	3.6

*Deaths are birth-related
**Deaths are method-related

RISKS OF TAKING ORAL CONTRACEPTIVES

1. Risk of developing blood clots

Blood clots and blockage of blood vessels are the most serious side effects of taking oral contraceptives. In particular, a clot in the legs can cause thrombophlebitis and a clot that travels to the lungs can cause a sudden blocking of the vessel carrying blood to the lungs. Rarely, clots occur in the blood vessels of the eye and may cause blindness, double vision, or impaired vision.

If you take oral contraceptives and need elective surgery, need to stay in bed for a prolonged illness or have recently delivered a baby, you may be at risk of developing blood clots. You should consult your doctor about stopping oral contraceptives three to four weeks before surgery and not taking oral contraceptives for two weeks after surgery or during bed rest. You should also not take oral contraceptives soon after delivery of a baby. It is advisable to wait for at least four weeks after delivery if you are not breast feeding. If you are breast feeding, you should wait until you have weaned your child before using the pill. (See also the section on Breast Feeding in General Precautions.)

The risk of circulatory disease in oral contraceptive users may be higher in users of high dose pills and may be greater with longer duration of oral contraceptive use. In addition, some of these increased risks may continue for a number of years after stopping oral contraceptives. The risk of abnormal blood clotting increases with age in both users and nonusers of oral contraceptives, but the increased risk from the oral contraceptive appears to be present at all ages. For women aged 20 to 44 it is estimated that about 1 in 2,000 using oral contraceptives will be hospitalized each year because of abnormal clotting. Among nonusers in the same age group, about 1 in 20,000 would be hospitalized each year. For oral contraceptive users in general, it has been estimated that in women between the ages of 15 and 34 the risk of death due to a circulatory disorder is about 1 in 12,000 per year, whereas for nonusers the rate is about 1 in 50,000 per year. In the age group 35 to 44, the risk is estimated to be about 1 in 2,500 per year for oral contraceptive users and about 1 in 10,000 per year for nonusers.

2. Heart attacks and strokes

Oral contraceptives may increase the tendency to develop strokes (stoppage or rupture of blood vessels in the brain) and angina pectoris and heart attacks (blockage of blood vessels in the heart). Any of these conditions can cause death or disability.

Smoking greatly increases the possibility of suffering heart attacks and strokes. Furthermore, smoking and the use of oral contraceptives greatly increase the chances of developing and dying of heart disease.

3. Gallbladder disease

Oral contraceptive users probably have a greater risk than nonusers of having gallbladder disease, although this risk may be related to pills containing high doses of estrogens.

4. Liver tumors

In rare cases, oral contraceptives can cause benign but dangerous liver tumors. These benign liver tumors can rupture and cause fatal internal bleeding. In addition, a possible but not definite association has been found with the pill and liver cancers in two studies, in which a few women who developed these very rare cancers were found to have used oral contraceptives for long periods. However, liver cancers are rare.

5. Cancer of the reproductive organs

There is conflict among studies regarding breast cancer and oral contraceptive use. Some studies have reported an increase in the risk of developing breast cancer, particularly at a younger age. This increased risk appears to be related to duration of use. The majority of studies have found no overall increase in the risk of developing breast cancer. Some studies have found an increase in the incidence of cancer of the cervix in women who use oral contraceptives. However, this finding may be related to factors other than the use of

oral contraceptives. There is insufficient evidence to rule out the possibility that pills may cause such cancers.

ESTIMATED RISK OF DEATH FROM A BIRTH CONTROL METHOD OR PREGNANCY

All methods of birth control and pregnancy are associated with a risk of developing certain diseases which may lead to disability or death. An estimate of the number of deaths associated with different methods of birth control and pregnancy has been calculated and is shown in the following table. [See table above.]

In the above table, the risk of death from any birth control method is less than the risk of childbirth, except for oral contraceptive users over the age of 35 who smoke and pill users over the age of 40 even if they do not smoke. It can be seen in the table that for women aged 15 to 39, the risk of death was highest with pregnancy (7–26 deaths per 100,000 women, depending on age). Among pill users who do not smoke, the risk of death was always lower than that associated with pregnancy for any age group, although over the age of 40, the risk increases to 32 deaths per 100,000 women, compared to 28 associated with pregnancy at that age. However, for pill users who smoke and are over the age of 35, the estimated number of deaths exceeds those for other methods of birth control. If a women is over the age of 40 and smokes, her estimated risk of death is four times higher (117/100,000 women) than the estimated risk associated with pregnancy (28/100,000 women) in that age group. Moreover, if you do not smoke and are under the age of 35, the possible risk of death from oral contraceptive use is extremely low when you consider the failure rate associated with other methods of contraception such as the condom or diaphragm and the resulting pregnancy-associated risk.

WARNING SIGNALS

If any of these adverse effects occur while you are taking oral contraceptives, call your doctor immediately.
- Sharp chest pain, coughing of blood, or sudden shortness of breath (indicating a possible clot in the lung)
- Pain in the calf (indicating a possible cloth in the leg)
- Crushing chest pain or heaviness in the chest (indicating a possible heart attack)
- Sudden severe headache or vomiting, dizziness or fainting, disturbances of vision or speech, weakness, or numbness in an arm or leg (indicating a possible stroke)
- Sudden partial or complete loss of vision (indicating a possible clot in the eye)
- Breast lumps (indicating possible breast cancer or fibrocystic disease of the breast; ask your doctor or health care provider to show you how to examine your breasts)
- Severe pain or tenderness in the stomach area (indicating a possibly ruptured liver tumor)
- Difficulty in sleeping, weakness, lack of energy, fatigue, or change in mood (possibly indicating severe depression)
- Jaundice or a yellowing of the skin or eyeballs, accompanied frequently by fever, fatigue, loss of appetite, dark colored urine, or light colored bowel movements (indicating possible liver problems)

SIDE EFFECTS OF ORAL CONTRACEPTIVES

1. Vaginal bleeding

Irregular vaginal bleeding or spotting may occur while you are taking the pills. Irregular bleeding may vary from slight staining between menstrual periods to breakthrough bleeding which is a flow much like a regular period. Irregular bleeding occurs most often during the first few months of oral contraceptive use, but may also occur after your have been taking the pill for some time. Such bleeding may be temporary and usually does not indicate any serious problems. It is important to continue taking your pills on schedule. If the bleeding occurs in more than one cycle or lasts for more than a few days, talk to your doctor or health care provider.

Continued on next page

Organon—Cont.

2. Contact lenses
If you wear contact lenses and notice a change in vision or an inability to wear your lenses, contact your doctor or health care provider.
3. Fluid retention
Oral contraceptives may cause edema (fluid retention) with swelling of the fingers or ankles and may raise your blood pressure. If you experience fluid retention, contact your doctor or health care provider.
4. Melasma
A spotty darkening of the skin is possible, particulary of the face, which may persist.
5. Other side effects
Other side may include nausea and vomiting, change in appetite, headache, nervousness, depression, dizziness, loss of scalp hair, rash, and vaginal infections.
If any of these side effects bother you, call your doctor or health care provider.

GENERAL PRECAUTIONS

1. Missed periods and use of oral contraceptives before or during early pregnancy
There may be times when you may not menstruate regularly after you have completed taking a cycle of pills. If you have taken your pills regularly and miss one menstrual period, continue taking your pills for the next cycle but be sure to inform your health care provider before doing so. If you have not taken the pills daily as instructed and missed a menstrual period, you may be pregnant. If you missed two consecutive menstrual periods, you may be pregnant. Check with your health care provider immediately to determine whether you are pregnant. Do not continue to take oral contraceptives until you are sure you are not pregnant, but continue to use another method of contraception.
There is no conclusive evidence that oral contraceptive use is associated with an increase in birth defects, when taken inadvertently during early pregnancy. Previously, a few studies had reported that oral contraceptives might be associated with birth defects, but these findings have not been seen in more recent studies. Nevertheless, oral contraceptives or any other drugs should not be used during pregnancy unless clearly necessary and prescribed by your doctor. You should check with your doctor about risks to your unborn child of any medication taken during pregnancy.
2. While breast feeding
If you are breast feeding, consult your doctor before starting oral contraceptives. Some of the drug will be passed on to the child in the milk. A few adverse effects on the child have been reported, including yellowing of the skin (jaundice) and breast enlargement. In addition, oral contraceptives may decrease the amount and quality of your milk. If possible, do not use oral contraceptives while breast feeding. You should use another method of contraception since breast feeding provides only partial protection from becoming pregnant and this partial protection decreases significantly as you breast feed for longer periods of time. You should consider starting oral contraceptives only after you have weaned your child completely.
3. Laboratory tests
If you are scheduled for any laboratory tests, tell your doctor you are taking birth control pills. Certain blood tests may be affected by birth control pills.
4. Drug interactions
Certain drugs may interact with birth control pills to make them less effective in preventing pregnancy or cause an increase in breakthrough bleeding. Such drugs include rifampin, drugs used for epilepsy such as barbiturates (for example, phenobarbital) and phenytoin (Dilantin is one brand of this drug), phenylbutazone (Butazolidin is one brand) and possibly certain antibiotics. You may need to use additional contraception when you take drugs which can make oral contraceptives less effective.

HOW TO TAKE ORAL CONTRACEPTIVES

1. General Instructions
You must take your pill every day according to the instructions. Oral contraceptives are most effective if taken no more than 24 hours apart. Take your pill at the same time every day so that you are less likely to forget to take it. You will then maintain an effective dose of the oral contraceptive in your body.
JENEST™-28—Sunday-Start Package:
28-Day Regimen: The first white tablet should be taken on the first Sunday after the menstrual period begins. If period begins on Sunday, begin taking tablets that day. If switching directly from another oral contraceptive, take the first white tablet on the first Sunday after your last ACTIVE tablet of the previous product. Take one white tablet at the same time each day for 7 consecutive days, take one peach tablet daily for 14 days, then take one green tablet daily for 7 days, during which time your period usually occurs. When newly starting oral contraceptives, if the Sunday you begin JENEST™-28 is more than 5 days from the start of your menstrual period, it is important that you use another method of birth control until you have taken a white tablet daily for seven consecutive days. After 28 tablets have been taken, (last green tablet will always be taken on a Saturday) take the first tablet (white) from your next package the following day (Sunday) whether or not you are still menstruating. With the 28-day regimen, pills are taken every day of the year.
If your doctor has scheduled you for surgery, or you need prolonged bed rest, he or she may suggest that you stop taking the pill four weeks before surgery to avoid an increased risk of blood clots. It is also advisable not to start oral contraceptives sooner than four weeks after delivery of a baby.
2. If you forget to take your pill
Combination Oral Contraceptives
If you miss only one combination pill in a cycle, the chance of becoming pregnant is small. Take the missed pill as soon as you realize that you have forgotten it and continue to take your tablets for the rest of that cycle as directed. Since the risk of pregnancy increases with each additional pill you skip, it is very important that you take one pill a day. If you should miss more than one tablet, do not take those tablets missed, but begin taking tablets again as soon as remembered and use another method of contraception for the balance of that tablet cycle.
3. Pregnancy due to pill failure
The incidence of pill failure resulting in pregnancy is approximately one percent (i.e., one pregnancy per 100 women per year) if taken every day as directed, but more typical failure rates are about 3%. If failure does occur, the risk to the fetus is minimal.
4. Pregnancy after stopping the pill
There may be some delay in becoming pregnant after you stop using oral contraceptives, especially if you had irregular menstrual cycles before you used oral contraceptives. It may be advisable to postpone conception until you begin menstruating regularly once you have stopped taking the pill and desire pregnancy.
There does not appear to be any increase in birth defects in newborn babies when pregnancy occurs soon after stopping the pill.
5. Overdosage
Serious ill effects have not been reported following ingestion of large doses of oral contraceptives by young children. Overdosage may cause nausea and withdrawal bleeding in females. In case of overdosage, contact your health care provider or pharmacist.
6. Other information
Your health care provider will take a medical and family history before prescribing oral contraceptives and will examine you. You should be reexamined at least once a year. Be sure to inform your health care provider if there is a family history of any of the conditions listed previously in this leaflet. Be sure to keep all appointments with your health care provider, because this is a time to determine if there are early signs of side effects of oral contraceptive use.
Do not use the drug for any condition other than the one for which it was prescribed. This drug has been prescribed specifically for you; do not give it to others who may want birth control pills.

HEALTH BENEFITS FROM ORAL CONTRACEPTIVES

In addition to preventing pregnancy, use of combination oral contraceptives may provide certain benefits. They are:
- menstrual cycles may become more regular
- blood flow during menstruation may be lighter and less iron may be lost. Therefore, anemia due to iron deficiency is less likely to occur.
- pain or other symptoms during menstruation may be encountered less frequently
- ectopic (tubal) pregnancy may occur less frequently
- noncancerous cysts or lumps in the breast may occur less frequently
- acute pelvic inflammatory disease may occur less frequently
- oral contraceptive use may provide some protection against developing two forms of cancer: cancer of the ovaries and cancer of the lining of the uterus.

If you want more information about birth control pills, ask your doctor or pharmacist. They have a more technical leaflet called the Professional Labeling, which you may wish to read. The Professional Labeling is also published in a book entitled *Physicians' Desk Reference,* available in many book stores and public libraries.
Manufactured for ORGANON INC.
W. Orange, NJ 07052
by
ORTHO PHARMACEUTICAL CORPORATION
Raritan, New Jersey 08869

631-10-791-2
REVISED FEBRUARY 1991
For JENEST™-28 inquiries call 1-800-544-7916.
Shown in Product Identification Section, page 421

LIQUAEMIN® Sodium ℞
(heparin sodium injection, USP)
from porcine intestinal mucosa

HOW SUPPLIED

1,000 USP Units/mL Vials, 10 mL and 30 mL
5,000 USP Units/mL Vials, 10 mL
20,000 USP Units/mL Vials, 1 mL, single use only, 2 mL and 5 mL
40,000 USP Units/mL Vials, 1 mL single use only

NORCURON® ℞
(vecuronium bromide) for injection

THIS DRUG SHOULD BE ADMINISTERED BY ADEQUATELY TRAINED INDIVIDUALS FAMILIAR WITH ITS ACTIONS, CHARACTERISTICS, AND HAZARDS.

DESCRIPTION

NORCURON® (vecuronium bromide) for injection is a nondepolarizing neuromuscular blocking agent of intermediate duration, chemically designated as piperidinium, 1-[(2β, 3α, 5α, 16β, 17β)-3, 17-bis(acetyloxy)-2-(1- piperidinyl) androstan-16-yl]-1-methyl-, bromide. The structural formula is:

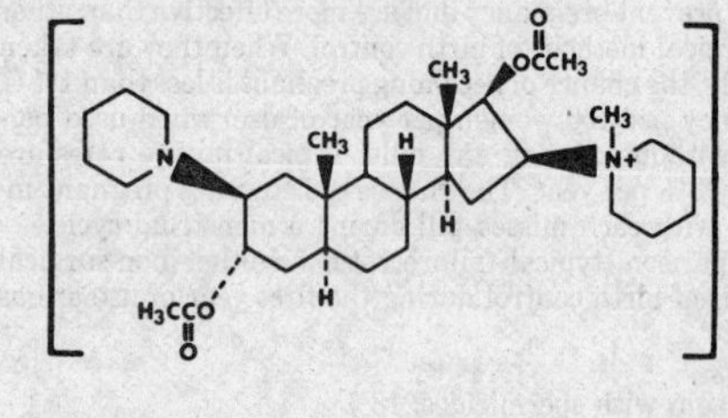

Its chemical formula is $C_{34}H_{57}BrN_2O_4$ with molecular weight 637.74.
Norcuron® is supplied as a sterile nonpyrogenic freeze-dried buffered cake of very fine microscopic crystalline particles for intravenous injection only. Each 10 mL vial contains 10 mg vecuronium bromide, 20.75 mg citric acid anhydrous, 16.25 mg sodium phosphate dibasic anhydrous, 97 mg mannitol (to adjust tonicity), sodium hydroxide and/or phosphoric acid to buffer and adjust to a pH of 4. Each 20 mL vial contains 20 mg of vecuronium bromide, 41.5 mg citric acid anhydrous, 32.5 mg sodium phosphate dibasic anhydrous, 194 mg mannitol (to adjust tonicity), sodium hydroxide and/or phosphoric acid to buffer and adjust to a pH of 4. Bacteriostatic water for injection, USP, when supplied, contains 0.9% w/v BENZYL ALCOHOL, WHICH IS NOT FOR USE IN NEWBORNS.

CLINICAL PHARMACOLOGY

Norcuron® (vecuronium bromide) for injection is a nondepolarizing neuromuscular blocking agent possessing all of the characteristic pharmacological actions of this class of drugs (curariform). It acts by competing for cholinergic receptors at the motor end-plate. The antagonism to acetylcholine is inhibited and neuromuscular block is reversed by acetylcholinesterase inhibitors such as neostigmine, edrophonium, and pyridostigmine. Norcuron® is about ⅓ more potent than pancuronium; the duration of neuromuscular blockade produced by Norcuron® is shorter than that of pancuronium at initially equipotent doses. The time to onset of paralysis decreases and the duration of maximum effect increases with increasing Norcuron® doses. The use of a peripheral nerve stimulator is recommended in assessing the degree of muscular relaxation with all neuromuscular blocking drugs. The ED_{90} (dose required to produce 90% suppression of the muscle twitch response with balanced anesthesia) has averaged 0.057 mg/kg (0.049 to 0.062 mg/kg in various studies). An initial Norcuron® dose of 0.08 to 0.10 mg/kg generally produces first depression of twitch in approximately 1 minute, good or excellent intubation conditions within 2.5 to 3 minutes, and maximum neuromuscular blockade within 3 to 5 minutes of injection in most patients. Under balanced anesthesia, the time to recovery to 25% of control (clinical duration) is approximately 25 to 40 minutes after injection and recovery is usually 95% complete approximately 45–65 minutes after injection of intubating dose. The neuromuscular blocking action of Norcuron® is slightly enhanced in the presence of potent inhalation anesthetics. If Norcuron® is first administered more than 5 minutes after the start of the inhalation of enflurane, isoflurane, or halothane, or when steady state has been achieved, the intubating dose of Norcuron® may be decreased by approximately 15% (see **DOSAGE AND ADMINISTRATION** section).
Prior administration of succinylcholine may enhance the

neuromuscular blocking effect of Norcuron® and its duration of action. With succinylcholine as the intubating agent, initial doses of 0.04–0.06 mg/kg of Norcuron® will produce complete neuromuscular block with clinical duration of action of 25–30 minutes. If succinylcholine is used prior to Norcuron®, the administration of Norcuron® should be delayed until the patient starts recovering from succinylcholine-induced neuromuscular blockade. The effect of prior use of other nondepolarizing neuromuscular blocking agents on the activity of Norcuron® has not been studied (see **Drug Interactions**).

Repeated administration of maintenance doses of Norcuron® has little or no cumulative effect on the duration of neuromuscular blockade. Therefore, repeat doses can be administered at relatively regular intervals with predictable results. After an initial dose of 0.08 to 0.10 mg/kg under balanced anesthesia, the first maintenance dose (suggested maintenance dose is 0.010 to 0.015 mg/kg) is generally required within 25 to 40 minutes; subsequent maintenance doses, if required, may be administered at approximately 12 to 15 minute intervals. Halothane anesthesia increases the clinical duration of the maintenance dose only slightly. Under enflurane a maintenance dose of 0.010 mg/kg is approximately equal to 0.015 mg/kg dose under balanced anesthesia.

The recovery index (time from 25% to 75% recovery) is approximately 15–25 minutes under balanced or halothane anesthesia. When recovery from Norcuron® neuromuscular blocking effect begins, it proceeds more rapidly than recovery from pancuronium. Once spontaneous recovery has started, the neuromuscular block produced by Norcuron® is readily reversed with various anticholinesterase agents, e.g. pyridostigmine, neostigmine, or edrophonium in conjunction with an anticholinergic agent such as atropine or glycopyrrolate. Rapid recovery is a finding consistent with Norcuron®'s short elimination half-life, although there have been occasional reports of prolonged neuromuscular blockade in patients in the intensive care unit (See **PRECAUTIONS**).

The administration of clinical doses of Norcuron® is not characterized by laboratory or clinical signs of chemically mediated histamine release. This does not preclude the possibility of rare hypersensitivity reactions (See ADVERSE REACTIONS).

Pharmacokinetics: At clinical doses of 0.04–0.10 mg/kg, 60–80% of Norcuron® is usually bound to plasma protein. The distribution half-life following a single intravenous dose (range 0.025–0.280 mg/kg) is approximately 4 minutes. Elimination half-life over this same dosage range is approximately 65–75 minutes in healthy surgical patients and in renal failure patients undergoing transplant surgery.

In late pregnancy, elimination half-life may be shortened to approximately 35–40 minutes. The volume of distribution at steady state is approximately 300–400 mL/kg; systemic rate of clearance is approximately 3–4.5 mL/minute/kg. In man, urine recovery of Norcuron® varies from 3–35% within 24 hours. Data derived from patients requiring insertion of a T-tube in the common bile duct suggests that 25–50% of a total intravenous dose of vecuronium may be excreted in bile within 42 hours. Only unchanged vecuronium has been detected in human plasma following use during surgery. In addition, one metabolite, 3-desacetyl vecuronium, has been rarely detected in human plasma following prolonged clinical use in the I.C.U. (See **PRECAUTIONS: Long Term Use in I.C.U.**). The 3-desacetyl vecuronium metabolite has been recovered in the urine of some patients in quantities that account for up to 10% of injected dose; 3-desacetyl vecuronium has also been recovered by T-tube in some patients accounting for up to 25% of the injected dose.

This metabolite has been judged by animal screening (dogs and cats) to have 50% or more of the potency of Norcuron®; equipotent doses are of approximately the same duration as Norcuron® in dogs and cats. Biliary excretion accounts for about half the dose of Norcuron® within 7 hours in the anesthetized rat. Circulatory bypass of the liver (cat preparation) prolongs recovery from Norcuron®. Limited data derived from patients with cirrhosis or cholestasis suggests that some measurements of recovery may be doubled in such patients. In patients with renal failure, measurements of recovery do not differ significantly from similar measurements in healthy patients.

Studies involving routine hemodynamic monitoring in good risk surgical patients reveal that the administration of Norcuron® in doses up to three times that needed to produce clinical relaxation (0.15 mg/kg) did not produce clinically significant changes in systolic, diastolic or mean arterial pressure. The heart rate, under similar monitoring, remained unchanged in some studies and was lowered by a mean of up to 8% in other studies. A large dose of 0.28 mg/kg administered during a period of no stimulation, while patients were being prepared for coronary artery bypass grafting, was not associated with alterations in rate-pressure-product or pulmonary capillary wedge pressure. Systemic vascular resistance was lowered slightly and cardiac output was increased insignificantly. (The drug has not been studied in patients with hemodynamic dysfunction secondary to cardiac valvular disease). Limited clinical experience with use of Norcuron® during surgery for pheochromocytoma has shown that administration of this drug is not associated with changes in blood pressure or heart rate.

Unlike other nondepolarizing skeletal muscle relaxants, Norcuron® has no clinically significant effects on hemodynamic parameters. Norcuron® will not counteract those hemodynamic changes or known side effects produced by or associated with anesthetic agents, other drugs or various other factors known to alter hemodynamics.

INDICATIONS AND USAGE

Norcuron® is indicated as an adjunct to general anesthesia, to facilitate endotracheal intubation and to provide skeletal muscle relaxation during surgery or mechanical ventilation.

CONTRAINDICATIONS

Norcuron® is contraindicated in patients known to have a hypersensitivity to it.

WARNINGS

NORCURON® SHOULD BE ADMINISTERED IN CAREFULLY ADJUSTED DOSAGE BY OR UNDER THE SUPERVISION OF EXPERIENCED CLINICIANS WHO ARE FAMILIAR WITH ITS ACTIONS AND THE POSSIBLE COMPLICATIONS THAT MIGHT OCCUR FOLLOWING ITS USE. THE DRUG SHOULD NOT BE ADMINISTERED UNLESS FACILITIES FOR INTUBATION, ARTIFICIAL RESPIRATION, OXYGEN THERAPY, AND REVERSAL AGENTS ARE IMMEDIATELY AVAILABLE. THE CLINICIAN MUST BE PREPARED TO ASSIST OR CONTROL RESPIRATION. TO REDUCE THE POSSIBILITY OF PROLONGED NEUROMUSCULAR BLOCKADE AND OTHER POSSIBLE COMPLICATIONS THAT MIGHT OCCUR FOLLOWING LONG-TERM USE IN THE ICU, NORCURON® OR ANY OTHER NEUROMUSCULAR BLOCKING AGENT SHOULD BE ADMINISTERED IN CAREFULLY ADJUSTED DOSES BY OR UNDER THE SUPERVISION OF EXPERIENCED CLINICIANS WHO ARE FAMILIAR WITH ITS ACTIONS AND WHO ARE FAMILIAR WITH APPROPRIATE PERIPHERAL NERVE STIMULATOR MUSCLE MONITORING TECHNIQUES (see **PRECAUTIONS**). In patients who are known to have myasthenia gravis or the myasthenic (Eaton-Lambert) syndrome, small doses of Norcuron® may have profound effects. In such patients, a peripheral nerve stimulator and use of a small test dose may be of value in monitoring the response to administration of muscle relaxants.

PRECAUTIONS

Renal Failure: Norcuron® is well tolerated without clinically significant prolongation of neuromuscular blocking effect in patients with renal failure who have been optimally prepared for surgery by dialysis. Under emergency conditions in anephric patients some prolongation of neuromuscular blockade may occur; therefore, if anephric patients cannot be prepared for non-elective surgery, a lower initial dose of Norcuron® should be considered.

Altered Circulation Time: Conditions associated with slower circulation time in cardiovascular disease, old age, edematous states resulting in increased volume of distribution may contribute to a delay in onset time, therefore, dosage should not be increased.

Hepatic Disease: Experience in patients with cirrhosis or cholestasis has revealed prolonged recovery time in keeping with the role the liver plays in Norcuron® metabolism and excretion (**see Pharmacokinetics**). Data currently available do not permit dosage recommendations in patients with impaired liver function.

Long-term Use in I.C.U.: In the intensive care unit, long-term use of neuromuscular blocking drugs to facilitate mechanical ventilation may be associated with prolonged paralysis and/or skeletal muscle weakness, that may be first noted during attempts to wean such patients from the ventilator. Typically, such patients receive other drugs such as broad spectrum antibiotics, narcotics and/or steroids and may have electrolyte imbalance and diseases which lead to electrolyte imbalance, hypoxic episodes of varying duration, acid-base imbalance and extreme debilitation, any of which may enhance the actions of a neuromuscular blocking agent. Additionally, patients immobilized for extended periods frequently develop symptoms consistent with disuse muscle atrophy. The recovery picture may vary from regaining movement and strength in all muscles to initial recovery of movement of the facial and small muscles of the extremities then to the remaining muscles. In rare cases recovery may be over an extended period of time and may even, on occasion, involve rehabilitation. Therefore, when there is a need for long-term mechanical ventilation, the benefits-to-risk ratio of neuromuscular blockade must be considered.

Continuous infusion or intermittent bolus dosing to support mechanical ventilation, has not been studied sufficiently to support dosage recommendations. IN THE INTENSIVE CARE UNIT, APPROPRIATE MONITORING, WITH THE USE OF A PERIPHERAL NERVE STIMULATOR TO ASSESS THE DEGREE OF NEUROMUSCULAR BLOCKADE IS RECOMMENDED TO HELP PRECLUDE POSSIBLE PROLONGATION OF THE BLOCKADE. WHENEVER THE USE OF NORCURON® OR ANY NEUROMUSCULAR BLOCKING AGENT IS CONTEMPLATED IN THE ICU, IT IS RECOMMENDED THAT NEUROMUSCULAR TRANSMISSION BE MONITORED CONTINUOUSLY DURING ADMINISTRATION AND RECOVERY WITH THE HELP OF A NERVE STIMULATOR. ADDITIONAL DOSES OF NORCURON® OR ANY OTHER NEUROMUSCULAR BLOCKING AGENT SHOULD NOT BE GIVEN BEFORE THERE IS A DEFINITE RESPONSE TO T_1 OR TO THE FIRST TWITCH. IF NO RESPONSE IS ELICITED, INFUSION ADMINISTRATION SHOULD BE DISCONTINUED UNTIL A RESPONSE RETURNS.

Severe Obesity or Neuromuscular Disease: Patients with severe obesity or neuromuscular disease may pose airway and/or ventilatory problems requiring special care before, during and after the use of neuromuscular blocking agents such as Norcuron®.

Malignant Hyperthermia: Many drugs used in anesthetic practice are suspected of being capable of triggering a potentially fatal hypermetabolism of skeletal muscle known as malignant hyperthermia. There are insufficient data derived from screening in susceptible animals (swine) to establish whether or not Norcuron® is capable of triggering malignant hyperthermia.

C.N.S.: Norcuron® has no known effect on consciousness, the pain threshold or cerebration. Administration must be accompanied by adequate anesthesia or sedation.

Drug Interactions: Prior administration of succinylcholine may enhance the neuromuscular blocking effect of Norcuron® (vecuronium bromide) for injection and its duration of action. If succinycholine is used before Norcuron® the administration of Norcuron® should be delayed until the succinylcholine effect shows signs of wearing off. With succinylcholine as the intubating agent, initial doses of 0.04–0.06 mg/kg of Norcuron® may be administered to produce complete neuromuscular block with clinical duration of action of 25–30 minutes (see **CLINICAL PHARMACOLOGY**). The use of Norcuron® before succinylcholine, in order to attenuate some of the side effects of succinylcholine, has not been sufficiently studied.

Other nondepolarizing neuromuscular blocking agents (pancuronium, d-tubocurarine, metocurine, and gallamine) act in the same fashion as does Norcuron®, therefore, these drugs and Norcuron® may manifest an additive effect when used together. There are insufficient data to support concomitant use of Norcuron® and other competitive muscle relaxants in the same patient.

Inhalational Anesthetics: Use of volatile inhalational anesthetics such as enflurane, isoflurane, and halothane with Norcuron® will enhance neuromuscular blockade. Potentiation is most prominent with use of enflurane and isoflurane. With the above agents the initial dose of Norcuron® may be the same as with balanced anesthesia unless the inhalational anesthetic has been administered for a sufficient time at a sufficient dose to have reached clinical equilibrium (see **CLINICAL PHARMACOLOGY**).

Antibiotics: Parenteral/intraperitoneal administration of high doses of certain antibiotics may intensify or produce neuromuscular block on their own. The following antibiotics have been associated with various degrees of paralysis: aminoglycosides (such as neomycin, streptomycin, kanamycin, gentamicin, and dihydrostreptomycin); tetracyclines; bacitracin; polymyxin B; colistin; and sodium colistimethate. If these or other newly introduced antibiotics are used in conjunction with Norcuron®, unexpected prolongation of neuromuscular block should be considered a possibility.

Other: Experience concerning injection of quinidine during recovery from use of other muscle relaxants suggests that recurrent paralysis may occur. This possibility must also be considered for Norcuron®. Norcuron® induced neuromuscular blockade has been counteracted by alkalosis and enhanced by acidosis in experimental animals (cat). Electrolyte imbalance and diseases which lead to electrolyte imbalance, such as adrenal cortical insufficiency, have been shown to alter neuromuscular blockade. Depending on the nature of the imbalance, either enhancement or inhibition may be expected. Magnesium salts, administered for the management of toxemia of pregnancy may enhance the neuromuscular blockade.

Drug/laboratory test interactions: None known

Carcinogenesis, Mutagensis, Impairment of Fertility: Long-term studies in animals have not been performed to evaluate carcinogenic or mutagenic potential or impairment of fertility.

Pregnancy: Pregnancy Category C: Animal reproduction studies have not been conducted with Norcuron®. It is also not known whether Norcuron® can cause fetal harm when administered to a pregnant woman or can affect reproduction capacity. Norcuron® should be given to a pregnant woman only if clearly needed.

Pediatric Use: Infants under 1 year of age but older than 7 weeks also tested under halothane anesthesia, are moderately more sensitive to Norcuron® on a mg/kg basis than

Continued on next page

Organon—Cont.

adults and take about 1½ times as long to recover. Information presently available does not permit recommendations for usage in neonates.

ADVERSE REACTIONS

The most frequent adverse reaction to nondepolarizing blocking agents as a class consists of an extension of the drug's pharmacological action beyond the time period needed. This may vary from skeletal muscle weakness to profound and prolonged skeletal muscle paralysis resulting in respiration insufficiency or apnea.

Inadequate reversal of the neuromuscular blockade is possible with Norcuron® as with all curariform drugs. These adverse reactions are managed by manual or mechanical ventilation until recovery is judged adequate. Little or no increase in intensity of blockade or duration of action with Norcuron® is noted from the use of thiobarbiturates, narcotic analgesics, nitrous oxide, or droperidol. See **OVERDOSAGE** for discussion of other drugs used in anesthetic practice which also cause respiratory depression.

Prolonged to profound extensions of paralysis and/or muscle weakness as well as muscle atrophy have been reported after long-term use to support mechanical ventilation in the intensive care unit (see **PRECAUTIONS**). The administration of Norcuron® has been associated with rare instances of hypersensitivity reactions (bronchospasm, hypotension and/or tachycardia, sometimes associated with acute urticaria or erythema); (see also **CLINICAL PHARMACOLOGY**).

OVERDOSAGE

The possibility of iatrogenic overdosage can be minimized by carefully monitoring muscle twitch response to peripheral nerve stimulation.

Excessive doses of Norcuron® produced enhanced pharmacological effects. Residual neuromuscular blockade beyond the time period needed may occur with Norcuron® as with other neuromuscular blockers. This may be manifested by skeletal muscle weakness, decreased respiratory reserve, low tidal volume, or apnea. A peripheral nerve stimulator may be used to assess the degree of residual neuromuscular blockade from other causes of decreased respiratory reserve.

Respiratory depression may be due either wholly or in part to other drugs used during the conduct of general anesthesia such as narcotics, thiobarbiturates and other central nervous system depressants. Under such circumstances the primary treatment is maintenance of a patent airway and manual or mechanical ventilation until complete recovery of normal respiration is assured. Regonol® (pyridostigmine bromide) injection, neostigmine, or edrophonium, in conjunction with atropine or glycopyrrolate will usually antagonize the skeletal muscle relaxant action of Norcuron®. Satisfactory reversal can be judged by adequacy of skeletal muscle tone and by adequacy of respiration. A peripheral nerve stimulator may also be used to monitor restoration of twitch height. Failure of prompt reversal (within 30 minutes) may occur in the presence of extreme debilitation, carcinomatosis, and with concomitant use of certain broad spectrum antibiotics, or anesthetic agents and other drugs which enhance neuromuscular blockade or cause respiratory depression of their own. Under such circumstances the management is the same as that of prolonged neuromuscular blockade. Ventilation must be supported by artificial means until the patient has resumed control of his respiration. Prior to the use of reversal agents, reference should be made to the specific package insert of the reversal agent.

DOSAGE AND ADMINISTRATION

Norcuron® (vecuronium bromide) for injection is for intravenous use only.

This drug should be administered by or under the supervision of experienced clinicians familar with the use of neuromuscular blocking agents. Dosage must be individualized in each case. The dosage information which follows is derived from studies based upon units of drug per unit of body weight and is intended to serve as a guide only, especially regarding enhancement of neuromuscular blockade of Norcuron® by volatile anesthetics and by prior use of succinylcholine (see **PRECAUTIONS/Drug Interactions**). Parenteral drug products should be inspected visually for particulate matter and discoloration prior to administration whenever solution and container permit.

To obtain maximum clinical benefits of Norcuron® and to minimize the possibility of overdosage, the monitoring of muscle twitch response to peripheral nerve stimulation is advised.

The recommended initial dose of Norcuron® is 0.08 to 0.10 mg/kg (1.4 to 1.75 times the ED_{90}) given as an intravenous bolus injection. This dose can be expected to produce good or excellent non-emergency intubation conditions in 2.5 to 3 minutes after injection. Under balanced anesthesia, clinically required neuromuscular blockade lasts approximately 25–30 minutes, with recovery to 25% of control achieved approximately 25 to 40 minutes after injection and recovery to 95% of control achieved approximately 45–65 minutes after injection. In the presence of potent inhalation anesthetics, the neuromuscular blocking effect of Norcuron® is enhanced. If Norcuron® is first administered more than 5 minutes after the start of inhalation agent or when steady-state has been achieved, the initial Norcuron® dose may be reduced by approximately 15%, i.e., 0.060 to 0.085 mg/kg.

Prior administration of succinylcholine may enhance the neuromuscular blocking effect and duration of action of Norcuron®. If intubation is performed using succinylcholine, a reduction of initial dose of Norcuron® to 0.04–0.06 mg/kg with inhalation anesthesia and 0.05–0.06 mg/kg with balanced anesthesia may be required.

During prolonged surgical procedures, maintenance doses of 0.010 to 0.015 mg/kg of Norcuron® are recommended; after the initial Norcuron® injection, the first maintenance dose will generally be required within 25 to 40 minutes. However, clinical criteria should be used to determine the need for maintenance doses.

Since Norcuron® lacks clinically important cumulative effects, subsequent maintenance doses, if required, may be administered at relatively regular intervals for each patient, ranging approximately from 12 to 15 minutes under balanced anesthesia, slightly longer under inhalation agents. (If less frequent administration is desired, higher maintenance doses may be administered.)

Should there be reason for the selection of larger doses in individual patients, initial doses ranging from 0.15 mg/kg up to 0.28 mg/kg have been administered during surgery under halothane anesthesia without ill effects to the cardiovascular system being noted as long as ventilation is properly maintained (see **CLINICAL PHARMACOLOGY**).

Use by Continuous Infusion: After an intubating dose of 80–100 μg/kg, a continuous infusion of 1 μg/kg/min can be initiated approximately 20–40 min later. Infusion of Norcuron® should be initiated only after early evidence of spontaneous recovery from the bolus dose. Long-term intravenous infusion to support mechanical ventilation in the intensive care unit has not been studied sufficiently to support dosage recommendations. (see **PRECAUTIONS**).

The infusion of Norcuron® should be individualized for each patient. The rate of administration should be adjusted according to the patient's twitch response as determined by peripheral nerve stimulation. An initial rate of 1 μg/kg/min is recommended, with the rate of the infusion adjusted thereafter to maintain a 90% suppression of twitch response. Average infusion rates may range from 0.8 to 1.2 μg/kg/min.

Inhalation anesthetics, particularly enflurane and isoflurane may enhance the neuromuscular blocking action of nondepolarizing muscle relaxants. In the presence of steady-state concentrations of enflurane or isoflurane, it may be necessary to reduce the rate of infusion 25–60 percent, 45–60 min after the intubating dose. Under halothane anesthesia it may not be necessary to reduce the rate of infusion.

Spontaneous recovery and reversal of neuromuscular blockade following discontinuation of Norcuron® infusion may be expected to proceed at rates comparable to that following a single bolus dose (see **CLINICAL PHARMACOLOGY**).

Infusion solutions of Norcuron® can be prepared by mixing Norcuron® with an appropriate infusion solution such as 5% glucose in water, 0.9% NaCl, 5% glucose in saline, or Lactated Ringers. Unused portions of infusion solutions should be discarded.

Infusion rates of Norcuron® can be individualized for each patient using the following table:

Drug Delivery Rate (μg/kg/min)	Infusion Delivery Rate (mL/kg/min) 0.1 mg/mL*	0.2 mg/mL†
0.7	0.007	0.0035
0.8	0.008	0.0040
0.9	0.009	0.0045
1.0	0.010	0.0050
1.1	0.011	0.0055
1.2	0.012	0.0060
1.3	0.013	0.0065

* 10 mg of Norcuron® in 100 mL solution
† 20 mg of Norcuron® in 100 mL solution

The following table is a guideline for mL/min delivery for a solution of 0.1 mg/mL (10 mg in 100 mL) with an infusion pump. [See table top of next column.]

NOTE: If a concentration of 0.2 mg/mL is used (20 mg in 100 mL), the rate should be decreased by one-half.

Dosage in Children: Older children (10 to 17 years of age) have approximately the same dosage requirements (mg/kg) as adults and may be managed the same way. Younger children (1 to 10 years of age) may require a slightly higher initial dose and may also require supplementation slightly more often than adults.

Infants under one year of age but older than 7 weeks are moderately more sensitive to Norcuron® on a mg/kg basis than adults and take about 1½ times as long to recover. See also subsection of **PRECAUTIONS** titled **Pediatric Use.** Information presently available does not permit recommendation on usage in neonates (see **PRECAUTIONS**). There are insufficient data concerning continuous infusion of vecuronium in children, therefore, no dosing recommendations can be made.

NORCURON® INFUSION RATE —mL/MIN

Amount of Drug μg/kg/min	Patient Weight—kg 40	50	60	70	80	90	100
0.7	0.28	0.35	0.42	0.49	0.56	0.63	0.70
0.8	0.32	0.40	0.48	0.56	0.64	0.72	0.80
0.9	0.36	0.45	0.54	0.63	0.72	0.81	0.90
1.0	0.40	0.50	0.60	0.70	0.80	0.90	1.00
1.1	0.44	0.55	0.66	0.77	0.88	0.99	1.10
1.2	0.48	0.60	0.72	0.84	0.96	1.08	1.20
1.3	0.52	0.65	0.78	0.91	1.04	1.17	1.30

COMPATIBILITY

Norcuron® is compatible in solution with:
0.9% NaCl solution
5% glucose in water
Sterile water for injection
5% glucose in saline
Lactated Ringers

Use within 24 hours of mixing with the above solutions. Parenteral drug products should be inspected visually for particulate matter and discoloration prior to administration whenever solution and container permit.

HOW SUPPLIED

10 mL vials (10 mg of vecuronium bromide) and 10 mL prefilled syringes of diluent (bacteriostatic water for injection, USP) 22g 1¼″ needle.
Boxes of 10 NDC No. 0052-0441-60
10 mL vials (10 mg vecuronium bromide) and 10 mL vials of diluent (bacteriostatic water for injection, USP).
Boxes of 10 NDC No. 0052-0441-17
10 mL vials (10 mg vecuronium bromide) only; DILUENT NOT SUPPLIED.
Boxes of 10 NDC No. 0052-0441-15
20 mL vials (20 mg vecuronium bromide) only; DILUENT NOT SUPPLIED.
Boxes of 10 NDC No. 0052-0442-46

STORAGE

15–30°C (59–86°F). Protect from light.

AFTER RECONSTITUTION

- When reconstituted with supplied bacteriostatic water for injection: CONTAINS BENZYL ALCOHOL, WHICH IS NOT INTENDED FOR USE IN NEWBORNS. Use within 5 days. May be stored at room temperature or refrigerated.
- When reconstituted with sterile water for injection or other compatible I.V. solutions: Refrigerate vial. Use within 24 hours. Single use only. Discard unused portion.

Caution: Federal law prohibits dispensing without prescription.

Manufactured for ORGANON INC.
By BEN VENUE LABORATORIES, INC.
BEDFORD OHIO 44146
or by
ORGANON INC.
WEST ORANGE, NEW JERSEY 07052
5310125 REVISED 1/92

PAVULON® ℞
[*pāv-u-lon*]
(pancuronium bromide) injection

HOW SUPPLIED

2 mL ampuls—2 mg/mL—boxes of 25—NDC-0052-0444-26
5 mL ampuls—2 mg/mL—boxes of 25—NDC-0052-0444-25
10 mL vials— 1 mg/mL—boxes of 25—NDC-0052-0443-25

PREGNYL® ℞
(chorionic gonadotropin for injection, U.S.P.)

DESCRIPTION

Human chorionic gonadotropin (HCG), a polypeptide hormone produced by the human placenta, is composed of an alpha and a beta sub-unit. The alpha sub-unit is essentially identical to the alpha sub-units of the human pituitary gonadotropins, luteinizing hormone (LH) and follicle-stimulating hormone (FSH), as well as to the alpha sub-unit of human

thyroid-stimulating hormone (TSH). The beta sub-units of these hormones differ in amino acid sequence.

PREGNYL® (chorionic gonadotropin for injection, USP) is a highly purified pyrogen free preparation obtained from the urine of pregnant females. It is standardized by a biological assay procedure. It is available for intramuscular injection in multiple dose vials containing 10,000 USP units of sterile dried powder with 5 mg. monobasic sodium phosphate and 4.4 mg. dibasic sodium phosphate. If required, pH is adjusted with sodium hydroxide and/or phosphoric acid. Each package also contains a 10 mL vial of solvent (water for injection with 0.56% sodium chloride and 0.9% benzyl alcohol). If required, pH is adjusted with sodium hydroxide and/or hydrochloric acid.

CLINICAL PHARMACOLOGY

The action of HCG is virtually identical to that of pituitary LH although HCG appears to have a small degree of FSH activity as well. It stimulates production of gonadal steroid hormones by stimulating the interstitial cells, (Leydig cells) of the testis to produce androgens and the corpus luteum of the ovary to produce progesterone.

Androgen stimulation in the male leads to the development of secondary sex characteristics and may stimulate testicular descent when no anatomical impediment to descent is present. This descent is usually reversible when HCG is discontinued. During the normal menstrual cycle, LH participates with FSH in the development and maturation of the normal ovarian follicle and the mid-cycle LH surge triggers ovulation. HCG can substitute for LH in this function. During a normal pregnancy, HCG secreted by the placenta maintains the corpus luteum after LH secretion decreases, supporting continued secretion of estrogen and progesterone and preventing menstruation. HCG HAS NO KNOWN EFFECT ON FAT MOBILIZATION, APPETITE OR SENSE OF HUNGER, OR BODY FAT DISTRIBUTION.

INDICATIONS

HCG HAS NOT BEEN DEMONSTRATED TO BE EFFECTIVE ADJUNCTIVE THERAPY IN THE TREATMENT OF OBESITY. THERE IS NO SUBSTANTIAL EVIDENCE THAT IT INCREASES WEIGHT LOSS BEYOND THAT RESULTING FROM CALORIC RESTRICTION, THAT IT CAUSES A MORE ATTRACTIVE OR "NORMAL" DISTRIBUTION OF FAT, OR THAT IT DECREASES THE HUNGER AND DISCOMFORT ASSOCIATED WITH CALORIE-RESTRICTED DIETS.

1. Prepubertal cryptorchidism not due to anatomical obstruction. In general, HCG is thought to induce testicular descent in situations when descent would have occurred at puberty. HCG thus may help predict whether or not orchiopexy will be needed in the future. Although, in some cases, descent following HCG administration is permanent, in most cases, the response is temporary. Therapy is usually instituted between the ages 4 and 9.
2. Selected cases of hypogonadotropic hypogonadism (hypogonadism secondary to a pituitary deficiency) in males.
3. Induction of ovulation and pregnancy in the anovulatory, infertile woman in whom the cause of anovulation is secondary and not due to primary ovarian failure and who has been appropriately pretreated with human menotropins.

CONTRAINDICATIONS

Precocious puberty, prostatic carcinoma or other androgen-dependent neoplasm, prior allergic reaction to HCG.

WARNINGS

HCG should be used in conjunction with human menopausal gonadotropins only by physicians experienced with infertility problems who are familiar with the criteria for patient selection, contraindications, warnings, precautions and adverse reactions described in the package insert for menotropins.

The principal serious adverse reactions during this use are: (1) Ovarian hyperstimulation, a syndrome of sudden ovarian enlargement, ascites with or without pain, and/or pleural effusion, (2) Rupture of ovarian cysts with resultant hemoperitoneum, (3) Multiple births, and (4) Arterial thromboembolism.

PRECAUTIONS

1. Induction of androgen secretion by HCG may induce precocious puberty in patients treated for cryptorchidism. Therapy should be discontinued if signs of precocious puberty occur.
2. Since androgens may cause fluid retention, HCG should be used with caution in patients with cardiac or renal disease, epilepsy, migraine, or asthma.

ADVERSE REACTIONS

Headache, irritability, restlessness, depression, fatigue, edema, precocious puberty, gynecomastia, pain at the site of injection.

DOSAGE AND ADMINISTRATION

(Intramuscular Use Only): The dosage regimen employed in any particular case will depend upon the indication for use, the age and weight of the patient, and the physician's prefer-

ence. The following regimens have been advocated by various authorities:

Prepubertal cryptorchidism not due to anatomical obstruction.
1. 4,000 U.S.P. Units three times weekly for three weeks.
2. 5,000 U.S.P. Units every second day for four injections.
3. 15 injections of 500 to 1,000 U.S.P. Units over a period of six weeks.
4. 500 U.S.P. Units three times weekly for four to six weeks. If this course of treatment is not successful, another series is begun one month later, giving 1,000 U.S.P. Units per injection.

Selected cases of hypogonadotropic hypogonadism in males.
1. 500 to 1,000 U.S.P. Units three times a week for three weeks, followed by the same dose twice a week for three weeks.
2. 4,000 U.S.P. Units three times weekly for six to nine months, following which the dosage may be reduced to 2,000 U.S.P. Units three times weekly for an additional three months.

Induction of ovulation and pregnancy in the anovulatory, infertile woman in whom the cause of anovulation is secondary and not due to primary ovarian failure and who has been appropriately pre-treated with human menotropins. (See prescribing information for menotropins for dosage and administration for that drug product). 5,000 to 10,000 U.S.P. Units one day following the last dose of menotropins. (A dosage of 10,000 U.S.P. Units is recommended in the labeling for menotropins).

IMPORTANT: USE COMPLETELY AFTER RECONSTITUTION. RECONSTITUTED SOLUTION IS STABLE FOR 60 DAYS WHEN REFRIGERATED.

HOW SUPPLIED

Two-vial package containing:
1–10 mL lyophilized multiple dose vial containing:
   10,000 USP Units chorionic gonadotropin per vial (NDC 0052-0315-10)
1–10 mL vial of solvent containing:
   water for injection with 0.56% sodium chloride and 0.9% benzyl alcohol (NDC 0052-0325-10.)
When reconstituted, each 10 mL vial contains:

Chorionic gonadotropin	10,000 USP Units
Monobasic sodium phosphate	5 mg.
Dibasic sodium phosphate	4.4 mg.
Sodium chloride	0.56%
Benzyl alcohol	0.9%

If required pH adjusted with sodium hydroxide and/or phosphoric acid.

CAUTION

Federal law prohibits dispensing without prescription.

STORAGE

Store at 15°–30°C (59°–86°F). Reconstituted material will remain stable for 60 days when refrigerated.

DIRECTIONS FOR RECONSTITUTION

Two vial package: Withdraw sterile air from lyophilized vial and inject into diluent vial. Remove 1–10 mL from diluent and add to lyophilized vial; agitate gently until powder is completely dissolved in solution.

Parenteral drug products should be inspected visually for particulate matter and discoloration prior to administration, whenever solution and container permit.

Revised 12/90

REGONOL®   ℞
[re-gō-nol]
(pyridostigmine bromide) injection, USP

HOW SUPPLIED

5 mg/mL: 2 mL ampuls—boxes of 25—NDC-0052-0460-02
5 mg/mL: 5 mL vials—   boxes of 25—NDC-0052-0460-05

REVERSOL®   ℞
(edrophonium chloride injection, USP)

HOW SUPPLIED

10 mL multidose vials-boxes of 25, NDC 0052-0466-34

SUCCINYLCHOLINE CHLORIDE INJECTION   ℞
USP

HOW SUPPLIED

20 mg/mL—10 mL vials, boxes of 25

TICE® BCG   ℞
BCG VACCINE, USP
(for intravesical or percutaneous use)

Distributed by Organon Inc.
(See page 1689 for complete product information.)

WIGRAINE®   ℞

DESCRIPTION

Wigraine® Tablet: Each tablet contains the following:

Ergotamine Tartrate, USP	1 mg
Caffeine, USP	100 mg

Each tablet also contains: Lactose, Magnesium Stearate, Microcrystalline Cellulose, Purified Water and Starch as inactive ingredients.
Wigraine® tablets are uncoated and prepared to insure rapid disintegration (by an exclusive manufacturing process) and facilitate quick absorption. Rapid onset of effect is important for the satisfactory treatment of acute attacks of vascular headaches.
Wigraine® Suppository: Each suppository contains the following:

Ergotamine tartrate, USP	2 mg
Caffeine, USP	100 mg
Tartaric Acid	21.5 mg

Wigraine® suppositories contain the active ingredients in a synthetic cocoa butter base which melts rapidly at room temperature.

CLINICAL PHARMACOLOGY

Ergotamine is an alpha adrenergic blocking agent with a direct stimulating effect on the smooth muscle of peripheral and cranial blood vessels and produces depression of central vasomotor centers. The compound also has the properties of serotonin antagonism. In comparison to hydrogenated ergotamine, the adrenergic blocking actions are less pronounced and vasoconstrictive actions are greater. Caffeine, also a cranial vasoconstrictor is added to further enhance the vasoconstrictive effect without the necessity of increasing ergotamine dosage.

INDICATIONS AND USAGE

Wigraine® is indicated as therapy to abort or prevent vascular headaches such as migraine, migraine variants, or so-called histamine cephalalgia.

CONTRAINDICATIONS

Wigraine® can cause fetal harm when administered to a pregnant women. It can produce prolonged uterine contractions which can result in abortion. Wigraine® is contraindicated in women who are or may become pregnant. If this is used during pregnancy, or if the patient becomes pregnant while taking this drug, the patient should be advised of the potential hazard to the fetus.

Peripheral vascular disease, coronary heart disease, hypertension, impaired hepatic or renal function, sepsis, and hypersensitivity to any of the components.

PRECAUTIONS

Although signs and symptoms of ergotism rarely develop even after long term intermittent use of the orally or rectally administered drugs, care should be exercised to remain within the limits of recommended dosage.
Pregnancy Category X. See Contraindications section.
Nursing Mothers. It is not known whether the ergotamine tartrate in Wigraine® is excreted in human milk. Because some ergot alkoids have been found in the milk of nursing mothers resulting in symptoms of ergotism in their children, a decision should be made whether to discontinue nursing or to discontinue the drug, taking into account the importance of the drug to the mother.
Pediatric Usage. Safety and effectiveness in children have not been established.

ADVERSE REACTIONS

In order of decreasing severity: precordial distress and pain, muscle pains in the extremities, numbness and tingling in fingers and toes, transient tachycardia or bradycardia, vomiting, nausea, weakness in the legs, diarrhea, localized edema and itching.

DOSAGE AND ADMINISTRATION

Best results are obtained if the tablets or suppositories are administered at the first sign of an attack. Wigraine® tablet: the average adult dose is 2 tablets at the start of a vascular headache (migraine) attack; followed by 1 additional tablet every ½ hour if needed, up to 6 tablets per attack. Total weekly dosage should not exceed 10 tablets. Wigraine® suppository: the maximum adult dose is 2 suppositories for an individual attack. In carefully selected patients, with due consideration of maximum dosage recommendations, administration of the drug at bedtime may be an appropriate short-term preventive measure.

Continued on next page

Organon—Cont.

OVERDOSAGE

The toxic effects of an acute overdosage of Wigraine® are due primarily to the ergotamine component. The amount of caffeine is such that its toxic effects will be overshadowed by those of ergotamine. Symptoms include vomiting, numbness, tingling, pain and cyanosis of the extremities associated with diminished or absent peripheral pulses, hypertension or hypotension, drowsiness, stupor, coma, convulsions and shock. Treatment consists of removal of the offending drug by induction of emesis, gastric lavage and catharsis. Maintenance of adequate pulmonary ventilation, correction of hypotension, and control of convulsions are important considerations. Treatment of peripheral vasospasm should consist of warmth, but not heat, and protection of the ischemic limbs. Vasodilators may be used with benefit but caution must be exercised to avoid aggravating an already existing hypotension. The LD50 limits of the various components as outlined in NIOSH 1978 Registry of Toxic Effects of Chemical Substances, published by U.S. Department of Health, Education and Welfare are as follows: Ergotamine Tartrate IV LD50 in rats = 80mg/Kg, Caffeine IV LD50 in rats = 105mg/Kg.

HOW SUPPLIED

Wigraine® tablets are white tablets embossed with "ORGANON 542" on one side. They are individually foil stripped and packaged in boxes of 20's NDC #0052-0542-20 and 100's NDC #0052-0542-91. Wigraine® suppositories are individuallly foil wrapped and packaged in boxes of 12. NDC #0052-0548-12.

STORAGE

Wigraine® tablets should be stored at a maximum of 30°C (86°F) and the suppositories should be refrigerated at 2°–8°C (36°–46°F).

CAUTION

Federal law prohibits dispensing without prescription.

Revised 9/91

Shown in Product Identification Section, page 421

ZYMASE™ ℞
(pancrelipase, USP)
enteric coated spheres

DESCRIPTION

Zymase capsules contain enteric coated spheres of pancrelipase, a substance containing enzymes, principally lipase, with amylase and protease obtained from the pancreas of the hog. Each capsule contains not less than:

Lipase—12,000 USP Units
Protease—24,000 USP Units
Amylase—24,000 USP Units

Each capsule also contains: Gelatin, purified water, starch, talc, titanium dioxide, FD&C Green #3, FD&C Yellow #10, and other inactive ingredients.

CLINICAL PHARMACOLOGY

Zymase is protected against inactivation by gastric acidity, and active enzymes are released in the duodenum. The enzymes promote hydrolysis of fats into glycerol and fatty acids, protein into proteases and derived substances, and starch into dextrans and sugars.

INDICATIONS AND USAGE

Zymase is indicated in conditions where pancreatic enzymes are either absent or deficient with resultant inadequate fat digestion. Such conditions include but are not limited to chronic pancreatitis, pancreatectomy, cystic fibrosis and steatorrhea of diverse etiologies.

CONTRAINDICATIONS

Known hypersensitivity to pork protein.

PRECAUTIONS

To maintain enteric coating integrity, do not chew or crush spheres.

ADVERSE REACTIONS

No adverse reactions have been reported. It should be noted, however, that extremely high does of exogenous pancreatic enzymes have been associated with hyperuricosuria and hyperuricemia.

DOSAGE AND ADMINISTRATION

One to two capsules with each meal or snack. Individual cases may require higher dosage and dietary adjustment. Where swallowing of capsules is difficult, capsules may be opened and the spheres taken with liquids or soft foods which do not require chewing.

STORAGE

Not to exceed 25°C (77°F). Store in dry place when opened.

DISPENSE

In tight container as defined in the USP.

Revised 1/92

Shown in Product Identification Section, page 421

Ortho Biotech
RARITAN, NJ 08869-0602

ORTHOCLONE OKT®3 Sterile Solution ℞
(muromonab-CD3)
For Intravenous Use Only

> **WARNING**
> Only physicians experienced in immunosuppressive therapy and management of renal transplant patients should use ORTHOCLONE OKT3 (muromonab-CD3).
> Patients receiving ORTHOCLONE OKT3 should be managed in facilities equipped and staffed for cardiopulmonary resuscitation.
> Patients with fluid overload have developed severe pulmonary edema upon treatment with ORTHOCLONE OKT3.

DESCRIPTION

ORTHOCLONE OKT3 (muromonab-CD3) Sterile Solution is a murine monoclonal antibody to the T3 (CD3) antigen of human T cells which functions as an immunosuppressant. It is for intravenous use only. The antibody is a biochemically purified IgG_{2a} immunoglobulin with a heavy chain of approximately 50,000 daltons and a light chain of approximately 25,000 daltons. It is directed to a glycoprotein with a molecular weight of 20,000 in the human T cell surface which is essential for T cell functions. Because it is a monoclonal antibody preparation, ORTHOCLONE OKT3 Sterile Solution is a homogeneous, reproducible antibody product with consistent, measurable reactivity to human T cells.

Each 5 ml ampule of ORTHOCLONE OKT3 Sterile Solution contains 5 mg (1 mg/ml) of muromonab-CD3 in a clear colorless solution which may contain a few fine translucent protein particles. Each ampule contains a buffered solution (pH 7.0 ±0.5) of monobasic sodium phosphate (2.25 mg), dibasic sodium phosphate (9.0 mg), sodium chloride (43 mg) and polysorbate 80 (1.0 mg) in water for injection.

The proper name, muromonab-CD3, is derived from the descriptive term murine monoclonal antibody. The CD3 designation identifies the specificity of the antibody as the Cell Differentiation (CD) cluster 3 defined by the First International Workshop on Human Leukocyte Differentiation Antigens.

CLINICAL PHARMACOLOGY

ORTHOCLONE OKT3 reverses graft rejection, most probably by blocking the function of all T cells which play a major role in acute renal rejection.

ORTHOCLONE OKT3 reacts with and blocks the function of a 20,000 dalton molecule (CD3) in the membrane of human T cells that has been associated *in vitro* with the antigen recognition structure of T cells and is essential for signal transduction. In *in vitro* cytolytic assays, ORTHOCLONE OKT3 blocks both the generation and function of effector cells. It is a potent mitogen *in vitro* in calf serum, but this mitogenicity is markedly reduced in human serum. ORTHOCLONE OKT3 thus blocks all known T cell functions.

In vivo, ORTHOCLONE OKT3 reacts with most peripheral blood T cells and T cells in body tissues, but has not been found to react with other hematopoietic elements or other tissues of the body.

In all patients studied, a rapid and concomitant decrease in the number of circulating CD3 positive, CD4 positive and CD8 positive T cells was observed within minutes after the administration of ORTHOCLONE OKT3. Between days two and seven increasing numbers of circulating CD4 positive and CD8 positive cells have been observed in patients although CD3 positive cells are not detectable. The presence of these CD4 and CD8 positive cells has not been found to affect the clinical course of the patient. CD3 positive cells reappear rapidly and reach pre-treatment levels within a week after termination of ORTHOCLONE OKT3 therapy. Increasing numbers of CD3 positive cells have been observed in some patients during the second week of ORTHOCLONE OKT3 therapy, possibly as a result of the development of neutralizing antibodies to ORTHOCLONE OKT3.

Antibodies to ORTHOCLONE OKT3 have been observed, occurring with an incidence of 21% (n=43) for IgM, 86% (n=43) for IgG and 29% (n=35) for IgE. The mean time of appearance of IgG antibodies was 20±2 (mean ±SD) days. Early IgG antibodies appeared towards the end of the second week of treatment in 3% (n=86) of the patients.

Serum levels of ORTHOCLONE OKT3 are measurable using an enzyme-linked immunosorbent assay (ELISA). During treatment with 5 mg per day for 14 days, mean serum trough levels of the drug rose over the first three days and then averaged 0.9 μg/ml on days 3 to 14. The levels obtained during therapy have been shown to block T cell effector functions *in vitro*.

Following administration of ORTHOCLONE OKT3 *in vivo*, leukocytes have been observed in cerebrospinal and peritoneal fluids. The mechanism for this effect is not understood.

INDICATIONS AND USAGE

ORTHOCLONE OKT3 is indicated for the treatment of acute allograft rejection in renal transplant patients.

In a controlled randomized clinical trial, ORTHOCLONE OKT3 was significantly more effective than conventional high dose steroid therapy in reversing acute renal allograft rejection. In this trial, 122 evaluable patients undergoing acute rejection of cadaveric renal transplants were treated either with ORTHOCLONE OKT3 daily for a mean of 14 days, with concomitant lowering of the dosage of azathioprine and maintenance steroids (62 patients), or with conventional high dose steroids (60 patients). ORTHOCLONE OKT3 reversed 94% of the rejections compared to a 75% reversal rate obtained with conventional high dose steroid treatment (p=0.006). The one year Kaplan-Meier (actuarial) estimates of graft survival rates for these patients who had acute rejection were 62% and 45% for ORTHOCLONE OKT3 and steroid treated patients, respectively (p=0.04). At two years the rates were 56% and 42%, respectively (p=0.06).

One- and two-year patient survivals were not significantly different between the two groups, being 85% and 75% for ORTHOCLONE OKT3 (muromonab-CD3) treated patients and 90% and 85% for steroid treated patients.

In additional open clinical trials, the observed rate of reversal of acute renal allograft rejection was 92% (n=126) for ORTHOCLONE OKT3 therapy. ORTHOCLONE OKT3 also was effective in reversing acute renal allograft rejections in 65% (n=225) of cases where steroids and lymphocyte immune globulin preparations were contraindicated or were not successful (rescue).

The dosage of other immunosuppressive agents used in conjunction with ORTHOCLONE OKT3 should be lowered to minimal levels (See DOSAGE AND ADMINISTRATION Section).

CONTRAINDICATIONS

ORTHOCLONE OKT3 should not be used in patients who are hypersensitive to this or any other product of murine origin nor in patients who are in fluid overload, as evidenced by chest x-ray or a greater than 3 percent weight gain within the week prior to planned ORTHOCLONE OKT3 administration.

WARNINGS

SEE BOXED WARNING

Immunosuppressive therapy can lead to increased susceptibility to infection. Further, lymphomas have been reported following immunosuppressive therapy, and data suggest that their occurrence is related to the intensity and duration of immunosuppression rather than being associated with the use of any one specific agent.

Significant adverse experiences including fever, chills, dyspnea, tachycardia, hypertension, hypotension, nausea, vomiting, abnormal chest sounds, headache, pruritus, hyperventilation, diarrhea, chest pains, tremor, wheezing, rigor, and malaise may occur within the first two days of ORTHOCLONE OKT3 (muromanob-CD3) treatment. Therefore, the administration of the first several doses of ORTHOCLONE OKT3 should be performed in a facility which is equipped and staffed for cardio-pulmonary resuscitation and where the patients can be closely monitored during the first 48 hours after the initial injection. In the initial renal rejection studies, the most serious first-dose reaction—potentially fatal severe pulmonary edema—occurred infrequently (4.7% of the initial 107 patients and 0.0% in the subsequent 311 patients treated with first-dose restrictions). In each case of severe pulmonary edema, fluid overload was present before treatment. Therefore, patients should be evaluated for fluid overload by chest x-ray or weight gain of greater than 3%. Weight should be reduced to a value less than or equal to 3% above the minimum weight reported during the week prior to ORTHOCLONE OKT3 administration. Reactions to the first dose may be minimized by using the recommended steroid regimen (See DOSAGE AND ADMINISTRATION Section).

This formulation of ORTHOCLONE OKT3 contains polysorbate 80 and must not be used for the *in vitro* treatment of bone marrow.

PRECAUTIONS

General

If the patient temperature exceeds 37.8°C (100°F), it should be lowered by antipyretics before administration of each dose of ORTHOCLONE OKT3.

Use a low protein-binding 0.2 or 0.22 micrometer (μm) filter to prepare the injections (See ADMINISTRATION INSTRUCTIONS).

ORTHOCLONE OKT3 is a heterologous protein and induces detectable antibodies in most patients. Limited data

are available regarding retreatment with ORTHOCLONE OKT3. The presence of antibodies to ORTHOCLONE OKT3 could limit its efficacy following re-administration and possibly cause serious adverse reactions. Caution should be used if retreatment is considered.

Physicians should be aware that in a post-marketing survey of 214 renal transplant patients, an aseptic meningitis syndrome was identified. The most commonly reported symptoms in this survey were: fever (89%), headache (44%), neck stiffness (14%) and photophobia (10%), which occurred most often during the first three days of ORTHOCLONE OKT3 therapy. Seizures were reported in two patients. A total of 13 patients were reported to have had symptoms of meningitis *and* had a documented lumbar puncture. The examination of cerebrospinal fluid in these thirteen patients showed leukocytosis (11/12)—(cells were mainly polymorphonuclear in 4 patients), elevated protein (8/10) and decreased glucose (4/10). One patient had a positive culture for enterovirus. All other viral, bacterial and fungal cultures were negative. One of the thirteen patients had a concomitant urinary tract infection. Although all patients had a benign course and recovered, infection must be considered in the differential diagnosis of an immunosuppressed transplant patient with any signs or symptoms of meningitis.

Information for patients: Patients should be informed of the expected first dose ORTHOCLONE OKT3 effects, which are markedly reduced on successive days of ORTHOCLONE OKT3 treatment. Patients should also be informed regarding the potential benefits and risks attendant to the use of ORTHOCLONE OKT3.

Laboratory tests: Chest x-ray taken within 24 hours before initiating ORTHOCLONE OKT3 (muromonab-CD3) treatment must be clear of fluid. WBCs and differentials should be monitored at intervals during treatment with ORTHOCLONE OKT3. The effect of ORTHOCLONE OKT3 on circulating T cells expressing the CD3 antigen should be monitored by an *in vitro* assay.

Carcinogenesis: Long term studies have not been performed in laboratory animals to evaluate the carcinogenic potential of ORTHOCLONE OKT3.

Pregnancy Category C: Animal reproductive studies have not been conducted with ORTHOCLONE OKT3. It is also not known whether ORTHOCLONE OKT3 can cause fetal harm when administered to a pregnant woman or can affect reproduction capacity. ORTHOCLONE OKT3 should be given to a pregnant woman only if clearly needed.

Pediatric use: Safety and effectiveness in children have not been established. Although no adequate controlled studies have been conducted in children, patients as young as two years of age have received ORTHOCLONE OKT3 with no unexpected adverse effects.

ADVERSE REACTIONS

ORTHOCLONE OKT3 for treatment of acute renal allograft rejection:
In clinical trials, when the incidence of adverse experiences reported by patients treated for rejection with ORTHOCLONE OKT3 plus concomitant low-dose immunosuppressive therapy (primarily azathioprine and corticosteroids) was compared to the incidence of adverse experiences reported by patients receiving conventional treatment, patients treated with ORTHOCLONE OKT3 were observed to have increased adverse experiences during the first two days of treatment. During this period the majority of patients experienced pyrexia (90%), (of which 19% were 40.0°C [104°F] or above) and chills (59%). In addition, other adverse experiences occurring in 8% or more of the patients during the first two days of ORTHOCLONE OKT3 therapy included dyspnea (21%), nausea (19%), vomiting (19%), chest pain (14%), diarrhea (14%), tremor (13%), wheezing (13%), headache (11%), tachycardia (10%), rigor (8%), and hypertension (8%). Similar advere effects were observed in the additional open clinical studies.

Potentially fatal severe pulmonary edema was reported following the first two doses in less than 2% of the cases and was always associated with fluid overload. It is, therefore, essential that patients receiving ORTHOCLONE OKT3 not be in fluid overload and remain under close medical supervision for 48 hours after the administration of the first dose. The first dose should be administered as detailed in the DOSAGE AND ADMINISTRATION Section.

In the controlled randomized renal rejection trial, the most common infections during the first 45 days of ORTHOCLONE OKT3 therapy were due to Herpes simplex (27%) and cytomegalovirus (19%). Other severe and life-threatening were*Staphylococcus epidermidis* (4.8%), *Pneumocystis carinii* (3.1%), Legionella (1.6%), Cryptococcus (1.6%), Serratia (1.6%) and gram-negative bacteria (1.6%). The incidence of infections was similar in patients treated with ORTHOCLONE OKT3 and in patients treated with high dose steroids.

ORTHOCLONE OKT3 in other clinical trials:
In additional clinical trials, the following adverse experiences were reported: hypotension, abnormal chest sounds, pruritus, and hyperventilation. The following clinically significant infections have also been reported: *Staphylococcus*

aureus, Staphylococcus faecalis, Escherichia coli, Cornyebacterium, *Pseudomonas aeruginosa,* and fungal infection. Additional clinically significant adverse experiences, whose causal relationship to ORTHOCLONE OKT3 therapy is unclear, include anaphylaxis (1 patient), serum sickness (2 patients) and lymphoma (2 patients).

A monoclonal B-cell-lymphoproliferative disorder, similar to Epstein-Barr virus (EBV) associated B-cell-lymphoproliferation, occurred in one of 22 bone marrow transplantation patients treated for graft-versus-host disease with ORTHOCLONE OKT3. One patient with acute renal rejection was diagnosed as having generalized lymphoma three weeks after receiving ORTHOCLONE OKT3 for three days. The patient received multi-drug immunosuppressive therapy prior to and during administration of ORTHOCLONE OKT3. The occurrence of potentially fatal lymphoproliferative disorders such as EBV-lymphoproliferative lesions, central nervous system lymphomas, polyclonal B-cell hyperplasia, and true malignant lymphomas are thought to be a result of the duration and intensity of immunosuppression rather than being associated with the use of any one specific agent. Long term risk for increased incidence of lymphoma or other malignancies has not been determined.

Post-marketing survey:
In a post-marketing survey of 214 renal transplant patients, an aseptic meningitis syndrome has been identified. The symptoms reported in the survey are fever (89%), headache (44%), neck stiffness (14%) and photophobia (10%). A combination of the above four symptoms occurred in 5% of the patients. This syndrome has been reported to occur usually during the first three days of ORTHOCLONE OKT3 (muromonab-CD3) therapy. All patients in the survey with the syndrome had a benign course and recovered.

In the first 3 years post-licensure, 34 patients (0.2%) of an estimated 18,900 patients treated with ORTHOCLONE OKT3 (muromonab-CD3) were reported to have had a seizure; twenty seizures were reported to have occurred during the first 3 days of ORTHOCLONE OKT3 therapy. Nine of the 20 patients had either known seizure disorder, hypoglycemia or were concurrently on dialysis. Cerebrospinal fluid in two of the patients, who had lumbar puncture, showed leukocytosis and elevated protein. One of the 34 patients was retreated with ORTHOCLONE OKT3 on two subsequent occasions without additional seizures. One patient with a past history of seizure disorder developed refractory generalized seizures two days after transplantation and initiation of prophylactic ORTHOCLONE OKT3 therapy and died one day later. The causal relationship between ORTHOCLONE OKT3 and seizure is unknown.

Although other immunosuppressives have been associated with CNS neurotoxicity, the following adverse experiences have also been reported and may bear a relationship to ORTHOCLONE OKT3 therapy: confusion, coma, lethargy, altered mental status, encephalopathy, hallucinations, and disorientation. Rash, arthralgia, arthritis amd myalgia have also been reported, but are of unknown causal relationship to ORTHOCLONE OKT3.

OVERDOSAGE

The maximum amount of ORTHOCLONE OKT3 that can safely be administered in single or multiple doses has not been determined.

DOSAGE AND ADMINISTRATION

The recommended dose of ORTHOCLONE OKT3 for the treatment of acute renal allograft rejection is 5 mg per day for 10 to 14 days. Treatment should begin once acute renal rejection is diagnosed.

Patients should be monitored closely for 48 hours after the first dose is administered. Intravenous methylprednisolone sodium succinate 1.0 mg/kg given prior to ORTHOCLONE OKT3 administration and intravenous hydrocortisone sodium succinate 100 mg given 30 minutes after ORTHOCLONE OKT3 administration is strongly recommended to decrease the incidence of reactions to the first dose which has been attributed in the literature to ORTHOCLONE OKT3 mediated cytokine release. Acetaminophen and antihistamines can be given concomitantly with ORTHOCLONE OKT3 to reduce early reactions. Patient temperature should not exceed 37.8°C (100°F) at the administration of each dose of ORTHOCLONE OKT3 (See TABLE I.)

Conventional concomitant immunosuppressive therapy should be lowered during ORTHOCLONE OKT3 (muromonab-CD3) administration to a daily dose of prednisone 0.5 mg/kg and azathioprine 25 mg. Retrospective analysis of open label studies suggest that cyclosporine should be discontinued at the start of ORTHOCLONE OKT3 therapy. Maintenance immunosuppression, including cyclosporine if indicated, should be resumed approximately three days prior to cessation of ORTHOCLONE OKT3 therapy.

ADMINISTRATION INSTRUCTIONS

1. Parenteral drug products should be inspected visually for particulate matter and discoloration prior to administration. Because ORTHOCLONE OKT3 is a protein solution, it may develop a few fine translucent particles which have been shown not to affect its potency.

TABLE I
Suggested Prevention And Treatment Of ORTHOCLONE OKT3 First Dose Effects

Adverse Reaction	Effective Prevention or Palliation	Supportive Treatment
1. Severe pulmonary edema	• Clear chest x-ray within 24 hrs. preinjection	• Prompt intubation and oxygenation
	• Weight restriction to ≤3% gain over 7 days pre-injection	• 24 hr. close observation
2. Fever, chills	• 1.0 mg/kg methylprednisolone sodium succinate preinjection	• Cooling blanket
	• Fever reduction below 37.8°C (100°F) preinjection	• Acetaminophen p.r.n.
3. Respiratory effects	• 100 mg hydrocortisone sodium succinate 30 min. post-injection	• Additional 100 mg hydrocortisone sodium succinate,p.r.n.

2. Prepare ORTHOCLONE OKT3 for injection by drawing solution into a syringe through a low protein-binding 0.2 or 0.22 micrometer (μm) filter. Discard filter and attach needle for IV bolus injection.
3. Administer ORTHOCLONE OKT3 as an IV bolus in less than one minute. Do not administer by intravenous infusion or in conjunction with other drug solutions.

HOW SUPPLIED

ORTHOCLONE OKT3 (muromonab-CD3) is supplied as a sterile solution in packages of 5 ampules (NDC 0062-7102-01). Each 5 ml ampule contains 5 mg of muromonab-CD3. **Storage:** Store in a refrigerator at 2 to 8°C (36 to 46°F). DO NOT FREEZE OR SHAKE.

REFERENCES

1. Kung, P.C., Goldstein, G., Reinherz, E.L. and Schlossman, S.F. (1979), "Monoclonal Antibodies Defining Distinctive Human T Cell Surface Antigens". *Science.* 206: 347–349.
2. ORTHO Multicenter Transplant Study Group (1985), "A Randomized Clinical Trial of OKT3 Monoclonal Antibody for Acute Rejection of Cadaveric Renal Transplants". *New England Journal of Medicine.* 313: 337–342.
3. Nomenclature Subcommittee, (1984), "Differentiation Human Leukocyte Antigens: A Proposed Nomenclature". *Immunology Today.* 5, No. 6.: 158–159.
4. Chatenoud, et al. (1990), "In Vivo Cell Activation Following OKT3 Administration". *Transplantation* 49: 697–702.

ORTHO BIOTECH DIVISION
ORTHO PHARMACEUTICAL CORPORATION
Raritan, New Jersey 08869, U.S.A.
©OPC 1986.   631-10-191-5
Revised March 1991

PROCRIT®   ℞
EPOETIN ALFA
PROCRIT registered trademark of distributor
For Injection

DESCRIPTION

Erythropoietin is a glycoprotein which stimulates red blood cell production. It is produced in the kidney and stimulates the division and differentiation of committed erythroid progenitors in the bone marrow. PROCRIT (Epoetin alfa), a 165 amino acid glycoprotein manufactured by recombinant DNA technology, has the same biological effects as endogenous erythropoietin.[1] It has a molecular weight of 30,400 daltons and is produced by mammalian cells into which the human erythropoietin gene has been introduced. The product contains the identical amino acid sequence of isolated natural erythropoietin.

PROCRIT is formulated as a sterile, colorless, preservative-free liquid for intravenous or subcutaneous administration. Each single-use vial contains 2,000, 3,000, 4,000, or 10,000 units of Epoetin alfa formulated in an isotonic sodium chloride/sodium citrate buffered solution (pH 6.9 ± 0.3) containing Albumin (Human) (2.5 mg), sodium citrate (5.8 mg), sodium chloride (5.8 mg), citric acid (0.06 mg) in Water for Injection, USP.

CLINICAL PHARMACOLOGY
Chronic Renal Failure Patients
Erythropoietin is a glycoprotein which stimulates red blood cell production. Endogenous production of erythropoietin is

Continued on next page

Ortho Biotech—Cont.

normally regulated by the level of tissue oxygenation. Hypoxia and anemia generally increase the production of erythropoietin, which in turn stimulates erythropoiesis.[2] In normal subjects, plasma erythropoietin levels range from 0.01 to 0.03 U/mL,[2,3] and increase up to 100- to 1000-fold during hypoxia or anemia.[2,3] In contrast, in patients with chronic renal failure (CRF), production of erythropoietin is impaired, and this erythropoietin deficiency is the primary cause of their anemia.[3,4]

Chronic renal failure is the clinical situation in which there is a progressive and usually irreversible decline in kidney function. Such patients may manifest the sequelae of renal dysfunction, including anemia, but do not necessarily require regular dialysis. Patients with end-stage renal disease (ESRD) are those patients with CRF who require regular dialysis or kidney transplantation for survival.

PROCRIT has been shown to stimulate erythropoiesis in anemic patients with CRF, including both patients on dialysis and those who do not require regular dialysis.[4-13] The first evidence of a response to the three times weekly (T.I.W.) administration of PROCRIT is an increase in the reticulocyte count within 10 days, followed by increases in the red cell count, hemoglobin, and hematocrit, usually within 2–6 weeks.[4,5] Because of the length of time required for erythropoiesis—several days for erythroid progenitors to mature and be released into the circulation—a clinically significant increase in hematocrit is usually not observed in less than 2 weeks and may require up to 6 weeks in some patients. Once the hematocrit reaches the target range (30–33%), that level can be sustained by PROCRIT therapy in the absence of iron deficiency and concurrent illnesses. The rate of hematocrit increase varies between patients and is dependent upon the dose of PROCRIT, within a therapeutic range of approximately 50–300 U/kg T.I.W.[4] a greater biologic response is not observed at doses exceeding 300 U/kg T.I.W.[6] Other factors affecting the rate and extent of response include availability of iron stores, the baseline hematocrit, and the presence of concurrent medical problems.

AZT-treated HIV-infected Patients
Responsiveness to PROCRIT in HIV-infected patients is dependent upon the endogenous serum erythropoietin level prior to treatment. Patients with endogenous serum erythropoietin levels ≤500 mU/mL and who are receiving a dose of AZT ≤4200 mg/week may respond to PROCRIT therapy. Patients with endogenous serum erythropoietin levels >500 mU/mL do not appear to respond to PROCRIT therapy. In a series of four clinical trials involving 255 patients, sixty to eighty percent of HIV-infected patients treated with Zidovudine (AZT) had endogenous serum erythropoietin levels ≤500 mU/mL.

Response to PROCRIT in AZT-treated HIV-infected patients is manifested by reduced transfusion requirements and increased hematocrit.

Pharmacokinetics
Intravenously administered PROCRIT (Epoetin alfa) is eliminated at a rate consistent with first order kinetics with a circulating half-life ranging from approximately 4 to 13 hours in patients with CRF. Within the therapeutic dose range, detectable levels of plasma erythropoietin are maintained for at least 24 hours.[7] After subcutaneous administration of PROCRIT to patients with CRF, peak serum levels are achieved within 5–24 hours after administration and decline slowly thereafter. There is no apparent difference in half-life between patients not on dialysis whose serum creatinine levels were greater than 3, and patients maintained on dialysis.

In normal volunteers, the half-life of intravenously administered PROCRIT is approximately 20% shorter than the half-life in CRF patients. The pharmacokinetics of PROCRIT have not been studied in HIV-infected patients.

INDICATIONS AND USAGE
Treatment of Anemia of Chronic Renal Failure Patients
PROCRIT is indicated in the treatment of anemia associated with chronic renal failure, including patients on dialysis (end-stage renal disease) and patients not on dialysis. PROCRIT is indicated to elevate or maintain the red blood cell level (as manifested by the hematocrit or hemoglobin determinations) and to decrease the need for transfusions in these patients.

PROCRIT is not intended for patients who require immediate correction of severe anemia. PROCRIT may obviate the need for maintenance transfusions but is not a substitute for emergency transfusion.

Prior to initiation of therapy, the patient's iron stores, including transferrin saturation and serum ferritin, should be evaluated. Transferrin saturation should be at least 20% and ferritin at least 100 ng/mL. Blood pressure should be adequately controlled prior to initiation of PROCRIT therapy, and must be closely monitored and controlled during therapy. Non-dialysis patients with symptomatic anemia considered for therapy should have a hematocrit less than 30%. All patients on PROCRIT therapy should be regu-

larly monitored (see "Laboratory Monitoring" and "Precautions").

PROCRIT should be administered under the guidance of a qualified physician (see "Dosage and Administration").

Treatment of Anemia in AZT-treated HIV-infected Patients
PROCRIT is indicated for the treatment of anemia related to therapy with Zidovudine (AZT) in HIV-infected patients. PROCRIT is indicated to elevate or maintain the red blood cell level (as manifested by the hematocrit or hemoglobin determinations) and to decrease the need for transfusions in these patients. PROCRIT is not indicated for the treatment of anemia in HIV-infected patients due to other factors such as iron or folate deficiencies, hemolysis or gastrointestinal bleeding which should be managed appropriately.

PROCRIT, at a dose of 100 U/kg three times per week, is effective in decreasing the transfusion requirement and increasing the red blood cell level of anemic, HIV-infected patients treated with AZT, when the endogenous serum erythropoietin level is ≤500 mU/mL and when patients are receiving a dose of AZT ≤4200 mg/week.

Clinical Experience: Response to PROCRIT
Chronic Renal Failure Patients
Response to PROCRIT was consistent across all studies. In the presence of adequate iron stores (see "Pre-Therapy Iron Evaluation"), the time to reach the target hematocrit is a function of the baseline hematocrit and the rate of hematocrit rise.

The rate of increase in hematocrit is dependent upon the dose of PROCRIT administered and individual patient variation. In clinical trials at starting doses of 50–150 U/kg T.I.W., patients responded with an average rate of hematocrit rise of:

HEMATOCRIT INCREASE

Starting Dose (T.I.W., IV)	Hematocrit Points/Day	Hematocrit Points/2 Weeks
50 U/kg	0.11	1.5
100 U/kg	0.18	2.5
150 U/kg	0.25	3.5

Over this dose range, approximately 95% of all patients respond with a clinically significant increase in hematocrit, and by the end of approximately two months of therapy virtually all patients were transfusion-independent. Once the target hematocrit was achieved, the maintenance dose was individualized for each patient.

Patients on Dialysis: Thirteen clinical studies were conducted, involving intravenous administration to a total of 1010 anemic patients on dialysis for 986 patient-years of PROCRIT (Epoetin alfa) therapy. In the three largest of these clinical trials, the median maintenance dose necessary to maintain the hematocrit between 30–36% was approximately 75 U/kg (T.I.W.). In the U.S. multicenter Phase III study, approximately 65% of the patients required doses of 100 U/kg T.I.W., or less, to maintain their hematocrit at approximately 35%. Almost 10% of patients required a dose of 25 U/kg, or less, and approximately 10% required a dose of more than 200 U/kg T.I.W. to maintain their hematocrit at this level.

Patients with CRF Not Requiring Dialysis: Four clinical trials were conducted in patients with CRF not on dialysis involving 181 PROCRIT-treated patients for approximately 67 patient-years of experience. These patients responded to PROCRIT therapy in a manner similar to that observed in patients on dialysis. Patients with CRF not on dialysis demonstrated a dose-dependent and sustained increase in hematocrit when PROCRIT was administered by either an intravenous (IV) or subcutaneous (SC) route, with similar rates of rise of hematocrit when PROCRIT was administered by either route. Moreover, PROCRIT doses of 75–150 U/kg per week have been shown to maintain hematocrits of 36–38% for up to six months.

Clinical Experience in AZT-treated HIV-infected Patients
PROCRIT has been studied in four placebo-controlled trials enrolling 297 anemic (hematocrit <30%) HIV-infected (AIDS) patients receiving concomitant therapy with Zidovudine (AZT), (all patients were treated with Epoetin alfa manufactured by Amgen Inc.). In the subgroup of patients (89/125 PROCRIT, and 88/130 placebo) with prestudy endogenous serum erythropoietin levels ≤500 mU/mL (normal endogenous serum erythropoietin levels are 4–26 mU/mL), PROCRIT reduced the mean cumulative number of units of blood transfused per patient by approximately 40%, as compared to the placebo group.[14] Among those patients who required transfusions at baseline, 43% of PROCRIT-treated patients versus 18% of placebo-treated patients were transfusion-independent during the second and third months of therapy. PROCRIT therapy also resulted in significant increases in hematocrit in comparison to placebo. When examining the results according to the weekly dose of AZT received during Month 3 of therapy, there was a statistically significant (p <0.003) reduction in transfusion requirements in PROCRIT-treated patients (N=51) compared to placebo-treated patients (N=54) whose mean weekly AZT dose was ≤4200 mg/week.[14] Approximately 17% of the patients with endogenous serum erythropoietin levels ≤500 mU/mL re-

ceiving PROCRIT in doses from 100–200 U/kg three times weekly (T.I.W.) achieved a hematocrit of 38% unrelated to transfusions or to a significant reduction in AZT dose. In the subgroup of patients whose prestudy endogenous serum erythropoietin levels were >500 mU/mL, PROCRIT therapy did not reduce transfusion requirements or increase hematocrit compared to the corresponding responses in placebo-treated patients.

Responsiveness to PROCRIT therapy may be blunted by intercurrent infectious/inflammatory episodes and by an increase in AZT dosage. Consequently, the dose of PROCRIT must be titrated based on these factors to maintain the desired erythropoietic response.

CONTRAINDICATIONS
PROCRIT is contraindicated in patients with:
1) Uncontrolled hypertension
2) Known hypersensitivity to mammalian cell-derived products
3) Known hypersensitivity to Albumin (Human).

WARNINGS
Chronic Renal Failure Patients
Hypertension: Patients with uncontrolled hypertension should not be treated with PROCRIT; blood pressure should be controlled adequately before initiation of therapy. Blood pressure may rise during PROCRIT therapy, often during the early phase of treatment when the hematocrit is increasing.

For patients who respond to PROCRIT with a rapid increase in hematocrit (e.g., more than 4 points in any two-week period), the dose of PROCRIT (Epoetin alfa) should be reduced because of the possible association of excessive rate of rise of hematocrit with an exacerbation of hypertension.

Seizures: Seizures have occurred in patients with CRF participating in PROCRIT clinical trials.

In patients on dialysis, there was a higher incidence of seizures during the first 90 days of therapy (occurring in approximately 2.5% of patients), as compared with later timepoints.

Given the potential for an increased risk of seizures during the first 90 days of therapy, blood pressure and the presence of premonitory neurologic symptoms should be monitored closely. Patients should be cautioned to avoid potentially hazardous activities such as driving or operating heavy machinery during this period.

Thrombotic Events: During hemodialysis, patients treated with PROCRIT may require increased anticoagulation with heparin to prevent clotting of the artificial kidney. Clotting of the vascular access (A-V shunt) has occurred at an annualized rate of about 0.25 events per patient-year on PROCRIT therapy.

Overall, for patients with CRF (whether on dialysis or not), other thrombotic events (e.g., myocardial infarction, cerebrovascular accident, transient ischemic attack) have occurred at an annualized rate of less than 0.04 events per patient-year of PROCRIT therapy. Patients with pre-existing vascular disease should be monitored closely.

AZT-treated HIV-infected Patients
In contrast to CFR patients, PROCRIT therapy has not been linked to exacerbation of hypertension, seizures, and thrombotic events in HIV-infected patients.

PRECAUTIONS
Chronic Renal Failure Patients and AZT-treated HIV-infected Patients
General: The parenteral administration of any biologic product should be attended by appropriate precautions in case allergic or other untoward reactions occur (see "Contraindications"). While transient rashes have occasionally been observed concurrently with PROCRIT therapy, no serious allergic or anaphylactic reactions have been reported.

The safety and efficacy of PROCRIT therapy have not been established in patients with a known history of a seizure disorder or underlying hematologic disease (e.g., sickle cell anemia, myelodysplastic syndromes, or hypercoagulable disorders).

In some female patients, menses have resumed following PROCRIT therapy; the possibility of potential pregnancy should be discussed and the need for contraception evaluated.

Hematology: Exacerbation of porphyria has been observed rarely in PROCRIT-treated patients with CRF. However, PROCRIT has not caused increased urinary excretion of prophyrin metabolites in normal volunteers, even in the presence of a rapid erythropoietic response. Nevertheless, PROCRIT should be used with caution in patients with known prophyria.

In pre-clinical studies in dogs and rats, but not in monkeys, PROCRIT therapy was associated with sub-clinical bone marrow fibrosis. Bone marrow fibrosis is a known complication of CRF in humans and may be related to secondary hyperparathyroidism or unknown factors. The incidence of bone marrow fibrosis was not increased in a study of patients on dialysis who were treated with PROCRIT for 12–19 months, compared to the incidence of bone marrow fibrosis

in a matched group of patients who had not been treated with PROCRIT.

Hematocrit in CRF patients should be measured twice a week; AZT-treated HIV-infected patients should have hematocrit measured once a week until hematocrit has been stabilized, and measured periodically thereafter.

Delayed or Diminished response: If the patient fails to respond or to maintain a response, the following etiologies should be considered and evaluated:

1) Iron deficiency: functional iron deficiency may develop with normal ferritin levels but low transferrin saturation (less than 20%), presumably due to the inability to mobilize iron stores rapidly enough to support increased erythropoiesis. Virtually all patients will eventually require supplemental iron therapy.

2) Underlying infectious, inflammatory, or malignant processes.

3) Occult blood loss.

4) Underlying hematologic diseases (i.e., thalassemia, refractory anemia, or other myelodysplastic disorders).

5) Vitamin deficiencies: folic acid or vitamin B_{12}.

6) Hemolysis.

7) Aluminum intoxication.

8) Osteitis fibrosa cystica.

Iron Evaluation: Prior to and during PROCRIT (Epoetin alfa) therapy, the patient's iron stores, including transferrin saturation (serum iron divided by iron binding capacity) and serum ferritin, should be evaluated. Transferrin saturation should be at least 20%, and ferritin should be at least 100 ng/mL. Supplemental iron may be required to increase and maintain transferrin saturation to levels that will adequately support PROCRIT-stimulated erythropoiesis.

Drug Interactions: No evidence of interaction of PROCRIT with other drugs was observed in the course of clinical trials.

Carcinogenesis, Mutagenesis, and Impairment of Fertility: Carcinogenic potential of PROCRIT has not been evaluated. PROCRIT does not induce bacterial gene mutation (Ames Test), chromosomal aberrations in mammalian cells, micronuclei in mice, or gene mutation at the HGPRT locus. In male and female rats treated intravenously with PROCRIT, there was a trend for slightly increased fetal wastage at doses of 100 and 500 U/kg.

Pregnancy Category C: PROCRIT has been shown to have adverse effects in rats when given in doses five times the human dose. There are no adequate and well-controlled studies in pregnant women. PROCRIT should be used during pregnancy only if potential benefit justifies the potential risk to the fetus.

In studies in female rats, there were decreases in body weight gain, delays in appearance of abdominal hair, delayed eyelid opening, delayed ossification, and decreases in the number of caudal vertebrae in the F1 fetuses of the 500 U/kg group. In female rats treated intravenously, there was a trend for slightly increased fetal wastage at doses of 100 and 500 U/kg. PROCRIT has not shown any adverse effect at doses as high as 500 U/kg in pregnant rabbits (from day 6 to 18 of gestation).

Nursing Mothers: Postnatal observations of the live offspring (F1 generation) of female rats treated with PROCRIT during gestation and lactation revealed no effect of PROCRIT at doses of up to 500 U/kg. There were, however, decreases in body weight gain, delays in appearance of abdominal hair, eyelid opening, and decreases in the number of caudal vertebrae in the F1 fetuses of the 500 U/kg group. There were no PROCRIT-related effects on the F2 generation fetuses.

It is not known whether PROCRIT is excreted in human milk. Because many drugs are excreted in human milk, caution should be exercised when PROCRIT is administered to a nursing woman.

Pediatric Use: The safety and effectiveness of PROCRIT in children have not been established.

Chronic Renal Failure Patients

Patients with CRF Not Requiring Dialysis: Blood pressure and hematocrit should be monitored no less frequently than for patients maintained on dialysis. Renal function and fluid and electrolyte balance should be closely monitored, as an improved sense of well-being may obscure the need to initiate dialysis in some patients.

Hematology: In order to avoid reaching the target hematocrit too rapidly, or exceeding the target range (hematocrit of 30–33%), the guidelines for dose and frequency of dose adjustments (see "Dosage and Administration") should be followed.

For patients who respond to PROCRIT with a rapid increase in hematocrit (e.g., more than 4 points in any two-week period), the dose of PROCRIT should be reduced because of the possible association of excessive rate of rise of hematocrit with an exacerbation of hypertension.

The elevated bleeding time characteristic of CRF decreases toward normal after correction of anemia in PROCRIT-treated patients. Reduction of bleeding time also occurs after correction of anemia by transfusion.

Sufficient time should be allowed to determine a patient's responsiveness to a dosage of PROCRIT before adjusting the dose. Because of the time required for erythropoiesis and the

red cell half-life, an interval of 2–6 weeks may occur between the time of a dose adjustment (initiation, increase, decrease, or discontinuation) and a significant change in hematocrit.

Laboratory Monitoring: The hematocrit should be determined twice a week until it has stabilized in the target range and the maintenance dose has been established. After any dose adjustment, the hematocrit should also be determined twice weekly for at least 2–6 weeks until it has been determined that the hematocrit has stabilized in response to the dose change. The hematocrit should then be monitored at regular intervals.

A complete blood count with differential and platelet count should be performed regularly. During clinical trials, modest increases were seen in platelets and white blood cell counts. While these changes were statistically significant, they were not clinically significant and the values remained within normal ranges.

In patients with CRF, serum chemistry values [including blood urea nitrogen (BUN), uric acid, creatinine, phosphorus, and potassium] should be monitored regularly. During clinical trials in patients on dialysis, modest increases were seen in BUN, creatinine, phosphorus, and potassium. In some patients with CRF not on dialysis, treated with PROCRIT (Epoetin alfa), modest increases in serum uric acid and phosphorus were observed. While changes were statistically significant, the values remained within the ranges normally seen in patients with CRF.

Hypertension: Patients with uncontrolled hypertension should not be treated with PROCRIT; blood pressure should be controlled adequately before initiation of therapy. Blood pressure may rise and episodes of hypertension may increase during PROCRIT therapy in all CRF patients, whether or not they require dialysis, often during the early phase of treatment when the hematocrit is increasing. To prevent hypertension and its sequelae, particular care needs to be taken in patients treated with PROCRIT to monitor and aggressively control blood pressure. During the period when hematocrit is increasing, approximately 25% of patients on dialysis may require initiation of, or increases in, antihypertensive therapy. Patients should be advised as to the importance of compliance with antihypertensive therapy and dietary restrictions. For patients who respond to PROCRIT with a rapid increase in hematocrit (e.g., more than 4 points in any two-week period), the dose of PROCRIT should be reduced because of the possible association of excessive rate of rise of hematocrit with an exacerbation of hypertension. If blood pressure is difficult to control, the dose of PROCRIT should be reduced; if clinically indicated, PROCRIT may be withheld until blood pressure control is re-established.

Seizures: Seizures have occurred in patients with CRF participating in PROCRIT clinical trials. In patients on dialysis, there was a higher incidence of seizures during the first 90 days of therapy (occurring in approximately 2.5% of patients), as compared with later timepoints.

Given the potential for an increased risk of seizures during the first 90 days of therapy, blood pressure and the presence of premonitory neurologic symptoms should be monitored closely. Patients should be cautioned to avoid potentially hazardous activities such as driving or operating heavy machinery during this period.

Thrombotic Events: During hemodialysis, patients treated with PROCRIT may require increased anticoagulation with heparin to prevent clotting of the artificial kidney. Clotting of the vascular access has occurred at an annualized rate of about 0.25 events per patient-year on PROCRIT therapy.

A relationship has not been established with statistical certainty between a rise in hematocrit and the rate of thrombotic events [including thrombosis of vascular access (A-V shunt)] in PROCRIT-treated patients. Overall, for patients with CRF (whether on dialysis or not), other thrombotic events (e.g., myocardial infarction, cerebrovascular accident, transient ischemic attack) have occurred at an annualized rate of less than 0.04 events per patient-year of PROCRIT therapy. Patients with pre-existing vascular disease should be monitored closely.

Diet: As the hematocrit increases and patients experience an improved sense of well-being and quality of life, the importance of compliance with dietary and dialysis prescriptions should be reinforced. In particular, hyperkalemia is not uncommon in patients with CRF. In U.S. studies in patients on dialysis, hyperkalemia has occurred at an annualized rate of approximately 0.11 episodes per patient-year of PROCRIT therapy, often in association with poor compliance to medication, dietary and/or dialysis prescriptions.

Dialysis Management: Therapy with PROCRIT (Epoetin alfa) results in an increase in hematocrit and a decrease in plasma volume which could affect dialysis efficiency. In studies to date, the resulting increase in hematocrit did not appear to adversely affect dialyzer function[9,10] or the efficiency of high flux hemodialysis.[11] During hemodialysis, patients treated with PROCRIT may require increased anticoagulation with heparin to prevent clotting of the artificial kidney. Patients who are marginally dialyzed may require adjustments in their dialysis prescription. As with all patients on dialysis, the serum chemistry values [including blood urea nitrogen (BUN), creatinine, phosphorus, and potassium] in

PROCRIT-treated patients should be monitored regularly to assure the adequacy of the dialysis prescription.

Renal Function: In patients with CRF not on dialysis, renal function and fluid and electrolyte balance should be closely monitored, as an improved sense of well-being may obscure the need to initiate dialysis in some patients. In patients with CRF not on dialysis, placebo-controlled studies of progression of renal dysfunction over periods of greater than one year have not been completed. In shorter-term trials in patients with CRF not on dialysis, changes in creatinine and creatinine clearance were not significantly different in PROCRIT-treated patients, compared with placebo-treated patients. Analysis of the slope of 1/serum creatinine vs. time plots in these patients indicates no significant change in the slope after the initiation of PROCRIT therapy.

AZT-treated HIV-infected Patients

Hypertension: Exacerbation of hypertension has not been observed in AZT-treated HIV-infected patients treated with PROCRIT. However, PROCRIT should be withheld in these patients if pre-existing hypertension is uncontrolled, and should not be started until blood pressure is controlled. In double-blind studies, a single seizure has been experienced by a PROCRIT-treated patient.[14]

ADVERSE REACTIONS

Chronic Renal Failure Patients

Studies analyzed to date indicate that PROCRIT is generally well-tolerated. The adverse events reported are frequent sequelae of CRF and are not necessarily attributable to PROCRIT therapy. In double-blind, placebo-controlled studies involving over 300 patients with CRF, the events reported in greater than 5% of PROCRIT-treated patients during the blinded phase were:

Event	Percent of Patients Reporting Event	
	PROCRIT-Treated Patients (n=200)	Placebo-Treated Patients (n=135)
Hypertension	24%	19%
Headache	16%	12%
Arthralgias	11%	6%
Nausea	11%	9%
Edema	9%	10%
Fatigue	9%	14%
Diarrhea	9%	6%
Vomiting	8%	5%
Chest Pain	7%	9%
Skin Reaction (Administration Site)	7%	12%
Asthenia	7%	12%
Dizziness	7%	13%
Clotted Access	7%	2%

Significant adverse events of concern in patients with CRF treated in double-blinded, placebo-controlled trials occurred in the following percent of patients during the blinded phase of the studies:

Seizure	1.1%	1.1%
CVA/TIA	0.4%	0.6%
MI	0.4%	1.1%
Death	0	1.7%

In the U.S. PROCRIT studies in patients on dialysis (over 567 patients) the incidence (number of events per patient-year) of the most frequently reported adverse events were: hypertension (0.75), headache (0.40), tachycardia (0.31), nausea/vomiting (0.26), clotted vascular access (0.25), shortness of breath (0.14), hyperkalemia (0.11), and diarrhea (0.11). Other reported events occurred at a rate of less than 0.10 events per patient per year.

Events reported to have occurred within several hours of administration of PROCRIT were rare, mild and transient, and included flu-like symptoms such as arthralgias and myalgias.

In all studies analyzed to date, PROCRIT administration was generally well tolerated, irrespective of the route of administration.

Allergic Reactions: There have been no reports of serious allergic reactions or anaphylaxis associated with PROCRIT (Epoetin alfa) administration. Skin rashes and urticaria have been observed rarely and when reported have been mild and transient in nature. There has been no evidence for development of antibodies to erythropoietin in patients tested to date, including those receiving intravenous PROCRIT for over two years. Nevertheless, if an anaphylactoid reaction occurs, PROCRIT should be immediately discontinued and appropriate therapy initiated.

Seizures: The relationship, if any, of PROCRIT therapy to seizures is uncertain. The baseline incidence of seizures in the untreated dialysis population is difficult to determine; it appears to be in the range of 5–10% per patient-year.[15–17] There have been 47 seizures in 1010 patients on dialysis treated with PROCRIT with an exposure of 986 patient-years

Continued on next page

Ortho Biotech—Cont.

for a rate of approximately 0.048 events per patient-year. However, there appeared to be a higher rate of seizures during the first 90 days of therapy (occurring in approximately 2.5% of patients), when compared to subsequent 90-day time periods. While the relationship between seizures and the rate of rise of hematocrit is uncertain, it is recommended that the dose of PROCRIT be decreased if the hematocrit increase exceeds 4 points in any two-week period.

Hypertension: Up to 80% of patients with CRF have a history of hypertension.[18] Blood pressure may rise during PROCRIT therapy in CRF patients whether or not maintained on dialysis; during the early phase of treatment when hematocrit is increasing, approximately 25% of patients on dialysis may require initiation or increases in antihypertensive therapy. Hypertensive encephalopathy and seizures have been observed in patients with CRF treated with PROCRIT. Increases in blood pressure may be associated with the rate of increase in hematocrit. It is recommended that the dose of PROCRIT be decreased if the hematocrit increase exceeds 4 points in any two-week period.

Increases in blood pressure have been reported in clinical trials, often during the first 90 days of therapy. When data from all patients in the U.S. Phase III multi-center trial were analyzed, there was an apparent trend of more reports of hypertensive adverse events in patients on dialysis with a faster rate of rise of hematocrit (greater than 4 hematocrit points in any two week period). However, in a double-blind, placebo-controlled trial, hypertensive adverse events were not reported at an increased rate in the PROCRIT-treated group (150 U/kg T.I.W.) relative to the placebo group. There do not appear to be any direct pressor effects of PROCRIT. Special care should be taken to closely monitor and control blood pressure in PROCRIT-treated patients.

Thrombotic Events: During hemodialysis, patients treated with PROCRIT may require increased anticoagulation with heparin to prevent clotting of the artificial kidney. Clotting of the vascular access has occurred at an annualized rate of about 0.25 events per patient-year on PROCRIT therapy.

A relationship has not been established with statistical certainty between a rise in hematocrit and the rate of thrombotic events [including thrombosis of vascular access (A-V shunt)] in PROCRIT-treated patients. Overall, for patients with CRF (whether on dialysis or not), other thrombotic events (e.g., myocardial infarction, cerebrovascular accident, transient ischemic attack) have occurred at an annualized rate of less than 0.04 events per patient-year of PROCRIT therapy. Patients with pre-existing vascular disease should be monitored closely.

AZT-treated HIV-infected Patients

Adverse experiences reported in clinical trials with PROCRIT in AZT-treated HIV-infected patients were consistent with the progression of HIV infection. In double-blind, placebo-controlled studies of 3-months duration involving approximately 300 AZT-treated HIV-infected patients, adverse events with an incidence of ≥ 10% in either PROCRIT-treated patients or placebo-treated patients were:

Event	Percent of Patients Reporting Event: PROCRIT-Treated Patients (n=144)	Placebo-Treated Patients (n=153)
Pyrexia	38%	29%
Fatigue	25%	31%
Headache	19%	14%
Cough	18%	14%
Diarrhea	16%	18%
Rash	16%	8%
Congestion, Respiratory	15%	10%
Nausea	15%	12%
Shortness of Breath	14%	13%
Asthenia	11%	14%
Skin Reaction, Medication Site	10%	7%
Dizziness	9%	10%

There were no statistically significant differences between treatment groups in the incidence of the above events.

In the 297 patients studied, PROCRIT (Epoetin alfa) was not associated with significant increases in opportunistic infections or mortality.[14] In 71 patients from this group treated with PROCRIT at 150 U/kg T.I.W., serum p24 antigen levels did not appear to increase.[14] Preliminary data showed no enhancement of HIV replication in infected cell lines *in vitro*.[14]

Peripheral white blood cell and platelet counts are unchanged following PROCRIT therapy.

Allergic Reactions: Two AZT-treated HIV-infected patients had urticarial reactions within 48 hours of their first exposure to study medication. One patient was treated with PROCRIT and one was treated with placebo (PROCRIT vehicle alone). Both patients had positive immediate skin tests against their study medication with a negative saline control. The basis for this apparent pre-existing hypersensitivity to components of the PROCRIT formulation is unknown, but may be related to HIV-induced immunosuppression or prior exposure to blood products.

Seizures: In double-blind and open label trials of PROCRIT in HIV-infected AZT-treated patients, 10 patients have experienced seizures.[14] In general, these seizures appear to be related to underlying pathology such as meningitis or cerebral neoplasms, not PROCRIT therapy.

OVERDOSAGE

The maximum amount of PROCRIT that can be safely administered in single or multiple doses has not been determined. Doses of up to 1500 U/kg T.I.W. for three to four weeks have been administered without any direct toxic effects of PROCRIT itself.[6]

Therapy with PROCRIT can result in polycythemia if the hematocrit is not carefully monitored and the dose appropriately adjusted. If the target range is exceeded, PROCRIT may be temporarily withheld until the hematocrit returns to the target range; PROCRIT therapy may then be resumed using a lower dose (see "Dosage and Administration"). If polycythemia is of concern, phlebotomy may be indicated to decrease the hematocrit.

DOSAGE AND ADMINISTRATION

Chronic Renal Failure Patients

Starting doses of PROCRIT over the range of 50–100 U/kg three times weekly (T.I.W.) have been shown to be safe and effective in increasing hematocrit and eliminating transfusion dependency in patients with CRF (see "Clinical Experience"). The dose of PROCRIT should be reduced when the hematocrit reaches the target range of 30–33% or increases by more than 4 points in any two-week period. The dosage of PROCRIT must be individualized to maintain the hematocrit within the target range. Dose changes should generally be in the range of 25 U/kg, T.I.W. The table below provides general therapeutic guidelines.

[See table at bottom of page.]

Starting Dose	Reduce Dose When:	Increase Dose If:	Maintenance Dose	Target Hct. Range
50–100 U/kg T.I.W.; IV: Dialysis Patients IV or SC: Non-dialysis CRF patients	1) Target range is reached or 2) Hct. increases >4 points in any 2-week period	Hct. does not increased by 5–6 points after 8 weeks of therapy, and hct. is below target range.	Individually titrate	30–33% (max: 36%)

In patients on dialysis, PROCRIT usually has been administered as an IV bolus T.I.W. While the administration of PROCRIT is independent of the dialysis procedure, PROCRIT may be administered into the venous line at the end of the dialysis procedure to obviate the need for additional venous access. In patients with CRF not on dialysis, PROCRIT may be given either as an intravenous or subcutaneous injection.

During therapy, hematological parameters should be monitored regularly (see "Laboratory Monitoring").

Pre-Therapy Iron Evaluation: Prior to and during PROCRIT (Epoetin alfa) therapy, the patient's iron stores, including transferrin saturation (serum iron divided by iron binding capacity) and serum ferritin, should be evaluated. Transferrin saturation should be at least 20%, and ferritin should be at least 100 ng/mL. Supplemental iron may be required to increase and maintain transferrin saturation to levels that will adequately support PROCRIT-stimulated erythropoiesis.

Dose Adjustment:

- When the hematocrit reaches 30–33%, the dosage should be decreased by approximately 25 U/kg T.I.W., to avoid exceeding the target range. Once the hematocrit is within the target range, the maintenance dose must be individualized for each patient (see "Maintenance Dose").
- At any time, if the hematocrit increases by more than 4 points in a two-week period, the dose should be immediately decreased. After the dose reduction, the hematocrit should be monitored twice weekly for 2–6 weeks, and further dose adjustments should be made as outlined in "Maintenance Dose".
- As the hematocrit approaches, or if it exceeds 36%, PROCRIT should be temporarily withheld until the hematocrit decreases to the target range of 30–33%; the dose should be reduced by approximately 25 U/kg T.I.W. upon re-initiation of therapy.
- If a hematocrit increase of 5–6 points is not achieved after an eight-week period and iron stores are adequate (see "Delayed or Diminished Response"), the dose of PROCRIT may be increased in increments of 25 U/kg T.I.W. Further increases of 25 U/kg T.I.W. may be made at 4–6 week intervals until the desired response is attained.

Maintenance Dose: The maintenance dose must be individualized for each patient. As the hematocrit approaches, or if it exceeds 36%, PROCRIT should be temporarily withheld until the hematocrit is 33% or less. Upon re-initiation of therapy, the dose should be reduced by approximately 25 U/kg T.I.W., or doses omitted, and an appropriate time interval (i.e., 2–6 weeks) allowed for stabilization of response.

If the hematocrit remains below, or falls below the target range, iron stores should be re-evaluated. If the transferrin saturation is less than 20%, supplemental iron should be administered. If the transferrin saturation is greater than 20%, the dose of PROCRIT may be increased by 25 U/kg T.I.W. Such dose increases should not be made more frequently than once a month, unless clinically indicated, as the response time of the hematocrit to a dose increase can be 2–6 weeks. Hematocrit should be measured twice weekly for 2–6 weeks following dose increases.

In the U.S. Phase III multicenter trial in patients on hemodialysis, the median maintenance dose was 75 U/kg T.I.W., with approximately 65% of the patients requiring doses of 100 U/kg T.I.W., or less, to maintain their hematocrit within the range of 32–38% (maintenance doses ranged from 12.5 to 525 U/kg T.I.W.). Almost 10% of the patients required a dose of 25 U/kg, or less, and approximately 10% of the patients required more than 200 U/kg T.I.W. to maintain their hematocrit in this range.

In patients with CRF not on dialysis, the maintenance dose must also be individualized. PROCRIT doses of 75–150 U/kg per week have been shown to maintain hematocrits of 36–38% for up to six months.

Delayed or Diminished Response: Over 95% of patients with CRF responded with clinically significant increases in hematocrit, and virtually all patients were transfusion-independent within approximately two months of initiation of PROCRIT therapy.

If a patient fails to respond or maintain a response, other etiologies should be considered and evaluated as clinically indicated. See "Precautions" section for discussion of delayed or diminished response.

AZT-treated HIV-infected Patients

Prior to beginning PROCRIT, it is recommended that the endogenous serum erythropoietin level be determined (prior to transfusion). Available evidence suggests that patients receiving AZT with endogenous serum erythropoietin levels >500 mU/mL are unlikely to respond to therapy with PROCRIT.

Starting Dose: For patients with serum erythropoietin levels ≤ 500 mU/mL who are receiving a dose of AZT ≤ 4200 mg/week, the recommended starting dose of PROCRIT is 100 U/kg as an intravenous or subcutaneous injection three times weekly (T.I.W.) for 8 weeks.

Increase Dose: During the dose adjustment phase of therapy, the hematocrit should be monitored weekly. If the response is not satisfactory in terms of reducing transfusions requirements or increasing hematocrit after 8 weeks of therapy, the dose of PROCRIT (Epoetin alfa) can be increased by 50–100 U/kg T.I.W. Response should be evaluated every 4–8 weeks thereafter and the dose adjusted accordingly by 50–100 U/kg increments T.I.W. If patients have not responded satisfactorily to a PROCRIT dose of 300 U/kg T.I.W., it is unlikely that they will respond to higher doses of PROCRIT.

Maintenance Dose: After attainment of the desired response (i.e., reduced transfusion requirements or increased hematocrit), the dose of PROCRIT should be titrated to maintain the response based on factors such as variations in AZT dose and the presence of intercurrent infectious or inflammatory episodes. If the hematocrit exceeds 40%, the dose should be discontinued until the hematocrit drops to 36%. The dose should be reduced by 25% when treatment is resumed and then titrated to maintain the desired hematocrit.

PREPARATION AND ADMINISTRATION OF PROCRIT

1. DO NOT SHAKE. Shaking may denature the glycoprotein, rendering it biologically inactive.
2. Parenteral drug products should be inspected visually for particulate matter and discoloration prior to administration. Do not use any vials exhibiting particulate matter or discoloration.
3. Using aseptic techniques, attach a sterile needle to a sterile syringe. Remove the flip top from the vial containing PROCRIT, and wipe the septum with a disinfectant. Insert the needle into the vial, and withdraw into the syringe an appropriate volume of solution.

4. Use only one dose per vial; do not re-enter the vial. Discard unused portions. Contains no preservative.
5. Do not administer in conjunction with other drug solutions.

HOW SUPPLIED

PROCRIT is available in vials containing 2,000 (NDC 0062-7402-01), 3,000 (NDC 0062-7405-01), 4,000 (NDC 0062-7400-03) or 10,000 (NDC 0062-7401-03) units of Epoetin alfa in 1.0 mL of a sterile, preservative-free solution. Each dosage form is supplied in boxes containing 6 single-use vials.

STORAGE

Store at 2° to 8°C (36° to 46°F). Do not freeze or shake.

REFERENCES

1. Egrie JC, Strickland TW, Lane J, Et Al., (1986). "Characterization and Biological Effects of Recombinant Human Erythropoietin." Immunobiol. 72: 213–224.
2. Graber SE, and Krantz SB, (1978). "Erythropoietin and the Control of Red Cell Production." Ann. Rev. Med. 29: 51–66.
3. Eschbach JW, and Adamson JW, (1985). "Anemia of End-Stage Renal Disease (ESRD)." Kidney Intl. 28: 1–5.
4. Eschbach JW, Egrie JC, Downing MR, Browne JK, and Adamson JW, (1987). "Correction of the Anemia of End-Stage Renal Disease with Recombinant Human Erythropoietin." NEJM 316: 73–78.
5. Eschbach JW, Adamson JW, and Cooperative Multicenter r-HuEPO Trial Group, (1988). "Correction of the Anemia of Hemodialysis (HD) Patients with Recombinant Human Erythropoietin (r-HuEPO): Results of a Multicenter Study." Kidney Intl. 33: 189.
6. Eschbach JW, Egrie JC, Downing MR, Browne JK, Adamson JW, (1989). "The use of Recombinant Human Erythropoietin (r-HuEPO): Effect in End-Stage Renal Disease (ESRD)." Prevention of Chronic Uremia (Friedman, Beyer, DeSanto, Giordano, eds.), Field and Wood Inc., Philadelphia, PA, pp 148–155.
7. Egrie JC, Eschbach JW, McGuire T, and Adamson JW, (1988). "Pharmacokinetics of Recombinant Human Erythropoietin (r-HuEPO) Administered to Hemodialysis (HD) Patients." Kidney Intl. 33: 262.
8. Lundin AP, Delano BG, Stein R, Quinn RM, and Friedman EA, (1988). "Recombinant Human Erythropoietin (r-HuEPO) Treatment Enhances Exercise Tolerance in Hemodialysis Patients." Kidney Intl. 33: 200.
9. Paganini E, Garcia J, Ellis P, Bodnar D, and Magnussen M, (1988). "Clinical Sequelae of Correction of Anemia with Recombinant Human Erythropoietin (r-HuEPO); Urea Kinetics, Dialyzer Function and Reuse." Am. J. Kid. Dis. 11: 16.
10. Delano BG, Lundin AP, Golansky R, Quinn RM, Rao TKS, and Friedman EA, (1988). "Dialyzer Urea and Creatinine Clearances Not Significantly Changed in r-HuEPO Treated Maintenance Hemodialysis (MD) Patients." Kidney Intl. 33: 219.
11. Stivelman J, Van Wyck D, and Ogden D, (1988). "Use of Recombinant Erythropoietin (r-HuEPO) with High Flux Dialysis (HFD) Does Not Worsen Azotemia or Shorten Access Survival." Kidney Intl. 33: 239.
12. Lim VS, DeGowin RL, Zavala D, Kirchner PT, Abels R, Perry P, and Fangman J, (1989). "Recombinant Human Erythropoietin Treatment in Pre-Dialysis Patients: A Double-Blind Placebo-Controlled Trial." Ann. Int. Med. 110: 108–114.
13. Stone WJ, Graber SE, Krantz SB, Et Al., (1988). "Treatment of the Anemia of Pre-Dialysis Patients with Recombinant Human Erythropoietin: A Randomized, Placebo-Controlled Trial." Am. J. Med. Sci. 296: 171–179.
14. Data on file, Ortho Biologics, Inc.
15. Raskin NH, and Fishman RA, (1976). "Neurologic Disorders in Renal Failure (First of Two Parts)." NEJM 294: 143–148.
16. Raskin NH, and Fishman RA, (1976). "Neurologic Disorders in Renal Failure (Second of Two Parts)." NEJM 294: 204–210.
17. Messing RO, and Simon RP, (1986). "Seizures as a Manifestation of Systemic Disease." Neurologic Clinics 4: 563–584.
18. Kerr DN, (1979). "Chronic Renal Failure." Cecil Textbook of Medicine, (Beeson PB, McDermott W, Wyngaarden JB, eds.), W.B. Saunders, Philadelphia, PA, pp 1351–1367.

Manufactured by:
Amgen Inc.
Amgen Center
Thousand Oaks, California 91320-1789
Distributed by:
Ortho Biotech Division
Ortho Pharmaceutical Corporation
Raritan, New Jersey 08869-0602

© OPC 1990 638-29-979-1

ISSUED DECEMBER 1990 7400G020

Shown in Product Identification Section, page 421

Ortho Diagnostic Systems Inc.
ROUTE 202
RARITAN, NEW JERSEY 08869

MICRhoGAM™ ℞

[mike'ro-gam]
Rh_o (D) Immune Globulin (Human)
For Intramuscular Injection Only

Micro-Dose for use *only* after spontaneous or induced abortion or termination of ectopic pregnancy up to and including 12 weeks' gestation.

DESCRIPTION

MICRhoGAM Rh_o(D) Immune Globulin (Human) is a sterile solution containing IgG anti-Rh_o(D) for use in preventing Rh immunization in Rh negative individuals exposed to Rh positive red blood cells. A single dose of MICRhoGAM contains sufficient anti-Rh_o(D) (approximately 50 μg)† to suppress the immune response to 2.5 mL (or less) of Rh positive red blood cells.

All donors are carefully screened to eliminate those in high risk groups for disease transmission. Fractionation of the plasma is done by a modification of the cold alcohol procedure. Glycine (15 mg/mL) is included in the final product as a stabilizer. The final product contains 5% ± 1% globulin, 2.9 mg/mL sodium chloride, 0.01% polysorbate 80 and 0.003% thimerosal (mercury derivative).

This product is for intramuscular injection only.

CLINICAL PHARMACOLOGY

Human immune globulins prepared by cold alcohol fractionation have not been reported to transmit hepatitis or other infectious diseases.

MICRhoGAM acts by suppressing the immune response of Rh negative women to Rh positive red blood cells. The risk of immunization is related to the number of Rh positive red cells received. The risk was found to be 3% when 0.1 mL of fetal red blood cells is present in the mother and 65% when 5 mL is present. In the first 12 weeks of gestation the total volume of red blood cells in the fetus is estimated at less than 2.5 mL.

Clinical studies demonstrated that administration of MICRhoGAM within three (3) hours following abortion was 100% effective in preventing Rh immunization. Studies in male volunteers showed MICRhoGAM to be effective when given as long as 72 hours after the infusion of Rh positive red cells. A lesser degree of protection is afforded if the antibody is administered beyond this time period.

INDICATIONS AND USAGE

MICRhoGAM is indicated for an Rh negative woman following spontaneous or induced abortion or termination of ectopic pregnancy up to and including 12 weeks' gestation, unless the father is conclusively shown to be Rh negative.

CONTRAINDICATIONS

MICRhoGAM must not be used for genetic amniocentesis at 15 to 18 weeks' gestation or antepartum prophylaxis at 28 weeks' gestation. RhoGAM™ Rh_o(D) Immune Globulin (Human) is recommended for any indication beyond 12 weeks' gestation.

Individuals known to have had an anaphylactic or severe systemic reaction to human globulin should not receive MICRhoGAM or any other Rh_o(D) Immune Globulin (Human).

WARNINGS

Do not inject intravenously.

PRECAUTIONS

Pregnancy Category C—Animal reproduction studies have not been conducted with MICRhoGAM. It is also not known whether Rh_o(D) Immune Globulin (Human) can cause fetal harm when administered to a pregnant woman or can affect reproduction capacity. Rh_o(D) Immune Globulin (Human) should be given to a pregnant woman only if clearly needed.

ADVERSE REACTIONS

Systemic reactions associated with administration of MICRhoGAM are extremely rare. Discomfort at the site of injection has been reported and a small number of women have noted a slight elevation in temperature.

† A full dose of Rh_o(D) Immune Globulin (Human) has traditionally been referred to as a "300 μg" dose and this usage is employed here for convenience in terminology. *It should not be construed as the actual anti-D content.* Each full dose of Rh_o(D) Immune Globulin (Human) must contain at least as much anti-D as 1 milliliter of the U.S. Reference Rh_o(D) Immune Globulin (Human). Studies performed at the Food and Drug Administration have shown that the U.S. Reference contains 820 international units (IU) of anti-D per milliliter. When the conversion factor determined for the International (WHO) Reference Preparation is used, 820 IU per milliliter is equivalent to 164 μg per milliliter of anti-D. MICRhoGAM contains approximately one-sixth the amount of anti-D contained in the full dose.

DOSAGE AND ADMINISTRATION

Parenteral drug products should be inspected visually for particulate matter and discoloration prior to administration, whenever solution and container permit.

A single dose (approximately 50 μg)† of MICRhoGAM will completely suppress the immune response to 2.5 mL of Rh positive red blood cells (packed cells, not whole blood).

Administer a single dose of MICRhoGAM intramuscularly as soon as possible after termination of a pregnancy up to and including 12 weeks' gestation. At or beyond 13 weeks' gestation it is recommended that a single dose of RhoGAM Rh_o(D) Immune Globulin (Human) (approximately 300 μg)† be given instead of MICRhoGAM.

Since there is no lot number and expiration date on the prefilled syringes, they should not be removed from the protective pouch until immediately before use.

HOW SUPPLIED

—5 prefilled single-dose syringes of MICRhoGAM (Product code 780800) NDC 0562-8080-80
—package insert
—5 control forms
—5 patient identification cards

and

—25 prefilled single-dose syringes of MICRhoGAM (Product code 780820) NDC 0562-8080-82
—package insert
—25 control forms
—25 patient identification cards

STORAGE

Store at 2 to 8°C. DO NOT FREEZE.

† See footnote under Description.

RhoGAM™ ℞

[ro'gam]
Rh_o (D) Immune Globulin (Human)
For Intramuscular Injection Only

DESCRIPTION

RhoGAM Rh_o(D) Immune Globulin (Human) is a sterile solution containing IgG anti-Rh_o(D) for use in preventing Rh immunization. Each single dose of RhoGAM contains sufficient anti-Rh_o(D) (approximately 300 μg)† to suppress the immune response to 15 mL (or less) of Rh positive red blood cells.

All donors are carefully screened to eliminate those in high risk groups for disease transmission. Fractionation of the plasma is done by a modification of the cold alcohol procedure. The final product contains 5% ± 1% globulin, 2.9 mg/mL sodium chloride, 0.01% polysorbate 80 and 0.003% thimerosal (mercury derivative), with glycine (15 mg/mL) as a stabilizer.

This product is for intramuscular injection only.

CLINICAL PHARMACOLOGY

Human immune globulins prepared by cold alcohol fractionation have not been reported to transmit hepatitis or other infectious diseases.

RhoGAM acts by suppressing the immune response of Rh negative individuals to Rh positive red blood cells.

The obstetrical patient may be exposed to red blood cells from her Rh positive fetus during the normal course of pregnancy. Clinical studies proved that the incidence of Rh immunization as a result of pregnancy was reduced to 1% to 2% from 12% to 13% when RhoGAM was given within 72 hours following delivery. Further studies in which patients received Rh immune globulin, antepartum at 28 to 32 weeks and postpartum, reduced the risk of immunization to less than 0.1%.

An Rh negative individual transfused with one unit of Rh positive red blood cells has about an 80% likelihood of producing anti-Rh_o(D). Protection from Rh immunization is accomplished by administering the appropriate dose of RhoGAM.

INDICATIONS AND USAGE

Pregnancy and Other Obstetric Conditions

RhoGAM is indicated whenever it is known or suspected that fetal red cells have entered the circulation of an Rh negative

† A full dose of Rh_o(D) Immune Globulin (Human) has traditionally been referred to as a "300 μg" dose and this usage is employed here for convenience in terminology. *It should not be construed as the actual anti-D content.* Each full dose of Rh_o(D) Immune Globulin (Human) must contain at least as much anti-D as 1 milliliter of the U.S. Reference Rh_o(D) Immune Globulin (Human). Studies performed at the Food and Drug Administration have shown that the U.S. Reference contains 820 international units (IU) of anti-D per milliliter. When the conversion factor determined for the International (WHO) Reference Preparation is used, 820 IU per milliliter is equivalent to 164 μg per milliliter of anti-D.

Continued on next page

Ortho Diagnostic—Cont.

mother unless the fetus or the father can be shown conclusively to be Rh negative.

Transfusion

RhoGAM is indicated for any Rh negative female of childbearing age who receives any Rh positive red blood cells or component such as platelets or granulocytes prepared from Rh positive blood.

CONTRAINDICATIONS

Individuals known to have had an anaphylactic or severe systemic reaction to human globulin should not receive RhoGAM or any other $Rh_o(D)$ Immune Globulin (Human).

WARNINGS

Do not inject intravenously.
Do not inject infant.

PRECAUTIONS

The presence of passively acquired anti-$Rh_o(D)$ in the maternal serum may cause a positive antibody screening test. This does not preclude further antepartum or postpartum prophylaxis.

Some babies born of women given $Rh_o(D)$ Immune Globulin (Human) antepartum have weakly positive direct antiglobulin tests at birth.

Late in pregnancy or following delivery there may be sufficient fetal red blood cells in the maternal circulation to cause a positive result if one tests for the $Rh_o(D)$ variant known as D^u. When there is any doubt as to the patient's Rh type, RhoGAM should be administered.

Pregnancy Category C

Animal reproduction studies have not been conducted with RhoGAM. It is also not known whether $Rh_o(D)$ Immune Globulin (Human) can cause fetal harm when administered to a pregnant woman or can affect reproduction capacity. $Rh_o(D)$ Immune Globulin (Human) should be given to a pregnant woman only if clearly needed. However, use of Rh antibody during the third trimester in full doses of antibody has been reported to produce no evidence of hemolysis in the infant.

ADVERSE REACTIONS

Systemic reactions associated with administration of RhoGAM are extremely rare. Discomfort at the site of injection has been reported and a small number of women have noted a slight elevation in temperature.

About one-quarter of a group of 22 individuals who were given multiple doses of RhoGAM to treat mismatched transfusions noted fever, myalgia and lethargy. Bilirubin levels of 0.4 to 6.8 mg/dL were observed in some of the treated individuals and one had splenomegaly.

DOSAGE AND ADMINISTRATION

Parenteral drug products should be inspected visually for particulate matter and discoloration prior to administration, whenever solution and container permit.

A single dose (approximately 300 µg)† is contained in each prefilled syringe of RhoGAM. This is the usual dose for the indications associated with pregnancy unless there is clinical or laboratory evidence of a fetal-maternal hemorrhage in excess of 15 mL of Rh positive red blood cells. The indications and recommended dosage for RhoGAM are summarized in the following table.

Indications and Recommended Dosage

Indication	Dose (approximately)
Threatened abortion at any stage of gestation with continuation of pregnancy	300 µg†
Abortion or termination of pregnancy at or beyond 13 weeks' gestation**	300 µg
Genetic amniocentesis, chorionic villus sampling (CVS) and percutaneous umbilical blood sampling (PUBS)	300 µg
Abdominal trauma	300 µg
Antepartum prophylaxis at 26 to 28 weeks' gestation††	300 µg
Postpartum (if newborn Rh positive)	300 µg

†See footnote under Description

**If abortion or termination of pregnancy occurs up to and including 12 weeks' gestation, a single dose of MICRhoGAM™ $Rh_o(D)$ Immune Globulin (Human) (approximately 50 µg)† may be used instead of RhoGAM.

††If antepartum prophylaxis is indicated, it is essential that the mother receive a postpartum dose if the infant is Rh positive.

If an adverse event requires the administration of RhoGAM early in the pregnancy, there is an obligation to maintain a level of passively acquired anti-$Rh_o(D)$ by administration of RhoGAM at 12-week intervals. RhoGAM should be given within 72 hours after delivery if the baby is Rh positive. If delivery occurs within three weeks after the last antepartum dose, the postpartum dose may be withheld, but a test for fetal-maternal hemorrhage (FMH) should still be performed

to determine a bleed greater than 15 mL of packed red blood cells.

Whenever there is a fetal-maternal hemorrhage in excess of 15 mL of Rh positive red blood cells, multiple doses of RhoGAM are required. A fetal-maternal hemorrhage of this magnitude is unlikely prior to the last trimester of pregnancy. Patients who may need multiple doses of RhoGAM can be identified by a fetal-maternal hemorrhage screening test. If the test is positive, the volume of the fetal-maternal hemorrhage should be determined by a quantitative method. A single dose of RhoGAM should be administered for every 15 mL of fetal red blood cells. If the dose calculation results in a fraction, administer the next number of whole syringes of RhoGAM.

Multiple doses of RhoGAM are usual for indications associated with transfusion. For every 15 mL of Rh positive red blood cells transfused, the patient should receive a single dose of RhoGAM. If multiple doses are required, consult your pharmacy for pooling directions.

Administer RhoGAM intramuscularly. Do not inject intravenously. Multiple doses may be administered at the same time or at spaced intervals, as long as the total dose is administered within three days of exposure.

Since there is no lot number and expiration date on the prefilled syringes, they should not be removed from the protective pouch until immediately before use.

HOW SUPPLIED

RhoGAM is available in packages containing:
—25 prefilled single-dose syringes of RhoGAM (Product code 780720) NDC 0562-8070-20
—25 package inserts
—25 control forms
—25 patient identification cards
           and
—100 prefilled single-dose syringes of RhoGAM (Product code 780790) NDC 0562-8070-90
—100 package inserts
—100 control forms
—100 patient identification cards

STORAGE

Store at 2 to 8°C. DO NOT FREEZE.

Ortho Pharmaceutical Corporation
RARITAN, NJ 08869-0602

ACI–JEL® Therapeutic Vaginal Jelly   ℞

DESCRIPTION

ACI-JEL Vaginal Jelly is a bland, non-irritating, water-dispersible, buffered acid jelly for intravaginal use. ACI-JEL is classified as a Vaginal Therapeutic Jelly. ACI-JEL contains 0.921% glacial acetic acid ($C_2H_4O_2$), 0.025% oxyquinoline sulfate ($C_{18}H_{16}N_2O_6S$), 0.7% ricinoleic acid ($C_{18}H_{34}O_3$), and 5% glycerin ($C_3H_8O_3$) compounded with tragacanth, acacia, propylparaben, potassium hydroxide, stannous chloride, egg albumen, potassium bitartrate, perfume and purified water. ACI-JEL is formulated to pH 3.9–4.1.

CLINICAL PHARMACOLOGY

ACI-JEL acts to restore and maintain normal vaginal acidity through its buffer action.

INDICATIONS AND USAGE

ACI-JEL is indicated as adjunctive therapy in those cases where restoration and maintenance of vaginal acidity are desirable.

CONTRAINDICATIONS

None known.

WARNINGS

No serious adverse reactions or potential safety hazards have been reported with the use of ACI-JEL.

PRECAUTIONS

General: No special care is required for the safe and effective use of ACI-JEL. *Drug Interactions:* No incidence of drug interactions have been reported with concomitant use of ACI-JEL and any other medications. *Laboratory Tests:* The monitoring of vaginal acidity (pH) may be helpful in following the patient's response. (The normal vaginal pH has been shown to be in the range of 4.0 to 5.0.) *Carcinogenesis:* No long-term studies in animals have been performed to evaluate carcinogenic potential. *Pregnancy:* Pregnancy Category C. Animal reproduction studies have not been conducted with ACI-JEL. It is also not known whether ACI-JEL can cause fetal harm when administered to a pregnant woman or can affect reproduction capacity. ACI-JEL should be given to a pregnant woman only if clearly needed. *Nursing Mothers:* It is not known whether this drug is excreted in human milk. Because many drugs are excreted in human milk, caution

should be exercised when ACI-JEL is administered to a nursing woman.

ADVERSE REACTIONS

Occasional cases of local stinging and burning have been reported.

DOSAGE AND ADMINISTRATION

The usual dose is one applicatorful, administered intravaginally, morning and evening. Duration of treatment may be determined by the patient's response to therapy.

HOW SUPPLIED

85g Tube (NDC 0062-5421-01) with ORTHO® Measured-Dose Applicator.

CONCEPTROL® Contraceptive Gel, Single Use Applicators   OTC

(See PDR For Nonprescription Drugs.)

CONCEPTROL® Contraceptive Inserts   OTC

(See PDR For Nonprescription Drugs.)

DELFEN® Contraceptive Foam   OTC

(See PDR For Nonprescription Drugs.)

DIENESTROL Cream   ℞

(See ORTHO® Dienestrol Cream.)

FLOXIN® I.V.   ℞
[*ofloxacin injection*]
for intravenous infusion

DESCRIPTION

FLOXIN® (ofloxacin injection) I.V. is a synthetic, broad-spectrum antimicrobial agent for intravenous administration. Chemically, ofloxacin, a fluorinated carboxyquinolone, is the racemate, ($\pm$)-9-fluoro-2,3-dihydro-3-methyl-10-(4-methyl-1-piperazinyl)-7-oxo-7H-pyrido[1,2,3-de]-1,4-benzoxazine-6-carboxylic acid. The chemical structure is:

Its empirical formula is $C_{18}H_{20}FN_3O_4$, and its molecular weight is 361.4. Ofloxacin is an off-white to pale yellow crystalline powder. The relative solubility characteristics of ofloxacin at room temperature, as defined by USP nomenclature, indicate that ofloxacin is considered to be *soluble* in aqueous solutions with pH between 2 and 5. It is *sparingly* to *slightly soluble* in aqueous solutions with pH 7 and *freely soluble* in aqueous solutions with pH above 9. Ofloxacin has the potential to form stable coordination compounds with many metal ions. This *in vitro* chelation potential has the following formation order: $Fe^{+3} > Al^{+3} > Cu^{+2} > Ni^{+2} > Pb^{+2} > Zn^{+2} > Mg^{+2} > Ca^{+2} > Ba^{+2}$.

FLOXIN I.V. IN SINGLE-USE VIALS is a sterile, preservative-free aqueous solution of ofloxacin with pH ranging from 3.5 to 5.5 FLOXIN I.V. IN PRE-MIXED BOTTLES and IN PRE-MIXED FLEXIBLE CONTAINERS are sterile, preservative-free aqueous solutions of ofloxacin with pH ranging from 3.8 to 5.8. The color of FLOXIN I.V. may range from light yellow to amber. This does not adversely affect product potency. FLOXIN I.V. IN SINGLE-USE VIALS contains ofloxacin in Water for Injection. FLOXIN I.V. IN PRE-MIXED BOTTLES and IN PRE-MIXED FLEXIBLE CONTAINERS are dilute, non-pyrogenic, nearly isotonic pre-mixed solutions that contain ofloxacin in 5% Dextrose (D_5W). Hydrochloric acid and sodium hydroxide may have been added to adjust the pH.

The flexible container is fabricated from a specially formulated non-plasticized, thermoplastic copolyester (CR3). The amount of water that can permeate from the container into the overwrap is insufficient to affect the solution significantly. Solutions in contact with the flexible container can leach out certain of the container's chemical components in very small amounts within the expiration period. The suitability of the container material has been confirmed by tests in animals according to USP biological tests for plastic containers.

CLINICAL PHARMACOLOGY

Following a single 60-minute intravenous infusion of 200 mg or 400 mg of ofloxacin to normal volunteers, the mean maximum plasma concentrations attained were 2.7 and 4.0 μg/mL, respectively; the concentrations at 12 hours (h) after dosing were 0.3 and 0.7 μg/mL, respectively.

Steady-state concentrations were attained after four doses, and the area under the curve (AUC) was approximately 40% higher than the AUC after a single dose. The mean peak and trough plasma steady-state levels attained following intravenous administration of 200 mg of ofloxacin q 12 h for seven days were 2.9 and 0.5 μg/mL, respectively. Following intravenous doses of 400 mg of ofloxacin q 12 h, the mean peak and trough plasma steady-state levels ranged, in two different studies, from 5.5 to 7.2 μg/mL and 1.2 to 1.9 μg/mL, respectively.

Following 7 days of intravenous administration, the elimination half-life of ofloxacin was 6 h (range 5 to 10 h). The total clearance and the volume of distribution were approximately 15 L/h and 120 L, respectively.

Elimination of ofloxacin is primarily by renal excretion. Approximately 65% of a dose is excreted renally within 48 h. Studies indicate that <5% of an administered dose is recovered in the urine as the desmethyl or N-oxide metabolites. Four to eight percent of an ofloxacin dose is excreted in the feces. This indicates a small degree of biliary excretion of ofloxacin.

In vitro, approximately 32% of the drug in plasma is protein bound.

The single dose and steady-state plasma profiles of ofloxacin injection were comparable in extent of exposure (AUC) to those of ofloxacin tablets when the injectable and tablet formulations of ofloxacin were administered in equal doses (mg/mg). The mean $AUC_{(0-12)}$ attained after the intravenous administration of 400 mg over 60 min was 43.5 $\mu g \cdot h$/mL; the mean $AUC_{(0-12)}$ attained after the oral administration of 400 mg was 41.2 $\mu g \cdot h$/mL (two one-sided t-test, 90% confidence interval was 103–109). [See following chart.]

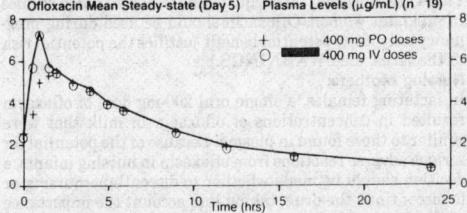

Ofloxacin Mean Steady-state (Day 5)   Plasma Levels (μg/mL) (n 19)

+ 400 mg PO doses
O 400 mg IV doses

Between 0 and 6 h following the administration of a single 200 mg oral dose of ofloxacin to 12 healthy volunteers, the average urine ofloxacin concentration was approximately 220 μg/mL. Between 12 and 24 h after administration, the average urine ofloxacin level was approximately 34 μg/mL. Following oral administration of recommended therapeutic doses, ofloxacin has been detected in blister fluid, cervix, lung tissue, ovary, prostatic fluid, prostatic tissue, skin, and sputum. The mean concentration of ofloxacin in each of these various body fluids and tissues after one or more doses was 0.8 to 1.5 times the concurrent plasma level. Inadequate data are presently available on the distribution or levels of ofloxacin in the cerebrospinal fluid or brain tissue.

Following the administration of oral doses of ofloxacin to healthy elderly volunteers (64–74 years of age) with normal renal function, the apparent half-life of ofloxacin was 7 to 8 h, compared to approximately 6 h in younger adults.

Clearance of ofloxacin is reduced in patients with impaired renal function (creatinine clearance ≤50 mL/min), and dosage adjustment is necessary. (See **DOSAGE AND ADMINISTRATION**.)

MICROBIOLOGY

Ofloxacin has *in vitro* activity against a broad-spectrum of gram-positive and gram-negative aerobic and anaerobic bacteria. Ofloxacin is often bactericidal at concentrations equal to or slightly greater than inhibitory concentrations. Ofloxacin is thought to exert a bactericidal effect on susceptible micro-organisms by inhibiting DNA gyrase, an essential enzyme that is a critical catalyst in the duplication, transcription, and repair of bacterial DNA.

Ofloxacin has been shown to be active against most strains of the following organisms both *in vitro* and in specific clinical infections: (See **INDICATIONS AND USAGE**.)

Chlamydia trachomatis
Citrobacter diversus
Enterobacter aerogenes
Escherichia coli
Haemophilus influenzae
Klebsiella pneumoniae
Neisseria gonorrhoeae
Proteus mirabilis
Pseudomonas aeruginosa
Staphylococcus aureus
Streptococcus pneumoniae
Streptococcus pyogenes

Beta-lactamase production should have no effect on ofloxacin activity.

The following *in vitro* data are available; **however, their clinical significance is unknown.**

Ofloxacin exhibits *in vitro* minimum inhibitory concentrations of 2 μg/mL or less against most strains of the following organisms; however, the safety and effectiveness of ofloxacin in treating clinical infections due to these organisms have not been established in adequate and well-controlled trials:

Gram-positive aerobes
Enterococcus faecalis
Staphylococcus epidermidis
  (including methicillin-resistant strains)
Staphylococcus saprophyticus
Streptococcus agalactiae (Group B)

Gram-negative aerobes
Acinetobacter calcoaceticus
Aeromonas hydrophila
Bordetella parapertussis
Bordetella pertussis
Campylobacter jejuni
Citrobacter freundii
Enterobacter cloacae
Haemophilus ducreyi
Klebsiella oxytoca
Moraxella (Branhamella)
  catarrhalis
Morganella morganii
Neisseria meningitidis
Plesiomonas shigelloides
Proteus vulgaris
Providencia rettgeri
Providencia stuartii
Pseudomonas fluorescens
Serratia marcescens

Anaerobes
Bacteroides fragilis
Bacteroides intermedius
Clostridium perfringens
Clostridium welchii
Eikenella corrodens
Gardnerella vaginalis
Peptococcus niger
Peptostreptococcus species

Other organisms
Chlamydia pneumoniae
Legionella pneumophila
Mycobacterium tuberculosis
Mycoplasma hominis
Mycoplasma pneumoniae
Ureaplasma urealyticum

Many strains of other streptococcal species, *Enterococcus* species, and anaerobes are resistant to ofloxacin.

Ofloxacin has not been shown to be active against *Treponema pallidum*. (See **WARNINGS**.)

Resistance to ofloxacin due to spontaneous mutation *in vitro* is a rare occurrence (range: 10^{-9} to 10^{-11}). To date, emergence of resistance has been relatively uncommon in clinical practice. With the exception of *Pseudomonas aeruginosa* (10%), less than a 4% rate of resistance emergence has been reported for most other species. Although cross-resistance has been observed between ofloxacin and other fluoroquinolones, some organisms resistant to other quinolones may be susceptible to ofloxacin.

SUSCEPTIBILITY TESTS

Diffusion techniques: Quantitative methods that require measurement of zone diameters give the most precise estimate of the susceptibility of bacteria to antimicrobial agents. One such standardized procedure[1] that has been recommended for use with disks to test the susceptibility of organisms to ofloxacin uses the 5-μg ofloxacin disk. Interpretation involves correlation of the diameter obtained in the disk test with the minimum inhibitory concentration (MIC) for ofloxacin.

Reports from the laboratory giving results of the standard single-disk susceptibility test with a 5-μg ofloxacin disk should be interpreted according to the following criteria:

Zone diameter (mm)	Interpretation
≥16	Susceptible
13–15	Intermediate
≤12	Resistant

A report of "Susceptible" indicates that the pathogen is likely to be inhibited by generally achievable drug concentrations. A report of "Intermediate" indicates that the result should be considered equivocal, and, if the organism is not fully susceptible to alternative, clinically feasible drugs, the test should be repeated. This category provides a buffer zone that prevents small uncontrolled technical factors from causing major discrepancies in interpretation. A report of "Resistant" indicates that achievable drug concentrations are unlikely to be inhibitory, and other therapy should be selected.

Standardized susceptibility test procedures require the use of laboratory control organisms. The 5-μg ofloxacin disk should give the following zone diameters:

Organism	Zone diameter (mm)
E. coli ATCC 25922	29–33
P. aeruginosa ATCC 27853	17–21
S. aureus ATCC 25923	24–28

Dilution techniques: Use a standardized dilution method[2] (broth, agar, or microdilution) or equivalent with ofloxacin powder. The MIC values obtained should be interpreted according to the following criteria:

MIC (μg/mL)	Interpretation
≤2	(S) Susceptible
4	(I) Intermediate
≥8	(R) Resistant

As with standard diffusion methods, dilution procedures require the use of laboratory control organisms. Standard ofloxacin powder should give the following MIC values:

Organism	MIC range (μg/mL)
E. coli ATCC 25922	0.015–0.120
E. faecalis ATCC 29212	1.000–4.000
P. aeruginosa ATCC 27853	1.000–8.000
S. aureus ATCC 25923	0.120–1.000

INDICATIONS AND USAGE

FLOXIN (ofloxacin injection) I.V. is indicated for the treatment of adults with mild to moderate infections caused by susceptible strains of the designated microorganisms in the infections listed below—when intravenous administration offers a route of administration advantageous to the patient, (i.e., patient cannot tolerate an oral dosage form, etc.). **The safety and effectiveness of the intravenous formulation in treating patients with severe infections have not been established.**

NOTE: IN THE ABSENCE OF VOMITING OR OTHER FACTORS INTERFERING WITH THE ABSORPTION OF ORALLY ADMINISTERED DRUG, PATIENTS RECEIVE ESSENTIALLY THE SAME SYSTEMIC ANTIMICROBIAL THERAPY AFTER EQUIVALENT DOSES OF OFLOXACIN ADMINISTERED BY EITHER THE ORAL OR THE INTRAVENOUS ROUTE. THEREFORE, THE INTRAVENOUS FORMULATION DOES NOT PROVIDE A HIGHER DEGREE OF EFFICACY OR MORE POTENT ANTIMICROBIAL ACTIVITY THAN AN EQUIVALENT DOSE OF THE ORAL FORMULATION OF OFLOXACIN.

Lower Respiratory Tract
Acute bacterial exacerbation of chronic bronchitis due to *Haemophilus influenzae* or *Streptococcus pneumoniae*.
Community-acquired Pneumonia due to *Haemophilus influenzae* or *Streptococcus pneumoniae*.

Skin and Skin Structures
Uncomplicated skin and skin structure infections due to *Staphylococcus aureus*, *Streptococcus pyogenes*, or *Proteus mirabilis**.

Sexually Transmitted Diseases (See **WARNINGS**.)
Acute, uncomplicated urethral and cervical gonorrhea due to *Neisseria gonorrhoeae*.
Nongonococcal urethritis and cervicitis due to *Chlamydia trachomatis*.
Mixed infections of the urethra and cervix due to *Chlamydia trachomatis* and *Neisseria gonorrhoeae*.

Urinary Tract
Uncomplicated cystitis due to *Citrobacter diversus*, *Enterobacter aerogenes*, *Escherichia coli*, *Klebsiella pneumoniae*, *Proteus mirabilis*, or *Pseudomonas aeruginosa*.
Complicated urinary tract infections due to *Escherichia coli*, *Klebsiella pneumoniae*, *Proteus mirabilis*, *Citrobacter diversus**, or *Pseudomonas aeruginosa**.

Prostate
Prostatitis due to *Escherichia coli*.

Beta-lactamase production should have no effect on ofloxacin activity.

Appropriate culture and susceptibility tests should be performed before treatment in order to isolate and identify organisms causing the infection and to determine their susceptibility to ofloxacin. Therapy with ofloxacin may be initiated before results of these tests are known; once results become available, appropriate therapy should be continued.

As with other drugs in this class, some strains of *Pseudomonas aeruginosa* may develop resistance fairly rapidly during treatment with ofloxacin. Culture and susceptibility testing

* = Although treatment of infections due to this organism in this infection demonstrated a clinically acceptable overall outcome, efficacy was demonstrated in fewer than 10 infections.

Continued on next page

Ortho—Cont.

performed periodically during therapy will provide information not only on the therapeutic effect of the antimicrobial agent but also on the possible emergence of bacterial resistance.

If anaerobic organisms are suspected of contributing to the infection, appropriate therapy for anaerobic pathogens should be administered.

CONTRAINDICATIONS

Ofloxacin is contraindicated in persons with a history of hypersensitivity to ofloxacin or members of the quinolone group of antimicrobial agents.

WARNINGS

THE SAFETY AND EFFICACY OF OFLOXACIN IN CHILDREN, ADOLESCENTS (UNDER THE AGE OF 18 YEARS), PREGNANT WOMEN, AND LACTATING WOMEN HAVE NOT BEEN ESTABLISHED. (SEE PEDIATRIC USE, USE IN PREGNANCY, AND NURSING MOTHERS SUBSECTIONS IN THE PRECAUTIONS SECTION.)

In the immature rat, the oral administrator of ofloxacin at 5 to 16 times the recommended maximum human dose based on mg/kg or 1–3 times based on mg/m^2 increased the incidence and severity of osteochondrosis. The lesions did not regress after 13 weeks of drug withdrawal. Other quinolones also produce similar erosions in the weight-bearing joints and other signs of arthropathy in immature animals of various species. (See ***ANIMAL PHARMACOLOGY.***)

Ofloxacin has not been shown to be effective in the treatment of syphilis. Antimicrobial agents used in high doses for short periods of time to treat gonorrhea may mask or delay the symptoms of incubating syphilis. All patients with gonorrhea should have a serologic test for syphilis at the time of diagnosis. Patients treated with ofloxacin should have a follow-up serologic test for syphilis after three months.

Serious and occasionally fatal hypersensitivity (anaphylactic) reactions, some following the first dose, have been reported in patients receiving therapy with quinolones, including ofloxacin. Some reactions were accompanied by cardiovascular collapse, loss of consciousness, tingling, angioedema (including laryngeal, pharyngeal or facial edema), airway obstruction, dyspnea, urticaria, and itching. If an allergic reaction to ofloxacin occurs, discontinue the drug. Serious acute hypersensitivity reactions may require treatment with epinephrine and other resuscitative measures, including oxygen, intravenous fluids, antihistamines, corticosteroids, pressor amines, and airway management, as clincially indicated.

Severe hypersensitivity reactions (generally following multiple doses) characterized by rash, fever, eosinophilia, jaundice and hepatic necrosis with a fatal outcome have also been reported extremely rarely in patients receiving another quinolone. Similar reactions may occur with ofloxacin. The drug should be discontinued at the first appearance of a skin rash or any other sign of hypersensitivity. (See **PRECAUTIONS** and **ADVERSE REACTIONS.**)

Convulsions, increased intracranial pressure, and toxic psychosis have been reported in patients receiving quinolones, including ofloxacin. Quinolones may also cause central nervous system stimulation, which may lead to tremors, restlessness, lightheadedness, confusion, and hallucinations. If these reactions occur in patients receiving ofloxacin, the drug should be discontinued and appropriate measures instituted. No evidence of an effect of ofloxacin on the electrical activity of the brain has been demonstrated. Ofloxacin does not alter the metabolism of glucose in the central nervous system based on positron emission tomography. It does not have effects upon the electrical patterns of brain function based on EEG's. However, until more information becomes available, ofloxacin, like all other quinolones, should be used with caution in patients with known or suspected CNS disorders, such as severe cerebral arteriosclerosis or epilepsy, or other factors (e.g., concomitant drug therapy) that predispose to seizures. (See **PRECAUTIONS** and **ADVERSE REACTIONS.**)

Pseudomembranous colitis has been reported with nearly all antibacterial agents, including ofloxacin, and may range in severity from mild to life-threatening. Therefore, it is important to consider this diagnosis in patients who present with diarrhea subsequent to the administration of any antibacterial agent.

Treatment with antibacterial agents alters the normal flora of the colon and may permit overgrowth of clostridia. Studies indicate a toxin produced by *Clostridium difficile* is one primary cause of "antibiotic-associated colitis".

After the diagnosis of pseudomembranous colitis has been established, therapeutic measures should be initiated. Mild cases of pseudomembranous colitis usually respond to drug discontinuation alone. In moderate to severe cases, consideration should be given to management with fluids and electrolytes, protein supplementation, and treatment with an oral antibacterial drug clinically effective against *C. difficile* colitis. (See **ADVERSE REACTIONS.**)

PRECAUTIONS

General:

Because a rapid or bolus intravenous injection may result in hypotension, **OFLOXACIN INJECTION SHOULD ONLY BE ADMINISTERED BY SLOW INTRAVENOUS INFUSION OVER A PERIOD OF 60 MINUTES.** (See **DOSAGE AND ADMINISTRATION.**)

Adequate hydration of patients receiving ofloxacin should be maintained to prevent the formation of highly concentrated urine.

In patients with impaired renal function (creatinine clearance $\leq$ 50 mg/mL), alteration of the dosage regimen is necessary. (See **DOSAGE AND ADMINISTRATION.**)

Moderate to severe phototoxicity reactions have been observed in patients exposed to direct sunlight while receiving some drugs in this class. Excessive sunlight should be avoided. Therapy should be discontinued if phototoxicity occurs.

As with any potent drug, periodic assessment of organ system functions, including renal, hepatic, and hematopoietic, is advisable during prolonged therapy.

Information for Patients

Patients should be advised:

—to drink fluids liberally if able to take fluids by the oral route.

—that ofloxacin can cause dizziness and lightheadedness and that patients should know how they react to ofloxacin before they operate an automobile or machinery and engage in activities requiring mental alertness and coordination. (See **WARNINGS** and **ADVERSE REACTIONS.**)

—that ofloxacin may be associated with hypersensitivity reactions, even following the first dose, and to discontinue the drug at the first sign of a skin rash, hives, rapid heartbeat, difficulty in swallowing or breathing, any swelling suggesting angioedema, or other symptom of an allergic reaction. (See **WARNINGS** and **ADVERSE REACTIONS.**)

—to avoid excessive sunlight or artificial ultraviolet light while receiving ofloxacin and to discontinue therapy if phototoxicity occurs.

Drug Interactions

Antacids, Sucralfate, Metal Cations, Multi-Vitamins:

There are no data concerning an interaction of **intravenous** quinolones with **oral** antacids, sucralfate, multi-vitamins, or metal cations. However, no quinolone should be co-administered with any solution containing multivalent cations, e.g., magnesium, through the same intravenous line. (See **DOSAGE AND ADMINISTRATION.**)

Caffeine: Interactions between ofloxacin and caffeine have not been detected.

Cimetidine: Cimetidine has demonstrated interference with the elimination of some quinolones. This interference has resulted in significant increases in half-life and AUC of some quinolones. The potential for interaction between ofloxacin and cimetidine has not been studied.

Cyclosporine: Elevated serum levels of cyclosporine have been reported with concomitant use of cyclosporine with some other quinolones. The potential for interaction between ofloxacin and cyclosporine has not been studied.

Non-steroidal anti-inflammatory drugs: Concomitant administration of the non-steroidal anti-inflammatory drug. fenbufen, with some quinolones, including ofloxacin, has been reported to increase the risk of CNS stimulation and convulsive seizures. Fenbufen is presently not an approved drug in the United States.

Probenecid: The concomitant use of probenecid with certain other quinolones has been reported to affect renal tubular secretion. The effect of probenecid on the elimination of ofloxacin has not been studied.

Theophylline: Although concurrent administration of some quinolones with theophylline may result in impaired elimination of theophylline, the extent of such impairment varies among different quinolones. Steady-state theophylline levels may increase when ofloxacin and theophylline are administered concurrently. In a pharmacokinetic study involving 15 healthy male subjects, steady-state peak theophylline concentration increased by an average of approximately 9%, and the AUC increased by an average of approximately 13% when oral ofloxacin and theophylline were administered concurrently. In clinical trials with intravenous ofloxacin, theophylline concentrations were determined in 41 patients who were treated with both drugs. In 38 patients, no apparent elevation in the serum theophylline was discernible. Marginal increases above the theophylline therapeutic range were reported in three patients; clinical toxicity was, however, not reported in these three patients. Generally, patients receiving theophylline in clinical trials of the intravenous formulation of ofloxacin reported nausea more frequently than those patients not receiving theophylline. As with some other quinolones, concomitant administration of ofloxacin may prolong the half-life of theophylline, elevate serum theophylline levels, and may increase the risk of theophylline-related adverse reactions. Theophylline levels should be closely monitored and theophylline dosage adjustments made, if appropriate, when ofloxacin is co-administered.

Warfarin: Some quinolones have been reported to enhance the effects of the oral anticoagulant warfarin or its derivatives. Therefore, if a quinolone antimicrobial is administered concomitantly with warfarin or its derivatives, the prothrombin time or other suitable coagulation test should be closely monitored.

Carcinogenesis, Mutagenesis, Impairment of Fertility:

Long term studies to determine the carcinogenic potential of ofloxacin have not been conducted.

Ofloxacin was not mutagenic in the Ames bacterial test, *in vitro* and *in vivo* cytogenetic assay, sister chromatid exchange (Chinese Hamster and Human Cell Lines), unscheduled DNA Repair (UDS) using human fibroblasts, dominant lethal assays, or mouse micronucleus assay. Ofloxacin was positive in the UDS test using rat hepatocytes and Mouse Lymphoma Assay.

Pregnancy: Teratogenic Effects. Pregnancy Category C.

Ofloxacin has not been shown to have any teratogenic effects at oral doses as high as 810 mg/kg/day (11 times the recommended maximum human dose based on mg/m^2 or 50 times based on mg/kg) and 160 mg/kg/day (4 times the recommended maximum human dose based on mg/m^2 or 10 times based on mg/kg) when administered to pregnant rats and rabbits, respectively. Additional studies in rats with oral doses up to 360 mg/kg/day (5 times the recommended maximum human dose based on mg/m^2 or 23 times based on mg/kg) demonstrated no adverse effect on late fetal development, labor, delivery, lactation, neonatal viability, or growth of the newborn. Doses equivalent to 50 and 10 times the recommended maximum human dose of ofloxacin (based on mg/kg) were fetotoxic (i.e., decreased fetal body weight and increased fetal mortality) in rats and rabbits, respectively. Minor skeletal variations were reported in rats receiving doses of 810 mg/kg/day, which is more than 10 times higher than the recommended maximum human dose based on mg/m^2.

There are, however, no adequate and well-controlled studies in pregnant women. Ofloxacin should be used during pregnancy only if the potential benefit justifies the potential risk to the fetus. (See **WARNINGS.**)

Nursing Mothers:

In lactating females, a single oral 200-mg dose of ofloxacin resulted in concentrations of ofloxacin in milk that were similar to those found in plasma. Because of the potential for serious adverse reactions from ofloxacin in nursing infants, a decision should be made whether to discontinue nursing or to discontinue the drug, taking into account the importance of the drug to the mother.

Pediatric Use:

Safety and effectiveness in children and adolescents below the age of 18 years have not been established. Ofloxacin causes arthropathy (arthrosis) and osteochondrosis in juvenile animals of several species. (See **WARNINGS.**)

ADVERSE REACTIONS

The following is a compilation of the data for ofloxacin based on clinical experience with both the oral and intravenous formulations. The incidence of drug-related adverse reactions in patients during Phase 2 and 3 clinical trials was 11%. Among patients receiving multiple-dose therapy, 4% discontinued ofloxacin due to adverse experiences.

In clinical trials, the following events were considered likely to be drug-related in patients receiving multiple doses of ofloxacin:

nausea 3%, insomnia 3%, headache 1%, dizziness 1%, diarrhea 1%, vomiting 1%, rash 1%, pruritus 1%, external genital pruritus in women 1%, vaginitis 1%, dysgeusia 1%.

Local injection site reactions (phlebitis, swelling, erythema) were reported in approximately 2% of patients treated with the 3.63 mg/mL final infusion concentration of intravenous ofloxacin used in the clinical safety trials. The final infusion concentration of intravenous ofloxacin in the commercially available intravenous preparations is 4.0 mg/mL. To date, individuals administered the 4.0 mg/mL concentration of the intravenous ofloxacin have demonstrated clinically acceptable rates of local injection site reactions. Due to the small difference in concentration, significant differences in local site reactions are unexpected with the 4.0 mg/mL concentration.

In clinical trials, the most frequently reported adverse events, regardless of relationship to drug were:

nausea 10%, headache 9%, insomnia 7%, external genital pruritus in women 6%, dizziness 5%, vaginitis 5%, diarrhea 4%, vomiting 4%.

In clinical trials, the following events, regardless of relationship to drug occurred in 1 to 3% of patients:

Abdominal pain and cramps, chest pain, decreased appetite, dry mouth, dysgeusia, fatigue, flatulence, gastrointestinal distress, nervousness, pharyngitis, pruritus, pyrexia, rash, sleep disorders, somnolence, trunk pain, vaginal discharge, visual disturbances, and constipation.

Additional events, occurring in clinical trials at a rate of less than 1%, regardless of relationship to drug, were:

Body as a whole:	asthenia, chills, malaise, extremity pain, pain, epistaxis
Cardiovascular System:	cardiac arrest, edema, hypertension, hypotension, palpitations, vasodilation
Gastrointestinal System:	dyspepsia
Genital/Reproductive System:	burning, irritation, pain and rash of the female genitalia; dysmenorrhea; menorrhagia; metrorrhagia
Musculoskeletal System:	arthralgia, myalgia
Nervous System:	seizures, anxiety, cognitive change, depression, dream abnormality, euphoria, hallucinations, paresthesia, syncope, vertigo, tremor, confusion
Nutritional/Metabolic:	thirst, weight loss
Respiratory System:	respiratory arrest, cough, rhinorrhea
Skin/Hypersensitivity:	angioedema, diaphoresis, urticaria, vasculitis
Special Senses:	decreased hearing acuity, tinnitus, photophobia
Urinary System:	dysuria, urinary frequency, urinary retention

The following laboratory abnormalities appeared in ≥ 1.0% of patients receiving multiple doses of ofloxacin. It is not known whether these abnormalities were caused by the drug or the underlying conditions being treated.

Hematopoietic:	anemia, leukopenia, leukocytosis, neutropenia, neutrophilia, increased band forms, lymphocytopenia, eosinophilia, lymphocytosis, thrombocytopenia, thrombocytosis, elevated ESR
Hepatic:	elevated alkaline phosphatase, elevated AST (SGOT), elevated ALT (SGPT)
Serum chemistry:	hyperglycemia, hypoglycemia, elevated creatinine, elevated BUN
Urinary:	glucosuria proteinuria, alkalinuria, hyposthenuria, hematuria, pyuria

Additional adverse events, regardless of relationship to drug, reported from marketing experience with including ofloxacin:

Clinical:

Cardiovascular System:	cerebral thrombosis, pulmonary edema
Gastrointestinal System:	hepatic dysfunction including: hepatic necrosis, jaundice, hepatitis; hiccough, intestinal perforation, painful oral mucosa, pseudomembranous colitis
Genitourinary System:	vaginal candidiasis
Nervous System:	psychotic reactions, ataxia, phobia, agitation, restlessness, aggressiveness, manic reaction, possible exacerbation of myasthenia gravis, dysphasia
Respiratory System:	dyspnea, bronchospasm
Skin/Hypersensitivity:	anaphylactic reactions; erythema multiforme/Stevens-Johnson syndrome, erythema nodosum, exfoliative dermatitis, hyperpigmentation, toxic epidermal necrolysis, laryngeal edema, photosensitivity
Special Senses:	diplopia, nystagmus
Urinary System:	polyuria, renal calculi, renal failure, urinary retention, interstitial nephritis (See **WARNINGS** and **PRECAUTIONS.**)

Laboratory:

Hematopoietic:	agranulocytosis, prolongation of prothrombin time
Serum chemistry:	acidosis, elevation of serum triglycerides, serum cholesterol, serum potassium
Urinary:	albuminuria, candiduria

In clinical trials using multiple-dose therapy, ophthalmologic abnormalities, including cataracts and multiple punctate lenticular opacities, have been noted in patients undergoing treatment with other quinolones. The relationship of the drugs to these events is not presently established. CRYSTALLURIA and CYLINDRURIA HAVE BEEN REPORTED with other quinolones.

Infection	Description*	Unit Dose	Frequency	Duration	Daily Dose
Lower Respiratory Tract	Exacerbation of Chronic Bronchitis	400 mg	q12h	10 days	800 mg
	Com. Acq. Pneumonia	400 mg	q12h	10 days	800 mg
Skin and Skin Structures	Uncomplicated infections	400 mg	q12h	10 days	800 mg
Sexually Transmitted Diseases	Acute, uncomplicated gonorrhea	400 mg	single dose	1 day	400 mg
	Cervicitis/ urethritis due to C. trachomatis	300 mg	q12h	7 days	600 mg
	Cervicitis/ urethritis due to C. trachomatis and N. gonorrhoeae	300 mg	q12h	7 days	600 mg
Urinary Tract	Cystitis due to E. coli or K. pneumoniae	200 mg	q12h	3 days	400 mg
	Cystitis due to other approved pathogens	200 mg	q12h	7 days	400 mg
	Complicated UTI's	200 mg	q12h	10 days	400 mg
Prostrate	Prostatitis due to E. coli	300 mg	q12h	6 wks**	600 mg

* DUE TO THE DESIGNATED PATHOGENS (See **INDICATIONS AND USAGE**.)

**BECAUSE THERE ARE NO SAFETY DATA PRESENTLY AVAILABLE TO SUPPORT THE USE OF THE INTRAVENOUS FORMULATION OF OFLOXACIN FOR MORE THAN 10 DAYS, THERAPY AFTER 10 DAYS SHOULD BE SWITCHED TO THE ORAL TABLET FORMULATION OR OTHER APPROPRIATE THERAPY.

OVERDOSAGE

Information on overdosage with ofloxacin is limited. One incident of accidental overdosage has been reported. In this case, an adult female received 3 grams of ofloxacin intravenously over 45 minutes. A blood sample obtained 15 minutes after the completion of the infusion revealed an ofloxacin level of 39.3 μg/mL. In 7 h, the level had fallen to 16.2 μg/mL, and by 24 h to 2.7 μg/mL. During the infusion, the patient developed drowsiness, nausea, dizziness, hot and cold flushes, subjective facial swelling and numbness, slurring of speech, and mild to moderate disorientation. All complaints except the dizziness subsided within 1 h after discontinuation of the infusion. The dizziness, most bothersome while standing, resolved in approximately 9 h. Laboratory testing reportedly revealed no clinically significant changes in routine parameters in this patient.

In the event of acute overdose, the patient should be observed and appropriate hydration maintained. Ofloxacin is not efficiently removed by hemodialysis or peritoneal dialysis.

DOSAGE AND ADMINISTRATION

FLOXIN I.V. should only be administered by **intravenous** infusion. It is not for intramuscular, intrathecal, intraperitoneal, or subcutaneous administration.

CAUTION: RAPID OR BOLUS INTRAVENOUS INFUSION MUST BE AVOIDED. Ofloxacin injection should be infused intravenously slowly over a period of not less than 60 minutes. (See **PRECAUTIONS**.)

Single-use vials require dilution prior to administration. (See **PREPARATION FOR ADMINISTRATION.**)

The usual dose of FLOXIN (ofloxacin injection) I.V. is 200 mg to 400 mg administered by slow infusion over 60 minutes every 12 h as described in the following dosing chart. These recommendations apply to patients with mild to moderate infection and normal renal function (i.e., creatinine clearance > 50 mL/min). For patients with altered renal function (i.e., creatinine clearance ≤50 mL/min), see the **DOSAGE ADJUSTMENT FOR RENAL IMPAIRMENT** subsection.

Patients with Normal Renal Function:
[See table above.]

Patients with Impaired Renal Function:
Dosage should be adjusted for patients with a creatinine clearance ≤ 50 mL/min. **After a normal initial dose,** dosage should be adjusted as follows:

Creatinine Clearance	Maintenance Dose	Frequency
10–50 mL/min	the usual recommended unit dose	q24h
< 10 mL/min	½ the usual recommended unit dose	q24h

When only the serum creatinine is known, the following formula may be used to estimate creatinine clearance.

Men: Creatinine clearance (mL/min) $= \dfrac{\text{Weight (kg)} \times (140\text{-age})}{72 \times \text{serum creatinine (mg/dL)}}$

Women: 0.85 × the value calculated for men.

The serum creatinine should represent a steady-state of renal function.

PREPARATION OF OFLOXACIN INJECTION FOR ADMINISTRATION:

FLOXIN I.V. IN SINGLE-USE VIALS:

FLOXIN I.V. is supplied in single-use vials. Each vial contains a concentrated ofloxacin solution with the equivalent of 400 mg of ofloxacin in Water for Injection. The 10 mL vials contain 40 mg of ofloxacin/mL, and the 20 mL vials contain 20 mg of ofloxacin/mL. **THESE FLOXIN I.V. SINGLE-USE VIALS MUST BE FURTHER DILUTED WITH AN APPROPRIATE SOLUTION PRIOR TO INTRAVENOUS ADMINISTRATION (See COMPATIBLE INTRAVENOUS SOLUTIONS.)** The concentration of the resulting diluted solution should be 4 mg/mL prior to administration.

This parenteral drug product should be inspected visually for discoloration and particulate matter prior to administration.

Because no preservative or bacteriostatic agent is present in this product, aseptic technique must be used. **Because the vials are for single use only, any unused portion should be discarded.**

Because only limited data are available on the compatibility of ofloxacin intravenous injection with other intravenous substances, **additives or other medications should not be added to FLOXIN I.V. or infused simultaneously through the same intravenous line.** If the same intravenous line is used for sequential infusion of several different drugs, the line should be flushed before and after infusion of FLOXIN I.V. with an infusion solution compatible with FLOXIN I.V. and with any other drug(s) administered via this common line.

Prepare the desired dosage of ofloxacin according to the following chart:

Desired Dosage Strength	From 10 mL Vial, Withdraw Volume	From 20 mL Vial, Withdraw Volume	Volume of Diluent	Infusion Time
200 mg	5 mL	10 mL	qs 50 mL	60 min
300 mg	7.5 mL	15 mL	qs 75 mL	60 min
400 mg	10 mL	20 mL	qs 100 mL	60 min

For example, to prepare a 200-mg dose using the 10 mL vial (40 mg/mL), withdraw 5 mL and dilute with a compatible intravenous solution to a total volume of 50 mL.

Compatible Intravenous Solutions
Any of the following intravenous solutions may be used to prepare a 4 mg/mL ofloxacin solution with the approximate pH values: [See table top of next page.]

FLOXIN I.V. PRE-MIXED IN BOTTLES:

FLOXIN I.V. is also supplied in 100 mL bottles containing a pre-mixed, ready-to-use ofloxacin solution in D_5W. **NO FURTHER DILUTION OF THIS PREPARATION IS NECESSARY.** Each 100 mL pre-mixed bottle already contains a dilute solution with the equivalent of 400 mg of ofloxacin (4 mg/mL) in 5% Dextrose (D_5W).

Continued on next page

Ortho—Cont.

Intravenous Fluids	pH of 4 mg/mL FLOXIN I.V. Solution
0.9% Sodium Chloride Injection, USP	4.69
5% Dextrose Injection, USP	4.57
5% Dextrose/0.9% NaCl Injection	4.56
5% Dextrose in Lactated Ringers	4.94
5% Sodium Bicarbonate Injection	7.95
Plasma-Lyte® 56/5% Dextrose Injection	5.02
5% Dextrose, 0.45% Sodium Chloride, and 0.15% Potassium Chloride Injection	4.64
Sodium Lactate Injection (M/6)	5.64
Water for Injection	4.66

This parenteral drug product should be inspected visually for discoloration and particulate matter prior to administration.

Because no preservative or bacteriostatic agent is present in this product, aseptic technique must be used. **Because the pre-mixed bottles are for single use only, any unused portion should be discarded.**

Because only limited data are available on the compatibility of ofloxacin intravenous injection with other intravenous substances, **additives or other medications should not be added to FLOXIN I.V. in pre-mixed bottles or infused simultaneously through the same intravenous line.** If the same intravenous line is used for sequential infusion of several different drugs, the line should be flushed before and after infusion of FLOXIN I.V. with an infusion solution compatible with FLOXIN I.V. and with any other drug(s) administered via this common line.

FLOXIN I.V. PRE-MIXED IN FLEXIBLE CONTAINERS:

FLOXIN I.V. is also supplied in 50 mL and 100 mL flexible containers. These are pre-mixed, ready-to-use ofloxacin solutions in D_5W for single-use. **NO FURTHER DILUTION OF THIS PREPARATION IS NECESSARY. Each 50 mL pre-mixed flexible container already contains a dilute solution with the equivalent of 200 mg of ofloxacin (4 mg/mL) in 5% Dextrose (D_5W). Each 100 mL pre-mixed flexible container already contains a dilute solution with the equivalent of 400 mg of ofloxacin (4 mg/mL) in 5% Dextrose (D_5W).**

This parenteral drug product should be inspected visually for discoloration and particulate matter prior to administration.

Because no preservative or bacteriostatic agent is present in this product, aseptic technique must be used. **Because the pre-mixed flexible containers are for single use only, any unused portion should be discarded.**

Because only limited data are available on the compatibility of ofloxacin intravenous injection with other intravenous substances, **additives or other medications should not be added to FLOXIN I.V. in flexible containers or infused simultaneously through the same intravenous line.** If the same intravenous line is used for sequential infusion of several different drugs, the line should be flushed before and after infusion of FLOXIN I.V. with an infusion solution compatible with FLOXIN I.V. and with any other drug(s) administered via this common line.

Instructions for the Use of FLOXIN I.V. PRE-MIXED IN FLEXIBLE CONTAINERS:

To open:

1. Tear outer wrap at the notch and remove solution container.
2. Check the container for minute leaks by squeezing the inner bag firmly. If leaks are found, or if the seal is not intact, discard the solution, as the sterility may be compromised.
3. Do not use if the solution is cloudy or a precipitate is present.
4. Use sterile equipment.
5. **WARNING: Do not use flexible containers in series connections.** Such use could result in air embolism due to residual air being drawn from the primary container before administration of the fluid from the secondary container is complete.

Preparation for administration:

1. Close flow control clamp of administration set.
2. Remove cover from port at bottom of container.
3. Insert piercing pin of administration set into port with a twisting motion until the pin is firmly seated. **NOTE: See full directions on administration set carton.**
4. Suspend container from hanger.
5. Squeeze and release drip chamber to establish proper fluid level in chamber during infusion of FLOXIN I.V. IN PRE-MIXED FLEXIBLE CONTAINERS.
6. Open flow control clamp to expel air from set. Close clamp.
7. Regulate rate of administration with flow control clamp.

Stability of FLOXIN I.V. as Supplied

When stored under recommended conditions, FLOXIN I.V., as supplied in 10 mL and 20 mL vials, 100 mL bottles, and 50 mL and 100 mL flexible containers, is stable through the expiration date on the label.

Stability of FLOXIN I.V. Following Dilution

FLOXIN I.V., when diluted in a compatible intravenous fluid to a concentration between 0.4 mg/mL and 4 mg/mL, is stable for 72 h when stored at or below 75°F (24°C) and for 14 days when stored under refrigeration at 41°F (5°C) in glass bottles or plastic intravenous containers. Solutions that are diluted in a compatible intravenous solution and frozen in glass bottles or plastic intravenous containers are stable for 6 months when stored at −20°C (−4°F). Once thawed, the solution is stable for up to 14 days, if refrigerated. **THAW FROZEN SOLUTIONS AT ROOM TEMPERATURE (25°C OR 77°F) OR IN A REFRIGERATOR (8°C OR 46°F). DO NOT FORCE THAW BY MICROWAVE IRRADIATION OR IMMERSION IN WATER BATHS. DO NOT RE-FREEZE AFTER INITIAL THAWING.**

HOW SUPPLIED

SINGLE-USE VIALS:

FLOXIN (ofloxacin injection) I.V. is supplied in single-use vials. Each vial contains a concentrated solution with the equivalent of 400 mg of ofloxacin.

40 mg/mL, 10 mL vials (NDC 0062-1550-01)
20 mg/mL, 20 mL vials (NDC 0062-1551-01)

FLOXIN I.V. Single-use Vials are manufactured for Ortho Pharmaceutical Corporation and McNeil Pharmaceutical by Ortho Pharmaceutical Corporation, Raritan, NJ 08869 and Schering-Plough Products, Inc., Manati, PR 00674.

PRE-MIXED IN BOTTLES:

FLOXIN (ofloxacin injection) I.V. PRE-MIXED IN BOTTLES is supplied in 100 mL, single-use, pre-mixed bottles. Each bottle contains a dilute solution with the equivalent of 400 mg of ofloxacin in 5% Dextrose (D_5W).

4 mg/mL, 100 mL bottle (NDC 0062-1552-01)

FLOXIN I.V. PRE-MIXED IN BOTTLES is manufactured for Ortho Pharmaceutical Corporation and McNeil Pharmaceutical by Schering-Plough Products, Inc., Manati, PR 00674.

PRE-MIXED IN FLEXIBLE CONTAINERS:

FLOXIN (ofloxacin injection) I.V. PRE-MIXED IN FLEXIBLE CONTAINERS is supplied as a single-use, pre-mixed solution in 50 mL and 100 mL flexible containers. Each contains a dilute solution with the equivalent of 200 mg or 400 mg of ofloxacin, respectively, in 5% Dextrose (D_5W).

4 mg/mL (200 mg), 50 mL flexible container (NDC 0062-1553-01)
4 mg/mL (400 mg), 100 mL flexible container (NDC 0062-1552-02)

FLOXIN I.V. PRE-MIXED IN FLEXIBLE CONTAINERS is manufactured for Ortho Pharmaceutical Corporation and McNeil Pharmaceutical by Abbott Laboratories, North Chicago, IL 60064.

FLOXIN (ofloxacin injection) I.V. in SINGLE-USE VIALS and PRE-MIXED IN BOTTLES should be stored at controlled room temperature 59° to 86°F (15° to 30°C) and protected from light. FLOXIN I.V. PRE-MIXED IN FLEXIBLE CONTAINERS should be stored at or below 77°F (25°C); however, brief exposure up to 104°F (40°C) does not adversely affect the product. Avoid excessive heat and protect from freezing and light.

Also available:

TABLETS

Ofloxacin is also available as FLOXIN TABLETS (ofloxacin tablets) 200, 300 and 400 mg.

ANIMAL PHARMACOLOGY:

Ofloxacin, as well as other drugs of the quinolone class, has been shown to cause arthropathies (arthrosis) in immature dogs and rats. In addition, these drugs are associated with an increased incidence of osteochondrosis in rats as compared to the incidence observed in vehicle-treated rats. (See **WARNINGS.**) There is no evidence of arthropathies in fully mature dogs at intravenous doses up to 3 times the recommended maximum human dose (on a mg/m^2 basis or 5 times based on a mg/kg basis) for a one-week exposure period.

Long-term, high-dose systemic use of other quinolones in experimental animals has caused lenticular opacities; however, this finding was not observed in any animal studies with ofloxacin.

Reduced serum globulin and protein levels were observed in animals treated with other quinolones. In one ofloxacin study, minor decreases in serum globulin and protein levels were noted in female cynomolgus monkeys dosed orally with 40 mg/kg ofloxacin daily for one year. These changes, however, were considered to be within normal limits for monkeys.

Crystalluria and ocular toxicity were not observed in any animals treated with ofloxacin.

Caution: Federal (U.S.A.) law prohibits dispensing without prescription.

FLOXIN® is a trademark of Ortho Pharmaceutical Corporation. U.S. Patent No. 4,382,892

REFERENCES

1. National Committee for Clinical Laboratory Standards, Performance Standards for Antimicrobial Disk Susceptibility Tests—Fourth Edition, Approved Standard NCCLS Document M2-A4, Vol. 10, No. 7, NCCLS, Villanova, PA, 1990.
2. National Committee for Clinical Laboratory Standards, Methods for Dilution Antimicrobial Susceptibility Tests for Bacteria that Grow Aerobically—Second Edition, Approved Standard NCCLS Document M7-A2, Vol. 10, No. 8, NCCLS, Villanova, PA, 1990.

Ortho Pharmaceutical Corporation
Raritan, NJ USA 08869, and
McNeil Pharmaceutical
Spring House, PA USA 19477

06-4723/R1-1/92
Issued April 1992
635-10-290-1
17028308

Shown in Product Identification Section, page 421

FLOXIN® Tablets ℞
(ofloxacin tablets)

Description

FLOXIN (ofloxacin) is a synthetic broad-spectrum antibacterial agent for oral administration. Chemically, ofloxacin, a fluorinated carboxyquinolone, is the racemate, 7H-pyrido[1,2,3-de]-1,4-benzoxazine-6-carboxylic acid, 9-fluoro-2,3-dihydro-3-methyl-10-(4-methyl-1-piperazinyl)-7-oxo,(±)-. The chemical structure is:

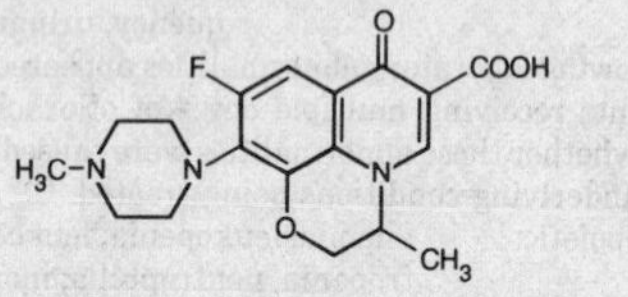

Its empirical formula is $C_{18}H_{20}FN_3O_4$, and its molecular weight is 361.4. Ofloxacin is a cream to pale yellow crystalline powder. The molecule exists as a zwitterion at the pH conditions in the small intestine. At room temperature, between pH 2 and 5, ofloxacin's aqueous solubility is 60 mg/mL. At pH 7, solubility falls to 4 mg/mL and increases to 303 mg/mL at pH 9.8. Ofloxacin has the potential to form stable coordination compounds with many metal ions. This *in vitro* chelation potential has the following formation order: $Fe^{+3} > Cu^{+2} > Ni^{+2} > Pb^{+2} > Zn^{+2} > Mg^{+2} > Ca^{+2} > Ba^{+2}$.

FLOXIN (ofloxacin) tablets contain the following inactive ingredients: anhydrous lactose, carboxymethylcellulose sodium, corn starch, hydroxypropyl cellulose, hydroxypropyl methylcellulose, magnesium stearate, polyethylene glycol, polysorbate 80, sodium starch glycolate, synthetic yellow iron oxide, and titanium dioxide.

CLINICAL PHARMACOLOGY

Following oral administration, the bioavailability of ofloxacin in the tablet formulation is approximately 98%. Maximum serum concentrations are achieved one to two hours after an oral dose. Absorption of ofloxacin after single or multiple doses of 200 to 400 mg is predictable, and the amount of drug absorbed increases proportionately with the dose.

Ofloxacin has biphasic elimination. The half-lives are approximately 4–5 hours and 20–25 hours. However, the longer half-life represents less than 5% of the total AUC. Accumulation at steady-state can be estimated using a half-life of 9 hours. The total clearance and volume of distribution are approximately similar after single or multiple doses. Elimination is mainly by renal excretion. The following are mean peak serum concentrations in healthy 70–80 kg male volunteers after single doses of 200, 300, or 400 mg of ofloxacin or after multiple doses of 400 mg.

Dose	Serum Concentration 2 hours after admin. (μg/mL)	Area Under the Curve (AUC) (μg×hr/mL)
200 mg single dose	1.5	14.1
300 mg single dose	2.4	21.2
400 mg single dose	2.9	31.4
400 mg steady state	4.6	61.0

Steady state concentrations are achieved after four doses and are, approximately, 50% higher than concentrations after single doses. Therefore, after multiple-dose administration of 200 mg and 300 mg doses, peak serum levels of 2.2 μg/mL and 3.6 μg/mL, respectively, are predicted at steady-state.

In vitro, approximately 32% of the drug in serum is protein bound.
Following administration of a single oral 200 mg dose of ofloxacin to 12 healthy volunteers, average urine concentrations were approximately 220 μg/mL 0 to 6 hours after administration. At 12 to 24 hours, urine levels were approximately 34 μg/mL.
Following oral administration of recommended doses, ofloxacin is widely distributed to body tissues and fluids. Ofloxacin has been detected in blister fluid, cervix, lung tissue, ovary, prostatic fluid, prostatic tissue, skin, and sputum. The mean concentration of ofloxacin in these various body fluids and tissues after one or more doses was 0.8 to 1.5 times the concurrent serum level. There is inadequate evidence to establish the extent of distribution to cerebrospinal fluid or brain tissue.
Ofloxacin has a pyridobenzoxazine ring that appears to decrease the extent of parent compound metabolism. Between 70% to 80% of an administered dose of ofloxacin is excreted unchanged via the kidneys within 36 hours of dosing. Studies indicate that less than 5% of an administered dose is recovered in the urine as the desmethyl or N-oxide metabolites. Four to eight percent is excreted in the feces. Mean peak fecal concentration of ofloxacin following multiple doses of 200 mg is approximately 300 μg/g.
The effect that food has on the absorption of ofloxacin tablets has not been studied.
In healthy elderly volunteers (64–74 years of age) with normal renal function, the apparent half-life of ofloxacin is 6 to 8 hours, compared to approximately 5 hours in younger adults. Drug absorption, however, appears to be unaffected by age.
Clearance of ofloxacin is reduced in patients with impaired renal function (creatinine clearance rate ≤50 mL/min), and dosage adjustment is necessary. (See DOSAGE & ADMINISTRATION.)

MICROBIOLOGY

Ofloxacin has *in vitro* activity against a broad range of gram-positive and gram-negative aerobic and anaerobic bacteria. Ofloxacin is bactericidal at concentrations equal to or slightly greater than inhibitory concentrations. Ofloxacin is thought to exert a bactericidal effect of susceptible bacterial cells by inhibiting DNA gyrase, an essential bacterial enzyme which is a critical catalyst in the duplication, transcription, and repair of bacterial DNA.
Ofloxacin has been shown to be active against most strains of the following organisms both *in vitro* and in clinical infections. (See *INDICATIONS AND USAGE*.):
Chlamydia trachomatis
Citrobacter diversus
Enterobacter aerogenes
Escherichia coli
Haemophilus influenzae
Klebsiella pneumoniae
Neisseria gonorrhoeae
Proteus mirabilis
Pseudomonas aeruginosa
Staphylococcus aureus
Streptococcus pneumoniae
Streptococcus pyogenes
Penicillinase production should have no effect on ofloxacin activity.
In addition, ofloxacin has also been shown to be active *in vitro* against most strains of the following organisms; however, *the clinical significance of these data is unknown:*

Gram-positive aerobes:
Enterococcus faecalis
Staphylococcus epidermidis
(including methicillin-resistant strains)
Staphylococcus saprophyticus
Streptococcus agalactiae

Gram-negative aerobes:
Acinetobacter species
Aeromonas hydrophila
Campylobacter jejuni
Citrobacter freundii
Enterobacter cloacae
Haemophilus parainfluenzae
Klebsiella oxytoca
Moraxella (Branhamella) catarrhalis
Morganella morganii
Neisseria meningitidis
Plesiomonas shigelloides
Proteus vulgaris
Providencia rettgeri
Providencia stuartii
Pseudomonas fluorescens
Salmonella species
Serratia marcescens
Shigella species
Vibrio cholerae
Xanthomonas (Pseudomonas) maltophilia
Yersinia enterocolitica

Anaerobes:
Bacteroides fragilis
Bacteroides intermedius
Clostridium perfringens
Clostridium welchii
Gardnerella vaginalis
Peptococcus niger
Peptostreptococcus species

Other organisms:
Chlamydia pneumoniae
Legionella pneumophila
Mycobacterium tuberculosis
Mycoplasma pneumoniae
Ureaplasma urealyticum
Many strains of other streptococcal species, *Enterococcus* species, and anaerobes are resistant to ofloxacin.
Ofloxacin has not been shown to be active against *Treponema pallidum*. (See *WARNINGS*.)
Resistance to ofloxacin due to spontaneous mutation *in vitro* is a rare occurrence (range: 10^{-9} to 10^{-11}). Although cross-resistance has been observed between ofloxacin and other fluoroquinolones, some oroganisms resistant to other quinolones may be susceptible to ofloxacin.

SUSCEPTIBILITY TESTING

Diffusion techniques: Quantitative methods that require measurement of zone diameters give the most precise estimates of antibiotic susceptibility. One such procedure is the National Committee for Clinical Laboratory Standards (NCCLS) approved procedure (M2-A4—Performance Standards for Antimicrobial Disk Susceptibility Tests 1990). This method has been recommended for use with the 5-μg ofloxacin disk to test susceptibility to ofloxacin.
Interpretation involves correlation of the diameters obtained in the disk test with minimum inhibitory concentrations (MIC) for ofloxacin. Other quinolone antibacterial disks should not be substituted when performing susceptibility tests for ofloxacin because of spectrum differences with ofloxacin. The 5-μg ofloxacin disk should be used for all *in vitro* testing of isolates using diffusion techniques.
Reports from the laboratory giving results of the standard single-disk susceptibility test with a 5-μg ofloxacin disk should be interpreted according to the following criteria:

Zone diameter (mm)	Interpretation
≥16	Susceptible
13–15	Moderately Susceptible
≤12	Resistant

A report of "susceptible" indicates that the pathogen is likely to be inhibited by generally achievable blood levels. A report of "moderately susceptible" suggests that the organism would be susceptible if high dosage is used or if the infection is confined to tissues and fluids in which ofloxacin levels are much higher than in plasma. A report of "resistant" indicates that achievable concentrations of ofloxacin are unlikely to be inhibitory and other therapy should be selected.
Standardized procedures require the use of laboratory control organisms. The 5-μg ofloxacin disk should give the following zone diameter:

Organism	Zone diameter (mm)
E. coli ATCC 25922	29–33
P. aeruginosa ATCC 27853	17–21
S. aureus ATCC 25923	24–28

Dilution Techniques: Broth and agar dilution methods, such as those recommended by the NCCLS (M7-A2—Methods for Dilution Antimicrobial Susceptibility Tests for Bacteria that Grow Aerobically 1990), may be used to determine the minimum inhibitory concentrations (MIC) of ofloxacin. MIC test results should be interpreted according to the following criteria:

MIC (μg/mL)	Interpretation
≤2	(S) Susceptible
4	(MS) Moderately Susceptible
≥8	(R) Resistant

As with standard diffusion methods, dilution procedures require the use of laboratory control organisms. Standard ofloxacin powder should give the following MIC values:

Organism	MIC range (μg/mL)
E. coli ATCC 25922	0.015–0.120
E. faecalis ATCC 29212	1.000–4.000
P. aeruginosa ATCC 27853	1.000–8.000
S. aureus ATCC 29213	0.120–1.000

INDICATIONS AND USAGE

FLOXIN (ofloxacin) is indicated for the treatment of adults with the following infections caused by susceptible strains of the designated microorganisms:

Lower Respiratory Tract Infections:
Acute bacterial exacerbations of chronic bronchitis due to *Haemophilus influenzae* or *Streptococcus pneumoniae*.
Pneumonia due to *Haemophilus influenzae* or *Streptococcus pneumoniae*.
Sexually Transmitted Diseases (See *WARNINGS*.):
Acute, uncomplicated urethral and cervical gonorrhea due to *Neisseria gonorrhoeae*.
Nongonococcal urethritis and cervicitis due to *Chlamydia trachomatis*.
Mixed infections of the urethra and cervix due to *Chlamydia trachomatis* and *Neisseria gonorrhoeae*.
Skin and Skin Structure Infections:
Mild to moderate skin and skin structure infections due to *Staphylococcus aureus, Streptococcus pyogenes,* or *Proteus mirabilis**.
Urinary Tract Infections:
Uncomplicated cystitis due to *Citrobacter diversus, Enterobacter aerogenes, Escherichia coli, Klebsiella pneumoniae, Proteus mirabilis, or Pseudomonas aeruginosa*.
Complicated urinary tract infections due to *Escherichia coli, Klebsiella pneumoniae, Proteus mirabilis, Citrobacter diversus**, or *Pseudomonas aeruginosa**.
Prostatitis due to *Escherichia coli*.
Penicillinase production should have no effect on ofloxacin activity.
Appropriate culture and susceptibility tests should be performed before treatment in order to isolate and identify organisms causing the infection and to determine their susceptibility to ofloxacin. Therapy with ofloxacin may be initiated before results of these tests are known; once results become available, appropriate therapy should be continued. Culture and susceptibility testing performed periodically during therapy will provide information not only on the therapeutic effect of the antimicrobial agent but also on the possible emergence of bacterial resistance.

CONTRAINDICATIONS

Ofloxacin is contraindicated in persons with a history of hypersensitivity to ofloxacin or members of the quinolone group of antibacterial agents.

WARNINGS

THE SAFETY AND EFFICACY OF OFLOXACIN IN CHILDREN, ADOLESCENTS (UNDER THE AGE OF 18 YEARS), PREGNANT WOMEN, AND LACTATING WOMEN HAVE NOT BEEN ESTABLISHED. (SEE PEDIATRIC USE, USE IN PREGNANCY, AND NURSING MOTHERS SUBSECTIONS IN THE PRECAUTIONS SECTION.)
In the immature rat, the oral administration of ofloxacin at 5–16 times the proposed therapeutic human dose increased the incidence and severity of osteochondrosis. The lesions did not regress after 13 weeks of drug withdrawal. Other quinolones also produce similar erosions in the weight-bearing joints and other signs of arthropathy in immature animals of various species. (See *ANIMAL PHARMACOLOGY*.)
Ofloxacin has not been shown to be effective in the treatment of syphilis. Antimicrobial agents used in high doses for short periods of time to treat gonorrhea may mask or delay the symptoms of incubating syphilis. All patients with gonorrhea should have a serologic test for syphilis at the time of diagnosis. Patients treated with ofloxacin should have a follow-up serologic test for syphilis after three months.
Serious and occasionally fatal hypersensitivity (anaphylactic) reactions, some following the first dose, have been reported in patients receiving therapy with quinolones including ofloxacin. Some reactions were accompanied by cardiovascular collapse, loss of consciousness, tingling, angioedema (including laryngeal, pharyngeal or facial edema), airway obstruction, dyspnea, urticaria, and itching. If an allergic reaction to ofloxacin occurs, discontinue the drug. Serious acute hypersensitivity reactions may require treatment with epinephrine and other resuscitative measures, including oxygen, intravenous fluids, antihistamines, corticosteroids, pressor amines, and airway management, as clinically indicated.
Severe hypersensitivity reactions (generally following multiple doses) characterized by rash, fever, eosinophilia, jaundice and hepatic necrosis with a fatal outcome have also been reported extremely rarely in patients receiving another quinolone. Similar reactions may occur with ofloxacin. The drug should be discontinued at the first appearance of a skin rash or any other sign of hypersensitivity. (See *PRECAUTIONS* and *ADVERSE REACTIONS*.)
Convulsions, increased intracranial pressure, and toxic psychosis have been reported in patients receiving quinolones, including ofloxacin. Quinolones may also cause central nervous system stimulation which may lead to tremors, restlessness, lightheadedness, confusion, and hallucinations. If these reactions occur in patients receiving ofloxacin, the drug should be discontinued and appropriate measures instituted. No evidence of an effect of ofloxacin on the electrical activity

*Efficacy for this organism in this organ system was studied in fewer than ten infections.

Continued on next page

Ortho—Cont.

of the brain has been demonstrated. Ofloxacin does not alter the metabolism of glucose in the central nervous system based on positron emission tomography. It does not have effects upon the electrical patterns of brain function based on EEGs. However, until more information becomes available, ofloxacin, like all other quinolones, should be used with caution in patients with known or suspected CNS disorders, such as severe cerebral arteriosclerosis or epilepsy, or other factors (e.g. concomitant drug therapy) which predispose to seizures. (See *PRECAUTIONS* and *ADVERSE REACTIONS.*)

Pseudomembranous colitis has been reported with nearly all antibacterial agents, including ofloxacin, and may range in severity from mild to life-threatening. Therefore, it is important to consider this diagnosis in patients who present with diarrhea subsequent to the administration of antibacterial agents. Treatment with antibacterial agents alters the normal flora of the colon and may permit overgrowth of clostridia. Studies indicate that a toxin produced by *Clostridium difficile* is one primary cause of "antibiotic-associated colitis". After the diagnosis of pseudomembranous colitis has been established, therapeutic measures should be initiated. Mild cases of pseudomembranous colitis usually respond to drug discontinuation alone. In moderate to severe cases, consideration should be given to management with fluids and electrolytes, protein supplementation, and treatment with an oral antibacterial drug effective against *C. difficile* (e.g. vancomycin). (See *ADVERSE REACTIONS.*)

PRECAUTIONS

General:
Alteration of the dosage regimen is necessary for patients with impairment of renal function. (See *DOSAGE AND ADMINISTRATION.*)
Moderate to severe phototoxicity reactions have been observed in patients who are exposed to direct sunlight while receiving some drugs in this class. Excessive sunlight should be avoided. Therapy should be discontinued if phototoxicity occurs.
As with any potent drug, periodic assessment of organ system functions, including renal, hepatic, and hematopoietic, is advisable during prolonged therapy.

Information for Patients
Patients should be advised:
—to drink fluids liberally.
—that mineral supplements, vitamins with iron or minerals, calcium-, aluminum- or magnesium-based antacids should not be taken within the two-hour period before or within the two-hour period after taking ofloxacin. (See *DRUG INTERACTIONS.*)
—that ofloxacin should not be taken with food.
—that ofloxacin can cause dizziness and lightheadedness and that, therefore, patients should know how they react to ofloxacin before they operate an automobile or machinery or engage in activities requiring mental alertness and coordination. (See *WARNINGS.*)
—that ofloxacin may be associated with hypersensitivity reactions, even following the first dose, and to discontinue the drug at the first sign of a skin rash, hives, rapid heartbeat, difficulty in swallowing or breathing, any swelling suggesting angioedema, or other allergic reaction. (See *WARNINGS* and *ADVERSE REACTIONS.*)

Drug Interactions
Theophylline: Although concurrent administration of quinolones with theophylline may result in impaired elimination of theophylline, the extent of such impairment varies among different quinolones. In normal volunteer trials, the concomitant administration of ofloxacin with theophylline resulted in either no effect or increases in serum theophylline levels of less than 10%. In a pharmacokinetic study involving 15 healthy male subjects, steady-state peak theophylline concentration increased by approximately 9%, and the AUC increased by approximately 13% when ofloxacin and theophylline were administered concurrently. In clinical trials with intravenous (I.V.) ofloxacin, theophylline concentrations were determined in 41 patients who were treated with both drugs. In 38 patients, no apparent interaction was discernible. However, marginal increases above the theophylline therapeutic range were reported in 3 patients; clinical toxicity was not reported. As with other quinolones, however, concomitant administration of ofloxacin may prolong the half-life of theophylline, elevate serum theophylline levels, and may increase the risk of theophylline-related adverse reactions. Theophylline levels should be closely monitored and theophylline dosage adjustments made, if appropriate, when any quinolone, including ofloxacin, is co-administered.

Antacids, Sucralfate, Metal Cations, Multi-Vitamins, etc.: Quinolones form chelates with alkaline earth and transition metal cations. Administration of quinolones with antacids containing calcium, magnesium, or aluminum, with sucralfate, with divalent or trivalent cations such as iron, or with multivitamins containing zinc may substantially interfere with the absorption of quinolones resulting in systemic levels considerably lower than desired. These agents should not be taken within the two-hour period before or within the two-hour period after ofloxacin administration. (See *DOSAGE AND ADMINISTRATION.*)

Warfarin: Some quinolones have been reported to enhance the effects of the oral anticoagulant warfarin or its derivatives. Therefore, if a quinolone antibiotic is administered concomitantly with warfarin or its derivatives, the prothrombin time (PT) (or other appropriate test(s) of coagulation) should be monitored and the dose of warfarin modified as appropriate.

Interactions between ofloxacin and caffeine have not been detected.

Carcinogenesis, Mutagenesis, Impairment of Fertility
Long-term studies to determine the carcinogenic potential of ofloxacin have not been conducted.
Ofloxacin was not mutagenic in the Ames bacterial test, *in vitro* and *in vivo* cytogenic assay, sister chromatid exchange (Chinese Hamster and Human Cell Lines), unscheduled DNA Repair or dominant lethal assays.

Pregnancy: Teratogenic Effects. Pregnancy Category C.
Ofloxacin has not been shown to have any teratogenic effects at doses as high as 810 mg/kg/day and 160 mg/kg/day when administered to pregnant rats and rabbits, respectively. Additional studies in rats with doses up to 360 mg/kg/day showed no adverse effect on late fetal development, labor, delivery, lactation, neonatal viability, or growth of the newborn. Doses equivalent to 50 and 10 times the maximum therapeutic dose of ofloxacin were fetotoxic (i.e., decreased fetal body weight and increased fetal mortality) in rats and rabbits, respectively. Minor skeletal variations were reported in rats receiving doses of 810 mg/kg/day, which is more than 50 times higher than the maximum intended human dose.
There are, however, no adequate and well-controlled studies in pregnant women. Ofloxacin should be used during pregnancy only if the potential benefit justifies the potential risk to the fetus. (See *WARNINGS.*)

Nursing Mothers
In nursing females, a single 200 mg dose resulted in concentrations of ofloxacin in milk which were similar to those found in plasma. Because of the potential for serious adverse reactions from ofloxacin in nursing infants, a decision should be made whether to discontinue nursing or to discontinue the drug, taking into account the importance of the drug to the mother.

Pediatric Use
Safety and effectiveness in children and adolescents below the age of 18 years have not been established. Ofloxacin causes arthropathy (arthrosis) and osteochondrosis in juvenile animals of several species. (See *WARNINGS.*)

ADVERSE REACTIONS

The incidence of patients reporting drug-related adverse reactions during Phase II and III clinical trials was 11%. Among patients receiving multiple-dose therapy, 4% discontinued the drug due to adverse experiences.
The following events were considered likely to be drug-related in clinical trials in patients receiving multiple doses of oral FLOXIN:
Nausea 3%, Insomnia 3%, Headache 1%, Dizziness 1%, Diarrhea 1%.
The most frequently reported events, regardless of relationship to drug, were:
Nausea 10%, Headache 9%, Insomnia 7%, External genital pruritus in women 6%, Dizziness 5%, Vaginitis 5%, Diarrhea 4%.
In clinical trials the following events, regardless of relationship to drug, were reported by 1 to 3% of patients: vomiting, gastrointestinal distress, pain and cramps, abdominal pain, flatulence, dysgeusia, dry mouth, decreased appetite; fatigue, somnolence, sleep disorders, visual disturbances, nervousness; vaginal discharge; rash, pruritus; pyrexia, chest pain, and trunk pain.
Additional events, occurring at a rate of less than 1%, regardless of relationship to drug, were:
Body as a whole: asthenia, chills, malaise, extremity pain, pain in the body as a whole
Nutritional/Metabolic: thirst, weight loss
Special Senses: decreased hearing acuity, tinnitus, photophobia
Nervous System: anxiety, cognitive change, depression, dream abnormality, euphoria, hallucinations, paresthesia, syncope, vertigo
Cardiovascular System: edema, hypertension, palpitations, vasodilation
Respiratory System: cough, rhinorrhea
Gastrointestinal System: constipation, dyspepsia
Genital/Reproductive System: burning, irritation, pain and rash of the female genitalia; dysmenorrhea; menorrhagia; metrorrhagia
Urinary System: dysuria, urinary frequency
Skin/Hypersensitivity: angioedema, diaphoresis, urticaria, vasculitis
Musculoskeletal System: arthralgia, myalgia

Adverse events reported from marketing experience with ofloxacin or other quinolones, include: anaphylactic reactions; erythema multiforme/Stevens-Johnson syndrome, exfoliative dermatitis, toxic epidermal necrolysis, photosensitivity; seizures, psychotic reactions, ataxia, tremor, agitation, restlessness, aggressiveness, confusion, possible exacerbation of myasthenia gravis, dysphasia; diplopia, nystagmus; dyspnea, bronchospasm, postural hypotension; hepatic dysfunction including: hepatic necrosis, jaundice, hepatitis, and abnormal liver function tests; pseudomembranous colitis; agranulocytosis, leukopenia, thrombocytopenia, prolongation of prothrombin time; vaginal candidiasis; elevation of serum triglycerides, serum cholesterol, blood glucose, serum potassium; albuminuria; candiduria; renal calculi. (See *WARNINGS* and *PRECAUTIONS.*)
In clinical trials using multiple-dose therapy, ophthalmologic abnormalities, including cataracts and multiple punctate lenticular opacities, have been noted in patients undergoing treatment with other quinolones. The relationship of the drugs to these events is not established.
The following laboratory abnormalities appeared in $\geq 1.0\%$ of patients receiving multiple doses of FLOXIN (ofloxacin). It is not known whether these abnormalities were caused by the drug or the underlying conditions.
  Hematopoietic: leukocytosis, lymphocytopenia, increased eosinophils, elevated ESR
  Hepatic: elevated SGPT, elevated SGOT
  Serum chemistry: hyperglycemia, hypoglycemia
  Urinary: glucosuria, proteinuria, hematuria, pyuria
CRYSTALLURIA, CYLINDRURIA AND HEMATURIA HAVE BEEN REPORTED with other quinolones.

OVERDOSAGE
In the event of acute overdose, the stomach should be emptied. The patient should be observed and appropriate hydration maintained. Ofloxacin is not efficiently removed by hemodialysis or peritoneal dialysis.

DOSAGE AND ADMINISTRATION
The usual daily dose of FLOXIN (ofloxacin) is 200 mg to 400 mg orally every 12 hours as described in the following chart. These recommendations apply to patients with normal renal function (i.e. creatinine clearance greater than 50 mL/min). For patients with altered renal function (i.e. creatinine clearance less than or equal to 50 mL/min) see the section **Dosage Adjustment for Renal Impairment.**
[See table on next page.]
Antacids containing calcium, magnesium, or aluminum sucralfate; divalent or trivalent cations such as iron; or multivitamins containing zinc should not be taken within the two-hour before, or within the two-hour period after ofloxacin administrations. (See *PRECAUTIONS.*)

Dosage Adjustment For Renal Impairment
Dosage should be adjusted for patients with a creatinine clearance value less than or equal to 50 mL/min. **After a normal initial dose,** dosage should be adjusted as follows:

Creatinine Clearance	Maintenance Unit Dose	Frequency
10–50 mL/min	As recommended in table above	q 24h
< 10 mL/min	½ dose recommended in table above	q 24h

When only the serum creatinine is known, the following formula may be used to estimate creatinine clearance.
Men: Creatinine clearance
$$(\text{mL/min}) = \frac{\text{Weight (kg)} \times (140 - \text{age})}{72 \times \text{serum creatinine (mg/dL)}}$$
Women: $0.85 \times$ the value calculated for men.
The serum creatinine should represent a steady state of renal function.

HOW SUPPLIED
FLOXIN (ofloxacin) is supplied as 200 mg, 300 mg, and 400 mg film-coated, pale gold tablets. Each tablet is printed with 'FLOXIN' and the appropriate strength. FLOXIN (ofloxacin) is packaged in bottles of 50 tablets and in unit-dose blister strips of 100 tablets in the following configurations:
200 mg tablets—bottles of 50 (NDC 0062-1540-02)
200 mg tablets—unit-dose/100 tablets (NDC 0062-1540-05)
300 mg tablets—bottles of 50 (NDC 0062-1541-02)
300 mg tablets—unit-dose/100 tablets (NDC 0062-1541-05)
400 mg tablets—bottles of 50 (NDC 0062-1542-02)
400 mg tablets—unit-dose/100 tablets (NDC 0062-1542-05)
FLOXIN (ofloxacin) tablets should be stored in well-closed containers. Store below 86°F (30°C).

ANIMAL PHARMACOLOGY
Ofloxacin and other drugs of the quinolone class have been shown to cause arthropathies (arthrosis) in immature dogs and rats, and, in addition, is associated with an increased incidence of osteochondrosis in rats as compared to the incidence observed in vehicle-treated rats. (See *WARNINGS.*) There is no evidence of arthropathies in fully

mature dogs at doses up to 5 times the recommended human clinical dose.
Long-term, high dose systemic use of other quinolones in experimental animals has caused lenticular opacities; however, this finding was not observed in any animal studies with ofloxacin.
Crystalluria and ocular toxicity were not observed in any animals treated with ofloxacin.
FLOXIN® is a trademark of Ortho Pharmaceutical Corporation.
U.S. Patent No. 4,382,982
Caution: Federal (U.S.A.) law prohibits dispensing without prescription.
Revised September 1991 633-10-270-4
Shown in Product Identification Section, page 421

Infection	Description	Unit Dose	Frequency	Duration	Daily Dose
Lower Respiratory Tract Infections	Exacerbation of Chronic Bronchitis	400 mg	q 12h	10 days	800 mg
	Pneumonia	400 mg	q 12h	10 days	800 mg
Sexually Transmitted Diseases	Acute, uncomplicated gonorrhea	400 mg	single dose	1 day	400 mg
	Cervicitis/urethritis due to *C. trachomatis*	300 mg	q 12h	7 days	600 mg
	Cervicitis/urethritis due to *C. trachomatis* and *N. gonorrhoeae*	300 mg	q 12h	7 days	600 mg
Skin and Skin Structure Infections	Mild to moderate	400 mg	q 12h	10 days	800 mg
Urinary Tract	Cystitis due to *E. Coli* or *K. pneumoniae*	200 mg	q 12h	3 days	400 mg
	Cystitis due to other organisms	200 mg	q 12h	7 days	400 mg
	Complicated UTI's	200 mg	q 12h	10 days	400 mg
Prostatitis		300 mg	q 12h	6 weeks	600 mg

GYNOL II® Contraceptive Jelly OTC

(See PDR For Nonprescription Drugs.)

GYNOL II® Extra Strength Contraceptive Jelly OTC

(See PDR For Nonprescription Drugs.)

LIPPES LOOP™ ℞
Intrauterine Device

DESCRIPTION
The LIPPES LOOP is made of polyethylene in the shape of a double S. Four different sizes are manufactured to allow for the variability in the size of the uterus. (See below.) A fine, double thread or "tail" made of polyethylene suture (monofilament) is attached to the lower end to facilitate removal. In addition, palpation of the tail through the cervix by the patient, or visualization by the physician, can assist in determining whether or not an undetected expulsion has occurred. A LIPPES LOOP comes prepackaged and sterilized with an introducer, together with an insertion tube in a polyethylene pouch. The insertion tube is equipped with a flange to aid in gauging the depth to which the insertion tube should be inserted through the cervical canal and into the uterine cavity. The four available sizes are as follows:

Loop A—22.2 mm. Blue thread. For those women who cannot tolerate a larger size device.

Loop B—27.5 mm. WITH REDUCED RADII. Black thread. Suggested for women who have had premature pregnancy losses and multiparous females whose uteri sound out less than 6 cm.

Loop C—30 mm. WITH REDUCED RADII. Yellow thread. Suggested for use when Loop D is removed for bleeding or pain. The physician is advised to wait two to four weeks between removing a loop for bleeding and reinserting a second loop.

Loop D—30 mm. White thread. Suggested for use in women with one or more children.

Mode of Action or Principles of IUD Design:
The exact mechanism of action of the LIPPES LOOP is not known. However, it is believed to interfere in some manner with nidation in the endometrium, probably through foreign body reaction in the uterus.

INDICATIONS AND USAGE
LIPPES LOOP is indicated for contraception.

CONTRAINDICATIONS
IUD's should not be inserted when the following conditions exist:

1. Pregnancy or suspicion of pregnancy.
2. Abnormalities of the uterus resulting in distortion of the uterine cavity.
3. Pelvic inflammatory disease or a history of repeated pelvic inflammatory disease.
4. Postpartum endometritis or infected abortion in the past three months.
5. Known or suspected uterine or cervical malignancy including unresolved, abnormal "Pap" smear.
6. Genital bleeding of unknown etiology.
7. Cervicitis until infection is controlled.

WARNINGS
1. Pregnancy. a. Long-term effects. Long-term effects on the offspring when pregnancy occurs with LIPPES LOOP in place are unknown.
b. Septic abortion. Reports have indicated an increased incidence of septic abortion associated in some instances with septicemia, septic shock, and death in patients becoming pregnant with an IUD in place. Most of these reports have been associated with the mid-trimester of pregnancy. In some cases, the initial symptoms have been insidious and not easily recognized. If pregnancy should occur with an IUD in place, the IUD should be removed if the string is visible or, if removal proves to be or would be difficult, termination of the pregnancy should be considered and offered the patient as an option, bearing in mind that the risks associated with an elective abortion increase with gestational age.
c. Continuation of pregnancy. If the patient chooses to continue the pregnancy, she must be warned of the increased risk of spontaneous abortion and of the increased risk of sepsis, including death, if the pregnancy continues with the IUD in place. The patient must be closely observed and she must be advised to report all abnormal symptoms, such as flu-like syndrome, fever, abdominal cramping and pain, bleeding, or vaginal discharge, immediately because generalized symptoms of septicemia may be insidious.
2. Ectopic pregnancy. a. A pregnancy that occurs with an IUD in place is more likely to be ectopic than a pregnancy occurring without an IUD in place. Accordingly, patients who become pregnant while using the IUD should be carefully evaluated for the possibility of an ectopic pregnancy.
b. Special attention should be directed to patients with delayed menses, slight metrorrhagia and/or unilateral pelvic pain, and to those patients who wish to terminate a pregnancy because of IUD failure, to determine whether ectopic pregnancy has occurred.
3. Pelvic infection. An increased risk of pelvic infection has been reported with the IUD in place. Although the etiology of this risk is not understood, it has been suggested that the tail may act as a mechanism for the passage of vaginal bacteria into the uterus. This, at times, may result in the development of bilateral or unilateral tubo-ovarian abscesses or general peritonitis. Pelvic infection may lead to hospitalization or surgery and infertility. Appropriate aerobic and anaerobic bacteriological studies should be done and antibiotic therapy initiated. The IUD should be removed and the continuing treatment reassessed based upon the results of culture and sensitivity tests.
Because of the increased risk of pelvic infection, the physician may wish each woman who has an IUD in place to have a periodic cervical vaginal "Pap" smear and pelvic exam. All "Pap" smears should include specific evaluation for actinomycosis.
4. Effect on future fertility. An increased risk of tubal infertility, with or without prior symptoms of pelvic infection, has been associated with the use of IUD's, particularly inert IUD's, including the LIPPES LOOP. This risk appears to be greatest for nulliparous women and those exposed to multiple sexual partners. The decision to use an IUD must be made by the physician and patient with appropriate regard for the possibility of future infertility. This consideration is especially important for women, particularly nulliparous women, who may wish to have children at a later date.
5. Embedment. Partial penetration or lodging of the IUD in the endometrium can result in difficult removals.
6. Perforation. Partial or total perforation of the uterine wall or cervix may occur with the use of IUDs. The possibility of perforation must be kept in mind during insertion and at the time of any subsequent examination. If perforation occurs, the IUD should be removed. Adhesions, foreign body reactions, and intestinal obstruction may result if an IUD is left in the peritoneal cavity. There are a few reports that there has been migration after insertion apparently in the absence of perforation at insertion. In any event, it is possible for the IUD to perforate outside the uterus.

PRECAUTIONS
1. Patient counseling. Prior to insertion, the physician, nurse or other trained health professional must provide the patient with the Patient Brochure. The patient should be given the opportunity to read the brochure and discuss fully any questions she may have concerning the IUD as well as other methods of contraception.
2. Patient evaluation and clinical considerations. a. A complete medical history should be obtained to determine conditions that might influence the selection of an IUD. Physical examination should include a pelvic examination, "Pap" smear, gonorrhea culture and, if indicated, appropriate tests for other forms of venereal disease. Papanicolaou smears should include specific evaluation for actinomycosis.
b. The uterus should be carefully sounded prior to insertion to determine the degree of patency of the endocervical canal and the internal os, and the direction and depth of the uterine cavity. In occasional cases, severe cervical stenosis may be encountered. Do not use excessive force to overcome this resistance.
c. The uterus should sound to a depth of 6 to 8 centimeters (cm). Insertion of an IUD into a uterine cavity measuring less than 6.5 cm by sounding may increase the incidence of expulsion, bleeding, pain and perforation.
d. The possibility of insertion in the presence of an existing undetermined pregnancy is reduced if insertion is performed during or shortly following a menstrual period. The IUD should not be inserted postpartum or postabortion until involution of the uterus is completed. The incidence of perforation and expulsion is greater if involution is not completed.
e. IUD's should be used with caution in those patients who have anemia or a history of menorrhagia or hypermenorrhea. Patients experiencing menorrhagia and/or metrorrhagia following IUD insertion may be at risk for the development of hypochromic microcytic anemia. Also, IUD's should be used with caution in patients receiving anticoagulants or having a coagulopathy.
f. Syncope, bradycardia, or other neurovascular episodes may occur during insertion or removal of IUD's especially in patients with a previous disposition to these conditions.
g. Patients with valvular or congenital heart disease are more prone to develop subacute bacterial endocarditis than patients who do not have valvular or congenital heart disease. Use of an IUD in these patients may represent a potential source of septic emboli.
h. Use of an IUD in those patients with cervicitis should be postponed until treatment has cured the infection (see CONTRAINDICATIONS Section).
i. Since an IUD may be expelled or displaced, patients should be reexamined and evaluated shortly after the first postinsertion menses, but definitely within three months after insertion. Thereafter, annual examination with appropriate medical and laboratory examination should be carried out.
j. The patient should be told that some bleeding and cramps may occur during the first few weeks after insertion, but if these symptoms continue or are severe, she should report them to her physician. The patient should be instructed on how to check to make certain that the thread still protrudes from the cervix, and she should be cautioned that there is no contraceptive protection if the IUD is expelled. She should be instructed to check the tail as often as possible, but at least after each menstrual period. The patient should be cautioned not to pull on the thread and displace the IUD. If partial expulsion occurs, removal is indicated and a new IUD may be inserted.
k. The use of medical diathermy (shortwave and microwave) in patients with metal-containing IUD's may cause heat injury to the surrounding tissue. Therefore, medical diathermy to the abdominal and sacral areas should not be used.
[LIPPES LOOP contains no metals. This section does not apply to LIPPES LOOP].

ADVERSE REACTIONS
These adverse reactions are not listed in any order of frequency or severity.

Continued on next page

Ortho—Cont.

TABLE I

LIPPES LOOP Size	Number Woman/Months	Woman/Months of Use 1st Year After Insertion	Woman/Months of Use 2nd Year After Insertion
A	13,453	8,751	4,702
B	12,463	9,660	2,803
C	50,775	31,032	19,743
D	121,566	72,046	49,520

Reported adverse reactions include: endometritis, spontaneous abortion, septic abortion, septicemia, perforation of the uterus and cervix, embedment, migration resulting in partial or complete perforation, fragmentation of the IUD, pelvic infection (pelvic inflammatory disease), future infertility, vaginitis, leukorrhea, cervical erosion, pregnancy, ectopic pregnancy, difficult removal, complete or partial expulsion of the IUD, intermenstrual spotting, prolongation of menstrual flow, anemia, pain and cramping, dysmenorrhea, backaches, dyspareunia, neurovascular episodes, including bradycardia and syncope secondary to insertion. Perforation into the abdomen has been followed by abdominal adhesions, intestinal penetration, intestinal obstruction, and cystic masses in the pelvis.

DIRECTIONS FOR USE
Preinsertion

1. It is imperative that sterile technique be maintained throughout the insertion procedure.

2. Perform a thorough pelvic examination to determine freedom from overt disease and to determine position and shape of the uterus. RULE OUT PREGNANCY AND OTHER CONTRAINDICATIONS.

3. With a speculum in place, gently insert a sterile sound to determine the depth and direction of the uterine canal. Be sure to determine the position of the uterus before insertion. Occasionally a tenaculum is required if the uterine canal needs to be straightened. If a stenotic cervix must be dilated, use a sterile Hank's dilator rather than a Hegar's; dilation to a Hank's 16 to 18 should be sufficient.

Insertion

Caution: It is generally felt that perforations are caused at the time of insertion, although the perforation may not be detected until some time later. The position of the uterus should be determined during the preinsertion examination. Great care must be exercised during the preinsertion sounding and subsequent insertion. No attempt should be made to force the insertion. There are a few reports, however, that there has been migration after insertion apparently in the absence of perforation at insertion. In any event, it is possible for the IUD to perforate outside the uterus.

1. How to prepare the LIPPES LOOP Intrauterine Double-S inserter.
Using sterile gloves, hold tube in one hand and with the other draw LOOP into inserter by pulling the push rod. As the LOOP is drawn into the inserter you will encounter some resistance. It is important to use a slow steady pulling action until all but the bulbous tip of the LOOP is entirely within the inserter. At this point, insure that both the flat surface of the bulbous tip and the inserter flange are in a horizontal plane.
Do this not more than one minute before insertion.

2. How to insert LIPPES LOOP Intrauterine Double-S.
Insert the loaded inserter gently through the endocervical canal, with the flange in a horizontal plane. DO NOT FORCE THE INSERTION. If resistance is encountered, do not proceed; perforation of the uterus may occur. If the flange makes contact with the cervix WITHOUT the inserter touching the fundal wall, withdraw ¼ inch before pressing the push rod to release the device in utero. Should the inserter touch the fundal wall BEFORE the flange makes contact, withdraw ½ inch prior to pressing the push rod to release the device in utero. With the inserter now in place, proceed, and WITHOUT UNDUE PRESSURE, push the rod slowly as far as it will go. LIPPES LOOP Intrauterine Double-S should now be in place. Withdraw the inserter tube and push rod from the cervical os until the tail is visible. Cut the tail leaving it as long as possible.

Time of Insertion
LIPPES LOOP Intrauterine Double-S should be inserted preferably the last one or two days of a normal menstrual period or the two days following the last day.
The expulsion and perforation rate may be increased when insertions are made before normal uterine involution occurs (usually four to six weeks postpartum or postabortion).

To Remove
To remove LIPPES LOOP Intrauterine Double-S, pull gently on the exposed tail. On those rare occasions that the tail is not available, the device should be carefully removed.

CLINICAL STUDIES
Different event rates have been recorded with the use of different IUD's. Inasmuch as these rates are usually derived from separate studies conducted by different investigators in several population groups, they cannot be compared with precision. Furthermore, event rates tend to be lower as clinical experience is expanded, possibly due to retention in the clinical study of those patients who accept the treatment regimen and do not discontinue due to adverse reactions or pregnancy. In clinical trials conducted by the Population Council with the LIPPES LOOP, use effectiveness was determined as follows for women, as tabulated by the life table method. (Rates are expressed as events per 100 women through 12 and 24 months of use). This experience is based on 198,257 woman/months of use, including 121,489 woman/months of use in first year after insertion, and 76,768 woman/months of use in second year after insertion. LIPPES LOOP Intrauterine Double-S devices are manufactured in four different sizes, and the figures given above represent the totals for the four sizes. The following table presents these figures individually for each size LOOP:
[See table above.]

Tables II–V below give the pregnancy, expulsion, medical removal and continuation rates for each individual size LOOP:

TABLE II
LOOP A
(Annual Rates Per 100 Users)

	12 Months	24 Months (cumulative)
Pregnancy	5.3	9.7
Expulsion	23.9	27.7
Medical Removal	12.2	20.0
Continuation Rate	75.2	63.6

TABLE III
LOOP B
(Annual Rates Per 100 Users)

	12 Months	24 Months (cumulative)
Pregnancy	3.4	6.3
Expulsion	18.9	24.9
Medical Removal	15.1	23.8
Continuation Rate	74.6	59.2

TABLE IV
LOOP C
(Annual Rates Per 100 Users)

	12 Months	24 Months (cumulative)
Pregnancy	3.0	4.8
Expulsion	19.1	24.6
Medical Removal	14.3	22.1
Continuation Rate	76.5	62.8

TABLE V
LOOP D
(Annual Rates Per 100 Users)

	12 Months	24 Months (cumulative)
Pregnancy	2.7	4.2
Expulsion	12.7	16.0
Medical Removal	15.2	23.3
Continuation Rate	77.4	65.6

LUTREPULSE® for Injection   ℞
(gonadorelin acetate)
Synthetic Gonadotropin-Releasing Hormone (GnRH)
For Pulsatile Intravenous Injection

DESCRIPTION
LUTREPULSE (gonadorelin acetate) for Injection is used for the induction of ovulation in women with primary hypothalamic amenorrhea. Gonadorelin acetate is a synthetic decapeptide that is identical in amino acid sequence to endogenous gonadotropin-releasing hormone (GnRH) synthesized in the human hypothalamus and in various neurons terminating in the hypothalamus. The molecular formula of gonadorelin acetate is:

$$C_{55}H_{75}N_{17}O_{13} \cdot xC_2H_4O_2 \cdot yH_2O$$

Its molecular weight is $1182.3 + x60 + y18$, where x and y represent a non-stoichiometric ratio of acetate and water

associated with the peptide, and x ranges from 1–2 and y ranges from 2–3. The amino acid sequence of GnRH is:
5-oxoPro-His-Trp-Ser-Tyr-Gly-Leu-Arg-Pro-Gly-NH₂

LUTREPULSE for Injection is a sterile, lyophilized powder intended for intravenous pulsatile injection after reconstitution. It is white and very soluble in water. Vials are available containing 0.8 mg or 3.2 mg gonadorelin acetate (expressed as the diacetate) and 10.0 mg mannitol as a carrier. After reconstituting with 8 mL of diluent (sterile 0.9% Sodium Chloride Solution and hydrochloric acid to adjust the pH) for LUTREPULSE for Injection, the concentration of gonadorelin acetate is 5 μg per 50 μl in each vial containing 0.8 mg lyophilized hormone, and 20 μg per 50 μl in each vial containing 3.2 mg lyophilized hormone. LUTREPULSE (gonadorelin acetate) for Injection is intended for use with the LUTREPULSE for Injection KITS. The volumes and concentrations are specific for use with the LUTREPULSE PUMP for appropriate dosing.

CLINICAL PHARMACOLOGY
Under physiologic conditions, gonadotropin-releasing hormone (GnRH) is released by the hypothalamus in a pulsatile fashion. The primary effect of GnRH is the synthesis and release of luteinizing hormone (LH) in the anterior pituitary gland. GnRH also stimulates the synthesis and release of follicle stimulating hormone (FSH), but this effect is less pronounced. LH and FSH subsequently stimulate the gonads to produce steroids which are instrumental in regulating reproductive hormonal status. Unlike human menopausal gonadotropin (hMG) which supplies pituitary hormones, pulsatile administration of LUTREPULSE for Injection replaces defective hypothalamic secretion of GnRH. The pulsatile administration of LUTREPULSE for Injection approximates the natural hormonal secretory pattern, causing pulsatile release of pituitary gonadotropins. Accordingly, LUTREPULSE for Injection is useful in treating conditions of infertility caused by defective GnRH stimulation from the hypothalamus (See INDICATIONS AND USAGE). The following information summarizes clinical efficacy of gonadorelin acetate administered by pulsatile intravenous injection to patients with primary hypothalamic amenorrhea.

44 patients with primary hypothalamic amenorrhea (HA)
93% (41/44) patients ovulatory with gonadorelin acetate therapy
62% (24/39)* patients pregnant
100% (7/7) of those failing past attempts at ovulation induction by other methods were ovulatory on gonadorelin acetate.

Following intravenous injection of GnRH into normal subjects and/or hypogonadotropic patients, plasma GnRH concentrations rapidly decline with initial and terminal half-lives of 2–10 min. and 10–40 min., respectively. In these studies, high clearance values (500–1500 L/day) and low volumes of distribution (10–15 L) were calculated. The pharmacokinetics of GnRH in normal subjects and in hypogonadotropic patients were similar. GnRH was rapidly metabolized to various biologically inactive peptide fragments which are readily excreted in urine. Renal failure, but not hepatic disease, prolonged the half-life and reduced the clearance of GnRH.

INDICATIONS AND USAGE
LUTREPULSE (gonadorelin acetate) for Injection is indicated in the treatment of primary hypothalamic amenorrhea.
DIFFERENTIAL DIAGNOSIS: Proper diagnosis is critical for successful treatment with LUTREPULSE for Injection. It must be established that hypothalamic amenorrhea or hypogonadism is, in fact, due to a deficiency in quantity or pulsing of endogenous GnRH. The diagnosis of hypothalamic amenorrhea or hypogonadism is based on the exclusion of other causes of the dysfunction, since there is currently no practical technique to directly assess hypothalamic function. Prior to initiation of therapy with LUTREPULSE (gonadorelin acetate) for Injection, the physician should rule out disorders of general health, reproductive organs, anterior pituitary, and central nervous system, other than abnormalities of GnRH secretion.

CONTRAINDICATIONS
LUTREPULSE for Injection is contraindicated in women with any condition that could be exacerbated by pregnancy. For example, pituitary prolactinoma should be considered one such condition. Additionally, any history of sensitivity to gonadorelin acetate, gonadorelin hydrochloride or any component of LUTREPULSE for Injection is a contraindication. Patients who have ovarian cysts or causes of anovulation other than those of hypothalamic origin should not receive LUTREPULSE for Injection.
LUTREPULSE for Injection is intended to initiate events including the production of reproductive hormones (e.g. estrogens and progestins). Therefore, any condition that may be worsened by reproductive hormones, such as hormonally-dependent tumor, is a contraindication to the use of LUTREPULSE for Injection.

*Five patients did not desire pregnancy.

WARNINGS

Therapy with LUTREPULSE (gonadorelin acetate) for Injection should be conducted by physicians familiar with pulsatile GnRH delivery and the clinical ramifications of ovulation induction. While there have been few cases of hyperstimulation(<1%) this possibility must be considered. If hyperstimulation should occur, therapy should be discontinued and spontaneous resolution can be expected. The preservation of the endogenous feedback mechanisms makes severe hyperstimulation (with ascites and pleural effusion) rare. However, the physician shoud be aware of the possibility and be alert for any evidence of ascites, pleural effusion, hemoconcentration, rupture of a cyst, fluid or electrolyte imbalance, or sepsis.

Multiple pregnancy is a possibility that can be minimized by careful attention to the recommended doses and ultrasonographic monitoring of the ovarian response to therapy. Following a baseline pelvic ultrasound, follow-up studies should be conducted at a minimum on day 7 and day 14 of therapy.

Serious hypersensitivity reactions (anaphylaxis) have been reported following gonadotropin-releasing hormone administration, including gonadorelin acetate. Clinical manifestations may include: cardiovascular collapse, hypotension, tachycardia, loss of consciousness, angioedema, bronchospasm, dyspnea, urticaria, flushing and pruritus. If any allergic reaction occurs, therapy with gonadorelin should be discontinued. Serious acute hypersensitivity reactions may require emergency medical treatment.

As with any intravenous medication, scrupulous attention to asepsis is important. The infusion area must be monitored as with all indwelling parenteral approaches. The cannula and IV site should be changed at 48-hour intervals.

PRECAUTIONS

GENERAL: Ovarian hyperstimulation has been reported. This may be related to pulse dosage or concomitant use of other ovulation stimulators. Hyperstimulation may be a greater risk in patients where spontaneous variations in endogenous GnRH secretion occur. Multiple follicle development, multiple pregnancy, and spontaneous termination of pregnancy have been reported. Multiple pregnancy can be minimized by appropriate monitoring of follicle formation; nonetheless, the patient and her partner should be advised of the frequency (12%) and potential risks of multiple pregnancy before starting treatment.

Ovarian hyperstimulation, a syndrome of sudden ovarian enlargement, ascites with or without pain, and/or pleural effusion, is rare with pulsatile GnRH therapy. Among 268 patients participating in clinical trials, one case of moderate hyperstimulation has been reported, but this cycle included the concomitant use of clomiphene citrate.

Antibody formation (IgE and IgG) has been reported following administration of gonadorelin. The safety and efficacy implication of antibody development are uncertain (see: **WARNINGS**).

LUTREPULSE (gonadorelin acetate) for Injection should be administered only with the LUTREPULSE PUMP. The patient should be provided with detailed oral and written instructions regarding infusion pump usage and potential sepsis in order to minimize the frequency of infusion pump malfunction and inflammation, infection, mild phlebitis, or hematoma at the catheter site.

INFORMATION FOR PATIENTS: The patient should be advised to discontinue the drug and seek medical attention at the first sign of skin rash, urticaria, rapid heart beat, difficulty in swallowing and breathing, or any swelling which may suggest angioedema (see: **WARNINGS** and **ADVERSE REACTIONS**).

LABORATORY TESTS: Following a diagnosis of primary hypothalamic amenorrhea, initiation of LUTREPULSE (gonadorelin acetate) for Injection therapy may be monitored by the following:

1) Ovarian ultrasound—baseline, therapy day 7, therapy day 14.
2) Mid-luteal phase serum progesterone.
3) Clinical observation of infusion site at each visit as needed.
4) Physical examination including pelvic at regularly scheduled visits.

DRUG INTERACTIONS: None are known. LUTREPULSE for Injection should not be used concomitantly with other ovulation stimulators.

DRUG/LABORATORY TEST INTERACTIONS: None are known.

CARCINOGENESIS, MUTAGENESIS, IMPAIRMENT OF FERTILITY: Since GnRH is a natural substance normally present in humans, long-term studies in animals have not been performed to evaluate carcinogenic potential. Mutagenicity testing was not done.

PREGNANCY: Pregnancy Category B

Reproduction studies (teratology and embryo-toxicity) performed in rats and rabbits have not revealed any evidence of harm to the fetus due to gonadorelin acetate. There was no evidence of teratogenicity when gonadorelin acetate was administered intravenously up to 120 μg/kg/day (>70 times the recommended human dose of 5 μg per pulse) in rats and rabbits.

Studies in pregnant women have shown that gonadorelin acetate does not increase the risk of abnormalities when administered during the first trimester of pregnancy. It appears that the possibility of fetal harm is remote, if the drug is used during pregnancy. In clinical studies, 47 pregnant patients have used gonadorelin acetate during the first trimester of pregnancy (51 pregnancies) and the drug had no apparent adverse effect on the course of pregnancy. Available follow-up reports on infants born to these women reveal no adverse effects or complications that were attributable to gonadorelin acetate. Nevertheless, because the studies in humans cannot rule out the possibility of harm, gonadorelin acetate should be used during pregnancy only for maintenance of the corpus luteum in ovulation induction cycles.

NURSING MOTHERS: It is not known whether this drug is excreted in human milk. There is no indication for use of LUTREPULSE (gonadorelin acetate) for Injection in a nursing woman.

PEDIATRIC USE: Safety and effectiveness in children under the age of 18 have not been established.

ADVERSE REACTIONS

Adverse reactions have been reported in approximately 10% of treatment regimens. Ten of 268 patients interrupted therapy because of an adverse reaction but subsequently resumed treatment. One other subject did not resume treatment.

In clinical studies involving 268 women, one case of moderate ovarian hyperstimulation has been reported. This cycle included concomitant use of clomiphene citrate. This low incidence of hyperstimulation appears to be due to the preservation of normal feedback mechanisms of the pituitary-ovarian axis.

Despite the preservation of feedback mechanisms, some incidents of multiple follicle development, multiple pregnancy, and spontaneous termination of pregnancy have been reported. Multiple pregnancy can be minimized by appropriate monitoring of follicle formation; nonetheless, the patient and her partner should be advised of the frequency and potential hazards of multiple pregnancy before starting treatment. In clinical studies involving 142 pregnancies, delivery information was available on 89 pregnancies. Eleven of these LUTREPULSE (gonadorelin acetate) for Injection-induced pregnancies (12%) were multiple (10 sets of twins, 1 set of triplets).

The following adverse reactions have occurred at the injection site: urticaria, pruritus, inflammation, infection, mild phlebitis, or hematoma at the catheter site. Additionally, infusion set malfunction and interruption of infusion may occur; this has no known adverse effect other than interruption of therapy. Acute generalized (anaphylaxis, angioedema, urticaria, etc.) hypersensitivity reactions have been reported (see: **WARNINGS** and **PRECAUTIONS**).

Anaphylaxis (bronchospasm, tachycardia, flushing, urticaria, induration at injection site) has also been reported with the related polypeptide hormone gonadorelin hydrochloride (FACTREL®).

® Registered trademark of Wyeth-Ayerst Laboratories.

OVERDOSAGE

Continuous, non-pulsatile exposure to gonadorelin acetate could temporarily reduce pituitary responsiveness. If the pump should malfunction and deliver the entire contents of the 3.2 mg system, no harmful effects would be expected. Bolus doses as high as 3000 μg of gonadorelin hydrochloride have not been harmful. Pituitary hyperstimulation and multiple follicle development can be minimized by adhering to recommended doses, and appropriate monitoring of follicle formation (see **PRECAUTIONS**).

Administration of 640 μg/kg in monkeys as a single intravenous bolus resulted in no compound-related effects in clinical observations or gross morphologic evaluations.

DOSAGE AND ADMINISTRATION

DOSAGE: Dosages between 1 and 20 μg have been successfully used in clinical studies. The recommended dose in primary hypothalamic amenorrhea is 5 μg every 90 minutes. This is delivered by LUTREPULSE PUMP using the 0.8 mg solution at 50 μl per pulse (see physician pump manual). Sixty-eight percent of the 5 μg every 90 minute regimens induced ovulation in patients with primary hypothalamic amenorrhea.

The LUTREPULSE PUMP is capable of delivering 2.5, 5, 10, or 20 μg of gonadorelin acetate every 90 minutes. Some women may require a reduction in the recommended dose of 5 μg should laboratory testing and patient monitoring indicate an inappropriate response. While most primary hypothalamic amenorrhea patients will ovulate during the first cycle of 5 μg therapy, some may be refractory to this dose. The recommended treatment interval is 21 days. It may be necessary to raise the dose cautiously, and in stepwise fashion if there is no response after three treatment intervals. All dose changes should be carefully monitored for inappropriate response.

The following table can be used to calculate the dose per pulse when individualizing treatment:

Vial	Diluent	Volume/pulse	Dose/pulse
0.8 mg	8 mL	25 μL	2.5 μg
0.8 mg	8 mL	50 μL	5 μg
3.2 mg	8 mL	25 μL	10 μg
3.2 mg	8 mL	50 μL	20 μg

The response to LUTREPULSE (gonadorelin acetate) for Injection usually occurs within two to three weeks after therapy initiation. When ovulation occurs with the LUTREPULSE PUMP in place, therapy should be continued for another two weeks to maintain the corpus luteum. A comparison of LUTREPULSE for Injection to hCG or hCG + LUTREPULSE for Injection for corpus luteum maintenance revealed the following information:

hCG

Delivered = $\frac{43}{63}$ = 68%

Aborted = $\frac{20}{63}$ = 32%

LUTREPULSE for Injection

Delivered = $\frac{19}{26}$ = 73%

Aborted = $\frac{7}{26}$ = 27%

hCG + LUTREPULSE for Injection

Delivered = $\frac{19}{25}$ = 76%

Aborted = $\frac{6}{25}$ = 24%

LUTREPULSE (gonadorelin acetate) for Injection alone was able to maintain the corpus luteum during pregnancy.

ADMINISTRATION: LUTREPULSE for Injection is to be reconstituted aseptically with 8 mL of diluent for LUTREPULSE for Injection. *The drug product should be reconstituted immediately prior to use and transferred to the plastic reservoir.* First withdraw 8 mL of the saline diluent and then inject it onto the lyophile (drug product) cake. The product is shaken for a few seconds to produce a solution which should be clear, colorless, and free of particulate matter. Parenteral drug products should be inspected visually for particulate matter and discoloration prior to administration, whenever solution and container permit. If particulate matter or discoloration are present, the solution should not be used. A presterilized reservoir (bag) with the infusion catheter set supplied with the LUTREPULSE for Injection is filled with the reconstituted solution, and administered intravenously using the LUTREPULSE PUMP. The pump should be set to deliver 25 or 50 μL of solution, based upon the dose selected, over a pulse period of one minute and at a pulse frequency of 90 minutes. The 8 mL of solution will supply 90 minute pulsatile doses for approximately 7 consecutive days.

HOW SUPPLIED

LUTREPULSE (gonadorelin acetate) for Injection is supplied in a LUTREPULSE for Injection 0.8 mg (NDC 55566-7212-1) or 3.2 mg (NDC 55566-7211-1) KIT. Each kit contains one 10 mL vial of 0.8 mg or 3.2 mg LUTREPULSE for Injection as a lyophilized, sterile powder which should be stored at controlled room temperature (15–30°C, 59–86°F). The following components are included in each kit:

10 mL diluent for LUTREPULSE for Injection
Sterile catheter tubing
Sterile reservoir catheter with double-female luer adaptor
Sterile IV cannula units (four supplied)
Sterile 10 mL syringe
Sterile syringe needle
Alcohol swabs (four supplied)
Elastic belt
9 V battery
Physician package insert, physician pump manual, and patient instructions

The LUTREPULSE PUMP kit contains the following components:

LUTREPULSE Pump
9 V batteries (two supplied)
3 V lithium battery
Physician pump manual
Physician package insert
Warranty card

Manufactured for
ORTHO PHARMACEUTICAL CORPORATION
RARITAN, NEW JERSEY 08869
by FERRING ARZNEIMITTEL GmbH, Kiel, W. Germany
Revised June 1991 632-10-600-4

Continued on next page

Ortho—Cont.

MONISTAT® 3   ℞
(miconazole nitrate, 200 mg)
Vaginal Suppositories

DESCRIPTION

MONISTAT 3 Vaginal Suppositories are white to off-white suppositories, each containing the antifungal agent, miconazole nitrate, 1-[2,4-Dichloro-β-[(2,4-dichlorobenzyl)oxy]phenethyl]- imidazole mononitrate, 200 mg, in a hydrogenated vegetable oil base. Miconazole nitrate for vaginal use is also available as MONISTAT 7 Vaginal Cream and MONISTAT 7 Vaginal Suppositories.

MICONAZOLE NITRATE

CLINICAL PHARMACOLOGY

Miconazole nitrate exhibits fungicidal activity *in vitro* against species of the genus *Candida*. The pharmacologic mode of action is unknown. Following intravaginal administration of miconazole nitrate, small amounts are absorbed. Administration of a single dose of miconazole nitrate suppositories (100mg) to healthy subjects resulted in a total recovery from the urine and feces of 0.85% (±0.43%) of the administered dose.

Animal studies indicate that the drug crossed the placenta and doses above those used in humans result in embryo- and fetotoxicity (80 mg/kg, orally), although this has not been reported in human subjects (See PRECAUTIONS).

In multi-center clinical trials in 440 women with vulvovaginal candidiasis, the efficacy of treatment with the MONISTAT 3 Vaginal Suppository for 3 days was compared with treatment for 7 days with MONISTAT 7 Vaginal Cream. The clinical cure rates (free of microbiological evidence and clinical signs and symptoms of candidiasis at 8–10 days and 30–35 days post-therapy) were numerically lower, although not statistically different, with the 3-Day Suppository when compared with the 7-Day Cream.

INDICATIONS AND USAGE

MONISTAT 3 Vaginal Suppositories are indicated for the local treatment of vulvovaginal candidiasis (moniliasis). Effectiveness in pregnancy and in diabetic patients has not been established. As MONISTAT is effective only for candidal vulvovaginitis, the diagnosis should be confirmed by KOH smear and/or cultures. Other pathogens commonly associated with vulvovaginitis (*Trichomonas* and *Haemophilus vaginalis* [*Gardnerella*]) should be ruled out by appropriate laboratory methods.

CONTRAINDICATIONS

Patients known to be hypersensitive to this drug.

PRECAUTIONS

General: Discontinue drug if sensitization or irritation is reported during use. The base contained in the suppository formulation may interact with certain latex products, such as that used in vaginal contraceptive diaphragms. Concurrent use is not recommended. MONISTAT 7 Vaginal Cream may be considered for use under these conditions.

Laboratory Tests: If there is a lack of response to MONISTAT 3 Vaginal Suppositories, appropriate microbiological studies (standard KOH smear and/or cultures) should be repeated to confirm the diagnosis and rule out other pathogens.

Carcinogenesis, Mutagenesis, Impairment of Fertility: Long-term animal studies to determine carcinogenic potential have not been performed.

Fertility (Reproduction): Oral administration of miconazole nitrate in rats has been reported to produce prolonged gestation. However, this effect was not observed in oral rabbit studies. In addition, signs of fetal and embryo toxicity were reported in rat and rabbit studies, and dystocia was reported in rat studies after oral doses at and above 80 mg per kg. Intravaginal administration did not produce these effects in rats.

Pregnancy: Since imidazoles are absorbed in small amounts from the human vagina, they should not be used in the first trimester of pregnancy unless the physician considers it essential to the welfare of the patient.

Clinical studies, during which miconazole nitrate vaginal cream and suppositories were used for up to 14 days, were reported to include 514 pregnant patients. Follow-up reports available in 471 of these patients reveal no adverse effects or complications attributable to miconazole nitrate therapy in infants born to these women.

Nursing Mothers: It is not known whether miconazole nitrate is excreted in human milk. Because many drugs are excreted in human milk, caution should be exercised when miconazole nitrate is administered to a nursing woman.

ADVERSE REACTIONS

During clinical studies with the MONISTAT 3 Vaginal Suppository (miconazole nitrate, 200 mg) 301 patients were treated. The incidence of vulvovaginal burning, itching or irritation was 2%. Complaints of cramping (2%) and headaches (1.3%) were also reported. Other complaints (hives, skin rash) occurred with less than a 0.5% incidence. The therapy-related dropout rate was 0.3%.

OVERDOSE

Overdose of miconazole nitrate in humans has not been reported to date. In mice, rats, guinea pigs and dogs, the oral LD 50 values were found to be 578.1, > 640, 275.9 and > 160 mg/kg, respectively.

DOSAGE AND ADMINISTRATION

MONISTAT 3 Vaginal Suppositories: One suppository (miconazole nitrate, 200 mg) is inserted intravaginally once daily at bedtime for three consecutive days. Before prescribing another course of therapy, the diagnosis should be reconfirmed by smears and/or cultures to rule out other pathogens.

HOW SUPPLIED

MONISTAT 3 Suppositories (miconazole nitrate, 200 mg) are available as 2.5 gm, elliptically shaped white to off-white suppositories in packages of three (NDC 0062-5437-01) with a vaginal applicator. Store at 59°–86° F (15–30° C).

Shown in Product Identification Section, page 421

MONISTAT®   ℞
(miconazole nitrate)
DUAL-PAK®

3 DAY SUPPOSITORY THERAPY
MONISTAT® 3
(miconazole nitrate, 200 mg)
Vaginal Suppositories

DESCRIPTION

MONISTAT 3 Vaginal Suppositories are white to off-white suppositories, each containing the antifungal agent, miconazole nitrate, 1-[2,4-Dichloro-β-[(2,4-dichlorobenzyl)oxy]phenethyl]-imidazole mononitrate, 200 mg., in a hydrogenated vegetable oil base. Miconazole nitrate for vaginal use is also available as MONISTAT 7 Vaginal Cream and MONISTAT 7 Vaginal Suppositories.

MICONAZOLE NITRATE

CLINICAL PHARMACOLOGY

Miconazole nitrate exhibits fungicidal activity *in vitro* against species of the genus *Candida*. The pharmacologic mode of action is unknown. Following intravaginal administration of miconazole nitrate, small amounts are absorbed. Administration of a single dose of miconazole nitrate suppositories (100 mg) to healthy subjects resulted in a total recovery from the urine and feces of 0.85% (±0.43%) of the administered dose.

Animal studies indicate that the drug crossed the placenta and doses above those used in humans result in embryo- and feto-toxicity (80 mg/kg, orally), although this has not been reported in human subjects (See PRECAUTIONS).

In multi-center clinical trials in 440 women with vulvovaginal candidiasis, the efficacy of treatment with the MONISTAT 3 Vaginal Suppository for 3 days was compared with treatment for 7 days with MONISTAT 7 Vaginal Cream. The clinical cure rates (free of microbiological evidence and clinical signs and symptoms of candidiasis at 8–10 days and 30–35 days post-therapy) were numerically lower, although not statistically different, with the 3-Day Suppository when compared with the 7-Day Cream.

INDICATIONS AND USAGE

MONISTAT 3 Vaginal Suppositories are indicated for the local treatment of vulvovaginal candidiasis (moniliasis). Effectiveness in pregnancy and in diabetic patients has not been established. As MONISTAT is effective only for candidal vulvovaginitis, the diagnosis should be confirmed by KOH smear and/or cultures. Other pathogens commonly associated with vulvovaginitis (*Trichomonas* and *Haemophilus vaginalis* [*Gardnerella*]) should be ruled out by appropriate laboratory methods.

CONTRAINDICATIONS

Patients known to be hypersensitive to this drug.

PRECAUTIONS

General: Discontinue drug if sensitization or irritation is reported during use. The base contained in the suppository formulation may interact with certain latex products, such as that used in vaginal contraceptive diaphragms. Concurrent use is not recommended. MONISTAT 7 Vaginal Cream may be considered for use under these conditions.

Laboratory Tests: If there is a lack of response to MONISTAT 3 Vaginal Suppositories, appropriate microbiological studies (standard KOH smear and/or cultures) should be repeated to confirm the diagnosis and rule out other pathogens.

Carcinogenesis, Mutagenesis, Impairment of Fertility: Long-term animal studies to determine carcinogenic potential have not been performed.

Fertility (Reproduction): Oral administration of miconazole nitrate in rats has been reported to produce prolonged gestation. However, this effect was not observed in oral rabbit studies. In addition, signs of fetal and embryo toxicity were reported in rat and rabbit studies; and dystocia was reported in rat studies after oral doses at and above 80 mg per kg. Intravaginal administration did not produce these effects in rats.

Pregnancy: Since imidazoles are absorbed in small amounts from the human vagina, they should not be used in the first trimester of pregnancy unless the physician considers it essential to the welfare of the patient.

Clinical studies, during which miconazole nitrate vaginal cream and suppositories were used for up to 14 days, were reported to include 514 pregnant patients. Follow-up reports available in 471 of these patients reveal no adverse effects or complications attributable to miconazole nitrate therapy in infants born to these women.

Nursing Mothers: It is not known whether miconazole nitrate is excreted in human milk. Because many drugs are excreted in human milk, caution should be exercised when miconazole nitrate is administered to a nursing woman.

ADVERSE REACTIONS

During clinical studies with the MONISTAT 3 Vaginal Suppository (miconazole nitrate, 200 mg) 301 patients were treated. The incidence of vulvovaginal burning, itching or irritation was 2%. Complaints of cramping (2%) and headaches (1.3%) were also reported. Other complaints (hives, skin rash) occurred with less than a 0.5% incidence. The therapy-related dropout rate was 0.3%.

OVERDOSE

Overdose of miconazole nitrate in humans has not been reported to date. In mice, rats, guinea pigs and dogs, the oral LD 50 values were found to be 578.1, > 640, 275.9 and > 160 mg/kg, respectively.

DOSAGE AND ADMINISTRATION

MONISTAT 3 Vaginal Suppositories: One suppository (miconazole nitrate, 200 mg) is inserted intravaginally once daily at bedtime for three consecutive days. Before prescribing another course of therapy, the diagnosis should be reconfirmed by smears and/or cultures to rule out other pathogens.

HOW SUPPLIED

MONISTAT 3 Suppositories (miconazole nitrate, 200 mg) are available as 2.5 gm, elliptically shaped white to off-white suppositories in packages of three (NDC 0062-5437-01) with a vaginal applicator. Store at 59–86°F (15–30°C).

7 DAY CREAM THERAPY
MONISTAT-DERM®
(miconazole nitrate 2%)
Cream
For Topical Use Only

DESCRIPTION

MONISTAT-DERM (miconazole nitrate 2%) Cream contains miconazole nitrate* 2%, formulated into a water-miscible base consisting of pegoxol 7 stearate, peglicol 5 oleate, mineral oil, benzoic acid, butylated hydroxyanisole and purified water.

ACTIONS

Miconazole nitrate is a synthetic antifungal agent which inhibits the growth of the common dermatophytes, *Trichophyton rubrum*, *Trichophyton mentagrophytes*, and *Epidermophyton floccosum*, the yeast-like fungus, *Candida albicans*, and the organism responsible for tinea versicolor (*Malassezia furfur*).

---

*Chemical name: 1-[2,4-dichloro-β-{(2,4- dichlorobenzyl) oxy}phenethyl] imidazole mononitrate.

Shown in Product Identification Section, page 421

INDICATIONS

For topical application in the treatment of tinea pedis (athlete's foot), tinea cruris, and tinea corporis caused by *Trichophyton rubrum, trichophyton mentagrophytes,* and *Epidermophyton floccosum,* in the treatment of cutaneous candidiasis (moniliasis), and in the treatment of tinea versicolor.

CONTRAINDICATIONS

MONISTAT-DERM (miconazole nitrate 2%) Cream has no known contraindications.

PRECAUTIONS

If a reaction suggesting sensitivity or chemical irritation should occur, use of the medication should be discontinued. For external use only. Avoid introduction of MONISTAT-DERM Cream into the eyes.

ADVERSE REACTIONS

There have been isolated reports of irritation, burning, maceration, and allergic contact dermatitis associated with the application of MONISTAT-DERM.

DOSAGE AND ADMINISTRATION

Sufficient MONISTAT-DERM Cream should be applied to cover affected areas twice daily (morning and evening) in patients with tinea pedis, tinea cruris, tinea corporis, and cutaneous candidiasis, and once daily in patients with tinea versicolor. If MONISTAT-DERM Cream is used in intertriginous areas, it should be applied sparingly and smoothed in well to avoid maceration effects.
Early relief of symptoms (2 to 3 days) is experienced by the majority of patients and clinical improvement may be seen fairly soon after treatment is begun; however, *Candida* infections and tinea cruris and corporis should be treated for two weeks and tinea pedis for one month in order to reduce the possibility of recurrence. If a patient shows no clinical improvement after a month of treatment, the diagnosis should be redetermined. Patients with tinea versicolor usually exhibit clinical and mycological clearing after two weeks of treatment.

HOW SUPPLIED

MONISTAT-DERM (miconazole nitrate 2%) Cream containing miconazole nitrate at 2% strength is supplied in 15 g. (NDC 0062-5434-02), 1 oz. (NDC 0062-5434-01) and 3 oz. (NDC 0062-5434-03) tubes.

ORTHO® DIAPHRAGM KITS ℞

DESCRIPTION

ORTHO Diaphragm Kits include three different types in a variety of sizes.
1. The ALL-FLEX® Arcing Spring Diaphragm is a molded, buff-colored, natural rubber vaginal diaphragm containing a distortion-free, dual spring-within-a-spring which provides unique arcing action no matter where the rim is compressed. It is appropriate not only where ordinary diaphragms are indicated, but also in patients with mild cystocele, rectocele or retroversion.
2. The ORTHO® Coil Spring Diaphragm is a molded natural rubber vaginal diaphragm. The rim encases a tension-adjusted, cadmium-plated coil spring.
3. The ORTHO-WHITE® Flat Spring Diaphragm is a molded, pure white, natural rubber vaginal diaphragm containing a flat, watch-type spring which allows compressibility in one plane only, thus facilitating insertion.
ORTHO Diaphragms are used in conjunction with spermicides, e.g., GYNOL II® Original Formula Contraceptive Jelly, ORTHO-GYNOL® Contraceptive Jelly or ORTHO-CREME® Contraceptive Cream in conception control.

ACTION

These Diaphragms when properly fitted serve two purposes:
a. To stop the sperm from entering the cervical canal;
b. To hold the spermicide.

INDICATIONS

ORTHO Diaphragms, in conjunction with an appropriate spermicide, are indicated for the prevention of pregnancy in women who elect to use diaphragms as a method of contraception.

CONTRAINDICATIONS

Known hypersensitivity to natural rubber products and prior history of Toxic Shock Syndrome (TSS).

WARNINGS

An association has been reported between diaphragm use and toxic shock syndrome (TSS), a serious condition which can be fatal.
For contraceptive effectiveness, the diaphragm should remain in place for six hours after intercourse and should be removed as soon as possible thereafter.
Continuous wearing of a contraceptive diaphragm for more than twenty-four hours is not recommended. Removal of the diaphragm before six hours may increase the risk of becoming pregnant. Retention of the diaphragm for any period of time may encourage the growth of certain bacteria in the vaginal tract. It has been suggested that under certain as yet unestablished conditions, overgrowth of these bacteria may lead to symptoms of toxic shock syndrome. Primary symptoms of TSS are sudden high fever (usually 102° or more), and vomiting, diarrhea, fainting or near fainting when standing up, dizziness or a rash that looks like sunburn. There may also be other signs of TSS such as aching of muscles and joints, redness of the eyes, sore throat and weakness. Patients should be instructed that if they experience sudden high fever and one or more of the other symptoms, they should remove the diaphragm and consult their physician immediately.

PRECAUTIONS

Diaphragm users should be instructed to consult their physician:
1. If they are not sure about the insertion and placement of the diaphragm.
2. If they or their partner feel or are made uncomfortable by the presence of the diaphragm.
3. If the diaphragm slips out of place when walking, coughing, or straining.
4. If the diaphragm no longer fits snugly above the pubic bone.
5. If at times other than menstruation there is blood on the diaphragm when it is removed.
6. If there are any holes, tears or other deterioration of the diaphragm.
7. If unable to remove the diaphragm.
8. IMPORTANT—For contraceptive effectiveness, the diaphragm should remain in place for six hours after intercourse and should be removed as soon as possible thereafter. Continuous wearing of a contraceptive diaphragm for more than twenty-four hours is not recommended. Removal of the diaphragm before six hours may increase the risk of becoming pregnant. Retention of the diaphragm for any period of time may encourage the growth of certain bacteria in the vaginal tract. It has been suggested that under certain as yet unestablished conditions, overgrowth of these bacteria may lead to symptoms of toxic shock syndrome. Primary symptoms of TSS are sudden high fever (usually 102° or more), and vomiting, diarrhea, fainting or near fainting when standing up, dizziness or a rash that looks like a sunburn. There may also be other signs of TSS such as aching of muscles and joints, redness of the eyes, sore throat and weakness. If the patient has a sudden high fever and one or more of the other symptoms, the diaphragm should be removed immediately and TSS should be considered.
9. Diaphragm users should have another diaphragm fitting if they have lost or gained more than ten pounds, have had the diaphragm for more than a year, or have had a baby or an abortion. As a matter of routine, each time a pelvic examination is performed, refitting should be done. The size and shape of the vagina changes and this may require a new size diaphragm. Even if the diaphragm size does not change, it is advisable to replace the diaphragm every two years or sooner.
10. Diaphragms may increase the risk of urinary tract infections especially if not properly fitted. Patients should be instructed to consult their physician if they experience any of the signs or symptoms of this type of infection which include pain on urination, blood in the urine, elevated temperature, frequent urination, or a sensation of obstruction while urinating.
11. Persons sensitive to natural rubber may have an allergic reaction to diaphragm use.

INSTRUCTIONS

1. Proper placement of the diaphragm is vital for effectiveness.
2. To be fully effective the diaphragm should never be used without contraceptive cream or jelly. The contraceptive cream or jelly must be spread around the inner surface of the diaphragm as well as around the rim.
3. To avoid pregnancy the diaphragm must be used every time there is intercourse.
4. The diaphragm may be inserted up to six hours before intercourse. If more than six hours has elapsed between insertion of the diaphragm and intercourse, additional contraceptive jelly or cream must be inserted. The diaphragm should not be removed to insert this additional cream or jelly.
The following Patient Instructions for insertion and removal are contained in the booklet "After Your Doctor Prescribes your Ortho Diaphragm" which is included in each Ortho Diaphragm Kit.
Preparing for insertion
1. It is recommended that you urinate and wash your hands before inserting the diaphragm.
2. Prior to inserting your diaphragm, put an applicatorful (about a teaspoon) of contraceptive jelly into the cup of the

dome of the diaphragm. You may elect to simply squeeze the tube or use the applicator provided with the starter kit of contraceptive cream or jelly.
3. Spread a small amount around the edge with your fingertip, (if the amount applied to the rim is excessive, it will be difficult to control the diaphragm during insertion) then insert.

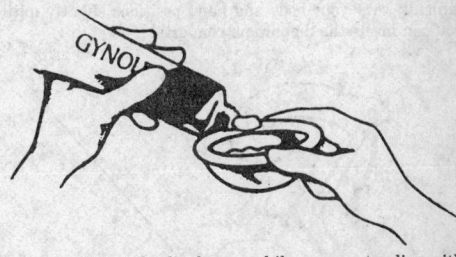

4. You can insert the diaphragm while you are standing with one leg up, squatting, or lying down. The position of the cervix and the walls of the vagina will be different depending on your position. If you are used to one position and then change to another, take extra care in positioning the diaphragm to be sure the cervix is covered.

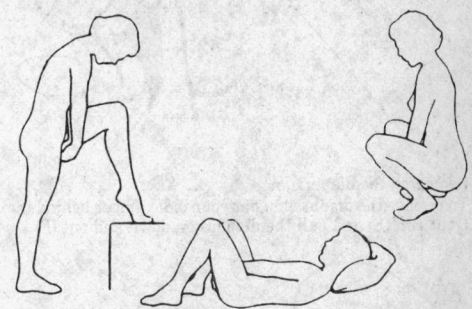

Inserting the diaphragm
1. Hold the diaphragm with the dome down (spermicide up) and press the opposite sides of the rim together between your thumb and third finger (A-1 and A-2). The diaphragm can be held from above or below.
2. Spread the lips of your vagina with your free hand. Hold the compressed diaphragm dome down (spermicide up) and push it gently inward along the rear wall of the vagina as far as it can go. Your index finger, kept on the outer rim of the diaphragm, helps you guide the diaphragm into place (B-1 and B-2).

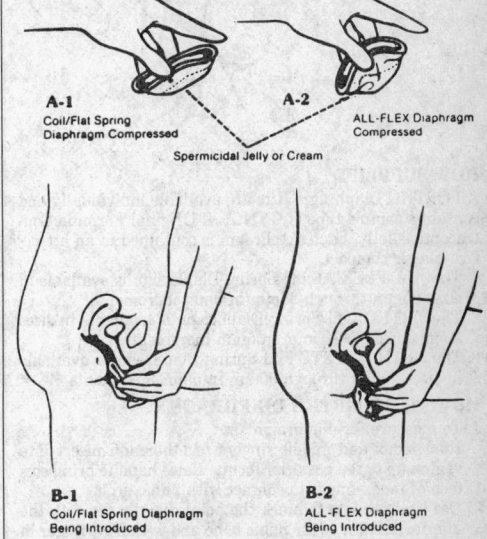

A-1 Coil/Flat Spring Diaphragm Compressed

A-2 ALL-FLEX Diaphragm Compressed

Spermicidal Jelly or Cream

B-1 Coil/Flat Spring Diaphragm Being Introduced

B-2 ALL-FLEX Diaphragm Being Introduced

3. With your index finger, push the front rim of the the diaphragm up until it is locked in place just above the pubic bone (C).
4. Check with your index finger to be sure the diaphragm is in place and is holding the contraceptive jelly or cream over the cervix. It is important that the cervix be covered by the diaphragm and spermicide and that the diaphragm be locked in place between the upper edge of the pubic bone and the rear wall of the vagina. You should be able to feel your cervix through the rubber shield. You can feel the front rim of the

Continued on next page

Ortho—Cont.

diaphragm above the pubic bone, but you may not be able to follow the rim all the way around since your fingers may not be long enough (D).

5. If, after some practice, you still find insertion awkward or difficult, vary your body and hand positions slightly until you can insert the diaphragm comfortably.

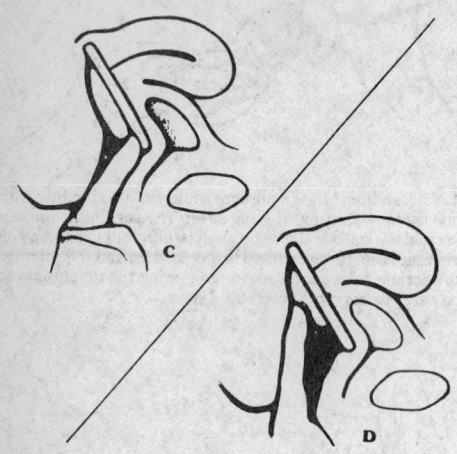

Removing the diaphragm
To remove the diaphragm, put your index finger behind the front rim (E) and pull the diaphragm down and out (F).

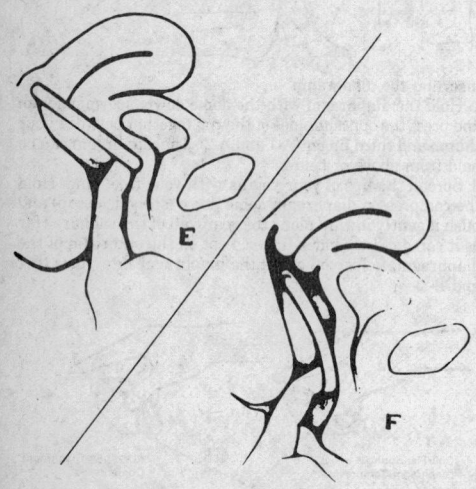

HOW SUPPLIED
All ORTHO Diaphragm Kits are available individually and contain a sample tube of GYNOL II Original Formula Contraceptive Jelly. Each diaphragm is contained in an attractive plastic compact.
1. The ALL-FLEX Arcing Spring Diaphragm is available in sizes 55mm through 95mm in 5mm increments.
2. The ORTHO Coil Spring Diaphragm is available in sizes 50mm through 105mm in 5mm increments.
3. The ORTHO-WHITE Flat Spring Diaphragm is available in sizes 55mm through 95mm in 5mm increments.

HOW TO FIT ORTHO DIAPHRAGMS
1. To measure for diaphragm size:
   Hold index and middle fingers together and insert into vagina up to the posterior fornix. Raise hand to bring surface of index finger to contact with pubic arch.
   Use tip of thumb to mark the point directly beneath the inferior margin of the pubic bone and withdraw finger in this position.
2. To determine diaphragm size:
   Place one end of rim of fitting diaphragm or ring on tip of middle finger. The opposite end should lie just in front of the thumb tip. This is the approximate diameter of the diaphragm needed.
   Insert a fitting diaphragm or ring of the appropriate size into the vagina.
   Try both a larger and a smaller size before making a decision.
3. The proper size will fit snugly in the posterior fornix and behind the pubic arch without undue pressure.

Shown in Product Identification Section, page 421

ORTHO® Dienestrol Cream   ℞

1. ESTROGENS HAVE BEEN REPORTED TO INCREASE THE RISK OF ENDOMETRIAL CARCINOMA.
Three independent case control studies have shown an increased risk of endometrial cancer in postmenopausal women exposed to exogenous estrogens for prolonged periods.[1-3] This risk was independent of the other known risk factors for endometrial cancer. These studies are further supported by the finding that incidence rates of endometrial cancer have increased sharply since 1969 in eight different areas of the United States with population-based cancer reporting systems, an increase which may be related to the rapidly expanding use of estrogens during the last decade.[4]
The three case control studies reported that the risk of endometrial cancer in estrogen users was about 4.5 to 13.9 times greater than in nonusers. The risk appears to depend on both duration of treatment[1] and on estrogen dose.[3] In view of these findings, when estrogens are used for the treatment of menopausal symptoms, the lowest dose that will control symptoms should be utilized and medication should be discontinued as soon as possible. When prolonged treatment is medically indicated, the patient should be reassessed on at least a semiannual basis to determine the need for continued therapy. Although the evidence must be considered preliminary, one study suggests that cyclic administration of low doses of estrogen may carry less risk than continuous administration;[3] it therefore appears prudent to utilize such a regimen.
Close clinical surveillance of all women taking estrogens is important. In all cases of undiagnosed persistent or recurring abnormal vaginal bleeding, adequate diagnostic measures should be undertaken to rule out malignancy.
There is no evidence at present that "natural" estrogens are more or less hazardous than "synthetic" estrogens at equiestrogenic doses.
2. AT THE PRESENT TIME ESTROGENS SHOULD NOT BE USED DURING PREGNANCY
The use of female sex hormones, both estrogens and progestogens, during early pregnancy may seriously damage the offspring. It has been shown that females exposed *in utero* to diethylstilbestrol, a non-steroidal estrogen, have an increased risk of developing in later life a form of vaginal or cervical cancer that ordinarily is extremely rare.[5,6] This risk has been estimated as not greater than 4 per 1000 exposures.[7] Furthermore, a high percentage of such exposed women (from 30 to 90 percent) have been found to have vaginal adenosis,[8-12] epithelial changes of the vagina and cervix. Although these changes are histologically benign, it is not known whether they are precursors of malignancy. Although similar data are not available with the use of other estrogens, it cannot be presumed they would not induce similar changes.
Several reports suggest an association between intrauterine exposure to female sex hormones and congenital anomalies, including congenital heart defects and limb reduction defects.[13-15] One case control study[16] estimated a 4.7 fold increased risk of limb reduction defects in infants exposed in utero to sex hormones (oral contraceptives, hormone withdrawal tests for pregnancy, or attempted treatment for threatened abortion). Some of these exposures were very short and involved only a few days of treatment. The data suggest that the risk of limb reduction defects in exposed fetuses is somewhat less than 1 per 1000.
In the past, female sex hormones have been used during pregnancy in an attempt to treat threatened or habitual abortion. There is considerable evidence that estrogens are ineffective for these indications, and there is no evidence from well controlled studies that progestogens are effective for these uses.
If ORTHO Dienestrol Cream is used during pregnancy, or if the patient becomes pregnant while using this drug, she should be apprised of the potential risks to the fetus, and the advisability of pregnancy continuation.

DESCRIPTION
ORTHO Dienestrol Cream
Cream for intravaginal use only
Active ingredient: Dienestrol 0.01%.
Dienestrol is a synthetic, non-steroidal estrogen. It is compounded in a cream base suitable for intravaginal use only. The cream base is composed of glyceryl monostearate, peanut oil, glycerin, benzoic acid, glutamic acid, butylated hydroxyanisole, citric acid, sodium hydroxide and water. The pH is approximately 4.3.
[See chemical structure at top of next column.]

4,4'-(Diethylideneethylene)diphenol

CLINICAL PHARMACOLOGY
Systemic absorption and mode of action of dienestrol are undetermined.

INDICATIONS AND USAGE
ORTHO Dienestrol Cream is indicated in the treatment of atrophic vaginitis and kraurosis vulvae.
ORTHO DIENESTROL CREAM HAS NOT BEEN SHOWN TO BE EFFECTIVE FOR ANY PURPOSE DURING PREGNANCY AND ITS USE MAY CAUSE SEVERE HARM TO THE FETUS (*SEE* BOXED WARNING).

CONTRAINDICATIONS
Estrogens may cause fetal harm when administered to a pregnant woman (see Boxed Warning). Estrogens are contraindicated in women who are or may become pregnant. If this drug is used during pregnancy, or if the patient becomes pregnant while using this drug, the patient should be apprised of the potential hazard to the fetus.
Estrogens should also not be used in women with any of the following conditions:
1. Known or suspected cancer of the breast.
2. Known or suspected estrogen-dependent neoplasia.
3. Undiagnosed abnormal genital bleeding.
4. Active thrombophlebitis or thromboembolic disorders.
5. A past history of thrombophlebitis, thrombosis, or thromboembolic disorders associated with previous estrogen use.

WARNINGS
1. *Induction of malignant neoplasms.* Long-term continuous administration of natural and synthetic estrogens in certain animal species increases the frequency of carcinomas of the breast, cervix, vagina, and liver. There is now evidence that estrogens increase the risk of carcinoma of the endometrium in humans. (*See* Boxed Warning.)
At the present time there is no satisfactory evidence that estrogens given to postmenopausal women increase the risk of cancer of the breast,[18] although a recent long-term followup of a single physician's practice has raised this possibility.[18a] Because of the animal data, there is a need for caution in prescribing estrogens for women with a strong family history of breast cancer or who have breast nodules, fibrocystic disease, or abnormal mammograms.
2. *Gallbladder disease.* A recent study has reported a 2- to 3-fold increase in the risk of surgically confirmed gall bladder disease in women receiving postmenopausal estrogens,[18] similar to the 2-fold increase previously noted in users of oral contraceptives.[19,24] In the case of oral contraceptives the increased risk appeared after two years of use.[24]
3. *Effects similar to those caused by estrogen-progestogen oral contraceptives.* There are several serious adverse effects of oral contraceptives, most of which have not, up to now, been documented as consequences of postmenopausal estrogen therapy. This may reflect the comparatively low doses of estrogen used in postmenopausal women. It would be expected that the larger doses of estrogen used to treat prostatic or breast cancer or postpartum breast engorgement are more likely to result in these adverse effects, and, in fact, it has been shown that there is an increased risk of thrombosis in men receiving estrogens for prostatic cancer and women for postpartum breast engorgement.[20-23]
a. *Thromboembolic disease.* It is now well established that users of oral contraceptives have an increased risk of various thromboembolic and thrombotic vascular diseases, such as thrombophlebitis, pulmonary embolism, stroke, and myocardial infarction.[24-31] Cases of retinal thrombosis, mesenteric thrombosis, and optic neuritis have been reported in oral contraceptive users. There is evidence that the risk of several of these adverse reactions is related to the dose of the drug.[32,33] An increased risk of postsurgery thromboembolic complications has also been reported in users of oral contraceptives.[34,35] If feasible, estrogen should be discontinued at least 4 weeks before surgery of the type associated with an increased risk of thromboembolism, or during periods of prolonged immobilization.
While an increased rate of thromboembolic and thrombotic disease in postmenopausal users of estrogens has not been found,[18,36] this does not rule out the possibility that such an increase may be present or that subgroups of women who have underlying risk factors or who are receiving relatively large doses of estrogens may have increased risk. Therefore estrogens should not be used in persons with active thrombophlebitis or thromboembolic disorders, and they should not be used (except in treatment of malignancy) in persons with a history of such disorders in association with estrogen use. They should be used with caution in patients with cerebral vascular or coronary artery disease and only for those in whom estrogens are clearly needed.

Large doses of estrogen (5 mg conjugated estrogens per day), comparable to those used to treat cancer of the prostate and breast, have been shown in a large prospective clinical trial in men to increase the risk of nonfatal myocardial infarction, pulmonary embolism and thrombophlebitis. When estrogen doses of this size are used, any of the thromboembolic and thrombotic adverse effects associated with oral contraceptive use should be considered a clear risk.

b. *Hepatic adenoma.* Benign hepatic adenomas appear to be associated with the use of oral contraceptives.[38–40] Although benign, and rare, these may rupture and may cause death through intra-abdominal hemorrhage. Such lesions have not yet been reported in association with other estrogen or progestogen preparations but should be considered in estrogen users having abdominal pain and tenderness, abdominal mass, or hypovolemic shock. Hepatocellular carcinoma has also been reported in women taking estrogen-containing oral contraceptives.[39] The relationship of this malignancy to these drugs is not known at this time.

c. *Elevated blood pressure.* Increased blood pressure is not uncommon in women using oral contraceptives. There is now a report that this may occur with use of estrogens during menopause.[41] Blood pressure should be monitored with estrogen use, especially if high doses are used.

d. *Glucose tolerance.* A worsening of glucose tolerance has been observed in a significant percentage of patients on estrogen-containing oral contraceptives. For this reason, diabetic patients should be carefully observed while receiving estrogen.

4. *Hypercalcemia.* Administration of estrogens may lead to severe hypercalcemia in patients with breast cancer and bone metastases. If this occurs, the drug should be stopped and appropriate measures taken to reduce the serum calcium level.

PRECAUTIONS

A. General

1. A complete medical and family history should be taken prior to the initiation of any estrogen therapy. The pretreatment and periodic physical examinations should include special reference to blood pressure, breasts, abdomen, and pelvic organs, and should include a Papanicolaou smear. As a general rule, estrogen should not be prescribed for longer than one year without another physical examination being performed.
2. Fluid retention—Because estrogens may cause some degree of fluid retention, conditions which might be influenced by this factor such as epilepsy, migraine, and cardiac or renal dysfunction, require careful observation.
3. Certain patients may develop undesirable manifestations of excessive estrogenic stimulation, such as abnormal or excessive uterine bleeding, mastodynia, etc.
4. Oral contraceptives appear to be associated with an increased incidence of mental depression.[24] Although it is not clear whether this is due to the estrogenic or progestogenic component of the contraceptive, patients with a history of depression should be carefully observed.
5. Preexisting uterine leiomyomata may increase in size during estrogen use.
6. The pathologist should be advised of estrogen therapy when relevant specimens are submitted.
7. Patients with a past history of jaundice during pregnancy have an increased risk of recurrence of jaundice while receiving estrogen-containing oral contraceptive therapy. If jaundice develops in any patient receiving estrogen, the medication should be discontinued while the cause is investigated.
8. Estrogens may be poorly metabolized in patients with impaired liver function and they should be administered with caution in such patients.
9. Because estrogens influence the metabolism of calcium and phosphorus, they should be used with caution in patients with metabolic bone diseases that are associated with hypercalcemia or in patients with renal insufficiency.
10. Because of the effects of estrogens on epiphyseal closure, they should be used judiciously in young patients in whom bone growth is not complete.
11. The lowest effective dose appropriate for the specific indication should be utilized. Studies of the addition of a progestin for seven or more days of a cycle of estrogen administration have reported a lowered incidence of endometrial hyperplasia. Morphological and biochemical studies of endometrium suggest that 10 to 13 days of progestin are needed to provide maximal maturation of the endometrium and to eliminate any hyperplastic changes. Whether this will provide protection from endometrial carcinoma has not been clearly established. There are possible additional risks which may be associated with the inclusion of progestin in estrogen replacement regimens.The potential risks include adverse effects on carbohydrate and lipid metabolism. The choice of progestin and dosage may be important in minimizing these adverse effects.

B. Information for Patients: See text of Patient Package Information which is reproduced below.

C. Drug/Laboratory Test Interactions

Certain endocrine and liver function tests may be affected by estrogen-containing oral contraceptives. The following similar changes may be expected with larger doses of estrogen:

1. Increased sulfobromophthalein retention.
2. Increased prothrombin and factors VII, VIII, IX and X; decreased antithrombin 3; increased norepinephrine-induced platelet aggregability.
3. Increased thyroid-binding globulin (TBG) leading to increased circulating total thyroid hormone, as measured by PBI, T4 by column, or T4 by radioimmunoassay. Free T3 resin uptake is decreased, reflecting the elevated TBG; free T4 concentration is unaltered.
4. Impaired glucose tolerance.
5. Decreased pregnanediol excretion.
6. Reduced response to metyrapone test.
7. Reduced serum folate concentration.
8. Increased serum triglyceride and phospholipid concentration.

D. Carcinogenesis, Mutagenesis, Impairment of Fertility: See "Warnings" section for information on carcinogenesis, mutagenesis and impairment of fertility.

E. Pregnancy:

Teratogenic Effects.

Pregnancy Category X.

See "Contraindications" section.

F. Nursing Mothers: It is not known whether this drug is excreted in human milk. Because many drugs are excreted in human milk, caution should be exercised when estrogens are administered to a nursing woman.

ADVERSE REACTIONS

(*See* Warnings regarding induction of neoplasia, adverse effects on the fetus, increased incidence of gall bladder disease, and adverse effects similar to those of oral contraceptives, including thromboembolism.) The following additional adverse reactions have been reported with estrogenic therapy, including oral contraceptives:

1. *Genitourinary system.*

Increase in size of uterine fibromyomata.
Vaginal candidiasis.
Breakthrough bleeding, spotting, change in menstrual flow.
Dysmenorrhea.
Premenstrual-like syndrome.
Amenorrhea during and after treatment.
Change in cervical eversion and in degree of cervical secretion.
Cystitis-like syndrome.

2. *Breasts.*

Tenderness, enlargement, secretion.

3. *Gastrointestinal.*

Cholestatic jaundice.
Nausea, vomiting.
Abdominal cramps, bloating.

4. *Skin.*

Erythema multiforme.
Erythema nodosum.
Hemorrhagic eruption.
Loss of scalp hair.
Hirsutism.
Chloasma or melasma which may persist when drug is discontinued.

5. *Eyes.*

Steepening of corneal curvature.
Intolerance to contact lenses.

6. *CNS.*

Mental depression.
Headache, migraine, dizziness.
Chorea.

7. *Miscellaneous.*

Reduced carbohydrate tolerance.
Aggravation of porphyria.
Edema.
Changes in libido.
Increase or decrease in weight.

OVERDOSAGE

Numerous reports of ingestion of large doses of estrogen-containing oral contraceptives by young children indicate that serious ill effects do not occur. Overdosage of estrogen may cause nausea, and withdrawal bleeding may occur in females.

DOSAGE AND ADMINISTRATION

Given cyclically for short term use only:

For treatment of atrophic vaginitis, or kraurosis vulvae associated with the menopause.

The lowest dose that will control symptoms should be chosen and medication should be discontinued as promptly as possible.

Attempts to discontinue or taper medication should be made at 3 to 6 month intervals.

The usual dosage range is one or two applicatorsful per day for one or two weeks, then gradually reduced to one half initial dosage for a similar period. A maintenance dosage of one applicatorful, one to three times a week, may be used after restoration of the vaginal mucosa has been achieved.

Treated patients with an intact uterus should be monitored closely for signs of endometrial cancer and appropriate diagnostic measures should be taken to rule out malignancy in the event of persistent or recurring abnormal vaginal bleeding.

HOW SUPPLIED

Available in 2.75 oz. (78g) tubes with or without ORTHO® Measured Dose Applicator.

With applicator: NDC 0062-5450-77

Without applicator: NDC 0062-5450-00

Store at controlled room temperature.

1. Ziel, H.K. and W.D. Finkle, "Increased Risk of Endometrial Carcinoma Among Users of Conjugated Estrogens," *New England Journal of Medicine,* 293:1167–1170, 1975.
2. Smith, D.C., R. Prentice, D.J. Thompson, and W.L. Hermann, "Association of Exogenous Estrogen and Endometrial Carcinoma," *New England Journal of Medicine,* 293:1164–1167, 1975.
3. Mack, T.M., M.C. Pike, B.E. Henderson, R.J. Pfeffer, V.R. Gerkins, M. Arthur, and S.E. Brown, "Estrogens and Endometrial Cancer in a Retirement Community," *New England Journal of Medicine,* 294:1267–1287, 1976.
4. Weiss, N.S., D.R. Szekely and D.F. Austin, "Increasing Incidence of Endometrial Cancer in the United States," *New England Journal of Medicine,* 294:1259–1262, 1976.
5. Herbst, A.L., H. Ulfelder and D.C. Poskanzer, "Adenocarcinoma of Vagina," *New England Journal of Medicine,* 284:878–881, 1971.
6. Greenwald, P., J. Barlow, P. Nasca, and W. Burnett, "Vaginal Cancer after Maternal Treatment with Synthetic Estrogens," *New England Journal of Medicine,* 285:390–392, 1971.
7. Lanier, A., K. Noller, D. Decker, L. Elveback, and L. Kurland, "Cancer and Stilbestrol. A Follow-up of 1719 Persons Exposed to Estrogens in Utero and Born 1943–1959," *Mayo Clinic Proceedings,* 48:793–799, 1973.
8. Herbst, A., R. Kurman, and R. Scully, "Vaginal and Cervical Abnormalities After Exposure to Stilbestrol In Utero," *Obstetrics and Gynecology,* 40:287–298, 1972.
9. Herbst, A., S. Robboy, G. Macdonald, and R. Scully, "The Effects of Local Progesterone on Stilbestrol-Associated Vaginal Adenosis," *American Journal of Obstetrics and Gynecology* 118:607–615, 1974.
10. Herbst, A., D. Poskanzer, S. Robboy, L. Friedlander, and R. Scully, "Prenatal Exposure to Stilbestrol, A Prospective Comparison of Exposed Female Offspring with Unexposed Controls," *New England Journal of Medicine,* 292:334–339, 1975.
11. Staffi, A., R. Mattingly, D. Foley, and W. Fetherston, "Clinical Diagnosis of Vaginal Adenosis," *Obstetrics and Gynecology,* 43:118–128, 1974.
12. Sherman, A.I., M. Goldrath, A. Berlin, V. Vakhariya, F. Banooni, W. Michaels, P. Goodman, S. Brown, "Cervical-Vaginal Adenosis After *In Utero* Exposure to Synthetic Estrogens," *Obstetrics and Gynecology,* 44:531–545, 1974.
13. Gal, I., B. Kirman, and J. Stern, "Hormone Pregnancy Tests and Congenital Malformation," *Nature,* 216:83, 1967.
14. Levy, E.P., A. Cohen, and F.C. Fraser, "Hormone Treatment During Pregnancy and Congenital Heart Defects," *Lancet,* 1:611, 1973.
15. Nora, J. and A. Nora, "Birth Defects and Oral Contraceptives," *Lancet,* 1:941–942, 1973.
16. Janerich, D.T., J.M. Piper, and D.M. Glebatis, "Oral Contraceptives and Congenital Limb-Reduction Defects," *New England Journal of Medicine,* 291:697–700, 1974.
17. "Estrogens for Oral or Parenteral Use," *Federal Register,* 40:8212, 1975.
18. Boston Collaborative Drug Surveillance Program, "Surgically Confirmed Gall Bladder Disease, Venous Thromboembolism and Breast Tumors in Relation to Post-Menopausal Estrogen Therapy," *New England Journal of Medicine,* 290:15–19, 1974.
18a. Hoover, R., L.A. Gray, Sr., P. Cole, and B. MacMahon, "Menopausal Estrogens and Breast Cancer," *New England Journal of Medicine,* 295:401–405, 1976.
19. Boston Collaborative Drug Surveillance Program, "Oral Contraceptives and Venous Thromboembolic Disease, Surgically Confirmed Gall Bladder Disease, and Breast Tumors," *Lancet* 1:1399–1404, 1973.
20. Daniel, D.G., H. Campbell, and A.C. Turnbull, "Puerperal Thromboembolism and Suppression of Lactation," *Lancet,* 2:287–289, 1967.
21. The Veterans Administration Cooperative Urological Research Group, "Carcinoma of the Prostate: Treatment Comparisons," *Journal of Urology,* 98:516–522, 1967.
22. Bailer, J.C., "Thromboembolism and Oestrogen Therapy," *Lancet,* 2:560, 1967.
23. Blackard, C., R. Doe, G. Mellinger, and D. Byar, "Incidence of Cardiovascular Disease and Death In Patients Receiving Diethylstilbestrol for Carcinoma of the Prostate," *Cancer,* 26:249–256, 1970.
24. Royal College of General Practitioners, "Oral Contraception and Thromboembolic Disease," *Journal of the Royal College of General Practitioners,* 13:267–279, 1967.

Continued on next page

Ortho—Cont.

25. Inman, W.H.W. and M.P. Vessey, "Investigation of Deaths from Pulmonary, Coronary, and Cerebral Thrombosis and Embolism in Women of Child-Bearing Age," *British Medical Journal,* 2:193–199, 1968.

26. Vessey, M.P. and R. Doll, "Investigation of Relation Between Use of Oral Contraceptives and Thromboembolic Disease, A Further Report," *British Medical Journal,* 2:651–657, 1969.

27. Sartwell, P.E., A.T. Masi, F.G. Arthes, G.R. Greene, and H.E. Smith, "Thromboembolism and Oral Contraceptives: An Epidemiological Case Control Study," *American Journal of Epidemiology,* 90:365–380, 1969.

28. Collaborative Group for the Study of Stroke In Young Women, "Oral Contraception and Increased Risk of Cerebral Ischemia or Thrombosis," *New England Journal of Medicine,* 288:871–878, 1973.

29. Collaborative Group for the Study of Stroke in Young Women, "Oral Contraceptives and Stroke in Young Women: Associated Risk Factors," *Journal of the American Medical Association,* 231:718–722, 1975.

30. Mann, J.I. and W.H.W. Inman, "Oral Contraceptives and Death from Myocardial Infarction," *British Medical Journal,* 2:245–248, 1975.

31. Mann, J.I., M.P. Vessey, M. Thorogood, and R. Doll., "Myocardial Infarction in Young Women with Special Reference to Oral Contraceptive Practice," *British Medical Journal,* 2:241–245, 1975.

32. Inman, W.H.W., V.P. Vessey, B. Westerholm, and A. Engelund, "Thromboembolic Disease and the Steroidal Content of Oral Contraceptives," *British Medical Journal,* 2:203–209, 1970.

33. Stolley, P.D., J.A. Tonascia, M.S. Tockman, P.E. Sartwell, A.H. Rutledge, and M.P. Jacobs, "Thrombosis with Low-Estrogen Oral Contraceptives," *American Journal of Epidemiology,* 102:197–208, 1975.

34. Vessey, M.P., R. Doll, A.S. Fairbairn, and G. Glober, "Post-Operative Thromboembolism and the Use of the Oral Contraceptives," *British Medical Journal,* 3:123–126, 1970.

35. Greene, G.R. and P.E. Sartwell, "Oral Contraceptive Use in Patients with Thromboembolism Following Surgery, Trauma or Infection," *American Journal of Public Health,* 62:680–685, 1972.

36. Rosenberg, L., M.B. Armstrong and H. Jick, "Myocardial Infarction and Estrogen Therapy in Postmenopausal Women," *New England Journal of Medicine,* 294:1256–1259, 1976.

37. Coronary Drug Project Research Group, "The Coronary Drug Project: Initial Findings Leading to Modifications of Its Research Protocol," *Journal of the American Medical Association,* 214:1303–1313, 1970.

38. Baum, J., F. Holtz, J.J. Bookstein, and E.W. Klein, "Possible Association between Benign Hepatomas and Oral Contraceptives," *Lancet,* 2:926–928, 1973.

39. Mays, E.T., W.M. Christopherson, M.M. Mahr, and H.C. Williams, "Hepatic Changes in Young Women Ingesting Contraceptive Steroids, Hepatic Hemorrhage and Primary Hepatic Tumors." *Journal of the American Medical Association,* 235:730–782, 1976.

40. Edmondson, H.A., B. Henderson, and B. Benton, "Liver Cell Adenomas Associated with the Use of Oral Contraceptives," *New England Journal of Medicine,* 294:470–472, 1976.

41. Pfeffer, R.I. and S. Van Den Noore, "Estrogen Use and Stroke Risk in Postmenopausal Women," *American Journal of Epidemiology,* 103:445–456, 1976.

PATIENT INFORMATION ABOUT ESTROGENS

Estrogens are female hormones produced by the ovaries. The ovaries make several different kinds of estrogens. In addition, scientists have been able to make a variety of synthetic estrogens. As far as we know, all these synthetic estrogens have similar properties and therefore much the same usefulness, side effects, and risks. This leaflet is intended to help you understand what estrogens are used for, some of the risks involved in their use, and to help minimize these risks. This leaflet includes important information about estrogens, but not all the information. If you want to know more, you can ask your doctor or pharmacist to let you read the package insert prepared for the doctor.

USES OF ESTROGEN

THERE IS NO PROPER USE OF ESTROGENS IN A PREGNANT WOMAN

Estrogens are prescribed by doctors for a number of purposes, including:

1. To provide estrogen during a period of adjustment when a woman's ovaries no longer produce it, in order to prevent certain uncomfortable symptoms of estrogen deficiency. (All women normally decrease the production of estrogens, generally between the ages of 45 and 55; this is called the menopause.)

2. To prevent symptoms of estrogen deficiency when a woman's ovaries have been removed surgically before the natural menopause.

3. To prevent pregnancy. (Estrogens are given along with a progestogen, another female hormone; these combinations are called oral contraceptives or birth control pills. Patient labeling is available to women taking oral contraceptives and they will not be discussed in this leaflet.)

4. To treat certain cancers in women and men.

5. To prevent painful swelling of the breasts after pregnancy in women who choose not to nurse their babies.

ESTROGENS IN THE MENOPAUSE

In the natural course of their lives, all women eventually experience a decrease in estrogen production. This usually occurs between ages 45 and 55 but may occur earlier or later. Sometimes the ovaries may need to be removed by an operation before natural menopause, producing a "surgical menopause."

When the amount of estrogen in the blood begins to decrease, many women may develop typical symptoms: Feelings of warmth in the face, neck, and chest or sudden intense episodes of heat and sweating throughout the body (called "hot flashes" or "hot flushes"). These symptoms are sometimes very uncomfortable. A few women eventually develop changes in the vagina (called "atrophic vaginitis") which cause discomfort, especially during and after intercourse. Estrogens can be prescribed to treat these symptoms of the menopause. It is estimated that considerably more than half of all women undergoing the menopause have only mild symptoms or no symptoms at all and therefore do not need estrogens. Other women may need estrogens for a few months, while their bodies adjust to lower estrogen levels. Sometimes the need will be for periods longer than six months. In an attempt to avoid over-stimulation of the uterus (womb), estrogens are usually given cyclically during each month of use, that is three weeks of pills followed by one week without pills.

Sometimes women experience nervous symptoms or depression during menopause. There is no evidence that estrogens are effective for such symptoms and they should not be used to treat them, although other treatment may be needed.

You may have heard that taking estrogens for long periods (years) after the menopause will keep your skin soft and supple and keep you feeling young. There is no evidence that this is so, however, and such long-term treatment carries important risks.

ESTROGENS TO PREVENT SWELLING OF THE BREASTS AFTER PREGNANCY

If you do not breast-feed your baby after delivery, your breasts may fill up with milk and become painful and engorged. This usually begins about three to four days after delivery and may last for a few days to up to a week or more. Sometimes the discomfort is severe, but usually it is not and can be controlled by pain-relieving drugs such as aspirin and by binding the breasts up tightly. Estrogens can be used to try to prevent the breasts from filling up. While this treatment is sometimes successful, in many cases the breasts fill up to some degree in spite of treatment. The dose of estrogens needed to prevent pain and swelling of the breasts is much larger than the dose needed to treat symptoms of the menopause and this may increase your chances of developing blood clots in the legs or lungs (see below). Therefore, it is important that you discuss the benefits and the risks of estrogen use with your doctor if you have decided not to breast-feed your baby.

SOME OF THE DANGERS OF ESTROGEN

1. *Cancer of the uterus.* If estrogens are used in the postmenopausal period for more than a year, there is an increased risk of *endometrial cancer* (cancer of the uterus). Women taking estrogens have roughly five to ten times as great a chance of getting this cancer as women who take no estrogens. To put this another way, while a postmenopausal woman not taking estrogens has one chance in 1,000 each year of getting cancer of the uterus, a woman taking estrogens has five to ten chances in 1,000 each year. For this reason *it is important to take estrogens only when you really need them.*

The risk of this cancer is greater the longer estrogens are used and also seems to be greater when larger doses are taken. For this reason *it is important to take the lowest dose of estrogen that will control symptoms and to take it only as long as it is needed.* If estrogens are needed for longer periods of time, your doctor will want to reevaluate your need for estrogens at least every six months.

Women using estrogens should report any irregular vaginal bleeding to their doctors; such bleeding may be of no importance, but it can be an early warning of cancer of the uterus. If you have undiagnosed vaginal bleeding, you should not use estrogens until a diagnosis is made and you are certain there is no cancer of the uterus.

If you have had your uterus completely removed (total hysterectomy), there is no danger of developing cancer of the uterus.

2. *Other possible cancers.* Estrogens can cause development of other tumors in animals, such as tumors of the breast, cervix, vagina, or liver, when given for a long time. At present there is no good evidence that women using estrogen in

the menopause have an increased risk of such tumors, but there is no way yet to be sure they do not; and one study raises the possibility that use of estrogens in the menopause may increase the risk of breast cancer many years later. This is a further reason to use estrogens only when clearly needed. While you are taking estrogens, it is important that you go to your doctor at least once a year for a physical examination. Also, if members of your family have had breast cancer or if you have breast nodules or abnormal mammograms (breast x-rays), your doctor may wish to carry out more frequent examinations of your breasts.

3. *Gall bladder disease.* Women who use estrogens after menopause are more likely to develop gall bladder disease needing surgery than women who do not use estrogens. Birth control pills have a similar effect.

4. *Abnormal blood clotting.* Oral contraceptives, some of which contain estrogens, increase the risk of blood clotting in various parts of the body. This can result in a stroke (if the clot is in the brain), a heart attack (clot in a blood vessel of the heart), or a pulmonary embolus (a clot which forms in the legs or pelvis, then breaks off and travels to the lungs). Any of these can be fatal. Blood clots may result in the loss of a limb, paralysis or loss of sight, depending on where the blood clot is formed or lodges if it breaks loose.

The larger doses of estrogen used to prevent swelling of the breasts after pregnancy have been reported to cause clotting in the legs and lungs.

It is recommended that if you have had any blood clotting disorders including clotting in the legs or lungs, or a heart attack or stroke, you should not use estrogens.

SPECIAL WARNING ABOUT PREGNANCY

You should not receive estrogen if you are pregnant. If this should occur, there is a greater than usual chance that the developing child will be born with a birth defect, although the possibility remains fairly small. A female child may have an increased risk of developing cancer of the vagina or cervix later in life (in the teens or twenties). Every possible effort should be made to avoid exposure to estrogens during pregnancy. If exposure occurs, see your doctor.

SOME OTHER EFFECTS OF ESTROGENS

In addition to the serious known risks of estrogens described above, estrogens have the following side effects and potential risks:

1. *Nausea and vomiting.* The most common side effect of estrogen therapy is nausea. Vomiting is less common.

2. *Effects on breasts.* Estrogens may cause breast tenderness or enlargement and may cause the breasts to secrete a liquid.

3. *Effects on the uterus.* Estrogens may cause benign fibroid tumors of the uterus to get larger.

Some women will have menstrual bleeding when estrogens are stopped. But if the bleeding occurs on days you are still taking estrogens you should report this to your doctor.

4. *Effects on liver.* Women taking estrogens develop on rare occasions a tumor of the liver which can rupture and bleed into the abdomen. You should report any swelling or unusual pain or tenderness in the abdomen to your doctor immediately.

Women with a past history of jaundice (yellowing of the skin and white parts of the eyes) may get jaundice again during estrogen use.

5. *Other effects.* Estrogens may cause excess fluid to be retained in the body. This may make some conditions worse, such as epilepsy, migraine, heart disease, or kidney disease. If any of the above occur, stop taking estrogens and call your doctor.

SUMMARY

Estrogens have important uses, but they have serious risks as well. You must decide, with your doctor, whether the risks are acceptable to you in view of the benefits of treatment. Except where your doctor has prescribed estrogens for use in special cases of cancer of the breast or prostate, you should not use estrogens if you have cancer of the breast or uterus, are pregnant, have undiagnosed abnormal vaginal bleeding, blood clotting disorders including clotting in the legs or lungs, or have had a stroke, heart attack or angina.

You must understand that your doctor will require regular physical examinations while you are taking them and will try to discontinue the drug as soon as possible and use the smallest dose possible. You can help minimize the risk by being alert for signs of trouble including:

1. Abnormal bleeding from the vagina.

2. Pains in the calves or chest or sudden shortness of breath, or coughing blood (indicating possible clots in the legs, heart or lungs).

3. Severe headache, dizziness, faintness, or changes in vision (indicating possible developing clots in the brain or eye).

4. Breast lumps (you should ask your doctor how to examine your own breasts).

5. Jaundice (yellowing of the skin).
6. Mental depression.
7. _Any_ other unusual condition or problem.

Based on his or her assessment of your medical needs, your doctor has prescribed this drug for you. Do not give the drug to anyone else.

HOW SUPPLIED

Available in 2.75 oz. (78g) tubes with or without ORTHO® Measured-Dose Applicator.
With applicator: NDC 0062-5450-77
Without applicator: NDC 0062-5450-00
Store at controlled room temperature.

ORTHO-GYNOL® Contraceptive Jelly   **OTC**

(See PDR For Nonprescription Drugs.)

ORTHO–NOVUM® Tablets   ℞
(norethindrone/mestranol) or
(norethindrone/ethinyl estradiol)
and
MODICON® Tablets   ℞
(norethindrone/ethinyl estradiol)
and
MICRONOR® Tablets   ℞
(norethindrone)

COMBINATION ORAL CONTRACEPTIVES

Each of the following products is a combination oral contraceptive containing the progestational compound norethindrone and the estrogenic compound ethinyl estradiol:
ORTHO-NOVUM 7/7/7 □ 21 Tablets and ORTHO-NOVUM 7/7/7 □ 28 Tablets: Each white tablet contains 0.5 mg of norethindrone and 0.035 mg of ethinyl estradiol. Inactive ingredients include lactose, magnesium stearate and pregelatinized starch. Each light peach tablet contains 0.75 mg of norethindrone and 0.035 mg of ethinyl estradiol. Inactive ingredients include FD&C Yellow No. 6, lactose, magnesium stearate and pregelatinized starch. Each peach tablet contains 1 mg of norethindrone and 0.035 mg of ethinyl estradiol. Inactive ingredients include FD&C Yellow No. 6, lactose, magnesium stearate and pregelatinized starch. Each green tablet in the ORTHO-NOVUM 7/7/7 □ 28 package contains only inert ingredients, as follows: D&C Yellow No. 10 Aluminum Lake, FD&C Blue No. 2 Aluminum Lake, lactose, magnesium stearate, microcrystalline cellulose and pregelatinized starch.
ORTHO-NOVUM 10/11 □ 21 Tablets and ORTHO-NOVUM 10/11 □ 28 Tablets: Each white tablet contains 0.5 mg of norethindrone and 0.035 mg of ethinyl estradiol. Inactive ingredients include lactose, magnesium stearate and pregelatinized starch. Each peach tablet contains 1 mg norethindrone and 0.035 mg of ethinyl estradiol. Inactive ingredients include FD&C Yellow No. 6, lactose, magnesium stearate and pregelatinized starch. Each green tablet in the ORTHO-NOVUM 10/11 □ 28 package contains only inert ingredients, as listed under green tablets in ORTHO-NOVUM 7/7/7 □ 28.
ORTHO-NOVUM 1/35 □ 21 Tablets and ORTHO-NOVUM 1/35 □ 28 Tablets: Each peach tablet contains 1 mg of norethindrone and 0.035 mg of ethinyl estradiol. Inactive ingredients include FD&C Yellow No. 6, lactose, magnesium stearate and pregelatinized starch. Each green tablet in the ORTHO-NOVUM 1/35 □ 28 package contains only inert ingredients, as listed under green tablets in ORTHO-NOVUM 7/7/7 □ 28.
MODICON 21 Tablets and MODICON 28 Tablets: Each white tablet contains 0.5 mg of norethindrone and 0.035 mg of ethinyl estradiol. Inactive ingredients include lactose, magnesium stearate and pregelatinized starch. Each green tablet in the MODICON 28 package contains only inert ingredients, as listed under green tablets in ORTHO-NOVUM 7/7/7 □ 28.
Each of the following products is a combination oral contraceptive containing the progestational compound norethindrone and the estrogenic compound mestranol:
ORTHO-NOVUM 1/50 □ 21 Tablets and ORTHO-NOVUM 1/50 □ 28 Tablets: Each yellow tablet contains 1 mg of norethindrone and 0.05 mg of mestranol. Inactive ingredients include D&C Yellow No. 10, lactose, magnesium stearate and pregelatinized starch. Each green tablet in the ORTHO-NOVUM 1/50 □ 28 package contains only inert ingredients, as listed under green tablets in ORTHO-NOVUM 7/7/7 □ 28.

PROGESTOGEN-ONLY ORAL CONTRACEPTIVE

The following product is a progestogen-only oral contraceptive containing the progestational compound norethindrone:
MICRONOR Tablets: Each tablet contains 0.35 mg of norethindrone. Inactive ingredients include D&C Green No. 5, D&C Yellow No. 10, lactose, magnesium stearate, povidone and starch.

The chemical name for norethindrone is 17-hydroxy-19-nor-17α-pregn-4-en-20-yn-3-one, for ethinyl estradiol is 19-nor-17α-pregna-1,3,5(10)-trien-20-yne-3,17-diol, and for mestranol is 3-methoxy-19-nor-17α-pregna-1,3,5(10)-trien-20-yn-17-ol. Their structural formulas are as follows:

norethindrone

ethinyl estradiol

mestranol

CLINICAL PHARMACOLOGY
COMBINATION ORAL CONTRACEPTIVES

Combination oral contraceptives act by suppression of gonadotropins. Although the primary mechanism of this action is inhibition of ovulation, other alterations include changes in the cervical mucus (which increase the difficulty of sperm entry into the uterus) and the endometrium (which reduce the likelihood of implantation).

CLINICAL PHARMACOLOGY
PROGESTOGEN-ONLY ORAL CONTRACEPTIVES

The primary mechanism through which MICRONOR prevents conception is not known, but progestogen-only contraceptives are known to alter the cervical mucus, exert a progestational effect on the endometrium, interfering with implantation, and, in some patients, suppress ovulation.

INDICATIONS AND USAGE

ORTHO-NOVUM 7/7/7 □ 21, ORTHO-NOVUM 7/7/7 □ 28, ORTHO-NOVUM 10/11 □ 21, ORTHO-NOVUM 10/11 □ 28, ORTHO-NOVUM 1/35 □ 21, ORTHO-NOVUM 1/35 □ 28, MODICON 21, MODICON 28, ORTHO-NOVUM 1/50 □ 21, ORTHO-NOVUM 1/50 □ 28, and MICRONOR are indicated for the prevention of pregnancy in women who elect to use this product as a method of contraception.
Oral contraceptives are highly effective. Table I lists the typical accidental pregnancy rates for users of combination oral contraceptives and other methods of contraception. The efficacy of these contraceptive methods, except sterilization, depends upon the reliability with which they are used. Correct and consistent use of methods can result in lower failure rates. [See Table 1 top of next column.]

CONTRAINDICATIONS

Oral contraceptives should not be used in women who currently have the following conditions:
• Thrombophlebitis or thromboembolic disorders
• A past history of deep vein thrombophlebitis or thromboembolic disorders
• Cerebral vascular or coronary artery disease
• Known or suspected carcinoma of the breast
• Carcinoma of the endometrium or other known or suspected estrogen-dependent neoplasia
• Undiagnosed abnormal genital bleeding
• Cholestatic jaundice of pregnancy or jaundice with prior pill use
• Hepatic adenomas or carcinomas
• Known or suspected pregnancy

WARNINGS

Cigarette smoking increases the risk of serious cardiovascular side effects from oral contraceptive use. This risk increases with age and with heavy smoking (15 or more cigarettes per day) and is quite marked in women over 35 years of age. Women who use oral contraceptives should be strongly advised not to smoke.

The use of oral contraceptives is associated with increased risks of several serious conditions including myocardial infarction, thromboembolism, stroke, hepatic neoplasia and gallbladder disease, although the risk of serious morbidity or mortality is very small in healthy women without underlying factors. The risk of morbidity and mortality increases

TABLE I: LOWEST EXPECTED AND TYPICAL FAILURE RATES DURING THE FIRST YEAR OF CONTINUOUS USE OF A METHOD
% of Women Experiencing an Accidental Pregnancy in the First Year of Continuous Use

Method	Lowest Expected*	Typical**
(No contraception)	(89)	(89)
Oral contraceptives		3
combined	0.1	N/A***
progestin only	0.5	N/A***
Diaphragm with spermicidal cream or jelly	3	18
Spermicides alone (foam, creams, jellies and vaginal suppositories)	3	21
Vaginal sponge		
nulliparous	5	18
multiparous	>8	>28
IUD (medicated)	1	6#
Condom without spermicides	2	12
Periodic abstinence (all methods)	2–10	20
Female sterilization	0.2	0.4
Male sterilization	0.1	0.15

Adapted from J. Trussell and K. Kost, Table II, ref. #1.
  * The authors' best guess of the percentage of women expected to experience an accidental pregnancy among couples who initiate a method (not necessarily for the first time) and who use it consistently and correctly during the first year if they do not stop for any other reason.
 ** This term represents "typical" couples who initiate use of a method (not necessarily for the first time), who experience an accidental pregnancy during the first year if they do not stop for any other reason.
*** N/A—Data not available
 # Combined typical rate for both medicated and nonmedicated IUD. The rate for medicated IUD alone is not available.

---

significantly in the presence of other underlying risk factors such as hypertension, hyperlipidemias, obesity and diabetes. Practitioners prescribing oral contraceptives should be familiar with the following information relating to these risks. The information contained in this package insert is principally based on studies carried out in patients who used oral contraceptives with higher formulations of estrogens and progestogens than those in common use today. The effect of long term use of the oral contraceptives with lower formulations of both estrogens and progestogens remains to be determined.
Throughout this labeling, epidemiological studies reported are of two types: retrospective or case control studies and prospective or cohort studies. Case control studies provide a measure of the relative risk of a disease, namely, a _ratio_ of the incidence of a disease among oral contraceptive users to that among nonusers. The relative risk does not provide information on the actual clinical occurrence of a disease. Cohort studies provide a measure of attributable risk, which is the _difference_ in the incidence of disease between oral contraceptive users and nonusers. The attributable risk does provide information about the actual occurrence of a disease in the population (adapted from refs. 2 and 3 with the author's permission). For further information, the reader is referred to a text on epidemiological methods.
1. THROMBOEMBOLIC DISORDERS AND OTHER VASCULAR PROBLEMS
a. Myocardial Infarction
An increased risk of myocardial infarction has been associated with oral contraceptive use. This risk is primarily in smokers or women with other underlying risk factors for coronary artery disease such as hypertension, hypercholesterolemia, morbid obesity, and diabetes. The relative risk of heart attack for current oral contraceptive users has been estimated to be two to six[4-10]. The risk is very low under the age of 30.
Smoking in combination with oral contraceptive use has been shown to contribute substantially to the incidence of myocardial infarctions in women in their mid-thirties or older with smoking accounting for the majority of excess cases[11]. Mortality rates associated with circulatory disease have been shown to increase substantially in smokers, especially in those 35 years of age and older among women who use oral contraceptives. [See graph next page.]
Oral contraceptives may compound the effects of well-known risk factors, such as hypertension, diabetes, hyperlipidemias, age and obesity[13]. In particular, some progestogens are known to decrease HDL cholesterol and cause glucose intolerance, while estrogens may create a state of hyperinsulin-

Continued on next page

Ortho—Cont.

CIRCULATORY DISEASE MORTALITY RATES PER 100,000 WOMAN-YEARS BY AGE, SMOKING STATUS AND ORAL CONTRACEPTIVE USE

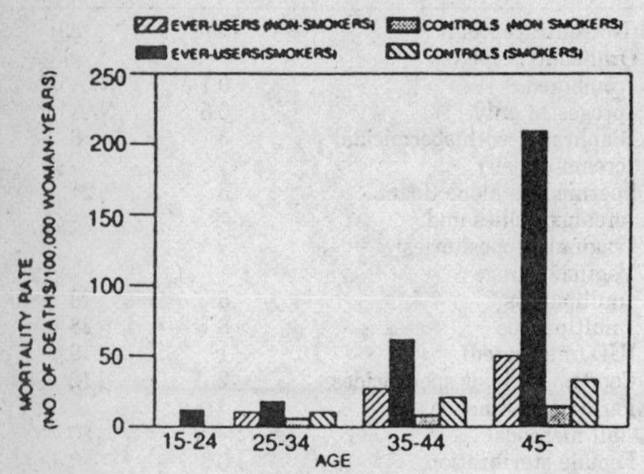

TABLE II. (Adapted from P.M. Layde and V. Beral, ref. #12.)

ism[14–18]. Oral contraceptives have been shown to increase blood pressure among users (see section 9 in WARNINGS). Similar effects on risk factors have been associated with an increased risk of heart disease. Oral contraceptives must be used with caution in women with cardiovascular disease risk factors.

b. Thromboembolism

An increased risk of thromboembolic and thrombotic disease associated with the use of oral contraceptives is well established. Case control studies have found the relative risk of users compared to non-users to be 3 for the first episode of superficial venous thrombosis, 4 to 11 for deep vein thrombosis or pulmonary embolism, and 1.5 to 6 for women with predisposing conditions for venous thromboembolic disease[2,3,19–24]. Cohort studies have shown the relative risk to be somewhat lower, about 3 for new cases and about 4.5 for new cases requiring hospitalization[25]. The risk of thromboembolic disease associated with oral contraceptives is not related to length of use and disappears after pill use is stopped[2].

A two- to four-fold increase in relative risk of post-operative thromboembolic complications has been reported with the use of oral contraceptives[9]. The relative risk of venous thrombosis in women who have predisposing conditions is twice that of women without such medical conditions[26]. If feasible, oral contraceptives should be discontinued at least four weeks prior to and for two weeks after elective surgery of a type associated with an increase in risk of thromboembolism and during and following prolonged immobilization. Since the immediate postpartum period is also associated with an increased risk of thromboembolism, oral contraceptives should be started no earlier than four weeks after delivery in women who elect not to breast feed.

c. Cerebrovascular diseases

Oral contraceptives have been shown to increase both the relative and attributable risks of cerebrovascular events (thrombotic and hemorrhagic strokes), although, in general, the risk is greatest among older (> 35 years), hypertensive women who also smoke. Hypertension was found to be a risk factor for both users and non-users, for both types of strokes, and smoking interacted to increase the risk of stroke[27–29].

In a large study, the relative risk of thrombotic strokes has been shown to range from 3 for normotensive users to 14 for users with severe hypertension[30]. The relative risk of hemorrhagic stroke is reported to be 1.2 for non-smokers who used oral contraceptives, 2.6 for smokers who did not use oral contraceptives, 7.6 for smokers who used oral contraceptives, 1.8 for normotensive users and 25.7 for users with severe hypertension[30]. The attributable risk is also greater in older women[3].

d. Dose-related risk of vascular disease from oral contraceptives

A positive association has been observed between the amount of estrogen and progestogen in oral contraceptives and the risk of vascular disease[31–33]. A decline in serum high density lipoproteins (HDL) has been reported with many progestational agents[14–16]. A decline in serum high density lipoproteins has been associated with an increased incidence of ischemic heart disease. Because estrogens increase HDL cholesterol, the net effect of an oral contraceptive depends on a balance achieved between doses of estrogen and progestogen and the activity of the progestogen used in the contraceptive. The activity and amount of both hormones should be considered in the choice of an oral contraceptive.

Minimizing exposure to estrogen and progestogen is in keeping with good principles of therapeutics. For any particular estrogen/progestogen combination, the dosage regimen prescribed should be one which contains the least amount of estrogen and progestogen that is compatible with a low failure rate and the needs of the individual patient. New acceptors of oral contraceptives agents should be started on preparations containing 0.035 mg or less of estrogen.

e. Persistence of risk of vascular disease

There are two studies which have shown persistence of risk of vascular disease for ever-users of oral contraceptives. In a study in the United States, the risk of developing myocardial infarction after discontinuing oral contraceptives persists for at least 9 years for women 40–49 years who had used oral contraceptives for five or more years, but this increased risk was not demonstrated in other age groups[8]. In another study in Great Britain, the risk of developing cerebrovascular disease persisted for at least 6 years after discontinuation of oral contraceptives, although excess risk was very small[34]. However, both studies were performed with oral contraceptive formulations containing 50 micrograms or higher of estrogens.

2. ESTIMATES OF MORTALITY FROM CONTRACEPTIVE USE

One study gathered data from a variety of sources which have estimated the mortality rate associated with different methods of contraception at different ages (Table III). These estimates include the combined risk of death associated with contraceptive methods plus the risk attributable to pregnancy in the event of method failure. Each method of contraception has its specific benefits and risks. The study concluded that with the exception of oral contraceptive users 35 and older who smoke and 40 and older who do not smoke, mortality associated with all methods of birth control is low and below that associated with childbirth. The observation of an increase in risk of mortality with age for oral contraceptive users is based on data gathered in the 1970's (35). Current clinical recommendation involves the use of lower estrogen dose formulations and a careful consideration of risk factors. In 1989, the Fertility and Maternal Health Drugs Advisory Committee was asked to review the use of oral contraceptives in women 40 years of age and older. The Committee concluded that although cardiovascular disease risks may be increased with oral contraceptive use after age 40 in healthy non-smoking women (even with the newer low-dose formulations), there are also greater potential health risks associated with pregnancy in older women and with the alternative surgical and medical procedures which may be necessary if such women do not have access to effective and acceptable means of contraception. The Committee recommended that the benefits of low-dose oral contraceptive use by healthy non-smoking women over 40 may outweigh the possible risks.

Of course, older women, as all women who take oral contraceptives, should take an oral contraceptive which contains the least amount of estrogen and progestogen that is compatible with a low failure rate and individual patient needs.

[See table below.]

TABLE III—ANNUAL NUMBER OF BIRTH-RELATED OR METHOD-RELATED DEATHS ASSOCIATED WITH CONTROL OF FERTILITY PER 100,000 NON-STERILE WOMEN, BY FERTILITY CONTROL METHOD ACCORDING TO AGE

Method of control and outcome	15–19	20–24	25–29	30–34	35–39	40–44
No fertility control methods*	7.0	7.4	9.1	14.8	25.7	28.2
Oral contraceptives non-smoker**	0.3	0.5	0.9	1.9	13.8	31.6
Oral contraceptives smoker**	2.2	3.4	6.6	13.5	51.1	117.2
IUD**	0.8	0.8	1.0	1.0	1.4	1.4
Condom*	1.1	1.6	0.7	0.2	0.3	0.4
Diaphragm/ spermacide*	1.9	1.2	1.2	1.3	2.2	2.8
Periodic abstinence*	2.5	1.6	1.6	1.7	2.9	3.6

* Deaths are birth-related
** Deaths are method-related

Adapted from H.W. Ory, ref. #35.

3. CARCINOMA OF THE REPRODUCTIVE ORGANS

Numerous epidemiological studies have been performed on the incidence of breast, endometrial, ovarian and cervical cancer in women using oral contraceptives. While there are conflicting reports most studies suggest that use of oral contraceptives is not associated with an overall increase in the risk of developing breast cancer. Some studies have reported an increased relative risk of developing breast cancer, particularly at a younger age. This increased relative risk appears to be related to duration of use[36–43,79–89].

Some studies suggest that oral contraceptive use has been associated with an increase in the risk of cervical intraepithelial neoplasia in some populations of women[45–48]. However, there continues to be controversy about the extent to which such findings may be due to differences in sexual behavior and other factors.

4. HEPATIC NEOPLASIA

Benign hepatic adenomas are associated with oral contraceptive use, although the incidence of benign tumors is rare in the United States. Indirect calculations have estimated the attributable risk to be in the range of 3.3 cases/100,000 for users, a risk that increases after four or more years of use especially with oral contraceptives of higher dose[49]. Rupture of benign, hepatic adenomas may cause death through intra-abdominal hemorrhage[50–51].

Studies from Britain have shown an increased risk of developing hepatocellular carcinoma[52–54] in long-term (> 8 years) oral contraceptive users. However, these cancers are rare in the U.S. and the attributable risk (the excess incidence) of liver cancers in oral contraceptive users approaches less than one per million users.

5. OCULAR LESIONS

There have been clincial case reports of retinal thrombosis associated with the use of oral contraceptives. Oral contraceptives should be discontinued if there is unexplained partial or complete loss of vision; onset of proptosis or diplopia; papilledema; or retinal vascular lesions. Appropriate diagnostic and therapeutic measures should be undertaken immediately.

6. ORAL CONTRACEPTIVE USE BEFORE OR DURING EARLY PREGNANCY

Extensive epidemiological studies have revealed no increased risk of birth defects in women who have used oral contraceptives prior to pregnancy[56,57]. The majority of recent studies also do not indicate a teratogenic effect, particularly in so far as cardiac anomalies and limb reduction defects are concerned[55,56,58,59], when taken inadvertently during early pregnancy.

The administration of oral contraceptives to induce withdrawal bleeding should not be used as a test for pregnancy. Oral contraceptives should not be used during pregnancy to treat threatened or habitual abortion.

It is recommended that for any patient who has missed two consecutive periods (or after 45 days from the last menstrual period if the progestogen-only oral contraceptives are used), pregnancy should be ruled out before continuing oral contraceptive use. If the patient has not adhered to the prescribed schedule, the possibility of pregnancy should be considered at the time of the first missed period or upon missing one MICRONOR Tablet. Oral contraceptive use should be discontinued until pregnancy is ruled out.

7. GALLBLADDER DISEASE

Earlier studies have reported an increased lifetime relative risk of gallbladder surgery in users of oral contraceptives and estrogens[60,61]. More recent studies, however, have shown that the relative risk of developing gallbladder disease among oral contraceptive users may be minimal[62–64]. The recent findings of minimal risk may be related to the use of oral contraceptive formulations containing lower hormonal doses of estrogens and progestogens.

8. CARBOHYDRATE AND LIPID METABOLIC EFFECTS

Oral contraceptives have been shown to cause a decrease in glucose tolerance in a significant percentage of users[17]. This effect has been shown to be directly related to estrogen dose[65]. Progestogens increase insulin secretion and create insulin resistance, this effect varying with different progestational agents[17,66]. However, in the non-diabetic woman, oral contraceptives appear to have no effect on fasting blood glucose[67]. Because of these demonstrated effects, prediabetic and diabetic women in particular should be carefully monitored while taking oral contraceptives.

A small proportion of women will have persistent hypertriglyceridemia while on the pill. As discussed earlier (see WARNINGS 1a and 1d), changes in serum triglycerides and

lipoprotein levels have been reported in oral contraceptive users.

9. ELEVATED BLOOD PRESSURE
An increase in blood pressure has been reported in women taking oral contraceptives[68] and this increase is more likely in older oral contraceptive users[69] and with extended duration of use[61]. Data from the Royal College of General Practitioners[12] and subsequent randomized trials have shown that the incidence of hypertension increases with increasing progestational activity.
Women with a history of hypertension or hypertension-related diseases, or renal disease[70] should be encouraged to use another method of contraception. If women elect to use oral contraceptives, they should be monitored closely and if significant elevation of blood pressure occurs, oral contraceptives should be discontinued. For most women, elevated blood pressure will return to normal after stopping oral contraceptives, and there is no difference in the occurrence of hypertension between former and never users[68-71].

10. HEADACHE
The onset or exacerbation of migraine or development of headache with a new pattern which is recurrent, persistent or severe requires discontinuation of oral contraceptives and evaluation of the cause.

11. BLEEDING IRREGULARITIES
Breakthrough bleeding and spotting are sometimes encountered in patients on oral contraceptives, especially during the first three months of use. Non-hormonal causes should be considered and adequate diagnostic measures taken to rule out malignancy or pregnancy in the event of breakthrough bleeding, as in the case of any abnormal vaginal bleeding. If pathology has been excluded, time or a change to another formulation may solve the problem. In the event of amenorrhea, pregnancy should be ruled out.
An alteration in menstrual patterns is likely to occur in women using progestogen-only contraceptives. The amount and duration of flow, cycle length, breakthrough bleeding, spotting and amenorrhea will probably be quite variable. Bleeding irregularities occur more frequently with the use of progestogen-only oral contraceptives than with the combinations and the dropout rate due to such conditions is higher.
Some women may encounter post-pill amenorrhea or oligomenorrhea, especially when such a condition was preexistent.

12. ECTOPIC PREGNANCY
Ectopic as well as intrauterine pregnancy may occur in contraceptive failures. However, in progestogen-only oral contraceptive failures, the ratio of ectopic to intrauterine pregnancies is higher than in women who are not receiving oral contraceptives, since the drugs are more effective in preventing intrauterine than ectopic pregnancies.

PRECAUTIONS

1. PHYSICAL EXAMINATION AND FOLLOW UP
A complete medical history and physical examination should be taken prior to the initiation or reinstitution of oral contraceptives and at least annually during use of oral contraceptives. These physical examinations should include special reference to blood pressure, breasts, abdomen and pelvic organs, including cervical cytology, and relevant laboratory tests. In case of undiagnosed, persistent or recurrent abnormal vaginal bleeding, appropriate diagnostic measures should be conducted to rule out malignancy. Women with a strong family history of breast cancer or who have breast nodules should be monitored with particular care.

2. LIPID DISORDERS
Women who are being treated for hyperlipidemias should be followed closely if they elect to use oral contraceptives. Some progestogens may elevate LDL levels and may render the control of hyperlipidemias more difficult.

3. LIVER FUNCTION
If jaundice develops in any woman receiving such drugs, the medication should be discontinued. Steroid hormones may be poorly metabolized in patients with impaired liver function.

4. FLUID RETENTION
Oral contraceptives may cause some degree of fluid retention. They should be prescribed with caution, and only with careful monitoring, in patients with conditions which might be aggravated by fluid retention.

5. EMOTIONAL DISORDERS
Women with a history of depression should be carefully observed and the drug discontinued if depression recurs to a serious degree.

6. CONTACT LENSES
Contact lens wearers who develop visual changes or changes in lens tolerance should be assessed by an ophthalmologist.

7. DRUG INTERACTIONS
Reduced efficacy and increased incidence of breakthrough bleeding and menstrual irregularities have been associated with concomitant use of rifampin. A similar assocation, though less marked, has been suggested with barbiturates, phenylbutazone, phenytoin sodium, and possibly with griseofulvin, ampicillin and tetracyclines[72].

8. INTERACTIONS WITH LABORATORY TESTS
Certain endocrine and liver function tests and blood components may be affected by oral contraceptives:
a. Increased prothrombin and factors VII, VIII, IX, and X; decreased antithrombin 3; increased norepinephrine-induced platelet aggregability.
b. Increased thyroid binding globulin (TBG) leading to increased circulating total thyroid hormone, as measured by protein-bound iodine (PBI), T4 by column or by radio-immunoassay. Free T3 resin uptake is decreased, reflecting the elevated TBG, free T4 concentration is unaltered.
c. Other binding proteins may be elevated in serum.
d. Sex-binding globulins are increased and result in elevated levels of total circulating sex steroids and corticoids; however, free or biologically active levels remain unchanged.
e. Triglycerides may be increased.
f. Glucose tolerance may be decreased.
g. Serum folate levels may be depressed by oral contraceptive therapy. This may be of clinical significance if a woman becomes pregnant shortly after discontinuing oral contraceptives.

9. CARCINOGENESIS
See WARNINGS section.

10. PREGNANCY
Pregnancy Category X. See CONTRAINDICATIONS and WARNINGS sections.

11. NURSING MOTHERS
Small amounts of oral contraceptive steroids have been identified in the milk of nursing mothers and a few adverse effects on the child have been reported, including jaundice and breast enlargement. In addition, oral contraceptives given in the postpartum period may interfere with lactation by decreasing the quantity and quality of breast milk. If possible, the nursing mother should be advised not to use oral contraceptives but to use other forms of contraception until she has completely weaned her child.

INFORMATION FOR THE PATIENT
See Patient Labeling Printed Below

ADVERSE REACTIONS
An increased risk of the following serious adverse reactions has been associated with the use of oral contraceptives (see WARNINGS section).
- Thrombophlebitis and venous thrombosis with or without embolism
- Arterial thromboembolism
- Pulmonary embolism
- Myocardial infarction
- Cerebral hemorrhage
- Cerebral thrombosis
- Hypertension
- Gallbladder disease
- Hepatic adenomas or benign liver tumors

The following adverse reactions have been reported in patients receiving oral contraceptives and are believed to be drug-related:
- Nausea
- Vomiting
- Gastrointestinal symptoms (such as abdominal cramps and bloating)
- Breakthrough bleeding
- Spotting
- Change in menstrual flow
- Amenorrhea
- Temporary infertility after discontinuance of treatment
- Edema
- Melasma which may persist
- Breast changes: tenderness, enlargement, secretion
- Change in weight (increase or decrease)
- Change in cervical erosion and secretion
- Diminution in lactation when given immediately postpartum
- Cholestatic jaundice
- Migraine
- Rash (allergic)
- Mental depression
- Reduced tolerance to carbohydrates
- Vaginal candidiasis
- Change in corneal curvature (steepening)
- Intolerance to contact lenses

The following adverse reactions have been reported in users of oral contraceptives and the association has been neither confirmed nor refuted:
- Pre-menstrual syndrome
- Cataracts
- Changes in appetite
- Cystitis-like syndrome
- Headache
- Nervousness
- Dizziness
- Hirsutism
- Loss of scalp hair
- Erythema multiforme
- Erythema nodosum
- Hemorrhagic eruption
- Vaginitis

- Porphyria
- Impaired renal function
- Hemolytic uremic syndrome
- Acne
- Changes in libido
- Colitis

OVERDOSAGE
Serious ill effects have not been reported following acute ingestion of large doses of oral contraceptives by young children. Overdosage may cause nausea, and withdrawal bleeding may occur in females.

NON-CONTRACEPTIVE HEALTH BENEFITS
The following non-contraceptive health benefits related to the use of combination oral contraceptives are supported by epidemiological studies which largely utilized oral contraceptive formulations containing estrogen doses exceeding 0.035 mg of estrogen[73-78].
Effects on menses:
- increased menstrual cycle regularity
- decreased blood loss and decreased incidence of iron deficiency anemia
- decreased incidence of dysmenorrhea
Effects related to inhibition of ovulation:
- decreased incidence of functional ovarian cysts
- decreased incidence of ectopic pregnancies
Other effects:
- decreased incidence of fibroadenomas and fibrocystic disease of the breast
- decreased incidence of acute pelvic inflammatory disease
- decreased incidence of endometrial cancer
- decreased incidence of ovarian cancer

DOSAGE AND ADMINISTRATION
To achieve maximum contraceptive effectiveness, ORTHO-NOVUM Tablets, MODICON Tablets and MICRONOR must be taken exactly as directed and at intervals not exceeding 24 hours.

21-Day Regimen (Sunday Start)
When taking ORTHO-NOVUM 7/7/7 □ 21, the first white tablet should be taken on the first Sunday after menstruation begins. If period begins on Sunday, the first white tablet is taken on that day. If switching directly from another oral contraceptive, the first white tablet should be taken on the first Sunday after the last ACTIVE tablet of the previous product. Tablets are taken as follows: One white tablet daily for 7 days, then one light peach tablet daily for 7 days, then one peach tablet daily for 7 days. For subsequent cycles, no tablets are taken for seven days, then a white tablet is taken the next day (Sunday), etc.
When taking ORTHO-NOVUM 10/11 □ 21, the first white tablet should be taken on the first Sunday after menstruation begins. If period begins on Sunday, the first white tablet is taken on that day. If switching directly from another oral contraceptive, the first white tablet shold be taken on the first Sunday after the last ACTIVE tablet of the previous product. Tablets are taken as follows: One white tablet daily for 10 days, then one peach tablet daily for 11 days. For subsequent cycles, no tablets are taken for 7 days, then a white tablet is taken the next day (Sunday), etc. If first starting oral contraceptives more than 5 days from the onset of menses, contraceptive reliance should not be placed on these products until after the first 7 consecutive days of administration. The use of ORTHO-NOVUM 7/7/7 □ 21 and ORTHO-NOVUM 10/11 □ 21 for contraception may be initiated postpartum. When the tablets are administered during the postpartum period, the increased risk of thromboembolic disease associated with the postpartum period must be considered. (See CONTRAINDICATIONS and WARNINGS concerning thromboembolic disease.) The possibility of ovulation and conception prior to initiation of medication should be considered. If the patient misses more than one tablet, the patient should begin taking tablets again as soon as remembered and another method of contraception used for the balance of that tablet cycle.

21-Day Regimen (21 days on, 7 days off)
The dosage of ORTHO-NOVUM 1/35 □ 21, MODICON 21, and ORTHO-NOVUM 1/50 □ 21 for the initial cycle of therapy is one tablet administered daily from the 5th day through the 25th day of the menstrual cycle, counting the first day of menstrual flow as "Day 1." The use of these products for contraception may be initiated postpartum. When the tablets are administered during the postpartum period, the increased risk of thromboembolic disease associated with the postpartum period must be considered. (See CONTRAINDICATIONS and WARNINGS concerning thromboembolic disease.) If ORTHO-NOVUM 1/35 □ 21, MODICON 21, and ORTHO-NOVUM 1/50 □ 21, are first taken later than the fifth day of the first menstrual cycle of medication or postpartum, contraceptive reliance should not be placed on these products until after the first seven consecutive days of administration. For subsequent cycles, no tablets are taken for 7 days, then a new course is started of one tablet a day for 21 days. The dosage regimen then continues with 7 days of no

Continued on next page

Ortho—Cont.

medication, followed by 21 days of medication, instituting a three-weeks-on, one-week-off dosage regimen. The possibility of ovulation and conception prior to initiation of medication should be considered. If the patient misses more than one tablet, the patient should begin taking tablets again as soon as remembered and another method of contraception used for the balance of that tablet cycle.

(See discussion of Dose-Related Risk of Vascular Disease from Oral Contraceptives.)

28-Day Regimen (Sunday Start)

When taking ORTHO-NOVUM 7/7/7 □ 28, the first white tablet should be taken on the first Sunday after menstruation begins. If period begins on Sunday, the first white tablet is taken on that day. If switching directly from another oral contraceptive, the first white tablet should be taken on the first Sunday after the last ACTIVE tablet of the previous product. Tablets are taken without interruption as follows: One white tablet daily for 7 days, one light peach tablet daily for 7 days, one peach tablet daily for 7 days, then one green tablet daily for 7 days. After 28 tablets have been taken, a white tablet is then taken the next day (Sunday), etc.

When taking ORTHO-NOVUM 10/11 □ 28, the first white tablet should be taken on the first Sunday after menstruation begins. If period begins on Sunday, the first white tablet is taken on that day. If switching directly from another oral contraceptive, the first white tablet should be taken on the first Sunday after the last ACTIVE tablet of the previous product. Tablets are taken without interruption as follows: one white tablet daily for 10 days, one peach tablet daily for 11 days, then one green tablet daily for 7 days. After 28 tablets have been taken, a white tablet is then taken the next day (Sunday), etc.

When taking ORTHO-NOVUM 1/35 □ 28, the first peach tablet should be taken on the first Sunday after mestruation begins. When taking MODICON 28, the first white tablet should be taken on the first Sunday after menstruation begins. When taking ORTHO-NOVUM 1/50 □ 28, the first yellow tablet should be taken on the first Sunday after menstruation begins. If period begins on Sunday, the first peach tablet, white tablet or yellow tablet is taken on that day. If switching directly from another oral contraceptive, the first peach, white or yellow tablet should be taken on the first Sunday after the last ACTIVE tablet of the previous product. Tablets are taken without interruption as follows: One peach, white or yellow tablet daily for 21 days, then one green tablet daily for 7 days. After 28 tablets have been taken, a peach, white or yellow tablet is then taken the next day (Sunday), etc. If first starting oral contraceptives more than 5 days from the onset of menses, contraceptive reliance should not be placed on these products until after the first 7 consecutive days of administration.

The use of ORTHO-NOVUM 7/7/7 □ 28, ORTHO-NOVUM 10/11 □ 28, ORTHO-NOVUM 1/35 □ 28, MODICON 28, and ORTHO-NOVUM 1/50 □ 28 for contraception may be initiated postpartum. When the tablets are administered during the postpartum period, the increased risk of thromboembolic disease associated with the postpartum period must be considered. (See CONTRAINDICATIONS and WARNINGS concerning thromboembolic disease.) The possibility of ovulation and conception prior to initiation of medication should be considered. If the patient misses more than one tablet, the patient should begin taking tablets again as soon as remembered and another method of contraception used for the balance of that tablet cycle.

MICRONOR (Continuous Regimen)

MICRONOR (norethindrone) is administered on a continuous daily dosage regimen starting on the first day of menstruation, i.e., one tablet each day, every day of the year. Tablets should be taken at the same time each day and continued daily. The patient should be advised that if prolonged bleeding occurs, she should consult her physician.

The use of MICRONOR for contraception may be initiated postpartum (see WARNINGS section). When MICRONOR is administered during the postpartum period, the increased risk of thromboembolic disease associated with the postpartum period must be considered. (See CONTRAINDICATIONS and WARNINGS concerning thromboembolic disease.)

If the patient misses one tablet, MICRONOR should be discontinued immediately and a method of nonhormonal contraception should be used until menses has appeared or pregnancy has been excluded.

Alternatively, if the patient has taken the tablets correctly, and if menses does not appear when expected, a nonhormonal method of contraception should be substituted until an appropriate diagnostic procedure is performed to rule out pregnancy.

All Oral Contraceptives

Breakthrough bleeding, spotting, and amenorrhea are frequent reasons for patients discontinuing oral contraceptives. In breakthrough bleeding, as in all cases of irregular bleeding from the vagina, nonfunctional causes should be borne in mind. In undiagnosed persistent or recurrent abnormal bleeding from the vagina, adequate diagnostic measures are indicated to rule out pregnancy or malignancy. If pathology has been excluded, time or a change to another formulation may solve the problem. Changing to an oral contraceptive with a higher estrogen content, while potentially useful in minimizing menstrual irregularity, should be done only if necessary since this may increase the risk of thromboembolic disease.

Use of oral contraceptives in the event of a missed menstrual period:

1. If the patient has not adhered to the prescribed schedule, the possibility of pregnancy should be considered at the time of the first missed period (or upon missing one MICRONOR Tablet) and oral contraceptive use should be discontinued until pregnancy is ruled out.
2. If the patient has adhered to the prescribed regimen and misses two consecutive periods (or after 45 days from the last menstrual period if the progestogen-only oral contraceptives are used), pregnancy should be ruled out before continuing oral contraceptive use.

HOW SUPPLIED

ORTHO-NOVUM 7/7/7 □ 21 Tablets are available in a DIALPAK* Tablet Dispenser (NDC 0062-1780-15) containing 21 tablets, as follows: 7 white tablets (0.5 mg norethindrone and 0.035 mg ethinyl estradiol), 7 light peach tablets (0.75 mg norethindrone and 0.035 mg ethinyl estradiol) and 7 peach tablets (1 mg norethindrone and 0.035 mg ethinyl estradiol). The white tablets are unscored with "Ortho" and "535" debossed on each side; the light peach tablets are unscored with "Ortho" and "75" debossed on each side; the peach tablets are unscored with "Ortho" and "135" debossed on each side.

ORTHO-NOVUM 7/7/7 □ 21 is available for clinic usage in a VERIDATE* Tablet Dispenser (unfilled) and VERIDATE Refills (NDC 0062-1780-20).

ORTHO-NOVUM 7/7/7 □ 28 Tablets are available in a DIALPAK Tablet Dispenser (NDC 0062-1781-15) containing 28 tablets as follows: 7 white, 7 light peach and 7 peach tablets as described under ORTHO-NOVUM 7/7/7 □ 21, and 7 green tablets containing inert ingredients.

ORTHO-NOVUM 7/7/7 □ 28 is available for clinic usage in a VERIDATE Tablet Dispenser (unfilled) and VERIDATE Refills (NDC 0062-1781-20).

ORTHO-NOVUM 10/11 □ 21 Tablets are available in a DIALPAK Tablet Dispenser (NDC 0062-1770-15) containing 21 tablets, as follows: 10 white tablets (0.5 mg norethindrone and 0.035 mg ethinyl estradiol) and 11 peach tablets (1 mg norethindrone and 0.035 mg ethinyl estradiol). The white tablets are unscored with "Ortho" and "535" debossed on each side; the peach tablets are unscored with "Ortho" and "135" debossed on each side.

ORTHO-NOVUM 10/11 □ 28 Tablets are available in a DIALPAK Tablet Dispenser (NDC 0062-1771-15) containing 28 tablets, as follows: 10 white and 11 peach tablets as described under ORTHO-NOVUM 10/11 □ 21, and 7 green tablets containing inert ingredients.

ORTHO-NOVUM 10/11 □ 28 is available for clinic usage in a VERIDATE Tablet Dispenser (unfilled) and VERIDATE Refills (NDC 0062-1771-20).

ORTHO-NOVUM 1/35 □ 21 Tablets are available in a DIALPAK Tablet Dispenser (NDC 0062-1760-15) containing 21 peach tablets (1 mg norethindrone and 0.035 mg ethinyl estradiol) which are unscored with "Ortho" and "135" debossed on each side.

ORTHO-NOVUM 1/35 □ 21 is available for clinic usage in a VERIDATE Tablet Dispenser (unfilled) and VERIDATE Refills (NDC 0062-1760-20).

ORTHO-NOVUM 1/35 □ 28 Tablets are available in a DIALPAK Tablet Dispenser (NDC 0062-1761-15) containing 28 tablets, as follows: 21 peach tablets as described under ORTHO-NOVUM 1/35 □ 21, and 7 green tablets containing inert ingredients.

ORTHO-NOVUM 1/35 □ 28 is available for clinic usage in a VERIDATE Tablet Dispenser (unfilled) and VERIDATE Refills (NDC 0062-1761-20).

MODICON 21 Tablets are available in a DIALPAK Tablet Dispenser (NDC 0062-1712-15) containing 21 white tablets (0.5 mg norethindrone and 0.035 mg ethinyl estradiol) which are unscored with "Ortho" and "535" debossed on each side.

MODICON 28 Tablets are available in a DIALPAK Tablet Dispenser (NDC 0062-1714-15) containing 28 tablets, as follows: 21 white tablets as described under MODICON 21, and 7 green tablets containing inert ingredients.

MODICON 28 is available for clinic usage in a VERIDATE Tablet Dispenser (unfilled) and VERIDATE Refills (NDC 0062-1714-20).

ORTHO-NOVUM 1/50 □ 21 Tablets are available in a DIALPAK Tablet Dispenser (NDC 0062-1331-15) containing 21 yellow tablets (1 mg norethindrone and 0.05 mg mestranol) which are unscored with "Ortho" and "150" debossed on each side.

ORTHO-NOVUM 1/50 □ 21 is available for clinic usage in a VERIDATE Tablet Dispenser (unfilled) and VERIDATE Refills (NDC 0062-1331-20).

ORTHO-NOVUM 1/50 □ 28 Tablets are available in a DIALPAK Tablet Dispenser (NDC 0062-1332-15) containing 28 tablets, as follows: 21 yellow tablets as described under ORTHO-NOVUM 1/50 □ 21, and 7 green tablets containing inert ingredients.

ORTHO-NOVUM 1/50 □ 28 is available for clinic usage in a VERIDATE Tablet Dispenser (unfilled) and VERIDATE Refills (NDC 0062-1332-20).

MICRONOR Tablets are available in a DIALPAK Tablet Dispenser (NDC 0062-1411-01) containing 28 lime tablets (0.35 mg norethindrone) which are unscored with "Ortho" and "0.35" debossed on each side.

MICRONOR is available for clinic usage in a VERIDATE Tablet Dispenser (unfilled) and VERIDATE Refills (NDC 0062-1411-23).

REFERENCES

1. Reproduced with permission of the Population Council from J. Trussell and K. Kost: Contraceptive failure in the United States: A critical review of the literature. Studies in Family Planning, 18 (5), September–October 1987. **2.** Stadel BV. Oral contraceptives and cardiovascular disease. (Pt. 1). N Engl J Med 1981; *305*:612–618. **3.** Stadel BV. Oral contraceptives and cardiovascular disease. (Pt. 2). N Engl J Med 1981; *305*:672–677. **4.** Adam SA, Thorogood M. Oral contraception and myocardial infarction revisted: the effects of new preparations and prescribing patterns. Br J Obstet Gynecol 1981; *88*:838–845. **5.** Mann JI, Inman WH. Oral contraceptives and death from myocardial infarction. Br Med J 1975; *2(5965)*:245–248. **6.** Mann JI, Vessel MP, Thorogood M, Doll R. Myocardial infarction in young women with special reference to oral contraceptive practice. Br Med J 1975; *2(5956)*:241–245. **7.** Royal College of General Practitioners' Oral Contraception Study: Further analyses of mortality in oral contraceptive users. Lancet 1981; *1*:541–546. **8.** Slone D, Shapiro S, Kaufman DW, Rosenberg L, Miettinen OS, Stolley PD. Risk of myocardial infarction in relation to current and discontinued use of oral contraceptives. N Engl J Med 1981; *305*:420–424. **9.** Vessey MP. Female hormones and vascular disease-an epidemiological overview. Br J Fam Plann 1980; *6(Supplement)*:1–12. **10.** Russell-Briefel RG, Ezzati TM, Fulwood R, Perlman JA, Murphy RS. Cardiovascular risk status and oral contraceptive use, United States, 1976–80. Prevent Med 1986; *15*:352–362. **11.** Goldbaum GM, Kendrick JS, Hogelin GC, Gentry EM. The relative impact of smoking and oral contraceptive use on women in the United States. JAMA 1987; *258*:1339–1342. **12.** Layde PM, Beral V. Further analyses of mortality in oral contraceptive users: Royal College of General Practitioners' Oral Contraception Study. (Table 5) Lancet 1981; *1*:541–546. **13.** Knopp RH. Arteriosclerosis risk: the roles of oral contraceptives and postmenopausal estrogens. J Reprod Med 1986; *31(9) (Supplement)*:913–921. **14.** Krauss RM, Roy S. Mishell DR, Casagrande J, Pike MC. Effects of two low-dose oral contraceptives on serum lipids and lipoproteins: Differential changes in high-density lipoproteins subclasses. Am J Obstet 1983; *145*:446–452. **15.** Wahl P, Walden C, Knopp R. Hoover J, Wallace R, Heiss G, Rifkind B. Effect of estrogen/progestin potency on lipid/lipoprotein cholesterol. N Engl J Med 1983; *308*:862–867. **16.** Wynn V. Niththyananthan R. The effect of progestin in combined oral contraceptives on serum lipids with special reference to high density lipoproteins. Am J Obstet Gynecol 1982; *142*:766–771. **17.** Wynn V, Godsland I. Effects of oral contraceptives on carbohydrate metabolism. J Reprod Med 1986; *31(9)(Supplement)*:892–897. **18.** La Rosa JC. Atherosclerotic risk factors in cardiovascular disease. J. Reprod Med 1986; *31(9)(Supplement)*:906–912. **19.** Inman WH, Vessey MP. Investigation of death from pulmonary, coronary, and cerebral thrombosis and embolism in women of child-bearing age. Br Med J 1968; *2(5599)*:193–199. **20.** Maquire MG, Tonascia J, Sartwell PE, Stolley PD, Tockman MS. Increased risk of thrombosis due to oral contraceptives: a further report. Am J Epidemiol 1979; *110(2)*:188–195. **21.** Petitti DB, Wingerd J, Pellegrin F, Ramacharan S. Risk of vascular disease in women: smoking, oral contraceptives, noncontraceptive estrogens, and other factors. JAMA 1979; *242*:1150–1154. **22.** Vessey MP, Doll R. Investigation of relation between use of oral contraceptives and thromboembolic disease. Br Med J 1968; *2(5599)*:199–205. **23.** Vessey MP, Doll R. Investigation of relation between use of oral contraceptives and thromboembolic disease. A further report. Br Med J 1969; *2(5658)*:651–657. **24.** Porter JB, Hunter JR, Danielson DA, Jick H. Stergachis A. Oral contraceptives and non-fatal vascular disease-recent experience. Obstet Gynecol 1982; *59(3)*:299–302. **25.** Vessey M, Doll R, Peto R, Johnson B, Wiggins P. A long-term follow-up study of women using different methods of contraception: an interim report. J Biosocial Sci 1976; *8*:375–427. **26.** Royal College of General Practitioners: Oral Contraceptives, venous thrombosis, and varicose veins. J Royal Coll Gen Pract 1978; *28*:393–399. **27.** Collaborative Group for the Study of Stroke in Young Women: Oral contraception and increased risk of cerebral ischemia or thrombosis. N Engl J Med 1973; *288*:871–878.

28. Petitti DB, Wingerd J. Use of oral contraceptives, cigarette smoking, and risk of subarachnoid hemorrhage. Lancet 1978; 2 :234–236. 29. Inman WH. Oral contraceptives and fatal subarachnoid hemorrhage. Br Med J 1979; 2(6203) :1468–1470. 30. Collaborative Group for the Study of Stroke in Young Women: Oral Contraceptives and stroke in young women: associated risk factors. JAMA 1975; 231 :718–722. 31. Inman WH, Vessey MP, Westerholm B, Engelund A. Thromboembolic disease and the steroidal content of oral contraceptives. A report to the Committee on Safety of Drugs. Br Med J 1970; 2 :203–209. 32. Meade TW, Greenberg G, Thompson SG. Progestogens and cardiovascular reactions associated with oral contraceptives and a comparison of the safety of 50- and 35-mcg oestrogen preparations. Br Med J 1980; 280(6224) :1157–1161. 33. Kay CR. Progestogens and arterial disease-evidence from the Royal College of General Practitioners' Study. Am J Obstet Gynecol 1982; 142 :762–765. 34. Royal College of General Practitioners: Incidence of arterial disease among oral contraceptive users. J Royal Coll Gen Pract 1983; 33 :75–82. 35. Ory HW. Mortality associated with fertility and fertility control: 1983. Family Planning Perspectives 1983; 15 :50–56. 36. The Cancer and Steroid Hormone Study of the Centers for Disease Control and the National Institute of Child Health and Human Development: Oral contraceptive use and the risk of breast cancer. N Engl J Med 1986; 315 :405–411. 37. Pike MC, Henderson BE, Krailo MD, Duke A, Roy S. Breast cancer in young women and use of oral contraceptives: possible modifying effect of formulation and age at use. Lancet 1983; 2 :926–929. 38. Paul C, Skegg DG, Spears GFS, Kaldor JM. Oral contraceptives and breast cancer: A national study. Br Med J 1986; 293 :723–725. 39. Miller DR, Rosenberg L, Kaufman DW, Schottenfeld D, Stolley PD, Shapiro S. Breast cancer risk in relation to early oral contraceptive use. Obstet Gynecol 1986; 68 :863–868. 40. Olson H, Olson KL, Moller TR, Ranstam J, Holm P. Oral contraceptive use and breast cancer in young women in Sweden (letter). Lancet 1985; 2 :748–749. 41. McPherson K, Vessey M, Neil A, Doll R, Jones L, Roberts M. Early contraceptive use and breast cancer: Results of another case-control study. Br J Cancer 1987; 56 :653–660. 42. Huggins GR, Zucker PF. Oral contraceptives and neoplasia: 1987 update. Fertil Steril 1987; 47 :733–761. 43. McPherson K, Drife JO. The pill and breast cancer: why the uncertainty? Br Med J 1986; 293 :709–710. 44. Shapiro S. Oral contraceptives-time to take stock. N Engl J Med 1987; 315 :450–451, 45. Ory H, Naib Z, Conger SB, Hatcher RA, Tyler CW. Contraceptive choice and prevalence of cervical dysplasia and carcinoma in situ. Am J Obstet Gynecol 1976; 124 : 573–577. 46. Vessey MP, Lawless M, McPherson K, Yeates D. Neoplasia of the cervix uteri and contraception: a possible adverse effect of the pill. Lancet 1983; 2 :930. 47. Brinton LA, Huggins GR, Lehman HF, Malli K, Savitz DA, Trapido E, Rosenthal J, Hoover R. Long term use of oral contraceptives and risk of invasive cervical cancer. Int J Cancer 1986; 38 :339–344. 48. WHO Collaborative Study of Neoplasia and Steroid Contraceptives: Invasive cervical cancer and combined oral contraceptives. Br Med J 1985; 290 :961–965. 49. Rooks JB, Ory HW, Ishak KG, Strauss LT, Greenspan JR, Hill AP, Tyler CW. Epidemiology of hepatocellular adenoma: the role of oral contraceptive use. JAMA 1979; 242 :644–648. 50. Bein NN, Goldsmith HS. Recurrent massive hemorrhage from benign hepatic tumors secondary to oral contraceptives. Br J Surg 1977; 64 :433–435. 51. Klatskin G, Hepatic tumors: possible relationship to use of oral contraceptives. Gastroenterology 1977; 73 :386–394. 52. Henderson BE, Preston-Martin S, Edmondson HA, Peters RL, Pike MC. Hepatocellular carcinoma and oral contraceptives. Br J Cancer 1983; 48 :437–440. 53. Neuberger J, Forman D, Doll R, Williams R. Oral contraceptives and hepatocellular carcinoma. Br Med J 1986; 292 :1355–1357. 54. Forman D, Vincent TJ, Doll R. Cancer of the liver and oral contraceptives. Br Med J 1986; 292 :1357–1361. 55. Harlap S, Eldor J. Births following oral contraceptive failures. Obstet Gynecol 1980; 55 : 447–452. 56. Savolainen E, Saksela E, Saxen L. Teratogenic hazards of oral contraceptives analyzed in a national malformation register. Am J Obstet Gynecol 1981: 140 :521–524. 57. Janerich DT, Piper JM, Glebatis DM. Oral contraceptives and birth defects. Am J Epidemiol 1980; 112 :73–79. 58. Ferencz C, Matanoski GM, Wilson PD, Rubin JD, Neill CA,Gutberlet R. Maternal hormone therapy and congenital heart disease. Teratology 1980; 21 :225–239. 59. Rothman KJ, Fyler DC, Goldblatt A, Kreidberg MB. Exogenous hormones and other drug exposures of children with congenital heart disease. Am J Epidemiol 1979; 109 :433–439. 60. Boston Collaborative Drug Surveillance Program: Oral contraceptives and venous thromboembolic disease, surgically confirmed gallbladder disease, and breast tumors. Lancet 1973; 1 :1399–1404. 61. Royal College of General Practitioners: Oral contraceptives and health. New York, Pittman 1974. 62. Layde PM, Vessey MP, Yeates D. Risk of gallbladder disease: a cohort study of young women attending family planning clinics. J Epidemiol Community Health 1982; 36 :274–278. 63. Rome Group for Epidemiology and Prevention of Cholelithiasis (GREPCO): Prevalence of gallstone disease in an Italian adult female population. Am J Epidemiol 1984; 119 :796–805. 64. Storm BL, Tamragouri RT, Morse ML, Lazar EL, West SL, Stolley PD, Jones JK. Oral contraceptives and other risk factors for gall bladder disease. Clin Pharmacol Ther 1986; 39 :335–341. 65. Wynn V, Adams PW, Godsland IF, Melrose J, Niththyananthan R, Oakley NW, Seedj A. Comparison of effects of different combined oral contraceptive formulations on carbohydrate and lipid metabolism. Lancet 1979; 1 :1045–1049. 66. Wynn V. Effect of progesterone and progestins on carbohydrate metabolism. In: Progesterone and Progestin. Bardin CW, Milgrom E, Mauvis-Jarvis P. eds. New York, Raven Press 1983; pp. 395–410. 67. Perlman JA, Roussell-Briefel RG, Ezzati TM, Lieberknecht G. Oral glucose tolerance and the potency of oral contraceptive progestogens. J Chronic Dis 1985:38 :857–864. 68. Royal College of General Practitioners' Oral Contraception Study: Effect on hypertension and benign breast disease of progestogen component in combined oral contraceptives. Lancet 1977; 1 :624. 69. Fisch IR, Frank J. Oral contraceptives and blood pressure. JAMA 1977; 237 :2499–2503. 70. Laragh AJ. Oral contraceptive induced hypertension-nine years later. Am J Obstet Gynecol 1976; 126 :141–147. 71. Ramcharan S, Peritz E, Pellegrin FA, Williams WT. Incidence of hypertension in the Walnut Creek Contraceptive Drug Study cohort: In: Pharmacology of steroid contraceptive drugs. Garattini S, Berendes HW. Eds. New York, Raven Press, 1977; pp. 277–288, (Monographs of the Mario Negri Institute for Pharmacological Research Milan). 72. Stockley I. Interactions with oral contraceptives. J Pharm 1976; 216 :140–143. 73. The Cancer and Steroid Hormone Study of the Centers for Disease Control and the National Institute of Child Health and Human Development: Oral contraceptive use and the risk of ovarian cancer. JAMA 1983; 249 :1596–1599. 74. The Cancer and Steroid Hormone Study of the Centers for Disease Control and the National Institute of Child Health and Human Development: Combination oral contraceptive use and the risk of endometrial cancer. JAMA 1987; 257 :796–800. 75. Ory HW. Functional ovarian cysts and oral contraceptives: negative association confirmed surgically. JAMA 1974; 228 :68–69. 76. Ory WH, Cole P, MacMahon B, Hoover R. Oral contraceptives and reduced risk of benign breast disease. N Engl J Med 1976; 294 :419–422. 77. Ory HW. The noncontraceptive health benefits from oral contraceptive use. Fam Plann Perspect 1982; 14 :182–184. 78. Ory HW, Forrest JD, Lincoln R. Making choices: Evaluating the health risks and benefits of birth control methods. New York, The Alan Guttmacher Institute, 1983; p. 1. 79. Schlesselman J, Stadel BV, Murray P, Lai S. Breast cancer in relation to early use of oral contraceptives. JAMA 1988; 259 :1828–1833. 80. Hennekens CH, Speizer FE, Lipnick RJ, Rosner B, Bain C, Belanger C, Stampfer MJ, Willett W, Peto R. A case-control study of oral contraceptive use and breast cancer. JNCI 1984; 72 :39–42. 81. LaVecchia C, DeCarli A, Fasoli M, Franceschi S, Gentile A, Negri E, Parazzini F, Tognoni G. Oral contraceptives and cancers of the breast and of the female genital tract. Interim results from a case-control study. Br J Cancer 1986; 54 :311–317. 82. Meirik O, Lund E, Adami H, Bergstrom R, Christoffersen T, Bergsjo P. Oral contraceptive use and breast cancer in young women. A Joint National Case-control study in Sweden and Norway. Lancet 1986; II :650–654. 83. Kay CR, Hannaford PC. Breast cancer and the pill-A further report from the Royal College of General Practitioners' oral contraception study. Br J Cancer 1988; 58 :675–680. 84. Stadel BV, Lai S, Schlesselman JJ, Murray P. Oral contraceptives and premenopausal breast cancer in nulliparous women. Contraception 1988; 38 :287–299. 85. Miller DR, Rosenberg L, Kaufman DW, Stolley P, Warshauer ME, Shapiro S. Breast cancer before age 45 and oral contraceptive use: New Findings. Am J Epidemiol 1989; 129 :269–280. 86. The UK National Case-Control Study Group, Oral contraceptive use and breast cancer risk in young women. Lancet 1989; 1 :973–982. 87. Schlesselman JJ. Cancer of the breast and reproductive tract in relation to use of oral contraceptives. Contraception 1989; 40 :1–38. 88. Vessey MP, McPherson K, Villard-Mackintosh L, Yeates D. Oral contraceptives and breast cancer; latest findings in a large cohort study. Br J Cancer 1989; 59 : 613–617. 89. Jick SS, Walker AM, Stergachis A, Jick H. Oral contraceptives and breast cancer. Br J Cancer 1989; 59 :618–621.

BRIEF SUMMARY PATIENT PACKAGE INSERT

Oral contraceptives, also known as "birth control pills" or "the pill", are taken to prevent pregnancy and when taken correctly, have a failure rate of less than 1% per year when used without missing any pills. The typical failure rate of large numbers of pill users is less than 3% per year when women who miss pills are included. For most women oral contraceptives are also free of serious or unpleasant side effects. However, forgetting to take pills considerably increases the chances of pregnancy.

For the majority of women, oral contraceptives can be taken safely. But there are some women who are at high risk of developing certain serious diseases that can be fatal or may cause temporary or permanent disability. The risks associated with taking oral contraceptives increase significantly if you:

- smoke
- have high blood pressure, diabetes, high cholesterol
- have or have had clotting disorders, heart attack, stroke, angina pectoris, cancer of the breast or sex organs, jaundice or malignant or benign liver tumors.

Although cardiovascular disease risks may be increased with oral contraceptive use after age 40 in healthy, non-smoking women (even with the newer low-dose formulations), there are also greater health risks associated with pregnancy in older women.

You should not take the pill if you suspect you are pregnant or have unexplained vaginal bleeding.

> **Cigarette smoking increases the risk of serious cardiovascular side effects from oral contraceptive use. This risk increases with age and with heavy smoking (15 or more cigarettes per day) and is quite marked in women over 35 years of age. Women who use oral contraceptives are strongly advised not to smoke.**

Most side effects of the pill are not serious. The most common such effects are nausea, vomiting, bleeding between menstrual periods, weight gain, breast tenderness, and difficulty wearing contact lenses. These side effects, especially nausea and vomiting, may subside within the first three months of use.

The serious side effects of the pill occur very infrequently, especially if you are in good health and are young. However, you should know that the following medical conditions have been associated with or made worse by the pill:

1. Blood clots in the legs (thrombophlebitis), lungs (pulmonary embolism), stoppage or rupture of a blood vessel in the brain (stroke), blockage of blood vessels in the heart (heart attack or angina pectoris) or other organs of the body. As mentioned above, smoking increases the risk of heart attacks and strokes and subsequent serious medical consequences.
2. Liver tumors, which may rupture and cause severe bleeding. A possible but not definite association has been found with the pill and liver cancer. However, liver cancers are extremely rare. The chance of developing liver cancer from using the pill is thus even rarer.
3. High blood pressure, although blood pressure usually returns to normal when the pill is stopped.

The symptoms associated with these serious side effects are discussed in the detailed leaflet given to you with your supply of pills. Notify your doctor or health care provider if you notice any unusual physical disturbances while taking the pill. In addition, drugs such as rifampin, as well as some anticonvulsants and some antibiotics may decrease oral contraceptive effectiveness.

There is conflict among studies regarding breast cancer and oral contraceptive use. Some studies have reported an increase in the risk of developing breast cancer, particularly at a younger age. This increased risk appears to be related to duration of use. The majority of studies have found no overall increase in the risk of developing breast cancer. Some studies have found an increase in the incidence of cancer of the cervix in women who use oral contraceptives. However, this finding may be related to factors other than the use of oral contraceptives. There is insufficient evidence to rule out the possibility pills may cause such cancers.

Taking the combination pill provides some important non-contraceptive benefits. These include less painful menstruation, less menstrual blood loss and anemia, fewer pelvic infections, and fewer cancers of the ovary and the lining of the uterus.

Be sure to discuss any medical condition you may have with your health care provider. Your health care provider will take a medical and family history before prescribing oral contraceptives and will examine you. You should be reexamined at least once a year while taking oral contraceptives. Your pharmacist should have given you the detailed patient information labeling which gives you further information which you should read and discuss with your health care provider.

DETAILED PATIENT LABELING

PLEASE NOTE: This labeling is revised from time to time as important new medical information becomes available. Therefore, please review this labeling carefully.

The following oral contraceptive products contain a combination of an estrogen and progestogen, the two kinds of female hormones:

ORTHO-NOVUM 7/7/7 ☐ 21 Day Regimen and ORTHO-NOVUM 7/7/7 ☐ 28 Day Regimen

Each white tablet contains 0.5 mg norethindrone and 0.035 mg ethinyl estradiol. Each light peach tablet contains 0.75 mg norethindrone and 0.035 mg ethinyl estradiol. Each peach tablet contains 1 mg norethindrone and 0.035 mg ethinyl estradiol. Each green tablet in ORTHO-NOVUM 7/7/7 ☐ 28 Day Regimen contains inert ingredients.

Continued on next page

Ortho—Cont.

ORTHO-NOVUM 10/11 ☐ 21 Day Regimen and ORTHO-NOVUM 10/11 ☐ 28 Day Regimen
Each white tablet contains 0.5 mg norethindrone and 0.035 mg ethinyl estradiol. Each peach tablet contains 1 mg norethindrone and 0.035 mg ethinyl estradiol. Each green tablet in ORTHO-NOVUM 10/11 ☐ 28 Day Regimen contains inert ingredients.
ORTHO-NOVUM 1/35 ☐ 21 Day Regimen and ORTHO-NOVUM 1/35 ☐ 28 Day Regimen
Each peach tablet contains 1 mg norethindrone and 0.035 mg ethinyl estradiol. Each green tablet in ORTHO-NOVUM 1/35 ☐ 28 Day Regimen contains inert ingredients.
MODICON 21 Day Regimen and MODICON 28 Day Regimen
Each white tablet contains 0.5 mg norethindrone and 0.035 mg ethinyl estradiol. Each green tablet in MODICON 28 Day Regimen contains inert ingredients.
ORTHO-NOVUM 1/50 ☐ 21 Day Regimen and ORTHO-NOVUM 1/50 ☐ 28 Day Regimen
Each yellow tablet contains 1 mg norethindrone and 0.05 mg mestranol. Each green tablet in ORTHO-NOVUM 1/50 ☐ 28 Day Regimen contains inert ingredients.
PROGESTOGEN-ONLY ORAL CONTRACEPTIVE
The following oral contraceptive product contains only a progestogen and is often called the "mini-pill":
MICRONOR 28 Day Regimen
Each tablet contains 0.35 mg norethindrone.

INTRODUCTION

Any woman who considers using oral contraceptives (the birth control pill or the pill) should understand the benefits and risks of using this form of birth control. This patient labeling will give you much of the information you will need to make this decision and will also help you determine if you are at risk of developing any of the serious side effects of the pill. It will tell you how to use the pill properly so that it will be as effective as possible. However, this labeling is not a replacement for a careful discussion between you and your health care provider. You should discuss the information provided in this labeling with him or her, both when you first start taking the pill and during your revisits. You should also follow your health care provider's advice with regard to regular check-ups while you are on the pill.

EFFECTIVENESS OF ORAL CONTRACEPTIVES

Oral contraceptives or "birth control pills" or "the pill" are used to prevent pregnancy and are more effective than other non-surgical methods of birth control. When they are taken correctly, the chance of becoming pregnant is less than 1% (1 pregnancy per 100 women per year of use) when used perfectly, without missing any pills. Typical failure rates are actually 3% per year. The chance of becoming pregnant increases with each missed pill during a menstrual cycle.
In comparison, typical failure rates for other non-surgical methods of birth control during the first year of use are as follows:
IUD: 6%
Diaphragm with spermicides: 18%
Spermicides alone: 21%
Vaginal sponge: 18% to 30%
Condom alone: 12%
Periodic abstinence: 20%
No methods: 89%

WHO SHOULD NOT TAKE ORAL CONTRACEPTIVES

Cigarette smoking increases the risk of serious cardiovascular side effects from oral contraceptive use. This risk increases with age and with heavy smoking (15 or more cigarettes per day) and is quite marked in women over 35 years of age. Women who use oral contraceptives are strongly advised not to smoke.

Some women should not use the pill. For example, you should not take the pill if you are pregnant or think you may be pregnant. You should also not use the pill if you have any of the following conditions:
- A history of heart attack or stroke
- Blood clots in the legs (thrombophlebitis), lungs (pulmonary embolism), or eyes
- A history of blood clots in the deep veins of your legs
- Chest pain (angina pectoris)
- Known or suspected breast cancer or cancer of the lining of the uterus, cervix or vagina
- Unexplained vaginal bleeding (until a diagnosis is reached by your doctor)
- Yellowing of the whites of the eyes or of the skin (jaundice) during pregnancy or during previous use of the pill
- Liver tumor (benign or cancerous)
- Known or suspected pregnancy

Tell your health care provider if you have ever had any of these conditions. Your health care provider can recommend a safer method of birth control.

OTHER CONSIDERATIONS BEFORE TAKING ORAL CONTRACEPTIVES

Tell your health care provider if you have or have had:
- Breast nodules, fibrocystic disease of the breast, an abnormal breast x-ray or mammogram
- Diabetes
- Elevated cholesterol or triglycerides
- High blood pressure
- Migraine or other headaches or epilepsy
- Mental depression
- Gallbladder, heart or kidney disease
- History of scanty or irregular menstrual periods

Women with any of these conditions should be checked often by their health care provider if they choose to use oral contraceptives.
Also, be sure to inform your doctor or health care provider if you smoke or are on any medications.

RISKS OF TAKING ORAL CONTRACEPTIVES

1. Risk of developing blood clots
Blood clots and blockage of blood vessels are the most serious side effects of taking oral contraceptives. In particular, a clot in the legs can cause thrombophlebitis and a clot that travels to the lungs can cause a sudden blocking of the vessel carrying blood to the lungs. Rarely, clots occur in the blood vessels of the eye and may cause blindness, double vision, or impaired vision.
If you take oral contraceptives and need elective surgery, need to stay in bed for a prolonged illness or have recently delivered a baby, you may be at risk of developing blood clots. You should consult your doctor about stopping oral contraceptives three to four weeks before surgery and not taking oral contraceptives for two weeks after surgery or during bed rest. You should also not take oral contraceptives soon after delivery of a baby. It is advisable to wait for at least four weeks after delivery if you are not breast feeding. If you are breast feeding, you should wait until you have weaned your child before using the pill. (See also the section on Breast Feeding in General Precautions.)
The risk of circulatory disease in oral contraceptive users may be higher in users of high dose pills and may be greater with longer duration of oral contraceptive use. In addition, some of these increased risks may continue for a number of years after stopping oral contraceptives. The risk of abnormal blood clotting increases with age in both users and nonusers of oral contraceptives, but the increased risk from the oral contraceptive appears to be present at all ages. For women aged 20 to 44 it is estimated that about 1 in 2,000 using oral contraceptives will be hospitalized each year because of abnormal clotting. Among nonusers in the same age group, about 1 in 20,000 would be hospitalized each year. For oral contraceptive users in general, it has been estimated that in women between the ages of 15 and 34 the risk of death due to a circulatory disorder is about 1 in 12,000 per year, whereas for nonusers the rate is about 1 in 50,000 per year. In the age group 35 to 44, the risk is estimated to be about 1 in 2,500 per year for oral contraceptive users and about 1 in 10,000 per year for nonusers.

2. Heart attacks and strokes
Oral contraceptives may increase the tendency to develop strokes (stoppage or rupture of blood vessels in the brain) and angina pectoris and heart attacks (blockage of blood vessels in the heart). Any of these conditions can cause death or disability.
Smoking greatly increases the possibility of suffering heart attacks and strokes. Furthermore, smoking and the use of oral contraceptives greatly increase the chances of developing and dying of heart disease.

3. Gallbladder disease
Oral contraceptive users probably have a greater risk than nonusers of having gallbladder disease, although this risk may be related to pills containing high doses of estrogens.

4. Liver tumors
In rare cases, oral contraceptives can cause benign but dangerous liver tumors. These benign liver tumors can rupture and cause fatal internal bleeding. In addition, a possible but not definite association has been found with the pill and liver cancers in two studies, in which a few women who developed these very rare cancers were found to have used oral contraceptives for long periods. However, liver cancers are rare.

5. Cancer of the reproductive organs
There is conflict among studies regarding breast cancer and oral contraceptive use. Some studies have reported an increase in the risk of developing breast cancer, particularly at a younger age. This increased risk appears to be related to duration of use. The majority of studies have found no overall increase in the risk of developing breast cancer. Some studies have found an increase in the incidence of cancer of the cervix in women who use oral contraceptives. However, this finding may be related to factors other than the use of oral contraceptives. There is insufficient evidence to rule out the possibility that pills may cause such cancers.

ESTIMATED RISK OF DEATH FROM A BIRTH CONTROL METHOD OR PREGNANCY

All methods of birth control and pregnancy are associated with a risk of developing certain diseases which may lead to disability or death. An estimate of the number of deaths associated with different methods of birth control and pregnancy has been calculated and is shown in the table below.

ANNUAL NUMBER OF BIRTH-RELATED OR METHOD-RELATED DEATHS ASSOCIATED WITH CONTROL OF FERTILITY PER 100,000 NONSTERILE WOMEN, BY FERTILITY CONTROL METHOD ACCORDING TO AGE

Method of control and outcome	15–19	20–24	25–29	30–34	35–39	40–44
No fertility control methods*	7.0	7.4	9.1	14.8	25.7	28.2
Oral contraceptives non-smoker**	0.3	0.5	0.9	1.9	13.8	31.6
Oral contraceptives smoker**	2.2	3.4	6.6	13.5	51.1	117.2
IUD**	0.8	0.8	1.0	1.0	1.4	1.4
Condom*	1.1	1.6	0.7	0.2	0.3	0.4
Diaphragm/ spermicide*	1.9	1.2	1.2	1.3	2.2	2.8
Periodic abstinence*	2.5	1.6	1.6	1.7	2.9	3.6

* Deaths are birth-related
** Deaths are method-related

In the above table, the risk of death from any birth control method is less than the risk of childbirth, except for oral contraceptive users over the age of 35 who smoke and pill users over the age of 40 even if they do not smoke. It can be seen in the table that for women aged 15 to 39, the risk of death was highest with pregnancy (7–26 deaths per 100,000 women, depending on age). Among pill users who do not smoke, the risk of death was always lower than that associated with pregnancy for any age group, although over the age of 40, the risk increases to 32 deaths per 100,000 women, compared to 28 associated with pregnancy at that age. However, for pill users who smoke and are over the age of 35, the estimated number of deaths exceeds those for other methods of birth control. If a woman is over the age of 40 and smokes, her estimated risk of death is four times higher (117/100,000 women) than the estimated risk associated with pregnancy (28/100,000 women) in that age group.
The suggestion that women over 40 who do not smoke should not take oral contraceptives is based on information from older higher-dose pills. An Advisory Committee of the FDA discussed this issue in 1989 and recommended that the benefits of low-dose oral contraceptive use by healthy, non-smoking women over 40 years of age may outweigh the possible risks.

WARNING SIGNALS

If any of these adverse effects occur while you are taking oral contraceptives, call your doctor immediately:
- Sharp chest pain, coughing of blood, or sudden shortness of breath (indicating a possible clot in the lung)
- Pain in the calf (indicating a possible clot in the leg)
- Crushing chest pain or heaviness in the chest (indicating a possible heart attack)
- Sudden severe headache or vomiting, dizziness or fainting, disturbances of vision or speech, weakness, or numbness in an arm or leg (indicating a possible stroke)
- Sudden partial or complete loss of vision (indicating a possible clot in the eye)
- Breast lumps (indicating possible breast cancer or fibrocystic disease of the breast; ask your doctor or health care provider to show you how to examine your breasts)
- Severe pain or tenderness in the stomach area (indicating a possibly ruptured liver tumor)
- Difficulty in sleeping, weakness, lack of energy, fatigue, or change in mood (possibly indicating severe depression)
- Jaundice or a yellowing of the skin or eyeballs, accompanied frequently by fever, fatigue, loss of appetite, dark colored urine, or light colored bowel movements (indicating possible liver problems)

SIDE EFFECTS OF ORAL CONTRACEPTIVES

1. Vaginal bleeding

Irregular vaginal bleeding or spotting may occur while you are taking the pills. Irregular bleeding may vary from slight staining between menstrual periods to breakthrough bleeding which is a flow much like a regular period. Irregular bleeding occurs most often during the first few months of oral contraceptive use, but may also occur after you have been taking the pill for some time. Such bleeding may be temporary and usually does not indicate any serious problems. It is important to continue taking your pills on schedule. If the bleeding occurs in more than one cycle or lasts for more than a few days, talk to your doctor or health care provider.

2. Contact lenses

If you wear contact lenses and notice a change in vision or an inability to wear your lenses, contact your doctor or health care provider.

3. Fluid retention

Oral contraceptives may cause edema (fluid retention) with swelling of the fingers or ankles and may raise your blood pressure. If you experience fluid retention, contact your doctor or health care provider.

4. Melasma

A spotty darkening of the skin is possible, particularly of the face, which may persist.

5. Other side effects

Other side effects may include nausea and vomiting, change in appetite, headache, nervousness, depression, dizziness, loss of scalp hair, rash, and vaginal infections.

If any of these side effects bother you, call your doctor or health care provider.

GENERAL PRECAUTIONS

1. Missed periods and use of oral contraceptives before or during early pregnancy

There may be times when you may not menstruate regularly after you have completed taking a cycle of pills. If you have taken your pills regularly and miss one menstrual period, continue taking your pills for the next cycle but be sure to inform your health care provider before doing so. If you have not taken the pills daily as instructed and missed a menstrual period, or if you are taking MICRONOR and missed one tablet, you may be pregnant. If you missed two consecutive menstrual periods, or if you are taking MICRONOR and it is 45 days or more from the start of your last menstrual period, you may be pregnant. Check with your health care provider immediately to determine whether you are pregnant. Do not continue to take oral contraceptives until you are sure you are not pregnant, but continue to use another method of contraception.

There is no conclusive evidence that oral contraceptive use is associated with an increase in birth defects, when taken inadvertently during early pregnancy. Previously, a few studies had reported that oral contraceptives might be associated with birth defects, but these findings have not been seen in more recent studies. Nevertheless, oral contraceptives or any other drugs should not be used during pregnancy unless clearly necessary and prescribed by your doctor. You should check with your doctor about risks to your unborn child of any medication taken during pregnancy.

2. While breast feeding

If you are breast feeding, consult your doctor before starting oral contraceptives. Some of the drug will be passed on to the child in the milk. A few adverse effects on the child have been reported, including yellowing of the skin (jaundice) and breast enlargement. In addition, oral contraceptives may decrease the amount and quality of your milk. If possible, do not use oral contraceptives while breast feeding. You should use another method of contraception since breast feeding provides only partial protection from becoming pregnant and this partial protection decreases significantly as you breast feed for longer periods of time. You should consider starting oral contraceptives only after you have weaned your child completely.

3. Laboratory tests

If you are scheduled for any laboratory tests, tell your doctor you are taking birth control pills. Certain blood tests may be affected by birth control pills.

4. Drug interactions

Certain drugs may interact with birth control pills to make them less effective in preventing pregnancy or cause an increase in breakthrough bleeding. Such drugs include rifampin, drugs used for epilepsy such as barbiturates (for example, phenobarbital) and phenytoin (Dilantin is one brand of this drug), phenylbutazone (Butazolidin is one brand) and possibly certain antibiotics. You may need to use additional contraception when you take drugs which can make oral contraceptives less effective.

HOW TO TAKE ORAL CONTRACEPTIVES

1. General Instructions

You must take your pill every day according to the instructions. Oral contraceptives are most effective if taken no more than 24 hours apart. Take your pill at the same time every day so that you are less likely to forget to take it. You will then maintain an effective dose of the oral contraceptive in your body.

ORTHO-NOVUM 7/7/7—Sunday-Start Package:

21-Day Regimen: The first white tablet should be taken on the first Sunday after the menstrual period begins. If period begins on Sunday, begin taking tablets that day. If switching directly from another oral contraceptive, take the first white tablet on the first Sunday after your last ACTIVE tablet of the previous product. Take one white tablet at the same time each day for 7 consecutive days, take one light peach tablet daily for 7 days, then take one peach tablet daily for 7 days. When newly starting oral contraceptives, if the Sunday you begin ORTHO-NOVUM 7/7/7 is more than 5 days from the start of your menstrual period, it is important that you use another method of birth control until you have taken a white tablet daily for seven consecutive days. After taking your last peach tablet, wait for seven days during which time a menstrual period usually occurs. After the seven-day waiting period, on Sunday, start taking a white tablet each day for the next 7 days; a light peach tablet for the next 7 days; then a peach tablet for the next 7 days, thus using a three-weeks-on, one-week-off regimen.

28-Day Regimen: The first white tablet should be taken on the first Sunday after the menstrual period begins. If period begins on Sunday, begin taking tablets that day. If switching directly from another oral contraceptive, take the first white tablet on the first Sunday after your last ACTIVE tablet of the previous product. Take one white tablet at the same time each day for 7 consecutive days, take one light peach tablet daily for 7 days, take one peach tablet daily for 7 days, then take one green tablet daily for 7 days, during which time your period usually occurs. When newly starting oral contraceptives, if the Sunday you begin ORTHO-NOVUM 7/7/7 is more than 5 days from the start of your menstrual period, it is important that you use another method of birth control until you have taken a white tablet daily for seven consecutive days. After 28 tablets have been taken, (last green tablet will always be taken on Saturday) take the first tablet (white) from your next package the following day (Sunday) whether or not you are still menstruating. With the 28-day regimen, tablets are taken every day of the year.

ORTHO-NOVUM 10/11—Sunday-Start Package:

21-Day Regimen: The first white tablet should be taken on the first Sunday after the menstrual period begins. If period begins on Sunday, begin taking tablets that day. If switching directly from another oral contraceptive, take the first white tablet on the first Sunday after your last ACTIVE tablet of the previous product. Take one white tablet at the same time each day for 10 consecutive days, then take one peach tablet daily for 11 days. When newly starting oral contraceptives, if the Sunday you begin ORTHO-NOVUM 10/11 is more than 5 days from the start of your menstrual period, it is important that you use another method of birth control until you have taken a white tablet daily for seven consecutive days. After taking your last peach tablet, wait for seven days during which time a menstrual period usually occurs. After the seven-day waiting period, on Sunday, start taking a white tablet each day for the next 10 days, then a peach tablet for the next 11 days, thus using a three-weeks-on, one-week-off regimen.

28-Day Regimen: The first white tablet should be taken on the first Sunday after the menstrual period begins. If period begins on Sunday, begin taking tablets that day. If switching directly from another oral contraceptive, take the first white tablet on the first Sunday after your last ACTIVE tablet of the previous product. Take one white tablet at the same time each day for 10 consecutive days, take one peach tablet daily for 11 days, then take one green tablet daily for 7 days, during which time your period usually occurs. When newly starting oral contraceptives, if the Sunday you begin ORTHO-NOVUM 10/11 is more than 5 days from the start of your menstrual period, it is important that you use another method of birth control until you have taken a white tablet daily for seven consecutive days. After 28 tablets have been taken, (last green tablet will always be taken on a Saturday) take the first tablet (white) from your next package the following day (Sunday) whether or not you are still menstruating. With the 28-day regimen, pills are taken every day of the year.

ORTHO-NOVUM 1/35, ORTHO-NOVUM 1/50 and MODICON

21-day Regimen: Counting the first day of menstrual flow as "Day 1," take one tablet daily from the 5th through the 25th day of the menstrual cycle. If the first tablet is taken later than the 5th day of the menstrual cycle or postpartum, contraceptive reliance should not be placed on ORTHO-NOVUM or MODICON until after the first seven consecutive days of administration. Take a tablet the same time each day, preferably at bedtime, for 21 days, then wait for 7 days during which time a menstrual period usually occurs. Following the 7-day waiting period, start taking a tablet each day for the next 21 days, thus using a three-weeks-on, one-week-off dosage regimen.

ORTHO-NOVUM 1/35, MODICON, and ORTHO-NOVUM 1/50

28-Day Regimen: The first white, yellow or peach tablet should be taken on the first Sunday after the menstrual period begins. If period begins on Sunday, begin taking tablets that day. If switching directly from another oral contraceptive, take the first white, yellow or peach tablet on the first Sunday after your last ACTIVE tablet of the previous product. Take one white, yellow or peach tablet at the same time each day for 21 consecutive days, then take one green tablet daily for 7 days during which time your menstrual period usually occurs. When newly starting oral contraceptives, if the Sunday you begin ORTHO-NOVUM 1/35, MODICON or ORTHO-NOVUM 1/50 is more than 5 days from the start of your menstrual period, it is important that you use another method of birth control until you have taken a white, yellow or peach tablet daily for seven consecutive days. After 28 tablets have been taken, (last green tablet will always be taken on a Saturday) take the first tablet (white, yellow or peach) from your next package the following day (Sunday) whether or not you are still menstruating. With the 28-day regimen, pills are taken every day of the year.

MICRONOR—Continuous Regimen

The first MICRONOR Tablet should be taken on the first day of the menstrual period. Take one tablet at the same time each day without interruption for as long as contraceptive protection is desired.

The effectiveness of progestogen-only oral contraceptives, such as MICRONOR, is lower than that of the combination oral contraceptives containing both estrogen and progestogen. If 100 women utilized an estrogen-containing oral contraceptive for a period of one year, generally less than one pregnancy would be expected to occur; however, if MICRONOR had been utilized, approximately three pregnancies might occur.

Women who participated in the clinical studies with MICRONOR and who had not taken other oral contraceptives before starting MICRONOR had a higher pregnancy rate (four women out of 100), particularly during the first six months of therapy, and to a large extent because they did not take their tablets correctly.

Of course, if you don't take your tablets as directed, or forget to take them every day, the chance you may become pregnant is naturally greater.

MICRONOR (norethindrone) will probably cause some changes in your menstrual pattern. Your cycle, that is the time between menstrual periods, will vary. For example, you might have a 28-day cycle, followed by a 17-day cycle, followed by a 35-day cycle, etc. This is common with MICRONOR.

While using MICRONOR, your period may be longer or shorter than before. If bleeding lasts more than eight days, be sure to let your doctor know.

If your doctor has scheduled you for surgery, or you need prolonged bed rest, he or she may suggest that you stop taking the pill four weeks before surgery to avoid an increased risk of blood clots. It is also advisable not to start oral contraceptives sooner than four weeks after delivery of a baby.

2. If you forget to take your pill

Combination Oral Contraceptives

If you miss only one combination pill in a cycle, the chance of becoming pregnant is small. Take the missed pill as soon as you realize that you have forgotten it and continue to take your tablets for the rest of that cycle as directed. Since the risk of pregnancy increases with each additional pill you skip, it is very important that you take one pill a day. If you should miss more than one tablet, do not take those tablets missed, but begin taking tablets again as soon as remembered and use another method of contraception for the balance of that tablet cycle.

MICRONOR Tablets

If you miss one MICRONOR Tablet in a cycle, you may become pregnant. Check with your doctor immediately. Oral contraceptives should not be taken by pregnant women.

3. Pregnancy due to pill failure

The incidence of pill failure resulting in pregnancy is approximately one percent (i.e., one pregnancy per 100 women per year) if taken every day as directed, but more typical failure rates are about 3%. If failure does occur, the risk to the fetus is minimal.

4. Pregnancy after stopping the pill

There may be some delay in becoming pregnant after you stop using oral contraceptives, especially if you had irregular menstrual cycles before you used oral contraceptives. It may be advisable to postpone conception until you begin menstruating regularly once you have stopped taking the pill and desire pregnancy.

There does not appear to be any increase in birth defects in newborn babies when pregnancy occurs soon after stopping the pill.

5. Overdosage

Serious ill effects have not been reported following ingestion of large doses of oral contraceptives by young children. Overdosage may cause nausea and withdrawal bleeding in

Continued on next page

Ortho—Cont.

females. In case of overdosage, contact your health care provider or pharmacist.

6. Other information

Your health care provider will take a medical and family history before prescribing oral contraceptives and will examine you. You should be reexamined at least once a year. Be sure to inform your health care provider if there is a family history of any of the conditions listed previously in this leaflet. Be sure to keep all appointments with your health care provider, because this is a time to determine if there are early signs of side effects of oral contraceptive use.

Do not use the drug for any condition other than the one for which it was prescribed. This drug has been prescribed specifically for you; do not give it to others who may want birth control pills.

HEALTH BENEFITS FROM ORAL CONTRACEPTIVES

In addition to preventing pregnancy, use of combination oral contraceptives may provide certain benefits. They are:

- menstrual cycles may become more regular
- blood flow during menstruation may be lighter and less iron may be lost. Therefore, anemia due to iron deficiency is less likely to occur.
- pain or other symptoms during menstruation may be encountered less frequently
- ectopic (tubal) pregnancy may occur less frequently
- noncancerous cysts or lumps in the breast may occur less frequently
- acute pelvic inflammatory disease may occur less frequently
- oral contraceptive use may provide some protection against developing two forms of cancer: cancer of the ovaries and cancer of the lining of the uterus.

If you want more information about birth control pills, ask your doctor or pharmacist. They have a more technical leaflet called the Professional Labeling, which you may wish to read. The Professional Labeling is also published in a book entitled *Physicians' Desk Reference,* available in many book stores and public libraries.

ORTHO PHARMACEUTICAL CORPORATION
Raritan, New Jersey 08869
Revised September 1991 TRADEMARK
631-10-030-5

Shown in Product Identification Section, page 421

PROTOSTAT®
(metronidazole) Tablets ℞

> **WARNING**
> Metronidazole has been shown to be carcinogenic in mice and rats. *(See Warnings.)* Unnecessary use of this drug should be avoided. Its use should be reserved for the conditions described in the *Indications And Usage* section below.

DESCRIPTION

PROTOSTAT (metronidazole) is a 1-(β-hydroxyethyl)-2-methyl-5-nitroimidazole. Both the 250 mg and 500 mg tablets include the following inactive ingredients: Lactose, magnesium stearate, microcrystalline cellulose, povidone, sodium starch glycolate, and stearic acid. Metronidazole is classified therapeutically as an antiprotozoal *(Trichomonas),* and antibacterial (antianaerobic) agent. It occurs as pale yellow crystals that are slightly soluble in water and alcohol. Metronidazole has the following structural formula:

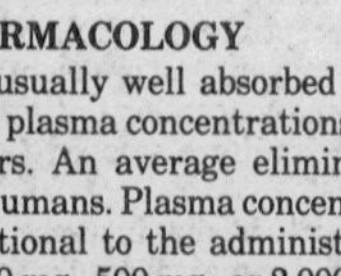

CLINICAL PHARMACOLOGY

Metronidazole is usually well absorbed after oral administration, with peak plasma concentrations occurring between one and two hours. An average elimination half-life is 8 hours in healthy humans. Plasma concentrations of metronidazole are proportional to the administered dose. Oral administration of 250 mg., 500 mg., or 2,000 mg. produced peak plasma concentrations of 6 mcg/ml, 12 mcg/ml, and 40 mcg/ml, respectively. Studies reveal no significant bioavailability differences between males and females; however, because of weight differences, the resulting plasma levels in males are generally lower.

Metronidazole is the major component appearing in the plasma, with lesser quantities of the 2-hydroxymethyl metabolite also being present. Less than 20% of the circulating metronidazole is bound to plasma proteins. Both the parent compound and the metabolite possess *in vitro* trichomonacidal activity and *in vitro* bactericidal activity against most strains of anaerobic bacteria.

The major route of elimination of metronidazole and its metabolites is via the urine (60-80% of the dose), with fecal excretion accounting for 6-15% of the dose. The metabolites that appear in the urine result primarily from side-chain oxidation [1-(β-hydroxyethyl)-2-hydroxymethyl-5-nitroimidazole and 2-methyl-5-nitroimidazole-1-yl-acetic acid] and glucuronide conjugation, with unchanged metronidazole accounting for approximately 20% of the total. Renal clearance of metronidazole is approximately 10 ml/min/1.73m^2.

Decreased renal function does not alter the single-dose pharmacokinetics of metronidazole. However, plasma clearance of metronidazole is decreased in patients with decreased liver function.

Metronidazole appears in cerebrospinal fluid, saliva, and breast milk in concentrations similar to those found in plasma. Bactericidal concentrations of metronidazole have also been detected in pus from hepatic abscesses.

Microbiology: Metronidazole possesses direct trichomonacidal and amoebicidal activity against *Trichomonas Vaginalis* and *Entamoeba histolytica.* The *in vitro* minimal inhibitory concentration (MIC) for most strains of these organisms is 1 mcg/ml or less. Metronidazole's mechanism of antiprotozoal action is unknown.

Anaerobic Bacteria: Metronidazole is active *in vitro* against obligate anaerobes, but does not appear to possess any clinically relevant activity against facultative anaerobes or obligate aerobes. Against susceptible organisms, metronidazole is generally bactericidal at concentrations equal to or slightly higher than the minimal inhibitory concentrations (MIC). Metronidazole has been shown to have *in vitro* and clinical activity against the following organisms:

Anaerobic gram-negative bacilli, including:
Bacteroides species, including the *Bacteroides fragilis* group *(B. fragilis, B. distasonis, B. ovatus, B. thetaiotaomicron, B. vulgatus)*
Fusobacterium species
Anaerobic gram-positive bacilli, including:
Clostridium species and susceptible strains of *Eubacterium*
Anaerobic gram-positive cocci, including:
Peptococcus species
Peptostreptococcus species

Susceptibility tests: Bacteriologic studies should be performed to determine the causative organisms and their susceptibility to metronidazole; however, the rapid, routine susceptibility testing of individual isolates of anaerobic bacteria is not always practical, and therapy may be started while awaiting these results.

Quantitative methods give the most precise estimates of susceptibility to antibacterial drugs. A standardized agar dilution method and a broth microdilution method are recommended.[1]

Control strains are recommended for standardized susceptibility testing. Each time the test is performed, one or more of the following strains should be included: *Clostridium perfringens* ATCC 13124, *Bacteroides fragilis* ATCC 25285, and *Bacteroides thetaiotaomicron* ATCC 29741. The mode metronidazole MIC's for those three strains are reported to be 0.25, 0.25, and 0.5 mcg/ml, respectively.

A clinical laboratory is considered under acceptable control if the results of the control strains are within one doubling dilution of the mode MIC's reported for metronidazole.

A bacterial isolate may be considered susceptible if the MIC value for metronidazole is not more than 16 mcg/ml. An organism is considered resistant if the MIC is greater than 16 mcg/ml. A report of "resistant" from the laboratory indicates that the infecting organism is not likely to respond to therapy.

INDICATIONS AND USAGE

Symptomatic Trichomoniasis: PROTOSTAT is indicated for the treatment of symptomatic trichomoniasis in females and males when the presence of trichomonad has been confirmed by appropriate laboratory procedures (wet smears and/or cultures).

Asymptomatic Trichomoniasis: PROTOSTAT is indicated in the treatment of asymptomatic females when the organism is associated with endocervicitis, cervicitis, or cervical erosion. Since there is evidence that presence of the trichomonad can interfere with accurate assessment of abnormal cytological smears, additional smears should be performed after eradication of the parasite.

Treatment of Asymptomatic Consorts: T. vaginalis infection is a venereal disease. Therefore, asymptomatic sexual partners of treated patients should be treated simultaneously if the organism has been found to be present in order to prevent reinfection of the partner. The decision as to whether to treat an asymptomatic male partner with a negative culture or one in whom no culture has been attempted is an individual one. In making this decision, it should be noted that there is evidence that women may become reinfected if the consort is not treated. Also, since there can be considerable difficulty in isolating the organism from the asymptomatic male carrier, negative smears and cultures cannot be relied upon in this regard. In any event, the consort should be treated with PROTOSTAT in cases of reinfection.

Amebiasis: PROTOSTAT is indicated in the treatment of acute intestinal amebiasis (amebic dysentery) and amebic liver abscess.

In amebic liver abscess, PROTOSTAT therapy does not obviate the need for aspiration or drainage of pus.

Anaerobic Bacterial Infections: PROTOSTAT is indicated in the treatment of serious infections caused by susceptible anaerobic bacteria. Indicated surgical procedures should be performed in conjunction with PROTOSTAT therapy. In a mixed aerobic and anaerobic infection, antibiotics appropriate for the treatment of aerobic infection should be used in addition to PROTOSTAT. In the treatment of most serious anaerobic infections the intravenous form of metronidazole is usually administered initially. This may be followed by oral therapy with PROTOSTAT at the discretion of the physician.

INTRA-ABDOMINAL INFECTION, including peritonitis, intra-abdominal abscess, and liver abscess, caused by *Bacteroides* species including the *B. fragilis* group *(B. fragilis, B. distasonis, B. ovatus, B. thetaiotaomicron, B. vulgatus), Clostridium* species, *Eubacterium* species, *Peptococcus* species, and *Peptostreptococcus* species.

SKIN AND SKIN STRUCTURE INFECTIONS caused by *Bacteroides* species including the *B. fragilis* group, *Clostridium* species, *Peptococcus* species, *Peptostreptococcus* species, and *Fusobacterium* species.

GYNECOLOGIC INFECTIONS, including endometritis, endomyometritis, tubo-ovarian abscess, and post-surgical vaginal cuff infection, caused by *Bacteroides* species including the *B. fragilis* group, *Clostridium* species, *Peptococcus* species, and *Peptostreptococcus* species.

BACTERIAL SEPTICEMIA caused by *Bacteroides* species including the *B. fragilis* group, and *Clostridium* species.

BONE AND JOINT INFECTIONS, as adjunctive therapy, caused by *Bacteroides* species including the *B. fragilis* group.

CENTRAL NERVOUS SYSTEM (CNS) INFECTIONS, including meningitis and brain abscess, caused by *Bacteroides* species including the *B. fragilis* group.

LOWER RESPIRATORY TRACT INFECTIONS, including pneumonia, empyema, and lung abscess, caused by *Bacteroides* species including the *B. fragilis* group.

ENDOCARDITIS caused by *Bacteroides* species including the *B. fragilis* group.

CONTRAINDICATIONS

PROTOSTAT is contraindicated in patients with a prior history of hypersensitivity to metronidazole or other nitroimidazole derivatives. PROTOSTAT is contraindicated during the first trimester of pregnancy. *(See Warnings.)*

WARNINGS

Convulsive Seizures and Peripheral Neuropathy: Convulsive seizures and peripheral neuropathy, the latter characterized mainly by numbness or paresthesia of an extremity, have been reported in patients treated with metronidazole. The appearance of abnormal neurologic signs demands the prompt discontinuation of PROTOSTAT therapy. PROTOSTAT should be administered with caution to patients with central nervous system diseases.

Tumorigenicity Studies in Rodents: Metronidazole has shown evidence of carcinogenic activity in a number of studies involving chronic, oral administration in mice and rats. Prominent among the effects in the mouse was the promotion of pulmonary tumorigenesis. This has been observed in all six reported studies in that species, including one study in which the animals were dosed on an intermittent schedule (administration during every fourth week only). At very high dose levels (approx. 500mg/kg/day) there was a statistically significant increase in the incidence of malignant liver tumors in males. Also, the published results of one of the mouse studies indicated an increase in the incidence of malignant lymphomas as well as pulmonary neoplasms associated with lifetime feeding of the drug. All these effects are statistically significant.

Several long-term oral dosing studies in the rats have been completed. There was a statistically significant increase in the incidence of various neoplasms, particularly in mammary and hepatic tumors, among female rats administered metronidazole over those noted in the concurrent female control groups.

Two lifetime tumorigenicity studies in hamsters have been performed and reported to be negative.

Mutagenicity Studies: Although metronidazole has shown mutagenic activity in a number of *in vitro* assay systems, studies in mammals (*in vivo*) have failed to demonstrate a potential for genetic damage.

PRECAUTIONS

General: Patients with severe hepatic disease metabolize metronidazole slowly, with resultant accumulation of metronidazole and its metabolites in the plasma. Accordingly, for

such patients, doses below those usually recommended should be administered cautiously.

Known or previously unrecognized candidiasis may present more prominent symptoms during therapy with PROTOSTAT and requires treatment with a candicidal agent.

Information for Patients: Alcoholic beverages should be avoided while taking metronidazole and at least one day afterward. (*See Drug Interactions.*)

Laboratory Tests: PROTOSTAT (metronidazole) is a nitroimidazole and should be used with care in patients with evidence of, or history of, blood dyscrasia. A mild leukopenia has been observed during its administration; however, no persistent hematologic abnormalities attributable to metronidazole have been observed in clinical studies. Total and differential leukocyte counts are recommended before and after therapy for trichomoniasis and amebiasis, especially if a second course of therapy is necessary, and before and after therapy for anaerobic infection.

Drug Interactions: Metronidazole has been reported to potentiate the anticoagulant effect of coumarin and warfarin resulting in a prolongation of prothrombin time. This possible drug interaction should be considered when PROTOSTAT is prescribed for patients on this type of anticoagulant therapy.

The simultaneous administration of drugs that induce microsomal liver enzymes, such as phenytoin or phenobarbital may accelerate the elimination of metronidazole, resulting in reduced plasma levels; impaired clearance of phenytoin has also been reported.

The simultaneous administration of drugs that decrease microsomal liver enzyme activity, such as cimetidine, may prolong the half-life and decrease plasma clearance of metronidazole. In patients stabilized on relatively high doses of lithium, short-term metronidazole therapy has been associated with elevation of serum lithium and, in a few cases, signs of lithium toxicity.

Alcoholic beverages should not be consumed during metronidazole therapy and for at least one day afterward because abdominal cramps, nausea, vomiting, headache, and flushing may occur.

Psychotic reactions have been reported in alcoholic patients who are using metronidazole and disulfiram concurrently. Metronidazole should not be given to patients who have taken disulfiram within the last two weeks.

Drug/Laboratory Test Interactions: Metronidazole may interfere with certain types of determinations of serum chemistry values, such as aspartate aminotransferase (AST, SGOT), alanine aminotransferase (ALT, SGPT), lactate dehydrogenase (LDH), triglycerides, and hexokinase glucose. Values of zero may be observed. All of the assays in which interference has been reported involve enzymatic coupling of the assay to oxidation-reduction of nicotine adenine dinucleotide (NAD NADH). Interference is due to the similarity in absorbance peaks of NADH (340 nm) and metronidazole (322 nm) at pH 7.

Carcinogenesis: (*See Warnings.*)

Pregnancy: Teratogenic Effects—Pregnancy Category B. Metronidazole crosses the placental barrier and enters the fetal circulation rapidly. Reproduction studies have been performed in rats at doses up to five times the human dose and have revealed no evidence of impaired fertility or harm to the fetus due to metronidazole. Metronidazole administered intraperitoneally to pregnant mice at approximately the human dose caused fetotoxicity; administered orally to pregnant mice, no fetotoxicity was observed. There are, however, no adequate and well-controlled studies in pregnant women. Because animal reproduction studies are not always predictive of human response, and because metronidazole is a carcinogen in rodents, this drug should be used during pregnancy only if clearly needed (see Contraindications).

Use of PROTOSTAT for trichomoniasis in the second and third trimesters should be restricted to those in whom local palliative treatment has been inadequate to control symptoms.

Nursing Mothers: Because of the potential for tumorigenicity shown for metronidazole in mouse and rat studies, a decision should be made whether to discontinue nursing or to discontinue the drug, taking into account the importance of the drug to the mother. Metronidazole is secreted in breast milk in concentrations similar to those found in plasma.

Pediatric Use: Safety and effectiveness in children have not been established, except for the treatment of amebiasis.

ADVERSE REACTIONS

The two most serious adverse reactions reported in patients treated with PROTOSTAT (metronidazole) have been convulsive seizures and peripheral neuropathy, the latter characterized mainly by numbness or paresthesia of an extremity. Since persistent peripheral neuropathy has been reported in some patients receiving prolonged administration of PROTOSTAT, patients should be specifically warned about these reactions and should be told to stop the drug and report immediately to their physicians if any neurologic symptoms occur.

The most common adverse reactions reported have been referable to the gastrointestinal tract, particularly nausea reported by about 12% of patients, sometimes accompanied by headache, anorexia, and occasionally vomiting; diarrhea; epigastric distress; and abdominal cramping. Constipation has also been reported.

The following reactions have also been reported during treatment with PROTOSTAT (metronidazole):

Mouth: A sharp, unpleasant metallic taste is not unusual. Furry tongue, glossitis, and stomatitis have occurred; these may be associated with a sudden overgrowth of *Candida* which may occur during effective therapy.

Hematopoietic: Reversible neutropenia (leukopenia); rarely, reversible thrombocytopenia.

Cardiovascular: Flattening of the T-wave may be seen in electrocardiographic tracings.

Central Nervous System: Convulsive seizures, peripheral neuropathy, dizziness, vertigo, incoordination, ataxia, confusion, irritability, depression, weakness, and insomnia.

Hypersensitivity: Urticaria, erythematous rash, flushing, nasal congestion, dryness of mouth (or vagina or vulva), and fever.

Renal: Dysuria, cystitis, polyuria, incontinence, and a sense of pelvic pressure. Instances of darkened urine have been reported by approximately one patient in 100,000. Although the pigment which is probably responsible for this phenomenon has not been positively identified, it is almost certainly a metabolite of metronidazole and seems to have no clinical significance.

Other: Proliferation of *Candida* in the vagina, dyspareunia, decrease of libido, proctitis, and fleeting joint pains sometimes resembling "serum sickness." If patients receiving PROTOSTAT drink alcoholic beverages, they may experience abdominal distress, nausea, vomiting, flushing, or headache. A modification of the taste of alcoholic beverages has also been reported.

Crohn's disease patients are known to have an increased incidence of gastrointestinal and certain extraintestinal cancers. There have been some reports in the medical literature of breast and colon cancer in Crohn's disease patients who have been treated with metronidazole at high doses for extended periods of time. A cause and effect relationship has not been established. Crohn's disease is not an approved indication for metronidazole.

OVERDOSAGE

Single oral doses of metronidazole, up to 15 g, have been reported in suicide attempts and accidental overdoses. Symptoms reported include nausea, vomiting, and ataxia. Oral metronidazole has been studied as a radiation sensitizer in the treating of malignant tumors. Neurotoxic effects, including seizures and peripheral neuropathy, have been reported after 5 to 7 days of doses of 6 to 10.4 g every other day.

Treatment: There is no specific antidote for PROTOSTAT overdose; therefore, management of the patient should consist of symptomatic and supportive therapy.

DOSAGE AND ADMINISTRATION

Trichomoniasis:

In The Female: One-day treatment—two grams of PROTOSTAT given either as a single dose or in two divided doses of one gram each given in the same day.

Seven-day course of treatment—250 mg three times daily for seven consecutive days. There is some indication from controlled comparative studies that cure rates as determined by vaginal smears, signs and symptoms, may be higher after a seven-day course of treatment than after a one-day treatment regimen.

The dosage regimen should be individualized. Single-dose treatment can assure compliance, especially if administered under supervision, in those patients who cannot be relied on to continue the seven-day regimen.

A seven-day course of treatment may minimize reinfection of the female long enough to treat sexual contacts. Further, some patients may tolerate one course of therapy better than the other.

Pregnant patients should not be treated during the first trimester with either regimen. If treated during the second or third trimester, the one-day course of therapy should not be used, as it results in higher serum levels which reach the fetal circulation. (*See Contraindications and Precautions.*)

When repeated courses of the drug are required, it is recommended that an interval of four to six weeks elapse between courses and that the presence of the trichomonad be reconfirmed by appropriate laboratory measures. Total and differential leukocyte counts should be made before and after treatment.

In The Male: Treatment should be individualized as for the female.

Amebiasis: Adults: For Acute Intestinal Amebiasis (Acute Amebic Dysentery):
750 mg. orally 3 times daily for 5 to 10 days.

For Amebic Liver Abscess: 500 mg or 750 mg orally 3 times daily for 5 to 10 days.

Children: 35 to 50 mg/kg of body weight/24 hours divided into 3 doses, orally for 10 days.

Anaerobic Bacterial Infections: In the treatment of most serious anaerobic infections the intravenous form of metronidazole is usually administered initially.

Following intravenous therapy, oral metronidazole may be used when conditions warrant based upon the severity of the disease and the response of the patient to intravenous treatment.

The usual adult *oral* dosage is 7.5 mg/kg every six hours (approximately 500 mg for a 70 kg adult). A maximum of 4.0 g should not be exceeded during a 24-hour period.

The usual duration of therapy is 7 to 10 days; however, infections of the bone and joint, lower respiratory tract, and endocardium may require longer treatment.

Patients with severe hepatic disease metabolize metronidazole slowly, with resultant accumulation of metronidazole and its metabolites in the plasma. Accordingly, for such patients, doses below those usually recommended should be administered cautiously. Close monitoring of plasma metronidazole levels[2] and toxicity is recommended.

The dose of PROTOSTAT should not be specifically reduced in anuric patients since accumulated metabolites may be rapidly removed by dialysis.

HOW SUPPLIED

Available in tablets containing 250 mg and 500 mg of metronidazole, USP. PROTOSTAT 250 mg is a white to off-white capsule-shaped, convex tablet. Each 250 mg PROTOSTAT Tablet is scored on one side and imprinted with ORTHO 1570 on the other side, packaged in a bottle of 100 tablets (NDC 0062-1570-01). PROTOSTAT 500 mg is a white to off-white capsule-shaped, convex tablet. Each 500 mg PROTOSTAT Tablet is scored on one side and imprinted with ORTHO 1571 on the other side, packaged in a bottle of 50 tablets (NDC 0062-1571-01).

Dispense in well-closed, light-resistant containers as defined in the USP.

Store below 86°F (30°C).

1. Proposed standard: PSM-11—Proposed Reference Dilution Procedure for Antimicrobic Susceptibility Testing of Anaerobic Bacteria, National Committee for Clinical Laboratory Standards, and Sutter, et al: Collaborative Evaluation of a Proposed Reference Dilution Method of Susceptibility Testing of Anaerobic Bacteria, Antimicrob. Agents Chemother. 16:495-502 (Oct.) 1979; and Talley, et al: In Vitro Activity of Thienamycin Antimicrob. Agents Chemother. 14:436-438 (Sept.) 1978.

2. Ralph, E.D., and Kirby, W.M.M.: Bioassay of Metronidazole With Either Anaerobic or Aerobic Incubation, J. Infect. Dis. 132:587-591 (Nov.) 1975; or Gulaid, et al: Determination of Metronidazole and Its Major Metabolites in Biological Fluids by High Pressure Liquid Chromatography, Br. J. Clin. Pharmacol. 6:430-432, 1978.

Revised January 1992
631-10-680-3

Shown in Product Identification Section, page 421

SULTRIN™ Triple Sulfa Cream ℞
(sulfathiazole/sulfacetamide/
sulfabenzamide)

SULTRIN™ Triple Sulfa ℞
Vaginal Tablets
(sulfathiazole/sulfacetamide/
sulfabenzamide)

DESCRIPTION

SULTRIN Cream contains sulfathiazole (Benzenesulfonamide,4-amino-N-2-thiazolyl-N¹-2-thiazolylsulfanilamide) 3.42%, sulfacetamide (Acetamide,N-[(4-aminophenyl) sulfonyl]-N-Sulfanilylacetamide) 2.86%, and sulfabenzamide (Benzamide,N-[(4-aminophenyl) sulfonyl]-N-Sulfanilylbenzamide) 3.7% with cetyl alcohol 2%, cholesterol, diethylaminoethyl stearamide, glyceryl monostearate, lanolin, lecithin, methylparaben, peanut oil, phosphoric acid, propylene glycol, propylparaben, purified water, stearic acid and urea.

Each SULTRIN Tablet contains sulfathiazole (Benzenesulfonamide,4-amino-N-2-thiazolyl-N¹-2-thiazolylsulfanilamide) 172.5 mg, sulfacetamide (Acetamide,N-[(4-aminophenyl)sulfonyl]-N-Sulfanilylacetamide) 143.75 mg and sulfabenzamide (Benzamide,N-[(4-aminophenyl)sulfonyl]-N-Sulfanilylbenzamide) 184.0 mg, compounded with guar gum, lactose, magnesium stearate, starch and urea.

SULTRIN Cream and SULTRIN Tablets are topical antibacterial preparations available for intravaginal administration.

[See chemical structures at top of next column.]

Continued on next page

Ortho—Cont.

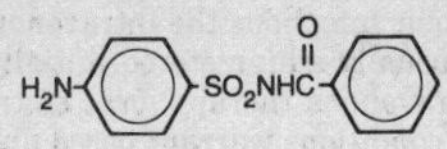

Sulfabenzamide

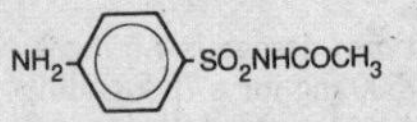

Sulfacetamide

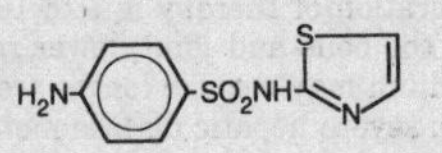

Sulfathiazole

CLINICAL PHARMACOLOGY

The mode of action of SULTRIN is not completely known. SULTRIN Cream and SULTRIN Tablets are topical antibacterial preparations used intravaginally against *Haemophilus (Gardnerella) vaginalis* bacteria. Indirect effects, such as lowering the vaginal pH, may be equally important mechanisms.

INDICATIONS AND USAGE

SULTRIN Cream and SULTRIN Tablets are indicated for the treatment of vaginitis caused by *Haemophilus (Gardnerella) vaginalis* bacteria.
The diagnosis of a *Haemophilus (Gardnerella) vaginalis* vaginitis should be firmly established before initiation of treatment with SULTRIN.

CONTRAINDICATIONS

SULTRIN is contraindicated in the following circumstances: kidney disease; hypersensitivity to sulfonamides; in pregnancy at term and during the nursing period because sulfonamides cross the placenta, are excreted in breast milk and may cause Kernicterus.

WARNINGS

Deaths associated with the administration of sulfonamides have been reported from hypersensitivity reactions, agranulocytosis, aplastic anemia and other blood dyscrasias.
The presence of clinical signs such as sore throat, fever, pallor, purpura or jaundice may be early indications of serious blood disorders.

PRECAUTIONS

Because sulfonamides may be absorbed from the vaginal mucosa, the usual precautions for oral sulfonamides apply. Patients should be observed for skin rash or evidence of systemic toxicity, and if these develop, the medications should be discontinued.
Laboratory tests: Standard office diagnostic procedures for vaginitis are usually sufficient to establish the diagnosis of *Haemophilus (Gardnerella) vaginalis* and to rule out a trichomonal or monilial infection. These include noting a fish-like odor upon addition of 10% KOH to vaginal discharge and microscopic identification of "clue cells" in a wet mount preparation. If cultures are obtained, care must be taken to use appropriate media and methods for *Haemophilus (Gardnerella) vaginalis.*
Carcinogenesis, mutagenesis, impairment of fertility: The sulfonamides bear certain chemical similarities to some goitrogens. Rats appear to be especially susceptible to the goitrogenic effects of sulfonamides, and long-term administration has produced thyroid malignancies in this species.
Pregnancy:
Teratogenic Effects: Pregnancy Category C: The safe use of sulfonamides in pregnancy has not been established. The teratogenicity potential of most sulfonamides has not been thoroughly investigated in either animals or humans. However, a significant increase in the incidence of cleft palate and other bony abnormalities of offspring has been observed when certain sulfonamides of the short, intermediate and long-acting types were given to pregnant rats and mice at high oral doses (7 to 25 times the human therapeutic dose).
Nursing Mothers: Because of the potential for serious adverse reactions in nursing infants from SULTRIN, a decision should be made whether to discontinue nursing or to discontinue the drug, taking into account the importance of the drug to the mother. See CONTRAINDICATIONS.
Pediatric use: Safety and effectiveness in children have not been established.

ADVERSE REACTIONS

There has been one reported case of Agranulocytosis in a patient receiving SULTRIN Cream. The most frequent adverse reactions to SULTRIN are localized irritation and/or allergy including rare reports of Stevens Johnson syndrome which may be fatal.

DOSAGE AND ADMINISTRATION

SULTRIN Cream. One full applicator intravaginally twice daily for four to six days. This course of therapy may be repeated if necessary; the dosage may be reduced one-half to one-quarter.
SULTRIN Vaginal Tablets. One tablet intravaginally before retiring and again in the morning for ten days. This course may be repeated, if necessary.

HOW SUPPLIED

Cream—78 g tubes with the ORTHO* Measured-Dose Applicator.
Vaginal Tablets (as white, capsule-shaped tablets with the Ortho Shield and the word "Ortho" debossed on one side)—Package of twenty foil-wrapped tablets with vaginal applicator.
NDC 0062-5440-77; SULTRIN Cream
NDC 0062-5441-64; SULTRIN Tablets
REVISED SEPTEMBER 1990 643-10-380-5

TERAZOL® 3 ℞
VAGINAL CREAM 0.8%
(terconazole)

DESCRIPTION

TERAZOL® 3 (terconazole) Vaginal Cream 0.8% is a white to off-white, water washable cream for intravaginal administration containing 0.8% of the antifungal agent terconazole, *cis*-1-[4-[[2-(2,4-dichlorophenyl)-2-(1H-1,2,4-triazol-1-ylmethyl)-1,3-dioxolan-4-yl] methoxy] phenyl]-4-(1-methylethyl) piperazine, compounded in a cream base consisting of butylated hydroxyanisole, cetyl alcohol, isopropyl myristate, polysorbate 60, polysorbate 80, propylene glycol, stearyl alcohol, and purified water.
The structural formula of terconazole is as follows:

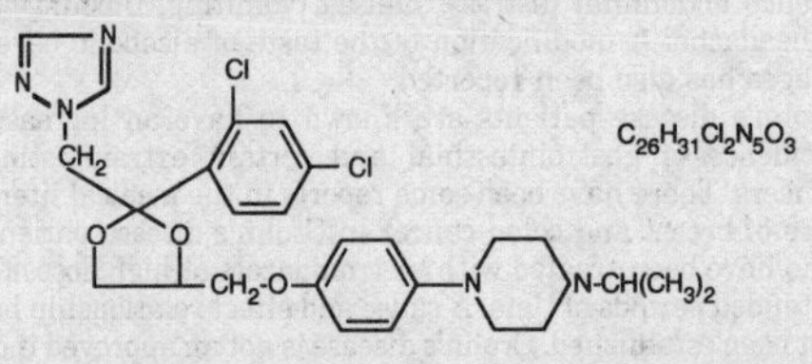
$C_{26}H_{31}Cl_2N_5O_3$

Terconazole, a triazole derivative, is a white to almost white powder with a molecular weight of 532.47. It is insoluble in water; sparingly soluble in ethanol; and soluble in butanol.

CLINICAL PHARMACOLOGY

Following daily intravaginal administration of 0.8% terconazole 40 mg (0.8% cream × 5 g) for seven days to normal humans, plasma concentrations were low and gradually rose to a daily peak (mean of 5.9 ng/mL or 0.006 mcg/mL) at 6.6 hours. Results from similar studies in patients with vulvovaginal candidiasis indicate that the slow rate of absorption, the lack of accumulation, and the mean peak plasma concentration of terconazole was not different from that observed in healthy women. The absorption characteristics of terconazole 0.8% in pregnant or non-pregnant patients with vulvovaginal candidiasis were also similar to those found in normal volunteers.
Following oral (30 mg) administration of ^{14}C-labelled terconazole, the harmonic half-life of elimination from the blood for the parent terconazole was 6.9 hours (range 4.0–11.3). Terconazole is extensively metabolized; the plasma AUC for terconazole compared to the AUC for total radioactivity was 0.6%. Total radioactivity was eliminated from the blood with a harmonic half-life of 52.2 hours (range 44–60). Excretion of radioactivity was both by renal (32–56%) and fecal (47–52%) routes.
In vitro, terconazole is highly protein bound (94.9%) and the degree of binding is independent of the drug concentration.
Photosensitivity reactions were observed in some normal volunteers following repeated dermal application of terconazole 2.0% and 0.8% creams under conditions of filtered artificial ultraviolet light. Photosensitivity reactions have not been observed in U.S. and foreign clinical trials in patients who were treated with terconazole 0.8% vaginal cream.
Microbiology: Terconazole exhibits fungicidal activity *in vitro* against *Candida albicans.* Antifungal activity also has been demonstrated against other fungi. The MIC values for terconazole against most species of lactic acid bacteria typically found in the human vagina were ≥128 mcg/mL. The exact pharmacologic mode of action of terconazole is uncertain; however, it may exert its antifungal activity by the disruption of normal fungal cell membrane permeability. No resistance to terconazole has developed during successive passages of *C. albicans.*

INDICATIONS AND USAGE

TERAZOL 3 Vaginal Cream is indicated for the local treatment of vulvovaginal candidiasis (moniliasis). As TERAZOL 3 Vaginal Cream is effective only for vulvovaginitis caused by the genus *Candida*, the diagnosis should be confirmed by KOH smears and/or cultures.

CONTRAINDICATIONS

Patients known to be hypersensitive to terconazole or to any of the components of the cream.

WARNINGS

None.

PRECAUTIONS

General: Discontinue use and do not retreat with terconazole if sensitization, irritation, fever, chills or flu-like symptoms are reported during use.
Laboratory Tests: If there is lack of response to TERAZOL 3 Vaginal Cream, appropriate microbiologic studies (standard KOH smear and/or cultures) should be repeated to confirm the diagnosis and rule out other pathogens.
Drug Interactions: The levels of estradiol (E2) and progesterone did not differ significantly when 0.8% terconazole vaginal cream was administered to healthy female volunteers established on a low dose oral contraceptive.
Carcinogenesis, Mutagenesis, Impairment of Fertility:
Carcinogenesis: Studies to determine the carcinogenic potential of terconazole have not been performed.
Mutagenicity: Terconazole was not mutagenic when tested *in vitro* for induction of microbial point mutations (Ames test) or for inducing cellular transformation, or *in vivo* for chromosome breaks (micronucleus test) or dominant lethal mutations in mouse germ cells.
Impairment of Fertility: No impairment of fertility occurred when female rats were administered terconazole orally up to 40 mg/kg/day for a three month period.

PREGNANCY: Teratogenic Effects.

Pregnancy Category C.
There was no evidence of teratogenicity when terconazole was administered orally up to 40 mg/kg/day or subcutaneously up to 20 mg/kg/day in rats. Dosages at or below 10 mg/kg/day produced no embryotoxicity; however, there was a delay in fetal ossification at 10 mg/kg/day in rats. There was some evidence of embryotoxicity in rabbits and rats at 20–40 mg/kg. In rats, this was reflected as a decrease in litter size and number of viable young and reduced fetal weight. There was also delay in ossification and an increased incidence of skeletal variants. The no-effect oral dose of 10/mg/kg/day resulted in a mean peak plasma level of terconazole in pregnant rats of 0.176 mcg/mL which exceeds by 30 times the mean peak plasma level (0.006 mcg/mL) seen in normal subjects after intravaginal administration of terconazole 0.8% vaginal cream. This safety assessment does not account for possible exposure of the fetus through direct transfer of terconazole from the irritated vagina by diffusion across amniotic membranes. Since terconazole is absorbed from the human vagina, it should not be used in the first trimester of pregnancy unless the physician considers it essential to the welfare of the patient.
Nursing Mothers: It is not known whether this drug is excreted in human milk. Animal studies have shown that rat offspring exposed via the milk of treated (40 mg/kg/orally) dams showed decreased survival during the first few postpartum days, but overall pup weight and weight gain were comparable to or greater than controls throughout lactation. Because many drugs are excreted in human milk, and because of the potential for adverse reaction in nursing infants from terconazole, a decision should be made whether to discontinue nursing or to discontinue the drug, taking into account the importance of the drug to the mother.
Pediatric Use: Safety and efficacy in children have not been established.

ADVERSE REACTIONS

During controlled clinical studies conducted in the United States, patients with vulvovaginal candidiasis were treated with terconazole 0.8% vaginal cream for three days. Based on comparative analyses with placebo and a standard agent, the adverse experiences considered most likely related to terconazole 0.8% vaginal cream were headache (21% vs. 16% with placebo) and dysmenorrhea (6% vs. 2% with placebo). Genital complaints in general, and burning and itching in particular, occurred less frequently in the terconazole 0.8% vaginal cream 3 day regimen (5% vs. 6%–9% with placebo). Other adverse experiences reported with terconazole 0.8% vaginal cream were abdominal pain (3.4% vs. 1% with placebo) and fever (1% vs. 0.3% with placebo). The therapy related dropout rate was 2.0% for the terconazole 0.8% vaginal cream. The adverse drug experience most frequently causing discontinuation of therapy was vulvovaginal itching, 0.7% with the terconazole 0.8% vaginal cream group and 0.3% with the placebo group.

OVERDOSAGE

Overdose of terconazole in humans has not been reported to date. In the rat, the oral LD 50 values were found to be 1741 and 849 mg/kg for the male and female, respectively. The oral LD 50 values for the male and female dog were ≃1280 and ≥640 mg/kg, respectively.

DOSAGE AND ADMINISTRATION

One full applicator (5 g) of TERAZOL 3 Vaginal Cream (40 mg terconazole) should be administered intravaginally once

daily at bedtime for three consecutive days. Before prescribing another course of therapy, the diagnosis should be reconfirmed by smears and/or cultures and other pathogens commonly associated with vulvovaginitis ruled out. The therapeutic effect of TERAZOL 3 Vaginal Cream is not affected by menstruation.

HOW SUPPLIED

TERAZOLE 3 (terconazole) Vaginal Cream 0.8% is available in 20 g (NDC 0062-5356-01) tubes with an ORTHO® Measured-Dose Applicator. Store at Controlled Room Temperature 15–30°C (59–86°F).

Caution: Federal (U.S.A.) law prohibits dispensing without prescription.

643-10-314-2 Revised February 1991

Shown in Product Identification Section, page 421

TERAZOL® 3 ℞
Vaginal Suppositories 80 mg
(terconazole)

DESCRIPTION

TERAZOL 3 Vaginal Suppositories are white to off-white suppositories for intravaginal administration containing 80 mg of the antifungal agent terconazole, *cis*-1-[4-[[2-(2,4-dichlorophenyl)-2-(1H-1,2,4-triazol-1-ylmethyl)-1,3-dioxolan-4-yl]methoxy]phenyl]-4-(1-methylethyl)piperazine, in triglycerides derived from coconut and/or palm kernel oil (a base of hydrogenated vegetable oils) and butylated hydroxyanisole.

TERCONAZOLE

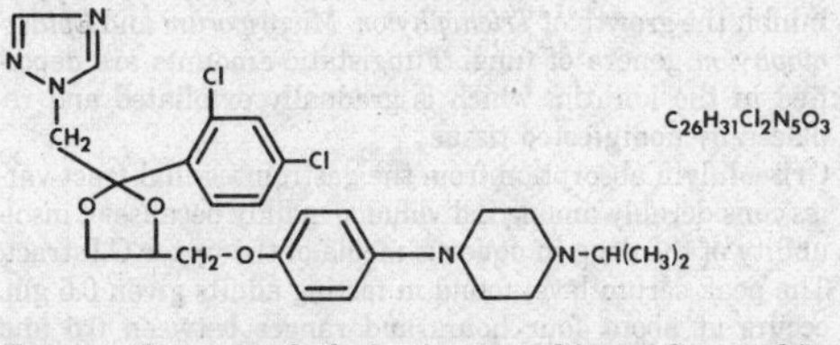
C26H31Cl2N5O3

Terconazole, a triazole derivative, is a white to almost white powder with a molecular weight of 532.47. It is insoluble in water; sparingly soluble in ethanol; and soluble in butanol.

CLINICAL PHARMACOLOGY

Microbiology: Terconazole exhibits fungicidal activity *in vitro* against *Candida albicans.* The MIC values for terconazole against most species of lactic acid bacteria typically found in the human vagina were ≥128 mcg/ml, therefore, these beneficial bacteria are not affected by drug treatment.

The exact pharmacologic mode of action of terconazole is uncertain; however, it may exert its antifungal activity by the disruption of normal fungal cell membrane permeability. No resistance to terconazole has developed during successive passages of *C. albicans.*

Human Pharmacology: Following intravaginal administration of terconazole in humans, absorption ranged from 5–8% in three hysterectomized subjects and 12–16% in two nonhysterectomized subjects with tubal ligations. Following oral (30 mg) administration of ^{14}C-labelled terconazole, the half-life of elimination from the blood for the parent terconazole was 6.9 hours (range 4.0–11.3). Terconazole is extensively metabolized; the plasma AUC for terconazole compared to the AUC for total radioactivity was 0.6%. Total radioactivity was eliminated from the blood with a half-life of 52.2 hours (range 44–60). Excretion of radioactivity was both by renal (32–56%) and fecal (47–52%) routes.

Photosensitivity reactions were observed in some normal volunteers following repeated dermal application of terconazole 2.0% and 0.8% creams under conditions of filtered artificial ultraviolet light.

Photosensitivity reactions have not been observed in U.S. and foreign clinical trials in patients who were treated vaginally with terconazole suppositories or cream.

INDICATIONS AND USAGE

TERAZOL 3 Vaginal Suppositories are indicated for the local treatment of vulvovaginal candidiasis (moniliasis). As TERAZOL 3 Vaginal Suppositories are effective only for vulvovaginitis caused by the genus *Candida,* the diagnosis should be confirmed by KOH smears and/or cultures.

CONTRAINDICATIONS

Patients known to be hypersensitive to terconazole or to any components of the suppository.

WARNINGS

None.

PRECAUTIONS

General: Discontinue use and do not retreat with terconazole if sensitization, irritation, fever, chills or flu-like symptoms are reported during use. The base contained in the suppository formulation may interact with certain rubber latex products, such as those used in vaginal contraceptive diaphragms, therefore concurrent use is not recommended. If there is lack of response to TERAZOL 3 Vaginal Suppositories, appropriate microbiological studies (standard KOH smear and/or cultures) should be repeated to confirm the diagnosis and rule out other pathogens.

Drug Interactions: The therapeutic effect of TERAZOL 3 Vaginal Suppositories is not affected by oral contraceptive usage.

Carcinogenesis, Mutagenesis, Impairment of Fertility

Carcinogenesis: Studies to determine the carcinogenic potential of terconazole have not been performed.

Mutagenicity: Terconazole was not mutagenic when tested *in vitro* for induction of microbial point mutations (Ames test), or for inducing cellular transformation, or *in vivo* for chromosome breaks (micronucleus test) or dominant lethal mutations in mouse germ cells.

Impairment of Fertility: No impairment of fertility occurred when female rats were administered terconazole orally up to 40 mg/kg/day.

Pregnancy: Pregnancy Category C

There was no evidence of teratogenicity when terconazole was administered orally up to 40 mg/kg/day (25 × the recommended intravaginal human dose) in rats, or 20 mg/kg/day in rabbits, or subcutaneously in rats up to 20 mg/kg/day. Dosages at or below 10 mg/kg/day produced no embryotoxicity; however, there was a delay in fetal ossification at 10 mg/kg/day in rats. There was some evidence of embryotoxicity in rabbits and rats at 20–40 mg/kg. In rats this was reflected as a decrease in litter size and number of viable young and reduced fetal weight. There was also delay in ossification and an increased incidence of skeletal variants.

The no-effect oral dose of 10 mg/kg/day resulted in a mean peak plasma level of terconazole in pregnant rats of 0.176 mcg/ml which exceeds by 44 times the mean peak plasma level (0.004 mcg/ml) seen in normal subjects after intravaginal administration of terconazole. This assessment does not account for possible exposure of the fetus through direct transfer of terconazole from the irritated vagina to the fetus by diffusion across amniotic membranes.

Since terconazole is absorbed from the human vagina, it should not be used in the first trimester of pregnancy unless the physician considers it essential to the welfare of the patient.

Nursing Mothers: It is not known whether terconazole is excreted in human milk. Animal studies have shown that rat off-spring exposed via the milk of treated (40 mg/kg/orally) dams showed decreased survival during the first few postpartum days. Because many drugs are excreted in human milk, and because of the potential for adverse reaction in nursing infants from terconazole, a decision should be made whether to discontinue nursing or to discontinue the drug, taking into account the importance of the drug to the mother.

Pediatric Use: Safety and efficacy in children have not been established.

ADVERSE REACTIONS

During controlled clinical studies conducted in the United States, 284 patients with vulvovaginal candidiasis were treated with terconazole 80 mg vaginal suppositories. Based on comparative analyses with placebo (295 patients) the adverse experiences considered adverse reactions most likely related to terconazole 80 mg vaginal suppositories were headache (30.3% vs 20.7% with placebo) and pain of the female genitalia (4.2% vs 0.7% with placebo). Adverse reactions that were reported but were not statistically significantly different from placebo were burning (15.2% vs 11.2% with placebo) and body pain (3.9% vs 1.7% with placebo). Fever (2.8% vs 1.4% with placebo) and chills (1.8% vs 0.7% with placebo) have also been reported. The therapy-related dropout rate was 3.5% and the placebo therapy-related dropout rate was 2.7%. The adverse drug experience on terconazole most frequently causing discontinuation was burning (2.5% vs 1.4% with placebo) and pruritus (1.8% vs 1.4% with placebo).

DOSAGE AND ADMINISTRATION

One TERAZOL 3 Vaginal Suppository (80 mg terconazole) is administered intravaginally once daily at bedtime for three consecutive days. Before prescribing another course of therapy, the diagnosis should be reconfirmed by smears and/or cultures and other pathogens commonly associated with vulvovaginitis ruled out. The therapeutic effect of TERAZOL 3 Vaginal Suppositories is not affected by menstruation.

HOW SUPPLIED

TERAZOL 3 (terconazole) Vaginal Suppositories 80 mg are available as 2.5 g, elliptically shaped white to off-white suppositories in packages of three (NDC 0062-5351-01) with a vaginal applicator. Store at Controlled Room Temperature (59°F–86°F or 15°C–30°C).

643-10-302-7 REVISED FEBRUARY 1990

Shown in Product Identification Section, page 421

TERAZOL® 7 ℞
Vaginal Cream 0.4%
(terconazole)

DESCRIPTION

TERAZOL 7 Vaginal Cream is a white to off-white, water washable cream for intravaginal administration containing 0.4% of the antifungal agent terconazole, *cis*-1-[4-[[2-(2,4-dichlorophenyl)-2-(1H-1, 2, 4-triazol-1-ylmethyl)-1,3-dioxolan-4-yl]methoxy]phenyl]-4-(1-methylethyl) piperazine, compounded in a cream base consisting of butylated hydroxyanisole, cetyl alcohol, isopropyl myristate, polysorbate 60, polysorbate 80, propylene glycol, stearyl alcohol, and purified water.

TERCONAZOLE

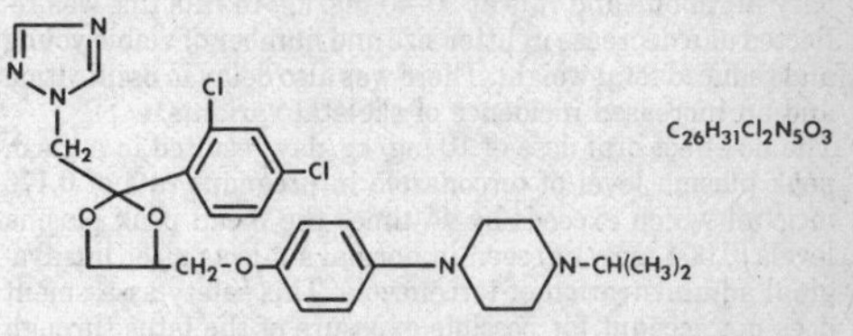
C26H31Cl2N5O3

Terconazole, a triazole derivative, is a white to almost white powder with a molecular weight of 532.47. It is insoluble in water; sparingly soluble in ethanol; and soluble in butanol.

CLINICAL PHARMACOLOGY

Microbiology: Terconazole exhibits fungicidal activity *in vitro* against *Candida albicans.* Antifungal activity also has been demonstrated against other fungi. The MIC values for terconazole against most species of lactic acid bacteria typically found in the human vagina were ≥128 mcg/ml, therefore these beneficial bacteria are not affected by drug treatment.

The exact pharmacologic mode of action of terconazole is uncertain; however, it may exert its antifungal activity by the disruption of normal fungal cell membrane permeability. No resistance to terconazole has developed during successive passages of *C. albicans.*

Human Pharmacology: Following intravaginal administration of terconazole in humans, absorption ranged from 5–8% in three hysterectomized subjects and 12–16% in two nonhysterectomized subjects with tubal ligations.

Following oral (30 mg) administration of ^{14}C-labelled terconazole, the half-life of elimination from the blood for the parent terconazole was 6.9 hours (range 4.0–11.3). Terconazole is extensively metabolized; the plasma AUC for terconazole compared to the AUC for total radioactivity was 0.6%. Total radioactivity was eliminated from the blood with a half-life of 52.2 hours (range 44–60). Excretion of radioactivity was both by renal (32–56%) and fecal (47–52%) routes.

Photosensitivity reactions were observed in some normal volunteers following repeated dermal application of terconazole, 2.0% and 0.8% creams under conditions of filtered artificial ultraviolet light. Photosensitivity reactions have not been observed in U.S. and foreign clinical trials in patients who were treated with terconazole 0.4% vaginal cream.

INDICATIONS AND USAGE

TERAZOL 7 Vaginal Cream is indicated for the local treatment of vulvovaginal candidiasis (moniliasis). As TERAZOL 7 Vaginal Cream is effective only for vulvovaginitis caused by the genus *Candida,* the diagnosis should be confirmed by KOH smears and/or cultures.

CONTRAINDICATIONS

Patients known to be hypersensitive to terconazole or to any of the components of the cream.

WARNINGS

None.

PRECAUTIONS

General: Discontinue use and do not retreat with terconazole if sensitization, irritation, fever, chills or flu-like symptoms are reported during use. If there is lack of response toTERAZOL 7 Vaginal Cream, appropriate microbiological studies (standard KOH smear and/or cultures) should be repeated to confirm the diagnosis and rule out other pathogens.

Drug Interactions: The therapeutic effect of TERAZOL 7 Vaginal Cream is not affected by oral contraceptive usage.

Carcinogenesis, Mutagenesis, Impairment of Fertility:

Carcinogenesis: Studies to determine the carcinogenic potential of terconazole have not been performed.

Mutagenicity: Terconazole was not mutagenic when tested *in vitro* for induction of microbial point mutations (Ames test) or for inducing cellular transformation, or *in vivo* for chromosome breaks (micronucleus test) or dominant lethal mutations in mouse germ cells.

Continued on next page

Ortho—Cont.

Impairment of Fertility: No impairment of fertility occurred when female rats were administered terconazole orally up to 40 mg/kg/day.

Pregnancy: Pregnancy Category C.

There was no evidence of teratogenicity when terconazole was administered orally up to 40 mg/kg/day (100 × the recommended intravaginal human dose) in rats, or 20 mg/kg/day in rabbits, or subcutaneously in rats up to 20 mg/kg/day.

Dosages at or below 10 mg/kg/day produced no embryotoxicity; however, there was a delay in fetal ossification at 10 mg/kg/day in rats. There was some evidence of embryotoxicity in rabbits and rats at 20–40 mg/kg. In rats this was reflected as a decrease in litter size and number of viable young and reduced fetal weight. There was also delay in ossification and an increased incidence of skeletal variants.

The no-effect oral dose of 10 mg/kg/day resulted in a mean peak plasma level of terconazole in pregnant rats of 0.176 mcg/ml which exceeds by 44 times the mean peak plasma levels (0.004 mcg/ml) seen in normal subjects after intravaginal administration of terconazole. This safety assessment does not account for possible exposure of the fetus through direct transfer of terconazole from the irritated vagina to the fetus by diffusion across amniotic membranes.

Since terconazole is absorbed from the human vagina, it should not be used in the first trimester of pregnancy unless the physician considers it essential to the welfare of the patient.

Nursing Mothers: It is not known whether this drug is excreted in human milk. Animal studies have shown that rat off-spring exposed via the milk of treated (40 mg/kg/orally) dams showed decreased survival during the first few postpartum days, but overall pup weight and weight gain were comparable to or greater than controls throughout lactation. Because many drugs are excreted in human milk, and because of the potential for adverse reaction in nursing infants from terconazole, a decision should be made whether to discontinue nursing or to discontinue the drug, taking into account the importance of the drug to the mother.

Pediatric Use: Safety and efficacy in children have not been established.

ADVERSE REACTIONS

During controlled clinical studies conducted in the United States, 521 patients with vulvovaginal candidiasis were treated with terconazole 0.4% vaginal cream. Based on comparative analyses with placebo, the adverse experiences considered most likely related to terconazole 0.4% vaginal cream were headaches (26% vs 17% with placebo) and body pain (2.1% vs 0% with placebo). Vulvovaginal burning (5.2%), itching (2.3%) or irritation (3.1%) occurred less frequently with terconazole 0.4% vaginal cream than with the vehicle placebo. Fever (1.7% vs 0.5% with placebo) and chills (0.4% vs 0.0% with placebo) have also been reported. The therapy-related dropout rate was 1.9%. The adverse drug experience on terconazole most frequently causing discontinuation was vulvovaginal itching (0.6%), which was lower than the incidence for placebo (0.9%).

OVERDOSAGE

Overdose of terconazole in humans has not been reported to date. In the rat, the oral LD 50 values were found to be 1741 and 849 mg/kg for the male and female, respectively. The oral LD 50 values for the male and female dog were ≃1280 and ≥640 mg/kg, respectively.

DOSAGE AND ADMINISTRATION

One full applicator (5 g) of TERAZOL 7 Vaginal Cream (20 mg terconazole) is administered intravaginally once daily at bedtime for seven consecutive days. Before prescribing another course of therapy, the diagnosis should be reconfirmed by smears and/or cultures and other pathogens commonly associated with vulvovaginitis ruled out. The therapeutic effect of TERAZOL 7 Vaginal Cream is not affected by menstruation.

HOW SUPPLIED

TERAZOL® 7 (terconazole) Vaginal Cream 0.4% is available in 45 g (NDC 0062-5350-01) tubes with an ORTHO™ Measured-Dose Applicator. Store at Controlled Room Temperature (59°F–86°F).

643-10-300-5   Revised January 1989

Shown in Product Identification Section, page 421

THE ORTHO FILM LIBRARY

Ortho Pharmaceutical Corporation can provide a number of educational films on a free-loan basis to hospitals, medical schools and health care professionals for use in training and educational programs.

These films, which are available directly from the distributor, KAROL MEDIA, 350 N. Pennsylvania Ave, Wilkes Barre, Pennsylvania 18773, or by calling (717) 822-8899 are:

Modern Obstetrics: Cesarean Section
Modern Obstetrics: Diabetes in Pregnancy
Modern Obstetrics: Fetal Evaluation
Modern Obstetrics: Normal Labor and Delivery—no printed narration available
Modern Obstetrics: Postpartum Hemorrhage
Modern Obstetrics: Pre-Eclampsia—Eclampsia
Chorionic Villi Sampling—no printed narration available

Printed narrations of these Modern Obstetrics films are available upon written request from: Medical Education Dept., Ortho Pharmaceutical Corporation, Route 202, P.O. Box 300, Raritan, New Jersey 08869-0602.

Ortho Pharmaceutical Corporation

DERMATOLOGICAL DIVISION
P.O. BOX 300
ROUTE 202
RARITAN, NJ 08869-0602

ERYCETTE®   ℞
[ə'ris-ət]
(erythromycin 2%)
TOPICAL SOLUTION

DESCRIPTION

Erythromycin is an antibiotic produced from a strain of *Streptomyces erythraeus*. It is basic and readily forms salts with acids. Each ml of ERYCETTE (erythromycin 2%) Topical Solution contains 20 mg of erythromycin base in a vehicle consisting of alcohol (66%) and propylene glycol. It may contain citric acid to adjust pH. Each pledget is filled to contain 0.8 ml. ERYCETTE is not USP with regard to minimum volume.

ACTIONS

Although the mechanism by which ERYCETTE Solution acts in reducing inflammatory lesions of acne vulgaris is unknown, it is presumably due to its antibiotic action.

INDICATIONS

ERYCETTE Solution is indicated for the topical control of acne vulgaris.

CONTRAINDICATIONS

ERYCETTE Solution is contraindicated in persons who have shown hypersensitivity to any of its ingredients.

PRECAUTIONS

General: The use of antibiotic agents may be associated with the overgrowth of antibiotic-resistant organisms. If this occurs, administration of this drug should be discontinued and appropriate measures taken.

Information for Patients: ERYCETTE Solution is for external use only and should be kept away from the eyes, nose, mouth, and other mucous membranes. Concomitant topical acne therapy should be used with caution because a cumulative irritant effect may occur, especially with the use of peeling, desquamating, or abrasive agents. Each pledget should be used once and discarded.

Carcinogenesis, Mutagenesis, Impairment of Fertility: Long-term animal studies to evaluate carcinogenic potential, mutagenicity, or the effect on fertility of erythromycin have not been performed.

Pregnancy: Pregnancy Category C. Animal reproduction studies have not been conducted with erythromycin. It is also not known whether erythromycin can cause fetal harm when administered to a pregnant woman or can affect reproduction capacity. Erythromycin should be given to a pregnant woman only if clearly needed.

Nursing Mothers: It is not known whether erythromycin is excreted in human milk after topical application. However, this is reported to occur with oral and parenteral administration. Therefore, caution should be exercised when erythromycin is administered to a nursing woman.

ADVERSE REACTIONS

Adverse conditions reported include dryness, tenderness, pruritis, desquamation, erythema, oiliness, and burning sensation. Irritation of the eyes has also been reported. A case of generalized urticarial reaction, possibly related to the drug, which required the use of systemic steroid therapy has been reported.

DOSAGE AND ADMINISTRATION

The ERYCETTE pledget should be rubbed over the affected area twice a day after the skin is thoroughly washed with warm water and soap and patted dry. Acne lesions on the face, neck, shoulders, chest and back may be treated in this manner. Additional pledgets may be used, if needed. Each pledget should be used once and discarded.

HOW SUPPLIED

ERYCETTE (erythromycin 2%) Topical Solution is supplied as foil-covered saturated pledgets (swabs) in boxes of 60 (NDC 0062-1185-01).

Store at controlled room temperature 15–30°C (59°–86°F).

Shown in Product Identification Section, page 421

GRIFULVIN® V   ℞
[gri'fulvən]
(griseofulvin microsize tablets)
(griseofulvin oral suspension)
Tablets/Suspension

DESCRIPTION

Griseofulvin is an antibiotic derived from a species of *Penicillium*. Each GRIFULVIN V Tablet contains either 250 mg or 500 mg of griseofulvin microsize, and also contains calcium stearate, colloidal silicon dioxide, starch, and wheat gluten. Additionally, the 250 mg tablet also contains dibasic calcium phosphate. Each 5 ml of GRIFULVIN V Suspension contains 125 mg of griseofluvin microsize and also contains alcohol 0.2%, docusate sodium, FD&C Red No. 40, FD&C Yellow No. 6, flavors, magnesium aluminium silicate, menthol, methylparaben, propylene glycol, propylparaben, saccharin sodium, simethicone emulsion, sodium alginate, sucrose, and purified water.

CLINICAL PHARMACOLOGY

GRIFULVIN V (griseofulvin microsize) acts systemically to inhibit the growth of *Trichophyton*, *Microsporum* and *Epidermophyton* genera of fungi. Fungistatic amounts are deposited in the keratin, which is gradually exfoliated and replaced by noninfected tissue.

Griseofulvin absorption from the gastrointestinal tract varies considerably among individuals, mainly because of insolubility of the drug in aqueous media of the upper G.I. tract. The peak serum level found in fasting adults given 0.5 gm. occurs at about four hours and ranges between 0.5 and 2.0 mcg./ml.

It should be noted that some individuals are consistently "poor absorbers" and tend to attain lower blood levels at all times. This may explain unsatisfactory therapeutic results in some patients. Better blood levels can probably be attained in most patients if the tablets are administered after a meal with a high fat content.

INDICATIONS AND USAGE

Major indications for GRIFULVIN V (griseofulvin microsize) are:

    Tinea capitis (ringworm of the scalp)
    Tinea corporis (ringworm of the body)
    Tinea pedis (athlete's foot)
    Tinea unguium (onychomycosis; ringworm of the nails)
    Tinea cruris (ringworm of the thigh)
    Tinea barbae (barber's itch)

GRIFULVIN V (griseofulvin microsize) inhibits the growth of those genera of fungi that commonly cause ringworm infections of the hair, skin, and nails, such as:

    Trichophyton rubrum
    Trichophyton tonsurans
    Trichophyton mentagrophytes
    Trichophyton interdigitalis
    Trichophyton verrucosum
    Trichophyton sulphureum
    Trichophyton schoenleini
    Microsporum audouini
    Microsporum canis
    Microsporum gypseum
    Epidermophyton floccosum
    Trichophyton megnini
    Trichophyton gallinae
    Trichophyton crateriform

Note: Prior to therapy, the type of fungi responsible for the infection should be identified. The use of the drug is not justified in minor or trivial infections which will respond to topical antifungal agents alone.

It is *not* effective in:
    Bacterial infections
    Candidiasis (Moniliasis)
    Histoplasmosis
    Actinomycosis
    Sporotrichosis
    Chromoblastomycosis
    Coccidioidomycosis
    North American Blastomycosis
    Cryptococcosis (Torulosis)
    Tinea versicolor
    Nocardiosis

CONTRAINDICATIONS

This drug is contraindicated in patients with porphyria, hepatocellular failure, and in individuals with a history of hypersensitivity to griseofulvin.

Two cases of conjoined twins have been reported in patients taking griseofulvin during the first trimester of pregnancy. Griseofulvin should not be prescribed to pregnant patients.

WARNINGS

Prophylactic Usage: Safety and efficacy of prophylactic use of this drug has not been established.

Chronic feeding of griseofulvin, at levels ranging from 0.5-2.5% of the diet, resulted in the development of liver tumors in several strains of mice, particularly in males. Smaller particle sizes result in an enhanced effect. Lower oral dosage levels have not been tested. Subcutaneous administration of relatively small doses of griseofulvin once a week during the first three weeks of life has also been reported to induce hepatomata in mice. Although studies in other animal species have not yielded evidence of tumorigenicity, these studies were not of adequate design to form a basis for conclusions in this regard.

In subacute toxicity studies, orally administered griseofulvin produced hepatocellular necrosis in mice, but this has not been seen in other species. Disturbances in porphyrin metabolism have been reported in griseofulvin-treated laboratory animals. Griseofulvin has been reported to have a colchicine-like effect on mitosis and cocarcinogenicity with methylcholanthrene in cutaneous tumor induction in laboratory animals.

Reports of animal studies in the Soviet literature state that a griseofulvin preparation was found to be embryotoxic and teratogenic on oral administration to pregnant Wistar rats. Rat reproduction studies done thus far in the United States and Great Britain have been inconclusive in this regard, and additional animal reproduction studies are underway. Pups with abnormalities have been reported in the litters of a few bitches treated with griseofulvin.

Suppression of spermatogenesis has been reported to occur in rats but investigation in man failed to confirm this.

PRECAUTIONS

Patients on prolonged therapy with any potent medication should be under close observation. Periodic monitoring of organ system function, including renal, hepatic and hemopoietic, should be done.

Since griseofulvin is derived from species of penicillin, the possibility of cross sensitivity with penicillin exists; however, known penicillin-sensitive patients have been treated without difficulty.

Since a photosensitivity reaction is occasionally associated with griseofulvin therapy, patients should be warned to avoid exposure to intense natural or artificial sunlight. Should a photosensitivity reaction occur, lupus erythematosus may be aggravated.

Drug Interactions: Patients on warfarin-type anticoagulant therapy may require dosage adjustment of the anticoagulant during and after griseofulvin therapy. Concomitant use of barbiturates usually depresses griseofulvin activity and may necessitate raising the dosage.

The concomitant administration of griseofulvin has been reported to reduce the efficacy of oral contraceptives and to increase the incidence of breakthrough bleeding.

ADVERSE REACTIONS

When adverse reactions occur, they are most commonly of the hypersensitivity type such as skin rashes, urticaria and rarely, angioneurotic edema, and may necessitate withdrawal of therapy and appropriate countermeasures. Paresthesias of the hands and feet have been reported rarely after extended therapy. Other side effects reported occasionally are oral thrush, nausea, vomiting, epigastric distress, diarrhea; headache, fatigue, dizziness, insomnia, mental confusion and impairment of performance of routine activities.

Proteinuria and leukopenia have been reported rarely. Administration of the drug should be discontinued if granulocytopenia occurs.

When rare, serious reactions occur with griseofulvin, they are usually associated with high dosages, long periods of therapy, or both.

DOSAGE AND ADMINISTRATION

Accurate diagnosis of the infecting organism is essential. Identification should be made either by direct microscopic examination of a mounting of infected tissue in a solution of potassium hydroxide or by culture on an appropriate medium.

Medication must be continued until the infecting organism is completely eradicated as indicated by appropriate clinical or laboratory examination. Representative treatment periods are tinea capitis, 4 to 6 weeks; tinea corporis, 2 to 4 weeks; tinea pedis, 4 to 8 weeks; tinea unguium—depending on rate of growth—fingernails, at least 4 months; toenails, at least 6 months.

General measures in regard to hygiene should be observed to control sources of infection or reinfection. Concomitant use of appropriate topical agents is usually required, particularly in treatment of tinea pedis since in some forms of athlete's foot, yeasts and bacteria may be involved. Griseofulvin will not eradicate the bacterial or monilial infection.

Adults: A daily dose of 500 mg. will give a satisfactory response in most patients with tinea corporis, tinea cruris, and tinea capitis.

For those fungus infections more difficult to eradicate such as tinea pedis and tinea unguium, a daily dose of 1.0 gram is recommended.

Children: Approximately 5 mg. per pound of body weight per day is an effective dose for most children. On this basis the following dosage schedule for children is suggested:

Children weighing 30 to 50 pounds—125 mg. to 250 mg. daily.

Children weighing over 50 pounds—250 mg. to 500 mg. daily.

HOW SUPPLIED

GRIFULVIN V (griseofulvin microsize) 250 mg. Tablets in bottles of 100 (NDC 0062-0211-60) (white, scored, imprinted "ORTHO 211").

GRIFULVIN V (griseofulvin microsize) 500 mg. Tablets in bottles of 100 (NDC 0062-0214-60) and 500 (NDC 0062-0214-70) (white, scored, imprinted "ORTHO 214").

Dispense GRIFULVIN V tablets in well-closed container as defined in the official compendia.

GRIFULVIN V (griseofulvin microsize) Suspension 125 mg. per 5 cc. in bottles of 4 fl. oz. (NDC 0062-0206-04).

Dispense GRIFULVIN V suspension in tight, light-resistant container as defined in the official compendia.

STORE AT ROOM TEMPERATURE

Shown in Product Identification Section, page 421

MECLAN® ℞

['mec-lan]

(meclocycline sulfosalicylate)

Cream 1%

For Topical Use Only

DESCRIPTION

MECLAN (meclocycline sulfosalicylate) Cream 1% is a homogeneous smooth yellow cream, each gram of which contains meclocycline sulfosalicylate equivalent to 10 mg. of meclocycline activity in an aqueous cream vehicle consisting of glyceryl stearate, propylene glycol stearate, caprylic/capric triglyceride, paraffin, trihydroxystearin, polysorbate 40, sorbitol solution, propyl gallate, sorbic acid, sodium formaldehyde sulfoxylate, perfume, and water. The vehicle is pharmaceutically compatible with both oil- and water-based systems.

Chemically meclocycline sulfosalicylate is [4S-(4α,4aα,5α,5aα,12aα)]-7-chloro-4-(dimethyl-amino)- 1,4,4a,5,5a,6,11,-12a-octahydro-3,5,10,12,12a-pentahydroxy- 6-methylene-1,-11- dioxo-2- naphthacenecarboxamide 5-sulfosalicylate. Its structure is as follows:

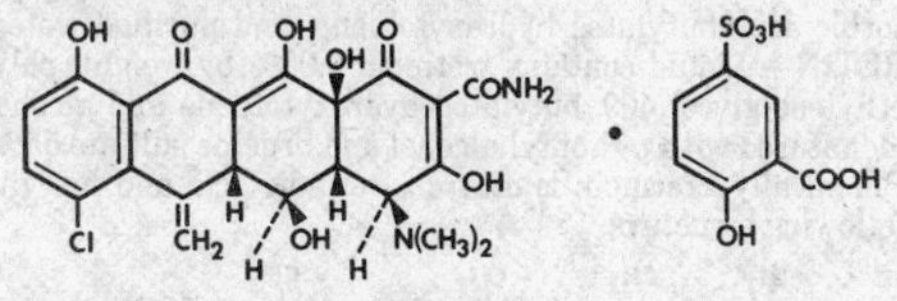

ACTIONS (Clinical Pharmacology)

The mode of action of MECLAN Cream in the treatment of acne is not fully understood. However, it appears that meclocycline possesses a localized effect, since it is not absorbed through the skin in sufficient quantities to be detected systemically. In subtotal body inunction studies, up to 40 times the average treatment dose was applied to 20 human subjects daily for 28 days. No measurable amounts of meclocycline appeared in the blood (0.1 microgram/ml. level of detectability) or urine (0.02 microgram/ml. level of detectability).

INDICATION

MECLAN Cream (meclocycline sulfosalicylate) is indicated for topical application in the treatment of acne vulgaris.

CONTRAINDICATIONS

MECLAN is contraindicated in persons who have shown hypersensitivity to any of its ingredients or to any of the other tetracyclines.

WARNINGS

Although no absorption has been demonstrated by 28-day inunction studies in humans, the possibility exists that significant percutaneous absorption may result from prolonged use. Therefore, caution is advised in administering MECLAN (meclocycline sulfosalicylate) to persons with hepatic or renal dysfunction.

Contains sodium formaldehyde sulfoxylate, a sulfite-producing agent that may cause allergic-type reactions including anaphylactic symptoms and life-threatening or less severe asthmatic episodes in certain susceptible people. The overall prevalence of sulfite sensitivity in the general population is unknown and probably low. Sulfite sensitivity is seen more frequently in asthmatic than in nonasthmatic people.

PRECAUTIONS

This drug is for external use only and should be kept out of the eyes, nose, and mouth. It should be used with caution by patients who are sensitive to formaldehyde.

Pregnancy: Pregnancy Category B. Reproduction studies have been performed in rats and rabbits at oral doses up to 1000 times the human dose (assuming the human dose to be one gram of cream per day) and have revealed no evidence of impaired fertility or harm to the fetus due to meclocycline sulfosalicylate. There was, however, a slight delay in ossification in rabbits when meclocycline was applied topically. There are no adequate and well-controlled studies in pregnant women. Because animal reproduction studies are not always predictive of human response, this drug should be used during pregnancy only if clearly needed.

Nursing Mothers: It is not known whether this drug is excreted in human milk. Because many drugs are excreted in human milk, caution should be exercised when meclocycline sulfosalicylate is administered to a nursing woman.

ADVERSE REACTIONS

MECLAN is well tolerated by the skin. In the clinical trials there was one report of acute contact dermatitis. There were isolated reports of skin irritation. Temporary follicular staining may occur with excessive application. Patch testing has demonstrated no photosensitivity or contact allergy potential.

DOSAGE AND ADMINISTRATION

It is recommended that MECLAN be applied to the affected area twice daily, morning and evening. Less frequent application may be used depending on patient response. Excessive use of MECLAN Cream may cause staining of some fabrics.

HOW SUPPLIED

MECLAN (meclocycline sulfosalicylate) Cream 1% is supplied in 20 gram (NDC 0062-0675-80) and 45 gram (NDC 0062-0675-01) sealed tubes.

Shown in Product Identification Section, page 421

MONISTAT-DERM® ℞

['män ə-stat-dərm]

(miconazole nitrate 2%)

Cream

For Topical Use Only

DESCRIPTION

MONISTAT-DERM (miconazole nitrate 2%) Cream contains miconazole nitrate* 2%, formulated into a water-miscible base consisting of pegoxol 7 stearate, peglicol 5 oleate, mineral oil, benzoic acid, and butylated hydroxyanisole and purified water.

ACTIONS

Miconazole nitrate is a synthetic antifungal agent which inhibits the growth of the common dermatophytes, *Trichophyton rubrum, Trichophyton mentagrophytes,* and *Epidermophyton floccosum,* the yeast-like fungus, *Candida albicans,* and the organism responsible for tinea versicolor *(Malassezia furfur).*

INDICATIONS

For topical application in the treatment of tinea pedis (athlete's foot), tinea cruris, and tinea corporis caused by *Trichophyton rubrum, Trichophyton mentagrophytes,* and *Epidermophyton floccosum,* in the treatment of cutaneous candidiasis (moniliasis), and in the treatment of tinea versicolor.

CONTRAINDICATIONS

MONISTAT-DERM (miconazole nitrate 2%) Cream has no known contraindications.

PRECAUTIONS

If a reaction suggesting sensitivity or chemical irritation should occur, use of the medication should be discontinued. For external use only. Avoid introduction of MONISTAT-DERM Cream into the eyes.

ADVERSE REACTIONS

There have been isolated reports of irritation, burning, maceration, and allergic contact dermatitis associated with application of MONISTAT-DERM.

DOSAGE AND ADMINISTRATION

Sufficient MONISTAT-DERM Cream should be applied to cover affected areas twice daily (morning and evening) in patients with tinea pedis, tinea cruris, tinea corporis, and cutaneous candidiasis, and once daily in patients with tinea

*Chemical name: 1-[2,4-dichloro-β-{(2,4-dichlorobenzyl)oxy} phenethyl] imidazole mononitrate.

Continued on next page

Ortho Dermatological—Cont.

versicolor. If MONISTAT-DERM Cream is used in intertriginous areas, it should be applied sparingly and smoothed in well to avoid maceration effects.
Early relief of symptoms (2 to 3 days) is experienced by the majority of patients and clinical improvement may be seen fairly soon after treatment is begun; however, *Candida* infections and tinea cruris and corporis should be treated for two weeks and tinea pedis for one month in order to reduce the possibility of recurrence. If a patient shows no clinical improvement after a month of treatment, the diagnosis should be redetermined. Patients with tinea versicolor usually exhibit clinical and mycological clearing after two weeks of treatment.

HOW SUPPLIED

MONISTAT-DERM (miconazole nitrate 2%) Cream containing miconazole nitrate at 2% strength is supplied in 15 g. (NDC 0062-5434-02), 1 oz. (NDC 0062-5434-01) and 3 oz. (NDC 0062-5434-03) tubes.

Shown in Product Identification Section, page 421

PERSA-GEL® 5% & 10% ℞
['pər-sə-jel]
(benzoyl peroxide)
acetone-base gel

PERSA-GEL® W 5% & 10% ℞
(benzoyl peroxide)
water-base gel

DESCRIPTION

PERSA-GEL and PERSA-GEL W 5% and 10% (benzoyl peroxide 5% and 10%) are topical gel preparations for use in the treatment of acne vulgaris. Benzoyl peroxide is an oxidizing agent which possesses antibacterial properties and is classified as a keratolytic. Benzoyl peroxide ($C_{14}H_{10}O_4$) is represented by the following chemical structure:

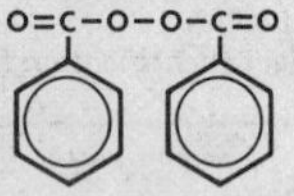

PERSA-GEL contains benzoyl peroxide 5% or 10% as the active ingredient in a gel base containing acetone, carbomer 940, trolamine, sodium lauryl sulfate, propylene glycol and purified water.
PERSA-GEL W contains benzoyl peroxide 5% or 10% as the active ingredient in a gel base containing purified water, carbomer 934P, sodium hydroxide, hydroxypropyl methylcellulose 2906, and laureth 4.

CLINICAL PHARMACOLOGY

The mechanism of action of benzoyl peroxide has not been determined but may be related to its antibacterial activity against **Propionibacterium acnes** and its ability to cause drying and peeling. Benzoyl peroxide reduces the concentration of free fatty acids in the sebum. Little is known about the percutaneous penetration, metabolism, and excretion of benzoyl peroxide, although it is likely that benzoic acid is a major metabolite. There is no evidence of systemic toxicity caused by benzoyl peroxide in humans.

INDICATIONS AND USAGE

These products are indicated for the topical treatment of acne vulgaris.

CONTRAINDICATIONS

These products are contraindicated in patients with a history of hypersensitivity to any of the components of the preparations.

PRECAUTIONS

General: For external use only. If severe irritation develops, discontinue use and institute appropriate therapy. After the reaction clears, treatment may often be resumed with less frequent application. This preparation should not be used in or near the eyes or on mucous membranes.
Information for Patients: Avoid contact with eyes, eyelids, lips and mucous membranes. If accidental contact occurs, rinse with water. May bleach hair and colored fabrics. If excessive irritation develops, discontinue use and consult your physician.
Carcinogenesis, Mutagenesis, Impairment of Fertility: Data from several studies using mice known to be highly susceptible to cancer suggest that benzoyl peroxide acts as a tumor promoter. The clinical significance of these findings to humans is unknown.
Pregnancy: Pregnancy Category C: Animal reproduction studies have not been conducted with benzoyl peroxide. It is also not known whether benzoyl peroxide can cause fetal harm when administered to a pregnant woman or can affect reproduction capacity. Benzoyl peroxide should be used by a pregnant woman only if clearly needed. There are no data available on the effect of benzoyl peroxide on the growth, development and functional maturation of the unborn child.
Nursing Mothers: It is not known whether this drug is excreted in human milk. Because many drugs are excreted in human milk, caution should be exercised when benzoyl peroxide is administered to a nursing woman.
Pediatric Use: Safety and effectiveness in children have not been established.

ADVERSE REACTIONS

Allergic contact dermatitis has been reported with topical benzoyl peroxide therapy.

DOSAGE AND ADMINISTRATION

PERSA-GEL or PERSA-GEL W 5% or 10% should be applied once or twice daily to affected areas after washing with a mild cleanser and water. The degree of drying and peeling can be adjusted by modification of the dosage schedule.

HOW SUPPLIED

PERSA-GEL 5%, 1.5 oz. tubes
(NDC 0062-8610-31)
PERSA-GEL 5%, 3 oz. tubes
(NDC 0062-8610-03)
PERSA-GEL 10%, 1.5 oz. tubes
(NDC 0062-8600-31)
PERSA-GEL 10%, 3 oz. tubes
(NDC 0062-8600-03)
PERSA-GEL W 5% 1.5 oz. tubes
(NDC 0062-8630-31)
PERSA-GEL W 5% 3.0 oz. tubes
(NDC 0062-8630-03)
PERSA-GEL W 10% 1.5 oz. tubes
(NDC 0062-8620-31)
PERSA-GEL W 10% 3.0 oz. tubes
(NDC 0062-8620-03)
Store at controlled room temperature (59°– 86°F).

Shown in Product Identification Section, page 421

RETIN-A® ℞
['ret in-ā]
(tretinoin)
Liquid
Creme • Gel • with DELCAP® unit dispensing cap
For Topical Use Only

DESCRIPTION

RETIN-A Gel, Cream and Liquid, containing tretinoin are used for the topical treatment of acne vulgaris. RETIN-A Gel contains tretinoin (retinoic acid, vitamin A acid) in either of two strengths. 0.025% or 0.01% by weight, in a gel vehicle of butylated hydroxytoluene, hydroxypropyl cellulose and alcohol (denatured with *tert*-butyl alcohol and brucine sulfate) 90% w/w. RETIN-A (tretinoin) Cream contains tretinoin in either of three strengths, 0.1%, 0.05%, or 0.025% by weight, in a hydrophilic cream vehicle of stearic acid, isopropyl myristate, polyoxyl 40 stearate, stearyl alcohol, xanthan gum, sorbic acid, butylated hydroxytoluene, and purified water. RETIN-A Liquid contains tretinoin 0.05% by weight, polyethylene glycol 400, butylated hydroxytoluene and alcohol (denatured with *tert*-butyl alcohol and brucine sulfate) 55%. Chemically, tretinoin is *all-trans*-retinoic acid and has the following structure:

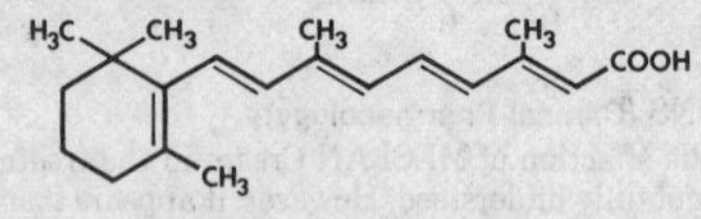

CLINICAL PHARMACOLOGY

Although the exact mode of action of tretinoin is unknown, current evidence suggests that topical tretinoin decreases cohesiveness of follicular epithelial cells with decreased microcomedo formation. Additionally, tretinoin stimulates mitotic activity and increased turnover of follicular epithelial cells causing extrusion of the comedones.

INDICATIONS AND USAGE

RETIN-A is indicated for topical application in the treatment of acne vulgaris. The safety and efficacy of the long-term use of this product in the treatment of other disorders have not been established.

CONTRAINDICATIONS

Use of the product should be discontinued if hypersensitivity to any of the ingredients is noted.

PRECAUTIONS

General: If a reaction suggesting sensitivity or chemical irritation occurs, use of the medication should be discontinued. Exposure to sunlight, including sunlamps, should be minimized during the use of RETIN-A, and patients with sunburn should be advised not to use the product until fully recovered because of heightened susceptibility to sunlight as a result of the use of tretinoin. Patients who may be required to have considerable sun exposure due to occupation and those with inherent sensitivity to the sun should exercise particular caution. Use of sunscreen products and protective clothing over treated areas is recommended when exposure cannot be avoided. Weather extremes, such as wind or cold, also may be irritating to patients under treatment with tretinoin.
RETIN-A (tretinoin) acne treatment should be kept away from the eyes, the mouth, angles of the nose, and mucous membranes. Topical use may induce severe local erythema and peeling at the site of application. If the degree of local irritation warrants, patients should be directed to use the medication less frequently, discontinue use temporarily, or discontinue use altogether. Tretinoin has been reported to cause severe irritation on eczematous skin and should be used with utmost caution in patients with this condition.
Drug Interactions: Concomitant topical medication, medicated or abrasive soaps and cleansers, soaps and cosmetics that have a strong drying effect, and products with high concentrations of alcohol, astringents, spices or lime should be used with caution because of possible interaction with tretinoin. Particular caution should be exercised in using preparations containing sulfur, resorcinol, or salicylic acid with RETIN-A. It also is advisable to "rest" a patient's skin until the effects of such preparations subside before use of RETIN-A is begun.
Carcinogenesis: Long-term animal studies to determine the carcinogenic potential of tretinoin have not been performed. Studies in hairless albino mice suggest that tretinoin may accelerate the tumorigenic potential of weakly carcinogenic light from a solar simulator. In other studies, when lightly pigmented hairless mice treated with tretinoin were exposed to carcinogenic doses of UVB light, the incidence and rate of development of skin tumors was reduced. Due to significantly different experimental conditions, no strict comparison of these disparate data is possible. Although the significance of these studies to man is not clear, patients should avoid or minimize exposure to sun.
Pregnancy: Teratogenic effects. Pregnancy Category C. *Oral* tretinoin has been shown to be teratogenic in rats when given in doses 1000 times the topical human dose. Oral tretinoin has been shown to be fetotoxic in rats when given in doses 500 times the topical human dose. *Topical* tretinoin has not been shown to be teratogenic in rats and rabbits when given in doses of 100 and 320 times the topical human dose, respectively (assuming a 50 kg adult applies 250 mg of 0.1% cream topically). However, at these topical doses, delayed ossification of a number of bones occurred in both species. These changes may be considered variants of normal development and are usually corrected after weaning. There are no adequate and well-controlled studies in pregnant women. Tretinoin should be used during pregnancy only if the potential benefit justifies the potential risk to the fetus.
Nursing mothers: It is not known whether this drug is excreted in human milk. Because many drugs are excreted in human milk, caution should be exercised when RETIN-A is administered to a nursing woman.

ADVERSE REACTIONS

The skin of certain sensitive individuals may become excessively red, edematous, blistered, or crusted. If these effects occur, the medication should either be discontinued until the integrity of the skin is restored, or the medication should be adjusted to a level the patient can tolerate. True contact allergy to topical tretinoin is rarely encountered. Temporary hyper- or hypopigmentation has been reported with repeated application of RETIN-A. Some individuals have been reported to have heightened susceptibility to sunlight while under treatment with RETIN-A. To date, all adverse effects of RETIN-A have been reversible upon discontinuance of therapy (see Dosage and Administration Section).

OVERDOSAGE

If medication is applied excessively, no more rapid or better results will be obtained and marked redness, peeling, or discomfort may occur. Oral ingestion of the drug may lead to the same side effects as those associated with excessive oral intake of Vitamin A.

DOSAGE AND ADMINISTRATION

RETIN-A Gel, Cream or Liquid should be applied once a day, before retiring, to the skin where acne lesions appear, using enough to cover the entire affected area lightly. Liquid: The liquid may be applied using a fingertip, gauze pad or cotton swab. If gauze or cotton is employed, care should be taken not to oversaturate it to the extent that the liquid would run into areas where treatment is not intended. Gel: Excessive application results in "pilling" of the gel, which minimizes the likelihood of overapplication by the patient.
Application may cause a transitory feeling of warmth or slight stinging. In cases where it has been necessary to temporarily discontinue therapy or to reduce the frequency of application, therapy may be resumed or frequency of application increased when the patients become able to tolerate the treatment.
Alterations of vehicle, drug concentration, or dose frequency should be closely monitored by careful observation of the clinical therapeutic response and skin tolerance.

During the early weeks of therapy, an *apparent* exacerbation of inflammatory lesions may occur. This is due to the action of the medication on deep, previously unseen lesions and should not be considered a reason to discontinue therapy. Therapeutic results should be noticed after two to three weeks but more than six weeks of therapy may be required before definite beneficial effects are seen.

Once the acne lesions have responded satisfactorily, it may be possible to maintain the improvement with less frequent applications, or other dosage forms.

Patients treated with RETIN-A (tretinoin) acne treatment may use cosmetics, but the areas to be treated should be cleansed thoroughly before the medication is applied. (See Precautions)

HOW SUPPLIED

RETIN-A (tretinoin) is supplied as:
RETIN-A Cream and Gel

NDC Code	RETIN-A Form/Strength	RETIN-A Qty.
0062-0165-01	0.025% Cream	20g
0062-0165-02	0.025% Cream	45g
0062-0175-12	0.05% Cream	20g
0062-0175-13	0.05% Cream	45g
0062-0275-23	0.1% Cream	20g
0062-0275-01	0.1% Cream	45g
0062-0575-44	0.01% Gel	15g
0062-0575-46	0.01% Gel	45g
0062-0475-42	0.025% Gel	15g
0062-0475-45	0.025% Gel	45g

RETIN-A Liquid

NDC Code	RETIN-A Form/Strength	RETIN-A Qty.
0062-0075-07	0.05% Liquid	28 ml

RETIN-A Gel and RETIN-A Cream tubes are supplied with DELCAP® unit dispensing cap and alternate cap.
Storage Conditions: RETIN-A Liquid, 0.05%, and RETIN-A Gel, 0.025% and 0.01%: store below 86°F. RETIN-A Cream, 0.1%, 0.5%, and 0.025%: store below 80°F.

Shown in Product Identification Section, page 421

SPECTAZOLE®   ℞
['spek-ti-zōl]
(econazole nitrate 1%)
Cream
For Topical Use Only

DESCRIPTION

SPECTAZOLE Cream contains the antifungal agent, econazole nitrate 1%, in a water-miscible base consisting of pegoxol 7 stearate, peglicol 5 oleate, mineral oil, benzoic acid, butylated hydroxyanisole, and purified water. The white to off-white soft cream is for topical use only.

Chemically, econazole nitrate is 1-[2-{(4-chlorophenyl) methoxy}-2-(2,4-dichlorophenyl)ethyl]-1H-imidazole mononitrate. Its structure is as follows:

CLINICAL PHARMACOLOGY

After topical application to the skin of normal subjects, systemic absorption of econazole nitrate is extremely low. Although most of the applied drug remains on the skin surface, drug concentrations were found in the stratum corneum which, by far, exceeded the minimum inhibitory concentration for dermatophytes. Inhibitory concentrations were achieved in the epidermis and as deep as the middle region of the dermis. Less than 1% of the applied dose was recovered in the urine and feces.

Microbiology: In *in vitro* studies, econazole nitrate exhibits broad-spectrum antifungal activity against the dermatophytes, *Trichophyton rubrum, Trichophyton mentagrophytes, Trichophyton tonsurans, Microsporum canis, Microsporum audouini, Microsporum gypseum,* and *Epidermophyton floccosum,* the yeasts, *Candida albicans* and *Pityrosporum orbiculare* (the organism responsible for tinea versicolor), and certain gram positive bacteria.

INDICATIONS AND USAGE

SPECTAZOLE Cream is indicated for topical application in the treatment of tinea pedis, tinea cruris, and tinea corporis caused by *Trichophyton rubrum, Trichophyton mentagrophytes, Trichophyton tonsurans, Microsporum canis, Microsporum audouini, Microsporum gypseum,* and *Epidermophy-*

---

ton floccosum, in the treatment of cutaneous candidiasis, and in the treatment of tinea versicolor.

CONTRAINDICATIONS

SPECTAZOLE Cream is contraindicated in individuals who have shown hypersensitivity to any of its ingredients.

WARNINGS

SPECTAZOLE is not for ophthalmic use.

PRECAUTIONS

General: If a reaction suggesting sensitivity or chemical irritation should occur, use of the medication should be discontinued.

For external use only. Avoid introduction of SPECTAZOLE Cream into the eyes.

Carcinogenicity Studies: Long-term animal studies to determine carcinogenic potential have not been performed.

Fertility (Reproduction): Oral administration of econazole nitrate in rats has been reported to produce prolonged gestation. Intravaginal administration in humans has not shown prolonged gestation or other adverse reproductive effects attributable to econazole nitrate therapy.

Pregnancy: Pregnancy Category C. Econazole nitrate has not been shown to be teratogenic when administered orally to mice, rabbits or rats. Fetotoxic or embryotoxic effects were observed in Segment I oral studies with rats receiving 10 to 40 times the human dermal dose. Similar effects were observed in Segment II or Segment III studies with mice, rabbits and/or rats receiving oral doses 80 or 40 times the human dermal dose.

Econazole nitrate should be used in the first trimester of pregnancy only when the physician considers it essential to the welfare of the patient. The drug should be used during the second and third trimesters of pregnancy only if clearly needed.

Nursing Mothers: It is not known whether econazole nitrate is excreted in human milk. Following oral administration of econazole nitrate to lactating rats, econazole and/or metabolites were excreted in milk and were found in nursing pups. Also, in lactating rats receiving large oral doses (40 or 80 times the human dermal dose), there was a reduction in postpartum viability of pups and survival to weaning; however, at these high doses, maternal toxicity was present and may have been a contributing factor. Caution should be exercised when econazole nitrate is administered to a nursing woman.

ADVERSE REACTIONS

During clinical trials, approximately 3% of patients treated with econazole nitrate 1% cream reported side effects thought possibly to be due to the drug, consisting mainly of burning, itching, stinging and erythema. One case of pruritic rash has also been reported.

OVERDOSE

Overdosage of econazole nitrate in humans has not been reported to date. In mice, rats, guinea pigs and dogs, the oral LD 50 values were found to be 462, 668, 272, and > 160 mg/kg, respectively.

DOSAGE AND ADMINISTRATION

Sufficient SPECTAZOLE Cream should be applied to cover affected areas once daily in patients with tinea pedis, tinea cruris, and tinea corporis, and tinea versicolor, and twice daily (morning and evening) in patients with cutaneous candidiasis.

Early relief of symptoms is experienced by the majority of patients and clinical improvement may be seen fairly soon after treatment is begun; however, candidal infections and tinea cruris and corporis should be treated for two weeks and tinea pedis for one month in order to reduce the possibility of recurrence. If a patient shows no clinical improvement after the treatment period, the diagnosis should be redetermined. Patients with tinea versicolor usually exhibit clinical and mycological clearing after two weeks of treatment.

HOW SUPPLIED

SPECTAZOLE (econazole nitrate 1%) Cream is supplied in tubes of 15 grams (NDC 0062-5460-02), 30 grams (NDC 0062-5460-01), and 85 grams (NDC 0062-5460-03).
Store SPECTAZOLE Cream below 86°F.

Shown in Product Identification Section, page 421

Products are cross-indexed by
generic and chemical names
in the
YELLOW SECTION.

Paddock Laboratories, Inc.
3101 LOUISIANA AVENUE NORTH
MINNEAPOLIS, MN 55427

ACTIDOSE with SORBITOL™   OTC
[act'ĭ-dose]
(Activated Charcoal with Sorbitol Suspension)

DESCRIPTION

Actidose with Sorbitol is supplied in bottles containing 25 grams and 50 grams activated charcoal suspension, with 48 grams and 96 grams sorbitol respectively. Each milliliter contains 208 mg (0.208 gram) activated charcoal and 400 mg (0.4 gram) sorbitol.

HOW SUPPLIED

120 ml unit-of-use bottle NDC 0574-0120-04
240 ml unit-of-use bottle NDC 0574-0120-08

ACTIDOSE-AQUA™   OTC
[act'ĭ'dose a-qua]
(Activated Charcoal Suspension)

DESCRIPTION

Actidose-Aqua is supplied in bottles containing 15 grams, 25 grams and 50 grams activated charcoal suspension. Each milliliter contains 208 mg (0.208 grams) activated charcoal in aqueous suspension.

HOW SUPPLIED

72 ml unit-of-use bottle NDC 0574-0121-25
120 ml unit-of-use bottle NDC 0574-0121-04
240 ml unit-of-use bottle NDC 0574-0121-08

ERYTHRA-DERM™ (Formerly ETS-2%)   ℞
(Erythromycin Topical Solution USP, 2%)

DESCRIPTION

Erythromycin is an antibiotic produced from a strain of Streptomyces erythraeus. It is basic and readily forms salts with acids. ERYTHRA-DERM contains 20 mg/ml erythromycin base in a clear solution vehicle of 66 percent alcohol, propylene glycol and citric acid.

HOW SUPPLIED

Bottles of 2 fl. oz. (60 ml). Store at controlled room temperature (59°F–86°F). NDC 0574-0014-02

GLUTOSE®   OTC
(Oral Glucose Gel)

DESCRIPTION

Glutose gel is a lemon-flavored, dye-free oral glucose gel for treatment of insulin reaction or hypoglycemia. Glutose gel contains Dextrose (D-Glucose) 40%.

HOW SUPPLIED

Three "unit-of-use" 25 gram tubes NDC 0574-0069-25
Multi-dose 80 gram tube NDC 0574-0069-80

GLUTOSE® Tablets   OTC
(Oral Glucose Chewable Tablets)

DESCRIPTION

Glutose tablets are a lemon-flavored chewable tablet for treatment of insulin reaction or hypoglycemia. Each tablet contains 5 grams of Dextrose.

HOW SUPPLIED

Box of 12 tablets NDC 0574-0068-12

NYSTATIN, USP   ℞
For Extemporaneous Preparation
of Oral Suspension

DESCRIPTION

Nystatin USP is an antifungal antibiotic obtained from *Streptomyces noursei.* It is known to be a mixture, but the composition has not been completely elucidated. Nystatin A_1 is closely related to amphotericin B. Each is a macrocyclic lactone containing a ketal ring, an all-trans polyene system, and a mycosamine (3-amino-3-deoxy-rhamnose) moiety. [See chemical structure at top of next page.]

Continued on next page

Paddock Laboratories—Cont.

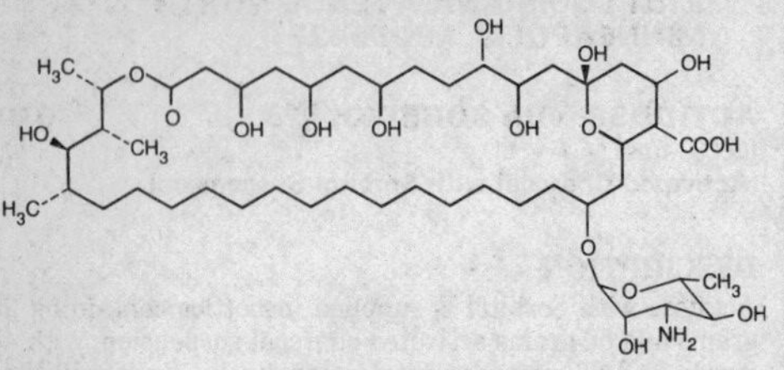

Nystatin A₁

Nystatin USP is a ready-to-use, non-sterile powder for oral administration which contains no excipients or preservatives. It is available in containers of 50 million, 150 million, 500 million, 1 billion, 2 billion, and 5 billion units. Each mg contains not less than 5,000 units.

CLINICAL PHARMACOLOGY
Nystatin probably acts by binding to sterols in the cell membrane of the fungus with a resultant change in membrane permeability allowing leakage of intracellular components. It is absorbed very sparingly following oral administration, with no detectable blood levels when given in the recommended doses. Most of the orally administered nystatin is passed unchanged in the stool.

INDICATIONS
For the treatment of intestinal and oral cavity infections caused by Candida (Monilia) albicans.

CONTRAINDICATIONS
Hypersensitivity to the drug.

ADVERSE REACTIONS
Large oral doses of nystatin have occasionally produced diarrhea, gastrointestinal distress, and possible irritation of the stomach that may result in nausea and vomiting.

DOSAGE AND ADMINISTRATION
General
Adults and older children: Add ⅛ teaspoonful (approximately 500,000 units) of Nystatin USP to about ½ cup of water and stir well. This product contains no preservatives and therefore should be used immediately after mixing and should not be stored. It is designed for extemporaneous preparation of a single dose at a time.
Infections of the oral cavity caused by Candida (Monilia) albicans:
Infants: 200,000 units four times daily.
Children and adults: 400,000 to 600,000 units four times daily (one-half dose in each side of mouth).
NOTE: Limited clinical studies in premature and low birthweight infants indicate that 100,000 units four times daily is effective.
Local treatment should be continued at least 48 hours after perioral symptoms have disappeared and cultures returned to normal.
It is recommended that the drug be retained in the mouth as long as possible before swallowing.
Intestinal candidiasis (moniliasis)
Usual dosage: 500,000 to 1 million units (approximately ⅛ to ¼ teaspoonful) three times daily. Treatment should generally be continued for at least 48 hours after clinical cure to prevent relapse.

HOW SUPPLIED
Containers of 50 million, 150 million, 500 million, 1 billion, 2 billion, and 5 billion units.

Product Code (NDC)	Size (units)	Approx. Weight (grams)
0574-0404-05	50 million	8.3 – 10
0574-0404-15	150 million	25 – 30
0574-0404-50	500 million	83 – 100
0574-0404-01	1 billion	167 – 200
5074-0404-02	2 billion	333 – 400
0574-0404-00	5 billion	833 – 1,000

Storage: Store under refrigeration 2°-8°C (36°–46°F) in a tight, light-resistant containers.

5/92

Products are
listed alphabetically
in the
PINK SECTION.

Palisades Pharmaceuticals, Inc.
219 COUNTY ROAD
TENAFLY, NEW JERSEY 07670

PALS™   OTC
['pals]
Internal Deodorant
Chlorophyllin Copper Complex

POD-BEN-25™   ℞
(podophyllum resin 25%)

DESCRIPTION
POD-BEN-25™ is a topical preparation containing podophyllum resin 25% in Tincture of Benzoin, U.S.P.

HOW SUPPLIED
NDC # 53159-025-30, 30 ml bottle
NDC # 53159-025-05, box of ten 0.5 ml ampules
NOTE
POD-BEN-25™ IS TO BE USED (APPLIED) ONLY BY THE DOCTOR. IT IS NOT TO BE DISPENSED TO THE PATIENT.

SCLEROMATE™   ℞
[skle "ro-māt]
MORRHUATE SODIUM INJECTION U.S.P.

DESCRIPTION
Morrhuate Sodium Injection, U.S.P. is a mixture of the sodium salts of the saturated and unsaturated fatty acids of Cod Liver Oil. SCLEROMATE Morrhuate Sodium Injection, U.S.P. is prepared by the saponification of selected Cod Liver Oils, it is overlaid with filtered Nitrogen to prevent discoloration that occurs on exposure to oxygen. Morrhuate Sodium occurs as a pale-yellowish, granular powder with a slight fishy odor and is soluble in water and in alcohol.
NOTE: Solid matter may develop a hazy appearance on standing and the injection should not be used if the solid matter does not dissolve completely on warming. The pH of the injection is adjusted to approximately 9.5.

CLINICAL PHARMACOLOGY
Morrhuate Sodium, when injected into the vein, causes inflammation of the intima and formation of a thrombus. This blood clot occludes the injected vein and fibrous tissue develops, resulting in the obliteration of the vein.

INDICATIONS AND USAGE
Morrhuate Sodium Injection is used for the obliteration of primary varicosed veins that consist of simple dilation with competent valves.
Sclerotherapy should not be used in patients with significant valvular or deep vein incompetence. (See Precautions.)
Although Morrhuate Sodium has been used as a sclerosing agent for the treatment of internal hemorrhoids, there is no substantial evidence that the drug is useful for this purpose. Most patients with symptomatic primary varicosed veins should be treated initially with compression stockings. If this treatment is inadequate, surgery may be required. Sclerosing agents may be useful as a supplement to venous ligation to obliterate residual varicosed veins or in patients who have conditions which increase the risk of surgery. However, many clinicians consider sclerotherapy if not effective may decrease the potential success of later surgery, should this be required.

CONTRAINDICATIONS
Morrhuate Sodium is contraindicated in patients who have shown a previous hypersensitivity reaction to the drug or to the fatty acids of cod liver oil. Continued administration of the drug is contraindicated when an unusual local reaction at the injection site or a systemic reaction occurs.
Thrombosis induced by Morrhuate Sodium may extend into the deep venous system in patients with significant valvular incompetence, therefore, valvular competency, deep vein patency, and deep vein competency should be determined by angiography and/or by tests such as the Trendelenberg and Perthes before injection of sclerosing agents. The drug is contraindicated for obliterations of superficial veins in patients with persistent occlusion of the deep veins. Morrhuate Sodium is also contraindicated in patients with acute superficial thrombophlebitis; underlying arterial disease; varicosities caused by abdominal and pelvic tumors, uncontrolled diabetes mellitus, thyrotoxicosis, tuberculosis, neoplasms, asthma, sepsis, blood dyscrasias, acute respiratory or skin disease; and in bedridden patients. Treatment with Morrhuate Sodium should be delayed in patients with acute local or systemic infections (including infected ulcers). Extensive therapy with the drug is inadvisable in patients who are severely debilitated or senile.

PRECAUTIONS
Burning or cramping sensations indicate local reactions. Urticaria may result. Sloughing and necrosis of tissue may occur with extravasation of the drug. Technique development is essential for optimal success in sclerotherapy, therefore the drug should be administered only by a physician familiar with proper injection technique. Drowsiness and headache may occur rarely. Pulmonary embolism has been reported.
Rarely, patients may have, or may develop hypersensitivity to Morrhuate Sodium, characterized by dizziness, weakness, vascular collapse, asthma, respiratory depression, gastrointestinal disturbances (i.e., nausea, vomiting), and urticaria. Anaphylactic reactions may occur within a few minutes after injection of the drug and are most likely to occur when therapy is reinstituted after an interval of several weeks. Morrhuate Sodium should only be administered when adequate facilities, drugs (i.e., epinephrine, antihistamines, corticosteroids), and personnel are available for the treatment of anaphylactic reactions.

PREGNANCY
Safety in use of Morrhuate Sodium during pregnancy has not been established.

DOSAGE
Morrhuate Sodium is administered only by INTRAVENOUS Injection. Care must be taken to avoid extravasation. (see Precautions.) Specialized references should be consulted for specific procedures and techniques of administration. When small veins are injected, or the injection solution is cold, or if solid matter has separated in the solution, the ampul or vial should be warmed by immersing in hot water. The solution should become clear on warming; only a clear solution should be used. Because the solution froths easily, a large bore needle should be used to fill the syringe, however, a small bore needle should be used for the injection.
To determine possible sensitivity to the drug, some clinicians recommend injection of 0.25–1 ml of 5% Morrhuate Sodium injection into a varicosity 24 hours before administration of a large dose.
Dosage of Morrhuate Sodium depends on the size and degree of varicosity. The usual adult dose for obliteration of small or medium veins is 50–100mg (1–2ml of the 5% injection). For large veins, 150–250 (3–5ml of the injection) is used. The drug may be given as multiple injections at one time or in single doses. Therapy may be repeated at 5–7 day intervals, according to the patient's response. Following injection of Morrhuate Sodium, the vein promptly becomes hard and swollen for 2–4 inches, depending on the size and response of the vein. After 24 hours, the vein is hard and slightly tender to the touch (with little or no periphlebitis). The skin around the injection becomes light-bronze; this color usually disappears shortly. An aching sensation and feeling of stiffness usually occur and last approximately 48 hours.

HOW SUPPLIED
MORRHUATE SODIUM INJECTION 5%
NDC-53159-003-01   30ml multiple use vials

STORAGE
Store below 40 degrees C. (104 degrees F.) preferably in a refrigerator, or between 15–30 degrees C. (59–86 degrees F.).
Rev. July 1985
Shown in Product Identification Section, page 422

VERR-CANTH™   ℞
(cantharidin 0.7%)

DESCRIPTION
Cantharidin 0.7% in an adherent-film-forming base of ethylcellulose, cellosolve, castor oil, penederm (octylphenylpolyethylene glycol), and acetone.

HOW SUPPLIED
7.5 ml bottle.
NDC # 53159-024-75

NOTE
VERR-CANTH™ IS TO BE USED (APPLIED) ONLY BY THE DOCTOR. IT IS NOT TO BE DISPENSED TO THE PATIENT.

For complete information on Pals and Palisades' line of wart-removal products (Lactisol, Lactisol-Forte, Pod-Ben-25, Verr-Canth, Verrex, and Verrusol) call 1-800-237-9083.

YOCON®   ℞

[yō′kon]

(brand of yohimbine hydrochloride)

DESCRIPTION

Yohimbine is a 3α-15α-20β-17α-hydroxy Yohimbine-16α-carboxylic acid methyl ester. The alkaloid is found in Rubaceae and related trees. Also in Rauwolfia Serpentina (L) Benth.

Yohimbine is an indolalkylamine alkaloid with chemical similarity to reserpine. It is a crystalline powder, odorless. Each compressed tablet contains (1/12 gr.) 5.4 mg of Yohimbine Hydrochloride.

ACTION

Yohimbine blocks presynaptic alpha-2 adrenergic receptors. Its action on peripheral blood vessels resembles that of reserpine, though it is weaker and of short duration. Yohimbine's peripheral autonomic nervous system effect is to increase parasympathetic (cholinergic) and decrease sympathetic (adrenergic) activity. It is to be noted that in male sexual performance, erection is linked to cholinergic activity and to alpha-2 adrenergic blockade which may theoretically result in increased penile inflow, decreased penile outflow or both. Yohimbine exerts a stimulating action on the mood and may increase anxiety. Such actions have not been adequately studied or related to dosage although they appear to require high doses of the drug. Yohimbine has a mild anti-diuretic action, probably via stimulation of hypothalmic centers and release of posterior pituitary hormone.

Reportedly, Yohimbine exerts no significant influence on cardiac stimulation and other effects mediated by β-adrenergic receptors, its effect on blood pressure, if any, would be to lower it; however, no adequate studies are at hand to quantitate this effect in terms of Yohimbine dosage.

INDICATIONS

YOCON is indicated as a sympathicolytic and mydriatic. It may have activity as an aphrodisiac.

CONTRAINDICATIONS

Renal diseases, and patients sensitive to the drug. In view of the limited and inadequate information at hand, no precise tabulation can be offered of additional contraindications.

WARNING

Generally, this drug is not proposed for use in females and certainly must not be used during pregnancy. Neither is this drug proposed for use in pediatric, geriatric or cardio-renal patients with gastric or duodenal ulcer history. Nor should it be used in conjunction with mood-modifying drugs such as antidepressants, or in psychiatric patients in general.

ADVERSE REACTIONS

Yohimbine readily penetrates the (CNS) and produces a complex pattern of responses in lower doses than required to produce peripheral α-adrenergic blockade. These include, anti-diuresis, a general picture of central excitation including elevation of blood pressure and heart rate increased motor activity, irritability and tremor. Sweating, nausea and vomiting are common after parenteral administration of the drug.[1,2] Also dizziness, headache, skin flushing reported when used orally[1,3].

DOSAGE AND ADMINISTRATION

Experimental dosage reported in treatment of erectile impotence:[1,3,4] 1 tablet (5.4 mg) 3 times a day, to adult males taken orally. Occasional side effects reported with this dosage are nausea, dizziness or nervousness. In the event of side effects dosage is to be reduced to ½ tablet 3 times a day, followed by gradual increases to 1 tablet 3 times a day. Reported therapy not more than 10 weeks[3].

HOW SUPPLIED

Oral tablets of Yocon® 1/12 gr 5.4 mg in bottles of 100's **NDC** 53159-001-01, 1000's **NDC** 53159-001-10, and blisterpaks of 30's **NDC** 53159-001-30.

REFERENCES

1. A. Morales et al., New England Journal of Medicine: 1221. November 12, 1981.
2. Goodman, Gilman —The Pharmacological basis of Therapeutics 6th ed., p. 176-188, McMillan
3. Weekly Urological Clinical letter, 27:2, July 4, 1983.
4. A. Morales et al., The Journal of Urology 128 : 45-47, 1982.
Rev. January 1985

Shown in Product Identification Section, page 422

Products are cross-indexed by
generic and chemical names in the
YELLOW SECTION.

Par Pharmaceutical, Inc.
ONE RAM RIDGE ROAD
SPRING VALLEY, NY 10977

COMPLETE LISTING OF PAR PRODUCTS

Par Pharmaceutical, Inc. manufactures tablets and capsules with an identification system that consists of the letters PAR and the NDC product numbers or product strength imprinted or embossed on the surface. To expedite product identification, an alphabetical listing of Par's products is provided below. Each product comes in a variety of packaging specifications, with the most common being 100's, 500's and 1000's.

Imprint numbers same as NDC numbers except where indicated otherwise.

NDC # 49884-	Product
104	Allopurinol Tablets 100 mg
105	Allopurinol Tablets 300 mg
117	Amiloride HCl Tablets 5 mg
128	Amiloride HCl and Hydrochlorothiazide 5 mg/50 mg
133	Amitriptyline HCl Tablets 10 mg
134	Amitriptyline HCl Tablets 25 mg
135	Amitriptyline HCl Tablets 50 mg
136	Amitriptyline HCl Tablets 75 mg
137	Amitriptyline HCl Tablets 100 mg
138	Amitriptyline HCl Tablets 150 mg
164	Benztropine Mesylate Tablets 0.5 mg
165	Benztropine Mesylate Tablets 1 mg
166	Benztropine Mesylate Tablets 2 mg
246	Carisoprodol and Aspirin Tablets 200 mg/325 mg
265	Chlordiazepoxide and Amitriptyline HCl Tablets 5 mg/12.5 mg
266	Chlordiazepoxide and Amitriptyline HCl Tablets 10 mg/25 mg
077	Chlorpropamide Tablets 100 mg
078	Chlorpropamide Tablets 250 mg
016	Chlorzoxazone Tablets 250 mg
110	Clonidine HCl Tablets 0.1 mg
111	Clonidine HCl Tablets 0.2 mg
112	Clonidine HCl Tablets 0.3 mg
113	Clonidine HCl and Chlorthalidone Tablets 0.1 mg/15 mg
115	Clonidine HCl and Chlorthalidone Tablets 0.2 mg/15 mg
116	Clonidine HCl and Chlorthalidone Tablets 0.3 mg/15 mg
043	Cyproheptadine HCl Tablets 4 mg
083	Dexamethasone Tablets 0.25 mg
084	Dexamethasone Tablets 0.5 mg
085	Dexamethasone Tablets 0.75 mg
086	Dexamethasone Tablets 1.5 mg
087	Dexamethasone Tablets 4 mg
129	Dexamethasone Tablets 6 mg
190	Diazepam Tablets 2 mg
191	Diazepam Tablets 5 mg
192	Diazepam Tablets 10 mg
153	Disulfiram Tablets 250 mg
154	Disulfiram Tablets 500 mg
217	Doxepin HCl Capsules 10 mg
218	Doxepin HCl Capsules 25 mg
219	Doxepin HCl Capsules 50 mg
220	Doxepin HCl Capsules 75 mg
221	Doxepin HCl Capsules 100 mg
222	Doxepin HCl Capsules 150 mg
018	Doxycycline Hyclate Capsules 50 mg
019	Doxycycline Hyclate Capsules 100 mg
287	Fenoprofen Calcium Capsules 200 mg
288	Fenoprofen Calcium Capsules 300 mg
286	Fenoprofen Calcium Tablets 600 mg
061	Fluphenazine HCl Tablets 1 mg
062	Fluphenazine HCl Tablets 2.5 mg
076	Fluphenazine HCl Tablets 5 mg
064	Fluphenazine HCl Tablets 10 mg
193	Flurazepam HCl Capsules 15 mg
194	Flurazepam HCl Capsules 30 mg
223	Haloperidol Tablets 0.5 mg
224	Haloperidol Tablets 1 mg
225	Haloperidol Tablets 2 mg
226	Haloperidol Tablets 5 mg
227	Haloperidol Tablets 10 mg
029	Hydralazine HCl Tablets 10 mg
027	Hydralazine HCl Tablets 25 mg
028	Hydralazine HCl Tablets 50 mg
121	Hydralazine HCl Tablets 100 mg
143	Hydra-Zide (Hydralazine HCl and Hydrochlorothiazide) Capsules 25 mg/25 mg
144	Hydra-Zide (Hydralazine HCl and Hydrochlorothiazide) Capsules 50 mg/50 mg
145	Hydra-Zide (Hydralazine HCl and Hydrochlorothiazide) Capsules 100 mg/50 mg
147	Hydroflumethiazide Tablets 50 mg
148	Reserpine and Hydroflumethiazide Tablets 0.125 mg/50 mg
012	Hydroxyzine HCl Tablets 10 mg
013	Hydroxyzine HCl Tablets 25 mg
014	Hydroxyzine HCl Tablets 50 mg
161	Ibuprofen Tablets 300 mg
162	Ibuprofen Tablets 400 mg
163	Ibuprofen Tablets 600 mg
216	Ibuprofen Tablets 800 mg
054	Imipramine HCl Tablets 10 mg
055	Imipramine HCl Tablets 25 mg
056	Imipramine HCl Tablets 50 mg
067	Indomethacin Capsules 25 mg
068	Indomethacin Capsules 50 mg
020	Isosorbide Dinitrate Tablets 5 mg
021	Isosorbide Dinitrate Tablets 10 mg
022	Isosorbide Dinitrate Tablets 20 mg
009	Isosorbide Dinitrate Tablets 30 mg
206	Lorazepam Tablets 0.5 mg
207	Lorazepam Tablets 1 mg
208	Lorazepam Tablets 2 mg
034	Meclizine HCl Tablets 12.5 mg
035	Meclizine HCl Tablets 25 mg
015	Meclizine HCl Tablets 50 mg
289	Megestrol Acetate Tablets 20 mg
290	Megestrol Acetate Tablets 40 mg
360	Metaproterenol Sulfate Inhalation Solution, 0.4%
361	Metaproterenol Sulfate Inhalation Solution, 0.6%
258	Metaproterenol Sulfate Tablets 10 mg
259	Metaproterenol Sulfate Tablets 20 mg
036	Methocarbamol Tablets 500 mg
037	Methocarbamol Tablets 750 mg
249	Methocarbamol and Aspirin Tablets 400 mg/325 mg
177	Methyclothiazide Tablets 2.5 mg
178	Methyclothiazide Tablets 5 mg
150	Methyldopa Tablets 125 mg
151	Methyldopa Tablets 250 mg
152	Methyldopa Tablets 500 mg
202	Methyldopa and Chlorothiazide Tablets 250 mg/150 mg
203	Methyldopa and Chlorothiazide Tablets 250 mg/250 mg
186	Methyldopa and Hydrochlorothiazide Tablets 250 mg/15 mg
187	Methyldopa and Hydrochlorothiazide Tablets 250 mg/25 mg
188	Methyldopa and Hydrochlorothiazide Tablets 500 mg/30 mg
189	Methyldopa and Hydrochlorothiazide Tablets 500 mg/50 mg
158	Methylprednisolone Tablets 16 mg
159	Methylprednisolone Tablets 24 mg
160	Methylprednisolone Tablets 32 mg
132	Metoclopramide HCl Tablets 10 mg
095	Metronidazole Compressed Tablets 250 mg
114	Metronidazole Compressed Tablets 500 mg
229	Metronidazole Film Coated Tablets 250 mg (I.D. Code #130)
230	Metronidazole Film Coated Tablets 500 mg (I.D. Code #131)
256	Minoxidil Tablets 2.5 mg
257	Minoxidil Tablets 10 mg
119	Nystatin Tablets 500,000 Units
900	Par-Glycerol Elixir (Iodinated Glycerol)
902	Par-Glycerol-C Ⓒ Liquid (Iodinated Glycerol with Codeine Phosphate)
903	Par-Glycerol DM Liquid (Iodinated Glycerol with Dextromethorphan)
181	Perphenazine and Amitriptyline HCl Tablets 2 mg/10 mg
182	Perphenazine and Amitriptyline HCl Tablets 2 mg/25 mg
183	Perphenazine and Amitriptyline HCl Tablets 4 mg/10 mg
184	Perphenazine and Amitriptyline HCl Tablets 4 mg/25 mg
185	Perphenazine and Amitriptyline HCl Tablets 4 mg/50 mg
118	Propantheline Bromide Tablets 15 mg
106	Propranolol HCl Tablets 10 mg
107	Propranolol HCl Tablets 20 mg
108	Propranolol HCl Tablets 40 mg
127	Propranolol Tablets 60 mg

Continued on next page

Par—Cont.

109	Propranolol HCl Tablets 80 mg
239	Propranolol 90 mg
247	Salsalate Tablets 500 mg
248	Salsalate Tablets 750 mg
521	Silver Sulfadiazine Cream, 1%
139	Sulfamethoxazole and Trimethoprim Tablets 400 mg/80 mg
140	Sulfamethoxazole and Trimethoprim Tablets 800 mg/160 mg
170	Sulfinpyrazone Tablets 100 mg
171	Sulfinpyrazone Capsules 200 mg
240	Temazepam Capsules 15 mg
241	Temazepam Capsules 30 mg
096	Thioridazine HCl Tablets 10 mg
097	Thioridazine HCl Tablets 15 mg
098	Thioridazine HCl Tablets 25 mg
099	Thioridazine HCl Tablets 50 mg
101	Thioridazine HCl Tablets 100 mg
122	Tolazamide Tablets 100 mg
123	Tolazamide Tablets 250 mg
124	Tolazamide Tablets 500 mg
039	Trichlormethiazide Tablets 4 mg
125	Valproic Acid Capsules 250 mg

Parke-Davis
Division of Warner-Lambert Company
201 TABOR ROAD
MORRIS PLAINS, NEW JERSEY 07950

PARCODE®
(Parke-Davis Accurate Recognition Code)

Code Number   Product Name

001   Peritrate® Tablets
Each tablet contains 20 mg pentaerythritol tetranitrate.

002-
003   Unassigned
004   Peritrate® SA Sustained Action Tablets
Each tablet contains 80 mg pentaerythritol tetranitrate (20 mg in the immediate release layer and 60 mg in the sustained release base).

005-
006   Unassigned
007   Dilantin® Infatabs®
Each tablet contains 50 mg phenytoin sodium, USP.

008   Peritrate® Tablets
Each tablet contains 40 mg pentaerythritol tetranitrate.

009-
012   Unassigned
013   Peritrate® Tablets
Each tablet contains 10 mg pentaerythritol tetranitrate.

014-
110   Unassigned
111   Ergostat® Sublingual Tablets
Each tablet contains 2 mg ergotamine tartrate.

112-
165   Unassigned
166   Mandelamine® Tablets
Each tablet contains 0.5 gram methenamine mandelate, USP.

167   Mandelamine® Tablets
Each tablet contains 1 gram methenamine mandelate, USP.

168-
176   Unassigned
177   Sinubid ® Tablets
Each tablet contains 600 mg acetaminophen, 100 mg phenylpropanolamine hydrochloride, and 66 mg phenyltoloxamine citrate.

178-
179   Unassigned
180   Pyridium® Tablets
Each tablet contains 100 mg phenazopyridine hydrochloride, USP.

181   Pyridium® Tablets
Each tablet contains 200 mg phenazopyridine hydrochloride, USP.

182   Pyridium® Plus Tablets
Each tablet contains 150 mg phenazopyridine hydrochloride (Pyridium®), 0.3 mg hyoscyamine hydrobromide, and 15 mg butabarbital.

183-
199   Unassigned
200   Brondecon® Tablets
Each tablet contains 200 mg oxtriphylline and 100 mg guaifenesin.

201   Unassigned
202   Procan® SR Tablets, 250 mg
Each sustained-release tablet contains 250 mg procainamide hydrochloride.

203   Unassigned
204   Procan® SR Tablets, 500 mg
Each sustained-release tablet contains 500 mg procainamide hydrochloride.

205   Procan® SR Tablets, 750 mg
Each sustained-release tablet contains 750 mg procainamide hydrochloride.

206   Unassigned
207   Procan® SR Tablets, 1000 mg
Each sustained-release tablet contains 1000 mg procainamide hydrochloride.

208-
209   Unassigned
210   Choledyl® Tablets
Each tablet contains 100 mg oxtriphylline, USP.

211   Choledyl® Tablets
Each tablet contains 200 mg oxtriphylline, USP.

212-
213   Unassigned
214   Choledyl® SA Tablets
Each sustained-action tablet contains 400 mg oxtriphylline, USP.

215-
220   Unassigned
221   Choledyl® SA Tablets
Each sustained-action tablet contains 600 mg oxtriphylline, USP.

222-
229   Unassigned
230   Tedral® Tablets
Each tablet contains 130 mg theophylline, 24 mg ephedrine hydrochloride, 8 mg phenobarbital.

231   Tedral® SA Tablets
Each sustained-action tablet contains 180 mg anhydrous theophylline (90 mg in the immediate release layer and 90 mg in the sustained-release layer); 48 mg ephedrine hydrochloride (16 mg in the immediate release layer and 32 mg in the sustained-release layer); 25 mg phenobarbital in the immediate release layer.

232-
236   Unassigned
237   Zarontin® Capsules
Each capsule contains 250 mg ethosuximide, USP.

238-
260   Unassigned
261   Euthroid®-1 Tablets
Each tablet contains 60 mcg levothyroxine sodium (T_4), 15 mcg liothyronine sodium (T_3).

262   Euthroid®-2 Tablets
Each tablet contains 120 mcg levothyroxine sodium (T_4), 30 mcg liothyronine sodium (T_3).

263   Euthroid®-3 Tablets
Each tablet contains 180 mcg levothyroxine sodium (T_4), 45 mcg liothyronine sodium (T_3).

264-
269   Unassigned
270   Nardil® Tablets
Each tablet contains 15 mg phenelzine sulfate, USP.

271-
281   Unassigned
282   Natafort® Filmseal®
Each tablet represents vitamin A (acetate), 6,000 IU; vitamin D 400 IU; folic acid, 1 mg; vitamin B_1 (thiamine mononitrate), 3 mg; vitamin B_2 (riboflavin), 2 mg; vitamin B_6 (pyridoxine hydrochloride), 15 mg; vitamin B_{12} (cyanocobalamin), crystalline, 6 mcg; vitamin C (ascorbic acid), 120 mg; nicotinamide (niacinamide), 20 mg; vitamin E (dl-alpha tocopheryl acetate), 30 IU; calcium (as calcium carbonate), 350 mg; magnesium (as magnesium oxide), 100 mg; iodine (as potassium iodide), 0.15 mg; iron (as ferrous fumarate), 65 mg; zinc (as zinc oxide), 25 mg.

283-
319   Unassigned
320   Parsidol® Tablets
Each tablet contains 10 mg ethopropazine hydrochloride, USP.

321   Parsidol® Tablets
Each tablet contains 50 mg ethopropazine hydrochloride, USP.

322-
336   Unassigned
337   Eldec® Kapseals®
Each capsule represents vitamin A (acetate), (0.5 mg) 1,667 IU; vitamin C (ascorbic acid), 66.7 mg; vitamin B_1 (thiamine mononitrate), 10 mg; vitamin B_2 (riboflavin), 0.87 mg; vitamin B_6 (pyridoxine hydrochloride), 0.67 mg; nicotinamide (niacinamide), 16.7 mg; dl-panthenol, 10 mg; ferrous sulfate, dried, 16.7 mg; iodine (as potassium iodide), 0.05 mg; calcium carbonate, 66.7 mg; vitamin E (dl-alpha tocopheryl acetate), (10 mg) 10 IU; vitamin B_{12} (cyanocobalamin), 2 mcg; folic acid, 0.33 mg. The Kapseal is a Dark Blue No. 1 capsule with Light Blue opaque band.

338-
361   Unassigned
362   Dilantin® Kapseals®
Each Kapseal contains 100 mg extended phenytoin sodium, USP. The Kapseal is a No. 3 capsule with Orange band. (The Orange band on White capsule is a trademark registered in the US Patent Office.)

363-
364   Unassigned
365   Dilantin® Kapseals®
Each Kapseal contains 30 mg extended phenytoin sodium, USP. The Kapseal is a No. 4 capsule with Pink opaque band.

366-
372   Unassigned
373   Benadryl® Kapseals®
Each Kapseal contains 50 mg diphenhydramine hydrochloride. The Kapseal is a Pink No. 4 capsule with White opaque band. (The White band on Pink capsule is a trademark registered in the US Patent Office.)

374   Unassigned
375   Dilantin® with Phenobarbital ($\frac{1}{4}$ grain) Kapseals®
Each Kapseal contains Dilantin (phenytoin sodium), 100 mg; phenobarbital, 16 mg ($\frac{1}{4}$ grain). The Kapseal is a No. 3 capsule with Garnet band.

376-
378   Unassigned
379   Chloromycetin® Kapseals®
Each Kapseal contains 250 mg chloramphenicol. The Kapseal is a White opaque No. 2 capsule with Gray opaque band. (The Gray band on White capsule is a trademark registered in the US Patent Office.)

380-
392   Unassigned
393   Milontin® Kapseals®
Each Kapseal contains 500 mg phensuximide, USP. The Kapseal is a Light Orange No. 0 capsule with Orange band.

394-
436   Unassigned
437   Estrovis® Tablets
Each tablet contains 100 mcg quinestrol.

438-
470   Unassigned
471   Benadryl® Capsules
Each capsule contains 25 mg diphenhydramine hydrochloride.

472-
489   Unassigned
490   Easprin® Enteric Coated Tablets
Each tablet contains 15 grains (975 mg) aspirin, USP.

491-
524   Unassigned
525   Celontin® Kapseals®
Each Kapseal contains 300 mg methsuximide, USP. The Kapseal is a Yellow Tint No. 2 capsule with Orange band.

526   Unassigned
527   Accupril® Tablets
Each tablet contains 5 mg quinapril hydrochloride.

528   Unassigned
529   Humatin® Capsules
Each capsule contains paromomycin sulfate, USP, equivalent to 250 mg paromomycin.

530   Accupril® Tablets
Each tablet contains 10 mg quinapril hydrochloride.

531   Dilantin® with Phenobarbital ($\frac{1}{2}$ grain) Kapseals®
Each Kapseal contains Dilantin (phenytoin sodium), 100 mg; phenobarbital, 32 mg ($\frac{1}{2}$ grain). The Kapseal is a No. 3 capsule with Black band.

532   Accupril® Tablets
Each tablet contains 20 mg quinapril hydrochloride.

533-
536   *Unassigned*
537   **Celontin® (Half Strength) Kapseals®**

Each Kapseal contains 150 mg methsuximide, USP. The Kapseal is a Yellow Tint No. 4 capsule with Brown opaque band.

538-
539   *Unassigned*
540   **Ponstel® Kapseals®**

Each Kapseal contains 250 mg mefenamic acid. The Kapseal is an Ivory opaque No. 1 capsule with Light Blue opaque band. The blue band on ivory capsule combination is a Parke-Davis trademark.

541-
543   *Unassigned*
544   **Geriplex-FS® Kapseals®**

Each Kapseal represents vitamin A (acetate), 5,000 IU; vitamin C (ascorbic acid), 50 mg; vitamin B₁ (thiamine mononitrate), 5 mg; vitamin B₂ (riboflavin), 5 mg; cyanocobalamin, 2 mcg; choline dihydrogen citrate, 20 mg; nicotinamide (niacinamide), 15 mg; vitamin E (*dl*-alpha tocopheryl acetate), 5 IU; ferrous sulfate, dried, 30 mg; copper sulfate (cupric sulfate anhydrous), 4 mg; manganese sulfate (monohydrate), 4 mg; zinc sulfate (monohydrate), 2 mg; calcium phosphate (dibasic), 200 mg; Taka-Diastase 3000%, 2½ gr; docusate sodium, 100 mg.

545-
546   *Unassigned.*
547   **Natabec ℞® Kapseals®**

Each Kapseal represents vitamin A (acetate) (1.2 mg); Vitamin D (10 mcg) 400 IU; ascorbic acid, 50 mg; thiamine mononitrate, 3 mg; riboflavin, 2 mg; pyridoxine hydrochloride, 3 mg; cyanocobalamin, 5 mcg; niacinamide, 10 mg; folic acid, 1 mg; calcium carbonate, precipitated, 600 mg; iron* 30 mg.

*Supplied as dried ferrous sulfate.

The Kapseal is a Blue opaque No. 0 capsule with Pink opaque band. The banded capsule is a Warner-Lambert trademark registered in the US Patent Office.

548-
551   *Unassigned*
552   **ℂℽCentrax® Capsules**

Each capsule contains 5 mg prazepam.

553   **ℂℽCentrax® Capsules**

Each capsule contains 10 mg prazepam.

554   **ℂℽCentrax® Capsules**

Each capsule contains 20 mg prazepam.

555-
617   *Unassigned*
618   **Placebo tablet in Norlestrin Ⓩ 1/50.**

619-
621   *Unassigned*
622   **Ferrous Fumarate Tablets**

Each tablet contains 75 mg ferrous fumarate, USP.

623-
637   *Unassigned*
638   **Tabron® Filmseal®**

Each tablet represents ferrous fumarate, 304.2 mg (represents 100 mg of elemental iron); vitamin C (ascorbic acid), 500 mg; vitamin B₁ (thiamine mononitrate), 6 mg; vitamin B₂ (riboflavin), 6 mg; vitamin B₆ (pyridoxine hydrochloride), 5 mg; vitamin B₁₂ (cyanocobalamin), crystalline, 25 mcg; folic acid, 1 mg; nicotinamide (niacinamide), 30 mg; calcium pantothenate, 10 mg; vitamin E (*dl*-alpha tocopheryl acetate), (30 mg), 30 IU; docusate sodium, 50 mg.

639-
695   *Unassigned*
696   **ERYC® Capsules**

Each capsule contains 250 mg erythromycin, USP.

697-
736   *Unassigned*
737   **Lopid® Tablets**

Each tablet contains 600 mg gemfibrozil.

738-
881   *Unassigned*
882   **Norlutin® Tablets**

Each tablet contains 5 mg norethindrone, USP.

883-
900   *Unassigned*
901   **Norlestrin® 2.5/50 Tablets**

Each tablet contains norethindrone acetate, 2.5 mg; ethinyl estradiol, 50 mcg.

902-
903   *Unassigned*
904   **Norlestrin® 1/50 Tablets**

Each tablet contains norethindrone acetate, 1 mg; ethinyl estradiol, 50 mcg.

905-
914   *Unassigned*
915   **Loestrin® 1/20 Tablets**

Each tablet contains norethindrone acetate, 1 mg; ethinyl estradiol, 20 mcg.

916   **Loestrin® 1.5/30 Tablets**

Each tablet contains norethindrone acetate, 1.5 mg; ethinyl estradiol, 30 mcg.

917
918   **Norlutate® Tablets**

Each tablet contains 5 mg norethindrone acetate.

919-
999   *Unassigned*

ACCUPRIL®   ℞
(Quinapril Hydrochloride Tablets)

USE IN PREGNANCY

When used in pregnancy during the second and third trimesters, ACE inhibitors can cause injury and even death to the developing fetus. When pregnancy is detected, ACCUPRIL should be discontinued as soon as possible. See Warnings: Fetal/Neonatal Morbidity and Mortality.

DESCRIPTION

ACCUPRIL® (quinapril hydrochloride) is the hydrochloride salt of quinapril, the ethyl ester of a nonsulfhydryl, angiotensin-converting enzyme (ACE) inhibitor, quinaprilat.

Quinapril hydrochloride is chemically described as [3S-[2[R*(R*)],   3R*]]-2-[2-[[1-(ethoxycarbonyl)-3-phenylpropyl]amino]-1-oxopropyl]-1,2,3,4-tetrahydro-3-isoquinolinecarboxylic acid, monohydrochloride. Its empirical formula is $C_{25}H_{30}N_2O_5 \cdot HCl$ and its structural formula is:

M.W. = 474.98

Quinapril hydrochloride is a white to off-white amorphous powder that is freely soluble in aqueous solvents.

ACCUPRIL tablets contain 5 mg, 10 mg, 20 mg, or 40 mg of quinapril for oral administration. Each tablet also contains candelilla wax, crospovidone, gelatin, lactose, magnesium carbonate, magnesium stearate, synthetic red iron oxide, and titanium dioxide.

CLINICAL PHARMACOLOGY

Mechanism of Action: Quinapril is deesterified to the principal metabolite, quinaprilat, which is an inhibitor of ACE activity in human subjects and animals. ACE is a peptidyl dipeptidase that catalyzes the conversion of angiotensin I to the vasoconstrictor, angiotensin II. The effect of quinapril in hypertension appears to result primarily from the inhibition of circulating and tissue ACE activity, thereby reducing angiotensin II formation. Quinapril inhibits the elevation in blood pressure caused by intravenously administered angiotensin I, but has no effect on the pressor response to angiotensin II, norepinephrine or epinephrine. Angiotensin II also stimulates the secretion of aldosterone from the adrenal cortex, thereby facilitating renal sodium and fluid reabsorption. Reduced aldosterone secretion by quinapril may result in a small increase in serum potassium. In controlled hypertension trials, treatment with ACCUPRIL alone resulted in mean increases in potassium of 0.07 mmol/L (see PRECAUTIONS). Removal of angiotensin II negative feedback on renin secretion leads to increased plasma renin activity (PRA).

While the principal mechanism of antihypertensive effect is thought to be through the renin-angiotensin-aldosterone system, quinapril exerts antihypertensive actions even in patients with low renin hypertension. ACCUPRIL was an effective antihypertensive in all races studied, although it was somewhat less effective in blacks (usually a predominantly low renin group) than in nonblacks. ACE is identical to kininase II, an enzyme that degrades bradykinin, a potent peptide vasodilator; whether increased levels of bradykinin play a role in the therapeutic effect of quinapril remains to be elucidated.

Pharmacokinetics and Metabolism: Following oral administration, peak plasma quinapril concentrations are observed within one hour. Based on recovery of quinapril and its metabolites in urine, the extent of absorption is at least 60%. The rate and extent of quinapril absorption are diminished moderately (approximately 25–30%) when ACCUPRIL tablets are administered during a high-fat meal. Following absorption, quinapril is deesterified to its major active metabolite, quinaprilat (about 38% of oral dose), and to other minor inactive metabolites. Following multiple oral dosing

of ACCUPRIL, there is an effective accumulation half-life of quinaprilat of approximately 3 hours, and peak plasma quinaprilat concentrations are observed approximately 2 hours post-dose. Quinaprilat is eliminated primarily by renal excretion, up to 96% of an IV dose, and has an elimination half-life in plasma of approximately 2 hours and a prolonged terminal phase with a half-life of 25 hours. The pharmacokinetics of quinapril and quinaprilat are linear over a single-dose range of 5–80 mg doses and 40–160 mg in multiple daily doses. Approximately 97% of either quinapril or quinaprilat circulating in plasma is bound to proteins.

In patients with renal insufficiency, the elimination half-life of quinaprilat increases as creatinine clearance decreases. There is a linear correlation between plasma quinaprilat clearance and creatinine clearance. In patients with end-stage renal disease, chronic hemodialysis or continuous ambulatory peritoneal dialysis has little effect on the elimination of quinapril and quinaprilat. Elimination of quinaprilat is reduced in elderly patients (≥65 years); this reduction is attributable to decrease in renal function (see DOSAGE AND ADMINISTRATION, and not to age itself. Quinaprilat concentrations are reduced in patients with alcoholic cirrhosis due to impaired deesterification of quinapril. Studies in rats indicate that quinapril and its metabolites do not cross the blood-brain barrier.

Pharmacodynamics and Clinical Effects: Single doses of 20 mg of ACCUPRIL provide over 80% inhibition of plasma ACE for 24 hours. Inhibition of the pressor response to angiotensin I is shorter-lived, with a 20 mg dose giving 75% inhibition for about 4 hours, 50% inhibition for about 8 hours, and 20% inhibition at 24 hours. With chronic dosing, however, there is substantial inhibition of angiotensin II levels at 24 hours by doses of 20–80 mg.

Administration of 10 to 80 mg of ACCUPRIL to patients with mild to severe hypertension results in a reduction of sitting and standing blood pressure to about the same extent with minimal effect on heart rate. Symptomatic postural hypotension is infrequent although it can occur in patients who are salt- and/or volume-depleted (see WARNINGS). Antihypertensive activity commences within 1 hour with peak effects usually achieved by 2 to 4 hours after dosing. During chronic therapy, most of the blood pressure lowering effect of a given dose is obtained in 1–2 weeks. In multiple-dose studies, 10–80 mg per day in single or divided doses lowered systolic and diastolic blood pressure throughout the dosing interval with a trough effect of about 5–11/3–7 mm Hg. The trough effect represents about 50% of the peak effect. While the dose-response relationship is relatively flat, doses of 40–80 mg were somewhat more effective at trough than 10–20 mg, and twice daily dosing tended to give a somewhat lower trough blood pressure than once daily dosing with the same total dose. The antihypertensive effect of ACCUPRIL continues during long-term therapy, with no evidence of loss of effectiveness.

Hemodynamic assessments in patients with hypertension indicate that blood pressure reduction produced by quinapril is accompanied by a reduction in total peripheral resistance and renal vascular resistance with little or no change in heart rate, cardiac index, renal blood flow, glomerular filtration rate, or filtration fraction.

Use of ACCUPRIL with a thiazide diuretic gives a blood-pressure lowering effect greater than that seen with either agent alone.

In patients with hypertension, ACCUPRIL 10–40 mg was similar in effectiveness to captopril, enalapril, propranolol, and thiazide diuretics.

Therapeutic effects appear to be the same for elderly (≥65 years of age) and younger adult patients given the same daily dosages, with no increase in adverse events in elderly patients.

INDICATIONS AND USAGE

ACCUPRIL is indicated for the treatment of hypertension. It may be used alone or in combination with thiazide diuretics.

In using ACCUPRIL, consideration should be given to the fact that another angiotensin converting enzyme inhibitor, captopril, has caused agranulocytosis, particularly in patients with renal impairment or collagen vascular disease. Available data are insufficient to show that ACCUPRIL does not have a similar risk (see WARNINGS).

CONTRAINDICATIONS

ACCUPRIL is contraindicated in patients who are hypersensitive to this product and in patients with a history of angioedema related to previous treatment with an ACE inhibitor.

Continued on next page

This product information was prepared in August 1992. On these and other Parke-Davis Products, information may be obtained by addressing PARKE-DAVIS, Division of Warner-Lambert Company, Morris Plains, New Jersey 07950.

Parke-Davis—Cont.

WARNINGS

Angioedema: Angioedema of the face, extremities, lips, tongue, glottis, and larynx has been reported in patients treated with ACE inhibitors and has been seen in 0.1% of patients receiving ACCUPRIL. Angioedema associated with laryngeal edema can be fatal. If laryngeal stridor or angioedema of the face, tongue, or glottis occurs, treatment with ACCUPRIL should be discontinued immediately, the patient treated in accordance with accepted medical care, and carefully observed until the swelling disappears. In instances where swelling is confined to the face and lips, the condition generally resolves without treatment; antihistamines may be useful in relieving symptoms. **Where there is involvement of the tongue, glottis, or larynx likely to cause airway obstruction, emergency therapy including, but not limited to, subcutaneous epinephrine solution 1:1000 (0.3 to 0.5 mL), should be promptly administered** (see ADVERSE REACTIONS).

Hypotension: Symptomatic hypotension was rarely seen in uncomplicated hypertensive patients treated with ACCUPRIL but, as with other ACE inhibitors, it is a possible consequence of therapy in salt/volume depleted patients, such as those previously treated with diuretics or dietary salt restriction or who are on dialysis (see PRECAUTIONS, DRUG INTERACTIONS, and ADVERSE REACTIONS). In controlled studies, syncope was observed in 0.4% of patients (N = 3203); this incidence was similar to that observed for captopril (1%) and enalapril (0.8%).

In patients with concomitant congestive heart failure, with or without associated renal insufficiency, ACE inhibitor therapy may cause excessive hypotension, which may be associated with oliguria or azotemia and, rarely, with acute renal failure and death. In such patients, ACCUPRIL therapy should be started at the recommended dose under close medical supervision. These patients should be followed closely for the first 2 weeks of treatment and whenever the dosage of antihypertensive medication is increased (see DOSAGE AND ADMINISTRATION).

If symptomatic hypotension occurs, the patient should be placed in the supine position and, if necessary, normal saline may be administered intravenously. A transient hypotensive response is not a contraindication to further doses; however, lower doses of ACCUPRIL or reduced concomitant diuretic therapy should be considered.

Neutropenia/Agranulocytosis: Another ACE inhibitor, captopril, has been shown to cause agranulocytosis and bone marrow depression rarely in patients with uncomplicated hypertension, but more frequently in patients with renal impairment, especially if they also have a collagen vascular disease, such as systemic lupus erythematosus or scleroderma. Agranulocytosis did occur during ACCUPRIL treatment in one patient with a history of neutropenia during previous captopril therapy. Available data from clinical trials of ACCUPRIL are insufficient to show that, in patients without prior reactions to other ACE inhibitors, ACCUPRIL does not cause agranulocytosis at similar rates. As with other ACE inhibitors, periodic monitoring of white blood cell counts in patients with collagen vascular disease and/or renal disease should be considered.

Fetal/Neonatal Morbidity and Mortality: ACE inhibitors can cause fetal and neonatal morbidity and death when administered to pregnant women. Several dozen cases have been reported in the world literature. When pregnancy is detected, ACE inhibitors should be discontinued as soon as possible.

The use of ACE inhibitors during the second and third trimesters of pregnancy has been associated with fetal and neonatal injury, including hypotension, neonatal skull hypoplasia, anuria, reversible or irreversible renal failure, and death. Oligohydramnios has also been reported, presumably resulting from decreased fetal renal function; oligohydramnios in this setting has been associated with fetal limb contractures, craniofacial deformation, and hypoplastic lung development. Prematurity, intrauterine growth retardation, and patent ductus arteriosis have also been reported, although it is not clear whether these occurrences were due to the ACE inhibitor exposure.

These adverse effects do not appear to have resulted from intrauterine ACE inhibitor exposure that has been limited to the first trimester. Mothers whose embryos and fetuses are exposed to ACE inhibitors only during the first trimester should be so informed. Nonetheless, when patients become pregnant, physicians should make every effort to discontinue the use of ACCUPRIL as soon as possible.

Rarely (probably less often than once in every thousand pregnancies), no alternative to ACE inhibitors will be found. In these rare cases, the mothers should be apprised of the potential hazards to their fetuses, and serial ultrasound examinations should be performed to assess the intraamniotic environment.

If oligohydramnios is observed, ACCUPRIL should be discontinued unless it is considered life-saving for the mother. Con-

traction stress testing (CST), a nonstress test (NST), or biophysical profiling (BPP) may be appropriate, depending upon the week of pregnancy. Patients and physicians should be aware, however, that oligohydramnios may not appear until after the fetus has sustained irreversible injury.

Infants with histories of *in utero* exposure to ACE inhibitors should be closely observed for hypotension, oliguria, and hyperkalemia. If oliguria occurs, attention should be directed toward support of blood pressure and renal perfusion. Exchange transfusion or dialysis may be required as a means of reversing hypotension and/or substituting for disordered renal function. Removal of ACCUPRIL, which crosses the placenta, from the neonatal circulation is not significantly accelerated by these means.

No teratogenic effects of ACCUPRIL were seen in studies of pregnant rats and rabbits. On a mg/kg basis, the doses used were up to 180 times (in rats) and one time (in rabbits) the maximum recommended human dose.

PRECAUTIONS

General

Impaired renal function: As a consequence of inhibiting the renin-angiotensin-aldosterone system, changes in renal function may be anticipated in susceptible individuals. In patients with severe heart failure whose renal function may depend on the activity of the renin-angiotensin-aldosterone system, treatment with ACE inhibitors, including ACCUPRIL, may be associated with oliguria and/or progressive azotemia and rarely acute renal failure and/or death.

In clinical studies in hypertensive patients with unilateral or bilateral renal artery stenosis, increases in blood urea nitrogen and serum creatinine have been observed in some patients following ACE inhibitor therapy. These increases were almost always reversible upon discontinuation of the ACE inhibitor and/or diuretic therapy. In such patients, renal function should be monitored during the first few weeks of therapy.

Some hypertensive patients with no apparent preexisting renal vascular disease have developed increases in blood urea and serum creatinine, usually minor and transient, especially when ACCUPRIL has been given concomitantly with a diuretic. This is more likely to occur in patients with preexisting renal impairment. Dosage reduction and/or discontinuation of any diuretic and/or ACCUPRIL may be required.

Evaluation of hypertensive patients should always include assessment of renal function (see DOSAGE AND ADMINISTRATION).

Hyperkalemia and potassium-sparing diuretics: In clinical trials, hyperkalemia (serum potassium ≥ 5.8 mmol/L) occurred in approximately 2% of patients receiving ACCUPRIL. In most cases, elevated serum potassium levels were isolated values which resolved despite continued therapy. Less than 0.1% of patients discontinued therapy due to hyperkalemia. Risk factors for the development of hyperkalemia include renal insufficiency, diabetes mellitus, and the concomitant use of potassium-sparing diuretics, potassium supplements, and/or potassium-containing salt substitutes, which should be used cautiously, if at all, with ACCUPRIL (see PRECAUTIONS, Drug Interactions).

Cough: Cough has been reported with the use of ACE inhibitors. Characteristically, the cough is nonproductive, persistent and resolves after discontinuation of therapy. ACE inhibitor-induced cough should be considered as part of the differential diagnosis of cough.

Surgery/anesthesia: In patients undergoing major surgery or during anesthesia with agents that produce hypotension, ACCUPRIL will block angiotensin II formation secondary to compensatory renin release. If hypotension occurs and is considered to be due to this mechanism, it can be corrected by volume expansion.

Information for Patients

Pregnancy: Female patients of childbearing age should be told about the consequences of second- and third-trimester exposure to ACE inhibitors, and they should also be told that these consequences do not appear to have resulted from intrauterine ACE-inhibitor exposure that has been limited to the first trimester. These patients should be asked to report pregnancies to their physicians as soon as possible.

Angioedema: Angioedema, including laryngeal edema can occur with treatment with ACE inhibitors, especially following the first dose. Patients should be so advised and told to report immediately any signs or symptoms suggesting angioedema (swelling of face, extremities, eyes, lips, tongue, difficulty in swallowing or breathing) and to stop taking the drug until they have consulted with their physician (see WARNINGS).

Symptomatic hypotension: Patients should be cautioned that lightheadedness can occur, especially during the first few days of ACCUPRIL therapy, and that it should be reported to a physician. If actual syncope occurs, patients should be told to not take the drug until they have consulted with their physician (see WARNINGS).

All patients should be cautioned that inadequate fluid intake or excessive perspiration, diarrhea, or vomiting can lead to an excessive fall in blood pressure because of reduction in

fluid volume, with the same consequences of lightheadedness and possible syncope.

Patients planning to undergo any surgery and/or anesthesia should be told to inform their physician that they are taking an ACE inhibitor.

Hyperkalemia: Patients should be told not to use potassium supplements or salt substitutes containing potassium without consulting their physician (see PRECAUTIONS).

Neutropenia: Patients should be told to report promptly any indication of infection (eg, sore throat, fever) which could be a sign of neutropenia.

NOTE: As with many other drugs, certain advice to patients being treated with ACCUPRIL is warranted. This information is intended to aid in the safe and effective use of this medication. It is not a disclosure of all possible adverse or intended effects.

Drug Interactions

Concomitant diuretic therapy: As with other ACE inhibitors, patients on diuretics, especially those on recently instituted diuretic therapy, may occasionally experience an excessive reduction of blood pressure after initiation of therapy with ACCUPRIL. The possibility of hypotensive effects with ACCUPRIL may be minimized by either discontinuing the diuretic or cautiously increasing salt intake prior to initiation of treatment with ACCUPRIL. If it is not possible to discontinue the diuretic, the starting dose of quinapril should be reduced (see DOSAGE AND ADMINISTRATION).

Agents increasing serum potassium: Quinapril can attenuate potassium loss caused by thiazide diuretics and increase serum potassium when used alone. If concomitant therapy of ACCUPRIL with potassium-sparing diuretics (e.g., spironolactone, triamterene, or amiloride), potassium supplements, or potassium-containing salt substitutes is indicated, they should be used with caution along with appropriate monitoring of serum potassium (see PRECAUTIONS).

Tetracycline and other drugs that interact with magnesium: Simultaneous administration of tetracycline with ACCUPRIL reduced the absorption of tetracycline by approximately 28% to 37%, possibly due to the high magnesium content in ACCUPRIL tablets. This interaction should be considered if coprescribing ACCUPRIL and tetracycline or other drugs that interact with magnesium.

Lithium: Increased serum lithium levels and symptoms of lithium toxicity have been reported in patients receiving concomitant lithium and ACE inhibitor therapy. These drugs should be coadministered with caution and frequent monitoring of serum lithium levels is recommended. If a diuretic is also used, it may increase the risk of lithium toxicity.

Other agents: Drug interaction studies of ACCUPRIL with other agents showed:

- Multiple dose therapy with propranolol or cimetidine has no effect on the pharmacokinetics of single doses of ACCUPRIL.
- The anticoagulant effect of a single dose of warfarin (measured by prothrombin time) was not significantly changed by quinapril coadministration twice-daily.
- ACCUPRIL treatment did not affect the pharmacokinetics of digoxin.
- No pharmacokinetic interaction was observed when single doses of ACCUPRIL and hydrochlorothiazide were administered concomitantly.

Carcinogenesis, Mutagenesis, Impairment of Fertility

Quinapril hydrochloride was not carcinogenic in mice or rats when given in doses up to 75 or 100 mg/kg/day (50 to 60 times the maximum human daily dose, respectively, on an mg/kg basis and 3.8 to 10 times the maximum human daily dose when based on an mg/m² basis) for 104 weeks. Female rats given the highest dose level had an increased incidence of mesenteric lymph node hemangiomas and skin/subcutaneous lipomas. Neither quinapril nor quinaprilat were mutagenic in the Ames bacterial assay with or without metabolic activation. Quinapril was also negative in the following genetic toxicology studies: *in vitro* mammalian cell point mutation, sister chromatid exchange in cultured mammalian cells, micronucleus test with mice, *in vitro* chromosome aberration with V79 cultured lung cells, and in an *in vivo* cytogenetic study with rat bone marrow. There were no adverse effects on fertility or reproduction in rats at doses up to 100 mg/kg/day (60 and 10 times the maximum daily human dose when based on mg/kg and mg/m², respectively).

Pregnancy

Pregnancy Category C (first trimester) and D (second and third trimesters): See WARNINGS, Fetal/Neonatal Morbidity and Mortality.

Nursing Mothers

It is not known if quinapril or its metabolites are secreted in human milk. Quinapril is secreted to a limited extent, however, in milk of lactating rats (5% or less of the plasma drug concentration was found in rat milk). Because many drugs are secreted in human milk, caution should be exercised when ACCUPRIL is given to a nursing mother.

Geriatric Use

Elderly patients exhibited increased area under the plasma concentration time curve (AUC) and peak levels for quinaprilat compared to values observed in younger patients; this

appeared to relate to decreased renal function rather than to age itself. In controlled and uncontrolled studies of ACCUPRIL where 918 (21%) patients were 65 years and older, no overall differences in effectiveness or safety were observed between older and younger patients. However, greater sensitivity of some older individual patients cannot be ruled out.

Pediatric Use

The safety and effectiveness of ACCUPRIL in children have not been established.

ADVERSE REACTIONS

ACCUPRIL has been evaluated for safety in 4960 subjects and patients. Of these, 3203 patients, including 655 elderly patients, participated in controlled clinical trials. ACCUPRIL has been evaluated for long-term safety in over 1400 patients treated for 1 year or more.

Adverse experiences were usually mild and transient.

Discontinuation of therapy because of adverse events was required in 4.7% of patients treated with ACCUPRIL in placebo-controlled hypertension trials.

Adverse experiences probably or possibly related to therapy or of unknown relationship to therapy occurring in 1% or more of the 1563 patients in placebo-controlled hypertension trials who were treated with ACCUPRIL are shown below.

Adverse Events in Placebo-Controlled Trials

	Accupril (N=1563) Incidence (Discontinuance)	Placebo (N=579) Incidence (Discontinuance)
Headache	5.6 (0.7)	10.9 (0.7)
Dizziness	3.9 (0.8)	2.6 (0.2)
Fatigue	2.6 (0.3)	1.0
Coughing	2.0 (0.5)	0.0
Nausea and/or Vomiting	1.4 (0.3)	1.9 (0.2)
Abdominal Pain	1.0 (0.2)	0.7

See PRECAUTIONS, Cough

Clinical adverse experiences probably or possibly related, or of uncertain relationship to therapy occurring in 0.5% to 1.0% (except as noted) of the patients treated with ACCUPRIL (with or without concomitant diuretic) in controlled or uncontrolled trials (N=4397) and less frequent, clinically significant events seen in clinical trials or post-marketing experience (the rarer events are in italics) include (listed by body system):

General: back pain, malaise

Cardiovascular: palpitation, vasodilation, tachycardia, *heart failure, hyperkalemia, myocardial infarction, cerebrovascular accident, hypertensive crisis, angina pectoris, orthostatic hypotension, cardiac rhythm disturbances*

Gastrointestinal: dry mouth or throat, constipation, *gastrointestinal hemorrhage, pancreatitis, abnormal liver function test*

Nervous/Psychiatric: somnolence, vertigo, syncope, nervousness, depression

Integumentary: increased sweating, pruritus, *exfoliative dermatitis, photosensitivity reaction*

Urogenital: *acute renal failure*

Other: amblyopia, pharyngitis, sinusitis, bronchitis, *agranulocytosis, thrombocytopenia*

Fetal/Neonatal Morbidity and Mortality

See WARNINGS, Fetal/Neonatal Morbidity and Mortality

Angioedema

Angioedema has been reported in patients receiving ACCUPRIL (0.1%). Angioedema associated with laryngeal edema may be fatal. If angioedema of the face, extremities, lips, tongue, glottis, and/or larynx occurs, treatment with ACCUPRIL should be discontinued and appropriate therapy instituted immediately. (See WARNINGS.)

Clinical Laboratory Test Findings

Hematology: (See WARNINGS)

Hyperkalemia: (See PRECAUTIONS)

Creatinine and Blood Urea Nitrogen: Increases (>1.25 times the upper limit of normal) in serum creatinine and blood urea nitrogen were observed in 2% and 2%, respectively, of patients treated with ACCUPRIL alone. Increases are more likely to occur in patients receiving concomitant diuretic therapy than in those on ACCUPRIL alone. These increases often remit on continued therapy.

OVERDOSAGE

No data are available with respect to overdosage in humans. Doses to 1440 to 4280 mg/kg of quinapril cause significant lethality in mice and rats.

The most likely clinical manifestation would be symptoms attributable to severe hypotension.

Laboratory determinations of serum levels of quinapril and its metabolites are not widely available, and such determinations have, in any event, no established role in the management of quinapril overdose.

No data are available to suggest physiological maneuvers (e.g., maneuvers to change pH of the urine) that might accelerate elimination of quinapril and its metabolites.

Hemodialysis and peritoneal dialysis have little effect on the elimination of quinapril and quinaprilat. Angiotensin II could presumably serve as a specific antagonist-antidote in the setting of quinapril overdose, but angiotensin II is essentially unavailable outside of scattered research facilities. Because the hypotensive effect of quinapril is achieved through vasodilation and effective hypovolemia, it is reasonable to treat quinapril overdose by infusion of normal saline solution.

DOSAGE AND ADMINISTRATION

Monotherapy: The recommended initial dosage of ACCUPRIL in patients not on diuretics is 10 mg once daily. Dosage should be adjusted according to blood pressure response measured at peak (2–6 hours after dosing) and trough (predosing). Generally, dosage adjustments should be made at intervals of at least 2 weeks. Most patients have required dosages of 20, 40, or 80 mg/day, given as a single dose or in 2 equally divided doses. In some patients treated once daily, the antihypertensive effect may diminish toward the end of the dosing interval. In such patients an increase in dosage or twice daily administration may be warranted. In general, doses of 40–80 mg and divided doses give a somewhat greater effect at the end of the dosing interval.

Concomitant Diuretics: If blood pressure is not adequately controlled with ACCUPRIL monotherapy, a diuretic may be added. In patients who are currently being treated with a diuretic, symptomatic hypotension occasionally can occur following the initial dose of ACCUPRIL. To reduce the likelihood of hypotension, the diuretic should, if possible, be discontinued 2 to 3 days prior to beginning therapy with ACCUPRIL (see WARNINGS). Then, if blood pressure is not controlled with ACCUPRIL alone, diuretic therapy should be resumed.

If the diuretic cannot be discontinued, an initial dose of 5 mg ACCUPRIL should be used with careful medical supervision for several hours and until blood pressure has stabilized.

The dosage should subsequently be titrated (as described above) to the optimal response (see WARNINGS, PRECAUTIONS, and Drug Interactions).

Renal Impairment: Kinetic data indicate that the apparent elimination half-life of quinaprilat increases as creatinine clearance decreases. Recommended starting doses, based on clinical and pharmacokinetic data from patients with renal impairment, are as follows:

Creatinine Clearance	Maximum Recommend Initial Dose
>60 mL/min	10 mg
30–60 mL/min	5 mg
10–30 mL/min	2.5 mg
<10 mL/min	Insufficient data for dosage recommendation

Patients should subsequently have their dosage titrated (as described above) to the optimal response.

Elderly (≥65 years): The recommended initial dosage of ACCUPRIL in elderly patients is 10 mg given once daily followed by titration (as described above) to the optimal response.

HOW SUPPLIED

ACCUPRIL tablets are supplied as follows:

5-mg tablets: brown, film-coated, elliptical, scored tablets, coded "PD 527" on one side and "5" on the other.

N0071-0527-23 bottles of 90 tablets

10-mg tablets: brown, film-coated, triangular, scored tablets, coded "PD 530" on one side and "10" on the other.

N0071-0530-23 bottles of 90 tablets

N0071-0530-40 10 × 10 unit dose blisters

20-mg tablets: brown, film-coated, round, scored tablets, coded "PD 532" on one side and "20" on the other.

N0071-0532-23 bottles of 90 tablets

N0071-0532-40 10 × 10 unit dose blisters

40-mg tablets: brown, film-coated, elliptical, scored tablets, coded "PD 535" on one side and "40" on the other.

N0071-0535-23 bottles of 90 tablets

N0071-0535-40 10 × 10 unit dose blisters

Dispense in well-closed containers as defined in the USP.

Storage: Store at controlled room temperature 15°–30°C (59°–86°F).

Caution—Federal law prohibits dispensing without prescription.

Revised November 1991 **0527G025**

Shown in Product Identification Section, page 422

ADRENALIN® CHLORIDE SOLUTION ℞

[ă-drĕn′ă-lĭn″ chlō′rīde]

(Epinephrine Injection, USP), 1:1000

DESCRIPTION

A sterile solution intended for subcutaneous or intramuscular injection. When diluted, it may also be administered intracardially or intravenously. Each milliliter contains 1 mg Adrenalin (epinephrine) as the hydrochloride dissolved in Water for Injection, USP, with sodium chloride added for isotonicity. The ampoules contain not more than 0.1% sodium bisulfite as an antioxidant, and the air in the ampoule has been displaced by nitrogen. The Steri-Vials® contain 0.5% Chloretone® (chlorobutanol) (chloroform derivative) as a preservative and not more than 0.15% sodium bisulfite as an antioxidant. Epinephrine is the active principle of the adrenal medulla, chemically described as (−)-3,4-Dihydroxy-α-[(methylamino) methyl] benzyl alcohol.

CLINICAL PHARMACOLOGY

Adrenalin (epinephrine) is a sympathomimetic drug. It activates an adrenergic receptive mechanism on effector cells and imitates all actions of the sympathetic nervous system except those on the arteries of the face and sweat glands. Epinephrine acts on both alpha and beta receptors and is the most potent alpha receptor activator.

INDICATIONS AND USAGE

In general, the most common uses of epinephrine are to relieve respiratory distress due to bronchospasm, to provide rapid relief of hypersensitivity reactions to drugs and other allergens, and to prolong the action of infiltration anesthetics. Its cardiac effects may be of use in restoring cardiac rhythm in cardiac arrest due to various causes, but it is not used in cardiac failure or in hemorrhagic, traumatic, or cardiogenic shock.

Epinephrine is used as a hemostatic agent. It is also used in treating mucosal congestion of hay fever, rhinitis, and acute sinusitis; to relieve bronchial asthmatic paroxysms; in syncope due to complete heart block or carotid sinus hypersensitivity; for symptomatic relief of serum sickness, urticaria, angioneurotic edema; for resuscitation in cardiac arrest following anesthetic accidents; in simple (open angle) glaucoma; for relaxation of uterine musculature and to inhibit uterine contractions. Epinephrine Injection can be utilized to prolong the action of intraspinal and local anesthetics (see Contraindications section).

CONTRAINDICATIONS

Epinephrine is contraindicated in narrow angle (congestive) glaucoma, shock, during general anesthesia with halogenated hydrocarbons or cyclopropane and in individuals with organic brain damage. Epinephrine is also contraindicated with local anesthesia of certain areas, eg, fingers, toes, because of the danger of vasoconstriction producing sloughing of tissue; in labor because it may delay the second stage; in cardiac dilatation and coronary insufficiency.

WARNINGS

Administer with caution to elderly people; to those with cardiovascular disease, hypertension, diabetes or hyperthyroidism; in psychoneurotic individuals, and in pregnancy.

Patients with long-standing bronchial asthma and emphysema who have developed degenerative heart disease should be administered the drug with extreme caution.

Overdosage or inadvertent intravenous injection of epinephrine may cause cerebrovascular hemorrhage resulting from the sharp rise in blood pressure.

Fatalities may also result from pulmonary edema because of the peripheral constriction and cardiac stimulation produced. Rapidly acting vasodilators such as nitrites, or alpha blocking agents may counteract the marked pressor effects of epinephrine.

Epinephrine is the preferred treatment for serious allergic or other emergency situations even though this product contains sodium bisulfite, a sulfite that may in other products cause allergic-type reactions including anaphylactic symptoms or life-threatening or less severe asthmatic episodes in certain susceptible persons. The alternatives to using epinephrine in a life-threatening situation may not be satisfactory. The presence of a sulfite in this product should not deter administration of the drug for treatment of serious allergic or other emergency situations.

PRECAUTIONS

General: Adrenalin (epinephrine injection) should be protected from exposure to light. Do not remove ampoules or vials from carton until ready to use. The solution should not

Continued on next page

This product information was prepared in August 1992. On these and other Parke-Davis Products, information may be obtained by addressing PARKE-DAVIS, Division of Warner-Lambert Company, Morris Plains, New Jersey 07950.

Parke-Davis—Cont.

be used if it is pinkish or darker than slightly yellow or if it contains a precipitate.
Epinephrine is readily destroyed by alkalies and oxidizing agents. In the latter category are oxygen, chlorine, bromine, iodine, permanganates, chromates, nitrites and salts of easily reducible metals, especially iron.
Drug Interactions: Use of epinephrine with excessive doses of digitalis, mercurial diuretics, or other drugs that sensitize the heart to arrhythmias is not recommended. Anginal pain may be induced when coronary insufficiency is present.
The effects of epinephrine may be potentiated by tricyclic antidepressants; certain antihistamines, eg, diphenhydramine, tripelennamine, d-chlorpheniramine; and sodium l-thyroxine.
Usage in Pregnancy: Pregnancy Category C. Adrenalin (epinephrine) has been shown to be teratogenic in rats when given in doses about 25 times the human dose. There are no adequate and well controlled studies in pregnant women. Adrenalin should be used during pregnancy only if the potential benefit justifies the potential risk to the fetus.

ADVERSE REACTIONS

Transient and minor side effects of anxiety, headache, fear and palpitations often occur with therapeutic doses, especially in hyperthyroid individuals. Repeated local injections can result in necrosis at sites of injection from vascular constriction. "Epinephrine-fastness" can occur with prolonged use.

DOSAGE AND ADMINISTRATION

Parenteral drug products should be inspected visually for particulate matter and discoloration whenever solution and container permit.
Subcutaneously or intramuscularly—0.2 to 1 ml (mg). Start with a small dose and increase if required.
Note: The subcutaneous is the preferred route of administration. If given intramuscularly, injection into the buttocks should be avoided.
For bronchial asthma and certain allergic manifestations, eg, angioedema, urticaria, serum sickness, anaphylactic shock, use epinephrine subcutaneously. For bronchial asthma in pediatric patients, administer 0.01 mg/kg or 0.3 mg/m^2 to a maximum of 0.5 mg subcutaneously, repeated every four hours if required.
For cardiac resuscitation—A dose of 0.5 ml (0.5 mg) diluted to 10 ml with sodium chloride injection can be administered intravenously or intracardially to restore myocardial contractility. External cardiac massage should follow intracardial administration to permit the drug to enter coronary circulation. The drug should be used secondarily to unsuccessful attempts with physical or electromechanical methods.
Ophthalmologic use (for producing conjunctival decongestion, to control hemorrhage, produce mydriasis and reduce intraocular pressure)—use a concentration of 1:10,000 (0.1 mg/ml) to 1:1,000 (1 mg/ml).
Intraspinal use (Amp 88)—Usual dose is 0.2 to 0.4 ml (0.2 to 0.4 mg) added to anesthetic spinal fluid mixture (may prolong anesthetic action by limiting absorption). For use with local anesthetic—Epinephrine 1:100,000 (0.01 mg /ml) to 1:20,000 (0.05 mg/ml) is the usual concentration employed with local anesthetics.

HOW SUPPLIED

N 0071-4188-03 (Amp 88) Sterile solution containing 1 mg Adrenalin (epinephrine) as the hydrochloride in each 1-ml ampoule (1:1000). For intramuscular or subcutaneous use. When diluted, it may also be administered intracardially, intravenously, or intraspinally. Supplied in packages of ten.
N 0071-4011-13 (S.V. 11) Sterile solution containing 1 mg Adrenalin (epinephrine) as the hydrochloride (1:1000). For intramuscular or subcutaneous use. When diluted, it may also be administered intracardially or intravenously. Supplied in a 30 ml Steri-Vial® (rubber-diaphragm-capped vial.)
Store between 59° and 77°F (15°-25°C). Protect from light and freezing.

4188G045

ANUSOL-HC® 2.5% ℞
(Hydrocortisone Cream, USP)

Caution—Federal law prohibits dispensing without prescription.

DESCRIPTION

The topical corticosteroids constitute a class of primarily synthetic steroids used as antiinflammatory and antipruritic agents. Anusol-HC 2.5% (Hydrocortisone Cream, USP) is a topical corticosteroid with hydrocortisone 2.5% (active ingredient) in a water-washable cream containing the following inactive ingredients: benzyl alcohol. petrolatum, stearyl alcohol, propylene glycol. isopropyl myristate, polyoxyl 40 stearate, carbomer 934, sodium lauryl sulfate, edetate disodium, sodium hydroxide to adjust the pH, and purified water.
Hydrocortisone has the chemical name Pregn-4-ene-3,20-dione, 11,17,21, trihydroxy-,(11β)- and the following chemical structure:

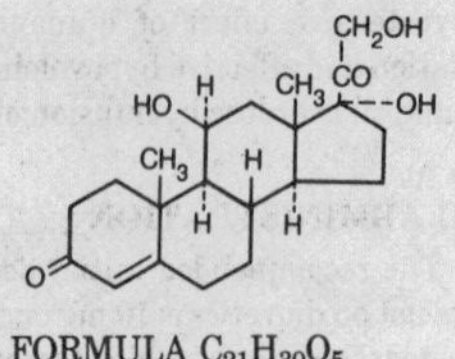

MOLECULAR FORMULA $C_{21}H_{30}O_5$
MOLECULAR WEIGHT 362.47
CAS REGISTRY NUMBER 50-23-7

CLINICAL PHARMACOLOGY

Topical corticosteroids share antiinflammatory, antipruritic and vasoconstrictive actions.
The mechanism of antiinflammatory activity of the topical corticosteroids is unclear. Various laboratory methods, including vasoconstrictor assays, are used to compare and predict potencies and/or clinical efficacies of the topical corticosteroids. There is some evidence to suggest that a recognizable correlation exists between vasoconstrictor potency and therapeutic efficacy in man.
Pharmacokinetics: The extent of percutaneous absorption of topical corticosteroids is determined by many factors including the vehicle, the integrity of the epidermal barrier, and the use of occlusive dressings.
Topical corticosteroids can be absorbed from normal intact skin. Inflammation and/or other disease processes in the skin increase percutaneous absorption. Occlusive dressings substantially increase the percutaneous absorption of topical corticosteroids. Thus, occlusive dressings may be a valuable therapeutic adjunct for treatment of resistant dermatoses (see DOSAGE AND ADMINISTRATION).
Once absorbed through the skin, topical corticosteroids are handled through pharmacokinetic pathways similar to systemically administered corticosteroids. Corticosteroids are bound to plasma proteins in varying degrees. Corticosteroids are metabolized primarily in the liver and are then excreted by the kidneys. Some of the topical corticosteroids and their metabolites are also excreted into the bile.

INDICATIONS AND USAGE

Topical corticosteroids are indicated for the relief of the inflammatory and pruritic manifestations of corticosteroid-responsive dermatoses.

CONTRAINDICATIONS

Topical corticosteroids are contraindicated in those patients with a history of hypersensitivity to any of the components of the preparation.

PRECAUTIONS

General: Systemic absorption of topical corticosteroids has produced reversible hypothalamic-pituitary-adrenal (HPA) axis suppression, manifestations of Cushing's syndrome, hyperglycemia, and glucosuria in some patients.
Conditions which augment systemic absorption include the application of the more potent steroids, use over large surface areas, prolonged use, and the addition of occlusive dressings.
If HPA axis suppression is noted (by using the urinary free cortisol and ACTH stimulation tests) an attempt should be made to withdraw the drug or to reduce the frequency of application.
Recovery of HPA axis function is generally prompt and complete upon discontinuation of the drug. Infrequently, signs and symptoms of steroid withdrawal may occur, requiring supplemental systemic corticosteroids.
Children may absorb proportionally larger amounts of topical corticosteroids and thus be more susceptible to systemic toxicity (see PRECAUTIONS—Pediatric Use).
If irritation develops, topical corticosteroids should be discontinued and appropriate therapy instituted. In the presence of dermatological infections, the use of an appropriate antifungal or antibacterial agent should be instituted. If a favorable response does not occur promptly, the corticosteroid should be discontinued until the infection has been adequately controlled.
Information for the Patient: Patients using topical corticosteroids should receive the following information and instructions:

1. This medication is to be used as directed by the physician. It is for external use only. Avoid contact with the eyes.
2. Patients should be advised not to use this medication for any disorder other than for which it has been prescribed.
3. The treated skin area should not be bandaged or otherwise covered or wrapped as to be occlusive unless directed by the physician.
4. Patients should report any signs of local adverse reactions especially under occlusive dressing.
5. Parents of pediatric patients should be advised not to use tight-fitting diapers or plastic pants on a child being treated in the diaper area, as these garments may constitute occlusive dressings.

Laboratory Tests: The urinary free cortisol test and the ACTH stimulation test may be helpful in evaluating the HPA axis suppression.
Carcinogenesis, Mutagenesis, and Impairment of Fertility: Long-term animal studies have not been performed to evaluate the carcinogenic potential or the effect on fertility of topical corticosteroids. Studies to determine mutagenicity with hydrocortisone have revealed negative results.
Pregnancy Category C: Corticosteroids are generally teratogenic in laboratory animals when administered systemically at relatively low dosage levels. The more potent corticosteroids have been shown to be teratogenic after dermal application in laboratory animals. There are no adequate and well-controlled studies in pregnant women on teratogenic effects from topically applied corticosteroids.
Therefore, topical corticosteroids should be used during pregnancy only if the potential benefit justifies the potential risk to the fetus. Drugs of this class should not be used extensively on pregnant patients, in large amounts, or for prolonged periods of time.
Nursing Mothers: It is not known whether topical administration of corticosteroids could result in sufficient systemic absorption to produce detectable quantities in breast milk. Systemically administered corticosteroids are secreted into breast milk in quantities not likely to have a deleterious effect on the infant. Nevertheless, caution should be exercised when topical corticosteroids are administered to a nursing woman.
Pediatric Use: PEDIATRIC PATIENTS MAY DEMONSTRATE GREATER SUSCEPTIBILITY TO TOPICAL CORTICOSTEROID-INDUCED HPA AXIS SUPPRESSION AND CUSHING'S SYNDROME THAN MATURE PATIENTS BECAUSE OF A LARGER SKIN SURFACE AREA TO BODY WEIGHT RATIO.
Hypothalamic-pituitary-adrenal (HPA) axis suppression, Cushing's syndrome, and intracranial hypertension have been reported in children receiving topical corticosteroids. Manifestations of adrenal suppression in children include linear growth retardation, delayed weight gain, low plasma cortisol levels, and absence of response to ACTH stimulation. Manifestations of intracranial hypertension include bulging fontanelles, headaches, and bilateral papilledema.
Administration of topical corticosteroids to children should be limited to the least amount compatible with an effective therapeutic regimen. Chronic corticosteroid therapy may interfere with the growth and development of children.

ADVERSE REACTIONS

The following local adverse reactions are reported infrequently with topical corticosteroids, but may occur more frequently with the use of occlusive dressings. These reactions are listed in an approximate decreasing order of occurrence:
Burning
Itching
Irritation
Dryness
Folliculitis
Hypertrichosis
Acneiform eruptions
Hypopigmentation
Perioral dermatitis
Allergic contact dermatitis
Maceration of the skin
Secondary infection
Skin atrophy
Striae
Miliaria

OVERDOSAGE

Topically applied corticosteroids can be absorbed in sufficient amounts to produce systemic effects. (See PRECAUTIONS).

DOSAGE AND ADMINISTRATION

Anusol-HC 25% (Hydrocortisone Cream, USP) should be applied to the affected area two to four times daily depending on the severity of the condition.
Occlusive dressings may be used for the management of psoriasis or recalcitrant conditions. If an infection develops, the use of occlusive dressings should be discontinued and appropriate antimicrobial therapy instituted.

HOW SUPPLIED

Anusol-HC 2.5% (Hydrocortisone Cream, USP) is supplied in 30 gram tubes (N 0071-3131-13).
Store at controlled room temperature 15°-30°C (59°-86°F).
Store away from heat. Protect from freezing.
Revised May 1991
Manufactured by
Herbert Laboratories
A Division of Allergan, Inc
Irvine, CA 92713 USA

Distributed by
PARKE-DAVIS
Div of Warner-Lambert Co　　　　　70221 30-6/S
Morris Plains, NJ 07950 USA　　　　　**3131G010**
Shown in Product Identification Section, page 422

ANUSOL–HC® 25–mg SUPPOSITORIES　　℞
[ăn 'ū-sŏl "]
(Hydrocortisone Acetate)

DESCRIPTION
Each Anusol-HC 25-mg Suppository contains 25 mg hydrocortisone acetate in a hydrogenated cocoglyceride base. Hydrocortisone acetate is a corticosteroid. Chemically, hydrocortisone acetate is pregn-4-ene-3,20-dione, 21-(acetyloxy)-11,17-dihydroxy-,(11β)-.

CLINICAL PHARMACOLOGY
In normal subjects, about 26 percent of hydrocortisone acetate is absorbed when the hydrocortisone acetate suppository is applied to the rectum. Absorption of hydrocortisone acetate may vary across abraded or inflamed surfaces. Topical steroids are primarily effective because of their antiinflammatory, antipruritic and vasoconstrictive action.

INDICATIONS AND USAGE
For use in inflamed hemorrhoids, post irradiation (factitial) proctitis, as an adjunct in the treatment of chronic ulcerative colitis, cryptitis, other inflammatory conditions of the anorectum, and pruritus ani.

CONTRAINDICATION
Anusol-HC suppositories are contraindicated in those patients with a history of hypersensitivity to any of the components.

PRECAUTIONS
Do not use unless adequate proctologic examination is made. If irritation develops, the product should be discontinued and appropriate therapy instituted.
In the presence of an infection, the use of an appropriate antifungal or antibacterial agent should be instituted. If a favorable response does not occur promptly, the corticosteroid should be discontinued until the infection has been adequately controlled.
No long-term studies in animals have been performed to evaluate the carcinogenic potential of corticosteroid suppositories.
Information for Patients
Staining of fabric may occur with use of the suppository. Precautionary measures are recommended.
Pregnancy Category C
In laboratory animals, topical steroids have been associated with an increase in the incidence of fetal abnormalities when gestating females have been exposed to rather low dosage levels. There are no adequate and well-controlled studies in pregnant women. Anusol-HC suppositories should only be used during pregnancy if the potential benefit justifies the risk to the fetus. Drugs of this class should not be used extensively on pregnant patients, in large amounts, or for prolonged periods of time.
It is not known whether this drug is excreted in human milk, and because many drugs are excreted in human milk and because of the potential for serious adverse reactions in nursing infants from Anusol-HC suppositories, a decision should be made whether to discontinue nursing or to discontinue the drug, taking into account the importance of the drug to the mother.

ADVERSE REACTIONS
The following local adverse reactions have been reported with corticosteroid suppositories:
1. Burning
2. Itching
3. Irritation
4. Dryness
5. Folliculitis
6. Hypopigmentation
7. Allergic Contact Dermatitis
8. Secondary infection

DRUG ABUSE AND DEPENDENCE
Drug abuse and dependence have not been reported in patients treated with Anusol-HC suppositories.

OVERDOSAGE
If signs and symptoms of systemic overdosage occur discontinue use.

DOSAGE AND ADMINISTRATION
Usual dosage: One suppository in the rectum morning and night for two weeks, in nonspecific proctitis. In more severe cases, one suppository three times daily; or two suppositories twice daily. In factitial proctitis, recommended therapy is six to eight weeks or less, according to response.

HOW SUPPLIED
Anusol-HC 25-mg Suppositories are off-white, smooth surfaced, rod shaped with one rounded end. Package of 12 suppositories (N-0071-1726-07) and package of 24 suppositories (N-0071-1726-13).
Store below 30° C (86° F). Protect from freezing.
Caution—Federal law prohibits dispensing without prescription.

1726G012
Shown in Product Identification Section, page 422

APLISOL®　　℞
[ă 'plĭ-sŏl "]
(tuberculin purified protein
derivative, diluted
[Stabilized Solution])

For complete product information, consult Diagnostic Product Information section.

APLITEST®　　℞
[ă 'plĭ-tĕst "]
(tuberculin purified protein
derivative)
Multiple-Puncture Device

For complete product information, consult Diagnostic Product Information section.

BENADRYL®　　℞
[bĕ 'nă-dril]
(Diphenhydramine Hydrochloride
Capsules, USP)

DESCRIPTION
Benadryl (diphenhydramine hydrochloride) is an antihistamine drug having the chemical name 2-(Diphenylmethoxy)-N, N-dimethylethylamine hydrochloride and has the empirical formula $C_{17}H_{21}NO \cdot HCl$ (molecular weight 291.82). It occurs as a white, crystalline powder and is freely soluble in water and alcohol.
Each Benadryl capsule contains 25 mg or 50 mg diphenhydramine hydrochloride for oral administration.
The 25-mg capsule also contains lactose, NF and magnesium stearate, NF. The capsule shell and/or band contains D&C red No. 28; FD&C blue No. 1; FD&C red No. 3; FD&C red No. 40; gelatin, NF; colloidal silicon dioxide, NF; and sodium lauryl sulfate, NF.
The 50-mg capsule also contains confectioner's sugar, NF and talc, USP. The capsule shell and/or band contains FD&C blue No. 1; FD&C red No. 3; gelatin, NF; glyceryl monooleate; colloidal silicon dioxide, NF; sodium lauryl sulfate, NF; and titanium dioxide, USP.

CLINICAL PHARMACOLOGY
Diphenhydramine hydrochloride is an antihistamine with anticholinergic (drying) and sedative effects. Antihistamines appear to compete with histamine for cell receptor sites on effector cells.
A single oral dose of diphenhydramine hydrochloride is quickly absorbed with maximum activity occurring in approximately one hour. The duration of activity following an average dose of Benadryl is from four to six hours. Diphenhydramine is widely distributed throughout the body, including the CNS. Little, if any, is excreted unchanged in the urine; most appears as the degradation products of metabolic transformation in the liver, which are almost completely excreted within 24 hours.

INDICATIONS AND USAGE
Benadryl in the oral form is effective for the following indications:
Antihistaminic: For allergic conjunctivitis due to foods; mild, uncomplicated allergic skin manifestations of urticaria and angioedema; amelioration of allergic reactions to blood or plasma; dermatographism; as therapy for anaphylactic reactions *adjunctive* to epinephrine and other standard measures after the acute manifestations have been controlled.
Motion sickness: For active and prophylactic treatment of motion sickness.
Antiparkinsonism: For parkinsonism (including drug-induced) in the elderly unable to tolerate more potent agents; mild cases of parkinsonism (including drug-induced) in other age groups; in other cases of parkinsonism (including drug-induced) in combination with centrally acting anticholinergic agents.

CONTRAINDICATIONS
Use in Newborn or Premature Infants
This drug should *not* be used in newborn or premature infants.
Use in Nursing Mothers
Because of the higher risk of antihistamines for infants generally, and for newborns and prematures in particular, antihistamine therapy is contraindicated in nursing mothers. Antihistamines are also contraindicated in the following conditions:
Hypersensitivity to diphenhydramine hydrochloride and other antihistamines of similar chemical structure.

WARNINGS
Antihistamines should be used with considerable caution in patients with narrow-angle glaucoma, stenosing peptic ulcer, pyloroduodenal obstruction, symptomatic prostatic hypertrophy, or bladder-neck obstruction.
Use in Children
In infants and children, especially, antihistamines in *overdosage* may cause hallucinations, convulsions, or death.
As in adults, antihistamines may diminish mental alertness in children. In the young child, particularly, they may produce excitation.
Use in the Elderly (approximately 60 years or older).
Antihistamines are more likely to cause dizziness, sedation, and hypotension in elderly patients.

PRECAUTIONS
General: Diphenhydramine hydrochloride has an atropine-like action and therefore should be used with caution in patients with a history of bronchial asthma, increased intraocular pressure, hyperthyroidism, cardiovascular disease or hypertension.
Information for Patients: Patients taking diphenhydramine hydrochloride should be advised that this drug may cause drowsiness and has an additive effect with alcohol. Patients should be warned about engaging in activities requiring mental alertness such as driving a car or operating appliances, machinery, etc.
Drug Interactions: Diphenhydramine hydrochloride has additive effects with alcohol and other CNS depressants (hypnotics, sedatives, tranquilizers, etc).
CAUTION—Patients taking monoamine oxidase inhibitors should not receive antihistamine therapy concurrently.
MAO inhibitors prolong and intensify the anticholinergic (drying) effects of antihistamines.
Carcinogenesis, Mutagenesis, Impairment of Fertility: Long-term studies in animals to determine mutagenic and carcinogenic potential have not been performed.
Pregnancy: Pregnancy Category B. Reproduction studies have been performed in rats and rabbits at doses up to 5 times the human dose and have revealed no evidence of impaired fertility or harm to the fetus due to diphenhydramine hydrochloride. There are, however, no adequate and well-controlled studies in pregnant women. Because animal reproduction studies are not always predictive of human response, this drug should be used during pregnancy only if clearly needed.

ADVERSE REACTIONS
The most frequent adverse reactions are underscored.
1. *General:* Urticaria, drug rash, anaphylactic shock, photosensitivity, excessive perspiration, chills, dryness of mouth, nose, and throat.
2. *Cardiovascular System:* Hypotension, headache, palpitations, tachycardia, extrasystoles.
3. *Hematologic System:* Hemolytic anemia, thrombocytopenia, agranulocytosis.
4. *Nervous System:* Sedation, sleepiness, dizziness, disturbed coordination, fatigue, confusion, restlessness, excitation, nervousness, tremor, irritability, insomnia, euphoria, paresthesia, blurred vision, diplopia, vertigo, tinnitus, acute labyrinthitis, neuritis, convulsions.
5. *GI System:* Epigastric distress, anorexia, nausea, vomiting, diarrhea, constipation.
6. *GU System:* Urinary frequency, difficult urination, urinary retention, early menses.
7. *Respiratory System:* Thickening of bronchial secretions, tightness of chest and wheezing, nasal stuffiness.

OVERDOSAGE
Antihistamine overdosage reactions may vary from central nervous system depression to stimulation. Stimulation is particularly likely in children. Atropine-like signs and symptoms, dry mouth; fixed, dilated pupils; flushing, and gastrointestinal symptoms may also occur.
If vomiting has not occurred spontaneously the patient should be induced to vomit. This is best done by having him drink a glass of water or milk after which he should be made to gag. Precautions against aspiration must be taken, especially in infants and children.
If vomiting is unsuccessful gastric lavage is indicated within 3 hours after ingestion and even later if large amounts of milk or cream were given beforehand. Isotonic or ½ isotonic saline is the lavage solution of choice.

Continued on next page

This product information was prepared in August 1992. On these and other Parke-Davis Products, information may be obtained by addressing PARKE-DAVIS, Division of Warner-Lambert Company, Morris Plains, New Jersey 07950.

Parke-Davis—Cont.

Saline cathartics, as milk of magnesia, by osmosis draw water into the bowel and therefore are valuable for their action in rapid dilution of food content.
Stimulants should not be used.
Vasopressors may be used to treat hypotension.

DOSAGE AND ADMINISTRATION
DOSAGE SHOULD BE INDIVIDUALIZED ACCORDING TO THE NEEDS AND THE RESPONSE OF THE PATIENT.
A single oral dose of diphenhydramine hydrochloride is quickly absorbed with maximum activity occurring in approximately one hour. The duration of activity following an average dose of Benadryl is from four to six hours.
ADULTS: 25 to 50 mg three or four times daily. The nighttime sleep-aid dosage is 50 mg at bedtime.
CHILDREN: (over 20 lb): 12.5 to 25 mg three to four times daily. Maximum daily dosage not to exceed 300 mg. For physicians who wish to calculate the dose on the basis of body weight or surface area, the recommended dosage is 5 mg/kg/24 hours or 150 mg/m²/24 hours.
Data are not available on the use of diphenhydramine hydrochloride as a nighttime sleep-aid in children under 12 years. The basis for determining the most effective dosage regimen will be the response of the patient to medication and the condition under treatment.
In motion sickness, full dosage is recommended for prophylactic use, the first dose to be given 30 minutes before exposure to motion and similar doses before meals and upon retiring for the duration of exposure.

HOW SUPPLIED
Benadryl 50 mg (P-D 373)—each banded capsule (Kapseals®) contains 50 mg diphenhydramine hydrochloride. Available as a pink capsule with white band in bottles of 100 (N 0071-0373-24), 1000 (N 0071-0373-32), and unit dose 100 (N 0071-0373-40).
Benadryl 25 mg (P-D 471)—each capsule contains 25 mg diphenhydramine hydrochloride. Available as a pink/white capsule in bottles of 100 (N 0071-0471-24), 1000 (N 0071-0471-32), and unit dose 100 (N 0071-0471-40).
Storage Conditions:
Store at controlled room temperature 15°–30°C (59°–86°F).
Protect from moisture.
Caution—Federal law prohibits dispensing without prescription.
Shown in Product Identification Section, page 422
0373G215

BENADRYL®
[*bĕ″nă-dril*]
(Diphenhydramine Hydrochloride Injection, USP)

℞

DESCRIPTION
Benadryl (diphenhydramine hydrochloride) is an antihistamine drug having the chemical name 2-(Diphenylmethoxy)-N,N-dimethylethylamine hydrochloride. It occurs as a white crystalline powder, is freely soluble in water and alcohol and has a molecular weight of 291.82. The molecular formula is $C_{17}H_{21}NO \cdot HCl$.
Benadryl in the parenteral form is a sterile, pyrogen-free solution available in two concentrations: 10 mg and 50 mg of diphenhydramine hydrochloride per mL. The solutions for parenteral use have been adjusted to a pH between 5.0 and 6.0 with either sodium hydroxide or hydrochloric acid. The multidose Steri-Vials® contain 0.1 mg/mL benzethonium chloride as a germicidal agent.

CLINICAL PHARMACOLOGY
Diphenhydramine hydrochloride is an antihistamine with anticholinergic (drying) and sedative side effects. Antihistamines appear to compete with histamine for cell receptor sites on effector cells.
Benadryl in the injectable form has a rapid onset of action. Diphenhydramine hydrochloride is widely distributed throughout the body, including the CNS. A portion of the drug is excreted unchanged in the urine, while the rest is metabolized via the liver. Detailed information on the pharmacokinetics of Diphenhydramine Hydrochloride Injection is not available.

INDICATIONS AND USAGE
Benadryl in the injectable form is effective for the following conditions when Benadryl in the oral form is impractical.
Antihistaminic: For amelioration of allergic reactions to blood or plasma, in anaphylaxis as an adjunct to epinephrine and other standard measures after the acute symptoms have been controlled, and for other uncomplicated allergic conditions of the immediate type when oral therapy is impossible or contraindicated.
Motion Sickness: For active treatment of motion sickness.
Antiparkinsonism: For use in parkinsonism, when oral therapy is impossible or contraindicated, as follows: parkin-

sonism in the elderly who are unable to tolerate more potent agents, mild cases of parkinsonism in other age groups, and in other cases of parkinsonism in combination with centrally acting anticholinergic agents.

CONTRAINDICATIONS
Use in Newborn or Premature Infants
This drug should *not* be used in newborn or premature infants.
Use in Nursing Mothers
Because of the higher risk of antihistamines for infants generally, and for newborns and prematures in particular, antihistamine therapy is contraindicated in nursing mothers.
Use as a Local Anesthetic
Because of the risk of local necrosis, this drug should not be used as a local anesthesia.
Antihistamines are also contraindicated in the following conditions:
Hypersensitivity to diphenhydramine hydrochloride and other antihistamines of similar chemical structure.

WARNINGS
Antihistamines should be used with considerable caution in patients with narrow-angle glaucoma, stenosing peptic ulcer, pyloroduodenal obstruction, symptomatic prostatic hypertrophy, or bladder-neck obstruction.
Use in Children
In infants and children, especially, antihistamines in *overdosage* may cause hallucinations, convulsions, or death.
As in adults, antihistamines may diminish mental alertness in children. In the young child, particularly, they may produce excitation.
Use in the Elderly (approximately 60 years or older)
Antihistamines are more likely to cause dizziness, sedation, and hypotension in elderly patients.

PRECAUTIONS
General: Diphenhydramine hydrochloride has an atropine-like action and therefore should be used with caution in patients with a history of bronchial asthma, increased intraocular pressure, hyperthyroidism, cardiovascular disease or hypertension. Use with caution in patients with lower respiratory disease, including asthma.
Information for Patients: Patients taking diphenhydramine hydrochloride should be advised that this drug may cause drowsiness and has an additive effect with alcohol. Patients should be warned about engaging in activities requiring mental alertness such as driving a car or operating appliances, machinery, etc.
Drug Interactions: Diphenhydramine hydrochloride has additive effects with alcohol and other CNS depressants (hypnotics, sedatives, tranquilizers, etc.).
MAO inhibitors prolong and intensify the anticholinergic (drying) effects of antihistamines.
Carcinogenesis, Mutagenesis, Impairment of Fertility: Long-term studies in animals to determine mutagenic and carcinogenic potential have not been performed.
Pregnancy: Pregnancy Category B. Reproduction studies have been performed in rats and rabbits at doses up to 5 times the human dose and have revealed no evidence of impaired fertility or harm to the fetus due to diphenhydramine hydrochloride. There are, however, no adequate and well-controlled studies in pregnant women. Because animal reproduction studies are not always predictive of human response, this drug should be used during pregnancy only if clearly needed.

ADVERSE REACTIONS
The most frequent adverse reactions are underscored.
1. *General:* Urticaria, drug rash, anaphylactic shock, photosensitivity, excessive perspiration, chills, dryness of mouth, nose, and throat
2. *Cardiovascular System:* Hypotension, headache, palpitations, tachycardia, extrasystoles
3. *Hematologic System:* Hemolytic anemia, thrombocytopenia, agranulocytosis
4. *Nervous System:* Sedation, <u>sleepiness</u>, <u>dizziness</u>, <u>disturbed coordination</u>, fatigue, confusion, restlessness, excitation, nervousness, tremor, irritability, insomnia, euphoria, paresthesia, blurred vision, diplopia, vertigo, tinnitus, acute labyrinthitis, neuritis, convulsions
5. *GI System:* <u>Epigastric distress</u>, anorexia, nausea, vomiting, diarrhea, constipation
6. *GU System:* Urinary frequency, difficult urination, urinary retention, early menses
7. *Respiratory System:* <u>Thickening of bronchial secretions</u>, tightness of chest and wheezing, nasal stuffiness

OVERDOSAGE
Antihistamine overdosage reactions may vary from central nervous system depression to stimulation. Stimulation is particularly likely in children. Atropine-like signs and symptoms, dry mouth; fixed, dilated pupils; flushing, and gastrointestinal symptoms may also occur.

Stimulants should not be used.
Vasopressors may be used to treat hypotension.

DOSAGE AND ADMINISTRATION
Benadryl in the injectable form is indicated when the oral form is impractical.
Parenteral drug products should be inspected visually for particulate matter and discoloration prior to administration, whenever solution and container permit.
DOSAGE SHOULD BE INDIVIDUALIZED ACCORDING TO THE NEEDS AND THE RESPONSE OF THE PATIENT.
Children: 5 mg/kg/24 hr or 150 mg/m²/24 hr. Maximum daily dosage is 300 mg. Divide into four doses, administered intravenously or deeply intramuscularly.
Adults: 10 to 50 mg intravenously or deeply intramuscularly; 100 mg if required; maximum daily dosage is 400 mg.

HOW SUPPLIED
Benadryl in parenteral form is supplied as:
Benadryl Steri-Vials®—sterile, pyrogen-free solution containing 10 mg diphenhydramine hydrochloride in each milliliter of solution with 0.1 mg/mL benzethonium chloride as a germicidal agent. Available in 10-mL (N 0071-4015-10) and 30-mL (N 0071-4015-13) Steri-Vials (rubber-diaphragm-capped vials).
Sterile, pyrogen-free solution containing 50 mg diphenhydramine hydrochloride in each milliliter of solution with 0.1 mg/mL benzethonium chloride as a germicidal agent. Available in 10-mL (N-0071-4402-10) Steri-Vials.
Benadryl Steri-Dose®—sterile, pyrogen-free solution containing 50 mg diphenhydramine hydrochloride in a 1-mL disposable syringe (Steri-Dose). Available in packages of ten individually cartoned syringes (N 0071-4259-40) and in packages of two trays of 5 syringes (N 0071-4259-41).
Benadryl Ampoule—sterile, pyrogen-free solution containing 50 mg diphenhydramine hydrochloride in a 1-mL ampoule. Available in packages of ten (N 0071-4259-03).

STORAGE CONDITIONS
Store at controlled room temperature 15°–30°C (59°–86°F). Protect from freezing and light.
Caution—Federal law prohibits dispensing without prescription.
4259G016

CELONTIN® KAPSEALS®
[*cĕ″lŏn′tĭn*]
(methsuximide capsules, USP)

℞

DESCRIPTION
Celontin (methsuximide) is an anticonvulsant succinimide, chemically designated as N,2-Dimethyl-2-phenylsuccinimide.
Each Celontin capsule contains 150 mg or 300 mg methsuximide, USP. Also contains starch, NF. The capsule and band contain citric acid, USP; colloidal silicon dioxide, NF; D&C yellow No. 10; FD&C red No. 3; FD&C yellow No. 6 (Sunset Yellow); gelatin, NF; glyceryl monooleate; sodium benzoate, NF; sodium lauryl sulfate NF. The 150-mg capsule and band also contain FD&C blue No. 1; titanium dioxide, USP. The 300-mg capsule and band also contain polyethylene glycol 200.

ACTION
Methsuximide suppresses the paroxysmal three-cycle-per-second spike and wave activity associated with lapses of consciousness which is common in absence (petit mal) seizures. The frequency of epileptiform attacks is reduced, apparently by depression of the motor cortex and elevation of the threshold of the central nervous system to convulsive stimuli.

INDICATION
Celontin is indicated for the control of absence (petit mal) seizures that are refractory to other drugs.

CONTRAINDICATION
Methsuximide should not be used in patients with a history of hypersensitivity to succinimides.

WARNINGS
Blood dyscrasias, including some with fatal outcome, have been reported to be associated with the use of succinimides; therefore, periodic blood counts should be performed. Should signs and/or symptoms of infection (eg sore throat, fever) develop, blood counts should be considered at that point.
It has been reported that succinimides have produced morphological and functional changes in animal liver. For this reason, methsuximide should be administered with extreme caution to patients with known liver or renal disease. Periodic urinalysis and liver function studies are advised for all patients receiving the drug.
Cases of systemic lupus erythematosus have been reported with the use of succinimides. The physician should be alert to this possibility.

USAGE IN PREGNANCY

The effects of Celontin in human pregnancy and nursing infants are unknown.

Recent reports suggest an association between the use of anticonvulsant drugs by women with epilepsy and an elevated incidence of birth defects in children born to these women. Data are more extensive with respect to phenytoin and phenobarbital, but these are also the most commonly prescribed anticonvulsants; less systematic or anecdotal reports suggest a possible similar association with the use of all known anticonvulsant drugs.

The reports suggesting an elevated incidence of birth defects in children of drug-treated epileptic women cannot be regarded as adequate to prove a definite cause-and-effect relationship. There are intrinsic methodologic problems in obtaining adequate data on drug teratogenicity in humans; the possibility also exists that other factors, eg, genetic factors or the epileptic condition itself, may be more important than drug therapy in leading to birth defects. The great majority of mothers on anticonvulsant medication deliver normal infants. It is important to note that anticonvulsant drugs should not be discontinued in patients in whom the drug is administered to prevent major seizures because of the strong possibility of precipitating status epilepticus with attendant hypoxia and threat to life. In individual cases where the severity and frequency of the seizure disorder are such that the removal of medication does not pose a serious threat to the patient, discontinuation of the drug may be considered prior to and during pregnancy, although it cannot be said with any confidence that even minor seizures do not pose some hazard to the developing embryo or fetus.

The prescribing physician will wish to weigh these considerations in treating or counseling epileptic women of childbearing potential.

Hazardous Activities: Methsuximide may impair the mental and/or physical abilities required for the performance of potentially hazardous tasks, such as driving a motor vehicle or other such activity requiring alertness; therefore, the patient should be cautioned accordingly.

PRECAUTIONS

General:
It is recommended that the physician withdraw the drug slowly on the appearance of unusual depression, aggressiveness, or other behavioral alterations.

As with other anticonvulsants, it is important to proceed slowly when increasing or decreasing dosage, as well as when adding or eliminating other medication. Abrupt withdrawal of anticonvulsant medication may precipitate absence (petit mal) status.

Methsuximide, when used alone in mixed types of epilepsy, may increase the frequency of grand mal seizures in some patients.

Information for Patients:
Methsuximide may impair the mental and/or physical abilities required for the performance of potentially hazardous tasks, such as driving a motor vehicle or other such activity requiring alertness, therefore, the patient should be cautioned accordingly.

Patients taking methsuximide should be advised of the importance of adhering strictly to the prescribed dosage regimen.

Patients should be instructed to promptly contact their physician if they develop signs and/or symptoms suggesting an infection (eg sore throat, fever).

ADVICE TO THE PHARMACIST AND PATIENT: Since methsuximide has a relatively low melting temperature (124°F), storage conditions which may promote high temperatures (closed cars, delivery vans, or storage near steam pipes) should be avoided. Do not dispense or use capsules that are not full or in which contents have melted. Effectiveness may be reduced. Protect from excessive heat (104°F).

Drug Interactions:
Since Celontin (methsuximide) may interact with concurrently administered antiepileptic drugs, periodic serum level determinations of these drugs may be necessary (eg methsuximide may increase the plasma concentrations of phenytoin and phenobarbital).

Pregnancy:
See WARNINGS.

ADVERSE REACTIONS

Gastrointestinal System: Gastrointestinal symptoms occur frequently and have included nausea or vomiting, anorexia, diarrhea, weight loss, epigastric and abdominal pain, and constipation.

Hemopoietic System: Hemopoietic complications associated with the administration of methsuximide have included eosinophilia, leukopenia, monocytosis, and pancytopenia.

Nervous System: Neurologic and sensory reactions reported during therapy with methsuximide have included drowsiness, ataxia or dizziness, irritability and nervousness, headache, blurred vision, photophobia, hiccups, and insomnia. Drowsiness, ataxia, and dizziness have been the most frequent side effects noted. Psychologic abnormalities have included confusion, instability, mental slowness, depression,

hypochondriacal behavior, and aggressiveness. There have been rare reports of psychosis, suicidal behavior, and auditory hallucinations.

Integumentary System: Dermatologic manifestations which have occurred with the administration of methsuximide have included urticaria, Stevens-Johnson syndrome, and pruritic erythematous rashes.

Cardiovascular: Hyperemia.

Genitourinary system: Proteinuria, microscopic hematuria

Body as a Whole: Periorbital edema.

OVERDOSAGE

Acute overdoses may produce nausea, vomiting, and CNS depression including coma with respiratory depression. Methsuximide poisoning may follow a biphasic course. Following an initial comatose state, patients have awakened and then relapsed into a coma within 24 hours. It is believed that an active metabolite of methsuximide, N-desmethylmethsuximide, is responsible for this biphasic profile. It is important to follow plasma levels of N-desmethylmethsuximide in methsuximide poisonings. Levels greater than 40 μg/mL have caused toxicity and coma has been seen at levels of 150 μg/mL.

Treatment:
Treatment should include emesis (unless the patient is or could rapidly become obtunded, comatose, or convulsing) or gastric lavage, activated charcoal, cathartics and general supportive measures. Charcoal hemoperfusion may be useful in removing the N-desmethyl metabolite of methsuximide. Forced diuresis and exchange transfusions are ineffective.

DOSAGE AND ADMINISTRATION

Optimum dosage of Celontin must be determined by trial. A suggested dosage schedule is 300 mg per day for the first week. If required, dosage may be increased thereafter at weekly intervals by 300 mg per day for the three weeks following to a daily dosage of 1.2 g. Because therapeutic effect and tolerance vary among patients, therapy with Celontin must be individualized according to the response of each patient. Optimal dosage is that amount of Celontin which is barely sufficient to control seizures so that side effects may be kept to a minimum. The smaller capsule (150 mg) facilitates administration to small children.

Celontin may be administered in combination with other anticonvulsants when other forms of epilepsy coexist with absence (petit mal.)

HOW SUPPLIED

N 0071-0525-24 (P-D 525)—Celontin Kapseals, #1 capsule each containing 300 mg methsuximide; bottles of 100.
N 0071-0537-24 (P-D 537)—Celontin Kapseals, Half Strength, #4 capsule each containing 150 mg methsuximide, bottles of 100.
Store at controlled room temperature 15°–30°C (59°–86°F). Protect from light and moisture.

0537G016

Shown in Product Identification Section, page 422

CENTRAX®   Ⓒ ℞
[cĕn 'trăx]
(prazepam capsules, USP)

DESCRIPTION

Centrax (prazepam) is a benzodiazepine derivative. Chemically, prazepam is 7-chloro-1-(cyclopropylmethyl)-1,3-dihydro-5-phenyl-2H-1,4-benzodiazepin-2-one, and has a molecular weight of 324.8.

Each Centrax capsule contains 5 mg, 10 mg, or 20 mg prazepam, USP. Also contains lactose, NF; magnesium stearate, NF; sodium lauryl sulfate, NF. The capsule contains colloidal silicon dioxide, NF; gelatin, NF; sodium lauryl sulfate, NF; titanium dioxide, USP. The Centrax 5-mg capsule also contains D&C yellow No. 10; FD&C blue No.1; FD&C yellow No. 6 (sunset yellow). The Centrax 10-mg capsule also contains FD&C blue No. 1; FD&C green No. 3. The Centrax 20-mg capsule also contains D&C yellow No. 10; FD&C yellow No. 6 (sunset yellow).

CLINICAL PHARMACOLOGY

Studies in normal subjects have shown that Centrax (prazepam) has depressant effects on the central nervous system. Oral administration of single doses as high as 60 mg and of divided doses up to 100 mg three times a day (300 mg total daily dosage) were without toxic effects.

Single, oral doses of Centrax (prazepam) in normal subjects produced average peak blood levels of the major metabolite norprazepam at 6 hours postadministration, with significant amounts still present after 48 hours. Prazepam was slowly absorbed over a prolonged period; rather constant blood levels were maintained on multiple-dose schedules; and excretion was prolonged. The mean half-life of norprazepam measured in subjects given 10 mg prazepam three times a day for one week was 63 (± 15 SD) hours before and 70 (± 10 SD) hours after multiple dosing—a nonsignificant difference.

Human metabolism studies showed that prior to elimination from the body, prazepam is metabolized in large part to 3-hydroxyprazepam and oxazepam.

INDICATIONS

Centrax is indicated for the management of anxiety disorders or for the short-term relief of the symptoms of anxiety. Anxiety or tension associated with the stress of everyday life usually does not require treatment with an anxiolytic.

The effectiveness of Centrax in long-term use, that is, more than 4 months, has not been assessed by systematic clinical studies. The physician should periodically reassess the usefulness of the drug for the individual patient.

CONTRAINDICATIONS

Centrax (prazepam) is contraindicated in patients with a known hypersensitivity to the drug and in those with acute narrow-angle glaucoma.

WARNINGS

Centrax (prazepam) is not recommended in psychotic states and in those psychiatric disorders in which anxiety is not a prominent feature.

Patients taking Centrax should be cautioned against engaging in hazardous occupations requiring mental alertness, such as operating dangerous machinery including motor vehicles.

Since Centrax has a central nervous system depressant effect, patients should be advised against the simultaneous ingestion of alcohol and other CNS-depressant drugs during Centrax therapy.

Physical and Psychological Dependence: Withdrawal symptoms, similar in character to those noted with barbiturates and alcohol (convulsions, tremor, abdominal and muscle cramps, vomiting and sweating), have occurred following abrupt discontinuance of benzodiazepines. The more severe withdrawal symptoms have usually been limited to those patients who received excessive doses over an extended period of time. Generally milder withdrawal symptoms (e.g., dysphoria and insomnia) have been reported following abrupt discontinuance of benzodiazepines taken continuously at therapeutic levels for several months. Consequently, after extended therapy, abrupt discontinuation should generally be avoided and a gradual dosage tapering schedule followed. Addiction-prone individuals (such as drug addicts or alcoholics) should be under careful surveillance when receiving prazepam or other psychotropic agents because of the predisposition of such patients to habituation and dependence.

PRECAUTIONS

Information for Patients:
To assure the safe and effective use of benzodiazepines, patients should be informed that since benzodiazepines may produce psychological and physical dependence, it is advisable that they consult with their physician before either increasing the dose or abruptly discontinuing this drug. Patients should also be advised to inform their physician if they are nursing, pregnant, planning to become pregnant or become pregnant while on this medication and about any alcohol consumption or medication they are taking. In addition, as with all CNS-acting agents, patients should be cautioned against driving or engaging in hazardous activities requiring mental alertness until they experience how this medication affects them.

Usage in Pregnancy and Lactation: An increased risk of congenital malformations associated with the use of minor tranquilizers (chlordiazepoxide, diazepam, and meprobamate) during the first trimester of pregnancy has been suggested in several studies. Prazepam, a benzodiazepine derivative, has not been studied adequately to determine whether it, too, may be associated with an increased risk of fetal abnormality. Because use of these drugs is rarely a matter of urgency, their use during this period should almost always be avoided. The possibility that a woman of childbearing potential may be pregnant at the time of institution of therapy should be considered. Patients should be advised that if they become pregnant during therapy or intend to become pregnant, they should communicate with their physicians about the desirability of discontinuing the drug. In view of their molecular size, prazepam and its metabolites are probably excreted in human milk. Therefore, this drug should not be given to nursing mothers.

In those patients in whom a degree of depression accompanies the anxiety, suicidal tendencies may be present and protective measures may be required. The least amount of drug that is feasible should be available to the patient at any one time.

Continued on next page

This product information was prepared in August 1992. On these and other Parke-Davis Products, information may be obtained by addressing PARKE-DAVIS, Division of Warner-Lambert Company, Morris Plains, New Jersey 07950.

Parke-Davis—Cont.

Patients taking Centrax (prazepam) for prolonged periods should have blood counts and liver function tests periodically. The usual precautions in treating patients with impaired renal or hepatic functions should also be observed. Hepatomegaly and cholestasis were observed in chronic toxicity studies in rats and dogs.
In elderly or debilitated patients, the initial dose should be small, and increments should be made gradually, in accordance with the response of the patient, to preclude ataxia or excessive sedation.
If Centrax is to be combined with other psychotropic agents or anticonvulsant drugs, careful consideration should be given to the pharmacology of the agents to be employed—particularly with known compounds which may potentiate the action of Centrax, such as phenothiazines, narcotics, barbiturates, MAO inhibitors and other antidepressants.
Pediatric Use: Safety and effectiveness in patients below the age of 18 have not been established.

ADVERSE REACTIONS

The side effects most frequently reported during double-blind, placebo-controlled trials employing a typical 30-mg divided total daily dosage and the percent incidence in the prazepam group were fatigue (11.6%), dizziness (8.7%), weakness (7.7%), drowsiness (6.8%), lightheadedness (6.8%), and ataxia (5.0%). Less frequently reported were headache, confusion, tremor, vivid dreams, slurred speech, palpitation, stimulation, dry mouth, diaphoresis, and various gastrointestinal complaints. Other side effects included pruritus, transient skin rashes, swelling of feet, joint pains, various genitourinary complaints, blurred vision, and syncope. Single, nightly dose, controlled trials of variable dosages showed a dose-related incidence of these same side effects. Transient and reversible aberrations of liver function tests have been reported, as have been slight decreases in blood pressure and increases in body weight.
These findings are characteristic of benzodiazepine drugs.

OVERDOSAGE

As in the management of overdosage with any drug, it should be borne in mind that multiple agents may have been taken. Vomiting should be induced if it has not occurred spontaneously. Immediate gastric lavage is also recommended. General supportive care, including frequent monitoring of vital signs and close observation of the patient, is indicated. Hypotension, though unlikely, may be controlled with Levophed® (levarterenol bitartrate), or Aramine® (metaraminol bitartrate).

DOSAGE AND ADMINISTRATION

Centrax (prazepam) is administered orally in divided doses. The usual daily dose is 30 mg. The dose should be adjusted gradually within the range of 20 mg to 60 mg daily in accordance with the response of the patient. In elderly or debilitated patients it is advisable to initiate treatment at a divided daily dose of 10 mg to 15 mg (see Precautions).
Centrax may also be administered as a single, daily dose at bedtime. The recommended starting nightly dose is 20 mg. The response of the patient to several days' treatment will permit the physician to adjust the dose upwards or, occasionally, downwards to maximize antianxiety effect with a minimum of daytime drowsiness. The optimum dosage will usually range from 20 mg to 40 mg.

DRUG INTERACTIONS

If Centrax (prazepam) is to be combined with other drugs acting on the central nervous system, careful consideration should be given to the pharmacology of the agents to be employed. The actions of the benzodiazepines may be potentiated by barbiturates, narcotics, phenothiazines, monoamine oxidase inhibitors, or other antidepressants.
If Centrax (prazepam) is used to treat anxiety associated with somatic disease states, careful attention must be paid to possible drug interaction with concomitant medication.

HOW SUPPLIED

Centrax 5 mg—Each capsule contains 5 mg prazepam. Available in bottles of 100 (N 0710-0552-24), and 500 (N 0710-0552-30). Centrax 10 mg—Each capsule contains 10 mg prazepam. Available in bottles of 100 (N 0710-0553-24), and 500 (N 0710-0553-30). Centrax 20 mg—Each capsule contains 20 mg prazepam. Available in bottles of 100 (N 0710-0554-24).

0552G127

Shown in Product Identification Section, page 422

CHLOROMYCETIN® CREAM, 1% ℞

[*chlō"rō-my-cē'tĭn*]
(chloramphenicol cream, USP) 1%

DESCRIPTION

Each gram of Chloromycetin Cream, 1%, contains 10 mg chloramphenicol with 0.1% propylparaben in a water-miscible ointment base of liquid petrolatum, cetyl alcohol, sodium lauryl sulfate, sodium phosphate buffer, and water.

CLINICAL PHARMACOLOGY

Chloramphenicol is a broad-spectrum antibiotic originally isolated from *Streptomyces venezuelae.* It is primarily bacteriostatic and acts by inhibition of protein synthesis by interfering with the transfer of activated amino acids from soluble RNA to ribosomes. Development of resistance to chloramphenicol can be regarded as minimal for staphylococci and many other species of bacteria.

INDICATIONS AND USAGE

Chloromycetin (chloramphenicol) Cream, 1%, is indicated for the treatment of surface skin infections caused by bacteria susceptible to chloramphenicol. Deeper cutaneous infections should be treated with appropriate systemic antibiotics.

CONTRAINDICATION

This product is contraindicated in persons sensitive to any of its components.

WARNINGS

Bone marrow hypoplasia, including aplastic anemia and death, has been reported following the local application of chloramphenicol.

PRECAUTIONS

The prolonged use of antibiotics may occasionally result in overgrowth of nonsusceptible organisms, including fungi. If new infections appear during medication, the drug should be discontinued and appropriate measures should be taken.
In all except very superficial infections, the topical use of chloramphenicol should be supplemented by appropriate systemic medication.
Not for ophthalmic use.

ADVERSE REACTIONS

Signs of local irritation with subjective symptoms of itching or burning, angioneurotic edema, urticaria, vesicular and maculopapular dermatitis have been reported in patients sensitive to chloramphenicol and are causes for discontinuing the medication. Similar sensitivity reactions to other materials in topical preparations may also occur. Blood dyscrasias have been reported in association with the use of chloramphenicol (See WARNINGS).

DOSAGE AND ADMINISTRATION

Apply to the infected area three or four times daily after cleansing.

HOW SUPPLIED

N 0071-3166-13
Chloromycetin Cream, 1% is supplied in 1 ounce tubes.
Store between 15°-30°C (59°-86°F).
Chloromycetin, brand of chloramphenicol. Reg US Pat Off
Caution—Federal law prohibits dispensing without prescription.

PARKE-DAVIS
Div of Warner-Lambert Co
Morris Plains, NJ 07950 USA **3166G015**
MADE IN CANADA

CHLOROMYCETIN® ℞

[*chlō"rō-my-cē'tĭn*]
HYDROCORTISONE OPHTHALMIC
(Chloramphenicol and Hydrocortisone Acetate for Suspension, USP)

> **WARNING**
> Bone marrow hypoplasia including aplastic anemia and death has been reported following local application of chloramphenicol. Chloramphenicol should not be used when less potentially dangerous agents would be expected to provide effective treatment.

DESCRIPTION

Chloromycetin® Hydrocortisone Ophthalmic (Chloramphenicol and Hydrocortisone Acetate for Suspension, USP) is a sterile, buffered antibiotic/antiinflammatory dry mixture for suspension for ophthalmic administration. Each vial of Chloromycetin Hydrocortisone Ophthalmic contains 12.5 mg chloramphenicol and 25 mg hydrocortisone acetate with boric acid-sodium borate buffer, cholesterol, methylcellulose, sodium chloride, and Phemerol® (benzethonium chloride), 0.1 mg per ml, in the suspension when prepared as directed. A 5 ml vial of Sterile Distilled Water is included in each package for use as a diluent in the preparation of a suspension of Chloromycetin Hydrocortisone suitable for ophthalmic use.
The chemical names for chloramphenicol are:
(1) Acetamide,2,2-dichloro-N-[2-hydroxy-1-(hydroxymethyl)-2-(4-nitrophenyl) ethyl]-, and
(2) D-*threo* -(–)-2,2-Dichloro-N-[β-hydroxy-α-(hydroxymethyl)-*p* -nitrophenethyl] acetamide
The chemical names for hydrocortisone acetate are:
(1) Pregn-4-ene-3,20-dione,21-(acetyloxy)-11,17-dihydroxy-,(11β)-, and
(2) 17-Hydroxycorticosterone 21-acetate

CLINICAL PHARMACOLOGY

Corticoids suppress the inflammatory response to a variety of agents and they probably delay or slow healing. Since corticoids may inhibit the body's defense mechanism against infection, a concomitant antimicrobial drug may be used when this inhibition is considered to be clinically significant in a particular case.
The antiinfective component in this combination is included to provide action against specific organisms susceptible to it. Chloramphenicol is considered active against a wide spectrum of gram-negative and gram-positive organisms such as *Escherichia coli, Hemophilus influenzae, Staphylococcus aureus, Streptococcus hemolyticus,* and *Moraxella lacunata* (Morax-Axenfeld bacillus). Development of resistance to chloramphenicol can be regarded as minimal for staphylococci and many other species of bacteria. Chloramphenicol is primarily bacteriostatic and acts by inhibition of protein synthesis by interfering with the transfer of activated amino acids from soluble RNA to ribosomes. It has been noted that chloramphenicol is found in measurable amounts in the aqueous humor following local application to the eye.
When a decision to administer both a corticoid and an antimicrobial is made, the administration of such drugs in combination has the advantage of greater patient compliance and convenience, with the added assurance that the appropriate dosage of both drugs is administered, plus assured compatibility of ingredients when both types of drug are in the same formulation and, particularly, that the correct volume of drug is delivered and retained.
The relative potency of corticosteroids depends on the molecular structure, concentration, and release from the vehicle.

INDICATIONS AND USAGE

Chloramphenicol should be used only in those serious infections for which less potentially dangerous drugs are ineffective or contraindicated. Bacteriological studies should be performed to determine the causative organisms and their sensitivity to chloramphenicol (See Box Warning).
For steroid-responsive inflammatory ocular conditions for which a corticosteroid is indicated and where bacterial infection or a risk of bacterial ocular infection exists.
Ocular steroids are indicated in inflammatory conditions of the palpebral and bulbar conjunctiva, cornea, and anterior segment of the globe where the inherent risk of steroid use in certain infective conjunctivitides is accepted to obtain a diminution in edema and inflammation. They are also indicated in chronic anterior uveitis and corneal injury from chemical radiation, thermal burns, or penetration of foreign bodies.
The use of a combination drug with an antiinfective component is indicated where the risk of infection is high or where there is an expectation that potentially dangerous numbers of bacteria will be present in the eye.
The particular antiinfective drug in this product is active against the following common bacterial eye pathogens:
Staphylococcus aureus
Streptococci, including *Streptococcus pneumoniae*
Escherichia coli
Hemophilus influenzae
Klebsiella/Enterobacter species
Moraxella lacunata (Morax-Axenfeld bacillus)
Neisseria species
The product does not provide adequate coverage against:
Pseudomonas aeruginosa
Serratia marcescens

CONTRAINDICATIONS

Epithelial herpes simplex keratitis (dendritic keratitis), vaccinia, varicella, and many other viral diseases of the cornea and conjunctiva. Mycobacterial infection of the eye. Fungal diseases of ocular structures. Hypersensitivity to a component of the medication. (Hypersensitivity to the antibiotic component occurs at a higher rate than for other components).
The use of these combinations is always contraindicated after uncomplicated removal of a corneal foreign body.

WARNINGS

SEE BOX WARNING
Prolonged use of steroids may result in glaucoma, with damage to the optic nerve, defects in visual acuity and fields of vision, and posterior subcapsular cataract formation. Prolonged use may suppress the host response and thus increase the hazard of secondary ocular infections. In those diseases causing thinning of the cornea or sclera, perforations have been known to occur with the use of topical steroids. In acute purulent conditions of the eye, steroids may mask infection or enhance existing infection. If these products are used for 10 days or longer, intraocular pressure should be routinely monitored even though it may be difficult in children and uncooperative patients.

Employment of steroid medication in the treatment of herpes simplex requires great caution.

PRECAUTIONS

The initial prescription and renewal of the medication order beyond 20 milliliters should be made by a physician only after examination of the patient with the aid of magnification, such as slit lamp biomicroscopy and, where appropriate, fluorescein staining.

The possibility of persistent fungal infections of the cornea should be considered after prolonged steroid dosing.

The prolonged use of antibiotics may occasionally result in overgrowth of nonsusceptible organisms, including fungi. If new infections appear during medication, the drug should be discontinued and appropriate measures should be taken.

In all serious infections the topical use of chloramphenicol should be supplemented by appropriate systemic medication.

ADVERSE REACTIONS

Blood dyscrasias have been reported in association with the use of chloramphenicol. (See **Warnings**).

Adverse reactions have occurred with steroid/antiinfective combination drugs which can be attributed to the steroid component, the antiinfective component, or the combination. Exact incidence figures are not available since no denominator of treated patients is available.

Reactions occurring most often from the presence of the antiinfective ingredient are allergic sensitizations. The reactions due to the steroid component in decreasing order of frequency are: elevation of intraocular pressure (IOP) with possible development of glaucoma, and infrequent optic nerve damage; posterior subcapsular cataract formation; and delayed wound healing.

Secondary Infection: The development of secondary infection has occurred after use of combinations containing steroids and antimicrobials. Fungal infections of the cornea are particularly prone to develop coincidentally with long-term applications of steroid. The possibility of fungal invasion must be considered in any persistent corneal ulceration where steroid treatment has been used.

Secondary bacterial ocular infection following suppression of host responses also occurs.

DOSAGE AND ADMINISTRATION

Two drops applied to the affected eye every three hours, or more frequently if deemed advisable by the prescribing physician. Administration should be continued day and night for the first 48 hours, after which the interval between applications may be increased. Treatment should be continued for at least 48 hours after the eye appears normal.

Directions for dispensing—Add 5 ml sterile distilled water to contents of vial under aseptic conditions. Shake to make uniform suspension. Place sterile dropper in vial. Each ml of suspension prepared as directed contains 2.5 mg Chloromycetin (chloramphenicol) and 5 mg Hydrocortisone Acetate.

Not more than 20 milliliters should be prescribed initially and the prescription should not be refilled without further evaluation as outlined in Precautions above.

HOW SUPPLIED

N 0071-3228-36 Chloromycetin Hydrocortisone Ophthalmic (Chloramphenicol and Hydrocortisone Acetate for Suspension, USP) is supplied in a package containing dry ingredients in a 5 ml vial and also a vial containing 5 ml of Sterile Distilled Water for use as a diluent in preparation of the ophthalmic suspension. After dispensing, the product may be stored at room temperature for a period of not more than 10 days. A sterilized dropper-cap assembly for use with the vial is included in the package.

Chloromycetin, brand of chloramphenicol, Reg US Pat Off.

3228G014

KAPSEALS®/CAPSULES CHLOROMYCETIN® ℞

[*chlō″rō-my-cē′tĭn*]

(chloramphenicol capsules, USP)

WARNING

Serious and fatal blood dyscrasias (aplastic anemia, hypoplastic anemia, thrombocytopenia, and granulocytopenia) are known to occur after the administration of chloramphenicol. In addition, there have been reports of aplastic anemia attributed to chloramphenicol which later terminated in leukemia. Blood dyscrasias have occurred after both short-term and prolonged therapy with this drug. Chloramphenicol must not be used when less potentially dangerous agents will be effective, as described in the Indications section. *It must not be used in the treatment of trivial infections or where it is not indicated, as in colds, influenza, infections of the throat; or as a prophylactic agent to prevent bacterial infections.*

Precautions: It is essential that adequate blood studies be made during treatment with the drug. While blood studies may detect early peripheral blood changes, such as leukopenia, reticulocytopenia, or granulocytopenia, before they become irreversible, such studies cannot be relied on to detect bone marrow depression prior to development of aplastic anemia. To facilitate appropriate studies and observation during therapy, it is desirable that patients be hospitalized.

DESCRIPTION

Chloramphenicol is an antibiotic that is clinically useful for, *and should be reserved for,* serious infections caused by organisms susceptible to its antimicrobial effects when less potentially hazardous therapeutic agents are ineffective or contraindicated. Sensitivity testing is essential to determine its indicated use, but may be performed concurrently with therapy initiated on clinical impression that one of the indicated conditions exists (see Indications and Usage section).

Each capsule contains 250 mg chloramphenicol. Also contains lactose, NF. The capsule shell and/or band contains gelatin, NF; colloidal silicon dioxide, NF; glyceryl monooleate; gray Opatint OD-7502; sodium lauryl sulfate, NF; titanium dioxide USP.

CLINICAL PHARMACOLOGY

In vitro chloramphenicol exerts mainly a bacteriostatic effect on a wide range of gram-negative and gram-positive bacteria and is active *in vitro* against rickettsiae, the lymphogranuloma psittacosis group, and *Vibrio cholerae.* It is particularly active against *Salmonella typhi* and *Hemophilus influenzae.* The mode of action is through interference or inhibition of protein synthesis in intact cells and in cell-free systems.

Chloramphenicol administered orally is absorbed rapidly from the intestinal tract. In controlled studies in adult volunteers using the recommended dosage of 50 mg/kg/day, a dosage of 1 g every 6 hours for 8 doses was given. Using the microbiological assay method, the average peak serum level was 11.2 mcg/ml one hour after the first dose. A cumulative effect gave a peak rise to 18.4 mcg/ml after the fifth dose of 1 g. Mean serum levels ranged from 8 to 14 mcg/ml over the 48-hour period. Total urinary excretion of chloramphenicol in these studies ranged from a low of 68% to a high of 99% over a three-day period. From 8 to 12% of the antibiotic excreted is in the form of free chloramphenicol; the remainder consists of microbiologically inactive metabolites, principally the conjugate with glucuronic acid. Since the glucuronide is excreted rapidly, most chloramphenicol detected in the blood is in the microbiologically active free form. Despite the small proportion of unchanged drug excreted in the urine, the concentration of free chloramphenicol is relatively high, amounting to several hundred mcg/ml in patients receiving divided doses of 50 mg/kg/day. Small amounts of active drug are found in bile and feces. Chloramphenicol diffuses rapidly, but its distribution is not uniform. Highest concentrations are found in liver and kidney, and lowest concentrations are found in brain and cerebrospinal fluid. Chloramphenicol enters cerebrospinal fluid even in the absence of meningeal inflammation, appearing in concentrations about half of those found in the blood. Measurable levels are also detected in pleural and in ascitic fluids, saliva, milk, and in the aqueous and vitreous humors. Transport across the placental barrier occurs with somewhat lower concentration in cord blood of newborn infants than in maternal blood.

INDICATIONS AND USAGE

In accord with the concepts in the warning box and this indications section, chloramphenicol must be used only in those serious infections for which less potentially dangerous drugs are ineffective or contraindicated. However, chloramphenicol may be chosen to initiate antibiotic therapy on the clinical impression that one of the conditions below is believed to be present; *in vitro* sensitivity tests should be performed concurrently so that the drug may be discontinued as soon as possible if less potentially dangerous agents are indicated by such tests. The decision to continue use of chloramphenicol rather than another antibiotic when both are suggested by *in vitro* studies to be effective against a specific pathogen should be based upon severity of the infection, susceptibility of the pathogen to the various antimicrobial drugs, efficacy of the various drugs in the infection, and the important additional concepts contained in the Warning Box above:

1. Acute infections caused by *Salmonella typhi*

Chloramphenicol is a drug of choice.* It is not recommended for the routine treatment of the typhoid carrier state.

2. Serious infections caused by susceptible strains in accordance with the concepts expressed above:

a. *Salmonella* species
b. *H influenzae,* specifically meningeal infections
c. Rickettsia
d. Lymphogranuloma-psittacosis group
e. Various gram-negative bacteria causing bacteremia, meningitis, or other serious gram-negative infections
f. Other susceptible organisms which have been demonstrated to be resistant to all other appropriate antimicrobial agents.

3. Cystic fibrosis regimens

CONTRAINDICATIONS

Chloramphenicol is contraindicated in individuals with a history of previous hypersensitivity and/or toxic reaction to it. *It must not be used in the treatment of trivial infections or where it is not indicated, as in colds, influenza, infections of the throat; or as a prophylactic agent to prevent bacterial infections.*

PRECAUTIONS

1. Baseline blood studies should be followed by periodic blood studies approximately every two days during therapy. The drug should be discontinued upon appearance of reticulocytopenia, leukopenia, thrombocytopenia, anemia, or any other blood study findings attributable to chloramphenicol. However, it should be noted that such studies do not exclude the possible later appearance of the irreversible type of bone marrow depression.

2. Repeated courses of the drug should be avoided if at all possible. Treatment should not be continued longer than required to produce a cure with little or no risk of relapse of the disease.

3. Concurrent therapy with other drugs that may cause bone marrow depression should be avoided.

4. Excessive blood levels may result from administration of the recommended dose to patients with impaired liver or kidney function, including that due to immature metabolic processes in the infant. The dosage should be adjusted accordingly or, preferably, the blood concentration should be determined at appropriate intervals.

5. There are no studies to establish the safety of this drug in pregnancy.

6. Since chloramphenicol readily crosses the placental barrier, caution in use of the drug is particularly important during pregnancy at term or during labor because of potential toxic effects on the fetus ("gray syndrome").

7. Precaution should be used in therapy of premature and full-term infants to avoid "gray syndrome" toxicity. (See Adverse Reactions.) Serum drug levels should be carefully followed during therapy of the newborn infant.

8. Precaution should be used in therapy during lactation because of the possibility of toxic effects on the nursing infant.

9. The use of this antibiotic, as with other antibiotics, may result in an overgrowth of nonsusceptible organisms, including fungi. If infections caused by nonsusceptible organisms appear during therapy, appropriate measures should be taken.

ADVERSE REACTIONS

1. Blood Dyscrasias

The most serious adverse effect of chloramphenicol is bone marrow depression. Serious and fatal blood dyscrasias (aplastic anemia, hypoplastic anemia, thrombocytopenia, and granulocytopenia) are known to occur after the administration of chloramphenicol. An irreversible type of marrow depression leading to aplastic anemia with a high rate of mortality is characterized by the appearance weeks or months after therapy of bone marrow aplasia or hypoplasia. Peripherally, pancytopenia is most often observed, but in a small number of cases only one or two of the three major cell types (erythrocytes, leukocytes, platelets) may be depressed.

A reversible type of bone marrow depression, which is dose-related, may occur. This type of marrow depression is characterized by vacuolization of the erythroid cells, reduction of reticulocytes, and leukopenia, and responds promptly to the withdrawal of chloramphenicol.

An exact determination of the risk of serious and fatal blood dyscrasias is not possible because of lack of accurate information regarding (1) the size of the population at risk, (2) the total number of drug-associated dyscrasias, and (3) the total number of nondrug-associated dyscrasias.

In a report to the California State Assembly by the California Medical Association and the State Department of Public Health in January 1967, the risk of fatal aplastic anemia was estimated at 1:24,200 to 1:40,500 based on two dosage levels.

There have been reports of aplastic anemia attributed to chloramphenicol which later terminated in leukemia.

Continued on next page

---

* In the treatment of typhoid fever, some authorities recommend that chloramphenicol be administered at therapeutic levels for 8 to 10 days after the patient has become afebrile to lessen the possibility of relapse.

This product information was prepared in August 1992. On these and other Parke-Davis Products, information may be obtained by addressing PARKE-DAVIS, Division of Warner-Lambert Company, Morris Plains, New Jersey 07950.

Parke-Davis—Cont.

Paroxysmal nocturnal hemoglobinuria has also been reported.

2. Gastrointestinal Reactions

Nausea, vomiting, glossitis and stomatitis, diarrhea, and enterocolitis may occur in low incidence.

3. Neurotoxic Reactions

Headache, mild depression, mental confusion, and delirium have been described in patients receiving chloramphenicol. Optic and peripheral neuritis have been reported, usually following long-term therapy. If this occurs, the drug should be promptly withdrawn.

4. Hypersensitivity Reactions

Fever, macular and vesicular rashes, angioedema, urticaria, and anaphylaxis may occur. Herxheimer reactions have occurred during therapy for typhoid fever.

5. "Gray Syndrome"

Toxic reactions including fatalities have occurred in the premature and newborn; the signs and symptoms associated with these reactions have been referred to as the "gray syndrome". One case of "gray syndrome" has been reported in an infant born to a mother having received chloramphenicol during labor. One case has been reported in a 3-month-old infant. The following summarizes the clinical and laboratory studies that have been made on these patients:

(a) In most cases, therapy with chloramphenicol had been instituted within the first 48 hours of life.

(b) Symptoms first appeared after 3 to 4 days of continued treatment with high doses of chloramphenicol.

(c) The symptoms appeared in the following order:
(1) abdominal distention with or without emesis;
(2) progressive pallid cyanosis;
(3) vasomotor collapse, frequently accompanied by irregular respiration;
(4) death within a few hours of onset of these symptoms.

(d) The progression of symptoms from onset to exitus was accelerated with higher dose schedules.

(e) Preliminary blood serum level studies revealed unusually high concentrations of chloramphenicol (over 90 mcg/ml after repeated doses).

(f) Termination of therapy upon early evidence of the associated symptomatology frequently reversed the process with complete recovery.

DOSAGE AND ADMINISTRATION

Dosage Recommendations For Oral Chloramphenicol Preparations

The majority of microorganisms susceptible to chloramphenicol will respond to a concentration between 5 and 20 mcg/ml. The desired concentration of active drug in blood should fall within this range over most of the treatment period. Dosage of 50 mg/kg/day divided into 4 doses at intervals of 6 hours will usually achieve and sustain levels of this magnitude.

Except in certain circumstances (eg, premature and newborn infants and individuals with impairment of hepatic or renal function), lower doses may not achieve these concentrations. Chloramphenicol, like other potent drugs, should be prescribed at recommended doses known to have therapeutic activity. Close observation of the patient should be maintained and in the event of any adverse reactions, dosage should be reduced or the drug discontinued, if other factors in the clinical situation permit.

Adults

Adults should receive 50 mg/kg/day (approximately one 250-mg capsule per each 10 lbs body weight) in divided doses at 6-hour intervals. In exceptional cases, patients with infections due to moderately resistant organisms may require increased dosage up to 100 mg/kg/day to achieve blood levels inhibiting the pathogen, but these high doses should be decreased as soon as possible. Adults with impairment of hepatic or renal function or both may have reduced ability to metabolize and excrete the drug. In instances of impaired metabolic processes, dosages should be adjusted accordingly. (See discussion under Newborn Infants.) Precise control of concentration of the drug in the blood should be carefully followed in patients with impaired metabolic processes by the available microtechniques (information available on request).

Children

Dosage of 50 mg/kg/day divided into 4 doses at 6-hour intervals yields blood levels in the range effective against most susceptible organisms. Severe infections (eg, bacteremia or meningitis), especially when adequate cerebrospinal fluid concentrations are desired, may require dosage up to 100 mg/kg/day; however, it is recommended that dosage be reduced to 50 mg/kg/day as soon as possible. Children with impaired liver or kidney function may retain excessive amounts of the drug.

Newborn Infants

(See section titled "Gray Syndrome" under Adverse Reactions.)

A total of 25 mg/kg/day in 4 equal doses at 6-hour intervals usually produces and maintains concentrations in blood and tissues adequate to control most infections for which the drug is indicated. Increased dosage in these individuals, demanded by severe infections, should be given only to maintain the blood concentration within a therapeutically effective range. After the first two weeks of life, full-term infants ordinarily may receive up to a total of 50 mg/kg/day equally divided into 4 doses at 6-hour intervals. **These dosage recommendations are extremely important because blood concentration in all premature infants and full-term infants under two weeks of age differs from that of other infants. This difference is due to variations in the maturity of the metabolic functions of the liver and the kidneys.**

When these functions are immature (or seriously impaired in adults), high concentrations of the drug are found which tend to increase with succeeding doses.

Infants and Children with Immature Metabolic Processes

In young infants and other children in whom immature metabolic functions are suspected, a dose of 25 mg/kg/day will usually produce therapeutic concentrations of the drug in the blood. In this group particularly, the concentration of the drug in the blood should be carefully following by microtechniques. (Information available on request.)

HOW SUPPLIED

Kapseals No. 379, Chloromycetin (Chloramphenicol Capsules), each contain 250 mg chloramphenicol.

N 0071-0379-24 Bottles of 100.

AHFS 8:12.08   0379G102

Chloromycetin, brand of chloramphenicol.

Reg. US Pat Off

STORAGE

Store at a room temperature below 86°F(30°C). Protect from moisture and excessive heat.

Caution—Federal law prohibits dispensing without prescription.

Shown in Product Identification Section, page 422

CHLOROMYCETIN® OPHTHALMIC   ℞

[chlō″rō-my-cē′tĭn]
(Chloramphenical for Ophthalmic Solution, USP)

> **WARNING**
>
> Bone marrow hypoplasia including aplastic anemia and death has been reported following local application of chloramphenicol. Chloramphenicol should not be used when less potentially dangerous agents would be expected to provide effective treatment.

DESCRIPTION

Each vial of Chloromycetin Ophthalmic contains 25 mg of Chloromycetin (chloramphenicol) with boric acid-sodium borate buffer. Sodium hydroxide may have been added for adjustment of pH. A 15 ml bottle of Sterile Distilled Water is included in each package for use as a diluent in the preparation of a solution of Chloromycetin suitable for ophthalmic use. By varying the quantity of diluent used solutions ranging in strength from 0.16% to 0.5% may be prepared. Both the powder for solution and the diluent contain no preservatives. Sterile powder.

The chemical names for chloramphenicol are:

(1) Acetamide,2,2-dichloro-*N*-[2-hydroxy-1-(hydroxymethyl)-2-(4-nitrophenyl) ethyl]-, and

(2) D-*threo*-(−)-2,2-Dichloro-*N*-[β-hydroxy-α-(hydroxymethyl)-*p*-nitrophenethyl] acetamide

CLINICAL PHARMACOLOGY

Chloramphenicol is a broad-spectrum antibiotic originally isolated from *Streptomyces venezuelae*. It is primarily bacteriostatic and acts by inhibition of protein synthesis by interfering with the transfer of activated amino acids from soluble RNA to ribosomes. It has been noted that chloramphenicol is found in measurable amounts in the aqueous humor following local application to the eye. Development of resistance to chloramphenicol can be regarded as minimal for staphylococci and many other species of bacteria.

INDICATIONS AND USAGE

Chloramphenicol should be used only in those serious infections for which less potentially dangerous drugs are ineffective or contraindicated. Bacteriological studies should be performed to determine the causative organisms and their sensitivity to chloramphenicol (See Box Warning).

Chloromycetin (chloramphenicol) Ophthalmic is indicated for the treatment of surface ocular infections involving the conjunctiva and/or cornea caused by chloramphenicol-susceptible organisms.

The particular antiinfective drug in this product is active against the following common bacterial eye pathogens:

Staphylococcus aureus
Streptococci, including *Streptococcus pneumoniae*
Escherichia coli
Haemophilus influenzae
Klebsiella/Enterobacter species
Moraxella lacunata (Morax-Axenfeld bacillus)
Neisseria species

The product does not provide adequate coverage against:
Pseudomonas aeruginosa
Serratia marcescens

CONTRAINDICATIONS

This product is contraindicated in persons sensitive to any of its components.

WARNINGS

SEE BOX WARNING

PRECAUTIONS

The prolonged use of antibiotics may occasionally result in overgrowth of nonsusceptible organisms, including fungi. If new infections appear during medication, the drug should be discontinued and appropriate measures should be taken. In all serious infections the topical use of chloramphenicol should be supplemented by appropriate systemic medication.

ADVERSE REACTIONS

Blood dyscrasias have been reported in association with the use of chloramphenicol (See WARNINGS). Transient burning or stinging sensations may occur with use of Chloromycetin Ophthalmic Solution.

DOSAGE AND ADMINISTRATION

Two drops applied to the affected eye every three hours, or more frequently if deemed advisable by the prescribing physician. Administration should be continued day and night for the first 48 hours, after which the interval between applications may be increased. Treatment should be continued for at least 48 hours after the eye appears normal.

Directions for dispensing—Prepare solution by adding sterile distilled water to the vial as follows:

Strength of solution desired	Add sterile distilled water
0.5%	5 ml
0.25%	10 ml
0.16%	15 ml

Solutions remain stable at room temperature for ten days.

HOW SUPPLIED

N 0071-3213-35 Chloromycetin (chloramphenicol) Ophthalmic is supplied in a package containing dry ingredients in a 15 ml vial and also a vial containing 15 ml of Sterile Distilled Water for use as a diluent in preparing the solution for ophthalmic use. A sterilized dropper-cap assembly for use on the vial of solution is included in the package.

Store below 30°C (86°F).

Chloromycetin, brand of chloramphenicol. Reg US Pat Off

3213G012

CHLOROMYCETIN®   ℞

[chlō″rō-my-cē′tĭn]
OPHTHALMIC OINTMENT, 1%
(chloramphenicol ophthalmic ointment, USP)

> **WARNING**
>
> Bone marrow hypoplasia including aplastic anemia and death has been reported following local application of chloramphenicol. Chloramphenicol should not be used when less potentially dangerous agents would be expected to provide effective treatment.

DESCRIPTION

Each gram of Chloromycetin Ophthalmic Ointment, 1% contains 10 mg chloramphenicol in a special base of liquid petrolatum and polyethylene. It contains no preservatives. Sterile ointment.

The chemical names for chloramphenicol are:

(1) Acetamide,2,2-dichloro-*N*-[2-hydroxy-1-(hydroxymethyl)-2-(4-nitrophenyl) ethyl]-, and

(2) D-*threo*-(−)-2,2-Dichloro-*N*-[β-hydroxy-α-(hydroxymethyl)-*p*-nitrophenethyl] acetamide

CLINICAL PHARMACOLOGY

Chloramphenicol is a broad-spectrum antibiotic originally isolated from *Streptomyces venezuelae*. It is primarily bacteriostatic and acts by inhibition of protein synthesis by interfering with the transfer of activated amino acids from soluble RNA to ribosomes. It has been noted that chloramphenicol is found in measurable amounts in the aqueous humor following local application to the eye. Development of resistance to

chloramphenicol can be regarded as minimal for staphylococci and many other species of bacteria.

INDICATIONS AND USAGE

Chloramphenicol should be used only in those serious infections for which less potentially dangerous drugs are ineffective or contraindicated. Bacteriological studies should be performed to determine the causative organisms and their sensitivity to chloramphenicol (See Box Warning).

Chloromycetin (chloramphenicol) Ophthalmic Ointment, 1% is indicated for the treatment of surface ocular infections involving the conjunctiva and/or cornea caused by chloramphenicol-susceptible organisms.

The particular antiinfective drug in this product is active against the following common bacterial eye pathogens:

Staphylococcus aureus
Streptococci, including *Streptococcus pneumoniae*
Escherichia coli
Haemophilus influenzae
Klebsiella/Enterobacter species
Moraxella lacunata (Morax-Axenfeld bacillus)
Neisseria species

The product does not provide adequate coverage against:
Pseudomonas aeruginosa
Serratia marcescens

CONTRAINDICATIONS

This product is contraindicated in persons sensitive to any of its components.

WARNINGS

SEE BOX WARNING

Ophthalmic ointments may retard corneal wound healing.

PRECAUTIONS

The prolonged use of antibiotics may occasionally result in overgrowth of nonsusceptible organisms, including fungi. If new infections appear during medication, the drug should be discontinued and appropriate measures should be taken.

In all serious infections the topical use of chloramphenicol should be supplemented by appropriate systemic medication.

ADVERSE REACTIONS

Blood dyscrasias have been reported in association with the use of chloramphenicol (See WARNINGS).

Allergic or inflammatory reactions due to individual hypersensitivity and occasional burning or stinging may occur with the use of Chloromycetin Ophthalmic Ointment. Blood dyscrasias have been reported in association with the use of chloramphenicol (See WARNINGS).

DOSAGE AND ADMINISTRATION

A small amount of ointment placed in the lower conjunctival sac every three hours, or more frequently if deemed advisable by the prescribing physician. Administration should be continued day and night for the first 48 hours, after which the interval between applications may be increased. Treatment should be continued for at least 48 hours after the eye appears normal.

HOW SUPPLIED

N 0071-3070-07

Chloromycetin Ophthalmic Ointment, 1% (Chloramphenicol Ophthalmic Ointment, USP) is supplied, sterile, in ophthalmic ointment tubes of 3.5 grams.

Chloromycetin, brand of chloramphenicol. Reg US Pat Off

AHFS Category 52:04.04 **3070G022**

CHLOROMYCETIN® OTIC ℞

[*chlō"rō-my-cē'tĭn ō'-tĭc*]
(chloramphenicol otic)

> **WARNING**
>
> Bone marrow hypoplasia including aplastic anemia and death has been reported following local application of chloramphenicol. Chloramphenicol should not be used when less potentially dangerous agents would be expected to provide effective treatment.

DESCRIPTION

Each milliliter of Chloromycetin Otic contains 5 mg (0.5%) chloramphenicol in propylene glycol. Sterile.

The chemical names for chloramphenicol are:

(1) Acetamide,2,2-dichloro -*N* - [2-hydroxy-1-(hydroxymethyl) -2- (4-nitrophenyl) ethyl]-, and

(2) D- *threo* - (—) -2,2 -Dichloro -*N* - [β-hydroxyα-(hydroxymethyl)-*p* -nitrophenethyl]acetamide

CLINICAL PHARMACOLOGY

Chloramphenicol is a broad-spectrum antibiotic originally isolated from *Streptomyces venezuelae*. It is primarily bacteriostatic and acts by inhibition of protein synthesis by interfering with the transfer of activated amino acids from soluble RNA to ribosomes. Development of resistance to chloramphenicol can be regarded as minimal for staphylococci and many other species of bacteria.

INDICATIONS AND USAGE

Chloromycetin (chloramphenicol) Otic is indicated for the treatment of surface infections of the external auditory canal caused by susceptible strains of various gram-positive and gram-negative organisms including:

Staphylococcus aureus, Escherichia coli, Hemophilus influenzae, Pseudomonas aeruginosa, Aerobacter aerogenes, Klebsiella pneumoniae and *Proteus* species.

Deeper infections should be treated with appropriate systemic antibiotics.

CONTRAINDICATIONS

This product is contraindicated in persons sensitive to any of its components.

Perforated tympanic membrance is considered a contraindication to the use of any medication in the external ear canal.

WARNINGS

SEE BOX WARNING.

Discontinue promptly if sensitization or irritation occurs.

PRECAUTIONS

The prolonged use of antibiotics may occasionally result in overgrowth of nonsusceptible organisms, including fungi. If new infections appear during medication, the drug should be discontinued and appropriate measures should be taken.

In all serious infections, the topical use of chloramphenicol should be supplemented by appropriate systemic medication.

The possibility of the occurrence of ototoxicity must be considered if this product is allowed to enter the middle ear.

ADVERSE REACTION

Signs of local irritation with subjective symptoms of itching or burning, angioneurotic edema, urticaria, vesicular and maculopapular dermatitis have been reported in patients sensitive to chloramphenicol and are causes for discontinuing the medication. Similar sensitivity reactions to other materials in topical preparations may also occur. Blood dyscrasias have been reported in association with the use of chloramphenicol (See WARNINGS).

DOSAGE AND ADMINISTRATION

Instill 2 or 3 drops into the affected ear three times daily.

HOW SUPPLIED

N0071-3313-35 Chloromycetin (chloramphenicol) Otic is supplied in 15 mL vials with droppers.

Store below 30°C (86°F).

Chloromycetin, brand of chloramphenicol, Reg US Pat Off.

Caution—Federal law prohibits dispensing without prescription.

3313G023

ORAL SUSPENSION

CHLOROMYCETIN® PALMITATE ℞

[*chlō"rō-my-ce'tĭn păl'mĭ-tāte"*]
(chloramphenicol palmitate oral suspension, USP)

> **WARNING**
>
> **Serious and fatal blood dyscrasias (aplastic anemia, hypoplastic anemia, thrombocytopenia, and granulocytopenia) are known to occur after the administration of chloramphenicol. In addition, there have been reports of aplastic anemia attributed to chloramphenicol which later terminated in leukemia. Blood dyscrasias have occurred after both short-term and prolonged therapy with this drug. Chloramphenicol must not be used when less potentially dangerous agents will be effective, as described in the Indications section. *It must not be used in the treatment of trivial infections or where it is not indicated, as in colds, influenza, infections of the throat; or as a prophylactic agent to prevent bacterial infections.***
>
> **Precautions: It is essential that adequate blood studies be made during treatment with the drug. While blood studies may detect early peripheral blood changes, such as leukopenia, reticulocytopenia, or granulocytopenia, before they become irreversible, such studies cannot be relied on to detect bone marrow depression prior to development of aplastic anemia. To facilitate appropriate studies and observation during therapy, it is desirable that patients be hospitalized.**

DESCRIPTION

Chloromycetin Palmitate Oral Suspension contains chloramphenicol palmitate equivalent to 150 mg chloramphenicol per 5 mL. Also contains alcohol, USP; carboxymethylcellulose sodium, USP; citric acid, USP; custard flavor, imitation; glycerin, USP; povidone, USP; propylene glycol, USP; sodium benzoate, NF; sorbitan monolaurate, NF; sucrose, NF; veegum, HV; purified water, USP.

Chloramphenicol is an antibiotic that is clinically useful for, *and should be reserved for,* serious infections caused by organisms susceptible to its antimicrobial effects when less potentially hazardous therapeutic agents are ineffective or contraindicated. Sensitivity testing is essential to determine its indicated use, but may be performed concurrently with therapy initiated on clinical impression that one of the indicated conditions exists (see Indications section).

CLINICAL PHARMACOLOGY

In vitro chloramphenicol exerts mainly a bacteriostatic effect on a wide range of gram-negative and gram-positive bacteria and is active *in vitro* against rickettsiae, the lymphogranuloma-psittacosis group and *Vibrio cholerae.* It is particularly active against *Salmonella typhi* and *Hemophilus influenzae.* The mode of action is through interference or inhibition of protein synthesis in intact cells and in cell-free systems.

Chloramphenicol administered orally is absorbed rapidly from the intestinal tract. In controlled studies in adult volunteers using the recommended dosage of 50 mg/kg/day, a dosage of 1 g every 6 hours for 8 doses was given. Using the microbiological assay method, the average peak serum level was 11.2 mcg/ml one hour after the first dose.

A cumulative effect gave a peak rise to 18.4 mcg/ml after the fifth dose of 1 g. Mean serum levels ranged from 8 to 14 mcg/ml over the 48-hour period. Total urinary excretion of chloramphenicol in these studies ranged from a low of 68% to a high of 99% over a three-day period. From 8% to 12% of the antibiotic excreted is in the form of free chloramphenicol; the remainder consists of microbiologically inactive metabolites, principally the conjugate with glucuronic acid. Since the glucuronide is excreted rapidly, most chloramphenicol detected in the blood is in the microbiologically active free form. Despite the small proportion of unchanged drug excreted in the urine, the concentration of free chloramphenicol is relatively high, amounting to several hundred mcg/ml in patients receiving divided doses of 50 mg/kg/day. Small amounts of active drug are found in bile and feces. Chloramphenicol diffuses rapidly, but its distribution is not uniform. Highest concentrations are found in liver and kidney, and lowest concentrations are found in brain and cerebrospinal fluid. Chloramphenicol enters cerebrospinal fluid even in the absence of meningeal inflammation, appearing in concentrations about half of those found in the blood. Measurable levels are also detected in pleural and in ascitic fluids, saliva, milk and in the aqueous and vitreous humors. Transport across the placental barrier occurs with somewhat lower concentration in cord blood of newborn infants than in maternal blood.

INDICATIONS AND USAGE

In accord with the concepts in the Warning Box and this Indications section, chloramphenicol must be used only in those serious infections for which less potentially dangerous drugs are ineffective or contraindicated. However, chloramphenicol may be chosen to initiate antibiotic therapy on the clinical impression that one of the conditions below is believed to be present; *in vitro* sensitivity tests should be performed concurrently *so* that the drug may be discontinued as soon as possible if less potentially dangerous agents are indicated by such tests. The decision to continue use of chloramphenicol rather than another antibiotic when both are suggested by *in vitro* studies to be effective against a specific pathogen should be based upon severity of the infection, susceptibility of the pathogen to the various antimicrobial drugs, efficacy of the various drugs in the infection, and the important additional concepts contained in the Warning Box above.

1. Acute infections caused by *Salmonella typhi*

Chloramphenicol is a drug of choice.* It is not recommended for the routine treatment of the typhoid carrier state.

2. Serious infections caused by susceptible strains in accordance with the concepts expressed above:

a. Salmonella species
b. *H influenzae,* specifically meningeal infections
c. Rickettsia
d. Lymphogranuloma-psittacosis group

*In the treatment of typhoid fever some authorities recommend that chloramphenicol be administered at therapeutic levels for 8 to 10 days after the patient has become afebrile to lessen the possibility of relapse.

Continued on next page

This product information was prepared in August 1992. On these and other Parke-Davis Products, information may be obtained by addressing PARKE-DAVIS, Division of Warner-Lambert Company, Morris Plains, New Jersey 07950.

Parke-Davis—Cont.

e. Various gram-negative bacteria causing bacteremia, meningitis or other serious gram-negative infections
f. Other susceptible organisms which have been demonstrated to be resistant to all other appropriate antimicrobial agents.

3. Cystic fibrosis regimens

CONTRAINDICATIONS

Chloramphenicol is contraindicated in individuals with a history of previous hypersensitivity and/or toxic reaction to it. *It must not be used in the treatment of trivial infections or where it is not indicated, as in colds, influenza, infections of the throat; or as a prophylactic agent to prevent bacterial infections.*

PRECAUTIONS

1. Baseline blood studies should be followed by periodic blood studies approximately every two days during therapy. The drug should be discontinued upon appearance of reticulocytopenia, leukopenia, thrombocytopenia, anemia, or any other blood study findings attributable to chloramphenicol. However, it should be noted that such studies do not exclude the possible later appearance of the irreversible type of bone marrow depression.
2. Repeated courses of the drug should be avoided if at all possible. Treatment should not be continued longer than required to produce a cure with little or no risk of relapse of the disease.
3. Concurrent therapy with other drugs that may cause bone marrow depression should be avoided.
4. Excessive blood levels may result from administration of the recommended dose to patients with impaired liver or kidney function, including that due to immature metabolic processes in the infant. The dosage should be adjusted accordingly or, preferably, the blood concentration should be determined at appropriate intervals.
5. There are no studies to establish the safety of this drug in pregnancy.
6. Since chloramphenicol readily crosses the placental barrier, caution in use of the drug is particularly important during pregnancy at term or during labor because of potential toxic effects on the fetus (gray syndrome).
7. Precaution should be used in therapy of premature and full-term infants to avoid "gray syndrome" toxicity. (See "Adverse Reactions.") Serum drug levels should be carefully followed during therapy of the newborn infant.
8. Precaution should be used in therapy during lactation because of the possibility of toxic effects on the nursing infant.
9. The use of this antibiotic, as with other antibiotics, may result in an overgrowth of nonsusceptible organisms, including fungi. If infections caused by nonsusceptible organisms appear during therapy, appropriate measures should be taken.

ADVERSE REACTIONS

1. Blood Dyscrasias

The most serious adverse effect of chloramphenicol is bone marrow depression. Serious and fatal blood dyscrasias (aplastic anemia, hypoplastic anemia, thrombocytopenia, and granulocytopenia) are known to occur after the administration of chloramphenicol. An irreversible type of marrow depression leading to aplastic anemia with a high rate of mortality is characterized by the appearance weeks or months after therapy of bone marrow aplasia or hypoplasia. Peripherally, pancytopenia is most often observed, but in a small number of cases only one or two of the three major cell types (erythrocytes, leukocytes, platelets) may be depressed.
A reversible type of bone marrow depression, which is dose related, may occur. This type of marrow depression is characterized by vacuolization of the erythroid cells, reduction of reticulocytes and leukopenia, and responds promptly to the withdrawal of chloramphenicol.
An exact determination of the risk of serious and fatal blood dyscrasias is not possible because of lack of accurate information regarding 1) the size of the population at risk, 2) the total number of drug-associated dyscrasias, and 3) the total number of nondrug associated dyscrasias.
In a report to the California State Assembly by the California Medical Association and the State Department of Public Health in January 1967, the risk of fatal aplastic anemia was estimated at 1:24,200 to 1:40,500 based on two dosage levels.
There have been reports of aplastic anemia attributed to chloramphenicol which later terminated in leukemia.
Paroxysmal nocturnal hemoglobinuria has also been reported.

2. Gastrointestinal Reactions

Nausea, vomiting, glossitis and stomatitis, diarrhea and enterocolitis may occur in low incidence.

3. Neurotoxic Reactions

Headache, mild depression, mental confusion and delirium have been described in patients receiving chloramphenicol. Optic and peripheral neuritis have been reported, usually following long-term therapy. If this occurs, the drug should be promptly withdrawn.

4. Hypersensitivity Reactions

Fever, macular and vesicular rashes, angioedema, urticaria and anaphylaxis may occur. Herxheimer reactions have occurred during therapy for typhoid fever.

5. "Gray Syndrome"

Toxic reactions including fatalities have occurred in the premature and newborn, the signs and symptoms associated with these reactions have been referred to as the gray syndrome. One case of gray syndrome has been reported in an infant born to a mother having received chloramphenicol during labor. One case has been reported in a 3-month-old infant. The following summarizes the clinical and laboratory studies that have been made on these patients.
(a) In most cases therapy with chloramphenicol had been instituted within the first 48 hours of life.
(b) Symptoms first appeared after 3 to 4 days of continued treatment with high doses of chloramphenicol
(c) The symptoms appeared in the following order:
1) abdominal distention with or without emesis;
2) progressive pallid cyanosis;
3) vasomotor collapse, frequently accompanied by irregular respiration;
4) death within a few hours of onset of these symptoms.
(d) The progression of symptoms from onset to exitus was accelerated with higher dose schedules.
(e) Preliminary blood serum level studies revealed unusually high concentrations of chloramphenicol (over 90 mcg/ml after repeated doses).
(f) Termination of therapy upon early evidence of the associated symptomatology frequently reversed the process with complete recovery.

DOSAGE AND ADMINISTRATION

Dosage Recommendations

The majority of microorganisms susceptible to chloramphenicol will respond to a concentration between 5 and 20 mcg/ml. The desired concentration of active drug in blood should fall within this range over most of the treatment period. Dosage of 50 mg/kg/day divided into 4 doses at intervals of 6 hours will usually achieve and sustain levels of this magnitude.
Except in certain circumstances (eg. premature and newborn infants and individuals with impairment of hepatic or renal function) lower doses may not achieve these concentrations. Chloramphenicol, like other potent drugs, should be prescribed at recommended doses known to have therapeutic activity. Close observation of the patient should be maintained and in the event of any adverse reactions, dosage should be reduced or the drug discontinued, if other factors in the clinical situation permit.

Adults

Adults should receive 50 mg/kg/day in divided doses at 6-hour intervals. In exceptional cases patients with infections due to moderately resistant organisms may require increased dosage up to 100 mg/kg/day to achieve blood levels inhibiting the pathogen, but these high doses should be decreased as soon as possible. Adults with impairment of hepatic or renal function or both may have reduced ability to metabolize and excrete the drug. In instances of impaired metabolic processes, dosages should be adjusted accordingly. (See discussion under Newborn Infants.) Precise control of concentration of the drug in the blood should be carefully followed in patients with impaired metabolic processes by the available microtechniques (information available on request).

Children

Dosage of 50 mg/kg/day divided into 4 doses at 6-hour intervals yields blood levels in the range effective against most susceptible organisms. Severe infections (eg. bacteremia or meningitis), especially when adequate cerebrospinal fluid concentrations are desired, may require dosage up to 100 mg/kg/day; however, it is recommended that dosage be reduced to 50 mg/kg/day as soon as possible. Children with impaired liver or kidney function may retain excessive amounts of the drug.

Newborn Infants

(See section titled "Gray Syndrome" under Adverse Reactions.)

A total of 25 mg/kg/day in 4 equal doses at 6-hour intervals usually produces and maintains concentrations in blood and tissues adequate to control most infections for which the drug is indicated. Increased dosage in these individuals, demanded by severe infections, should be given only to maintain the blood concentration within a therapeutically effective range. After the first two weeks of life, full-term infants ordinarily may receive up to a total of 50 mg/kg/day equally divided into 4 doses at 6-hour intervals. *These dosage recommendations are extremely important because blood concentration in all premature infants and full-term infants under two weeks of age differs from that of other infants.* This difference is due to variations in the maturity of the metabolic functions of the liver and the kidneys.
When these functions are immature (or seriously impaired in adults), high concentrations of the drug are found which tend to increase with succeeding doses.

Infants and Children with Immature Metabolic Processes

In young infants and other children in whom immature metabolic functions are suspected, a dose of 25 mg/kg/day will usually produce therapeutic concentrations of the drug in the blood. In this group particularly, the concentration of the drug in the blood should be carefully followed by microtechniques. (Information available on request.)

HOW SUPPLIED

N 0071-2310-15

Oral Suspension Chloromycetin Palmitate (Chloramphenicol Palmitate Oral Suspension, USP), each 5 ml contains chloramphenicol palmitate equivalent to 150 mg chloramphenicol with 0.5% sodium benzoate as preservative, in bottles of 60 ml.
Chloramphenicol Palmitate is hydrolyzed to chloramphenicol before absorption. Resulting blood concentration is similar to that produced by the oral administration of chloramphenicol.
Chloromycetin, brand of chloramphenicol. Reg. US Pat Off

2310G042

Caution—Federal law prohibits dispensing without prescription.

CHLOROMYCETIN® ℞

[chlō"rō-my-cē'tĭn sŭc'cĭ-nāte"]

SODIUM SUCCINATE

(sterile chloramphenicol sodium succinate, USP)

FOR INTRAVENOUS ADMINISTRATION

WARNING

Serious and fatal blood dyscrasias (aplastic anemia, hypoplastic anemia, thrombocytopenia, and granulocytopenia) are known to occur after the administration of chloramphenicol. In addition, there have been reports of aplastic anemia attributed to chloramphenicol which later terminated in leukemia. Blood dyscrasias have occurred after both short-term and prolonged therapy with this drug. Chloramphenicol must not be used when less potentially dangerous agents will be effective, as described in the Indications section. *It must not be used in the treatment of trivial infections or where it is not indicated, as in colds, influenza, infections of the throat; or as a prophylactic agent to prevent bacterial infections.*

Precautions: It is essential that adequate blood studies be made during treatment with the drug. While blood studies may detect early peripheral blood changes, such as leukopenia, reticulocytopenia, or granulocytopenia, before they become irreversible, such studies cannot be relied on to detect bone marrow depression prior to development of aplastic anemia. To facilitate appropriate studies and observation during therapy, it is desirable that patients be hospitalized.

IMPORTANT CONSIDERATIONS IN PRESCRIBING INJECTABLE CHLORAMPHENICOL SODIUM SUCCINATE CHLORAMPHENICOL SODIUM SUCCINATE IS INTENDED FOR INTRAVENOUS USE ONLY. IT HAS BEEN DEMONSTRATED TO BE INEFFECTIVE WHEN GIVEN INTRAMUSCULARLY.

1. Chloramphenicol sodium succinate must be hydrolyzed to its microbiologically active form and there is a lag in achieving adequate blood levels compared with the base given intravenously.
2. The oral form of chloramphenicol is readily absorbed and adequate blood levels are achieved and maintained on the recommended dosage.
3. Patients started on intravenous chloramphenicol sodium succinate should be changed to the oral form as soon as practicable.

DESCRIPTION

Chloramphenicol is an antibiotic that is clinically useful for, *and should be reserved for,* serious infections caused by organisms susceptible to its antimicrobial effects when less potentially hazardous therapeutic agents are ineffective or contraindicated. Sensitivity testing is essential to determine its indicated use, but may be performed concurrently with therapy initiated on clinical impression that one of the indicated conditions exists (see Indications section).
Each gram (10 ml of a 10% solution) of chloramphenicol sodium succinate contains approximately 52 mg (2.25 mEq) of sodium.

ACTIONS AND PHARMACOLOGY

In vitro chloramphenicol exerts mainly a bacteriostatic effect on a wide range of gram-negative and gram-positive bacteria and is active *in vitro* against rickettsiae, the lymphogranuloma-psittacosis group, and *Vibrio cholerae.* It is partic-

ularly active against *Salmonella typhi* and *Hemophilus influenzae.* The mode of action is through interference or inhibition of protein synthesis in intact cells and in cell-free systems.

Chloramphenicol administered orally is absorbed rapidly from the intestinal tract. In controlled studies in adult volunteers using the recommended dosage of 50 mg/kg/day, a dosage of 1 g every 6 hours for 8 doses was given. Using the microbiological assay method, the average peak serum level was 11.2 mcg/ml one hour after the first dose. A cumulative effect gave a peak rise to 18.4 mcg/ml after the fifth dose of 1 g. Mean serum levels ranged from 8 to 14 mcg/ml over the 48-hour period. Total urinary excretion of chloramphenicol in these studies ranged from a low of 68% to a high of 99% over a three-day period. From 8 to 12% of the antibiotic excreted is in the form of free chloramphenicol; the remainder consists of microbiologically inactive metabolites, principally the conjugate with glucuronic acid. Since the glucuronide is excreted rapidly, most chloramphenicol detected in the blood is in the microbiologically active free form. Despite the small proportion of unchanged drug excreted in the urine, the concentration of free chloramphenicol is relatively high, amounting to several hundred mcg/ml in patients receiving divided doses of 50 mg/kg/day. Small amounts of active drug are found in bile and feces. Chloramphenicol diffuses rapidly, but its distribution is not uniform. Highest concentrations are found in liver and kidney, and lowest concentrations are found in brain and cerebrospinal fluid. Chloramphenicol enters cerebrospinal fluid even in the absence of meningeal inflammation, appearing in concentrations about half of those found in the blood. Measurable levels are also detected in pleural and in ascitic fluids, saliva, milk, and in the aqueous and vitreous humors. Transport across the placental barrier occurs with somewhat lower concentration in cord blood of newborn infants than in maternal blood.

INDICATIONS

In accord with the concepts in the warning box and this Indications section, chloramphenicol must be used only in those serious infections for which less potentially dangerous drugs are ineffective or contraindicated. However, chloramphenicol may be chosen to initiate antibiotic therapy on the clinical impression that one of the conditions below is believed to be present; *in vitro* sensitivity tests should be performed concurrently so that the drug may be discontinued as soon as possible if less potentially dangerous agents are indicated by such tests. The decision to continue use of chloramphenicol rather than another antibiotic when both are suggested by *in vitro* studies to be effective against a specific pathogen should be based upon severity of the infection, susceptibility of the pathogen to the various antimicrobial drugs, efficacy of the various drugs in the infection, and the important additional concepts contained in the Warning Box above:

1. Acute infections caused by *S typhi**

It is not recommended for the routine treatment of the typhoid carrier state.

2. Serious infections caused by susceptible strains in accordance with the concepts expressed above:

a. *Salmonella* species
b. *H influenzae,* specifically meningeal infections
c. Rickettsia
d. Lymphogranuloma-psittacosis group
e. Various gram-negative bacteria causing bacteremia, meningitis, or other serious gram-negative infections
f. Other susceptible organisms which have been demonstrated to be resistant to all other appropriate antimicrobial agents.

3. Cystic fibrosis regimens

CONTRAINDICATIONS

Chloramphenicol is contraindicated in individuals with a history of previous hypersensitivity and/or toxic reaction to it. *It must not be used in the treatment of trivial infections or where it is not indicated, as in colds, influenza, infections of the throat; or as a prophylactic agent to prevent bacterial infection.*

PRECAUTIONS

1. Baseline blood studies should be followed by periodic blood studies approximately every two days during therapy. The drug should be discontinued upon appearance of reticulocytopenia, leukopenia, thrombocytopenia, anemia, or any other blood study findings attributable to chloramphenicol. However, it should be noted that such studies do not exclude the possible later appearance of the irreversible type of bone marrow depression.

2. Repeated courses of the drug should be avoided if at all possible. Treatment should not be continued longer than required to produce a cure with little or no risk of relapse of the disease.

3. Concurrent therapy with other drugs that may cause bone marrow depression should be avoided.

4. Excessive blood levels may result from administration of the recommended dosage to patients with impaired liver or kidney function, including that due to immature metabolic processes in the infant. The dosage should be adjusted accordingly or, preferably, the blood concentration should be determined at appropriate intervals.

5. There are no studies to establish the safety of this drug in pregnancy.

6. Since chloramphenicol readily crosses the placental barrier, caution in use of the drug is particularly important during pregnancy at term or during labor because of potential toxic effects on the fetus (gray syndrome).

7. Precaution should be used in therapy of premature and full-term infants to avoid gray syndrome toxicity (see Adverse Reactions). Serum drug levels should be carefully followed during therapy of the newborn infant.

8. Precaution should be used in therapy during lactation because of the possibility of toxic effects on the nursing infant.

9. The use of this antibiotic, as with other antibiotics, may result in an overgrowth of nonsusceptible organisms, including fungi. If infections caused by nonsusceptible organisms appear during therapy, appropriate measures should be taken.

*In the treatment of typhoid fever, some authorities recommend that chloramphenicol be administered at therapeutic levels for 8 to 10 days after the patient has become afebrile to lessen the possibility of relapse.

ADVERSE REACTIONS

1. Blood Dyscrasias

The most serious adverse effect of chloramphenicol is bone marrow depression. Serious and fatal blood dyscrasias (aplastic anemia, hypoplastic anemia, thrombocytopenia, and granulocytopenia) are known to occur after the administration of chloramphenicol. An irreversible type of marrow depression leading to aplastic anemia with a high rate of mortality is characterized by the appearance weeks or months after therapy of bone marrow aplasia or hypoplasia. Peripherally, pancytopenia is most often observed, but in a small number of cases only one or two of the three major cell types (erythrocytes, leukocytes, platelets) may be depressed.

A reversible type of bone marrow depression, which is dose-related, may occur. This type of marrow depression is characterized by vacuolization of the erythroid cells, reduction of reticulocytes, and leukopenia, and responds promptly to the withdrawal of chloramphenicol.

An exact determination of the risk of serious and fatal blood dyscrasias is not possible because of lack of accurate information regarding (1) the size of the population at risk, (2) the total number of drug-associated dyscrasias, and (3) the total number of nondrug-associated dyscrasias.

In a report to the California State Assembly by the California Medical Association and the State Department of Public Health in January 1967, the risk of fatal aplastic anemia was estimated at 1:24,200 to 1:40,500 based on two dosage levels.

There have been reports of aplastic anemia attributed to chloramphenicol which later terminated in leukemia.

Paroxysmal nocturnal hemoglobinuria has also been reported.

2. Gastrointestinal Reactions

Nausea, vomiting, glossitis and stomatitis, diarrhea, and enterocolitis may occur in low incidence.

3. Neurotoxic Reactions

Headache, mild depression, mental confusion, and delirium have been described in patients receiving chloramphenicol. Optic and peripheral neuritis have been reported, usually following long-term therapy. If this occurs, the drug should be promptly withdrawn.

4. Hypersensitivity Reactions

Fever, macular and vesicular rashes, angio- edema, urticaria, and anaphylaxis may occur. Herxheimer reactions have occurred during therapy for typhoid fever.

5. "Gray Syndrome"

Toxic reactions including fatalities have occurred in the premature and newborn; the signs and symptoms associated with these reactions have been referred to as the gray syndrome. One case of gray syndrome has been reported in an infant born to a mother having received chloramphenicol during labor. One case has been reported in a 3-month-old infant. The following summarizes the clinical and laboratory studies that have been made on these patients:

a) In most cases, therapy with chloramphenicol had been instituted within the first 48 hours of life.
b) Symptoms first appeared after 3 to 4 days of continued treatment with high doses of chloramphenicol.
c) The symptoms appeared in the following order:
 (1) abdominal distention with or without emesis;
 (2) progressive pallid cyanosis;
 (3) vasomotor collapse, frequently accompanied by irregular respiration;
 (4) death within a few hours of onset of these symptoms.
d) The progression of symptoms from onset to exitus was accelerated with higher dose schedules.
e) Preliminary blood serum level studies revealed unusually high concentrations of chloramphenicol (over 90 mcg/ml after repeated doses).
f) Termination of therapy upon early evidence of the associated symptomatology frequently reversed the process with complete recovery.

ADMINISTRATION

Chloramphenicol, like other potent drugs, should be prescribed at recommended doses known to have therapeutic activity. Administration of 50 mg/kg/day in divided doses will produce blood levels of the magnitude to which the majority of susceptible microorganisms will respond.

As soon as feasible, an oral dosage form of chloramphenicol should be substituted for the intravenous form because adequate blood levels are achieved with chloramphenicol by mouth.

The following method of administration is recommended:

Intravenously as a 10% (100 mg/ml) solution to be injected over at least a one-minute interval. This is prepared by the addition of 10 ml of an aqueous diluent, such as water for injection or 5% dextrose injection.

DOSAGE

Adults

Adults should receive 50 mg/kg/day in divided doses at 6-hour intervals. In exceptional cases, patients with infections due to moderately resistant organisms may require increased dosage up to 100 mg/kg/day to achieve blood levels inhibiting the pathogen, but these high doses should be decreased as soon as possible. Adults with impairment of hepatic or renal function or both may have reduced ability to metabolize and excrete the drug. In instances of impaired metabolic processes, dosages should be adjusted accordingly. (See discussion under Newborn Infants.) Precise control of concentration of the drug in the blood should be carefully followed in patients with impaired metabolic processes by the available microtechniques (information available on request).

Children

Dosage of 50 mg/kg/day divided into 4 doses at 6-hour intervals yields blood levels in the range effective against most susceptible organisms. Severe infections (eg, bacteremia or meningitis), especially when adequate cerebrospinal fluid concentrations are desired, may require dosage up to 100 mg/kg/day; however, it is recommended that dosage be reduced to 50 mg/kg/day as soon as possible. Children with impaired liver or kidney function may retain excessive amounts of the drug.

Newborn Infants

(See section titled Gray Syndrome under Adverse Reactions.)

A total of 25 mg/kg/day in 4 equal doses at 6-hour intervals usually produces and maintains concentrations in blood and tissues adequate to control most infections for which the drug is indicated. Increased dosage in these individuals, demanded by severe infections, should be given only to maintain the blood concentration within a therapeutically effective range. After the first two weeks of life, full-term infants ordinarily may receive up to a total of 50 mg/kg/day equally divided into 4 doses at 6-hour intervals. *These dosage recommendations are extremely important because blood concentration in all premature infants and full-term infants under two weeks of age differs from that of other infants.* This difference is due to variations in the maturity of the metabolic functions of the liver and the kidneys.

When these functions are immature (or seriously impaired in adults), high concentrations of the drug are found which tend to increase with succeeding doses.

Infants and Children with Immature Metabolic Processes

In young infants and other children in whom immature metabolic functions are suspected, a dose of 25 mg/kg/day will usually produce therapeutic concentrations of the drug in the blood. In this group particularly, the concentration of the drug in the blood should be carefully followed by microtechniques. (Information available on request.)

HOW SUPPLIED

N 0071-4057-03—(Steri-Vial® No. 57) Chloromycetin Sodium Succinate (Chloramphenicol Sodium Succinate for Injection, USP) is freeze-dried in the vial and supplied in Steri-Vials (rubber diaphragm-capped vials). When reconstituted as directed, each vial contains a sterile solution equivalent to 100 mg of chloramphenicol per milliliter (1 g/10 ml). Available in packages of 10 vials.

Chloromycetin, brand of chloramphenicol, Reg US Pat Off

AHFS 8:12.08 **4057G020**

Continued on next page

This product information was prepared in August 1992. On these and other Parke-Davis Products, information may be obtained by addressing PARKE-DAVIS, Division of Warner-Lambert Company, Morris Plains, New Jersey 07950.

Parke-Davis—Cont.

CHOLEDYL® ℞
[*kō 'lĕ-dyl"*]
(oxtriphylline, USP)
Delayed-release Tablets, USP

DESCRIPTION

Choledyl Delayed-release tablets contain oxtriphylline which is the choline salt of theophylline. Theophylline is a bronchodilator structurally classified as a xanthine derivative. It occurs as a white, odorless, crystalline powder having a bitter taste. Theophylline anhydrous has the chemical name 1*H*-Purine-2,6-dione, 3,7-dihydro-1,3-dimethyl-. The molecular formula is $C_{12}H_{21}N_5O_3$. The molecular weight is 283.33.
Choledyl tablets are available as enteric, sugar-coated tablets intended for oral administration, containing 100 mg or 200 mg oxtriphylline (64 mg and 127 mg of theophylline anhydrous, respectively). Each tablet also contains acacia, NF; precipitated calcium carbonate, USP; tribasic calcium phosphate, NF; carnauba wax; confectioner's sugar, NF; gelatin, NF; kaolin, USP; magnesium stearate, NF; pharmaceutical glaze; starch, NF; sucrose, NF; talc, USP; titanium dioxide, USP; tragacanth, NF; and white wax, NF. The 100-mg tablet also contains D&C red No. 7 Lake and FD&C yellow No. 6 Lake. The 200-mg tablet also contains D&C yellow No. 10.

CLINICAL PHARMACOLOGY

Theophylline directly relaxes the smooth muscle of the bronchial airways and pulmonary blood vessels, thus acting mainly as a bronchodilator and smooth muscle relaxant. It has also been demonstrated that aminophylline has a potent effect on diaphragmatic contractility in normal persons and may then be capable of reducing fatigability and thereby improve contractility in patients with chronic obstructive airways disease. The exact mode of action remains unsettled.
Although theophylline does cause inhibition of phosphodiesterase with a resultant increase in intracellular cyclic AMP, other agents similarly inhibit the enzyme producing a rise of cyclic AMP but are unassociated with any demonstrable bronchodilation. Other mechanisms proposed include an effect on translocation of intracellular calcium; prostaglandin antagonism; stimulation of catecholamines endogenously; inhibition of cyclic guanosine monophosphate metabolism and adenosine receptor antagonism. None of these mechanisms has been proved, however.
In vitro, theophylline has been shown to act synergistically with beta agonists, and there are now available data which do demonstrate an additive effect in vivo with combined use.

Pharmacokinetics:
The half-life of theophylline is influenced by a number of known variables. It may be prolonged in chronic alcoholics, particularly those with liver disease (cirrhosis or alcoholic liver disease), in patients with congestive heart failure, and in those patients taking certain other drugs (see PRECAUTIONS, Drug Interactions). Newborns and neonates have extremely slow clearance rates compared to older infants and children, ie, those over 1 year. Older children have rapid clearance rates while most nonsmoking adults have clearance rates between these two extremes. In premature neonates, the decreased clearance is related to oxidative pathways that have yet to be established.

Theophylline Elimination Characteristics

	Range	Half-Life (in hours) *Mean*
Children	1–9	3.7
Adults	3–15	7.7

In cigarette smokers (1–2 packs/day) the mean half-life is 4–5 hours, much shorter than in nonsmokers. The increase in clearance associated with smoking is presumably due to stimulation of the hepatic metabolic pathway by components of cigarette smoke. The duration of this effect after cessation of smoking is unknown but may require 6 months to 2 years before the rate approaches that of the nonsmoker.

INDICATIONS AND USAGE

Choledyl (oxtriphylline) is indicated for relief and/or prevention of symptoms from asthma and reversible bronchospasm associated with chronic bronchitis and emphysema.

CONTRAINDICATIONS

Choledyl is contraindicated in individuals who have shown hypersensitivity to its components. It is also contraindicated in patients with active peptic ulcer disease, and in individuals with underlying seizure disorders (unless receiving appropriate anticonvulsant medication).

WARNINGS

Serum levels above 20 μg/mL are rarely found after appropriate administration of the recommended doses. However, in individuals in whom theophylline plasma clearance is reduced *for any reason,* even conventional doses may result in increased serum levels and potential toxicity. Reduced theophylline clearance has been documented in the following readily identifiable groups: 1) patients with impaired liver function; 2) patients over 55 years of age, particularly males and those with chronic lung disease; 3) those with cardiac failure from any cause; 4) patients with sustained high fever; 5) neonates and infants under 1 year of age; and 6) those patients taking certain drugs (see PRECAUTIONS, Drug Interactions). Frequently, such patients have markedly prolonged theophylline serum levels following discontinuation of the drug.
Reduction of dosage and laboratory monitoring is especially appropriate in the above individuals.
Serious side effects such as ventricular arrhythmias, convulsions or even death may appear as the first sign of toxicity without any previous warning. Less serious signs of theophylline toxicity (ie, nausea and restlessness) may occur frequently when initiating therapy, but are usually transient; when such signs are persistent during maintenance therapy, they are often associated with serum concentrations above 20 μg/mL. Stated differently; *serious toxicity is not reliably preceded by less severe side effects.* A serum concentration measurement is the only reliable method of predicting potentially life-threatening toxicity.
Many patients who require theophylline exhibit tachycardia due to their underlying disease process so that the cause/effect relationship to elevated serum theophylline concentrations may not be appreciated.
Theophylline products may cause dysrhythmia and/or worsen preexisting arrhythmias and any significant change in rate and/or rhythm warrants monitoring and further investigation.
Studies in laboratory animals (minipigs, rodents, and dogs) recorded the occurrence of cardiac arrhythmias and sudden death (with histologic evidence of myocardial necrosis) when beta-agonists and methylxanthines were administered concurrently. The significance of these findings when applied to humans is currently unknown.

PRECAUTIONS

General:
On the average, theophylline half-life is shorter in cigarette and marijuana smokers than in nonsmokers, but smokers can have half-lives as long as nonsmokers. Theophylline should not be administered concurrently with other xanthines. Use with caution in patients with hypoxemia, hypertension, or those with history of peptic ulcer. Theophylline may occasionally act as a local irritant to the GI tract although gastrointestinal symptoms are more commonly centrally mediated and associated with serum drug concentrations over 20 μg/mL.

Information for Patients:
Tablets should not be chewed, or crushed or dissolved.
The importance of taking only the prescribed dose and time interval between doses should be reinforced.

Laboratory Tests:
Serum levels should be monitored periodically to determine the theophylline level associated with observed clinical response and as the method of predicting toxicity. For such measurements, the serum sample should be obtained at the time of peak concentration, 1 to 2 hours after administration for immediate release products. It is important that the patient will not have missed or taken additional doses during the previous 48 hours and that dosing intervals will have been reaonably equally spaced. DOSAGE ADJUSTMENT BASED ON SERUM THEOPHYLLINE MEASUREMENTS WHEN THESE INSTRUCTIONS HAVE NOT BEEN FOLLOWED MAY RESULT IN RECOMMENDATIONS THAT PRESENT RISK OF TOXICITY TO THE PATIENT.

Drug Interactions:
Toxic synergism with ephedrine has been documented and may occur with other sympathomimetic bronchodilators. In addition, the following drug interactions have been demonstrated: [See table at top of next column.]

Theophylline with:	
Allopurinol (high-dose)	Increased serum theophylline levels
Cimetidine	Increased serum theophylline levels
Erythromycin, Troleandomycin	Increased serum theophylline levels
Lithium Carbonate	Increased renal excretion of lithium
Oral Contraceptives	Increased serum theophylline levels
Phenytoin	Decreased theophylline and phenytoin serum levels
Rifampin	Decreased serum theophylline levels

Drug-Laboratory Test Interactions:
Currently available analytical methods, including high pressure liquid chromatography and immunoassay techniques, for measuring serum theophylline levels are specific. Metabolites and other drugs generally do not affect the results. Other new analytic methods are also now in use. The physician should be aware of the laboratory method used and whether other drugs will interfere with the assay for theophylline.

Carcinogenesis, Mutagenesis, and Impairment of Fertility:
Long-term carcinogenicity studies have not been performed with theophylline.
Chromosome-breaking activity was detected in human cell cultures at concentrations of theophylline up to 50 times the therapeutic serum concentration in humans. Theophylline was not mutagenic in the dominant lethal assay in male mice given theophylline intraperitoneally in doses up to 30 times the maximum daily oral dose.
Studies to determine the effect on fertility have not been performed with theophylline.

Pregnancy:
Category C—Animal reproduction studies have not been conducted with oxtriphylline. It is not known whether theophylline can cause fetal harm when administered to a pregnant woman or can affect reproduction capacity. Oxtriphylline should be given to a pregnant woman only if clearly needed.

Nursing Mothers:
Theophylline is distributed into breast milk and may cause irritability or other signs of toxicity in nursing infants. Because of the potential for serious adverse reactions in nursing infants from theophylline, a decision should be made whether to discontinue nursing or to discontinue the drug, taking into account the importance of the drug to the mother.

Pediatric Use:
Sufficient numbers of infants under the age of 1 year have not been studied in clinical trials to support use in this age group; however, there is evidence recorded that the use of dosage recomendations for older infants and young children (16 mg/kg/24 hours) may result in the development of toxic serum levels. Such findings very probably reflect differences in the metabolic handling of the drug related to absent or undeveloped enzyme systems. Consequently, the use of the drug in this age group should carefully consider the associated benefits and risks. If used, the maintenance dose must be conservative and in accord with the following guidelines:

Initial Theophylline Maintenance Dosage:
Premature Infants:
Up to 24 days postnatal age—1.0 mg/kg q 12h
Beyond 24 days postnatal age—1.5 mg/kg q 12h
Infants 6 to 52 Weeks:
$[(0.2 \times \text{age in weeks}) + 5.0] \times \text{kg body wt} = 24$ hour dose in mg.
Up to 26 weeks, divide into q 8h dosing intervals.
From 26–52 weeks, divide into q 6h dosing intervals.
Final dosage should be guided by serum concentration after a steady state (no further accumulation of drug) has been achieved.

ADVERSE REACTIONS

The following adverse reactions have been observed, but there has not been enough systematic collection of data to support an estimate of their frequency. The most consistent adverse reactions are usually due to overdosage.
1. **Gastrointestinal:** nausea, vomiting, epigastric pain, hematemesis, diarrhea.
2. **Central nervous system:** headaches, irritability, restlessness, insomnia, reflex hyperexcitability, muscle twitching, clonic and tonic generalized convulsions.
3. **Cardiovascular:** palpitation, tachycardia, extrasystoles, flushing, hypotension, circulatory failure, ventricular arrhythmias.
4. **Respiratory:** tachypnea.
5. **Renal:** potentiation of diuresis.
6. **Others:** alopecia, hyperglycemia, inappropriate ADH syndrome, rash.

OVERDOSAGE

Management:
It is suggested that the management principles (consistent with the clinical status of the patient when first seen) outlined below be instituted and that simultaneous contact with a Regional Poison Control Center be established. In this way both updated information and individualization regarding required therapy may be provided.
1. When potential oral overdose is established and seizure has not occurred:
   a. If patient is alert and seen within the early hours after ingestion, induction of emesis may be of value. Gastric lavage has been demonstrated to be of no value in influ-

encing outcome in patients who present more than 1 hour after ingestion.

b. Administer a cathartic. Sorbitol solution is reported to be of value.

c. Administer repeated doses of activated charcoal and monitor theophylline serum levels.

d. Prophylactic administration of phenobarbital has been shown to increase the seizure threshold in laboratory animals, and administration of this drug can be considered.

2. If patient presents with a seizure:

a. Establish an airway.

b. Administer oxygen.

c. Treat the seizure with intravenous diazepam, 0.1 to 0.3 mg/kg up to 10 mg. If seizures cannot be controlled, the use of general anesthesia should be considered.

d. Monitor vital signs, maintain blood pressure and provide adequate hydration.

3. If postseizure coma is present:

a. Maintain airway and oxygenation.

b. If a result of oral medication, follow above recommendations to prevent absorption of the drug, but intubation and lavage will have to be performed instead of inducing emesis, and the cathartic and charcoal will need to be introduced via large bore gastric lavage tube.

c. Continue to provide full supportive care and adequate hydration until the drug is metabolized. In general, drug metabolism is sufficiently rapid so as not to warrant dialysis. If repeated oral activated charcoal is ineffective (as noted by stable or rising serum levels), charcoal hemoperfusion may be indicated.

DOSAGE AND ADMINISTRATION

Tablets should not be chewed, or crushed or dissolved.

Effective use of theophylline (ie, the concentration of drug in the serum associated with optimal benefit and minimal risk of toxicity) is considered to occur when the theophylline concentration is maintained from 10 to 20 μg/mL. The early studies from which these levels were derived were carried out in patients immediately or shortly after recovery from acute exacerbations of their disease (some hospitalized with status asthmaticus).

Although the 20 μg/mL level remains appropriate as a critical value (above which toxicity is more likely to occur) for safety purposes, additional data are now available which indicate that the serum theophylline concentrations required to produce maximum physiologic benefit may, in fact, fluctuate with the degree of bronchospasm present and are variable. Therefore, the physician should individualize the range appropriate to the patient's requirements, based on both symptomatic response and improvement in pulmonary function. It should be stressed that serum theophylline concentrations maintained at the upper level of the 10 to 20 μg/mL range may be associated with potential toxicity when factors known to reduce theophylline clearance are operative. (See WARNINGS).

If it is not possible to obtain serum level determinations, restriction of the daily dose (in otherwise healthy adults) to not greater than 13 mg/kg/day (of anhydrous theophylline), to a maximum of 900 mg, in divided doses will result in relatively few patients exceeding serum levels of 20 μg/mL and the resultant greater risk of toxicity.

Caution should be exercised for younger children who cannot complain of minor side effects. Older adults, those with cor pulmonale, congestive heart failure, and/or liver disease may have unusually low dosage requirements and thus may experience toxicity at the maximal dosage recommended below.

Theophylline does not distribute into fatty tissue. Dosage should be calculated on the basis of lean (ideal) body weight where mg/kg doses are presented.

Frequency of Dosing:

When immediate release products with rapid absorption are used, dosing to maintain serum levels generally requires administration every 6 hours. This is particularly true in children, but dosing intervals up to 8 hours may be satisfactory in adults since they eliminate the drug at a slower rate. Some children and adults requiring higher than average doses (those having rapid rates of clearance, eg, half-lives of under 6 hours) may benefit and be more effectively controlled during chronic therapy when given products with sustained release characteristics since these provide longer dosing intervals and/or less fluctuation in serum concentration between dosing.

Dosage guidelines are approximations only and the wide range of theophylline clearance between individuals (particularly those with concomitant disease) make indiscriminate usage hazardous.

Dosage Guidelines:

The following dosage information relates to initiation and titration of daily dosage requirements utilizing a nonsustained action form of Choledyl (eg, Choledyl Tabs, Elixir).

I. Acute symptoms of bronchospasm requiring rapid attainment of theophylline serum levels for bronchodilation.

NOTE: Status asthmaticus should be considered a medical emergency and is defined as that degree of bronchospasm which is not rapidly responsive to usual doses of conven-

Choledyl Dosage	Oral Loading	Maintenance
Children age 1 to 9 years	7.8 mg/kg *(5 mg/kg)	6.2 mg/kg q 6 hours *(4 mg/kg q 6 hours)
Children age 9 to 16 years and smokers	7.8 mg/kg *(5 mg/kg)	4.7 mg/kg q 6 hours *(3 mg/kg q 6 hours)
Otherwise healthy nonsmoking adults	7.8 mg/kg *(5 mg/kg)	4.7 mg/kg q 8 hours *(3 mg/kg q 8 hours)
Older patients and patients with cor pulmonale	7.8 mg/kg *(5 mg/kg)	3.1 mg/kg q 8 hours *(2 mg/kg q 8 hours)
Patients with congestive heart failure	7.8 mg/kg *(5 mg/kg)	1.6–3.1 mg/kg q 12 hours *(1–2 mg/kg q 12 hours)

* Anhydrous theophylline included in ( ).

tional bronchodilators. Optimal therapy for such patients frequently requires both *additional medication*, parenterally administered, and *close monitoring*, preferably in an intensive care setting.

A. Patients not currently receiving theophylline products. [See table above.]

B. Patients currently receiving theophylline products: Determine, where possible, the time, amount, dosage form, and route of administration of the last dose the patient received.

The loading dose for theophylline will be based on the principle that each 0.8 mg/kg oxtriphylline (equivalent to 0.5 mg/kg of theophylline) administered as a loading dose will result in a 1.0 μg/mL increase in serum theophylline concentration. Ideally, the loading dose should be deferred if a serum theophylline concentration can be obtained rapidly.

If this is not possible, the clinician must exercise judgment in selecting a dose based on the potential for benefit and risk. When there is sufficient respiratory distress to warrant a small risk, then 4 mg/kg of oxtriphylline (equivalent to 2.5 mg/kg of theophylline) administered in rapidly absorbed form is likely to increase the serum concentration by approximately 5 μg/mL. If the patient is not experiencing theophylline toxicity, this is unlikely to result in dangerous adverse effects.

Subsequent to the decision regarding use of a loading dose for this group of patients, the maintenance dosage recommendations are the same as those described above.

II. Chronic Therapy

Theophylline is a treatment for the management of reversible bronchospasm (asthma, chronic bronchitis and emphysema) to prevent symptoms and maintain patent airways. A dosage form which allows small incremental doses is desirable for initiating therapy. A liquid preparation should be considered for children to permit both greater ease of and more accurate dosage adjustment. Slow clinical titration is generally preferred to assure acceptance and safety of the medication, and to allow the patient to develop tolerance to transient caffeine-like side effects.

Initial Dose: 25mg*/kg/24 hours or 625 mg/24 hours (whichever is less) of oxtriphylline in divided doses at 6- or 8-hour intervals.

Increasing Dose: The above dosage may be increased in approximately 25-percent increments at 3-day intervals as long as the drug is tolerated; until clinical response is satisfactory or the maximum dose as indicated in section III (below) is reached. The serum concentration may be checked at these intervals, but at a minimum, should be determined at the end of this adjustment period.

It is important that no patient be maintained on any dosage that is not tolerated. When instructing patients to increase dosage according to the schedule above, they should be told not to take a subsequent dose if apparent side effects occur and to resume therapy at a lower dose once adverse effects have disappeared.

III. Maximum Dose of Choledyl (oxtriphylline) Where the Serum Concentration is Not Measured

WARNING: DO NOT ATTEMPT TO MAINTAIN ANY DOSE THAT IS NOT TOLERATED.

Not to exceed the following: [or 1400 mg** (900 mg) whichever is less]

Age 1–9 years	37.5 mg/kg/day	**(24 mg/kg/day)
Age 9–12 years	31 mg/kg/day	**(20 mg/kg/day)
Age 12–16 years	28 mg/kg/day	**(18 mg/kg/day)
Age 16 years and older	20 mg/kg/day	**(13 mg/kg/day)

**Anhydrous theophylline indicated in ( ).

* 25 mg oxtriphylline = 16 mg anhydrous theophylline.

IV. Measurement of Serum Theophylline Concentrations During Chronic Therapy.

If the above maximum doses are to be maintained or exceeded, serum theophylline measurement is essential (see PRECAUTIONS, Laboratory Tests, for guidance).

V. Final Adjustment of Dosage

Dosage adjustment after serum theophylline measurement:

If serum theophylline is:		Directions:
Within desired range		Maintain dosage if tolerated.
Too high	20 to 25 μg/mL	Decrease doses by about 10% and recheck serum level after 3 days.
	25 to 30 μg/mL	Skip the next dose and decrease subsequent doses by about 25%. Recheck serum level after 3 days.
	Over 30 μg/mL	Skip next 2 doses and decrease subsequent doses by 50%. Recheck serum level after 3 days.
Too low		Increase dosage by 25% at 3-day intervals until either the desired serum concentration and/or clinical response is achieved. The total daily dose may need to be administered at more frequent intervals if symptoms occur repeatedly at the end of a dosing interval.

The serum concentration may be rechecked at appropriate intervals, but at least at the end of any adjustment period. When the patient's condition is otherwise clinically stable and none of the recognized factors which alter elimination are present, measurement of serum levels need be repeated only every 6 to 12 months.

HOW SUPPLIED

Choledyl (oxtriphylline) 100 mg is supplied as round, red, enteric, sugar-coated tablets, coded PD 210, in bottles of 100 (N 0071-0210-24).

Choledyl (oxtriphylline) 200 mg is supplied as round, yellow, enteric, sugar-coated tablets, coded PD 211, in bottles of 100 (N 0071-0211-24), 1000 (N 0071-0211-32) and Unit Dose—10 × 10 strips (N 0071-0211-40).

Store between 15°–30°C (59°–86°F).

Caution—Federal law prohibits dispensing without prescription.

0210G055

Shown in Product Identification Section, page 422

Continued on next page

This product information was prepared in August 1992. On these and other Parke-Davis Products, information may be obtained by addressing PARKE-DAVIS, Division of Warner-Lambert Company, Morris Plains, New Jersey 07950.

Parke-Davis—Cont.

CHOLEDYL® SA   ℞
[kō'lĕ-dyl"]
(Oxtriphylline Extended-release Tablets, USP)

DESCRIPTION

Choledyl (oxtriphylline) is a xanthine bronchodilator—the choline salt of theophylline.

Each film-coated Choledyl SA tablet contains 400 mg or 600 mg oxtriphylline (equivalent to 254 mg or 382 mg anhydrous theophylline, respectively). Each tablet also contains, candelilla wax, confectioner's sugar, NF; magnesium stearate, NF; Opaseal pharmaceutical sealant; talc, USP and other ingredients. The 400-mg tablet also contains Opaspray pink and triethyl citrate. The 600-mg tablet also contains Opaspray tan.

Each tablet of Choledyl SA contains oxtriphylline in a tablet matrix specially designed for the prolonged release of the drug in the gastrointestinal tract. Following release of the drug, the expended wax tablet matrix, which is not absorbed, may be detected in the stool.

CLINICAL PHARMACOLOGY

Choledyl (oxtriphylline), the choline salt of theophylline, effects significant improvement in pulmonary function parameters which have been impaired by bronchospasm. It is more soluble than either aminophylline or theophylline. Film-coated Choledyl SA tablets are less irritating to the gastric mucosa than aminophylline.

Choledyl SA tablets have been formulated to provide therapeutic serum levels when administered every 12 hours and minimize the peaks and valleys of serum levels commonly found with shorter acting theophylline products.

The sustained action characteristic of Choledyl SA tablets has been demonstrated in studies in human subjects. Single and multiple dose studies have shown equivalent steady-state theophylline plasma levels of Choledyl SA tablets given every 12 hours when compared with an equal total daily dose of (the nonsustained action) Choledyl Elixir given every six hours.

Theophylline directly relaxes the smooth muscle of the bronchial airways and pulmonary blood vessels, thus acting mainly as a bronchodilator, pulmonary vasodilator and smooth muscle relaxant. The drug also possesses other actions typical of the xanthine derivatives: coronary vasodilator, diuretic, cardiac stimulant, cerebral stimulant and skeletal muscle stimulant. The actions of theophylline may be mediated through inhibition of phosphodiesterase and a resultant increase in intracellular cyclic AMP which could mediate smooth muscle relaxation. At concentrations higher than attained *in vivo*, theophylline also inhibits the release of histamine by mast cells.

Theophylline has been shown to react synergistically with beta agonists that increase intracellular cyclic AMP through the stimulation of adenyl cyclase (isoproterenol).

Apparently, the development of tolerance does not occur with chronic use of theophylline.

The half-life is shortened with cigarette smoking. The half-life is prolonged in alcoholism, reduced hepatic or renal function, congestive heart failure, and in patients receiving antibiotics such as TAO (troleandomycin), erythromycin and clindamycin. High fever for prolonged periods may decrease theophylline elimination.

Theophylline Elimination Characteristics

	Theophylline Clearance Rates (mean ± S.D.)	Half-Life Average (mean ± S.D.)
Children (over 6 months of age)	1.45 ± .58 ml/kg/min	3.7 ± 1.1 hours
Adult non-smokers with uncomplicated asthma	.65 ± .19 ml/kg/min	8.7 ± 2.2 hours

Newborn infants have extremely slow clearance and half-lives exceeding 24 hours, which approach those seen for older children after about 3–6 months.

Older adults with chronic obstructive pulmonary disease, and patients with cor pulmonale or other causes of heart failure, and patients with liver pathology may have much lower clearances with half-lives that may exceed 24 hours. The half-life of theophylline is prolonged in patients with congestive heart failure, in those with reduced hepatic or renal function, and in alcoholism. The half-life of theophylline may also be prolonged by concurrent use of various drugs such as phenobarbital, and certain antibiotics, including troleandomycin, erythromycin, and lincomycin.

Theophylline half-life is shortened in cigarette smokers (1 to 2 packs/day) as compared to nonsmokers. The increase in theophylline clearance caused by smoking is probably the result of induction of drug metabolizing enzymes that do not readily normalize after cessation of smoking. It appears that between 3 months and 2 years may be necessary for normalization of the effect of smoking on theophylline pharmacokinetics.

INDICATIONS

Choledyl (oxtriphylline) is indicated for relief of acute and chronic bronchial asthma and for reversible bronchospasm associated with chronic bronchitis and emphysema.

CONTRAINDICATIONS

Choledyl is contraindicated in individuals who have shown hypersensitivity to theophylline or to Choledyl (oxtriphylline) or any of its components.

WARNINGS

Status asthmaticus is a medical emergency. Optimal therapy frequently requires additional medication including corticosteroids when the patient is not rapidly responsive to bronchodilators.

Excessive theophylline doses may be associated with toxicity, and serum theophylline levels are recommended to assure maximal benefit without excessive risk; incidence of toxicity increases at levels greater than 20 mcg theophylline/ml. Morphine, curare, and stilbamidine should be used with caution in patients with airflow obstruction since they stimulate histamine release and can induce asthmatic attacks. These drugs may also suppress respiration leading to respiratory failure. Alternative drugs should be chosen whenever possible.

There is an excellent correlation between high blood levels of theophylline resulting from conventional doses and associated clinical manifestations of toxicity in patients with liver dysfunction or chronic obstructive lung disease.

There is excellent correlation between high serum levels of theophylline (over 20 mcg/ml) and the clinical manifestations of toxicity. Careful reduction of dosage and monitoring of serum levels are especially important in patients manifesting a decrease in total body theophylline clearance rate, including those with generalized debility, acute hypoxia, cardiac decompensation, hepatic dysfunction, or renal failure. Dosage reduction may also be necessary in patients who are older than 55 years of age, particularly males.

Serious toxic effects may occur suddenly and are not invariably preceded by minor adverse effects such as nausea, vomiting, and restlessness. Convulsions, tachycardia, or ventricular arrhythmias may be the first sign of toxicity.

Children have a marked sensitivity to the CNS stimulant action of theophylline. Serious toxic effects, including fatalities have been reported in children as well as adults.

Theophylline products may worsen pre-existing arrhythmias.

USAGE IN PREGNANCY

Safe use of Choledyl (oxtriphylline) in pregnancy and lactation has not been established relative to possible adverse effects on fetal or neonatal development. Therefore Choledyl (oxtriphylline) should not be used in patients who are pregnant or who may become pregnant, or during lactation unless, in the judgment of the physician, the potential benefits outweigh the possible hazards.

PRECAUTIONS

Mean half-life in smokers is shorter than nonsmokers, therefore, smokers may require larger doses of theophylline. Theophylline should not be administered concurrently with other xanthine medications or with xanthine-containing beverages or foods. Use with caution in patients with severe cardiac disease, severe hypoxemia, hypertension, hyperthyroidism, acute myocardial injury, cor pulmonale, congestive heart failure, or liver disease, and in the elderly (especially males) and in neonates. Great caution should especially be used in giving theophylline to patients in congestive heart failure. Such patients have shown markedly prolonged theophylline blood level curves with theophylline persisting in serum for long periods following discontinuation of the drug. Use theophylline cautiously in patients with a history of peptic ulcer. Theophylline may occasionally act as a local irritant to the GI tract although gastrointestinal symptoms are more commonly central and associated with serum theophylline concentrations over 20 mcg/ml.

ADVERSE REACTIONS

The most consistent adverse reactions are usually due to overdose and are:

1. Gastrointestinal: nausea, vomiting, epigastric pain, hematemesis, diarrhea.
2. Central nervous system: headaches, irritability, restlessness, insomnia, reflex hyperexcitability, muscle twitching, clonic and tonic generalized convulsions.
3. Cardiovascular: palpitation, tachycardia, extrasystoles, flushing, hypotension, circulatory failure, life-threatening ventricular arrhythmias.
4. Respiratory: tachypnea.
5. Renal: albuminuria, increased excretion of renal tubular cells and red blood cells, diuresis.
6. Others: hyperglycemia and inappropriate antidiuretic hormone (ADH) syndrome.

Drug Interactions: Theophylline-containing preparations have exhibited interaction with the following drugs:

Drug	Effect
Lithium carbonate	Increased excretion of lithium carbonate.
Propranolol	Antagonism of propranolol effect.
Furosemide	Increased furosemide diuresis.
Hexamethonium	Decreased hexamethonium-induced chronotropic effect
Reserpine	Reserpine-induced tachycardia.
Chlordiazepoxide	Chlordiazepoxide-induced fatty acid mobilization.
Troleandomycin, erythromycin or lincomycin	Increased theophylline plasma levels.

DOSAGE AND ADMINISTRATION

Therapy should be initiated and daily dosage requirements established utilizing a nonsustained-action form of Choledyl (oxtriphylline) (eg, Choledyl Tablets, Elixir).

If the total daily maintenance dosage requirement of the Choledyl (oxtriphylline) nonsustained preparation is established at approximately 1200 mg, Choledyl SA 600 mg Sustained Action Tablets, one every 12 hours, may be substituted to provide smoother steady-state theophylline levels and the convenience of bid dosage. Similarly, if the total daily maintenance dosage is established at approximately 800 mg, Choledyl SA 400 mg Sustained Action Tablets, one every 12 hours, may be substituted.

Therapeutic serum levels associated with optimal likelihood of benefit and minimal risk of toxicity are considered to be between 10 mcg/ml and 20 mcg/ml. Levels above 20 mcg/ml may produce toxic effects.

There is great variation from patient to patient in dosage needed in order to achieve a therapeutic blood level because of variable rates of elimination. Because of this wide variation from patient to patient and the relatively narrow therapeutic blood level range, dosage must be individualized; monitoring of theophylline serum levels is highly recommended. Dosage should be calculated on the basis of lean (ideal) body weight—mg/kg. Theophylline does not distribute into fatty tissue.

Giving Choledyl (oxtriphylline) with food may prevent the rare case of stomach irritation, and although absorption may be slower, it is still complete.

When rapidly absorbed products such as solutions are used, dosing to maintain "around the clock" blood levels generally requires administration every 6 hours to obtain the greatest efficacy for use in children, dosing intervals up to 8 hours may be satisfactory for adults because of their slower elimination. Children and adults requiring higher than average doses may benefit from products with slower absorption. This may allow longer dosing intervals and/or less fluctuation in serum concentration over a dosing interval during chronic therapy. In patients receiving concurrent bronchodilator therapy, eg, beta agonists, downward adjustment of Choledyl (oxtriphylline) dosage is necessary.

The following dosage information relates to initiation and titration of daily dosage requirements utilizing a nonsustained action form of Choledyl (eg Choledyl Tabs, Elixir).
[See table on next page.]

II. *Those currently receiving theophylline products:*

Determine where possible, the time, amount, route of administration and form of the patient's last dose.

The loading dose for theophylline will be based on the principle that each 0.8 mg/kg of Choledyl (oxtriphylline) (0.5 mg/kg of theophylline) administered as a loading dose will result in a 1 mcg/ml increase in serum theophylline concentration. Ideally, then, the loading dose should be deferred if a serum theophylline concentration can be rapidly obtained. If this is not possible, the clinician must exercise his judgment in selecting a dose based on the potential for benefit and risk. When there is sufficient respiratory distress to warrant a small risk, 4 mg/kg Choledyl (oxtriphylline) (2.5 mg/kg of theophylline) is likely to increase the serum concentration when administered as a loading dose in rapidly absorbed form by only about 5 mcg/ml. If the patient is not already experiencing theophylline toxicity, this is unlikely to result in dangerous adverse effect.

Following the decision regarding loading dose in this group of patients, the subsequent maintenance dosage recommendations are the same as those described above.

To achieve optimal therapeutic theophylline dosage, monitoring of serum theophylline concentrations is recom-

CHOLEDYL (OXTRIPHYLLINE) DOSAGE FOR PATIENT POPULATION

Acute Symptoms of Asthma Requiring Rapid Theophyllinization:

1. *Not currently receiving theophylline products:*

GROUP	ORAL LOADING DOSE CHOLEDYL	MAINTENANCE DOSE FOR NEXT 12 HOURS CHOLEDYL	MAINTENANCE DOSE BEYOND 12 HOURS CHOLEDYL
1. Children 6 months to 9 years	9.4 mg/kg *(6 mg/kg)	6.2 mg/kg q4 hrs *(4 mg/kg q4 hrs)	6.2 mg/kg q6 hrs *(4 mg/kg q6 hrs)
2. Children age 9–16 and young adult smokers	9.4 mg/kg *(6 mg/kg)	4.7 mg/kg q4 hrs *(3 mg/kg q4 hrs)	4.7 mg/kg q6 hrs *(3 mg/kg q6 hrs)
3. Otherwise healthy nonsmoking adults	9.4 mg/kg *(6 mg/kg)	4.7 mg/kg q6 hrs *(3 mg/kg q6 hrs)	4.7 mg/kg q8 hrs *3 mg/kg q8 hrs)
4. Older patients and patients with cor pulmonale	9.4 mg/kg *(6 mg/kg)	3.1 mg/kg q6 hrs *(2 mg/kg q6 hrs)	3.1 mg/kg q8 hrs *(2 mg/kg q8 hrs)
5. Patients with congestive heart failure, liver failure	9.4 mg/kg *(6 mg/kg)	3.1 mg/kg q8 hrs *(2 mg/kg q8 hrs)	1.6–3.1 mg/kg q12 hrs *(1–2 mg/kg q12 hrs)

*Anhydrous theophylline indicated in ( ).

mended. However, it is not always possible or practical to obtain a serum theophylline level.
Patients should be closely monitored for signs of toxicity. The present data suggests that the above dosage recommendations will achieve therapeutic serum concentrations with minimal risk of toxicity for most patients. However, some risk of toxic serum concentrations is still present.
Adverse reactions to theophylline often occur when serum theophylline levels exceed 20 mcg/ml.

Chronic Asthma
Theophyllinization is a treatment of first choice for the management of chronic asthma (to prevent symptoms and maintain patent airways). Slow clinical titration is generally preferred to assure acceptance and safety of the medication. [See table below.]

Maximum dose of Choledyl (oxtriphylline) without measurement of serum theophylline concentration:
Not to exceed the following: (WARNING: DO NOT ATTEMPT TO MAINTAIN ANY DOSE THAT IS NOT TOLERATED)

Age <9 years	—37.5 mg/kg/day **(24 mg/kg/day)
Age 9–12 years	—31 mg/kg/day **(20 mg/kg/day)
Age 12–16 years	—28 mg/kg/day **(18 mg/kg/day)
Age >16 years	—20 mg/kg/day or 1400 mg/day (WHICHEVER IS LESS) **(13 mg/kg/day or 900 mg/day) (WHICHEVER IS LESS)

Note: Use ideal body weight for obese patients.
**Anhydrous theophylline indicated in ( ).

If the total daily maintenance dosage requirement of the Choledyl (oxtriphylline) nonsustained preparation is established at approximately 1200 mg, Choledyl SA 600 mg Sustained Action Tablets, one every 12 hours, may be substituted to provide smoother steady-state theophylline levels and the convenience of bid dosage. Similarly, if the total daily maintenance dosage is established at approximately 800 mg, Choledyl SA 400 mg Sustained Action Tablets, one every 12 hours, may be substituted.

Measurement of serum theophylline concentration during chronic therapy
If the above maximum dosages are to be maintained or exceeded, serum theophylline measurement is recommended. This should be obtained at the approximate time of peak absorption (1 to 2 hours after dosing) during chronic therapy. It is important that the patient will have missed *no* doses during the previous 48 hours and that dosing intervals will have been reasonably typical, with no added doses during that period of time.

DOSAGE ADJUSTMENT BASED ON SERUM THEOPHYLLINE MEASUREMENTS IF THE ABOVE INSTRUCTIONS HAVE NOT BEEN FOLLOWED MAY RESULT IN RISK OF TOXICITY TO THE PATIENT.
Caution should be exercised for younger children who cannot complain of minor side effects. Older adults, those with cor

pulmonale, congestive heart failure, and/or liver disease, may have unusually low dosage requirements and thus may experience toxicity at the maximal dosage recommended above.
It is important that no patient be maintained on any dosage that he is not tolerating. In instructing patients to increase dosage according to the schedule above, they should be instructed to not take a subsequent dose if apparent side effects occur and to resume therapy at a lower dose once adverse effects have disappeared.

OVERDOSAGE
Serious toxic effects due to overdosage may occur suddenly and are not invariably preceded by minor adverse effects. Therefore, careful observation of the patient and prompt institution of appropriate therapeutic measures are essential in all cases of overdosage. All patients suspected of overdosage should be hospitalized.

Signs and symptoms of overdosage are related primarily to the cardiovascular, gastrointestinal, and central nervous systems.
Cardiovascular symptoms include precordial pain, tachycardia, ventricular and other arrhythmias; also varying degrees of hypotension including, in extreme cases, severe shock, cardiovascular collapse and death.
Gastrointestinal symptoms include abdominal pain, nausea, persistent vomiting, and hematemesis.
Central nervous system symptoms include headache, dizziness, restlessness, irritability, tremors, hyperactivity, and agitation followed, in severe cases, by convulsions, drowsiness, coma and death.

Treatment of overdosage should be directed toward minimizing absorption and supporting vital functions.
In the alert patient emesis should be induced, followed by appropriate additional measures, as listed below.
In the obtunded patient, the airway should be secured immediately by means of an endotracheal tube with cuff inflated. After the airway has been secured, lavage should be carried out, and activated charcoal slurry and a cathartic should be administered.
CNS stimulation may be controlled with diazepam, 0.1–0.3 mg/kg intravenously in children, and 10 mg intravenously in adults. Respiration should be supported by appropriate means. Hypotension and shock should be treated with appropriate fluid replacement, avoiding the use of vasopressors, if possible. Additional supportive measures should be carried out as required.
Serial serum theophylline levels are of value in following the patient's course and in guiding further management.
Forced diuresis is of no value because of the small amount of theophylline excreted unchanged by the kidney. There has been a single report of survival with the use of an activated charcoal column (hemoperfusion) in massive theophylline overdosage.

HOW SUPPLIED
Choledyl SA 400 mg—each sustained action tablet contains 400 mg oxtriphylline. Available as pink film-coated tablets

in bottles of 100 (N 0071-0214-24), and unit-dose 100's (N 0071-0214-40).
Choledyl SA 600 mg—each sustained action tablet contains 600 mg oxtriphylline. Available as tan film-coated tablets in bottles of 100 (N 0071-0221-24), and unit-dose 100's (N 0071-0221-40).

0214G093
Shown in Product Identification Section, page 422

COLY-MYCIN® M PARENTERAL   ℞
[cō"ly-my'cĭn pă"rĕn'tĕr-ăl]
(sterile colistimethate sodium, USP)
for intramuscular and intravenous use

DESCRIPTION
Coly-Mycin M Parenteral (sterile colistimethate sodium) contains the sodium salt of colistimethate. Colistimethate sodium is a polypeptide antibiotic with an approximate molecular weight of 1750; the empirical formula is $C_{58}H_{105}N_{16}Na_5O_{28}S_5$.

CLINICAL PHARMACOLOGY
Microbiology
Coly-Mycin M Parenteral has bactericidal activity against the following gram-negative bacilli: *Enterobacter aerogenes, Escherichia coli, Klebsiella pneumoniae,* and *Pseudomonas aeruginosa.*

Human Pharmacology
Typical serum and urine levels following a single 150 mg dose of Coly-Mycin M Parenteral IM or IV in normal adult subjects are shown in Figure 1.

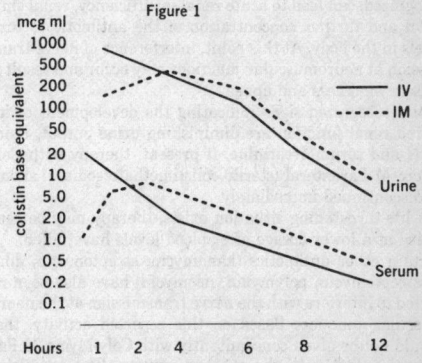

Figure 1. Urine and serum values in adults following parenteral (IM or IV) administration of Coly-Mycin M Parenteral Higher serum levels were obtained at 10 minutes following IV administration. Serum concentration declined with a half-life of 2-3 hours following either intravenous or intramuscular administration in adults and children, including premature infants.
Colistimethate sodium is transferred across the placental barrier, and blood levels of about 1 mcg/ml are obtained in the fetus following intravenous administration to the mother.
Average urine levels ranged from about 270 mcg/ml at 2 hours to about 15 mcg/ml at 8 hours after intravenous administration and from about 200 to about 25 mcg/ml during a similar period following intramuscular administration.

INDICATIONS AND USAGE
Coly-Mycin M Parenteral (sterile colistimethate sodium) is indicated for the treatment of acute or chronic infections due to sensitive strains of certain gram-negative bacilli. It is particularly indicated when the infection is caused by sensitive strains of *Pseudomonas aeruginosa.* This antibiotic is not indicated for infections due to *Proteus* or *Neisseria.* Coly-Mycin M Parenteral has proven clinically effective in treatment of infections due to the following gram-negative organisms: *Enterobacter aerogenes, Escherichia coli, Klebsiella pneumoniae,* and *Pseudomonas aeruginosa.*
Pending results of appropriate bacteriologic cultures and sensitivity tests, Coly-Mycin M Parenteral may be used to initiate therapy in serious infections that are suspected to be due to gram-negative organisms.

CONTRAINDICATIONS
The use of Coly-Mycin M Parenteral is contraindicated for patients with a history of sensitivity to the drug.

Continued on next page

This product information was prepared in August 1992. On these and other Parke-Davis Products, information may be obtained by addressing PARKE-DAVIS, Division of Warner-Lambert Company, Morris Plains, New Jersey 07950.

Choledyl (oxtriphylline)

Initial dose:	25 mg*/kg/day or 625 mg/day (whichever is lower) in 3 to 4 divided doses at 6–8 hour intervals.
Increased dose:	The above dosage may be increased in approximately 25 percent increments at 2 to 3 day intervals so long as no intolerance is observed until the maximum indicated below is reached.

*25 mg Choledyl = 16 mg anhydrous theophylline.

Parke-Davis—Cont.

WARNING

Maximum daily dose should not exceed 5 mg/kg/day (2.3 mg/lb) with normal renal function.

Transient neurological disturbances may occur. These include circumoral paresthesias or numbness, tingling or formication of the extremities, generalized pruritus, vertigo, dizziness, and slurring of speech. For these reasons, patients should be warned not to drive vehicles or use hazardous machinery while on therapy. Reduction of dosage may alleviate symptoms. Therapy need not be discontinued, but such patients should be observed with particular care. Overdosage can result in renal insufficiency, muscle weakness and apnea. See PRECAUTIONS for use concomitantly with curariform drugs, and DOSAGE and ADMINISTRATION Section for use in renal impairment.

PRECAUTIONS

Since Coly-Mycin M Parenteral (sterile colistimethate sodium) is eliminated mainly by renal excretion, it should be used with caution when the possibility of impaired renal function exists. The decline in renal function with advanced age should be considered.

When actual renal impairment is present, Coly-Mycin M Parenteral may be used, but the greatest caution should be exercised and the dosage should be reduced in proportion to the extent of the impairment. Administration of amounts of Coly-Mycin M Parenteral in excess of renal excretory capacity will lead to high serum levels and can result in further impairment of renal function, initiating a cycle which, if not recognized, can lead to acute renal insufficiency, renal shutdown and further concentration of the antibiotic to toxic levels in the body. At this point, interference of nerve transmission at neuromuscular junctions may occur and result in muscle weakness and apnea.

Easily recognized signs indicating the development of impaired renal function are diminishing urine output, rising BUN and serum creatinine. If present, therapy with Coly-Mycin M Parenteral (sterile colistimethate sodium) should be discontinued immediately.

If a life-threatening situation exists, therapy may be reinstated at a lower dosage after blood levels have fallen.

Certain other antibiotics (kanamycin, streptomycin, dihydrostreptomycin, polymyxin, neomycin) have also been reported to interfere with the nerve transmission at the neuromuscular junction. Based on this reported activity, they should not be given concomitantly with Coly-Mycin M Parenteral except with the greatest caution. The antibiotics with a gram-positive antimicrobial spectrum, e.g., penicillin, tetracycline, sodium cephalothin, have not been reported to interfere with nerve transmission and, accordingly, would not be expected to potentiate this activity of Coly-Mycin M Parenteral.

Other drugs, including curariform muscle relaxants (ether, tubocurarine, succinylcholine, gallamine, decamethonium and sodium citrate), potentiate the neuromuscular blocking effect and should be used with extreme caution in patients being treated with Coly-Mycin M Parenteral.

If apnea occurs, it may be treated with assisted respiration, oxygen, and calcium chloride injections.

USE IN PREGNANCY

The safety of colistimethate sodium during human pregnancy has not been established.

ADVERSE REACTIONS

Respiratory arrest has been reported following intramuscular administration of colistimethate sodium. Impaired renal function increases the possibility of apnea and neuromuscular blockade following administration of colistimethate sodium. This has been generally due to failure to follow recommended guidelines, usually overdosage, failure to reduce dose commensurate with degree of renal impairment, and/or concomitant use of other antibiotics or drugs with neuromuscular blocking potential.

A decrease in urine output or increase in blood urea nitrogen or serum creatinine can be interpreted as signs of nephrotoxicity, which is probably a dose-dependent effect of colistimethate sodium. These manifestations of nephrotoxicity are reversible following discontinuation of the antibiotic.

Increases of blood urea nitrogen have been reported for patients receiving Coly-Mycin M Parenteral (sterile colistimethate sodium) at dose levels of 1.6-5 mg/kg per day. The BUN values returned to normal following cessation of Coly-Mycin M Parenteral administration.

Paresthesia, tingling of the extremities or tingling of the tongue and generalized itching or urticaria have been reported by patients who received Coly-Mycin M Parenteral by intravenous or intramuscular injection. In addition, the following adverse reactions have been reported for colistimethate sodium: drug fever and gastrointestinal upset, vertigo, and slurring of speech. The subjective symptoms reported by the adult may not be manifest in infants or young children, thus requiring close attention to renal function.

DOSAGE AND ADMINISTRATION

Important: Coly-Mycin M Parenteral (sterile colistimethate sodium) is supplied in vials containing colistimethate sodium equivalent to 150 mg colistin base activity per vial.

Reconstitution: The *150-mg* vial should be reconstituted with *2.0 ml* Sterile Water for Injection USP. The reconstituted solution provides colistimethate sodium at a concentration of 75 mg/ml.

During reconstitution swirl *gently* to avoid frothing.

DOSAGE

Adults and children—intravenous or intramuscular administration—Coly-Mycin M Parenteral should be given in 2 to 4 divided doses at dose levels of 2.5 to 5 mg/kg per day for patients with normal renal function, depending on the severity of the infection.

The daily dose should be reduced in the presence of any renal impairment, which can often be anticipated from the history.

Modifications of dosage in the presence of renal impairment are presented in Table 1.

INTRAVENOUS ADMINISTRATION
1.   Direct Intermittent Administration — slowly inject one-half of the total daily dose over a period of 3 to 5 minutes every 12 hours.
2.   Continuous Infusion — slowly inject one-half the total daily dose over 3 to 5 minutes. Add the remaining half of the total daily dose of Coly-Mycin M Parenteral to one of the following: 0.9% NaCl;

5% dextrose in 0.9% NaCl; 5% dextrose in water; 5% dextrose in 0.45% NaCl; 5% dextrose in 0.225% NaCl; lactated Ringer's solution, or 10% invert sugar solution. There are not sufficient data to recommend usage of Coly-Mycin M Parenteral with other drugs or with other than the above listed infusion solutions.

Administer by slow intravenous infusion starting 1 to 2 hours after the initial dose at a rate of 5-6 mg/hr in the presence of normal renal function. In the presence of impaired renal function, reduce the infusion rate depending on the degree of renal impairment.

The choice of intravenous solution and the volume to be employed are dictated by the requirements of fluid and electrolyte management.

Any infusion solution containing colistimethate sodium should be freshly prepared and used for no longer than 24 hours.

HOW SUPPLIED

Coly-Mycin M Parenteral (sterile colistimethate sodium) is supplied in vials containing colistimethate sodium (150 mg colistin base equivalent per vial) as a white to slightly yellow lyophilized cake and is available as one vial per carton (N 0071-4145-01) or as 50 vials per carton (N 0071-4145-47).

STORE AT CONTROLLED ROOM TEMPERATURE (15° to 30°C) (59° to 86°F).

STORE RECONSTITUTED SOLUTION IN REFRIGERATOR (2° to 8°C) (36° to 46°F) OR AT CONTROLLED ROOM TEMPERATURE (15° to 30°C) (59° to 86°F), and use within 7 days.

Toxicology and Animal Pharmacology:

Acute Toxicity: The intravenous LD$_{50}$ was 41.5 mg/kg in the dog and 739 mg/kg in the mouse; intramuscular toxicity was 42 mg/kg in the dog and 267 mg/kg in the mouse.

Subacute Toxicity: In albino rabbits and beagle dogs, IV doses of 5, 10 and 20 mg/kg/day for 28 days resulted in elevated blood urea nitrogen in the dog (10 mg/kg/day dose group) and in both 20 mg/kg dose groups.

Clinical Studies: Clinically, Coly-Mycin M Parenteral (sterile colistimethate sodium) has been of particular therapeutic value in acute and chronic urinary tract infections caused by sensitive strains of *Pseudomonas aeruginosa*. Colistimethate sodium is clinically effective in the treatment of infections due to other sensitive gram-negative pathogenic bacilli that have become resistant to broad-spectrum antibiotics.

Colistimethate sodium has been used to treat bacteriuria and overt urinary infections in pregnant women during the third trimester. However, in view of the evidence of possible embryotoxic and teratogenic effects of colistimethate sodium in pregnant rabbits, caution should be exercised in use of this drug in women of childbearing potential.

4145G014

COLY-MYCIN® S OTIC   ℞

[cō"ly-my'cin s ō'tic]

with Neomycin and Hydrocortisone (colistin sulfate—neomycin sulfate—thonzonium bromide—hydrocortisone acetate otic suspension)

DESCRIPTION

Coly-Mycin S Otic with Neomycin and Hydrocortisone (colistin sulfate-neomycin sulfate-thonzonium bromide-hydrocortisone acetate otic suspension) is a sterile aqueous suspension containing in each ml: Colistin base activity, 3 mg (as the sulfate); Neomycin base activity, 3.3 mg (as the sulfate); Hydrocortisone acetate, 10 mg (1%); Thonzonium bromide, 0.5 mg (0.05%); Polysorbate 80, acetic acid, and sodium acetate in a buffered aqueous vehicle. Thimerosal (mercury derivative), 0.002%, added as a preservative. It is a nonviscous liquid, buffered at pH 5, for instillation into the canal of the external ear or direct application to the affected aural skin.

CLINICAL PHARMACOLOGY

1. Colistin sulfate—an antibiotic with bactericidal action against most gram-negative organisms, notably *Pseudomonas aeruginosa*, *E. coli.*, and *Klebsiella-Aerobacter*.
2. Neomycin sulfate—a broad-spectrum antibiotic, bactericidal to many pathogens, notably *Staph aureus* and *Proteus* sp.
3. Hydrocortisone acetate—a corticosteroid that controls inflammation, edema, pruritus and other dermal reactions.
4. Thonzonium bromide—a surface-active agent that promotes tissue contact by dispersion and penetration of the cellular debris and exudate.

INDICATIONS AND USAGE

For the treatment of superficial bacterial infections of the external auditory canal, caused by organisms susceptible to the action of the antibiotics; and for the treatment of infec-

---

Table 1

SUGGESTED MODIFICATION OF DOSAGE SCHEDULES OF COLY-MYCIN M PARENTERAL (STERILE COLISTIMETHATE SODIUM) FOR ADULTS WITH IMPAIRED RENAL FUNCTION

RENAL FUNCTION	Normal	DEGREE OF IMPAIRMENT		
		Mild	Moderate	Considerable
Plasma creatinine, (mg/100 ml)	0.7–1.2	1.3–1.5	1.6–2.5	2.6–4.0
Urea clearance, % of normal	80–100	40–70	25–40	10–25
DOSAGE				
Unit dose of Coly-Mycin M, mg	100–150	75–115	66–150	100–150
Frequency, times/day	4 to 2	2	2 or 1	every 36 hr
Total daily dose, mg	300	150–230	133–150	100
Approximate daily dose, mg/kg/day	5.0	2.5–3.8	2.5	1.5

NOTE

The suggested unit dose is 2.5–5 mg/kg; however, the time INTERVAL between injections should be increased in the presence of impaired renal function.

tions of mastoidectomy and fenestration cavities, caused by organisms susceptible to the antibiotics.

CONTRAINDICATIONS

This product is contraindicated in those individuals who have shown hypersensitivity to any of its components, and in herpes simplex, vaccinia and varicella.

WARNINGS

As with other antibiotic preparations, prolonged treatment may result in overgrowth of nonsusceptible organisms and fungi.

If the infection is not improved after one week, cultures and susceptibility tests should be repeated to verify the identity of the organism and to determine whether therapy should be changed.

Patients who prefer to warm the medication before using should be cautioned against heating the solution above body temperature, in order to avoid loss of potency.

PRECAUTIONS

General: If sensitization or irritation occurs, medication should be discontinued promptly.

This drug should be used with care in cases of perforated eardrum and in longstanding cases of chronic otitis media because of the possibility of ototoxicity caused by neomycin. Treatment should not be continued for longer than ten days. Allergic cross-reactions may occur which could prevent the use of any or all of the following antibiotics for the treatment of future infections: kanamycin, paromomycin, streptomycin, and possibly gentamicin.

ADVERSE REACTIONS

Neomycin is a not uncommon cutaneous sensitizer. There are articles in the current literature that indicate an increase in the prevalence of persons sensitive to neomycin.

DOSAGE AND ADMINISTRATION

The external auditory canal should be thoroughly cleansed and dried with a sterile cotton applicator.

When using the calibrated dropper:

For adults, 5 drops of the suspension should be instilled into the affected ear 3 or 4 times daily. For infants and children, 4 drops are suggested because of the smaller capacity of the ear canal.

This dosage correlates to the 4 drops (for adults) and 3 drops (for children) recommended when using the dropper-bottle container for this product.

The patient should lie with the affected ear upward and then the drops should be instilled. This position should be maintained for 5 minutes to facilitate penetration of the drops into the ear canal. Repeat, if necessary, for the opposite ear. If preferred, a cotton wick may be inserted into the canal and then the cotton may be saturated with the solution. This wick should be kept moist by adding further solution every 4 hours. The wick should be replaced at least once every 24 hours.

HOW SUPPLIED

Coly-Mycin S Otic is supplied as:
N 0071-3141-35—5-mL bottle with dropper
N 0071-3141-36—10-mL bottle with dropper
Each ml contains: Colistin sulfate equivalent to 3 mg of colistin base, Neomycin sulfate equivalent to 3.3 mg neomycin base, Hydrocortisone acetate 10 mg (1%), Thonzonium bromide 0.5 mg (0.05%), and Polysorbate 80 in an aqueous vehicle buffered with acetic acid and sodium acetate. Thimerosal (mercury derivative) 0.002% added as a preservative.
Shake well before using.
Store at controlled room temperature 15°–30°C (59°–86°F). Stable for 18 months at room temperature; prolonged exposure to higher temperatures should be avoided.

3141G033

Caution—Federal law prohibits dispensing without prescription.

KAPSEALS®
DILANTIN® ℞
[dī-lăn'tĭn"]
(Extended Phenytoin Sodium Capsules, USP)

DESCRIPTION

Phenytoin Sodium is an antiepileptic drug. Phenytoin sodium is related to the barbiturates in chemical structure, but has a five-membered ring. The chemical name is sodium 5,5-diphenyl-2,4-imidazolidinedione.

Each Dilantin—*Extended Phenytoin Sodium Capsule* USP contains 30 mg or 100 mg phenytoin sodium USP. Also contains lactose, NF; sucrose, NF; talc, USP; and other ingredients. The capsule shell and band contain colloidal silicon dioxide, NF; FD&C red No. 3; gelatin, NF; glyceryl monooleate; sodium lauryl sulfate, NF. The Dilantin 30-mg capsule shell and band also contain citric acid, USP; FD&C blue No. 1; sodium benzoate, NF; titanium dioxide, USP. The Dilantin 100-mg capsule shell and band also contain FD&C yellow No. 6; hydrogen peroxide 3%; polyethylene glycol 200. Prod-

uct *in vivo* performance is characterized by a slow and extended rate of absorption with peak blood concentrations expected in 4 to 12 hours as contrasted to *Prompt Phenytoin Sodium Capsules* USP with a rapid rate of absorption with peak blood concentration expected in 1½ to 3 hours.

CLINICAL PHARMACOLOGY

Phenytoin is an antiepileptic drug which can be useful in the treatment of epilepsy. The primary site of action appears to be *the motor cortex* where spread of seizure activity is inhibited. Possibly by promoting sodium efflux from neurons, phenytoin tends to *stabilize* the threshold against hyperexcitability caused by excessive stimulation or environmental changes capable of reducing membrane sodium gradient. This includes the reduction of posttetanic potentiation at synapses. Loss of posttetanic potentiation prevents cortical seizure foci from detonating adjacent cortical areas. Phenytoin reduces the maximal activity of brain stem centers responsible for the tonic phase of tonic-clonic (grand mal) seizures.

The plasma half-life in man after oral administration of phenytoin averages 22 hours, with a range of 7 to 42 hours. Steady-state therapeutic levels are achieved 7 to 10 days after initiation of therapy with recommended doses of 300 mg/day.

When serum level determinations are necessary, they should be obtained at least 5-7 half-lives after treatment initiation, dosage change, or addition or subtraction of another drug to the regimen so that equilibrium or steady-state will have been achieved. Trough levels provide information about clinically effective serum level range and confirm patient compliance and are obtained just prior to the patient's next scheduled dose. Peak levels indicate an individual's threshold for emergence of dose-related side effects and are obtained at the time of expected peak concentration. For Dilantin Kapseals peak serum levels occur 4-12 hours after administration.

Optimum control without clinical signs of toxicity occurs more often with serum levels between 10 and 20 mcg/ml, although some mild cases of tonic-clonic (grand mal) epilepsy may be controlled with lower-serum levels of phenytoin.

In most patients maintained at a steady dosage, stable phenytoin serum levels are achieved. There may be wide interpatient variability in phenytoin serum levels with equivalent dosages. Patients with unusually low levels may be noncompliant or hypermetabolizers of phenytoin. Unusually high levels result from liver disease, congenital enzyme deficiency or drug interactions which result in metabolic interference. The patient with large variations in phenytoin plasma levels, despite standard doses, presents a difficult clinical problem. Serum level determinations in such patients may be particularly helpful. As phenytoin is highly protein bound, free phenytoin levels may be altered in patients whose protein binding characteristics differ from normal.

Most of the drug is excreted in the bile as inactive metabolites which are then reabsorbed from the intestinal tract and excreted in the urine. Urinary excretion of phenytoin and its metabolites occurs partly with glomerular filtration but more importantly, by tubular secretion. Because phenytoin is hydroxylated in the liver by an enzyme system which is saturable, small incremental doses may produce very substantial increases in serum levels, when these are in the upper range. The steady-state level may be disproportionately increased, with resultant intoxication, from an increase in dosage of 10% or more.

INDICATIONS AND USAGE

Dilantin is indicated for the control of tonic-clonic and psychomotor (grand mal and temporal lobe) seizures and prevention and treatment of seizures occurring during or following neurosurgery.

Phenytoin serum level determinations may be necessary for optimal dosage adjustments (see Dosage and Administration).

CONTRAINDICATIONS

Phenytoin is contraindicated in those patients who are hypersensitive to phenytoin or other hydantoins.

WARNINGS

Abrupt withdrawal of phenytoin in epileptic patients may precipitate status epilepticus. When, in the judgment of the clinician, the need for dosage reduction, discontinuation, or substitution of alternative antiepileptic medication arises, this should be done gradually. However, in the event of an allergic or hypersensitivity reaction, rapid substitution of alternative therapy may be necessary. In this case, alternative therapy should be an antiepileptic drug not belonging to the hydantoin chemical class.

There have been a number of reports suggesting a relationship between phenytoin and the development of lymphadenopathy (local or generalized) including benign lymph node hyperplasia, pseudolymphoma, lymphoma, and Hodgkin's Disease.

Although a cause and effect relationship has not been established, the occurrence of lymphadenopathy indicates the need to differentiate such a condition from other types of

lymph node pathology. Lymph node involvement may occur with or without symptoms and signs resembling serum sickness eg, fever, rash and liver involvement.

In all cases of lymphadenopathy, follow-up observation for an extended period is indicated and every effort should be made to achieve seizure control using alternative antiepileptic drugs.

Acute alcoholic intake may increase phenytoin serum levels while chronic alcoholic use may decrease serum levels.

In view of isolated reports associating phenytoin with exacerbation of porphyria, caution should be exercised in using this medication in patients suffering from this disease.

Usage in Pregnancy:

A number of reports suggests an association between the use of antiepileptic drugs by women with epilepsy and a higher incidence of birth defects in children born to these women. Data are more extensive with respect to phenytoin and phenobarbital, but these are also the most commonly prescribed antiepileptic drugs; less systematic or anecdotal reports suggest a possible similar association with the use of all known antiepileptic drugs.

The reports suggesting a higher incidence of birth defects in children of drug-treated epileptic women cannot be regarded as adequate to prove a definite cause and effect relationship. There are intrinsic methodologic problems in obtaining adequate data on drug teratogenicity in humans; genetic factors or the epileptic condition itself may be more important than drug therapy in leading to birth defects. The great majority of the mothers on antiepileptic medication deliver normal infants. It is important to note that antiepileptic drugs should not be discontinued in patients in whom the drug is administered to prevent major seizures, because of the strong possibility of precipitating status epilepticus with attendant hypoxia and threat to life. In individual cases where the severity and frequency of the seizure disorder are such that the removal of medication does not pose a serious threat to the patient, discontinuation of the drug may be considered prior to and during pregnancy, although it cannot be said with any confidence that even minor seizures do not pose some hazards to the developing embryo or fetus. The prescribing physician will wish to weigh these considerations in treating and counseling epileptic women of childbearing potential.

In addition to the reports of increased incidence of congenital malformation, such as cleft lip/palate and heart malformations in children of women receiving phenytoin and other antiepileptic drugs, there have more recently been reports of a fetal hydantoin syndrome. This consists of prenatal growth deficiency, microcephaly and mental deficiency in children born to mothers who have received phenytoin, barbiturates, alcohol, or trimethadione. However, these features are all interrelated and are frequently associated with intrauterine growth retardation from other causes.

There have been isolated reports of malignancies, including neuroblastoma, in children whose mothers received phenytoin during pregnancy.

An increase in seizure frequency during pregnancy occurs in a high proportion of patients, because of altered phenytoin absorption or metabolism. Periodic measurement of serum phenytoin levels is particularly valuable in the management of a pregnant epileptic patient as a guide to an appropriate adjustment of dosage. However, postpartum restoration of the original dosage will probably be indicated.

Neonatal coagulation defects have been reported within the first 24 hours in babies born to epileptic mothers receiving phenobarbital and/or phenytoin. Vitamin K_1 has been shown to prevent or correct this defect and has been recommended to be given to the mother before delivery and the neonate after birth.

PRECAUTIONS

General:

The liver is the chief site of biotransformation of phenytoin; patients with impaired liver function, elderly patients, or those who are gravely ill may show early signs of toxicity.

A small percentage of individuals who have been treated with phenytoin have been shown to metabolize the drug slowly. Slow metabolism may be due to limited enzyme availability and lack of induction; it appears to be genetically determined.

Phenytoin should be discontinued if a skin rash appears (see "Warnings" section regarding drug discontinuation). If the rash is exfoliative, purpuric, or bullous or if lupus erythematosus or Stevens-Johnson syndrome or toxic epidermal necrolysis is suspected, use of the drug should not be resumed. (See Adverse Reactions.) If the rash is of a milder type (measles-like or scarlatiniform), therapy may be resumed after

Continued on next page

This product information was prepared in August 1992. On these and other Parke-Davis Products, information may be obtained by addressing PARKE-DAVIS, Division of Warner-Lambert Company, Morris Plains, New Jersey 07950.

Parke-Davis—Cont.

the rash has completely disappeared. If the rash recurs upon reinstitution of therapy, further phenytoin medication is contraindicated.
Phenytoin and other hydantoins are contraindicated in patients who have experienced phenytoin hypersensitivity. Additionally, caution should be exercised if using structurally similar compounds (eg, barbiturates, succinimides, oxazolidinediones and other related compounds) in these same patients.
Hyperglycemia, resulting from the drug's inhibitory effects on insulin release, has been reported. Phenytoin may also raise the serum glucose level in diabetic patients.
Osteomalacia has been associated with phenytoin therapy and is considered to be due to phenytoin's interference with Vitamin D metabolism.
Phenytoin is not indicated for seizures due to hypoglycemic or other causes. Appropriate diagnostic procedures should be performed as indicated.
Phenytoin is not effective for absence (petit mal) seizures. If tonic-clonic (grand-mal) and absence (petit mal) seizures are present, combined drug therapy is needed.
Serum levels of phenytoin sustained above the optimal range may produce confusional states referred to as "delirium," "psychosis," or "encephalopathy," or rarely irreversible cerebellar dysfunction. Accordingly, at the first sign of acute toxicity, plasma levels are recommended. Dose reduction of phenytoin therapy is indicated if plasma levels are excessive; if symptoms persist, termination is recommended. (See Warnings.)

Information for Patients:
Patients taking phenytoin should be advised of the importance of adhering strictly to the prescribed dosage regimen, and of informing the physician of any clinical condition in which it is not possible to take the drug orally as prescribed, eg, surgery, etc.
Patients should also be cautioned on the use of other drugs or alcoholic beverages without first seeking the physician's advice.
Patients should be instructed to call their physician if skin rash develops.
The importance of good dental hygiene should be stressed in order to minimize the development of gingival hyperplasia and its complications.

Laboratory Tests:
Phenytoin serum level determinations may be necessary to achieve optimal dosage adjustments.

Drug Interactions:
There are many drugs which may increase or decrease phenytoin levels or which phenytoin may affect. Serum level determinations for phenytoin are especially helpful when possible drug interactions are suspected. The most commonly occurring drug interactions are listed below.

1. Drugs which may increase phenytoin serum levels include: acute alcohol intake, amiodarone, chloramphenicol, chlordiazepoxide, diazepam, dicumarol, disulfiram, estrogens, H_2-antagonists, halothane, isoniazid, methylphenidate, phenothiazines, phenylbutazone, salicylates, succinimides, sulfonamides, tolbutamide, trazodone.
2. Drugs which may decrease phenytoin levels include: carbamazepine, chronic alcohol abuse, reserpine, and sucralfate. Moban® brand of molindone hydrochloride contains calcium ions which interfere with the absorption of phenytoin. Ingestion times of phenytoin and antacid preparations containing calcium should be staggered in patients with low serum phenytoin levels to prevent absorption problems.
3. Drugs which may either increase or decrease phenytoin serum levels include: phenobarbital, sodium valproate, and valproic acid. Similarly, the effect of phenytoin on phenobarbital, valproic acid and sodium valproate serum levels is unpredictable.
4. Although not a true drug interaction, tricyclic antidepressants may precipitate seizures in susceptible patients and phenytoin dosage may need to be adjusted.
5. Drugs whose efficacy is impaired by phenytoin include: corticosteroids, coumarin anticoagulants, digitoxin, doxycycline, estrogens, furosemide, oral contraceptives, quinidine, rifampin, theophylline, vitamin D.

Drug/Laboratory Test Interactions:
Phenytoin may cause decreased serum levels of protein-bound iodine (PBI). It may also produce lower than normal values for dexamethasone or metyrapone tests. Phenytoin may cause raised serum levels of glucose, alkaline phosphatase, and gamma glutamyl transpeptidase (GGT).

Carcinogenesis:
See 'Warnings' section for information on carcinogenesis.

Pregnancy:
See Warnings

Nursing Mothers:
Infant breast feeding is not recommended for women taking this drug because phenytoin appears to be secreted in low concentrations in human milk.

ADVERSE REACTIONS

Central Nervous System: The most common manifestations encountered with phenytoin therapy are referable to this system and are usually dose-related. These include nystagmus, ataxia, slurred speech, and mental confusion. Dizziness, insomnia, transient nervousness, motor twitchings, and headaches have also been observed. There have also been rare reports of phenytoin induced dyskinesias, including chorea, dystonia, tremor and asterixis, similar to those induced by phenothiazine and other neuroleptic drugs.
A predominantly sensory peripheral polyneuropathy has been observed in patients receiving long-term phenytoin therapy.
Gastrointestinal System: Nausea, vomiting, constipation, toxic hepatitis and liver damage.
Integumentary System: Dermatological manifestations sometimes accompanied by fever have included scarlatiniform or morbilliform rashes. A morbilliform rash (measles-like) is the most common; other types of dermatitis are seen more rarely. Other more serious forms which may be fatal have included bullous, exfoliative or purpuric dermatitis, lupus erythematosus, Stevens-Johnson syndrome, and toxic epidermal necrolysis (see Precautions).
Hemopoietic System: Hemopoietic complications, some fatal, have occasionally been reported in association with administration of phenytoin. These have included thrombocytopenia, leukopenia, granulocytopenia, agranulocytosis, and pancytopenia. While macrocytosis and megaloblastic anemia have occurred, these conditions usually respond to folic acid therapy. Lymphadenopathy including benign lymph node hyperplasia, pseudolymphoma, lymphoma, and Hodgkin's Disease have been reported (see Warnings).
Connective Tissue System: Coarsening of the facial features, enlargement of the lips, gingival hyperplasia, hirsutism, and Peyronie's Disease.
Cardiovascular: Periarteritis nodosa.
Immunologic: Hypersensitivity syndrome (which may include, but is not limited to, symptoms such as arthralgias, eosinophilia, fever, liver dysfunction, lymphadenopathy or rash), systemic lupus erythematosus, immunoglobulin abnormalities.

OVERDOSAGE

The lethal dose in children is not known. The lethal dose in adults is estimated to be 2 to 5 grams. The initial symptoms are nystagmus, ataxia, and dysarthria. Other signs are tremor, hyperflexia, lethargy, slurred speech, nausea, vomiting. The patient may become comatose and hypotensive. Death is due to respiratory and circulatory depression.
There are marked variations among individuals with respect to phenytoin plasma levels where toxicity may occur. Nystagmus, on lateral gaze, usually appears at 20 mcg/ml, ataxia at 30 mcg/ml, dysarthria and lethargy appear when the plasma concentration is over 40 mcg/ml, but as high a concentration as 50 mcg/ml has been reported without evidence of toxicity. As much as 25 times the therapeutic dose has been taken to result in a serum concentration over 100 mcg/ml with complete recovery.

Treatment:
Treatment is nonspecific since there is no known antidote. The adequacy of the respiratory and circulatory systems should be carefully observed and appropriate supportive measures employed. Hemodialysis can be considered since phenytoin is not completely bound to plasma proteins. Total exchange transfusion has been used in the treatment of severe intoxication in children.
In acute overdosage the possibility of other CNS depressants, including alcohol, should be borne in mind.

DOSAGE AND ADMINISTRATION

Serum concentrations should be monitored in changing from extended Phenytoin Sodium Capsules USP (Dilantin) to Prompt Phenytoin sodium capsules USP, and from the sodium salt to the free acid form.
Dilantin® Kapseals,® Dilantin Parenteral, and Dilantin with Phenobarbital are formulated with the sodium salt of phenytoin. The free acid form of phenytoin is used in Dilantin-30 Pediatric and Dilantin-125 Suspensions and Dilantin Infatabs. Because there is approximately an 8% increase in drug content with the free acid form over that of the sodium salt, dosage adjustments and serum level monitoring may be necessary when switching from a product formulated with the free acid to a product formulated with the sodium salt and vice versa.

General:
Dosage should be individualized to provide maximum benefit. In some cases serum blood level determinations may be necessary for optimal dosage adjustments—the clinically effective serum level is usually 10-20 mcg/ml. With recommended dosage, a period of seven to ten days may be required to achieve steady-state blood levels with phenytoin and changes in dosage (increase or decrease) should not be carried out at intervals shorter than seven to ten days.

Adult Dosage:
Divided Daily Dosage
Patients who have received no previous treatment may be started on one 100 mg Dilantin (Extended Phenytoin Sodium Capsule) three times daily and the dosage then adjusted to suit individual requirements. For most adults, the satisfactory maintenance dosage will be one capsule three to four times a day. An increase up to two capsules three times a day may be made, if necessary.

Once-a-Day Dosage:
In adults, if seizure control is established with divided doses of three 100 mg Dilantin capsules daily, once-a-day dosage with 300 mg of extended phenytoin sodium capsules may be considered. Studies comparing divided doses of 300 mg with a single daily dose of this quantity indicated absorption, peak plasma levels, biologic half-life, difference between peak and minimum values, and urinary recovery were equivalent. Once-a-day dosage offers a convenience to the individual patient or to nursing personnel for institutionalized patients and is intended to be used only for patients requiring this amount of drug daily. A major problem in motivating noncompliant patients may also be lessened when the patient can take this drug once a day. However, patients should be cautioned not to miss a dose, inadvertently.
Only extended phenytoin sodium capsules are recommended for once-a-day dosing. Inherent differences in dissolution characteristics and resultant absorption rates of phenytoin due to different manufacturing procedures and/or dosage forms preclude such recommendation for other phenytoin products. When a change in the dosage form or brand is prescribed, careful monitoring of phenytoin serum levels should be carried out.

Loading Dose:
Some authorities have advocated use of an oral loading dose of phenytoin in adults who require rapid steady-state serum levels and where intravenous administration is not desirable. This dosing regimen should be reserved for patients in a clinic or hospital setting where phenytoin serum levels can be closely monitored. Patients with a history of renal or liver disease should not receive the oral loading regimen.
Initially, one gram of phenytoin capsules is divided into 3 doses (400 mg, 300 mg, 300 mg) and administered at two-hourly intervals. Normal maintenance dosage is then instituted 24 hours after the loading dose, with frequent serum level determinations.

Pediatric Dosage:
Initially, 5 mg/kg/day in two or three equally divided doses, with subsequent dosage individualized to a maximum of 300 mg daily. A recommended daily maintenance dosage is usually 4 to 8 mg/kg. Children over 6 years old may require the minimum adult dose (300 mg/day).

HOW SUPPLIED

N 0071-0362 (Kapseal 362, transparent #3 capsule with an orange band)—Dilantin 100 mg; in 100's, 1,000's, and unit dose 100's.
N 0071-0365 (Kapseal 365, transparent #4 capsule with a pink band)—Dilantin 30 mg; in 100's.
Store below 30°C (86°F). Protect from light and moisture.
Also available as:
N 0071-2214—Dilantin-125® Suspension 125 mg phenytoin/5 ml with a maximum alcohol content not greater than 0.6 percent, available in 8-oz bottles and individual unit dose foil pouches which deliver 5 ml (125 mg phenytoin). The minimum sales unit is 100 pouches.
N 0071-2315—Dilantin-30® Pediatric Suspension 30 mg phenytoin/5 ml with a maximum alcohol content not greater than 0.6 percent; available in 8-oz bottles.
N 0071-0375 (Kapseal 375)—Dilantin with Phenobarbital each contain 100 mg phenytoin sodium with 16 mg (1/4 gr) phenobarbital; in 100's.
N 0071-0531 (Kapseal 531)—Dilantin with Phenobarbital each contain 100 mg phenytoin sodium with 32 mg (1/2 gr) phenobarbital; in 100's.
N 0071-0007 (Tablet 7)—Dilantin Infatabs® each contain 50 mg phenytoin, 100's and unit dose 100's.
For Parenteral Use:
N 0071-4488-05 (Ampoule 1488) Dilantin ready-mixed solution containing 50 mg phenytoin sodium per milliliter is supplied in 2-mL ampoules. Package of ten.
N 0071-4488-41 (Steri-Dose® 4488)—Dilantin ready-mixed solution containing 50 mg phenytoin sodium per milliliter is supplied in a 2-mL sterile disposable syringe (22 gauge × 1¼ inch needle). Packages of ten individually cartoned syringes.
N 0071-4475-08 (Ampoule 1475)—Dilantin ready-mixed solution containing 50 mg phenytoin sodium per milliliter is supplied in packages of ten 5-mL ampoules without syringes.
N 0071-4488-45 Dilantin ready-mixed solution containing 50 mg phenytoin sodium per milliliter is supplied in 2-mL Steri-Vials.® Packages of twenty-five.
N 0071-4475-45 Dilantin ready-mixed solution containing 50 mg phenytoin sodium per milliliter is supplied in 5-mL Steri-Vials.® Packages of twenty-five.

Store below 30°C (86°F). Protect from light and moisture.
0362G282

Shown in Product Identification Section, page 422

INFATABS®
DILANTIN® ℞
[*dī-lăn'tĭn" ĭn'fă-tăbs"*]
(Phenytoin Tablets, USP)

NOT FOR ONCE A DAY DOSING

DESCRIPTION

Dilantin is an antiepileptic drug.
Dilantin (phenytoin) is related to the barbiturates in chemical structure, but has a five-membered ring. The chemical name is 5,5-diphenyl-2,4-imidazolidinedione.
Each Dilantin Infatab, for oral administration, contains 50 mg phenytoin, USP. Also contains: D&C yellow No. 10, Al lake; FD&C yellow No. 6, Al lake flavor; saccharin sodium, USP; sucrose, NF; talc, USP; and other ingredients.

CLINICAL PHARMACOLOGY

Phenytoin is an antiepileptic drug which can be useful in the treatment of epilepsy. The primary site of action appears to be the motor cortex where spread of seizure activity is inhibited. Possibly by promoting sodium efflux from neurons, phenytoin tends to stabilize the threshold against hyperexcitability caused by excessive stimulation or environmental changes capable of reducing membrane sodium gradient. This includes the reduction of posttetanic potentiation at synapses. Loss of posttetanic potentiation prevents cortical seizure foci from detonating adjacent cortical areas. Phenytoin reduces the maximal activity of brain stem centers responsible for the tonic phase of tonic-clonic (grand mal) seizures.
Clinical studies using Dilantin Infatabs have shown an average plasma half-life of 14 hours with a range of 7 to 29 hours. Steady-state therapeutic levels are achieved at least 7 to 10 days (5-7 half-lives) after initiation of therapy with recommended doses of 300 mg/day.
When serum level determinations are necessary, they should be obtained at least 5-7 half-lives after treatment initiation, dosage change, or addition or subtraction of another drug to the regimen so that equilibrium or steady-state will have been achieved. Trough levels provide information about clinically effective serum level range and confirm patient compliance and are obtained just prior to the patient's next scheduled dose. Peak levels indicate an individual's threshold for emergence of dose-related side effects and are obtained at the time of expected peak concentration. For Dilantin Infatabs peak levels occur 1½-3 hours after administration.
Optimum control without clinical signs of toxicity occurs more often with serum levels between 10 and 20 mcg/ml, although some mild cases of tonic-clonic (grand mal) epilepsy may be controlled with lower-serum levels of phenytoin.
In most patients maintained at a steady dosage, stable phenytoin serum levels are achieved. There may be wide interpatient variability in phenytoin serum levels with equivalent dosages. Patients with unusually low levels may be noncompliant or hypermetabolizers of phenytoin. Unusually high levels result from liver disease, congenital enzyme deficiency or drug interactions which result in metabolic interference. The patient with large variations in phenytoin plasma levels, despite standard doses, presents a difficult clinical problem. Serum level determinations in such patients may be particularly helpful. As phenytoin is highly protein bound, free phenytoin levels may be altered in patients whose protein binding characteristics differ from normal.
Most of the drug is excreted in the bile as inactive metabolites which are then reabsorbed from the intestinal tract and excreted in the urine. Urinary excretion of phenytoin and its metabolites occurs partly with glomerular filtration but more importantly, by tubular secretion. Because phenytoin is hydroxylated in the liver by an enzyme system which is saturable at high plasma levels small incremental doses may increase the half-life and produce very substantial increases in serum levels, when these are in the upper range. The steady-state level may be disproportionately increased, with resultant intoxication, from an increase in dosage of 10% or more.
Clinical studies show that chewed and unchewed Dilantin Infatabs are bioequivalent, yield approximately equivalent plasma levels, and are more rapidly absorbed than 100-mg Dilantin Kapseals.®

INDICATIONS AND USAGE

Dilantin Infatabs (Phenytoin Tablets, USP) are indicated for the control of generalized tonic-clonic (grand mal) and complex partial (psychomotor, temporal lobe) seizures and prevention and treatment of seizures occurring during or following neurosurgery. Phenytoin serum level determinations may be necessary for optimal dosage adjustments (see Dosage and Administration and Clinical Pharmacology).

CONTRAINDICATIONS

Phenytoin is contraindicated in those patients who are hypersensitive to phenytoin or other hydantoins.

WARNINGS

Abrupt withdrawal of phenytoin in epileptic patients may precipitate status epilepticus. When, in the judgment of the clinician, the need for dosage reduction, discontinuation, or substitution of alternative antiepileptic medication arises, this should be done gradually. However, in the event of an allergic or hypersensitivity reaction, rapid substitution of alternative therapy may be necessary. In this case, alternative therapy should be an antiepileptic drug not belonging to the hydantoin chemical class.
There have been a number of reports suggesting a relationship between phenytoin and the development of lymphadenopathy (local or generalized) including benign lymph node hyperplasia, pseudolymphoma, lymphoma, and Hodgkin's Disease. Although a cause and effect relationship has not been established, the occurrence of lymphadenopathy indicates the need to differentiate such a condition from other types of lymph node pathology. Lymph node involvement may occur with or without symptoms and signs resembling serum sickness eg, fever, rash and liver involvement. In all cases of lymphadenopathy, follow-up observation for an extended period is indicated and every effort should be made to achieve seizure control using alternative antiepileptic drugs.
Acute alcoholic intake may increase phenytoin serum levels while chronic alcoholic use may decrease serum levels.
In view of isolated reports associating phenytoin with exacerbation of porphyria, caution should be exercised in using this medication in patients suffering from this disease.

Usage in Pregnancy

A number of reports suggest an association between the use of antiepileptic drugs by women with epilepsy and a higher incidence of birth defects in children born to these women. Data are more extensive with respect to phenytoin and phenobarbital, but these are also the most commonly prescribed antiepileptic drugs; less systematic or anecdotal reports suggest a possible similar association with the use of all known antiepileptic drugs.
The reports suggesting a higher incidence of birth defects in children of drug-treated epileptic women cannot be regarded as adequate to prove a definite cause and effect relationship. There are intrinsic methodologic problems in obtaining adequate data on drug teratogenicity in humans: genetic factors or the epileptic condition itself, may be more important than drug therapy in leading to birth defects. The great majority of mothers on antiepileptic medication deliver normal infants. It is important to note that antiepileptic drugs should not be discontinued in patients in whom the drug is administered to prevent major seizures, because of the strong possibility of precipitating status epilepticus with attendant hypoxia and threat to life. In individual cases where the severity and frequency of the seizure disorder are such that the removal of medication does not pose a serious threat to the patient, discontinuation of the drug may be considered prior to and during pregnancy, although it cannot be said with any confidence that even minor seizures do not pose some hazard to the developing embryo or fetus. The prescribing physician will wish to weigh these considerations in treating or counseling epileptic women of childbearing potential.
In addition to the reports of increased incidence of congenital malformations, such as cleft lip/palate and heart malformations in children of women receiving phenytoin and other antiepileptic drugs, there have more recently been reports of a fetal hydantoin syndrome. This consists of prenatal growth deficiency, microcephaly and mental deficiency in children born to mothers who have received phenytoin, barbiturates, alcohol, or trimethadione. However, these features are all interrelated and are frequently associated with intrauterine growth retardation from other causes.
There have been isolated reports of malignancies, including neuroblastoma, in children whose mothers received phenytoin during pregnancy.
An increase in seizure frequency during pregnancy occurs in a high proportion of patients, because of altered phenytoin absorption or metabolism. Periodic measurement of serum phenytoin levels is particularly valuable in the management of a pregnant epileptic patient as a guide to an appropriate adjustment of dosage. However, postpartum restoration of the original dosage will probably be indicated.
Neonatal coagulation defects have been reported within the first 24 hours in babies born to epileptic mothers receiving phenobarbital and/or phenytoin. Vitamin K has been shown to prevent or correct this defect and has been recommended to be given to the mother before delivery and to the neonate after birth.

PRECAUTIONS

General

The liver is the chief site of biotransformation of phenytoin; patients with impaired liver function, elderly patients, or those who are gravely ill may show early signs of toxicity.
A small percentage of individuals who have been treated with phenytoin have been shown to metabolize the drug slowly. Slow metabolism may be due to limited enzyme availability and lack of induction; it appears to be genetically determined.
Phenytoin should be discontinued if a skin rash appears (see "Warnings" section regarding drug discontinuation). If the rash is exfoliative, purpuric, or bullous or if lupus erythematosus, Stevens-Johnson syndrome, or toxic epidermal necrolysis is suspected, use of the drug should not be resumed, and alternative therapy should be considered (see Adverse Reactions). If the rash is of a milder type (measles-like or scarlatiniform), therapy may be resumed after the rash has completely disappeared. If the rash recurs upon reinstitution of therapy, further phenytoin medication is contraindicated.
Phenytoin and other hydantoins are contraindicated in patients who have experienced phenytoin hypersensitivity. Additionally, caution should be exercised if using structurally similar compounds (eg barbiturates, succinimides, oxazolidinediones and other related compounds) in these same patients.
Hyperglycemia, resulting from the drug's inhibitory effects on insulin release, has been reported. Phenytoin may also raise the serum glucose level in diabetic patients.
Osteomalacia has been associated with phenytoin therapy and is considered to be due to phenytoin's interference with Vitamin D metabolism.
Phenytoin is not indicated for seizures due to hypoglycemic or other metabolic causes. Appropriate diagnostic procedures should be performed as indicated.
Phenytoin is not effective for absence (petit mal) seizures. If tonic-clonic (grand-mal) and absence (petit mal) seizures are present, combined drug therapy is needed.
Serum levels of phenytoin sustained above the optimal range may produce confusional states referred to as "delirium," "psychosis," or "encephalopathy," or rarely irreversible cerebellar dysfunction. Accordingly, at the first sign of acute toxicity, plasma levels are recommended. Dose reduction of phenytoin therapy is indicated if plasma levels are excessive, if symptoms persist, termination is recommended. (See Warnings).

Information for Patients

Patients taking phenytoin should be advised of the importance of adhering strictly to the prescribed dosage regimen, and of informing the physician of any clinical condition in which it is not possible to take the drug orally as prescribed, eg, surgery, etc.
Patients should also be cautioned on the use of other drugs or alcoholic beverages without first seeking the physician's advice.
Patients should be instructed to call their physician if skin rash develops.
The importance of good dental hygiene should be stressed in order to minimize the development of gingival hyperplasia and its complications.

Laboratory Tests

Phenytoin serum level determinations may be necessary to achieve optimal dosage adjustments.

Drug Interactions

There are many drugs which may increase or decrease phenytoin levels or which phenytoin may affect. Serum level determinations for phenytoin are especially helpful when possible drug interactions are suspected. The most commonly occurring drug interactions are listed below.

1. Drugs which may increase phenytoin serum levels include: acute alcohol intake, amiodarone, chloramphenicol, chlordiazepoxide, diazepam, dicumarol, disulfiram, estrogens, H_2 -antagonists, halothane, isoniazid, methylphenidate, phenothiazines, phenylbutazone, salicylates, succinimides, sulfonamides, tolbutamide, trazodone.
2. Drugs which may decrease phenytoin levels include: carbamazepine, chronic alcohol abuse, reserpine, and sucralfate . Moban® brand of molindone hydrochloride contains calcium ions which interfere with the absorption of phenytoin. Ingestion times of phenytoin and antacid preparations containing calcium should be staggered in patients with low serum phenytoin levels to prevent absorption problems.
3. Drugs which may either increase or decrease phenytoin serum levels include: phenobarbital, sodium valproate, and valproic acid. Similarly, the effect of phenytoin on phenobarbital, valproic acid and sodium valproate serum levels is unpredictable.
4. Although not a true drug interaction, tricyclic antidepressants may precipitate seizures in susceptible patients and phenytoin dosage may need to be adjusted.
5. Drugs whose efficacy is impaired by phenytoin include: corticosteroids, coumarin anticoagulants, digitoxin, doxycy-

Continued on next page

This product information was prepared in August 1992. On these and other Parke-Davis Products, information may be obtained by addressing PARKE-DAVIS, Division of Warner-Lambert Company, Morris Plains, New Jersey 07950.

Parke-Davis—Cont.

cline, estrogens, furosemide, oral contraceptives, quinidine, rifampin, theophylline, vitamin D.

Drug/Laboratory Test Interactions

Phenytoin may cause decreased serum levels of protein-bound iodine (PBI). It may also produce lower than normal values for dexamethasone or metyrapone tests. Phenytoin may cause increased serum levels of glucose, alkaline phosphatase, and gamma glutamyl transpeptidase (GGT).

Carcinogenesis

See 'Warnings' section for information on carcinogenesis.

Pregnancy

See Warnings

Nursing Mothers

Infant breast-feeding is not recommended for women taking this drug because phenytoin appears to be secreted in low concentrations in human milk.

ADVERSE REACTIONS

Central Nervous System: The most common manifestations encountered with phenytoin therapy are referable to this system and are usually dose-related. These include nystagmus, ataxia, slurred speech, decreased coordination and mental confusion. Dizziness, insomnia, transient nervousness, motor twitchings, and headache have also been observed.

There have also been rare reports of phenytoin induced dyskinesias, including chorea, dystonia, tremor and asterixis, similar to those induced by phenothiazine and other neuroleptic drugs.

A predominantly sensory peripheral polyneuropathy has been observed in patients receiving long-term phenytoin therapy.

Gastrointestinal System: Nausea, vomiting, constipation, toxic hepatitis and liver damage.

Integumentary System: Dermatological manifestations sometimes accompanied by fever have included scarlatiniform or morbilliform rashes. A morbilliform rash (measles-like) is the most common; other types of dermatitis are seen more rarely. Other more serious forms which may be fatal have included bullous, exfoliative or purpuric dermatitis, lupus erythematosus, Stevens-Johnson syndrome, and toxic epidermal necrolysis (see Precautions).

Hemopoietic System: Hemopoietic complications, some fatal, have occasionally been reported in association with administration of phenytoin. These have included thrombocytopenia, leukopenia, granulocytopenia, agranulocytosis, and pancytopenia with or without bone marrow suppression. While macrocytosis and megaloblastic anemia have occurred, these conditions usually respond to folic acid therapy. Lymphadenopathy including benign lymph node hyperplasia, pseudolymphoma, lymphoma, and Hodgkin's Disease have been reported (see Warnings).

Connective Tissue System: Coarsening of the facial features, enlargement of the lips, gingival hyperplasia, hypertrichosis, and Peyronie's Disease.

Cardiovascular: Periarteritis nodosa.

Immunologic: Hypersensitivity syndrome (which may include, but is not limited to, symptoms such as arthralgias, eosinophilia, fever, liver dysfunction, lymphadenopathy or rash), systemic lupus erythematosus, and immunoglobulin abnormalities.

OVERDOSAGE

The lethal dose in children is not known. The lethal dose in adults is estimated to be 2 to 5 grams. The initial symptoms are nystagmus, ataxia, and dysarthria. Other signs are tremor, hyperflexia, lethargy, slurred speech, nausea, vomiting. The patient may become comatose and hypotensive. Death is due to respiratory and circulatory depression.

There are marked variations among individuals with respect to phenytoin plasma levels where toxicity may occur. Nystagmus on lateral gaze usually appears at 20 mcg/ml, ataxia at 30 mcg/ml, dysarthria and lethargy appear when the plasma concentration is over 40 mcg/ml, but as high a concentration as 50 mcg/ml has been reported without evidence of toxicity. As much as 25 times the therapeutic dose has been taken to result in a serum concentration over 100 mcg/ml with complete recovery.

Treatment

Treatment is nonspecific since there is no known antidote. The adequacy of the respiratory and circulatory systems should be carefully observed and appropriate supportive measures employed. Hemodialysis can be considered since phenytoin is not completely bound to plasma proteins. Total exchange transfusion has been used in the treatment of severe intoxication in children.

In acute overdosage the possibility of other CNS depressants, including alcohol, should be borne in mind.

DOSAGE AND ADMINISTRATION

When given in equal doses, Dilantin Infatabs yield higher plasma levels than Dilantin Kapseals.® For this reason serum concentrations should be monitored and care should be taken when switching a patient from the sodium salt to the free acid form.

Dilantin® Kapseals,® Dilantin Parenteral, and Dilantin with Phenobarbital are formulated with the sodium salt of phenytoin. The free acid form of phenytoin is used in Dilantin-30 Pediatric and Dilantin-125 Suspensions and Dilantin Infatabs. Because there is approximately an 8% increase in drug content with the free acid form over that of the sodium salt, dosage adjustments and serum level monitoring may be necessary when switching from a product formulated with the free acid to a product formulated with the sodium salt and vice versa.

General

Not for once a day dosing.

Dosage should be individualized to provide maximum benefit. In some cases, serum blood level determinations may be necessary for optimal dosage adjustments—the clinically effective serum level is usually 10–20 mcg/ml. With recommended dosage, a period of seven to ten days may be required to achieve steady-state blood levels with phenytoin and changes in dosage (increase or decrease) should not be carried out at intervals shorter than seven to ten days.

Dilantin Infatabs can be either chewed thoroughly before being swallowed or swallowed whole.

Adult Dosage

Patients who have received no previous treatment may be started on two Infatabs three times daily, and the dose is then adjusted to suit individual requirements. For most adults, the satisfactory maintenance dosage will be six to eight Infatabs daily; an increase to twelve Infatabs daily may be made, if necessary.

Pediatric Dosage

Initially, 5 mg/kg/day in two or three equally divided doses, with subsequent dosage individualized to a maximum of 300 mg daily. A recommended daily maintenance dosage is usually 4 to 8 mg/kg. Children over 6 years old may require the minimum adult dose (300 mg/day). If the daily dosage cannot be divided equally, the larger dose should be given before retiring.

HOW SUPPLIED

Dilantin Infatabs are supplied as:

N 0071-0007-24—Bottle of 100.

Store at a room temperature below 30°C (86°F).

N 0071-0007-40—Unit dose (10/10's).

Store at controlled room temperature 15°–30°C (59°–86°F). Protect from moisture.

Each tablet contains 50 mg phenytoin in a yellow triangular scored chewable tablet.

Shown in Product Identification Section, page 422

Dilantin is also supplied in the following forms:

N 0071-0362-24—Bottle of 100.

N 0071-0362-32—Bottle of 1000.

N 0071-0362-40—Unit dose (10/10's).

Each capsule contains 100 mg phenytoin sodium.

N 0071-0365-24—Bottle of 100.

Each capsule contains 30 mg phenytoin sodium.

N 0071-2214-20—8 oz bottle.

N 0071-2214-40—Unit dose pouches (5 ml × 100).

Each 5 ml of suspension contains 125 mg phenytoin with a maximum alcohol content not greater than 0.6 percent.

N 0071-2315-20—8 oz bottle.

Each 5 ml of suspension contains 30 mg phenytoin with a maximum alcohol content not greater than 0.6 percent.

N 0071-0375-24—Bottle of 100.

Each capsule contains phenytoin sodium 100 mg and phenobarbital 16 mg (1/4 gr).

N 0071-0531-24—Bottle of 100.

Each capsule contains phenytoin sodium 100 mg and phenobarbital 32 mg (1/2 gr).

N 0071-4488-05—2-ml ampoules.

A sterile solution for parenteral use containing 50 mg phenytoin sodium per ml. Supplied in packages of ten.

N 0071-4488-41—2-ml prefilled syringes.

A sterile solution for parenteral use containing 50 mg phenytoin sodium per ml in an individually cartoned disposable syringe (22 gauge × 1 1/4 inch needle). Supplied in packages of ten.

N 0071-4475-08—5-ml ampoules.

A sterile solution for parenteral use containing 50 mg phenytoin sodium per ml. Supplied in packages of ten.

N 0071-4488-45 Dilantin ready-mixed solution containing 50 mg phenytoin sodium per milliliter is supplied in 2-mL Steri-Vials.® Packages of twenty-five.

N 0071-4475-45 Dilantin ready-mixed solution containing 50 mg phenytoin sodium per milliliter is supplied in 5 mL Steri-Vials.® Packages of twenty-five.

0007G049

Storage: Store below 30°C (86°F).

Caution—Federal law prohibits dispensing without prescription.

Parenteral

DILANTIN® ℞

[dī-lăn' tĭn"]

(Phenytoin Sodium Injection, USP)

> **IMPORTANT NOTE**
> **This drug must be administered slowly. In adults do not exceed 50 mg per minute intravenously. In neonates, the drug should be administered at a rate not exceeding 1–3 mg/kg/min.**

DESCRIPTION

Dilantin (phenytoin sodium injection, USP) is a ready-mixed solution of phenytoin sodium in a vehicle containing 40% propylene glycol and 10% alcohol in water for injection, adjusted to pH 12 with sodium hydroxide. Phenytoin sodium is related to the barbiturates in chemical structure, but has a five-membered ring. The chemical name is sodium 5,5-diphenyl-2,4-imidazolidinedione.

CLINICAL PHARMACOLOGY

Phenytoin is an anticonvulsant which may be useful in the treatment of status epilepticus of the grand mal type. The primary site of action appears to be the motor cortex where spread of seizure activity is inhibited. Possibly by promoting sodium efflux from neurons, phenytoin tends to stabilize the threshold against hyperexcitability caused by excessive stimulation or environmental changes capable of reducing membrane sodium gradient. This includes the reduction of posttetanic potentiation at synapses. Loss of posttetanic potentiation prevents cortical seizure foci from detonating adjacent cortical areas. Phenytoin reduces the maximal activity of brain stem centers responsible for the tonic phase of grand mal seizures.

The plasma half-life in man after intravenous administration ranges from 10 to 15 hours. Optimum control without clinical signs of toxicity occurs most often with serum levels between 10 and 20 mcg/mL.

A fall in plasma levels may occur when patients are changed from oral to intramuscular administration. The drop is caused by slower absorption, as compared to oral administration, due to the poor water solubility of phenytoin. Intravenous administration is the preferred route for producing rapid therapeutic serum levels.

There are occasions when intramuscular administration may be required, ie, postoperatively, in comatose patients, for GI upsets. During these periods, a sufficient dose must be administered intramuscularly to maintain the plasma level within the therapeutic range. Where oral dosage is resumed following intramuscular usage, the oral dose should be properly adjusted to compensate for the slow, continuing IM absorption to avoid toxic symptoms.

Patients stabilized on a daily oral regimen of Dilantin experience a drop in peak blood levels to 50–60 percent of stable levels if crossed over to an equal dose administered intramuscularly. However, the intramuscular depot of poorly soluble material is eventually absorbed, as determined by urinary excretion of 5-(p-hydroxyphenyl)-5-phenylhydantoin (HPPH), the principal metabolite, as well as the total amount of drug eventually appearing in the blood.

A short-term (one week) study indicates that patients do not experience the expected drop in blood levels when crossed over to the intramuscular route if the Dilantin IM dose is increased by 50 percent over the previously established oral dose. To avoid drug cumulation due to absorption from the muscle depots, it is recommended that for the first week back on oral Dilantin, the dose be reduced to half of the original oral dose (one third of the IM dose). Experience for periods greater than one week is lacking and blood level monitoring is recommended. For administration of Dilantin in patients who cannot take oral medication for periods greater than a week, gastric intubation may be considered.

INDICATIONS

Parenteral Dilantin is indicated for the control of status epilepticus of the grand mal type, and prevention and treatment of seizures occurring during neurosurgery.

CONTRAINDICATIONS

Phenytoin is contraindicated in patients with a history of hypersensitivity to hydantoin products.

Because of its effect on ventricular automaticity, phenytoin is contraindicated in sinus bradycardia, sino-atrial block, second and third degree A-V block, and patients with Adams-Stokes syndrome.

WARNINGS

Intravenous administration should not exceed 50 mg per minute in adults. In neonates, the drug should be administered at a rate not exceeding 1–3mg/kg/min.

Severe cardiotoxic reactions and fatalities have been reported with atrial and ventricular conduction depression and ventricular fibrillation. Severe complications are most commonly encountered in elderly or gravely ill patients.

Phenytoin should be used with caution in patients with hypotension and severe myocardial insufficiency.

Hypotension usually occurs when the drug is administered rapidly by the intravenous route.

The intramuscular route is not recommended for the treatment of status epilepticus since blood levels of phenytoin in the therapeutic range cannot be readily achieved with doses and methods of administration ordinarily employed.

There have been a number of reports suggesting a relationship between phenytoin and the development of lymphadenopathy (local or generalized) including benign lymph node hyperplasia, pseudolymphoma, lymphoma, and Hodgkin's Disease. Although a cause and effect relationship has not been established, the occurrence of lymphadenopathy indicates the need to differentiate such a condition from other types of lymph node pathology. Lymph node involvement may occur with or without symptoms and signs resembling serum sickness eg, fever, rash and liver involvement.

In all cases of lymphadenopathy, follow-up observation for an extended period is indicated and every effort should be made to achieve seizure control using alternative antiepileptic drugs.

Acute alcoholic intake may increase phenytoin serum levels while chronic alcoholic use may decrease serum levels.

Usage in Pregnancy: A number of reports suggests an association between the use of antiepileptic drugs by women with epilepsy and a higher incidence of birth defects in children born to these women. Data are more extensive with respect to phenytoin and phenobarbital, but these are also the most commonly prescribed antiepileptic drugs; less systematic or anecdotal reports suggest a possible similar association with the use of all known antiepileptic drugs.

The reports suggesting a higher incidence of birth defects in children of drug-treated epileptic women cannot be regarded as adequate to prove a definite cause and effect relationship. There are intrinsic methodologic problems in obtaining adequate data on drug teratogenicity in humans; genetic factors or the epileptic condition itself may be more important than drug therapy in leading to birth defects. The great majority of mothers on antiepileptic medication deliver normal infants. It is important to note that antiepileptic drugs should not be discontinued in patients in whom the drug is administered to prevent major seizures, because of the strong possibility of precipitating status epilepticus with attendant hypoxia and threat to life. In individual cases where the severity and frequency of the seizure disorder are such that the removal of medication does not pose a serious threat to the patient, discontinuation of the drug may be considered prior to and during pregnancy, although it cannot be said with any confidence that even minor seizures do not pose some hazard to the developing embryo or fetus. The prescribing physician will wish to weigh these considerations in treating or counseling epileptic women of childbearing potential.

In addition to the reports of increased incidence of congenital malformation, such as cleft lip/palate and heart malformations in children of women receiving phenytoin and other antiepileptic drugs, there have more recently been reports of a fetal hydantoin syndrome. This consists of prenatal growth deficiency, microcephaly and mental deficiency in children born to mothers who have received phenytoin, barbiturates, alcohol, or trimethadione. However, these features are all interrelated and are frequently associated with intrauterine growth retardation from other causes.

There have been isolated reports of malignancies, including neuroblastoma, in children whose mothers received phenytoin during pregnancy.

An increase in seizure frequency during pregnancy occurs in a high proportion of patients, because of altered phenytoin absorption or metabolism. Periodic measurement of serum phenytoin levels is particularly valuable in the management of a pregnant epileptic patient as a guide to an appropriate adjustment of dosage. However, postpartum restoration of the original dosage will probably be indicated.

Neonatal coagulation defects have been reported within the first 24 hours in babies born to epileptic mothers receiving phenobarbital and/or phenytoin. Vitamin K has been shown to prevent or correct this defect and has been recommended to be given to the mother before delivery and the neonate after birth.

PRECAUTIONS

General: The addition of Dilantin solution to intravenous infusion is not recommended due to lack of solubility and resultant precipitation.

Parenteral Dilantin should be injected slowly (not exceeding 50 mg per minute in adults), directly into a large vein through a large-gauge needle or intravenous catheter. Each injection of intravenous Dilantin should be followed by an injection of sterile saline through the same needle or intravenous catheter to avoid local venous irritation due to the alkalinity of the solution. Continuous infusion should be avoided.

Soft tissue irritation and inflammation has occurred at the site of injection with and without extravasation of intravenous phenytoin. Soft tissue irritation may vary from slight tenderness to extensive necrosis, sloughing, and in rare instances has led to amputation. Improper administration including subcutaneous or perivascular injection should be avoided to help prevent possibility of the above.

The liver is the site of biotransformation. Patients with impaired liver function, elderly patients, or those who are gravely ill may show early toxicity.

A small percentage of individuals who have been treated with phenytoin have been shown to metabolize the drug slowly. Slow metabolism may be due to limited enzyme availability and lack of induction; it appears to be genetically determined.

Phenytoin should be discontinued if a skin rash appears (see "Warnings" section regarding drug discontinuation). If the rash is exfoliative, purpuric, or bullous or if lupus erythematosus, Stevens-Johnson syndrome, or toxic epidermal necrolysis is suspected, use of this drug should not be resumed and alternative therapy should be considered. (See Adverse Reactions.) If the rash is of a milder type (measles-like or scarlatiniform), therapy may be resumed after the rash has completely disappeared. If the rash recurs upon reinstitution of therapy, further phenytoin medication is contraindicated.

Hyperglycemia, resulting from the drug's inhibitory effects on insulin release, has been reported. Phenytoin may also raise the serum glucose level in diabetic patients.

Phenytoin is not indicated for seizures due to hypoglycemic or other metabolic causes. Appropriate diagnostic procedures should be performed as indicated.

Phenytoin is not effective for absence (petit mal) seizures. If tonic-clonic (grand-mal) and absence (petit mal) seizures are present, combined drug therapy is needed.

Serum levels of phenytoin sustained above the optimal range may produce confusional states referred to as "delirium," "psychosis," or "encephalopathy," or rarely irreversible cerebellar dysfunction. Accordingly, at the first sign of acute toxicity, plasma levels are recommended. Dose reduction of phenytoin therapy is indicated if plasma levels are excessive; if symptoms persist, termination is recommended. (See Warnings)

Laboratory Tests: Phenytoin serum level determinations may be necessary to achieve optimal dosage adjustments.

Drug Interactions: There are many drugs which may increase or decrease phenytoin levels or which phenytoin may affect. The most commonly occurring drug interactions are listed below:

1. Drugs which may increase phenytoin serum levels include: chloramphenicol, dicumarol, disulfiram, tolbutamide, isoniazid, phenylbutazone, acute alcohol intake, salicylates, chlordiazepoxide, phenothiazines, diazepam, estrogens, ethosuximide, halothane, methylphenidate, sulfonamides, cimetidine, trazodone.
2. Drugs which may decrease phenytoin levels include: carbamazepine, chronic alcohol abuse, reserpine. Moban® brand of Molindone Hydrochloride contains calcium ions which interfere with the absorption of phenytoin. Ingestion times of phenytoin and antacid preparations containing calcium should be staggered in patients with low serum phenytoin levels to prevent absorption problems.
3. Drugs which may either increase or decrease phenytoin serum levels include: phenobarbital, valproic acid, and sodium valproate. Similarly, the effect of phenytoin on phenobarbital, valproic acid and sodium valproate serum levels is unpredictable.
4. Although not a true drug interaction, tricyclic antidepressants may precipitate seizures in susceptible patients and phenytoin dosage may need to be adjusted.
5. Drugs whose efficacy is impaired by phenytoin include: corticosteroids, coumarin anticoagulants, oral contraceptives, quinidine, vitamin D, digitoxin, rifampin, doxycycline, estrogens, furosemide.

Serum level determinations are especially helpful when possible drug interactions are suspected.

Drug/Laboratory Test Interactions: Phenytoin may cause decreased serum levels of protein-bound iodine (PBI). It may also produce lower than normal values for dexamethasone or metyrapone tests. Phenytoin may cause increased serum levels of glucose, alkaline phosphatase, and gamma glutamyl transpeptidase (GGT).

Carcinogenesis: See 'Warnings' section for information on carcinogenesis.

Pregnancy: See Warnings

Nursing Mothers: Infant breast feeding is not recommended for women taking this drug because phenytoin appears to be secreted in low concentrations in human milk.

ADVERSE REACTIONS

The most notable signs of toxicity associated with the intravenous use of this drug are cardiovascular collapse and/or central nervous system depression. Hypotension does occur when the drug is administered rapidly by the intravenous route. The *rate* of administration is very important; it should not exceed 50 mg per minute in adults, and 1–3 mg/kg/min in neonates. At this rate, toxicity should be minimized.

Cardiovascular: Severe cardiotoxic reactions and fatalities have been reported with atrial and ventricular conduction depression and ventricular fibrillation. Severe complications are most commonly encountered in elderly or gravely ill patients.

Central Nervous System: The most common manifestations encountered with phenytoin therapy are referable to this system and are usually dose-related. These include nystagmus, ataxia, slurred speech, decreased coordination and mental confusion. Dizziness, insomnia, transient nervousness, motor twitchings, and headaches have also been observed. There have also been rare reports of phenytoin induced dyskinesias, including chorea, dystonia, tremor and asterixis, similar to those induced by phenothiazine and other neuroleptic drugs.

A predominantly sensory peripheral polyneuropathy has been observed in patients receiving long-term phenytoin therapy.

Gastrointestinal System: Nausea, vomiting, and constipation.

Integumentary System: Dermatological manifestations sometimes accompanied by fever have included scarlatiniform or morbilliform rashes. A morbilliform rash (measles-like) is the most common; other types of dermatitis are seen more rarely. Other more serious forms which may be fatal have included bullous, exfoliative or purpuric dermatitis, lupus erythematosus, Stevens-Johnson syndrome, and toxic epidermal necrolysis (see Precautions).

Hemopoietic System: Hemopoietic complications, some fatal, have occasionally been reported in association with administration of phenytoin. These have included thrombocytopenia, leukopenia, granulocytopenia, agranulocytosis, and pancytopenia with or without bone marrow suppression. While macrocytosis and megaloblastic anemia have occurred, these conditions usually respond to folic acid therapy. Lymphadenopathy including benign lymph node hyperplasia, pseudolymphoma, lymphoma, and Hodgkin's Disease have been reported (see Warnings).

Connective Tissue System: Coarsening of the facial features, enlargement of the lips, gingival hyperplasia, hypertrichosis, and Peyronie's Disease.

Injection Site: Local irritation, inflammation, tenderness, necrosis, and sloughing have been reported with or without extravasation of intravenous phenytoin.

Other: Systemic lupus erythematosus, periarteritis nodosa, toxic hepatitis, liver damage, and immunoglobulin abnormalities may occur.

OVERDOSAGE

The lethal dose in children is not known. The lethal dose in adults is estimated to be 2 to 5 grams. The initial symptoms are nystagmus, ataxia and dysarthria. Other signs are tremor, hyperflexia, lethargy, slurred speech, nausea, vomiting. The patient may become comatose and hypertensive. Death is due to respiratory and circulatory depression.

There are marked variations among individuals with respect to phenytoin plasma levels where toxicity may occur. Nystagmus, on lateral gaze, usually appears at 20 mcg/mL, ataxia at 30 mcg/mL, dysarthria and lethargy appear when the plasma concentration is over 40 mcg/mL, but as high a concentration as 50 mcg/mL has been reported without evidence of toxicity. As much as 25 times the therapeutic dose has been taken to result in a serum concentration over 100 mcg/mL with complete recovery.

Treatment: Treatment is nonspecific since there is no known antidote.

The adequacy of the respiratory and circulatory systems should be carefully observed and appropriate supportive measures employed. Hemodialysis can be considered since phenytoin is not completely bound to plasma proteins. Total exchange transfusion has been used in the treatment of severe intoxication in children.

In acute overdosage the possibility of other CNS depressants, including alcohol, should be borne in mind.

DOSAGE AND ADMINISTRATION

The addition of Dilantin solution to intravenous infusion is not recommended due to lack of solubility and resultant precipitation.

Not to exceed 50 mg per minute, intravenously in adults, and not exceeding 1–3 mg/kg/min in neonates There is a relatively small margin between full therapeutic effect and minimally toxic doses of this drug.

The solution is suitable for use as long as it remains free of haziness and precipitate. Upon refrigeration or freezing, a precipitate might form; this will dissolve again after the solution is allowed to stand at room temperature. The product is still suitable for use. Only a clear solution should be used. A faint yellow coloration may develop; however, this has no effect on the potency of the solution.

Continued on next page

This product information was prepared in August 1992. On these and other Parke-Davis Products, information may be obtained by addressing PARKE-DAVIS, Division of Warner-Lambert Company, Morris Plains, New Jersey 07950.

Parke-Davis—Cont.

In the treatment of status epilepticus, the intravenous route is preferred because of the delay in absorption of phenytoin when administered intramuscularly.
Serum concentrations should be monitored and care should be taken when switching a patient from the sodium salt to the free acid form.
Dilantin® Kapseals®, Dilantin Parenteral, and Dilantin with Phenobarbital are formulated with the sodium salt of phenytoin. The free acid form of phenytoin is used in Dilantin-30 Pediatric and Dilantin-125 Suspensions and Dilantin Infatabs. Because there is approximately an 8% increase in drug content with the free acid form over that of the sodium salt, dosage adjustments and serum level monitoring may be necessary when switching from a product formulated with the free acid to a product formulated with the sodium salt and vice versa.
Status Epilepticus: In adults, a loading dose of 10 to 15 mg/kg should be administered slowly intravenously, at a rate not exceeding 50 mg per minute (this will require approximately 20 minutes in a 70-kg patient). The loading dose should be followed by maintenance doses of 100 mg orally or intravenously every 6–8 hours.
Recent work in neonates and children has shown that absorption of phenytoin is unreliable after oral administration, but a loading dose of 15–20 mg/kg of Dilantin intravenously will usually produce plasma concentrations of phenytoin within the generally accepted therapeutic range (10–20 mcg/mL). The drug should be injected slowly intravenously at a rate not exceeding 1–3 mg/kg/min.
Parenteral Dilantin should be injected *slowly* and directly into a large vein through a large-gauge needle or intravenous catheter. Each injection of intravenous Dilantin should be followed by an injection of sterile saline through the same needle or catheter to avoid local venous irritation due to alkalinity of the solution. Continuous infusion should be avoided; the addition of Parenteral Dilantin to intravenous infusion fluids is not recommended because of the likelihood of precipitation.
Continuous monitoring of the electrocardiogram and blood pressure is essential. The patient should be observed for signs of respiratory depression. Determination of phenytoin plasma levels is advised when using Dilantin in the management of status epilepticus and in the subsequent establishment of maintenance dosage.
Other measures, including concomitant administration of an intravenous benzodiazepine such as diazepam, or an intravenous short-acting barbiturate, will usually be necessary for rapid control of seizures because of the required slow rate of administration of Dilantin.
If administration of Parenteral Dilantin does not terminate seizures, the use of other anticonvulsants, intravenous barbiturates, general anesthesia, and other appropriate measures should be considered.
Intramuscular administration should not be used in the treatment of status epilepticus because the attainment of peak plasma levels may require up to 24 hours.
Neurosurgery: Prophylactic dosage—100 to 200 mg (2 to 4 mL) intramuscularly at approximately 4-hour intervals during surgery and continued during the postoperative period.
When intramuscular administration is required for a patient previously stabilized orally, compensating dosage adjustments are necessary to maintain therapeutic plasma levels. An intramuscular dose 50% greater than the oral dose is necessary to maintain these levels. When returned to oral administration, the dose should be reduced by 50% of the original oral dose for one week to prevent excessive plasma levels due to sustained release from intramuscular tissue sites.
If the patient requires more than a week of IM Dilantin, alternative routes should be explored, such as gastric intubation. For time periods less than one week, the patient shifted back from IM administration should receive one half the original oral dose for the same period of time the patient received IM Dilantin. Monitoring plasma levels would help prevent a fall into the subtherapeutic range. Serum blood level determinations are especially helpful when possible drug interactions are suspected.

HOW SUPPLIED

N 0071-4488-05 (Ampoule 1488) Dilantin ready-mixed solution containing 50 mg phenytoin sodium per milliliter is supplied in 2-mL ampoules. Packages of ten.
N 0071-4488-41 (Steri-Dose® 4488) Dilantin ready-mixed solution containing 50 mg phenytoin sodium per milliliter is supplied in a 2-mL sterile disposable syringe (22 gauge × $1\frac{1}{4}$ inch needle). Packages of ten individually cartoned syringes.
N 0071-4475-08 (Ampoule 1475) Dilantin ready-mixed solution contaning 50 mg phenytoin sodium per milliliter is supplied in packages of ten 5-mL ampoules without syringes.
N 0071-4488-45 Dilantin ready-mixed solution containing 50 mg phenytoin sodium per milliliter is supplied in 2-mL sterivials. Packages of twenty-five.
N 0071-4475-45 Dilantin ready-mixed solution containing 50 mg phenytoin sodium per milliliter is supplied in 5-mL sterivials. Packages of twenty-five.
Caution—Federal law prohibits dispensing without prescription.

4475G028

DILANTIN-30® PEDIATRIC/ DILANTIN-125® ℞

[*dī-lăn'tĭn*]
(Phenytoin Oral Suspension, USP)

DESCRIPTION

Dilantin (phenytoin) is related to the barbiturates in chemical structure, but has a five-membered ring. The chemical name is 5,5-diphenyl-2,4 imidazolidinedione.
Each teaspoonful of suspension contains 30 mg or 125 mg of phenytoin, USP with a maximum alcohol content not greater than 0.6 percent. Also contains carboxymethylcellulose sodium, USP; citric acid; anhydrous, USP; flavors; glycerin, USP; magnesium aluminum silicate, NF; polysorbate 40, NF; purified water, USP; sodium benzoate, NF; sucrose, NF; vanillin NF. The 30 mg per teaspoonful suspension also contains D&C red No. 33; FD&C red No. 40. The 125 mg per teaspoonful suspension also contains FD&C yellow No. 6.

CLINICAL PHARMACOLOGY

Phenytoin is an antiepileptic drug which can be useful in the treatment of epilepsy. The primary site of action appears to be *the motor cortex* where spread of seizure activity is inhibited. Possibly by promoting sodium efflux from neurons, phenytoin tends to *stabilize* the threshold against hyperexcitability caused by excessive stimulation or environmental changes capable of reducing membrane sodium gradient. This includes the reduction of posttetanic potentiation at synapses. Loss of posttetanic potentiation prevents cortical seizure foci from detonating adjacent cortical areas. Phenytoin reduces the maximal activity of brain stem centers responsible for the tonic phase of tonic-clonic (grand mal) seizures.
The plasma half-life in man after oral administration of phenytoin averages 22 hours, with a range of 7 to 42 hours. Steady-state therapeutic levels are achieved at least 7 to 10 days (5–7 half-lives) after initiation of therapy with recommended doses of 300 mg/day.
When serum level determinations are necessary, they should be obtained at least 5–7 half-lives after treatment initiation, dosage change, or addition or subtraction of another drug to the regimen so that equilibrium or steady-state will have been achieved. Trough levels provide information about clinically effective serum level range and confirm patient compliance and are obtained just prior to the patient's next scheduled dose. Peak levels indicate an individual's threshold for emergence of dose-related side effects and are obtained at the time of expected peak concentration. For Dilantin-30 Pediatric and Dilantin-125 Suspensions peak levels occur $1\frac{1}{2}$–3 hours after administration.
Optimum control without clinical signs of toxicity occurs more often with serum levels between 10 and 20 mcg/mL, although some mild cases of tonic-clonic (grand mal) epilepsy may be controlled with lower serum levels of phenytoin.
In most patients maintained at a steady dosage, stable phenytoin serum levels are achieved. There may be wide interpatient variability in phenytoin serum levels with equivalent dosages. Patients with unusually low levels may be noncompliant or hypermetabolizers of phenytoin. Unusally high levels result from liver disease, congenital enzyme deficiency or drug interactions which result in metabolic interference. The patient with large variations in phenytoin plasma levels, despite standard doses, presents a difficult clinical problem. Serum level determinations in such patients may be particularly helpful. As phenytoin is highly protein bound, free phenytoin levels may be altered in patients whose protein binding characteristics differ from normal.
Most of the drug is excreted in the bile as inactive metabolites which are then reabsorbed from the intestinal tract and excreted in the urine. Urinary excretion of phenytoin and its metabolites occurs partly with glomerular filtration but more importantly, by tubular secretion. Because phenytoin is hydroxylated in the liver by an enzyme system which is saturable at high plasma levels small incremental doses may increase the half-life and produce very substantial increases in serum levels, when these are in the upper range. The steady-state level may be disproportionately increased, with resultant intoxication, from an increase in dosage of 10% or more.

INDICATIONS AND USAGE

Dilantin (phenytoin) is indicated for the control of tonic-clonic (grand mal) and psychomotor (temporal lobe) seizures.
Phenytoin serum level determinations may be necessary for optimal dosage adjustments (see Dosage and Administration and Clinical Pharmacology)

CONTRAINDICATIONS

Dilantin is contraindicated in those patients with a history of hypersensitivity to phenytoin or other hydantoins.

WARNINGS

Abrupt withdrawal of phenytoin in epileptic patients may precipitate status epilepticus. When in the judgment of the clinician the need for dosage reduction, discontinuation, or substitution of alternative anticonvulsant medication arises, this should be done gradually. In the event of an allergic or hypersensitivity reaction, more rapid substitution of alternative therapy may be necessary. In this case, alternative therapy should be an anticonvulsant not belonging to the hydantion chemical class.
There have been a number of reports suggesting a relationship between phenytoin and the development of lymphadenopathy (local or generalized) including benign lymph node hyperplasia, pseudolymphoma, lymphoma, and Hodgkin's Disease. Although a cause and effect relationship has not been established, the occurrence of lymphadenopathy indicates the need to differentiate such a condition from other types of lymph node pathology. Lymph node involvement may occur with or without symptoms and signs resembling serum sickness eg, fever, rash and liver involvement.
In all cases of lymphadenopathy, follow-up observation for an extended period is indicated and every effort should be made to achieve seizure control using alternative antiepileptic drugs. Acute alcoholic intake may increase phenytoin serum levels while chronic alcoholic use may decrease serum levels.
In view of isolated reports associating phenytoin with exacerbation of porphyria, caution should be exercised in using this medication in patients suffering from this disease.
Usage in Pregnancy: A number of reports suggests an association between the use of antiepileptic drugs by women with epilepsy and a higher incidence of birth defects in children born to these women. Data are more extensive with respect to phenytoin and phenobarbital, but these are also the most commonly prescribed antiepileptic drugs; less systematic or anecdotal reports suggest a possible similar association with the use of all known antiepileptic drugs.
The reports suggesting a higher incidence of birth defects in children of drug-treated epileptic women cannot be regarded as adequate to prove a definite cause and effect relationship. There are intrinsic methodologic problems in obtaining adequate data on drug teratogenicity in humans; genetic factors or the epileptic condition itself may be more important than drug therapy in leading to birth defects. The great majority of mothers on antiepileptic medication deliver normal infants. It is important to note that antiepileptic drugs should not be discontinued in patients in whom the drug is administered to prevent major seizures, because of the strong possibility of precipitating status epilepticus with attendant hypoxia and threat to life. In individual cases where the severity and frequency of the seizure disorder are such that the removal of medication does not pose a serious threat to the patient, discontinuation of the drug may be considered prior to and during pregnancy, although it cannot be said with any confidence that even minor seizures do not pose some hazards to the developing embryo or fetus. The prescribing physician will wish to weigh these considerations in treating and counseling epileptic women of childbearing potential.
In addition to the reports of increased incidence of congenital malformation, such as cleft lip/palate and heart malformations in children of women receiving phenytoin and other antiepileptic drugs, there have more recently been reports of a fetal hydantoin syndrome. This consists of prenatal growth deficiency, microcephaly and mental deficiency in children born to mothers who have received phenytoin, barbiturates, alcohol, or trimethadione. However, these features are all interrelated and are frequently associated with intrauterine growth retardation from other causes.
There have been isolated reports of malignancies, including neuroblastoma, in children whose mothers received phenytoin during pregnancy.
An increase in seizure frequency during pregnancy occurs in a high proportion of patients, because of altered phenytoin absorption or metabolism. Periodic measurement of serum phenytoin levels is particularly valuable in the management of a pregnant epileptic patient as a guide to an appropriate adjustment of dosage. However, postpartum restoration of the original dosage will probably be indicated.
Neonatal coagulation defects have been reported within the first 24 hours in babies born to epileptic mothers receiving phenobarbital and/or phenytoin. Vitamin K has been shown to prevent or correct this defect and has been recommended to be given to the mother before delivery and the neonate after birth.

PRECAUTIONS

General: The liver is the chief site of biotransformation of phenytoin; patients wth impaired liver function, elderly patients, or those who are gravely ill may show early signs of toxicity.
A small percentage of individuals who have been treated with phenytoin have been shown to metabolize the drug

slowly. Slow metabolism may be due to limited enzyme availability and lack of induction; it appears to be genetically determined.

Phenytoin should be discontinued if a skin rash appears (see "Warnings" section regarding drug discontinuation). If the rash is exfoliative, purpuric, or bullous or if lupus erythematosus, Stevens-Johnson syndrome, or toxic epidermal necrolysis is suspected, use of this drug should not be resumed and alternative therapy should be considered. (See Adverse Reactions). If the rash is of a milder type (measles-like or scarlatiniform), therapy may be resumed after the rash has completely disappeared. If the rash recurs upon reinstitution of therapy, further phenytoin medication is contraindicated. Phenytoin and other hydantoins are contraindicated in patients who have experienced phenytoin hypersensitivity. Additionally, caution should be exercised if using structurally similar (eg, barbiturates, succinamides, oxazolidinediones and other related compounds) in these same patients. Hyperglycemia, resulting from the drug's inhibitory effects on insulin release, has been reported. Phenytoin may also raise the serum glucose level in diabetic patients.

Osteomalacia has been associated with phenytoin therapy and is considered to be due to phenytoin's interference with Vitamin D metabolism.

Phenytoin is not indicated for seizures due to hypoglycemic or other metabolic causes. Appropriate diagnostic procedures should be performed as indicated.

Phenytoin is not effective for absence (petit mal) seizures. If tonic-clonic (grand mal) and absence (petit mal) seizures are present, combined drug therapy is needed.

Serum levels of phenytoin sustained above the optimal range may produce confusional states referred to as "delirium," "psychosis" or "encephalopathy," or rarely irreversible cerebellar dysfunction. Accordingly, at the first sign of acute toxicity, plasma levels are recommended. Dose reduction of phenytoin therapy is indicated if plasma levels are excessive; if symptoms persist, termination is recommended. (See Warnings).

Information for Patients: Patients taking phenytoin should be advised of the importance of adhering strictly to the prescribed dosage regimen, and of informing the physician of any clinical condition in which it is not possible to take the drug orally as prescribed, eg, surgery, etc.

Patients should also be cautioned on the use of other drugs or alcoholic beverages without first seeking the physician's advice.

Patients should be instructed to call their physician if skin rash develops.

The importance of good dental hygiene should be stressed in order to minimize the development of gingival hyperplasia and its complications.

Laboratory Tests: Phenytoin serum level determinations may be necessary to achieve optimal dosage adjustments.

Drug Interactions: There are many drugs which may increase or decrease phenytoin levels or which phenytoin may affect. Serum level determinations for phenytoin are especially helpful when possible drug interactions are suspected. The most commonly occurring drug interactions are listed below.

1. Drugs which may increase phenytoin serum levels include: acute alcohol intake, amiodarone, chloramphenicol, chlordiazepoxide, diazepam, dicumarol, disulfiram, estrogens, ethosuximide, H_2-antagonists, halothane, isoniazid, methylphenidate, phenothiazines, phenylbutazone, salicylates, succinimides, sulfonamides, tolbutamide, trazodone.

2. Drugs which may decrease phenytoin levels include: carbamazepine, chronic alcohol abuse, reserpine and sucralfate. Moban® brand of molindone hydrochloride contains calcium ions which interfere with the absorption of phenytoin. Ingestion times of phenytoin and antacid preparations containing calcium should be staggered in patients with low serum phenytoin levels to prevent absorption problems.

3. Drugs which may either increase or decrease phenytoin serum levels include: phenobarbital, sodium valproate, and valproic acid. Similarly, the effect of phenytoin on phenobarbital, valproic acid and sodium valproate serum levels is unpredictable.

4. Although not a true drug interaction, tricyclic antidepressants may precipitate seizures in susceptible patients and phenytoin dosage may need to be adjusted.

5. Drugs whose efficacy is impaired by phenytoin include: corticosteroids, coumarin anticoagulants, digitoxin, doxycycline, estrogens, furosemide, oral contraceptives, quinidine, rifampin, theophylline, vitamin D.

Drug/Laboratory Test Interactions: Phenytoin may cause decreased serum levels of protein-bound iodine (PBI). It may also produce lower than normal values for dexamethasone or metyrapone tests. Phenytoin may cause increased serum levels of glucose, alkaline phosphatase, and gamma glutamyl transpeptidase (GGT).

Carcinogenesis: See 'Warnings' section for information on carcinogenesis.

Pregnancy: See Warnings

Nursing Mothers: Infant breast feeding is not recommended for women taking this drug because phenytoin appears to be secreted in low concentrations in human milk.

ADVERSE REACTIONS

Central Nervous System: The most common manifestations encountered with phenytoin therapy are referable to this system and are usually dose-related. These include nystagmus, ataxia, slurred speech, decreased coordination, and mental confusion. Dizziness, insomnia, transient nervousness, motor twitchings, and headaches have also been observed. There have also been rare reports of phenytoin induced dyskinesias, including chorea, dystonia, tremor and asterixis, similar to those induced by phenothiazine and other neuroleptic drugs.

A predominantly sensory peripheral polyneuropathy has been observed in patients receiving long-term phenytoin therapy.

Gastrointestinal System: Nausea, vomiting, constipation, toxic hepatitis and liver damage.

Integumentary System: Dermatological manifestations sometimes accompanied by fever have included scarlatiniform or morbilliform rashes. A morbilliform rash (measles-like) is the most common; other types of dermatitis are seen more rarely. Other more serious forms which may be fatal have included bullous, exfoliative or purpuric dermatitis, lupus erythematosus, Stevens-Johnson syndrome, and toxic epidermal necrolysis (see Precautions).

Hemopoietic System: Hemopoietic complications, some fatal, have occasionally been reported in association with administration of phenytoin. These have included thrombocytopenia, leukopenia, granulocytopenia, agranulocytosis, and pancytopenia with or without bone marrow suppression. While macrocytosis and megaloblastic anemia have occurred, these conditions usually respond to folic acid therapy. Lymphadenopathy including benign lymph node hyperplasia, pseudolymphoma, lymphoma, and Hodgkin's Disease have been reported (see Warnings).

Connective Tissue System: Coarsening of the facial features, enlargement of the lips, gingival hyperplasia, hypertrichosis, and Peyronie's Disease.

Cardiovascular: Periarteritis nodosa.

Immunologic: Hypersensitivity syndrome (which may include, but is not limited to, symptoms such as arthralgias, eosinophilia, fever, liver dysfunction, lymphadenopathy or rash), systemic lupus erythematosus, and immunoglobulin abnormalities.

OVERDOSAGE

The lethal dose in children is not known. The lethal dose in adults is estimated to be 2 to 5 grams. The initial symptoms are nystagmus, ataxia, and dysarthria. Other signs are tremor, hyperflexia, lethargy, slurred speech, nausea, vomiting. The patient may become comatose and hypotensive. Death is due to respiratory and circulatory depression.

There are marked variations among individuals with respect to phenytoin plasma levels where toxicity may occur. Nystagmus, on lateral gaze, usually appears at 20 mcg/mL, ataxia at 30 mcg/mL, dysarthria and lethargy appear when the plasma concentration is over 40 mcg/mL, but as high a concentration as 50 mcg/mL has been reported without evidence of toxicity. As much as 25 times the therapeutic dose has been taken to result in a serum concentration over 100 mcg/mL with complete recovery.

Treatment: Treatment is nonspecific since there is no known antidote.

The adequacy of the respiratory and circulatory systems should be carefully observed and appropriate supportive measures employed. Hemodialysis can be considered since phenytoin is not completely bound to plasma proteins. Total exchange transfusion has been used in the treatment of severe intoxication in children.

In acute overdosage the possibility of other CNS depressants, including alcohol, should be borne in mind.

DOSAGE AND ADMINISTRATION

Serum concentrations should be monitored and care should be taken when switching a patient from the sodium salt to the free acid form.

Dilantin® Kapseals®, Dilantin Parenteral, and Dilantin with Phenobarbital are formulated with the sodium salt of phenytoin. The free acid form of phenytoin is used in Dilantin-30 Pediatric and Dilantin-125 Suspensions and Dilantin Infatabs. Because there is approximately an 8% increase in drug content with the free acid form over that of the sodium salt, dosage adjustments and serum level monitoring may be necessary when switching from a product formulated with the free acid to a product formulated with the sodium salt and vice versa.

General: Dosage should be individualized to provide maximum benefit. In some cases serum blood level determinations may be necessary for optimal dosage adjustments—the clinically effective serum level is usually 10–20 mcg/mL. With recommended dosage, a period of seven to ten days may be required to achieve steady-state blood levels with phenytoin and changes in dosage (increase or decrease) should not be carried out at intervals shorter than seven to ten days.

Adult Dose: Patients who have received no previous treatment may be started on one teaspoonful (5 mL) of Dilantin-125 Suspension three times daily, and the dose is then adjusted to suit individual requirements. An increase to five teaspoonfuls daily may be made, if necessary.

Pediatric Dose: Initially, 5 mg/kg/day in two or three equally divided doses, with subsequent dosage individualized to a maximum of 300 mg daily. A recommended daily maintenance dosage is usually 4 to 8 mg/kg. Children over 6 years may require the minimum adult dose (300 mg/day).

HOW SUPPLIED

N 0071-2214—Dilantin-125® Suspension (phenytoin oral suspension, USP), 125 mg phenytoin/5 mL with a maximum alcohol content not greater than 0.6 percent, an orange suspension with an orange-vanilla flavor; available in 8-oz bottles and individual unit dose foil pouches which deliver 5 mL (125 mg phenytoin). The minimum sales unit is 100 pouches.

N 0071-2315—Dilantin-30® Pediatric Suspension (phenytoin oral suspension, USP), 30 mg phenytoin/5 mL with a maximum alcohol content not greater than 0.6 percent, a red suspension with a banana-orange-vanilla flavor; available in 8-oz bottles.

Store below 30°C (86°F). Protect from freezing and light.

Also available as:

N 0071-0362 (Kapseal® 362)—Dilantin (extended phenytoin sodium capsules, USP) 100 mg; in 100's, 1000's, unit dose 100's.

N 0071-0365 (Kapseal 365)—Dilantin (extended phenytoin sodium capsules, USP) 30 mg, in 100's.

N 0071-0375 (Kapseal 375)—Dilantin with Phenobarbital each contain 100 mg phenytoin sodium with 16 mg (¼ gr) phenobarbital; in 100's.

N 0071-0531 (Kapseal 531)—Dilantin with Phenobarbital each contain 100 mg phenytoin sodium with 32 mg (½ gr) phenobarbital; in 100's.

N 0071-0007 (Tablet 7)—Dilantin Infatabs® (phenytoin tablets, USP) each contain 50 mg phenytoin; 100's and unit dose 100's.

For Parenteral Use:

N 0071-4488-05 (Ampoule 1488)—Dilantin ready-mixed solution containing 50 mg phenytoin sodium per milliliter is supplied in 2-mL ampoules. Packages of ten.

N 0071-4475-08 (Ampoule 1475)—Dilantin ready-mixed solution containing 50 mg phenytoin sodium per milliliter is supplied in packages of ten 5-mL ampoules without syringes.

N 0071-4488-41 (Steri-Dose® 4488)—Dilantin ready-mixed solution containing 50 mg phenytoin sodium per milliliter is supplied in a 2-mL sterile disposable syringe (22 gauge × 1¼ inch needle). Packages of ten individually cartoned syringes.

N 0071-4488-45 Dilantin ready-mixed solution containing 50 mg phenytoin sodium per milliliter is supplied in 2 mL Steri-Vials.® Packages of twenty-five.

N 0071-4475-45 Dilantin ready-mixed solution containing 50 mg phenytoin sodium per milliliter is supplied in 5 mL Steri-Vials.® Packages of twenty-five.

Storage: Store below 30° C (86° F).

Caution—Federal law prohibits dispensing without prescription.

                                              2214G109

KAPSEALS®
DILANTIN®   ℞
[di-lăn'tĭn]
(Phenytoin Sodium) with Phenobarbital

DESCRIPTION

Dilantin (phenytoin sodium) is related to the barbiturates in chemical structure, but has a five-membered ring. The chemical name is sodium 5,5-diphenyl-2,4-imidazolidinedione.

Phenobarbital is a derivative of barbituric acid and is chemically described as 5-ethyl-5-phenylbarbituric acid.

Each Dilantin® with ¼ gr Phenobarbital Kapseal® contains:

Dilantin (phenytoin sodium) .... 100 mg
Phenobarbital .... 16 mg (¼ gr)
(Warning—May be habit forming)

Each Dilantin with ½ gr Phenobarbital Kapseal contains:
Dilantin (phenytoin sodium) .... 100 mg
Phenobarbital .... 32 mg (½ gr)
(Warning—May be habit forming)

Continued on next page

This product information was prepared in August 1992. On these and other Parke-Davis Products, information may be obtained by addressing PARKE-DAVIS, Division of Warner-Lambert Company, Morris Plains, New Jersey 07950.

Parke-Davis—Cont.

Also contains confectioner's sugar NF, magnesium stearate, NF; talc, USP. The capsule shell and band contain citric acid, USP; colloidal silicon dioxide, NF; FD&C blue No. 1; FD&C red No. 40; gelatin NF; glyceryl monooleate; polyethylene glycol 200; sodium benzoate, NF; sodium lauryl sulfate, NF. The Dilantin with Phenobarbital ¼ gr capsule shell and band also contain FD&C red No. 3; hydrogen peroxide 3%. The Dilantin with Phenobarbital ½ gr capsule shell and band also contain FD&C yellow No. 6.

CLINICAL PHARMACOLOGY

Phenytoin—Phenytoin is an antiepileptic drug which can be useful in the treatment of epilepsy. The primary site of action appears to be the *motor cortex* where spread of seizure activity is inhibited. Possibly by promoting sodium efflux from neurons, phenytoin tends to *stabilize* the threshold against hyperexcitability caused by excessive stimulation or environmental changes capable of reducing membrane sodium gradient. This includes the reduction of posttetanic potentiation at synapses. Loss of posttetanic potentiation prevents cortical seizure foci from detonating adjacent cortical areas. Phenytoin reduces the maximal activity of brain stem centers responsible for the tonic phase of tonic-clonic (grand mal) seizures.

The plasma half-life in man after oral administration of phenytoin averages 22 hours, with a range of 7 to 42 hours. Steady-state therapeutic levels are achieved at least 7 to 10 days (5–7 half-lives) after initiation of therapy with recommended doses of 300 mg/day.

When serum level determinations are necessary, they should be obtained at least 5–7 half-lives after treatment initiation, dosage change, or addition or subtraction of another drug to the regimen so that equilibrium or steady-state will have been achieved. Trough levels provide information about clinically effective serum level range and confirm patient compliance and are obtained just prior to the patient's next scheduled dose. Peak levels indicate an individual's threshold for emergence of dose-related side effects and are obtained at the time of expected peak concentration. For Dilantin with Phenobarbital Kapseals peak serum levels occur 1½–3 hours after administration.

Optimum control without clinical signs of toxicity occurs more often with serum levels between 10 and 20 mcg/mL, although some mild cases of tonic-clonic (grand mal) epilepsy may be controlled with lower serum levels of phenytoin.

In most patients maintained at a steady dosage, stable phenytoin serum levels are achieved. There may be wide interpatient variability in phenytoin serum levels with equivalent dosages. Patients with unusually low levels may be noncompliant or hypermetabolizers of phenytoin. Unusually high levels result from liver disease, congenital enzyme deficiency or drug interactions which result in metabolic interference. The patient with large variations in phenytoin plasma levels, despite standard doses, presents a difficult clinical problem. Serum level determinations in such patients may be particularly helpful. As phenytoin is highly protein bound, free phenytoin levels may be altered in patients whose protein binding characteristics differ from normal.

Most of the drug is excreted in the bile as inactive metabolites which are then reabsorbed from the intestinal tract and excreted in the urine. Urinary excretion of phenytoin and its metabolites occurs partly with glomerular filtration, but more importantly, by tubular secretion. Because phenytoin is hydroxylated in the liver by an enzyme system which is saturable at high plasma levels small incremental doses may increase the half-life and produce very substantial increases in serum levels, when these are in the upper range. The steady-state level may be disproportionately increased, with resultant intoxication, from an increase in dosage of 10% or more.

Phenobarbital—Phenobarbital produces its anticonvulsant effect by depressing the motor cortex and raising the seizure threshold.

Phenobarbital is absorbed completely, although slowly, following oral administration and undergoes partial biotransformation in the liver by hydroxylation. Phenobarbital is excreted via the kidneys, 10% to 25% as free drug and the reminder primarily as the inactive para-hydroxyphenyl metabolite. The plasma half-life is long, approximately two to six days in adults, and shorter and more variable in children. In adults, the oral anticonvulsant dose of 1 to 3 mg/kg will produce therapeutic concentrations of 10 to 30 mcg/mL in the serum, the levels usually necessary for seizure control. At this dose, approximately three weeks may be required for the serum levels to achieve steady-state.

High serum levels occur when liver disease, diminished urinary flow, acidosis, or obesity is present. Low serum levels in adults may be due to poor patient compliance.

When used as an anticonvulsant, the clinical phenomenon of breakthrough seizures has been seen. Whether this is a case of true pharmacologic tolerance or some form of spontaneous variation is not known. Physical dependence does develop and may produce accentuation of seizures in epileptics when the drug is abruptly withdrawn.

INDICATIONS AND USAGE

Dilantin with Phenobarbital is indicated for the control of generalized tonic-clonic (grand mal) and complex partial (psychomotor, temporal lobe) seizures, only in those patients who require both drugs for seizure control and who previously have had their daily anticonvulsant requirements determined by the administration of the two drugs separately. Combinations should not be used to initiate anticonvulsant therapy and are provided as a convenience for epileptic patients.

Phenytoin serum level determinations may be necessary for optimal dosage adjustments (see Dosage and Administration and Clinical Pharmacology).

CONTRAINDICATIONS

Phenytoin is contraindicated in those patients with a history of hypersensitivity to phenytoin or other hydantoins.

Phenobarbital is contraindicated in the following conditions: latent or manifest porphyria or familial history of intermittent porphyria, history of confusion or restlessness from hypnotics, history of abnormal reaction or known hypersensitivity to barbital and its derivatives, including phenobarbital, or a known previous addiction to sedative-hypnotics. Other contraindications include renal and hepatic impairment and severe pulmonary insufficiency.

WARNINGS

Warning—Phenobarbital may be habit forming. Abrupt withdrawal of phenytoin in epileptic patients may precipitate status epilepticus. When, in the judgment of the clinician, the need for dosage reduction, discontinuation, or substitution of alternative anticonvulsant medication arises, this should be done gradually. In the event of an allergic or hypersensitivity reaction, more rapid substitution of alternative therapy may be necessary. In this case, alternative therapy should be an anticonvulsant not belonging to the hydantoin chemical class.

There have been a number of reports suggesting a relationship between phenytoin and the development of lymphadenopathy (local or generalized) including benign lymph node hyperplasia, pseudolymphoma, lymphoma, and Hodgkin's Disease. Although a cause and effect relationship has not been established, the occurrence of lymphadenopathy indicates the need to differentiate such a condition from other types of lymph node pathology. Lymph node involvement may occur with or without symptoms and signs resembling serum sickness eg, fever, rash and liver involvement.

In all cases of lymphadenopathy, follow-up observation for an extended period is indicated and every effort should be made to achieve seizure control using alternative antiepileptic drugs.

Acute alcoholic intake may increase phenytoin serum levels while chronic alcoholic use may decrease serum levels.

In view of isolated reports associating phenytoin with exacerbation of porphyria, caution should be exercised in using this medication in patients suffering from this disease.

Usage in Pregnancy: A number of reports suggests an association between the use of antiepileptic drugs by women with epilepsy and a higher incidence of birth defects in children born to these women. Data are more extensive with respect to phenytoin and phenobarbital, but these are also the most commonly prescribed antiepileptic drugs; less systematic or anecdotal reports suggest a possible similar association with the use of all known antiepileptic drugs.

The reports suggesting a higher incidence of birth defects in children of drug-treated epileptic women cannot be regarded as adequate to prove a definite cause and effect relationship. There are intrinsic methodologic problems in obtaining adequate data on drug teratogenicity in humans; genetic factors or the epileptic condition itself may be more important than drug therapy in leading to birth defects. The great majority of mothers on antiepileptic medication deliver normal infants. It is important to note that antiepileptic drugs should not be discontinued in patients in whom the drug is administered to prevent major seizures, because of the strong possibility of precipitating status epilepticus with attendant hypoxia and threat to life. In individual cases where the severity and frequency of the seizure disorder are such that the removal of medication does not pose a serious threat to the patient, discontinuation of the drug may be considered prior to and during pregnancy, although it cannot be said with any confidence that even minor seizures do not pose some hazards to the developing embryo or fetus. The prescribing physician will wish to weigh these considerations in treating and counseling epileptic women of childbearing potential.

In addition to the reports of increased incidence of congenital malformation, such as cleft lip/palate and heart malformations in children of women receiving phenytoin and other antiepileptic drugs, there have more recently been reports of a fetal hydantoin syndrome. This consists of prenatal growth deficiency, microcephaly and mental deficiency in children born to mothers who have received phenytoin, barbiturates, alcohol, or trimethadione. However, these features are all interrelated and are frequently associated with intrauterine growth retardation from other causes.

There have been isolated reports of malignancies, including neuroblastoma, in children whose mothers received phenytoin during pregnancy.

An increase in seizure frequency during pregnancy occurs in a high proportion of patients, because of altered phenytoin absorption or metabolism. Periodic measurement of serum phenytoin levels is particularly valuable in the management of a pregnant epileptic patient as a guide to an appropriate adjustment of dosage. However, postpartum restoration of the original dosage will probably be indicated.

Neonatal coagulation defects have been reported within the first 24 hours in babies born to epileptic mothers receiving phenobarbital and/or phenytoin. Vitamin K has been shown to prevent or correct this defect and has been recommended to be given to the mother before delivery and the neonate after birth.

PRECAUTIONS

Phenytoin

General: The liver is the chief site of biotransformation of phenytoin; patients with impaired liver function may show early signs of toxicity. Elderly patients or those who are gravely ill may show early signs of toxicity.

A small percentage of indiviauals who have been treated with phenytoin have been shown to metabolize the drug slowly. Slow metabolism may be due to limited enzyme availability and lack of induction; it appears to be genetically determined.

Phenytoin should be discontinued if a skin rash appears (see "Warnings" section regarding drug discontinuation). If the rash is exfoliative, purpuric, or bullous or if lupus erythematosus, Stevens-Johnson syndrome, or toxic epidermal necrolysis is suspected, use of this drug should not be resumed and alternative therapy should be considered. (See Adverse Reactions.) If the rash is of a milder type (measles-like or scarlatiniform), therapy may be resumed after the rash has completely disappeared. If the rash recurs upon reinstitution of therapy, further phenytoin medication is contraindicated.

Phenytoin and other hydantoins are contraindicated in patients who have experienced phenytoin hypersensitivity. Additionally, caution should be exercised if using structurally similar compounds (eg barbiturates, succinimides, oxazolidinediones and other related compounds) in these same patients.

Hyperglycemia, resulting from the drug's inhibitory effects on insulin release, has been reported. Phenytoin may also raise the serum glucose level in diabetic patients.

Osteomalacia has been associated with phenytoin therapy and is considered to be due to phenytoin's interference with Vitamin D metabolism.

Phenytoin is not indicated for seizures due to hypoglycemic or other metabolic causes. Appropriate diagnostic procedures should be performed as indicated.

Phenytoin is not effective for absence (petit mal) seizures. If tonic-clonic (grand mal) and absence (petit mal) seizures are present, combined drug therapy is needed.

Serum levels of phenytoin sustained above the optimal range may produce confusional states referred to as "delirium," "psychosis," or "encephalopathy," or rarely irreversible cerebellar dysfunction. Accordingly, at the first sign of acute toxicity, plasma levels are recommended. Dose reduction of phenytoin therapy is indicated if plasma levels are excessive; if symptoms persist termination is recommended. (See Warnings)

Information for Patients: Patients taking phenytoin should be advised of the importance of adhering strictly to the prescribed dosage regimen, and of informing the physician of any clinical condition in which it is not possible to take the drug orally as prescribed, eg, surgery, etc.

Patients should also be cautioned on the use of other drugs or alcoholic beverages without first seeking the physician's advice.

Patients should be instructed to call their physician if skin rash develops.

The importance of good dental hygiene should be stressed in order to minimize the development of gingival hyperplasia and its complications.

Laboratory Tests: Phenytoin serum level determinations may be necessary to achieve optimal dosage adjustments.

Drug Interactions: There are many drugs which may increase or decrease phenytoin levels or which phenytoin may affect. Serum level determinations for phenytoin are especially helpful when possible drug interactions are suspected. The most commonly occurring drug interactions are listed below:

1. Drugs which may increase phenytoin serum levels include: acute alcohol intake, amiodarone, chloramphenicol, chlordiazepoxide, diazepam, dicumarol, disulfiram, estrogens, H₂-antagonists, halothane, isoniazid, methylphenidate, phenothiazines, phenylbutazone, salicylates, succinimides, sulfonamides, tolbutamide, trazodone.
2. Drugs which may decrease phenytoin levels include: carbamazepine, chronic alcohol abuse, reserpine, and sucralfate. Moban® brand of molindone hydrochloride contains

calcium ions which interfere with the absorption of phenytoin. Ingestion times of phenytoin and antacid preparations containing calcium should be staggered in patients with low serum phenytoin levels to prevent absorption problems.

3. Drugs which may either increase or decrease phenytoin serum levels include: phenobarbital, sodium valproate, and valproic acid. Similarly, the effect of phenytoin on phenobarbital, valproic acid and sodium valproate serum levels is unpredictable.

4. Although not a true drug interaction, tricyclic antidepressants may precipitate seizures in susceptible patients and phenytoin dosage may need to be adjusted.

5. Drugs whose efficacy is impaired by phenytoin include: corticosteroids, coumarin anticoagulants, digitoxin, doxycycline, estrogens, furosemide, oral contraceptives, quinidine, rifampin, theophylline, vitamin D.

Drug/Laboratory Test Interactions: Phenytoin may cause decreased serum levels of protein-bound iodine (PBI). It may also produce lower than normal values for dexamethasone or metyrapone tests. Phenytoin may cause increased serum levels of glucose, alkaline phosphatase, and gamma glutamyl transpeptidase (GGT).

Carcinogenesis: See 'Warnings' section for information on carcinogenesis.

Pregnancy: See Warnings.

Nursing Mothers: Infant breast-feeding is not recommended for women taking this drug because phenytoin appears to be secreted in low concentrations in human milk.

Phenobarbital

Withdrawal symptoms, including convulsions and delirium, may occur upon discontinuance of phenobarbital in patients with chronic intoxication. Analgesics, if used with phenobarbital, should be prescribed with caution because of possible additive effects. Caution should be exercised in prescribing this drug to patients with suicidal tendencies or with a predilection to abusive use of barbiturates.

Phenobarbital should be used with caution in debilitating and pulmonary diseases.

Phenobarbital should be used with caution in patients with severely impaired liver function, severe anemia, congestive heart failure, fever, neuroses, hyperthyroidism, diabetes mellitus, and any conditions in which respiratory depression may be characteristic. Marked excitement rather than depression may occur in aged or debilitated patients, particularly those with cerebral arteriosclerosis.

Confusion or euphoria may result from use of this drug. Symptoms in mentally ill, phobic, and emotionally disturbed patients may be accentuated. Prolonged usage may produce psychological habituation. Sudden discontinuation or radical reduction of dosage may precipitate withdrawal symptoms in patients who have taken the drug for prolonged periods; dosage should be gradually reduced to the point of complete discontinuation.

Barbiturates should be prescribed with extreme caution for persons known or suspected of routinely or periodically consuming large quantities of alcoholic beverages. Potentiation of effect, even to the extent of causing death, may result from consumption of barbiturates by patients with a high serum alcohol level.

Information for Patients: Phenobarbital may impair the mental and/or physical abilities required for the performance of potentially hazardous tasks, such as driving a motor vehicle or other such activity requiring alertness; therefore, the patient should be cautioned accordingly.

Drug Interactions: The effects of phenobarbital may be increased by many drugs, including antihistamines, tranquilizers, corticosteroids, monoamine oxidase inhibitors, narcotic analgesics, amitriptyline, imipramine, and rauwolfia alkaloids.

Pregnancy

See WARNINGS

Nursing Mothers: Evidence that phenobarbital is secreted in human milk is inadequate. The drug appears to be secreted in low concentrations which are unlikely to affect the infant. If the mother is receiving large doses of phenobarbital, however, the drug concentration in milk might increase. For this reason, artificial feeding of the infant is recommended for women taking this drug.

Labor and Delivery: Barbiturates readily cross the placental barrier and, if administered during labor, may have a depressant effect on the fetus; infants born of mothers receiving barbiturates may have difficulty breathing spontaneously.

ADVERSE REACTIONS

Phenytoin

Central Nervous System: The most common manifestations encountered with phenytoin therapy are referable to this system and are usually dose-related. These include nystagmus, ataxia, slurred speech, decreased coordination and mental confusion. Dizziness, insomnia, transient nervousness, motor twitchings, and headaches have also been observed. There have also been rare reports of phenytoin induced dyskinesias, including chorea, dystonia, tremor and

asterixis, similar to those induced by phenothiazine and other neuroleptic drugs.

A predominantly sensory peripheral polyneuropathy has been observed in patients receiving long-term phenytoin therapy.

Gastrointestinal System: Nausea, vomiting, constipation, toxic hepatitis and liver damage.

Integumentary System: Dermatological manifestations sometimes accompanied by fever have included scarlatiniform or morbilliform rashes. A morbilliform rash (measles-like) is the most common; other types of dermatitis are seen more rarely. Other more serious forms which may be fatal have included bullous, exfoliative, or purpuric dermatitis, lupus erythematosus, Stevens-Johnson syndrome, and toxic epidermal necrolysis (see Precautions).

Hemopoietic System: Hemopoietic complications, some fatal, have occasionally been reported in association with administration of phenytoin. These have included thrombocytopenia, leukopenia, granulocytopenia, agranulocytosis, and pancytopenia with or without bone marrow suppression. While macrocytosis and megaloblastic anemia have occurred, these conditions usually respond to folic acid therapy. Lymphadenopathy including benign lymph node hyperplasia, pseudolymphoma, lymphoma, and Hodgkin's Disease have been reported (see Warnings).

Connective Tissue System: Coarsening of the facial features, enlargement of the lips, gingival hyperplasia, hypertrichosis, and Peyronie's Disease.

Cardiovascular: Periarteritis nodosa.

Immunologic: Hypersensitivity syndrome (which may include, but is not limited to, symptoms such as arthralgias, eosinophilia, fever, liver dysfunction, lymphadenopathy or rash), systemic lupus erythematosus, and immunoglobulin abnormalities.

Phenobarbital

Central Nervous System: With larger doses, the most common manifestations relate to this system. These include drowsiness, vertigo, ataxia, hebetude, headache, delirium and stupor.

Gastrointestinal System: Phenobarbital may cause gastrointestinal discomfort and nausea.

Integumentary System: Hypersensitivity reactions are rare. Cutaneous eruptions are principally due to idiosyncrasy. Fatalities from exfoliative dermatitis and cutaneous eruptions have been reported. There are two syndromes associated with phenobarbital administration: Stevens-Johnson and a phenobarbital sensitivity syndrome. The phenobarbital sensitivity syndrome, which has resulted in fatalities, is characterized by an erythematous rash, high fever, jaundice, mental confusion, and toxic damage of "parenchymatous organs."

Hemopoietic System: Megaloblastic anemia has been reported; this condition usually responds to folic acid therapy.

OVERDOSAGE

The therapeutic ranges for phenytoin and phenobarbital in adults are 10 to 20 mcg/mL and 10 to 30 mcg/mL, respectively. Following acute overdosage of this combination, the patient at steady-state may experience evidence of phenytoin toxicity ahead of phenobarbital toxicity because phenytoin plasma levels rise more rapidly than phenobarbital levels. Phenytoin also has a narrower margin between therapeutic and toxic levels than does phenobarbital.

Phenytoin

The lethal dose in children is not known. The lethal dose in adults is estimated to be 2 to 5 grams. The initial symptoms are nystagmus, ataxia, and dysarthria. Other signs are tremor, hyperflexia, lethargy, slurred speech, nausea, vomiting. The patient may become comatose and hypotensive. Death is due to respiratory and circulatory depression.

There are marked variations among individuals with respect to phenytoin plasma levels where toxicity may occur. Nystagmus, on lateral gaze, usually appears at 20 mcg/mL, ataxia at 30 mcg/mL, dysarthria and lethargy appear when the plasma concentration is over 40 mcg/mL, but as high a concentration as 50 mcg/mL has been reported without evidence of toxicity. As much as 25 times the therapeutic dose has been taken to result in a serum concentration over 100 mcg/mL with complete recovery.

Treatment is nonspecific since there is no known antidote. The adequacy of the respiratory and circulatory systems should be carefully observed and appropriate supportive measures employed. Hemodialysis can be considered since phenytoin is not completely bound to plasma proteins. Total exchange transfusion has been used in the treatment of severe intoxication in children.

In acute overdosage the possibility of other CNS depressants, including alcohol, should be borne in mind.

Phenobarbital

The lethal dose of phenobarbital is believed to be 5 grams. The highest known blood level from which a patient recovered was 580 mcg/mL. An overdose of phenobarbital will include the classical picture of progressive central nervous system depression. In its severest form this syndrome leads to respiratory arrest as a result of general reflex paralysis. The milder forms of this syndrome may mimic any stage of

clinical anesthesia. Except for a rapid (and weak) pulse, vital signs are characteristically reduced. In addition to direct inhibition of the cardiac contractile mechanism with consequent hypotension, circulatory insufficiency may be aggravated by hypoxia from inadequate pulmonary ventilation. Early deaths are usually due to respiratory arrest, but delayed fatalities may arise from one or any combination of the following complications: hypostatic pneumonia, bronchopneumonia, lung abscess, pulmonary edema, cerebral edema, circulatory collapse, and irreversible renal shutdown. The treatment of barbiturate poisoning consists in removing any unabsorbed drug from the stomach, supporting the respiration and circulation, and expediting elimination of the drug which has been absorbed.

DOSAGE AND ADMINISTRATION

Serum concentrations should be monitored and care should be taken when switching a patient from the sodium salt to the free acid form.

Dilantin® Kapseals®, Dilantin Parenteral, and Dilantin with Phenobarbital are formulated with the sodium salt of phenytoin. The free acid form of phenytoin is used in Dilantin-30 Pediatric and Dilantin-125 Suspensions and Dilantin Infatabs. Because there is approximately an 8% increase in drug content with the free acid form over that of the sodium salt, dosage adjustments and serum level monitoring may be necessary when switching from a product formulated with the free acid to a product formulated with the sodium salt and vice versa.

The combination of Dilantin with Phenobarbital Kapseals is provided as a convenience for epileptic patients who require both drugs for seizure control. Anticonvulsant therapy should be initiated with either phenytoin or phenobarbital and, if indicated, the other drug can then be added. If the total daily doses of the two drugs used separately are within those given below, the combination of Dilantin with Phenobarbital Kapseals can then be substituted in equivalent amounts. When plasma level determinations are necessary for optimal dosage adjustments, the clinically effective level of Dilantin is usually 10 to 20 mcg/mL and for phenobarbital 10 to 30 mcg/mL in adults. Serum blood level determinations are especially helpful when possible drug interactions are suspected.

If either the phenytoin or phenobarbital dosage requires adjustment, this should be done by switching the patient to separate phenytoin and phenobarbital dosage forms in order to enable subsequent dosage adjustment of either or both drugs.

The recommended starting phenobarbital dose for children is 2 to 3 mg/kg/day in two or three equally divided doses. The recommended starting Dilantin dose for children is 5 mg/kg/day in two or three equally divided doses.

Adult Dosage: For maintenance (see above)—usually three or four capsules daily. An increase to six capsules daily may be made, if necessary.

Pediatric Dosage: For maintenance (see above)—individualized to a maximum of 300 mg Dilantin daily.

HOW SUPPLIED

N 0071-0375 (Kapseal 375, transparent #3 capsule with a garnet band)—Dilantin with Phenobarbital each contain 100 mg phenytoin sodium with 16 mg ($\frac{1}{4}$ gr) phenobarbital; in 100's.

N 0071-0531 (Kapseal 531, transparent #3 capsule with a black band)—Dilantin with Phenobarbital each contain 100 mg phenytoin sodium with 32 mg ($\frac{1}{2}$ gr) phenobarbital in 100's.

Store at room temperature below 30°C (86°F).

Protect from moisture and light.

Also Available As:

N 0071-0362 (Kapseal 362)—Dilantin (phenytoin sodium) 100 mg; in 100's.

N 0071-0365 (Kapseal 365)—Dilantin (phenytoin sodium) 30 mg in 100's.

N 0071-0007 (Tablet 7)—Dilantin Infatabs® each contain 50 mg phenytoin; 100's, and unit dose 100's.

N 0071-2214—Dilantin-125® Suspension (phenytoin oral suspension USP.) 125 mg phenytoin/5 mL with a maximum alcohol content not greater than 0.6 percent; available in 8-oz bottles and individual dose foil pouches which deliver 5 mL (125 mg phenytoin). The minimum sales unit is 100 pouches.

N 0071-2315—Dilantin-30® Pediatric Suspension (phenytoin oral suspension, USP.) 30 mg phenytoin/5 mL with a maximum alcohol content not greater than 0.6 percent; available in 8-oz bottles.

Continued on next page

This product information was prepared in August 1992. On these and other Parke-Davis Products, information may be obtained by addressing PARKE-DAVIS, Division of Warner-Lambert Company, Morris Plains, New Jersey 07950.

Parke-Davis—Cont.

For Parenteral Use:
N 0071-4488-05 (Ampoule 1488)—Dilantin ready-mixed solution containing 50 mg phenytoin sodium per milliliter is supplied in 2-mL ampoules. Packages of ten.
N 0071-4488-41 (Steri-Dose® 4488)—Dilantin ready-mixed solution containing 50 mg phenytoin sodium per milliliter is supplied in a 2-mL sterile disposable syringe (22 gauge × 1¼ inch needle).
Packages of ten individually cartoned syringes.
N 0071-4475-08 (Ampoule 1475)—Dilantin ready-mixed solution containing 50 mg phenytoin sodium per milliliter is supplied in packages of ten 5-mL ampoules without syringes.
N 0071-4488-45 Dilantin ready-mixed solution containing 50 mg phenytoin sodium per milliliter is supplied in 2-mL Steri-Vials.® Packages of twenty-five.
N 0071-4475-45 Dilantin ready-mixed solution containing 50 mg phenytoin sodium per milliliter is supplied in 5-mL Steri-Vials.® Packages of twenty-five.

REFERENCES

1. Woodbury, DM and Fingl, E. "Drugs Effective in the Therapy of the Epilepsies," in Goodman, LS and Gilman, A(eds): The Pharmacological Basis of Therapeutics ed 5. New York, Macmillan Publishing Co, Inc, 1975, pp 201–226.
2. Henn, K. "Diphenylhydantoin: Relation of Plasma Levels to Clinical Control," in Woodbury, DM, Penry, JK, and Schmidt, RP, (eds): Antiepileptic Drugs, New York, Raven Press, Publishers, 1972, pp 211–218.

Caution—Federal law prohibits dispensing without prescription.

0375G121

Shown in Product Identification Section, page 422

DORYX® ℞
(Coated Doxycycline Hyclate Pellets)

DESCRIPTION

DORYX® Capsules contain specially coated pellets of doxycycline hyclate for oral administration. Also contains lactose, NF; microcrystalline cellulose, NF; povidone, USP. The capsule shell and/or band contains FD and C blue No. 1; FD and C yellow No. 6; D and C yellow No. 10; gelatin, NF; silicon dioxide; sodium lauryl sulfate, NF; titanium dioxide, USP. Doxycycline is a broad-spectrum antibiotic synthetically derived from oxytetracycline and available as doxycycline hyclate. The chemical designation of this light-yellow crystalline powder is alpha-6-desoxy-5-oxytetracycline. Doxycycline has a high degree of lipoid solubility and a low affinity for calcium binding. It is highly stable in normal human serum. Doxycycline will not degrade into an epianhydro form.

CLINICAL PHARMACOLOGY

Tetracyclines are readily absorbed and are bound to plasma proteins in varying degree. They are concentrated by the liver in the bile, and excreted in the urine and feces at high concentrations and in a biologically active form.
Doxycycline is virtually completely absorbed after oral administration. Following a 200 mg dose, normal adult volunteers averaged peak serum levels of 2.6 mcg/mL of doxycycline at 2 hours decreasing to 145 mcg/mL at 24 hours. Excretion of doxycycline by the kidney is about 40%/72 hours in individuals with normal function (creatinine clearance about 75 mL/min). This percentage excretion may fall as low as 1–5%/72 hours in individuals with severe renal insufficiency (creatinine clearance below 10 mL/min). Studies have shown no significant difference in serum half-life of doxycycline (range 18–22 hours) in individuals with normal and severely impaired renal function.
Hemodialysis does not alter serum half-life.
Microbiology: Doxycycline is primarily bacteriostatic and is thought to exert its antimicrobial effect by the inhibition of protein synthesis. Doxycycline is active against a wide range of gram-positive and gram-negative organisms. The drugs in the tetracycline class have closely similar antimicrobial spectra and cross resistance among them is common.
Susceptibility Tests: Diffusion Techniques: The use of antibiotic disc susceptibility test methods which measure zone diameter gives an accurate estimation of susceptibility of organisms to DORYX: One such standard procedure[1] has been recommended for use with discs for testing antimicrobials. Doxycycline 30 mcg discs should be used for the determination of the susceptibility of organisms to doxycycline.
With this type of procedure, a report of "susceptible" from the laboratory indicates that the infecting organism is likely to respond to therapy. A report of "intermediate susceptibility" suggests that the organism would be susceptible if high dosage is used or if the infection is confined to tissue and fluids (e.g., urine) in which high antibiotic levels are obtained. A report of "resistant" indicates that the infecting organism is not likely to respond to therapy. With the doxycycline disc, a zone of 16 mm or greater indicates susceptibility, zone sizes of 12 mm or less indicate resistance, and zone sizes of 13 to 15 mm indicate intermediate susceptibility.
Standardized procedures require the use of laboratory control organisms. The 30 mcg tetracycline disc should give zone diameters between 19 and 28 mm for *S.aureus* ATCC 25923 and between 18 and 25 mm for *E.coli* ATCC 25922. The 30 mcg doxycycline disc should give zone diameters between 23 and 29 mm for *S.aureus* ATCC 25923, and between 18 and 24 mm for *E.coli* ATCC 25922.
Dilution Techniques: A bacterial isolate may be considered susceptible if the MIC (minimal inhibitory concentration) value for doxycycline is less than 4 mcg/mL. Organisms are considered resistant if the MIC is greater than 12.5 mcg/mL. MICs greater than 4.0 mcg/mL and less than 12.5 mcg/mL indicate intermediate susceptibility.
As with standard diffusion methods, dilution procedures require the use of laboratory control mechanisms. Standard doxycycline powder should give MIC values in the range of 0.25 mcg/mL and 1.0 mcg/mL for *S.aureus* ATCC 25923. For *E.coli* ATCC 25922 the MIC range should be between 1.0 mcg/mL and 4.0 mcg/mL.

INDICATIONS AND USAGE

Doxycycline is indicated in infections caused by the following microorganisms:
- Rickettsiae (Rocky Mountain spotted fever, typhus fever and the typhus group, Q fever, rickettsialpox and tick fevers).
- *Mycoplasma pneumoniae* (PPLO, Eaton's agent).
- Agents of psittacosis and ornithosis.
- Agents of lymphogranuloma venereum and granuloma inguinale.

The following gram-negative microorganisms:
- *Haemophilus ducreyi* (chancroid)
- *Yersinia pestis* (formerly *Pasteurella pestis*)
- *Francisella tularensis* (formerly *Pasteurella tularensis*)
- *Bartonella bacilliformis*
- *Bacteroides* species
- *Vibrio cholerae* (formerly *Vibrio comma*)
- *Campylobacter fetus* (formerly *Vibrio fetus*)
- *Brucella* species (in conjunction with streptomycin)

Because many strains of the following groups of microorganisms have been shown to be resistant to tetracyclines, culture and susceptibility testing are recommended.
Doxycycline is indicated for treatment of infections caused by the following gram-negative microorganisms, when bacteriological testing indicates appropriate susceptibility to the drug:
- *Escherichia coli*
- *Enterobacter aerogenes* (formerly *Aerobacter aerogenes*)
- *Shigella* species
- *Mima* species and *Herellea* species
- *Haemophilus influenzae* (respiratory infections)
- *Klebsiella* species (respiratory and urinary infections)

Doxycycline is indicated for treatment of infections caused by the following gram-positive microorganisms when bacteriological testing indicates appropriate susceptibility to the drug:
Streptococcus species:
Up to 44 percent of strains of *Streptococcus pyogenes* and 74 percent of *Streptococcus faecalis* have been found to be resistant to tetracycline drugs. Therefore, tetracyclines should not be used for streptococcal disease unless the organism has been demonstrated to be susceptible.
For upper respiratory infections due to group A beta-hemolytic streptococci, penicillin is the usual drug of choice, including prophylaxis of rheumatic fever.
Diplococcus pneumoniae.
Staphylococcus aureus, (respiratory, skin and soft-tissue infections). Tetracyclines are not the drug of choice in the treatment of any type of staphylococcal infection.
When penicillin is contraindicated, doxycycline is an alternative drug in the treatment of infections due to:
- *Treponema pallidum* and *Treponema pertenue* (syphilis and yaws)
- *Listeria monocytogenes*
- *Clostridium* species
- *Bacillus anthracis*
- *Fusobacterium fusiforme* (Vincent's infection)
- *Actinomyces* species

In acute intestinal amebiasis doxycycline may be a useful adjunct to amebicides.
In severe acne doxycycline may be useful adjunctive therapy.
Doxycycline is indicated in the treatment of trachoma, although the infectious agent is not always eliminated, as judged by immunofluorescence.
Inclusion conjunctivitis may be treated with oral doxycycline alone, or with a combination of topical agents.
Doxycycline is indicated for the treatment of uncomplicated urethral, endocervical or rectal infections in adults caused by *Chlamydia trachomatis.*[2]
Doxycycline is indicated for the treatment of nongonococcal urethritis caused by *Chlamydia trachomatis* and *Ureaplasma urealyticum* and for the treatment of acute epididymo-orchitis caused by *Chlamydia trachomatis.*[2]
Doxycycline is indicated for the treatment of uncomplicated gonococcal infections in adults (except for anorectal infections in men), the gonococcal arthritis-dermatitis syndrome and acute epididymo-orchitis caused by *N. gonorrhoeae.*[2]

CONTRAINDICATIONS

The drug is contraindicated in persons who have shown hypersensitivity to any of the tetracyclines.

WARNINGS

THE USE OF DRUGS OF THE TETRACYCLINE CLASS DURING TOOTH DEVELOPMENT (LAST HALF OF PREGNANCY, INFANCY AND CHILDHOOD TO THE AGE OF 8 YEARS) MAY CAUSE PERMANENT DISCOLORATION OF THE TEETH (YELLOW-GRAY-BROWN). This adverse reaction is more common during long term use of the drugs but has been observed following repeated short term courses. Enamel hypoplasia has also been reported. TETRACYCLINE DRUGS, THEREFORE, SHOULD NOT BE USED IN THIS AGE GROUP UNLESS OTHER DRUGS ARE NOT LIKELY TO BE EFFECTIVE OR ARE CONTRAINDICATED.
Results of animal studies indicate that tetracyclines cross the placenta, are found in fetal tissues and can have toxic effects on the developing fetus (often related to retardation of skeletal development). Evidence of embryotoxicity has been noted in animals treated early in pregnancy. If any tetracycline is used during pregnancy or if the patient becomes pregnant while taking these drugs, the patient should be apprised of potential hazard to the fetus.
As with other tetracyclines, doxycycline forms a stable calcium complex in any bone-forming tissue. A decrease in the fibula growth rate has been observed in prematures given oral tetracycline in doses of 25 mg/kg every six hours. This reaction was shown to be reversible when the drug was discontinued.
Photosensitivity manifested by an exaggerated sunburn reaction has been observed in some individuals taking tetracyclines. Patients apt to be exposed to direct sunlight or ultraviolet light should be advised that this reaction can occur with tetracycline drugs, and treatment should be discontinued at the first evidence of skin erythema.
The antianabolic action of the tetracyclines may cause an increase in BUN. Studies to date indicate that this does not occur with the use of doxycycline in patients with impaired renal function.

PRECAUTIONS

As with other antibiotic preparations, use of this drug may result in overgrowth of nonsusceptible organisms, including fungi. If superinfection occurs, the antibiotic should be discontinued and appropriate therapy instituted.
All infections due to group A beta-hemolytic streptococci should be treated for at least 10 days.
Laboratory tests: In venereal disease when coexistent syphilis is suspected, dark-field examination should be done before treatment is started and the blood serology repeated monthly for at least 4 months.
In long term therapy, periodic laboratory evaluation of organ systems, including hematopoietic, renal and hepatic studies should be performed.
Drug interactions: Because tetracyclines have been shown to depress plasma prothrombin activity, patients who are on anticoagulant therapy may require downward adjustment of their anticoagulant dosage.
Since bacteriostatic drugs may interfere with the bactericidal action of penicillin, it is advisable to avoid giving tetracyclines in conjunction with penicillin.
For concomitant therapy with antacids or iron-containing preparations and food see "Dosage and Administration" section.
Carcinogenesis, mutagenesis, impairment of fertility: Long term studies are currently being conducted to determine whether tetracyclines have carcinogenic potential. Animal studies conducted in rats and mice have not provided conclusive evidence that tetracyclines may be carcinogenic or that they impair fertility. In two mammalian cell assays (L51784 mouse lymphoma and Chinese hamster lung cells *in vitro*) positive responses for mutagenicity occurred at concentrations of 60 and 10 mcg/mL respectively. In humans no association between tetracyclines and these effects have been made.
Pregnancy: Pregnancy Category D (See Warnings section).
Nursing mothers: Tetracyclines are present in the milk of lactating women who are taking a drug in this class. Because of the potential for serious adverse reactions in nursing infants from the tetracyclines, a decision should be made whether to discontinue nursing or discontinue the drug, taking into account the importance of the drug to the mother (see Warnings section).
Pediatric use: See Warnings and Dosage and Administration sections.

ADVERSE REACTIONS

Due to oral doxycycline's virtually complete absorption, side effects to the lower bowel, particularly diarrhea, have been infrequent. The following adverse reactions have been observed in patients receiving tetracyclines:

Gastrointestinal: Anorexia, nausea, vomiting, diarrhea, glossitis, dysphagia, enterocolitis, and inflammatory lesions (with monilial overgrowth) in the anogenital region. These reactions have been caused by both the oral and parenteral administration of tetracyclines. Rare instances of esophagitis and esophageal ulcerations have been reported in patients receiving capsule and tablet forms of drugs in the tetracycline class. Most of these patients took medications immediately before going to bed. (See Dosage and Administration).

Skin: Maculopapular and erythematous rashes. Exfoliative dermatitis has been reported but is uncommon. Photosensitivity is discussed above (see Warnings).

Renal toxicity: Rise in BUN has been reported and is apparently dose related. (See Warnings).

Hypersensitivity reactions: Urticaria, angioneurotic edema, anaphylaxis, anaphylactoid purpura, pericarditis, and exacerbation of systemic lupus erythematosus.

Bulging fontanels in infants and benign intracranial hypertension in adults have been reported in individuals receiving tetracyclines. These conditions disappeared when the drug was discontinued.

Blood: Hemolytic anemia, thrombocytopenia, neutropenia, and eosinophilis have been reported with tetracyclines.

When given over prolonged periods, tetracyclines have been reported to produce brown-black microscopic discoloration of thyroid glands. No abnormalities of thyroid function are known to occur.

DOSAGE AND ADMINISTRATION

THE USUAL DOSAGE AND FREQUENCY OF ADMINISTRATION OF DOXYCYCLINE DIFFERS FROM THAT OF THE OTHER TETRACYCLINES. EXCEEDING THE RECOMMENDED DOSAGE MAY RESULT IN AN INCREASED INCIDENCE OF SIDE EFFECTS.

Adults: The usual dose of oral doxycycline is 200 mg on the first day of treatment (administered 100 mg every 12 hours) followed by a maintenance dose of 100 mg/day. The maintenance dose may be administered as a single dose or as 50 mg every 12 hours. In the management of more severe infections (particularly chronic infections of the urinary tract), 100 mg every 12 hours is recommended.

For children above eight years of age: The recommended dosage schedule for children weighing 100 pounds or less is 2 mg/lb of body weight divided into two doses on the first day of treatment, followed by 1 mg/lb of body weight given as a single daily dose or divided into two doses on subsequent days. For more severe infections up to 2 mg/lb of body weight may be used. For children over 100 pounds, the usual adult dose should be used.

Uncomplicated gonococcal infections in adults (except anorectal infections in men): 100 mg, by mouth, twice-a-day for 7 days.[2] As an alternate single visit dose, administer 300 mg stat followed in one hour by a second 300 mg dose. The dose may be administered with food, including milk or carbonated beverage, as required.

Acute epididymo-orchitis caused by *N. gonorrhoeae:* 100 mg, by mouth, twice-a-day for at least 10 days.[2]

Primary and secondary syphilis: 300 mg a day in divided doses for at least 10 days.

Uncomplicated urethral, endocervical, or rectal infection in adults caused by *Chlamydia trachomatis:* 100 mg by mouth, twice-a-day for at least 7 days.[2]

Nongonococcal urethritis caused by *C. trachomatis* and *U. urealyticum:* 100 mg, by mouth, twice-a-day for at least 7 days.[2]

Acute epididymo-orchitis caused by *C. trachomatis:* 100 mg, by mouth, twice-a-day for at least 10 days.[2]

The therapeutic antibacterial serum activity will usually persist for 24 hours following recommended dosage.

When used in streptococcal infections, therapy should be continued for 10 days.

Administration of adequate amounts of fluid along with capsule and tablet forms of drugs in the tetracycline class is recommended to wash down the drugs and reduce the risk of esophageal irritation and ulceration (see Adverse Reactions).

If gastric irritation occurs, it is recommended that doxycycline be given with food or milk. The absorption of doxycycline is not markedly influenced by simultaneous ingestion of food or milk.

Concomitant therapy: Antacids containing aluminum, calcium or magnesium, sodium bicarbonate, and iron-containing preparations should not be given to patients taking oral tetracyclines.

Studies to date have indicated that administration of doxycycline at the usual recommended doses does not lead to excessive accumulation of the antibiotic in patients with renal impairment.

HOW SUPPLIED

DORYX® Capsules have a yellow transparent body with light blue opaque cap; the capsule bearing the inscription "DORYX" in white. Pellets are colored yellow. Each capsule contains specially coated pellets of doxycycline hyclate equivalent to 100 mg of doxycycline, supplied in:

Bottles of 50 capsules ....N 0071-0838-19

STORAGE CONDITIONS

Store at controlled room temperature below 25° C (77° F).

References:

1. NCCLS Approved Standard: M2-A3, Vol. 4, Performance Standards for Antimicrobial Disk Susceptibility Tests, Third Edition: available from the National Committee for Clinical Laboratory Standards, 771 East Lancaster Avenue, Villanova, Pa. 19085
2. CDC Sexually Transmitted Diseases Treatment Guidelines 1982

Caution—Federal law prohibits dispensing without prescription.

Manufactured by
Faulding International
129 Dew Street,
Thebarton, South Australia, 5031
Distributed by
PARKE-DAVIS
Div of Warner-Lambert Co
Morris Plains, NJ 07950 USA

0838G023

Shown in Product Identification Section, page 422

EASPRIN® ℞

[ēas'prĭn"]
(Aspirin Delayed-release Tablets, USP)
Enteric Coated Tablets

Caution—Federal law prohibits dispensing without prescription.

DESCRIPTION

Easprin (Aspirin Delayed-release Tablets, USP) enteric coated tablets contain 15 grains (975 mg) aspirin for oral administration. Also contains: candelilla wax; colloidal silicon dioxide, NF; corn starch 1500; dusty rose Opaspray; hydroxypropyl methylcellulose, USP (15 cps); methylparaben, NF; microcrystalline cellulose, NF; mistron spray talc; polyethylene glycol 3350, NF; propylparaben, NF; stearic acid powder; vanillin, NF; zinc stearate, USP. The enteric coating is designed to prevent the release of aspirin in the stomach and thereby reduce gastric irritation and total occult blood loss. The pharmacologic effects of aspirin include analgesia, antipyresis, antiinflammatory activity, and antirheumatic activity.

CLINICAL PHARMACOLOGY

Aspirin is a salicylate that has demonstrated antiinflammatory, analgesic, antipyretic, and antirheumatic activity.

Aspirin's mode of action as an antiinflammatory and antirheumatic agent may be due to inhibition of synthesis and release of prostaglandins.

Aspirin appears to produce analgesia by virtue of both a peripheral and CNS effect. Peripherally, aspirin acts by inhibiting the synthesis and release of prostaglandins. Acting centrally, it would appear to produce analgesia at a hypothalamic site in the brain, although the mode of action is not known.

Aspirin also acts on the hypothalamus to produce antipyresis; heat dissipation is increased as a result of vasodilation and increased peripheral blood flow. Aspirin's antipyretic activity may also be related to inhibition of synthesis and release of prostaglandins.

In a crossover study, Easprin at a dose of one tablet (15 grains) three times a day produced an average fecal blood loss of 1.54 ml per day. Uncoated aspirin at a dosage of three 5 grain tablets given three times a day caused an average fecal blood loss of 4.33 ml per day.

Easprin Tablets are enteric coated. This coating acts to prevent the release of aspirin in the stomach but permits the tablet to dissolve with resultant absorption in the upper portion of the small intestine. This reduces any gastric irritation that may occur with uncoated aspirin but does delay the onset of action. Aspirin is rapidly hydrolyzed primarily in the liver to salicylic acid, which is conjugated with glycine (forming salicyluric acid) and glucuronic acid and excreted largely in the urine. As a result of the rapid hydrolysis, plasma concentrations of aspirin are always low and rarely exceed 20 mcg/ml at ordinary therapeutic doses. The peak salicylate level for uncoated aspirin occurs in about 2 hours; however with enteric coated aspirin tablets this is delayed. A direct correlation between salicylate plasma levels and clinical analgesic effectiveness has not been definitely established, but effective analgesia is usually achieved at plasma levels of 15 to 30 mg per 100 ml. Effective antiinflammatory activity is usually achieved at salicylate plasma levels of 20 to 30 mg per 100 ml. There is also poor correlation between toxic symptoms and plasma salicylate concentrations, but most patients exhibit symptoms of salicylism at plasma salicylate levels of 35 mg per 100 ml. The plasma half-life for aspirin is approximately 15 minutes; that for salicylate lengthens as the dose increases: Doses of 300 to 650 mg have a half-life of 3.1 to 3.2 hours; with doses of 1 gram, the half-life is increased to 5 hours and with 2 grams it is increased to about 9 hours.

Salicylates are excreted mainly by the kidney. Studies in man indicate that salicylate is excreted in the urine as free salicylic acid (10%), salicyluric acid (75%), salicylic phenolic (10%), and acyl (5%) glucuronides and gentisic acid.

INDICATIONS AND USAGE

Easprin is indicated in patients who need the higher 15 grain dose of aspirin in the long-term palliative treatment of mild to moderate pain and inflammation of arthritic and other inflammatory conditions.

CONTRAINDICATIONS

Easprin should not be used in patients who have previously exhibited hypersensitivity to aspirin and/or nonsteroidal antiinflammatory agents.

Easprin should not be given to patients with a recent history of gastrointestinal bleeding or in patients with bleeding disorders (eg, hemophilia).

WARNINGS

Easprin Tablets should be used with caution when anticoagulants are prescribed concurrently, for aspirin may depress the concentration of prothrombin in plasma and thereby increase bleeding time. Large doses of salicylates have a hypoglycemic action and may enhance the effect of the oral hypoglycemics. Consequently, they should not be given concomitantly; if however, this is necessary, the dosage of the hypoglycemic agent must be reduced while the salicylate is given. This hypoglycemic action may also affect the insulin requirements of diabetics.

Although salicylates in large doses are uricosuric agents, smaller amounts may decrease the uricosuric effects of probenecid, sulfinpyrazone, and phenylbutazone.

PRECAUTIONS

General: Easprin Tablets should be administered with caution to patients with asthma, nasal polyps, or nasal allergies. In patients receiving large doses of aspirin and/or prolonged therapy, mild salicylate intoxication (salicylism) may develop that may be reversed by reduction in dosage.

Although the fecal blood loss with Easprin is less than that with uncoated aspirin tablets, Easprin Tablets should be administered with caution to patients with a history of gastric distress, ulcer, or bleeding problems. Occult gastrointestinal bleeding occurs in many patients but is not correlated with gastric distress. The amount of blood lost is usually insignificant clinically, but with prolonged administration, it may result in iron deficiency anemia.

Sodium excretion produced by spironolactone may be decreased in the presence of salicylates.

Salicylates can produce changes in thyroid function tests.

Salicylates should be used with caution in patients with severe hepatic damage, preexisting hypoprothrombinemia, or Vitamin K deficiency, and in those undergoing surgery.

DRUG INTERACTIONS

Anticoagulants: See Warnings.

Hypoglycemic Agents: See Warnings.

Uricosuric Agents: Aspirin may decrease the effects of probenecid, sulfinpyrazone, and phenylbutazone.

Spironolactone: See general precautions above.

Alcohol: Has a synergistic effect with aspirin in causing gastrointestinal bleeding.

Corticosteroids: Concomitant administration with aspirin may increase the risk of gastrointestinal ulceration and may reduce serum salicylate levels.

Pyrazolone Derivatives (phenylbutazone, oxyphenbutazone, and possibly dipyrone): Concomitant administration with aspirin may increase the risk of gastrointestinal ulceration.

Nonsteroidal Antiinflammatory Agents: Aspirin is contraindicated in patients who are hypersensitive to nonsteroidal antiinflammatory agents.

Urinary Alkalinizers: Decrease aspirin effectiveness by increasing the rate of salicylate renal excretion.

Phenobarbital: Decreases aspirin effectiveness by enzyme induction.

Phenytoin: Serum phenytoin levels may be increased by aspirin.

Propranolol: May decrease aspirin's antiinflammatory action by competing for the same receptors.

Continued on next page

This product information was prepared in August 1992. On these and other Parke-Davis Products, information may be obtained by addressing PARKE-DAVIS, Division of Warner-Lambert Company, Morris Plains, New Jersey 07950.

Parke-Davis—Cont.

Antacids: Easprin should not be given concurrently with antacids, since an increase in the pH of the stomach may affect the enteric coating of the tablets.
Usage in Pregnancy: It has been reported that adverse effects were increased in the mother and fetus following chronic ingestion of aspirin. Prolonged pregnancy and labor with increased bleeding before and after delivery, as well as decreased birth weight and increased rate of stillbirth were correlated with high blood salicylate levels. Because of possible adverse effects on the neonate and the potential for increased maternal blood loss, aspirin should be avoided during the last three months of pregnancy.

ADVERSE REACTIONS

Gastrointestinal: Dyspepsia, thirst, nausea, vomiting, diarrhea, acute reversible heptatotoxicity, gastrointestinal bleeding, and/or ulceration.
Special Senses: Tinnitus, vertigo, reversible hearing loss and dimness of vision.
Hematologic: Prolongation of bleeding time, leukopenia, thrombocytopenia, purpura, decreased plasma iron concentration and shortened erythrocyte survival time.
Dermatologic and Hypersensitivity: Urticaria, angioedema, pruritus, sweating, various skin eruptions, asthma, and anaphylaxis.
Neurologic: Mental confusion, drowsiness and dizziness.
Body as a whole: Headache and fever.

OVERDOSAGE

Overdosage of 200 to 500 mg/kg is in the fatal range. Early symptoms are CNS stimulation with vomiting, hyperpnea, hyperactivity, and possibly convulsions. This progresses quickly to depression, coma, respiratory failure, and collapse. These symptoms are accompanied by severe electrolyte disturbances.
In the treatment of salicylate overdosage, intensive supportive therapy should be instituted immediately. Plasma salicylate levels should be measured in order to determine the severity of the poisoning and to provide a guide for therapy. Emptying of the stomach should be accomplished as soon as possible with ipecac syrup unless the patient is depressed. In depressed patients use airway protected gastric lavage. Delay absorption with activated charcoal and give a saline cathartic. Proceed according to Standard Reference Procedures for Salicylate Intoxication.

DOSAGE AND ADMINISTRATION

Usual Adult Dosage: One tablet 3 to 4 times daily.
Patients who have displayed no significant adverse effects on a long term qid regimen and who receive a total daily dosage of aspirin no greater than 3.9 grams may be considered for a bid regimen (2 tablets of Easprin twice daily). Patients on the bid Easprin regimen should be closely monitored for serum salicylate levels, increased incidence of CNS-related adverse effects, increased fecal blood loss, or any other signs or symptoms suggestive of significant blood loss.
If necessary, dosage may be increased until relief is obtained, but dosage should be maintained slightly below that which produces tinnitus. Plasma salicylate levels may also be helpful in determining proper dosage (see CLINICAL PHARMACOLOGY section).

HOW SUPPLIED

Easprin enteric coated tablets each containing 15 grains (975 mg) aspirin are available:
N 0071-0490-24—Bottles of 100
Storage: Store at controlled room temperature 15° to 30°C (59° to 86°F).
AHFS Category 28:08 **0490G016**
Shown in Product Identification Section, page 422

ERGOSTAT® ℞
(Ergotamine Tartrate Tablets, USP) SUBLINGUAL

DESCRIPTION

Each sublingual tablet contains 2 mg ergotamine tartrate. Also contains hydroxypropyl cellulose, NF; FD&C yellow No. 6 Al lake; lactose, NF; magnesium stearate, NF; mannitol, USP; artificial peppermint flavor; pregelatinized starch, NF; saccharin, NF; saccharin sodium, USP; and corn starch, NF.
Pharmacological Category: Vasoconstrictor, uterine stimulant, alpha adrenoreceptor antagonist.
Therapeutic Class: Antimigraine.
Chemical Name: Ergotaman-3′,6′,18-trione,12′-hydroxy-2′-methyl-5′-(phenylmethyl)-,(5′α)-,[R-(R*, R*)]-2,3-dihydroxybutanedioate (2:1) salt.

CLINICAL PHARMACOLOGY

The pharmacological properties of ergotamine are extremely complex; some of its actions are unrelated to each other, and even mutually antagonistic. The drug has partial agonist and/or antagonist activity against tryptaminergic, dopaminergic and alpha adrenergic receptors depending upon their site, and it is a highly active uterine stimulant. It causes constriction of peripheral and cranial blood vessels and produces depression of central vasomotor centers. The pain of a migraine attack is believed to be due to greatly increased amplitude of pulsations in the cranial arteries, especially the meningeal branches of the external carotid artery. Ergotamine reduces extracranial blood flow, causes a decline in the amplitude of pulsation in the cranial arteries, and decreases hyperperfusion of the territory of the basilar artery. It does not reduce cerebral hemispheric blood flow. Long-term usage has established the fact that ergotamine tartrate is effective in controlling up to 70% of acute migraine attacks, so that it is now considered specific for the treatment of this headache syndrome. Ergotamine produces constriction of both arteries and veins. In doses used in the treatment of vascular headaches, ergotamine usually produces only small increases in blood pressure, but it does increase peripheral resistance and decrease blood flow in various organs. Small doses of the drug increase the force and frequency of uterine contraction; larger doses increase the resting tone of the uterus also. The gravid uterus is particularly sensitive to these effects of ergotamine. Although specific teratogenic effects attributable to ergotamine have not been found, the fetus suffers if ergotamine is given to the mother. Retarded fetal growth and an increase in intrauterine death and resorption have been seen in animals. These are thought to result from ergotamine-induced increases in uterine motility and vasoconstriction in the placental vascular bed.
The bioavailability of sublingually administered ergotamine has not been determined.
Ergotamine is metabolized in the liver by largely undefined pathways, and 90% of the metabolites are excreted in the bile. The unmetabolized drug is erratically secreted in the saliva, and only traces of unmetabolized drug appear in the urine and feces. Ergotamine is secreted into breast milk. The elimination half-life of ergotamine from plasma is about 2 hours, but the drug may be stored in some tissues, which would account for its long-lasting therapeutic and toxic actions.

INDICATIONS AND USAGE

Ergotamine tartrate is indicated as therapy to abort or prevent vascular headache, e.g., migraine, migraine variants, or so called "histaminic cephalalgia".

CONTRAINDICATIONS

Ergotamine is contraindicated in peripheral vascular disease (thromboangiitis obliterans, luetic arteritis, severe arteriosclerosis, thrombophlebitis, Raynaud's disease), coronary heart disease, hypertension, impaired hepatic or renal function, severe pruritus, and sepsis. It is also contraindicated in patients who are hypersensitive to any of its components. Ergotamine may cause fetal harm when administered to a pregnant woman by virtue of its powerful uterine stimulant actions. It is contraindicated in women who are, or may become, pregnant.

PRECAUTIONS

General: Although signs and symptoms of ergotism rarely develop even after long-term intermittent use of ergotamine, care should be exercised to remain within the limits of recommended dosage.
Drug Interactions: The effects of ergotamine tartrate may be potentiated by triacetyloleandomycin which inhibits the metabolism of ergotamine. The pressor effects of ergotamine and other vasoconstrictor drugs can combine to cause dangerous hypertension.
Carcinogenesis: No studies have been performed to investigate ergotamine tartrate for carcinogenic effects.
Pregnancy: Pregnancy Category X—See CONTRAINDICATIONS.
Nursing Mothers: Ergotamine is secreted into human milk. It can reach the breast-fed infant by this route and exert pharmacologic effects in it. Caution should be exercised when ergotamine is administered to a nursing woman. Excessive dosing or prolonged administration of ergotamine may inhibit lactation.

ADVERSE REACTIONS

Nausea and vomiting occur in up to 10% of patients after ingestion of therapeutic doses of ergotamine. Weakness of the legs and pain in limb muscles are also frequent complaints. Numbness and tingling of the fingers and toes, precordial pain, transient changes in heart rate and localized edema and itching may also occur, particularly in patients who are sensitive to the drug.

DRUG ABUSE AND DEPENDENCE

Patients who take ergotamine for extended periods of time may become dependent upon it and require progressively increasing doses for relief of vascular headaches, and for prevention of dysphoric effects which follow withdrawal of the drug.

OVERDOSAGE

Overdosage with ergotamine causes nausea, vomiting, weakness of the legs, pain in limb muscles, numbness and tingling of the fingers and toes, precordial pain, tachycardia or bradycardia, hypertension or hypotension and localized edema and itching together with signs and symptoms of ischemia due to vasconstriction of peripheral arteries and arterioles. The feet and hands become cold, pale and numb. Muscle pain occurs while walking and later at rest also. Gangrene may ensue. Confusion, depression, drowsiness, and convulsions are occasional signs of ergotamine toxicity. Overdosage is particularly likely to occur in patients with sepsis or impaired renal or hepatic function. Patients with peripheral vascular disease are especially at risk of developing peripheral ischemia following treatment with ergotamine. Some cases of ergotamine poisoning have been reported in patients who have taken less than 5 mg of the drug. Usually, however, toxicity is seen at doses of ergotamine tartrate in excess of about 15 mg in 24 hours or 40 mg in a few days.
Treatment of ergotamine overdosage consists of the withdrawal of the drug followed by symptomatic measures including attempts to maintain an adequate circulation in the affected parts. Anticoagulant drugs, low molecular weight dextran and potent vasodilator drugs may all be beneficial. Intravenous infusion of sodium nitroprusside has also been reported to be successful. Vasodilators must be used with special care in the presence of hypotension.
Nausea and vomiting may be relieved by atropine or antiemetic compounds of the phenothiazine group. Ergotamine is dialyzable.

DOSAGE AND ADMINISTRATION

All efforts should be made to initiate therapy as soon as possible after the first symptoms of the attack are noted, because success is proportional to rapidity of treatment, and lower dosages will be effective. At the first sign of an attack or to relieve the symptoms of the full-blown attack, one sublingual tablet (2 mg) is placed under the tongue. Another sublingual tablet (2 mg) should be placed under the tongue at half-hourly intervals thereafter, if necessary, for a total of three tablets (6 mg). Dosage must not exceed three tablets (6 mg) in any 24-hour period. Limit dosage to not more than five tablets (10 mg) in any one week.

HOW SUPPLIED

Ergostat (Ergotamine Tartrate Tablets, USP) sublingual, 2 mg (round, orange, coded P-D 111), is supplied as follows:
N 0071-0111-13 Packages of 24 unit-dose tablets.
Store at controlled room temperature 15°–30°C (59°–86°F).
Caution—Federal law prohibits dispensing without prescription.
Protect from moisture and light.
AHFS Category 12:16 **0111G018**
Shown in Product Identification Section, page 422

ERYC® ℞
[ĕ′ryc]
(Erythromycin Delayed-Release Capsules, USP)

DESCRIPTION

ERYC Capsules contain enteric-coated pellets of erythromycin base for oral administration. Erythromycin is produced by a strain of *Streptomyces erythraeus* and belongs to the macrolide group of antibiotics. It is basic and readily forms salts with acids, but it is the base which is microbiologically active. Each ERYC Capsule contains 250 milligrams of erythromycin base. Also contains: lactose NF; povidone USP; FD&C Yellow #6. The capsule shell contains gelatin NF; titanium dioxide USP; FD&C Yellow #6. Erythromycin base is (3*R**,4*S**,5*S**,6*R**,7*R**,9*R**, 11*R**,12*R**,13*S**,14*R**)-4-[(2,6-Dideoxy-3- *C* -methyl-3- *O* -methyl- α -*L- ribo* -hexopyranosyl)-oxy]-14-ethyl-7,12,13-trihydroxy-3,5,7,9,11,13-hexamethyl-6-[[3,4,6-trideoxy-3-(dimethylamino)-β-D- *xylo* -hexopyranosyl]oxy]oxacyclotetradecane-2,10-dione.

CLINICAL PHARMACOLOGY

Orally administered erythromycin base and its salts are readily absorbed in the microbiologically active form. Interindividual variations in the absorption of erythromycin are, however, observed, and some patients do not achieve acceptable serum levels. Erythromycin is largely bound to plasma proteins, and the freely dissociating bound fraction after administration of erythromycin base represents 90% of the total erythromycin absorbed. After absorption erythromycin diffuses readily into most body fluids. In the absence of meningeal inflammation, low concentrations are normally achieved in the spinal fluid but the passage of the drug across the blood-brain barrier increases in meningitis. Erythromycin is excreted in breast milk. The drug crosses the placental barrier but fetal plasma levels are low.
In the presence of normal hepatic function erythromycin is concentrated in the liver and is excreted in the bile; the effect of hepatic dysfunction on biliary excretion of erythromycin is not known. After oral administration less than 5% of the administered dose can be recovered in the active form in the urine.
The enteric coating of pellets in ERYC Capsules protects the erythromycin base from inactivation by gastric acidity. Be-

cause of their small size and enteric coating, the pellets readily pass intact from the stomach to the small intestine and dissolve efficiently to allow absorption of erythromycin in a uniform manner. After administration of a single dose of a 250 mg ERYC capsule, peak serum levels in the range of 1.13 to 1.68 mcg/ml are attained in approximately 3 hours and decline to 0.30-0.42 mcg/ml in 6 hours. Optimal conditions for stability in the presence of gastric secretion and for complete absorption are attained when ERYC is taken on an empty stomach.

Microbiology Erythromycin acts by inhibition of protein synthesis by binding 50 S ribosomal subunits of susceptible organisms. It does not affect nucleic acid synthesis. Antagonism has been demonstrated between clindamycin and erythromycin. Resistance to erythromycin by some strains of *Haemophilus influenzae* and staphylococci has been demonstrated. Specimens should be obtained for culture and susceptibility testing.

Erythromycin is usually active against the following organisms in *vitro* and in clinical infections:

Streptococcus pyogenes
Alpha hemolytic streptococci (viridans group)
Staphylococcus aureus (Resistant organisms may emerge during treatment.)
Streptococcus pneumoniae
Mycoplasma pneumoniae (Eaton's Agent)
Haemophilus influenzae (Many strains are resistant to erythromycin alone, but are susceptible to erythromycin and sulfonamides together.)
Treponema pallidum
Corynebacterium diphtheriae
Corynebacterium minutissimum
Entamoeba histolytica
Listeria monocytogenes
Neisseria gonorrhoeae
Bordetella pertussis
Legionella pneumophila (agent of Legionnaires' Disease)

Susceptibility Testing Quantitative methods that require measurement of zone diameters give the most precise estimates of antibiotic susceptibility. One such standardized single disc procedure has been recommended for use with discs to test susceptibility to erythromycin.[1] Interpretation involves correlation of the zone diameters obtained in the disc test with minimum inhibitory concentration (MIC) values for erythromycin.

Reports from the laboratory giving results of the standardized single-disc susceptibility test using a 15 mcg erythromycin disc should be interpreted according to the following criteria:

Susceptible organisms produce zones of 18 mm or greater indicating that the tested organism is likely to respond to therapy.

Resistant organisms produce zones of 13 mm or less, indicating that other therapy should be selected.

Organisms of intermediate susceptibility produce zones of 14 to 17 mm. The "intermediate" category provides a "buffer zone" which should prevent small uncontrolled technical factors from causing major discrepancies in interpretations, thus when a zone diameter falls within the "intermediate" range, the results may be considered equivocal. If alternate drugs are not available, confirmation by dilution tests may be indicated.

A bacterial isolate may be considered susceptible if the MIC value[2] (minimal inhibitory concentration) for erythromycin is not more than 2 mcg/ml. Organisms are considered resistant if the MIC is 8 mcg/ml or higher.

INDICATIONS AND USAGE

ERYC is indicated in children and adults for the treatment of the following conditions:

Upper respiratory tract infections of mild to moderate degree caused by *Streptococcus pyogenes* (group A beta hemolytic streptococci); *Streptococcus pneumoniae (Diplococcus pneumoniae): Haemophilus influenzae* (when used concomitantly with adequate doses of sulfonamides, since not all strains of *H influenzae* are susceptible at the erythromycin concentrations ordinarily achieved). (See appropriate sulfonamide labeling for prescribing information.)

Lower respiratory tract infections of mild to moderate severity caused by *Streptococcus pyogenes* (group A beta hemolytic streptococci): *Streptococcus pneumoniae (Diplococcus pneumoniae).*

Respiratory tract infections due to *Mycoplasma pneumoniae (Eaton's agent).*

Pertussis (whooping cough) caused by *Bordetella pertussis.* Erythromycin is effective in eliminating the organism from the nasopharynx of infected individuals, rendering them noninfectious. Some clinical studies suggest that erythromycin may be helpful in the prophylaxis of pertussis in exposed susceptible individuals.

Diphtheria—As an adjunct to antitoxin in infections due to *Corynebacterium diphtheriae,* to prevent establishment of carriers and to eradicate the organism in carriers.

Erythrasma—In the treatment of infections due to *Corynebacterium minutissimum.*

Intestinal amebiasis caused by *Entamoeba histolytica* (oral erythromycins only). Extraenteric amebiasis requires treatment with other agents.

Infections due to *Listeria monocytogenes.*

Skin and soft tissue infections of mild to moderate severity caused by *Streptococcus pyogenes* and *Staphylococcus aureus* (Resistant staphylococci may emerge during treatment.)

Primary syphilis caused by *Treponema pallidum.* Erythromycin (oral forms only) is an alternate choice of treatment for primary syphilis in patients allergic to the penicillins. In treatment of primary syphilis, spinal fluid should be examined before treatment and as part of the follow-up after therapy. The use of erythromycin for the treatment of *in utero* syphilis is not recommended (See CLINICAL PHARMACOLOGY).

Erythromycins are indicated for treatment of the following infections caused by *Chlamydia trachomatis:* conjunctivitis of the newborn, pneumonia of infancy, urogenital infections during pregnancy. When tetracyclines are contraindicated or not tolerated, erythromycin is indicated for the treatment of uncomplicated urethral, endocervical, or rectal infections in adults due to *Chlamydia trachomatis*[4].

Legionnaires' disease caused by *Legionella pneumophila.* Although no controlled clinical efficacy studies have been conducted, *in vitro* and limited preliminary clinical data suggest that erythromycin may be effective in treating Legionnaires' disease.

Therapy with erythromycin should be monitored by bacteriological studies and by clinical response (See CLINICAL PHARMACOLOGY—Microbiology).

Injectable benzathine penicillin G is considered by the American Heart Association to be the drug of choice in the treatment and prevention of streptococcal pharyngitis and in long-term prophylaxis of rheumatic fever. When oral medication is preferred for treatment of the above conditions, penicillin G, V, or erythromycin are alternate drugs of choice.

Although no controlled clinical efficacy trials have been conducted, erythromycin has been suggested by the American Heart Association and the American Dental Association for use in a regimen for prophylaxis against bacterial endocarditis in patients allergic to penicillin who have congenital and/or rheumatic or other acquired valvular heart disease when they undergo dental procedures and surgical procedures of the upper respiratory tract.[3] (Erythromycin is not suitable prior to genitourinary surgery where the organisms likely to lead to bacteremia are gram-negative bacilli or the enterococcal group of streptococci).

NOTE: When selecting antibiotics for the prevention of bacterial endocarditis the physician or dentist should read the full joint 1984 statement of the American Heart Association and the American Dental Association.[3]

CONTRAINDICATION

ERYC is contraindicated in patients with known hypersensitivity to this antibiotic.

WARNING

There have been a few reports of hepatic dysfunction, with or without jaundice, occurring in patients receiving erythromycin ethylsuccinate, base, and stearate products.

PRECAUTIONS

General: Erythromycin is principally excreted by the liver. Caution should be exercised when erythromycin is administered to patients with impaired hepatic function. (See CLINICAL PHARMACOLOGY and WARNING sections).

Prolonged or repeated use of erythromycin may result in an overgrowth of nonsusceptible bacteria or fungi. If superinfection occurs, erythromycin should be discontinued and appropriate therapy instituted.

When indicated, incision and drainage or other surgical procedures should be performed in conjunction with antibiotic therapy.

Laboratory Tests: Erythromycin interferes with the fluorometric determination of urinary catecholamines.

Drug Interactions: Recent data from studies of erythromycin reveal that its use in patients who are receiving high doses of theophylline may be associated with an increase of serum theophylline levels and potential theophylline toxicity. In cases of theophylline toxicity and/or elevated serum theophylline levels, the dose of theophylline should be reduced while the patient is receiving concomitant erythromycin therapy.

Erythromycin administration in children receiving carbamazepine has been reported to cause increased blood levels of carbamazepine with subsequent development of signs of carbamazepine toxicity (ataxia, dizziness, vomiting).

Erythromycin has been reported to decrease the clearance of triazolam and thus may increase pharmacologic effect of triazolam. Erythromycin has been reported to decrease the clearance of cyclosporine causing elevated cyclosporine levels and associated increased serum creatinine. Renal function as well as serum concentration of cyclosporine should be closely monitored when both drugs are administered concomitantly. An interaction between erythromycin and ergotamine has been reported to increase the vasospasm associated with ergotamine.

Concomitant administration of erythromycin and digoxin has been reported to result in elevated digoxin serum levels.

There have been reports of increased anticoagulant effects when erythromycin and oral anticoagulants were used concomitantly.

Carcinogenesis, Mutagenesis and Impairment of Fertility: Long-term (2-year) oral studies conducted in rats with erythromycin base did not provide evidence of tumorigenicity. Mutagenicity studies have not been conducted. There was no apparent effect on male or female fertility in rats fed erythromycin (base) at levels up to 0.25 percent of diet.

Pregnancy: Pregnancy Category B: There is no evidence of teratogenicity or any other adverse effect on reproduction in female rats fed erythromycin base (up to 0.25 percent of diet) prior to and during mating, during gestation, and through weaning of two successive litters. There are, however, no adequate and well-controlled studies in pregnant women. Because animal reproduction studies are not always predictive of human response, this drug should be used during pregnancy only if clearly needed. Erythromycin has been reported to cross the placental barrier in humans, but fetal plasma levels are generally low.

Labor and Delivery: The effect of erythromycin on labor and delivery is unknown.

Nursing Mothers: Erythromycin is excreted in breast milk, therefore, caution should be exercised when erythromycin is administered to a nursing woman.

Pediatric Use: See INDICATIONS AND USAGE and DOSAGE AND ADMINISTRATION sections.

ADVERSE REACTIONS

The most frequent side effects of oral erythromycin preparations are gastrointestinal and are dose-related. They include nausea, vomiting, abdominal pain, diarrhea and anorexia. Symptoms of hepatic dysfunction and/or abnormal liver function test results may occur (see WARNING).

Mild allergic reactions such as rashes with or without pruritus, urticaria, bullous fixed eruptions, and eczema have been reported with erythromycin. Serious allergic reactions, including anaphylaxis have been reported.

A few cases of transient deafness have been reported with high doses of erythromycin.

DOSAGE AND ADMINISTRATION

ERYC is well absorbed and may be given without regard to meals. Optimum blood levels are obtained in a fasting state (administration at least one half hour and preferably two hours before or after a meal); however, blood levels obtained upon administration of enteric-coated erythromycin products in the presence of food are still above minimal inhibitory concentrations (MICs) of most organisms for which erythromycin is indicated.

ADULTS: The usual dose is 250 mg every 6 hours taken one hour before meals. If twice-a-day dosage is desired, the recommended dose is 500 mg every 12 hours. Dosage may be increased up to 4 grams per day, according to the severity of infection. Twice-a-day dosing is not recommended when doses larger than 1 gram daily are administered.

CHILDREN: Age, weight, and severity of the infection are important factors in determining the proper dosage. The usual dosage is 30 to 50 mg/kg/day in divided doses. For the treatment of more severe infections, this dose may be doubled.

Streptococcal infections: A therapeutic dosage of oral erythromycin should be administered for at least 10 days. For continuous prophylaxis against recurrences of streptococcal infections in persons with a history of rheumatic heart disease, the dose is 250 mg twice a day.

For the prevention of bacterial endocarditis in penicillin-allergic patients with valvular heart disease who are to undergo dental procedures or surgical procedures of the upper respiratory tract, the adult dose is 1 gram orally (20 mg/kg for children) one hour prior to the procedure and then 500 mg (10 mg/kg for children) orally 6 hours later.[3] (See Indications and Usage).

Primary syphilis: 30-40 grams given in divided doses over a period of 10-15 days.

Intestinal amebiasis: 250 mg four times daily for 10 to 14 days for adults; 30 to 50 mg/kg/day in divided doses for 10 to 14 days for children.

Legionnaires' Disease: Although optimal doses have not been established, doses utilized in reported clinical data were

Continued on next page

This product information was prepared in August 1992. On these and other Parke-Davis Products, information may be obtained by addressing PARKE-DAVIS, Division of Warner-Lambert Company, Morris Plains, New Jersey 07950.

Parke-Davis—Cont.

those recommended above (1 to 4 grams daily in divided doses).

Urogenital infections during pregnancy due to *Chlamydia trachomatis*: Although the optimal dose and duration of therapy have not been established, the suggested treatment is erythromycin 500 mg, by mouth, 4 times a day on an empty stomach for at least 7 days. For women who cannot tolerate this regimen, a decreased dose of 250 mg, by mouth, 4 times a day should be used for at least 14 days[4].

For adults with uncomplicated urethral, endocervical, or rectal infections caused by *Chlamydia trachomatis* in whom tetracyclines are contraindicated or not tolerated: 500 mg. by mouth, 4 times a day for at least 7 days[4].

Pertussis: Although optimum dosage and duration of therapy have not been established, doses of erythromycin utilized in reported clinical studies were 40-50 mg/kg/day, given in divided doses for 5 to 14 days.

HOW SUPPLIED

ERYC (Capsule 696), clear and orange opaque capsules, each containing 250 mg erythromycin as enteric coated pellets, are available as follows:

N 0071-0696-16 Bottles of 40
N 0071-0696-24 Bottles of 100
N 0071-0696-30 Bottles of 500
N 0071-0696-40 Unit dose package of 100 (10 strips of 10 capsules each).

Storage Conditions: Store at a room temperature below 30°C (86°F). Protect from moisture and light.

REFERENCES

1. Approved Standard ASM-2 "Performance Standards for Anti-microbial Disc Susceptibility Test." National Committee for Clinical Laboratory Standards. 771 East Lancaster Avenue, Villanova. PA 19085.
2. Ericson, H.M. and Sherris, J.C.: "Antibiotic Sensitivity Testing Report of an International Collaborative Study." *Acta Pathologica et Microbiologica Scandinavica.* Section B. Supp. 217, 1971, pp. 1-90.
3. Am. Heart Assoc. and Am. Dental Assoc. "Prevention of Bacterial Endocarditis." *Circulation:* Vol. 70, No. 6, December, 1984, 1123A-1127A.
4. CDC Sexually Transmitted Diseases Treatment Guidelines 1982.

0696G187

Shown in Product Identification Section, page 422

ESTROVIS® ℞

[ĕs-trō′vĭs″]
(Quinestrol tablets, USP)

WARNING

1. Estrogens Have Been Reported to Increase the Risk of Endometrial Carcinoma.

Three independent case control studies have shown an increased risk of endometrial cancer in postmenopausal women exposed to exogenous estrogens for prolonged periods.[1–3] This risk was independent of the other known risk factors for endometrial cancer. These studies are further supported by the finding that incidence rates of endometrial cancer have increased sharply since 1969 in eight different areas of the United States with population-based cancer reporting systems, an increase which may be related to the rapidly expanding use of estrogens during the last decade.[4]

The three case control studies reported that the risk of endometrial cancer in estrogen users was about 4.5 to 13.9 times greater than in nonusers. The risk appears to depend on both duration of treatment[1] and on estrogen dose.[3] In view of these findings, when estrogens are used for the treatment of menopausal symptoms, the lowest dose that will control symptoms should be utilized and medication should be discontinued as soon as possible. When prolonged treatment is medically indicated, the patient should be reassessed on at least a semiannual basis to determine the need for continued therapy. Although the evidence must be considered preliminary, one study suggests that cyclic administration of low doses of estrogen may carry less risk than continuous administration.[3] Therefore, while it appears prudent to utilize such a regimen with other orally administered estrogens, Estrovis may be administered, following a seven-day priming schedule, on a once weekly maintenance dosage beginning two weeks after the start of treatment.

Close clinical surveillance of all women taking estrogens is important. In all cases of undiagnosed persistent or recurring abnormal vaginal bleeding, adequate diagnostic measures should be undertaken to rule out malignancy.

There is no evidence at present that "natural" estrogens are more or less hazardous than "synthetic" estrogens at equiestrogenic doses.

2. Estrogens Should not be Used During Pregnancy.

The use of female sex hormones, both estrogens and progestogens, during early pregnancy may seriously damage the offspring. It has been shown that females exposed *in utero* to diethylstilbestrol, a nonsteroidal estrogen, have an increased risk of developing in later life a form of vaginal or cervical cancer that is ordinarily extremely rare.[5–6] This risk has been estimated as not greater than 4 per 1,000 exposures.[7] Furthermore, a high percentage of such exposed women (from 30 to 90%) have been found to have vaginal adenosis,[8–12] epithelial changes of the vagina and cervix. Although these changes are histologically benign, it is not known whether they are precursors of malignancy. Although similar data are not available with the use of other estrogens, it cannot be presumed they would not induce similar changes.

Several reports suggest an association between intrauterine exposure to female sex hormones and congenital anomalies, including congenital heart defects and limb-reduction defects.[13–16] One case control study[16] estimated a 4.7-fold increased risk of limb-reduction defects in infants exposed *in utero* to sex hormones (oral contraceptives, hormone withdrawal tests for pregnancy, or attempted treatment for threatened abortion). Some of these exposures were very short and involved only a few days of treatment. The data suggest that the risk of limb-reduction defects in exposed fetuses is somewhat less than 1 per 1,000.

In the past, female sex hormones have been used during pregnancy in an attempt to treat threatened or habitual abortion. There is considerable evidence that estrogens are ineffective for these indications, and there is no evidence from well-controlled studies that progestogens are effective for these uses.

If Estrovis (quinestrol) is used during pregnancy, or if the patient becomes pregnant while taking this drug, she should be apprised of the potential risks to the fetus and the advisability of pregnancy continuation.

DESCRIPTION

Estrovis is the 3-cyclopentylether of ethinyl estradiol. It is an estrogenic agent for oral administration. Each tablet contains 100 mcg quinestrol, USP. Estrovis also contains: FD&C blue No. 1 Al lake; lactose, NF; and magnesium stearate, NF. The chemical name is 3-cyclopentyloxy-17α-ethynylestra-1,3,5(10)-trien-17β-ol.

It is a white, essentially odorless powder, insoluble in water and soluble in alcohol, chloroform, and ether.

CLINICAL PHARMACOLOGY

Estrovis (quinestrol) is an orally effective estrogen as judged by conventional assay procedures employing vagina and uterine end-points in mice, rats and rabbits.

The estrogenic effects of Estrovis have been demonstrated in clinical studies by its effects on the endometrium, maturation of the vaginal epithelium, thinning of cervical mucus, suppression of pituitary gonadotropin, inhibition of ovulation, and prevention of postpartum breast discomfort.

INDICATIONS

Estrovis (quinestrol) is indicated in the treatment of:

1. Moderate to severe vasomotor symptoms associated with the menopause. (There is no evidence that estrogens are effective for nervous symptoms or depression which might occur during menopause, and they should not be used to treat these conditions.)
2. Atrophic vaginitis
3. Kraurosis vulvae
4. Female hypogonadism
5. Female castration
6. Primary ovarian failure

Estrovis (Quinestrol) Has Not Been Shown to be Effective for any Purpose during Pregnancy and Its Use May Cause Severe Harm to the Fetus (See Boxed Warning).

CONTRAINDICATIONS

Estrogens should not be used in women (or men) with any of the following conditions:

1. Known or suspected cancer of the breast except in appropriately selected patients being treated for metastatic disease
2. Known or suspected estrogen-dependent neoplasia
3. Known or suspected pregnancy (See Boxed Warning)
4. Undiagnosed abnormal genital bleeding
5. Active thrombophlebitis or thromboembolic disorders
6. A past history of thrombophlebitis, thrombosis, or thromboembolic disorders associated with previous estrogen use (except when used in treatment of breast or prostatic malignancy)

WARNINGS

1. *Induction of malignant neoplasms.* Long-term continuous administration of natural and synthetic estrogens in certain animal species increases the frequency of carcinomas of the breast, cervix, vagina, and liver. There is now evidence that estrogens increase the risk of carcinoma of the endometrium in humans. (See Boxed Warning.)

At the present time, there is no satisfactory evidence that estrogens given to postmenopausal women increase the risk of cancer of the breast,[18] although a recent long-term follow up of a single physician's practice has raised this possibility.[18a] Because of the animal data, there is a need for caution in prescribing estrogens for women with a strong family history of breast cancer or who have breast nodules, fibrocystic disease, or abnormal mammograms.

2. *Gallbladder disease.* A recent study has reported a 2- to 3-fold increase in the risk of surgically confirmed gallbladder disease in women receiving postmenopausal estrogens,[18] similar to the 2-fold increase previously noted in users of oral contraceptives.[19–24] In the case of oral contraceptives, the increased risk appeared after two years of use.[24]

3. *Effects similar to those caused by estrogen-progestogen oral contraceptives.* There are several serious adverse effects of oral contraceptives, most of which have not, up to now, been documented as consequences of postmenopausal estrogen therapy. This may reflect the comparatively low doses of estrogen used in postmenopausal women. It would be expected that the larger doses of estrogen used to treat prostatic or breast cancer or postpartum breast engorgement are more likely to result in these adverse effects, and, in fact, it has been shown that there is an increased risk of thrombosis in men receiving estrogens for prostatic cancer and women for postpartum breast engorgement.[20-23]

a. *Thromboembolic disease.* It is now well established that users of oral contraceptives have an increased risk of various thromboembolic and thrombotic vascular diseases, such as thrombophlebitis, pulmonary embolism, stroke, and myocardial infarction.[24–31] Cases of retinal thrombosis, mesenteric thrombosis, and optic neuritis have been reported in oral contraceptive users. There is evidence that the risk of several of these adverse reactions is related to the dose of the drug.[32,33] An increased risk of postsurgery thromboembolic complications has also been reported in users of oral contraceptives.[34,35] If feasible, estrogen should be discontinued at least 4 weeks before surgery of the type associated with an increased risk of thromboembolism, or during periods of prolonged immobilization.

While an increased rate of thromboembolic and thrombotic disease in postmenopausal users of estrogens has not been found,[18,36] this does not rule out the possibility that such an increase may be present or that subgroups of women who have underlying risk factors or who are receiving relatively large doses of estrogens may have increased risk. Therefore, estrogens should not be used in persons with active thrombophlebitis or thromboembolic disorders, and they should not be used (except in treatment of malignancy) in persons with a history of such disorders in association with estrogen use. They should be used with caution in patients with cerebral vascular or coronary artery disease and only for those in whom estrogens are clearly needed.

Large doses of estrogen (5 mg conjugated estrogens per day), comparable to those used to treat cancer of the prostate and breast, have been shown in a large prospective clinical trial in men[37] to increase the risk of nonfatal myocardial infarction, pulmonary embolism, and thrombophlebitis. When estrogen doses of this size are used, any of the thromboembolic and thrombotic adverse effects associated with oral contraceptive use should be considered a clear risk.

b. *Hepatic adenoma.* Benign hepatic adenomas appear to be associated with the use of oral contraceptives.[38–40] Although benign, and rare, these may rupture and may cause death through intra-abdominal hemorrhage. Such lesions have not yet been reported in association with other estrogen or progestogen preparations but should be considered in estrogen users having abdominal pain and tenderness, abdominal mass, or hypovolemic shock. Hepatocellular carcinoma has also been reported in women taking estrogen-containing oral contraceptives.[39] The relationship of this malignancy to these drugs is not known at this time.

c. *Elevated blood pressure.* Increased blood pressure is not uncommon in women using oral contraceptives. There is now a report that this may occur with use of estrogens in the menopause[11] and blood pressure should be monitored with estrogen use, especially if high doses are used.

d. *Glucose tolerance.* A worsening of glucose tolerance has been observed in a significant percentage of patients on estrogen-containing oral contraceptives. For this reason, diabetic patients should be carefully observed while receiving estrogen.

4. *Hypercalcemia.* Administration of estrogens may lead to severe hypercalcemia in patients with breast cancer and bone metastases. If this occurs, the drug should be stopped and appropriate measures taken to reduce the serum calcium level.

PRECAUTIONS

A. General Precautions

1. A complete medical and family history should be taken prior to the initiation of any estrogen therapy. The pretreat-

ment and periodic physical examinations should include special reference to blood pressure, abdomen, and pelvic organs, and should include a Papanicolaou smear. As a general rule, estrogen should not be prescribed for longer than one year without another physical examination being performed.

2. Fluid retention—Because estrogens may cause some degree of fluid retention, conditions which might be influenced by this factor, such as epilepsy, migraine, and cardiac or renal dysfunction, require careful observation.

3. Certain patients may develop undesirable manifestations of excessive estrogenic stimulation, such as abnormal or excessive uterine bleeding, mastodynia, etc.

4. Oral contraceptives appear to be associated with an increased incidence of mental depression.[24] Although it is not clear whether this is due to the estrogenic or progestogenic component of the contraceptive, patients with a history of depression should be carefully observed.

5. Preexisting uterine leiomyomata may increase in size during estrogen use.

6. The pathologist should be advised of estrogen therapy when relevant specimens are submitted.

7. Patients with a past history of jaundice during pregnancy have an increased risk of recurrence of jaundice while receiving estrogen-containing oral contraceptive therapy. If jaundice develops in any patient receiving estrogen, the medication should be discontinued while the cause is investigated.

8. Estrogens may be poorly metabolized in patients with impaired liver function and they should be administered with caution in such patients.

9. Because estrogens influence the metabolism of calcium and phosphorus, they should be used with caution in patients with metabolic bone diseases that are associated with hypercalcemia or in patients with renal insufficiency.

10. Because of the effects of estrogens on epiphyseal closure, they should be used judiciously in young patients in whom bone growth is not complete.

11. Certain endocrine and liver function tests may be affected by estrogen-containing oral contraceptives. The following similar changes may be expected with larger doses of estrogen:

a. Increased sulfobromophthalein retention.

b. Increased prothrombin and factors VII, VIII, IX, and X; decreased antithrombin 3; increased norepinephrine-induced platelet aggregability.

c. Increased thyroid binding globulin (TBG) leading to increased circulating total thyroid hormone, as measured by PHI, T4 by column, or T4 by radioimmunoassay. Free T3 resin uptake is decreased, reflecting the elevated TBG; free T4 concentration is unaltered.

d. Impaired glucose tolerance.

e. Decreased pregnanediol excretion.

f. Reduced response to metyrapone test.

g. Reduced serum folate concentration.

h. Increased serum triglyceride and phospholipid concentration.

B. Concomitant Progestin Use
The lowest effective dose appropriate for the specific indication should be utilized. Studies of the addition of a progestin for seven or more days of a cycle of estrogen administration have reported a lowered incidence of endometrial hyperplasia. Morphological and biochemical studies of endometrium suggest that 10 to 13 days of progestin are needed to provide maximal maturation of the endometrium and to eliminate any hyperplastic changes. Whether this will provide protection from endometrial carcinoma has not been clearly established. There are possible additional risks which may be associated with the inclusion of progestin in estrogen replacement regimens. The potential risks include adverse effects on carbohydrate and lipid metabolism. The choice of progestin and dosage may be important in minimizing these adverse effects.

C. Information for the patient. See text of Patient Package Insert.

D. Pregnancy. See Contraindications and Boxed Warning.

E. Nursing Mothers. As a general principle, the administration of any drug to nursing mothers should be done only when clearly necessary because many drugs are excreted in human milk.

ADVERSE REACTIONS
(See Warnings regarding induction of neoplasia, adverse effects on the fetus, increased incidence of gallbladder disease, and adverse effects similar to those of oral contraceptives, including thromboembolism.) The following additional adverse reactions have been reported with estrogenic therapy, including oral contraceptives:

1. *Genitourinary system.*
Breakthrough bleeding, spotting, change in menstrual flow
Dysmenorrhea
Premenstrual-like syndrome
Amenorrhea during and after treatment

Increase in size of uterine fibromyomata
Vaginal candidiasis
Change in cervical eversion and in degree of cervical secretion
Cystitis-like syndrome

2. *Breasts.*
Tenderness, enlargement, secretion

3. *Gastrointestinal.*
Nausea, vomiting
Abdominal cramps, bloating
Cholestatic jaundice

4. *Skin.*
Chloasma or melasma which may persist when drug is discontinued
Erythema multiforme
Erythema nodosum
Hemorrhagic eruption
Loss of scalp hair
Hirsutism

5. *Eyes.*
Steepening of corneal curvature
Intolerance to contact lenses

6. *CNS.*
Headache, migraine, dizziness
Mental depression
Chorea

7. *Miscellaneous.*
Increase or decrease in weight
Reduced carbohydrate tolerance
Aggravation of porphyria
Edema
Changes in libido

ACUTE OVERDOSAGE
Numerous reports of ingestion of large doses of estrogen-containing oral contraceptives by young children indicate that serious ill effects do not occur. Overdosage of estrogen may cause nausea, and withdrawal bleeding may occur in females.

DOSAGE AND ADMINISTRATION
For treatment of moderate to severe vasomotor symptoms associated with the menopause, and for atrophic vaginitis, kraurosis vulvae, female hypogonadism, female castration, and primary ovarian failure.
One Estrovis (quinestrol) 100-mcg tablet once daily for seven days, followed by one 100-mcg tablet weekly as a maintenance schedule, commencing two weeks after inception of treatment. The dosage may be increased to 200 mcg weekly if the therapeutic response is not that which may be desirable or considered optimal.
The lowest maintenance dose that will control symptoms should be chosen and medication should be discontinued as promptly as possible.
Attempts to discontinue or taper medication should be made at three- to six-month intervals.
Treated patients with an intact uterus should be monitored closely for signs of endometrial cancer and appropriate diagnostic measures should be taken to rule out malignancy in the event of persistent or recurring abnormal vaginal bleeding.

HOW SUPPLIED
N 0071-0437-24 (P-D 437) Estrovis (quinestrol) 100-mcg tablets are supplied in bottles of 100.

PHYSICIAN REFERENCES
1. Ziel, H.K. and W.D. Finkle, "Increased Risk of Endometrial Carcinoma Among Users of Conjugated Estrogens." *New England Journal of Medicine,* 293:1167–1170, 1975.
2. Smith, D.C., R. Prentic, D.J. Thompson, and W.L. Hermann, "Association of Exogenous Estrogen and Endometrial Carcinoma." *New England Journal of Medicine,* 293:1164–1167, 1975.
3. Mack, T.M., M.C. Pike, B.E. Henderson, R.I. Pfeffer, V.R. Gerkins, M. Arthur, and S.E. Brown, "Estrogens and Endometrial Cancer in a Retirement Community." *New England Journal of Medicine,* 294:1262–1267, 1976.
4. Weiss, N.D., D.R. Szekely and D.F. Austin, "Increasing Incidence of Endometrial Cancer in the United States." *New England Journal of Medicine,* 294:1259–1262, 1976.
5. Herbst, A.L., H. Ulfelder and D.C. Poskanzer, "Adenocarcinoma of Vagina." *New England Journal of Medicine,* 284:878–881, 1971.
6. Greenwald, P., J. Barlow, P. Nasca, and W. Burnett, "Vaginal Cancer after Maternal Treatment with Synthetic Estrogens." *New England Journal of Medicine,* 285:390–392, 1971.
7. Lanier, A., K. Noller, D. Decker, L. Elveback, and L. Kurland, "Cancer and Stilbestrol, A Follow-Up of 1719 Persons Exposed to Estrogens in *Utero* and Born 1943–1959." *Mayo Clinic Proceedings,* 48:793–799, 1973.
8. Herbst, A., R. Kurman, and R. Scully, "Vaginal and Cervical Abnormalities After Exposure to Stilbestrol in Utero." *Obstetrics and Gynecology,* 40:287–298, 1972.
9. Herbst, A., S. Robboy, G. Macdonald, and R. Scully, "The Effects of Local Progesterone on Stilbestrol-Associated Vagi-

nal Adenosis." *American Journal of Obstetrics and Gynecology,* 118:607–615, 1974.
10. Herbst, A., D. Poskanzer, S. Robboy, L. Friedlander, and R. Scully, "Prenatal Exposure to Stilbestrol, A Prospective Comparison of Exposed Female Offspring with Unexpected Controls." *New England Journal of Medicine,* 292:334–339, 1975.
11. Stafl, A., R. Mattingly, D. Foley, and W. Fetherston, "Clinical Diagnosis of Vaginal Adenosis." *Obstetrics and Gynecology,* 43:118–128, 1974.
12. Sherman, A.I., M. Goldrath, A. Berlin, V. Vakhariya, F. Banooni, W. Michaels, P. Goodman, S. Brown, "Cervical-Vaginal Adenosis After *In Utero* Exposure to Synthetic Estrogens," *Obstetrics and Gynecology,* 44:531–545, 1974.
13. Gal, I., B. Kirman, and J. Stern, "Hormone Pregnancy Tests and Congenital Malformation," *Nature,* 216:83, 1967.
14. Levy, E.P., A. Cohen, and F.C. Fraser, "Hormone Treatment During Pregnancy and Congenital Heart Defects," *Lancet,* 1:611, 1973.
15. Nora, J. and A. Nora, "Birth Defects and Oral Contraceptives," *Lancet,* 1:941–942, 1973.
16. Janerich, D.T., J.M. Piper, and D.M. Glebatis, "Oral Contraceptives and Congenital Limb-Reduction Defects," *New England Journal of Medicine,* 291:697–700, 1974.
17. "Estrogens for Oral or Parenteral Use," *Federal Register,* 40:8212, 1975.
18. Boston Collaborative Drug Surveillance Program "Surgically Confirmed Gallbladder Disease, Venous Thromboembolism and Breast Tumors in Relation to Post-Menopausal Estrogen Therapy," *New England Journal of Medicine,* 210:15–19, 1974.
18a. Hoover, R., L.A. Gray, Sr., P. Cole, and B. MacMahon, "Menopausal Estrogens and Breast Cancer." *New England Journal of Medicine,* 295:401–405, 1976.
19. Boston Collaborative Drug Surveillance Program, "Oral Contraceptives and Venous Thromboembolic Disease, Surgically Confirmed Gallbladder Disease, and Breast Tumors," *Lancet,* 1:1399–1404, 1973.
20. Daniel, D.G., H. Campbell, and A.C. Turnbull, "Puerperal Thromboembolism and Suppression of Lactation." *Lancet,* 2:287–289, 1967.
21. The Veterans Administration Cooperative Urological Research Group, "Carcinoma of the Prostate: Treatment Comparisons," *Journal of Urology,* 98:516–522, 1967.
22. Ballar, J.C., "Thromboembolism and Oestrogen Therapy," *Lancet,* 2, 560. 1967.
23. Blackard, C., R. Doe, G. Mellinger, and D. Byar, "Incidence of Cardiovascular Disease and Death in Patients Receiving Diethylstilbestrol for Carcinoma of the Prostate," *Cancer,* 26:249–256, 1970.
24. Royal College of General Practitioners, "Oral Contraception and Thromboembolic Disease," *Journal of the Royal College of General Practitioners,* 13, 267–279, 1967.
25. Inman, W.H.W. and M.P. Vessey, "Investigation of Deaths from Pulmonary, Coronary, and Cerebral Thrombosis and Embolism in Women of Child-Bearing Age." *British Medical Journal,* 2:193–199, 1968.
26. Vessey, M.P. and R. Doll, "Investigation of Relation Between Use of Oral Contraceptives and Thromboembolic Disease, A Further Report," *British Medical Journal,* 2:651–657, 1969.
27. Sartwell, P.E., A.T. Masi, F.G. Arthes, G.R. Greene and H.E. Smith, "Thromboembolism and Oral Contraceptives: An Epidemiological Case Control Study." *American Journal of Epidemiology,* 90:365–380, 1969.
28. Collaborative Group for the Study of Stroke in Young Women, "Oral Contraception and Increased Risk of Cerebral Ischemia or Thrombosis," *New England Journal of Medicine,* 288:871–878, 1973.
29. Collaborative Group for the Study of Stroke in Young Women: "Oral Contraceptives and Stroke in Young Women: Associated Risk Factors," 231:718–722, 1975. *Journal of the American Medical Assoc.* 231:718–722, 1975.
30. Mann, J.I. and W.H.W. Inman, "Oral Contraceptives and Death from Myocardial Infarction," *British Medical Journal,* 2:245–248, 1975.
31. Mann, J.I., M.P. Vessey, M. Thorogood, and R. Doll, "Myocardial Infarction in Young Women with Special Reference to Oral Contraceptive Practice," *British Medical Journal,* 2:241–245, 1975.
32. Inman, W.H.W., M.P. Vessey, B. Westerholm, and A. Engelund. "Thromboembolic Disease and the Steroidal Content of Oral Contraceptives," *British Medical Journal,* 2:203–209, 1970.
33. Stolley, P.D., J.A. Tonascia, M.S. Tockman, P.E. Sartwell, A.H. Rutledge, and M.P. Jacobs, "Thrombosis with

Continued on next page

This product information was prepared in August 1992. On these and other Parke-Davis Products, information may be obtained by addressing PARKE-DAVIS, Division of Warner-Lambert Company, Morris Plains, New Jersey 07950.

Parke-Davis—Cont.

Low-Estrogen Oral Contraceptives," *American Journal of Epidemiology,* 102:197–208, 1975.
34. Vessey, M.P., R. Doll, A.S. Fairbairn, and G. Glober, "Post-Operative Thromboembolism and the use of the Oral Contraceptives," *British Medical Journal,* 3:123–126, 1970.
35. Greene, G.R. and P.E. Sartwell, "Oral Contraceptive Use in Patients with Thromboembolism Following Surgery, Trauma or Infection," *American Journal of Public Health,* 62:680–685, 1972.
36. Rosenberg, L., M.B. Armstrong and H. Jick "Myocardial Infarction and Estrogen Therapy in Post-menopausal Women," *New England Journal of Medicine,* 294:1256–1259, 1976.
37. Coronary Drug Project Research Group, "The Coronary Drug Project: Initial Findings Leading to Modifications of Its Research Protocol," *Journal of the American Medical Association,* 214:1303–1313, 1970.
38. Baum, J., F. Holtz, J.J. Bookstein, and E.W. Klein, "Possible Association between Benign Hepatomas and Oral Contraceptives," *Lancet,* 2:926–928, 1973.
39. Mays, E.T., W.M. Christopherson, M.M. Mahr, and H.C. Williams, "Hepatic Changes in Young Women Ingesting Contraceptive Steroids, Hepatic Hemorrhage and Primary Hepatic Tumors," *Journal of the American Medical Association,* 235:780–782, 1976.
40. Edmondson, H.A., B. Henderson, and B. Benton, "Liver Cell Adenomas Association with the Use of Oral Contraceptives," *New England Journal of Medicine,* 294:470–472, 1976.
41. Pfeffer, A.I. and S. Van Den Noore, "Estrogen use and Stroke Risk in Post-menopausal Women," *American Journal of Epidemiology,* 103:545–546, 1976.

Patient Labeling for Estrogens

WHAT YOU SHOULD KNOW ABOUT ESTROGENS

Estrogens are female hormones produced by the ovaries. The ovaries make several different kinds of estrogens. In addition, scientists have been able to make a variety of synthetic estrogens. As far as we know, all these estrogens have similar properties and, therefore, much the same usefulness, side effects, and risks. This leaflet is intended to help you understand what estrogens are used for, the risks involved in their use, and how to use them as safely as possible.

This leaflet includes the most important information about estrogens, but not all the information. If you want to know more, you can ask your doctor or pharmacist to let you read the package insert prepared for the doctor.

USES OF ESTROGEN

Estrogens are prescribed by doctors for a number of purposes, including the following:

1. To provide estrogen during a period of adjustment when a woman's ovaries no longer produce estrogen, in order to prevent certain uncomfortable symptoms of estrogen deficiency. (All women normally stop producing estrogens, generally between the ages of 45 and 55; this is called the menopause.)
2. To prevent symptoms of estrogen deficiency when a woman's ovaries have been removed surgically before the natural menopause.
3. To prevent pregnancy. (Estrogens are given along with a progestogen, another female hormone; these combinations are called oral contraceptives or birth control pills. Patient labeling is available to women taking oral contraceptives and they will not be discussed in this leaflet.)
4. To treat certain cancers in women and men.
5. To prevent painful swelling of the breasts after pregnancy in women who choose not to nurse their babies.

THERE IS NO PROPER USE OF ESTROGENS IN A PREGNANT WOMAN.

ESTROGENS IN THE MENOPAUSE

In the natural course of their lives, all women eventually experience a decrease in estrogen production. This usually occurs between ages 45 and 55 but may occur earlier or later. Sometimes the ovaries may need to be removed before natural menopause by an operation, producing a "surgical menopause."

When the amount of estrogen in the blood begins to decrease, many women may develop typical symptoms: feelings of warmth in the face, neck, and chest; or sudden intense episodes of heat and sweating throughout the body (called "hot flashes" or "hot flushes"). These symptoms are sometimes very uncomfortable. A few women eventually develop changes in the vagina (called "atrophic vaginitis") which cause discomfort, especially during and after intercourse.

Estrogens can be prescribed to treat these symptoms of the menopause. It is estimated that considerably more than half of all women undergoing the menopause have only mild symptoms or no symptoms at all and, therefore, do not need estrogens. Other women may need estrogens for a few months, while their bodies adjust to lower estrogen levels. Sometimes the need will be for periods longer than six months. In an attempt to avoid overstimulation of the uterus (womb), estrogens are usually given cyclically during each month of use, that is, three weeks of pills followed by one week without pills. However, Estrovis (quinestrol tablets, USP) is given once daily for seven days, followed by once weekly use beginning two weeks after the start of treatment.

Sometimes, women experience nervous symptoms or depression during menopause. There is no evidence that estrogens are effective for such symptoms and they should not be used to treat them, although other treatment may be needed.

You may have heard that taking estrogens for long periods (years) after the menopause will keep your skin soft and supple and keep you feeling young. There is no evidence that this is so, however, and such long-term treatment carries important risks.

THE DANGERS OF ESTROGEN

1. *Cancer of the uterus.* If estrogens are used in the postmenopausal period for more than a year, there is an increased risk of *endometrial cancer* (cancer of the uterus). Women taking estrogens have roughly 5 to 10 times as great a chance of getting this cancer as women who take no estrogens. To put this another way, while a postmenopausal woman not taking estrogens has 1 chance in 1,000 each year of getting cancer of the uterus, a woman taking estrogens has 5 to 10 chances in 1,000 each year. For this reason *it is important to take estrogens only when you really need them.*

The risk of this cancer is greater the longer estrogens are used and also seems to be greater when larger doses are taken. For this reason *it is important to take the lowest dosage of estrogens that will control symptoms and to take it only as long as it is needed.* If estrogens are needed for longer periods of time, your doctor will want to reevaluate your need for estrogens at least every six months.

Women using estrogens should report any irregular vaginal bleeding to their doctors; although such bleeding may be of no importance, it can be an early warning of cancer of the uterus. If you have undiagnosed vaginal bleeding, you should not use estrogens until a diagnosis is made and you are certain there is no cancer of the uterus.

If you have had your uterus completely removed (total hysterectomy), there is no danger of developing cancer of the uterus.

2. *Other possible cancers.* Estrogens can cause development of other tumors in animals, such as tumors of the breast, cervix, vagina, or liver, when given for a long time. At present, there is no good evidence that women using estrogen in the menopause have an increased risk of such tumors, but there is no way yet to be sure they do not. One study raises the possibility that use of estrogen in the menopause may increase the risk of breast cancer many years later. This is a further reason to use estrogens only when clearly needed. While you are taking estrogens, it is important that you go to your doctor at least once a year for a physical examination. Also, if members of your family have had breast cancer or if you have breast nodules or abnormal mammograms (breast x-rays), your doctor may wish to carry out more frequent examinations of your breasts.

3. *Gallbladder disease.* Women who use estrogens after menopause are more likely to develop gallbladder disease requiring surgery than women who do not use estrogens. Birth control pills have a similar effect.

4. *Abnormal blood clotting.* Oral contraceptives increase the risk of blood clotting in various parts of the body. This can result in a stroke (if the clot is in the brain), a heart attack (a clot in a blood vessel of the heart), or a pulmonary embolus (a clot which forms in the legs or pelvis, then breaks off and travels to the lungs.) Any of these can be fatal.

At this time use of estrogens in the menopause is not known to cause such blood clotting, but this has not been fully studied and there could still prove to be such a risk. It is recommended that if you have had clotting in the legs or lungs or a heart attack or stroke while you were using estrogens or birth control pills, you should not use estrogens (unless they are being used to treat cancer of the breast or prostate.) If you have had a stroke or heart attack or if you have angina pectoris, estrogens should be used with great caution and only if clearly needed (for example, if you have severe symptoms of the menopause).

The larger dosages of estrogen used to prevent swelling of the breasts after pregnancy have been reported to cause clotting in the legs and lungs.

SPECIAL WARNING ABOUT PREGNANCY

You should not receive estrogen if you are pregnant. If this should occur, there is a greater than usual chance that the developing child will be born with a birth defect, although the possibility remains fairly small. A female child may have an increased risk of developing cancer of the vagina or cervix later in life (in the teens or twenties). Every possible effort should be made to avoid exposure to estrogens during pregnancy. If exposure occurs, see your doctor.

OTHER EFFECTS OF ESTROGENS

In addition to the serious known risks of estrogens previously described, estrogens have the following side effects and potential risks:

1. *Nausea and vomiting.* The most common side effect of estrogen therapy is nausea. Vomiting is less common.
2. *Effects on the breasts.* Estrogens may cause breast tenderness or enlargement and may cause the breasts to secrete a liquid. These effects are not dangerous.
3. *Effects on the uterus.* Estrogens may cause benign fibroid tumors of the uterus to enlarge.

Some women will have menstrual bleeding when estrogens are stopped. However, if the bleeding occurs on days you are still taking estrogens, you should report this to your doctor.

4. *Effects on the liver.* On rare occasions, women taking oral contraceptives develop a tumor of the liver which can rupture and bleed into the abdomen. So far, these tumors have not been reported in women using estrogens in the menopause, but you should report to your doctor immediately any swelling or unusual pain or tenderness in the abdomen.

Women with a past history of jaundice (yellowing of the skin and white parts of the eyes) may get jaundice again during estrogen use. If this occurs, stop taking estrogens and see your doctor.

5. *Other effects.* Estrogens may cause excess fluid to be retained in the body. This may make some conditions worse, such as epilepsy, migraine, heart disease, or kidney disease.

SUMMARY

Estrogens have important uses, but they have serious risks as well. You must decide, with your doctor, whether the risks are acceptable to you in view of the benefits of treatment. Except where your doctor has prescribed estrogens for use in special cases of cancer of the breast or prostate, you should not use estrogens if you have cancer of the breast or uterus, are pregnant, have undiagnosed abnormal vaginal bleeding, clotting in the legs or lungs, or have had a stroke, heart attack or angina, or clotting in the legs or lungs in the past while you were taking estrogens.

You can use estrogens as safely as possible by understanding that your doctor will require regular physical examinations while you are taking them and will try to use the smallest dosage possible and discontinue the drug as soon as possible.

Be alert for signs of trouble including:

1. Abnormal bleeding from the vagina
2. Pains in the calves or chest or sudden shortness of breath, or coughing blood (indicating possible clots in the legs, heart, or lungs)
3. Severe headache, dizziness, faintness, or changes in vision (indicating possible developing clots in the brain or eye)
4. Breast lumps (you should ask you doctor how to examine your own breasts)
5. Jaundice (yellowing of the skin)
6. Mental depression

Based on his or her assessment of your medical needs, your doctor has prescribed this drug for you. Do not give this drug to anyone else.

Storage—Store between 15°–30°C (59°–86°F).

Caution—Federal law prohibits dispensing without prescription

0437G027

Shown in Product Identification Section, page 422

EUTHROID® ℞

[*ūth 'roid*]

(Liotrix Tablets, USP)

DESCRIPTION

Euthroid (Liotrix Tablets, USP) is synthetic microcrystalline levothyroxine sodium (T_4) USP and synthetic microcrystalline liothyronine sodium (T_3) USP combined in a constant 4:1 ratio. Each Euthroid-1 tablet contains 60 mcg levothyroxine (T_4) and 15 mcg liothyronine (T_3).

Each Euthroid-1 tablet will give a dose benefit approximately equivalent to 1 grain of desiccated thryoid, 100 mcg T_4 (levothyroxine sodium), 25 mcg T_3 (liothyronine sodium), or 60 mcg T_4/15 mcg T_3 (liotrix). See Conversion Table at end of insert.

Euthroid tablets also contain calcium phosphate, USP; cellulose, NF; corn starch, NF; hydrogenated vegetable oil, NF; magnesium stearate, NF; mannitol, USP; and silicon dioxide, NF. Euthroid-1 and Euthroid-3 contain D&C red No. 30 lake, FD&C blue No. 2 lake, and FD&C yellow No. 5 lake. Euthroid-2 contains D&C red No. 30 lake and FD&C blue No. 2 lake.

Thyroid hormone drugs are natural or synthetic preparations containing tetraiodothyronine (T_4 levothyroxine) sodium or triiodothyronine (T_3, liothyronine) sodium or both. T_4 and T_3 are produced in the human thyroid gland by the iodination and coupling of the amino acid tyrosine. T_4 contains four iodine atoms and is formed by the coupling of two molecules of diiodotyrosine (DIT). T_3 contains three atoms of iodine and is formed by the coupling of one molecule of DIT with one molecule of monoiodotyrosine (MIT). Both hormones are stored in the thyroid colloid as thyroglobulin.

Thyroid hormone preparations belong to two categories: (1) natural hormonal preparations derived from animal thyroid, and (2) synthetic preparations. Natural preparations include desiccated thyroid and thyroglobulin. Desiccated thyroid is derived from domesticated animals that are used

for food by man (either beef or hog thyroid), and thyroglobulin is derived from thyroid glands of the hog.
There are five (5) preparations in the USP. They are: (1) Thyroid Tablets, (2) Thyroglobulin Tablets, (3) Levothyroxine Sodium Tablets, (4) Liothyronine Sodium Tablets, and (5) Liotrix Tablets (a ratio, by weight, of 4 to 1, of the sodium salts of T_4 and T_3, respectively).

CLINICAL PHARMACOLOGY

The steps in the synthesis of the thyroid hormones are controlled by thyrotropin (Thyroid Stimulating Hormone, TSH) secreted by the anterior pituitary. This hormone's secretion is in turn controlled by a feedback mechanism effected by the thyroid hormones themselves and by thyrotropin releasing hormone (TRH), a tripeptide of hypothalamic origin. Endogenous thyroid hormone secretion is suppressed when exogenous thyroid hormones are administered to euthyroid individuals in excess of the normal gland's secretion.
The mechanisms by which thyroid hormones exert their physiologic action are not well understood. These hormones enhance oxygen consumption by most tissues of the body, increase the basal metabolic rate, and the metabolism of carbohydrates, lipids, and proteins. Thus, they exert a profound influence on every organ system in the body and are of particular importance in the development of the central nervous system.
The normal thyroid gland contains approximately 200 mcg of levothyroxine (T_4) per gram of gland, and 15 mcg of triiodothyronine (T_3) per gram. The ratio of these two hormones in the circulation does not represent the ratio in the thyroid gland, since about 80 percent of peripheral triiodothyronine comes from monodeiodination of levothyroxine. Peripheral monodeiodination of levothyroxine at the 5 position (inner ring) also results in the formation of reverse triiodothyronine (rT_3), which is calorigenically inactive. These facts would seem to advocate levothyroxine as the treatment of choice for the hypothyroid patient and to militate against the administration of hormone combinations, which while normalizing thyroxine levels may produce triiodothyronine levels in the thyrotoxic range.
Triiodothyronine (T_3) level is low in the fetus and newborn, in old age, in chronic caloric deprivation, hepatic cirrhosis, renal failure, surgical stress, and chronic illnesses representing what has been called the "low triiodothyronine syndrome."
Pharmacokinetics: Animal studies have shown that T_4 is only partially absorbed from the gastrointestinal tract. The degree of absorption is dependent on the vehicle used for its administration and by the character of the intestinal contents, the intestinal flora, including plasma protein, soluble dietary factors, all of which bind thyroid and thereby make it unavailable for diffusion. Only 41 percent is absorbed when given in a gelatin capsule as opposed to a 74 percent absorption when given with an albumin carrier.
Depending on other factors, absorption has varied from 48 to 79 percent of the administered dose. Fasting increases absorption. Malabsorption syndromes, as well as dietary factors (children's soybean formula, concomitant use of anionic exchange resins such as cholestyramine), cause excessive fecal loss. T_3 is almost totally absorbed, 95 percent in 4 hours. The hormones contained in the natural preparations are absorbed in a manner similar to the synthetic hormones.
More than 99 percent of circulating hormones are bound to serum proteins, including thyroid-binding globulin (TB_g), thyroid-binding prealbumin (TBPA), and albumin (TB_a), whose capacities and affinities vary for the hormones. The higher affinity of levothyroxine (T_4) for both TB_g and TBPA as compared to triiodothyronine (T_3) partially explains the higher serum levels and longer half-life of the former hormone. Both protein-bound hormones exist in reverse equilibrium with minute amounts of free hormone, the latter accounting for the metabolic activity.
Deiodination of levothyroxine (T_4) occurs at a number of sites, including liver, kidney, and other tissues. The conjugated hormone, in the form of glucuronide or sulfate, is found in the bile and gut where it may complete an enterohepatic circulation. Eighty-five percent of levothyroxine (T_4) metabolized daily is deiodinated.

INDICATIONS AND USAGE

Thyroid hormone drugs are indicated:
As replacement or supplemental therapy in patients with hypothyroidism of any etiology, except transient hypothyroidism during the recovery phase of subacute thyroiditis. This category includes cretinism, myxedema, and ordinary hypothyroidism in patients of any age (children, adults, the elderly), or state (including pregnancy); primary hypothyroidism resulting from functional deficiency, primary atrophy, partial or total absence of thyroid gland, or the effects of surgery, radiation, or drugs, with or without the presence of goiter; and secondary (pituitary) or tertiary (hypothalamic) hypothyroidism (See WARNINGS).

CONTRAINDICATIONS

Thyroid hormone preparations are generally contraindicated in patients with diagnosed but as yet uncorrected adrenal cortical insufficiency, untreated thyrotoxicosis, and apparent hypersensitivity to any of their active or extraneous constituents. There is no well documented evidence from the literature, however, of true allergic or idiosyncratic reactions to thyroid hormone.

WARNINGS

Drugs with thyroid hormone activity, alone or together with other therapeutic agents, have been used for the treatment of obesity. In euthyroid patients, doses within the range of daily hormonal requirements are ineffective for weight reduction. Larger doses may produce serious or even life-threatening manifestations of toxicity, particularly when given in association with sympathomimetic amines such as those used for their anorectic effects.

The use of thyroid hormones in the therapy of obesity, alone or combined with other drugs, is unjustified and has been shown to be ineffective. Neither is their use justified for the treatment of male or female infertility unless this condition is accompanied by hypothyroidism.

PRECAUTIONS

General: Thyroid hormones should be used with great caution in a number of circumstances where the integrity of the cardiovascular system, particularly the coronary arteries, is suspect. These include patients with angina pectoris or the elderly, in whom there is a greater likelihood of occult cardiac disease. In these patients, therapy should be initiated with low doses, ie, 25–50 mcg levothyroxine (T_4) or its isocaloric equivalents (see Conversion Table at end of insert). When, in such patients, a euthyroid state can only be reached at the expense of an aggravation of the cardiovascular disease, thyroid hormone dosage should be reduced.
Thyroid hormone therapy in patients with concomitant diabetes mellitus or insipidus or adrenal cortical insufficiency aggravates the intensity of their symptoms. Appropriate adjustments of the various therapeutic measures directed at these concomitant endocrine diseases are required. The therapy of myxedema coma requires simultaneous administration of glucocorticoids (See DOSAGE AND ADMINISTRATION).
Hypothyroidism decreases and hyperthyroidism increases the sensitivity to oral anticoagulants. Prothrombin time should be closely monitored in thyroid-treated patients on oral anticoagulants and dosage of the latter agents adjusted on the basis of frequent prothrombin time determination. In infants, excessive doses of thyroid hormone preparations may produce craniosynostosis.
Euthroid-½, -1, -3 contains FD&C Yellow No 5 (tartrazine) which may cause allergic-type reactions (including bronchial asthma) in certain susceptible individuals. Although the overall incidence of FD&C Yellow No 5 (tartrazine) sensitivity in the population is low, it is frequently seen in patients who also have aspirin hypersensitivity.
Information for the Patient: Patients on thyroid hormone preparations and parents of children on thyroid therapy should be informed that:
1. Replacement therapy is to be taken essentially for life, with the exception of cases of transient hypothyroidism, usually associated with thyroiditis, and in those patients receiving a therapeutic trial of the drug.
2. They should immediately report during the course of therapy any signs or symptoms of thyroid hormone toxicity, eg, chest pain, increased pulse rate, palpitations, excessive sweating, heat intolerance, nervousness, or any other unusual event.
3. In case of concomitant diabetes mellitus, the daily dosage of antidiabetic medication may need readjustment as thyroid hormone replacement is achieved. If thyroid medication is stopped, a downward readjustment of the dosage of insulin or oral hypoglycemic agent may be necessary to avoid hypoglycemia. At all times, close monitoring of urinary glucose levels is mandatory in such patients.
4. In case of concomitant oral anticoagulant therapy, the prothrombin time should be measured frequently to determine if the dosage of oral anticoagulants is to be readjusted.
5. Partial loss of hair may be experienced by children in the first few months of thyroid therapy, but this is usually a transient phenomenon and later recovery is usually the rule.
Laboratory Tests: Treatment of patients with thyroid hormones requires the periodic assessment of thyroid status by means of appropriate laboratory tests besides the full clinical evaluation. The TSH suppression test can be used to test the effectiveness of any thyroid preparation, bearing in mind the relative insensitivity of the infant pituitary to the negative feedback effect of thyroid hormones. Serum T_4 levels can be used to test the effectiveness of all thyroid medications except T_3. When the total serum T_4 is low but TSH is normal, a test specific to assess unbound (free) T_4 levels is warranted. Specific measurements of T_4 and T_3 by competitive protein binding or radioimmunoassay are not influenced by blood levels of organic or inorganic iodine and have essentially replaced older tests of thyroid hormone measurements, ie, PBI, BEI, and T_4 by column.
Drug Interactions: Oral Anticoagulants—Thyroid hormones appear to increase catabolism of vitamin K-dependent clotting factors. If oral anticoagulants are also being given, compensatory increases in clotting factor synthesis are impaired. Patients stabilized on oral anticoagulants who are found to require thyroid replacement therapy should be watched very closely when thyroid is started. If a patient is truly hypothyroid, it is likely that a reduction in anticoagulant dosage will be required. No special precautions appear to be necessary when oral anticoagulant therapy is begun in a patient already stabilized on maintenance thyroid replacement therapy.
Insulin or Oral Hypoglycemics—Initiating thyroid replacement therapy may cause increases in insulin or oral hypoglycemic requirements. The effects seen are poorly understood and depend upon a variety of factors such as dosage and type of thyroid preparations and endocrine status of the patient. Patients receiving insulin or oral hypoglycemics should be closely watched during initiation of thyroid replacement therapy.
Cholestyramine—Cholestyramine binds both T_4 and T_3 in the intestine, thus impairing absorption of these thyroid hormones. *In vitro* studies indicate that the binding is not easily removed. Therefore, four to five hours should elapse between administration of cholestyramine or similar resins, such as colestipol, and thyroid hormones.
Estrogen, Oral Contraceptives—Estrogens tend to increase serum thyroxine-binding globulin (TB_g). In a patient with a nonfunctioning thyroid gland who is receiving thyroid replacement therapy, free levothyroxine may be decreased when estrogens are started thus increasing thyroid requirements. However, if the patient's thyroid gland has sufficient function, the decreased free thyroxine will result in a compensatory increase in thyroxine output by the thyroid. Therefore, patients without a functioning thyroid gland who are on thyroid replacement therapy may need to increase their thyroid dose if estrogens or estrogen-containing oral contraceptives are given.
Drug/Laboratory Test Interactions: The following drugs or moieties are known to interfere with laboratory tests performed in patients on thyroid hormone therapy: androgens, corticosteroids, estrogens, oral contraceptives containing estrogens, iodine-containing preparations, and the numerous preparations containing salicylates.
1. Changes in TB_g concentration should be taken into consideration in the interpretation of T_4 and T_3 values. In such cases, the unbound (free) hormone should be measured. Pregnancy, estrogens, and estrogen-containing oral contraceptives increase TB_g concentrations. TB_g may also be increased during infectious hepatitis. Decreases in TB_g concentrations are observed in nephrosis, acromegaly, and after androgen or corticosteroid therapy. Familial hyper- or hypo-thyroxine binding globulinemias have been described. The incidence of TB_g deficiency approximates 1 in 9000. The binding of thyroxine by TBPA is inhibited by salicylates.
2. Medicinal or dietary iodine interferes with all *in vivo* tests of radioiodine uptake, producing low uptakes which may not be reflective of a true decrease in hormone synthesis.
3. The persistence of clinical and laboratory evidence of hypothyroidism in spite of adequate dosage replacement indicates poor patient compliance, poor absorption, excessive fecal loss, or inactivity of the preparation. Intracellular resistance to thyroid hormone is quite rare.
Carcinogenesis, Mutagenesis, and Impairment of Fertility: A reportedly apparent association between prolonged thyroid therapy and breast cancer has not been confirmed and patients on thyroid for established indications should not discontinue therapy. No confirmatory long-term studies in animals have been performed to evaluate carcinogenic potential, mutagenicity, or impairment of fertility in either males or females.
Pregnancy—Category A: Thyroid hormones do not readily cross the placental barrier. The clinical experience to date does not indicate any adverse effect on fetuses when thyroid hormones are administered to pregnant women. On the basis of current knowledge, thyroid replacement therapy to hypothyroid women should not be discontinued during pregnancy.
Nursing Mothers: Minimal amounts of thyroid hormones are excreted in human milk. Thyroid is not associated with serious adverse reactions and does not have a known tumorigenic potential. However, caution should be exercised when thyroid is administered to a nursing woman.
Pediatric Use: Pregnant mothers provide little or no thyroid hormone to the fetus. The incidence of congenital hypo-

Continued on next page

This product information was prepared in August 1992. On these and other Parke-Davis Products, information may be obtained by addressing PARKE-DAVIS, Division of Warner-Lambert Company, Morris Plains, New Jersey 07950.

Parke-Davis—Cont.

thyroidism is relatively high (1:4,000) and the hypothyroid fetus would not derive any benefit from the small amounts of hormone crossing the placental barrier. Routine determinations of serum T_4 and/or TSH are strongly advised in neonates in view of the deleterious effects of thyroid deficiency on growth and development.

Treatment should be initiated immediately upon diagnosis and maintained for life, unless transient hypothyroidism is suspected; in which case, therapy may be interrupted for 2 to 8 weeks after the age of 3 years to reassess the condition. Cessation of therapy is justified in patients who have maintained a normal TSH during those 2 to 8 weeks.

ADVERSE REACTIONS

Adverse reactions other than those indicative of hyperthyroidism because of therapeutic overdosage, either initially or during the maintenance period, are rare (See OVERDOSAGE).

OVERDOSAGE

Signs and Symptoms: Excessive doses of thyroid result in a hypermetabolic state resembling in every respect the condition of endogenous origin. The condition may be self-induced.

Treatment of Overdosage: Dosage should be reduced or therapy temporarily discontinued if signs and symptoms of overdosage appear. Treatment may be reinstituted at a lower dosage. In normal individuals, normal hypothalamic-pituitary-thyroid axis function is restored in 6 to 8 weeks after thyroid suppression.

Treatment of acute massive thyroid hormone overdosage is aimed at reducing gastrointestinal absorption of the drugs and counteracting central and peripheral effects, mainly those of increased sympathetic activity. Vomiting may be induced initially if further gastrointestinal absorption can reasonably be prevented and barring contraindications such as coma, convulsions, or loss of the gagging reflex. Treatment is symptomatic and supportive. Oxygen may be administered and ventilation maintained. Cardiac glycosides may be indicated if congestive heart failure develops. Measures to control fever, hypoglycemia, or fluid loss should be instituted if needed. Antiadrenergic agents, particularly propranolol, have been used advantageously in the treatment of increased sympathetic activity. Propranolol may be administered intravenously at a dosage of 1 to 3 mg over a 10 minute period or orally, 80 to 160 mg/day initially, especially when no contraindications exist for its use.

DOSAGE AND ADMINISTRATION

The dosage of thyroid hormones is determined by the indication and must in every case be individualized according to patient response and laboratory findings.

Thyroid hormones are given orally. In acute, emergency conditions, injectable sodium levothyroxine may be given intravenously when oral administration is not feasible or desirable, as in the treatment of myxedema coma, or during total parenteral nutrition. Injectable sodium liothyronine is also available upon request from the manufacturer, under investigational status, for the treatment of myxedema coma. Intramuscular administration of these two preparations is not advisable because of reported poor absorption.

Hypothyroidism: Therapy is usually instituted using low doses, with increments which depend on the cardiovascular status of the patient. The usual starting dose is 50 mcg of levothyroxine (T_4) or its isocaloric equivalent (Euthroid-½), with increments of 25 mcg every 2 to 3 weeks. A lower starting dosage, 25 mcg/day of levothyroxine (T_4) or its isocaloric equivalent, is recommended in patients with longstanding myxedema, particularly if cardiovascular impairment is suspected, in which case extreme caution is recommended. The appearance of angina is an indication for a reduction in dosage. The 200 to 400 mcg levothyroxine (T_4) recommended in the early trials are now considered excessive and most patients require 100 to 200 mcg/day or the caloric equivalent. Failure to respond to doses of 300 mcg suggests lack of compliance or malabsorption. Maintenance dosages of 100–200 mcg/day (Euthroid-1 or Euthroid-2) usually result in normal serum levothyroxine (T_4) and triiodothyronine (T_3) levels. Adequate therapy usually results in normal TSH and T_4 levels after 2 to 3 weeks of therapy.

Readjustment of thyroid hormone dosage should be made within the first four weeks of therapy, after proper clinical and laboratory evaluations, including serum levels of T_4, bound and free, and TSH.

The rapid onset and dissipation of action of sodium liothyronine (T_3), as compared with sodium levothyroxine (T_4), has led some clinicians to prefer its use in patients who might be more susceptible to the untoward effects of thyroid medication. However, the wide swings in serum T_3 levels that follow its administration and the possibility of more pronounced cardiovascular side effects tend to counterbalance the stated advantages. Many physicians continue to use thyroid tablets, USP, a T_3/T_4 combination, or a newer synthetic combination.

Table 2 Conversion Table

Euthroid (liotrix tablets, USP)			Natural	Synthetic	
Tablet	T_4*/T_3** mcg	Color	Thyroid USP	T_4*	T_3**
Euthroid-1	(60/15)	light brown	1 grain	0.1 mg	25.0 mcg
Euthroid-2	(120/30)	violet	2 grains	0.2 mg	50.0 mcg
Euthroid-3	(180/45)	gray	3 grains	0.3 mg	75.0 mcg

*T_4= levothyroxine sodium (*l*-thyroxine) **T_3= liothyronine sodium (*l*-triiodothyronine)

T_3 may be used in preference to levothyroxine (T_4) during radioisotope scanning procedures, since induction of hypothyroidism in those cases is more abrupt and can be of shorter duration. It may also be preferred when impairment of peripheral conversion of T_4 and T_3 is suspected.

Myxedema Coma: Myxedema coma is usually precipitated in the hypothyroid patient of long standing by intercurrent illness or drugs such as sedatives and anesthetics and should be considered a medical emergency. Therapy should be directed to the correction of electrolyte disturbances and possible infection besides the administration of thyroid hormones. Corticosteroids should be administered routinely. T_4 and T_3 may be administered via nasogastric tube, but the preferred route of administration of both hormones is intravenous. Sodium levothyroxine (T_4) is given at a starting dose of 400 mcg (100 mcg/mL) given rapidly and is usually well tolerated, even in the elderly. This initial dose is followed by daily supplements of 100 to 200 mcg given IV. Normal T_4 levels are achieved in 24 hours followed in 3 days by threefold elevation of T_3. Triiodothyronine (T_3) (which is obtained only by special request from the manufacturer) is given at doses of 200 mcg IV followed by 25 mcg supplements at 8-hour intervals. Oral therapy with either hormone would be resumed as soon as the clinical situation has been stabilized and the patient is able to take oral medication.

Thyroid Cancer: Exogenous thyroid hormone may produce regression of metastases from follicular and papillary carcinoma of the thyroid and is used as ancillary therapy of these conditions with radioactive iodine. TSH should be suppressed to low or undetectable levels. Therefore, larger amounts of thyroid hormone than those used for replacement therapy are required. Medullary carcinoma of the thyroid is usually unresponsive to this therapy.

Thyroid Suppression Therapy: Administration of thyroid hormone in doses higher than those produced physiologically by the gland results in suppression of the production of endogenous hormone. This is the basis for the thyroid suppression test and is used as an aid in the diagnosis of patients with signs of mild hyperthyroidism in whom baseline laboratory tests appear normal or to demonstrate thyroid gland autonomy in patients with Graves' ophthalmopathy. 131_1 uptake is determined before and after the administration of the exogenous hormone. A fifty percent or greater suppression of uptake indicates a normal thyroid-pituitary axis and thus rules out thyroid gland autonomy.

For adults, the usual suppressive dose of levothyroxine (T_4) is 2.6 mcg/kg of body weight per day given for 7 to 10 days. These doses usually yield normal serum T_4 and T_3 levels and lack of response to TSH.

T_3 is given in doses of 75–100 mcg/day for 7 days and radioactive iodine uptake is determined before and after administration of the hormone. If thyroid function is under normal control, the radioiodine uptake will drop significantly after treatment with either hormone.

Either hormone or combination therapy should be administered cautiously to patients in whom there is a strong suspicion of thyroid gland autonomy, in view of the fact that the exogenous hormone effects will be additive to the endogenous source.

Pediatric Dosage: Pediatric dosage should follow the recommendations summarized in Table 1. In infants with congenital hypothyroidism, therapy with full doses should be instituted as soon as the diagnosis has been made.

Table 1 Recommended Pediatric Dosage for Congenital Hypothyroidism

	Tetraiodothyronine (T_4, levothyroxine) sodium	
Age	Dose per day	Daily dose per kg of body weight
0–6 mos	25–50 mcg	8–10 mcg
6–12 mos	50–75 mcg	6– 8 mcg
1–5 yrs	75–100 mcg	5– 6 mcg
6–12 yrs	100–150 mcg	4– 5 mcg
over 12 yrs	over 150 mcg	2– 3 mcg

[See Table 2 above.]

Following a change from one type of thyroid preparation to another, patients may still require fine adjustment of dosage because the equivalents are only estimates.

HOW SUPPLIED

Square monogrammed scored tablets of four potencies, each identified by a different color (see Table 2).

Euthroid-1 is supplied as: N 0071-0261-24—Bottles of 100.
Euthroid-2 is supplied as: N 0071-0262-24—Bottles of 100.
Euthroid-3 is supplied as: N 0071-0263-24—Bottles of 100.

Store at controlled room temperature 15°-25°C (59°-77°F).

Licensed under US Patent 2,823,164

Caution—Federal law prohibits dispensing without prescription.

0260G026

Shown in Product Identification Section, page 422

FLUOGEN® ℞

[flŭ 'ō-jĕn "]
(influenza virus vaccine)

The formulation of influenza virus vaccine for use during each season is established by the Office of Biologics, Food and Drug Administration, Public Health Service. For information regarding the current formulation, please refer to the product package insert, contact your Parke-Davis representative, or call (800) 223-0432.

HUMATIN® ℞

(Paromomycin Sulfate, USP)

DESCRIPTION

Humatin is a broad spectrum antibiotic produced by *Streptomyces rimosus* var. *paromomycinus*. It is a white, amorphous, stable, water-soluble product supplied as capsules containing the equivalent of 250 mg paromomycin. The capsule contains D&C yellow No. 10; FD&C blue No. 1; FD&C red No. 3; FD&C yellow No. 6; gelatin, NF; and titanium dioxide, USP.

ACTION

The *in vitro* and *in vivo* antibacterial action of paromomycin closely parallels that of neomycin. It is poorly absorbed after oral administration, with almost 100% of the drug recoverable in the stool.

INDICATIONS

Humatin is indicated for intestinal amebiasis—acute and chronic (NOTE—It is not effective in extra-intestinal amebiasis); management of hepatic coma—as adjunctive therapy.

CONTRAINDICATIONS

Paromomycin sulfate is contraindicated in individuals with a history of previous hypersensitivity reactions to it. It is also contraindicated in intestinal obstruction.

PRECAUTIONS

The use of this antibiotic, as with other antibiotics, may result in an overgrowth of nonsusceptible organisms, including fungi. Constant observation of the patient is essential. If new infections caused by nonsusceptible organisms appear during therapy, appropriate measures should be taken.

The drug should be used with caution in individuals with ulcerative lesions of the bowel to avoid renal toxicity through inadvertent absorption.

ADVERSE REACTIONS

Nausea, abdominal cramps, and diarrhea have been reported in patients on doses over 3 g daily.

DOSAGE AND ADMINISTRATION

Intestinal amebiasis: Adults and Children: Usual dose—25 to 35 mg/kg body weight daily, administered in three doses with meals, for five to ten days.

Management of hepatic coma: Adults: Usual dose—4 g daily in divided doses, given at regular intervals for five to six days.

HOW SUPPLIED

N 0071-0529-09

Humatin Capsules, each containing paromomycin sulfate equivalent to 250 mg paromomycin, are supplied in bottles of 16.

Caution—Federal law prohibits dispensing without prescription.

0529G031

Shown in Product Identification Section, page 422

KETALAR® ℞
[kē'tă-lär"]
(Ketamine Hydrochloride Injection, USP)

SPECIAL NOTE
EMERGENCE REACTIONS HAVE OCCURRED IN APPROXIMATELY 12 PERCENT OF PATIENTS.
THE PSYCHOLOGICAL MANIFESTATIONS VARY IN SEVERITY BETWEEN PLEASANT DREAM-LIKE STATES, VIVID IMAGERY, HALLUCINATIONS, AND EMERGENCE DELIRIUM. IN SOME CASES THESE STATES HAVE BEEN ACCOMPANIED BY CONFUSION, EXCITEMENT, AND IRRATIONAL BEHAVIOR WHICH A FEW PATIENTS RECALL AS AN UNPLEASANT EXPERIENCE. THE DURATION ORDINARILY IS NO MORE THAN A FEW HOURS; IN A FEW CASES, HOWEVER, RECURRENCES HAVE TAKEN PLACE UP TO 24 HOURS POSTOPERATIVELY. NO RESIDUAL PSYCHOLOGICAL EFFECTS ARE KNOWN TO HAVE RESULTED FROM USE OF KETALAR.
THE INCIDENCE OF THESE EMERGENCE PHENOMENA IS LEAST IN THE YOUNG (15 YEARS OF AGE OR LESS) AND ELDERLY (OVER 65 YEARS OF AGE) PATIENT. ALSO, THEY ARE LESS FREQUENT WHEN THE DRUG IS GIVEN INTRAMUSCULARLY AND THE INCIDENCE IS REDUCED AS EXPERIENCE WITH THE DRUG IS GAINED.
THE INCIDENCE OF PSYCHOLOGICAL MANIFESTATIONS DURING EMERGENCE, PARTICULARLY DREAM-LIKE OBSERVATIONS AND EMERGENCE DELIRIUM, MAY BE REDUCED BY USING LOWER RECOMMENDED DOSAGES OF KETALAR IN CONJUNCTION WITH INTRAVENOUS DIAZEPAM DURING INDUCTION AND MAINTENANCE OF ANESTHESIA. (See Dosage and Administration.) ALSO, THESE REACTIONS MAY BE REDUCED IF VERBAL, TACTILE AND VISUAL STIMULATION OF THE PATIENT IS MINIMIZED DURING THE RECOVERY PERIOD. THIS DOES NOT PRECLUDE THE MONITORING OF VITAL SIGNS.
IN ORDER TO TERMINATE A SEVERE EMERGENCE REACTION THE USE OF A SMALL HYPNOTIC DOSE OF A SHORT-ACTING OR ULTRASHORT-ACTING BARBITURATE MAY BE REQUIRED.
WHEN KETALAR IS USED ON AN OUTPATIENT BASIS, THE PATIENT SHOULD NOT BE RELEASED UNTIL RECOVERY FROM ANESTHESIA IS COMPLETE AND THEN SHOULD BE ACCOMPANIED BY A RESPONSIBLE ADULT.

DESCRIPTION
Ketalar is a nonbarbiturate anesthetic, chemically designated *dl* 2-(o-chlorophenyl)-2-(methylamino) cyclohexanone hydrochloride. It is formulated as a slightly acid (pH 3.5-5.5) sterile solution for intravenous or intramuscular injection in concentrations containing the equivalent of either 10, 50 or 100 mg ketamine base per milliliter and contains not more than 0.1 mg/ml Phemerol® (benzethonium chloride) added as a preservative. The 10 mg/ml solution has been made isotonic with sodium chloride.

CLINICAL PHARMACOLOGY
Ketalar is a rapid-acting general anesthetic producing an anesthetic state characterized by profound analgesia, normal pharyngeal-laryngeal reflexes, normal or slightly enhanced skeletal muscle tone, cardiovascular and respiratory stimulation, and occasionally a transient and minimal respiratory depression.
A patent airway is maintained partly by virtue of unimpaired pharyngeal and laryngeal reflexes. (See Warnings and Precautions.)
The biotransformation of Ketalar includes N-dealkylation (metabolite I), hydroxylation of the cyclohexone ring (metabolites III and IV), conjugation with glucuronic acid and dehydration of the hydroxylated metabolites to form the cyclohexene derivative (metabolite II).
Following intravenous administration, the ketamine concentration has an initial slope (alpha phase) lasting about 45 minutes with a half-life of 10 to 15 minutes. This first phase corresponds clinically to the anesthetic effect of the drug. The anesthetic action is terminated by a combination of redistribution from the CNS to slower equilibrating peripheral tissues and by hepatic biotransformation to metabolite I. This metabolite is about ⅓ as active as ketamine in reducing halothane requirements (MAC) of the rat. The later half-life of ketamine (beta phase) is 2.5 hours.
The anesthetic state produced by Ketalar has been termed "dissociative anesthesia" in that it appears to selectively interrupt association pathways of the brain before producing somesthetic sensory blockade. It may selectively depress the thalamoneocortical system before significantly obtunding

the more ancient cerebral centers and pathways (reticular-activating and limbic systems).
Elevation of blood pressure begins shortly after injection, reaches a maximum within a few minutes and usually returns to preanesthetic values within 15 minutes after injection. In the majority of cases, the systolic and diastolic blood pressure peaks from 10% to 50% above preanesthetic levels shortly after induction of anesthesia, but the elevation can be higher or longer in individual cases (see Contraindications).
Ketamine has a wide margin of safety; several instances of unintentional administration of overdoses of Ketalar (up to ten times that usually required) have been followed by prolonged but complete recovery.
Ketalar has been studied in over 12,000 operative and diagnostic procedures, involving over 10,000 patients from 105 separate studies. During the course of these studies Ketalar was administered as the sole agent, as induction for other general agents, or to supplement low-potency agents.
Specific areas of application have included the following:
1. debridement, painful dressings, and skin grafting in burn patients, as well as other superficial surgical procedures.
2. neurodiagnostic procedures such as pneumoencephalograms, ventriculograms, myelograms, and lumbar punctures. See also Precaution concerning increased intracranial pressure.
3. diagnostic and operative procedures of the eye, ear, nose, and mouth, including dental extractions.
4. diagnostic and operative procedures of the pharynx, larynx, or bronchial tree. NOTE: Muscle relaxants, with proper attention to respiration, may be required (see Precautions).
5. sigmoidoscopy and minor surgery of the anus and rectum, and circumcision.
6. extraperitoneal procedures used in gynecology such as dilatation and curettage.
7. orthopedic procedures such as closed reductions, manipulations, femoral pinning, amputations, and biopsies.
8. as an anesthetic in poor-risk patients with depression of vital functions.
9. in procedures where the intramuscular route of administration is preferred.
10. in cardiac catheterization procedures.
In these studies, the anesthesia was rated either "excellent" or "good" by the anesthesiologist and the surgeon at 90% and 93%, respectively; rated "fair" at 6% and 4%, respectively; and rated "poor" at 4% and 3%, respectively. In a second method of evaluation, the anesthesia was rated "adequate" in at least 90%, and "inadequate" in 10% or less of the procedures.

INDICATIONS AND USAGE
Ketalar is indicated as the sole anesthetic agent for diagnostic and surgical procedures that do not require skeletal muscle relaxation. Ketalar is best suited for short procedures but it can be used, with additional doses, for longer procedures. Ketalar is indicated for the induction of anesthesia prior to the administration of other general anesthetic agents.
Ketalar is indicated to supplement low-potency agents, such as nitrous oxide.
Specific areas of application are described in the Clinical Pharmacology section.

CONTRAINDICATIONS
Ketamine hydrochloride is contraindicated in those in whom a significant elevation of blood pressure would constitute a serious hazard and in those who have shown hypersensitivity to the drug.

WARNINGS
Cardiac function should be continually monitored during the procedure in patients found to have hypertension or cardiac decompensation.
Postoperative confusional states may occur during the recovery period. (See Special Note.)
Respiratory depression may occur with overdosage or too rapid a rate of administration of Ketalar, in which case supportive ventilation should be employed. Mechanical support of respiration is preferred to administration of analeptics.

PRECAUTIONS
General
Ketalar should be used by or under the direction of physicians experienced in administering general anesthetics and in maintenance of an airway and in the control of respiration.
Because pharyngeal and laryngeal reflexes are usually active, Ketalar should not be used alone in surgery or diagnostic procedures of the pharynx, larynx, or bronchial tree. Mechanical stimulation of the pharynx should be avoided, whenever possible, if Ketalar is used alone. Muscle relaxants, with proper attention to respiration, may be required in both of these instances.
Resuscitative equipment should be ready for use.
The incidence of emergence reactions may be reduced if verbal and tactile stimulation of the patient is minimized during

the recovery period. This does not preclude the monitoring of vital signs (see Special Note).
The intravenous dose should be administered over a period of 60 seconds. More rapid administration may result in respiratory depression or apnea and enhanced pressor response.
In surgical procedures involving visceral pain pathways, Ketalar should be supplemented with an agent which obtunds visceral pain.
Use with caution in the chronic alcoholic and the acutely alcohol-intoxicated patient.
An increase in cerebrospinal fluid pressure has been reported following administration of ketamine hydrochloride. Use with extreme caution in patients with preanesthetic elevated cerebrospinal fluid pressure.
Information for Patients
As appropriate, especially in cases where early discharge is possible, the duration of Ketalar and other drugs employed during the conduct of anesthesia should be considered. The patients should be cautioned that driving an automobile, operating hazardous machinery or engaging in hazardous activities should not be undertaken for 24 hours or more (depending upon the dosage of Ketalar and consideration of other drugs employed) after anesthesia.
Drug Interactions
Prolonged recovery time may occur if barbiturates and/or narcotics are used concurrently with Ketalar.
Ketalar is clinically compatible with the commonly used general and local anesthetic agents when an adequate respiratory exchange is maintained.
Usage in Pregnancy
Since the safe use in pregnancy, including obstetrics (either vaginal or abdominal delivery), has not been established, such use is not recommended (see Animal Reproduction).

ADVERSE REACTIONS
Cardiovascular: Blood pressure and pulse rate are frequently elevated following administration of Ketalar alone. However, hypotension and bradycardia have been observed. Arrhythmia has also occurred.
Respiration: Although respiration is frequently stimulated, severe depression of respiration or apnea may occur following rapid intravenous administration of high doses of Ketalar. Laryngospasms and other forms of airway obstruction have occurred during Ketalar anesthesia.
Eye: Diplopia and nystagmus have been noted following Ketalar administration.
It also may cause a slight elevation in intraocular pressure measurement.
Psychological: (See Special Note).
Neurological: In some patients, enhanced skeletal muscle tone may be manifested by tonic and clonic movements sometimes resembling seizures (see Dosage and Administration).
Gastrointestinal: Anorexia, nausea and vomiting have been observed; however this is not usually severe and allows the great majority of patients to take liquids by mouth shortly after regaining consciousness (see Dosage and Administration).
General: Local pain and exanthema at the injection site have infrequently been reported. Transient erythema and/or morbilliform rash have also been reported.

OVERDOSAGE
Respiratory depression may occur with overdosage or too rapid a rate of administration of Ketalar, in which case supportive ventilation should be employed. Mechanical support of respiration is preferred to administration of analeptics.

DOSAGE AND ADMINISTRATION
Note: Barbiturates and Ketalar, being chemically incompatible because of precipitate formation, *should not* be injected from the same syringe.
If the Ketalar dose is augmented with diazepam, the two drugs must be given separately. Do not mix Ketalar and diazepam in syringe or infusion flask. For additional information on the use of diazepam, refer to the Warnings and Dosage and Administration Sections of the diazepam insert.
Preoperative Preparations:
1. While vomiting has been reported following Ketalar administration, some airway protection may be afforded because of active laryngeal-pharyngeal reflexes. However, since aspiration may occur with Ketalar and since protective reflexes may also be diminished by supplementary anesthetics and muscle relaxants, the possibility of aspiration must be considered. Ketalar is recommended for use in the patient whose stomach is not empty when, in the judgment of the practitioner, the benefits of the drug outweigh the possible risks.

Continued on next page

This product information was prepared in August 1992. On these and other Parke-Davis Products, information may be obtained by addressing PARKE-DAVIS, Division of Warner-Lambert Company, Morris Plains, New Jersey 07950.

Parke-Davis—Cont.

2. Atropine, scopolamine, or another drying agent should be given at an appropriate interval prior to induction.

Onset and Duration:

Because of rapid induction following the initial intravenous injection, the patient should be in a supported position during administration.

The onset of action of Ketalar is rapid; an intravenous dose of 2 mg/kg (1 mg/lb) of body weight usually produces surgical anesthesia within 30 seconds after injection, with the anesthetic effect usually lasting five to ten minutes. If a longer effect is desired, additional increments can be administered intravenously or intramuscularly to maintain anesthesia without producing significant cumulative effects.

Intramuscular doses, from experience primarily in children, in a range of 9 to 13 mg/kg (4 to 6 mg/lb) usually produce surgical anesthesia within 3 to 4 minutes following injection, with the anesthetic effect usually lasting 12 to 25 minutes.

Dosage:

As with other general anesthetic agents, the individual response to Ketalar is somewhat varied depending on the dose, route of administration, and age of patient, so that dosage recommendation cannot be absolutely fixed. The drug should be titrated against the patient's requirements.

Induction:

Intravenous Route: The initial dose of Ketalar administered intravenously may range from 1 mg/kg to 4.5 mg/kg (0.5 to 2 mg/lb). The average amount required to produce five to ten minutes of surgical anesthesia has been 2 mg/kg (1 mg/lb).

Alternatively, in adult patients an induction dose of 1.0 mg to 2.0 mg/kg intravenous ketamine at a rate of 0.5 mg/kg/min may be used for induction of anesthesia. In addition, diazepam in 2 mg to 5 mg doses, administered in a separate syringe over 60 seconds, may be used. In most cases, 15.0 mg of intravenous diazepam *or less* will suffice. The incidence of psychological manifestations during emergence, particularly dream-like observations and emergence delirium, may be reduced by this induction dosage program.

Note: The 100 mg/ml concentration of Ketalar *should not* be injected intravenously without proper dilution. It is recommended the drug be diluted with an equal volume of either Sterile Water for Injection, USP, Normal Saline, or 5% Dextrose in Water.

Rate of Administration: It is recommended that Ketalar be administered slowly (over a period of 60 seconds). More rapid administration may result in respiratory depression and enhanced pressor response.

Intramuscular Route: The initial dose of Ketalar administered intramuscularly may range from 6.5 to 13 mg/kg (3 to 6 mg/lb). A dose of 10 mg/kg (5 mg/lb) will usually produce 12 to 25 minutes of surgical anesthesia.

Maintenance of Anesthesia:

The maintenance dose should be adjusted according to the patient's anesthetic needs and whether an additional anesthetic agent is employed.

Increments of one-half to the full induction dose may be repeated as needed for maintenance of anesthesia. However, it should be noted that purposeless and tonic-clonic movements of extremities may occur during the course of anesthesia. These movements do not imply a light plane and are not indicative of the need for additional doses of the anesthetic.

It should be recognized that the larger the total dose of Ketalar administered, the longer will be the time to complete recovery.

Adult patients induced with Ketalar augmented with intravenous diazepam may be maintained on Ketalar given by slow microdrip infusion technique at a dose of 0.1 to 0.5 mg/minute, augmented with diazepam 2 to 5 mg administered intravenously as needed. In many cases 20 mg *or less* of intravenous diazepam total for combined induction and maintenance will suffice. However, slightly more diazepam may be required depending on the nature and duration of the operation, physical status of the patient, and other factors. The incidence of psychological manifestations during emergence, particularly dream-like observations and emergence delirium, may be reduced by this maintenance dosage program.

Dilution: To prepare a dilute solution containing 1 mg of ketamine per ml, aseptically transfer 10 ml (50 mg per ml Steri-Vial) or 5 ml (100 mg per ml Steri-Vial) to 500 ml of 5% Dextrose Injection, USP or Sodium Chloride (0.9%) Injection, USP (Normal Saline) and mix well. The resultant solution will contain 1 mg of ketamine per ml.

The fluid requirements of the patient and duration of anesthesia must be considered when selecting the appropriate dilution of Ketalar. If fluid restriction is required, Ketalar can be added to a 250 ml infusion as described above to provide a Ketalar concentration of 2 mg/ml.

Ketalar Steri-Vials, 10 mg/ml are not recommended for dilution.

Supplementary Agents:

Ketalar is clinically compatible with the commonly used general and local anesthetic agents when an adequate respiratory exchange is maintained.

The regimen of a reduced dose of Ketalar supplemented with diazepam can be used to produce balanced anesthesia by combination with other agents such as nitrous oxide and oxygen.

HOW SUPPLIED

Ketalar is supplied as the hydrochloride in concentrations equivalent to ketamine base.

N 0071-4581-15—Each 50-ml vial contains 10 mg/ml. Supplied in cartons of 10.

N 0071-4581-12—Each 20-ml vial contains 10 mg/ml. Supplied in cartons of 10.

N 0071-4582-10—Each 10-ml vial contains 50 mg/ml. Supplied in cartons of 10.

N 0071-4585-08—Each 5-ml vial contains 100 mg/ml. Supplied in cartons of 10.

Animal Pharmacology and Toxicology:

Toxicity: The acute toxicity of Ketalar has been studied in several species. In mature mice and rats, the intraperitoneal LD_{50} values are approximately 100 times the average human intravenous dose and approximately 20 times the average human intramuscular dose. A slightly higher acute toxicity observed in neonatal rats was not sufficiently elevated to suggest an increased hazard when used in children. Daily intravenous injections in rats of five times the average human intravenous dose and intramuscular injections in dogs at four times the average human intramuscular dose demonstrated excellent tolerance for as long as 6 weeks. Similarly, twice weekly anesthetic sessions of one, three, or six hours' duration in monkeys over a four-to six-week period were well tolerated.

Interaction With Other Drugs Commonly Used For Preanesthetic Medication: Large doses (three or more times the equivalent effective human dose) of morphine, meperidine, and atropine increased the depth and prolonged the duration of anesthesia produced by a standard anesthetizing dose of Ketalar in Rhesus monkeys. The prolonged duration was not of sufficient magnitude to contraindicate the use of these drugs for preanesthetic medication in human clinical trials.

Blood Pressure: Blood pressure responses to Ketalar vary with the laboratory species and experimental conditions. Blood pressure is increased in normotensive and renal hypertensive rats with and without adrenalectomy and under pentobarbital anesthesia.

Intravenous Ketalar produces a fall in arterial blood pressure in the Rhesus monkey and a rise in arterial blood pressure in the dog. In this respect the dog mimics the cardiovascular effect observed in man. The pressor response to Ketalar injected into intact, unanesthetized dogs is accompanied by a tachycardia, rise in cardiac output and a fall in total peripheral resistance. It causes a fall in perfusion pressure following a large dose injected into an artificially perfused vascular bed (dog hindquarters), and it has little or no potentiating effect upon vasoconstriction responses of epinephrine or norepinephrine. The pressor response to Ketalar is reduced or blocked by chlorpromazine (central depressant and peripheral α-adrenergic blockade), by β-adrenergic blockade, and by ganglionic blockade. The tachycardia and increase in myocardial contractile force seen in intact animals does not appear in isolated hearts (Langendorff) at a concentration of 0.1 mg of Ketalar nor in Starling dog heart-lung preparations at a Ketalar concentration of 50 mg/kg of HLP. These observations support the hypothesis that the hypertension produced by Ketalar is due to selective activation of central cardiac stimulating mechanisms leading to an increase in cardiac output. The dog myocardium is not sensitized to epinephrine and Ketalar appears to have a weak antiarrhythmic activity.

Metabolic Disposition: Ketalar is rapidly absorbed following parenteral administration. Animal experiments indicated that Ketalar was rapidly distributed into body tissues, with relatively high concentrations appearing in body fat, liver, lung, and brain; lower concentrations were found in the heart, skeletal muscle, and blood plasma. Placental transfer of the drug was found to occur in pregnant dogs and monkeys. No significant degree of binding to serum albumin was found with Ketalar.

Balance studies in rats, dogs, and monkeys resulted in the recovery of 85% to 95% of the dose in the urine, mainly in the form of degradation products. Small amounts of drug were also excreted in the bile and feces. Balance studies with tritium-labeled Ketalar in human subjects (1 mg/lb given intravenously) resulted in the mean recovery of 91% of the dose in the urine and 3% in the feces. Peak plasma levels averaged about 0.75 μg/ml, and CSF levels were about 0.2 μg/ml, 1 hour after dosing.

Ketalar undergoes N-demethylation and hydroxylation of the cyclohexanone ring, with the formation of water-soluble conjugates which are excreted in the urine. Further oxidation also occurs with the formation of a cyclohexanone derivative. The unconjugated N-demethylated metabolite was found to be less than one-sixth as potent as Ketalar. The unconjugated demethyl cyclohexanone derivative was found to be less than one-tenth as potent as Ketalar. Repeated doses of Ketalar administered to animals did not produce any detectable increase in microsomal enzyme activity.

Reproduction: Male and female rats, when given five times the average human intravenous dose of Ketalar for three consecutive days about one week before mating, had a reproductive performance equivalent to that of saline-injected controls. When given to pregnant rats and rabbits intramuscularly at twice the average human intramuscular dose during the respective periods of organogenesis, the litter characteristics were equivalent to those of saline-injected controls. A small group of rabbits was given a single large dose (six times the average human dose) of Ketalar on Day 6 of pregnancy to simulate the effect of an excessive clinical dose around the period of nidation. The outcome of pregnancy was equivalent in control and treated groups.

To determine the effect of Ketalar on the perinatal and postnatal period, pregnant rats were given twice the average human intramuscular dose during Days 18 to 21 of pregnancy. Litter characteristics at birth and through the weaning period were equivalent to those of the control animals. There was a slight increase in incidence of delayed parturition by one day in treated dams of this group. Three groups each of mated beagle bitches were given 2.5 times the average human intramuscular dose twice weekly for the three weeks of the first, second, and third trimesters of pregnancy, respectively, without the development of adverse effects in the pups.

4581G032

LOESTRIN® 21 ℞
(Norethindrone Acetate and Ethinyl Estradiol Tablets, USP)

LOESTRIN® 21 1/20 ℞
(Each white tablet contains 1 mg norethindrone acetate and 20 mcg ethinyl estradiol.)

LOESTRIN® 21 1.5/30 ℞
(Each green tablet contains 1.5 mg norethindrone acetate and 30 mcg ethinyl estradiol.)

LOESTRIN® Fe ℞
(Norethindrone Acetate and Ethinyl Estradiol Tablets, USP and Ferrous Fumarate Tablets, USP)

LOESTRIN® Fe 1/20 ℞
(Each white tablet contains 1 mg norethindrone acetate and 20 mcg ethinyl estradiol. Each brown tablet contains 75 mg ferrous fumarate, USP)

LOESTRIN® Fe 1.5/30 ℞
(Each green tablet contains 1.5 mg norethindrone acetate and 30 mcg ethinyl estradiol. Each brown tablet contains 75 mg ferrous fumarate)

Each white tablet contains norethindrone acetate (17 alpha-ethinyl-19-nortestosterone acetate), 1 mg; ethinyl estradiol (17 alpha-ethinyl-1,3,5(10)-estratriene-3,17 beta-diol), 20 mcg. Also contains acacia, NF; lactose, NF; magnesium stearate, NF; starch, NF; confectioner's sugar, NF; talc, USP.

Each green tablet contains norethindrone acetate (17 alpha-ethinyl-19-nortestosterone acetate), 1.5 mg; ethinyl estradiol (17 alpha-ethinyl-1,3,5(10)-estratriene-3, 17 beta-diol), 30 mcg. Also contains acacia, NF; lactose, NF; magnesium stearate, NF; starch, NF; confectioner's sugar, NF; talc, USP; D&C yellow No. 10; FD&C yellow No. 6; FD&C blue No. 1.

Each brown tablet contains microcrystalline cellulose, NF; ferrous fumarate, USP; magnesium stearate, NF; povidone, USP; sodium starch glycolate, NF; sucrose with modified dextrins.

DESCRIPTION

Loestrin **21** and Loestrin **Fe** are progestogen-estrogen combinations.

Loestrin **Fe** 1/20 and 1.5/30: Each provides a continuous dosage regimen consisting of 21 oral contraceptive tablets and seven ferrous fumarate tablets. The ferrous fumarate tablets are present to facilitate ease of drug administration via a 28-day regimen and are not intended to serve any therapeutic purpose.

CLINICAL PHARMACOLOGY

Combination oral contraceptives act by suppression of gonadotropins. Although the primary mechanism of this action is inhibition of ovulation, other alterations include changes in the cervical mucus (which increase the difficulty of sperm entry into the uterus) and the endometrium (which reduce the likelihood of implantation).

INDICATIONS AND USAGE

Loestrin **21** and Loestrin **Fe** are indicated for the prevention of pregnancy in women who elect to use oral contraceptives as a method of contraception.

Oral contraceptives are highly effective. Table I lists the typical accidental pregnancy rates for users of combination oral contraceptives and other methods of contraception. The efficacy of these contraceptive methods, except sterilization, depends upon the reliability with which they are used. Correct and consistent use of methods can result in lower failure rates. [See Table I below.]

CONTRAINDICATIONS

Oral contraceptives should not be used in women who currently have the following conditions:

- Thrombophlebitis or thromboembolic disorders
- A past history of deep vein thrombophlebitis or thromboembolic disorders
- Cerebral vascular or coronary artery disease
- Known or suspected carcinoma of the breast
- Carcinoma of the endometrium or other known or suspected estrogen-dependent neoplasia
- Undiagnosed abnormal genital bleeding
- Cholestatic jaundice of pregnancy or jaundice with prior pill use
- Hepatic adenomas or carcinomas
- Known or suspected pregnancy

WARNINGS

> Cigarette smoking increases the risk of serious cardiovascular side effects from oral contraceptive use. This risk increases with age and with heavy smoking (15 or more cigarettes per day) and is quite marked in women over 35 years of age. Women who use oral contraceptives should be strongly advised not to smoke.

The use of oral contraceptives is associated with increased risks of several serious conditions including myocardial infarction, thromboembolism, stroke, hepatic neoplasia, and gallbladder disease, although the risk of serious morbidity or mortality is very small in healthy women without underlying risk factors. The risk of morbidity and mortality increases significantly in the presence of other underlying risk factors such as hypertension, hyperlipidemias, obesity and diabetes.

Practitioners prescribing oral contraceptives should be familiar with the following information relating to these risks. The information contained in this package insert is principally based on studies carried out in patients who used oral contraceptives with higher formulations of estrogens and progestogens than those in common use today. The effect of long-term use of the oral contraceptives with lower formulations of both estrogens and progestogens remains to be determined.

Throughout this labeling, epidemiological studies reported are of two types: retrospective or case control studies and prospective or cohort studies. Case control studies provide a measure of the relative risk of a disease, namely, a *ratio* of the incidence of a disease among oral contraceptive users to that among nonusers. The relative risk does not provide information on the actual clinical occurrence of a disease. Cohort studies provide a measure of attributable risk, which is the *difference* in the incidence of disease between oral contraceptive users and nonusers. The attributable risk does provide information about the actual occurrence of a disease in the population (adapted from refs. 2 and 3 with the author's permission). For further information, the reader is referred to a text on epidemiological methods.

1. Thromboembolic Disorders And Other Vascular Problems.

a. Myocardial infarction

An increased risk of myocardial infarction has been attributed to oral contraceptive use. This risk is primarily in smokers or women with other underlying risk factors for coronary artery disease such as hypertension, hypercholesterolemia, morbid obesity, and diabetes. The relative risk of heart attack for current oral contraceptive users has been estimated to be two to six (4–10). The risk is very low under the age of 30.

Smoking in combination with oral contraceptive use has been shown to contribute substantially to the incidence of myocardial infarctions in women in their mid-thirties or older with smoking accounting for the majority of excess cases (11). Mortality rates associated with circulatory disease have been shown to increase substantially in smokers over the age of 35 and nonsmokers over the age of 40 (Table II) among women who use oral contraceptives.

[See table above.]

Oral contraceptives may compound the effects of well-known risk factors, such as hypertension, diabetes, hyperlipidemias, age and obesity (13). In particular, some progestogens are known to decrease HDL cholesterol and cause glucose intolerance, while estrogens may create a state of hyperinsulinism (14–18). Oral contraceptives have been shown to increase blood pressure among users (see section 9 in WARNINGS). Similar effects on risk factors have been associated with an increased risk of heart disease. Oral contraceptives must be used with caution in women with cardiovascular disease risk factors.

b. Thromboembolism

An increased risk of thromboembolic and thrombotic disease associated with the use of oral contraceptives is well established. Case control studies have found the relative risk of users compared to non-users to be 3 for the first episode of superficial venous thrombosis, 4 to 11 for deep vein thrombosis or pulmonary embolism, and 1.5 to 6 for women with predisposing conditions for venous thromboembolic disease (2,3,19–24). Cohort studies have shown the relative risk to be somewhat lower, about 3 for new cases and about 4.5 for new cases requiring hospitalization (25). The risk of thromboembolic disease due to oral contraceptives is not related to length of use and disappears after pill use is stopped (2).

A two- to four-fold increase in relative risk of postoperative thromboembolic complications has been reported with the use of oral contraceptives (9,26). The relative risk of venous thrombosis in women who have predisposing conditions is twice that of women without such medical conditions (9,26). If feasible, oral contraceptives should be discontinued at least four weeks prior to and for two weeks after elective surgery of a type associated with an increase in risk of thromboembolism and during and following prolonged immobilization. Since the immediate post partum period is also associated with an increased risk of thromboembolism, oral contraceptives should be started no earlier than four to six weeks after delivery in women who elect not to breast feed.

c. Cerebrovascular diseases

Oral contraceptives have been shown to increase both the relative and attributable risks of cerebrovascular events (thrombotic and hemorrhagic strokes), although, in general, the risk is greatest among older (> 35 years), hypertensive women who also smoke. Hypertension was found to be a risk factor for both users and non-users, for both types of strokes, while smoking interacted to increase the risk for hemorrhagic strokes (27–29).

In a large study, the relative risk of thrombotic strokes has been shown to range from 3 for normotensive users to 14 for users with severe hypertension (30). The relative risk of hemorrhagic stroke is reported to be 1.2 for non-smokers who used oral contraceptives, 2.6 for smokers who did not use oral contraceptives, 7.6 for smokers who used oral contraceptives, 1.8 for normotensive users and 25.7 for users with severe hypertension (30). The attributable risk is also greater in older women (3).

d. Dose-related risk of vascular disease from oral contraceptives

A positive association has been observed between the amount of estrogen and progestogen in oral contraceptives and the risk of vascular disease. (31–33). A decline in serum high density lipoproteins (HDL) has been reported with

Continued on next page

This product information was prepared in August 1992. On these and other Parke-Davis Products, information may be obtained by addressing PARKE-DAVIS, Division of Warner-Lambert Company, Morris Plains, New Jersey 07950.

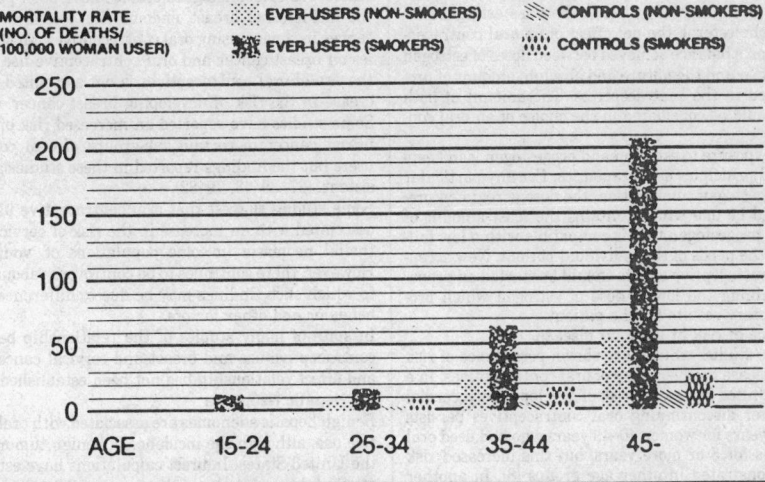

TABLE II
CIRCULATORY DISEASE MORTALITY RATES PER 100,000 WOMAN YEARS BY AGE, SMOKING STATUS AND ORAL CONTRACEPTIVE USE

Adapted from P.M. Layde and V. Beral, ref #12.

TABLE I
LOWEST EXPECTED AND TYPICAL FAILURE RATES DURING THE FIRST YEAR OF CONTINUOUS USE OF A METHOD
% of Women Experiencing an Accidental Pregnancy in the First Year of Continuous Use

Method	Lowest Expected*	Typical**
(No contraception)	(89)	(89)
Oral contraceptives		3
combined	0.1	N/A***
progestin only	0.5	N/A***
Diaphragm with spermicidal cream or jelly	3	18
Spermicides alone (foam, creams, jellies and vaginal suppositories)	3	21
Vaginal sponge		
nulliparous	5	18
multiparous	>8	>28
IUD (medicated)	1	6†
Condom without spermicides	2	12
Periodic abstinence (all methods)	2–10	20
Female sterilization	0.2	0.4
Male sterilization	0.1	0.15

Adapted from J. Trussell and K. Kost, Table 11, ref. #1.

* The authors' best guess of the percentage of women expected to experience an accidental pregnancy among couples who initiate a method (not necessarily for the first time) and who use it consistently and correctly during the first year if they do not stop for any other reason.
** This term represents "typical" couples who initiate use of a method (not necessarily for the first time), who experience an accidental pregnancy during the first year if they do not stop use for any other reason.
*** N/A—Data not available
† Combined typical rate for both medicated and non-medicated IUD. The rate for medicated IUD alone is not available.

Parke-Davis—Cont.

many progestational agents (14–16). A decline in serum high density lipoproteins has been associated with an increased incidence of ischemic heart disease. Because estrogens increase HDL cholesterol, the net effect of an oral contraceptive depends on a balance achieved between doses of estrogen and progestogen and the nature and absolute amount of progestogens used in the contraceptives. The amount of both hormones should be considered in the choice of an oral contraceptive.

Minimizing exposure to estrogen and progestogen is in keeping with good principles of therapeutics. For any particular estrogen/progestogen combination, the dosage regimen prescribed should be one which contains the least amount of estrogen and progestogen that is compatible with a low failure rate and the needs of the individual patient. New acceptors of oral contraceptive agents should be started on preparations containing the lowest dose of estrogen which produces satisfactory results for the patient.

e. Persistence of risk of vascular disease

There are two studies which have shown persistence of risk of vascular disease for ever users of oral contraceptives. In a study in the United States, the risk of developing myocardial infarction after discontinuing oral contraceptives persists for at least 9 years for women 40–49 years who had used oral contraceptives for 5 or more years, but this increased risk was not demonstrated in other age groups (8). In another study in Great Britain, the risk of developing cerebrovascular disease persisted for at least 6 years after discontinuation of oral contraceptives, although excess risk was very small (34). However, both studies were performed with oral contraceptive formulations containing 50 micrograms or higher of estrogens.

2. Estimates Of Mortality From Contraceptive Use

One study gathered data from a variety of sources which have estimated the mortality rate associated with different methods of contraception at different ages (Table III). These estimates include the combined risk of death associated with contraceptive methods plus the risk attributable to pregnancy in the event of method failure. Each method of contraception has its specific benefits and risks. The study concluded that with the exception of oral contraceptive users 35 and older who smoke and 40 and older who do not smoke, mortality associated with all methods of birth control is low and below that associated with childbirth. The observation of a possible increase in risk of mortality with age for oral contraceptive users is based on data gathered in the 1970's—but not reported until 1983 (35). However, current clinical practice involves the use of lower estrogen dose formulations combined with careful restriction of oral contraceptive use to women who do not have the various risk factors listed in this labeling.

Because of these changes in practice and, also, because of some limited new data which suggest that the risk of cardiovascular disease with the use of oral contraceptives may now be less than previously observed (Porter JB, Hunter J, Jick H, et al. Oral contraceptives and nonfatal vascular disease. Obstet Gynecol 1985;66:1–4 and Porter JB, Hershel J, Walker AM. Mortality among oral contraceptive users. Obstet Gynecol 1987; 70:29–32), the Fertility and Maternal Health Drugs Advisory Committee was asked to review the topic in 1989. The Committee concluded that although cardiovascular disease risks may be increased with oral contraceptive use after age 40 in healthy non-smoking women (even with the newer low-dose formulations), there are greater potential health risks associated with pregnancy in older women and with the alternative surgical and medical procedures which may be necessary if such women do not have access to effective and acceptable means of contraception.

Therefore, the Committee recommended that the benefits of oral contraceptive use by healthy non-smoking women over 40 may outweigh the possible risks. Of course, older women, as all women who take oral contraceptives, should take the lowest possible dose formulation that is effective. (See Table I.)

[See also Table III below.]

3. Carcinoma Of The Reproductive Organs

Numerous epidemiological studies have been performed on the incidence of breast, endometrial, ovarian and cervical cancer in women using oral contraceptives. Most of the studies on breast cancer and oral contraceptive use report that the use of oral contraceptives is not associated with an increase in the risk of developing breast cancer. (36, 38, 83). Some studies have reported an increased risk of developing breast cancer in certain sub-groups of oral contraceptive users but the findings reported in these studies are not consistent. (37, 39–43, 79–82).

Some studies suggest that oral contraceptive use has been associated with an increase in the risk of cervical intraepithelial neoplasia in some populations of women (45–48). However, there continues to be controversy about the extent to which such findings may be due to differences in sexual behavior and other factors.

In spite of many studies of the relationship between oral contraceptive use and breast and cervical cancers, a cause and effect relationship has not been established.

4. Hepatic Neoplasia

Benign hepatic adenomas are associated with oral contraceptive use, although the incidence of benign tumors is rare in the United States. Indirect calculations have estimated the attributable risk to be in the range of 3.3 cases/100,000 for users, a risk that increases after four or more years of use (49). Rupture of rare, benign, hepatic adenomas may cause death through intra-abdominal hemorrhage (50,51).

Studies from Britain have shown an increased risk of developing hepatocellular carcinoma (52–54) in long-term (>8 years) oral contraceptive users. However, these cancers are extremely rare in the U.S., and the attributable risk (the excess incidence) of liver cancers in oral contraceptive users approaches less than one per million users.

5. Ocular Lesions

There have been clinical case reports of retinal thrombosis associated with the use of oral contraceptives. Oral contraceptives should be discontinued if there is unexplained partial or complete loss of vision; onset of proptosis or diplopia; papilledema; or retinal vascular lesions. Appropriate diagnostic and therapeutic measures should be undertaken immediately.

6. Oral Contraceptive Use Before Or During Early Pregnancy: Risk Of Birth Defects

Extensive epidemiological studies have revealed no increased risk of birth defects in women who have used oral contraceptives prior to pregnancy (55–57). Studies also do not suggest a teratogenic effect, particularly insofar as cardiac anomalies and limb reduction defects are concerned (55,56,58,59), when taken inadvertently during early pregnancy.

The administration of oral contraceptives to induce withdrawal bleeding should not be used as a test for pregnancy. Oral contraceptives should not be used during pregnancy to treat threatened or habitual abortion.

It is recommended that for any patient who has missed two consecutive periods, pregnancy should be ruled out before continuing oral contraceptive use. If the patient has not adhered to the prescribed schedule, the possibility of pregnancy should be considered at the time of the first missed period. Oral contraceptive use should be discontinued if pregnancy is confirmed.

7. Gallbladder Disease

Earlier studies have reported an increased lifetime relative risk of gallbladder surgery in users of oral contraceptives and estrogens (60,61). More recent studies, however, have shown that the relative risk of developing gallbladder disease among oral contraceptive users may be minimal (62–64). The recent findings of minimal risk may be related to the use of oral contraceptive formulations containing lower hormonal doses of estrogens and progestogens.

TABLE III
ANNUAL NUMBER OF BIRTH-RELATED OR METHOD-RELATED DEATHS ASSOCIATED WITH CONTROL OF FERTILITY PER 100,000 NONSTERILE WOMEN, BY FERTILITY CONTROL METHOD ACCORDING TO AGE

Method of control and outcome	15–19	20–24	25–29	30–34	35–39	40–44
No fertility control methods*	7.0	7.4	9.1	14.8	25.7	28.2
Oral contraceptives non-smoker**	0.3	0.5	0.9	1.9	13.8	31.6
Oral contraceptives smoker**	2.2	3.4	6.6	13.5	51.1	117.2
IUD**	0.8	0.8	1.0	1.0	1.4	1.4
Condom*	1.1	1.6	0.7	0.2	0.3	0.4
Diaphragm/spermicide*	1.9	1.2	1.2	1.3	2.2	2.8
Periodic abstinence*	2.5	1.6	1.6	1.7	2.9	3.6

* Deaths are birth related
** Deaths are method related

Adapted from HW Ory, ref. #35.

8. Carbohydrate And Lipid Metabolic Effects

Oral contraceptives have been shown to cause glucose intolerance in a significant percentage of users (17). Oral contraceptives containing greater than 75 micrograms of estrogens cause hyperinsulinism, while lower doses of estrogen cause less glucose intolerance (65). Progestogens increase insulin secretion and create insulin resistance, this effect varying with different progestational agents (17, 66). However, in the non-diabetic woman, oral contraceptives appear to have no effect on fasting blood glucose (67). Because of these demonstrated effects, prediabetic and diabetic women should be carefully observed while taking oral contraceptives.

A small proportion of women will have persistent hypertriglyceridemia while on the pill. As discussed earlier (see WARNINGS 1a. and 1d.), changes in serum triglycerides and lipoprotein levels have been reported in oral contraceptive users.

9. Elevated Blood Pressure

An increase in blood pressure has been reported in women taking oral contraceptives (68) and this increase is more likely in older oral contraceptive users (69) and with continued use (68). Data from the Royal College of General Practitioners (12) and subsequent randomized trials have shown that the incidence of hypertension increases with increasing concentrations of progestogens.

Women with a history of hypertension or hypertension-related diseases, or renal disease (70) should be encouraged to use another method of contraception. If women elect to use oral contraceptives, they should be monitored closely and if significant elevation of blood pressure occurs, oral contraceptives should be discontinued. For most women, elevated blood pressure will return to normal after stopping oral contraceptives (69), and there is no difference in the occurrence of hypertension among ever and never users (68,70,71).

10. Headache.

The onset or exacerbation of migraine or development of headache of a new pattern which is recurrent, persistent or severe requires discontinuation of oral contraceptives and evaluation of the cause.

11. Bleeding Irregularities

Breakthrough bleeding and spotting are sometimes encountered in patients on oral contraceptives, especially during the first three months of use. Non-hormonal causes should be considered and adequate diagnostic measures taken to rule out malignancy or pregnancy in the event of breakthrough bleeding, as in the case of any abnormal vaginal bleeding. If pathology has been excluded, time or a change to another formulation may solve the problem. In the event of amenorrhea, pregnancy should be ruled out.

Some women may encounter post-pill amenorrhea or oligomenorrhea, especially when such a condition was preexistent.

PRECAUTIONS

1. Physical Examination And Follow-Up

A complete medical history and physical examination should be taken prior to the initiation or reinstitution of oral contraceptives and at least annually during use of oral contraceptives. These physical examinations should include special reference to blood pressure, breasts, abdomen and pelvic organs, including cervical cytology, and relevant laboratory tests. In case of undiagnosed, persistent or recurrent abnormal vaginal bleeding, appropriate diagnostic measures should be conducted to rule out malignancy. Women with a strong family history of breast cancer or who have breast nodules should be monitored with particular care.

2. Lipid Disorders

Women who are being treated for hyperlipidemias should be followed closely if they elect to use oral contraceptives. Some progestogens may elevate LDL levels and may render the control of hyperlipidemias more difficult.

3. Liver Function

If jaundice develops in any woman receiving such drugs, the medication should be discontinued. Steroid hormones may be poorly metabolized in patients with impaired liver function.

4. Fluid Retention

Oral contraceptives may cause some degree of fluid retention. They should be prescribed with caution, and only with careful monitoring, in patients with conditions which might be aggravated by fluid retention.

5. Emotional Disorders

Women with a history of depression should be carefully observed and the drug discontinued if depression recurs to a serious degree.

6. Contact Lenses

Contact lens wearers who develop visual changes or changes in lens tolerance should be assessed by an ophthalmologist.

7. Drug Interactions

Reduced efficacy and increased incidence of breakthrough bleeding and menstrual irregularities have been associated with concomitant use of rifampin. A similar association though less marked, has been suggested with barbiturates, phenylbutazone, phenytoin sodium, and possibly with griseofulvin, ampicillin and tetracyclines (72).

8. Interactions With Laboratory Tests

Certain endocrine and liver function tests and blood components may be affected by oral contraceptives:

a. Increased prothrombin and factors VII, VIII, IX, and X; decreased antithrombin 3; increased norepinephrine-induced platelet aggregability.

b. Increased thyroid binding globulin (TBG) leading to increased circulating total thyroid hormone, as measured by protein-bound iodine (PBI), T4 by column, or by radioimmunoassay. Free T3 resin uptake is decreased, reflecting the elevated TBG; free T4 concentration is unaltered.

c. Other binding proteins may be elevated in serum.

d. Sex-binding globulins are increased and result in elevated levels of total circulating sex steroids and corticoids; however, free or biologically active levels remain unchanged.

e. Triglycerides may be increased.

f. Glucose tolerance may be decreased.

g. Serum folate levels may be depressed by oral contraceptive therapy. This may be of clinical significance if a woman becomes pregnant shortly after discontinuing oral contraceptives.

9. Carcinogenesis

See **WARNINGS** section.

10. Pregnancy

Pregnancy Category X. See **CONTRAINDICATIONS** and **WARNINGS** sections.

11. Nursing Mothers

Small amounts of oral contraceptive steroids have been identified in the milk of nursing mothers and a few adverse effects on the child have been reported, including jaundice and breast enlargement. In addition, oral contraceptives given in the postpartum period may interfere with lactation by decreasing the quantity and quality of breast milk. If possible, the nursing mother should be advised not to use oral contraceptives but to use other forms of contraception until she has completely weaned her child.

INFORMATION FOR THE PATIENT

See patient labeling printed below.

ADVERSE REACTIONS

An increased risk of the following serious adverse reactions has been associated with the use of oral contraceptives (see WARNINGS section).

- Thrombophlebitis
- Arterial thromboembolism
- Pulmonary embolism
- Myocardial infarction
- Cerebral hemorrhage
- Cerebral thrombosis
- Hypertension
- Gallbladder disease
- Hepatic adenomas or benign liver tumors

There is evidence of an association between the following conditions and the use of oral contraceptives, although additional confirmatory studies are needed:

- Mesenteric thrombosis
- Retinal thrombosis

The following adverse reactions have been reported in patients receiving oral contraceptives and are believed to be drug related:

- Nausea
- Vomiting
- Gastrointestinal symptoms (such as abdominal cramps and bloating)
- Breakthrough bleeding
- Spotting
- Change in menstrual flow
- Amenorrhea
- Temporary infertility after discontinuation of treatment
- Edema
- Melasma which may persist
- Breast changes: tenderness, enlargement, secretion
- Change in weight (increase or decrease)
- Change in cervical erosion and secretion
- Diminution in lactation when given immediately postpartum
- Cholestatic jaundice
- Migraine
- Rash (allergic)
- Mental depression
- Reduced tolerance to carbohydrates
- Vaginal candidiasis
- Change in corneal curvature (steepening)
- Intolerance to contact lenses

The following adverse reactions have been reported in users of oral contraceptives and the association has been neither confirmed nor refuted:

- Pre-menstrual syndrome
- Cataracts
- Changes in appetite
- Cystitis-like syndrome
- Headache
- Nervousness
- Dizziness
- Hirsutism

- Loss of scalp hair
- Erythema multiforme
- Erythema nodosum
- Hemorrhagic eruption
- Vaginitis
- Porphyria
- Impaired renal function
- Hemolytic uremic syndrome
- Budd-Chiari syndrome
- Acne
- Changes in libido
- Colitis

While the following adverse reactions or conditions have been reported to be associated with the use of oral contraceptives, no causal relationship has been established:

- Congenital anomalies
- Raynaud's disease
- Sickle cell disease
- Mitral valve prolapse
- Increased risk of developing venous thromboembolic disease among women with blood types A, B, or AB, as opposed to women with blood type O.

OVERDOSAGE

Serious ill effects have not been reported following acute ingestion of large doses of oral contraceptives by young children. Overdosage may cause nausea, and withdrawal bleeding may occur in females.

NON-CONTRACEPTIVE HEALTH BENEFITS

The following non-contraceptive health benefits related to the use of oral contraceptives are supported by epidemiological studies which largely utilized oral contraceptive formulations containing estrogen doses exceeding 0.05 mg of estrogen (73–78).

Effects on menses:

- Increased menstrual cycle regularity
- Decreased blood loss and decreased incidence of iron deficiency anemia
- Decreased incidence of dysmenorrhea

Effects related to inhibition of ovulation:

- Decreased incidence of functional ovarian cysts
- Decreased incidence of ectopic pregnancies

Effects from long-term use:

- Decreased incidence of fibroadenomas and fibrocystic disease of the breast
- Decreased incidence of acute pelvic inflammatory disease
- Decreased incidence of endometrial cancer
- Decreased incidence of ovarian cancer

DOSAGE AND ADMINISTRATION

The tablet dispenser has been designed to make oral contraceptive dosing as easy and as convenient as possible. The tablets are arranged in either three or four rows of seven tablets each, with the days of the week appearing on the tablet dispenser above the first row of tablets.

Important Notes: The patient should be instructed to use an additional method of protection until after the first week of administration in the initial cycle if utilizing the Sunday-Start Regimen.

The possibility of ovulation and conception prior to initiation of use should be considered.

Dosage And Administration For 21-Day Dosage Regimen

To achieve maximum contraceptive effectiveness, Loestrin 21 must be taken exactly as directed and at intervals not exceeding 24 hours. Loestrin 21 provides the patient with a convenient tablet schedule of "3 weeks on—1 week off." Two dosage regimens are described, one of which may be more convenient or suitable than the other for an individual patient. For the initial cycle of therapy, the patient begins her tablets according to the Day-5 or Sunday-Start Regimen. With either regimen, the patient takes one tablet daily for 21 consecutive days followed by one week of no tablets.

A. Sunday-Start Regimen: The patient begins taking tablets from the top row on the first Sunday after menstrual flow begins. When menstrual flow begins on Sunday, the first tablet is taken on the same day. The last tablet in the dispenser will then be taken on a Saturday, followed by no tablets for a week (7 days). For all subsequent cycles the patient then begins a new 21-tablet regimen on the eighth day, Sunday, after taking her last tablet. Following this regimen, of 21 days on—7 days off, the patient will start all subsequent cycles on a Sunday.

B. Day-5 Regimen: The first day of menstrual flow is Day 1. On Day 5 of her menstrual flow, the patient starts taking 1 tablet daily, beginning with the tablet in the top row that corresponds to Day 5 of her flow. After the last tablet (Saturday) has been taken, if any tablets remain in the top row, the patient completes her 21-tablet regimen starting with the Sunday tablet in the top row, followed by no tablets for a week (7 days). For all subsequent cycles, the patient begins a new 21 tablet regimen on the eighth day after taking her last tablet, again beginning on the same day of the week on which she began her first course. Following this regimen of 21 days on—7 days off, the patient will start all subsequent cycles on the same day of the week as the first course. Likewise, the

interval of no tablets will always start on the same day of the week.

Whether utilizing the Sunday-Start or Day-5 Regimen, all tablets should be taken regularly with a meal or at bedtime. It should be stressed that efficacy of medication depends on strict adherence to the dosage schedule.

Special Notes on Administration

Menstruation usually begins two or three days, but may begin as late as the fourth or fifth day, after discontinuing medication. Because of the relatively low estrogenic content, Loestrin **21** is not a good cyclic regulator. There are patients whose inherent hormone balance will require larger amounts of estrogen to achieve cyclic regularity than that contained in Loestrin **21**. These patients experience altered bleeding patterns, which do not conform to treatment schedules, while taking Loestrin **21** tablets. However, it is important that patients adhere to the dosage schedule regardless of when bleeding occurs.

The occurrence of altered bleeding is highest in Cycle 1. The majority of patients will have seven days or less of total bleeding during the 28-day cycle (including both withdrawal bleeding and breakthrough bleeding and spotting). Should irregular bleeding occur, patients should be reassured and instructed to continue taking the tablets as directed. If by the third cycle the irregular patterns are unacceptable, consideration should be given to changing the medication to a product with a higher estrogen content (Norlestrin* **21** 1/50 or Norlestrin **21** 2.5/50). The physician should be alert to the fact that the irregular bleeding patterns could mask an organic cause, and appropriate diagnostic measures should be taken if the bleeding persists or continues after changing to a higher estrogen-content product.

If a patient forgets to take one or more tablets, the following is suggested: If one tablet is missed, take it as soon as remembered, or take two tablets the next day. If two consecutive tablets are missed, take two tablets daily for the next two days, then resume the regular schedule. While there is little likelihood of pregnancy occurring if the patient misses only one or two tablets, the possibility of pregnancy increases with each successive day that tablets are missed. *However if the patient is taking* Loestrin 21 1/20, *in addition to taking two* white *tablets a day for two days, the patient should use an additional means of contraception for seven consecutive days.* If three consecutive tablets are missed, the patient starts a new course of tablets in the following manner: If the patient is on the Sunday-Start Regimen, a new course of tablets is started on the first Sunday following the last missed tablet, whether or not she is still menstruating. If the patient is on the Day 5-Regimen, a new course of tablets is started on the eighth day after the last tablet was taken. For example, if the patient took her last tablet on Monday, she should start her new course of tablets the following Monday. The patient should also use an additional method of birth control during the seven days without tablets, and until she has taken a tablet daily for seven consecutive days.

The possibility of ovulation occurring increases with each successive day that scheduled tablets are missed. While there is little likelihood of ovulation occurring if only one tablet is missed, the possibility of spotting or bleeding is increased. This is particularly likely to occur if two or more consecutive tablets are missed.

Dosage And Administration For 28-Day Dosage Regimen

To achieve maximum contraceptive effectiveness, Loestrin Fe must be taken exactly as directed and at intervals not exceeding 24 hours.

Loestrin Fe provides a continuous administration regimen consisting of 21 *light-colored* (white or green) tablets of Loestrin and 7 *brown* tablets of ferrous fumarate. The ferrous fumarate tablets are present to facilitate ease of drug administration via a 28-day regimen and do not serve any therapeutic purpose. There is no need for the patient to count days between cycles because there are no "off-tablet days."

The patient begins taking *light-colored* tablets from the top row on the first Sunday after menstrual flow begins. When menstrual flow begins on Sunday, the first *light-colored* tablet is taken on the same day. The patient takes one *light-colored* tablet daily for 21 days. The last *light-colored* tablet taken is the Saturday tablet. Upon completion of all 21 tablets, and without interruption, the patient takes one *brown* tablet daily for 7 days. Upon completion of this first course of tablets, the patient begins a second course of 28 tablets without interruption, the next day, Sunday, starting with the Sunday *light-colored* tablet in the top row. Adhering to this

*Norlestrin (Norethindrone Acetate and Ethinyl Estradiol Tablets, USP)

Continued on next page

This product information was prepared in August 1992. On these and other Parke-Davis Products, information may be obtained by addressing PARKE-DAVIS, Division of Warner-Lambert Company, Morris Plains, New Jersey 07950.

Parke-Davis—Cont.

regimen, of one *light-colored* tablet daily for 21 days, followed without interruption by one *brown* tablet daily for seven days, the patient will start all subsequent cycles on a Sunday.

Tablets should be taken regularly with a meal or at bedtime. It should be stressed that efficacy of medication depends on strict adherence to the dosage schedule.

Special Notes on Administration

Menstruation usually begins two or three days, but may begin as late as the fourth or fifth day, after the *brown* tablets have been started. Because of the relatively low estrogenic content, Loestrin **Fe** is not a good cyclic regulator. There are patients whose inherent hormone balance will require larger amounts of estrogen to achieve cyclic regularity than that contained in Loestrin **Fe**. These patients experience altered bleeding patterns, which do not conform to treatment schedules, while taking the *light-colored* Loestrin **Fe** tablets. However, it is important that patients adhere to the dosage schedule regardless of when bleeding occurs.

The occurrence of altered bleeding is highest in Cycle 1. The majority of patients will have seven days or less of total bleeding during the 28-day cycle (including both withdrawal bleeding and breakthrough bleeding and spotting). Should irregular bleeding occur, patients should be reassured and instructed to continue taking the tablets as directed. If by the third cycle the irregular patterns are unacceptable, consideration should be given to changing the medication to a product with a higher estrogen content (Norlestrin* **Fe** 1/50 or Norlestrin **Fe** 2.5/50). The physician should be alert to the fact that the irregular bleeding patterns could mask bleeding from organic causes, and appropriate diagnostic measures should be taken if the bleeding persists or continues after changing to a higher estrogen-content product.

If a patient forgets to take one or more *light-colored* tablets, the following is suggested. If one *light-colored* tablet is missed, take it as soon as remembered, or take two *light-colored* tablets the next day. If two consecutive *light-colored* tablets are missed, take two *light-colored* tablets daily for the next two days, then resume the regular schedule. While there is little likelihood of pregnancy occurring if the patient misses only one or two *light-colored* tablets, the possibility of pregnancy increases with each successive day that *light-colored* tablets are missed. *However, if the patient is taking* **Loestrin Fe 1/20**, *in addition to taking two white tablets a day for two days, the patient should use an additional means of contraception for seven consecutive days.* If three consecutive *light-colored* tablets are missed, the patient starts a new course of tablets the first Sunday following the last missed tablet, whether or not she is still menstruating. The patient should also use an additional method of birth control during the days without tablets, and until she has taken a tablet for seven consecutive days.

The possibility of ovulation occurring increases with each successive day that scheduled *light-colored* tablets are missed. While there is little likelihood of ovulation occurring if only one *light-colored* tablet is missed, the possibility of spotting or bleeding is increased. This is particularly likely to occur if two or more consecutive *light-colored* tablets are missed.

If one or more *brown* tablets are missed, the *light-colored* tablets should be started no later than the eighth day after the last *light-colored* tablet was taken. The possibility of conception occurring is not increased if *brown* tablets are missed.

Use Of Oral Contraceptives In The Event Of A Missed Menstrual Period

1. If the patient has not adhered to the prescribed dosage regimen, the possibility of pregnancy should be considered after the first missed period and oral contraceptives should be withheld until pregnancy has been ruled out.
2. If the patient has adhered to the prescribed regimen and misses two consecutive periods, pregnancy should be ruled out before continuing the contraceptive regimen.

After several months on treatment, bleeding may be reduced to a point of virtual absence. This reduced flow may occur as a result of medication, in which event it is not indicative of pregnancy.

HOW SUPPLIED

Loestrin **21** 1/20 is available in dispensers each containing 21 tablets. Each tablet contains 1 mg of norethindrone acetate and 20 mcg of ethinyl estradiol. Available in packages of five dispensers.

Loestrin **Fe** 1/20 is available in dispensers each containing 21 white tablets and 7 brown tablets. Each white tablet contains 1 mg of norethindrone acetate and 20 mcg of ethinyl estradiol. Each brown tablet contains 75 mg ferrous fumarate. Available in packages of five dispensers.

Loestrin **21** 1.5/30 is available in dispensers each containing 21 tablets. Each tablet contains 1.5 mg of norethindrone acetate and 30 mcg of ethinyl estradiol. Available in packages of five dispensers.

Loestrin **Fe** 1.5/30 is available in dispensers each containing 21 green tablets and 7 brown tablets. Each green tablet contains 1.5 mg of norethindrone acetate and 30 mcg of ethinyl estradiol. Each brown tablet contains 75 mg ferrous fumarate. Available in packages of five dispensers.

*Norlestrin (Norethindrone Acetate and Ethinyl Estradiol Tablets, USP)

REFERENCES

1. Reproduced with permission of the Population Council from J. Trussell and K. Kost: Contraceptive failure in the United States: A critical review of the literature. *Studies in Family Planning,* 18 (5), September–October 1987.
2. Stadel, BV: Oral contraceptives and cardiovascular disease. (Pt. 1). *New England Journal of Medicine,* 305:612–618, 1981.
3. Stadel, B.V.: Oral contraceptives and cardiovascular disease. (Pt. 2.). *New England Journal of Medicine,* 305:672–677, 1981.
4. Adam, S.A., and M. Thorogood: Oral contraception and myocardial infarction revisited: The effects of new preparations and prescribing patterns. *Brit. J. Obstet. and Gynec.,* 88:838–845, 1981.
5. Mann, J.I., and W.H. Inman: Oral contraceptives and death from myocardial infarction. *Brit. Med. J.,* 2(5965): 245–248, 1975.
6. Mann, J.I., M.P. Vessey, M. Thorogood, and R. Doll: Myocardial infarction in young women with special reference to oral contraceptive practice. *Brit. Med. J.,* 2(5956):241–245, 1975.
7. Royal College of General Practitioners' Oral Contraception Study: Further analyses of mortality in oral contraceptive users. *Lancet* 1:541–546, 1981.
8. Slone, D., S. Shapiro, D.W. Kaufman, L. Rosenberg, O.S. Miettinen, and P.D. Stolley: Risk of myocardial infarction in relation to current and discontinued use of oral contraceptives. *N.E.J.M.,* 305:420–424, 1981.
9. Vessey, M.P.: Female hormones and vascular disease: An epidemiological overview, *Brit. J. Fam. Plann.,* 6:1–12, 1980.
10. Russell-Brief, R.G., T.M. Ezzati, R. Fulwood, J.A. Perlman, and R.S. Murphy: Cardiovascular risk status and oral contraceptive use, United States, 1976–80. *Preventive Medicine,* 15:352–362, 1986.
11. Goldbaum, G.M., J.S. Kendrick, G.C. Hogelin, and E.M. Gentry: The relative impact of smoking and oral contraceptive use on women in the United States. *J.A.M.A.,* 258:1339–1342, 1987.
12. Layde, P.M., and V. Beral: Further analyses of mortality in oral contraceptive users: Royal College General Practitioners' Oral Contraception Study. (Table 5) *Lancet,* 1:541–546, 1981.
13. Knopp, R.H.: Arteriosclerosis risk: The roles of oral contraceptives and postmenopausal estrogens. *J. of Reprod. Med.,* 31(9)(Supplement): 913–921, 1986.
14. Krauss, R.M., S. Roy, D.R. Mishell, J. Casagrande, and M.C. Pike: Effects of two low-dose oral contraceptives on serum lipids and lipoproteins: Differential changes in high-density lipoproteins subclasses. *Am. J. Obstet. Gyn.,* 145:446–452, 1983.
15. Wahl, P., C. Walden, R. Knopp, J. Hoover, R. Wallace, G. Heiss, and B. Rifkind: Effect of estrogen/progestin potency on lipid/lipoprotein cholesterol, *N.E.J.M.,* 308:862–867, 1983.
16. Wynn, V., and R. Niththyananthan: The effect of progestin in combined oral contraceptives on serum lipids with special reference to high-density lipoproteins. *Am. J. Obstet. and Gyn.,* 142:766–771, 1982.
17. Wynn, V., and I. Godsland: Effects of oral contraceptives on carbohydrate metabolism. *J. Reprod. Medicine,* 31(9)(Supplement): 892–897, 1986.
18. LaRosa, J.C.: Atherosclerotic risk factors in cardiovascular disease. *J. Reprod. Med.,* 31(9)(Supplement): 906–912, 1986.
19. Inman, W.H., and M.P. Vessey: Investigations of death from pulmonary, coronary, and cerebral thrombosis and embolism in women of child-bearing age. *Brit. Med. J.,* 2(5599): 193–199, 1968.
20. Maguire, M.G., J. Tonascia, P.E. Sartwell, P.D. Stolley, and M.S. Tockman: Increased risk of thrombosis due to oral contraceptives: A further report. *Am. J. Epidemiology,* 110(2):188–195, 1979.
21. Pettiti, D.B., J. Wingerd, F. Pellegrin, and S. Ramacharan: Risk of vascular disease in women: Smoking, oral contraceptives, noncontraceptive estrogens, and other factors, *J.A.M.A.,* 242:1150–1154, 1979.
22. Vessey, M.P., and R. Doll: Investigation of relation between use of oral contraceptives and thromboembolic disease. *Brit. Med. J.,* 2(5599): 199–205, 1968.
23. Vessey, M.P., and R. Doll: Investigation of relation between use of oral contraceptives and thromboembolic disease: A further report. *Brit. Med. J.,* 2(5658): 651–657, 1969.
24. Porter, J.B., J.R. Hunter, D.A. Danielson, H. Jick, and A. Stergachis: Oral contraceptives and non-fatal vascular disease: Recent experience. *Obstet. and Gyn.,* 59(3):299–302, 1982.
25. Vessey, M., R. Doll, R. Peto, B. Johnson, and P. Wiggins: A long-term follow-up study of women using different methods of contraception: An interim report. *J. Biosocial. Sci.,* 8:375–427, 1976.
26. Royal College of General Practitioners: Oral contraceptives, venous thrombosis, and varicose veins. *J. of Royal College of General Practitioners,* 28:393–399, 1978.
27. Collaborative Group for the study of stroke in young women: Oral contraception and increased risk of cerebral ischemia or thrombosis. *N.E.J.M.,* 288:871–878, 1973.
28. Petitti, D.B., and J. Wingerd: Use of oral contraceptives, cigarette smoking, and risk of subarachnoid hemorrhage. *Lancet,* 2:234–236, 1978.
29. Inman, W.H.: Oral contraceptives and fatal subarachnoid hemorrhage. *Brit. Med. J.,* 2(6203): 1468–70, 1979.
30. Collaborative Group for the study of stroke in young women: Oral contraceptives and stroke in young women: Associated risk factors. *J.A.M.A.,* 231:718–722, 1975.
31. Inman, W.H., M.P. Vessey, B. Westerholm, and A. Engelund: Thromboembolic disease and the steroidal content of oral contraceptives. A report to the Committee on Safety of Drugs. *Brit. Med. J.,* 2:203–209, 1970.
32. Meade, T.W., G. Greenberg, and S.G. Thompson: Progestogens and cardiovascular reactions associated with oral contraceptives and a comparison of the safety of 50- and 35-mcg oestrogen preparations. *Brit. Med. J.,* 280(6224): 1157–1161, 1980.
33. Kay, C.R.: Progestogens and arterial disease: Evidence from the Royal College of General Practitioners' study. *Amer. J. Obstet. Gyn.,* 142:762–765, 1982.
34. Royal College of General Practitioners: Incidence of arterial disease among oral contraceptive users. *J. Coll. Gen. Pract.,* 33:75–82, 1983.
35. Ory, H.W.: Mortality associated with fertility and fertility control: 1983. *Family Planning Perspectives,* 15:50–56, 1983.
36. The Cancer and Steroid Hormone Study of the Centers for Disease Control and the National Institute of Child Health and Human Development: Oral-contraceptive use and the risk of breast cancer. *N.E.J.M.,* 315:405–411, 1986.
37. Pike, M.C., B.E. Henderson, M.D. Krailo, A. Duke, and S. Roy: Breast cancer in young women and use of oral contraceptives: Possible modifying effect of formulation and age at use. *Lancet,* 2:926–929. 1983.
38. Paul, C., D.G. Skegg, G.F.S. Spears, and J.M. Kaldor: Oral contraceptives and breast cancer: A national study. *Brit. Med. J.,* 293:723–725, 1986.
39. Miller, D.R., L. Rosenberg, D.W. Kaufman, D. Schottenfeld, P.D. Stolley, and S. Shapiro: Breast cancer risk in relation to early oral contraceptive use. *Obstet. Gynec.,* 68:863–868, 1986.
40. Olson, H., K.L. Olson, T.R. Moller, J. Ranstam, P. Holm: Oral contraceptive use and breast cancer in young women in Sweden (letter). *Lancet,* 2:748–749, 1985.
41. McPherson, K., M. Vessey, A. Neil, R. Doll, L. Jones, and M. Roberts: Early contraceptive use and breast cancer: Results of another case-control study. *Brit. J. Cancer,* 56: 653–660, 1987.
42. Huggins, G.R., and P.F. Zucker: Oral contraceptives and neoplasia: 1987 update. Fertil. *Steril.,* 47:733–761, 1987.
43. McPherson, K., and J.O. Drife: The pill and breast cancer: Why the uncertainty? *Brit. Med. J.,* 293:709–710, 1986.
44. Shapiro, S.: Oral contraceptives: Time to take stock. *N.E.J.M.,* 315:450–451, 1987.
45. Ory, I.I., Z. Naib, S.B. Conger, R.A. Hatcher, and C.W. Tyler: Contraceptive choice and prevalence of cervical dysplasia and carcinoma in situ. *Am. J. Obstet. Gynec.,* 124:573–577, 1976.
46. Vessey, M.P., M. Lawless, K. McPherson, D. Yeates: Neoplasia of the cervix uteri and contraception: A possible adverse effect of the pill. *Lancet,* 2:930, 1983.
47. Brinton, L.A., G.R. Huggins, H.F. Lehman, K. Malli, D.A. Savitz, E. Trapido, J. Rosenthal, and R. Hoover: Long-term use of oral contraceptives and risk of invasive cervical cancer. *Int. J. Cancer,* 38:339–344, 1986.
48. WHO Collaborative Study of Neoplasia and Steroid Contraceptives: Invasive cervical cancer and combined oral contraceptives. *Brit. Med. J.,* 290:961–965, 1985.
49. Rooks, J.B., H.W. Ory, K.G. Ishak, L.T. Strauss, J.R. Greenspan, A.P. Hill, and C.W. Tyler: Epidemiology of hepatocellular adenoma: The role of oral contraceptive use. *J.A.M.A.,* 242:644–648, 1979.
50. Bein, N.N., and H.S. Goldsmith: Recurrent massive hemorrhage from benign hepatic tumors secondary to oral contraceptives. *Brit. J. Surg.,* 64:433–435, 1977.
51. Klatskin, G.: Hepatic tumors: Possible relationship to use of oral contraceptives. *Gastroenterology,* 73:386–394, 1977.
52. Henderson, B.E., S. Preston-Martin, H.A. Edmondson, R.L. Peters, and M.C. Pike: Hepatocellular carcinoma

and oral contraceptives. *Brit. J. Cancer,* 48:437–440, 1983.
53. Neuberger, J., D. Forman, R. Doll, and R. Williams: Oral contraceptives and hepatocellular carcinoma, *Brit. Med. J.,* 292:1355–1357, 1986.
54. Forman, D., T.J. Vincent, and R. Doll: Cancer of the liver and oral contraceptives. *Brit. Med. J.,* 292:1357–1361, 1986.
55. Harlap, S., and J. Eldor: Births following oral contraceptive failures. *Obstet. Gynec.,* 55:447–452, 1980.
56. Savolainen, E., E. Saksela, and L. Saxen: Teratogenic hazards of oral contraceptives analyzed in a national malformation register. *Amer. J. Obstet. Gynec.,* 140:521–524, 1981.
57. Janerich, D.T., J.M. Piper, and D.M. Glebatis: Oral contraceptives and birth defects. *Am. J. Epidemiology,* 112:73–79, 1980.
58. Ferencz, C., G.M. Matanoski, P.D. Wilson, J.D. Rubin, C.A. Neill, and R. Gutberlet: Maternal hormone therapy and congenital heart disease. *Teratology,* 21:225–239, 1980.
59. Rothman, K.J., D.C. Fyler, A. Goldbatt, and M.B. Kreidberg: Exogenous hormones and other drug exposures of children with congenital heart disease. *Am. J. Epidemiology,* 109:433–439, 1979.
60. Boston Collaborative Drug Surveillance Program: Oral contraceptives and venous thromboembolic disease, surgically confirmed gallbladder disease, and breast tumors. *Lancet,* 1:1399–1404, 1973.
61. Royal College of General Practitioners: *Oral Contraceptives and Health.* New York, Pittman, 1974, 100p.
62. Layde, P.M., M.P. Vessey, and D. Yeates: Risk of gallbladder disease: A cohort study of young women attending family planning clinics. *J. of Epidemiol. and Comm. Health,* 36: 274–278, 1982.
63. Rome Group for the Epidemiology and Prevention of Cholelithiasis (GREPCO): Prevalence of gallstone disease in an Italian adult female population, *Am. J. Epidemiol.,* 119:796–805, 1984.
64. Strom, B.L., R.T. Tamragouri, M.L. Morse, E.L. Lazar, S.L. West, P.D. Stolley, and J.K. Jones: Oral contraceptives and other risk factors for gallbladder disease. *Clin. Pharmacol. Ther.,* 39:335–341, 1986.
65. Wynn, V., P.W. Adams, I.F. Godsland, J. Melrose, R. Niththyananthan, N.W. Oakley, and A. Seedj: Comparison of effects of different combined oral-contraceptive formulations on carbohydrate and lipid metabolism. *Lancet,* 1:1045–1049, 1979.
66. Wynn, V.: Effect of progesterone and progestins on carbohydrate metabolism. In Progesterone and Progestin. Edited by C.W. Bardin, E. Milgrom, P. Mauvis-Jarvis. New York, *Raven Press,* pp. 395–410, 1983.
67. Perlman, J.A., R.G. Roussell-Briefel, T.M. Ezzati, and G. Lieberknecht: Oral glucose tolerance and the potency of oral contraceptive progestogens. *J. Chronic Dis.,* 38:857–864, 1985.
68. Royal College of General Practitioners' Oral Contraception Study: Effect on hypertension and benign breast disease of progestogen component in combined oral contraceptives. *Lancet,* 1:624, 1977.
69. Fisch, I.R., and J. Frank. Oral contraceptives and blood pressure. *J.A.M.A.* 237:2499–2503, 1977.
70. Laragh, A.J.: Oral contraceptive induced hypertension: Nine years later. *Amer. J. Obstet. Gynecol.,* 126:141–147, 1976.
71. Ramcharan, S., E. Peritz, F.A. Pellegrin, and W.T. Williams: Incidence of hypertension in the Walnut Creek Contraceptive Drug Study cohort. In Pharmacology of Steroid Contraceptive Drugs. Edited by S. Garattini and H.W. Berendes, New York. *Raven Press,* pp. 277–288, 1977. (Monographs of the Mario Negri Institute for Pharmacological Research, Milan).
72. Stockley, I.: Interactions with oral contraceptives. *Pharm. J.* 216:140–143, 1976.
73. The Cancer and Steroid Hormone Study of the Centers for Disease Control and the National Institute of Child Health and Human Development: Oral contraceptive use and the risk of ovarian cancer. *J.A.M.A.,* 249:1596–1599, 1983.
74. The Cancer and Steroid Hormone Study of the Centers for Disease Control and the National Institute of Child Health and Human Development: Combination oral contraceptive use and the risk of endometrial cancer. *J.A.M.A.,* 257:796–800, 1987.
75. Ory, H.W.: Functional ovarian cysts and oral contraceptives: Negative association confirmed surgically. *J.A.M.A.,* 228:68–69, 1974.
76. Ory, H.W., P. Cole, B. Macmahon, and R. Hoover: Oral contraceptives and reduced risk of benign breast disease. *N.E.J.M.,* 294:41–422, 1976.
77. Ory, H.W.: The noncontraceptive health benefits from oral contraceptive use. *Fam. Plann. Perspectives,* 14:182–184, 1982.
78. Ory, H.W., J.D. Forrest, and R. Lincoln: Making Choices: Evaluating the health risks and benefits of birth control methods. New York, The Alan Guttmacher Institute, p.1, 1983.
79. Miller, D. R., L. Rosenberg, D. W. Kaufman, P. Stolley, M.E. Warshauer, and S. Shapiro: Breast Cancer Before Age 45 and Oral Contraceptive Use: New Findings. *Am. J. Epidemiol.,* 129:269–280, 1989.
80. Kay, C. R. and P.C. Hannaford: Breast Cancer and the Pill; A Further Report from The Royal College of General Practitioners Oral Contraception Study *Br. J. Cancer,* 48:675–680, 1988.
81. Stadel, B.V., S. Lai, J.J. Schlesselman and P. Murray: Oral Contraceptives and Premenopausal Breast Cancer in Nulliparous Women. *Contraception.* 38:287–299, 1988.
82. UK National Case - Control Study Group: Oral Contraceptive Use and Breast Cancer Risk in Young Women. *Lancet,* 973–982, 1989.
83. Romieu, I., W.C. Willett, G.A. Colditz, M.J. Stampfer, B. Rosner, C.H. Hennekens, F.E. Speizer Prospective Study of Oral Contraceptive Use and Risk of Breast Cancer in Women. *J. Natl. Cancer Inst.* 81;1313–1321, 1989.

The patient labeling for oral contraceptive drug products is set forth below:

BRIEF SUMMARY PATIENT PACKAGE INSERT

Oral contraceptives, also known as "birth control pills" or "the pill," are taken to prevent pregnancy and when taken correctly, have a failure rate of about 1% per year when used without missing any pills. The typical failure rate of large numbers of pill users is less than 3% per year when women who miss pills are included. For most women oral contraceptives are also free of serious or unpleasant side effects. However, forgetting to take pills considerably increases the chances of pregnancy.

For the majority of women, oral contraceptives can be taken safely. But there are some women who are at high risk of developing certain serious diseases that can be life-threatening or may cause temporary or permanent disability. The risks associated with taking oral contraceptives increase significantly if you:

- Smoke
- Are over the age of 40
- Have high blood pressure, diabetes, high cholesterol
- Have or have had clotting disorders, heart attack, stroke, angina pectoris, cancer of the breast or sex organs, jaundice or malignant or benign liver tumors.

You should not take the pill if you suspect you are pregnant or have unexplained vaginal bleeding.

> Cigarette smoking increases the risk of serious cardiovascular side effects from oral contraceptive use. This risk increases with age and with heavy smoking (15 or more cigarettes per day) and is quite marked in women over 35 years of age. Women who use oral contraceptives are strongly advised not to smoke.

Most side effects of the pill are not serious. The most common side effects are nausea, vomiting, bleeding between menstrual periods, weight gain, and breast tenderness, and difficulty wearing contact lenses. These side effects, especially nausea and vomiting, may subside within the first three months of use.

The serious side effects of the pill occur very infrequently, especially if you are in good health and are young. However, you should know that the following medical conditions have been associated with or made worse by the pill:

1. Blood clots in the legs (thrombophlebitis), lungs (pulmonary embolism), stoppage or rupture of a blood vessel in the brain (stroke), blockage of blood vessels in the heart (heart attack or angina pectoris) or other organs of the body. As mentioned above, smoking increases the risk of heart attacks and strokes and subsequent serious medical consequences.
2. Liver tumors, which may rupture and cause severe bleeding. A possible but not definite association has been found with the pill and liver cancer. However, liver cancers are extremely rare. The chance of developing liver cancer from using the pill is thus even rarer.
3. High blood pressure, although blood pressure usually returns to normal when the pill is stopped.

The symptoms associated with these serious side effects are discussed in the detailed leaflet given to you with your supply of pills. Notify your doctor or health care provider if you notice any unusual physical disturbances while taking the pill. In addition, drugs such as rifampin, as well as some anticonvulsants and some antibiotics may decrease oral contraceptive effectiveness.

Most of the studies to date on breast cancer and pill use have found no increase in the risk of developing breast cancer although some studies have reported an increased risk of developing breast cancer in certain groups of women. However, some studies have found an increase in the risk of developing cancer of the cervix in women taking the pill, but this finding may be related to differences in sexual behavior or other factors not related to use of the pill. Therefore, there is insufficient evidence to rule out the possibility that the pill may cause cancer of the breasst or cervix.

Taking the pill provides some important non-contraceptive benefits. These include less painful menstruation, less menstrual blood loss and anemia, fewer pelvic infections, and fewer cancers of the ovary and the lining of the uterus.

Be sure to discuss any medical condition you may have with your health care provider. Your health care provider will take a medical and family history and examine you before prescribing oral contraceptives. You should be reexamined at least once a year while taking oral contraceptives. The detailed patient information leaflet gives you further information which you should read and discuss with your health care provider.

Caution: Oral contraceptives are of no value in the prevention or treatment of venereal disease.

INSTRUCTIONS TO PATIENTS

TABLET DISPENSER

The tablet dispenser has been designed to make oral contraceptive dosing as easy and as convenient as possible. The tablets are arranged in either three or four rows of seven tablets each, with the days of the week appearing on the tablet dispenser above the first row of tablets.

If your tablet dispenser contains:	You are taking:
21 white tablets	LOESTRIN 21 1/20
21 green tablets	LOESTRIN 21 1.5/30
21 white tablets and 7 brown tablets	LOESTRIN Fe 1/20
21 green tablets and 7 brown tablets	LOESTRIN Fe 1.5/30

Each *white* tablet contains 1 mg norethindrone acetate and 20 mcg ethinyl estradiol.

Each *green* tablet contains 1.5 mg norethindrone acetate and 30 mcg ethinyl estradiol.

Each *brown* tablet contains 75 mg ferrous fumarate, and is intended to help you remember to take the tablets correctly. These brown tablets are not intended to have any health benefit.

To remove a tablet, press down on it with your thumb or finger. The tablet will drop through the back of the tablet dispenser. Do not press on the tablet with your thumbnail or fingernail or any other sharp object.

LOESTRIN 21-DAY DOSAGE REGIMEN

If your tablet dispenser contains 21 tablets (3 rows of 7), you are on a 21-day regimen and should follow either the Sunday-Start or Day-5 Start directions.

A. Sunday-Start Regimen

1. Unless your physician or health care provider has instructed you differently, begin taking tablets on the first Sunday after your menstrual period begins whether or not you are still bleeding. If your period begins on Sunday, take your first tablet that very same day. START WITH THE SUNDAY TABLET IN THE TOP ROW.

Note: During the first cycle, it is important that you use another method of birth control until you have taken a tablet daily for seven consecutive days.

2. Take all the tablets in the top row first, followed by the second row. Continue to take one tablet every day until you finish all 21 tablets. Your last tablet should be on Saturday.
3. After you have taken all 21 tablets, stop, and don't take any tablets for the next seven days. You should have a menstrual period one to three days after you stop taking tablets; sometimes it may take a day or so longer.
4. After the seven days during which you take no tablets, obtain a new course of tablets. Begin the new course of 21 tablets on Sunday, the 8th day after you took your last tablet, starting with the Sunday tablet in the top row.
5. Continue to take one tablet daily until you finish all 21 tablets. If you follow the schedule properly, you will always take the last tablet in the dispenser on a Saturday, and always start each new course of 21 tablets 8 days later, on the following Sunday.
6. If, in any cycle, you start your tablets later than the proper day, you should also use another method of birth control until you have taken seven consecutive tablets.

Continued on next page

This product information was prepared in August 1992. On these and other Parke-Davis Products, information may be obtained by addressing PARKE-DAVIS, Division of Warner-Lambert Company, Morris Plains, New Jersey 07950.

Parke-Davis—Cont.

B. Day 5 Regimen

If your physician or health care provider has directed you to begin taking your first cycle of tablets using the Day-5 Regimen, you should start taking your tablets on Day 5 after the start of your period.

1. The first day of your period is Day 1. On the 5th day (Day 5), start taking one tablet daily, beginning with the tablet in the top row that corresponds to Day 5 after your flow began.

If your period begins on:	Start taking tablets in the top row on:
Sunday	Thursday
Monday	Friday
Tuesday	Saturday
Wednesday	Sunday
Thursday	Monday
Friday	Tuesday
Saturday	Wednesday

Note: During the first cycle, if you start taking tablets later than Day 5 of your menstrual period, you should use another method of birth control until you have taken a tablet daily for seven consecutive days.

2. Continue to take one tablet daily. After the last Saturday tablet has been taken, if any tablets remain in the first row, complete your 21-day regimen by taking one tablet daily starting with the Sunday tablet in the top row.

3. After you have taken all 21 tablets, stop and don't take any tablets for the next seven days. You should have a menstrual period one to three days after you stop taking tablets, sometimes it may take a day or so longer.

4. After the seven days during which you take no tablets, obtain a new course of tablets. Begin a new course of 21-day tablets, the 8th day after you took your last tablet, starting with the tablet in the top row that corresponds to that day.

5. Continue to take one tablet daily until you finish all 21 tablets. If you follow the schedule properly, you will always take the last tablet in the dispenser on the same day of the week, and always start each new course of 21 tablets the same day of the week on which you began the previous cycle of tablets.

6. If, in any cycle, you start your tablets later than the proper day, you should also use another method of birth control until you have taken seven consecutive tablets.

Whether you started your tablets using the Sunday-Start or Day-5 Regimen, the following directions apply:

1. Continue taking your tablets whether or not your period has occurred or is still in progress. Your period will usually occur during the seven days you are taking no tablets.

2. If spotting should occur at an unexpected time, continue to take your tablets as directed. Spotting is usually temporary and without significance. However, if bleeding should occur at an unexpected time, consult your physician or health care provider. Call your physician or health care provider regarding any problem or change in your general health that may concern you.

LOESTRIN 28-DAY DOSAGE REGIMEN

If your tablet dispenser contains 28 tablets (3 rows of 7 *light-colored* (white or green) tablets and 1 row of 7 *brown* tablets), you are on a 28-day regimen and should follow these directions. Each *brown* tablet contains 75 mg ferrous fumarate and is intended to help you remember to take the tablets correctly. These brown tablets are not intended to have any health benefits.

Sunday-Start Regimen:

1. Begin taking tablets on the first Sunday after your menstrual period begins whether or not you are still bleeding. If your period begins on Sunday, take your first tablet that very same day. START WITH THE SUNDAY TABLET IN THE TOP ROW.

Note: During the first cycle, it is important that you use another method of birth control until you have taken a *light-colored* tablet daily for seven consecutive days.

2. Take all the tablets in the top row first, followed by the second row and so on.

3. Continue to take one tablet every day until you finish all 21 *light-colored* tablets. On the day after taking the last *light-colored* tablet, begin taking one *brown* tablet daily until all the tablets have been taken.

4. When the last tablet has been taken, obtain a new course of tablets and, without interruption, begin a new course of 28-day tablets, the next day, starting with the Sunday

tablet in the top row. There should never be a day when you are not taking a tablet.

5. If, in any cycle, you start your tablets later than the proper day, you should also use another method of birth control until you have taken seven *light-colored* tablets.

6. Continue taking *light-colored* tablets without interruption whether or not your period has occurred or is still in progress. Your period will usually occur during the time you are taking *brown* tablets.

7. If spotting should occur at an unexpected time, continue to take your tablets as directed. Spotting is usually temporary and without significance. However, if bleeding should occur at an unexpected time, consult your physician or health care provider. Call your physician or health care provider regarding any problem or change in your general health that may concern you.

In Case You Forget (21-Day and 28-Day Regimens)

The following instructions apply only to missing the white 1/20 tablets or the green 1.5/30 tablets.

If you forget to take one tablet, take it as soon as you remember, even if it is the next day. Then take the next scheduled tablet at the usual time. If you miss two consecutive tablets, take two tablets daily for the next two days. Then resume the regular schedule. While there is little likelihood of pregnancy occurring if you miss only one or two tablets, the possibility of pregnancy increases with each successive day that tablets are missed.

If you are taking Loestrin 21 1/20 or Loestrin Fe 1/20, in addition to taking two *white* tablets a day for two days, you should use an additional means of contraception until you've taken a *white* tablet every day for seven days.

21-Day Regimen: If you miss three consecutive tablets, discard any tablets remaining in the tablet dispenser and follow these instructions.

If you are on the Sunday-Start Regimen, start a new course of tablets the first Sunday following the last missed tablet, whether or not you are still menstruating.

If you are on the Day-5 Regimen, begin a new course of tablets on the 8th day after the last tablet was taken. For example, if you took your last tablet on a Monday, you should begin your new course of tablets the following Monday.

During the seven days without tablets, and until you have taken a tablet daily for seven consecutive days from your course of tablets, you should also use another method of birth control.

28-Day Regimen: If you miss three consecutive *light-colored* tablets, discard any tablets remaining in the tablet dispenser and begin a new course of tablets the first Sunday following the last missed tablet, whether or not you are still menstruating. During the days without tablets and until you have taken a tablet daily for seven consecutive days from your new course of tablets, you should also use another method of birth control.

If you miss one or more *brown* tablets discard the remainder and begin a new course of tablets on the next Sunday (which should be the 8th day after you took your last *light-colored* tablet). Start with the *light-colored* tablets in the top row. Skipping one or more *brown* tablets contained in the 28-day regimen products won't increase the risk of pregnancy. They are there to help keep you on a schedule and to eliminate the need for counting days. *Under no circumstances* should you substitute a *brown* tablet for a *light-colored* tablet nor should a *brown* tablet be taken until you have finished all the *light-colored* tablets, unless your physician or health care provider advises you to do so.

Remembering to take tablets according to schedule is stressed because of its importance in providing you the greatest degree of protection.

MISSED MENSTRUAL PERIODS FOR BOTH DOSAGE REGIMENS

At times there may be no menstrual period after a cycle of pills. Therefore, if you miss one menstrual period but have taken the pills *exactly as your were supposed to*, continue as usual into the next cycle. If you have not taken the pills correctly and miss a menstrual period, *you may be pregnant* and should stop taking oral contraceptives until your doctor or health care provider determines whether or not you are pregnant. Until you can get to your doctor or health care provider, use another form of contraception. If two consecutive menstrual periods are missed, you should stop taking pills until it is determined whether or not you are pregnant. Although there does not appear to be any increase in birth defects in newborn babies if you become pregnant while using oral contraceptives, if you do become pregnant, you should discuss the situation with your doctor or health care provider.

Periodic Examination

Your doctor or health care provider will take a complete medical and family history before prescribing oral contraceptives. At that time and about once a year thereafter, he will generally examine your blood pressure, breasts, abdomen, and pelvic organs (including a Papanicolaou smear, ie, test for cancer).

SUMMARY

Oral contraceptives are the most effective method, except sterilization, for preventing pregnancy. Other methods, when used conscientiously, are also very effective and have fewer risks. Although the serious risks of oral contraceptives are uncommon, some of the risks may persist after you stop using the pill. On the other hand, the "pill" is a very convenient method of preventing pregnancy.

If you have certain conditions or have had these conditions in the past, you should not use oral contraceptives because the risk is too great. These conditions are listed in this leaflet. If you do not have these conditions, and decide to use the "pill," please read this leaflet carefully so that you can use the "pill" most safely and effectively.

Based on his or her assessment of your medical needs, your doctor or health care provider has prescribed this drug for you. Do not give this drug to anyone else.

Keep this and all drugs out of the reach of children.

Caution—Federal law prohibits dispensing without prescription.

DETAILED PATIENT PACKAGE INSERT

What You Should Know About Oral Contraceptives

Any woman who considers using oral contraceptives (the "birth control pill" or the "pill") should understand the benefits and risks of using this form of birth control. This leaflet will give you much of the information you will need to make this decision and will also help you determine if you are at risk of developing any of the serious side effects of the pill. It will tell you how to use the pill properly so that it will be as effective as possible. However, this leaflet is not a replacement for a careful discussion between you and your health care provider. You should discuss the information provided in this leaflet with him or her, both when you first start taking the pill and during your revisits. You should also follow your health care provider's advice with regard to regular check-ups while you are on the pill.

EFFECTIVENESS OF ORAL CONTRACEPTIVES

Oral contraceptives or "birth control pills" or "the pill" are used to prevent pregnancy and are more effective than other non-surgical methods of birth control. When they are taken correctly, the chance of becoming pregnant is less than 1% (1 pregnancy per 100 women per year of use) when used perfectly, without missing pills. Typical failure rates are actually 3% per year. The chance of becoming pregnant increases with each missed pill during a menstrual cycle.

In comparison, typical failure rates for other methods of birth control during the first year of use are as follows:

IUD: 6%
Diaphragm with spermicides: 18%
Spermicides alone: 21%
Vaginal sponge: 18 to 30%
Condom alone: 12%
Periodic abstinence: 20%
No method: 89%.

WHO SHOULD NOT TAKE ORAL CONTRACEPTIVES

> Cigarette smoking increases the risk of serious cardiovascular side effects from oral contraceptives use. This risk increases with age and with heavy smoking (15 or more cigarettes per day) and is quite marked in women over 35 years of age. Women who use oral contraceptives are strongly advised not to smoke.

Some women should not use the pill. For example, you should not take the pill if you are pregnant or think you may be pregnant. You should also not use the pill if you have any of the following conditions:

- A history of heart attack or stroke
- Blood clots in the legs (thrombophlebitis), lungs (pulmonary embolism), or eyes
- A history of blood clots in the deep veins of your legs
- Chest pain (angina pectoris)
- Known or suspected breast cancer or cancer of the lining of the uterus, cervix or vagina
- Unexplained vaginal bleeding (until a diagnosis is reached by your doctor)
- Yellowing of the whites of the eyes or of the skin (jaundice) during pregnancy or during previous use of the pill
- Liver tumor (benign or cancerous)
- Known or suspected pregnancy

Tell your health care provider if you have ever had any of these conditions. Your health care provider can recommend a safer method of birth control.

OTHER CONSIDERATIONS BEFORE TAKING ORAL CONTRACEPTIVES

Tell your health care provider if you have:

- Breast nodules, fibrocystic disease of the breast, an abnormal breast x-ray or mammogram
- Diabetes
- Elevated cholesterol or triglycerides
- High blood pressure
- Migraine or other headaches or epilepsy
- Mental depression

- Gallbladder, heart or kidney disease
- History of scanty or irregular menstrual periods

Women with any of these conditions should be checked often by their health care provider if they choose to use oral contraceptives.

Also, be sure to inform your doctor or health care provider if you smoke or are on any medications.

RISKS OF TAKING ORAL CONTRACEPTIVES

1. Risk Of Developing Blood Clots

Blood clots and blockage of blood vessels are the most serious side effects of taking oral contraceptives. In particular, a clot in the legs can cause thrombophlebitis and a clot that travels to the lungs can cause a sudden blocking of the vessel carrying blood to the lungs. Rarely, clots occur in the blood vessels of the eye and may cause blindness, double vision, or impaired vision.

If you take oral contraceptives and need elective surgery, need to stay in bed for a prolonged illness or have recently delivered a baby, you may be at risk of developing blood clots. You should consult your doctor or health care provider about stopping oral contraceptives three to four weeks before surgery and not taking oral contraceptives for two weeks after surgery or during bed rest. You should also not take oral contraceptives soon after delivery of a baby. It is advisable to wait for at least four weeks after delivery if you are not breast feeding. If you are breast feeding, you should wait until you have weaned your child before using the pill. (See also the section on Breast Feeding in GENERAL PRECAUTIONS.)

2. Heart Attacks And Strokes

Oral contraceptives may increase the tendency to develop strokes (stoppage or rupture of blood vessels in the brain) and angina pectoris and heart attacks (blockage of blood vessels in the heart). Any of these conditions can cause death or disability.

Smoking greatly increases the possibility of suffering heart attacks and strokes. Furthermore, smoking and the use of oral contraceptives greatly increase the chances of developing and dying of heart disease.

3. Gallbladder Disease

Oral contraceptive users probably have a greater risk than nonusers of having gallbladder disease, although this risk may be related to pills containing high doses of estrogens.

4. Liver Tumors

In rare cases, oral contraceptives can cause benign but dangerous liver tumors. These benign liver tumors can rupture and cause fatal internal bleeding. In addition, a possible but not definite association has been found with the pill and liver cancers in two studies, in which a few women who developed these very rare cancers were found to have used oral contraceptives for long periods. However, liver cancers are extremely rare. The chance of developing liver cancer from using the pill is thus even rarer.

5. Cancer Of The Reproductive Organs

There is, at present, no confirmed evidence that oral contraceptive use increases risk of developing cancer of the reproductive organs. Studies to date of women taking the pill have reported conflicting findings on whether pill use increases the risk of developng cancer of the breast or cervix. Most of the studies on breast cancer and pill use have found no increase in the risk of developing breast cancer although some studies have reported an increased risk of developing breast cancer in certain groups of women. Women who use oral contraceptives and have a strong family history of breast cancer or who have breast nodules or abnormal mammograms should be closely followed by their doctors.

Some studies have found an increase in the incidence of cancer of the cervix in women who use oral contraceptives. However, this finding may be related to factors other than the use of oral contraceptives.

ESTIMATED RISK OF DEATH FROM A BIRTH CONTROL METHOD OR PREGNANCY

All methods of birth control and pregnancy are associated with a risk of developing certain diseases which may lead to disability or death. An estimate of the number of deaths associated with different methods of birth control and pregnancy has been calculated and is shown in the table above.

In the above table, the risk of death from any birth control method is less than the risk of childbirth, except for oral contraceptive users over the age of 35 who smoke and pill users over the age of 40 even if they do not smoke. It can be seen in the table that for women aged 15 to 39, the risk of death was highest with pregnancy (7-26 deaths per 100,000 women, depending on age). Among pill users who do not smoke, the risk of death was always lower than that associated with pregnancy for any age group, although over the age of 40, the risk increases to 32 deaths per 100,000 women, compared to 28 associated with pregnancy at that age. However, for pill users who smoke and are over the age of 35, the estimated number of deaths exceeds those for other methods of birth control. If a woman is over the age of 40 and smokes, her estimated risk of death is four times higher (117/100,000 women) than the estimated risk associated with pregnancy (28/100,000 women) in that age group.

ANNUAL NUMBER OF BIRTH-RELATED OR METHOD-RELATED DEATHS ASSOCIATED WITH CONTROL OF FERTILITY PER 100,000 NONSTERILE WOMEN, BY FERTILITY CONTROL METHOD ACCORDING TO AGE

Method of control and outcome	15–19	20–24	25–29	30–34	35–39	40–44
No fertility control methods*	7.0	7.4	9.1	14.8	25.7	28.2
Oral contraceptives non-smoker**	0.3	0.5	0.9	1.9	13.8	31.6
Oral contraceptives smoker**	2.2	3.4	6.6	13.5	51.1	117.2
IUD**	0.8	0.8	1.0	1.0	1.4	1.4
Condom*	1.1	1.6	0.7	0.2	0.3	0.4
Diaphragm/spermicide*	1.9	1.2	1.2	1.3	2.2	2.8
Periodic abstinence*	2.5	1.6	1.6	1.7	2.9	3.6

* Deaths are birth related
** Deaths are method related

The suggestion that women over 40 who don't smoke should not take oral contraceptives is based on information from older high-dose pills and less selective use of pills than is practiced today. An Advisory Committee of the FDA discussed this issue in 1989 and recommended that the benefits of oral contraceptive use by healthy, non-smoking women over 40 years of age may outweigh the possible risks. However, all women, especially older women, are cautioned to use the lowest dose pill that is effective.

WARNING SIGNALS

If any of these adverse effects occur while you are taking oral contraceptives, call your doctor immediately:

- Sharp chest pain, coughing of blood, or sudden shortness of breath (indicating a possible clot in the lung)
- Pain in the calf (indicating a possible clot in the leg)
- Crushing chest pain or heaviness in the chest (indicating a possible heart attack)
- Sudden severe headache or vomiting, dizziness or fainting, disturbances of vision or speech, weakness, or numbness in an arm or leg (indicating a possible stroke)
- Sudden partial or complete loss of vision (indicating a possible clot in the eye)
- Breast lumps (indicating possible breast cancer or fibrocystic disease of the breast; ask your doctor or health care provider to show you how to examine your breasts)
- Severe pain or tenderness in the stomach area (indicating a possibly ruptured liver tumor)
- Difficulty in sleeping, weakness, lack of energy, fatigue, or change in mood (possibly indicating severe depression)
- Jaundice or a yellowing of the skin or eyeballs, accompanied frequently by fever, fatigue, loss of appetite, dark colored urine, or light colored bowel movements (indicating possible liver problems)

SIDE EFFECTS OF ORAL CONTRACEPTIVES

1. Vaginal Bleeding

Irregular vaginal bleeding or spotting may occur while you are taking the pills. Irregular bleeding may vary from slight staining between menstrual periods to breakthrough bleeding which is a flow much like a regular period. Irregular bleeding occurs most often during the first few months of oral contraceptive use, but may also occur after you have been taking the pill for some time. Such bleeding may be temporary and usually does not indicate any serious problems. It is important to continue taking your pills on schedule. If the bleeding occurs in more than one cycle or lasts for more than a few days, talk to your doctor or health care provider.

2. Contact Lenses

If you wear contact lenses and notice a change in vision or an inability to wear your lenses, contact your doctor or health care provider.

3. Fluid Retention

Oral contraceptives may cause edema (fluid retention) with swelling of the fingers or ankles and may raise your blood pressure. If you experience fluid retention, contact your doctor or health care provider.

4. Melasma

A spotty darkening of the skin is possible, particularly on the face.

5. Other Side Effects

Other side effects include change in appetite, headache, nervousness, depression, dizziness, loss of scalp hair, rash, and vaginal infections.

If any of these side effects bother you, call your doctor or health care provider.

GENERAL PRECAUTIONS

1. Missed Periods And Use Of Oral Contraceptives Before Or During Early Pregnancy

There may be times when you may not menstruate regularly after you have completed taking a cycle of pills. If you have taken your pills regularly and miss one menstrual period, continue taking your pills for the next cycle but be sure to inform your health care provider before doing so. If you have not taken the pills daily as instructed and missed a menstrual period, or if you missed two consecutive menstrual periods, you may be pregnant. Check with your health care provider immediately to determine whether you are pregnant. Do not continue to take oral contraceptives until you are sure you are not pregnant, but continue to use another method of contraception.

There is no conclusive evidence that oral contraceptive use is associated with an increase in birth defects, when taken inadvertently during early pregnancy. Previously, a few studies had reported that oral contraceptives might be associated with birth defects, but these studies have not been confirmed. Nevertheless, oral contraceptives or any other drugs should not be used during pregnancy unless clearly necessary and prescribed by your doctor. You should check with your doctor about risks to your unborn child of any medication taken during pregnancy.

2. While Breast Feeding

If you are breast feeding consult your doctor before starting oral contraceptives. Some of the drug will be passed on to the child in the milk. A few adverse effects on the child have been reported, including yellowing of the skin (jaundice) and breast enlargement. In addition, oral contraceptives may decrease the amount and quality of your milk. If possible, do not use oral contraceptives while breast feeding. You should use another method of contraception since breast feeding provides only partial protection from becoming pregnant and this partial protection decreases significantly as you breast feed for longer periods of time. You should consider starting oral contraceptives only after you have weaned your child completely.

3. Laboratory Tests

If you are scheduled for any laboratory tests, tell your doctor you are taking birth control pills. Certain blood tests may be affected by birth control pills.

4. Drug Interactions

Certain drugs may interact with birth control pills to make them less effective in preventing pregnancy or cause an increase in breakthrough bleeding. Such drugs include rifampin, drugs used for epilepsy such as barbiturates (for example, phenobarbital) and phenytoin (Dilantin® is one brand of this drug), phenylbutazone (Butazolidin® is one brand) and possibly certain antibiotics. You may need to use additional contraception when you take drugs which can make oral contraceptives less effective.

HOW TO TAKE ORAL CONTRACEPTIVES

1. General Instructions

You must take your pill every day according to the instructions. Oral contraceptives are most effective if taken no more than 24 hours apart. Take your pill at the same time every day so that you are less likely to forget to take it. You will then maintain an effective dose of oral contraceptive in your body.

If your doctor has scheduled you for surgery, or you need prolonged bed rest, he or she may suggest that you stop taking the pill four weeks before surgery to avoid an increased risk of blood clots. It is also advisable not to start oral contraceptives sooner than four weeks after delivery of a baby.

2. If You Forget To Take Your Pill

If you miss only one pill in a cycle, the chance of becoming pregnant is small. Take the missed pill as soon as you realize that you have forgotten it. Since the risk of pregnancy increases with each additional pill you skip, it is very important that you take one pill a day.

3. Pregnancy Due To Pill Failure

The incidence of pill failure resulting in pregnancy is approximately 1% (i.e., one pregnancy per 100 women per year) if taken every day as directed, but more typical failure rates

Continued on next page

This product information was prepared in August 1992. On these and other Parke-Davis Products, information may be obtained by addressing PARKE-DAVIS, Division of Warner-Lambert Company, Morris Plains, New Jersey 07950.

Parke-Davis—Cont.

are about 3%. If failure does occur, the risk to the fetus is minimal.

4. Pregnancy After Stopping The Pill

There may be some delay in becoming pregnant after you stop using oral contraceptives, especially if you had irregular menstrual cycles before you used oral contraceptives. It may be advisable to postpone conception until you begin menstruating regularly once you have stopped taking the pill and desire pregnancy.

There does not appear to be any increase in birth defects in newborn babies when pregnancy occurs soon after stopping the pill.

5. Overdosage

Serious ill effects have not been reported following ingestion of large doses of oral contraceptives by young children. Overdosage may cause nausea and withdrawal bleeding in females. In case of overdosage, contact your health care provider or pharmacist.

6. Other Information

Your health care provider will take a medical and family history and examine you before prescribing oral contraceptives. You should be reexamined at least once a year. Be sure to inform your health care provider if there is a family history of any of the conditions listed previously in this leaflet. Be sure to keep all appointments with your health care provider, because this is a time to determine if there are early signs of side effects of oral contraceptive use.

Do not use the drug for any condition other than the one for which it was prescribed. This drug has been prescribed specifically for you; do not give it to others who may want birth control pills.

HEALTH BENEFITS FROM ORAL CONTRACEPTIVES

In addition to preventing pregnancy, use of oral contraceptives may provide certain benefits.

They are:

- Menstrual cycles may become more regular
- Blood flow during menstruation may be lighter and less iron may be lost. Therefore, anemia due to iron deficiency is less likely to occur
- Pain or other symptoms during menstruation may be encountered less frequently
- Ectopic (tubal) pregnancy may occur less frequently
- Noncancerous cysts or lumps in the breast may occur less frequently
- Acute pelvic inflammatory disease may occur less frequently
- Oral contraceptive use may provide some protection against developing two forms of cancer: cancer of the ovaries and cancer of the lining of the uterus.

If you want more information about birth control pills, ask your doctor or pharmacist. They have a more technical leaflet called the "Physician Insert," which you may wish to read.

INSTRUCTIONS TO PATIENT

TABLET DISPENSER

The tablet dispenser has been designed to make oral contraceptive dosing as easy and as convenient as possible. The tablets are arranged in either three or four rows of seven tablets each, with the days of the week appearing on the tablet dispenser above the first row of tablets.

If your tablet dispenser contains:	You are taking:
21 white tablets	LOESTRIN 21 1/20
21 green tablets	LOESTRIN 21 1.5/30
21 white tablets and 7 brown tablets	LOESTRIN Fe 1/20
21 green tablets and 7 brown tablets	LOESTRIN Fe 1.5/30

Each *white* tablet contains 1 mg norethindrone acetate and 20 mcg ethinyl estradiol.

Each *green* tablet contains 1.5 mg norethindrone acetate and 30 mcg ethinyl estradiol.

Each *brown* tablet contains 75 mg ferrous fumarate, and is intended to help you remember to take the tablets correctly. These brown tablets are not intended to have any health benefit.

To remove a tablet, press down on it with your thumb or finger. The tablet will drop through the back of the tablet dispenser. Do not press on the tablet with your thumbnail or fingernail or any other sharp object.

LOESTRIN 21-DAY DOSAGE REGIMEN

If your tablet dispenser contains 21 tablets (3 rows of 7), you are on a 21-day regimen and should follow either the Sunday-Start or Day-5 Start directions.

A. Sunday-Start Regimen

1. Unless your physician or health care provider has instructed you differently, begin taking tablets on the first Sunday after your menstrual period begins whether or not you are still bleeding. If your period begins on Sunday, take your first tablet that very same day. START WITH THE SUNDAY TABLET IN THE TOP ROW.

Note: During the first cycle, it is important that you use another method of birth control until you have taken a tablet daily for seven consecutive days.

2. Take all the tablets in the top row first, followed by the second row. Continue to take one tablet every day until you finish all 21 tablets. Your last tablet should be on Saturday.
3. After you have taken all 21 tablets, stop, and don't take any tablets for the next seven days. You should have a menstrual period one to three days after you stop taking tablets; sometimes it may take a day or so longer.
4. After the seven days during which you take no tablets, obtain a new course of tablets. Begin the new course of 21 day tablets on Sunday, the 8th day after you took your last tablet, starting with the Sunday tablet in the top row.
5. Continue to take one tablet daily until you finish all 21 tablets. If you follow the schedule properly, you will always take the last tablet in the dispenser on a Saturday, and always start each new course of 21 tablets 8 days later, on the following Sunday.
6. If, in any cycle, you start your tablets later than the proper day, you should also use another method of birth control until you have taken seven consecutive tablets.

B. Day-5 Regimen

If your physician or health care provider has directed you to begin taking your first cycle of tablets using the Day-5 Regimen, you should start taking your tablets on Day 5 after the start of your period.

1. The first day of your period is Day 1. On the 5th day (Day 5), start taking one tablet daily, beginning with the tablet in the top row that corresponds to Day 5 after your flow began.

If your period begins on:	Start taking tablets in the top row on:
Sunday	Thursday
Monday	Friday
Tuesday	Saturday
Wednesday	Sunday
Thursday	Monday
Friday	Tuesday
Saturday	Wednesday

Note: During the first cycle, if you start taking tablets later than Day 5 of your menstrual period, you should use another method of birth control until you have taken a tablet daily for seven consecutive days.

2. Continue to take one tablet daily. After the last Saturday tablet has been taken, if any tablets remain in the first row, complete your 21-day regimen by taking one tablet daily starting with the Sunday tablet in the top row.
3. After you have taken all 21 tablets, stop, and don't take any tablets for the next seven days. You should have a menstrual period one to three days after you stop taking tablets; sometimes it may take a day or so longer.
4. After the seven days during which you take no tablets, obtain a new course of tablets. Begin a new course of 21-day tablets, the 8th day after you took your last tablet, starting with the tablet in the top row that corresponds to that day.
5. Continue to take one tablet daily until you finish all 21 tablets. If you follow the schedule properly, you will always take the last tablet in the dispenser on the same day of the week, and always start each new course of 21 tablets the same day of the week on which you began the previous cycle of tablets.
6. If, in any cycle, you start your tablets later than the proper day, you should also use another method of birth control until you have taken seven consecutive tablets.

Whether you started your tablets using the Sunday-Start or Day-5 Regimen, the following directions apply:

1. Continue taking your tablets whether or not your period has occurred or is still in progress. Your period will usually occur during the seven days you are taking no tablets.
2. If spotting should occur at an unexpected time, continue to take your tablets as directed. Spotting is usually temporary and without significance. However, if bleeding should occur at an unexpected time, consult your physician or health care provider. Call your physician or health care provider regarding any problem or change in your general health that may concern you.

LOESTRIN 28-DAY DOSAGE REGIMEN

If your tablet dispenser contains 28 tablets (3 rows of 7 *light-colored* (white or green) tablets and 1 row of 7 *brown* tablets), you are on a 28-day regimen and should follow these directions.

Sunday-Start Regimen:

1. Begin taking tablets on the first Sunday after your menstrual period begins whether or not you are still bleeding. If your period begins on Sunday, take your first tablet that very same day. START WITH THE SUNDAY TABLET IN THE TOP ROW.

Note: During the first cycle, it is important that you use another method of birth control until you have taken a *light-colored* tablet daily for seven consecutive days.

2. Take all the tablets in the top row first, followed by the second row and so on.
3. Continue to take one tablet every day until you finish all 21 *light-colored* tablets. On the day after taking the last *light-colored* tablet, begin taking one *brown* tablet daily until all the tablets have been taken.
4. When the last tablet has been taken, obtain a new course of tablets and, without interruption, begin a new course of 28-day tablets, the next day, starting with the Sunday tablet in the top row. There should never be a day when you are not taking a tablet.
5. If, in any cycle, you start your tablets later than the proper day, you should also use another method of birth control until you have taken seven *light-colored* tablets.
6. Continue taking *light-colored* tablets without interruption whether or not your period has occurred or is still in progress. Your period will usually occur during the time you are taking *brown* tablets.
7. If spotting should occur at an unexpected time, continue to take your tablets as directed. Spotting is usually temporary and without significance. However, if bleeding should occur at an unexpected time, consult your physician or health care provider. Call your physician regarding any problem or change in your general health that may concern you.

In Case You Forget (21-Day and 28-Day Regimens)

The following instructions apply only to missing the white 1/20 tablets or the green 1.5/30 tablets.

If you forget to take one tablet, take it as soon as you remember, even if it is the next day. Then take the next scheduled tablet at the usual time. If you miss two consecutive tablets, take two tablets daily for the next two days. Then resume the regular schedule. While there is little likelihood of pregnancy occurring if you miss only one or two tablets, the possibility of pregnancy increases with each successive day that tablets are missed.

If you are taking Loestrin **21** 1/20 or Loestrin **Fe** 1/20, in addition to taking two *white* tablets a day for two days, you should use an additional means of contraception until you've taken a *white* tablet every day for seven days.

21-Day Regimen: If you miss three consecutive tablets, discard any tablets remaining in the tablet dispenser and follow these instructions.

If you are on the Sunday-Start Regimen, start a new course of tablets the first Sunday following the last missed tablet, whether or not you are still menstruating.

If you are on the Day-5 Regimen, begin a new course of tablets on the 8th day after the last tablet was taken. For example, if you took your last tablet on a Monday, you should begin your new course of tablets the following Monday.

During the seven days without tablets, and until you have taken a tablet daily for seven consecutive days from your course of tablets, you should also use another method of birth control.

28-Day Regimen: If you miss three consecutive *light-colored* tablets, discard any tablets remaining in the tablet dispenser and begin a new course of tablets the first Sunday following the last missed tablet, whether or not you are still menstruating. During the days without tablets and until you have taken a tablet daily for seven consecutive days from your new course of tablets, you should also use another method of birth control.

If you miss one or more *brown* tablets discard the remainder and begin a new course of tablets on the next Sunday (which should be the 8th day after you took your last *light-colored* tablet). Start with the *light-colored* tablets in the top row. Skipping one or more *brown* tablets contained in the 28-day regimen products won't increase the risk of pregnancy. They are there to help keep you on schedule and to eliminate the need for counting days. *Under no circumstances* should you

substitute a *brown* tablet for a *light-colored* tablet nor should a *brown* tablet be taken until you have finished all the *light-colored* tablets, unless your physician or health care provider advises you to do so.

Remembering to take tablets according to schedule is stressed because of its importance in providing you the greatest degree of protection.

MISSED MENSTRUAL PERIODS FOR BOTH DOSAGE REGIMENS

At times there may be no menstrual period after a cycle of pills. Therefore, if you miss one menstrual period but have taken the pills *exactly as you were supposed to*, continue as usual into the next cycle. If you have not taken the pills correctly and miss a menstrual period, *you may be pregnant* and should stop taking oral contraceptives until your doctor or health care provider determines whether or not you are pregnant. Until you can get to your doctor or health care provider, use another form of contraception. If two consecutive menstrual periods are missed, you should stop taking pills until it is determined whether or not you are pregnant. Although there does not appear to be any increase in birth defects in newborn babies if you become pregnant while using oral contraceptives, if you do become pregnant, you should discuss the situation with your doctor or health care provider.

Periodic Examination

Your doctor will take a complete medical and family history before prescribing oral contraceptives. At that time and about once a year thereafter, he will generally examine your blood pressure, breasts, abdomen, and pelvic organs (including a Papanicolaou smear, ie, test for cancer).

SUMMARY

Oral contraceptives are the most effective method, except sterilization, for preventing pregnancy. Other methods, when used conscientiously, are also very effective and have fewer risks. Although the serious risks of oral contraceptives are uncommon, some of the risks may persist after you stop using the pill. On the other hand, the "pill" is a very convenient method of preventing pregnancy.

If you have certain conditions or have had these conditions in the past, you should not use oral contraceptives because the risk is too great. These conditions are listed in this leaflet. If you do not have these conditions, and decide to use the "pill," please read this leaflet carefully so that you can use the "pill" most safely and effectively.

Based on his or her assessment of your medical needs, your doctor or health care provider has prescribed this drug for you. Do not give this drug to anyone else.

Keep this and all drugs out of the reach of children.

Caution—Federal law prohibits dispensing without prescription.

January 1990 **0913G156**

Shown in Product Identification Section, page 422

LOPID® ℞
[lō′pĭd]
(Gemfibrozil Tablets)

DESCRIPTION

Lopid® (gemfibrozil tablets) is a lipid regulating agent. It is available as tablets for oral administration. Each tablet contains 600 mg gemfibrozil. Each also contains calcium stearate, NF; candelilla wax FCC; microcrystalline cellulose, NF; hydroxypropyl cellulose, NF: hydroxypropyl methylcellulose, USP; methylparaben, NF; Opaspray white; polyethylene glycol, NF; polysorbate 80, NF; propylparaben, NF; colloidal silicon dioxide, NF; pregelatinized starch, NF. The chemical name is 5-(2,5-dimethylphenoxy)-2,2-dimethylpentanoic acid.

The empirical formula is $C_{15}H_{22}O_3$ and the molecular weight is 250.35; the solubility in water and acid is 0.0019% and in dilute base it is greater than 1%. The melting point is 58°–61°C. Gemfibrozil is a white solid which is stable under ordinary conditions.

CLINICAL PHARMACOLOGY

LOPID (gemfibrozil tablets) is a lipid regulating agent which decreases serum triglycerides and very low density lipoprotein (VLDL) cholesterol, and increases high density lipoprotein (HDL) cholesterol. While modest decreases in total and low density lipoprotein (LDL) cholesterol may be observed with Lopid therapy, treatment of patients with elevated triglycerides due to Type IV hyperlipoproteinemia often results in a rise in LDL-cholesterol. LDL-cholesterol levels in Type IIb patients with elevations of both serum LDL-cholesterol and triglycerides are, in general, minimally affected by Lopid treatment; however, Lopid usually raises HDL-cholesterol significantly in this group. Lopid increases levels of high density lipoprotein (HDL) subfractions HDL_2 and HDL_3, as well as apolipoproteins AI and AII. Epidemiological studies have shown that both low HDL-cholesterol and high LDL-cholesterol are independent risk factors for coronary heart disease.

Table I
Reduction in CHD Rates (events per 1000 patients) by Baseline Lipids[1] in the Helsinki Heart Study, Years 0–5[2]

	All Patients			LDL-C > 175; HDL-C > 46.4			LDL-C > 175; TG > 177			LDL-C > 175; TG > 200; HDL-C < 35		
	P	L	Dif[3]	P	L	Dif	P	L	Dif	P	L	Dif
Incidence of Evidents[4]	41	27	14	32	29	3	71	44	27	149	64	85

[1] lipid values in mg/dL at baseline
[2] P=placebo group; L=Lopid group
[3] difference in rates between placebo and Lopid groups
[4] fatal and nonfatal myocardial infarctions plus sudden cardiac deaths (events per 1000 patients over 5 years)

In the primary prevention component of the Helsinki Heart Study (refs. 1,2), in which 4081 male patients between the ages of 40 and 55 were studied in a randomized, double-blind, placebo-controlled fashion, Lopid therapy was associated with significant reductions in total plasma triglycerides and a significant increase in high density lipoprotein cholesterol. Moderate reductions in total plasma cholesterol and low density lipoprotein cholesterol were observed for the Lopid treatment group as a whole, but the lipid response was heterogeneous, especially among different Fredrickson types. The study involved subjects with serum non-HDL-cholesterol of over 200 mg/dL and no previous history of coronary heart disease. Over the 5-year study period, the Lopid group experienced a 1.4% absolute (34% relative) reduction in the rate of serious coronary events (sudden cardiac deaths plus fatal and nonfatal myocardial infarctions) compared to placebo, p = 0.04 (see Table I). There was a 37% relative reduction in the rate of nonfatal myocardial infarction compared to placebo, equivalent to a treatment-related difference of 13.1 events per thousand persons. Deaths from any cause during the double-blind portion of the study totaled 44 (2.2%) in the Lopid randomization group and 43 (2.1%) in the placebo group.

Among Fredrickson types, during the 5-year double-blind portion of the primary prevention component of the Helsinki Heart Study, the greatest reduction in the incidence of serious coronary events occurred in Type IIb patients who had elevations of both LDL-cholesterol and total plasma triglycerides. This subgroup of Type IIb gemfibrozil group patients had a lower mean HDL-cholesterol level at baseline than the Type IIa subgroup that had elevations of LDL-cholesterol and normal plasma triglycerides. The mean increase in HDL-cholesterol among the Type IIb patients in this study was 12.6% compared to placebo. The mean change in LDL-cholesterol among Type IIb patients was −4.1% with Lopid compared to a rise of 3.9% in the placebo subgroup. The Type IIb subjects in the Helsinki Heart Study had 26 fewer coronary events per thousand persons over 5 years in the gemfibrozil group compared to placebo. The difference in coronary events was substantially greater between Lopid and placebo for that subgroup of patients with the triad of LDL-cholesterol >175 mg/dL (>4.5 mmol), triglycerides >200 mg/dL (>2.2 mmol), and HDL-cholesterol <35 mg/dL (<0.90 mmol) (see Table I).

Further information is available from a 3.5 year (8.5 year cumulative) follow-up of all subjects who had participated in the Helsinki Heart Study. At the completion of the Helsinki Heart study, subjects could choose to start, stop, or continue to receive Lopid; without knowledge of their own lipid values or double-blind treatment, 60% of patients originally randomized to placebo began therapy with Lopid and 60% of patients originally randomized to Lopid continued medication. After approximately 6.5 years following randomization, all patients were informed of their original treatment group and lipid values during the 5 years of the double-blind treatment. After further elective changes in Lopid treatment status, 61% of patients in the group originally randomized to Lopid were taking drug; in the group originally randomized to placebo, 65% were taking Lopid. The event rate per 1000 occurring during the open-label follow-up period is detailed in Table II.

Cumulative mortality through 8.5 years showed a 20% relative excess of deaths in the group originally randomized to Lopid versus the originally randomized placebo group and a 20% relative decrease in cardiac events in the group originally randomized to Lopid versus the originally randomized placebo group (see Table III). This analysis of the originally randomized "intent-to-treat" population neglects the possible complicating effects of treatment switching during the open-label phase. Adjustment of hazard ratios taking into account open-label treatment status from years 6.5 to 8.5 could change the reported hazard ratios for mortality toward unity.

Table II
Cardiac Events and All-Cause Mortality (events per 1000 patients) Occurring during the 3.5 Year Open-Label Follow-up to the Helsinki Heart Study[1]

Group:	PDrop N=215	PN N=494	PL N=1283	LDrop N=221	LN N=574	LL N=1207
Cardiac Events	38.8	22.9	22.5	37.2	28.3	25.4
All-Cause Mortality	41.9	22.3	15.6	72.3	19.2	24.9

[1] The six open-label groups are designated first by the original randomization (P = placebo, L = Lopid) and then by the drug taken in the follow-up period (N = Attend clinic but took no drug, L = Lopid, Drop = No attendance at clinic during open-label).

Table III
Cardiac Events, Cardiac Deaths, Non-Cardiac Deaths and All-Cause Mortality in the Helsinki Heart Study, Year 5.0–8.5.[1]

Event	Lopid at Study Start	Placebo at Study Start	Lopid: Placebo Hazard Ratio[2]	Cl Hazard Ratio
Cardiac Events[4]	10	131	0.80	0.62–1.03
Cardiac Deaths	36	38	0.98	0.63–1.54
Non-Cardiac Deaths	65	45	1.40	0.95–2.05
All-Cause Mortality	101	83	1.20	0.90–1.61

[1] Intention-to-Treat Analysis of originally randomized patients neglecting the open-label treatment switches and exposure to study conditions.
[2] Hazard ratio for risk of event in the group originally randomized to Lopid compared to the group originally randomized to placebo neglecting open-label treatment switch and exposure to study condition.
[3] 95% confidence intervals of Lopid:placebo group hazard ratio.
[4] Fatal and non-fatal myocardial infarctions plus sudden cardiac deaths over the 8.5 year period.

It is not clear to what extent the findings of the primary prevention component of the Helsinki Heart Study can be extrapolated to other segments of the dyslipidemic population not studied (such as women, younger or older males, or those with lipid abnormalities limited solely to HDL-cholesterol) or to other lipid-altering drugs.

The secondary prevention component of the Helsinki Heart Study was conducted over 5 years in parallel and at the same centers in Finland in 628 middle-aged males excluded from the primary prevention component of the Helsinki Heart Study because of a history of angina, myocardial infarction or unexplained ECG changes. The primary efficacy endpoint of the study was cardiac events (the sum of fatal and non-

Continued on next page

This product information was prepared in August 1992. On these and other Parke-Davis Products, information may be obtained by addressing PARKE-DAVIS, Division of Warner-Lambert Company, Morris Plains, New Jersey 07950.

Parke-Davis—Cont.

fatal myocardial infarctions and sudden cardiac deaths). The hazard ratio (Lopid:placebo) for cardiac events was 1.47 (95% confidence limits 0.88–2.48, p = 0.14). Of the 35 patients in the Lopid group who experienced cardiac events, 12 patients suffered events after discontinuation from the study. Of the 24 patients in the placebo group with cardiac events, 4 patients suffered events after discontinuation from the study. There were 17 cardiac deaths in the Lopid group and 8 in the placebo group (hazard ratio 2.18; 95% confidence limits 0.94–5.05, p = 0.06). Ten of these deaths in the Lopid group and 3 in the placebo group occurred after discontinuation from therapy. In this study of patients with known or suspected coronary heart disease, no benefit from Lopid treatment was observed in reducing cardiac events or cardiac deaths. Thus, Lopid has shown benefit only in selected dyslipidemic patients *without* suspected or established coronary heart disease. Even in patients with coronary heart disease and the triad of elevated LDL-cholesterol, elevated triglycerides, plus low HDL-cholesterol, the possible effect of Lopid on coronary events has not been adequately studied.

No efficacy in the patients with established coronary heart disease was observed during the Coronary Drug Project with the chemically and pharmacologically related drug, clofibrate. The Coronary Drug Project was a 6-year randomized, double-blind study involving 1000 clofibrate, 1000 nicotinic acid, and 3000 placebo patients with known coronary heart disease. A clinically and statistically significant reduction in myocardial infarctions was seen in the concurrent nicotinic acid group compared to placebo; no reduction was seen with clofibrate.

The mechanism of action of gemfibrozil has not been definitely established. In man, Lopid has been shown to inhibit peripheral lipolysis and to decrease the hepatic extraction of free fatty acids, thus reducing hepatic triglyceride production. Lopid inhibits synthesis and increases clearance of VLDL carrier apolipoprotein B, leading to a decrease in VLDL production.

Animal studies suggest that gemfibrozil may, in addition to elevating HDL-cholesterol, reduce incorporation of long-chain fatty acids into newly formed triglycerides, accelerate turnover and removal of cholesterol from the liver, and increase excretion of cholesterol in the feces. Lopid is well absorbed from the gastrointestinal tract after oral administration. Peak plasma levels occur in 1 to 2 hours with a plasma half-life of 1.5 hours following multiple doses. Plasma levels appear proportional to dose and do not demonstrate accumulation across time following multiple doses.

Lopid mainly undergoes oxidation of a ring methyl group to successively form a hydroxymethyl and a carboxyl metabolite. Approximately seventy percent of the administered human dose is excreted in the urine, mostly as the glucuronide conjugate, with less than 2% excreted as unchanged gemfibrozil. Six percent of the dose is accounted for in the feces.

INDICATIONS AND USAGE

Lopid (gemfibrozil tablets) is indicated as adjunctive therapy to diet for:

1. Treatment of adult patients with very high elevations of serum triglyceride levels (Types IV and V hyperlipidemia) who present a risk of pancreatitis and who do not respond adequately to a determined dietary effort to control them. Patients who present such risk typically have serum triglycerides over 2000 mg/dL and have elevations of VLDL-cholesterol as well as fasting chylomicrons (Type V hyperlipidemia). Subjects who consistently have total serum or plasma triglycerides below 1000 mg/dL are unlikely to present a risk of pancreatitis. Lopid therapy may be considered for those subjects with triglyceride elevations between 1000 and 2000 mg/dL who have a history of pancreatitis or of recurrent abdominal pain typical of pancreatitis. It is recognized that some Type IV patients with triglycerides under 1000 mg/dL may, through dietary or alcoholic indiscretion, convert to a Type V pattern with massive triglyceride elevations accompanying fasting chylomicronemia, but the influence of Lopid therapy on the risk of pancreatitis in such situations has not been adequately studied. Drug therapy is not indicated for patients with Type I hyperlipoproteinemia, who have elevations of chylomicrons and plasma triglycerides, but who have normal levels of very low density lipoprotein (VLDL). Inspection of plasma refrigerated for 14 hours is helpful in distinguishing Types I, IV, and V hyperlipoproteinemia (ref. 3).

2. Reducing the risk of developing coronary heart disease **only** in Type IIb patients without history of or symptoms of existing coronary heart disease who have had an inadequate response to weight loss, dietary therapy, exercise, and other pharmacologic agents (such as bile acid sequestrants and nicotinic acid, known to reduce LDL- and raise HDL-cholesterol **and** who have the following triad of lipid abnormalities: low HDl-cholesterol levels in addition to elevated LDL-cholesterol and elevated triglycerides (see

WARNINGS, PRECAUTIONS, and CLINICAL PHARMACOLOGY). The National Cholesterol Education Program has defined a serum HDL-cholesterol value that is consistently below 35 mg/dL as constituting an independent risk factor for coronary heart disease (ref. 4). Patients with significantly elevated triglycerides should be closely observed when treated with gemfibrozil. In some patients with high triglyceride levels, treatment with gemfibrozil is associated with a significant increase in LDL-cholesterol. BECAUSE OF POTENTIAL TOXICITY SUCH AS MALIGNANCY, GALLBLADDER DISEASE, ABDOMINAL PAIN LEADING TO APPENDECTOMY AND OTHER ABDOMINAL SURGERIES, AN INCREASED INCIDENCE IN NONCORONARY MORTALITY, AND THE 44% RELATIVE INCREASE DURING THE TRIAL PERIOD IN AGE-ADJUSTED ALL-CAUSE MORTALITY SEEN WITH THE CHEMICALLY AND PHARMACOLOGICALLY RELATED DRUG, CLOFIBRATE, THE POTENTIAL BENEFIT OF GEMFIBROZIL IN TREATING TYPE IIA PATIENTS WITH ELEVATIONS OF LDL-CHOLESTEROL ONLY IS NOT LIKELY TO OUTWEIGH THE RISKS. LOPID IS ALSO NOT INDICATED FOR THE TREATMENT OF PATIENTS WITH LOW HDL-CHOLESTEROL AS THEIR ONLY LIPID ABNORMALITY.

In a subgroup analysis of patients in the Helsinki Heart Study with above-median HDL-cholesterol values at baseline (greater than 46.4 mg/dL), the incidence of serious coronary events was similar for gemfibrozil and placebo subgroups (see Table I).

The initial treatment for dyslipidemia is dietary therapy specific for the type of lipoprotein abnormality. Excess body weight and excess alcohol intake may be important factors in hypertriglyceridemia and should be managed prior to any drug therapy. Physical exercise can be an important ancillary measure, and has been associated with rises in HDL-cholesterol. Diseases contributory to hyperlipidemia such as hypothyroidism or diabetes mellitus should be looked for and adequately treated. Estrogen therapy is sometimes associated with massive rises in plasma triglycerides, especially in subjects with familial hypertriglyceridemia. In such cases, discontinuation of estrogen therapy may obviate the need for specific drug therapy of hypertriglyceridemia. The use of drugs should be considered only when reasonable attempts have been made to obtain satisfactory results with nondrug methods. If the decision is made to use drugs, the patient should be instructed that this does not reduce the importance of adhering to diet.

CONTRAINDICATIONS

1. Hepatic or severe renal dysfunction, including primary biliary cirrhosis.
2. Preexisting gallbladder disease (see WARNINGS).
3. Hypersensitivity to gemfibrozil.

WARNINGS

1. Because of chemical, pharmacological, and clinical similarities between gemfibrozil and clofibrate, the adverse findings with clofibrate in two large clinical studies may also apply to gemfibrozil. In the first of those studies, the Coronary Drug Project, 1000 subjects with previous myocardial infarction were treated for 5 years with clofibrate. There was no difference in mortality between the clofibrate-treated subjects and 3000 placebo-treated subjects, but twice as many clofibrate-treated subjects developed cholelithiasis and cholecystitis requiring surgery. In the other study, conducted by the World Health Organization (WHO), 5000 subjects without known coronary heart disease were treated with clofibrate for 5 years and followed one year beyond. There was a statistically significant, 44%, higher age-adjusted total mortality in the clofibrate-treated than in a comparable placebo-treated control group during the trial period. The excess mortality was due to a 33% increase in noncardiovascular causes, including malignancy, post-cholecystectomy complications, and pancreatitis. The higher risk of clofibrate-treated subjects for gallbladder disease was confirmed.

Because of the more limited size of the Helsinki Heart Study, the observed difference in mortality from any cause between the Lopid and placebo group is not statistically significantly different from the 29% excess mortality reported in the clofibrate group in the separate WHO study at the 9 year follow-up (see CLINICAL PHARMACOLOGY). Noncoronary heart disease related mortality showed an excess in the group originally randomized to Lopid primarily due to cancer deaths observed during the open-label extension.

During the 5 year primary prevention component of the Helsinki Heart Study mortality from any cause was 44 (2.2%) in the Lopid group and 43 (2.1%) in the placebo group; including the 3.5 year follow-up period since the trial was completed, cumulative mortality from any cause was 101 (4.9%) in the Lopid group and 83 (4.1%) in the group originally randomized to placebo (hazard ratio 1.20 in favor of placebo). Because of the more limited size of the Helsinki Heart Study, the observed difference in mortality

from any cause between the Lopid and placebo groups at year-5 or at year-8.5 is not statistically significantly different from the 29% excess mortality reported in the clofibrate group in the separate WHO study at the 9 year follow-up. Noncoronary heart disease related mortality showed an excess in the group originally randomized to Lopid at the 8.5 year follow-up (65 Lopid versus 45 placebo noncoronary deaths).

The incidence of cancer (excluding basal cell carcinoma) discovered during the trial and in the 3.5 years after the trial was completed was 51 (2.5%) in both originally randomized groups. In addition, there were 16 basal cell carcinomas in the group originally randomized to Lopid and 9 in the group randomized to placebo (p = 0.22). There were 30 (1.5%) deaths attributed to cancer in the group originally randomized to Lopid and 18 (0.9%) in the group originally randomized to placebo (p = 0.11). Adverse outcomes, including coronary events, were higher in gemfibrozil patients in a corresponding study in men with a history of known or suspected coronary heart disease in the secondary prevention component of the Helsinki Heart Study. (See CLINICAL PHARMACOLOGY.)

2. A gallstone prevalence substudy of 450 Helsinki Heart Study participants showed a trend toward a greater prevalence of gallstones during the study within the Lopid treatment group (7.5% vs 4.9% for the placebo group, a 55% excess for the gemfibrozil group). A trend toward a greater incidence of gallbladder surgery was observed for the Lopid group (17 vs 11 subjects, a 54% excess). This result did not differ statistically from the increased incidence of cholecystectomy observed in the WHO study in the group treated with clofibrate. Both clofibrate and gemfibrozil may increase cholesterol excretion into the bile leading to cholelithiasis. If cholelithiasis is suspected, gallbladder studies are indicated. Lopid therapy should be discontinued if gallstones are found.

3. Since a reduction of mortality from coronary artery disease has not been demonstrated and because liver and interstitial cell testicular tumors were increased in rats, Lopid should be administered only to those patients described in the INDICATIONS AND USAGE section. If a significant serum lipid response is not obtained, Lopid should be discontinued.

4. Concomitant Anticoagulants—Caution should be exercised when anticoagulants are given in conjunction with Lopid. The dosage of the anticoagulant should be reduced to maintain the prothrombin time at the desired level to prevent bleeding complications. Frequent prothrombin determinations are advisable until it has been definitely determined that the prothrombin level has stabilized.

5. Concomitant therapy with Lopid and Mevacor® (lovastatin) has been associated with rhabdomyolysis, markedly elevated creatine kinase (CK) levels and myoglobinuria, leading in a high proportion of cases to acute renal failure. IN VIRTUALLY ALL PATIENTS WHO HAVE HAD AN UNSATISFACTORY LIPID RESPONSE TO EITHER DRUG ALONE, ANY POTENTIAL LIPID BENEFIT OF COMBINED THERAPY WITH LOVASTATIN AND GEMFIBROZIL DOES NOT OUTWEIGH THE RISKS OF SEVERE MYOPATHY, RHABDOMYOLYSIS, AND ACUTE RENAL FAILURE (see Drug Interactions). The use of fibrates alone, including Lopid, may occasionally be associated with myositis. Patients receiving Lopid and complaining of muscle pain, tenderness, or weakness should have prompt medical evaluation for myositis, including serum creatine kinase level determination. If myositis is suspected or diagnosed, Lopid therapy should be withdrawn.

6. Cataracts—Subcapsular bilateral cataracts occurred in 10% and unilateral in 6.3% of male rats treated with gemfibrozil at 10 times the human dose.

PRECAUTIONS

1. **Initial Therapy**—Laboratory studies should be done to ascertain that the lipid levels are consistently abnormal. Before instituting Lopid therapy, every attempt should be made to control serum lipids with appropriate diet, exercise, weight loss in obese patients, and control of any medical problems such as diabetes mellitus and hypothryroidism that are contributing to the lipid abnormalities.

2. **Continued Therapy**—Periodic determination of serum lipids should be obtained, and the drug withdrawn if lipid response is inadequate after 3 months of therapy.

3. **Drug Interactions**—(A) **HMG-CoA reductase inhibitors:** Rhabdomyolysis has occurred with combined gemfibrozil and lovastatin therapy. It may be seen as early as 3 weeks after initiation of combined therapy or after several months. In most subjects who have had an unsatisfactory lipid response to either drug alone, the possible benefit of combined therapy with lovastatin (or other HMG-CoA reductase inhibitors) and gemfibrozil does not outweigh the risks of severe myopathy, rhabdomyolysis, and acute renal failure. There is no assurance that periodic monitoring of creatine kinase will prevent the occurrence of severe myopathy and kidney damage.

(B) Anticoagulants: CAUTION SHOULD BE EXERCISED WHEN ANTICOAGULANTS ARE GIVEN IN CONJUNCTION WITH LOPID. THE DOSAGE OF THE ANTICOAGULANT SHOULD BE REDUCED TO MAINTAIN THE PROTHROMBIN TIME AT THE DESIRED LEVEL TO PREVENT BLEEDING COMPLICATIONS. FREQUENT PROTHROMBIN DETERMINATIONS ARE ADVISABLE UNTIL IT HAS BEEN DEFINITELY DETERMINED THAT THE PROTHROMBIN LEVEL HAS STABILIZED.

4. **Carcinogenesis, Mutagenesis, Impairment of Fertility**—Long-term studies have been conducted in rats at 0.2 and 2 times the human dose (based on surface area, mg/meter^2). The incidence of benign liver nodules and liver carcinomas was significantly increased in high dose male rats. The incidence of liver carcinomas increased also in low dose males, but this increase was not statistically significant (p=0.1). Male rats had a dose-related and statistically significant increase of benign Leydig cell tumors. The higher dose female rats had a significant increase in the combined incidence of benign and malignant liver neoplasms.

Long-term studies have been conducted in mice at 0.1 and 1 times the human dose (based on surface area). There were no statistically significant differences from controls in the incidence of liver tumors, but the doses tested were lower than those shown to be carcinogenic with other fibrates.

Electron microscopy studies have demonstrated a florid hepatic peroxisome proliferation following Lopid administration to the male rat. An adequate study to test for peroxisome proliferation has not been done in humans, but changes in peroxisome morphology have been observed. Peroxisome proliferation has been shown to occur in humans with either of two other drugs of the fibrate class when liver biopsies were compared before and after treatment in the same individual.

Administration of approximately 0.6 and 2 times the human dose (based on surface area) to male rats for 10 weeks resulted in a dose-related decrease of fertility. Subsequent studies demonstrated that this effect was reversed after a drug-free period of about eight weeks, and it was not transmitted to the offspring.

5. **Pregnancy Category C**—Lopid has been shown to produce adverse effects in rats and rabbits at doses between 0.5 and 3 times the human dose (based on surface area) but no developmental toxicity or teratogenicity among offspring of either species. There are no adequate and well-controlled studies in pregnant women. Lopid should be used during pregnancy only if the potential benefit justifies the potential risk to the fetus.

Administration of Lopid to female rats at 0.6 and 2 times the human dose (based on surface area) before and throughout gestation caused a dose-related decrease in conception rate and, at the high dose, an increase in stillborns and a slight reduction in pup weight during lactation. There were also dose-related increased skeletal variations. Anophthalmia occurred, but rarely.

Administration of 0.6 and 2 times the human dose (based on surface area) of Lopid to female rats from gestation day 15 through weaning caused dose-related decreases in birth weight and suppressions of pup growth during lactation.

Administration of 1 and 3 times the human dose (based on surface area) of Lopid to female rabbits during organogenesis caused a dose-related decrease in litter size and, at the high dose, an increased incidence of parietal bone variations.

6. **Nursing Mothers**—It is not known whether this drug is excreted in human milk. Because many drugs are excreted in human milk and because of the potential for tumorigenicity shown for Lopid in animal studies, a decision should be made whether to discontinue nursing or to discontinue the drug, taking into account the importance of the drug to the mother.

7. **Hematologic Changes**—Mild hemoglobin, hematocrit and white blood cell decreases have been observed in occasional patients following initiation of Lopid therapy. However, these levels stabilize during long-term administration. Rarely, severe anemia, leukopenia, thrombocytopenia, and bone marrow hypoplasia have been reported. Therefore, periodic blood counts are recommended during the first 12 months of Lopid administration.

8. **Liver Function**—Abnormal liver function tests have been observed occasionally during Lopid administration, including elevations of AST (SGOT), ALT (SGPT), LDH, bilirubin, and alkaline phosphatase. These are usually reversible when Lopid is discontinued. Therefore periodic liver function studies are recommended and Lopid therapy should be terminated if abnormalities persist.

9. **Kidney Function**—There have been reports of worsening renal insufficiency upon the addition of Lopid therapy in individuals with baseline plasma creatinine > 2.0 mg/dL. In such patients, the use of alternative therapy should be considered against the risks and benefits of a lower dose of Lopid.

10. **Use in Children**—Safety and efficacy in children have not been established.

ADVERSE REACTIONS

In the double-blind controlled phase of the primary prevention component of the Helsinki Heart Study, 2046 patients received Lopid for up to 5 years. In that study, the following adverse reactions were statistically more frequent in subjects in the Lopid group:

	LOPID (N=2046)	PLACEBO (N=2035)
	Frequency in percent of subjects	
Gastrointestinal reactions	34.2	23.8
Dyspepsia	19.6	11.9
Abdominal pain	9.8	5.6
Acute appendicitis (histologically confirmed in most cases where data were available)	1.2	0.6
Atrial fibrillation	0.7	0.1

Adverse events reported by more than 1% of subjects, but without a significant difference between groups:

Diarrhea	7.2	6.5
Fatigue	3.8	3.5
Nausea/Vomiting	2.5	2.1
Eczema	1.9	1.2
Rash	1.7	1.3
Vertigo	1.5	1.3
Constipation	1.4	1.3
Headache	1.2	1.1

Gallbladder surgery was performed in 0.9% of Lopid and 0.5% of placebo subjects in the primary prevention component, a 64% excess, which is not statistically different from the excess of gallbladder surgery observed in the clofibrate compared to the placebo group of the WHO study. Gallbladder surgery was also performed more frequently in the Lopid group compared to placebo (1.9% vs 0.3%, p = 0.07) in the secondary prevention component. A statistically significant increase in appendectomy in the gemfibrozil group was seen also in the secondary prevention component (6 on gemfibrozil vs 0 on placebo, p = 0.014).

Nervous system and special senses adverse reactions were more common in the Lopid group. These included hypesthesia, paresthesias, and taste perversion. Other adverse reactions that were more common among Lopid treatment group

	CAUSAL RELATIONSHIP PROBABLE	CAUSAL RELATIONSHIP NOT ESTABLISHED
General:		weight loss
Cardiac:		extrasystoles
Gastrointestinal:	cholestatic jaundice	pancreatitis
		hepatoma
		colitis
Central Nervous System:	dizziness	confusion
	somnolence	convulsions
	paresthesia	syncope
	peripheral neuritis	
	decreased libido	
	depression	
	headache	
Eye:	blurred vision	retinal edema
Genitourinary:	impotence	decreased male fertility
		renal dysfunction
Musculoskeletal:	myopathy	
	myasthenia	
	myalgia	
	painful extremities	
	arthralgia	
	synovitis	
	rhabdomyolysis (see WARNINGS and Drug Interactions under PRECAUTIONS)	
Clinical Laboratory:	increased creatine phosphokinase	positive antinuclear antibody
	increased bilirubin	
	increased liver transaminases (AST [SGOT], ALT [SGPT])	
	increased alkaline phosphatase	
Hematopoietic:	anemia	thrombocytopenia
	leukopenia	
	bone marrow hypoplasia	
	eosinophilia	
Immunologic:	angioedema	anaphylaxis
	laryngeal edema	Lupus-like syndrome
	urticaria	vasculitis
Integumentary:	exfoliative dermatitis	alopecia
	rash	
	dermatitis	
	pruritus	

subjects but where a causal relationship was not established include cataracts, peripheral vascular disease, and intracerebral hemorrhage.

From other studies it seems probable that Lopid is causally related to the occurrence of MUSCULOSKELETAL SYMPTOMS (see WARNINGS), and to ABNORMAL LIVER FUNCTION TESTS and HEMATOLOGIC CHANGES (see PRECAUTIONS).

Reports of viral and bacterial infections (common cold, cough, urinary tract infections) were more common in gemfibrozil treated patients in other controlled clinical trials of 805 patients. Additional adverse reactions that have been reported for gemfibrozil are listed above by system. These are categorized according to whether a causal relationship to treatment with Lopid is probable or not established:

DOSAGE AND ADMINISTRATION

The recommended dose for adults is 1200 mg administered in two divided doses 30 minutes before the morning and evening meal.

OVERDOSE

While there has been no reported case of overdosage, symptomatic supportive measures should be taken should it occur.

HOW SUPPLIED

Lopid (Tablet 737), white, elliptical, film-coated, scored tablets, each containing 600 mg gemfibrozil, are available as follows:

N 0071-0737-20: Bottles of 60
N 0071-0737-30: Bottles of 500
N 0071-0737-40: Unit dose packages of 100 (10 strips of 10 tablets each)
Parcode No. 737
Storage: Store below 30°C (86°F).

REFERENCES

1. Frick MH, Elo O, Haapa K, et al: Helsinki Heart Study: Primary prevention trial with gemfibrozil in middle-aged men with dyslipidemia. *N Engl J Med* 1987; 317:1237-1245.

Continued on next page

This product information was prepared in August 1992. On these and other Parke-Davis Products, information may be obtained by addressing PARKE-DAVIS, Division of Warner-Lambert Company, Morris Plains, New Jersey 07950.

Parke-Davis—Cont.

2. Manninen V, Elo O, Frick MH, et al: Lipid alterations and decline in the incidence of coronary heart disease in the Helsinki Heart Study. *JAMA* 1988; 260:641-651.
3. Nikkila EA: Familial lipoprotein lipase deficiency and related disorders of chylomicron metabolism. In Stanbury J.B. et al. (eds.): *The Metabolic Basis of Inherited Disease*, 5th ed., McGraw-Hill, 1983, Chap. 30, pp. 622-642.
4. Report of the National Cholesterol Education Program Expert Panel on Detection, Evaluation, and Treatment of High Blood Cholesterol. *Arch Int Med* 1988;148:36-69.
Caution—Federal law prohibits dispensing without prescription.

0737G015

Shown in Product Identification Section, page 422

MANDELAMINE® TABLETS   ℞
[măn"dĕ'lă-mı̄ne]
(methenamine mandelate tablets, USP)

MANDELAMINE SUSPENSION FORTE,   ℞
500 mg/5ml

MANDELAMINE SUSPENSION,   ℞
250 mg/5ml
(methenamine mandelate
oral suspension, USP)

MANDELAMINE GRANULES   ℞
(methenamine mandelate)

DESCRIPTION

Mandelamine (methenamine mandelate, USP), a urinary antibacterial agent, is the chemical combination of mandelic acid with methenamine. Mandelamine is available for oral use as film-coated tablets, suspension, and granules.
Each tablet contains 0.5 g or 1 g of methenamine mandelate, USP; and also contains calcium stearate, NF; candelilla wax; colloidal silicon dioxide, NF; croscarmellose sodium, NF; hydroxypropylmethylcellulose; Opaspray brown (0.5 g tablet) or Opaspray purple (1 g tablet); povidone, USP; propylene glycol, USP; and silica gel.
Each teaspoonful of suspension contains 250 mg or 500 mg of methenamine mandelate, USP; and also contains flavors; propylparaben, NF; saccharin sodium, USP; sesame oil, NF and thixcin. The 500 mg per teaspoonful suspension also contains D&C red No. 6 Ba Lake.
Each packet of granules contains 0.5 g or 1 g of methenamine mandelate, USP; and also contains colloidal silicon dioxide, NF; D&C yellow No. 10; FD&C yellow No. 6 (sunset yellow); flavors; povidone, USP; saccharin sodium, USP; and sucrose, NF.

CLINICAL PHARMACOLOGY

Mandelamine is readily absorbed but remains essentially inactive until it is excreted by the kidney and concentrated in the urine. An acid urine is essential for antibacterial action, with maximum efficacy occurring at pH 5.5 or less. In an acid urine, mandelic acid exerts its antibacterial action and also contributes to the acidification of the urine. Mandelic acid is excreted by both glomerular filtration and tubular excretion. The methenamine component, in an acid urine, is hydrolyzed to ammonia and to the bactericidal agent formaldehyde. There is equally effective antibacterial activity against both gram-positive and gram-negative organisms, since the antibacterial action of mandelic acid and formaldehyde is nonspecific. There are reports that Mandelamine is ineffective in some infections with *Proteus vulgaris* and urea-splitting strains of *Pseudomonas aeruginosa* and *A aerogenes*. Since urea-splitting strains may raise the pH of the urine, particular attention to supplementary acidification is required. However, results in any single case will depend to a large extent on the underlying pathology and the overall management.

INDICATIONS AND USAGE

Mandelamine is indicated for the suppression or elimination of bacteriuria associated with pyelonephritis, cystitis, and other chronic urinary tract infections; also for infected residual urine sometimes accompanying neurologic diseases. When used as recommended, Mandelamine is particularly suitable for long-term therapy because of its safety and because resistance to the nonspecific bactericidal action of formaldehyde does not develop. Pathogens resistant to other antibacterial agents may respond to Mandelamine because of the non-specific effect of formaldehyde formed in an acid urine.
Prophylactic use rationale: Urine is a good culture medium for many urinary pathogens. Inoculation by a few organisms (relapse or reinfection) may lead to bacteriuria in susceptible individuals. Thus, the rationale of management in recurring urinary tract infection (bacteriuria) is to change the urine from a growth-supporting to a growth-inhibiting medium. There is a growing body of evidence that long-term adminis-

DOSAGES

Dosage

	Adults	Children
Tablets and Granules		
1 gram	1 tablet qid	
	1 packet qid	
0.5 gram	2 tablets qid	(Ages 6–12) 1 tablet qid
	—	(Ages 6–12) 1 packet qid
Suspension Forte		
500 mg/ 5 ml teasp.	2 teaspoonfuls (10 ml) qid	(Ages 6–12) 1 teaspoonful (5 ml) qid
Suspension		
250 mg/5 ml teasp.	—	(Age under 6) 1 teaspoonful (5 ml) per 30 lb body weight qid

tration of Mandelamine can prevent the recurrence of bacteriuria in patients with chronic pyelonephritis.
Therapeutic use rationale: Mandelamine helps to sterilize the urine, and in some situations in which underlying pathologic conditions prevent sterilization by any means, it can help to suppress the bacteriuria. Mandelamine should not be used alone for acute infections with parenchymal involvement causing systemic symptoms such as chills and fever. A thorough diagnostic investigation as a part of the overall management of the urinary tract infection should accompany the use of Mandelamine.

CONTRAINDICATIONS

Contraindicated in renal insufficiency.
Mandelamine should not be used in patients who have previously exhibited hypersensitivity to it.

PRECAUTIONS

General: Dysuria may occur (usually at higher than recommended dosage). This can be controlled by reducing the dosage and the acidification. When urine acidification is contraindicated or unattainable (as with some urea-splitting bacteria), the drug is not recommended.
To avoid inducing lipid pneumonia, administer Mandelamine Suspension Forte and Mandelamine Suspension with care to elderly, debilitated or otherwise susceptible patients.
Drug Interactions: Formaldehyde and sulfamethizole form an insoluble precipitate in acid urine; therefore, Mandelamine should not be administered concurrently with sulfamethizole.
Drug/Laboratory Test Interactions: Formaldehyde interferes with fluorometric procedures for determination of urinary catecholamines and vanilmandelic acid (VMA) causing erroneously high results. Formaldehyde also causes falsely decreased urine estriol levels by reacting with estriol when acid hydrolysis techniques are used; estriol determinations which use enzymatic hydrolysis are unaffected by formaldehyde. Formaldehyde causes falsely elevated 17-hydroxycorticosteroid levels when the Porter-Silber method is used and falsely decreased 5-hydroxy-indoleacetic acid (5HIAA) levels by inhibiting color development when nitrosonaphthol methods are used.
Pregnancy Category C. Animal reproduction studies have not been conducted with Mandelamine. It is also not known whether Mandelamine can cause fetal harm when administered to a pregnant woman or can affect reproduction capacity. Mandelamine should be given to a pregnant woman only if clearly needed.
Since introduction, published reports on the use of Mandelamine in pregnant women have not shown an increased risk of fetal abnormalities from use during pregnancy.

ADVERSE REACTIONS

An occasional patient may experience gastrointestinal disturbance or a generalized skin rash. Microscopic and rarely gross hematuria have been described.

DOSAGE AND ADMINISTRATION

Directions for using Granules: dissolve contents of packet in 2–4 oz of water immediately before using. Solution formed may remain turbid.
Suspensions: Shake well before using.
The average adult dosage is 4 grams daily given as 1 gram after each meal and at bedtime. Children 6 to 12 should re-

ceive half the adult dose and children under 6 years of age should receive 250 mg per 30 lb body weight, four times daily. (See chart.) Since an acid urine is essential for antibacterial activity, with maximum efficacy occurring at pH 5.5 or below, restriction of alkalinizing foods and medication is thus desirable. If testing of urine pH reveals the need, supplemental acidification should be given.

HOW SUPPLIED

Mandelamine Tablets are supplied as:
N 0071-0166-24 0.5 g—Bottles of 100
Each tablet is film coated, brown, and bears the P-D 166 monogram.
N 0071-0167-24 1 g—Bottles of 100
Each tablet is film coated, and bears the P-D 167 monogram.
Mandelamine Granules are supplied as:
N 0071-2176-03 1 g—Cartons of 56 individual packets.
Granules are orange flavored.
Mandelamine Suspension is supplied as:
N 0071-2173-23 250 mg/5 ml—Bottles of 16 fl oz
Suspension is cream colored, coconut flavored, and in vegetable oil.
Mandelamine Suspension Forte is supplied as:
N 0071-2174-23 500 mg/5 ml—Bottles of 16 fl oz
Suspension is rosy pink, cherry flavored, and in vegetable oil.
Store between 15°–30°C (59°–86°F).

0166G039

Shown in Product Identification Section, page 422

MECLOMEN®   ℞
[mĕ'clō"mĕn]
(Meclofenamate Sodium Capsules, USP)

DESCRIPTION

Meclomen (meclofenamate sodium) is N-(2, 6-dichloro-m-tolyl) anthranilic acid, sodium salt, monohydrate. It is an antiinflammatory drug for oral administration. Meclomen capsules contain 50 mg or 100 mg meclofenamic acid as the sodium salt. Also contains lactose, NF; magnesium stearate, NF; silica gel, NF; sodium lauryl sulfate, NF. The capsule shell contains colloidal silicon dioxide, NF; FD&C yellow No. 6; gelatin, NF; sodium lauryl sulfate, NF; titanium dioxide, USP.
The structural formula of Meclomen is below:

$$CO_2Na \cdot H_2O$$

It is a white powder with melting point 287° to 291°C, molecular weight 336.15, and water solubility greater than 250 mg/mL.

CLINICAL PHARMACOLOGY
PHARMACODYNAMICS

Meclomen is a nonsteroidal agent which has demonstrated antiinflammatory, analgesic, and antipyretic activity in laboratory animals. The mode of action, like that of other nonsteroidal antiinflammatory agents, is not known. Therapeutic action does not result from pituitary-adrenal stimulation. In animal studies, Meclomen was found to inhibit prostaglandin synthesis and to compete for binding at the prostaglandin receptor site. In vitro, Meclomen was found to be an inhibitor of human leukocyte 5-lipoxygenase activity. These properties may be responsible for the antiinflammatory action of Meclomen. There is no evidence that Meclomen alters the course of the underlying disease.
In several human isotope studies, Meclomen, at a dosage of 300 mg/day, produced a fecal blood loss of 1 to 2 ml per day and 2 to 3 ml per day at 400 mg/day. Aspirin, at a dosage of 3.6 g/day, caused a fecal blood loss of 6 ml per day.
In a multiple-dose, one-week study in normal human volunteers, Meclomen had little or no effect on collagen-induced platelet aggregation, platelet count, or bleeding time. In comparison, aspirin suppressed collagen-induced platelet aggregation and increased bleeding time. The concomitant administration of antacids (aluminum and magnesium hydroxides) does not interfere with absorption of Meclomen.
PHARMACOKINETICS

Meclomen is rapidly absorbed in man following single and multiple oral doses with peak plasma concentrations occurring in 0.5 to 2 hours. Based on a comparison to a suspension of meclofenamic acid, Meclomen is completely bioavailable. The plasma concentrations of meclofenamic acid decline monoexponentially following oral administration. In a study in 10 healthy subjects following a single oral dose the apparent elimination half-life ranged from 0.8 to 5.3 hours. After the administration of Meclomen for 14 days every 8 hours, the apparent elimination half-life ranged from 0.8 to 2.1

hours with no evidence of accumulation of meclofenamic acid in plasma (see Table).

Meclofenamic acid is extensively metabolized to an active metabolite (Metabolite I; 3-hydroxymethyl metabolite of meclofenamic acid) and at least six other less well characterized minor metabolites.

Only this Metabolite I has been shown *in vitro* to inhibit cyclooxygenase activity with approximately one fifth the activity of Meclomen. Metabolite I (3-hydroxymethyl metabolite of meclofenamic acid) with a mean half-life of approximately 15 hours did accumulate following multiple dosing. After the administration of 100 mg Meclomen for 14 days every 8 hours, Metabolite I reached a peak plasma concentration of only 1 μg/mL. By contrast, the peak concentration was 4.8 μg/mL for the parent compound on both days 1 and 14. Therefore, the accumulation of Metabolite I is probably not clinically significant.

Approximately 70% of the administered dose is excreted by the kidneys with 8–35% excreted as predominantly conjugated species of meclofenamic acid and Metabolite I (see Table). Other metabolites, whose excretion rates are unknown, account for the remaining 35–62% of the dose excreted in the urine. The remainder of the administered dose (approximately 30%) is eliminated in the feces (apparently through biliary excretion). There is insufficient experience to know if Meclomen or its metabolites accumulate in patients with compromised renal or hepatic function. Therefore, Meclomen should be used with caution in these patients. (See PRECAUTIONS.) Trace amounts of Meclomen are excreted in human breast milk.

Meclofenamic acid is greater than 99% bound to plasma proteins over a wide drug concentration range.

Unlike most NSAIDs, which when administered with food have a decrease in rate but not in extent of absorption, meclofenamic acid is decreased in both. Following the administration of Meclomen capsules one half-hour after a meal, the average extent of bioavailability decreased by 26%, the average peak concentration (Cmax) decreased 4 fold and the time to Cmax was delayed by 3 hours.

CLINICAL STUDIES

Controlled clinical trials comparing Meclomen with aspirin demonstrated comparable efficacy in rheumatoid arthritis. The Meclomen-treated patients had fewer reactions involving the special senses, specifically tinnitus, but more gastrointestinal reactions, specifically diarrhea.

The incidence of patients who discontinued therapy due to adverse reactions was similar for both the Meclomen and aspirin-treated groups.

The improvement with Meclomen reported by patients and the reduction of the disease activity as evaluated by both physicians and patients with rheumatoid arthritis are associated with a significant reduction in number of tender joints, severity of tenderness, and duration of morning stiffness.

The improvement reported by patients and as evaluated by physicians in patients treated with Meclomen for osteoarthritis is associated with a significant reduction in night pain, pain on walking, degree of starting pain, and pain on passive motion. The function of knee joints also improved significantly.

Meclomen has been used in combination with gold salts or corticosteroids in patients with rheumatoid arthritis. Studies have demonstrated that Meclomen contributes to the improvement of patients' conditions while maintained on gold salts or corticosteroids. Data are inadequate to demonstrate that Meclomen in combination with salicylates produces greater improvement than that achieved with Meclomen alone.

In controlled clinical trials of patients with mild to moderate pain, Meclomen 50 mg provided significant pain relief. In these studies of episiotomy and dental pain, Meclomen 100 mg demonstrated additional benefit in some patients. The onset of analgesic effect was generally within one hour and the duration of action was 4 to 6 hours.

In controlled clinical trials of patients with dysmenorrhea, Meclomen 100 mg t.i.d. provided significant reduction in the symptoms associated with dysmenorrhea.

In randomized double-blind crossover trials of Meclomen 100 mg t.i.d. versus placebo in women with heavy menstrual blood loss (MBL), Meclomen treatment was usually associated with a reduction in menstrual flow.

The graph above is a scatter plot of menstrual flow from the average of two menstrual periods on Meclomen treatments (x-axis) versus two menstrual periods on placebo (y-axis) for 55 women. Of note, although the amount of reduction in MBL was variable, some degree of reduction occurred in 90% of women in this study.

The points on the graph represent the mean MBL for each subject when treated for two periods with placebo and two periods with Meclomen. To ease in interpretation, the following examples may be helpful. Point A represents a woman who had MBL of 459 mL while on placebo, and 405 mL on Meclomen. Point B represents a woman who had MBL of 472 mL while on placebo, and 64 mL when treated with Meclomen.

TABLE
SUMMARY OF MECLOMEN PHARMACOKINETIC PARAMETERS
Mean (Range) Parameter Values (n = 10)

	Meclofenamic Acid		Metabolite I[a]	
	100-mg[c]			
Cmax μg/mL[1]	4.8	(1.8–7.2)	1.0	(0.5–1.5)
tmax hr[2]	0.9	(0.5–1.5)	2.4	(0.5–4.0)
Cmin μg/mL[3]	0.2	(0.5–1.5)	0.4	(0.2–1.1)
Cl/F mL/min[4]	206.0	(126–342)	–	
Vd/F liters[5]	23.3	(9.1–43.2)	–	
t₁/₂ hr[6]	1.3	(0.8–2.1)	15.3[b]	
% of Dose in Urine				
Unconjugated	0.0	–	0.5	(0–1.2)
Total	2.7	(0–4.5)	21.6	(7.5–32.6)

[a] 3-Hydroxymethyl metabolite of meclofenamic acid with 20% activity of Meclomen *in vitro*
[b] Estimated from mean data
[c] Administered every 8 hours for 14 days
[1] Peak plasma concentration
[2] Time to peak plasma concentration
[3] Trough plasma concentration
[4] Oral clearance
[5] Oral distribution volume
[6] Elimination half-life

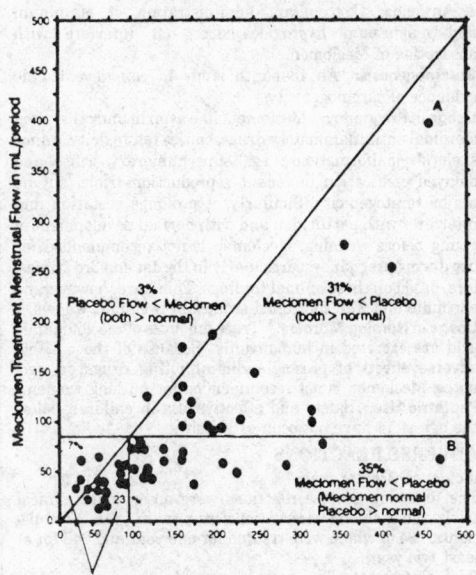

Scattergram of Menstrual Flow Average of Two Periods on Each Treatment of 55 Women from Three Clinical Trials

Placebo Treatment Menstrual Flow in mL/period
Placebo - Meclomen (both within normal range)

In association with this reduction in menstrual blood loss, the duration of menses was decreased by 1 day, tampon/pad usage was decreased by an average of 2 per day on the two days of heaviest flow, and symptoms of dysmenorrhea were significantly reduced.

INDICATIONS AND USAGE

Meclomen is indicated for the relief of mild to moderate pain. Meclomen is also indicated for the treatment of primary dysmenorrhea and for the treatment of idiopathic heavy menstrual blood loss. (See CLINICAL PHARMACOLOGY and PRECAUTIONS sections.)

Meclomen is also indicated for relief of the signs and symptoms of acute and chronic rheumatoid arthritis and osteoarthritis. As with all nonsteroidal antiinflammatory drugs, selection of Meclomen requires a careful assessment of the benefit/risk ratio. (See WARNINGS, PRECAUTIONS and ADVERSE REACTIONS sections.)

Meclomen is not recommended in children because adequate studies to demonstrate safety and efficacy have not been carried out.

CONTRAINDICATIONS

Meclomen should not be used in patients who have previously exhibited hypersensitivity to it.

Because the potential exists for cross-sensitivity to aspirin or other nonsteroidal antiinflammatory drugs, Meclomen should not be given to patients in whom these drugs induce symptoms of bronchospasm, allergic rhinitis, or urticaria.

WARNINGS

Risk of GI Ulceration, Bleeding and Perforation with NSAID Therapy: Serious gastrointestinal toxicity, such as bleeding, ulceration, and perforation, can occur at any time, with or without warning symptoms, in patients treated chroni-

cally with NSAID therapy. Although minor upper gastrointestinal problems, such as dyspepsia, are common, usually developing early in therapy, physicians should remain alert for ulceration and bleeding in patients treated chronically with NSAIDs even in the absence of previous GI tract symptoms. In patients observed in clinical trials of several months to two years' duration, symptomatic upper GI ulcers, gross bleeding or perforation appear to occur in approximately 1% of patients treated for 3–6 months, and in about 2–4% of patients treated for one year. Physicians should inform patients about the signs and/or symptoms of serious GI toxicity and what steps to take if they occur.

Studies to date have not identified any subset of patients not at risk of developing peptic ulceration and bleeding. Except for a prior history of serious GI events and other risks factors known to be associated with peptic ulcer disease, such as alcoholism, smoking, etc, no risk factors (eg, age, sex) have been associated with increased risk. Elderly or debilitated patients seem to tolerate ulceration or bleeding less well than other individuals, and most spontaneous reports of fatal GI events are in this population. Studies to date are inconclusive concerning the relative risk of various NSAIDs in causing such reactions. High doses of any NSAID probably carry a greater risk of these reactions, although controlled clinical trials showing this do not exist in most cases. In considering the use of relatively large doses (within the recommended dosage range), sufficient benefit should be anticipated to offset the potential increased risk of GI toxicity.

PRECAUTIONS

General: Patients receiving nonsteroidal antiinflammatory agents, such as Meclomen, should be evaluated periodically to insure that the drug is still necessary and well tolerated. (See other PRECAUTIONS, WARNINGS, and ADVERSE REACTIONS.)

Diarrhea, gastrointestinal irritation and abdominal pain may be associated with Meclomen therapy. Dosage reduction or temporarily stopping the drug have generally controlled these symptoms. (See ADVERSE REACTIONS and DOSAGE AND ADMINISTRATION sections.)

Decreases in hemoglobin and/or hematocrit levels have occurred in approximately 1 of 6 patients, but rarely required discontinuation of Meclomen therapy. The clinical data revealed no evidence of increased chronic blood loss, bone-marrow suppression, or hemolysis to account for the decreases in hemoglobin or hematocrit levels. Patients who are receiving long-term Meclomen therapy should have hemoglobin and hematocrit values determined if anemia is suspected on clinical grounds.

If a patient develops visual symptoms (see ADVERSE REACTIONS) during Meclomen therapy, the drug should be discontinued and the patient should have a complete ophthalmologic examination.

When Meclomen is used in combination with steroid therapy, any reduction in steroid dosage should be gradual to avoid the possible complications of sudden steroid withdrawal.

Elderly: Adverse effects are seen more commonly in the elderly; therefore, a lower starting dose and careful follow-up are advised.

Continued on next page

This product information was prepared in August 1992. On these and other Parke-Davis Products, information may be obtained by addressing PARKE-DAVIS, Division of Warner-Lambert Company, Morris Plains, New Jersey 07950.

Parke-Davis—Cont.

Evaluation of Patients with Heavy Menstrual Blood Loss: Prior to prescribing Meclomen for heavy blood flow and primary dysmenorrhea, a thorough risk/benefit assessment should be made that takes into account the results described in the CLINICAL PHARMACOLOGY section. It is recommended that Meclomen treatment not be prescribed for heavy menstrual flow without establishing its idiopathic nature. Spotting or bleeding between cycles should be evaluated fully and not treated with Meclomen. Worsening of menstrual blood loss or excessive blood loss failing to respond to Meclomen should also be evaluated by an appropriate work-up and not treated with Meclomen.

Hepatic Reactions: As with other nonsteroidal antiinflammatory drugs, borderline evalutions of one or more liver tests may occur in some patients. These abnormalities may progress, may remain essentially unchanged, or may be transient with continued therapy. The SGPT (ALT) test is probably the most sensitive indicator of liver dysfunction. Meaningful (3 times the upper limit of normal) elevations of SGPT or SGOT (AST) occurred in controlled clinical trials in less than 1% of patients. A patient with symptoms and/or signs suggesting liver dysfunction, or in whom an abnormal liver test has occurred, should be evaluated for evidence of the development of more severe hepatic reaction while on therapy with Meclomen. Severe hepatic reactions, including jaundice and cases of fatal hepatitis, have been reported with other nonsteroidal antiinflammatory drugs. Although such reactions are rare, if abnormal liver tests persist or worsen, if clinical signs and symptoms consistent with liver disease develop, or if systemic manifestations occur (eg, eosinophilia, rash), Meclomen should be discontinued.

Renal Effects: As with other nonsteroidal antiinflammatory drugs, long-term administration of meclofenamate sodium to animals has resulted in renal papillary necrosis and other abnormal renal pathology. In humans, there have been reports of acute interstitial nephritis with hematuria, proteinuria, and occasionally nephrotic syndrome.

A second form of renal toxicity has been seen in patients with prerenal conditions leading to a reduction in renal blood flow or blood volume, where the renal prostaglandins have a supportive role in the maintenance of renal perfusion. In these patients administration of an NSAID may cause a dose-dependent reduction in prostaglandin formation and may precipitate overt renal decompensation. Patients at greatest risk of this reaction are those with impaired renal function, heart failure, liver dysfunction, those taking diuretics, and the elderly. Discontinuation of NSAID therapy is typically followed by recovery to the pretreatment state.

Since Meclomen metabolites are eliminated primarily by the kidneys, patients with significantly impaired renal function should be closely monitored; a lower daily dosage should be employed to avoid excessive drug accumulation.

Information for Patients: Patients should be advised that nausea, vomiting, diarrhea, and abdominal pain have been associated with the use of Meclomen. The patient should be made aware of a possible drug connection and accordingly should consider discontinuing the drug and contacting his or her physician if any of these conditions are severe.

Women who are taking Meclomen for heavy menstrual flow should be advised to consult their doctor if they have spotting or bleeding between cycles or worsening of their menstrual blood flow. These symptoms may be signs of the development of a more serious condition that is not appropriately treated with Meclomen.

Meclomen may be taken with meals or milk to control gastrointestinal complaints. Concomitant administration of an antacid (specifically, aluminum and magnesium hydroxides) does not interfere with the absorption of the drug.

Meclomen, like other drugs of its class, is not free of side effects. The side effects of these drugs can cause discomfort and, rarely, there are more serious side effects, such as gastrointestinal bleeding, which may result in hospitalization and even fatal outcomes.

NSAIDs (nonsteroidal antiinflammatory drugs) are often essential agents in the management of arthritis and have a major role in the treatment of pain, but they also may be commonly employed for conditions which are less serious. Physicians may wish to discuss with their patients the potential risks (see WARNINGS, PRECAUTIONS, and ADVERSE REACTIONS sections) and likely benefits of NSAID treatment, particularly when the drugs are used for less serious conditions where treatment without NSAIDs may represent an acceptable alternative to both the patient and physician.

Laboratory Tests: Patients receiving long-term Meclomen therapy should have hemoglobin and hematocrit values determined if signs or symptoms of anemia occur.

Low white blood cell counts were rarely observed in clinical trials. These low counts were transient and usually returned to normal while the patient continued on Meclomen therapy. Persistent leukopenia, granulocytopenia, or thrombocytopenia warrant further clinical evaluation and may require discontinuation of the drug.

When abnormal blood chemistry values are obtained, follow-up studies are indicated.

Elevations of serum transaminase levels and of alkaline phosphatase levels occurred in approximately 4% of patients. An occasional patient had elevations of serum creatinine or BUN levels.

Because serious GI tract ulceration and bleeding can occur without warning symptoms, physicians should follow chronically treated patients for the signs and symptoms of ulceration and bleeding and should inform them of the importance of this follow-up (see Risk of GI Ulcerations, Bleeding and Perforation with NSAID Therapy).

Drug Interactions

1. **Warfarin:** Meclomen enhances the effect of warfarin. Therefore, when Meclomen is given to a patient receiving warfarin, the dosage of warfarin should be reduced to prevent excessive prolongation of the prothrombin time.

2. **Aspirin:** Concurrent administration of aspirin may lower Meclomen plasma levels, possibly by competing for protein-binding sites. The urinary excretion of Meclomen is unaffected by aspirin, indicating no change in Meclomen absorption. Meclomen does not affect serum salicylate levels. Greater fecal blood loss results from concomitant administration of both drugs than from either drug alone.

3. **Propoxyphene:** The concurrent administration of propoxyphene hydrochloride does not affect the bioavailability of Meclomen.

4. **Antacids:** Concomitant administration of aluminum and magnesium hydroxides does not interfere with absorption of Meclomen.

Carcinogenesis: An 18-month study in rats revealed no evidence of carcinogenicity.

Usage in Pregnancy: Meclomen, like aspirin and other nonsteroidal antiinflammatory drugs, causes fetotoxicity, minor skeletal malformations, eg, supernumerary ribs, and delayed ossification in rodent reproduction trials, but no major teratogenicity. Similarly, it prolongs gestation and interferes with parturition and with normal development of young before weaning. Meclomen is not recommended for use during pregnancy, particularly in the 1st and 3rd trimesters, based on these animal findings. There are, however, no adequate and well-controlled studies in pregnant women.

Usage in Nursing Mothers: Trace amounts of meclofenamic acid are excreted in human milk. Because of the possible adverse effects of prostaglandin-inhibiting drugs on neonates, Meclomen is not recommended for nursing women.

Pediatric Use: Safety and effectiveness in children below the age of 14 have not been established.

ADVERSE REACTIONS

Incidence Greater than 1%

The following adverse reactions were observed in clinical trials and included observations from more than 2,700 patients, 594 of whom were treated for one year and 248 for at least two years.

Gastrointestinal: The most frequently reported adverse reactions associated with Meclomen involve the gastrointestinal system. In controlled studies of up to six months duration, these disturbances occurred in the following decreasing order of frequency with the approximate incidences in parentheses: diarrhea (10–33%), nausea with or without vomiting (11%), other gastrointestinal disorders (10%), and abdominal pain.* In long-term uncontrolled studies of up to four years duration, one third of the patients had at least one episode of diarrhea some time during Meclomen therapy.

In approximately 4% of the patients in controlled studies, diarrhea was severe enough to require discontinuation of Meclomen. The occurrence of diarrhea is dose related, generally subsides with dose reduction, and clears with termination of therapy. The incidence of diarrhea in patients with osteoarthritis is generally lower than that reported in patients with rheumatoid arthritis.

Other reactions less frequently reported were pyrosis,* flatulence,* anorexia, constipation, stomatitis, and peptic ulcer. The majority of the patients with peptic ulcer had either a history of ulcer disease or were receiving concomitant antiinflammatory drugs, including corticosteroids, which are known to produce peptic ulceration.

Cardiovascular: edema

Dermatologic: rash,* urticaria, pruritus

Central Nervous System: headache,* dizziness*

Special Senses: tinnitus

Incidence Less than 1%

Probably Causally Related

The following adverse reactions were reported less frequently than 1% during controlled clinical trials and through voluntary reports since marketing. The probability of a causal relationship exists between the drug and these adverse reactions.

Gastrointestinal: bleeding and/or perforation with or without obvious ulcer formation, colitis, cholestatic jaundice

*Incidence between 3% and 9%. Those reactions occurring in 1% to 3% of patients are not marked with an asterisk.

Renal: renal failure.

Hematologic: neutropenia, thrombocytopenic purpura, leukopenia, agranulocytosis, hemolytic anemia, eosinophilia, decrease in hemoglobin and /or hematocrit

Dermatologic: erythema multiforme, Stevens-Johnson syndrome, exfoliative dermatitis

Hepatic: alteration of liver function tests

Allergic: lupus and serum sickness-like symptoms

Incidence Less than 1%

Causal Relationship Unknown

Other reactions have been reported but under conditions where a causal relationship could not be established. However, in these rarely reported events, that possibility cannot be excluded. Therefore, these observations are listed to alert physicians.

Cardiovascular: palpitations

Central Nervous System: malaise, fatigue, paresthesia, insomnia, depression

Special Senses: blurred vision, taste disturbances, decreased visual acuity, temporary loss of vision, reversible loss of color vision, retinal changes including macular fibrosis, macular and perimacular edema, conjunctivitis, iritis

Renal: nocturia

Gastrointestinal: paralytic ileus

Dermatologic: erythema nodosum, hair loss

OVERDOSAGE

The following is based on the little information available concerning overdosage with Melcomen and related compounds. After a massive overdose, CNS stimulation may be manifested by irrational behavior, marked agitation and generalized seizures. Following this phase, renal toxicity (falling urine output, rising creatinine, abnormal urinary cellular elements) may be noted with possible oliguria or anuria and azotemia. A 24-year-old male was anuric for approximately 1 week after ingesting an overdose of 6–7 grams of Meclomen. Spontaneous diuresis and recovery subsequently occurred.

Management consists of emptying the stomach by emesis or lavage and instilling an ample dose of activated charcoal into the stomach. There is some evidence that charcoal will actively absorb Meclomen, but dialysis or hemoperfusion may be less effective because of plasma protein binding. The seizures should be controlled by an appropriate anticonvulsant regimen. Attention should be directed throughout, by careful monitoring, to the preservation of vital functions and fluid-electrolyte balance. Dialysis may be required to correct serious azotemia or electrolyte imbalance.

DOSAGE AND ADMINISTRATION

Usual Dosage: *For mild to moderate pain,* the recommended dose is 50 mg every 4 to 6 hours. Doses of 100 mg may be needed in some patients for optimal pain relief. (See CLINICAL PHARMACOLOGY section.) However, the daily dose should not exceed 400 mg. (See ADVERSE REACTIONS section.)

For excessive menstrual blood loss and primary dysmenorrhea, the recommended dose of Meclomen is 100 mg three times a day, for up to six days, starting at the onset of menstrual flow.

For rheumatoid arthritis and osteoarthritis, including acute exacerbations of chronic disease, the dosage is 200 to 400 mg per day, administered in three or four equal doses.

Therapy should be initiated at the lower dosage, then increased as necessary to improve clinical response. The dosage should be individually adjusted for each patient depending on the severity of the symptoms and the clinical response. The daily dosage should not exceed 400 mg per day. The smallest dosage of Meclomen that yields clinical control should be employed.

Although improvement may be seen in some patients in a few days, two to three weeks of treatment may be required to obtain the optimum therapeutic benefit.

After a satisfactory response has been achieved, the dosage should be adjusted as required. A lower dosage may suffice for long-term administration.

If gastrointestinal complaints occur, see WARNINGS and PRECAUTIONS. Meclomen may be administered with meals or with milk. (See CLINICAL PHARMACOLOGY for a description of food effects.) If intolerance occurs, the dosage may need to be reduced. Therapy should be terminated if any severe adverse reactions occur.

HOW SUPPLIED

(Capsule 268) Meclomen Capsules, each containing meclofenamate sodium monohydrate equivalent to 50 mg meclofenamic acid, are available:

N 0071-0268-24—bottles of 100

N 0071-0268-40—Uni/Use® 100's (10×10)

(Capsule 269) Meclomen Capsules, each containing meclofenamate sodium monohydrate equivalent to 100 mg meclofenamic acid, are available:

N 0071-0269-24—bottles of 100

N 0071-0269-30—bottles of 500

N 0071-0269-40—Uni/Use 100's (10×10)

Storage: Store at room temperature below 30°C (86°F). Protect from moisture and light.

Caution: Federal law prohibits dispensing without prescription.

0268G313

Shown in Product Identification Section, page 422

MILONTIN®   ℞
[mĭ"lŏn'tĭn]
(phensuximide, USP)

DESCRIPTION

Milontin (phensuximide) is an anticonvulsant succinimide, chemically designated as N-methyl-2-phenylsuccinimide. Each Milontin capsule contains 500 mg phensuximide USP. The capsule and band contain citric acid, USP; colloidal silicon dioxide, NF; D&C yellow No. 10, FD&C red No. 3, FD&C yellow No. 6, gelatin, NF; glyceryl monooleate, polyethylene glycol 200, sodium benzoate, NF; sodium lauryl sulfate, NF.

CLINICAL PHARMACOLOGY

Phensuximide suppresses the paroxysmal three-cycle-per-second spike and wave activity associated with lapses of consciousness which is common in absence (petit mal) seizures. The frequency of epileptiform attacks is reduced, apparently by depression of the motor cortex and elevation of the threshold of the central nervous system to convulsive stimuli.

INDICATIONS AND USAGE

Milontin is indicated for the control of absence (petit mal) seizures.

CONTRAINDICATION

Phensuximide should not be used in patients with a history of hypersensitivity to succinimides.

WARNINGS

Blood dyscrasias, including some with fatal outcome, have been reported to be associated with the use of succinimides; therefore, periodic blood counts should be performed. Should signs and/or symptoms of infection (eg sore throat, fever) develop, blood counts should be considered at that point.

It has been reported that succinimides have produced morphological and functional changes in animal liver. For this reason, phensuximide should be administered with extreme caution to patients with known liver or renal diseases. Periodic urinalysis and liver function studies are advised for all patients receiving the drug.

Cases of systemic lupus erythematosus have been reported with the use of succinimides. The physician should be alert to this possibility.

Usage in pregnancy: The effects of Milontin in human pregnancy and nursing infants are unknown.

Recent reports suggest an association between the use of anticonvulsant drugs by women with epilepsy and an elevated incidence of birth defects in children born to these women. Data is more extensive with respect to phenytoin and phenobarbital, but these are also the most commonly prescribed anticonvulsants; less systematic or anecdotal reports suggest a possible similar association with the use of all known anticonvulsant drugs.

The reports suggesting an elevated incidence of birth defects in children of drug-treated epileptic women cannot be regarded as adequate to prove a definite cause-and-effect relationship. There are intrinsic methodologic problems in obtaining adequate data on drug teratogenicity in humans; the possibility also exists that other factors, eg, genetic factors or the epileptic condition itself, may be more important than drug therapy in leading to birth defects. The great majority of mothers on anticonvulsant medication deliver normal infants. It is important to note that anticonvulsant drugs should not be discontinued in patients in whom the drug is administered to prevent major seizures because of the strong possibility of precipitating status epilepticus with attendant hypoxia and threat to life. In individual cases where the severity and frequency of the seizure disorder are such that the removal of medication does not pose a serious threat to the patient, discontinuation of the drug may be considered prior to and during pregnancy, although it cannot be said with any confidence that even minor seizures do not pose some hazard to the developing embryo or fetus.

The prescribing physician will wish to weigh these considerations in treating or counseling epileptic women of childbearing potential.

Hazardous activities: Phensuximide may impair the mental and/or physical abilities required for the performance of potentially hazardous tasks, such as driving a motor vehicle or other such activity requiring alertness; therefore, the patient should be cautioned accordingly.

PRECAUTIONS

General:
Phensuximide, when used alone in mixed types of epilepsy, may increase the frequency of grand mal seizures in some patients.

As with other anticonvulsants, it is important to proceed slowly when increasing or decreasing dosage, as well as when adding or eliminating other medication. Abrupt withdrawal

---

of anticonvulsant medication may precipitate absence (petit mal) status.

Information for Patients:
Phensuximide may impair the mental and/or physical abilities required for the performance of potentially hazardous tasks, such as driving a motor vehicle or other such activity requiring alertness, therefore, the patient should be cautioned accordingly.

Patients taking phensuximide should be advised of the importance of adhering strictly to the prescribed regimen. Patients should be instructed to promptly contact their physician if they develop signs and/or symptoms suggesting an infection (eg sore throat, fever).

Drug Interactions:
Since Milontin (phensuximide), as a member of the succinimide class, may interact with concurrently administered antiepileptic drugs, periodic serum level determinations of these drugs may be necessary.

Pregnancy:
See WARNINGS.

ADVERSE REACTIONS

Gastrointestinal System: Gastrointestinal symptoms, such as nausea, vomiting, and anorexia, occur frequently, but may be the result of overdosage.

Nervous System: Neurologic and sensory reactions reported during therapy with phensuximide have included drowsiness, dizziness, ataxia, headache, dreamlike state, and lethargy. Side effects, such as drowsiness and dizziness, may be relieved by a reduction in total dosage.

Integumentary System: Dermatologic manifestations reported to be associated with the administration of phensuximide have included pruritus, skin eruptions, erythema multiforme, erythematous rashes, Stevens-Johnson syndrome, and alopecia.

Genitourinary System: Genitourinary complications which have been reported include urinary frequency, renal damage, and hematuria.

Hemopoietic System: Hemopoietic complications associated with the administration of phensuximide include granulocytopenia, transient leukopenia, and pancytopenia with or without bone marrow suppression.

Musculoskeletal System: Muscular weakness.

OVERDOSAGE

Acute overdoses may produce nausea, vomiting, and CNS depression including coma with respiratory depression.

Treatment:
Treatment should include emesis (unless the patient is, or could rapidly become, obtunded, comatose, or convulsing) or gastric lavage, activated charcoal, cathartics and general supportive measures. Forced diuresis and exchange transfusions are ineffective.

DOSAGE AND ADMINISTRATION

Milontin (phensuximide capsules, USP) is administered by the oral route in doses of 500 mg to 1 g two or three times daily. As with other anticonvulsant medication, the dosage should be adjusted to suit individual requirements. The total dosage, irrespective of age, may, therefore, vary between 1 and 3 g per day, the average being 1.5 g.

Milontin may be administered in combination with other anticonvulsants when other forms of epilepsy coexist with absence (petit mal).

HOW SUPPLIED

N 0071-0393-24 (Kapseal® 393)—Milontin Kapseals, each containing 0.5 g phensuximide; bottles of 100.

0393G013

Shown in Product Identification Section, page 422

NARDIL®   ℞
[när'dĭl"]
(Phenelzine Sulfate Tablets, USP)

DESCRIPTION

Nardil (phenelzine sulfate) belongs to the class of drugs known as monoamine oxidase (MAO) inhibitors.
Chemically it is phenethylhydrazine sulfate, a hydrazine derivative with the following structural formula:

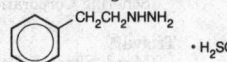

Molecular weight: 234.27

Each Nardil tablet for oral administration contains phenelzine sulfate equivalent to 15 mg of phenelzine base. Also contains acacia, NF; calcium carbonate, carnauba wax, NF; corn starch, NF; FD and C yellow No. 6; gelatin, NF; kaolin, USP; magnesium stearate, NF; mannitol, USP; pharmaceutical glaze, NF; povidone, USP; sucrose, NF; talc, USP; white wax, NF; white wheat flour.

ACTIONS

Monoamine oxidase is a complex enzyme system, widely distributed throughout the body. Drugs that inhibit monoamine oxidase in the laboratory are associated with a number of clinical effects. Thus, it is unknown whether MAO inhibition *per se*, other pharmacologic actions, or an interaction of both is responsible for the clinical effects observed. Therefore, the physician should become familiar with all the effects produced by drugs of this class.

All the currently employed MAO inhibitors are readily absorbed when given by mouth. They are not given parenterally. These drugs produce maximal inhibition of MAO in biopsy samples from man within 5 to 10 days. There is little information on their pharmacokinetics. However, their biological activity is prolonged due to the characteristics of their interaction with the enzyme.

INDICATIONS

Nardil has been found to be effective in depressed patients clinically characterized as "atypical," "nonendogenous," or "neurotic." These patients often have mixed anxiety and depression and phobic or hypochondriacal features. There is less conclusive evidence of its usefulness with severely depressed patients with endogenous features.

Nardil should rarely be the first antidepressant drug used. Rather, it is more suitable for use with patients who have failed to respond to the drugs more commonly used for these conditions.

CONTRAINDICATIONS

Nardil is contraindicated in patients with known sensitivity to the drug, pheochromocytoma, congestive heart failure, a history of liver disease, or abnormal liver function tests.

The potentiation of sympathomimetic substances and related compounds by MAO inhibitors may result in hypertensive crises (See WARNINGS). Therefore, patients being treated with Nardil should not take sympathomimetic drugs (including amphetamines, cocaine, methylphenidate, dopamine, epinephrine and norepinephrine) or related compounds (including methyldopa, L-dopa, L-tryptophan, L-tyrosine, and phenylalanine). Hypertensive crises during Nardil therapy may also be caused by the ingestion of foods with a high concentration of tyramine or dopamine. Therefore, patients being treated with Nardil should avoid high protein food that has undergone protein breakdown by aging, fermentation, pickling, smoking, or bacterial contamination; patients should also avoid cheeses (especially aged varieties), pickled herring, beer, wine, liver, yeast extract (including brewer's yeast in large quantities), dry sausage (including Genoa salami, hard salami, pepperoni, and Lebanon bologna), pods of broad beans (Fava beans), and yogurt. Excessive amounts of caffeine and chocolate may also cause hypertensive reactions.

Nardil should not be used in combination with dextromethorphan or with CNS depressants such as alcohol and certain narcotics. Excitation, seizures, delirium, hyperpyrexia, circulatory collapse, coma, and death have been reported in patients receiving MAOI therapy who have been given a single dose of meperidine. Nardil should not be administered together with or in rapid succession to other MAO inhibitors because HYPERTENSIVE CRISES and convulsive seizures, fever, marked sweating, excitation, delirium, tremor, coma, and circulatory collapse may occur.

List of MAO Inhibitors

Generic Name	Trademark
pargyline hydrochloride	Eutonyl® (Abbott Laboratories)
pargyline hydrochloride and methyclothiazide	Eutron® (Abbott Laboratories)
furazolidone	Furoxone® (Eaton Laboratories)
isocarboxazid	Marplan® (Roche)
procarbazine	Matulane® (Roche)
tranylcypromine	Parnate® (Smith Kline & French Laboratories)

Nardil should also not be used in combination with buspirone HCl, since several cases of elevated blood pressure have been reported in patients taking MAO inhibitors who were then given buspirone HCl. At least 10 days should elapse between the discontinuation of Nardil and the institution of another antidepressant or buspirone HCl, or the discontinuation of another MAO inhibitor and the institution of Nardil.

There have been reports of serious reactions (including hyperthermia, rigidity, myoclonic movements and death) when

Continued on next page

This product information was prepared in August 1992. On these and other Parke-Davis Products, information may be obtained by addressing PARKE-DAVIS, Division of Warner-Lambert Company, Morris Plains, New Jersey 07950.

Parke-Davis—Cont.

fluoxetine has been combined with an MAO inhibitor. Therefore, Nardil should not be used in combination with fluoxetine. Allow at least five weeks between discontinuation of fluoxetine and initiation of Nardil and at least 10 days between discontinuation of Nardil and initiation of fluoxetine.
The combination of MAO inhibitors and tryptophan has been reported to cause behavioral and neurologic syndromes including disorientation, confusion, amnesia, delirium, agitation, hypomanic signs, ataxia, myoclonus, hyperreflexia, shivering, ocular oscillations and Babinski signs.
The concurrent administration of an MAO inhibitor and bupropion hydrochloride (Wellbutrin®) is contraindicated. At least 14 days should elapse between discontinuation of an MAO inhibitor and initiation of treatment with bupropion hydrochloride.
Patients taking Nardil should not undergo elective surgery requiring general anesthesia. Also, they should not be given cocaine or local anesthesia containing sympathomimetic vasoconstrictors. The possible combined hypotensive effects of Nardil and spinal anesthesia should be kept in mind. Nardil should be discontinued at least 10 days prior to elective surgery.
MAO inhibitors including Nardil are contraindicated in patients receiving guanethidine.

WARNINGS

The most serious reactions to Nardil involve changes in blood pressure.
Hypertensive Crises: The most important reaction associated with Nardil administration is the occurrence of hypertensive crises, which have sometimes been fatal.
These crises are characterized by some or all of the following symptoms: occipital headache which may radiate frontally, palpitation, neck stiffness or soreness, nausea, vomiting, sweating (sometimes with fever and sometimes with cold, clammy skin), dilated pupils, and photophobia. Either tachycardia or bradycardia may be present and can be associated with constricting chest pain.
NOTE: Intracranial bleeding has been reported in association with the increase in blood pressure.
Blood pressure should be observed frequently to detect evidence of any pressor response in all patients receiving Nardil. Therapy should be discontinued immediately upon the occurrence of palpitation or frequent headaches during therapy.
Recommended treatment in hypertensive crisis: If a hypertensive crisis occurs, Nardil should be discontinued immediately and therapy to lower blood pressure should be instituted immediately. On the basis of present evidence, phentolamine is recommended. (The dosage reported for phentolamine is 5 mg intravenously.) Care should be taken to administer this drug slowly in order to avoid producing an excessive hypotensive effect. Fever should be managed by means of external cooling.
Warning to the patient: All patients should be warned that the following foods, beverages and medications must be avoided while taking Nardil, and for two weeks after discontinuing use.

Foods and Beverages To Avoid
Meat and Fish
Pickled herring
Liver
Dry sausage (including Genoa salami, hard salami, pepperoni, and Lebanon bologna)
Vegetables
Broad bean pods (fava bean pods)
Sauerkraut
Dairy Products
Cheese (cottage cheese and cream cheese are allowed)
Yogurt
Beverages
Beer and wine
Alcohol-free and reduced-alcohol beer and wine products
Miscellaneous
Yeast extract (including brewer's yeast in large quantities)
Meat extract
Excessive amounts of chocolate and caffeine
Also, any spoiled or improperly refrigerated, handled or stored protein-rich foods such as meats, fish, and dairy products, including foods that may have undergone protein changes by aging, pickling, fermentation, or smoking to improve flavor should be avoided.
OTC Medications To Avoid
Cold and cough preparations (including those containing dextromethorphan)
Nasal decongestants (tablets, drops or spray)
Hay-fever medications
Sinus medications
Asthma inhalant medications
Antiappetite medicines
Weight-reducing preparations
"Pep" pills
L-tryptophan containing preparations
Also, certain prescription drugs should be avoided. Therefore, patients under the care of another physician or dentist, should inform him/her they are taking Nardil.
Patients should be warned that the use of the above foods, beverages or medications may cause a reaction characterized by headache and other serious symptoms due to a rise in blood pressure, with the exception of dextromethorphan which may cause reactions similar to those seen with meperidine. Also, there has been a report of an interaction between Nardil and dextromethorphan (ingested as a lozenge) causing drowsiness and bizarre behavior.
Patients should be instructed to report promptly the occurrence of headache or other unusual symptoms.

PRECAUTIONS

General:
In depressed patients, the possibility of suicide should always be considered and adequate precautions taken. It is recommended that careful observations of patients undergoing Nardil treatment be maintained until control of depression is achieved. If necessary, additional measures (ECT, hospitalization, etc.) should be instituted.
All patients undergoing treatment with Nardil should be closely followed for symptoms of postural hypotension. Hypotensive side effects have occurred in hypertensive as well as normal and hypotensive patients. Blood pressure usually returns to pretreatment levels rapidly when the drug is discontinued or the dosage is reduced.
Because the effect of Nardil on the convulsive threshold may be variable, adequate precautions should be taken when treating epileptic patients.
Of the more severe side effects that have been reported with any consistency, hypomania has been the most common. This reaction has been largely limited to patients in whom disorders characterized by hyperkinetic symptoms coexist with, but are obscured by, depressive affect; hypomania usually appeared as depression improved. If agitation is present, it may be increased with Nardil. Hypomania and agitation have also been reported at higher than recommended doses, or following long-term therapy.
Nardil may cause excessive stimulation in schizophrenic patients; in manic-depressive states it may result in a swing from a depressive to a manic phase.
MAO inhibitors, including Nardil potentiate hexobarbital hypnosis in animals. Therefore, barbiturates should be given at a reduced dose with Nardil.
MAO inhibitors inhibit the destruction of serotonin and norepinephrine, which are believed to be released from tissue stores by rauwolfia alkaloids. Accordingly, caution should be exercised when rauwolfia is used concomitantly with an MAO inhibitor, including Nardil.
There is conflicting evidence as to whether or not MAO inhibitors affect glucose metabolism or potentiate hypoglycemic agents. This should be kept in mind if Nardil is administered to diabetics.
Nardil, as with other hydrazine derivatives, has been reported to induce pulmonary and vascular tumors in an uncontrolled lifetime study in mice.
Information for Patients: See to the Patient in the WARNING section.
Drug Interactions:
See CONTRAINDICATIONS and WARNINGS sections for additional drug interactions.
Nardil should be used with caution in combination with antihypertensive drugs, including thiazide diuretics and β-blockers, since exaggerated hypotensive effects may result.
Concomitant Use with Dibenzazepine Derivative Drugs
If the decision is made to administer Nardil concurrently with other antidepressant drugs, or within less than 10 days after discontinuation of antidepressant therapy, the patient should be cautioned by the physician regarding the possibility of adverse drug interaction.
List of Dibenzazepine Derivative Drugs

Generic Name	*Trademark*
nortriptyline hydrochloride	Aventyl® (Eli Lilly & Co.)
amitriptyline hydrochloride	Elavil® (Merck Sharp & Dohme)
amitriptyline hydrochloride	Endep® (Roche)
perphenazine and amitriptyline hydrochloride	Etrafon® (Schering Corporation)
perphenazine and amitriptyline hydrochloride	Triavil® (Merck Sharp & Dohme)
clomipramine hydrochloride	Anafranil® (CIBA-Geigy)
desipramine hydrochloride	Norpramin® (Merrell-National)
desipramine hydrochloride	Pertofrane® (USV)
imipramine hydrochloride	Tofranil® (Geigy)
doxepin	Adapin® (Pennwalt)
doxepin	Sinequan® (Pfizer)
carbamazepine	Tegretol® (Geigy)
cyclobenzaprine HCl	Flexeril® (Merck Sharp & Dohme)
amoxapine	Asendin® (Lederle)
maprotiline HCl	Ludiomil® (CIBA)
trimipramine maleate	Surmontil® (Wyeth)
protriptyline HCl	Vivactil® (Merck Sharp & Dohme)

Pregnancy Category C: Nardil has been shown to have an adverse effect in mice when given in doses well exceeding the maximum recommended human dose. There are no adequate and well-controlled studies in pregnant women. Nardil should be used during pregnancy only if the potential benefit justifies the potential risk to the fetus.
Doses of Nardil in pregnant mice well exceeding the maximum recommended human dose have caused a significant decrease in the number of viable offspring per mouse. In addition, the growth of young dogs and rats has been retarded by doses exceeding the maximum human dose.
Nursing Mothers: It is not known whether this drug is excreted in human milk. Because many drugs are excreted in human milk and because of the potential for serious adverse reactions in nursing infants from Nardil, a decision should be made whether to discontinue the drug, taking into account the importance of the drug to the mother.
Pediatric Use: Nardil is not recommended for patients under 16 years of age, since there are no controlled studies of safety in this age group.

ADVERSE REACTIONS

Nardil is a potent inhibitor of monoamine oxidase. Because this enzyme is widely distributed throughout the body, diverse pharmacologic effects can be expected to occur. When they occur, such effects tend to be mild or moderate in severity (see below), often subside as treatment continues, and can be minimized by adjusting dosage; rarely is it necessary to institute counteracting measures or to discontinue Nardil.
Common side effects include:
Nervous System—Dizziness, headache, drowsiness, sleep disturbances (including insomnia and hypersomnia), fatigue, weakness, tremors, twitching, myoclonic movements, hyperreflexia.
Gastrointestinal—Constipation, dry mouth, gastrointestinal disturbances, elevated serum transaminases (without accompanying signs and symptoms).
Metabolic—Weight gain.
Cardiovascular—Postural hypotension, edema.
Genitourinary—Sexual disturbances, ie, anorgasmia and ejaculatory disturbances.
Less common mild to moderate side effects (some of which have been reported in a single patient or by a single physician) include:
Nervous System—Jitteriness, palilalia, euphoria, nystagmus, paresthesias.
Genitourinary—Urinary retention.
Metabolic—Hypernatremia.
Dermatologic—Skin rash, sweating.
Special senses—Blurred vision, glaucoma.
Although reported less frequently, and sometimes only once, additional severe side effects include:
Nervous System—Ataxia, shock-like coma, toxic delirium, manic reaction, convulsions, acute anxiety reaction, precipitation of schizophrenia, transient respiratory and cardiovascular depression following ECT.
Gastrointestinal—To date, fatal progressive necrotizing hepatocellular damage has been reported in a very few patients. Reversible jaundice.
Hematologic—Leukopenia.
Metabolic—Hypermetabolic syndrome (which may include, but is not limited to, hyperpyrexia, tachycardia, tachypnea, muscular rigidity, elevated CK levels, metabolic acidosis, hypoxia, coma and may resemble an overdose).
Respiratory—Edema of the glottis.
Withdrawal may be associated with nausea, vomiting and malaise.
General: Fever associated with increased muscle tone.
An uncommon withdrawal syndrome following abrupt withdrawal of Nardil has been infrequently reported. Signs and symptoms of this syndrome generally commence 24 to 72 hours after drug discontinuation and may range from vivid nightmares with agitation to frank psychosis and convulsions. This syndrome generally responds to reinstitution of low-dose Nardil therapy followed by cautious downward titration and discontinuation.

DOSAGE AND ADMINISTRATION

Initial dose: the usual starting dose of Nardil is one tablet (15 mg) three times a day.
Early phase treatment: Dosage should be increased to at least 60 mg per day at a fairly rapid pace consistent with

patient tolerance. It may be necessary to increase dosage up to 90 mg per day to obtain sufficient MAO inhibition. Many patients do not show a clinical response until treatment at 60 mg has been continued for at least 4 weeks.

Maintenance dose: After maximum benefit from Nardil is achieved, dosage should be reduced slowly over several weeks. Maintenance dose may be as low as 1 tablet, 15 mg, a day or every other day, and should be continued for as long as is required.

OVERDOSAGE

Note—For management of *hypertensive crises* see WARNINGS section.

Accidental or intentional overdosage may be more common in patients who are depressed. It should be remembered that multiple drugs and/or alcohol may have been ingested.

Depending on the amount of overdosage with Nardil, a varying and mixed clinical picture may develop, involving signs and symptoms of central nervous system and cardiovascular stimulation and/or depression. Signs and symptoms may be absent or minimal during the initial 12-hour period following ingestion and may develop slowly thereafter, reaching a maximum in 24–48 hours. Death has been reported following overdosage. Therefore, immediate hospitalization, with continuous patient observation and monitoring throughout this period, is essential.

Signs and symptoms of overdosage may include, alone or in combination, any of the following: drowsiness, dizziness, faintness, irritability, hyperactivity, agitation, severe headache, hallucinations, trismus, opisthotonus, convulsions and coma; rapid and irregular pulse, hypertension, hypotension and vascular collapse; precordial pain, respiratory depression and failure, hyperpyrexia, diaphoresis, and cool, clammy skin.

Intensive symptomatic and supportive treatment may be required. Induction of emesis or gastric lavage with instillation of charcoal slurry may be helpful in early poisoning, provided the airway has been protected against aspiration. Signs and symptoms of central nervous system stimulation, including convulsions, should be treated with diazepam, given slowly intravenously. Phenothiazine derivatives and central nervous system stimulants should be avoided. Hypotension and vascular collapse should be treated with intravenous fluids and, if necessary, blood pressure titration with an intravenous infusion of dilute pressor agent. It should be noted that adrenergic agents may produce a markedly increased pressor response.

Respiration should be supported by appropriate measures, including management of the airway, use of supplemental oxygen, and mechanical ventilatory assistance, as required. Body temperature should be monitored closely. Intensive management of hyperpyrexia may be required. Maintenance of fluid and electrolyte balance is essential.

There are no data on the lethal dose in man. The pathophysiologic effects of massive overdosage may persist for several days, since the drug acts by inhibiting physiologic enzyme systems. With symptomatic and supportive measures, recovery from *mild* overdosage may be expected within 3 to 4 days. Hemodialysis, peritoneal dialysis, and charcoal hemoperfusion may be of value in massive overdosage, but sufficient data are not available to recommend their routine use in these cases.

Toxic blood levels of phenelzine have not been established, and assay methods are not practical for clinical or toxicological use.

HOW SUPPLIED

Each Nardil tablet is orange, biconvex, glossy, sugar-coated and imprinted with 'P-D 270' in brown ink and contains phenelzine sulfate equivalent to 15 mg of phenelzine base. N 0071-0270-24 Bottles of 100

Store between 15°–30° C (59°–86°F).

Caution: Federal law prohibits dispensing without prescription.

0270G051

Shown in Product Identification Section, page 422

NICOTROL™   ℞
(Nicotine Transdermal System)

Systemic delivery of 15, 10, or 5 mg/day over 16 hours.

DESCRIPTION

Nicotrol transdermal system provides systemic delivery of nicotine for up to 24 hours following its application to intact skin (see CLINICAL PHARMACOLOGY, Pharmacokinetics).

Nicotine is a tertiary amine composed of a pyridine and a pyrrolidine ring. It is a colorless to pale yellow, freely water-soluble, strongly alkaline, oily, volatile, hygroscopic liquid obtained from the tobacco plant. Nicotine has a characteristic pungent odor and turns brown on exposure to air or light. Of its two stereoisomers, S(-)nicotine is the more active. It is the prevalent form in tobacco, and is the form in the Nicotrol

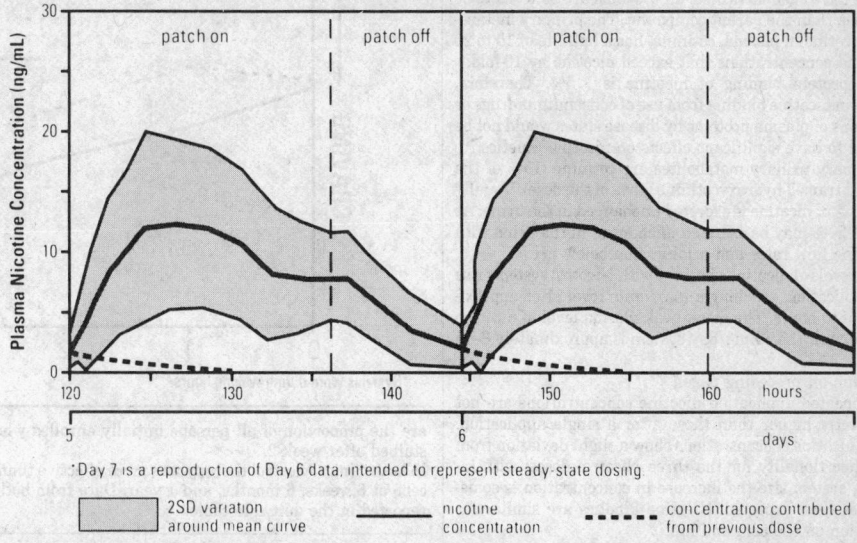

Plasma Nicotine Concentrations after Two Consecutive Days' Application of Nicotrol 15 mg for 16 Hours per Day (Mean ± 2SD, N=12)

† Day 7 is a reproduction of Day 6 data, intended to represent steady-state dosing

2SD variation around mean curve	nicotine concentration · · · · · concentration contributed from previous dose

---

system. The free alkaloid is absorbed rapidly through the skin and respiratory tract.

Chemical Name: S-3-(1-methyl-2-pyrrolidinyl) pyridine
Molecular Formula: $C_{10}H_{14}N_2$
Molecular Weight: 162.23
Ionization Constants: $pKa_1 = 7.84$, $pKa_2 = 3.04$ at 15°C
Octanol-Water Partition Coefficient: 15:1 at pH 7

The Nicotrol systems are a multilayered, rectangular, thin film laminated units containing nicotine as the active agent. For the treatment and the weaning doses the composition per unit area is identical.

Proceeding from the visible surface toward the surface attached to the skin, there are 3 distinct layers:

1) an outer backing layer composed of a laminated polyester film,
2) a middle layer containing rate-controlling adhesive, a structural nonwoven material and nicotine, and
3) a disposable liner that protects the system and must be removed prior to use.

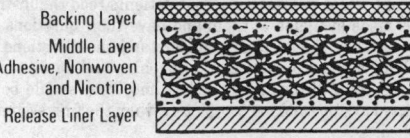

Backing Layer
Middle Layer
(Adhesive, Nonwoven and Nicotine)
Release Liner Layer

Cross Section View Not to Scale

Nicotine is the active ingredient; other components of the system are pharmacologically inactive.

The average amount of nicotine delivered to the patient from each system (31 mcg/cm²/hr) is approximately proportional to the surface area. About 40% of the total amount of nicotine remains in the system 16 hours after application. Nicotrol systems ae labeled with the average amount of nicotine absorbed by the patient over 16 hours. The dose of nicotine absorbed from the Nicotrol systems represents approximately 95% of the amount released in 16 hours. The remainder of the nicotine is lost via evaportion from the edge.

	Dose Absorbed in 16 Hours (mg/day)	System Area (cm²)	Total Nicotine Content (mg)
Treatment Dose	15	30	24.9
First Weaning Dose	10	20	16.6
Second Weaning Dose	5	10	8.3

CLINICAL PHARMACOLOGY
Pharmacologic Action

Nicotine, the chief alkaloid in tobacco products, binds stereoselectively to acetylcholine receptors at the autonomic ganglia, in the adrenal medulla, at neuromuscular junc-

---

tions, and in the brain. Two types of central nervous system effects are believed to be the basis of nicotine's positively reinforcing properties. A stimulating effect, exerted mainly in the cortex via the locus ceruleus, produces increased alertness and cognitive performance. A "reward" effect via the "pleasure system" in the brain is exerted in the limbic system. At low doses the stimulant effects predominate while at high doses the reward effects predominate. Intermittent intravenous administration of nicotine activates neurohormonal pathways, releasing acetylcholine, norepinephrine, dopamine, serotonin, vasopressin, beta-endorphin, growth hormone, and ACTH.

Pharmacodynamics

The cardiovascular effects of nicotine include peripheral vasoconstriction, tachycardia, and elevated blood pressure. Acute and chronic tolerance to nicotine develops from smoking tobacco or ingesting nicotine preparations. Acute tolerance (a reduction in response for a given dose) develops rapidly (less than 1 hour), but not at the same rate for different physiologic effects (skin temperature, heart rate, subjective effects). Withdrawal symptoms such as cigarette craving can be reduced in some individuals by plasma nicotine levels lower than those from smoking.

Withdrawal from nicotine in addicted individuals can be characterized by craving, nervousness, restlessness, irritability, mood lability, anxiety, drowsiness, sleep disturbances, impaired concentration, increased appetite, minor somatic complaints (headache, myalgia, constipation, fatigue), and weight gain. Nicotine toxicity is characterized by nausea, abdominal pain, vomiting, diarrhea, diaphoresis, flushing, dizziness, disturbed hearing and vision, confusion, weakness, palpitations, altered respiration, and hypotension.

Both smoking and nicotine can increase circulating cortisol and catecholamines, and tolerance does not develop to the catecholamine-releasing effects of nicotine. Changes in the response to a concomitantly administered adrenergic agonist or antagonist should be watched for when nicotine intake is altered during Nicotrol therapy and/or smoking cessation (see PRECAUTIONS, Drug Interactions).

Pharmacokinetics

Following application of the Nicotrol system to the upper arm or hip, approximately 95% of the nicotine released from the system enters the systemic circulation. The remainder of the nicotine released from the system is lost via evaporation from the edge. All Nicotrol systems are labeled by the average amount of nicotine absorbed by the average patient over 16 hours.

The volume of distribution following i.v. administration of nicotine is approximately 2 to 3 L/kg and the half-life ranges from 1 to 2 hours. The major eliminating organ is the liver, and average plasma clearance is about 1.2 L/min; the kidney and lung also metabolize nicotine. There is no significant skin metabolism of nicotine. More than 20 metabolites of

Continued on next page

This product information was prepared in August 1992. On these and other Parke-Davis Products, information may be obtained by addressing PARKE-DAVIS, Division of Warner-Lambert Company, Morris Plains, New Jersey 07950.

Parke-Davis—Cont.

nicotine have been identified, all of which are believed to be less active than the parent compound. The primary metabolite of nicotine in plasma, cotinine, has a half-life of 15 to 20 hours and concentrations that exceed nicotine by 10-fold. Plasma protein binding of nicotine is <5%. Therefore, changes in nicotine binding from use of concomitant drugs or alterations of plasma proteins by disease states would not be expected to have significant effects on nicotine kinetics.

The primary urinary metabolites are cotinine (15% of the dose) and trans-3-hydroxycotinine (45% of the dose). Usually about 10% of nicotine is excreted unchanged in the urine. As much as 30% may be excreted unchanged in the urine with high urine flow rates and acidification below pH 5.

Plasma levels of nicotine obtained with Nicotrol systems rise after application, reaching a maximum level after approximately 5–10 hours. The mean peak plasma level of nicotine achieved with the 15 mg/day system is approximately 9–15 ng/mL.

[See graph on preceding page.]

After repeated application nicotine concentrations are not significantly higher than those after a single application. Plasma nicotine concentrations show a slight deviation from dose proportionality for the three Nicotrol doses; with increasing system size the increase in concentration is somewhat less than expected. Nicotine kinetics are similar for application on the arm and hip.

Following removal of the Nicotrol system after 16 hours of wear, plasma nicotine concentrations decline in an apparently exponential fashion. The half-life after removal was about twice that observed after intravenous infusion, suggesting continued absorption from the skin depot. Patients had nondetectable nicotine concentrations within 10 to 12 hours after removing the system.

Steady State Nicotine Pharmacokinetic Parameters for Nicotrol Systems Applied for 16 Hours
[Mean±SD (Range), N=12]

	Delivery Rate (mg/day)		
	15* Mean±SD (Range)	10 Mean±SD (Range)	5 Mean±SD (Range)
C_{max} (ng/mL)	13.0±3.1 (7.8–17.9)	6.9±2.0 (4.8–10.0)	3.5±0.7 (2.7–4.7)
C_{avg}, 16 (ng/mL)	9.4±2.4 (5.3–13.3)	4.9±1.2 (3.0–6.8)	2.7±0.5 (2.0–3.6)
C_{avg}, 24 (ng/mL)	8.7±2.1 (5.2–11.8)	4.8±1.0 (3.3–6.3)	2.7±0.4 (2.1–3.3)
C_{min} (ng/mL)	2.5±0.8 (1.2–4.1)	1.4±0.5 (0.5–2.4)	0.8±0.3 (0.3–1.2)
T_{max} (hrs)	8±3 (4–16)	9±4 (6–16)	9±4 (3–16)

C_{max}: maximum observed plasma concentration
C_{avg}, 16: estimated average plasma concentration during the 0 to 16 hour period, calculated as AUC (0–16)/16
C_{avg}, 24: average plasma concentration calculated over 24 hrs
C_{min}: minimum observed plasma concentration
T_{max}: time of maximum plasma concentration
* Data for 15 mg/day system are derived from a different study than the 5 and 10 mg/day systems.

If the 15 mg/day Nicotrol system is left on for 24 hours, as opposed to 16 hours, plasma levels of nicotine decline from a mean of 7.2 to 5.6 ng/mL over the last 8 hours. The smaller systems may be expected to follow a similar pattern at proportionally lower plasma levels.

There are no differences in nicotine kinetics between men and women using Nicotrol systems. Linear regression of both AUC and C_{max} vs. total body weight shows the expected inverse relationship. Men and women having low body weight are expected to have higher AUC and C_{max} values.

CLINICAL TRIALS

The efficacy of Nicotrol therapy as an aid to smoking cessation was demonstrated in two single-center, placebo-controlled, double-blind trials in smokers, smoking ≥10 cigarettes per day (N=509), who were healthy or had diseases in their past medical history such as chronic obstructive pulmonary disease, hypertension, or myocardial infarction.

In both clinics Nicotrol systems were applied on awakening and removed at bedtime each day. They were used with only limited behavioral support. Patients in both clinics were treated for 12 weeks followed by a 4 to 6 week weaning period. The subjects were followed for 12 months. Quitting was defined as total abstinence from smoking. The "quit rates"

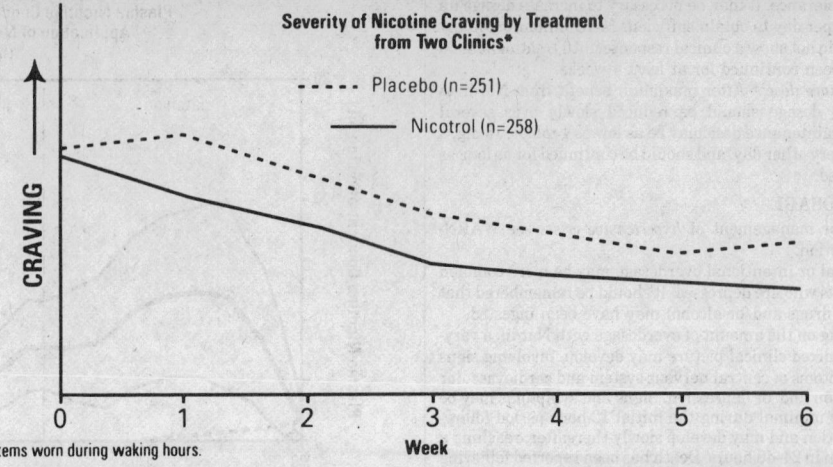

Severity of Nicotine Craving by Treatment from Two Clinics*

- - - - - Placebo (n=251)
——— Nicotrol (n=258)

CRAVING

Week: 0 1 2 3 4 5 6

*Systems worn during waking hours.

are the proportion of all persons initially enrolled who abstained after week 2.

In both clinics Nicotrol therapy was more effective than placebo at 6 weeks, 6 months, and 1 year. Data from both are reported in the quit rate table.

Quit Rates by Treatment
(N=509 smokers in 2 clinics)*

Treatment Group	Number of Patients	At 6 Weeks	At 6 Months	At 1 Year
Nicotrol	258	35–61%	19–35%	12–25%
Placebo	251	7–35%	3–12%	3–9%

* Trials involved 2 clinics; the number of patients per treatment ranged from 107 to 145.

Patients who used Nicotrol systems had a significant reduction in craving for cigarettes, a major nicotine withdrawal symptom, compared with placebo-treated patients (see figure). The effect on withdrawal symptoms, as with quit rate, is quite variable and is presumed to be due to inherent differences in patient populations, e.g., patient motivation, concomitant illness, number of cigarettes smoked per day, number of years smoking, exposure to other smokers, socioeconomic status, etc., as well as differences between the clinics themselves (one Danish, one U.S.). [See table above.]

Patients using Nicotrol systems withdrew from the trials less frequently than did patients receiving placebo. Quit rates for the 79 patients over age 60 were comparable to the quit rates for the 430 patients aged 60 and under.

Individualization of Dosage

It is important to make sure that patients read the instructions made available to them and have their questions answered. They should clearly understand the directions for applying a Nicotrol system on awakening and for removing and disposing of the system at bedtime. They should be instructed to stop smoking completely when the first system is applied.

The success or failure of smoking cessation is influenced by the quality, intensity, and frequency of supportive care. Patients are more likely to quit smoking if they are seen frequently and participate in formal smoking cessation programs.

The goal of Nicotrol therapy is complete abstinence. If a patient is unable to stop smoking by the fourth week of therapy, treatment probably should be discontinued. Patients who have not stopped smoking after 4 weeks of Nicotrol therapy are unlikely to quit on that attempt.

Patients who fail to quit on any attempt may benefit from interventions to improve their chances for success on subsequent attempts. Patients who were unsuccessful should be counselled to determine why they failed. Patients should then probably be given a "therapy holiday" before the next attempt. A new quit attempt should be encouraged when the factors that contributed to failure can be eliminated or reduced, and conditions are more favorable.

Based on the clinical trials, a reasonable approach to assisting patients in their attempt to quit smoking is to begin initial treatment using the recommended dosage schedule (see DOSAGE AND ADMINISTRATION). The need for dose adjustment should be assessed during the first 2 weeks in those patients who have signs or symptoms of nicotine excess. Patients should continue on the dose selected over the treatment period. Those who have successfully stopped smoking during that time should be supported during the 4 to 8 weeks of weaning after which treatment should be terminated. Therapy should begin with the Nicotrol 15 mg/day dose (see dosing schedule below). If the patient has signs or symptoms

suggesting nicotine excess, the 10 mg/day system may be tried.

The symptoms of nicotine withdrawal and excess overlap (see Pharmacodynamics and ADVERSE REACTIONS sections). Since patients using Nicotrol treatment may also smoke intermittently, it may be difficult to determine if patients are experiencing nicotine withdrawal or nicotine excess. The controlled clinical trials suggest that dizziness, rash, and sweating are more often symptoms of nicotine excess whereas anxiety and irritability are more often symptoms of nicotine withdrawal.

Dosing Schedule

Initial/Starting Dose	15 mg/day
Duration of Treatment	4–12 weeks
First Weaning Dose	10 mg/day
Duration of Treatment	2–4 weeks
Second Weaning Dose	5 mg/day
Duration of Treatment	2–4 weeks

INDICATIONS AND USAGE

Nicotrol systems, applied while patients are awake, are indicated as an aid to smoking cessation for the relief of nicotine withdrawal symptoms. Nicotrol therapy is recommended for use as part of a comprehensive behavioral smoking cessation program.

The use of Nicotrol systems beyond 5 months has not been studied.

CONTRAINDICATIONS

Use of Nicotrol systems is contraindicated in patients with known hypersensitivity or allergy to nicotine or to any component of Nicotrol transdermal systems.

WARNINGS

Nicotine from any source can be toxic and addictive. Smoking causes lung cancer, heart disease, emphysema, and may adversely affect the fetus and the pregnant woman. For any smoker, with or without concomitant disease or pregnancy, the risk of nicotine replacement in a smoking cessation program should be weighed against the hazard of continued smoking while using Nicotrol systems, and the likelihood of achieving cessation of smoking without nicotine replacement.

Pregnancy, Warning

Tobacco smoke, which has been shown to be harmful to the fetus, contains nicotine, hydrogen cyanide, and carbon monoxide. Nicotine has been shown in animal studies to cause fetal harm. It is therefore presumed that Nicotrol systems can cause fetal harm when administered to a pregnant woman. The effect of nicotine delivery by Nicotrol systems has not been examined in pregnancy (see PRECAUTIONS). Therefore, pregnant smokers should be encouraged to attempt cessation using educational and behavioral interventions before using pharmacological approaches. If Nicotrol therapy is used during pregnancy, or if the patient becomes pregnant while using Nicotrol systems, the patient should be apprised of the potential hazard to the fetus.

Safety Note Concerning Children

The amounts of nicotine that are tolerated by adult smokers can produce symptoms of poisoning and could prove fatal if a Nicotrol system is applied or ingested by children or pets. Used 15 mg/day systems contain about 40% (10 mg) of its initial drug content. Therefore, patients should be cautioned to keep both the used and unused Nicotrol systems out of the reach of children and pets.

PRECAUTIONS

The patient should be urged to stop smoking completely when initiating Nicotrol therapy (see DOSAGE AND ADMINISTRATION). Patients should be informed that if they

continue to smoke while using Nicotrol systems, they may experience adverse effects due to peak nicotine levels higher than those experienced from smoking alone. If there is a clinically significant increase in cardiovascular or other effects attributable to nicotine, the treatment should be discontinued (see WARNINGS). Physicians should anticipate that concomitant medications may need dosage adjustment (see Drug Interactions).

Use of Nicotrol systems beyond 5 months by patients who stop smoking should be discouraged because the chronic consumption of nicotine by any route can be harmful and addicting.

Allergic Reactions

In a 3-week open-label dermal irritation and sensitization study of Nicotrol systems applied 23 hours per day, 3 of 215 patients (1.4%) exhibited definite erythema at 24 hours after application. Upon rechallenge, none of the subjects exhibited any contact allergy. In the efficacy trials erythema following system removal was typically seen in 7% of patients, edema was seen in 3%, and dropouts due to skin reactions were reported in 1% of patients. Severe skin reactions were not observed in either of the trials.

Patients who exhibit contact sensitization should be cautioned that a serious reaction could occur from exposure to other nicotine containing products or smoking.

Patients should be instructed to discontinue promptly the use of Nicotrol systems and contact their physicians in the case of severe or persistent local skin reactions at the site of application (e.g., severe erythema, pruritus, or edema) or a generalized skin reaction (e.g., urticaria, hives, or generalized rashes).

Skin Disease

The Nicotrol system is usually well tolerated by patients with normal skin, but may be irritating for patients with some skin disorders (psoriasis, atopic or eczematous dermatitis).

Cardiovascular or Peripheral Vascular Diseases

The risks of nicotine replacement in patients with certain cardiovascular and peripheral vascular diseases should be weighed against the benefits of including nicotine replacement in a smoking cessation program for them. Specifically, patients with coronary heart disease (history of myocardial infarction and/or angina pectoris), serious cardiac arrhythmias, or vasospastic diseases (Buerger's disease, Prinzmetal's variant angina) should be carefully screened and evaluated before nicotine replacement is prescribed.

Tachycardia occurring in association with the use of Nicotrol therapy was reported occasionally. If serious cardiovascular symptoms occur with the use of Nicotrol systems, the therapy should be discontinued.

Nicotrol therapy should generally not be used in patients during the immediate post-myocardial infarction period or in patients with serious arrhythmias or with severe or worsening angina pectoris.

Renal or Hepatic Insufficiency

The pharmacokinetics of nicotine have not been studied in the elderly or in patients with renal or hepatic impairment. However, given that nicotine is extensively metabolized and that its total system clearance is dependent on liver blood flow, some influence of hepatic impairment on drug kinetics (reduced clearance) should be anticipated. Only severe renal impairment would be expected to affect the clearance of nicotine or its metabolites from the circulation (see Pharmacokinetics).

Endocrine Diseases

Nicotrol therapy should be used with caution in patients with hyperthyroidism, pheochromocytoma or insulin-dependent diabetes, since nicotine causes the release of catecholamines by the adrenal medulla.

Peptic Ulcer Disease

Nicotine delays healing in peptic ulcer disease; therefore, Nicotrol therapy should be used with caution in patients with active peptic ulcers and only when the benefits of including nicotine replacement in a smoking cessation program outweigh the risks.

Accelerated Hypertension

Nicotine therapy constitutes a risk factor for development of malignant hypertension in patients with accelerated hypertension; therefore, Nicotrol therapy should be used with caution in these patients and only when the benefits of including nicotine replacement in a smoking cessation program outweigh the risks.

Information for Patient

A patient instruction sheet is included in the package of Nicotrol systems dispensed to the patient. It contains important information and instructions on how to use and dispose of Nicotrol systems properly. Patients should be encouraged to ask questions of the physician and pharmacist.

Patients must be advised to keep both used and unused systems out of the reach of children and pets.

Drug Interactions

Smoking cessation, with or without nicotine replacement, may alter the pharmacokinetics of certain concomitant medications.

May Require a Decrease in Dose at Cessation of Smoking	Possible Mechanism
Acetaminophen, caffeine, imipramine, oxazepam, pentazocine, propranolol, theophylline	Deinduction of hepatic enzymes on smoking cessation.
Insulin	Increase of subcutaneous insulin absorption with smoking cessation.
Adrenergic antagonists (e.g., prazosin, labetalol)	Decrease in circulating catecholamines with smoking cessation.

May Require an Increase in Dose at Cessation of Smoking	Possible Mechanism
Adrenergic agonists (e.g., isoproterenol, phenylephrine)	Decrease in circulating catecholamines with smoking cessation.

Carcinogenesis, Mutagenesis, Impairment of Fertility

Nicotine itself does not appear to be a carcinogen in laboratory animals. However, nicotine and its metabolites increased the incidences of tumors in the cheek pouches of hamsters and forestomach of F344 rats, respectively, when given in combination with tumor-initiators. One study, which could not be replicated, suggested that cotinine, the primary metabolite of nicotine, may cause lymphoreticular sarcoma in the large intestine in rats.

Neither nicotine nor cotinine were mutagenic in the Ames *Salmonella* test. Nicotine induced repairable DNA damage in an *E. coli* test system. Nicotine was shown to be genotoxic in a test system using Chinese hamster ovary cells. In rats and rabbits, implantation can be delayed or inhibited by a reduction in DNA synthesis that appears to be caused by nicotine. Studies have shown a decrease in litter size in rats treated with nicotine during gestation.

PREGNANCY

Pregnancy Category D (see WARNINGS section).

The harmful effects of cigarette smoking on maternal and fetal health are clearly established. These include low birth weight, an increased risk of spontaneous abortion, and increased perinatal mortality. The specific effects of Nicotrol therapy on fetal development are unknown. Therefore, pregnant smokers should be encouraged to attempt cessation using educational and behavioral interventions before using pharmacological approaches.

Spontaneous abortion during nicotine replacement therapy has been reported; as with smoking, nicotine as a contributing factor cannot be excluded.

Nicotrol systems should be used during pregnancy only if the likelihood of smoking cessation justifies the potential risk of using Nicotrol systems by the pregnant patient, who might continue to smoke.

Teratogenicity

Animal Studies: Nicotine was shown to produce skeletal abnormalities in the offspring of mice when given doses toxic to the dams (25 mg/kg IP or SC).

Human Studies: Nicotine teratogenicity has not been studied in humans except as a component of cigarette smoke (each cigarette smoked delivers about 1 mg of nicotine). It has not been possible to conclude whether cigarette smoking is teratogenic to humans.

Other Effects

Animal Studies: A nicotine bolus (up to 2 mg/kg) to pregnant rhesus monkeys caused acidosis, hypercarbia, and hypotension (fetal and maternal concentrations were about 20 times those achieved after smoking one cigarette in 5 minutes). Fetal breathing movements were reduced in the fetal lamb after intravenous injection of 0.25 mg/kg nicotine to the ewe (equivalent to smoking 1 cigarette every 20 seconds for 5 minutes). Uterine blood flow was reduced about 30% after infusion of 0.1 μg/kg/min nicotine to pregnant rhesus monkeys (equivalent to smoking about six cigarettes every minute for 20 minutes).

Human Experience: Cigarette smoking during pregnancy is associated with an increased risk of spontaneous abortion, low birth weight infants, and perinatal mortality. Nicotine and carbon monoxide are considered the most likely mediators of these outcomes. The effects of cigarette smoking on fetal cardiovascular parameters have been studied near term. Cigarettes increased fetal aortic blood flow and heart rate and decreased uterine blood flow and fetal breathing movements. Nicotrol systems have not been tested in pregnant women.

Labor and Delivery

Nicotrol systems are not recommended for use during labor and delivery. The effects of nicotine on a mother or the fetus during labor is unknown.

Use in Nursing Mothers

Caution should be exercised when Nicotrol systems are administered to nursing women. The safety of Nicotrol therapy in nursing infants has not been examined. Nicotine passes freely into breast milk; the milk to plasma ratio averages 2.9. Nicotine is absorbed orally. An infant has the ability to clear nicotine by hepatic first pass clearance; however the efficiency of removal is probably lowest at birth. Nicotine concentrations in milk can be expected to be lower with Nicotrol systems when used while awake than with cigarette smoking, as maternal plasma nicotine concentrations are generally reduced with nicotine replacement. The risk of exposure of the infant to nicotine from Nicotrol therapy should be weighed against the risks associated with the infant's exposure to nicotine from continued smoking by the mother (passive smoking exposure and contaimination of breast milk with other components of tobacco smoke) and from Nicotrol therapy alone or in combination with continued smoking.

Pediatric Use

Nicotrol therapy is not recommended for use in children because the safety and effectiveness of Nicotrol therapy in children and adolescents who smoke have not been evaluated.

Geriatric Use

Seventy-nine patients over the age of 60 participated in clinical trials of Nicotrol therapy. Nicotrol therapy appeared to be as effective in this age group as in younger smokers.

ADVERSE REACTIONS

Assessment of adverse events in the 509 subjects who participated in controlled clinical trials is complicated by the occurrence of GI and CNS effects of nicotine withdrawal as well as nicotine excess. The actual incidences of both are confounded by the smoking of many patients. When reporting adverse events in the trials the investigators did not attempt to identify the cause of the symptom. No serious adverse events were reported during the trials.

Topical Adverse Events

The most common adverse event associated with topical nicotine is a mild and short-lived erythema, pruritus, or burning at the application site, which was seen at least once in 47% of patients on Nicotrol systems in the efficacy trials. Local erythema after system removal was noted at least once in 7% of patients and local edema in 3%. Erythema generally resolved within 24 hours. About 1% of patients dropped out of clinical trials due to skin reactions; none had classical contact sensitization (see PRECAUTIONS, Allergic Reactions).

In the clinical trials performed (one Danish and one U.S. clinic), fewer total patients were used than in trials of other nicotine transdermal systems, and fewer adverse reactions were reported than in U.S. trials with other systems achieving comparable blood levels. Therefore, the systemic adverse event rates in the two sections below are based in part on 1200 patients treated with systems delivering comparable rates of nicotine per hour.

Probably Causally Related

The following adverse events are believed related to Nicotrol treatment based on experience in clinical trials.

Nervous system
Dizziness*
Musculoskeletal system
Arthralgia†
Skin and appendages
Rash,† sweating†

Complaints occurring in fewer than 1% are not listed.

Causal Relationship UNKNOWN

Adverse events reported in active- and placebo-treated patients at about the same frequency in clinical trials are listed below. The clinical significance of the association between Nicotrol treatment and the following events is unknown, but they are reported as alerting information for the clinician.

Body as a whole
Back pain,† pain†
Digestive system
Abdominal pain,† constipation,* diarrhea,† dyspepsia,† flatulence,† nausea,* vomiting†
Musculoskeletal system
Myalgia†
Nervous system
Concentration impairment,† depression,† headache,* insomnia,† nervousness†
Respiratory system
Cough increased,† sinusitis†
Special senses
Taste perversion†
Urogenital system
Dysmenorrhea†

* reported in 3% to 9% of patients.
† reported in 1% to 3% of patients.
Complaints occurring in fewer than 1% are not listed.

Continued on next page

This product information was prepared in August 1992. On these and other Parke-Davis Products, information may be obtained by addressing PARKE-DAVIS, Division of Warner-Lambert Company, Morris Plains, New Jersey 07950.

Parke-Davis—Cont.

DRUG ABUSE AND DEPENDENCE

The Nicotrol system is likely to have a low abuse potential based on differences between it and cigarettes in four characteristics commonly considered important in contributing to abuse: much slower absorption, much smaller fluctuations in blood levels, lower blood levels of nicotine, and less frequent use (once daily).

Dependence on nicotine polacrilex chewing gum replacement therapy has been reported, and such dependence might also occur from transference of tobacco-based nicotine dependence to Nicotrol systems. The use of the system beyond 5 months has not been evaluated and should be discouraged.

To minimize the risk of dependence, patients should be encouraged to withdraw gradually from Nicotrol treatment after 12 weeks of usage. Dose reduction can be achieved by progressively decreasing the dose every 2 to 4 weeks (see DOSAGE AND ADMINISTRATION).

OVERDOSAGE

The effects of applying several Nicotrol systems simultaneously or of swallowing Nicotrol systems are unknown (see WARNINGS, Safety Note Concerning Children).

The oral LD_{50} for nicotine in rodents varies with species, but is in excess of 24 mg/kg; death is due to respiratory paralysis. The oral minimum lethal dose of nicotine in dogs is greater than 5 mg/kg. The oral minimum acute lethal dose for nicotine in human adults is reported to be 40 to 60 mg (< 1 mg/kg).

Signs and Symptoms of Nicotine Toxicity

Signs and symptoms of an overdose of Nicotrol systems would be expected to be the same as those of acute nicotine poisoning including: pallor, cold sweat, nausea, salivation, vomiting, abdominal pain, diarrhea, headache, dizziness, disturbed hearing and vision, tremor, mental confusion, and weakness. Prostration, hypotension, and respiratory failure may ensue with large overdoses. Lethal doses produce convulsions quickly, and death follows as a result of peripheral or central respiratory paralysis or, less frequently, cardiac failure.

Overdose from Topical Exposure

The Nicotrol system should be removed immediately if the patient shows signs of overdosage, and the patient should seek immediate medical care. The skin surface may be flushed with water and dried. No soap should be used, since it may increase nicotine absorption. Nicotine will continue to be delivered into the bloodstream for several hours (see Pharmacokinetics) after removal of the system because of a depot of nicotine in the skin.

Overdose from Ingestion

Persons ingesting Nicotrol systems should be referred to a health care facility for management. Due to the possibility of nicotine-induced seizures, activated charcoal should be administered. In unconscious patients with a secure airway, instill activated charcoal via a nasogastric tube. A saline cathartic or sorbitol added to the first dose of activated charcoal may speed gastrointestinal passage of the system. Repeated doses of activated charcoal should be administered as long as the system remains in the gastrointestinal tract since it will continue to release nicotine for many hours.

Management of Nicotine Poisoning

Other supportive measures include diazepam or barbiturates for seizures, atropine for excessive bronchial secretions or diarrhea, respiratory support for respiratory failure, and vigorous fluid support for hypotension and cardiovascular collapse.

DOSAGE AND ADMINISTRATION

Patients must desire to stop smoking and should be instructed to *stop smoking immediately* as they begin using Nicotrol therapy during waking hours. The patient should read the patient instruction sheet on Nicotrol therapy and be encouraged to ask any questions. Treatment should be initiated with the Nicotrol 15 mg/day system. The patients should continue the treatment (one system each day) for 4–12 weeks of therapy. The patient should stop smoking cigarettes completely during this period. If the patient is unable to stop cigarette smoking within 4 weeks, Nicotrol therapy should be stopped, since few additional patients in clinical trials were able to abstain after this time.

Recommended Dosing Schedule

Dose	Duration
Nicotrol 15 mg/day	First 12 weeks
Nicotrol 10 mg/day	Next 2 weeks[a]
Nicotrol 5 mg/day	Last 2 weeks[b]

[a] Patients who have successfully abstained from smoking should have their dose of nicotine reduced after each 2–4 weeks of treatment until the Nicotrol 5 mg/day dose has been used for 2–4 weeks.

[b] The entire course of nicotine substitution and gradual withdrawal should take 14–20 weeks. The use of Nicotrol therapy beyond 5 months has not been studied.

The Nicotrol system should be applied promptly upon its removal from the protective pouch to prevent loss of nicotine from the system. The Nicotrol system should be used only when the pouch is intact to assure the product has not been tampered with.

A Nicotrol system should be applied only once a day to a non-hairy, clean, and dry skin site on the upper arm or the hip. Each day a Nicotrol system should be applied upon waking and removed at bedtime.

SAFETY AND HANDLING

Nicotrol systems can be a dermal irritant and can cause contact sensitization. Although exposure of health care workers to nicotine from Nicotrol systems should be minimal, care should be taken to avoid unnecessary contact with active systems. If you do handle active systems, wash with water alone, since soap may increase nicotine absorption. Do not touch your eyes.

Disposal

When the used system is removed from the skin, it should be folded over and placed in its pouch. The used system should immediately be disposed of in such a way as to prevent its access by children or pets. See patient information for further directions on handling and disposal.

HOW SUPPLIED

NDC 0071-9854-08
—Nicotrol 15 mg/day system, 14 systems per box.
NDC 0071-9853-08
—Nicotrol 10 mg/day system, 14 systems per box.
NDC 0071-9852-08
—Nicotrol 5 mg/day system, 14 systems per box.

HOW TO STORE

Do not store above 86°F (30°C) because nicotine is sensitive to heat. A slight discoloration of the system is insignificant. Do not store unpouched. Once removed from the protective pouch, Nicotrol systems should be applied promptly since nicotine is volatile and the system may lose strength.

Caution—Federal law prohibits dispensing without prescription.

9854G010

Shown in Product Identification Section, page 422

NIPENT™ ℞
(Pentostatin for Injection)

> **WARNING**
>
> NIPENT should be administered under the supervision of a physician qualified and experienced in the use of cancer chemotherapeutic agents. The use of higher doses than those specified (see DOSAGE AND ADMINISTRATION) is not recommended. Dose-limiting severe renal, liver, pulmonary, and CNS toxicities occurred in Phase 1 studies that used NIPENT at higher doses (20–50 mg/m^2 in divided doses over 5 days) than recommended.
>
> In a clinical investigation in patients with refractory chronic lymphocytic leukemia using NIPENT at the recommended dose in combination with fludarabine phosphate, 4 of 6 patients entered in the study had severe or fatal pulmonary toxicity. The use of NIPENT in combination with fludarabine phosphate is not recommended.

DESCRIPTION

NIPENT (pentostatin for injection) is supplied as a sterile, apyrogenic, lyophilized powder in single-dose vials for intravenous administration. Each vial contains 10 mg of pentostatin and 50 mg of mannitol USP. The pH of the final product is maintained between 7.0 and 8.5 by addition of sodium hydroxide or hydrochloric acid.

Pentostatin, also known as 2′-deoxycoformycin (DFC), is a potent inhibitor of the enzyme adenosine deaminase and is isolated from fermentation cultures of *Streptomyces antibioticus.* Pentostatin is known chemically as (R)-3-(2-deoxy-β-D-*erythro*-pentofuranosyl)-3, 6, 7, 8-tetrahydroimidazo[4,5-d][1,3]diazephin-8-ol with a molecular formula of $C_{11}H_{16}N_4O_4$ and a molecular weight of 268.27.

The molecular structure of pentostatin is:

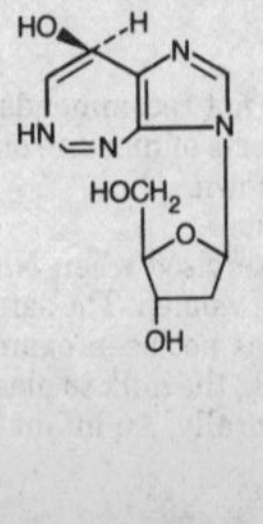

Pentostatin is a white to off-white solid, freely soluble in distilled water.

CLINICAL PHARMACOLOGY

Mechanism of Action

Pentostatin is a potent transition state inhibitor of the enzyme adenosine deaminase (ADA). The greatest activity of ADA is found in cells of the lymphoid system with T-cells having higher activity than B-cells and T-cell malignancies higher ADA activity than B-cell malignancies. Pentostatin inhibition of ADA, particularly in the presence of adenosine or deoxyadenosine, leads to cytotoxicity, and this is believed to be due to elevated intracellular levels of dATP which can block DNA synthesis through inhibition of ribonucleotide reductase. Pentostatin can also inhibit RNA synthesis as well as cause increased DNA damage. In addition to elevated dATP, these mechanisms may contribute to the overall cytotoxic effect of pentostatin. The precise mechanism of pentostatin's antitumor effect, however, in hairy cell leukemia is not known.

Pharmacokinetics/Drug Metabolism

A tissue distribution and whole-body autoradiography study in the rat revealed that radioactivity concentrations were highest in the kidneys with very little central nervous system penetration.

In man, following a single dose of 4 mg/m^2 of pentostatin infused over 5 minutes, the distribution half-life was 11 minutes, the mean terminal half-life was 5.7 hours, the mean plasma clearance was 68 mL/min/m^2, and approximately 90% of the dose was excreted in the urine as unchanged pentostatin and/or metabolites as measured by adenosine deaminase inhibitory activity. The plasma protein binding of pentostatin is low, approximately 4%.

A positive correlation was observed between pentostatin clearance and creatinine clearance (CrCl) in patients with creatinine clearance values ranging from 60 mL/min to 130 mL/min.[1] Pentostatin half-life in patients with renal impairment (CrCl < 50 mL/min, n = 2) was 18 hours, which was much longer than that observed in patients with normal renal function (CrCl > 60 mL/min, n = 14), about 6 hours.

CLINICAL STUDIES

One hundred thirty-three patients with hairy cell leukemia previously treated with alpha-interferon were treated with NIPENT in five clinical studies. Forty-four of these patients were established to be refractory to alpha-interferon and were evaluable for response to NIPENT. The majority of these patients were treated during studies conducted at the M.D. Anderson Hospital and by the Cancer and Leukemia Group B (CALGB). At M.D. Anderson NIPENT was administered at a dose of 4 mg/m^2 every other week for 3 months and responding patients received 3 additional months. CALGB patients received 4 mg/m^2 of NIPENT every other week for 3 months and responding patients were treated monthly for up to 9 additional months. A complete response required clearing of the peripheral blood and bone marrow of hairy cells, normalization of organomegaly and lymphadenopathy, and recovery of the hemoglobin to at least 12 g/dL, platelet count to at least 100,000/mm^3, and granulocyte count to at least 1500/mm^3. A partial response required that the percentage of hairy cells in the blood and bone marrow decrease by more than 50%, enlarged organs and lymph nodes had to decrease by more than 50%, and hematologic parameters had to meet the same criteria as for a complete response. For those patients who were clearly refractory to alpha-interferon, the complete response rate was 58% and the partial response rate was 28% giving a total response rate (complete plus partial responses) of 86%. The median time to achieve a response was 4.7 months with a range of 2.9 to 24.1 months. Occasionally a complete response has occurred after discontinuation of treatment. The duration of response ranged from 1.4 months to 35.1+ months in the CALGB study (median > 7.7 months) and from 1.3+ months to 31.2+ months for the M.D. Anderson study (median > 15.2 months). The median duration of follow-up ranged from 3.9 months in the CALGB study to 19.3 months in the M.D. Anderson study. Only 4 of 20 and 2 of 13 responding patients had relapsed, respectively.

Responding patients with abnormal peripheral blood counts at the start of therapy showed increases in their hemoglobin, granulocyte count, and platelet count in response to treatment with NIPENT.

INDICATIONS AND USAGE

NIPENT is indicated as single agent treatment for adult patients with alpha-interferon-refractory hairy cell leukemia (HCL). Alpha-interferon-refractory disease is defined as progressive disease after a minimum of 3 months of alpha-interferon treatment or no response after a minimum of 6 months of alpha-interferon treatment.

CONTRAINDICATIONS

NIPENT is contraindicated in patients who have demonstrated hypersensitivity to NIPENT.

WARNINGS

See Boxed Warning.

Patients with hairy cell leukemia may experience myelosuppression primarily during the first few courses of treatment. Patients with infections prior to NIPENT treatment have in some cases developed worsening of their condition leading to death, whereas others have achieved complete response. Patients with infection should be treated only when the potential benefit of treatment justifies the potential risk to the patient. Efforts should be made to control the infection before treatment is initiated or resumed.

In patients with progressive hairy cell leukemia, the initial courses of NIPENT treatment were associated with worsening of neutropenia. Therefore, frequent monitoring of complete blood counts during this time is necessary. If severe neutropenia continues beyond the initial cycles, patients should be evaluated for disease status, including a bone marrow examination.

Elevations in liver function tests occurred during treatment with NIPENT and were generally reversible.

Renal toxicity was observed at higher doses in early studies; however, in patients treated at the recommended dose, elevations in serum creatinine were usually minor and reversible. There were some patients who began treatment with normal renal function who had evidence of mild to moderate toxicity at a final assessment. (See DOSAGE AND ADMINISTRATION.)

Rashes, occasionally severe, were commonly reported and may worsen with continued treatment. Withholding of treatment may be required. (See DOSAGE AND ADMINISTRATION.)

Pregnancy Category D:

Pentostatin can cause fetal harm when administered to a pregnant woman. Pentostatin was administered intravenously at doses of 0, 0.01, 0.1, or 0.75 mg/kg/day (0, 0.06, 0.6, and 4.5 mg/m^2) to pregnant rats on days 6 through 15 of gestation. Drug-related maternal toxicity occurred at doses of 0.1 and 0.75 mg/kg/day (0.6 and 4.5 mg/m^2). Teratogenic effects were observed at 0.75 mg/kg/day (4.5 mg/m^2) manifested by increased incidence of various skeletal malformations. In a dose range-finding study, pentostatin was administered intravenously to rats at doses of 0, 0.05, 0.1, 0.5, 0.75, or 1 mg/kg/day (0, 0.3, 0.6, 3, 4.5, 6 mg/m^2) on days 6 through 15 of gestation. Fetal malformations that were observed were an omphalocele at 0.05 mg/kg (0.3 mg/m^2), gastroschisis at 0.75 mg/kg and 1 mg/kg (4.5 and 6 mg/m^2), and a flexure defect of the hindlimbs at 0.75 mg/kg (4.5 mg/m^2). Pentostatin was also shown to be teratogenic in mice when administered as a single 2 mg/kg (6 mg/m^2) intraperitoneal injection on day 7 of gestation. Pentostatin was not teratogenic in rabbits when administered intravenously on days 6 through 18 of gestation at doses of 0, 0.005, 0.01, or 0.02 mg/kg/day (0, 0.015, 0.03, or 0.06 mg/m^2); however maternal toxicity, abortions, early deliveries, and deaths occurred in all drug-treated groups. There are no adequate and well-controlled studies in pregnant women. If NIPENT is used during pregnancy, or if the patient becomes pregnant while taking (receiving) this drug, the patient should be apprised of the potential hazard to the fetus. Women of childbearing potential receiving NIPENT should be advised to avoid becoming pregnant.

PRECAUTIONS

General

Therapy with NIPENT requires regular patient observation and monitoring of hematologic parameters and blood chemistry values. If severe adverse reactions occur, the drug should be withheld (see DOSAGE AND ADMINISTRATION), and appropriate corrective measures should be taken according to the clinical judgment of the physician.

NIPENT treatment should be withheld or discontinued in patients showing evidence of nervous system toxicity.

Information for Patients

Patients should be advised of the signs and symptoms of adverse events associated with NIPENT therapy. (See ADVERSE REACTIONS.)

Laboratory Tests

Prior to initiating therapy with NIPENT, renal function should be assessed with a serum creatinine and/or a creatinine clearance assay. (See CLINICAL PHARMACOLOGY and DOSAGE AND ADMINISTRATION.) Complete blood counts and serum creatinine should be performed before each dose of NIPENT and at other appropriate periods during therapy (see DOSAGE AND ADMINISTRATION). Severe neutropenia has been observed following the early courses of treatment with NIPENT and therefore frequent monitoring of complete blood counts is recommended during this time. If hematologic parameters do not improve with subsequent courses, patients should be evaluated for disease status, including a bone marrow examination. Periodic monitoring of the peripheral blood for hairy cells should be performed to assess the response to treatment.

In addition, bone marrow aspirates and biopsies may be required at 2 to 3 month intervals to assess the response to treatment.

TABLE 1

Adverse Event*	Number (%) of Patients (N=197)	Adverse Event*	Number (%) of Patients (N=197)
Leukopenia	118 (60)	Skin Disorder	34 (17)
Nausea and Vomiting	104 (53)	Increased Cough	33 (17)
Fever	83 (42)	Upper Respiratory Infection	31 (16)
Infection	70 (36)	Anorexia	32 (16)
Anemia	68 (35)	Genitourinary Disorder	30 (15)
Thrombocytopenia	64 (32)	Diarrhea	29 (15)
Fatigue	57 (29)	Headache	25 (13)
Rash	52 (26)	Lung Disorder	24 (12)
Nausea	43 (22)	Allergic Reaction	22 (11)
Pain	40 (20)	Chills	22 (11)
Hepatic Disorder/Elevated		Myalgia	22 (11)
Liver Function Tests	38 (19)	Neurologic Disorder, CNS	21 (11)

*Occurring in at least 11% of patients

Drug Interactions

Allopurinol and NIPENT are both associated with skin rashes. Based on clinical studies in 25 refractory patients who received both NIPENT and allopurinol, the combined use of NIPENT and allopurinol did not appear to produce a higher incidence of skin rashes than observed with NIPENT alone. There has been a report of one patient who received both drugs and experienced a hypersensitivity vasculitis that resulted in death. It was unclear whether this adverse event and subsequent death resulted from the drug combination.

Biochemical studies have demonstrated that pentostatin enhances the effects of vidarabine, a purine nucleoside with antiviral activity. The combined use of vidarabine and NIPENT may result in an increase in adverse reations associated with each drug. The therapeutic benefit of the drug combination has not been established.

The combined use of NIPENT and fludarabine phosphate is not recommended because it may be associated with an increased risk of fatal pulmonary toxicity (see WARNINGS).

Carcinogenesis, Mutagenesis, Impairment of Fertility

Carcinogenesis: No animal carcinogenicity studies have been conducted with pentostatin.

Mutagenesis: Pentostatin was nonmutagenic when tested in *Salmonella typhimurium* strains TA-98, TA-1535, TA-1537, and TA-1538. When tested with strain TA-100, a repeatable statistically significant response trend was observed with and without metabolic activation. The response was 2.1 to 2.2 fold higher than the background at 10 mg/plate, the maximum possible drug concentration. Formulated pentostatin was clastogenic in the *in vivo* mouse bone marrow micronucleus assay at 20, 120, and 240 mg/kg. Pentostatin was not mutagenic to V79 Chinese hamster lung cells at the HGPRT locus exposed 3 hours to concentrations of 1 to 3 mg/mL, with or without metabolic activation. Pentostatin did not significantly increase chromosomal aberrations in V79 Chinese hamster lung cells exposed 3 hours to 1 to 3 mg/mL in the presence or absence of metabolic activation.

Impairment of Fertility: No fertility studies have been conducted in animals; however, in a 5-day intravenous toxicity study in dogs, mild seminiferous tubular degeneration was observed with doses of 1 and 4 mg/kg. The possible adverse effects on fertility in humans have not been determined.

Pregnancy

Pregnancy Category D: (See WARNINGS)

Nursing Mothers

It is not known whether NIPENT is excreted in human milk. Because many drugs are excreted in human milk, and because of the potential for serious adverse reactions in nursing infants from pentostatin, a decision should be made whether to discontinue nursing or discontinue the drug, taking into account the importance of NIPENT to the mother.

Pediatric Use

Safety and effectiveness in children or adolescents have not been established.

ADVERSE REACTIONS

The following adverse events were reported during clinical studies with NIPENT in patients with hairy cell leukemia who were refractory to alpha-interferon therapy. Most patients experienced an adverse event. The drug association of these adverse events in particular cases is uncertain as they may be associated with the disease itself (e.g., fever, infection, anemia), but other events, such as the gastrointestinal symptoms, hematologic suppression, rashes, and abnormal liver function tests, can in many cases be attributed to the drug. Most adverse events that were assessed for severity were either mild (52% of reports) or moderate (26% of reports) and diminished in frequency with continued therapy. Eleven percent of patients withdrew from treatment due to an adverse event.

The following table lists adverse events that occurred in at least 21 (11%) of 197 alpha-interferon refractory patients with hairy cell leukemia:

[See table above.]

Adverse events that occurred in 3% to 10% of alpha-interferon-refractory patients are as follows. The drug relatedness of many of these adverse events is uncertain.

Body as a Whole

Death, sepsis, chest pain, abdominal pain, back pain, flu syndrome, asthenia, malaise, and neoplasm

Cardiovascular System

Arrhythmia, abnormal electrocardiogram, thrombophlebitis, and hemorrhage

Digestive System

Constipation, flatulence, and stomatitis

Hemic and Lymphatic System

Ecchymosis, lymphadenopathy, and petechia

Metabolic and Nutritional System

Weight loss, peripheral edema, increased lactate dehydrogenase (LDH)

Musculoskeletal System

Arthralgia

Nervous System

Anxiety, confusion, depression, dizziness, insomnia, nervousness, paresthesia, somnolence, and abnormal thinking

Respiratory System

Bronchitis, dyspnea, epistaxis, lung edema, pneumonia, pharyngitis, rhinitis, and sinusitis

Skin and Appendages

Eczema, dry skin, herpes simplex, herpes zoster, maculopapular rash, pruritus, seborrhea, skin discoloration, sweating, and vesiculobullous rash

Special Senses

Abnormal vision, conjunctivitis, ear pain, and eye pain

Urogenital System

Hematuria and dysuria, increased BUN, and increased creatinine

The remaining adverse events occurred in less than 3% of patients; their relationship to pentostatin is uncertain; **Body as a Whole**—abscess, enlarged abdomen, ascites, cellulitis, cyst, face edema, fibrosis, granuloma, hernia, injection-site hemorrhage, injection-site inflammation, moniliasis, neck rigidity, pelvic pain, photosensitivity reaction, anaphylactoid reaction, immune system disorder, mucous membrane disorder, neck pain; **Cardiovascular System**—aortic stenosis, arterial anomaly, cardiomegaly, congestive heart failure, flushing, cardiac arrest, hypertension, myocardial infarct, palpitation, shock, and varicose vein; **Digestive System**—colitis, dysphagia, eructation, gastritis, gastrointestinal hemorrhage, gum hemorrhage, hepatitis, hepatomegaly, intestinal obstruction, jaundice, leukoplakia, melena, periodontal abscess, proctitis, abnormal stools, dyspepsia, esophagitis, gingivitis, hepatic failure, mouth disorder; **Hemic and Lymphatic System**—abnormal erythrocytes, leucocytosis, pancytopenia, purpura, splenomegaly, eosinophilia, hematologic disorder, hemolysis, lymphoma-like reaction, thrombocythemia; **Metabolic and Nutritional System**—acidosis, increased creatine phosphokinase, dehydration, diabetes mellitus, increased gamma globulins, gout, abnormal healing, hypocholesterolemia, weight gain, hyponatremia; **Musculoskeletal System**—arthritis, bone pain, osteomyelitis, pathological fracture; **Nervous System**—agitation, amnesia, apathy, ataxia, central nervous system depression, coma, convulsion, abnormal dreams, depersonalization, emotional lability, facial paralysis, abnormal gait, hyperesthesia, hyp-

Continued on next page

This product information was prepared in August 1992. On these and other Parke-Davis Products, information may be obtained by addressing PARKE-DAVIS, Division of Warner-Lambert Company, Morris Plains, New Jersey 07950.

Parke-Davis—Cont.

esthesia, hypertonia, incoordination, decreased libido, neuropathy, postural dizziness, decreased reflexes, stupor, tremor, vertigo; **Respiratory System**—asthma, atelectasis, hemoptysis, hyperventilation, hypoventilation, laryngitis, larynx edema, lung fibrosis, pleural effusion, pneumothorax, pulmonary embolus, increased sputum; **Skin and Appendages**—acne, alopecia, contact dermatitis, exfoliative dermatitis, fungal dermatitis, psoriasis, benign skin neoplasm, subcutaneous nodule, skin hypertrophy, urticaria; **Special Senses**—blepharitis, cataract, deafness, diplopia, exophthalmos, lacrimation disorder, optic neuritis, otitis media, parosmia, retinal detachment, taste perversion, tinnitus; **Urogenital System**—albuminuria, fibrocystic breast, glycosuria, gynecomastia, hydronephrosis, kidney failure, oliguria, polyuria, pyuria, toxic nephropathy, urinary frequency, urinary retention, urinary tract infection, urinary urgency, impaired urination, urolithiasis, and vaginitis.

One patient with hairy cell leukemia treated with NIPENT during another clinical study developed unilateral uveitis with vision loss.

OVERDOSAGE

No specific antidote for NIPENT overdose is known. NIPENT administered at higher doses (20–50 mg/m² in divided doses over 5 days) than recommended was associated with deaths due to severe renal, hepatic, pulmonary, and CNS toxicity. In case of overdose, management would include general supportive measures through any period of toxicity that occurs.

DOSAGE AND ADMINISTRATION

It is recommended that patients receive hydration with 500 to 1,000 mL of 5% Dextrose in 0.5 Normal Saline or equivalent before NIPENT administration. An additional 500 mL of 5% Dextrose or equivalent should be administered after NIPENT is given.

The recommended dosage of NIPENT for the treatment of alpha-interferon-refractory hairy cell leukemia is 4 mg/m² every other week. NIPENT may be administered intravenously by bolus injection or diluted in a larger volume and given over 20 to 30 minutes. (See PREPARATION OF INTRAVENOUS SOLUTION.)

Higher doses are not recommended.

No extravasation injuries were reported in clinical studies. The optimal duration of treatment has not been determined. In the absence of major toxicity and with observed continuing improvement, the patient should be treated until a complete response has been achieved. Although not established as required, the administration of two additional doses has been recommended following the achievement of a complete response.

All patients receiving NIPENT at 6 months should be assessed for response to treatment. If the patient has not achieved a complete or partial response, treatment with NIPENT should be discontinued.

If the patient has achieved a partial response, NIPENT treatment should be continued in an effort to achieve a complete response. At any time thereafter that a complete response is achieved, two additional doses of NIPENT are recommended. NIPENT treatment should then be stopped. If the best response to treatment at the end of 12 months is a partial response, it is recommended that treatment with NIPENT be stopped.

Withholding or discontinuation of individual doses may be needed when severe adverse reactions occur. Drug treatment should be withheld in patients with severe rash, and withheld or discontinued in patients showing evidence of nervous system toxicity.

NIPENT treatment should be withheld in patients with active infection occurring during the treatment but may be resumed when the infection is controlled.

Patients who have elevated serum creatinine should have their dose withheld and a creatinine clearance determined. There are insufficient data to recommend a starting or a subsequent dose for patients with impaired renal function (creatinine clearance <60 mL/min).

Patients with impaired renal function should be treated only when the potential benefit justifies the potential risk. Two patients with impaired renal function (creatinine clearances 50 to 60 mL/min) achieved complete response without unusual adverse events when treated with 2 mg/m².

No dosage reduction is recommended at the start of therapy with NIPENT in patients with anemia, neutropenia, or thrombocytopenia. In addition, dosage reductions are not recommended during treatment in patients with anemia and thrombocytopenia if patients can be otherwise supported hematologically. NIPENT should be temporarily withheld if the absolute neutrophil count falls during treatment below 200 cells/mm³ in a patient who had an initial neutrophil count greater than 500 cells/mm³ and may be resumed when the count returns to predose levels.

Preparation of Intravenous Solution

1. Procedures for proper handling and disposal of anticancer drugs should be followed. Several guidelines on this subject have been published.[2-7] There is no general agreement that all of the procedures recommended in the guidelines are necessary or appropriate. Spills and wastes should be treated with a 5% sodium hypochlorite solution prior to disposal.
2. Protective clothing including polyethylene gloves must be worn.
3. Transfer 5 mL of Sterile Water for Injection USP to the vial containing NIPENT and mix thoroughly to obtain complete dissolution of a solution yielding 2 mg/mL. Parenteral drug products should be inspected visually for particulate matter and discoloration prior to administration.
4. NIPENT may be given intravenously by bolus injection or diluted in a larger volume (25 to 50 mL) with 5% Dextrose Injection USP or 0.9% Sodium Chloride Injection USP. Dilution of the entire contents of a reconstituted vial with 25 mL or 50 mL provides a pentostatin concentration of 0.33 mg/mL or 0.18 mg/mL respectively for the diluted solutions.
5. NIPENT solution when diluted for infusion with 5% Dextrose Injection USP or 0.9% Sodium Chloride Injection USP does not interact with PVC infusion containers or administration sets at concentrations of 0.18 mg/mL to 0.33 mg/mL.

Stability

NIPENT vials are stable at refrigerated storage temperature 2° to 8°C (36°to 46°F) for the period stated on the package. Vials reconstituted or reconstituted and further diluted as directed may be stored at room temperature and ambient light but should be used within 8 hours because NIPENT contains no preservatives.

HOW SUPPLIED

NIPENT (pentostatin for injection) is supplied as a sterile lyophilized white to off-white powder in single-dose vials containing 10 mg of pentostatin. The vials are packed in individual cartons. N0071-4243-01 is supplied in packages of ten single-dose vials.

Storage: Store NIPENT vials under refrigerated storage conditions 2° to 8°C (36° to 46°F).

Caution—Federal law prohibits dispensing without prescription.

REFERENCES

1. Malspeis L, et. al. Clinical Pharmacokinetics of 2'-Deoxycoformycin. Cancer Treatment Symposia 2:7–15, 1984.
2. Recommendations for the safe handling of parenteral antineoplastic drugs. NIH publication 83-2621. For sale by the Superintendent of Documents, US Government Printing Office, Washington, DC 20402.
3. AMA council report. Guidelines for handling parenteral antineoplastics. JAMA 25:590–2, 1985.
4. National Study Commission on Cytotoxic Exposure—Recommendations for handling cytotoxic agents. Director of Pharmacy Services, Rhode Island Hospital, 593 Eddy Street, Providence, RI 02902.
5. Clinical Oncological Society of Australia: Guidelines and recommendations for safe handling of antineoplastic agents. Med J Australia 1:426–8, 1983.
6. Jones RB, et. al. Safe handling of chemotherapeutic agents: A report from the Mount Sinai Medical Center. CA: A Cancer Journal for Clinicians 33:258–63, 1983.
7. American Society of Hospital Pharmacists technical assistance bulletin on handling cytotoxic and hazardous drugs. Am J Hosp Pharm 47:1033–49, 1990.

Issued Date: Oct. 1991

PARKE-DAVIS
Div of Warner-Lambert Co © 1991   4243G030
Morris Plains, NJ 07950 USA

Shown in Product Identification Section, page 422

NITROSTAT® ℞
[nī'trō"stăt]
(nitroglycerin tablets, USP)

DESCRIPTION

Nitrostat is a stabilized sublingual nitroglycerin tablet manufactured by a patented process* which prevents the migration of nitroglycerin by adding the nonvolatile fixing agent polyethylene glycol 3350. This stabilized formulation has been shown to be more stable and more uniform than conventional molded tablets. Nitrostat tablets contain 0.15 mg (1/400 grain), 0.3 mg (1/200 grain), 0.4 mg (1/150 grain) and 0.6 mg (1/100 grain) nitroglycerin. Also contains lactose, NF; polyethylene glycol 3350, NF; sucrose, NF.

Nitroglycerin, an organic nitrate, is a vasodilating agent. The chemical name for nitroglycerin is 1,2,3-propanetriol trinitrate.

---

*US Patent No. 3,789,119

CLINICAL PHARMACOLOGY

Relaxation of vascular smooth muscle is the principal pharmacologic action of nitroglycerin. The mechanism by which nitroglycerin produces relaxation of smooth muscle is unknown. Although venous effects predominate, nitroglycerin produces, in a dose-related manner, dilation of both arterial and venous beds. Dilation of the postcapillary vessels, including large veins, promotes peripheral pooling of blood and decreases venous return to the heart, reducing left ventricular end-diastolic pressure (preload). Arteriolar relaxation reduces systemic vascular resistance and arterial pressure (afterload). Myocardial oxygen consumption or demand (as measured by the pressure-rate product, tension-time index and stroke-work index) is decreased by both the arterial and venous effects of nitroglycerin, and a more favorable supply-demand ratio can be achieved.

Therapeutic doses of nitroglycerin may reduce systolic, diastolic and mean arterial blood pressure. Effective coronary perfusion pressure is usually maintained, but can be compromised if blood pressure falls excessively or increased heart rate decreases diastolic filling time.

Elevated central venous and pulmonary capillary wedge pressures, pulmonary vascular resistance and systemic vascular resistance are also reduced by nitroglycerin therapy. Heart rate is usually slightly increased, presumably a reflex response to the fall in blood pressure. Cardiac index may be increased, decreased, or unchanged. Patients with elevated left ventricular filling pressure and systemic vascular resistance values in conjunction with a depressed cardiac index are likely to experience an improvement in cardiac index. On the other hand, when filling pressures and cardiac index are normal, cardiac index may be slightly reduced by intravenous nitroglycerin.

Nitroglycerin is rapidly absorbed following sublingual administration. Its onset of action is approximately one to three minutes. Significant pharmacologic effects are present for 30 to 60 minutes following administration by the above route.

Nitroglycerin is rapidly metabolized to dinitrates and mononitrates, with a short half-life, estimated at 1 to 4 minutes. At plasma concentrations of between 50 and 500 ng/ml, the binding of nitroglycerin to plasma proteins is approximately 60%, while that of 1,2 dinitroglycerin and 1,3 dinitroglycerin is 60% and 30% respectively. The activity and half-life of 1,2 dinitroglycerin and 1,3 dinitroglycerin are not well characterized. The mononitrate is not active.

INDICATIONS AND USAGE

Nitroglycerin is indicated for the prophylaxis, treatment and management of patients with angina pectoris.

CONTRAINDICATIONS

Sublingual nitroglycerin therapy is contraindicated in patients with early myocardial infarction, severe anemia, increased intracranial pressure, and those with a known hypersensitivity to nitroglycerin.

PRECAUTIONS

General: Only the smallest dose required for effective relief of the acute anginal attack should be used. Excessive use may lead to the development of tolerance. Nitrostat tablets are intended for sublingual or buccal administration and should not be swallowed. The drug should be discontinued if blurring of vision or drying of the mouth occurs. Excessive dosage of nitroglycerin may produce severe headaches.

Information for Patients: If possible, patients should sit down when taking Nitrostat tablets. This eliminates the possibility of falling due to lightheadedness or dizziness.

Drug Interactions: Concomitant use of nitrates and alcohol may cause hypotension. Patients receiving antihypertensive drugs, beta-adrenergic blockers, or phenothiazines and nitrates should be observed for possible additive hypotensive effects.

Drug/Laboratory Test Interactions: Nitrates may interfere with the Zlatkis-Zak color reaction causing a false report of decreased serum cholesterol.

Carcinogenesis, Mutagenesis, Impairment of Fertility: No long-term studies in animals were performed to evaluate the carcinogenic potential of nitroglycerin.

Pregnancy Category C: Animal reproduction studies have not been conducted with nitroglycerin. It is also not known whether nitroglycerin can cause fetal harm when administered to a pregnant woman or can affect reproduction capacity. Nitroglycerin should be given to a pregnant woman only if clearly needed.

Nursing Mother: It is not known whether nitroglycerin is excreted in human milk. Because many drugs are excreted in human milk, caution should be exercised when intravenous nitroglycerin is administered to a nursing woman.

Pediatric Use: The safety and effectiveness of nitroglycerin in children have not been established.

ADVERSE REACTIONS

Transient headache may occur immediately after use. Vertigo, weakness, palpitation, and other manifestations of pos-

tural hypotension may develop occasionally, particularly in erect, immobile patients. Syncope due to nitrate vasodilation has been reported.

DOSAGE AND ADMINISTRATION

One tablet should be dissolved under the tongue or in the buccal pouch at the first sign of an acute anginal attack. The dose may be repeated approximately every five minutes until relief is obtained. If the pain persists after a total of 3 tablets in a 15-minute period, the physician should be notified. Nitrostat may be used prophylactically five to ten minutes prior to engaging in activities which might precipitate an acute attack.

HOW SUPPLIED

Nitrostat is supplied in four strengths in bottles containing 100 tablets each, with color-coded labels, and in color-coded Patient Convenience Packages of four bottles of 25 tablets each.

0.15 mg (1/400 grain):
N 0071-0568-24—Bottle of 100 tablets
N 0071-0568-13—Convenience Package
0.3 mg (1/200 grain):
N 0071-0569-24—Bottle of 100 tablets
0.4 mg (1/150 grain):
N 0071-0570-24—Bottle of 100 tablets
N 0071-0570-13—Convenience Package
0.6 mg (1/100 grain):
N 0071-0571-24—Bottle of 100 tablets

Store at controlled room temperature 15°–30°C (59°–86°F). Protect from moisture.

0568G065

Shown in Product Identification Section, page 422

NITROSTAT® IV ℞

[nī′trō″stăt]
(Nitroglycerin Injection, USP)
FOR INTRAVENOUS USE ONLY

NOT FOR DIRECT INTRAVENOUS INJECTION. NITROSTAT IV IS A CONCENTRATED, POTENT DRUG WHICH MUST BE DILUTED IN DEXTROSE (5%) INJECTION, USP OR SODIUM CHLORIDE (0.9%) INJECTION, USP PRIOR TO ITS INFUSION. THE CONTAINER AND ADMINISTRATION SET USED FOR INFUSION MAY AFFECT THE AMOUNT OF INTRAVENOUS NITROGLYCERIN DELIVERED TO THE PATIENT. (SEE WARNINGS AND DOSAGE AND ADMINISTRATION SECTIONS.)

CAUTION: SEVERAL PREPARATIONS OF NITROGLYCERIN INJECTION ARE AVAILABLE. THEY DIFFER IN CONCENTRATION AND/OR VOLUME PER VIAL. WHEN SWITCHING FROM ONE PRODUCT TO ANOTHER, ATTENTION MUST BE PAID TO THE DILUTION AND DOSAGE AND ADMINISTRATION INSTRUCTIONS.

DESCRIPTION

Nitrostat IV is a clear, practically colorless additive solution for intravenous infusion after dilution. Nitrostat IV is available in three strengths, an 8 mg per ampoule, a 50 mg per ampoule or vial, and a 100 mg per ampoule or vial. Each milliliter of Nitrostat IV 8 mg per ampoule contains 0.8 mg nitroglycerin, with citric acid, USP, anhydrous and sodium citrate, USP, hydrous as buffers, and 5% alcohol in Water for Injection, USP. Each milliliter of Nitrostat IV 50 mg per ampoule or vial contains 5 mg nitroglycerin, 30% propylene glycol, USP and 30% alcohol, USP (28.5% alcohol) in Water for Injection, USP. Each milliliter of Nitrostat IV 100 mg per ampoule or vial contains 10 mg of nitroglycerin in 50% propylene glycol, USP and 50% alcohol. The solutions are sterile, nonpyrogenic, and nonexplosive. Intravenous nitroglycerin, an organic nitrate, is a vasodilator. The chemical name for nitroglycerin is 1,2,3-propanetriol trinitrate and its chemical structure is:

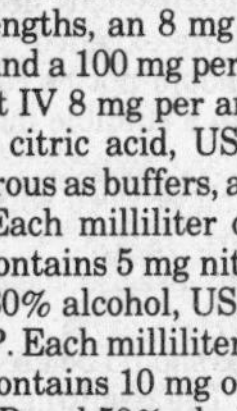

H2C-O-NO2
HC-O-NO2
H2C-O-NO2

$C_3H_5N_3O_9$ MOL WT 227.09

CLINICAL PHARMACOLOGY

Relaxation of vascular smooth muscle is the principal pharmacologic action of intravenous nitroglycerin. Although venous effects predominate, nitroglycerin produces, in a dose-related manner, dilation of both arterial and venous beds. Dilation of the postcapillary vessels, including large veins, promotes peripheral pooling of blood and decreases venous return to the heart, reducing left ventricular end-diastolic pressure (preload). Arteriolar relaxation reduces systemic vascular resistance and arterial pressure (afterload). Myocardial oxygen consumption or demand (as measured by the pressure-rate product, tension-time index and stroke-work index) is decreased by both the arterial and venous effects of nitroglycerin, and a more favorable supply-demand ratio can be achieved.

Therapeutic doses of intravenous nitroglycerin reduce systolic, diastolic and mean arterial blood pressure. Effective coronary perfusion pressure is usually maintained, but can be compromised if blood pressure falls excessively or increased heart rate decreases diastolic filling time.

Elevated central venous and pulmonary capillary wedge pressures, pulmonary vascular resistance and systemic vascular resistance are also reduced by nitroglycerin therapy. Heart rate is usually slightly increased, presumably a reflex response to the fall in blood pressure. Cardiac index may be increased, decreased, or unchanged. Patients with elevated left ventricular filling pressure and systemic vascular resistance values in conjunction with a depressed cardiac index are likely to experience an improvement in cardiac index. On the other hand, when filling pressures and cardiac index are normal, cardiac index may be slightly reduced by intravenous nitroglycerin.

Nitroglycerin is widely distributed in the body with an apparent volume of distribution of approximately 200 liters in adult male subjects, and is rapidly metabolized to dinitrates and mononitrates with a short half-life, estimated at 1 to 4 minutes. This results in a low plasma concentration after intravenous infusion. At plasma concentrations of between 50 and 500 mg/mL, the binding of nitroglycerin to plasma proteins is approximately 60%, while that of 1,2 dinitroglycerin and 1,3 dinitroglycerin is 60% and 30% respectively. The activity and half-life of 1,2 dinitroglycerin and 1,3 dinitroglycerin are not well characterized. The mononitrate is not active.

INDICATIONS AND USAGE

Nitrostat IV is indicated for:

1. *Control of blood pressure in perioperative hypertension*, ie, hypertension associated with surgical procedures, especially cardiovascular procedures, such as the hypertension seen during intratracheal intubation, anesthesia, skin incision, sternotomy, cardiac bypass, and in the immediate postsurgical period.
2. *Congestive heart failure associated with acute myocardial infarction.*
3. *Treatment of angina pectoris* in patients who have not responded to recommended doses of organic nitrates and/or a beta blocker.
4. *Production of controlled hypotension during surgical procedures.*

CONTRAINDICATIONS

Nitrostat IV should not be administered to individuals with:

1. A known hypersensitivity to nitroglycerin or a known idiosyncratic reaction to organic nitrates.
2. Hypotension or uncorrected hypovolemia, as the use of Nitrostat IV in such states could produce severe hypotension or shock.
3. Increased intracranial pressure (eg, head trauma or cerebral hemorrhage).
4. Constrictive pericarditis and pericardial tamponade.
5. Inadequate cerebral circulation.

WARNINGS

1. Nitroglycerin readily migrates into many plastics. To avoid absorption of nitroglycerin into plastic parenteral solution containers, the dilution and storage of nitroglycerin injection should be made only in glass parenteral solution bottles.
2. Some filters also absorb nitroglycerin; they should be avoided.
3. Forty to 80% of the total amount of nitroglycerin in the final diluted solution for infusion is absorbed by the polyvinyl chloride (PVC) tubing of the intravenous administration sets currently in general use. The higher rates of absorption occur when flow rates are low, nitroglycerin concentrations are high, and tubing is long. Although the rate of loss is highest during the early phase of administration (when flow rates are lowest), the loss is neither constant nor self-limiting; consequently no simple calculation or correction can be performed to convert the theoretical infusion rate (based on the concentration of the infusion solution) to the actual delivery rate.

   Because of this problem, Parke-Davis, Division of Warner-Lambert Company has developed a nonabsorbing infusion set, Nitrostat IV intravenous infusion set, in which the loss of nitroglycerin is minimal (less than 5%). The Nitrostat IV intravenous infusion set or a similar infusion set is recommended for infusions of intravenous nitroglycerin. Dosage instructions must be followed with care. It should be noted that when these infusion sets are used, the calculated dose will be delivered to the patient because the loss of nitroglycerin due to absorption in standard PVC tubing will be kept to a minimum. Note that the dosages commonly used in published studies utilized general-use PVC infusion sets and recommended doses based on this experience are too high if the new infusion sets are used.
4. A potential safety problem exists with the combined use of some infusion pumps and some nonPVC infusion sets. Because the special tubing required to prevent the absorption of nitroglycerin tends to be less pliable than the conventional PVC tubing normally used with such infusion pumps, the pumps may fail to occlude the infusion sets completely. The results may be excessive flow at low infusion rate settings, causing alarms, or unregulated gravity flow when the infusion pump is stopped; this could lead to over-infusion of nitroglycerin. All infusion pumps should be tested with the infusion sets to ensure their ability to deliver nitroglycerin accurately at low flow rates, and to occlude the infusion sets properly when the infusion is stopped.

PRECAUTIONS

Nitrostat IV should be used with caution in patients who have severe hepatic or renal disease.

Excessive hypotension, especially for prolonged periods of time, must be avoided because of possible deleterious effects on the brain, heart, liver and kidney from poor perfusion and the attendant risk of ischemia, thrombosis, and altered function of these organs. Paradoxical bradycardia and increased angina pectoris may accompany nitroglycerin-induced hypotension. Patients with normal or low pulmonary capillary wedge pressure are especially sensitive to the hypotensive effects of intravenous nitroglycerin. If pulmonary capillary wedge pressure is being monitored, it will be noted that a fall in wedge pressure precedes the onset of arterial hypotension, and the pulmonary capillary wedge pressure is thus a useful guide to safe titration of the drug.

NITROSTAT IV CONTAINS ALCOHOL. SAFETY FOR INTRACORONARY INJECTION HAS NOT BEEN SHOWN.

Carcinogenesis, Mutagenesis, Impairment of Fertility:
No long-term studies in animals were performed to evaluate the carcinogenic potential of nitroglycerin.

Pregnancy:
Category C: Animal reproduction studies have not been conducted with nitroglycerin. It is also not known whether nitroglycerin can cause fetal harm when administered to a pregnant woman or can affect reproduction capacity. Nitroglycerin should be given to a pregnant woman only if clearly needed.

Nursing Mother:
It is not known whether nitroglycerin is excreted in human milk. Because many drugs are excreted in human milk, caution should be exercised when intravenous nitroglycerin is administered to a nursing woman.

Pediatric Use:
The safety and effectiveness of nitroglycerin in children have not been established.

ADVERSE REACTIONS

The most frequent adverse reaction in patients treated with nitroglycerin is headache, which occurs in approximately 2% of patients. Other adverse reactions occurring in less than 1% of patients are the following: tachycardia, nausea, vomiting, apprehension, restlessness, muscle twitching, retrosternal discomfort, palpitations, dizziness and abdominal pain.

The following additional adverse reactions have been reported with the oral and/or topical use of nitroglycerin: cutaneous flushing, weakness, and occasionally drug rash or exfoliative dermatitis.

OVERDOSAGE

Accidental overdosage of nitroglycerin may result in severe hypotension and reflex tachycardia which can be treated by elevating the legs and decreasing or temporarily terminating the infusion until the patient's condition stabilizes. Since the duration of the hemodynamic effects following nitroglycerin administration is quite short, additional corrective measures are usually not required. However, if further therapy is indicated, administration of an intravenous alpha adrenergic agonist (eg, methoxamine or phenylephrine) should be considered.

DOSAGE AND ADMINISTRATION

NOT FOR DIRECT INTRAVENOUS INJECTION

NITROSTAT IV IS A CONCENTRATED, POTENT DRUG WHICH MUST BE DILUTED IN DEXTROSE (5%) INJECTION, USP OR SODIUM CHLORIDE (0.9%) INJECTION, USP PRIOR TO ITS INFUSION.

NITROSTAT IV SHOULD NOT BE ADMIXED WITH OTHER DRUGS.

Continued on next page

This product information was prepared in August 1992. On these and other Parke-Davis Products, information may be obtained by addressing PARKE-DAVIS, Division of Warner-Lambert Company, Morris Plains, New Jersey 07950.

Parke-Davis—Cont.

Parenteral drug products should be inspected visually for particulate matter and discoloration prior to administration, whenever solution and container permit. [See table below.]
Dilution: Aseptically transfer the desired amount of Nitrostat IV (as noted in the preceding tables) into a glass IV bottle containing the stated volume of 5% Dextrose Injection, USP or 0.9% Sodium Chloride Injection, USP and mix well. The resultant solution is stable for at least 96 hours at controlled room temperature (15°–30°C) or under refrigeration. It is important to consider the fluid requirements of the patient as well as the expected duration of infusion in selecting the appropriate dilution of nitroglycerin. The preceding tables give the nitroglycerin concentrations at various dilutions.
After the initial dosage titration, the concentration of the admixture may be increased, if necessary, to limit fluids given to the patient. The concentration of the infusion solution should not exceed 400 mcg/mL of nitroglycerin.
NOTE: If the concentration is adjusted, it is imperative to flush or replace the Nitrostat IV infusion set before a new concentration is utilized. The dead space of the set is approximately 20 mL and, depending on the flow rate, it could take from 6 minutes to 13 hours for the new concentration to reach the patient if the set were not flushed or replaced.
Dosage: *IMPORTANT NOTICE:* Dosage is affected by the type of container used as well as the type of infusion set used (See Warnings). Although the usual starting adult dose

range reported in clinical studies was 25 mcg/min or more, those studies used *PVC TUBING. The use of nonabsorbing tubing will result in the need to use reduced doses.*
The recommended dosage when using the nonabsorbing Nitrostat IV Intravenous Infusion Set should initially be 5 mcg/min delivered through an infusion pump capable of exact and constant delivery of the drug. Subsequent titration must be adjusted to the clinical situation, with dose increments becoming more cautious as partial response is seen. Initial titration should be 5 mcg/min increments, with increases every 3 to 5 minutes until some response is noted. If no response is seen at 20 mcg/min, increments of 10 and later 20 mcg/min can be used. Once a partial blood pressure response is observed, the dose increase should be reduced and the interval between increments should be lengthened. Patients with normal or low left ventricular filling pressure or pulmonary capillary wedge pressure (eg, angina patients without other complications) may be hypersensitive to the effects of nitroglycerin and may respond fully to doses as small as 5 mcg/min. These patients require especially careful titration and monitoring.
There is no fixed optimum dose of nitroglycerin. Due to variations in the responsiveness of individual patients to the drug, each patient must be titrated to the desired level of hemodynamic function. Therefore, continuous monitoring of physiologic parameters (blood pressure and heart rate in all patients, other measurements such as pulmonary capillary wedge pressure, as appropriate) MUST BE PERFORMED to achieve the correct dose. Adequate systemic blood pressure and coronary perfusion pressure must be maintained.

DILUTION AND ADMINISTRATION TABLES
(60 microdrops=1 milliliter)

Nitrostat IV 8 mg per ampoule

Concentration	1 amp in 250 mL approx 30 mcg/mL	2 amp in 250 mL approx 60 mcg/mL	3 amp in 250 mL approx 85 mcg/mL
Dose (mcg/min)	Flow Rate mL/hour (microdrops/minute)		
5	10	5	3
10	20	10	7
15	30	15	10
20	40	20	14
30	60	30	21
40	80	40	28
50	100	50	35
60	120	60	42
80	160	80	56
100	200	100	71

Nitrostat IV 50 mg per ampoule or vial

Concentration	1 amp/vial in 500 mL approx 100 mcg/mL	2 amp/vial in 500 mL approx 200 mcg/mL
Dose (mcg/min)	Flow Rate mL/hour (microdrops/minute)	
5	3	1.5
10	6	3
15	9	4.5
20	12	6
30	18	9
40	24	12
50	30	15
60	36	18
80	48	24
100	60	30
120	72	36
160	96	48
200	120	60

Nitrostat IV 100 mg per ampoule or vial

Concentration	1 amp/vial in 500 mL approx 200 mcg/mL	2 amp/vial in 500 mL approx 400 mcg/mL
Dose (mcg/min)	Flow Rate mL/hour (microdrops/minute)	
5	1.5	0.75
10	3	1.5
15	4.5	2.25
20	6	3
30	9	4.5
40	12	6
50	15	7.5
60	18	9
80	24	12
100	30	15
120	36	18
160	48	24
200	60	30

DIRECTIONS FOR PREPARING NITROSTAT IV INFUSION SET

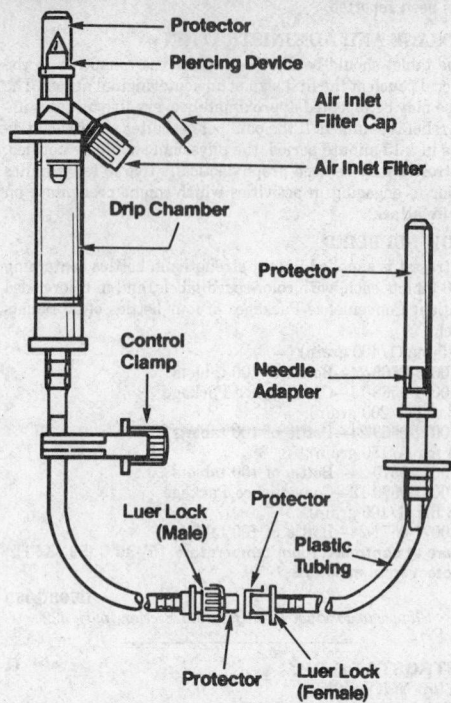

Caution—The fluid path and areas under the protectors of the intravenous infusion set are sterile. Do not use if damaged or if end protectors are not in place.
1. Position control clamp 6 to 8 inches from the Male Luer Lock connector, then close clamp. (To close clamp, rotate screw stem clockwise.)
2. Remove plastic protector from each Luer Lock end and connect the Luer Lock attachment.
3. With IV solution bottle in the upright position.
   a) remove plastic protector from the piercing device;
   b) THRUST the piercing device STRAIGHT DOWN through the CENTER of the target area in the rubber stopper (push straight down, do not twist).
   c) squeeze drip chamber and hold.
4. Invert the bottle and suspend from suitable stand.
5. Release pressure from drip chamber.
6. Remove needle adapter protector by pulling straight off (do not twist off). If required, place needle on needle adapter. Hold this end of the tubing above the level of the nitroglycerin solution in the bottle. Loosen the control clamp and allow the solution to run in and fill the tubing and needle. Displace the air in the entire injection set by raising or lowering the intravenous needle end of tubing until all the air bubbles are expelled.
   (NOTE: Drip chamber should not be completely filled.)
7. Attach the infusion set to a suitable mechanical infusion control device.
8. Tighten control clamp and proceed with venipuncture or connect to needle.
9. Adjust control device for precise measurement of flow rate.
NOTE: Only glass IV bottles should be used in preparing the Nitrostat IV admixture. The resulting solution should be administered using the intravenous infusion set supplied in the Nitrostat IV infusion kit.
If a Volumetric infusion pump is used: Follow step 1, then aseptically remove plastic protector from each Luer Lock end and attach both Luer Lock ends to the cassette of the infusion pump. Install cassette and close door of pump. Follow steps 3, 4, and 5. Remove needle adapter protector, prime set, and purge out air. Set rate and volume and start infusion. [See illustration next page.]
Directions for using the Spike-Adapter (use with McGaw LVP bottles): Remove the plastic protector from the piercing device on the drip chamber. Aseptically insert the piercing device on the drip chamber into the spike adapter tubing coupler as far as it will go. Remove the end plastic protector from the spike adapter and proceed with the above directions for preparing the infusion set depending on what pump/controller is used.

HOW SUPPLIED
N0071-4572-10 Carton of 10 x 10-mL ampoules of Nitrostat IV, 8 mg (0.8 mg/mL).
N0071-4575-45 Carton of 10 x 10-mL vials of Nitrostat IV, 50 mg (5 mg/mL).
N0071-4579-45 Carton of 10 x 10-mL vials of Nitrostat IV, 100 mg (10 mg/mL).

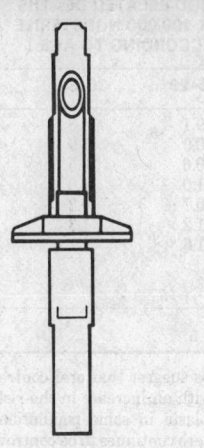

Spike-Adapter

Store at controlled room temperature 15°–30°C (59°–86°F). **Caution**—Federal law prohibits dispensing without prescription.

4572G027

Shown in Product Identification Section, page 422

NORLESTRIN® 21   ℞
(Norethindrone Acetate and Ethinyl Estradiol Tablets, USP)

NORLESTRIN® 21 1/50   ℞
(Each tablet contains 1 mg norethindrone acetate and 50 mcg ethinyl estradiol.)

NORLESTRIN® 21 2.5/50   ℞
(Each tablet contains 2.5 mg norethindrone acetate and 50 mcg ethinyl estradiol.)

NORLESTRIN® Fe   ℞
(Norethindrone Acetate and Ethinyl Estradiol Tablets, USP and Ferrous Fumarate Tablets.)

NORLESTRIN® Fe 1/50   ℞
(Each yellow tablet contains 1 mg norethindrone acetate and 50 mcg ethinyl estradiol. Each brown tablet contains 75 mg ferrous fumarate.)

NORLESTRIN® Fe 2.5/50   ℞
(Each pink tablet contains 2.5 mg norethindrone acetate and 50 mcg ethinyl estradiol. Each brown tablet contains 75 mg ferrous fumarate.)

Each yellow tablet contains norethindrone acetate (17 alpha-ethinyl-19-nortestosterone acetate), 1 mg; ethinyl estradiol (17 alpha-ethinyl-1,3,5(10)-estratriene-3, 17 beta-diol), 50 mcg. Also contains acacia, NF; lactose, NF; magnesium stearate, NF; starch, NF; confectioner's sugar, NF; talc, USP; D&C yellow No. 10; FD&C yellow No. 6.
Each pink tablet contains norethindrone acetate (17 alpha-ethinyl-19-nortestosterone acetate), 2.5 mg; ethinyl estradiol (17 alpha-ethinyl-1,3,5(10)-estratriene-3, 17 beta-diol), 50 mcg. Also contains acacia, NF; lactose, NF; magnesium stearate, NF; starch, NF; confectioner's sugar, NF; talc, USP; FD&C red No. 40.
Each brown tablet contains microcrystalline cellulose, NF; ferrous fumarate, USP; magnesium stearate, NF; povidone, USP; sodium starch glycolate, NF; sucrose with modified dextrins.

DESCRIPTION
Norlestrin **21** and Norlestrin **Fe** are progestogen-estrogen combinations.
Norlestrin **Fe** 1/50 and 2.5/50 provide a continuous dosage regimen consisting of 21 oral contraceptive tablets and seven ferrous fumarate tablets. The ferrous fumarate tablets are present to facilitate ease of drug administration via a 28-day regimen and are not intended to serve any therapeutic purpose.

CLINICAL PHARMACOLOGY
Combination oral contraceptives act by suppression of gonadotropins. Although the primary mechanism of this action is inhibition of ovulation, other alterations include changes in the cervical mucus (which increase the difficulty of sperm entry into the uterus) and the endometrium (which reduce the likelihood of implantation).

TABLE I
LOWEST EXPECTED AND TYPICAL FAILURE RATES DURING THE FIRST YEAR
OF CONTINUOUS USE OF A METHOD
% of Women Experiencing an Accidental Pregnancy in the First Year of Continuous Use

Method	Lowest Expected*	Typical**
(No contraception)	(89)	(89)
Oral contraceptives		3
combined	0.1	N/A***
progestin only	0.5	N/A***
Diaphragm with spermicidal cream or jelly	3	18
Spermicides alone (foam, creams, jellies and vaginal suppositories)	3	21
Vaginal sponge		
nulliparous	5	18
multiparous	>8	>28
IUD (medicated)	1	6†
Condom without spermicides	2	12
Periodic abstinence (all methods)	2–10	20
Female sterilization	0.2	0.4
Male sterilization	0.1	0.15

Adapted from J. Trussell and K. Kost, Table 11, ref #1.
  * The authors' best guess of the percentage of women expected to experience an accidental pregnancy among couples who initiate a method (not necessarily for the first time) and who use it consistently and correctly during the first year if they do not stop for any other reason.
 ** This term represents "typical" couples who initiate use of a method (not necessarily for the first time), who experience an accidental pregnancy during the first year if they do not stop use for any other reason.
*** N/A—Data not available
  † Combined typical rate for both medicated and non-medicated IUD. The rate for medicated IUD alone is not available.

INDICATIONS AND USAGE
Norlestrin **21** and Norlestrin **Fe** are indicated for the prevention of pregnancy in women who elect to use oral contraceptives as a method of contraception.
Oral contraceptives are highly effective. Table I lists the typical accidental pregnancy rates for users of combination oral contraceptives and other methods of contraception. The efficacy of these contraceptive methods, except sterilization, depends upon the reliability with which they are used. Correct and consistent use of methods can result in lower failure rates.
[See table above.]

CONTRAINDICATIONS
Oral contraceptives should not be used in women who currently have the following conditions:
● Thrombophlebitis or thromboembolic disorders
● A past history of deep vein thrombophlebitis or thromboembolic disorders
● Cerebral vascular or coronary artery disease
● Known or suspected carcinoma of the breast
● Carcinoma of the endometrium or other known or suspected estrogen-dependent neoplasia
● Undiagnosed abnormal genital bleeding
● Cholestatic jaundice of pregnancy or jaundice with prior pill use
● Hepatic adenomas or carcinomas
● Known or suspected pregnancy

WARNINGS

> **Cigarette smoking increases the risk of serious cardiovascular side effects from oral contraceptive use. This risk increases with age and with heavy smoking (15 or more cigarettes per day) and is quite marked in women over 35 years of age. Women who use oral contraceptives should be strongly advised not to smoke.**

The use of oral contraceptives is associated with increased risks of several serious conditions including myocardial infarction, thromboembolism, stroke, hepatic neoplasia, and gallbladder disease, although the risk of serious morbidity or mortality is very small in healthy women without underlying risk factors. The risk of morbidity and mortality increases significantly in the presence of other underlying risk factors such as hypertension, hyperlipidemias, obesity and diabetes.
Practitioners prescribing oral contraceptives should be familiar with the following information relating to these risks.
The information contained in this package insert is principally based on studies carried out in patients who used oral contraceptives with higher formulations of estrogens and progestogens than those in common use today. The effect of long-term use of the oral contraceptives with lower formulations of both estrogens and progestogens remains to be determined.
Throughout this labeling, epidemiological studies reported are of two types: retrospective or case control studies and prospective or cohort studies. Case control studies provide a measure of the relative risk of a disease, namely, a *ratio of* the incidence of a disease among oral contraceptive users to that among nonusers. The relative risk does not provide in-

formation on the actual clinical occurrence of a disease. Cohort studies provide a measure of attributable risk, which is the *difference* in the incidence of disease between oral contraceptive users and nonusers. The attributable risk does provide information about the actual occurrence of a disease in the population (adapted from refs. 2 and 3 with the author's permission). For further information, the reader is referred to a text on epidemiological methods.

1. Thromboembolic Disorders And Other Vascular Problems.
a. Myocardial infarction
An increased risk of myocardial infarction has been attributed to oral contraceptive use. This risk is primarily in smokers or women with other underlying risk factors for coronary artery disease such as hypertension, hypercholesterolemia, morbid obesity, and diabetes. The relative risk of heart attack for current oral contraceptive users has been estimated to be two to six (4–10). The risk is very low under the age of 30.
Smoking in combination with oral contraceptive use has been shown to contribute substantially to the incidence of myocardial infarctions in women in their mid-thirties or older with smoking accounting for the majority of excess cases (11). Mortality rates associated with circulatory disease have been shown to increase substantially in smokers over the age of 35 and nonsmokers over the age of 40 (Table II) among women who use oral contraceptives.
[See Table II on next page.]
Oral contraceptives may compound the effects of well-known risk factors, such as hypertension, diabetes, hyperlipidemias, age and obesity (13). In particular, some progestogens are known to decrease HDL cholesterol and cause glucose intolerance, while estrogens may create a state of hyperinsulinism (14–18). Oral contraceptives have been shown to increase blood pressure among users (see section 9 in WARNINGS). Similar effects on risk factors have been associated with an increased risk of heart disease. Oral contraceptives must be used with caution in women with cardiovascular disease risk factors.
b. Thromboembolism
An increased risk of thromboembolic and thrombotic disease associated with the use of oral contraceptives is well established. Case control studies have found the relative risk of users compared to non-users to be 3 for the first episode of superficial venous thrombosis, 4 to 11 for deep vein thrombosis or pulmonary embolism, and 1.5 to 6 for women with predisposing conditions for venous thromboembolic disease (2,3,19–24). Cohort studies have shown the relative risk to be somewhat lower, about 3 for new cases and about 4.5 for new cases requiring hospitalization (25). The risk of thromboembolic disease due to oral contraceptives is not related to length of use and disappears after pill use is stopped (2).

Continued on next page

This product information was prepared in August 1992. On these and other Parke-Davis Products, information may be obtained by addressing PARKE-DAVIS, Division of Warner-Lambert Company, Morris Plains, New Jersey 07950.

Parke-Davis—Cont.

A two- to four-fold increase in relative risk of postoperative thromboembolic complications has been reported with the use of oral contraceptives (9,26). The relative risk of venous thrombosis in women who have predisposing conditions is twice that of women without such medical conditions (9,26). If feasible, oral contraceptives should be discontinued at least four weeks prior to and for two weeks after elective surgery of a type associated with an increase in risk of thromboembolism and during and following prolonged immobilization. Since the immediate post partum period is also associated with an increased risk of thromboembolism, oral contraceptives should be started no earlier than four to six weeks after delivery in women who elect not to breast feed.

c. Cerebrovascular diseases

Oral contraceptives have been shown to increase both the relative and attributable risks of cerebrovascular events (thrombotic and hemorrhagic strokes), although, in general, the risk is greatest among older (> 35 years), hypertensive women who also smoke. Hypertension was found to be a risk factor for both users and non-users, for both types of strokes, while smoking interacted to increase the risk for hemorrhagic strokes (27–29).

In a large study, the relative risk of thrombotic strokes has been shown to range from 3 for normotensive users to 14 for users with severe hypertension (30). The relative risk of hemorrhagic stroke is reported to be 1.2 for non-smokers who used oral contraceptives, 2.6 for smokers who did not use oral contraceptives, 7.6 for smokers who used oral contraceptives, 1.8 for normotensive users and 25.7 for users with severe hypertension (30). The attributable risk is also greater in older women (3).

d. Dose-related risk of vascular disease from oral contraceptives

A positive association has been observed between the amount of estrogen and progestogen in oral contraceptives and the risk of vascular disease. (31–33). A decline in serum high density lipoproteins (HDL) has been reported with many progestational agents (14–16). A decline in serum high density lipoproteins has been associated with an increased incidence of ischemic heart disease. Because estrogens increase HDL cholesterol, the net effect of an oral contraceptive depends on a balance achieved between doses of estrogen and progestogen and the nature and absolute amount of progestogens used in the contraceptives. The amount of both hormones should be considered in the choice of an oral contraceptive.

Minimizing exposure to estrogen and progestogen is in keeping with good principles of therapeutics. For any particular estrogen/progestogen combination, the dosage regimen prescribed should be one which contains the least amount of estrogen and progestogen that is compatible with a low failure rate and the needs of the individual patient. New acceptors of oral contraceptive agents should be started on preparations containing the lowest dose of estrogen which produces satisfactory results for the patient.

e. Persistence of risk of vascular disease

There are two studies which have shown persistence of risk of vascular disease for ever users of oral contraceptives. In a study in the United States, the risk of developing myocardial infarction after discontinuing oral contraceptives persists for at least 9 years for women 40–49 years who had used oral

TABLE III
ANNUAL NUMBER OF BIRTH-RELATED OR METHOD-RELATED DEATHS ASSOCIATED WITH CONTROL OF FERTILITY PER 100,000 NONSTERILE WOMEN, BY FERTILITY CONTROL METHOD ACCORDING TO AGE

Method of control and outcome	15–19	20–24	25–29	30–34	35–39	40–44
No fertility control methods*	7.0	7.4	9.1	14.8	25.7	28.2
Oral contraceptives non-smoker**	0.3	0.5	0.9	1.9	13.8	31.6
Oral contraceptives smoker**	2.2	3.4	6.6	13.5	51.1	117.2
IUD**	0.8	0.8	1.0	1.0	1.4	1.4
Condom*	1.1	1.6	0.7	0.2	0.3	0.4
Diaphragm/spermicide*	1.9	1.2	1.2	1.3	2.2	2.8
Periodic abstinence*	2.5	1.6	1.6	1.7	2.9	3.6

* Deaths are birth related
** Deaths are method related

Adapted from HW Ory, ref. #35.

contraceptives for 5 or more years, but this increased risk was not demonstrated in other age groups (8). In another study in Great Britain, the risk of developing cerebrovascular disease persisted for at least 6 years after discontinuation of oral contraceptives, although excess risk was very small (34). However, both studies were performed with oral contraceptive formulations containing 50 micrograms or higher of estrogens.

2. Estimates Of Mortality From Contraceptive Use

One study gathered data from a variety of sources which have estimated the mortality rate associated with different methods of contraception at different ages (Table III). These estimates include the combined risk of death associated with contraceptive methods plus the risk attributable to pregnancy in the event of method failure. Each method of contraception has its specific benefits and risks. The study concluded that with the exception of oral contraceptive users 35 and older who smoke and 40 and older who do not smoke, mortality associated with all methods of birth control is low and below that associated with childbirth. However, smokers 35 and older and non-smokers 40 and older who use oral contraceptives have an increase in mortality higher than those using other methods of birth control. These facts must be weighed in conjunction with failure rates for other methods and the risk associated with subsequent pregnancy. (See Table I.)

[See also Table III above.]

3. Carcinoma Of The Reproductive Organs

Numerous epidemiological studies have been performed on the incidence of breast, endometrial, ovarian and cervical cancer in women using oral contraceptives. The overwhelming evidence in the literature suggests that use of oral contraceptives is not associated with an increase in the risk of developing breast cancer, regardless of the age and parity of first use or with most of the marketed brands and doses (36, 38). The Cancer and Steroid Hormone (CASH) study (36) also showed no latent effect on the risk of breast cancer for at least a decade following long-term use. A few studies have shown a slightly increased relative risk of developing breast cancer (37, 39–41), although the methodology of these studies, which included differences in examination of users and nonusers and differences in age at start of use, has been questioned (41–43).

Some studies suggest that oral contraceptive use has been associated with an increase in the risk of cervical intraepithelial neoplasia in some populations of women (45–48). However, there continues to be controversy about the extent to which such findings may be due to differences in sexual behavior and other factors.

In spite of many studies of the relationship between oral contraceptive use and breast and cervical cancers, a cause and effect relationship has not been established.

4. Hepatic Neoplasia

Benign hepatic adenomas are associated with oral contraceptive use, although the incidence of benign tumors is rare in the United States. Indirect calculations have estimated the attributable risk to be in the range of 3.3 cases/100,000 for users, a risk that increases after four or more years of use (49). Rupture of rare, benign, hepatic adenomas may cause death through intra-abdominal hemorrhage (50,51).

Studies from Britain have shown an increased risk of developing hepatocellular carcinoma (52–54) in long-term (> 8 years) oral contraceptive users. However, these cancers are extremely rare in the U.S., and the attributable risk (the excess incidence) of liver cancers in oral contraceptive users approaches less than one per million users.

5. Ocular Lesions

There have been clinical case reports of retinal thrombosis associated with the use of oral contraceptives. Oral contraceptives should be discontinued if there is unexplained partial or complete loss of vision; onset of proptosis or diplopia; papilledema; or retinal vascular lesions. Appropriate diagnostic and therapeutic measures should be undertaken immediately.

6. Oral Contraceptive Use Before Or During Early Pregnancy: Risk Of Birth Defects

Extensive epidemiological studies have revealed no increased risk of birth defects in women who have used oral contraceptives prior to pregnancy (55–57). Studies also do not suggest a teratogenic effect, particularly insofar as cardiac anomalies and limb reduction defects are concerned (55,56,58,59), when taken inadvertently during early pregnancy.

The administration of oral contraceptives to induce withdrawal bleeding should not be used as a test for pregnancy. Oral contraceptives should not be used during pregnancy to treat threatened or habitual abortion.

It is recommended that for any patient who has missed two consecutive periods, pregnancy should be ruled out before continuing oral contraceptive use. If the patient has not adhered to the prescribed schedule, the possibility of pregnancy should be considered at the time of the first missed period. Oral contraceptive use should be discontinued if pregnancy is confirmed.

7. Gallbladder Disease

Earlier studies have reported an increased lifetime relative risk of gallbladder surgery in users of oral contraceptives and estrogens (60,61). More recent studies, however, have shown that the relative risk of developing gallbladder disease among oral contraceptive users may be minimal (62–64). The recent findings of minimal risk may be related to the use of oral contraceptive formulations containing lower hormonal doses of estrogens and progestogens.

8. Carbohydrate And Lipid Metabolic Effects

Oral contraceptives have been shown to cause glucose intolerance in a significant percentage of users (17). Oral contraceptives containing greater than 75 micrograms of estrogens cause hyperinsulinism, while lower doses of estrogen cause less glucose intolerance (65). Progestogens increase insulin secretion and create insulin resistance, this effect varying with different progestational agents (17, 66). However, in the non-diabetic woman, oral contraceptives appear to have no effect on fasting blood glucose (67). Because of these demonstrated effects, prediabetic and diabetic women should be carefully observed while taking oral contraceptives.

A small proportion of women will have persistent hypertriglyceridemia while on the pill. As discussed earlier (see WARNINGS 1a. and 1d.), changes in serum triglycerides and

TABLE II
CIRCULATORY DISEASE MORTALITY RATES PER 100,000 WOMAN YEARS BY AGE, SMOKING STATUS AND ORAL CONTRACEPTIVE USE

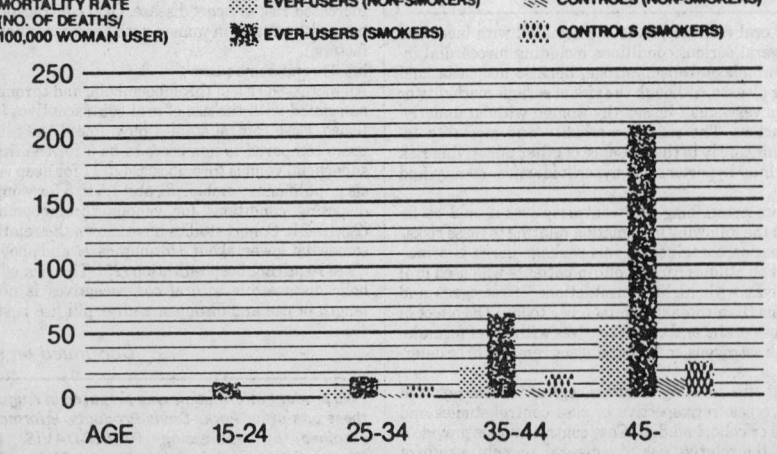

Adapted from P.M. Layde and V. Beral, ref #12.

lipoprotein levels have been reported in oral contraceptive users.

9.　Elevated Blood Pressure

An increase in blood pressure has been reported in women taking oral contraceptives (68) and this increase is more likely in older oral contraceptive users (69) and with continued use (68). Data from the Royal College of General Practitioners (12) and subsequent randomized trials have shown that the incidence of hypertension increases with increasing concentrations of progestogens.

Women with a history of hypertension or hypertension-related diseases, or renal disease (70) should be encouraged to use another method of contraception. If women elect to use oral contraceptives, they should be monitored closely and if significant elevation of blood pressure occurs, oral contraceptives should be discontinued. For most women, elevated blood pressure will return to normal after stopping oral contraceptives (69), and there is no difference in the occurrence of hypertension among ever and never users (68,70,71).

10.　Headache

The onset or exacerbation of migraine or development of headache of a new pattern which is recurrent, persistent or severe requires discontinuation of oral contraceptives and evaluation of the cause.

11.　Bleeding Irregularities

Breakthrough bleeding and spotting are sometimes encountered in patients on oral contraceptives, especially during the first three months of use. Non-hormonal causes should be considered and adequate diagnostic measures taken to rule out malignancy or pregnancy in the event of breakthrough bleeding, as in the case of any abnormal vaginal bleeding. If pathology has been excluded, time or a change to another formulation may solve the problem. In the event of amenorrhea, pregnancy should be ruled out.

Some women may encounter post-pill amenorrhea or oligomenorrhea, especially when such a condition was preexistent.

PRECAUTIONS

1.　Physical Examination And Follow Up

A complete medical history and physical examination should be taken prior to the initiation or reinstitution of oral contraceptives and at least annually during use of oral contraceptives. These physical examinations should include special reference to blood pressure, breasts, abdomen and pelvic organs, including cervical cytology, and relevant laboratory tests. In case of undiagnosed, persistent or recurrent abnormal vaginal bleeding, appropriate diagnostic measures should be conducted to rule out malignancy. Women with a strong family history of breast cancer or who have breast nodules should be monitored with particular care.

2.　Lipid Disorders

Women who are being treated for hyperlipidemias should be followed closely if they elect to use oral contraceptives. Some progestogens may elevate LDL levels and may render the control of hyperlipidemias more difficult.

3.　Liver Function

If jaundice develops in any woman receiving such drugs, the medication should be discontinued. Steroid hormones may be poorly metabolized in patients with impaired liver function.

4.　Fluid Retention

Oral contraceptives may cause some degree of fluid retention. They should be prescribed with caution, and only with careful monitoring, in patients with conditions which might be aggravated by fluid retention.

5.　Emotional Disorders

Women with a history of depression should be carefully observed and the drug discontinued if depression recurs to a serious degree.

6.　Contact Lenses

Contact lens wearers who develop visual changes or changes in lens tolerance should be assessed by an ophthalmologist.

7.　Drug Interactions

Reduced efficacy and increased incidence of breakthrough bleeding and menstrual irregularities have been associated with concomitant use of rifampin. A similar association though less marked, has been suggested with barbiturates, phenylbutazone, phenytoin sodium, and possibly with griseofulvin, ampicillin and tetracyclines (72).

8.　Interactions With Laboratory Tests

Certain endocrine and liver function tests and blood components may be affected by oral contraceptives:

a. Increased prothrombin and factors VII, VIII, IX, and X; decreased antithrombin 3; increased norepinephrine-induced platelet aggregability.

b. Increased thyroid binding globulin (TBG) leading to increased circulating total thyroid hormone, as measured by protein-bound iodine (PBI), T4 by column, or by radioimmunoassay. Free T3 resin uptake is decreased, reflecting the elevated TBG; free T4 concentration is unaltered.

c. Other binding proteins may be elevated in serum.

d. Sex-binding globulins are increased and result in elevated levels of total circulating sex steroids and corticoids; however, free or biologically active levels remain unchanged.

e. Triglycerides may be increased.

f. Glucose tolerance may be decreased.

g. Serum folate levels may be depressed by oral contraceptive therapy. This may be of clinical significance if a woman becomes pregnant shortly after discontinuing oral contraceptives.

9.　Carcinogenesis

See **WARNINGS** section.

10.　Pregnancy

Pregnancy Category X. See **CONTRAINDICATIONS** and **WARNINGS** sections.

11.　Nursing Mothers

Small amounts of oral contraceptive steroids have been identified in the milk of nursing mothers and a few adverse effects on the child have been reported, including jaundice and breast enlargement. In addition, oral contraceptives given in the postpartum period may interfere with lactation by decreasing the quantity and quality of breast milk. If possible, the nursing mother should be advised not to use oral contraceptives but to use other forms of contraception until she has completely weaned her child.

INFORMATION FOR THE PATIENT

See patient labeling printed below.

ADVERSE REACTIONS

An increased risk of the following serious adverse reactions has been associated with the use of oral contraceptives (see WARNINGS section).

- Thrombophlebitis
- Arterial thromboembolism
- Pulmonary embolism
- Myocardial infarction
- Cerebral hemorrhage
- Cerebral thrombosis
- Hypertension
- Gallbladder disease
- Hepatic adenomas or benign liver tumors

There is evidence of an association between the following conditions and the use of oral contraceptives, although additional confirmatory studies are needed:

- Mesenteric thrombosis
- Retinal thrombosis

The following adverse reactions have been reported in patients receiving oral contraceptives and are believed to be drug related:

- Nausea
- Vomiting
- Gastrointestinal symptoms (such as abdominal cramps and bloating)
- Breakthrough bleeding
- Spotting
- Change in menstrual flow
- Amenorrhea
- Temporary infertility after discontinuation of treatment
- Edema
- Melasma which may persist
- Breast changes: tenderness, enlargement, secretion
- Change in weight (increase or decrease)
- Change in cervical erosion and secretion
- Diminution in lactation when given immediately postpartum
- Cholestatic jaundice
- Migraine
- Rash (allergic)
- Mental depression
- Reduced tolerance to carbohydrates
- Vaginal candidiasis
- Change in corneal curvature (steepening)
- Intolerance to contact lenses

The following adverse reactions have been reported in users of oral contraceptives and the association has been neither confirmed nor refuted:

- Pre-menstrual syndrome
- Cataracts
- Changes in appetite
- Cystitis-like syndrome
- Headache
- Nervousness
- Dizziness
- Hirsutism
- Loss of scalp hair
- Erythema multiforme
- Erythema nodosum
- Hemorrhagic eruption
- Vaginitis
- Porphyria
- Impaired renal function
- Hemolytic uremic syndrome
- Budd-Chiari syndrome
- Acne
- Changes in libido
- Colitis

While the following adverse reactions or conditions have been reported to be associated with the use of oral contraceptives, no causal relationship has been established:

- Congenital anomalies
- Raynaud's disease
- Sickle cell disease
- Mitral valve prolapse
- Increased risk of developing venous thromboembolic disease among women with blood types A, B, or AB, as opposed to women with blood type O.

OVERDOSAGE

Serious ill effects have not been reported following acute ingestion of large doses of oral contraceptives by young children. Overdosage may cause nausea, and withdrawal bleeding may occur in females.

NON-CONTRACEPTIVE HEALTH BENEFITS

The following non-contraceptive health benefits related to the use of oral contraceptives are supported by epidemiological studies which largely utilized oral contraceptive formulations containing estrogen doses exceeding 0.05 mg of estrogen (73–78).

Effects on menses:

- Increased menstrual cycle regularity
- Decreased blood loss and decreased incidence of iron deficiency anemia
- Decreased incidence of dysmenorrhea

Effects related to inhibition of ovulation:

- Decreased incidence of functional ovarian cysts
- Decreased incidence of ectopic pregnancies

Effects from long-term use:

- Decreased incidence of fibroadenomas and fibrocystic disease of the breast
- Decreased incidence of acute pelvic inflammatory disease
- Decreased incidence of endometrial cancer
- Decreased incidence of ovarian cancer

DOSAGE AND ADMINISTRATION

The tablet dispenser has been designed to make oral contraceptive dosing as easy and as convenient as possible. The tablets are arranged in either three or four rows of seven tablets each, with the days of the week appearing on the tablet dispenser above the first row of tablets.

Important Notes:　The patient should be instructed to use an additional method of protection until after the first week of administration in the initial cycle if utilizing the Sunday-Start Regimen.

The possibility of ovulation and conception prior to initiation of use should be considered.

Dosage And Administration For 21-Day Dosage Regimen

To achieve maximum contraceptive effectiveness, Norlestrin 21 must be taken exactly as directed and at intervals not exceeding 24 hours. Norlestrin 21 provides the patient with a convenient tablet schedule of "3 weeks on—1 week off." Two dosage regimens are described, one of which may be more convenient or suitable than the other for an individual patient. For the initial cycle of therapy, the patient begins her tablets according to the Day-5 or Sunday-Start Regimen. With either regimen, the patient takes one tablet daily for 21 consecutive days followed by one week of no tablets.

A. Sunday-Start Regimen:　The patient begins taking tablets from the top row on the first Sunday after menstrual flow begins. When menstrual flow begins on Sunday, the first tablet is taken on the same day. The last tablet in the dispenser will then be taken on a Saturday, followed by no tablets for a week (7 days). For all subsequent cycles the patient then begins a new 21-tablet regimen on the eighth day, Sunday, after taking her last tablet. Following this regimen, of 21 days on—7 days off, the patient will start all subsequent cycles on a Sunday.

B. Day-5 Regimen:　The first day of menstrual flow is Day 1. On Day 5 of her menstrual flow, the patient starts taking 1 tablet daily, beginning with the tablet in the top row that corresponds to Day 5 of her flow. After the last tablet (Saturday) has been taken, if any tablets remain in the top row, the patient completes her 21-tablet regimen starting with the Sunday tablet in the top row, followed by no tablets for a week (7 days). For all subsequent cycles, the patient begins a new 21 tablet regimen on the eighth day after taking her last tablet, again beginning on the same day of the week on which she began her first course. Following this regimen of 21 days on—7 days off, the patient will start all subsequent cycles on the same day of the week as the first course. Likewise, the interval of no tablets will always start on the same day of the week.

Whether utilizing the Sunday-Start or Day-5 Regimen, all tablets should be taken regularly with a meal or at bedtime. It should be stressed that efficacy of medication depends on strict adherence to the dosage schedule.

Continued on next page

This product information was prepared in August 1992. On these and other Parke-Davis Products, information may be obtained by addressing PARKE-DAVIS, Division of Warner-Lambert Company, Morris Plains, New Jersey 07950.

Parke-Davis—Cont.

Special Notes on Administration

Menstruation usually begins two or three days, but may begin as late as the fourth or fifth day, after discontinuing medication. If spotting occurs while on the usual regimen of one tablet daily, the patient should continue medication without interruption.

If a patient forgets to take one or more tablets, the following is suggested: If one tablet is missed, take it as soon as remembered, or take two tablets the next day. If two consecutive tablets are missed, take two tablets daily for the next two days, then resume the regular schedule. While there is little likelihood of pregnancy occurring if the patient misses only one or two tablets, the possibility of pregnancy increases with each successive day that tablets are missed. If three consecutive tablets are missed, the patient starts a new course of tablets in the following manner: If the patient is on the Sunday-Start Regimen, a new course of tablets is started on the first Sunday following the last missed tablet, whether or not she is still menstruating. If the patient is on the Day-5 Regimen, a new course of tablets is started on the eighth day after the last tablet was taken. For example, if the patient took her last tablet on Monday, she should start her new course of tablets the following Monday. The patient should also use an additional method of birth-control during the seven days without tablets, and until she has taken a tablet daily for seven consecutive days.

The possibility of ovulation occurring increases with each successive day that scheduled tablets are missed. While there is little likelihood of ovulation occurring if only one tablet is missed, the possibility of spotting or bleeding is increased. This is particularly likely to occur if two or more consecutive tablets are missed.

In the rare case of bleeding which resembles menstruation, the patients should be advised to discontinue medication and then begin taking tablets from a dispenser on the next Sunday or the fifth day (Day 5) depending on their regimen. Persistent bleeding which is not controlled by this method indicates the need for reexamination of the patient at which time nonfunctional causes should be borne in mind.

Dosage And Administration For 28-Day Dosage Regimen

To achieve maximum contraceptive effectiveness, Norlestrin Fe must be taken exactly as directed and at intervals not exceeding 24 hours.

Norlestrin Fe provides a continuous administration regimen consisting of 21 *light-colored* (yellow or pink) tablets of Norlestrin and 7 *brown* tablets of ferrous fumarate. The ferrous fumarate tablets are present to facilitate ease of drug administration via a 28-day regimen and do not serve any therapeutic purpose. There is no need for the patient to count days between cycles because there are no off-tablet days.

The patient begins taking *light-colored* tablets from the top row on the first Sunday after menstrual flow begins. When menstrual flow begins on Sunday, the first *light-colored* tablet is taken on the same day. The patient takes one *light-colored* tablet daily for 21 days. The last *light-colored* tablet taken is the Saturday tablet. Upon completion of all 21 tablets, and without interruption, the patient takes one *brown* tablet daily for 7 days. Upon completion of this first course of tablets, the patient begins a second course of 28 tablets without interruption, the next day, Sunday, starting with the Sunday *light-colored* tablet in the top row. Adhering to this regimen, of one *light-colored* tablet daily for 21 days, followed without interruption by one *brown* tablet daily for seven days, the patient will start all subsequent cycles on a Sunday.

Tablets should be taken regularly with a meal or at bedtime. It should be stressed that efficacy of medication depends on strict adherence to the dosage schedule.

Special Notes on Administration

Menstruation usually begins two or three days, but may begin as late as the fourth or fifth day, after the *brown* tablets have been started. In any event, the next course of tablets should be started without interruption. There should never be a day when the patient is not taking a tablet.

If spotting occurs while the patient is taking *light-colored* tablets, continue medication without interruption.

If a patient forgets to take one or more *light-colored* tablets, the following is suggested: If one *light-colored* tablet is missed, take it as soon as remembered, or take two *light-colored* tablets the next day. If two consecutive *light-colored* tablets are missed, take two *light-colored* tablets daily for the next two days, then resume the regular schedule. While there is little likelihood of pregnancy occurring if the patient misses only one or two *light-colored* tablets, the possibility of pregnancy increases with each successive day that *light-colored* tablets are missed. If three consecutive tablets are missed, the patient starts a new course of tablets the first Sunday following the last missed tablet, whether or not she is still menstruating. The patient should also use an additional method of birth-control during the days without tab-

lets, and until she has taken a tablet daily for seven consecutive days.

The possibility of ovulation occurring increases with each successive day that scheduled *light-colored* tablets are missed. While there is little likelihood of ovulation occurring if only one *light-colored* tablet is missed, the possibility of spotting or bleeding is increased. This is particularly likely to occur if two or more consecutive *light-colored* tablets are missed.

If one or more *brown* tablets are missed, the *light-colored* tablets should be started no later than the eighth day after the last *light-colored* tablet was taken. The possibility of conception occurring is not increased if *brown* tablets are missed.

Use Of Oral Contraceptives In The Event Of A Missed Menstrual Period

1. If the patient has not adhered to the prescribed dosage regimen, the possibility of pregnancy should be considered after the first missed period and oral contraceptives should be withheld until pregnancy has been ruled out.
2. If the patient has adhered to the prescribed regimen and misses two consecutive periods, pregnancy should be ruled out before continuing the contraceptive regimen.

After several months on treatment, bleeding may be reduced to a point of virtual absence.

This reduced flow may occur as a result of medication, in which event it is not indicative of pregnancy.

HOW SUPPLIED

Norlestrin 21 1/50 is available in dispensers each containing 21 tablets. Each tablet contains 1 mg of norethindrone acetate and 50 mcg of ethinyl estradiol. Available in packages of five dispensers.

Norlestrin 21 2.5/50 is available in dispensers each containing 21 tablets. Each tablet contains 2.5 mg of norethindrone acetate and 50 mcg of ethinyl estradiol. Available in packages of five dispensers.

Norlestrin Fe 1/50 is available in dispensers each containing 21 yellow tablets and 7 brown tablets. Each yellow tablet contains 1 mg of norethindrone acetate and 50 mcg of ethinyl estradiol. Each brown tablet contains 75 mg ferrous fumarate. Available in packages of five dispensers.

Norlestrin Fe 2.5/50 is available in dispensers each containing 21 pink tablets and 7 brown tablets. Each pink tablet contains 2.5 mg of norethindrone acetate and 50 mcg of ethinyl estradiol. Each brown tablet contains 75 mg ferrous fumarate. Available in packages of five dispensers.

REFERENCES

1. Reproduced with permission of the Population Council from J. Trussell and K. Kost: Contraceptive failure in the United States: A critical review of the literature. *Studies in Family Planning*, 18 (5), September–October 1987.
2. Stadel, BV: Oral contraceptives and cardiovascular disease. (Pt. 1). *New England Journal of Medicine*, 305:612–618, 1981.
3. Stadel, B.V.: Oral contraceptives and cardiovascular disease. (Pt. 2). *New England Journal of Medicine*, 305:672–677, 1981.
4. Adam, S.A., and M. Thorogood: Oral contraception and myocardial infarction revisited: The effects of new preparations and prescribing patterns. *Brit. J. Obstet. and Gynec.*, 88:838–845, 1981.
5. Mann, J.I., and W.H. Inman: Oral contraceptives and death from myocardial infarction. *Brit. Med. J.*, 2(5965): 245–248, 1975.
6. Mann, J.I., M.P. Vessey, M. Thorogood, and R. Doll: Myocardial infarction in young women with special reference to oral contraceptive practice. *Brit. Med. J.*, 2(5956):241–245, 1975.
7. Royal College of General Practitioners' Oral Contraception Study: Further analyses of mortality in oral contraceptive users. *Lancet*, 1:541–546, 1981.
8. Slone, D., S. Shapiro, DW. Kaufman, L. Rosenberg, O.S. Miettinen, and P.D. Stolley: Risk of myocardial infarction in relation to current and discontinued use of oral contraceptives. *N.E.J.M.*, 305:420–424, 1981.
9. Vessey, M.P.: Female hormones and vascular disease: an epidemiological overview, *Brit. J. Fam. Plann.*, 6:1–12, 1980.
10. Russell-Briefel, R.G., T.M. Ezzati, R. Fulwood, J.A. Perlman, and R.S. Murphy: Cardiovascular risk status and oral contraceptive use, United States, 1976–80. *Preventive Medicine*, 15:352–362, 1986.
11. Goldbaum, G.M., J.S. Kendrick, G.C. Hogelin, and E.M. Gentry: The relative impact of smoking and oral contraceptive use on women in the United States. *J.A.M.A.*, 258:1339–1342, 1987.
12. Layde, P.M., and V. Beral: Further analyses of mortality in oral contraceptive users: Royal College General Practitioners' Oral Contraception Study. (Table 5) *Lancet*, 1:541–546, 1981.
13. Knopp, R.H.: Arteriosclerosis risk: the roles of oral contraceptives and postmenopausal estrogens. *J. of Reprod. Med.*, 31(9)(Supplement): 913–921, 1986.

14. Krauss, R.M., S. Roy, D.R. Mishell, J. Casagrande, and M.C. Pike: Effects of two low-dose oral contraceptives on serum lipids and lipoproteins: Differential changes in high-density lipoproteins subclasses. *Am. J. Obstet. Gyn.*, 145:446–452, 1983.
15. Wahl, P., C. Walden, R. Knopp, J. Hoover, R. Wallace, G. Heiss, and B. Rifkind: Effect of estrogen/progestin potency on lipid/lipoprotein cholesterol, *N.E.J.M.*, 308:862–867, 1983.
16. Wynn, V., and R. Niththyananthan: The effect of progestin in combined oral contraceptives on serum lipids with special reference to high-density lipoproteins. *Am. J. Obstet. and Gyn.*, 142:766–771, 1982.
17. Wynn, V., and I. Godsland: Effects of oral contraceptives on carbohydrate metabolism. *J. Reprod. Medicine*, 31(9)(Supplement): 892–897, 1986.
18. LaRosa, J.C.: Atherosclerotic risk factors in cardiovascular disease. *J. Reprod. Med.*, 31(9)(Supplement): 906–912, 1986.
19. Inman, W.H., and M.P. Vessey: Investigations of death from pulmonary, coronary, and cerebral thrombosis and embolism in women of child-bearing age. *Brit. Med. J.*, 2(5599): 193–199, 1968.
20. Maguire, M.G., J. Tonascia, P.E. Sartwell, P.D. Stolley, and M.S. Tockman: Increased risk of thrombosis due to oral contraceptives: A further report. *Am. J. Epidemiology*, 110(2):188–195, 1979.
21. Pettiti, D.B., J. Wingerd, F. Pellegrin, and S. Ramacharan: Risk of vascular disease in women: smoking, oral contraceptives, noncontraceptive estrogens, and other factors, *J.A.M.A.*, 242:1150–1154, 1979.
22. Vessey, M.P., and R. Doll: Investigation of relation between use of oral contraceptives and thromboembolic disease. *Brit. Med. J.*, 2(5599): 199–205, 1968.
23. Vessey, M.P., and R. Doll: Investigation of relation between use of oral contraceptives and thromboembolic disease: A further report. *Brit. Med. J.*, 2(5658): 651–657, 1969.
24. Porter, J.B., J.R. Hunter, D.A. Danielson, H. Jick, and A. Stergachis: Oral contraceptives and non-fatal vascular disease: Recent experience. *Obstet. and Gyn.*, 59(3):299–302, 1982.
25. Vessey, M., R. Doll, R. Peto, B. Johnson, and P. Wiggins: A long-term follow-up study of women using different methods of contraception: An interim report. *J. Biosocial. Sci.*, 8:375–427, 1976.
26. Royal College of General Practitioners: Oral contraceptives, venous thrombosis, and varicose veins. *J. of Royal College of General Practitioners*, 28:393–399, 1978.
27. Collaborative Group for the study of stroke in young women: Oral contraception and increased risk of cerebral ischemia or thrombosis. *N.E.J.M.*, 288:871–878, 1973.
28. Petitti, D.B., and J. Wingerd: Use of oral contraceptives, cigarette smoking, and risk of subarachnoid hemorrhage. *Lancet*, 2:234–236, 1978.
29. Inman, W.H.: Oral contraceptives and fatal subarachnoid hemorrhage. *Brit. Med. J.*, 2(6203): 1468–70, 1979.
30. Collaborative Group for the study of stroke in young women: Oral contraceptives and stroke in young women: associated risk factors. *J.A.M.A.*, 231:718–722, 1975.
31. Inman, W.H., M.P. Vessey, B. Westerholm, and A. Engelund: Thromboembolic disease and the steroidal content of oral contraceptives. A report to the Committee on Safety of Drugs. *Brit. Med. J.*, 2:203–209, 1970.
32. Meade, T.W., G. Greenberg, and S.G. Thompson: Progestogens and cardiovascular reactions associated with oral contraceptives and a comparison of the safety of 50- and 35-mcg oestrogen preparations. *Brit. Med. J.*, 280(6244): 1157–1161, 1980.
33. Kay, C.R.: Progestogens and arterial disease-evidence from the Royal College of General Practitioners' study. *Amer. J. Obstet. Gyn.*, 142:762–765, 1982.
34. Royal College of General Practitioners: Incidence of arterial disease among oral contraceptive users. *J. Coll. Gen. Pract.*, 33:75–82, 1983.
35. Ory, H.W.: Mortality associated with fertility and fertility control: 1983. *Family Planning Perspectives*, 15:50–56, 1983.
36. The Cancer and Steroid Hormone Study of the Centers for Disease Control and the National Institute of Child Health and Human Development: Oral-contraceptive use and the risk of breast cancer. *N.E.J.M.*, 315:405–411, 1986.
37. Pike, M.C., B.E. Henderson, M.D. Krailo, A. Duke, and S. Roy: Breast cancer in young women and use of oral contraceptives: possible modifying effect of formulation and age at use. *Lancet*, 2:926–929. 1983.
38. Paul, C., D.G. Skegg, G.F.S. Spears, and J.M. Kaldor: Oral contraceptives and breast cancer: A national study. *Brit. Med. J.*, 293:723–725, 1986.
39. Miller, D.R., L. Rosenberg, D.W. Kaufman, D. Schottenfeld, P.D. Stolley, and S. Shapiro: Breast cancer risk in relation to early oral contraceptive use. *Obstet. Gynec.*, 68:863–868, 1986.

40. Olson, H., K.L. Olson, T.R. Moller, J. Ranstam, P. Holm: Oral contraceptive use and breast cancer in young women in Sweden (letter). *Lancet,* 2:748–749, 1985.
41. McPherson, K., M. Vessey, A. Neil, R. Doll, L. Jones, and M. Roberts: Early contraceptive use and breast cancer: Results of another case-control study. *Brit. J. Cancer,* 56: 653–660, 1987.
42. Huggins, G.R., and P.F. Zucker: Oral contraceptives and neoplasia: 1987 update. *Fertil. Steril.,* 47:733–761, 1987.
43. McPherson, K., and J.O. Drife: The pill and breast cancer: why the uncertainty? *Brit. Med. J.,* 293:709–710, 1986.
44. Shapiro, S.: Oral contraceptives: time to take stock. *N.E.J.M.,* 315:450–451, 1987.
45. Ory, H., Z. Naib, S.B. Conger, R.A. Hatcher, and C.W. Tyler: Contraceptive choice and prevalence of cervical dysplasia and carcinoma in situ. *Am. J. Obstet. Gynec.,* 124:573–577, 1976.
46. Vessey, M.P., M. Lawless, K. McPherson, D. Yeates: Neoplasia of the cervix uteri and contraception: a possible adverse effect of the pill. *Lancet,* 2:930, 1983.
47. Brinton, L.A., G.R. Huggins, H.F. Lehman, K. Malli, D.A. Savitz, E. Trapido, J. Rosenthal, and R. Hoover: Long term use of oral contraceptives and risk of invasive cervical cancer. *Int. J. Cancer,* 38:339–344, 1986.
48. WHO Collaborative Study of Neoplasia and Steroid Contraceptives: Invasive cervical cancer and combined oral contraceptives. *Brit. Med. J.,* 290:961–965, 1985.
49. Rooks, J.B., H.W. Ory, K.G. Ishak, L.T. Strauss, J.R. Greenspan, A.P. Hill, and C.W. Tyler: Epidemiology of hepatocellular adenoma: The role of oral contraceptive use. *J.A.M.A.,* 242:644–648, 1979.
50. Bein, N.N., and H.S. Goldsmith: Recurrent massive hemorrhage from benign hepatic tumors secondary to oral contraceptives. *Brit. J. Surg.,* 64:433–435, 1977.
51. Klatskin, G.: Hepatic tumors: possible relationship to use of oral contraceptives. *Gastroenterology,* 73:386–394, 1977.
52. Henderson, B.E., S. Preston-Martin, H.A. Edmondson, R.L. Peters, and M.C. Pike: Hepatocellular carcinoma and oral contraceptives. *Brit. J. Cancer,* 48:437–440, 1983.
53. Neuberger, J., D. Forman, R. Doll, and R. Williams: Oral contraceptives and hepatocellular carcinoma, *Brit. Med. J.,* 292:1355–1357, 1986.
54. Forman, D., T.J. Vincent, and R. Doll: Cancer of the liver and oral contraceptives. *Brit. Med. J.,* 292:1357–1361, 1986.
55. Harlap, S., and J. Eldor: Births following oral contraceptive failures. *Obstet. Gynec.,* 55:447–452, 1980.
56. Savolainen, E., E. Saksela, and L. Saxen: Teratogenic hazards of oral contraceptives analyzed in a national malformation register. *Amer. J. Obstet. Gynec.,* 140:521–524, 1981.
57. Janerich, D.T., J.M. Piper, and D.M. Glebatis: Oral contraceptives and birth defects. *Am. J. Epidemiology,* 112:73–79, 1980.
58. Ferencz, C., G.M. Matanoski, P.D. Wilson, J.D. Rubin, C.A. Neill, and R. Gutberlet: Maternal hormone therapy and congenital heart disease. *Teratology,* 21:225–239, 1980.
59. Rothman, K.J., D.C. Fyler, A. Goldbatt, and M.B. Kreidberg: Exogenous hormones and other drug exposures of children with congenital heart disease. *Am. J. Epidemiology,* 109:433–439, 1979.
60. Boston Collaborative Drug Surveillance Program: Oral contraceptives and venous thromboembolic disease, surgically confirmed gallbladder disease, and breast tumors. *Lancet,* 1:1399–1404, 1973.
61. Royal College of General Practitioners: *Oral contraceptives and health.* New York, Pittman, 1974, 100p.
62. Layde, P.M., M.P. Vessey, and D. Yeates: Risk of gallbladder disease: a cohort study of young women attending family planning clinics. *J. of Epidemiol. and Comm. Health,* 36: 274–278, 1982.
63. Rome Group for the Epidemiology and Prevention of Cholelithiasis (GREPCO): Prevalence of gallstone disease in an Italian adult female population, *Am. J. Epidemiol.,* 119:796–805, 1984.
64. Strom, B.L., R.T. Tamragouri, M.L. Morse, E.L. Lazar, S.L. West, P.D. Stolley, and J.K. Jones: Oral contraceptives and other risk factors for gallbladder disease. *Clin. Pharmacol. Ther.,* 39:335–341, 1986.
65. Wynn, V., P.W. Adams, I.F. Godsland, J. Melrose, R. Niththyananthan, N.W. Oakley, and A. Seedj: Comparison of effects of different combined oral-contraceptive formulations on carbohydrate and lipid metabolism. *Lancet,* 1:1045–1049, 1979.
66. Wynn, V.: Effect of progesterone and progestins on carbohydrate metabolism. In Progesterone and Progestin. Edited by C.W. Bardin, E. Milgrom, P. Mauvis-Jarvis. New York, Raven Press, pp. 395–410, 1983.
67. Perlman, J.A., R.G. Roussell-Briefel, T.M. Ezzati, and G. Lieberknecht: Oral glucose tolerance and the potency of oral contraceptive progestogens. *J. Chronic Dis.,* 38:857–864, 1985.
68. Royal College of General Practitioners' Oral Contraception Study: Effect on hypertension and benign breast disease of progestogen component in combined oral contraceptives. *Lancet,* 1:624, 1977.
69. Fisch, I.R., and J. Frank. Oral contraceptives and blood pressure. *J.A.M.A.* 237:2499–2503, 1977.
70. Laragh, A.J.: Oral contraceptive induced hypertension: Nine years later. *Amer. J. Obstet. Gynecol.,* 126:141–147, 1976.
71. Ramcharan, S., E. Peritz, F.A. Pellegrin, and W.T. Williams: Incidence of hypertension in the Walnut Creek Contraceptive Drug Study cohort. In Pharmacology of Steroid Contraceptive Drugs. Edited by S. Garattini and H.W. Berendes, New York. Raven Press, pp. 277–288, 1977. (Monographs of the Mario Negri Institute for Pharmacological Research, Milan).
72. Stockley, I.: Interactions with oral contraceptives. *Pharm. J.* 216:140–143, 1976.
73. The Cancer and Steroid Hormone Study of the Centers for Disease Control and the National Institute of Child Health and Human Development: Oral contraceptive use and the risk of ovarian cancer. *J.A.M.A.,* 249:1596–1599, 1983.
74. The Cancer and Steroid Hormone Study of the Centers for Disease Control and the National Institute of Child Health and Human Development: Combination oral contraceptive use and the risk of endometrial cancer. *J.A.M.A.,* 257:796–800, 1987.
75. Ory, H.W.: Functional ovarian cysts and oral contraceptives: negative association confirmed surgically. *J.A.M.A.,* 228:68–69, 1974.
76. Ory, H.W., P. Cole, B. Macmahon, and R. Hoover: Oral contraceptives and reduced risk of benign breast disease. *N.E.J.M.,* 294:41–422, 1976.
77. Ory, H.W.: The noncontraceptive health benefits from oral contraceptive use. *Fam. Plann. Perspectives,* 14:182–184, 1982.
78. Ory, H.W., J.D. Forrest, and R. Lincoln: Making Choices: Evaluating the health risks and benefits of birth control methods. New York, The Alan Guttmacher Institute, p.1, 1983.

The patient labeling for oral contraceptive drug products is set forth below:

BRIEF SUMMARY PATIENT PACKAGE INSERT

Oral contraceptives, also known as "birth control pills" or "the pill," are taken to prevent pregnancy and when taken correctly, have a failure rate of about 1% per year when used without missing any pills. The typical failure rate of large numbers of pill users is less than 3% per year when women who miss pills are included. For most women oral contraceptives are also free of serious or unpleasant side effects. However, forgetting to take pills considerably increases the chances of pregnancy.

For the majority of women, oral contraceptives can be taken safely. But there are some women who are at high risk of developing certain serious diseases that can be life-threatening or may cause temporary or permanent disability. The risks associated with taking oral contraceptives increase significantly if you:

- Smoke
- Are over the age of 40
- Have high blood pressure, diabetes, high cholesterol
- Have or have had clotting disorders, heart attack, stroke, angina pectoris, cancer of the breast or sex organs, jaundice or malignant or benign liver tumors.

You should not take the pill if you suspect you are pregnant or have unexplained vaginal bleeding.

> Cigarette smoking increases the risk of serious cardiovascular side effects from oral contraceptive use. This risk increases with age and with heavy smoking (15 or more cigarettes per day) and is quite marked in women over 35 years of age. Women who use oral contraceptives are strongly advised not to smoke.

Most side effects of the pill are not serious. The most common side effects are nausea, vomiting, bleeding between menstrual periods, weight gain, and breast tenderness, and difficulty wearing contact lenses. These side effects, especially nausea and vomiting, may subside within the first three months of use.

The serious side effects of the pill occur very infrequently, especially if you are in good health and are young. However, you should know that the following medical conditions have been associated with or made worse by the pill:

1. Blood clots in the legs (thrombophlebitis), lungs (pulmonary embolism), stoppage or rupture of a blood vessel in the brain (stroke), blockage of blood vessels in the heart (heart attack or angina pectoris) or other organs of the body. As mentioned above, smoking increases the risk of heart attacks and strokes and subsequent serious medical consequences.
2. Liver tumors, which may rupture and cause severe bleeding. A possible but not definite association has been found with the pill and liver cancer. However, liver cancers are extremely rare. The chance of developing liver cancer from using the pill is thus even rarer.
3. High blood pressure, although blood pressure usually returns to normal when the pill is stopped.

The symptoms associated with these serious side effects are discussed in the detailed leaflet given to you with your supply of pills. Notify your doctor or health care provider if you notice any unusual physical disturbances while taking the pill. In addition, drugs such as rifampin, as well as some anticonvulsants and some antibiotics may decrease oral contraceptive effectiveness.

Studies to date of women taking the pill have not shown an increase in the incidence of cancer of the breast or cervix. There is, however, insufficient evidence to rule out the possibility that pills may cause such cancers.

Taking the pill provides some important non-contraceptive benefits. These include less painful menstruation, less menstrual blood loss and anemia, fewer pelvic infections, and fewer cancers of the ovary and the lining of the uterus.

Be sure to discuss any medical condition you may have with your health care provider. Your health care provider will take a medical and family history and examine you before prescribing oral contraceptives. You should be reexamined at least once a year while taking oral contraceptives. The detailed patient information leaflet gives you further information which you should read and discuss with your health care provider.

Caution: Oral contraceptives are of no value in the prevention or treatment of venereal disease.

INSTRUCTIONS TO PATIENTS

TABLET DISPENSER

The tablet dispenser has been designed to make oral contraceptive dosing as easy and as convenient as possible. The tablets are arranged in either three or four rows of seven tablets each, with the days of the week appearing on the tablet dispenser above the first row of tablets.

If your tablet dispenser contains:	You are taking:
21 yellow tablets	NORLESTRIN 21 1/50
21 pink tablets	NORLESTRIN 21 2.5/50
21 yellow tablets and 7 brown tablets	NORLESTRIN Fe 1/50
21 pink tablets and 7 brown tablets	NORLESTRIN Fe 2.5/50

Each *yellow* tablet contains 1 mg norethindrone acetate and 50 mcg ethinyl estradiol.

Each *pink* tablet contains 2.5 mg norethindrone acetate and 50 mcg ethinyl estradiol.

Each *brown* tablet contains 75 mg ferrous fumarate, and is intended to help you remember to take the tablets correctly. These brown tablets are not intended to have any health benefit.

To remove a tablet, press down on it with your thumb or finger. The tablet will drop through the back of the tablet dispenser. Do not press on the tablet with your thumbnail or fingernail or any other sharp object.

NORLESTRIN 21-DAY DOSAGE REGIMEN

If your tablet dispenser contains 21 tablets (3 rows of 7), you are on a 21-day regimen and should follow either the Sunday-Start or Day-5 Start directions.

A. Sunday-Start Regimen

1. Unless your physician or health care provider has instructed you differently, begin taking tablets on the first Sunday after your menstrual period begins whether or not you are still bleeding. If your period begins on Sunday, take your first tablet that very same day. START WITH THE SUNDAY TABLET IN THE TOP ROW.

Note: During the first cycle, it is important that you use another method of birth control until you have taken a tablet daily for seven consecutive days.

2. Take all the tablets in the top row first, followed by the second row. Continue to take one tablet every day until you finish all 21 tablets. Your last tablet should be on Saturday.
3. After you have taken all 21 tablets, stop, and don't take any tablets for the next seven days. You should have a menstrual period one to three days after you stop taking tablets; sometimes it may take a day or so longer.

Continued on next page

This product information was prepared in August 1992. On these and other Parke-Davis Products, information may be obtained by addressing PARKE-DAVIS, Division of Warner-Lambert Company, Morris Plains, New Jersey 07950.

Parke-Davis—Cont.

4. After the seven days during which you take no tablets, obtain a new course of tablets. Begin the new course of 21 tablets on Sunday, the 8th day after you took your last tablet, starting with the Sunday tablet in the top row.
5. Continue to take one tablet daily until you finish all 21 tablets. If you follow the schedule properly, you will always take the last tablet in the dispenser on a Saturday, and always start each new course of 21 tablets 8 days later, on the following Sunday.
6. If, in any cycle, you start your tablets later than the proper day, you should also use another method of birth control until you have taken seven consecutive tablets.

B. Day-5 Regimen

If your physician or health care provider has directed you to begin taking your first cycle of tablets using the Day-5 Regimen, you should start taking your tablets on Day 5 after the start of your period.

1. The first day of your period is Day 1. On the 5th day (Day 5), start taking one tablet daily, beginning with the tablet in the top row that corresponds to Day 5 after your flow began.

If your period begins on:	Start taking tablets in the top row on:
Sunday	Thursday
Monday	Friday
Tuesday	Saturday
Wednesday	Sunday
Thursday	Monday
Friday	Tuesday
Saturday	Wednesday

Note: During the first cycle, if you start taking tablets later than Day 5 of your menstrual period, you should use another method of birth control until you have taken a tablet daily for seven consecutive days.

2. Continue to take one tablet daily. After the last Saturday tablet has been taken, if any tablets remain in the first row, complete your 21-day regimen by taking one tablet daily starting with the Sunday tablet in the top row.
3. After you have taken all 21 tablets, stop, and don't take any tablets for the next seven days. You should have a menstrual period one to three days after you stop taking tablets; sometimes it may take a day or so longer.
4. After the seven days during which you take no tablets, obtain a new course of tablets. Begin a new course of 21-day tablets, the 8th day after you took your last tablet, starting with the tablet in the top row that corresponds to that day.
5. Continue to take one tablet daily until you finish all 21 tablets. If you follow the schedule properly, you will always take the last tablet in the dispenser on the same day of the week, and always start each new course of 21 tablets the same day of the week on which you began the previous cycle of tablets.
6. If, in any cycle, you start your tablets later than the proper day, you should also use another method of birth control until you have taken seven consecutive tablets.

Whether you started your tablets using the Sunday-Start or Day-5 Regimen, the following directions apply:

1. Continue taking your tablets whether or not your period has occurred or is still in progress. Your period will usually occur during the seven days you are taking no tablets.
2. If spotting should occur at an unexpected time, continue to take your tablets as directed. Spotting is usually temporary and without significance. However, if bleeding should occur at an unexpected time, consult your physician or health care provider. Call your physician or health care provider regarding any problem or change in your general health that may concern you.

NORLESTRIN 28-DAY DOSAGE REGIMEN

If your tablet dispenser contains 28 tablets (3 rows of 7 *light-colored* (yellow or pink) tablets and 1 row of 7 *brown* tablets), you are on a 28-day regimen and should follow these directions. Each *brown* tablet contains 75 mg ferrous fumarate and is intended to help you remember to take the tablets correctly. These brown tablets are not intended to have any health benefit.

Sunday-Start Regimen:

1. Begin taking tablets on the first Sunday after your menstrual period begins whether or not you are still bleeding. If your period begins on Sunday, take your first tablet that very same day. START WITH THE SUNDAY TABLET IN THE TOP ROW.

Note: During the first cycle, it is important that you use another method of birth control until you have taken a *light-colored* tablet daily for seven consecutive days.

2. Take all the tablets in the top row first, followed by the second row and so on.
3. Continue to take one tablet every day until you finish all 21 *light-colored* tablets. On the day after taking the last *light-colored* tablet, begin taking one *brown* tablet daily until all the tablets have been taken.
4. When the last tablet has been taken, obtain a new course of tablets and, without interruption, begin a new course of 28-day tablets, the next day, starting with the Sunday tablet in the top row. There should never be a day when you are not taking a tablet.
5. If, in any cycle, you start your tablets later than the proper day, you should also use another method of birth control until you have taken seven *light-colored* tablets.
6. Continue taking *light-colored* tablets without interruption whether or not your period has occurred or is still in progress. Your period will usually occur during the time you are taking *brown* tablets.
7. If spotting should occur at an unexpected time, continue to take your tablets as directed. Spotting is usually temporary and without significance. However, if bleeding should occur at an unexpected time, consult your physician or health care provider. Call your physician or health care provider regarding any problem or change in your general health that may concern you.

In Case You Forget (21-Day and 28-Day Regimens)

The following instructions apply only to missing the yellow 1/50 tablets or the pink 2.5/50 tablets.

If you forget to take one tablet, take it as soon as you remember, even if it is the next day. Then take the next scheduled tablet at the usual time. If you miss two consecutive tablets, take two tablets daily for the next two days. Then resume the regular schedule. While there is little likelihood of pregnancy occurring if you miss only one or two tablets, the possibility of pregnancy increases with each successive day that tablets are missed.

21-Day Regimen: If you miss three consecutive tablets, discard any tablets remaining in the tablet dispenser and follow these instructions.

If you are on the Sunday-Start Regimen, start a new course of tablets the first Sunday following the last missed tablet, whether or not you are still menstruating.

If you are on the Day-5 Regimen, begin a new course of tablets on the 8th day after the last tablet was taken. For example, if you took your last tablet on a Monday, you should begin your new course of tablets the following Monday.

During the seven days without tablets, and until you have taken a tablet daily for seven consecutive days from your new course of tablets, you should also use another method of birth control.

28-Day Regimen: If you miss three consecutive *light-colored* tablets, discard any tablets remaining in the tablet dispenser and begin a new course of tablets the first Sunday following the last missed tablet, whether or not you are still menstruating. During the days without tablets and until you have taken a tablet daily for seven consecutive days from your new course of tablets, you should also use another method of birth control.

If you miss one or more *brown* tablets discard the remainder and begin a new course of tablets on the next Sunday (which should be the 8th day after you took your last *light-colored* tablet). Start with the *light-colored* tablets in the top row. Skipping one or more *brown* tablets contained in the 28-day regimen products won't increase the risk of pregnancy. They are there to help keep you on a schedule and to eliminate the need for counting days. *Under no circumstances* should you substitute a *brown* tablet for a *light-colored* tablet nor should a *brown* tablet be taken until you have finished all the *light-colored* tablets, unless your physician or health care provider advises you to do so.

Remembering to take tablets according to schedule is stressed because of its importance in providing you the greatest degree of protection.

MISSED MENSTRUAL PERIODS FOR BOTH DOSAGE REGIMENS

At times there may be no menstrual period after a cycle of pills. Therefore, if you miss one menstrual period but have taken the pills *exactly as you were supposed to,* continue as usual into the next cycle. If you have not taken the pills correctly and miss a menstrual period, *you may be pregnant* and should stop taking oral contraceptives until your doctor or health care provider determines whether or not you are pregnant. Until you can get to your doctor or health care provider, use another form of contraception. If two consecutive menstrual periods are missed, you should stop taking pills until it is determined whether or not you are pregnant. Although there does not appear to be any increase in birth defects in newborn babies if you become pregnant while using oral contraceptives, if you do become pregnant, you should discuss the situation with your doctor or health care provider.

Periodic Examination

Your doctor or health care provider will take a complete medical and family history before prescribing oral contraceptives. At that time and about once a year thereafter, he will generally examine your blood pressure, breasts, abdomen, and pelvic organs (including a Papanicolaou smear, ie, test for cancer).

SUMMARY

Oral contraceptives are the most effective method, except sterilization, for preventing pregnancy. Other methods, when used conscientiously, are also very effective and have fewer risks. Although the serious risks of oral contraceptives are uncommon, some of the risks may persist after you stop using the pill. On the other hand, the "pill" is a very convenient method of preventing pregnancy.

If you have certain conditions or have had these conditions in the past, you should not use oral contraceptives because the risk is too great. These conditions are listed in this leaflet. If you do not have these conditions, and decide to use the "pill," please read this leaflet carefully so that you can use the "pill" most safely and effectively.

Based on his or her assessment of your medical needs, your doctor or health care provider has prescribed this drug for you. Do not give this drug to anyone else.

Keep this and all drugs out of the reach of children.

Caution—Federal law prohibits dispensing without prescription.

DETAILED PATIENT PACKAGE INSERT

What You Should Know About Oral Contraceptives

Any woman who considers using oral contraceptives (the "birth control pill" or the "pill") should understand the benefits and risks of using this form of birth control. This leaflet will give you much of the information you will need to make this decision and will also help you determine if you are at risk of developing any of the serious side effects of the pill. It will tell you how to use the pill properly so that it will be as effective as possible. However, this leaflet is not a replacement for a careful discussion between you and your health care provider. You should discuss the information provided in this leaflet with him or her, both when you first start taking the pill and during your revisits. You should also follow your health care provider's advice with regard to regular check-ups while you are on the pill.

EFFECTIVENESS OF ORAL CONTRACEPTIVES

Oral contraceptives or "birth control pills" or "the pill" are used to prevent pregnancy and are more effective than other non-surgical methods of birth control. When they are taken correctly, the chance of becoming pregnant is less than 1% (1 pregnancy per 100 women per year of use) when used perfectly, without missing pills. Typical failure rates are actually 3% per year. The chance of becoming pregnant increases with each missed pill during a menstrual cycle.

In comparison, typical failure rates for other methods of birth control during the first year of use are as follows:

IUD: 6%
Diaphragm with spermicides: 18%
Spermicides alone: 21%
Vaginal sponge: 18 to 30%
Condom alone: 12%
Periodic abstinence: 20%
No method: 89%

WHO SHOULD NOT TAKE ORAL CONTRACEPTIVES

Cigarettes smoking increases the risk of serious cardiovascular side effects from oral contraceptives use. This risk increases with age and with heavy smoking (15 or more cigarettes per day) and is quite marked in women over 35 years of age. Women who use oral contraceptives are strongly advised not to smoke.

Some women should not use the pill. For example, you should not take the pill if you are pregnant or think you may be pregnant. You should also not use the pill if you have any of the following conditions:

- A history of heart attack or stroke
- Blood clots in the legs (thrombophlebitis), lungs (pulmonary embolism), or eyes
- A history of blood clots in the deep veins of your legs
- Chest pain (angina pectoris)
- Known or suspected breast cancer or cancer of the lining of the uterus, cervix or vagina
- Unexplained vaginal bleeding (until a diagnosis is reached by your doctor)
- Yellowing of the whites of the eyes or of the skin (jaundice) during pregnancy or during previous use of the pill
- Liver tumor (benign or cancerous)
- Known or suspected pregnancy

Tell your health care provider if you have ever had any of these conditions. Your health care provider can recommend a safer method of birth control.

OTHER CONSIDERATIONS BEFORE TAKING ORAL CONTRACEPTIVES

Tell your health care provider if your have:

- Breast nodules, fibrocystic disease of the breast, an abnormal breast x-ray or mammogram
- Diabetes
- Elevated cholesterol or triglycerides
- High blood pressure
- Migraine or other headaches or epilepsy
- Mental depression
- Gallbladder, heart or kidney disease
- History of scanty or irregular menstrual periods

Women with any of these conditions should be checked often by their health care provider if they choose to use oral contraceptives.

Also, be sure to inform your doctor or health care provider if you smoke or are on any medications.

RISKS OF TAKING ORAL CONTRACEPTIVES

1. Risk Of Developing Blood Clots

Blood clots and blockage of blood vessels are the most serious side effects of taking oral contraceptives. In particular, a clot in the legs can cause thrombophlebitis and a clot that travels to the lungs can cause a sudden blocking of the vessel carrying blood to the lungs. Rarely, clots occur in the blood vessels of the eye and may cause blindness, double vision, or impaired vision.

If you take oral contraceptives and need elective surgery, need to stay in bed for a prolonged illness or have recently delivered a baby, you may be at risk of developing blood clots. You should consult your doctor about stopping oral contraceptives three to four weeks before surgery and not taking oral contraceptives for two weeks after surgery or during bed rest. You should also not take oral contraceptives soon after delivery of a baby. It is advisable to wait for at least four weeks after delivery if you are not breast feeding. If you are breast feeding, you should wait until you have weaned your child before using the pill. (See also the section on Breast Feeding in GENERAL PRECAUTIONS.)

2. Heart Attacks And Strokes

Oral contraceptives may increase the tendency to develop strokes (stoppage or rupture of blood vessels in the brain) and angina pectoris and heart attacks (blockage of blood vessels in the heart). Any of these conditions can cause death or disability.

Smoking greatly increases the possibility of suffering heart attacks and strokes. Furthermore, smoking and the use of oral contraceptives greatly increase the chances of developing and dying of heart disease.

3. Gallbladder Disease

Oral contraceptive users probably have a greater risk than nonusers of having gallbladder disease, although this risk may be related to pills containing high doses of estrogens.

4. Liver Tumors

In rare cases, oral contraceptives can cause benign but dangerous liver tumors. These benign liver tumors can rupture and cause fatal internal bleeding. In addition, a possible but not definite association has been found with the pill and liver cancers in two studies, in which a few women who developed these very rare cancers were found to have used oral contraceptives for long periods. However, liver cancers are extremely rare. The chance of developing liver cancer from using the pill is thus even rarer.

5. Cancer Of The Reproductive Organs

There is, at present, no confirmed evidence that oral contraceptives increase the risk of cancer of the reproductive organs in human studies. Several studies have found no overall increase in the risk of developing breast cancer. However, women who use oral contraceptives and have a strong family history of breast cancer or who have breast nodules or abnormal mammograms should be closely followed by their doctors.

Some studies have found an increase in the incidence of cancer of the cervix in women who use oral contraceptives. However, this finding may be related to factors other than the use of oral contraceptives.

ESTIMATED RISK OF DEATH FROM A BIRTH CONTROL METHOD OR PREGNANCY

All methods of birth control and pregnancy are associated with a risk of developing certain diseases which may lead to disability or death. An estimate of the number of deaths associated with different methods of birth control and pregnancy has been calculated and is shown in the table above.

In the above table, the risk of death from any birth control method is less than the risk of childbirth, except for oral contraceptive users over the age of 35 who smoke and pill users over the age of 40 even if they do not smoke. It can be seen in the table that for women aged 15 to 39, the risk of death was highest with pregnancy (7–26 deaths per 100,000 women, depending on age). Among pill users who do not smoke, the risk of death was always lower than that associated with pregnancy for any age group, although over the age of 40, the risk increases to 32 deaths per 100,000 women, compared to 28 associated with pregnancy at that age. However, for pill users who smoke and are over the age of 35, the estimated number of deaths exceeds those for other methods of birth control. If a woman is over the age of 40 and smokes, her estimated risk of death is four times higher (117/100,000 women) than the estimated risk associated with pregnancy (28/100,000 women) in that age group.

Moreover, if you do not smoke and are under the age of 35, the possible risk of death from oral contraceptive use is extremely low when you consider the failure rate associated with other methods of contraception such as the condom or diaphragm and the resulting pregnancy-associated risk.

ANNUAL NUMBER OF BIRTH-RELATED OR METHOD-RELATED DEATHS ASSOCIATED WITH CONTROL OF FERTILITY PER 100,000 NONSTERILE WOMEN, BY FERTILITY CONTROL METHOD ACCORDING TO AGE

Method of control and outcome	15–19	20–24	25–29	30–34	35–39	40–44
No fertility control methods*	7.0	7.4	9.1	14.8	25.7	28.2
Oral contraceptives non-smoker**	0.3	0.5	0.9	1.9	13.8	31.6
Oral contraceptives smoker**	2.2	3.4	6.6	13.5	51.1	117.2
IUD**	0.8	0.8	1.0	1.0	1.4	1.4
Condom*	1.1	1.6	0.7	0.2	0.3	0.4
Diaphragm/spermicide*	1.9	1.2	1.2	1.3	2.2	2.8
Periodic abstinence*	2.5	1.6	1.6	1.7	2.9	3.6

* Deaths are birth related
** Deaths are method related

WARNING SIGNALS

If any of these adverse effects occur while you are taking oral contraceptives, call your doctor immediately:

- Sharp chest pain, coughing of blood, or sudden shortness of breath (indicating a possible clot in the lung)
- Pain in the calf (indicating a possible clot in the leg)
- Crushing chest pain or heaviness in the chest (indicating a possible heart attack)
- Sudden severe headache or vomiting, dizziness or fainting, disturbances of vision or speech, weakness, or numbness in an arm or leg (indicating a possible stroke)
- Sudden partial or complete loss of vision (indicating a possible clot in the eye)
- Breast lumps (indicating possible breast cancer or fibrocystic disease of the breast; ask your doctor or health care provider to show you how to examine your breasts)
- Severe pain or tenderness in the stomach area (indicating a possibly ruptured liver tumor)
- Difficulty in sleeping, weakness, lack of energy, fatigue, or change in mood (possibly indicating severe depression)
- Jaundice or a yellowing of the skin or eyeballs, accompanied frequently by fever, fatigue, loss of appetite, dark colored urine, or light colored bowel movements (indicating possible liver problems)

SIDE EFFECTS OF ORAL CONTRACEPTIVES

1. Vaginal Bleeding

Irregular vaginal bleeding or spotting may occur while you are taking the pills. Irregular bleeding may vary from slight staining between menstrual periods to breakthrough bleeding which is a flow much like a regular period. Irregular bleeding occurs most often during the first few months of oral contraceptive use, but may also occur after you have been taking the pill for some time. Such bleeding may be temporary and usually does not indicate any serious problems. It is important to continue taking your pills on schedule. If the bleeding occurs in more than one cycle or lasts for more than a few days, talk to your doctor or health care provider.

2. Contact Lenses

If you wear contact lenses and notice a change in vision or an inability to wear your lenses, contact your doctor or health care provider.

3. Fluid Retention

Oral contraceptives may cause edema (fluid retention) with swelling of the fingers or ankles and may raise your blood pressure. If you experience fluid retention, contact your doctor or health care provider.

4. Melasma

A spotty darkening of the skin is possible, particularly on the face.

5. Other Side Effects

Other side effects include change in appetite, headache, nervousness, depression, dizziness, loss of scalp hair, rash, and vaginal infections.

If any of these side effects bother you, call your doctor or health care provider.

GENERAL PRECAUTIONS

1. Missed Periods And Use Of Oral Contraceptives Before Or During Early Pregnancy

There may be times when you may not menstruate regularly after you have completed taking a cycle of pills. If you have taken your pills regularly and miss one menstrual period, continue taking your pills for the next cycle but be sure to inform your health care provider before doing so. If you have not taken the pills daily as instructed and missed a menstrual period, or if you missed two consecutive menstrual periods, you may be pregnant. Check with your health care provider immediately to determine whether you are pregnant. Do not continue to take oral contraceptives until you are sure you are not pregnant, but continue to use another method of contraception.

There is no conclusive evidence that oral contraceptive use is associated with an increase in birth defects, when taken inadvertently during early pregnancy. Previously, a few studies had reported that oral contraceptives might be associated with birth defects, but these studies have not been confirmed. Nevertheless, oral contraceptives or any other drugs should not be used during pregnancy unless clearly necessary and prescribed by your doctor. You should check with your doctor about risks to your unborn child of any medication taken during pregnancy.

2. While Breast Feeding

If you are breast feeding consult your doctor before starting oral contraceptives. Some of the drug will be passed on to the child in the milk. A few adverse effects on the child have been reported, including yellowing of the skin (jaundice) and breast enlargement. In addition, oral contraceptives may decrease the amount and quality of your milk. If possible, do not use oral contraceptives while breast feeding. You should use another method of contraception since breast feeding provides only partial protection from becoming pregnant and this partial protection decreases significantly as you breast feed for longer periods of time. You should consider starting oral contraceptives only after you have weaned your child completely.

3. Laboratory Tests

If you are scheduled for any laboratory tests, tell your doctor you are taking birth control pills. Certain blood tests may be affected by birth control pills.

4. Drug Interactions

Certain drugs may interact with birth control pills to make them less effective in preventing pregnancy or cause an increase in breakthrough bleeding. Such drugs include rifampin, drugs used for epilepsy such as barbiturates (for example, phenobarbital) and phenytoin (Dilantin® is one brand of this drug), phenylbutazone (Butazolidin® is one brand) and possibly certain antibiotics. You may need to use additional contraception when you take drugs which can make oral contraceptives less effective.

HOW TO TAKE ORAL CONTRACEPTIVES

1. General Instructions

You must take your pill every day according to the instructions. Oral contraceptives are most effective if taken no more than 24 hours apart. Take your pill at the same time every day so that you are less likely to forget to take it. You will then maintain an effective dose of oral contraceptive in your body.

If your doctor has scheduled you for surgery, or you need prolonged bed rest, he or she may suggest that you stop taking the pill four weeks before surgery to avoid an increased risk of blood clots. It is also advisable not to start oral contraceptives sooner than four weeks after delivery of a baby.

2. If You Forget To Take Your Pill

If you miss only one pill in a cycle, the chance of becoming pregnant is small. Take the missed pill as soon as you realize that you have forgotten it. Since the risk of pregnancy increases with each additional pill you skip, it is very important that you take one pill a day.

3. Pregnancy Due To Pill Failure

The incidence of pill failure resulting in pregnancy is approximately 1% (i.e., one pregnancy per 100 women per year) if taken every day as directed, but more typical failure rates are about 3%. If failure does occur, the risk to the fetus is minimal.

4. Pregnancy After Stopping The Pill

There may be some delay in becoming pregnant after you stop using oral contraceptives, especially if you had irregular

Continued on next page

This product information was prepared in August 1992. On these and other Parke-Davis Products, information may be obtained by addressing PARKE-DAVIS, Division of Warner-Lambert Company, Morris Plains, New Jersey 07950.

Parke-Davis—Cont.

menstrual cycles before you used oral contraceptives. It may be advisable to postpone conception until you begin menstruating regularly once you have stopped taking the pill and desire pregnancy.
There does not appear to be any increase in birth defects in newborn babies when pregnancy occurs soon after stopping the pill.

5. Overdosage
Serious ill effects have not been reported following ingestion of large doses of oral contraceptives by young children. Overdosage may cause nausea and withdrawal bleeding in females. In case of overdosage, contact your health care provider or pharmacist.

6. Other Information
Your health care provider will take a medical and family history and examine you before prescribing oral contraceptives. You should be reexamined at least once a year. Be sure to inform your health care provider if there is a family history of any of the conditions listed previously in this leaflet. Be sure to keep all appointments with your health care provider, because this is a time to determine if there are early signs of side effects of oral contraceptive use.
Do not use the drug for any condition other than the one for which it was prescribed. This drug has been prescribed specifically for you; do not give it to others who may want birth control pills.

HEALTH BENEFITS FROM ORAL CONTRACEPTIVES

In addition to preventing pregnancy, use of oral contraceptives may provide certain benefits.
They are:

- Menstrual cycles may become more regular
- Blood flow during menstruation may be lighter and less iron may be lost. Therefore, anemia due to iron deficiency is less likely to occur
- Pain or other symptoms during menstruation may be encountered less frequently
- Ectopic (tubal) pregnancy may occur less frequently
- Noncancerous cysts or lumps in the breast may occur less frequently
- Acute pelvic inflammatory disease may occur less frequently
- Oral contraceptive use may provide some protection against developing two forms of cancer: cancer of the ovaries and cancer of the lining of the uterus.

If you want more information about birth control pills, ask your doctor or pharmacist. They have a more technical leaflet called the "Physician Insert," which you may wish to read.

INSTRUCTIONS TO PATIENTS

TABLET DISPENSER
The tablet dispenser has been designed to make oral contraceptive dosing as easy and as convenient as possible. The tablets are arranged in either three or four rows of seven tablets each, with the days of the week appearing on the tablet dispenser above the first row of tablets.

If your tablet dispenser contains:	You are taking:
21 yellow tablets	NORLESTRIN 21 1/50
21 pink tablets	NORLESTRIN 21 2.5/50
21 yellow tablets and 7 brown tablets	NORLESTRIN Fe 1/50
21 pink tablets and 7 brown tablets	NORLESTRIN Fe 2.5/50
21 yellow tablets and 7 white tablets	NORLESTRIN 28 1/50

Each *yellow* tablet contains 1 mg norethindrone acetate and 50 mcg ethinyl estradiol.
Each *pink* tablet contains 2.5 mg norethindrone acetate and 50 mcg ethinyl estradiol.
Each *brown* tablet contains 75 mg ferrous fumarate and is intended to help you remember to take the tablets correctly. These brown tablets are not intended to have any health benefit.
To remove a tablet, press down on it with your thumb or finger. The tablet will drop through the back of the tablet dispenser. Do not press on the tablet with your thumbnail or fingernail or any other sharp object.

NORLESTRIN 21-DAY DOSAGE REGIMEN

If your tablet dispenser contains 21 tablets (3 rows of 7), you are on a 21-day regimen and should follow either the Sunday-Start or Day-5 Start directions.

A. Sunday-Start Regimen

1. Unless your physician or health care provider has instructed you differently, begin taking tablets on the first Sunday after your menstrual period begins whether or not you are still bleeding. If your period begins on Sunday, take your first tablet that very same day. START WITH THE SUNDAY TABLET IN THE TOP ROW.

Note: During the first cycle, it is important that you use another method of birth control until you have taken a tablet daily for seven consecutive days.

2. Take all the tablets in the top row first, followed by the second row. Continue to take one tablet every day until you finish all 21 tablets. Your last tablet should be on Saturday.
3. After you have taken all 21 tablets, stop, and don't take any tablets for the next seven days. You should have a menstrual period one to three days after you stop taking tablets; sometimes it may take a day or so longer.
4. After the seven days during which you take no tablets, obtain a new course of tablets. Begin the new course of 21 day tablets on Sunday, the 8th day after you took your last tablet, starting with the Sunday tablet in the top row.
5. Continue to take one tablet daily until you finish all 21 tablets. If you follow the schedule properly, you will always take the last tablet in the dispenser on a Saturday, and always start each new course of 21 tablets 8 days later, on the following Sunday.
6. If, in any cycle, you start your tablets later than the proper day, you should also use another method of birth control until you have taken seven consecutive tablets.

B. Day-5 Regimen
If your physician or health care provider has directed you to begin taking your first cycle of tablets using the Day-5 Regimen, you should start taking your tablets on Day 5 after the start of your period.

1. The first day of your period is Day 1. On the 5th day (Day 5), start taking one tablet daily, beginning with the tablet in the top row that corresponds to Day 5 after your flow began.

If your period begins on:	Start taking tablets in the top row on:
Sunday	Thursday
Monday	Friday
Tuesday	Saturday
Wednesday	Sunday
Thursday	Monday
Friday	Tuesday
Saturday	Wednesday

Note: During the first cycle, if you start taking tablets later than Day 5 of your menstrual period, you should use another method of birth control until you have taken a tablet daily for seven consecutive days.

2. Continue to take one tablet daily. After the last Saturday tablet has been taken, if any tablets remain in the first row, complete your 21-day regimen by taking one tablet daily starting with the Sunday tablet in the top row.
3. After you have taken all 21 tablets, stop, and don't take any tablets for the next seven days. You should have a menstrual period one to three days after you stop taking tablets; sometimes it may take a day or so longer.
4. After the seven days during which you take no tablets, obtain a new course of tablets. Begin a new course of 21-day tablets, the 8th day after you took your last tablet, starting with the tablet in the top row that corresponds to that day.
5. Continue to take one tablet daily until you finish all 21 tablets. If you follow the schedule properly, you will always take the last tablet in the dispenser on the same day of the week, and always start each new course of 21 tablets the same day of the week on which you began the previous cycle of tablets.
6. If, in any cycle, you start your tablets later than the proper day, you should also use another method of birth control until you have taken seven consecutive tablets.

Whether you started your tablets using the Sunday-Start or Day-5 Regimen, the following directions apply:

1. Continue taking your tablets whether or not your period has occurred or is still in progress. Your period will usually occur during the seven days you are taking no tablets.
2. If spotting should occur at an unexpected time, continue to take your tablets as directed. Spotting is usually temporary and without significance. However, if bleeding should occur at an unexpected time, consult your physician or health care provider. Call your physician or health care provider regarding any problem or change in your general health that may concern you.

NORLESTRIN 28-DAY DOSAGE REGIMEN

If your tablet dispenser contains 28 tablets (3 rows of 7 *light-colored* (yellow or pink) tablets and 1 row of 7 *brown* tablets), you are on a 28-day regimen and should follow these directions.

Sunday-Start Regimen:

1. Begin taking tablets on the first Sunday after your menstrual period begins whether or not you are still bleeding. If your period begins on Sunday, take your first tablet that very same day. START WITH THE SUNDAY TABLET IN THE TOP ROW.

Note: During the first cycle, it is important that you use another method of birth control until you have taken a *light-colored* tablet daily for seven consecutive days.

2. Take all the tablets in the top row first, followed by the second row and so on.
3. Continue to take one tablet every day until you finish all 21 *light-colored* tablets. On the day after taking the last *light-colored* tablet, begin taking one *brown* tablet daily until all the tablets have been taken.
4. When the last tablet has been taken, obtain a new course of tablets and, without interruption, begin a new course of 28-day tablets, the next day, starting with the Sunday tablet in the top row. There should never be a day when you are not taking a tablet.
5. If, in any cycle, you start your tablets later than the proper day, you should also use another method of birth control until you have taken seven *light-colored* tablets.
6. Continue taking *light-colored* tablets without interruption whether or not your period has occurred or is still in progress. Your period will usually occur during the time you are taking *brown* tablets.
7. If spotting should occur at an unexpected time, continue to take your tablets as directed. Spotting is usually temporary and without significance. However, if bleeding should occur at an unexpected time, consult your physician or health care provider. Call your physician or health care provider regarding any problem or change in your general health that may concern you.

In Case You Forget (21-Day And 28-Day Regimens)
The following instructions apply only to missing the yellow 1/50 tablets or the pink 2.5/50 tablets.
If you forget to take one tablet, take it as soon as you remember, even if it is the next day. Then take the next scheduled tablet at the usual time. If you miss two consecutive tablets, take two tablets daily for the next two days. Then resume the regular schedule. While there is little likelihood of pregnancy occurring if you miss only one or two tablets, the possibility of pregnancy increases with each successive day that tablets are missed.
21-Day Regimen: If you miss three consecutive tablets, discard any tablets remaining in the tablet dispenser and follow these instructions.
If you are on the Sunday-Start Regimen, start a new course of tablets the first Sunday following the last missed tablet, whether or not you are still menstruating.
If you are on the Day-5 Regimen, begin a new course of tablets on the 8th day after the last tablet was taken. For example, if you took your last tablet on a Monday, you should begin your new course of tablets the following Monday.
During the seven days without tablets, and until you have taken a tablet daily for seven consecutive days from your new course of tablets, you should also use another method of birth control.
28-Day Regimen: If you miss three consecutive *light-colored* tablets, discard any tablets remaining in the tablet dispenser and begin a new course of tablets the first Sunday following the last missed tablet, whether or not you are still menstruating. During the days without tablets and until you have taken a tablet daily for seven consecutive days from your new course of tablets, you should also use another method of birth control.
If you miss one or more *brown* tablets discard the remainder and begin a new course of tablets on the next Sunday (which should be the 8th day after you took your last *light-colored* tablet). Start with the *light-colored* tablets in the top row. Skipping one or more *brown* tablets contained in the 28-day regimen products won't increase the risk of pregnancy. They are there to help keep you on schedule and to eliminate the need for counting days. *Under no circumstances* should you substitute a *brown* tablet for a *light-colored* tablet nor should a *brown* tablet be taken until you have finished all the *light-colored* tablets, unless your physician or health care provider advises you to do so.
Remembering to take tablets according to schedule is stressed because of its importance in providing you the greatest degree of protection.

MISSED MENSTRUAL PERIODS FOR BOTH DOSAGE REGIMENS

At times there may be no menstrual period after a cycle of pills. Therefore, if you miss one menstrual period but have taken the pills *exactly as you were supposed to,* continue as usual into the next cycle. If you have not taken the pills correctly and miss a menstrual period, *you may be pregnant* and

should stop taking oral contraceptives until your doctor or health care provider determines whether or not you are pregnant. Until you can get to your doctor, use another form of contraception. If two consecutive menstrual periods are missed, you should stop taking pills until it is determined whether or not you are pregnant. Although there does not appear to be any increase in birth defects in newborn babies if you become pregnant while using oral contraceptives, if you do become pregnant, you should discuss the situation with your doctor or health care provider.

Periodic Examination

Your doctor or health care provider will take a complete medical and family history before prescribing oral contraceptives. At that time and about once a year thereafter, he will generally examine your blood pressure, breasts, abdomen, and pelvic organs (including a Papanicolaou smear, ie, test for cancer).

SUMMARY

Oral contraceptives are the most effective method, except sterilization, for preventing pregnancy. Other methods, when used conscientiously, are also very effective and have fewer risks. Although the serious risks of oral contraceptives are uncommon, some of the risks may persist after you stop using the pill. On the other hand, the "pill" is a very convenient method of preventing pregnancy.

If you have certain conditions or have had these conditions in the past, you should not use oral contraceptives because the risk is too great. These conditions are listed in this leaflet. If you do not have these conditions, and decide to use the "pill," please read this leaflet carefully so that you can use the "pill" most safely and effectively.

Based on his or her assessment of your medical needs, your doctor or health care provider has prescribed this drug for you. Do not give this drug to anyone else.

Keep this and all drugs out of the reach of children.

Caution—Federal law prohibits dispensing without prescription.

0901G137

Shown in Product Identification Section, pages 422 and 423

NORLUTATE® ℞

[nōr″lū′tāte]

(norethindrone acetate tablets, USP)

DESCRIPTION

Norlutate is the acetic acid ester of norethindrone, which is the 17 alpha-ethinyl derivative of 19-nortestosterone. It is a progestational agent for oral administration. Each tablet contains 5 mg of norethindrone acetate, USP. Norlutate also contains: acacia, NF; confectioner's sugar, NF; D&C red No. 30 Al lake; FD&C yellow No. 6 Al lake; lactose, NF; light mineral oil, NF; magnesium stearate, NF; corn starch, NF; and talc, USP. The chemical name is 17-Hydroxy-19-nor-17α-pregn-4-en-20-yn-3-one acetate.

CLINICAL PHARMACOLOGY

Transforms proliferative endometrium into secretory endometrium. Inhibits (at the usual dose range) the secretion of pituitary gonadotropins, which in turn prevents follicular maturation and ovulation.

May also demonstrate some estrogenic, anabolic or androgenic activity but should not be relied upon.

INDICATIONS AND USAGE

Norlutate is indicated in amenorrhea; in abnormal uterine bleeding due to hormonal imbalance in the absence of organic pathology, such as submucous fibroids or uterine cancer; and in endometriosis.

CONTRAINDICATIONS

1. Current or past history of thrombophlebitis, thromboembolic disorders, or cerebral apoplexy.
2. Liver dysfunction or disease.
3. Known or suspected malignancy of breast or genital organs.
4. Undiagnosed vaginal bleeding.
5. Missed abortion.
6. As a diagnostic test for pregnancy.
7. Known sensitivity to norethindrone acetate.

WARNINGS

1. The use of progestational drugs during the first four months of pregnancy is not recommended. Progestational agents have been used beginning with the first trimester of pregnancy in attempts to prevent abortion but there is no evidence that such use is effective. Furthermore, the use of progestational agents, with their uterine-relaxant properties, in patients with fertilized defective ova may cause a delay in spontaneous abortion.
2. Several reports suggest an association between intrauterine exposure to progestational drugs in the first trimester of pregnancy and genital abnormalities in male and female fetuses. The risk of hypospadias (5 to 8 per 1,000 male births in the general population) may be approximately doubled with exposure to these drugs. There are insufficient data to quantify the risk to exposed female fetuses, but insofar as some of these drugs induce mild virilization of the external genitalia of the female fetus, and because of the increased association of hypospadias in the male fetus, it is prudent to avoid the use of these drugs during the first trimester of pregnancy.
3. The physician should be alert to the earliest manifestations of thrombotic disorders (thrombophlebitis, cerebrovascular disorders, pulmonary embolism, and retinal thrombosis). Should any of these occur or be suspected, the drug should be discontinued immediately.
4. Medication should be discontinued pending examination if there is a sudden partial or complete loss of vision, or if there is a sudden onset of proptosis, diplopia or migraine. If examination reveals papilledema or retinal vascular lesions, medication should be withdrawn.
5. Detectable amounts of drug have been identified in the milk of mothers receiving progestational drugs. The effect of this on the nursing infant has not been determined.

PRECAUTIONS

1. The pretreatment physical examination should include special reference to breast and pelvic organs, as well as a Papanicolaou smear.
2. Because progestational drugs may cause some degree of fluid retention, conditions which might be influenced by this condition, such as epilepsy, migraine, asthma, cardiac or renal dysfunction, require careful observation.
3. In cases of breakthrough bleeding, as in all cases of irregular bleeding per vaginum, nonfunctional causes should be borne in mind and adequate diagnostic measures undertaken.
4. Patients who have a history of psychic depression should be carefully observed and the drug discontinued if the depression recurs to a serious degree.
5. The age of the patient constitutes no absolute limiting factor although treatment with progestin may mask the onset of the climacteric.
6. The pathologist should be advised of progestin therapy when relevant specimens are submitted.
7. Studies of the addition of a progestin product to an estrogen replacement regimen for seven or more days of a cycle of estrogen administration have reported a lowered incidence of endometrial hyperplasia. Morphological and biochemical studies of endometria suggest that 10–13 days of a progestin are needed to provide maximal maturation of the endometrium and to eliminate any hyperplastic changes. Whether, this will provide protection from endometrial carcinoma has not been clearly established.
8. There are possible risks which may be associated with the inclusion of progestin in estrogen replacement regimen, including adverse effects on carbohydrate and lipid metabolism. The dosage used may be important in minimizing these adverse effects.
9. A decrease in glucose tolerance has been observed in a small percentage of patients on estrogen-progestin combination treatment. The mechanism of this decrease is obscure. For this reason, diabetic patients should be carefully observed while receiving such therapy.

CARCINOGENESIS, MUTAGENESIS, IMPAIRMENT OF FERTILITY

Long-term intramuscular administration of Medroxyprogesterone acetate (MPA) has been shown to produce mammary tumors in beagle dogs. There is no evidence of a carcinogenic effect associated with the oral administration of MPA to rats and mice. Medroxyprogesterone acetate was not mutagenic in a battery of *in vitro* or *in vivo* genetic toxicity assays.

Norlutate at high doses is an antifertility drug and high doses would be expected to impair fertility until the cessation of treatment.

INFORMATION FOR THE PATIENT

See Patient Information at end of insert.

ADVERSE REACTIONS

—(See WARNINGS for possible adverse effects on the fetus)
—breakthough bleeding
—spotting
—change in menstrual flow
—amenorrhea
—edema
—change in weight (increase or decrease)
—changes in cervical erosion and cervical secretions
—cholestatic jaundice
—breast tenderness and galactorrhea
—skin sensitivity reactions consisting of urticaria, pruritus, edema and generalized rash
—acne, alopecia and hirsutism
—rash (allergic) with and without pruritus
—anaphylactoid reactions
—mental depression
—pyrexia
—insomnia
—nausea
—somnolence

A statistically significant association has been demonstrated between use of estrogen-progestin combination drugs and pulmonary embolism and cerebral thrombosis and embolism. For this reason patients on progestin therapy should be carefully observed. There is also evidence suggestive of an association with neuro-ocular lesions, eg, retinal thrombosis and optic neuritis.

The following adverse reactions have been observed in patients receiving estrogen-progestin combination drugs:
—rise in blood pressure in susceptible individuals
—premenstrual syndrome
—changes in libido
—changes in appetite
—cystitis-like syndrome
—headache
—nervousness
—fatigue
—backache
—hirsutism
—loss of scalp hair
—erythema multiforme
—erythema nodosum
—hemorrhagic eruption
—itching
—dizziness

The following laboratory results may be altered by the use of estrogen-progestin combination drugs:
—increased sulfobromophthalein retention and other hepatic function tests
—coagulation tests: increase in prothrombin factors VII, VIII, IX, and X
—metyrapone test
—pregnanediol determinations
—thyroid function: increase in PBI, and butanol extractable protein bound iodine and decrease in T^3 uptake values.

DOSAGE AND ADMINISTRATION

Therapy with Norlutate must be adapted to the specific indications and therapeutic response of the individual patient.

This dosage schedule assumes the interval between menses to be 28 days.

Amenorrhea, abnormal uterine bleeding due to hormonal imbalance in the absence of organic pathology: 2.5 to 10 mg Norlutate starting with the fifth day of the menstrual cycle and ending on the 25th day.

Endometriosis: Initial daily dose of 5 mg Norlutate for two weeks with increments of 2.5 mg per day of Norlutate every two weeks until 15 mg per day of Norlutate is reached. Therapy may be held at this level for from six to nine months or until annoying breakthrough bleeding demands temporary termination.

HOW SUPPLIED

N 0071-0918-19—Norlutate is supplied as 5-mg pink, scored, cup-shaped tablets, debossed with P-D 918 in bottles of 50.

PATIENT INFORMATION

Norlutate is a progestational drug. The information below is required by the U.S. Food and Drug Administration to be provided to all patients taking such products. This information relates only to the risk to the unborn child associated with use of progestational drugs during pregnancy. For further information on the use, side effects, and other risks associated with this product, ask your doctor.

WARNING FOR WOMEN

Progesterone or progesterone-like drugs have been used to prevent miscarriage in the first few months of pregnancy. No adequate evidence is available to show that they are effective for this purpose. Furthermore, most cases of early miscarriage are due to causes which could not be helped by these drugs.

There is an increased risk of minor birth defects in children whose mothers take this drug during the first 4 months of pregnancy. Several reports suggest an association between mothers who take these drugs in the first trimester of pregnancy and genital abnormalities in male and female babies. The risk to the male baby is the possibility of being born with a condition in which the opening of the penis is on the underside rather than the tip of the penis (hypospadias). Hypospadias occurs in about 5 to 8 per 1000 male births and is about doubled with exposure to these drugs. There is not enough information to quantify the risk to exposed female fetuses, but enlargement of the clitoris and fusion of the labia may occur, although rarely.

Therefore, since drugs of this type may induce mild masculinization of the external genitalia of the female fetus, as well as hypospadias in the male fetus, it is wise to avoid using the drug during the first trimester of pregnancy.

Continued on next page

This product information was prepared in August 1992. On these and other Parke-Davis Products, information may be obtained by addressing PARKE-DAVIS, Division of Warner-Lambert Company, Morris Plains, New Jersey 07950.

Parke-Davis—Cont.

These drugs have been used as a test for pregnancy but such use is no longer considered safe because of possible damage to a developing baby. Also more rapid methods for testing for pregnancy are now available.

If you take Norlutate and later find you were pregnant when you took it, be sure to discuss this with your doctor as soon as possible.

0918G038

Shown in Product Identification Section, page 423

NORLUTIN®   ℞
[nŏr″lū′tĭn]
(norethindrone tablets, USP)

DESCRIPTION

Norlutin is the 17 alpha-ethinyl derivative of 19-nortestosterone. It is a progestational agent for oral administration. Each tablet contains 5 mg of norethindrone, USP. Norlutin also contains: acacia, NF; confectioner's sugar, NF; lactose, NF; magnesium stearate, NF; starch potato, NF; and talc, USP. The chemical name is 17-Hydroxy-19-nor-17α-pregn-4-en-20-yn-3-one.

CLINICAL PHARMACOLOGY

Transforms proliferative endometrium into secretory endometrium.

Inhibits (at the usual dosage range) the secretion of pituitary gonadotropins, which in turn prevents follicular maturation and ovulation.

May also demonstrate some estrogenic, anabolic, or androgenic activity but should not be relied upon.

INDICATIONS AND USAGE

Norlutin is indicated in amenorrhea; in abnormal uterine bleeding due to hormonal imbalance in the absence of organic pathology, such as submucous fibroids or uterine cancer; and in endometriosis.

CONTRAINDICATIONS

1. Current or past history of thrombophlebitis, thromboembolic disorders, or cerebral apoplexy.
2. Liver dysfunction or disease.
3. Known or suspected malignancy of breast or genital organs.
4. Undiagnosed vaginal bleeding.
5. Missed abortion.
6. As a diagnostic test for pregnancy.
7. Known sensitivity to norethindrone.

WARNINGS

1. The use of progestational drugs during the first four months of pregnancy is not recommended. Progestational agents have been used beginning with the first trimester of pregnancy in attempts to prevent abortion but there is no evidence that such use is effective. Furthermore, the use of progestational agents, with their uterine-relaxant properties, in patients with fertilized defective ova may cause a delay in spontaneous abortion.
2. Several reports suggest an association between intrauterine exposure to progestational drugs in the first trimester of pregnancy and genital abnormalities in male and female fetuses. The risk of hypospadias (5 to 8 per 1,000 male births in the general population) may be approximately doubled with exposure to these drugs. There are insufficient data to quantify the risk to exposed female fetuses, but insofar as some of these drugs induce mild virilization of the external genitalia of the female fetus, and because of the increased association of hypospadias in the male fetus, it is prudent to avoid the use of these drugs during the first trimester of pregnancy.
3. The physician should be alert to the earliest manifestations of thrombotic disorders (thrombophlebitis, cerebrovascular disorders, pulmonary embolism, and retinal thrombosis). Should any of these occur or be suspected, the drug should be discontinued immediately.
4. Medication should be discontinued pending examination if there is sudden partial or complete loss of vision, or if there is a sudden onset of proptosis, diplopia or migraine. If examination reveals papilledema or retinal vascular lesions, medication should be withdrawn.
5. Detectable amounts of drug have been identified in the milk of mothers receiving progestational drugs. The effect of this on the nursing infant has not been determined.

PRECAUTIONS

1. The pretreatment physical examination should include special reference to breasts and pelvic organs, as well as a Papanicolaou smear.
2. Because progestational drugs may cause some degree of fluid retention, conditions which might be influenced by this condition, such as epilepsy, migraine, asthma, cardiac or renal dysfunction, require careful observation.

3. In cases of breakthrough bleeding, as in all cases of irregular bleeding per vaginum, nonfunctional causes should be borne in mind and adequate diagnostic measures undertaken.
4. Patients who have a history of psychic depression should be carefully observed and the drug discontinued if the depression recurs to a serious degree.
5. The age of the patient constitutes no absolute limiting factor although treatment with progestin may mask the onset of the climacteric.
6. The pathologist should be advised of progestin therapy when relevant specimens are submitted.
7. Studies of the addition of a progestin product to an estrogen replacement regimen for seven or more days of a cycle of estrogen administration have reported a lowered incidence of endometrial hyperplasia. Morphological and biochemical studies of endometria suggest that 10–13 days of a progestin are needed to provide maximal maturation of the endometrium and to eliminate any hyperplastic changes. Whether this will provide protection from endometrial carcinoma has not been clearly established.
8. There are possible risks which may be associated with the inclusion of progestin in estrogen replacement regimen, including adverse effects on carbohydrate and lipid metabolism. The dosage used may be important in minimizing these adverse effects.
9. A decrease in glucose tolerance has been observed in a small percentage of patients on estrogen-progestin combination treatment. The mechanism of this decrease is obscure. For this reason, diabetic patients should be carefully observed while receiving such therapy.

CARCINOGENESIS, MUTAGENESIS, IMPAIRMENT OF FERTILITY

Long-term intramuscular administration of Medroxyprogesterone acetate (MPA) has been shown to produce mammary tumors in beagle dogs. There is no evidence of a carcinogenic effect associated with the oral administration of MPA to rats and mice. Medroxyprogesterone acetate was not mutagenic in a battery of *in vitro* or *in vivo* genetic toxicity assays. Norlutin at high doses is an antifertility drug and high doses would be expected to impair fertility until the cessation of treatment.

INFORMATION FOR THE PATIENT

See Patient Information at end of insert.

ADVERSE REACTIONS

—(See WARNINGS for possible adverse effects on the fetus)
—breakthrough bleeding
—spotting
—change in menstrual flow
—amenorrhea
—edema
—change in weight (increase or decrease)
—changes in cervical erosion and cervical secretions
—cholestatic jaundice
—breast tenderness and galactorrhea
—skin sensitivity reactions consisting of urticaria, pruritus, edema and generalized rash
—acne, alopecia and hirsutism
—rash (allergic) with and without pruritus
—anaphylactoid reactions
—mental depression
—pyrexia
—insomnia
—nausea
—somnolence

A statistically significant association has been demonstrated between use of estrogen-progestin combination drugs and pulmonary embolism and cerebral thrombosis and embolism. For this reason patients on progestin therapy should be carefully observed. There is also evidence suggestive of an association with neuro-ocular lesions, eg, retinal thrombosis and optic neuritis.

The following adverse reactions have been observed in patients receiving estrogen-progestin combination drugs:
—rise in blood pressure in susceptible individuals
—premenstrual syndrome
—changes in libido
—changes in appetite
—cystitis-like syndrome
—headache
—nervousness
—fatigue
—backache
—hirsutism
—loss of scalp hair
—erythema multiforme
—erythema nodosum
—hemorrhagic eruption
—itching
—dizziness

The following laboratory results may be altered by the use of estrogen-progestin combination drugs:
—increased sulfobromophthalein retention and other hepatic function tests

—coagulation tests: increase in prothrombin factors VII, VIII, IX, and X
—metyrapone test
—pregnanediol determinations
—thyroid function: increase in PBI, and butanol extractable protein bound iodine and decrease in T³ uptake values

PATIENT INFORMATION

Norlutin is a progestational drug. The information below is required by the U.S. Food and Drug Administration to be provided to all patients taking such products. This information relates only to the risk to the unborn child associated with use of progestational drugs during pregnancy. For further information on the use, side effects, and other risks associated with this product, ask your doctor.

WARNING FOR WOMEN

Progesterone or progesterone-like drugs have been used to prevent miscarriage in the first few months of pregnancy. No adequate evidence is available to show that they are effective for this purpose. Furthermore, most cases of early miscarriages are due to causes which could not be helped by these drugs.

There is an increased risk of minor birth defects in children whose mothers take this drug during the first 4 months of pregnancy. Several reports suggest an association between mothers who take these drugs in the first trimester of pregnancy and genital abnormalities in male and female babies. The risk to the male baby is the possibility of being born with a condition in which the opening of the penis is on the underside rather than the tip of the penis (hypospadias). Hypospadias occurs in about 5 to 8 per 1000 male births and is about doubled with exposure to these drugs. There is not enough information to quantify the risk to exposed female fetuses, but enlargement of the clitoris and fusion of the labia may occur, although rarely.

Therefore, since drugs of this type may induce mild masculinization of the external genitalia of the female fetus, as well as hypospadias in the male fetus, it is wise to avoid using the drug during the first trimester of pregnancy.

These drugs have been used as a test for pregnancy but such use is no longer considered safe because of possible damage to a developing baby. Also, more rapid methods for testing for pregnancy are now available.

If you take Norlutin and later find you were pregnant when you took it, be sure to discuss this with your doctor as soon as possible.

DOSAGE AND ADMINISTRATION

Therapy with Norlutin must be adapted to the specific indications and therapeutic response of the individual patient.

This dosage schedule assumes the interval between menses to be 28 days.

Amenorrhea, abnormal uterine bleeding due to hormonal imbalance in the absence of organic pathology: 5 to 20 mg Norlutin starting with the fifth day of the menstrual cycle and ending on the 25th day.

Endometriosis: Initial daily dose of 10 mg Norlutin for two weeks with increments of 5 mg per day of Norlutin every two weeks until 30 mg per day of Norlutin is reached. Therapy may be held at this level for from six to nine months or until annoying breakthrough bleeding demands temporary termination.

HOW SUPPLIED

N 0071-0882-19—Norlutin is supplied as 5-mg white, scored, cup-shaped tablets, debossed with P-D 882 in bottles of 50.
Storage—Store below 30°C (86°F).
Caution—Federal law prohibits dispensing without prescription.

0882G014

Shown in Product Identification Section, page 423

PERITRATE® SA   ℞
[pĕ′rĭ-trāte″]
(pentaerythritol tetranitrate tablets)
Sustained Action

PERITRATE®   ℞
(pentaerythritol tetranitrate tablets, USP)

DESCRIPTION

Each tablet of Peritrate 40 mg contains pentaerythritol tetranitrate 40 mg.
Each tablet of Peritrate 20 mg contains pentaerythritol tetranitrate 20 mg.
Each tablet of Peritrate 10 mg contains pentaerythritol tetranitrate 10 mg.

Pentaerythritol tetranitrate is a nitric acid ester of a tetrahydric alcohol (pentaerythritol).

Peritrate 10 mg and 20 mg contain alginic acid, NF; D&C yellow No. 10; FD&C blue No. 1; gelatin, NF; lactose, NF; methylcellulose, USP; propylparaben, NF; corn starch, NF; stearic acid, NF; and may also contain magnesium stearate, NF. Peritrate 40 mg contains D&C yellow No. 10 Al lake; D&C red No. 30 Al lake; lactose, NF; povidone, USP; silicon

dioxide, NF; corn starch, NF; stearic acid, NF; and confectioner's sugar, NF.

Each tablet of Peritrate SA Sustained Action contains: pentaerythritol tetranitrate 80 mg (20 mg in immediate release layer and 60 mg in sustained release base). Pentaerythritol tetranitrate is a nitric acid ester of a tetrahydric alcohol (pentaerythritol).

Peritrate SA 80 mg also contains D&C yellow No. 10; FD&C blue No. 1; lactose, NF; magnesium stearate, NF; silicon dioxide, NF; confectioner's sugar, NF; and other ingredients.

CLINICAL PHARMACOLOGY

The exact cause of angina pectoris (that is, the pain associated with coronary artery disease) remains obscure, despite the numerous and often conflicting hypotheses concerning its pathophysiology. Therapy at the present time, therefore, remains essentially empirical. Customarily, clinical improvement has been measured by: reduction in (1) number, intensity and duration of angina pectoris attacks and (2) necessity for glyceryl trinitrate intake for prevention or relief of anginal attacks. Peritrate SA (pentaerythritol tetranitrate) Sustained Action and Peritrate (pentaerythritol tetranitrate) have been reported in clinical usage to reduce in number and severity the incidence of angina pectoris attacks, with concomitant reduction in glyceryl trinitrate intake.

In the evaluation of Peritrate and Peritrate SA in angina pectoris, clinical improvement has been customarily measured subjectively by: reduction in number and severity of attacks and necessity for glyceryl trinitrate intake for prevention or abortion of anginal attacks. Individual patterns of angina pectoris differ widely as does the symptomatic response to antianginal agents such as pentaerythritol tetranitrate. The published literature contains both favorable and unfavorable clinical reports. In conjunction with total management of the patient with angina pectoris, Peritrate and Peritrate SA have been accepted as safe for prolonged administration and widely regarded as useful.

INDICATIONS AND USAGE

Based on a review of this drug by the National Academy of Sciences—National Research Council and/or other information, FDA has classified the indications as follows:

"Possibly" effective: Peritrate is indicated for the relief of angina pectoris (pain associated with coronary artery disease). It is not intended to abort the acute anginal episode but is widely regarded as useful in the prophylactic treatment of angina pectoris.

Final classification of the less-than-effective indications requires further investigation.

CONTRAINDICATIONS

Peritrate SA and Peritrate are contraindicated in patients who have a history of sensitivity to the drug.

WARNINGS

Data supporting the use of Peritrate or Peritrate SA during the early days of the acute phase of myocardial infarction (the period during which clinical and laboratory findings are unstable) are insufficient to establish safety.

This drug can act as a physiological antagonist to norepinephrine, acetylcholine, histamine, and many other agents.

PRECAUTIONS

Should be used with caution in patients who have glaucoma. Tolerance to this drug and cross-tolerance to other nitrites and nitrates may occur.

ADVERSE REACTIONS

Side effects reported to date have been predominantly related to rash (which requires discontinuation of medication) and headache and gastrointestinal distress, which are usually mild and transient with continuation of medication. In some cases severe persistent headaches may occur. In addition, the following adverse reactions to nitrates such as pentaerythritol tetranitrate have been reported in the literature:

(a) Cutaneous vasodilatation with flushing.
(b) Transient episodes of dizziness and weakness, as well as other signs of cerebral ischemia associated with postural hypotension, may occasionally develop.
(c) An occasional individual exhibits marked sensitivity to the hypotensive effects of nitrite and severe responses (nausea, vomiting, weakness, restlessness, pallor, perspiration and collapse) can occur, even with the usual therapeutic doses. Alcohol may enhance this effect.

DOSAGE AND ADMINISTRATION

Peritrate may be administered in individualized doses up to 160 mg a day. Dosage can be initiated at one 10 mg or 20 mg tablet q.i.d. and titrated upward to 40 mg (two 20 mg tablets or one 40 mg tablet) q.i.d. one-half hour before or one hour after meals and at bedtime. Tablets can be chewed or swallowed whole. Alternatively, Peritrate SA can be administered on a convenient b.i.d. (on an empty stomach) dosage

schedule. One tablet immediately on arising and 1 tablet 12 hours later. Tablets should not be chewed.

HOW SUPPLIED

Peritrate SA double layer, biconvex, dark green/light green tablets in bottles of 100 (N 0071-0004-24) and 1000 (N 0071-0004-32).

Also supplied as:

Peritrate 40 mg—coral, scored tablets in bottles of 100 (N 0071-0008-24).

Peritrate 20 mg—light green, scored tablets in bottles of 100 (N 0071-0001-24).

Peritrate 10 mg—light green, unscored tablets in bottles of 100 (N 0071-0013-24) and 1000 (N 0071-0013-32.)

For full prescribing information, see specific package insert. Store at controlled room temperature 15°–30°C (59°–86°F).

ANIMAL PHARMACOLOGY

In a series of carefully designed studies in pigs, Peritrate was administered for 48 hours before an artificially induced occlusion of a major coronary artery and for seven days thereafter. The pigs were sacrificed at various intervals for periods up to six weeks. The result showed a significantly larger number of survivors in the drug-treated group. Damage to myocardial tissue in the drug-treated survivors was less extensive than in the untreated group. Studies in dogs subjected to oligemic shock through progressive bleeding have demonstrated that Peritrate is vasoactive at the postarteriolar level, producing increased blood flow and better tissue perfusion. These animal experiments cannot be translated to the drug's actions in humans.

0004G013/0001G013

Shown in Product Identification Section, page 423

PITOCIN®   ℞
[pĭ″tō′cĭn]
(oxytocin injection, USP) synthetic

DESCRIPTION

Pitocin (oxytocin injection, USP) is a sterile, clear, colorless aqueous solution of synthetic oxytocin, for intravenous infusion or intramuscular injection. Pitocin is a nonapeptide found in pituitary extracts from mammals. It is standardized to contain 10 units of oxytocic hormone/mL and contains 0.5% Chloretone® (chlorobutanol, a chloroform derivative) as a preservative, with the pH adjusted with acetic acid. The hormone is prepared synthetically to avoid possible contamination with vasopressin (ADH) and other small polypeptides with biologic activity. Pitocin has the empirical formula $C_{43}H_{66}N_{12}O_{12}S_2$ (molecular weight 1007.19). The structural formula is as follows:

$$H-Cys-Tyr-Ile-Glu(NH_2)-Asp(NH_2)-Cys-Pro-Leu-Gly-NH_2$$
$$1 \quad 2 \quad 3 \quad 4 \qquad 5 \qquad 6 \quad 7 \quad 8 \quad 9$$

CLINICAL PHARMACOLOGY

Uterine motility depends on the formation of the contractile protein actomyosin under the influence of the Ca^{2+}-dependent phosphorylating enzyme myosin light-chain kinase. Oxytocin promotes contractions by increasing the intracellular Ca^{2+}. Oxytocin has specific receptors in the myometrium and the receptor concentraton increases greatly during pregnancy, reaching a maximum in early labor at term. The response to a given dose of oxytocin is very individualized and depends on the sensitivity of the uterus, which is determined by the oxytocin receptor concentration. However, the physician should be aware of the fact that oxytocin even in its pure form has inherent pressor and antidiuretic properties which may become manifest when large doses are administered. These properties are thought to be due to the fact that oxytocin and vasopressin differ in regard to only two of the eight amino acids. (See PRECAUTIONS)

Oxytocin is distributed throughout the extracellular fluid. Small amounts of the drug probably reach the fetal circulation. Oxytocin has a plasma half-life of about 1 to 6 minutes which is decreased in late pregnancy and during lactation. Following intravenous administration of oxytocin, uterine response occurs almost immediately and subsides within 1 hour. Following intramuscular injection of the drug, uterine response occurs within 3 to 5 minutes and persists for 2 to 3 hours. Its rapid removal from plasma is accomplished largely by the kidney and the liver. Only small amounts are excreted in urine unchanged.

INDICATIONS AND USAGE

IMPORTANT NOTICE

Elective induction of labor is defined as the initiation of labor in a pregnant individual who has no medical indications for induction. Since the available data are inadequate to evaluate the benefits-to-risks considerations, Pitocin is not indicated for elective induction of labor.

Antepartum: Pitocin is indicated for the initiation or improvement of uterine contractions, where this is desirable and considered suitable for reasons of fetal or maternal concern, in order to achieve vaginal delivery. It is indicated for (1) induction of labor in patients with a medical indication for the initiation of labor, such as Rh problems, maternal diabetes, preeclampsia at or near term, when delivery is in the best interest of mother and fetus or when membranes are prematurely ruptured and delivery is indicated; (2) stimulation or reinforcement of labor, as in selected cases of uterine inertia; (3) as adjunctive therapy in the management of incomplete or inevitable abortion. In the first trimester curettage is generally considered primary therapy. In second trimester abortion, oxytocin infusion will often be successful in emptying the uterus. Other means of therapy, however, may be required in such cases.

Postpartum: Pitocin is indicated to produce uterine contractions during the third stage of labor and to control postpartum bleeding or hemorrhage.

CONTRAINDICATIONS

Antepartum use of Pitocin is contraindicated in any of the following circumstances:

1. Where there is significant cephalopelvic disproportion;
2. In unfavorable fetal positions or presentations, such as transverse lies, which are undeliverable without conversion prior to delivery;
3. In obstetrical emergencies where the benefit-to-risk ratio for either the fetus or the mother favors surgical intervention;
4. In fetal distress where delivery is not imminent;
5. Where adequate uterine activity fails to achieve satisfactory progress;
6. Where the uterus is already hyperactive or hypertonic;
7. In cases where vaginal delivery is contraindicated, such as invasive cervical carcinoma, active herpes genitalis, total placenta previa, vasa previa, and cord presentation or prolapse of the cord;
8. In patients with hypersensitivity to the drug.

WARNINGS

Pitocin, when given for induction of labor or augmentation of uterine activity, should be administered only by the intravenous route and with adequate medical supervision in a hospital.

PRECAUTIONS

General

1. All patients receiving intravenous oxytocin must be under continuous observation by trained personnel who have a thorough knowledge of the drug and are qualified to identify complications. A physician qualified to manage any complications should be immediately available. Electronic fetal monitoring provides the best means for early detection of overdosage (see OVERDOSAGE section). However, it must be borne in mind that only intrauterine pressure recording can accurately measure the intrauterine pressure during contractions. A fetal scalp electrode provides a more dependable recording of the fetal heart rate than any external monitoring system.

2. When properly administered, oxytocin should stimulate uterine contractions comparable to those seen in normal labor. Overstimulation of the uterus by improper administration can be hazardous to both mother and fetus. Even with proper administration and adequate supervision, hypertonic contractions can occur in patients whose uteri are hypersensitive to oxytocin. This fact must be considered by the physician in exercising his judgment regarding patient selection.

3. Except in unusual circumstances, oxytocin should not be administered in the following conditions: fetal distress, partial placenta previa, prematurity, borderline cephalopelvic disproportion, and any condition in which there is a predisposition for uterine rupture, such as previous major surgery on the cervix or uterus including cesarean section, overdistention of the uterus, grand multiparity, or past history of uterine sepsis or of traumatic delivery. Because of the variability of the combinations of factors which may be present in the conditions listed above, the definition of "unusual circumstances" must be left to the judgment of the physician. The decision can be made only by carefully weighing the potential benefits which oxytocin can provide in a given case against rare but definite potential for the drug to produce hypertonicity or tetanic spasm.

4. Maternal deaths due to hypertensive episodes, subarachnoid hemorrhage, rupture of the uterus, and fetal deaths due to various causes have been reported associated with

Continued on next page

This product information was prepared in August 1992. On these and other Parke-Davis Products, information may be obtained by addressing PARKE-DAVIS, Division of Warner-Lambert Company, Morris Plains, New Jersey 07950.

Parke-Davis—Cont.

the use of parenteral oxytocic drugs for induction of labor or for augmentation in the first and second stages of labor.

5. Oxytocin has been shown to have an intrinsic antidiuretic effect, acting to increase water reabsorption from the glomerular filtrate. Consideration should, therefore, be given to the possibility of water intoxication, particularly when oxytocin is administered continuously by infusion and the patient is receiving fluids by mouth.
6. When oxytocin is used for induction or reinforcement of already existent labor, patients should be carefully selected. Pelvic adequacy must be considered and maternal and fetal conditions evaluated before use of the drug.

Drug Interactions

Severe hypertension has been reported when oxytocin was given three to four hours following prophylactic administration of a vasoconstrictor in conjunction with caudal block anesthesia. Cyclopropane anesthesia may modify oxytocin's cardiovascular effects, so as to produce unexpected results such as hypotension. Maternal sinus bradycardia with abnormal atrioventricular rhythms has also been noted when oxytocin was used concomitantly with cyclopropane anesthesia.

Carcinogenesis, Mutagenesis, Impairment of Fertility

There are no animal or human studies on the carcinogenicity and mutagenicity of this drug, nor is there any information on its effect on fertility.

Pregnancy

Teratogenic Effects

Animal reproduction studies have not been conducted with oxytocin. There are no known indications for use in the first trimester of pregnancy other than in relation to spontaneous or induced abortion. Based on the wide experience with this drug and its chemical structure and pharmacological properties, it would not be expected to present a risk of fetal abnormalities when used as indicated.

Nonteratogenic Effects

See ADVERSE REACTIONS in the fetus or infant.

Labor and Delivery

See "INDICATIONS AND USAGE"

ADVERSE REACTIONS

The following adverse reactions have been reported in the mother:

Anaphylactic reaction
Postpartum hemorrhage
Cardiac arrhythmia
Fatal afibrinogenemia
Nausea
Vomiting
Premature ventricular contractions
Pelvic hematoma

Excessive dosage or hypersensitivity to the drug may result in uterine hypertonicity, spasm, tetanic contraction, or rupture of the uterus.

The possibility of increased blood loss and afibrinogenemia should be kept in mind when administering the drug.

Severe water intoxication with convulsions and coma has occurred, associated with a slow oxytocin infusion over a 24-hour period. Maternal death due to oxytocin-induced water intoxication has been reported.

The following adverse reactions have been reported in the fetus or infant:

Due to induced uterine motility:
Bradycardia
Premature ventricular contractions and other arrhythmias
Permanent CNS or brain damage
Fetal death

Due to use of oxytocin in the mother:
Low Apgar scores at five minutes
Neonatal jaundice
Neonatal retinal hemorrhage

OVERDOSAGE

Overdosage with oxytocin depends essentially on uterine hyperactivity whether or not due to hypersensitivity to this agent. Hyperstimulation with strong (hypertonic) or prolonged (tetanic) contractions, or a resting tone of 15 to 20 mmH_2O or more between contractions can lead to tumultuous labor, uterine rupture, cervical and vaginal lacerations, postpartum hemorrhage, uteroplacental hypoperfusion, and variable deceleration of fetal heart, fetal hypoxia, hypercapnia or death. Water intoxication with convulsions, which is caused by the inherent antidiuretic effect of oxytocin is a serious complication that may occur if large doses (40 to 50 milliunits/minute) are infused for long periods. Management consists of immediate discontinuation of oxytocin and symptomatic and supportive therapy.

DOSAGE AND ADMINISTRATION

Parenteral drug products should be inspected visually for particulate matter and discoloration prior to administration whenever solution and container permit.

The dosage of oxytocin is determined by the uterine response and must therefore be individualized and initiated at a very low level. The following dosage information is based upon various regimens and indications in general use.

A. Induction or Stimulation of Labor

Intravenous infusion (drip method) is the only acceptable method of parenteral administration of Pitocin for the induction or stimulation of labor. Accurate control of the rate of infusion is essential and is best accomplished by an infusion pump. It is convenient to piggyback the Pitocin infusion on a physiologic electrolyte solution, permitting the Pitocin infusion to be stopped abruptly without interrupting the electrolyte infusion. This is done in the following way:

1. Preparation

a. The standard solution for infusion of Pitocin is prepared by adding the contents of one 1-mL ampoule containing 10 units of oxytocin to 1,000 mL of 0.9% aqueous sodium chloride or Ringer's lactate. The combined solution containing 10 milliunits (mU) of oxytocin/mL is rotated in the infusion bottle for thorough mixing. The same concentration can be obtained by mixing the contents of one 0.5-mL ampoule, containing 5 units of oxytocin, with 500 mL of electrolyte solution.
b. Establish the infusion with a separate bottle of physiologic electrolyte solution not containing Pitocin.
c. Attach (piggyback) the Pitocin-containing bottle with the infusion pump to the infusion line as close to the infusion site as possible.

2. Administration

The initial dose should be 0.5–1 mU/min (equal to 3–6 mL of the dilute oxytocin solution per hour). At 30–60 minute intervals the dose should be gradually increased in increments of 1–2 mU/min until the desired contraction pattern has been established.

Once the desired frequency of contractions has been reached and labor has progressed to 5–6 cm dilation, the dose may be reduced by similar increments.

Studies of the concentrations of oxytocin in the maternal plasma during Pitocin infusion have shown that infusion rates up to 6 mU/min give the same oxytocin levels that are found in spontaneous labor. At term, higher infusion rates should be given with great care, and rates exceeding 9-10 mU/min are rarely required. Before term, when the sensitivity of the uterus is lower because of a lower concentration of oxytocin receptors, a higher infusion rate may be required.

3. Monitoring

a. Electronically monitor the uterine activity and the fetal heart rate throughout the infusion of Pitocin. Attention should be given to tonus, amplitude and frequency of contractions and to the fetal heart rate in relation to uterine contractions. If uterine contractions become too powerful, the infusion can be abruptly stopped, and oxytocic stimulation of the uterine musculature will soon wane (See PRECAUTIONS section).
b. Discontinue the infusion of Pitocin immediately in the event of uterine hyperactivity and/or fetal distress. Administer oxygen to the mother, who preferably should be put in a lateral position. The condition of mother and fetus should immediately be evaluated by the responsible physician and appropriate steps taken.

B. Control of Postpartum Uterine Bleeding

1. **Intravenous infusion (drip method).** If the patient has an intravenous infusion running, 10 to 40 units of oxytocin may be added to the bottle, depending on the amount of electrolyte or dextrose solution remaining (maximum 40 units to 1000 mL). Adjust the infusion rate to sustain uterine contraction and control uterine atony.
2. **Intramuscular administration.** (One mL) Ten (10) units of Pitocin can be given after the delivery of the placenta.

C. Treatment of Incomplete, Inevitable or Elective Abortion

Intravenous infusion of 10 units of Pitocin added to 500 mL of a physiologic saline solution or 5% dextrose-in-water solution may help the uterus contract after a suction or sharp curettage for an incomplete, inevitable or elective abortion.

Subsequent to intra-amniotic injection of hypertonic saline, prostaglandins, urea, etc, for midtrimester elective abortion, the injection-to-abortion time may be shortened by infusion of Pitocin at the rate of 10 to 20 milliunits (20 to 40 drops) per minute. The total dose should not exceed 30 units in a 12-hour period due to the risk of water intoxication.

HOW SUPPLIED

Pitocin (Oxytocin Injection, USP) Synthetic is available as follows:

N 0071-4160-02 Packages of ten 0.5-mL ampoules, each containing 5 units of oxytocin.

N 0071-4160-03 Packages of ten 1-mL ampoules, each containing 10 units of oxytocin.

N 0071-4160-10 A 10-mL multiple-dose Steri-Vial® containing 10 units of oxytocin per mL (total = 100 units of oxytocin).

N 0071-4160-40 Packages of ten sterile disposable 1-mL syringes, each containing 10 units of oxytocin.

N 0071-4160-45 Packages of twenty-five oversized 1-mL Steri-Vials®, each containing 10 units of oxytocin.

STORAGE

Store between 59° and 77°F (15° and 25°C. Protect from freezing.

REFERENCES

1. Seitchik J. Castillo M: Oxytocin augmentation of dysfunctional labor. I. Clinical data. *Am J Obstet Gynecol* 1982; 144:899–905.
2. Seitchik J. Castillo M: Oxytocin augmentation of dysfunctional labor. II. Multiparous patients. *Am J Obstet Gynecol* 1983; 145:777–780.
3. Fuchs A, Goeschen K, Husslein P, et al: Oxytocin and the initiation of human parturition. III. Plasma concentrations of oxytocin and 13, 14-dihydro-15-keto-prostaglandin $F_{2\alpha}$ in spontaneous and oxytocin-induced labor at term. *Am J Obstet Gynecol* 1983; 145:497–502.
4. Seitchik J, Amico J, et al: Oxytocin augmentation of dysfunctional labor. IV. Oxytocin Pharmacokinetics. *Am J Obstet Gynecol.* 1984; 150:225–228.
5. American College of Obstetricians and Gynecologists: ACOG Technical Bulletin Number 110, November 1987: Induction and augmentation of labor.

Caution—Federal law prohibits dispensing without prescription.

4160G334

PITRESSIN® ℞

[pĭ″trĕ′ssĭn]

(vasopressin injection, USP)

synthetic

DESCRIPTION

Pitressin (Vasopressin Injection, USP) Synthetic is a sterile, aqueous solution of synthetic vasopressin (8-Arginine vasopressin) of the posterior pituitary gland. It is substantially free from the oxytocic principle and is standardized to contain 20 pressor units/ml. The solution contains 0.5% Chloretone (chlorobutanol) (chloroform derivative) as a preservative. The acidity of the solution is adjusted with acetic acid.

CLINICAL PHARMACOLOGY

The antidiuretic action of vasopressin is ascribed to increasing reabsorption of water by the renal tubules.

Vasopressin can cause contraction of smooth muscle of the gastrointestinal tract and of all parts of the vascular bed, especially the capillaries, small arterioles and venules with less effect on the smooth musculature of the large veins. The direct effect on the contractile elements is neither antagonized by adrenergic blocking agents nor prevented by vascular denervation.

Following subcutaneous or intramuscular administration of vasopressin injection, the duration of antidiuretic activity is variable but effects are usually maintained for 2–8 hours.

The majority of a dose of vasopressin is metabolized and rapidly destroyed in the liver and kidneys. Vasopressin has a plasma half-life of about 10 to 20 minutes. Approximately 5% of a subcutaneous dose of vasopressin is excreted in urine unchanged after four hours.

CONTRAINDICATION

Anaphylaxis or hypersensitivity to the drug or its components.

INDICATIONS AND USAGE

Pitressin is indicated for prevention and treatment of postoperative abdominal distention, in abdominal roentgenography to dispel interfering gas shadows, and in diabetes insipidus.

WARNINGS

This drug should not be used in patients with vascular disease, especially disease of the coronary arteries, except with extreme caution. In such patients, even small doses may precipitate anginal pain, and with larger doses, the possibility of myocardial infarction should be considered.

Vasopressin may produce water intoxication. The early signs of drowsiness, listlessness, and headaches should be recognized to prevent terminal coma and convulsions.

PRECAUTIONS

General:

Vasopressin should be used cautiously in the presence of epilepsy, migraine, asthma, heart failure or any state in which a rapid addition to extracellular water may produce hazard for an already overburdened system.

Chronic nephritis with nitrogen retention contraindicates the use of vasopressin until reasonable nitrogen blood levels have been attained.

Information for Patients: Side effects such as blanching of skin, abdominal cramps, and nausea may be reduced by taking 1 or 2 glasses of water at the time of vasopressin administration. These side effects are usually not serious and probably will disappear within a few minutes.

Laboratory Tests: Electrocardiograms (ECG) and fluid and electrolyte status determinations are recommended at periodic intervals during therapy.

Drug Interactions: 1) The following drugs may potentiate the antidiuretic effect of vasopressin when used concurrently: carbamazepine; chlorpropamide; clofibrate; urea; fludrocortisone; tricyclic antidepressants. 2) The following drugs may decrease the antidiuretic effect of vasopressin when used concurrently: demeclocycline; norepinephrine; lithium; heparin; alcohol. 3) Ganglionic blocking agents may produce a marked increase in sensitivity to the pressor effects of vasopressin.

Pregnancy Category C: Animal reproduction studies have not been conducted with Pitressin. It is also not known whether Pitressin can cause fetal harm when administered to a pregnant woman or can affect reproduction capacity. Pitressin should be given to a pregnant woman only if clearly needed.

Labor and Delivery: Doses of vasopressin sufficient for an antidiuretic effect are not likely to produce tonic uterine contractions that could be deleterious to the fetus or threaten the continuation of the pregnancy.

Nursing Mothers: Caution should be exercised when Pitressin is administered to a nursing woman.

ADVERSE REACTIONS

Local or systemic allergic reactions may occur in hypersensitive individuals. The following side effects have been reported following the administration of vasopressin:

Body as a Whole: anaphylaxis (cardiac arrest and/or shock) have been observed shortly after injection of vasopressin.

Cardiovascular: cardiac arrest, circumoral pallor, arrhythmias, decreased cardiac output, angina, myocardial ischemia, peripheral vasoconstriction and gangrene.

Gastrointestinal: abdominal cramps, nausea, vomiting, passage of gas.

Nervous System: tremor, vertigo, "pounding" in head.

Respiratory: bronchial constriction.

Skin and Appendages: sweating, urticaria, cutaneous gangrene.

Overdosage:

Water intoxication may be treated with water restriction and temporary withdrawal of vasopressin until polyuria occurs. Severe water intoxication may require osmotic diuresis with mannitol, hypertonic dextrose, or urea alone or with furosemide.

DOSAGE AND ADMINISTRATION

Pitressin may be administered subcutaneously or intramuscularly.

Ten units of Pitressin (0.5 mL) will usually elicit full physiologic response in adult patients; 5 units will be adequate in many cases. Pitressin should be given intramuscularly at three- or four-hour intervals as needed. The dosage should be proportionately reduced for children. (For an additional discussion of dosage, consult the sections below.)

When determining the dose of Pitressin for a given case, the following should be kept in mind:

It is particularly desirable to give a dose not much larger than is just sufficient to elicit the desired physiologic response. Excessive doses may cause undesirable side effects—blanching of the skin, abdominal cramps, nausea—which, though not serious, may be alarming to the patient. Spontaneous recovery from such side effects occurs in a few minutes. It has been found that one or two glasses of water given at the time Pitressin is administered reduce such symptoms.

Abdominal Distention: In the average postoperative adult patient, give 5 units (0.25 mL) initially, increase to 10 units (0.5 mL) at subsequent injections if necessary. It is recommended that Pitressin be given intramuscularly and that injections be repeated at three- or four-hour intervals as required. Dosage to be reduced proportionately for children. Pitressin used in this manner will frequently prevent or relieve postoperative distention. These recommendations apply also to distention complicating pneumonia or other acute toxemias.

Abdominal Roentgenography: For the average case two injections of 10 units each (0.5 mL) are suggested. These should be given two hours and one-half hour, respectively, before films are exposed. Many roentgenologists advise giving an enema prior to the first dose of Pitressin.

Diabetes Insipidus: Pitressin may be given by injection or administered intranasally on cotton pledgets, by nasal spray, or by dropper. The dose by injection is 5 to 10 units (0.25 to 0.5 mL) repeated two or three times daily as needed. When Pitressin is administered intranasally by spray or on pledgets, the dosage and interval between treatments must be determined for each patient.

HOW SUPPLIED

Pitressin (Vasopressin Injection, USP) Synthetic is supplied in ampoules and vials as follows:

N 0071-4200-02
0.5 mL ampoule (10 pressor units). Packages of 10 ampoules.
N 0071-4200-03
1 mL ampoule (20 pressor units). Packages of 10 ampoules.
N 0071-4200-45
0.5 mL vial (10 pressor units). Packages of 25 Steri-Vials®
N 0071-4200-46
1 mL vial (20 pressor units). Packages of 25 Steri-Vials®

STORAGE

Store between 15° AND 25°C (59° AND 77°F).

Caution—Federal law prohibits dispensing without a prescription.

4200G143

PONSTEL® ℞
[pŏn 'stĕl"]
(mefenamic acid)

DESCRIPTION

Ponstel (mefenamic acid) is N-(2,3-xylyl)-anthranilic acid. It is an analgesic agent for oral administration. Ponstel is available in capsules containing 250 mg of mefenamic acid. Each capsule also contains lactose, NF. The capsule shell and/or band contains citric acid, USP; D&C yellow No. 10; FD&C blue No. 1; FD&C red No. 3; FD&C yellow No. 6; gelatin, NF; glycerol monooleate; silicon dioxide, NF; sodium benzoate, NF; sodium lauryl sulfate, NF; titanium dioxide, USP.

It is a white powder with a melting point of 230–231° C, molecular weight 241.28, and water solubility of 0.004% at pH 7.1.

CLINICAL PHARMACOLOGY

Ponstel is a nonsteroidal agent with demonstrated antiinflammatory, analgesic, and antipyretic activity in laboratory animals.[1,2] The mode of action is not known. In animal studies, Ponstel was found to inhibit prostaglandin synthesis and to compete for binding at the prostaglandin receptor site.[3]

Pharmacologic studies show Ponstel did not relieve morphine abstinence signs in abstinent, morphine-habituated monkeys.[1]

Following a single 1-gram oral dose, peak plasma levels of 10 μg/ml occurred in 2 to 4 hours with a half-life of 2 hours. Following multiple doses, plasma levels are proportional to dose with no evidence of drug accumulation. One gram of Ponstel given four times daily produces peak blood levels of 20 μg/ml by the second day of administration.[4]

Following a single dose, sixty-seven percent of the total dose is excreted in the urine as unchanged drug or as one of two metabolites. Twenty to twenty-five percent of the dose is excreted in the feces during the first three days.[4]

In controlled, double-blind, clinical trials, Ponstel was evaluated for the treatment of primary spasmodic dysmenorrhea. The parameters used in determining efficacy included pain assessment by both patient and investigator; the need for concurrent analgesic medication; and evaluation of change in frequency and severity of symptoms characteristic of spasmodic dysmenorrhea. Patients received either Ponstel, 500 mg (2 capsules) as an initial dose and 250 mg every 6 hours, or placebo at onset of bleeding or of pain, whichever began first. After three menstrual cycles, patients were crossed over to the alternate treatment for an additional three cycles. Ponstel was significantly superior to placebo in all parameters, and both treatments (drug and placebo) were equally tolerated.

INDICATIONS AND USAGE

Ponstel is indicated for the relief of moderate pain[5] when therapy will not exceed one week. Ponstel is also indicated for the treatment of primary dysmenorrhea.[5,6]

Studies in children under 14 years of age have been inadequate to evaluate the safety and effectiveness of Ponstel.

CONTRAINDICATIONS

Ponstel should not be used in patients who have previously exhibited hypersensitivity to it.

Because the potential exists for cross-sensitivity to aspirin or other nonsteroidal antiinflammatory drugs, Ponstel should not be given to patients in whom these drugs induce symptoms of bronchospasm, allergic rhinitis, or urticaria.

Ponstel is contraindicated in patients with active ulceration or chronic inflammation of either the upper or lower gastrointestinal tract.

Ponstel should be avoided in patients with preexisting renal disease.

WARNINGS

If diarrhea occurs, the dosage should be reduced or temporarily suspended (see Adverse Reactions and Dosage and Administration). Certain patients who develop diarrhea may be unable to tolerate the drug because of recurrence of the symptoms on subsequent exposure.

Risk of GI Ulceration, Bleeding and Perforation with NSAID Therapy: Serious gastrointestinal toxicity such as bleeding, ulceration, and perforation, can occur at any time, with or without warning symptoms, in patients treated chronically with NSAID therapy. Although minor upper gastrointestinal problems, such as dyspepsia, are common, usually developing early in therapy, physicians should remain alert for ulceration and bleeding in patients treated chronically with NSAIDs even in the absence of previous GI tract symptoms. In patients observed in clinical trials of several months to two years duration, symptomatic upper GI ulcers, gross bleeding or perforation appear to occur in approximately 1% of patients treated for 3–6 months, and in about 2–4% of patients treated for one year. Physicians should inform patients about the signs and/or symptoms of serious GI toxicity and what steps to take if they occur.

Studies to date have not identified any subset of patients not at risk of developing peptic ulceration and bleeding. Except for a prior history of serious GI events and other risk factors known to be associated with peptic ulcer disease, such as alcoholism, smoking, etc., no risk factors (eg, age, sex) have been associated with increased risk. Elderly or debilitated patients seem to tolerate ulceration or bleeding less well than other individuals and most spontaneous reports of fatal GI events are in this population. Studies to date are inconclusive concerning the relative risk of various NSAIDs in causing such reactions. High doses of any NSAID probably carry a greater risk of these reactions, although controlled clinical trials showing this do not exist in most cases. In considering the use of relatively large doses (within the recommended dosage range), sufficient benefit should be anticipated to offset the potential increased risk of GI toxicity.

PRECAUTIONS

If rash occurs, administration of the drug should be stopped.

A false-positive reaction for urinary bile, using the diazo tablet test, may result after mefenamic acid administration. If biliuria is suspected, other diagnostic procedures, such as the Harrison spot test, should be performed.

Renal Effects: As with other nonsteroidal antiinflammatory drugs, long-term administration of mefenamic acid to animals has resulted in renal papillary necrosis and other abnormal renal pathology. In humans, there have been reports of acute interstitial nephritis with hematuria, proteinuria and occasionally nephrotic syndrome.

A second form of renal toxicity has been seen in patients with prerenal conditions leading to a reduction in renal blood flow or blood volume, where the renal prostaglandins have a supportive role in the maintenance of renal perfusion. In these patients administration of an NSAID may cause a dose-dependent reduction in prostaglandin formation and may precipitate overt renal decompensation. Patients at greatest risk of this reaction are those with impaired renal function, heart failure, liver dysfunction, those taking diuretics, and the elderly Discontinuation of NSAID therapy is typically followed by recovery to the pretreatment state.

Since Ponstel is eliminated primarily by the kidneys, the drug should not be administered to patients with significantly impaired renal functions.

As with other nonsteroidal antiinflammatory drugs, borderline elevations of one or more liver tests may occur in some patients. These abnormalities may progress, may remain essentially unchanged, or may be transient with continued therapy. The SGPT (ALT) test is probably the most sensitive indicator of liver dysfunction. Meaningful (3 times the upper limit of normal) elevations of SGPT or SGOT (AST) occurred in controlled clinical trials in less than 1% of patients. A patient with symptoms and/or signs suggesting liver dysfunction, or in whom an abnormal liver test has occurred, should be evaluated for evidence of the development of more severe hepatic reaction while on therapy with Ponstel. Severe hepatic reactions, including jaundice and cases of fatal hepatitis, have been reported with other nonsteroidal antiinflammatory drugs. Although such reactions are rare, if abnormal liver tests persist or worsen, if clinical signs and symptoms consistent with liver disease develop, or if systemic manifestations occur (eg eosinophilia, rash, etc), Ponstel should be discontinued.

Information for Patients: Patients should be advised that if rash, diarrhea or other digestive problems arise, they should stop the drug and consult their physician.

Patients in whom aspirin or other nonsteroidal antiinflammatory drugs induce symptoms of bronchospasm, allergic rhinitis, or urticaria should be made aware that the potential exists for cross-sensitivity to Ponstel.

The long-term effects, if any, of intermittent Ponstel therapy for dysmenorrhea are not known. Women on such therapy should consult their physician if they should decide to become pregnant.

Ponstel, like other drugs of its class, is not free of side effects. The side effects of these drugs can cause discomfort and, rarely, there are more serious side effects, such as gastrointestinal bleeding, which may result in hospitalization and even fatal outcomes.

NSAIDs (nonsteroidal antiinflammatory drugs) are often essential agents in the management of arthritis and have a

Continued on next page

This product information was prepared in August 1992. On these and other Parke-Davis Products, information may be obtained by addressing PARKE-DAVIS, Division of Warner-Lambert Company, Morris Plains, New Jersey 07950.

Parke-Davis—Cont.

major role in the treatment of pain, but they also may be commonly employed for conditions which are less serious. Physicians may wish to discuss with their patients the potential risks (see WARNINGS, PRECAUTIONS, and ADVERSE REACTIONS sections) and likely benefits of NSAID treatment, particularly when the drugs are used for less serious conditions where treatment without NSAIDs may represent an acceptable alternative to both the patient and physician.

Laboratory Tests: Because serious GI tract ulceration and bleeding can occur without warning symptoms, physicians should follow chronically treated patients for the signs and symptoms of ulceration and bleeding and should inform them of the importance of this follow-up (see Risk of GI Ulcerations, Bleeding and Perforation with NSAID Therapy).

Drug Interactions: Ponstel may prolong prothrombin time.[5] Therefore, when the drug is administered to patients receiving oral anticoagulant drugs, frequent monitoring of prothrombin time is necessary.

Use in Pregnancy: Pregnancy Category C. Reproduction studies have been performed in rats, rabbits and dogs. Rats given up to 10 times the human dose showed decreased fertility, delay in parturition, and a decreased rate of survival to weaning. Rabbits at 2.5 times the human dose showed an increase in the number of resorptions. There were no fetal anomalies observed in these studies nor in dogs at up to 10 times the human dose.[5]

There are no adequate and well-controlled studies in pregnant women. Because animal reproduction studies are not always predictive of human response, this drug should be used only if clearly needed.

The use of Ponstel in late pregnancy is not recommended because of the effects on the fetal cardiovascular system of drugs of this class.

Nursing Mothers: Trace amounts of Ponstel may be present in breast milk and transmitted to the nursing infant[7]; thus Ponstel should not be taken by the nursing mother because of the effects on the infant cardiovascular system of drugs of this class.

Use in Children: Safety and effectiveness in children below the age of 14 have not been established.

ADVERSE REACTIONS

Gastrointestinal: The most frequently reported adverse reactions associated with the use of Ponstel involve the gastrointestinal tract. In controlled studies for up to eight months, the following disturbances were reported in decreasing order of frequency: diarrhea (approximately 5% of patients), nausea with or without vomiting, other gastrointestinal symptoms, and abdominal pain.

In certain patients, the diarrhea was of sufficient severity to require discontinuation of medication. The occurrence of the diarrhea is usually dose related, generally subsides on reduction of dosage, and rapidly disappears on termination of therapy.

Other gastrointestinal reactions less frequently reported were anorexia, pyrosis, flatulence, and constipation. Gastrointestinal ulceration with and without hemorrhage has been reported.

Hematopoietic: Cases of autoimmune hemolytic anemia have been associated with the continuous administration of Ponstel for 12 months or longer. In such cases the Coombs test results are positive with evidence of both accelerated RBC production and RBC destruction. The process is reversible upon termination of Ponstel administration.

Decreases in hematocrit have been noted in 2–5% of patients and primarily in those who have received prolonged therapy. Leukopenia, eosinophilia, thrombocytopenic purpura, agranulocytosis, pancytopenia, and bone marrow hypoplasia have also been reported on occasion.

Nervous System: Drowsiness, dizziness, nervousness, headache, blurred vision, and insomnia have occurred.

Integumentary: Urticaria, rash, and facial edema have been reported.

Renal: As with other nonsteroidal antiinflammatory agents, renal failure, including papillary necrosis, has been reported. In elderly patients renal failure has occurred after taking Ponstel for 2–6 weeks. The renal damage may not be completely reversible. Hematuria and dysuria have also been reported with Ponstel.

Other: Eye irritation, ear pain, perspiration, mild hepatic toxicity, and increased need for insulin in a diabetic have been reported. There have been rare reports of palpitation, dyspnea, and reversible loss of color vision.

OVERDOSAGE

Although doses up to 6000 mg/day have been given, no specific information is available on the management of acute massive overdosage.

Should accidental overdosage occur, the stomach should be emptied by inducing emesis or by careful gastric lavage followed by the administration of activated charcoal.[8] Laboratory studies indicate that Ponstel should be adsorbed from the gastrointestinal tract by activated charcoal.[4] Vital func-

tions should be monitored and supported. Because mefenamic acid and its metabolites are firmly bound to plasma proteins, hemodialysis and peritoneal dialysis may be of little value.[4]

DOSAGE AND ADMINISTRATION

Administration is by the oral route, preferably with food. The recommended regimen in acute pain for adults and children over 14 years of age is 500 mg as an initial dose followed by 250 mg every six hours as needed, usually not to exceed one week.[5]

For the treatment of primary dysmenorrhea, the recommended dosage is 500 mg as an initial dose followed by 250 mg every 6 hours, starting with the onset of bleeding and associated symptoms. Clinical studies indicate that effective treatment can be initiated with the start of menses and should not be necessary for more than 2 to 3 days.[6]

HOW SUPPLIED

N 0071-0540-24 (P-D 540) Ponstel (mefenamic acid) is available as 250 mg capsules in bottles of 100.

REFERENCES

1. Winder CV, et al: Antiinflammatory, antipyretic and antinociceptive properties of N-(2,3-xylyl) anthranilic acid (mefenamic acid). *J Pharmacol Exp Ther* 138: 405–413, 1962.
2. Wax J, et al: Comparative activities, tolerances and safety of nonsteroidal antiinflammatory agents in rats. *J Pharmacol Exp Ther* 192: 172–178, 1975.
3. Ferreira SH, Vane JR: Aspirin and prostaglandins, in *The Prostaglandins*, Ramwell PW Ed, Plenum Press, NY, vol. 2, 1974, pp 1–47.
4. Glazko AJ: Experimental observations of flufenamic, mefenamic, and meclofenamic acids. Part III. Metabolic disposition, in *Fenamates in Medicine.* A Symposium, London 1966; *Annals of Physical Medicine,* supplement, pp 23–36, 1967.
5. Data on file, Medical Affairs Dept, Parke-Davis.
6. Budoff PW: Use of mefenamic acid in the treatment of primary dysmenorrhea. *JAMA* 241: 2713–2716, 1979.
7. Buchanan RA, et al: The breast milk excretion of mefenamic acid. *Curr Ther Res* 10:592, 1968.
8. Corby DG, Decker WJ: Management of acute poisoning with activated charcoal. *Pediatrics* 54:324, 1974.

                 0540G150

Caution—Federal law prohibits dispensing without prescription.

Shown in Product Identification Section, page 423

PROCAN® SR   **℞**
[prō'căn″]
(procainamide hydrochloride extended-release tablets, USP)
SUSTAINED RELEASE

> **WARNING**
>
> Positive ANA Titer: The prolonged administration of procainamide often leads to the development of a positive antinuclear antibody (ANA) test, with or without symptoms of a lupus erythematosus-like syndrome. If a positive ANA titer develops, the benefits versus risks of continued procainamide therapy should be assessed.

DESCRIPTION

Procan SR (procainamide hydrochloride), a Group 1A cardiac antiarrhythmic drug, is p-amino-N(2-(diethylamino)ethyl)-benzamide monohydrochloride, molecular weight 271.79.

Procainamide hydrochloride differs from procaine which is the p-aminobenzoyl ester of 2-(diethylamino)-ethanol. Procainamide as the free base has a pk_a of 9.23; the monohydrochloride is very soluble in water.

Procan SR (Procainamide Hydrochloride Extended-release Tablets, USP) Sustained Release is available for oral administration as green, film-coated tablets containing 250 mg procainamide hydrochloride; as yellow, scored, film-coated tablets containing 500 mg procainamide hydrochloride; as orange, scored, film-coated tablets containing 750 mg procainamide hydrochloride; and as red, scored, film-coated tablets containing 1000 mg procainamide hydrochloride.

All strengths of Procan SR contain candelilla wax, FCC; colloidal silicon dioxide, NF; magnesium stearate, NF; titanium dioxide; vanillin, NF; and other ingredients. The individual strengths contain additional ingredients as follows:
250 mg: D&C yellow No. 10 Al lake; FD&C blue No. 1 Al lake; FD&C yellow No. 6 Al lake; lactose, NF; may also contain methylparaben, NF; and propylparaben, NF; or simethicone emulsion and polysorbate 80, NF.
500 mg: D&C yellow No. 10 Al lake; FD&C blue No. 2 Al lake; FD&C yellow No. 6 Al lake; sucrose, NF; may also contain methylparaben, NF; and propylparaben, NF; or simethicone emulsion and polysorbate 80, NF.

750 mg: FD&C yellow No. 6 Al lake; may also contain propylene glycol, USP; or simethicone emulsion and polysorbate 80, NF.
1000 mg: FD&C red No. 3 Al lake; FD&C yellow No. 6 Al lake; propylene glycol, USP.

CLINICAL PHARMACOLOGY

Procainamide (PA) increases the effective refractory period of the atria, and to a lesser extent the bundle of His-Purkinje system and ventricles of the heart. It reduces impulse conduction velocity in the atria, His-Purkinje fibers, and ventricular muscle, but has variable effects on the atrioventricular (A-V) node, a direct slowing action and a weaker vagolytic effect which may speed A-V conduction slightly. Myocardial excitability is reduced in the atria, Purkinje fibers, papillary muscles, and ventricles by an increase in the threshold for excitation, combined with inhibition of ectopic pacemaker activity by retardation of the slow phase of diastolic depolarization, thus decreasing automaticity especially in ectopic sites. Contractility of the undamaged heart is usually not affected by therapeutic concentrations, although slight reduction of cardiac output may occur, and may be significant in the presence of myocardial damage. Therapeutic levels of PA may exert vagolytic effects and produce slight acceleration of heart rate, while high or toxic concentrations may prolong A-V conduction time or induce A-V block, or even cause abnormal automaticity and spontaneous firing, by unknown mechanisms.

Procainamide Hydrochloride Extended-release Tablets, USP, are designed to provide the biopharmaceutic characteristics of a sustained and relatively constant rate of release and absorption, independent of dose, primarily from the small intestine.

The electrocardiogram may reflect these effects by showing slight sinus tachycardia (due to the anticholinergic action) and widened QRS complexes and, less regularly, prolonged Q-T and P-R intervals (due to longer systole and slower conduction), as well as some decrease in QRS and T wave amplitude. These direct effects of PA on electrical activity, conduction, responsiveness, excitability and automaticity are characteristic of a Group 1A antiarrhythmic agent, the prototype for which is quinidine; PA effects are very similar. However, PA has weaker vagal blocking action than does quinidine, does not induce alpha-adrenergic blockade, and is less depressing to cardiac contractility.

Ingested PA is resistant to digestive hydrolysis, and the drug is well absorbed from the entire small intestinal surface, but individual patients vary in their completeness of absorption of PA. Following oral administration every six hours procainamide hydrochloride sustained-release tablets achieve a mean steady state of procainamide (as well as procainamide N-acetylprocainamide) serum concentrations approximately equivalent to those from a comparable dose of an immediate-release dosage form given every three hours. Procainamide hydrochloride sustained-release tablets have a half-life which is significantly longer than that of procainamide immediate-release dosage forms. About 15 to 20 percent of PA is reversibly bound to plasma proteins, and considerable amounts are more slowly and reversibly bound to tissues of the heart, liver, lung, and kidney. The apparent volume of distribution eventually reaches about 2 liters per kilogram body weight with a half-time of approximately five minutes. While PA has been shown in the dog to cross the blood-brain barrier, it did not concentrate in the brain at levels higher than in plasma. It is not known if PA crosses the placenta. Plasma esterases are far less active in hydrolysis of PA than of procaine. The half-time for elimination is three to four hours in patients with normal renal function, but reduced creatinine clearance and advancing age each prolong the half-time of elimination of PA.

A significant fraction of the circulating PA may be metabolized in hepatocytes of N-acetylprocainamide (NAPA), ranging from 16 to 21 percent of an administered dose in "slow acetylators" to 24 to 33 percent in "fast acetylators." Since NAPA also has significant antiarrhythmic activity and somewhat slower renal clearance than PA, both hepatic acetylation rate capability and renal function, as well as age, have significant effects on the effective biologic half-time of therapeutic action of administered PA and the NAPA derivative. Trace amounts may be excreted in the urine as free and conjugated p-aminobenzoic acid, 30 to 60 percent as unchanged PA, and 6 to 52 percent as the NAPA derivative. Both PA and NAPA are eliminated by active tubular secretion as well as by glomerular filtration. Action of PA on the central nervous system is not prominent, but high plasma concentrations may cause tremors. While therapeutic plasma levels for PA have been reported to be 3 to 10 μg/mL certain patients such as those with sustained ventricular tachycardia, may need higher levels for adequate control. This may justify the increased risk of toxicity (see OVERDOSAGE). Where programmed ventricular stimulation has been used to evaluate efficacy of PA in preventing recurrent ventricular tachyarrhythmias, higher plasma levels (mean, 13.6 μg/mL) of PA were found necessary for adequate control.

INDICATIONS AND USAGE

Procan SR tablets are indicated for the treatment of documented ventricular arrhythmias, such as sustained ventricular tachycardia, that, in the judgment of the physician, are life-threatening. Because of the proarrhythmic effects of procainamide, its use with lesser arrhythmias is generally not recommended. Treatment of patients with asymptomatic ventricular premature contractions should be avoided.

Initiation of procainamide treatment, as with other antiarrhythmic agents used to treat life-threatening arrhythmias, should be carried out in the hospital.

Antiarrhythmic drugs have not been shown to enhance survival in patients with ventricular arrhythmias.

Because procainamide has the potential to produce serious hematological disorders (0.5 percent) particularly leukopenia or agranulocytosis (sometimes fatal), its use should be reserved for patients in whom, in the opinion of the physician, the benefits of treatment clearly outweight the risks. (See WARNINGS,and Boxed Warning.)

CONTRAINDICATIONS

Complete heart block: Procainamide should not be administered to patients with complete heart block because of its effects in suppressing nodal or ventricular pacemakers and the hazard of asystole. It may be difficult to recognize complete heart block in patients with ventricular tachycardia, but if significant slowing of ventricular rate occurs during PA treatment without evidence of A-V conduction appearing; PA should be stopped. In cases of second degree A-V block or various types of hemiblock, PA should be avoided or discontinued because of the possibility of increased severity of block, unless the ventricular rate is controlled by an electrical pacemaker.

Idiosyncratic hypersensitivity: In patients sensitive to procaine or other ester-type local anesthetics, cross sensitivity to PA is unlikely; however, it should be borne in mind, and PA should not be used if it produces acute allergic dermatitis, asthma, or anaphylactic symptoms.

Lupus Erythematosus: An established diagnosis of systemic lupus erythematosus is a contraindication to PA therapy, since aggravation of symptoms is highly likely.

Torsades de Pointes: In the unusual ventricular arrhythmia called "les torsades de pointes" (twisting of the points), characterized by alternation of one or more ventricular premature beats in the directions of the QRS complexes on ECG in persons with prolonged Q-T and often enhanced U waves, Group 1A antiarrhythmic drugs are contraindicated. Administration of PA in such cases may aggravate this special type of ventricular extrasystole or tachycardia instead of suppressing it.

WARNINGS

Mortality: In the National Heart, Lung and Blood Institute's Cardiac Arrhythmia Suppression Trial (CAST), a long-term, multi-centered, randomized, double-blind study in patients with asymptomatic non-life-threatening ventricular arrhythmias who had had myocardial infarctions more than six days but less than two years previously, an excessive mortality or non-fatal cardiac arrest rate was seen in patients treated with encainide or flecainide (56/730) compared with that seen in patients assigned to matched, placebo-treated groups (22/725). The average duration of treatment with encainide or flecainide in this study was ten months.

The applicability of these results to other populations (e.g., those without recent myocardial infarctions) or to other antiarrhythmic drugs is uncertain, but at present it is prudent to consider any antiarrhythmic agent to have a significant risk in patients with structural heart disease.

Blood Dyscrasias: Agranulocytosis, bone marrow depression, neutropenia, hypoplastic anemia and thrombocytopenia have been reported in patients receiving procainamide hydrochloride. Most of these patients received procainamide hydrochloride within the recommended dosage range. Fatalities have occurred (with approximately 20-25 percent mortality in reported cases of agranulocytosis). Since most of these events have been noted during the first 12 weeks of therapy, it is recommended that complete blood counts including white cell, differential and platelet counts be performed at weekly intervals for the first three months of therapy; and periodically thereafter. Complete blood counts should be performed promptly if the patient develops any signs of infection (such as fever, chills, sore throat, or stomatitis), bruising, or bleeding. If any of these hematologic disorders are identified, procainamide hydrochloride should be discontinued. Blood counts usually return to normal within one month of discontinuation. Caution should be used in patients with preexisting marrow failure or cytopenia of any type (see ADVERSE REACTIONS).

Digitalis Intoxication: Caution should be exercised in the use of procainamide in arrhythmias associated with digitalis intoxication. Procainamide can suppress digitalis-induced arrhythmias; however, if there is concomitant marked disturbance of atrioventricular conduction, additional depression of conduction and ventricular asystole or fibrillation may result. Therefore, use of procainamide should be considered only if discontinuation of digitalis, and therapy with potassium, lidocaine, or phenytoin are ineffective.

First Degree Heart Block: Caution should be exercised also if the patient exhibits or develops first degree heart block while taking PA, and dosage reduction is advised in such cases. If the block persists despite dosage reduction, continuation of PA administration must be evaluated on the basis of current benefit versus risk of increased heart block.

Predigitalization for Atrial Flutter or Fibrillation: Patients with atrial flutter or fibrillation should be cardioverted or digitalized prior to PA administration to avoid enhancement of A-V conduction which may result in ventricular rate acceleration beyond tolerable limits. Adequate digitalization reduces but does not eliminate the possibility of sudden increase in ventricular rate as the atrial rate is slowed by PA in these arrhythmias.

Congestive Heart Failure: For patients in congestive heart failure, and those with acute ischemic heart disease or cardiomyopathy, caution should be used in PA therapy, since even slight depression of myocardial contractility may further reduce the cardiac output of the damaged heart.

Concurrent Other Antiarrhythmic Agents: Concurrent use of PA with other Group 1A antiarrhythmic agents such as quinidine or disopyramide may produce enhanced prolongation of conduction or depression of contractility and hypotension, especially in patients with cardiac decompensation. Such use should be reserved for patients with serious arrhythmias unresponsive to a single drug and employed only if close observation is possible.

Renal Insufficiency: Renal insufficiency may lead to accumulation of high plasma levels from conventional oral doses of PA, with effects similar to those of overdosage (see OVERDOSAGE), unless dosage is adjusted for the individual patient.

Myasthenia Gravis: Patients with myasthenia gravis may show worsening of symptoms from PA due to its procaine-like effect on diminishing acetylcholine release at skeletal muscle motor nerve endings, so that PA administration may be hazardous without optimal adjustment of anticholinesterase medications or other precautions.

PRECAUTIONS

General: Immediately after initiation of PA therapy, patients should be closely observed for possible hypersensitivity reactions, especially if procaine or local anesthetic sensitivity is suspected, and for muscular weakness if myasthenia gravis is a possibility.

In conversion of arterial fibrillation to normal sinus rhythm by any means, dislodgment of mural thrombi may lead to embolization, which should be kept in mind.

After approximately two days, steady state plasma PA levels are produced following regular oral administration of a given dose of Procan SR tablets at set intervals. After achieving and maintaining therapeutic plasma concentrations and satisfactory electrocardiographic and clinical responses, continued frequent periodic monitoring of vital signs and electrocardiograms is advised. If evidence of QRS widening of more than 25 percent or marked prolongation of the Q-T interval occurs, concern for overdosage is appropriate, and reduction in dosage is advisable if a 50 percent increase occurs. Elevated serum creatinine or urea nitrogen, reduced creatinine clearance, or history of renal insufficiency, as well as use in older patients (over age 50), provide grounds to anticipate that less than the usual dosage and longer time intervals between doses may suffice, since the urinary elimination of PA and NAPA may be reduced, leading to gradual accumulation beyond normally predicted amounts. If facilities are available for measurement of plasma PA and NAPA, or acetylation capability, individual dose adjustment for optimal therapeutic levels may be easier, but close observation of clinical effectiveness is the most important criterion. In the longer term, period complete blood counts are useful to detect possible idiosyncratic hematologic effects of PA on neutrophil, platelet or red cell homeostasis; agranulocytosis has been reported to occur occasionally in patients on long-term PA therapy. A rising titer of serum ANA may precede clinical symptoms of the lupoid syndrome (see Boxed Warnings and ADVERSE REACTIONS). If the lupus erythematosus-like syndrome develops in a patient with recurrent life-threatening arrhythmias not controlled by other agents, corticosteroid suppressive therapy may be used concomitantly with PA. Since the PA-induced lupoid syndrome rarely includes the dangerous pathologic renal changes, PA therapy may not necessarily have to be stopped unless the symptoms of serositis and the possibility of further lupoid effects are of greater risk than the benefit of PA in controlling arrhythmias. Patients with rapid acetylation capability are less likely to develop the lupoid syndrome after prolonged PA therapy.

Information for Patients: The physician is advised to explain to the patient that the close cooperation in adhering to the prescribed dosage schedule is of great importance in controlling the cardiac arrhythmia safely. The patient should understand clearly that more medication is not necessarily better and may be dangerous, that skipping doses or increasing intervals between doses to suit personal convenience may lead to loss of control of the heart problem, and that "making up" missed doses by doubling up later may be hazardous.

The patient should be encouraged to disclose any past history of drug sensitivity, especially to procaine or other local anesthetic agents, or aspirin, and to report any history of kidney disease, congestive heart failure, myasthenia gravis, liver disease, or lupus erythematosus.

The patient should be counseled to report promptly any symptoms of arthralgia, myalgia, fever, chills, skin rash, easy bruising, sore throat or sore mouth, infections, dark urine or icterus, wheezing, muscular weakness, chest or abdominal pain, palpitations, nausea, vomiting, anorexia, diarrhea, hallucinations, dizziness, or depression.

The patient should be advised not to break or chew the tablet as this would interfere with designed dissolution characteristics. The tablet matrix of Procan SR may be seen in the stool since it does not disintegrate following release of procainamide.

Laboratory Tests: Laboratory tests such as complete blood count (CBC), electrocardiogram, and serum creatinine or urea nitrogen may be indicated, depending on the clinical situation, and periodic rechecking of the CBC and ANA may be helpful in early detection of untoward reactions.

Drug Interactions: If other antiarrhythmic drugs are being used, additive effects on the heart may occur with PA administration, and dosage reduction may be necessary (see WARNINGS).

Anticholinergic drugs administered concurrently with PA may produce additive antivagal effects on A-V nodal conduction, although this is not as well documented for PA as for quinidine.

Patients taking PA who require neuromuscular blocking agents such as succinylcholine may require less than usual doses of the latter, due to PA effects of reducing acetylcholine release.

Of 10,867 patients treated with mexiletine in a compassionate use program, six cases of agranulocytosis were reported. Five of the six cases involved patients who were concomitantly receiving PA.

Drug/Laboratory Test Interactions: Suprapharmacologic concentrations of lidocaine and meprobamate may inhibit fluorescence of PA and NAPA and propranolol shows a native fluorescence close to the PA/NAPA peak wavelengths, so that tests which depend on fluorescence measurement may be affected.

Carcinogenesis, Mutagenesis, Impairment of Fertility: Long term studies in animals have not been performed.

Teratogenic Effects: Pregnancy Category C: Animal reproduction studies have not been conducted with PA. It also is not known whether PA can cause fetal harm when administered to a pregnant woman or can affect reproduction capacity. PA should be given to a pregnant woman only if clearly needed.

Nursing Mothers: Both PA and NAPA are excreted in human milk, and absorbed by the nursing infant. Because of the potential for serious adverse reactions in nursing infants, a decision to discontinue nursing or the drug should be made, taking into account the importance of the drug to the mother.

Pediatric Use: Safety and effectiveness in children have not been established.

ADVERSE REACTIONS

Cardiovascular System: Hypotension following oral PA administration is rare. Hypotension and serious disturbances of cardiorhythm such as ventricular asystole or fibrillation are more common after intravenous administration (see OVERDOSAGE, WARNINGS). Second degree heart block has been reported in 2 of almost 500 patients taking PA orally.

Multisystem Effects: A lupus erythematosus-like syndrome of arthralgia, pleural or abdominal pain, and sometime arthritis, pleural effusion, pericarditis, fever, chills, myalgia, and possibly related hematologic or skin lesions (see below) is fairly common after prolonged PA administration, perhaps more often in patients who are slow acetylators (See Boxed Warnings and PRECAUTIONS). While some series have reported less than 1 in 500, others have reported the syndrome in up to 30 percent of long term oral PA therapy. If discontinuation of PA does not reverse the lupoid symptoms, corticosteroid treatment may be effective.

Continued on next page

This product information was prepared in August 1992. On these and other Parke-Davis Products, information may be obtained by addressing PARKE-DAVIS, Division of Warner-Lambert Company, Morris Plains, New Jersey 07950.

Hematologic System: Neutropenia, thrombocytopenia, or hemolytic anemia may rarely be encountered. Agranulocytosis has occurred after repeated use of PA, and deaths have been reported (see WARNINGS and Boxed Warnings).
Skin: Angioneurotic edema, urticaria, pruritus, flushing, and maculopapular rash have also occurred occasionally.
Gastrointestinal System: Anorexia, nausea, vomiting, abdominal pain, bitter taste, or diarrhea may occur in 3 to 4 percent of patients taking oral procainamide. Hepatomegaly with increased serum aminotransferase activity has been reported after a single oral dose.
Nervous System: Dizziness or giddiness, weakness, mental depression, and psychosis with hallucinations have been reported occasionally.

OVERDOSAGE

Progressive widening of the QRS complex, prolonged Q-T and P-R intervals, lowering of the R and T waves, as well as increasing A-V block, may be seen with doses which are excessive for a given patient, increased ventricular extrasystoles, or even ventricular tachycardia or fibrillation may occur. After intravenous administration but seldom after oral therapy, transient high plasma levels of PA may induce hypotension, affecting systolic more than diastolic pressures, especially in hypertensive patients. Such high levels may also produce central nervous depression, tremor, and even respiratory depression.

Plasma levels above 10 μg/mL are increasingly associated with toxic findings, which are seen occasionally in the 10 to 12 μg/mL range, more often in the 12 to 15 μg/mL range, and commonly in patients with plasma levels greater than 15 μg/mL. A single oral dose of 2 g may produce overdosage symptoms, while 3 g may be dangerous, especially if the patient is a slow acetylator, has decreased renal function, or underlying organic heart disease.

Treatment of overdosage or toxic manifestations includes general supportive measures, close observation, monitoring of vital signs and possibly intravenous pressor agents and mechanical cardiorespiratory support. If available, PA and NAPA plasma levels may be helpful in assessing the potential degree of toxicity and response to therapy. Both PA and NAPA are removed from the circulation by hemodialysis but not peritoneal dialysis. No specific antidote for PA is known.

DOSAGE AND ADMINISTRATION

The oral dose and interval of administration should be adjusted for the individual patient, based on clinical assessment of the degree of underlying myocardial disease, the patient's age, and renal function.

As a general guide, for younger patients with normal renal function, an initial total daily oral dose of up to 50 mg/kg of body weight of Procan SR Tablets may be used, given in divided doses, every six hours, to maintain therapeutic blood levels. For older patients, especially those over 50 years of age, or for patients with renal, hepatic or cardiac insufficiency, lesser amounts or longer intervals may produce adequate blood levels, and decrease the probability of occurrence of dose related adverse reactions.

To provide up to 50 mg per kg of body weight per day*	
Patients weighing	
88–110 (40–50 kg)	500 mg q6 hrs
132–154 (60–70 kg)	750 mg q6 hrs
176–198 (80–90 kg)	1 g q6 hrs
>220 lb (> 100 kg)	1.25 g q6 hrs

*Initial dosage schedule guide only, to be adjusted for each patient individually, based on age, cardiorenal function, blood level (if available), and clinical response.

HOW SUPPLIED

Procan SR 250 mg (elliptical, green, scored, film-coated, coded PD 202) is a sustained-release tablet that contains 250 mg of procainamide hydrochloride. It is supplied as follows:

N 0071-0202-24	Bottles of 100
N 0071-0202-30	Bottles of 500
N 0071-0202-40	Unit-dose packages of 100 (10 strips of 10 tablets each)

Procan SR 500 mg (elliptical, yellow, scored, film-coated, coded PD 204) is a sustained-release tablet that contains 500 mg of procainamide hydrochloride. It is supplied as follows:

N 0071-0204-24	Bottles of 100
N 0071-0204-30	Bottles of 500
N 0071-0204-40	Unit-dose packages of 100 (10 strips of 10 tablets each)

Procan SR 750 mg (elliptical, orange, scored, film-coated, coded PD 205) is a sustained-release tablet that contains 750 mg of procainamide hydrochloride. It is supplied as follows:

N 0071-0205-24	Bottles of 100
N 0071-0205-30	Bottles of 500
N 0071-0205-40	Unit-dose packages of 100 (10 strips of 10 tablets each)

Procan SR 1000 mg (elliptical, red, scored, film-coated, coded PD 207) is a sustained-release tablet that contains 1000 mg of procainamide hydrochloride. It is supplied as follows:

N 0071-0207-24	Bottle of 100
N 0071-0207-40	Unit-dose packages of 100 (10 strips of 10 tablets each)

0207G076

Shown in Product Identification Section, page 423

PYRIDIUM® ℞

[py″rĭ′dĭ-ŭm]

(Phenazopyridine Hydrochloride Tablets, USP)

DESCRIPTION

Pyridium (phenazopyridine hydrochloride) is chemically designated 2,6-Pyridinediamine, 3-(phenylazo), monohydrochloride. It is a urinary tract analgesic agent for oral administration. Pyridium tablets contain 100 mg or 200 mg phenazopyridine hydrochloride. Also contains carnauba wax, NF; corn starch, NF; D and C red No. 7; FD and C blue No. 2; FD and C yellow No. 6; gelatin, NF; lactose, NF; magnesium stearate, NF; methylcellulose, USP; sodium starch glycolate, NF; sucrose, NF; titanium dioxide, USP; white wax. NF.

CLINICAL PHARMACOLOGY

Pyridium is excreted in the urine where it exerts a topical analgesic effect on the mucosa of the urinary tract. This action helps to relieve pain, burning, urgency and frequency. The precise mechanism of action is not known.

The pharmacokinetic properties of Pyridium have not been determined. Phenazopyridine is rapidly excreted by the kidneys, with as much as 65% of an oral dose being excreted unchanged in the urine.

INDICATIONS AND USAGE

Pyridium is indicated for the symptomatic relief of pain, burning, urgency, frequency, and other discomforts arising from irritation of the lower urinary tract mucosa caused by infection, trauma, surgery, endoscopic procedures, or the passage of sounds or catheters. The use of Pyridium for relief of symptoms should not delay definitive diagnosis and treatment of causative conditions. Because it provides only symptomatic relief, prompt appropriate treatment of the cause of pain must be instituted and Pyridium should be discontinued when symptoms are controlled.

The analgesic action may reduce or eliminate the need for systemic analgesics or narcotics. It is, however, compatible with antibacterial therapy and can help to relieve pain and discomfort during the interval before antibacterial therapy controls the infection. Treatment of a urinary tract infection with Pyridium should not exceed 2 days because there is a lack of evidence that the combined administration of Pyridium and an antibacterial provides greater benefit than administration of the antibacterial alone after 2 days. (See Dosage and Administration Section.)

CONTRAINDICATIONS

Pyridium should not be used in patients who have previously exhibited hypersensitivity to it. The use of Pyridium is contraindicated in patients with renal insufficiency.

PRECAUTIONS

General: A yellowish tinge of the skin or sclera may indicate accumulation due to impaired renal excretion and the need to discontinue therapy.

The decline in renal function associated with advanced age should be kept in mind.

Information for Patients: Pyridium produces an orange to red color in the urine and may stain fabric. Staining of contact lenses has been reported.

Laboratory Test Interactions: Due to its properties as an azo dye, Pyridium may interfere with urinalysis based on spectrometry or color reactions.

Carcinogenesis, Mutagenesis, Impairment of Fertility: Long-term administration of phenazopyridine hydrochloride has induced neoplasia in rats (large intestine) and mice (liver). Although no association between phenazopyridine hydrochloride and human neoplasia has been reported, adequate epidemiological studies along these lines have not been conducted.

Pregnancy Category B: Reproduction studies have been performed in rats at doses up to 50 mg/kg/day and have revealed no evidence of impaired fertility or harm to the fetus due to Pyridium. There are, however, no adequate and well controlled studies in pregnant women. Because animal reproduction studies are not always predictive of human response, this drug should be used during pregnancy only if clearly needed.

Nursing Mothers: No information is available on the appearance of Pyridium or its metabolites in human milk.

ADVERSE REACTIONS

Headache, rash, pruritus and occasional gastrointestinal disturbance. An anaphylactoid-like reaction has been described. Methemoglobinemia, hemolytic anemia, renal and hepatic toxicity have been described, usually at overdose levels (see Overdosage section). Staining of contact lenses has been reported.

OVERDOSAGE

Exceeding the recommended dose in patients with good renal function or administering the usual dose to patients with impaired renal function (common in elderly patients), may lead to increased serum levels and toxic reactions. Methemoglobinemia generally follows a massive, acute overdose. Methylene blue, 1 to 2 mg/kg body weight intravenously, or ascorbic acid 100 to 200 mg given orally should cause prompt reduction of the methemoglobinemia and disappearance of the cyanosis which is an aid in diagnosis. Oxidative Heinz body hemolytic anemia may also occur, and "bite cells" (degmacytes) may be present in a chronic overdosage situation. Red blood cell G-6-PD deficiency may predispose to hemolysis. Renal and hepatic impairment and occasional failure, usually due to hypersensitivity, may also occur.

DOSAGE AND ADMINISTRATION

100 mg tablets: Adult dosage is two tablets 3 times a day after meals. 200 mg tablets: Adult dosage is one tablet 3 times a day after meals.

When used concomitantly with an antibacterial agent for the treatment of a urinary tract infection, the administration of Pyridium should not exceed 2 days.

HOW SUPPLIED

N 0071-0180-24 100 mg tablets
Bottles of 100
N 0071-0180-32 100 mg tablets
Bottles of 1000
N 0071-0180-40 100 mg tablets Unit dose packages of 100
(10 strips of 10)

Tablets are dark maroon, coated, round and coded P-D 180.

N 0071-0181-24 200 mg tablets
Bottles of 100
N 0071-0181-32 200 mg tablets
Bottles of 1000
N 0071-0181-40 200 mg tablets Unit dose packages of 100
(10 strips of 10)

Tablets are dark maroon, coated, round and coded P-D 181.

Store at controlled room temperature 15° to 30° C (59° to 86° F).

AHFS Category 84:08 0180G015

Shown in Product Identification Section, page 423

PYRIDIUM® PLUS Tablets ℞

[py″rĭ′dĭ-ŭm]

DESCRIPTION

Each Pyridium Plus tablet contains:
150 mg phenazopyridine hydrochloride (Pyridium®)
0.3 mg hyoscyamine hydrobromide
15 mg butabarbital

Also contains: carnauba wax, NF; corn starch, NF; D&C Red No. 7 Lake; FD&C Blue No. 2 Lake; FD&C Yellow No. 8 Lake; gelatin, NF; lactose, NF; magnesium stearate, NF; sodium starch glycolate, NF; sucrose, NF; titanium dioxide, USP; white wax, NF.

CLINICAL PHARMACOLOGY

Pyridium Plus relieves lower urinary symptoms of pain, frequency, urgency, burning and dysuria arising from inflammation of the urothelium, the mucosal lining of the lower urinary tract.

Lower urinary tract pain can cause reflex spasm of the detrusor. Pain and spasm are often aggravated by apprehension to promote a pain-spasm-apprehension cycle. Each of the three pharmacologic components of Pyridium Plus acts against a phase of this cycle.

Phenazopyridine hydrochloride (Pyridium), excreted in the urine, is a topical analgesic to relieve pain and discomfort. Hyoscyamine hydrobromide, a parasympatholytic, acts to relieve detrusor muscle spasm. Butabarbital, a short-to-intermediate-acting sedative, helps to allay associated anxiety and apprehension.

INDICATIONS AND USAGE

Pyridium Plus is indicated for the symptomatic relief of pain, burning, frequency, urgency, and dysuria, particularly when accompanied by detrusor muscle spasm and apprehension.

These symptoms may arise from infection, trauma, surgery, endoscopic procedures, or passage of sounds or catheters.

Therapy with Pyridium Plus does not interfere with antibacterial therapy and can help to relieve symptoms of pain and discomfort before definitive treatment is effective. The use of Pyridium Plus for symptomatic relief should not delay definitive diagnosis and treatment. Treatment of a urinary tract

infection with Pyridium Plus should not exceed 2 days because there is a lack of evidence that the combined administration of phenazopyridine hydrochloride and an antibacterial provides greater benefit than administration of the antibacterial alone after 2 days. (See Dosage and Administration Section.)

In the absence of infection, Pyridium Plus may be the only medication required.

CONTRAINDICATIONS

Pyridium Plus should not be used in patients who have previously exhibited hypersensitivity to any component. The use of Pyridium Plus is contraindicated in patients with renal or hepatic insufficiency, glaucoma, bladder neck obstruction, porphyria.

WARNING

BUTABARBITAL MAY BE HABIT-FORMING. Drowsiness or dizziness may occur. Patients should be instructed to use caution in driving or operating machinery.

PRECAUTIONS

General: A yellowish tinge of the skin or sclera may indicate accumulation due to impaired renal excretion of phenazopyridine (Pyridium) and the need to discontinue therapy.

The decline in renal function asssociated with advanced age should be kept in mind.

Information for Patients: Phenazopyridine hydrochloride produces an orange to red color in the urine and may stain fabric. Staining of contact lenses has been reported. Butabarbital may cause drowsiness or dizziness, patients should be instructed to use caution in driving or operating machinery.

Laboratory Test Interactions: Due to its properties as an azo dye, phenazopyridine hydrochloride may interfere with urinalysis based on spectrometry or color reactions.

Carcinogenesis, Mutagenesis, Impairment of Fertility: Pyridium Plus has not undergone adequate studies relating to carcinogenesis, mutagenesis, or impairment of fertility; however, the component phenazopyridine hydrochloride has induced neoplasia in rats (large intestine) and mice (liver). Although no association between phenazopyridine hydrochloride and human neoplasia has been reported, adequate epidemiological studies along these lines have not been conducted.

Pregnancy Category C: Animal reproduction studies have not been conducted with Pyridium Plus. It is also not known whether Pyridium Plus can cause fetal harm when administered to a pregnant woman or can affect reproduction capacity. Pyridium Plus should be given to a pregnant woman only if clearly needed.

Nursing Mothers: No information is available on the appearance of the components of Pyridium Plus in human milk.

ADVERSE REACTIONS

Methemoglobinemia, hemolytic anemia, and renal and hepatic toxicity have been described for phenazopyridine, usually at overdosage levels (see Overdosage Section). Headache, rash, pruritus and occasional gastrointestinal disturbance. An anaphylactoid-like reaction has been described.

Hyoscyamine hydrobromide is an atropinic drug that may produce adverse effects characteristic of this class of drugs. Dry mouth, drowsiness, or dizziness is noted in more than one third of patients (and may occur in half of the patients of older age groups). Other atropine-like effects, such as blurred vision, may occur. There may be occasional gastrointestinal disturbances.

Butabarbital is a short- to intermediate-acting barbiturate which has the potential for adverse reactions attributable to barbiturates.

OVERDOSAGE

Pyridium Plus is a combination of three active drugs, and overdosage can be expected to show the effects related to each ingredient. Management includes the usual measures to empty the stomach by emesis or lavage, administration of a charcoal slurry, and supportive measures as needed.

Toxicity and management suggestions relating to the individual ingredients are as follows:

Phenazopyridine Hydrochloride (Pyridium): Exceeding the recommended dose in patients with good renal function or administering the usual dose to patients with impaired renal function (common in elderly patients), may lead to increased serum levels and toxic reactions. Methemoglobinemia generally follows a massive, acute overdose. Methylene blue, 1 to 2 mg/kg body weight intravenously or ascorbic acid 100 to 200 mg given orally should cause prompt reduction of the methemoglobinemia and disappearance of cyanosis which is an aid in diagnosis. Oxidative Heinz body hemolytic anemia may also occur, and "bite cells" (degmacytes) may be present in a chronic overdosage situation. Red blood cell G-6-PD deficiency may predispose to hemolysis. Renal and hepatic impairment and occasional failure, usually due to hypersensitivity, may also occur.

Hyoscyamine Hydrobromide: Overdosage of hyoscyamine, a form of atropine, will cause dilated pupils, blurred vision, rapid pulse, increased intraocular tension, hot, dry, red skin,

dry mouth, disorientation, delirium, fever, convulsions, and coma. As an antidote, physostigmine salicylate may be given IV slowly. Dilute 1 mg in 5 ml of saline and use 1 ml of this dilution in children. Repeat every five minutes as needed up to a total of 2 mg in children, or 6 mg in adults every 30 minutes.

Butabarbital: This drug may produce sedation and respiratory depression progressing to coma, depending on the amount ingested. General and supportive measures should be instituted.

DOSAGE AND ADMINISTRATION

Adult Dosage: One tablet four times a day (after meals and at bedtime).

When used concomitantly with an antibacterial agent for the treatment of a urinary tract infection, the administration of Pyridium Plus should not exceed 2 days.

HOW SUPPLIED

N 0071-0182-24 Bottles of 100. Tablets are dark maroon, coated, square and coded P-D 182.

Store at controlled room temperature 15° to 30°C (59° to 86°F).

AHFS Category 8:12.24   0182G065

Shown in Product Identification Section, page 423

SINUBID®   ℞

[sĭn ′ū-bĭd]
(Acetaminophen, Phenylpropanolamine Hydrochloride, and Phenyltoloxamine Citrate)
Extended-release Tablets

DESCRIPTION

Sinubid is an analgesic/decongestant/antihistamine combination product for oral administration. Each two layer extended-release tablet contains:

600 mg acetaminophen
100 mg phenylpropanolamine hydrochloride
66 mg phenyltoloxamine citrate

Phenylpropanolamine hydrochloride is present in Sinubid as the racemic mixture.

Also contains calcium sulfate, NF; carnauba wax; confectioners sugar, NF; D and C red No. 30 lake; ethylcellulose, NF, 45 cps; FD and C blue No. 2 lake; FD and C yellow No. 6 lake; hydrogenated vegetable oil; hydroxypropyl methylcellulose, USP, 2910; lactose, USP; locust bean gum; magnesium stearate, NF; stearic acid, NF; syloid 244 silica gel; talc, USP; titanium dioxide, USP.

CLINICAL PHARMACOLOGY

Sinubid is designed to provide symptomatic relief of coryza and nasal congestion when given twice a day (every 12 hours). Sinubid can provide symptomatic relief of headache, fever, and other symptoms associated with mucosal congestion (nasopharyngeal), general malaise, and irritability associated with the common cold, allergic and vasomotor disorders, sinusitis, and rhinitis.

Sinubid contains an analgesic-antipyretic (acetaminophen) to relieve the pain of sinus headache and nasal congestion. This analgesic-antipyretic is rapidly absorbed and as effective as aspirin in raising the pain threshold, but has the advantage of causing little or no gastric irritation. Sinubid, because it contains no salicylates, can be used by patients who are allergic to aspirin.

Decongestion of the nasopharyngeal mucosa is provided by phenylpropanolamine hydrochloride, a sympathomimetic amine which provides symptomatic relief. Because its vasoconstrictor activity is similar to that of ephedrine, but less likely to cause CNS stimulation, Sinubid may eliminate the need for topical decongestants.

Phenyltoloxamine citrate is a mild antihistamine which may provide symptomatic relief of seasonal and perennial allergic rhinitis, vasomotor rhinitis, nasal and sinus symptoms of sinusitis, and adjunctive therapy for bacterial sinusitis in uncomplicated upper respiratory infections.

INDICATIONS AND USAGE

Sinubid is indicated for the rapid, prolonged, symptomatic relief of nasal congestion in sinus or other frontal headache; allergic and vasomotor manifestations of upper respiratory disorders such as sinusitis, allergic rhinitis, vasomotor rhinitis, coryza; facial pain and "pressure" of acute and chronic sinusitis; and for the relief of accompanying fever. Sinubid is indicated only for intermittent treatment of the above noted acute symptoms.

CONTRAINDICATIONS

This compound should not be used in patients whose oversensitivity to small doses of sympathomimetic amines produces sleeplessness, dizziness, light-headedness, weakness, tremulousness, or cardiac arrhythmias. The drug is contraindicated in any patient hypersensitive to any of the ingredients of the formulation.

WARNINGS

Instruct patients not to drive or operate machinery if drowsiness occurs. Individuals should not ingest alcoholic beverages, monoamine oxidase inhibitors, or barbiturates while taking this medication.

PRECAUTIONS

General: Individuals with high blood pressure, heart disease, diabetes mellitus, chronic renal disease, or thyroid disease should use only as directed by a physician.

Information for Patients: Patients taking this medication should be instructed not to operate heavy machinery, drive an auto, or ingest alcoholic beverages, sedatives, or monoamine oxidase inhibitors.

Drug Interactions: See WARNINGS

Carcinogenesis, Mutagenesis, Teratogenesis and Impairment of Reproduction: No long-term studies have been conducted with Sinubid.

Pregnancy: Pregnancy Category C. Animal reproduction studies have not been conducted with Sinubid. It is also not known whether Sinubid can cause fetal harm when administered to a pregnant woman or can affect reproduction capacity. Sinubid should be given to a pregnant woman only if clearly needed.

Nursing Mothers: This drug should not be used in nursing mothers.

ADVERSE REACTIONS

The following adverse reactions have been reported for each of the individual or combinations of ingredients: Acetaminophen—urticaria, epigastric distress, dizziness, and palpitation. Phenylpropanolamine HCl—anxiety, restlessness, tension, insomnia, tremor, weakness, headache, vertigo, sweating, arrhythmia, nausea, and vomiting. Phenyltoloxamine Citrate—urticaria, drowsiness, disturbed coordination, inability to concentrate, dizziness, insomnia, tremors, nervousness, palpitation, convulsions, muscular weakness, gastric distress, diarrhea, intestinal cramps, blurred vision, hypotension, urinary retention, and dryness of mouth, throat, and nose.

OVERDOSAGE

Antihistamine overdosage reactions may vary from CNS depression to stimulation. There is no specific therapy for acute overdosage with antihistamines. The latent period from ingestion to appearance of toxic effects is short (1½–2 hours). General symptomatic and supportive measures should be instituted and maintained for as long as necessary.

DOSAGE AND ADMINISTRATION

Adults: One tablet twice daily (every 12 hours).
Children (6–12 years of age): One half tablet twice daily (every 12 hours).
Not to be given to children under the age of 12.
Tablets should not be chewed, or crushed, or dissolved.

HOW SUPPLIED

Sinubid (P-D 177) is an ellipsoid, bilayered (light pink/pink), scored tablet, supplied in bottles of 100 (N 0071-0177-24). Each Sinubid tablet contains:

600 mg acetaminophen
100 mg phenylpropanolamine hydrochloride
66 mg phenyltoloxamine citrate

0177G023

SURITAL®   Ⓒ ℞

[sŭ ′rĭ-tăl ″]
(thiamylal sodium for injection, USP)

DESCRIPTION

Surital (thiamylal sodium for injection, USP) is sodium-5-allyl-5-(1-methylbutyl)-2-thiobarbiturate.

ACTIONS

Thiamylal sodium is a rapid, ultra-short-acting barbiturate, intravenous, anesthetic agent.

INDICATIONS

Surital is indicated for induction of anesthesia, for supplementing other anesthetic agents, as intravenous anesthesia for short surgical procedures with minimal painful stimuli, or as an agent for inducing a hypnotic state.

CONTRAINDICATIONS

Thiamylal sodium is contraindicated when general anesthesia is contraindicated, in patients with latent or manifest porphyria, or in patients with a known hypersensitivity to barbiturates.

Continued on next page

This product information was prepared in August 1992. On these and other Parke-Davis Products, information may be obtained by addressing PARKE-DAVIS, Division of Warner-Lambert Company, Morris Plains, New Jersey 07950.

Parke-Davis—Cont.

PREPARING *SURITAL* SOLUTIONS

Surital (g)	Amount of solvent required (in ml) for percentage solutions shown								
	0.2%	0.3%	0.4%	2%	2.5%	3%	4%	5%	10%
1	500	333	250	50	40	33.3	25	20	10
5	2,500	1,670	1,250	250	200	167	125	100	50
10	5,000	3,333	2,500	500	400	333	250	200	100

WARNINGS

RESUSCITATIVE EQUIPMENT AND DRUGS SHOULD BE IMMEDIATELY AVAILABLE. This drug should be administered by persons qualified in the use of intravenous anesthetics.

Repeated and continuous infusion may cause cumulative effects resulting in prolonged somnolence, and respiratory and circulatory depression.

Usage in pregnancy: Safe use of thiamylal sodium has not been established with respect to adverse effects upon fetal development. Therefore, thiamylal sodium should not be used in women of childbearing potential, and particularly during early pregnancy, unless, in the judgment of the physician, the expected benefits outweigh the potential hazards.

PRECAUTIONS

Respiratory depression, apnea, or hypotension may occur due to variations in tolerance from individual to individual or to physical status of patient. Caution should be exercised in debilitated patients, or those with impaired function of respiratory, circulatory, renal, hepatic, and endocrine systems.

Thiamylal sodium should be used with extreme caution in patients in status asthmaticus.

Extravascular injection may cause pain, swelling, ulceration, and necrosis. Intra-arterial injection is dangerous and may produce gangrene of an extremity.

ADVERSE REACTIONS

The following adverse reactions have been reported: circulatory depression, thrombophlebitis, pain at injection site, and respiratory depression, including apnea, laryngospasm, bronchospasm, salivation, hiccups, emergence delirium, headache, injury to nerves adjacent to injection site, skin rashes, urticaria, nausea, and emesis.

DOSAGE AND ADMINISTRATION

The dosage is individualized according to the patient's response.

A 2.5% solution is recommended for induction of anesthesia as well as for maintenance by intermittent intravenous injection. A dilute solution (0.3%) may be used by continuous drip for maintenance. The rate of injection during induction should be approximately 1 ml of 2.5% solution every five seconds; an initial injection of 3 to 6 ml of 2.5% solution is generally sufficient to produce short periods of surgical anesthesia.

Sterile Water for Injection is the preferred solvent for preparing Surital (thiamylal sodium for injection, USP) solutions. Initially, Surital solutions are clear, but they may become cloudy on aging. Thiamylal sodium cannot be reconstituted with Ringer's Solution or solutions containing bacteriostatic or buffer agents, because they may tend to cause precipitation. In preparing dilute solutions for continuous drip maintenance, either 5% dextrose or isotonic sodium chloride should be used instead of sterile water for injection to avoid extreme hypotonicity. Dextrose solutions are occasionally sufficiently acid, however, to cause precipitation. Injection of air into the solution should be avoided because this may hasten the development of cloudiness.

Solutions of atropine sulfate, *d*-tubocurarine, or succinylcholine may be given concurrently with Surital, but they should not be mixed prior to administration.

Thiamylal sodium solutions should be prepared under aseptic conditions. Solutions cannot be heated for sterilization. The solutions should be stored in a refrigerator and used within six days. If kept at room temperature, the solution should be used within 24 hours. Only clear solutions should be used; discard if cloudiness or precipitate form. Refrigeration of the reconstituted Surital contributes to the maintenance of a clear solution.

[See table above.]

HOW SUPPLIED

Surital is supplied as follows.

N 0071-4064-03 (35-64-25)
1 g, in packages of 25 (Steri-Vial® 64)
N 0071-4122-08 (35-122-10)
5 g, in packages of 10 (Steri-Vial 122)
N 0071-4123-10 (35-123-10)
10 g, in packages of 10 (Steri-Vial 123)
AHFS 28:24   4064G020

TEDRAL®SA   ℞
[*tĕd 'ral*]

DESCRIPTION

Tedral SA: Each tablet contains 180 mg anhydrous theophylline (90 mg in the immediate release layer and 90 mg in the sustained release layer); 48 mg ephedrine hydrochloride (16 mg in the immediate release layer and 32 mg in the sustained release layer); 25 mg phenobarbital in the immediate release layer.

Also contains: D&C red No. 30 and yellow No. 10 Lake; lactose, NF; magnesium stearate, NF; starch; sucrose and other ingredients.

ACTIONS

Tedral SA combines theophylline and ephedrine—widely accepted oral bronchodilators with differing modes of action. From experimental evidence,[1] it appears that a combination of a sympathomimetic and methylxanthine is more effective than either drug alone in inhibiting the release of bronchoconstricting mediators (histamine and slow-reacting substance of anaphylaxis) produced by antigen-antibody (IgE) interaction on sensitive cells. Th β-adrenergic stimulation by the sympathomimetics produces cyclic 3'5'-adenosine monophosphate (cAMP), and the degradation of cAMP by the specific enzyme, phosphodiesterase, is inhibited by methylxanthines. Thus, at present, the principal action of Tedral SA in the relief or prevention of bronchoconstriction appears to be involved with the cAMP system.

Phenobarbital is incorporated into Tedral SA to counteract possible stimulation by ephedrine and to provide a mild, long-acting sedative for the apprehensive asthmatic patient. Tedral SA provides sustained as well as immediate bronchodilatation for the asthmatic patient, with the convenience of bid dosage.

INDICATIONS

Tedral SA is indicated for the symptomatic relief of bronchial asthma, asthmatic bronchitis, and other bronchospastic disorders. It may also be used prophylactically to abort or minimize asthmatic attacks and is of value in managing occasional, seasonal, or perennial asthma.

Tedral SA (Sustained Action) offers the convenience of bid dosage.

This Tedral formulation is an adjunct in the total management of the asthmatic patient. Acute or severe asthmatic attacks may necessitate supplemental therapy with other drugs by inhalation or other parenteral routes.

CONTRAINDICATIONS

Sensitivity to any of the ingredients; porphyria.

WARNINGS

Drowsiness may occur. Phenobarbital may be habit forming.

PRECAUTIONS

Use with caution in the presence of cardiovascular disease, severe hypertension, hyperthyroidism, prostatic hypertrophy, or glaucoma.

ADVERSE REACTIONS

Mild epigastric distress, palpitation, tremulousness, insomnia, difficulty of micturition, and CNS stimulation have been reported.

DOSAGE AND ADMINISTRATION

Adults—one tablet on arising and one tablet 12 hours later. Tablets should not be chewed.
Children—not established for children under 12.

HOW SUPPLIED

Tedral SA is supplied as double-layered, uncoated, coral/mottled white tablets in bottles of 100 (N 0071-0231-24) and 1000 (N 0071-0231-32).

Store between 15°–30°C (59°–86°F).

Reference: 1. Koopman WJ, Orange RP, Austen KF. *J Immunol* 105:1096, November 1970.

0231G114

THROMBOSTAT®   ℞
(Thrombin, USP) Bovine Origin

Thrombostat must not be injected! Apply on the surface of bleeding tissue as a solution or powder.

DESCRIPTION

Thrombostat (Thrombin, USP) is a protein substance produced through a conversion reaction in which prothrombin of bovine origin is activated by tissue thromboplastin in the presence of calcium chloride. It is supplied as a sterile powder that has been freeze-dried in the final container. Also contained in this preparation are calcium chloride, sodium chloride, and aminoacetic acid (glycine) as follows: calcium chloride—5 mg per 5000 unit vial, 10 mg per 10,000 unit vial, and 21 mg per 20,000 unit vial; sodium chloride—8 mg per 5000 unit vial, 15 mg per 10,000 unit vial, and 30 mg per 20,000 unit vial; aminoacetic acid—39 mg per 5000 unit vial, 78 mg per 10,000 unit vial, and 156 mg per 20,000 unit vial. Glycine is included to make the dried product friable and more readily soluble.

A 5 mL, 10 mL, or 20 mL vial of Isotonic Saline is enclosed to be used as a diluent with the 5 mL, 5000 unit; 10 mL, 10,000 unit; or 20 mL, 20,000 unit vial, respectively, of Thrombostat. Isotonic Saline is a sterile, isotonic solution of sodium chloride in Water For Injection, USP. It contains Phemerol® (benzethonium chloride) 0.02 mg per mL as a preservative. (See Dosage and Administration for additional information on diluents which may be used.)

This product is prepared under rigid assay control. A unit is defined as the amount required to clot 1 mL of standardized fibrinogen solution in 15 seconds.

Approximately 2 units are required to clot 1 mL of oxalated human plasma in the same period of time.

CLINICAL PHARMACOLOGY

Thrombostat requires no intermediate physiological agent for its action. It clots the fibrinogen of the blood directly. Failure to clot blood occurs in the rare case where the primary clotting defect is the absence of fibrinogen itself. The speed with which thrombin clots blood is dependent upon its concentration. For example, the contents of a 5000 unit vial of Thrombostat dissolved in 5 mL of saline diluent is capable of clotting an equal volume of blood in less than a second, or 1000 mL in less than a minute.

INDICATIONS AND USAGE

Thrombostat (Thrombin, USP) is indicated as an aid in hemostasis wherever oozing blood from capillaries and small venules is accessible.

In various types of surgery solutions of Thrombostat may be used in conjunction with Absorbable Gelatin Sponge, USP for hemostasis.

CONTRAINDICATIONS

Thrombostat is contraindicated in persons known to be sensitive to any of its components and/or to material of bovine origin.

WARNING

Because of its action in the clotting mechanism, Thrombostat must not be injected or otherwise allowed to enter large blood vessels. Extensive intravascular clotting and even death may result. Thrombostat is an antigenic substance and has caused sensitivity and allergic reactions when injected into animals.

PRECAUTIONS

General: Consult the absorbable gelatin sponge product labeling for complete information for use prior to utilizing the thrombin-saturated sponge procedure.

Pregnancy—
Teratogenic effects: Pregnancy Category C. Animal reproduction studies have not been conducted with Thrombin, USP. It is also not known whether Thrombin, USP can cause fetal harm when administered to a pregnant woman or can affect reproduction capacity. Thrombin, Topical (Bovine) should be given to a pregnant woman only if clearly indicated.

Pediatric Use: Safety and effectiveness in children have not been established.

ADVERSE REACTIONS

An allergic type reaction following the use of Thrombostat for treatment of epistaxis has been reported. Febrile reactions have also been observed following the use of Thrombostat in certain surgical procedures but no cause-effect relationship has been established.

DOSAGE AND ADMINISTRATION

General: Solutions of Thrombostat may be prepared in sterile distilled water or isotonic saline. The intended use determines the strength of the solution to prepare. For general use in plastic surgery, dental extractions, skin grafting, neurosurgery, etc, solutions containing approximately 100 units per mL are frequently used. For this, an appropriate dilution of Thrombostat should be prepared to yield a concentration of 100 units per mL. Where bleeding is profuse, as from cut surfaces of liver and spleen, concentrations as high as 1000 to 2000 units per mL may be required. For this the 5000 unit vial dissolved in 5 mL or 2.5 mL, respectively, of the diluent supplied in the package is convenient. Intermediate strengths to suit the needs of the case may be prepared by selecting the proper strength package and dissolving the contents in an appropriate volume of diluent. In many situations, it may be advantageous to use Thrombostat in dry form on oozing surfaces.

Caution:
Solutions should be used immediately upon reconstitution. If necessary, refrigerate the solution and use within 3 hours of reconstitution.
The following techniques are suggested for the topical application of Thrombostat.
1. The recipient surface should be sponged (not wiped) free of blood before Thrombostat is applied.
2. A spray may be used or the surface may be flooded using a sterile syringe and small gauge needle. The most effective hemostasis results when the Thrombostat mixes freely with the blood as soon as it reaches the surface.
3. In instances where Thrombostat in dry form is needed, the vial is opened by removing the metal ring by flipping up the plastic cap and tearing counterclockwise. The rubber-diaphragm cap may be easily removed and the dried Thrombostat is then broken up into a powder by means of a sterile glass rod or other suitable sterile instrument.
4. Sponging of treated surfaces should be avoided in order that the clot remain securely in place.
Thrombostat may be used in conjunction with Absorbable Gelatin Sponge, USP as follows:
1. Prepare Thrombostat solution of the desired strength.
2. Immerse sponge strips of the desired size in the Thrombostat solution. Knead the sponge strips vigorously with moistened gloved fingers to remove trapped air, thereby facilitating saturation of the sponge.
3. Apply saturated sponge to bleeding area. Hold in place for 10 to 15 seconds with a pledget of cotton or a small gauze sponge.

Sterile Packages
Thrombostat Sterile Packages are available in two strengths, 5000 units and 10,000 units. A Sterile Package contains one sterile vial of Thrombostat, one sterile vial of Isotonic Saline Diluent, and one sterile transfer device. The Sterile Package may be used as follows:
1. Remove the Tyvek® blister lid by pulling up at the indicated corner. The sterile inner tray can be lifted out or introduced into the operating field.
2. The cover to the sterile inner tray is removed by pulling up on the finger tab, exposing the sterile contents.
3. Thrombostat solution of the desired strength is prepared using the transfer device.
4. Alternatively, when Thrombostat in dry form is needed, the vial is opened as described above and the dried Thrombostat broken up into a powder by means of a sterile glass rod or other suitable sterile instrument.

Kits
Thrombostat Kits are available in two strengths, 10,000 units and 20,000 units. The 10,000 unit kit contains one sterile 10,000 unit vial of Thrombostat, one sterile vial of Isotonic Saline Diluent, one sterile transfer device, and one sterile pump sprayer cap. The 20,000 unit kit contains one sterile 20,000 unit vial of Thrombostat, one sterile vial of Isotonic Saline Diluent, one sterile transfer device, and one sterile pump sprayer cap. The kit may be used as follows:
1. Remove the Tyvek® blister lid by pulling up at the indicated corner. The sterile inner tray can be lifted out or introduced into the operating field.
2. The cover to the sterile inner tray is removed by pulling up on the finger tab, exposing the sterile contents.
3. Thrombostat solution of the desired strength is prepared using the transfer device. See directions above. After reconstitution, the pump sprayer cap is inserted and seated on the Thrombostat solution vial. Note: Several strokes of the pump sprayer will be required before the Thrombostat solution is expelled.
4. Alternatively, when Thrombostat in dry form is needed, the vial is opened as described above and the dried Thrombostat broken up into a powder by means of a sterile glass rod or other suitable sterile instrument.

HOW SUPPLIED

Thrombostat is supplied as:
N 0071-4173-35—Package contains one 5000 unit vial of Thrombostat and one 5 mL vial of Isotonic Saline Diluent with Phemerol, 0.02 mg per mL, as a preservative.
N 0071-4176-35—Package contains one 10,000 unit vial of Thrombostat and one 10 mL vial of Isotonic Saline Diluent with Phemerol, 0.02 mg per mL, as a preservative.
N 0071-4180-35—Package contains one 20,000 unit vial of Thrombostat and one 20 mL vial of Isotonic Saline Diluent with Phemerol, 0.02 mg per mL, as a preservative.
N 0071-4173-36—Sterile Package contains one sterile 5000 unit vial of Thrombostat, one sterile 5 mL vial of Isotonic Saline Diluent with Phemerol, 0.02 mg per mL, as a preservative, and one sterile transfer device in a sterile tray with a Tyvek lid.
N 0071-4176-36—Sterile Package contains one sterile 10,000 unit vial of Thrombostat, one sterile 10 mL vial of Isotonic Saline Diluent with Phemerol, 0.02 mg per mL, as a preservative, and one sterile transfer device in a sterile tray with a Tyvek lid.
N 0071-4176-37—Kit contains one sterile 10,000 unit vial of Thrombostat, one sterile 10 mL vial of Isotonic Saline Diluent with Phemerol, 0.02 mg per mL, as a preservative, one sterile transfer device, and one sterile pump sprayer cap in a sterile tray with a Tyvek lid.
N 0071-4180-36—Kit contains one sterile 20,000 unit vial of Thrombostat, one sterile 20 mL vial of Isotonic Saline Diluent with Phemerol, 0.02 mg per mL, as a preservative, one sterile transfer device, and one sterile pump sprayer cap in a sterile tray with a Tyvek lid.

STORAGE

Store at room temperature 15 to 30°C (59 to 86°F).
Caution—Federal law prohibits dispensing without prescription.
Tyvek is a registered trademark of E. I. du Pont de Nemours & Co.

4173G200

VIRA-A® ℞

[vī″ră ā′]
(vidarabine concentrate for injection, USP)

DESCRIPTION

Vira-A is the trade name for vidarabine (also known as adenine arabinoside and Ara-A), an antiviral drug. Vira-A is a purine nucleoside obtained from fermentation cultures of *Streptomyces antibioticus*. Each milliliter of sterile suspension contains 200 milligrams of vidarabine monohydrate equivalent to 187.4 milligrams of vidarabine. Each milliliter contains 0.1 milligrams Phemerol® (benzethonium chloride) as a preservative; sodium phosphate, USP, 1.8 milligrams, and sodium biphosphate, USP, 4.8 milligrams as buffering agents. Hydrochloric acid may have been added to adjust pH. Vira-A is a white, crystalline solid with this empirical formula: $C_{10}H_{13}N_5O_4.H_2O$. The molecular weight is 285.2; the solubility is 0.45 mg/ml at 25°C; and the melting point ranges from 260° to 270°C. The chemical name is 9-β-D-arabinofuranosyladenine monohydrate.

CLINICAL PHARMACOLOGY

Following intravenous administration, Vira-A is rapidly deaminated into arabinosylhypoxanthine (Ara-Hx), the principal metabolite, which is promptly distributed into the tissues. In adults peak Ara-Hx and vidarabine plasma levels ranging from 3 to 6 μg/ml and 0.2 to 0.4 μg/ml, respectively, are attained after slow intravenous infusion of Vira-A doses of 10 mg/kg of body weight. These levels reflect the rate of infusion and show no accumulation across time. The mean half-life of Ara-Hx is 3.3 hours. Ara-Hx penetrates into the cerebrospinal fluid (CSF) to give a CSF/plasma ratio of approximately 1:3.
Excretion of Vira-A is principally via the kidneys. Urinary excretion is constant over 24 hours. Forty-one percent to 53% of the daily dose is recovered in the urine as Ara-Hx with 1% to 3% appearing as the parent compound. There is no evidence of fecal excretion of drug or metabolites. In patients with impaired renal function Ara-Hx may accumulate in the plasma and reach levels several-fold higher than those described above.
Vira-A possesses *in vitro* and *in vivo* antiviral activity against Herpes simplex virus types 1 and 2 (HSV-1 and HSV-2), and *in vitro* activity against varicella-zoster virus (VZV).
The antiviral mechanism of action has not yet been established. Vidarabine is converted into nucleotides which inhibit viral DNA polymerase. In KB cells infected with Herpes simplex virus type 1, Vira-A inhibits viral DNA synthesis. Vira-A is rapidly deaminated to Ara-Hx, the principal metabolite, in cell cultures, laboratory animals, and humans.
Ara-Hx also possesses *in vitro* antiviral activity but this activity is significantly less than the activity of Vira-A.

INDICATIONS AND USAGE

Herpes Simplex Virus Encephalitis—Vira-A is indicated for the treatment of Herpes simplex virus encephalitis. Controlled studies indicated that Vira-A therapy will reduce the mortality caused by Herpes simplex virus encephalitis from 70 to 28% 30 days following onset. In a larger uncontrolled study of 75 patients with biopsy-proven herpes simplex encephalitis, the mortality 6 months from onset was 39%, similar to 44% in the initial controlled study at 6 months.
Morbidity from both studies one year after onset was: normal 53%, moderately debilitated 29%, and severely damaged 18%. Vira-A does not appear to alter morbidity and resulting serious neurological sequelae in the comatose patient. Therefore early diagnosis and treatment are essential.
Herpes simplex virus encephalitis should be suspected in patients with a history of an acute febrile encephalopathy associated with disordered mentation, altered level of consciousness and focal cerebral signs.
Studies which may support the suspected diagnosis include examination of cerebrospinal fluid and localization of an intra-cerebral lesion by brain scan, electroencephalography or computerized axial tomography (CAT).
Brain biopsy is required in order to confirm the etiological diagnosis by means of viral isolation in cell cultures.
Detection of Herpes simplex virus in the biopsied brain tissue can also be reliably done by specific fluorescent antibody techniques. Detection of Herpes virus-like particles by electron microscopy or detection of intranuclear inclusions by histopathologic techniques only provides a presumptive diagnosis.
Neonatal Herpes Simplex Virus Infections—Vira-A is also indicated for the treatment of Herpes simplex infections in the newborn, including disseminated infection with visceral involvement, encephalitis, and infections of the skin, eyes and mouth. Controlled studies indicated that Vira-A therapy reduced mortality in encephalitis and disseminated infection from 74% to 38%. Following Vira-A therapy the incidence of neurological abnormalities at one year of age was 44% in infants with localized CNS infection and 67% in infants with disseminated infection. Therefore, early diagnosis and treatment are essential to reduce both mortality and morbidity.
Herpes simplex virus infections should be suspected in babies born to mothers with a history of genital or nongenital Herpes simplex virus infections during gestation or prior to the onset of labor or to mothers with a sexual partner with a history of genital Herpes simplex virus infections. A sick newborn suspected of having a herpes virus infection may present with fever, lethargy, poor feeding or seizures. Most of the infected newborns will develop skin vesicles (about 70%) with or without signs and symptoms of CNS infection or visceral dissemination (hepatitis, pneumonitis, intravascular coagulopathy). The etiological diagnosis is established by isolation of HSV from skin vesicles, mouth, conjunctivae, cerebrospinal fluid, blood, or brain biopsy.
Herpes zoster—Vira-A is indicated for the treatment of herpes zoster (shingles) due to reactivated varicella-zoster virus infections in immunosuppressed patients. Placebo-controlled studies have shown that Vira-A significantly reduced the severity of acute pain, new vesicle formation, time to pustulation and scabbing, cutaneous dissemination inside and outside the primary dermatome(s), and the overall frequency of visceral complications (uveitis or keratitis, hepatitis, encephalitis and peripheral neuropathy). To be effective, Vira-A therapy should be initiated as early as possible, within 72 hours after the appearance of vesicular lesions.
Herpes zoster is recognized by the formation of clear skin vesicles progressing to pustules and scabs along a sensory nerve distribution. The appearance of vesicles may be preceded by fever, local pain and erythema. Varicella-zoster virus can be isolated from vesicular lesions or detected by fluorescent antibody techniques.

CONTRAINDICATIONS

Vira-A is contraindicated in patients who develop hypersensitivity reactions to it.

WARNINGS

Vira-A should not be administered by the intramuscular or subcutaneous route because of its low solubility and poor absorption.
There are no reports available to indicate that Vira-A for infusion is effective in the management of encephalitis due to varicella-zoster or vaccinia viruses. Vira-A is not effective against infections caused by adenovirus or RNA viruses. It is also not effective against bacterial or fungal infections. There are no data to support efficacy of Vira-A against cytomegalovirus, vaccinia virus, or smallpox virus.

PRECAUTIONS

General—Treatment should be discontinued in adult or pediatric patients with a clinical diagnosis of suspected encephalitis if the brain biopsy specimen is negative for Herpes simplex virus in cell cultures.
Special care should be exercised when administering Vira-A to patients susceptible to fluid overloading or cerebral edema. Examples are patients with CNS infections and impaired renal function.
Patients with impaired renal function, such as post-operative renal transplant recipients, may have a slower rate of renal excretion of Ara-Hx. Therefore, the dose of Vira-A may need to be adjusted according to the severity of impairment. These patients should be carefully monitored.
Patients with impaired liver function should also be observed for possible adverse effects.
Patients with Herpes simplex encephalitis or newborns with Herpes simplex infections should be managed by physicians skilled in the treatment of these diseases.
Although clear evidence of adverse experience in humans from simultaneous Vira-A and allopurinol administration has not been reported, laboratory studies indicate that allopurinol may interfere with Vira-A metabolism. Therefore,

Continued on next page

This product information was prepared in August 1992. On these and other Parke-Davis Products, information may be obtained by addressing PARKE-DAVIS, Division of Warner-Lambert Company, Morris Plains, New Jersey 07950.

Parke-Davis—Cont.

caution is recommended when administering Vira-A to patients receiving allopurinol.

Laboratory Tests—Appropriate hematologic tests are recommended during Vira-A administration since hemoglobin, hematocrit, white blood cells, and platelets may be depressed during therapy.

Some degree of immunocompetence must be present in order for Vira-A to achieve clinical response.

Carcinogenesis—Chronic parenteral (IM) studies of vidarabine have been conducted in mice and rats.

In the mouse study, there was a statistically significant increase in liver tumor incidence among the vidarabine-treated females. In the same study, some vidarabine-treated male mice developed kidney neoplasia. No renal tumors were found in the vehicle-treated control mice or the vidarabine-treated female mice.

In the rat study, intestinal, testicular, and thyroid neoplasia occurred with greater frequency among the vidarabine-treated animals than in the vehicle-treated controls. The increases in thyroid adenoma incidence in the high-dose (50 mg/kg) males and the low-dose (30 mg/kg) females were statistically significant.

Hepatic megalocytosis, associated with vidarabine treatment, has been found in short- and long-term rodent (rat and mouse) studies. It is not clear whether or not this represents a preneoplastic change.

In the Balb/3T3 *in vitro* neoplastic transformation assay, used to provide preliminary assessment of potential oncogenicity, vidarabine induced a significant and dose-related increase in transformed foci over the concentration range of 0.5–3.0 μg/ml.

Mutagenesis—Results of *in vitro* experiments indicate that vidarabine can be incorporated into mammalian DNA and can induce mutation in mammalian cells (mouse L5178Y cell line). In the Ames/Salmonella/microsome plate assay, vidarabine elicited a positive response for mutagenicity in *Salmonella typhimurium*, strain TA 1537, at high doses (2500 μg/plate). Thus far, *in vivo* studies have not been as conclusive, but there is some evidence (dominant lethal assay in mice) that vidarabine may be capable of producing mutagenic effects in male germ cells.

It has also been reported that vidarabine causes chromosome breaks and gaps when added to human leukocytes *in vitro*. Vidarabine also induced significant dose-related increases in chromosome aberrations (breaks and exchange aberrations) in Chinese hamster ovary cells *in vitro*. While the significance of these effects in terms of mutagenicity is not fully understood, there is a well-known correlation between the ability of various agents to produce such effects and their ability to produce heritable genetic damage.

Pregnancy Category C—Vira-A given parenterally is teratogenic in rats and rabbits. Doses of 5 mg/kg or higher given intramuscularly to pregnant rabbits during organogenesis induced fetal abnormalities. Doses of 3 mg/kg or less did not induce teratogenic changes in pregnant rabbits. Vira-A doses ranging from 30 to 250 mg/kg were given intramuscularly to pregnant rats during organogenesis; signs of maternal toxicity were induced at doses of 100 mg/kg or higher and frank fetal anomalies were found at doses of 150 to 250 mg/kg.

A safe dose for the human embryo or fetus has not been established.

There are no adequate and well controlled studies in pregnant women. Vira-A should be used during pregnancy only if the potential benefit justifies the potential risk to the fetus.

Nursing Mothers—It is not known whether Vira-A is excreted in human milk. Because many drugs are excreted in human milk and because of the potential tumorigenicity shown for Vira-A in animal studies, a decision should be made whether to discontinue nursing or to discontinue the drug, taking into account the importance of the drug to the mother.

ADVERSE REACTIONS

The principal adverse reactions in adults involve the gastrointestinal tract and are anorexia, nausea, vomiting, and diarrhea. These reactions are mild to moderate, and seldom require termination of Vira-A therapy.

CNS disturbances have been reported at therapeutic doses. These are tremor, dizziness, hallucinations, confusion, psychosis, ataxia, headache and encephalopathy. These adverse drug reactions have occurred mostly in patients with impaired hepatic or renal function.

Hematologic clinical laboratory changes noted in controlled and uncontrolled studies were a decrease in hemoglobin or hematocrit, white blood cell count, and platelet count. Elevations of aspartate aminotransferase (SGOT) were also observed. Other changes occasionally observed were decreases in reticulocyte count and elevated total bilirubin. In newborns with HSV infections, no clear evidence of hematologic, renal, or hepatic toxicity was noted at the recommended doses.

Other symptoms which have been reported are weight loss, malaise, pruritus, rash, hematemesis, and pain at the injection site.

OVERDOSAGE

Acute massive overdose of the intravenous form has been reported without any serious evidence of adverse effect. Because of the low solubility of Vira-A, acute water overloading would pose a greater threat to the patient than Vira-A. Doses of Vira-A over 20 mg/kg/day can produce bone marrow depression with concomitant thrombocytopenia and leukopenia. If a massive overdose of the intravenous form occurs, hematologic, liver, and renal functions should be carefully monitored.

DOSAGE AND ADMINISTRATION

CAUTION—1) THE CONTENTS OF THE VIAL MUST BE DILUTED IN AN APPROPRIATE INTRAVENOUS SOLUTION PRIOR TO ADMINISTRATION. RAPID OR BOLUS INJECTION MUST BE AVOIDED. THE DOSE DEPENDS ON THE DISEASE BEING TREATED.

2) SEE SPECIAL INSTRUCTIONS FOR PREPARATION OF VIRA-A FOR ADMINISTRATION TO NEWBORNS.

Dosage— Herpes simplex virus encephalitis—15 mg/kg/day for 10 days.

Neonatal Herpes simplex virus infections—15 mg/kg/day for 10 days.

Herpes zoster—10 mg/kg/day for 5 days.

Method of Preparation—Each 5-ml vial contains 1 gram of Vira-A (200 mg per ml of suspension). The solubility of Vira-A in intravenous infusion fluids is limited. Each one mg of Vira-A requires 2.22 ml of intravenous infusion fluid for complete solubilization. Therefore, each one liter of intravenous infusion fluid will solubilize a maximum of 450 mg of Vira-A.

Any appropriate intravenous solution is suitable for use as a diluent *EXCEPT* biologic or colloidal fluids (e.g., blood products, protein solutions, etc.).

Shake the Vira-A vial well to obtain a homogeneous suspension before measuring and transferring.

Prepare the Vira-A solution for intravenous administration by aseptically transferring the proper dose of Vira-A into an appropriate intravenous infusion fluid. The intravenous infusion fluid used to prepare the Vira-A solution should be prewarmed to 35° to 40°C (95° to 100°F) to facilitate solution of the drug following its transference. Depending on the dose to be given, more than one liter of intravenous infusion fluid may be required. Thoroughly agitate the prepared admixture until *completely* clear. Complete solubilization of the drug, as indicated by a completely clear solution, is ascertained by careful visual inspection. Final filtration with an in-line membrane filter (0.45 μ pore size or smaller) is necessary.

Dilution should be made just prior to administration and used at least within 48 hours. Subsequent agitation, shaking, or inversion of the bottle is unnecessary once the drug is completely in solution. DO NOT REFRIGERATE THE DILUTION.

Administration—Using aseptic technique, slowly infuse the total daily dose by intravenous infusion (prepared as discussed above) at a constant rate over a 12- to 24-hour period.

Administration to Newborns—Due to the small quantity required by the infant, 1 ml of Vira-A (200 mg per ml of suspension) should be aseptically added to 9 ml of sterile normal saline or sterile water for injection to provide a suspension of 20 mg per ml. Then prepare the Vira-A solution for intravenous infusion, as described above, by transferring the proper dose to the MINIMUM VOLUME of an appropriate intravenous fluid required to assure complete solubilization of the drug. Each 1 mg of Vira-A requires 2.22 ml of intravenous infusion fluid for complete solubilization. EXTREME CARE MUST BE EXERCISED TO MAKE CERTAIN THAT THE DRUG SOLUTION IS ADMINISTERED SLOWLY.

HOW SUPPLIED

N 0071-4150-08 (Steri-Vial® 4150) Vira-A (Vidarabine Concentrate for Injection, USP), a sterile suspension containing 200 mg/ml, is supplied in 5 ml Steri-Vials; packages of 10.

ANIMAL PHARMACOLOGY AND ANIMAL TOXICITY

Acute Toxicity: The intraperitoneal LD_{50} for Vira-A ranged from 3,890 to 4,500 mg/kg in mice, and from 2,239 to 2,512 mg/kg in rats, suggesting a low order of toxicity to a single parenteral dose. Hepatic megalocytosis was observed in rats after single, intraperitoneal injections at doses near and exceeding the LD_{50} value. The hepatic megalocytosis appeared to regress completely over several months. Acute intravenous LD_{50} values could not be obtained because of the limited solubility of Vira-A.

Subacute Toxicity: Rats, dogs, and monkeys have been given daily intramuscular injections of Vira-A as a 20% suspension for 28 days. These animal species showed dose related decreases in hemoglobin, hematocrit, and lymphocytes. Bone marrow depression was also observed in monkeys. Except for localized, injection-site injury and weight gain inhibition or loss, rats tolerated daily doses up to 150 mg/kg, and dogs tolerated daily doses up to 50 mg/kg. Megalocytosis was not seen in the rats dosed by the intramuscular route for 28 days. Rhesus monkeys were particularly sensitive to Vira-A. Daily intramuscular doses of 15 mg/kg were tolerable, but doses of 25 mg/kg or higher induced progressively severe clinical signs of CNS toxicity. Three monkeys given slow intravenous infusions of Vira-A in solution at a dose of 15 mg/kg daily for 28 days had no significant adverse reactions.

4150G022

VIRA-A® ℞

[*vī″rā ā′*]

(vidarabine ophthalmic ointment, USP), 3%

DESCRIPTION

VIRA-A is the trade name for vidarabine (also known as adenine arabinoside and Ara-A), an antiviral drug for the topical treatment of epithelial keratitis caused by Herpes simplex virus. The chemical name is 9-β-D-arabinofuranosyladenine. Each gram of the ophthalmic ointment contains 30 mg of vidarabine monohydrate equivalent to 28.11 mg of vidarabine in a sterile, inert, petrolatum base.

CLINICAL PHARMACOLOGY

Vira-A is a purine nucleoside obtained from fermentation cultures of *Streptomyces antibioticus*. Vira-A possesses *in vitro* and *in vivo* antiviral activity against Herpes simplex types 1 and 2, Varicella-Zoster, and Vaccinia viruses. Except for Rhabdovirus and Oncornavirus, Vira-A does not display *in vitro* antiviral activity against other RNA or DNA viruses, including Adenovirus.

The antiviral mechanism of action has not been established. Vira-A appears to interfere with the early steps of viral DNA synthesis. Vira-A is rapidly deaminated to arabinosyl-hypoxanthine (Ara-Hx), the principal metabolite. Ara-Hx also possesses *in vitro* antiviral activity but this activity is less than that of Vira-A. Because of the low solubility of Vira-A, trace amounts of both Vira-A and Ara-Hx can be detected in the aqueous humor only if there is an epithelial defect in the cornea. If the cornea is normal, only trace amounts of Ara-Hx can be recovered from the aqueous humor.

Systemic absorption of Vira-A should not be expected to occur following ocular administration and swallowing lacrimal secretions. In laboratory animals, Vira-A is rapidly deaminated in the gastrointestinal tract to Ara-Hx.

In contrast to topical idoxuridine, Vira-A demonstrated less cellular toxicity in the regenerating corneal epithelium in the rabbit.

INDICATIONS AND USAGE

Vira-A Ophthalmic Ointment, 3%, is indicated for the treatment of acute keratoconjunctivitis and recurrent epithelial keratitis due to Herpes simplex virus types 1 and 2. It is also effective in superficial keratitis caused by Herpes simplex virus which has not responded to topical idoxuridine or when toxic or hypersensitivity reactions to idoxuridine have occurred. The effectiveness of Vira-A Ophthalmic Ointment, 3%, against stromal keratitis and uveitis due to Herpes simplex virus has not been established.

The clinical diagnosis of keratitis caused by Herpes simplex virus is usually established by the presence of typical dendritic or geographic lesions on slit-lamp examination.

In controlled and uncontrolled clinical trials, an average of seven and nine days of continuous Vira-A Ophthalmic Ointment, 3%, therapy was required to achieve corneal re-epithelialization. In the controlled trials, 70 of 81 subjects (86%) re-epithelialized at the end of three weeks of therapy. In the uncontrolled trials, 101 of 142 subjects (71%) re-epithelialized at the end of three weeks. Seventy-five percent of the subjects in these uncontrolled trials had either not healed previously or had developed hypersensitivity to topical idoxuridine therapy.

The following topical antibiotics: gentamicin, erythromycin, and chloramphenicol; or topical steroids: prednisolone or dexamethasone, have been administered concurrently with Vira-A Ophthalmic Ointment, 3%, without an increase in adverse reactions.

CONTRAINDICATION

Vira-A Ophthalmic Ointment, 3%, is contraindicated in patients who develop hypersensitivity reactions to it.

WARNINGS

Normally, corticosteroids alone are contraindicated in Herpes simplex virus infections of the eye. If Vira-A Ophthalmic Ointment, 3%, is administered concurrently with topical corticosteroid therapy, corticosteroid-induced ocular side effects must be considered. These include corticosteroid-induced glaucoma or cataract formation and progression of a bacterial or viral infection.

Vira-A is not effective against RNA virus or adenoviral ocular infections. It is also not effective against bacterial, fungal, or chlamydial infections of the cornea or nonviral trophic ulcers.

Although viral resistance to VIRA-A has not been observed, this possibility may exist.

PRECAUTIONS

General—The diagnosis of keratoconjunctivitis due to Herpes simples virus should be established clinically prior to prescribing VIRA-A Ophthalmic Ointment, 3%.

Patients should be forewarned that VIRA-A Ophthalmic Ointment, 3%, like any ophthalmic ointment, may produce a temporary visual haze.

Carcinogenesis—Chronic parenteral (IM) studies of vidarabine have been conducted in mice and rats.

In the mouse study, there was a statistically significant increase in liver tumor incidence among the vidarabine-treated females. In the same study some vidarabine-treated male mice developed kidney neoplasia. No renal tumors were found in the vehicle-treated control mice or the vidarabine-treated female mice.

In the rat study, intestinal, testicular, and thyroid neoplasia occurred with greater frequency among the vidarabine-treated animals than in the vehicle-treated controls. The increases in thyroid adenoma incidence in the high dose (50 mg/kg) males and the low dose (30 mg/kg) females were statistically significant.

Hepatic megalocytosis, associated with vidarabine treatment, has been found in short- and long-term rodent (rat and mouse) studies. It is not clear whether or not this represents a preneoplastic change.

The recommended frequency and duration of administration should not be exceeded (See Dosage and Administration).

Mutagenesis—Results of *in vitro* experiments indicate that vidarabine can be incorporated into mammalian DNA and can induce mutation in mammalian cells (mouse L5178Y cell line). Thus far, *in vivo* studies have not been as conclusive, but there is some evidence (dominant lethal assay in mice) that vidarabine may be capable of producing mutagenic effects in male germ cells.

It has also been reported that vidarabine causes chromosome breaks and gaps when added to human leukocytes *in vitro*. While the significance of these effects in terms of mutagenicity is not fully understood, there is a well-known correlation between the ability of various agents to produce such effects and their ability to produce heritable genetic damage.

Pregnancy Category C—VIRA-A parenterally is teratogenic in rats and rabbits. Ten percent VIRA-A ointment applied to 10% of the body surface during organogenesis induced fetal abnormalities in rabbits. When 10% VIRA-A ointment was applied to 2% to 3% of the body surface of rabbits, no fetal abnormalities were found. This dose greatly exceeds the total recommended ophthalmic dose in humans. The possibility of embryonic or fetal damage in pregnant women receiving VIRA-A Ophthalmic Ointment, 3%, is remote. The topical ophthalmic dose is small, and the drug relatively insoluble. Its ocular penetration is very low. However, a safe dose for a human embryo or fetus has not been established. There are no adequate and well controlled studies in pregnant women. VIRA-A should be used during pregnancy only if the potential benefit justifies the potential risk to the fetus.

Nursing Mothers—It is not known whether VIRA-A is secreted in human milk. Because many drugs are excreted in human milk and because of the potential for tumorigenicity shown for VIRA-A in animal studies, a decision should be made whether to discontinue nursing or to discontinue the drug, taking into account the importance of the drug to the mother. However, breast milk excretion is unlikely because VIRA-A is rapidly deaminated in the gastrointestinal tract.

ADVERSE REACTIONS

Lacrimation, foreign body sensation, conjunctival injection, burning, irritation, superficial punctate keratitis, pain, photophobia, punctal occlusion, and sensitivity have been reported with VIRA-A Ophthalmic Ointment, 3%. The following have also been reported but appear disease-related: uveitis, stromal edema, secondary glaucoma, trophic defects, corneal vascularization, and hyphema.

OVERDOSAGE

Acute massive overdosage by oral ingestion of the ophthalmic ointment has not occurred. However, the rapid deamination to arabinosylhypoxanthine should preclude any difficulty. The oral LD_{50} for vidarabine is greater than 5020 mg/kg in mice and rats. No untoward effects should result from ingestion of the entire contents of a tube.

Overdosage by ocular instillation is unlikely because any excess should be quickly expelled from the conjunctival sac. Too frequent administration should be avoided.

DOSAGE AND ADMINISTRATION

Administer approximately one half inch of VIRA-A Ophthalmic Ointment, 3%, into the lower conjunctival sac five times daily at three-hour intervals.

If there are no signs of improvement after 7 days, or complete re-epithelialization has not occurred by 21 days, other forms of therapy should be considered. Some severe cases may require longer treatment.

After re-epithelialization has occurred, treatment for an additional seven days at a reduced dosage (such as twice daily) is recommended in order to prevent recurrence.

HOW SUPPLIED

N 0071-3677-07 (Stock 18-1677-139)

VIRA-A Ophthalmic Ointment, 3%, is supplied sterile in ophthalmic ointment tubes of 3.5 g. The base is a 60:40 mixture of solid and liquid petrolatum.

3677G020

ZARONTIN® ℞

[ză″rŏn′tĭn]

(ethosuximide, USP)

Capsules

DESCRIPTION

Zarontin (ethosuximide) is an anticonvulsant succinimide, chemically designated as alpha-ethyl-alpha-methyl-succinimide, with the following structural formula:

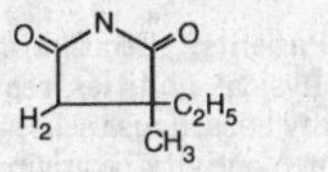

Each Zarontin capsule contains 250 mg ethosuximide, USP. Also contains: polyethylene glycol 400, NF. The capsule contains D&C yellow No. 10; FD&C red No. 3; gelatin, NF; glycerin, USP; and sorbitol.

CLINICAL PHARMACOLOGY

Ethosuximide suppresses the paroxysmal three cycle per second spike and wave activity associated with lapses of consciousness which is common in absence (petit mal) seizures. The frequency of epileptiform attacks is reduced, apparently by depression of the motor cortex and elevation of the threshold of the central nervous system to convulsive stimuli.

INDICATIONS AND USAGE

Zarontin is indicated for the control of absence (petit mal) epilepsy.

CONTRAINDICATION

Ethosuximide should not be used in patients with a history of hypersensitivity to succinimides.

WARNINGS

Blood dyscrasias, including some with fatal outcome, have been reported to be associated with the use of ethosuximide; therefore, periodic blood counts should be performed. Should signs and/or symptoms of infection (eg, sore throat, fever) develop, blood counts should be considered at that point.

Ethosuximide is capable of producing morphological and functional changes in the animal liver. In humans, abnormal liver and renal function studies have been reported.

Ethosuximide should be administered with extreme caution to patients with known liver or renal diseases. Periodic urinalysis and liver function studies are advised for all patients receiving the drug.

Cases of systemic lupus erythematosus have been reported with the use of ethosuximide. The physician should be alert to this possibility.

Usage in Pregnancy: Reports suggest an association between the use of anticonvulsant drugs by women with epilepsy and an elevated incidence of birth defects in children born to these women. Data are more extensive with respect to phenytoin and phenobarbital, but these are also the most commonly prescribed anticonvulsants; less systematic or anecdotal reports suggest a possible similar association with the use of all known anticonvulsant drugs.

The reports suggesting an elevated incidence of birth defects in children of drug-treated epileptic women cannot be regarded as adequate to prove a definite cause and effect relationship. There are intrinsic methodological problems in obtaining adequate data on drug teratogenicity in humans; the possibility also exists that other factors, eg, genetic factors or the epileptic condition itself, may be more important than drug therapy in leading to birth defects. The great majority of mothers on anticonvulsant medication deliver normal infants. It is important to note that anticonvulsant drugs should not be discontinued in patients in whom the drug is administered to prevent major seizures because of the strong possibility of precipitating status epilepticus with attendant hypoxia and threat to life. In individual cases where the severity and frequency of the seizure disorder are such that the removal of medication does not pose a serious threat to the patient, discontinuation of the drug may be considered prior to and during pregnancy, although it cannot be said with any confidence that even minor seizures do not pose some hazard to the developing embryo or fetus.

The prescribing physician will wish to weigh these considerations in treating or counseling epileptic women of childbearing potential.

PRECAUTIONS

General

Ethosuximide, when used alone in mixed types of epilepsy, may increase the frequency of grand mal seizures in some patients.

As with other anticonvulsants, it is important to proceed slowly when increasing or decreasing dosage, as well as when adding or eliminating other medication. Abrupt withdrawal of anticonvulsant medication may precipitate absence (petit mal) status.

Information for Patients

Ethosuximide may impair the mental and/or physical abilities required for the performance of potentially hazardous tasks, such as driving a motor vehicle or other such activity requiring alertness; therefore, the patient should be cautioned accordingly.

Patients taking ethosuximide should be advised of the importance of adhering strictly to the prescribed dosage regimen.

Patients should be instructed to promptly contact their physician if they develop signs and/or symptoms (eg, sore throat, fever) suggesting an infection.

Drug Interactions

Since Zarontin (ethosuximide) may interact with concurrently administered antiepileptic drugs, periodic serum level determinations of these drugs may be necessary (eg, ethosuximide may elevate phenytoin serum levels and valproic acid has been reported to both increase and decrease ethosuximide levels).

Pregnancy

See WARNINGS.

ADVERSE REACTIONS

Gastrointestinal System: Gastrointestinal symptoms occur frequently and include anorexia, vague gastric upset, nausea and vomiting, cramps, epigastric and abdominal pain, weight loss, and diarrhea. There have been reports of gum hypertrophy and swelling of the tongue.

Hemopoietic System: Hemopoietic complications associated with the administration of ethosuximide have included leukopenia, agranulocytosis, pancytopenia, with or without bone marrow suppression, and eosinophilia.

Nervous System: Neurologic and sensory reactions reported during therapy with ethosuximide have included drowsiness, headache, dizziness, euphoria, hiccups, irritability, hyperactivity, lethargy, fatigue, and ataxia. Psychiatric or psychological aberrations associated with ethosuximide administration have included disturbances of sleep, night terrors, inability to concentrate, and aggressiveness. These effects may be noted particularly in patients who have previously exhibited psychological abnormalities. There have been rare reports of paranoid psychosis, increased libido, and increased state of depression with overt suicidal intentions.

Integumentary System: Dermatologic manifestations which have occurred with the administration of ethosuximide have included urticaria, Stevens-Johnson syndrome, systemic lupus erythematosus, pruritic erythematous rashes, and hirsutism.

Special Senses: Myopia.

Genitourinary System: Vaginal bleeding, microscopic hematuria.

OVERDOSAGE

Acute overdoses may produce nausea, vomiting, and CNS depression including coma with respiratory depression. A relationship between ethosuximide toxicity and its plasma levels has not been established. The therapeutic range of serum levels is 40 mcg/mL to 100 mcg/mL, although levels as high as 150 mcg/mL have been reported without signs of toxicity.

Treatment:

Treatment should include emesis (unless the patient is or could rapidly become obtunded, comatose, or convulsing) or gastric lavage, activated charcoal, cathartics and general supportive measures. Hemodialysis may be useful to treat ethosuximide overdose. Forced diuresis and exchange transfusions are ineffective.

DOSAGE AND ADMINISTRATION

Zarontin is administered by the oral route. The *initial* dose for patients 3 to 6 years of age is one capsule (250 mg) per day; for patients 6 years of age and older, 2 capsules (500 mg) per day. The dose thereafter must be individualized according to the patient's response. Dosage should be increased by small increments. One useful method is to increase the daily dose by 250 mg every four to seven days until control is achieved with minimal side effects. Dosages exceeding 1.5 g daily, in divided doses, should be administered only under

Continued on next page

This product information was prepared in August 1992. On these and other Parke-Davis Products, information may be obtained by addressing PARKE-DAVIS, Division of Warner-Lambert Company, Morris Plains, New Jersey 07950.

Parke-Davis—Cont.

the strictest supervision of the physician. The *optimal* dose for most children is 20 mg/kg/day. This dose has given average plasma levels within the accepted therapeutic range of 40 to 100 mcg/mL. Subsequent dose schedules can be based on effectiveness and plasma level determinations.

Zarontin may be administered in combination with other anticonvulsants when other forms of epilepsy coexist with absence (petit mal). The *optimal* dose for most children is 20 mg/kg/day.

HOW SUPPLIED

Zarontin is supplied as:
N 0071-0237-24 Bottles of 100. Each capsule contains 250 mg ethosuximide.
Store below 30°C (86°F).
Zarontin is also supplied as:
N 0071-2418-23—1 pint bottles. Each 5 mL of syrup contains 250 mg ethosuximide in a raspberry flavored base.
Caution—Federal law prohibits dispensing without prescription.

0237G024

Shown in Product Identification Section, page 423

ZARONTIN®   ℞
[ză″rŏn′tĭn]
(ethosuximide)
Syrup

DESCRIPTION

Zarontin (ethosuximide) is an anticonvulsant succinimide, chemically designated as alpha-ethyl-alpha-methyl-succinimide, with the following structural formula:

Each teaspoonful (5 mL), for oral administration, contains 250 mg ethosuximide, USP. Also contains citric acid; anhydrous, USP; FD&C red No. 40; FD&C yellow No. 6; flavor; glycerin, USP; purified water, USP; saccharin sodium, USP; sodium benzoate, NF; sodium citrate, USP; sucrose, NF.

CLINICAL PHARMACOLOGY

Ethosuximide suppresses the paroxysmal three cycle per second spike and wave activity associated with lapses of consciousness which is common in absence (petit mal) seizures. The frequency of epileptiform attacks is reduced, apparently by depression of the motor cortex and elevation of the threshold of the central nervous system to convulsive stimuli.

INDICATION AND USAGE

Zarontin is indicated for the control of absence (petit mal) epilepsy.

CONTRAINDICATIONS

Ethosuximide should not be used in patients with a history of hypersensitivity to succinimides.

WARNINGS

Blood dyscrasias, including some with fatal outcome, have been reported to be associated with the use of ethosuximide; therefore, periodic blood counts should be performed. Should signs and/or symptoms of infection (eg, sore throat, fever) develop, blood counts should be considered at that point. Ethosuximide is capable of producing morphological and functional change in the animal liver. In humans, abnormal liver and renal function studies have been reported. Ethosuximide should be administered with extreme caution to patients with known liver or renal disease. Periodic urinalysis and liver function studies are advised for all patients receiving the drug.

Cases of systemic lupus erythematosus have been reported with the use of ethosuximide. The physician should be alert to this possibility.

Usage in Pregnancy: Reports suggest an association between the use of anticonvulsant drugs by women with epilepsy and an elevated incidence of birth defects in children born to these women. Data are more extensive with respect to phenytoin and phenobarbital, but these are also the most commonly prescribed anticonvulsants; less systematic or anecdotal reports suggest a possible similar association with the use of all known anticonvulsant drugs.

The reports suggesting an elevated incidence of birth defects in children of drug-treated epileptic women cannot be regarded as adequate to prove a definite cause and effect relationship. There are intrinsic methodologic problems in obtaining adequate data on drug teratogenicity in humans; the possibility also exists that other factors, eg. genetic factors or the epileptic condition itself, may be more important than drug therapy in leading to birth defects. The great majority of mothers on anticonvulsant medication deliver normal

infants. It is important to note that anticonvulsant drugs should not be discontinued in patients in whom the drug is administered to prevent major seizures because of the strong possibility of precipitating status epilepticus with attendant hypoxia and threat to life. In individual cases where the severity and frequency of the seizure disorder are such that the removal of medication does not pose a serious threat to the patient, discontinuation of the drug may be considered prior to and during pregnancy, although it cannot be said with any confidence that even minor seizures do not pose some hazard to the developing embryo or fetus.

The prescribing physician will wish to weigh these considerations in treating or counseling epileptic women of childbearing potential.

PRECAUTIONS

General: Ethosuximide, when used alone in mixed types of epilepsy, may increase the frequency of grand mal seizures in some patients.

As with other anticonvulsants, it is important to proceed slowly when increasing or decreasing dosage, as well as when adding or eliminating other medication. Abrupt withdrawal of anticonvulsant medication may precipitate absence (petit mal) status.

Information for Patients: Ethosuximide may impair the mental and/or physical abilities required for the performance of potentially hazardous tasks such as driving a motor vehicle or other such activity requiring alertness; therefore, the patient should be cautioned accordingly.

Patients taking ethosuximide should be advised of the importance of adhering strictly to the prescribed dosage regimen. Patients should be instructed to promptly contact their physician when they develop signs and/or symptoms suggesting an infection (eg, sore throat, fever).

Drug Interactions: Since Zarontin (ethosuximide) may interact with concurrently administered antiepileptic drugs, periodic serum level determinations of both drugs are recommended (ethosuximide may elevate phenytoin serum levels and valproic acid has been reported to both increase and decrease ethosuximide levels).

Pregnancy: See WARNINGS

ADVERSE REACTIONS

Gastrointestinal System: Gastrointestinal symptoms occur frequently and include anorexia, vague gastric upset, nausea and vomiting, cramps, epigastric and abdominal pain, weight loss, and diarrhea. There have been reports of gum hypertrophy and swelling of the tongue.

Hemopoietic System: Hemopoietic complications associated with the administration of ethosuximide have included leukopenia, agranulocytosis, pancytopenia with or without bone marrow suppression, and eosinophilia.

Nervous System: Neurologic and sensory reactions reported during therapy with ethosuximide have included drowsiness, headache, dizziness, euphoria, hiccups, irritability, hyperactivity, lethargy, fatigue, and ataxia.

Psychiatric or psychological aberrations associated with ethosuximide administration have included disturbances of sleep, night terrors, inability to concentrate, and aggressiveness. These effects may be noted particularly in patients who have previously exhibited psychological abnormalities. There have been rare reports of paranoid psychosis, increased libido, and increased state of depression with overt suicidal intentions.

Integumentary System: Dermatologic manifestations which have occurred with the administration of ethosuximide have included urticaria, Stevens-Johnson syndrome, systemic lupus erythematosus, pruritic erythematous rashes, and hirsutism.

Special Senses: Myopia.

Genitourinary System: Vaginal bleeding, microscopic hematuria.

DOSAGE AND ADMINISTRATION

Zarontin is administered by the oral route. The *initial* dose for patients 3 to 6 years of age is one teaspoonful (250 mg) per day; for patients 6 years of age and older, 2 teaspoonfuls (500 mg) per day. The dose thereafter must be individualized according to the patient's response. Dosage should be increased by small increments. One useful method is to increase the daily dose by 250 mg every four to seven days until control is achieved with minimal side effects. Dosages exceeding 1.5 g daily, in divided doses, should be administered only under the strictest supervision of the physician. The *optimal* dose for most children is 20 mg/kg/day. This dose has given average plasma levels within the accepted therapeutic range of 40 to 100 mcg/mL. Subsequent dose schedules can be based on effectiveness and plasma level determinations.

Zarontin may be administered in combination with other anticonvulsants when other forms of epilepsy coexist with absence (petit mal). The optimal dose for most children is 20 mg/kg/day.

OVERDOSAGE

Acute overdoses produce CNS depression including coma with respiratory depression. A relationship between ethosuximide toxicity and its plasma levels has not been estab-

lished. The therapeutic range of serum levels is 40 mcg/mL to 100 mcg/mL, although levels as high as 150 mcg/mL have been reported without signs of toxicity.

Treatment: Treatment should include emesis (unless the patient is, or could rapidly become, obtunded, comatose, or convulsing) or gastric lavage, activated charcoal, cathartics, and general supportive measures. Hemodialysis may be useful to treat ethosuximide overdose. Forced diuresis and exchange transfusions are ineffective.

HOW SUPPLIED

Zarontin is supplied as:
N0071-2418-23—1 pint bottles. Each 5 ml of syrup contains 250 mg ethosuximide in a raspberry flavored base.
Store below 30°C (86°F). Protect from freezing and light.
Zarontin is also supplied in the following form:
N0071-0237-24—Bottles of 100. Each capsule contains 250 mg ethosuximide.
Store below 30°C (86°F).
Caution—Federal law prohibits dispensing without prescription.

2418G024

Pedinol Pharmacal Inc.
30 BANFI PLAZA NORTH
FARMINGDALE, N.Y. 11735

BREEZEE MIST® FOOT POWDER   OTC

COMPOSITION

Actives: Aluminum Chlorhydrate, Menthol, Undecylenic Acid. **Inactives:** Talc, Isobutane, Isopropyl Myristate, Bentone, Propylene Carbonate, Fragrance. Contains no Fluorocarbons.

INDICATIONS

Topical treatment for hyperhidrosis, bromidrosis and tinea pedis (athlete's foot).

HOW SUPPLIED

4 oz. (113g) aerosol can. NDC 00884 0659-04

CASTELLANI PAINT   ℞
CASTELLANI PAINT–Colorless   ℞

COMPOSITION

Actives: 10% Resorcinol, 4.5% Phenol **Inactives:** Alcohol, Acetone, Basic Fuchsin. Purified Water. COLORLESS—Without Basic Fuchsin.

INDICATIONS

Topical antifungal agent for macerations and ulcerations.

PRECAUTIONS

If irritation or sensitivity develops, discontinue treatment and consult podiatrist or physician. **Keep out of reach of children.** Care should be taken to avoid spilling and guard against staining.

ADMINISTRATION

Apply to affected areas once or twice a day.

HOW SUPPLIED

	Bottle Size 1 oz. (29.57 mL)	1 pt. (453.6 mL)
Color	NDC 00884-2878-01	NDC 00884-2878-16
Colorless	NDC 00884-2978-01	NDC 00884-2978-16

CAUTION

Federal law prohibits dispensing without a prescription.

FORMALYDE-10® SPRAY   ℞

INGREDIENTS

Active: 10% Formaldehyde **Inactives:** Water, FDA-40 Alcohol, Polysorbate 20, Fragrance.

INDICATIONS

Anti-perspirant for treatment of hyperhidrosis and bromidrosis. Drying agent for pre and post surgical removal of warts or for non-surgical laser treatment of warts.

CONTRAINDICATIONS

Do not use in patients known to be sensitive to any ingredients in FORMALYDE-10 SPRAY.

PRECAUTION

Check skin for sensitivity to Formaldehyde prior to application since it may be irritating and sensitizing to the skin of some patients. If redness or irritation persists, consult your PODIATRIST, DERMATOLOGIST or PHYSICIAN. **Keep out of reach of children. For external use only.** Avoid contact with eyes or mucous membranes.

DIRECTIONS

Spray on to affected areas once a day or as directed by a PODIATRIST, DERMATOLOGIST or PHYSICIAN. Keep cap tightly closed when not in use.

HOW SUPPLIED

Available in 2 oz. (59.14 mL) plastic spray bottle. NDC 00884 4789-02

CAUTION

Federal law prohibits dispensing without a prescription.

FUNGOID® CREME   ℞
FUNGOID® HC CREME   ℞

COMPOSITION

FUNGOID CREME Actives: 1.0% Triacetin, 1.25% Chloroxylenol, 0.5% Cetyl Pyridinium Chloride; **Inactive:** Vanishing Creme Base
FUNGOID-HC CREME Actives: 1.0% Triacetin, 1.25% Chloroxylenol, 0.5% Cetyl Pyridinium Chloride, 0.5% Hydrocortisone; **Inactive:** Vanishing Creme Base

INDICATIONS

Topical treatment for fungus, yeast, bacterial infections of the skin and anti-inflammatory.

CONTRAINDICATIONS

Do not use on patients known to be sensitive to any ingredients in Fungoid HC Creme.

WARNING

Not for Ophthalmic use.

PRECAUTION

It is prudent to use with clinical caution on patients with diabetes or impaired circulation.
If irritation or sensitivity develops, discontinue treatment and consult your PODIATRIST, DERMATOLOGIST, or PHYSICIAN. **Keep out of the reach of children. For External Use Only.**

ADMINISTRATION

Apply to affected areas twice a day.

HOW SUPPLIED

Available in 1 oz. (28.35g) and 2oz. (56.7g) plastic tubes.
Fungoid Creme—NDC 00884 2448-01 NDC 00884 2448-02
Fungoid-HC Creme—NDC 00884 4187-01 NDC 00884 4187-02

CAUTION

Federal law prohibits dispensing without a prescription.

FUNGOID® SOLUTION   ℞

COMPOSITION

Actives: 12.0% Triacetin, 1.0% Chloroxylenol, 0.2% Cetyl Pyridinium Chloride
Inactive: Oil Base Solution

INDICATIONS

Topical treatment for fungus, yeast and bacterial infections of the skin.

CONTRAINDICATIONS

Do not use on patients sensitive to any of the ingredients in this product.

WARNING

Not for Ophthalmic use.

PRECAUTIONS

It is prudent to use with clinical caution on patients with diabetes or impaired circulation.
If irritation or sensitivity develops, discontinue treatment and consult podiatrist or physician.
Keep out of the reach of children. FOR EXTERNAL USE ONLY.

ADMINISTRATION

Apply to affected areas twice a day.

HOW SUPPLIED

0.5 fl. oz (15 mL) plastic bottle with controlled dropper. NDC 00884 3149-15

CAUTION

Federal law prohibits dispensing without a prescription.

FUNGOID® TINCTURE   ℞

COMPOSITION

Actives: 12.0% Triacetin, 0.5% Chloroxylenol, 1.0% Cetyl Pyridinium Chloride; **Inactives:** Sodium Propionate, Benzalkonium Chloride, Glacial Acetic Acid, Acetone, Alcohol.

INDICATIONS

Topical treatment for fungus infections of the nails, tinea unguium (onychomycosis).

CONTRAINDICATIONS

Do not use on patients sensitive to any of the ingredients in this product.

WARNING

Not for Opthalmic use.

PRECAUTIONS

It is prudent to use with clinical caution on patients with diabetes or impaired circulation.
If irritation or sensitivity develops, discontinue treatment and consult podiatrist or physician.
Keep out of the reach of children. FOR EXTERNAL USE ONLY.

ADMINISTRATION

Debride or avulse nail before applying Fungoid Tincture. Cleanse and dry affected areas. Apply twice a day to affected nail surface, beds, edges and undersurface of the nail using attached brush. Continued usage may be necessary for several months before results are seen.
POST SURGICAL APPLICATION: Apply one week postoperatively and continue for at least four months.

HOW SUPPLIED

1 oz. (29.57 mL) bottle with brush applicator NDC 00884-0248-01, 1 pt. (473.12 mL) bottle NDC 00884 0248-16.
FUNGOID TINCTURE NAIL TREATMENT KIT includes: 1 oz. (29.57 mL) FUNGOID TINCTURE, 2 oz. (56.7g) nail scrub, nail brush. NDC 00884-5490-01.

CAUTION

Federal law prohibits dispensing without a prescription.

G-MYTICIN® CREME and   ℞
OINTMENT 0.1%
(gentamicin sulfate 0.1%)

COMPOSITION

Active: Creme and ointment—each gram contains gentamicin sulfate equivalent to 1 mg. of gentamicin base.

INDICATIONS

Topical wide-spectrum antibiotic provides highly effective treatment in primary and secondary bacterial infections of the skin. *NOTE:* G-myticin Creme/Ointment is not effective against viruses or fungal skin infections.

ADVERSE REACTIONS

In patients with dermatoses treated with G-myticin erythema and pruritis that did not usually require discontinuance of treatment has been reported in a small percentage of cases.

CONTRAINDICATIONS

G-myticin creme/ointment, is contraindicated in those patients with a history of hypersensitivity to any of the components of this preparation.

PRECAUTIONS

The overgrowth of nonsusceptible organisms, including fungi, occasionally occurs with the use of topical antibiotics. If this occurs, or if irritation, sensitization, or superinfection develops, treatment with G-myticin should be discontinued and consult podiatrist or physician.

ADMINISTRATION

Apply 3 to 4 times daily.

HOW SUPPLIED

G-myticin Creme/Ointment—15 gm tubes.
Creme NDC 00884-3684-15
Ointment NDC 00884-3784-15

CAUTION

Federal law prohibits dispensing without a prescription.

HYDRISALIC™ GEL   ℞

COMPOSITION

Active: 60 mg Salicyclic Acid, **Inactives:** Isopropanol, Propylene Glycol, Hydroxypropyl Cellulose.

INDICATIONS

Topical treatment for hyperkeratotic skin.

PRECAUTIONS

Use should be limited in children under 12 years of age. If irritation or sensitivity develops, discontinue treatment and consult podiatrist or physician. For External Use Only.

ADMINISTRATION

Apply to affected area in the evening. Wash hands thoroughly following application. The medication is washed off the following morning.

HOW SUPPLIED

1 oz. (28.35g) plastic tubes. NDC 00884-2242-01

CAUTION

Federal law prohibits dispensing without a prescription.

HYDRISINOL® CREME and LOTION   OTC

COMPOSITION

Active: Sulfonated Hydrogenated Castor Oil, N.F. IX; **Inactive:** Hydrogenated Vegetable Oil.

INDICATIONS

Topical emollient to soften dry, cracked, calloused skin.

ADMINISTRATION

Apply as needed.

HOW SUPPLIED

4 oz. (113.4g) NDC 00884 0142-04 and 1 lb. (453.6g) jars NDC 00884-0142-16;
8 oz. (226.8g) plastic bottle NDC 00884-3042-08.

LACTINOL-E® CREME   ℞
LACTINOL® LOTION   ℞

COMPONENTS

Lactinol-E Creme: Actives: 10% Lactic Acid, Vitamin E 3500 u/oz. **Inactives:** Water, Glyceryl Stearate (and) PEG-100 Stearate, Cetyl Alcohol, Glycerine, PEG-40 Stearate, Caprylic Capric Triglyceride, Lecithin, Dimethicone, EDTA, Methyl Paraben, Propyl Paraben, Diazolidinyl Urea. Sodium Benzoate.
Lactinol Lotion: Active: 10% Lactic Acid. **Inactives:** Water, Isopropyl Palmitate, Cetyl Alcohol, Glyceryl Stearate (and) PEG-100 Stearate, Glycerine, PEG-40 Stearate, Lecithin, Caprylic Capric Triglyceride, Dimethicone, EDTA, Methyl Paraben, Propyl Paraben, Diazolidinyl Urea, Sodium Benzoate.

ACTION

Lactic Acid is reported as an effective naturally occurring humectant in the skin. It has beneficial effects on dry skin and on severe hyperkeratotic conditions. The Vitamin E in Lactinol-E Creme is a healing aid for lesions, keratosis and drying of the skin, enhances regeneration of the skin and revitalizes tissue.

INDICATIONS

Lactinol-E Creme and Lactinol Lotion are indicated for moisturizing and softening dry, scaly skin (xerosis), ichthyosis vulgaris and itching associated with these conditions.

DIRECTIONS

Rub thoroughly twice a day to affected areas or as prescribed by your PODIATRIST, DERMATOLOGIST or PHYSICIAN.

CONTRAINDICATIONS

Not to be used in patients known to be sensitive to any ingredient in Lactinol E Creme or Lactinol Lotion.

PRECAUTIONS

For external use only. Keep out of the reach of children. Avoid contact with eyes, lips, or mucous membranes. A mild, stinging, burning or peeling may occur on sensitive, inflamed or irritated skin areas. If symptoms persist, consult your PODIATRIST, DERMATOLOGIST or PHYSICIAN.

HOW SUPPLIED

Lactinol-E Creme is available in a 2 oz. (56.7g) plastic jar. NDC 00884-4990-02
Lactinol Lotion is available in an 8 oz. (226.8g) bottle. NDC 00884-5292-08
Store at controlled room temperature 15°–30°C (59°–86°F).

CAUTION

Federal law prohibits dispensing without a prescription.

LAZER® CREME   OTC

COMPOSITION

Vitamin E, 3,500 u/oz., Vitamin A, 100,000 u/oz.

INDICATIONS

To aid post surgical regeneration of skin, revitalize lasered tissue, healing aid for post surgical lesions, keratosis and dryness of the skin.

Continued on next page

Pedinol Pharmacal—Cont.

CAUTION

FOR EXTERNAL USE ONLY. Keep out of reach of children. Keep in cool place.

ADMINISTRATION

Apply topically to affected area as often as needed or as directed by your podiatrist or physician.

HOW SUPPLIED

Available in 2 oz. (56.7g) plastic jar. NDC 00884 3886-02

LAZERFORMALYDE® SOLUTION   ℞

COMPOSITION

Active: 10% Formaldehyde. **Inactives:** Polysorbate 20, Mint Fragrance, Hydroxyethyl Cellulose, Water.

INDICATIONS

Drying Agent for pre and post surgical removal of warts or for non-surgical laser treatment of warts. Anti-perspirant for treatment of hyperhidrosis and bromidosis of the feet.

CONTRAINDICATIONS

Do not use in patients known to be sensitive to any ingredients in LazerFormalyde Solution.

PRECAUTION

Check skin for sensitivity to Formaldehyde prior to application since it may be irritating and sensitizing to the skin of some patients. Keep out of the reach of children. FOR EXTERNAL USE ONLY. Avoid contact with eyes or mucous membranes.
If redness or irritation persists, consult your podiatrist or physician. **Keep out of reach of children. For external use only. Avoid contact with eyes or mucous membranes.**

ADMINISTRATION

Apply with **roll-on** applicator once a day to affected areas or as directed by your podiatrist or physician.

HOW SUPPLIED

Available in 3 oz. (88.71 mL) plastic bottle with **roll-on** applicator. NDC 00884 3986-03

CAUTION

Federal law prohibits dispensing without a prescription.

LAZERSPORIN-C® SOLUTION   ℞

COMPOSITION

Actives: Neomycin Sulfate equivalent to 3.5 mg., Polymyxin B Sulfate 10,000 U, Hydrocortisone 1%.

INDICATIONS AND USAGE

For the treatment of superficial bacterial infections of the external auditory canal caused by organisms susceptible to the action of the antibiotics.

CONTRAINDICATIONS

Do not use in patients known to be sensitive to any ingredients in LazerSporin-C Solution.

WARNINGS

As with other antibiotic preparations, prolonged treatment may result in overgrowth of nonsusceptible organisms and fungi. If the infection is not improved after one week, cultures and susceptibility test should be repeated to verify the identity of the organism and to determine whether therapy should be changed.

PRECAUTION

If redness, irritation or pain and swelling persist, discontinue use and consult your physician. **Keep out of reach of children. For external use only.**

ADMINISTRATION

Apply to affected area 3 or 4 times a day or as directed by your physician.

HOW SUPPLIED

10cc bottle with sterile dropper. NDC 00884 4086-10

CAUTION

Federal law prohibits dispensing without a prescription.

NAIL SCRUB™   OTC

INGREDIENTS

Active: 2–6% Sodium Hypochlorite. **Inactives:** Water, Isopropyl Palmitate, Isopropyl Myristate, Mineral Oil, Glyceryl Stearate SE, Propylene Glycol, Lanolin Alcohol, Cetyl Esters, Stearic Acid, Calcium Carbonate, Propylene Glycol

Monostearate, Triethanolamine, Methyl Paraben, Propyl Paraben, DMDM Hydantoin, Diazolidinyl Urea.

INDICATIONS

To cleanse, bleach, debride nail surface prior to use of Fungoid Tincture or Ony-Clear Nail Spray.

DIRECTIONS

Apply to nail surface, scrub briskly with nail brush. Wash off nail, dry and apply Fungoid Tincture or Ony-Clear Nail Spray.

PRECAUTION

If diabetic or have impaired blood circulation, consult your PODIATRIST, DERMATOLOGIST or PHYSICIAN before using. Do not use if sensitive to any of the ingredients.

CAUTION

For external use only. Keep out of reach of children. If redness or irritation occurs, discontinue use and consult your PODIATRIST, DERMATOLOGIST or PHYSICIAN.

HOW SUPPLIED

Available in 2 oz. (56.7g) plastic bottle with applicator tip. NDC 00884 4891-02

ONY–CLEAR® NAIL SPRAY   ℞

INGREDIENTS

Actives: 12.0% Triacetin, 0.5% Chloroxylenol, 1.0% Cetyl Pyridinium Chloride.
Inactives: Glacial Acetic Acid, Sodium Propionate, Propionic Acid, Benzalkonium Chloride, Acetone, Alcohol, Water.

INDICATIONS

A topical spray for treatment of nail fungus, onychomycosis, helps removal of hyperkeratotic or mycotic tissue before debriding nail groove.

CONTRAINDICATIONS

Do not use on patients sensitive to any of the ingredients in this product.

WARNING: Flammable

WARNING: Avoid prolonged contact with skin, or spraying in eyes. Use only as directed. Contents under pressure. Do not store at temperatures above 120°F. Intentional misuse by inhaling the contents can be harmful or fatal.

PRECAUTION

Not to be used by patients known to be sensitive to any ingredient of ONY-CLEAR SPRAY. If signs of irritation appear, discontinue use and consult your PODIATRIST, DERMATOLOGIST or PHYSICIAN. **Keep out of reach of children. For external use only.**

DIRECTIONS

Debride or avulse nail before applying Ony-Clear Nail Spray. Shake Well. Dry affected areas, hold spray 1 or 2 inches away from affected nail, spray for 1 or 2 seconds under the top of the nail, on the nail plate and nail borders twice a day. Wipe excess from surrounding skin. Continued usage may be necessary for several months before results are seen.

HOW SUPPLIED

ONY-CLEAR NAIL SPRAY: 1.5 oz. (42.5g) NDC 00884 4889-45.
ONY-CLEAR NAIL SPRAY KIT includes: Ony-Clear nail spray 1.5 oz (42.5g), nail scrub 2 oz. (56.7g), nail brush NDC 00884 5590-45.

CAUTION

Federal law prohibits dispensing without a prescription.

OSTI–DERM®   OTC

COMPOSITION

Actives: Aluminum Sulfate 14.5 mg, Phenol 10 mg.
Inactives: Glycerin, Sorbitol, Zinc Oxide, Magnesium Carbonate, Bentonite, Silica, Acetic Acid, Polysorbate 20, Propylene Glycol Alginate, Calcium Carbonate, Camphor, Iron Oxides, Fragrance and Purified Water.

INDICATIONS

Topical treatment for bromidosis, hyperhidrosis, decubitus ulcers, blisters, itching, poison ivy and dermatitis.

PRECAUTIONS

Check skin sensitivity to phenol. If irritation or sensitivity develops, discontinue treatment and consult podiatrist or physician. **For External Use Only.**

ADMINISTRATION

Apply 2–3 times a day.

HOW SUPPLIED

1.5 oz. (42.5g) jar. NDC 00884 2051-45

PEDI–BORO® SOAK PAKS   OTC

COMPOSITION

Active: Each pak, 2.7 gm contains 220.5 mg AL (Aluminum SULFATE).
325.3 mg Ca (Calcium Acetate), Coloring Agent.

ACTIONS

A soothing astringent wet dressing of a modified Burow's Solution, buffered.

DOSAGE AND ADMINISTRATION

Dissolve 1 or 2 paks in a pint of water. Prepare fresh daily.

HOW SUPPLIED

Box of 12's NDC 00884 1773-27
Box of 100's NDC 00884 1773-10

PEDI–DRI® FOOT POWDER   ℞

COMPOSITION

Actives: 2.5% Aluminum Chlorhydroxide, 1.0% Menthol, 0.5% Zinc Undecylenate, 0.5% Formaldehyde.
Inactives: Corn starch, micro kaolin.

INDICATIONS

Topical treatment for hyperhidrosis, bromidrosis and tinea pedis (athlete's foot).

CONTRAINDICATIONS

Do not use in patients known to be sensitive to any ingredients in Pedi-Dri Foot Powder.

PRECAUTIONS

External use only. Keep out of reach of children. Check for skin sensitivity to formaldehyde. If irritation or sensitivity develops, discontinue treatment and consult podiatrist or physician.

ADMINISTRATION

Apply twice a day.

HOW SUPPLIED

2 oz. (56.7g) plastic bottle. NDC 00884 0349-02

CAUTION

Federal law prohibits dispensing without a prescription.

PEDI–PRO® FOOT POWDER   OTC

COMPOSITION

Actives: 2.5% Aluminum Chlorhydroxide, 1.0% Chloroxylenol, 0.5% Zinc Undecylenate, 1.0% Menthol
Inactives: Micro-Kaolin, Starch

INDICATIONS

Athlete's Foot: Aids in temporary relief of burning, itching and cracking skin in athlete's foot.

CONTRAINDICATIONS

Do not use in patients known to be sensitive to any ingredients in Pedi-Pro Foot Powder.

CAUTION

External use only. Do not use near eyes or mucous membranes. **Keep out of reach of children.** Persons with impaired circulation, including diabetes, should consult a podiatrist or physician before using medication. If symptoms persist consult your podiatrist or physician.

ADMINISTRATION

Apply twice a day as needed.

HOW SUPPLIED

2 oz. (56.7g) plastic bottle. NDC 00884 3584-02

SALACTIC® FILM
SAL–PLANT® GEL   OTC

INGREDIENTS

Actives: Salicylic Acid U.S.P. 17.0% in flexible collodion.
Inactives: Coloring Agent.

INDICATIONS

For the removal of common warts. The common wart is easily recognized by the rough cauliflower-like appearance of the surface.
For the removal of plantar warts on the bottom of the foot. The plantar wart is recognized by its location only on the bottom of the foot, its tenderness and the interruption of the footprint pattern.

WARNINGS

FOR EXTERNAL USE ONLY. Do not use this product on irritated skin, on any area that is infected or reddened, if you are a diabetic, or if you have poor blood circulation. If discom-

fort persists, consult your PODIATRIST, DERMATOLOGIST or PHYSICIAN. Do not use on moles, birthmarks, warts with hair growing from them, genital warts, or warts on the face or mucous membranes. **Keep out of the reach of children.**

If product gets into the eye, flush with water for 15 minutes. Avoid inhaling vapors.

FLAMMABLE.

Extremely Flammable. Keep away from fire or flame. Cap tube tightly and store at room temperature away from heat.

DIRECTIONS

Soak wart in warm water for 5 minutes. Dry area thoroughly. Apply one drop at a time to sufficiently cover each wart. Let dry. Repeat this procedure once or twice daily as needed (until wart is removed) for up to 12 weeks.

HOW SUPPLIED

Salactic Film available in 0.5 oz (15 mL) bottle with brush applicator. NDC 00884-2592-15

Sal-Plant Gel available in a 0.5 oz (14g) tube with tip applicator. NDC 00884 5192-15

UREACIN®–10 LOTION   OTC
UREACIN®–20 CREME   OTC
UREACIN®–40 CREME   ℞

COMPOSITION

Ureacin-10 Lotion: Active: 10% Urea, **Inactives:** Mineral Oil, Propylene Glycol, Stearate SE, Cetyl Esters, Magnesium Aluminum Silicate, Petrolatum, Beeswax, Hydrogenated Vegetable Oil, Lanolin, Triethanolamine, Propyl Paraben, Sodium Borate, Methyl Paraben. Lactic Acid.

Ureacin-20 Creme: Active: 20% Urea, **Inactives:** Water, Lactic Acid, TEA-Stearate, Mineral Oil, Peg-2 Stearate, Glycerin, Sodium Borate, Methyl Paraben, Propyl Paraben, EDTA.

Ureacin-40 Creme: Active: 40% Urea (400 mg). **Inactives:** Glyceryl Stearate SE, Glycerin, Octyldodecyl Stearoyl Stearate, Cetyl Esters, Myristyl Myristate. **Preservatives:** Methylparaben and Propylparaben.

INDICATIONS

Ureacin-10 Lotion, Ureacin-20 Creme is a topical treatment for rough, dry, cracked, calloused skin. Ureacin-40 Creme is indicated for the treatment of nail destruction and dissolution.

CONTRAINDICATIONS

Do not use on patients known to be sensitive to any ingredients in Ureacin-10, -20, or -40.

PRECAUTIONS

If irritation or sensitivity develops, discontinue treatment and consult podiatrist or physician. **For External Use Only. Keep out of the reach of children.**

ADMINISTRATION

Rub in gently twice a day to affected area. **Ureacin-40 Creme to be applied to diseased nail surface only by a podiatrist or physician.**

HOW SUPPLIED

Ureacin®-10, 8 oz. (226.8g) plastic bottle NDC 00884 3249-08, Ureacin®-20, 2½ oz. (70.875g) plastic jar NDC 00884-0449-03, Ureacin®-40, 1 oz. (28.35g) plastic jar NDC 00884-3349-01.

For further product information please contact Pedinol Pharmacal Inc.

CAUTION

For Ureacin-40 Creme—Federal law prohibits dispensing without a prescription.

Persōn & Covey, Inc.
P.O. Box 25018
GLENDALE, CA 91221-5018

AQUANIL™ LOTION   OTC
Lipid-free cleanser for sensitive skin
Non-comedogenic

DIRECTIONS

Apply a generous amount of Aquanil to the skin and gently rub, resulting in a lather. Remove the excess with a soft tissue or cloth.

CONTAINS

Purified Water, U.S.P., Glycerin, Cetyl Alcohol, Stearyl Alcohol, Benzyl Alcohol, Sodium Laureth Sulfate, Xanthan Gum.

INDICATIONS

AQUANIL™ provides gentle, complete cleansing for sensitive skin which cannot tolerate the irritating action of soaps.

Aquanil is specially formulated to be free of oils and is particularly useful in such conditions as atopic dermatitis, atopic eczema, diaper dermatitis and other eczemas. Aquanil, with its emollient effect, provides a softening action to sensitive, traumatized skin, as it cleanses. Aquanil contains no fats of any type.

HOW SUPPLIED

Plastic bottles, 8 and 16 fl oz. (NDC 0096-0724-08, 0096-0724-16).

DHS™ HAIR CARE PRODUCTS   OTC

Formulated for the therapeutic needs of the dermatologist.

DHS™ Conditioning Rinse•†

Helps make hair easier to comb and manage, while adding lustre and body.

DIRECTIONS

Shampoo and rinse well (We suggest DHS™ Shampoo). Apply a generous amount of DHS™ Conditioning Rinse and work evenly through the hair for 60 seconds. Rinse with warm water for 30 seconds.

CONTAINS

Purified water, U.S.P., glyceryl stearate, quaternium-31, panthenol, cetearyl alcohol, dimethicone copolyol, fragrance, FD&C Yellow #6.

HOW SUPPLIED

Plastic bottle, 8 fl. oz. (NDC 0096-0726-08).

DHS™ Shampoo•†

For routine daily hair and scalp cleansing.

DIRECTIONS

Wet hair thoroughly; apply a liberal supply of DHS™ Shampoo, and massage into a lather. Rinse thoroughly and repeat application. Repeat as necessary, or as directed by your physician.

CONTAINS

Purified water, U.S.P., TEA-lauryl sulfate, sodium chloride, PEG-8 distearate, cocamide DEA, cocamide MEA, fragrance and FD&C yellow #6.

HOW SUPPLIED

Plastic bottles, 8 and 16 fl. oz. (NDC 0096-0727-08 and 0096-0727-16).

DHS™ Clear Shampoo•†

A fragrance-free and color-free shampoo designed for routine, gentle, daily hair and scalp cleansing for patients with sensitive skin.

DIRECTIONS

Wet hair thoroughly; apply DHS Clear, lather and rinse. Repeat as necessary, or as directed by your physician.

CONTAINS

Purified Water, U.S.P., TEA-Lauryl Sulfate, Sodium Chloride, PEG-8 Distearate, Cocamide DEA and Cocamide MEA.

HOW SUPPLIED

Plastic bottles, 8 and 16 fl. oz. (NDC 0096-0725-08 and 0096-0725-16).

DHS™ Tar Shampoo and
DHS™ Tar Gel Shampoo (Scented)•†

Aids in the control of the scaling of seborrhea (dandruff) and psoriasis of the scalp.

DIRECTIONS

Wet hair thoroughly; apply a liberal quantity of DHS™ Tar Shampoo and massage into a lather. Rinse thoroughly and repeat application. Allow lather to remain on scalp for about 5 minutes. Use DHS™ Tar Shampoo once or twice weekly, or as directed by your physician.

CONTAINS

Tar, equivalent to 0.5% Coal Tar U.S.P., TEA-lauryl sulfate, purified water, U.S.P., sodium chloride, PEG-8 distearate, cocamide DEA, cocamide MEA, citric acid. DHS™ Tar Gel Shampoo also contains: Hydroxypropyl methylcellulose and fragrance.

HOW SUPPLIED

Plastic bottles. DHS™ Tar Shampoo, 4, 8 and 16 fl. oz. (NDC 0096-0728-04, 0096-0728-08, 0096-0728-16). DHS™ Tar Gel Shampoo 8 fl. oz. (NDC 0096-0730-08).

DHS™ Zinc Dandruff Shampoo•†
2% Zinc Pyrithione

Aids in the control of dandruff/seborrheic dermatitis of the scalp.

---

* Caution: Avoid contact with the eyes. In case of contact, wash out with water. If irritation occurs, discontinue use and consult physician.

† Warning: For external use only. Keep out of the reach of children.

DIRECTIONS

Shake well before using. Wet hair thoroughly; apply a liberal quantity of DHS™ Zinc Shampoo and massage into a lather. Rinse thoroughly and repeat application. Allow lather to remain on scalp for about 5 minutes. Use DHS™ Zinc Shampoo at least twice weekly for the first two weeks, then regularly thereafter, or as directed by your physician.

CONTAINS

2% zinc pyrithione, purified water, U.S.P., TEA-lauryl sulfate, PEG-8 distearate, sodium chloride, cocamide DEA, cocamide MEA, magnesium aluminum silicate, hydroxypropyl methylcellulose, fragrance and FD&C yellow #6.

HOW SUPPLIED

Plastic bottles, 6 and 12 fl. oz. (NDC 0096-0729-06, 0096-0729-12).

DML™ FACIAL MOISTURIZER   OTC
Moisturizer with Sunscreen (SPF 15)
Hyaluronic Acid
Non-comedogenic
Fragrance Free

INDICATION

Soothes and heals dry, sensitive skin. Helps to relieve itching and irritation resulting from environmental toxins and the use of chemicals on the face. Contains sunscreen agents with an SPF of 15 to protect from damaging effects of sunlight (UVA & UVB).

DIRECTIONS

Apply to face as needed or as directed by your dermatologist. It acts as a base for makeup.

CAUTION

For external use only. Avoid contact with eyes. Keep out of reach of children.

CONTENTS

Octyl Methoxycinnamate 8%, Oxybenzone USP 4%, Purified Water, Propylene Glycol Dioctanoate, Petrolatum USP, Glycerin, Cetyl Phosphate (and) DEA-Cetyl Phosphate, Glyceryl Stearate (and) PEG-100 Stearate, Stearic Acid, Hyaluronic Acid, Benzyl Alcohol, Dimethicone, PVP/Eicosene Copolymer, Sodium Carbomer 941, Disodium EDTA, Magnesium Aluminum Silicate.

HOW SUPPLIED

Plastic tube, 1½ oz.   (NDC 0096-0721-45)

DML™   OTC
Moisturizer and Skin Lubricant
Fragrance Free
Non-comedogenic

CONTAINS

Purified water U.S.P., petrolatum, glycerin, methyl glucose sesquistearate, dimethicone, methyl gluceth-20 sesquistearate, benzyl alcohol, volatile silicone, glyceryl stearate, stearic acid, palmitic acid, cetyl alcohol, xanthan gum, magnesium aluminum silicate, carbomer 941, sodium hydroxide.

HOW SUPPLIED

Plastic bottles, 8 and 16 fl. oz.
(NDC 0096-0722-08, 0096-0722-16).

DIRECTIONS

Apply as often as needed, or as directed by physician.

CAUTION

Avoid contact with the eyes. In case of contact, wash out with water. If irritation occurs, discontinue use and consult physician.

WARNING

For external use only. Keep out of the reach of children.

DML™ FORTE Cream   OTC

A fragrance-free formulation to treat severe, recalcitrant dry skin.

DIRECTIONS

Apply as often as needed, or as directed by physician.

HOW SUPPLIED

Plastic tube, 4 oz. NDC 0096-0720-04

CONTAINS

Purified Water, U.S.P., Petrolatum U.S.P., PPG-2 Myristyl Ether Propionate; Glyceryl Stearate; Glycerin; Stearic Acid; D-Panthenol; DEA-Cetyl Phosphate; Simethicone U.S.P.; PVP Eicosene Copolymer; Benzyl Alcohol; Cetyl Alcohol;

Continued on next page

Persōn & Covey—Cont.

Silica; Disodium EDTA; BHA; Magnesium Aluminum Silicate; Sodium Carbomer 1342.

CAUTION
Avoid contact with the eyes. In case of contact, wash out with water. If irritation occurs, discontinue use and consult physician.

WARNING
For external use only. Keep out of the reach of children.

DRYSOL™   ℞

A Solution of:
Aluminum Chloride (Hexahydrate) 20% w/v in Anhydrous Ethyl Alcohol (S.D. Alcohol 40) 93% v/v.

INDICATION
An aid in the management of hyperhidrosis.

DIRECTIONS
Apply Drysol™ to the affected area once a day, **only at bedtime.** To help prevent irritation, the area should be completely dry prior to application. Do not apply Drysol to broken, irritated or recently shaved skin.

FOR MAXIMUM EFFECT
Your doctor may instruct you to cover the treated area with saran wrap held in place by a snug fitting "T" or body shirt, mitten or sock. (Never hold saran in place with tape.) Wash the treated area the following morning. Excessive sweating may be stopped after two or more treatments. Thereafter, apply Drysol™ once or twice weekly or as needed.

NOTICE
Drysol™ may produce a burning or prickling sensation. Keep cap tightly closed when not in use to prevent evaporation.

WARNING
For external use only. Keep out of the reach of children. Avoid contact with the eyes. If irritation or sensitization occurs, discontinue use or consult with a physician. Drysol™ may be harmful to certain metals and fabrics. Keep away from open flame.

HOW SUPPLIED
37.5 cc polyethylene bottle (NDC 0096-0707-37) and 35 cc bottle with Dab-O-Matic applicator head (NDC 0096-0707-35).

SOLBAR® SPF 15 SUNSCREENS   OTC

SOLBAR® SPF 15 Sunscreens are specially formulated to provide maximum protection from the sun's burning and tanning rays. Provides substantial broad spectrum protection from UVA and UVB light for sun sensitive and fair skinned persons. Fragrance-free formula. Liberal and regular use of these products over the years may help reduce the chance of premature aging of the skin and skin cancer.

SOLBAR® PF 15 LIQUID†*+

CONTAINS
Octyl methoxycinnamate 7.5%, Oxybenzone USP 6%, SD alcohol 40, 76%.

HOW SUPPLIED
Plastic bottle, 4 oz. (NDC 0096-0684-04).

WARNING
Keep away from open flame.

SOLBAR® PF 15 CREAM†*+

CONTAINS
Octyl methoxycinnamate 7.5%, Oxybenzone USP 5%.

HOW SUPPLIED
Plastic tube, 2.5 oz. (NDC 0096-0682-75).

SOLBAR® PLUS 15 CREAM†*+

CONTAINS
Oxybenzone USP 4%, Dioxybenzone USP 2%, Octyl dimethyl PABA 6%.

HOW SUPPLIED
Plastic tube, 4 oz. (NDC 0096-0681-04).

† Directions: Apply liberally on all exposed skin. To ensure maximum protection, reapply after swimming or exercise.
* Caution: If irritation or sensitization occurs, discontinue use and consult a physician. Avoid contact with the eyes.
+ Warning: For external use only. Keep out of the reach of children.

SOLBAR® PF ULTRA CREAM SPF 50   OTC
Ultra protection sunscreen
Broad Spectrum UVA and UVB protection

DIRECTIONS
Apply liberally to all exposed areas before sun exposure. Massage in gently. Reapply to dry skin after prolonged sunning, swimming, excessive perspiration or towel drying. Repeated applications during prolonged sun exposure are recommended.

CONTAINS
Oxybenzone USP, Octyl Methoxycinnamate, Octocrylene

INDICATIONS
SOLBAR® PF 50 Cream is specially formulated for ultra protection from the sun's burning and tanning rays. Oxybenzone enhances protection from UVA and UVB light which is particularly important to photosensitive or photoallergic people. Waterproof formula maintains sunburn protection up to 80 minutes in water. Liberal and regular use of this product over the years may help reduce the chance of premature aging of the skin and skin cancer.

CAUTION
For external use only, not to be swallowed. If irritation or sensitization occurs, discontinue use and consult a physician. Avoid contact with the eyes. In case of contact, rinse eyes with water. Keep this and all drugs out of reach of children.

HOW SUPPLIED
Plastic bottle, 4oz. (NDC 0096-0686-04).

SOLBAR® PF ULTRA LIQUID SPF 30   OTC
Ultra protection sunscreen
Broad Spectrum UVA and UVB protection

DIRECTIONS
Apply liberally by spreading to all exposed areas before sun exposure. To ensure maximum protection, reapply to dry skin after prolonged sunning, swimming, excessive perspiration or towel drying. Repeated applications during prolonged sun exposure are recommended.

CONTAINS
Octocrylene, Octyl Methoxycinnamate, Oxybenzone and SD Alcohol 40.

INDICATIONS
SOLBAR PF 30 LIQUID is specially formulated for ultra protection from the sun's burning and tanning rays. Oxybenzone enhances the protection from long wave ultraviolet which is particularly important to photosensitive or photoallergic people.

FRAGRANCE FREE
Liberal and regular use of this product over the years may help reduce the chance of premature aging of the skin and skin cancer.

CAUTION
For external use only, not to be swallowed. If irritation or sensitization occurs, discontinue use and consult a physician. Avoid contact with the eyes. In case of contact, rinse eyes with water. Keep away from open flame. Keep this and all drugs out of reach of children. Use on children under two years of age only with the advice of a physician.

HOW SUPPLIED
Plastic bottle, 3.8 oz. (NDC 0096-0685-04)

XERAC™ AC   ℞
Aluminum Chloride Hexahydrate in
Anhydrous Ethyl Alcohol

DESCRIPTION
A solution of Aluminum Chloride (Hexahydrate) 6.25% (w/v) in Anhydrous Ethyl Alcohol (S.D. Alcohol 40) 96% (v/v).

INDICATION
For topical application as an antiperspirant (anhidrotic).

DIRECTIONS
Apply Xerac™ AC to the axillae at bedtime or as directed by physician. To help prevent irritation, the area should be completely dry prior to application. Do not apply Xerac AC to broken or irritated skin. Keep container tightly closed.

ADVERSE REACTIONS
Transient stinging or itching may occur. It is not evidence of contact sensitivity and may be prevented or reduced by applying Xerac™ AC only to skin which is completely dry or by removing the solution with soap and water.

WARNING
For External Use Only. Some users of this product will experience skin irritation. If this occurs, discontinue use. Avoid contact with the eyes. This product may be harmful to certain metals and fabrics. Keep the container tightly closed when not in use to prevent evaporation. Keep this and all medication out of the reach of children. Do not use near open flame.

HOW SUPPLIED
In bottles with Dab-O-Matic applicator head. 35 cc (NDC 0096-0709-35) and 60 cc (NDC 0096-0709-60).

XERAC™ BP5   OTC
XERAC™ BP10
(benzoyl peroxide water gel)

For the treatment of acne. XERAC™ BP5 and XERAC™ BP10 help dry and clear acne blemishes, reduce blackheads and prevent the development of new acne lesions.

XERAC™ BP5†*+

CONTAINS
5% benzoyl peroxide, laureth-4, carbomer-934, triethanolamine, disodium EDTA, purified water U.S.P.

HOW SUPPLIED
Plastic tubes, 1½ oz. and 3 oz. (NDC 0096-0790-45 and 0096-0790-90)

XERAC™ BP10†*+

CONTAINS
10% benzoyl peroxide, laureth-4, carbomer-934, triethanolamine, disodium EDTA.

HOW SUPPLIED
Plastic tubes, 1½ oz. and 3 oz. (NDC 0096-0791-45 and 0096-0791-90).

† Directions: Cleanse the skin thoroughly before applying medication. Cover the entire affected area with a thin layer one to three times daily. Because excessive drying of the skin may occur, start with one application daily, then gradually increase to two or three times daily, or as directed by a physician.
* Caution: Persons with very sensitive skin, or known allergy to benzoyl peroxide should not use this medication. If uncomfortable irritation, or excessive dryness and/or peeling occurs, reduce frequency of use. If excessive itching, redness, burning or swelling occurs, discontinue use and consult a physician. Keep away from eyes, lips and other mucous membranes. May bleach hair or dyed fabrics.
+ Warning: For external use only. Keep out of the reach of children.

Pfizer Consumer Health Care
Division of Pfizer Inc
100 JEFFERSON ROAD
PARSIPPANY, NJ 07054

BEN-GAY® EXTERNAL   OTC
[ben-gā¹]
ANALGESIC PRODUCTS

(See PDR For Nonprescription Drugs.)

BONINE®   OTC
(Meclizine hydrochloride)
Chewable Tablets

ACTION
BONINE (meclizine) is an H_1 histamine receptor blocker of the piperazine side chain group. It exhibits its action by an effect on the Central Nervous System (CNS), possibly by its ability to block muscarinic receptors in the brain.

INDICATIONS
BONINE is effective in the management of nausea, vomiting and dizziness associated with motion sickness.

CONTRAINDICATIONS
Asthma, glaucoma, emphysema, chronic pulmonary disease, shortness of breath, difficulty in breathing, or difficulty in urination due to enlargement of the prostate gland unless directed by a doctor.

WARNINGS
May cause drowsiness; alcohol, sedatives and tranquilizers may increase the drowsiness effect. Avoid alcoholic beverages while taking this product. Do not take this product if you are taking sedatives or tranquilizers without first con-

sulting your doctor. Do not drive or operate dangerous machinery while taking this medication.

Usage in Children:

Clinical studies establishing safety and effectiveness in children have not been done; therefore, usage is not recommended in children under 12 years of age.

Usage in Pregnancy:

As with any drug, if you are pregnant or nursing a baby, seek advice of a health care professional before taking this product.

ADVERSE REACTIONS

Drowsiness, dry mouth, and on rare occasions, blurred vision have been reported.

DOSAGE AND ADMINISTRATION

For motion sickness, take one or two tablets of BONINE once daily, one hour before travel starts, for up to 24 hours of protection against motion sickness. The tablet can be chewed with or without water or swallowed whole with water. Thereafter, the dose may be repeated every 24 hours for the duration of the travel.

HOW SUPPLIED

BONINE (meclizine HCl) is available in convenient packets of 8 chewable tablets of 25 mg. meclizine HCl.

INACTIVE INGREDIENTS

FD&C Red #40, Lactose, Magnesium Stearate, Purified Siliceous Earth, Raspberry Flavor, Saccharin Sodium, Starch, Talc.

DESITIN® OINTMENT   OTC

[des "i-tin ']

(See PDR For Nonprescription Drugs.)

RHEABAN®Maximum Strength   OTC
TABLETS

[rē 'ă-ban]

(attapulgite)

(See PDR For Nonprescription Drugs.)

RID® Spray   OTC
Lice Control Spray

PRODUCT OVERVIEW

KEY FACTS

Rid Lice Control Spray is a pediculicide spray for controlling lice and louse eggs on inanimate objects, to help prevent reinfestation. It contains a highly active synthetic pyrethroid that kills lice and their eggs on inanimate objects.

MAJOR USES

Rid Lice Control Spray effectively kills lice and louse eggs on garments, bedding, furniture and other inanimate objects that cannot be either laundered or dry cleaned.

SAFETY INFORMATION

Rid Lice Control Spray is intended for use on inanimate objects only; it is not for use on humans or animals. It is harmful if swallowed. It should not be sprayed in the eyes or on the skin and should not be inhaled. The product should be used only in well ventilated areas; room(s) should be vacated after treatment and ventilated before reoccupying.

PRESCRIBING INFORMATION

RID® Spray
Lice Control Spray

THIS PRODUCT IS NOT FOR USE ON HUMANS OR ANIMALS

ACTIVE INGREDIENT

Permethrin*	0.5%
Inert Ingredients	99.5%
	100.00%

*(3-phenoxyphenol)methyl ± cis/trans 3-(2,2-dichloroethenyl) 2,2-dimethylcyclopropane-carboxylate, cis/trans ratio: Minimum 35% (± cis) and maximum 65% (± trans).

ACTIONS

A highly active synthetic pyrethroid for the control of lice and louse eggs on garments, bedding, furniture and other inanimate objects.

WARNINGS

Avoid contamination of feed and foodstuffs. Cover or remove fishbowls. HARMFUL IF SWALLOWED. This product is not for use on humans or animals. If lice infestations should occur on humans, consult either your physician or pharmacist for a product for use on humans.

PHYSICAL AND CHEMICAL HAZARDS

Contents under pressure. Do not use or store near heat or open flame. Do not puncture or incinerate container. Exposure to temperatures above 130° F may cause bursting. Store in cool, dry area. Do not store below 32° F.

CAUTION: Avoid spraying in eyes. Avoid breathing spray mist. Use only in well ventilated areas. Avoid contact with skin. In case of contact wash immediately with soap and water. Vacate room after treatment and ventilate before reoccupying.

Statement of Practical Treatment:

If inhaled: Remove affected person to fresh air. Apply artificial respiration if indicated.

If in eyes: Flush with plenty of water. Contact physician if irritation persists.

If on skin: Wash affected areas immediately with soap and water.

DIRECTION FOR USE

It is a violation of Federal law to use this product in a manner inconsistent with its labeling.

Shake well before each use. Remove protective cap. Aim spray opening away from person. Push button to spray.

To kill lice and louse eggs: Spray in an inconspicuous area to test for possible staining or discoloration. Inspect again after drying, then proceed to spray entire area to be treated. Hold container upright with nozzle away from you. Depress valve and spray from a distance of 8 to 10 inches.

Spray each square foot for 3 seconds. Spray only those garments, parts of bedding, including mattresses and furniture that cannot be either laundered or dry cleaned.

Allow all sprayed articles to dry thoroughly before use. Repeat treatment as necessary.

Buyer assumes all risks of use, storage or handling of this material not in strict accordance with direction given herewith.

DISPOSAL OF CONTAINER

Wrap container and dispose of in trash. Do not incinerate or puncture.

HOW SUPPLIED

5 ounce aerosol can.

Also available in combination with RID® Lice Killing Shampoo as the RID® Lice Elimination Kit.

RID®   OTC
Lice Killing Shampoo

PRODUCT OVERVIEW

KEY FACTS

The Rid Lice Killing Shampoo contains a liquid pediculicide effective against head, body, and pubic lice and their eggs. The active ingredients in Rid are pyrethrins, which attack the louse's nervous system and piperonyl butoxide, a synergist. Rid rinses out completely after treatment and its active ingredients are poorly absorbed through the skin. Each Rid Lice Killing Shampoo package also contains an exclusive nit removal comb that removes all nits.

MAJOR USES

Rid has proved to be clinically effective in treating infestations of head lice, body lice, and pubic (crab) lice and their eggs.

SAFETY INFORMATION

Rid should be used with caution by ragweed sensitized persons. It is intended for external use only and is harmful if swallowed. It should not be inhaled or allowed to come in contact with the eyes or mucous membranes. Contamination of feed or foodstuffs should be avoided.

PRESCRIBING INFORMATION

RID®
Lice Killing Shampoo

DESCRIPTION

Rid contains a liquid pediculicide whose active ingredients are: pyrethrins 0.3% and piperonyl butoxide, technical 3.00%, equivalent to 2.4% (butylcarbityl) (6-propylpiperonyl) ether and to 0.6% related compounds. Inert ingredients 96.7%.

ACTIONS

RID kills head lice (*Pediculus humanus capitis*), body lice (*Pediculus humanus humanus*), and pubic or crab lice (*Phthirus pubis*), and their eggs.

The pyrethrins act as a contact poison and affect the parasite's nervous system, resulting in paralysis and death. The efficacy of the pyrethrins is enhanced by the synergist, piperonyl butoxide. Rid rinses out completely after treatment and is not designed to leave long-acting residues. The active ingredients in RID are poorly absorbed through the skin. Of the relatively minor amounts that are absorbed, they are rapidly metabolized to water-soluble compounds and elimi-

nated from the body without ill effects. RID works faster than other OTC pediculicides.

INDICATIONS

RID is indicated for the treatment of infestations of head lice, body lice and pubic (crab) lice and their eggs.

WARNING

RID should be used with caution by ragweed sensitized persons.

PRECAUTIONS

This product is for external use only. It is harmful if swallowed. It should not be inhaled. It should be kept out of the eyes and contact with mucous membranes should be avoided. If accidental contact with eyes occurs, flush immediately with water. In case of infection or skin irritation, discontinue use and consult a physician. Consult a physician if infestation of eyebrows or eyelashes occurs. Avoid contamination of feed or foodstuffs.

STORAGE AND DISPOSAL

Do not store below 32°F (0°C). Do not reuse empty container. Wrap in several layers of newspaper and discard in trash.

DOSAGE AND ADMINISTRATION

(1) Shake well. Apply undiluted RID to dry hair and scalp or to any other infested area until entirely wet. Do not use on eyelashes or eyebrows. (2) Allow RID to remain on area for 10 minutes but no longer. (3) Wash thoroughly with warm water and soap or shampoo. (4) Dead lice and eggs should be removed with special nit comb provided. (5) Repeat treatment in 7 to 10 days to kill any newly hatched lice. Do not exceed two consecutive applications within 24 hours.

Since lice infestations are spread by contact, each family member should be examined carefully. If infested, he or she should be treated promptly to avoid spread or reinfestation of previously treated individuals. Contaminated clothing and other articles, such as hats, etc., should be dry cleaned, boiled or otherwise treated until decontaminated to prevent reinfestation or spread.

HOW SUPPLIED

In 2, 4 and 8 fl. oz. plastic bottles. Exclusive nit removal comb that removes all the nits and patient instruction booklet (English and Spanish) are included in each package of RID. Also available in combination with RID Lice Control Spray as the RID Lice Elimination Kit.

UNISOM WITH PAIN RELIEF®   OTC

[yu 'na-som]
(previously marketed as
Unisom Dual Relief)
Nighttime Sleep Aid and Pain Reliever

PRODUCT OVERVIEW

KEY FACTS

Unisom With Pain Relief (diphenhydramine sleep aid/acetaminophen pain relief formula) is a product with a dual antihistamine sleep aid/analgesic action to utilize the sedative effects of an antihistamine and relieve mild to moderate pain that may disturb normal sleep patterns. If patients have difficulty in falling asleep but are not experiencing pain at the same time, regular Unisom Sleep Aid which contains doxylamine succinate is indicated.

MAJOR USES

One Unisom With Pain Relief is indicated 30 minutes before retiring to help reduce difficulty in falling asleep while relieving accompanying minor aches and pains, such as headache, muscle aches or menstrual discomfort.

SAFETY INFORMATION

Unisom With Pain Relief is contraindicated in patients with asthma, glaucoma, emphysema, chronic pulmonary disease, shortness of breath, difficulty in breathing, or difficulty in urination due to enlargement of the prostate gland unless directed by a doctor, or in pregnancy or in nursing mothers. Excessive dosing may lead to liver damage. Product is intended for patients 12 years and older. Alcoholic beverages should be avoided while taking this product. This product should not be taken without first consulting a physician if sedatives or tranquilizers are being taken.

PRESCRIBING INFORMATION

UNISOM WITH PAIN RELIEF®

[yu 'na-som]
Nighttime Sleep Aid and Pain Reliever

DESCRIPTION

Unisom With Pain Relief® is a pale blue, capsule-shaped, coated tablet.

ACTIVE INGREDIENTS

650 mg. acetaminophen and 50 mg. diphenhydramine HCl per tablet.

Continued on next page

Pfizer Consumer—Cont.

INDICATIONS

Unisom With Pain Relief (diphenhydramine sleep aid formula) is indicated to help reduce difficulty in falling asleep while relieving accompanying minor aches and pains such as headache, muscle ache or menstrual discomfort. If there is difficulty in falling asleep, but pain is not being experienced at the same time, regular Unisom sleep aid is indicated which contains doxylamine succinate as its active ingredient.

ADMINISTRATION AND DOSAGE

One tablet at bedtime if needed, or as directed by a physician.

CONTRAINDICATIONS

Do not take this product if you have asthma, glaucoma, emphysema, chronic pulmonary disease, shortness or breath, difficulty in breathing, or difficulty in urination due to enlargement of the prostate gland except under the advice and supervision of a physician. Do not take this product if pregnant or nursing a baby.

Do not take this product for treatment of arthritis except under the advice and supervision of a physician.

WARNINGS

Do not exceed recommended dosage because severe liver damage may occur. If symptoms persist continuously for more than ten days, consult your physician. Insomnia may be a symptom of serious underlying medical illness. Avoid alcoholic beverages while taking this product. Do not take this product if you are taking sedatives or tranquilizers, without first consulting your doctor. For adults only. Do not give to children under 12 years of age. Keep this and all medications out of reach of children. IN CASE OF ACCIDENTAL OVERDOSE SEEK PROFESSIONAL ADVICE OR CONTACT A POISON CONTROL CENTER IMMEDIATELY.

CAUTION

This product contains an antihistamine and will cause drowsiness. It should be used only at bedtime.

DRUG INTERACTION

Monoamine oxidase (MAO) inhibitors prolong and intensify the anticholinergic effects of antihistamines. The CNS depressant effect is heightened by alcohol and other CNS depressant drugs.

ATTENTION

Use only if tablet blister seals are unbroken. Child resistant packaging.

HOW SUPPLIED

Boxes of 8 and 16 tablets in child resistant blisters.

INACTIVE INGREDIENTS

Corn starch, FD&C Blue #1 Aluminum Lake, FD&C Blue #2 Aluminum Lake, Hydroxypropyl Methylcellulose, Magnesium Stearate, Polyethylene Glycol, Polysorbate 80, Povidone, Stearic Acid, Titanium Dioxide.

UNISOM®   OTC
[yu'na-som]
Nighttime Sleep Aid
(doxylamine succinate)

PRODUCT OVERVIEW

KEY FACTS

Unisom is an ethanolamine antihistamine (doxylamine) which characteristically shows a high incidence of sedation. It produces a reduced latency to end of wakefulness and early onset of sleep.

MAJOR USES

Unisom has been shown to be clinically effective as a sleep aid when 1 tablet is given 30 minutes before retiring.

SAFETY INFORMATION

Unisom is contraindicated in pregnancy and nursing mothers. It is also contraindicated in patients with asthma, glaucoma, and enlargement of the prostate. Caution should be used if taken when alcohol is being consumed. Caution is also indicated when taken concurrently with other medications due to the anticholinergic properties of antihistamines.

PRESCRIBING INFORMATION

UNISOM®   OTC
[yu'na-som]
Nighttime Sleep Aid
(doxylamine succinate)

DESCRIPTION

Pale blue oval scored tablets containing 25 mg. of doxylamine succinate, 2-[α-(2-dimethylaminoethoxy)α-methylbenzyl]pyridine succinate.

ACTION AND USES

Doxylamine succinate is an antihistamine of the ethanolamine class, which characteristically shows a high incidence of sedation. In a comparative clinical study of over 20 antihistamines on more than 3000 subjects, doxylamine succinate 25 mg. was one of the three most sedating antihistamines, producing a significantly reduced latency to end of wakefulness and comparing favorably with established hypnotic drugs such as secobarbital and pentobarbital in sedation activity. It was chosen as the antihistamine, based on dosage, causing the earliest onset of sleep. In another clinical study, doxylamine succinate 25 mg. scored better than secobarbital 100 mg. as a nighttime hypnotic. Two additional, identical clinical studies, involving a total of 121 subjects demonstrated that doxylamine succinate 25 mg. reduced the sleep latency period by a third, compared to placebo. Duration of sleep was 26.6% longer with doxylamine succinate, and the quality of sleep was rated higher with the drug than with placebo. An EEG study on 6 subjects confirmed the results of these studies. In yet another study, no statistically significant difference was found between doxylamine succinate and flurazepam in the average time required for 200 patients with mild to moderate insomnia to fall asleep over 5 nights following a nightly dose of doxylamine succinate 25 mg. or flurazepam 30 mg., nor was any statistically significant difference found in the total time the 200 patients slept. Patients on doxylamine succinate awoke an average of 1.2 times per night while those on flurazepam awoke an average of 0.9 times per night. In either case the patients awoke rested the following morning. On a rating scale of 1 to 5, doxylamine succinate was given a 3.0, flurazepam a 3.4 by patients rating the degree of restfulness provided by their medication (5 represents "very well rested"). Although statistically significant, the difference between doxylamine succinate 25 mg. and flurazepam 30 mg. in the number of awakenings and degree of restfulness is clinically insignificant.

ADMINISTRATION AND DOSAGE

One tablet 30 minutes before retiring. Not for children under 12 years of age.

SIDE EFFECTS

Occasional anticholinergic effects may be seen.

PRECAUTIONS

Unisom® should be taken only at bedtime.

CONTRAINDICATIONS

Asthma, glaucoma, enlargement of the prostate gland. This product should not be taken by pregnant women or those who are nursing a baby.

WARNINGS

Should be taken with caution if alcohol is being consumed. Product should not be taken if patient is concurrently on any other drug, without prior consultation with physician. Should not be taken for longer than two weeks unless approved by physician.

HOW SUPPLIED

Boxes of 8, 16, 32 or 48 tablets.

INACTIVE INGREDIENTS

Dibasic Calcium Phosphate, FD&C Blue #1 Aluminum Lake, Magnesium Stearate, Microcrystalline Cellulose, Sodium Starch Glycolate.

VISINE®   OTC
Tetrahydrozoline Hydrochloride
Redness Reliever Eye Drops

(See PDR For Nonprescription Drugs.)

VISINE A.C.®   OTC
Astringent/Redness Reliever Eye
Drops

(See PDR For Nonprescription Drugs.)

VISINE EXTRA®   OTC
Redness Reliever/Lubricant Eye
Drops

(See PDR For Nonprescription Drugs.)

VISINE L.R.™   OTC
Oxymetazoline Hydrochloride
Redness Reliever Eye Drops

(See PDR For Nonprescription Drugs.)

Pfizer Labs Division
Pfizer Inc
235 EAST 42ND STREET
NEW YORK, NY 10017-5755

Full prescribing information for all Pfizer Labs products is available from your Pfizer Labs representative.

Product Identification Codes

To provide quick and positive identification of Pfizer Labs Division products, we have imprinted the product identification number of the National Drug Code on all tablets and capsules.

In order that you may quickly identify a product by its code number, we have compiled below a numerical list of code numbers with their corresponding product names. We are also listing the code numbers by alphabetical order of products.

NUMERICAL PRODUCT INDEX

Product Identification Code	Product
094	Vibramycin® Hyclate (doxycycline hyclate) Capsules 50 mg
095	Vibramycin® Hyclate (doxycycline hyclate) Capsules 100 mg
099	Vibra-Tabs® (doxycycline hyclate) Film Coated Tablets 100 mg
152	Norvasc® (amlodipine besylate) Tablets 2.5 mg
153	Norvasc® (amlodipine besylate) Tablets 5 mg
154	Norvasc® (amlodipine besylate) Tablets 10 mg
260	Procardia® (nifedipine) Capsules 10 mg
261	Procardia® (nifedipine) Capsules 20 mg
265	Procardia XL® (nifedipine) Extended Release Tablets 30 mg GITS
266	Procardia XL® (nifedipine) Extended Release Tablets 60 mg GITS
267	Procardia XL® (nifedipine) Extended Release Tablets 90 mg GITS
305	Zithromax® (azithromycin) Capsules 250 mg
322	Feldene® (piroxicam) Capsules 10 mg
323	Feldene® (piroxicam) Capsules 20 mg
393	Diabinese® (chlorpropamide) Tablets 100 mg
394	Diabinese® (chlorpropamide) Tablets 250 mg
430	Minizide® 1 Capsules (1 mg prazosin HCl and 0.5 mg polythiazide)
431	Minipress® (prazosin HCl) Capsules 1 mg
432	Minizide® 2 Capsules (2 mg prazosin HCl and 0.5 mg polythiazide)
436	Minizide® 5 Capsules (5 mg prazosin HCl and 0.5 mg polythiazide)
437	Minipress® (prazosin HCl) Capsules 2 mg
438	Minipress® (prazosin HCl) Capsules 5 mg
541	Vistaril® (hydroxyzine pamoate) Capsules 25 mg
542	Vistaril® (hydroxyzine pamoate) Capsules 50 mg
543	Vistaril® (hydroxyzine pamoate) Capsules 100 mg

ALPHABETICAL PRODUCT INDEX

Product	Product Identification Code
Diabinese® (chlorpropamide) Tablets 100 mg	393
Diabinese® (chlorpropamide) Tablets 250 mg	394
Feldene® (piroxicam) Capsules 10 mg	322
Feldene® (piroxicam) Capsules 20 mg	323
Minipress® (prazosin HCl) Capsules 1 mg	431
Minipress® (prazosin HCl) Capsules 2 mg	437
Minipress® (prazosin HCl) Capsules 5 mg	438
Minizide® 1 Capsules (1 mg prazosin HCl and 0.5 mg polythiazide)	430

Minizide® 2 Capsules (2 mg prazosin HCl and 0.5 mg polythiazide)	432
Minizide® 5 Capsules (5 mg prazosin HCl and 0.5 mg polythiazide)	436
Norvasc® (amlodipine besylate) Tablets 2.5 mg	152
Norvasc® (amlodipine besylate) Tablets 5 mg	153
Norvasc® (amlodipine besylate) Tablets 10 mg	154
Procardia® (nifedipine) Capsules 10 mg	260
Procardia® (nifedipine) Capsules 20 mg	261
Procardia XL® (nifedipine) Extended Release Tablets 30 mg GITS	265
Procardia XL® (nifedipine) Extended Release Tablets 60 mg GITS	266
Procardia XL® (nifedipine) Extended Release Tablets 90 mg GITS	267
Vibramycin® Hyclate (doxycycline hyclate) Capsules 50 mg	094
Vibramycin® Hyclate (doxycycline hyclate) Capsules 100 mg	095
Vibra-Tabs® (doxycycline hyclate) Film Coated Tablets 100 mg	099
Vistaril® (hydroxyzine pamoate) Capsules 25 mg	541
Vistaril® (hydroxyzine pamoate) Capsules 50 mg	542
Vistaril® (hydroxyzine pamoate) Capsules 100 mg	543
Zithromax® (azithromycin) Capsules 250 mg	305

DIABINESE® ℞

[dī-ab 'in-ees]
(chlorpropamide)
Tablets, USP
For Oral Use

DESCRIPTION

DIABINESE (chlorpropamide), is an oral blood-glucose-lowering drug of the sulfonylurea class. Chlorpropamide is 1-[(p-Chlorophenyl) sulfonyl]-3-propylurea, $C_{10}H_{13}ClN_2O_3S$.

Chlorpropamide is a white crystalline powder, that has a slight odor. It is practically insoluble in water at pH 7.3 (solubility at pH 6 is 2.2 mg/ml). It is soluble in alcohol and moderately soluble in chloroform. The molecular weight of chlorpropamide is 276.74. DIABINESE is available as 100 mg and 250 mg tablets.

Inert ingredients are: alginic acid; Blue 1 Lake; hydroxypropyl cellulose; magnesium stearate; precipitated calcium carbonate; sodium lauryl sulfate; starch.

CLINICAL PHARMACOLOGY

DIABINESE appears to lower the blood glucose acutely by stimulating the release of insulin from the pancreas, an effect dependent upon functioning beta cells in the pancreatic islets. The mechanism by which DIABINESE lowers blood glucose during long-term administration has not been clearly established. Extra-pancreatic effects may play a part in the mechanism of action of oral sulfonylurea hypoglycemic drugs. While chlorpropamide is a sulfonamide derivative, it is devoid of antibacterial activity.

DIABINESE may also prove effective in controlling certain patients who have experienced primary or secondary failure to other sulfonylurea agents.

A method developed which permits easy measurement of the drug in blood is available on request.

Chlorpropamide does not interfere with the usual tests to detect albumin in the urine.

DIABINESE is absorbed rapidly from the gastrointestinal tract. Within one hour after a single oral dose, it is readily detectable in the blood, and the level reaches a maximum within two to four hours. It undergoes metabolism in humans and it is excreted in the urine as unchanged drug and as hydroxylated or hydrolyzed metabolites. The biological half-life of chlorpropamide averages about 36 hours. Within 96 hours, 80–90% of a single oral dose is excreted in the urine. However, long-term administration of therapeutic doses does not result in undue accumulation in the blood, since absorption and excretion rates become stabilized in about 5 to 7 days after the initiation of therapy.

DIABINESE exerts a hypoglycemic effect in normal humans within one hour, becoming maximal at 3 to 6 hours and persisting for at least 24 hours. The potency of chlorpropamide is approximately six times that of tolbutamide. Some experimental results suggest that its increased duration of action may be the result of slower excretion and absence of significant deactivation.

INDICATIONS AND USAGE

DIABINESE is indicated as an adjunct to diet to lower the blood glucose in patients with non-insulin-dependent diabetes mellitus (type II) whose hyperglycemia cannot be controlled by diet alone.

In initiating treatment for non-insulin-dependent diabetes, diet should be emphasized as the primary form of treatment. Caloric restriction and weight loss are essential in the obese diabetic patient. Proper dietary management alone may be effective in controlling the blood glucose and symptoms of hyperglycemia. The importance of regular physical activity should also be stressed, and cardiovascular risk factors should be identified and corrective measures taken where possible.

If this treatment program fails to reduce symptoms and/or blood glucose, the use of an oral sulfonylurea or insulin should be considered. Use of DIABINESE must be viewed by both the physician and patient as a treatment in addition to diet, and not as a substitute for diet or as a convenient mechanism for avoiding dietary restraint. Furthermore, loss of blood glucose control on diet alone may be transient, thus requiring only short-term administration of DIABINESE.

During maintenance programs, DIABINESE should be discontinued if satisfactory lowering of blood glucose is no longer achieved. Judgments should be based on regular clinical and laboratory evaluations.

In considering the use of DIABINESE in asymptomatic patients, it should be recognized that controlling the blood glucose in non-insulin-dependent diabetes, has not been definitely established to be effective in preventing the long-term cardiovascular or neural complications of diabetes.

CONTRAINDICATIONS

DIABINESE is contraindicated in patients with:

1. Known hypersensitivity to the drug.
2. Diabetic ketoacidosis, with or without coma. This condition should be treated with insulin.

WARNINGS

SPECIAL WARNING ON INCREASED RISK OF CARDIOVASCULAR MORTALITY

The administration of oral hypoglycemic drugs has been reported to be associated with increased cardiovascular mortality as compared to treatment with diet alone or diet plus insulin. This warning is based on the study conducted by the University Group Diabetes Program (UGDP), a long-term prospective clinical trial designed to evaluate the effectiveness of glucose-lowering drugs in preventing or delaying vascular complications in patients with non-insulin-dependent diabetes. The study involved 823 patients who were randomly assigned to one of four treatment groups (*Diabetes,* 19 (supp. 2): 747–830, 1970.)

UGDP reported that patients treated for 5 to 8 years with diet plus a fixed dose of tolbutamide (1.5 grams per day) had a rate of cardiovascular mortality approximately 2½ times that of patients treated with diet alone. A significant increase in total mortality was not observed, but the use of tolbutamide was discontinued based on the increase in cardiovascular mortality, thus limiting the opportunity for the study to show an increase in over-all mortality. Despite controversy regarding the interpretation of these results, the findings of the UGDP study provide an adequate basis for this warning. The patient should be informed of the potential risks and advantages of DIABINESE and of alternative modes of therapy.

Although only one drug in the sulfonylurea class (tolbutamide) was included in this study, it is prudent from a safety standpoint to consider that this warning may also apply to other oral hypoglycemic drugs in this class, in view of their close similarities in mode of action and chemical structure.

PRECAUTIONS

General

Hypoglycemia: All sulfonylurea drugs are capable of producing severe hypoglycemia. Proper patient selection, dosage, and instructions are important to avoid hypoglycemic episodes. Renal or hepatic insufficiency may cause elevated blood levels of DIABINESE and the latter may also diminish gluconeogenic capacity, both of which increase the risk of serious hypoglycemic reactions. Elderly, debilitated or malnourished patients, and those with adrenal or pituitary insufficiency are particularly susceptible to the hypoglycemic action of glucose-lowering drugs. Hypoglycemia may be difficult to recognize in the elderly, and in people who are taking beta-adrenergic blocking drugs. Hypoglycemia is more likely to occur when caloric intake is deficient, after severe or prolonged exercise, when alcohol is ingested, or when more than one glucose-lowering drug is used.

Because of the long half-life of chlorpropamide, patients who become hypoglycemic during therapy require careful supervision of the dose and frequent feedings for at least 3 to 5 days. Hospitalization and intravenous glucose may be necessary.

Loss of control of blood glucose: When a patient stabilized on any diabetic regimen is exposed to stress such as fever, trauma, infection, or surgery, a loss of control may occur. At such times, it may be necessary to discontinue DIABINESE and administer insulin.

The effectiveness of any oral hypoglycemic drug, including DIABINESE, in lowering blood glucose to a desired level decreases in many patients over a period of time, which may be due to progression of the severity of the diabetes or to diminished responsiveness to the drug. This phenomenon is known as secondary failure, to distinguish it from primary failure in which the drug is ineffective in an individual patient when first given.

INFORMATION FOR PATIENTS

Patients should be informed of the potential risks and advantages of DIABINESE and of alternative modes of therapy. They should also be informed about the importance of adherence to dietary instructions, of a regular exercise program, and of regular testing of urine and/or blood glucose.

The risks of hypoglycemia, its symptoms and treatment, and conditions that predispose to its development should be explained to patients and responsible family members. Primary and secondary failure should also be explained.

Patients should be instructed to contact their physician promptly if they experience symptoms of hypoglycemia or other adverse reactions.

LABORATORY TESTS

Blood and urine glucose should be monitored periodically. Measurement of glycosylated hemoglobin may be useful.

DRUG INTERACTIONS

The hypoglycemic action of sulfonylurea may be potentiated by certain drugs including nonsteroidal anti-inflammatory agents and other drugs that are highly protein bound, salicylates, sulfonamides, chloramphenicol, probenecid, coumarins, monoamine oxidase inhibitors, and beta-adrenergic blocking agents. When such drugs are administered to a patient receiving DIABINESE, the patient should be observed closely for hypoglycemia. When such drugs are withdrawn from a patient receiving DIABINESE, the patient should be observed closely for loss of control.

Certain drugs tend to produce hyperglycemia and may lead to loss of control. These drugs include the thiazides and other diuretics, corticosteroids, phenothiazines, thyroid products, estrogens, oral contraceptives, phenytoin, nicotinic acid, sympathomimetics, calcium channel blocking drugs, and isoniazid. When such drugs are administered to a patient receiving DIABINESE, the patient should be closely observed for loss of control. When such drugs are withdrawn from a patient receiving DIABINESE, the patient should be observed closely for hypoglycemia.

Since animal studies suggest that the action of barbiturates may be prolonged by therapy with chlorpropamide, barbiturates should be employed with caution. In some patients, a disulfiram-like reaction may be produced by the ingestion of alcohol.

A potential interaction between oral miconazole and oral hypoglycemic agents leading to severe hypoglycemia has been reported. Whether this interaction also occurs with the intravenous, topical, or vaginal preparations of miconazole is not known.

Carcinogenesis, Mutagenesis, Impairment of Fertility: Chronic toxicity studies have been carried out in dogs and rats. Dogs treated for 6, 13, or 20 months with doses of DIABINESE greater than 20 times the human dose, have not shown any gross histological or pathological abnormalities. After treatment with 100 mg/kg of DIABINESE for 20 months, a dog showed no histopathological liver changes.

Rats treated with continuous DIABINESE therapy for 6 to 12 months showed varying degrees of suppression of spermatogenesis at higher dosage levels (up to 125 mg/kg). The extent of suppression seemed to follow that of growth retardation associated with chronic administration of high-dose DIABINESE in rats.

Pregnancy

Teratogenic Effects:

Pregnancy Category C. Animal reproductive studies have not been conducted with DIABINESE. It is also not known whether DIABINESE can cause fetal harm when administered to a pregnant woman or can affect reproduction capacity. DIABINESE should be given to a pregnant woman only if clearly needed.

Because recent information suggests that abnormal blood glucose levels during pregnancy are associated with a higher incidence of congenital abnormalities, many experts recommend that insulin be used during pregnancy to maintain blood glucose levels as close to normal as possible.

Nonteratogenic Effects:

Prolonged severe hypoglycemia (4 to 10 days) has been reported in neonates born to mothers who were receiving a sulfonylurea drug at the time of delivery. This has been reported more frequently with the use of agents with prolonged half-lives. If DIABINESE is used during pregnancy, it should be discontinued at least one month before the expected delivery date.

Continued on next page

Pfizer—Cont.

Nursing Mothers: An analysis of a composite of two samples of human breast milk, each taken five hours after ingestion of 500 mg of chlorpropamide by a patient, revealed a concentration of 5 mcg/ml. For reference, the normal peak blood level of chlorpropamide after a single 250 mg dose is 30 mcg/ml. Therefore, it is not recommended that a woman breast feed while taking this medication.
Use in Children: Safety and effectiveness in children have not been established.

ADVERSE REACTIONS

Hypoglycemia: See PRECAUTIONS and OVERDOSAGE sections.
Gastrointestinal Reactions: Cholestatic jaundice may occur rarely; DIABINESE should be discontinued if this occurs. Gastrointestinal disturbances are the most common reactions; nausea has been reported in less than 5% of patients, and diarrhea, vomiting, anorexia, and hunger in less than 2%. Other gastrointestinal disturbances have occurred in less than 1% of patients including proctocolitis. They tend to be dose related and may disappear when dosage is reduced.
Dermatologic Reactions: Pruritus has been reported in less than 3% of patients. Other allergic skin reactions, e.g., urticaria and maculopapular eruptions, have been reported in approximately 1% or less of patients. These may be transient and may disappear despite continued use of DIABINESE; if skin reactions persist the drug should be discontinued.
Porphyria cutanea tarda and photosensitivity reactions have been reported with sulfonylureas.
Skin eruptions rarely progressing to erythema multiforme and exfoliative dermatitis have also been reported.
Hematologic Reactions: Leukopenia, agranulocytosis, thrombocytopenia, hemolytic anemia, aplastic anemia, pancytopenia, and eosinophilia have been reported with sulfonylureas.
Metabolic Reactions: Hepatic porphyria and disulfiram-like reactions have been reported with DIABINESE. See DRUG INTERACTIONS section.
Endocrine Reactions: On rare occasions, chlorpropamide has caused a reaction identical to the syndrome of inappropriate antidiuretic hormone (ADH) secretion. The features of this syndrome result from excessive water retention and include hyponatremia, low serum osmolality, and high urine osmolality. This reaction has also been reported for other sulfonylureas.

OVERDOSAGE

Overdose of sulfonylureas including DIABINESE can produce hypoglycemia. Mild hypoglycemic symptoms without loss of consciousness or neurologic findings should be treated aggressively with oral glucose and adjustments in drug dosage and/or meal patterns. Close monitoring should continue until the physician is assured that the patient is out of danger. Severe hypoglycemic reactions with coma, seizure, or other neurological impairment occur infrequently, but constitute medical emergencies requiring immediate hospitalization. If hypoglycemic coma is diagnosed or suspected, the patient should be given a rapid intravenous injection of concentrated (50%) glucose solution. This should be followed by a continuous infusion of a more dilute (10%) glucose solution at a rate that will maintain the blood glucose at a level above 100 mg/dL. Patients should be closely monitored for a minimum of 24 to 48 hours since hypoglycemia may recur after apparent clinical recovery.

DOSAGE AND ADMINISTRATION

There is no fixed dosage regimen for the management of diabetes mellitus with DIABINESE or any other hypoglycemic agent. In addition to the usual monitoring of urinary glucose, the patient's blood glucose must also be monitored periodically to determine the minimum effective dose for the patient; to detect primary failure, i.e., inadequate lowering of blood glucose at the maximum recommended dose of medication; and to detect secondary failure, i.e., loss of an adequate blood glucose lowering response after an initial period of effectiveness. Glycosylated hemoglobin levels may also be of value in monitoring the patient's response to therapy.
Short-term administration of DIABINESE may be sufficient during periods of transient loss of control in patients usually controlled well on diet.
The total daily dosage is generally taken at a single time each morning with breakfast. Occasionally cases of gastrointestinal intolerance may be relieved by dividing the daily dosage. A LOADING OR PRIMING DOSE IS NOT NECESSARY AND SHOULD NOT BE USED.
Initial Therapy: 1. The mild to moderately severe, middle-aged, stable, non-insulin-dependent diabetic patient should be started on 250 mg daily. In elderly patients, debilitated or malnourished patients, and patients with impaired renal or hepatic function, the initial and maintenance dosing should be conservative to avoid hypoglycemic reactions (see PRECAUTIONS section). Older patients should be started on smaller amounts of DIABINESE, in the range of 100 to 125 mg daily.
2. No transition period is necessary when transferring patients from other oral hypoglycemic agents to DIABINESE. The other agent may be discontinued abruptly and chlorpropamide started at once. In prescribing chlorpropamide, due consideration must be given to its greater potency.
Many mild to moderately severe, middle-aged, stable non-insulin-dependent diabetic patients receiving insulin can be placed directly on the oral drug and their insulin abruptly discontinued. For patients requiring more than 40 units of insulin daily, therapy with DIABINESE may be initiated with a 50 per cent reduction in insulin for the first few days, with subsequent further reductions dependent upon the response.
During the initial period of therapy with chlorpropamide, hypoglycemic reactions may occasionally occur, particularly during the transition from insulin to the oral drug. Hypoglycemia within 24 hours after withdrawal of the intermediate or long-acting types of insulin will usually prove to be the result of insulin carry-over and not primarily due to the effect of chlorpropamide.
During the insulin withdrawal period, the patient should test his urine for sugar and ketone bodies at least three times daily and report the results frequently to his physician. If they are abnormal, the physician should be notified immediately. In some cases, it may be advisable to consider hospitalization during the transition period.
Five to seven days after the initial therapy, the blood level of chlorpropamide reaches a plateau. Dosage may subsequently be adjusted upward or downward by increments of not more than 50 to 125 mg at intervals of three to five days to obtain optimal control. More frequent adjustments are usually undesirable.
Maintenance Therapy: Most moderately severe, middle-aged, stable non-insulin-dependent diabetic patients are controlled by approximately 250 mg daily. Many investigators have found that some milder diabetics do well on daily doses of 100 mg or less. Many of the more severe diabetics may require 500 mg daily for adequate control. PATIENTS WHO DO NOT RESPOND COMPLETELY TO 500 MG DAILY WILL USUALLY NOT RESPOND TO HIGHER DOSES. MAINTENANCE DOSES ABOVE 750 mg DAILY SHOULD BE AVOIDED.

HOW SUPPLIED

[See table below.]

RECOMMENDED STORAGE

Store below 86°F (30°C).

CAUTION

Federal law prohibits dispensing without prescription.
69-2141-37-0 Revised Dec. 1986
Literature Available: Yes.
Shown in Product Identification Section, page 423

Strength	Tablet Description	Tablet Code	NDC	Package Size
DIABINESE (chlorpropamide) 100 mg	Blue, D-shaped, scored	393	0663-3930-66 0663-3930-73 0663-3930-41	100's 500's 100 (10 × 10) unit dose
DIABINESE (chlorpropamide) 250 mg	Blue, D-shaped, scored	394	0663-3940-66 0663-3940-71 0663-3940-82 0663-3940-41	100's 250's 1000's 100 (10 × 10) unit dose

FELDENE® ℞

[fĕl 'deen]
(piroxicam)
CAPSULES
For Oral Use

DESCRIPTION

FELDENE (piroxicam) is 4-Hydroxy-2-methyl-*N*-2-pyridinyl-2*H*-1,2-benzothiazine-3-carboxamide 1,1-dioxide, an oxicam. Members of the oxicam family are not carboxylic acids, but they are acidic by virtue of the enolic 4-hydroxy substituent. FELDENE occurs as a white crystalline solid, sparingly soluble in water, dilute acid and most organic solvents. It is slightly soluble in alcohols and in aqueous alkaline solution. It exhibits a weakly acidic 4-hydroxy proton (pKa 5.1) and a weakly basic pyridyl nitrogen (pKa 1.8). Inert ingredients in the formulations are: hard gelatin capsules (which may contain Blue 1, Red 3, and other inert ingredients); lactose; magnesium stearate; sodium lauryl sulfate; starch.

CLINICAL PHARMACOLOGY

FELDENE has shown anti-inflammatory, analgesic and antipyretic properties in animals. Edema, erythema, tissue proliferation, fever, and pain can all be inhibited in laboratory animals by the administration of FELDENE. It is effective regardless of the etiology of the inflammation. The mode of action of FELDENE is not fully established at this time. However, a common mechanism for the above effects may exist in the ability of FELDENE to inhibit the biosynthesis of prostaglandins, known mediators of inflammation.
It is established that FELDENE does not act by stimulating the pituitary-adrenal axis.
FELDENE is well absorbed following oral administration. Drug plasma concentrations are proportional for 10 and 20 mg doses, generally peak within three to five hours after medication, and subsequently decline with a mean half-life of 50 hours (range of 30 to 86 hours; although values outside of this range have been encountered).
This prolonged half-life results in the maintenance of relatively stable plasma concentrations throughout the day on once daily doses and to significant drug accumulation upon multiple dosing. A single 20 mg dose generally produces peak piroxicam plasma levels of 1.5 to 2 mcg/ml, while maximum drug plasma concentrations, after repeated daily ingestion of 20 mg FELDENE, usually stabilize at 3–8 mcg/ml. Most patients approximate steady state plasma levels within 7 to 12 days. Higher levels, which approximate steady state at two to three weeks, have been observed in patients in whom longer plasma half-lives of piroxicam occurred.
FELDENE and its biotransformation products are excreted in urine and feces, with about twice as much appearing in the urine as the feces. Metabolism occurs by hydroxylation at the 5 position of the pyridyl side chain and conjugation of this product; by cyclodehydration; and by a sequence of reactions involving hydrolysis of the amide linkage, decarboxylation, ring contraction, and N-demethylation. Less than 5% of the daily dose is excreted unchanged.
Concurrent administration of aspirin (3900 mg/day) and FELDENE (20 mg/day), resulted in a reduction of plasma levels of piroxicam to about 80% of their normal values. The use of FELDENE in conjunction with aspirin is not recommended because data are inadequate to demonstrate that the combination produces greater improvement than that achieved with aspirin alone and the potential for adverse reactions is increased. Concomitant administration of antacids had no effect on FELDENE plasma levels. The effects of impaired renal function or hepatic disease on plasma levels have not been established.
FELDENE, like salicylates and other nonsteroidal anti-inflammatory agents, is associated with symptoms of gastrointestinal tract irritation (see ADVERSE REACTIONS). However, in a study utilizing ^{51}Cr-tagged red blood cells, 20 mg of FELDENE administered as a single dose for four days did not result in a significant increase in fecal blood loss and did not detectably affect the gastric mucosa. In the same study a total daily dose of 3900 mg of aspirin, i.e., 972 mg q.i.d., caused a significant increase in fecal blood loss and mucosal lesions as demonstrated by gastroscopy.
In controlled clinical trials, the effectiveness of FELDENE (piroxicam) has been established for both acute exacerbations and long-term management of rheumatoid arthritis and osteoarthritis.
The therapeutic effects of FELDENE are evident early in the treatment of both diseases with a progressive increase in response over several (8–12) weeks. Efficacy is seen in terms of pain relief and, when present, subsidence of inflammation.
Doses of 20 mg/day FELDENE display a therapeutic effect comparable to therapeutic doses of aspirin, with a lower incidence of minor gastrointestinal effects and tinnitus.
FELDENE has been administered concomitantly with fixed doses of gold and corticosteroids. The existence of a "steroid-sparing" effect has not been adequately studied to date.

INDICATIONS AND USAGE

FELDENE is indicated for acute or long-term use in the relief of signs and symptoms of the following:

1. osteoarthritis
2. rheumatoid arthritis

Dosage recommendations for use in children have not been established.

CONTRAINDICATIONS

FELDENE should not be used in patients who have previously exhibited hypersensitivity to it, or in individuals with the syndrome comprised of bronchospasm, nasal polyps, and angioedema precipitated by aspirin or other nonsteroidal anti-inflammatory drugs.

WARNINGS

Risk of GI Ulceration, Bleeding and Perforation with NSAID Therapy

Serious gastrointestinal toxicity such as bleeding, ulceration, and perforation can occur at any time, with or without warning symptoms, in patients treated chronically with NSAID therapy. Although minor upper gastrointestinal problems, such as dyspepsia, are common, usually developing early in therapy, physician should remain alert for ulceration and bleeding in patients treated chronically with NSAIDs even in the absence of previous GI tract symptoms. In patients observed in clinical trials of several months to two years duration, symptomatic upper GI ulcers, gross bleeding or perforation appear to occur in approximately 1% of patients treated for 3–6 months, and in about 2–4% of patients treated for one year. Physicians should inform patients about the signs and/or symptoms of serious GI toxicity and what steps to take if they occur.

Studies to date have not identified any subset of patients not at risk of developing peptic ulceration and bleeding. Except for a prior history of serious GI events and other risk factors known to be associated with peptic ulcer disease, such as alcoholism, smoking, etc., no risk factors (e.g., age, sex) have been associated with increased risk. Elderly or debilitated patients seem to tolerate ulceration or bleeding less well than other individuals and most spontaneous reports of fatal GI events are in this population. Studies to date are inconclusive concerning the relative risk of various NSAIDs in causing such reactions. High doses of any NSAID probably carry a greater risk of these reactions, although controlled clinical trials showing this do not exist in most cases. In considering the use of relatively large doses (within the recommended dosage range), sufficient benefit should be anticipated to offset the potential increased risk of GI toxicity.

PRECAUTIONS

Renal Effects: As with other nonsteroidal anti-inflammatory drugs, long-term administration of piroxicam to animals has resulted in renal papillary necrosis and other abnormal renal pathology. In humans, there have been reports of acute interstitial nephritis with hematuria, proteinuria, and occasionally, nephrotic syndrome.

A second form of renal toxicity has been seen in patients with prerenal conditions leading to a reduction in renal blood flow or blood volume, where the renal prostaglandins have a supportive role in the maintenance of renal perfusion. In these patients administration of an NSAID may cause a dose-dependent reduction in prostaglandin formation and may precipitate overt renal decompensation. Patients at greatest risk of this reaction are those with impaired renal function, heart failure, liver dysfunction, those taking diuretics, and the elderly. Discontinuation of NSAID therapy is typically followed by recovery to the pretreatment state.

Because of extensive renal excretion of piroxicam and its biotransformation products (less than 5% of the daily dose excreted unchanged, see CLINICAL PHARMACOLOGY), lower doses of piroxicam should be anticipated in patients with impaired renal function, and they should be carefully monitored.

Although other nonsteroidal anti-inflammatory drugs do not have the same direct effects on platelets that aspirin does, all drugs inhibiting prostaglandin biosynthesis do interfere with platelet function to some degree; therefore, patients who may be adversely affected by such an action should be carefully observed when FELDENE is administered.

Because of reports of adverse eye findings with nonsteroidal anti-inflammatory agents, it is recommended that patients who develop visual complaints during treatment with FELDENE have ophthalmic evaluation.

As with other nonsteroidal anti-inflammatory drugs, borderline elevations of one or more liver tests may occur in up to 15% of patients. These abnormalities may progress, may remain essentially unchanged, or may be transient with continued therapy. The SGPT (ALT) test is probably the most sensitive indicator of liver dysfunction. Meaningful (3 times the upper limit of normal) elevations of SGPT or SGOT (AST) occurred in controlled clinical trials in less than 1% of patients. A patient with symptoms and/or signs suggesting liver dysfunction, or in whom an abnormal liver test has occurred, should be evaluated for evidence of the development of more severe hepatic reaction while on therapy with

FELDENE. Severe hepatic reactions, including jaundice and cases of fatal hepatitis, have been reported with FELDENE. Although such reactions are rare, if abnormal liver tests persist or worsen, if clinical signs and symptoms consistent with liver disease develop, or if systemic manifestations occur (e.g. eosinophilia, rash, etc.), FELDENE should be discontinued. (See also ADVERSE REACTIONS.)

Although at the recommended dose of 20 mg/day of FELDENE increased fecal blood loss due to gastrointestinal irritation did not occur (see CLINICAL PHARMACOLOGY), in about 4% of the patients treated with FELDENE alone or concomitantly with aspirin, reductions in hemoglobin and hematocrit values were observed. Therefore, these values should be determined if signs or symptoms of anemia occur. Peripheral edema has been observed in approximately 2% of the patients treated with FELDENE. Therefore, as with other nonsteroidal anti-inflammatory drugs, FELDENE should be used with caution in patients with heart failure, hypertension or other conditions predisposing to fluid retention, since its usage may be associated with a worsening of these conditions.

A combination of dermatological and/or allergic signs and symptoms suggestive of serum sickness have occasionally occurred in conjunction with the use of FELDENE. These include arthralgias, pruritus, fever, fatigue, and rash including vesiculo bullous reactions and exfoliative dermatitis.

Information for Patients

FELDENE, like other drugs of its class, is not free of side effects. The side effects of these drugs can cause discomfort and, rarely, there are more serious side effects, such as gastrointestinal bleeding, which may result in hospitalization and even fatal outcomes.

NSAIDs (Nonsteroidal Anti-Inflammatory Drugs) are often essential agents in the management of arthritis, but they also may be commonly employed for conditions which are less serious.

Physicians may wish to discuss with their patients the potential risks (see WARNINGS, PRECAUTIONS, and ADVERSE REACTIONS sections) and likely benefits of NSAID treatment, particularly when the drugs are used for less serious conditions where treatment without NSAIDs may represent an acceptable alternative to both the patient and physician.

Laboratory Tests

Because serious GI tract ulceration and bleeding can occur without warning symptoms, physicians should follow chronically treated patients for the signs and symptoms of ulceration and bleeding and should inform them of the importance of this follow-up (see Risk of GI Ulceration, Bleeding and Perforation with NSAID Therapy).

Drug Interactions

FELDENE is highly protein bound, and, therefore, might be expected to displace other protein-bound drugs. Although this has not occurred in in vitro studies with coumarin-type anticoagulants, interactions with coumarin-type anticoagulants have been reported with FELDENE since marketing, therefore, physicians should closely monitor patients for a change in dosage requirements when administering FELDENE to patients in coumarin-type anticoagulants and other highly protein-bound drugs.

Plasma levels of piroxicam are depressed to approximately 80% of their normal values when FELDENE is administered in conjunction with aspirin (3900 mg/day), but concomitant administration of antacids has no effect on piroxicam plasma levels (see CLINICAL PHARMACOLOGY).

Nonsteroidal anti-inflammatory agents, including FELDENE, have been reported to increase steady state plasma lithium levels. It is recommended that plasma lithium levels be monitored when initiating, adjusting and discontinuing FELDENE.

Carcinogenesis, Chronic Animal Toxicity and Impairment of Fertility

Subacute and chronic toxicity studies have been carried out in rats, mice, dogs, and monkeys.

The pathology most often seen was that characteristically associated with the animal toxicology of anti-inflammatory agents: renal papillary necrosis (see PRECAUTIONS) and gastrointestinal lesions.

In classical studies in laboratory animals piroxicam did not show any teratogenic potential.

Reproductive studies revealed no impairment of fertility in animals.

Pregnancy and Nursing Mothers

Like other drugs which inhibit the synthesis and release of prostaglandins, piroxicam increased the incidence of dystocia and delayed parturition in pregnant animals when piroxicam administration was continued late into pregnancy. Gastrointestinal tract toxicity was increased in pregnant females in the last trimester of pregnancy compared to nonpregnant females or females in earlier trimesters of pregnancy.

FELDENE is not recommended for use in nursing mothers or in pregnant women because of the animal findings and since safety for such use has not been established in humans.

Use in Children

Dosage recommendations and indications for use in children have not been established.

ADVERSE REACTIONS

The incidence of adverse reactions to piroxicam is based on clinical trials involving approximately 2300 patients, about 400 of whom were treated for more than one year and 170 for more than two years. About 30% of all patients receiving daily doses of 20 mg of FELDENE experienced side effects. Gastrointestinal symptoms were the most prominent side effects—occurring in approximately 20% of the patients, which in most instances did not interfere with the course of therapy. Of the patients experiencing gastrointestinal side effects, approximately 5% discontinued therapy with an overall incidence of peptic ulceration of about 1%.

Other than the gastrointestinal symptoms, edema, dizziness, headache, changes in hematological parameters, and rash have been reported in a small percentage of patients. Routine ophthalmoscopy and slit-lamp examinations have revealed no evidence of ocular changes in 205 patients followed from 3 to 24 months while on therapy.

Incidence Greater Than 1%. The following adverse reactions occurred more frequently than 1 in 100.

Gastrointestinal: stomatitis, anorexia, epigastric distress*, nausea*, constipation, abdominal discomfort, flatulence, diarrhea, abdominal pain, indigestion

Hematological: decreases in hemoglobin* and hematocrit* (see PRECAUTIONS), anemia, leucopenia, eosinophilia

Dermatologic: pruritus, rash

Central Nervous System: dizziness, somnolence, vertigo

Urogenital: BUN and creatinine elevations (see PRECAUTIONS)

Body as a Whole: headache, malaise

Special Senses: tinnitus

Cardiovascular/Respiratory: edema (see PRECAUTIONS)

Incidence Less Than 1% (Causal Relationship Probable)

The following adverse reactions occurred less frequently than 1 in 100. The probability exists that there is a causal relationship between FELDENE and these reactions.

Gastrointestinal: liver function abnormalities, jaundice, hepatitis (see PRECAUTIONS), vomiting, hematemesis, melena, gastrointestinal bleeding, perforation and ulceration (see WARNINGS), dry mouth

Hematological: thrombocytopenia, petechial rash, ecchymosis, bone marrow depression including aplastic anemia, epistaxis

Dermatologic: sweating, erythema, bruising, desquamation, exfoliative dermatitis, erythema multiforme, toxic epidermal necrolysis, Stevens-Johnson syndrome, vesiculo bullous reaction, photoallergic skin reactions

Central Nervous System: depression, insomnia, nervousness

Urogenital: hematuria, proteinuria, interstitial nephritis, renal failure, hyperkalemia, glomerulitis, papillary necrosis, nephrotic syndrome (see PRECAUTIONS)

Body as a Whole: pain (colic), fever, flu-like syndrome (see PRECAUTIONS)

Special Senses: swollen eyes, blurred vision, eye irritations

Cardiovascular/Respiratory: hypertension, worsening of congestive heart failure (see PRECAUTIONS), exacerbation of angina

Metabolic: hypoglycemia, hyperglycemia, weight increase, weight decrease

Hypersensitivity: anaphylaxis, bronchospasm, urticaria/angioedema, vasculitis, "serum sickness" (see PRECAUTIONS)

Incidence Less Than 1% (Causal Relationship Unknown)

Other adverse reactions were reported with a frequency of less than 1 in 100, but a causal relationship between FELDENE and the reaction could not be determined.

Gastrointestinal: pancreatitis

Dermatologic: onycholysis, loss of hair

Central Nervous System: akathisia, hallucinations, mood alterations, dream abnormalities, mental confusion, paresthesias

Urogenital System: dysuria

Body as a Whole: weakness

Cardiovascular/Respiratory: palpitations, dyspnea

Hypersensitivity: positive ANA

Special Senses: transient hearing loss

Hematological: hemolytic anemia

OVERDOSAGE

In the event treatment for overdosage is required the long plasma half-life (see CLINICAL PHARMACOLOGY) of piroxicam should be considered. The absence of experience with acute overdosage precludes characterization of sequelae and recommendation of specific antidotal efficacy at this time. It is reasonable to assume, however, that the standard measures of gastric evacuation and general supportive therapy would apply. In addition to supportive measures, the use of activated charcoal may effectively reduce the absorption and reabsorption of piroxicam. Experiments in dogs have demonstrated that the use of multiple-dose treatments with

---

*Reactions occurring in 3% to 9% of patients treated with FELDENE. Reactions occurring in 1–3% of patients are unmarked.

Continued on next page

Pfizer—Cont.

activated charcoal could reduce the half-life of piroxicam elimination from 27 hours (without charcoal) to 11 hours and reduce the systemic bioavailability of piroxicam by as much as 37% when activated charcoal is given as late as 6 hours after administration of piroxicam.

ADMINISTRATION AND DOSAGE

Rheumatoid Arthritis, Osteoarthritis

It is recommended that FELDENE therapy be initiated and maintained at a single daily dose of 20 mg. If desired the daily dose may be divided. Because of the long half-life of FELDENE, steady-state blood levels are not reached for 7–12 days. Therefore although the therapeutic effects of FELDENE are evident early in treatment, there is a progressive increase in response over several weeks and the effect of therapy should not be assessed for two weeks.

Dosage recommendations and indications for use in children have not been established.

HOW SUPPLIED

FELDENE Capsules for oral administration

Bottles of 100: 10 mg (NDC 0663-3220-66) maroon and blue #322

20 mg (NDC 0069-3230-66) maroon #323

Bottles of 500: 20 mg (NDC 0663-3230-73) maroon #323

Unit dose packages of 100: 20 mg (NDC 0663-3230-41) maroon #323

65-4100-00-3   Revised July 1990

LITERATURE AVAILABLE

Yes.

Shown in Product Identification Section, page 423

MINIPRESS® CAPSULES   ℞
[mĭn 'ē-prĕs]
(prazosin hydrochloride)
For Oral Use

DESCRIPTION

MINIPRESS (prazosin hydrochloride), a quinazoline derivative, is the first of a new chemical class of antihypertensives. It is the hydrochloride salt of 1-(4-amino-6,7-dimethoxy-2-quinazolinyl)-4-(2-furoyl) piperazine.

It is a white, crystalline substance, slightly soluble in water and isotonic saline, and has a molecular weight of 419.87.

Each 1 mg capsule of MINIPRESS for oral use contains drug equivalent to 1 mg free base.

Inert ingredients in the formulations are: hard gelatin capsules (which may contain Blue 1, Red 3, Red 28, Red 40, and other inert ingredients); magnesium stearate; sodium lauryl sulfate; starch; sucrose.

CLINICAL PHARMACOLOGY

The exact mechanism of the hypotensive action of prazosin is unknown. Prazosin causes a decrease in total peripheral resistance and was originally thought to have a direct relaxant action on vascular smooth muscle. Recent animal studies, however, have suggested that the vasodilator effect of prazosin is also related to blockade of postsynaptic *alpha*-adrenoceptors. The results of dog forelimb experiments demonstrate that the peripheral vasodilator effect of prazosin is confined mainly to the level of the resistance vessels (arterioles). Unlike conventional *alpha*-blockers, the antihypertensive action of prazosin is usually not accompanied by a reflex tachycardia. Tolerance has not been observed to develop in long term therapy.

Hemodynamic studies have been carried out in man following acute single dose administration and during the course of long term maintenance therapy. The results confirm that the therapeutic effect is a fall in blood pressure unaccompanied by a clinically significant change in cardiac output, heart rate, renal blood flow and glomerular filtration rate. There is no measurable negative chronotropic effect. In clinical studies to date, MINIPRESS has not increased plasma renin activity.

In man, blood pressure is lowered in both the supine and standing positions. This effect is most pronounced on the diastolic blood pressure.

Following oral administration, human plasma concentrations reach a peak at about three hours with a plasma half-life of two to three hours. The drug is highly bound to plasma protein. Bioavailability studies have demonstrated that the total absorption relative to the drug in a 20% alcoholic solution is 90%, resulting in peak levels approximately 65% of that of the drug in solution. Animal studies indicate that MINIPRESS is extensively metabolized, primarily by demethylation and conjugation, and excreted mainly via bile and feces. Less extensive human studies suggest similar metabolism and excretion in man.

In clinical studies in which lipid profiles were followed, there were generally no adverse changes noted between pre- and post-treatment lipid levels.

INDICATIONS AND USAGE

MINIPRESS (prazosin hydrochloride) is indicated in the treatment of hypertension. It can be used alone or in combination with other antihypertensive drugs such as diuretics or beta-adrenergic blocking agents.

CONTRAINDICATIONS

None known.

WARNINGS

MINIPRESS may cause syncope with sudden loss of consciousness. In most cases this is believed to be due to an excessive postural hypotensive effect, although occasionally the syncopal episode has been preceded by a bout of severe tachycardia with heart rates of 120–160 beats per minute. Syncopal episodes have usually occurred within 30 to 90 minutes of the initial dose of the drug; occasionally they have been reported in association with rapid dosage increases or the introduction of another antihypertensive drug into the regimen of a patient taking high doses of MINIPRESS. The incidence of syncopal episodes is approximately 1% in patients given an initial dose of 2 mg or greater. Clinical trials conducted during the investigational phase of this drug suggest that syncopal episodes can be minimized by limiting the initial dose of the drug to 1 mg, by subsequently increasing the dosage slowly, and by introducing any additional antihypertensive drugs into the patient's regimen with caution (see DOSAGE AND ADMINISTRATION). Hypotension may develop in patients given MINIPRESS who are also receiving a beta-blocker such as propranolol.

If syncope occurs, the patient should be placed in the recumbent position and treated supportively as necessary. This adverse effect is self-limiting and in most cases does not recur after the initial period of therapy or during subsequent dose titration.

Patients should always be started on the 1 mg capsules of MINIPRESS. The 2 and 5 mg capsules are not indicated for initial therapy.

More common than loss of consciousness are the symptoms often associated with lowering of the blood pressure, namely, dizziness and lightheadedness. The patient should be cautioned about these possible adverse effects and advised what measures to take should they develop. The patient should also be cautioned to avoid situations where injury could result should syncope occur during the initiation of MINIPRESS therapy.

PRECAUTIONS

Information for Patients: Dizziness or drowsiness may occur after the first dose of this medicine. Avoid driving or performing hazardous tasks for the first 24 hours after taking this medicine or when the dose is increased. Dizziness, lightheadedness or fainting may occur, especially when rising from a lying or sitting position. Getting up slowly may help lessen the problem. These effects may also occur if you drink alcohol, stand for long periods of time, exercise, or if the weather is hot. While taking MINIPRESS, be careful in the amount of alcohol you drink. Also, use extra care during exercise or hot weather, or if standing for long periods. Check with your physician if you have any questions.

Drug Interactions

MINIPRESS has been administered without any adverse drug interaction in limited clinical experience to date with the following: (1) cardiac glycosides—digitalis and digoxin; (2) hypoglycemics—insulin, chlorpropamide, phenformin, tolazamide, and tolbutamide; (3) tranquilizers and sedatives—chlordiazepoxide, diazepam, and phenobarbital; (4) antigout—allopurinol, colchicine, and probenecid; (5) antiarrhythmics—procainamide, propranolol (see WARNINGS however), and quinidine; and (6) analgesics, antipyretics and anti-inflammatories—propoxyphene, aspirin, indomethacin and phenylbutazone.

Addition of a diuretic or other antihypertensive agent to MINIPRESS has been shown to cause an additive hypotensive effect. This effect can be minimized by reducing the MINIPRESS dose to 1 to 2 mg three times a day, by introducing additional antihypertensive drugs cautiously and then by retitrating MINIPRESS based on clinical response.

Drug/Laboratory Test Interactions

In a study on five patients given from 12 to 24 mg of prazosin per day for 10 to 14 days, there was an average increase of 42% in the urinary metabolite of norepinephrine and an average increase in urinary VMA of 17%. Therefore, false positive results may occur in screening tests for pheochromocytoma in patients who are being treated with prazosin. If an elevated VMA is found, prazosin should be discontinued and the patient retested after a month.

Laboratory Tests

In clinical studies in which lipid profiles were followed, there were generally no adverse changes noted between pre- and post-treatment lipid levels.

Carcinogenesis, Mutagenesis, Impairment of Fertility: No carcinogenic potential was demonstrated in an 18 month study in rats with MINIPRESS at dose levels more than 225 times the usual maximum recommended human dose of 20 mg per day. MINIPRESS was not mutagenic in *in vivo* genetic toxicology studies. In a fertility and general reproduc-

tive performance study in rats, both males and females, treated with 75 mg/kg (225 times the usual maximum recommended human dose), demonstrated decreased fertility while those treated with 25 mg/kg (75 times the usual maximum recommended human dose) did not.

In chronic studies (one year or more) of MINIPRESS in rats and dogs, testicular changes consisting of atrophy and necrosis occurred at 25 mg/kg/day (75 times the usual maximum recommended human dose). No testicular changes were seen in rats or dogs at 10 mg/kg/day (30 times the usual maximum recommended human dose). In view of the testicular changes observed in animals, 105 patients on long term MINIPRESS therapy were monitored for 17-ketosteroid excretion and no changes indicating a drug effect were observed. In addition, 27 males on MINIPRESS for up to 51 months did not have changes in sperm morphology suggestive of drug effect.

Usage in Pregnancy: Pregnancy Category C. MINIPRESS has been shown to be associated with decreased litter size at birth, 1, 4, and 21 days of age in rats when given doses more than 225 times the usual maximum recommended human dose. No evidence of drug-related external, visceral, or skeletal fetal abnormalities were observed. No drug-related external, visceral, or skeletal abnormalities were observed in fetuses of pregnant rabbits and pregnant monkeys at doses more than 225 times and 12 times the usual maximum recommended human dose respectively.

The use of prazosin and a beta-blocker for the control of severe hypertension in 44 pregnant women revealed no drug-related fetal abnormalities or adverse effects. Therapy with prazosin was continued for as long as 14 weeks.[1]

Prazosin has also been used alone or in combination with other hypotensive agents in severe hypertension of pregnancy by other investigators. No fetal or neonatal abnormalities have been reported with the use of prazosin.[2]

There are no adequate and well controlled studies which establish the safety of MINIPRESS (prazosin HCl) in pregnant women. MINIPRESS should be used during pregnancy only if the potential benefit justifies the potential risk to the mother and fetus.

Nursing Mothers: MINIPRESS has been shown to be excreted in small amounts in human milk. Caution should be exercised when MINIPRESS is administered to a nursing woman.

Usage in Children: Safety and effectiveness in children have not been established.

ADVERSE REACTIONS

Clinical trials were conducted on more than 900 patients. During these trials and subsequent marketing experience, the most frequent reactions associated with MINIPRESS therapy are: dizziness 10.3%, headache 7.8%, drowsiness 7.6%, lack of energy 6.9%, weakness 6.5%, palpitations 5.3%, and nausea 4.9%. In most instances side effects have disappeared with continued therapy or have been tolerated with no decrease in dose of drug.

Less frequent adverse reactions which are reported to occur in 1–4% of patients are:

Gastrointestinal: vomiting, diarrhea, constipation.

Cardiovascular: edema, orthostatic hypotension, dyspnea, syncope.

Central Nervous System: vertigo, depression, nervousness.

Dermatologic: rash.

Genitourinary: urinary frequency.

EENT: blurred vision, reddened sclera, epistaxis, dry mouth, nasal congestion.

In addition, fewer than 1% of patients have reported the following (in some instances, exact causal relationships have not been established):

Gastrointestinal: abdominal discomfort and/or pain, liver function abnormalities, pancreatitis.

Cardiovascular: tachycardia.

Central Nervous System: paresthesia, hallucinations.

Dermatologic: pruritus, alopecia, lichen planus.

Genitourinary: incontinence, impotence, priapism.

EENT: tinnitus.

Other: diaphoresis, fever, positive ANA titer, arthralgia.

Single reports of pigmentary mottling and serous retinopathy, and a few reports of cataract development or disappearance have been reported. In these instances, the exact causal relationship has not been established because the baseline observations were frequently inadequate.

In more specific slit-lamp and funduscopic studies, which included adequate baseline examinations, no drug-related abnormal ophthalmological findings have been reported. Literature reports exist associating MINIPRESS therapy with a worsening of pre-existing narcolepsy. A causal relationship is uncertain in these cases.

OVERDOSAGE

Accidental ingestion of at least 50 mg of MINIPRESS (prazosin hydrochloride) in a two year old child resulted in profound drowsiness and depressed reflexes. No decrease in blood pressure was noted. Recovery was uneventful.

Strength	Capsule Color	Capsule Code	NDC	Package Size
MINIPRESS 1 mg	White	431	0069-4310-71 0663-4310-82 0663-4310-41	250's 1000's 100 (10×10) Unit Dose
MINIPRESS 2 mg	Pink and White	437	0663-4370-71 0663-4370-82 0663-4370-41	250's 1000's 100 (10×10) Unit Dose
MINIPRESS 5 mg	Blue and White	438	0663-4380-71 0663-4380-73 0663-4380-41	250's 500's 100 (10×10) Unit Dose

Should overdosage lead to hypotension, support of the cardiovascular system is of first importance. Restoration of blood pressure and normalization of heart rate may be accomplished by keeping the patient in the supine position. If this measure is inadequate, shock should first be treated with volume expanders. If necessary, vasopressors should then be used. Renal function should be monitored and supported as needed. Laboratory data indicate MINIPRESS is not dialysable because it is protein bound.

DOSAGE AND ADMINISTRATION

The dose of MINIPRESS should be adjusted according to the patient's individual blood pressure response. The following is a guide to its administration:

Initial Dose

1 mg two or three times a day. (See WARNINGS)

Maintenance Dose

Dosage may be slowly increased to a total daily dose of 20 mg given in divided doses. The therapeutic dosages most commonly employed have ranged from 6 mg to 15 mg daily given in divided doses. Doses higher than 20 mg usually do not increase efficacy, however a few patients may benefit from further increases up to a daily dose of 40 mg given in divided doses. After initial titration some patients can be maintained adequately on a twice daily dosage regimen.

Use With Other Drugs

When adding a diuretic or other antihypertensive agent, the dose of MINIPRESS should be reduced to 1 mg or 2 mg three times a day and retitration then carried out.

HOW SUPPLIED

[See table above.]

References

1. Lubbe, WF, and Hodge, JV: *New Zealand Med J* **94** (691) 169–172, 1981.
2. Davey, DA, and Dommisse, J: *S.A. Med J,* Oct 4, 1980 (551–556).

77-2318-00-1   Revised July 1990

Shown in Product Identification Section, page 423

MINIZIDE® CAPSULES   ℞

[mĭn 'ē-zīd]

(prazosin hydrochloride and polythiazide)

FOR ORAL ADMINISTRATION

This fixed combination drug is not indicated for initial therapy of hypertension. Hypertension requires therapy titrated to the individual patient. If the fixed combination represents the dose so determined, its use may be more convenient in patient management. The treatment of hypertension is not static, but must be re-evaluated as conditions in each patient warrant.

DESCRIPTION

MINIZIDE is a combination of MINIPRESS® (prazosin hydrochloride) plus RENESE® (polythiazide).

MINIPRESS (prazosin hydrochloride), a quinazoline derivative, is the first of a new chemical class of antihypertensives. It is the hydrochloride salt of 1-(4-amino-6,7-dimethoxy-2-quinazolinyl)-4-(2-furoyl) piperazine and its structural formula is:

It is a white, crystalline substance, slightly soluble in water and isotonic saline, and has a molecular weight of 419.87. Each 1 mg capsule of MINIPRESS (prazosin hydrochloride) contains drug equivalent to 1 mg free base.

RENESE (polythiazide) is an orally effective, nonmercurial diuretic, saluretic, and antihypertensive agent.

It is designated chemically as 2 *H*-1,2,4-Benzothiadiazine-7-sulfonamide, 6-chloro-3,4-dihydro-2-methyl-3-[[(2,2,2-trifluoroethyl)thio]methyl]-,1,1-dioxide, and has the following structural formula:

It is a white, crystalline substance insoluble in water, but readily soluble in alkaline solution.

Inert ingredients in the formulations are: hard gelatin capsules (which may contain Blue 1, Green 3, Red 3 and other inert ingredients); magnesium stearate; sodium lauryl sulfate; starch; sucrose.

CLINICAL PHARMACOLOGY

MINIZIDE (prazosin hydrochloride/polythiazide)

Minizide produces a more pronounced antihypertensive response than occurs after either prazosin hydrochloride or polythiazide alone in equivalent doses.

MINIPRESS (prazosin hydrochloride)

The exact mechanism of the hypotensive action of prazosin is unknown. Prazosin causes a decrease in total peripheral resistance and was originally thought to have a direct relaxant action on vascular smooth muscle. Recent animal studies, however, have suggested that the vasodilator effect of prazosin is also related to blockade of postsynaptic *alpha*-adrenoceptors. The results of dog forelimb experiments demonstrate that the peripheral vasodilator effect of prazosin is confined mainly to the level of the resistance vessels (arterioles). Unlike conventional *alpha*-blockers, the antihypertensive action of prazosin is usually not accompanied by a reflex tachycardia. Tolerance has not been observed to develop in long term therapy.

Hemodynamic studies have been carried out in man following acute single dose administration and during the course of long term maintenance therapy. The results confirm that the therapeutic effect is a fall in blood pressure unaccompanied by a clinically significant change in cardiac output, heart rate, renal blood flow, and glomerular filtration rate. There is no measurable negative chronotropic effect.

In clinical studies to date, MINIPRESS has not increased plasma renin activity.

In man, blood pressure is lowered in both the supine and standing positions. This effect is most pronounced on the diastolic blood pressure.

Following oral administration, human plasma concentrations reach a peak at about three hours with a plasma half-life of two to three hours. The drug is highly bound to plasma protein. Bioavailability studies have demonstrated that the total absorption relative to the drug in a 20% alcoholic solution is 90%, resulting in peak levels approximately 65% of that of the drug in solution. Animal studies indicate that MINIPRESS is extensively metabolized, primarily by demethylation and conjugation, and excreted mainly via bile and feces. Less extensive human studies suggest similar metabolism and excretion in man.

MINIPRESS has been administered without any adverse drug interaction in limited clinical experience to date with the following: (1) cardiac glycosides—digitalis and digoxin; (2) hypoglycemics—insulin, chlorpropamide, phenformin, tolazamide, and tolbutamide; (3) tranquilizers and sedatives—chlordiazepoxide, diazepam, and phenobarbital; (4) antigout—allopurinol, colchicine, and probenecid; (5) antiarrhythmics—procainamide, propranolol (see WARNINGS however), and quinidine; and (6) analgesics, antipyretics and anti-inflammatories—propoxyphene, aspirin, indomethacin, and phenylbutazone.

RENESE (polythiazide)

RENESE is a member of the benzothiadiazine (thiazide) family of diuretic/antihypertensive agents. Its mechanism of action results in an interference with the renal tubular mechanism of electrolyte reabsorption. At maximal therapeutic dosage all thiazides are approximately equal in their diuretic potency. The mechanism whereby thiazides function in the control of hypertension is unknown. Renese is well absorbed, giving peak human plasma concentrations about 5 hours after oral administration. Drug is removed slowly thereafter with a plasma elimination half-life of approximately 27 hours. One fifth of the drug is recovered unchanged in human urine; the remainder is cleared via feces and as metabolites. Animal studies indicate metabolism occurs by rupture of the thiadiazine ring and loss of the side chain.

INDICATIONS AND USAGE

MINIZIDE is indicated in the treatment of hypertension. (See box warning.)

CONTRAINDICATIONS

RENESE (polythiazide) is contraindicated in patients with anuria, and in patients known to be sensitive to thiazides or to other sulfonamide derivatives.

WARNINGS

MINIPRESS (prazosin hydrochloride)

MINIPRESS may cause syncope with sudden loss of consciousness. In most cases this is believed to be due to an excessive postural hypotensive effect, although occasionally the syncopal episode has been preceded by a bout of severe tachycardia with heart rates of 120–160 beats per minute. Syncopal episodes have usually occurred within 30 to 90 minutes of the initial dose of the drug; occasionally they have been reported in association with rapid dosage increases or the introduction of another antihypertensive drug into the regimen of a patient taking high doses of MINIPRESS. The incidence of syncopal episodes is approximately 1% in patients given an initial dose of 2 mg or greater. Clinical trials conducted during the investigational phase of this drug suggest that syncopal episodes can be minimized by limiting the initial dose of the drug to 1 mg, by subsequently increasing the dosage slowly, and by introducing any additional antihypertensive drugs into the patient's regimen with caution (see DOSAGE AND ADMINISTRATION). Hypotension may develop in patients given MINIPRESS who are also receiving a beta-blocker such as propranolol.

If syncope occurs, the patient should be placed in the recumbent position and treated supportively as necessary. This adverse effect is self-limiting and in most cases does not recur after the initial period of therapy or during subsequent dose titration.

Patients should always be started on the 1 mg capsules of MINIPRESS (prazosin hydrochloride). The 2 and 5 mg capsules are not indicated for initial therapy.

More common than loss of consciousness are the symptoms often associated with lowering of the blood pressure, namely, dizziness and lightheadedness. The patient should be cautioned about these possible adverse effects and advised what measures to take should they develop. The patient should also be cautioned to avoid situations where injury could result should syncope occur during the initiation of MINIPRESS therapy.

RENESE (polythiazide)

RENESE should be used with caution in severe renal disease. In patients with renal disease, thiazides may precipitate azotemia. Cumulative effects of the drug may develop in patients with impaired renal function.

Thiazides should be used with caution in patients with impaired hepatic function or progressive liver disease, since minor alterations of fluid and electrolyte balance may precipitate hepatic coma.

Sensitivity reactions may occur in patients with a history of allergy or bronchial asthma.

The possibility of exacerbation or activation of systemic lupus erythematosus has been reported.

Thiazides may be additive or potentiative of the action of other antihypertensive drugs.

Potentiation occurs with ganglionic or peripheral adrenergic blocking drugs.

Periodic determinations of serum electrolytes to detect possible electrolyte imbalance should be performed at appropriate intervals.

All patients receiving thiazide therapy should be observed for clinical signs of fluid or electrolyte imbalance, namely, hyponatremia, hypochloremic alkalosis, and hypokalemia. Serum and urine electrolyte determinations are particularly important when the patient is vomiting excessively or receiving parenteral fluids. Medications such as digitalis may also influence serum electrolytes. Warning signs, irrespective of cause, are: dryness of mouth, thirst, weakness, lethargy, drowsiness, restlessness, muscle pains or cramps, muscular fatigue, hypotension, oliguria, tachycardia, and gastrointestinal disturbances such as nausea and vomiting.

Continued on next page

Pfizer—Cont.

Hypokalemia may develop with thiazides as with any potent diuretic, especially with brisk diuresis, when severe cirrhosis is present, or during concomitant use of corticosteroids or ACTH.
Interference with adequate oral electrolyte intake will also contribute to hypokalemia. Digitalis therapy may exaggerate the metabolic effects of hypokalemia, especially with reference to myocardial activity.
Any chloride deficit is generally mild and usually does not require specific treatment except under extraordinary circumstances (as in hepatic or renal disease). Dilutional hyponatremia may occur in edematous patients in hot weather; appropriate therapy is water restriction rather than administration of salt, except in rare instances when the hyponatremia is life-threatening. In actual salt depletion, appropriate replacement is the therapy of choice.
Hyperuricemia may occur or frank gout may be precipitated in certain patients receiving thiazide therapy.
Insulin requirements in diabetic patients may be either increased, decreased, or unchanged. Latent diabetes mellitus may become manifest during thiazide administration.
Thiazide drugs may increase responsiveness to tubocurarine.
The antihypertensive effects of the drug may be enhanced in the post-sympathectomy patient.
Thiazides may decrease arterial responsiveness to norepinephrine. This diminution is not sufficient to preclude effectiveness of the pressor agent for therapeutic use.
If progressive renal impairment becomes evident, as indicated by a rising nonprotein nitrogen or blood urea nitrogen, a careful reappraisal of therapy is necessary with consideration given to withholding or discontinuing diuretic therapy.
Thiazides may decrease serum protein-bound iodine levels without signs of thyroid disturbance.

PRECAUTIONS

Drug/Laboratory Test Interactions: In a study on five patients given from 12 to 24 mg of prazosin per day for 10 to 14 days, there was an average increase of 42% in the urinary metabolite of norepinephrine and an average increase in urinary VMA of 17%. Therefore, false positive results may occur in screening tests for pheochromocytoma in patients who are being treated with prazosin. If an elevated VMA is found, prazosin should be discontinued and the patient retested after a month.
Carcinogenesis, Mutagenesis, Impairment of Fertility: No carcinogenic or mutagenic studies have been conducted with MINIZIDE. However, no carcinogenic potential was demonstrated in 18 month studies in rats with either MINIPRESS or RENESE at dose levels more than 100 times the usual maximum human doses. MINIPRESS was not mutagenic in *in vivo* genetic toxicology studies.
MINIZIDE produced no impairment of fertility in male or female rats at 50 and 25 mg/kg/day of MINIPRESS and RENESE respectively. In chronic studies (one year or more) of MINIPRESS in rats and dogs, testicular changes consisting of atrophy and necrosis occurred at 25 mg/kg/day (60 times the usual maximum recommended human dose). No testicular changes were seen in rats or dogs at 10 mg/kg/day (24 times the usual maximum recommended human dose). In view of the testicular changes observed in animals, 105 patients on long term MINIPRESS therapy were monitored for 17-ketosteroid excretion and no changes indicating a drug effect were observed. In addition, 27 males on MINIPRESS alone for up to 51 months did not have changes in sperm morphology suggestive of drug effect.
Use in Pregnancy: Pregnancy Category C. MINIZIDE was not teratogenic in either rats or rabbits when administered in oral doses more than 100 times the usual maximum human dose. Studies in rats indicated that the combination of RENESE (40 times the usual maximum recommended human dose) and MINIPRESS (8 times the usual maximum recommended human dose) caused a greater number of stillbirths, a more prolonged gestation, and a decreased survival of pups to weaning than that caused by MINIPRESS alone. There are no adequate and well controlled studies in pregnant women. Therefore, MINIZIDE should be used in pregnancy only if the potential benefit justifies the potential risk to the fetus.
Nursing Mothers: It is not known whether MINIPRESS or RENESE are excreted in human milk. Thiazides appear in breast milk. Thus, if use of the drug is deemed essential the patient should stop nursing.
Pediatric Use: Safety and effectiveness in children has not been established.

ADVERSE REACTIONS

MINIPRESS (prazosin hydrochloride)
The most common reactions associated with MINIPRESS therapy are: dizziness 10.3%, headache 7.8%, drowsiness 7.6%, lack of energy 6.9%, weakness 6.5%, palpitations 5.3%, and nausea 4.9%. In most instances side effects have disappeared with continued therapy or have been tolerated with no decrease in dose of drug.
The following reactions have been associated with MINIPRESS, some of them rarely. (In some instances exact causal relationships have not been established.)

Gastrointestinal: vomiting, diarrhea, constipation, abdominal discomfort and/or pain, liver function abnormalities, pancreatitis.
Cardiovascular: edema, dyspnea, syncope, tachycardia.
Central Nervous System: nervousness, vertigo, depression, paresthesia, hallucinations.
Dermatologic: rash, pruritus, alopecia, lichen planus.
Genitourinary: urinary frequency, incontinence, impotence, priapism.
EENT: blurred vision, reddened sclera, epistaxis, tinnitus, dry mouth, nasal congestion.
Other: diaphoresis, fever.

Single reports of pigmentary mottling and serous retinopathy, and a few reports of cataract development or disappearance have been reported. In these instances, the exact causal relationship has not been established because the baseline observations were frequently inadequate.
In more specific slit-lamp and funduscopic studies, which included adequate baseline examinations, no drug-related abnormal ophthalmological findings have been reported.
Literature reports exist associating MINIPRESS therapy with a worsening of pre-existing narcolepsy. A causal relationship is uncertain in these cases.
RENESE (polythiazide)

Gastrointestinal: anorexia, gastric irritation, nausea, vomiting, cramping, diarrhea, constipation, jaundice (intrahepatic cholestatic jaundice), pancreatitis.
Central Nervous System: dizziness, vertigo, paresthesia, headache, xanthopsia.
Hematologic: leukopenia, agranulocytosis, thrombocytopenia, aplastic anemia.
Dermatologic: purpura, photosensitivity, rash, urticaria, necrotizing angiitis, (vasculitis) (cutaneous vasculitis).
Cardiovascular: Orthostatic hypotension may occur and be aggravated by alcohol, barbiturates, or narcotics.
Other: hyperglycemia, glycosuria, hyperuricemia, muscle spasm, weakness, restlessness.

OVERDOSAGE

MINIPRESS (prazosin hydrochloride)
Accidental ingestion of at least 50 mg of MINIPRESS in a two year old child resulted in profound drowsiness and depressed reflexes. No decrease in blood pressure was noted. Recovery was uneventful.
Should overdosage lead to hypotension, support of the cardiovascular system is of first importance. Restoration of blood pressure and normalization of heart rate may be accomplished by keeping the patient in the supine position. If this measure is inadequate, shock should first be treated with volume expanders. If necessary, vasopressors should then be used. Renal function should be monitored and supported as needed. Laboratory data indicate that MINIPRESS is not dialyzable because it is protein bound.
RENESE (polythiazide)
Should overdosage with RENESE occur, electrolyte balance and adequate hydration should be maintained. Gastric lavage is recommended, followed by supportive treatment. Where necessary, this may include intravenous dextrose and saline with potassium and other electrolyte therapy, administered with caution as indicated by laboratory testing at appropriate intervals.

DOSAGE AND ADMINISTRATION

MINIZIDE (prazosin hydrochloride/polythiazide)
Dosage: as determined by individual titration of MINIPRESS (prazosin hydrochloride) and RENESE (polythiazide). (See box warning.)
Usual MINIZIDE dosage is one capsule two or three times daily, the strength depending upon individual requirement following titration.
The following is a general guide to the administration of the individual components of MINIZIDE:
MINIPRESS (prazosin hydrochloride)
Initial Dose: 1 mg two or three times a day. (See WARNINGS.)
Maintenance Dose: Dosage may be slowly increased to a total daily dose of 20 mg given in divided doses. The therapeutic dosages most commonly employed have ranged from 6 mg to 15 mg daily given in divided doses. Doses higher than 20 mg usually do not increase efficacy, however a few patients may benefit from further increases up to a daily dose of 40 mg given in divided doses. After initial titration some patients can be maintained adequately on a twice daily dosage regimen.
Use With Other Drugs: When adding a diuretic or other antihypertensive agent, the dose of MINIPRESS should be reduced to 1 mg or 2 mg three times a day and retitration then carried out.
RENESE (polythiazide)
The usual dose of RENESE for antihypertensive therapy is 2 to 4 mg daily.
[See table below.]

Revised Dec. 1988
Shown in Product Identification Section, page 423

HOW SUPPLIED

STRENGTH	COMPONENTS	COLOR	CAPSULE CODE	PKG. SIZE
MINIZIDE 1	1 mg prazosin + 0.5 mg polythiazide (NDC 0663-4300-66)	Blue-Green	430	100's
MINIZIDE 2	2 mg prazosin + 0.5 mg polythiazide (NDC 0663-4320-66)	Blue-Green/Pink	432	100's
MINIZIDE 5	5 mg prazosin + 0.5 mg polythiazide (NDC 0663-4360-66)	Blue-Green/Blue	436	100's

NORVASC® ℞
(amlodipine besylate)
Tablets

DESCRIPTION

NORVASC® is the besylate salt of amlodipine, a long-acting calcium channel blocker.
NORVASC is chemically described as (R.S.) 3-ethyl-5-methyl -2- (2-aminoethoxymethyl) -4- (2-chlorophenyl) -1,4-dihydro-6-methyl-3,5-pyridinedicarboxylate benzenesulphonate. Its empirical formula is $C_{20}H_{25}ClN_2O_5 \cdot C_6H_6O_3S$, and its structural formula is:

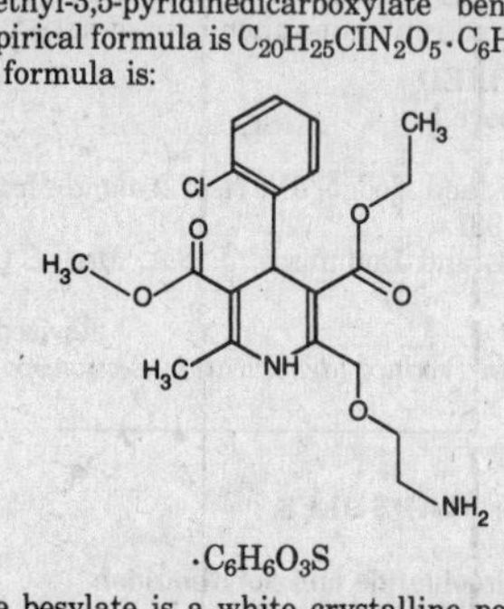

$\cdot C_6H_6O_3S$

Amlodipine besylate is a white crystalline powder with a molecular weight of 567.1. It is slightly soluble in water and sparingly soluble in ethanol. NORVASC (amlodipine besylate) tablets are formulated as white tablets equivalent to 2.5, 5 and 10 mg of amlodipine for oral administration. In addition to the active ingredient, amlodipine besylate, each tablet contains the following inactive ingredients: microcrystalline cellulose, dibasic calcium phosphate anhydrous, sodium starch glycolate, and magnesium stearate.

CLINICAL PHARMACOLOGY

Mechanism of Action: NORVASC is a dihydropyridine calcium antagonist (calcium ion antagonist or slow channel blocker) that inhibits the transmembrane influx of calcium ions into vascular smooth muscle and cardiac muscle. Experimental data suggest that NORVASC binds to both dihydropyridine and nondihydropyridine binding sites. The contractile processes of cardiac muscle and vascular smooth muscle are dependent upon the movement of extracellular calcium ions into these cells through specific ion channels. NORVASC inhibits calcium ion influx across cell membranes selectively, with a greater effect on vascular smooth muscle cells than on cardiac muscle cells. Negative inotropic effects can be detected *in vitro* but such effects have not been seen in intact animals at therapeutic doses. Serum calcium concentration is not affected by NORVASC. Within the physiologic pH range, NORVASC is an ionized compound (pKa = 8.6), and its kinetic interaction with the calcium channel receptor is characterized by a gradual rate of association and dissociation with the receptor binding site, resulting in a gradual onset of effect.
NORVASC is a peripheral arterial vasodilator that acts directly on vascular smooth muscle to cause a reduction

in peripheral vascular resistance and reduction in blood pressure.

The precise mechanisms by which NORVASC relieves angina have not been fully delineated, but are thought to include the following:

Exertional Angina: In patients with exertional angina, NORVASC reduces the total peripheral resistance (afterload) against which the heart works and reduces the rate pressure product, and thus myocardial oxygen demand, at any given level of exercise.

Vasospastic Angina: NORVASC has been demonstrated to block constriction and restore blood flow in coronary arteries and arterioles in response to calcium, potassium epinephrine, serotonin, and thromboxane A_2 analog in experimental animal models and in human coronary vessels *in vitro*. This inhibition of coronary spasm is responsible for the effectiveness of NORVASC in vasospastic (Prinzmetal's or variant) angina.

Pharmacokinetics and Metabolism: After oral administration of therapeutic doses of NORVASC, absorption produces peak plasma concentrations between 6 and 12 hours. Absolute bioavailability has been estimated to be between 64 and 90%. The bioavailability of NORVASC is not altered by the presence of food.

NORVASC is extensively (about 90%) converted into inactive metabolites via hepatic metabolism with 10% of the parent compound and 60% of the metabolites excreted in the urine. *Ex vivo* studies have shown that approximately 93% of the circulating drug is bound to plasma proteins in hypertensive patients. Elimination from the plasma is biphasic with a terminal elimination half-life of about 30–50 hours. Steady state plasma levels of NORVASC are reached after 7 to 8 days of consecutive daily dosing.

The pharmacokinetics of NORVASC are not significantly influenced by renal impairment. Patients with renal failure may therefore receive the usual initial dose.

Elderly patients and patients with hepatic insufficiency have decreased clearance of amlodipine with a resulting increase in AUC of approximately 40–60%, and a lower initial dose may be required.

Pharmacodynamics: *Hemodynamics* Following administration of therapeutic doses to patients with hypertension, NORVASC produces vasodilation resulting in a reduction of supine and standing blood pressures. These decreases in blood pressure are not accompanied by a significant change in heart rate or plasma catecholamine levels with chronic dosing. Although the acute intravenous administration of amlodipine decreases arterial blood pressure and increases heart rate in hemodynamic studies of patients with chronic stable angina, chronic administration of oral amlodipine in clinical trials did not lead to clinically significant changes in heart rate or blood pressures in normotensive patients with angina.

With chronic once daily oral administration, antihypertensive effectiveness is maintained for at least 24 hours. Plasma concentrations correlate with effect in both young and elderly patients. The magnitude of reduction in blood pressure with NORVASC is also correlated with the height of pretreatment elevation; thus, individuals with moderate hypertension (diastolic pressure 105–114 mmHg) had about a 50% greater response than patients with mild hypertension (diastolic pressure 90–104 mmHg). Normotensive subjects experienced no clinically significant change in blood pressures (+ 1/− 2 mmHg).

As with other calcium channel blockers, hemodynamic measurements of cardiac function at rest and during exercise (or pacing) in patients with normal ventricular function treated with NORVASC have generally demonstrated a small increase in cardiac index without significant influence on dP/dt or on left ventricular end diastolic pressure or volume. In hemodynamic studies, NORVASC has not been associated with a negative inotropic effect when administered in the therapeutic dose range to intact animals and man, even when co-administered with beta-blockers to man. Similar findings, however, have been observed in normals or well-compensated patients with heart failure with agents possessing significant negative inotropic effects.

In a double-blind, placebo-controlled clinical trial involving 118 patients with well compensated heart failure (NYHA Class II and Class III), treatment with NORVASC did not lead to worsened heart failure, based on measures of exercise tolerance, left ventricular ejection fraction and clinical symptomatology. Studies in patients with NYHA Class IV heart failure have not been performed and, in general, all calcium channel blockers should be used with caution in any patient with heart failure.

In hypertensive patients with normal renal function, therapeutic doses of NORVASC resulted in a decrease in renal vascular resistance and an increase in glomerular filtration rate and effective renal plasma flow without change in filtration fraction or proteinuria.

Electrophysiologic Effects: NORVASC does not change sinoatrial nodal function or atrioventricular conduction in intact animals or man. In patients with chronic stable angina, intravenous administration of 10 mg did not significantly alter A-H and H-V conduction and sinus node recovery time after pacing. Similar results were obtained in patients receiving NORVASC and concomitant beta blockers. In clinical studies in which NORVASC was administered in combination with beta-blockers to patients with either hypertension or angina, no adverse effects on electrocardiographic parameters were observed. In clinical trials with angina patients alone, NORVASC therapy did not alter electrocardiographic intervals or produce higher degrees of AV blocks.

Effects in Hypertension: The antihypertensive efficacy of NORVASC has been demonstrated in a total of 15 double-blind, placebo-controlled, randomized studies involving 800 patients on NORVASC and 538 on placebo. Once daily administration produced statistically significant placebo-corrected reductions in supine and standing blood pressures at 24 hours postdose, averaging about 12/6 mmHg in the standing position and 13/7 mmHg in the supine position in patients with mild to moderate hypertension. Maintenance of the blood pressure effect over the 24 hour dosing interval was observed, with little difference in peak and trough effect. Tolerance was not demonstrated in patients studied for up to 1 year. The 3 parallel, fixed dose, dose response studies showed that the reduction in supine and standing blood pressures was dose-related within the recommended dosing range. Effects on diastolic pressure were similar in young and older patients. The effect on systolic pressure was greater in older patients, perhaps because of greater baseline systolic pressure. Effects were similar in black and white patients.

Effects in Chronic Stable Angina: The effectiveness of 5–10 mg/day of NORVASC in exercise-induced angina has been evaluated in 8 placebo-controlled, double-blind clinical trials of up to 6 weeks duration involving 1038 patients (684 NORVASC, 354 placebo) with chronic stable angina. In 5 of the 8 studies significant increases in exercise time (bicycle or treadmill) were seen with the 10 mg dose. Increases in symptom-limited exercise time averaged 12.8% (63 sec) for NORVASC 10 mg. and averaged 7.9% (38 sec) for NORVASC 5 mg. NORVASC 10 mg also increased time to 1 mm ST segment deviation in several studies and decreased angina attack rate. The sustained efficacy of NORVASC in angina patients has been demonstrated over long-term dosing. In patients with angina there were no clinically significant reductions in blood pressures (4/1 mmHg) or changes in heart rate (+0.3 bpm).

Effects in Vasospastic Angina: In a double-blind, placebo-controlled clinical trial of 4 weeks duration in 50 patients. NORVASC therapy decreased attacks by approximately 4/week compared with a placebo decrease of approximately 1/week ($p < 0.01$). Two of 23 NORVASC and 7 of 27 placebo patients discontinued from the study due to lack of clinical improvement.

INDICATIONS AND USAGE

1. Hypertension

NORVASC is indicated for the treatment of hypertension. It may be used alone or in combination with other antihypertensive agents.

2. Chronic Stable Angina

NORVASC is indicated for the treatment of chronic stable angina. NORVASC may be used alone or in combination with other antianginal agents.

3. Vasospastic Angina (Prinzmetal's or Variant Angina)

NORVASC is indicated for the treatment of confirmed or suspected vasospastic angina. NORVASC may be used as monotherapy or in combination with other antianginal drugs.

CONTRAINDICATIONS

NORVASC is contraindicated in patients with known sensitivity to amlodipine.

WARNINGS

Increased Angina and/or Myocardial Infarction: Rarely, patients, particulary those with severe obstructive coronary artery disease, have developed documented increased frequency, duration and/or severity of angina or acute myocardial infarction on starting calcium channel blocker therapy or at the time of dosage increase. The mechanism of this effect has not been elucidated.

PRECAUTIONS

General: Since the vasodilation induced by NORVASC is gradual in onset, acute hypotension has rarely been reported after oral administration of NORVASC. Nonetheless, caution should be exercised when administering NORVASC as with any other peripheral vasodilator particularly in patients with severe aortic stenosis.

Use in Patients with Congestive Heart Failure: Although hemodynamic studies and a controlled trial in NYHA Class II–III heart failure patients have shown that NORVASC did not lead to clinical deterioration as measured by exercise tolerance, left ventricular ejection fraction, and clinical symptomatology, studies have not been performed in patients with NYHA Class IV heart failure. In general, all calcium channel blockers should be used with caution in patients with heart failure.

Beta-Blocker Withdrawal: NORVASC is not a beta-blocker and therefore gives no protection against the dangers of abrupt beta-blocker withdrawal; any such withdrawal should be by gradual reduction of the dose of beta-blocker.

Patients with Hepatic Failure: Since NORVASC is extensively metabolized by the liver and the plasma elimination half-life ($t_{1/2}$) is 56 hours in patients with impaired hepatic function, caution should be exercised when administering NORVASC to patients with severe hepatic impairment.

Drug Interactions: *In vitro* data in human plasma indicate that NORVASC has no effect on the protein binding of drugs tested (digoxin, phenytoin, warfarin, and indomethacin). Special studies have indicated that the co-administration of NORVASC with digoxin did not change serum digoxin levels or digoxin renal clearance in normal volunteers; that co-administration with cimetidine did not alter the pharmacokinetics of amlodipine; and that co-administration with warfarin did not change the warfarin prothrombin response time.

In clinical trials, NORVASC has been safely administered with thiazide diuretics, beta-blockers, angiotensin converting enzyme inhibitors, long-acting nitrates, sublingual nitroglycerin, digoxin, warfarin, non-steroidal anti-inflammatory drugs, antibiotics, and oral hypoglycemic drugs.

Drug/Laboratory Test Interactions: None known.

Carcinogenesis, Mutagenesis, Impairment of Fertility: Rats and mice treated with amlodipine in the diet for two years, at concentrations calculated to provide daily dosage levels of 0.5, 1.25, and 2.5 mg/kg/day showed no evidence of carcinogenicity. The highest dose (for mice, similar to, and for rats twice* the maximum recommended clinical dose of 10 mg on a mg/m^2 basis), was close to the maximum tolerated dose for mice but not for rats.

Mutagenicity studies revealed no drug related effects at either the gene or chromosome levels.

There was no effect on the fertility of rats treated with amlodipine (males for 64 days and females 14 days prior to mating) at doses up to 10 mg/kg/day (8 times* the maximum recommended human dose of 10 mg on a mg/m^2 basis).

Pregnancy Category C: No evidence of teratogenicity or other embryo/fetal toxicity was found when pregnant rats or rabbits were treated orally with up to 10 mg/kg amlodipine (respectively 8 times* and 23 times* the maximum recommended human dose of 10 mg on a mg/m^2 basis) during their respective periods of major organogenesis. However, litter size was significantly decreased (by about 50%) and the number of intrauterine deaths was significantly increased (about 5-fold) in rats administered 10 mg/kg amlodipine for 14 days before mating and throughout mating and gestation. Amlodipine has been shown to prolong both the gestation period and the duration of labor in rats at this dose. There are no adequate and well-controlled studies in pregnant women. Amlodipine should be used during pregnancy only if the potential benefit justifies the potential risk to the fetus.

Nursing Mothers: It is not known whether amlodipine is excreted in human milk. In the absence of this information, it is recommended that nursing be discontinued while NORVASC is administered.

Pediatric Use: Safety and effectiveness of NORVASC in children have not been established.

ADVERSE REACTIONS

NORVASC has been evaluated for safety in more than 11,000 patients in U.S. and foreign clinical trials. In general, treatment with NORVASC was well-tolerated at doses up to 10 mg daily. Most adverse reactions reported during therapy with NORVASC were of mild or moderate severity. In controlled clinical trials directly comparing NORVASC (N=1730) in doses up to 10 mg to placebo (N=1250), discontinuation of NORVASC due to adverse reactions was required in only about 1.5% of patients and was not significantly different from placebo (about 1%). The most common side effects are headache and edema. The incidence (%) of side effects which occurred in a dose related manner are as follows:

Adverse Event	2.5 mg N=275	5.0 mg N=296	10.0 mg N=268	Placebo N=520
Edema	1.8	3.0	10.8	0.6
Dizziness	1.1	3.4	3.4	1.5
Flushing	0.7	1.4	2.6	0.0
Palpitation	0.7	1.4	4.5	0.6

Other adverse experiences which were not clearly dose related but which were reported with an incidence greater than 1.0% in placebo-controlled clinical trials include the following:

Placebo Controlled Studies

	NORVASC (%) (N=1730)	PLACEBO (%) (N=1250)
Headache	7.3	7.8
Fatigue	4.5	2.8
Nausea	2.9	1.9
Abdominal Pain	1.6	0.3
Somnolence	1.4	0.6

* Based on patient weight of 50 kg.

Continued on next page

Pfizer—Cont.

For several adverse experiences that appear to be drug and dose related, there was a greater incidence in women than men associated with amlodipine treatment as shown in the following table:

ADR	NORVASC M=% (N=1218)	NORVASC F=% (N=512)	PLACEBO M=% (N=914)	PLACEBO F=% (N=336)
Edema	5.6	14.6	1.4	5.1
Flushing	1.5	4.5	0.3	0.9
Palpitations	1.4	3.3	0.9	0.9
Somnolence	1.3	1.6	0.8	0.3

The following events occurred in ≤1% but >0.1% of patients in controlled clinical trials or under conditions of open trials or marketing experience where a causal relationship is uncertain; they are listed to alert the physician to a possible relationship:

Cardiovascular: arrhythmia, bradycardia, chest pain, hypotension, peripheral ischemia, syncope, tachycardia, postural dizziness, postural hypotension.

Central and Peripheral Nervous System: hypoesthesia, paresthesia, tremor, vertigo.

Gastrointestinal: anorexia, constipation, dyspepsia,** dysphagia, diarrhea, flatulence, vomiting.

General: asthenia,** back pain, hot flushes, malaise, pain, rigors, weight gain.

Musculo-skeletal System: arthralgia, arthrosis, muscle cramps,** myalgia.

Psychiatric: sexual dysfunction (male** and female), insomnia, nervousness, depression, abnormal dreams, anxiety, depersonalization.

Respiratory System: dyspnea,** epistaxis.

Skin and Appendages: pruritus,** rash,** rash erythematous, rash maculopapular.

Special Senses: abnormal vision, conjunctivitis, diplopia, eye pain, tinnitus.

Urinary System: micturition frequency, micturition disorder, nocturia.

Autonomic Nervous System: dry mouth, sweating increased.

Metabolic and Nutritional: thirst.

Hemopoietic: purpura.

The following events occurred in ≤0.1% of patients: cardiac failure, pulse irregularity, extrasystoles, skin discoloration, urticaria, skin dryness, alopecia, dermatitis, muscle weakness, twitching, ataxia, hypertonia, migraine, cold and clammy skin, apathy, agitation, amnesia, gastritis, increased appetite, loose stools, coughing, rhinitis, dysuria, polyuria, parosmia, taste perversion, abnormal visual accommodation, and xerophthalmia.

Other reactions occurred sporadically in single patients and cannot be distinguished from concurrent disease states or medications.

NORVASC therapy has not been associated with clinically significant changes in routine laboratory tests. No clinically relevant changes were noted in serum potassium, serum glucose, total triglycerides, total cholesterol, HDL cholesterol, uric acid, blood urea nitrogen, creatinine or liver function tests.

NORVASC has been used safely in patients with chronic obstructive pulmonary disease, well compensated congestive heart failure, peripheral vascular disease, diabetes mellitus, and abnormal lipid profiles.

OVERDOSAGE

Single oral doses of 40 mg/kg and 100 mg/kg in mice and rats, respectively, caused deaths. A single oral dose of 4 mg/kg or higher in dogs caused a marked peripheral vasodilation and hypotension.

Overdosage might be expected to cause excessive peripheral vasodilation with marked hypotension and possibly a reflex tachycardia. In humans, experience with intentional overdosage of NORVASC is limited. Reports of intentional overdosage include a patient who ingested 250 mg and was asymptomatic and was not hospitalized; another (120 mg) was hospitalized, underwent gastric lavage and remained normotensive; the third (105 mg) was hospitalized and had hypotension (90/50 mmHg) which normalized following plasma expansion. A patient who took 70 mg amlodipine and an unknown quantity of benzodiazepine in a suicide attempt, developed shock which was refractory to treatment and died the following day with abnormally high benzodiazepine plasma concentration. A case of accidental drug overdose has been documented in a 19 month old male who ingested 30 mg amlodipine (about 2 mg/kg). During the emergency room presentation, vital signs were stable with no evidence of hypotension, but a heart rate of 180 bpm. Ipecac was administered 3.5 hours after ingestion and on subsequent observation (overnight) no sequelae were noted.

** These events occurred in less than 1% in placebo controlled trials, but the incidence of these side effects was between 1% and 2% in all multiple dose studies.

If massive overdose should occur, active cardiac and respiratory monitoring should be instituted. Frequent blood pressure measurements are essential. Should hypotension occur, cardiovascular support including elevation of the extremities and the judicious administration of fluids should be initiated. If hypotension remains unresponsive to these conservative measures, administration of vasopressors (such as phenylephrine), should be considered with attention to circulating volume and urine output. Intravenous calcium gluconate may help to reverse the effects of calcium entry blockade. As NORVASC is highly protein bound, hemodialysis is not likely to be of benefit.

DOSAGE AND ADMINISTRATION

The usual initial antihypertensive oral dose of NORVASC is 5 mg once daily with a maximum dose of 10 mg once daily. Small, fragile, or elderly individuals, or patients with hepatic insufficiency may be started on 2.5 mg once daily and this dose may be used when adding NORVASC to other antihypertensive therapy.

Dosage should be adjusted according to each patient's need. In general, titration should proceed over 7 to 14 days so that the physician can fully assess the patient's response to each dose level. Titration may proceed more rapidly, however, if clinically warranted, provided the patient is assessed frequently.

The recommended dose for chronic stable or vasospastic angina is 5–10 mg, with the lower dose suggested in the elderly and in patients with hepatic insufficiency. Most patients will require 10 mg for adequate effect. See Adverse Reactions section for information related to dosage and side effects.

Co-administration with Other Antihypertensive and/or Antianginal Drugs: NORVASC has been safely administered with thiazides, ACE inhibitors, beta-blockers, long-acting nitrates, and/or sublingual nitroglycerin.

HOW SUPPLIED

NORVASC® —2.5 mg Tablets (amlodipine besylate equivalent to 2.5 mg of amlodipine per tablet) are supplied as white, diamond, flat-faced, beveled edged engraved with "NORVASC" on one side and "2.5" on the other side and supplied as follows:

NDC 0069-1520-66—Bottle of 100

NORVASC® —5 mg Tablets (amlodipine besylate equivalent to 5 mg of amlodipine per tablet) are white, elongated octagon, flat-faced, beveled edged engraved with both "NORVASC" and "5" on one side and plain on the other side and supplied as follows:

NDC 0069-1530-66—Bottle of 100

NORVASC® —10 mg Tablets (amlodipine besylate equivalent to 10 mg of amlodipine per tablet) are white, round, flat-faced, beveled edged engraved with both "NORVASC" and "10" on one side and plain on the other side and supplied as follows:

NDC 0069-1540-66—Bottle of 100

Store bottles at controlled room temperature, 59° to 86°F (15° to 30°C) and dispense in tight, light-resistant containers (USP).

© 1992 PFIZER INC.

65-4782-00-0   Issued August 1992

PROCARDIA®   ℞
[pro-car'dē-ă]
(nifedipine)
CAPSULES
For Oral Use

DESCRIPTION

PROCARDIA (nifedipine) is an antianginal drug belonging to a new class of pharmacological agents, the calcium channel blockers. Nifedipine is 3,5-pyridinedicarboxylic acid, 1,4-dihydro-2,6-dimethyl-4-(2-nitrophenyl)-, dimethyl ester, $C_{17}H_{18}N_2O_6$.

Nifedipine is a yellow crystalline substance, practically insoluble in water but soluble in ethanol. It has a molecular weight of 346.3. PROCARDIA CAPSULES are formulated as soft gelatin capsules for oral administration each containing 10 mg or 20 mg nifedipine.

Inert ingredients in the formulations are: glycerin; peppermint oil; polyethylene glycol; soft gelatin capsules (which contain Yellow 6, and may contain Red Ferric Oxide and other inert ingredients), and water. The 10 mg capsules also contain saccharin sodium.

CLINICAL PHARMACOLOGY

PROCARDIA is a calcium ion influx inhibitor (slow channel blocker or calcium ion antagonist) and inhibits the transmembrane influx of calcium ions into cardiac muscle and smooth muscle. The contractile processes of cardiac muscle and vascular smooth muscle are dependent upon the movement of extracellular calcium ions into these cells through specific ion channels. PROCARDIA selectively inhibits calcium ion influx across the cell membrane of cardiac muscle

and vascular smooth muscle without changing serum calcium concentrations.

Mechanism of Action

The precise means by which this inhibition relieves angina has not been fully determined, but includes at least the following two mechanisms:

1) Relaxation and prevention of coronary artery spasm

PROCARDIA dilates the main coronary arteries and coronary arterioles, both in normal and ischemic regions, and is a potent inhibitor of coronary artery spasm, whether spontaneous or ergonovine-induced. This property increases myocardial oxygen delivery in patients with coronary artery spasm, and is responsible for the effectiveness of PROCARDIA in vasospastic (Prinzmetal's or variant) angina. Whether this effect plays any role in classical angina is not clear, but studies of exercise tolerance have not shown an increase in the maximum exercise rate-pressure product, a widely accepted measure of oxygen utilization. This suggests that, in general, relief of spasm or dilation of coronary arteries is not an important factor in classical angina.

2) Reduction of oxygen utilization

PROCARDIA regularly reduces arterial pressure at rest and at a given level of exercise by dilating peripheral arterioles and reducing the total peripheral resistance (afterload) against which the heart works. This unloading of the heart reduces myocardial energy consumption and oxygen requirements and probably accounts for the effectiveness of PROCARDIA in chronic stable angina.

Pharmacokinetics and Metabolism

PROCARDIA is rapidly and fully absorbed after oral administration. The drug is detectable in serum 10 minutes after oral administration, and peak blood levels occur in approximately 30 minutes. Bioavailability is proportional to dose from 10 to 30 mg; half-life does not change significantly with dose. There is little difference in relative bioavailability when PROCARDIA capsules are given orally and either swallowed whole; bitten and swallowed; or, bitten and held sublingually. However, biting through the capsule prior to swallowing does result in slightly earlier plasma concentrations (27 ng/ml 10 minutes after 10 mg) than if capsules are swallowed intact. It is highly bound by serum proteins. PROCARDIA is extensively converted to inactive metabolites and approximately 80 percent of PROCARDIA and metabolites are eliminated via the kidneys. The half-life of nifedipine in plasma is approximately two hours. There is no information on the effects of renal or hepatic impairment on excretion or metabolism of PROCARDIA.

Hemodynamics

Like other slow channel blockers, PROCARDIA exerts a negative inotropic effect on isolated myocardial tissue. This is rarely, if ever, seen in intact animals or man, probably because of reflex responses to its vasodilating effects. In man, PROCARDIA causes decreased peripheral vascular resistance and a fall in systolic and diastolic pressure, usually modest (5–10mm Hg systolic), but sometimes larger. There is usually a small increase in heart rate, a reflex response to vasodilation. Measurements of cardiac function in patients with normal ventricular function have generally found a small increase in cardiac index without major effects on ejection fraction, left ventricular end diastolic pressure (LVEDP) or volume (LVEDV). In patients with impaired ventricular function, most acute studies have shown some increase in ejection fraction and reduction in left ventricular filling pressure.

Electrophysiologic Effects

Although like other members of its class, PROCARDIA decreases sinoatrial node function and atrioventricular conduction in isolated myocardial preparations, such effects have not been seen in studies in intact animals or in man. In formal electrophysiologic studies, predominantly in patients with normal conduction systems, PROCARDIA has had no tendency to prolong atrioventricular conduction, prolong sinus node recovery time, or slow sinus rate.

INDICATIONS AND USAGE

I. Vasospastic Angina

PROCARDIA (nifedipine) is indicated for the management of vasospastic angina confirmed by any of the following criteria: 1) classical pattern of angina at rest accompanied by ST segment elevation, 2) angina or coronary artery spasm provoked by ergonovine, or 3) angiographically demonstrated coronary artery spasm. In those patients who have had angiography, the presence of significant fixed obstructive disease is not incompatible with the diagnosis of vasospastic angina, provided that the above criteria are satisfied. PROCARDIA may also be used where the clinical presentation suggests a possible vasospastic component but where vasospasm has not been confirmed, e.g., where pain has a variable threshold on exertion or in unstable angina where electrocardiographic findings are compatible with intermittent vasospasm, or when angina is refractory to nitrates and/or adequate doses of beta blockers.

II. Chronic Stable Angina (Classical Effort-Associated Angina)

PROCARDIA is indicated for the management of chronic stable angina (effort-associated angina) without evidence of vasospasm in patients who remain symptomatic despite adequate doses of beta blockers and/or organic nitrates or who cannot tolerate those agents.

In chronic stable angina (effort-associated angina) PROCARDIA has been effective in controlled trials of up to eight weeks duration in reducing angina frequency and increasing exercise tolerance, but confirmation of sustained effectiveness and evaluation of long term safety in these patients are incomplete.

Controlled studies in small numbers of patients suggest concomitant use of PROCARDIA and beta blocking agents may be beneficial in patients with chronic stable angina, but available information is not sufficient to predict with confidence the effects of concurrent treatment, especially in patients with compromised left ventricular function or cardiac conduction abnormalities. When introducing such concomitant therapy, care must be taken to monitor blood pressure closely since severe hypotension can occur from the combined effects of the drugs. (See WARNINGS.)

CONTRAINDICATIONS

Known hypersensitivity reaction to PROCARDIA.

WARNINGS

Excessive Hypotension

Although in most patients, the hypotensive effect of PROCARDIA is modest and well tolerated, occasional patients have had excessive and poorly tolerated hypotension. These responses have usually occurred during initial titration or at the time of subsequent upward dosage adjustment, and may be more likely in patients on concomitant beta blockers.

Severe hypotension and/or increased fluid volume requirements have been reported in patients receiving PROCARDIA together with a beta blocking agent who underwent coronary artery bypass surgery using high dose fentanyl anesthesia. The interaction with high dose fentanyl appears to be due to the combination of PROCARDIA and a beta blocker, but the possibility that it may occur with PROCARDIA alone, with low doses of fentanyl, in other surgical procedures, or with other narcotic analgesics cannot be ruled out. In PROCARDIA treated patients where surgery using high dose fentanyl anesthesia is contemplated, the physician should be aware of these potential problems and, if the patient's condition permits, sufficient time (at least 36 hours) should be allowed for PROCARDIA to be washed out of the body prior to surgery.

Increased Angina and/or Myocardial Infarction

Rarely, patients, particularly those who have severe obstructive coronary artery disease, have developed well documented increased frequency, duration and/or severity of angina or acute myocardial infarction on starting PROCARDIA or at the time of dosage increase. The mechanism of this effect is not established.

Beta Blocker Withdrawal

Patients recently withdrawn from beta blockers may develop a withdrawal syndrome with increased angina, probably related to increased sensitivity to catecholamines. Initiation of PROCARDIA treatment will not prevent this occurrence and might be expected to exacerbate it by provoking reflex catecholamine release. There have been occasional reports of increased angina in a setting of beta blocker withdrawal and PROCARDIA initiation. It is important to taper beta blockers if possible, rather than stopping them abruptly before beginning PROCARDIA.

Congestive Heart Failure

Rarely, patients, usually receiving a beta blocker, have developed heart failure after beginning PROCARDIA. Patients with tight aortic stenosis may be at greater risk for such an event, as the unloading effect of PROCARDIA would be expected to be of less benefit to these patients, owing to their fixed impedance to flow across the aortic valve.

PRECAUTIONS

General: Hypotension: Because PROCARDIA decreases peripheral vascular resistance, careful monitoring of blood pressure during the initial administration and titration of PROCARDIA is suggested. Close observation is especially recommended for patients already taking medications that are known to lower blood pressure. (See WARNINGS.)

Peripheral edema: Mild to moderate peripheral edema, typically associated with arterial vasodilation and not due to left ventricular dysfunction, occurs in about one in ten patients treated with PROCARDIA. This edema occurs primarily in the lower extremities and usually responds to diuretic therapy. With patients whose angina is complicated by congestive heart failure, care should be taken to differentiate this peripheral edema from the effects of increasing left ventricular dysfunction.

Laboratory tests: Rare, usually transient, but occasionally significant elevations of enzymes such as alkaline phosphatase, CPK, LDH, SGOT and SGPT have been noted. The relationship to PROCARDIA therapy is uncertain in most cases,

but probable in some. These laboratory abnormalities have rarely been associated with clinical symptoms, however, cholestasis with or without jaundice has been reported. Rare instances of allergic hepatitis have been reported.

PROCARDIA, like other calcium channel blockers, decreases platelet aggregation *in vitro*. Limited clinical studies have demonstrated a moderate but statistically significant decrease in platelet aggregation and increase in bleeding time in some PROCARDIA patients. This is thought to be a function of inhibition of calcium transport across the platelet membrane. No clinical significance for these findings has been demonstrated.

Positive direct Coombs test with/without hemolytic anemia has been reported.

Although PROCARDIA has been used safely in patients with renal dysfunction and has been reported to exert a beneficial effect in certain cases, rare, reversible elevations in BUN and serum creatinine have been reported in patients with pre-existing chronic renal insufficiency. The relationship to PROCARDIA therapy is uncertain in most cases but probable in some.

Drug interactions: Beta-adrenergic blocking agents: (See INDICATIONS and WARNINGS.) Experience in over 1400 patients in a non-comparative clinical trial has shown that concomitant administration of PROCARDIA and beta-blocking agents is usually well tolerated, but there have been occasional literature reports suggesting that the combination may increase the likelihood of congestive heart failure, severe hypotension or exacerbation of angina.

Long acting nitrates: PROCARDIA may be safely co-administered with nitrates, but there have been no controlled studies to evaluate the antianginal effectiveness of this combination.

Digitalis: Administration of PROCARDIA with digoxin increased digoxin levels in nine of twelve normal volunteers. The average increase was 45%. Another investigator found no increase in digoxin levels in thirteen patients with coronary artery disease. In an uncontrolled study of over two hundred patients with congestive heart failure during which digoxin blood levels were not measured, digitalis toxicity was not observed. Since there have been isolated reports of patients with elevated digoxin levels, it is recommended that digoxin levels be monitored when initiating, adjusting, and discontinuing PROCARDIA to avoid possible over- or under-digitalization.

Coumarin anticoagulants: There have been rare reports of increased prothrombin time in patients taking coumarin anticoagulants to whom PROCARDIA was administered. However, the relationship to PROCARDIA therapy is uncertain.

Cimetidine: A study in six healthy volunteers has shown a significant increase in peak nifedipine plasma levels (80%) and area-under-the-curve (74%) after a one week course of cimetidine at 1000 mg per day and nifedipine at 40 mg per day. Ranitidine produced smaller, non-significant increases. The effect may be mediated by the known inhibition of cimetidine on hepatic cytochrome P-450, the enzyme system probably responsible for the first-pass metabolism of nifedipine. If nifedipine therapy is initiated in a patient currently receiving cimetidine, cautious titration is advised.

Carcinogenesis, mutagenesis, impairment of fertility: Nifedipine was administered orally to rats for two years and was not shown to be carcinogenic. When given to rats prior to mating, nifedipine caused reduced fertility at a dose approximately 30 times the maximum recommended human dose. *In vivo* mutagenicity studies were negative.

Pregnancy: Pregnancy category C. Nifedipine has been shown to be teratogenic in rats when given in doses 30 times the maximum recommended human dose. Nifedipine was embryotoxic (increased fetal resorptions, decreased fetal weight, increased stunted forms, increased fetal deaths, decreased neonatal survival) in rats, mice and rabbits at doses of from 3 to 10 times the maximum recommended human dose. In pregnant monkeys, doses 2/3 and twice the maximum recommended human dose resulted in small placentas and underdeveloped chorionic villi. In rats, doses three times maximum human dose and higher caused prolongation of pregnancy. There are no adequate and well controlled studies in pregnant women. PROCARDIA should be used during pregnancy only if the potential benefit justifies the potential risk to the fetus.

ADVERSE REACTIONS

In multiple-dose U.S. and foreign controlled studies in which adverse reactions were reported spontaneously, adverse effects were frequent but generally not serious and rarely required discontinuation of therapy or dosage adjustment. Most were expected consequences of the vasodilator effects of PROCARDIA. [See table top of next column.]

There is also a large uncontrolled experience in over 2100 patients in the United States. Most of the patients had vasospastic or resistant angina pectoris, and about half had concomitant treatment with beta-adrenergic blocking agents. The most common adverse events were:

Adverse Effect	PROCARDIA (%) (N = 226)	Placebo (%) (N = 235)
Dizziness, lightheadedness, giddiness	27	15
Flushing, heat sensation	25	8
Headache	23	20
Weakness	12	10
Nausea, heartburn	11	8
Muscle cramps, tremor	8	3
Peripheral edema	7	1
Nervousness, mood changes	7	4
Palpitation	7	5
Dyspnea, cough, wheezing	6	3
Nasal congestion, sore throat	6	8

Incidence Approximately 10% *Cardiovascular:* peripheral edema
Central Nervous System: dizziness or lightheadedness
Gastrointestinal: nausea
Systemic: headache and flushing, weakness

Incidence Approximately 5% *Cardiovascular:* transient hypotension

Incidence 2% or Less *Cardiovascular:* palpitation
Respiratory: nasal and chest congestion, shortness of breath
Gastrointestinal: diarrhea, constipation, cramps, flatulence
Musculoskeletal: inflammation, joint stiffness, muscle cramps
Central Nervous System: shakiness, nervousness, jitteriness, sleep disturbances, blurred vision, difficulties in balance
Other: dermatitis, pruritus, urticaria, fever, sweating, chills, sexual difficulties.

Incidence Approximately 0.5% *Cardiovascular:* syncope. Syncopal episodes did not recur with reduction in the dose of PROCARDIA or concomitant antianginal medication.

Incidence Less Than 0.5% *Hematologic:* thrombocytopenia, anemia, leukopenia, purpura
Gastrointestinal: allergic hepatitis
Oral: gingival hyperplasia
CNS: depression, paranoid syndrome
Special Senses: transient blindness at the peak of plasma level
Other: erythromelalgia, arthritis with ANA (+)

Several of these side effects appear to be dose related. Peripheral edema occurred in about one in 25 patients at doses less than 60 mg per day and in about one patient in eight at 120 mg per day or more. Transient hypotension, generally of mild to moderate severity and seldom requiring discontinuation of therapy, occurred in one of 50 patients at less than 60 mg per day and in one of 20 patients at 120 mg per day or more. Very rarely, introduction of PROCARDIA therapy was associated with an increase in anginal pain, possibly due to associated hypotension.

In addition, more serious adverse events were observed, not readily distinguishable from the natural history of the disease in these patients. It remains possible, however, that some or many of these events were drug related. Myocardial infarction occurred in about 4% of patients and congestive heart failure or pulmonary edema in about 2%. Ventricular arrhythmias or conduction disturbances each occurred in fewer than 0.5% of patients.

In a subgroup of over 1000 patients receiving PROCARDIA with concomitant beta blocker therapy, the pattern and incidence of adverse experiences was not different from that of the entire group of PROCARDIA treated patients. (See PRECAUTIONS.)

In a subgroup of approximately 250 patients with a diagnosis of congestive heart failure as well as angina, dizziness or lightheadedness, peripheral edema, headache or flushing each occurred in one in eight patients. Hypotension occurred in about one in 20 patients. Syncope occurred in approximately one patient in 250. Myocardial infarction or symptoms of congestive heart failure each occurred in about one patient in 15. Atrial or ventricular dysrhythmias each occurred in about one patient in 150.

OVERDOSAGE

Although there is no well documented experience with PROCARDIA overdosage, available data suggest that gross overdosage could result in excessive peripheral vasodilation with subsequent marked and probably prolonged systemic hypotension. Clinically significant hypotension due to PROCARDIA overdosage calls for active cardiovascular support including monitoring of cardiac and respiratory function, elevation of extremities, and attention to circulating fluid volume and urine output. A vasoconstrictor (such as norepinephrine) may be helpful in restoring vascular tone and blood pressure, provided that there is no contraindication to its use. Clearance of PROCARDIA would be expected to be prolonged in patients with impaired liver function. Since PROCARDIA is highly protein-bound, dialysis is not likely to be of benefit.

Continued on next page

Pfizer—Cont.

DOSAGE AND ADMINISTRATION

The dosage of PROCARDIA needed to suppress angina and that can be tolerated by the patient must be established by titration. Excessive doses can result in hypotension.

Therapy should be initiated with the 10 mg capsule. The starting dose is one 10 mg capsule, swallowed whole, 3 times/day. The usual effective dose range is 10–20 mg three times daily. Some patients, especially those with evidence of coronary artery spasm, respond only to higher doses, more frequent administration, or both. In such patients, doses of 20–30 mg three or four times daily may be effective. Doses above 120 mg daily are rarely necessary. More than 180 mg per day is not recommended.

In most cases, PROCARDIA titration should proceed over a 7–14 day period so that the physician can assess the response to each dose level and monitor the blood pressure before proceeding to higher doses.

If symptoms so warrant, titration may proceed more rapidly provided that the patient is assessed frequently. Based on the patient's physical activity level, attack frequency, and sublingual nitroglycerin consumption, the dose of PROCARDIA may be increased from 10 mg t.i.d to 20 mg t.i.d and then to 30 mg t.i.d over a three-day period.

In hospitalized patients under close observation, the dose may be increased in 10 mg increments over four to six-hour periods as required to control pain and arrhythmias due to ischemia. A single dose should rarely exceed 30 mg.

No "rebound effect" has been observed upon discontinuation of PROCARDIA. However, if discontinuation of PROCARDIA is necessary, sound clinical practice suggests that the dosage should be decreased gradually with close physician supervision.

Co-Administration with Other Antianginal Drugs

Sublingual nitroglycerin may be taken as required for the control of acute manifestations of angina, particularly during PROCARDIA titration. See **Precautions, Drug Interactions,** for information on co-administration of PROCARDIA with beta blockers or long acting nitrates.

HOW SUPPLIED

PROCARDIA soft gelatin capsules are supplied in:
Bottles of 100: 10 mg (NDC 0069-2600-66) orange #260;
20 mg (NDC 0069-2610-66) orange and light brown #261
Bottles of 300: 10 mg (NDC 0069-2600-72) orange #260;
20 mg (NDC 0069-2610-72) orange and light brown #261
Unit dose packages of 100: 10 mg (NDC 0069-2600-41) orange #260; 20 mg (NDC 0069-2610-41) orange and light brown #261

The capsules should be protected from light and moisture and stored at controlled room temperature 59° to 77°F (15° to 25°C) in the manufacturer's original container.

69-4052-00-0 Revised July 1987

LITERATURE AVAILABLE

Yes.

Shown in Product Identification Section, page 423

PROCARDIA XL® ℞

[pro-car 'dē-ă]
(nifedipine)
Extended Release Tablets
For Oral Use

DESCRIPTION

Nifedipine is a drug belonging to a class of pharmacological agents known as the calcium channel blockers. Nifedipine is 3,5-pyridinedicarboxylic acid, 1,4-dihydro-2,6-dimethyl-4-(2-nitrophenyl)-, dimethyl ester, $C_{17}H_{18}N_2O_6$, and has the structural formula:

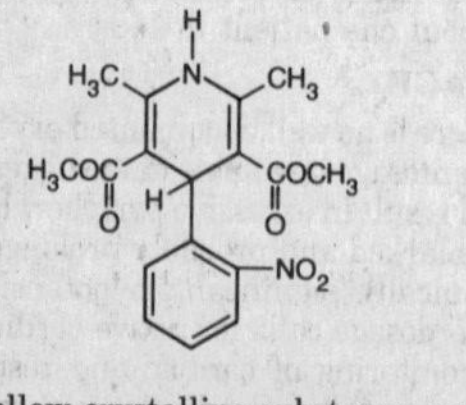

Nifedipine is a yellow crystalline substance, practically insoluble in water but soluble in ethanol. It has a molecular weight of 346.3. PROCARDIA XL is a trademark for Nifedipine GITS. Nifedipine GITS (Gastrointestinal Therapeutic System) Tablet is formulated as a once-a-day controlled-release tablet for oral administration designed to deliver 30, 60, or 90 mg of nifedipine.

Inert ingredients in the formulations are: cellulose acetate; hydroxypropyl cellulose; hydroxypropyl methylcellulose; magnesium stearate; polyethylene glycol; polyethylene oxide; red ferric oxide; sodium chloride; titanium dioxide.

System Components and Performance

PROCARDIA XL Extended Release Tablet is similar in appearance to a conventional tablet. It consists, however, of a semipermeable membrane surrounding an osmotically active drug core. The core itself is divided into two layers: an "active" layer containing the drug, and a "push" layer containing pharmacologically inert (but osmotically active) components. As water from the gastrointestinal tract enters the tablet, pressure increases in the osmotic layer and "pushes" against the drug layer, releasing drug through the precision laser-drilled tablet orifice in the active layer.

PROCARDIA XL Extended Release Tablet is designed to provide nifedipine at an approximately constant rate over 24 hours. This controlled rate of drug delivery into the gastrointestinal lumen is independent of pH or gastrointestinal motility. PROCARDIA XL depends for its action on the existence of an osmotic gradient between the contents of the bilayer core and fluid in the GI tract. Drug delivery is essentially constant as long as the osmotic gradient remains constant, and then gradually falls to zero. Upon swallowing, the biologically inert components of the tablet remain intact during GI transit and are eliminated in the feces as an insoluble shell.

CLINICAL PHARMACOLOGY

Nifedipine is a calcium ion influx inhibitor (slow-channel blocker or calcium ion antagonist) and inhibits the transmembrane influx of calcium ions into cardiac muscle and smooth muscle. The contractile processes of cardiac muscle and vascular smooth muscle are dependent upon the movement of extracellular calcium ions into these cells through specific ion channels. Nifedipine selectively inhibits calcium ion influx across the cell membrane of cardiac muscle and vascular smooth muscle without altering serum calcium concentrations.

Mechanism of Action

A) Angina

The precise mechanisms by which inhibition of calcium influx relieves angina has not been fully determined, but includes at least the following two mechanisms:

1) Relaxation and Prevention of Coronary Artery Spasm

Nifedipine dilates the main coronary arteries and coronary arterioles, both in normal and ischemic regions, and is a potent inhibitor of coronary artery spasm, whether spontaneous or ergonovine-induced. This property increases myocardial oxygen delivery in patients with coronary artery spasm, and is responsible for the effectiveness of nifedipine in vasospastic (Prinzmetal's or variant) angina. Whether this effect plays any role in classical angina is not clear, but studies of exercise tolerance have not shown an increase in the maximum exercise rate-pressure product, a widely accepted measure of oxygen utilization. This suggests that, in general, relief of spasm or dilation of coronary arteries is not an important factor in classical angina.

2) Reduction of Oxygen Utilization

Nifedipine regularly reduces arterial pressure at rest and at a given level of exercise by dilating peripheral arterioles and reducing the total peripheral resistance (afterload) against which the heart works. This unloading of the heart reduces myocardial energy consumption and oxygen requirements, and probably accounts for the effectiveness of nifedipine in chronic stable angina.

B) Hypertension

The mechanism by which nifedipine reduces arterial blood pressure involves peripheral arterial vasodilatation and the resulting reduction in peripheral vascular resistance. The increased peripheral vascular resistance that is an underlying cause of hypertension results from an increase in active tension in the vascular smooth muscle. Studies have demonstrated that the increase in active tension reflects an increase in cytosolic free calcium.

Nifedipine is a peripheral arterial vasodilator which acts directly on vascular smooth muscle. The binding of nifedipine to voltage-dependent and possibly receptor-operated channels in vascular smooth muscle results in an inhibition of calcium influx through these channels. Stores of intracellular calcium in vascular smooth muscle are limited and thus dependent upon the influx of extracellular calcium for contraction to occur. The reduction in calcium influx by nifedipine causes arterial vasodilation and decreased peripheral vascular resistance which results in reduced arterial blood pressure.

Pharmacokinetics and Metabolism

Nifedipine is completely absorbed after oral administration. Plasma drug concentrations rise at a gradual, controlled rate after a PROCARDIA XL Extended Release Tablet dose and reach a plateau at approximately six hours after the first dose. For subsequent doses, relatively constant plasma concentrations at this plateau are maintained with minimal fluctuations over the 24 hour dosing interval. About a four-fold higher fluctuation index (ratio of peak to trough plasma concentration) was observed with the conventional immediate release Procardia® capsule at t.i.d. dosing than with once daily PROCARDIA XL Extended Release Tablet. At steady-state the bioavailability of the PROCARDIA XL Extended Release Tablet is 86% relative to Procardia capsules. Administration of the PROCARDIA XL Extended Release Tablet in the presence of food slightly alters the early rate of drug absorption, but does not influence the extent of drug bioavailability. Markedly reduced GI retention time over prolonged periods (i.e., short bowel syndrome), however, may influence the pharmacokinetic profile of the drug which could potentially result in lower plasma concentrations. Pharmacokinetics of PROCARDIA XL Extended Release Tablets are linear over the dose range of 30 to 180 mg in that plasma drug concentrations are proportional to dose administered. There was no evidence of dose dumping either in the presence or absence of food for over 150 subjects in pharmacokinetic studies.

Nifedipine is extensively metabolized to highly water-soluble, inactive metabolites accounting for 60 to 80% of the dose excreted in the urine. The elimination half-life of nifedipine is approximately two hours. Only traces (less than 0.1% of the dose) of unchanged form can be detected in the urine. The remainder is excreted in the feces in metabolized form, most likely as a result of biliary excretion. Thus, the pharmacokinetics of nifedipine are not significantly influenced by the degree of renal impairment. Patients in hemodialysis or chronic ambulatory peritoneal dialysis have not reported significantly altered pharmacokinetics of nifedipine. Since hepatic biotransformation is the predominant route for the disposition of nifedipine, the pharmacokinetics may be altered in patients with chronic liver disease. Patients with hepatic impairment (liver cirrhosis) have a longer disposition half-life and higher bioavailability of nifedipine than healthy volunteers. The degree of serum protein binding of nifedipine is high (92–98%). Protein binding may be greatly reduced in patients with renal or hepatic impairment.

Hemodynamics

Like other slow-channel blockers, nifedipine exerts a negative inotropic effect on isolated myocardial tissue. This is rarely, if ever, seen in intact animals or man, probably because of reflex responses to its vasodilating effects. In man, nifedipine decreases peripheral vascular resistance which leads to a fall in systolic and diastolic pressures, usually minimal in normotensive volunteers (less than 5–10 mm Hg systolic), but sometimes larger. With PROCARDIA XL Extended Release Tablets, these decreases in blood pressure are not accompanied by any significant change in heart rate. Hemodynamic studies in patients with normal ventricular function have generally found a small increase in cardiac index without major effects on ejection fraction, left ventricular end diastolic pressure (LVEDP) or volume (LVEDV). In patients with impaired ventricular function, most acute studies have shown some increase in ejection fraction and reduction in left ventricular filling pressure.

Electrophysiologic Effects

Although, like other members of its class, nifedipine causes a slight depression of sinoatrial node function and atrioventricular conduction in isolated myocardial preparations, such effects have not been seen in studies in intact animals or in man. In formal electrophysiologic studies, predominantly in patients with normal conduction systems, nifedipine has had no tendency to prolong atrioventricular conduction or sinus node recovery time, or to slow sinus rate.

INDICATIONS AND USAGE

I. Vasospastic Angina

PROCARDIA XL is indicated for the management of vasospastic angina confirmed by any of the following criteria: 1) classical pattern of angina at rest accompanied by ST segment elevation, 2) angina or coronary artery spasm provoked by ergonovine, or 3) angiographically demonstrated coronary artery spasm. In those patients who have had angiography, the presence of significant fixed obstructive disease is not incompatible with the diagnosis of vasospastic angina, provided that the above criteria are satisfied. PROCARDIA XL may also be used where the clinical presentation suggests a possible vasospastic component but where vasospasm has not been confirmed, e.g., where pain has a variable threshold on exertion or in unstable angina where electrocardiographic findings are compatible with intermittent vasospasm, or when angina is refractory to nitrates and/or adequate doses of beta blockers.

II. Chronic Stable Angina (Classical Effort-Associated Angina)

PROCARDIA XL is indicated for the management of chronic stable angina (effort-associated angina) without evidence of vasospasm in patients who remain symptomatic despite adequate doses of beta blockers and/or organic nitrates or who cannot tolerate those agents.

In chronic stable angina (effort-associated angina) nifedipine has been effective in controlled trials of up to eight weeks duration in reducing angina frequency and increasing exercise tolerance, but confirmation of sustained effectiveness and evaluation of long term safety in these patients are incomplete.

Controlled studies in small numbers of patients suggest concomitant use of nifedipine and beta blocking agents may be beneficial in patients with chronic stable angina, but avail-

able information is not sufficient to predict with confidence the effects of concurrent treatment, especially in patients with compromised left ventricular function or cardiac conduction abnormalities. When introducing such concomitant therapy, care must be taken to monitor blood pressure closely since severe hypotension can occur from the combined effects of the drugs. (See WARNINGS.)

III. Hypertension

PROCARDIA XL is indicated for the treatment of hypertension. It may be used alone or in combination with other antihypertensive agents.

CONTRAINDICATIONS

Known hypersensitivity reaction to nifedipine.

WARNINGS

Excessive Hypotension

Although in most angina patients the hypotensive effect of nifedipine is modest and well tolerated, occasional patients have had excessive and poorly tolerated hypotension. These responses have usually occurred during initial titration or at the time of subsequent upward dosage adjustment, and may be more likely in patients on concomitant beta blockers. Severe hypotension and/or increased fluid volume requirements have been reported in patients receiving nifedipine together with a beta-blocking agent who underwent coronary artery bypass surgery using high dose fentanyl anesthesia. The interaction with high dose fentanyl appears to be due to the combination of nifedipine and a beta blocker, but the possibility that it may occur with nifedipine alone, with low doses of fentanyl, in other surgical procedures, or with other narcotic analgesics cannot be ruled out. In nifedipine-treated patients where surgery using high dose fentanyl anesthesia is contemplated, the physician should be aware of these potential problems and if the patient's condition permits, sufficient time (at least 36 hours) should be allowed for nifedipine to be washed out of the body prior to surgery. The following information should be taken into account in those patients who are being treated for hypertension as well as angina:

Increased Angina and/or Myocardial Infarction

Rarely, patients, particularly those who have severe obstructive coronary artery disease, have developed well documented increased frequency, duration and/or severity of angina or acute myocardial infarction on starting nifedipine or at the time of dosage increase. The mechanism of this effect is not established.

Beta Blocker Withdrawal

It is important to taper beta blockers if possible, rather than stopping them abruptly before beginning nifedipine. Patients recently withdrawn from beta blockers may develop a withdrawal syndrome with increased angina, probably related to increased sensitivity to catecholamines. Initiation of nifedipine treatment will not prevent this occurrence and on occasion has been reported to increase it.

Congestive Heart Failure

Rarely, patients, usually receiving a beta blocker, have developed heart failure after beginning nifedipine. Patients with tight aortic stenosis may be at greater risk for such an event, as the unloading effect of nifedipine would be expected to be of less benefit to those patients, owing to their fixed impedance to flow across the aortic valve.

PRECAUTIONS

General—Hypotension

Because nifedipine decreases peripheral vascular resistance, careful monitoring of blood pressure during the initial administration and titration of nifedipine is suggested. Close observation is especially recommended for patients already taking medications that are known to lower blood pressure. (See WARNINGS.)

Peripheral Edema

Mild to moderate peripheral edema occurs in a dose dependent manner with an incidence ranging from approximately 10% to about 30% at the highest dose studied (180 mg). It is a localized phenomenon thought to be associated with vasodilation of dependent arterioles and small blood vessels and not due to left ventricular dysfunction or generalized fluid retention. With patients whose angina or hypertension is complicated by congestive heart failure, care should be taken to differentiate this peripheral edema from the effects of increasing left ventricular dysfunction.

Other

As with any other non-deformable material, caution should be used when administering PROCARDIA XL in patients with preexisting severe gastrointestinal narrowing (pathologic or iatrogenic). There have been rare reports of obstructive symptoms in patients with known strictures in association with the ingestion of PROCARDIA XL.

Information for Patients

PROCARDIA XL Extended Release Tablets should be swallowed whole. Do not chew, divide or crush tablets. Do not be concerned if you occasionally notice in your stool something that looks like a tablet. In PROCARDIA XL, the medication is contained within a nonabsorbable shell that has been specially designed to slowly release the drug for your body to

absorb. When this process is completed, the empty tablet is eliminated from your body.

Laboratory Tests

Rare, usually transient, but occasionally significant elevations of enzymes such as alkaline phosphatase, CPK, LDH, SGOT and SGPT have been noted. The relationship to nifedipine therapy is uncertain in most cases, but probable in some. These laboratory abnormalities have rarely been associated with clinical symptoms; however, cholestasis with or without jaundice has been reported. A small (5.4%) increase in mean alkaline phosphatase was noted in patients treated with PROCARDIA XL. This was an isolated finding not associated with clinical symptoms and it rarely resulted in values which fell outside the normal range. Rare instances of allergic hepatitis have been reported. In controlled studies, PROCARDIA XL did not adversely affect serum uric acid, glucose, or cholesterol. Serum potassium was unchanged in patients receiving PROCARDIA XL in the absence of concomitant diuretic therapy, and slightly decreased in patients receiving concomitant diuretics.

Nifedipine, like other calcium channel blockers, decreases platelet aggregation *in vitro*. Limited clinical studies have demonstrated a moderate but statistically significant decrease in platelet aggregation and increase in bleeding time in some nifedipine patients. This is thought to be a function of inhibition of calcium transport across the platelet membrane. No clinical significance for these findings has been demonstrated.

Positive direct Coombs test with/without hemolytic anemia has been reported but a causal relationship between nifedipine administration and positivity of this laboratory test, including hemolysis, could not be determined.

Although nifedipine has been used safely in patients with renal dysfunction and has been reported to exert a beneficial effect in certain cases, rare reversible elevations in BUN and serum creatinine have been reported in patients with preexisting chronic renal insufficiency. The relationship to nifedipine therapy is uncertain in most cases but probable in some.

Drug Interactions

Beta-adrenergic blocking agents: (See INDICATIONS and WARNINGS) Experience in over 1400 patients with Procardia capsules in a noncomparative clinical trial has shown that concomitant administration of nifedipine and beta-blocking agents is usually well tolerated but there have been occasional literature reports suggesting that the combination may increase the likelihood of congestive heart failure, severe hypotension, or exacerbation of angina.

Long Acting Nitrates: Nifedipine may be safely co-administered with nitrates, but there have been no controlled studies to evaluate the antianginal effectiveness of this combination.

Digitalis: Administration of nifedipine with digoxin increased digoxin levels in nine of twelve normal volunteers. The average increase was 45%. Another investigator found no increase in digoxin levels in thirteen patients with coronary artery disease. In an uncontrolled study of over two hundred patients with congestive heart failure during which digoxin blood levels were not measured, digitalis toxicity was not observed. Since there have been isolated reports of patients with elevated digoxin levels, it is recommended that digoxin levels be monitored when initiating, adjusting, and discontinuing nifedipine to avoid possible over- or under-digitalization.

Coumarin Anticoagulants: There have been rare reports of increased prothrombin time in patients taking coumarin anticoagulants to whom nifedipine was administered. However, the relationship to nifedipine therapy is uncertain.

Cimetidine: A study in six healthy volunteers has shown a significant increase in peak nifedipine plasma levels (80%) and area-under-the-curve (74%) after a one week course of cimetidine at 1000 mg per day and nifedipine at 40 mg per day. Ranitidine produced smaller, non-significant increases. The effect may be mediated by the known inhibition of cimetidine on hepatic cytochrome P-450, the enzyme system probably responsible for the first-pass metabolism of nifedipine. If nifedipine therapy is initiated in a patient currently receiving cimetidine, cautious titration is advised.

Carcinogenesis, Mutagenesis, Impairment of Fertility

Nifedipine was administered orally to rats for two years and was not shown to be carcinogenic. When given to rats prior to mating, nifedipine caused reduced fertility at a dose approximately 30 times the maximum recommended human dose. *In vivo* mutagenicity studies were negative.

Pregnancy

Pregnancy Category C. Nifedipine has been shown to be teratogenic in rats when given in doses 30 times the maximum recommended human dose. Nifedipine was embryotoxic (increased fetal resorptions, decreased fetal weight, increased stunted forms, increased fetal deaths, decreased neonatal survival) in rats, mice and rabbits at doses of from 3 to 10 times the maximum recommended human dose. In pregnant monkeys, doses 2/3 and twice the maximum recommended human dose resulted in small placentas and underdeveloped chorionic villi. In rats, doses three times maximum human dose and higher caused prolongation of preg-

nancy. There are no adequate and well controlled studies in pregnant women. PROCARDIA XL Extended Release Tablets should be used during pregnancy only if the potential benefit justifies the potential risk to the fetus.

ADVERSE EXPERIENCES

Over 1000 patients from both controlled and open trials with PROCARDIA XL Extended Release Tablets in hypertension and angina were included in the evaluation of adverse experiences. All side effects reported during PROCARDIA XL Extended Release Tablet therapy were tabulated independent of their causal relation to medication. The most common side effect reported with PROCARDIA XL was edema which was dose related and ranged in frequency from approximately 10% to about 30% at the highest dose studied (180 mg). Other common adverse experiences reported in placebo-controlled trials include:

Adverse Effect	PROCARDIA XL (%) (N = 707)	Placebo (%) (N = 266)
Headache	15.8	9.8
Fatigue	5.9	4.1
Dizziness	4.1	4.5
Constipation	3.3	2.3
Nausea	3.3	1.9

Of these, only edema and headache were more common in PROCARDIA XL patients than placebo patients.

The following adverse reactions occurred with an incidence of less than 3.0%. With the exception of leg cramps, the incidence of these side effects was similar to that of placebo alone.

Body as a Whole/Systemic: asthenia, flushing, pain
Cardiovascular: palpitations
Central Nervous System: insomnia, nervousness, paresthesia, somnolence
Dermatologic: pruritus, rash
Gastrointestinal: abdominal pain, diarrhea, dry mouth, dyspepsia, flatulence
Musculoskeletal: arthralgia, leg cramps
Respiratory: chest pain (nonspecific), dyspnea
Urogenital: impotence, polyuria

Other adverse reactions were reported sporadically with an incidence of 1.0% or less. These include:

Body as a Whole/Systemic: face edema, fever, hot flashes, malaise, periorbital edema, rigors
Cardiovascular: arrhythmia, hypotension, increased angina, tachycardia, syncope
Central Nervous System: anxiety, ataxia, decreased libido, depression, hypertonia, hypoesthesia, migraine, paroniria, tremor, vertigo
Dermatologic: alopecia, increased sweating, urticaria, purpura
Gastrointestinal: eructation, gastroesophageal reflux, gum hyperplasia, melena, vomiting, weight increase
Musculoskeletal: back pain, gout, myalgias
Respiratory: coughing, epistaxis, upper respiratory tract infection, respiratory disorder, sinusitis
Special Senses: abnormal lacrimation, abnormal vision, taste perversion, tinnitus
Urogenital/Reproductive: breast pain, dysuria, hematuria, nocturia

Adverse experiences which occurred in less than 1 in 1000 patients cannot be distinguished from concurrent disease states or medications.

The following adverse experiences, reported in less than 1% of patients, occurred under conditions (e.g., open trials, marketing experience) where a causal relationship is uncertain: gastrointestinal irritation, gastrointestinal bleeding.

In multiple-dose U.S. and foreign controlled studies with nifedipine capsules in which adverse reactions were reported spontaneously, adverse effects were frequent but generally not serious and rarely required discontinuation of therapy or dosage adjustment. Most were expected consequences of the vasodilator effects of PROCARDIA.

Adverse Effect	PROCARDIA CAPSULES (%) (N = 226)	Placebo (%) (N = 235)
Dizziness, lightheadedness, giddiness	27	15
Flushing, heat sensation	25	8
Headache	23	20
Weakness	12	10
Nausea, heartburn	11	8
Muscle cramps, tremor	8	3
Peripheral edema	7	1
Nervousness, mood changes	7	4
Palpitation	7	5
Dyspnea, cough, wheezing	6	3
Nasal congestion, sore throat	6	8

There is also a large uncontrolled experience in over 2100 patients in the United States. Most of the patients had vasospastic or resistant angina pectoris, and about half had concomitant treatment with beta-adrenergic blocking agents.

Continued on next page

Pfizer—Cont.

The relatively common adverse events were similar in nature to those seen with PROCARDIA XL.

In addition, more serious adverse events were observed, not readily distinguishable from the natural history of the disease in these patients. It remains possible, however, that some or many of these events were drug related. Myocardial infarction occurred in about 4% of patients and congestive heart failure or pulmonary edema in about 2%. Ventricular arrhythmias or conduction disturbances each occurred in fewer than 0.5% of patients.

In a subgroup of over 1000 patients receiving PROCARDIA with concomitant beta blocker therapy, the pattern and incidence of adverse experiences was not different from that of the entire group of PROCARDIA (nifedipine) treated patients. (See PRECAUTIONS.)

In a subgroup of approximately 250 patients with a diagnosis of congestive heart failure as well as angina, dizziness or lightheadedness, peripheral edema, headache or flushing each occurred in one in eight patients. Hypotension occurred in about one in 20 patients. Syncope occurred in approximately one patient in 250. Myocardial infarction or symptoms of congestive heart failure each occurred in about one patient in 15. Atrial or ventricular dysrhythmias each occurred in about one patient in 150.

In post-marketing experience, there have been rare reports of exfoliative dermatitis caused by nifedipine.

OVERDOSAGE

Experience with nifedipine overdosage is limited. Generally, overdosage with nifedipine leading to pronounced hypotension calls for active cardiovascular support including monitoring of cardiovasular and respiratory function, elevation of extremities, judicious use of calcium infusion, pressor agents and fluids. Clearance of nifedipine would be expected to be prolonged in patients with impaired liver function. Since nifedipine is highly protein-bound, dialysis is not likely to be of any benefit.

There has been one reported case of massive overdosage with PROCARDIA XL Extended Release Tablets. The main effect of ingestion of approximately 4800 mg of PROCARDIA XL in a young man attempting suicide as a result of cocaine-induced depression was initial dizziness, palpitations, flushing, and nervousness. Within several hours of ingestion, nausea, vomiting, and generalized edema developed. No significant hypotension was apparent at presentation, 18 hours post-ingestion. Electrolyte abnormalities consisted of a mild, transient elevation of serum creatinine, and modest elevations of LDH and CPK, but normal SGOT. Vital signs remained stable, no electrocardiographic abnormalities were noted and renal function returned to normal with 24 to 48 hours with routine supportive measures alone. No prolonged sequelae were observed.

The effect of a single 900 mg ingestion of PROCARDIA capsules in a depressed anginal patient also on tricyclic antidepressants was a loss of consciousness within 30 minutes of ingestion, and profound hypotension, which responded to calcium infusion, pressor agents, and fluid replacement. A variety of ECG abnormalities were seen in this patient with a history of bundle branch block, including sinus bradycardia and varying degrees of AV block. These dictated the prophylactic placement of a temporary ventricular pacemaker, but otherwise resolved spontaneously. Significant hyperglycemia was seen initially in this patient, but plasma glucose levels rapidly normalized without further treatment.

A young hypertensive patient with advanced renal failure ingested 280 mg of PROCARDIA capsules at one time, with resulting marked hypotension responding to calcium infusion and fluids. No AV conduction abnormalities, arrhythmias, or pronounced changes in heart rate were noted, nor was there any further deterioration in renal function.

DOSAGE AND ADMINISTRATION

Dosage must be adjusted to each patient's needs. Therapy for either hypertension or angina should be initiated with 30 or 60 mg once daily. PROCARDIA XL Extended Release Tablets should be swallowed whole and should not be bitten or divided. In general, titration should proceed over a 7–14 day period so that the physician can fully assess the response to each dose level and monitor blood pressure before proceeding to higher doses. Since steady-state plasma levels are achieved on the second day of dosing, if symptoms so warrant, titration may proceed more rapidly provided the patient is assessed frequently. Titration to doses above 120 mg is not recommended.

Angina patients controlled on PROCARDIA capsules alone or in combination with other antianginal medications may be safely switched to PROCARDIA XL Extended Release Tablets at the nearest equivalent total daily dose (e.g., 30 mg t.i.d. of PROCARDIA capsules may be changed to 90 mg once daily of PROCARDIA XL Extended Release Tablets). Subsequent titration to higher or lower doses may be necessary and should be initiated as clinically warranted. Experience with doses greater than 90 mg in patients with angina is limited. Therefore, doses greater than 90 mg should be used with caution and only when clinically warranted.

No "rebound effect" has been observed upon discontinuation of PROCARDIA XL Extended Release Tablets. However, if discontinuation of nifedipine is necessary, sound clinical practice suggests that the dosage should be decreased gradually with close physician supervision.

Care should be taken when dispensing PROCARDIA XL to assure that the extended release dosage form has been prescribed.

Co-Administration with Other Antianginal Drugs

Sublingual nitroglycerin may be taken as required for the control of acute manifestations of angina, particularly during nifedipine titration. See PRECAUTIONS, Drug Interactions, for information on co-administration of nifedipine with beta blockers or long acting nitrates.

HOW SUPPLIED

PROCARDIA XL® Extended Release Tablets are supplied as 30 mg, 60 mg and 90 mg round biconvex, rose-pink, film-coated tablets in:

Bottles of 100: 30 mg (NDC 0069-2650-66)
 60 mg (NDC 0069-2660-66)
 90 mg (NDC 0069-2670-66)
Bottles of 300: 30 mg (NDC 0069-2650-72)
 60 mg (NDC 0069-2660-72)
Unit dose packages of 100: 30 mg (NDC 0069-2650-41)
 60 mg (NDC 0069-2660-41)

The tablets should be protected from moisture and humidity and stored below 86°F (30°C).

77-4467-00-6 Revised August 1990

Shown in Product Identification Section, page 423

VIBRAMYCIN® Calcium ℞
doxycycline calcium
oral suspension
SYRUP

VIBRAMYCIN® Hyclate
doxycycline hyclate
CAPSULES

VIBRAMYCIN® Monohydrate
doxycycline monohydrate
for ORAL SUSPENSION

VIBRA-TABS®
doxycycline hyclate
FILM COATED TABLETS

DESCRIPTION

Vibramycin is a broad-spectrum antibiotic synthetically derived from oxytetracycline, and is available as Vibramycin Monohydrate (doxycycline monohydrate); Vibramycin Hyclate and Vibra-Tabs (doxycycline hydrochloride hemiethanolate hemihydrate); and Vibramycin Calcium (doxycycline calcium) for oral administration.

The structural formula of doxycycline monohydrate is

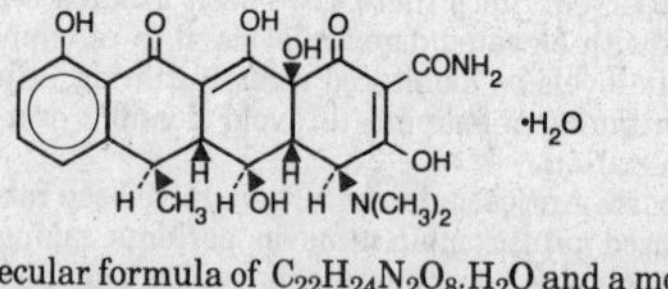

with a molecular formula of $C_{22}H_{24}N_2O_8.H_2O$ and a molecular weight of 462.46. The chemical designation for doxycycline is 4-(Dimethylamino)-1, 4, 4a, 5, 5a, 6, 11, 12a-octahydro-3, 5, 10, 12, 12a-pentahydroxy-6-methyl-1, 11-dioxo-2-naphthacenecarboxamide monohydrate. The molecular formula for doxycycline hydrochloride hemiethanolate hemihydrate is $(C_{22}H_{24}N_2O_8.HCl)_2.C_2H_6O.H_2O$ and the molecular weight is 1025.89. Doxycycline is a light-yellow crystalline powder. Doxycycline hyclate is soluble in water, while doxycycline monohydrate is very slightly soluble in water. Doxycycline has a high degree of lipoid solubility and a low affinity for calcium binding. It is highly stable in normal human serum. Doxycycline will not degrade into an epianhydro form.

Inert ingredients in the syrup formulation are: apple flavor; butylparaben; calcium chloride; carmine; glycerin; hydrochloric acid; magnesium aluminum silicate; povidone; propylene glycol; propylparaben; raspberry flavor; simethicone emulsion; sodium hydroxide; sodium metabisulfite; sorbitol solution; water.

Inert ingredients in the capsule formulations are: hard gelatin capsules (which may contain Blue 1 and other inert ingredients); magnesium stearate; microcrystalline cellulose; sodium lauryl sulfate.

Inert ingredients for the oral suspension formulation are: carboxymethylcellulose sodium; Blue 1; methylparaben; microcrystalline cellulose; propylparaben; raspberry flavor; Red 28; simethicone emulsion; sucrose.

Inert ingredients for the tablet formulation are: ethylcellulose; hydroxypropyl methylcellulose; magnesium stearate; microcrystalline cellulose; propylene glycol; sodium lauryl sulfate; talc; titanium dioxide; Yellow 6 Lake.

CLINICAL PHARMACOLOGY

Tetracyclines are readily absorbed and are bound to plasma proteins in varying degree. They are concentrated by the liver in the bile, and excreted in the urine and feces at high concentrations and in a biologically active form. Doxycycline is virtually completely absorbed after oral administration.

Following a 200 mg dose, normal adult volunteers averaged peak serum levels of 2.6 mcg/mL of doxycycline at 2 hours decreasing to 1.45 mcg/mL at 24 hours. Excretion of doxycycline by the kidney is about 40%/72 hours in individuals with normal function (creatinine clearance about 75 mL/min.). This percentage excretion may fall as low as 1–5%/72 hours in individuals with severe renal insufficiency (creatinine clearance below 10 mL/min.). Studies have shown no significant difference in serum half-life of doxycycline (range 18–22 hours) in individuals with normal and severely impaired renal function.

Hemodialysis does not alter serum half-life.

Results of animal studies indicate that tetracyclines cross the placenta and are found in fetal tissues.

MICROBIOLOGY

The tetracyclines are primarily bacteriostatic and are thought to exert their antimicrobial effect by the inhibition of protein synthesis. The tetracyclines, including doxycycline, have a similar antimicrobial spectrum of activity against a wide range of gram-positive and gram-negative organisms. Cross-resistance of these organisms to tetracyclines is common.

Gram-Negative Bacteria

Neisseria gonorrhoeae
Calymmatobacterium granulomatis
Haemophilus ducreyi
Haemophilus influenzae
Yersinia pestis (formerly *Pasteurella pestis*)
Francisella tularensis (formerly *Pasteurella tularensis*)
Vibrio cholera (formerly *Vibrio comma*)
Bartonella bacilliformis
Brucella species

Because many strains of the following groups of gram-negative microorganisms have been shown to be resistant to tetracyclines, culture and susceptibility testing are recommended:

Escherichia coli
Klebsiella species
Enterobacter aerogenes
Shigella species
Acinetobacter species (formerly *Mima* species and *Herellea* species)
Bacteroides species

Gram-Positive Bacteria

Because many strains of the following groups of gram-positive microorganisms have been shown to be resistant to tetracycline, culture and susceptibility testing are recommended. Up to 44 percent of strains of *Streptococcus pyogenes* and 74 percent of *Streptococcus faecalis* have been found to be resistant to tetracycline drugs. Therefore, tetracycline should not be used for streptococcal disease unless the organism has been demonstrated to be susceptible.

Streptococcus pyogenes
Streptococcus pneumoniae
Enterococcus group (*Streptococcus faecalis* and *Streptococcus faecium*)
Alpha-hemolytic streptococci (viridans group)

Other Microorganisms

Rickettsiae
Chlamydia psittaci
Chlamydia trachomatis
Mycoplasma pneumoniae
Ureaplasma urealyticum
Borrelia recurrentis
Treponema pallidum
Treponema pertenue
Clostridium species
Fusobacterium fusiforme
Actinomyces species
Bacillus anthracis
Propionbacterium acnes
Entamoeba species
Balantidium coli

Susceptibility tests: Diffusion techniques: Quantitative methods that require measurement of zone diameters give the most precise estimate of the susceptibility of bacteria to antimicrobial agents. One such standard procedure[1] which has been recommended for use with disks to test susceptibility of organisms to doxycycline, uses the 30-mcg tetracycline-class disk or the 30-mcg doxycycline disk. Interpretation involves the correlation of the diameter obtained in the disk test with the minimum inhibitory concentration (MIC) for tetracycline or doxycycline, respectively.

Reports from the laboratory giving results of the standard single-disk susceptibility test with a 30-mcg tetracycline-

class disk or the 30-mcg doxycycline disk should be interpreted according to the following criteria:

Zone Diameter (mm)		Interpretation
tetracycline	doxycycline	
≥19	≥16	Susceptible
15–18	13–15	Intermediate
≤14	≤12	Resistant

A report of "susceptible" indicates that the pathogen is likely to be inhibited by generally achievable blood levels. A report of "intermediate" suggests that the organism would be susceptible if a high dosage is used or if the infection is confined to tissues and fluids in which high antimicrobial levels are attained. A report of "resistant" indicates that achievable concentrations are unlikely to be inhibitory, and other therapy should be selected.

Standardized procedures require the use of laboratory control organisms. The 30-mcg tetracycline-class disk or the 30-mcg doxycycline disk should give the following zone diameters:

Organism	Zone Diameter (mm)	
	tetracycline	doxycycline
E. coli ATCC 25922	18–25	18–24
S. aureus ATCC 25923	19–28	23–29

Dilution techniques: Use a standardized dilution method[2] (broth, agar, microdilution) or equivalent with tetracycline powder. The MIC values obtained should be interpreted according to the following criteria:

MIC (mcg mL)	Interpretation
≤4	Susceptible
8	Intermediate
≥16	Resistant

As with standard diffusion techniques, dilution methods require the use of laboratory control organisms. Standard tetracycline powder should provide the following MIC values:

Organism	MIC (mcg/mL)
E. coli ATCC 25922	1.0–4.0
S. aureus ATCC 29213	0.25–1.0
E. faecalis ATCC 29212	8–32
P. aeruginosa ATCC 27853	8–32

INDICATIONS AND USAGE

Doxycycline is indicated for the treatment of the following infections:

Rocky mountain spotted fever, typhus fever and the typhus group, Q fever, rickettsialpox, and tick fevers caused by Rickettsiae.

Respiratory tract infections caused by Mycoplasma pneumoniae.

Lymphogranuloma venereum caused by Chlamydia trachomatis.

Psittacosis (ornithosis) caused by Chlamydia psittaci.

Trachoma caused by Chlamydia trachomatis, although the infectious agent is not always eliminated as judged by immunofluorescence.

Inclusion conjunctivitis caused by Chlamydia trachomatis.

Uncomplicated urethral, endocervical or rectal infections in adults caused by Chlamydia trachomatis.

Nongonococcal urethritis caused by Ureaplasma urealyticum.

Relapsing fever due to Borrelia recurrentis.

Doxycycline is also indicated for the treatment of infections caused by the following gram-negative microorganisms:

Chancroid caused by Haemophilus ducreyi.

Plague due to Yersinia pestis (formerly Pasteurella pestis).

Tuleremia due to Francisella tulerensis (formerly Pasteurella tulerensis).

Cholera caused by Vibrio cholerae (formerly Vibrio comma).

Campylobacter fetus infections caused by Campylobacter fetus (formerly Vibrio fetus).

Brucellosis due to Brucella species (in conjunction with streptomycin).

Bartonellosis due to Bartonella bacilliformis.

Granuloma inguinale caused by Calymmatobacterium granulomatis.

Because many strains of the following groups of microorganisms have been shown to be resistant to doxycycline, culture and susceptibility testing are recommended.

Doxycycline is indicated for treatment of infections caused by the following gram-negative microorganisms, when bacteriologic testing indicates appropriate susceptibility to the drug:

Escherichia coli.

Enterobacter aerogenes (formerly Aerobacter aerogenes).

Shigella species.

Acinetobacter species (formerly Mima species and Herellea species).

Respiratory tract infections caused by Haemophilus influenzae.

Respiratory tract and urinary tract infections caused by Klebsiella species.

Doxycycline is indicated for treatment of infections caused by the following gram-positive microorganisms when bacteriologic testing indicates appropriate susceptibility to the drug:

Upper respiratory infections caused by Streptococcus pneumoniae (formerly Diplococcus pneumoniae).

When penicillin is contraindicated, doxycycline is an alternative drug in the treatment of the following infections:

Uncomplicated gonorrhea caused by Neisseria gonorrhoeae.

Syphilis caused by Treponema pallidum.

Yaws caused by Treponema pertenue.

Listeriosis due to Listeria monocytogenes.

Anthrax due to Bacillus anthracis.

Vincent's infection caused by Fusobacterium fusiforme.

Actinomycosis caused by Actinomyces israelii.

Infections caused by Clostridium species.

In acute intestinal amebiasis, doxycycline may be a useful adjunct to amebicides.

In severe acne, doxycycline may be useful adjunctive therapy.

CONTRAINDICATIONS

This drug is contraindicated in persons who have shown hypersensitivity to any of the tetracyclines.

WARNINGS

THE USE OF DRUGS OF THE TETRACYCLINE CLASS DURING TOOTH DEVELOPMENT (LAST HALF OF PREGNANCY, INFANCY AND CHILDHOOD TO THE AGE OF 8 YEARS) MAY CAUSE PERMANENT DISCOLORATION OF THE TEETH (YELLOW-GRAY-BROWN). This adverse reaction is more common during long-term use of the drugs, but has been observed following repeated short-term courses. Enamel hypoplasia has also been reported. TETRACYCLINE DRUGS, THEREFORE, SHOULD NOT BE USED IN THIS AGE GROUP UNLESS OTHER DRUGS ARE NOT LIKELY TO BE EFFECTIVE OR ARE CONTRAINDICATED.

All tetracyclines form a stable calcium complex in any bone-forming tissue. A decrease in fibula growth rate has been observed in prematures given oral tetracycline in doses of 25 mg/kg every 6 hours. This reaction was shown to be reversible when the drug was discontinued.

Results of animal studies indicate that tetracyclines cross the placenta, are found in fetal tissues, and can have toxic effects on the developing fetus (often related to retardation of skeletal development). Evidence of embryotoxicity has also been noted in animals treated early in pregnancy. If any tetracycline is used during pregnancy or if the patient becomes pregnant while taking this drug, the patient should be apprised of the potential hazard to the fetus.

The antianabolic action of the tetracyclines may cause an increase in BUN. Studies to date indicate that this does not occur with the use of doxycycline in patients with impaired renal function.

Photosensitivity manifested by an exaggerated sunburn reaction has been observed in some individuals taking tetracyclines. Patients apt to be exposed to direct sunlight or ultraviolet light should be advised that this reaction can occur with tetracycline drugs, and treatment should be discontinued at the first evidence of skin erythema.

Vibramycin Syrup contains sodium metabisulfite, a sulfite that may cause allergic-type reactions including anaphylactic symptoms and life-threatening or less severe asthmatic episodes in certain susceptible people. The over-all prevalence of sulfite sensitivity in the general population is unknown and probably low. Sulfite sensitivity is seen more frequently in asthmatic than in non-asthmatic people.

PRECAUTIONS

General

As with other antibiotic preparations, use of this drug may result in overgrowth of nonsusceptible organisms, including fungi. If superinfection occurs, the antibiotic should be discontinued and appropriate therapy instituted.

Bulging fontanels in infants and benign intracranial hypertension in adults have been reported in individuals receiving tetracyclines. These conditions disappeared when the drug was discontinued.

Incision and drainage of other surgical procedures should be performed in conjunction with antibiotic therapy, when indicated.

Laboratory Tests

In venereal disease, when co-existent syphilis is suspected, dark field examinations should be done before treatment is started and the blood serology repeated monthly for at least 4 months.

In long-term therapy, periodic laboratory evaluation of organ systems, including hematopoietic, renal, and hepatic studies, should be performed.

Drug Interactions

Because tetracyclines have been shown to depress plasma prothrombin activity, patients who are on anticoagulant therapy may require downward adjustment of their anticoagulant dosage.

Since bacteriostatic drugs may interfere with the bactericidal action of penicillin, it is advisable to avoid giving tetracyclines in conjunction with penicillin.

Absorption of tetracyclines is impaired by antacids containing aluminum, calcium, or magnesium, and iron-containing preparations.

Barbiturates, carbamazepine, and phenytoin decrease the half-life of doxycycline.

The concurrent use of tetracycline and Penthrane (methoxyflurane) has been reported to result in fatal renal toxicity.

Concurrent use of tetracycline may render oral contraceptives less effective.

Drug/Laboratory Test Interactions

False elevations of urinary catecholamine levels may occur due to interference with the fluorescence test.

Carcinogenesis, Mutagenesis, Impairment of Fertility

Long-term studies in animals to evaluate carcinogenic potential of doxycycline have not been conducted. However, there has been evidence of oncogenic activity in rats in studies with the related antibiotics, oxytetracycline (adrenal and pituitary tumors), and minocycline (thyroid tumors). Likewise, although mutagenicity studies of doxycycline have not been conducted, positive results in in vitro mammalian cell assays have been reported for related antibiotics (tetracycline, oxytetracycline).

Doxycycline administered orally at dosage levels as high as 250 mg/kg/day had no apparent effect on the fertility of female rats. Effect on male fertility has not been studied.

Pregnancy Category

Teratogenic effects: Category "D" — (See WARNINGS).

Nonteratogenic effects: (See WARNINGS).

Labor and Delivery

The effect of tetracyclines on labor and delivery is unknown.

Nursing Mothers

Tetracyclines are excreted in human milk. Because of the potential for serious adverse reactions in nursing infants from doxycycline, a decision should be made whether to discontinue nursing or to discontinue the drug, taking into account the importance of the drug to the mother. (See WARNINGS).

Pediatric Use

See WARNINGS and DOSAGE AND ADMINISTRATION.

ADVERSE REACTIONS

Due to oral doxycycline's virtually complete absorption, side effects of the lower bowel, particularly diarrhea, have been infrequent. The following adverse reactions have been observed in patients receiving tetracyclines:

Gastrointestinal: anorexia, nausea, vomiting, diarrhea, glossitis, dysphagia, enterocolitis, and inflammatory lesions (with monilial overgrowth) in the anogenital region. Hepatotoxicity has been reported rarely. These reactions have been caused by both the oral and parenteral administration of tetracyclines. Rare instances of esophagitis and esophageal ulcerations have been reported in patients receiving capsule and tablet forms of the drugs in the tetracycline class. Most of these patients took medications immediately before going to bed. (See DOSAGE AND ADMINISTRATION.)

Skin: maculopapular and erythematous rashes. Exfoliative dermatitis has been reported but is uncommon. Photosensitivity is discussed above. (See WARNINGS.)

Renal toxicity: Rise in BUN has been reported and is apparently dose related. (See WARNINGS.)

Hypersensitivity reactions: urticaria, angioneurotic edema, anaphylaxis, anaphylactoid purpura, serum sickness, pericarditis, and exacerbation of systemic lupus erythematosus.

Blood: Hemolytic anemia, thrombocytopenia, neutropenia, and eosinophilia have been reported.

Other: bulging fontanels in infants and intracranial hypertension in adults. (See PRECAUTIONS—General.)

When given over prolonged periods, tetracyclines have been reported to produce brown-black microscopic discoloration of the thyroid gland. No abnormalities of thyroid function studies are known to occur.

OVERDOSAGE

In case of overdosage, discontinue medication, treat symptomatically and institute supportive measures. Dialysis does not alter serum half-life and thus would not be of benefit in treating cases of overdosage.

DOSAGE AND ADMINISTRATION

THE USUAL DOSAGE AND FREQUENCY OF ADMINISTRATION OF DOXYCYCLINE DIFFERS FROM THAT OF THE OTHER TETRACYCLINES. EXCEEDING THE RECOMMENDED DOSAGE MAY RESULT IN AN INCREASED INCIDENCE OF SIDE EFFECTS. Adults: The usual dose of oral doxycycline is 200 mg on the first day of treatment (administered 100 mg every 12 hours) followed by a maintenance dose of 100 mg/day. The maintenance dose may be administered as a single dose or as 50 mg every 12 hours.

In the management of more severe infections (particularly chronic infections of the urinary tract), 100 mg every 12 hours is recommended.

For children above eight years of age: The recommended dosage schedule for children weighing 100 pounds or less is 2 mg/lb of body weight divided into two doses on the first day of treatment, followed by 1 mg/lb of body weight given as a single daily dose or divided into two doses, on subsequent days. For more severe infections up to 2 mg/lb of body weight

Continued on next page

Pfizer—Cont.

may be used. For children over 100 lb the usual adult dose should be used.

The therapeutic antibacterial serum activity will usually persist for 24 hours following recommended dosage.

When used in streptococcal infections, therapy should be continued for 10 days.

Administration of adequate amounts of fluid along with capsule and tablet forms of drugs in the tetracycline class is recommended to wash down the drugs and reduce the risk of esophageal irritation and ulceration. (See ADVERSE REACTIONS.)

If gastric irritation occurs, it is recommended that doxycycline be given with food or milk. The absorption of doxycycline is not markedly influenced by simultaneous ingestion of food or milk.

Studies to date have indicated that administration of doxycycline at the usual recommended doses does not lead to excessive accumulation of the antibiotic in patients with renal impairment.

Uncomplicated gonococcal infections in adults (except anorectal infections in men): 100 mg, by mouth, twice a day for 7 days. As an alternate single visit dose, administer 300 mg stat followed in one hour by a second 300 mg dose. The dose may be administered with food, including milk or carbonated beverage, as required.

Uncomplicated urethral, endocervical, or rectal infection in adults caused by *Chlamydia trachomatis*: 100 mg by mouth twice a day for 7 days.

Nongonococcal urethritis (NGU) caused by *C. trachomatis* or *U. urealyticum*: 100 mg by mouth twice a day for 7 days.

Syphilis—early: Patients who are allergic to penicillin should be treated with doxycycline 100 mg by mouth twice a day for 2 weeks.

Syphilis of more than one year's duration: Patients who are allergic to penicillin should be treated with doxycycline 100 mg by mouth twice a day for 4 weeks.

Acute epididymo-orchitis caused by *N. gonorrhoeae*: 100 mg, by mouth, twice a day for at least 10 days.

Acute epididymo-orchitis caused by *C. trachomatis*: 100 mg, by mouth, twice a day for at least 10 days.

HOW SUPPLIED

Vibramycin Hyclate (doxycycline hyclate) is available in capsules containing doxycycline hyclate equivalent to:

50 mg doxycycline

bottles of 50 (NDC 0069-0940-50),

unit-dose pack of 100 (10 × 10's) (NDC 0069-0940-41).

The capsules are white and light blue and are imprinted with "VIBRA" on one half and "PFIZER 094" on the other half.

100 mg doxycycline

bottles of 50 (NDC 0069-0950-50) and 500 (NDC 0069-0950-73),

unit-dose pack of 100 (10 × 10's) (NDC 0069-0950-41).

The capsules are light blue and are imprinted with "VIBRA" on one half and "PFIZER 095" on the other half.

Vibra-Tabs (doxycycline hyclate) is available in salmon colored film-coated tablets containing doxycycline hyclate equivalent to:

100 mg doxycycline

bottles of 50 (NDC 0069-0990-50) and 500 (NDC 0069-0990-73),

unit-dose pack of 100 (10 × 10's) (NDC 0069-0990-41).

The tablets are imprinted on one side with "VIBRA-TABS" and "PFIZER 099" on the other side.

Vibramycin Calcium Syrup (doxycycline calcium oral suspension) is available as a raspberry-apple flavored oral suspension. Each teaspoonful (5 mL) contains doxycycline calcium equivalent to 50 mg of doxycycline: bottles of 1 oz (30 mL) (NDC 0069-0971-51), and 1 pint (473 mL) (NDC 0069-0971-93).

Vibramycin Monohydrate (doxycycline monohydrate) for Oral Suspension is available as a raspberry-flavored, dry powder for oral suspension. When reconstituted, each teaspoonful (5 mL) contains doxycycline monohydrate equivalent to 25 mg of doxycycline: 2 oz (60 mL) bottles (NDC 0069-0970-65).

All products are to be stored below 86°F (30°C) and dispensed in tight, light-resistant containers (USP). The unit dose packs should also be stored in a dry place.

ANIMAL PHARMACOLOGY AND ANIMAL TOXICOLOGY

Hyperpigmentation of the thyroid has been produced by members of the tetracycline class in the following species: in rats by oxytetracycline, doxycycline, tetracycline PO₄, and methacycline; in minipigs by doxycycline, minocycline, tetracycline PO₄, and methacycline; in dogs by doxycycline and minocycline; in monkeys by minocycline.

Minocycline, tetracycline PO₄, methacycline, doxycycline, tetracycline base, oxytetracycline HCl, and tetracycline HCl were goitrogenic in rats fed a low iodine diet. This goitrogenic effect was accompanied by high radioactive iodine uptake. Administration of minocycline also produced a large

goiter with high radioiodine uptake in rats fed a relatively high iodine diet.

Treatment of various animal species with this class of drugs has also resulted in the induction of thyroid hyperplasia in the following: in rats and dogs (minocycline); in chickens (chlortetracycline); and in rats and mice (oxytetracycline). Adrenal gland hyperplasia has been observed in goats and rats treated with oxytetracycline.

REFERENCES

1. National Committee for Clinical Laboratory Standards, *Performance Standards for Antimicrobial Disk Susceptibility Tests*, Fourth Edition. Approved Standard NCCLS Document M2-A4, Vol. 10, No. 7 NCCLS, Villanova, PA, April 1990.
2. National Committee for Clinical Laboratory Standards, *Methods for Dilution Antimicrobial Susceptibility Tests for Bacteria that Grow Aerobically*, Second Edition. Approved Standard NCCLS Document M7-A2, Vol. 10, No. 8 NCCLS, Villanova, PA, April 1990.

65-1680-00-4 Revised Oct. 1991

Shown in Product Identification Section, page 423

VISTARIL® ℞
[vĭs'tăr-ĭl]
(hydroxyzine pamoate)
Capsules and Oral Suspension

DESCRIPTION

Hydroxyzine pamoate is designated chemically as 1-(p-chlorobenzhydryl) 4-[2-(2-hydroxyethoxy) ethyl] diethylenediamine salt of 1,1'-methylene bis (2 hydroxy-3-naphthalene carboxylic acid).

Inert ingredients for the capsule formulations are: hard gelatin capsules (which may contain Yellow 10, Green 3, Yellow 6, Red 33, and other inert ingredients); magnesium stearate; sodium lauryl sulfate; starch; sucrose.

Inert ingredients for the oral suspension formulation are: carboxymethylcellulose sodium; lemon flavor; propylene glycol; sorbic acid; sorbitol solution; water.

CLINICAL PHARMACOLOGY

Vistaril (hydroxyzine pamoate) is unrelated chemically to the phenothiazines, reserpine, meprobamate, or the benzodiazepines.

Vistaril is not a cortical depressant, but its action may be due to a suppression of activity in certain key regions of the subcortical area of the central nervous system. Primary skeletal muscle relaxation has been demonstrated experimentally. Bronchodilator activity, and antihistaminic and analgesic effects have been demonstrated experimentally and confirmed clinically. An antiemetic effect, both by the apomorphine test and the veriloid test, has been demonstrated. Pharmacological and clinical studies indicate that hydroxyzine in therapeutic dosage does not increase gastric secretion or acidity and in most cases has mild antisecretory activity. Hydroxyzine is rapidly absorbed from the gastrointestinal tract and Vistaril's clinical effects are usually noted within 15 to 30 minutes after oral administration.

INDICATIONS

For symptomatic relief of anxiety and tension associated with psychoneurosis and as an adjunct in organic disease states in which anxiety is manifested.

Useful in the management of pruritus due to allergic conditions such as chronic urticaria and atopic and contact dermatoses, and in histamine-mediated pruritus.

As a sedative when used as premedication and following general anesthesia, **Hydroxyzine may potentiate meperidine (Demerol®) and barbiturates,** so their use in pre-anesthetic adjunctive therapy should be modified on an individual basis. Atropine and other belladonna alkaloids are not affected by the drug. Hydroxyzine is not known to interfere with the action of digitalis in any way and it may be used concurrently with this agent.

The effectiveness of hydroxyzine as an antianxiety agent for long term use, that is more than 4 months, has not been assessed by systematic clinical studies. The physician should reassess periodically the usefulness of the drug for the individual patient.

CONTRAINDICATIONS

Hydroxyzine, when administered to the pregnant mouse, rat, and rabbit, induced fetal abnormalities in the rat and mouse at doses substantially above the human therapeutic range. Clinical data in human beings are inadequate to establish safety in early pregnancy. Until such data are available, hydroxyzine is contraindicated in early pregnancy.

Hydroxyzine pamoate is contraindicated for patients who have shown a previous hypersensitivity to it.

WARNINGS

Nursing Mothers: It is not known whether this drug is excreted in human milk. Since many drugs are so excreted, hydroxyzine should not be given to nursing mothers.

PRECAUTIONS

THE POTENTIATING ACTION OF HYDROXYZINE MUST BE CONSIDERED WHEN THE DRUG IS USED IN CONJUNCTION WITH CENTRAL NERVOUS SYSTEM DEPRESSANTS SUCH AS NARCOTICS, NON-NARCOTIC ANALGESICS AND BARBITURATES. Therefore, when central nervous system depressants are administered concomitantly with hydroxyzine their dosage should be reduced. Since drowsiness may occur with use of the drug, patients should be warned of this possibility and cautioned against driving a car or operating dangerous machinery while taking Vistaril (hydroxyzine pamoate). Patients should be advised against the simultaneous use of other CNS depressant drugs, and cautioned that the effect of alcohol may be increased.

ADVERSE REACTIONS

Side effects reported with the administration of Vistaril are usually mild and transitory in nature.

Anticholinergic: Dry mouth.

Central Nervous System: Drowsiness is usually transitory and may disappear in a few days of continued therapy or upon reduction of the dose. Involuntary motor activity including rare instances of tremor and convulsions has been reported, usually with doses considerably higher than those recommended. Clinically significant respiratory depression has not been reported at recommended doses.

OVERDOSAGE

The most common manifestation of overdosage of Vistaril is hypersedation. As in the management of overdosage with any drug, it should be borne in mind that multiple agents may have been taken.

If vomiting has not occurred spontaneously, it should be induced. Immediate gastric lavage is also recommended. General supportive care, including frequent monitoring of the vital signs and close observation of the patient, is indicated. Hypotension, though unlikely, may be controlled with intravenous fluids and Levophed® (levarterenol) or Aramine® (metaraminol). Do not use epinephrine as Vistaril counteracts its pressor action. Caffeine and Sodium Benzoate Injection, U.S.P., may be used to counteract central nervous system depressant effects.

There is no specific antidote. It is doubtful that hemodialysis would be of any value in the treatment of overdosage with hydroxyzine. However, if other agents such as barbiturates have been ingested concomitantly, hemodialysis may be indicated. There is no practical method to quantitate hydroxyzine in body fluids or tissue after its ingestion or administration.

DOSAGE

For symptomatic relief of anxiety and tension associated with psychoneurosis and as an adjunct in organic disease states in which anxiety is manifested: in adults, 50–100 mg q.i.d.; children under 6 years, 50 mg daily in divided doses and over 6 years, 50–100 mg daily in divided doses.

For use in the management of pruritus due to allergic conditions such as chronic urticaria and atopic and contact dermatoses, and in histamine-mediated pruritus: in adults, 25 mg t.i.d. or q.i.d.; children under 6 years, 50 mg daily in divided doses and over 6 years, 50–100 mg daily in divided doses.

As a sedative when used as a premedication and following general anesthesia: 50–100 mg in adults, and 0.6 mg/kg in children.

When treatment is initiated by the intramuscular route of administration, subsequent doses may be administered orally.

As with all medications, the dosage should be adjusted according to the patient's response to therapy.

SUPPLY

Vistaril Capsules (hydroxyzine pamoate equivalent to hydroxyzine hydrochloride)

25 mg:	100's (NDC 0069-5410-66), 500's (NDC 0069-5410-73), and Unit Dose (10 × 10's) (NDC 0069-5410-41) two-tone green capsules
50 mg:	100's (NDC 0069-5420-66), 500's (NDC 0069-5420-73), and Unit Dose (10 × 10's) (NDC 0069-5420-41) green and white capsules
100 mg:	100's (NDC 0069-5430-66), 500's (NDC 0069-5430-73), and Unit Dose (10 × 10's) (NDC 0069-5430-41) green and gray capsules

Vistaril Oral Suspension (hydroxyzine pamoate equivalent to 25 mg hydroxyzine hydrochloride per teaspoonful-5 ml): 1 pint bottles (NDC 0069-5440-93) and 4 ounce (120 ml) bottles (NDC 0069-5440-97) in packages of 4.

BIBLIOGRAPHY

Available on request.

69-0846-00-0 Revised November 1986

Shown in Product Identification Section, page 423

ZITHROMAX®   ℞
(azithromycin)
Capsules

DESCRIPTION

ZITHROMAX® (azithromycin) is an azalide, a subclass of macrolide antibiotics, for oral administration. Azithromycin has the chemical name $(2R,3S,4R,5R,8R,10R,11R,12S, 13S,14R)$-13-[(2,6- dideoxy-3-C -methyl-3-O -methyl-α-L -ribo - hexopyranosyl) oxy] -2-ethyl-3,4,10-trihydroxy- 3,5,6,8,10,12, 14-heptamethyl -11- [[3,4,6-trideoxy-3-(dimethylamino)-β-D - xylo-hexopyranosyl]oxy]-1-oxa-6-azacyclopentadecan-15-one. The structural formula is:

Azithromycin, as the dihydrate, is a white crystalline powder with a chemical formula of $C_{38}H_{72}N_2O_{12}·2H_2O$ and a molecular weight of 785.0. ZITHROMAX® is supplied in red hard gelatin capsules (containing FD&C red #40) containing azithromycin dihydrate equivalent to 250 mg azithromycin and the following inactive ingredients: anhydrous lactose, corn starch, magnesium stearate, and sodium lauryl sulfate.

CLINICAL PHARMACOLOGY

Following oral administration, azithromycin is rapidly absorbed and widely distributed throughout the body. Rapid distribution of azithromycin into tissues and high concentration within cells result in significantly higher azithromycin concentrations in tissues than in plasma or serum.

The pharmacokinetic parameters of azithromycin in plasma after dosing as per labeled recommendations (i.e., 500 mg loading dose on day 1 followed by 250 mg q. d. on days 2 through 5) in healthy young adults (age 18–40 years old) are portrayed in the following chart:

PK Parameter (Mean)	Total n = 12	
	Day 1	Day 5
$C_{max}(\mu g/mL)$	0.41	0.24
$T_{max}(h)$	2.5	3.2
AUC 0–24 $(\mu g·h/mL)$	2.6	2.1
$C_{min}(\mu g/mL)$	0.05	0.05
Urinary Excret. (% dose)	4.5	6.5

In this study, there was no significant difference in the disposition of azithromycin between male and female subjects. Plasma concentrations of azithromycin declined in a polyphasic pattern resulting in an average terminal half-life of 68 hours. On the recommended dosing regimen, C_{min} and C_{max} remained essentially unchanged from day 2 through day 5 of therapy. However, without a loading dose, azithromycin C_{min} levels required 5 to 7 days to reach steady-state. When studied in healthy elderly subjects from age 65 to 85 years, the pharmacokinetic parameters of azithromycin in elderly men were similar to those in young adults; however, in elderly women, although higher peak concentrations (increased by 30 to 50%) were observed, no significant accumulation occurred.

The high values for apparent steady-state volume of distribution (31.1 L/kg) and plasma clearance (630 mL/min) suggest that the prolonged half-life is due to extensive uptake and subsequent release of drug from tissues. Selected tissue (or fluid) to plasma/serum concentration ratios are shown in the following table:

[See table above.]

The extensive tissue distribution was confirmed by examination of additional tissues and fluids (bone, ejaculum, prostate, ovary, uterus, salpinx, stomach, liver, and gallbladder). As there are no data from adequate and well-controlled studies of azithromycin treatment of infections in these additional body sites, the clinical significance of these tissue concentration data is unknown.

Only very low concentrations were noted in cerebrospinal fluid (less than 0.01 $\mu g/mL$) in the presence of non-inflamed meninges.

The serum protein binding of azithromycin is variable in the concentration range approximating human exposure, decreasing from 51% at 0.02 $\mu g/mL$ to 7% at 2 $\mu g/mL$.

Biliary excretion of azithromycin, predominantly as unchanged drug, is a major route of elimination. Over the course of a week, approximately 6% of the administered dose appears as unchanged drug in urine.

There are no pharmacokinetic data available from studies in hepatically- or renally-impaired individuals.

Food decreases the absorption of azithromycin, reducing the C_{max} by 52% and the AUC by 43%.

The AUC of azithromycin was unaffected by co-administration of an aluminum and magnesium hydroxide antacid on ZITHROMAX® (azithromycin); however, the C_{max} was reduced by 24%. Administration of cimetidine (800 mg) two hours prior to azithromycin had no effect on azithromycin absorption.

The effect of azithromycin on the plasma levels or pharmacokinetics of theophylline administered in multiple doses adequate to reach therapeutic steady-state plasma levels is not known. (See PRECAUTIONS.)

Microbiology:

Azithromycin acts by binding to the 50S ribosomal subunit of susceptible organisms and thus interfering with microbial protein synthesis. Nucleic acid synthesis is not affected.

Azithromycin concentrates in phagocytes and fibroblasts as demonstrated by in vitro incubation techniques. Using such methodology, the ratio of intracellular to extracellular concentration was > 30 after one hour incubation. In vivo studies suggest that concentration in phagocytes may contribute to drug distribution to inflamed tissues.

Azithromycin has been shown to be active against most strains of the following organisms—both in vitro and in clinical infections: (See INDICATIONS AND USAGE.)

Gram-positive aerobes

Staphylococcus aureus   Streptococcus pneumoniae
Streptococcus agalactiae   Streptococcus pyogenes
NOTE: Azithromycin demonstrates cross-resistance with erythromycin-resistant gram-positive strains. Most strains of Enterococcus faecalis and methicillin-resistant staphylococci are resistant to azithromycin.

Gram-negative aerobes   **Other organisms**
Haemophilus influenzae   Chlamydia trachomatis
Moraxella catarrhalis
Beta-lactamase production should have no effect on azithromycin activity.

Azithromycin exhibits in vitro minimum inhibitory concentrations of 2.0 $\mu g/mL$ or less against most strains of the following organisms. The safety and efficacy of azithromycin in treating infections due to these organisms have not been established in adequate and well-controlled trials. The following in vitro data are available; however, their clinical significance is unknown.

Gram-positive aerobes   **Anaerobic bacteria**
Streptococci (Groups C, F, G)   Bacteroides bivius
Viridans group streptococci   Clostridium perfringens
    Peptostreptococcus species

Gram-negative aerobes   **Other organisms**
Bordetella pertussis   Borrelia burgdorferi
Campylobacter jejuni   Mycoplasma pneumoniae
Haemophilus ducreyi   Treponema pallidum
Legionella pneumophila   Ureaplasma urealyticum

SUSCEPTIBILITY TESTS

Diffusion Techniques: Quantitative methods that require measurement of zone diameters give the most precise estimate of the susceptibility of bacteria to antimicrobial agents. One such standard procedure[1] which has been recommended for use with disks to test susceptibility of organisms to azithromycin uses the 15-μg azithromycin disk. Interpretation involves the correlation of the diameter obtained in the disk test with the minimum inhibitory concentration (MIC) for azithromycin.

Reports from the laboratory giving results of the standard single-disk susceptibility test with a 15-μg azithromycin disk should be interpreted according to the following criteria:

Zone Diameter (mm)	Interpretation
≥ 18	(S) Susceptible
14–17	(I) Intermediate
≤ 13	(R) Resistant

A report of "Susceptible" indicates that the pathogen is likely to respond to monotherapy with azithromycin. A report of "Intermediate" indicates that the result be considered equivocal, and, if the organism is not fully susceptible to alternative clinically feasible drugs, the test should be repeated. This category provides a buffer zone which prevents small uncontrolled technical factors from causing major discrepancies in interpretations. A report of "Resistant" indicates that achievable drug concentrations are unlikely to be inhibitory and other therapy should be selected.

Standardized procedures require the use of laboratory control organisms. The 15-μg azithromycin disk should give the following zone diameter:

Organism	Zone diameter (mm)
S. aureus ATCC 25923	21–26

Dilution Techniques: Use a standardized dilution method[2] (broth, agar, microdilution) or equivalent with azithromycin powder. The MIC values obtained should be interpreted according to the following criteria:

MIC $(\mu g/mL)$	Interpretation
≤ 2	(S) Susceptible
4	(I) Intermediate
≥ 8	(R) Resistant

The in vitro potency of azithromycin is markedly affected by the pH of the microbiological growth medium during incubation. Incubation in CO_2 atmosphere will result in lowering of media pH (7.2 to 6.6, 18 hours in 10% CO_2) and an apparent reduction in in vitro potency of azithromycin. Thus, the initial pH of the growth medium should be 7.2–7.4, and the CO_2 content of the incubation atmosphere should be as low as practical.

Azithromycin can be solubilized for in vitro testing by dissolving in a minimum amount of 95% ethanol and diluting to working concentration with water.

As with standard diffusion methods, dilution methods require the use of laboratory control organisms. Standard azithromycin powder should provide the following MIC values:

Organism	MIC $(\mu g/mL)$
E. coli ATCC 25922	2.0–8.0
E. faecalis ATCC 29212	1.0–4.0
S. aureus ATCC 29213	0.25–1.0

INDICATIONS AND USAGE

ZITHROMAX® (azithromycin) is indicated for the treatment of individuals 16 years of age and older with mild to moderate infections (pneumonia: see WARNINGS) caused by susceptible strains of the designated microorganisms in the specific conditions listed below:

Lower Respiratory Tract
Acute bacterial exacerbations of chronic obstructive pulmonary disease due to Haemophilus influenzae, Moraxella catarrhalis, or Streptococcus pneumoniae.

AZITHROMYCIN CONCENTRATIONS FOLLOWING RECOMMENDED CLINICAL DOSAGE REGIMEN

TISSUE OR FLUID	TIME AFTER DOSE (h)	TISSUE OR FLUID CONCENTRATION $(\mu g/g$ or $\mu g/mL)$[1]	CORRESPONDING PLASMA OR SERUM LEVEL $(\mu g/mL)$	TISSUE (FLUID) PLASMA (SERUM) RATIO[1]
SKIN	72–96	0.4	0.012	35
LUNG	72–96	4.0	0.012	> 100
SPUTUM*	2–4	1.0	0.64	2
SPUTUM**	10–12	2.9	0.1	30
TONSIL***	9–18	4.5	0.03	> 100
TONSIL***	180	0.9	0.006	> 100
CERVIX****	19	2.8	0.04	70

[1] High tissue concentrations should not be interpreted to be quantitatively related to clinical efficacy. The antimicrobial activity of azithromycin is pH related. Azithromycin is concentrated in cell lysosomes which have a low intraorganelle pH, at which the drug's activity is reduced. However, the extensive distribution of drug to tissues may be relevant to clinical activity.

* Sample was obtained 2–4 hours after the first dose.
** Sample was obtained 10–12 hours after the first dose.
*** Dosing regimen of 2 doses of 250 mg each, separated by 12 hours.
**** Sample was obtained 19 hours after a single 500 mg dose.

Continued on next page

Pfizer—Cont.

Community-acquired pneumonia of mild severity due to *Streptococcus pneumoniae* or *Haemophilus influenzae* in patients appropriate for outpatient oral therapy.

NOTE: Azithromycin should not be used in patients with pneumonia who are judged to be inappropriate for outpatient oral therapy because of moderate to severe illness or risk factors such as any of the following:

patients with nosocomially acquired infections,

patients with known or suspected bacteremia,

patients requiring hospitalization,

elderly or debilitated patients, or

patients with significant underlying health problems that may compromise their ability to respond to their illness (including immunodeficiency or functional asplenia).

Upper Respiratory Tract

Streptococcal pharyngitis/tonsillitis—As an alternative to first line therapy of acute pharyngitis/tonsillitis due to *Streptococcus pyogenes* occurring in individuals who cannot use first line therapy.

NOTE: Penicillin is the usual drug of choice in the treatment of *Streptococcus pyogenes* infections and the prophylaxis of rheumatic fever. ZITHROMAX® is often effective in the eradication of susceptible strains of *Streptococcus pyogenes* from the nasopharynx. Because some strains are resistant to ZITHROMAX®, susceptibility tests should be performed when patients are treated with ZITHROMAX®. Data establishing efficacy of azithromycin in subsequent prevention of rheumatic fever are not available.

Skin and Skin Structure

Uncomplicated skin and skin structure infections due to *Staphylococcus aureus*, *Streptococcus pyogenes*, or *Streptococcus agalactiae*. Abscesses usually require surgical drainage.

Sexually Transmitted Diseases

Non-gonococcal urethritis and cervicitis due to *Chlamydia trachomatis*.

ZITHROMAX®, at the recommended dose, should not be relied upon to treat gonorrhea or syphilis. Antimicrobial agents used in high doses for short periods of time to treat non-gonococcal urethritis may mask or delay the symptoms of incubating gonorrhea or syphilis. All patients with sexually-transmitted urethritis or cervicitis should have a serologic test for syphilis and appropriate cultures for gonorrhea performed at the time of diagnosis. Appropriate antimicrobial therapy and follow-up tests for these diseases should be initiated if infection is confirmed.

Appropriate culture and susceptibility tests should be performed before treatment to determine the causative organism and its susceptibility to azithromycin. Therapy with ZITHROMAX® may be initiated before results of these tests are known; once the results become available, antimicrobial therapy should be adjusted accordingly.

CONTRAINDICATIONS

ZITHROMAX® is contraindicated in patients with known hypersensitivity to azithromycin, erythromycin, or any macrolide antibiotic.

WARNINGS

In the treatment of pneumonia, azithromycin has only been shown to be safe and effective in the treatment of community-acquired pneumonia of mild severity due to *Streptococcus pneumoniae* or *Haemophilus influenzae* in patients appropriate for outpatient oral therapy. Azithromycin should not be used in patients with pneumonia who are judged to be inappropriate for outpatient oral therapy because of moderate to severe illness or risk factors such as any of the following:

patients with nosocomially acquired infections,

patients with known or suspected bacteremia,

patients requiring hospitalization,

elderly or debilitated patients, or

patients with significant underlying health problems that may compromise their ability to respond to their illiness (including immunodeficiency or functional asplenia).

Pseudomembranous colitis has been reported with nearly all antibacterial agents and may range in severity from mild to life-threatening. Therefore, it is important to consider this diagnosis in patients who present with diarrhea subsequent to the administration of antibacterial agents.

Treatment with antibacterial agents alters the normal flora of the colon and may permit overgrowth of clostridia. Studies indicate that a toxin produced by *Clostridium difficile* is a primary cause of "antibiotic-associated colitis."

After the diagnosis of pseudomembranous colitis has been established, therapeutic measures should be initiated. Mild cases of pseudomembranous colitis usually respond to discontinuation of the drug alone. In moderate to severe cases, consideration should be given to management with fluids and electrolytes, protein supplementation, and treatment with an antibacterial drug clinically effective against *Clostridium difficile* colitis.

PRECAUTIONS

General: Because azithromycin is principally eliminated via the liver, caution should be exercised when azithromycin is administered to patients with impaired hepatic function. There are no data regarding azithromycin usage in patients with renal impairment; thus, caution should be exercised when prescribing azithromycin in these patients.

The following adverse event has not been reported in clinical trials with azithromycin, an azalide. However, it has been reported with macrolide products: ventricular arrhythmias, including ventricular tachycardia and *torsades de pointes*, in individuals with prolonged QT intervals.

Information for patients: Patients should be cautioned to take this medication at least one hour prior to a meal or at least two hours after a meal. This medication should not be taken with food.

Patients should also be cautioned not to take aluminum- and magnesium-containing antacids and azithromycin simultaneously.

Drug Interactions: Aluminum- and magnesium-containing antacids reduce the peak serum levels (rate) but not the A.U.C. (extent) of azithromycin absorption.

Administration of cimetidine (800 mg) two hours prior to azithromycin had no effect on azithromycin absorption.

Azithromycin did not affect the plasma levels or pharmacokinetics of theophylline administered as a single intravenous dose. The effect of azithromycin on the plasma levels or pharmacokinetics of theophylline administered in multiple doses resulting in therapeutic steady state levels of theophylline is not known. However, concurrent use of macrolides and theophylline has been associated with increases in the serum concentrations of theophylline. Therefore, until further data are available, prudent medical practice dictates careful monitoring of plasma theophylline levels in patients receiving azithromycin and theophylline concomitantly.

Azithromycin did not affect the prothrombin time response to a single dose of warfarin. However, prudent medical practice dictates careful monitoring of prothrombin time in all patients treated with azithromycin and warfarin concomitantly. Concurrent use of macrolides and warfarin in clinical practice has been associated with increased anticoagulant effects.

The following drug interactions have not been reported in clinical trials with azithromycin; however, no specific drug interaction studies have been performed to evaluate potential drug-drug interaction. Nonetheless, they have been observed with macrolide products. Until further data are developed regarding drug interactions when azithromycin and these drugs are used concomitantly, careful monitoring of patients is advised:

Digoxin—elevated digoxin levels.

Ergotamine or dihydroergotamine—acute ergot toxicity characterized by severe peripheral vasospasm and dysesthesia.

Triazolam—decrease the clearance of triazolam and thus may increase the pharmacologic effect of triazolam.

Drugs metabolized by the cytochrome P450 system—elevations of serum carbamazepine, cyclosporine, hexobarbital, and phenytoin levels.

Laboratory Test Interactions: There are no reported laboratory test interactions.

Carcinogenesis, mutagenesis, impairment of fertility: Long-term studies in animals have not been performed to evaluate carcinogenic potential. Azithromycin has shown no mutagenic potential in standard laboratory tests: mouse lymphoma assay, human lymphocyte clastogenic assay, and mouse bone marrow clastogenic assay.

Pregnancy: Teratogenic Effects. Pregnancy Category B: Reproduction studies have been performed in rats and mice at doses up to moderately maternally toxic dose levels (i.e., 200 mg/kg/day). These doses, based on a mg/m^2 basis, are estimated to be 4 and 2 times, respectively, the human daily dose of 500 mg. No evidence of impaired fertility or harm to the fetus due to azithromycin was found. There are, however, no adequate and well-controlled studies in pregnant women. Because animal reproduction studies are not always predictive of human response, azithromycin should be used during pregnancy only if clearly needed.

Nursing Mothers: It is not known whether azithromycin is excreted in human milk. Because many drugs are excreted in human milk, caution should be exercised when azithromycin is administered to a nursing woman.

Pediatric Use: Safety and effectiveness in children or adolescents under 16 years of age have not been established.

Geriatric Use: Pharmacokinetic parameters in older volunteers (65–85 years old) were similar to those in younger volunteers (18–40 years old) for the 5-day therapeutic regimen. Dosage adjustment does not appear to be necessary for older patients with normal renal and hepatic function receiving treatment with this dosage regimen. (See CLINICAL PHARMACOLOGY.)

ADVERSE REACTIONS

In clinical trials most of the reported side effects were mild to moderate in severity and were reversible upon discontinu-

ation of the drug. Approximately 0.7% of the patients from the multiple-dose clinical trials discontinued ZITHROMAX® (azithromycin) therapy because of treatment-related side effects. Most of the side effects leading to discontinuation were related to the gastrointestinal tract, e.g., nausea, vomiting, diarrhea, or abdominal pain. Rare, but potentially serious side effects, were angioedema (1 case) and cholestatic jaundice (1 case).

Clinical:

Multiple-dose regimen: Overall, the most common side effects in patients receiving the multiple-dose regimen of ZITHROMAX® were related to the gastrointestinal system with diarrhea/loose stools (5%), nausea (3%), and abdominal pain (3%) being the most frequently reported.

No other side effects occurred in patients on the multiple-dose regimen of ZITHROMAX® with a frequency greater than 1%. Side effects that occurred with a frequency of 1% or less included the following:

Cardiovascular: Palpitations, chest pain.

Gastrointestinal: Dyspepsia, flatulence, vomiting, melena, and cholestatic jaundice.

Genitourinary: Monilia, vaginitis, and nephritis.

Nervous System: Dizziness, headache, vertigo, and somnolence.

General: Fatigue.

Allergic: Rash, photosensitivity, and angioedema.

Single 1-gram dose regimen: Overall, the most common side effects in patients receiving a single-dose regimen of 1 gram of ZITHROMAX® were related to the gastrointestinal system and were more frequently reported than in patients receiving the multiple-dose regimen.

Side effects that occurred in patients on the single one-gram dosing regimen of ZITHROMAX® with a frequency of 1% or greater included diarrhea/loose stools (7%), nausea (5%), vomiting (2%), and vaginitis (2%).

Laboratory Abnormalities: Significant abnormalities (irrespective of drug relationship) occurring during the clinical trials were reported as follows:

With an incidence of 1–2%, elevated serum creatinine phosphokinase, potassium, ALT (SGPT), GGT, and AST (SGOT).

With an incidence of less than 1%, leukopenia, neutropenia, decreased platelet count, elevated serum alkaline phosphatase, bilirubin, BUN, creatinine, blood glucose, LDH, and phosphate.

When follow-up was provided, changes in laboratory tests appeared to be reversible.

In multiple-dose clinical trials involving more than 3000 patients, 3 patients discontinued therapy because of treatment-related liver enzyme abnormalities and 1 because of a renal function abnormality.

DOSAGE AND ADMINISTRATION

(See INDICATIONS AND USAGE.)

ZITHROMAX® *(azithromycin) should be given at least 1 hour before or 2 hours after a meal.*

The recommended dose of ZITHROMAX® for the treatment of individuals 16 years of age and older with mild to moderate acute bacterial exacerbations of chronic obstructive pulmonary disease, pneumonia, pharyngitis/tonsillitis (as second-line therapy), and uncomplicated skin and skin structure infections due to the indicated organisms is: 500 mg as a single dose on the first day followed by 250 mg once daily on days 2 through 5 for a total dose of 1.5 grams of ZITHROMAX®.

The recommended dose of ZITHROMAX® for the treatment of non-gonococcal urethritis and cervicitis due to *C. trachomatis* is: a single 1 gram (1000 mg) dose of ZITHROMAX®.

HOW SUPPLIED

ZITHROMAX® (azithromycin) capsules are provided as red opaque hard-gelatin capsules containing azithromycin dihydrate equivalent to 250 mg of azithromycin. These are packaged in bottles. Capsules should be stored below 86°F (30°C). Capsules are imprinted with "PFIZER 305."

ZITHROMAX® capsules are supplied as follows:

NDC 0069-3050-50 Bottles of 50

ANIMAL TOXICOLOGY

Phospholipidosis (intracellular phospholipid binding) has been observed in some tissues of mice, rats, and dogs given multiple doses of azithromycin. It has been demonstrated in numerous organ systems (e.g., eye, dorsal root ganglia, liver, gallbladder, kidney, spleen, and pancreas) in dogs administered doses which, based on pharmacokinetics, are as low as 2 times greater than the recommended human dose and in rats at doses comparable to the recommended human dose. This effect has been reversible after cessation of azithromycin treatment. The significance of these findings for humans is unknown.

REFERENCES

1. National Committee for Clinical Laboratory Standards, Performance Standards for Antimicrobial Disk Susceptibility Tests—Fourth Edition. Approved Standard NCCLS Document M2-A4, Vol. 10, No. 7, NCCLS, Villanova, PA, 1990.

2. National Committee for Clinical Laboratory Standards, Methods for Dilution Antimicrobial Susceptibility Tests for Bacteria that Grow Aerobically—Second Edition. Approved Standard NCCLS Document M7-A2, Vol. 10, No. 8, NCCLS, Villanova, PA, 1990.

Licensed from Pliva
70-4763-00-1
Issued February 1992
Shown in Product Identification Section, page 423

Porton Products Limited
30401 AGOURA ROAD #102
AGOURA HILLS, CA 91301

HYATE:C® ℞
Antihemophilic Factor (Porcine)

DESCRIPTION

Antihemophilic Factor (Porcine)—HYATE:C® is a highly purified sterile freeze-dried concentrate of porcine antihemophilic factor (Factor VIII:C) in the form of a white lyophilized powder for reconstitution.

HOW SUPPLIED

Antihemophilic Factor (Porcine)—HYATE:C® is supplied in vials containing between 400–700 porcine units of Factor VIII:C, to be reconstituted with 20mL Sterile Water for Injection U.S.P. (not supplied).

1 Vial NDC 55688-106-02

Manufactured by:
Porton Speywood Limited
Ash Road, Wrexham Industrial Estate
Wrexham, Clwyd LL13 9UF
United Kingdom
Tel. 978 661181
US License #1014

Distributed by:
Porton Products Limited
30401 Agoura Road #102
Agoura Hills, CA 91301
Tel. 818-879-2200
FAX 818-879-2208

EDUCATIONAL MATERIAL

Educational Information concerning Factor VIII Inhibitors or Acquired Hemophilia is available free of charge. Please call or write Porton Products Limited.

Pratt Pharmaceuticals Division Pfizer Inc
235 EAST 42ND STREET
NEW YORK, NY 10017-5755

Full prescribing information for all Pratt Pharmaceuticals products is available from your Pratt Pharmaceuticals representative.

Product Identification Codes

To provide quick and positive identification of Pratt Pharmaceuticals Division products, we have imprinted the product identification number of the National Drug Code on all tablets and capsules.

In order that you may quickly identify a product by its code number, we have compiled below a numerical list of code numbers with their corresponding product names. We are also listing the code numbers by alphabetical order of products.

NUMERICAL PRODUCT INDEX

Product Identification Code	Product
260	Procardia® (nifedipine) Capsules, 10 mg
261	Procardia® (nifedipine) Capsules, 20 mg
265	Procardia XL® (nifedipine) Extended Release Tablets, 30 mg GITS
266	Procardia XL® (nifedipine) Extended Release Tablets, 60 mg GITS
267	Procardia XL® (nifedipine) Extended Release Tablets, 90 mg GITS
322	Feldene® (piroxicam) Capsules, 10 mg
323	Feldene® (piroxicam) Capsules, 20 mg
411	Glucotrol® (glipizide) Tablets, 5 mg
412	Glucotrol® (glipizide) Tablets, 10 mg
490	Zoloft™ (sertraline HCl) Tablets, 50 mg
491	Zoloft™ (sertraline HCl) Tablets, 100 mg

ALPHABETICAL PRODUCT INDEX

Product	Product Identification Code
Feldene® (piroxicam) Capsules, 10 mg	322
Feldene® (piroxicam) Capsules, 20 mg	323
Glucotrol® (glipizide) Tablets, 5 mg	411
Glucotrol® (glipizide) Tablets, 10 mg	412
Procardia® (nifedipine) Capsules, 10 mg	260
Procardia® (nifedipine) Capsules, 20 mg	261
Procardia XL® (nifedipine) Extended Release Tablets, 30 mg GITS	265
Procardia XL® (nifedipine) Extended Release Tablets, 60 mg GITS	266
Procardia XL® (nifedipine) Extended Release Tablets, 90 mg GITS	267
Zoloft™ (sertraline HCl) Tablets, 50 mg	490
Zoloft™ (sertraline HCl) Tablets, 100 mg	491

FELDENE® ℞
[fēl 'deen]
(piroxicam)
CAPSULES
For Oral Use

DESCRIPTION

FELDENE (piroxicam) is 4-Hydroxy-2-methyl-*N*-2-pyridinyl-2*H*-1,2-benzothiazine-3-carboxamide 1,1-dioxide, an oxicam. Members of the oxicam family are not carboxylic acids, but they are acidic by virtue of the enolic 4-hydroxy substituent. FELDENE occurs as a white crystalline solid, sparingly soluble in water, dilute acid and most organic solvents. It is slightly soluble in alcohols and in aqueous alkaline solution. It exhibits a weakly acidic 4-hydroxy proton (pKa 5.1) and a weakly basic pyridyl nitrogen (pKa 1.8). Inert ingredients in the formulations are: hard gelatin capsules (which may contain Blue 1, Red 3, and other inert ingredients); lactose; magnesium stearate; sodium lauryl sulfate; starch.

CLINICAL PHARMACOLOGY

FELDENE has shown anti-inflammatory, analgesic and antipyretic properties in animals. Edema, erythema, tissue proliferation, fever, and pain can all be inhibited in laboratory animals by the administration of FELDENE. It is effective regardless of the etiology of the inflammation. The mode of action of FELDENE is not fully established at this time. However, a common mechanism for the above effects may exist in the ability of FELDENE to inhibit the biosynthesis of prostaglandins, known mediators of inflammation.

It is established that FELDENE does not act by stimulating the pituitary-adrenal axis.

FELDENE is well absorbed following oral administration. Drug plasma concentrations are proportional for 10 and 20 mg doses, generally peak within three to five hours after medication, and subsequently decline with a mean half-life of 50 hours (range of 30 to 86 hours; although values outside of this range have been encountered).

This prolonged half-life results in the maintenance of relatively stable plasma concentrations throughout the day on once daily doses and to significant drug accumulation upon multiple dosing. A single 20 mg dose generally produces peak piroxicam plasma levels of 1.5 to 2 mcg/ml, while maximum drug plasma concentrations, after repeated daily ingestion of 20 mg FELDENE, usually stabilize at 3–8 mcg/ml. Most patients approximate steady state plasma levels within 7 to 12 days. Higher levels, which approximate steady state at two to three weeks, have been observed in patients in whom longer plasma half-lives of piroxicam occurred.

FELDENE and its biotransformation products are excreted in urine and feces, with about twice as much appearing in the urine as the feces. Metabolism occurs by hydroxylation at the 5 position of the pyridyl side chain and conjugation of this product; by cyclodehydration; and by a sequence of reactions involving hydrolysis of the amide linkage, decarboxylation, ring contraction, and N-demethylation. Less than 5% of the daily dose is excreted unchanged.

Concurrent administration of aspirin (3900 mg/day) and FELDENE (20 mg/day), resulted in a reduction of plasma levels of piroxicam to about 80% of their normal values. The use of FELDENE in conjunction with aspirin is not recommended because data are inadequate to demonstrate that the combination produces greater improvement than that achieved with aspirin alone and the potential for adverse reactions is increased. Concomitant administration of antacids had no effect on FELDENE plasma levels. The effects of impaired renal function or hepatic disease on plasma levels have not been established.

FELDENE, like salicylates and other nonsteroidal anti-inflammatory agents, is associated with symptoms of gastrointestinal tract irritation (see ADVERSE REACTIONS). However, in a study utilizing ^{51}Cr-tagged red blood cells, 20 mg of FELDENE administered as a single dose for four days did not result in a significant increase in fecal blood loss and did not detectably affect the gastric mucosa. In the same study a total daily dose of 3900 mg of aspirin, i.e., 972 mg q.i.d., caused a significant increase in fecal blood loss and mucosal lesions as demonstrated by gastroscopy.

In controlled clinical trials, the effectiveness of FELDENE (piroxicam) has been established for both acute exacerbations and long-term management of rheumatoid arthritis and osteoarthritis.

The therapeutic effects of FELDENE are evident early in the treatment of both diseases with a progressive increase in response over several (8–12) weeks. Efficacy is seen in terms of pain relief and, when present, subsidence of inflammation.

Doses of 20 mg/day FELDENE display a therapeutic effect comparable to therapeutic doses of aspirin, with a lower incidence of minor gastrointestinal effects and tinnitus.

FELDENE has been administered concomitantly with fixed doses of gold and corticosteroids. The existence of a "steroid-sparing" effect has not been adequately studied to date.

INDICATIONS AND USAGE

FELDENE is indicated for acute or long-term use in the relief of signs and symptoms of the following:

1. osteoarthritis
2. rheumatoid arthritis

Dosage recommendations for use in children have not been established.

CONTRAINDICATIONS

FELDENE should not be used in patients who have previously exhibited hypersensitivity to it, or in individuals with the syndrome comprised of bronchospasm, nasal polyps, and angioedema precipitated by aspirin or other nonsteroidal anti-inflammatory drugs.

WARNINGS

Risk of GI Ulceration, Bleeding and Perforation with NSAID Therapy

Serious gastrointestinal toxicity such as bleeding, ulceration, and perforation can occur at any time, with or without warning symptoms, in patients treated chronically with NSAID therapy. Although minor upper gastrointestinal problems, such as dyspepsia, are common, usually developing early in therapy, physician should remain alert for ulceration and bleeding in patients treated chronically with NSAIDs even in the absence of previous GI tract symptoms. In patients observed in clinical trials of several months to two years duration, symptomatic upper GI ulcers, gross bleeding or perforation appear to occur in approximately 1% of patients treated for 3–6 months, and in about 2–4% of patients treated for one year. Physicians should inform patients about the signs and/or symptoms of serious GI toxicity and what steps to take if they occur.

Studies to date have not identified any subset of patients not at risk of developing peptic ulceration and bleeding. Except for a prior history of serious GI events and other risk factors known to be associated with peptic ulcer disease, such as alcoholism, smoking, etc., no risk factors (e.g., age, sex) have been associated with increased risk. Elderly or debilitated patients seem to tolerate ulceration or bleeding less well than other individuals and most spontaneous reports of fatal GI events are in this population. Studies to date are inconclusive concerning the relative risk of various NSAIDs in causing such reactions. High doses of any NSAID probably carry a greater risk of these reactions, although controlled clinical trials showing this do not exist in most cases. In considering the use of relatively large doses (within the recommended dosage range), sufficient benefit should be anticipated to offset the potential increased risk of GI toxicity.

PRECAUTIONS

Renal Effects: As with other nonsteroidal anti-inflammatory drugs, long-term administration of piroxicam to animals has resulted in renal papillary necrosis and other abnormal renal pathology. In humans, there have been reports of acute interstitial nephritis with hematuria, proteinuria, and occasionally, nephrotic syndrome.

A second form of renal toxicity has been seen in patients with prerenal conditions leading to a reduction in renal blood flow or blood volume, where the renal prostaglandins have a supportive role in the maintenance of renal perfusion. In these patients administration of an NSAID may cause a dose-dependent reduction in prostaglandin formation and may precipitate overt renal decompensation. Patients at greatest risk of this reaction are those with impaired renal function, heart failure, liver dysfunction, those taking diuretics, and the elderly. Discontinuation of NSAID therapy is typically followed by recovery to the pretreatment state.

Because of extensive renal excretion of piroxicam and its biotransformation products (less than 5% of the daily dose excreted unchanged, see CLINICAL PHARMACOLOGY), lower doses of piroxicam should be anticipated in patients

Continued on next page

Pratt—Cont.

with impaired renal function, and they should be carefully monitored.

Although other nonsteroidal anti-inflammatory drugs do not have the same direct effects on platelets that aspirin does, all drugs inhibiting prostaglandin biosynthesis do interfere with platelet function to some degree; therefore, patients who may be adversely affected by such an action should be carefully observed when FELDENE is administered.

Because of reports of adverse eye findings with nonsteroidal anti-inflammatory agents, it is recommended that patients who develop visual complaints during treatment with FELDENE have ophthalmic evaluation.

As with other nonsteroidal anti-inflammatory drugs, borderline elevations of one or more liver tests may occur in up to 15% of patients. These abnormalities may progress, may remain essentially unchanged, or may be transient with continued therapy. The SGPT (ALT) test is probably the most sensitive indicator of liver dysfunction. Meaningful (3 times the upper limit of normal) elevations of SGPT or SGOT (AST) occurred in controlled clinical trials in less than 1% of patients. A patient with symptoms and/or signs suggesting liver dysfunction, or in whom an abnormal liver test has occurred, should be evaluated for evidence of the development of more severe hepatic reaction while on therapy with FELDENE. Severe hepatic reactions, including jaundice and cases of fatal hepatitis, have been reported with FELDENE. Although such reactions are rare, if abnormal liver tests persist or worsen, if clinical signs and symptoms consistent with liver disease develop, or if systemic manifestations occur (e.g. eosinophilia, rash, etc.), FELDENE should be discontinued. (See also ADVERSE REACTIONS.)

Although at the recommended dose of 20 mg/day of FELDENE increased fecal blood loss due to gastrointestinal irritation did not occur (see CLINICAL PHARMACOLOGY), in about 4% of the patients treated with FELDENE alone or concomitantly with aspirin, reductions in hemoglobin and hematocrit values were observed. Therefore, these values should be determined if signs or symptoms of anemia occur.

Peripheral edema has been observed in approximately 2% of the patients treated with FELDENE. Therefore, as with other nonsteroidal anti-inflammatory drugs, FELDENE should be used with caution in patients with heart failure, hypertension or other conditions predisposing to fluid retention, since its usage may be associated with a worsening of these conditions.

A combination of dermatological and/or allergic signs and symptoms suggestive of serum sickness have occasionally occurred in conjunction with the use of FELDENE. These include arthralgias, pruritus, fever, fatigue, and rash including vesiculo bullous reactions and exfoliative dermatitis.

Information for Patients

FELDENE, like other drugs of its class, is not free of side effects. The side effects of these drugs can cause discomfort and, rarely, there are more serious side effects, such as gastrointestinal bleeding, which may result in hospitalization and even fatal outcomes.

NSAIDs (Nonsteroidal Anti-Inflammatory Drugs) are often essential agents in the management of arthritis, but they also may be commonly employed for conditions which are less serious.

Physicians may wish to discuss with their patients the potential risks (see WARNINGS, PRECAUTIONS, and ADVERSE REACTIONS sections) and likely benefits of NSAID treatment, particularly when the drugs are used for less serious conditions where treatment without NSAIDs may represent an acceptable alternative to both the patient and physician.

Laboratory Tests

Because serious GI tract ulceration and bleeding can occur without warning symptoms, physicians should follow chronically treated patients for the signs and symptoms of ulceration and bleeding and should inform them of the importance of this follow-up (see Risk of GI Ulceration, Bleeding and Perforation with NSAID Therapy).

Drug Interactions

FELDENE is highly protein bound, and, therefore, might be expected to displace other protein-bound drugs. Although this has not occurred in *in vitro* studies with coumarin-type anticoagulants, interactions with coumarin-type anticoagulants have been reported with FELDENE since marketing, therefore, physicians should closely monitor patients for a change in dosage requirements when administering FELDENE to patients in coumarin-type anticoagulants and other highly protein-bound drugs.

Plasma levels of piroxicam are depressed to approximately 80% of their normal values when FELDENE is administered in conjunction with aspirin (3900 mg/day), but concomitant administration of antacids has no effect on piroxicam plasma levels (see CLINICAL PHARMACOLOGY).

Nonsteroidal anti-inflammatory agents, including FELDENE, have been reported to increase steady state plasma lithium levels. It is recommended that plasma lithium levels be monitored when initiating, adjusting and discontinuing FELDENE.

Carcinogenesis, Chronic Animal Toxicity and Impairment of Fertility

Subacute and chronic toxicity studies have been carried out in rats, mice, dogs, and monkeys.

The pathology most often seen was that characteristically associated with the animal toxicology of anti-inflammatory agents: renal papillary necrosis (see PRECAUTIONS) and gastrointestinal lesions.

In classical studies in laboratory animals piroxicam did not show any teratogenic potential.

Reproductive studies revealed no impairment of fertility in animals.

Pregnancy and Nursing Mothers

Like other drugs which inhibit the synthesis and release of prostaglandins, piroxicam increased the incidence of dystocia and delayed parturition in pregnant animals when piroxicam administration was continued late into pregnancy. Gastrointestinal tract toxicity was increased in pregnant females in the last trimester of pregnancy compared to nonpregnant females or females in earlier trimesters of pregnancy.

FELDENE is not recommended for use in nursing mothers or in pregnant women because of the animal findings and since safety for such use has not been established in humans.

Use in Children

Dosage recommendations and indications for use in children have not been established.

ADVERSE REACTIONS

The incidence of adverse reactions to piroxicam is based on clinical trials involving approximately 2300 patients, about 400 of whom were treated for more than one year and 170 for more than two years. About 30% of all patients receiving daily doses of 20 mg of FELDENE experienced side effects. Gastrointestinal symptoms were the most prominent side effects—occurring in approximately 20% of the patients, which in most instances did not interfere with the course of therapy. Of the patients experiencing gastrointestinal side effects, approximately 5% discontinued therapy with an overall incidence of peptic ulceration of about 1%.

Other than the gastrointestinal symptoms, edema, dizziness, headache, changes in hematological parameters, and rash have been reported in a small percentage of patients. Routine ophthalmoscopy and slit-lamp examinations have revealed no evidence of ocular changes in 205 patients followed from 3 to 24 months while on therapy.

Incidence Greater Than 1%. The following adverse reactions occurred more frequently than 1 in 100.

Gastrointestinal: stomatitis, anorexia, epigastric distress*, nausea*, constipation, abdominal discomfort, flatulence, diarrhea, abdominal pain, indigestion

Hematological: decreases in hemoglobin* and hematocrit* (see PRECAUTIONS), anemia, leucopenia, eosinophilia

Dermatologic: pruritus, rash

Central Nervous System: dizziness, somnolence, vertigo

Urogenital: BUN and creatinine elevations (see PRECAUTIONS)

Body as a Whole: headache, malaise

Special Senses: tinnitus

Cardiovascular/Respiratory: edema (see PRECAUTIONS)

Incidence Less Than 1% (Causal Relationship Probable)

The following adverse reactions occurred less frequently than 1 in 100. The probability exists that there is a causal relationship between FELDENE and these reactions.

Gastrointestinal: liver function abnormalities, jaundice, hepatitis (see PRECAUTIONS), vomiting, hematemesis, melena, gastrointestinal bleeding, perforation and ulceration (see WARNINGS), dry mouth

Hematological: thrombocytopenia, petechial rash, ecchymosis, bone marrow depression including aplastic anemia, epistaxis

Dermatologic: sweating, erythema, bruising, desquamation, exfoliative dermatitis, erythema multiforme, toxic epidermal necrolysis, Stevens-Johnson syndrome, vesiculo bullous reaction, photoallergic skin reactions

Central Nervous System: depression, insomnia, nervousness

Urogenital: hematuria, proteinuria, interstitial nephritis, renal failure, hyperkalemia, glomerulitis, papillary necrosis, nephrotic syndrome (see PRECAUTIONS)

Body as a Whole: pain (colic), fever, flu-like syndrome (see PRECAUTIONS)

Special Senses: swollen eyes, blurred vision, eye irritations

Cardiovascular/Respiratory: hypertension, worsening of congestive heart failure (see PRECAUTIONS), exacerbation of angina

Metabolic: hypoglycemia, hyperglycemia, weight increase, weight decrease

Hypersensitivity: anaphylaxis, bronchospasm, urticaria/angioedema, vasculitis, "serum sickness" (see PRECAUTIONS)

*Reactions occurring in 3% to 9% of patients treated with FELDENE. Reactions occurring in 1–3% of patients are unmarked.

Incidence Less Than 1% (Causal Relationship Unknown)

Other adverse reactions were reported with a frequency of less than 1 in 100, but a causal relationship between FELDENE and the reaction could not be determined.

Gastrointestinal: pancreatitis

Dermatologic: onycholysis, loss of hair

Central Nervous System: akathisia, hallucinations, mood alterations, dream abnormalities, mental confusion, paresthesias

Urogenital System: dysuria

Body as a Whole: weakness

Cardiovascular/Respiratory: palpitations, dyspnea

Hypersensitivity: positive ANA

Special Senses: transient hearing loss

Hematological: hemolytic anemia

OVERDOSAGE

In the event treatment for overdosage is required the long plasma half-life (see CLINICAL PHARMACOLOGY) of piroxicam should be considered. The absence of experience with acute overdosage precludes characterization of sequelae and recommendation of specific antidotal efficacy at this time. It is reasonable to assume, however, that the standard measures of gastric evacuation and general supportive therapy would apply. In addition to supportive measures, the use of activated charcoal may effectively reduce the absorption and reabsorption of piroxicam. Experiments in dogs have demonstrated that the use of multiple-dose treatments with activated charcoal could reduce the half-life of piroxicam elimination from 27 hours (without charcoal) to 11 hours and reduce the systemic bioavailability of piroxicam by as much as 37% when activated charcoal is given as late as 6 hours after administration of piroxicam.

ADMINISTRATION AND DOSAGE

Rheumatoid Arthritis, Osteoarthritis

It is recommended that FELDENE therapy be initiated and maintained at a single daily dose of 20 mg. If desired the daily dose may be divided. Because of the long half-life of FELDENE, steady-state blood levels are not reached for 7–12 days. Therefore although the therapeutic effects of FELDENE are evident early in treatment, there is a progressive increase in response over several weeks and the effect of therapy should not be assessed for two weeks.

Dosage recommendations and indications for use in children have not been established.

HOW SUPPLIED

FELDENE Capsules for oral administration

Bottles of 100: 10 mg (NDC 0663-3220-66) maroon and blue #322

20 mg (NDC 0069-3230-66) maroon #323

Bottles of 500: 20 mg (NDC 0663-3230-73) maroon #323

Unit dose packages of 100: 20 mg (NDC 0663-3230-41) maroon #323

65-4100-00-3 Revised July 1990

LITERATURE AVAILABLE

Yes.

Shown in Product Identification Section, page 423

GLUCOTROL® ℞

[glū'kă-trōl]

(glipizide)

TABLETS

For Oral Use

DESCRIPTION

GLUCOTROL (glipizide) is an oral blood-glucose-lowering drug of the sulfonylurea class.

The Chemical Abstracts name of glipizide is 1-cyclohexyl-3-[[p-[2-(5-methylpyrazinecarboxamido)ethyl]phenyl]sulfonyl]urea. The molecular formula is $C_{21}H_{27}N_5O_4S$; the molecular weight is 445.55; the structural formula is shown below:

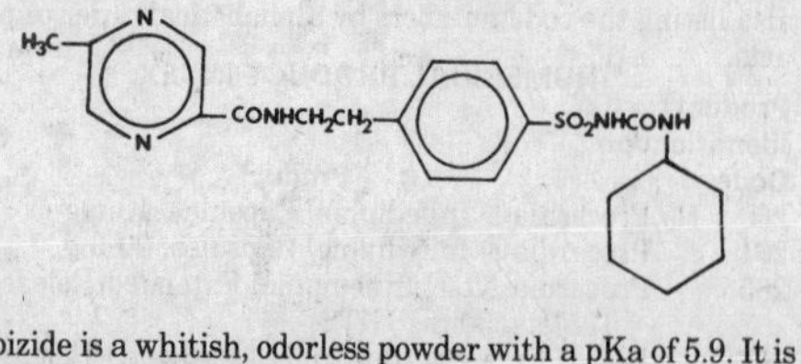

Glipizide is a whitish, odorless powder with a pKa of 5.9. It is insoluble in water and alcohols, but soluble in 0.1 *N* NaOH; it is freely soluble in dimethylformamide. GLUCOTROL tablets for oral use are available in 5 and 10 mg strengths. Inert ingredients are: colloidal silicon dioxide; lactose; microcrystalline cellulose; starch; stearic acid.

CLINICAL PHARMACOLOGY

Mechanism of Action: The primary mode of action of GLUCOTROL in experimental animals appears to be the stimulation of insulin secretion from the beta cells of pancre-

atic islet tissue and is thus dependent on functioning beta cells in the pancreatic islets. In humans GLUCOTROL appears to lower the blood glucose acutely by stimulating the release of insulin from the pancreas, an effect dependent upon functioning beta cells in the pancreatic islets. The mechanism by which GLUCOTROL lowers blood glucose during long-term administration has not been clearly established. In man, stimulation of insulin secretion by GLUCOTROL in response to a meal is undoubtedly of major importance. Fasting insulin levels are not elevated even on long-term GLUCOTROL administration, but the postprandial insulin response continues to be enhanced after at least 6 months of treatment. The insulinotropic response to a meal occurs within 30 minutes after an oral dose of GLUCOTROL in diabetic patients, but elevated insulin levels do not persist beyond the time of the meal challenge. Extrapancreatic effects may play a part in the mechanism of action of oral sulfonylurea hypoglycemic drugs.

Blood sugar control persists in some patients for up to 24 hours after a single dose of GLUCOTROL, even though plasma levels have declined to a small fraction of peak levels by that time (see Pharmacokinetics below).

Some patients fail to respond initially, or gradually lose their responsiveness to sulfonylurea drugs, including GLUCOTROL. Alternatively, GLUCOTROL may be effective in some patients who have not responded or have ceased to respond to other sulfonylureas.

Other Effects: It has been shown that GLUCOTROL therapy was effective in controlling blood sugar without deleterious changes in the plasma lipoprotein profiles of patients treated for NIDDM.

In a placebo-controlled, crossover study in normal volunteers, GLUCOTROL had no anti-diuretic activity, and, in fact, led to a slight increase in free water clearance.

Pharmacokinetics: Gastrointestinal absorption of GLUCOTROL in man is uniform, rapid, and essentially complete. Peak plasma concentrations occur 1–3 hours after a single oral dose. The half-life of elimination ranges from 2–4 hours in normal subjects, whether given intravenously or orally. The metabolic and excretory patterns are similar with the two routes of administration, indicating that first-pass metabolism is not significant. GLUCOTROL does not accumulate in plasma on repeated oral administration. Total absorption and disposition of an oral dose was unaffected by food in normal volunteers, but absorption was delayed by about 40 minutes. Thus GLUCOTROL was more effective when administered about 30 minutes before, rather than with, a test meal in diabetic patients. Protein binding was studied in serum from volunteers who received either oral or intravenous GLUCOTROL and found to be 98–99% one hour after either route of administration. The apparent volume of distribution of GLUCOTROL after intravenous administration was 11 liters, indicative of localization within the extracellular fluid compartment. In mice no GLUCOTROL or metabolites were detectable autoradiographically in the brain or spinal cord of males or females, nor in the fetuses of pregnant females. In another study, however, very small amounts of radioactivity were detected in the fetuses of rats given labelled drug.

The metabolism of GLUCOTROL is extensive and occurs mainly in the liver. The primary metabolites are inactive hydroxylation products and polar conjugates and are excreted mainly in the urine. Less than 10% unchanged GLUCOTROL is found in the urine.

INDICATIONS AND USAGE

GLUCOTROL is indicated as an adjunct to diet for the control of hyperglycemia and its associated symptomatology in patients with non-insulin-dependent diabetes mellitus (NIDDM; type II), formerly known as maturity-onset diabetes, after an adequate trial of dietary therapy has proved unsatisfactory.

In initiating treatment for non-insulin-dependent diabetes, diet should be emphasized as the primary form of treatment. Caloric restriction and weight loss are essential in the obese diabetic patient. Proper dietary management alone may be effective in controlling the blood glucose and symptoms of hyperglycemia. The importance of regular physical activity should also be stressed, and cardiovascular risk factors should be identified, and corrective measures taken where possible.

If this treatment program fails to reduce symptoms and/or blood glucose, the use of an oral sulfonylurea or insulin should be considered. Use of GLUCOTROL must be viewed by both the physician and patient as a treatment in addition to diet, and not as a substitute for diet or as a convenient mechanism for avoiding dietary restraint. Furthermore, loss of blood glucose control on diet alone also may be transient, thus requiring only short-term administration of GLUCOTROL.

During maintenance programs, GLUCOTROL should be discontinued if satisfactory lowering of blood glucose is no longer achieved. Judgments should be based on regular clinical and laboratory evaluations.

In considering the use of GLUCOTROL in asymptomatic patients, it should be recognized that controlling blood glucose in non-insulin-dependent diabetes has not been definitely established to be effective in preventing the long-term cardiovascular or neural complications of diabetes.

CONTRAINDICATIONS

GLUCOTROL is contraindicated in patients with:

1. Known hypersensitivity to the drug.
2. Diabetic ketoacidosis, with or without coma. This condition should be treated with insulin.

WARNINGS

SPECIAL WARNING ON INCREASED RISK OF CARDIOVASCULAR MORTALITY: The administration of oral hypoglycemic drugs has been reported to be associated with increased cardiovascular mortality as compared to treatment with diet alone or diet plus insulin. This warning is based on the study conducted by the University Group Diabetes Program (UGDP), a long-term prospective clinical trial designed to evaluate the effectiveness of glucose-lowering drugs in preventing or delaying vascular complications in patients with non-insulin-dependent diabetes. The study involved 823 patients who were randomly assigned to one of four treatment groups (*Diabetes,* 19, supp. 2: 747–830, 1970).

UGDP reported that patients treated for 5 to 8 years with diet plus a fixed dose of tolbutamide (1.5 grams per day) had a rate of cardiovascular mortality approximately 2½ times that of patients treated with diet alone. A significant increase in total mortality was not observed, but the use of tolbutamide was discontinued based on the increase in cardiovascular mortality, thus limiting the opportunity for the study to show an increase in overall mortality. Despite controversy regarding the interpretation of these results, the findings of the UGDP study provide an adequate basis for this warning. The patient should be informed of the potential risks and advantages of GLUCOTROL and of alternative modes of therapy.

Although only one drug in the sulfonylurea class (tolbutamide) was included in this study, it is prudent from a safety standpoint to consider that this warning may also apply to other oral hypoglycemic drugs in this class, in view of their close similarities in mode of action and chemical structure.

PRECAUTIONS

General

Renal and Hepatic Disease: The metabolism and excretion of GLUCOTROL may be slowed in patients with impaired renal and/or hepatic function. If hypoglycemia should occur in such patients, it may be prolonged and appropriate management should be instituted.

Hypoglycemia: All sulfonylurea drugs are capable of producing severe hypoglycemia. Proper patient selection, dosage, and instructions are important to avoid hypoglycemic episodes. Renal or hepatic insufficiency may cause elevated blood levels of GLUCOTROL and the latter may also diminish gluconeogenic capacity, both of which increase the risk of serious hypoglycemic reactions. Elderly, debilitated or malnourished patients, and those with adrenal or pituitary insufficiency are particularly susceptible to the hypoglycemic action of glucose-lowering drugs. Hypoglycemia may be difficult to recognize in the elderly, and in people who are taking beta-adrenergic blocking drugs. Hypoglycemia is more likely to occur when caloric intake is deficient, after severe or prolonged exercise, when alcohol is ingested, or when more than one glucose-lowering drug is used.

Loss of Control of Blood Glucose: When a patient stabilized on any diabetic regimen is exposed to stress such as fever, trauma, infection, or surgery, a loss of control may occur. At such times, it may be necessary to discontinue GLUCOTROL and administer insulin.

The effectiveness of any oral hypoglycemic drug, including GLUCOTROL, in lowering blood glucose to a desired level decreases in many patients over a period of time, which may be due to progression of the severity of the diabetes or to diminished responsiveness to the drug. This phenomenon is known as secondary failure, to distinguish it from primary failure in which the drug is ineffective in an individual patient when first given.

Laboratory Tests: Blood and urine glucose should be monitored periodically. Measurement of glycosylated hemoglobin may be useful.

Information for Patients: Patients should be informed of the potential risks and advantages of GLUCOTROL and of alternative modes of therapy. They should also be informed about the importance of adhering to dietary instructions, of a regular exercise program, and of regular testing of urine and/or blood glucose.

The risks of hypoglycemia, its symptoms and treatment, and conditions that predispose to its development should be explained to patients and responsible family members. Primary and secondary failure should also be explained.

Drug Interactions: The hypoglycemic action of sulfonylureas may be potentiated by certain drugs including nonsteroidal anti-inflammatory agents and other drugs that are highly protein bound, salicylates, sulfonamides, chloramphenicol, probenecid, coumarins, monoamine oxidase inhibitors, and beta-adrenergic blocking agents. When such drugs are administered to a patient receiving GLUCOTROL, the patient should be observed closely for hypoglycemia. When such drugs are withdrawn from a patient receiving GLUCOTROL, the patient should be observed closely for loss of control. *In vitro* binding studies with human serum proteins indicate that GLUCOTROL binds differently than tolbutamide and does not interact with salicylate or dicumarol. However, caution must be exercised in extrapolating these findings to the clinical situation and in the use of GLUCOTROL with these drugs.

Certain drugs tend to produce hyperglycemia and may lead to loss of control. These drugs include the thiazides and other diuretics, corticosteroids, phenothiazines, thyroid products, estrogens, oral contraceptives, phenytoin, nicotinic acid, sympathomimetics, calcium channel blocking drugs, and isoniazid. When such drugs are administered to a patient receiving GLUCOTROL, the patient should be closely observed for loss of control. When such drugs are withdrawn from a patient receiving GLUCOTROL, the patient should be observed closely for hypoglycemia.

A potential interaction between oral miconazole and oral hypoglycemic agents leading to severe hypoglycemia has been reported. Whether this interaction also occurs with the intravenous, topical, or vaginal preparations of miconazole is not known.

Carcinogenesis, Mutagenesis, Impairment of Fertility: A twenty month study in rats and an eighteen month study in mice at doses up to 75 times the maximum human dose revealed no evidence of drug-related carcinogenicity. Bacterial and *in vivo* mutagenicity tests were uniformly negative. Studies in rats of both sexes at doses up to 75 times the human dose showed no effects on fertility.

Pregnancy: Pregnancy Category C: GLUCOTROL (glipizide) was found to be mildly fetotoxic in rat reproductive studies at all dose levels (5–50 mg/kg). This fetotoxicity has been similarly noted with other sulfonylureas, such as tolbutamide and tolazamide. The effect is perinatal and believed to be directly related to the pharmacologic (hypoglycemic) action of GLUCOTROL. In studies in rats and rabbits no teratogenic effects were found. There are no adequate and well controlled studies in pregnant women. GLUCOTROL should be used during pregnancy only if the potential benefit justifies the potential risk to the fetus.

Because recent information suggests that abnormal blood glucose levels during pregnancy are associated with a higher incidence of congenital abnormalities, many experts recommend that insulin be used during pregnancy to maintain blood glucose levels as close to normal as possible.

Nonteratogenic Effects: Prolonged severe hypoglycemia (4 to 10 days) has been reported in neonates born to mothers who were receiving a sulfonylurea drug at the time of delivery. This has been reported more frequently with the use of agents with prolonged half-lives. If GLUCOTROL is used during pregnancy, it should be discontinued at least one month before the expected delivery date.

Nursing Mothers: Although it is not known whether GLUCOTROL is excreted in human milk, some sulfonylurea drugs are known to be excreted in human milk. Because the potential for hypoglycemia in nursing infants may exist, a decision should be made whether to discontinue nursing or to discontinue the drug, taking into account the importance of the drug to the mother. If the drug is discontinued and if diet alone is inadequate for controlling blood glucose, insulin therapy should be considered.

Pediatric Use: Safety and effectiveness in children have not been established.

ADVERSE REACTIONS

In U.S. and foreign controlled studies, the frequency of serious adverse reactions reported was very low. Of 702 patients, 11.8% reported adverse reactions and in only 1.5% was GLUCOTROL discontinued.

Hypoglycemia: See PRECAUTIONS and OVERDOSAGE sections.

Gastrointestinal: Gastrointestinal disturbances are the most common reactions. Gastrointestinal complaints were reported with the following approximate incidence: nausea and diarrhea, one in seventy; constipation and gastralgia, one in one hundred. They appear to be dose-related and may disappear on division or reduction of dosage. Cholestatic jaundice may occur rarely with sulfonylureas: GLUCOTROL should be discontinued if this occurs.

Dermatologic: Allergic skin reactions including erythema, morbilliform or maculopapular eruptions, urticaria, pruritus, and eczema have been reported in about one in seventy patients. These may be transient and may disappear despite continued use of GLUCOTROL; if skin reactions persist, the drug should be discontinued. Porphyria cutanea tarda and photosensitivity reactions have been reported with sulfonylureas.

Hematologic: Leukopenia, agranulocytosis, thrombocytopenia, hemolytic anemia, aplastic anemia, and pancytopenia have been reported with sulfonylureas.

Continued on next page

Pratt—Cont.

Metabolic: Hepatic porphyria and disulfiram-like reactions have been reported with sulfonylureas. In the mouse, GLUCOTROL pretreatment did not cause an accumulation of acetaldehyde after ethanol administration. Clinical experience to date has shown that GLUCOTROL has an extremely low incidence of disulfiram-like alcohol reactions.

Endocrine Reactions: Cases of hyponatremia and the syndrome of inappropriate antidiuretic hormone (SIADH) secretion have been reported with this and other sulfonylureas.

Miscellaneous: Dizziness, drowsiness, and headache have each been reported in about one in fifty patients treated with GLUCOTROL. They are usually transient and seldom require discontinuance of therapy.

Laboratory Tests: The pattern of laboratory test abnormalities observed with GLUCOTROL was similar to that for other sulfonylureas. Occasional mild to moderate elevations of SGOT, LDH, alkaline phosphatase, BUN and creatinine were noted. One case of jaundice was reported. The relationship of these abnormalities to GLUCOTROL is uncertain, and they have rarely been associated with clinical symptoms.

OVERDOSAGE

There is no well documented experience with GLUCOTROL overdosage. The acute oral toxicity was extremely low in all species tested (LD_{50} greater than 4 g/kg).

Overdosage of sulfonylureas including GLUCOTROL can produce hypoglycemia. Mild hypoglycemic symptoms without loss of consciousness or neurologic findings should be treated aggressively with oral glucose and adjustments in drug dosage and/or meal patterns. Close monitoring should continue until the physician is assured that the patient is out of danger. Severe hypoglycemic reactions with coma, seizure, or other neurological impairment occur infrequently, but constitute medical emergencies requiring immediate hospitalization. If hypoglycemic coma is diagnosed or suspected, the patient should be given a rapid intravenous injection of concentrated (50%) glucose solution. This should be followed by a continuous infusion of a more dilute (10%) glucose solution at a rate that will maintain the blood glucose at a level above 100 mg/dL. Patients should be closely monitored for a minimum of 24 to 48 hours since hypoglycemia may recur after apparent clinical recovery. Clearance of GLUCOTROL from plasma would be prolonged in persons with liver disease. Because of the extensive protein binding of GLUCOTROL, dialysis is unlikely to be of benefit.

DOSAGE AND ADMINISTRATION

There is no fixed dosage regimen for the management of diabetes mellitus with GLUCOTROL or any other hypoglycemic agent. In addition to the usual monitoring of urinary glucose, the patient's blood glucose must also be monitored periodically to determine the minimum effective dose for the patient; to detect primary failure, i.e., inadequate lowering of blood glucose at the maximum recommended dose of medication; and to detect secondary failure, i.e., loss of an adequate blood-glucose-lowering response after an initial period of effectiveness. Glycosylated hemoglobin levels may also be of value in monitoring the patient's response to therapy.

Short-term administration of GLUCOTROL may be sufficient during periods of transient loss of control in patients usually controlled well on diet.

In general, GLUCOTROL should be given approximately 30 minutes before a meal to achieve the greatest reduction in postprandial hyperglycemia.

Initial Dose: The recommended starting dose is 5 mg, given before breakfast. Geriatric patients or those with liver disease may be started on 2.5 mg.

Titration: Dosage adjustments should ordinarily be in increments of 2.5–5 mg, as determined by blood glucose response. At least several days should elapse between titration steps. If response to a single dose is not satisfactory, dividing that dose may prove effective. The maximum recommended once daily dose is 15 mg. Doses above 15 mg should ordinarily be divided and given before meals of adequate caloric content. The maximum recommended total daily dose is 40 mg.

Maintenance: Some patients may be effectively controlled on a once-a-day regimen, while others show better response with divided dosing. Total daily doses above 15 mg should ordinarily be divided. Total daily doses above 30 mg have been safely given on a b.i.d. basis to long-term patients.

In elderly patients, debilitated or malnourished patients, and patients with impaired renal or hepatic function, the initial and maintenance dosing should be conservative to avoid hypoglycemic reactions (see PRECAUTIONS section).

Patients Receiving Insulin: As with other sulfonylurea-class hypoglycemics, many stable non-insulin-dependent diabetic patients receiving insulin may be safely placed on GLUCOTROL. When transferring patients from insulin to GLUCOTROL, the following general guidelines should be considered:

For patients whose daily insulin requirement is 20 units or less, insulin may be discontinued and GLUCOTROL ther-

apy may begin at usual dosages. Several days should elapse between GLUCOTROL titration steps.

For patients whose daily insulin requirement is greater than 20 units, the insulin dose should be reduced by 50% and GLUCOTROL therapy may begin at usual dosages. Subsequent reductions in insulin dosage should depend on individual patient response. Several days should elapse between GLUCOTROL titration steps.

During the insulin withdrawal period, the patient should test urine samples for sugar and ketone bodies at least three times daily. Patients should be instructed to contact the prescriber immediately if these tests are abnormal. In some cases, especially when patient has been receiving greater than 40 units of insulin daily, it may be advisable to consider hospitalization during the transition period.

Patients Receiving Other Oral Hypoglycemic Agents: As with other sulfonylurea-class hypoglycemics, no transition period is necessary when transferring patients to GLUCOTROL. Patients should be observed carefully (1–2 weeks) for hypoglycemia when being transferred from longer half-life sulfonylureas (e.g., chlorpropamide) to GLUCOTROL due to potential overlapping of drug effect.

HOW SUPPLIED

GLUCOTROL tablets are white, dye-free, scored, diamond-shaped, and imprinted as follows:

　5 mg—Pfizer 411; 10 mg—Pfizer 412.
　5 mg Bottles: 100's (NDC 0049-4110-66); 500's (NDC 0049-4110-73); Unit Dose 100's (NDC 0049-4110-41);
　10 mg Bottles: 100's (NDC 0049-4120-66); 500's (NDC 0049-4120-73); Unit Dose 100's (NDC 0049-4120-41)

Recommended Storage: Store below 86°F (30°C).

Caution: Federal law prohibits dispensing without prescription.

69-4856-00-8

Shown in Product Identification Section, page 423

PROCARDIA®　　　　　　　　　　　　　　　　　　℞
[pro-car ′dē-ă]
(nifedipine)
CAPSULES
For Oral Use

DESCRIPTION

PROCARDIA (nifedipine) is an antianginal drug belonging to a new class of pharmacological agents, the calcium channel blockers. Nifedipine is 3,5-pyridinedicarboxylic acid, 1,4-dihydro-2,6-dimethyl-4-(2-nitrophenyl)-, dimethyl ester, $C_{17}H_{18}N_2O_6$.

Nifedipine is a yellow crystalline substance, practically insoluble in water but soluble in ethanol. It has a molecular weight of 346.3. PROCARDIA CAPSULES are formulated as soft gelatin capsules for oral administration each containing 10 mg or 20 mg nifedipine.

Inert ingredients in the formulations are: glycerin; peppermint oil; polyethylene glycol; soft gelatin capsules (which contain Yellow 6, and may contain Red Ferric Oxide and other inert ingredients); and water. The 10 mg capsules also contain saccharin sodium.

CLINICAL PHARMACOLOGY

PROCARDIA is a calcium ion influx inhibitor (slow channel blocker or calcium ion antagonist) and inhibits the transmembrane influx of calcium ions into cardiac muscle and smooth muscle. The contractile processes of cardiac muscle and vascular smooth muscle are dependent upon the movement of extracellular calcium ions into these cells through specific ion channels. PROCARDIA selectively inhibits calcium ion influx across the cell membrane of cardiac muscle and vascular smooth muscle without changing serum calcium concentrations.

Mechanism of Action

The precise means by which this inhibition relieves angina has not been fully determined, but includes at least the following two mechanisms:

1) Relaxation and prevention of coronary artery spasm

PROCARDIA dilates the main coronary arteries and coronary arterioles, both in normal and ischemic regions, and is a potent inhibitor of coronary artery spasm, whether spontaneous or ergonovine-induced. This property increases myocardial oxygen delivery in patients with coronary artery spasm, and is responsible for the effectiveness of PROCARDIA in vasospastic (Prinzmetal's or variant) angina. Whether this effect plays any role in classical angina is not clear, but studies of exercise tolerance have not shown an increase in the maximum exercise rate-pressure product, a widely accepted measure of oxygen utilization. This suggests that, in general, relief of spasm or dilation of coronary arteries is not an important factor in classical angina.

2) Reduction of oxygen utilization

PROCARDIA regularly reduces arterial pressure at rest and at a given level of exercise by dilating peripheral arterioles and reducing the total peripheral resistance (afterload) against which the heart works. This unloading of the heart

reduces myocardial energy consumption and oxygen requirements and probably accounts for the effectiveness of PROCARDIA in chronic stable angina.

Pharmacokinetics and Metabolism

PROCARDIA is rapidly and fully absorbed after oral administration. The drug is detectable in serum 10 minutes after oral administration, and peak blood levels occur in approximately 30 minutes. Bioavailability is proportional to dose from 10 to 30 mg; half-life does not change significantly with dose. There is little difference in relative bioavailability when PROCARDIA capsules are given orally and either swallowed whole; bitten and swallowed; or, bitten and held sublingually. However, biting through the capsule prior to swallowing does result in slightly earlier plasma concentrations (27 ng/ml 10 minutes after 10 mg) than if capsules are swallowed intact. It is highly bound by serum proteins. PROCARDIA is extensively converted to inactive metabolites and approximately 80 percent of PROCARDIA and metabolites are eliminated via the kidneys. The half-life of nifedipine in plasma is approximately two hours. There is no information on the effects of renal or hepatic impairment on excretion or metabolism of PROCARDIA.

Hemodynamics

Like other slow channel blockers, PROCARDIA exerts a negative inotropic effect on isolated myocardial tissue. This is rarely, if ever, seen in intact animals or man, probably because of reflex responses to its vasodilating effects. In man, PROCARDIA causes decreased peripheral vascular resistance and a fall in systolic and diastolic pressure, usually modest (5–10mm Hg systolic), but sometimes larger. There is usually a small increase in heart rate, a reflex response to vasodilation. Measurements of cardiac function in patients with normal ventricular function have generally found a small increase in cardiac index without major effects on ejection fraction, left ventricular end diastolic pressure (LVEDP) or volume (LVEDV). In patients with impaired ventricular function, most acute studies have shown some increase in ejection fraction and reduction in left ventricular filling pressure.

Electrophysiologic Effects

Although like other members of its class, PROCARDIA decreases sinoatrial node function and atrioventricular conduction in isolated myocardial preparations, such effects have not been seen in studies in intact animals or in man. In formal electrophysiologic studies, predominantly in patients with normal conduction systems, PROCARDIA has had no tendency to prolong atrioventricular conduction, prolong sinus node recovery time, or slow sinus rate.

INDICATIONS AND USAGE

I. Vasospastic Angina

PROCARDIA (nifedipine) is indicated for the management of vasospastic angina confirmed by any of the following criteria: 1) classical pattern of angina at rest accompanied by ST segment elevation, 2) angina or coronary artery spasm provoked by ergonovine, or 3) angiographically demonstrated coronary artery spasm. In those patients who have had angiography, the presence of significant fixed obstructive disease is not incompatible with the diagnosis of vasospastic angina, provided that the above criteria are satisfied. PROCARDIA may also be used where the clinical presentation suggests a possible vasospastic component but where vasospasm has not been confirmed, e.g., where pain has a variable threshold on exertion or in unstable angina where electrocardiographic findings are compatible with intermittent vasospasm, or when angina is refractory to nitrates and/or adequate doses of beta blockers.

II. Chronic Stable Angina (Classical Effort-Associated Angina)

PROCARDIA is indicated for the management of chronic stable angina (effort-associated angina) without evidence of vasospasm in patients who remain symptomatic despite adequate doses of beta blockers and/or organic nitrates or who cannot tolerate those agents.

In chronic stable angina (effort-associated angina) PROCARDIA has been effective in controlled trials of up to eight weeks duration in reducing angina frequency and increasing exercise tolerance, but confirmation of sustained effectiveness and evaluation of long term safety in these patients are incomplete.

Controlled studies in small numbers of patients suggest concomitant use of PROCARDIA and beta blocking agents may be beneficial in patients with chronic stable angina, but available information is not sufficient to predict with confidence the effects of concurrent treatment, especially in patients with compromised left ventricular function or cardiac conduction abnormalities. When introducing such concomitant therapy, care must be taken to monitor blood pressure closely since severe hypotension can occur from the combined effects of the drugs. (See WARNINGS.)

CONTRAINDICATIONS

Known hypersensitivity reaction to PROCARDIA.

WARNINGS

Excessive Hypotension

Although in most patients, the hypotensive effect of PROCARDIA is modest and well tolerated, occasional patients have had excessive and poorly tolerated hypotension. These responses have usually occurred during initial titration or at the time of subsequent upward dosage adjustment, and may be more likely in patients on concomitant beta blockers.

Severe hypotension and/or increased fluid volume requirements have been reported in patients receiving PROCARDIA together with a beta blocking agent who underwent coronary artery bypass surgery using high dose fentanyl anesthesia. The interaction with high dose fentanyl appears to be due to the combination of PROCARDIA and a beta blocker, but the possibility that it may occur with PROCARDIA alone, with low doses of fentanyl, in other surgical procedures, or with other narcotic analgesics cannot be ruled out. In PROCARDIA treated patients where surgery using high dose fentanyl anesthesia is contemplated, the physician should be aware of these potential problems and, if the patient's condition permits, sufficient time (at least 36 hours) should be allowed for PROCARDIA to be washed out of the body prior to surgery.

Increased Angina and/or Myocardial Infarction

Rarely, patients, particularly those who have severe obstructive coronary artery disease, have developed well documented increased frequency, duration and/or severity of angina or acute myocardial infarction on starting PROCARDIA or at the time of dosage increase. The mechanism of this effect is not established.

Beta Blocker Withdrawal

Patients recently withdrawn from beta blockers may develop a withdrawal syndrome with increased angina, probably related to increased sensitivity to catecholamines. Initiation of PROCARDIA treatment will not prevent this occurrence and might be expected to exacerbate it by provoking reflex catecholamine release. There have been occasional reports of increased angina in a setting of beta blocker withdrawal and PROCARDIA initiation. It is important to taper beta blockers if possible, rather than stopping them abruptly before beginning PROCARDIA.

Congestive Heart Failure

Rarely, patients, usually receiving a beta blocker, have developed heart failure after beginning PROCARDIA. Patients with tight aortic stenosis may be at greater risk for such an event, as the unloading effect of PROCARDIA would be expected to be of less benefit to these patients, owing to their fixed impedance to flow across the aortic valve.

PRECAUTIONS

General: Hypotension: Because PROCARDIA decreases peripheral vascular resistance, careful monitoring of blood pressure during the initial administration and titration of PROCARDIA is suggested. Close observation is especially recommended for patients already taking medications that are known to lower blood pressure. (See WARNINGS.)

Peripheral edema: Mild to moderate peripheral edema, typically associated with arterial vasodilation and not due to left ventricular dysfunction, occurs in about one in ten patients treated with PROCARDIA. This edema occurs primarily in the lower extremities and usually responds to diuretic therapy. With patients whose angina is complicated by congestive heart failure, care should be taken to differentiate this peripheral edema from the effects of increasing left ventricular dysfunction.

Laboratory tests: Rare, usually transient, but occasionally significant elevations of enzymes such as alkaline phosphatase, CPK, LDH, SGOT and SGPT have been noted. The relationship to PROCARDIA therapy is uncertain in most cases, but probable in some. These laboratory abnormalities have rarely been associated with clinical symptoms, however, cholestasis with or without jaundice has been reported. Rare instances of allergic hepatitis have been reported.

PROCARDIA, like other calcium channel blockers, decreases platelet aggregation *in vitro*. Limited clinical studies have demonstrated a moderate but statistically significant decrease in platelet aggregation and increase in bleeding time in some PROCARDIA patients. This is thought to be a function of inhibition of calcium transport across the platelet membrane. No clinical significance for these findings has been demonstrated.

Positive direct Coombs test with/without hemolytic anemia has been reported.

Although PROCARDIA has been used safely in patients with renal dysfunction and has been reported to exert a beneficial effect in certain cases, rare, reversible elevations in BUN and serum creatinine have been reported in patients with pre-existing chronic renal insufficiency. The relationship to PROCARDIA therapy is uncertain in most cases but probable in some.

Drug interactions: Beta-adrenergic blocking agents: (See INDICATIONS and WARNINGS.) Experience in over 1400 patients in a non-comparative clinical trial has shown that concomitant administration of PROCARDIA and beta-blocking agents is usually well tolerated, but there have been occasional literature reports suggesting that the combination may increase the likelihood of congestive heart failure, severe hypotension or exacerbation of angina.

Long acting nitrates: PROCARDIA may be safely co-administered with nitrates, but there have been no controlled studies to evaluate the antianginal effectiveness of this combination.

Digitalis: Administration of PROCARDIA with digoxin increased digoxin levels in nine of twelve normal volunteers. The average increase was 45%. Another investigator found no increase in digoxin levels in thirteen patients with coronary artery disease. In an uncontrolled study of over two hundred patients with congestive heart failure during which digoxin blood levels were not measured, digitalis toxicity was not observed. Since there have been isolated reports of patients with elevated digoxin levels, it is recommended that digoxin levels be monitored when initiating, adjusting, and discontinuing PROCARDIA to avoid possible over- or under-digitalization.

Coumarin anticoagulants: There have been rare reports of increased prothrombin time in patients taking coumarin anticoagulants to whom PROCARDIA was administered. However, the relationship to PROCARDIA therapy is uncertain.

Cimetidine: A study in six healthy volunteers has shown a significant increase in peak nifedipine plasma levels (80%) and area-under-the-curve (74%) after a one week course of cimetidine at 1000 mg per day and nifedipine at 40 mg per day. Ranitidine produced smaller, non-significant increases. The effect may be mediated by the known inhibition of cimetidine on hepatic cytochrome P-450, the enzyme system probably responsible for the first-pass metabolism of nifedipine. If nifedipine therapy is initiated in a patient currently receiving cimetidine, cautious titration is advised.

Carcinogenesis, mutagenesis, impairment of fertility: Nifedipine was administered orally to rats for two years and was not shown to be carcinogenic. When given to rats prior to mating, nifedipine caused reduced fertility at a dose approximately 30 times the maximum recommended human dose. *In vivo* mutagenicity studies were negative.

Pregnancy: Pregnancy category C. Nifedipine has been shown to be teratogenic in rats when given in doses 30 times the maximum recommended human dose. Nifedipine was embryotoxic (increased fetal resorptions, decreased fetal weight, increased stunted forms, increased fetal deaths, decreased neonatal survival) in rats, mice and rabbits at doses of from 3 to 10 times the maximum recommended human dose. In pregnant monkeys, doses ⅔ and twice the maximum recommended human dose resulted in small placentas and underdeveloped chorionic villi. In rats, doses three times maximum human dose and higher caused prolongation of pregnancy. There are no adequate and well controlled studies in pregnant women. PROCARDIA should be used during pregnancy only if the potential benefit justifies the potential risk to the fetus.

ADVERSE REACTIONS

In multiple-dose U.S. and foreign controlled studies in which adverse reactions were reported spontaneously, adverse effects were frequent but generally not serious and rarely required discontinuation of therapy or dosage adjustment. Most were expected consequences of the vasodilator effects of PROCARDIA.

Adverse Effect	PROCARDIA (%) (N = 226)	Placebo (%) (N = 235)
Dizziness, lightheadedness, giddiness	27	15
Flushing, heat sensation	25	8
Headache	23	20
Weakness	12	10
Nausea, heartburn	11	8
Muscle cramps, tremor	8	3
Peripheral edema	7	1
Nervousness, mood changes	7	4
Palpitation	7	5
Dyspnea, cough, wheezing	6	3
Nasal congestion, sore throat	6	8

There is also a large uncontrolled experience in over 2100 patients in the United States. Most of the patients had vasospastic or resistant angina pectoris, and about half had concomitant treatment with beta-adrenergic blocking agents. The most common adverse events were:

Incidence Approximately 10% *Cardiovascular:* peripheral edema

Central Nervous System: dizziness or lightheadedness

Gastrointestinal: nausea

Systemic: headache and flushing, weakness

Incidence Approximately 5% *Cardiovascular:* transient hypotension

Incidence 2% or Less *Cardiovascular:* palpitation

Respiratory: nasal and chest congestion, shortness of breath

Gastrointestinal: diarrhea, constipation, cramps, flatulence

Musculoskeletal: inflammation, joint stiffness, muscle cramps

Central Nervous System: shakiness, nervousness, jitteriness, sleep disturbances, blurred vision, difficulties in balance

Other: dermatitis, pruritus, urticaria, fever, sweating, chills, sexual difficulties.

Incidence Approximately 0.5% *Cardiovascular:* syncope. Syncopal episodes did not recur with reduction in the dose of PROCARDIA or concomitant antianginal medication.

Incidence Less Than 0.5% *Hematologic:* thrombocytopenia, anemia, leukopenia, purpura

Gastrointestinal: allergic hepatitis

Oral: gingival hyperplasia

CNS: depression, paranoid syndrome

Special Senses: transient blindness at the peak of plasma level

Other: erythromelalgia, arthritis with ANA (+)

Several of these side effects appear to be dose related. Peripheral edema occurred in about one in 25 patients at doses less than 60 mg per day and in about one patient in eight at 120 mg per day or more. Transient hypotension, generally of mild to moderate severity and seldom requiring discontinuation of therapy, occurred in one of 50 patients at less than 60 mg per day and in one of 20 patients at 120 mg per day or more. Very rarely, introduction of PROCARDIA therapy was associated with an increase in anginal pain, possibly due to associated hypotension.

In addition, more serious adverse events were observed, not readily distinguishable from the natural history of the disease in these patients. It remains possible, however, that some or many of these events were drug related. Myocardial infarction occurred in about 4% of patients and congestive heart failure or pulmonary edema in about 2%. Ventricular arrhythmias or conduction disturbances each occurred in fewer than 0.5% of patients.

In a subgroup of over 1000 patients receiving PROCARDIA with concomitant beta blocker therapy, the pattern and incidence of adverse experiences was not different from that of the entire group of PROCARDIA treated patients. (See PRECAUTIONS.)

In a subgroup of approximately 250 patients with a diagnosis of congestive heart failure as well as angina, dizziness or lightheadedness, peripheral edema, headache or flushing each occurred in one in eight patients. Hypotension occurred in about one in 20 patients. Syncope occurred in approximately one patient in 250. Myocardial infarction or symptoms of congestive heart failure each occurred in about one patient in 15. Atrial or ventricular dysrhythmias each occurred in about one patient in 150.

OVERDOSAGE

Although there is no well documented experience with PROCARDIA overdosage, available data suggest that gross overdosage could result in excessive peripheral vasodilation with subsequent marked and probably prolonged systemic hypotension. Clinically significant hypotension due to PROCARDIA overdosage calls for active cardiovascular support including monitoring of cardiac and respiratory function, elevation of extremities, and attention to circulating fluid volume and urine output. A vasoconstrictor (such as norepinephrine) may be helpful in restoring vascular tone and blood pressure, provided that there is no contraindication to its use. Clearance of PROCARDIA would be expected to be prolonged in patients with impaired liver function. Since PROCARDIA is highly protein-bound, dialysis is not likely to be of benefit.

DOSAGE AND ADMINISTRATION

The dosage of PROCARDIA needed to suppress angina and that can be tolerated by the patient must be established by titration. Excessive doses can result in hypotension.

Therapy should be initiated with the 10 mg capsule. The starting dose is one 10 mg capsule, swallowed whole, 3 times/day. The usual effective dose range is 10–20 mg three times daily. Some patients, especially those with evidence of coronary artery spasm, respond only to higher doses, more frequent administration, or both. In such patients, doses of 20–30 mg three or four times daily may be effective. Doses above 120 mg daily are rarely necessary. More than 180 mg per day is not recommended.

In most cases, PROCARDIA titration should proceed over a 7–14 day period so that the physician can assess the response to each dose level and monitor the blood pressure before proceeding to higher doses.

If symptoms so warrant, titration may proceed more rapidly provided that the patient is assessed frequently. Based on the patient's physical activity level, attack frequency, and sub-

Continued on next page

Pratt—Cont.

lingual nitroglycerin consumption, the dose of PROCARDIA may be increased from 10 mg t.i.d to 20 mg t.i.d and then to 30 mg t.i.d over a three-day period.

In hospitalized patients under close observation, the dose may be increased in 10 mg increments over four to six-hour periods as required to control pain and arrhythmias due to ischemia. A single dose should rarely exceed 30 mg.

No "rebound effect" has been observed upon discontinuation of PROCARDIA. However, if discontinuation of PROCARDIA is necessary, sound clinical practice suggests that the dosage should be decreased gradually with close physician supervision.

Co-Administration with Other Antianginal Drugs

Sublingual nitroglycerin may be taken as required for the control of acute manifestations of angina, particularly during PROCARDIA titration. See **Precautions, Drug Interactions**, for information on co-administration of PROCARDIA with beta blockers or long acting nitrates.

HOW SUPPLIED

PROCARDIA soft gelatin capsules are supplied in:
Bottles of 100: 10 mg (NDC 0069-2600-66) orange #260;
20 mg (NDC 0069-2610-66) orange and light brown #261
Bottles of 300: 10 mg (NDC 0069-2600-72) orange #260;
20 mg (NDC 0069-2610-72) orange and light brown #261
Unit dose packages of 100: 10 mg (NDC 0069-2600-41) orange #260; 20 mg (NDC 0069-2610-41) orange and light brown #261

The capsules should be protected from light and moisture and stored at controlled room temperature 59° to 77°F (15° to 25°C) in the manufacturer's original container.

69-4052-00-0 Revised July 1987

LITERATURE AVAILABLE

Yes.

Shown in Product Identification Section, page 423

PROCARDIA XL® ℞

[pro-car'dē-ă]
(nifedipine)
Extended Release Tablets
For Oral Use

DESCRIPTION

Nifedipine is a drug belonging to a class of pharmacological agents known as the calcium channel blockers. Nifedipine is 3,5-pyridinedicarboxylic acid, 1,4-dihydro-2,6-dimethyl-4-(2-nitrophenyl)-, dimethyl ester, $C_{17}H_{18}N_2O_6$, and has the structural formula:

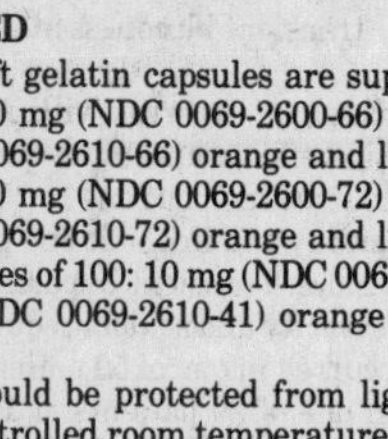

Nifedipine is a yellow crystalline substance, practically insoluble in water but soluble in ethanol. It has a molecular weight of 346.3. PROCARDIA XL is a trademark for Nifedipine GITS. Nifedipine GITS (Gastrointestinal Therapeutic System) Tablet is formulated as a once-a-day controlled-release tablet for oral administration designed to deliver 30, 60, or 90 mg of nifedipine.

Inert ingredients in the formulations are: cellulose acetate; hydroxypropyl cellulose; hydroxypropyl methylcellulose; magnesium stearate; polyethylene glycol; polyethylene oxide; red ferric oxide; sodium chloride; titanium dioxide.

System Components and Performance

PROCARDIA XL Extended Release Tablet is similar in appearance to a conventional tablet. It consists, however, of a semipermeable membrane surrounding an osmotically active drug core. The core itself is divided into two layers: an "active" layer containing the drug, and a "push" layer containing pharmacologically inert (but osmotically active) components. As water from the gastrointestinal tract enters the tablet, pressure increases in the osmotic layer and "pushes" against the drug layer, releasing drug through the precision laser-drilled tablet orifice in the active layer.

PROCARDIA XL Extended Release Tablet is designed to provide nifedipine at an approximately constant rate over 24 hours. This controlled rate of drug delivery into the gastrointestinal lumen is independent of pH or gastrointestinal motility. PROCARDIA XL depends for its action on the existence of an osmotic gradient between the contents of the bi-layer core and fluid in the GI tract. Drug delivery is essentially constant as long as the osmotic gradient remains constant, and then gradually falls to zero. Upon swallowing, the biologically inert components of the tablet remain intact during GI transit and are eliminated in the feces as an insoluble shell.

CLINICAL PHARMACOLOGY

Nifedipine is a calcium ion influx inhibitor (slow-channel blocker or calcium ion antagonist) and inhibits the transmembrane influx of calcium ions into cardiac muscle and smooth muscle. The contractile processes of cardiac muscle and vascular smooth muscle are dependent upon the movement of extracellular calcium ions into these cells through specific ion channels. Nifedipine selectively inhibits calcium ion influx across the cell membrane of cardiac muscle and vascular smooth muscle without altering serum calcium concentrations.

Mechanism of Action

A) Angina

The precise mechanisms by which inhibition of calcium influx relieves angina has not been fully determined, but includes at least the following two mechanisms:

1) Relaxation and Prevention of Coronary Artery Spasm

Nifedipine dilates the main coronary arteries and coronary arterioles, both in normal and ischemic regions, and is a potent inhibitor of coronary artery spasm, whether spontaneous or ergonovine-induced. This property increases myocardial oxygen delivery in patients with coronary artery spasm, and is responsible for the effectiveness of nifedipine in vasospastic (Prinzmetal's or variant) angina. Whether this effect plays any role in classical angina is not clear, but studies of exercise tolerance have not shown an increase in the maximum exercise rate-pressure product, a widely accepted measure of oxygen utilization. This suggests that, in general, relief of spasm or dilation of coronary arteries is not an important factor in classical angina.

2) Reduction of Oxygen Utilization

Nifedipine regularly reduces arterial pressure at rest and at a given level of exercise by dilating peripheral arterioles and reducing the total peripheral resistance (afterload) against which the heart works. This unloading of the heart reduces myocardial energy consumption and oxygen requirements, and probably accounts for the effectiveness of nifedipine in chronic stable angina.

B) Hypertension

The mechanism by which nifedipine reduces arterial blood pressure involves peripheral arterial vasodilatation and the resulting reduction in peripheral vascular resistance. The increased peripheral vascular resistance that is an underlying cause of hypertension results from an increase in active tension in the vascular smooth muscle. Studies have demonstrated that the increase in active tension reflects an increase in cytosolic free calcium.

Nifedipine is a peripheral arterial vasodilator which acts directly on vascular smooth muscle. The binding of nifedipine to voltage-dependent and possibly receptor-operated channels in vascular smooth muscle results in an inhibition of calcium influx through these channels. Stores of intracellular calcium in vascular smooth muscle are limited and thus dependent upon the influx of extracellular calcium for contraction to occur. The reduction in calcium influx by nifedipine causes arterial vasodilation and decreased peripheral vascular resistance which results in reduced arterial blood pressure.

Pharmacokinetics and Metabolism

Nifedipine is completely absorbed after oral administration. Plasma drug concentrations rise at a gradual, controlled rate after a PROCARDIA XL Extended Release Tablet dose and reach a plateau at approximately six hours after the first dose. For subsequent doses, relatively constant plasma concentrations at this plateau are maintained with minimal fluctuations over the 24 hour dosing interval. About a four-fold higher fluctuation index (ratio of peak to trough plasma concentration) was observed with the conventional immediate release Procardia® capsule at t.i.d. dosing than with once daily PROCARDIA XL Extended Release Tablet. At steady-state the bioavailability of the PROCARDIA XL Extended Release Tablet is 86% relative to Procardia capsules. Administration of the PROCARDIA XL Extended Release Tablet in the presence of food slightly alters the early rate of drug absorption, but does not influence the extent of drug bioavailability. Markedly reduced GI retention time over prolonged periods (i.e., short bowel syndrome), however, may influence the pharmacokinetic profile of the drug which could potentially result in lower plasma concentrations. Pharmacokinetics of PROCARDIA XL Extended Release Tablets are linear over the dose range of 30 to 180 mg in that plasma drug concentrations are proportional to dose administered. There was no evidence of dose dumping either in the presence or absence of food for over 150 subjects in pharmacokinetic studies.

Nifedipine is extensively metabolized to highly water-soluble, inactive metabolites accounting for 60 to 80% of the dose excreted in the urine. The elimination half-life of nifedipine is approximately two hours. Only traces (less than 0.1% of the dose) of unchanged form can be detected in the urine. The remainder is excreted in the feces in metabolized form, most likely as a result of biliary excretion. Thus, the pharmacokinetics of nifedipine are not significantly influenced by the degree of renal impairment. Patients in hemodialysis or chronic ambulatory peritoneal dialysis have not reported significantly altered pharmacokinetics of nifedipine. Since hepatic biotransformation is the predominant route for the disposition of nifedipine, the pharmacokinetics may be altered in patients with chronic liver disease. Patients with hepatic impairment (liver cirrhosis) have a longer disposition half-life and higher bioavailability of nifedipine than healthy volunteers. The degree of serum protein binding of nifedipine is high (92–98%). Protein binding may be greatly reduced in patients with renal or hepatic impairment.

Hemodynamics

Like other slow-channel blockers, nifedipine exerts a negative inotropic effect on isolated myocardial tissue. This is rarely, if ever, seen in intact animals or man, probably because of reflex responses to its vasodilating effects. In man, nifedipine decreases peripheral vascular resistance which leads to a fall in systolic and diastolic pressures, usually minimal in normotensive volunteers (less than 5–10 mm Hg systolic), but sometimes larger. With PROCARDIA XL Extended Release Tablets, these decreases in blood pressure are not accompanied by any significant change in heart rate. Hemodynamic studies in patients with normal ventricular function have generally found a small increase in cardiac index without major effects on ejection fraction, left ventricular end diastolic pressure (LVEDP) or volume (LVEDV). In patients with impaired ventricular function, most acute studies have shown some increase in ejection fraction and reduction in left ventricular filling pressure.

Electrophysiologic Effects

Although, like other members of its class, nifedipine causes a slight depression of sinoatrial node function and atrioventricular conduction in isolated myocardial preparations, such effects have not been seen in studies in intact animals or in man. In formal electrophysiologic studies, predominantly in patients with normal conduction systems, nifedipine has had no tendency to prolong atrioventricular conduction or sinus node recovery time, or to slow sinus rate.

INDICATIONS AND USAGE

I. Vasospastic Angina

PROCARDIA XL is indicated for the management of vasospastic angina confirmed by any of the following criteria: 1) classical pattern of angina at rest accompanied by ST segment elevation, 2) angina or coronary artery spasm provoked by ergonovine, or 3) angiographically demonstrated coronary artery spasm. In those patients who have had angiography, the presence of significant fixed obstructive disease is not incompatible with the diagnosis of vasospastic angina, provided that the above criteria are satisfied. PROCARDIA XL may also be used where the clinical presentation suggests a possible vasospastic component but where vasospasm has not been confirmed, e.g., where pain has a variable threshold on exertion or in unstable angina where electrocardiographic findings are compatible with intermittent vasospasm, or when angina is refractory to nitrates and/or adequate doses of beta blockers.

II. Chronic Stable Angina
(Classical Effort-Associated Angina)

PROCARDIA XL is indicated for the management of chronic stable angina (effort-associated angina) without evidence of vasospasm in patients who remain symptomatic despite adequate doses of beta blockers and/or organic nitrates or who cannot tolerate those agents.

In chronic stable angina (effort-associated angina) nifedipine has been effective in controlled trials of up to eight weeks duration in reducing angina frequency and increasing exercise tolerance, but confirmation of sustained effectiveness and evaluation of long term safety in these patients are incomplete.

Controlled studies in small numbers of patients suggest concomitant use of nifedipine and beta blocking agents may be beneficial in patients with chronic stable angina, but available information is not sufficient to predict with confidence the effects of concurrent treatment, especially in patients with compromised left ventricular function or cardiac conduction abnormalities. When introducing such concomitant therapy, care must be taken to monitor blood pressure closely since severe hypotension can occur from the combined effects of the drugs. (See WARNINGS.)

III. Hypertension

PROCARDIA XL is indicated for the treatment of hypertension. It may be used alone or in combination with other antihypertensive agents.

CONTRAINDICATIONS

Known hypersensitivity reaction to nifedipine.

WARNINGS

Excessive Hypotension

Although in most angina patients the hypotensive effect of nifedipine is modest and well tolerated, occasional patients have had excessive and poorly tolerated hypotension. These responses have usually occurred during initial titration or at the time of subsequent upward dosage adjustment, and may be more likely in patients on concomitant beta blockers.

Severe hypotension and/or increased fluid volume requirements have been reported in patients receiving nifedipine together with a beta-blocking agent who underwent coronary artery bypass surgery using high dose fentanyl anesthesia. The interaction with high dose fentanyl appears to be due to the combination of nifedipine and a beta blocker, but the possibility that it may occur with nifedipine alone, with low doses of fentanyl, in other surgical procedures, or with other narcotic analgesics cannot be ruled out. In nifedipine-treated patients where surgery using high dose fentanyl anesthesia is contemplated, the physician should be aware of these potential problems and if the patient's condition permits, sufficient time (at least 36 hours) should be allowed for nifedipine to be washed out of the body prior to surgery.

The following information should be taken into account in those patients who are being treated for hypertension as well as angina:

Increased Angina and/or Myocardial Infarction

Rarely, patients, particularly those who have severe obstructive coronary artery disease, have developed well documented increased frequency, duration and/or severity of angina or acute myocardial infarction on starting nifedipine or at the time of dosage increase. The mechanism of this effect is not established.

Beta Blocker Withdrawal

It is important to taper beta blockers if possible, rather than stopping them abruptly before beginning nifedipine. Patients recently withdrawn from beta blockers may develop a withdrawal syndrome with increased angina, probably related to increased sensitivity to catecholamines. Initiation of nifedipine treatment will not prevent this occurrence and on occasion has been reported to increase it.

Congestive Heart Failure

Rarely, patients, usually receiving a beta blocker, have developed heart failure after beginning nifedipine. Patients with tight aortic stenosis may be at greater risk for such an event, as the unloading effect of nifedipine would be expected to be of less benefit to those patients, owing to their fixed impedance to flow across the aortic valve.

PRECAUTIONS

General—Hypotension

Because nifedipine decreases peripheral vascular resistance, careful monitoring of blood pressure during the initial administration and titration of nifedipine is suggested. Close observation is especially recommended for patients already taking medications that are known to lower blood pressure. (See WARNINGS.)

Peripheral Edema

Mild to moderate peripheral edema occurs in a dose dependent manner with an incidence ranging from approximately 10% to about 30% at the highest dose studied (180 mg). It is a localized phenomenon thought to be associated with vasodilation of dependent arterioles and small blood vessels and not due to left ventricular dysfunction or generalized fluid retention. With patients whose angina or hypertension is complicated by congestive heart failure, care should be taken to differentiate this peripheral edema from the effects of increasing left ventricular dysfunction.

Other

As with any other non-deformable material, caution should be used when administering PROCARDIA XL in patients with preexisting severe gastrointestinal narrowing (pathologic or iatrogenic). There have been rare reports of obstructive symptoms in patients with known strictures in association with the ingestion of PROCARDIA XL.

Information for Patients

PROCARDIA XL Extended Release Tablets should be swallowed whole. Do not chew, divide or crush tablets. Do not be concerned if you occasionally notice in your stool something that looks like a tablet. In PROCARDIA XL, the medication is contained within a nonabsorbable shell that has been specially designed to slowly release the drug for your body to absorb. When this process is completed, the empty tablet is eliminated from your body.

Laboratory Tests

Rare, usually transient, but occasionally significant elevations of enzymes such as alkaline phosphatase, CPK, LDH, SGOT and SGPT have been noted. The relationship to nifedipine therapy is uncertain in most cases, but probable in some. These laboratory abnormalities have rarely been associated with clinical symptoms; however, cholestasis with or without jaundice has been reported. A small (5.4%) increase in mean alkaline phosphatase was noted in patients treated with PROCARDIA XL. This was an isolated finding not associated with clinical symptoms and it rarely resulted in values which fell outside the normal range. Rare instances of allergic hepatitis have been reported. In controlled studies, PROCARDIA XL did not adversely affect serum uric acid, glucose, or cholesterol. Serum potassium was unchanged in patients receiving PROCARDIA XL in the absence of concomitant diuretic therapy, and slightly decreased in patients receiving concomitant diuretics.

Nifedipine, like other calcium channel blockers, decreases platelet aggregation *in vitro*. Limited clinical studies have demonstrated a moderate but statistically significant decrease in platelet aggregation and increase in bleeding time in some nifedipine patients. This is thought to be a function of inhibition of calcium transport across the platelet membrane. No clinical significance for these findings has been demonstrated.

Positive direct Coombs test with/without hemolytic anemia has been reported but a causal relationship between nifedipine administration and positivity of this laboratory test, including hemolysis, could not be determined.

Although nifedipine has been used safely in patients with renal dysfunction and has been reported to exert a beneficial effect in certain cases, rare reversible elevations in BUN and serum creatinine have been reported in patients with preexisting chronic renal insufficiency. The relationship to nifedipine therapy is uncertain in most cases but probable in some.

Drug Interactions

Beta-adrenergic blocking agents: (See INDICATIONS and WARNINGS) Experience in over 1400 patients with Procardia capsules in a noncomparative clinical trial has shown that concomitant administration of nifedipine and beta-blocking agents is usually well tolerated but there have been occasional literature reports suggesting that the combination may increase the likelihood of congestive heart failure, severe hypotension, or exacerbation of angina.

Long Acting Nitrates: Nifedipine may be safely co-administered with nitrates, but there have been no controlled studies to evaluate the antianginal effectiveness of this combination.

Digitalis: Administration of nifedipine with digoxin increased digoxin levels in nine of twelve normal volunteers. The average increase was 45%. Another investigator found no increase in digoxin levels in thirteen patients with coronary artery disease. In an uncontrolled study of over two hundred patients with congestive heart failure during which digoxin blood levels were not measured, digitalis toxicity was not observed. Since there have been isolated reports of patients with elevated digoxin levels, it is recommended that digoxin levels be monitored when initiating, adjusting, and discontinuing nifedipine to avoid possible over- or under-digitalization.

Coumarin Anticoagulants: There have been rare reports of increased prothrombin time in patients taking coumarin anticoagulants to whom nifedipine was administered. However, the relationship to nifedipine therapy is uncertain.

Cimetidine: A study in six healthy volunteers has shown a significant increase in peak nifedipine plasma levels (80%) and area-under-the-curve (74%) after a one week course of cimetidine at 1000 mg per day and nifedipine at 40 mg per day. Ranitidine produced smaller, non-significant increases. The effect may be mediated by the known inhibition of cimetidine on hepatic cytochrome P-450, the enzyme system probably responsible for the first-pass metabolism of nifedipine. If nifedipine therapy is initiated in a patient currently receiving cimetidine, cautious titration is advised.

Carcinogenesis, Mutagenesis, Impairment of Fertility

Nifedipine was administered orally to rats for two years and was not shown to be carcinogenic. When given to rats prior to mating, nifedipine caused reduced fertility at a dose approximately 30 times the maximum recommended human dose. *In vivo* mutagenicity studies were negative.

Pregnancy

Pregnancy Category C. Nifedipine has been shown to be teratogenic in rats when given in doses 30 times the maximum recommended human dose. Nifedipine was embryotoxic (increased fetal resorptions, decreased fetal weight, increased stunted forms, increased fetal deaths, decreased neonatal survival) in rats, mice and rabbits at doses of from 3 to 10 times the maximum recommended human dose. In pregnant monkeys, doses ⅔ and twice the maximum recommended human dose resulted in small placentas and underdeveloped chorionic villi. In rats, doses three times maximum human dose and higher caused prolongation of pregnancy. There are no adequate and well controlled studies in pregnant women. PROCARDIA XL Extended Release Tablets should be used during pregnancy only if the potential benefit justifies the potential risk to the fetus.

ADVERSE EXPERIENCES

Over 1000 patients from both controlled and open trials with PROCARDIA XL Extended Release Tablets in hypertension and angina were included in the evaluation of adverse experiences. All side effects reported during PROCARDIA XL Extended Release Tablet therapy were tabulated independent of their causal relation to medication. The most common side effect reported with PROCARDIA XL was edema which was dose related and ranged in frequency from approximately 10% to about 30% at the highest dose studied (180 mg). Other common adverse experiences reported in placebo-controlled trials include: [See top of next column.]

Adverse Effect	PROCARDIA XL (%) (N=707)	Placebo (%) (N=266)
Headache	15.8	9.8
Fatigue	5.9	4.1
Dizziness	4.1	4.5
Constipation	3.3	2.3
Nausea	3.3	1.9

Of these, only edema and headache were more common in PROCARDIA XL patients than placebo patients.

The following adverse reactions occurred with an incidence of less than 3.0%. With the exception of leg cramps, the incidence of these side effects was similar to that of placebo alone.

Body as a Whole/Systemic: asthenia, flushing, pain
Cardiovascular: palpitations
Central Nervous System: insomnia, nervousness, paresthesia, somnolence
Dermatologic: pruritus, rash
Gastrointestinal: abdominal pain, diarrhea, dry mouth, dyspepsia, flatulence
Musculoskeletal: arthralgia, leg cramps
Respiratory: chest pain (nonspecific), dyspnea
Urogenital: impotence, polyuria

Other adverse reactions were reported sporadically with an incidence of 1.0% or less. These include:

Body as a Whole/Systemic: face edema, fever, hot flashes, malaise, periorbital edema, rigors
Cardiovascular: arrhythmia, hypotension, increased angina, tachycardia, syncope
Central Nervous System: anxiety, ataxia, decreased libido, depression, hypertonia, hypoesthesia, migraine, paroniria, tremor, vertigo
Dermatologic: alopecia, increased sweating, urticaria, purpura
Gastrointestinal: eructation, gastroesophageal reflux, gum hyperplasia, melena, vomiting, weight increase
Musculoskeletal: back pain, gout, myalgias
Respiratory: coughing, epistaxis, upper respiratory tract infection, respiratory disorder, sinusitis
Special Senses: abnormal lacrimation, abnormal vision, taste perversion, tinnitus
Urogenital/Reproductive: breast pain, dysuria, hematuria, nocturia

Adverse experiences which occurred in less than 1 in 1000 patients cannot be distinguished from concurrent disease states or medications.

The following adverse experiences, reported in less than 1% of patients, occurred under conditions (e.g., open trials, marketing experience) where a causal relationship is uncertain: gastrointestinal irritation, gastrointestinal bleeding.

In multiple-dose U.S. and foreign controlled studies with nifedipine capsules in which adverse reactions were reported spontaneously, adverse effects were frequent but generally not serious and rarely required discontinuation of therapy or dosage adjustment. Most were expected consequences of the vasodilator effects of PROCARDIA.

Adverse Effect	PROCARDIA CAPSULES (%) (N=226)	Placebo (%) (N=235)
Dizziness, lightheadedness, giddiness	27	15
Flushing, heat sensation	25	8
Headache	23	20
Weakness	12	10
Nausea, heartburn	11	8
Muscle cramps, tremor	8	3
Peripheral edema	7	1
Nervousness, mood changes	7	4
Palpitation	7	5
Dyspnea, cough, wheezing	6	3
Nasal congestion, sore throat	6	8

There is also a large uncontrolled experience in over 2100 patients in the United States. Most of the patients had vasospastic or resistant angina pectoris, and about half had concomitant treatment with beta-adrenergic blocking agents. The relatively common adverse events were similar in nature to those seen with PROCARDIA XL.

In addition, more serious adverse events were observed, not readily distinguishable from the natural history of the disease in these patients. It remains possible, however, that some or many of these events were drug related. Myocardial infarction occurred in about 4% of patients and congestive heart failure or pulmonary edema in about 2%. Ventricular arrhythmias or conduction disturbances each occurred in fewer than 0.5% of patients.

In a subgroup of over 1000 patients receiving PROCARDIA with concomitant beta blocker therapy, the pattern and incidence of adverse experiences was not different from that of the entire group of PROCARDIA (nifedipine) treated patients. (See PRECAUTIONS.)

In a subgroup of approximately 250 patients with a diagnosis of congestive heart failure as well as angina, dizziness or lightheadedness, peripheral edema, headache or flushing each occurred in one in eight patients. Hypotension occurred in about one in 20 patients. Syncope occurred in approximately one patient in 250. Myocardial infarction or symptoms of congestive heart failure each occurred in about one

Continued on next page

Pratt—Cont.

patient in 15. Atrial or ventricular dysrhythmias each occurred in about one patient in 150.
In post-marketing experience, there have been rare reports of exfoliative dermatitis caused by nifedipine.

OVERDOSAGE

Experience with nifedipine overdosage is limited. Generally, overdosage with nifedipine leading to pronounced hypotension calls for active cardiovascular support including monitoring of cardiovasular and respiratory function, elevation of extremities, judicious use of calcium infusion, pressor agents and fluids. Clearance of nifedipine would be expected to be prolonged in patients with impaired liver function. Since nifedipine is highly protein-bound, dialysis is not likely to be of any benefit.
There has been one reported case of massive overdosage with PROCARDIA XL Extended Release Tablets. The main effect of ingestion of approximately 4800 mg of PROCARDIA XL in a young man attempting suicide as a result of cocaine-induced depression was initial dizziness, palpitations, flushing, and nervousness. Within several hours of ingestion, nausea, vomiting, and generalized edema developed. No significant hypotension was apparent at presentation, 18 hours post-ingestion. Electrolyte abnormalities consisted of a mild, transient elevation of serum creatinine, and modest elevations of LDH and CPK, but normal SGOT. Vital signs remained stable, no electrocardiographic abnormalities were noted and renal function returned to normal with 24 to 48 hours with routine supportive measures alone. No prolonged sequelae were observed.
The effect of a single 900 mg ingestion of PROCARDIA capsules in a depressed anginal patient also on tricyclic antidepressants was a loss of consciousness within 30 minutes of ingestion, and profound hypotension, which responded to calcium infusion, pressor agents, and fluid replacement. A variety of ECG abnormalities were seen in this patient with a history of bundle branch block, including sinus bradycardia and varying degrees of AV block. These dictated the prophylactic placement of a temporary ventricular pacemaker, but otherwise resolved spontaneously. Significant hyperglycemia was seen initially in this patient, but plasma glucose levels rapidly normalized without further treatment.
A young hypertensive patient with advanced renal failure ingested 280 mg of PROCARDIA capsules at one time, with resulting marked hypotension responding to calcium infusion and fluids. No AV conduction abnormalities, arrhythmias, or pronounced changes in heart rate were noted, nor was there any further deterioration in renal function.

DOSAGE AND ADMINISTRATION

Dosage must be adjusted to each patient's needs. Therapy for either hypertension or angina should be initiated with 30 or 60 mg once daily. PROCARDIA XL Extended Release Tablets should be swallowed whole and should not be bitten or divided. In general, titration should proceed over a 7–14 day period so that the physician can fully assess the response to each dose level and monitor blood pressure before proceeding to higher doses. Since steady-state plasma levels are achieved on the second day of dosing, if symptoms so warrant, titration may proceed more rapidly provided the patient is assessed frequently. Titration to doses above 120 mg is not recommended.
Angina patients controlled on PROCARDIA capsules alone or in combination with other antianginal medications may be safely switched to PROCARDIA XL Extended Release Tablets at the nearest equivalent total daily dose (e.g., 30 mg t.i.d. of PROCARDIA capsules may be changed to 90 mg once daily of PROCARDIA XL Extended Release Tablets). Subsequent titration to higher or lower doses may be necessary and should be initiated as clinically warranted. Experience with doses greater than 90 mg in patients with angina is limited. Therefore, doses greater than 90 mg should be used with caution and only when clinically warranted.
No "rebound effect" has been observed upon discontinuation of PROCARDIA XL Extended Release Tablets. However, if discontinuation of nifedipine is necessary, sound clinical practice suggests that the dosage should be decreased gradually with close physician supervision.
Care should be taken when dispensing PROCARDIA XL to assure that the extended release dosage form has been prescribed.

Co-Administration with Other Antianginal Drugs
Sublingual nitroglycerin may be taken as required for the control of acute manifestations of angina, particularly during nifedipine titration. See PRECAUTIONS, Drug Interactions, for information on co-administration of nifedipine with beta blockers or long acting nitrates.

HOW SUPPLIED

PROCARDIA XL® Extended Release Tablets are supplied as 30 mg, 60 mg and 90 mg round biconvex, rose-pink, film-coated tablets in:
Bottles of 100: 30 mg (NDC 0069-2650-66)
60 mg (NDC 0069-2660-66)
90 mg (NDC 0069-2670-66)
Bottles of 300: 30 mg (NDC 0069-2650-72)
60 mg (NDC 0069-2660-72)
Unit dose packages of 100: 30 mg (NDC 0069-2650-41)
60 mg (NDC 0069-2660-41)
The tablets should be protected from moisture and humidity and stored below 86°F (30°C).
77-4467-00-6 Revised August 1990
Shown in Product Identification Section, page 423

ZOLOFT™ ℞
(sertraline hydrochloride)
Tablets

DESCRIPTION

ZOLOFT™ (sertraline hydrochloride) is an antidepressant for oral administration. It is chemically unrelated to tricylic, tetracyclic, or other available antidepressant agents. It has a molecular weight of 342.7. Sertraline hydrochloride has the following chemical name: (1S-cis)-4-(3-4-dichlorophenyl)-1,2,3,4-tetrahydro-N-methyl-1-naphthalenamine hydrochloride. The empirical formula $C_{17}H_{17}NCl_2 \cdot HCl$ is represented by the following structural formula:

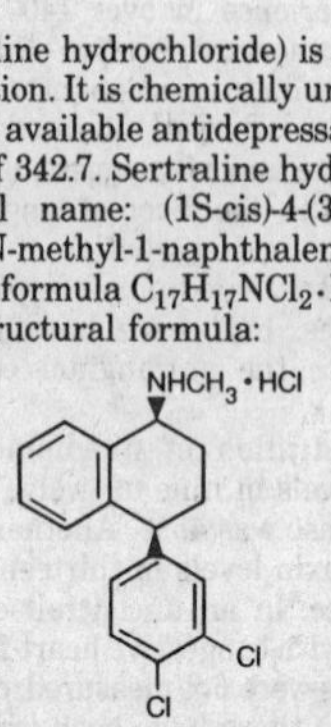

Sertraline hydrochloride is a white crystalline powder that is slightly soluble in water and isopropyl alcohol, and sparingly soluble in ethanol.
ZOLOFT is supplied for oral administration as scored tablets containing sertraline hydrochloride equivalent to 50 and 100 mg of sertraline and the following inactive ingredients: dibasic calcium phosphate dihydrate, FD&C Blue #2 aluminum lake (in 50 mg tablet), hydroxypropyl cellulose, hydroxypropyl methylcellulose, magnesium stearate, microcrystalline cellulose, polyethylene glycol, polysorbate 80, sodium starch glycolate, synthetic yellow iron oxide (in 100 mg tablet), and titanium dioxide.

CLINICAL PHARMACOLOGY

Pharmacodynamics
The mechanism of action of sertraline is presumed to be linked to its inhibition of CNS neuronal uptake of serotonin (5HT). Studies at clinically relevant doses in man have demonstrated that sertraline blocks the uptake of serotonin into human platelets. *In vitro* studies in animals also suggest that sertraline is a potent and selective inhibitor of neuronal serotonin reuptake and has only very weak effects on norepinephrine and dopamine neuronal reuptake. *In vitro* studies have shown that sertraline has no significant affinity for adrenergic ($alpha_1$, $alpha_2$, beta), cholinergic, GABA, dopaminergic, histaminergic, serotonergic ($5HT_{1A}$, $5HT_{1B}$, $5HT_2$), or benzodiazepine receptors; antagonism of such receptors has been hypothesized to be associated with various anticholinergic, sedative, and cardiovascular effects for other psychotropic drugs. The chronic administration of sertraline was found in animals to downregulate brain norepinephrine receptors, as has been observed with other clinically effective antidepressants. Sertraline does not inhibit monoamine oxidase.

Pharmacokinetics
Systemic Bioavailability—In man, following oral once-daily dosing over the range of 50 to 200 mg for 14 days, mean peak plasma concentrations (Cmax) of sertraline occurred between 4.5 to 8.4 hours postdosing. The average terminal elimination half-life of plasma sertraline is about 26 hours. Based on this pharmacokinetic parameter, steady-state sertraline plasma levels should be achieved after approximately one week of once-daily dosing. Linear dose-proportional pharmacokinetics were demonstrated in a single dose study in which the Cmax and area under the plasma concentration time curve (AUC) of sertraline were proportional to dose over a range of 50 to 200 mg. Consistent with the terminal elimination half-life, there is an approximately two-fold accumulation, compared to a single dose, of sertraline with repeated dosing over a 50 to 200 mg dose range. The single-dose bioavailability of sertraline tablets is approximately equal to an equivalent dose of solution.
The effects of food on the bioavailability of sertraline were studied in subjects administered a single-dose with and without food. AUC was slightly increased when drug was administered with food but the Cmax was 25% greater, while the time to reach peak plasma concentration decreased from 8 hours post-dosing to 5.5 hours.

Metabolism—Sertraline undergoes extensive first pass metabolism. The principal initial pathway of metabolism for sertraline is N-demethylation. N-desmethylsertraline has a plasma terminal elimination half-life of 62 to 104 hours. Both *in vitro* biochemical and *in vivo* pharmacological testing have shown N-desmethylsertraline to be substantially less active than sertraline. Both sertraline and N-desmethylsertraline undergo oxidative deamination and subsequent reduction, hydroxylation, and glucuronide conjugation. In a study of radiolabeled sertraline involving two healthy male subjects, sertraline accounted for less than 5% of the plasma radioactivity. About 40–45% of the administered radioactivity was recovered in urine in 9 days. Unchanged sertraline was not detectable in the urine. For the same period, about 40–45% of the administered radioactivity was accounted for in feces, including 12–14% unchanged sertraline.
Desmethylsertraline exhibits time-related, dose dependent increases in AUC (0–24 hour), Cmax and Cmin, with about a 5–9 fold increase in these pharmacokinetic parameters between day 1 and day 14.

Protein Binding—*In vitro* protein binding studies performed with radiolabeled ^{3}H-sertraline showed that sertraline is highly bound to serum proteins (98%) in the range of 20 to 500 ng/mL. However, at up to 300 and 200 ng/mL concentrations, respectively, sertraline and N-desmethylsertraline did not alter the plasma protein binding of two other highly protein bound drugs, viz., warfarin and propranolol (see Precautions).

Age—Sertraline plasma clearance in a group of 16 (8 male, 8 female) elderly patients treated for 14 days at dose of 100 mg/day was approximately 40% lower than in a similarly studied group of younger (25 to 32 y.o.) individuals. Steady state, therefore, should be achieved after 2 to 3 weeks in older patients. The same study showed a decreased clearance of desmethylsertraline in older males, but not in older females.

Liver Disease and Renal Disease—The pharmacokinetics of sertraline in patients with significant hepatic or renal dysfunction have not been determined.

INDICATIONS AND USAGE

ZOLOFT (sertraline hydrochloride) is indicated for the treatment of depression. The efficacy of ZOLOFT in the treatment of a major depressive episode was established in six to eight week controlled trials of outpatients whose diagnoses corresponded most closely to the DSM-III category of major depressive disorder.
A major depressive episode implies a prominent and relatively persistent depressed or dysphoric mood that usually interferes with daily functioning (nearly every day for at least 2 weeks); it should include at least 4 of the following 8 symptoms: change in appetite, change in sleep, psychomotor agitation or retardation, loss of interest in usual activities or decrease in sexual drive, increased fatigue, feelings of guilt or worthlessness, slowed thinking or impaired concentration, and a suicide attempt or suicidal ideation.
The antidepressant action of ZOLOFT in hospitalized depressed patients has not been adequately studied.
A study of depressed outpatients who had responded to ZOLOFT during an initial eight-week open treatment phase and were then randomized to continuation on ZOLOFT or placebo demonstrated a significantly lower relapse rate over the next eight weeks for patients taking ZOLOFT compared to those on placebo. However, the effectiveness of ZOLOFT in long-term use, that is, for more than 16 weeks, has not been systematically evaluated in controlled trials. Therefore, the physician who elects to use ZOLOFT for extended periods should periodically reevaluate the long-term usefulness of the drug for the individual patient.

CONTRAINDICATIONS

None known.

WARNINGS

In patients receiving another serotonin reuptake inhibitor drug in combination with a monoamine oxidase inhibitor (MAOI), there have been reports of serious, sometimes fatal, reactions including hyperthermia, rigidity, myoclonus, autonomic instability with possible rapid fluctuations of vital signs, and mental status changes that include extreme agitation progressing to delirium and coma. These reactions have also been reported in patients who have recently discontinued that drug and have been started on an MAOI. Some cases presented with features resembling neuroleptic malignant syndrome. Therefore, it is recommended that ZOLOFT (sertraline hydrochloride) not be used in combination with an MAOI, or within 14 days of discontinuing treatment with an MAOI. Similarly, at least 14 days should be allowed after stopping ZOLOFT before starting an MAOI.

PRECAUTIONS

General
Activation of Mania/Hypomania—During premarketing testing, hypomania or mania occurred in approximately 0.4% of ZOLOFT (sertraline hydrochloride) treated patients. Activation of mania/hypomania has also been reported in a

small proportion of patients with Major Affective Disorder treated with other marketed antidepressants.

Weight Loss—Significant weight loss may be an undesirable result of treatment with sertraline for some patients, but on average, patients in controlled trials had minimal, 1 to 2 pound weight loss, versus smaller changes on placebo. Only rarely have sertraline patients been discontinued for weight loss.

Seizure—ZOLOFT has not been evaluated in patients with a seizure disorder. These patients were excluded from clinical studies during the product's premarket testing. Accordingly, like other antidepressants, ZOLOFT should be introduced with care in epileptic patients.

Suicide—The possibility of a suicide attempt is inherent in depression and may persist until significant remission occurs. Close supervision of high risk patients should accompany initial drug therapy. Prescriptions for ZOLOFT should be written for the smallest quantity of tablets consistent with good patient management, in order to reduce the risk of overdose.

Weak Uricosuric Effect—ZOLOFT is associated with a mean decrease in serum uric acid of approximately 7%. The clinical significance of this weak uricosuric effect is unknown, and there have been no reports of acute renal failure with ZOLOFT.

Use in Patients with Concomitant Illness—Clinical experience with ZOLOFT in patients with certain concomitant systemic illness is limited. Caution is advisable in using ZOLOFT in patients with diseases or conditions that could affect metabolism or hemodynamic responses.

ZOLOFT has not been evaluated or used to any appreciable extent in patients with a recent history of myocardial infarction or unstable heart disease. Patients with these diagnoses were excluded from clinical studies during the product's premarket testing. However, the electrocardiograms of 774 patients who received ZOLOFT in double-blind trials were evaluated and the data indicate that ZOLOFT is not associated with the development of significant ECG abnormalities. ZOLOFT is extensively metabolized by the liver. The pharmacokinetics of ZOLOFT have not been studied in patients with significant hepatic dysfunction nor have patients with significant hepatic dysfunction been evaluated during treatment with ZOLOFT. Accordingly, ZOLOFT should be used with caution in such patients.

Since ZOLOFT is extensively metabolized, excretion of unchanged drug in urine is a minor route of elimination. However, until the pharmacokinetics of ZOLOFT have been studied in patients with renal impairment and until adequate numbers of patients with severe renal impairment have been evaluated during chronic treatment with ZOLOFT, it should be used with caution in such patients.

Interference with Cognitive and Motor Performance—In controlled studies, ZOLOFT did not cause sedation and did not interfere with psychomotor performance.

Information for Patients

Physicians are advised to discuss the following issues with patients for whom they prescribe ZOLOFT:

Patients should be told that although ZOLOFT has not been shown to impair the ability of normal subjects to perform tasks requiring complex motor and mental skills in laboratory experiments, drugs that act upon the central nervous system may affect some individuals adversely.

Patients should be told that although ZOLOFT has not been shown in experiments with normal subjects to increase the mental and motor skill impairments caused by alcohol, the concomitant use of ZOLOFT and alcohol in depressed patients is not advised.

Patients should be told that while no adverse interaction of ZOLOFT with over-the-counter (OTC) drug products is known to occur, the potential for interaction exists. Thus, the use of any OTC product should be initiated cautiously according to the directions of use given for the OTC product.

Patients should be advised to notify their physician if they become pregnant or intent to become pregnant during therapy.

Patients should be advised to notify their physician if they are breast feeding an infant.

Laboratory Tests

None.

Drug Interactions

Potential Effects of Coadministration of Drugs Highly Bound to Plasma Proteins—Because sertraline is tightly bound to plasma protein, the administration of ZOLOFT (sertraline hydrochloride) to a patient taking another drug which is tightly bound to protein, (e.g., warfarin, digitoxin) may cause a shift in plasma concentrations potentially resulting in an adverse effect. Conversely, adverse effects may result from displacement of protein bound ZOLOFT by other tightly bound drugs.

In a study comparing prothrombin time AUC (0–120 hr) following dosing with warfarin (0.75 mg/kg) before and after 21 days of dosing with either ZOLOFT (50–200 mg/day) or placebo, there was a mean increase in prothrombin time of 8% relative to baseline for ZOLOFT compared to a 1% decrease for placebo (p < 0.02). The normalization of prothrombin time for the ZOLOFT group was delayed compared to the

placebo group. The clinical significance of this change is unknown. Accordingly, prothrombin time should be carefully monitored when ZOLOFT therapy is initiated or stopped.

CNS Active Drugs—In a study comparing the disposition of intravenously administered diazepam before and after 21 days of dosing with either ZOLOFT (50 to 200 mg/day escalating dose) or placebo, there was a 32% decrease relative to baseline in diazepam clearance for the ZOLOFT group compared to a 19% decrease relative to baseline for the placebo group (p < 0.03). There was a 23% increase in Tmax for desmethyldiazepam in the ZOLOFT group compared to a 20% decrease in the placebo group (p < 0.03). The clinical significance of these changes is unknown.

In a placebo-controlled trial in normal volunteers, the administration of two doses of ZOLOFT did not significantly alter steady-state lithium levels or the renal clearance of lithium.

Nonetheless, at this time, it is recommended that plasma lithium levels be monitored following initiation of ZOLOFT therapy with appropriate adjustments to the lithium dose. The risk of using ZOLOFT in combination with other CNS active drugs has not been systematically evaluated. Consequently, caution is advised if the concomitant administration of ZOLOFT and such drugs is required.

Hypoglycemic Drugs—In a placebo-controlled trial in normal volunteers, administration of ZOLOFT for 22 days (including 200 mg/day for the final 13 days) caused a statistically significant 16% decrease from baseline in the clearance of tolbutamide following an intravenous 1000 mg dose. ZOLOFT administration did not noticeably change either the plasma protein binding or the apparent volume of distribution of tolbutamide, suggesting that the decreased clearance was due to a change in the metabolism of the drug. The clinical significance of this decrease in tolbutamide clearance is unknown.

Atenolol—ZOLOFT (100 mg) when administered to 10 healthy male subjects had no effect on the beta-adrenergic blocking ability of atenolol.

Microsomal Enzyme Induction—Preclinical studies have shown ZOLOFT to induce hepatic microsomal enzymes. In clinical studies, ZOLOFT was shown to induce hepatic enzymes minimally as determined by a small (5%) but statistically significant decrease in antipyrine half-life following administration of 200 mg/day for 21 days. This small change in antipyrine half-life reflects a clinically insignificant change in hepatic metabolism.

Electroconvulsive Therapy—There are no clinical studies establishing the risks or benefits of the combined use of electroconvulsive therapy (ECT) and ZOLOFT.

Alcohol—Although ZOLOFT did not potentiate the cognitive and psychomotor effects of alcohol in experiments with normal subjects, the concomitant use of ZOLOFT and alcohol in depressed patients is not recommended.

Carcinogenesis, Mutagenesis, Impairment of Fertility

Lifetime carcinogenicity studies were carried out in CD-1 mice and Long-Evans rats at doses up to 40 mg/kg in mice (10 times, on a mg/kg basis, and the same, on a mg/m^2 basis, as the maximum recommended human dose) and at doses up to 40 mg/kg in rats (10 times, on a mg/kg basis, and 2 times, on a mg/m^2 basis, the maximum recommended human dose). There was a dose-related increase in the incidence of liver adenomas in male mice receiving sertraline at 10–40 mg/kg. No increase was seen in female mice or in rats of either sex receiving the same treatments, nor was there an increase in hepatocellular carcinomas. Liver adenomas have a variable rate of spontaneous occurrence in the CD-1 mouse and are of unknown significance to humans. There was an increase in follicular adenomas of the thyroid in female rats receiving sertraline at 40 mg/kg; this was not accompanied by thyroid hyperplasia. While there was an increase in uterine adenocarcinomas in rats receiving sertraline at 10–40 mg/kg compared to placebo controls, this effect was not clearly drug related.

Sertraline had no genotoxic effects, with or without metabolic activation, based on the following assays: bacterial mutation assay; mouse lymphoma mutation assay; and tests for cytogenetic aberrations in vivo in mouse bone marrow and in vitro in human lymphocytes.

A decrease in fertility was seen in one of two rat studies at a dose of 80 mg/kg (20 times the maximum human dose on a mg/kg basis and 4 times on a mg/m^2 basis).

Pregnancy-Pregnancy Category B

Teratogenic Effects—Reproduction studies have been performed in rats and rabbits at doses up to approximately 20 times and 10 times the maximum daily human mg/kg dose (4 to 4.5 times the mg/m^2 dose), respectively.

There was no evidence of teratogenicity at any dose level. At doses approximately 2.5–10 times the maximum daily human mg/kg dose, sertraline was associated with delayed ossification in fetuses, probably secondary to effects on the dams.

There are no adequate and well-controlled studies in pregnant women. Because animal reproduction studies are not always predictive of human response, this drug should be used during pregnancy only if clearly needed.

Non-teratogenic Effects—There was also decreased neonatal survival following maternal administration of sertraline at doses as low as approximately 5 times the maximum human mg/kg dose. The decrease in pup survival was shown to be most probably due to in utero exposure to sertraline. The clinical significance of these effects is unknown.

Labor and Delivery—The effect of ZOLOFT on labor and delivery in humans is unknown.

Nursing Mothers—It is not known whether, and if so in what amount, sertraline or its metabolites are excreted in human milk. Because many drugs are excreted in human milk, caution should be exercised when ZOLOFT is administered to a nursing woman.

Pediatric Use—Safety and effectivenesss in children have not been established.

Geriatric Use—Several hundred elderly patients have participated in clinical studies with ZOLOFT. The pattern of adverse reactions in the elderly was similar to that in younger patients.

ADVERSE REACTIONS

Commonly Observed—The most commonly observed adverse events associated with the use of ZOLOFT (sertraline hydrochloride) and not seen at an equivalent incidence among placebo treated patients were: gastrointestinal complaints, including nausea, diarrhea/loose stools and dyspepsia; tremor; dizziness; insomnia; somnolence; increased sweating; dry mouth; and male sexual dysfunction (primarily ejaculatory delay).

Associated with Discontinuation of Treatment—Fifteen percent of 2710 subjects who received ZOLOFT in premarketing multiple dose clinical trials discontinued treatment due to an adverse event. The more common events (reported by at least 1% of subjects) associated with discontinuation included agitation, insomnia, male sexual dysfunction (primarily ejaculatory delay), somnolence, dizziness, headache, tremor, anorexia, diarrhea/loose stools, nausea, and fatigue.

Incidence in Controlled Clinical Trials—The table that follows enumerates adverse events that occurred at a frequency of 1% or more among ZOLOFT patients who participated in controlled trials comparing titrated ZOLOFT with placebo. Most patients received doses of 50 to 200 mg per day. The prescriber should be aware that these figures cannot be used to predict the incidence of side effects in the course of usual medical practice where patient characteristics and other factors differ from those which prevailed in the clinical trials. Similarly, the cited frequencies cannot be compared with figures obtained from other clinical investigations involving different treatments, uses, and investigators. The cited figures, however, do provide the prescribing physician with some basis for estimating the relative contribution of drug and non-drug factors to the side effect incidence rate in the population studied. [See table next page.]

Other Events Observed During the Premarketing Evaluation of ZOLOFT (sertraline hydrochloride): During its premarketing assessment, multiple doses of ZOLOFT were administered to approximately 2700 subjects. The conditions and duration of exposure to ZOLOFT varied greatly, and included (in overlapping categories) clinical pharmacology studies, open and double-blind studies, uncontrolled and controlled studies, inpatient and outpatient studies, fixed-dose and titration studies, and studies for indications other than depression. Untoward events associated with this exposure were recorded by clinical investigators using terminology of their own choosing. Consequently, it is not possible to provide a meaningful estimate of the proportion of individuals experiencing adverse events without first grouping similar types of untoward events into a smaller number of standardized event categories.

In the tabulations that follow, a World Health Organization dictionary of terminology has been used to classify reported adverse events. The frequencies presented, therefore, represent the proportion of the approximately 2700 individuals exposed to multiple doses of ZOLOFT who experienced an event of the type cited on at least one occasion while receiving ZOLOFT. All events are included except those already listed in the previous table and those reported in terms so general as to be uninformative. It is important to emphasize that although the events reported occurred during treatment with ZOLOFT, they were not necessarily caused by it. Events are further categorized by body system and listed in order of decreasing frequency according to the following definitions: frequent adverse events are those occurring on one or more occasions in at least 1/100 patients (only those not already listed in the tabulated results from placebo controlled trials appear in this listing); infrequent adverse events are those occurring in 1/100 to 1/1000 patients; rare events are those occurring in fewer than 1/1000 patients. Events of major clinical importance are also described in the PRECAUTIONS section.

Autonomic Nervous System Disorders—*Infrequent:* flushing, mydriasis, increased saliva, cold clammy skin; *Rare:* pallor.

Continued on next page

Pratt—Cont.

Treatment-Emergent Adverse Experience Incidence in Placebo-Controlled Clinical Trials*

Adverse Experience	(Percent of Patients Reporting)	
	Zoloft (N=861)	Placebo (N=853)
Autonomic Nervous System Disorders		
Mouth Dry	16.3	9.3
Sweating Increased	8.4	2.9
Cardiovascular		
Palpitations	3.5	1.6
Chest Pain	1.0	1.6
Centr. & Periph. Nerv. System Disorders		
Headache	20.3	19.0
Dizziness	11.7	6.7
Tremor	10.7	2.7
Paresthesia	2.0	1.8
Hypoesthesia	1.7	0.6
Twitching	1.4	0.1
Hypertonia	1.3	0.4
Disorders of Skin and Appendages		
Rash	2.1	1.5
Gastrointestinal Disorders		
Nausea	26.1	11.8
Diarrhea/Loose Stools	17.7	9.3
Constipation	8.4	6.3
Dyspepsia	6.0	2.8
Vomiting	3.8	1.8
Flatulence	3.3	2.5
Anorexia	2.8	1.6
Abdominal Pain	2.4	2.2
Appetite Increased	1.3	0.9
General		
Fatigue	10.6	8.1
Hot Flushes	2.2	0.5
Fever	1.6	0.6
Back Pain	1.5	0.9
Metabolic and Nutritional Disorders		
Thirst	1.4	0.9
Musculoskeletal System Disorders		
Myalgia	1.7	1.5
Psychiatric Disorders		
Insomnia	16.4	8.8
Sexual Dysfunction-Male (1)	15.5	2.2
Somnolence	13.4	5.9
Agitation	5.6	4.0
Nervousness	3.4	1.9
Anxiety	2.6	1.3
Yawning	1.9	0.2
Sexual Dysfunction-Female (2)	1.7	0.2
Concentration Impaired	1.3	0.5
Reproductive		
Menstrual Disorder (2)	1.0	0.5
Respiratory System Disorders		
Rhinitis	2.0	1.5
Pharyngitis	1.2	0.9
Special Senses		
Vision Abnormal	4.2	2.1
Tinnitus	1.4	1.1
Taste Perversion	1.2	0.7
Urinary System Disorders		
Micturition Frequency	2.0	1.2
Micturition Disorder	1.4	0.5

*Events reported by at least 1% of patients treated with ZOLOFT are included.

(1)—% based on male patients only: 271 ZOLOFT (primarily ejaculatory delay) and 271 placebo patients.

(2)—% based on female patients only: 590 ZOLOFT and 582 placebo patients.

Cardiovascular—*Infrequent:* postural dizziness, hypertension, hypotension, postural hypotension, edema, dependent edema, periorbital edema, peripheral edema, peripheral ischemia, syncope, tachycardia; *Rare:* precordial chest pain, substernal chest pain, aggravated hypertension, myocardial infarction, varicose veins.

Central and Peripheral Nervous System Disorders—*Frequent:* confusion; *Infrequent:* ataxia, abnormal coordination, abnormal gait, hyperesthesia, hyperkinesia, hypokinesia, migraine, nystagmus, vertigo; *Rare:* local anesthesia, coma, convulsions, dyskinesia, dysphonia, hyporeflexia, hypotonia, ptosis.

Disorders of Skin and Appendages—*Infrequent:* acne, alopecia, pruritus, erythematous rash, maculopapular rash, dry skin; *Rare:* bullous eruption, dermatitis, erythema multiforme, abnormal hair texture, hypertrichosis, photosensitivity reaction, follicular rash, skin discoloration, abnormal skin odor, urticaria.

Endocrine Disorders—*Rare:* exophthalmos, gynecomastia.

Gastrointestinal Disorders—*Infrequent:* dysphagia, eructation; *Rare:* diverticulitis, fecal incontinence, gastritis, gastroenteritis, glossitis, gum hyperplasia, hemorrhoids, hiccup, melena, hemorrhagic peptic ulcer, proctitis, stomatitis, ul-

cerative stomatitis, tenesmus, tongue edema, tongue ulceration.

General—*Frequent:* asthenia; *Infrequent:* malaise, generalized edema, rigors, weight decrease, weight increase; *Rare:* enlarged abdomen, halitosis, otitis media, aphthous stomatitis.

Hematopoietic and Lymphatic—*Infrequent:* lymphadenopathy, purpura; *Rare:* anemia, anterior chamber eye hemorrhage.

Metabolic and Nutritional Disorders—*Rare:* dehydration, hypercholesterolemia, hypoglycemia.

Musculoskeletal System Disorders—*Infrequent:* arthralgia, arthrosis, dystonia, muscle cramps, muscle weakness; *Rare:* hernia.

Psychiatric Disorders—*Infrequent:* abnormal dreams, aggressive reaction, amnesia, apathy, delusion, depersonalization, depression, aggravated depression, emotional lability, euphoria, hallucination, neurosis, paranoid reaction, suicide ideation and attempt, teeth-grinding, abnormal thinking; *Rare:* hysteria, somnambulism, withdrawal syndrome.

Reproductive—*Infrequent:* dysmenorrhea (2), intermenstrual bleeding (2); *Rare:* amenorrhea (2), balanoposthitis (1), breast enlargement (2), female breast pain (2), leukorrhea (2), menorrhagia (2), atrophic vaginitis (2).

(1)—% based on male subjects only: 1005.

(2)—% based on female subjects only: 1705.

Respiratory System Disorders—*Infrequent:* bronchospasm, coughing, dyspnea, epistaxis; *Rare:* bradypnea, hyperventilation, sinusitis, stridor.

Special Senses—*Infrequent:* abnormal accommodation, conjunctivitis, diplopia, earache, eye pain, xerophthalmia; *Rare:* abnormal lacrimation, photophobia, visual field defect.

Urinary System Disorders—*Infrequent:* dysuria, face edema, nocturia, polyuria, urinary incontinence; *Rare:* oliguria, renal pain, urinary retention.

Laboratory Tests—In man, asymptomatic elevations in serum transaminases (SGOT [or AST] and SGPT [or ALT]) have been reported infrequently (approximately 0.8%) in association with ZOLOFT administration. These hepatic enzyme elevations usually occurred within the first 1 to 9 weeks of drug treatment and promptly diminished upon drug discontinuation.

ZOLOFT therapy was associated with small mean increases in total cholesterol (approximately 3%) and triglycerides (approximately 5%), and a small mean decrease in serum uric acid (approximately 7%) of no apparent clinical importance.

DRUG ABUSE AND DEPENDENCE

Controlled Substance Class—ZOLOFT (sertraline hydrochloride) is not a controlled substance.

Physical and Psychological Dependence—ZOLOFT has not been systematically studied, in animals or humans, for its potential for abuse, tolerance, or physical dependence. However, the premarketing clinical experience with ZOLOFT did not reveal any tendency for a withdrawal syndrome or any drug-seeking behavior. As with any new CNS active drug, physicians should carefully evaluate patients for history of drug abuse and follow such patients closely, observing them for signs of ZOLOFT misuse or abuse (e.g., development of tolerance, incrementation of dose, drug-seeking behavior).

OVERDOSAGE

Human Experience—There have been 3 cases of ZOLOFT (sertraline hydrochloride) overdosage (approximately 750-2,100 mg). No specific therapy was required for any of the 3 patients, all of whom recovered completely.

Management of Overdoses—Establish and maintain an airway, insure adequate oxygenation and ventilation. Activated charcoal, which may be used with sorbitol, may be as or more effective than emesis or lavage, and should be considered in treating overdose.

Cardiac and vital signs monitoring is recommended along with general symptomatic and supportive measures.

There are no specific antidotes for ZOLOFT.

Due to the large volume of distribution of ZOLOFT, forced diuresis, dialysis, hemoperfusion, and exchange transfusion are unlikely to be of benefit.

In managing overdosage, consider the possibility of multiple drug involvement. The physician should consider contacting a poison control center on the treatment of any overdose.

DOSE AND ADMINISTRATION

Initial Treatment—ZOLOFT (sertraline hydrochloride) treatment should be initiated with a dose of 50 mg once daily. While a relationship between dose and antidepressant effect has not been established, patients were dosed in a range of 50–200 mg/day in the clinical trials demonstrating the antidepressant effectiveness of ZOLOFT. Consequently, patients not responding to a 50 mg dose may benefit from dose increases up to a maximum of 200 mg/day. Given the 24 hour elimination half-life of ZOLOFT, dose changes should not occur at intervals of less than 1 week.

ZOLOFT should be administered once daily, either in the morning or evening.

As indicated under Precautions, particular care should be used in patients with hepatic and/or renal impairment.

Maintenance/Continuation/Extended Treatment—There is evidence to suggest that depressed patients responding during an initial 8 week treatment phase will continue to benefit during an additional 8 weeks of treatment. While there are insufficient data regarding any benefits from treatment beyond 16 weeks, it is generally agreed among expert psychopharmacologists that acute episodes of depression require several months or longer of sustained pharmacological therapy. Whether the dose of antidepressant needed to induce remission is identical to the dose needed to maintain and/or sustain euthymia is unknown.

HOW SUPPLIED

ZOLOFT™ capsular-shaped scored tablets, containing sertraline hydrochloride equivalent to 50 and 100 mg of sertraline, are packaged in bottles.

ZOLOFT™ 50 mg Tablets: light blue film coated tablets engraved on the front with ZOLOFT and on the back scored and engraved with 50 mg.

NDC 0049-4900-50   Bottles of 50

ZOLOFT™ 100 mg Tablets: light yellow film coated tablets engraved on the front with ZOLOFT and on the back scored and engraved with 100 mg.

NDC 0049-4910-50   Bottles of 50

Store at controlled room temperature of 59°F to 86°F (15° to 30°C).

65-4721-00-0   Issued Jan. 1992

Shown in Product Identification Section, page 423

Princeton Pharmaceutical Products

A Bristol-Myers Squibb Company
P. O. BOX 4500
PRINCETON, NJ 08543-4500

BUSPAR®   ℞
[būspăr]
(buspirone HCl)

Tablets, 5 mg, bottles of 100	NSN 6505-01-253-2832 (M)
Tablets, 10 mg, bottles of 100	NSN 6505-01-267-3449 (M)

PRODUCT OVERVIEW

KEY FACTS

BuSpar® (buspirone hydrochloride) is an antianxiety agent that is neither chemically nor pharmacologically related to the benzodiazepines, barbiturates, or other sedative/anxiolytic drugs. BuSpar is less sedating than other anxiolytics. BuSpar has shown no potential for abuse or diversion and there is no evidence that it causes either physical or psychological dependence. BuSpar is not a controlled substance.

MAJOR USES

BuSpar is clinically effective for the management of anxiety disorders or the short-term relief of symptoms of anxiety, even in the presence of coexisting symptoms. The recommended initial dose is 5 mg three times a day, with divided doses of 20 to 30 mg per day commonly employed after titration in 5-mg increments.

SAFETY INFORMATION

BuSpar is contraindicated in patients hypersensitive to buspirone hydrochloride. It is recommended that BuSpar not be used concomitantly with a monoamine oxidase inhibitor. Because BuSpar will not block the withdrawal syndrome often seen with benzodiazepines and other common sedative/hypnotic drugs, it is advisable to withdraw such patients gradually from their prior treatment before starting BuSpar therapy.

PRESCRIBING INFORMATION

BUSPAR®   ℞
[būspăr]
(buspirone HCl)

DESCRIPTION

BuSpar® (buspirone hydrochloride) is an antianxiety agent that is not chemically or pharmacologically related to the benzodiazepines, barbiturates, or other sedative/anxiolytic drugs.

Buspirone hydrochloride is a white crystalline, water soluble compound with a molecular weight of 422.0. Chemically, buspirone hydrochloride is 8-[4-[4-(2-pyrimidinyl)-1-piperazinyl]butyl]-8-azaspiro[4.5]decane-7,9-dione monohydrochloride. The empirical formula $C_{21}H_{31}N_5O_2 \cdot HCl$ is represented by the following structural formula:

BuSpar is supplied for oral administration in 5 mg and 10 mg white, ovoid-rectangular, scored tablets. BuSpar tablets, 5

mg and 10 mg, contain the following inactive ingredients: colloidal silicon dioxide, lactose, magnesium stearate, microcrystalline cellulose, and sodium starch glycolate.

CLINICAL PHARMACOLOGY

The mechanism of action of buspirone is unknown. Buspirone differs from typical benzodiazepine anxiolytics in that it does not exert anticonvulsant or muscle relaxant effects. It also lacks the prominent sedative effect that is associated with more typical anxiolytics. *In vitro* preclinical studies have shown that buspirone has a high affinity for serotonin ($5\text{-}HT_{1A}$) receptors. Buspirone has no significant affinity for benzodiazepine receptors and does not affect GABA binding *in vitro* or *in vivo* when tested in preclinical models.

Buspirone has moderate affinity for brain D_2-dopamine receptors. Some studies do suggest that buspirone may have indirect effects on other neurotransmitter systems.

BuSpar is rapidly absorbed in man and undergoes extensive first pass metabolism. In a radiolabeled study, unchanged buspirone in the plasma accounted for only about 1% of the radioactivity in the plasma. Following oral administration, plasma concentrations of unchanged buspirone are very low and variable between subjects. Peak plasma levels of 1 to 6 ng/mL have been observed 40 to 90 minutes after single oral doses of 20 mg. The single-dose bioavailability of unchanged buspirone when taken as a tablet is on the average about 90% of an equivalent dose of solution, but there is large variability.

The effects of food upon the bioavailability of BuSpar have been studied in eight subjects. They were given a 20-mg dose with and without food; the area under the plasma concentration-time curve (AUC) and peak plasma concentration (Cmax) of unchanged buspirone increased by 84% and 116% respectively, but the total amount of buspirone immunoreactive material did not change. This suggests that food may decrease the extent of presystemic clearance of buspirone, but the clinical significance of these findings is unknown.

A multiple-dose study conducted in 15 subjects suggests that buspirone has nonlinear pharmacokinetics. Thus, dose increases and repeated dosing may lead to somewhat higher blood levels of unchanged buspirone than would be predicted from results of single-dose studies.

In man, approximately 95% of buspirone is plasma protein bound, but other highly bound drugs, eg, phenytoin, propranolol, and warfarin are not displaced by buspirone from plasma protein *in vitro*. However, *in vitro* binding studies show that buspirone does displace digoxin.

Buspirone is metabolized primarily by oxidation producing several hydroxylated derivatives and a pharmacologically active metabolite, 1-pyrimidinylpiperazine (1-PP). In animal models predictive of anxiolytic potential, 1-PP has about one quarter of the activity of buspirone, but is present in up to 20-fold greater amounts. However, this is probably not important in humans: blood samples from humans chronically exposed to BuSpar do not exhibit high levels of 1-PP; mean values are approximately 3 ng/mL and the highest human blood level recorded among 108 chronically dosed patients was 17 ng/mL, less than 1/200th of 1-PP levels found in animals given large doses of buspirone without signs of toxicity.

In a single-dose study using 14C-labeled buspirone, 29% to 63% of the dose was excreted in the urine within 24 hours, primarily as metabolites; fecal excretion accounted for 18 to 38% of the dose. The average elimination half-life of unchanged buspirone after single doses of 10 to 40 mg is about 2 to 3 hours.

The pharmacokinetics of BuSpar in patients with hepatic or renal dysfunction has not been determined, nor has the effect of age. The effect of BuSpar on drug metabolism or concomitant drug disposition has not been investigated.

INDICATIONS AND USAGE

BuSpar is indicated for the management of anxiety disorders or the short-term relief of the symptoms of anxiety. Anxiety or tension associated with the stress of everyday life usually does not require treatment with an anxiolytic.

The efficacy of BuSpar has been demonstrated in controlled clinical trials of outpatients whose diagnosis roughly corresponds to Generalized Anxiety Disorder (GAD). Many of the patients enrolled in these studies also had coexisting depressive symptoms and BuSpar relieved anxiety in the presence of these coexisting depressive symptoms. The patients evaluated in these studies had experienced symptoms for periods of 1 month to over 1 year prior to the study, with an average symptom duration of 6 months. Generalized Anxiety Disorder (300.02) is described in the American Psychiatric Association's Diagnostic and Statistical Manual, III[1] as follows: Generalized, persistent anxiety (of at least 1 month continual duration), manifested by symptoms from three of the four following categories:

1. Motor tension: shakiness, jitteriness, jumpiness, trembling, tension, muscle aches, fatigability, inability to relax, eyelid twitch, furrowed brow, strained face, fidgeting, restlessness, easy startle.
2. Autonomic hyperactivity: sweating, heart pounding or racing, cold, clammy hands, dry mouth, dizziness, lightheadedness, paresthesias (tingling in hands or feet), upset stomach, hot or cold spells, frequent urination, diarrhea, discomfort in the pit of the stomach, lump in the throat, flushing, pallor, high resting pulse, and respiration rate.
3. Apprehensive expectation: anxiety, worry, fear, rumination, and anticipation of misfortune to self or others.
4. Vigilance and scanning: hyperattentiveness resulting in distractibility, difficulty in concentrating, insomnia, feeling "on edge," irritability, impatience.

The above symptoms would not be due to another mental disorder, such as a depressive disorder or schizophrenia. However, mild depressive symptoms are common in GAD. The effectiveness of BuSpar in long-term use, that is, for more than 3 to 4 weeks, has not been demonstrated in controlled trials. There is no body of evidence available that systematically addresses the appropriate duration of treatment for GAD. However, in a study of long-term use, 264 patients were treated with BuSpar for 1 year without ill effect. Therefore, the physician who elects to use BuSpar for extended periods should periodically reassess the usefulness of the drug for the individual patient.

CONTRAINDICATIONS

BuSpar is contraindicated in patients hypersensitive to buspirone hydrochloride.

WARNINGS

The administration of BuSpar to a patient taking a monoamine oxidase inhibitor (MAOI) may pose a hazard. There have been reports of the occurrence of elevated blood pressure when BuSpar has been added to a regimen including an MAOI. Therefore, it is recommended that BuSpar not be used concomitantly with an MAOI.

Because BuSpar has no established antipsychotic activity, it should not be employed in lieu of appropriate antipsychotic treatment.

PRECAUTIONS

General:

Interference with cognitive and motor performance:
Studies indicate that BuSpar is less sedating than other anxiolytics and that it does not produce significant functional impairment. However, its CNS effects in any individual patient may not be predictable. Therefore, patients should be cautioned about operating an automobile or using complex machinery until they are reasonably certain that buspirone treatment does not affect them adversely.

While formal studies of the interaction of BuSpar with alcohol indicate that buspirone does not increase alcohol-induced impairment in motor and mental performance, it is prudent to avoid concomitant use of alcohol and buspirone.

Potential for withdrawal reactions in sedative/hypnotic/anxiolytic drug-dependent patients:
Because BuSpar does not exhibit cross-tolerance with benzodiazepines and other common sedative/hypnotic drugs, it will not block the withdrawal syndrome often seen with cessation of therapy with these drugs. Therefore, before starting therapy with BuSpar, it is advisable to withdraw patients gradually, especially patients who have been using a CNS-depressant drug chronically, from their prior treatment. Rebound or withdrawal symptoms may occur over varying time periods, depending in part on the type of drug, and its effective half-life of elimination.

The syndrome of withdrawal from sedative/hypnotic/anxiolytic drugs can appear as any combination of irritability, anxiety, agitation, insomnia, tremor, abdominal cramps, muscle cramps, vomiting, sweating, flu-like symptoms without fever, and occasionally, even as seizures.

Possible concerns related to buspirone's binding to dopamine receptors:
Because buspirone can bind to central dopamine receptors, a question has been raised about its potential to cause acute and chronic changes in dopamine-mediated neurological function (eg, dystonia, pseudoparkinsonism, akathisia, and tardive dyskinesia). Clinical experience in controlled trials has failed to identify any significant neuroleptic-like activity; however, a syndrome of restlessness, appearing shortly after initiation of treatment, has been reported in some small fraction of buspirone-treated patients. The syndrome may be explained in several ways. For example, buspirone may increase central noradrenergic activity; alternatively, the effect may be attributable to dopaminergic effects (ie, represent akathisia). Obviously, the question cannot be totally resolved at this point in time. Generally, long-term sequelae of any drug's use can be identified only after several years of marketing.

Information for Patients:
To assure safe and effective use of BuSpar, the following information and instructions should be given to patients:

1. Inform your physician about any medications, prescription or nonprescription, alcohol, or drugs that you are now taking or plan to take during your treatment with BuSpar.
2. Inform your physician if you are pregnant, or if you are planning to become pregnant, or if you become pregnant while you are taking BuSpar.
3. Inform your physician if you are breastfeeding an infant.
4. Until you experience how this medication affects you, do not drive a car or operate potentially dangerous machinery.

Laboratory Tests:
There are no specific laboratory tests recommended.

Drug Interactions:
Because the effects of concomitant administration of BuSpar with most other psychotropic drugs have not been studied, the concomitant use of BuSpar with other CNS-active drugs should be approached with caution (see WARNINGS).

There is one report suggesting that the concomitant use of Desyrel® (trazodone hydrochloride) and BuSpar may have caused 3- to 6-fold elevations on SGPT (ALT) in a few patients. In a similar study, attempting to replicate this finding, no interactive effect on hepatic transaminases was identified.

In a study in normal volunteers, concomitant administration of BuSpar and haloperidol resulted in increased serum haloperidol concentrations. The clinical significance of this finding is not clear.

In vitro, buspirone does not displace tightly bound drugs like phenytoin, propranolol, and warfarin from serum proteins. However, there has been one report of prolonged prothrombin time when buspirone was added to the regimen of a patient treated with warfarin. The patient was also chronically receiving phenytoin, phenobarbital, digoxin, and Synthroid. *In vitro*, buspirone may displace less firmly bound drugs like digoxin. The clinical significance of this property is unknown.

Drug/Laboratory Test Interactions:
Buspirone is not known to interfere with commonly employed clinical laboratory tests.

Carcinogenesis, Mutagenesis, Impairment of Fertility:
No evidence of carcinogenic potential was observed in rats during a 24-month study at approximately 133 times the maximum recommended human oral dose; or in mice, during an 18-month study at approximately 167 times the maximum recommended human oral dose.

With or without metabolic activation, buspirone did not induce point mutations in five strains of *Salmonella typhimurium* (Ames Test) or mouse lymphoma L5178YTK⁺ cell cultures, nor was DNA damage observed with buspirone in Wi-38 human cells. Chromosomal aberrations or abnormalities did not occur in bone marrow cells of mice given one or five daily doses of buspirone.

Pregnancy: Teratogenic effects:
Pregnancy Category B: No fertility impairment or fetal damage was observed in reproduction studies performed in rats and rabbits at buspirone doses of approximately 30 times the maximum recommended human dose. In humans, however, adequate and well-controlled studies during pregnancy have *not* been performed. Because animal reproduction studies are not always predictive of human response, this drug should be used during pregnancy only if clearly needed.

Labor and Delivery:
The effect of BuSpar on labor and delivery in women is unknown. No adverse effects were noted in reproduction studies in rats.

Nursing Mothers:
The extent of the excretion in human milk of buspirone or its metabolites is not known. In rats, however, buspirone and its metabolites are excreted in milk. BuSpar administration to nursing women should be avoided if clinically possible.

Pediatric Use:
The safety and effectiveness of BuSpar have not been determined in individuals below 18 years of age.

Use in the Elderly:
BuSpar has not been systematically evaluated in older patients; however, several hundred elderly patients have participated in clinical studies with BuSpar and no unusual adverse age-related phenomena have been identified. In 87 elderly patients for whom dosage data were available, the modal total daily dose of BuSpar was 15 mg per day, the same as that in the total sample of patients treated with BuSpar.

Use in Patients with Impaired Hepatic or Renal Function:
Since BuSpar is metabolized by the liver and excreted by the kidneys, its administration to patients with severe hepatic or renal impairment cannot be recommended.

ADVERSE REACTIONS (See also PRECAUTIONS)

Commonly Observed:
The more commonly observed untoward events associated with the use of BuSpar not seen at an equivalent incidence among placebo-treated patients include dizziness, nausea, headache, nervousness, lightheadedness, and excitement.

Associated with Discontinuation of Treatment:
One guide to the relative clinical importance of adverse events associated with BuSpar is provided by the frequency with which they caused drug discontinuation during clinical testing. Approximately 10% of the 2200 anxious patients who participated in the BuSpar premarketing clinical efficacy trials in anxiety disorders lasting 3 to 4 weeks discontin-

Continued on next page

Princeton—Cont.

ued treatment due to an adverse event. The more common events causing discontinuation included: central nervous system disturbances (3.4%), primarily dizziness, insomnia, nervousness, drowsiness and lightheaded feeling; gastrointestinal disturbances (1.2%), primarily nausea; and miscellaneous disturbances (1.1%), primarily headache and fatigue. In addition, 3.4% of patients had multiple complaints, none of which could be characterized as primary.

Incidence in Controlled Clinical Trials:
The table that follows enumerates adverse events that occurred at a frequency of 1% or more among BuSpar patients who participated in 4-week, controlled trials comparing BuSpar with placebo. The frequencies were obtained from pooled data for 17 trials. The prescriber should be aware that these figures cannot be used to predict the incidence of side effects in the course of usual medical practice where patient characteristics and other factors differ from those which prevailed in the clinical trials. Similarly, the cited frequencies cannot be compared with figures obtained from other clinical investigations involving different treatments, uses, and investigators. Comparison of the cited figures, however, does provide the prescribing physician with some basis for estimating the relative contribution of drug and nondrug factors to the side-effect incidence rate in the population studied.

TREATMENT-EMERGENT ADVERSE EXPERIENCE INCIDENCE IN PLACEBO-CONTROLLED CLINICAL TRIALS*
(Percent of Patients Reporting)

Adverse Experience	BuSpar (n=477)	Placebo (n=464)
Cardiovascular		
Tachycardia/Palpitations	1	1
CNS		
Dizziness	12	3
Drowsiness	10	9
Nervousness	5	1
Insomnia	3	3
Lightheadedness	3	—
Decreased Concentration	2	2
Excitement	2	—
Anger/Hostility	2	—
Confusion	2	—
Depression	2	2
EENT		
Blurred Vision	2	—
Gastrointestinal		
Nausea	8	5
Dry Mouth	3	4
Abdominal/Gastric Distress	2	2
Diarrhea	2	—
Constipation	1	2
Vomiting	1	2
Musculoskeletal		
Musculoskeletal Aches/Pains	1	—
Neurological		
Numbness	2	—
Paresthesia	1	—
Incoordination	1	—
Tremor	1	—
Skin		
Skin Rash	1	—
Miscellaneous		
Headache	6	3
Fatigue	4	4
Weakness	2	—
Sweating/Clamminess	1	—

* Events reported by at least 1% of BuSpar patients are included.
—Incidence less than 1%.

Other Events Observed During the Entire Premarketing Evaluation of BuSpar:
During its premarketing assessment, BuSpar was evaluated in over 3500 subjects. This section reports event frequencies for adverse events occurring in approximately 3000 subjects from this group who took multiple doses of BuSpar in the dose range for which BuSpar is being recommended (ie, the modal daily dose of BuSpar fell between 10 and 30 mg for 70% of the patients studied) and for whom safety data were systematically collected. The conditions and duration of exposure to BuSpar varied greatly, involving well-controlled studies as well as experience in open and uncontrolled clinical settings. As part of the total experience gained in clinical studies, various adverse events were reported. In the absence of appropriate controls in some of the studies, a causal relationship to BuSpar treatment cannot be determined. The list includes all undesirable events reasonably associated with the use of the drug.
The following enumeration by organ system describes events in terms of their relative frequency of reporting in this data base. Events of major clinical importance are also described in the PRECAUTIONS section.

The following definitions of frequency are used: Frequent adverse events are defined as those occurring in at least 1/100 patients. Infrequent adverse events are those occurring in 1/100 to 1/1000 patients, while rare events are those occurring in less than 1/1000 patients.

Cardiovascular:
Frequent was nonspecific chest pain; infrequent were syncope, hypotension and hypertension; rare were cerebrovascular accident, congestive heart failure, myocardial infarction, cardiomyopathy and bradycardia.

Central Nervous System:
Frequent were dream disturbances; infrequent were depersonalization, dysphoria, noise intolerance, euphoria, akathisia, fearfulness, loss of interest, dissociative reaction, hallucinations, suicidal ideation and seizures; rare were feelings of claustrophobia, cold intolerance, stupor, and slurred speech and psychosis.

EENT:
Frequent were tinnitus, sore throat, and nasal congestion. Infrequent were redness and itching of the eyes, altered taste, altered smell, and conjunctivitis; rare were inner ear abnormality, eye pain, photophobia, and pressure on eyes.

Endocrine:
Rare were galactorrhea and thyroid abnormality.

Gastrointestinal:
Infrequent were flatulence, anorexia, increased appetite, salivation, irritable colon and rectal bleeding; rare was burning of the tongue.

Genitourinary:
Infrequent were urinary frequency, urinary hesitancy, menstrual irregularity and spotting, and dysuria; rare were amenorrhea, pelvic inflammatory disease, enuresis, and nocturia.

Musculoskeletal:
Infrequent were muscle cramps, muscle spasms, rigid/stiff muscles, and arthralgias.

Neurological:
Infrequent were involuntary movements and slowed reaction time; rare was muscle weakness.

Respiratory:
Infrequent were hyperventilation, shortness of breath, and chest congestion; rare was epistaxis.

Sexual Function:
Infrequent were decreased or increased libido; rare were delayed ejaculation and impotence.

Skin:
Infrequent were edema, pruritus, flushing, easy bruising, hair loss, dry skin, facial edema and blisters; rare were acne and thinning of nails.

Clinical Laboratory:
Infrequent were increases in hepatic aminotransferases (SGOT, SGPT); rare were eosinophilia, leukopenia, and thrombocytopenia.

Miscellaneous:
Infrequent were weight gain, fever, roaring sensation in the head, weight loss, and malaise; rare were alcohol abuse, bleeding disturbance, loss of voice, and hiccoughs.

POSTINTRODUCTION CLINICAL EXPERIENCE
Postmarketing experience has shown an adverse experience profile similar to that given above. Voluntary reports since introduction have included rare occurrences of allergic reactions, cogwheel rigidity, dystonic reactions, ecchymosis, emotional lability, tunnel vision, and urinary retention. Because of the uncontrolled nature of these spontaneous reports, a causal relationship to BuSpar treatment has not been determined.

DRUG ABUSE AND DEPENDENCE
Controlled Substance Class:
BuSpar is not a controlled substance.
Physical and Psychological Dependence:
In human and animal studies, buspirone has shown no potential for abuse or diversion and there is no evidence that it causes tolerance, or either physical or psychological dependence. Human volunteers with a history of recreational drug or alcohol usage were studied in two double-blind clinical investigations. None of the subjects were able to distinguish between BuSpar and placebo. By contrast, subjects showed a statistically significant preference for methaqualone and diazepam. Studies in monkeys, mice, and rats have indicated that buspirone lacks potential for abuse.
Following chronic administration in the rat, abrupt withdrawal of buspirone did not result in the loss of body weight commonly observed with substances that cause physical dependency.
Although there is no direct evidence that BuSpar causes physical dependence or drug-seeking behavior, it is difficult to predict from experiments the extent to which a CNS-active drug will be misused, diverted, and/or abused once marketed. Consequently, physicians should carefully evaluate patients for a history of drug abuse and follow such patients closely, observing them for signs of BuSpar misuse or abuse (eg, development of tolerance, incrementation of dose, drug-seeking behavior).

OVERDOSAGE
Signs and Symptoms:
In clinical pharmacology trials, doses as high as 375 mg/day were administered to healthy male volunteers. As this dose was approached, the following symptoms were observed: nausea, vomiting, dizziness, drowsiness, miosis, and gastric distress. No deaths have been reported in humans either with deliberate or accidental overdosage of BuSpar. Toxicology studies of buspirone yielded the following LD_{50} values: mice, 655 mg/kg; rats, 196 mg/kg; dogs, 586 mg/kg; and monkeys, 356 mg/kg. These dosages are 160–550 times the recommended human daily dose.
Recommended Overdose Treatment:
General symptomatic and supportive measures should be used along with immediate gastric lavage. Respiration, pulse, and blood pressure should be monitored as in all cases of drug overdosage. No specific antidote is known to buspirone, and dialyzability of buspirone has not been determined.

DOSAGE AND ADMINISTRATION
The recommended initial dose is 15 mg daily (5 mg three times a day). To achieve an optimal therapeutic response, at intervals of 2 to 3 days the dosage may be increased 5 mg per day, as needed. The maximum daily dosage should not exceed 60 mg per day. In clinical trials allowing dose titration, divided doses of 20 to 30 mg per day were commonly employed.

HOW SUPPLIED
BuSpar® (buspirone hydrochloride)
Tablets, 5 mg and 10 mg (white, ovoid-rectangular with score, MJ logo, strength, and the name BuSpar embossed) are available in bottles of 100 and 500, and in cartons containing 100 individually packaged tablets.

NDC 0087-0818-41 5 mg tablet	Bottles of 100
NDC 0087-0818-44 5 mg tablet	Bottles of 500
NDC 0087-0818-43 5 mg tablet	Cartons of 100 unit dose
NDC 0087-0819-41 10 mg tablet	Bottles of 100
NDC 0087-0819-44 10 mg tablet	Bottles of 500
NDC 0087-0819-43 10 mg tablet	Cartons of 100 unit dose

U.S. Patent No. 4,182,763
Store at room temperature. Protect from temperatures greater than 86° F (30° C). Dispense in a tight, light-resistant container (USP).

REFERENCE
1. American Psychiatric Association, Ed.: Diagnostic and Statistical Manual of Mental Disorders—III, American Psychiatric Association, May 1980.
Shown in Product Identification Section, page 423

CAPOTEN® TABLETS   ℞
[kap 'o-ten ″]
Captopril Tablets

> **USE IN PREGNANCY**
> When used in pregnancy during the second and third trimesters, ACE inhibitors can cause injury and even death to the developing fetus. When pregnancy is detected, CAPOTEN should be discontinued as soon as possible. See WARNINGS: Fetal/Neonatal Morbidity and Mortality.

DESCRIPTION
CAPOTEN (captopril) is the first of a new class of antihypertensive agents, a specific competitive inhibitor of angiotensin I-converting enzyme (ACE), the enzyme responsible for the conversion of angiotensin I to angiotensin II. Captopril is also effective in the management of heart failure.
CAPOTEN (captopril) is designated chemically as 1-[(2S)-3-mercapto-2-methylpropionyl]-L-proline [MW 217.29].
Captopril is a white to off-white crystalline powder that may have a slight sulfurous odor; it is soluble in water (approx. 160 mg/mL), methanol, and ethanol and sparingly soluble in chloroform and ethyl acetate.
CAPOTEN (captopril) is available in potencies of 12.5 mg, 25 mg, 50 mg, and 100 mg as scored tablets for oral administration. Inactive ingredients: microcrystalline cellulose, corn starch, lactose, and stearic acid.

CLINICAL PHARMACOLOGY
Mechanism of Action
The mechanism of action of CAPOTEN (captopril) has not yet been fully elucidated. Its beneficial effects in hypertension and heart failure appear to result primarily from suppression of the renin-angiotensin-aldosterone system. How-

ever, there is no consistent correlation between renin levels and response to the drug. Renin, an enzyme synthesized by the kidneys, is released into the circulation where it acts on a plasma globulin substrate to produce angiotensin I, a relatively inactive decapeptide. Angiotensin I is then converted by angiotensin converting enzyme (ACE) to angiotensin II, a potent endogenous vasoconstrictor substance. Angiotensin II also stimulates aldosterone secretion from the adrenal cortex, thereby contributing to sodium and fluid retention.

CAPOTEN (captopril) prevents the conversion of angiotensin I to angiotensin II by inhibition of ACE, a peptidyldipeptide carboxy hydrolase. This inhibition has been demonstrated in both healthy human subjects and in animals by showing that the elevation of blood pressure caused by exogenously administered angiotensin I was attenuated or abolished by captopril. In animal studies, captopril did not alter the pressor responses to a number of other agents, including angiotensin II and norepinephrine, indicating specificity of action.

ACE is identical to "bradykininase", and CAPOTEN (captopril) may also interfere with the degradation of the vasodepressor peptide, bradykinin. Increased concentrations of bradykinin or prostaglandin E_2 may also have a role in the therapeutic effect of CAPOTEN.

Inhibition of ACE results in decreased plasma angiotensin II and increased plasma renin activity (PRA), the latter resulting from loss of negative feedback on renin release caused by reduction in angiotensin II. The reduction of angiotensin II leads to decreased aldosterone secretion, and, as a result, small increases in serum potassium may occur along with sodium and fluid loss.

The antihypertensive effects persist for a longer period of time than does demonstrable inhibition of circulating ACE. It is not known whether the ACE present in vascular endothelium is inhibited longer than the ACE in circulating blood.

Pharmacokinetics

After oral administration of therapeutic doses of CAPOTEN (captopril), rapid absorption occurs with peak blood levels at about one hour. The presence of food in the gastrointestinal tract reduces absorption by about 30 to 40 percent; captopril therefore should be given one hour before meals. Based on carbon-14 labeling, average minimal absorption is approximately 75 percent. In a 24-hour period, over 95 percent of the absorbed dose is eliminated in the urine; 40 to 50 percent is unchanged drug; most of the remainder is the disulfide dimer of captopril and captopril-cysteine disulfide.

Approximately 25 to 30 percent of the circulating drug is bound to plasma proteins. The apparent elimination half-life for total radioactivity in blood is probably less than 3 hours. An accurate determination of half-life of unchanged captopril is not, at present, possible, but it is probably less than 2 hours. In patients with renal impairment, however, retention of captopril occurs (see DOSAGE AND ADMINISTRATION).

Pharmacodynamics

Administration of CAPOTEN (captopril) results in a reduction of peripheral arterial resistance in hypertensive patients with either no change, or an increase, in cardiac output. There is an increase in renal blood flow following administration of CAPOTEN (captopril) and glomerular filtration rate is usually unchanged.

Reductions of blood pressure are usually maximal 60 to 90 minutes after oral administration of an individual dose of CAPOTEN (captopril). The duration of effect is dose related. The reduction in blood pressure may be progressive, so to achieve maximal therapeutic effects, several weeks of therapy may be required. The blood pressure lowering effects of captopril and thiazide-type diuretics are additive. In contrast, captopril and beta-blockers have a less than additive effect.

Blood pressure is lowered to about the same extent in both standing and supine positions. Orthostatic effects and tachycardia are infrequent but may occur in volume-depleted patients. Abrupt withdrawal of CAPOTEN has not been associated with a rapid increase in blood pressure.

In patients with heart failure, significantly decreased peripheral (systemic vascular) resistance and blood pressure (afterload), reduced pulmonary capillary wedge pressure (preload) and pulmonary vascular resistance, increased cardiac output, and increased exercise tolerance time (ETT) have been demonstrated. These hemodynamic and clinical effects occur after the first dose and appear to persist for the duration of therapy. Placebo controlled studies of 12 weeks duration in patients who did not respond adequately to diuretics and digitalis show no tolerance to beneficial effects on ETT; open studies, with exposure up to 18 months in some cases, also indicate that ETT benefit is maintained. Clinical improvement has been observed in some patients where acute hemodynamic effects were minimal.

Studies in rats and cats indicate that CAPOTEN (captopril) does not cross the blood-brain barrier to any significant extent.

INDICATIONS AND USAGE

Hypertension: CAPOTEN (captopril) is indicated for the treatment of hypertension.

In using CAPOTEN, consideration should be given to the risk of neutropenia/agranulocytosis (see WARNINGS).

CAPOTEN may be used as initial therapy for patients with normal renal function, in whom the risk is relatively low. In patients with impaired renal function, particularly those with collagen vascular disease, captopril should be reserved for hypertensives who have either developed unacceptable side effects on other drugs, or have failed to respond satisfactorily to drug combinations.

CAPOTEN is effective alone and in combination with other antihypertensive agents, especially thiazide-type diuretics. The blood pressure lowering effects of captopril and thiazides are approximately additive.

Heart Failure: CAPOTEN is indicated in the treatment of congestive heart failure in patients who have not responded adequately to treatment with diuretics and digitalis. Although the beneficial effect of captopril in heart failure does not require the presence of digitalis, most controlled clinical trial experience with captopril has been in patients receiving digitalis, as well as diuretic treatment. Consequently, CAPOTEN should generally be added to both of these agents except when digitalis use is poorly tolerated or otherwise not feasible.

CONTRAINDICATIONS

CAPOTEN is contraindicated in patients who are hypersensitive to this product or any other angiotensin-converting enzyme inhibitor (e.g., a patient who has experienced angioedema during therapy with any other ACE inhibitor).

WARNINGS

Angioedema

Angioedema involving the extremities, face, lips, mucous membranes, tongue, glottis or larynx has been seen in patients treated with ACE inhibitors, including captopril. If angioedema involves the tongue, glottis or larynx, airway obstruction may occur and be fatal. Emergency therapy, including but not necessarily limited to, subcutaneous administration of a 1:1000 solution of epinephrine should be promptly instituted.

Swelling confined to the face, mucous membranes of the mouth, lips and extremities has usually resolved with discontinuation of captopril; some cases required medical therapy. (See PRECAUTIONS: Information for Patients and ADVERSE REACTIONS.)

Neutropenia/Agranulocytosis

Neutropenia ($<1000/mm^3$) with myeloid hypoplasia has resulted from use of captopril. About half of the neutropenic patients developed systemic or oral cavity infections or other features of the syndrome of agranulocytosis.

The risk of neutropenia is dependent on the clinical status of the patient:

In clinical trials in patients with hypertension who have normal renal function (serum creatinine less than 1.6 mg/dL and no collagen vascular disease), neutropenia has been seen in one patient out of over 8,600 exposed.

In patients with some degree of renal failure (serum creatinine at least 1.6 mg/dL) but no collagen vascular disease, the risk of neutropenia in clinical trials was about 1 per 500, a frequency over 15 times that for uncomplicated hypertension. Daily doses of captopril were relatively high in these patients, particularly in view of their diminished renal function. In foreign marketing experience in patients with renal failure, use of allopurinol concomitantly with captopril has been associated with neutropenia but this association has not appeared in U.S. reports.

In patients with collagen vascular diseases (e.g., systemic lupus erythematosus, scleroderma) and impaired renal function, neutropenia occurred in 3.7 percent of patients in clinical trials.

While none of the over 750 patients in formal clinical trials of heart failure developed neutropenia, it has occurred during the subsequent clinical experience. About half of the reported cases had serum creatinine $\geq$ 1.6 mg/dL and more than 75 percent were in patients also receiving procainamide. In heart failure, it appears that the same risk factors for neutropenia are present.

The neutropenia has usually been detected within three months after captopril was started. Bone marrow examinations in patients with neutropenia consistently showed myeloid hypoplasia, frequently accompanied by erythroid hypoplasia and decreased numbers of megakaryocytes (e.g., hypoplastic bone marrow and pancytopenia); anemia and thrombocytopenia were sometimes seen.

In general, neutrophils returned to normal in about two weeks after captopril was discontinued, and serious infections were limited to clinically complex patients. About 13 percent of the cases of neutropenia have ended fatally, but almost all fatalities were in patients with serious illness, having collagen vascular disease, renal failure, heart failure

or immunosuppressant therapy, or a combination of these complicating factors.

Evaluation of the hypertensive or heart failure patient should always include assessment of renal function.

If captopril is used in patients with impaired renal function, white blood cell and differential counts should be evaluated prior to starting treatment and at approximately two-week intervals for about three months, then periodically.

In patients with collagen vascular disease or who are exposed to other drugs known to affect the white cells or immune response, particularly when there is impaired renal function, captopril should be used only after an assessment of benefit and risk, and then with caution.

All patients treated with captopril should be told to report any signs of infection (e.g., sore throat, fever). If infection is suspected, white cell counts should be performed without delay.

Since discontinuation of captopril and other drugs has generally led to prompt return of the white count to normal, upon confirmation of neutropenia (neutrophil count $< 1000/mm^3$) the physician should withdraw captopril and closely follow the patient's course.

Proteinuria

Total urinary proteins greater than 1 g per day were seen in about 0.7 percent of patients receiving captopril. About 90 percent of affected patients had evidence of prior renal disease or received relatively high doses of captopril (in excess of 150 mg/day), or both. The nephrotic syndrome occurred in about one-fifth of proteinuric patients. In most cases, proteinuria subsided or cleared within six months whether or not captopril was continued. Parameters of renal function, such as BUN and creatinine, were seldom altered in the patients with proteinuria.

Since most cases of proteinuria occurred by the eighth month of therapy with captopril, patients with prior renal disease or those receiving captopril at doses greater than 150 mg per day, should have urinary protein estimations (dipstick on first morning urine) prior to treatment, and periodically thereafter.

Hypotension

Excessive hypotension was rarely seen in hypertensive patients but is a possible consequence of captopril use in salt/volume depleted persons (such as those treated vigorously with diuretics), patients with heart failure or those patients undergoing renal dialysis. (See PRECAUTIONS: Drug Interactions.)

In heart failure, where the blood pressure was either normal or low, transient decreases in mean blood pressure greater than 20 percent were recorded in about half of the patients. This transient hypotension is more likely to occur after any of the first several doses and is usually well tolerated, producing either no symptoms or brief mild lightheadedness, although in rare instances it has been associated with arrhythmia or conduction defects. Hypotension was the reason for discontinuation of drug in 3.6 percent of patients with heart failure.

BECAUSE OF THE POTENTIAL FALL IN BLOOD PRESSURE IN THESE PATIENTS, THERAPY SHOULD BE STARTED UNDER VERY CLOSE MEDICAL SUPERVISION. A starting dose of 6.25 or 12.5 mg tid may minimize the hypotensive effect. Patients should be followed closely for the first two weeks of treatment and whenever the dose of captopril and/or diuretic is increased.

Hypotension is not *per se* a reason to discontinue captopril. Some decrease of systemic blood pressure is a common and desirable observation upon initiation of CAPOTEN (captopril) treatment in heart failure. The magnitude of the decrease is greatest early in the course of treatment; this effect stabilizes within a week or two, and generally returns to pretreatment levels, without a decrease in therapeutic efficacy, within two months.

Fetal/Neonatal Morbidity and Mortality

ACE inhibitors can cause fetal and neonatal morbidity and death when administered to pregnant women. Several dozen cases have been reported in the world literature. When pregnancy is detected, ACE inhibitors should be discontinued as soon as possible.

The use of ACE inhibitors during the second and third trimesters of pregnancy has been associated with fetal and neonatal injury, including hypotension, neonatal skull hypoplasia, anuria, reversible or irreversible renal failure, and death. Oligohydramnios has also been reported, presumably resulting from decreased fetal renal function; oligohydramnios in this setting has been associated with fetal limb contractures, craniofacial deformation, and hypoplastic lung development. Prematurity, intrauterine growth retardation, and patent ductus arteriosus have also been reported, although it is not clear whether these occurrences were due to the ACE-inhibitor exposure.

These adverse effects do not appear to have resulted from intrauterine ACE-inhibitor exposure that has been limited to the first trimester. Mothers whose embryos and fetuses are exposed to ACE inhibitors only during the first trimester

Continued on next page

Princeton—Cont.

should be so informed. Nonetheless, when patients become pregnant, physicians should make every effort to discontinue the use of captopril as soon as possible.

Rarely (probably less often than once in every thousand pregnancies), no alternative to ACE inhibitors will be found. In these rare cases, the mothers should be apprised of the potential hazards to their fetuses, and serial ultrasound examinations should be performed to assess the intraamniotic environment.

If oligohydramnios is observed, captopril should be discontinued unless it is considered life-saving for the mother. Contraction stress testing (CST), a non-stress test (NST), or biophysical profiling (BPP) may be appropriate, depending upon the week of pregnancy. Patients and physicians should be aware, however, that oligohydramnios may not appear until after the fetus has sustained irreversible injury.

Infants with histories of *in utero* exposure to ACE inhibitors should be closely observed for hypotension, oliguria, and hyperkalemia. If oliguria occurs, attention should be directed toward support of blood pressure and renal perfusion. Exchange transfusion or dialysis may be required as a means of reversing hypotension and/or substituting for disordered renal function. While captopril may be removed from the adult circulation by hemodialysis, there is inadequate data concerning the effectiveness of hemodialysis for removing it from the circulation of neonates or children. Peritoneal dialysis is not effective for removing captopril; there is no information concerning exchange transfusion for removing captopril from the general circulation.

When captopril was given to rabbits at doses about 0.8 to 70 times (on a mg/kg basis) the maximum recommended human dose, low incidences of craniofacial malformations were seen. No teratogenic effects of captopril were seen in studies of pregnant rats and hamsters. On a mg/kg basis, the doses used were up to 150 times (in hamsters) and 625 times (in rats) the maximum recommended human dose.

PRECAUTIONS
General
Impaired Renal Function
Hypertension—Some patients with renal disease, particularly those with severe renal artery stenosis, have developed increases in BUN and serum creatinine after reduction of blood pressure with captopril. Captopril dosage reduction and/or discontinuation of diuretic may be required. For some of these patients, it may not be possible to normalize blood pressure and maintain adequate renal perfusion.

Heart Failure—About 20 percent of patients develop stable elevations of BUN and serum creatinine greater than 20 percent above normal or baseline upon long-term treatment with captopril. Less than 5 percent of patients, generally those with severe preexisting renal disease, required discontinuaton of treatment due to progressively increasing creatinine; subsequent improvement probably depends upon the severity of the underlying renal disease.

See CLINICAL PHARMACOLOGY, DOSAGE AND ADMINISTRATION, ADVERSE REACTIONS: Altered Laboratory Findings.
Hyperkalemia: Elevations in serum potassium have been observed in some patients treated with ACE inhibitors, including captopril. When treated with ACE inhibitors, patients at risk for the development of hyperkalemia include those with: renal insufficiency; diabetes mellitus; and those using concomitant potassium-sparing diuretics, potassium supplements or potassium-containing salt substitutes; or other drugs associated with increases in serum potassium. (See PRECAUTIONS: Information for Patients and Drug Interactions; ADVERSE REACTIONS: Altered Laboratory Findings.)
Cough: Cough has been reported with the use of ACE inhibitors. Characteristically, the cough is nonproductive, persistent and resolves after discontinuation of therapy. ACE inhibitor-induced cough should be considered as part of the differential diagnosis of cough.
Valvular Stenosis: There is concern, on theoretical grounds, that patients with aortic stenosis might be at particular risk of decreased coronary perfusion when treated with vasodilators because they do not develop as much afterload reduction as others.
Surgery/Anesthesia: In patients undergoing major surgery or during anesthesia with agents that produce hypotension, captopril will block angiotensin II formation secondary to compensatory renin release. If hypotension occurs and is considered to be due to this mechanism, it can be corrected by volume expansion.
Information for Patients
Patients should be advised to immediately report to their physician any signs or symptoms suggesting angioedema (e.g., swelling of face, eyes, lips, tongue, larynx and extremities; difficulty in swallowing or breathing; hoarseness) and to discontinue therapy. (See WARNINGS.)

Patients should be told to report promptly any indication of infection (e.g., sore throat, fever), which may be a sign of neu-

tropenia, or of progressive edema which might be related to proteinuria and nephrotic syndrome.

All patients should be cautioned that excessive perspiration and dehydration may lead to an excessive fall in blood pressure because of reduction in fluid volume. Other causes of volume depletion such as vomiting or diarrhea may also lead to a fall in blood pressure; patients should be advised to consult with the physician.

Patients should be advised not to use potassium-sparing diuretics, potassium supplements or potassium-containing salt substitutes without consulting their physician. (See PRECAUTIONS: General and Drug Interactions; ADVERSE REACTIONS.)

Patients should be warned against interruption or discontinuation of medication unless instructed by the physician. Heart failure patients on captopril therapy should be cautioned against rapid increases in physical activity.

Patients should be informed that CAPOTEN (captopril) should be taken one hour before meals (see DOSAGE AND ADMINISTRATION).

Pregnancy. Female patients of childbearing age should be told about the consequences of second- and third-trimester exposure to ACE inhibitors, and they should also be told that these consequences do not appear to have resulted from intrauterine ACE-inhibitor exposure that has been limited to the first trimester. These patients should be asked to report pregnancies to their physicians as soon as possible.

Drug Interactions
Hypotension—Patients on Diuretic Therapy: Patients on diuretics and especially those in whom diuretic therapy was recently instituted, as well as those on severe dietary salt restriction or dialysis, may occasionally experience a precipitous reduction of blood pressure usually within the first hour after receiving the initial dose of captopril.

The possibility of hypotensive effects with captopril can be minimized by either discontinuing the diuretic or increasing the salt intake approximately one week prior to initiation of treatment with CAPOTEN (captopril) or initiating therapy with small doses (6.25 or 12.5 mg). Alternatively, provide medical supervision for at least one hour after the initial dose. If hypotension occurs, the patient should be placed in a supine position and, if necessary, receive an intravenous infusion of normal saline. This transient hypotensive response is not a contraindication to further doses which can be given without difficulty once the blood pressure has increased after volume expansion.

Agents Having Vasodilator Activity: Data on the effect of concomitant use of other vasodilators in patients receiving CAPOTEN for heart failure are not available; therefore, nitroglycerin or other nitrates (as used for management of angina) or other drugs having vasodilator activity should, if possible, be discontinued before starting CAPOTEN. If resumed during CAPOTEN therapy, such agents should be administered cautiously, and perhaps at lower dosage.

Agents Causing Renin Release: Captopril's effect will be augmented by antihypertensive agents that cause renin release. For example, diuretics (e.g., thiazides) may activate the renin-angiotensin-aldosterone system.

Agents Affecting Sympathetic Activity: The sympathetic nervous system may be especially important in supporting blood pressure in patients receiving captopril alone or with diuretics. Therefore, agents affecting sympathetic activity (e.g., ganglionic blocking agents or adrenergic neuron blocking agents) should be used with caution. Beta-adrenergic blocking drugs add some further antihypertensive effect to captopril, but the overall response is less than additive.

Agents Increasing Serum Potassium: Since captopril decreases aldosterone production, elevation of serum potassium may occur. Potassium-sparing diuretics such as spironolactone, triamterene, or amiloride, or potassium supplements should be given only for documented hypokalemia, and then with caution, since they may lead to a significant increase of serum potassium. Salt substitutes containing potassium should also be used with caution.

Inhibitors Of Endogenous Prostaglandin Synthesis: It has been reported that indomethacin may reduce the antihypertensive effect of captopril, especially in cases of low renin hypertension. Other nonsteroidal anti-inflammatory agents (e.g., aspirin) may also have this effect.

Lithium: Increased serum lithium levels and symptoms of lithium toxicity have been reported in patients receiving concomitant lithium and ACE inhibitor therapy. These drugs should be coadministered with caution and frequent monitoring of serum lithium levels is recommended. If a diuretic is also used, it may increase the risk of lithium toxicity.

Drug/Laboratory Test Interaction
Captopril may cause a false-positive urine test for acetone.
Carcinogenesis, Mutagenesis and Impairment of Fertility
Two-year studies with doses of 50 to 1350 mg/kg/day in mice and rats failed to show any evidence of carcinogenic potential.

Studies in rats have revealed no impairment of fertility.
Animal Toxicology
Chronic oral toxicity studies were conducted in rats (2 years), dogs (47 weeks; 1 year), mice (2 years), and monkeys (1 year).

Significant drug related toxicity included effects on hematopoiesis, renal toxicity, erosion/ulceration of the stomach, and variation of retinal blood vessels.

Reductions in hemoglobin and/or hematocrit values were seen in mice, rats, and monkeys at doses 50 to 150 times the maximum recommended human dose (MRHD). Anemia, leukopenia, thrombocytopenia, and bone marrow suppression occurred in dogs at doses 8 to 30 times MRHD. The reductions in hemoglobin and hematocrit values in rats and mice were only significant at 1 year and returned to normal with continued dosing by the end of the study. Marked anemia was seen at all dose levels (8 to 30 times MRHD) in dogs, whereas moderate to marked leukopenia was noted only at 15 and 30 times MRHD and thrombocytopenia at 30 times MRHD. The anemia could be reversed upon discontinuation of dosing. Bone marrow suppression occurred to a varying degree, being associated only with dogs that died or were sacrificed in a moribund condition in the 1 year study. However, in the 47-week study at a dose 30 times MRHD, bone marrow suppression was found to be reversible upon continued drug administration.

Captopril caused hyperplasia of the juxtaglomerular apparatus of the kidneys at doses 7 to 200 times the MRHD in rats and mice, at 20 to 60 times MRHD in monkeys, and at 30 times the MRHD in dogs.

Gastric erosions/ulcerations were increased in incidence at 20 and 200 times MRHD in male rats and at 30 and 65 times MRHD in dogs and monkeys, respectively. Rabbits developed gastric and intestinal ulcers when given oral doses approximately 30 times MRHD for only 5 to 7 days.

In the two-year rat study, irreversible and progressive variations in the caliber of retinal vessels (focal sacculations and constrictions) occurred at all dose levels (7 to 200 times MRHD) in a dose-related fashion. The effect was first observed in the 88th week of dosing, with a progressively increased incidence thereafter, even after cessation of dosing.

Pregnancy Categories C (first trimester) and D (second and third trimesters)

See WARNINGS: Fetal/Neonatal Morbidity and Mortality.
Nursing Mothers
Concentrations of captopril in human milk are approximately one percent of those in maternal blood. Because of the potential for serious adverse reactions in nursing infants from captopril, a decision should be made whether to discontinue nursing or to discontinue the drug, taking into account the importance of CAPOTEN to the mother. (See PRECAUTIONS: Pediatric Use.)
Pediatric Use
Safety and effectiveness in children have not been established. There is limited experience reported in the literature with the use of captopril in the pediatric population; dosage, on a weight basis, was generally reported to be comparable to or less than that used in adults.

Infants, especially newborns, may be more susceptible to the adverse hemodynamic effects of captopril. Excessive, prolonged and unpredictable decreases in blood pressure and associated complications, including oliguria and seizures, have been reported.

CAPOTEN (captopril) should be used in children only if other measures for controlling blood pressure have not been effective.

ADVERSE REACTIONS
Reported incidences are based on clinical trials involving approximately 7000 patients.
Renal: About one of 100 patients developed proteinuria (see WARNINGS).

Each of the following has been reported in approximately 1 to 2 of 1000 patients and are of uncertain relationship to drug use: renal insufficiency, renal failure, nephrotic syndrome, polyuria, oliguria, and urinary frequency.
Hematologic: Neutropenia/agranulocytosis has occurred (see WARNINGS). Cases of anemia, thrombocytopenia, and pancytopenia have been reported.
Dermatologic: Rash, often with pruritus, and sometimes with fever, arthralgia, and eosinophilia, occurred in about 4 to 7 (depending on renal status and dose) of 100 patients, usually during the first four weeks of therapy. It is usually maculopapular, and rarely urticarial. The rash is usually mild and disappears within a few days of dosage reduction, short-term treatment with an antihistaminic agent, and/or discontinuing therapy; remission may occur even if captopril is continued. Pruritus, without rash, occurs in about 2 of 100 patients. Between 7 and 10 percent of patients with skin rash have shown an eosinophilia and/or positive ANA titers. A reversible associated pemphigoid-like lesion, and photosensitivity, have also been reported.

Flushing or pallor has been reported in 2 to 5 of 1000 patients.
Cardiovascular: Hypotension may occur; see WARNINGS and PRECAUTIONS [Drug Interactions] for discussion of hypotension with captopril therapy.

Tachycardia, chest pain, and palpitations have each been observed in approximately 1 of 100 patients.

Angina pectoris, myocardial infarction, Raynaud's syndrome, and congestive heart failure have each occurred in 2 to 3 of 1000 patients.
Dysgeusia: Approximately 2 to 4 (depending on renal status and dose) of 100 patients developed a diminution or loss of taste perception. Taste impairment is reversible and usually self-limited (2 to 3 months) even with continued drug administration. Weight loss may be associated with the loss of taste.
Angioedema: Angioedema involving the extremities, face, lips, mucous membranes, tongue, glottis or larynx has been reported in approximately one in 1000 patients. Angioedema involving the upper airways has caused fatal airway obstruction. (See WARNINGS and PRECAUTIONS: Information for Patients.)
Cough: Cough has been reported in 0.5–2% of patients treated with captopril in clinical trials (see PRECAUTIONS: General, Cough).
The following have been reported in about 0.5 to 2 percent of patients but did not appear at increased frequency compared to placebo or other treatments used in controlled trials: gastric irritation, abdominal pain, nausea, vomiting, diarrhea, anorexia, constipation, aphthous ulcers, peptic ulcer, dizziness, headache, malaise, fatigue, insomnia, dry mouth, dyspnea, alopecia, paresthesias.
Other clinical adverse effects reported since the drug was marketed are listed below by body system. In this setting, an incidence or causal relationship cannot be accurately determined.
General: Asthenia, gynecomastia.
Cardiovascular: Cardiac arrest, cerebrovascular accident/insufficiency, rhythm disturbances, orthostatic hypotension, syncope.
Dermatologic: Bullous pemphigus, erythema multiforme (including Stevens-Johnson syndrome), exfoliative dermatitis.
Gastrointestinal: Pancreatitis, glossitis, dyspepsia.
Hematologic: Anemia, including aplastic and hemolytic.
Hepatobiliary: Jaundice, hepatitis, including rare cases of necrosis, cholestasis.
Metabolic: Symptomatic hyponatremia.
Musculoskeletal: Myalgia, myasthenia.
Nervous/Psychiatric: Ataxia, confusion, depression, nervousness, somnolence.
Respiratory: Bronchospasm, eosinophilic pneumonitis, rhinitis.
Special Senses: Blurred vision.
Urogenital: Impotence.
As with other ACE inhibitors, a syndrome has been reported which may include: fever, myalgia, arthralgia, interstitial nephritis, vasculitis, rash or other dermatologic manifestations, eosinophilia and an elevated ESR.

Fetal/Neonatal Morbidity and Mortality
See WARNINGS: Fetal/Neonatal Morbidity and Mortality.

Altered Laboratory Findings
Serum Electrolytes: Hyperkalemia: small increases in serum potassium, especially in patients with renal impairment (see PRECAUTIONS).
Hyponatremia: particularly in patients receiving a low sodium diet or concomitant diuretics.
BUN/Serum Creatinine: Transient elevations of BUN or serum creatinine especially in volume or salt depleted patients or those with renovascular hypertension may occur. Rapid reduction of longstanding or markedly elevated blood pressure can result in decreases in the glomerular filtration rate and, in turn, lead to increases in BUN or serum creatinine.
Hematologic: A positive ANA has been reported.
Liver Function Tests: Elevations of liver transaminases, alkaline phosphatase, and serum bilirubin have occurred.

OVERDOSAGE

Correction of hypotension would be of primary concern. Volume expansion with an intravenous infusion of normal saline is the treatment of choice for restoration of blood pressure.
While captopril may be removed from the adult circulation by hemodialysis, there is inadequate data concerning the effectiveness of hemodialysis for removing it from the circulation of neonates or children. Peritoneal dialysis is not effective for removing captopril; there is no information concerning exchange transfusion for removing captopril from the general circulation.

DOSAGE AND ADMINISTRATION

CAPOTEN (captopril) should be taken one hour before meals. Dosage must be individualized.
Hypertension—Initiation of therapy requires consideration of recent antihypertensive drug treatment, the extent of blood pressure elevation, salt restriction, and other clinical circumstances. If possible, discontinue the patient's previous antihypertensive drug regimen for one week before starting CAPOTEN.
The initial dose of CAPOTEN (captopril) is 25 mg bid or tid. If satisfactory reduction of blood pressure has not been achieved after one or two weeks, the dose may be increased to 50 mg bid or tid. Concomitant sodium restriction may be beneficial when CAPOTEN is used alone.
The dose of CAPOTEN in hypertension usually does not exceed 50 mg tid. Therefore, if the blood pressure has not been satisfactorily controlled after one to two weeks at this dose, (and the patient is not already receiving a diuretic), a modest dose of a thiazide-type diuretic (e.g., hydrochlorothiazide, 25 mg daily), should be added. The diuretic dose may be increased at one- to two-week intervals until its highest usual antihypertensive dose is reached.
If CAPOTEN is being started in a patient already receiving a diuretic, CAPOTEN therapy should be initiated under close medical supervision (see WARNINGS and PRECAUTIONS [Drug Interactions] regarding hypotension), with dosage and titration of CAPOTEN as noted above.
If further blood pressure reduction is required, the dose of CAPOTEN may be increased to 100 mg bid or tid and then, if necessary, to 150 mg bid or tid (while continuing the diuretic). The usual dose range is 25 to 150 mg bid or tid. A maximum daily dose of 450 mg CAPOTEN should not be exceeded.
For patients with severe hypertension (e.g., accelerated or malignant hypertension), when temporary discontinuation of current antihypertensive therapy is not practical or desirable, or when prompt titration to more normotensive blood pressure levels is indicated, diuretic should be continued but other current antihypertensive medication stopped and CAPOTEN dosage promptly initiated at 25 mg bid or tid, under close medical supervision.
When necessitated by the patient's clinical condition, the daily dose of CAPOTEN may be increased every 24 hours or less under continuous medical supervision until a satisfactory blood pressure response is obtained or the maximum dose of CAPOTEN is reached. In this regimen, addition of a more potent diuretic, e.g., furosemide, may also be indicated. Beta-blockers may also be used in conjunction with CAPOTEN therapy (see PRECAUTIONS: Drug Interactions), but the effects of the two drugs are less than additive.
Heart Failure—Initiation of therapy requires consideration of recent diuretic therapy and the possibility of severe salt/volume depletion. In patients with either normal or low blood pressure, who have been vigorously treated with diuretics and who may be hyponatremic and/or hypovolemic, a starting dose of 6.25 or 12.5 mg tid may minimize the magnitude or duration of the hypotensive effect (see WARNINGS: Hypotension); for these patients, titration to the usual daily dosage can then occur within the next several days.
For most patients the usual initial daily dosage is 25 mg tid. After a dose of 50 mg tid is reached, further increases in dosage should be delayed, where possible, for at least two weeks to determine if a satisfactory response occurs. Most patients studied have had a satisfactory clinical improvement at 50 or 100 mg tid. A maximum daily dose of 450 mg of CAPOTEN (captopril) should not be exceeded.
CAPOTEN should generally be used in conjunction with a diuretic and digitalis. CAPOTEN therapy must be initiated under very close medical supervision.
Dosage Adjustment in Renal Impairment—Because CAPOTEN (captopril) is excreted primarily by the kidneys, excretion rates are reduced in patients with impaired renal function. These patients will take longer to reach steady-state captopril levels and will reach higher steady-state levels for a given daily dose than patients with normal renal function. Therefore, these patients may respond to smaller or less frequent doses.
Accordingly, for patients with significant renal impairment, initial daily dosage of CAPOTEN (captopril) should be reduced, and smaller increments utilized for titration, which should be quite slow (one- to two-week intervals). After the desired therapeutic effect has been achieved, the dose should be slowly back-titrated to determine the minimal effective dose. When concomitant diuretic therapy is required, a loop diuretic (e.g., furosemide), rather than a thiazide diuretic, is preferred in patients with severe renal impairment.

HOW SUPPLIED

12.5 mg tablets in bottles of 100 (NDC 0003-0450-54) and 1000 (NDC 0003-0450-75), **25 mg tablets** in bottles of 100 (NDC 0003-0452-50) and 1000 (NDC 0003-0452-75), **50 mg tablets** in bottles of 100 (NDC 0003-0482-50) and 1000 (NDC 0003-0482-75), and **100 mg tablets** in bottles of 100 (NDC 0003-0485-50). Bottles contain a desiccant-charcoal canister.
Unimatic® unit-dose packs containing 100 tablets are also available for each potency: **12.5 mg** (NDC 0003-0450-51), **25 mg** (NDC 0003-0452-51), **50 mg** (NDC 0003-0482-51), and **100 mg** (NDC 0003-0485-51).
The **12.5 mg tablet** is a biconvex oval with a partial bisect bar; the **25 mg tablet** is a biconvex rounded square with a quadrisect bar; the **50 and 100 mg tablets** are biconvex ovals with a bisect bar.
All captopril tablets are white and may exhibit a slight sulfurous odor.

Storage
Do not store above 86°F. Keep bottles tightly closed (protect from moisture).
(J3-658Z)

Shown in Product Identification Section, page 423

DURICEF® ℞
[dur′ĭ-sef]
(cefadroxil monohydrate, USP)

Capsules, 500 mg, bottles of 100
NSN 6505-01-096-3886 (M)

DESCRIPTION

DURICEF® (cefadroxil monohydrate, USP) is a semisynthetic cephalosporin antibiotic intended for oral administration. It is a white to yellowish-white crystalline powder. It is soluble in water and it is acid-stable. It is chemically designated as 5-Thia-1-azabicyclo[4.2.0]oct-2-ene-2-carboxylic acid, 7-[[amino(4-hydroxyphenyl)acetyl]amino]-3-methyl-8-oxo, monohydrate, [6R-[6α,7β(R*)]]-. It has the formula $C_{16}H_{17}N_3O_5S \cdot H_2O$ and the molecular weight of 381.40.
DURICEF® film-coated tablets, 1 g, contain the following inactive ingredients: microcrystalline cellulose, hydroxypropyl methylcellulose, magnesium stearate, polyethylene glycol, polysorbate 80, simethicone emulsion, and titanium dioxide.
DURICEF® for Oral Suspension contains the following inactive ingredients: FD&C Yellow No. 6, flavors (natural and artificial), polysorbate 80, sodium benzoate, sucrose, and xanthan gum.
DURICEF® capsules contain the following inactive ingredients: D&C Red No. 28, FD&C Blue No. 1, FD&C Red No. 40, gelatin, magnesium stearate, and titanium dioxide.

Clinical Pharmacology—DURICEF is rapidly absorbed after oral administration. Following single doses of 500 and 1000 mg, average peak serum concentrations were approximately 16 and 28 μg/mL, respectively. Measurable levels were present 12 hours after administration. Over 90% of the drug is excreted unchanged in the urine within 24 hours. Peak urine concentrations are approximately 1800 μg/mL during the period following a single 500-mg oral dose. Increases in dosage generally produce a proportionate increase in DURICEF urinary concentration. The urine antibiotic concentration, following a 1-g dose, was maintained well above the MIC of susceptible urinary pathogens for 20 to 22 hours.

Microbiology: *In vitro* tests demonstrate that the cephalosporins are bactericidal because of their inhibition of cell-wall synthesis. Cefadroxil has been shown to be active against the following organisms both *in vitro* and in clinical infections (see INDICATIONS AND USAGE):
Beta- hemolytic streptococci
Staphylococci, including
penicillinase-producing strains
Streptococcus (Diplococcus) pneumoniae
Escherichia coli.
Proteus mirabilis
Klebsiella species
Moraxella (Branhamella) catarrhalis

Note: Most strains of *Enterococci faecalis* (formerly *Streptococcus faecalis)* and *Enterococcus faecium* (formerly *Streptococcus faecium)* are resistant to DURICEF. It is not active against most strains of *Enterobacter* species, *Morganella morganii* (formerly *Proteus morganii*), and *P. vulgaris.* It has no activity against *Pseudomonas* species and *Acinetobacter calcoaceticus* (formerly *Mima* and *Herellea* species.)

Susceptibility tests: Diffusion techniques
The use of antibiotic disk susceptibility test methods which measure zone diameter give an accurate estimation of antibiotic susceptibility. One such standard procedure[1] which has been recommended for use with disks to test susceptibility of organisms to cefadroxil uses the cephalosporin class (cephalothin) disk. Interpretation involves the correlation of the diameters obtained in the disk test with the minimum inhibitory concentration (MIC) for cefadroxil.
Reports from the laboratory giving results of the standard single-disk susceptibility test with a 30 μg cephalothin disk should be interpreted according to the following criteria:

Zone diameter (mm)	Interpretation
≥18	(S) Susceptible
15–17	(I) Intermediate
≤14	(R) Resistant

A report of "Susceptible" indicates that the pathogen is likely to be inhibited by generally achievable blood levels. A report of "Intermediate susceptibility" suggests that the organism would be susceptible if high dosage is used or if the infection is confined to tissue and fluid (eg, urine) in which high antibiotic levels are attained. A report of "Resistant" indicates that achievable concentrations of the antibiotic are unlikely to be inhibitory and other therapy should be selected.

Continued on next page

Princeton—Cont.

Standardized procedures require the use of laboratory control organisms. The 30 μg cephalothin disk should give the following zone diameters:

Organism	Zone Diameter (mm)
Staphylococcus aureus ATCC 25923	29–37
Escherichia coli ATCC 25922	17–22

Dilution Techniques

When using the NCCLS agar dilution or broth dilution (including microdilution) method[2] or equivalent, a bacterial isolate may be considered susceptible if the MIC (minimum inhibitory concentration) value for cephalothin is 8 μg/mL or less. Organisms are considered resistant if the MIC is 32 μg/mL or greater. Organisms with an MIC value of less than 32 μg/mL but greater than 8 μg/mL are intermediate.

As with standard diffusion methods, dilution procedures require the use of laboratory control organisms. Standard cephalothin powder should give MIC values in the range of 0.12 μg/mL and 0.5 μg/mL for *Staphylococcus aureus* ATCC 29213. For *Escherichia coli* ATCC 25922, the MIC range should be between 4.0 μg/mL and 16.0 μg/mL. For *Streptococcus faecalis* ATCC 29212, the MIC range should be between 8.0 and 32.0 μg/mL.

INDICATIONS AND USAGE

DURICEF is indicated for the treatment of patients with infection caused by susceptible strains of the designated organisms in the following diseases:

Urinary tract infections caused by *E. coli, P. mirabilis,* and *Klebsiella* species.

Skin and skin structure infections caused by staphylococci and/or streptococci.

Pharyngitis and tonsillitis caused by group A beta-hemolytic streptococci. (Penicillin is the usual drug of choice in the treatment and prevention of streptococcal infections, including the prophylaxis of rheumatic fever. DURICEF is generally effective in the eradication of streptococci from the nasopharynx; however, substantial data establishing the efficacy of DURICEF in the subsequent prevention of rheumatic fever are not available at present.)

Note: Culture and susceptibility tests should be initiated prior to and during therapy. Renal function studies should be performed when indicated.

CONTRAINDICATIONS

DURICEF is contraindicated in patients with known allergy to the cephalosporin group of antibiotics.

WARNINGS

BEFORE THERAPY WITH DURICEF IS INSTITUTED, CAREFUL INQUIRY SHOULD BE MADE TO DETERMINE WHETHER THE PATIENT HAS HAD PREVIOUS HYPERSENSITIVITY REACTIONS TO CEFADROXIL, CEPHALOSPORINS, PENICILLINS OR OTHER DRUGS. IF THIS PRODUCT IS TO BE GIVEN TO PENICILLIN-SENSITIVE PATIENTS, CAUTION SHOULD BE EXERCISED BECAUSE CROSS-SENSITIVITY AMONG BETA-LACTAM ANTIBIOTICS HAS BEEN CLEARLY DOCUMENTED AND MAY OCCUR IN UP TO 10% OF PATIENTS WITH A HISTORY OF PENICILLIN ALLERGY.

IF AN ALLERGIC REACTION TO DURICEF OCCURS, DISCONTINUE THE DRUG. SERIOUS ACUTE HYPERSENSITIVITY REACTIONS MAY REQUIRE TREATMENT WITH EPINEPHRINE AND OTHER EMERGENCY MEASURES, INCLUDING OXYGEN, INTRAVENOUS FLUIDS, INTRAVENOUS ANTIHISTAMINES, CORTICOSTEROIDS, PRESSOR AMINES, AND AIRWAY MANAGEMENT, AS CLINICALLY INDICATED.

Pseudomembranous colitis has been reported with nearly all antibacterial agents, including cefadroxil, and may range from mild to life-threatening. Therefore, it is important to consider this diagnosis in patients who present with diarrhea subsequent to the administration of antibacterial agents.

Treatment with antibacterial agents alters the normal flora of the colon and may permit overgrowth of clostridia. Studies indicate that a toxin produced by *Clostridium difficile* is a primary cause of "antibiotic-associated colitis".

After the diagnosis of pseudomembranous colitis has been established, therapeutic measures should be initiated. Mild cases of pseudomembranous colitis usually repond to discontinuation of the drug alone. In moderate to severe cases, consideration should be given to management with fluids and electrolytes, protein supplementation and treatment with an antibacterial drug effective against *Clostridium difficile.*

PRECAUTIONS

General: DURICEF should be used with caution in the presence of markedly impaired renal function (creatinine clearance rate of less than 50 mL/min/1.73 M^2) (See DOSAGE AND ADMINISTRATION.) In patients with known or suspected renal impairment, careful clinical observation and appropriate laboratory studies should be made prior to and during therapy.

Prolonged use of DURICEF may result in the overgrowth of nonsusceptible organisms. Careful observation of the patient is essential. If superinfection occurs during therapy, appropriate measures should be taken.

DURICEF should be prescribed with caution in individuals with history of gastrointestinal disease, particularly colitis.

Drug/Laboratory Test Interactions

Positive direct Coombs' tests have been reported during treatment with the cephalosporin antibiotics. In hematologic studies or in transfusion cross-matching procedures when antiglobulin tests are performed on the minor side or in Coombs' testing of newborns whose mothers have received cephalosporin antibiotics before parturition, it should be recognized that a positive Coombs' test may be due to the drug.

Carcinogenesis, Mutagenesis, and Impairment of Fertility: No long-term studies have been performed to determine carcinogenic potential. No genetic toxicity tests have been performed.

Pregnancy: Pregnancy Category B: Reproduction studies have been performed in mice and rats at doses up to 11 times the human dose and have revealed no evidence of impaired fertility or harm to the fetus due to cefadroxil monohydrate. There are, however, no adequate and well-controlled studies in pregnant women. Because animal reproduction studies are not always predictive of human response, this drug should be used during pregnancy only if clearly needed.

Labor and Delivery: DURICEF® (cefadroxil monohydrate, USP) has not been studied for use during labor and delivery. Treatment should only be given if clearly needed.

Nursing Mothers: Caution should be exercised when cefadroxil monohydrate is administered to a nursing mother.

Pediatric Use: (See DOSAGE AND ADMINISTRATION).

ADVERSE REACTIONS

Gastrointestinal—Onset of pseudomembranous colitis symptoms may occur during or after antibiotic treatment (See WARNINGS). Nausea and vomiting have been reported rarely. Diarrhea has also occurred.

Hypersensitivity—Allergies (in the form of rash, urticaria, and angioedema) have been observed. These reactions usually subsided upon discontinuation of the drug.

Other reactions have included genital pruritus, genital moniliasis, vaginitis, moderate transient neutropenia, and minor elevations in serum transaminase. Stevens-Johnson syndrome has been rarely reported.

In addition to the adverse reactions listed above which have been observed in patients treated with cefadroxil, the following adverse reactions and altered laboratory tests have been reported for cephalosporin-class antibiotics:

Anaphylaxis, erythema multiforme, toxic epidermal necrolysis, fever, abdominal pain, superinfection, renal dysfunction, toxic nephropathy, hepatic dysfunction including cholestasis, aplastic anemia, hemolytic anemia, hemorrhage, prolonged prothrombin time, positive Coombs' test, increased BUN, increased creatinine, elevated alkaline phosphatase, elevated aspartate aminotransferase (AST), elevated alanine aminotransferase (ALT), elevated bilirubin, elevated LDH, eosinophilia, pancytopenia, neutropenia, agranlocytosis, thrombocytopenia.

Several cephalosporins have been implicated in triggering seizures, particularly in patients with renal impairment, when the dosage was not reduced (see DOSAGE AND ADMINISTRATION and OVERDOSAGE). If seizures associated with drug therapy occur, the drug should be discontinued. Anticonvulsant therapy can be given if clinically indicated.

OVERDOSAGE

A study of children under six years of age suggested that ingestion of less than 250 mg/kg of cephalosporins is not associated with significant outcomes. No action is required other than general support and observation. For amounts greater than 250 mg/kg, induce gastric emptying.

In five anuric patients. it was demonstrated that an average of 63% of a 1 g oral dose is extracted from the body during a 6–8 hour hemodialysis session.

DOSAGE AND ADMINISTRATION

DURICEF is acid-stable and may be administered orally without regard to meals. Administration with food may be helpful in diminishing potential gastrointestinal complaints occasionally associated with oral cephalosporin therapy.

Adults

Urinary Tract Infections: For uncomplicated lower urinary tract infections (ie, cystitis) the usual dosage is 1 or 2 g per day in single (q.d.) or divided doses (b.i.d.).

For all other urinary tract infections the usual dosage is 2 g per day in divided doses (b.i.d.).

Skin and Skin Structure Infections: For skin and skin structure infections the usual dosage is 1 g per day in single (q.d.) or divided doses (b.i.d.).

Pharyngitis and Tonsillitis: Treatment of group A beta-hemolytic streptococcal pharyngitis and tonsillitis—1 g per day in single (q.d.) or divided doses (b.i.d.) for 10 days.

Children

For urinary tract infections, the recommended daily dosage for children is 30 mg/kg/day in divided doses every 12 hours. For pharyngitis, tonsillitis, and impetigo, the recommended daily dosage for children is 30 mg/kg/day in a single dose or in equally divided doses every 12 hours. For other skin and skin structure infections, the recommended daily dosage is 30 mg/kg/day in equally divided doses every 12 hours. In the treatment of beta-hemolytic streptococcal infections, a therapeutic dosage of DURICEF should be administered for at least 10 days. See chart for total daily dosage for children.

In patients with renal impairment, the dosage of cefadroxil monohydrate should be adjusted according to creatinine clearance rates to prevent drug accumulation. The following schedule is suggested. In adults, the initial dose is 1000 mg of DURICEF and the maintenance dose (based on the creatinine clearance rate [(mL/min/1.73 M^2)] is 500 mg at the time intervals listed below.

Creatinine Clearances	Dosage Interval
0–10 mL/min	36 hours
10–25 mL/min	24 hours
25–50 mL/min	12 hours

Patients with creatinine clearance rates over 50 mL/min may be treated as if they were patients having normal renal function.

Reconstitution Directions for Oral Suspension

Bottle Size	Reconstitution Directions
100 mL	Suspend in a total of 66 mL water. Method: Tap bottle lightly to loosen powder. Add 66 mL of water in two portions. Shake well after each addition.
50 mL	Suspend in a total of 33 mL water. Method: Tap bottle lightly to loosen powder. Add 33 mL of water in two portions. Shake well after each addition.

After reconstitution, store in refrigerator. Shake well before using. Keep container tightly closed. Discard unused portion after 14 days.

HOW SUPPLIED

DURICEF® Capsules, 500 mg are supplied as follows:

NDC 0087-0784-46 Bottle of 50
NDC 0087-0784-42 Bottle of 100
NDC 0087-0784-44 10 strips of 10 individually labeled blisters with 1 capsule per blister

Store at controlled room temperature (15°–30°C).

DURICEF® Tablets, 1 g, are supplied as follows:

NDC 0087-0785-43 Bottle of 50
NDC 0087-0785-42 Bottle of 100
NDC 0087-0785-44 10 strips of 10 individually labeled blisters with 1 tablet per blister
NDC 0087-0785-45 4 packs of 10 individually labeled blisters with 1 tablet per blister

Store at controlled room temperature (15°–30°C).

DURICEF® for Oral Suspension is orange-pineapple flavored, and is supplied as follows:

125 mg/5 ml **NDC** 0087-0786-42 50 mL Bottle
NDC 0087-0786-41 100 mL Bottle
250 mg/5mL **NDC** 0087-0782-42 50 mL Bottle
NDC 0087-0782-41 100 mL Bottle
500 mg/5mL **NDC** 0087-0783-42 50 mL Bottle
NDC 0087-0783-41 100 mL Bottle

Prior to reconstitution: Store at controlled room temperature (15°–30°C).

8/91 U.S. Patent Nos. 4,160,863
4,504,657

Child's Weight		Daily Dosage of DURICEF® Suspension		
lbs	kg	125 mg/5 mL	250 mg/5 mL	500 mg/5mL
10	4.5	1 tsp	—	
20	9.1	2 tsp	1 tsp	
30	13.6	3 tsp	$1\frac{1}{2}$ tsp	
40	18.2	4 tsp	2 tsp	1 tsp
50	22.7	5 tsp	$2\frac{1}{2}$ tsp	$1\frac{1}{4}$ tsp
60	27.3	6 tsp	3 tsp	$1\frac{1}{2}$ tsp
70 & above	31.8+	—	—	2 tsp

REFERENCES

1. National Committee for Clinical Laboratory Standards, Approved Standard, *Performance Standards for Antimicrobial Disk Susceptibility Test,* 4th Edition, Vol. 10(7):M2-A4, Villanova, PA, April, 1990.
2. National Committee for Clinical Laboratory Standards, Approved Standard: *Methods for Dilution Antimicrobial Susceptibility Tests for Bacteria that Grow Aerobically,* 2nd Edition, Vol. 10(8):M7-A2, Villanova, PA, April, 1990.

Shown in Product Identification Section, page 423

PRAVACHOL® ℞

[*prăv 'a-cōl*]

Pravastatin Sodium Tablets

DESCRIPTION

PRAVACHOL (pravastatin sodium) is one of a new class of lipid-lowering compounds, the HMG-CoA reductase inhibitors, which reduce cholesterol biosynthesis. These agents are competitive inhibitors of 3-hydroxy-3-methylglutaryl-coenzyme A (HMG-CoA) reductase, the enzyme catalyzing the early rate-limiting step in cholesterol biosynthesis, conversion of HMG-CoA to mevalonate.

Pravastatin sodium is designated chemically as 1-Naphthalene-heptanoic acid, 1,2,6,7,8,8a-hexahydro-β,Δ,6-trihydroxy-2-methyl-8-(2-methyl-1-oxobutoxy)-, monosodium salt, [1*S* -[1α(β*S**,ΔS*),2α,6α,8β(R*),8aα]]-.

Pravastatin sodium is an odorless, white to off-white, fine or crystalline powder. It is a relatively polar hydrophilic compound with a partition coefficient (octanol/water) of 0.59 at a pH of 7.0. It is soluble in methanol and water (> 300 mg/mL), slightly soluble in isopropanol, and practically insoluble in acetone, acetonitrile, chloroform, and ether.

PRAVACHOL is available for oral administration as 10 mg and 20 mg tablets. Inactive ingredients include: croscarmellose sodium, lactose, magnesium stearate, microcrystalline cellulose, and povidone.

CLINICAL PHARMACOLOGY

Mechanism of Action

Cholesterol and triglycerides in the bloodstream circulate as part of lipoprotein complexes. These complexes can be separated by density ultracentrifugation into high (HDL), intermediate (IDL), low (LDL), and very low (VLDL) density lipoprotein fractions. Triglycerides (TG) and cholesterol synthesized in the liver are incorporated into very low density lipoproteins (VLDLs) and released into the plasma for delivery to peripheral tissues. In a series of subsequent steps, VLDLs are transformed into intermediate density lipoproteins (IDLs), and cholesterol-rich low density lipoproteins (LDLs). High density lipoproteins (HDLs), containing apolipoprotein A, are hypothesized to participate in the reverse transport of cholesterol from tissues back to the liver.

PRAVACHOL produces its lipid-lowering effect in two ways. First, as a consequence of its reversible inhibition of HMG-CoA reductase activity, it effects modest reductions in intracellular pools of cholesterol. This results in an increase in the number of LDL-receptors on cell surfaces and enhanced receptor-mediated catabolism and clearance of circulating LDL. Second, pravastatin inhibits LDL production by inhibiting hepatic synthesis of VLDL, the LDL precursor.

Clinical and pathologic studies have shown that elevated levels of total cholesterol (Total-C), low density lipoprotein cholesterol (LDL-C), and apolipoprotein B (a membrane transport complex for LDL) promote human atherosclerosis. Similarly, decreased levels of HDL-cholesterol (HDL-C) and its transport complex, apolipoprotein A, are associated with the development of atherosclerosis. Epidemiologic investigations have established that cardiovascular morbidity and mortality vary directly with the level of Total-C and LDL-C and inversely with the level of HDL-C. In multicenter clinical trials, those pharmacologic and/or non-pharmacologic interventions that simultaneously lowered LDL-C and increased HDL-C reduced the rate of cardiovascular events (both fatal and nonfatal myocardial infarctions). In both normal volunteers and patients with hypercholesterolemia, treatment with PRAVACHOL reduced Total-C, LDL-C, and apolipoprotein B. PRAVACHOL also modestly reduced VLDL-C and TG while producing increases of variable magnitude in HDL-C and apolipoprotein A. The effects of pravastatin on Lp(a), fibrinogen, and certain other independent biochemical risk markers for coronary heart disease are unknown. The effect of pravastatin-induced changes in lipoprotein levels on the evolution of atherosclerosis is also unknown. Although pravastatin is relatively more hydrophilic than other HMG-CoA reductase inhibitors, the effect of relative hydrophilicity, if any, on either efficacy or safety has not been established.

Pharmacokinetics/Metabolism

PRAVACHOL (pravastatin sodium) is administered orally in the active form. In clinical pharmacology studies in man, pravastatin is rapidly absorbed, with peak plasma levels of parent compound attained 1 to 1.5 hours following ingestion. Based on urinary recovery of radiolabeled drug, the average oral absorption of pravastatin is 34% and absolute bioavailability is 17%. While the presence of food in the gastrointestinal tract reduces systemic bioavailability, the lipid-lowering effects of the drug are similar whether taken with, or 1 hour prior, to meals.

Pravastatin undergoes extensive first-pass extraction in the liver (extraction ratio 0.66), which is its primary site of action, and the primary site of cholesterol synthesis and of LDL-C clearance. *In vitro* studies demonstrated that pravastatin is transported into hepatocytes with substantially less uptake into other cells. In view of pravastatin's apparently extensive first-pass hepatic metabolism, plasma levels may not necessarily correlate perfectly with lipid-lowering efficacy. Pravastatin plasma concentrations [including: area under the concentration-time curve (AUC), peak (Cmax), and steady-state minimum (Cmin)] are directly proportional to administered dose. Systemic bioavailability of pravastatin administered following a bedtime dose was decreased 60% compared to that following an AM dose. Despite this decrease in systemic bioavailability, the efficacy of pravastatin administered once daily in the evening, although not statistically significant, was marginally more effective than that after a morning dose. This finding of lower systemic bioavailability suggests greater hepatic extraction of the drug following the evening dose. Steady-state AUCs, Cmax and Cmin plasma concentrations showed no evidence of pravastatin accumulation following once or twice daily administration of PRAVACHOL tablets. Approximately 50% of the circulating drug is bound to plasma proteins. Following single dose administration of ^{14}C-pravastatin, the elimination half-life ($t_{1/2}$) for total radioactivity (pravastatin plus metabolites) in humans is 77 hours.

Pravastatin, like other HMG-CoA reductase inhibitors, has variable bioavailability. The coefficient of variation, based on between-subject variability, was 50% to 60% for AUC.

Approximately 20% of a radiolabeled oral dose is excreted in urine and 70% in the feces. After intravenous administration of radiolabeled pravastatin to normal volunteers, approximately 47% of total body clearance was via renal excretion and 53% by non-renal routes (i.e., biliary excretion and biotransformation). Since there are dual routes of elimination, the potential exists both for compensatory excretion by the alternate route as well as for accumulation of drug and/or metabolites in patients with renal or hepatic insufficiency.

In a study comparing the kinetics of pravastatin in patients with biopsy confirmed cirrhosis (N=7) and normal subjects (N=7), the mean AUC varied 18-fold in cirrhotic patients and 5-fold in healthy subjects. Similarly, the peak pravastatin values varied 47-fold for cirrhotic patients compared to 6-fold for healthy subjects.

Biotransformation pathways elucidated for pravastatin include: (a) isomerization to 6-epi pravastatin and the 3α-hydroxyisomer of pravastatin (SQ 31,906), (b) enzymatic ring hydroxylation to SQ 31,945, (c) -1 oxidation of the ester side chain, (d) β-oxidation of the carboxy side chain, (e) ring oxidation followed by aromatization, (f) oxidation of a hydroxyl group to a keto group, and (g) conjugation. The major degradation product is the 3α-hydroxy isomeric metabolite, which has one-tenth to one-fortieth the HMG-CoA reductase inhibitory activity of the parent compound.

Clinical Studies

PRAVACHOL (pravastatin sodium) is highly effective in reducing Total-C and LDL-C in patients with heterozygous familial, presumed familial combined, and non-familial (non-FH) forms of primary hypercholesterolemia. A therapeutic response is seen within 1 week, and the maximum response usually is achieved within 4 weeks. This response is maintained during extended periods of therapy.

A single daily dose administered in the evening (the recommended dosing) is as effective as the same total daily dose given twice a day. Once daily administration in the evening appears to be marginally more effective than once daily administration in the morning, perhaps because hepatic cholesterol is synthesized mainly at night. In multicenter, double-blind, placebo-controlled studies of patients with primary hypercholesterolemia, treatment with pravastatin in daily doses ranging from 10 mg to 40 mg consistently and significantly decreased Total-C, LDL-C, and Total-C/HDL-C and LDL-C/HDL-C ratios; modestly decreased VLDL-C and plasma TG levels; and produced increases in HDL-C of variable magnitude.

Primary Hypercholesterolemia Study
Dose Response of PRAVACHOL*
Once Daily Administration At Bedtime

Dose	Total-C	LDL-C	HDL-C	TG
10 mg	−16%	−22%	+7%	−15%
20 mg	−24%	−32%	+2%	−11%
40 mg	−25%	−34%	+12%	−24%

*Mean percent change from baseline after 8 weeks

In another clinical trial, patients treated with pravastatin in combination with cholestyramine (70% of patients were taking cholestyramine 20 or 24 g per day) had reductions equal to or greater than 50% in LDL-C. Furthermore, pravastatin attenuated cholestyramine-induced increases in TG levels (which are themselves of uncertain clinical significance).

INDICATIONS AND USAGE

Therapy with lipid-altering agents should be considered a component of multiple risk factor intervention in those individuals at increased risk for atherosclerotic vascular disease. PRAVACHOL (pravastatin sodium) is indicated as an adjunct to diet for the reduction of elevated total and LDL-cholesterol levels in patients with primary hypercholesterolemia (Type IIa and IIb)[1] when the response to a diet restricted in saturated fat and cholesterol has not been adequate.

Prior to initiating therapy with pravastatin, secondary causes for hypercholesterolemia (e.g., poorly controlled diabetes mellitus, hypothyroidism, nephrotic syndrome, dysproteinemias, obstructive liver disease, other drug therapy, alcoholism) should be excluded, and a lipid profile performed to measure Total-C, HDL-C, and TG. For patients with triglycerides (TG) < 400 mg/dL (< 4.5 mmol/L), LDL-C can be estimated using the following equation:

$$\text{LDL-C} = \text{Total-C} - \text{HDL-C} - \tfrac{1}{5}\,\text{TG}$$

For TG levels > 400 mg/dL (> 4.5 mmol/L), this equation is less accurate and LDL-C concentrations should be determined by ultracentrifugation.

Lipid determinations should be performed at intervals of no less than four weeks and dosage adjusted according to the patient's response to therapy.

The National Cholesterol Education Program's Treatment Guidelines† are summarized below:

[See table at top of next page.]

Since the goal of treatment is to lower LDL-C, the NCEP recommends that LDL-C levels be used to initiate and assess treatment response. Only if LDL-C levels are not available, should the Total-C be used to monitor therapy.

As with other lipid-lowering therapy, PRAVACHOL (pravastatin sodium) is not indicated when hypercholesterolemia is due to hyperalphalipoproteinemia (elevated HDL-C). The efficacy of pravastatin has not been evaluated in patients with combined elevated Total-C and hypertriglyceridemia [> 500 mg/dL (> 5.7 mmol/L)] or in patients with elevated intermediate density lipoproteins as their primary lipid abnormality.

CONTRAINDICATIONS

Hypersensitivity to any component of this medication.

Active liver disease or unexplained, persistent elevations in liver function tests (see WARNINGS).

Pregnancy and lactation. Atherosclerosis is a chronic process and discontinuation of lipid-lowering drugs during pregnancy should have little impact on the outcome of long-term therapy of primary hypercholesterolemia. Cholesterol and other products of cholesterol biosynthesis are essential components for fetal development (including synthesis of steroids and cell membranes). Since HMG-CoA reductase inhibitors decrease cholesterol synthesis and possibly the synthesis of other biologically active substances derived from cholesterol, they may cause fetal harm when administered to pregnant women. Therefore, HMG-CoA reductase inhibitors

[1]Classification of Hyperlipoproteinemias

Type		Lipoproteins Elevated	Lipid Elevations major	minor
I	(rare)	chylomicrons	TG	↑→C
IIa		LDL	C	—
IIb		LDL, VLDL	C	TG
III	(rare)	IDL	C/TG	—
IV		VLDL	TG	↑→C
V	(rare)	chylomicrons, VLDL	TG	↑→C

C = cholesterol, TG = triglycerides,
LDL = low density lipoprotein,
VLDL = very low density lipoprotein,
IDL = intermediate density lipoprotein.

[1] Fredrickson classification: Type IIa—elevation of LDL; Type IIb—elevation of LDL and VLDL. Type III (familial dysbetalipoproteinemia)-elevation of IDL. Fredrickson, DS, Fat transport in lipoproteins—an integrated approach to mechanism and disorders, *N Eng J Med* 276:34, 1967.

†For adult diabetic subjects, a modification of these guidelines is recommended—see: American Diabetes Association Consensus Statement: Role of Cardiovascular Risk Factors in Prevention and Treatment of Macrovascular Disease in Diabetes. *Diabetes Care* 12(8):573–579, 1989.

Continued on next page

Princeton—Cont.

are contraindicated during pregnancy and in nursing mothers. **Pravastatin should be administered to women of childbearing age only when such patients are highly unlikely to conceive and have been informed of the potential hazards.** If the patient becomes pregnant while taking this class of drug, therapy should be discontinued and the patient apprised of the potential hazard to the fetus.

WARNINGS

Liver Enzymes

HMG-CoA reductase inhibitors, like some other lipid-lowering therapies, have been associated with biochemical abnormalities of liver function. Increases of serum transaminase (ALT, AST) values to more than 3 times the upper limit of normal occurring on 2 or more (not necessarily sequential) occasions have been reported in 1.3% of patients treated with pravastatin in the US over an average period of 18 months. These abnormalities were not associated with cholestasis and did not appear to be related to treatment duration. In those patients in whom these abnormalities were believed to be related to pravastatin and who were discontinued from therapy, the transaminase levels usually fell slowly to pretreatment levels. These biochemical findings are usually asymptomatic although worldwide experience indicates that anorexia, weakness, and/or abdominal pain may also be present in rare patients.

As with other lipid-lowering agents, liver function tests should be performed during therapy with pravastatin. Serum aminotransferases, including ALT (SGPT), should be monitored before treatment begins, every six weeks for the first three months, every eight weeks during the remainder of the first year, and periodically thereafter (e.g., at about six-month intervals). Special attention should be given to patients who develop increased transaminase levels. Liver function tests should be repeated to confirm an elevation and subsequently monitored at more frequent intervals. If increases in AST and ALT equal or exceed three times the upper limit of normal and persist, then therapy should be discontinued. Persistence of significant aminotransferase elevations following discontinuation of therapy may warrant consideration of liver biopsy.

Active liver disease or unexplained transaminase elevations are contraindications to the use of pravastatin (see CONTRAINDICATIONS). Caution should be exercised when pravastatin is administered to patients with a history of liver disease or heavy alcohol ingestion (see CLINICAL PHARMACOLOGY: Pharmacokinetics/Metabolism). Such patients should be closely monitored, started at the lower end of the recommended dosing range, and titrated to the desired therapeutic effect.

Skeletal Muscle

Rhabdomyolysis with renal dysfunction secondary to myoglobinuria has been reported with pravastatin and other drugs in this class. Uncomplicated myalgia has been reported in pravastatin-treated patients (see ADVERSE REACTIONS). Myopathy, defined as muscle aching or muscle weakness in conjunction with increases in creatine phosphokinase (CPK) values to greater than 10 times the upper limit of normal was reported to be possibly due to pravastatin in only one patient in clinical trials (<0.1%). Myopathy should be considered in any patient with diffuse myalgias, muscle tenderness or weakness, and/or marked elevation of CPK. Patients should be advised to report promptly unexplained muscle pain, tenderness or weakness, particularly if accompanied by malaise or fever. **Pravastatin therapy should be discontinued if markedly elevated CPK levels occur or myopathy is diagnosed or suspected. Pravastatin therapy should also be temporarily withheld in any patient experiencing an acute or serious condition predisposing to the development of renal failure secondary to rhabdomyolysis, e.g., sepsis; hypotension; major surgery; trauma; severe metabolic, endocrine, or electrolyte disorders; or uncontrolled epilepsy.**

The risk of myopathy during treatment with lovastatin is increased if therapy with either cyclosporine, gemfibrozil, erythromycin, or niacin is administered concurrently. There is no experience with the use of pravastatin together with cyclosporine. Myopathy has not been observed in clinical trials involving small numbers of patients who were treated with pravastatin together with niacin. One trial of limited size involving combined therapy with pravastatin and gemfibrozil showed a trend toward more frequent CPK elevations and patient withdrawals due to musculoskeletal symptoms in the group receiving combined treatment as compared with the groups receiving placebo, gemfibrozil, or pravastatin monotherapy. Myopathy was not reported in this trial (see PRECAUTIONS: Drug Interactions). One patient developed myopathy when clofibrate was added to a previously well tolerated regimen of pravastatin; the myopathy resolved when clofibrate therapy was stopped and pravastatin treatment continued. **The use of fibrates alone may occasionally be associated with myopathy. The combined use of pravastatin and fibrates should generally be avoided.**

	LDL-Cholesterol mg/dL (mmol/L) Initiation Level	LDL-Cholesterol mg/dL (mmol/L) Minimum Goal	Total-Cholesterol mg/dL (mmol/L) Minimum Goal
Without Definite CHD or Two Other Risk Factors*	≥190 (≥4.9)	<160 (<4.1)	<240 (<6.2)
With Definite CHD or Two Other Risk Factors*	≥160 (≥4.1)	<130 (<3.4)	<200 (<5.2)

* Other risk factors for coronary heart disease (CHD) include: male sex, family history of premature CHD, cigarette smoking, hypertension, confirmed HDL-C <35 mg/dL (<0.91 mmol/L), diabetes mellitus, definite cerebrovascular or peripheral vascular disease, or severe obesity.

PRECAUTIONS

General

Pravastatin may elevate creatine phosphokinase and transaminase levels (see ADVERSE REACTIONS). This should be considered in the differential diagnosis of chest pain in a patient on therapy with pravastatin.

Homozygous Familial Hypercholesterolemia. Pravastatin has not been evaluated in patients with rare homozygous familial hypercholesterolemia. In this group of patients, it has been reported that HMG-CoA reductase inhibitors are less effective because the patients lack functional LDL receptors.

Renal Insufficiency. A single 20 mg oral dose of pravastatin was administered to 24 patients with varying degrees of renal impairment (as determined by creatinine clearance). No effect was observed on the pharmacokinetics of pravastatin or its 3α-hydroxy isomeric metabolite (SQ 31,906). A small increase was seen in mean AUC values and half-life ($t^{1/2}$) for the inactive enzymatic ring hydroxylation metabolite (SQ 31,945). Given this small sample size, the dosage administered, and the degree of individual variability, patients with renal impairment who are receiving pravastatin should be closely monitored.

Information for Patients

Patients should be advised to report promptly unexplained muscle pain, tenderness or weakness, particularly if accompanied by malaise or fever.

Drug Interactions

Immunosuppressive Drugs, Gemfibrozil, Niacin (Nicotinic Acid), Erythromycin: See WARNINGS: Skeletal Muscle.

Antipyrine: Clearance by the cytochrome P450 system was unaltered by concomitant administration of pravastatin. Since pravastatin does not appear to induce hepatic drug-metabolizing enzymes, it is not expected that any significant interaction of pravastatin with other drugs (e.g., phenytoin, quinidine) metabolized by the cytochrome P450 system will occur.

Cholestyramine/Colestipol: Concomitant administration resulted in an approximately 40 to 50% decrease in the mean AUC of pravastatin. However, when pravastatin was administered 1 hour before or 4 hours after cholestyramine or 1 hour before colestipol and a standard meal, there was no clinically significant decrease in bioavailability or therapeutic effect. (See DOSAGE AND ADMINISTRATION: Concomitant Therapy.)

Warfarin: In a study involving 10 healthy male subjects given pravastatin and warfarin concomitantly for 6 days, bioavailability parameters at steady state for pravastatin (parent compound) were not altered. Pravastatin did not alter the plasma protein-binding of warfarin. Concomitant dosing did increase the AUC and Cmax of warfarin but did not produce any changes in its anticoagulant action (i.e., no increase was seen in mean prothrombin time after 6 days of concomitant therapy). However, bleeding and extreme prolongation of prothrombin time has been reported with another drug in this class. Patients receiving warfarin-type anticoagulants should have their prothrombin times closely monitored when pravastatin is initiated or the dosage of pravastatin is changed.

Cimetidine: The AUC_{0-12hr} for pravastatin when given with cimetidine was not significantly different from the AUC for pravastatin when given alone. A significant difference was observed between the AUC's for pravastatin when given with cimetidine compared to when administered with antacid.

Digoxin: In a crossover trial involving 18 healthy male subjects given pravastatin and digoxin concurrently for 9 days, the bioavailability parameters of digoxin were not affected. The AUC of pravastatin tended to increase, but the overall bioavailability of pravastatin plus its metabolites SQ 31,906 and SQ 31,945 was not altered.

Gemfibrozil: In a crossover study in 20 healthy male volunteers given concomitant single doses of pravastatin and gemfibrozil, there was a significant decrease in urinary excretion and protein binding of pravastatin. In addition, there was a significant increase in AUC, Cmax, and Tmax for the pravastatin metabolite SQ 31,906. Combination therapy with pravastatin and gemfibrozil is generally not recommended.

In interaction studies with *aspirin, antacids* (1 hour prior to PRAVACHOL), *cimetidine, nicotinic acid,* or *probucol,* no statistically significant differences in bioavailability were seen when PRAVACHOL (pravastatin sodium) was administered.

Other Drugs: During clinical trials, no noticeable drug interactions were reported when PRAVACHOL was added to: diuretics, antihypertensives, digitalis, converting-enzyme inhibitors, calcium channel blockers, beta-blockers, or nitroglycerin.

Endocrine Function

HMG-CoA reductase inhibitors interfere with cholesterol synthesis and lower circulating cholesterol levels and, as such, might theoretically blunt adrenal or gonadal steroid hormone production. Results of clinical trials with pravastatin in males and post-menopausal females were inconsistent with regard to possible effects of the drug on basal steroid hormone levels. In a study of 21 males, the mean testosterone response to human chorionic gonadotropin was significantly reduced ($p<0.004$) after 16 weeks of treatment with 40 mg of pravastatin. However, the percentage of patients showing a ≥50% rise in plasma testosterone after human chorionic gonadotropin stimulation did not change significantly after therapy in these patients. The effects of HMG-CoA reductase inhibitors on spermatogenesis and fertility have not been studied in adequate numbers of patients. The effects, if any, of pravastatin on the pituitary-gonadal axis in pre-menopausal females are unknown. Patients treated with pravastatin who display clinical evidence of endocrine dysfunction should be evaluated appropriately. Caution should be exercised if an HMG-CoA reductase inhibitor or other agent used to lower cholesterol levels is administered to patients also receiving other drugs (e.g., ketoconazole, spironolactone, cimetidine) that may diminish the levels or activity of steroid hormones.

CNS Toxicity

CNS vascular lesions, characterized by perivascular hemorrhage and edema and mononuclear cell infiltration of perivascular spaces, were seen in dogs treated with pravastatin at a dose of 25 mg/kg/day, a dose that produced a plasma drug level about 50 times higher than the mean drug level in humans taking 40 mg/day. Similar CNS vascular lesions have been observed with several other drugs in this class.

A chemically similar drug in this class produced optic nerve degeneration (Wallerian degeneration of retinogeniculate fibers) in clinically normal dogs in a dose-dependent fashion starting at 60 mg/kg/day, a dose that produced mean plasma drug levels about 30 times higher than the mean drug level in humans taking the highest recommended dose (as measured by total enzyme inhibitory activity). This same drug also produced vestibulocochlear Wallerian-like degeneration and retinal ganglion cell chromatolysis in dogs treated for 14 weeks at 180 mg/kg/day, a dose which resulted in a mean plasma drug level similar to that seen with the 60 mg/kg dose.

Carcinogenesis, Mutagenesis, Impairment of Fertility

In a 2-year study in rats fed pravastatin at doses of 10, 30, or 100 mg/kg body weight, there was an increased incidence of hepatocellular carcinomas in males at the highest dose ($p<0.01$). Although rats were given up to 125 times the human dose (HD) on a mg/kg body weight basis, their serum drug levels were only 6 to 10 times higher than those measured in humans given 40 mg pravastatin as measured by AUC.

The oral administration of 10, 30, or 100 mg/kg (producing plasma drug levels approximately 0.5 to 5.0 times the human drug levels at 40 mg) of pravastatin to mice for 22 months resulted in a statistically significant increase in the incidence of malignant lymphomas in treated females when all treatment groups were pooled and compared to controls ($p<0.05$). The incidence was not dose-related and male mice were not affected.

A chemically similar drug in this class was administered to mice for 72 weeks at 25, 100, and 400 mg/kg body weight, which resulted in mean serum drug levels approximately 3, 15, and 33 times higher than the mean human serum drug concentration (as total inhibitory activity) after a 40 mg oral dose. Liver carcinomas were significantly increased in high-dose females and mid- and high-dose males, with a maximum incidence of 90 percent in males. The incidence of adenomas of the liver was significantly increased in mid- and high-dose females. Drug treatment also significantly increased the

incidence of lung adenomas in mid- and high-dose males and females. Adenomas of the eye Harderian gland (a gland of the eye of rodents) were significantly higher in high-dose mice than in controls.

No evidence of mutagenicity was observed *in vitro*, with or without rat-liver metabolic activation, in the following studies: microbial mutagen tests, using mutant strains of *Salmonella typhimurium* or *Escherichia coli;* a forward mutation assay in L5178YTK +/− mouse lymphoma cells; a chromosomal aberration test in hamster cells; and a gene conversion assay using *Saccharomyces cerevisiae.* In addition, there was no evidence of mutagenicity in either a dominant lethal test in mice or a micronucleus test in mice.

In a study in rats, with daily doses up to 500 mg/kg, pravastatin did not produce any adverse effects on fertility or general reproductive performance. However, in a study with another HMG-CoA reductase inhibitor, there was decreased fertility in male rats treated for 34 weeks at 25 mg/kg body weight, although this effect was not observed in a subsequent fertility study when this same dose was administered for 11 weeks (the entire cycle of spermatogenesis, including epididymal maturation). In rats treated with this same reductase inhibitor at 180 mg/kg/day, seminiferous tubule degeneration (necrosis and loss of spermatogenic epithelium) was observed. Although not seen with pravastatin, two similar drugs in this class caused drug-related testicular atrophy, decreased spermatogenesis, spermatocytic degeneration, and giant cell formation in dogs. The clinical significance of these findings is unclear.

Pregnancy
Pregnancy Category X.
See CONTRAINDICATIONS.
Safety in pregnant women has not been established. Pravastatin was not teratogenic in rats at doses up to 1000 mg/kg daily or in rabbits at doses of up to 50 mg/kg daily. These doses resulted in 20× (rabbit) or 240× (rat) the human exposure based on surface area (mg/meter^2). However, in studies with another HMG-CoA reductase inhibitor, skeletal malformations were observed in rats and mice. PRAVACHOL (pravastatin sodium) should be administered to women of child-bearing potential only when such patients are highly unlikely to conceive and have been informed of the potential hazards. If the woman becomes pregnant while taking PRAVACHOL (pravastatin sodium), it should be discontinued and the patient advised again as to the potential hazards to the fetus.

Nursing Mothers
A small amount of pravastatin is excreted in human breast milk. Because of the potential for serious adverse reactions in nursing infants, women taking PRAVACHOL (pravastatin sodium) should not nurse (see CONTRAINDICATIONS).

Pediatric Use
Safety and effectiveness in individuals less than 18 years old have not been established. Hence, treatment in patients less than 18 years old is not recommended at this time. See also PRECAUTIONS: General.

ADVERSE REACTIONS
Pravastatin is generally well tolerated; adverse reactions have usually been mild and transient. In 4-month long placebo-controlled trials, 1.7% of pravastatin-treated patients and 1.2% of placebo-treated patients were discontinued from treatment because of adverse experiences attributed to study drug therapy; this difference was not statistically significant. In long-term studies, the most common reasons for discontinuation were asymptomatic serum transaminase increases and mild, non-specific gastrointestinal complaints. During clinical trials the overall incidence of adverse events in the elderly was not different than the incidence observed in younger patients.

Adverse Clinical Events
All adverse clinical events (regardless of attribution) reported in more than 2% of pravastatin-treated patients in the placebo-controlled trials are identified in the table above; also shown are the percentages of patients in whom these medical events were believed to be related or possibly related to the drug.

The following effects have been reported with drugs in this class:
Skeletal: myopathy, rhabdomyolysis.
Neurological: dysfunction of certain cranial nerves (including alteration of taste, impairment of extra-ocular movement, facial paresis), tremor, vertigo, memory loss, paresthesia, peripheral neuropathy, peripheral nerve palsy.
Hypersensitivity Reactions: An apparent hypersensitivity syndrome has been reported rarely which has included one or more of the following features: anaphylaxis, angioedema, lupus erythematous-like syndrome, polymyalgia rheumatica, vasculitis, purpura, thrombocytopenia, leukopenia, hemolytic anemia, positive ANA, ESR increase, arthritis, arthralgia, urticaria, asthenia, photosensitivity, fever, chills, flushing, malaise, dyspnea, toxic epidermal necrolysis, erythema multiforme, including Stevens-Johnson syndrome.
Gastrointestinal: pancreatitis, hepatitis, including chronic active hepatitis, cholestatic jaundice, fatty change in liver,

Body System/ Event	All Events		Events Attributed to Study Drug	
	Pravastatin (N = 900) %	Placebo (N = 411) %	Pravastatin (N = 900) %	Placebo (N = 411) %
Cardiovascular				
Cardiac Chest Pain	4.0	3.4	0.1	0.0
Dermatologic				
Rash	4.0*	1.1	1.3	0.9
Gastrointestinal				
Nausea/Vomiting	7.3	7.1	2.9	3.4
Diarrhea	6.2	5.6	2.0	1.9
Abdominal Pain	5.4	6.9	2.0	3.9
Constipation	4.0	7.1	2.4	5.1
Flatulence	3.3	3.6	2.7	3.4
Heartburn	2.9	1.9	2.0	0.7
General				
Fatigue	3.8	3.4	1.9	1.0
Chest Pain	3.7	1.9	0.3	0.2
Influenza	2.4*	0.7	0.0	0.0
Musculoskeletal				
Localized Pain	10.0	9.0	1.4	1.5
Myalgia	2.7	1.0	0.6	0.0
Nervous System				
Headache	6.2	3.9	1.7*	0.2
Dizziness	3.3	3.2	1.0	0.5
Renal/Genitourinary				
Urinary Abnormality	2.4	2.9	0.7	1.2
Respiratory				
Common Cold	7.0	6.3	0.0	0.0
Rhinitis	4.0	4.1	0.1	0.0
Cough	2.6	1.7	0.1	0.0

*Statistically significantly different from placebo.

and, rarely, cirrhosis, fulminant hepatic necrosis, and hepatoma; anorexia, vomiting.
Reproductive: gynecomastia, loss of libido, erectile dysfunction.
Eye: progression of cataracts (lens opacities), ophthalmoplegia.

Laboratory Test Abnormalities
Increases in serum transaminase (ALT, AST) values and CPK have been observed (see WARNINGS).
Transient, asymptomatic eosinophilia has been reported. Eosinophil counts usually returned to normal despite continued therapy. Anemia, thrombocytopenia, and leukopenia have been reported with other HMG-CoA reductase inhibitors.

Concomitant Therapy
Pravastatin has been administered concurrently with cholestyramine, colestipol, nicotinic acid, probucol and gemfibrozil. Preliminary data suggest that the addition of either probucol or gemfibrozil to therapy with lovastatin or pravastatin is **not** associated with greater reduction in LDL-cholesterol than that achieved with lovastatin or pravastatin alone. No adverse reactions unique to the combination or in addition to those previously reported for each drug alone have been reported. Myopathy and rhabdomyolysis (with or without acute renal failure) have been reported when another HMG-CoA reductase inhibitor was used in combination with immunosuppressive drugs, gemfibrozil, erythromycin, or lipid-lowering doses of nicotinic acid. Concomitant therapy with HMG-CoA reductase inhibitors and these agents is generally not recommended. (See WARNINGS: **Skeletal Muscle** and PRECAUTIONS: **Drug Interactions.**)

OVERDOSAGE
There have been no reports of overdoses with pravastatin. Should an accidental overdose occur, treat symptomatically and institute supportive measures as required.

DOSAGE AND ADMINISTRATION
Prior to initiating PRAVACHOL (pravastatin sodium), the patient should be placed on a standard cholesterol-lowering diet (AHA Phase I or NCEP Step 1) for a minimum of 3 to 6 months, depending upon the severity of the lipid elevation. Dietary therapy should be continued during treatment.
The recommended starting dose is 10 or 20 mg once daily at bedtime. In primary hypercholesterolemic patients with significant renal or hepatic dysfunction, and in the elderly, a starting dose of 10 mg daily at bedtime is recommended. PRAVACHOL may be taken without regard to meals.
Since the maximal effect of a given dose is seen within 4 weeks, periodic lipid determinations should be performed at this time and dosage adjusted according to the patient's response to therapy and established treatment guidelines. The recommended dosage range is generally 10 to 40 mg administered once a day at bedtime. In the elderly, maximum reductions in LDL-cholesterol may be achieved with daily doses of 20 mg or less.

Concomitant Therapy
The lipid-lowering effects of PRAVACHOL (pravastatin sodium) on total and LDL cholesterol are enhanced when combined with a bile-acid-binding resin. When administering a bile-acid-binding resin (e.g., cholestyramine, colestipol) and pravastatin, PRAVACHOL should be given either 1 hour or more before or at least 4 hours following the resin. See also ADVERSE REACTIONS: **Concomitant Therapy.**

HOW SUPPLIED
10 mg tablets: bottles of 100 (NDC 0003-0154-50)
20 mg tablets: bottles of 100 (NDC 0003-0178-50)
Bottles contain a desiccant canister.
Unimatic® unit-dose packs are also available for each potency: **10 mg** (NDC 0003-0154-51), **20 mg** (NDC 0003-0178-51).
Tablets are white to off white, round and biconvex. Tablet identification numbers: **10 mg** 154 and **20 mg** 178.
Storage
Do not store above 86°F (30°C). Keep tightly closed (protect from moisture). Protect from light.

(J4-422A)
Shown in Product Identification Section, page 423

Procter & Gamble
P. O. BOX 5516
CINCINNATI, OH 45201

HEAD & SHOULDERS®   OTC
DANDRUFF SHAMPOO

(See PDR For Nonprescription Drugs.)

HEAD & SHOULDERS® DRY SCALP   OTC
DANDRUFF SHAMPOO

(See PDR For Nonprescription Drugs.)

HEAD & SHOULDERS®   OTC
INTENSIVE TREATMENT DANDRUFF SHAMPOO

(See PDR For Nonprescription Drugs.)

Continued on next page

Procter & Gamble—Cont.

METAMUCIL®　　　　　　　　　　OTC
[met 'uh-mū 'sil]
(psyllium hydrophilic mucilloid)

DESCRIPTION
Metamucil is a bulk forming natural therapeutic fiber for restoring and maintaining regularity. It contains hydrophilic mucilloid, a highly efficient dietary fiber derived from the husk of the psyllium seed (*Plantago ovata*). Metamucil contains no chemical stimulants and is nonaddictive. Each dose contains approximately 3.4 grams of psyllium hydrophilic mucilloid. Inactive ingredients, sodium, potassium,

calories, carbohydrate, fat and phenylalanine content are shown in Table 1 for all forms and flavors. Sugar-Free forms contain NutraSweet®* brand sweetener (aspartame). Phenylketonurics should be aware that Sugar Free forms of Metamucil contain phenylalanine. Metamucil in powdered forms is gluten-free. Wafers contain gluten: Apple Crisp 0.7 g/dose, Cinnamon Spice 0.5 g/dose.

ACTIONS
Metamucil provides bulk that promotes elimination. The product is uniform, palatable, and nonirritative in the gastrointestinal tract. Metamucil powder is instantly miscible.

---
*NutraSweet® is a registered trademark of the NutraSweet Company.

INDICATIONS
Metamucil is indicated in the management of chronic constipation, in irritable bowel syndrome, as adjunctive therapy in the constipation of diverticular disease, in the bowel management of patients with hemorrhoids, and for constipation during pregnancy, convalescence, and senility.

CONTRAINDICATIONS
Intestinal obstruction, fecal impaction.

WARNING
Patients are advised they should not use the product without consulting a doctor when abdominal pain, nausea, or vomiting are present, if they have noticed a sudden change in bowel habits that persists over a period of 2 weeks, or rectal bleeding, or if they have been diagnosed with esophageal narrowing or have difficulty in swallowing.

Table 1 — METAMUCIL

FORMS/FLAVORS	INACTIVE INGREDIENTS	SODIUM mg/DOSE	POTASSIUM mg/DOSE	CALORIES PER DOSE	CARBO-HYDRATE g/DOSE	FAT g/DOSE	PHENYL-ALANINE mg/DOSE	DOSAGE 1–3 TIMES DAILY. EACH DOSE CONTAINS 3.4 g PSYLLIUM HYDROPHILIC MUCILLOID	HOW SUPPLIED
Regular Flavor METAMUCIL Powder	Dextrose	<5	30	14	6	—	—	1 rounded teaspoonful 7 g	Canisters: 13, 19 and 29 ozs.
Orange Flavor METAMUCIL Powder	Citric acid, FD&C Yellow No. 6, Flavoring, Sucrose	<5	35	30	10	—	—	1 rounded tablespoonful 11 g	Canisters: 13, 19 and 29 ozs.
Sugar-Free Lemon-Lime Flavor METAMUCIL Effervescent Powder	Aspartame, Calcium carbonate, Citric acid, Flavoring, Potassium bicarbonate, Silicon dioxide, Sodium bicarbonate	10	280	6	4	—	30	1 packet 5.4 g	Cartons: 30 single-dose packets (OTC), 100 single-dose packets (Institutional)
Sugar-Free Orange Flavor METAMUCIL Effervescent Powder	Aspartame, Citric acid, FD&C Yellow No. 6, Flavoring, Potassium bicarbonate, Silicon dioxide, Sodium bicarbonate	5	280	6	4	—	28	1 packet 5.2 g	Cartons: 30 single-dose packets (OTC)
Sunrise Smooth Orange Flavor METAMUCIL Powder	Citric acid, D&C Yellow No. 10, FD&C Yellow No. 6, Flavoring, Sucrose	<5	30	35	12	—	—	1 rounded tablespoonful 12 g	Canisters: 13, 19 and 29 ozs.; Cartons: 30 single-dose packets (OTC)
Sunrise Smooth Citrus Flavor METAMUCIL Powder	Citric acid, D&C Yellow No. 10, FD&C Yellow No. 6, Flavoring, Sucrose	<5	40	35	12	—	—	1 rounded tablespoonful 12 g	Canisters: 13, 19 and 29 ozs.; Cartons: 30 single-dose packets (OTC) 100 single-dose packets (Institutional)
Sunrise Smooth Sugar-Free Orange Flavor METAMUCIL Powder	Aspartame, Citric acid, D&C Yellow No. 10, FD&C Yellow No. 6, Flavoring, Maltodextrin	<5	30	10	5	—	25	1 rounded teaspoonful 5.8 g	Canisters: 10, 15 and 23 ozs.; Cartons: 30 single-dose packets (OTC), 100 single-dose packets (Institutional)
Sunrise Smooth Sugar-Free Citrus Flavor METAMUCIL Powder	Aspartame, Citric acid, D&C Yellow No. 10, FD&C Yellow No. 6, Flavoring, Maltodextrin	<5	30	10	5	—	25	1 rounded teaspoonful 5.8 g	Canisters: 10, 15 and 23 ozs.; Cartons: 30 single-dose packets (OTC)
Apple Crisp METAMUCIL Wafers	Ascorbic acid, Brown sugar, Cinnamon, Corn oil, Flavors, Fructose, Lecithin, Modified food starch, Molasses, Oat hull fiber, Sodium bicarbonate, Sucrose, Water, Wheat flour	20	50	100	19	5	—	2 wafers 25 g	Cartons: 12 doses; 24 doses
Cinnamon Spice METAMUCIL Wafers	Ascorbic acid, Cinnamon, Corn oil, Flavors, Fructose, Lecithin, Modified food starch, Molasses, Nutmeg, Oat hull fiber, Oats, Sodium bicarbonate, Sucrose, Water, Wheat flour	20	45	100	18	5	—	2 wafers 25 g	Cartons: 12 doses; 24 doses,

PRECAUTION

May cause allergic reaction in people sensitive to inhaled or ingested psyllium. Notice to Health Care Professionals: To minimize the potential for allergic reaction, health care professionals who frequently dispense powdered psyllium products should avoid inhaling airborne dust while dispensing these products. Handling and Dispensing: To minimize generating airborne dust, spoon product from the canister into a glass according to label directions.

DOSAGE AND ADMINISTRATION

The usual adult dosage is 1 rounded teaspoonful or tablespoonful of powder, depending on the flavor, measured into a standard 8-oz glass which is then filled with cool water, fruit juice, milk or other beverage, or 2 wafers with an 8-oz glass of beverage. See Table 1. With effervescent forms, the contents of a packet are poured into an 8-oz glass and the glass is slowly filled with liquid. An additional glass of liquid after each dose is helpful. The product should be taken with enough liquid or it may obstruct the throat. For children (6 to 12 years old), use $\frac{1}{2}$ the adult dose in/with 8-oz of liquid, 1 to 3 times daily.

Metamucil can be taken orally one to three times a day, depending on the need and response. The product generally produces an effect in 12 to 72 hours.

NEW USERS

(Label statement)

Your doctor can recommend the right dosage of Metamucil to best meet your needs. In general, start by taking one dose each day. Gradually increase to three doses per day, if needed or recommended by your doctor. If minor gas or bloating occurs when you increase doses, try slightly reducing the amount you are taking.

HOW SUPPLIED

Powder: canisters (OTC) and cartons of single-dose packets (OTC and Institutional). Wafers: cartons of single-dose packets (OTC). (See Table 1).

PEPTO-BISMOL® ORIGINAL LIQUID AND ORIGINAL AND CHERRY TABLETS — OTC

For diarrhea, heartburn, indigestion, upset stomach and nausea.

DESCRIPTION

Each Pepto-Bismol Tablet contains 262 mg bismuth subsalicylate and each tablespoonful (15 ml) of Pepto-Bismol Liquid contains 262 mg bismuth subsalicylate. Each tablet contains 102 mg salicylate (99 mg salicylate for Cherry) and each tablespoonful of liquid contains 130 mg salicylate. Liquid and tablets contain no sugar. Tablets are very low in sodium (less than 2 mg/tablet) and Liquid is low in sodium (less than 3 mg/tablespoonful). Inactive ingredients include (Tablets): adipic acid (in Cherry only), calcium carbonate, D&C Red No. 27, FD&C Red No. 40 (in Cherry only), flavors, magnesium stearate, mannitol, povidone, saccharin sodium and talc; (Liquid): benzoic acid, D&C Red No. 22, D&C Red No. 28, flavor, magnesium aluminum silicate, methylcellulose, saccharin sodium, salicylic acid, sodium salicylate, sorbic acid and water.

INDICATIONS

Pepto-Bismol controls diarrhea within 24 hours, relieving associated abdominal cramps; soothes heartburn and indigestion without constipating; and relieves nausea and upset stomach.

WARNINGS

Children and teenagers who have or are recovering from chicken pox or flu should not use this medicine to treat nausea or vomiting. If nausea or vomiting is present, patients are advised to consult a doctor because this could be an early sign of Reye Syndrome, a rare but serious illness.

This product contains salicylates. If taken with aspirin and ringing in the ears occurs, discontinue use. This product does not contain aspirin, but should not be administered to those patients who have a known allergy to aspirin or salicylates. Caution is advised in the administration to patients taking medication for anticoagulation, diabetes and gout.

If diarrhea is accompanied by a high fever or continues more than 2 days, patients are advised to consult a physician. As with any drug, caution is advised in the administration to pregnant or nursing women.

Note: This medication may cause a temporary and harmless darkening of the tongue and/or stool. Stool darkening should not be confused with melena.

OVERDOSAGE

In case of overdose, patients are advised to contact a physician or Poison Control Center. Emesis induced by ipecac syrup is indicated in large ingestions provided ipecac can be administered within one hour of ingestion. Activated charcoal should be administered after gastric emptying. Patients should be evaluated for signs and symptoms of salicylate toxicity.

DOSAGE AND ADMINISTRATION

Tablets:

Adults—Two tablets

Children (according to age)—

9–12 yrs. 1 tablet

6–9 yrs. $\frac{2}{3}$ tablet

3–6 yrs. $\frac{1}{3}$ tablet

Chew or dissolve in mouth. Repeat every $\frac{1}{2}$ to 1 hour as needed, to a maximum of 8 doses in a 24-hour period.

Liquid: Shake well before using.

Adults—2 tablespoonsful (1 dose cup)

Children (according to age)—

9–12 yrs. 1 tablespoonful ($\frac{1}{2}$ dose cup)

6–9 yrs. 2 teaspoonsful ($\frac{1}{3}$ dose cup)

3–6 yrs. 1 teaspoonful ($\frac{1}{6}$ dose cup)

Repeat dosage every $\frac{1}{2}$ to 1 hour, if needed, to a maximum of 8 doses in a 24-hour period.

For children under 3 years, dose according to weight.

18–28 lbs. 1 teaspoonful

14–18 lbs. $\frac{1}{2}$ teaspoonful

Repeat every 4 hours, if needed, to a maximum of 6 doses in a 24-hour period.

HOW SUPPLIED

Pepto-Bismol Liquid is available in: 4 fl. oz. bottle, 8 fl. oz. bottle, 12 fl. oz. bottle, 16 fl. oz. bottle. Pepto-Bismol Tablets are pink, round, chewable tablets imprinted with "Pepto-Bismol" on one side. Tablets are available in: box of 30, box of 48 and roll pack of 12 (cherry only).

PEPTO-BISMOL® MAXIMUM STRENGTH LIQUID — OTC

For diarrhea, heartburn, indigestion, upset stomach and nausea.

DESCRIPTION

Each tablespoonful (15 ml) of Maximum Strength Pepto-Bismol Liquid contains 525 mg bismuth subsalicylate (236 mg salicylate). Maximum Strength Pepto-Bismol Liquid contains no sugar and is low in sodium (less than 3 mg/tablespoonful). Inactive ingredients include: benzoic acid, D&C Red No. 22, D&C Red No. 28, flavor, magnesium aluminum silicate, methylcellulose, saccharin sodium, salicylic acid, sodium salicylate, sorbic acid and water.

INDICATIONS

Maximum Strength Pepto-Bismol controls diarrhea within 24 hours, relieving associated abdominal cramps; soothes heartburn and indigestion without constipating; and relieves nausea and upset stomach.

WARNINGS

Children and teenagers who have or are recovering from chicken pox or flu should NOT use this medicine to treat nausea or vomiting. If nausea or vomiting is present, patients are advised to consult a doctor because this could be an early sign of Reye Syndrome, a rare but serious illness.

This product contains salicylates. If taken with aspirin and ringing in the ears occurs, discontinue use. This product does not contain aspirin, but should not be administered to those patients who have a known allergy to aspirin or salicylates. Caution is advised in the administration to patients taking medication for anticoagulation, diabetes, and gout.

If diarrhea is accompanied by a high fever or continues more than 2 days, patients are advised to consult a physician. As with any drug, caution is advised in the administration to pregnant or nursing women.

Note: This medication may cause a temporary and harmless darkening of the tongue and/or stool. Stool darkening should not be confused with melena.

OVERDOSAGE

In case of overdose, patients are advised to contact a physician or Poison Control Center. Emesis induced by ipecac syrup is indicated in large ingestions provided ipecac can be administered within one hour of ingestion. Activated charcoal should be administered after gastric emptying. Patients should be evaluated for signs and symptoms of salicylate toxicity.

DOSAGE AND ADMINISTRATION

Shake well before using.

Adults—2 tablespoonfuls (1 dose cup)

Children (according to age)—

9–12 yrs. 1 tablespoonful ($\frac{1}{2}$ dose cup)

6–9 yrs. 2 teaspoonful ($\frac{1}{3}$ dose cup)

3–6 yrs. 1 teaspoonful ($\frac{1}{6}$ dose cup)

Repeat dosage every hour, if needed, to a maximum of 4 doses in a 24 hour period.

HOW SUPPLIED

Maximum Strength Pepto-Bismol is available in:

4 fl. oz. bottle

8 fl. oz. bottle

12 fl. oz. bottle

PERIDEX® — ℞

[per-i-dex]

(chlorhexidine gluconate)

Oral Rinse

PRODUCT OVERVIEW

KEY FACTS

Peridex is an antimicrobial oral rinse containing 0.12% chlorhexidine gluconate. Peridex has been shown to achieve significant reductions in gingivitis as characterized by gingival inflammation and associated bleeding which can complicate certain dental procedures. Approximately 30% of the active ingredient is retained in the oral cavity following a single rinsing. This retained active is slowly released into the oral fluids.

MAJOR USES

Peridex has proved to be clinically effective for use between dental visits as part of a professional program for the treatment of gingivitis as characterized by gingival bleeding and inflammation. Therapy should be initiated directly following an oral prophylaxis. Patients using Peridex should be reevaluated and given a thorough prophylaxis at intervals no longer than six months. Recommended use is a 30-second rinse of $\frac{1}{2}$ fluid ounce (marked in cap) twice daily.

SAFETY INFORMATION

The most common side effects associated with chlorhexidine oral rinses are (1) an increase in staining of teeth and other oral surfaces on certain individuals, (2) an increase in supragingival calculus formation, and (3) an alteration in taste perception. Not all patients will experience a visually significant increase in tooth staining. Staining can be removed from most tooth surfaces by a conventional professional prophylaxis. No serious systemic adverse reactions associated with use of Peridex were observed in clinical testing.

PRESCRIBING INFORMATION

PERIDEX® — ℞

(chlorhexidine gluconate)

Oral Rinse

DESCRIPTION

Peridex is an oral rinse containing 0.12% chlorhexidine gluconate (1,1′ -hexamethylene bis [5-(p-chlorophenyl) biguanide] di-D-gluconate) in a base containing water, 11.6% alcohol, glycerin, PEG-40 sorbitan diisostearate, flavor, sodium saccharin, and FD&C Blue No. 1. Peridex is a near-neutral solution (pH range 5–7). Chlorhexidine gluconate is a salt of chlorhexidine and gluconic acid. Its chemical structure is:

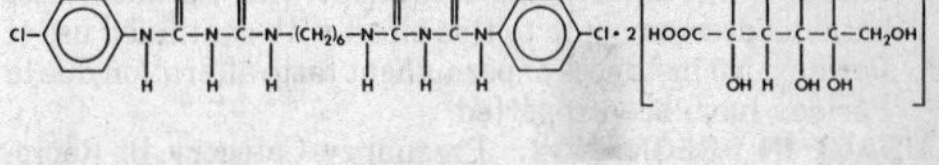

CLINICAL PHARMACOLOGY

Peridex provides microbicidal activity during oral rinsing. The clinical significance of Peridex's antimicrobial activities is not clear. Microbiological sampling of plaque has shown a general reduction of counts of certain assayed bacteria, both aerobic and anaerobic, ranging from 54–97% through six months' use.

Use of Peridex in a six-month clinical study did not result in any significant changes in bacterial resistance, overgrowth of potentially opportunistic organisms or other adverse changes in the oral microbial ecosystem. Three months after Peridex use was discontinued the number of bacteria in plaque had returned to baseline levels and resistance of plaque bacteria to chlorhexidine gluconate was equal to that at baseline.

PHARMACOKINETICS

Pharmacokinetic studies with Peridex indicate approximately 30% of the active ingredient, chlorhexidine gluconate, is retained in the oral cavity following rinsing. This retained drug is slowly released into the oral fluids. Studies conducted on human subjects and animals demonstrate that any ingested chlorhexidine gluconate is poorly absorbed from the gastrointestinal tract. The mean plasma level of chlorhexidine gluconate reached a peak of 0.206 μg/g in humans 30 minutes after they ingested a 300-mg dose of the drug. Detectable levels of chlorhexidine gluconate were not present in the plasma of these subjects 12 hours after the compound was administered. Excretion of chlorhexidine gluconate occurred primarily through the feces (~90%). Less than 1% of the chlorhexidine gluconate ingested by these subjects was excreted in the urine.

INDICATION

Peridex is indicated for use between dental visits as part of a professional program for the treatment of gingivitis as characterized by redness and swelling of the gingivae, including gingival bleeding upon probing. Peridex has not been tested

Continued on next page

Procter & Gamble—Cont.

among patients with acute necrotizing ulcerative gingivitis (ANUG). For patients having coexisting gingivitis and periodontitis, see PRECAUTIONS.

CONTRAINDICATIONS

Peridex should not be used by persons who are known to be hypersensitive to chlorhexidine gluconate.

WARNINGS

The effect of Peridex on periodontitis has not been determined. An increase in supragingival calculus was noted in clinical testing in Peridex users compared with control users. It is not known if Peridex use results in an increase in subgingival calculus. Calculus deposits should be removed by a dental prophylaxis at intervals no greater than six months. Rare hypersensitivity and generalized allergic reactions have also been reported. Peridex should not be used by persons who have a sensitivity to it or its components.

PRECAUTIONS

GENERAL:

1. For patients having coexisting gingivitis and periodontitis, the presence or absence of gingival inflammation following treatment with Peridex should not be used as a major indicator of underlying periodontitis.
2. Peridex can cause staining of oral surfaces, such as tooth surfaces, restorations, and the dorsum of the tongue. Not all patients will experience a visually significant increase in toothstaining. In clinical testing, 56% of Peridex users exhibited a measurable increase in facial anterior stain, compared to 35% of control users after six months; 15% of Peridex users developed what was judged to be heavy stain, compared to 1% of control users after six months. Stain will be more pronounced in patients who have heavier accumulations of unremoved plaque.
   Stain resulting from use of Peridex does not adversely affect health of the gingivae or other oral tissues. Stain can be removed from most tooth surfaces by conventional professional prophylactic techniques. Additional time may be required to complete the prophylaxis.
   Discretion should be used when prescribing to patients with anterior facial restorations with rough surfaces or margins. If natural stain cannot be removed from these surfaces by a dental prophylaxis, patients should be excluded from Peridex treatment if permanent discoloration is unacceptable. Stain in these areas may be difficult to remove by dental prophylaxis and on rare occasions may necessitate replacement of these restorations.
3. Some patients may experience an alteration in taste perception while undergoing treatment with Peridex. Most patients accommodate to this effect with continued use of Peridex. No instances of permanent taste alteration due to Peridex have been reported.

USAGE IN PREGNANCY: Pregnancy Category B. Reproduction and fertility studies with chlorhexidine gluconate have been conducted. No evidence of impaired fertility was observed in rats at doses up to 100 mg/kg/day, and no evidence of harm to the fetus was observed in rats and rabbits at doses up to 300 mg/kg/day and 40 mg/kg/day, respectively. These doses are approximately 100, 300, and 40 times that which would result from a person's ingesting 30 ml (2 capfuls) of Peridex per day. Since controlled studies in pregnant women have not been conducted, the benefits of the drug in pregnant women should be weighed against possible risk to the fetus.

NURSING MOTHERS: It is not known whether this drug is excreted in human milk. Because many drugs are excreted in human milk, caution should be exercised when Peridex is administered to a nursing woman.

In parturition and lactation studies with rats, no evidence of impaired parturition or of toxic effects to suckling pups was observed when chlorhexidine gluconate was administered to dams at doses that were over 100 times greater than that which would result from a person's ingesting 30 ml (2 capfuls) of Peridex per day.

PEDIATRIC USE: Clinical effectiveness and safety of Peridex have not been established in children under the age of 18.

CARCINOGENESIS, MUTAGENESIS: In a drinking water study in rats, carcinogenesis was not observed. The highest dose of chlorhexidine gluconate used in this study, 38 mg/kg/day, is at least 500 times the amount that would be ingested from the recommended daily dose of Peridex.

In two mammalian *in vivo* mutagenic studies with chlorhexidine gluconate, mutagenesis was not observed. The highest dose of chlorhexidine gluconate used in a mouse dominant lethal assay was 1000 mg/kg/day and in a hamster cytogenetics test was 250 mg/kg/day, i.e. > 3200 times the amount that would be ingested from the recommended daily dose of Peridex.

ADVERSE REACTIONS

The most common side effects associated with chlorhexidine gluconate oral rinses are (1) an increase in staining of teeth and other oral surfaces, (2) an increase in calculus formation, and (3) an alteration in taste perception; see WARNINGS and PRECAUTIONS. No serious systemic adverse reactions associated with use of Peridex were observed in clinical testing.

Minor irritation and superficial desquamation of the oral mucosa have been noted in patients using Peridex, particularly among children.

Although there have been no reports of parotitis (inflammation or swelling of salivary glands) among Peridex users in controlled clinical studies, transient parotitis has been reported in research studies with chlorhexidine-containing mouthrinses.

OVERDOSAGE

Ingestion of 1 or 2 ounces of Peridex by a small child (~10 kg body weight) might result in gastric distress, including nausea, or signs of alcohol intoxication. Medical attention should be sought if more than 4 ounces of Peridex is ingested by a small child or if signs of alcohol intoxication develop.

DOSAGE AND ADMINISTRATION

Peridex therapy should be initiated directly following a dental prophylaxis and periodontal examination. Patients using Peridex should be reevaluated and given a thorough prophylaxis at intervals no longer than six months.

Recommended use is twice daily oral rinsing for 30 seconds, morning and evening after toothbrushing. Usual dosage is ½ fl. oz. (marked in cap) of undiluted Peridex. Peridex is not intended for ingestion and should be expectorated after rinsing.

HOW SUPPLIED

Peridex is supplied as a blue liquid in dispenser packs of three 1-pint amber plastic bottles with child-resistant dispensing closures. Store above freezing (32°F).

NDC 37000-007- 01

Military-6505-01-253-8138

Procter & Gamble Pharmaceuticals, Inc.

13-27 EATON AVENUE
NORWICH, NY 13815-1799

Formerly Norwich Eaton Pharmaceuticals, Inc.
(Also see Procter & Gamble and Richardson-Vicks, Inc.)

Literature on Procter & Gamble Pharmaceuticals products sent to physicians on request.

Information on these Procter & Gamble Pharmaceuticals products is based on labeling in effect June 1, 1992. Further information on these and other Procter & Gamble Pharmaceuticals products may be obtained by direct inquiry to Medical Department, Procter & Gamble Pharmaceuticals, P.O. Box 191, Norwich, N.Y. 13815-0191, or phone 800, 448-4878.

ASACOL® ℞

[*āce 'ah-kol*]
(mesalamine)
Delayed-Release Tablets

DESCRIPTION

Each **Asacol** delayed-release tablet for oral administration contains 400 mg of mesalamine, an anti-inflammatory drug. The **Asacol** delayed-release tablets are coated with acrylic based resin, Eudragit S (methacrylic acid copolymer B, NF), which dissolves at pH 7 or greater, releasing mesalamine in the terminal ileum and beyond for topical anti-inflammatory action in the colon. Mesalamine has the chemical name 5-amino-2-hydroxybenzoic acid; its structural formula is:

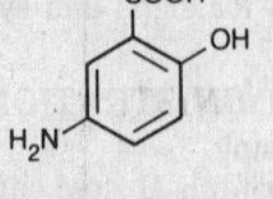

Molecular Weight: 153.1
Molecular Formula: $C_7H_7NO_3$

Inactive Ingredients: Each tablet contains colloidal silicon dioxide, dibutyl phthalate, edible black ink, iron oxide red, iron oxide yellow, lactose, magnesium stearate, methacrylic acid copolymer B (Eudragit S), polyethylene glycol, povidone, sodium starch glycolate, and talc.

CLINICAL PHARMACOLOGY

Mesalamine is thought to be the major therapeutically active part of the sulfasalazine molecule in the treatment of ulcerative colitis. Sulfasalazine is converted to equimolar amounts of sulfapyridine and mesalamine by bacterial action in the colon. The usual oral dose of sulfasalazine for active ulcerative colitis is 3 to 4 grams daily in divided doses, which provides 1.2 to 1.6 grams of mesalamine to the colon.

The mechanism of action of mesalamine (and sulfasalazine) is unknown, but appears to be topical rather than systemic. Mucosal production of arachidonic acid (AA) metabolites, both through the cyclooxygenase pathways, *i.e.*, prostanoids, and through the lipoxygenase pathways, *i.e.*, leukotrienes (LTs) and hydroxyeicosatetraenoic acids (HETEs), is increased in patients with chronic inflammatory bowel disease, and it is possible that mesalamine diminishes inflammation by blocking cyclooxygenase and inhibiting prostaglandin (PG) production in the colon.

Pharmacokinetics: Asacol tablets are coated with an acrylic-based resin that delays release of mesalamine until it reaches the terminal ileum and beyond. This has been demonstrated in human studies conducted with radiological and serum markers. Approximately 28% of the mesalamine in **Asacol** tablets is absorbed after oral ingestion, leaving the remainder available for topical action and excretion in the feces. Absorption of mesalamine is similar in fasted and fed subjects. The absorbed mesalamine is rapidly acetylated in the gut mucosal wall and by the liver. It is excreted mainly by the kidney as N-acetyl-5-amino-salicylic acid.

Mesalamine from orally administered **Asacol** tablets appears to be more extensively absorbed than the mesalamine released from sulfasalazine. Maximum plasma levels of mesalamine and N-acetyl-5-aminosalicylic acid following multiple **Asacol** doses are about 1.5 to 2 times higher than those following an equivalent dose of mesalamine in the form of sulfasalazine. Combined mesalamine and N-acetyl-5-aminosalicylic acid AUC's and urine drug dose recoveries following multiple doses of **Asacol** tablets are about 1.3 to 1.5 times higher than those following an equivalent dose of mesalamine in the form of sulfasalazine.

The t_{max} for mesalamine and its metabolite, N-acetyl-5-aminosalicylic acid, is usually delayed, reflecting the delayed release, and ranges from 4 to 12 hours. The half-lives of elimination ($t½_{elm}$) for mesalamine and N-acetyl-5-aminosalicylic acid are usually about 12 hours, but are variable, ranging from 2 to 15 hours. There is a large inter-subject variability in the plasma concentrations of mesalamine and N-acetyl-5-aminosalicyclic acid and in their elimination half-lives following administration of **Asacol** tablets.

Clinical Studies: Two placebo-controlled studies have demonstrated the efficacy of **Asacol** tablets in patients with mildly to moderately active ulcerative colitis. In one randomized, double-blind, multicenter trial of 158 patients, **Asacol** doses of 1.6 g/day and 2.4 g/day were compared to placebo. At the dose of 2.4 g/day, **Asacol** tablets reduced the disease activity, with 21 of 43 (49%). **Asacol** patients showing improvement in sigmoidoscopic appearance of the bowel compared to 12 of 44 (27%) placebo patients ($p=0.048$). In addition, significantly more patients in the **Asacol** 2.4 g/day group showed improvement in rectal bleeding and stool frequency. The 1.6 g/day dose did not produce consistent evidence of effectiveness.

In a second randomized, double-blind, placebo-controlled clinical trial of 6 weeks duration in 87 ulcerative colitis patients, **Asacol** tablets, at a dose of 4.8 g/day, gave sigmoidoscopic improvement in 28 of 38 (74%) patients compared to 10 of 38 (26%) placebo patients ($p<0.001$). Also, more patients in the **Asacol** 4.8 g/day group showed improvement in overall symptoms.

The effect of **Asacol** (mesalamine) on sulfasalazine-induced impairment of male fertility was examined in an open-label study. Nine patients (age < 40 years) with chronic ulcerative colitis in clinical remission on sulfasalazine 2–3 g/day were crossed over to an equivalent **Asacol** dose (0.8–1.2 g/day) for 3 months. Improvement in sperm count ($p<0.02$) and morphology ($p<0.02$) occurred in all cases. Improvement in sperm motility ($p<0.001$) occurred in 8 of the 9 patients.

INDICATIONS AND USAGE

Asacol tablets are indicated for the treatment of mildly to moderately active ulcerative colitis.

CONTRAINDICATIONS

Asacol tablets are contraindicated in patients with hypersensitivity to salicylates or to any of the components of the **Asacol** tablet.

PRECAUTIONS

General: Patients with pyloric stenosis may have prolonged gastric retention of **Asacol** tablets which could delay release of mesalamine in the colon.

Exacerbation of the symptoms of colitis, thought to have been caused by mesalamine or sulfasalazine has been reported in 3% of patients in controlled clinical trials. This acute reaction, characterized by cramping, abdominal pain, bloody diarrhea, and occasionally by fever, headache, malaise, pruritus, rash, and conjunctivitis, has been reported after the initiation of **Asacol** tablets as well as other mesalamine products. Symptoms usually abate when **Asacol** tablets are discontinued.

Renal: Renal impairment, including minimal change nephropathy, and acute and chronic interstitial nephritis, has been reported in patients taking **Asacol** tablets as well as in patients taking other mesalamine products. In animal studies (rats, dogs), the kidney is the principal target organ for toxicity. At doses of approximately 750–1000 mg/kg [15–20 times the administered recommended human dose (based on a 50 kg person) on a mg/kg basis and 3–4 times on a mg/m² basis], mesalamine causes renal papillary necrosis. **Therefore, caution should be exercised when using Asacol (mesalamine) or other compounds converted to mesalamine or its metabolites in patients with known renal dysfunction or history of renal disease. It is recommended that all patients have an evaluation of renal function prior to initiation of Asacol tablets and periodically while on Asacol therapy.**
Information for Patients: Patients should be instructed to swallow the **Asacol** tablets whole, taking care not to break the outer coating. The outer coating is designed to remain intact to protect the active ingredient and thus ensure mesalamine availability for action in the colon. In 2–3% of patients in clinical studies, intact or partially intact tablets have been reported in the stool. If this occurs repeatedly, patients should contact their physician.
Drug Interactions: There are no known drug interactions.
Carcinogenesis, Mutagenesis, Impairment of Fertility: Long-term studies in animals have not been performed to evaluate the carcinogenicity potential of mesalamine. Mesalamine was not mutagenic in fluctuation assay in *K. pneumoniae* and Ames assay in *S. typhimurium*. Mesalamine, at oral doses up to 480 mg/kg/day, had no adverse effect on fertility or reproductive performance of male and female rats. The oligospermia and infertility in men associated with sulfasalazine have not been reported with **Asacol** delayed-release tablets.
Pregnancy: Teratogenic Effects: Pregnancy Category B: Reproduction studies in rats and rabbits at oral doses up to 480 mg/kg/day have revealed no evidence of teratogenic effects or fetal toxicity due to mesalamine. There are, however, no adequate and well-controlled studies in pregnant women. Because animal reproduction studies are not always predictive of human response, this drug should be used during pregnancy only if clearly needed.
Nursing Mothers: Low concentrations of mesalamine and higher concentrations of its N-acetyl metabolite have been detected in human breast milk. While the clinical significance of this has not been determined, caution should be exercised when mesalamine is administered to a nursing woman.
Pediatric Use: Safety and effectiveness of **Asacol** tablets in children have not been established.

ADVERSE REACTIONS

Asacol tablets have been evaluated in about 1830 inflammatory bowel disease patients (most patients with ulcerative colitis) in controlled and open-label studies. Adverse events seen in clinical trials with **Asacol** tablets have generally been mild and reversible. In two short-term (6 weeks) placebo-controlled clinical studies involving 245 patients, 155 of whom were randomized to **Asacol** tablets, five (3.2%) of the **Asacol** patients discontinued **Asacol** therapy because of adverse events as compared to two (2.2%) of the placebo patients. Adverse reactions leading to withdrawal of **Asacol** tablets included (each in one patient): diarrhea and colitis flare; dizziness, nausea, joint pain, and headache; rash, lethargy and constipation; dry mouth, malaise, lower back discomfort, mild disorientation, mild indigestion and cramping; headache, nausea, malaise, aching, vomiting, muscle cramps, a stuffy head, plugged ears, and fever.
Adverse events occurring at a frequency of 2% or greater in the two short-term, double-blind, placebo-controlled trials mentioned above are listed in Table 1 above. Overall, the incidence of adverse events seen with **Asacol** tablets was similar to placebo.
Of these adverse events, only rash showed a consistently higher frequency with increasing **Asacol** dose in these studies. In uncontrolled data, fever, flu syndrome, and headache also seemed dose-related.
In addition, the following adverse reactions were seen in 1–2% of the patients in the controlled studies: malaise, arthritis, increased cough, acne, and conjunctivitis.
Over 1800 patients have been treated with **Asacol** tablets in clinical studies. In addition to the adverse events listed above, the following adverse events also have been reported in controlled clinical studies, open-label studies, or foreign marketing experience. The relationship of the reported events to **Asacol** administration is unclear in many cases. Some complaints, including anorexia, joint pains, pyoderma gangrenosum, oral ulcers, and anemia could be part of the clinical presentation of inflammatory bowel disease.
Body as a Whole: Weakness, neck pain, abdominal enlargement, facial edema, edema.
Cardiovascular: Pericarditis (rare), myocarditis (rare), vasodilation, migraine.
Digestive: Anorexia, hepatitis (rare), pancreatitis, gastroenteritis, gastritis, increased appetite, cholecystitis, dry

Table 1
Frequency (%) of Common Adverse Events
Reported in Ulcerative Colitis Patients
Treated with **Asacol** Tablets or Placebo in
Double-Blind Controlled Studies

	Percent of Patients with Adverse Events	
Event	Placebo (n=89)	Asacol tablets (n=152)
Headache	35	35
Abdominal pain	12	18
Eructation	13	16
Pain	8	14
Nausea	15	13
Pharyngitis	9	11
Dizziness	8	8
Asthenia	15	7
Diarrhea	9	7
Back pain	5	7
Fever	8	7
Rash	3	6
Dyspepsia	1	6
Rhinitis	5	5
Arthralgia	3	5
Vomiting	2	5
Constipation	1	5
Hypertonia	4	5
Flatulence	7	3
Flu syndrome	2	3
Chills	2	3
Colitis exacerbation	0	3
Chest pain	2	3
Peripheral edema	2	3
Myalgia	1	3
Pruritus	0	3
Sweating	1	3
Dysmenorrhea	3	3

mouth, oral ulcers, perforated peptic ulcer (rare), bloody diarrhea, tenesmus.
Hematologic: Agranulocytosis (rare), thrombocytopenia, eosinophilia, leukopenia, anemia, lymphadenopathy.
Musculoskeletal: Gout.
Nervous: Anxiety, insomnia, depression, somnolence, emotional lability, hyperesthesia, vertigo, nervousness, confusion, paresthesia, tremor, peripheral neuropathy (rare), transverse myelitis (rare), Guillain-Barre syndrome (rare).
Respiratory/Pulmonary: Sinusitis, interstitial pneumonitis, asthma exacerbation.
Skin: Alopecia, psoriasis (rare), pyoderma gangrenosum (rare), dry skin, erythema nodosum, urticaria.
Special Senses: Ear pain, eye pain, taste perversion, blurred vision, tinnitus.
Urogenital: Interstitial nephritis (See also Renal subsection in PRECAUTIONS), minimal change nephropathy (See also Renal subsection in PRECAUTIONS), dysuria, urinary urgency, hematuria, epididymitis, menorrhagia.
Laboratory Abnormalities: Elevated AST (SGPT) or ALT (SGOT), elevated alkaline phosphatase, elevated serum creatinine and BUN.
Hepatitis has been reported to occur rarely with **Asacol** tablets. More commonly, asymptomatic elevations of liver enzymes have occurred which usually resolve during continued use or with discontinuation of the drug.

DRUG ABUSE AND DEPENDENCY
Abuse: None reported.
Dependency: Drug dependence has not been reported with chronic administration of mesalamine.

OVERDOSAGE
One case of overdosage has been reported. A 3-year-old male ingested 2 grams of **Asacol** tablets. He was treated with ipecac and activated charcoal. No adverse events occurred. Oral doses of mesalamine in mice and rats of 5000 mg/kg and 4595 mg/kg, respectively, cause significant lethality.

DOSAGE AND ADMINISTRATION
The usual dosage in adults is two 400-mg tablets to be taken three times a day for a total daily dose of 2.4 grams for a duration of 6 weeks.

HOW SUPPLIED
Asacol tablets are available as red-brown, capsule-shaped tablets containing 400 mg mesalamine and imprinted "Asacol NE" in black.
NDC 0149-0752-02 Bottle of 100
Store at controlled room temperature (59°–86°F or 15°–30°C).

CAUTION
Federal law prohibits dispensing without prescription.
Manufactured by:
Röhm Pharma, G.m.b.H.
D-6108 Weiterstadt 1
Germany

for:
Procter & Gamble Pharmaceuticals
Norwich, New York 13815
Under license from Tillotts Pharma AG, the registered trademark owner.
©1992 P&GP
JANUARY 1992
ASACOL-P2

COMHIST® LA   ℞
[kŏm'hist]

DESCRIPTION
Each COMHIST LA yellow and clear capsule for oral administration contains:

chlorpheniramine maleate .... 4 mg
phenyltoloxamine citrate .... 50 mg
phenylephrine hydrochloride .... 20 mg

in a special base to provide a prolonged therapeutic effect. This product contains ingredients of the following therapeutic classes: antihistamine and decongestant.
Chlorpheniramine maleate is an antihistamine having the chemical name γ-(4-chlorophenyl)-N,N-dimethyl-2-pyridine-propanamine,(Z)-2-butenedioate(1:1) with the following structure:

Phenyltoloxamine citrate is an antihistamine having the chemical name N,N-dimethyl-2-(α-phenyl-o-tolyloxy) ethylamine dihydrogen citrate with the following structure:

Phenylephrine hydrochloride is a decongestant having the chemical name 3-hydroxy-α[(methylamino)methyl]benzenemethanol hydrochloride with the following structure:

INACTIVE INGREDIENTS
Each capsule contains FD&C Blue #2, edible black ink, gelatin, sugar spheres, D&C Yellow #10, FD&C Yellow #6, and other ingredients.

CLINICAL PHARMACOLOGY
Chlorpheniramine maleate is an alkylamine-type antihistamine while phenyltoloxamine citrate belongs to the ethanolamine chemical class. The antihistamines in COMHIST LA act by competing with histamine for H_1 histamine receptor sites, thereby preventing the action of histamine on the cell. Clinically, chlorpheniramine and phenyltoloxamine suppress the histamine-mediated symptoms of allergic rhinitis, relieving sneezing, rhinorrhea, and itching of the eyes, nose, and throat.
Phenylephrine hydrochloride is an α-adrenergic receptor agonist (sympathomimetic) which produces vasoconstriction by stimulating α-receptors within the mucosa of the respiratory tract. Clinically, phenylephrine shrinks swollen mucous membranes, reduces tissue hyperemia, edema, and nasal congestion, and increases nasal airway patency.

INDICATIONS AND USAGE
COMHIST LA is indicated for the relief of rhinorrhea and congestion associated with seasonal and/or perennial allergic rhinitis and vasomotor rhinitis.

CONTRAINDICATIONS
COMHIST LA is contraindicated in persons hypersensitive to any of its components. It should not be administered to children under 12 years of age, patients with severe hypertension, narrow angle glaucoma, or asthmatic symptoms, or patients taking monoamine oxidase inhibitors.

WARNINGS
Chlorpheniramine maleate and phenyltoloxamine citrate should be used with extreme caution in patients with stenosing peptic ulcer, pyloroduodenal obstruction, prostatic hypertrophy, or bladder neck obstruction. These compounds have an atropine-like action and therefore should be used with caution in patients with a history of bronchial asthma, increased intraocular pressure, cardiovascular disease, or

Continued on next page

Procter & Gamble Pharm.—Cont.

hypertension. Sympathomimetic amines should be used with caution in patients with hypertension, diabetes mellitus, heart disease, increased intraocular pressure, hyperthyroidism, or prostatic hypertrophy.

PRECAUTIONS

Information for Patients: This product may cause sedation. Patients should be cautioned against engaging in activities requiring mental alertness, such as driving a car or operating machinery.

Drug Interactions: The sedative effects of chlorpheniramine maleate and phenyltoloxamine citrate are additive to the CNS depressant effects of alcohol, hypnotics, sedatives, and tranquilizers. COMHIST LA should not be used in patients taking monoamine oxidase inhibitors.

Pregnancy: Pregnancy Category C. Animal reproduction studies have not been conducted with COMHIST LA. It is also not known whether COMHIST LA can cause fetal harm when administered to a pregnant woman or can affect reproduction capacity. COMHIST LA should be given to pregnant woman only if clearly needed.

Nursing Mothers: It is not known whether the drugs in COMHIST LA are excreted in human milk. Because many drugs are excreted in human milk and because of the potential for serious adverse reactions in nursing infants, a decision should be made whether to discontinue nursing or to discontinue the product, taking into account the importance of the drug to the mother.

Pediatric Use: Safety and effectiveness of COMHIST LA in children below the age of 12 have not been established.

ADVERSE REACTIONS

General: Urticaria, drug rash, dryness of mouth, nose, and throat.

Cardiovascular System: Hypotension, headache, palpitations.

Hematologic System: Thrombocytopenia, agranulocytosis, leukopenia.

Nervous System: Sedation, dizziness, excitation (especially in children), nervousness, insomnia, blurred vision, convulsions.

Gastrointestinal System: Epigastric distress, anorexia, nausea, vomiting, diarrhea, constipation.

Genitourinary System: Urinary frequency, urinary retention.

Respiratory System: Thickening of bronchial secretions, tightness of chest and wheezing, nasal stuffiness.

OVERDOSAGE

The treatment of overdosage should provide symptomatic and supportive care. If the amount ingested is considered dangerous or excessive, induce vomiting with ipecac syrup unless the patient is convulsing, comatose, or has lost the gag reflex, in which case perform gastric lavage using a large-bore tube. If indicated, follow with activated charcoal and a saline cathartic. Since the effects of COMHIST LA may last up to 12 hours, treatment should be continued for at least that length of time.

DOSAGE AND ADMINISTRATION

Adults and children 12 years of age and older—1 capsule every 8 to 12 hours; not recommended for children under 12 years of age.

HOW SUPPLIED

COMHIST LA is available as a yellow and clear capsule imprinted "COMHIST LA" and "01490446".

NDC 0149-0446-01 Bottle of 100

CAUTION

Federal law prohibits dispensing without prescription.

Manufactured for
Norwich Eaton Pharmaceuticals, Inc.
by **KV Pharmaceutical Company**
St. Louis, Missouri 63144
REVISED SEPTEMBER 1985 COMLA-X7

DANTRIUM® ℞

[dan 'trē-um]
(dantrolene sodium)
CAPSULES

Dantrium (dantrolene sodium) has a potential for hepatotoxicity, and should not be used in conditions other than those recommended. Symptomatic hepatitis (fatal and non-fatal) has been reported at various dose levels of the drug. The incidence reported in patients taking up to 400 mg/day is much lower than in those taking doses of 800 mg or more per day. Even sporadic short courses of these higher dose levels within a treatment regimen markedly increased the risk of serious hepatic injury. Liver dysfunction as evidenced by blood chemical abnormalities alone (liver enzyme elevations) has been observed in patients exposed to **Dantrium** for varying periods of time. Overt hepatitis has occurred at varying intervals after initiation of therapy, but has been most frequently observed between the third and twelfth month of therapy. The risk of hepatic injury appears to be greater in females, in patients over 35 years of age, and in patients taking other medication(s) in addition to **Dantrium** (dantrolene sodium). **Dantrium** should be used only in conjunction with appropriate monitoring of hepatic function including frequent determination of SGOT or SGPT. If no observable benefit is derived from the administration of **Dantrium** after a total of 45 days, therapy should be discontinued. The lowest possible effective dose for the individual patient should be prescribed.

DESCRIPTION

The chemical formula of **Dantrium** (dantrolene sodium) is hydrated 1-[[[5-(4-nitrophenyl)-2-furanyl]methylene]amino]-2, 4-imidazolidinedione sodium salt. It is an orange powder, slightly soluble in water, but due to its slightly acidic nature the solubility increases somewhat in alkaline solution. The anhydrous salt has a molecular weight of 336. The hydrated salt contains approximately 15% water (3½ moles) and has a molecular weight of 399. The structural formula for the hydrated salt is:

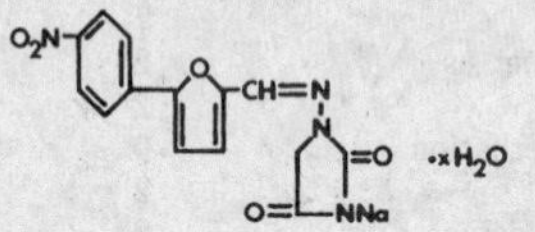

Dantrium is supplied in capsules of 25 mg, 50 mg, and 100 mg.

Inactive Ingredients: Each capsule contains edible black ink, FD&C Yellow No. 6, gelatin, lactose, magnesium stearate, starch, synthetic iron oxide red, synthetic iron oxide yellow, talc, and titanium dioxide.

CLINICAL PHARMACOLOGY

In isolated nerve-muscle preparation, **Dantrium** has been shown to produce relaxation by affecting the contractile response of the skeletal muscle at a site beyond the myoneural junction, directly on the muscle itself. In skeletal muscle, **Dantrium** dissociates the excitation-contraction coupling, probably by interfering with the release of Ca^{++} from the sarcoplasmic reticulum. This effect appears to be more pronounced in fast muscle fibers as compared to slow ones, but generally affects both. A central nervous system effect occurs, with drowsiness, dizziness, and generalized weakness occasionally present. Although **Dantrium** does not appear to directly affect the CNS, the extent of its indirect effect is unknown. The absorption of **Dantrium** after oral administration in humans is incomplete and slow but consistent, and dose-related blood levels are obtained. The duration and intensity of skeletal muscle relaxation is related to the dosage and blood levels. The mean biologic half-life of **Dantrium** in adults is 8.7 hours after a 100-mg dose. Specific metabolic pathways in the degradation and elimination of **Dantrium** in human subjects have been established. Metabolic patterns are similar in adults and children. In addition to the parent compound, dantrolene, which is found in measurable amounts in blood and urine, the major metabolites noted in body fluids are the 5-hydroxy analog and the acetamido analog. Since **Dantrium** is probably metabolized by hepatic microsomal enzymes, enhancement of its metabolism by other drugs is possible. However, neither phenobarbital nor diazepam appears to affect **Dantrium** metabolism.

Clinical experience in the management of fulminant human malignant hyperthermia, as well as experiments conducted in malignant hyperthermia susceptible swine, have revealed that the administration of intravenous dantrolene, combined with indicated supportive measures, is effective in reversing the hypermetabolic process of malignant hyperthermia. Known differences between human and swine malignant hyperthermia are minor. The prophylactic administration of oral or intravenous dantrolene to malignant hyperthermia susceptible swine will attenuate or prevent the development of signs of malignant hyperthermia in a manner dependent upon the dosage of dantrolene administered and the intensity of the malignant hyperthermia triggering stimulus. Limited clinical experience with the administration of oral dantrolene to patients judged malignant hyperthermia susceptible, when combined with clinical experience in the use of intravenous dantrolene for the treatment of malignant hyperthermia and data derived from the above cited animal model experiments, suggests that oral dantrolene will also attenuate or prevent the development of signs of human malignant hyperthermia, provided that currently accepted practices in the management of such patients are adhered to (see INDICATIONS AND USAGE); intravenous dantrolene should also be available for use should the signs of malignant hyperthermia appear.

INDICATIONS AND USAGE

In Chronic Spasticity:

Dantrium is indicated in controlling the manifestations of clinical spasticity resulting from upper motor neuron disorders (*e.g.,* spinal cord injury, stroke, cerebral palsy, or multiple sclerosis). It is of particular benefit to the patient whose functional rehabilitation has been retarded by the sequelae of spasticity. Such patients must have presumably reversible spasticity where relief of spasticity will aid in restoring residual function. **Dantrium** is not indicated in the treatment of skeletal muscle spasm resulting from rheumatic disorders.

If improvement occurs, it will ordinarily occur within the dosage titration (see DOSAGE AND ADMINISTRATION), and will be manifested by a decrease in the severity of spasticity and the ability to resume a daily function not quite attainable without **Dantrium.**

Occasionally, subtle but meaningful improvement in spasticity may occur with **Dantrium** therapy. In such instances, information regarding improvement should be solicited from the patient and those who are in constant daily contact and attendance with him. Brief withdrawal of **Dantrium** for a period of 2 to 4 days will frequently demonstrate exacerbation of the manifestations of spasticity and may serve to confirm a clinical impression.

A decision to continue the administration of **Dantrium** on a long-term basis is justified if introduction of the drug into the patient's regimen:

produces a significant reduction in painful and/or disabling spasticity such as clonus, or

permits a significant reduction in the intensity and/or degree of nursing care required, or

rids the patient of any annoying manifestation of spasticity considered important by the patient himself.

In Malignant Hyperthermia:

Oral **Dantrium** is also indicated preoperatively to prevent or attenuate the development of signs of malignant hyperthermia in known, or strongly suspect, malignant hyperthermia susceptible patients who require anesthesia and/or surgery. Currently accepted clinical practices in the management of such patients must still be adhered to (careful monitoring for early signs of malignant hyperthermia, minimizing exposure to triggering mechanisms and prompt use of intravenous dantrolene sodium and indicated supportive measures should signs of malignant hyperthermia appear); see also the package insert for **Dantrium** (dantrolene sodium) Intravenous.

Oral **Dantrium** should be administered following a malignant hyperthermic crisis to prevent recurrence of the signs of malignant hyperthermia.

CONTRAINDICATIONS

Active hepatic disease, such as hepatitis and cirrhosis, is a contraindication for use of **Dantrium. Dantrium** is contraindicated where spasticity is utilized to sustain upright posture and balance in locomotion or whenever spasticity is utilized to obtain or maintain increased function.

WARNINGS

It is important to recognize that fatal and non-fatal liver disorders of an idiosyncratic or hypersensitivity type may occur with **Dantrium** therapy.

At the start of **Dantrium** therapy, it is desirable to do liver function studies (SGOT, SGPT, alkaline phosphatase, total bilirubin) for a baseline or to establish whether there is preexisting liver disease. If baseline liver abnormalities exist and are confirmed, there is a clear possibility that the potential for **Dantrium** hepatotoxicity could be enhanced, although such a possibility has not yet been established.

Liver function studies (*e.g.,* SGOT or SGPT) should be performed at appropriate intervals during **Dantrium** therapy. If such studies reveal abnormal values, therapy should generally be discontinued. Only where benefits of the drug have been of major importance to the patient, should reinitiation or continuation of therapy be considered. Some patients have revealed a return to normal laboratory values in the face of continued therapy while others have not.

If symptoms compatible with hepatitis, accompanied by abnormalities in liver function tests or jaundice appear, **Dantrium** should be discontinued. If caused by **Dantrium** and detected early, the abnormalities in liver function characteristically have reverted to normal when the drug was discontinued.

Dantrium therapy has been reinstituted in a few patients who have developed clinical and/or laboratory evidence of hepatocellular injury. If such reinstitution of therapy is done, it should be attempted only in patients who clearly need **Dantrium** and only after previous symptoms and laboratory abnormalities have cleared. The patient should be hospitalized and the drug should be restarted in very small and gradually increasing doses. Laboratory monitoring should be frequent and the drug should be withdrawn immediately if there is any indication of recurrent liver involvement. Some patients have reacted with unmistakable signs of liver abnormality upon administration of a challenge dose, while others have not.

Dantrium should be used with particular caution in females and in patients over 35 years of age in view of apparent greater likelihood of drug-induced, potentially fatal, hepatocellular disease in these groups.

Long-term safety of **Dantrium** in humans has not been established. Chronic studies in rats, dogs, and monkeys at dosages greater than 30 mg/kg/day showed growth or weight depression and signs of hepatopathy and possible occlusion nephropathy, all of which were reversible upon cessation of treatment. Sprague-Dawley female rats fed dantrolene sodium for 18 months at dosage levels of 15, 30, and 60 mg/kg/day showed an increased incidence of benign and malignant mammary tumors compared with concurrent controls and, at the highest dosage, an increase in the incidence of hepatic lymphangiomas and hepatic angiosarcomas. These effects were not seen in 2½-year studies in Sprague-Dawley or Fischer 344 rats or in 2-year studies in mice of the HaM/ICR strain. Carcinogenicity in humans cannot be fully excluded, so that this possible risk of chronic administration must be weighed against the benefits of the drug (*i.e.,* after a brief trial) for the individual patient.

USAGE IN PREGNANCY

The safety of **Dantrium** for use in women who are or who may become pregnant has not been established. **Dantrium** should not be used in nursing mothers.

Usage in Children: The long-term safety of **Dantrium** in children under the age of 5 years has not been established. Because of the possibility that adverse effects of the drug could become apparent only after many years, a benefit-risk consideration of the long-term use of **Dantrium** is particularly important in pediatric patients.

Drug Interactions: While a definite drug interaction with estrogen therapy has not yet been established, caution should be observed if the two drugs are to be given concomitantly. Hepatotoxicity has occurred more often in women over 35 years of age receiving concomitant estrogen therapy.

There are very rare reports of cardiovascular collapse in patients treated simultaneously with verapamil and dantrolene sodium. The combination of therapeutic doses of intravenous dantrolene sodium and verapamil in halothane/α-chloralose anesthetized swine has resulted in ventricular fibrillation and cardiovascular collapse in association with marked hyperkalemia. Until the relevance of these findings to humans is established, the combination of dantrolene sodium and verapamil is not recommended during the management of malignant hyperthermia.

PRECAUTIONS

Dantrium should be used with caution in patients with impaired pulmonary function, particularly those with obstructive pulmonary disease, and in patients with severely impaired cardiac function due to myocardial disease. It should be used with caution in patients with a history of previous liver disease or dysfunction (see WARNINGS).

Patients should be cautioned against driving a motor vehicle or participating in hazardous occupations while taking **Dantrium.** Caution should be exercised in the concomitant administration of tranquilizing agents.

Dantrium might possibly evoke a photosensitivity reaction; patients should be cautioned about exposure to sunlight while taking it.

ADVERSE REACTIONS

The most frequently occurring side effects of **Dantrium** have been drowsiness, dizziness, weakness, general malaise, fatigue, and diarrhea. These are generally transient, occurring early in treatment, and can often be obviated by beginning with a low dose and increasing dosage gradually until an optimal regimen is established. Diarrhea may be severe and may necessitate temporary withdrawal of **Dantrium** therapy. If diarrhea recurs upon readministration of **Dantrium,** therapy should probably be withdrawn permanently.

Other less frequent side effects, listed according to system, are:

Gastrointestinal: Constipation, GI bleeding, anorexia, swallowing difficulty, gastric irritation, abdominal cramps.
Hepatobiliary: Hepatitis (see WARNINGS).
Neurologic: Speech disturbance, seizure, headache, lightheadedness, visual disturbance, diplopia, alteration of taste, insomnia.
Cardiovascular: Tachycardia, erratic blood pressure, phlebitis.
Psychiatric: Mental depression, mental confusion, increased nervousness.
Urogenital: Increased urinary frequency, crystalluria, hematuria, difficult erection, urinary incontinence and/or nocturia, difficult urination and/or urinary retention.
Integumentary: Abnormal hair growth, acne-like rash, pruritus, urticaria, eczematoid eruption, sweating.
Musculoskeletal: Myalgia, backache.
Respiratory: Feeling of suffocation.
Special Senses: Excessive tearing.
Hypersensitivity: Pleural effusion with pericarditis.
Other: Chills and fever.

DOSAGE AND ADMINISTRATION

For Use in Chronic Spasticity:

Prior to the administration of **Dantrium,** consideration should be given to the potential response to treatment. A decrease in spasticity sufficient to allow a daily function not otherwise attainable should be the therapeutic goal of treatment with **Dantrium.** Refer to INDICATIONS AND USAGE section for description of response to be anticipated.

It is important to establish a therapeutic goal (regain and maintain a specific function such as therapeutic exercise program, utilization of braces, transfer maneuvers, etc.) before beginning **Dantrium** therapy. Dosage should be increased until the maximum performance compatible with the dysfunction due to underlying disease is achieved. No further increase in dosage is then indicated.

Usual Dosage: It is important that the dosage be titrated and individualized for maximum effect. The lowest dose compatible with optimal response is recommended.

In view of the potential for liver damage in long-term **Dantrium** *use, therapy should be stopped if benefits are not evident within 45 days.*

Adults: Begin therapy with 25 mg once daily; increase to 25 mg two, three, or four times daily and then by increments of 25 mg up to as high as 100 mg two, three, or four times daily if necessary. As most patients will respond to a dose of 400 mg/day or less, rarely should doses higher than 400 mg/day be used (see Box Warning).

Each dosage level should be maintained for four to seven days to determine the patient's response. The dose should not be increased beyond, and may even have to be reduced to, the amount at which the patient received maximal benefit without adverse effects.

Children: A similar approach should be utilized starting with 0.5 mg/kg of body weight twice daily; this is increased to 0.5 mg/kg three or four times daily and then by increments of 0.5 mg/kg up to as high as 3.0 mg/kg two, three, or four times daily, if necessary. Doses higher than 100 mg four times daily should not be used in children.

For Malignant Hyperthermia:

Preoperatively: Administer 4 to 8 mg/kg/day of oral **Dantrium** in 3 or 4 divided doses for one or two days prior to surgery, with the last dose being given approximately 3 to 4 hours before scheduled surgery with a minimum of water. This dosage will usually be associated with skeletal muscle weakness and sedation (sleepiness or drowsiness); adjustment can usually be made within the recommended dosage range to avoid incapacitation or excessive gastrointestinal irritation (including nausea and/or vomiting).

Post Crisis Follow-up:

Oral **Dantrium** should also be administered following a malignant hyperthermia crisis, in doses of 4 to 8 mg/kg per day in four divided doses, for a one to three day period to prevent recurrence of the manifestations of malignant hyperthermia.

OVERDOSAGE

For acute overdosage, general supportive measures should be employed along with immediate gastric lavage.

Intravenous fluids should be administered in fairly large quantities to avert the possibility of crystalluria. An adequate airway should be maintained and artificial resuscitation equipment should be at hand. Electrocardiographic monitoring should be instituted, and the patient carefully observed. To date, no experience has been reported with dialysis and its value in **Dantrium** overdosage is not known.

HOW SUPPLIED

Dantrium (dantrolene sodium) is available in:
25-mg opaque, orange and tan capsules:
NDC 0149-0030-05 bottle of 100
NDC 0149-0030-66 bottle of 500
NDC 0149-0030-77 hospital unit-dose strips in boxes of 100
50-mg opaque, orange and tan capsules:
NDC 0149-0031-05 bottle of 100
100-mg opaque, orange and tan capsules:
NDC 0149-0033-05 bottle of 100
NDC 0149-0033-77 hospital unit-dose strips in boxes of 100
Address medical inquiries to Procter & Gamble Pharmaceuticals, Medical Department, Norwich, NY 13815-0191.

CAUTION

Federal law prohibits dispensing without prescription.

Procter & Gamble Pharmaceuticals
Norwich, New York 13815-0191
REVISED SEPTEMBER 1991 DANTCAPS-U2

DANTRIUM® Intravenous ℞

[*dan 'trē-um*]
(dantrolene sodium for injection)

DESCRIPTION

Dantrium Intravenous is a sterile, non-pyrogenic, lyophilized formulation of dantrolene sodium for injection. **Dantrium Intravenous** is supplied in 70 ml vials containing 20 mg dantrolene sodium, 3000 mg mannitol, and sufficient sodium hydroxide to yield a pH of approximately 9.5 when reconstituted with 60 ml sterile water for injection USP (without a bacteriostatic agent).

Dantrium is classified as a direct-acting skeletal muscle relaxant. Chemically, **Dantrium** is hydrated 1-[[[5-(4-nitrophenyl)-2-furanyl]methylene]amino]-2,4-imidazolidinedione sodium salt. The structural formula for the hydrated salt is:

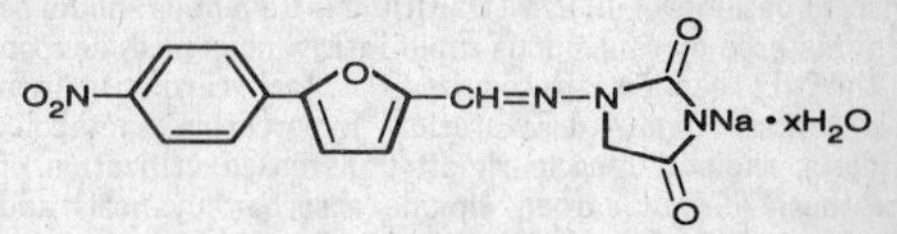

The hydrated salt contains approximately 15% water (3-½ moles) and has a molecular weight of 399. The anhydrous salt (dantrolene) has a molecular weight of 336.

CLINICAL PHARMACOLOGY

In isolated nerve-muscle preparation, **Dantrium** produces skeletal muscle relaxation by directly affecting the contractile response of the muscle at a site beyond the myoneural junction. In skeletal muscle, **Dantrium** dissociates excitation-contraction coupling, probably by interfering with the release of Ca^{++} from the sarcoplasmic reticulum. The administration of intravenous **Dantrium** to human volunteers is associated with loss of grip strength and weakness in the legs, as well as subjective CNS complaints (see also PRECAUTIONS, Information for Patients). Information concerning the passage of **Dantrium** across the blood-brain barrier is not available.

In the anesthetic-induced malignant hyperthermia (MH) syndrome, evidence points to an intrinsic abnormality of skeletal muscle tissue. In affected humans, it has been postulated that "triggering agents" (*e.g.,* general anesthetics and depolarizing neuromuscular blocking agents) produce a change within the cell which results in an elevated myoplasmic calcium. This elevated myoplasmic calcium activates acute cellular catabolic processes that cascade to the MH crisis.

It is hypothesized that addition of **Dantrium** to the "triggered" malignant hyperthermic muscle cell reestablishes a normal level of ionized calcium in the myoplasm. Inhibition of calcium release from the sarcoplasmic reticulum by **Dantrium** reestablishes the myoplasmic calcium equilibrium, increasing the percentage of bound calcium. In this way, physiologic, metabolic, and biochemical changes associated with the MH crisis may be reversed or attenuated. Experimental results in malignant hyperthermia susceptible (MHS) swine show that prophylactic administration of intravenous or oral dantrolene prevents or attentuates the development of vital sign and blood gas changes characteristic of malignant hyperthermia (MH) in a dose related manner.

The efficacy of intravenous dantrolene in the treatment of human and porcine MH crisis, when considered along with prophylactic experiments in MHS swine, lends support to prophylactic use of oral or intravenous dantrolene in MHS humans. When prophylactic intravenous dantrolene is administered as directed, whole blood concentrations remain at a near steady state level for 3 or more hours after the infusion is completed. Clinical experience has shown that early vital sign and/or blood gas changes characteristic of MH may appear during or after anesthesia and surgery despite the prophylactic use of dantrolene and adherence to currently accepted patient management practices. These signs are compatible with attenuated MH and respond to the administration of additional i.v. dantrolene (see DOSAGE AND ADMINISTRATION). The administration of the recommended prophylactic dose of intravenous dantrolene to healthy volunteers was not associated with clinically significant cardiorespiratory changes.

Specific metabolic pathways for the degradation and elimination of **Dantrium** in humans have been established. Dantrolene is found in measurable amounts in blood and urine. Its major metabolites in body fluids are 5-hydroxy dantrolene and an acetylamino metabolite of dantrolene. Another metabolite with an unknown structure appears related to the latter. **Dantrium** may also undergo hydrolysis and subsequent oxidation forming nitrophenylfuroic acid.

The mean biologic half-life of **Dantrium** after intravenous administration is variable, between 4 to 8 hours under most experimental conditions. Based on assays of whole blood and plasma, slightly greater amounts of dantrolene are associated with red blood cells than with the plasma fraction of blood. Significant amounts of dantrolene are bound to plasma proteins, mostly albumin, and this binding is readily reversible.

Cardiopulmonary depression has not been observed in MHS swine following the administration of up to 7.5 mg/kg i.v. dantrolene. This is twice the amount needed to maximally diminish twitch response to single supramaximal peripheral nerve stimulation (95% inhibition). A transient, inconsis-

Continued on next page

Procter & Gamble Pharm.—Cont.

tent, depressant effect on gastrointestinal smooth muscles has been observed at high doses.

INDICATIONS AND USAGE

Dantrium Intravenous is indicated, along with appropriate supportive measures, for the management of the fulminant hypermetabolism of skeletal muscle characteristic of MH crisis in patients of all ages. **Dantrium Intravenous** should be administered by continuous rapid intravenous push as soon as the MH reaction is recognized (*i.e.*, tachycardia, tachypnea, central venous desaturation, hypercarbia, metabolic acidosis, skeletal muscle rigidity, increased utilization of anesthesia circuit carbon dioxide absorber, cyanosis and mottling of the skin, and, in many cases, fever).

Dantrium Intravenous is also indicated preoperatively, and sometimes postoperatively, to prevent or attenuate the development of clinical and laboratory signs of malignant hyperthermia in individuals judged to be malignant hyperthermia susceptible.

CONTRAINDICATIONS

None.

WARNINGS

*The use of **Dantrium Intravenous** in the management of MH crisis is not a substitute for previously known supportive measures. These measures must be individualized, but it will usually be necessary to discontinue the suspect triggering agents, attend to increased oxygen requirements, manage the metabolic acidosis, institute cooling when necessary, monitor urinary output, and monitor for electrolyte imbalance.*

Since the effect of disease state and other drugs on the consequences of **Dantrium** related skeletal muscle weakness, including possible respiratory depression, cannot be predicted, patients who receive i.v. **Dantrium** preoperatively should have vital signs monitored.

If patients judged malignant hyperthermia susceptible are administered intravenous or oral **Dantrium** preoperatively, anesthetic preparation must still follow a standard MHS regimen, including the avoidance of known triggering agents. Monitoring for early clinical and metabolic signs of MH is indicated because attenuation of MH, rather than prevention, is possible. These signs usually call for the administration of additional i.v. dantrolene.

PRECAUTIONS

General: Care must be taken to prevent extravasation of **Dantrium** solution into the surrounding tissues due to the high pH of the intravenous formulation.

When mannitol is used for prevention or treatment of late renal complications of MH, the 3 g of mannitol needed to dissolve each 20 mg vial of i.v. **Dantrium** should be taken into consideration.

Information for Patients: Based upon data in human volunteers, it will sometimes be appropriate to tell patients who receive **Dantrium Intravenous** that decrease in grip strength and weakness of leg muscles, especially walking down stairs, can be expected postoperatively. In addition, symptoms such as "lightheadedness" may be noted. Since some of these symptoms may persist for up to 48 hours, patients must not operate an automobile or engage in other hazardous activity during this time. Caution is also indicated at meals on the day of administration because difficulty swallowing and choking has been reported.

Drug Interactions: **Dantrium** is metabolized by the liver, and it is theoretically possible that its metabolism may be enhanced by drugs known to induce hepatic microsomal enzymes. However, neither phenobarbital nor diazepam appears to affect **Dantrium** metabolism. Binding to plasma protein is not significantly altered by diazepam, diphenylhydantoin, or phenylbutazone. Binding to plasma proteins is reduced by warfarin and clofibrate and increased by tolbutamide.

The combination of therapeutic doses of intravenous dantrolene sodium and verapamil in halothane/α-chloralose anesthetized swine has resulted in ventricular fibrillation and cardiovascular collapse in association with marked hyperkalemia. It is recommended that the combination of intravenous dantrolene sodium and calcium channel blockers, such as verapamil, not be used together during the management of malignant hyperthermia crisis until the relevance of these findings to humans is established.

Carcinogenesis, Mutagenesis, and Impairment of Fertility: Studies of **Dantrium** in animals to evaluate mutagenic potential and the effect on fertility have not been conducted. Sprague-Dawley female rats fed **Dantrium** for 18 months at dosage levels of 15, 30, and 60 mg/kg/day showed an increased incidence of benign and malignant mammary tumors compared with concurrent controls. At the highest dosage, there was an increase in the incidence of hepatic lymphangiomas and hepatic angiosarcomas. These effects were not seen in 30-month studies in Sprague-Dawley or Fischer-344 rats or in 24-month studies in mice of the HaM/ICR strain. Although the possibility that the drug may be carcinogenic in humans cannot be fully excluded, the risks

associated with administration of **Dantrium Intravenous** in a life-threatening crisis would appear to be minimal.

Usage In Pregnancy: Pregnancy Category C: **Dantrium** has been shown to be embryocidal in the rabbit and has been shown to decrease pup survival in the rat when given at doses seven times the human oral dose. There are no adequate and well-controlled studies in pregnant women. **Dantrium Intravenous** should be used during pregnancy only if the potential benefit justifies the potential risk to the fetus.

Labor and Delivery: In one uncontrolled study, 100 mg per day of prophylactic oral **Dantrium** was administered to term pregnant patients awaiting labor and delivery. Dantrolene readily crossed the placenta, with maternal and fetal whole blood levels approximately equal at delivery; neonatal levels then fell approximately 50% per day for 2 days before declining sharply. No neonatal respiratory and neuromuscular side effects were detected at low dose. More data, at higher doses, are needed before more definitive conclusions can be made.

ADVERSE REACTIONS

There have been occasional reports of death following MH crisis even when treated with intravenous dantrolene; incidence figures are not available (the pre-dantrolene mortality of MH crisis was approximately 50%). Most of these deaths can be accounted for by late recognition, delayed treatment, inadequate dosage, lack of supportive therapy, intercurrent disease and/or the development of delayed complications such as renal failure or disseminated intravascular coagulopathy. In some cases there are insufficient data to completely rule out therapeutic failure of dantrolene.

There are rare reports of fatality in MH crisis, despite initial satisfactory response to i.v. dantrolene, which involve patients who could not be weaned from dantrolene after initial treatment.

The following adverse reactions are in approximate order of severity:

There are rare reports of pulmonary edema developing during the treatment of MH crisis in which the diluent volume and mannitol needed to deliver i.v. dantrolene possibly contributed.

There have been reports of thrombophlebitis following administration of intravenous dantrolene; actual incidence figures are not available.

There have been rare reports of urticaria and erythema possibly associated with the administration of i.v. **Dantrium**. There has been one case of anaphylaxis.

None of the serious reactions occasionally reported with long-term oral **Dantrium** use, such as hepatitis, seizures, and pleural effusion with pericarditis, have been reasonably associated with short-term **Dantrium Intravenous** therapy.

The following events have been reported in patients receiving oral dantrolene: aplastic anemia, leukopenia, lymphocytic lymphoma, and heart failure. (See package insert for **Dantrium Capsules** for a complete listing of adverse reactions.)

The published literature has included some reports of **Dantrium** use in patients with Neuroleptic Malignant Syndrome (NMS). **Dantrium Intravenous** is not indicated for the treatment of NMS and patients may expire despite treatment with **Dantrium Intravenous**.

OVERDOSAGE

Because **Dantrium Intravenous** must be administered at a low concentration in a large volume of fluid, acute toxicity of **Dantrium** could not be assessed in animals. In 14-day (subacute) studies, the intravenous formulation of **Dantrium** was relatively non-toxic to rats at doses of 10 mg/kg/day and 20 mg/kg/day. While 10 mg/kg/day in dogs for 14 days evoked little toxicity, 20 mg/kg/day for 14 days caused hepatic changes of questionable biologic significance.

No data are available to define the symptomatology of an overdose of **Dantrium Intravenous**. If an overdose is suspected, treatment is symptomatic and supportive. There is no known antidote.

DOSAGE AND ADMINISTRATION

As soon as the MH reaction is recognized, all anesthetic agents should be discontinued; the administration of 100% oxygen is recommended. **Dantrium Intravenous** should be administered by continuous rapid intravenous push beginning at a minimum dose of 1 mg/kg, and continuing until symptoms subside or the maximum cumulative dose of 10 mg/kg has been reached.

If the physiologic and metabolic abnormalities reappear, the regimen may be repeated. It is important to note that administration of **Dantrium Intravenous** should be continuous until symptoms subside. The effective dose to reverse the crisis is directly dependent upon the individual's degree of susceptibility to MH, the amount and time of exposure to the triggering agent, and the time elapsed between onset of the crisis and initiation of treatment.

Children's Dose: Experience to date indicates that the dose of **Dantrium Intravenous** for children is the same as for adults.

Preoperatively: **Dantrium Intravenous** and/or **Dantrium Capsules** may be administered preoperatively to patients judged MH susceptible as part of the overall patient management to prevent or attenuate the development of clinical and laboratory signs of MH.

Dantrium Intravenous: The recommended prophylactic dose of **Dantrium Intravenous** is 2.5 mg/kg, starting approximately 1¼ hours before anticipated anesthesia and infused over approximately 1 hour. This dose should prevent or attenuate the development of clinical and laboratory signs of MH provided that the usual precautions, such as avoidance of established MH triggering agents, are followed.

Additional **Dantrium Intravenous** may be indicated during anesthesia and surgery because of the appearance of early clinical and/or blood gas signs of MH or because of prolonged surgery (see also CLINICAL PHARMACOLOGY, WARNINGS, and PRECAUTIONS). Additional doses must be individualized.

Oral administration of Dantrium Capsules: Administer 4 to 8 mg/kg/day of oral **Dantrium** in 3 or 4 divided doses for one or two days prior to surgery, with the last dose being given with a minimum of water approximately 3 to 4 hours before scheduled surgery. Adjustment can usually be made within the recommended dosage range to avoid incapacitation (weakness, drowsiness, etc.) or excessive gastrointestinal irritation (nausea and/or vomiting). See also the package insert for **Dantrium** (dantrolene sodium) **Capsules**.

Post Crisis Follow-up: **Dantrium Capsules**, 4 to 8 mg/kg/day, in four divided doses should be administered for one to three days following a malignant hyperthermia crisis to prevent recurrence of the manifestations of malignant hyperthermia.

Intravenous **Dantrium** may be used postoperatively to prevent or attenuate the recurrence of signs of MH when oral **Dantrium** administration is not practical. The i.v. dose of **Dantrium** in the postoperative period must be individualized, starting with 1 mg/kg or more as the clinical situation dictates.

PREPARATION

Each vial of **Dantrium Intravenous** should be reconstituted by adding 60 ml of *sterile water for injection USP (without a bacteriostatic agent), and the vial shaken until the solution is clear*. 5% Dextrose Injection USP, 0.9% Sodium Chloride Injection USP, and other acidic solutions are not compatible with **Dantrium Intravenous** and should not be used. The contents of the vial must be *protected from direct light* and *used within 6 hours* after reconstitution. Store reconstituted solutions at controlled room temperature (59°F to 86°F or 15°C to 30°C).

Reconstituted **Dantrium Intravenous** should <u>not</u> be transferred to large glass bottles for prophylactic infusion due to precipitate formation observed with the use of some glass bottles as reservoirs.

For prophylactic infusion, the required number of individual vials of **Dantrium Intravenous** should be reconstituted as outlined above. The contents of individual vials are then transferred to a larger volume sterile intravenous plastic bag. Stability data on file at Procter & Gamble Pharmaceuticals indicate commercially available sterile plastic bags are acceptable drug delivery devices. However, it is recommended that the prepared infusion be inspected carefully for cloudiness and/or precipitation prior to dispensing and administration. Such solutions should not be used. While stable for 6 hours, it is recommended that the infusion be prepared immediately prior to the anticipated dosage administration time.

Parenteral drug products should be inspected visually for particulate matter and discoloration prior to administration.

HOW SUPPLIED

Dantrium Intravenous (NDC 0149-0734-02) is available in vials containing a sterile lyophilized mixture of 20 mg dantrolene sodium, 3000 mg mannitol, and sufficient sodium hydroxide to yield a pH of approximately 9.5 when reconstituted with 60 ml sterile water for injection USP (without a bacteriostatic agent).

Store unreconstituted product at controlled room temperature (59°F to 86°F or 15°C to 30°C) and avoid prolonged exposure to light.

Address medical inquiries to Procter & Gamble Pharmaceuticals, Medical Department, P.O. Box 191, Norwich, NY 13815-0191.

CAUTION

Federal law prohibits dispensing without prescription.

Procter & Gamble Pharmaceuticals
Norwich, New York 13815
©1992 NEPI
REVISED MAY 1992   DANTIV-P7

DIDRONEL® ℞
[*dī'drō-nel*]
(etidronate disodium)

DESCRIPTION

Didronel tablets contain either 200 mg or 400 mg of etidronate disodium, the disodium salt of (1-hydroxyethylidene) diphosphonic acid, for oral administration. This compound, also known as EHDP, regulates bone metabolism. It is a white powder, highly soluble in water, with a molecular weight of 250 and the following structural formula:

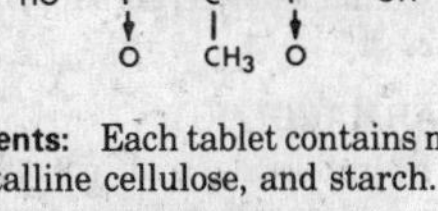

Inactive Ingredients: Each tablet contains magnesium stearate, microcrystalline cellulose, and starch.

CLINICAL PHARMACOLOGY

Didronel acts primarily on bone. It can inhibit the formation, growth and dissolution of hydroxyapatite crystals and their amorphous percursors by chemisorption to calcium phosphate surfaces. Inhibition of crystal resorption occurs at lower doses than are required to inhibit crystal growth. Both effects increase as the dose increases.

Didronel is not metabolized. Absorption averages about 1% of an oral dose of 5 mg/kg body weight/day. This increases to about 2.5% at 10 mg/kg/day and 6% at 20 mg/kg/day. Most of the absorbed drug is cleared from the blood within 6 hours. Within 24 hours about half of the absorbed dose is excreted in the urine. The remainder is chemically adsorbed to bone, especially to areas of elevated osteogenesis, and is slowly eliminated. Unabsorbed drug is excreted intact in the feces.

Didronel therapy does not adversely affect serum levels of parathyroid hormone or calcium. Hyperphosphatemia has been observed in **Didronel** patients, usually in association with doses of 10–20 mg/kg/day. No adverse effects have been traced to this, and it is not a contraindication for therapy. It is apparently due to drug-related increased tubular reabsorption of phosphate by the kidney. Serum phosphate levels generally return to normal 2–4 weeks posttherapy.

PAGET'S DISEASE: Paget's disease of bone (osteitis deformans) is an idiopathic, progressive disease characterized by abnormal and accelerated bone metabolism in one or more bones. Signs and symptoms may include bone pain and/or deformity, neurologic disorders, elevated cardiac output and other vascular disorders, and increased serum alkaline phosphatase and/or urinary hydroxyproline levels. Bone fractures are common in patients with Paget's disease.

Didronel slows accelerated bone turnover (resorption and accretion) in pagetic lesions and, to a lesser extent, in normal bone. This has been demonstrated histologically, scintigraphically, biochemically, and through calcium kinetic and balance studies. Reduced bone turnover is often accompanied by symptomatic improvement, including reduced bone pain. Also, the incidence of pagetic fractures may be reduced, and elevated cardiac output and other vascular disorders may be improved by **Didronel** therapy.

HETEROTOPIC OSSIFICATION: Heterotopic ossification, also referred to as myositis ossificans (circumscripta, progressiva or traumatica), ectopic calcification, periarticular ossification, or paraosteoarthropathy, is characterized by metaplastic osteogenesis. It usually presents with signs of localized inflammation or pain, elevated skin temperature, and redness. When tissues near joints are involved, functional loss may also be present.

Heterotopic ossification may occur for no known reason as in myositis ossificans progressiva or may follow a wide variety of surgical, occupational, and sports trauma (e.g., hip arthroplasty, spinal cord injury, head injury, burns and severe thigh bruises). Heterotopic ossification has also been observed in non-traumatic conditions (e.g., infections of the central nervous system, peripheral neuropathy, tetanus, biliary cirrhosis, Peyronie's disease, as well as in association with a variety of benign and malignant neoplasms).

Clinical trials have demonstrated the efficacy of **Didronel** in heterotopic ossification following total hip replacement, or due to spinal cord injury.

—*Heterotopic ossification complicating total hip replacement* typically develops radiographically 3–8 weeks postoperatively in the pericapsular area of the affected hip joint. The overall incidence is about 50%; about one-third of these cases are clinically significant.

—*Heterotopic ossification due to spinal cord injury* typically develops radiographically 1–4 months after injury. It occurs below the level of injury, usually at major joints. The overall incidence is about 40%; about one-half of these cases are clinically significant.

Didronel chemisorbs to calcium hydroxyapatite crystals and their amorphous precursors, blocking the aggregation, growth and mineralization of these crystals. This is thought to be the mechanism by which **Didronel** prevents or retards heterotopic ossification. There is no evidence **Didronel** affects mature heterotopic bone.

INDICATIONS AND USAGE

PAGET'S DISEASE: **Didronel** is indicated for the treatment of symptomatic Paget's disease of bone. **Didronel** therapy usually arrests or significantly impedes the disease process as evidenced by:

—Symptomatic relief, including decreased pain and/or increased mobility (experienced by 3 out of 5 patients).
—Reductions in serum alkaline phosphatase and urinary hydroxyproline levels (30% or more in 4 out of 5 patients).
—Histomorphometry showing reduced numbers of osteoclasts and osteoblasts, and more lamellar bone formation.
—Bone scans showing reduced radionuclide uptake at pagetic lesions.

In addition, reductions in pagetically elevated cardiac output and skin temperature have been observed in some patients. Also, the incidence of pagetic fractures may be reduced when **Didronel** is administered intermittently over a period of years.

In many patients, the disease process will be suppressed for a period of at least one year following cessation of therapy. The upper limit of this period has not been determined.

The effects of the **Didronel** treatment in patients with asymptomatic Paget's disease have not been studied. However, **Didronel** treatment of such patients may be warranted if extensive involvement threatens irreversible neurologic damage, major joints, or major weight-bearing bones.

HETEROTOPIC OSSIFICATION: **Didronel** is indicated in the prevention and treatment of heterotopic ossification following total hip replacement or due to spinal cord injury.

Didronel reduces the incidence of clinically important heterotopic bone by about two-thirds. Among those patients who form heterotopic bone, **Didronel** retards the progression of immature lesions and reduces the severity by at least half. Follow-up data (at least nine months posttherapy) suggest these benefits persist.

In total hip replacement patients, **Didronel** does not promote loosening of the prosthesis or impede trochanteric reattachment.

In spinal cord injury patients, **Didronel** does not inhibit fracture healing or stabilization of the spine.

CONTRAINDICATIONS

None known.

WARNINGS

In Paget's patients the response to therapy may be of slow onset and continue for months after **Didronel** therapy is discontinued. Dosage should not be increased prematurely. A 90-day drug-free interval should be provided between courses of therapy.

Heterotopic ossification: No specific warnings.

PRECAUTIONS

General: Patients should maintain an adequate nutritional status, particularly an adequate intake of calcium and vitamin D.

Therapy has been withheld from some patients with enterocolitis since diarrhea may be experienced, particularly at higher doses.

Didronel is not metabolized and is excreted intact via the kidney. There is no experience to specifically guide treatment in patients with impaired renal function. **Didronel** dosage should be reduced when reductions in glomerular filtration rates are present. Patients with renal impairment should be closely monitored.

Didronel suppresses bone turnover, and may retard mineralization of osteoid laid down during the bone accretion process. These effects are dose and time dependent. Osteoid, which may accumulate noticeably at doses of 10–20 mg/kg/day, mineralizes normally posttherapy. In patients with fractures, especially of long bones, it may be advisable to delay or interrupt treatment until callus is evident.

In Paget's patients, treatment regimens exceeding the recommended (see DOSAGE AND ADMINISTRATION) daily maximum dose of 20 mg/kg or continuous administration of medication for periods greater than 6 months may be associated with an increased risk of fracture.

Long bones predominantly affected by lytic lesions, particularly in those patients unresponsive to **Didronel** therapy, may be especially prone to fracture. Patients with predominantly lytic lesions should be monitored radiographically and biochemically to permit termination of **Didronel** in those patients unresponsive to treatment.

Carcinogenesis: Long-term studies in rats have indicated that **Didronel** is not carcinogenic.

Pregnancy: Teratogenic Effects: Pregnancy Category C. In teratology ande developmental toxicity studies conducted in rats and rabbits treated with dosages up to 100 mg/kg (5–20 times the clinical dose), no adverse or teratogenic effects have been observed in the offspring. Etidronate disodium has been shown to cause skeletal abnormalities in rats when given at oral dose levels of 300 mg/kg (15–60 times the human dose). Other effects on the offspring (including decreased live births) are at dosages that cause significant toxicity in the parent generation and are 25 to 200 times the human dose. The skeletal effects are thought to be the result of the pharmacological effects of the drug on bone.

There are no adequate, well-controlled studies in pregnant women. **Didronel** (etidronate disodium) should be used in pregnancy only if the potential benefit justifies the potential risk to the fetus.

Nursing Mothers: It is not known whether this drug is excreted in human milk. Because many drugs are excreted in human milk, caution should be exercised when **Didronel** is administered to a nursing woman.

Pediatric Use: Safety and effectiveness in children have not been established. Children have been treated with **Didronel,** at doses recommended for adults, to prevent heterotopic ossifications or soft tissue calcifications. A rachitic syndrome has been reported infrequently at doses of 10 mg/kg/day and more for prolonged periods approaching or exceeding a year. The epiphyseal radiologic changes associated with retarded mineralization of new osteoid and cartilage, and occasional symptoms reported, have been reversible when medication is discontinued.

ADVERSE REACTIONS

The incidence of gastrointestinal complaints (diarrhea, nausea) is the same for **Didronel** at 5 mg/kg/day as for placebo, about 1 patient in 15. At 10–20 mg/kg/day the incidence may increase to 2 or 3 in 10. These complaints are often alleviated by dividing the total daily dose.

Hypersensitivity reactions, including angioedema/urticaria, rash and/or pruritis have been reported rarely.

In Paget's patients, increased or recurrent bone pain at pagetic sites, and/or the onset of pain at previously asymptomatic sites has been reported. At 5 mg/kg/day about 1 patient in 10 (verus 1 in 15 in the placebo group) report these phenomena. At higher doses the incidence rises to about 2 in 10. When therapy continues, pain resolves in some patients but persists in others.

Heterotopic ossification: No specific adverse reactions.

OVERDOSAGE

Clinical experience with **Didronel** overdosage is extremely limited. Decreases in serum calcium following substantial overdosage may be expected in some patients. Signs and symptoms of hypocalcemia also may occur in some of these patients. In one event, an 18–year–old female who ingested an estimated single dose of 4,000–6,000 mg (67–100 mg/kg) of **Didronel** was reported to be mildly hypocalcemic (7.52 mg/dl) and experienced paresthesia of the fingers. Some patients may develop vomiting and expel the drug.

Gastric lavage may remove unabsorbed drug. Standard procedures for treating hypocalcemia, including the administration of Ca^{++} intravenously, would be expected to restore physiologic amounts of ionized calcium and relieve signs and symptoms of hypocalcemia. Such treatment has been effective.

DOSAGE AND ADMINISTRATION

Didronel should be taken as a single, oral dose. However, should gastrointestinal discomfort occur, the dose may be divided. To maximize absorption, patients should avoid taking the following items within two hours of dosing:

—Food, especially those high in calcium, such as milk or milk products.
—Vitamins with mineral supplements or antacids which are high in metals such as calcium, iron, magnesium or aluminum.

PAGET'S DISEASE

Initial Treatment Regimens: 5–10 mg/kg/day, not to exceed 6 months, or 11–20 mg/kg/day, not to exceed 3 months.

The recommended initial dose is 5 mg/kg/day for a period not to exceed six months. Doses above 10 mg/kg/day should be reserved for when 1) lower doses are ineffective or 2) there is an overriding need to suppress rapid bone turnover (especially when irreversible neurologic damage is possible) or reduce elevated cardiac output. Doses in excess of 20 mg/kg/day are not recommended.

Retreatment Guidelines: Retreatment should be initiated only after: 1) a **Didronel**-free period of at least 90 days and 2) there is biochemical, symptomatic or other evidence of active disease process. It is advisable to monitor patients every 3–6 months although some patients may go drug free for extended periods. Retreatment regimens are the same as for initial treatment. For most patients the original dose will be adequate for retreatment. If not, consideration should be given to increasing the dose within the recommended guidelines.

HETEROTOPIC OSSIFICATION: The following treatment regimens have been shown to be effective:

—Total Hip Replacement Patients: 20 mg/kg/day for 1 month before and 3 months after surgery (4 months total).
—Spinal Cord Injured Patients: 20 mg/kg/day for 2 weeks followed by 10 mg/kg/day for 10 weeks (12 weeks total). **Didronel** therapy should begin as soon as medically feasible following the injury, preferably prior to evidence of heterotopic ossification.

Retreatment has not been studied.

Continued on next page

Procter & Gamble Pharm.—Cont.

HOW SUPPLIED

Didronel is available as 200-mg, white, rectangular tablets with "P&G" on one face and "402" on the other.
NDC 0149-0405-60   bottle of 60
400-mg, white, scored, capsule-shaped tablets with "N E" on one face and "406" on the other.
NDC 0149-0406-60   bottle of 60

CAUTION

Federal law prohibits dispensing without prescription.

Norwich Eaton Pharmaceuticals, Inc.
A Procter & Gamble Company
Norwich, New York 13815
© 1990 NEPI
REVISED OCTOBER 1990

                          DID-P1
Shown in Product Identification Section, page 423

ENTEX®   ℞
[n'tex]
(phenylephrine hydrochloride/phenylpropanolamine hydrochloride/guaifenesin)

DESCRIPTION

Each ENTEX orange and white capsule for oral administration contains
phenylephrine hydrochloride .... 5 mg
phenylpropanolamine hydrochloride .... 45 mg
guaifenesin .... 200 mg
This product contains ingredients of the following therapeutic classes: decongestant and expectorant.
Phenylephrine hydrochloride is a decongestant having the chemical name, 3-hydroxy-α-[(methylamino)methyl]benzenemethanol hydrochloride, with the following structure:

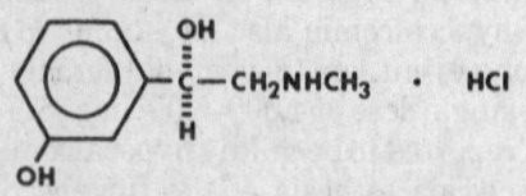

Phenylpropanolamine hydrochloride is a decongestant having the chemical name, benzenemethanol, α-(1-aminoethyl)-, hydrochloride (R*, S*), (±), with the following structure:

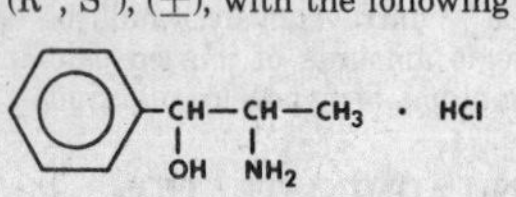

Guaifenesin is an expectorant having the chemical name, 1,2-propanediol, 3-(2-methoxyphenoxy)-, with the following structure:

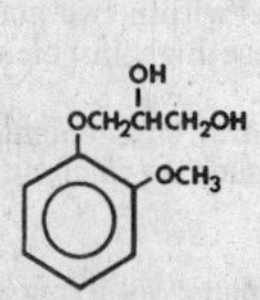

Inactive Ingredients: Each capsule contains D&C Red No. 28, D&C Yellow No. 10, edible black ink, FD&C Red No, 40, gelatin, silica gel, starch, titanium dioxide, zinc stearate.

CLINICAL PHARMACOLOGY

Phenylephrine hydrochloride and phenylpropanolamine hydrochloride are α-adrenergic receptor agonists (sympathomimetics) which produce vasoconstriction by stimulating α-receptors within the mucosa of the respiratory tract. Clinically, phenylephrine and phenylpropanolamine shrink swollen mucous membranes, reduce tissue hyperemia, edema, and nasal congestion, and increase nasal airway patency. Guaifenesin promotes lower respiratory tract drainage by thinning bronchial secretions, lubricates irritated respiratory tract membranes through increased mucous flow, and facilitates removal of viscous, inspissated mucus. As a result of these drugs, sinus and bronchial drainage is improved, and dry, nonproductive coughs become more productive and less frequent.

INDICATIONS AND USAGE

ENTEX is indicated for the symptomatic relief of sinusitis, bronchitis, pharyngitis, and coryza when these conditions are associated with nasal congestion and viscous mucus in the lower respiratory tract.

CONTRAINDICATIONS

ENTEX is contraindicated in individuals with known hypersensitivity to sympathomimetics, severe hypertension, or in patients receiving monoamine oxidase inhibitors.

WARNINGS

Sympathomimetic amines should be used with caution in patients with hypertension, diabetes mellitus, heart disease, peripheral vascular disease, increased intraocular pressure, hyperthyroidism, or prostatic hypertrophy.

PRECAUTIONS

Drug Interactions: ENTEX should not be used in patients taking monoamine oxidase inhibitors or other sympathomimetics.
Drug/Laboratory Test Interactions: Guaifenesin has been reported to interfere with clinical laboratory determinations of urinary 5-hydroxyindoleacetic acid (5-HIAA) and urinary vanillylmandelic acid (VMA).
Pregnancy: Pregnancy Category C. Animal reproduction studies have not been conducted with ENTEX. It is also not known whether ENTEX can cause fetal harm when administered to a pregnant woman or can affect reproduction capacity. ENTEX should be given to a pregnant woman only if clearly needed.
Nursing Mothers: It is not known whether the drugs in ENTEX are excreted in human milk. Because many drugs are excreted in human milk and because of the potential for serious adverse reactions in nursing infants, a decision should be made whether to discontinue nursing or to discontinue the product, taking into account the importance of the drug to the mother.
Pediatric Use: Safety and effectiveness of ENTEX capsules in children below the age of 12 have not been established.

ADVERSE REACTIONS

Possible adverse reactions include nervousness, insomnia, restlessness, headache, nausea, or gastric irritation. These reactions seldom, if ever, require discontinuation of therapy. Urinary retention may occur in patients with prostatic hypertrophy.

OVERDOSAGE

The treatment of overdosage should provide symptomatic and supportive care. If the amount ingested is considered dangerous or excessive, induce vomiting with ipecac syrup unless the patient is convulsing, comatose, or has lost the gag reflex, in which case perform gastric lavage using a large-bore tube. If indicated, follow with activated charcoal and a saline cathartic.

DOSAGE AND ADMINISTRATION

Adults and children 12 years of age and older—one capsule four times daily (every 6 hours) with food or fluid. ENTEX is not recommended for children under 12 years of age.

HOW SUPPLIED

ENTEX orange and white capsules are imprinted "ENTEX" and "0149 0412".
NDC 0149-0412-01 Bottle of 100
NDC 0149-0412-05 Bottle of 500

CAUTION

Federal law prohibits dispensing without prescription.

Norwich Eaton Pharmaceuticals, Inc.
A Procter & Gamble Company
Norwich, New York 13815
© 1991 NEPI
REVISED MARCH 1991

                          ENXCP-P8

ENTEX® LIQUID   ℞
[n'tex]
(phenylephrine hydrochloride/phenylpropanolamine hydrochloride/guaifenesin)

DESCRIPTION

Each 5 ml (one teaspoonful) for oral administration contains
phenylephrine hydrochloride .... 5 mg
phenylpropanolamine hydrochloride .... 20 mg
guaifenesin .... 100 mg
alcohol 5%
This product contains ingredients of the following therapeutic classes: decongestant and expectorant.
Phenylephrine hydrochloride is a decongestant having the chemical name, 3-hydroxy-α-[(methylamino)methyl]benzenemethanol hydrochloride, with the following structure:

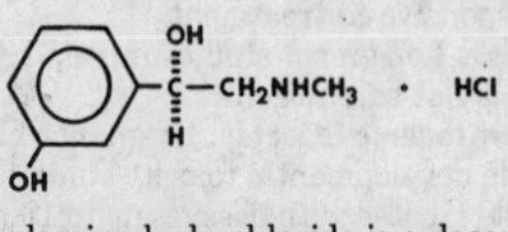

Phenylpropanolamine hydrochloride is a decongestant having the chemical name, benzenemethanol, α-(1-aminoethyl)-, hydrochloride (R*, S*), (±), with the following structure:

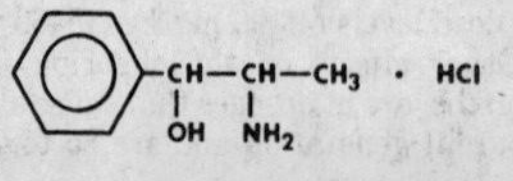

Guaifenesin is an expectorant having the chemical name, 1,2-propanediol, 3-(2-methoxyphenoxy)-, with the following structure:

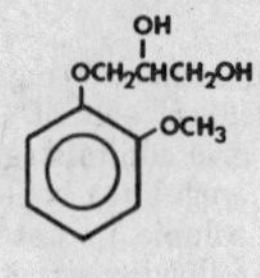

Inactive Ingredients: ENTEX LIQUID contains citric acid, flavoring, glycerin, purified water, saccharin sodium, sodium benzoate, sodium chloride, sorbitol solution, sucrose, and FD&C Yellow #6.

CLINICAL PHARMACOLOGY

Phenylephrine hydrochloride and phenylpropanolamine hydrochloride are α-adrenergic receptor agonists (sympathomimetics) which produce vasoconstriction by stimulating α-receptors within the mucosa of the respiratory tract. Clinically, phenylephrine and phenylpropanolamine shrink swollen mucous membranes, reduce tissue hyperemia, edema, and nasal congestion, and increase nasal airway patency. Guaifenesin promotes lower respiratory tract drainage by thinning bronchial secretions, lubricates irritated respiratory tract membranes through increased mucous flow, and facilitates removal of viscous, inspissated mucus. As a result, sinus and bronchial drainage is improved, and dry, nonproductive coughs become more productive and less frequent.

INDICATIONS AND USAGE

ENTEX LIQUID is indicated for the symptomatic relief of sinusitis, bronchitis, pharyngitis, and coryza when these conditions are associated with nasal congestion and inspissated mucus in the lower respiratory tract.

CONTRAINDICATIONS

ENTEX LIQUID is contraindicated in individuals with hypersensitivity to sympathomimetics, severe hypertension, or in patients receiving monoamine oxidase inhibitors.

WARNINGS

Sympathomimetic amines should be used with caution in patients with hypertension, diabetes mellitus, heart disease, peripheral vascular disease, increased intraocular pressure, hyperthyroidism, or prostatic hypertrophy.

PRECAUTIONS

Drug Interactions: ENTEX LIQUID should not be used in patients taking monoamine oxidase inhibitors or other sympathomimetics.
Drug/Laboratory Test Interactions: Guaifenesin has been reported to interfere with clinical laboratory determinations of urinary 5-hydroxyindoleacetic acid (5-HIAA) and urinary vanillylmandelic acid (VMA).
Pregnancy: Pregnancy Category C. Animal reproduction studies have not been conducted with ENTEX LIQUID. It is also not known whether ENTEX LIQUID can cause fetal harm when administered to a pregnant woman or can affect reproduction capacity. ENTEX LIQUID should be given to a pregnant woman only if clearly needed.
Nursing Mothers: It is not known whether the drugs in EXTEX LIQUID are excreted in human milk. Because many drugs are excreted in human milk and because of the potential for serious adverse reactions in nursing infants, a decision should be made whether to discontinue nursing or to discontinue the product, taking into account the importance of the drug to the mother.
Pediatric Use: Safety and effectiveness of ENTEX LIQUID in children below the age of 2 have not been established.

ADVERSE REACTIONS

Possible adverse reactions include nervousness, insomnia, restlessness, headache, nausea, or gastric irritation. These reactions seldom, if ever, require discontinuation of therapy. Urinary retention may occur in patients with prostatic hypertrophy.

OVERDOSAGE

The treatment of overdosage should provide symptomatic and supportive care. If the amount ingested is considered dangerous or excessive, induce vomiting with ipecac syrup unless the patient is convulsing, comatose, or has lost the gag reflex, in which case perform gastric lavage using a large-bore tube. If indicated, follow with activated charcoal and a saline cathartic.

DOSAGE AND ADMINISTRATION

All dosage should be administered four times daily (every 6 hours).

Children:
2 to under 4 years .... ½ teaspoonful (2.5 ml)
4 to under 6 years .... 1 teaspoonful (5.0 ml)
6 to under 12 years .... 1½ teaspoonfuls (7.5 ml)
Adults and children 12 years of age and older: 2 teaspoonfuls (10.0 ml)

HOW SUPPLIED

ENTEX LIQUID is available as an orange-colored, pleasant-tasting liquid.
NDC 0149-0414-16 16 FL. OZ. (1 Pint) bottle

CAUTION

Federal law prohibits dispensing without prescription.
REVISED SEPTEMBER 1985 ENXLQ-P5

ENTEX® LA ℞

[n'tex]
(phenylpropanolamine hydrochloride/guaifenesin)

DESCRIPTION

Each **Entex LA** orange, scored, long-acting tablet for oral administration contains
phenylpropanolamine hydrochloride .... 75 mg
guaifenesin .... 400 mg
in a special base to provide a prolonged therapeutic effect.
This product contains ingredients of the following therapeutic classes: decongestant and expectorant.
Phenylpropanolamine hydrochloride is a decongestant having the chemical name, benzenemethanol, α-(1-aminoethyl)-, hydrochloride (R*, S*), (±), with the following structure:

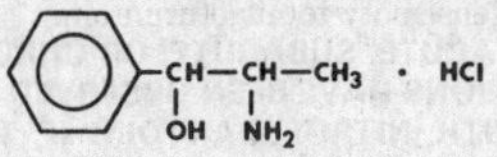

Guaifenesin is an expectorant having the chemical name, 1,2-propanediol, 3-(2-methoxyphenoxy)-, with the following structure:

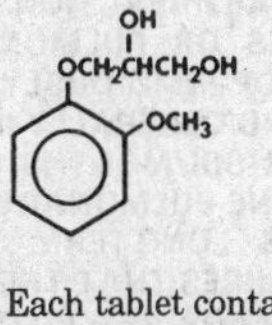

Inactive Ingredients: Each tablet contains carbomer 934 P, compressible sugar, docusate sodium, FD&C Yellow No. 6 Aluminum Lake, hydroxypropyl cellulose, hydroxypropyl methylcellulose, polyethylene glycol, silicon dioxide, stearic acid, titanium dioxide, and zinc stearate.

CLINICAL PHARMACOLOGY

Phenylpropanolamine hydrochloride is an α-adrenergic receptor agonist (sympathomimetic) which produces vasoconstriction by stimulating α-receptors within the mucosa of the respiratory tract. Clinically, phenylpropanolamine shrinks swollen mucous membranes, reduces tissue hyperemia, edema, and nasal congestion, and increases nasal airway patency. Guaifenesin promotes lower respiratory tract drainage by thinning bronchial secretions, lubricates irritated respiratory tract membranes through increased mucous flow, and facilitates removal of viscous, inspissated mucus. As a result of these drugs, sinus and bronchial drainage is improved, and dry, nonproductive coughs become more productive and less frequent.

INDICATIONS AND USAGE

Entex LA is indicated for the symptomatic relief of sinusitis, bronchitis, pharyngitis, and coryza when these conditions are associated with nasal congestion and viscous mucus in the lower respiratory tract.

CONTRAINDICATIONS

Entex LA is contraindicated in individuals with known hypersensitivity to sympathomimetics, severe hypertension, or in patients receiving monoamine oxidase inhibitors.

WARNINGS

Sympathomimetic amines should be used with caution in patients with hypertension, diabetes mellitus, heart disease, peripheral vascular disease, increased intraocular pressure, hyperthyroidism, or prostatic hypertrophy.

PRECAUTIONS

Information for Patients: Do not crush or chew **Entex LA** tablets prior to swallowing.
Drug Interactions: **Entex LA** should not be used in patients taking monoamine oxidase inhibitors or other sympathomimetics.
Drug/Laboratory Test Interactions: Guaifenesin has been reported to interfere with clinical laboratory determinations of urinary 5-hydroxyindoleacetic acid (5-HIAA) and urinary vanillylmandelic acid (VMA).
Pregnancy: Pregnancy Category C. Animal reproduction studies have not been conducted with **Entex LA**. It is also not known whether **Entex LA** can cause fetal harm when administered to a pregnant woman or can affect reproduction capacity. **Entex LA** should be given to a pregnant woman only if clearly needed.
Nursing Mothers: It is not known whether the drugs in **Entex LA** are excreted in human milk. Because many drugs are excreted in human milk and because of the potential for serious adverse reactions in nursing infants, a decision should be made whether to discontinue nursing or to discontinue the product, taking into account the importance of the drug to the mother.
Pediatric Use: Safety and effectiveness of **Entex LA** tablets in children below the age of 6 have not been established.

ADVERSE REACTIONS

Possible adverse reactions include nervousness, insomnia, restlessness, headache, nausea, or gastric irritation. These reactions seldom, if ever, require discontinuation of therapy. Urinary retention may occur in patients with prostatic hypertrophy.

OVERDOSAGE

The treatment of overdosage should provide symptomatic and supportive care. If the amount ingested is considered dangerous or excessive, induce vomiting with ipecac syrup unless the patient is convulsing, comatose, or has lost the gag reflex, in which case perform gastric lavage using a large-bore tube. If indicated, follow with activated charcoal and a saline cathartic. Since the effects of **Entex LA** may last up to 12 hours, treatment should be continued for at least that length of time.

DOSAGE AND ADMINISTRATION

Adults and children 12 years of age and older: one tablet twice daily (every 12 hours),
Children 6 to under 12 years: one-half (½) tablet twice daily (every 12 hours). **Entex LA** is not recommended for children under 6 years of age.
Tablets may be broken in half for ease of administration without affecting release of medication but should not be crushed or chewed prior to swallowing.

HOW SUPPLIED

Entex LA is available as an orange, scored tablet coded with "ENTEX LA" on one side and "0149 0436" on the scored side.
NDC 0149-0436-01 bottle of 100
NDC 0149-0436-05 bottle of 500
Store below 86°F (30°C).

CAUTION

Federal law prohibits dispensing without prescription.
Proctor & Gamble Pharmaceuticals
Norwich, New York 13815
REVISED JULY 1988
ENXLA-P2
Shown in Product Identification Section, page 423

ENTEX® PSE ℞

[n'tex P-S-E]
(pseudoephedrine hydrochloride/guaifenesin)

DESCRIPTION

Each **Entex PSE** yellow coated, scored, long-acting tablet for oral administration contains
pseudoephedrine hydrochloride .... 120 mg
guaifenesin .... 600 mg
in a special base to provide a prolonged therapeutic effect.
This product contains ingredients of the following therapeutic classes: decongestant and expectorant.
Pseudoephedrine hydrochloride is a decongestant having the chemical name, benzenemethanol,α-(1-(methylamino)ethyl)-[S-(R*,R*)]-, hydrochloride, with the following structure:

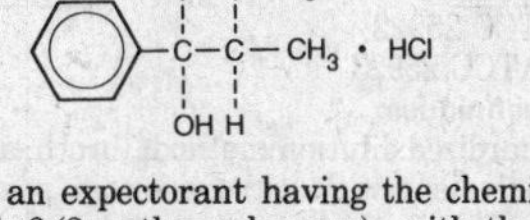

Guaifenesin is an expectorant having the chemical name, 1,2-propanediol, 3-(2-methoxyphenoxy)-, with the following structure:

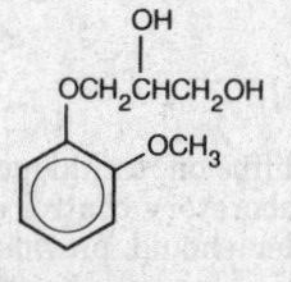

Inactive Ingredients: Each tablet contains compressible sugar, D&C Yellow No. 10 Aluminum Lake, dioctyl sodium sulfosuccinate, FD&C Yellow No. 6 Aluminum Lake, hydroxypropyl cellulose, hydroxypropyl methylcellulose, magnesium stearate, polyethylene glycol, purified water, silicon dioxide, sodium citrate, stearic acid, and titanium dioxide.

CLINICAL PHARMACOLOGY

Pseudoephedrine hydrochloride is an α-adrenergic receptor agonist (sympathomimetic) which produces vasoconstriction by stimulating α-receptors within the mucosa of the respiratory tract. Clinically, pseudoephedrine shrinks swollen mucous membranes, reduces tissue hyperemia, edema, and nasal congestion, and increases nasal airway patency. Guaifenesin promotes lower respiratory tract drainage by thinning bronchial secretions, lubricates irritated respiratory tract membranes through increased mucus flow, and facilitates removal of viscous, inspissated mucus. As a result of these drugs, sinus and bronchial drainage is improved, and dry, nonproductive coughs become more productive and less frequent.

INDICATIONS AND USAGE

Entex PSE tablets are indicated for the relief of nasal congestion due to the common cold, hay fever or other upper respiratory allergies, and nasal congestion associated with sinusitis. To promote nasal or sinus drainage; for the symptomatic relief of respiratory conditions characterized by dry nonproductive cough and in the presence of tenacious mucus and/or mucous plugs in the respiratory tract.

CONTRAINDICATIONS

Entex PSE tablets are contraindicated in patients with a known hypersensitivity to any of its ingredients, in nursing mothers, or in patients with severe hypertension, severe coronary artery disease, prostatic hypertrophy, or in patients on MAO inhibitor therapy.

WARNINGS

Sympathomimetic amines should be used with caution in patients with hypertension, diabetes mellitus, heart disease, peripheral vascular disease, increased intraocular pressure, hyperthyroidism, or prostatic hypertrophy.

PRECAUTIONS

General: Hypertensive patients should use **Entex PSE** tablets only with medical advice, as they may experience a change in blood pressure due to added vasoconstriction.
Information for Patients: Persistent cough may indicate a serious condition. If cough persists for more than one week, tends to recur, or is accompanied by a high fever, rash, or persistent headache, consult a physician.
Drug Interactions: MAO inhibitors and beta adrenergic blockers increase effects of sympathomimetics. Sympathomimetics may reduce the antihypertensive effects of methyldopa, guanethidine, mecamylamine, reserpine and veratrum alkaloids.
Drug/Laboratory Test Interactions: Guaifenesin has been reported to interfere with clinical laboratory determinations of urinary 5-hydroxyindoleacetic acid (5-HIAA) and urinary vanillylmandelic acid (VMA).
Pregnancy: Pregnancy Category C. Animal reproduction studies have not been conducted with **Entex PSE** tablets. It is also not known whether **Entex PSE** tablets can cause fetal harm when administered to a pregnant woman or can affect reproduction capacity. **Entex PSE** tablets should be given to a pregnant woman only if clearly needed.
Nursing Mothers: Entex PSE tablets are contraindicated in the nursing mother because of the higher than usual risks to infants from sympathomimetic agents.
Usage in Elderly: Patients 60 years and older are more likely to experience adverse reactions to sympathomimetics. Overdose may cause hallucinations, convulsions, CNS depression and death. Demonstrate safe use of a short-acting sympathomimetic before use of a sustained action formulation in elderly patients.
Pediatric Use: Safety and effectiveness of **Entex PSE** tablets in children below the age of 6 have not been established.

ADVERSE REACTIONS

Gastrointestinal: nausea and vomiting.
Central Nervous System: nervousness, dizziness, sleeplessness, lightheadedness, tremor, hallucinations, convulsions, CNS depression, fear, anxiety, headache, increased irritability or excitement.
Cardiovascular: palpitations, tachycardia, cardiovascular collapse and death.
General: weakness.
Respiratory: respiratory difficulties.

OVERDOSAGE

Symptoms: Overdosage may cause hallucinations, convulsions, CNS depression, cardiovascular collapse and death.
Treatment: Treatment of overdosage should provide symptomatic care. If the amount ingested is considered dangerous or excessive, induce vomiting with ipecac syrup unless the patient is convulsing, comatose, or has lost the gag reflex, in which case, perform gastric lavage using a large-bore tube. If indicated, follow with activated charcoal and a saline cathartic. Since the effects of **Entex PSE** tablets may last up to 12

Continued on next page

Procter & Gamble Pharm.—Cont.

hours, treatment should be continued for at least that length of time.

DOSAGE AND ADMINISTRATION

Adults and children 12 years of age and older: one tablet twice daily (every 12 hours).

Children 6 to under 12 years: one-half (½) tablet twice daily (every 12 hours). **Entex PSE** tablets are not recommended for children under 6 years of age.

Tablets may be broken in half for ease of administration without affecting release of medication but should not be crushed or chewed prior to swallowing.

HOW SUPPLIED: Entex PSE tablets are coated yellow, scored and coded with "**Entex PSE**" on one side and "NE" on the scored side.

NDC 0149-0427-02 bottle of 100

Store at controlled room temperature (59°–86°F or 15°–30°C).

Dispense in tight, light-resistant containers as defined in USP.

CAUTION: Federal law prohibits dispensing without prescription.

Proctor & Gamble Pharmaceuticals
Norwich, New York 13815
NOVEMBER 1991 ENXPSE-P2

Shown in Product Identification Section, page 423

MACROBID® ℞

[mak' ró bid]
(nitrofurantoin monohydrate/
macrocrystals)
Capsules

DESCRIPTION

Nitrofurantoin is an antibacterial agent specific for urinary tract infections. The Macrobid® brand of nitrofurantoin is a hard gelatin capsule shell containing the equivalent of 100 mg of nitrofurantoin in the form of 25 mg of nitrofurantoin macrocrystals and 75 mg of nitrofurantoin monohydrate.

The chemical name of nitrofurantoin macrocrystals is 1-[[[5-nitro-2-furanyl]methylene]amino]-2,4-imidazolidinedione. The chemical structure is the following:

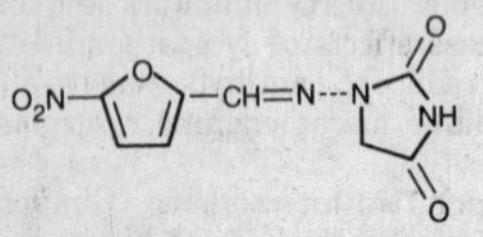

Molecular Weight: 238.16

The chemical name of nitrofurantoin monohydrate is 1-[[[5-nitro-2-furanyl]methylene]amino]-2,4-imidazolidinedione monohydrate. The chemical structure is the following:

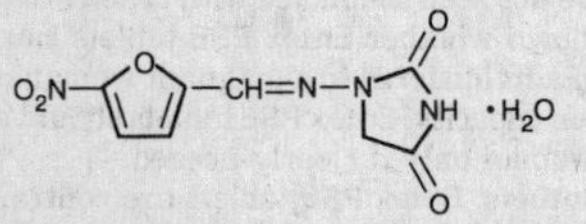

Molecular Weight: 256.17

Inactive Ingredients: Each capsule contains carbomer 934P, corn starch, compressible sugar, D&C Yellow No. 10, edible gray ink, FD&C Blue No. 1, FD&C Red No. 40, gelatin, lactose, magnesium stearate, povidone, talc, and titanium dioxide.

CLINICAL PHARMACOLOGY

Each Macrobid capsule contains two forms of nitrofurantoin. Twenty-five percent is macrocrystalline nitrofurantoin, which has slower dissolution and absorption than nitrofurantoin monohydrate. The remaining 75% is nitrofurantoin monohydrate contained in a powder blend which, upon exposure to gastric and intestinal fluids, forms a gel matrix that releases nitrofurantoin over time. Based on urinary pharmacokinetic data, the extent and rate of urinary excretion of nitrofurantoin from the 100-mg Macrobid capsule are similar to those of the 50-mg or 100-mg Macrodantin® (nitrofurantoin macrocrystals) capsule. Approximately 20–25% of a single dose of nitrofurantoin is recovered from the urine unchanged over 24 hours.

Plasma nitrofurantoin concentrations after a single oral dose of the 100-mg Macrobid capsule are low, with peak levels usually less than 1 mcg/mL. Nitrofurantoin is highly soluble in urine, to which it may impart a brown color. When Macrobid is administered with food, the bioavailability of nitrofurantoin is increased by approximately 40%.

Microbiology: Nitrofurantoin is bactericidal in urine at therapeutic doses. The mechanism of the antimicrobial action of nitrofurantoin is unusual among antibacterials. Nitrofurantoin is reduced by bacterial flavoproteins to reactive intermediates which inactivate or alter bacterial ribosomal proteins and other macromolecules. As a result of such inactivations, the vital biochemical processes of protein synthesis, aerobic energy metabolism, DNA synthesis, RNA synthesis, and cell wall synthesis are inhibited. The broad-based nature of this mode of action may explain the lack of acquired bacterial resistance to nitrofurantoin, as the necessary multiple and simultaneous mutations of the target macromolecules would likely be lethal to the bacteria. Development of resistance to nitrofurantoin has not been a significant problem since its introduction in 1953. Cross-resistance with antibiotics and sulfonamides has not been observed, and transferable resistance is, at most, a very rare phenomenon.

Nitrofurantoin, in the form of Macrobid, has been shown to be active against most strains of the following bacteria both *in vitro* and in clinical infections: (See **INDICATIONS AND USAGE.**)

Gram-Positive Aerobes
Staphylococcus saprophyticus
Gram-Negative Aerobes
Escherichia coli

Nitrofurantoin also demonstrates *in vitro* activity against the following microorganisms, although the clinical significance of these data with respect to treatment with Macrobid is unknown:

Gram-Positive Aerobes
Coagulase-negative staphylococci
(including *Staphylococcus epidermidis*)
Enterococcus faecalis
Staphylococcus aureus
Streptococcus agalactiae
Group D streptococci
Viridans group streptococci
Gram-Negative Aerobes
Citrobacter amalonaticus
Citrobacter diversus
Citrobacter freundii
Klebsiella oxytoca
Klebsiella ozaenae

Nitrofurantoin is not active against most strains of *Proteus* species or *Serratia* species. It has no activity against *Pseudomonas* species.

Antagonism has been demonstrated *in vitro* between nitrofurantoin and quinolone antimicrobials. The clinical significance of this finding is unknown.

Susceptibility Tests:
Diffusion Techniques:

Quantitative methods that require measurement of zone diameters give the most precise estimate of the susceptibility of bacteria to antimicrobial agents. One such standard procedure,[1] which has been recommended for use with disks to test susceptibility of organisms to nitrofurantoin, uses the 300-mcg nitrofurantoin disk. Interpretation involves the correlation of the diameter obtained in the disk test with the minimum inhibitory concentration (MIC) for nitrofurantoin. Reports from the laboratory giving results of the standard single-disk susceptibility test with a 300-mcg nitrofurantoin disk should be interpreted according to the following criteria:

Zone Diameter (mm)	Interpretation
≥17	Susceptible
15–16	Intermediate
≤14	Resistant

A report of "susceptible" indicates that the pathogen is likely to be inhibited by generally achievable urinary levels. A report of "intermediate" indicates that the result be considered equivocal and, if the organism is not fully susceptible to alternative clinically feasible drugs, the test should be repeated. This category provides a buffer zone which prevents small uncontrolled technical factors from causing major discrepancies in interpretations. A report of "resistant" indicates that achievable concentrations are unlikely to be inhibitory, and other therapy should be selected.

Standardized procedures require the use of laboratory control organisms. The 300-mcg nitrofurantoin disk should give the following zone diameters:

Organism	Zone Diameter (mm)
E. coli ATCC 25922	20–25
S. aureus ATCC 25923	18–22

Dilution Techniques:

Use a standardized dilution method[2] (broth, agar, microdilution) or equivalent with nitrofurantoin powder. The MIC values obtained should be interpreted according to the following criteria:

MIC (mcg/mL)	Interpretation
≤32	Susceptible
64	Intermediate
≥128	Resistant

As with standard diffusion techniques, dilution methods require the use of laboratory control organisms. Standard nitrofurantoin powder should provide the following MIC values:

Organism	MIC (mcg/mL)
E. coli ATCC 25922	4–16
S. aureus ATCC 29213	8–32
E. faecalis ATCC 29212	4–16

INDICATIONS AND USAGE

Macrobid is indicated only for the treatment of acute uncomplicated urinary tract infections (acute cystitis) caused by susceptible strains of *Escherichia coli* or *Staphylococcus saprophyticus.*

Nitrofurantoin is not indicated for the treatment of pyelonephritis or perinephric abscesses.

Nitrofurantoins lack the broader tissue distribution of other therapeutic agents approved for urinary tract infections. Consequently, many patients who are treated with Macrobid are predisposed to persistence or reappearance of bacteriuria. (See CLINICAL STUDIES.) Urine specimens for culture and susceptibility testing should be obtained before and after completion of therapy. If persistence or reappearance of bacteriuria occurs after treatment with Macrobid, other therapeutic agents with broader tissue distribution should be selected. In considering the use of Macrobid, lower eradication rates should be balanced against the increased potential for systemic toxicity and for the development of antimicrobial resistance when agents with broader tissue distribution are utilized.

CONTRAINDICATIONS

Anuria, oliguria, or significant impairment of renal function (creatinine clearance under 60 mL per minute or clinically significant elevated serum creatinine) are contraindications. Treatment of this type of patient carries an increased risk of toxicity because of impaired excretion of the drug.

Because of the possibility of hemolytic anemia due to immature erythrocyte enzyme systems (glutathione instability), the drug is contraindicated in pregnant patients at term (38–42 weeks gestation), during labor and delivery, or when the onset of labor is imminent. For the same reason, the drug is contraindicated in neonates under one month of age.

Macrobid is also contraindicated in those patients with known hypersensitivity to nitrofurantoin.

WARNINGS: ACUTE, SUBACUTE, OR CHRONIC PULMONARY REACTIONS HAVE BEEN OBSERVED IN PATIENTS TREATED WITH NITROFURANTOIN. IF THESE REACTIONS OCCUR, MACROBID SHOULD BE DISCONTINUED AND APPROPRIATE MEASURES TAKEN. REPORTS HAVE CITED PULMONARY REACTIONS AS A CONTRIBUTING CAUSE OF DEATH.

CHRONIC PULMONARY REACTIONS (DIFFUSE INTERSTITIAL PNEUMONITIS OR PULMONARY FIBROSIS, OR BOTH) CAN DEVELOP INSIDIOUSLY. THESE REACTIONS OCCUR RARELY AND GENERALLY IN PATIENTS RECEIVING THERAPY FOR SIX MONTHS OR LONGER. CLOSE MONITORING OF THE PULMONARY CONDITION OF PATIENTS RECEIVING LONG-TERM THERAPY IS WARRANTED AND REQUIRES THAT THE BENEFITS OF THERAPY BE WEIGHED AGAINST POTENTIAL RISKS. (SEE RESPIRATORY REACTIONS.)

Hepatic reactions, including hepatitis, cholestatic jaundice, and chronic active hepatitis, occur rarely. Fatalities have been reported. The onset of chronic active hepatitis may be insidious, and patients should be monitored periodically for changes in liver function. If hepatitis occurs, the drug should be withdrawn immediately and appropriate measures should be taken.

Peripheral neuropathy, which may become severe or irreversible, has occurred. Fatalities have been reported. Conditions such as renal impairment (creatinine clearance under 60 mL per minute or clinically significant elevated serum creatinine), anemia, diabetes mellitus, electrolyte imbalance, vitamin B deficiency, and debilitating disease may enhance the occurrence of peripheral neuropathy. Patients receiving long-term therapy should be monitored periodically for changes in renal function.

Cases of hemolytic anemia of the primaquine-sensitivity type have been induced by nitrofurantoin. Hemolysis appears to be linked to a glucose-6-phosphate dehydrogenase deficiency in the red blood cells of the affected patients. This deficiency is found in 10 percent of Blacks and a small percentage of ethnic groups of Mediterranean and Near-Eastern origin. Hemolysis is an indication for discontinuing Macrobid; hemolysis ceases when the drug is withdrawn.

PRECAUTIONS

Information for Patients: Patients should be advised to take Macrobid with food (ideally breakfast and dinner) to further enhance tolerance and improve drug absorption. Patients should be instructed to complete the full course of therapy; however, they should be advised to contact their physician if any unusual symptoms occur during therapy.

Patients should be advised not to use antacid preparations containing magnesium trisilicate while taking Macrobid.

Drug Interactions: Antacids containing magnesium trisilicate, when administered concomitantly with nitrofurantoin, reduce both the rate and extent of absorption. The mechanism for this interaction probably is adsorption of nitrofurantoin onto the surface of magnesium trisilicate.

Uricosuric drugs, such as probenecid and sulfinpyrazone, can inhibit renal tubular secretion of nitrofurantoin. The resulting increase in nitrofurantoin serum levels may increase toxicity, and the decreased urinary levels could lessen its efficacy as a urinary tract antibacterial.

Drug/Laboratory Test Interactions: As a result of the presence of nitrofurantoin, a false-positive reaction for glucose in the urine may occur. This has been observed with Benedict's and Fehling's solutions but not with the glucose enzymatic test.

Carcinogenesis, Mutagensis, Impairment of Fertility: Nitrofurantoin was not carcinogenic when fed to female Holtzman rats for 44.5 weeks or to female Sprague-Dawley rats for 75 weeks. Two chronic rodent bioassays utilizing male and female Sprague-Dawley rats and two chronic bioassays in Swiss mice and in BDF_1 mice revealed no evidence of carcinogenicity.

Nitrofurantoin presented evidence of carcinogenic activity in female $B6C3F_1$ mice as shown by increased incidences of tubular adenomas, benign mixed tumors, and granulosa cell tumors of the ovary. In male F344/N rats, there were increased incidences of uncommon kidney tubular cell neoplasms, osteosarcomas of the bone, and neoplasms of the subcutaneous tissue. In one study involving subcutaneous administration of 75 mg/kg nitrofurantoin to pregnant female mice, lung papillary adenomas of unknown significance were observed in the F1 generation.

Nitrofurantoin has been shown to induce point mutations in certain strains of *Salmonella typhimurium* and forward mutations in L5178Y mouse lymphoma cells. Nitrofurantoin induced increased numbers of sister chromatid exchanges and chromosomal aberrations in Chinese hamster ovary cells but not in human cells in culture. Results of the sex-linked recessive lethal assay in Drosophila were negative after administration of nitrofurantoin by feeding or by injection. Nitrofurantoin did not induce heritable mutation in the rodent models examined.

The significance of the carcinogenicity and mutagenicity findings relative to the therapeutic use of nitrofurantoin in humans is unknown.

The administration of high doses of nitrofurantoin to rats causes temporary spermatogenic arrest; this is reversible on discontinuing the drug. Doses of 10 mg/kg/day or greater in healthy human males may, in certain unpredictable instances, produce a slight to moderate spermatogenic arrest with a decrease in sperm count.

Pregnancy:

Teratogenic effects: Pregnancy Category B. Several reproduction studies have been performed in rabbits and rats at doses up to six times the human dose and have revealed no evidence of impaired fertility or harm to the fetus due to nitrofurantoin. In a single published study conducted in mice at 68 times the human dose (based on mg/kg administered to the dam), growth retardation and a low incidence of minor and common malformations were observed. However, at 25 times the human dose, fetal malformations were not observed; the relevance of these findings to humans is uncertain. There are, however, no adequate and well-controlled studies in pregnant women. Because animal reproduction studies are not always predictive of human response, this drug should be used during pregnancy only if clearly needed.

Non-teratogenic effects: Nitrofurantoin has been shown in one published transplacental carcinogenicity study to induce lung papillary adenomas in the F1 generation mice at doses 19 times the human dose on a mg/kg basis. The relationship of this finding to potential human carcinogenesis is presently unknown. Because of the uncertainty regarding the human implications of these animal data, this drug should be used during pregnancy only if clearly needed.

Labor and Delivery: See CONTRAINDICATIONS.

Nursing Mothers: Nitrofurantoin has been detected in human breast milk in trace amounts. Because of the potential for serious adverse reactions from nitrofurantoin in nursing infants under one month of age, a decision should be made whether to discontinue nursing or to discontinue the drug, taking into account the importance of the drug to the mother. (See CONTRAINDICATIONS.)

Pediatric Use: Macrobid is contraindicated in infants below the age of one month. (See CONTRAINDICATIONS.) Safety and effectiveness in children below the age of twelve years have not been established.

ADVERSE REACTIONS

In clinical trials of Macrobid, the most frequent clinical adverse events that were reported as possibly or probably drug-related were nausea (8%), headache (6%), and flatulence (1.5%). Additional clinical adverse events reported as possibly or probably drug-related occurred in less than 1% of patients studied and are listed below within each body system in order of decreasing frequency:

Gastrointestinal: Diarrhea, dyspepsia, abdominal pain, constipation, emesis

Neurologic: Dizziness, drowsiness, amblyopia

Respiratory: Acute pulmonary hypersensitivity reaction (see WARNINGS)

Allergic: Pruritus, urticaria

Dermatologic: Alopecia

Miscellaneous: Fever, chills, malaise

The following additional clinical adverse events have been reported with the use of nitrofurantoin:

Gastrointestinal: Sialadenitis, pancreatitis

Neurologic: Peripheral neuropathy, which may become severe or irreversible, has occurred. Fatalities have been reported. Conditions such as renal impairment (creatinine clearance under 60 mL per minute or clinically significant elevated serum creatinine), anemia, diabetes mellitus, electrolyte imbalance, vitamin B deficiency, and debilitating diseases may increase the possibility of peripheral neuropathy. (See WARNINGS.)

Asthenia, vertigo, and nystagmus also have been reported with the use of nitrofurantoin.

Respiratory:

CHRONIC, SUBACUTE, OR ACUTE PULMONARY HYPERSENSITIVITY REACTIONS MAY OCCUR WITH THE USE OF NITROFURANTOIN.

CHRONIC PULMONARY REACTIONS GENERALLY OCCUR IN PATIENTS WHO HAVE RECEIVED CONTINUOUS TREATMENT FOR SIX MONTHS OR LONGER. MALAISE, DYSPNEA ON EXERTION, COUGH, AND ALTERED PULMONARY FUNCTION ARE COMMON MANIFESTATIONS WHICH CAN OCCUR INSIDIOUSLY. RADIOLOGIC AND HISTOLOGIC FINDINGS OF DIFFUSE INTERSTITIAL PNEUMONITIS OR FIBROSIS, OR BOTH, ARE ALSO COMMON MANIFESTATIONS OF THE CHRONIC PULMONARY REACTION. FEVER IS RARELY PROMINENT.

THE SEVERITY OF CHRONIC PULMONARY REACTIONS AND THEIR DEGREE OF RESOLUTION APPEAR TO BE RELATED TO THE DURATION OF THERAPY AFTER THE FIRST CLINICAL SIGNS APPEAR. PULMONARY FUNCTION MAY BE IMPAIRED PERMANENTLY, EVEN AFTER CESSATION OF THERAPY. THE RISK IS GREATER WHEN CHRONIC PULMONARY REACTIONS ARE NOT RECOGNIZED EARLY.

In subacute pulmonary reactions, fever and eosinophilia occur less than in the acute form. Upon cessation of therapy, recovery may require several months. If the symptoms are not recognized as being drug-related and nitrofurantoin therapy is not stopped, the symptoms may become more severe.

Acute pulmonary reactions are commonly manifested by fever, chills, cough chest pain, dyspnea, pulmonary infiltration with consolidation or pleural effusion on x-ray, and eosinophilia. Acute reactions usually occur within the first week of treatment and are reversible with cessation of therapy. Resolution often is dramatic. (See WARNINGS.)

Hepatic: Hepatic reactions, including hepatitis, cholestatic jaundice, and chronic active hepatitis, occur rarely. (See WARNINGS.)

Allergic: Lupus-like syndrome associated with pulmonary reaction to nitrofurantoin has been reported. Also, angioedema; maculopapular, erythematous, or eczematous eruptions; anaphylaxis; arthralgia; myalgia; drug fever; and chills have been reported.

Dermatologic: Exfoliative dermatitis and erythema multiforme (including Stevens-Johnson Syndrome) have been reported rarely.

Miscellaneous: As with other antimicrobial agents, superinfections with resistant organisms, *e.g., Pseudomonas* species or *Candida* species, may occur with the use of nitrofurantoin. Superinfections have been limited to the genitourinary tract.

In clinical trials of Macrobid, the most frequent laboratory adverse events (1–5%), without regard to drug relationship, were as follows: eosinophilia, increased AST (SGOT), increased ALT (SGPT), decreased hemoglobin, increased serum phosphorus. The following laboratory adverse events also have been reported with the use of nitrofurantoin: glucose-6-phosphate dehydrogenase deficiency anemia (see WARNINGS), agranulocytosis, leukopenia, granulocytopenia, hemolytic anemia, thrombocytopenia, megaloblastic anemia. In most cases, these hematologic abnormalities resolved following cessation of therapy. Aplastic anemia has been reported rarely.

OVERDOSAGE

Occasional incidents of acute overdosage of nitrofurantoin have not resulted in any specific symptoms other than vomiting. Induction of emesis is recommended. There is no specific antidote, but a high fluid intake should be maintained to promote urinary excretion of the drug. Nitrofurantoin is dialyzable.

DOSAGE AND ADMINISTRATION

Macrobid capsules should be taken with food.

Adults and Children Over 12 Years: One 100-mg capsule every 12 hours for seven days.

HOW SUPPLIED

Macrobid is available as 100-mg opaque black and yellow capsules imprinted "Macrobid" on the black portion and "Norwich Eaton" on the yellow portion.

NDC 0149-0710-01 bottle of 100

Store at controlled room temperature (59° to 86°F or 15° to 30°C).

CAUTION: Federal law prohibits dispensing without prescription.

REFERENCES:

1. National Committee for Clinical Laboratory Standards. Performance Standards for Antimicrobial Disk Susceptibility Tests—Fourth Edition. Approved Standard NCCLS Document M2-A4, Vol. 10, No. 7, NCCLS, Villanova, PA, 1990.
2. National Committee for Clinical Laboratory Standards. Methods for Dilution Antimicrobial Susceptibility Tests for Bacteria that Grow Aerobically—Second Edition. Approved Standard NCCLS Document M7-A2, Vol. 10, No. 8, NCCLS, Villanova, PA, 1990.

CLINICAL STUDIES

Controlled clinical trials comparing Macrobid 100 mg p.o. q12h and Macrodantin® 50 mg p.o. q6h in the treatment of acute uncomplicated urinary tract infections demonstrated approximately 75% microbiologic eradication of susceptible pathogens in each treatment group.

MACROBID-P2

Procter & Gamble Pharmaceuticals
Norwich, New York 13815

December 10, 1991

Shown in Product Identification Section, page 423

MACRODANTIN® CAPSULES ℞

[*mak"rō-dan'tĭn*]

(nitrofurantoin macrocrystals)

DESCRIPTION

Macrodantin (nitrofurantoin macrocrystals) is a synthetic chemical of controlled crystal size. It is a stable, yellow crystalline compound. Macrodantin is an antibacterial agent for specific urinary tract infections. It is available in 25-mg, 50-mg, and 100-mg capsules for oral administration.

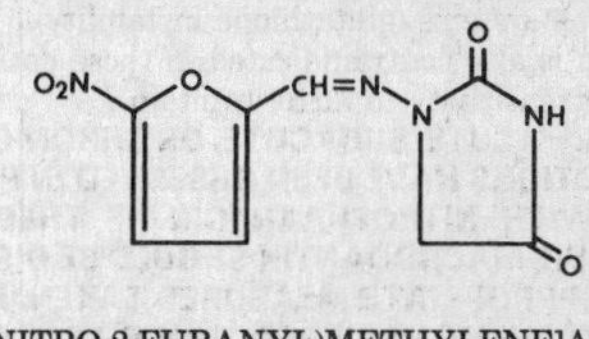

1-[[(5-NITRO-2-FURANYL)METHYLENE]AMINO]-2,4-IMIDAZOLIDINEDIONE

INACTIVE INGREDIENTS: Each capsule contains edible black ink, gelatin, lactose, starch, talc, titanium dioxide, and may contain FD&C Yellow #6 and and D&C Yellow #10.

CLINICAL PHARMACOLOGY

Macrodantin is a larger crystal form of Furadantin® (nitrofurantoin). The absorption of Macrodantin is slower and its excretion somewhat less when compared to Furandantin. Blood concentrations at therapeutic dosage are usually low. Many patients who cannot tolerate microcrystalline nitrofurantoin are able to take Macrodantin without nausea. It is highly soluble in urine, to which it may impart a brown color.

Following a dose regimen of 100 mg q.i.d. for 7 days, average urinary drug recoveries (0-24 hours) on day 1 and day 7 were 37.9% and 35.0%.

Unlike many drugs, the presence of food or agents delaying gastric emptying can increase the bioavailability of Macrodantin, presumably by allowing better dissolution in gastric juices.

Microbiology: Macrodantin, *in vitro,* is bacteriostatic in low concentrations (5-10 mcg/ml) and is considered bactericidal in higher concentrations. Its mode of action is presumed to be interference with several bacterial enzyme systems. Bacteria develop only a limited resistance to furan derivatives.

While *in vitro* studies have demonstrated the susceptibility of most strains of the following organisms, clinical efficacy for infections other than those included in the INDICATIONS AND USAGE section has not been documented: *Escherichia coli,* enterococci (e.g., *Streptococcus faecalis*), *Staphylococcus aureus, Staphylococcus epidermidis.*

Note: Some strains of *Enterobacter* species and *Klebsiella* species are resistant to Macrodantin. It is not active against most strains of *Proteus* and *Serratia* species. It has no activity against *Pseudomonas* species.

Antagonism has been demonstrated between nitrofurantoin and both nalidixic acid and oxolinic acid *in vitro.*

Susceptibility Tests—Quantitative methods that require measurement of zone diameters give the most precise estimates of antimicrobial susceptibility. One recommended

Continued on next page

Procter & Gamble Pharm.—Cont.

procedure, (NCCLS, ASM-2)*, uses a disc containing 300 micrograms for testing susceptibility; interpretations correlate zone diameters of this disc test with MIC values for nitrofurantoin. Reports from the laboratory should be interpreted according to the following criteria:

Susceptible organisms produce zones of 17 mm or greater, indicating that the tested organism is likely to respond to therapy.

Organisms of intermediate susceptibility produce zones of 15 to 16 mm, indicating that the tested organism would be susceptible if high dosage is used.

Resistant organisms produce zones of 14 mm or less, indicating that other therapy should be selected.

A bacterial isolate may be considered susceptible if the MIC value for nitrofurantoin is 25 micrograms per ml or less. Organisms are considered resistant if the MIC is not less than 100 micrograms per ml or more.

NOTE

Specimens for culture and susceptibility testing should be obtained prior to and during the drug administration.

INDICATIONS AND USAGE

Macrodantin is specifically indicated for the treatment of urinary tract infections when due to susceptible strains of *E. coli*, enterococci, *S. aureus* (it is not indicated for the treatment of associated renal cortical or perinephric abscesses), and certain susceptible strains of *Klebsiella, Enterobacter* and *Proteus* species.

CONTRAINDICATIONS

Anuria, oliguria, or significant impairment of renal function (creatinine clearance under 40 ml per minute) are contraindications. Treatment of this type of patient carries an increased risk of toxicity and is much less effective because of impaired excretion of the drug.

The drug is contraindicated in pregnant patients at term (during labor and delivery) as well as in infants under one month of age because of the possibility of hemolytic anemia in the fetus or in the newborn infant due to immature erythrocyte enzyme systems (glutathione instability).

Macrodantin is also contraindicated in those patients with known hypersensitivity to nitrofurantoin.

WARNINGS: ACUTE, SUBACUTE, OR CHRONIC PULMONARY REACTIONS HAVE BEEN OBSERVED IN PATIENTS TREATED WITH NITROFURANTOIN. IF THESE REACTIONS OCCUR, MACRODANTIN SHOULD BE DISCONTINUED AND APPROPRIATE MEASURES TAKEN. REPORTS HAVE CITED PULMONARY REACTIONS AS A CONTRIBUTING CAUSE OF DEATH.

CHRONIC PULMONARY REACTIONS (DIFFUSE INTERSTITIAL PNEUMONITIS OR PULMONARY FIBROSIS, OR BOTH) CAN DEVELOP INSIDIOUSLY. THESE REACTIONS OCCUR RARELY AND GENERALLY IN PATIENTS RECEIVING THERAPY FOR SIX MONTHS OR LONGER. CLOSE MONITORING OF THE PULMONARY CONDITION OF PATIENTS RECEIVING LONG-TERM THERAPY IS WARRANTED AND REQUIRES THAT THE BENEFITS OF THERAPY BE WEIGHED AGAINST POTENTIAL RISKS. (SEE RESPIRATORY REACTIONS.)

Hepatitis, including chronic active hepatitis, occurs rarely. Fatalities have been reported. The onset of chronic active hepatitis may be insidious, and patients receiving long-term therapy should be monitored periodically for changes in liver function. If hepatitis occurs, the drug should be withdrawn immediately and appropriate measures taken.

Peripheral neuropathy, which may become severe or irreversible, has occurred. Fatalities have been reported. Conditions such as renal impairment (creatinine clearance under 40 ml per minute), anemia, diabetes mellitus, electrolyte imbalance, vitamin B deficiency, and debilitating disease may enhance the occurence of peripheral neuropathy.

Cases of hemolytic anemia of the primaquine sensitivity type have been induced by nitrofurantoin. Hemolysis appears to be linked to a glucose-6-phosphate dehydrogenase deficiency in the red blood cells of the affected patients. This deficiency is found in 10 percent of Negroes and a small percentage of ethnic groups of Mediterranean and Near Eastern origin. Hemolysis is an indication for discontinuing Macrodantin; hemolysis ceases when the drug is withdrawn.

PRECAUTIONS

Drug Interactions: Magnesium trisilicate, when administered concomitantly with Macrodantin, reduces both the rate and extent of absorption. The mechanism for this interaction probably is adsorption of drug onto the surface of magnesium trisilicate.

Uricosuric drugs such as probenecid and sulfinpyrazone may inhibit renal tubular secretion of Macrodantin. The resulting increase in serum levels may increase toxicity and the

*National Committee for Clinical Laboratory Standards. Approved Standard: ASM-2, Performance Standards for Antimicrobial Disc Susceptibility Tests, July, 1975.

decreased urinary levels could lessen its efficacy as a urinary tract antibacterial.

Carcinogensis, Mutagenesis: Nitrofurantoin, when fed to female Holzman rats at levels of 0.3% in a commercial diet for up to 44.5 weeks, was not carcinogenic. Nitrofurantoin was not carcinogenic when female Sprague-Dawley rats were fed a commercial diet with nitrofurantoin levels at 0.1% to 0.187% (total cumulative, 9.25 g) for 75 weeks. Further studies of the effects chronic administration to rodents are in progress.

Results of microbial *in vitro* tests using *Escherichia coli, Salmonella typhimurium*, and *Aspergillus nidulans* suggest that nitrofurantoin is a weak mutagen. Results of a dominant lethal assay in the mouse were negative.

Impairment of Fertility: The administration of high doses of nitrofurantoin to rats causes temporary spermatogenic arrest; this is reversible on discontinuing the drug. Doses of 10 mg/kg or greater in healthy human males may, in certain unpredictable instances, produce slight to moderate spermatogenic arrest with a decrease in sperm count.

Pregnancy: The safety of Macrodantin during pregnancy and lactation has not been established. Use of this drug in women of childbearing potential requires that the anticipated benefit be weighed against the possible risks.

Labor and Delivery: See CONTRAINDICATIONS.

Nursing Mothers: Nitrofurantoin has been detected in breast milk, in trace amounts. Caution should be exercised when Macrodantin is administered to a nursing woman, especially if the infant is known or suspected to have a glucose-6-phosphate dehydrogenase deficiency.

Pediatric Use: Contraindicated in infants under one month of age. (See CONTRAINDICATIONS.)

ADVERSE REACTIONS

Respiratory:
CHRONIC, SUBACUTE, OR ACUTE PULMONARY HYPERSENSITIVITY REACTIONS MAY OCCUR.

CHRONIC PULMONARY REACTIONS OCCUR GENERALLY IN PATIENTS WHO HAVE RECEIVED CONTINUOUS TREATMENT FOR SIX MONTHS OR LONGER. MALAISE, DYSPNEA ON EXERTION, COUGH, AND ALTERED PULMONARY FUNCTION ARE COMMON MANIFESTATIONS WHICH CAN OCCUR INSIDIOUSLY. RADIOLOGIC AND HISTOLOGIC FINDINGS OF DIFFUSE INTERSTITIAL PNEUMONITIS OR FIBROSIS, OR BOTH, ARE ALSO COMMON MANIFESTATIONS OF THE CHRONIC PULMONARY REACTION. FEVER IS RARELY PROMINENT.

THE SEVERITY OF CHRONIC PULMONARY REACTIONS AND THEIR DEGREE OF RESOLUTION APPEAR TO BE RELATED TO THE DURATION OF THERAPY AFTER THE FIRST CLINICAL SIGNS APPEAR. PULMONARY FUNCTION MAY BE IMPAIRED PERMANENTLY, EVEN AFTER CESSATION OF THERAPY. THE RISK IS GREATER WHEN CHRONIC PULMONARY REACTIONS ARE NOT RECOGNIZED EARLY.

In subacute pulmonary reactions, fever and eosinophilia occur less often than in the acute form. Upon cessation of therapy, recovery may require several months. If the symptoms are not recognized as being drug-related and nitrofurantoin therapy is not stopped, the symptoms may become more severe.

Acute pulmonary reactions are commonly manifested by fever, chills, cough, chest pain, dyspnea, pulmonary infiltration with consolidation or pleural effusion on x-ray, and eosinophilia. Acute reactions usually occur within the first week of treatment and are reversible with cessation of therapy. Resolution often is dramatic. (See WARNINGS.)

Gastrointestinal: Hepatitis, including chronic active hepatitis, and cholestatic jaundice occur rarely.

Nausea, emesis, and anorexia occur most often. Abdominal pain and diarrhea are less common gastrointestinal reactions. These dose-related reactions can be minimized by reduction of dosage.

Neurologic: Peripheral neuropathy, which may become severe or irreversible, has occurred. Fatalities have been reported. Conditions such as renal impairment (creatinine clearance under 40 ml per minute), anemia, diabetes mellitus, electrolyte imbalance, vitamin B deficiency, and debilitating diseases may increase the possibility of peripheral neuropathy.

Less frequent reactions, of unknown causal relationship, are nystagmus, vertigo, dizziness, asthenia, headache, and drowsiness.

Dermatologic: Exfoliative dermititis and erythema multiforme (including Stevens-Johnson Syndrome) have been reported rarely. Transient alopecia also has been reported.

Allergic Reactions: Lupus-like syndrome associated with pulmonary reaction to nitrofurantoin has been reported. Also, angioedema, maculopapular, erythematous or eczematous eruptions, urticaria, rash, and pruritus have occurred. Anaphylaxis, sialadentitis, pancreatitis, arthralgia, myalgia, drug fever, and chills or chills and fever have been reported.

Hematologic: Agranulocytosis, leukopenia, granulocytopenia, hemolytic anemia, thrombocytopenia, glucose-6-phosphate dehydrogenase deficiency anemia, megaloblastic

anemia, and eosinophilia have occurred. Cessation of therapy has returned the blood picture to normal. Aplastic anemia has been reported rarely.

Miscellaneous reactions: As with other antimicrobial agents, superinfections by resistant organisms, e.g., *Pseudomonas*, may occur. However, these are limited to the genitourinary tract because suppression of normal bacterial flora does not occur elsewhere in the body.

OVERDOSAGE

Occasional incidents of acute overdosage of Macrodantin have not resulted in any specific symptoms other than vomiting. In case vomiting does not occur soon after an excessive dose, induction of emesis is recommended. There is no specific antidote, but a high fluid intake should be maintained to promote urinary excretion of the drug.

DOSAGE AND ADMINISTRATION

Macrodantin should be given with food to improve drug absorption and, in some patients, tolerance.

Adults: 50–100 mg four times a day—the lower dosage level is recommended for uncomplicated urinary tract infections.

Children: 5–7 mg/kg of body weight per 24 hours, given in four divided doses (contraindicated under one month of age). Therapy should be continued for one week or for at least 3 days after sterility of the urine is obtained. Continued infection indicates the need for reevaluation.

For long-term suppressive therapy in adults, a reduction of dosage to 50–100 mg at bedtime may be adequate. For long-term suppressive therapy in children, doses as low as 1 mg/kg per 24 hours, given in a single or in two divided doses, may be adequate. SEE WARNINGS SECTION REGARDING RISKS ASSOCIATED WITH LONG-TERM THERAPY.

HOW SUPPLIED

Macrodantin is available as follows:

25-mg opaque, white capsule imprinted with one black line encircling the capsule and coded "Macrodantin 25 mg" and "0149-0007".

NDC 0149-0007-05	bottle of 100

50-mg opaque, yellow and white capsule imprinted with two black lines encircling the capsule and coded "Macrodantin 50 mg" and "0149-0008".*

NDC 0149-0008-05	bottle of 100
NDC 0149-0008-25	MACPAC® ,box of 7 DAYCARD® blisters, 4 capsules each.
NDC 0149-0008-66	bottle of 500
NDC 0149-0008-67	bottle of 1000
NDC 0149-0008-77	hospital unit-dose strips in box of 100

100-mg opaque, yellow capsule imprinted with three black lines encircling the capsule and coded "Macrodantin 100 mg" and "0149 0009".*

NDC 0149-0009-05	bottle of 100
NDC 0149-0009-23	MACPAC® , box of 7 DAYCARD® blisters, 4 capsules each.
NDC 0149-0009-66	bottle of 500
NDC 0149-0009-67	bottle of 1000
NDC 0149-0009-77	hospital unit-dose strips in box of 100

Furadantin/Macrodantin Sensi-Discs for the laboratory determination of bacterial sensitivity are available from BBL, Division of BioQuest. For information on nitrofurantoin assays in blood, serum, and urine, write or call the Medical Department. Literature sent to physicians on request. Address medical inquires to Norwich Eaton Pharmaceuticals, Inc. Medical Department, P.O. Box 191, Norwich, NY 13815-0191.

CAUTION

Federal law prohibits dispensing without prescription.
Procter & Gamble Pharmaceuticals

*capsule design, registered trademark of Eaton Laboratories, Inc.

REVISED MAY 1988   MACRO-U1

Shown in Product Identification Section, page 424

EDUCATIONAL MATERIAL

Procter & Gamble Pharmaceuticals offers a wide range of educational services to the medical profession. Please write to Manager, Professional Services, Procter & Gamble Pharmaceuticals. Norwich, NY 13815-1799 for further information.

- AUA/Procter & Gamble Video Library—more than 100 videotape programs are available for free-loan or purchase (Directory available upon request).
- Professional Speaker Bureaus (Urology, Ulcerative Colitis, and Clinical Disorder of Bone)
- Patient Education Booklets and Videos in Urology
- Resident/Fellow Conferences
- Newsletters

The Purdue Frederick Company

100 CONNECTICUT AVENUE
NORWALK, CT 06850-3590

ALFERON® N INJECTION ℞

Interferon alfa-n3
(Human Leukocyte Derived)

DESCRIPTION

Alferon® N Injection [Interferon alfa-n3 (Human Leukocyte Derived)] is a sterile aqueous formulation of purified, natural, human interferon alpha proteins for use by injection. Alferon® N Injection consists of interferon alpha proteins comprising approximately 166 amino acids ranging in molecular weights from 16,000 to 27,000 daltons. The specific activity of Interferon alfa-n3 is approximately equal to, or greater than, 2×10^8 IU/mg of protein.

Alferon® N Injection is manufactured from pooled units of human leukocytes which have been induced by incomplete infection with an avian virus (Sendai virus) to produce Interferon alfa-n3. The manufacturing process includes immunoaffinity chromatography with a murine monoclonal antibody, acidification (pH 2) for 5 days at 4°C, and gel filtration chromatography.

Since Alferon® N Injection is manufactured using source leukocytes, human, donor screening is performed to minimize the risk that the leukocytes could contain infectious agents. In addition, the manufacturing process contains steps which have been shown to inactivate viruses, and there has been no evidence of infection transmission to recipients in clinical trials. The laboratory and clinical data obtained support the conclusion that Alferon® N Injection is equivalent to other products derived from human blood or plasma which are free of risk of transmission of infectious agents, such as immunoglobulin and albumin.

The Alferon® N Injection manufacturing process was evaluated for quantitative removal or inactivation of model pathogenic viruses. The viruses were deliberately added to the leukocytes in amounts far exceeding those present in contaminated blood, i.e., $\geq 10^9$ infectious units per milliliter. The manufacturing process yielded a cumulative reduction of $\geq 10^{14}$ of infectious HIV-1, i.e., $\geq 10^{6.5}$ removal by acid inactivation and $\geq 10^{7.9}$ removal by the purification process. In the validation studies, there was 10^8 reduction in the titer of hepatitis B virus as determined by HBsAg assay, and a 10^9 reduction in the infectious titer of herpes simplex virus-1 (HSV-1). Cultivation of Alferon® N Injection Purified Drug Concentrate with human indicator cells, i.e., MRC-5 cells, peripheral blood leukocytes in the presence of Cyclosporin A, and fetal cord blood cells, did not detect the presence of infectious viruses.

As part of a validation study, Alferon® N Injection [Interferon alfa-n3 (Human Leukocyte Derived)] was examined for the presence of the following viruses; Sendai virus (SV), HIV-1, HTLV-1, HBV, HSV-1, CMV, and EBV. Alferon® N Injection contained no detectable quantities of these viruses. In addition other studies, i.e., Polymerase Chain Reaction (PCR) and Dot Blot Hybridization (DBH), have shown no detectable genetic material from these viruses in Alferon® N Injection. The sensitivity of the PCR was 10 copies for HIV-1 (env gene probe) and 10 copies for HBV (S/P gene probe). The sensitivity of the DBH was 1 pg for EBV, < 10 pg for CMV, < 10 pg for HSV-1, and < 2 pg for SV. Furthermore, sera from 105 patients treated with Alferon® N Injection (95 with condylomata acuminata and 10 with cancer) were tested for antibody HIV-1 and HIV p24 antigen. There was no evidence to suggest transmission of HIV-1 by Alferon® N Injection. Sera from 135 patients with condylomata, acuminata treated with Alferon® N Injection were tested to determine abnormal SGOT laboratory values. There was no evidence to suggest transmission of hepatitis by Alferon® N Injection based on both SGOT results and patient data collected during clinical trials.

Alferon® N Injection has been extensively purified using immunoaffinity chromatography with a murine monoclonal antibody, acidifcation (pH 2) for 5 days at 4°C, and gel filtration chromatography. Alferon® N Injection has been subjected to the acid treatment for five days during its manufacture in order to reduce the risk of viral transmission. Subsequent analyses of the Alferon® N Injection Purified Drug Concentrate confirm the absence of detectable infectious or non-infectious viral particles.

The leukocyte nutrient medium contains the antibotic neomycin sulfate at a concentration of 35 mg/L; however, neomycin sulfate is not detectable in the final product, i.e., < 0.64 μg/ml.

Murine immunoglobulin (IgG) is detected in the Alferon® N Injection Purified Drug Concentrate at levels below 0.15% of the Interferon alfa-n3 protein. This equates to levels less than 8 ng of murine IgG per million IU Interferon alfa-n3 (range of 0.9 to 5.6 ng typically found).

Table 1
Degree of Resolution as Measured By Total Wart Volume per Patient

	Percent of Patients with: Complete Resolution	Partial Resolution (≥ 50% resolution)	Minor Resolution (< 50% resolution)	Progression/ No change
Alferon® (n = 81)	54%	26%	15%	5%
Placebo (n = 75)	20%	24%	13%	43%

Alferon® N Injection [Interferon alfa-n3 (Human Leukocyte Derived)] is available in an injectable solution containing 5 million IU Alferon® N Injection per vial for intralesional injection. The solution is clear and colorless. Each milliliter (ml) contains five million IU of Interferon alfa-n3 in phosphate buffered saline (8.0 mg sodium chloride, 1.74 mg sodium phosphate dibasic, 0.20 mg potassium phosphate monobasic, and 0.20 mg potassium chloride) containing 3.3 mg phenol as a preservative and 1 mg Albumin (Human) as a stabilizer.

CLINICAL PHARMACOLOGY

General Interferons are naturally occuring proteins with both antiviral and antiproliferative properties. They are produced and secreted in response to viral infections and to a variety of other synthetic and biological inducers. Three major families of interferons have been identified: alpha, beta, and gamma. The interferon alpha family contains at least 15 different molecular species. Their molecular weights range from 16,000 to 27,000 daltons.

Interferons bind to specific membrane receptors on cell surfaces. Interferon alfa-n3 has been shown to bind to the same receptors as Interferon alfa-2b. The receptors have a high degree of selectivity for the binding of human but not mouse interferon. This correlates with the high species specificity found in laboratory studies.

Binding of interferon to membrane receptors initiates a series of events including induction of protein synthesis. These actions are followed by a variety of cellular responses, including inhibition of virus replication and suppression of cell proliferation. Immunomodulation, including enhancement of phagocytosis by macrophages, augmentation of the cytotoxicity of lymphocytes and enhancement of human leukocyte antigen expression occurs in response to exposure to interferons. One or more of these activities may contribute to the therapeutic effect of interferon.

Pharmacokinetics In a study of intralesional use of Alferon® N Injection [Interferon alfa-n3 (Human Leukocyte Derived)] for the treatment of condylomata acuminata, plasma concentrations of interferon were below the detection limit of the assay, i.e., ≤ 3 IU/ml. Minor systemic effects (e.g., myalgias, fever, and headaches) were noted, indicating that some of the injected interferon entered the systemic circulation (See ADVERSE REACTIONS).

Condylomata Acuminata Condylomata acuminata (venereal or genital warts) are associated with infections of human papilloma virus (HPV), especially HPV type-6 and possibly type-11. Given the antiviral and antiproliferative activities of interferons and the viral etiology of condylomata, a placebo-controlled clinical trial was conducted to evaluate the safety and efficacy of intralesional injection of Alferon® N Injection in the treatment of condylomata acuminata.

In a multicenter randomized double-blind, placebo-controlled clinical trial, intralesional administration of Alferon® N Injection was an effective treatment for condylomata acuminata.[1–4] One hundred fifty-six patients were evaluable for efficacy (81 Alferon® N Injection patients and 75 placebo patients). Patients had a mean of five warts (range was 2-14) and all warts were treated. Patients were injected intralesionally with a mean of 225,000 IU of Alferon® N Injection per wart 2 times a week for up to 8 weeks. Overall, 80% ($^{65}/_{81}$) of patients treated with Alferon® N Injection had a complete or partial resolution of warts compared with 44% ($^{33}/_{75}$) of placebo-treated patients ($p < 0.001$). Alferon® N Injection was significantly more effective than placebo in producing a complete resolution of warts ($p < 0.001$), as shown by the table above.

Of the patients who had a complete resolution of warts, approximately half ($^{21}/_{44}$) the patients had complete resolution of warts by the end of treatment, and half ($^{23}/_{44}$) had complete resolution of warts during the three months after the cessation of treatment. Patients with complete resolution of warts were followed for a median of 48 weeks. Overall, 76% ($^{31}/_{41}$) of Alferon® N Injection [Infereon alfa-n3 (Human Leukocyte Derived)]-treated patients who achieved complete resolution of warts remained clear of all treated lesions during follow-up, while 79% ($^{11}/_{14}$) of the placebo-treated patients remained clear of all treated lesions during follow-up.

A total of 762 evaluable warts were injected in this trial. Of the 407 Alferon® N Injection-treated warts, 73% ($^{297}/_{407}$) completely resolved, as compared to 35% ($^{125}/_{355}$) of the placebo-treated warts ($p < 0.0001$). Alferon® N Injection was effective in treating lesions of all sizes, and there was no difference in resolution for perianal, penile, or vulvar lesions.

There was no difference in resolution for patients who had received prior treatment of their warts and for those who had not. Among patients with recalcitrant warts (i.e., warts that were refractory to previous treatment or recurring), 82% ($^{58}/_{71}$) of the evaluable patients had complete or partial resolution of warts due to intralesional administration of Alferon® N Injection as compared to 43% ($^{29}/_{67}$) of placebo patients ($p < 0.001$). Fifty-four percent ($^{38}/_{71}$) of the evaluable Alferon® N Injection patients had complete resolution of warts as compared to 18% ($^{12}/_{67}$) of placebo patients ($p < 0.001$). Patients with primary occurrence of genital warts (i.e., no prior treatment of warts) had a similar resolution rate compared to the patients with recalcitrant warts: 70% ($^{7}/_{10}$) had complete or partial resolution of warts due to Alferon® N Injection treatment at 60% ($^{6}/_{10}$) had complete resolution of warts, as compared to 50% ($^{4}/_{8}$) of placebo recipients who had complete or partial resolution of warts and 38% ($^{3}/_{8}$) who had complete resolution. Overall, 83% ($^{5}/_{6}$) of Alferon® Injection [Interferon alfa-n3 (Human Leukocyte Derived)]- treated patients with primary occurrence, who achieved complete resolution of warts, remained clear of all treated lesions during a median follow-up of 52 weeks. Because the number of patients with primary occurrence of warts was small (10 Alferon® N Injection recipients and 8 placebo recipients), the difference between Alferon® N Injection and placebo treatment was not statistically significant. However, when the resolution of primary warts was examined, 75% ($^{33}/_{44}$) of the Alferon® N Injection-treated primary warts resolved completely as compared to 39% ($^{11}/_{28}$) of the placebo-treated primary warts ($p = 0.003$).

In an open clinical trial using a once a week treatment schedule for up to 16 weeks, 28 patients were evaluable for efficacy. Eighty-nine percent ($^{25}/_{28}$) of patients had a complete or partial resolution of warts following treatment with Alferon® N Injection. The condylomata acuminata resolved completely in 46% ($^{13}/_{28}$) of the patients. Of the 154 warts treated, 77% ($^{118}/_{154}$) resolved completely.

After injections of Alferon® N Injection, side effects were minor and transient. After 4 weeks of treatment, the frequency of adverse reactions was similar in Alferon® N Injection and placebo treatment groups. The most frequent side effects were myalgias, fever, and headache (See ADVERSE REACTIONS).

Antigenicity

1. Alferon® Injection
One hundred and five (105) patients treated with Alferon® N Injection during clinical trials were tested for the presence of anti-interferon antibodies using three different antibody assays: Immunoradiometric Assay (IRMA), Enzyme Linked Immunosorbent Assay (ELISA), and neutralization by the Cytopathic Effect Assay (CPE). To date, no antibodies to Interferon alfa-n3 have been detected in any of the patients.
2. Mouse Proteins
No hypersensitivity reactions to the components in Alferon® N Injection [Interferon alfa-n3 (Human Leukocyte Derived)] have been observed. Alferon® N Injection uses a murine monoclonal antibody in one of the purification procedures. A possibility exists that patients treated with Alferon® N Injection may develop hypersensitivity to the mouse proteins. However, none of the patients receiving Alferon® N Injection during clinical trials developed antibodies or hypersensitivity to mouse proteins (See CONTRAINDICATIONS).
3. Egg Protein
The initial stage in the manufacture of Alferon® N Injection uses Sendai virus which was grown in chicken eggs as the specific Interferon alfa-n3 inducer. Although no egg protein (ovalbumin) has been detected in the initial stage of interferon manufacture using an ELISA (sensitivity of 16 ng/ml), a possibility exists that patients treated with Alferon® N Injection may develop hypersensitivity to egg protein (See CONTRAINDICATIONS).

INDICATIONS AND USAGE

Alferon® N Injection is indicated for the intralesional treatment of refractory or recurring external condylomata acu-

Continued on next page

Purdue Frederick—Cont.

minata in patients 18 years of age or older (See DOSAGE AND ADMINISTRATION).
The physician should select patients for treatment with Alferon® N Injection after consideration of a number of factors: the locations and sizes of the lesions, past treatment and response thereto, and the patient's ability to comply with the treatment regimen. Alferon® N Injection is particularly useful for patients who have not responded satisfactorily to other treatment modalities, e.g., podophyllin resin, surgery, laser or cryotherapy.
There have been no studies with this product in adolescents. This product is not recommended for use in patients less than 18 years of age.

CONTRAINDICATIONS

Alferon® N Injection is contraindicated in patients with known hypersensitivity to human interferon alpha or any component of the product. The product also is contraindicated in patients who have anaphylactic sensitivity to mouse immunoglobulin (IgG), egg protein or neomycin.

WARNINGS

Because of the fever and other "flu-like" symptoms associated with Alferon® N Injection [Interferon alfa-n3 (Human Leukocyte Derived)] (See ADVERSE REACTIONS), it should be used cautiously in patients with debilitating medical conditions such as cardiovascular disease (e.g., unstable angina and uncontrolled congestive heart failure), severe pulmonary disease (e.g., chronic obstructive pulmonary disease), or diabetes mellitus with ketoacidosis. Alferon® N Injection should be used cautiously in patients with coagulation disorders (e.g., thrombophlebitis, pulmonary embolism and hemophilia), severe myelosuppression, or seizure disorders. Acute, serious hypersensitivity reactions (e.g., urticaria, angioedema, bronchoconstriction, and anaphylaxis) have not been observed in patients receiving Alferon® N Injection. However, if such reactions develop, drug administration should be discontinued immediately and appropriate medical therapy should be instituted.

PRECAUTIONS

General Patients being treated with Alferon® N Injection should be informed of the benefits and risks associated with the treatment. Because the manufacturing process, strength, and type of interferon (e.g., natural, human leukocyte interferon versus single-subspecies recombinant interferon) may vary for different interferon formulations, changing brands may require a change in dosage. Therefore, physicians are cautioned not to change from one interferon product to another without considering these factors.
Information for Patients Patients should be informed of the early signs of hypersensitivity reactions including hives, generalized urticaria, tightness of the chest, wheezing, hypotension, and anaphylaxis, and should be advised to contact their physician if these symptoms occur.
Patients being treated with Alferon® N Injection should be informed of benefits and risks associated with treatment.
Patients should be cautioned not to change brands of interferon without medical consultation, as a change in dosage may occur.
Carcinogenesis, Mutagenesis, Impairment of Fertility Studies with Alferon® N Injection [Interferon alfa-n3 (Human Leukocyte Derived)] have not been performed to determine carcinogenicity, mutagenicity, or the effect on fertility. In studies with adult females, interferon alpha has been shown to affect the menstrual cycle and decrease serum estradiol and progesterone levels[5].
Alferon® N Injection should be used with caution in fertile men. Fertile women should be cautioned to use effective contraception while being treated with Alferon® N Injection.
Changes in the menstrual cycle and abortions have been reported to occur in non-human primates given extremely high doses of recombinant interferon alpha[6]. In these studies, Macaca mulatta (rhesus monkeys) were given interferon daily by intramuscular injection. When given at daily intramuscular doses 326 times the average intralesional dose of Alferon® N Injection (120 times the maximum recommended dose), this recombinant interferon formulation produced menstrual cycle changes in the monkeys.
In human clinical trials with Alferon® N Injection, menstrual cycle data were reported by 51 patients (36 Alferon® N Injection and 15 placebo). There was no significant difference between Alferon® N Injection and placebo treatment groups with regard to menstrual cycle changes.
PREGNANCY Pregnancy Category C Animal reproduction studies have not been conducted with Alferon® N Injection. It is also not known whether Alferon® N Injection can cause fetal harm when administered to a pregnant woman or can affect reproductive capacity. Alferon® N Injection should be given to a pregnant woman only if clearly needed.
Changes in the menstrual cycle and abortions have been reported to occur in non-human primates given extremely high doses of recombinant interferon alpha. In these studies, Macaca mulatta (rhesus monkeys) were given interferon daily by intramuscular injection. Abortifacient effects were noted when the recombinant interferon alpha was given daily during early to mid-gestation at intramuscular doses of 978 times the average intralesional dose of Alferon® N Injection [Interferon alfa-n3 (Human Leukocyte Derived)] (360 times the maximum recommended dose).
Nursing Mothers It is not known whether Alferon® N Injection is excreted in human milk. Studies in mice have shown that mouse interferons are excreted in milk[7]. Because many drugs are excreted in human milk and because of the potential for serious adverse rections in nursing infants, a decision should be made whether to discontinue nursing or to not initiate drug treatment, taking into account the importance of the drug to the mother and the potential risk to the infant.
Pediatric Use Safety and effectiveness have not been established in patients below the age of 18 years.

ADVERSE REACTIONS

Adverse reactions were evaluated in 202 patients with condylomata acuminata receiving Alferon® N Injection by intralesional administration and in 31 patients with cancer receiving Alferon® N Injection by systemic administration. In the double-blind efficacy trial for the treatment of condylomata acuminata, 104 patients were treated with doses of Alferon® N Injection of 0.05 million to 2.5 million IU per treatment session (average dose = 0.92 million IU per treatment session) by intralesional injection. In open trials, an additional 98 patients received a dose range of 0.05 to 4.6 million IU of Alferon® N Injection per treatment session (average dose = 1.12 million IU per treatment session). Patients with cancer were given doses of Alferon® N Injection of 3 million, 9 million, or 15 million IU per day for ten days by intramuscular injection.
Adverse Reactions in Patients with Condylomata Acuminata A total of 104 patients with condylomata acuminata was treated with Alferon® N Injection during the double-blind clinical trial. Adverse reactions were reported to be likely, unlikely, or not known to be related to Alferon® N Injection. Adverse reactions consisted primarily of "flu-like" symptoms (myalgias, fever, and/or headache) which were in most cases mild or moderate, and transient, and did not interfere with treatment.
The "flu-like" adverse reactions, consisting of fever myalgias, and/or headache, occurred primarily after the first treatment session and were reported by 30% of the patients. The frequency of "flu-like" adverse reactions abated with repeated dosing of Alferon® N Injection [Interferon alfa-n3 (Human Leukocyte Derived)] so that the incidences due to Alferon® N Injection and placebo were similar after three to four weeks of treatment (after six to eight treatment sessions). "Flu-like" symptoms were relieved by administration of acetominophen.
Adverse reactions were reported at least once during the course of treatment in the following percentages of patients in each treatment group. [See table above.]
Most of the systemic adverse reactions were mild or moderate. Severe systemic adverse reactions were reported by 18% of Alferon® N Injection [Interferon alfa-n3 (Human Leukocyte Derived)]-treated patients and 13% of placebo-treated patients (not a statistically significant difference). Most of the severe systemic adverse reactions reported were "flu-like". Other severe systemic adverse reactions included back pain, insomnia, and sensitivity to allergens. Those adverse reactions which were reported by 1% of patients treated with Alferon® N Injection in the double-blind trial include: left groin lymph node swelling, tongue hyperaesthesia, thirst, tingling of legs/feet, hot sensation on bottom of feet, strange taste in mouth, increased salivation, heat intolerance, visual disturbances, pharyngitis, sensitivity to allergens, muscle cramps, nose bleed, throat tightness, and papular rash on neck. Additional adverse reactions which were reported by 1% of patients treated with placebo include: pharyngitis, oral pain, penile discharge, cold, knuckle stiffness, herpes outbreak, cough, disorientation, and weight/appetitite loss.
Additional adverse reactions which occurred only in open clinical trials of intralesional use of Alferon® N Injection for treatment of condylomata acuminata were herpes labialis, hot flashes, nervousness, decrease in concentration, dysuria, photosensitivity, and swollen lymph nodes. These reactions occurred in 1% of the patients. One patient with a history of epilepsy, who was not taking anticonvulsant medication, had a grand mal seizure while being treated with Alferon® N Injection; this seizure was judged to be unrelated to Alferon® Injection administration.
Application Site Disorders The frequency of application site disorders (such as itching and pain) for patients treated with Alferon® N Injection was significantly less than that reported with placebo (12% versus 26%). No severe application site disorders were reported by patients treated with Alferon® N Injection, while 7% of placebo-treated patients reported severe disorders.
Labortory Test Values Abnormalities were seen with statistically equivalent frequencies in both the Alferon® N Injection and placebo groups. None of the laboratory abnormalities were considered clinically significant. The abnormalities

Table 2
Percent of Patients with Adverse Reactions

Adverse Reactions:	Alferon® (n = 104)	Placebo (n = 85)
Autonomic Nervous System		
Sweating	2%	1%
Vasovagal Reaction	2%	0%
Body as a Whole		
Fever	40%	19%
Chills	14%	2%
Fatigue	14%	6%
Malaise	9%	9%
Skin		
Generalized Pruritis	2%	0%
Central & Peripheral Nervous System		
Dizziness	9%	4%
Insomnia	2%	1%
Gastrointestinal System		
Nausea	4%	7%
Vomiting	3%	0%
Dyspepsia/ Heartburn	3%	1%
Diarrhea	2%	2%
Musculoskeletal System		
Arthralgia	5%	1%
Back Pain	4%	1%
Myalgias	45%	15%
Headache	31%	15%
Psychiatric Disorders		
Depression	2%	1%
Nasopharyngeal		
Nose/sinus drainage	2%	2%

in the Alferon® N Injection [Interferon alfa-n3 (Human Leukocyte Derived)]-treated patients consisted primarily of deceased WBC (11%). Decreases also occurred in 4% of the placebo patients (not a statistically significant difference). The abnormalities in Alferon® N Injection-treated patients involved increases of only one WHO grade.
Adverse Reactions in Patients with Cancer Thirty-one patients with cancer were treated with a maximum of ten intramuscular injections of Alferon® N Injection in doses of 3 million IU, 9 million IU, or 15 million IU per treatment session. The occurrence of adverse reactions was judged to be unrelated to the dose of Alferon® N Injection. The following adverse reactions were reported at least once (the percentage of patients experiencing the reaction is indicated in parentheses): chills (87%), fever (81%), anorexia (68%), malaise (65%), nausea (48%), vomiting (29%), myalgias (16%), arthralgia (10%), chest pains (10%), soreness at injection site (10%), sleepiness (10%), headache (10%), diarrhea (6%), fatigue (6%), low blood pressure (6%), sore mouth/stomatitis (6%), and blurred vision (6%). Those adverse reactions which were each reported by only one patient treated with Alferon® N Injection include: stiff shoulders, face flushed, edema, dry mouth, mucositis, coughing, numbness, numbness in hands, numbness in fingers, pain on ocular rotation, shakes/shivers, ringing in ears, cramps, constipation, muscle soreness, confusion, light-headedness, depression, upset stomach, and sweating. The following adverse reactions were reported as severe by at least one patient (the percentage of patients experiencing the reaction is indicated in parentheses): fever (55%), malaise (54%), anorexia (45%), chills (45%), nausea (16%), myalgias (13%), vomiting (10%), fatigue (6%), low blood pressure (6%), chest pains (6%), sore mouth/stomatitis (6%), headache (3%), diarrhea (3%), sleepiness (3%), arthralgia (3%), blurred vision (3%), stiff shoulders (3%), numbness (3%), pain on ocular rotation (3%), muscle soreness (3%), confusion (3%), light-headedness (3%), depression (3%), and sweating (3%).

The number and percentge of patients with cancer who experiencd a significant abnormal laboratory test value (values that changed from WHO Grades 0, 1, or 2 at baseline to WHO Grades 3 or 4 during or after treatment) at least once during the trials are shown in the following table:

Table 3
Abnormal Laboratory Test Values

	Cancer (n = 31)
Hemoglobin Level	2 (7%)
White Blood Cell Count	1 (3%)
Platelet Count	1 (3%)
GGT	1 (6%)
SGOT	1 (3%)
Alkaline Phosphatase	2 (8%)
Total Bilirubin	1 (4%)

DOSAGE AND ADMINISTRATION

The recommended dose of Alferon® N Injection [Interferon alfa-n3 (Human Leukocyte Derived)] for the treatment of condylomata acuminata is 0.05 ml (250,000 IU) per wart. Alferon® N Injection should be administered twice weekly for up to 8 weeks. The maximum recommended dose per treatment session is 0.5 ml (2.5 million IU). Alferon® N Injection should be injected into the base of each wart, preferably using a 30 gauge needle. For large warts, Alferon® N Injection may be injected at several points around the periphery of the wart, using a total dose of 0.05 ml per wart. The minimum effective dose of Alferon® N Injection for the treatment of condylomata acuminata has not been established. Moderate to severe adverse experiences may require modification of the dosage regimen or, in some cases, termination of therapy with Alferon® N Injection.
Genital warts usually begin to disappear after several weeks of treatment with Alferon® N Injection. Treatment should continue for a maximum of 8 weeks. In clinical trials with Alferon® N Injection, many patients who had partial resolution of warts during treatment experienced further resolution of their warts after cessation of treatment. Of the patients who had complete resolution of warts due to treatment, half the patients had complete resolution of warts by the end of the treatment and half had complete resolution of warts during the 3 months after cessation of treatment. Thus, it is recommended that no further therapy (Alferon® N Injection or conventional therapy) be administered for 3 months after the initial 8-week course of treatment unless the warts enlarge or new warts appear. Studies to determine the safety and efficacy of a second course of treatment with Alferon® N Injection [Interferon alfa-n3 (Human Leukocyte Derived)] have not been conducted.
Parenteral drug products should be inspected visually for particulate matter and discoloration prior to administration, whenever solution and container permit.

HOW SUPPLIED

Injectable Solution: 5 Million IU Alferon® N Injection per vial. Each vial contains 1 ml of Alferon® N Injection. Each ml of Alferon® N Injection contains 5 million IU of Interferon alfa-n3, 3.3. mg of phenol, and 1 mg of Albumin (Human) in a pH 7.4 phosphate buffered saline solution (8.0 mg/ml sodium chloride, 1.74 mg/ml sodium phosphate dibasic, 0.20 mg/ml potassium phosphate monobasic, and 0.20 mg/ml potassium chloride). One vial per box. (NDC 0034-1019-01).

STORAGE

Alferon® N Injection should be stored at 2° to 8°C (36° to 46°F). Do not freeze. Do not shake.
CAUTION: FEDERAL (U.S.A.) LAW PROHIBITS DISPENSING WITHOUT PRESCRIPTION.

REFERENCES

1. Friedman-Kien, AE, Eron, LJ, Conant, M, et al., *JAMA*, 259: 533–538, 1988.
2. Kirby, P. (editorial comment), *JAMA*, 259: 570–572, 1988.
3. Friedman-Kien, AE, Plasse, TF, et al., *Papilloma Viruses: Molecular and Clinical Aspects* [Howley, PM, Broker, TR (eds)], New York, Alan R. Liss, Inc., 1986, pp. 217–233.
4. Geffen, JR, Klein, RJ, Friedman-Kien, AE, *J Infect. Dis.*, 150: 612–615, 1984.
5. Kauppila, A, et al., *Int. J. Cancer*, 29: 291–294, 1982.
6. Trown, PW, et al., *Cancer*, 57 (Suppl): 1648–1656, 1986.
7. Schafer, TW, et al., *Science*, 176: 1326–1327, 1972.

Manufactured by:
Interferon Sciences, Inc.
783 Jersey Avenue
New Brunswick, NJ 08901
U.S. Lic. No. 930
Distributed by:
The Purdue Frederick Company
100 Connecticut Avenue
Norwalk, CT 06850-3590
Copyright © 1989, 1990 Interferon Sciences, Inc.
New Brunswick, NJ 08901.

01-B-01   8/90   B3126
Shown in Product Identification Section, page 424

BETADINE® Microbicides   OTC
[ba̅ʹtăh-dīn]
(povidone-iodine)

BETADINE Microbicides (povidone-iodine) are available in 23 product forms—more than any other antiseptic agent. BETADINE Microbicides are designed especially to meet the varied antiseptic needs of physicians, nurses and patients in the hospital, office and home. Of all antiseptic preparations, only povidone-iodine, as in BETADINE Microbicides, is capable of killing all classes of pathogens encountered in nosocomial infections: gram-positive bacteria and gram-negative bacteria (including antibiotic-resistant strains and mycobacteria), fungi/yeasts, viruses, and protozoa. It is the only microbicide with this broad spectrum of activity.
Other advantages: Most bacteria are killed in 15 to 30 seconds in-vitro. Resistance has not been reported. Microbicidal activity is retained in the presence of moderate quantities of blood, pus, mucosal secretions, and soap and water. More frequent application of BETADINE Microbicides is indicated in the presence of excessive amount of blood, pus, or mucosal secretions. When used as a surgical scrub, the effect lasts 6 to 8 hours. Virtually nonirritating when used as directed; washes easily off skin and natural fabrics. BETADINE® Solution and BETADINE® Aerosol Spray are film-forming and may be applied with or without bandages. BETADINE® First Aid Cream and BETADINE® Ointment may be bandaged or covered with gauze.
WARNINGS: Read the "WARNINGS" section for each BETADINE product before use.
BETADINE® Microbicides are available for hospital use and home healthcare.
BETADINE® Aerosol Spray (povidone-iodine, 5%)
BETADINE® Antiseptic Gauze Pad (povidone-iodine, 10%)
BETADINE® Antiseptic Lubricating Gel (povidone-iodine, 5%)
BETADINE® First Aid Cream (povidone-iodine, 5%)
BETADINE® Medicated Disposable Douche (povidone-iodine, 10%)
BETADINE® Medicated Douche (povidone-iodine, 10%)
BETADINE® Medicated Douche Kit (povidone-iodine, 10%)
BETADINE® Medicated Gel (povidone-iodine, 10%)
BETADINE® Medicated Vaginal Suppositories (povidone-iodine, 10%)
BETADINE® Mouthwash/Gargle (povidone-iodine, 0.5%)
BETADINE® Ointment (povidone-iodine, 10%)
BETADINE® Perineal Wash Concentrate Kit (povidone-iodine,10%)
BETADINE® Pre-Mixed Medicated Disposable Douche (povidone-iodine, .30%)
BETADINE® Shampoo (povidone-iodine, 7.5%)
BETADINE® Skin Cleanser (povidone-iodine, 7.5%)
BETADINE® Skin Cleanser Foam (povidone-iodine, 7.5%)
BETADINE® Solution (povidone-iodine, 10%)
BETADINE® Solution Swab Aid® (povidone-iodine, 10%)
BETADINE® Solution Swabsticks (povidone-iodine, 10%)
BETADINE® Surgical Scrub (povidone-iodine, 7.5%)
BETADINE® Surgi-Prep Sponge-Brush (povidone-iodine, 7.5%)
BETADINE® Viscous Formula Antiseptic Gauze Pad (povidone-iodine, 10%)
BETADINE® Whirlpool Concentrate (povidone-iodine, 10%)
Copyright 1991, The Purdue Frederick Company
Norwalk, CT 06850-3590

BETADINE® FIRST AID CREAM   OTC
[ba̅ʹtăh-dīn]
(povidone-iodine, 5%)

ACTION AND USES

BETADINE First Aid Cream is a topical antiseptic containing 5% povidone-iodine (PVP-I) in an oil-in-water emulsion. It combines the essential microbicidal properties of povidone-iodine with the ease of application and comfort of a cream formulation. BETADINE First Aid Cream is virtually nonirritating, nonstinging and nonburning when applied to open cuts, burns, or scrapes. BETADINE First Aid Cream kills most bacteria and other pathogens virtually on contact. It enhances healing of minor wounds and has a very broad spectrum of microbicidal activity.
BETADINE First Aid Cream is easy to apply and remove. Oil-in-water creams mix with exudates and are particularly suitable for weeping or wounded surfaces. BETADINE First Aid Cream has shown no phototoxic or contact sensitizing potential and has exhibited no photocontact allergenicity when tested on humans. BETADINE First Aid Cream is preservative-free.

ADMINISTRATION

Apply directly to affected area as needed. May be bandaged.

WARNINGS

For External Use Only. In case of deep or puncture wounds or serious burns, consult physician. If redness, irritation, swelling or pain persists or increases, or if infection occurs, discontinue use and consult physician. Keep out of reach of children.

SUPPLIED

½ oz. plastic tube, with an applicator tip for easy and economical application.
Copyright 1991, The Purdue Frederick Company
Norwalk, CT 06850-3590

BETADINE® MEDICATED GEL   OTC
[ba̅ʹtăh-dīn]
(povidone-iodine, 10%)

ACTION AND USES

BETADINE Medicated Gel provides prompt, soothing, symptomatic relief of minor vaginal irritation, itching and soreness associated with vaginitis due to *Candida albicans*, *Trichomonas vaginalis*, and *Gardnerella vaginalis*. Offers relief from annoying vaginal symptoms and odor.

ADVANTAGES

Its gel formulation is convenient for evening application to irritated vaginal tissue. BETADINE Medicated Gel is gentle and virtually nonirritating to delicate vaginal tissue. It is nongreasy and nonsticky. Its active ingredient—the broadspectrum microbicide povidone-iodine—significantly and rapidly reduces the aerobic and anaerobic bacterial count.

DIRECTIONS FOR USE

Insert one applicatorful of BETADINE Medicated Gel. A sanitary napkin should be worn. When external irritation is present, BETADINE Medicated Gel may be applied manually to the affected area. Treatment should be continued for seven days.

WARNINGS

Do not use during pregnancy or while nursing except with the approval of your physician. If symptoms persist after seven days of treatment, or redness, pain or swelling develops, discontinue use and consult physician. Women with iodine sensitivity should not use this product. Keep out of reach of children.

HOW SUPPLIED

18 g tubes (approximately 1 use) and 3 oz. tubes (approximately 14 uses), each packaged with a convenient, easy-to-use vaginal applicator.
Copyright 1991, The Purdue Frederick Company
Norwalk, CT 06850-3590

BETADINE® MEDICATED DOUCHE   OTC
[ba̅ʹtăh-dīn]
(povidone-iodine, 10%)

A pleasantly scented solution, BETADINE Medicated Douche is indicated for the prompt symptomatic relief of minor vaginal irritation, itching, and soreness associated with vaginitis due to *Candida albicans*, *Trichomonas vaginalis*, and *Gardnerella vaginalis*. May be used as a cleansing douche.

ADVANTAGES

Low surface tension, with uniform wetting action to assist penetration into vaginal crypts and crevices. Microbicidal activity is retained in the presence of moderate quantities of blood, pus, mucosal secretions, and soap and water. Virtually nonirritating to vaginal mucosa. Will not stain skin or natural fabrics.

DIRECTIONS FOR USE

Professional Labeling
Suggested Regimen For Therapeutic Use: In the office, swab the cervix and vulvovaginal area with BETADINE Solution. Prescribe BETADINE Medicated Douche: Two tablespoonfuls of BETADINE Douche Concentrate or two ½ fl. oz. packets to a quart of lukewarm water once daily for five days. If further therapy is warranted, douching should be continued through the next cycle. The patient may be instructed to return for an office visit following two weeks of therapy.
As a Routine Cleansing Douche: Two (2) tablespoonfuls of BETADINE Douche Concentrate to a quart of lukewarm water once or twice per week.
As a douche for prompt symptomatic relief of minor vaginal irritation and itching: Two (2) tablespoonfuls of BETADINE Douche Concentrate to a quart of lukewarm water once daily

Continued on next page

Purdue Frederick—Cont.

for five days. Treatment should continue for the full five days, even if symptoms are relieved earlier.

WARNINGS

Douching does not prevent pregnancy. Do not use during pregnancy or while nursing except with the approval of physician. If symptoms persist after five days of use, or redness, swelling or pain develops, discontinue use and consult a physician. As a cleansing and deodorizing douche, do not use more often than twice weekly. Women with iodine sensitivity should not use this product. Douching is reported to be associated with Pelvic Inflammatory Disease, a serious infection of the reproductive system. Keep out of reach of children.

HOW SUPPLIED

1 oz. and 8 oz. plastic bottles. Disposable $\frac{1}{2}$ oz. (1 tablespoonful) packets. Also available: BETADINE Medicated Douche Kit 8 oz. (approximately 20 uses), BETADINE Medicated Disposable Douche (single- and twin-pack) and BETADINE Pre-Mixed Medicated Disposable Douche, which requires no measuring or mixing (single- and twin-pack).
Copyright 1991, The Purdue Frederick Company
Norwalk, CT 06850-3590

BETADINE® OINTMENT　　　　　　　　　　　　OTC
[bā'tăh-dīn"]
(povidone-iodine, 10%)

ACTION

BETADINE Ointment, in a water-soluble base, is a topical microbicide active against organisms commonly encountered in skin and wound infections.

INDICATIONS

Therapeutically, BETADINE Ointment may be used as an adjunct to systemic therapy where indicated; for primary or secondary topical infections, infected surgical incisions, infected decubitus or stasis ulcers, pyodermas, secondarily infected dermatoses, and infected traumatic lesions.
Prophylactically: BETADINE Ointment may be used to prevent microbial contamination in burns, incisions and other topical lesions; for degerming skin in hyperalimentation and catheter care. The use of BETADINE Ointment for abrasions, minor cuts, and wounds, may prevent the development of infections and permit wound healing.

ADMINISTRATION

Apply directly to affected area as needed. May be bandaged.

WARNINGS

For External Use Only. In case of deep or puncture wounds or serious burns, consult physician. If redness, irritation, swelling or pain persists or increases, or if infection occurs, discontinue use and consult physician. Keep out of reach of children.

SUPPLIED

$\frac{1}{32}$ oz. and $\frac{1}{8}$ oz. packettes; 1 oz. tubes; 16 oz. (1 lb.).
Copyright 1991, The Purdue Frederick Company
Norwalk, CT 06850-3590

BETADINE® SKIN CLEANSER　　　　　　　　　　OTC
[bā'tăh-dīn"]
(povidone-iodine, 7.5%)

BETADINE Skin Cleanser is a sudsing, antiseptic bactericidal, virucidal liquid cleanser which forms a rich, golden lather.

INDICATIONS

BETADINE Skin Cleanser aids in degerming the skin of patients with common pathogens, including *Staphylococcus aureus.* To help prevent the recurrence of acute inflammatory skin infections caused by iodine-susceptible pyogenic bacteria. In pyodermas, as a topical adjunct to systemic antimicrobial therapy. To help prevent spread of infection in acne pimples. Also kills three organisms often associated with acne vulgaris: *Staph. epidermidis, Corynebacterium acnes* and Pityrosporon. To clean superficial wounds. Aids in removal of foreign material such as dirt and debris.

DIRECTIONS FOR USE

Wet the skin and apply a sufficient amount of Skin Cleanser to work up a rich golden lather. Allow lather to remain about 3 minutes. Then rinse thoroughly with water. Repeat 2–3 times a day or as needed.

WARNINGS

For External Use Only. In case of deep or puncture wounds or serious burns, consult physician. If redness, irritation, swelling or pain persists or increases, or if infection occurs,

discontinue use and consult physician. Keep out of reach of children.

HOW SUPPLIED

1 fl. oz. and 4 fl. oz. plastic bottles.

NOTE

Blue stains on starched linen will wash off with soap and water.
Copyright 1991, The Purdue Frederick Company
Norwalk, CT 06850-3590

BETADINE® SOLUTION　　　　　　　　　　　　OTC
[bā'tăh-dīn"]
(povidone-iodine, 10%)
Topical Antiseptic Bactericide/Virucide

INDICATIONS

For preoperative prepping of operative site, including the vagina, and as a general topical bactericide/virucide for: disinfection of wounds; emergency treatment of lacerations and abrasions; second- and third-degree burns; as a prophylactic anti-infective agent in hospital and office procedures, including postoperative application to incisions to help prevent infection; oral moniliasis (thrush); bacterial and mycotic skin infections; decubitus and stasis ulcers; as a preoperative swab in the mouth and throat.

ADMINISTRATION

Apply full strength as often as needed as a paint, spray, or wet soak. May be bandaged.

WARNINGS

For External Use Only. In preoperative prepping, avoid "pooling" beneath the patient. Prolonged exposure to wet solution may cause irritation or rarely, severe skin reactions. Do not heat prior to application. In case of deep or puncture wounds or serious burns, consult physician. If redness, irritation, swelling or pain persists or increases, or if infection occurs, discontinue use and consult physician. Keep out of reach of children.

HOW SUPPLIED

$\frac{1}{2}$ oz., 8 oz., 16 oz. (1 pt.), 32 oz. (1 qt.) and 1 gal. plastic bottles and 1 oz. packettes.

ALSO AVAILABLE

BETADINE® Solution Swab Aid® Pads for degerming small areas of skin or mucous membranes prior to injections, aspirations, catheterization and surgery; boxes of 100 packettes. Also: disposable BETADINE® Solution Swabsticks, in packettes of 1's and 3's.
Copyright 1991, The Purdue Frederick Company
Norwalk, CT 06850-3590

BETADINE® SURGICAL SCRUB　　　　　　　　　OTC
[bā'tăh-dīn"]
(povidone-iodine, 7.5%)
Topical Antiseptic Bactericide/Virucide

INDICATIONS

A broad-spectrum antiseptic, bactericidal, virucidal sudsing skin cleanser for pre- and postoperative scrubbing or washing by hospital operating room personnel; for preoperative use on patients; and general use as an antiseptic microbicide in physician's office. Forms rich, golden lather.

DIRECTIONS FOR USE

A.　For Preoperative Washing by Operating Personnel
1.　Wet hands and forearms with water. Pour about 5 cc. (1 teaspoonful) of BETADINE Surgical Scrub on the palm of the hand and spread over both hands and forearms. Without adding more water, rub the Scrub thoroughly over all areas for about five minutes. Use a brush if desired. Clean thoroughly under fingernails. Add a little water and develop copious suds. Rinse thoroughly under running water.
2.　Complete the wash by scrubbing with another 5 cc. of BETADINE Surgical Scrub in the same way.

B.　For Preoperative Use on Patients
After the skin area is shaved, wet it with water. Apply BETADINE Surgical Scrub (1 cc. is sufficient to cover an area of 20-30 square inches), develop lather and scrub thoroughly for about five minutes. Rinse off by aid of sterile gauze saturated with water. The area may then be painted with BETADINE Solution or sprayed with BETADINE Aerosol Spray and allowed to dry.

C.　For Use in the Physician's Office
Use for washing whenever a bactericidal/virucidal detergent is required. For maximum degerming of the hands proceed as under (A). To prepare the patient's skin proceed as under (B).

Note: Blue stains on starched linen will wash off with soap and water.

WARNINGS

For External Use Only. Do not heat prior to application. In rare instances of local irritation or sensitivity, discontinue use. Keep out of reach of children.

SUPPLIED

16 oz. (1 pint) plastic bottle with and without pump, 32 oz. (1 quart) and 1 gal. plastic bottles, and $\frac{1}{2}$ oz. packettes.
Copyright 1991, The Purdue Frederick Company
Norwalk, CT 06850-3590

BETADINE® MEDICATED VAGINAL　　　　　　　OTC
SUPPOSITORIES
[bā'tăh-dīn"]
(povidone-iodine, 10%)

ACTION AND USES

BETADINE Medicated Vaginal Suppositories provide prompt symptomatic relief of minor vaginal irritation, itching and soreness associated with vaginitis due to *Candida albicans, Trichomonas vaginalis, and Gardnerella vaginalis*. Its active ingredient—the broad-spectrum microbicide povidone-iodine—significantly and rapidly reduces the aerobic and anaerobic microbial count. Offers soothing relief from annoying vaginal symptoms and odor.

ADVANTAGES

Each measured-dose BETADINE Medicated Vaginal Suppository is convenient for application to irritated vaginal tissue in the evening or at night. BETADINE Medicated Vaginal Suppositories are gentle and virtually nonirritating to delicate vaginal tissue. Nonstaining to skin and natural fabrics, color can be washed off with soap and water.

DIRECTIONS FOR USE

Unwrap a suppository and gently insert its smaller end into the applicator. Insert the applicator into the vagina and push plunger to release the suppository. A sanitary napkin should be worn. Treatment should be continued for seven days.

WARNINGS

Do not use during pregnancy or while nursing except with the approval of your physician. If symptoms persist after seven days of treatment, or redness, pain or swelling develops, discontinue use and consult your physician. Women with iodine sensitivity should not use this product. Keep out of reach of children.

HOW SUPPLIED

7 Suppositories packaged with a convenient, easy-to-use applicator and patient instruction booklet.
Copyright 1991, The Purdue Frederick Company
Norwalk, CT 06850-3590

CARDIOQUIN® TABLETS　　　　　　　　　　　　℞
[car'dē"ō-quin"]
(quinidine polygalacturonate)
275 mg
In the treatment of cardiac arrhythmias

DESCRIPTION

Quinidine Polygalacturonate, an antiarrhythmic, is a polymer of quinidine and polygalacturonic acid which occurs as a creamy white, amorphous powder and is sparingly soluble in water, and freely soluble in hot 40% alcohol.
Chemically, quinidine polygalacturonate is $C_{20}H_{24}N_2O_2C_6H_{10}O_7H_2O$ and has the following structural formula:

CARDIOQUIN Tablets, for oral administration, contain 275 mg quinidine polygalacturonate equivalent in content to 200 mg (3 grains) of quinidine sulfate.
Inactive components include: Corn starch, Lactose, Magnesium stearate, Povidone and Talc.

ACTIONS

The quinidine component slows conduction time, prolongs the refractory period, and depresses the excitability of heart

muscle. Polygalacturonate slows ionization of the drug and protects the gastrointestinal tract by its demulcent effect.

INDICATIONS

CARDIOQUIN Tablets are indicated as maintenance therapy after spontaneous and electrical conversion of atrial tachycardia, flutter or fibrillation and in the treatment of:

- Premature atrial and ventricular contractions.
- Paroxysmal atrial tachycardia.
- Paroxymal A-V junctional rhythm.
- Atrial flutter.
- Paroxysmal atrial fibrillation.
- Established atrial fibrillation when therapy is appropriate.
- Paroxysmal ventricular tachycardia when not associated with complete heartblock.

CONTRAINDICATIONS

1. History of hypersensitivity to quinidine manifested by thrombocytopenia, skin eruptions, febrile reactions, etc.
2. Complete A-V block.
3. Complete bundle branch block or other severe intraventricular conduction defects exhibiting marked QRS widening or bizarre complexes.
4. Myasthenia gravis.
5. Arrhythmias associated with digitalis toxicity.

WARNINGS

1. In the treatment of atrial fibrillation with rapid ventricular response, ventricular rate should be controlled with digitalis glycosides prior to administration of quinidine.
2. In the treatment of atrial flutter with quinidine, reversion to sinus rhythm may be preceded by progressive reduction in the degree of A-V block to a 1:1 ratio resulting in an extremely high ventricular rate. This potential hazard may be reduced by digitalization prior to administration of quinidine.
   Recent reports have described increased, potentially toxic, digoxin plasma levels when quinidine is administered concurrently. When concurrent use is necessary, digoxin dosage should be reduced and plasma concentration should be monitored and patients observed closely for digitalis intoxication.
3. Quinidine cardiotoxicity may be manifested by increased P-R and Q-T intervals, 50% widening of QRS, and/or ventricular ectopic beats or tachycardia. Appearance of these toxic signs during quinidine administration mandates immediate discontinuation of the drug, and/or close clinical and electrocardiographic monitoring. Note: Quinidine effect is enhanced by potassium and reduced in the presence of hypokalemia.
4. Quinidine syncope may occur as a complication of long-term therapy. It is manifested by sudden loss of consciousness and by ventricular arrhythmias with bizarre QRS complexes. This syndrome does not appear to be related to dose or plasma levels, but occurs more often with prolonged Q-T intervals.
5. Because quinidine antagonizes the effect of vagal excitation upon the atrium and the A-V node, the administration of parasympathomimetic drugs (choline esters) or the use of any other procedure to enhance vagal activity may fail to terminate paroxysmal supraventricular tachycardia in patients receiving quinidine.
6. Quinidine should be used with extreme caution in:
   a) The presence of incomplete A-V block, since a complete block and asystole may result.
   b) Quinidine may cause unpredictable abnormalities of rhythm in digitalized hearts. Therefore, it should be used with caution in the presence of digitalis intoxication (see 2 above).
   c) Partial bundle branch block.
   d) Severe congestive heart failure and hypotensive states due to the depressant effects of quinidine on myocardial contractility and arterial pressure.
   e) Poor renal function, especially renal tubular acidosis, because of the potential accumulation of quinidine in plasma leading to toxic concentrations.

PRECAUTIONS

1. **Test Dose**—A preliminary test dose of a single tablet of quinidine *sulfate* should be administered prior to the initiation of treatment with CARDIOQUIN Tablets to determine whether the patient has an idiosyncrasy to the quinidine molecule.
2. **Hypersensitivity**—During the first weeks of therapy, hypersensitivity to quinidine, although rare, should be considered (e.g., angioedema, purpura, acute asthmatic episode, vascular collapse).
3. **Long-Term Therapy**—Periodic blood counts and liver and kidney function tests should be performed during long-term therapy, and the drug should be discontinued if blood dyscrasias or signs of hepatic or renal disorders occur.
4. **Large Doses**—ECG monitoring and determination of plasma quinidine levels are recommended when doses greater than 2.5 g/day are administered.
5. **Usage in Pregnancy**—The use of quinidine in pregnancy should be reserved only for those cases where the benefits outweigh the possible hazards to the patient and fetus.
6. **Nursing Mothers**—The drug should be used with extreme caution in nursing mothers because the drug is excreted in breast milk.
7. **General**—In patients exhibiting asthma, muscle weakness and infection with fever *prior* to quinidine administration, hypersensitivity reactions to the drug may be masked.

DRUG INTERACTIONS

1. Caution should be used when quinidine and its analogs are administered concurrently with coumarin anticoagulants. This combination may reduce prothrombin levels and cause bleeding.
2. Quinidine, a weak base, may have its half-life prolonged in patients who are concurrently taking drugs that can alkalize the urine, such as thiazide diuretics, sodium bicarbonate, and carbonic anhydrase inhibitors. Quinidine and drugs which alkalize the urine should be used together cautiously.
3. Quinidine exhibits a distinct anticholinergic activity in the myocardial tissues. An additive vagolytic effect may be seen when quinidine and drugs having anticholinergic blocking activity are used together. Drugs having cholinergic activity may be antagonized by quinidine.
4. Quinidine and other antiarrhythmic agents may produce additive cardiac depressant effects when administered together.
5. Quinidine interaction with cardiac glycosides (digoxin). See **WARNINGS**.
6. Antacids may delay absorption of quinidine but appear unlikely to cause incomplete absorption.
7. Phenobarbital and phenytoin may reduce plasma half-life of quinidine by 50%.
8. Quinidine may potentiate the neuromuscular blocking effect in ventilatory depression of patients receiving decamethonium, tubocurare or succinylcholine.

ADVERSE REACTIONS

Symptoms of cinchonism (ringing in the ears, headache, disturbed vision) may appear in sensitive patients after a single dose of the drug.

Gastrointestinal:
The most common side effects encountered with quinidine are referable to this system. Diarrhea frequently occurs, but it rarely necessitates withdrawal of the drug. Nausea, vomiting and abdominal pain also occur. Some of these effects may be minimized by administering the drug with meals.

Cardiovascular:
Widening of QRS complex, cardiac asystole, ventricular ectopic beats, idioventricular rhythms including ventricular tachycardia and fibrillation; paradoxical tachycardia, arterial embolism, and hypotension.

Hematologic:
Acute hemolytic anemia, hypoprothrombinemia, thrombocytopenic purpura, agranulocytosis.

CNS:
Headache, fever, vertigo, apprehension, excitement, confusion, delirium, and syncope, disturbed hearing (tinnitus, decreased auditory acuity), disturbed vision (mydriasis, blurred vision, disturbed color perception, photophobia, diplopia, night blindness, scotomata), optic neuritis.

Dermatologic:
Cutaneous flushing with intense pruritus.

Hypersensitivity Reactions:
Angioedema, acute asthmatic episode, vascular collapse, respiratory arrest, hepatic dysfunction.

DOSAGE AND ADMINISTRATION

Each CARDIOQUIN Tablet contains 275 mg quinidine polygalacturonate, equivalent to a 3-grain tablet of quinidine sulfate. Dosage must be adjusted to individual patient's needs, both for conversion and maintenance. An initial dose of 1 to 3 tablets may be used to terminate arrhythmia, and may be repeated in 3–4 hours. If normal sinus rhythm is not restored after 3 or 4 equal doses, the dose may be increased by ½ to 1 tablet (137.5 to 275 mg) and administered three to four times before any further dosage increase. For maintenance, one tablet may be used two or three times a day; generally, one tablet morning and night will be adequate.

OVERDOSAGE

Cardiotoxic effects of quinidine may be reversed in part by molar sodium lactate; the hypotension may be reversed by vasoconstrictors and by catecholamines (since vasodilation is partly due to alpha-adrenergic blockage).

HOW SUPPLIED

CARDIOQUIN (quinidine polygalacturonate) 275 mg scored, uncoated tablets are supplied in white-opaque plastic bottles containing 100 tablets (NDC #0034-5470-80) and 500 tablets (NDC #0034-5470-90). Each round tablet bears the symbol "PF" on one side and is marked "C275" on the other.
Store tablets at controlled room temperature 15° to 30°C (59°–86°F).

CAUTION

Federal law prohibits dispensing without prescription.

REFERENCES

1. Schwartz, G.: *Angiology* 10:115 (Apr.) 1959.
2. Tricot, R., Nogrette, P.: *Presse med.* 68:1085 (June 4) 1960.
3. Shaftel, N., Halpern, A.: *Am. J. Med. Sci.* 236:184 (Aug.) 1958.

Copyright © 1989, 1990
The Purdue Frederick Company
Norwalk, CT 06850-3590
December 17, 1990 J8038

Shown in Product Identification Section, page 424

CERUMENEX® EARDROPS ℞
[sĕ-rū ′mĕn-ĕx″]
(triethanolamine polypeptide oleate-condensate)

DESCRIPTION

CERUMENEX Eardrops contain Triethanolamine Polypeptide Oleate-Condensate (10%). Inactive Ingredients: Chlorobutanol 0.5%, Propylene Glycol and Water. Triethanolamine Polypeptide Oleate is a hygroscopic-miscible solution with low surface tension and optimal viscosity of 50–90 cps. It also has a slightly acid pH range (5.0–6.0) to approximate the surface of a normal ear canal.

CLINICAL PHARMACOLOGY

CERUMENEX Eardrops emulsify and disperse excess or impacted earwax. The triethanolamine polypeptide oleate, a surfactant, in a hygroscopic vehicle lyses cerumen to facilitate removal by subsequent water irrigation.

INDICATIONS AND USAGE

For removal of impacted cerumen prior to ear examination, otologic therapy and/or audiometry.

CONTRAINDICATIONS

Perforated tympanic membrane or otitis media is considered a contraindication to the use of this medication in the external ear canal.
A history of hypersensitivity to CERUMENEX Eardrops or to any of its components is also a contraindication to the use of this medication.

WARNINGS

Discontinue promptly if sensitization or irritation occurs.

PRECAUTIONS

General
It is recommended that the following precautions be observed in prescribing and administration of this agent:

1. Extreme caution is indicated in patients with demonstrable dermatologic idiosyncrasies or with history of allergic reactions in general.
2. Exposure of the ear canal to the CERUMENEX Eardrops should be limited to 15–30 minutes.
3. When administering CERUMENEX Eardrops, care must be taken to avoid undue exposure of the skin outside the ear during the instillation and the flushing out of the medication. If the medication comes in contact with the skin, the area should be washed with soap and water. Use of proper technique (see Dosage and Administration) will help avoid such undue exposure.
4. CERUMENEX Eardrops should be used only with caution in external otitis.

Information for Patients

1. Patients should be cautioned to avoid placing the applicator tip into the ear canal.
2. Patients should be cautioned to gently flush the ear with lukewarm water.
3. Patients should be warned to use CERUMENEX Eardrops in ears only. Surrounding skin should be promptly rinsed of any excess drops.
4. Patients should be instructed not to leave CERUMENEX Eardrops in the ear for longer than 30 minutes. A second application may be made, if needed, but more frequent use must be indicated by the physician.
5. Patients must be instructed not to exceed the time of exposure, nor to use the medication more frequently than directed by the physician.
6. Patients should be advised to discontinue the use of the medication in case of a possible reaction and to consult their physician promptly.

Carcinogenesis, Mutagenesis, Impairment of Fertility
Long-term animal studies have not been performed to evaluate the carcinogenic potential or the effect on fertility of CERUMENEX Eardrops.

Pregnancy
Teratogenic Effects: Pregnancy Category C. Animal reproduction studies have not yet been conducted with CERUMENEX Eardrops. It is also not known whether CERUMENEX Eardrops can cause fetal harm when administered to a preg-

Continued on next page

Purdue Frederick—Cont.

nant woman or can affect reproduction capacity. CERUMENEX Eardrops should be given to a pregnant woman only if clearly needed.

Nursing Mother
It is not known whether this drug is excreted in human milk. Because many drugs are excreted in human milk, caution should be exercised when CERUMENEX Eardrops are administered to a nursing mother.

Pediatric Use
Safety and effectiveness in children have not been established.

ADVERSE REACTIONS

Clinical Reactions of Possible Allergic Origin
Localized dermatitis reactions were reported in about 1% of 2,700 patients treated, ranging from a very mild erythema and pruritus of the external canal to a severe eczematoid reaction involving the external ear and periauricular tissue, generally with duration of 2–10 days. Other reactions which have been reported in connection with the use of CERUMENEX Eardrops include allergic contact dermatitis, skin ulcerations, burning and pain at the application site and skin rash.

DOSAGE AND ADMINISTRATION

1. Fill ear canal with CERUMENEX Eardrops with the patient's head tilted at a 45° angle.
2. Insert cotton plug and allow to remain 15–30 minutes.
3. Then gently flush with lukewarm water, using a soft rubber syringe (avoid excessive pressure). Exposure of skin outside the ear to the drug should be avoided. The procedure may be repeated if the first application fails to clear the impaction.

CAUTION: Federal Law Prohibits Dispensing Without a Prescription.

FOR EXTERNAL USE IN THE EAR ONLY

HOW SUPPLIED

CERUMENEX Eardrops (triethanolamine polypeptide oleate-condensate) are supplied in 6 ml (NDC 0034-5490-06) and 12 ml (NDC 0034-5490-12) bottles with a cellophane wrapped dropper.
Store at Controlled Room Temperature 15–30°C (59–86°F).
Copyright 1991, THE PURDUE FREDERICK COMPANY
Norwalk, Connecticut 06850-3590
May 15, 1991 L8037

MS CONTIN® 15 mg Tablets Ⓒ II
MS CONTIN® 30 mg Tablets Ⓒ II
MS CONTIN® 60 mg Tablets Ⓒ II
MS CONTIN® 100 mg Tablets Ⓒ II
[em es"kŏn'tĕn]
Morphine Sulfate Controlled-Release
WARNING: May be habit forming.

DESCRIPTION

Chemically, morphine sulfate is 7,8-didehydro-4,5α-epoxy-17- methylmorphinan-3,6 α-diol sulfate (2:1) (salt) pentahydrate and has the following structural formula:

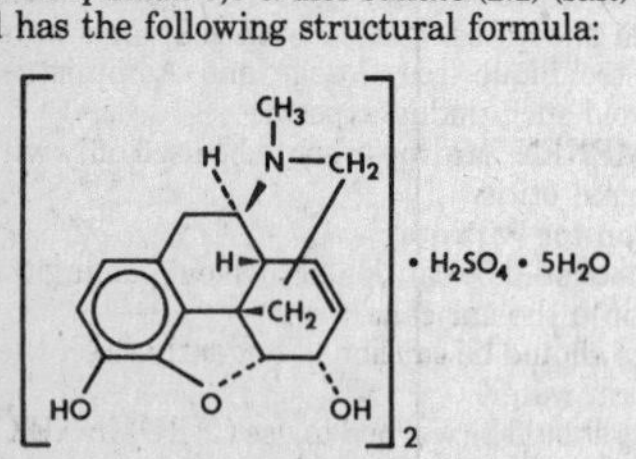

Each MS CONTIN 15 mg Controlled-Release Tablet contains: 15 mg Morphine Sulfate U.S.P. Inactive ingredients: Cetostearyl Alcohol, FD&C Blue No. 2, Hydroxyethyl Cellulose, Hydroxypropyl Methylcellulose, Lactose, Magnesium Stearate, Talc, Titanium Dioxide and other ingredients.
Each MS CONTIN 30 mg Controlled-Release Tablet contains: 30 mg Morphine Sulfate U.S.P. Inactive ingredients: Cetostearyl Alcohol, D&C Red No. 7, FD&C Blue No. 1, Hydroxyethyl Cellulose, Hydroxypropyl Methylcellulose, Lactose, Magnesium Stearate, Talc, Titanium Dioxide, and other ingredients.
Each MS CONTIN 60 mg Controlled-Release Tablet contains: 60 mg Morphine Sulfate U.S.P. Inactive ingredients: Cetostearyl Alcohol, D&C Red No. 30, D&C Yellow No. 10, Hydroxyethyl Cellulose, Hydroxypropyl Methylcellulose, Lactose, Magnesium Stearate, Talc, Titanium dioxide, and other ingredients.
Each MS CONTIN 100 mg Controlled-Release Tablet contains: 100 mg Morphine Sulfate U.S.P. Inactive ingredients: Cetostearyl Alcohol, Hydroxyethyl Cellulose, Hydroxypropyl Methylcellulose, Magnesium Stearate, Synthetic Black Iron Oxide, Talc, Titanium Dioxide and other ingredients.

CLINICAL PHARMACOLOGY

Metabolism and Pharmacokinetics
MS CONTIN is a controlled-release tablet containing morphine sulfate. Following oral administration of a given dose of morphine, the amount ultimately absorbed is essentially the same whether the source is MS CONTIN or a conventional formulation. Morphine is released from MS CONTIN somewhat more slowly than from conventional oral preparations. Because of pre-systemic elimination (i.e., metabolism in the gut wall and liver) only about 40% of the administered dose reaches the central compartment.
Once absorbed, morphine is distributed to skeletal muscle, kidneys, liver, intestinal tract, lungs, spleen and brain. Morphine also crosses the placental membranes and has been found in breast milk.
Although a small fraction (less than 5%) of morphine is demethylated, for all practical purposes, virtually all morphine is converted to glucuronide metabolites; among these, morphine-3-glucuronide is present in the highest plasma concentration following oral administration.
The glucuronide system has a very high capacity and is not easily saturated even in disease. Therefore, rate of delivery of morphine to the gut and liver should not influence the total and, probably, the relative quantities of the various metabolites formed. Moreover, even if rate affected the relative amounts of each metabolite formed, it should be unimportant clinically because morphine's metabolites are ordinarily inactive.
The following pharmacokinetic parameters show considerable inter-subject variation but are representative of average values reported in the literature. The volume of distribution (Vd) for morphine is 4 liters per kilogram, and its terminal elimination half-life is normally 2 to 4 hours.
Following the administration of conventional oral morphine products, approximately fifty percent of the morphine that will reach the central compartment intact reaches it within 30 minutes. Following the administration of an equal amount of MS CONTIN to normal volunteers, however, this extent of absorption occurs, on average, after 1.5 hours.
The possible effect of food upon the systemic bioavailability of MS CONTIN has not been evaluated.
Variation in the physical/mechanical properties of a formulation of an oral morphine drug product can affect both its absolute bioavailability and its absorption rate constant (k_a). The formulation employed in MS CONTIN has not been shown to affect morphine's oral bioavailability, but does decrease its apparent k_a. Other basic pharmacokinetic parameters (e.g., volume of distribution [Vd], elimination rate constant [k_e], clearance [Cl]), are unchanged as they are fundamental properties of morphine in the organism. However, in chronic use, the possibility that shifts in metabolite to parent drug ratios may occur cannot be excluded.
When immediate-release oral morphine or MS CONTIN is given on a fixed dosing regimen, steady state is achieved in about a day.
For a given dose and dosing interval, the AUC and average blood concentration of morphine at steady state (Css) will be independent of the specific type of oral formulation administered so long as the formulations have the same absolute bioavailability. The absorption rate of a formulation will, however, affect the maximum (Cmax) and minimum (Cmin) blood levels and the times of their occurrence.
While there is no predictable relationship between morphine blood levels and analgesic response, effective analgesia will not occur below some minimum blood level in a given patient. The minimum effective blood level for analgesia will, of course, vary among patients, especially among patients who have been previously treated with potent mu agonist opioids. Similarly, there is no predictable relationship between blood morphine concentration and untoward clinical responses; again, however, higher concentrations are more likely to be toxic than lower ones.
For any fixed dose and dosing interval, MS CONTIN will have at steady state, a lower Cmax and a higher Cmin than conventional morphine. This is a potential advantage; a reduced fluctuation in morphine concentration during the dosing interval should keep morphine blood levels more centered within the theoretical "therapeutic window." (Fluctuation for a dosing interval is defined as [Cmax-Cmin]/[Css-average].) On the other hand, the degree of fluctuation in serum morphine concentration might conceivably affect other phenomena. For example, reduced fluctuations in blood morphine concentrations might influence the rate of tolerance induction.
The elimination of morphine occurs primarily as renal excretion of 3-morphine glucuronide. A small amount of the glucuronide conjugate is excreted in the bile, and there is some minor enterohepatic recycling. Because morphine is primarily metabolized to inactive metabolites, the effects of renal disease on morphine's elimination are not likely to be pronounced. However, as with any drug, caution should be taken to guard against unanticipated accumulation if renal and/or hepatic function is seriously impaired.

PHARMACODYNAMICS

The effects described below are common to all morphine-containing products.

Central Nervous System
The principal actions of therapeutic value of morphine are analgesia and sedation (i.e., sleepiness and anxiolysis).
The precise mechanism of the analgesic action is unknown. However, specific CNS opiate receptors and endogenous compounds with morphine-like activity have been identified throughout the brain and spinal cord and are likely to play a role in the expression of analgesic effects.
Morphine produces respiratory depression by direct action on brain stem respiratory centers. The mechanism of respiratory depression involves a reduction in the responsiveness of the brain stem respiratory centers to increases in carbon dioxide tension, and to electrical stimulation.
Morphine depresses the cough reflex by direct effect on the cough center in the medulla. Antitussive effects may occur with doses lower than those usually required for analgesia.
Morphine causes miosis, even in total darkness. Pinpoint pupils are a sign of narcotic overdose but are not pathognomonic (e.g., pontine lesions of hemorrhagic or ischemic origins may produce similar findings). Marked mydriasis rather than miosis may be seen with worsening hypoxia.

Gastrointestinal Tract and Other Smooth Muscle
Gastric, biliary and pancreatic secretions are decreased by morphine. Morphine causes a reduction in motility associated with an increase in tone in the antrum of the stomach and duodenum. Digestion of food in the small intestine is delayed and propulsive contractions are decreased. Propulsive peristaltic waves in the colon are decreased, while tone is increased to the point of spasm. The end result is constipation. Morphine can cause a marked increase in biliary tract pressure as a result of spasm of sphincter of Oddi.

Cardiovascular System
Morphine produces peripheral vasodilation which may result in orthostatic hypotension. Release of histamine can occur and may contribute to narcotic-induced hypotension. Manifestations of histamine release and/or peripheral vasodilation may include pruritis, flushing, red eyes and sweating.

INDICATIONS AND USAGE

MS CONTIN is a controlled-release oral morphine formulation indicated for the relief of moderate to severe pain. It is intended for use in patients who require repeated dosing with potent opioid analgesics over periods of more than a few days.

CONTRAINDICATIONS

MS CONTIN is contraindicated in patients with known hypersensitivity to the drug, in patients with respiratory depression in the absence of resuscitative equipment, and in patients with acute or severe bronchial asthma.
MS CONTIN is contraindicated in any patient who has or is suspected of having a paralytic ileus.

WARNINGS

(See also: CLINICAL PHARMACOLOGY)

Impaired Respiration
Respiratory depression is the chief hazard of all morphine preparations. Respiratory depression occurs most frequently in the elderly and debilitated patients, as well as in those suffering from conditions accompanied by hypoxia or hypercapnia when even moderate therapeutic doses may dangerously decrease pulmonary ventilation.
Morphine should be used with extreme caution in patients with chronic obstructive pulmonary disease or cor pulmonale, and in patients having a substantially decreased respiratory reserve, hypoxia, hypercapnia, or preexisting respiratory depression. In such patients, even usual therapeutic doses of morphine may decrease respiratory drive while simultaneously increasing airway resistance to the point of apnea.

Head Injury and Increased Intracranial Pressure
The respiratory depressant effects of morphine with carbon dioxide retention and secondary elevation of cerebrospinal fluid pressure may be markedly exaggerated in the presence of head injury, other intracranial lesions, or preexisting increase in intracranial pressure. Morphine produces effects which may obscure neurologic signs of further increases in pressure in patients with head injuries.

Hypotensive Effect
MS CONTIN, like all opioid analgesics, may cause severe hypotension in an individual whose ability to maintain his blood pressure has already been compromised by a depleted blood volume, or a concurrent administration of drugs such as phenothiazines or general anesthetics. (See also: PRECAUTIONS: Drug Interactions.) MS CONTIN may produce orthostatic hypotension in ambulatory patients.
MS CONTIN, like all opioid analgesics, should be administered with caution to patients in circulatory shock, since vasodilation produced by the drug may further reduce cardiac output and blood pressure.

Interactions with other CNS Depressants

MS CONTIN, like all opioid analgesics, should be used with great caution and in reduced dosage in patients who are concurrently receiving other central nervous system depressants including sedatives or hypnotics, general anesthetics, phenothiazines, other tranquilizers and alcohol because respiratory depression, hypotension and profound sedation or coma may result.

Interactions with Mixed Agonist/Antagonist Opioid Analgesics

From a theoretical perspective, agonist/antagonist analgesics (i.e., pentazocine, nalbuphine, butorphanol and buprenorphine) should NOT be administered to a patient who has received or is receiving a course of therapy with a pure opioid agonist analgesic. In these patients, mixed agonist/antagonist analgesics may reduce the analgesic effect or may precipitate withdrawal symptoms.

Drug Dependence

Morphine can produce drug dependence and has a potential for being abused. Tolerance as well as psychological and physical dependence may develop upon repeated administration. Physical dependence, however, is not of paramount importance in the management of terminally ill patients or any patients in severe pain. Abrupt cessation or a sudden reduction in dose after prolonged use may result in withdrawal symptoms. After prolonged exposure to opioid analgesics, if withdrawal is necessary, it must be undertaken gradually. (See DRUG ABUSE AND DEPENDENCE.)

Infants born to mothers physically dependent on opioid analgesics may also be physically dependent and exhibit respiratory depression and withdrawal symptoms. (See DRUG ABUSE AND DEPENDENCE.)

PRECAUTIONS

(See also: CLINICAL PHARMACOLOGY)

General

MS CONTIN is intended for use in patients who require more than several days continuous treatment with a potent opioid analgesic. The controlled-release nature of the formulation allows it to be administered on a more convenient schedule than conventional immediate-release oral morphine products. (See CLINICAL PHARMACOLOGY: "Metabolism and Pharmacokinetics".) However, MS CONTIN does not release morphine continuously over the course of a dosing interval. The administration of single doses of MS CONTIN on a q12 hour dosing schedule will result in higher peak and lower trough plasma levels than those that occur when an identical daily dose of morphine is administered using conventional oral formulations on a q4h regimen. The clinical significance of greater fluctuations in morphine plasma level has not been systematically evaluated. (See DOSAGE AND ADMINISTRATION)

As with any potent opioid, it is critical to adjust the dosing regimen for each patient individually, taking into account the patient's prior analgesic treatment experience. Although it is clearly impossible to enumerate every consideration that is important to the selection of the initial dose and dosing interval of MS CONTIN, attention should be given to 1) the daily dose, potency, and characteristics of the opioid the patient has been taking previously (e.g., whether it is a pure agonist or mixed agonist/antagonist), 2) the reliability of the relative potency estimate used to calculate the dose of morphine needed [N.B. potency estimates may vary with the route of administration], 3) the degree of opioid tolerance, if any, and 4) the general condition and medical status of the patient.

Selection of patients for treatment with MS CONTIN should be governed by the same principles that apply to the use of morphine or other potent opioid analgesics. Specifically, the increased risks associated with its use in the following populations should be considered: the elderly or debilitated and those with severe impairment of hepatic, pulmonary or renal function; myxedema or hypothyroidism; adrenocortical insufficiency (e.g., Addison's Disease); CNS depression or coma; toxic psychosis; prostatic hypertrophy or urethral stricture; acute alcoholism; delirium tremens; kyphoscoliosis, or inability to swallow.

The administration of morphine, like all opioid analgesics, may obscure the diagnosis or clinical course in patients with acute abdominal conditions. Morphine may aggravate preexisting convulsions in patients with convulsive disorders.

Morphine should be used with caution in patients about to undergo surgery of the biliary tract since it may cause spasm of the sphincter of Oddi. Similarly, morphine should be used with caution in patients with acute pancreatitis secondary to biliary tract disease.

Information for Patients

If clinically advisable, patients receiving MS CONTIN should be given the following instructions by the physician:

1. Morphine may produce psychological and/or physical dependence. For this reason, the dose of the drug should not be adjusted without consulting a physician.
2. Morphine may impair mental and/or physical ability required for the performance of potentially hazardous tasks (e.g., driving, operating machinery).

3. Morphine should not be taken with alcohol or other CNS depressants (sleep aids, tranquilizers) because addictive effects including CNS depression may occur. A physician should be consulted if other prescription medications are currently being used or are prescribed for future use.
4. For women of childbearing potential who become or are planning to become pregnant, a physician should be consulted regarding analgesics and other drug use.

Drug Interactions (See WARNINGS)

The concomitant use of other central nervous system depressants including sedatives or hypnotics, general anesthetics, phenothiazines, tranquilizers and alcohol may produce additive depressant effects. Respiratory depression, hypotension and profound sedation or coma may occur. When such combined therapy is contemplated, the dose of one or both agents should be reduced. Opioid analgesics, including MS CONTIN, may enhance the neuromuscular blocking action of skeletal muscle relaxants and produce an increased degree of respiratory depression.

Carcinogenicity/Mutagenicity/Impairment of Fertility

Studies of morphine sulfate in animals to evaluate the drug's carcinogenic and mutagenic potential or the effect on fertility have not been conducted.

Pregnancy

Teratogenic effects—CATEGORY C: Adequate animal studies on reproduction have not been performed to determine whether morphine affects fertility in males or females. There are no well-controlled studies in women, but marketing experience does not include any evidence of adverse effects on the fetus following routine (short-term) clinical use of morphine sulfate products. Although there is no clearly defined risk, such experience can not exclude the possibility of infrequent or subtle damage to the human fetus.

MS CONTIN should be used in pregnant women only when clearly needed. (See also: PRECAUTIONS: Labor and Delivery, and DRUG ABUSE AND DEPENDENCE.)

Nonteratogenic effects: Infants born from mothers who have been taking morphine chronically may exhibit withdrawal symptoms.

Labor and Delivery

MS CONTIN is not recommended for use in women during and immediately prior to labor. Occasionally, opioid analgesics may prolong labor through actions which temporarily reduce the strength, duration and frequency of uterine contractions. However, this effect is not consistent and may be offset by an increased rate of cervical dilatation which tends to shorten labor.

Neonates whose mothers received opioid analgesics during labor should be observed closely for signs of respiratory depression. A specific narcotic antagonist, naloxone, should be available for reversal of narcotic-induced respiratory depression in the neonate.

Nursing Mothers

Low levels of *morphine* have been detected in the breast milk. Withdrawal symptoms can occur in breast-feeding infants when maternal administration of morphine sulfate is stopped. Ordinarily, nursing should not be undertaken while a patient is receiving MS CONTIN since morphine may be excreted in the milk.

Pediatric Use

MS CONTIN has not been evaluated systematically in children.

ADVERSE REACTIONS

The adverse reactions caused by morphine are essentially those observed with other opioid analgesics. They include the following major hazards: respiratory depression, apnea, and to a lesser degree, circulatory depression; respiratory arrest, shock and cardiac arrest.

Most Frequently Observed

Constipation, lightheadedness, dizziness, sedation, nausea, vomiting, sweating, dysphoria and euphoria.

Some of these effects seem to be more prominent in ambulatory patients and in those not experiencing severe pain. Some adverse reactions in ambulatory patients may be alleviated if the patient lies down.

Less Frequently Observed Reactions

Central Nervous System: Weakness, headache, agitation, tremor, uncoordinated muscle movements, seizure, alterations of mood (nervousness, apprehension, depression, floating feelings), dreams, muscle rigidity, transient hallucinations and disorientation, visual disturbances, insomnia and increased intracranial pressure.

Gastrointestinal: Dry mouth, constipation, biliary tract spasm, laryngospasm, anorexia, diarrhea, cramps and taste alterations.

Cardiovascular: Flushing of the face, chills, tachycardia, bradycardia, palpitation, faintness, syncope, hypotension and hypertension.

Genitourinary: Urine retention or hesitance, reduced libido and/or potency.

Dermatologic: Pruritis, urticaria, other skin rashes, edema and diaphoresis.

Other: Antidiuretic effect, paresthesia, muscle tremor, blurred vision, nystagmus, diplopia and miosis.

DRUG ABUSE AND DEPENDENCE

Opioid analgesics may cause psychological and physical dependence (see WARNINGS). Physical dependence results in withdrawal symptoms in patients who abruptly discontinue the drug or may be precipitated through the administration of drugs with narcotic antagonist activity, e.g., naloxone or mixed agonist/antagonist analgesics (pentazocine, etc.; See also OVERDOSAGE). Physical dependence usually does not occur to a clinically significant degree until after several weeks of continued narcotic usage. Tolerance, in which increasingly large doses are required in order to produce the same degree of analgesia, is initially manifested by a shortened duration of analgesic effect, and, subsequently, by decreases in the intensity of analgesia.

In chronic pain patients, and in narcotic-tolerant cancer patients, the administration of MS CONTIN should be guided by the degree of tolerance manifested. Physical dependence, per se, is not ordinarily a concern when one is dealing with opioid-tolerant patients whose pain and suffering is associated with an irreversible illness.

If MS CONTIN is abruptly discontinued, a moderate to severe abstinence syndrome may occur. The opioid agonist abstinence syndrome is characterized by some or all of the following: restlessness, lacrimation, rhinorrhea, yawning, perspiration, gooseflesh, restless sleep or "yen" and mydriasis during the first 24 hours. These symptoms often increase in severity and over the next 72 hours may be accompanied by increasing irritability, anxiety, weakness, twitching and spasms of muscles; kicking movements; severe backache, abdominal and leg pains; abdominal and muscle cramps; hot and cold flashes, insomnia; nausea, anorexia, vomiting, intestinal spasm, diarrhea; coryza and repetitive sneezing; increase in body temperature, blood pressure, respiratory rate and heart rate. Because of excessive loss of fluids through sweating, vomiting and diarrhea, there is usually marked weight loss, dehydration, ketosis, and disturbances in acid-base balance. Cardiovascular collapse can occur. Without treatment most observable symptoms disappear in 5–14 days; however, there appears to be a phase of secondary or chronic abstinence which may last for 2–6 months characterized by insomnia, irritability, and muscular aches.

If treatment of physical dependence of patients on MS CONTIN is necessary, the patient may be detoxified by gradual reduction of the dosage. Gastrointestinal disturbances or dehydration should be treated accordingly.

OVERDOSAGE

Acute overdosage with morphine is manifested by respiratory depression, somnolence progressing to stupor or coma, skeletal muscle flaccidity, cold and clammy skin, constricted pupils, and, sometimes, bradycardia and hypotension.

In the treatment of overdosage, primary attention should be given to the re-establishment of a patent airway and institution of assisted or controlled ventilation. The pure opioid antagonist, naloxone, is a specific antidote against respiratory depression which results from opioid overdose. Naloxone (usually 0.4 to 2.0 mg) should be administered intravenously; however, because its duration of action is relatively short, the patient must be carefully monitored until spontaneous respiration is reliably re-established. If the response to naloxone is suboptimal or not sustained, additional naloxone may be re-administered, as needed, or given by continuous infusion to maintain alertness and respiratory function; however, there is no information available about the cumulative dose of naloxone that may be safely administered.

Naloxone should not be administered in the absence of clinically significant respiratory or circulatory depression secondary to morphine overdose. Naloxone should be administered cautiously to persons who are known, or suspected to be physically dependent on MS CONTIN. In such cases, an abrupt or complete reversal of narcotic effects may precipitate an acute abstinence syndrome.

Note: In an individual physically dependent on opioids, administration of the usual dose of the antagonist will precipitate an acute withdrawal syndrome. The severity of the withdrawal syndrome produced will depend on the degree of physical dependence and the dose of the antagonist administered. Use of a narcotic antagonist in such a person should be avoided. If necessary to treat serious respiratory depression in the physically dependent patient, the antagonist should be administered with extreme care and by titration with smaller than usual doses of the antagonist.

Supportive measures (including oxygen, vasopressors) should be employed in the management of circulatory shock and pulmonary edema accompanying overdose as indicated. Cardiac arrest or arrhythmias may require cardiac massage or defibrillation.

DOSAGE AND ADMINISTRATION

(See also: CLINICAL PHARMACOLOGY, WARNINGS AND PRECAUTIONS sections)

MS CONTIN TABLETS ARE TO BE TAKEN WHOLE, AND ARE NOT TO BE BROKEN, CHEWED OR CRUSHED.

Continued on next page

Purdue Frederick—Cont.

TAKING BROKEN, CHEWED OR CRUSHED MS CONTIN TABLETS COULD LEAD TO THE RAPID RELEASE AND ABSORPTION OF A POTENTIALLY TOXIC DOSE OF MORPHINE.

MS CONTIN is intended for use in patients who require more than several days continuous treatment with a potent opioid analgesic. The controlled-release nature of the formulation allows it to be administered on a more convenient schedule than conventional immediate-release oral morphine products. (See CLINICAL PHARMACOLOGY: "Metabolism and Pharmacokinetics".) However, MS CONTIN does not release morphine continuously over the course of the dosing interval. The administration of single doses of MS CONTIN on a q12h dosing schedule will result in higher peak and lower trough plasma levels than those that occur when an identical daily dose of morphine is administered using conventional oral formulations on a q4h regimen. The clinical significance of greater fluctuations in morphine plasma level has not been systematically evaluated.

As with any potent opioid drug product, it is critical to adjust the dosing regimen for each patient individually, taking into account the patient's prior analgesic treatment experience. Although it is clearly impossible to enumerate every consideration that is important to the selection of initial dose and dosing interval of MS CONTIN, attention should be given to 1) the daily dose, potency and precise characteristics of the opioid the patient has been taking previously (e.g., whether it is a pure agonist or mixed agonist/antagonist), 2) the reliability of the relative potency estimate used to calculate the dose of morphine needed [N.B. potency estimates may vary with the route of administration], 3) the degree of opioid tolerance, if any, and 4) the general condition and medical status of the patient.

The following dosing recommendations, therefore, can only be considered suggested approaches to what is actually a series of clinical decisions in the management of the pain of an individual patient.

Conversion from Conventional Oral Morphine to MS CONTIN
A patient's daily morphine requirement is established using immediate-release oral morphine (dosing every 4 to 6 hours). The patient is then converted to MS CONTIN in either of two ways: 1) by administering one-half of the patient's 24-hour requirement as MS CONTIN on an every 12-hour schedule; or, 2) by administering one-third of the patient's daily requirement as MS CONTIN on an every eight hour schedule. With either method, dose and dosing interval is then adjusted as needed (see discussion below.) The 15 mg tablet should be used for initial conversion for patients whose total daily requirement is expected to be less than 60 mg. The 30 mg tablet strength is recommended for patients with a daily morphine requirement of 60 to 120 mg. When the total daily dose is expected to be greater than 120 mg, the appropriate combination of tablet strengths should be employed.

Conversion from Parenteral Morphine or Other Opioids (Parenteral or Oral) to MS CONTIN
MS CONTIN can be administered as the initial oral morphine drug product; in this case, however, particular care must be exercised in the conversion process. Because of uncertainty about, and intersubject variation in, relative estimates of opioid potency and cross tolerance, initial dosing regimens should be conservative; that is, an underestimation of the 24 hour oral morphine requirement is preferred to an overestimate. To this end, initial individual doses of MS CONTIN should be estimated conservatively. In patients whose daily morphine requirements are expected to be less than or equal to 120 mg per day, the 30 mg tablet strength is recommended for the initial titration period. Once a stable dose regimen is reached, the patient can be converted to the 60 mg or 100 mg tablet strength, or appropriate combination of tablet strengths, if desired.

Estimates of the relative potency of opioids are only approximate and are influenced by route of administration, individual patient differences, and possibly, by an individual's medical condition. Consequently, it is difficult to recommend any fixed rule for converting a patient to MS CONTIN directly. The following general points should be considered, however.

1. *Parenteral to oral morphine ratio:* Estimates of the oral to parenteral potency of morphine vary. Some authorities suggest that a dose of oral morphine only three times the daily parenteral morphine requirement may be sufficient in chronic use settings.

2. *Other parenteral or oral opioids to oral morphine:* Because there is lack of systemic evidence bearing on these types of analgesic substitutions, specific recommendations are not possible. Physicians are advised to refer to published relative potency data, keeping in mind that such ratios are only approximate. In general, it is safer to underestimate the daily dose of MS CONTIN required and rely upon ad hoc supplementation to deal with inadequate analgesia. (See discussion which follows.)

Use of MS CONTIN as the First Opioid Analgesic
There has been no systematic evaluation of MS CONTIN as an initial opioid analgesic in the management of pain. Because it may be more difficult to titrate a patient using a controlled-release morphine, it is ordinarily advisable to begin treatment using an immediate-release formulation.

Considerations in the Adjustment of Dosing Regimens
Whatever the approach, if signs of excessive opioid effects are observed early in a dosing interval, the next dose should be reduced. If this adjustment leads to inadequate analgesia, that is, 'breakthrough' pain occurs late in the dosing interval, the dosing interval may be shortened. Alternatively, a supplemental dose of a short-acting analgesic may be given. As experience is gained, adjustments can be made to obtain an appropriate balance between pain relief, opioid side effects, and the convenience of the dosing schedule.

In adjusting dosing requirements, it is recommended that the dosing interval never be extended beyond 12 hours because the administration of very large single doses may lead to acute overdose. (N.B. MS CONTIN is a controlled-release formulation; it does not release morphine continuously over the dosing interval.)

For patients with low daily morphine requirements, the 15 mg tablet should be used.

Conversion from MS CONTIN to parenteral opioids:
When converting a patient from MS CONTIN to parenteral opioids, it is best to assume that the parenteral to oral potency is high. NOTE THAT THIS IS THE CONVERSE OF THE STRATEGY USED WHEN THE DIRECTION OF CONVERSION IS FROM THE PARENTERAL TO ORAL FORMULATIONS. IN BOTH CASES, HOWEVER, THE AIM IS TO ESTIMATE THE NEW DOSE CONSERVATIVELY. For example, to estimate the required 24-hour dose of morphine for IM use, one could employ a conversion of 1 mg of morphine IM for every 6 mg of morphine as MS CONTIN. Of course, the IM 24-hour dose would have to be divided by six and administered on a q4h regimen. This approach is recommended because it is least likely to cause overdose.

HOW SUPPLIED

NDC 0034-0514-10: MS CONTN (morphine sulfate controlled-release tablets) 15 mg are supplied in opaque plastic bottles containing 100 tablets.
NDC 0034-0514-90: MS CONTIN (morphine sulfate controlled-release tablets) 15 mg are supplied in opaque plastic bottles containing 500 tablets.
NDC 0034-0514-25: MS CONTIN (morphine sulfate controlled-release tablets) 15 mg are supplied in unit dose packaging with 25 individually numbered tablets per card (numbered in descending order for easier counting) and shrink-wrapped in inner packs of 100 tablets (4 cards of 25 tablets per card). One shipper contains 300 tablets (3 inner packs of 100 tablets each). Each individual tablet-unit is labeled "MS CONTIN CII, 15 mg."
NDC 0034-0515-50: MS CONTIN (morphine sulfate controlled-release tablets) 30 mg are supplied in opaque plastic bottles containing 50 tablets.
NDC 0034-0515-10: MS CONTIN (morphine sulfate controlled-release tablets) 30 mg are supplied in opaque plastic bottles containing 100 tablets.
NDC 0034-0515-45: MS CONTIN (morphine sulfate controlled-release tablets) 30 mg are supplied in opaque plastic bottles containing 250 tablets.
NDC 0034-0515-90: MS CONTIN (morphine sulfate controlled-release tablets) 30 mg are supplied in opaque plastic bottles containing 500 tablets.
NDC 0034-0515-25: MS CONTIN (morphine sulfate controlled-release tablets) 30 mg supplied in unit dose packaging with 25 individually-numbered tablets per card (numbered in descending order for easier counting) and shrink-wrapped in inner packs of 100 tablets (4 cards of 25 tablets per card). One shipper contains 300 tablets (3 inner packs of 100 tablets each). Each individual tablet-unit is labeled "MS CONTIN CII, 30 mg."
NDC 0034-0516-10: MS CONTIN (morphine sulfate controlled-release tablets) 60 mg are supplied in opaque plastic bottles containing 100 tablets.
NDC 0034-0516-90: MS CONTIN (morphine sulfate controlled-release tablets) 60 mg are supplied in opaque plastic bottles containing 500 tablets.
NDC 0034-0516-25: MS CONTIN (morphine sulfate controlled-release tablets) 60 mg supplied in unit dose packaging with 25 individually numbered tablets per card (numbered in descending order for easier counting) and shrink-wrapped in inner packs of 100 tablets (4 cards of 25 tablets per card). One shipper contains 300 tablets (3 inner packs of 100 tablets each). Each individual tablet-unit is labeled "MS CONTIN CII, 60 mg".
NDC 0034-0517-10: MS CONTIN (morphine sulfate controlled-release tablets) 100 mg are supplied in opaque plastic bottles containing 100 tablets.
NDC 0034-0517-90: MS CONTIN (morphine sulfate controlled-release tablets) 100 mg are supplied in opaque plastic bottles containing 500 tablets.

NDC 0034-0517-25: MS CONTIN (morphine sulfate controlled-release tablets) 100 mg are supplied with unit dose packaging with 25 individually numbered tablets per card (numbered in descending order for easier counting) and shrink-wrapped in inner packs of 100 tablets (4 cards of 25 tablets per card). One shipper contains 300 tablets (3 inner packs of 100 tablets each). Each individual tablet-unit is labeled "MS CONTIN CII, 100 mg."

15 mg: Each round, blue-colored tablet bears the symbol PF on one side and M15 on the other side.
30 mg: Each round, lavender-colored tablet bears the symbol PF on one side and M30 on the other side.
60 mg: Each round, orange-colored tablet bears the symbol PF on one side and M60 on the other side.
100 mg: Each round, gray-colored tablet bears the symbol PF on one side and 100 on the other side.
Store tablets at controlled room temperature 15°–30°C (59°–86°F).
Dispense in tight, light-resistant container.

CAUTION
DEA Order Form Required.
Federal law prohibits dispensing without prescription.
THE PURDUE FREDERICK COMPANY
Norwalk, CT 06850-3590
Copyright © 1987, 1991, The Purdue Frederick Company
U.S. Patent Numbers 3965256 and 4235870
September 3, 1991   E3220 2003
Shown in Product Identification Section, page 424

MSIR® Oral Solution   ℞
[em ′es ĭ ″ahr]
(morphine sulfate)
   (WARNING: May be habit forming)
MSIR® Oral Solution Concentrate   ℞
(morphine sulfate)
   (WARNING: May be habit forming)
MSIR® Immediate Release Oral Tablets   ℞
(morphine sulfate)
   (WARNING: May be habit forming)

DESCRIPTION
Chemically, morphine sulfate is 7,8 didehydro-4,5-α-epoxy-17-methyl-morphinian-3,6 α-diol sulfate (2:1) (salt) pentahydrate and has the following structural formula:

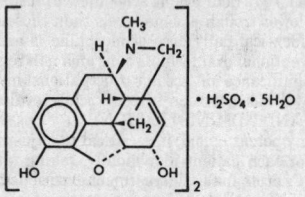

Each 5 ml of MSIR Oral Solution contains:
Morphine Sulfate .... 10 or 20 mg
Inactive Ingredients: Edetate disodium, FD&C Red. No. 40, Glycerin, Invert Sugar, Sodium benzoate, Sodium chloride, Sucrose, Artificial & Natural Flavors, and other ingredients.
Each 1 ml of MSIR Oral Solution Concentrate contains:
Morphine Sulfate .... 20 mg
Inactive Ingredients: Edetate disodium, Sodium benzoate, and other ingredients.
Each MSIR Tablet for oral administration contains:
Morphine Sulfate .... 15 or 30 mg
Inactive Ingredients: Corn starch, Lactose, Magnesium stearate, and Talc.
   (WARNING: May be habit forming)

CLINICAL PHARMACOLOGY

Metabolism and Pharmacokinetics
MSIR Solutions and Tablets containing morphine sulfate are for oral administration and are conventional immediate release products. Only about 40% of the administered dose reaches the central compartment because of pre-systemic elimination (i.e., metabolism in the gut wall and liver).
Once absorbed, morphine is distributed in skeletal muscle, kidneys, liver, intestinal tract, lungs, spleen and brain. Morphine also crosses the placental membranes and has been found in breast milk.
Although a small fraction (less than 5%) of morphine is demethylated, for all practical purposes, virtually all morphine is converted to glucuronide metabolites; among these, morphine-3-glucuronide is present in the highest plasma concentration following oral administration.
The glucuronide system has a very high capacity and is not easily saturated even in disease. Therefore, the rate of delivery of morphine to the gut and liver does not influence the total and/or the relative quantities of the various metabolites formed.
The following pharmacokinetic parameters show considerable inter-subject variation but are representative of average values reported in the literature. The volume of distribu-

tion (Vd) for morphine is 4 liters per kilogram, and the terminal elimination half-life is approximately 2 to 4 hours. Fifty percent of the morphine that will reach the central compartment intact, reaches it within 30 minutes following the administration of conventional oral morphine products.

Variation in the physical/mechanical properties of a formulation of an oral morphine drug product can affect both its absolute bioavailability and its absorption rate constant (k_a). The basic pharmacokinetic parameters (e.g., volume of distribution [Vd], elimination rate constant [k_e], clearance [Cl]) are fundamental properties of morphine in the organism. While there is no predictable relationship between morphine blood levels and analgesic response, effective analgesia probably will not occur below some minimum blood level in a given patient. The minimum effective blood level for analgesia will vary among patients, especially among patients who have or have not been previously treated with potent mu (μ) agonist opioids. Similarly, there is no predictable relationship between blood morphine concentration and untoward clinical responses; but higher concentrations are more likely to be toxic.

The elimination of morphine occurs primarily as renal excretion of 3-morphine glucuronide. A small amount of the glucuronide conjugate is excreted in the bile, and there is some minor enterohepatic recycling.

The elimination half-life of morphine is reported to vary between 2 and 4 hours. Thus, steady state is probably achieved on most regimens within a day. Because morphine is primarily metabolized to inactive metabolites, the effects of renal disease on morphine's elimination are not likely to be pronounced. However, as with any drug, caution should be taken to guard against unanticipated accumulation if renal and/or hepatic function is seriously impaired.

Individual differences in the metabolism of morphine suggest that MSIR Oral Solutions and Tablets be dosed conservatively according to the dosing initiation and titration recommendations in the Dosage and Administration section.

PHARMACODYNAMICS

The effects described below are common to all morphine-containing products.

Central Nervous System

The principal actions of therapeutic value of morphine are analgesia and sedation.

The precise mechanism of analgesic action is unknown. However, specific CNS opiate receptors and endogenous compounds with morphine-like activity have been identified throughout the brain and spinal cord and are likely to play a role in the expression of analgesic effects.

Morphine produces respiratory depression by direct action on brain stem respiratory centers. The mechanism of respiratory depression involves a reduction in the responsiveness of the brain stem respiratory centers to increases in carbon dioxide tension, and to electrical stimulation.

Morphine depresses the cough reflex by direct effect on the cough center in the medulla. Antitussive effects may occur with doses lower than those usually required for analgesia. Morphine causes miosis, even in total darkness. Pinpoint pupils are a sign of narcotic overdose but are not pathognomonic (e.g., pontine lesions hemorrhagic or ischemic origins may produce similar findings). Marked mydriasis rather than miosis may be seen with worsening hypoxia.

Gastrointestinal Tract and Other Smooth Muscle

Gastric, biliary and pancreatic secretions are decreased by morphine. Morphine causes a reduction in motility associated with an increase in tone in the antrum of the stomach and duodenum. Digestion of food in the small intestine is delayed and propulsive contractions are decreased. In addition propulsive peristaltic waves in the colon are decreased, while tone is increased to the point of spasm. The end result is constipation. Morphine can cause a marked increase in biliary tract pressure as a result of spasm of the sphincter of Oddi.

Cardiovascular System

Morphine produces peripheral vasodilation which may result in orthostatic hypotension. Release of histamine can occur and may contribute to narcotic-induced hypotension. Manifestations of histamine release and/or peripheral vasodilation may include pruritus, flushing, red eyes and sweating.

INDICATIONS AND USAGE

MSIR Oral Solutions and Tablets are indicated for the relief of moderate to severe pain.

CONTRAINDICATIONS

MSIR Oral Solutions and Tablets are contraindicated in patients with known hypersensitivity to the drug, in patients with respiratory depression in the absence of resuscitative equipment, and in patients with acute or severe bronchial asthma.

MSIR Oral Solutions and Tablets are contraindicated in any patient who has or is suspected of having a paralytic ileus.

WARNINGS

(see also: CLINICAL PHARMACOLOGY)

Impaired Respiration

Respiratory depression is the chief hazard of all morphine preparations although mitigated in the presence of pain. Respiratory depression occurs most frequently in elderly and debilitated patients, and those suffering from conditions accompanied by hypoxia or hypercapnia when even moderate therapeutic doses may dangerously decrease pulmonary ventilation.

Morphine should be used with extreme caution in patients with chronic obstructive pulmonary disease or cor pulmonale, and in patients having a substantially decreased respiratory reserve, hypoxia, hypercapnia, or preexisting respiratory depression. In such patients, even usual therapeutic doses of morphine may decrease respiratory drive while simultaneously increasing airway resistance to the point of apnea.

Head Injury and Increased Intracranial Pressure

The respiratory depressant effects of morphine with carbon dioxide retention and secondary elevation of cerebrospinal fluid pressure may be markedly exaggerated in the presence of head injury, other intracranial lesions, or preexisting increase in intracranial pressure. Morphine produces effects which may obscure neurologic signs of further increase in pressure in patients with head injuries.

Hypotensive Effects

MSIR Oral Solutions and Tablets, like all opioid analgesics, may cause severe hypotension in an individual whose ability to maintain his blood pressure has already been compromised by a depleted blood volume, or a concurrent administration of drugs such as phenothiazines, or general anesthetics. (See also: PRECAUTIONS: Drug Interactions.) MSIR Oral Solutions and Tablets may produce orthostatic hypotension in ambulatory patients.

MSIR Oral Solutions and Tablets, like all opioid analgesics, should be administered with caution to patients in circulatory shock, since vasodilation produced by the drug may further reduce cardiac output and blood pressure.

Interactions with Other CNS Depressants

MSIR Oral Solutions and Tablets, like all opioid analgesics, should be used with great caution and in reduced dosage in patients who are concurrently receiving other central nervous system depressants including sedatives or hypnotics, general anesthetics, phenothiazines, other tranquilizers and alcohol, because respiratory depression, hypotension and profound sedation or coma may result.

Interactions with Mixed Agonist/Antagonist Opioid Analgesics

From a theoretical perspective, agonist/antagonist analgesics (i.e., pentazocine, nalbuphine, butorphanol and buprenorphine) should NOT be administered to a patient who has received or is receiving a course of therapy with a pure agonist opioid analgesic: In these patients, mixed agonist-antagonist analgesics may reduce the analgesic effect or may precipitate withdrawal symptoms.

Drug Dependence

Morphine can produce drug dependence and has a potential for being abused. Tolerance and psychological and physical dependence may develop upon repeated administration. Physical dependence, however, is not of paramount importance in the management of any patient in severe pain. Abrupt cessation or a sudden reduction in dose after prolonged use may result in withdrawal symptoms. After prolonged exposure to opioid analgesics, if withdrawal is necessary, it must be undertaken gradually. (See DRUG ABUSE AND DEPENDENCE.)

Infants born to mothers physically dependent on opioid analgesics may also be physically dependent and exhibit respiratory depression and withdrawal symptoms. (See DRUG ABUSE AND DEPENDENCE.)

The development of psychological dependence is relatively rare when morphine is used under medically supervised conditions.

PRECAUTIONS

(See also: CLINICAL PHARMACOLOGY.)

General

MSIR Oral Solutions and Tablets are intended for use in patients who require a potent opioid analgesic for relief of moderate to severe pain.

Selection of patients for treatment with MSIR Oral Solutions and Tablets should be governed by the same principles that apply to the use of morphine and other potent opioid analgesics which take into account: the elderly or debilitated and those with the following—severe impairment of hepatic, pulmonary or renal function; myxedema or hypothyroidism; adrenocortical insufficiency (e.g., Addison's Disease); CNS depression or coma; toxic psychoses; prostatic hypertrophy or urethral stricture; acute alcoholism; delirium tremens; kyphoscoliosis.

The administration of morphine, like all opioid analgesics, may obscure the diagnosis or clinical course in patients with acute abdominal conditions.

Morphine may aggravate preexisting convulsions in patients with convulsive disorders.

Morphine should be used with caution in patients about to undergo surgery of the biliary tract, since it may cause spasm of the sphincter of Oddi. Similarly, morphine should be used with caution in patients with acute pancreatitis secondary to biliary tract disease.

Information for Patients

If clinically advisable, patients receiving MSIR Oral Solutions and Tablets should be given the following instructions by the physician.

1. Morphine may produce physical dependence and may be associated with the development of psychological dependence. For this reason, the dose of the drug should not be adjusted without consulting a physician.
2. Morphine may impair mental and/or physical ability required for the performance of potentially hazardous tasks (e.g., driving, operating machinery).
3. Morphine should not be taken with alcohol or other CNS depressants (sleep aids, tranquilizers) because additive effects including CNS depression may occur. A physician should be consulted if other prescription medications are currently being used or are prescribed for future use.
4. For women of childbearing potential who become or are planning to become pregnant, a physician should be consulted regarding analgesics and other drug use.

Drug Interactions (See also WARNINGS.)

The concomitant use of other central nervous system depressants including sedatives or hypnotics, general anesthetics, phenothiazines, tranquilizers and alcohol may produce additive depressant effects. Respiratory depression, hypotension and profound sedation or coma may occur. When such combined therapy is contemplated, the dose of one or both agents should be reduced. Opioid analgesics, including MSIR Oral Solutions and Tablets, may enhance the neuromuscular blocking action of skeletal muscle relaxants and produce an increased degree of respiratory depression.

Carcinogenicity/Mutagenicity/Impairment of Fertility

Studies of morphine sulfate in animals to evaluate the drug's carcinogenic and mutagenic potential or the effect on fertility have not been conducted.

Pregnancy

Teratogenic effects—CATEGORY C: There are no well-controlled studies in women, but marketing experience does not include any evidence of adverse effects on the fetus following routine (short-term) clinical use of morphine sulfate products. Although there is no clearly defined risk, such experience cannot exclude the possibility of infrequent or subtle damage to the human fetus. MSIR Oral Solutions and Tablets should be used in pregnant women only when clearly needed. (See also: PRECAUTIONS: Labor and Delivery, and DRUG ABUSE AND DEPENDENCE.)

Nonteratogenic effects: Infants born from mothers who have been taking morphine chronically may exhibit withdrawal symptoms.

Labor and Delivery

MSIR Oral Solutions and Tablets are not recommended for use in women during and immediately prior to labor. Occasionally, opioid analgesics may prolong labor through actions which temporarily reduce the strength, duration and frequency of uterine contractions. However, this effect is not consistent and may be offset by an increased rate of cervical dilatation which tends to shorten labor.

Neonates whose mothers receive opioid analgesics during labor should be observed closely for signs of respiratory depression. A specific narcotic antagonist, naloxone, should be available for reversal of narcotic-induced respiratory depression in the neonate.

Nursing Mothers

Low levels of morphine sulfate have been detected in human milk. Withdrawal symptoms can occur in breast-feeding infants when maternal administration of morphine sulfate is stopped. Nursing should not be undertaken while a patient is receiving MSIR Oral Solutions and Tablets since morphine may be excreted in the milk.

ADVERSE REACTIONS

The adverse reactions caused by morphine are essentially the same as those observed with other opioid analgesics. They include the following major hazards: respiratory depression, apnea, and to a lesser degree, circulatory depression; respiratory arrest, shock, and cardiac arrest.

Most Frequently Observed

Constipation, lightheadedness, dizziness, sedation, nausea, vomiting, and sweating.

Some of these effects seem to be more prominent in ambulatory patients and in those not experiencing severe pain. Some adverse reactions in ambulatory patients may be alleviated if the patient lies down.

Less Frequently Observed Reactions

Central Nervous System: Weakness, headache, agitation, tremor, uncoordinated muscle movements, seizure, alterations of mood (dysphoria, euphoria, nervousness, apprehension, depression, floating feelings), dreams, muscle rigidity,

Continued on next page

Purdue Frederick—Cont.

transient hallucinations and disorientation, visual disturbances, insomnia and increased intracranial pressure.
Gastrointestinal: Dry mouth, biliary tract spasm, anorexia, diarrhea, cramps and taste alterations.
Cardiovascular: Flushing of the face, chills, tachycardia, bradycardia, palpitation, faintness, syncope, hypotension and hypertension.
Genitourinary: Urinary retention or hesitance, reduced libido, and/or impotence.
Dermatologic: Pruritus, urticaria, other skin rashes, and edema.
Other: Antidiuretic effect, paresthesia, muscle tremor, blurred vision, nystagmus, diplopia, miosis and laryngospasm.

DRUG ABUSE AND DEPENDENCE

Opioid analgesics may cause physical dependence and be associated with the development of psychological dependence. (See WARNINGS.) Physical dependence results in withdrawal symptoms in patients who abruptly discontinue the drug or may be precipitated through the administration of drugs with narcotic antagonist activity, e.g., naloxone or mixed agonist/antagonist analgesics (pentazocine, etc.; see also OVERDOSE). Physical dependence usually does not occur to a clinically significant degree until after several weeks of continued narcotic usage. Tolerance, in which increasingly large doses are required in order to produce the same degree of analgesia, is initially manifested by a shortened duration of analgesic effect, and, subsequently, by decreases in the intensity of analgesia. In chronic-pain patients and in narcotic-tolerant cancer patients, the administration of MSIR Oral Solutions and Tablets should be guided by the degree of tolerance manifested. Physical dependence, per se, is not a concern when one is dealing with the cancer patient with moderate to severe pain. The primary objective in this situation is to relieve the patient's pain.
If MSIR Oral Solutions and Tablets are abruptly discontinued, a moderate to severe abstinence syndrome may occur. The opioid agonist abstinence syndrome is characterized by some or all of the following: restlessness, lacrimation, rhinorrhea, yawning, perspiration, cutis anserina, restless sleep known as the "yen" and mydriasis during the first 24 hours. These symptoms often increase in severity and over the next 72 hours may be accompanied by increasing irritability, anxiety, weakness, twitching and spasms of muscles; kicking movements; severe backache, abdominal and leg pains; abdominal and muscle cramps; hot and cold flashes; insomnia; nausea, anorexia, vomiting, intestinal spasm, diarrhea; coryza and repetitive sneezing; and increase in body temperature, blood pressure, respiratory rate and heart rate. Because of excessive loss of fluids through sweating, vomiting and diarrhea, there is usually marked weight loss, dehydration, ketosis, and disturbances in acid-base balance. Cardiovascular collapse can occur. Without treatment, most observable symptoms disappear in 5–14 days; however, there appears to be a phase of secondary or chronic abstinence which may last for 2–6 months, characterized by insomnia, irritability, and muscular aches.
If treatment of physical dependence on MSIR Oral Solutions and Tablets is necessary, the patient may be detoxified by gradual reduction of the dosage. If abstinence symptoms become severe, the patient may be given methadone. Temporary administration of tranquilizers and sedatives may aid in reducing patient anxiety and narcotic craving. Gastrointestinal disturbances or dehydration should be treated accordingly.

OVERDOSE

Acute overdosage with morphine is manifested by respiratory depression, somnolence progressing to stupor or coma, skeletal muscle flaccidity, cold and clammy skin, constricted pupils, and, sometimes, bradycardia and hypotension.
In the treatment of overdosage, primary attention should be given to the re-establishment of a patent airway and institution of assisted or controlled ventilation. The pure opioid antagonist, naloxone, is a specific antidote against respiratory depression which results from opioid overdose. Naloxone (usually 0.4 to 2.0 mg) should be administered intravenously; however, because its duration of action is relatively short, the patient must be carefully monitored until spontaneous respiration is reliably reestablished. If the response to naloxone is suboptimal or not sustained, additional naloxone may be re-administered, as needed, or given by continuous infusion to maintain alertness and respiratory function; however, there is no information available about the cumulative dose of naloxone that may be safely administered.
Naloxone should not be administered in the absence of clinically significant respiratory or circulatory depression secondary to morphine overdose. Naloxone should be administered cautiously to persons who are known or suspected to be physically dependent on morphine. In such cases, an abrupt or complete reversal of narcotic effects may precipitate an acute abstinence syndrome.
Note: In an individual physically dependent on opioids, administration of the usual dose of the antagonist will precipitate an acute withdrawal syndrome. The severity of the withdrawal syndrome produced will depend on the degree of physical dependence and the dose of the antagonist administered. Use of a narcotic antagonist in such a person should be avoided. If necessary to treat serious respiratory depression in the physically dependent patient, the antagonist should be administered with extreme care and by titration with smaller than usual doses of the antagonist.
Supportive measures (including oxygen, vasopressors) should be employed in the management of circulatory shock and pulmonary edema accompanying overdose as indicated. Cardiac arrest or arrhythmias may require cardiac massage or defibrillation.

CAUTION

DEA Order Form Required.
Federal law prohibits dispensing without prescription.

DOSAGE AND ADMINISTRATION: (See also: CLINICAL PHARMACOLOGY, WARNINGS AND PRECAUTIONS sections)

Dosage of morphine is a patient-dependent variable, which must be individualized according to patient metabolism, age and disease state and also response to morphine. Each patient should be maintained at the lowest dosage level that will produce acceptable analgesia. As the patient's well-being improves after successful relief of moderate to severe pain, periodic reduction of dosage and/or extension of dosing interval should be attempted to minimize exposure to morphine.
Usual Adult Oral Dose: 5 to 30 mg every four (4) hours or as directed by physician administered either as MSIR Oral Solutions or MSIR Oral Tablets. For control of pain in terminal illness, it is recommended that the appropriate dose of MSIR Oral Solutions or MSIR Oral Tablets be given on a regularly scheduled basis every four hours at the minimum dose to achieve acceptable analgesia. If converting a patient from another narcotic to morphine sulfate on the basis of standard equivalence tables, a 1 to 3 ratio of parenteral to oral morphine equivalence is suggested. This ratio is conservative and may underestimate the amount of morphine required. If this is the case, the dose of MSIR Oral Solutions or MSIR Oral Tablets should be gradually increased to achieve acceptable analgesia and tolerable side effects.
For those liquids in a bottle, use a calibrated cup or dropper to measure dosage accurately.

HOW SUPPLIED

MSIR (morphine sulfate) Oral Solution:
(pleasantly flavored)
10 mg per 5 ml.
NDC 0034-0521-01: 5 ml polypropylene unit dose cups, 10 cups per single tray, ten trays per shipper carton.
NDC 0034-0521-02: high density polyethylene plastic bottle of 120 ml with child-resistant closure.
NDC 0034-0521-03: high density polyethylene plastic bottle of 500 ml with child-resistant closure.
20 mg per 5 ml.
NDC 0034-0522-01: 5 ml polypropylene unit dose cups, 10 cups per single tray, ten trays per shipper carton.
NDC 0034-0522-02: high density polyethylene plastic bottle of 120 ml with child-resistant closure.
NDC 0034-0522-03: high density polyethylene plastic bottle of 500 ml with child-resistant closure.

MSIR (morphine sulfate) Oral Solution Concentrate:
(unflavored)
20 mg per 1 ml.
NDC 0034-0523-01: high density polyethylene plastic, child-resistant closure bottle with child-resistant dropper in 30 ml size.
NDC 0034-0523-02: high density polyethylene plastic, child-resistant closure bottle with child-resistant dropper in 120 ml size.
Discard opened bottle of Oral Solution after 90 days. Protect from light.

MSIR (morphine sulfate) Tablets:
15 mg round, white scored tablets
NDC 0034-0518-15: opaque plastic bottle, containing 50 tablets. Each tablet bears the symbol *PF* on the scored side and *MI* 15 on the other side.
30 mg capsule-shaped, white scored tablets
NDC 0034-0519-30: opaque plastic bottle containing tablets. Each tablet bears the symbol *PF* on the scored side and *MI* 30 on the other side.

Store Oral Solutions and Tablets at controlled room temperature 15°to 30°C (59°–86°F).
Copyright © 1985, 1990, 1991
The Purdue Frederick Company
Norwalk, CT 06850-3590
8/20/91 E1966-TAB/SOL
Shown in Product Identification Section, page 424

SENOKOT® TABLETS/GRANULES OTC

[sen'o-kot]
SenokotXTRA® Tablets
(standardized senna concentrate)

INDICATIONS

Indicated for relief of functional constipation (chronic* or occasional). SENOKOT Tablets/Granules and Double-Strength SenokotXTRA Tablets contain a natural vegetable derivative, standardized for uniform action. Each Double-Strength SenokotXTRA Tablet contains twice the active ingredient in one SENOKOT Tablet; patients may take one Double-Strength SenokotXTRA Tablet instead of two SENOKOT Tablets.
Senokot Laxatives provide a virtually colon-specific action which is gentle, effective and predictable, generally producing bowel movement in 6 to 12 hours. SENOKOT has been found to be effective even in many previously intractable cases of functional constipation. SENOKOT preparations may aid in rehabilitation of the constipated patient by facilitating regular elimination. At proper dosage levels, SENOKOT preparations are virtually free of adverse reactions (such as loose stools or abdominal discomfort) and enjoy high patient acceptance. Numerous and extensive clinical studies show their high degree of effectiveness in several types of functional constipation: chronic, geriatric, and postpartum, drug-induced, pediatric, as well as in functional constipation concurrent with heart disease or anorectal surgery.

DESCRIPTION

SENOKOT Tablets: Each tablet contains 8.6 mg sennosides.
Active Ingredient: Standardized Senna Concentrate.
Inactive Ingredients: Corn starch, Glycerin, Lactose, Magnesium Stearate, Talc, and other ingredients.
SENOKOT Granules: (deliciously cocoa-flavored): Each teaspoonful contains 15 mg sennosides.
Active Ingredient: Standardized Senna Concentrate.
Inactive Ingredients: Cocoa, Malt extract, Sodium lauryl sulfate, Sucrose, Vanillin, and other ingredients.
SenokotXTRA Tablets: Each tablet contains 17 mg sennosides.
Active Ingredients: Standardized Senna Concentrate.
Inactive Ingredients: Corn Starch, Glycerin, Lactose, Magnesium stearate, Talc, and other ingredients.

ADMINISTRATION AND DOSAGE

SENOKOT Granules: **Recommended Dosage (or as directed by a doctor):** Take preferably at bedtime. Adults and children 12 years of age and over: 1 teaspoon once a day (maximum: 2 teaspoons twice a day, not to exceed 4 teaspoons in a day). Children 6 to under 12 years of age: ½ teaspoon once a day (maximum: 1 teaspoon twice a day, not to exceed 2 teaspoons in a day). Children 2 to under 6 years of age: ¼ teaspoon once a day (maximum: ½ teaspoon twice a day, not to exceed 1 teaspoon in a day). For children under 2 years of age, consult a doctor. For older, debilitated, and OB/GYN patients, the physician may consider prescribing ½ the initial adult dose.
SENOKOT Tablets: **Recommended Dosage (or as directed by a doctor):** Take preferably at bedtime. Adults and children 12 years of age and over: 2 tablets once a day (maximum: 4 tablets twice a day, not to exceed 8 tablets in a day). Children 6 to under 12 years of age: 1 tablet once a day (maximum: 2 tablets twice a day, not to exceed 4 tablets in a day). Children 2 to under 6 years of age: ½ tablet once a day (maximum: 1 tablet twice a day, not to exceed 2 tablets in a day). For children under 2 years of age, consult a doctor. For older, debilitated, and OB/GYN patients, the physician may consider prescribing ½ the initial dose.
Double-Strength SenokotXTRA Tablets: **Recommended Dosage (or as directed by a doctor):** Take preferably at bedtime. Adults and children 12 years of age and over: 1 tablet once a day (maximum: 2 tablets twice a day, not to exceed 4 tablets in a day). For children 6 to under 12 years of age: ½ tablet once a day (maximum: 1 tablet twice a day, not to exceed 2 tablets in a day). Senokot Tablets and Granules are available for children under 6 years of age. For children under 2 years of age, consult a doctor. For older, debilitated, and OB/GYN patients, the physician may consider prescribing ½ the initial adult dose. [Note: One Double-Strength SenokotXTRA Tablet is equal to two SENOKOT Tablets.]

WARNINGS

Do not use laxative products when abdominal pain, nausea or vomiting are present unless directed by a doctor. If you have noticed a sudden change in bowel movements that persists over a period of 2 weeks, consult a doctor before using a laxative. Laxative products should not be used for a period longer than 1 week unless directed by a doctor. Rectal bleeding or failure to have a bowel movement after use of a laxative may indicate a serious condition. Discontinue use and consult your doctor. As with any drug, if you are pregnant or

*Regarding chronic constipation, refer to the "WARNINGS" section.

nursing a baby, seek the advice of a health professional before using this product. In case of accidental overdose, seek professional assistance or contact a Poison Control Center immediately. Keep out of children's reach.

HOW SUPPLIED

Granules: 2, 6, and 12 oz. plastic containers. Tablets: Boxes of 10 and 20; bottles of 50, 100 and 1000. Unit Strip Packs in boxes of 100 tablets: each tablet individually sealed. Double-Strength SenokotXTRA Tablets: Boxes of 12 and 36.

ALSO AVAILABLE

SENOKOT Syrup (standardized extract of senna fruit) in bottles of 2 and 8 fl. oz. Each teaspoon of SENOKOT Syrup contains 8.8 mg sennosides.

Active Ingredient: Standardized Concentrate Senna Fruit.

Inactive Ingredients: Alcohol 7% by volume, Methyl paraben, Potassium sorbate, Propyl paraben, Sodium lauryl sulfate, Sucrose, Water, Natural and Artificial Flavors and other ingredients.

ADMINISTRATION AND DOSAGE

Recommended dosage (or as directed by a doctor): Take preferably at bedtime. Adults and children 12 years of age and over: 2–3 teaspoons once a day (maximum: 3 teaspoons twice a day, not to exceed 6 teaspoons in a day). Children 6 to under 12 years of age: 1–1½ teaspoons once a day (maximum: 1½ teaspoons twice a day, not to exceed 3 teaspoons in a day). Children 2 to under 6 years of age: ½–¾ teaspoons once a day (maximum: ¾ teaspoon twice a day, not to exceed 1½ teaspoons in a day). For children under 2 years of age, consult a doctor.

Copyright 1991, The Purdue Frederick Company
Norwalk, CT 06850-3590

SENOKOT-S® Tablets OTC

[sĕn′ō-kŏt-ĕs″]

(standardized senna concentrate and docusate sodium)

Natural Laxative/Stool Softener Combination

INDICATIONS

SENOKOT-S Tablets are designed to relieve both aspects of functional constipation—bowel inertia and hard, dry stools. They provide a natural neuroperistaltic stimulant combined with a classic stool softener: standardized senna concentrate gently stimulates the colon while docusate sodium softens the stool for smoother and easier evacuation. This coordinated dual action of the two ingredients results in colon-specific, predictable laxative effect, generally producing bowel movement in 6 to 12 hours. Administering the tablets at bedtime allows the patient an uninterrupted night's sleep, with a comfortable evacuation in the morning. Flexibility of dosage permits fine adjustment to individual requirements. At proper dosage levels, SENOKOT-S Tablets are virtually free from side effects. SENOKOT-S Tablets are highly suitable for relief of postsurgical and postpartum constipation, and effectively counter-act drug-induced constipation. They facilitate regular elimination in impaction-prone and elderly patients, and are indicated in the presence of cardiovascular disease where straining must be avoided, as well as in the presence of hemorrhoids and anorectal disease.

DESCRIPTION

Each tablet contains 8.6 mg sennosides and 50 mg of docusate sodium. Active Ingredients: Docusate Sodium and Standardized Senna Concentrate.

Inactive Ingredients: Cellulose polymers, Corn starch, FD&C Yellow No. 10, FD&C Yellow No. 6 (Sunset Yellow), Guar Gum, Lactose, Polyethylene glycol, Talc, Titanium dioxide, and other ingredients.

ADMINISTRATION AND DOSAGE

Recommended Dosage (or as directed by a doctor): Take preferably at bedtime. Adults and children 12 years of age and over: 2 tablets once a day (maximum: 4 tablets twice a day, not to exceed 8 tablets in a day). Children 6 to under 12 years of age: 1 tablet once a day (maximum: 2 tablets twice a day, not to exceed 4 tablets in a day). Children 2 to under 6 years of age: ½ tablet once a day (maximum: 1 tablet twice a day, not to exceed 2 tablets in a day). For children under 2 years of age, consult a doctor.

WARNINGS

Do not use laxative products when abdominal pain, nausea, or vomiting are present unless directed by a doctor. If you have noticed a sudden change in bowel movements that persists over a period of 2 weeks, consult a doctor before using a laxative. Laxative products should not be used for a period longer than 1 week unless directed by a doctor. Rectal bleeding or failure to have a bowel movement after use of a laxative may indicate a serious condition. Discontinue use and consult your doctor. As with any drug, if you are pregnant or nursing a baby, seek the advice of a health professional before using this product. In case of accidental overdose, seek professional assistance or contact a Poison Control Center immediately. Keep out of children's reach.

SUPPLIED

Bottles of 30, 60 and 1000 tablets, and Unit Strip Boxes of 100 tablets.

Copyright 1991, The Purdue Frederick Company
Norwalk, CT 06850-3590

T-PHYL® ℞

(theophylline)

200 mg Tablets

UNICONTIN®

Controlled-Release System

DESCRIPTION

Each T-Phyl Tablet, for oral administration, contains 200 mg of anhydrous theophylline in a controlled-release system. Theophylline is a bronchodilator structurally classified as a xanthine derivative. It occurs as a white, odorless, crystalline powder having a bitter taste. Theophylline anhydrous has the chemical name, 1 *H* Purine-2,6-dione, 3,7-dihydro-1,3 dimethyl-, with a molecular formula of $C_7H_8N_4O_2$ and molecular weight of 180.18, and is represented by the following structural formula:

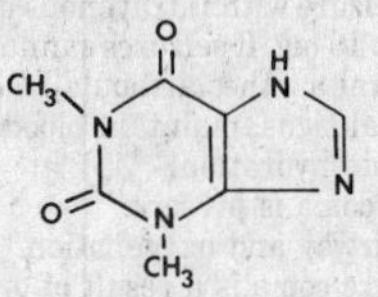

Inactive Ingredients: Cetostearyl alcohol, Hydroxyethyl cellulose, Magnesium stearate, Povidone, Talc, and other ingredients.

CLINICAL PHARMACOLOGY

Theophylline directly relaxes the smooth muscle of the bronchial airways and pulmonary blood vessels, thus acting mainly as bronchodilator and smooth muscle relaxant. It has also been demonstrated that aminophylline has a potent effect on diaphragmatic contractility in normal persons and may then be capable of reducing fatigability and thereby improve contractility in patients with chronic obstructive airways disease. The exact mode of action remains unsettled. Although theophylline does cause inhibition of phosphodiesterase with a resultant increase in intracellular cyclic AMP, other agents similarly inhibit the enzyme producing a rise of cyclic AMP but are unassociated with any demonstrable bronchodilation. Other mechanisms proposed include an effect on translocation of intracellular calcium; prostaglandin antagonism; stimulation of catecholamines endogenously; inhibition of cyclic guanosine monophosphate metabolism and adenosine receptor antagonism. None of these mechanisms have been proven, however.

In vitro, theophylline has been shown to act synergistically with beta agonists and there are now available data which do demonstrate an additive effect *in vivo* with combined use.

Pharmacokinetics:

The half-life of theophylline is influenced by a number of known variables. It may be prolonged in chronic alcoholics, particularly those with liver disease (cirrhosis or alcoholic liver disease), in patients with congestive heart failure, and in those patients taking certain other drugs (See PRECAUTIONS, Drug Interactions). Newborns and neonates have extremely slow clearance rates compared to older infants and children, i.e., those over 1 year. Older children have rapid clearance rates while most non-smoking adults have clearance rates between the two extremes. In premature neonates the decreased clearance is related to oxidative pathways that have yet to be established.

Theophylline Elimination Characteristics

Half-Life (in hours)

	Range	Mean
Children	1–9	3.7
Adults	3–15	7.7

In cigarette smokers (1–2 packs/day) the mean half-life is 4–5 hours, much shorter than in non-smokers. The increase in clearance associated with smoking is presumably due to stimulation of the hepatic metabolic pathway by components of cigarette smoke. The duration of this effect after cessation of smoking is unknown but may require 6 months to 2 years before the rate approaches that of a non-smoker.

In a single-dose bioavailability study, thirteen normal adult nonsmoking subjects were given 400 mg (2 × 200 mg) of T-Phyl under fasting conditions. The mean peak serum concentration (C_{max}) was about 3 mcg/mL at 5.7 hours (Mean T_{max}) following administration.

INDICATIONS AND USAGE

T-Phyl Tablets are indicated for relief and/or prevention of symptoms from asthma and reversible bronchospasm associated with chronic bronchitis and emphysema.

CONTRAINDICATIONS

This product is contraindicated in individuals who have shown hypersensitivity to its components. It is also contraindicated in patients with active peptic ulcer disease, and in individuals with underlying seizure disorders (unless receiving appropriate anticonvulsant medication).

WARNINGS

Serum levels above 20 mcg/mL are rarely found after appropriate administration of the recommended doses. However, in individuals in whom theophylline plasma clearance is reduced for any reason, even conventional doses may result in increased serum levels and potential toxicity. Reduced theophylline clearance has been documented in the following readily identifiable groups: 1) patients with impaired liver function; 2) patients over 55 years of age, particularly males and those with chronic lung disease; 3) those with cardiac failure from any cause; 4) patients with sustained high fever; 5) neonates and infants under 1 year of age; and 6 those patients taking certain drugs (see PRECAUTIONS, Drug Interactions). Frequently, such patients have markedly prolonged theophylline serum levels following discontinuation of the drug. Decreased theophylline clearance may occur following immunization for influenza, with active influenza, or other viral illnesses, and also with high fever for prolonged periods. This may be specially true in infants and the elderly.

Reduction of dosage and laboratory monitoring are especially appropriate in the above individuals.

Serious side effects such as ventricular arrhythmias, convulsions or even death may appear as the first sign of toxicity without any previous warning. Elderly patients with serum concentrations above 20 μg/mL are more likely to experience serious side effects such as ventricular arrhythmias or convulsions than are younger patients. Less serious signs of theophylline toxicity (i.e., nausea and restlessness) may occur frequently when initiating therapy, but are usually transient; when such signs are persistent during maintenance therapy, they are often associated with serum concentrations above 20 mcg/mL. Stated differently: *serious toxicity is not reliably preceded by less severe side effects.* A serum concentration measurement is the only reliable method of predicting potentially life-threatening toxicity.

Many patients who require theophylline exhibit tachycardia due to their underlying disease process so that the cause/effect relationship to elevated serum theophylline concentrations may not be appreciated.

Theophylline products may cause or worsen arrhythmias and any significant change in rate and/or rhythm warrants monitoring and further investigation.

Studies in laboratory animals (minipigs, rodents and dogs) recorded the occurrence of cardiac arrhythmias and sudden death (with histologic evidence of myocardial necrosis) when beta-agonists and methylxanthines were administered concurrently. The significance of these findings when applied to humans is currently unknown.

PRECAUTIONS

General:

On the average, theophylline half-life is shorter in cigarette and marijuana smokers than in non-smokers, but smokers can have half-lives as long as non-smokers. Theophylline should not be administered concurrently with other xanthines. Use with caution in patients with hypoxemia, hypertension, or those with history of peptic ulcer. Theophylline may occasionally act as a local irritant to G.I. tract although gastrointestinal symptoms are more commonly centrally mediated and associated with serum drug concentrations over 20 mcg/mL.

Information for Patients:

The importance of taking only the prescribed dose and time interval between doses should be reinforced. T-Phyl Tablets are not to be chewed or crushed. The patient should alert the physician if symptoms occur repeatedly, especially near the end of a dosing interval.

Laboratory Tests:

Serum levels should be monitored periodically to determine the theophylline level associated with observed clinical response and as the method of predicting toxicity. For such measurements, the serum sample should be obtained at the time of peak concentration, approximately 6–8 hours after administration of T-Phyl Tablets. It is important that the patient will not have missed or taken additional doses during the previous 48 hours and that dosing intervals will have been reasonably equally spaced. DOSAGE ADJUSTMENT BASED ON SERUM THEOPHYLLINE MEASUREMENTS WHEN THESE INSTRUCTIONS HAVE NOT BEEN FOLLOWED MAY RESULT IN RECOMMENDATIONS THAT PRESENT RISK OF TOXICITY TO THE PATIENT.

Drug-Drug Interactions:

Toxic synergism with ephedrine has been documented and may occur with other sympathomimetic bronchodilators. In addition, the following drug interactions have been demonstrated:

Continued on next page

Purdue Frederick—Cont.

Theophylline with:

Allopurinol (high-dose)	Increased serum theophylline levels
Cimetidine	Increased serum theophylline levels
Ciprofloxacin	Increased serum theophylline levels
Erythromycin, Troleandomycin	Increased serum theophylline levels
Lithium carbonate	Increased renal excretion of lithium
Norfloxacin	Increased serum theophylline levels
Oral Contraceptives	Increased serum theophylline levels
Phenytoin	Decreased theophylline and phenytoin serum levels
Propranolol	Increased serum theophylline levels
Rifampin	Decreased serum theophylline levels

Drug-Food Interactions:
T-Phyl has not been adequately studied to determine the extent of alteration of bioavailability when it is given with food as compared to the fasting state.
However, there is data to indicate that drug administration at the time of food ingestion will result in an increase (less than 20%) in the extent of bioavailability, and an increase in the rate (greater C_{max}) of absorption.
The influence of the type and amount of food, as well as the time interval between drug and food, on performance of T-Phyl tablets is under study.

Drug-Laboratory Test Interactions:
Currently available analytical methods, including high pressure liquid chromatography and immunoassay techniques, for measuring serum theophylline levels are specific. Metabolites and other drugs generally do not affect the results. Other new analytic methods are also now in use. The physician should be aware of the laboratory method used and whether other drugs will interfere with the assay for theophylline.

Carcinogenesis, Mutagenesis, and Impairment of Fertility:
Long-term carcinogenicity studies have not been performed with theophylline. Chromosome-breaking activity was detected in human cell cultures at concentrations of theophylline up to 50 times the therapeutic serum concentrations in humans. Theophylline was not mutagenic in the dominant lethal assay in male mice given theophylline intraperitoneally in doses up to 30 times the maximum daily human oral dose.
Studies to determine the effect on fertility have not been performed with theophylline.

Pregnancy:
Category C—Animal reproduction studies have not been conducted with theophylline. It is also not known whether theophylline can cause fetal harm when administered to a pregnant woman or can affect reproduction capacity. Xanthines should be given to a pregnant woman only if clearly needed.

Nursing Mothers:
Theophylline is distributed into breast milk and may cause irritability or other signs of toxicity in nursing infants. Because of the potential for serious adverse reactions in nursing infants from theophylline, a decision should be made whether to discontinue nursing or to discontinue the drug, taking into account the importance of the drug to the mother.

Pediatric Use:
Safety and effectiveness of T-Phyl Tablets in children under 6 years of age have not been established.

ADVERSE REACTIONS

The following adverse reactions have been observed, but there has not been enough systematic collection of data to support an estimate of their frequency. The most consistent adverse reactions are usually due to overdosage.

1. **Gastrointestinal:** nausea, vomiting, epigastric pain, hematemesis, diarrhea.
2. **Central nervous system:** headaches, irritability, restlessness, insomnia, reflex hyperexcitability, muscle twitching, clonic and tonic generalized convulsions.
3. **Cardiovascular:** palpitation, tachycardia, extrasystoles, flushing, hypotension, circulatory failure, ventricular arrhythmias.
4. **Respiratory:** tachypnea.
5. **Renal:** potentiation of diuresis.
6. **Others:** alopecia, hyperglycemia, inappropriate ADH syndrome, rash, Stevens-Johnson Syndrome.

OVERDOSAGE

Management:
It is suggested that the management principles (consistent with the clinical status of the patient when first seen) outlined below be instituted and that simultaneous contact with a Regional Poison Control Center be established. In this way, both updated information and individualization regarding required therapy may be provided.

1. When potential oral overdose is established and seizure has not occurred:
   a) If patient is alert and seen within the early hours after ingestion, induction of emesis may be of value. Gastric lavage has been demonstrated to be of no value in influencing outcome in patients who present more than 1 hour after ingestion.
   b) Administer a cathartic. Sorbitol solution is reported to be of value.
   c) Administer repeated doses of activated charcoal and monitor theophylline serum levels.
   d) Prophylactic administration of phenobarbital has been shown to increase the seizure threshold in laboratory animals, and administration of this drug can be considered.
2. If patient presents with a seizure:
   a) Establish an airway.
   b) Administer oxygen.
   c) Treat the seizure with intravenous diazepam, 0.1 to 0.3 mg/kg up to 10 mg. If seizures cannot be controlled, the use of general anethesia should be considered.
   d) Monitor vital signs, maintain blood pressure and provide adequate hydration.
3. If post-seizure coma is present:
   a) Maintain airway and oxygenation.
   b) If post-seizure coma is a result of oral medication, follow above recommendations to prevent absorption of the drug, but intubation and lavage will have to be performed instead of inducing emesis, and the cathartic and charcoal will need to be introduced via a large bore gastric lavage tube.
   c) Continue to provide full supportive care and adequate hydration until the drug is metabolized. In general, drug metabolism is sufficiently rapid so as not to warrant dialysis. If repeated oral activated charcoal is ineffective (as noted by stable or rising serum levels) charcoal hemoperfusion may be indicated.

DOSAGE AND ADMINISTRATION

Taking T-Phyl tablets with food may increase the rate (C_{max}) and extent of absorption when compared to the fasting state. The prescriber should consider this information in determining a dosing schedule.
Effective use of theophylline (i.e., the concentration of drug in the serum associated with optimal benefit and minimal risk of toxicity) is considered to occur when the theophylline concentration is maintained from 10 to 20 mcg/mL. The early studies from which these levels were derived were carried out in patients immediately or shortly after recovery from acute exacerbations of their disease (some hospitalized with status asthmaticus).
Although the 20 mcg/mL level remains appropriate as a critical value (above which toxicity is more likely to occur) for safety purposes, additional data are now available which indicate that the serum theophylline concentration required to produce maximum physiologic benefit may, in fact, fluctuate with the degree of bronchospasm present and are variable. Therefore, the physician should individualize the range appropriate to the patient's requirements, based on both symptomatic response and improvement in pulmonary function. It should be stressed that serum theophylline concentrations maintained at the upper level of the 10 to 20 mcg/mL range may be associated with potential toxicity when factors known to reduce theophylline clearance are operative. (See WARNINGS).
If it is not possible to obtain serum level determinations, restriction of the daily dose (in otherwise healthy adults) to not greater than 13 mg/kg/day, to a maximum of 900 mg, in divided doses, will result in relatively few patients exceeding serum levels of 20 mcg/mL and the resultant greater risk of toxicity.
Caution should be exercised for younger children who cannot complain of minor side effects. Older adults, those with cor pulmonale, congestive heart failure, and/or liver disease may have unusually low dosage requirements and thus may experience toxicity at the maximal dosage recommended below.
Theophylline does not distribute to fatty tissue. Dosage should be calculated on the basis of lean (ideal) body weight where mg/kg doses are presented.

Frequency of Dosing:
When immediate release products with rapid absorption are used, dosing to maintain serum levels generally requires administration every 6 hours. This is particularly true in children, but dosing intervals up to 8 hours may be satisfactory in adults since they eliminate the drug at a slower rate. Some children, and adults requiring higher than average

doses (those having rapid rates of clearance, e.g, half-lives of under 6 hours), may benefit and be more effectively controlled during chronic therapy when given products with sustained-release characteristics since these provide longer dosing intervals and/or less fluctuation in serum concentration between dosing.

DOSAGE GUIDELINES

WARNING: DO NOT ATTEMPT TO MAINTAIN ANY DOSE THAT IS NOT WELL TOLERATED.
Dosage guidelines are approximations only and the wide range of theophylline clearance between individuals (particularly those with concomitant disease) makes indiscriminate usage hazardous. When appropriate dosage should be calculated on the basis of lean body weight where mg/kg doses are to be prescribed, since theophylline does not distribute into fatty tissue.

I. ACUTE SYMPTOMS
T-Phyl Tablets are not intended for patients experiencing an acute episode of bronchospasm (associated with asthma, chronic bronchitis, or emphysema). Such patients require **rapid** relief of symptoms and should be treated with an immediate-release or intravenous theophylline preparation (or other bronchodilators) and not with controlled-release products.

II. CHRONIC THERAPY
Initiating Therapy with an Immediate-Release Product:
It is recommended that the appropriate dosage be established using an immediate-release preparation. Children weighing less than 25 kg should have their daily dosage requirements established with a liquid preparation to permit small dosage increments. Slow clinical titration is generally performed to help assure acceptance and safety of this medication. Then, if the total 24 hour dose can be given by use of the available strengths of this product, the patient can usually be switched to T-Phyl Tablets giving one-half of the daily dose at 12 hour intervals. Patients who metabolize theophylline rapidly, such as the young, smokers, and some non-smoking adults are the most likely candidates for dosing at 8 hour intervals. Such patients can generally be identified as having trough serum concentration lower than desired or repeatedly exhibiting symptoms near the end of a dosing interval.

III. TITRATION AND DOSE ADJUSTMENT
A. Maximum Dose of Theophylline Where the Serum Concentration is Not Measured: WARNING: DO NOT ATTEMPT TO MAINTAIN ANY DOSE THAT IS NOT TOLERATED.
Not to exceed the following: (or 900 mg, whichever is less).

DOSE PER 12 HOURS

Age 6–under 9 years	24 mg/kg/day	12 mg/kg
Age 9–under 12 years	20 mg/kg/day	10 mg/kg
Age 12–under 16 years	18 mg/kg/day	9 mg/kg
Age 16 years and older	13 mg/kg/day	6.5 mg/kg

B. Measurement of Serum Theophylline Concentration During Chronic Therapy:
If the above maximum doses are to be maintained or exceeded, serum theophylline measurement is recommended. The serum sample should be obtained at the time of peak absorption, 6 to 8 hours after administration of T-Phyl Tablets. It is important that the patient will have missed *no* doses during the previous 48 hours and that dosing intervals will have been reasonably typical with no added doses during that period of time. DOSAGE ADMINISTRATION BASED ON SERUM THEOPHYLLINE MEASUREMENTS WHEN THESE INSTRUCTIONS HAVE NOT BEEN FOLLOWED MAY RESULT IN RECOMMENDATIONS THAT PRESENT RISK OF TOXICITY TO THE PATIENT.
C. Final Adjustment of Dosage
Dosage adjustment after serum theophylline measurement [See table at top of next page.]
When the patient's condition is otherwise clinically stable and none of the recognized factors which alter elimination are present, measurement of serum levels need to be repeated only every 6 to 12 months.
Caution should be exercised for younger children who cannot complain of minor side effects. Older adults, those with cor pulmonale, congestive heart failure, and/or liver disease may have unusually low dosage requirements and thus may experience toxicity at the maximal dosage recommended above. It is important that no patient be maintained on any dosage that is not tolerated. In instructing the patients to increase dosage according to the schedule above, they should be instructed not to take a subsequent dose if apparent side effects occur and to resume therapy at a lower dose once adverse effects have disappeared.

WARNING

DO NOT MAINTAIN ANY DOSE THAT IS NOT TOLERATED.

HOW SUPPLIED

T-Phyl (theophylline, anhydrous) 200 mg Controlled-Release Tablets supplied in white-opaque plastic bottles containing 100 tablets (NDC 0034-7102-80). Each round, white, scored

If serum theophylline level is:		Directions:
Within desired range		Maintain dosage if tolerated.
Too high	20 to 25 mcg/mL	Decrease doses by about 10% and recheck serum level after 3 days.
	25 to 30 mcg/mL	Skip the next dose and decrease subsequent doses by about 25%. Recheck serum level after 3 days.
	Over 30 mcg/mL	Skip next 2 doses and decrease subsequent doses by 50%. Recheck serum level after 3 days.
Too low		Increase dosage at 3 day intervals by 25%. The serum concentration may be rechecked at appropriate intervals, but at least at the end of the adjustment period. The total daily dose may need to be administered at more frequent intervals if symptoms occur repeatedly at the end of a dosing interval.

tablet bears the symbol PF on one side and is marked U200 on the other side.
Store at controlled room temperature 15°–30° C (59°–86° F).
CAUTION:Federal law prohibits dispensing without prescription.
THE PURDUE FREDERICK COMPANY
Norwalk, CT 06850–3590
Copyright© 1983, 1987, 1991, 1992,
The Purdue Frederick Company
U.S. Patent Numbers 4,235,870 and 4,366,310
February 18, 1992 I1494
Shown in Product Identification Section, page 424

TRILISATE® TABLETS/LIQUID ℞
[trĭl ′ĭ-sāt ″]
(choline magnesium trisalicylate)
500 mg, 750 mg, or 1000 mg
salicylate content

DESCRIPTION

TRILISATE Tablets/Liquid are nonsteroidal, anti-inflammatory preparations containing choline magnesium trisalicylate which is freely soluble in water. The absolute structure of choline magnesium trisalicylate is not known at this time. Choline magnesium trisalicylate has a molecular formula of $C_{26}H_{29}O_{10}NMg$, a molecular weight of 539.8, and it may be represented in the solid form as:

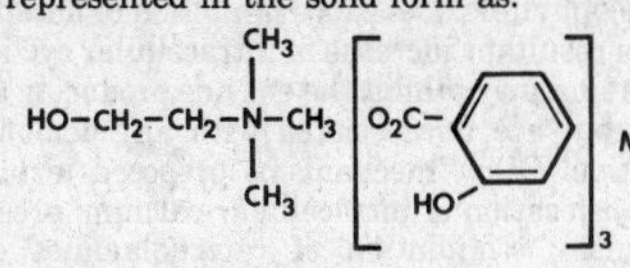

This substance when dissolved in water would appear to form 5 ions (1 choline ion, 1 magnesium ion and 3 salicylate ions) which may be represented as:

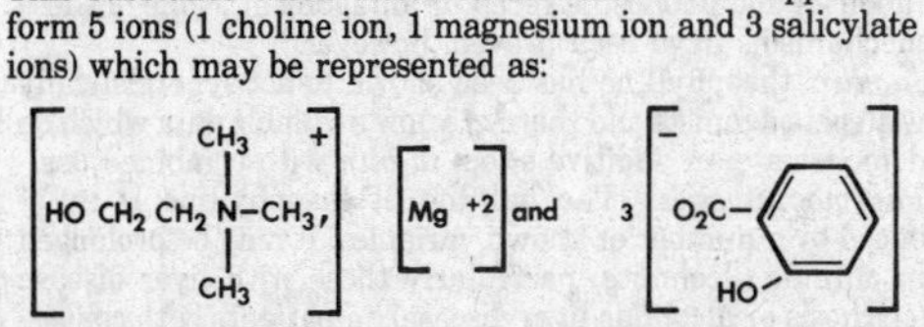

TRILISATE Tablets/Liquid are available in scored, pale pink 500 mg tablets; in scored, white film-coated 750 mg tablets, and in scored, red, film-coated 1000 mg tablets. TRILISATE Liquid is a cherry cordial-flavored liquid providing 500 mg salicylate content per teaspoonful (5 ml) for oral administration.
Each 500 mg tablet contains 293 mg of choline salicylate combined with 362 mg of magnesium salicylate to provide 500 mg salicylate content. Each 750 mg tablet contains 440 mg of choline salicylate combined with 544 mg of magnesium salicylate to provide 750 mg salicylate content. Each 1000 mg tablet contains 587 mg of choline salicylate combined with 725 mg magnesium salicylate to provide 1000 mg salicylate content. TRILISATE Liquid contains 293 mg of choline salicylate combined with 362 mg of magnesium salicylate to provide 500 mg salicylate per teaspoonful (5 ml) in a clear amber, cherry cordial-flavored vehicle.
Inactive Ingredients: Each 500 mg tablet contains Carboxymethylcellulose sodium, Corn starch, Edetate disodium, FD&C Yellow No. 6, Stearic acid, and other ingredients.
Each 750 mg tablet contains Carboxymethylcellulose sodium, Edetate disodium, Hydroxypropyl methylcellulose, Polyethylene glycol, Polysorbate 20, Polysorbate 80, Stearic acid, Talc, Titanium doixide, and other ingredients.
Each 1000 mg tablet contains Carboxymethylcellulose sodium, Edetate disodium, FD&C Red No. 40, FD&C Yellow No. 6, FD&C Blue No. 2, Hydroxypropyl methylcellulose, Polyethylene glycol, Polysorbate 20, Polysorbate 80, Stearic acid, Talc, Titanium dioxide and other ingredients.
Each teaspoonful (5 ml) of Liquid contains: Caramel, Carboxymethylcellulose sodium, Edetate disodium, FD&C Yellow No. 6, Glycerin, High fructose corn syrup, Potassium sorbate, Water, and Artificial flavors.

CLINICAL PHARMACOLOGY

TRILISATE Tablets/Liquid contain salicylate with anti-inflammatory, analgesic and antipyretic action. On ingestion of TRILISATE Tablets/Liquid, the salicylate moiety is absorbed rapidly and reaches peak blood levels within an average of one to two hours after single doses of the tablets of liquid. The primary route of excretion is renal: the excretion products are chiefly the glycine and glucuronide conjugates. At higher serum salicylate concentrations, the glycine conjugation pathway becomes rapidly saturated. Thus, the slower glucuronide conjugation pathway becomes the rate limiting step for salicylate excretion. In addition, salicylate excreted in the bile as glucuronide conjugate may be re-absorbed. These factors account for the prolongation of salicylate half-life and the nonlinear increase in plasma salicylate level as the salicylate dose is increased. The serum concentration of salicylate is increased by conditions that decrease glomerular filtration rate or proximal tubular secretion.
The bioequivalence of TRILISATE Liquid and Tablets 500 mg/ 750 mg/1000 mg has been established. With the tablets, a steady-state condition is usually reached after 4 to 5 doses, and the half-life of elimination, on repeated administration of tablets, is 9 to 17 hours. This permits a maintenance dosage schedule of once or twice daily. Unlike aspirin and certain other non-steroidal anti-inflammatory agents, such as arylpropionic acid derivatives and arylacetic acid derivatives, choline magnesium trisalicylate, at therapeutic dosage levels, does not affect platelet aggregation, as shown by in-vitro and in-vivo studies.

INDICATIONS AND USAGE

Osteoarthritis, Rheumatoid Arthritis and Acute Painful Shoulder: Salicylates are considered the base therapy of choice in the arthritides; and TRILISATE preparations are indicated for the relief of the signs and symptoms of rheumatoid arthritis, osteoarthritis and other arthritides. TRILISATE Tablets or Liquid are indicated in the long-term management of these diseases and especially in the acute flare of rheumatoid arthritis. TRILISATE Tablets or Liquid are also indicated for the treatment of acute painful shoulder.
TRILISATE preparations are effective and generally well tolerated, and are logical choices whenever salicylate treatment is indicated. They are particularly suitable when a once-a-day or b.i.d. dosage regimen is important to patient compliance; when gastrointestinal intolerance to aspirin is encountered; when gastrointestinal microbleeding or hematologic effects of aspirin are considered a patient hazard; and when interference (or the risk of interference) with normal platelet function by aspirin or by propionic acid derivatives is considered to be clinically undesirable. Use of TRILISATE Liquid is appropriate when a liquid dosage form is preferred, as in the elderly patient.
The efficacy of TRILISATE preparations has not been studied in those patients who are designated by the American Rheumatism Association as belonging in Functional Class IV (incapacitated, largely or wholly bedridden or confined to a wheelchair, with little or no self-care). Analgesic and Antipyretic Action: TRILISATE Tablets/Liquid are also indicated for the relief of mild to moderate pain and for antipyresis. **In children,** TRILISATE preparations are indicated for conditions requiring anti-inflammatory or analgesic action—such as juvenile rheumatoid arthritis and other appropriate conditions.

CONTRAINDICATIONS

Patients who are hypersensitive to non-acetylated salicylates should not take TRILISATE Tablets or Liquid.

WARNINGS

Reye Syndrome is a rare but serious disease which may develop in children and teenagers who have chicken pox, influenza, or flu symptoms. While the cause of Reye Syndrome is unknown, some studies suggest a possible association between the development of Reye Syndrome and the use of medicines containing acetylated salicylates or aspirin. TRILISATE Tablets and Liquid are a combination of choline salicylate and magnesium salicylate which are nonacetylated salicylates, and there have been no reported cases associating TRILISATE with Reye Syndrome. Nevertheless, TRILISATE, as a salicylate-containing product, is not recommended for use in children and teenagers with chicken pox, influenza or flu symptoms.

PRECAUTIONS

General Precautions: As with other salicylates and non-steroidal anti-inflammatory drugs, TRILISATE preparations should be used with caution in patients with acute or chronic renal insufficiency, with acute or chronic hepatic dysfunction, or with gastritis or peptic ulcer disease.
Although reports exist of cross reactivity, including bronchospasm, with the use of non-acetylated salicylate products in aspirin-sensitive patients, TRILISATE preparations were found to be well tolerated with regard to pulmonary function and respiratory symptoms when these parameters were monitored in a group of documented aspirin-sensitive asthmatics dosed with TRILISATE in both controlled and open label studies.[1]
Concurrent use of other salicylate-containing products and TRILISATE preparations can lead to an increase in plasma salicylate concentration and may result in potentially toxic salicylate levels.
Laboratory Tests: Plasma salicylate levels can be periodically assessed during treatment with TRILISATE preparations to determine whether a therapeutically effective anti-inflammatory concentration of 15 to 30 mg/100 ml (150–300 micrograms/ml) is being maintained. Manifestations of systemic salicylate intoxication are usually not seen until the concentration exceeds 30 mg/100 ml. However, such tests rarely differentiate between the active free and inactive protein bound salicylate components. Since protein binding of salicylate is affected by age, nutritional status, competitive binding of other drugs, and underlying disease (e.g. rheumatoid arthritis), plasma salicylate level determinations may not always accurately reflect efficacious or toxic levels of active free salicylate. Acidification of the urine can significantly diminish the renal clearance of salicylate and increase plasma salicylate concentrations.
Drug Interactions: Foods and drugs that alter urine pH may affect renal clearance of salicylate and plasma salicylate concentrations. Raising urine pH, as with chronic antacid use, can enhance renal salicylate clearance and diminish plasma salicylate concentration; urine acidification can decrease urinary salicylate excretion and increase plasma levels.
When salicylate drug products are concurrently dosed with other plasma protein bound drug products, adverse effects may result. Although TRILISATE preparations are a rational choice for anti-inflammatory and analgesic therapy in patients on oral anticoagulants due to their demonstrated lack of effect in vivo and in vitro on platelet aggregation, bleeding time, platelet count, prothrombin time, and serum thromboxane B2 generation[1–7], the potential exists for increased levels of unbound warfarin with their concurrent use. Prothrombin time should be closely monitored and warfarin dose appropriately adjusted when therapy with TRILISATE preparations is initiated. The effect of TRILISATE on blood prothrombin levels has not been established.
Salicylates may increase the therapeutic as well as toxic effects of methotrexate, particularly when administered in chemotherapeutic doses, but inhibition of renal methotrexate excretion and by displacement of plasma protein bound methotrexate. Caution should be exercised in administering TRILISATE to rheumatoid arthritis patients on methotrexate. When sulfonylurea oral hypoglycemic agents are co-administered with salicylates, the hypoglycemic effect may be enhanced via increased insulin secretion or by displacement of sulfonylurea agents from binding sites. Insulin-treated diabetics on high doses of salicylates should also be closely monitored for a similar hypoglycemic response. Other drugs with which salicylate competes for protein binding sites, and whose plasma concentration or free fraction may be altered by concurrent salicylate administration, include the following: phenytoin, valproic acid, and carbonic anhydrase inhibitors.
The efficacy of uricosuric agents may be decreased when administered with salicylate products. Although low doses of salicylate (1 to 2 grams per day) have been reported to decrease urate excretion and elevate plasma urate concentrations, intermediate doses (2 to 3 grams per day) usually do not alter urate excretion. Larger salicylate doses (over 5 grams per day) can induce uricosuria and lower plasma urate levels.
Corticosteroids can reduce plasma salicylate levels by increasing renal elimination and perhaps by also stimulating hepatic metabolism of salicylates. By monitoring plasma salicylate levels, salicylate dosage may be titrated to accommodate changes in corticosteroid dose or to avoid salicylate toxicity during corticosteroid taper.
Drug/Laboratory Test Interactions: Free T4 values may be increased in patients on salicylate drug products due to competitive plasma protein binding; a concurrent decrease in total plasma T4 may be observed. Thyroid function is not affected.
Carcinogenesis: No long-term animal studies have been performed with TRILISATE to evaluate its carcinogenic potential.

Continued on next page

Purdue Frederick—Cont.

Use in Pregnancy: Pregnancy Category C. Animal reproduction studies have not been conducted with TRILISATE preparations. It is also not known whether TRILISATE can cause fetal harm when administered to a pregnant woman or can affect reproduction capacity. TRILISATE should be given to a pregnant woman only if clearly needed. Because of the known effects of other salicylate drug products on the fetal cardiovascular system (closure of ductus arteriosus), use during late pregnancy should be avoided.

Labor and Delivery: The effects of TRILISATE on labor and delivery in pregnant women are unknown. Since prolonged gestation and prolonged labor due to prostaglandin inhibition have been reported with the use of other salicylate products, the use of TRILISATE preparations near term is not recommended. Other salicylate products have also been associated with alterations in maternal and neonatal hemostasis mechanisms and with perinatal mortality.

Nursing Mothers: Salicylate is excreted in human milk. Peak milk salicylate levels are delayed, occurring as long as 9 to 12 hours post dose, and the milk:plasma ratio has been reported to be as high as 0.34. Because of the potential for significant salicylate absorption by the nursing infant, caution should be exercised when TRILISATE is administered to a nursing woman.

Pediatric Use: In a four-week open label pilot study of patients with juvenile rheumatoid arthritis, children from 6 to 16 years of age previously on aspirin received weight adjusted doses (50–60 mg/kg) of TRILISATE 500 mg tablets on a divided BID schedule with subsequent dose titration to achieve therapeutic serum salicylate levels. Eighty-three percent (83%) of the patients rated the therapeutic effect of TRILISATE as good or excellent. Tinnitus was reported by one patient and elevated SGOT levels at Week 1, which decreased during the trial, were detected in two patients. (See WARNINGS section).

ADVERSE REACTIONS

The most frequent adverse reactions observed with TRILISATE preparations in clinical trials[8–12] are tinnitus and gastrointestinal complaints (including nausea, vomiting, gastric upset, indigestion, heartburn, diarrhea, constipation and epigastric pain). These occur in less than twenty percent (20%) of patients. Should tinnitus develop, reduction of daily dosage is recommended until the tinnitus is resolved. Less frequent adverse reactions, occurring in less than two percent (2%) of patients, are: hearing impairment, headache, lightheadedness, dizziness, drowsiness, and lethargy. Adverse reactions occurring in less than one percent (1%) of patients are: gastric ulceration, positive fecal occult blood, elevation in serum BUN and creatinine, rash, pruritus, anorexia, weight gain, edema, epistaxis and dysgeusia.

Spontaneous reporting has yielded isolated or rare reports of the following adverse experiences: duodenal ulceration, elevated hepatic transaminases, hepatitis, esophagitis, asthma, erythema multiforme, urticaria, ecchymoses, irreversible hearing loss and/or tinnitus, mental confusion, hallucinations.

DRUG ABUSE AND DEPENDENCE

Drug abuse and dependence have not been reported with TRILISATE preparations.

OVERDOSAGE

Death in adults has been reported following ingestion of doses of from 10 to 30 grams of salicylate; however, larger doses have been taken without resulting fatality.

Symptoms: Salicylate intoxication, known as salicylism, may occur with large doses or extended therapy. Common symptoms of salicylism include headache, dizziness, tinnitus, hearing impairment, confusion, drowsiness, sweating, vomiting, diarrhea, and hyperventilation. A more severe degree of salicylate intoxication can lead to CNS disturbances, alteration in electrolyte balance, respiratory and metabolic acidosis, hyperthermia, and dehydration.

Treatment: Reduction of further absorption of salicylate from the gastrointestinal tract can be achieved via emesis, gastric lavage, use of activated charcoal, or a combination of the above. Appropriate I.V. fluids should be administered to correct dehydration, electrolyte imbalance, and acidosis and to maintain adequate renal function. To accelerate salicylate excretion, forced diuresis with alkalinizing solution is recommended. In extreme cases, peritoneal dialysis or hemodialysis should be considered for effective salicylate removal.

DOSAGE AND ADMINISTRATION

ADULTS: In rheumatoid arthritis, osteoarthritis, the more severe arthritides, and acute painful shoulder, the recommended starting dosage is 1500 mg given b.i.d. Some patients may be treated with 3000 mg given once per day (h.s.) In the elderly patient, a daily dosage of 2250 mg given as 750 mg t.i.d. may be efficacious and well tolerated. Dosage should be adjusted in accordance with the patient's response. In patients with renal dysfunction, monitor salicylate levels and adjust dose accordingly.

For mild to moderate pain or for antipyresis, the usual dosage is 2000 mg to 3000 mg daily in divided doses (b.i.d.). Based on patient response or salicylate blood levels, dosage may be adjusted to achieve optimum therapeutic effect. Salicylate blood levels should be in the range of 15 to 30 mg/100 ml for anti-inflammatory effect and 5 to 15 mg/100 ml for analgesia and antipyresis.

Each 500 mg tablet or teaspoonful is equivalent in salicylate content to 10 gr of aspirin; each 750 mg tablet, to 15 gr of aspirin; and each 1000 mg tablet, to 20 gr of aspirin.

If the physician prefers, the recommended daily dosage may be administered on a t.i.d. schedule.

As with other therapeutic agents, individual dosage adjustment is advisable, and a number of patients may require higher or lower dosages than those recommended. Certain patients require 2 to 3 weeks of therapy for optimal effect.

CHILDREN: Usual daily dose for children for anti-inflammatory or analgesic action:

TRILISATE 500 mg Tablets/Liquid and TRILISATE 750 mg and 1000 mg Tablets, 50 mg/kg/day.

Weight (kg)	Total daily dose
12–13	500 mg
14–17	750 mg
18–22	1000 mg
23–27	1250 mg
28–32	1500 mg
33–37	1750 mg

Total daily doses should be administered in divided doses (b.i.d.). Doses of TRILISATE preparations are calculated as the total daily dose of 50 mg/kg/day for children of 37 kg body weight or less and 2250 mg/day for heavier children. TRILISATE Liquid is available for greater convenience in treating younger patients and those adult patients unable to swallow a solid dosage form.

CAUTION

Federal law prohibits dispensing without a prescription.

HOW SUPPLIED

NDC 0034-0500-80: TRILISATE 500 mg Tablets (pale pink, scored) supplied in bottles of 100 tablets.

NDC 0034-0500-50: TRILISATE 500 mg Tablets (pale pink, scored) supplied in bottles of 500 tablets.

NDC 0034-0500-10: TRILISATE 500 mg Tablets (pale pink, scored) supplied in unit dose packaging with 10 tablets per card. Ten cards are packed in each carton; 10 cartons are packed in each shipper.

NDC 0034-0505-80: TRILISATE 750 mg Tablets (scored, white, film-coated) in bottles of 100 tablets.

NDC 0034-0505-50: TRILISATE 750 mg Tablets (scored, white, film-coated) in bottles of 500 tablets.

NDC 0034-0505-10: TRILISATE 750 mg Tablets (scored, white, film-coated) supplied in unit dose packaging with 10 tablets per card. Ten cards are packed in each carton; 10 cartons are packed in each shipper.

NDC 0034-0510-60: TRILISATE 1000 mg Tablets (scored, red, film-coated) in bottles of 60 tablets.

NDC 0034-0510-80: TRILISATE 1000 mg Tablets (scored, red, film-coated) in bottles of 100 tablets.

NDC 0034-0520-80: TRILISATE Liquid in bottles of 8 fl. oz. (237 ml).

Store at controlled room temperature 59° to 86°F (15° to 30°C).

REFERENCES

1. Szczeklik, A et al; Choline magnesium trisalicylate in patients with aspirin-induced asthma; *Eur Respir J*; 3:535–539, 1990.
2. Zucker, MB and Rothwell KB; Differential influences of salicylate compounds on platelet aggregation and serotonin release; *Current Therapeutic Research*; 23(2), Feb 1987.
3. Stuart, JJ and Pisko, EJ; Choline magnesium trisalicylate does not impair platelet aggregation; *Pharmatherapeutica*; 2(8):547, 1981.
4. Danesh, BJZ, Saniabadi, AR, Russel, RI et al; Therapeutic potential of choline magnesium trisalicylate as an alternative to aspirin for patients with bleeding tendencies; *Scottish Medical Journal*; 32:167–168, 1987.
5. Danesh, BJZ, McLaren, M. Russell, RI et al; Does non-acetylated salicylate inhibit thromboxane biosynthesis in human platelets? *Scottish Medical Journal*; 33: 315–316, 1988.
6. Danesh, BJZ, McLaren, M, Russell, RI et al; Comparison of the effect of aspirin and choline magnesium trisalicylate on thromboxane biosynthesis in human platelets: role of the acetyl moiety; *Haemostasis*; 19:169–173, 1989.
7. Data on file. Medical Department. The Purdue Frederick Company, 1989.
8. Blechman, WJ, and Lechner, BL; Clinical comparative evaluation of choline magnesium trisalicylate and acetylsalicylic acid in rheumatoid arthritis; *Rheumatology and Rehabilitation*; 18:119–124, 1979.
9. McLaughlin, G; Choline magnesium trisalicylate vs. naproxen in rheumatoid arthritis; *Current Therapeutic Research*; 32(4):579–585, 1982.
10. Ehrlich, GE; Miller, SB; and Zeiders, RS; Choline magnesium trisalicylate vs. ibuprofen in rheumatoid arthritis; *Rheumatology and Rehabilitation*; 19:30–41, 1980.
11. Goldenberg, A; Rudnicki, RD, and Koonce, ML; Clinical comparison of efficacy and safety of choline magnesium trisalicylate and indomethacin in treating osteoarthritis; *Current Therapeutic Research*; 24(3):245–260, 1978.
12. Guerin, BK and Burnstein, SL; Conservative therapy of acute painful shoulder; *Orthopedic Review*; XI(7):29–37, 1982.

The Purdue Frederick Company, Norwalk, CT 06850-3590
Copyright©1982, 1991 The Purdue Frederick Company
U.S. Patent Number 4067974
July 24, 1991   Q145

Shown in Product Identification Section, page 424

UNIPHYL® Tablets   ℞
[ū'nĭ-fĭl]
(theophylline)
400 mg

UNICONTIN®
Controlled-Release System

DESCRIPTION

Uniphyl Tablets for oral administration contain 400 mg anhydrous theophylline in a controlled-release system which allows a 24-hour dosing interval for appropriate patients. Theophylline anhydrous, a xanthine bronchodilator, is a white, odorless crystalline powder having a bitter taste. Theophylline has a molecular weight of 180.18, represented by $C_7H_8N_4O_2$ and is depicted as:

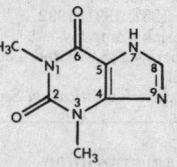

Inactive Ingredients: Cetostearyl alcohol, Hydroxyethyl cellulose, Magnesium stearate, Povidone, Talc, and other ingredients.

CLINICAL PHARMACOLOGY

Theophylline directly relaxes the smooth muscle of the bronchial airways and pulmonary blood vessels, thus acting mainly as a bronchodilator and smooth muscle relaxant. It has also been demonstrated that aminophylline has a potent effect on diaphragmatic contractility in normal persons and may then be capable of reducing fatigability and thereby improve contractility in patients with chronic obstructive airways disease. The exact mode of action remains unsettled. Although theophylline does cause inhibition of phosphodiesterase with a resultant increase in intracellular cyclic AMP, other agents similarly inhibit the enzyme producing a rise of cyclic AMP but are unassociated with any demonstrable bronchodilation. Other mechanisms proposed included an effect on translocation of intracellular calcium; prostaglandin antagonism; stimulation of catecholamines endogenously; inhibition of cyclic guanosine monophosphate metabolism and adenosine receptor antagonism. None of these mechanisms have been proven, however.

In vitro, theophylline has been shown to act synergistically with beta agonists and there are now available data which do demonstrate an additive effect *in vivo* with combined use.

Pharmacokinetics: The half-life of theophylline is influenced by a number of known variables. It may be prolonged in chronic alcoholics, partcularly those with liver disease (cirrhosis or alcoholic liver disease), in patients with congestive heart failure, and in those patients taking certain other drugs (see PRECAUTIONS, Drug Interactions). Newborns and neonates have extremely slow clearance rates compared to older infants and children, i.e., those over 1 year. Older children have rapid clearance rates while most non-smoking adults have clearance rates between these two extremes. In premature neonates the decreased clearance is related to oxidative pathways that have yet to be established.

Conventional Theophylline
Immediate-Release
Elimination Characteristics
Half-Life (in hours)

	Range	Mean
Children	1–9	3.7
Adults	3–15	7.7

In cigarette smokers (1–2 packs/day) the mean half-life is 4–5 hours, much shorter than in non-smokers. The increase in clearance associated with smoking is presumably due to stimulation of the hepatic metabolic pathways by components of cigarette smoke. The duration of this effect after cessation of smoking is unknown but may require 6 months to 2 years before the rate approaches that of a non-smoker.

A single-dose study in 15 normal fasting male volunteers whose theophylline inherent mean elimination half-life was verified by a liquid theophylline product to be 6.9 ± 2.5 (S.D.) hours were administered two or three 400 mg Uniphyl Tablets. The relative bioavailability of Uniphyl given in the fasting state in comparison to an immediate-release product was 59%. Peak serum theophylline levels occurred at 6.9 ± 5.2 (S.D.) hours, with a normalized (to 800 mg) peak level being 6.2 ± 2.1 (S.D.). The apparent elimination half-life for the 400 mg Uniphyl Tablets was 17.2 ± 5.8 (S.D.) hours.

Steady-state pharmacokinetics were determined in a study in 12 fasted patients with chronic reversible obstructive pulmonary disease. All were dosed with two 400 mg Uniphyl Tablets given once-daily in the morning and a widely-used approved controlled-release BID product administered as two 200 mg tablets given 12 hours apart. The pharmacokinetic parameters obtained for Uniphyl Tablets given at doses of 800 mg once-daily in the morning were virtually identical to the corresponding parameters for the reference drug when given as 400 mg BID. In particular, the AUC, Cmax and Cmin values obtained in this study were as follows:

	Uniphyl Tablets 800 mg O 24 h ± S.D.	Reference Drug 400 mg O 12 h ± S.D.
AUC, (0–24 hours), mcg hr/ml	288.9 ± 21.5	283.5 ± 38.4
Cmax, mcg/ml	15.7 ± 2.8	15.2 ± 2.1
Cmin, mcg/ml	7.9 ± 1.6	7.8 ± 1.7
Cmax-Cmin diff.	7.7 ± 1.5	7.4 ± 1.5

Bioavailability was calculated to be 104 ± 18% (S.D.) for the 24-hour period with Uniphyl Tablets once-daily as compared with the reference drug given twice daily, as shown above.

In a single-dose crossover study, two 400 mg Uniphyl Tablets were administered to 19 normal volunteers in the morning or evening immediately following the same standardized meal (769 calories consisting of 97 grams carbohydrates, 33 grams protein and 27 grams fat). There was no evidence of dose dumping nor were there any significant differences in pharmacokinetic parameters attributable to time of drug administration. On the morning arm, the pharmacokinetic parameters were AUC = 241.9 ± 83.0 mcg hr/ml, Cmax = 9.3 ± 2.0 mcg/ml, Tmax = 12.8 ± 4.2 hours. On the evening arm, the pharmacokinetic parameters were AUC = 219.7 ± 83.0 mcg hr/ml, Cmax = 9.2 ± 2.0 mcg/ml, Tmax = 12.5 ± 4.2 hours.

A study in which Uniphyl was administered to 17 fed adult asthmatics produced similar theophylline level-time curves when administered in the morning or evening. Serum levels were generally higher in the evening regimen but there were no statistically significant differences between the two regimens.

	MORNING	*EVENING*
AUC (0–24 hrs) (mcg hr/ml)	236.0 ± 76.7	256.0 ± 80.4
Cmax (mcg/ml)	14.5 ± 4.1	16.3 ± 4.5
Cmin (mcg/ml)	5.5 ± 2.9	5.0 ± 2.5
Tmax (hours)	8.1 ± 3.7	10.1 ± 4.1

The absorption characteristics of Uniphyl Tablets (theophylline, anhydrous) have been extensively studied. A steady-state crossover bioavailability study in 22 normal males compared two Uniphyl 400 mg Tablets administered O24h at 8 a.m. immediately after breakfast with a reference controlled-release theophylline product administered BID in fed subjects at 8 a.m. immediately after breakfast and 8 p.m. immediately after dinner (769 calories, consisting of 97 grams carbohydrates, 33 grams protein and 27 grams fat).

The pharmacokinetic parameters for Uniphyl 400 mg Tablets under these steady-state conditions were AUC = 203.3 ± 87.1 mcg hr/ml, Cmax = 12.1 ± 3.8 mcg/ml, Cmin = 4.50 ± 3.6, Tmax = 8.8 ± 4.6 hours. For the reference BID product, the pharmacokinetic parameters were AUC = 219.2 ± 88.4 mcg hr/ml, Cmax = 11.0 ± 4.1 mcg/ml, Cmin = 7.28 ± 3.5, Tmax = 6.9 ± 3.4 hours. The mean percent fluctuation [(Cmax-Cmin/Cmin) ×100] = 169% for the once-daily regimen and 51% for the reference product BID regimen.

Single-dose studies in which subjects were fasted for twelve (12) hours prior and an additional four (4) hours following dosing, demonstrated reduced bioavailability as compared to dosing with food. One single-dose study in 20 normal volunteers dosed with two 400 mg tablets in the morning, compared dosing under these fasting conditions with dosing immediately prior to a standardized breakfast (769 calories, consisting of 97 grams carbohydrates, 33 grams protein and 27 grams fat). Under fed conditions, the pharmacokinetic parameters were: AUC = 231.7 ± 92.4 mcg hr/ml, Cmax = 8.4 ± 2.6 mcg/ml, Tmax = 17.3 ± 6.7 hours. Under fasting conditions, these parameters were AUC = 141.2 ± 65.3 mcg hr/ml, Cmax = 5.5 ± 1.5 mcg/ml, Tmax = 6.5 ± 2.1 hours.

Another single-dose study in 21 normal male volunteers, dosed in the evening, compared fasting to a standardized high calorie, high fat meal (870–1,020 calories, consisting of 33 grams protein, 55–75 grams fat, 58 grams carbohydrates). In the fasting arm subjects received one Uniphyl 400 mg Tablet at 8 p.m. after an eight hour fast followed by a further four hour fast. In the fed arm, subjects were again dosed with one 400 mg Uniphyl Tablet, but at 8 p.m. immediately after the high fat content standardized meal cited above. The pharmacokinetic parameters (normalized to 800 mg) fed were AUC = 221.8 ± 40.9 mcg hr/ml, Cmax = 10.9 ± 1.7 mcg/ml, Tmax = 11.8 ± 2.2 hours. In the fasting arm, the pharmacokinetic parameters (normalized to 800 mg) were AUC = 146.4 ± 40.9 mcg hr/ml, Cmax = 6.7 ± 1.7 mcg/ml, Tmax = 7.3 ± 2.2 hours.

Thus, it has been established that while there is reduced bioavailability with fasting there is no failure of the delivery system leading to a sudden and unexpected release of a large quantity of theophylline with Uniphyl Tablets even when they are administered with a high fat, high calorie meal.

These studies demonstrate that as long as subjects were either consistently fed or consistently fasted, there is similar bioavailability with once-daily administration of Uniphyl Tablets, whether dosed in the morning or evening.

The AUC and Cmax are dose-dependent and will increase by upward dosage adjustment with Uniphyl Tablets. Patients who are fast theophylline metabolizers (clearance-greater than 5 L/hr) may not be suitable candidates for once-daily dosing. Those patients who are not well-maintained on recommended once-a-day therapy are likely to be better controlled when theophylline is administered in divided doses.

INDICATIONS AND USAGE

For relief and/or prevention of symptoms from asthma and reversible bronchospasm associated with chronic bronchitis and emphysema.

CONTRAINDICATIONS

This product is contraindicated in individuals who have shown hypersensitivity to its components. It is also contraindicated in patients with active peptic ulcer disease, and in individuals with underlying seizure disorders (unless receiving appropriate anticonvulsant medication).

WARNINGS

Serum levels above 20 mcg/ml are rarely found after appropriate administration of the recommended doses. However, in individuals in whom theophylline plasma clearance is reduced for any reason, even conventional doses may result in increased serum levels and potential toxicity. Reduced theophylline clearance has been documented in the following readily identifiable groups: 1) patients with impaired liver function; 2) patients over 55 years of age, particularly males and those with chronic lung disease; 3) those with cardiac failure from any cause; 4) patients with sustained high fever; 5) neonates and infants under 1 year of age; and 6) those patients taking certain drugs (see PRECAUTIONS, Drug Interactions). Frequently, such patients have markedly prolonged theophylline serum levels following discontinuation of the drug. Decreased theophylline clearance may occur following immunization for influenza, with active influenza, or other viral illnesses, and also with high fever for prolonged periods. This may be specially true in infants and the elderly.

Reduction of dosage and laboratory monitoring are especially appropriate in the above individuals.

Serious side effects such as ventricular arrhythmias, convulsions or even death may appear as the first sign of toxicity without any previous warning. Elderly patients with serum concentrations above 20 μg/ml are more likely to experience serious side effects such as ventricular arrhythmias or convulsions than are younger patients. Less serious signs of theophylline toxicity (i.e., nausea and restlessness) may occur frequently when initiating therapy, but are usually transient; when such signs are persistent during maintenance therapy, they are often associated with serum concentrations above 20 mcg/ml. Stated differently: *serious toxicity is not reliably preceded by less severe side effects.* A serum concentration measurement is the only reliable method of predicting potentially life-threatening toxicity.

Many patients who require theophylline exhibit tachycardia due to their underlying disease process so that the cause/effect relationship to elevated serum theophylline concentrations may not be appreciated.

Theophylline products may cause or worsen arrhythmias and any significant change in rate and/or rhythm warrants monitoring and further investigation.

Studies in laboratory animals (minipigs, rodents and dogs) recorded the occurrence of cardiac arrhythmias and sudden death (with histologic evidence of myocardial necrosis) when beta-agonists and methylxanthines were administered concurrently. The significance of these findings when applied to humans is currently unknown.

PRECAUTIONS

General: On the average, theophylline half-life is shorter in cigarette and marijuana smokers than in non-smokers, but smokers can have half-lives as long as non-smokers. Theophylline should not be administered concurrently with other xanthines. Use with caution in patients with hypoxemia, hypertension, or those with history of peptic ulcer. Theophylline may occasionally act as a local irritant to G.I. tract although gastrointestinal symptoms are more commonly centrally mediated and associated with serum drug concentrations over 20 mcg/ml.

Information for Patients: The physician should reinforce the importance of taking only the prescribed dose and observing the time interval between doses. Information relating to taking Uniphyl in relation to meals or fasting should be provided. All patients should be asked to report side effects which occur at any time or recurrence of symptoms, especially toward the end of a 24-hour dosing interval. Uniphyl Tablets are not to be chewed or crushed.

Laboratory Tests: Serum levels should be monitored periodically to determine the theophylline level associated with observed clinical response and as the method of predicting toxicity. For such measurements, the serum sample should be obtained at the approximate time of the expected peak concentration, i.e., about 9 hours after administration in the morning or about 12 hours after administration in the evening. It is important that the patient will not have missed or taken additional doses during the previous 48 hours and that dosing intervals will have been reasonably equally spaced. DOSAGE ADJUSTMENT BASED ON SERUM THEOPHYLLINE MEASUREMENTS WHEN THESE INSTRUCTIONS HAVE NOT BEEN FOLLOWED MAY RESULT IN RECOMMENDATIONS THAT PRESENT RISK OF TOXICITY TO THE PATIENT.

Drug Interactions: Toxic synergism with ephedrine has been documented and may occur with other sympathomimetic bronchodilators. In addition, the following drug interactions have been demonstrated:

Theophylline with:	
Allopurinol (high-dose)	Increased serum theophylline levels
Cimetidine	Increased serum theophylline levels
Ciprofloxacin	Increased serum theophylline levels
Erythromycin, Troleandomycin	Increased serum theophylline levels
Lithium carbonate	Increased renal excretion of lithium
Norfloxacin	Increased serum theophylline levels
Oral Contraceptives	Increased serum theophylline levels
Phenytoin	Decreased theophylline and phenytoin serum levels
Propranolol	Increased serum theophylline levels
Rifampin	Decreased serum theophylline levels

Drug-Food Interactions: The absorption characteristics of Uniphyl® Tablets (theophylline, anydrous) have been studied and are enhanced by co-administration with food. In two single-dose studies in which subjects were given Uniphyl with either a standardized breakfast or a high fat content meal, bioavailability under the fasting conditions were 61% and 66% respectively in comparison to under the fed condition. (SEE CLINICAL PHARMACOLOGY, Pharmacokinetics).

A drug-free effect, if any, would likely have its greatest clinical significance when high theophylline serum levels are being maintained and/or when large single doses (greater than 13 mg/kg or 900 mg) of a controlled-release theophylline product are given.

Drug-Laboratory Test Interactions: Currently available analytical methods, including high pressure liquid chromatography and immunoassay techniques, for measuring serum theophylline levels are specific. Metabolites and other drugs generally do not affect the results. Other new analytic methods are also now in use. The physician should be aware of the laboratory method used and whether other drugs will interfere with the assay for theophylline.

Carcinogenesis, Mutagenesis, and Impairment of Fertility: Long-term carcinogenicity studies have not been performed with theophylline.

Chromosome-breaking activity was detected in human cell cultures at concentrations of theophylline up to 50 times the therapeutic serum concentrations in humans. Theophylline was not mutagenic in the dominant lethal assay in male mice given theophylline intraperitoneally in doses up to 30 times the maximum daily human oral dose.

Studies to determine the effect on fertility have not been performed with theophylline.

Pregnancy: Category C—Animal reproduction studies have not been conducted with theophylline. It is also not known whether theophylline can cause fetal harm when administered to a pregnant woman or can affect reproduction capacity. Xanthines should be given to a pregnant woman only if clearly needed.

Nursing Mothers: Theophylline is distributed into breast milk and may cause irritability or other signs of toxicity in nursing infants. Because of the potential for serious adverse reactions in nursing infants from theophylline, a decision

Continued on next page

Purdue Frederick—Cont.

should be made whether to discontinue nursing or to discontinue the drug, taking into account the importance of the drug to the mother.

Pediatric Use: Safety and effectiveness in children under 12 years of age have not been established with 400 mg Uniphyl Tablets.

ADVERSE REACTIONS

The following adverse reactions have been observed, but there has not been enough systematic collection of data to support an estimate of their frequency. The most consistent adverse reactions are usually due to overdosage.

1. *Gastrointestinal:* nausea, vomiting, epigastric pain, hematemesis, diarrhea.
2. *Central nervous system:* headaches, irritability, restlessness, insomnia, reflex hyperexcitability, muscle twitching, clonic and tonic generalized convulsions.
3. *Cardiovascular:* palpitation, tachycardia, extrasystoles, flushing, hypotension, circulatory failure, ventricular arrhythmias.
4. *Respiratory:* tachypnea.
5. *Renal:* potentiation of diuresis.
6. *Others:* alopecia, hyperglycemia, inappropriate ADH syndrome, rash, Stevens-Johnson syndrome.

OVERDOSAGE

Management: It is suggested that the management principles (consistent with the clinical status of the patient when first seen) outlined below be instituted and that simultaneous contact with a Regional Poison Control Center be established. In this way, both updated information and individualization regarding required therapy may be provided.

1. When potential oral overdose is established and seizure has not occurred:
   a) If patient is alert and seen within the early hours after ingestion, induction of emesis may be of value. Gastric lavage has been demonstrated to be of no value in influencing outcome in patients who present more than 1 hour after ingestion.
   b) Administer a cathartic. Sorbitol solution is reported to be of value.
   c) Administer repeated doses of activated charcoal and monitor theophylline serum levels.
   d) Prophylactic administration of phenobarbital has been shown to increase the seizure threshold in laboratory animals, and administration of this drug can be considered.
2. If patient presents with a seizure:
   a) Establish an airway.
   b) Administer oxygen.
   c) Treat the seizure with intravenous diazepam, 0.1 to 0.3 mg/kg up to 10 mg. If seizure cannot be controlled, the use of general anesthesia should be considered.
   d) Monitor vital signs, maintain blood pressure and provide adequate hydration.
3. If post-seizure coma is present:
   a) Maintain airway and oxygenation.
   b) If post-seizure coma is a result of oral medication, follow above recommendations to prevent absorption of the drug, but intubation and lavage will have to be performed instead of inducing emesis, and the cathartic and charcoal will need to be introduced via a large bore gastric lavage tube.
   c) Continue to provide full supportive care and adequate hydration until the drug is metabolized. In general, drug metabolism is sufficiently rapid so as not to warrant dialysis. If repeated oral activated charcoal is ineffective (as noted by stable or rising serum levels) charcoal hemoperfusion may be indicated.

DOSAGE AND ADMINISTRATION

Uniphyl 400 mg Tablets can be taken once a day in the morning or evening. Until further data are available, evening dosing is limited to patients whose daily dose is 800 mg or less. It is recommended that Uniphyl be taken with meals. Patients should be advised that if they choose to take Uniphyl with food it should be taken consistently with food and if they take it in a fasted condition it should routinely be taken fasted. It is important that the product whenever dosed be dosed consistently with or without food.

Effective use of theophylline (i.e., the concentration of drug in the serum associated with optimal benefit and minimal risk of toxicity) is considered to occur when the theophylline concentration is maintained from 10 to 20 mcg/ml. The early studies from which these levels were derived were carried out in patients immediately or shortly after recovery from acute exacerbations of their disease (some hospitalized with status asthmaticus).

Although the 20 mcg/ml level remains appropriate as a critical value (above which toxicity is more likely to occur) for safety purposes, additional data are now available which indicate that the serum theophylline concentrations required to produce maximum physiologic benefit may, in fact, fluctuate with the degree of bronchospasm present and are variable. Therefore, the physician should individualize the range appropriate to the patient's requirements, based on both symptomatic response and improvement in pulmonary function.

As with all sustained-release theophylline products, Uniphyl Tablets are for chronic or long-term use and are not intended for initial treatment in a patient with acute symptoms.

If it is not possible to obtain serum level determinations, restriction of the daily dose (in otherwise healthy adults) to not greater than 13 mg/kg/day, to a maximum of 900 mg, in divided doses will result in relatively few patients exceeding serum levels of 20 mcg/ml and the resultant greater risk of toxicity.

Caution should be exercised in younger children who cannot complain of minor side effects. Older adults, those with cor pulmonale, congestive heart failure, and/or liver disease may have unusually low dosage requirements and thus may experience toxicity at the maximal dosage recommended below.

Theophylline does not distribute to fatty tissue. Dosage should be calculated on the basis of lean (ideal) body weight where mg/kg doses are presented.

Frequency of Dosing: Patients who clear theophylline normally or relatively slowly, e.g., non-smokers, may be reasonable candidates for taking Uniphyl Tablets once-daily. However, certain patients, such as the young, smokers and some non-smoking adults are likely to metabolize theophylline more rapidly and may require dosing at 12 hour intervals. Such patients may experience symptoms of bronchospasm toward the end of a once-daily dosing interval and/or require a high daily dose (higher than those recommended in labeling) and are more likely to experience relatively wide peak to trough differences in serum theophylline concentrations.

Dosage Guidelines: WARNING: DO NOT ATTEMPT TO MAINTAIN ANY DOSE THAT IS NOT WELL TOLERATED. Dosage guidelines are approximations only, and the wide range of clearance of theophylline among individuals (particularly those with concomitant disease) makes indiscriminate usage hazardous. When appropriate, dosage should be calculated on the basis of lean body weight where mg/kg doses are to be prescribed since theophylline does not distribute into fatty tissue.

I. *Initiation of Therapy with Uniphyl Tablets*
   a. *Stabilized Patients (12 years of age or older)*
   Individuals who are taking an immediate-release or controlled-release theophylline product may be transferred to once-daily administration of 400 mg Uniphyl Tablets on a mg-for-mg basis. For example, a patient stabilized on 400 mg twice daily (800 mg total daily dose) should be given two 400 mg Uniphyl Tablets as a single daily dose of 800 mg in either the morning or the evening. However, until further data are available, evening dosing is limited to patients whose total daily dose is 800 mg or less.
   It must be recognized that the peak and trough serum theophylline levels produced by the once-daily dosage may vary from those produced by the previous product and/or regimen.
   b. *Initiation of Theophylline Dosing*
   Adult patients and children 12 years of age and over not currently receiving theophylline may be titrated using an immediate or sustained-release theophylline product, which can be adjusted in small dosage increments. Patients titrated to a total daily dose of approximately 400, 600, 800, 1,000 or 1,200 mg may be transferred to once-daily dosage with 400 mg Uniphyl Tablets as is described in (a) above. However, until further data are available, evening dosing is limited to patients whose total daily dose is 800 mg or less.

II. *Titration and Dose Adjustment*
   a. *When Serum Levels Are Measured*
   After 4 days therapy with Uniphyl Tablets, steady-state should have been achieved, and approximate peak serum theophylline concentration samples should be determined from blood samples obtained about 9 hours after administration in the morning or about 12 hours after administration in the evening. When taken in the evening with supper it may not be possible to get blood levels within 12 hours following the daily dose. Under these circumstances blood levels should be measured as early in the morning as practical, recognizing that such levels may be somewhat lower than the actual peak achieved. Trough concentration should be taken just prior to the administration of the next dose. It is important that the patient not have missed or added any dose during the previous 72 hours, and that the dosing intervals remain relatively constant. DOSAGE ADJUSTMENT BASED ON MEASUREMENTS WHEN THESE INSTRUCTIONS HAVE NOT BEEN FOLLOWED RESULT IN TOXICITY.
   b. *When Serum Levels Are Not Measured*
   In the absence of laboratory facilities for determining serum theophylline concentration levels, clinical judgment should be followed. The original total

once-daily dose should continue if it is well tolerated and the clinical response is satisfactory.

If adverse reactions occur, decrease the dose as stated below.

If a patient is better controlled on another regimen than on a once-daily regimen, the patient should be maintained on the more effective regimen.

   c. *Increasing the Dose of Uniphyl Tablets*
   If patient response with Uniphyl Tablets is unsatisfactory and/or the observed serum theophylline concentration range is too low, the patient should be transferred to an immediate or controlled-release (BID) theophylline schedule and dosage increased at recommended intervals as follows:

Serum Theophylline (mcg/ml)	Directions
Too low	Increase dosage at 3 day intervals by 25%. The serum concentration may be rechecked at appropriate intervals, but at least at the end of the adjustment period.*

When the patient's condition is otherwise clinically stable and none of the recognized factors which alter elimination are present, measurement of serum levels need be repeated only every 6 to 12 months.

*The total daily dose may need to be administered at more frequent intervals if symptoms occur repeatedly at the end of a dosing interval.

   d. *Decreasing the Dose of Uniphyl Tablets*
   Serum theophylline values above 20 mcg/ml require decreasing the daily dose unless such dose is required to maintain the patient and is well-tolerated. Dosage may be reduced by transferring the patient to an immediate or controlled-release (BID) theophylline product and making adjustments. Peak and trough measurements should be taken 3 days after each decrease in dosage.

Serum Theophylline (mcg/ml)	Directions
20 to 25	Decrease dose by about 10%
25 to 30	Skip next dose and decrease subsequent doses by about 25%
Over 30	Skip next 2 doses and decrease subsequent doses by 50%

Finer adjustments in dosage may be needed for some patients.

III. *Maintenance Therapy*
   Careful clinical titration is important to assure patient acceptance and safety of the medication. Patients, when stabilized as established by serum theophylline concentration or respiratory function, usually remain controlled without further dosage adjustment. It should be borne in mind, however, that for reasons stated in the PRECAUTIONS and WARNINGS sections, dosage adjustments may be necessary. Serum theophylline levels should be measured periodically (at 6 to 12-month intervals) even in clinically controlled patients.
   The elderly as well as patients with congestive heart failure, cor pulmonale, and/or liver disease may have unusually low dosage requirements and thus may experience toxicity even at the dosages recommended above.

WARNING

DO NOT MAINTAIN ANY DOSE THAT IS NOT TOLERATED.

HOW SUPPLIED

Uniphyl (theophylline, anhydrous) 400 mg scored Controlled-Release Tablets are supplied in white-opaque plastic bottles, containing 100 tablets [NDC #0034-7004-80] or 500 tablets [NDC #0034-7004-70] or in unit dose packaging with 10 tablets per card [NDC #0034-7004-10]; ten cards are packed in each carton; 10 cartons are packed in each shipper. Each round, white tablet bears the symbols PF on one side and is marked U400 on the other side.

Store tablets at controlled room temperature 15° to 30°C (59°–86°F).

CAUTION

Federal law prohibits dispensing without prescription.
Copyright © 1983, 1990
The Purdue Frederick Company
Norwalk, CT 06850-3590
U.S. Patent Numbers 3965256 and 4235870
March 11, 1991   L1374
Shown in Product Identification Section, page 424

EDUCATIONAL MATERIAL

Audio Visuals—Booklets—Samples
Q & A: "Genital Warts—More Common Than You Think" booklet (Alferon N Injection)
Pain Assessment Kit (Pain Assessment Tools) (MS Contin)
Pain Assessment Program (medical forms and patient booklets) (MS Contin)
Cancer Pain Management Slide Program (MS Contin)
"Up-To-Date Answers About Pain Medications" booklet for patient education. (MS Contin)
"Home Care of the Hospice Patient"—Guide to caring for cancer patients. (English/Spanish) (MS Contin)
Pain Assessment Questionnaire (MS Contin)
Dosing Conversion Reference (MS Contin)
Controlling Cancer Pain—Video film (MS Contin)
Arthritis Exercise Pads (English and Spanish) (Trilisate)
Arthritis Assessment Questionnaire (Trilisate)
"Nocturnal Asthma"—Understanding and Managing the Disease at night" (Uniphyl)
Respiratory Assessment Questionnaire (English and Spanish) (Uniphyl)
Patient Dosing Instructions Sheets (English and Spanish) (Uniphyl)
Asthma—A Nocturnal Video Film (Uniphyl)
"Protect Your Family From Germs" patient-aid booklet (English and Spanish) (Betadine)
Samples of Betadine First Aid and Betadine Feminine Hygiene Products.
"Fem-Facts®" booklets (Facts about Vaginitis Symptoms for Patients) (Betadine)
"Betadine Microbicides and the AIDS Virus" brochure
"How You Can Make It Feel Better"—Guide to Caring for Cuts, Burns and Scrapes (Betadine)
"Helping Your Wounds Heal"—Care of Cuts, Scrapes, Minor Burns (Betadine)
Spanning the Spectrum in Hospital Infection Control Videotape film (Betadine)
"Fiber and Your Health" booklet (Fibermed)
Senokot Constipation Assessment In-Service Training Videotape "Current Concepts in Constipation Management"
Senokot Family Dosage Card (Senokot)
Senokot Patient Information Booklet "When a common side effect of many medications becomes a problem—Drug-Induced Constipation" (Senokot)
Senokot Laxative Protocal Pad (Senokot)

R&D Laboratories, Inc.
4204 GLENCOE AVENUE
MARINA DEL REY, CA 90292

Products for use primarily with Renal Disease.

CALCI–CHEW™   OTC

1.25 gm USP grade calcium carbonate chewable tablets—500 mg elemental calcium. Packaged as four separate flavors—cherry, lemon, orange, peppermint.
DESCRIPTION
Tablets supplying 1.25 gm USP grade calcium carbonate. No oyster shell.
INDICATIONS
For use as calcium supplementation and in the treatment of hypocalcemia.
DOSAGE
For hypocalcemia, use as necessary to restore calcium to normal levels. For patients with impaired calcium absorption or on a calcium restricted diet, give under a physician's guidance.
SUPPLIED
Plastic bottles of 100 tablets. NDC Nos. 54391-0(0,2,3,4)25-2

CALCI–MIX®   OTC

1.25 gm USP grade calcium carbonate in capsules. 500 mg of elemental calcium. Premeasured to swallow or sprinkle on food or drink. Conforms 94% with USP dissolution standards.
DESCRIPTION
Capsules providing 1.25 gm USP grade calcium carbonate. No oyster shell.

INDICATIONS
For use as calcium supplementation and in the treatment of hypocalcemia.
DOSAGE
For hypocalcemia, use as necessary to restore calcium to normal levels. For patients with impaired calcium absorption or on a calcium restricted diet, give under a physician's guidance.
SUPPLIED
Plastic bottles of 100 tablets. NDC No. 54391-0027-3.

NEPHRO–CALCI™   OTC

1.5 gm U.S.P. grade calcium carbonate tablets—600 mg elemental calcium. Conforms 97% with USP dissolution standards.
DESCRIPTION
Tablets supplying 1.5 gm of calcium carbonate. USP grade—no oyster shell.
INDICATIONS
For use as calcium supplementation and in the treatment of hypocalcemia.
DOSAGE
For hypocalcemia, use as necessary to restore calcium to normal levels. For patients with impaired calcium absorption and patients on a calcium restricted diet give under a physician's guidance.
SUPPLIED
Plastic bottles of 100 tablets. NDC 54391-0026-3.

NEPHRO–DERM®   OTC
NDC 54391-2000-4, 2000-5

OTC skin cream for the relief of uremic itching. Nephro-Derm® contains Eucerin®, camphor, and menthol as its active ingredients and is formulated to help relieve general and uremic itching. This product is supplied in 4 oz jars and 1 oz jars.

®Beiersdorf, Inc., Norwalk, CT

NEPHRO–FER™   OTC

An OTC ferrous fumarate preparation for oral iron supplementation in patients particularly those undergoing therapy with erythropoietin.
DESCRIPTION
Each tablet supplies 350 mg of ferrous fumarate—115 mg of elemental iron.
INDICATIONS
Patients taking EPO requiring oral iron supplementation—particularly patients who experience gastric problems with ferrous sulfate. Appropriate for any iron supplementation. (See Nephro-Fer™ Rx for side effects.)
DOSAGE
One to three tablets daily as required, under the supervision of a physician.
SUPPLIED
Plastic bottles of 100 tablets only. NDC 54391-0013-9.

NEPHRO-FER™ Rx   ℞

Oral iron supplement containing 324 mg ferrous fumarate and 1 mg folic acid. For any patient needing iron supplementation for documented iron deficiency. Suitable for certain patients undergoing therapy with erythropoietin.
DESCRIPTION
Each tablet contains 324 mg ferrous fumarate—106.5 mg elemental iron—and 1 mg folic acid. Product does not contain any coloring agents/dyes. The product has been formulated to disintegrate quickly at stomach and upper intestinal pHs to optimize available iron at the sites of absorption. Ferrous fumarate may be better tolerated than ferrous sulfate in some patients.
INDICATIONS
Renal failure patients and patients not on dialysis who have documented iron deficiency. Patients undergoing erythropoietin therapy who risk iron deficiency as reflected by low transferrin saturation and low serum ferritin.
DOSAGE
One to three tablets daily between meals in increments throughout the day, as required to correct iron deficiency

condition. The total amount of elemental iron prescribed should be titrated to the amount of iron assessed to provide adequate iron for red blood cell synthesis and replacement of iron body stores, particularly preceding or during erythropoietin therapy.
SIDE EFFECTS
Transient bloating, flatulence, constipation, and diarrhea. Ingestion of greater than 400 mg per day of elemental iron can result in nausea and vomiting.
PRECAUTION
Folic acid can mask the symptoms of anemia. A careful assessment of the patient should precede prescribing this medication.
SUPPLIED
Brown, oval tablets marked RD33.
Plastic bottles of 120 tablets. NDC 54391-1313-6.

NEPHRO–VITE®Rx   ℞
Renal Patient Vitamin Replacement Formulation

DESCRIPTION
The process of hemodialysis and CAPD causes vitamin losses necessitating the regular replacement of the water soluble vitamins. It is important not to over supplement some vitamins. VITAMIN A SHOULD NOT BE SUPPLEMENTED AND VITAMIN C SUPPLEMENTATION SHOULD BE LIMITED TO 60 MG PER DAY TO AVOID THE RISK OF INCREASED OXALATE FORMATION*.
Each (film coat) tablet provides*:

Vitamin	Nephro-Vite®℞	Nephro-Vite® (OTC)
Vitamin C(mg)	60	60
Vitamin B$_1$(mg)	1.5	1.5
Vitamin B$_2$(mg)	1.7	1.7
Niacinamide(mg)	20	20
Vitamin B$_6$(mg)	10	10
Vitamin B$_{12}$(mcg)	6	6
Folic Acid(mcg)	1000	800
Pantothenic Acid(mg)	10	10
Biotin(mcg)	300	300

* Formulated to provide optimum one-a-day vitamin replacement amounts daily as suggested by latest literature on the subject. Please ask for R & D's review of the literature on this subject.

INDICATIONS
Dialysis patients; Azotemic patients not on dialysis who eat poorly.
DOSAGE
One tablet daily.
SUPPLIED
Small yellow tablets marked RD 12.
Plastic bottles of 100. NDC 54391-1002-1.

NEPHRO–VITE®   OTC

OTC Renal vitamin replacement formulation—see table for description. Same dosage as Nephro-Vite®℞.
Supplied in plastic bottles of 100. NDC 54391-0002-1.

Reckitt & Colman Pharmaceuticals Inc.
1901 HUGUENOT ROAD
RICHMOND, VA 23235

BUPRENEX®   Ⓒ ℞
[būp 'rĕn-ex]
(buprenorphine hydrochloride)
INJECTABLE

DESCRIPTION
Buprenex (buprenorphine hydrochloride) is a narcotic under the Controlled Substances Act due to its chemical derivation from thebaine. Chemically, it is 17-(cyclopropylmethyl)-α-(1,1-dimethylethyl)-4, 5-epoxy-18, 19-dihydro-3-hydroxy-6-methoxy-α-methyl-6, 14-ethenomorphinan-7-methanol, hydrochloride [5α, 7α(S)]. Buprenorphine hydrochloride is a white powder, weakly acidic and with limited solubility in water. Buprenex is a clear, sterile, injectable agonist-antagonist analgesic intended for intravenous or intramuscular administration. Each ml of Buprenex contains 0.324 mg buprenorphine hydrochloride (equivalent to 0.3 mg buprenor-

Continued on next page

Reckitt & Colman—Cont.

phine), 50 mg anhydrous dextrose, water for injection and HCl to adjust pH. Buprenorphine hydrochloride has the molecular formula, $C_{29}H_{41}NO_4\text{-}HCl$, and the following structure:

Molecular weight: 504.09

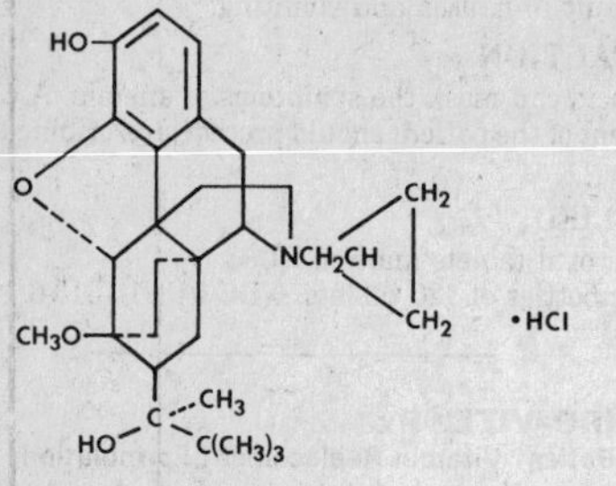

CLINICAL PHARMACOLOGY

Buprenex is a parenteral opioid analgesic with 0.3 mg Buprenex being approximately equivalent to 10 mg morphine sulfate in analgesic and respiratory depressant effects. Pharmacological effects occur as soon as 15 minutes after intramuscular injection and persist for 6 hours or longer. Peak pharmacologic effects usually are observed at 1 hour. When used intravenously, the times to onset and peak effect are shortened.

The limits of sensitivity of available analytical methodology precluded demonstration of bioequivalence between intramuscular and intravenous routes of administration. In postoperative patients, pharmacokinetic studies have shown elimination half-lives ranging from 1.2–7.2 hours (mean 2.2 hours) after intravenous administration of 0.3 mg of buprenorphine.

Buprenorphine, in common with morphine and other phenolic opioid analgesics, is metabolized by the liver and its clearance is related to hepatic blood flow. Studies in patients anesthetized with 0.5% halothane have shown that this anesthetic decreases hepatic blood flow by about 30%.

Mechanism of Analgesic Action: Buprenex exerts its analgesic effect via high affinity binding to μ subclass opiate receptors in the central nervous system. Although Buprenex may be classified as a partial agonist, under the conditions of recommended use it behaves very much like classical μ agonists such as morphine. One unusual property of Buprenex observed in *in vitro* studies is its very slow rate of dissociation from its receptor. This could account for its longer duration of action than morphine, the unpredictability of its reversal by opioid antagonists, and its low level of manifest physical dependence.

Narcotic Antagonist Activity: Buprenorphine demonstrates narcotic antagonist activity and has been shown to be equipotent with naloxone as an antagonist of morphine in the mouse tail flick test.

Cardiovascular Effects: Buprenex may cause a decrease or, rarely, an increase in pulse rate and blood pressure in some patients.

Effects on Respiration: Under usual conditions of use, both Buprenex and morphine show similar dose-related respiratory depressant effects. A therapeutic dose of Buprenex (0.3 mg buprenorphine) can decrease respiratory rate in an equivalent manner to an equianalgesic dose of morphine (10 mg). (See WARNINGS.)

INDICATIONS AND USAGE

Buprenex is indicated for the relief of moderate to severe pain.

CONTRAINDICATIONS

Buprenex should not be administered to patients who have been shown to be hypersensitive to the drug.

WARNINGS

Impaired Respiration: As with other potent opioids, clinically significant respiratory depression may occur within the recommended dose range in patients receiving therapeutic doses of buprenorphine. Buprenex should be used with caution in patients with compromised respiratory function (e.g., chronic obstructive pulmonary disease, cor pulmonale, decreased respiratory reserve, hypoxia, hypercapnia, or preexisting respiratory depression). Particular caution is advised if Buprenex is administered to patients taking or recently receiving drugs with CNS/respiratory depressant effects. In patients with the physical and/or pharmacological risk factors above, the dose should be reduced by approximately one-half.

NALOXONE MAY NOT BE EFFECTIVE IN REVERSING THE RESPIRATORY DEPRESSION PRODUCED BY BUPRENEX. THEREFORE, AS WITH OTHER POTENT OPIOIDS, THE PRIMARY MANAGEMENT OF OVERDOSE SHOULD BE THE REESTABLISHMENT OF ADEQUATE VENTILATION WITH MECHANICAL ASSISTANCE OF RESPIRATION, IF REQUIRED.

Interaction with Other Central Nervous System Depressants: Patients receiving Buprenex in the presence of other narcotic analgesics, general anesthetics, antihistamines, benzodiazepines, phenothiazines, other tranquilizers, sedative/hypnotics or other CNS depressants (including alcohol) may exhibit increased CNS depression. When such combined therapy is contemplated, it is particularly important that the dose of one or both agents be reduced.

Head Injury and Increased Intracranial Pressure: Buprenex, like other potent analgesics, may itself elevate cerebrospinal fluid pressure and should be used with caution in head injury, intracranial lesions and other circumstances where cerebrospinal pressure may be increased. Buprenex can produce miosis and changes in the level of consciousness which may interfere with patient evaluation.

Use in Ambulatory Patients: Buprenex may impair the mental or physical abilities required for the performance of potentially dangerous tasks such as driving a car or operating machinery. Therefore, Buprenex should be administered with caution to ambulatory patients who should be warned to avoid such hazards.

Use in Narcotic-Dependent Patients: Because of the narcotic antagonist activity of Buprenex, use in the physically dependent individual may result in withdrawal effects.

PRECAUTIONS

General: Buprenex should be administered with caution in the elderly or debilitated and those with severe impairment of hepatic, pulmonary, or renal function; myxedema or hypothyroidism; adrenal cortical insufficiency (e.g., Addison's disease); CNS depression or coma; toxic psychoses; prostatic hypertrophy or urethral stricture; acute alcoholism, delirium tremens; or kyphoscoliosis.

Because Buprenex is metabolized by the liver, the activity of Buprenex may be increased and/or extended in those individuals with impaired hepatic function or those receiving other agents known to decrease hepatic clearance.

Buprenex has been shown to increase intracholedochal pressure to a similar degree as other opioid analgesics, and thus should be administered with caution to patients with dysfunction of the biliary tract.

Information for Patients: The effects of Buprenex, particularly drowsiness, may be potentiated by other centrally acting agents such as alcohol or benzodiazepines. It is particularly important that in these circumstances patients must not drive or operate machinery. Buprenex has some pharmacologic effects similar to morphine which in susceptible patients may lead to self-administration of the drug when pain no longer exists. Patients must not exceed the dosage of Buprenex prescribed by their physician. Patients should be urged to consult their physician if other prescription medications are currently being used or are prescribed for future use.

Drug Interactions: Drug interactions common to other potent opioid analgesics also may occur with Buprenex. Particular care should be taken when Buprenex is used in combination with central nervous system depressant drugs (see WARNINGS). Although specific information is not presently available, caution should be exercised when Buprenex is used in combination with MAO inhibitors. There have been reports of respiratory and cardiovascular collapse in patients who received therapeutic doses of diazepam and Buprenex. A suspected interaction between Buprenex and phenprocoumon resulting in purpura has been reported.

Carcinogenesis, Mutagenesis, Impairment of Fertility: The effects of Buprenex on fertility and gestation indices were investigated in rats by the subcutaneous and intramuscular routes at doses 10 to 1,000 times the proposed human doses. Dystocia was noted in dams treated with 1,000 times the human dose. No effects on fertility or gestation were noted in these Segment 1 studies.

Pregnancy: Pregnancy Category C. Reproduction studies have been performed in the rat at doses which ranged from 10 to 1,000 times the proposed human dose by the subcutaneous and intramuscular routes and 160 times the proposed human dose by the intravenous routes. By the intramuscular route, Buprenex produced mild but statistically significant ($p < 0.05$) post-implantation losses and early fetal deaths at 10 and 100 but not 1,000 times the proposed human dose. No fetal malformations were noted in rats at any dose when Buprenex was administered by subcutaneous, intramuscular, or intravenous routes. In rabbits, intramuscularly administered Buprenex produced a dose-related trend for extra rib formation which attained statistical significance ($p < 0.01$) at 1,000 times the proposed human dose. By the intravenous route, doses in rats of 40 and 160 times the proposed human dose of Buprenex caused a slight increase in post-implantation losses that may have been treatment-related. No major fetal malformations were noted in drug treated groups when administered by intramuscular or intravenous routes.

There are no adequate and well-controlled studies in pregnant women. Buprenex should be used during pregnancy only if the potential benefit justifies the potential risk to the fetus.

Labor and Delivery: The safety of Buprenex given during labor and delivery has not been established.

Nursing Mothers: An apparent lack of milk production during general reproduction studies with Buprenex in rats caused decreased viability and lactation indices. It is unknown at this time whether or not Buprenex is excreted in human milk. Despite the lack of specific knowledge on this issue, it is reasonable to assume that Buprenex will enter human milk and caution should be exercised in the use of Buprenex when it is administered to nursing mothers.

Pediatric Use: Safety and effectiveness in children have not been established.

ADVERSE REACTIONS

The most frequent side effect in clinical studies involving 1,133 patients was sedation which occurred in approximately two-thirds of the patients. Although sedated, these patients could easily be aroused to an alert state.

Other less frequent adverse reactions occurring in 5–10% of the patients were:

Nausea	Dizziness/Vertigo

Occurring in 1–5% of the patients:

Sweating	Headache
Hypotension	Nausea/Vomiting
Vomiting	Hypoventilation
Miosis	

The following adverse reactions were reported to have occurred in less than 1% of the patients:

CNS Effect: confusion, blurred vision, euphoria, weakness/fatigue, dry mouth, nervousness, depression, slurred speech, paresthesia.

Cardiovascular: hypertension, tachycardia, bradycardia.

Gastrointestinal: constipation.

Respiratory: dyspnea, cyanosis.

Dermatological: pruritus.

Ophthalmological: diplopia, visual abnormalities.

Miscellaneous: injection site reaction, urinary retention, dreaming, flushing/warmth, chills/cold, tinnitus, conjunctivitis, Wenckebach block, and psychosis.

Other effects observed infrequently include malaise, hallucinations, depersonalization, coma, dyspepsia, flatulence, apnea, rash, amblyopia, tremor, and pallor.

The following reactions have been reported to occur rarely: loss of appetite, dysphoria/agitation, diarrhea, urticaria, and convulsions/lack of muscle coordination.

In the United Kingdom, buprenorphine hydrochloride was made available under monitored release regulation during the first year of sale, and yielded data from 1,736 physicians on 9,123 patients (17,120 administrations). No important new adverse effects attributable to buprenorphine hydrochloride were observed.

DRUG ABUSE AND DEPENDENCE

Buprenorphine hydrochloride is a partial agonist of the morphine type: *i.e.,* it has certain opioid properties which may lead to psychic dependence of the morphine type due to an opiate-like euphoric component of the drug. Direct dependence studies have shown little physical dependence upon withdrawal of the drug. However, caution should be used in prescribing to individuals who are known to be drug abusers or ex-narcotic addicts. The drug may not substitute in acutely dependent narcotic addicts due to its antagonist component and may induce withdrawal symptoms.

OVERDOSAGE

Manifestations: Clinical experience with Buprenex overdosage has been insufficient to define the signs of this condition at this time. Although the antagonist activity of buprenorphine may become manifest at doses somewhat above the recommended therapeutic range, doses in the recommended therapeutic range may produce clinically significant respiratory depression in certain circumstances. (See WARNINGS.)

Treatment: The respiratory and cardiac status of the patients should be monitored carefully. Primary attention should be given to the reestablishment of adequate respiratory exchange through provision of a patent airway and institution of assisted or controlled ventilation. Oxygen, intravenous fluids, vasopressors, and other supportive measures should be employed as indicated. Doxapram, a respiratory stimulant, may be used. **NALOXONE MAY NOT BE EFFECTIVE IN REVERSING THE RESPIRATORY DEPRESSION PRODUCED BY BUPRENEX. THEREFORE, AS WITH OTHER POTENT OPIOIDS, THE PRIMARY MANAGEMENT OF OVERDOSE SHOULD BE THE REESTABLISHMENT OF ADEQUATE VENTILATION WITH MECHANICAL ASSISTANCE OF RESPIRATION, IF REQUIRED.**

DOSAGE AND ADMINISTRATION

The usual dosage for persons 13 years of age and over is 1 ml Buprenex (0.3 mg buprenorphine) given by deep intramuscular or slow (over at least 2 minutes) intravenous injection at up to 6-hour intervals, as needed. Repeat once (up to 0.3 mg) if required, 30 to 60 minutes after initial dosage, giving consideration to previous dose pharmacokinetics, and thereafter only as needed. In high-risk patients (e.g., elderly, debili-

tated, presence of respiratory disease, etc.) and or in patients where other CNS depressants are present, such as in the immediate postoperative period, the dose should be reduced by approximately one-half. Extra caution should be exercised with the intravenous route of administration, particularly with the initial dose.

Occasionally, it may be necessary to administer single doses of up to 0.6 mg depending on the severity of the pain and the response of the patient. This dose should only be given I.M. and only to patients who are not in a high risk category (see WARNINGS and PRECAUTIONS). At this time, there are insufficient data to recommend single doses greater than 0.6 mg for long-term use.

Parenteral drug products should be inspected visually for particulate matter and discoloration prior to administration, whenever solution and container permit.

HOW SUPPLIED
Buprenex (buprenorphine hydrochloride) is supplied in clear glass snap-ampuls of 1 ml (0.3 mg buprenorphine).
NDC 12496-0757-1
Avoid excessive heat (over 104°F or 40°C). Protect from prolonged exposure to light.

CAUTION
Federal law prohibits dispensing without prescription.
Manufactured by:
Reckitt & Colman Products,
Hull, England HU8 7DS.

Distributed by:
Reckitt & Colman Pharmaceuticals Inc.,
Richmond, VA 23235.
Buprenex® is a trademark of Reckitt & Colman (Overseas) Limited.
REVISED NOVEMBER 1987

562647

Shown in Product Identification Section, page 424

Reed & Carnrick
DIVISION OF BLOCK DRUG COMPANY, INC
257 CORNELISON AVENUE
JERSEY CITY, NJ 07302-9988

COLYTE® and COLYTE®-FLAVORED ℞
(PEG-3350 & Electrolytes) For Oral Solution
For Gastrointestinal Lavage

DESCRIPTION
COLYTE® and COLYTE®-FLAVORED are colon lavage preparations provided as water-soluble components for solution. In solution each COLYTE® and COLYTE®-FLAVORED preparation delivers the following, in grams per liter.

Polyethylene glycol 3350	60.00
Sodium chloride	1.46
Potassium chloride	0.745
Sodium bicarbonate	1.68
Sodium sulfate	5.68
Flavor ingredients (COLYTE®-FLAVORED)	0.483

When dissolved in sufficient water to make 4 liters, the final solution contains 125 mEq/L sodium, 10 mEq/L potassium, 20 mEq/L bicarbonate, 80 mEq/L sulfate, 35 mEq/L chloride and 18 mEq/L polyethylene glycol 3350. The reconstituted solution is isosmotic and has a mildly salty taste. COLYTE® and COLYTE®-FLAVORED are administered orally or via nasogastric tube.

CLINICAL PHARMACOLOGY
COYLTE® and COLYTE®-FLAVORED cleanse the bowel by induction of diarrhea. The osmotic activity of Polyethylene Glycol 3350, in combination with the electrolyte concentration, results in virtually no net absorption or excretion of ions or water. Accordingly, large volumes may be administered without significant changes in fluid and electrolyte balance.

INDICATIONS AND USAGE
COLYTE® and COLYTE®-FLAVORED are indicated for bowel cleansing prior to colonoscopy or barium enema X-ray examination.

CONTRAINDICATIONS
COLYTE® and COLYTE®-FLAVORED are contraindicated in patients with ileus, gastric retention, gastrointestinal obstruction, bowel perforation, toxic colitis and toxic megacolon.

WARNINGS
No additional ingredients (e.g., flavorings) should be added to the solution. COLYTE® and COLYTE®-FLAVORED should be used with caution in patients with severe ulcerative colitis.

PRECAUTIONS
General: Patients with impaired gag reflex, unconscious or semiconscious patients and patients prone to regurgitation or aspiration should be observed during the administration of COLYTE® or COLYTE®-FLAVORED, especially if it is administered via nasogastric tube.
If gastrointestinal obstruction or perforation is suspected appropriate studies should be performed to rule out these conditions before administration of COLYTE® or COLYTE®-FLAVORED.

INFORMATION FOR PATIENTS
COLYTE® and COLYTE®-FLAVORED (PEG-3350 & Electrolytes) for Oral Solution produce a watery stool which cleanses the bowel prior to examination.
For best results, no solid food should be ingested during the 3 to 4 hour period prior to the initiation of COLYTE® or COLYTE®-FLAVORED administration. In no case should solid foods be eaten within 2 hours of drinking COLYTE® or COLYTE®-FLAVORED.
The rate of administration is 240 ml (8 fl. oz.) every 10 minutes. Rapid drinking of each portion is preferred rather than drinking small amounts continuously. The first bowel movement should occur approximately one hour after the start of COLYTE® or COLYTE®-FLAVORED administration. Administration of COLYTE® or COLYTE®-FLAVORED should be continued until the watery stool is clear and free of solid matter. This normally requires the consumption of approximately 3–4 liters (3–4 quarts), although more or less may be required in some patients. The unused portion should be discarded.

DRUG INTERACTIONS
Oral medication administered within one hour of the start of administration of COLYTE® or COLYTE®-FLAVORED may be flushed from the gastrointestinal tract and not absorbed.

CARCINOGENESIS, MUTAGENESIS, IMPAIRMENT OF FERTILITY
Studies to evaluate carcinogenic or mutagenic potential or potential to adversely affect male or female fertility have not been performed.

PREGNANCY
Category C. Animal reproduction studies have not been conducted with COLYTE® or COLYTE®-FLAVORED, and it is not known whether COLYTE® or COLYTE®-FLAVORED can affect reproductive capacity or harm the fetus when administered to a pregnant patient. COLYTE® or COLYTE®-FLAVORED should be given to a pregnant patient only if clearly needed.

PEDIATRIC USE
Safety and effectiveness in children have not been established.

ADVERSE REACTIONS
Nausea, abdominal fullness and bloating are the most frequent adverse reactions, occurring in up to 50% of patients. Abdominal cramps, vomiting and anal irritation occur less frequently. These adverse reactions are transient. Isolated cases of urticaria, rhinorrhea and dermatitis have been reported which may represent allergic reactions.

DOSAGE AND ADMINISTRATION
COLYTE® or COLYTE®-FLAVORED can be administered orally or by nasogastric tube. Patients should fast at least 3 hours prior to administration. A one hour waiting period after the appearance of clear liquid stool should be allowed prior to examination to complete bowel evacuation. No foods except clear liquids should be permitted prior to examination after COLYTE® or COLYTE®-FLAVORED administration.

ORAL
The recommended adult oral dose is 240 ml (8 fl. oz.) every 10 minutes (see INFORMATION FOR PATIENTS). Lavage is complete when fecal discharge is clear. Lavage is usually complete after the ingestion of 3–4 liters.

NASOGASTRIC TUBE
COLYTE® or COLYTE®-FLAVORED (PEG-3350 & Electrolytes For Oral Solution) administered at a rate of 20–30 ml per minute (1.2–1.8 L/hour).

PREPARATION OF COLYTE® OR COLYTE®-FLAVORED SOLUTION:
4 Liter: Add tap water to FILL line. Replace cap tightly and mix or shake well until all ingredients have dissolved. (No additional ingredients, e.g., flavoring, should be added to the solution.)
One Gallon: The preparation is made by dissolving the contents of the bottle in a food-grade container, in a sufficient quantity of water to produce the final volume according to package directions. (No additional ingredients, e.g., flavoring, should be added to the solution.) Mix well.

HOW SUPPLIED
COLYTE® and COLYTE®-FLAVORED are supplied in 4 liter (NDC 0021-4401-23 and NDC 0021-4403-05, respectively) and 18 oz. (NDC 0021-4401-49 and NDC 0021-4403-13, respectively) bottles in powdered form, for oral administration as a solution. Each contains the following:
4 liter, (NDC 0021-4401-23 and NDC 0021-4403-05): polyethylene glycol 3350 240 g, sodium chloride 5.84 g, potassium chloride 2.98 g, sodium bicarbonate 6.72 g, sodium sulfate (anhydrous) 22.72 g, flavor ingredients (COLYTE®-FLAVORED only) 1.93 g, in a bottle.
18 oz., (NDC 0021-4401-49 and NDC 0021-4403-13): polyethylene glycol 3350 227.10 g, sodium chloride 5.53 g, potassium chloride 2.82 g, sodium bicarbonate 6.36 g, sodium sulfate (anhydrous) 21.50 g, flavor ingredients (COLYTE®-FLAVORED only) 1.83 g, in a bottle.
Store powder at controlled room temperature 15°–30°C (59°–86°F).

CAUTION
Federal law prohibits dispensing without a prescription.
KEEP RECONSTITUTED SOLUTION REFRIGERATED. USE WITHIN 48 HOURS. DISCARD UNUSED PORTION.
NOVEMBER 1991

Reed & Carnrick
Division of Block Drug Company, Inc.
Jersey City, New Jersey 07302-9988
© 1991 Block Drug Company, Inc.
Shown in Product Identification Section, page 424

CORTIFOAM® ℞
(hydrocortisone acetate) 10%
Rectal Foam

DESCRIPTION
Contains hydrocortisone acetate 10% as the sole active ingredient in 20 g of a foam containing propylene glycol, emulsifying wax, polyoxyethylene-10-stearyl ether, cetyl alcohol, methylparaben and propylparaben, trolamine, purified water and inert propellants, dichlorodifluoromethane and dichlorotetrafluoroethane.
Each application delivers approximately 900 mg of foam containing 80 mg of hydrocortisone (90 mg of hydrocortisone acetate).
Molecular weight: Hydrocortisone acetate 404.50
Solubility of hydrocortisone acetate in water: 1 mg/100 ml
Chemical name: Pregn-4-ene-3,20-dione, 21-(acetyloxy)-11,17-dihydroxy-, (11β)-.

CLINICAL PHARMACOLOGY
CORTIFOAM provides effective topical administration of an anti-inflammatory corticosteroid as adjunctive therapy of ulcerative proctitis.

INDICATIONS
CORTIFOAM is indicated as adjunctive therapy in the topical treatment of ulcerative proctitis of the distal portion of the rectum in patients who cannot retain hydrocortisone or other corticosteroid enemas. Direct observations of methylene blue-containing foam have shown staining about 10 centimeters into the rectum.

CONTRAINDICATIONS
Local contraindications to the use of intrarectal steroids include obstruction, abscess, perforation, peritonitis, fresh intestinal anastomoses, extensive fistulas and sinus tracts. Tuberculosis (active, latent or questionably healed), ocular herpes simplex and acute psychosis are usually considered absolute contraindications to the use of corticosteroids. Relative contraindications include active peptic ulcer, acute glomerulonephritis, myasthenia gravis, osteoporosis, diverticulitis, thrombophlebitis, psychic disturbances, pregnancy, diabetes, hyperthyroidism, acute coronary disease, hypertension, limited cardiac reserve, and local or systemic infections, including fungal or exanthematous diseases. Where these conditions exist, the expected benefits from steroid therapy must be weighed against the risks involved in its use. Pregnancy is a relative contraindication to corticosteroids, particularly during third trimester. If corticosteroids must be administered in pregnancy, watch newborn infant closely for signs of hypoadrenalism, and administer appropriate therapy if needed.

Continued on next page

Reed & Carnrick—Cont.

WARNINGS

Do not insert any part of the aerosol container into the anus. Contents of the container are under pressure, but not flammable. Do not burn or puncture the aerosol container. Store at room temperature and not over 120° F. Because CORTIFOAM is not expelled, systemic hydrocortisone absorption may be greater from CORTIFOAM than from corticosteroid enema formulations. If there is not evidence of clinical or proctologic improvement within two or three weeks after starting CORTIFOAM therapy, or if the patient's condition worsens, discontinue the drug.

Children who are on immunosuppressant drugs are more susceptible to infections than healthy children. Chickenpox and measles, for example, can have a more serious or even fatal course in children on immunosuppressant corticosteroids. In such children, or in adults who have not had these diseases, particular care should be taken to avoid exposure. If exposed, therapy with varicella zoster immune globulin (VZIG) or pooled intravenous immunoglobulin (IVIG), as appropriate, may be indicated. If chickenpox develops, treatment with antiviral agents may be considered.

PRECAUTIONS

Steroid therapy should be administered with caution in patients with severe ulcerative disease because these patients are predisposed to perforation of the bowel wall. Where surgery is imminent, it is hazardous to wait more than a few days for a satisfactory response to medical treatment. General precautions common to all corticosteroid therapy should be observed during treatment with CORTIFOAM. These include gradual withdrawal of therapy to allow for possible adrenal insufficiency and awareness to possible growth suppression in children. Patients should be kept under close observation, for, as with all drugs, rare individuals may react unfavorably under certain conditions. If severe reactions or idiosyncrasies occur, steroids should be discontinued immediately and appropriate measures instituted. Do not employ in immediate or early postoperative period following ileorectostomy.

Information for patients: Patients who are on immunosuppressant doses of corticosteroids should be warned to avoid exposure to chickenpox or measles and, if exposed, to obtain medical advice.

ADVERSE REACTIONS

Corticosteroid therapy may produce side effects which include moon face, fluid retention, excessive appetite and weight gain, abnormal fat deposits, mental symptoms, hypertrichosis, acne, ecchymosis, increased sweating, pigmentation, dry scaly skin, thinning scalp hair, thrombophlebitis, decreased resistance to infection, negative nitrogen balance with delayed bone and wound healing, menstrual disorders, neuropathy, peptic ulcer, decreased glucose tolerance, hypopotassemia, adrenal insufficiency, necrotizing angiitis, hypertension, pancreatitis and increased intraocular pressure. In children, suppression of growth may occur. Increased intracranial pressure may occur and possibly account for headache, insomnia and fatigue. Subcapsular cataracts may result from prolonged usage. Long-term use of all corticosteroids results in catabolic effects characterized by negative protein and calcium balance. Osteoporosis, spontaneous fractures and aseptic necrosis of the hip and humerus may occur as part of this catabolic phenomenon. Where hypopotassemia and other symptoms associated with fluid and electrolyte imbalance call for potassium supplementation and salt poor or salt-free diets, these may be instituted and are compatible with diet requirements for ulcerative proctitis.

ADMINISTRATION AND DOSAGE

NOTE: SEE INNER PACKAGE FOR FULL DIRECTIONS FOR USE.)

Usual dose is one applicatorful once or twice daily for two or three weeks, and every second day thereafter, administered rectally. The patient direction package with the applicator describes how to use the aerosol container and applicator. Satisfactory response usually occurs within five to seven days marked by a decrease in symptoms. Symptomatic improvement in ulcerative proctitis should not be used as the sole criterion for evaluating efficacy. Sigmoidoscopy is also recommended to judge dosage adjustment, duration of therapy and rate of improvement.

DIRECTIONS FOR USE

1) Shake foam container vigorously before use. Hold container upright and insert into the opening of the tip of the applicator. **Be sure applicator plunger is drawn all the way out.** Container must be held upright to obtain proper flow of medication. 2) To fill, press down slowly on container cap. When foam reaches fill line in the applicator, it is ready for use. **Caution:** The aerosol container should never be inserted directly into the anus. 3) Remove applicator from container. Allow some foam to remain on the applicator tip. Hold applicator by barrel and gently insert tip into the anus. With applicator in place, push plunger in order to expel foam, then withdraw applicator. (Applicator parts should be pulled apart for thorough cleaning with warm water.)

CAUTION

Federal law prohibits dispensing without prescription.

HOW SUPPLIED

CORTIFOAM (NDC 0021-0695-20) is supplied in an aerosol container with a special rectal applicator. Each applicator delivers approximately 900 mg of foam containing approximately 80 mg of hydrocortisone as 90 mg of hydrocortisone acetate. The aerosol container will deliver a minimum of 14 applications.

Store upright at controlled room temperature 15°-30°C (59°-86°F).

December 1991
Reed & Carnrick
Division of Block Drug Company, Inc.
Jersey City, New Jersey 07302-9988

Shown in Product Identification Section, page 424

DILATRATE®-SR ℞

[*dī'lă-trāt*]
(isosorbide dinitrate)
Sustained Release Capsules
40 mg

DESCRIPTION

Isosorbide dinitrate, an organic nitrate, is a vasodilator with effects on both arteries and veins. Isosorbide dinitrate is available as a 40 mg sustained release capsule. The chemical name for isosorbide dinitrate is D-Glucitol, 1,4:3,6-dianhydro, dinitrate, and the compound has the following structural formula:

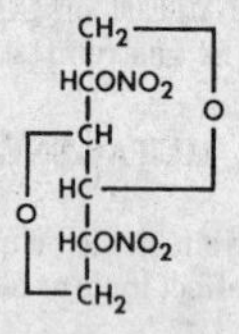

Molecular Weight: 236.14

Isosorbide dinitrate is a white, crystalline, odorless compound which is stable in air and in solution, has a melting point of 70°C and has an optical rotation of +134° (c=1.0, alcohol, 20°C). Isosorbide dinitrate is freely soluble in organic solvents such as acetone, alcohol, and ether, but is only sparingly soluble in water.

CLINICAL PHARMACOLOGY

The principal pharmacological action of isosorbide dinitrate is relaxation of vascular smooth muscle, producing a vasodilatory effect on both peripheral arteries and veins, with predominant effects on the latter. Dilation of the postcapillary vessels, including large veins, promotes peripheral pooling of blood and decreases venous return to the heart, thereby reducing left-ventricular end-diastolic pressure (preload). Arteriolar relaxation reduces systemic vascular resistance and arterial pressure (after-load).

The mechanism by which isosorbide dinitrate relieves angina pectoris is not fully understood. Myocardial oxygen consumption or demand (as measured by the pressure-rate product, tension-time index, and stroke work index) is decreased by both the arterial and venous effects of isosorbide dinitrate and, presumably, a more favorable supply-demand ratio is achieved. While the large epicardial coronary arteries are also dilated by isosorbide dinitrate, the extent to which this contributes to relief of exertional angina is unclear.

Therapeutic doses of isosorbide dinitrate may reduce systolic, diastolic, and mean arterial blood pressures, especially in the upright posture. Effective coronary perfusion is usually maintained. The decrease in systemic blood pressure may result in reflex tachycardia, an effect which results in an unfavorable influence on myocardial oxygen demand. Hemodynamic studies indicate that isosorbide dinitrate may reduce the abnormally elevated left ventricular end-diastolic and pulmonary capillary wedge pressures that occur during an acute episode of angina pectoris.

Isosorbide dinitrate is metabolized by enzymatic denitration to the intermediate products isosorbide-2-mononitrate and isosorbide-5-mononitrate. Both metabolites have biological activity, especially the 5-mononitrate which is also the principal metabolite. The liver is a principal site of metabolism and isosorbide dinitrate is subject to a large first pass effect. The systemic clearance of the drug following intravenous infusion is about 3.4 liters/min. Since the clearance exceeds hepatic blood flow, considerable extra hepatic metabolism must also occur.

The average bioavailability of isosorbide dinitrate is 59 and 22 percent following sublingual and oral administration, respectively. The terminal half-life is about 20 minutes, 60 minutes, and 4 hours following IV, sublingual, and oral administration, respectively. The dependence of half-life on the route of administration is not understood. Over limited ranges of IV dosing, the pharmacokinetics of isosorbide dinitrate appear linear. However, both the 2- and 5-mononitrate metabolites have been shown to decrease the rate of disappearance of the dinitrate from the blood and the half-lives of isosorbide-5-mononitrate and isosorbide-2-mononitrate range from 4.0–5.6 and 1.5–3.1 hours, respectively.

The pharmacokinetics and/or bioavailability of isosorbide dinitrate during multiple dosing have not been well-studied. Because the metabolites influence the clearance of isosorbide dinitrate, prediction of blood levels of parent compound or metabolites from single-dose studies is uncertain.

INDICATIONS AND USAGE

Isosorbide dinitrate is indicated for the treatment and prevention of angina pectoris. Controlled clinical trials have demonstrated that the sublingual, chewable, immediate release, and controlled-release oral dosage forms of isosorbide dinitrate are effective in improving exercise tolerance in patients with angina pectoris. When single sublingual or chewable doses (5mg) of isosorbide dinitrate were administered prophylactically to patients with angina pectoris in various clinical studies, duration of exercise until chest pain or fatigue was significantly improved for at least 45 minutes (and as long as 2 hours in some studies) following dosing. Similar studies after single oral (15 to 120 mg) and oral controlled-released (40 to 80 mg) doses of isosorbide dinitrate have shown significant improvement in exercise tolerance for up to 8 hours following dosing. The exercise electrocardiographic evidence suggests that improved exercise tolerance with isosorbide dinitrate is not at the expense of greater myocardial ischemia. All dosage forms of isosorbide dinitrate may therefore be used prophylactically to decrease frequency and severity of anginal attacks and can be expected to decrease the need for sublingual nitroglycerin.

The sublingual and chewable forms of the drug are indicated for acute prophylaxis of angina pectoris when taken a few minutes before situations likely to provoke anginal attacks. Because of a slower onset of effect, the oral forms of isosorbide dinitrate are not indicated for acute prophylaxis.

In controlled clinical trials chewable and sublingual isosorbide dinitrate were effective in relieving an acute attack of angina pectoris. Relief occurred with a mean time of 2.9 and 3.4 minutes (chewable and sublingual, respectively) compared to relief of angina with a mean time of 1.9 minutes following sublingual nitroglycerin. Because of the more rapid relief of chest pain with sublingual nitroglycerin, the use of sublingual or chewable isosorbide dinitrate for aborting an acute anginal attack should be limited to patients intolerant or unresponsive to sublingual nitroglycerin.

CONTRAINDICATIONS

Isosorbide dinitrate is contraindicated in patients who have shown purported hypersensitivity or idiosyncrasy to it or other nitrates or nitrites.

WARNINGS

The benefits of isosorbide dinitrate during the early days of an acute myocardial infarction have not been established. If one elects to use organic nitrates in early infarction, hemodynamic monitoring and frequent clinical assessment should be used because of the potential deleterious effects of hypotension.

PRECAUTIONS

General: Severe hypotensive response, particularly with upright posture, may occur with even small doses of isosorbide dinitrate. The drug should therefore be used with caution in subjects who may have blood volume depletion from diuretic therapy or in subjects who have low systolic blood pressure (e.g., below 90 mm Hg). Paradoxical bradycardia and increased angina pectoris may accompany nitrate-induced hypotension.

Nitrate therapy may aggravate the angina caused by hypertrophic cardiomyopathy. Tolerance to this drug and cross-tolerance to other nitrates and nitrites may occur.

Marked symptomatic, orthostatic hypotension has been reported when calcium channel blockers and organic nitrates were used in combination. Dose adjustment of either class of agents may be necessary.

Tolerance to the vascular and antianginal effects of isosorbide dinitrate or nitroglycerin has been demonstrated in clinical trials, experience through occupational exposure, and in isolated tissue experiments in the laboratory. The importance of tolerance to the appropriate use of isosorbide dinitrate in the management of patients with angina pectoris has not been determined. However, one clinical trial using treadmill exercise tolerance (as an endpoint) found an 8 hour duration of action of oral isosorbide dinitrate following the first dose (after a 2 week placebo washout) and only a 2 hour duration of effect of the same dose after 1 week of repetitive dosing at conventional dosing intervals. On the other hand, several trials have been able to differentiate isosorbide dinitrate from placebo after 4 weeks of therapy,

and in open trials an effect seems detectable for as long as several months.

Tolerance clearly occurs in industrial workers continuously exposed to nitroglycerin. Moreover, physical dependence also occurs since chest pain, acute myocardial infarction, and even sudden death have occurred during temporary withdrawal of nitroglycerin from the workers. In clinical trials in angina patients, there are reports of anginal attacks being more easily provoked and of rebound in the hemodynamic effects soon after nitrate withdrawal. The relative importance of these observations to the routine, clinical use of isosorbide dinitrate is not known. However, it seems prudent to gradually withdraw patients from isosorbide dinitrate when the therapy is being terminated, rather than stopping the drug abruptly.

Information for Patients: Headache may occur during initial therapy with isosorbide dinitrate. Headache is usually relieved by the use of standard headache remedies, or by lowering the dose, and tends to disappear after the first week or two of use.

Drug Interactions: Alcohol may enhance any marked sensitivity to the hypotensive effect of nitrates. Isosorbide dinitrate acts directly on vascular smooth muscle; therefore, any other agent that depends on vascular smooth muscle as the final common path can be expected to have decreased or increased effect depending on the agent.

Carcinogenesis, Mutagenesis, Impairment of Fertility: No long-term studies in animals have been performed to evaluate the carcinogenic potential of this drug. A modified two-litter reproduction study in rats fed isosorbide dinitrate at 25 or 100 mg/kg/day did not reveal any effects on fertility or gestation or any remarkable growth pathology in any parent or offspring fed isosorbide dinitrate as compared with rats fed a basal controlled diet.

Pregnancy Category C: Isosorbide dinitrate has been shown to cause a dose-related increase in embryotoxicity (increase in mummified pups) in rabbits at oral doses 35 and 150 times the maximum recommended human daily dose. There are no adequate and well-controlled studies in pregnant women. Isosorbide dinitrate should be used during pregnancy only if the potential benefit justifies the potential risk to the fetus.

Nursing Mothers: It is not known whether this drug is excreted in human milk. Because many drugs are excreted in human milk, caution should be exercised when isosorbide dinitrate is administered to a nursing woman.

Pediatric Use: The safety and effectiveness of isosorbide dinitrate in children has not been established.

ADVERSE REACTIONS

Adverse reactions, particularly headache and hypotension, are dose related. In clinical trials at various doses, the following have been observed.

Headache is the most common (reported incidence varies widely, apparently being dose related, with an average occurrence of about 25%) adverse reaction and may be severe and persistent. Cutaneous vasodilation wth flushing may occur. Transient episodes of dizziness and weakness, as well as other signs of cerebral ischemia associated with postural hypotension, may occasionally develop (the incidence of reported symptomatic hypotension ranges from 2% to 36%). An occasional individual will exhibit marked sensitivity to the hypotensive effects of nitrates and severe responses (nausea, vomiting, weakness, restlessness, pallor, perspiration, and collapse) may occur even with the usual therapeutic dose. Drug rash and/or exfoliative dermatitis may occasionally occur. Nausea and vomiting appear to be uncommon.

OVERDOSAGE

Signs and Symptoms: These may include the following: a prompt fall in blood pressure, persistent and throbbing headache, vertigo, palpitation, visual disturbances, flushed and perspiring skin (later becoming cold and cyanotic), nausea and vomiting (possibly with colic and even bloody diarrhea), syncope (especially in the upright position), methemoglobinemia with cyanosis and anoxia, initial hyperpnea, dyspnea and slow breathing, slow pulse (dicrotic and intermittent), heart block, increased intracranial pressure with cerebral symptoms of confusion and moderate fever, paralysis and coma followed by clonic convulsions and possibly death due to circulatory collapse.

It is not known what dose of the drug is associated with symptoms of overdosing or what dose of the drug would be life-threatening. The acute oral LD50 of isosorbide dinitrate in rats was found to be approximately 1100 mg/kg of body weight. These animal experiments indicate that approximately 500 times the usual therapeutic dose would be required to produce such toxic symptoms in humans. It is not known whether the drug is dialyzable.

Treatment of Overdosage: Prompt removal of the ingested material by gastric lavage is reasonable but not documented to be useful. Keep the patient recumbent in a shock position and comfortably warm. Passive movements of the extremities may aid venous return. Administer oxygen and artificial respiration if necessary. If methemoglobinemia is present, administer methylene blue (1% solution), 1 to 2 mg/kg intravenously.

Methemoglobin: Case reports of clinically significant methemoglobinemia are rare at conventional doses of organic nitrates. The formation of methemoglobin is dose related and in the case of genetic abnormalities of hemoglobin that favor methemoglobin formation, even conventional doses of organic nitrate could produce harmful concentrations of methemoglobin.

WARNING

Epinephrine is ineffective in reversing the severe hypotensive events associated with overdose. It and related compounds are contraindicated in this situation.

DOSAGE AND ADMINISTRATION

Because of a slower onset of effect, the oral forms of isosorbide dinitrate are not indicated for acute prophylaxis or for the treament of acute anginal attacks.

Isosorbide dinitrate should be titrated upward until angina is relieved or side effects limit the dose. In ambulatory patients, the magnitude of the incremental dose increase should be guided by measurements of standing blood pressure.

For the treatment of chronic stable angina pectoris, the usual starting dose for controlled-release forms is 40 mg. For maintenance therapy, oral controlled-release doses of 40 to 80 mg given every 8 to 12 hours is generally recommended. The extent to which development of tolerance should modify the dosage program has not been defined. The oral controlled release forms of isosorbide dinitrate should not be chewed.

HOW SUPPLIED

Bottles of 60 and 100 opaque pink and colorless capsules.

STORAGE

Store at controlled room temperature 15°–30°C (59°–86°F) in a dry place.

WARNING

KEEP OUT OF REACH OF CHILDREN.

CAUTION

Federal law prohibits dispensing without prescription.

Manufactured for
Reed & Carnrick
Division of Block Drug Company, Inc.
Jersey City, N.J. 07302-9988
by Eon Labs Manufacturing, Inc.
Laurelton, NY 11413

Date of Revision
May 1992

Shown in Product Identification Section, page 424

EPIFOAM® ℞

topical aerosol
(hydrocortisone acetate 1% and pramoxine hydrochloride 1%)

DESCRIPTION

A topical corticosteroid in an aerosol foam containing hydrocortisone acetate 1% and pramoxine hydrochloride 1% in a base containing: propylene glycol, cetyl alcohol, glyceryl stearate, PEG-100 stearate, laureth-23, polyoxyl-40 stearate, methylparaben, propylparaben, trolamine or hydrochloric acid to adjust pH, purified water and propellants (inert): butane and propane.

EPIFOAM contains a synthetic steroid used as an anti-inflammatory and antipruritic agent, and a local anesthetic.

Hydrocortisone acetate

Molecular weight: 404.50. Solubility of hydrocortisone acetate in water: 1 mg/100 ml. Chemical name: Pregn-4-ene-3,20-dione, 21-(acetyloxy)-11, 17-dihydroxy-, (11β).

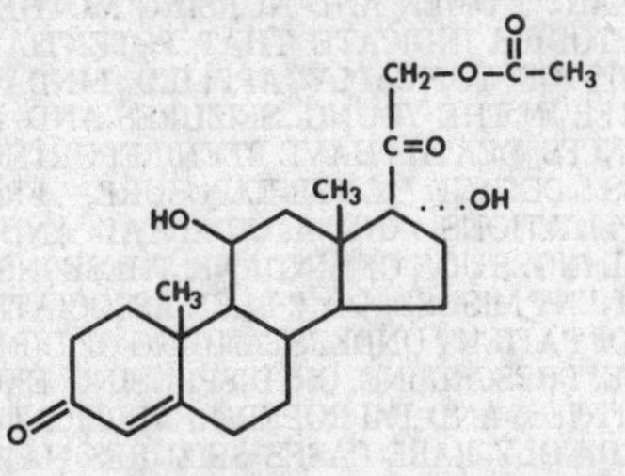

Pramoxine hydrochloride

Molecular weight: 329.87. Pramoxine hydrochloride is freely soluble in water. Chemical name: Morpholine, 4-[3-(4-butoxyphenoxy) propyl]-, hydrochloride, 4-[3-(p-butoxyphenoxy)-propyl] morpholine hydrochloride.

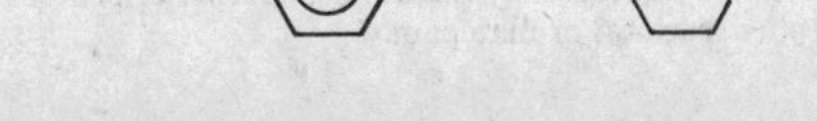

CLINICAL PHARMACOLOGY

Topical corticosteroids share anti-inflammatory, antipruritic and vascoconstrictive actions.

The mechanism of anti-inflammatory activity of the topical corticosteroids is unclear. Various laboratory methods, including vasoconstrictor assays, are used to compare and predict potencies and/or clinical efficacies of the topical corticosteroids. There is some evidence to suggest that a recognizable correlation exists between vasoconstrictor potency and therapeutic efficacy in man.

Pramoxine hydrochloride: A surface or local anesthetic which is not chemically related to the "caine" types of local anesthetics. Its unique chemical structure is likely to minimize the danger of cross-sensitivity reactions in patients allergic to other local anesthetics.

Pharmacokinetics: The extent of percutaneous absorption of topical corticosteroids is determined by many factors including the vehicle, the integrity of the epidermal barrier, and the use of occlusive dressings.

Topical corticosteroids can be absorbed from normal intact skin. Inflammation and/or disease processes in the skin increase the percutaneous absorption of topical corticosteroids. Occlusive dressings substantially increase the percutaneous absorption of topical corticosteroids. Thus, occlusive dressings may be a valuable therapeutic adjunct for treatment of resistant dermatoses. (See DOSAGE AND ADMINISTRATION.)

Once absorbed through the skin, topical corticosteroids are handled through pharmacokinetic pathways similar to systemically administered corticosteroids. Corticosteroids are bound to plasma proteins in varying degrees. Corticosteroids are metabolized primarily in the liver and are then excreted by the kidneys. Some of the topical corticosteroids and their metabolites are also excreted in the bile.

INDICATIONS AND USAGE

Topical corticosteroids are indicated for the relief of the inflammatory and pruritic manifestations of corticosteroid-responsive dermatoses.

CONTRAINDICATIONS

Topical corticosteroid products are contraindicated in those patients with a history of hypersensitivity to any of the components of the preparation.

WARNINGS

Not for prolonged use. If redness, pain, irritation or swelling persists, discontinue use and consult a physician. Contents of the container are under pressure, but not flammable. Do not burn or puncture the aerosol container. Store at temperatures below 120°F. Keep this and all medicines out of the reach of children.

PRECAUTIONS

General: Systemic absorption of topical corticosteroids has produced reversible hypothalamic-pituitary-adrenal (HPA) axis suppression, manifestations of Cushing's syndrome, hyperglycemia and glucosuria in some patients.

Conditions which augment systemic absorption include the application of the more potent steroids, use over large surface areas, prolonged use and the addition of occlusive dressings.

Therefore, patients receiving a large dose of a potent topical steroid applied to a large surface area or under an occlusive dressing should be evaluated periodically for evidence of HPA axis suppression by using the urinary free cortisol and ACTH stimulation tests. If HPA axis suppression is noted, an attempt should be made to withdraw the drug to reduce the frequency of application, or to substitute a less potent steroid.

Recovery of HPA axis function is generally prompt and complete upon discontinuation of the drug. Infrequently, signs and symptoms of steroid withdrawal may occur, requiring supplemental systemic corticosteroids.

In children, absorption may result in higher blood levels and thus more susceptibility to systemic toxicity. (See PRECAUTIONS—Pediatric Use.)

If irritation develops, topical corticosteroids should be discontinued and appropriate therapy instituted.

In the presence of dermatological infections, the use of an appropriate antifungal or antibacterial agent should be instituted. If a favorable response does not occur promptly, the corticosteroid should be discontinued until the infection has been adequately controlled.

Information for the Patient: Patients using topical corticosteroids should receive the following information and instructions:

1. This medication is to be used as directed by the physician. It is for external use only. Avoid contact with the eyes.
2. Do not use this medication for any disorder other than for which it has been prescribed.
3. The treated skin area should not be bandaged or otherwise covered or wrapped as to be occlusive unless directed by the physician.

Continued on next page

Reed & Carnrick—Cont.

4. Report any signs of local adverse reactions especially under occlusive dressings.
5. Do not use any tight fitting diapers or plastic pants on a child being treated in the diaper area, as these garments may constitute occlusive dressings.

Laboratory Tests: The following test may be helpful in evaluating the HPA axis suppression:
Urinary free cortisol test
ACTH stimulation test

Carcinogenesis, Mutagenesis, and Impairment of Fertility: Long-term animal studies have not been performed to evaluate carcinogenic potential or the effect on fertility of topical corticosteroids.

Studies to determine mutagenicity with prednisolone and hydrocortisone have revealed negative results.

Pregnancy Category C: Corticosteroids are generally teratogenic in laboratory animals when administered systemically at relatively low dosage levels. The more potent corticosteroids have been shown to be teratogenic after dermal application in laboratory animals. There are no adequate and well-controlled studies in pregnant women of teratogenic effects from topically applied corticosteroids. Therefore, topical corticosteroids should be used during pregnancy only if the potential benefit justifies the potential risk to the fetus. Drugs of this class should not be used extensively on pregnant patients, in large amounts, or for prolonged periods of time.

Nursing Mothers: It is not known whether topical administration of corticosteroids could result in sufficient systemic absorption to produce detectable quantities in breast milk. Systemically administered corticosteroids are secreted into breast milk in quantities not likely to have a deleterious effect on the infant. Caution should be exercised when any topical corticosteroids are administered to a nursing woman.

Pediatric Use: *Pediatric patients may demonstrate greater susceptibility to topical corticosteroid-induced HPA axis suppression and Cushing's syndrome than mature patients because of a larger skin surface area to body weight ratio.*

Hypothalamic-pituitary-adrenal (HPA) axis suppression, Cushing's syndrome and intracranial hypertension have been reported in children receiving topical corticosteroids. Manifestations of adrenal suppression in children include linear growth retardation, delayed weight gain, low plasma cortisone levels and absence of response to ACTH stimulation. Manifestations of intracranial hypertension include bulging fontanelles, headaches and bilateral papilledema. Administration of topical corticosteroids to children should be limited to the least amount compatible with an effective therapeutic regimen. Chronic corticosteroid therapy may interfere with the growth and development of children.

ADVERSE REACTIONS

The following local adverse reactions are reported infrequently with topical corticosteroids, but may occur more frequently with the use of occlusive dressings. These reactions are listed in an approximately decreasing order of occurrence:
Burning
Itching
Irritation
Dryness
Folliculitis
Hypertrichosis
Acneiform eruptions
Hypopigmentation
Perioral dermatitis
Allergic contact dermatitis
Maceration of the skin
Secondary infection
Skin atrophy
Striae
Miliaria

OVERDOSAGE

Topically applied corticosteroids can be absorbed in sufficient amounts to produce systemic effects. (See PRECAUTIONS.)

DOSAGE AND ADMINISTRATION

Apply to affected area 3 or 4 times daily.
(NOTE: Refer to the enclosed Directions for Use.):

DIRECTIONS FOR USE

1. Shake foam container vigorously before use.
2. Hold container upright and apply only a small amount directly to affected areas. Alternatively, dispense a small amount onto a pad and apply to affected areas.
3. The container and cap should be disassembled and rinsed with warm water after use.
NOTE: The aerosol container should never be inserted into the vagina or anus.

HOW SUPPLIED

EPIFOAM® topical aerosol (hydrocortisone acetate 1% and pramoxine hydrochloride 1%) (NDC-0021-0740-10) available in 10g pressurized cans.
Store upright at controlled room temperature 15°–30°C (59°–86°F).

CAUTION

FEDERAL LAW PROHIBITS DISPENSING WITHOUT PRESCRIPTION.
Revised December 1991
Reed & Carnrick
Division of Block Drug Company, Inc.
Jersey City, N.J. 07302-9988
Shown in Product Identification Section, page 424

KWELL® Cream　　　　　　　　　　　　　　　　℞
(lindane) 1%

DESCRIPTION

KWELL Cream (lindane) 1% is an ectoparasiticide and ovicide effective against Sarcoptes scabiei (scabies) and their ova. Inert ingredients: 99% in a pleasantly scented water dispersible cream containing stearic acid, glycerin, lanolin, 2-amino-2-methyl-1-propanol, perfume and purified water. Lindane, which is the highly purified gamma isomer of 1, 2, 3, 4, 5, 6, hexachlorocyclohexane, has the following chemical structure.

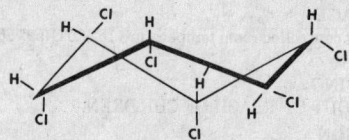

CLINICAL PHARMACOLOGY

KWELL Cream exerts its parasiticidal action by being directly absorbed into the parasites and their ova. Feldmann and Maibach[1] reported approximately 10% absorption of a lindane acetone solution applied to the forearm and left in place to 24 hours. Dale, et al[2] reported a blood level of 290ng/ml associated with convulsions following the accidental ingestion of a lindane containing product. Ginsburg[3] found a mean peak blood level of 28ng/ml 6 hours after total body application of KWELL Lotion to scabietic infants and children. The half-life was determined to be 18 hours.

INDICATIONS AND USAGE

KWELL Cream is indicated for the treatment of patients infested with Sarcoptes scabiei (scabies).

CONTRAINDICATIONS

KWELL Cream is contraindicated for premature neonates because their skin may be more permeable and their liver enzymes may not be sufficiently developed. It is also contraindicated for patients with Norwegian (crusted) scabies due to a possible increased absorption. It is also contraindicated for patients with known seizure disorders and for individuals with a known sensitivity to the product or any of its components.

WARNINGS

LINDANE PENETRATES HUMAN SKIN AND HAS THE POTENTIAL FOR CNS TOXICITY (SEE CLINICAL PHARMACOLOGY SECTION). KWELL CREAM SHOULD BE USED ACCORDING TO RECOMMENDED DOSAGE (SEE DIRECTIONS FOR USE) ESPECIALLY ON INFANTS, PREGNANT WOMEN AND NURSING MOTHERS. ANIMAL STUDIES INDICATE THAT POTENTIAL TOXIC EFFECTS OF TOPICALLY APPLIED LINDANE ARE GREATER IN THE YOUNG. SEIZURES AND, IN RARE INSTANCES, DEATHS HAVE BEEN REPORTED AFTER EXCESS DOSAGE, OVER-EXPOSURE, FREQUENT REAPPLICATIONS, AND ACCIDENTAL AND INTENTIONAL INGESTION OF LINDANE. THESE INSTANCES OF PATIENT MISUSE HAVE BEEN ASSOCIATED WITH LACK OF PATIENT UNDERSTANDING OF DIRECTIONS OF USE, PRESCRIBING OR DISPENSING EXCESSIVE QUANTITIES, AND IMPROPER REAPPLICATIONS. IN EXCEEDINGLY RARE CASES SEIZURES HAVE BEEN REPORTED WHEN USED ACCORDING TO DIRECTIONS. NO RESIDUAL EFFECTS OF KWELL® (LINDANE) 1% TREATMENT HAVE BEEN DEMONSTRATED. THEREFORE, THIS PRODUCT SHOULD NOT BE USED TO WARD OFF A POSSIBLE INFESTATION.

If accidental ingestion occurs prompt gastric lavage is indicated. Because oils may enhance absorption, saline rather than oily cathartics should be used. Central nervous excitation can be controlled by the administration of pentobarbital, phenobarbital or diazepam.

PRECAUTIONS

General
Care should be taken to avoid contact with the eyes. If such contact occurs, eyes should be immediately flushed with water. If irritation or sensitization occurs, the patient should be advised to consult a physician.
Geriatric
Dosage may have to be reduced due to the possibility of increased absorption through elderly skin.
Information to Patients
Patients must be instructed on the proper use of this medication, especially as to the amount applied and duration of use. Patient Directions for Use must accompany the product.

LABORATORY TESTS

No laboratory tests are needed for the proper use of this medication.

DRUG INTERACTIONS

Oils may enhance absorption, therefore, simultaneous use of creams, ointments or oils should be avoided.

CARCINOGENESIS

Although no studies have been conducted with KWELL Cream, numerous long term feeding studies have been conducted on mice and rats to evaluate the carcinogenic potential of the technical grade of hexachlorocyclohexane (BHC) as well as the alpha, beta, gamma (lindane) and delta isomers. Both oral and topical applications have been evaluated. Nagasaki, et al[4], Goto et al[5] and Hanada et al[6] found varying amounts of benign and malignant hepatomas associated with BHC and the alpha, delta and epsilon isomers. None reported a carcinogenic potential for lindane. Tumors were found only in the animals which had received the alpha isomer. Weisse and Herbst[7] also evaluated the carcinogenic potential of lindane in mice but could find no evidence of lindane carcinogenicity. The National Cancer Institute[8] also found no evidence of carcinogenicity.

Thorpe and Walker[9] compared beta BHC with lindane, dieldrin, DDT and hexabarbital in mice. Despite the unusually high incidence of tumors in the control group, they concluded that 600 ppm of lindane was associated with a significant increase of hepatoma and thus considered it a tumorigen.

Orr[10] and Kashyap, et al[11] evaluated the carcinogenic potential in mice of topically applied BHC. In neither study was there any evidence of a tumorigenic or carcinogenic potential associated with topical application of BHC.

Mutagenicity tests have been used as predictive information about the carcinogenicity of various chemical compounds. Numerous types of mutagenicity tests have been performed with lindane. The results of these tests do not indicate that lindane is mutagenic.

PREGNANCY

Teratogenic Effects

Pregnancy category B: Reproduction, including multigeneration, studies have been performed in mice, rats, rabbits, pigs, and dogs at doses up to 10 times the human dose and have revealed no evidence of impaired fertility or harm to the fetus due to orally administered lindane. There are, however, no adequate and well controlled studies in pregnant women. Because animal reproduction studies are not always predictive of human response, the recommended dosage should not be exceeded on pregnant women. They should be treated no more than twice during a pregnancy.

NURSING MOTHERS

Lindane is secreted in human milk in low concentrations. Studies conducted in the United States as well as Europe and South America found levels of lindane in human milk ranging from 0 to 113 ppb, as the result of ingestion of foods which had been treated with lindane. There appeared to be no difference in concentrations between country and urban dwellers. Although the levels of lindane found in blood after topical application with KWELL® Cream (lindane) 1% make it unlikely that amounts of lindane sufficient to cause serious adverse reactions will be excreted in the milk of nursing mothers who have used KWELL Cream, if there is any concern, an alternate method of feeding may be used for 4 days if there is any concern.

PEDIATRIC USE

Refer to the Contraindications and Warnings sections.

ADVERSE REACTIONS

Lindane has been reported to cause central nervous stimulation ranging from dizziness to convulsions. Cases of convulsions have been reported in connection with KWELL Cream therapy. However, these incidents were almost always associated with accidental oral ingestion or misuse of the product. In exceedingly rare cases, seizures have been reported when used according to directions. Eczematous eruptions due to irritation from this product have also been reported. Incidence of these adverse reactions is relatively infrequent, occurring in less than 1 in 100,000 patients.

DRUG ABUSE AND DEPENDENCE
KWELL Cream is not subject to abuse, nor is there any dependence on the drug.

OVERDOSAGE
Overdosage or oral ingestion of KWELL Cream can cause central nervous system excitation and, if taken in sufficient quantities, convulsions may occur.

If accidental ingestion occurs, prompt gastric lavage should be instituted. However, since oils favor absorption, saline cathartics for intestinal evacuation should be given rather than oil laxatives. If central nervous system manifestations occur they can be antagonized by the administration of pentobarbital, phenobarbital or diazepam.

DOSAGE AND ADMINISTRATION
CAUTION: USE ONLY AS DIRECTED. DO NOT EXCEED RECOMMENDED DOSAGE

No residual effects of KWELL® (lindane) 1% treatment have been demonstrated, therefore, this product should not be used to ward off a possible infestation. However sexual contacts should be treated simultaneously.

NOTE: PLEASE READ CAREFULLY.

DIRECTIONS FOR USE

WARNING:
THIS PRODUCT CAN BE POISONOUS IF MISUSED. CHILDREN MUST NOT BE ALLOWED TO APPLY THIS DRUG WITHOUT DIRECT ADULT SUPERVISION. USE CREAM FOR SCABIES ONLY. APPLY ONLY ONCE. USE ONLY ENOUGH TO COVER THE BODY IN A THIN LAYER. 1 OUNCE (HALF OF A 2 OUNCE CONTAINER) SHOULD BE ALL THAT IS NEEDED FOR CHILDREN UNDER 6 YEARS OF AGE; USE 1 TO 2 OUNCES FOR OLDER CHILDREN AND ADULTS. DO NOT LEAVE ON FOR MORE THAN 12 HOURS. DO NOT INGEST. KEEP AWAY FROM MOUTH AND EYES. COVER INFANT'S HANDS AND FEET DURING TREATMENT TO PREVENT SUCKING AND LICKING OF CREAM. DO NOT USE IF OPEN WOUNDS, CUTS OR SORES ARE PRESENT, UNLESS DIRECTED BY YOUR PHYSICIAN.

1. APPLY THIS PREPARATION TO DRY SKIN IN A THIN LAYER AND RUB IN THOROUGHLY.
2. TRIM NAILS AND APPLY UNDER NAILS WITH TOOTHBRUSH (THROW AWAY TOOTHBRUSH AFTER USE).
3. IF A WARM BATH IS TAKEN BEFORE APPLICATION ALLOW THE SKIN TO DRY AND COOL COMPLETELY BEFORE APPLYING THE MEDICATION.
4. A TOTAL BODY APPLICATION SHOULD BE MADE FROM THE NECK DOWN, INCLUDING SOLES OF FEET, UNLESS OTHERWISE DIRECTED BY YOUR PHYSICIAN.
5. THE CREAM SHOULD BE LEFT ON FOR 8 TO 12 HOURS (USUALLY OVERNIGHT) AND THEN REMOVED BY THOROUGH WASHING (BATH OR SHOWER).
6. AVOID UNNECESSARY CONTACT WITH YOUR SKIN IF YOU ARE APPLYING TO ANOTHER PERSON. IF TREATING MORE THAN ONE PERSON, THE PERSON APPLYING CREAM (ESPECIALLY PREGNANT OR NURSING WOMEN) SHOULD WEAR RUBBER GLOVES.
7. ALL RECENTLY WORN CLOTHING, UNDERWEAR AND PAJAMAS, AND USED SHEETS, PILLOW CASES AND TOWELS SHOULD BE WASHED IN VERY HOT WATER OR DRY-CLEANED.

AFTER ONE APPLICATION, ITCHING WILL CONTINUE FOR SEVERAL WEEKS. THIS IS NORMAL AND DOES NOT REQUIRE REAPPLICATION.

IF YOU HAVE ANY QUESTIONS OR CONCERNS ABOUT YOUR CONDITION OR USE OF THE CREAM, CONTACT YOUR PHYSICIAN.

CAUTION
Federal law prohibits dispensing without prescription.

HOW SUPPLIED
KWELL® Cream (lindane) 1% in tubes of 60 grams.

REFERENCES
1. Feldmann, R.J. and Maibach, H.I., *Toxicol. Applied. Pharmacol.* 28:126, 1974.
2. Dale, W.E., Curly, A. and Cueto, C., *Life Sci.* 5:47, 1966.
3. Ginsburg, C.M., et al., *J. Pediatr.* 91:6, 998, 1977.
4. Nagasaki, T., Tomii, S., Mega, T., Marugami, M. and Ito, N. *Gann* (Cancer) 63:393, 1972.
5. Goto, M. Hattori, M., Miyagawa, T. and Enomoto, M., *Chemosphere* 6:279, 1972.
6. Hanada, M., Yatani, C., and Miyaji, T., *Gann* 64:511, 1973.
7. Weisse, I. and Herbst, M., *Toxicol* 7:233, 1977.
8. Technical Report Series, NCI-CG-TR-14, *HEW PUBLICATIONS*, No. (NIH) 77-814.
9. Thorpe, E., and Walker, A.I.T., *Food Cosmetic Toxicol.* 11:433, 1973.
10. Orr, J.W., *Nature* 162:189, 1948.
11. Kashyap, S.K. et al., *J. Environ, Sci. Health* 14:305, 1979.

Revised April 1992

Manufactured for
Reed & Carnrick
Division of Block Drug Company, Inc.
Jersey City, NJ 07302-9988
By Reedco Inc., Humacao, P.R. 00791

Shown in Product Identification Section, page 424

KWELL® Lotion ℞
(lindane) 1%

DESCRIPTION
KWELL Lotion (lindane) 1% is an ectoparasiticide and ovicide effective against Sarcoptes scabiei (scabies). In addition to the active ingredient, lindane, it contains glyceryl monostearate, cetyl alcohol, stearic acid, trolamine, 2-amino-2-methyl-1 propanol, methyl p-hydroxybenzoate, butyl p-hydroxybenzoate, carrageenan, perfume and purified water to form a non-greasy lotion. Lindane, which is the highly purified gamma isomer of 1, 2, 3, 4, 5, 6, hexachlorocyclohexane, has the following chemical structure:

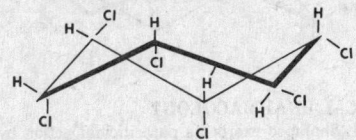

CLINICAL PHARMACOLOGY
KWELL Lotion exerts its parasiticidal action by being directly absorbed into the parasites and their ova. Feldman and Maibach[1] reported approximately 10% absorption of a lindane acetone solution applied to the forearm and left in place to 24 hours. Dale, et al[2] reported a blood level of 290ng/ml associated with convulsions following the accidental ingestion of a lindane-containing product. Ginsburg[3] found a mean peak blood level of 28ng/ml 6 hours after total body application of KWELL Lotion to scabietic infants and children. The half-life was determined to be 18 hours.

INDICATIONS AND USAGE
KWELL Lotin is indicated for the treatment of patients infested with Sarcoptes scabiei (scabies).

CONTRAINDICATIONS
KWELL Lotion is contraindicated for premature neonates because their skin may be more permeable than full term infants and their liver enzymes may not be sufficiently developed. It is also contraindicated for patients with known seizure disorders and for individuals with a known sensitivity to the product or any of its components.

WARNINGS
LINDANE PENETRATES HUMAN SKIN AND HAS THE POTENTIAL FOR CNS TOXICITY (SEE CLINICAL PHARMACOLOGY SECTION). KWELL LOTION SHOULD BE USED ACCORDING TO RECOMMENDED DOSAGE (SEE DIRECTIONS FOR USE) ESPECIALLY ON INFANTS, PREGNANT WOMEN AND NURSING MOTHERS. ANIMAL STUDIES INDICATE THAT POTENTIAL TOXIC EFFECTS OF TOPICALLY APPLIED LINDANE ARE GREATER IN THE YOUNG. SEIZURES AND, IN RARE INSTANCES, DEATHS HAVE BEEN REPORTED AFTER EXCESS DOSAGE, OVER-EXPOSURE, FREQUENT REAPPLICATIONS, AND ACCIDENTAL AND INTENTIONAL INGESTION OF LINDANE. THESE INSTANCES OF PATIENT MISUSE HAVE BEEN ASSOCIATED WITH LACK OF PATIENT UNDERSTANDING OF DIRECTIONS OF USE, PRESCRIBING OR DISPENSING EXCESSIVE QUANTITIES, AND IMPROPER REAPPLICATIONS. IN EXCEEDINGLY RARE CASES SEIZURES HAVE BEEN REPORTED WHEN USED ACCORDING TO DIRECTIONS. NO RESIDUAL EFFECTS OF KWELL® (lindane) 1% TREATMENT HAVE BEEN DEMONSTRATED; THEREFORE, THIS PRODUCT SHOULD NOT BE USED TO WARD OFF A POSSIBLE INFESTATION.

If accidental ingestion occurs prompt gastric lavage is indicated. Because oils may enhance absorption, saline rather than oily cathartics should be used. Central nervous excitation can be controlled by the administration of pentobarbital, phenobarbital or diazepam.

PRECAUTIONS
General
Care should be taken to avoid contact with the eyes. If such contact occurs, eyes should be immediately flushed with water. If irritation or sensitization occurs, the patient should be advised to consult a physician.

Geriatric
Dosage may have to be reduced due to the possibility of increased absorption through elderly skin.

Information to Patients
Patients must be instructed on the proper use of this medication, especially as to amount applied and duration of use. Patient Directions for Use must accompany the product.

LABORATORY TESTS
No laboratory tests are needed for the proper use of this medication.

DRUG INTERACTIONS
Oils may enhance absorption, therefore, simultaneous use of creams, ointments or oils should be avoided.

CARCINOGENESIS
Although no studies have been conducted with KWELL Lotion, numerous long term feeding studies have been conducted in mice and rats to evaluate the carcinogenic potential of the technical grade of hexachlorocyclohexane (BHC) as well as the alpha, beta, gamma (lindane) and delta isomers. Both oral and topical applications have been evaluated. Nagasaki, et al[4], Goto, et al [5] and Hanada, et al[6] found varying amounts of benign and malignant hepatomas associated with BHC and the alpha, delta and epsilon isomers. None reported a carcinogenic potential for lindane. Tumors were found only in the animals which had received the alpha isomer. Weisse and Herbst[7] also evaluated the carcinogenic potential of lindane in mice but could find no evidence of lindane carcinogenicity. The National Cancer Institute[8] also found no evidence of carcinogenicity.

Thorpe and Walker[9] compared beta BHC with lindane, dieldrin, DDT and hexabarbital in mice. Despite the unusually high incidence of tumors in the control group, they concluded that 600 ppm of lindane was associated with a significant increase of hepatoma and thus considered it a tumorigen.

Orr[10] and Kashyap, et al[11] evaluated the carcinogenic potential in mice of topically applied BHC. In neither study was there any evidence of a tumorigenic or carcinogenic potential associated with topical application of BHC.

Mutagenicity tests have been used as predictive information about the carcinogenicity of various chemical compounds. Numerous types of mutagenicity tests have been performed with lindane. The results of these tests do not indicate that lindane is mutagenic.

PREGNANCY
Teratogenic Effects
Pregnancy category B: Reproduction, including multigeneration, studies have been performed in mice, rats, rabbits, pigs, and dogs at doses up to 10 times the human dose and have revealed no evidence of impaired fertility or harm to the fetus due to orally administered lindane. There are, however, no adequate and well controlled studies in pregnant women. Because animal reproduction studies are not always predictive of human response, the recommended dosage should not be exceeded on pregnant women. They should be treated no more than twice during a pregnancy.

NURSING MOTHERS
Lindane is secreted in human milk in low concentrations. Studies conducted in the United States as well as Europe and South America found levels of lindane in human milk range from 0 to 113 ppb, as the result of ingestion of foods which had been treated with lindane. There appeared to be no difference in concentrations between country and urban dwellers. Although the levels of lindane found in blood after topical application with KWELL Lotion make it unlikely that amounts of lindane sufficient to cause serious adverse reactions will be excreted in the milk of nursing mothers who have used KWELL® Lotion (lindane) 1%, an alternate method of feeding may be used for 4 days if there is any concern.

PEDIATRIC USE
Refer to the Contraindications and Warnings section.

ADVERSE REACTIONS
Lindane has been reported to cause central nervous stimulation ranging from dizziness to convulsions. Cases of convulsions have been reported in connection with KWELL Lotion therapy. However, these incidents were almost always associated with accidental oral ingestion or misuse of the product. In exceedingly rare cases, seizures have been reported when used according to directions. Eczematous eruptions due to irritation from this product have also been reported. Incidence of these adverse reactions is relatively infrequent, occurring in less than 1 in 100,000 patients.

DRUG ABUSE AND DEPENDENCE
KWELL Lotion is not subject to abuse, nor is there any dependence on the drug.

OVERDOSAGE
Overdosage or oral ingestion of KWELL Lotion can cause central nervous system excitation and, if taken in sufficient quantities, convulsions may occur.

If accidental ingestion occurs, prompt gastric lavage should be instituted. However, since oils favor absorption, saline

Continued on next page

Reed & Carnrick—Cont.

cathartics for intestinal evacuation should be given rather than oil laxatives. If central nervous system manifestations occur they can be antagonized by the administration of pentobarbital, phenobarbital or diazepam.

DOSAGE AND ADMINISTRATION
CAUTION: USE ONLY AS DIRECTED. DO NOT EXCEED RECOMMENDED DOSAGE

No residual effects of KWELL® (lindane) 1% treatment have been demonstrated, therefore, this product should not be used to ward off a possible infestation. However, sexual contacts should be treated simultaneously.
NOTE: PLEASE READ CAREFULLY.

DIRECTIONS FOR USE

WARNING:

THIS PRODUCT CAN BE POISONOUS IF MISUSED. CHILDREN MUST NOT BE ALLOWED TO APPLY THIS DRUG WITHOUT DIRECT ADULT SUPERVISION. USE LOTION FOR SCABIES ONLY. APPLY ONLY ONCE. USE ONLY ENOUGH TO COVER THE BODY IN A THIN LAYER. 1 OUNCE (HALF OF A 2 OUNCE CONTAINER) SHOULD BE ALL THAT IS NEEDED FOR CHILDREN UNDER 6 YEARS OF AGE; 1 TO 2 OUNCES FOR OLDER CHILDREN AND ADULTS. DO NOT LEAVE ON FOR MORE THAN 12 HOURS. DO NOT INGEST. KEEP AWAY FROM MOUTH AND EYES. COVER INFANT'S HANDS AND FEET DURING TREATMENT TO PREVENT SUCKING AND LICKING OF LOTION. DO NOT USE IF OPEN WOUNDS, CUTS OR SORES ARE PRESENT, UNLESS DIRECTED BY YOUR PHYSICIAN.
(LOTION: SHAKE WELL)
1. APPLY THIS PREPARATION TO DRY SKIN IN A THIN LAYER AND RUB IN THOROUGHLY.
2. TRIM NAILS AND APPLY UNDER NAILS WITH TOOTHBRUSH (THROW AWAY TOOTHBRUSH AFTER USE).
3. IF A WARM BATH IS TAKEN BEFORE APPLICATION ALLOW THE SKIN TO DRY AND COOL COMPLETELY BEFORE APPLYING THE MEDICATION.
4. A TOTAL BODY APPLICATION SHOULD BE MADE FROM THE NECK DOWN, INCLUDING SOLES OF FEET, UNLESS OTHERWISE DIRECTED BY YOUR PHYSICIAN.
5. THE LOTION SHOULD BE LEFT ON FOR 8 TO 12 HOURS (USUALLY OVERNIGHT) AND THEN REMOVED BY THOROUGH WASHING (BATH OR SHOWER).
6. AVOID UNNECESSARY CONTACT WITH YOUR SKIN IF YOU ARE APPLYING TO ANOTHER PERSON. IF TREATING MORE THAN ONE PERSON, PERSON APPLYING LOTION (ESPECIALLY PREGNANT OR NURSING WOMEN) SHOULD WEAR RUBBER GLOVES.
7. ALL RECENTLY WORN CLOTHING, UNDERWEAR AND PAJAMAS, AND USED SHEETS, PILLOW CASES, AND TOWELS SHOULD BE WASHED IN VERY HOT WATER OR DRY-CLEANED.
AFTER ONE APPLICATION, ITCHING WILL CONTINUE FOR SEVERAL WEEKS. THIS IS NORMAL AND DOES NOT REQUIRE REAPPLICATION.
IF YOU HAVE ANY QUESTIONS OR CONCERNS ABOUT YOUR CONDITION OR USE OF THE LOTION, CONTACT YOUR PHYSICIAN.

CAUTION
Federal law prohibits dispensing without prescription.

HOW SUPPLIED
KWELL® Lotion (lindane) 1% in bottles of patient-size 2 fl. oz. (59 ml), pharmacy-size only 16 fl. oz. (473 ml) and pharmacy-size only 1 gallon (3.8 liters).

REFERENCES
1. Feldmann, R.J. and Maibach, H.I., *Toxicol. Appl. Pharmacol.* 28:126, 1974.
2. Dale, W.E., Curley, A. and Cueto, C. *Life Sci.* 5:47, 1966.
3. Ginsburg, C.M., et al., *J. Pediatr.* 91:6, 998, 1977.
4. Nagasaki, T., Tomii, S., Mepa, T., Marugami, M. and Ito, N. *Gann* (Cancer) 63:393, 1972.
5. Goto, M., Hattori, M., Miyagawa, T. and Enomoto, M., *Chemosphere* 6:279, 1972.
6. Hanada, M., Yatani, C., Miyaji, T., *Gann* 64:511, 1973.
7. Weisse, I. and Herbst, M., *Toxicol.* 7:233, 1977.
8. Technical Report Series, NCI-CG-TR-14, *HEW PUBLICATIONS,* No. (NIH) 77–814.
9. Thorpe, E., and Walker, A.I.T., *Food Cosmetic Toxicol.* 11:433, 1973.
10. Orr, J.W., *Nature* 162:189, 1948.
11. Kashyap, S.K. et al., *J. Environ. Sci. Health* 14:305,318, 1979.

Revised April 1992
Manufactured For
Reed & Carnick
Division of Block Drug Company, Inc.
Jersey City, New Jersey 07302-9988
By Reedco Inc., Humacao, PR 00791
Shown in Product Identification Section, page 424

KWELL® Shampoo   ℞
(lindane) 1%

DESCRIPTION
KWELL Shampoo (lindane) 1% is an ectoparasiticide and ovicide effective against Pediculosis capitis (head lice), Pediculosis pubis (crab lice) and their ova. In addition to the active ingredient, lindane, it contains trolamine lauryl sulfate, polysorbate 60, acetone and purified water to form a cosmetically pleasant shampoo. Lindane, which is the highly purified gamma isomer of 1, 2, 3, 4, 5, 6, hexachlorocyclohexane, has the following chemical structure:

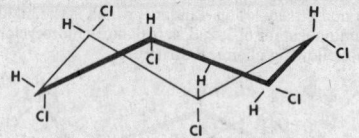

CLINICAL PHARMACOLOGY
KWELL Shampoo exerts its parasiticidal action by being directly absorbed into the parasites and their ova. Dale et al.[1] reported a blood level of 290ng/ml associated with convulsions following the accidental ingestion of a lindane containing product. Analysis of blood taken from subjects before and after the use of KWELL Shampoo showed a mean peak blood level of only 3ng/ml which appeared at six hours and disappeared at eight hours after the shampoo was applied.[2]

INDICATIONS AND USAGE
KWELL Shampoo is indicated for the treatment of patients infested with Pediculus capitis (head lice), Pediculus pubis (crab lice) and their ova.

CONTRAINDICATIONS
KWELL Shampoo is contraindicated for premature neonates because their skin may be more permeable than full term infants and their liver enzymes may not be sufficiently developed. It is also contraindicated for patients with known seizure disorders and for individuals with a known sensitivity to the product or any of its components.

WARNINGS
LINDANE PENETRATES HUMAN SKIN AND HAS THE POTENTIAL FOR CNS TOXICITY (SEE CLINICAL PHARMACOLOGY SECTION). KWELL SHAMPOO SHOULD BE USED ACCORDING TO RECOMMENDED DOSAGE (SEE DIRECTIONS FOR USE) ESPECIALLY ON INFANTS, PREGNANT WOMEN AND NURSING MOTHERS. ANIMAL STUDIES INDICATE THAT POTENTIAL TOXIC EFFECTS OF TOPICALLY APPLIED LINDANE ARE GREATER IN THE YOUNG. SEIZURES, AND, IN RARE INSTANCES, DEATHS HAVE BEEN REPORTED AFTER EXCESS DOSAGE, OVER-EXPOSURE, FREQUENT REAPPLICATIONS, AND ACCIDENTAL AND INTENTIONAL INGESTION OF LINDANE. THESE INSTANCES OF PATIENT MISUSE HAVE BEEN ASSOCIATED WITH LACK OF PATIENT UNDERSTANDING OF DIRECTIONS FOR USE, PRESCRIBING OR DISPENSING EXCESSIVE QUANTITIES, AND IMPROPER REAPPLICATIONS. IN EXCEEDINGLY RARE CASES SEIZURES HAVE BEEN REPORTED WHEN USED ACCORDING TO DIRECTIONS. NO RESIDUAL EFFECTS OF KWELL® TREATMENT HAVE BEEN DEMONSTRATED; THEREFORE, THIS PRODUCT SHOULD NOT BE USED TO WARD OFF A POSSIBLE INFESTATION.
If accidental ingestion occurs prompt gastric lavage is indicated. Because oils may enhance absorption, saline rather than oily cathartics should be used. Central nervous excitation can be controlled by the administration of pentobarbital, phenobarbital or diazepam.

PRECAUTIONS
General
Care should be taken to avoid contact with the eyes. If such contact occurs, eyes should be immediately flushed with water. If irritation or sensitization occurs, the patient should be advised to consult a physician.
Information to Patients
Patients should be instructed on the proper use of this medication, especially as to amount applied and duration of use. Patient Directions For Use must accompany the product.

LABORATORY TESTS
No laboratory tests are needed for the proper use of this medication.

DRUG INTERACTIONS
Oils may enhance absorption, therefore, avoid using oil treatments, or oil based hair dressings or conditioners immediately before and after applying KWELL® Shampoo (lindane) 1%.

CARCINOGENESIS
Although no studies have been conducted with KWELL Shampoo, numerous long term feeding studies have been conducted in mice and rats to evaluate the carcinogenic potential of the technical grade of hexachlorocyclohexane (BHC) as well as the alpha, beta, gamma (lindane) and delta isomers. Both oral and topical applications have been evaluated. Nagasaki, et al[3], Goto, et al[4] and Hanada, et al[5] found varying amounts of benign and malignant hepatomas associated with BHC and the alpha, delta and epsilon isomers. None reported a carcinogenic potential for lindane. Tumors were found only in the animals which had received the alpha isomer. Weisse and Herbst[6] also evaluated the carcinogenic potential of lindane in mice but could find no evidence of lindane carcinogenicity. The National Cancer Institute[7] had also found no evidence of carcinogenicity.
Thorpe and Walker[8] compared beta BHC with lindane, dieldrin, DDT and hexabarbital in mice. Despite the unusually high incidence of tumors in the control group, they concluded that 600 ppm of lindane was associated with a significant increase in the incidence of hepatoma and, thus, considered it a tumorigen.
Orr[9] and Kashyap, et al[10] evaluated the carcinogenic potential in mice of topically applied BHC. In neither study was there any evidence of a tumorigenic or carcinogenic potential associated with topical application of BHC.
Mutagenicity tests have been used as predictive information about the carcinogenicity of various chemical compounds. Numerous types of mutagenicity tests have been performed with lindane. The results of these tests do not indicate that lindane is mutagenic.

PREGNANCY
Teratogenic Effects
Pregnancy category B: Reproduction, including multigeneration, studies have been performed in mice, rats, rabbits, pigs, and dogs at doses up to 10 times the human dose and have revealed no evidence of impaired fertility or harm to the fetus due to orally administered lindane. There are, however, no adequate and well controlled studies in pregnant women. Because animal reproduction studies are not always predictive of human response, the recommended dosage should not be exceeded on pregnant women. They should be treated no more than twice during a pregnancy.

NURSING MOTHERS
Lindane is secreted in human milk in low concentrations. Studies conducted in the United States as well as Europe and South America found levels of lindane in human milk ranging from 0 to 113 ppb, as the result of ingestion of foods which had been treated with lindane. There appeared to be no difference in concentrations between country and urban dwellers. Although the levels of lindane found in blood after topical application with KWELL® Shampoo (lindane) 1% make it unlikely that amounts of lindane sufficient to cause serious adverse reactions will be excreted in the milk of nursing mothers who have used KWELL Shampoo, an alternate method of feeding may be used for 4 days if there is any concern.

PEDIATRIC USE
Refer to the Contraindications and Warnings sections.

ADVERSE REACTIONS
Lindane has been reported to cause central nervous stimulation ranging from dizziness to convulsions. Cases of convulsions have been reported in connection with KWELL Shampoo therapy. However, these incidents were almost always associated with accidental oral ingestion or misuse of the product. In exceedingly rare cases, seizures have been reported when used according to directions. Eczematous eruptions due to irritation from this product have also been reported. Incidence of these adverse reactions is relatively infrequent, occurring in less than 1 in 100,000 patients.

DRUG ABUSE AND DEPENDENCE
KWELL Shampoo is not subject to abuse nor is there any dependence on the drug.

OVERDOSAGE
Overdosage or oral ingestion of KWELL Shampoo can cause central nervous system excitation and, if taken in sufficient quantities, convulsions may occur.
If accidental ingestion occurs, prompt gastric lavage should be instituted. However, since oils favor absorption, saline cathartics for intestinal evacuation should be given rather than oil laxatives. If central nervous system manifestations occur, they can be antagonized by the administration of pentobarbital, phenobarbital and diazepam.

DOSAGE AND ADMINISTRATION
CAUTION: USE ONLY AS DIRECTED. DO NOT EXCEED RECOMMENDED DOSAGE.

No residual effects of KWELL® Shampoo (lindane) 1% treatment have been demonstrated, therefore, this product should not be used to ward off a possible infestation. However, sexual contacts should be treated simultaneously.

NOTE: PLEASE READ CAREFULLY

DIRECTIONS FOR USE

WARNING:

THIS PRODUCT CAN BE POISONOUS IF MISUSED. CHILDREN MUST NOT BE ALLOWED TO APPLY THIS DRUG WITHOUT DIRECT ADULT SUPERVISION. USE SHAMPOO FOR HEAD AND PUBIC LICE ONLY. DO NOT USE FOR SCABIES. USE ONLY IN AMOUNTS DIRECTED BELOW. IN NO CASE SHOULD MORE THAN 2 OUNCES BE USED BY ONE PERSON IN ONE APPLICATION. DO NOT INGEST. KEEP AWAY FROM MOUTH AND EYES. DO NOT USE IF OPEN WOUNDS, CUTS OR SORES ARE PRESENT ON SCALP OR GROIN, UNLESS DIRECTED BY YOUR PHYSICIAN.

AVOID USING OIL TREATMENTS, OIL BASED HAIR DRESSINGS OR CONDITIONERS IMMEDIATELY BEFORE OR AFTER APPLYING KWELL SHAMPOO.

(SHAKE WELL)

1. BEFORE APPLYING KWELL SHAMPOO, USE REGULAR SHAMPOO (WITHOUT CONDITIONERS), RINSE AND COMPLETELY DRY HAIR.
2. USE 1 OUNCE (HALF OF A 2 OUNCE BOTTLE) FOR SHORT HAIR; 1.5 OUNCES (THREE-QUARTERS OF A 2 OUNCE BOTTLE) FOR MEDIUM LENGTH HAIR; AND FULL 2 OUNCE BOTTLE FOR LONG HAIR.
3. APPLY SHAMPOO DIRECTLY TO DRY HAIR WITHOUT ADDING WATER. WORK THOROUGHLY INTO THE HAIR AND ALLOW TO REMAIN IN PLACE FOR 4 MINUTES ONLY.
4. AFTER 4 MINUTES, ADD SMALL QUANTITIES OF WATER TO HAIR UNTIL A GOOD LATHER FORMS.
5. IMMEDIATELY RINSE ALL LATHER AWAY. AVOID UNNECESSARY CONTACT OF LATHER WITH OTHER BODY SURFACES.
6. TOWEL BRISKLY AND REMOVE NITS WITH NIT COMB OR TWEEZERS.
7. AVOID UNNECESSARY CONTACT WITH YOUR SKIN IF YOU ARE APPLYING SHAMPOO TO ANOTHER PERSON. IF TREATING MORE THAN ONE PERSON, PERSON APPLYING SHAMPOO (ESPECIALLY PREGNANT AND/OR NURSING WOMEN) SHOULD WEAR RUBBER GLOVES.

RE-TREATMENT IS USUALLY NOT NECESSARY, BUT PRESENCE OF LIVING LICE IN HAIR 7 DAYS AFTER TREATMENT INDICATES THAT RE-TREATMENT MAY BE NECESSARY. DO NOT RETREAT WITHOUT THE ADVICE OF A PHYSICIAN.

CAUTION

Federal law prohibits dispensing without prescription.

HOW SUPPLIED

KWELL® Shampoo (lindane) 1% in bottles of patient-size 2 fl. oz. (59 ml), and pharmacy-size only 16 fl. oz. (473 ml).

REFERENCES

1. Dale, W.E., Curly, A. and Cueto, C. *Life Sci* 5:47, 1966.
2. Data on File at Reed & Carnrick.
3. Nagasaki, T., Tomii, S., Mega, T., Marugami, M. and Ito, N. *Gann* (Cancer) 63(3):393, 1972.
4. Goto, M., Hattori, M., Miyagawa, T. and Enomoto, M., *Chemosphere* 6:279, 1972.
5. Hanada, M., Yatani, C., Miyaji, T., *Gann* 64:511, 1973.
6. Weisse, I. and Herbst, M., *Toxicol.* 7:233, 1977.
7. Technical Report Series, NCI-CG-TR-14, *HEW PUBLICATIONS,* No. (NIH) 77–814.
8. Thorpe, E., and Walker, A.I.T., *Food Cosmetic Toxicol.* 11:433, 1973.
9. Orr, J.W., *Nature* 162:189, 1948.
10. Kashyap, S.K., et al, *J. Environ. Sci. Health* 14:305,318, 1979.

MANUFACTURED FOR
REED & CARNRICK
Division of Block Drug Company, Inc.
Jersey City, N.J. 07302-9988
By Reedco Inc., Humacao, P.R. 00791

Date of Revision
Revised March 1992

Shown in Product Identification Section, page 424

LEVATOL® ℞
[lev'a-tol]
(penbutolol sulfate) 20 mg
TABLETS

DESCRIPTION

Levatol® (penbutolol sulfate) is a synthetic β-receptor antagonist for oral administration. The chemical name of penbutolol sulfate is (S)-1-tert-butylamino-3-(o-cyclopentylphenoxy)-2-propanol sulfate. It is provided as the levorotatory isomer. The empirical formula for penbutolol sulfate is $C_{36}H_{60}N_2O_8S$. Its molecular weight is 680.94. A dose of 20 mg is equivalent to 29.4 μmol. The structural formula is as follows:

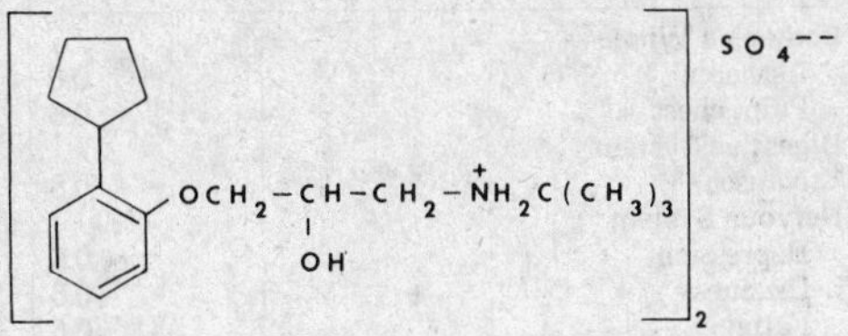

Penbutolol is a white, odorless, crystalline powder. Levatol is available as tablets for oral administration. Each tablet contains 20 mg of penbutolol sulfate. It also contains corn starch, D&C Yellow No. 10, lactose, magnesium stearate, povidone, silicon dioxide, talc, titanium dioxide, and other inactive ingredients.

CLINICAL PHARMACOLOGY

Penbutolol is a β-1, β-2 (nonselective) adrenergic receptor antagonist. Experimental studies showed a dose-dependent increase in heart rate in reserpinized (norepinephrine-depleted) rats given penbutolol intravenously at doses of 0.25 to 1.0 mg/kg, suggesting that penbutolol has some intrinsic sympathomimetic activity. In human studies, however, heart rate decreases have been similar to those seen with propranolol.

Penbutolol antagonizes the heart rate effects of exercise and infused isoproterenol. The β-blocking potency of penbutolol is approximately 4 times that of propranolol. An oral dose of less than 10 mg will reduce exercise-induced tachycardia to one-half its usual level; maximum antagonism follows doses of 10 to 20 mg. The peak effect is between 1.5 and 3 hours after oral administration. The duration of effect exceeds 20 hours during a once-daily dosing regimen. During chronic administration of penbutolol, the duration of antihypertensive effects permits a once-daily dosage schedule.

Acute hemodynamic effects of penbutolol have been studied following single intravenous doses between 0.1 and 4 mg. The cardiovascular responses included significant reductions in heart rate, left ventricular maximum dP/dt, cardiac output, stroke volume index, stroke work, and stroke work index. Systolic pressure and mean arterial pressure were reduced, and total peripheral resistance was increased.

Chronic administration of penbutolol to hypertensive patients results in the hemodynamic pattern typical of β-adrenergic blocking drugs: a reduction in cardiac index, heart rate, systolic and diastolic blood pressures, and the product of heart rate and mean arterial pressure both at rest and with all levels of exercise, without significant change in total peripheral resistance. Penbutolol causes a reduction in left ventricular contractility. Penbutolol decreases glomerular filtration rate, but not significantly.

Clinical trial doses of 10 to 80 mg per day in single daily doses have reduced supine and standing systolic and diastolic blood pressures. In most studies, effects were small, generally a change in blood pressure 5 to 8/3 to 5 mm Hg greater than seen with a placebo measured 24 hours after dosing. It is not clear whether this relatively small effect reflects a characteristic of penbutolol or the particular population studied (the population had relatively mild hypertension but did not appear unusual in others respects). In a direct comparison of penbutolol with adequate doses of twice daily propranolol, no difference in blood pressure effect was seen. In a comparison of placebo and 10-, 20- and 40-mg single daily doses of penbutolol, no significant dose-related difference was seen in response to active drug at 6 weeks, but compared to the 10-mg dose, the two larger doses showed greater effects at 2 and 4 weeks and reached their maximum effect at 2 weeks. In several studies, dose increases from 40 to 80 mg were without additional effect on blood pressure. Response rates to penbutolol are unaffected by sex or age but are greater in caucasians than blacks.

Penbutolol decreases plasma renin activity in normal subjects and in patients with essential and renovascular hypertension. The mechanisms of the antihypertensive actions of β-receptor antagonists have not been established. However, factors that may be involved are: (1) competitive antagonism of catecholamines at peripheral adrenergic receptor sites (especially cardiac) that leads to decreased cardiac output; (2) a central-nervous-system (CNS) action that results in a decrease in tonic sympathetic neural outflow to the periphery; and (3) a reduction of renin secretion through blockade of β-receptors involved in release of renin from the kidneys.

Penbutolol dose dependently increases the RR and QT intervals. There is no influence on the PR, QRS or QT c (corrected) intervals.

Pharmacokinetics—Following oral administration, penbutolol is rapidly and completely absorbed. Peak plasma concentrations of penbutolol occur between 2 and 3 hours after oral administration and are proportional to single and multiple doses between 10 and 40 mg once a day. The average plasma elimination half-life of penbutolol is approximately 5 hours in normal subjects. There is no significant difference in the plasma half-life of penbutolol in healthy elderly persons or patients on renal dialysis. Twelve to 24 hours after oral administration of doses up to 120 mg, plasma concentrations of parent drug are 0% to 10% of the peak level. No accumulation of penbutolol is observed in hypertensive patients after 8 days of therapy at doses of 40 mg daily or 20 mg twice a day. Penbutolol is approximately 80% to 98% bound to plasma proteins.

The metabolism of penbutolol in humans involves conjugation and oxidation. The metabolites are excreted principally in the urine. When radiolabeled penbutolol was administered to humans, approximately 90% of the radioactivity was excreted in the urine. Approximately $\frac{1}{6}$ of the dose of penbutolol was recovered as penbutolol conjugate, while the remaining fraction was not identified. Conjugated penbutolol has a plasma elimination half-life of approximately 20 hours in healthy persons, 25 hours in healthy elderly persons and 100 hours in patients on renal dialysis. Thus, accumulation of penbutolol conjugate may be expected upon multiple-dosing in renal insufficiency. An oxidative metabolite of penbutolol, 4-hydroxy penbutolol, has been identified in small quantities in plasma and urine. It is $\frac{1}{8}$ to $\frac{1}{15}$ times as active as the parent compound in blocking isoproterenol-induced β-adrenergic receptor responses in isolated guinea-pig trachea and is $\frac{1}{8}$ to 1 times as potent in anesthetized dogs.

INDICATIONS AND USAGE

Levatol® (penbutolol sulfate) 20 mg is indicated in the treatment of mild to moderate arterial hypertension. It may be used alone or in combination with other antihypertensive agents, especially thiazide-type diuretics.

CONTRAINDICATIONS

Levatol is contraindicated in patients with cardiogenic shock, sinus bradycardia, second and third degree atrioventricular conduction block, bronchial asthma, and those with known hypersensitivity to this product (*see* WARNINGS).

WARNINGS

Cardiac Failure—Sympathetic stimulation may be essential for supporting circulatory function in patients with heart failure, and its inhibition by β-adrenergic receptor blockade may precipitate more severe failure. Although β-blockers should be avoided in overt congestive heart failure, Levatol can, if necessary, be used with caution in patients with a history of cardiac failure who are well compensated, on treatment with vasodilators, digitalis and/or diuretics. Both digitalis and penbutolol slow AV conduction. Beta-adrenergic receptor antagonists do not inhibit the inotropic action of digitalis on heart muscle. If cardiac failure persists, treatment with Levatol should be discontinued.

Patients Without History of Cardiac Failure—Continued depression of the myocardium with β-blocking agents over a period of time can, in some cases, lead to cardiac failure. At the first evidence of heart failure, patients receiving Levatol should be given appropriate treatment, and the response should be closely observed. If cardiac failure continues despite adequate intervention with appropriate drugs, Levatol should be withdrawn (gradually, if possible).

Exacerbation of Ischemic Heart Disease Following Abrupt Withdrawal—Hypersensitivity to catecholamines has been observed in patients who were withdrawn from therapy with β-blocking agents; exacerbation of angina, and, in some cases, myocardial infarction have occurred after abrupt discontinuation of such therapy. When discontinuing Levatol, particularly in patients with ischemic heart disease, the dosage should be reduced gradually over a period of 1 to 2 weeks and the patient should be monitored carefully. If angina becomes more pronounced or acute coronary insufficiency develops, administration of Levatol should be reinstated promptly, at least on a temporary basis, and appropriate measures should be taken for the management of unstable angina. Patients should be warned against interruption or discontinuation of therapy without the physician's advice. Because coronary artery disease is common and may not be recognized, it may not be prudent to discontinue Levatol® (penbutolol sulfate) 20 mg abruptly, even in patients who are being treated only for hypertension.

Nonallergic Bronchospasm (e.g., chronic bronchitis, emphysema)—Levatol is contraindicated in bronchial asthma. In general, patients with bronchospastic diseases should not receive β-blockers. Levatol should be administered with caution because it may block bronchodilation produced by endogenous catecholamine stimulation of β-2 receptors.

Anesthesia and Major Surgery—The necessity, or desirability, of withdrawal of a β-blocking therapy prior to major surgery is controversial. Beta-adrenergic receptor blockade impairs the ability of the heart to respond to β-adrenergically mediated reflex stimuli. Although this might be of benefit in preventing arrhythmic response, the risk of excessive myocardial depression during general anesthesia may be

Continued on next page

Reed & Carnrick—Cont.

enhanced and difficulty in restarting and maintaining the heartbeat has been reported with β-blockers. If treatment is continued, particular care should be taken when using anesthetic agents that depress the myocardium, such as ether, cyclopropane, and trichloroethylene, and it is prudent to use the lowest possible dose of Levatol. Levatol like other β-blockers, is a competitive inhibitor of β-receptor agonists, and its effect on the heart can be reversed by cautious administration of such agents (e.g., dobutamine or isoproterenol—see Overdose). Manifestations of excessive vagal tone (e.g., profound bradycardia, hypotension) may be corrected with atropine 1 to 3 mg IV in divided doses.

Diabetes Mellitus and Hypoglycemia —Beta-adrenergic receptor blockade may prevent the appearance of signs and symptoms of acute hypoglycemia, such as tachycardia and blood pressure changes. This is especially important in patients with labile diabetes. Beta-blockade also reduces the release of insulin in response to hyperglycemia; therefore, it may be necessary to adjust the dose of hypoglycemic drugs. Beta-adrenergic blockade may also impair the homeostatic response to hypoglycemia; in that event, the spontaneous recovery from hypoglycemia may be delayed during treatment with β-adrenergic receptor antagonists.

Thyrotoxicosis —Beta-adrenergic blockade may mask certain clinical signs (e.g., tachycardia) of hyperthyrodism. Patients suspected of developing thyrotoxicosis should be managed carefully to avoid abrupt withdrawal of β-adrenergic receptor blockers that might precipitate a thyroid storm.

PRECAUTIONS

Information for Patients —Patients, especially those with evidence of coronary artery insufficiency, should be warned against interruption or discontinuation of Levatol without the physician's advice. Although cardiac failure rarely occurs in properly selected patients, those being treated with β-adrenergic receptor antagonists should be advised of the symptoms of heart failure and to report such symptoms immediately, should they develop.

Drug Interactions —Levatol has been used in combination with hydrochlorothiazide in at least 100 patients without unexpected adverse reactions.

In one study, the combination of penbutolol and alcohol increased the number of errors in the eye-hand psychomotor function test.

Penbutolol increases the volume of distribution of lidocaine in normal subjects. This could result in a requirement for higher loading doses of lidocaine.

Cimetidine has no effect on the clearance of penbutolol. The major metabolite of penbutolol is a glucuronide, and it has been shown that cimetidine does not inhibit glucuronidation.

Synergistic hypotensive effects, bradycardia, and arrhythmias have been reported in some patients receiving β-adrenergic blocking agents when an oral calcium antagonist was added to the treatment regimen.

Generally, Levatol® (penbutolol sulfate) 20 mg should not be used in patients receiving catecholamine-depleting drugs.

Risk of Anaphylactic Reaction —While taking beta-blockers, patients with a history of severe anaphylactic reaction to a variety of allergens may be more reactive to repeated challenge, either accidental, diagnostic, or therapeutic. Such patients may be unresponsive to the usual doses of epinephrine used to treat allergic reaction.

Carcinogenesis, Mutagenesis, and Impairment of Fertility —There was no evidence of carcinogenicity observed in a 21-month study in mice or a 2-year study in rats. Mice were given penbutolol in the diet for 18 months at doses up to 395 mg/kg/day (about 500 times the maximum recommended dose of 40 mg in a 50 kg person). Rats were given 141 mg/kg/day for the same length of time. Mice were observed for 3 months and rats for 5.5 to 7 months after termination of treatment before necropsy was performed.

No evidence of mutagenic activity of penbutolol was seen in the *Salmonella* mutagenicity test (Ames test), the point mutation induction test (*Saccharomyces*) and the micronucleus test.

Penbutolol had no adverse effects on fertility or general reproductive performance in mice and rats at oral doses up to 172 mg/kg/day.

Pregnancy—Teratogenic Effects: Pregnancy Category C —Teratology studies in rats and rabbits revealed no teratogenic effects related to treatment with penbutolol at oral doses up to 200 mg/kg/day (250 times the maximum recommended human dose). In rabbits, a slight increase in the intrauterine fetal mortality and a reduced 24-hour offspring survival rate were observed in the groups treated with 125 mg/kg/day (156 times the maximum recommended dose) but not in the groups treated with 0.2 and 5 mg (0.25 to 6 times the maximum recommended dose).

There are no adequate and well-controlled studies in pregnant women. Levatol should be used during pregnancy only if the potential benefit justifies the potential risk to the fetus.

Nonteratogenic Effects —In a perinatal and postnatal study in rats, the pup body weight and pup survival rate were reduced at the highest dose level of 160 mg/kg/day (200 times the maximum recommended dose).

Nursing Mothers —It is not known whether Levatol is excreted in human milk. Because many drugs are excreted in human milk, caution should be exercised when Levatol is administered to a nursing woman.

Usage in Children —Safety and effectiveness of Levatol in children have not been established.

ADVERSE REACTIONS

Levatol® (penbutolol sulfate) 20 mg is usually well tolerated in properly selected patients. Most adverse effects observed during clinical trials have been mild and reversible.

Table 1 lists the adverse reactions reported from 4 controlled studies conducted in the United States involving once-a-day administration of Levatol (at doses ranging from 10 to 120 mg) as monotherapy or in combination with hydrochlorothiazide. Levatol doses above 40 mg/day are not, however, recommended. The table includes only those events where the prevalence rate in the Levatol group was at least 1.5%, or where the reaction is of particular interest.

Over a dose range from 10 to 40 mg, once a day, fatigue, nausea, and sexual impotence occurred at a greater frequency as the dose was increased.

[See table below.]

In a double-blind clinical trial comparing Levatol (40 mg and greater once a day) and propranolol (40 mg or more twice a day), heart rates of less than 60 beats/min were recorded at least once in 25% of the patients in the group receiving Levatol and in 37% of the patients in the propranolol group. Corresponding figures for heart rates of less than 50 beats/min were 1.2% and 6%, respectively. No symptoms associated with bradycardia were reported.

Discontinuations of Levatol because of adverse reactions has ranged between 2.4% and 6.9% of patients in double-blind, parallel, controlled clinical trials, as compared to 1.8% to 4.1% in the corresponding control groups that were given placebo. The frequency and severity of adverse reactions have not increased during long-term administration of Levatol® (penbutolol sulfate) 20 mg. The prevalence of adverse reactions reported from 4 controlled clinical trials (referred to in Table 1) as reasons for discontinuation of therapy by ≥ 0.5% of the Levatol group is listed in Table 2.

[See table above.]

Potential Adverse Effects —In addition, certain adverse effects not listed above have been reported with other β-blocking agents and should also be considered as potential adverse effects of Levatol.

Central Nervous System —Reversible mental depression progressing to catatonia (an acute syndrome characterized by disorientation for time and place), short-term memory loss, emotional lability, slightly clouded sensorium, and decreased performance (neuropsychometrics).

Cardiovascular —Intensification of AV block (see CONTRAINDICATIONS).

Allergic —Erythematous rash, fever combined with aching and sore throat, laryngospasm, and respiratory distress.

Hematologic —Agranulocytosis, nonthrombocytopenic, and thrombocytopenic purpura.

Gastrointestinal —Mesenteric arterial thrombosis and ischemic colitis.

Miscellaneous —Reversible alopecia and Peyronie's disease. The oculomucocutaneous syndrome associated with the β-blocker practolol has not been reported with Levatol during investigational use and extensive foreign clinical experience.

OVERDOSAGE

There is no actual experience with Levatol overdose. The signs and symptoms that would be expected with overdosage of β-adrenergic receptor antagonists are symptomatic bradycardia, hypotension, bronchospasm, and acute cardiac failure. In addition to discontinuation of Levatol, gastric emptying, and close observation of the patient, the following measures might be considered as appropriate:

Excessive Bradycardia —Administer atropine sulfate to induce vagal blockade. If bradycardia persists, intravenous isoproterenol hydrochloride may be administered cautiously; larger than usual doses may be needed. In refractory cases, the use of a transvenous cardiac pacemaker may be necessary.

Hypotension —Sympathomimetic drug therapy, such as dopamine, dobutamine, or levarterenol, may be considered if hypotension persists despite correction of bradycardia. In refractory cases, administration of glucagon hydrochloride has been reported to be useful.

Bronchospasm —A β-2-agonist or isoproterenol hydrochloride may be administered. Additional therapy with aminophylline may be considered.

Acute Cardiac Failure —Institute conventional therapy immediately. Intravenous administration of dobutamine and glucagon hydrochloride have been reported to be useful.

Heart Block (Second or Third Degree) —Isoproterenol hydrochloride or a transvenous cardiac pacemaker may be used.

DOSAGE AND ADMINISTRATION

The usual starting and maintenance dose of Levatol® (penbutolol sulfate) 20 mg, used alone or in combination with

Table 2.
DISCONTINUATIONS DURING CONTROLLED U.S. STUDIES

Body System Experience	Penbutolol (N = 628) %	Placebo (N = 212) %	Propranolol (N = 266) %
Body as a Whole			
Asthenia	0.6	0.0	0.4
Pain, chest	0.6	1.4	0.4
Digestive System			
Nausea	0.8	0.0	0.8
Nervous System			
Depression	0.6	0.5	0.8
Dizziness	0.6	0.0	0.4
Fatigue	0.5	0.5	0.0
Headache	0.6	0.5	0.4

Table 1.
ADVERSE REACTIONS DURING CONTROLLED U.S. STUDIES

Body System Experience	Penbutolol (N = 628) %	Placebo (N = 212) %	Propranolol (N = 266) %
Body as a Whole			
Asthenia	1.6	0.9	4.9
Pain, chest	2.4	2.8	2.3
Pain, limb	2.4	1.4	1.5
Digestive System			
Diarrhea	3.3	1.9	2.6
Nausea	4.3	0.9	2.3
Dyspepsia	2.7	1.4	5.3
Nervous System			
Dizziness	4.9	2.4	4.2
Fatigue	4.4	1.9	2.6
Headache	7.8	6.1	7.5
Insomnia	1.9	0.9	2.6
Respiratory System			
Cough	2.1	0.5	1.1
Dyspnea	2.1	1.4	3.4
Upper respiratory infection	2.5	3.3	4.9
Skin and Appendages			
Sweating, excessive	1.6	0.5	2.3
Urogenital System			
Impotence, sexual	0.5	0.0	0.8

other antihypertensive agents, such as thiazide-type diuretics, is 20 mg given once daily.

Doses of 40 mg and 80 mg have been well-tolerated but have not been shown to give a greater antihypertensive effect. The full effect of a 20- or 40-mg dose is seen by the end of 2 weeks. A dose of 10 mg also lowers blood pressure, but the full effect is not seen for 4 to 6 weeks.

HOW SUPPLIED

Tablets, yellow, scored capsule-shaped, engraved RC 22
20 mg—(100s) NDC 0021-4500-15.
Store at controlled room temperature 15°–30°C (59°–86°F).
Keep tightly closed and protect from light.

ANIMAL TOXICOLOGY

Studies in rats indicated that the combination of penbutolol, triamterene, and hydrochlorothiazide (up to 40, 50 and 25 mg/kg, respectively) increased the incidence and severity of renal tubular dilation and regeneration when compared to that in rats treated only with triamterene and hydrochlorothiazide. Dogs administered the same doses of triamterene and hydrochlorothiazide alone and in combination with penbutolol had an increase in serum alkaline phosphatase and serum alanine transferase, but there were no gross or microscopic abnormalities observed. No significant toxicologic findings were observed in rats and dogs treated with a combination of penbutolol and hydrochlorothiazide.

Revised December 1991

Manufactured For:
REED & CARNRICK
Division of Block Drug Company, Inc.
Jersey City, N.J. 07302-9988
By: ELI LILLY AND COMPANY
Indianapolis, IN 46285 USA

Shown in Product Identification Section, page 424

PHAZYME® Drops   OTC
[fā ′zīm]
(simethicone/antiflatulent)

(See PDR For Nonprescription Drugs.)

PHAZYME®–95 Tablets   OTC
[fā ′zīm]

(See PDR For Nonprescription Drugs.)

PHAZYME®–125 Softgels   OTC
[fā ′zīm]

(See PDR For Nonprescription Drugs.)

PROCTOCREAM®–HC   ℞
(hydrocortisone acetate 1% and
pramoxine hydrochloride 1%)

DESCRIPTION

PROCTOCREAM®-HC is a topical preparation containing hydrocortisone acetate 1.0% and pramoxine hydrochloride 1.0% in a hydrophilic cream base containing stearic acid, cetyl alcohol, aquaphor, isopropyl palmitate, polyoxyl-40 stearate, propylene glycol, potassium sorbate 0.1%, sorbic acid 0.1%, triethanolamine lauryl sulfate and water.
Topical corticosteroids are anti-inflammatory and antipruritic agents. The chemical structural formulae for the active ingredients are presented below.

Hydrocortisone acetate
(Pregn-4-ene-3,20-dione, 21-(acetyloxy)-11, 17-dihydroxy-, (11β).

Pramoxine hydrochloride
(4-(3-(p-butoxyphenoxy)propyl)morpholine hydrochloride)

CLINICAL PHARMACOLOGY

Topical corticosteroids share anti-inflammatory, antipruritic and vasoconstrictive actions.
The mechanism of anti-inflammatory activity of the topical corticosteroids is unclear. Various laboratory methods, including vasoconstrictor assays, are used to compare and predict potencies and/or clinical efficacies of the topical corticosteroids. There is some evidence to suggest that a recognizable correlation exists between vasoconstrictor potency and therapeutic efficacy in man.
Pramoxine hydrochloride is a topical anesthetic agent which provides temporary relief from itching and pain. It acts by stabilizing the neuronal membrane of nerve endings with which it comes into contact.

PHARMACOKINETICS

The extent of percutaneous absorption of topical corticosteroids is determined by many factors including the vehicle, the integrity of the epidermal barrier, and the use of occlusive dressings.
Topical corticosteroids can be absorbed from normal intact skin. Inflammation and/or other disease processes in the skin increase the percutaneous absorption. Occlusive dressings substantially increase the percutaneous absorption of topical corticosteroids. Thus, occlusive dressings may be a valuable therapeutic adjunct for treatment of resistant dermatoses. (See DOSAGE AND ADMINISTRATION).
Once absorbed through the skin, topical corticosteroids are handled through pharmacokinetic pathways similar to systemically administered corticosteroids. Corticosteroids are bound to plasma proteins in varying degress. Corticosteroids are metabolized primarily in the liver and are then excreted by the kidneys. Some of the topical corticosteroids and their metabolites are also excreted into the bile.

INDICATIONS AND USAGE

Topical corticosteroids are indicated for the relief of the inflammatory and pruritic manifestations of corticosteroid-responsive dermatoses.

CONTRAINDICATIONS

Topical corticosteroids are contraindicated in those patients with a history of hypersensitivity to any of the components of the preparation.

PRECAUTIONS

General: Systemic absorption of topical corticosteroids has produced reversible hypothalamic-pituitary-adrenal (HPA) axis suppression, manifestations of Cushing's syndrome, hyperglycemia, and glucosuria in some patients.
Conditions which augment systemic absorption include the applications of the more potent steroids, use over large surface areas, prolonged use, and the addition of occlusive dressings.
Therefore, patients receiving a large dose of a potent topical steroid applied to a large surface area and under an occlusive dressing should be evaluated periodically for evidence of HPA axis suppression by using the urinary free cortisol and ACTH stimulation tests. If HPA axis suppression is noted, an attempt should be made to withdraw the drug, to reduce the frequency of application, or to substitute a less potent steroid.
Recovery of HPA axis function is generally prompt and complete upon discontinuation of the drug. Infrequently, signs and symptoms of steroid withdrawal may occur, requiring supplemental systemic corticosteroids.
Children may absorb proportionally larger amounts of topical corticosteroids and, thus, be more susceptible to systemic toxicity. (See PRECAUTIONS—Pediatric Use.)
If irritation develops, topical corticosteroids should be discontinued and appropriate therapy instituted.
In the presence of dermatological infections, the use of an appropriate antifungal or antibacterial agent should be instituted. If a favorable response does not occur promptly, the corticosteroid should be discontinued until the infection has been adequately controlled.

Information for the Patient: Patients using topical corticosteroids should receive the following information and instructions.
1. The medication is to be used as directed by the physician. It is for external use only. Avoid contact with the eyes.
2. Patients should be advised not to use this medication for any disorder other than for which it was prescribed.
3. The treated skin area should not be bandaged or otherwise covered or wrapped as to be occlusive unless directed by the physician.
4. Patients should report any signs of local adverse reactions especially under occlusive dressing.
5. Parents of pediatric patients should be advised not to use tight-fitting diapers or plastic pants on a child being treated in the diaper area, as these garments may constitute occlusive dressings.

Laboratory Tests: The following tests may be helpful in evaluating the HPA axis suppression:
Urinary free cortisol test
ACTH stimulation test

Carcinogenesis, Mutagenesis, and Impairment of Fertility:
Long-term animal studies have not been performed to evaluate the carcinogenic potential or the effect on fertility of topical corticosteroids.
Studies to determine mutagenicity with prednisolone and hydrocortisone have revealed negative results.
Pregnancy Category C: Corticosteroids are genrally teratogenic in laboratory animals when administered systemically at relatively low dosage levels. The more potent corticosteroids have been shown to be teratogenic after dermal application in laboratory animals. There are no adequate and well-controlled studies in pregnant women on teratogenic effects from topically applied corticosteroids. Therefore, topical corticosteroids should be used during pregnancy only if the potential benefit justifies the potential risk to the fetus. Drugs of this class should not be used extensively on pregnant patients, in large amounts, or for prolonged periods of time.
Nursing Mothers: It is not known whether topical administration of corticosteroids could result in sufficient systemic absorption to produce detectable amounts in breast milk. Systemically administered corticosteroids are secreted into breast milk in quantities NOT likely to have a deleterious effect on the infant. Nevertheless, caution should be exercised when topical corticosteroids are administered to a nursing woman.
Pediatric Use: Pediatric patients may demonstrate greater susceptibility to topical corticosteroid-induced HPA axis suppression and Cushing's syndrome than mature patients because of a large skin surface area to body weight ratio. Hypothalamic-pituitary-adrenal (HPA) axis suppression, Cushing's syndrome, and intracranial hypertension have been reported in children receiving topical corticosteroids. Manifestations of adrenal suppression in children include linear growth retardation, delayed weight gain, low plasma cortisol levels, and absence of response of ACTH stimulation. Manifestations of intracranial hypertension include bulging fontanelles, headaches, and bilateral papilledema. Administration of topical corticosteroids to children should be limited to the least amount compatible with an effective therapeutic regimen. Chronic corticosteroid therapy may interfere with the growth and development of children.

ADVERSE REACTIONS

The following local adverse reactions are reported infrequently with topical corticosteroids, but may occur more frequently with the use of occlusive dressings. These reactions are listed in an approximate decreasing order of occurrence:
Burning
Itching
Irritation
Dryness
Folliculitis
Hypertrichosis
Acneiform eruptions
Hypopigmentation
Perioral dermatitis
Allergic contact dermatitis
Maceration of the skin
Secondary infection
Skin Atrophy
Striae
Miliaria

OVERDOSAGE

Topically applied corticosteroids can be absorbed in sufficient amounts to produce systemic effects (See PRECAUTIONS).

DOSAGE AND ADMINISTRATION

Topical corticosteroids are generally applied to the affected area as a thin film three or four times daily depending on the severity of the condition.
Occlusive dressings may be used for the management of psoriasis or recalcitrant conditions.
If an infection develops, the use of occlusive dressings should be discontinued and appropriate antimicrobial therapy instituted.

HOW SUPPLIED

1 oz. tube. (NDC 0021-4620-10)
Store at controlled room temperature 15°–30°C (59°–86°F).

CAUTION

Federal law prohibits dispensing without prescription.

Revised November 1991

Manufactured for
REED & CARNRICK
Division of Block Drug Company, Inc.
Jersey City, New Jersey 07302-9988
By FERNDALE LABORATORIES, INC.
Ferndale, Michigan 48220

Shown in Product Identification Section, page 424

Continued on next page

Reed & Carnrick—Cont.

PROCTOFOAM®-HC ℞
(hydrocortisone acetate 1%
and pramoxine hydrochloride 1%)
TOPICAL AEROSOL

DESCRIPTION
A topical corticosteroid aerosol foam for anal use containing hydrocortisone acetate 1% and pramoxine hydrochloride 1% in a hydrophilic base of: propylene glycol, ethoxylated cetyl and stearyl alcohols, steareth-10, cetyl alcohol, methylparaben, propylparaben, trolamine, purified water and propellants (inert): dichlorodifluoromethane and dichlorotetrafluoroethane.
PROCTOFOAM®-HC contains a synthetic steroid used as an anti-inflammatory and antipruritic agent, and a local anesthetic.
Hydrocortisone acetate
Molecular weight: 404.50. Solubility of hydrocortisone acetate in water: 1 mg/100ml.
Chemical name: Pregn-4-ene,3,20-dione, 21-(acetyloxy)-11, 17-dihydroxy-,(11β).

Pramoxine hydrochloride
Molecular weight: 329.87. Pramoxine hydrochloride is freely soluble in water. Chemical name: Morpholine, 4-[3-(4-butoxyphenoxy) propyl]-, hydrochloride, 4-[3(p-Butoxyphenoxy) propyl] morpholine hydrochloride.

CLINICAL PHARMACOLOGY
Topical corticosteroids share anti-inflammatory, antipruritic and vasoconstrictive actions.
The mechanism of anti-inflammatory activity of the topical corticosteroids is unclear. Various laboratory methods, including vasoconstrictor assays, are used to compare and predict potencies and/or clinical efficacies of the topical corticosteroids. There is some evidence to suggest that a recognizable correlation exists between vasoconstrictor potency and therapeutic efficacy in man.
Pramoxine hydrochloride: A surface or local anesthetic which is not chemically related to the "caine" types of local anesthetics. Its unique chemical structure is likely to minimize the danger of cross-sensitivity reactions in patients allergic to other local anesthetics.
Pharmacokinetics: The extent of percutaneous absorption of topical corticosteroids is determined by many factors including the vehicle, the integrity of the epidermal barrier, and the use of occlusive dressings.
Topical corticosteroids can be absorbed through normal intact skin. Inflammation and/or other disease processes in the skin increase the percutaneous absorption of topical corticosteroids. Occlusive dressings substantially increase the percutaneous absorption of topical corticosteroids. Thus, occlusive dressings may be a valuable therapeutic adjunct for treatment of resistant dermatoses. (See DOSAGE AND ADMINISTRATION.)
Once absorbed through the skin, topical corticosteroids are handled through pharmacokinetic pathways similar to systemically administered corticosteroids. Corticosteroids are bound to plasma proteins in varying degrees. Corticosteroids are metabolized primarily in the liver and are then excreted by the kidneys. Some of the topical corticosteroids and their metabolites are also excreted in the bile.

INDICATIONS AND USAGE
Topical corticosteroids are indicated for the relief of the inflammatory and pruritic manifestations of corticosteroid-responsive dermatoses of the anal region.

CONTRAINDICATIONS
Topical corticosteroid products are contraindicated in those patients with a history of hypersensitivity to any of the components of the preparation.

WARNINGS
Do not insert any part of the aerosol container into the anus. Contents of the container are under pressure. Do not burn or puncture the aerosol container. Store at temperatures below 120°F. If there is no evidence of clinical or proctologic improvement within two or three weeks after therapy, or if the patient's condition worsens, discontinue the drug. Keep this and all medicines out of the reach of children.

PRECAUTIONS
General: Systemic absorption of topical corticosteroids has produced reversible hypothalamic-pituitary-adrenal (HPA) axis suppression, manifestations of Cushing's syndrome, hyperglycemia and glucosuria in some patients.
Conditions which augment systemic absorption include the application of the more potent steroids, use over large surface areas, prolonged use and the addition of occlusive dressings.
Therefore, patients receiving a large dose of a potent topical steroid applied to a large surface area or under an occlusive dressing should be evaluated periodically for evidence of HPA axis suppression by using the urinary free cortisol and ACTH stimulation tests. If HPA axis suppression is noted, an attempt should be made to withdraw the drug, to reduce the frequency of application, or to substitute a less potent steroid.
Recovery of HPA axis function is generally prompt and complete upon discontinuation of the drug. Infrequently, signs and symptoms of steroid withdrawal may occur, requiring supplemental systemic corticosteroids.
In children, absorption may result in higher blood levels and thus more susceptibility to systemic toxicity. (See PRECAUTIONS—Pediatric Use.)
If irritation develops, topical corticosteroids should be discontinued and appropriate therapy instituted.
In the presence of dermatological infections, the use of an appropriate antifungal or antibacterial agent should be instituted. If a favorable response does not occur promptly, the corticosteroid should be discontinued until the infection has been adequately controlled.
Information for the Patient
Patients using topical corticosteroids should receive the following information and instructions:
1. This medication is to be used as directed by the physician. It is for anal or perianal use only. Avoid contact with the eyes.
2. Be advised not to use this medication for any disorder other than for which it has been prescribed.
3. Report any signs of adverse reactions.
Laboratory Tests
The following tests may be helpful in evaluating the HPA axis suppression:
  Urinary free cortisol test
  ACTH stimulation test
Carcinogenesis, Mutagenesis, and Impairment of Fertility
Long-term animal studies have not been performed to evaluate carcinogenic potential or the effect on fertility of topical corticosteroids.
Studies to determine mutagenicity with prednisolone and hydrocortisone have revealed negative results.
Pregnancy Category C
Corticosteroids are generally teratogenic in laboratory animals when administered systemically at relatively low dosage levels. The more potent corticosteroids have been shown to be teratogenic after dermal application in laboratory animals. There are no adequate and well-controlled studies in pregnant women of teratogenic effects from topically applied corticosteroids. Therefore, topical corticosteroids should be used during pregnancy only if the potential benefit justifies the potential risk to the fetus. Drugs of this class should not be used extensively on pregnant patients, in large amounts, or for prolonged periods of time.
Nursing Mothers
It is not known whether topical administration of corticosteroids could result in sufficient systemic absorption to produce detectable quantities in breast milk. Systemically administered corticosteroids are secreted into breast milk in quantities not likely to have a deleterious effect on the infant. Caution should be exercised when any topical corticosteroids are administered to a nursing woman.
Pediatric Use
Pediatric patients may demonstrate greater susceptibility to topical corticosteroid-induced HPA axis suppression and Cushing's syndrome than mature patients because of a larger skin surface area to body weight ratio.
Hypothalamic-pituitary-adrenal (HPA) axis suppression, Cushing's syndrome and intracranial hypertension have been reported in children receiving topical corticosteroids. Manifestations of adrenal suppression in children include linear growth retardation, delayed weight gain, low plasma cortisone levels and absense of response to ACTH stimulation. Manifestations of intracranial hypertension include bulging fontanelles, headaches and bilateral papilledema. Administration of topical corticosteroids to children should be limited to the least amount compatible with an effective therapeutic regimen. Chronic corticosteroid therapy may interfere with the growth and development of children.

ADVERSE REACTIONS
The following local adverse reactions are reported infrequently with topical corticosteroids, but may occur more frequently with the use of occlusive dressings. These reactions are listed in an approximate decreasing order of occurrence.

Burning	Perioral dermatitis
Itching	Allergic contact
Irritation	dermatitis
Dryness	Maceration of the skin
Folliculitis	Secondary infection
Hypertrichosis	Skin atrophy
Acneiform eruptions	Striae
Hypopigmentation	Miliaria

OVERDOSAGE
Topically applied corticosteroids can be absorbed in sufficient amounts to produce systemic effects. (See PRECAUTIONS.)

DOSAGE AND ADMINISTRATION
(NOTE: SEE PACKAGE FOR FULL DIRECTIONS FOR USE.)
Apply to affected areas 3 or 4 times daily. Use the applicator supplied for anal administration. For perianal use, transfer a small quantity to a tissue and rub in gently.
1. Shake foam container vigorously before use. Hold container upright and insert into opening of the tip of the applicator. Be sure applicator plunger is drawn all the way out. **CONTAINER MUST BE HELD UPRIGHT TO OBTAIN PROPER FLOW OF MEDICATION.**
2. To fill, press down slowly on container cap. Repeat until foam reaches fill line in the applicator. CAUTION: The aerosol container should never be inserted directly into the anus.
3. Remove applicator from container. Allow some foam to remain on the applicator tip. Hold applicator by barrel and gently insert tip into the anus. With applicator in place, push plunger in order to expel foam, then withdraw applicator. (Applicator parts should be pulled apart for thorough cleaning with warm water.)

HOW SUPPLIED
PROCTOFOAM®-HC (hydrocortisone acetate 1% and pramoxine hydrochloride 1%) topical aerosol (NDC 0021-0690-10) is supplied in 10 gram aerosol container with a special anal applicator. **Store upright at controlled room temperature 15°-30°C (59°-86°F).**
When used correctly, the aerosol container will deliver a minimum of 14 applications.

CAUTION
FEDERAL LAW PROHIBITS DISPENSING WITHOUT PRESCRIPTION.
Revised May 1992
Reed & Carnrick
Division of Block Drug Company, Inc.
Jersey City, N.J. 07302-9988
Shown in Product Identification Section, page 424

Regency Medical Research, Ltd.
2401 S. 24TH ST.
PHOENIX, AZ 85034

MEDI-MIST Intra-Oral Spray   OTC
Dietary Supplements

DESCRIPTION
Medi-Mist spray is a patented Intra-Oral application of vitamin and mineral supplementation. A 50 microliter spray delivers high concentrations of nutrients directly into the mouth's sensitive tissue. The buccal mucosa transfers the nutrients into the bloodstream, bypassing the G.I. tract.

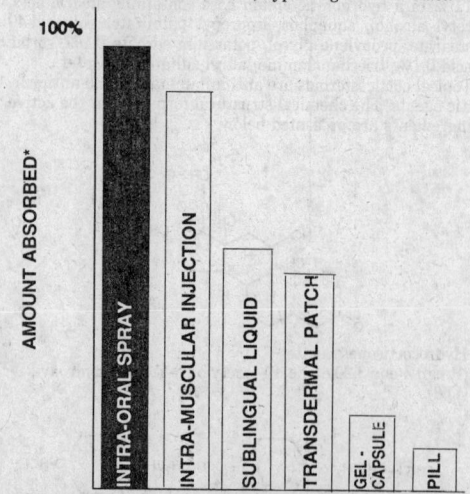

METHOD OF DELIVERY
*Representative of the product class.

PRODUCT FORMULATIONS AND COMPOSITION

Multiple 11 vitamins and 72 trace minerals in adult/child doses

Vitamin C, E + Zinc with lysine and bioflavonoids

Stress double compounded B-complex vitamins in a herbal base

Vitamin B-12 1000% of USRDA per dose

Vitamin A high concentration 25,000 I.U. per spray

PMS supplements the nutrient needs during syndrome

Smoke-less herbal combination with Ascorbic Acid and D-Alpha Tocopheryl supplement nutrient needs, aid smoking cessation

Nutra-lean dietary snack replacements with a combination of Amino Acids, B-6, B-12 and Chromium Polynicotinate

DOSAGE AND ADMINISTRATION

8 sprays = 1 dose (except Vit. A formula, 1 spray = 1 dose). Spray directly into mouth 2 sprays 4 times per day.

HOW SUPPLIED

Medi-Mist Intra-Oral sprays are supplied in a 13.3 ml vial containing approximately 240 metered sprays from a non-aerosol pump

---

EDUCATIONAL MATERIAL

If desired, additional literature on oral absorption will be provided upon request to Regency Medical Research.

Research Industries Corporation
Pharmaceutical Division
6864 SOUTH 300 WEST
MIDVALE, UTAH 84047

RIMSO®–50   ℞
[rĭm 'sō-50]
(brand of dimethyl sulfoxide)

PRODUCT OVERVIEW

KEY FACTS

The active component of Rimso®-50 is sterile and pyrogen-free dimethyl sulfoxide.

MAJOR USES

Rimso®-50 has been proved to be clinically effective for the symptomatic relief of patients with interstitial cystitis.

SAFETY INFORMATION

Intravesical instillation of Rimso®-50 may be harmful to patients with urinary tract malignancy because of dimethyl sulfoxide-induced vasodilation.

Dimethyl sulfoxide can initiate the liberation of histamine and there have been occasional hypersensitivity reactions with topical administration.

Dimethyl sulfoxide should be used during pregnancy only if the potential benefit justifies the potential risk to the fetus.

PRESCRIBING INFORMATION

RIMSO®–50   ℞
[rĭm 'sō-50]
(brand of dimethyl sulfoxide)

DESCRIPTION

RIMSO®-50, brand of dimethyl sulfoxide ((DMSO) 50% w/w Aqueous Solution for intravesical instillation. Each ml contains 0.54 gm dimethyl sulfoxide STERILE AND PYROGEN-FREE.

Intravesical instillation for the treatment of interstitial cystitis.

NOT FOR I.M. OR I.V. INJECTION

CAUTION

Federal law prohibits dispensing without a prescription. The active component of RIMSO®-50 is dimethyl sulfoxide which has the empirical formula C_2H_6OS.

Dimethyl sulfoxide is a clear, colorless and essentially odorless liquid which is miscible with water and most organic solvents. Other physical characteristics include: molecular weight 78.13, melting point 18.4°C, and a specific gravity of 1.096.

CLINICAL PHARMACOLOGY

Dimethyl sulfoxide is metabolized in man by oxidation to dimethyl sulfone or by reduction to dimethyl sulfide. Dimethyl sulfoxide and dimethyl sulfone are excreted in the urine and feces. Dimethyl sulfide is eliminated through the breath and skin and is responsible for the characteristic odor from patients on dimethyl sulfoxide medication. Dimethyl sulfone can persist in serum for longer than two weeks after a single intravesical instillation. No residual accumulation of dimethyl sulfoxide has occurred in man or lower animals who have received treatment for protracted periods of time.

Following topical application, dimethyl sulfoxide is absorbed and generally distributed in the tissues and body fluids.

INDICATIONS AND USAGE

RIMSO®-50 (dimethyl sulfoxide) is indicated for the symptomatic relief of patients with interstitial cystitis. RIMSO®-50 has not been approved as being safe and effective for any other indication. There is no clinical evidence of effectiveness of dimethyl sulfoxide in the treatment of bacterial infections of the urinary tract.

CONTRAINDICATIONS

None known.

WARNINGS

Dimethyl sulfoxide can initiate the liberation of histamine and there has been an occasional hypersensitivity reaction with topical administration of dimethyl sulfoxide. This hypersensitivity has been reported in one patient receiving intravesical RIMSO®-50. The physician should be cognizant of this possibility in prescribing RIMSO®-50. If anaphylactoid symtoms develop, appropriate therapy should be instituted.

PRECAUTIONS

Changes in the refractive index and lens opacities have been seen in monkeys, dogs and rabbits given high doses of dimethyl sulfoxide chronically. Since lens changes were noted in animals, full eye evaluations, including slit lamp examinations are recommended prior to and periodically during treatment.

Approximately every six months patients receiving dimethyl sulfoxide should have a biochemical screening, particularly liver and renal function tests, and complete blood count. Intravesical instillation of RIMSO®-50 may be harmful to patients with urinary tract malignancy because of dimethyl sulfoxide-induced vasodilation.

Some data indicate that dimethyl sulfoxide potentiates other concomitantly administered medications.

Pregnancy Category C. Dimethyl sulfoxide caused teratogenic responses in hamsters, rats and mice when administered intraperitoneally at high doses (2.5–12 gm/kg). Oral or topical doses of dimethyl sulfoxide did not cause problems of reproduction in rats, mice and hamsters. Topical doses (5 gm/kg first two days, then 2.5 gm/kg-last eight days) produced terata in rabbits, but in another study, topical doses of 1.1 gm/kg days 3 through 16 of gestation failed to produce any abnormalities. There are no adequate and well controlled studies in pregnant women. Dimethyl sulfoxide should be used during pregnancy only if the potential benefit justifies the potential risk to the fetus. It is not known whether this drug is excreted in human milk. Because many drugs are excreted in human milk, caution should be exercised when dimethyl sulfoxide is administered to a nursing woman.

Safety and effectiveness in children has been established.

Information available to be given to the patient is reprinted at the end of this text.

ADVERSE REACTIONS

A garlic-like taste may be noted by the patient within a few minutes after instillation of RIMSO®-50 (dimethyl sulfoxide). This taste may last several hours and because of the presence of metabolites an odor on the breath and skin may remain for 72 hours.

Transient chemical cystitis has been noted following instillation of dimethyl sulfoxide.

The patient may experience moderately severe discomfort on administration. Usually this becomes less prominent with repeated administration.

DRUG ABUSE AND DEPENDENCE

None known.

OVERDOSAGE

The oral LD_{50} of dimethyl sulfoxide in the dog is greater than 10 gm/kg. It is improbable that this dosage level could be obtained with intravesical instillation of RIMSO®-50 in the patient.

In case of accidental oral ingestion, specific measures should be taken to induce emesis. Additional measures which may be considered are gastric lavage, activated charcoal and forced diuresis.

DOSAGE AND ADMINISTRATION

Instillation of 50 ml of RIMSO®-50 (dimethyl sulfoxide) directly into the bladder may be accomplished by catheter or asepto syringe and allowed to remain for 15 minutes. Application of an analgesic lubricant gel such as lidocaine jelly to the urethra is suggested prior to insertion of the catheter to avoid spasm. The medication is expelled by spontaneous voiding. It is recommended that the treatment be repeated every two weeks until maximum symptomatic relief is obtained. Thereafter, time intervals between therapy may be increased appropriately.

Administration of oral analgesic medication or suppositories containing belladonna and opium prior to the instillation of RIMSO®-50 can reduce bladder spasm.

In patients with severe interstitial cystitis with very sensitive bladders, the initial treatment, and possibly the second and third (depending on patient response) should be done under anesthesia. (Saddle block has been suggested).

HOW SUPPLIED

Bottles contain 50 ml of sterile and pyrogen-free RIMSO®-50 (50% w/w dimethyl sulfoxide aqueous solution).

Dimethyl sulfoxide is clear and colorless

Protect from strong light

Store at room temperature (59° to 86°F) (15° to 30°C)

Do not autoclave

NDC #0433-0433-05

For additional information concerning RIMSO®-50, contact the Pharmaceutical Division, Research Industries Corporation. Salt Lake City, Utah

RIMSO®-50 is manufactured by Tera Pharmaceuticals, Inc., Buena Park, California, for the Pharmaceutical Division, Research Industries Corp., Salt Lake City, Utah.

Rexar Pharmacal Corp.
396 ROCKAWAY AVENUE
VALLEY STREAM, NY 11581

OBETROL™ Tablets   ℃II

DESCRIPTION

A single entity amphetamine product combining the neutral sulfate salts of dextroamphetamine and amphetamine, with the dextro isomer of amphetamine saccharate and d,l amphetamine aspartate.

EACH TABLET CONTAINS:	10 mg.	20 mg.
Dextroamphetamine Saccharate	2.5 mg.	5 mg.
Amphetamine Aspartate	2.5 mg.	5 mg.
Dextroamphetamine Sulfate	2.5 mg.	5 mg.
Amphetamine Sulfate	2.5 mg.	5 mg.

Inactive Ingredients: Sucrose, Lactose, Cornstarch, Acacia and Magnesium Stearate.

Colors: Obetrol 10 contains FD&C Blue #1

Colors: Obetrol 20 contains FD&C Yellow #6 as a color additive

HOW SUPPLIED

Obetrol 10 mg Blue scored tablet IMPRINTED OP-32
   NDC 0477-5432-01   for 100's
   NDC 0477-5432-05   for 500's
   NDC 0477-5432-10   for 1000's
Obetrol 20 mg Orange scored tablet IMPRINTED 0P-33
   NDC 0477-5433-01   for 100's
   NDC 0477-5433-05   for 500's
   NDC 0477-5433-10   for 1000's

Dispense in a tight container as defined in the USP.

Store at controlled room Temperature 15-30°C (59°–86°F).

Shown in Product Identification Section, page 424

DEXTROAMPHETAMINE SULFATE, USP   ℃II
5 mg and 10 mg Tablets

Shown in Product Identification Section, page 424

OBY-TRIM Capsules   ℞
Phentermine Hydrochloride, USP, 30 mg
(equivalent to 24 mg phentermine base)

REXATAL Tablets   ℞
Phenobarbital, USP, (¼ gr) 16.2 mg
Hyoscyamine Sulfate, USP, 0.1037 mg
Atropine Sulfate, USP, 0.0194 mg
Scopolamine Hydrobromide, USP, 0.0065 mg

X-TROZINE Tablets   ℞
X-TROZINE Capsules
Phendimetrazine Tartrate, USP, 35 mg

X-TROZINE L.A. Extended Release Capsules   ℞
Phendimetrazine Tartrate, USP, 105 mg

Rhône-Poulenc Rorer Pharmaceuticals Inc.
500 ARCOLA ROAD
COLLEGEVILLE, PA 19426-0107

Following is a list of Rhône-Poulenc Rorer Pharmaceuticals Inc. products. Full prescribing information is provided on the following pages for those products indicated by an asterisk. For further information, please call the Rhône-Poulenc Rorer Medical Affairs Information Line at (215) 454-8110 (8:15 a.m. to 4:45 p.m., Eastern Time). After hours, please call (919) 967-8090.

ACTHAR® for Injection   ℞
25 USP Units and 40 USP Units
Corticotropin for injection available as a lyophilized powder in vials containing 25 USP Units or 40 USP Units per vial.

H.P. ACTHAR® GEL
40 USP Units/mL and 80 USP Units/mL
Repository corticotropin injection available in strengths of 40 USP Units or 80 USP units per mL.

*AZMACORT® Oral Inhaler   ℞
Each metered-dose inhaler contains 60 mg triamcinolone acetonide. Each oral inhaler unit delivers 240 actuations of approximately 100 mcg of triamcinolone acetonide.
Pictured in Product Identification Section, page 424

BAROTRAST®   ℞
This radiopaque contrast medium contains 92.5% barium sulfate, suspending agents, and sodium saccharin.

*CALCIMAR® Injection, Synthetic   ℞
Each 2-mL vial contains 400 I.U. (200 I.U. per mL) calcitonin-salmon as a sterile solution for subcutaneous or intramuscular injection.
Pictured in Product Identification Section, page 424

CALEL-D® Tablets
Each tablet provides 500 mg of elemental Calcium (50% of U.S. RDA) from calcium carbonate and 200 I.U. of Vitamin D₃ (Cholecalciferol) (50% of U.S. RDA).

CLYSODRAST®   ℞
Clysodrast is supplied in packets containing 1.5 mg bisacodyl and 2.5 gm of tannic acid.

*DDAVP® Injection   ℞
Each mL of sterile, aqueous solution for injection provides 4.0 mcg desmopressin acetate.
Pictured in Product Identification Section, page 424

*DDAVP® Nasal Spray 5 mL   ℞
*DDAVP® Rhinal Tube 2.5 mL   ℞
Each mL of sterile, aqueous solution for intranasal use provides 0.1 mg desmopressin acetate.
Pictured in Product Identification Section, page 424

DEMI-REGROTON® Tablets
See Regroton® Tablets.

*DILACOR™ XR Extended-release Capsules ℞
Each capsule contains multiple units of diltiazem HCl 60 mg in a Geomatrix™ controlled-release system, resulting in 180-mg and 240-mg dosage strengths.
Pictured in Product Identification Section, page 424

ESOPHOTRAST® Cream   ℞
This radiopaque contrast medium contains 560 mg per gm (100% w/v) barium sulfate, suspending agent, and fruit flavoring.

HYGROTON® Tablets   ℞
25 mg, 50 mg, and 100 mg
Each tablet contains 25 mg, 50 mg, or 100 mg chlorthalidone, USP.
Pictured in Product Identification Section, page 424

*LOZOL® Tablets   ℞
Each tablet contains 2.5 mg indapamide.
Pictured in Product Identification Section, page 424

*NASACORT® Nasal Inhaler   ℞
This metered-dose aerosol unit delivers 100 actuations of approximately 55 mcg of triamcinolone acetonide.
Pictured in Product Identification Section, page 425

*NICOBID® Tempules®   ℞
125 mg, 250 mg, and 500 mg
Each timed-release capsule contains 125 mg, 250 mg, or 500 mg of niacin (nicotinic acid).

*NICOLAR® Tablets   ℞
Each tablet contains 500 mg of niacin (nicotinic acid).

*NITROLINGUAL® SPRAY   ℞
A 200-dose metered lingual aerosol delivering 0.4 mg of nitroglycerin per actuation.
Pictured in Product Identification Section, page 425

ORATRAST®   ℞
This radiopaque contrast medium contains 92% barium sulfate, suspending agents, and lime flavoring.

PARATHAR™ Injection, Synthetic   ℞
Teriparatide acetate synthetic injection is supplied in a 10-mL vial as a sterile, lyophilized powder containing 200 units hPTH activity with a 10-mL vial of diluent.

PAREPECTOLIN® Suspension
Each tablespoon contains 600 mg
attapulgite in a pleasant-tasting suspension. (OTC)

*PENETREX™ Tablets   ℞
Each 200-mg and 400-mg film-coated tablet contains enoxacin sesquihydrate equivalent to 200 mg and 400 mg of anhydrous enoxacin, respectively.
Pictured in Product Identification Section, page 425

REGROTON® Tablets   ℞
DEMI-REGROTON® Tablets   ℞
Each Regroton tablet provides 50 mg chlorthalidone, USP, and 0.25 mg reserpine, USP.
Each Demi-Regroton tablet provides 25 mg chlorthalidone, USP, and 0.125 mg reserpine, USP.
Pictured in Product Identification Section, page 425

*SLO-BID™ Gyrocaps®   ℞
50 mg, 75 mg, 100 mg, 125 mg, 200 mg, and 300 mg
Each extended-release capsule contains theophylline, anhydrous, USP.
Pictured in Product Identification Section, page 425

SLO-PHYLLIN® GYROCAPS®   ℞
60 mg, 125 mg, and 250 mg
Each extended-release capsule contains 60 mg, 125 mg, or 250 mg theophylline, anhydrous, USP.
Pictured in Product Identification Section, page 425

SLO-PHYLLIN® Tablets   ℞
100 mg and 200 mg
Each tablet contains 100 mg or 200 mg theophylline, anhydrous, USP.
Pictured in Product Identification Section, page 425

SLO-PHYLLIN® Syrup   ℞
Each 15 mL contains 80 mg theophylline, anhydrous, USP.

SLO-PHYLLIN® GG Capsules, Syrup   ℞
Each capsule or 15 mL of syrup contains 150 mg of theophylline, anhydrous, and 90 mg of guaifenesin.

THYRAR® Tablets   ℞
30 mg (½ gr), 60 mg (1 gr), and 120 mg (2 gr)
Thyroid tablets, bovine, provide 35 mcg levothyroxine (T₄) and 5 mcg liothyronine (T₃) per grain of thyroid.

THYTROPAR®   ℞
Thyrotropin for Injection is supplied as a sterile, lyophilized powder containing 10 IU of thyrotropic activity. Each package contains one vial of Thytropar and one vial of Thytropar Diluent (sodium chloride injection).

TUSSAR® DM Syrup   ℞
Each 5 mL contains 15 mg dextromethorphan hydrobromide, USP; 2 mg chlorpheniramine maleate, USP; and 30 mg psuedoephedrine HCl, USP.

TUSSAR®-2 Syrup   ℂ
Each 5 mL contains 10 mg codeine phosphate, USP; 30 mg pseudoephedrine HCl, USP; 100 mg guaifenesin, USP; and 2.5% alcohol.
(Warning: May be habit-forming.)

TUSSAR® SF Syrup   ℂ
(Sugar Free)
Formulation identical to Tussar-2, except Tussar SF contains saccharin-sorbitol base for patients who must limit sugar intake. Alcohol content 2.5%.
(Warning: May be habit-forming.)

* Please see full prescribing information on the following pages.

AZMACORT®   ℞
[ăz 'ma-kort]
(triamcinolone acetonide)
Oral Inhaler

FOR ORAL INHALATION ONLY
PRODUCT OVERVIEW
KEY FACTS
Azmacort® is an anti-inflammatory steroid in a metered-dose aerosol unit containing at least 240 actuations. Each actuation releases approximately 200 mcg triamcinolone acetonide, of which approximately 100 mcg are delivered from the unit. Azmacort provides effective local steroid activity with minimal systemic effect. Triamcinolone acetonide is a very potent derivative of triamcinolone.

MAJOR USES
Azmacort® inhaler is indicated only for patients who require chronic treatment with corticosteroids for the control of symptoms of bronchial asthma. Azmacort® Oral Inhaler is not to be regarded as a bronchodilator and is not indicated for rapid relief of bronchospasm.

SAFETY INFORMATION
Azmacort® Oral Inhaler is contraindicated in the primary treatment of status asthmaticus or other acute episodes of asthma requiring intensive measures. Particular care is needed in patients transferred from systemically active corticosteroids to Azmacort® inhaler because deaths due to adrenal insufficiency have occurred in asthmatic patients during and after such a transfer. Patients who are on immunosuppressant doses of corticosteroids should be warned to avoid exposure to chickenpox or measles and, if exposed, to obtain medical advice.

PRESCRIBING INFORMATION

AZMACORT®   ℞
[ăz 'ma-kort]
(triamcinolone acetonide)
Oral Inhaler

For Oral Inhalation Only
Shake Well Before Using
DESCRIPTION
Triamcinolone acetonide, USP, the active ingredient in Azmacort® Oral Inhaler, is a glucocorticosteroid with a molecular weight of 434.5 and with the chemical designation 9-Fluoro-11β, 16α, 17, 21-tetrahydroxypregna-1,4-diene-3, 20-dione cyclic 16, 17-acetal with acetone. ($C_{24}H_{31}FO_6$).

Azmacort Oral Inhaler is a metered-dose aerosol unit containing a microcrystalline suspension of triamcinolone acetonide in the propellant dichlorodifluoromethane and dehydrated alcohol USP 1% w/w. Each canister contains 60 mg triamcinolone acetonide. Each actuation releases approximately 200 mcg triamcinolone acetonide, of which approximately 100 mcg are delivered from the unit (in-vitro testing). There are at least 240 actuations in one Azmacort aerosol canister. After 240 actuations, the amount delivered per actuation may not be consistent and the unit should be discarded.

CLINICAL PHARMACOLOGY
The precise mechanism of the action of the inhaled drug is unknown. However, use of the inhaler makes it possible to provide effective local steroid activity with minimal systemic effect.
Triamcinolone acetonide is a very potent derivative of triamcinolone. Although triamcinolone itself is one to two times as potent as prednisone in animal models of inflammation, triamcinolone acetonide is approximately 8 times more potent than prednisone.
Pharmacokinetic studies with radiolabeled triamcinolone acetonide have been carried out by the oral route and intravenous route in several species. The pharmacokinetic behavior of the triamcinolone acetonide was similar in all species within each route of administration. The major portion of the dose was eliminated in the feces irrespective of route of administration with only one species (rabbit) showing significant urinary excretion of radioactivity.
The results of studies in which triamcinolone acetonide was administered as an aerosol showed rapid disappearance of radioactivity from the lungs comparable to that observed following oral administration with peak blood levels occurring in one to two hours. Virtually no radioactivity was present in the lung and trachea 24 hours after dosing.
Based upon intravenous dosing of triamcinolone acetonide phosphate ester, the half-life of triamcinolone acetonide was reported to be 88 minutes. The volume of distribution (Vd) reported was 99.5 L (SD ± 27.5) and clearance was 45.2 L/hour (SD ± 9.1) for triamcinolone acetonide. The plasma half-life of corticoids does not correlate well with the biologic half-life.
Three metabolites of triamcinolone acetonide have been identified. They are 6β-hydroxytriamcinolone acetonide, 21-carboxytriamcinolone acetonide and 21-carboxy-6β-hydroxytriamcinolone acetonide. All three metabolites are expected to be substantially less active than the parent compound due to (a) the dependence of anti-inflammatory activity on the presence of a 21-hydroxyl group, (b) the decreased activity observed upon 6-hydroxylation, and (c) the markedly increased water solubility favoring rapid elimination. There

appeared to be some quantitative differences in the metabolites among species. No differences were detected in metabolic pattern as a function of route of administration.

INDICATIONS

Azmacort (triamcinolone acetonide) Oral Inhaler is indicated only for patients who require chronic treatment with corticosteroids for the control of the symptoms of bronchial asthma. Such patients would include those already receiving systemic corticosteroids and selected patients who are inadequately controlled on a non-steroid regimen and in whom steroid therapy has been withheld because of concern over potential adverse effects.

Azmacort Oral Inhaler is *NOT* indicated:

1. For relief of asthma which can be controlled by bronchodilators and other non-steroid medications.
2. In patients who require systemic corticosteroid treatment infrequently.
3. In the treatment of non-asthmatic bronchitis.

CONTRAINDICATIONS

Azmacort Oral Inhaler is contraindicated in the primary treatment of status asthmaticus or other acute episodes of asthma where intensive measures are required.

Hypersensitivity to any of the ingredients of this preparation contraindicates its use.

WARNINGS

Particular care is needed in patients who are transferred from systemically active corticosteroids to **Azmacort** Oral Inhaler because deaths due to adrenal insufficiency have occurred in asthmatic patients during and after transfer from systemic corticosteroids to aerosolized steroids in recommended doses. After withdrawal from systemic corticosteroids, a number of months is usually required for recovery of hypothalamic-pituitary-adrenal (HPA) function. For some patients who have received large doses of oral steroids for long periods of time before therapy with **Azmacort** Oral Inhaler is initiated, recovery may be delayed for one year or longer. During this period of HPA suppression, patients may exhibit signs and symptoms of adrenal insufficiency when exposed to trauma, surgery or infections, particularly gastroenteritis or other conditions with acute electrolyte loss. Although **Azmacort** Oral Inhaler may provide control of asthmatic symptoms during these episodes, in recommended doses it supplies only normal physiological amounts of corticosteroid systemically and does NOT provide the increased systemic steroid which is necessary for coping with these emergencies.

During periods of stress or a severe asthmatic attack, patients who have been recently withdrawn from systemic corticosteroids should be instructed to resume systemic steroids (in large doses) immediately and to contact their physician for further instruction. These patients should also be instructed to carry a warning card indicating that they may need supplementary systemic steroids during periods of stress or a severe asthma attack.

Localized infections with *Candida albicans* have occurred infrequently in the mouth and pharynx. These areas should be examined by the treating physician at each patient visit. The percentage of positive mouth and throat cultures for *Candida albicans* did not change during a year of continuous therapy. The incidence of clinically apparent infection is low (2.5%). These infections may disappear spontaneously or may require treatment with appropriate antifungal therapy or discontinuance of treatment with **Azmacort** Oral Inhaler.

Children who are on immunosuppressant drugs are more susceptible to infections than healthy children. Chickenpox and measles, for example, can have a more serious or even fatal course in children on immunosuppressant doses of corticosteroids. In such children, or in adults who have not had these diseases, particular care should be taken to avoid exposure. If exposed, therapy with varicella zoster immune globulin (VZIG) or pooled intravenous immunoglobulin (IVIG), as appropriate, may be indicated. If chickenpox develops, treatment with antiviral agents may be considered.

Azmacort Oral Inhaler is not to be regarded as a bronchodilator and is not indicated for rapid relief of bronchospasm.

Patients should be instructed to contact their physician immediately when episodes of asthma which are not responsive to bronchodilators occur during the course of treatment with **Azmacort** Oral Inhaler. During such episodes, patients may require therapy with systemic corticosteroids.

There is no evidence that control of asthma can be achieved by the administration of **Azmacort** Oral Inhaler in amounts greater than the recommended doses, which appear to be the therapeutic equivalent of approximately 10 mg/day of oral prednisone.

The use of **Azmacort** Oral Inhaler with alternate-day systemic prednisone could increase the likelihood of HPA suppression compared to a therapeutic dose of either one alone. Therefore, **Azmacort** Oral Inhaler should be used with caution in patients already receiving alternate-day prednisone treatment for any disease.

Transfer of patients from systemic steroid therapy to **Azmacort** Oral Inhaler may unmask allergic conditions previously suppressed by the systemic steroid therapy, e.g., rhinitis, conjunctivitis, and eczema.

PRECAUTIONS

During withdrawal from oral steroids, some patients may experience symptoms of systemically active steroid withdrawal, e.g., joint and/or muscular pain, lassitude and depression, despite maintenance or even improvement of respiratory function (see DOSAGE AND ADMINISTRATION for details). Although steroid withdrawal effects are usually transient and not severe, severe and even fatal exacerbation of asthma can occur if the previous daily oral corticosteroid requirement had significantly exceeded 10 mg/day of prednisone or equivalent.

In responsive patients, inhaled corticosteroids will often permit control of asthmatic symptoms with less suppression of HPA function than therapeutically equivalent oral doses of prednisone. Since triamcinolone acetonide is absorbed into the circulation and can be systemically active, the beneficial effects of **Azmacort** Oral Inhaler in minimizing or preventing HPA dysfunction may be expected only when recommended dosages are not exceeded.

Suppression of HPA function has been reported in volunteers who received 4000 mcg daily of triamcinolone acetonide. In addition, suppression of HPA function has been reported in some patients who have received recommended doses for as little as 6–12 weeks. Since the response of HPA function to inhaled corticosteroids is highly individualized, the physician should consider this information when treating patients.

Because of the possibility of systemic absorption of inhaled corticosteroids, patients treated with these drugs should be observed carefully for any evidence of systemic corticosteroid effects including suppression of growth in children. Particular care should be taken in observing patients postoperatively or during periods of stress for evidence of a decrease in adrenal function.

The long-term effects of triamcinolone acetonide inhaler in human subjects are not completely known, although patients have received **Azmacort** Oral Inhaler on a continuous basis for periods of two years or longer. While there has been no clinical evidence of adverse experiences, the local effects of the agent on developmental or immunologic processes in the mouth, pharynx, trachea and lung are also unknown.

Azmacort Oral Inhaler should be used with caution, if at all, in patients with active or quiescent tuberculous infections of the respiratory tract or in patients with untreated fungal, bacterial, or systemic viral infections or ocular herpes simplex. The potential effects of long-term administration of **Azmacort** Oral Inhaler on lung or other tissues are unknown. However, pulmonary infiltrates with eosinophilia have occurred in patients receiving other inhaled corticosteroids.

When used at excessive doses, systemic corticosteroid effects such as hypercorticism and adrenal suppression may appear. If such changes occur, **Azmacort** Oral Inhaler should be discontinued slowly, consistent with accepted procedures for discontinuing oral steroid therapy.

Information for Patients: Patients who are on immunosuppressant doses of corticosteroids should be warned to avoid exposure to chickenpox or measles and, if exposed, to obtain medical advice.

Carcinogenesis, Mutagenesis: Animal studies of triamcinolone acetonide to tests its carcinogenic potential are underway.

Impairment of Fertility: Male and female rats which were administered oral triamcinolone acetonide at doses as high as 15 mcg/kg/day (110 mcg/m^2/day, as calculated on a surface area basis) exhibited no evidence of impaired fertility. The maximum human dose, for comparison, is 22.9 mcg/kg/day (889 mcg/m^2/day). However, a few female rats which received maternally toxic doses of 8 or 15 mcg/kg/day (60 mcg/m^2/day or 110 mcg/m^2/day, respectively, as calculated on a surface area basis) exhibited dystocia and prolonged delivery. Developmental toxicity, which included increases in fetal resorptions and stillbirths and decreases in pup body weight and survival, also occurred at the maternally toxic doses (2.5–15.0 mcg/kg/day or 20–110 mcg/m^2/day, as calculated on a surface area basis). Reproductive performance of female rats and effects on fetuses and offspring were comparable between groups that received placebo and non-toxic or marginally toxic doses (0.5 and 1.0 mcg/kg/day or 3.8 mcg/m^2/day and 7.0 mcg/m^2/day).

Pregnancy: Pregnancy Category C. Like other corticoids, triamcinolone acetonide has been shown to be teratogenic in rats and rabbits. Teratogenic effects, which occurred in both species at 0.02, 0.04 and 0.08 mg/kg/day (approximately 135, 270 and 540 mcg/m^2/day in the rat and 320, 640 and 1280 mcg/m^2/day in the rabbit, as calculated on a surface area basis), included a low incidence of cleft palate and/or internal hydrocephaly and axial skeletal defects. Teratogenic effects, including CNS and cranial malformations, have also been observed in non-human primates at 0.5 mg/kg/day (approximately 6.7 mg/m^2/day). Administration of aerosol by inhalation to pregnant rats and rabbits produced embryotoxic and fetotoxic effects which were comparable to those produced by administration by other routes. There are no adequate and well-controlled studies in pregnant women. Triamcinolone acetonide should be used during pregnancy only if the potential benefit justifies the potential risk to the fetus.

Experience with oral corticoids since their introduction in pharmacologic as opposed to physiologic doses suggests that rodents are more prone to teratogenic effects from corticoids than humans. In addition, because there is a natural increase in glucocorticoid production during pregnancy, most women will require a lower exogenous steroid dose and many will not need corticoid treatment during pregnancy.

Nonteratogenic Effects: Hypoadrenalism may occur in infants born of mothers receiving corticosteroids during pregnancy. Such infants should be carefully observed.

Nursing Mothers: It is not known whether triamcinolone acetonide is excreted in human milk. Because other corticosteroids are excreted in human milk, caution should be exercised when **Azmacort** Oral Inhaler is administered to nursing women.

Pediatric Use: Safety and effectiveness have not been established in children below the age of 6. Oral corticoids have been shown to cause growth suppression in children and teenagers, particularly with higher doses over extended periods. If a child or teenager on any corticoid appears to have growth suppression, the possibility that they are particularly sensitive to this effect of steroids should be considered.

ADVERSE REACTIONS

A few cases of oral candidiasis have been reported (see WARNINGS). In addition, some patients receiving **Azmacort** Oral Inhaler have experienced hoarseness, dry throat, irritated throat and dry mouth. Increased wheezing and cough have been reported infrequently as has facial edema. These adverse effects have generally been mild and transient.

DOSAGE AND ADMINISTRATION

All patients should be instructed that the **Azmacort** Oral Inhaler must be used on a regular daily basis rather than *prn*. Reliable dosage delivery cannot be assured after 240 actuations and patients should be cautioned against longer use of individual canisters.

Good oral hygiene including rinsing of the mouth after inhalation is recommended.

Adults: The usual dosage is two inhalations (approximately 200 mcg) given three to four times a day. The maximal daily intake should not exceed 16 inhalations (1600 mcg) in adults. Higher initial doses (12–16 inhalations per day) may be advisable in patients with more severe asthma, the dosage then being adjusted downward according to the response of the patient. In some patients maintenance can be accomplished when the total daily dose is given on a twice a day schedule.

Children 6 to 12 years of age: The usual dosage is one or two inhalations (100 to 200 mcg) given three to four times a day according to the response of the patient. The maximal daily intake should not exceed 12 inhalations (1200 mcg) in children 6 to 12 years of age. Insufficient clinical data exist with respect to the administration of **Azmacort** Oral Inhaler in children below the age of 6. The long-term effects of inhaled steroids on growth are still under evaluation.

Patients receiving bronchodilators by inhalation should be advised to use the bronchodilator before **Azmacort** Oral Inhaler in order to enhance penetration of triamcinolone acetonide into the bronchial tree. After use of an aerosol bronchodilator, several minutes should elapse before use of the **Azmacort** Oral Inhaler to reduce the potential toxicity from the inhaled fluorocarbon propellants in the two aerosols.

Different considerations must be given to the following groups of patients in order to obtain the full therapeutic benefit of **Azmacort** Oral Inhaler:

Patients not receiving systemic steroids: The use of **Azmacort** Oral Inhaler is straightforward in patients who are inadequately controlled with non-steroid medications but in whom systemic steroid therapy has been withheld because of concern over potential adverse reactions. In patients who respond to **Azmacort**, an improvement in pulmonary function is usually apparent within one to two weeks after the start of **Azmacort** Oral Inhaler.

Patients receiving systemic steroids: In those patients dependent on systemic steroids, transfer to **Azmacort** Oral Inhaler and subsequent management may be more difficult because recovery from impaired adrenal function is usually slow. Such suppression has been known to last for up to 12 months or longer. Clinical studies, however, have demonstrated that **Azmacort** Oral Inhaler may be effective in the management of these asthmatic patients and may permit

Continued on next page

replacement or significant reduction in the dosage of systemic corticosteroids.
The patient's asthma should be reasonably stable before treatment with **Azmacort** Oral Inhaler is started. Initially, the inhaler should be used concurrently with the patient's usual maintenance dose of systemic steroid. After approximately one week, gradual withdrawal of the systemic steroid is started by reducing the dose. The next reduction is made after an interval of one or two weeks, depending on the response of the patient. Generally, these decrements should not exceed 2.5 mg of prednisone or its equivalent. A slow rate of withdrawal cannot be overemphasized. During withdrawal, some patients may experience symptoms of systemically active steroid withdrawal, e.g., joint and/or muscular pain, lassitude and depression, despite maintenance or even improvement of respiratory function. Such patients should be encouraged to continue with the inhaler but should be watched carefully for objective signs of adrenal insufficiency, such as hypotension and weight loss. If evidence of adrenal insufficiency occurs, the systemic steroid dose should be boosted temporarily and thereafter further withdrawal should continue more slowly. No clinical studies have been conducted evaluating **Azmacort** with alternate day prednisone regimens. However, based on the results of such a study with another inhaled corticosteroid, inhaled corticosteroids generally are not recommended for chronic use with alternate day prednisone regimens (see WARNINGS).
During periods of stress or a severe asthma attack, transfer patients will require supplementary treatment with systemic steroids. Exacerbations of asthma which occur during the course of treatment with **Azmacort** Oral Inhaler should be treated with a short course of systemic steroid which is gradually tapered as these symptoms subside. There is no evidence that control of asthma can be achieved by administration of **Azmacort** Oral Inhaler in amounts greater than the recommended doses.

Directions for Use: An illustrated leaflet of patient instructions for proper use accompanies each package of **Azmacort** Oral Inhaler.

Contents Under Pressure: Do not puncture. Do not use or store near heat or open flame. Exposure to temperatures above 120°F may cause bursting. Never throw container into fire or incinerator. Keep out of reach of children.

HOW SUPPLIED

Azmacort Oral Inhaler contains 60 mg triamcinolone acetonide in a 20 gram package which delivers at least 240 actuations. It is supplied with an oral adapter and patient's leaflet of instructions: box of one.
NDC 0075-0060-37

Military and Veterans Administration: 20 gram inhaler (NSN 6505-01-206-9233).

STORE AT ROOM TEMPERATURE.

CAUTION

Federal (U.S.A.) law prohibits dispensing without prescription.

Rev. 11/91 IN-0367C

Marketed by
RHÔNE-POULENC RORER PHARMACEUTICALS INC.
Collegeville, PA, U.S.A. 19426-0107

Shown in Product Identification Section, page 424

CALCIMAR® ℞

[*kal'sĭ-mar*]
(calcitonin-salmon)
INJECTION, SYNTHETIC

PRODUCT OVERVIEW

KEY FACTS

Calcimar® Injection, Synthetic is a synthetic polypeptide of 32 amino acids in the same linear sequence found in calcitonin of salmon origin. It is provided as a sterile solution in 2 mL vials containing 400 I.U. (200 I.U. per mL) for subcutaneous or intramuscular injection.

MAJOR USES

Calcimar® Injection, Synthetic is indicated for the relief of bone pain and other symptoms of Paget's disease, for the treatment of hypercalcemia, and for the treatment of postmenopausal osteoporosis (PMO) to prevent the progressive loss of bone mass. Adequate calcium and Vitamin D intake in conjunction with Calcimar is essential to prevent the progressive loss of bone mass in PMO.

SAFETY INFORMATION

Skin testing should be considered prior to treatment with calcitonin because of its protein nature. Careful instruction in sterile injection technique should be given to the patient and to other persons who may administer Calcimar.

PRESCRIBING INFORMATION

CALCIMAR® ℞

[*kal'sĭ-mar*]
(calcitonin-salmon)
INJECTION, SYNTHETIC

DESCRIPTION

Calcitonin is a polypeptide hormone secreted by the parafollicular cells of the thyroid gland in mammals and by the ultimobranchial gland of birds and fish.
CALCIMAR® (calcitonin-salmon) Injection, Synthetic is a synthetic polypeptide of 32 amino acids in the same linear sequence that is found in calcitonin of salmon origin. This is shown by the following graphic formula:

Cys - Ser - Asn - Leu - Ser - Thr - Cys - Val - Leu - Gly - Lys -
1 2 3 4 5 6 7 8 9 10 11
Leu - Ser - Gln - Glu - Leu - His - Lys - Leu - Gln - Thr - Tyr -
12 13 14 15 16 17 18 19 20 21 22
Pro - Arg - Thr - Asn - Thr - Gly - Ser - Gly - Thr - Pro - NH_2
23 24 25 26 27 28 29 30 31 32

It is provided in sterile solution for subcutaneous or intramuscular injection. Each milliliter contains 200 I.U. (MRC) of calcitonin-salmon, 5 mg phenol (as preservative), with sodium chloride, sodium acetate, acetic acid, and sodium hydroxide to adjust tonicity and pH.
The activity of CALCIMAR is stated in International Units (equal to MRC or Medical Research Council units) based on bio-assay in comparison with the International Reference Preparation of Calcitonin, Salmon for Bioassay, distributed by the National Institute for Biological Standards and Control, Holly Hill, London.

CLINICAL PHARMACOLOGY

Calcitonin acts primarily on bone, but direct renal effects and actions on the gastrointestinal tract are also recognized. Calcitonin-salmon appears to have actions essentially identical to calcitonins of mammalian origin, but its potency per mg is greater and it has a longer duration of action. The actions of calcitonin on bone and its role in normal human bone physiology are still incompletely understood.
Bone—Single injections of calcitonin cause a marked transient inhibition of the ongoing bone resorptive process. With prolonged use, there is a persistent, smaller decrease in the rate of bone resorption. Histologically this is associated with a decreased number of osteoclasts and an apparent decrease in their resorptive activity. Decreased osteocytic resorption may also be involved. There is some evidence that initially bone formation may be augmented by calcitonin through increased osteoblastic activity. However, calcitonin will probably not induce a long-term increase in bone formation.
Animal studies indicate that endogenous calcitonin, primarily through its action on bone, participates with parathyroid hormone in the homeostatic regulation of blood calcium. Thus, high blood calcium levels cause increased secretion of calcitonin which, in turn, inhibits bone resorption. This reduces the transfer of calcium from bone to blood and tends to return blood calcium to the normal level. The importance of this process in humans has not been determined. In normal adults, who have a relatively low rate of bone resorption, the administration of exogenous calcitonin results in only a slight decrease in serum calcium. In normal children and in patients with generalized Paget's disease, bone resorption is more rapid and decreases in serum calcium are more pronounced in response to calcitonin.
Paget's Disease of Bone (osteitis deformans)—Paget's disease is a disorder of uncertain etiology characterized by abnormal and accelerated bone formation and resorption in one or more bones. In most patients only small areas of bone are involved and the disease is not symptomatic. In a small fraction of patients, however, the abnormal bone may lead to bone pain and bone deformity, cranial and spinal nerve entrapment, or spinal cord compression. The increased vascularity of the abnormal bone may lead to high output congestive heart failure.
Active Paget's disease involving a large mass of bone may increase the urinary hydroxyproline excretion (reflecting breakdown of collagen-containing bone matrix) and serum alkaline phosphatase (reflecting increased bone formation).
Calcitonin-salmon, presumably by an initial blocking effect on bone resorption, causes a decreased rate of bone turnover with a resultant fall in the serum alkaline phosphatase and urinary hydroxyproline excretion in approximately ⅔ of patients treated. These biochemical changes appear to correspond to changes toward more normal bone, as evidenced by a small number of documented examples of: 1) radiologic regression of Pagetic lesions, 2) improvement of impaired auditory nerve and other neurologic function, 3) decreases (measured) in abnormally elevated cardiac output. These improvements occur extremely rarely, if ever, spontaneously (elevated cardiac output may disappear over a period of years when the disease slowly enters a sclerotic phase; in the cases treated with calcitonin, however, the decreases were seen in less than one year).
Some patients with Paget's disease who have good biochemical and/or symptomatic responses initially, later relapse. Suggested explanations have included the formation of neutralizing antibodies and the development of secondary hyperparathyroidism, but neither suggestion appears to explain adequately the majority of relapses.
Although the parathyroid hormone levels do appear to rise transiently during each hypocalcemic response to calcitonin, most investigators have been unable to demonstrate persistent hypersecretion of parathyroid hormone in patients treated chronically with calcitonin.
Circulating antibodies to calcitonin after 2–18 months' treatment have been reported in about half of the patients with Paget's disease in whom antibody studies were done, but calcitonin treatment remained effective in many of these cases. Occasionally patients with high antibody titers are found. These patients usually will have suffered a biochemical relapse of Paget's disease and are unresponsive to the acute hypocalcemic effects of calcitonin.
Hypercalcemia—In clinical trials, CALCIMAR has been shown to lower the elevated serum calcium of patients with carcinoma (with or without demonstrated metastases), multiple myeloma or primary hyperparathyroidism (lesser response). Patients with higher values for serum calcium tend to show greater reduction during CALCIMAR therapy. The decrease in calcium occurs about 2 hours after the first injection and lasts for about 6-8 hours. CALCIMAR given every 12 hours maintained a calcium lowering effect for about 5-8 days, the time period evaluated for most patients during the clincal studies. The average reduction of 8-hour post-injection serum calcium during this period was about 9 percent.
Kidney—Calcitonin increases the excretion of filtered phosphate, calcium, and sodium by decreasing their tubular reabsorption. In some patients the inhibition of bone resorption by calcitonin is of such magnitude that the consequent reduction of filtered calcium load more than compensates for the decrease in tubular reabsorption of calcium. The result in these patients is a decrease rather than an increase in urinary calcium.
Transient increases in sodium and water excretion may occur after the initial injection of calcitonin. In most patients these changes return to pre-treatment levels with continued therapy.
Gastrointestinal tract—Increasing evidence indicates that calcitonin has significant actions on the gastrointestinal tract. Short-term administration results in marked transient decreases in the volume and acidity of gastric juice and in the volume and the trypsin and amylase content of pancreatic juice. Whether these effects continue to be elicited after each injection of calcitonin during chronic therapy has not been investigated.
Metabolism—The metabolism of calcitonin-salmon has not yet been studied clinically. Information from animal studies with calcitonin-salmon and from clinical studies with calcitonins of porcine and human origin suggest that calcitonin-salmon is rapidly metabolized by conversion to smaller inactive fragments, primarily in the kidneys, but also in the blood and peripheral tissues. A small amount of unchanged hormone and its inactive metabolites are excreted in the urine.
It appears that calcitonin-salmon cannot cross the placental barrier and its passage to the cerebrospinal fluid or to breast milk has not been determined.

INDICATIONS AND USAGE

CALCIMAR is indicated for the treatment of symptomatic Paget's disease of bone, the treatment of hypercalcemia, and the treatment of postmenopausal osteoporosis.
Paget's Disease—At the present time effectiveness has been demonstrated principally in patients with moderate to severe disease characterized by polyostotic involvement with elevated serum alkaline phosphatase and urinary hydroxyproline excretion.
In these patients, the biochemical abnormalities were substantially improved (more than 30% reduction) in about ⅔ of patients studied, and bone pain was improved in a similar fraction. A small number of documented instances of reversal of neurologic deficits has occurred, including improvement in the basilar compression syndrome, and improvement of spinal cord and spinal nerve lesions. At present there is too little experience to predict the likelihood of improvement of any given neurologic lesion. Hearing loss, the most common neurologic lesion of Paget's disease, is improved infrequently (4 of 29 patients studied audiometrically).
Patients with increased cardiac output due to extensive Paget's disease have had measured decreases in cardiac output while receiving calcitonin. The number of treated patients in this category is still too small to predict how likely such a result will be.
The large majority of patients with localized, especially monostotic disease do not develop symptoms and most patients with mild symptoms can be managed with analgesics. There is no evidence that the prophylactic use of calcitonin is beneficial in asymptomatic patients, although treatment may be considered in exceptional circumstances in which there is extensive involvement of the skull or spinal cord with the possibility of irreversible neurologic damage. In these in-

stances treatment would be based on the demonstrated effect of calcitonin on Pagetic bone, rather than on clinical studies in the patient population in question.

Hypercalcemia —CALCIMAR is indicated for early treatment of hypercalcemic emergencies, along with other appropriate agents, when a rapid decrease in serum calcium is required, until more specific treatment of the underlying disease can be accomplished. It may also be added to existing therapeutic regimens for hypercalcemia such as intravenous fluids and furosemide, oral phosphate or corticosteroids, or other agents.

Postmenopausal Osteoporosis —CALCIMAR is indicated for the treatment of postmenopausal osteoporosis in conjunction with an adequate calcium and vitamin D intake to prevent the progressive loss of bone mass. No evidence currently exists to indicate whether or not CALCIMAR decreases the risk of vertebral crush fractures or spinal deformity. A recent controlled study, which was discontinued prior to completion because of questions regarding its design and implementation, failed to demonstrate any benefit of CALCIMAR on fracture rate. No adequate controlled trials have examined the effect of calcitonin-salmon injection on vertebral bone mineral density beyond one year of treatment. Two controlled studies with CALCIMAR have shown an increase in total body calcium at one year, followed by a trend to decreasing total body calcium (still above baseline) at two years. It has been suggested that those postmenopausal patients having increased rates of bone turnover may be more likely to respond to antiresorptive agents such as CALCIMAR.

CONTRAINDICATIONS
Clinical allergy to synthetic calcitonin-salmon.

WARNINGS
Allergic Reactions
Because calcitonin is protein in nature, the possibility of a systemic allergic reaction exists. Administration of calcitonin-salmon has been reported in a few cases to cause serious allergic-type reaction (e.g. bronchospasms, swelling of the tongue or throat, and anaphylactic shock), and in one case, death due to anaphylaxis. The usual provisions should be made for the emergency treatment of such a reaction should it occur. Allergic reactions should be differentiated from generalized flushing and hypotension.

Skin testing should be considered prior to treatment with calcitonin, particularly for patients with suspected sensitivity to calcitonin. The following procedure is suggested: Prepare a dilution at 10 I.U. per mL by withdrawing $\frac{1}{20}$ mL (0.05 mL) in a tuberculin syringe and filling it to 1.0 mL with Sodium Chloride Injection, USP. Mix well, discard 0.9 mL and inject intracutaneously 0.1 mL (approximately 1 I.U.) on the inner aspect of the forearm. Observe the injection site 15 minutes after injection. The appearance of more than mild erythema or wheal constitutes a positive response.

General.
The incidence of osteogenic sarcoma is known to be increased in Paget's disease. Pagetic lesions, with or without therapy, may appear by X-ray to progress markedly, possibly with some loss of definition of periosteal margins. Such lesions should be evaluated carefully to differentiate these from osteogenic sarcoma.

PRECAUTIONS
1. General
The administration of calcitonin possibly could lead to hypocalcemic tetany under special circumstances. Provisions for parenteral calcium administration should be available during the first several administrations of calcitonin.

2. Laboratory Tests
Periodic examinations of urine sediment of patients on chronic therapy are recommended.

Coarse granular casts and casts containing renal tubular epithelial cells were reported in young adult volunteers at bed rest who were given calcitonin-salmon to study the effect on immobilization osteoporosis. There was no other evidence of renal abnormality and the urine sediment became normal after calcitonin was stopped. Urine sediment abnormalities have not been reported by other investigators.

3. Instructions for the patient
Careful instruction in sterile injection technique should be given to the patient, and to other persons who may administer CALCIMAR.

4. Carcinogenesis, Mutagenesis, and Impairment of Fertility
An increased incidence of pituitary adenomas has been observed in one-year toxicity studies in Sprague-Dawley rats administered calcitonin salmon at dosages of 20 and 80 I.U./kg/day and in Fisher 344 rats given 80 I.U./kg/day. The relevance of these findings to humans is unknown. Calcitonin-salmon was not mutagenic in tests using *Salmonella typhimurium, Escherichia coli,* and Chinese Hamster V79 cells.

5. Pregnancy: Teratogenic effects. Category C.
Calcitonin-salmon has been shown to cause a decrease in fetal birth weights in rabbits when given in doses 14–56 times the dose recommended for human use. Since calcitonin does not cross the placental barrier, this finding may be due to metabolic effect of calcitonin on the pregnant animal. There are no adequate and well-controlled studies in preg-

nant women. CALCIMAR should be used during pregnancy only if the potential benefit justifies the potential risk to the fetus.

6. Nursing Mothers
It is not known whether this drug is excreted in human milk. As a general rule, nursing should not be undertaken while a patient is on this drug since many drugs are excreted in human milk. Calcitonin has been shown to inhibit lactation in animals.

7. Pediatric Use
Disorders of bone in children referred to as juvenile Paget's disease have been reported rarely. The relationship of these disorders to adult Paget's disease has not been established and experience with the use of calcitonin in these disorders is very limited. There are no adequate data to support the use of CALCIMAR in children.

ADVERSE REACTIONS
Gastrointestinal System —Nausea with or without vomiting has been noted in about 10% of patients treated with calcitonin. It is most evident when treatment is first initiated and tends to decrease or disappear with continued administration.

Dermatologic/Hypersensitivity —Local inflammatory reactions at the site of subcutaneous or intramuscular injection have been reported in about 10% of patients. Flushing of face or hands occurred in about 2% to 5% of patients. Skin rashes have been reported occasionally. Administration of calcitonin-salmon has been reported in a few cases to cause serious allergic-type reactions (e.g. bronchospasms, swelling of the tongue or throat, and anaphylactic shock), and in one case, death due to anaphylaxis. (SEE WARNINGS.)

OVERDOSAGE
A dose of 1000 I.U. subcutaneously may produce nausea and vomiting as the only adverse effects. Doses of 32 units per kg per day for one or two days demonstrate no other adverse effects.
Data on chronic high dose administration are insufficient to judge toxicity.

DOSAGE AND ADMINISTRATION
Paget 's Disease —The recommended starting dose of calcitonin in Paget's disease is 100 I.U. (0.5 mL) per day administered subcutaneously (preferred for outpatient self-administration) or intramuscularly. Drug effect should be monitored by periodic measurement of serum alkaline phosphatase and 24-hour urinary hydroxyproline (if available) and evaluation of symptoms. A decrease toward normal of the biochemical abnormalities is usually seen, if it is going to occur, within the first few months. Bone pain may also decrease during that time. Improvement of neurologic lesions, when it occurs, requires a longer period of treatment, often more than one year.

In many patients doses of 50 I.U. (0.25 mL) per day or every other day are sufficient to maintain biochemical and clinical improvement. At the present time, however, there are insufficient data to determine whether this reduced dose will have the same effect as the higher dose on forming more normal bone structure. It appears preferable, therefore, to maintain the higher dose in any patient with serious deformity or neurological involvement.

In any patient with a good response initially who later relapses, either clinically or biochemically, the possibility of antibody formation should be explored. The patient may be tested for antibodies by an appropriate specialized test or evaluated for the possibility of antibody formation by critical clinical evaluation.
Patient compliance should also be assessed in the event of relapse.

In patients who relapse, whether because of antibodies or for unexplained reasons, a dosage increase beyond 100 I.U. per day does not usually appear to elicit an improved response.

Hypercalcemia —The recommended starting dose of CALCIMAR in hypercalcemia is 4 I.U./kg body weight every 12 hours by subcutaneous or intramuscular injection. If the response to this dose is not satisfactory after one or two days, the dose may be increased to 8 I.U./kg every 12 hours. If the response remains unsatisfactory after two more days, the dose may be further increased to a maximum of 8 I.U./kg every 6 hours.

Postmenopausal Osteoporosis —The recommended dose of calcitonin is 100 I.U. per day administered subcutaneously or intramuscularly. Patients should also receive supplemental calcium such as calcium carbonate 1.5 g daily and an adequate vitamin D intake (400 units daily). An adequate diet is also essential.
If the volume of CALCIMAR to be injected exceeds 2 mL, intramuscular injection is preferable and multiple sites of injection should be used.
The minimum effective dose of CALCIMAR for the prevention of vertebral bone mineral density loss has not been established. Data from a single one-year placebo-controlled study with calcitonin-salmon injection suggested that 100 IU every other day might be effective in preserving vertebral bone mineral density. Baseline and interval monitoring of biochemical markers of bone resorption/turnover (*e.g.,* fast-

ing A.M., urine hydroxyproline to creatinine ratio) and of bone mineral density may be useful in achieving the minimum effective dose.
Parenteral drug products should be inspected visually for particulate matter and discoloration prior to administration whenever solution and container permit.

HOW SUPPLIED
CALCIMAR is available as a sterile solution in 2 mL vials containing 200 I.U. per mL (NDC 0075-1306-01).
Store in refrigerator, 2°–8°C (36°–46°F).
Military: NSN 6505-01-079-2635.
CAUTION: FEDERAL (U.S.A.) LAW PROHIBITS DISPENSING WITHOUT PRESCRIPTION.
Rev. 5/92   IN-4001G
RHÔNE-POULENC RORER PHARMACEUTICALS INC.
Collegeville, PA, U.S.A. 19426-0107
Shown in Product Identification Section, page 424

DDAVP® Injection   ℞
(desmopressin acetate)

DESCRIPTION
DDAVP® Injection (desmopressin acetate) is an antidiuretic hormone affecting renal water conservation and is a synthetic analogue of 8-arginine vasopressin. It is chemically defined as follows:
Mol. Wt. 1183.2
Empirical Formula: $C_{48}H_{74}N_{14}O_{17}S_2$
SCH$_2$CH$_2$CO-Tyr-Phe-Gln-Asn-Cys-Pro-D-Arg-Gly-NH$_2$·

$$C_2H_4O_2 \cdot 3H_2O$$

1-(3-mercaptopropionic acid)-8-D-arginine
vasopressin monoacetate (salt) trihydrate

DDAVP Injection is provided as a sterile, aqueous solution for injection.
Each mL provides: Desmopressin acetate   4.0 mcg
                    Sodium chloride   9.0 mg
                    Hydrochloric acid to adjust pH to 4.0
The 10-mL vial contains chlorobutanol as a preservative (5.0 mg/mL).

CLINICAL PHARMACOLOGY
DDAVP Injection contains as active substance, 1-(3-mercaptopropionic acid)-8-D-arginine vasopressin, a synthetic analogue of the natural hormone arginine vasopressin. One mL (4 mcg) of DDAVP (desmopressin acetate) solution has an antidiuretic activity of about 16 IU; 1 mcg of DDAVP is equivalent to 4 IU.
DDAVP has been shown to be more potent than arginine vasopressin in increasing plasma levels of factor VIII activity in patients with hemophilia and von Willebrand's disease Type I.
Dose-response studies were performed in healthy persons, using doses of 0.1 to 0.4 mcg/kg body weight, infused over a 10-minute period. Maximal dose response occurred at 0.3 to 0.4 mcg/kg. The response to DDAVP of factor VIII activity and plasminogen activator is dose-related, with maximal plasma levels of 300 to 400 percent of initial concentrations obtained after infusion of 0.4 mcg/kg body weight. The increase is rapid and evident within 30 minutes, reaching a maximum at a point ranging from 90 minutes to two hours. The factor VIII related antigen and ristocetin cofactor activity were also increased to a smaller degree, but still are dose-dependent.
1. The biphasic half-lives of DDAVP were 7.8 and 75.5 minutes for the fast and slow phases, respectively, compared with 2.5 and 14.5 minutes for lysine vasopressin, another form of the hormone. As a result, DDAVP (desmopressin acetate) provides a prompt onset of antidiuretic action with a long duration after each administration.
2. The change in structure of arginine vasopressin to DDAVP has resulted in a decreased vasopressor action and decreased actions on visceral smooth muscle relative to the enhanced antidiuretic activity, so that clinically effective antidiuretic doses are usually below threshold levels for effects on vascular or visceral smooth muscle.
3. When administered by injection, DDAVP has an antidiuretic effect about ten times that of an equivalent dose administered intranasally.
4. The bioavailability of the subcutaneous route of administration was determined qualitatively using urine output data. The exact fraction of drug absorbed by that route of administration has not been quantitatively determined.
5. The percentage increase of factor VIII levels in patients with mild hemophilia A and von Willebrand's disease was not significantly different from that observed in normal healthy individuals when treated with 0.3 mcg/kg of DDAVP infused over 10 minutes.
6. Plasminogen activator activity increases rapidly after DDAVP infusion, but there has been no clinically significant fibrinolysis in patients treated with DDAVP.

Continued on next page

Rhône-Poulenc Rorer—Cont.

7. The effect of repeated DDAVP administration when doses were given every 12 to 24 hours has generally shown a gradual diminution of the factor VIII activity increase noted with a single dose. The initial response is reproducible in any particular patient if there are 2 or 3 days between administrations.

INDICATIONS AND USAGE

Hemophilia A

DDAVP Injection is indicated for patients with hemophilia A with factor VIII coagulant activity levels greater than 5%. DDAVP will often maintain hemostasis in patients with hemophilia A during surgical procedures and postoperatively when administered 30 minutes prior to scheduled procedure.

DDAVP will also stop bleeding in hemophilia A patients with episodes of spontaneous or trauma-induced injuries such as hemarthroses, intramuscular hematomas or mucosal bleeding.

DDAVP is not indicated for the treatment of hemophilia A with factor VIII coagulant activity levels equal to or less than 5%, or for the treatment of hemophilia B, or in patients who have factor VIII antibodies.

In certain clinical situations, it may be justified to try DDAVP in patients with factor VIII levels between 2%–5%; however, these patients should be carefully monitored.

von Willebrand's Disease (Type I)

DDAVP Injection is indicated for patients with mild to moderate classic von Willebrand's disease (Type I) with factor VIII levels greater than 5%. DDAVP will often maintain hemostasis in patients with mild to moderate von Willebrand's disease during surgical procedures and postoperatively when administered 30 minutes prior to the scheduled procedure.

DDAVP will usually stop bleeding in mild to moderate von Willebrand's patients with episodes of spontaneous or trauma-induced injuries such as hemarthroses, intramuscular hematomas or mucosal bleeding.

Those von Willebrand's disease patients who are least likely to respond are those with severe homozygous von Willebrand's disease with factor VIII coagulant activity and factor VIII von Willebrand factor antigen levels less than 1%. Other patients may respond in a variable fashion depending on the type of molecular defect they have. Bleeding time and factor VIII coagulant activity, ristocetin cofactor activity, and von Willebrand factor antigen should be checked during administration of DDAVP to ensure that adequate levels are being achieved.

DDAVP is not indicated for the treatment of severe classic von Willebrand's disease (Type I) and when there is evidence of an abnormal molecular form of factor VIII antigen. See Warning.

Diabetes Insipidus

DDAVP Injection is indicated as antidiuretic replacement therapy in the management of central (cranial) diabetes insipidus and for the management of the temporary polyuria and polydipsia following head trauma or surgery in the pituitary region. DDAVP is ineffective for the treatment of nephrogenic diabetes insipidus.

DDAVP is also available as an intranasal preparation. However, this means of delivery can be compromised by a variety of factors that can make nasal insufflation ineffective or inappropriate. These include poor intranasal absorption, nasal congestion and blockage, nasal discharge, atrophy of nasal mucosa, and severe atrophic rhinitis. Intranasal delivery may be inappropriate where there is an impaired level of consciousness. In addition, cranial surgical procedures, such as transphenoidal hypophysectomy, create situations where an alternative route of administration is needed as in cases of nasal packing or recovery from surgery.

CONTRAINDICATION

Known hypersensitivity to DDAVP.

WARNINGS

Patients who do not have need of antidiuretic hormone for its antidiuretic effect, in particular those who are young or elderly, should be cautioned to ingest only enough fluid to satisfy thirst, in order to decrease the potential occurrence of water intoxication and hyponatremia.

Fluid intake should be adjusted, particularly in very young and elderly patients, in order to decrease the potential occurrence of water intoxication and hyponatremia.

Particular attention should be paid to the possibility of the rare occurrence of an extreme decrease in plasma osmolality and resulting seizures.

DDAVP should not be used to treat patients with Type IIB von Willebrand's disease since platelet aggregation may be induced.

PRECAUTIONS

GENERAL: For injection use only.
DDAVP Injection (desmopressin acetate) has infrequently produced changes in blood pressure causing either a slight

elevation in blood pressure or a transient fall in blood pressure and a compensatory increase in heart rate. The drug should be used with caution in patients with coronary artery insufficiency and/or hypertensive cardiovascular disease.

DDAVP Injection should be used with caution in patients with conditions associated with fluid and electrolyte imbalance, such as cystic fibrosis, because these patients are prone to hyponatremia.

There have been rare reports of thrombotic events following DDAVP Injection in patients predisposed to thrombus formation. No causality has been determined, however, the drug should be used with caution in these patients.

Severe allergic reactions have not been reported with DDAVP Injection (desmopressin acetate). It is not known whether antibodies to DDAVP Injection (desmopressin acetate) are produced after repeated injections.

Hemophilia A

Laboratory tests for assessing patient status include levels of factor VIII coagulant, factor VIII antigen and factor VIII ristocetin cofactor (von Willebrand factor) as well as activated partial thromboplastin time. Factor VIII coagulant activity should be determined before giving DDAVP for hemostasis. If factor VIII coagulant activity is present at less than 5% of normal, DDAVP should not be relied on.

von Willebrand's Disease

Laboratory tests for assessing patient status include levels of factor VIII coagulant activity, factor VIII ristocetin cofactor activity, and factor VIII von Willebrand factor antigen. The skin bleeding time may be helpful in following these patients.

Diabetes Insipidus

Laboratory tests for monitoring the patient include urine volume and osmolality. In some cases, plasma osmolality may be required.

DRUG INTERACTIONS: Although the pressor activity of DDAVP is very low compared with the antidiuretic activity, use of doses as large as 0.3 mcg/kg of DDAVP with other pressor agents should be done only with careful patient monitoring.

DDAVP has been used with epsilon aminocaproic acid without adverse effects.

CARCINOGENICITY, MUTAGENICITY, IMPAIRMENT OF FERTILITY: Teratology studies in rats have shown no abnormalities. No further data are available.

PREGNANCY CATEGORY B: Reproduction studies performed in rats and rabbits with subcutaneous doses up to 12.5 times the human dose when used for factor VIII stimulation and 125 times the human dose when used in diabetes insipidus have revealed no evidence of harm to the fetus due to DDAVP. There are several publications of management of diabetes insipidus in pregnant women with no harm to the fetus reported; however, there are no adequate and well-controlled studies in pregnant women. Published reports stress that, as opposed to preparations containing the natural hormones, DDAVP in antidiuretic doses has no uterotonic action, but the physician will have to weigh possible therapeutic advantages against possible danger in each case.

NURSING MOTHERS: It is not known whether this drug is excreted in human milk. Because many drugs are excreted in human milk, caution should be exercised when DDAVP is administered to a nursing woman.

PEDIATRIC USE: Use in infants and children will require careful fluid intake restriction to prevent possible hyponatremia and water intoxication. *DDAVP Injection should not be used in infants younger than three months* in the treatment of hemophilia A or von Willebrand's disease; safety and effectiveness in children under 12 years of age with diabetes insipidus have not been established.

ADVERSE REACTIONS

Infrequently, DDAVP has produced transient headache, nausea, mild abdominal cramps and vulval pain. These symptoms disappeared with reduction in dosage. Occasionally, injection of DDAVP has produced local erythema, swelling or burning pain. Occasional facial flushing has been reported with the administration of DDAVP.

DDAVP Injection has infrequently produced changes in blood pressure causing either a slight elevation or a transient fall and a compensatory increase in heart rate.

See WARNING for the possibility of water intoxication and hyponatremia.

There have been rare reports of thrombotic events (acute cerebrovascular thrombosis, acute myocardial infarction) following DDAVP Injection in patients predisposed to thrombus formation.

OVERDOSAGE

See ADVERSE REACTIONS above. In case of overdosage, the dosage should be reduced, frequency of administration decreased, or the drug withdrawn according to the severity of the condition.

There is no known specific antidote for DDAVP.
An oral LD_{50} has not been established. An intravenous dose of 2 mg/kg in mice demonstrated no effect.

DOSAGE AND ADMINISTRATION

Hemophilia A and von Willebrand's Disease (Type I)

DDAVP Injection is administered as an intravenous infusion at a dose of 0.3 mcg DDAVP/kg body weight diluted in sterile physiological saline and infused slowly over 15 to 30 minutes. In adults and children weighing more than 10 kg, 50 mL of diluent is used; in children weighing 10 kg or less, 10 mL of diluent is used. Blood pressure and pulse should be monitored during infusion. If DDAVP Injection is used preoperatively, it should be administered 30 minutes prior to the scheduled procedure.

The necessity for repeat administration of DDAVP or use of any blood products for hemostasis should be determined by laboratory response as well as the clinical condition of the patient. The tendency toward tachyphylaxis (lessening of response) with repeated administration given more frequently than every 48 hours should be considered in treating each patient.

Diabetes Insipidus

This formulation is administered subcutaneously or by direct intravenous injection. DDAVP Injection (desmopressin acetate) dosage must be determined for each patient and adjusted according to the pattern of response. Response should be estimated by two parameters: adequate duration of sleep and adequate, not excessive, water turnover.

The usual dosage range in adults is 0.5 mL (2.0 mcg) to 1 mL (4.0 mcg) daily, administered intravenously or subcutaneously, usually in two divided doses. The morning and evening doses should be separately adjusted for an adequate diurnal rhythm of water turnover. For patients who have been controlled on intranasal DDAVP and who must be switched to the injection form, either because of poor intranasal absorption or because of the need for surgery, the comparable antidiuretic dose of the injection is about one-tenth the intranasal dose.

Parenteral drug products should be inspected visually for particulate matter and discoloration prior to administration whenever solution and container permit.

HOW SUPPLIED

DDAVP Injection (desmopressin acetate) is available as a sterile solution in cartons of ten 1 mL single-dose ampules (NDC 0075-2451-01) and in 10 mL multiple-dose vials (NDC 0075-2451-53), each containing 4.0 mcg DDAVP per mL. Keep refrigerated at about 4°C.
Caution: Federal (U.S.A.) law prohibits dispensing without prescription.
Rev. 10/91   IN-4708F
Manufactured for
RHÔNE-POULENC RORER PHARMACEUTICALS INC.
Collegeville, PA, U.S.A. 19426-0107
By Ferring Pharmaceuticals, Malmö, Sweden
Shown in Product Identification section, page 424

DDAVP® Nasal Spray   ℞
(desmopressin acetate)
DDAVP® Rhinal Tube   ℞
(desmopressin acetate)

COMBINED PRODUCT OVERVIEW

KEY FACTS

DDAVP® is an antidiuretic hormone affecting renal water conservation and is a synthetic analogue of 8-arginine vasopressin. DDAVP Nasal Spray and DDAVP Rhinal Tube are each provided as a sterile, aqueous solution for intranasal use only.

MAJOR USES

DDAVP is indicated for the management of primary nocturnal enuresis. It may be used alone or adjunctive to behavioral conditioning or other nonpharmacological intervention. It has been shown to be effective in some cases that are refractory to conventional therapies.

DDAVP is also indicated as antidiuretic replacement therapy in the management of central cranial diabetes insipidus and for management of the temporary polyuria and polydipsia following head trauma or surgery in the pituitary region. DDAVP is not effective for the treatment of nephrogenic diabetes insipidus.

SAFETY INFORMATION

Patients who do not have need of antidiuretic hormone for its antidiuretic effect (i.e. those who are young or elderly) should be cautioned to ingest only enough fluid to satisfy thirst, in order to decrease the potential occurrence of water intoxication and hyponatremia.

DDAVP® Nasal Spray ℞
(desmopressin acetate)
DDAVP® Rhinal Tube ℞
(desmopressin acetate)

COMBINED PRESCRIBING INFORMATION

DESCRIPTION

DDAVP (desmopressin acetate) is an antidiuretic hormone affecting renal water conservation and a synthetic analogue of 8-arginine vasopressin. It is chemically defined as follows:
Mol. wt. 1183.2
Empirical formula: $C_{48}H_{74}N_{14}O_{17}S_2$

SCH_2CH_2CO-Tyr-Phe-Gln-Asn-Cys-Pro-D-Arg-Gly-NH_2·

$C_2H_4O_2 \cdot 3H_2O$

1-(3-mercaptopropionic acid)-8-D-arginine vasopressin monoacetate (salt) trihydrate

DDAVP Nasal Spray (desmopressin acetate) and DDAVP Rhinal Tube (desmopressin acetate) are each provided as a sterile, aqueous solution for intranasal use. Each mL contains:

Desmopressin acetate	0.1 mg
Chlorobutanol	5.0 mg
Sodium Chloride	9.0 mg

Hydrochloric acid to adjust pH to approximately 4
The DDAVP Nasal Spray compression pump delivers 0.1 mL (10 mcg) of DDAVP per spray.

CLINICAL PHARMACOLOGY

DDAVP contains as active substance 1-(3-mercaptopropionic acid)-8-D-arginine vasopressin, which is a synthetic analogue of the natural hormone arginine vasopressin. One mL (0.1 mg) of DDAVP has an antidiuretic activity of about 400 IU; 10 mcg of desmopressin acetate is equivalent to 40 IU.

1. The biphasic half-lives for DDAVP were 7.8 and 75.5 minutes for the fast and slow phases, compared with 2.5 and 14.5 minutes for lysine vasopressin, another form of the hormone used in this condition. As a result, DDAVP provides a prompt onset of antidiuretic action with a long duration after each administration.
2. The change in structure of arginine vasopressin to DDAVP has resulted in a decreased vasopressor action and decreased actions on visceral smooth muscle relative to the enhanced antidiuretic activity, so that clinically effective antidiuretic doses are usually below threshold levels for effects on vascular or visceral smooth muscle.
3. DDAVP administered intranasally has an antidiuretic effect about one-tenth that of an equivalent dose administered by injection.

INDICATIONS AND USAGE

Primary Nocturnal Enuresis: DDAVP Nasal Spray and DDAVP Rhinal Tube are indicated for the management of primary nocturnal enuresis. It may be used alone or adjunctive to behavioral conditioning or other nonpharmacological intervention. It has been shown to be effective in some cases that are refractory to conventional therapies.

Central Cranial Diabetes Insipidus: DDAVP Nasal Spray and DDAVP Rhinal Tube are indicated as antidiuretic replacement therapy in the management of central cranial diabetes insipidus and for management of the temporary polyuria and polydipsia following head trauma or surgery in the pituitary region. It is ineffective for the treatment of nephrogenic diabetes insipidus.

The use of DDAVP Nasal Spray or DDAVP Rhinal Tube in patients with an established diagnosis will result in a reduction in urinary output with increase in urine osmolality and a decrease in plasma osmolality. This will allow the resumption of a more normal life-style with a decrease in urinary frequency and nocturia.

There are reports of an occasional change in response to DDAVP Nasal Spray or DDAVP Rhinal Tube with time, usually greater than 6 months. Some patients may show a decreased responsiveness, others a shortened duration of effect. There is no evidence this effect is due to the development of binding antibodies but may be due to a local inactivation of the peptide.

Patients are selected for therapy by establishing the diagnosis by means of the water deprivation test, the hypertonic saline infusion test, and/or the response to antidiuretic hormone. Continued response to DDAVP can be monitored by urine volume and osmolality.

DDAVP is also available as a solution for injection when the intranasal route may be compromised. These situations include nasal congestion and blockage, nasal discharge, atrophy of nasal mucosa, and severe atrophic rhinitis. Intranasal delivery may also be inappropriate where there is an impaired level of consciousness. In addition, cranial surgical procedures, such as transphenoidal hypophysectomy create situations where an alternative route of administration is needed as in cases of nasal packing or recovery from surgery.

CONTRAINDICATION

Known hypersensitivity to DDAVP.

WARNINGS

1. For intranasal use only.
2. In very young and elderly patients in particular, fluid intake should be adjusted in order to decrease the potential occurrence of water intoxication and hyponatremia. Particular attention should be paid to the possibility of the rare occurrence of an extreme decrease in plasma osmolality and resulting seizures.

PRECAUTIONS

General: DDAVP Nasal Spray and DDAVP Rhinal Tube at high dosage have infrequently produced a slight elevation of blood pressure, which disappeared with a reduction in dosage. The drug should be used with caution in patients with coronary artery insufficiency and/or hypertensive cardiovascular disease because of possible rise in blood pressure.

DDAVP should be used with caution in patients with conditions associated with fluid and electrolyte imbalance, such as cystic fibrosis, because these patients are prone to hyponatremia.

Central Cranial Diabetes Insipidus: Since DDAVP is used intranasally, changes in the nasal mucosa such as scarring, edema, or other disease may cause erratic, unreliable absorption in which case intranasal DDAVP should not be used. For such situations, DDAVP Injection should be considered.

Primary Nocturnal Enuresis: If changes in the nasal mucosa have occurred, unreliable absorption may result. DDAVP intranasal solution should be discontinued until the nasal problems resolve.

INFORMATION FOR PATIENTS: Patients should be informed that the DDAVP Nasal Spray bottle accurately delivers 50 doses of 10 mcg each. Any solution remaining after 50 doses should be discarded since the amount delivered thereafter may be substantially less than 10 mcg of drug. No attempt should be made to transfer remaining solution to another bottle. Patients should be instructed to read accompanying directions on use of the spray pump carefully before use.

LABORATORY TESTS: Laboratory tests for following the patient with central cranial diabetes insipidus or post-surgical or head trauma-related polyuria and polydipsia include urine volume and osmolality. In some cases plasma osmolality may be required. For the healthy patient with primary nocturnal enuresis, serum electrolytes should be checked at least once if therapy is continued beyond 7 days.

DRUG INTERACTIONS: Although the pressor activity of DDAVP is very low compared to the antidiuretic activity, use of large doses of DDAVP with other pressor agents should only be done with careful patient monitoring.

CARCINOGENESIS, MUTAGENESIS, IMPAIRMENT OF FERTILITY: Teratology studies in rats have shown no abnormalities. No further information is available.

PREGNANCY—CATEGORY B: Reproduction studies performed in rats and rabbits with doses up to 12.5 times the human intranasal dose (i.e. about 125 times the total adult human dose given systemically) have revealed no evidence of harm to the fetus due to desmopressin acetate. There are several publications of management of diabetes insipidus in pregnant women with no harm to the fetus reported; however, no controlled studies in pregnant women have been carried out. Published reports stress that, as opposed to preparations containing the natural hormones, DDAVP (desmopressin acetate) in antidiuretic doses has no uterotonic action, but the physician will have to weigh possible therapeutic advantages against possible dangers in each individual case.

NURSING MOTHERS: There have been no controlled studies in nursing mothers. A single study in a postpartum woman demonstrated a marked change in plasma, but little if any change in assayable DDAVP in breast milk following an intranasal dose of 10 mcg.

PEDIATRIC USE:

Primary Nocturnal Enuresis: DDAVP has been used in childhood nocturnal enuresis. Short-term (4–8 weeks) DDAVP administration has been shown to be safe and modestly effective in children aged 6 years or older with severe childhood nocturnal enuresis. Adequately controlled studies with intranasal DDAVP in primary nocturnal enuresis have not been conducted beyond 4–8 weeks. The dose should be individually adjusted to achieve the best results.

Central Cranial Diabetes Insipidus: DDAVP Nasal Spray and DDAVP Rhinal Tube have been used in children with diabetes insipidus. Use in infants and children will require careful fluid intake restriction to prevent possible hyponatremia and water intoxication. The dose must be individually adjusted to the patient with attention in the very young to the danger of an extreme decrease in plasma osmolality with resulting convulsions. Dose should start at 0.05 mL or less.

Since the spray cannot deliver less than 0.1 mL (10 mcg), smaller doses should be administered using the rhinal tube delivery system. Do not use the nasal spray in pediatric patients requiring less than 0.1 mL (10 mcg) per dose.

There are reports of an occasional change in response to DDAVP Nasal Spray or DDAVP Rhinal Tube with time, usually greater than 6 months. Some patients may show a decreased responsiveness, others a shortened duration of effect. There is no evidence this effect is due to the development of binding antibodies but may be due to a local inactivation of the peptide.

ADVERSE REACTIONS

Infrequently, high dosages of DDAVP Nasal Spray or DDAVP Rhinal Tube have produced transient headache and nausea. Nasal congestion, rhinitis and flushing have also been reported occasionally along with mild abdominal cramps. These symptoms disappeared with reduction in dosage. Nosebleed, sore throat, cough and upper respiratory infections have also been reported.

The following table lists the percent of patients having adverse experiences without regard to relationship to study drug from the pooled pivotal study data for nocturnal enuresis.

ADVERSE REACTION	PLACEBO (N=59) %	DDAVP 20 mcg (N=60) %	DDAVP 40 mcg (N=61) %
BODY AS A WHOLE			
Abdominal Pain	0	2	2
Asthenia	0	0	2
Chills	0	0	2
Headache	0	2	5
Throat Pain	2	0	0
NERVOUS SYSTEM			
Depression	2	0	0
Dizziness	0	0	3
RESPIRATORY SYSTEM			
Epistaxis	2	3	0
Nostril Pain	0	2	0
Respiratory Infection	2	0	0
Rhinitis	2	8	3
CARDIOVASCULAR SYSTEM			
Vasodilation	2	0	0
DIGESTIVE SYSTEM			
Gastrointestinal Disorder	0	2	0
Nausea	0	0	2
SKIN & APPENDAGES			
Leg Rash	2	0	0
Rash	2	0	0
SPECIAL SENSES			
Conjunctivitis	0	2	0
Edema Eyes	0	2	0
Lachrymation Disorder	0	0	2

OVERDOSAGE

See ADVERSE REACTIONS above. In case of overdosage, the dose should be reduced, frequency of administration decreased, or the drug withdrawn according to the severity of the condition. There is no known specific antidote for DDAVP.

An oral LD_{50} has not been established. An intravenous dose of 2 mg/kg in mice demonstrated no effect.

DOSAGE AND ADMINISTRATION

Primary Nocturnal Enuresis: Dosage should be adjusted according to the individual. The recommended initial dose for those 6 years of age and older is 20 mcg or 0.2 mL solution intranasally at bedtime. Adjustment up to 40 mcg is suggested if the patient does not respond. Some patients may respond to 10 mcg and adjustment to that lower dose may be done if the patient has shown a response to 20 mcg. It is recommended that one-half of the dose be administered per nostril. Adequately controlled studies with intranasal DDAVP in primary nocturnal enuresis have not been conducted beyond 4–8 weeks.

Central Cranial Diabetes Insipidus: DDAVP dosage must be determined for each individual patient and adjusted according to the diurnal pattern of response. Response should be estimated by two parameters: adequate duration of sleep and adequate, not excessive, water turnover. Patients with nasal congestion and blockage have often responded well to DDAVP. The nasal spray pump can only deliver doses of 0.1 mL (10 mcg) or multiples of 0.1 mL. If doses other than these are required, the rhinal tube delivery system may be used. DDAVP Rhinal Tube is administered into the nose through a soft, flexible plastic rhinal tube that has four graduation marks on it that measure 0.2, 0.15, 0.1, and 0.05 mL. The usual dosage range in adults is 0.1 to 0.4 mL daily, either as a single dose or divided into two or three doses. Most adults require 0.2 mL daily in two divided doses. The morning and evening doses should be separately adjusted for an adequate diurnal rhythm of water turnover. For children aged 3 months to 12 years, the usual dosage range is 0.05 to 0.3 mL daily, either as a single dose or divided into two doses. About ¼ to ⅓ of patients can be controlled by a single daily dose of DDAVP administered intranasally.

HOW SUPPLIED

DDAVP Nasal Spray is available in a 5-mL bottle with spray pump delivering 50 doses of 10 mcg (NDC 0075-2450-02).

Continued on next page

Rhône-Poulenc Rorer—Cont.

Keep refrigerated at 2°–8°C (36°–46°F). When traveling, product will maintain stability for up to 3 weeks when stored at room temperature, 22°C (72°F).
DDAVP Rhinal Tube 2.5 mL per vial is packaged with two rhinal tube applicators per carton (NDC 0075-2450-01). **Keep refrigerated at about 4°C (39°F).** When traveling—controlled room temperature 22°C (72°F) closed sterile bottles will maintain stability for 3 weeks.
Military: DDAVP Rhinal Tube, 1 × 2.5 mL (NSN 6505-01-145-6338).

CAUTION

Federal (U.S.A.) law prohibits dispensing without prescription.
Rev. 6/91 M-0370C and M-0369 C
Manufactured for:
RHÔNE-POULENC RORER PHARMACEUTICALS INC.
Collegeville, PA, U.S.A. 19426-0107
By: Ferring Pharmaceuticals, Malmö, Sweden
Shown in Product Identification Section, page 424

DILACOR™ XR ℞

[*dĭl 'a-kor*]
(diltiazem HCl)
Extended-release Capsules

KEY FACTS

Dilacor™ XR capsules contain multiple units of diltiazem HCl Extended-release 60 mg, resulting in 180 mg or 240 mg dosage strengths.
Dilacor™ XR capsules contain a degradable controlled-release tablet formulation designed to release diltiazem over a 24-hour period. Geomatrix™, a registered trademark of Jago Research AG, Zollikon, Switzerland, is a patented controlled-release system incorporated in the tablets.

MAJOR USES

Dilacor™ XR is indicated for the treatment of hypertension. Diltiazem hydrochloride may be used alone or in combination with other antihypertensive medications, such as diuretics.
Dosages must be adjusted to each patient's needs, starting with 180 or 240 mg once-daily. Based on the antihypertensive effect, the dose may be adjusted as needed. The usual dosage range studied in clinical trials was 180 to 480 mg once daily. Although current clinical experience with the 540 mg dose is limited, the dose may be increased to 540 mg with little or no increased risk of adverse reactions.

SAFETY INFORMATION

Diltiazem hydrochloride is contraindicated in: (1) patients with sick sinus syndrome except in the presence of a functioning ventricular pacemaker; (2) patients with second or third degree AV block except in the presence of a functioning ventricular pacemaker; (3) patients with hypotension (less than 90 mmHg systolic); (4) patients who have demonstrated hypersensitivity to the drug; and (5) patients with acute myocardial infarction and pulmonary congestion as documented by X-ray on admission.

DILACOR™ XR

(diltiazem HCl)
Extended-release Capsules

DESCRIPTION

Dilacor™ XR (diltiazem hydrochloride) is a calcium ion influx inhibitor (slow channel blocker or calcium antagonist). Chemically, diltiazem hydrochloride is 1,5-Benzothiazepin-4(5H)one,3- (acetyloxy) -5- [2-(dimethylamino) ethyl]-2,3-dihydro-2-(4-methoxyphenyl)-,monohydrochloride, (+)-cis-. Its molecular formula is $C_{22}H_{26}N_2O_4S$ HCl and its molecular weight is 450.98. Its structural formula is as follows:

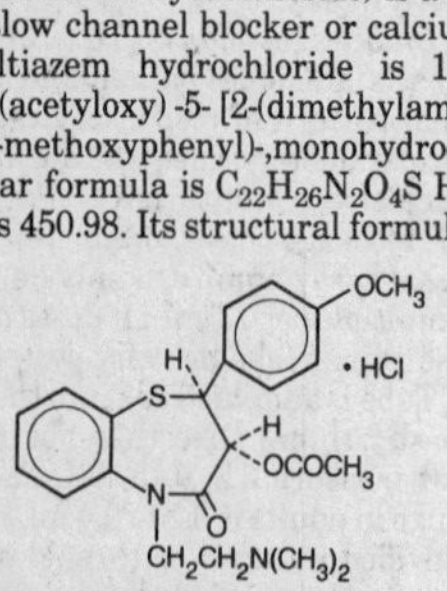

Diltiazem hydrochloride is a white to off-white crystalline powder with a bitter taste. It is soluble in water, methanol, and chloroform.
Dilacor™ XR capsules contain multiple units of diltiazem HCl Extended-release 60 mg, resulting in 180 mg or 240 mg dosage strengths.
Inactive Ingredients: Dilacor™ XR capsules also contain mannitol, ethyl cellulose, hydroxypropylmethyl cellulose, hydrogenated castor oil, ferric oxides, silicon dioxide, magnesium stearate, gelatin, D&C Yellow No. 10, FD&C Red No. 40, D&C Red No. 28, and titanium dioxide.
For oral administration.

CLINICAL PHARMACOLOGY

The therapeutic benefits of diltiazem hydrochloride are believed to be related to its ability to inhibit the influx of calcium ions during membrane depolarization of cardiac and vascular smooth muscle.
Mechanisms of Action. Dilacor™ XR produces its antihypertensive effect primarily by relaxation of vascular smooth muscle with a resultant decrease in peripheral vascular resistance. The magnitude of blood pressure reduction is related to the degree of hypertension; thus hypertensive individuals experience an antihypertensive effect, whereas there is only a modest fall in blood pressure in normotensives.
Hemodynamic and Electrophysiologic Effects. Like other calcium antagonists, diltiazem decreases sinoatrial and atrioventricular conduction in isolated tissues and has a negative inotropic effect in isolated preparations. In the intact animal, prolongation of the AH interval can be seen at higher doses.
In man, diltiazem prevents spontaneous and ergonovine-provoked coronary artery spasm. It causes a decrease in peripheral vascular resistance and a modest fall in blood pressure in normotensive individuals. Studies to date, primarily in patients with good ventricular function, have not revealed evidence of a negative inotropic effect. Cardiac output, ejection fraction and left ventricular end diastolic pressure have not been affected. Increased heart failure has, however, been reported in occasional patients with preexisting impairment of ventricular function. There are as yet few data on the interaction of diltiazem and beta-blockers in patients with poor ventricular function. Resting heart rate is usually slightly reduced by diltiazem.
Dilacor™ XR produces antihypertensive effects both in the supine and standing positions. Postural hypotension is infrequently noted upon suddenly assuming an upright position. Diltiazem decreases vascular resistance, increases cardiac output (by increasing stroke volume), and produces a slight decrease or no change in heart rate. No reflex tachycardia is associated with the chronic antihypertensive effects.
During dynamic exercise, increases in diastolic pressure are inhibited while maximum achievable systolic pressure is usually reduced. Heart rate at maximum exercise does not change or is slightly reduced.
Diltiazem antagonizes the renal and peripheral effects of angiotensin II. No increased activity of the renin-angiotensin-aldosterone axis has been observed. Chronic therapy with diltiazem produces no change or an increase in plasma catecholamines. Hypertensive animal models respond to diltiazem with reductions in blood pressure and increased urinary output and natriuresis without a change in the urinary sodium/potassium ratio. In man, transient natriuresis and kaliuresis have been reported, but only in high intravenous doses of 0.5 mg/kg of body weight.
Diltiazem-associated prolongation of the AH interval is not more pronounced in patients with first-degree heart block. In patients with sick sinus syndrome, diltiazem significantly prolongs sinus cycle length (up to 50% in some cases). Intravenous diltiazem in doses of 20 mg prolongs AH conduction time and AV node functional and effective refractory periods approximately 20%.
In two short-term, double-blind, placebo-controlled studies, 303 hypertensive patients were treated with once-daily Dilacor™ XR in doses of up to 540 mg. There were no instances of greater than first-degree atrioventricular block, and the maximum increase in the PR interval was .08 seconds. No patients were prematurely discontinued from the medication due to symptoms related to prolongation of the PR interval.
Pharmacodynamics. In one short-term, double-blind, placebo-controlled study, Dilacor™ XR 120, 240, 360 and 480 mg/day demonstrated a dose-related antihypertensive response among patients with mild to moderate hypertension. Statistically significant decreases in trough mean supine diastolic blood pressure were seen through four weeks of treatment: 120 mg/day (−5.1 mmHg); 240 mg/day (−6.9 mmHg); 360 mg/day (−6.9 mmHg); and 480 mg/day (−10.6 mmHg). Statistically significant decreases in trough mean supine systolic blood pressure were also seen through four weeks of treatment: 120 mg/day (−2.6 mmHg); 240 mg/day (−6.5 mmHg); 360 mg/day (−4.8 mmHg); and 480 mg/day (−10.6 mmHg). The proportion of evaluable patients exhibiting a therapeutic response (supine diastolic blood pressure <90 mmHg or decrease >10 mmHg) was greater as the dose increased: 31%, 42%, 48% and 69% with the 120, 240, 360 and 480 mg/day diltiazem groups, respectively. Similar findings were observed for standing systolic and diastolic blood pressures. The trough (24 hours after a dose) antihypertensive effect of Dilacor™ XR retained more than one-half of the response seen at peak (3–6 hours after administration).
Significant reductions of mean supine blood pressure (at trough) in patients with mild to moderate hypertension were also seen in a short-term, double-blind, dose-escalation, placebo-controlled study after 2 weeks of once-daily Dilacor™ XR 180 mg/day (diastolic: −6.1 mmHg; systolic: −4.7 mmHg) and again, 2 weeks after escalation to 360 mg/day (diastolic: −9.3 mmHg; systolic: −7.2 mmHg). However, a further increase in dose to 540 mg/day for 2 weeks provided only a minimal further increase in the antihypertensive effect (diastolic: −10.2 mmHg; systolic: −6.7 mmHg).
Pharmacokinetics and Metabolism. Diltiazem is well-absorbed from the gastrointestinal tract, and is subject to an extensive first-pass effect. When given as an immediate release oral formulation, the absolute bioavailability (compared to intravenous administration) of diltiazem is approximately 40%. Diltiazem undergoes extensive hepatic metabolism in which 2% to 4% of the unchanged drug appears in the urine. Total radioactivity measurement following short IV administration in healthy volunteers suggests the presence of other unidentified metabolites which attain higher concentrations than those of diltiazem and are more slowly eliminated; half-life of total radioactivity is about 20 hours compared to 2 to 5 hours for diltiazem. *In-vitro* binding studies show diltiazem HCl is 70% to 80% bound to plasma proteins. Competitive *in-vitro* ligand binding studies have also shown diltiazem HCl binding is not altered by therapeutic concentrations of digoxin, HCTZ, phenylbutazone, propranolol, salicylic acid, or warfarin. The plasma elimination half-life of diltiazem is approximately 3.0 to 4.5 hours. Desacetyl-diltiazem, the major metabolite of diltiazem, which is also present in the plasma at concentrations of 10% to 20% of the parent drug, is approximately 25% to 50% as potent a coronary vasodilator as diltiazem. Therapeutic blood levels of diltiazem hydrochloride appear to be in the range of 40–200 ng/mL. There is a departure from linearity when dose strengths are increased; the half-life is slightly increased with dose.
A study that compared patients with normal hepatic function to patients with cirrhosis found an increase in half-life and a 69% increase in bioavailability in the hepatically impaired patients. A single study in patients with severely impaired renal function showed no difference in the pharmacokinetic profile of diltiazem compared to patients with normal renal function.
Dilacor™ XR capsules contain a degradable controlled-release tablet formulation designed to release diltiazem over a 24-hour period. Geomatrix™, a registered trademark of Jago Research AG, Zollikon, Switzerland, is a patented controlled-release system incorporated in the tablets. Controlled absorption of diltiazem begins within 1 hour, with maximum plasma concentrations being achieved 4 to 6 hours after administration. The apparent steady-state half-life of diltiazem following once-daily administration of Dilacor™ XR capsules ranges from 5 to 10 hours. This prolongation of half-life is attributed to continued absorption of diltiazem rather than to alterations in its elimination.
Neither the absolute bioavailability of Dilacor™ XR capsules nor its relative bioavailability compared to immediate release products has been definitively determined. No information is currently available as to the relative bioavailability of Dilacor™ XR capsules compared to other approved controlled-release diltiazem products.
As the dose of Dilacor™ XR capsules is increased from a daily dose of 120 mg to 240 mg, there is an increase in the AUC of 2.3 fold. When the dose is increased from 240 mg to 360 mg, AUC increases 1.6 fold and when increased from 240 mg to 480 mg, AUC increases 2.4 fold.
In-vivo release of diltiazem occurs throughout the gastrointestinal tract, with controlled release still occurring for up to 24 hours after administration, as determined by radiolabelled methods. As the once-daily dose of Dilacor™ XR was increased, departures from linearity were noted. There were disproportionate increases in area under the curve for doses from 120 mg to 480 mg.
The presence of food did not affect the ability of Dilacor™ XR to maintain a continuous release of drug for up to 24 hours after administration. Simultaneous administration of Dilacor™ XR with a high-fat breakfast had a modest effect on diltiazem bioavailability with AUC increasing by 13% and C_{max} by 37%.

INDICATIONS AND USAGE

Dilacor™ XR is indicated for the treatment of hypertension. Diltiazem hydrochloride may be used alone or in combination with other antihypertensive medications, such as diuretics.

CONTRAINDICATIONS

Diltiazem hydrochloride is contraindicated in: (1) patients with sick sinus syndrome except in the presence of a functioning ventricular pacemaker; (2) patients with second or third degree AV block except in the presence of a functioning ventricular pacemaker; (3) patients with hypotension (less than 90 mmHg systolic); (4) patients who have demonstrated hypersensitivity to the drug; and (5) patients with acute myocardial infarction and pulmonary congestion as documented by X-ray on admission.

WARNINGS

1. **Cardiac Conduction.** Diltiazem hydrochloride prolongs AV node refractory periods without significantly prolonging sinus node recovery time, except in patients with sick sinus syndrome. This effect may rarely result in abnormally slow heart rates (particularly in patients with sick sinus syndrome) or second, or third degree AV block (22 of

10,119 patients, or 0.2%); 41% of these 22 patients were receiving concomitant β-adrenoceptor antagonists versus 17% of the total group. Concomitant use of diltiazem with beta-blockers or digitalis may result in additive effects on cardiac conduction. A patient with Prinzmetal's angina developed periods of asystole (2 to 5 seconds) after a single 60 mg dose of diltiazem.

2. **Congestive Heart Failure.** Although diltiazem has a negative inotropic effect in isolated animal tissue preparations, hemodynamic studies in humans with normal ventricular function have not shown a reduction in cardiac index nor consistent negative effects on contractility (dp/dt). An acute study of oral diltiazem in patients with impaired ventricular function (ejection fraction of 24% ± 6%) showed improvement in indices of ventricular function without significant decrease in contractile function (dp/dt). Worsening of congestive heart failure has been reported in patients with preexisting impairment of ventricular function. Experience with the use of diltiazem hydrochloride in combination with beta-blockers in patients with impaired ventricular function is limited. Caution should be exercised when using this combination.
3. **Hypotension.** Decreases in blood pressure associated with diltiazem hydrochloride therapy may occasionally result in symptomatic hypotension.
4. **Acute Hepatic Injury.** Mild elevations of serum transaminases with and without concomitant elevation in alkaline phosphatase and bilirubin have been observed in clinical studies. Such elevations were usually transient and frequently resolved even with continued diltiazem treatment. In rare instances, significant elevations in alkaline phosphatase, LDH, SGOT, SGPT, and other phenomena consistent with acute hepatic injury have been noted. These reactions tended to occur early after therapy initiation (1 to 6 weeks) and have been reversible upon discontinuation of drug therapy. The relationship to diltiazem is uncertain in some cases, but probable in some others (see PRECAUTIONS).

PRECAUTIONS

General. Diltiazem hydrochloride is extensively metabolized by the liver and is excreted by the kidneys and in bile. As with any drug given over prolonged periods, laboratory parameters should be monitored at regular intervals. The drug should be used with caution in patients with impaired renal or hepatic function. In subacute and chronic dog and rat studies designed to produce toxicity, high doses of diltiazem were associated with hepatic damage. In special subacute hepatic studies, oral doses of 125 mg/kg and higher in rats were associated with histological changes in the liver which were reversible when the drug was discontinued. In dogs, doses of 20 mg/kg were also associated with hepatic changes; however, these changes were reversible with continued dosing.

Dermatological events (see ADVERSE REACTIONS) may be transient and may disappear despite continued use of diltiazem hydrochloride. However, skin eruptions progressing to erythema multiforme and/or exfoliative dermatitis have also been infrequently reported. Should a dermatologic reaction persist, the drug should be discontinued.

Although Dilacor™ XR utilizes a slowly disintegrating matrix, caution should still be used in patients with preexisting severe gastrointestinal narrowing (pathologic or iatrogenic). There have been no reports of obstructive symptoms in patients with known strictures in association with the ingestion of Dilacor™ XR.

Information for Patients. Dilacor™ XR capsules should be taken on an empty stomach. Patients should be cautioned that the Dilacor™ XR capsules should not be opened, chewed or crushed, and should be swallowed whole.

Drug Interaction. Due to the potential for additive effects, caution and careful titration are warranted in patients receiving diltiazem hydrochloride concomitantly with any agents known to affect cardiac contractility and/or conduction (see WARNINGS). Pharmacologic studies indicate that there may be additive effects in prolonging AV conduction when using beta-blockers or digitalis concomitantly with diltiazem hydrochloride (see WARNINGS). As with all drugs, care should be exercised when treating patients with multiple medications. Diltiazem hydrochloride undergoes biotransformation by cytochrome P-450 mixed function oxidase. Co-administration of diltiazem hydrochloride with other agents which follow the same route of biotransformation may result in the competitive inhibition of metabolism. Dosages of similarly metabolized drugs such as cyclosporin, particularly those of low therapeutic ratio or in patients with renal and/or hepatic impairment, may require adjustment when starting or stopping concomitantly administered diltiazem hydrochloride to maintain optimum therapeutic blood levels.

Beta-Blockers: Controlled and uncontrolled domestic studies suggest that concomitant use of diltiazem hydrochloride and beta-blockers is usually well-tolerated, but available data are not sufficient to predict the effects of concomitant treatment in patients with left ventricular dysfunction or cardiac conduction abnormalities. Administration of diltiazem hydrochloride concomitantly with propranolol in five normal volunteers resulted in increased propranolol levels in all subjects and the bioavailability of propranolol was increased approximately 50%. If combination therapy is initiated or withdrawn in conjunction with propranolol, an adjustment in the propranolol dose may be warranted (see WARNINGS).

Cimetidine: A study in six healthy volunteers has shown a significant increase in peak diltiazem plasma levels (58%) and area-under-the-curve (53%) after a 1-week course of cimetidine at 1,200 mg per day and diltiazem 60 mg per day. Ranitidine produced smaller, nonsignificant increases. The effect may be mediated by cimetidine's known inhibition of hepatic cytochrome P-450, the enzyme system responsible for the first-pass metabolism of diltiazem. Patients currently receiving diltiazem therapy should be carefully monitored for a change in pharmacological effect when initiating and discontinuing therapy with cimetidine. An adjustment in the diltiazem dose may be warranted.

Digitalis: Administration of diltiazem hydrochloride with digoxin in 24 healthy male subjects increased plasma digoxin concentrations approximately 20%. Another investigator found no increase in digoxin levels in 12 patients with coronary artery disease. Since there have been conflicting results regarding the effect of digoxin levels, it is recommended that digoxin levels be monitored when initiating, adjusting, and discontinuing diltiazem hydrochloride therapy to avoid possible over- or under-digitalization (see WARNINGS).

Anesthetics: The depression of cardiac contractility, conductivity, and automaticity as well as the vascular dilation associated with anesthetics may be potentiated by calcium channel blockers. When used concomitantly, anesthetics and calcium channel blockers should be titrated carefully.

Carcinogenesis, Mutagenesis, Impairment of Fertility. A 24-month study in rats and an 18-month study in mice showed no evidence of carcinogenicity. There was also no mutagenic response *in-vitro* or *in-vivo* in mammalian cell assays or *in-vitro* in bacteria. No evidence of impaired fertility was observed in male or female rats at oral doses of up to 100 mg/kg/day.

Pregnancy. Category C. Reproduction studies have been conducted in mice, rats, and rabbits. Administration of doses ranging from 4 to 6 times (depending on species) the upper limit of the optimum dosage range in clinical trials (480 mg q.d. or 8 mg/kg q.d. for a 60 kg patient) has resulted in embryo and fetal lethality. These studies have revealed, in one species or another, a propensity to cause abnormalities of the skeleton, heart, retina, and tongue. Also observed were reductions in early individual pup weights and pup survival, prolonged delivery and increased incidence of stillbirths. There are no well-controlled studies in pregnant women; therefore, use diltiazem hydrochloride in pregnant women only if the potential benefit justifies the potential risk to the fetus.

Nursing Mothers. Diltiazem is excreted in human milk. One report suggests that concentrations in breast milk may approximate serum levels. If use of diltiazem hydrochloride is deemed essential, an alternative method of infant feeding should be instituted.

Pediatric Use. Safety and effectiveness in children have not been established.

ADVERSE REACTIONS

Serious adverse reactions to diltiazem hydrochloride have been rare in studies with other formulations, as well as with Dilacor™ XR. It should be recognized, however, that patients with impaired ventricular function and cardiac conduction abnormalities have usually been excluded from these studies.

The most common adverse events (frequency ≥1%) in placebo-controlled, clinical hypertension studies with Dilacor™ XR using daily doses up to 540 mg are listed in the table below with placebo-treated patients included for comparison.

MOST COMMON ADVERSE EVENTS IN DOUBLE-BLIND, PLACEBO-CONTROLLED HYPERTENSION TRIALS*

Adverse Events (COSTART Term)	Dilacor™ XR n=303 # pts (%)	Placebo n=87 # pts (%)
rhinitis	29 (9.6)	7 (8.0)
headache	27 (8.9)	12 (13.8)
pharyngitis	17 (5.6)	4 (4.6)
constipation	11 (3.6)	2 (2.3)
cough increase	9 (3.0)	2 (2.3)
flu syndrome	7 (2.3)	1 (1.1)
edema, peripheral	7 (2.3)	0 (0.0)
myalgia	7 (2.3)	0 (0.0)
diarrhea	6 (2.0)	0 (0.0)
vomiting	6 (2.0)	0 (0.0)
sinusitis	6 (2.0)	1 (1.1)
asthenia	5 (1.7)	0 (0.0)
pain, back	5 (1.7)	2 (2.3)
nausea	5 (1.7)	1 (1.1)
dyspepsia	4 (1.3)	0 (0.0)
vasodilatation	4 (1.3)	0 (0.0)
injury, accident	4 (1.3)	0 (0.0)
pain, abdominal	3 (1.0)	0 (0.0)
arthrosis	3 (1.0)	0 (0.0)
insomnia	3 (1.0)	0 (0.0)
dyspnea	3 (1.0)	0 (0.0)
rash	3 (1.0)	1 (1.1)
tinnitus	3 (1.0)	0 (0.0)

* Adverse events occurring in 1% or more of patients receiving Dilacor™ XR.

The following additional events (COSTART Terms), listed by body system, were reported infrequently in all subjects and hypertensive patients who received Dilacor™ XR (n = 425):

Cardiovascular: First-degree AV block, arrhythmia, postural hypotension, tachycardia, pallor, palpitations, phlebitis, ECG abnormality, ST elevation.

Nervous System: Vertigo, hypertonia, paresthesia, dizziness, somnolence.

Digestive System: Dry mouth, anorexia, tooth disorder, eructation.

Skin and Appendages: Sweating, urticaria, skin hypertrophy (nevus).

Respiratory System: Epistaxis, bronchitis, respiratory disorder.

Urogenital System: Cystitis, kidney calculus, impotence, dysmenorrhea, vaginitis, prostate disease.

Metabolic and Nutritional Disorders: Gout, edema.

Musculoskeletal System: Arthralgia, bursitis, bone pain.

Hemic and Lymphatic System: Lymphadenopathy.

Body as a Whole: Pain, unevaluable reaction, neck pain, neck rigidity, fever, chest pain, malaise.

Special Senses: Amblyopia (blurred vision), ear pain.

OVERDOSAGE OR EXAGGERATED RESPONSE

Overdosage experience with oral diltiazem hydrochloride has been limited. The administration of ipecac to induce vomiting and activated charcoal to reduce drug absorption have been advocated as initial means of intervention. In addition to gastric lavage, the following measures should also be considered:

Bradycardia: Administer atropine (0.60 mg to 1.0 mg). If there is no response to vagal blockade, administer isoproterenol cautiously.

High-Degree AV Block: Treat as for bradycardia above. Fixed high-degree AV block should be treated with cardiac pacing.

Cardiac Failure: Administer inotropic agents (dopamine or dobutamine) and diuretics.

Hypotension: Vasopressors (*e.g.* dopamine or levarterenol bitartrate).

Actual treatment and dosage should depend on the severity of the clinical situation as well as the judgment and experience of the treating physician.

Strength	Size	NDC 0075-	Color	Markings
180 mg	Bottles of 100	0251-00	orange cap white body	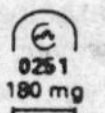 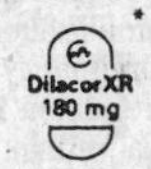 *
	Unit Dose 100	0251-62		
240 mg	Bottles of 100	0252-00	brown cap white body	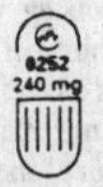 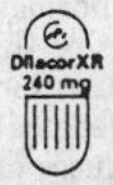 *
	Unit Dose 100	0252-62		

* Revised markings to be implemented in 1992.

Continued on next page

Rhône-Poulenc Rorer—Cont.

Due to extensive metabolism, plasma concentrations after a standard dose of diltiazem can vary over tenfold, which significantly limits their value in evaluating cases of overdosage.
Charcoal hemoperfusion has been used successfully as an adjunct therapy to hasten drug elimination. Overdoses with as much as 10.8 gm of oral diltiazem have been successfully treated using appropriate supportive care.

DOSAGE AND ADMINISTRATION

Dosage: Dosages must be adjusted to each patient's needs, starting with 180 mg or 240 mg once-daily. Based on the antihypertensive effect, the dose may be adjusted as needed. The usual dosage range studied in clinical trials was 180 mg to 480 mg once daily. Although current clinical experience with the 540 mg dose is limited, the dose may be increased to 540 mg with little or no increased risk of adverse reactions.
While a dose of Dilacor™ XR given once-daily may produce an antihypertensive effect similar to the same total daily dose given in divided doses, individual dose adjustment may be needed.
Administration: Studies have shown a slight increase in the rate of absorption of Dilacor™ XR, when ingested with a high-fat breakfast; therefore, administration in the morning on an empty stomach is recommended.
Patients should be cautioned that the Dilacor™ XR capsules should not be opened, chewed or crushed, and should be swallowed whole.

HOW SUPPLIED

[See table on preceding page.]

National Stock Number

Strength	Size	NSN
180 mg	Bottles of 100	6505-01-355-3602
240 mg	Bottles of 100	6505-01-355-3601

STORE AT CONTROLLED ROOM TEMPERATURE, 15°–30°C (59°–86°F).
CAUTION: FEDERAL (U.S.A.) LAW PROHIBITS DISPENSING WITHOUT PRESCRIPTION.
Rev. 6/92 IN-1005B, 14161
RHÔNE-POULENC RORER PHARMACEUTICALS INC.
Collegeville, PA, U.S.A. 19426-0107
Shown in Product Identification Section, page 424

LOZOL® ℞
[lō 'zôl]
(indapamide)
2.5 mg tablets

PRODUCT OVERVIEW

KEY FACTS

Lozol® (indapamide) is the first of a new class of oral antihypertensive/diuretics, the indolines. In addition to its diuretic effect, the drug decreases peripheral resistance with little or no effect on cardiac output, rate or rhythm. Chronic administration of indapamide has little or no effect on glomerular filtration rate or renal plasma flow. Mean changes in potassium, sodium, chloride and uric acid are slight.

MAJOR USES

Lozol is indicated for the treatment of hypertension, alone or in combination with other antihypertensive drugs. Lozol is also indicated for the treatment of salt and fluid retention associated with congestive heart failure. The adult starting dose for hypertension or edema of congestive heart failure is 2.5 mg as a single daily dose taken in the morning. Higher doses (5.0 mg and larger) provide little additional antihypertensive effect, yet may produce greater electrolyte shifts.

SAFETY INFORMATION

Hypokalemia occurs commonly with diuretics, and electrolyte monitoring is essential. Diuretics should not be given concomitantly with lithium. Lozol is contraindicated in anuria as well as in known hypersensitivity to indapamide or to other sulfonamide-derived drugs.

PRESCRIBING INFORMATION

LOZOL® ℞
[lō 'zôl]
indapamide
2.5 mg tablets

DESCRIPTION

LOZOL® (indapamide) is an oral antihypertensive/diuretic. Its molecule contains both a polar sulfamoyl chlorobenzamide moiety and a lipid-soluble methylindoline moiety. It differs chemically from the thiazides in that it does not possess the thiazide ring system and contains only one sulfonamide group. The chemical name of LOZOL is 1-(4-chloro-3-sulfamoylbenzamido)-2-methylindoline, and its molecular weight is 365.84. The compound is a weak acid, $pK_a = 8.8$, and is soluble in aqueous solutions of strong bases. It is a white to yellow-white crystalline (tetragonal) powder.

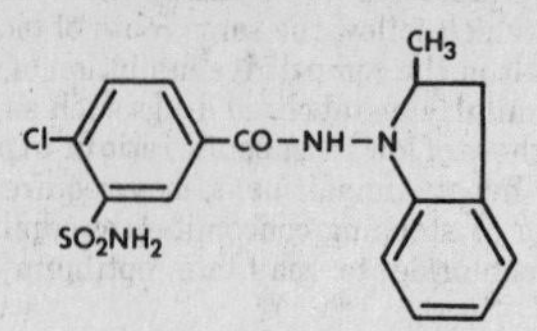

The tablets also contain microcrystalline cellulose, coloring agent, cornstarch, hydroxypropyl methylcellulose, lactose, magnesium stearate, polyethylene glycol, and talc.

CLINICAL PHARMACOLOGY

Indapamide is the first of a new class of antihypertensive/diuretics, the indolines. The oral administration of 5 mg (two 2.5-mg tablets) of indapamide to healthy male subjects produced peak concentrations of approximately 260 ng/mL of the drug in the blood within two hours. A minimum of 70% of a single oral dose is eliminated by the kidneys and an additional 23% by the gastrointestinal tract, probably including the biliary route. The half-life of LOZOL in whole blood is approximately 14 hours.
LOZOL is preferentially and reversibly taken up by the erythrocytes in the peripheral blood. The whole blood/plasma ratio is approximately 6:1 at the time of peak concentration and decreases to 3.5:1 at eight hours. From 71 to 79% of the LOZOL in plasma is reversibly bound to plasma proteins.
LOZOL is an extensively metabolized, unchanged drug accounting for approximately 7% of the total dose recovered in the urine during the first 48 hours after administration. The urinary elimination of ^{14}C-labeled indapamide and metabolites is biphasic with a terminal half-life of excretion of total radioactivity of 26 hours.
In parallel design, dose-ranging clinical trials in hypertension and edema, daily doses of indapamide between 0.5 and 5.0 mg produced dose-related effects. Generally, doses of 2.5 and 5.0 mg were not distinguishable from each other although each was differentiated from placebo and from 0.5 or 1.0 mg indapamide. At daily doses of 2.5 and 5.0 mg a mean decrease of serum potassium of 0.5 and 0.6 mEq/Liter, respectively, was observed and uric acid increased by about 1.0 mg/100 mL.
Thus, at these doses, the effects of indapamide on blood pressure and edema are approximately equal to those obtained with conventional doses of other antihypertensive/diuretics.
In hypertensive patients, daily doses of 2.5 and 5.0 mg of indapamide have no appreciable cardiac inotropic or chronotropic effect. The drug decreases peripheral resistance, with little or no effect on cardiac output, rate or rhythm. Chronic administration of indapamide to hypertensive patients has little or no effect on glomerular filtration rate or renal plasma flow.
LOZOL had an antihypertensive effect in patients with varying degrees of renal impairment, although in general, diuretic effects declined as renal function decreased.
In limited controlled studies, adding LOZOL to other antihypertensive drugs such as hydralazine, propranolol, guanethidine, and methyldopa, indapamide appeared to have the additive effect typical of thiazide-type diuretics.

INDICATIONS

LOZOL is indicated for the treatment of hypertension, alone or in combination with other antihypertensive drugs.
LOZOL is also indicated for the treatment of salt and fluid retention associated with congestive heart failure.
Usage in Pregnancy: The routine use of diuretics in an otherwise healthy woman is inappropriate and exposes mother and fetus to unnecessary hazard (see PRECAUTIONS below).
Diuretics do not prevent development of toxemia of pregnancy, and there is no satisfactory evidence that they are useful in the treatment of developed toxemia.
Edema during pregnancy may arise from pathological causes or from the physiologic and mechanical consequences of pregnancy. Indapamide is indicated in pregnancy when edema is due to pathologic causes, just as it is in the absence of pregnancy (however, see PRECAUTIONS below). Dependent edema in pregnancy, resulting from restriction of venous return by the expanded uterus, is properly treated through elevation of the lower extremities and use of support hose; use of diuretics to lower intravascular volume in this case is illogical and unnecessary. There is hypervolemia during normal pregnancy which is not harmful to either the fetus or the mother (in the absence of cardiovascular disease), but which is associated with edema, including generalized edema in the majority of pregnant women. If this edema produces discomfort, increased recumbency will often provide relief. In rare instances, this edema may cause extreme discomfort which is not relieved by rest. In these cases, a short course of diuretics may provide relief and may be appropriate.

CONTRAINDICATIONS

Anuria. Known hypersensitivity to indapamide or to other sulfonamide-derived drugs.

WARNINGS

Infrequent cases of severe hyponatremia, accompanied by hypokalemia, have been reported with the use of recommended doses of indapamide primarily in elderly females. Symptoms were reversed by electrolyte replenishment (see PRECAUTIONS).
Hypokalemia occurs commonly with diuretics (**see ADVERSE REACTIONS, hypokalemia**), and electrolyte monitoring is essential, particularly in patients who would be at increased risk from hypokalemia, such as those with cardiac arrhythmias or who are receiving concomitant cardiac glycosides.
In general, diuretics should not be given concomitantly with lithium because they reduce its renal clearance and add a high risk of lithium toxicity. Read prescribing information for lithium preparations before use of such concomitant therapy.

PRECAUTIONS

General:

1. *Hypokalemia, Hyponatremia, and Other Fluid and Electrolyte Imbalances:* Periodic determinations of serum electrolytes should be performed at appropriate intervals. In addition, patients should be observed for clinical signs of fluid or electrolyte imbalance, such as hyponatremia, hypochloremic alkalosis, or hypokalemia. Warning signs include dry mouth, thirst, weakness, fatigue, lethargy, drowsiness, restlessness, muscle pains or cramps, hypotension, oliguria, tachycardia, and gastrointestinal disturbance. Electrolyte determinations are particularly important in patients who are vomiting excessively or receiving parenteral fluids, in patients subject to electrolyte imbalance (including those with heart failure, kidney disease, and cirrhosis), and in patients on a salt-restricted diet.
   The risk of hypokalemia secondary to diuresis and natriuresis is increased when larger doses are used, when the diuresis is brisk, when severe cirrhosis is present and during concomitant use of corticosteroids or ACTH. Interference with adequate oral intake of electrolytes will also contribute to hypokalemia. Hypokalemia can sensitize or exaggerate the response of the heart to the toxic effects of digitalis, such as increased ventricular irritability.
   Dilutional hyponatremia may occur in edematous patients; the appropriate treatment is restriction of water rather than administration of salt, except in rare instances when the hyponatremia is life threatening. However, in actual salt depletion, appropriate replacement is the treatment of choice. Any chloride deficit that may occur during treatment is generally mild and usually does not require specific treatment except in extraordinary circumstances as in liver or renal disease.
2. *Hyperuricemia and Gout:* Serum concentrations of uric acid increased by an average of 1.0 mg/100 mL in patients treated with indapamide, and frank gout may be precipitated in certain patients receiving indapamide (see ADVERSE REACTIONS below). Serum concentrations of uric acid should therefore be monitored periodically during treatment.
3. *Renal Impairment:* Indapamide, like the thiazides, should be used with caution in patients with severe renal disease, as reduced plasma volume may exacerbate or precipitate azotemia. If progressive renal impairment is observed in a patient receiving indapamide, withholding or discontinuing diuretic therapy should be considered. Renal function tests should be performed periodically during treatment with indapamide.
4. *Impaired Hepatic Function:* Indapamide, like the thiazides, should be used with caution in patients with impaired hepatic function or progressive liver disease, since minor alterations of fluid and electrolyte balance may precipitate hepatic coma.
5. *Glucose Tolerance:* Latent diabetes may become manifest and insulin requirements in diabetic patients may be altered during thiazide administration. Serum concentrations of glucose should be monitored routinely during treatment with LOZOL.
6. *Calcium Excretion:* Calcium excretion is decreased by diuretics pharmacologically related to indapamide. In long-term studies of hypertensive patients, however, serum concentrations of calcium increased only slightly with indapamide. Prolonged treatment with drugs pharmacologically related to indapamide may in rare instances be associated with hypercalcemia and hypophosphatemia secondary to physiologic changes in the parathyroid gland; however, the common complications of hyperparathyroidism, such as renal lithiasis, bone resorption, and peptic ulcer, have not been seen. Treatment should be discontinued before tests for parathyroid function are performed. Like the thiazides, indapamide may decrease serum PBI levels without signs of thyroid disturbance.

7. *Interaction With Systemic Lupus Erythematosus:* Thiazides have exacerbated or activated systemic lupus erythematosus and this possibility should be considered with indapamide as well.

DRUG INTERACTIONS

1. *Other Antihypertensives:* LOZOL (indapamide) may add to or potentiate the action of other antihypertensive drugs. In limited controlled trials that compared the effect of indapamide combined with other antihypertensive drugs with the effect of the other drugs administered alone, there was no notable change in the nature or frequency of adverse reactions associated with the combined therapy.
2. *Lithium:* See WARNINGS.
3. *Post-Sympathectomy Patient:* The antihypertensive effect of the drug may be enhanced in the postsympathectomized patient.
4. *Norepinephrine:* Indapamide, like the thiazides, may decrease arterial responsiveness to norepinephrine, but this diminution is not sufficient to preclude effectiveness of the pressor agent for therapeutic use.

CARCINOGENESIS, MUTAGENESIS, IMPAIRMENT OF FERTILITY: Both mouse and rat lifetime carcinogenicity studies were conducted. There was no significant difference in the incidence of tumors between the indapamide-treated animals and the control groups.

Pregnancy/Teratogenic Effects: Pregnancy Category B. Reproduction studies have been performed in rats, mice, and rabbits at doses up to 6,250 times the therapeutic human dose and have revealed no evidence of impaired fertility or harm to the fetus due to LOZOL. Postnatal development in rats and mice was unaffected by pretreatment of parent ani-

Incidence ≥ 5%	Incidence < 5%
CENTRAL NERVOUS SYSTEM/ NEUROMUSCULAR	
Headache	Lightheadedness
Dizziness	Drowsiness
Fatigue, weakness, loss of energy, lethargy, tiredness, or malaise	Vertigo Insomnia Depression
Muscle cramps or spasm, or numbness of the extremities	Blurred Vision
Nervousness, tension, anxiety, irritability, or agitation	
GASTROINTESTINAL SYSTEM	
	Constipation
	Nausea
	Vomiting
	Diarrhea
	Gastric irritation
	Abdominal pain or cramps
	Anorexia
CARDIOVASCULAR SYSTEM	
	Orthostatic hypotension
	Premature ventricular contractions
	Irregular heart beat
	Palpitations
GENITOURINARY SYSTEM	
	Frequency of urination
	Nocturia
	Polyuria
DERMATOLOGIC/ HYPERSENSITIVITY	
	Rash
	Hives
	Pruritus
	Vasculitis
OTHER	
	Impotence or reduced libido
	Rhinorrhea
	Flushing
	Hyperuricemia
	Hyperglycemia
	Hyponatremia
	Hypochloremia
	Increase in serum urea nitrogen (BUN) or creatinine
	Glycosuria
	Weight loss
	Dry mouth
	Tingling of extremities

mals during gestation. There are, however, no adequate and well-controlled studies in pregnant women. Moreover, diuretics are known to cross the placental barrier and appear in cord blood. Because animal reproduction studies are not always predictive of human response, this drug should be used during pregnancy only if clearly needed. There may be hazards associated with this use such as fetal or neonatal jaundice, thrombocytopenia, and possibly other adverse reactions that have occurred in the adult.

Nursing Mothers: It is not known whether this drug is excreted in human milk. Because most drugs are excreted in human milk, if use of this drug is deemed essential, the patient should stop nursing.

ADVERSE REACTIONS

Most adverse effects have been mild and transient.

The clinical adverse reactions listed in the table at left. represent data from Phase II placebo-controlled studies and long-term controlled clinical trials (426 patients given LOZOL 2.5 mg or 5.0 mg). The reactions are arranged into two groups: 1) a cumulative incidence equal to or greater than 5%; 2) a cumulative incidence less than 5%. Reactions are counted regardless of relation to drug.[See table at left.] Because most of these data are from long-term studies (up to 40 weeks of treatment), it is probable that many of the adverse experiences reported are due to causes other than the drug. Approximately 10% of patients given indapamide discontinued treatment in long-term trials because of reactions either related or unrelated to the drug.

Hypokalemia with concomitant clinical signs or symptoms occurred in 3% of patients receiving indapamide 2.5 mg q.d. and 7% of patients receiving indapamide 5 mg q.d. In long-term controlled clinical trials comparing the hypokalemic effects of daily doses of indapamide and hydrochlorothiazide, however, 47% of patients receiving indapamide 2.5 mg, 72% of patients receiving indapamide 5 mg, and 44% of patients receiving hydrochlorothiazide 50 mg had at least one potassium value (out of a total of 11 taken during the study) below 3.5 mEq/L. In the indapamide 2.5 mg group, over 50% of those patients returned to normal serum potassium values without intervention.

As expected in long-term clinical trials, many patients experienced single instances of abnormal clinical laboratory test results. However, over time, the mean changes in selected values are slight, as shown in the table above.

[See top table above.]

Other adverse reactions reported with antihypertensive/diuretics are jaundice (intrahepatic cholestatic jaundice), sialadenitis, xanthopsia, photosensitivity, purpura, bullous eruptions, Stevens-Johnson Syndrome, necrotizing angiitis, fever, respiratory distress (including pneumonitis), and anaphylactic reactions; also, agranulocytosis, leukopenia, thrombocytopenia, and aplastic anemia. These reactions should be considered as possible occurrences with clinical usage of LOZOL.

OVERDOSAGE

Symptoms of overdosage include nausea, vomiting, weakness, gastrointestinal disorders and disturbances of electrolyte balance. In severe instances, hypotension and depressed respiration may be observed. If this occurs, support of respiration and cardiac circulation should be instituted. There is no specific antidote. An evacuation of the stomach is recommended by emesis and gastric lavage after which the electrolyte and fluid balance should be evaluated carefully.

DOSAGE AND ADMINISTRATION

Hypertension and edema of congestive heart failure: The adult starting dose for hypertension or edema of congestive heart failure is 2.5 mg as a *single daily dose* taken in the morning. If the response to 2.5 mg is not satisfactory after one (edema) to four (hypertension) weeks, the daily dose may be increased to 5.0 mg taken once daily.

If the antihypertensive response to indapamide is insufficient, LOZOL may be combined with other antihypertensive drugs, with careful monitoring of blood pressure. It is recommended that the usual dose of other agents be reduced by 50% during initial combination therapy. As the blood pres-

Mean Changes from Baseline after 40 Weeks of Treatment

	Serum Electrolytes (mEq/L) Potassium Sodium Chloride			Serum Uric Acid (mg/dL)	BUN (mg/dL)
Indapamide 2.5 mg (n=76)	−0.4	−0.6	−3.6	0.7	−0.1
Indapamide 5.0 mg (n=81)	−0.6	−0.7	−5.1	1.1	1.4

Strength	Size	NDC 0075-	Color	Shape	Markings
2.5 mg	Bottles of 100	0082-00	White film-coated	Octagon Shaped*	R and 8
"	Bottles of 1000	0082-99			
"	Unit Dose 100	0082-62			

*The distinctive design of the Lozol tablet is patented by Rhone-Poulenc Rorer Pharmaceuticals Inc. U.S. Pat. No. Des. 300,673.

sure response becomes evident, further dosage adjustments may be necessary.

In general, doses of 5.0 mg and larger have not appeared to provide additional effects on blood pressure or heart failure, but are associated with a greater degree of hypokalemia. There is little clinical trial experience in patients with doses greater than 5.0 mg once a day.

HOW SUPPLIED

[See second table above.]

Military: 100s (NSN 6505-01-216-4975), 1000s (NSN 6505-01-187-0109).

Veterans Administration: 100s (NSN 6505-01-216-4975).

CAUTION

Federal (U.S.A.) law prohibits dispensing without prescription.

Keep tightly closed. Store at room temperature. Avoid excessive heat. Dispense in tight containers as defined in USP.

Revised: 3/92   IN-4182E

RHÔNE-POULENC RORER PHARMACEUTICALS INC. Collegeville, PA, U.S.A. 19426-0107

Shown in Product Identification Section, page 424

NASACORT®   ℞

[na 'za-cort]
(triamcinolone acetonide)
Nasal Inhaler

For Intranasal Use Only
Shake Well Before Using

PRODUCT OVERVIEW

Nasacort Nasal Inhaler is a metered-dose aerosol unit containing a microcrystalline suspension of triamcinolone acetonide in dichlorodifluoromethane and dehydrated alcohol USP 0.7% w/w. Each actuation releases approximately 55 mcg triamcinolone acetonide from the nasal actuator to the patient. There are at least 100 actuations in one Nasacort Nasal Inhaler canister. Triamcinolone acetonide is a very potent derivative of triamcinolone.

MAJOR USE

Nasacort Nasal Inhaler is indicated for the nasal treatment of seasonal and perennial allergic rhinitis symptoms.

Adults and Children 12 years of age and older: The recommended starting dose of Nasacort Nasal Inhaler is 220 mcg per day given as two sprays (approximately 55 mcg/spray) in each nostril once a day.

SAFETY INFORMATION

Hypersensitivity to any of the ingredients of this preparation contraindicates its use. Patients previously treated for prolonged periods with systemic corticosteroids and transferred to topical corticoids should be carefully monitored for acute adrenal insufficiency in response to stress.

NASACORT®   ℞

[na 'za-cort]
(triamcinolone acetonide)
Nasal Inhaler

For Intranasal Use Only
Shake Well Before Using

DESCRIPTION

Triamcinolone acetonide, USP, the active ingredient in **Nasacort®** Nasal Inhaler, is a glucocorticosteroid with a molecular weight of 434.5 and with the chemical designation 9-Fluoro-11 β,16 α,17,21-tetrahydroxypregna-1,4-diene-3,20-dione cyclic 16,17-acetal with acetone. ($C_{24}H_{31}FO_6$).

[See chemical structure at top of next column.]

Nasacort Nasal Inhaler is a metered-dose aerosol unit containing a microcrystalline suspension of triamcinolone acetonide in dichlorodifluoromethane and dehydrated alcohol USP 0.7% w/w. Each canister contains 15 mg triamcinolone acetonide. Each actuation releases approximately 55 mcg triamcinolone acetonide from the nasal actuator to the

Continued on next page

Rhône-Poulenc Rorer—Cont.

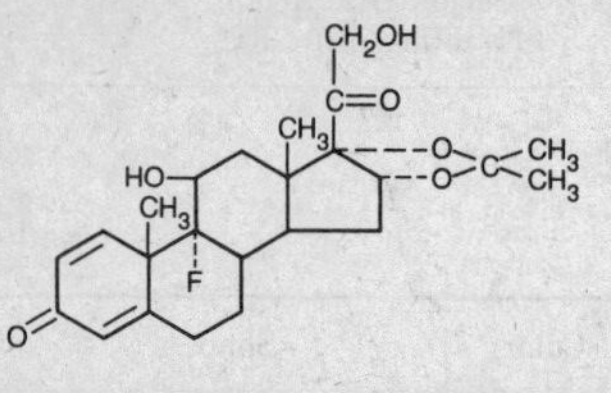

patient (estimated from *in vitro* testing). There are at least 100 actuations in one **Nasacort** Nasal Inhaler canister. After 100 actuations, the amount delivered per actuation may not be consistent and the unit should be discarded. Patients are provided with a check-off card to track usage as part of the Information for Patients tear-off sheet.

CLINICAL PHARMACOLOGY

Triamcinolone acetonide is a more potent derivative of triamcinolone. Although triamcinolone itself is approximately one to two times as potent as prednisone in animal models of inflammation, triamcinolone acetonide is approximately 8 times more potent than prednisone.

Although the precise mechanism of glucocorticoid antiallergic action is unknown, glucocorticoids are very effective. However, when allergic symptoms are very severe, local treatment with recommended doses (microgram) of any available aerosolized corticoid are not as effective as treatment with larger doses (milligram) of oral or parenteral formulations.

Corticoids do not have an immediate effect on allergic signs and symptoms. Treatment effects may be observed as early as 12 hours after onset of treatment and, generally, it takes 3–4 days to reach maximum benefit. Similarly when corticoids are prematurely discontinued symptoms may not recur for several days.

Based upon intravenous dosing of triamcinolone acetonide phosphate ester, the half-life of triamcinolone acetonide was reported to be 88 minutes. The volume of distribution (Vd) reported was 99.5 L (SD ± 27.5) and clearance was 45.2 L/hour (SD ± 9.1) for triamcinolone acetonide. The plasma half-life of corticoids does not correlate well with the biologic half-life.

When administered intranasally to man at 440 mcg/day dose, the peak plasma concentration was <1 ng/mL and occurred on average at 3.4 hours (range 0.5–8.0 hours) post dosing. The apparent half-life was 4.0 hours (range 1.0–7.0 hours); however, this value probably reflects lingering absorption. Intranasal doses below 440 mcg/day gave sparse data and did not allow for the calculation of meaningful pharmacokinetic parameters.

Three metabolites of triamcinolone acetonide have been identified. They are 6β-hydroxytriamcinolone acetonide, 21-carboxytriamcinolone acetonide and 21-carboxy-6β-hydroxytriamcinolone acetonide. All three metabolites are expected to be substantially less active than the parent compound due to (a) the dependence of anti-inflammatory activity on the presence of a 21-hydroxyl group, (b) the decreased activity observed upon 6-hydroxylation, and (c) the markedly increased water solubility favoring rapid elimination. There appeared to be some quantitative differences in the metabolites among species. No differences were detected in metabolic pattern as a function of route of administration.

CLINICAL TRIALS

In double-blind, parallel, placebo-controlled clinical trials of seasonal and perennial allergic rhinitis, in fixed total daily doses of 110, 220 and 440 mcg per day, the responses to aerosolized triamcinolone acetonide demonstrated a statistically significant improvement over placebo. In open label trials where the doses were sometimes adjusted according to patients' signs and symptoms, the daily doses and regimens varied. The most commonly used dose was 110 mcg per day.

In attempting to determine if systemic absorption played a role in the response to **Nasacort**, a clinical study comparing intranasal and depot intramuscular triamcinolone acetonide was conducted. The doses used were based on bioavailability studies of each formulation. The final doses of **Nasacort** 440 mcg once a day and Kenalog®-40, 4 mg intramuscularly once a week, were chosen to deliver comparable total amounts of weekly triamcinolone acetonide. However, the weekly injection yielded sustained plasma levels throughout the dosing interval while the daily **Nasacort** application resulted in daily peak and trough concentrations, the mean of which was 3.5 times below the Kenalog plasma levels. Both topical **Nasacort** and intramuscular Kenalog-40 were clinically effective. In addition, in some studies there was evidence of improvement of eye symptoms. This suggests that **Nasacort**, at least to some degree is acting by a systemic mechanism.

In order to evaluate the effects of systemic absorption on the Hypothalamic-Pituitary-Adrenal (HPA) axis, **Nasacort** in doses of 440 mcg once a day was compared to placebo and 42 days of a single morning dose of prednisone 10 mg. Adrenal response to a six-hour cosyntropin stimulation test suggests that intranasal **Nasacort** 440 mcg/day for six weeks did not measurably affect adrenal activity. Conversely, oral prednisone at 10 mg/day significantly reduced the response to ACTH.

INDIVIDUALIZATION OF DOSAGE

Individual patients will experience a variable time to onset and degree of symptom relief when using **Nasacort**. It is recommended that dosing be started at 220 mcg once a day and the effect be assessed in four–seven days. Some relief can be expected in approximately two-thirds of patients within that time. If greater effect is desired an increase of dose to 440 mcg once a day can be tried. If adequate relief has not been obtained by the third week of **Nasacort** treatment, consideration to alternate forms of treatment should be given.

A dose-response between 110 mcg/day (one spray/nostril/day) and 440 mcg/day (four sprays/nostril/day) is not clearly discernible. In general, in the clinical trials the highest dose tended to provide relief sooner. This suggests an alternative approach to starting therapy with **Nasacort**, *e.g.*, starting treatment with 440 mcg (four sprays/nostril/day) and then, depending on the patient's response, decreasing the dose by one spray per day every four to seven days.

Although **Nasacort** may be used at 220 mcg/day or 440 mcg/day divided into two or four times a day, the degree of relief does not seem to be significantly different compared to once-a-day dosing. As with other nasal corticoids, the vehicle used to deliver the corticoid may cause symptoms that are difficult to distinguish from the patient's rhinitis symptoms. Thus, depending upon the balance between these vehicle side effects and the benefits of treatment, in determining the optimal dose for the relief of symptoms, individual patients may need to have a trial of high and low doses.

After symptoms have been brought under control, reducing the daily dose to 110 mcg has been shown to be effective in control of symptoms in approximately one-half of patients being treated long term for allergic rhinitis. It is always desirable to titrate an individual patient to the minimum effective dose to reduce the possibility of side effects (see PRECAUTIONS, WARNINGS, INFORMATION FOR PATIENTS and ADVERSE REACTIONS sections).

INDICATIONS AND USAGE

Nasacort Nasal Inhaler is indicated for the nasal treatment of seasonal and perennial allergic rhinitis symptoms.

CONTRAINDICATIONS

Hypersensitivity to any of the ingredients of this preparation contraindicates its use.

WARNINGS

The replacement of a systemic corticosteroid with a topical corticoid can be accompanied by signs of adrenal insufficiency and, in addition, some patients may experience symptoms of withdrawal, *e.g.*, joint and/or muscular pain, lassitude and depression. Patients previously treated for prolonged periods with systemic corticosteroids and transferred to topical corticoids should be carefully monitored for acute adrenal insufficiency in response to stress. In those patients who have asthma or other clinical conditions requiring long-term systemic corticosteroid treatment, too rapid a decrease in systemic corticosteroids may cause a severe exacerbation of their symptoms.

Children who are on immunosuppressant drugs are more susceptible to infections than healthy children. Chickenpox and measles, for example, can have a more serious or even fatal course in children on immunosuppressant doses of corticosteroids. In such children, or in adults who have not had these diseases, particular care should be taken to avoid exposure. If exposed, therapy with varicella zoster immune globulin (VZIG) or pooled intravenous immunoglobulin (IVIG), as appropriate, may be indicated. If chickenpox develops, treatment with antiviral agents may be considered.

The use of **Nasacort** Nasal Inhaler with alternate-day systemic prednisone could increase the likelihood of hypothalamic-pituitary-adrenal (HPA) suppression compared to a therapeutic dose of either one alone. Therefore, **Nasacort** Nasal Inhaler should be used with caution in patients already receiving alternate-day prednisone treatment for any disease.

PRECAUTIONS

General: In clinical studies with triamcinolone acetonide administered intranasally, the development of localized infections of the nose and pharynx with *Candida albicans* has rarely occurred. When such an infection develops it may require treatment with appropriate local therapy and discontinuance of treatment with **Nasacort** Nasal Inhaler.

Triamcinolone acetonide administered intranasally has been shown to be absorbed into the systemic circulation in humans. Patients with active rhinitis showed absorption similar to that found in normal volunteers. **Nasacort** at 440 mcg/day for 42 days did not measurably affect adrenal response to a six hour cosyntropin test. In the same study prednisone 10 mg/day significantly reduced adrenal response to ACTH over the same period (see CLINICAL TRIALS section).

Nasacort Nasal Inhaler should be used with caution, if at all, in patients with active or quiescent tuberculous infections of the respiratory tract or in patients with untreated fungal, bacterial, or systemic viral infections or ocular herpes simplex.

Because of the inhibitory effect of corticosteroids on wound healing in patients who have experienced recent nasal septal ulcers, nasal surgery or trauma, a corticosteroid should be used with caution until healing has occurred.

When used at excessive doses, systemic corticosteroid effects such as hypercorticism and adrenal suppression may appear. If such changes occur, **Nasacort** Nasal Inhaler should be discontinued slowly, consistent with accepted procedures for discontinuing oral steroid therapy.

Information for Patients: Patients being treated with **Nasacort** Nasal Inhaler should receive the following information and instructions.

Patients who are on immunosuppressant doses of corticosteroids should be warned to avoid exposure to chickenpox or measles and, if exposed, to obtain medical advice.

Patients should use **Nasacort** Nasal Inhaler at regular intervals since its effectiveness depends on its regular use. A decrease in symptoms may occur as soon as 12 hours after starting steroid therapy and generally can be expected to occur within a few days of initiating therapy in allergic rhinitis. The patient should take the medication as directed and should not exceed the prescribed dosage. The patient should contact the physician if symptoms do not improve after three weeks, or if the condition worsens. Nasal irritation and/or burning or stinging after use of the spray occur only rarely with this product. The patient should contact the physician if they occur.

For the proper use of this unit and to attain maximum improvement, the patient should read and follow the accompanying patient instructions carefully. Because the amount dispensed per puff may not be consistent, it is important to shake the canister well. Also, the canister should be discarded after 100 actuations.

Carcinogenesis, Mutagenesis: Animal studies of triamcinolone acetonide to test its carcinogenic potential are underway.

Impairment of Fertility: Male and female rats which were administered oral triamcinolone acetonide at doses as high as 15 mcg/kg/day (110 mcg/m^2/day, as calculated on a surface area basis) exhibited no evidence of impaired fertility. The maximum human dose, for comparison, is 6.3 mcg/kg/day (240 mcg/m^2/day). However, a few female rats which received maternally toxic doses of 8 or 15 mcg/kg/day (60 mcg/m^2/day or 110 mcg/m^2/day, respectively, as calculated on a surface area basis) exhibited dystocia and prolonged delivery. Developmental toxicity, which included increases in fetal resorptions and stillbirths and decreases in pup body weight and survival, also occurred at the maternally toxic doses (2.5–15.0 mcg/kg/day or 20–110 mcg/m^2/day, as calculated on a surface area basis). Reproductive performance of female rats and effects on fetuses and offspring were comparable between groups that received placebo and non-toxic or marginally toxic doses (0.5 and 1.0 mcg/kg/day or 3.8 mcg/m^2/day and 7.0 mcg/m^2/day).

Pregnancy: Pregnancy Category C. Like other corticoids, triamcinolone acetonide has been shown to be teratogenic in rats and rabbits. Teratogenic effects, which occurred in both species at 0.02, 0.04 and 0.08 mg/kg/day (approximately 135, 270 and 540 mcg/m^2/day in the rat and 320, 640 and 1280 mcg/m^2/day in the rabbit, as calculated on a surface area basis), included a low incidence of cleft palate and/or internal hydrocephaly and axial skeletal defects. Teratogenic effects, including CNS and cranial malformations, have also been observed in non-human primates at 0.5 mg/kg/day (approximately 6.7 mg/m^2/day). The doses of 0.02, 0.04, 0.08, and 0.5 mg/kg/day used in these toxicology studies are approximately 12.8, 25.5, 51, and 318.7 times the minimum recommended dose of 110 mcg of **Nasacort** per day and 3.2, 6.4, 12.7, and 80 times the maximum recommended dose of 440 mcg of **Nasacort** per day based on a patient body weight of 70 kg. Administration of aerosol by inhalation to pregnant rats and rabbits produced embryotoxic and fetotoxic effects which were comparable to those produced by administration by other routes. There are no adequate and well-controlled studies in pregnant women. Triamcinolone acetonide should be used during pregnancy only if the potential benefit justifies the potential risk to the fetus.

Experience with oral corticoids since their introduction in pharmacologic as opposed to physiologic doses suggests that rodents are more prone to teratogenic effects from corticoids than humans. In addition, because there is a natural increase in glucocorticoid production during pregnancy, most women will require a lower exogenous steroid dose and many will not need corticoid treatment during pregnancy.

Nonteratogenic Effects: Hypoadrenalism may occur in infants born of mothers receiving corticosteroids during pregnancy. Such infants should be carefully observed.

Nursing Mothers: It is not known whether triamcinolone acetonide is excreted in human milk. Because other corticosteroids are excreted in human milk, caution should be exer-

cised when **Nasacort** Nasal Inhaler is administered to nursing women.

Pediatric Use: Safety and effectiveness have not been established in children below the age of 12. Oral corticoids have been shown to cause growth suppression in children and teenagers, particularly with higher doses over extended periods. If a child or teenager on any corticoid appears to have growth suppression, the possibility that they are particularly sensitive to this effect of steroids should be considered.

ADVERSE REACTIONS

In controlled and uncontrolled studies, 1257 patients received treatment with intranasal triamcinolone acetonide. Adverse reactions are based on the 567 patients who received a product similar to the marketed **Nasacort** canister. These patients were treated for an average of 48 days (range 1 to 117 days). The 145 patients enrolled in uncontrolled studies received treatment from 1 to 820 days (average 332 days). The most prevalent adverse experience was headache, being reported by approximately 18% of the patients who received **Nasacort**. Nasal irritation was reported by 2.8% of the patients receiving **Nasacort**. Other nasopharyngeal side effects were reported by fewer than 5% of the patients who received **Nasacort** and included: dry mucous membranes, naso-sinus congestion, throat discomfort, sneezing, and epistaxis. The complaints do not usually interfere with treatment and in the controlled and uncontrolled studies approximately 1% of patients have discontinued because of these nasal adverse effects.

In the event of accidental overdose, an increased potential for these adverse experiences may be expected, but systemic adverse experiences are unlikely (see OVERDOSAGE section).

DOSAGE AND ADMINISTRATION

A decrease in symptoms may occur as soon as 12 hours after starting steroid therapy and generally can be expected to occur within a few days of initiating therapy in allergic rhinitis.

If improvement is not evident after 2–3 weeks, the patient should be re-evaluated. (See INDIVIDUALIZATION OF DOSAGE section.)

Adults and Children 12 years of age and older: The recommended starting dose of **Nasacort** Nasal Inhaler is 220 mcg per day given as two sprays (approximately 55 mcg/spray) in each nostril once a day. If needed, the dose may be increased to 440 mcg per day (approximately 55 mcg/spray) either as once a day dosage or divided up to four times a day, *i.e.*, twice a day (two sprays/nostril), or four times a day (one spray/nostril). After the desired effect is obtained, some patients may be maintained on a dose of as little as one spray (approximately 55 mcg) in each nostril once a day (total daily dose 110 mcg per day).

Directions for Use: Illustrated Patient's Instructions for use accompany each package of **Nasacort** Nasal Inhaler.

OVERDOSAGE

Acute overdosage with this dosage form is unlikely. The acute topical application of the entire 15 mg of the canister would most likely cause nasal irritation and headache. It would be unlikely to see acute systemic adverse effects if the nasal application of the 15 mg of triamcinolone acetonide was administered all at once.

HOW SUPPLIED

Nasacort Nasal Inhaler is supplied as an aerosol canister which will provide 100 actuations. It is supplied with a nasal adapter and patient instructions.
NDC 0075-1505-43.
Caution: Federal (U.S.A.) law prohibits dispensing without prescription.

CONTENTS UNDER PRESSURE

Do not puncture. Do not use or store near heat or open flame. Exposure to temperatures above 120°F may cause bursting. Never throw container into fire or incinerator. Keep out of reach of children.
Store at controlled room temperature, 15°–30°C (59°–86°F).
Rev. 1/92   IN-0479B
Marketed by
RHÔNE-POULENC RORER PHARMACEUTICALS INC.
Collegeville, PA, U.S.A. 19426-0107
Shown in Product Identification Section, page 425

NICOBID® Tempules®   OTC
(niacin)
TIMED-RELEASE NICOTINIC ACID SUPPLEMENT

DESCRIPTION

Each black-and-clear Tempule® (timed-release capsule) contains 125 mg niacin (nicotinic acid); each green-and-clear Tempule (timed-release capsule) contains 250 mg niacin (nicotinic acid); and each opaque blue and white Tempule (timed-release capsule) contains 500 mg niacin (nicotinic acid). Nicobid® Tempules® provide the full actions of niacin (nicotinic acid). Portions of the pellets contained in the Tempule

STRENGTH	SIZE	COLOR	MARKINGS	
125 mg	Bottles of 100	black (cap) clear (body)	RORER NICOBID 125	* ℞ NICOBID 125 mg
250 mg	Bottles of 100	green (cap) clear (body)	RORER NICOBID 250	* ℞ NICOBID 250 mg
500 mg	Bottles of 100 Bottles of 500	opaque blue (cap) opaque white (body)	RORER NICOBID 500	* ℞ NICOBID 500 mg

* To be implemented beginning 1992

are released immediately. The remainder is released over several hours.

INDICATIONS AND USAGE

Nicobid (niacin) is used in all those conditions in which niacin (nicotinic acid) supplementation is indicated. It has the advantage of a slower release of niacin (nicotinic acid) than conventional tablet dosage forms. This may permit its use by those who do not tolerate the tablets.

PRECAUTIONS

Nicobid should not be used by persons with a known sensitivity to niacin (nicotinic acid) and by persons with heart or gallbladder disease, gout, arterial bleeding, glaucoma, diabetes, impaired liver function, peptic ulcer, or by pregnant women. Patients taking antihypertensive drugs should consult a physician before taking Nicobid. **Abnormal liver function tests have been reported in patients taking daily doses of 500 mg and above of timed-release niacin. Patients should consult their doctor before using daily doses of 500 mg or more of timed-release niacin.**

ADVERSE REACTIONS

Temporary flushing and feeling of warmth may be expected. These seldom reach levels so as to necessitate discontinuance. If these symptoms persist, discontinue use and consult a physician. Temporary headache, itching and tingling, gastric disturbances, skin rash, allergies, and impaired liver function may occur. Peptic ulcer disease, glucose intolerance and gout may also occur.

DOSAGE

Usual Adult Dose:
125 mg and 250 mg Tempules—one Tempule morning and evening.
500 mg Tempules—one Tempule in the morning *or* evening. Before using or exceeding 500 mg daily, consult a physician.
NOTE: See **PRECAUTIONS**.
KEEP OUT OF THE REACH OF CHILDREN

HOW SUPPLIED

[See table above.]
Revised: 8/91   IN 3930C
RHÔNE-POULENC RORER PHARMACEUTICALS INC.
Collegeville, PA, U.S.A. 19426-0107

NICOLAR®   ℞
[nic'ō-lär'']
(niacin tablets)

DESCRIPTION

Nicolar® (niacin tablets) is a scored yellow-colored tablet containing 500 mg of niacin (nicotinic acid).
The tablets also contain microcrystalline cellulose, FD&C yellow No. 5 (tartrazine) (see PRECAUTIONS), magnesium stearate, povidone, and colloidal silica.

ACTIONS

Niacin functions in the body as a component of two hydrogen transporting coenzymes: Coenzyme I (Nicotinamide Adenine Dinucleotide [NAD], sometimes called Diphosphopyridine Nucleotide [DPN]) and Coenzyme II (Nicotinamide Adenine Dinucleotide Phosphate [NADP], sometimes called Triphosphopyridine Nucleotide [TPN]). Niacin, in addition to its functions as a vitamin, exerts several distinctive pharmacologic effects which vary according to the dosage level employed.
Niacin, in large doses, causes a reduction in serum lipids. The exact mechanism of this action is unknown.

INDICATIONS

Since no drug is innocuous, strict attention should be paid to the indications and contraindications, particularly when selecting drugs for long-term use.
Nicolar® (niacin tablets) is indicated as adjunctive therapy in patients with significant hyperlipidemia (elevated cholesterol and/or triglycerides) who do not respond adequately to diet and weight loss.
Notice: It has not been established whether the drug-induced lowering of serum cholesterol or triglyceride levels has a bene-

ficial effect, no effect, or a detrimental effect on the morbidity or mortality due to atherosclerosis including coronary heart disease. Investigations now in progress may yield an answer to this question.

CONTRAINDICATIONS

Niacin is contraindicated in patients with a known idiosyncrasy to niacin, with hepatic dysfunction, with active peptic ulcer or with arterial bleeding.

WARNINGS

Use of this drug in pregnancy, lactation or in women of childbearing age requires that the potential benefits of the drug be weighed against its possible hazards to the mother and child. Although fetal abnormalities have not been reported with this drug, its use as an antilipidemic agent requires high dosages, and animal reproduction or teratology studies have not been done. There are insufficient studies done for usage in children.
Keep out of reach of children.

PRECAUTIONS

Great caution must be exercised when niacin is used in patients with coronary disease, in particular unstable angina and recent myocardial infarction. Great caution must be also taken in patients with gallbladder disease. Patients with a past history of jaundice, liver disease or peptic ulcer should be observed closely while taking the medication.
Frequent monitoring of liver function tests and blood glucose should be performed during therapy to ascertain that the drug has no adverse effects on these organ systems.
Antihypertensive drugs of the adrenergic-blocking type may have an additive vasodilating effect and produce postural hypotension.
Elevated uric acid levels have occurred, therefore use with caution in patients predisposed to gout.
Drug Interactions: Antihypertensive drugs may have an additive vasodilating effect and produce postural hypotension.
Diabetic or potential diabetic patients should be observed closely in the event of decreased glucose tolerance. Adjustment of diet and/or hypoglycemic therapy may be necessary.
Rare cases of rhabdomyolysis have been associated with co-administration of lipid-lowering doses of niacin (greater than 1 g/day) and lovastatin. No cases have been reported with niacin use without lovastatin.
Physicians contemplating combined therapy of niacin and lovastatin should weigh the potential benefits and risks and should monitor patients for any signs of muscle pain, tenderness or weakness, particularly during initial dosing or periods of upward dose titration of either drug.
Periodic CPK and plasma potassium monitoring should be considered in such situations, but there is no assurance that such monitoring will prevent the occurrence of severe myopathy.
This product contains FD&C Yellow No. 5 (tartrazine) which may cause allergic-type reactions (including bronchial asthma) in certain susceptible persons. Although the overall incidence of FD&C Yellow No. 5 (tartrazine) sensitivity in the general population is low, it is frequently seen in patients who also have aspirin hypersensitivity.

ADVERSE REACTIONS

Atrial fibrillation and other cardiac arrhythmias
Severe generalized flushing
Decreased glucose tolerance
Activation of peptic ulcers
Abnormalities of hepatic
    functional tests
Jaundice
Gastrointestinal disorders
Dryness of the skin
Acanthosis Nigricans
Pruritus
Hyperuricemia
Toxic amblyopia
Hypotension
Transient headache

Continued on next page

Rhône-Poulenc Rorer—Cont.

OVERDOSAGE
High doses of nicotinic acid may produce temporary flushing, pruritus, and gastrointestinal distress.

DOSAGE AND ADMINISTRATION
Usually Recommended Adult Dosage—1 to 2 grams three times a day. The dosage must be adjusted to the response of the patient.

Start with two tablets (1 g) three times a day with food or after meals, taken with cold liquids, if necessary, to facilitate swallowing. Since low doses may control hyperlipidemia in some patients, the dosage should be individualized according to the effect on serum lipid levels. If the plasma cholesterol and/or triglyceride level does not show a decrease after a reasonable time at this dosage, an increase in dosage may be considered but requires careful titration and observation of the patient for unwanted effects. The dosage may be increased every 2 to 4 weeks, but in no case should the dosage exceed 6 grams/day.

Since flushing, pruritus and gastrointestinal distress appear frequently and tend to be dose-related, increase the dosage gradually in increments of 500 mg (1 tablet) while carefully observing the patient and monitoring the plasma cholesterol and/or triglyceride level for therapeutic response and for adverse effects.

Where the observed adverse reactions or potential hazards exceed the benefits of use, dosage should be reduced to the minimum recommended dosage and, where necessary, discontinued entirely.

HOW SUPPLIED
Nicolar® (niacin tablets) is available in bottles of 100 scored tablets, (NDC 0075-2850-01). Each tablet contains 500 mg of nicotinic acid (identified by the code NE).

Dispense in a tight container as defined in the USP. Store at controlled room temperature, 59°–86°F (15°–30°C).

Caution: Federal (U.S.A.) law prohibits dispensing without prescription.

Rev. 3/92

RHÔNE-POULENC RORER PHARMACEUTICALS INC.
Collegeville, PA, U.S.A. 19426-0107

NITROLINGUAL® SPRAY   ℞
(nitroglycerin lingual aerosol)
0.4 mg/metered dose

PRODUCT OVERVIEW

KEY FACTS
Nitrolingual® Spray is a metered-dose aerosol containing 200 doses of nitroglycerin. Each metered dose of Nitrolingual Spray delivers 0.4 mg of nitroglycerin per actuation. Nitrolingual Spray offers guaranteed potency for 3 years from date of manufacture.

MAJOR USES
Nitrolingual® Spray is indicated for acute relief of an attack or prophylaxis of angina pectoris due to coronary artery disease.

SAFETY INFORMATION
Nitrolingual® Spray is contraindicated in patients who have shown purported hypersensitivity or idiosyncrasy to it or to other nitrates or nitrites.
NOTE: THE SPRAY SHOULD NOT BE INHALED.

PRESCRIBING INFORMATION

NITROLINGUAL® SPRAY   ℞
(nitroglycerin lingual aerosol)
0.4 mg/metered dose

DESCRIPTION
Nitroglycerin, an organic nitrate, is a vasodilator which has effects on both arteries and veins. The chemical name for nitroglycerin is 1,2,3-propanetriol trinitrate ($C_3H_5N_3O_9$). The compound has a molecular weight of 227.09. The chemical structure is:

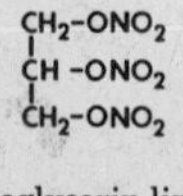

$$CH_2-ONO_2$$
$$CH\ -ONO_2$$
$$CH_2-ONO_2$$

Nitrolingual Spray (nitroglycerin lingual aerosol 0.4 mg) is a metered dose aerosol containing nitroglycerin in propellants (dichlorodifluoromethane and dichlorotetrafluoroethane). Each metered dose of Nitrolingual Spray delivers 0.4 mg of nitroglycerin per spray emission. This product delivers nitroglycerin in the form of spray droplets onto or under the tongue. Inactive ingredients: caprylic/capric/diglyceryl succinate, ether, flavors.

CLINICAL PHARMACOLOGY
The principal pharmacological action of nitroglycerin is relaxation of vascular smooth muscle, producing a vasodilator effect on both peripheral arteries and veins with more prominent effects on the latter. Dilation of the post-capillary vessels, including large veins, promotes peripheral pooling of blood and decreases venous return to the heart, thereby reducing left ventricular end-diastolic pressure (preload). Arteriolar relaxation reduces systemic vascular resistance and arterial pressure (after-load).

The mechanism by which nitroglycerin relieves angina pectoris is not fully understood. Myocardial oxygen consumption or demand (as measured by the pressure-rate product, tension-time index, and stroke-work index) is decreased by both the arterial and venous effects of nitroglycerin and presumably, a more favorable supply-demand ratio is achieved. While the large epicardial coronary arteries are also dilated by nitroglycerin, the extent to which this action contributes to relief of exertional angina is unclear.

Nitroglycerin is rapidly metabolized *in vivo*, with a liver reductase enzyme having primary importance in the formation of glycerol nitrate metabolites and inorganic nitrate. Two active major metabolites, 1, 2- and 1,3-dinitroglycerols, the products of hydrolysis, although less potent as vasodilators, have longer plasma half-lives than the parent compound. The dinitrates are further metabolized to mononitrates (considered biologically inactive with respect to cardiovascular effects) and ultimately glycerol and carbon dioxide.

Therapeutic doses of nitroglycerin may reduce systolic, diastolic, and mean arterial blood pressure. Effective coronary perfusion pressure is usually maintained, but can be compromised if blood pressure falls excessively or increased heart rate decreases diastolic filling time.

Elevated central venous and pulmonary capillary wedge pressures, pulmonary vascular resistance and systemic vascular resistance are also reduced by nitroglycerin therapy. Heart rate is usually slightly increased, presumably a reflex response to the fall in blood pressure. Cardiac index may be increased, decreased, or unchanged. Patients with elevated left ventricular filling pressure and systemic vascular resistance values in conjunction with a depressed cardiac index are likely to experience an improvement in cardiac index. On the other hand, when filling pressures and cardiac index are normal, cardiac index may be slightly reduced.

A pharmacokinetic study in 13 healthy men showed no statistically significant differences between the mean values for maximum plasma concentration and time to achieve maximum plasma level with equal doses (0.8 mg) of Nitrolingual Spray and sublingual nitroglycerin tablets. Peak plasma concentration after 0.8 mg of Nitrolingual occurred within 4 minutes and the apparent plasma half-life was approximately 5 minutes. In a randomized, double-blind study in patients with exertional angina pectoris dose-related increases in exercise tolerance were seen following doses of 0.2, 0.4, and 0.8 mg delivered by metered spray.

INDICATIONS AND USAGE
Nitrolingual Spray is indicated for acute relief of an attack or prophylaxis of angina pectoris due to coronary artery disease.

CONTRAINDICATIONS
Nitrolingual Spray is contraindicated in patients who have shown purported hypersensitivity or idiosyncrasy to it or other nitrates or nitrites.

WARNINGS
The use of any form of nitroglycerin during the early days of acute myocardial infarction requires particular attention to hemodynamic monitoring and clinical status.

PRECAUTIONS
General—Severe hypotension, particularly with upright posture, may occur even with small doses of nitroglycerin. The drug, therefore, should be used with caution in subjects who may have volume depletion from diuretic therapy or in patients who have low systolic blood pressure (e.g. below 90 mm Hg). Paradoxical bradycardia and increased angina pectoris may accompany nitroglycerin-induced hypotension.

Nitrate therapy may aggravate the angina caused by hypertrophic cardiomyopathy.

Tolerance to this drug and cross-tolerance to other nitrates and nitrites may occur. Tolerance to the vascular and antianginal effects of nitrates has been demonstrated in clinical trials, experience through occupational exposure, and in isolated tissue experiments in the laboratory.

In industrial workers continuously exposed to nitroglycerin, tolerance clearly occurs. Moreover, physical dependence also occurs since chest pain, acute myocardial infarction, and even sudden death have occurred during temporary withdrawal of nitroglycerin from the workers. In various clinical trials in angina patients, there are reports of anginal attacks being more easily provoked and of rebound in the hemodynamic effects soon after nitrate withdrawal. The relative importance of these observations to the routine, clinical use of nitroglycerin is not known.

Drug Interactions: Alcohol may enhance sensitivity to the hypotensive effects of nitrates. Nitroglycerin acts directly on vascular muscle. Therefore, any other agents that depend on vascular smooth muscle as the final common path can be expected to have decreased or increased effect depending upon the agent.

Marked symptomatic orthostatic hypotension has been reported when calcium channel blockers and oral controlled-release nitroglycerin were used in combination. Dose adjustments of either class of agents may be necessary.

Carcinogenesis, Mutagenesis, Impairment of Fertility: No long-term studies in animals have been performed to evaluate carcinogenic potential of Nitrolingual Spray.

Pregnancy: Pregnancy Category C—Animal reproduction studies have not been conducted with Nitrolingual Spray. It is not known whether nitroglycerin can cause fetal harm when administered to a pregnant woman or can affect reproduction capacity. Nitroglycerin should be given to a pregnant woman only if clearly needed.

Nursing Mothers: It is not known whether nitroglycerin is excreted in human milk. Because many drugs are excreted in human milk, caution should be exercised when Nitrolingual Spray is administered to a nursing woman.

Pediatric Use: The safety and effectiveness of nitroglycerin in children have not been established.

ADVERSE REACTIONS
Adverse reaction to Nitrolingual Spray, particularly headache and hypotension, is generally dose-related. In clinical trials at various doses of nitroglycerin, the following adverse effects have been observed:

Headache, which may be severe and persistent, is the most commonly reported side effect of nitroglycerin with an incidence on the order of about 50% in some studies. Cutaneous vasodilation with flushing may occur. Transient episodes of dizziness and weakness, as well as other signs of cerebral ischemia associated with postural hypotension, may occasionally develop. An occasional individual may exhibit marked sensitivity to the hypotensive effects of nitrates and severe responses (nausea, vomiting, weakness, restlessness, pallor, perspiration, and collapse) may occur even with therapeutic doses. Drug rash and/or exfoliative dermatitis have been reported in patients receiving nitrate therapy. Nausea and vomiting appear to be uncommon.

OVERDOSAGE
Signs and Symptoms:
Nitrate overdosage may result in: severe hypotension, persistent throbbing headache, vertigo, palpitation, visual disturbance, flushing and perspiring skin (later becoming cold and cyanotic), nausea and vomiting (possibly with colic and even bloody diarrhea), syncope (especially in the upright posture), methemoglobinemia with cyanosis and anorexia, initial hypernea, dyspnea, and slow breathing, slow pulse (dicrotic and intermittent), heart block, increased intracranial pressure with cerebral symptoms of confusion and moderate fever, paralysis and coma followed by clonic convulsions, and possibly death due to circulatory collapse.

Treatment of Overdosage:
Keep the patient recumbent in a shock position and comfortably warm. Gastric lavage may be of use if the medication has only recently been swallowed. Passive movement of the extremities may aid venous return. Administer oxygen and artificial ventilation, if necessary. If methemoglobinemia is present, administration of methylene blue (1% solution), 1–2 mg per kilogram of body weight intravenously, may be required.

Methemoglobinemia:
Case reports of clinically significant methemoglobinemia are rare at conventional doses of organic nitrates. The formation of methemoglobin is dose-related and in the case of genetic abnormalities of hemoglobin that favor methemoglobin formation, even conventional doses of organic nitrates could produce harmful concentrations of methemoglobin.

WARNING
Epinephrine is ineffective in reversing the severe hypotensive events associated with overdosage. It and related compounds are contraindicated in this situation.

DOSAGE AND ADMINISTRATION
At the onset of an attack, one or two metered doses should be sprayed onto or under the tongue. No more than three metered doses are recommended within a 15-minute period. If the chest pain persists, prompt medical attention is recommended. Nitrolingual Spray may be used prophylactically five to ten minutes prior to engaging in activities which might precipitate an acute attack.

During application the patient should rest, ideally in the sitting position. The canister should be held vertically with the valve head uppermost and the spray orifice as close to the mouth as possible. The dose should preferably be sprayed onto the tongue by pressing the button firmly and the mouth should be closed immediately after each dose. THE SPRAY SHOULD NOT BE INHALED. Patients should be instructed to familiarize themselves with the position of the spray orifice, which can be identified by the finger rest on top of the

valve, in order to facilitate orientation for administration at night.

HOW SUPPLIED

Nitrolingual Spray, 14.49 g (Net Contents) containing 200 metered doses, box of one (NDC 0075-0850-84).
Store at room temperature. Do not expose to temperatures exceeding 50°C (122°F).

CAUTION

Federal (U.S.A.) law prohibits dispensing without prescription.
Rev. 1/91 J-3997F
Manufactured by:
G. Pohl-Boskamp GmbH & Co.,
D-2214 Hohenlockstedt
Fed. Rep. of Germany
Distributed by:
RHÔNE-POULENC RORER PHARMACEUTICALS INC.
Collegeville, PA, U.S.A. 19426-0107
Shown in Product Identification Section, page 425

PENETREX™ ℞
(enoxacin) Tablets

KEY FACTS

Penetrex is available in 200-mg and 400-mg film-coated tablets. Each "200" and "400" Penetrex tablet contains enoxacin sesquihydrate equivalent to 200 mg and 400 mg of anhydrous enoxacin, respectively.
Following oral administration to healthy subjects, peak plasma enoxacin concentrations were achieved within 1 to 3 hours. Absolute oral bioavailability of enoxacin is approximately 90%. Maximum plasma concentrations of enoxacin average 0.93 mcg/mL and 2.0 mcg/mL after single 200-mg and 400-mg doses, respectively. Enoxacin plasma half-life is 3 to 6 hours.

MAJOR USES

INDICATIONS AND USAGE

Penetrex (enoxacin) is indicated for the treatment of adults (≥18 years of age) with the following infections caused by susceptible strains of the designated microorganisms:
Sexually Transmitted Diseases (See **WARNINGS.**) **Uncomplicated urethral or cervical gonorrhea** due to *Neisseria gonorrhoeae.*
Urinary Tract: **Uncomplicated urinary tract infections** (cystitis) due to *Escherichia coli, Staphylococcus epidermidis,* or *Staphylococcus saprophyticus.*
Complicated urinary tract infections due to *Escherichia coli, Klebsiella pneumoniae, Proteus mirabilis, Pseudomonas aeruginosa, Staphylococcus epidermidis,* or *Enterobacter cloacae.*

DOSAGE AND ADMINISTRATION

Sexually Transmitted Diseases
Uncomplicated urethral or cervical gonorrhea: 400 mg single dose
Urinary Tract Infections
Uncomplicated urinary tract infections: 200 mg q12h for 7 days
Complicated urinary tract infections: 400 mg q12h for 14 days

SAFETY INFORMATION

Enoxacin is contraindicated for individuals with a history of hypersensitivity to enoxacin or to any of the other members of the quinolone class of antimicrobial agents.
The safety and effectiveness of enoxacin in children, adolescents (under the age of 18 years), pregnant women, and lactating women have not been established.
Serious and occasionally fatal hypersensitivity (anaphylactoid or anaphylactic) reactions, some following the first dose, have been reported in patients receiving quinolone therapy.
Pseudomembranous colitis has been reported with nearly all antibacterial agents, including enoxacin, and may range in severity from mild to life-threatening. Therefore, it is important to consider this diagnosis in patients who present with diarrhea subsequent to the administration of antibacterial agents.

PENETREX™ ℞
(enoxacin) Tablets

DESCRIPTION

Penetrex™ (enoxacin) is a broad-spectrum azafluoroquinolone antibacterial agent for oral administration. Enoxacin is 1-ethyl-6-fluoro-1,4-dihydro-4-oxo-7-(1-piperazinyl)-1,8-naphthyridine-3-carboxylic acid sesquihydrate. The chemical structure of enoxacin is:

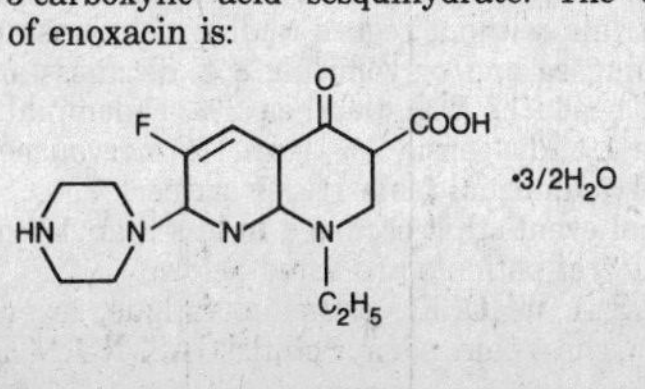

Its empirical formula is $C_{15}H_{17}N_4O_3F \cdot 1\frac{1}{2}\ H_2O$, and its molecular weight is 320.32 (anhydrous). Enoxacin is an ivory-to-slightly yellow powder. In dilute aqueous solution, it is unstable in strong sunlight.
Penetrex is available in 200-mg and 400-mg film-coated tablets. Each "200" and "400" Penetrex tablet contains enoxacin sesquihydrate equivalent to 200 mg and 400 mg of anhydrous enoxacin, respectively. Each Penetrex 200-mg and 400-mg tablet contains the following inactive ingredients: cellulose microcrystalline NF, colloidal silicon dioxide NF, croscarmellose sodium NF, FD&C Blue No. 2 aluminum lake, hydroxypropyl cellulose NF, hydroxypropyl methylcellulose, magnesium stearate USP, polyethylene glycol, simethicone, sorbic acid, stearate emulsifiers, and titanium dioxide.

CLINICAL PHARMACOLOGY

Following oral administration to healthy subjects, peak plasma enoxacin concentrations were achieved within 1 to 3 hours. Absolute oral bioavailability of enoxacin is approximately 90%. Maximum plasma concentrations of enoxacin average 0.93 mcg/mL and 2.0 mcg/mL after single 200-mg and 400-mg doses, respectively. Enoxacin plasma half-life is 3 to 6 hours. Enoxacin is excreted primarily via the kidney. After a single dose, greater than 40% was recovered in urine by 48 hours as unchanged drug. In elderly patients, the mean peak enoxacin plasma concentration was 50% higher than that in young adult volunteers receiving comparable single doses of enoxacin. This appears to correspond to age-associated reduction of renal function in the elderly population.
Five metabolites of enoxacin have been identified in human urine and account for 15% to 20% of the administered dose.
Enoxacin diffuses into cervix, fallopian tube, and myometrium at levels approximately 1–2 times those achieved in plasma, and into kidney and prostate at levels approximately 2–4 times those achieved in plasma. Studies have not been conducted to assess the penetration of enoxacin into human cerebrospinal fluid.
Enoxacin is approximately 40% bound to plasma proteins in healthy subjects and is approximately 14% bound to plasma proteins in patients with impaired renal function.
The effect of food on the absorption of enoxacin from the tablet formulation has not been studied.
Some isozymes of the cytochrome P-450 hepatic microsomal enzyme system are inhibited by enoxacin. This inhibition results in significant drug/drug interactions with theophylline and caffeine. Enoxacin interferes with the metabolism of theophylline, resulting in a dose-related decrease in theophylline clearance. Elevated serum theophylline concentrations may increase the risk of theophylline-related adverse reactions. (See **Drug Interactions.**)
Clearance of enoxacin is reduced in patients with impaired renal function (creatinine clearance ≤30 mL/min/1.73 m^2), and dosage adjustment is necessary. (See **DOSAGE AND ADMINISTRATION.**)

MICROBIOLOGY

Enoxacin is an inhibitor of the bacterial enzyme DNA gyrase and is a bactericidal agent. Enoxacin may be active against pathogens resistant to drugs that act by different mechanisms.
Enoxacin has been shown to be active against most strains of the following organisms both *in vitro* and in clinical infections: (See **INDICATIONS AND USAGE.**)
Gram-positive aerobes: *Staphylococcus epidermidis, Staphylococcus saprophyticus.*
Gram-negative aerobes: *Enterobacter cloacae, Escherichia coli, Klebsiella pneumoniae, Neisseria gonorrhoeae, Proteus mirabilis, Pseudomonas aeruginosa.*
The following *in vitro* data are available but their clinical significance is unknown.
In addition, enoxacin exhibits *in vitro* minimum inhibitory concentrations (MICs) of 2.0 mcg/mL or less against most strains of the following organisms; however, the safety and effectiveness of enoxacin in treating clinical infections due to these organisms have not been established in adequate and well-controlled trials.
Gram-negative aerobes: *Aeromonas hydrophila, Citrobacter diversus, Citrobacter freundii, Citrobacter koseri, Enterobacter aerogenes, Haemophilus ducreyi, Klebsiella oxytoca, Klebsiella ozaenae, Morganella morganii, Proteus vulgaris, Providencia stuartii, Providencia alcalifaciens, Serratia marcescens, Serratia proteomaculans* (formerly *S. liquefaciens*).
Many strains of *Streptococcus* species and anaerobes are usually resistant to enoxacin.
The activity of enoxacin against *Treponema pallidum* has not been evaluated; however, other quinolones are not active against *T. pallidum.* (See **WARNINGS.**)
Cross-resistance with other quinolones has been demonstrated.
The addition of human serum has no effect on the *in vitro* MIC values; however, enoxacin activity is decreased in acidic (pH 5.5) environments.

SUSCEPTIBILITY TESTING

Diffusion Techniques: Quantitative methods that require measurement of zone diameters give the most precise estimate of susceptibility of bacteria to antimicrobial agents. One such standardized procedure[1] that has been recommended for use with disks to test susceptibility of organisms to enoxacin uses the 10-mcg enoxacin disk.
Interpretation involves the correlation of the diameter obtained in the disk test with the minimum inhibitory concentration (MIC) for enoxacin.
Reports from the laboratory giving results of the standard single-disk susceptibility test with a 10-mcg enoxacin disk should be interpreted according to the following criteria:

Zone Diameter (mm)	Interpretation
≥18	(S) Susceptible
15–17	(MS) Moderately susceptible
≤14	(R) Resistant

A report of "susceptible" indicates that the pathogen is likely to be inhibited by generally achievable blood concentrations. A report of "moderately susceptible" suggests that the organism would be susceptible if high dosage is used or if the infection is confined to tissues or fluids in which high antimicrobial levels are attained. A report of "resistant" indicates that achievable drug concentrations are unlikely to be inhibitory, and other therapy should be selected.
Standardized susceptibility test procedures require the use of laboratory control organisms. The 10-mcg enoxacin disk should give the following zone diameters:

Organism	Zone Diameter (mm)
Escherichia coli (ATCC 25922)	28–36
Neisseria gonorrhoeae (ATCC 49226)	43–51
Pseudomonas aeruginosa (ATCC 27853)	22–28
Staphylococcus aureus (ATCC 25923)	22–28

Other quinolone antibacterial disks should not be substituted when performing susceptibility tests for enoxacin because of spectrum differences. The 10-mcg enoxacin disk should be used for all *in vitro* testing of isolates for enoxacin susceptibility using diffusion techniques.
Dilution Techniques: Use a standardized dilution method[2] (broth, agar, or microdilution) or equivalent with enoxacin powder. The MIC values obtained should be interpreted according to the following criteria:

MIC (mcg/mL)	Interpretation
≤2	(S) Susceptible
4	(MS) Moderately susceptible
≥8	(R) Resistant

As with standard diffusion methods, dilution procedures require the use of laboratory control organisms. Standard enoxacin powder should give the following MIC values:

Organism	MIC (mcg/mL)
Enterococcus faecalis (ATCC 29212)	2–16
Escherichia coli (ATCC 25922)	0.06–0.25
Neisseria gonorrhoeae (ATCC 49226)	0.015–0.06
Pseudomonas aeruginosa (ATCC 27853)	2–8
Staphylococcus aureus (ATCC 29213)	0.5–2

INDICATIONS AND USAGE

Penetrex™ (enoxacin) is indicated for the treatment of adults (≥18 years of age) with the following infections caused by susceptible strains of the designated microorganisms:
Sexually Transmitted Diseases (See **WARNINGS.**) **Uncomplicated urethral or cervical gonorrhea** due to *Neisseria gonorrhoeae.*
Urinary Tract: **Uncomplicated urinary tract infections** (cystitis) due to *Escherichia coli, Staphylococcus epidermidis**, or *Staphylococcus saprophyticus**.
Complicated urinary tract infections due to *Escherichia coli, Klebsiella pneumoniae, Proteus mirabilis, Pseudomonas aeruginosa, Staphylococcus epidermidis,* or *Enterobacter cloacae**.
The dosage regimens for complicated and uncomplicated urinary tract infections are different. (See **DOSAGE AND ADMINISTRATION.**)
Penicillinase production should have no effect on enoxacin activity.
Appropriate culture and susceptibility tests should be performed before treatment in order to isolate and identify organisms causing the infection and to determine their susceptibility to enoxacin. Therapy with enoxacin may be initiated while awaiting the results of these studies; therapy should be adjusted if necessary once the results are known. Culture and susceptibility testing performed periodically during therapy will provide information not only on the therapeutic

*Efficacy for this organism in this organ system at the recommended dose was studied in fewer than ten infections.

Continued on next page

Rhône-Poulenc Rorer—Cont.

effect of the antimicrobial agent but also on the possible emergence of bacterial resistance.

CONTRAINDICATIONS

Enoxacin is contraindicated for individuals with a history of hypersensitivity to enoxacin or to any of the other members of the quinolone class of antimicrobial agents.

WARNINGS

THE SAFETY AND EFFECTIVENESS OF ENOXACIN IN CHILDREN, ADOLESCENTS (UNDER THE AGE OF 18 YEARS), PREGNANT WOMEN, AND LACTATING WOMEN HAVE NOT BEEN ESTABLISHED. (See PRECAUTIONS—Pregnancy, Nursing Mothers, and Pediatric Use.) Enoxacin has been shown to cause arthropathy in immature rats and dogs when given in oral doses approximately 1.5 and 3.8 times, respectively, the highest human clinical dose based on a mg/m^2 basis after a four-week dosage regimen. Gross and histopathological examination of the weight-bearing joints of the dogs revealed lesions of the cartilage. Other quinolones also produce erosions of cartilage of weight-bearing joints and other signs of arthropathy in immature animals of various species. (See **ANIMAL PHARMACOLOGY.**)

Enoxacin has not been shown to be effective in the treatment of syphilis. Antimicrobial agents used in high doses for short periods of time to treat gonorrhea may mask or delay the symptoms of incubating syphilis. All patients with gonorrhea should have a serologic test for syphilis at the time of diagnosis. Patients treated with enoxacin should have a follow-up serologic test for syphilis after 3 months.

Serious and occasionally fatal hypersensitivity (anaphylactoid or anaphylactic) reactions, some following the first dose, have been reported in patients receiving quinolone therapy. Some reactions were accompanied by cardiovascular collapse, loss of consciousness, tingling, pharyngeal or facial edema, dyspnea, urticaria, or itching. Only a few patients had a history of previous hypersensitivity reactions. Serious hypersensitivity reactions have also been reported following treatment with enoxacin. If an allergic reaction to enoxacin occurs, discontinue the drug. Serious acute hypersensitivity reactions may require immediate treatment with epinephrine. Oxygen, intravenous fluids, antihistamines, corticosteroids, pressor amines, and airway management, including intubation, should be administered as indicated.

Convulsions and abnormal electroencephalograms have been reported in some patients receiving enoxacin. Convulsions, increased intracranial pressure, and/or toxic psychoses have also been reported in patients receiving other drugs in this class. Quinolones may also cause central nervous system (CNS) stimulation which may lead to tremors, restlessness, lightheadedness, confusion, or hallucinations. If these reactions occur in patients receiving enoxacin, the drug should be discontinued and appropriate measures instituted. Enoxacin, as well as other quinolones, should be used with caution in patients with known or suspected CNS disorders, such as severe cerebral arteriosclerosis, epilepsy, and other factors that predispose to seizures. (See **ADVERSE REACTIONS.**)

Pseudomembranous colitis has been reported with nearly all antibacterial agents, including enoxacin, and may range in severity from mild to life-threatening. Therefore, it is important to consider this diagnosis in patients who present with diarrhea subsequent to the administration of antibacterial agents.

Treatment with broad-spectrum antibacterial agents alters the normal flora of the colon and may permit overgrowth of clostridia. Studies indicate that a toxin produced by *Clostridium difficile* is a primary cause of "antibiotic-associated colitis."

After the diagnosis of pseudomembranous colitis has been established, therapeutic measures should be initiated.

Mild cases of pseudomembranous colitis usually respond to discontinuation of the drug alone. In moderate to severe cases, consideration should be given to management with fluids and electrolytes, protein supplementation, and treatment with an antibacterial drug clinically effective against *C. difficile* colitis.

Enoxacin is a potent inhibitor of the hepatic microsomal enzyme system, resulting in significant drug/drug interactions with theophylline and caffeine. (See **DRUG INTERACTIONS.**)

PRECAUTIONS

General: Alteration of the dosage regimen is necessary for patients with impaired renal function (creatinine clearance ≤30 mL/min/1.73 m^2). (See **DOSAGE AND ADMINISTRATION.**)

Moderate-to-severe phototoxicity reactions have been observed in patients exposed to direct sunlight while receiving enoxacin or some other drugs in this class. Excessive sunlight should be avoided. Therapy should be discontinued if phototoxicity occurs.

Ophthalmologic abnormalities, including cataracts and multiple punctate lenticular opacities, have been noted in patients undergoing treatment with enoxacin, as well as with some other quinolones, but have also been observed in patients receiving placebo in comparative trials. In clinical trials using multiple-dose therapy, ophthalmic tissue levels of enoxacin and other quinolones were significantly higher than respective plasma concentrations. The causal relationship, if any, of quinolones to lenticular abnormalities has not been established.

Decreased spermatogenesis and subsequent decreased fertility were noted in rats and dogs treated with doses of enoxacin that produced plasma levels in the animals three times higher than those produced in humans at the recommended therapeutic dosage. The potential for enoxacin to affect spermatogenesis in male patients is unknown.

Information for Patients: Patients should be advised:

- not to take magnesium-, aluminum-, or calcium-containing antacids, bismuth subsalicylate, products containing iron, or multivitamins containing zinc for 8 hours prior to enoxacin or for 2 hours after enoxacin administration (see **PRECAUTIONS—Drug Interactions**);
- to drink fluids liberally;
- to avoid consumption of caffeine-containing products (certain drugs, coffee, tea, chocolate, certain carbonated beverages) during enoxacin therapy (see **PRECAUTIONS—Drug Interactions**);
- that enoxacin may cause dizziness and lightheadedness and, therefore, patients should know how they react to enoxacin before they operate an automobile or machinery or engage in activities requiring mental alertness and coordination;
- that enoxacin may be associated with hypersensitivity reaction, even following the first dose, and to discontinue the drug at the first sign of a skin rash or other allergic reaction;
- to avoid undue exposure to excessive sunlight while receiving enoxacin and to discontinue therapy if phototoxicity occurs.

Drug Interactions

Bismuth: Bismuth subsalicylate, given concomitantly with enoxacin or 60 minutes following enoxacin administration, decreased enoxacin bioavailability by approximately 25%. Thus, concomitant administration of enoxacin and bismuth subsalicylate should be avoided.

Caffeine: Enoxacin is a potent inhibitor of the cytochrome P-450 isozymes responsible for the metabolism of methylxanthines. In a multiple-dose study, enoxacin caused a dose-related increase in the mean elimination half-life of caffeine, thereby decreasing the clearance of caffeine by up to 80% and leading to a five-fold increase in the AUC and the half-life of caffeine. Trough plasma enoxacin levels were also 20% higher when caffeine and enoxacin were administered concomitantly. Caffeine-related adverse effects have occurred in patients consuming caffeine while on therapy with enoxacin. (See **WARNINGS.**)

Cyclosporine: Elevated serum levels of cyclosporine have been reported with concomitant use of cyclosporine with other members of the quinolone class.

Digoxin: Enoxacin may raise serum digoxin levels in some individuals. If signs and symptoms suggestive of digoxin toxicity occur when enoxacin and digoxin are given concomitantly, physicians are advised to obtain serum digoxin levels and adjust digoxin doses appropriately.

Nonsteroidal anti-inflammatory agents: Seizures have been reported in patients taking enoxacin concomitantly with the nonsteroidal anti-inflammatory drug fenbufen. Animal studies also suggest an increased potential for seizures when these two drugs are given concomitantly. Fenbufen is not approved in the United States at this time.

Sucralfate and antacids: Quinolones form chelates with metal cations. Therefore, administration of quinolones with antacids containing calcium, magnesium, or aluminum; with sucralfate; with divalent or trivalent cations such as iron; or with multivitamins containing zinc may substantially interfere with drug absorption and result in insufficient plasma and tissue quinolone concentrations. Antacids containing aluminum hydroxide and magnesium hydroxide reduce the oral absorption of enoxacin by 75%. The oral bioavailability of enoxacin is reduced by 60% with coadministration of ranitidine. These agents should not be taken for 8 hours before or for 2 hours after enoxacin administration.

Theophylline: Enoxacin is a potent inhibitor of the cytochrome P-450 isozymes responsible for the metabolism of methylxanthines. Enoxacin interferes with the metabolism of theophylline resulting in a 42% to 74% dose-related decrease in theophylline clearance and a subsequent 260% to 350% increase in serum theophylline levels. Theophylline-related adverse effects have occurred in patients when theophylline and enoxacin were coadministered. (See **WARNINGS.**)

Warfarin: Quinolones, including enoxacin, decrease the clearance of R-warfarin, the less active isomer of racemic warfarin. Enoxacin does not affect the clearance of the active S-isomer, and changes in clotting time have not been observed when enoxacin and warfarin were coadministered. Nevertheless, the prothrombin time or other suitable coagulation test should be monitored when warfarin or its derivatives and enoxacin are given concomitantly.

Carcinogenesis, Mutagenesis, Impairment of Fertility: Long-term studies in animals to determine the carcinogenic potential of enoxacin have not been conducted.

Genetic toxicology tests included *in vitro* mutagenicity and cytogenetic assays and *in vivo* cytogenetic and micronucleus tests. Enoxacin did not induce point mutations in bacterial cells or mitotic gene conversion in yeast cells, with or without metabolic activation. Enoxacin did not induce sister chromatid exchanges or structural chromosomal aberrations in mammalian cells *in vitro*, with or without metabolic activation. In addition, enoxacin did not induce chromosomal aberrations in mice.

There was a minimal, dose-related, statistically significant increase in micronuclei at high doses in mice. The significance of these findings, in the absence of effects in other test systems, is not established.

Enoxacin produced no consistent effects on fertility and reproductive parameters in female rats given oral doses of enoxacin at levels up to 1000 mg/kg. Decreased spermatogenesis and subsequent impaired fertility was noted in male rats given oral doses of 1000 mg/kg. This dose is approximately 13-fold greater than the highest human clinical daily oral dose of 16 mg/kg, assuming a 50 kg person and based on a mg/m^2 basis.

Pregnancy: Teratogenic effects. Pregnancy Category C. Studies with enoxacin given orally to mice and rats have shown no evidence of teratogenic potential. The intravenous infusion of enoxacin into pregnant rabbits at doses of 10 to 50 mg/kg caused dose-related maternal toxicity (venous irritation, body weight loss, and reduced food intake) and, at 50 mg/kg, fetal toxicity (increased post-implantation loss and stunted fetuses).

At 50 mg/kg, the incidence of fetal malformations was significantly increased in the presence of overt maternal and fetal toxicity. There are no adequate and well-controlled studies in pregnant women. Enoxacin should be used during pregnancy only if the potential benefit justifies the potential risk to the fetus. (See **WARNINGS.**)

Nursing mothers: It is not known whether enoxacin is excreted in human milk. Enoxacin is excreted in the milk of lactating rats. Because drugs of this class are excreted in human milk and because of the potential for serious adverse reactions from enoxacin in nursing infants, a decision should be made whether to discontinue nursing or to discontinue the drug, taking into account the importance of the drug to the mother.

Pediatric use: Safety and effectiveness in children and adolescents below the age of 18 years have not been established. Enoxacin causes arthropathy in juvenile animals. (See **WARNINGS** and **ANIMAL PHARMACOLOGY.**)

Geriatric use: In multiple-dose clinical trials of enoxacin, elderly patients (≥65 years of age) experienced significantly more overall adverse events than patients under 65 years of age. However, the incidence of drug-related adverse reactions was comparable between age groups.

ADVERSE REACTIONS

Single-Dose Studies: During clinical trials, approximately 9% of patients treated with a single dose of 400 mg of enoxacin for uncomplicated urethral or endocervical gonorrhea reported adverse events.

The most frequently reported events in single-dose trials, without regard to drug relationship, were nausea and vomiting (2%). Events that occurred in less than 1% of patients are listed below.

CENTRAL NERVOUS SYSTEM: headache, dizziness, somnolence; GASTROINTESTINAL: abdominal pain; GYNECOLOGIC: vaginal moniliasis; SKIN/HYPERSENSITIVITY: rash; LABORATORY ABNORMALITIES: increased AST (SGOT), decreased hemoglobin, decreased hematocrit, eosinophilia, leukocytosis, leukopenia, thrombocytosis, increased urinary protein, increased alkaline phosphatase, increased ALT (SGPT), increased bilirubin, hyperkalemia.

Multiple-Dose Studies: The incidence of adverse events reported by patients in multiple-dose clinical trials, without regard to drug relationship, was 23%. The incidence of drug-related adverse reactions in multiple-dose clinical trials was 16%. Among patients receiving multiple-dose therapy, enoxacin was discontinued because of an adverse event in 3.8% of patients.

The following events were considered likely to be drug-related in patients receiving multiple doses of enoxacin in clinical trials: nausea and/or vomiting 6%, dizziness 2%, headache 1%, abdominal pain 1%, diarrhea 1%, dyspepsia 1%.

The most frequently reported events in all multiple-dose clinical trials, without regard to drug relationship, were as follows: nausea and/or vomiting 8%, dizziness and/or vertigo 3%, headache 2%, diarrhea 2%, abdominal pain 2%, insomnia 1%, dyspepsia 1%, rash 1%, nervousness and/or anxiety 1%, unusual taste 1%, pruritus 1%.

Additional events that occurred in less than 1% of patients but >0.1% of patients are listed below.

BODY AS A WHOLE: asthenia, fatigue, fever, malaise, back pain, chest pain, edema, chills; GASTROINTESTINAL:

Strength	Size	NDC 0075-	Color	Markings
200 mg	Bottles of 50	5100-50	light blue	5100
400 mg	Bottles of 50	5140-50	dark blue	5140

flatulence, constipation, dry mouth/throat, stomatitis, anorexia, gastritis, bloody stools; CENTRAL NERVOUS SYSTEM: somnolence, tremor, convulsions, paresthesia, confusion, agitation, depression, syncope, myoclonus, depersonalization, hypertonia; SKIN/HYPERSENSITIVITY: photosensitivity reaction, urticaria, hyperhidrosis, mycotic infection, erythema multiforme, toxic epidermal necrolysis, Stevens-Johnson syndrome; SPECIAL SENSES: tinnitus, conjunctivitis, visual disturbances including amblyopia; MUSCULOSKELETAL: myalgia, arthralgia; CARDIOVASCULAR: palpitations, tachycardia, vasodilation; RESPIRATORY: dyspnea, cough, epistaxis; HEMIC AND LYMPHATIC: purpura; UROGENITAL: vaginal moniliasis, vaginitis, urinary incontinence, renal failure.

The following adverse events occurred in less than 0.1% of patients in multiple-dose clinical trials but were considered significant: pseudomembranous colitis, hyperkinesia, amnesia, ataxia, hypotonia, psychosis, emotional lability, hallucination, schizophrenic reaction.

LABORATORY CHANGES: The following laboratory abnormalities appeared in ≥ 1.0% of patients receiving multiple doses of enoxacin: elevated AST (SGOT), elevated ALT (SGPT). It is not known whether these abnormalities were caused by the drug or the underlying conditions.

Worldwide Post-Marketing Experience: The most frequent spontaneously-reported adverse events in the worldwide post-marketing experience with multiple- and single-dose enoxacin use have been rashes, seizures/convulsions, and photosensitivity reactions; however, there is no evidence that the incidences of these events were larger than those observed in the clinical trials population.

Quinolone-class adverse reactions: Although not reported in completed clinical studies with enoxacin, a variety of adverse events have been reported with other quinolones.

Clinical adverse events include: erythema nodosum, hepatic necrosis, possible exacerbation of myasthenia gravis, nystagmus, intestinal perforation, hyperpigmentation, interstitial nephritis, polyuria, urinary retention, renal calculi, cardiopulmonary arrest, cerebral thrombosis, and laryngeal or pulmonary edema.

Laboratory adverse events include: agranulocytosis, elevation of serum triglycerides and/or serum cholesterol, prolongation of the prothrombin time, candiduria, and crystalluria.

OVERDOSAGE: In the event of acute overdosage, the stomach should be emptied by inducing vomiting or by gastric lavage and the patient carefully observed and given supportive treatment. Enoxacin is poorly removed (<5% over 4 hours) by hemodialysis.

DOSAGE AND ADMINISTRATION

Penetrex™ (enoxacin) should be taken at least one hour before or at least two hours after a meal. See **INDICATIONS AND USAGE** for information on appropriate pathogens and patient populations.

Sexually Transmitted Diseases

Uncomplicated urethral or cervical gonorrhea: 400 mg single dose

Urinary Tract Infections

Uncomplicated urinary tract infections: 200 mg q12h for 7 days

Complicated urinary tract infections: 400 mg q12h for 14 days

Dosage Adjustment for Renal Impairment: Dosage should be adjusted in patients with a creatinine clearance value of 30 mL/min/1.73 m^2 or less. After a normal initial dose, the dosing interval should be adjusted as follows:

Creatinine Clearance	Dosage Adjustment	Dosage Interval
> 30 mL/min/1.73 m^2	None	12 hours
≤ 30 mL/min/1.73 m^2	½ recommended dose	12 hours

When only the serum creatinine is known, the following formula may be used to estimate creatinine clearance.

Men:

$$\text{creatinine clearance (mL/min)} = \frac{\text{Weight (kg)} \times (140 - \text{age})}{72 \times \text{serum creatinine (mg/dL)}}$$

Women: 0.85 × the value calculated for men.

The serum creatinine should represent a steady state of renal function.

Dosage adjustment is not necessary in elderly patients with normal renal function, but dose should be adjusted according to the previous guidelines in elderly patients with compromised renal function.

HOW SUPPLIED

[See table above.]

Store at controlled room temperature, 15°C to 30°C (59°F to 86°F).

ANIMAL PHARMACOLOGY

Enoxacin and other members of the quinolone class have been shown to cause arthropathy in immature animals of most species tested. (See **WARNINGS.**)

REFERENCES

1. National Committee for Clinical Laboratory Standards, Performance Standards for Antimicrobial Disk Susceptibility Tests—Fourth Edition. Approved Standard NCCLS Document M2-A4, Vol. 10, No. 7, NCCLS, Villanova, PA, 1990.
2. National Committee for Clinical Laboratory Standards, Methods for Dilution Antimicrobial Susceptibility Tests for Bacteria that Grow Aerobically—Second Edition. Approved Standard NCCLS Document M7-A2, Vol. 10, No. 8, NCCLS, Villanova, PA, 1990.

CAUTION: Federal (U.S.A.) law prohibits dispensing without a prescription.

Rev. 4/92 IN-0898

Distributed by

RHÔNE-POULENC RORER PHARMACEUTICALS INC.

Collegeville, PA, U.S.A. 19426-0107

Shown in Product Identification Section, page 425

SLO-BID™ ℞

[slō 'bid ")

(Theophylline, Extended-release Capsules, USP)

50 mg, 75 mg, 100 mg, 125 mg, 200 mg, and 300 mg Gyrocaps®

PRODUCT OVERVIEW

KEY FACTS

Slo-bid™ Gyrocaps® contain theophylline, anhydrous in the form of long-acting beads within a dye-free hard gelatin capsule for oral administration (intact or sprinkled). Theophylline is a bronchodilator and is a member of the xanthine class of chemical compounds.

MAJOR USES

Slo-bid™ is indicated for relief and/or prevention of symptoms of asthma and reversible bronchospasm associated with chronic bronchitis and emphysema.

SAFETY INFORMATION

Slo-bid™ is contraindicated in persons who have shown hypersensitivity to any of the components of this product. It is not intended for patients experiencing an acute episode of bronchospasm. Such patients require *rapid* relief of symptoms and should be treated with an immediate-release or intravenous theophylline preparation. Status asthmaticus should be considered a medical emergency. Adverse reactions are usually due to overdose.

PRESCRIBING INFORMATION

SLO-BID™ ℞

[slō 'bid ")

(Theophylline, Extended-release Capsules, USP)

50 mg, 75 mg, 100 mg, 125 mg, 200 mg, and 300 mg Gyrocaps®

DESCRIPTION

Slo-bid™ Gyrocaps® contain 50 mg, 75 mg, 100 mg, 125 mg, 200 mg, or 300 mg theophylline, anhydrous in the form of long-acting beads within a dye-free hard gelatin capsule and are intended for oral administration. Theophylline is a bronchodilator structurally classified as a xanthine derivative.

Slo-bid Gyrocaps can be administered with a 12-hour dosing interval for a majority of patients and a 24-hour dosing interval for selected patients (see DOSAGE AND ADMINISTRATION section for description of appropriate patient population).

Theophylline is *1H*-Purine-2, 6-dione,3, 7-dihydro-1,3-dimethyl represented by the following structural formula:

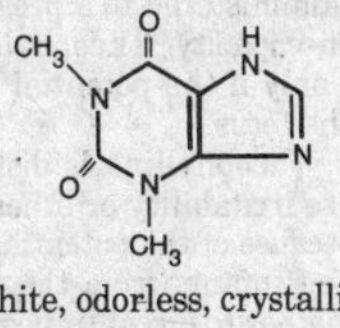

Theophylline is a white, odorless, crystalline powder having a bitter taste.

CLINICAL PHARMACOLOGY

Theophylline directly relaxes the smooth muscle of the bronchial airways and pulmonary blood vessels, thus acting as a bronchodilator and smooth muscle relaxant. It has also been demonstrated that aminophylline has a potent effect on diaphragmatic contractility in normal persons and may then be capable of reducing fatigability and thereby improve contractility in patients with chronic obstructive airways disease. The exact mode of action remains unsettled. Although theophylline does cause inhibition of phosphodiesterase with a resultant increase in intracellular cyclic AMP, other agents similarly inhibit the enzyme producing a rise of cyclic AMP but are unassociated with any demonstrable bronchodilation. Other mechanisms proposed include an effect on translocation of intracellular calcium; prostaglandin antagonism; stimulation of catecholamines endogenously; inhibition of cyclic guanosine monophosphate metabolism and adenosine receptor antagonism. None of these mechanisms has been proved, however.

In vitro, theophylline has been shown to act synergistically with beta agonists, and there are now available data that do demonstrate an additive effect *in vivo* with combined use.

Pharmacokinetics:

The half-life of theophylline is influenced by a number of known variables. It may be prolonged in chronic alcoholics, particularly those with liver disease (cirrhosis or alcoholic liver disease), in patients with congestive heart failure and in those patients taking certain other drugs (See PRECAUTIONS, Drug Interactions).

Newborns and neonates have extremely slow clearance rates compared to older infants and children, i.e., those over one year. Older children have rapid clearance rates while most nonsmoking adults have clearance rates between these two extremes. In premature neonates the decreased clearance is related to oxidative pathways that have yet to be established.

Theophylline Elimination Characteristics
Half-life (in hours)

	Range	Mean
Children	1–9	3.7
Adults	3–15	7.7

In cigarette smokers (1–2 packs/day) the mean half-life is 4–5 hours, much shorter than in nonsmokers. The increase in clearance associated with smoking is presumably due to stimulation of the hepatic metabolic pathway by components of cigarette smoke. The duration of this effect after cessation of smoking is unknown but may require 6 months to 2 years before the rate approaches that of the nonsmoker.

In a single-dose bioavailability study in 18 normal subjects, 300 mg sustained-release Slo-bid Gyrocaps produced mean peak serum concentrations of 3.5 ± 0.7 μg/mL at a mean time of 7.8 ± 1.8 hours after dosing. Subjects fasted overnight before dosing and four hours after the dose. When compared to a syrup dosage form, relative bioavailability of Slo-bid Gyrocaps was about 91%. At steady state in a multiple-dose bioavailability study in 18 normal subjects with q12h dosing (600–1000 mg/day), the mean peak-trough variation was 3.5 ± 0.9 μg/mL. The mean C_{max} and C_{min} were 12.9 ± 3.0 and 9.4 ± 2.5 μg/mL, respectively. The mean percent fluctuation [$(C_{max}$-$C_{min}/C_{min}) \times 100$] was 40 ± 15%. Subjects fasted 12 hours before the dose and 4 hours after the dose was administered on the days that the blood samples were drawn. A multiple-dose bioequivalence study with 15 asthmatic children, ages 9–16, comparing Slo-bid Gyrocaps administered as intact capsules and as the beaded contents sprinkled on applesauce with b.i.d. dosing (150–600 mg/dose) indicated no significant differences in maximum and minimum theophylline concentrations, time to achieve peak concentration, and peak-trough differences. The bioavailability as measured by comparing area under the curves ($AUC_{0-12\ hours}$ granules/$AUC_{0-12\ hours}$ capsules) was 0.990 ± 0.214.

Taking Slo-bid immediately after a high-fat content meal may result in a decrease in the rate of absorption (lower C_{max} and later T_{max}) but with no significant difference in the extent of absorption (see PRECAUTIONS, Drug-Food Interactions). In a single-dose bioavailability study, 24 normal adult nonsmoking subjects were given 900 mg extended-release Slo-bid Gyrocaps with food and under fasting conditions. Results (mean ± S.D.) showed:

	Food	Fasting
$AUC0 \rightarrow \infty$ (μg-hr/mL)	260.5±60.6	280.5±68.7
C_{max} (μg/mL)	10.57±2.00	12.49±2.15
T_{max} (hr)	9.8±2.1	7.0±1.4

Steady-state pharmacokinetics were determined in 26 normal male volunteers (with theophylline clearance rates less than or equal to 5.0 L/hr and/or a theophylline elimination half-life of 6 to 12 hours) who received 900 mg of theophylline per day for five days. Twenty-six were dosed with three 300 mg extended-release Slo-bid Gyrocaps administered 24 hours apart immediately after the consumption of breakfast, and seventeen were dosed with one 300 mg, one 100 mg, and one 50 mg Slo-bid Gyrocap administered 12 hours apart (immediately after consuming breakfast and two hours after the consumption of dinner).

Continued on next page

Rhône-Poulenc Rorer—Cont.

The pharmacokinetic parameters obtained for the extended-release Slo-bid Gyrocaps given as 900 mg once daily in the morning after a high-fat content breakfast were essentially the same as those parameters obtained after Slo-bid Gyrocaps administered in the widely-acceptable, approved manner of twice-daily. In particular, the area-under-the-curve values were 238 ± 27 (S.D.) and 251 ± 29 μg-hr/mL for the products administered q24h and q12h, respectively. Mean C_{max} values of 13.2 ± 2.0 μg/mL and 12.2 ± 2.2 μg/mL and C_{min} values of 5.9 ± 1.0 μg/mL and 8.6 ± 1.1 μg/mL were obtained after q24h and q12h administration, respectively. The mean percent fluctuation $[(C_{max}-C_{min})/C_{min} \times 100)]$ was 140 ± 66% (S.D.) and 40 ± 15% (S.D.) when Slo-bid was given once- or twice-daily, respectively.

INDICATIONS AND USAGE

For relief and/or prevention of symptoms from asthma and reversible bronchospasm associated with chronic bronchitis and emphysema.

CONTRAINDICATIONS

Slo-bid is contraindicated in individuals who have shown hypersensitivity to any of the components of this product or to xanthine derivatives. It is also contraindicated in patients with active peptic ulcer disease and in individuals with underlying seizure disorders (unless receiving appropriate anticonvulsant medication).

WARNINGS

Serum levels above 20 μg/mL are rarely found after appropriate administration of the recommended doses. However, in individuals in whom theophylline plasma clearance is reduced *for any reason,* even conventional doses may result in increased serum levels and potential toxicity. Reduced theophylline clearance has been documented in the following readily identifiable groups: 1) patients with impaired renal or liver function; 2) patients over 55 years of age, particularly males and those with chronic lung disease; 3) those with cardiac failure from any cause; 4) patients with sustained high fever; 5) neonates and infants under 1 year of age; and 6) those patients taking certain drugs (see PRECAUTIONS, Drug Interactions). Frequently, such patients have markedly prolonged theophylline serum levels following discontinuation of the drug.

Decreased clearance of theophylline may be associated with either influenza immunization or active influenza, and with other viral infections.

It is important to consider reduction of dosage and measurement of serum theophylline levels in the above individuals.

Serious side effects such as ventricular arrhythmias, convulsions or even death may appear as the first sign of toxicity without any previous warning. Less serious signs of theophylline toxicity (i.e., nausea and restlessness) may occur frequently when initiating therapy but are usually transient; when such signs are persistent during maintenance therapy, they are often associated with serum concentrations above 20 μg/mL. Stated differently, *serious toxicity is not reliably preceded by less severe side effects.* A serum concentration measurement is the only reliable method of identifying a potential for life-threatening toxicity.

Many patients who require theophylline exhibit tachycardia due to their underlying disease process, so the cause/effect relationship to elevated serum theophylline concentrations may not be appreciated.

Theophylline products may cause or worsen arrhythmias and any significant change in rate and/or rhythm warrants monitoring and further investigation.

Studies in laboratory animals (minipigs, rodents and dogs) recorded the occurrence of cardiac arrhythmias and sudden death (with histologic evidence of myocardial necrosis) when beta agonists and methylxanthines were administered concurrently. The significance of these findings when applied to humans is currently unknown.

PRECAUTIONS

General: On the average, theophylline half-life is shorter in cigarette and marijuana smokers than in nonsmokers, but smokers can have half-lives as long as nonsmokers. Theophylline should not be administered concurrently with other xanthine preparations. Use with caution in patients with hypoxemia, hypertension or with a history of peptic ulcer. Theophylline may occasionally act as a local irritant to the GI tract, although GI symptoms are more commonly centrally mediated and associated with serum drug concentrations over 20 μg/mL.

Xanthines can potentiate hypokalemia resulting from $beta_2$ agonist therapy, steroids, diuretics, other xanthines and hypoxia. Particular caution is advised in severe asthma. It is recommended that serum potassium levels be monitored in such situations.

Information for Patients:

The physician should reinforce the importance of taking only the prescribed dose at the prescribed time intervals. The patient should alert the physician if symptoms occur repeatedly, especially near the end of a dosing interval. When prescribing administration by the sprinkle method, details of the proper technique should be explained to the patient.

Laboratory Test: Serum levels should be monitored periodically to determine the theophylline levels associated with observed clinical response and to identify the potential for toxicity. For such measurements, the serum sample should be obtained at the time of peak concentration, approximately 5–9 hours after the morning dose. It is important that the patient has not missed or taken additional doses during the previous 48 hours and that dosing intervals have been reasonably equally spaced.

DOSE ADJUSTMENT BASED ON SERUM THEOPHYLLINE MEASUREMENTS WHEN THESE INSTRUCTIONS HAVE NOT BEEN FOLLOWED MAY RESULT IN RECOMMENDATIONS THAT PRESENT RISK OF TOXICITY TO THE PATIENT.

Drug Interactions:

Drug-Drug: Toxic synergism with ephedrine has been documented and may occur with some other sympathomimetic bronchodilators. In addition, the following drug interactions have been demonstrated:

Drug	Effect
Theophylline with:	
Allopurinol (high dose)	Increased serum theophylline levels
Cimetidine	Increased serum theophylline levels
Ciprofloxacin	Increased serum theophylline levels
Erythromycin, Troleandomycin	Increased serum theophylline levels
Lithium carbonate	Increased renal excretion of lithium
Oral contraceptives	Increased serum theophylline levels
Propranolol	Increased serum theophylline levels
Phenytoin	Decreased theophylline and phenytoin serum levels
Rifampin	Decreased serum theophylline levels

Drug-Food: Taking Slo-bid immediately after a high-fat content meal such as 8 ounces whole milk, 2 fried eggs, 2 strips bacon, one bran muffin with butter, 2 ounces hash brown potatoes (about 789 calories, including approximately 49 g of fat) may result in a decrease in the rate of absorption, but with no significant difference in the extent of absorption (see CLINICAL PHARMACOLOGY, Pharmacokinetics). The influence of the type and amount of other foods, as well as the time interval between drug and food, has not been studied.

Drug/Laboratory Test Interactions: Currently available analytic methods, including high-pressure liquid chromatography and immunoassay techniques, for measuring serum theophylline levels are specific. Metabolites and other drugs generally do not affect the results. Other new analytic methods are also now in use. The physician should be aware of the laboratory method used and whether other drugs will interfere with the assay for theophylline.

Carcinogenesis, Mutagenesis, Impairment of Fertility: Long-term carcinogenicity studies have not been performed with theophylline.

Chromosome-breaking activity was detected in human cell cultures at concentrations of theophylline up to 50 times the therapeutic serum concentrations in humans. Theophylline was not mutagenic in the dominant lethal assay in male mice given theophylline intraperitoneally in doses up to 30 times the maximum daily human oral dose.

Studies to determine the effect on fertility have not been performed with theophylline.

Pregnancy: Pregnancy Category C—Reproduction studies performed in mice and rats at oral doses from 7 to 17 times the human dose (maximum human dose for adults assumed to be 13 mg/kg/day) have indicated that theophylline may cause malformations, but these effects only occurred at or near doses that were toxic to the maternal animals.

There are no adequate and well-controlled studies in pregnant women. It is not known whether theophylline can cause fetal harm when administered to a pregnant woman or can affect reproduction capacity. Theophylline should be used during pregnancy only if the potential benefit justifies the potential risk to the fetus.

Nursing Mothers: Theophylline is distributed into breast milk and may cause irritability or other signs of toxicity in nursing infants. Because of the potential for serious adverse reactions in nursing infants from theophylline, a decision should be made whether to discontinue nursing or to discontinue the drug, taking into account the importance of the drug to the mother.

Pediatric Use: Safety and effectiveness of Slo-bid Gyrocaps administered:

1. Every 24 hours in children under 12 years of age, have not been established.
2. Every 12 hours in children under 6 years of age, have not been established.

ADVERSE REACTIONS

The following adverse reactions have been observed, but there has not been enough systematic collection of data to support an estimate of their frequency. The most consistent adverse reactions are usually due to overdosage.

Gastrointestinal: nausea, vomiting, epigastric pain, hematemesis, diarrhea.

Central Nervous System: headaches, irritability, restlessness, insomnia, reflex hyperexcitability, muscle twitching, clonic and tonic generalized convulsions.

Cardiovascular: palpitation, tachycardia, extrasystoles, flushing, hypotension, circulatory failure, ventricular arrhythmias.

Respiratory: tachypnea.

Renal: potentiation of diuresis.

Other: alopecia, hyperglycemia, inappropriate ADH syndrome, rash.

OVERDOSAGE:

Management: It is suggested that the management principles (consistent with the clinical status of the patient when first seen) outlined below be instituted and that simultaneous contact with a Regional Poison Control Center be established. In this way both updated information and individualization regarding therapy may be provided.

1. When potential oral overdose is established and seizure has not occurred:
   a) If patient is alert and seen soon after ingestion, induction of emesis may be of value. Gastric lavage has been demonstrated to be of no value in influencing outcome in patients who present more than 1 hour after ingestion.
   b) Administer a cathartic. Sorbitol solution is reported to be of value.
   c) Administer repeated doses of activated charcoal and monitor theophylline serum levels.
   d) Prophylactic administration of phenobarbital has been shown to increase the seizure threshold in laboratory animals, and administration of this drug may be of value.
   e) Monitor serum potassium.
2. If patient presents with a seizure:
   a) Establish an airway.
   b) Administer oxygen.
   c) Treat the seizure with intravenous diazepam 0.1 to 0.3 mg/kg up to 10 mg. If seizures cannot be controlled, the use of general anesthesia should be considered.
   d) Monitor vital signs, maintain blood pressure and provide adequate hydration.
3. Postseizure Coma:
   a) Maintain airway and oxygenation.
   b) If a result of oral medication, follow above recommendations to prevent absorption of drug, but intubation and lavage will have to be performed instead of inducing emesis and the cathartic and charcoal will need to be introduced via a large-bore gastric lavage tube.
   c) Continue to provide full supportive care and adequate hydration until the drug is metabolized. In general, drug metabolism is sufficiently rapid so as not to warrant dialysis. If repeated oral activated charcoal is ineffective (as noted by stable or rising serum levels), charcoal hemoperfusion may be indicated.

DOSAGE AND ADMINISTRATION

Taking Slo-bid immediately after a high-fat-content meal may alter its rate of absorption (see CLINICAL PHARMACOLOGY and PRECAUTIONS, Drug-Food Interactions). However, the differences are usually small and Slo-bid may normally be administered without regard to meals.

Effective use of theophylline (i.e., the concentration of drug in the serum associated with optimal benefit and minimal risk of toxicity) is considered to occur when the theophylline concentration is maintained from 10 to 20 μg/mL. The early studies from which these levels were derived were carried out in patients immediately or shortly after recovery from acute exacerbations of their disease (some hospitalized with status asthmaticus).

Although the 20 μg/mL level remains appropriate as a critical value (above which toxicity is more likely to occur) for safety purposes, additional data are now available that indicate that the serum theophylline concentrations required to produce maximum physiologic benefit may, in fact, fluctuate with the degree of bronchospasm present and are variable. Therefore, the physician should individualize the range appropriate to the patient's requirements, based on both symptomatic response and improvement in pulmonary function. It should be stressed that serum theophylline concentrations maintained at the upper level of the 10 to 20 μg/mL range may be associated with potential toxicity when factors known to reduce theophylline clearance are operative. (See WARNINGS.)

		Dose per 8 hours	Dose per 12 hours
Age 6–under 9 years	24 mg/kg/day	8.0 mg/kg	12.0 mg/kg
Age 9–under 12 years	20 mg/kg/day	6.7 mg/kg	10.0 mg/kg
Age 12–under 16 years	18 mg/kg/day	6.0 mg/kg	9.0 mg/kg
Age over 16 years	13 mg/kg/day	4.3 mg/kg	6.5 mg/kg
	OR 900 mg		
	(WHICHEVER IS LESS)		

If it is not possible to obtain serum level determinations, restriction of the daily dose (in otherwise healthy adults) to not greater than 13 mg/kg/day, to a maximum of 900 mg, in divided doses will result in relatively few patients exceeding serum levels of 20 µg/mL and the resultant greater risk of toxicity.

Caution should be exercised for younger children who cannot complain of minor side effects. Older adults, those with cor pulmonale, congestive heart failure, and/or liver disease may have unusually low dosage requirements and thus may experience toxicity at the maximal dosage recommended below.

Theophylline does not distribute into fatty tissue. Dosage should be calculated on the basis of lean (ideal) body weight where mg/kg doses are presented.

Frequency of Dosing: When immediate-release products with rapid absorption are used, dosing to maintain serum levels generally requires administration every 6 hours. This is particularly true in children, but dosing intervals up to 8 hours may be satisfactory in adults since they eliminate the drug at a slower rate. Some children, and adults requiring higher than average doses (those having rapid rates of clearance, e.g., half-lives of under 6 hours) may benefit and be more effectively controlled during chronic therapy when given products with extended-release characteristics since these provide longer dosing intervals and/or less fluctuation in serum concentration between dosing. Those extended-release products which provide flexibility in dosage through formulations of varying strengths are also helpful in controlling serum levels. Dosage guidelines are approximations only and the wide range of theophylline clearance between individuals (particularly those with concomitant disease) make indiscriminate usage hazardous.

Dosage Guidelines:

I. Acute Symptoms

NOTE: Status asthmaticus should be considered a medical emergency and is defined as that degree of bronchospasm that is not rapidly responsive to usual doses of conventional bronchodilators. Optimal therapy for such patients frequently requires both *additional medication* parenterally administered, and *close monitoring*, preferably in an intensive care setting.

Slo-bid is not intended for patients experiencing an acute episode of bronchospasm (associated with asthma, chronic bronchitis, or emphysema). Such patients require *rapid* relief of symptoms and should be treated with an immediate-release or intravenous theophylline preparation (or other bronchodilators) and not with extended-release products.

II. Chronic Therapy

A. Initiating Therapy with an Immediate-Release Product

It is recommended that the appropriate dosage be established using an immediate-release preparation. A dosage form that allows small incremental doses is desirable for initiating therapy. A liquid preparation should be considered for children to permit easier and more accurate dosage adjustment. Slow clinical titration is generally preferred to help assure acceptance and safety of the medication and to allow the patient to develop tolerance to transient caffeine-like side effects. Then, if the total 24-hour dose can be given by use of the available strengths of this product, the patient can usually be switched to Slo-bid, giving one third of the daily dose at 8-hour intervals or one half the daily dose at 12-hour intervals. Patients who metabolize theophylline rapidly, such as the young, smokers, and some nonsmoking adults are the most likely candidates for dosing at 8-hour intervals. Such patients can generally be identified as having trough serum concentrations lower than desired or repeatedly exhibiting symptoms near the end of a dosing interval.

B. Initiating Therapy with Slo-bid Gyrocaps

Alternatively, therapy can be initiated with Slo-bid Gyrocaps since they are available in dosage strengths that permit titration and adjustments of dosage (in adults and older children). Children weighing less than 25 kg should have their daily dosage requirements established with Slo-Phyllin® 80 mg Syrup to permit small dosage increments.

Initial Dose: 16 mg/kg/24 hours or 400 mg/24 hours (whichever is less) of anhydrous theophylline in 2 or 3 divided doses at 8- or 12-hour intervals.

Increasing Dose: The above dosage may be increased in approximately 25-percent increments at 3-day intervals so long as the drug is tolerated. Following each adjustment, if the clinical response is satisfactory and serum levels can be measured, then such measurements should be obtained as directed under section IV (below). If serum levels cannot be obtained, then that dosage level should be maintained. Dosage increases may be made in this manner until the maximum dose indicated in section III (below) is reached.

It is important that no patient be maintained on any dosage that is not tolerated. When instructing patients to increase dosage according to the schedule above, they should be told not to take a subsequent dose if apparent side effects occur and to resume therapy at a lower dose once adverse effects have disappeared.

C. Sprinkling Contents on Food

Slo-bid Gyrocaps may be administered by carefully opening the capsule and sprinkling the beaded contents on a spoonful of soft food such as applesauce or pudding; the soft food should be swallowed immediately without chewing and followed with a glass of cool water or juice to ensure complete swallowing of the beads. It is recommended that the food used should not be hot and should be soft enough to be swallowed without chewing. Any bead/food mixture should be used immediately and not stored for future use. SUBDIVIDING THE CONTENTS OF A CAPSULE IS NOT RECOMMENDED.

D. Once-Daily Dosing

The slow absorption rate of this preparation may allow once-daily administration in adult non-smokers with appropriate total body clearance and other patients with low dosage requirements. Once-daily dosing should be considered only after the patient has been gradually and satisfactorily titrated to therapeutic levels with q12h dosing. Once-daily dosing should be based on twice the q12h dose and should be initiated at the end of the last q12h dosing interval. The trough concentration (C_{min}) obtained following conversion to once-daily dosing may be lower (especially in high clearance patients) and the peak concentration (C_{max}) may be higher (especially in low clearance patients) than that obtained with q12h dosing. If symptoms recur, or signs of toxicity appear during the once-daily dosing interval, dosing on the q12h basis should be reinstituted.

It is essential that serum theophylline concentrations be monitored before and after transfer to once-daily dosing. Food and posture, along with changes associated with circadian rhythm, may influence the rate of absorption and/or clearance rates of theophylline from extended-release dosage forms administered at night. The exact relationship of these and other factors to nighttime serum concentrations and the clinical significance of such findings require additional study. Therefore, it is not recommended that Slo-bid, when used as a once-a-day product, be administered at night.

III. Maximum Dose of Theophylline Where the Serum Concentration is Not Measured:

WARNING: DO NOT ATTEMPT TO MAINTAIN ANY DOSE THAT IS NOT TOLERATED.

Not to exceed the following: [See table above.]

IV. Measurement of Serum Theophylline Concentrations During Chronic Therapy: If the above maximum doses are to be maintained or exceeded, serum theophylline measurement is essential (See PRECAUTIONS, Laboratory Tests for guidance).

V. Final Adjustment of Dosage:

Dosage adjustment after serum theophylline measurement

If serum theophylline is:		Directions:
Within desired range		Maintain dosage if tolerated.
Too high	20 to 25 µg/mL	Decrease doses by about 10% and recheck serum level after 3 days.
	25 to 30 µg/mL	Skip next dose and decrease subsequent doses by about 25%. Recheck serum level after 3 days.
	Over 30 µg/mL	Skip next 2 doses and decrease subsequent doses by 50%. Recheck serum level after 3 days.
Too low		Increase dosage by 25% at 3-day intervals until either the desired serum concentration and/or clinical response is achieved. The total daily dose may need to be administered at more frequent intervals if symptoms occur repeatedly at the end of a dosing interval.

The serum concentration may be rechecked at appropriate intervals, but at least at the end of any adjustment period. When the patient's condition is otherwise clinically stable and none of the recognized factors which alter elimination are present, measurement of serum levels need be repeated only every 6 to 12 months.

STORAGE CONDITIONS

Store at room temperature. Protect from excessive heat, light and moisture.

CAUTION

Federal (U.S.A.) law prohibits dispensing without prescription. Keep this and all medications out of the reach of children.

HOW SUPPLIED

[See table at left.]

Military: 50 mg—100s (NSN 6505-01-172-2852), 50 mg—1000s (NSN 6505-01-178-3942), 100 mg—100s (NSN 6505-01-166-9018), 100 mg—1000s (NSN 6505-01-180-3221), 200 mg—100s (NSN 6505-01-166-8989), 200 mg—1000s (NSN 6505-01-173-1906), 300 mg—100s (NSN 6505-01-164-8736), 300 mg—1000s (NSN 6505-01-172-1054).

Slo-bid Gyrocaps are manufactured by:

RHÔNE-POULENC RORER PHARMACEUTICALS INC.
Collegeville, PA, U.S.A. 19426-0107
Rev. 7/91

Shown in Product Identification Section, page 425

Strength	Size	NDC 0075-	Color	Markings
50 mg	Bottles of 100	0057-00	Clear (Cap)*	
	Bottles of 1000	0057-99	and opaque	50 printed
	Unit Dose 100	0057-62	white (body)	in red
75 mg	Bottles of 100	1075-00	Opaque* white (cap)	75 printed
	Unit Dose 100	1075-62	and clear (body)	in red
100 mg	Bottles of 100	0100-00	Opaque	
	Bottles of 1000	0100-99	white	100 printed
	Unit Dose 100	0100-62	capsule	in red
125 mg	Bottles of 100	1125-00	Opaque white	125 printed
	Unit Dose 100	1125-62	capsule	in red
200 mg	Bottles of 100	0200-00	Opaque	
	Bottles of 1000	0200-99	white	200 printed
	Unit Dose 100	0200-62	capsule	in red
300 mg	Bottles of 100	0300-00	Opaque	
	Bottles of 1000	0300-99	white	300 printed
	Unit Dose 100	0300-62	capsule	in red

*These capsules are being converted to all-white opaque color.

Products are cross-indexed by
generic and chemical names in the
YELLOW SECTION.

Rhône-Poulenc Rorer Pharmaceuticals Inc.
Consumer Pharmaceutical Products
500 VIRGINIA DRIVE
FORT WASHINGTON, PA 19034

Regular Strength   OTC
ASCRIPTIN®
[ă"skrĭp'tin]
Analgesic
Aspirin buffered with Maalox®

ACTIVE INGREDIENTS
Each tablet contains Aspirin (325 mg), buffered with Maalox (Alumina-Magnesia) and Calcium Carbonate.

INACTIVE INGREDIENTS
Hydroxypropyl Methylcellulose, Magnesium Stearate, Microcrystalline Cellulose, Starch, Talc, Titanium Dioxide, and other ingredients.

DESCRIPTION
Ascriptin is an excellent analgesic, antipyretic, and anti-inflammatory agent for general use, particularly where there is concern over aspirin-induced gastric distress. Coated tablets make swallowing easy.

INDICATIONS
As an analgesic for the relief of pain in such conditions as headache, neuralgia, minor injuries, and dysmenorrhea. As an analgesic and antipyretic in colds and influenza. As an analgesic and anti-inflammatory agent in arthritis and other rheumatic diseases. As an inhibitor of platelet aggregation, see MI's and TIA's indications.

USUAL ADULT DOSE
Two or three tablets, four times daily. Do not exceed 12 tablets in a 24-hour period. For children under twelve, consult a doctor.
WARNINGS: Children and teenagers should not use this medicine for chicken pox or flu symptoms before a doctor is consulted about Reye syndrome, a rare but serious illness reported to be associated with aspirin. Keep this and all medicines out of children's reach. If pain persists more than 10 days, redness or swelling is present, fever persists more than 3 days, or symptoms worsen, consult a doctor immediately. If you are under medical care or have a history of stomach, kidney, or bleeding disorders or asthma, consult a doctor before using. Do not use if allergic to aspirin. As with any drug, if you are pregnant or nursing a baby, consult a doctor before using. **IT IS ESPECIALLY IMPORTANT NOT TO USE ASPIRIN DURING THE LAST 3 MONTHS OF PREGNANCY UNLESS SPECIFICALLY DIRECTED TO DO SO BY A DOCTOR BECAUSE IT MAY CAUSE PROBLEMS IN THE UNBORN CHILD OR COMPLICATIONS DURING DELIVERY.** If ringing in the ears or loss of hearing occurs, consult a doctor before taking any more of this product. In case of accidental overdose, contact a doctor immediately. *Drug interaction precaution:* Do not use if taking a prescription drug for anticoagulation (blood thinning), diabetes, gout or arthritis, or a tetracycline antibiotic unless directed by a doctor.

PROFESSIONAL LABELING
ASCRIPTIN FOR MYOCARDIAL INFARCTION
INDICATION
Aspirin is indicated to reduce the risk of death and/or nonfatal myocardial infarction in patients with a previous infarction or unstable angina pectoris.

DOSAGE AND ADMINISTRATION
Although most of the studies used dosages exceeding 300 mg, two trials used only 300 mg, and pharmacologic data indicate that this dose inhibits platelet function fully. Therefore, 300 mg or a conventional 325-mg aspirin dose is a reasonable, routine dose that would minimize gastrointestinal adverse reactions. This use of aspirin applies to both solid, oral dosage forms (buffered and plain aspirin), and buffered aspirin in solution. *Note:* Complete information and references available.

ASCRIPTIN FOR RECURRENT TIA's IN MEN
Clinical Trials:
The indication is supported by the results of a Canadian study (1) in which 585 patients with threatened stroke were followed in a randomized clincial trial for an average of 26 months to determine whether aspirin or sulfinpyrazone, singly or in combination was superior to placebo in preventing transient ischemic attacks, stroke, or death. The study showed that, although sulfinpyrazone had no statistically significant effect, aspirin reduced the risk of continuing transient ischemic attacks, stroke, or death by 19 percent and reduced the risk of stroke or death by 31 percent. Another aspirin study carried out in the United States with 178 patients, showed a statistically significant number of "favorable outcomes" including reduced transient ischemic attacks, stroke, and death (2).

INDICATIONS
For reducing the risk of recurrent transient ischemic attacks (TIA's) or stroke in men who have had transient ischemia of the brain due to fibrin platelet emboli. There is inadequate evidence that aspirin or buffered aspirin is effective in reducing TIA's in women at the recommended dosage. There is no evidence that aspirin or buffered aspirin is of benefit in the treatment of completed strokes in men or women.

PRECAUTIONS
(1) Patients presenting with signs and symptoms of TIA's should have a complete medical and neurologic evaluation. Consideration should be given to other disorders which resemble TIA's. **(2)** Attention should be given to risk factors; it is important to evaluate and treat, if appropriate, other diseases associated with TIA's and stroke such as hypertension and diabetes. **(3)** Concurrent administration of absorbable antacids at therapeutic doses may increase the clearance of salicylates in some individuals. The concurrent administration of nonabsorbable antacids may alter the rate of absorption of aspirin, thereby resulting in a decreased acetylsalicylic acid/salicylate ratio in plasma. The clinical significance on TIA's of these decreases in available aspirin is unknown.
Aspirin at dosages of 1,000 milligrams per day has been associated with small increases in blood pressure, blood urea nitrogen, and serum uric acid levels. It is recommended that patients placed on long-term aspirin treatment be seen at regular intervals to assess changes in these measurements.
Adverse Reactions:
At dosages of 1,000 milligrams or higher of aspirin per day, gastrointestinal side effects include stomach pain, heartburn, nausea and/or vomiting, as well as increased rates of gross gastrointestinal bleeding."

DOSAGE
Adults dosage for men is 1300 mg a day, in divided doses of 650 mg twice a day or 325 mg four times a day.
References
(1) The Canadian Cooperative Study Group. "A Randomized Trial of Aspirin and Sulfinpyrazone in Threatened Stroke," *New England Journal of Medicine,* 299:53–59, 1978.
(2) Fields, W.S., et al., "Controlled Trial of Aspirin in Cerebral Ischemia." *Stroke* 8:301–316, 1977."

HOW SUPPLIED
Bottles of 60 tablets (NDC 0067-0145-60), 100 Tablets (NDC 0067-0145-68), 160 (NDC 0067-0145-30) and 225 Tablets (NDC 0067-0145-77).
Bottles of 500 tablets (NDC 0067-0145-74) without child-resistant closures (for arthritic patients). Military Stock #NSN 6505-00-135-2783 V.A. Stock #6505-00-890-1979 (bottles of 500).

ASCRIPTIN® A/D for arthritis pain   OTC
Analgesic
Aspirin buffered with extra Maalox® for pain relief with extra stomach comfort

ACTIVE INGREDIENTS
Each caplet contains Aspirin (325 mg), buffered with Maalox (Alumina-Magnesia) and Calcium Carbonate.

INACTIVE INGEDIENETS
Hydroxypropyl Methylcellulose, Magnesium Stearate, Microcrystalline Cellulose, Starch, Talc, Titanium Dioxide, and other ingredients.

DESCRIPTION
Ascriptin A/D is a highly buffered analgesic, anti-inflammatory, and antipyretic agent for use in the treatment of rheumatoid arthritis, osteoarthritis, and other arthritic conditions. It is formulated with 50% more Maalox than Regular Strength Ascriptin to provide increased neutralization of gastric acid thus reducing the likelihood of GI disturbance when large antiarthritic doses of aspirin are used. Coated caplets make swallowing easy.

INDICATIONS
As an analgesic, anti-inflammatory, and antipyretic agent in rheumatoid arthritis, osteoarthritis, and other arthritic conditions.

USUAL ADULT DOSE
Two or three caplets, four times daily, or as directed by the physician for arthritis therapy. For children under twelve, at the discretion of the physician.
WARNINGS: Children and teenagers should not use this medicine for chicken pox or flu symptoms before a doctor is consulted about Reye syndrome, a rare but serious illness reported to be associated with aspirin. Keep this and all medicines out of children's reach. If pain persists more than 10 days, redness or swelling is present, fever persists more than 3 days, or symptoms worsen, consult a doctor immediately. If you are under medical care or have a history of stomach, kidney, or bleeding disorders or asthma, consult a doctor

before using. Do not use if allergic to aspirin. As with any drug, if you are pregnant or nursing a baby, consult a doctor before using. **IT IS ESPECIALLY IMPORTANT NOT TO USE ASPIRIN DURING THE LAST 3 MONTHS OF PREGNANCY UNLESS SPECIFICALLY DIRECTED TO DO SO BY A DOCTOR BECAUSE IT MAY CAUSE PROBLEMS IN THE UNBORN CHILD OR COMPLICATIONS DURING DELIVERY.** If ringing in the ears or loss of hearing occurs, consult a doctor before taking any more of this product. **In case of accidental overdose, contact a doctor immediately.** *Drug interaction precaution:* Do not use if taking a prescription drug for anticoagulation (blood thinning), diabetes, gout or arthritis, or if taking a tetracycline antibiotic, unless directed by a doctor.

HOW SUPPLIED
Available in bottles of 60 Caplets (NDC 0067-0147-60), 100 caplets (NDC 0067-0147-68), and 225 caplets (NDC 0067-0147-77) with child-resistant caps and in special bottles of 500 caplets (without child-resistant closures) for arthritic patients (NDC 0067-0147-74).

MAALOX® Suspension and Tablets   OTC

(See PDR For Nonprescription Drugs.)

MAALOX® HRF   OTC
Heartburn Relief Formula™
Suspension
Rhone-Poulenc Rorer

DESCRIPTION
Maalox HRF provides symptomatic relief of heartburn, acid indigestion and/or sour stomach. Each 10 ml (2 teaspoonfuls) contains aluminum hydroxide-magnesium carbonate co-dried gel 280 mg and magnesium carbonate USP 350 mg. It is formulated in a pleasant, cool mint flavor to help provide a cooling and soothing sensation as it goes down the esophagus.

INACTIVE INGREDIENTS
Calcium carbonate, calcium saccharin, FD&C Blue No. 1, Yellow No. 5 (tartrazine) as a color additive, flavors, magnesium alginate, methyl and propyl parabens, potassium bicarbonate, purified water, sorbitol and other ingredients.

DIRECTIONS FOR USE
Maalox HRF—two to four teaspoonfuls after meals and at bedtime, or as directed by a physician.

PATIENT WARNINGS
Do not take more than 16 teaspoonfuls in a 24-hour period or use the maximum dosage for more than 2 weeks or use if you have kidney disease except under the advice and supervision of a physician. Keep this and all drugs out of the reach of children.

DRUG INTERACTION PRECAUTION
Do not use if you are taking a prescription antibiotic drug containing any form of tetracycline.

PROFESSIONAL LABELING: WARNINGS
Prolonged use of aluminum-containing antacids in patients with renal failure may result in or worsen dialysis osteomalacia. Elevated tissue aluminum levels contribute to the development of the dialysis encephalopathy and osteomalacia syndromes. Small amounts of aluminum are absorbed from the gastrointestinal tract and renal excretion of aluminum is impaired in renal failure. Aluminum is not well removed by dialysis because it is bound to albumin and transferrin, which do not cross dialysis membranes. As a result, aluminum is deposited in bone, and dialysis osteomalacia may develop when large amounts of aluminum are ingested orally by patients with impaired renal function.
Aluminum forms insoluble complexes with phosphate in the gastrointestinal tract, thus decreasing phosphate absorption. Prolonged use of antacids containing aluminum by normophosphatemic patients may result in hypophosphatemia if phosphate intake is not adequate. In its more severe forms, hypophosphatemia can lead to anorexia, malaise, muscle weakness, and osteomalacia.

HOW SUPPLIED
Maalox HRF is available in 12 fl oz (NDC 0067-0350-71).

MAALOX® Plus   OTC
Alumina, Magnesia and Simethicone Tablets
Antacid/Anti-Gas
Rhône-Poulenc Rorer

Tablets
    Lemon Swiss Creme
    Cherry Creme
    ... the flavors preferred by the physician and patient.

- Physician-proven Maalox® formula for antacid effectiveness.
- Simethicone, at a recognized clinical dose, for antiflatulent action.

DESCRIPTION
Maalox® Plus, a balanced combination of magnesium and aluminum hydroxides plus simethicone, is a non-constipating antacid/anti-gas which comes in pleasant tasting flavors.

COMPOSITION
To provide symptomatic relief of hyperacidity plus alleviation of gas symptoms, each tablet contains:

Active Ingredients	Maalox® Plus Per Tablet
Magnesium Hydroxide	200 mg
Aluminum Hydroxide (equivalent to dried gel, USP)	200 mg
Simethicone	25 mg

INACTIVE INGREDIENTS
Maalox® Plus Tablets: Citric acid, confectioners' sugar, artificial colors, dextrose, flavors, glycerin, magnesium stearate, mannitol, saccharin sodium, sorbitol, starch, talc and may also contain hydrogenated vegetable oil.
To aid in establishing proper dosage schedules, the following information is provided:

	Minimum Recommended Dosage: Per Tablet
Acid neutralizing capacity	10.65 mEq
Sodium content*	<1 mg
Sugar content	0.57 g
Lactose content	None

*Dietetically insignificant.

INDICATIONS
As an antacid for symptomatic relief of hyperacidity associated with the diagnosis of peptic ulcer, gastritis, peptic esophagitis, gastric hyperacidity, heartburn, or hiatal hernia. As an antiflatulent to alleviate the symptoms of gas, including postoperative gas pain.

Professional Labeling

WARNINGS
Prolonged use of aluminum-containing antacids in patients with renal failure may result in or worsen dialysis osteomalacia. Elevated tissue aluminum levels contribute to the development of the dialysis encephalopathy and osteomalacia syndromes. Small amounts of aluminum are absorbed from the gastrointestinal tract and renal excretion of aluminum is impaired in renal failure. Aluminum is not well removed by dialysis because it is bound to albumin and transferrin, which do not cross dialysis membranes. As a result, aluminum is deposited in bone, and dialysis osteomalacia may develop when large amounts of aluminum are ingested orally by patients with impaired renal function.
Aluminum forms insoluble complexes with phosphate in the gastrointestinal tract, thus decreasing phosphate absorption. Prolonged use of aluminum-containing antacids by normophosphatemic patients may result in hypophosphatemia if phosphate intake is not adequate. In its more severe forms, hypophosphatemia can lead to anorexia, malaise, muscle weakness, and osteomalacia.

ADVANTAGES
Maalox® Plus Tablets are uniquely palatable—an important feature which encourages patients to follow your dosage directions. Maalox® Plus Tablets have the time-proven, nonconstipating, sodium-free* Maalox® formula—useful for those patients suffering from the problems associated with hyperacidity. Additionally, Maalox® Plus Tablets contain simethicone to alleviate discomfort associated with entrapped gas.

DIRECTIONS FOR USE
One to four tablets, well chewed, four times a day, taken twenty minutes to one hour after meals and at bedtime, or as directed by a physician.

PATIENT WARNINGS
Do not take more than 16 tablets in a 24-hour period or use the maximum dosage for more than 2 weeks or use if you have kidney disease except under the advice and supervision of a physician. Keep this and all drugs out of the reach of children.

DRUG INTERACTION PRECAUTION
Do not use with patients taking a prescription antibiotic containing any form of tetracycline. As with all aluminum-containing antacids, Maalox® Plus may prevent the proper absorption of the tetracycline.

HOW SUPPLIED
Maalox® Plus Lemon Swiss Creme Tablets are available in bottles of 50 tablets (NDC 0067-0339-50) and 100 tablets (NDC 0067-0339-67), convenience packs of 12 tablets (NDC 0067-0339-19), Roll Packs of 12 tablets (NDC 0067-0339-23). **Maalox Plus Cherry Creme Tablets** are available in bottles of 50 tablets (NDC 0067-0341-50) and 100 tablets (NDC 0067-0341-68), roll packs of 12 tablets (NDC 0067-0341-23) and 3 roll packs of 36 tablets (NDC 0067-0341-33).

EXTRA STRENGTH   OTC
MAALOX® Plus (Reformulated Maalox Plus)
Alumina, Magnesia and Simethicone Oral Suspension and Tablets, Antacid/Anti-Gas
Rhône-Poulenc Rorer

Liquids	Tablets
☐ Lemon Swiss Creme	Mint Creme
Cherry Creme	
Mint Creme	

... the flavors preferred by the physician and patient.
- Physician-proven Maalox® formula for antacid effectiveness.
- Simethicone, at a recognized clinical dose, for antiflatulent action.

DESCRIPTION
Extra Strength Maalox® Plus, a balanced combination of magnesium and aluminum hydroxides plus simethicone, is a non-constipating antacid/anti-gas product to provide symptomatic relief of hyperacidity plus alleviation of gas symptoms. Available in liquid form in Cherry Creme, Mint Creme or Lemon Swiss Creme flavors, and in tablet form in the Mint Creme flavor.

COMPOSITION
To provide symptomatic relief of hyperacidity plus alleviation of gas symptoms, each teaspoonful/tablet contains:

Active Ingredients	Extra Strength Maalox® Plus Per Tsp. (5 mL)	Extra Strength Maalox® Plus Per Tablet
Magnesium Hydroxide	450 mg	350 mg
Aluminum Hydroxide (equivalent to dried gel, USP)	500 mg	350 mg
Simethicone	40 mg	30 mg

INACTIVE INGREDIENTS
Extra Strength Maalox® Plus Suspension: Citric acid, flavors, methylparaben, propylparaben, purified water, saccharin sodium, sorbitol, and other ingredients.
Extra Strength Maalox® Plus Tablets: Citric acid, confectioners' sugar, D&C yellow No. 10, dextrose, FD&C Blue No. 1, flavors, glycerin, hydrogenated vegetable oil, magnesium stearate, mannitol, saccharin sodium, sorbitol, starch, talc.
To aid in establishing proper dosage schedules, the following information is provided: [See box above.]

INDICATIONS
As an antacid for symptomatic relief of hyperacidity associated with the diagnosis of peptic ulcer, gastritis, peptic esophagitis, gastric hyperacidity, heartburn, or hiatal hernia. As an antiflatulent to alleviate the symptoms of gas, including postoperative gas pain.

ADVANTAGES
Among antacids, Extra Strength Maalox® Plus Suspension and Extra Strength Maalox® Plus Tablets are uniquely palatable—an important feature which encourages patients to follow your dosage directions. Extra Strength Maalox® Plus Suspension and Extra Strength Maalox® Plus Tablets have the time-proven, nonconstipating, sodium-free* Maa-

	Minimum Recommended Dosage: Extra Strength Maalox Plus	
	Per 2 Tsp. (10 mL)	Per Tablet
Acid neutralizing capacity	58.1 mEq	18.6 mEq
Sodium content*	<2.5 mg	<1.7 mg
Sugar content	None	0.72 g
Lactose content	None	None

*Dietetically insignificant.

lox® formula—useful for those patients suffering from the problems associated with hyperacidity. Additionally, Extra Strength Maalox® Plus Suspension and Extra Strength Maalox® Plus Tablets contain simethicone to alleviate discomfort associated with entrapped gas.

PROFESSIONAL LABELING

WARNINGS
(i) Prolonged use of aluminum-containing antacids in patients with renal failure may result in or worsen dialysis osteomalacia. Elevated tissue aluminum levels contribute to the development of the dialysis encephalopathy and osteomalacia syndromes. Small amounts of aluminum are absorbed from the gastrointestinal tract and renal excretion of aluminum is impaired in renal failure. Aluminum is not well removed by dialysis because it is bound to albumin and transferrin, which do not cross dialysis membranes. As a result, aluminum is deposited in bone, and dialysis osteomalacia may develop when large amounts of aluminum are ingested orally by patients with impaired renal function.
(ii) Aluminum forms insoluble complexes with phosphate in the gastrointestinal tract, thus decreasing phosphate absorption. Prolonged use of aluminum-containing antacids by normophosphatemic patients may result in hypophosphatemia if phosphate intake is not adequate. In its more severe forms, hypophosphatemia can lead to anorexia, malaise, muscle weakness, and osteomalacia.

EXTRA STRENGTH MAALOX® PLUS SUSPENSION

DIRECTIONS FOR USE
Two to four teaspoonfuls, four times a day, taken twenty minutes to one hour after meals and at bedtime, or as directed by a physician. Stomach pain and discomfort should always be evaluated by a physician for proper diagnosis.

PATIENT WARNINGS
Do not take more than 12 teaspoonfuls in a 24-hour period or use the maximum dosage for more than 2 weeks or use if you have kidney disease except under the advice and supervision of a physician. Keep this and all drugs out of the reach of children.

EXTRA STRENGTH MAALOX® PLUS TABLETS

DIRECTIONS FOR USE
Chew one to three tablets twenty minutes to one hour after meals and at bedtime, or as directed by a physician.

PATIENT WARNINGS
Do not take more than 12 tablets in a 24-hour period or use the maximum dosage for more than two weeks or use if you have kidney disease except under the advice and supervision of a physician. Keep this and all drugs out of the reach of children.

DRUG INTERACTION PRECAUTION
Do not use with patients taking a prescription antibiotic containing any form of tetracycline. As with all aluminum-containing antacids, Extra Strength Maalox® Plus may prevent the proper absorption of the tetracycline.

HOW SUPPLIED
Extra Strength Maalox® Plus Suspension
Available in Lemon Swiss Creme in the following sizes: 5 fl. oz. (148 mL) (NDC 0067-0333-62), 12 fl. oz. (355 mL) (NDC 0067-0333-71), and 26 fl. oz. (769 mL) (NDC 0067-0333-44).
Cherry Creme is available in plastic bottles of 5 fl. oz. (148 mL) (NDC 0067-0336-62), 12 fl. oz. (355 mL) (NDC 0067-0336-71), and 26 fl. oz. (769 mL) (NDC 0067-0336-44).
Mint Creme is available in plastic bottles of 5 fl. oz. (148 mL) (NDC 0067-0338-62), 12 fl. oz. (355 mL) (NDC 0067-0338-71) and 26 fl. oz. (769 mL) (NDC 0067-0338-44).
Extra Strength Maalox® Plus Mint Creme Tablets are available in flip-top bottles of 38 tablets (NDC 0067-0345-38) and 75 tablets (NDC 0067-0345-75).

Continued on next page

Rhône-Poulenc Rorer Consumer—Cont.

MAALOX® TC Suspension OTC
Therapeutic Concentrate Antacid
Magnesium & Aluminum Hydroxides Oral Suspension

DESCRIPTION
Maalox® TC Suspension is a potent, concentrated, balanced formulation of 300 mg magnesium hydroxide and 600 mg aluminum hydroxide (equivalent to dried gel, USP) per teaspoonful (5 mL). This formulation produces a therapeutically concentrated antacid that exceeds standard antacids in acid neutralizing capacity. Maalox® TC Suspension is formulated to reduce the need to alter therapy due to treatment-induced changes in bowel habits. Palatability is enhanced by a pleasant-tasting peppermint flavor.

INACTIVE INGREDIENTS
Citric acid, flavor, guar gum, methylparaben, propylparaben, sorbitol solution, purified water.

Acid Neutralizing Capacity
Maalox® TC Suspension—27.2 mEq/5 mL
Sodium Content:
Maalox® TC Suspension—< 1 mg/5 mL *

* Dietetically insignificant.

INDICATIONS
Maalox® TC Suspension is indicated for the symptomatic relief of hyperacidity associated with the diagnosis of peptic ulcer and other gastrointestinal conditions where a high degree of acid neutralization is desired.

DIRECTIONS FOR USE
Maalox® TC Suspension—one or two teaspoonfuls four times a day, taken 20 minutes to 1 hour after meals and at bedtime, or as directed by a physician. Higher dosage regimens may be employed under the direct supervision of a physician in the treatment of active peptic ulcer disease.
Stomach pain and discomfort should be evaluated by a physician for the proper diagnosis.

PATIENT WARNING
Do not take more than 8 teaspoonfuls of the suspension in a 24-hour period, or use the maximum dosage of this product for more than two weeks except under the advice and supervision of a physician. Also, if you have kidney disease, do not use except under the advice and supervision of a physician. Keep this and all drugs out of the reach of children.

DRUG INTERACTION PRECAUTION
Do not use with patients taking a prescription antibiotic drug containing any form of tetracycline. As with all aluminum-containing antacids, Maalox® TC may prevent the proper absorption of the tetracycline.

PROFESSIONAL LABELING

INDICATIONS
Maalox® TC is indicated for the prevention of stress-induced upper gastrointestinal hemorrhage. As an antacid, for the symptomatic relief of hyperacidity associated with the diagnosis of peptic ulcer and other gastrointestinal conditions where a high degree of acid neutralization is desired.

DIRECTIONS FOR USE
PREVENTION OF STRESS-INDUCED UPPER GASTROINTESTINAL HEMORRHAGE: 1) Aspirate stomach via nasogastric tube* and record pH. 2) Instill 10 mL of Maalox® TC followed by 30 mL of water via nasogastric tube. Clamp tube. 3) Wait one hour. Aspirate stomach and record pH. 4a) If pH equals or exceeds 4.0, apply drainage or intermittent suction for one hour, then repeat the cycle. 4b) If pH is less than 4.0, instill double (20 mL) Maalox® TC followed by 30 mL of water. Clamp tube. 5) Wait one hour. If pH equals or exceeds 4.0, see number 7. If pH is still less than 4.0, instill double (40 mL) Maalox® TC followed by 30 mL of water. Clamp tube. 6) Wait one hour. If pH equals or exceeds 4.0, see number 7. If pH is still less than 4.0, instill double (80 mL)** Maalox® TC followed by 30 mL of water. 7) Drain for one hour and repeat cycle with the effective dosage of Maalox® TC. IN HYPERACID STATES FOR SYMPTOMATIC RELIEF: One or two teaspoonfuls as needed between meals and at bedtime or as directed by a physician. Higher dosage regimens may be employed under the direct supervision of a physician in the treatment of active peptic ulcer disease.

* If nasogastric tube is not in place, administer 20 mL of Maalox® TC orally q2h.
** In a recent clinical study,[1] 20 mL of Maalox® TC, q2h, was sufficient in more than 85 percent of the patients. No patient studied required more than 80 mL of Maalox® TC q2h.

WARNINGS
Prolonged use of aluminum-containing anatacids in patients with renal failure may result in or worsen dialysis osteomalacia. Elevated tissue aluminum levels contribute to the development of the dialysis encephalopathy and osteomalacia syndromes. Small amounts of aluminum are absorbed from the gastrointestinal tract and renal excretion of aluminum is impaired in renal failure. Aluminum is not well removed by dialysis because it is bound to albumin and tranferrin, which do not cross dialysis membranes. As a result, aluminum is depositied in bone, and dialysis osteomalacia may develop when large amounts of aluminum are ingested orally by patients with impaired renal function.
Aluminum forms insoluble complexes with phosphate in the gastrointestinal tract, thus decreasing phosphate absorption. Prolonged use of aluminum-containing antacids by normophosphatemic patients may result in hypophosphatemia if phosphate intake is not adequate. In its more severe forms, hypophosphatemia can lead to anorexia, malaise, muscle weakness, and osteomalacia.

ADVERSE EFFECTS
Occasional regurgitation and mild diarrhea have been reported with the dosage recommended for the prevention of stress-induced upper gastrointestinal hemorrhage.

REFERENCES
1. Zinner MJ, Zuidema GD, Smith PL, Mignosa M: The prevention of upper gastrointestinal tract bleeding in patients in an intensive care unit. *Surg Gynec & Obstet* 153:214–220, 1981. 2. Lucas CE, Sugawa C, Riddle J et al.: Natural history and surgical dilemma of "stress" gastric bleeding. *Arch Surg* 102:266–273, 1971. 3. Hastings PR, Skillman JJ, Bushnell LS, Silen W: Antacid titration in the prevention of acute gastrointestinal bleeding: a controlled, randomized trial in 100 critically ill patients. *New England J Med* 298:1042–1045, 1978. 4. Day SB, MacMillan BG, Altemeier WA: Curling's Ulcer, An Experiment of Nature. Springfield, IL, Charles C. Thomas Co., 1972, p 205. 5. Skillman JJ, Bushnell LS, Goldman H, Silen W: Respiratory failure, hypotension, sepsis, and jaundice. A clinical syndrome associated with lethal hemorrhage from acute stress ulceration of the stomach. *Am J Surg* 117:523–530, 1969. 6. Priebe HJ, Skillman JJ, Bushnell LS et al.: Antacid versus cimetidine in preventing acute gastrointestinal bleeding. *New England J Med* 302:426–430, 1980. 7. Silen W: The prevention and management of stress ulcers. *Hospital Practice* 15:93–97, 1980. 8. Herrmann V, Kaminski DL: Evaluation of intragastric pH in acutely ill patients. *Arch Surg* 114:511–514, 1979. 9. Martin LF, Staloch DK, Simonowitz DA et al.: Failure of cimetidine prophylaxis in the critically ill. *Arch Surg* 114:492–496, 1979. 10. Zinner MJ, Turtinen L, Gurll N, Reynolds DG: The effect of metiamide on gastric mucosal injury in rat restraint. *Clin Res* 23:484A, 1975. 11. Zinner M, Turtinen BA, Gurll NJ: The role of acid and ischemia in production of stress ulcers during canine hemorrhagic shock. *Surgery* 77:807–816, 1975. 12. Winans CS: Prevention and treatment of stress ulcer bleeding: Antacids or cimetidine? *Drug Therapy* (hospital) 12:37–45, 1981.

HOW SUPPLIED
Maalox® TC Suspension is available in a 12-fluid ounce (355 mL) plastic bottle (NDC 0067-0334-71).

PERDIEM® OTC
[*pĕr"dē'ŭm*]
Bulk-Forming Laxative

INDICATION
For relief of constipation.

ACTIONS
Perdiem®, with its 100% natural, gentle action provides comfortable relief from constipation. Perdiem® is a unique combination of bulk-forming fiber and natural stimulant. The vegetable mucilages of Perdiem® soften the stool and provide pain-free evacuation of the bowel with no chemical stimulants. Perdiem® is effective as an aid to elimination for the hemorrhoid or fissure patient prior to and following surgery.

COMPOSITION
Perdiem® contains as its active ingredients, 82% psyllium (Plantago Hydrocolloid) a natural grain and 18% senna (Cassia Pod Concentrate) a natural vegetable derivative. Each rounded teaspoonful (6.0 g) contains 3.25 g psyllium, 0.74 g senna, 1.8 mg of sodium, 35.5 mg of potassium, and 4 calories. Perdiem® is "Dye-Free" and contains no artificial sweeteners.

INACTIVE INGREDIENTS
Acacia, iron oxides, natural flavors, paraffin, sucrose, talc.

PATIENT WARNING
Should not be used in the presence of undiagnosed abdominal pain. Frequent or prolonged use without the direction of a physician is not recommended, as it may lead to laxative dependence. Do not use in patients with a history of psyllium allergy. Psyllium allergy is rare but can be severe. If an allergic reaction occurs, discontinue use and consult a physician immediately.
Bulk-forming agents have the potential to obstruct the esophagus, particularly in the presence of esophageal narrowing or when consumed with insufficient fluid. Patients should be made aware of the symptoms of esophageal obstruction, including chest pain/pressure, regurgitation, and difficulty swallowing. Patients experiencing these symptoms should seek immediate medical attention. Patients with esophageal narrowing or dysphagia should not use Perdiem®.
As with any drug, if you are pregnant or nursing a baby, seek the advice of a health professional before using this product. Keep this and all drugs out of the reach of children. In case of accidental overdose, seek professional assistance or contact a poison control center immediately.

DIRECTIONS FOR USE
Perdiem must be taken with at least 8 ounces of cool liquid.
Adults and children 12 years and older: In the evening and/or before breakfast, 1–2 rounded teaspoonfuls of Perdiem® granules (in single or partial teaspoon doses) should be placed in the mouth and swallowed with at least 8 fl oz of cool beverage after the dose. Additional liquid would be helpful. Perdiem® granules should not be chewed.
Children 7 to 11 years: One (1) rounded teaspoon one to two times daily with at least 8 ounches of cool liquid.
Perdiem® generally takes effect within 12 hours. Subsequent doses may be adjusted after adequate laxation is obtained.

NOTE
It is extremely important that Perdiem® be taken with at least 8 fl oz of cool liquid.
WARNING: TAKE THIS PRODUCT WITH AT LEAST 8 OUNCHES [A FULL GLASS] OF WATER OR OTHER FLUID. TAKING THIS PRODUCT WITHOUT ADEQUATE FLUID MAY CAUSE IT TO SWELL AND BLOCK YOUR THROAT OR ESOPHAGUS AND MAY CAUSE CHOKING. DO NOT TAKE THIS PRODUCT IF YOU HAVE EVER HAD DIFFICULTY IN SWALLOWING OR HAVE ANY THROAT PROBLEMS. IF YOU EXPERIENCE CHEST PAIN, VOMITING, OR DIFFICULTY IN SWALLOWING OR BREATHING AFTER TAKING THIS PRODUCT, SEEK IMMEDIATE MEDICAL ATTENTION.

IN SEVERE CASES OF CONSTIPATION
Perdiem® may be taken more frequently, up to 2 rounded teaspoonfuls every 6 hours not to exceed 5 teaspoonfuls in a 24-hour period. In severe cases, 24 to 72 hours may be required for optimal relief.

FOR PATIENTS HABITUATED TO STRONG PURGATIVES
Two rounded teaspoonfuls of Perdiem® in the morning and evening may be required along with half the usual dose of the purgative being used. The purgative should be discontinued as soon as possible and the dosage of Perdiem® granules reduced when and if bowel tone shows lessened laxative dependence.

FOR COLOSTOMY PATIENTS
To ensure formed stools, give one to two rounded teaspoonfuls of Perdiem® in the evening.

FOR CLINICAL REGULATION
For patients confined to bed, for those of inactive habits, and in the presence of cardiovascular disease where straining must be avoided, one rounded teaspoonful of Perdiem® taken once or twice daily will provide regular bowel habits.

HOW SUPPLIED
Granules: 100-gram (3.5 oz) (NDC 0067-0690-68) and 250-gram (8.8 oz) (NDC 0067-0690-70) canisters.
6-6 g individual packets (NDC 0067-0690-16) and 20-6 g individual packets (NDC 0067-0690-17).

PERDIEM® FIBER OTC
[*pĕr"dē'ŭm*]
Bulk Forming Laxative

INDICATIONS
Perdiem® Fiber provides gentle relief from simple, chronic, and spastic constipation. In addition, it relieves constipation associated with convalescence, pregnancy, and advanced age. Perdiem® Fiber is also indicated for use in special diets lacking in residue fiber to aid regularity and in the management of constipation associated with irritable bowel syndrome, diverticular disease, hemorrhoids, and anal fissures.

ACTION
Perdiem® Fiber, is a 100% natural bulk-forming fiber that gently helps maintain regularity and prevents constipation. Perdiem® Fiber's unique form is easy to swallow and requires no mixing but must be followed by at least 8 ounces of cool liquid. Perdiem Fiber contains no chemical stimulants and may be used daily by those who may lack sufficient di-

etary fiber. When recommended by a doctor, Perdiem Fiber is also useful for the treatment of bowel disorders other than constipation.

COMPOSITION
Perdiem® Fiber contains as its active ingredient 100% psyllium (Plantago Hydrocolloid), a natural grain with no chemical stimulants. Each rounded teaspoonful (6.0 g) contains 4.03 g of psyllium, 1.8 mg of sodium, 36.1 mg of potassium and 4 calories. Perdiem® Fiber is "Dye-Free" and contains no artificial sweeteners.

INACTIVE INGREDIENTS
Acacia, iron oxides, natural flavors, paraffin, sucrose, talc, titanium dioxide.

DIRECTIONS FOR USE
Perdiem Fiber must be taken with at least 8 ounces of cool liquid. Additional liquid is helpful.
Adults and children 12 years and older: In the evening and/or before breakfast, 1 to 2 rounded teaspoonfuls (6.0 to 12.0 g) of Perdiem® Fiber granules (in full or partial teaspoon doses) should be placed in the mouth and swallowed with at least 8 fl oz of cool beverage after the dose. Perdiem® Fiber granules should not be chewed.
During Pregnancy: Because of its natural ingredients and bulking action, Perdiem Fiber is effective for expectant mothers—follow directions.
Children 7 to 11 years: One (1) rounded teaspoonful one to two times daily with at least 8 ounces of cool liquid.

PATIENT WARNING
Should not be used in the presence of undiagnosed abdominal pain. Frequent or prolonged use without the direction of a physician is not recommended.
Do not use in patients with a history of psyllium allergy. Psyllium allergy is rare but can be severe. If an allergic reaction occurs, discontinue use.
Bulk-forming agents have the potential to obstruct the esophagus, particularly in the presence of esophageal narrowing or when combined with insufficient fluid. Patients should be made aware of the symptoms of esophageal obstruction, including chest pain/pressure, regurgitation, and difficulty swallowing. Patients experiencing these symptoms should seek immediate medical attention. Patients with esophageal narrowing or dysphagia should not use Perdiem® Fiber.
Keep this and all drugs out of the reach of children. In case of accidental overdose, seek professional assistance or contact a poison control center immediately.

IN SEVERE CASES OF CONSTIPATION
Perdiem® Fiber may be taken more frequently, up to 2 rounded teaspoonfuls every 6 hours depending upon need and response not to exceed 5 teaspoonfuls in a 24-hour period. Perdiem Fiber generally takes effect after 24 hours; in severe cases 48 to 72 hours may be required to provide optimal benefit.
WARNING: TAKE THIS PRODUCT WITH AT LEAST 8 OUNCES [A FULL GLASS] OF WATER OR OTHER FLUID. TAKING THIS PRODUCT WITHOUT ADEQUATE FLUID MAY CAUSE IT TO SWELL AND BLOCK YOUR THROAT OR ESOPHAGUS AND MAY CAUSE CHOCKING. DO NOT TAKE THIS PRODUCT IF YOU HAVE EVER HAD DIFFICULTY IN SWALLOWING OR HAVE ANY THROAT PROBLEMS. IF YOU EXPERIENCE CHEST PAIN, VOMITING, OR DIFFICULTY IN SWALLOWING OR BREATHING AFTER TAKING THIS PRODUCT, SEEK IMMEDIATE MEDICAL ATTENTION.

AFTER RECTAL SURGERY
The vegetable mucilages of Perdiem® Fiber soften the stool and ensure pain-free evacuation of the bowel. Perdiem® Fiber is effective as an aid to elimination for the hemorrhoid or fissure patient prior to and following surgery.

FOR CLINICAL REGULATION
For patients confined to bed—after an operation for example—and for those of inactive habits, 1 rounded teaspoonful of Perdiem® Fiber taken 1–2 times daily will ensure regular bowel habits.

HOW SUPPLIED
Granules: 100-gram (3.5 oz) (NDC 0067-0795-68) and 250-gram (8.8 oz) (NDC 0067-0795-70) canisters, 42-gram (1.4 oz) (NDC 0067-0795-42) and 42-gram sample (1.4 oz) (NDC 0067-0795-52).
6-6 g individual packets (NDC 0067-0795-09) and 20-6 g individual packets (NDC 0067-0795-10).

Products are cross-indexed by
generic and chemical names in the
YELLOW SECTION.

Richardson-Vicks Inc.
P.O. Box 5516
CINCINNATI, OH 45201

CHILDREN'S   OTC
CHLORASEPTIC®
LOZENGES
Benzocaine/Oral Anesthetic

(See PDR For Nonprescription Drugs.)

CHILDREN'S CHLORASEPTIC® SPRAY   OTC
Phenol/Oral
Anesthetic/Antiseptic

(See PDR For Nonprescription Drugs.)

CHLORASEPTIC® LIQUID   OTC
Phenol/oral anesthetic/antiseptic
Cherry, Menthol and Cool Mint
Flavors

(See PDR For Nonprescription Drugs.)

CHLORASEPTIC® LOZENGES   OTC
Cherry, Menthol & Cool Mint
Flavor
Menthol/Benzocaine
Oral Anesthetic

(See PDR For Nonprescription Drugs.)

OIL OF OLAY®—Daily UV Protectant   OTC
SPF 15 Beauty Fluid—Regular &
Fragrance Free
(Olay Co., Inc.)

(See PDR For Nonprescription Drugs.)

OIL OF OLAY®—Daily UV Protectant   OTC
SPF 15 Moisture Replenishing
Cream—Regular & Fragrance Free
(Olay Co., Inc.)

(See PDR For Nonprescription Drugs.)

OIL OF OLAY®—Foaming Face Wash   OTC
Regular & Sensitive Skin
(Olay Co., Inc.)

(See PDR For Nonprescription Drugs.)

PERCOGESIC®   OTC
[pĕr 'kō-gē-sĭk]
Analgesic Tablets
Pain Reliever/Fever Reducer

(See PDR For Nonprescription Drugs.)

VICKS® CHILDREN'S COUGH SYRUP   OTC
Cough Suppressant, Expectorant

(See PDR For Nonprescription Drugs.)

VICKS CHILDREN'S NYQUIL®   OTC
[nĭ 'quil]
NIGHTTIME COLD/COUGH MEDICINE
ANTIHISTAMINE, NASAL DECONGESTANT/COUGH
SUPPRESSANT

(See PDR For Nonprescription Drugs.)

VICKS CHILDREN'S NYQUIL®   OTC
Nighttime Head Cold/Allergy
Medicine
Antihistamine/Nasal Decongestant

(See PDR For Nonprescription Drugs.)

VICKS COUGH DROPS   OTC
Menthol Cough Suppressant/Oral
Anesthetic

(See PDR For Nonprescription Drugs.)

EXTRA STRENGTH VICKS®   OTC
COUGH DROPS
Menthol Cough Suppressant/Oral
Anesthetic

(See PDR For Nondescription Drugs.)

VICKS DAYQUIL®   OTC
VICKS DAYQUIL® LIQUICAPS   OTC
Non-Drowsy Colds/Flu Medicine
Nasal Decongestant/Pain
Reliever-Fever Reducer
Cough Suppressant/Expectorant

(See PDR For Nonprescription Drugs.)

VICKS FORMULA 44®   OTC
COUGH MEDICINE
Dextromethorphan HBr/
Cough Suppressant

(See PDR For Nonprescription Drugs.)

VICKS FORMULA 44D®   OTC
Cough & Decongestant
Medicine
Cough Suppressant/
Nasal Decongestant

(See PDR For Nonprescription Drugs.)

VICKS FORMULA 44E®   OTC
Cough & Expectorant Medicine
Cough Suppressant/Expectorant

(See PDR For Nonprescription Drugs.)

VICKS FORMULA 44M®   OTC
Multi-symptom Cough &
Cold Medicine
Cough Suppressant/Nasal
Decongestant/Antihistamine/
Pain Reliever-Fever Reducer

(See PDR For Nonprescription Drugs.)

VICKS® INHALER   OTC
with decongestant action
l-Desoxypehedrine/Nasal
Decongestant

(See PDR For Nonprescription Drugs.)

VICKS NYQUIL®   OTC
Adult Nighttime Colds/Flu
Medicine
Original and Cherry Flavor
Nasal Decongestant/Antihistamine/
Cough Suppressant/Pain
Reliever, Fever Reducer

(See PDR For Nonprescription Drugs.)

VICKS NYQUIL® LIQUICAPS   OTC
Adult Nighttime Colds/Flu Medicine
Nasal Decongestant/Antihistamine/
Cough Suppressant/Pain
Reliever-Fever Reducer

(See PDR For Nonprescription Drugs.)

Continued on next page

Richardson-Vicks—Cont.

VICKS PEDIATRIC FORMULA 44®   OTC
Cough Medicine
Dextromethorphan HBr/Cough
Suppressant

(See PDR For Nonprescription Drugs.)

VICKS PEDIATRIC FORMULA 44d®   OTC
Cough & Decongestant
Medicine

(See PDR For Nonprescription Drugs.)

VICKS PEDIATRIC FORMULA 44e®   OTC
Cough & Expectorant Medicine

(See PDR For Nonprescription Drugs.)

VICKS PEDIATRIC FORMULA 44m®   OTC
Multi-Symptom Cough &
Cold Medicine
Cough Suppressant/Nasal
Decongestant/Antihistamine

(See PDR For Nonprescription Drugs.)

VICKS SINEX®   OTC
[sī'něx]
Decongestant Nasal Spray and
Ultra Fine Mist

(See PDR For Nonprescription Drugs.)

VICKS SINEX® LONG–ACTING   OTC
12-hour Formula Decongestant
Nasal Spray and Ultra Fine Mist

(See PDR For Nonprescription Drugs.)

VICKS VAPORUB®   OTC
[vā pō-rub]
Nasal Decongestant/Cough
Suppresssant

(See PDR For Nonprescription Drugs.)

VICKS VAPOSTEAM®   OTC
[vā'pō"stēm]
Liquid Medication for
Hot Steam Vaporizers.
Nasal Decongestant/Cough
Suppressant

(See PDR For Nonprescription Drugs.)

VICKS VATRONOL®   OTC
[vā'trō"nŏl]
Ephedrine Sulfate/Nasal
Decongestant
Nose Drops

(See PDR For Nonprescription Drugs.)

IDENTIFICATION PROBLEM?
Consult PDR's
Product Identification Section
where you'll find over 1700
products pictured actual size
and in full color.

Richwood Pharmaceutical Company Inc.
P.O. BOX 6497
FLORENCE, KENTUCKY 41022

ACUPRIN®—81 mg Adult Low Dose Aspirin.   OTC

81 mg 100's NDC 58521-081-01
81 mg 500's NDC 58521-081-05

ANEMATRINSIC   ℞
Hematinic Concentrate
with Intrinsic Factor
A Highly Potent Oral Antianemia Preparation

DESCRIPTION
Each AnemaTrinsic capsule contains:
Special liver-stomach concentrate
  (containing intrinsic factor) .... 240 mg
Vitamin B$_{12}$
  (activity equivalent) .... 15 mcg
Iron, elemental
  (as ferrous fumarate) .... 110 mg
Ascorbic acid
  (Vitamin C) .... 75 mg
Folic Acid .... 0.5 mg
with other factors of Vitamin B complex present in the liver-stomach concentrate. Each capsule also contains the inert ingredients: Dicalcium Phosphate, Cellulose, Magnesium Stearate, Gelatin, FD&C Blue #1, FD&C Red #3, FD&C Red #40 and Titanium Dioxide.

DOSAGE AND ADMINISTRATION
One capsule of AnemaTrinsic twice a day. (Two capsules daily produce a standard response in the average uncomplicated case of pernicious anemia.)

HOW SUPPLIED
Bottles of 100, red clear capsules with scarlet opaque body. Imprinted: B121 (NDC 58521-121-01).

HYDROSTAT   Ⓒ ℞
Hydromorphone Hydrochloride

WARNING—MAY BE HABIT FORMING
DESCRIPTION
Oral tablets contain 1, 2, 3, or 4 mg of hydromorphone hydrochloride.

HOW SUPPLIED
Oral Color coded Tablets (NOT FOR INJECTION)
1 mg tablet (green) —Bottle of 100-NDC 58521-001-01 embossed RW/1
2 mg tablet (orange) —Bottle of 100-NDC 58521-002-01 embossed RW/2
3 mg tablet (blue) —Bottle of 100-NDC 58521-003-01 embossed RW/3
4 mg tablet (yellow) —Bottle of 100-NDC 58521-004-01 embossed RW/4

MS/S Suppositories   Ⓒ ℞
Rectal Morphine Sulfate

WARNING—MAY BE HABIT FORMING
DESCRIPTION
Suppositories contain 5, 10, 20, or 30 mg of morphine sulfate.

HOW SUPPLIED
MS/S Suppositories are individually sealed in unit dose packets of 12 suppositories per carton.
5 mg Red carton   NDC 58521-005-12
10 mg Light blue carton   NDC 58521-010-12
20 mg Light green carton   NDC 58521-020-12
30 mg Purple carton   NDC 58521-030-12

VERIN—500 mg of Constant Release   OTC
Rate Aspirin.

Products are cross-indexed by
generic and chemical names in the
YELLOW SECTION.

Roberts Pharmaceutical Corp.
6 G INDUSTRIAL WAY WEST
EATONTOWN, NJ 07724

CEVI–FER™ CAPSULES   ℞
Hematinic with 300 mg Vitamin C
SUSTAINED RELEASE BY
MICRO-DIALYSIS DIFFUSION

DESCRIPTION
Each capsule contains:
- Ascorbic Acid   300 mg
- Ferrous Fumarate   60 mg. (Equivalent to 20 mg. elemental iron)
- Folic Acid   1 mg.
- Prepared in a special base for prolonged therapeutic effect.

INDICATIONS
Cevi-Fer Capsules is a high potency formulation of Iron, Ascorbic Acid, and Folic Acid and is intended for use as:
1) intensive therapy for the acute and/or severe iron deficiency anemia where a high intake of elemental iron is required.
2) a maintenance hematinic for those patients needing a daily iron supplement to maintain normal hemoglobin levels.
3) prevention of concomitant folic acid deficiency in adults.
4) especially indicated in geriatric patients who are on special diets or suffer from nutritional anemias.
5) folic acid is effective in the treatment of megaloblastic anemias due to a deficiency of folic acid (as may be seen in tropical or nontropical sprue) and in anemias of nutritional origin, pregnancy, infancy, or childhood.

ACTIONS AND USES
The Ferrous form of iron is better absorbed and utilized than the ferric form. Absorption of iron can occur along the entire length of the alimentary tract, but is greatest in the duodenum and becomes progressively less distal.
The stomach, being acid, keeps the iron salts in Ferrous state. Reducing agents such as Ascorbic Acid increase iron absorption.
In Cevi-Fer's special sustained release pattern, Ferrous Fumerate and the Ascorbic Acid will be released over a 12 hour period.
The advantage of having Ferrous Fumarate present in a Sustained Release pellet formulation is that it provides high levels of elemental iron with a low incidence of gastric distress.
300 mg. of Sustained Release Ascorbic-Acid serves to maintain the iron in a more absorbable Ferrous state.
Studies have found that large doses of Ascorbic Acid tend to enhance iron absorption

CONTRAINDICATIONS
Folic acid (pteroylglutamic acid) is contraindicated in patients with untreated and uncomplicated pernicious anemia, and in those with anaphylactic sensitivity to folic acid. Iron therapy is contraindicated in patients with hemochromatosis, iron storage disease or the potential for iron storage disease due to chronic hemolytic anemia (e.g., inherited anomalies of hemoglobin structure or synthesis and/or red cell enzyme deficiencies, etc.) pyriodoxine responsive anemia, or cirrhosis of the liver.

WARNINGS
Pernicious anemia should be ruled out before starting treatment. While folic acid corrects the blood picture of pernicious anemia, it does not ameliorate the attendant neurologic involvement.
Resistance to treatment may be due to depressed hematopoiesis, alcoholism, the presence of antimetabolic drugs and to deficiencies of vitamins.
Iron deficiency anemia may be due to occult blood loss, the cause of which should be determined and treated appropriately. Prolonged therapeutic use of iron salts may produce iron storage disease.

PRECAUTIONS
Folic acid in doses above 0.1 mg. daily may obscure pernicious anemia, in that hematologic remission may occur while neurological manifestations remain progressive.
Folic acid (pteroylglutamic acid) microbiological blood assays are invalidated by the administration of most antibiotics, methotrexate, and pyrimethamine. Folic acid is not effective in reversing the toxic effects of methotrexate. Folinic acid (5-formyl-5,6,7,8-tetrahydrofolic acid) must be used in this situation. Black tarry stools may be due to either occult G.I. bleeding or iron therapy, or both.

ADVERSE REACTIONS
Allergic sensitivity reactions and gastrointestinal disturbances may occur.

DOSAGE AND ADMINISTRATION

One capsule after breakfast and supper for two weeks in severe anemias, then one capsule a day. Not to be administered to children under 12 years of age.

OVERDOSAGE

The average human lethal dose of iron is about 200 to 250 mg. iron/kg. body weight. In the case of a 4 kg. infant, this is about 800 mg. iron or about 2 grams anhydrous ferrous sulfate or ferrous fumarate.

WARNING

Keep out of the reach of children. In case of accidental overdose, seek professional assitance or contact a poison control center immediately. Protect from heat and moisture.

HOW SUPPLIED

Available in bottles of 30, NDC 54092-134-30 and 100 capsules NDC 54092-134-01.

CAUTION

Federal law prohibits dispensing without a prescription.
Issued 1/82
Manufactured for:
Roberts Laboratories, Inc.
a wholly owned subsidiary of
Roberts Pharmaceutical Corporation
Eatontown, New Jersey 07724

CHERACOL®Cough Syrup   ℂ
Exempt Narcotic Cough
suppressant/expectorant

DESCRIPTION

CHERACOL® syrup's an exempt narcotic cough suppressant/expectorant cough formula which combines two important medicines in a fast acting, pleasant tasting liquid.

INDICATIONS

CHERACOL® syrup temporarily relieves cough due to common cold and minor throat and bronchial irritation. The antitussive, codeine, calms the cough control center and relieves coughing. The expectorant, guaifenesin, increases the flow of natural secretions making a dry cough more productive.

DOSAGE AND ADMINISTRATION

Adults and children 12 years of age and over: Oral dosage is 2 teaspoonfuls every 4 to 6 hours, not to exceed 12 teaspoonfuls in 24 hours, or as directed by a doctor. Children 6 to under 12 years of age: Oral dosage is 1 teaspoonful every 4 to 6 hours, not to exceed 6 teaspoonfuls in 24 hours, or as directed by a doctor. Children under 6 years of age: consult a doctor. A special measuring device should be used to give an accurate dose of this product to children under 6 years of age. Giving a higher dose than recommended by a doctor could result in serious side effects for your child.
Each teaspoonful (5ml) contains: Codeine phosphate, 10 mg **(Warning: May be habit forming)**; Guaifenesin, 100 mg; Alcohol, 4.75%. Also contains benzoic acid, flavors, fragrances, fructose, glycerin, propylene glycol, FD&C Red #40, sodium chloride, sucrose, and purified water. Warnings: Do not give this product to children under 2 years or to children taking other drugs except under the advice and supervision of a physician. Do not take this product for persistent or chronic cough such as occurs with smoking, asthma, emphysema, or where cough is accompanied by excessive secretions, or if you have a chronic pulmonary disease or shortness of breath, except under the advice and supervision of a physician. May cause or aggravate constipation. As with any drug, if you are pregnant or nursing a baby, seek the advice of a health professional before using this product. Caution: A persistent cough may be a sign of a serious condition. If cough persists for more than 1 week, tends to recur or is accompanied by high fever, rash, or persistent headache, consult a physician. Keep this and all drugs out of the reach of children. In case of accidental overdose, seek professional assistance or contact a poison control center immediately. Store at controlled room temperature, 15°–30°C (59°–86°F).

HOW SUPPLIED

Available in 2 fl oz (NDC 54092-402-60), 4 fl oz (NDC 54092-402-04), and 16 fl oz (NDC 54092-402-16).
Revised May 1991
Manufactured for:
Roberts Laboratories, Inc.
a wholly owned subsidiary of
Roberts Pharmaceutical Corporation
Eatontown, New Jersey 07724

Shown in Product Identification Section, page 425

CHLORAFED® H.S. TIMECELLES   ℞
(CHLORAFED® HALF-STRENGTH)

DESCRIPTION

Each capsule contains:
Chlorpheniramine maleate .... **4 mg**
Pseudoephedrine hydrocloride........................... **60 mg**
in a specially prepared base to provide prolonged action.
Inactive Ingredients:
Gelatin, pharmaceutical glaze, starch, sucrose and other ingredients. This product contains ingredients of the following therapeutic classes: antihistamine and decongestant.

CLINICAL PHARMACOLOGY

Chlorpheniramine maleate is an alkylamine type antihistamine. This group of antihistamines are among the most active histamine antagonists and are generally effective in relatively low doses. The drugs are not so prone to produce drowsiness and are among the most suitable agents for daytime use; but again, a significant proportion of patients do experience this effect. Pseudoephedrine hydrochloride is a sympathomimetic which acts predominantly on alpha receptors and has little action on beta receptors. It therefore functions as an oral nasal decongestant with minimal CNS stimulation.

INDICATIONS

For the temporary relief of symptoms of the common cold, allergic rhinitis (hay fever) and sinusitis.

CONTRAINDICATIONS

Hypersensitivity to any of the ingredients. Also contraindicated in patients with severe hypertension, severe coronary artery disease, patients on MAO inhibitor therapy, patients with narrow-angle glaucoma, urinary retention, peptic ulcer and during an asthmatic attack. Should not be used in nursing mothers.

WARNINGS

Considerable caution should be exercised in patients with hypertension, diabetes mellitus, ischemic heart disease, hyperthyroidism, increased intraocular pressure and prostatic hypertrophy. The elderly (60 years or older) are more likely to exhibit adverse reactions. Antihistamines may cause excitability especially in children. At dosages higher than the recommended dose, nervousness, dizziness or sleeplessness may occur.
General: Caution should be exercised in patients with high blood pressure, heart disease, diabetes or thyroid disease. The antihistamine in this product may exhibit additive effects with other CNS depressants including alcohol.
Information for Patients: Antihistamine may cause drowsiness, and ambulatory patients who operate machinery or motor vehicles should be cautioned accordingly.
Drug Interactions: MAO inhibitors and beta adrenergic blockers increase the effects of sympathomimetics. Sympathomimetics may reduce the antihypertensive effects of methyldopa, mecamylamine, reserpine and veratrum alkaloids. Concomitant use of antihistamines with alcohol and other CNS depressants may have an additive effect.
Pregnancy Category C: Animal reproduction studies have not been conducted with Chlorafed® H.S. Timecelles. It is also not known whether Chlorafed® H.S. Timecelles can cause fetal harm when administered to a pregnant woman or can affect reproduction capacity. Chlorafed® H.S. Timecelles should be given to a pregnant woman only if clearly needed.

ADVERSE REACTIONS

Adverse reactions include drowsiness, lassitude, nausea, giddiness, dryness of mouth, blurred vision, cardiac palpitations, flushing, increased irritability or excitement (especially in children).

DOSAGE AND ADMINISTRATION

Adults and children over 12 years: 1 or 2 capsules orally every 12 hours. Children 6 to 12 years of age: 1 capsule orally every 12 hours. Do not give to children under 6 years of age.

HOW SUPPLIED

Clear, dye-free imprinted capsules. Bottles of 100 NDC 54092-135-01.
STORE AT CONTROLLED ROOM TEMPERATURE BETWEEN 15°–30°C (59°–86°F).
DISPENSE IN A TIGHT CONTAINER AS DEFINED IN USP/NF WITH A CHILD-RESISTANT CLOSURE.
Distributed by:
Roberts/Hauck Pharmaceuticals, Inc.
a wholly owned subsidiary of
Roberts Pharmaceutical Corporation
Eatontown, New Jersey 07724

Revised 5/91

CHLORAFED® LIQUID   OTC
(Corn, Dye, Alcohol, Sugar Free)

DESCRIPTION

Each 5 ml. (teaspoonful) of dye-free CHLORAFED® LIQUID contains Chlorpheniramine Maleate 2 mg and Pseudoephedrine HCl 30 mg.

HOW SUPPLIED

CHLORAFED LIQUID is available as a clear liquid that is free of corn, dye, alcohol and sugar.
NDC 54092-435-04 Bottle of 4 fl. oz.
NDC 54092-435-16 Bottle of 16 fl. oz.

CHLORAFED® TIMECELLES   ℞

DESCRIPTION

Each extended-release capsule contains:
Chlorpheniramine
Maleate.. 8 mg
Pseudoephedrine
Hydrochloride .... 120 mg
in a specially prepared base to provide prolonged action. This product contains ingredients of the following therapeutic classes: antihistamine and nasal decongestant.

CAUTION

Federal law prohibits dispensing without prescription.

CLINICAL PHARMACOLOGY

Chlorpheniramine maleate is an alkylamine type antihistamine. This group of antihistamines is among the most active histamine antagonists and are generally effective in relatively low doses. The drugs are not so prone to produce drowsiness and are among the most suitable agents for day time use: but again, a significant proportion of patients do experience this effect. Pseudoephedrine hydrochloride is a sympathomimetic which acts predominantly on alpha receptors and has little action on beta receptors. It therefore functions as an oral nasal decongestant with minimal CNS stimulation.

INDICATIONS

For the temporary relief of symptoms of the common cold, allergic rhinitis (hay fever) and sinusitis.

CONTRAINDICATIONS

Hypersensitivity to any of the ingredients. Also contraindicated in patients with severe hypertension, severe coronary artery disease, patients on MAO inhibitor therapy, patients with narrow-angle glaucoma, urinary retention, peptic ulcer and during an asthmatic attack.
Should not be used in children under 12 years or in nursing mothers.

WARNINGS

Considerable caution should be exercised in patients with hypertension, diabetes mellitus, ischemic heart disease, hyperthyroidism, increased intraocular pressure and prostatic hypertrophy. The elderly (60 years or older) are more likely to exhibit adverse reactions.
Antihistamines may cause excitability, especially in children. At dosages higher than the recommended dose, nervousness, dizziness or sleeplessness may occur.

PRECAUTIONS

General: Caution should be exercised in patients with high blood pressure, heart disease, diabetes or thyroid disease. The antihistamine in this product may exhibit additive effects with other CNS depressants, including alcohol.
Information for Patients: Antihistamine may cause drowsiness and ambulatory patients who operate machinery or motor vehicles should be cautioned accordingly.
Drug Interactions: MAO inhibitors and beta adrenergic blockers increase the effects of sympathomimetics. Sympathomimetics may reduce the antihypertensive effects of methyldopa, mecamylamine, reserpine and veratrum alkaloids. Concomitant use of antihistamines with alcohol and other CNS depressants may have an additive effect.
Use in pregnancy: Pregnancy Category C: There are no adequate and well-controlled studies in pregnant women. Chlorafed® Timecelles should be used during pregnancy only if the potential benefit justifies the potential risk to the fetus.

ADVERSE REACTIONS

Adverse reactions include drowsiness, lassitude, nausea, giddiness, dryness of mouth, blurred vision, cardiac palpitations, flushing, increased irritability or excitement (especially in children).

DOSAGE AND ADMINISTRATION

Adults and children over 12 years of age - 1 capsule orally every 12 hours.

Continued on next page

Roberts—Cont.

HOW SUPPLIED
Imprinted DYE FREE Clear Capsules
Bottles of 100 NDC 54092-136-01
DISPENSE IN A TIGHT CONTAINER AS DEFINED IN THE USP/NF WITH A CHILD-RESISTANT CLOSURE.
STORE AT CONTROLLED ROOM TEMPERATURE 15°–30°C (59°–86°F)
Distributed by:
Roberts/Hauck Pharmaceuticals, Inc.
a wholly owned subsidiary of
Roberts Pharmaceutical Corporation
Eatontown, New Jersey 07724 Rev. 9/91

DOPAR® ℞
(levodopa)

Toward reducing the high incidence of adverse reactions, it is necessary to individualize the therapy and to gradually increase the dosage to the desired therapeutic level.

DESCRIPTION
Chemically, levodopa is 3-hydroxy-L-tyrosine. It is a colorless, crystalline compound, slightly soluble in water and insoluble in alcohol, with a molecular weight of 197.2 and the following structural formula:

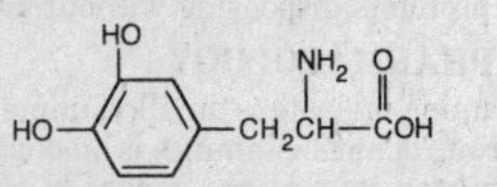

Inactive Ingredients: Each capsule contains edible black ink, FD&C Blue #1, gelatin, lactose, talc, titanium dioxide, and FD&C Yellow #5.

ACTIONS
Evidence indicates the the symptoms of Parkinson's disease are related to depletion of striatal dopamine. Since dopamine apparently does not cross the blood-brain barrier, its administration is ineffective in the treatment of Parkinson's disease. However, levodopa, the levorotatory isomer of dihydroxyphenylalanine (dopa) which is the metabolic precursor of dopamine, does cross the blood-brain barrier. Presumably it is converted into dopamine in the basal ganglia. This is generally thought to be the mechanism whereby oral levodopa acts in relieving the symptoms of Parkinson's disease.
The major uninary metabolites of levodopa in man appear to be dopamine and homovanillic acid (HVA). In 24-hour urine samples, HVA accounts for 13 to 42 percent of the ingested dose of levodopa.

INDICATIONS
Levodopa is indicated in the treatment of idiopathic Parkinson's disease (Paralysis Agitans), post encephalitic parkinsonism, symptomatic parkinsonism which may follow injury to the nervous system by carbon monoxide intoxication, and manganese intoxication. It is indicated in those elderly patients believed to develop parkinsonism in association with cerebral arteriosclerosis.

CONTRAINDICATIONS
Monoamine oxidase (MAO) inhibitors and levodopa should not be given concomitantly and these inhibitors must be discontinued two weeks prior to initiating therapy with levodopa. Levodopa is contraindicated in patients with known hypersensitivity to the drug and in narrow angle glaucoma. Because levodopa may activate a malignant melanoma, it should not be used in patients with suspicious, undiagnosed skin lesions or a history of melanoma.

WARNINGS
Levodopa should be administered cautiously to patients with severe cardiovascular or pulmonary disease, bronchial asthma, renal, hepatic or endocrine disease.
Care should be exercised in administering levodopa to patients with a history of myocardial infarction who have residual atrial, nodal or ventricular arrhythmias. If levodopa is necessary in this type of patient, it should be done in a facility with a coronary care unit or an intensive care unit.
One must be on the alert for the possibility of upper gastrointestinal hemorrhage in those patients with a past history of active peptic ulcer disease.
All patients should be carefully observed for the development of depression with concomitant suicidal tendencies. Psychotic patients should be treated with caution.
Pyridoxine hydrochloride (vitamin B6) in oral doses of 10 or 25 mg rapidly reverses the toxic and therapeutic effect of levodopa. This should be considered before recommending vitamin preparations containing pyridoxine hydrochloride (vitamin B6).
Usage in Pregnancy: The safety of levodopa in women who are or who may become pregnant has not been established; hence it should be given only when the potential benefits have been weighed against possible hazards to mother and child. Studies in rodents have shown that levodopa at dosages in excess of 200 mg/kg/day has an adverse effect on fetal and post-natal growth and viability.
Levodopa should not be used in nursing mothers.
Usage in Children: The safety of levodopa under the age of 12 have not been established.

PRECAUTIONS
Periodic evaluations of hepatic, hematopoietic, cardiovascular and renal function are recommended during extended therapy in all patients.
Patients with chronic wide angle glaucoma may be treated cautiously with levodopa, provided the intraocular pressure is well-controlled and the patient monitored carefully for changes in intraocular pressure during therapy.
Postural hypotensive episodes have been reported as adverse reactions. Therefore, levodopa should be administered to patients on antihypertensive drugs cautiously (for patients reciving pargyline, see note on MAO inhibitors under contraindications), and it may be necessary to adjust the dosage of the antihypertensive drugs.
This product contains FD&C Yellow No. 5 (tartrazine) which may cause allergic-type reactions (including bronchial asthma) in certain susceptible individuals. Although the overall incidence of FD&C Yellow No. 5 (tartrazine) sensitivity in the general population is low, it is frequently seen in patients who also have aspirin hypersensitivity.

ADVERSE REACTIONS
The most serious adverse reactions associated with the administration of levodopa having frequent occurrences are: adventitious movements such as choreiform and/or dystonic movements. Other serious adverse reactions with a lower incidence are: cardiac irregularities and/or palpitations, orthostatic hypotensive episodes, bradykinetic episodes (the "on-off" phenomena), mental changes including paranoid ideation and psychotic episodes, depression with or without the development of suicidal tendencies, dementia, and urinary retention.
Rarely gastrointestinal bleeding, development of duodenal ulcer, hypertension, phlebitis, hemolytic anemia, agranulocytosis, and convulsions have been observed. (The causal relationship between convulsions and levodopa has not been established.)
Adverse reactions of a less serious nature having a relatively frequent occurrence are the following: anorexia, nausea, and vomiting with or without abdominal pain and distress, dry mouth, dysphagia, sialorrhea, ataxia, increased hand tremor, headache, dizziness, numbness, weakness and faintness, bruxism, confusion, insomnia, nightmares, hallucinations and delusions, agitation and anxiety, malaise, fatigue, and euphoria. Occurring with a lesser order of frequency are the following: muscle twitching and blepharospasm, trismus, burning sensation of the tongue, bitter taste, diarrhea, constipation, flatulence, flushing, skin rash, increased sweating, bizarre breathing patterns, urinary incontinence, diplopia, blurred vision, dilated pupils, hot flashes, weight gain or loss, dark sweat and/or urine.
Rarely, oculogyric crises, sense of stimulation hiccups, development of edema, loss of hair, hoarseness, priapism, and activation of latent Horner's syndrome have been observed.
Elevations of blood urea nitrogen, SGOT, SGPT, LDH, bilirubin, alkaline phosphatase or protein bound iodine have been reported; and the significance of this is not known. Occasional reductions in WBC, hemoglobin, and hematocrit have been noted.
Leukopenia has occurred and requires cessation at least temporarily, of levodopa administration. The Coomb's test has occasionally become positive during extended therapy. Elevations of uric acid have been noted when colorimetric method was used but not when uricase method was used.

OVERDOSAGE
For acute overdosage, general supportive measures should be employed, along with immediate gastric lavage. Intravenous fluids should be administered judiciously and an adequate airway maintained.
Electrocardiographic monitoring should be insituted and the patient carefully observed for the possible development of arrhythmias; if required, appropriate antiarrhythmic therapy should be given. Consideration should be given to the possibilty of multiple drug ingestion by the patient. To date, no experience has been reported with dialysis; hence its value in levodopa overdosage is not known. Although pyridoxine hydrochloride (vitamin B6) has been reported to reverse the anti-parkinson effects of levodopa, its usefulness in the management of acute overdosage has not been established.

DOSAGE AND ADMINISTRATION
The optimal daily dose of levodopa, i.e., the dose producing maximal improvement with tolerated side effects, must be determined and carefully titrated for each individual patient. The usual initial dosage is 0.5 to 1 g daily, divided in two or more doses with food.
The total daily dosage is then increased gradually in increments of not more than 0.75 g every three to seven days as tolerated. The usual optimal therapeutic dosage should not exceed 8 g. The exceptional patient may carefully be given more than 8 g as required. In some patients, a significant therapeutic response may not be obtained until six months of treatment.
In the event general anesthesia is required, levodopa therapy may be continued as long as the patient is able to take fluids and medication by mouth. If therapy is temporarily interrupted, the usual daily dosage may be administered as soon as the patient is able to take oral medication. Whenever therapy has been interrupted for longer periods, dosage should again be adjusted gradually; however, in many cases the patient can be rapidly titrated to his previous therapeutic dosage.

HOW SUPPLIED
Dopar is available as follows:
100 mg: opaque, green capsule imprinted "Eaton 013"
NDC 54092-060-01 bottle of 100.
250 mg: opaque green and white capsule imprinted "Eaton 014"
NDC 54092-061-01 bottle of 100
500 mg: opaque green capsule imprinted "Eaton 015"
NDC 54092-062-01 bottle of 100
Manufactured for:
Roberts Laboratories, Inc.
a wholly owned subsidiary of
Roberts Pharmaceutical Corporation
Eatontown, New Jersey 07724
Shown in Product Identification Section, page 425

DUVOID® ℞
(bethanechol chloride tablets, USP)

DESCRIPTION
Duvoid (bethanechol chloride), a cholinergic agent, is a synthetic ester which is structurally and pharmacologically related to acetylcholine. Its chemical name is 2-[(aminocarbonyl)oxy] -N.N.N- trimethyl -1- propanaminium chloride. Bethanechol chloride is a white, hygroscopic, crystalline powder having a slight amine-like odor and is freely soluble in water. The structural formula is:

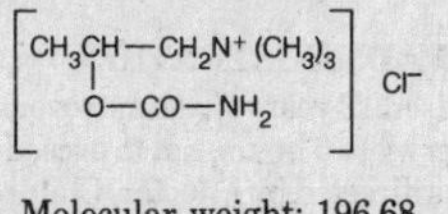

Molecular weight: 196.68
Molecular formula: $C_7H_{17}ClN_2O_2$
Duvoid is available as 10mg, 25mg, and 50mg scored tablets intended for oral use.
Inactive Ingredients: Each tablet contains calcium pyrophosphate, magnesium stearate, microcrystalline cellulose, corn starch and may contain one or more of the following: FD&C Blue #2. FD&C Yellow #6.

CLINICAL PHARMACOLOGY
Bethanechol chloride acts principally by producing the effects of stimulation of the parasympathetic nervous system. It increases the tone of the detrusor urinae muscle. Usually producing a contraction sufficiently strong to initiate micturition and empty the bladder. It stimulates gastric motility, increases gastric tone and often restores impaired rhythmic peristalsis. Stimulation of the parasympathetic nervous system releases acetylcholine at the nerve endings. When spontaneous stimulation is reduced and therapeutic intervention is required, acetylcholine can be given, but is rapidly hydrolyzed by cholinesterase, and its effect are transient. Bethanechol chloride is not destroyed by cholinesterase and its effects are more prolonged than those of acetylcholine. Effects on the g.I. and urinary tracts sometimes appear within 30 minutes after oral administration of bethanechol chloride, but more often 60–90 minutes are required to reach maximum effectiveness. Following oral administration the usual duration of action of bethanechol is one hours, although large doses (300–400 mg) have been reported to produce effects for up to six hours. Subcutaneous injection produces a more intense action on bladder muscle than does oral administration of the drug. Because of the selective action of bethanechol, nicotinic symptoms of cholinergic stimulation are usually absent or minimal when orally or subcutaneously administered in therapeutic doses, while muscarinic effects are prominent. Muscarinic effects usually occur within 5–15 minutes after subcutaneous injection, reach a maximum in 15–30 minutes, and disappear within two hours. Doses that stimulate micturition and defecation and increase peristalsis do not ordinarily stimulate ganglia or voluntary muscles. Therapeutic test does in normal human subjects have little effect on heart rate, blood pressure, or peripheral circulation.

Bethanechol chloride does not cross the blood-brain barrier because of its charged quaternary amine moiety. The metabolic fate and mode of excretion of the drug have not been elucidated.
A clinical study was conducted on the relative effectiveness of oral and subcutaneous doses of bethanechol chloride on the stretch response of bladder muscle in patients with urinary retention. Results showed that 5 mg of the drug given subcutaneously stimulated a response that was more rapid in onset and of a large magnitude than an oral dose of 50 mg, 100 mg or 200 mg. All the oral doses, however, had a longer duration of effect than the subcutaneous dose. Although the 50 mg oral dose caused little change in intravesical pressure in this study, this dose has been found in other studies to be clinically effective in the rehabilitation of patients with decompensated bladders.

INDICATIONS AND USAGE

Duvoid is indicated for the treatment of acute postoperative and postpartum nonobstructive (functional) urinary retention, and neurogenic atony of the urinary bladder with retention.

CONTRAINDICATIONS

Bethanechol chloride is contraindicated in individuals with hypersensitivity to bethanechol chloride tablets, hyperthyroidism peptic ulcer, latent or active bronchial asthma, pronounced bradycardia or hypotension, vasomotor instability, coronary artery disease, epilepsy and parkinsonism. Bethanechol chloride should not be employed when the strength or integrity of the gastrointestinal or bladder wall is in question, or in the presence of mechanical obstruction: when increased muscular activity of the gastrointestinal tract or urinary bladder might prove harmful, as following recent urinary bladder surgery, gastrointestinal resection and anastomosis, or when there is possible gastrointestinal obstruction: in bladder neck obstruction, spastic gastrointestinal disturbances, acute inflammatory lesions of the gastrointestinal tract or peritonitis: or in marked vagotonia.

PRECAUTIONS

General: In urinary retention, if the sphincter fails to relax as bethanechol contracts the bladder, urine may be forced up the ureter into the kidney pelvis. If there is bacteriuria, this may case a reflux infection.
Information for Patients: Bethanechol chloride tablets should preferably be taken one hour before or two hours after meals to avoid nausea or vomiting. Dizziness, light-headedness or fainting may occur especially when getting up from a lying or sitting position.
Drug Interactions: Special care is required if this drug is given to patients receiving ganglion blocking compounds because a critical fall in blood pressure may occur. Usually, severe abdominal symptoms appear before there is such a fall in the blood pressure.
Carcinogensis, Mutagenesis, Impairment or Fertility: Long-term studies in animals have not been performed to evaluate the effects upon fertility, mutagenic or carcinogenic potential of bethanechol chloride.
Pregnancy: Pregnancy Category C. Animal reproduction studies have not been conducted with bethanechol chloride. It is also not known whether bethanechol can cause fetal harm when administered to a pregnant woman or can affect reproduction capacity. Bethanechol should be given to a pregnant woman only if clearly needed.
Nursing Mothers: It is not known whether this drug is excreted in human milk. Because many drugs are excreted in human milk and because of the potential for serious adverse reactions from bethanechol chloride in nursing infants a decision should be made whether to discontinue nursing or to discontinue the drug, taking into account the importance of the drug to the mother.
Pediatric Use: Safety and effectiveness in children have not been established.

ADVERSE REACTIONS

Adverse reactions are infrequent with bethanechol chloride. Reactions are more likely to occur when dosage is increased. The following may occur:
Body as a Whole: Malaise
Cardiovascular: Fall in blood pressure with reflex tachycardia, vasomotor response.
Digestive: Colicky pain, abdominal cramps or discomfort diarrhea, nausea and belching, salivation and borborygmi.
Skin: Flushing producing a feeling of warmth sensation of heat about the face sweating.
Respiratory: Asthmatic attacks and dyspnea.
Nervous System: Headache.
Renal: Urinary urgency.
Special Senses: Lacrimation miosis.

OVERDOSAGE

Early signs of overdosage are abdominal discomfort, salivation, flushing of the skin ("hot feeling"), sweating, nausea and vomiting Atropine sulfate is a specific antidote. The recommended dose for adults is 0.6 mg. Repeat doses can be given every two hours, according to clinical response. The recommended dosage in infants and children up to 12 years of age is 0.01 mg kg (to a maximum single dose of 0.4 mg) repeated every two hours as needed until the desired effect is obtained, or adverse effects of atropine preclude further usage. Subcutaneous injection of atropine is preferred except in emergencies when the intravenous route may be employed. The oral LD_{50} of bethanechol chloride is 1510 mg kg in the mouse.

DOSAGE AND ADMINISTRATION

Dosage must be individualized, depending on type and severity of the condition to be treated. Preferably give the drug when the stomach is empty. If taken soon after eating, nausea and vomiting may occur. The usual adult oral dose ranges from 10 to 50 mg three or four times a day. The minimum effective dose is determined by giving 5 or 10 mg initially, and repeating the same amount at hourly intervals until satisfactory response occurs, or until a maximum of 50 mg has been given. The effects of the drug sometimes appear within 30 minutes, and are usually maximal within 90 minutes. The drug's effects persist for about one hour. If necessary, the effects of the drug can be abolished promptly by atropine (see OVERDOSAGE).

HOW SUPPLIED

Duvoid is available as follows: 10mg: pale orange, scored tablet coded "Eaton 045" on smooth side and "10" on scored side, NDC 54092-101-01 bottle of 100. NDC 54092-101-52 hospital unit dose strips on box of 100. 25 mg: white, scored tablet coded "Eaton 046" on smooth side and "25" on scored side. NDC 54092-102-01 bottle of 100. NDC 54092-102-52 hospital unit dose strips in box of 100. 50 mg: tan, scored tablet coded "Eaton 047" on smooth side and "50" on scored side, NDC 54092-103-01 bottle of 100. NDC 54092-103-52 hospital unit dose strips in box of 100.

CAUTION

Federal law prohibits dispensing without prescription. Keep container tightly closed. Avoid excessive heat (over 104°F or 40°C).
Revised May 1991
Manufactured for:
Roberts Laboratories, Inc.
a wholly owned subsidiary of
Roberts Pharmaceutical Corporation
Eatontown, New Jersey 07724
Shown in Product Identification Section, page 425

ENTUSS EXPECTORANT ℂ℞

DESCRIPTION

A light amber color, apricot sweet-tasting syrup for oral administration, which is ALCOHOL FREE, CORN FREE, TARTRAZINE FREE and SUGAR FREE.

Each teaspoonful (5 ml.) contains:

Hydrocodone Bitartrate .... 5 mg.
WARNING—May be habit forming
Potassium Guaiacolsulfonate .... 300 mg.

This product contains ingredients of the following therapeutic classes: antitussive and expectorant.

CLINICAL PHARMACOLOGY

Hydrocodone bitartrate is a potent antitussive which causes suppression of the cough reflex by direct action on the cough center. Hydrocodone is approximately three times as potent as codeine on a weight basis and has a higher addiction potential also. Potassium guaiacolsulfonate has been used empirically for many decades as an expectorant.

INDICATIONS

For the temporary relief of dry, non-productive cough due to colds, pertussis or influenza.

CONTRAINDICATIONS

Hypersensitivity to any of the ingredients.

WARNINGS

Hydrocodone can produce drug dependence and therefore has the potential for being abused. Entuss should be prescribed and administered with the degree of caution appropriate for this type product.

PRECAUTIONS

General: The hydrocodone in this product may exhibit additive effects with other CNS depressants, including alcohol. Respiratory depression can be a real hazard so caution should be used, especially in patients with chronic obstructive pulmonary disease.
Information for Patients: The hydrocodone may cause drowsiness and ambulatory patients who operate machinery or motor vehicles should be cautioned accordingly.
Drug Interactions: Concommitant use of hydrocodone with alcohol and/or other CNS depressants may have an additive effect.
Pregnancy: The safety of use of the product in pregnancy has not been established, therefore pregnant women should consult a physician before taking this medication.

ADVERSE REACTIONS

Adverse reactions include drowsiness, lassitude, nausea, giddiness, constipation, respiratory depression and addiction.

DRUG ABUSE AND DEPENDENCE

This product is a Schedule III Controlled Substance. Because of the hydrocodone content, some abuse might be expected. Psychic dependence, physical dependence and tolerance may develop upon repeated administration. It should be prescribed and administered with the degree of caution appropriate for this type product.

DOSAGE AND ADMINISTRATION

Adults and older children - 1 to 1 ½ teaspoonfuls; children, 6 to 12 years of age ½ to 1 teaspoonful; children, 3 to 6 years of age - ¼ to ½ teaspoonful. These doses may be given four times daily as needed. Not recommended for children under 3 years of age.

OVERDOSAGE

Symptoms of overdosage include respiratory depression, extreme somnolence progressing to stupor or coma, skeletal muscle flaccidity, cold and clammy skin and other symptoms common with narcotic overdosage.
Primary treatment consists of insuring adequate respiration through provision of a patent airway and the institution of assisted or controlled ventilation. Naloxone hydrochloride should be administered in small intravenous doses (consult specific product labeling before use). In addition, oxygen, intravenous fluids, vasopressors and other supportive measures should be employed as indicated. Gastric emptying may be useful in removing unabsorbed drug. Activated charcoal may also be of benefit.

HOW SUPPLIED

Bottles of 4 oz. - NDC 54092-437-04
Bottles of 1 pint - NDC 54092-437-16
STORE AND DISPENSE IN TIGHT CONTAINERS AS DEFINED IN USP/NF.
STORE BETWEEN 15°-30°C (59°-86°F)
DISPENSE IN CHILD-RESISTANT CONTAINERS

Manufactured for:
Roberts Laboratories, Inc.
a wholly owned subsidiary of
ROBERTS PHARMACEUTICAL CORP.
Eatontown, New Jersey 07724

ENTUSS TABLETS ℂ℞

Each tablet contains:
Hydrocodone Bitartrate .... 5 mg.
(Warning — May be habit forming)
Guaifenesin .... 300 mg.

CLINICAL PHARMACOLOGY

Hydrocodone bitartrate is a potent antitussive which causes suppression of the cough reflex by direct action on the cough center. Hydrocodone is approximately six times as potent as codeine on a weight basis and has a higher addiction potential. Guaifenesin is an expectorant which increases respiratory tract fluid secretions and helps to loosen phlegm and bronchial secretions. By reducing the viscosity of secretions, guaifenesin increases the efficiency of the cough reflex and of ciliary action in removing accumulated secretions from the trachea and bronchi.

INDICATIONS

For the temporary relief of dry, non-productive cough due to colds, pertussis or influenza.

CONTRAINDICATIONS

Hypersensitivity to any of the ingredients.

WARNINGS

Hydrocodone can produce drug dependence and therefore has the potential for being abused. ENTUSS should be prescribed and administered with the degree of caution appropriate for this type of product.

PRECAUTIONS

General: The hydrocodone in this product may exhibit additive effects with other CNS depressants, including alcohol. Respiratory depression can be a real hazard so caution should be used, especially in patients with chronic obstructive pulmonary disease.

INFORMATION FOR PATIENTS

The hydrocodone may cause drowsiness and ambulatory patients who operate machinery or motor vehicles should be cautioned accordingly.

DRUG INTERACTIONS

Concommitant use of hydrocodone with alcohol and/or other CNS depressants may have an additive effect.

Continued on next page

Roberts—Cont.

PREGNANCY
The safety of use of the product in pregnancy has not been established.

ADVERSE REACTIONS
Adverse reactions include drowsiness, lassitude, nausea, giddiness, constipation, respiratory depression and addiction.

DRUG ABUSE AND DEPENDENCE
This product is a Schedule III Controlled Substance. Because of the hydrocodone content, some abuse might be expected. Psychic dependence, physical dependence and tolerance may develop upon repeated administration. It should be prescribed and administerd with the degree of caution appropriate for this type of product.

DOSAGE AND ADMINISTRATION
Adults and older children - 1 to 1½ tablets; children, 6 to 12 years of age ½ to 1 tablets. These doses may be given up to 4 times daily as needed.

OVERDOSE
Symptoms of overdosage include respiratory depression, extreme somnolence progressing to stupor or coma, skeletal muscle flaccidity, cold and clammy skin and other symptoms common with narcotic overdosage.
Primary treatment consists of insuring adequate respiration through provision of a patent airway and the institution of assisted or controlled ventilation. Naloxone hydrochloride should be administered in small intravenous doses (consult specific product labeling before use). In addition, oxygen, intravenous fluids, vasopressors and other supportive measures should be employed as indicated. Gastric emptying may be useful in removing unabsorbed drug. Activated charcoal may also be of benefit.

HOW SUPPLIED
Bottles of 100 - (NDC 54092-141-01). Light orange scored tablets imprinted Blansett.
STORE AND DISPENSE IN TIGHT CONTAINERS AS DEFINED IN USP/NF.
STORE BETWEEN 15°–30°C (59°–89°F)
DISPENSE IN CHILD-RESISTANT CONTAINERS

CAUTION
Federal law prohibits dispensing without prescription.
　　　　　　　　　　　　　　　　　　　Rev. 2/90

Manufactured for:
Roberts/Hauck Pharmaceuticals, Inc.
a wholly owned subsidiary of
Roberts Pharmaceutical Corporation
Eatontown, New Jersey 07724

ENTUSS–D LIQUID and TABLETS　　Ⓒ Ⓡ
(Sugar, Dye, Corn, Alcohol Free)

DESCRIPTION
Each tablet contains Hydrocodone Bitartrate (WARNING: May be habit forming) 5 mg., Guaifenesin 300 mg. and Pseudoephedrine Hydrochloride 30 mg. Each 5 mL teaspoonful contains Hydrocodone Bitartrate (WARNING: May be habit forming) 5 mg., Pseudoephedrine Hydrochloride 30 mg. and Potassium Guaiacolsulfonate 300 mg.

HOW SUPPLIED
Each ENTUSS-D TABLET is white, dye-free, scored and imprinted HAUCK 258.
NDC 54092-142-01 Bottle of 100.
ENTUSS-D LIQUID is a clear, dye-free liquid.
NDC 54092-438-16 Bottle of 16 oz.

ENTUSS–D JR. LIQUID　　　　　Ⓒ

DESCRIPTION
Each mL teaspoonful contains Hydrocodone Bitartrate (WARNING: may be habit forming) 2.5 mg, Pseudoephedrine Hydrochloride 30 mg. and Guaifenesin 100 mg.

HOW SUPPLIED
ENTUSS-D JR. LIQUID is a red, tropical fruit punch flavor.
NDC 54092-439-04 Bottle of 4 fl. oz.
NDC 54092-439-16 Bottle of 16 fl. oz.

FURACIN® SOLUBLE DRESSING　　　Ⓡ
[fewr 'a-sin]
(nitrofurazone)

DESCRIPTION
Chemically, Furacin is nitrofurazone, 2-[(5-nitro-2- furanyl)-methylene]hydrazinecarboxamide, with the following structure:

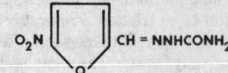

Furacin Soluble Dressing is a preparation containing 0.2% nitrofurazone in Solubase® (a water-soluble base of polyethylene glycols 3350, 900, and 300).
Furacin Soluble Dressing is an antibacterial agent for topical use.

CLINICAL PHARMACOLOGY
Furacin Soluble Dressing (nitrofurazone) is a nitrofuran that is bactericidal for most pathogens commonly causing surface infections, including *Staphylococcus aureus, Streptococcus, Escherichia coli, Clostridium perfringens, Aerobacter aerogenes,* and *Proteus.*
Furacin Soluble Dressing inhibits a number of bacterial enzymes, especially those involved in the aerobic and anaerobic degradation of glucose and pyruvate. The activity appears to involve the pyruvate dehydrogenase system as well as citrate synthetase, malate dehydrogenase, glutathione reductase, and pyruvate decarboxylase. Glutathione reductase inhibition may be caused by control of pentose phosphate metabolism. Although Furacin Soluble Dressing inhibits a variety of enzymes, it is not considered to be a general enzyme inactivator since many enzymes are not inhibited by this compound.

INDICATIONS AND USAGE
Furacin Soluble Dressing is a topical antibacterial agent indicated for adjunctive therapy of patients with second- and third-degree burns when bacterial resistance to other agents is a real or potential problem.
It is also indicated in skin grafting where bacterial contamination may cause graft rejection and/or donor site infection particularly in hospitals with historical resistant-bacteria epidemics.
There is no known evidence of effectiveness of this product in the treatment of minor burns or surface bacterial infections involving wounds, cutaneous ulcers, or the various pyodermas.

CONTRAINDICATIONS
Known sensitization to any of the components of this preparation is a contraindication for use.

WARNINGS
Nitrofurazone has been shown to produce mammary tumors when fed at high doses to female Sprague-Dawley rats. The relevance of this to topical use in humans is unknown.
Furacin Soluble Dressing should be used with caution in patients with known or suspected renal impairment. The polyethylene glycols in the base can be absorbed through denuded skin and may not be excreted normally by the compromised kidney. This may lead to symptoms of progressive renal impairment such as increased BUN, anion gap, and metabolic acidosis. (NOTE: Furacin (nitrofurazone) Topical Cream does not contain polyethylene glycols.)

PRECAUTIONS
General: Use of topical antimicrobials occasionally allows overgrowth of nonsusceptible organisms including fungi. If this occurs, or if irritation, sensitization or superinfection develops, treatment with Furacin Soluble Dressing should be discontinued and appropriate therapy instituted.
Carcinogenesis, mutagenesis, and impairment of fertility: Nitrofurazone has been shown to produce mammary tumors when fed at high doses to female Sprague-Dawley rats. The relevance of this to topical use in humans is unknown. Dietary dosage levels of 60 and 30 mg/kg/day shortened the onset time of the typical mammary gland tumors associated with older female rats. These tumors exhibited the same histological characteristics seen in the spontaneously occurring tumors, and were seen only in the female animals. No mammary tumors were seen in rats treated with nitrofurazone orally in the diet for 1 year at levels of approximately 11 mg/kg/day. Spermatogenic arrest was noted in the male rats in dietary dosage levels of 30 mg/kg/day and above, after one year on test.
Pregnancy: Pregnancy Category C: Nitrofurazone has been shown to have an embryocidal effect in rabbits when given in oral doses thirty times the human dose. There are no adequate and well controlled studies in pregnant women. Furacin Soluble Dressing should be used during pregnancy only if the potential benefit justifies the potential risk to the fetus.
Nursing mothers: It is not known whether this drug is excreted in human milk. Because many drugs are excreted in human milk and because of the potential for tumorigenicity shown for nitrofurazone in animal studies, a decision should

---

be made whether to discontinue nursing or to discontinue the drug, taking into account the importance of the drug to the mother.
Pediatric use: Safety and effectiveness in children have not been established.

ADVERSE REACTIONS
Instances of clinical skin reactions have been reported for patients treated with Furacin formulations. Symptoms appear as varying degrees of contact dermatitides such as rash, pruritus, and local edema. Although the exact incidence such reactions is difficult to determine, historically, a survey of world literature and clinical trials data indicates an overall incidence of approximately 1%. Allergic reactions to Furacin Soluble Dressing should be treated symptomatically.

DOSAGE AND ADMINISTRATION
Burns: Apply directly to the lesion with a spatula, or first place on gauze. Impregnated gauze may be used. Reapply depending on the preferred dressing technique. Flushing the dressing with sterile saline facilitates its removal.

PREPARATION OF IMPREGNATED GAUZE
Sterile gauze strips are placed in a tray and covered with Furacin Soluble Dressing. Repeat the procedure, adding several layers of gauze for each layer of Furacin Soluble Dressing. Sprinkling a little sterile water on each layer of dressing will minimize any color change from autoclaving. Cover the tray very loosely and autoclave at 121°C for 30 minutes at 15 to 20 pounds pressure. To impregnate bandage rolls, place some Furacin Soluble Dressing in the bottom of a glass jar. Stand rolls on end. Place more Furacin Soluble Dressing on top. Cover top of jar with aluminum foil. Autoclave at 121°C for 45 minutes to 20 pounds pressure. Do not store impregnated bandage rolls for more than 24 hours. Autoclaving more than once is not recommended.

HOW SUPPLIED
Furacin Soluble Dressing is available in:
NDC 54092-310-28 tube of 28 grams
NDC 54092-310-56 tube of 56 grams
NDC 54092-310-16 jar of 454 grams

ANIMAL TOXICOLOGY
The oral administration of nitrofurazone for 7 days to rats at extremely high dosage levels of 240 mg/kg/day produced severe hepatorenal lesions whereas only renal changes were seen when the dosage level was reduced to 60 mg/kg/day for 60 days. Dogs treated orally with nitrofurazone for 400 days at levels of 11 mg/kg/day showed no toxic effects related to drug treatment. The single intravenous administration in dogs of 20, 35, or 75 mg/kg nitrofurazone produced clinical signs of lacrimation, salivation, emesis, diarrhea, excitation, weakness, ataxia, and weight loss, whereas 100 mg/kg/day produced convulsions and death. There was no evidence of toxicosis in rhesus monkeys treated with doses of nitrofurazone as high as 58 mg/kg/day for 10 weeks and 23 mg/kg/day for 63 weeks. The peroral LD 50 of nitrofurazone in mice and rats is 747 and 590 mg/kg/respectively. For bacterial sensitivity tests: Furacin Sensi-Discs are available from BBL, Division of BioQuest.
Revised May 1991
Manufactured for:
Roberts Laboratories, Inc.
a wholly owned subsidiary of
Roberts Pharmaceutical Corporation
Eatontown, New Jersey 07724
　　Shown in Product Identification Section, page 425

FURACIN® TOPICAL CREAM　　　　　Ⓡ
[fewr 'a-sin]
(nitrofurazone)

DESCRIPTION
Chemically, Furacin is nitrofurazone, 2-[(5-nitro-2- furanyl) methylene]hydrazinecarboxamide, with the following structure:

$$O_2N \quad \quad CH = NNHCONH_2$$

Furacin Topical Cream is a preparation containing 0.2% Furacin in a water-miscible base consisting of glycerin, cetyl alcohol, mineral oil, an ethoxylated fatty alcohol, methylparaben, propylparaben, and purified water.
Furacin Topical Cream is an antibacterial agent for topical use.

CLINICAL PHARMACOLOGY
Furacin Topical Cream is a nitrofuran that is bactericidal for most pathogens commonly causing surface infections, including *Staphylococcus aureus, Streptococcus, Escherichia coli, Clostridium perfringens, Aerobacter aerogenes,* and *Proteus.*

Furacin Topical Cream inhibits a number of bacterial enzymes, especially those involved in the aerobic and anaerobic degradation of glucose and pyruvate. The activity appears to involve the pyruvate dehydrogenase system as well as citrate synthetase, malate dehydrogenase, glutathione reductase, and pyruvate decarboxylase. Glutathion reductase inhibition may be caused by control of pentose phosphate metabolism. Although Furacin Topical Cream inhibits a variety of enzymes, it is not considered to be a general enzyme inactivator since many enzymes are not inhibited by this compound.

INDICATIONS AND USAGE

Furacin Topical Cream is a topical antibacterial agent indicated for adjunctive therapy of patients with second- and third-degree burns when bacterial resistance to other agents is a real or potential problem.

It is also indicated in skin grafting where bacterial contamination may cause graft rejection and/or donor site infection particularly in hospitals with historical resistant-bacteria epidemics.

There is no known evidence of effectiveness of this product in the treatment of minor burns or surface bacterial infections involving wounds, cutaneous ulcers or the various pyodermas.

CONTRAINDICATIONS

Known sensitization to any of the components of this preparation is a contraindication for use.

WARNINGS

None

PRECAUTIONS

General: Use of Furacin Topical Cream occasionally allows overgrowth of nonsusceptible organisms including fungi and *Pseudomonas*. If this occurs, or if irritation, sensitization or superinfection develops, treatment with Furacin Topical Cream should be discontinued and appropriate therapy instituted.

Information for Patients: Patients should be told to use Furacin Topical Cream only as directed by a physician. Patients should be advised to discontinue the drug and contact a physician should rash or irritation occur.

Carcinogenesis, Mutagenesis, and Impairment of Fertility: Nitrofurazone has been shown to produce mammary tumors when fed at high doses to female Sprague-Dawley rats. The relevance of this to topical use in humans is unknown.

Dietary dosage levels of 60 and 30 mg/kg/day shortened the onset time of the typical mammary gland tumors associated with older female rats. These tumors exhibited the same histological characteristics seen in the spontaneously occurring tumors, and were seen only in the female animals. No mammary tumors were seen in rats treated with nitrofurazone orally in the diet for 1 year at levels approximately 11 mg/kg/day. Spermatogenic arrest was noted in the male rats in dietary dosage levels of 30 mg/kg/day and above, after one year on test.

Pregnancy: Pregnancy Category C: Nitrofurazone, when administered orally to pregnant rabbits, caused a slight increase in the frequency of still-births when given in doses thirty times the human dose. There are no adequate and well controlled studies in pregnant women. Furacin Topical Cream should be used during pregnancy only if the potential benefit justifies the potential risk to the fetus.

Nursing Mothers: It is not known whether this drug is excreted in human milk. Because many drugs are excreted in human milk and because of the potential for tumorigenicity shown for nitrofurazone in animal studies, a decision should be made whether to discontinue nursing or to discontinue the drug, taking into account the importance of the drug to the mother.

ADVERSE REACTIONS

Instances of clinical skin reactions have been reported for patients treated with Furacin formulations. Symptoms appear as varying degrees of contact dermatitides such as rash, pruritus, and local edema. Although the exact incidence of such reactions is difficult to determine, historically, a survey of world literature and clinical trials data indicates an overall incidence of approximately 1%. Allergic reactions to Furacin Topical Cream should be treated symptomatically.

DOSAGE AND ADMINISTRATION

Apply Furacin Topical Cream directly to the lesion, or first place on gauze. Reapply once daily or every few days, depending on the usual dressing technique.

HOW SUPPLIED

Furacin Topical Cream is available in:
NDC 54092-311-28 tube of 28 grams

Storage: Avoid exposure to direct sunlight, strong fluorescent lighting, alkaline materials, and excessive heat (over 104°F or 40°C).

ANIMAL TOXICOLOGY

The oral administration of nitrofurazone for 7 days to rats at extremely high dosage levels of 240 mg/kg/day produced severe hepatorenal lesions whereas only renal changes were seen when the dosage level was reduced to 60 mg/kg/day for 60 days. Dogs treated orally with nitrofurazone for 400 days at levels of 11 mg/kg/day showed no toxic effects related to drug treatment. There was no evidence of toxicosis in rhesus monkeys treated with doses of nitrofurazone as high as 58 mg/kg/day 10 weeks and 23 mg/kg/day for 63 weeks. The peroral LD_{50} of nitrofurazone in mice and rats is 747 and 590 mg/kg respectively. For bacterial sensitivity tests: Furacin Sensi-Discs are available from BBL, Division of BioQuest.

CAUTION

Federal law prohibits dispensing without prescription.
Revised May 1991
Manufactured for:
Roberts Laboratories, Inc.
or wholly owned subsidiary of
Roberts Pharmaceutical Corporation
Eatontown, New Jersey 07724

FURACIN® Topical Solution 0.2%, USP ℞

Furacin® Topical Solution is a preparation containing 0.2% nitrofurazone in polyethylene glycol 400, polyethylene glycol 4000, octoxynol-9 and purified water.

Chemically, nitrofurazone is 5 Nitro-2-furaldehyde semicarbazone. The structural formula is as follows:

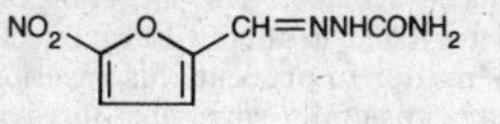

NO2
O
CH=NNHCONH2

M.W.—198.14
$C_6H_6N_4O_4$

Furazone solution is an antibacterial agent for topical use.

CLINICAL PHARMACOLOGY

Nitrofurazone is a nitrofuran that is bactericidal for most pathogens commonly causing surface infections, including Staphylococcus aureus, Streptococcus, Escherichia coli, Clostridium perfringens, Aerobacter aerogenes, and Proteus.

Furacin® solution inhibits a number of bacterial enzymes, especially those involved in the aerobic and anaerobic degradation of glucose and pyruvate. The activity appears to involve the pyruvate dehydrogenase system as well as citrate synthetase, malate dehydrogenase, glutathione reductase, and pyruvate decarboxylase. Glutathione reductase inhibition may be caused by control of pentose phosphate metabolism.

Although Furacin solution inhibits a variety of enzymes, it is not considered to be a general enzyme inactivator since many enzymes are not inhibited by this compound.

INDICATIONS AND USAGE

Furacin solution is a topical antibacterial agent indicated for adjunctive therapy of patients with second-and third- degree burns when bacterial resistance to other agents is a real or potential problem. It is also indicated in skin grafting where bacterial contamination may cause graft rejection and/or donor site infection particularly in hospitals with historical resistant-bacteria epidemics. There is no known evidence of effectivemess of this product in the treatment of minor burns or surface bacterial infections involving wounds, cutaneous ulcers, or the various pyodermas.

CONTRAINDICATIONS

Known sensitization to any of the components of this preparation is a contraindication for use.

WARNINGS

Nitrofurazone has been shown to produce mammary tumors when fed at high doses to female Sprague-Dawley rats. The relevance of this to topical use in humans is unknown. Nitrofurazone preparations should be used with caution in patients with known or suspected renal impairment. The polyethylene glycols in the base can be absorbed through denuded skin and may not be excreted normally by the compromised kidney. This may lead to symptoms of progressive renal impairment such as increased BUN, anion gap, and metabolic acidosis.

PRECAUTIONS

General: Use of topical antimicrobials occasionally allows overgrowth of nonsusceptible organisms including fungi. If this occurs, or if irritation sensitization or superinfection develops, treatment with furazone preparations should be discontinued and appropriate therapy instituted.

Carcinogensis, Mutagenesis, and Impairment of Fertility: Nitrofurazone has been shown to produce mammary tumors when fed at high doses to female Sprague-Dawley rats. The relevance of this to topical use in humans is unknown. Dietary dosage levels of 60 and 30 mg/kg/day shortened the onset time of the typical mammary gland tumors associated with other female rats. These tumors exhibited the same histological characteristics seen in the spontaneously occurring tumors, and were seen only in the female animals. No mammary tumors were seen in rats treated with furazone orally in the diet for 1 year at levels of approximately 11 mg/kg/day. Spermatogenic arrest was noted in the male rats in dietary dosage levels of 30 mg/kg/day and above, after one year on test.

Usage in Pregnancy: Pregnancy Category C: Nitrofurazone has been shown to have an embryocidal effect in rabbits when given in oral doses thirty times the human dose. There are no adequate and well controlled studies in pregnant women. Nitrofurazone preparations should be used during pregnancy only if the potential benefit justifies the potential risk to the fetus. **Nursing Mothers:** It is not known whether this drug is excreted in human milk. Because many drugs are excreted in human milk and because of the potential for tumorigenicity shown for nitrofurazone in animal studies, a decision should be made whether to discontinue nursing or to discontinue the drug, taking into account the importance of the drug to the mother. **Pediatric Use:** Safety and effectiveness in children have not been established.

ADVERSE REACTIONS

In quantitative studies published during the period 1945–70, 206 instances of clinical skin reaction were reported out of 18,249 patients (an incidence of 1.1%) treated with nitrofurazone formulations. Symptoms appeared as varying degrees of contact dermatitides such as rash, pruritus, and local edema. Allergic reactions to nitrofurazone preparations should be treated symptomatically.

DOSAGE AND ADMINISTRATION

Burns: Apply Furacin Topical Solution directly to the lesion, or first place on gauze. Impregnated gauze may be used. Reapply depending on the preferred dressing technique. Flushing the dressing with sterile saline facilitates its removal. Preparation of Impregnated Gauze: Sterile gauze strips are placed in a tray and covered with Furacin® Solution. Repeat the procedure, adding several layers of gauze for each layer of Furacin® Solution. Sprinkling a little sterile water on each layer of dressing will minimize any color change from autoclaving. Cover the tray very loosely and autoclave at 121°C for 30 minutes at 15 to 20 pounds pressure. To impregnate bandage rolls, place some Furacin® Solution in the Bottom of a glass jar. Stand rolls on end. Place more Furacin Solution on top. Cover top of jar with aluminum foil. Autoclave at 121°C for 45 minutes at 15 to 20 pounds pressure. Do not store impregnated bandage rolls for more than 24 hours. Autoclaving more than once is not recommended.

ANIMAL TOXICOLOGY

The oral administration of nitrofurazone for 7 days to rats at extremely high dosage levels of 240 mg/kg/day produced severe hepatorenal lesions whereas only renal changes were seen when the dosage level was reduced to 60 mg/kg/days for 60 days. Dogs treated orally with nitrofurazone for 400 days at levels of 11 mg/kg/day showed no toxic effects related to drug treatment. The single intravenous administration in dogs of 20, 35 and 75 mg/kg nitrofurazone produced clinical signs of lacrimation, salivation, emesis, diarrhea, excitation, weakness, ataxia, and weight loss, whereas 100 mg/kg/day for 10 weeks and 23 mg/kg/day for 63 weeks. The peroral LD_{50} of nitrofurazone in mice and rats is 747 and 590 mg/kg respectively.

CAUTION

Federal law prohibits dispensing without prescription.

HOW SUPPLIED

Furacin® Topical Solution 0.2%: 16 oz. bottles, NDC 54092-312-16.

FOR EXTERNAL USE ONLY
KEEP OUT OF REACH OF CHILDREN
KEEP AWAY FROM EXCESSIVE HEAT AND SUNLIGHT

Manufactured for:
Roberts Laboratories, Inc.
a wholly owned subsidiary of
Roberts Pharmaceutical Corporation
Eatontown, New Jersey 07724

FUROXONE® ℞

[fewr-ox 'ōne]
(furazolidone)
Tablets and Liquid

DESCRIPTION

Furoxone (furazolidone) is one of the synthetic antimicrobial nitrofurans. It is a stable, yellow, crystalline compound with the following structure:

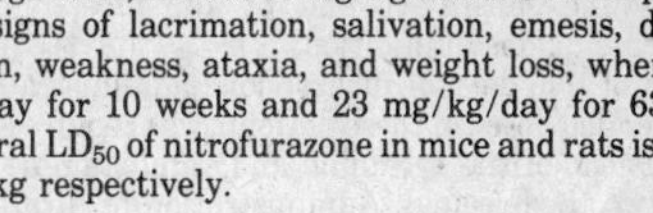

O2N
O
CH=N—N
C=O
O
H2C
CH2

3-(5-nitrofurfurylideneamino)-2-oxazolidinone

Inactive Ingredients: Furoxone tablets contain calcium pyrophosphate, FD&C Blue #2, magnesium stearate, starch, and sucrose. Furoxone liquid contains carboxymethylcellu-

Continued on next page

Roberts—Cont.

lose sodium, flavors, glycerin, magnesium aluminum silicate, methylparaben, propylparaben, purified water, and saccharin sodium.

ACTION

Furoxone has a broad antibacterial spectrum covering the majority of gastrointestinal tract pathogens including *E. coli*, staphylococci, *Salmonella, Shigella, Proteus, Aerobacter aerogenes, Vibrio cholerae* [9,10,11] and *Giardia lamblia*. [5,6] Its bactericidal activity is based upon its interference with several bacterial enzyme systems; this antimicrobial action minimizes the development of resistant organisms. It neither significantly alters the normal bowel flora nor results in fungal overgrowth. The brown color found in the urine with adequate dosage is of no clinical significance.

INDICATIONS

Indicated in the specific and symptomatic treatment of bacterial or protozoal diarrhea and enteritis caused by susceptible organisms. Furoxone products are well tolerated, have a very low incidence of adverse reactions.

CONTRAINDICATIONS

Furoxone is contraindicated in patients with known hypersensitivity to furazolidine and in patients with glucose and phosphate dehydrogenase deficiency. It is contraindicated in infants under one month.

WARNINGS

Use In Pregnancy: The safety of Furoxone during the childbearing age has not been established; as with any potent antibacterial, Furoxone must be administered with caution during the childbearing age. However, animal breeding studies have revealed no evidence of teratogenicity following the administration of Furoxone for long periods of time and at doses far in excess of those recommended for the human. There have been no clinical reports regarding this possible adverse effect on the fetus or the newborn infant.

Furoxone concentration in breast milk of lactating mothers has not been established, therefore safety of this drug in this circumstance has not been established. Caution should be exercised while prescribing Furoxone to nursing mothers.

PRECAUTIONS AND DRUG INTERACTIONS

A disulfiram like reaction may occur in patients ingesting alcohol while taking Furoxone. Alcohol should be avoided during or within four days after Furoxone therapy.

Monoamine Oxidase Inhibition:[7] Effective inhibition of monoamine oxidase by furazolidone has been demonstrated experimentally in man by the enhancement of tyramine and amphetamine sensitivity and by the directly measured monoamine oxidase inhibition.

A period of five days of furazolidone administration in the recommended doses in these patients was required to give an enhancement of the tyramine and amphetamine sensitivities by two to threefold. Administration of furazolidone in the recommended dose of 400 mg/day for a period of five days should not subject the adult patient to an undue hazard of hypertensive crisis due to monoamine oxidase inhibition. Hypertensive crises have never been reported even after the peroral administration of larger doses and/or for longer periods of time. Controlled studies reveal no signs or symptoms of hypertensive crisis even after the peroral administration of Furoxone in doses of 400 mg/day in excessive of 48 consecutive months.[8]

If administered in doses larger than recommended or in excess of five days, the indications must be weighed against the possible hazards of hypertensive crisis related to the accumulation of monoamine oxidase inhibition. If indications are sufficient, the patients should be informed of drugs and foods which predispose to hypertensive crises:

(A) Other known MAOI drugs; however, when indicated they should be prescribed with caution and at a reduced dosage.

(B) Tyramine-containing foods such as broad beans, yeast extracts, strong unpasteurized cheeses, beer, wine, pickled herring, chicken livers, and fermented products are contraindicated.

(C) Indirectly-acting sympathomimetic amines such as those found in nasal decongestants (phenylephrine, ephedrine) and anorectics (amphetamines) are contraindicated.

(D) Likewise, sedatives, antihistamines, tranquilizers, and narcotics should be used in reduced dosages and with caution.

Orthostatic hypotension and hypoglycemia may occur.

Carcinogenesis, Mutagenesis, Impairment of Fertility: Furazolidone has shown evidence of tumorigenic activity in several studies involving chronic, high-dose oral administration to rodents. Promotion of the development of mammary neoplasia has been demonstrated in rats of two strains. Prominent among the findings in mice was that furazolidone caused significant increases in malignant lung tumors. The relevance of these animal findings, particularly in relationship to short-term therapy in humans, is not established.

ADVERSE REACTIONS

A few hypersensitivity reactions to Furoxone have been reported including a fall in blood pressure, urticaria, fever, arthralgia, and a vesicular morbilliform rash. These reactions subsided following withdrawal of the drug.

Nausea, emesis, headache, or malaise occur occasionally and may be minimized or eliminated by reduction in dosage or withdrawal of the drug.

Rarely, individuals receiving Furoxone have exhibited an Antabuse® (disulfiram)-like reaction to alcohol characterized by flushing, slight temperature elevation, dyspnea, and in some instances, a sense of constriction within the chest. All symptomatology disappeared within 24 hours with no lasting ill effects. During nine years of clinical use and approximately 3.5 million courses of therapy (in the U.S.A. alone) in the published literature and documented case reports 43 cases have been reported—of which 14 were produced under experimental conditions with planned doses of the compound in excess of those recommended.

Three of these experienced a fall in blood pressure necessitating active therapy. Indications are that levarterenol (Levophed®) may be used to combat such hypotensive episodes since human studies show that this drug is not potentiated in patients treated with Furoxone. (Indirectly acting pressor agents should be avoided.) The ingestion of alcohol in any form should be avoided during Furoxone therapy and for four days thereafter to prevent this reaction.

Furoxone may cause mild reversible intravascular hemolysis in certain ethnic groups of Mediterranean and Near-Eastern origin, and Negroes.[1,3] This is due to an intrinsic defect of red blood cell metabolism in a small percentage of these ethnic groups, making them unusually susceptible to hemolysis by numerous compounds.[2] It is necessary to observe such patients closely while receiving Furoxone and to discontinue its use if there is any indication of hemolysis.

Should not be administered to infants under 1 month of age because of the possibility of producing a hemolytic anemia due to immature enzyme systems (glutathione instability) in the early neonatal period.[4]

Colitis, proctitis, anal pruritus, staphylococcic enteritis, renal or hepatic toxicity have not been a significant problem with Furoxone.

DOSAGE AND ADMINISTRATION

FUROXONE TABLETS, 100 mg each, are green and scored to facilitate adjustment of dosage.

Average Adult Dosage: One 100-mg tablet four times daily.

Average Dosage for Children: Those 5 years of age or older should receive 25 to 50 mg (¼ to ½ tablet) four times daily. The tablet dosage may be crushed and given in a spoonful of corn syrup.

FUROXONE LIQUID composition: each 15 ml tablespoonful contains Furoxone 50 mg per 15 ml (3.33 mg per ml) in a light-yellow aqueous vehicle. Suitable flavoring, suspending and preservative agents complete the formulation. (See Inactive Ingredients.) It is stable in storage. Prior to administering Furoxone Liquid shake the bottle vigorously. It should be dispensed in amber bottles.

Average Adult Dosage: Two tablespoonfuls four times daily.

Average Dosage for Children:

5 years or older—½ to 1 tablespoonful four times daily (7.5–15.0 ml)

1 to 4 years old—1 to 1½ teaspoonfuls four times daily (5.0–7.5 ml)

1 month to 1 year—½ to 1 teaspoonful four times daily (2.5–5.0 ml)

In Giardiasis the usual adult dose is 100mg four times daily for 7 to 10 days. Children may be given 1.25mg/Kg body weight four times daily.

This dosage is based on an average dose of 5 mg of Furoxone per Kg (2.3 mg per lb) of body weight given in four equally divided doses during 24 hours. The maximal dose of 8.8 mg of Furoxone per Kg (4 mg per lb) of body weight per 24 hours should probably not be exceeded because of the possibility of producing nausea or emesis. If these are severe, the dosage should be reduced.

The average case of diarrhea treated with Furoxone will respond within 2 to 5 days of therapy. Occasional patients may require a longer term of therapy. If satisfactory clinical response is not obtained within 7 days it indicates that the pathogen is refractory to Furoxone and the drug should be discontinued. Adjunctive therapy with other antibacterial agents or bismuth salts is not contraindicated. (N.B. Refer to WARNINGS.)

In order to administer furazolidone in doses larger than recommended or in excess of five days the indications must be weighed against the possible hazards of hypertensive crisis related to the accumulation of monoamine oxidase inhibition. If indications are sufficient, the patient should be informed of drugs and foods which predispose to hypertensive crises. (See PRECAUTIONS.)

OVERDOSE

In case of accidental overdosage, supportive and or symptomatic therapy should be provided. Induction of vomiting or gastric laverage may be required. Vomiting should not be induced in unconscious patients or in children under one year of age.

HOW SUPPLIED

Furoxone Tablets, 100mg each, codes "Eaton 072", are supplied in amber bottles containing 20 tablets NDC 54092–130–20 and 100 tablets NDC 54092–130–01. (Should be dispensed in amber bottles.)

Furoxone Liquid is supplied in amber bottles containing 60 ml NDC 54092–430–60 and 473 ml NDC 54092–430–16. (Should be dispensed in amber bottles.)

REFERENCES

1 Kellermeyer, R.S., Tarlov, A.R., Schrier, S.L., and Alving, A.S.J. Lab. Clin. Med. 52:827–828 (Nov) 1958.
2 Tarlov et al. Arch. Int. Med. 109:209–204, 1962.
3 Kellermeyer et al. J.A.M.A. 180: No. 5, 388–394, 1962.
4 Zinkham, Pediatrics 23:18–32, 1959; Gross & Hurwitz, Pediatrics 22:453, 1958.
5 Fallas Vargas, M.un Nuevo Tratamiento para la Giardiasis (A New Treatment for Giardiasis). Rev. Med. Costa Rica 19:269–284 (July) 1962.
6 Webster, B. H. Furazolidone in the Treatment of Giardiasis. Amer. J. Dig. Diseases 5:618–622 (July) 1960.
7 Oates, J.A., Pettinger, W.A. Inhibition of Monoamine Oxidase by Furazolidone in Man. Data on file: Office of the Medical Director, Roberts Pharmaceutical, Corp. Available upon request.
8 Kirsner, Joseph B., M.D., Ph.D. Data on file: Office of the Medical Director, Roberts Pharmaceutical, Corp. Available upon request.
9 Neogy, K.N., et al. Furazolidone in Cholera, Journ. Indian Med. Assoc. 48:137, 1967.
10 Chaudhuri, R.N. et al. Furazolidone in Cholera, Lancet 2:909 (Oct 30) 1965.
11 Curlin, G. Comparison of Antibiotic Regimens in Cholera. Abstracts of papers, Epidemiological Intelligence Service Conference, Atlanta, Ga., April 11–14, 1967, p. 11.

FUROXONE (FURAZOLIDONE) SENSI-DISCS for laboratory determination of bacterial sensitivity are available from BBL, division of BioQuest.

CAUTION

Federal law prohibits dispensing without prescription.
Revised May 1991
Manufactured for:
Roberts Laboratories, Inc.
a wholly owned subsidiary of
Roberts Pharmaceutical Corporation
Eatontown, New Jersey 07724

Shown in Product Identification Section, page 425

ROMYCIN™ (erythromycin)　　　　　　　　　　　　℞
Topical Solution USP, 2%

DESCRIPTION

Erythromycin is an antibiotic produced from a strain of Streptomyces erytheus. It is basic and readily forms salts with acids.

Contains: erythromycin USP 2% (20mg/ml)
with SD Alcohol 40-A (66%), propylene glycol, and citric acid to adjust pH.

CLINICAL PHARMACOLOGY

Although the mechanism by which Romycin (erythromycin) Topical Solution acts in reducing inflammatory lesions of acne vulgaris is unknown, it is presumably due to its antibiotic action.

INDICATIONS AND USAGE

Romycin™ (erythromycin) Topical Solution is indicated for the topical control of acne vulgaris.

CONTRAINDICATIONS

Romycin™ (erythromycin) Topical Solution is contraindicated in persons who have shown hypersensitivity to erythromycin or any of the other listed ingredients.

WARNING

The safe use of Romycin™ (erythromycin) Topical Solution during pregnancy or lactation has not been established.

PRECAUTIONS

General: The use of antibiotic agents may be associated with the overgrowth of antibiotic-resistant organisms. If this occurs, administration of this drug should be discontinued and appropriate measures taken.

Information for patients: Romycin™ (erythromycin) Topical Solution is for external use only and should be kept away from the eyes, nose, mouth and other mucous membranes. Concomitant topical acne therapy should be used with caution because a cumulative irritant effect may occur, especially with the use of peeling, desquamating or abrasive agents.

Carcinogenesis, Mutagenesis, Impairment of Fertility: Long-term animal studies to evaluate carcinogenic potential, mu-

tagenicity or the effect on fertility of erythromycin have not been performed.

Pregnancy: Pregnancy Category C. Animal reproduction studies have not been conducted with erythromycin. It is also not known whether erythromycin can cause fetal harm when administered to a pregnant woman or can effect reproduction capacity. Erythromycin should be given to a pregnant woman only if clearly needed.

Nursing Mothers: Erythromycin is excreted in breast milk. Caution should be exercised when erythromycin is administered to a nursing woman.

ADVERSE REACTIONS

Adverse conditions reported with the use of erythromycin topical solutions include dryness, tenderness, pruritus, desquamation, erythema, oiliness, and burning sensation. Irritation of the eyes has also been reported. A case of generalized urticarial reaction, possibly related to the drug, which required the use of systemic steroid therapy had been reported.

DOSAGE AND ADMINISTRATION

Romycin (erythromycin) Topical Solution should be applied to the affected area(s) each morning and evening after the skin is thoroughly washed with warm water and soap and patted dry. Use enough solution to thoroughly wet the affected area(s). The hands should be washed after application. When using the Dab-O-Matic applicator to apply Romycin (erythromycin) Topical Solution, it should be moistened first by holding the bottle upside down and pressing once on the applicator surface with a clean finger. Then, Romycin (erythromycin) Topical Solution can be applied with the applicator to the affected area(s) using a dabbing motion. The bottle should be closed tightly after each use.

HOW SUPPLIED

Romycin (erythromycin) Topical Solution USP, 2% is supplied in a 60ml plastic bottle with optional Dab-O-Matic applicator. NDC 54092-316-60.

Note: FLAMMABLE. Keep away from heat and flame. Store in tight, light-resistant container at controlled room temperature, 15° to 30°C (59° to 86°).

CAUTION

Federal law prohibits dispensing without prescription.
Manufactured for:
Roberts Laboratories, Inc.
a wholly owned subsidiary of
ROBERTS PHARMACEUTICAL CORPORATION
Eatontown, New Jersey 07724
Copyright °1992 Roberts Laboratories, Inc.

SINUFED TIMECELLES   ℞

DESCRIPTION

Each capsule contains:
Pseudoephedrine hydrochloride .... 60 mg.
  in a specially prepared base to provide
  prolonged action
Guaifenesin ....300 mg.
  designed for immediate release to provide rapid action.
CAUTION: Federal law prohibits dispensing without prescription.
This product contains ingredients of the following therapeutic classes: decongestant and expectorant.

CLINICAL PHARMACOLOGY

Pseudoephedrine hydrochloride is a sympathomimetic which acts predominantly on alpha receptors and has little action on beta receptors. It therefore functions as an oral nasal decongestant with minimal CNS stimulation. This product is designed to release the pseudoephedrine hydrochloride gradually over a period of 5 to 7 hours resulting in activity up to 10 to 12 hours. Guaifenesin is an expectorant which thins the mucous in the bronchial tract due to a reflex action in the stomach. The guaifenesin, therefore, is not in sustained release form. It is available immediately to trigger the reflex action.

INDICATIONS

For temporary relief of nasal congestion and dry non-productive cough associated with the common cold and other respiratory allergies.

CONTRAINDICATIONS

This product is contraindicated in patients with a known hypersensitivity to any of its ingredients. Also contraindicated in patients with severe hypertension, severe coronary artery disease and patients on MAO inhibitor therapy. Should not be used in nursing mothers.

WARNINGS

Considerable caution should be exercised in patients with hypertension, diabetes mellitus, ischemic heart disease, hyperthyroidism and prostatic hypertrophy. The elderly (60 years or older) are more likely to exhibit adverse reactions.

At doses higher than the recommended dose, nervousness, dizziness or sleeplessness may occur.

PRECAUTIONS

General: Caution should be exercised in patients with high blood pressure, heart disease, diabetes or thyroid disease.
Drug Interactions: MAO inhibitors and beta adrenergic blockers increase the effects of sympathomimetics. Sympathomimetics may reduce the antihypertensive effect of methyldopa, mecamylamine, reserpine and veratrum alkaloids.
Guaifenesin has been shown to produce a color interference with certain clinical laboratory determinations of 5 hydroxyindoleacetic acid (5-H1AA) and vanillyl mandelic acid (VMA).
Pregnancy: The safety of use of this product in pregnancy has not been established, however, pregnant women should seek the advice of a physician before taking this product.

ADVERSE REACTIONS

Adverse reactions include nausea, cardiac palpitations, increased irritability or excitement, headache, dizziness and tachycardia.

DOSAGE AND ADMINISTRATION

Adults and children over 12 years of age: 1 or 2 capsules orally every 12 hours. Children 6 to 12 years of age: one capsule orally every 12 hours.

HOW SUPPLIED

Imprinted Green and clear capsule in Bottles of 100 NDC 54092-151-01
STORE AND DISPENSE IN TIGHT CONTAINERS AND DEFINED IN THE USP/NF.
STORE BETWEEN 15–30°C (59–86°F)
DISPENSE IN CHILD RESISTANT CONTAINERS.

Manufactured for:
Roberts Laboratories, Inc.
a wholly owned subsidiary of
Roberts Pharmaceutical Corporation
Eatontown, New Jersey 07724

SINUMIST–SR CAPSULETS®   ℞
(Guaifenesin)

DESCRIPTION

Each green speckled capsule-shaped sustained release Capsulet® provides 600 mg guaifenesin.

HOW SUPPLIED

Each SINUMIST-SR CAPSULET® is imprinted HAUCK 048.
NDC 54092-152-01 Bottle of 100.

SUPPRELIN™ (histrelin acetate) INJECTION   ℞

DESCRIPTION

SUPPRELIN™ (histrelin acetate) Injection contains a synthetic nonapeptide agonist of the naturally occurring gonadotropin releasing hormone (GnRH or LHRH). The analog possesses a greater potency than the natural sequence hormone. The amino acid sequence and chemical name of histrelin acetate is:
5-oxo-L-prolyl-L-histidyl-L-tryptophyl-L-seryl-L-tyrosyl-N^t-benzyl-D-histidyl-L-leucyl-L-arginyl-N-ethyl-L-prolinamide acetate (salt) $[C_{66}H_{86}N_{18}O_{12} \cdot (1.7–2.8 \text{ moles}) CH_3COOH \cdot (0.6–7.0 \text{ moles}) H_2O]$.
The molecular weight of the peptide base is 1323.52.
SUPPRELIN™ Injection is a sterile, aqueous solution for subcutaneous administration available in single-use vials of 0.6 mL. It contains histrelin equivalent to either 200 mcg/mL, 500 mcg/mL, or 1000 mcg/mL peptide base with 0.9% sodium chloride and 10% mannitol. The pH of the 200 mcg/mL solution is 4.5–6.5 and the pH of the 500 mcg/mL and 1000 mcg/mL solutions is 4.5–6.0. All solutions are unbuffered, hypertonic and contain no preservative.

CLINICAL PHARMACOLOGY

SUPPRELIN™ Injection, a GnRH agonist, is a potent inhibitor of gonadotropin secretion when administered daily in therapeutic doses. Both animal and human studies indicate that following an initial stimulatory phase, chronic, subcutaneous administration of histrelin acetate desensitizes responsiveness of the pituitary gonadotropin which, in turn, causes a reduction in ovarian and testicular steroidogenesis. Although animal studies have shown that *acute* administration of SUPPRELIN™ (histrelin acetate) Injection results in stimulation of the reproductive system, *chronic* SUPPRELIN™ Injection administration in the rat delays sexual development, inhibits estrous cyclicity and pregnancy, reduces reproductive organ weight and inhibits ovarian and testicular steroidogenesis in a reversible fashion. In the rabbit, chronic administration of SUPPRELIN Injection resulted in decreased reproductive organ weights.

In human studies, chronic administration of SUPPRELIN™ Injection controls the secretion of pituitary gonadotropins resulting in decreased sex steroid levels and in the regression of secondary sexual characteristics in children with precocious puberty. In girls, menses cease, serum estradiol levels are decreased to prepubertal levels, linear growth velocities decrease, skeletal maturation is slowed and adult height predictions increase. In boys, testicular steroidogenesis is inhibited and testicular volume is reduced.

Continuous SUPPRELIN™ Injection administration to patients with central precocious puberty can be monitored by standard GnRH testing and by serial determinations of sex steroid levels. The decreases in LH, FSH, and sex steroid levels are evident within three months of the initiation of therapy. These effects have been demonstrated in the 10 female patients who were studied for periods up to eighteen months. The metabolism, distribution, and excretion of SUPPRELIN™ Injection in humans have not been determined.

INDICATIONS AND USAGE

SUPPRELIN™ Injection is indicated for the control of the biochemical and clinical manifestations of central precocious puberty.
Selection of Patients

1. Only patients with centrally mediated precocious puberty (either idiopathic or neurogenic and occurring before age 8 years in girls or 9.5 years in boys) should receive SUPPRELIN™ Injection treatment.
2. Before treatment with SUPPRELIN™ (histrelin acetate) Injection is instituted, a thorough physical and endocrinologic evaluation should be performed. This should include:
a. Height and weight as baseline for serial monitoring.
b. Hand and wrist x-ray for bone age determination, to document advanced skeletal age and as baseline for serially monitoring predicted height.
c. Total sex steriod level (estradiol or testosterone).
d. Adrenal steroid level, to exclude congenital adrenal hyperplasia.
e. Beta-Human Chorionic Gonadotropin level, to rule out a chorionic gonadotropin-secreting tumor.
f. GnRH stimulation test, to demonstrate activation of the Hypothalamic-Pituitary-Gonadal (HPG) axis.
g. Pelvic/adrenal/testicular ultrasound, to rule out a steroid-secreting tumor and to document gonadal size for serial monitoring.
h. Computerized tomography of the head, to rule out previously undiagnosed intracranial tumor.
3. Patients must be able to maintain compliance with a *daily* regimen of injections.

CONTRAINDICATIONS

SUPPRELIN™ Injection should not be administered to patients known to be hypersensitive to any of its components.
SUPPRELIN™ Injection is contraindicated in women who are or may become pregnant while receiving the drug and in nursing mothers. There was increased fetal size and mortality in rats and increased fetal mortality in rabbits but not in mice after SUPPRELIN™ Injection administration. Other responses to SUPPRELIN™ Injection included dystocia, a greater incidence of unilateral hydroureter, and incomplete ossification in rat fetuses in all treated groups. When administered to rabbits on days 6–18 of pregnancy at doses of 20 to 80 mcg/kg/day (2 to 8 times the human dose), SUPPRELIN™ Injection produced early termination of pregnancy and increased fetal death. In rats administered SUPPRELIN Injection on days 7–20 of pregnancy at doses of 1 to 15 mcg/kg/day (0.1 to 1.5 times the human dose) there was an increase in fetal resorptions. In mice treated on days 6–15 of pregnancy at 10 to 100 times the human dose, Supprelin Injection had no adverse effects. The effects on fetal mortality are expected consequences of the alterations in hormonal levels brought about by the drug. If this drug is inadvertently used during pregnancy or in the rare event that a patient becomes pregnant while taking this drug, she should be apprised of the potential hazard to the fetus.
It is not known if this drug is excreted in human milk, but because many drugs are excreted in human milk and because of the potential for serious adverse reactions in nursing infants from SUPPRELIN™, the drug should not be given to nursing mothers.

WARNINGS

Non-compliance with drug regimen or inadequate dosing may result in inadequate control of the pubertal process. The consequences of poor control include the return of pubertal signs such as menses, breast development, and testicular growth. The long-term consequences of inadequate control of gonadal steroid secretion are unknown, but may include a further compromise of adult stature.
Serious hypersensitivity reactions (angioedema, urticaria) have been reported following SUPPRELIN™ (histrelin acetate) Injection administration. Clinical manifestations may include: cardiovascular collapse, hypotension, tachycardia, loss of consciousness, angioedema, bronchospasm, dyspnea,

Continued on next page

Roberts—Cont.

urticaria, flushing and pruritus. If any allergic reaction occurs, therapy with SUPPRELIN™ should be discontinued. Serious acute hypersensitivity reactions may require emergency medical treatment.

PRECAUTIONS

General: Studies in rats and monkeys have indicated that all of the known biochemical and antifertility effects of SUPPRELIN™ Injection are reversible. Because animal studies are not always predictive of human response, and because children who have received SUPPRELIN™ Injection have not been followed sufficiently long to ensure reactivation of the HPG axis following long-term therapy, this drug should be used only when the benefits to the patient outweigh the potential risks. In addition, the patient (and/or guardian) should be advised that hypogonadism may result if the HPG axis fails to reactivate after the drug is discontinued.

Information to patient: Prior to SUPPRELIN™ Injection therapy, patients and their families should be informed of the importance of complying with the schedule of single, daily injections, given at approximately the same time each day. If injections are not given daily, the pubertal process may be reactivated. SUPPRELIN™ Injection contains no preservative. Patients should be informed that vials are to be used once and any unused solution is to be discarded. Medication should be allowed to reach room temperature before injecting. Daily injections should be rotated through different body sites (upper arms, thighs, abdomen).

Patients should be made aware of the required monitoring of their condition and of the potential risks of therapy. Within the first month of therapy, girls being treated with SUPPRELIN™ (histrelin acetate) Injection may experience a light menstrual flow. This menstrual flow is common and likely is related to the lower estrogen levels brought about by treatment, and the withdrawal of estrogen support from the endometrium.

Irritation, redness, or swelling at the injection sites may occur. If these reactions are severe, or do not go away, the patient's doctor should be notified.

The patients and their families should be advised to discontinue the drug and seek medical attention at the first sign of skin rash, urticaria, rapid heartbeat, difficulty in swallowing and breathing, or any swelling which may suggest angioedema (See Warnings and Adverse Reactions).

Clinical Evaluations/Laboratory Tests: An initial pelvic ultrasound should be performed to exclude other conditions before treating with SUPPRELIN™ Injection. The patient should be monitored carefully after 3 months and every 6 to 12 months thereafter by serial clinical evaluations, repeated height measurements, bone age determinations (yearly), and serial GnRH testing to document that gonadotropin responsiveness of the pituitary remains prepubertal while on therapy. During the initial agonistic phase of treatment, the patient may demonstrate transient increases in breast tissue, moodiness, vaginal secretions, or testicular volume. After this initial agonistic phase (usually one to three weeks), control of the biochemical and physical manifestations of puberty should remain as long as chronic therapy is in effect. Treatment should be discontinued when the onset of puberty is desired. Following the discontinuation of SUPPRELIN™ Injection treatment, the onset of normal puberty should be documented. In addition, patients should be monitored to assess menstrual cyclicity, reproductive function, and ultimate adult height.

Carcinogenesis, Mutagenesis, and Impairment of Fertility: Carcinogenicity studies were conducted in rats for 2 years at doses of 5, 25 or 150 mcg/kg/day (up to 15 times the human dose) and in mice for 18 months at doses of 20, 200, or 2000 mcg/kg/day (up to 200 times the human dose). As seen with other GnRH agonists, SUPPRELIN™ (histrelin acetate) Injection administration was associated with an increase in tumors of hormonally responsive tissues. There was a significant increase in pituitary adenomas in rats. There was an increase in pancreatic islet-cell adenomas in treated female rats and a non-dose-related increase in testicular Leydig-cell tumors (highest incidence in the low-dose group). In mice, there was a significant increase in mammary-gland adenocarcinomas in all treated females. In addition, there were increases in stomach papillomas in male rats given high doses, and an increase in histiocytic sarcomas in female mice at the highest dose.

Mutagenicity studies have not been performed. Fertility studies have been conducted in rats and monkeys given subcutaneous daily doses of SUPPRELIN™ Injection up to 180 mcg/kg for 6 months and full reversibility of fertility suppression was demonstrated. The development and reproductive performance of offspring from parents treated with SUPPRELIN Injection has not been investigated.

Pregnancy, Teratogenic effects: Pregnancy Category X. See "CONTRAINDICATIONS" section.

Nursing Mothers: See "CONTRAINDICATIONS" section.

Pediatric Use: Safety and effectiveness in children below the age of two years have not been established.

ADVERSE REACTIONS

At least one adverse experience was reported for 139 of the 183 (76%) children in clinical studies of central precocious puberty. Three of the 183 children (2%) stopped therapy due to a hypersensitivity reaction.

Adverse experience considered related or probably related to drug therapy included:

skin reactions at the medication site (redness, swelling, and itching)	45%
vaginal bleeding (usually only one episode within 1 to 3 weeks of starting therapy lasting several days)	22%
urticaria	4%
purpura	2%
convulsions (increased frequency)	2%
visual disturbances	2%
hot flashes/flushes	2%
edema (other than at medication site)	2%
mood changes	2%
erythema (other than at medication site)	1%
conduct disorder	1%

Other adverse experiences considered possibly related to drug therapy and reported in at least 1% of patients are as follows:

Cardiovascular: (1–3%)—palpitations, tachycardia, epistaxis, hypertension, migraine headache, pallor.

Endocrine: (6%)—leukorrhea; (1%)—goiter, hyperlipidemia, anemia, breast edema, breast pain, breast discharge, glycosuria

Gastrointestinal: (3–10%)—gastrointestinal pain, abdominal pain, nausea, vomiting, diarrhea; (1–3%)—GI cramps, GI distress, constipation, appetite decreased, thirsty

Miscellaneous: (14%)—pyrexia; (6%)—extremity pain; (1–3%)—fatigue, chills, malaise, neck or chest or trunk pain, viral infection

Musculoskeletal:(4%)—arthralgia; (1%)—pain, hypotonia

Nervous System: (22%)—headache; 1–3%)—somnolence, lethergy, dizziness impaired consciousness, syncope, tremor, hyperkinesia, nervousness, anxiety, depression

Respiratory: (3–10%)—cough, pharyngitis; (1–3%)—hyperventilation, upper respiratory infection

Skin: (7%)—rash; (1–3%—pruritus, dyschromia, keratoderma, alopecia, sweating

Special Senses: (1–3%)—abnormal pupillary function, otalgia, hearing loss, polyopia, photophobia

Urogenital: (1–3%)—irritation or odor or pruritus or infections of the female genitalia, polyuria, dysuria, urinary frequency, incontinence, hematuria, nocturia

Acute generalized (angioedema, urticaria) hypersensitivity reactions have been reported (See: Warnings and Precautions).

Other Patients

SUPPRELIN™ (histrelin acetate) injection has been studied in other patients for various indications (N=196). Adverse experiences occurring in 2% or more of the study population are:

Cardiovascular: (35%)—vasodilation; (3%)—edema, migraine headache, hypertension

Endocrine: (12%)—vaginal dryness; (3–10%)—metrorrhagia, breast pain, breast edema; (2–3%)—leukorrhea, breast discharge, decreased breast size, tenderness of female genitalia

Gastrointestinal: (3–10%)—nausea, GI pain, flatulence, decreased appetitie, dyspepsia; (2–3%)—vomiting, constipation, diarrhea, GI cramps, gastritis

Miscellaneous: (12%)—abdominal pain; (3–10%)—pain in trunk, body, or extremities, fatigue, pyrexia, weight gain, chest pain, viral infection; (2–3%)—chills, malaise, head/face pain, neck pain, purpura

Musculoskeletal: (3–10%)—arthralgia, joint stiffness, muscle crampl (2–3%)—muscle stiffness, myalgia

Nervous System: (22%)—headache; (3–10%)—mood changes, nervousness, dizziness, depression, libido changes, insomnia, anxiety; (2–3%)—paresthesia, cognitive changes, syncope

Respiratory: (3–10%)—upper respiratory infection, pharyngitis, respiratory congestion; (2–3%)—cough, asthma, breathing disorder, rhinorrhea, bronchitis, sinusitis

Skin: (12%)—skin reaction at the medication site; (3–10%)—acne, rash, sweating; (2–3%)—keratoderma, pruritus, pain

Special Senses: (6%)—visual disturbances; (2–3%)—ear congestion, otalgia

Urogenital: (3–10%)—pain of female genitalia, vaginitis, dysemenorrhea; (2–3%)—dyspareunia, dysuria, hypertrophy of female genitalia, pruritus of external female genitalia

Urticaria which was reported by less than 2% of the population, may be clinically significant.

DRUG ABUSE AND DEPENDENCE

No instances of drug abuse or dependence have been reported.

OVERDOSAGE

SUPPRELIN™ (histrelin acetate) injection of up to 200 mcg/kg (rats, rabbits), or 2000 mcg/kg (mice) resulted in no systemic toxicity. This represents 20 to 200 times the maximial recommended human dose of 10 mcg/kg/day.

DOSAGE AND ADMINISTRATION

The dose of SUPPRELIN™ Injection that is recommended for the treatment of central precocious puberty is 10 mcg/kg of body weight administered as a single, daily subcutaneous injection. If prepubertal levels of sex steroids and/or a prepubertal gonadotropin response to GnRH testing are not achieved within the first 3 months of treatment, the patient should be reevaluated. Doses greater than 10 mcg/kg/day have not been evaluated in clinical trials. The injection site should be varied daily.

NOTE: Parenteral drug products should be inspected visually for discoloration and particulate matter before use. SUPPRELIN™ contains no preservative. Vials are to be used once. Any unused solution is to be discarded.

HOW SUPPLIED

SUPPRELIN™ Injection is supplied in a 7-day kit of single-use vials that deliver 0.6 mL of a sterile, preservative-free solution. Each kit contains 7 vials of the same strength of SUPPRELIN™ Injection, expressed as mcg of peptide base, 7 syringes with needles, prescribing information and patient information.

NDC#	SUPPRELIN™ Injection Strength (mcg peptide base)	SUPPRELIN™ *Injection per Vial (0.6 mL)
54092-637-75	200 mcg/mL	120 mcg
54092-638-75	500 mcg/mL	300 mcg
54092-639-75	1000 mcg/mL	600 mcg

Store refrigerated at 2–8°C (36–46°F) and protect from light. Remove vial from packaging only at time of use. Allow vial to reach room temperature before injecting contents. Discard unused portion of the vial after administration.

CAUTION

Federal (U.S.A.) law prohibits dispensing without prescription.

U.S. patent No. 4,244,946.

Manufactured for:

Roberts Laboratories, Inc.
a wholly owned subsidiary of
Roberts Pharmaceutical Corporation
Eatontown, New Jersey 07724

TOPICYCLINE® ℞

(tetracycline hydrochloride)
for Topical Solution

DESCRIPTION

TOPICYCLINE is a topical antibiotic preparation containing 2.2 mg. of tetracyline hydrochloride per ml as the active ingredient, as well as 4-epitetracycline hydrochloride and sodium bisulfite in an aqueous base of 40% ethanol, citric acid and n-decyl methyl sulfoxide. Tetracycline is 4-(dimethylamino)-1,4,4a,5,5a,6,11,12a-octahydro-3,6,10,12a-pentahydroxy-6-methyl-1,11-dioxo-2-naphthacenecarboxamide, the structural formula of which is

Tetracycline Structure

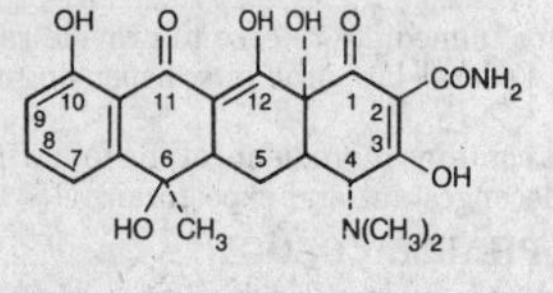

CLINICAL PHARMACOLOGY

Topicycline delivers tetracycline to the pilosebaceous apparatus and the adjacent tissues. Topicycline on the face and neck twice daily delivered to the skin an average dose of 2.9 mg of tetracycline hydrochloride per day. Patients who used the medication twice daily on other acne-involved areas in addition to the face and neck applied an average dose of 4.8 mg of tetracycline hydrochloride per day. Topicycline has been formulated such that the recrystallization properties of the tetracyclines on the skin greatly reduce or eliminate the yellow color often associated with topical tetracycline.

INDICATIONS AND USAGE

Topicycline is indicated in the treatment of acne vulgaris.

CONTRAINDICATIONS

Topicycline is contraindicated in persons who have shown hypersensitivity to any of its ingredients or to any of the other tetracyclines.

WARNINGS

Contains sodium bisulfite, a sulfite that may cause allergic type reactions including anaphylactic symptoms and life threatening or less severe asthmatic episodes in certain susceptible people. The overall prevalence of sulfite sensitivity in the general population is unknown and probably low. Sulfite sensitivity is seen more frequently in asthmatic than in nonasthmatic people.

PRECAUTIONS

General: This drug is for external use only and care should be taken to keep it out of the eyes, nose and mouth.

Carcinogenesis, Mutagenesis, and Impairment of Fertility: A two-year dermal study in mice has been performed with Topicycline and indicates there is no carcinogenic potential with this drug.

Pregnancy: Pregnancy Category B. Reproduction studies have been performed in rats and rabbits at doses of up to 246 times the human dose (assuming the human dose to be 1.3 ml/40kg/day) and have revealed no evidence of impaired fertility or harm to the fetus from Topicycline. There are, however, no adequate and well-controlled studies in pregnant women. Because animal reproduction studies are not always predictive of human response, this drug should be used during pregnancy only if clearly needed.

Nursing Mothers: It is not known whether tetracycline or any other component of Topicycline administered in this topical form is excreted in human milk. Because many drugs are excreted in human milk, caution should be exercised when Topicycline is administered to a nursing woman.

Pediatric Use: Safety and effectiveness in children below the age of eleven have not been established.

ADVERSE REACTIONS

Among the 838 patients treated with Topicycline under normal usage conditions during clinical evaluation, there was one instance of severe dermatitis requiring systemic steroid therapy. About one-third of patients are likely to experience a stinging or burning sensation upon application of Topicycline. The sensation ordinarily lasts no more than a few minutes, and does not occur at every application. There has been no indication that patients experience sufficient discomfort to reduce the frequency of use or to discontinue use of the product. The kinds of side effects often associated with oral or parenteral administration of tetracyclines (e.g., various gastrointestinal complaints, vainitis, hematologic abnormalities, manifestations of systemic hypersensitivity reactions, and dental and skeletal disorders) have not been observed with Topicycline. Because of Topicycline's topical form of administration, it is highly unlikely that such side effects will occur from its use.

DOSAGE AND ADMINISTRATION

It is recommended that Topicycline be applied generously twice daily to the entire affected area (not just to individual lesions) until the skin is thoroughly wet. Instructions to the patient for proper application are provided on the Topicycline bottle label. Patients may continue their normal use of cosmetics. Concomitant use with benzoyl peroxide or oral tetracycline has been reported without observed problems.

HOW SUPPLIED

Topicycline is supplied in a single carton containing a powder and a liquid which must be combined prior to using. Complete instructions for mixing are provided on the carton. Once combined, the Topicycline bottle contains 70 ml of medication. This constitutes about an eight-week supply for treating the face and neck, or about a four-week supply for treating the face, neck and additional acne involved areas. Differences in individual usage habits will result in variation from these averages.

NDC 54092-316-70, 70 ml as dispensed.

TOPICYCLINE should be kept at controlled room temperature 59°F–86°F (15°C-30°C) or below.

CAUTION

Federal law prohibits dispensing without prescription.

Revised May 1991

Manufactured for:
Roberts Laboratories, Inc.
a wholly owned subsidiary of
Roberts Pharmaceutical Corporation
Eatontown, New Jersey 07724

Shown in Product Identification Section, page 425

Important Notice
Before prescribing or administering any product described in PHYSICIANS' DESK REFERENCE always consult the PDR Supplement for possible new or revised information.

A. H. Robins Company

1407 CUMMINGS DRIVE
RICHMOND, VA 23220

For prescribing information for products of Elkins-Sinn Incorporated, see page 984 of the 1993 PDR, and page 2537 for products of Wyeth-Ayerst Laboratories. Information for these products can also be obtained by writing to Professional Service, Wyeth-Ayerst Laboratories, P.O. Box 8299, Philadelphia, PA 19101, or by contacting your local Wyeth-Ayerst representative.

DIMETANE®-DC CV ℞

[*di′mĕ-tāne*]
COUGH SYRUP
SUGAR-FREE

DESCRIPTION

Dimetane-DC Cough Syrup is a light bluish-pink syrup with a raspberry flavor.

Each 5 mL (1 teaspoonful) contains:

Brompheniramine Maleate, USP	2.0 mg
Phenylpropanolamine Hydrochloride, USP	12.5 mg
Codeine Phosphate, USP	10.0 mg
(Warning: May be habit forming)	
Alcohol 0.95 percent	

In a palatable aromatic vehicle.

Inactive Ingredients: Citric Acid, FD&C Blue 1, FD&C Red 40, Flavors, Glycerin, Sodium Benzoate, Sorbitol, Water.

Antihistamine/Nasal Decongestant/Antitussive syrup for oral administration.

CLINICAL PHARMACOLOGY

Brompheniramine maleate is a histamine antagonist, specifically an H_1-receptor-blocking agent belonging to the alkylamine class of antihistamines. Antihistamines appear to compete with histamine for receptor sites on effector cells. Brompheniramine also has anticholinergic (drying) and sedative effects. Among the antihistaminic effects, it antagonizes the allergic response (vasodilatation, increased vascular permeability, increased mucus secretion) of nasal tissue. Brompheniramine is well absorbed from the gastrointestinal tract, with peak plasma concentration after a single oral dose of 4 mg reached in 5 hours; urinary excretion is the major route of elimination, mostly as products of biodegradation; the liver is assumed to be the main site of metabolic transformation.

Phenylpropanolamine hydrochloride is a sympathomimetic drug which is readily absorbed from the gastrointestinal tract and produces nasal vasoconstriction (decongestion). Phenylpropanolamine stimulates both α and β-adrenergic receptors, similar to ephedrine. Part of its peripheral action is indirect and is due to the displacement of norepinephrine from storage sites, but it also has direct effect on the adrenergic receptors.

Codeine is an opiate analgesic and antitussive. Codeine calms the cough control center.

INDICATIONS AND USAGE

For relief of coughs and upper respiratory symptoms, including nasal congestion, associated with allergy or the common cold.

CONTRAINDICATIONS

Hypersensitivity to any of the ingredients. Do not use in the newborn, in premature infants, in nursing mothers, in patients with severe hypertension or severe coronary artery disease, or in those receiving monoamine oxidase (MAO) inhibitors.

Antihistamines should not be used to treat lower respiratory tract conditions including asthma.

WARNINGS

Especially in infants and small children, antihistamines in overdosage may cause hallucinations, convulsions, death. Codeine may cause or aggravate constipation.

Antihistamines may diminish mental alertness. In the young child, they may produce excitation.

PRECAUTIONS

General: Because of its antihistamine component, Dimetane-DC Cough Syrup should be used with caution in patients with a history of bronchial asthma, narrow angle glaucoma, gastrointestinal obstruction, or urinary bladder neck obstruction. Because of its sympathomimetic component, Dimetane-DC Cough Syrup should be used with caution in patients with diabetes, hypertension, heart disease, or thyroid disease.

Information for Patients: Patients should be warned about engaging in activities requiring mental alertness, such as driving a car or operating dangerous machinery.

Drug Interactions: Antihistamines have additive effects with alcohol and other CNS depressants (hypnotics, sedatives, tranquilizers, antianxiety agents, etc.). MAO inhibitors prolong and intensify the anticholinergic (drying) effects of antihistamines. MAO inhibitors may enhance the effect of phenylpropanolamine. Sympathomimetics may reduce the effects of antihypertensive drugs.

Carcinogenesis, Mutagenesis: Long-term studies in animals to evaluate carcinogenic and mutagenic potential have not been performed.

Pregnancy Category C: Animal reproduction studies have not been conducted with Dimetane-DC Cough Syrup. It is also not known whether Dimetane-DC Cough Syrup can cause fetal harm when administered to a pregnant woman or can affect reproduction capacity. Dimetane-DC Cough Syrup should be given to a pregnant woman only if clearly needed. Reproduction studies of brompheniramine maleate (one of the components of the Dimetane formulations) in rats and mice at doses up to 16 times the maximum human dose have revealed no evidence of impaired fertility or harm to the fetus.

Nursing Mothers: Because of the higher risk of intolerance of antihistamines in small infants generally, and in newborns and prematures in particular, and the fact that codeine appears in human milk, Dimetane-DC Cough Syrup is contraindicated in nursing mothers.

ADVERSE REACTIONS

The most frequent adverse reactions to Dimetane-DC Cough Syrup are: sedation; dryness of mouth, nose and throat; thickening of bronchial secretions; dizziness. Other adverse reactions may include:

Dermatologic: Urticaria, drug rash, photosensitivity, pruritus.

Cardiovascular System: Hypotension, hypertension, cardiac arrhythmias.

CNS: Disturbed coordination, tremor, irritability, insomnia, visual disturbances, weakness, nervousness, convulsions, headache, euphoria, and dysphoria.

G. U. System: Urinary frequency, difficult urination.

G. I. System: Epigastric discomfort, anorexia, nausea, vomiting, diarrhea, constipation.

Respiratory System: Tightness of chest and wheezing, shortness of breath. At higher doses, codeine has most of the disadvantages of morphine including respiratory depression.

Hematologic System: Hemolytic anemia, thrombocytopenia, agranulocytosis.

DRUG ABUSE AND DEPENDENCE

Codeine can produce drug dependence of the morphine type, and therefore has the potential for being abused. Psychic dependence, physical dependence and tolerance may develop upon repeated administration of this drug, and it should be prescribed and administered with the same degree of caution appropriate to the use of other oral narcotic medications. Dimetane-DC Cough Syrup is subject to the Federal Controlled Substances Act (Schedule V).

OVERDOSAGE

Signs and Symptoms: Serious overdose with codeine is characterized by respiratory depression, extreme somnolence progressing to stupor or coma. In severe overdosage, apnea, circulatory collapse, cardiac arrest and death may occur. The central nervous system effects from overdosage of brompheniramine may vary from depression to stimulation. Anticholinergic effects may also occur. Overdosage of phenylpropanolamine may be associated with tachycardia, hypertension and cardiac arrhythmias.

Toxic Doses: Doses of 800 mg or more of codeine have caused partial loss of consciousness, delirium, restlessness, excitement, tremors, convulsions and collapse; or respiratory paralysis with such sequelae as mydriasis, marked vasodilatation, and finally death. A 2½-year-old child survived a dose of 300–900 mg of brompheniramine; the lethal dose of phenylpropanolamine is in the range of 50 mg/kg.

Treatment: Respiratory depression should be treated promptly. Oxygen, intravenous fluids, vasopressors and other supportive measures should be employed as indicated. If necessary, reestablishment of adequate respiratory exchange through provision of a patent airway and the institution of assisted or controlled ventilation must be provided. The narcotic antagonist, naloxone, is a specific antidote to codeine-induced respiratory depression, and should be administered by the intravenous route if appropriate (see package insert for naloxone). Since the duration of action of codeine may exceed that of the antagonist, the patient should be kept under constant surveillance.

Gastric emptying may be useful in removing unabsorbed drug, either by inducing emesis or lavage; precautions against aspiration must be taken. Stimulants or depressants should be used cautiously and only when specifically indi-

Continued on next page

Prescribing information on A. H. Robins products listed here is based on official labeling in effect June 1, 1992, with Indications, Contraindications, Warnings, Precautions, Adverse Reactions, and Dosage stated in full.

A. H. Robins—Cont.

cated. If marked excitement is present, one of the short-acting barbiturates or chloral hydrate may be used.

DOSAGE AND ADMINISTRATION

Adults and children 12 years of age and over: 2 teaspoonfuls every 4 hours. Children 6 to under 12 years: 1 teaspoonful every 4 hours. Children 2 to under 6 years: ½ teaspoonful every 4 hours. Children 6 months to under 2 years: Dosage to be established by physician.
Do not exceed 6 doses during a 24-hour period.

HOW SUPPLIED

Dimetane-DC Cough Syrup is a light bluish-pink syrup containing in each 5 mL (1 teaspoonful): brompheniramine maleate 2 mg, phenylpropanolamine HCl 12.5 mg, and codeine phosphate 10 mg; available in pints (NDC 0031-1833-25) and gallons (NDC 0031-1833-29).
Store at controlled room temperature, between 15°C and 30°C (59°F and 86°F).
Dispense in tight, light-resistant container.

DIMETANE®-DX ℞

[di 'mĕ-tāne]
COUGH SYRUP
SUGAR-FREE

DESCRIPTION

Dimetane-DX Cough Syrup is a light-red syrup with a butterscotch flavor.
Each 5 mL (1 teaspoonful) contains:

Brompheniramine Maleate, USP	2 mg
Pseudoephedrine Hydrochloride, USP	30 mg
Dextromethorphan Hydrobromide, USP	10 mg

Alcohol 0.95 percent
In a palatable, aromatic vehicle.
Inactive Ingredients: Citric Acid, FD&C Red 40, FD&C Yellow 6, Flavors, Glycerin, Saccharin Sodium, Sodium Benzoate, Sorbitol, Water.
Antihistamine/Nasal Decongestant/Antitussive syrup for oral administration.

CLINICAL PHARMACOLOGY

Brompheniramine maleate is a histamine antagonist, specifically an H_1-receptor-blocking agent belonging to the alkylamine class of antihistamines. Antihistamines appear to compete with histamine for receptor sites on effector cells. Brompheniramine also has anticholinergic (drying) and sedative effects. Among the antihistaminic effects, it antagonizes the allergic response (vasodilatation, increased vascular permeability, increased mucus secretion) of nasal tissue. Brompheniramine is well absorbed from the gastrointestinal tract, with peak plasma concentration after single, oral dose of 4 mg reached in 5 hours; urinary excretion is the major route of elimination, mostly as products of biodegradation; the liver is assumed to be the main site of metabolic transformation.
Pseudoephedrine acts on sympathetic nerve endings and also on smooth muscle, making it useful as a nasal decongestant. The nasal decongestant effect is mediated by the action of pseudoephedrine on α-sympathetic receptors, producing vasoconstriction of the dilated nasal arterioles. Following oral administration, effects are noted within 30 minutes with peak activity occurring at approximately one hour.
Dextromethorphan acts centrally to elevate the threshold for coughing. It has no analgesic or addictive properties. The onset of antitussive action occurs in 15 to 30 minutes after administration and is of long duration.

INDICATIONS AND USAGE

For relief of coughs and upper respiratory symptoms, including nasal congestion, associated with allergy or the common cold.

CONTRAINDICATIONS

Hypersensitivity to any of the ingredients. Do not use in the newborn, in premature infants, in nursing mothers, in patients with severe hypertension or severe coronary artery disease, or in those receiving monoamine oxidase (MAO) inhibitors.
Antihistamines should not be used to treat lower respiratory tract conditions including asthma.

WARNINGS

Especially in infants and small children, antihistamines in overdosage may cause hallucinations, convulsions, and death.
Antihistamines may diminish mental alertness. In the young child, they may produce excitation.

PRECAUTIONS

General: Because of its antihistamine component, Dimetane-DX Cough Syrup should be used with caution in patients with a history of bronchial asthma, narrow angle glaucoma, gastrointestinal obstruction, or urinary bladder neck obstruction. Because of its sympathomimetic component, Dimetane-DX Cough Syrup should be used with caution in patients with diabetes, hypertension, heart disease, or thyroid disease.
Information for Patients: Patients should be warned about engaging in activities requiring mental alertness, such as driving a car or operating dangerous machinery.
Drug Interactions: Antihistamines have additive effects with alcohol and other CNS depressants (hypnotics, sedatives, tranquilizers, antianxiety agents, etc.). MAO inhibitors prolong and intensify the anticholinergic (drying) effects of antihistamines. MAO inhibitors may enhance the effect of pseudoephedrine. Sympathomimetics may reduce the effects of antihypertensive drugs.
Carcinogenesis, Mutagenesis, Impairment of Fertility
Animal studies of Dimetane-DX Cough Syrup to assess the carcinogenic and mutagenic potential or the effect on fertility have not been performed.
Pregnancy
Teratogenic Effects—Pregnancy Category C
Animal reproduction studies have not been conducted with Dimetane-DX Cough Syrup. It is also not known whether Dimetane-DX Cough Syrup can cause fetal harm when administered to a pregnant woman or can affect reproduction capacity. Dimetane-DX Cough Syrup should be given to a pregnant woman only if clearly needed.
Reproduction studies of brompheniramine maleate (a component of Dimetane-DX Cough Syrup) in rats and mice at doses up to 16 times the maximum human dose have revealed no evidence of impaired fertility or harm to the fetus.
Nursing Mothers: Because of the higher risk of intolerance of antihistamines in small infants generally, and in newborns and prematures in particular, Dimetane-DX Cough Syrup is contraindicated in nursing mothers.

ADVERSE REACTIONS

The most frequent adverse reactions to Dimetane-DX Cough Syrup are: sedation; dryness of mouth, nose and throat; thickening of bronchial secretions; dizziness. Other adverse reactions may include:
Dermatologic: Urticaria, drug rash, photosensitivity, pruritus.
Cardiovascular System: Hypotension, hypertension, cardiac arrhythmias, palpitation.
CNS: Disturbed coordination, tremor, irritability, insomnia, visual disturbances, weakness, nervousness, convulsions, headache, euphoria, and dysphoria.
G. U. System: Urinary frequency, difficult urination.
G. I. System: Epigastric discomfort, anorexia, nausea, vomiting, diarrhea, constipation.
Respiratory System: Tightness of chest and wheezing, shortness of breath.
Hematologic System: Hemolytic anemia, thrombocytopenia, agranulocytosis.

OVERDOSAGE

Signs and Symptoms: Central nervous system effects from overdosage of brompheniramine may vary from depression to stimulation, especially in children. Anticholinergic effects may be noted. Toxic doses of pseudoephedrine may result in CNS stimulation, tachycardia, hypertension, and cardiac arrhythmias; signs of CNS depression may occasionally be seen. Dextromethorphan in toxic doses will cause drowsiness, ataxia, nystagmus, opisthotonos, and convulsive seizures.
Toxic Doses: Data suggest that individuals may respond in an unexpected manner to apparently small amounts of a particular drug. A 2½-year-old child survived the ingestion of 21 mg/kg of dextromethorphan exhibiting only ataxia, drowsiness, and fever, but seizures have been reported in 2 children following the ingestion of 13–17 mg/kg. Another 2½-year-old child survived a dose of 300–900 mg of brompheniramine. The toxic dose of pseudoephedrine should be less than that of ephedrine, which is estimated to be 50 mg/kg.
Treatment: Induce emesis if patient is alert and is seen prior to 6 hours following ingestion. Precautions against aspiration must be taken, especially in infants and small children. Gastric lavage may be carried out, although in some instances tracheostomy may be necessary prior to lavage. Naloxone hydrochloride 0.005 mg/kg intravenously may be of value in reversing the CNS depression that may occur from an overdose of dextromethorphan. CNS stimulants may counter CNS depression. Should CNS hyperactivity or convulsive seizures occur, intravenous short-acting barbiturates may be indicated. Hypertensive responses and/or tachycardia should be treated appropriately. Oxygen, intravenous fluids, and other supportive measures should be employed as indicated.

DOSAGE AND ADMINISTRATION

Adults and children 12 years of age and over: 2 teaspoonfuls every 4 hours. Children 6 to under 12 years: 1 teaspoonful every 4 hours. Children 2 to under 6 years: ½ teaspoonful every 4 hours. Children 6 months to under 2 years: Dosage to be established by physician.
Do not exceed 6 doses during a 24-hour period.

HOW SUPPLIED

Dimetane-DX Cough Syrup is a light-red syrup containing in each 5 mL (1 teaspoonful) brompheniramine maleate 2 mg, pseudoephedrine hydrochloride 30 mg and dextromethorphan hydrobromide 10 mg, available in pints (NDC 0031-1836-25) and gallons (NDC 0031-1836-29).
Store at controlled room temperature, between 15°C and 30°C (59°F and 86°F).
Dispense in tight, light-resistant container.

DONNATAL® TABLETS ℞
DONNATAL® CAPSULES ℞
DONNATAL® ELIXIR ℞

[don 'nă-tal]

DESCRIPTION

Each Donnatal tablet, capsule or 5 mL (teaspoonful) of elixir (23% alcohol) contains:

Phenobarbital, USP (¼ gr)	16.2 mg
(Warning: May be habit forming)	
Hyoscyamine Sulfate, USP	0.1037 mg
Atropine Sulfate, USP	0.0194 mg
Scopolamine Hydrobromide, USP	0.0065 mg

Inactive Ingredients:
TABLETS: Dibasic Calcium Phosphate, Magnesium Stearate, Microcrystalline Cellulose, Silicon Dioxide, Sodium Starch Glycolate, Stearic Acid, Sucrose. May contain Corn Starch, Dextrose, or Invert Sugar.
CAPSULES: Corn Starch, Edible Ink, D&C Yellow 10 and FD&C Green 3 or FD&C Blue 1 and FD&C Yellow 6, FD&C Blue 2 Aluminum Lake, Gelatin, Lactose, Sucrose. May contain FD&C Red 40 and Yellow 6 Aluminum Lakes.
ELIXIR: D&C Yellow 10, FD&C Blue 1, FD&C Yellow 6, Flavors, Glucose, Saccharin Sodium, Water.

ACTIONS

This drug combination provides natural belladonna alkaloids in a specific, fixed ratio combined with phenobarbital to provide peripheral anticholinergic/antispasmodic action and mild sedation.

Indications

Based on a review of this drug by the National Academy of Sciences—National Research Council and/or other information, FDA has classified the following indications as "possibly" effective:
For use as adjunctive therapy in the treatment of irritable bowel syndrome (irritable colon, spastic colon, mucous colitis) and acute enterocolitis.
May also be useful as adjunctive therapy in the treatment of duodenal ulcer. IT HAS NOT BEEN SHOWN CONCLUSIVELY WHETHER ANTICHOLINERGIC/ANTISPASMODIC DRUGS AID IN THE HEALING OF A DUODENAL ULCER, DECREASE THE RATE OF RECURRENCES OR PREVENT COMPLICATIONS.

CONTRAINDICATIONS

Glaucoma, obstructive uropathy (for example, bladder neck obstruction due to prostatic hypertrophy); obstructive disease of the gastrointestinal tract (as in achalasia, pyloroduodenal stenosis, etc.); paralytic ileus, intestinal atony of the elderly or debilitated patient; unstable cardiovascular status in acute hemorrhage; severe ulcerative colitis especially if complicated by toxic megacolon; myasthenia gravis; hiatal hernia associated with reflux esophagitis.
Donnatal is contraindicated in patients with known hypersensitivity to any of the ingredients. Phenobarbital is contraindicated in acute intermittent porphyria and in those patients in whom phenobarbital produces restlessness and/or excitement.

WARNINGS

In the presence of a high environmental temperature, heat prostration can occur with belladonna alkaloids (fever and heatstroke due to decreased sweating).
Diarrhea may be an early symptom of incomplete intestinal obstruction, especially in patients with ileostomy or colostomy. In this instance treatment with this drug would be inappropriate and possibly harmful.
Donnatal may produce drowsiness or blurred vision. The patient should be warned, should these occur, not to engage in activities requiring mental alertness, such as operating a motor vehicle or other machinery, and not to perform hazardous work.
Phenobarbital may decrease the effect of anticoagulants, and necessitate larger doses of the anticoagulant for optimal effect. When the phenobarbital is discontinued, the dose of the anticoagulant may have to be decreased.
Phenobarbital may be habit forming and should not be administered to individuals known to be addiction prone or to

those with a history of physical and/or psychological dependence upon drugs.
Since barbiturates are metabolized in the liver, they should be used with caution and initial doses should be small in patients with hepatic dysfunction.

PRECAUTIONS
Use with caution in patients with: autonomic neuropathy, hepatic or renal disease, hyperthyroidism, coronary heart disease, congestive heart failure, cardiac arrhythmias, tachycardia, and hypertension.
Belladonna alkaloids may produce a delay in gastric emptying (antral stasis) which would complicate the management of gastric ulcer.
Theoretically, with overdosage, a curare-like action may occur.
Carcinogenesis, mutagenesis. Long-term studies in animals have not been performed to evaluate carcinogenic potential.
Pregnancy Category C. Animal reproduction studies have not been conducted with Donnatal. It is not known whether Donnatal can cause fetal harm when administered to a pregnant woman or can affect reproduction capacity. Donnatal should be given to a pregnant woman only if clearly needed.
Nursing mothers. It is not known whether this drug is excreted in human milk. Because many drugs are excreted in human milk, caution should be exercised when Donnatal is administered to a nursing mother.

ADVERSE REACTIONS
Adverse reactions may include xerostomia; urinary hesitancy and retention; blurred vision; tachycardia; palpitation; mydriasis; cycloplegia; increased ocular tension; loss of taste sense; headache; nervousness; drowsiness; weakness; dizziness; insomnia; nausea; vomiting; impotence; suppression of lactation; constipation; bloated feeling; musculoskeletal pain; severe allergic reaction or drug idiosyncrasies, including anaphylaxis, urticaria and other dermal manifestations; and decreased sweating. Elderly patients may react with symptoms of excitement, agitation, drowsiness, and other untoward manifestations to even small doses of the drug.
Phenobarbital may produce excitement in some patients, rather than a sedative effect. In patients habituated to barbiturates, abrupt withdrawal may produce delirium or convulsions.

DOSAGE AND ADMINISTRATION
The dosage of Donnatal should be adjusted to the needs of the individual patient to assure symptomatic control with a minimum of adverse effects.
Donnatal Tablets or Capsules. Adults: One or two Donnatal tablets or capsules three or four times a day according to condition and severity of symptoms.
Donnatal Elixir. Adults: One or two teaspoonfuls of elixir three or four times a day according to conditions and severity of symptoms.
Children (Elixir)—may be dosed every 4 or 6 hours.:

Body Weight	Starting Dosage q4h	Starting Dosage q6h
10 lb (4.5 kg)	0.5 mL	0.75 mL
20 lb (9.1 kg)	1.0 mL	1.5 mL
30 lb (13.6 kg)	1.5 mL	2.0 mL
50 lb (22.7 kg)	½ tsp	¾ tsp
75 lb (34.0 kg)	¾ tsp	1 tsp
100 lb (45.4 kg)	1 tsp	1½ tsp

OVERDOSAGE
The signs and symptoms of overdose are headache, nausea, vomiting, blurred vision, dilated pupils, hot and dry skin, dizziness, dryness of the mouth, difficulty in swallowing, CNS stimulation. Treatment should consist of gastric lavage, emetics, and activated charcoal. If indicated, parenteral cholinergic agents such as physostigmine or bethanechol chloride, should be added.

HOW SUPPLIED
Donnatal Tablets. White, compressed, scored and embossed "R"; in bottles of 100 (NDC 0031-4250-63), 1000 (NDC 0031-4250-74) and Dis-Co® Unit Dose Packs of 100 (NDC 0031-4250-64).
Donnatal Capsules. Green and white, monogrammed "AHR" and "4207"; in bottles of 100 (NDC 0031-4207-63) and 1000 (NDC 0031-4207-74).
Donnatal Elixir. Green, citrus flavored, in 4 fl. oz. (NDC 0031-4221-12), pints (NDC 0031-4221-25), gallons (NDC 0031-4221-29) and 5 mL Dis-Co® Unit Dose Packs (4 × 25s) (NDC 0031-4221-13).
Store at controlled room temperature, between 15°C and 30°C (59°F and 86°F).
Dispense in tight, light-resistant container.
Shown in Product Identification Section, page 425

DONNATAL EXTENTABS® ℞
[don'nă-tal ĕks"tĕn'tabs]

DESCRIPTION
Each Donnatal Extentabs tablet contains:

Phenobarbital, USP (¾ gr)	48.6 mg
(Warning: May be habit forming)	
Hyoscyamine Sulfate, USP	0.3111 mg
Atropine Sulfate, USP	0.0582 mg
Scopolamine Hydrobromide, USP	0.0195 mg

Each Donnatal Extentabs tablet contains the equivalent of three Donnatal tablets. Extentabs are designed to release the ingredients gradually to provide effects for up to twelve (12) hours.
Inactive Ingredients: Acacia, Acetylated Monoglycerides, Calcium Sulfate, Carnauba Wax, D&C Yellow 10, Edible Ink, FD&C Blue 1, FD&C Blue 2 Aluminum Lake, FD&C Yellow 6, Gelatin, Guar Gum, Magnesium Stearate, Polysorbates, Shellac, Sodium Phosphate, Sucrose, Titanium Dioxide, Wheat Flour, White Wax and other ingredients, one of which is a corn derivative. May include FD&C Red 40 and Yellow 6 Aluminum Lakes.

ACTIONS
This drug combination provides natural belladonna alkaloids in a specific, fixed ratio combined with phenobarbital to provide peripheral anticholinergic/antispasmodic action and mild sedation.

INDICATIONS
Based on a review of this drug by the National Academy of Sciences—National Research Council and/or other information, FDA has classified the following indications as "possibly" effective:
For use as adjunctive therapy in the treatment of irritable bowel syndrome (irritable colon, spastic colon, mucous colitis) and acute enterocolitis.
May also be useful as adjunctive therapy in the treatment of duodenal ulcer. IT HAS NOT BEEN SHOWN CONCLUSIVELY WHETHER ANTICHOLINERGIC/ANTISPASMODIC DRUGS AID IN THE HEALING OF A DUODENAL ULCER, DECREASE THE RATE OF RECURRENCES OR PREVENT COMPLICATIONS.

CONTRAINDICATIONS
Glaucoma, obstructive uropathy (for example, bladder neck obstruction due to prostatic hypertrophy); obstructive disease of the gastrointestinal tract (as in achalasia, pyloroduodenal stenosis, etc.); paralytic ileus, intestinal atony of the elderly or debilitated patient; unstable cardiovascular status in acute hemorrhage; severe ulcerative colitis especially if complicated by toxic megacolon; myasthenia gravis, hiatal hernia associated with reflux esophagitis.
Donnatal is contraindicated in patients with known hypersensitivity to any of the ingredients. Phenobarbital is contraindicated in acute intermittent porphyria and in those patients in whom phenobarbital produces restlessness and/or excitement.

WARNINGS
In the presence of a high environmental temperature, heat prostration can occur with belladonna alkaloids (fever and heatstroke due to decreased sweating).
Diarrhea may be an early symptom of incomplete intestinal obstruction, especially in patients with ileostomy or colostomy. In this instance treatment with this drug would be inappropriate and possibly harmful.
Donnatal may produce drowsiness or blurred vision. The patient should be warned, should these occur, not to engage in activities requiring mental alertness, such as operating a motor vehicle or other machinery, and not to perform hazardous work.
Phenobarbital may decrease the effect of anticoagulants and necessitate larger doses of the anticoagulant for optimal effect. When the phenobarbital is discontinued, the dose of the anticoagulant may have to be decreased.
Phenobarbital may be habit forming and should not be administered to individuals known to be addiction prone or to those with a history of physical and/or psychological dependence upon drugs.
Since barbiturates are metabolized in the liver, they should be used with caution and initial doses should be small in patients with hepatic dysfunction.

PRECAUTIONS
Use with caution in patients with: autonomic neuropathy, hepatic or renal disease, hyperthyroidism, coronary heart disease, congestive heart failure, cardiac arrhythmias, tachycardia, and hypertension.
Belladonna alkaloids may produce a delay in gastric emptying (antral stasis) which would complicate the management of gastric ulcer.
Theoretically, with overdosage, a curare-like action may occur.
Carcinogenesis, mutagenesis. Long-term studies in animals have not been performed to evaluate carcinogenic potential.
Pregnancy Category C. Animal reproduction studies have not been conducted with Donnatal. It is not known whether Donnatal can cause fetal harm when administered to a pregnant woman or can affect reproduction capacity. Donnatal should be given to a pregnant woman only if clearly needed.
Nursing mothers. It is not known whether this drug is excreted in human milk. Because many drugs are excreted in human milk, caution should be exercised when Donnatal is administered to a nursing mother.

ADVERSE REACTIONS
Adverse reactions may include xerostomia; urinary hesitancy and retention; blurred vision; tachycardia; palpitation; mydriasis; cycloplegia; increased ocular tension; loss of taste sense; headache; nervousness; drowsiness; weakness; dizziness; insomnia; nausea; vomiting; impotence; suppression of lactation; constipation; bloated feeling; musculoskeletal pain; severe allergic reaction or drug idiosyncrasies, including anaphylaxis, urticaria and other dermal manifestations; and decreased sweating. Elderly patients may react with symptoms of excitement, agitation, drowsiness, and other untoward manifestations to even small doses of the drug.
Phenobarbital may produce excitement in some patients, rather than a sedative effect. In patients habituated to barbiturates, abrupt withdrawal may produce delirium or convulsions.

DOSAGE AND ADMINISTRATION
The dosage of Donnatal Extentabs should be adjusted to the needs of the individual patient to assure symptomatic control with a minimum of adverse reactions. The usual dose is one tablet every twelve (12) hours. If indicated, one tablet every eight (8) hours may be given.

OVERDOSAGE
The signs and symptoms of overdose are headache, nausea, vomiting, blurred vision, dilated pupils; hot and dry skin, dizziness, dryness of the mouth, difficulty in swallowing, CNS stimulation. Treatment should consist of gastric lavage, emetics, and activated charcoal. If indicated, parenteral cholinergic agents such as physostigmine or bethanechol chloride should be added.

HOW SUPPLIED
Pale green, coated tablets, monogrammed AHR and Donnatal Extentab in bottles of 100 (NDC 0031-4235-63) and 500 (NDC 0031-4235-70); and Dis-Co® Unit Dose Packs of 100 (NDC 0031-4235-64).
Store at controlled room temperature, between 15°C and 30°C (59°F and 86°F).
Dispense in well-closed, light-resistant container.
Shown in Product Identification Section, page 425

DONNAZYME® Tablets ℞
[don'nă" zīm]
Pancreatic Enzyme Replacement

DESCRIPTION
Donnazyme tablets are available for oral administration.
Each tablet contains:
Pancreatin, USP equivalent .... 500 mg
which provides not less than the following enzymatic activity—

Lipase	1,000 USP Units
Protease	12,500 USP Units
Amylase	12,500 USP Units

Inactive Ingredients: Acacia, Acetylated Monoglycerides, Calcium Sulfate, Carnauba Wax, Cellulose Acetate Phthalate, Corn Starch, D&C Yellow 10 Aluminum Lake, Diethyl Phthalate, Edible Ink, FD&C Blue 1 Aluminum Lake, FD&C Yellow 6 Aluminum Lake, Gelatin, Methylparaben, Microcrystalline Cellulose, Polysorbates, Povidone, Propylparaben, Shellac, Sodium Benzoate, Stearic Acid, Sucrose, Titanium Dioxide, Wheat Flour, White Wax. May contain Docusate Sodium.

CLINICAL PHARMACOLOGY
The outer layer of Donnazyme tablets is gastric-soluble. The core of the tablet contains pancreatin. It is designed to disintegrate in the alkaline medium of the duodenum where it releases the active enzyme components of pancreatin (trypsin, amylase and lipase). Trypsin breaks down larger protein fractions into peptides; amylase converts starch into maltose; lipase splits fat into fatty acids and glycerin.

Continued on next page

Prescribing information on A. H. Robins products listed here is based on official labeling in effect June 1, 1992, with Indications, Contraindications, Warnings, Precautions, Adverse Reactions, and Dosage stated in full.

A. H. Robins—Cont.

INDICATIONS AND USAGE

Donnazyme is indicated for the treatment of exocrine pancreatic insufficiency.

CONTRAINDICATIONS

Donnazyme is contraindicated in patients with known hypersensitivity to the drug.

WARNINGS

Do not take this product if you are allergic to pork.
Do not take this product unless directed by a physician.
Do not exceed the labeled dose unless directed by a physician.
Do not chew tablets.
Swallow tablets quickly to lessen potential for mouth irritation.

PRECAUTIONS

Carcinogenesis, mutagenesis: Long-term studies in animals have not been performed to evaluate carcinogenic potential.
Pregnancy Category C. Animal reproduction studies have not been conducted with Donnazyme. It is not known whether Donnazyme can cause fetal harm when administered to a pregnant woman or can affect reproduction capacity. Donnazyme should be given to a pregnant woman only if clearly needed.
Nursing mothers: It is not known whether this drug is excreted in human milk. Because many drugs are excreted in human milk, caution should be exercised when Donnazyme is administered to a nursing mother.
Pediatric Use: Safety and effectiveness in children have not been established.

ADVERSE REACTIONS

Skin rash is the most frequently reported adverse reaction to Donnazyme and appears to be associated with hypersensitivity to pork protein in the pancreatin. At high doses, a laxative effect may occur.

OVERDOSAGE

Excessive dosage may produce a laxative effect. Systemic toxicity does not occur.

DOSAGE AND ADMINISTRATION

Two tablets with each meal and 2 tablets taken with food eaten between meals or as directed by a physician. Donnazyme tablets should be swallowed whole and not crushed or chewed.

HOW SUPPLIED

Kelly green tablets in bottles of 100 (NDC 0031-4650-63). Store at controlled room temperature, between 15°C and 30°C (59°F and 86°F). Dispense in tight container.
Shown in Product Identification Section, page 425

DOPRAM® INJECTABLE   ℞
[*do'pram*]
brand of Doxapram Hydrochloride Injection, USP

DESCRIPTION

Dopram Injectable (Doxapram Hydrochloride Injection, USP) is a clear, colorless, sterile, non-pyrogenic, aqueous solution with pH 3.5—5.0, for intravenous administration.
Each 1 mL contains:
Doxapram Hydrochloride, USP..................................... 20 mg.
Benzyl Alcohol, NF (as preservative)............................ 0.9%
Water for Injection, USP..................................... q.s.
Due to its benzyl alcohol content, Dopram Injectable should not be used in newborns.
Dopram Injectable is a respiratory stimulant.
Doxapram hydrochloride is a white to off-white, crystalline powder, sparingly soluble in water, alcohol and chloroform. It has the following chemical name:
1-ethyl-4-[2-(4-morpholinyl)ethyl]-3,3-diphenyl-2-pyrrolidinone monohydrochloride, monohydrate.

CLINICAL PHARMACOLOGY

Doxapram hydrochloride produces respiratory stimulation mediated through the peripheral carotid chemoreceptors. As the dosage level is increased, the central respiratory centers in the medulla are stimulated with progressive stimulation of other parts of the brain and spinal cord.
The onset of respiratory stimulation following the recommended single intravenous injection of doxapram hydrochloride usually occurs in 20–40 seconds with peak effect at 1–2 minutes. The duration of effect may vary from 5–12 minutes. The respiratory stimulant action is manifested by an increase in tidal volume associated with a slight increase in respiratory rate.
A pressor response may result following doxapram administration. Provided there is no impairment of cardiac function, the pressor effect is more marked in hypovolemic than in normovolemic states. The pressor response is due to the improved cardiac output rather than peripheral vasoconstric-

tion. Following doxapram administration an increased release of catecholamines has been noted.
Although opiate induced respiratory depression is antagonized by doxapram, the analgesic effect is not affected.

INDICATIONS

1. *Postanesthesia.*
   a. When the possibility of airway obstruction and/or hypoxia have been eliminated, doxapram may be used to stimulate respiration in patients with drug-induced postanesthesia respiratory depression or apnea other than that due to muscle relaxant drugs.
   b. To pharmacologically stimulate deep breathing in the so-called "stir-up" regimen in the postoperative patient. (Simultaneous administration of oxygen is desirable.)
2. *Drug-induced central nervous system depression.*
   Exercising care to prevent vomiting and aspiration, doxapram may be used to stimulate respiration, hasten arousal, and to encourage the return of laryngopharyngeal reflexes in patients with mild to moderate respiratory and CNS depression due to drug overdosage.
3. *Chronic pulmonary disease associated with acute hypercapnia.*
   Doxapram is indicated as a temporary measure in hospitalized patients with acute respiratory insufficiency superimposed on chronic obstructive pulmonary disease. Its use should be for a short period of time (approximately 2 hours) as an aid in the prevention of elevation of arterial CO_2 tension during the administration of oxygen. It should not be used in conjuction with mechanical ventilation.

CONTRAINDICATIONS

Due to its benzyl alcohol content, Dopram Injectable should not be used in newborns.
Doxapram should not be used in patients with epilepsy or other convulsive disorders.
Doxapram is contraindicated in patients with mechanical disorders of ventilation such as mechanical obstruction, muscle paresis, flail chest, pneumothorax, acute bronchial asthma, pulmonary fibrosis or other conditions resulting in restriction of chest wall, muscles of respiration or alveolar expansion.
Doxapram is contraindicated in patients with evidence of head injury or cerebral vascular accident and in those with significant cardiovascular impairment, severe hypertension, or known hypersensitivity to the drug.

WARNINGS

1. *In postanesthetic use.*
   a. Doxapram is neither an antagonist to muscle relaxant drugs nor a specific narcotic antagonist. Adequacy of airway and oxygenation must be assured prior to doxapram administration.
   b. Doxapram should be administered with great care and only under careful supervision to patients with hypermetabolic states such as hyperthyroidism or pheochromocytoma.
   c. Since narcosis may recur after stimulation with doxapram, care should be taken to maintain close observation until the patient has been fully alert for ½ to 1 hour.
2. *In drug-induced CNS and respiratory depression.*
   Doxapram alone may not stimulate adequate spontaneous breathing or provide sufficient arousal in patients who are *severely* depressed either due to respiratory failure or to CNS depressant drugs, but should be used as an adjunct to established supportive measures and resuscitative techniques.
3. *In chronic obstructive pulmonary disease.*
   a. Because of the associated increased work of breathing, do not increase the rate of infusion of doxapram in severely ill patients in an attempt to lower pCO_2.
   b. Doxapram should not be used in conjunction with mechanical ventilation.

PRECAUTIONS

1. *General.*
   a. An adequate airway is essential.
   b. Recommended dosages of doxapram should be employed and maximum total dosages should not be exceeded. In order to avoid side effects, it is advisable to use the minimum effective dosage.
   c. Monitoring of the blood pressure and deep tendon reflexes is recommended to prevent overdosage.
   d. Vascular extravasation or use of a single injection site over an extended period should be avoided since either may lead to thrombophlebitis or local skin irritation.
   e. Rapid infusion may result in hemolysis.
   f. Lowered pCO_2 induced by hyperventilation produces cerebral vasoconstriction and slowing of the cerebral circulation. This should be taken into consideration on an individual basis.
   g. Intravenous short-acting barbiturates, oxygen and resuscitative equipment should be readily available to manage overdosage manifested by excessive central nervous system stimulation. Slow administration of

the drug, and careful observation of the patient during administration and for some time subsequently are advisable. These precautions are to assure that the protective reflexes have been restored and to prevent possible post-hyperventilation hypoventilation.
   h. Doxapram should be administered cautiously to patients receiving sympathomimetic or monoamine oxidase inhibiting drugs, since an additive pressor effect may occur.
   i. Blood pressure increases are generally modest but significant increases have been noted in some patients. Because of this doxapram is not recommended for use in severe hypertension (see Contraindications).
   j. If sudden hypotension or dyspnea develops, doxapram should be stopped.
2. *In postanesthetic use.*
   a. The same consideration to pre-existing disease states should be exercised as in non-anesthetized individuals. See Contraindications and Warnings covering use in hypertension, asthma, disturbances of respiratory mechanics including airway obstruction, CNS disorders including increased cerebrospinal fluid pressure, convulsive disorders, acute agitation, and profound metabolic disorders.
   b. See Drug Interactions.
3. *In chronic obstructive pulmonary disease.*
   a. Arrhythmias seen in some patients in acute respiratory failure secondary to chronic obstructive pulmonary disease are probably the result of hypoxia. Doxapram should be used with caution in these patients.
   b. Arterial blood gases should be drawn prior to the initiation of doxapram infusion and oxygen administration, then at least every ½ hour. Doxapram administration does not diminish the need for careful monitoring of the patient or the need for supplemental oxygen in patients with acute respiratory failure. Doxapram should be stopped if the arterial blood gases deteriorate, and mechanical ventilation initiated.

Drug Interactions: Administration of doxapram to patients who are receiving sympathomimetic or monoamine oxidase inhibiting drugs may result in an additive pressor effect. (See Precautions).
In patients who have received muscle relaxants, doxapram may temporarily mask the residual effects of muscle relaxant drugs.
In patients who have received anesthetics known to sensitize the myocardium to catecholamines, such as halothane, cyclopropane and enflurane, initiation of doxapram therapy should be delayed for at least 10 minutes following discontinuance of anesthesia, since an increase in epinephrine release has been noted with doxapram.
Carcinogenesis, mutagenesis, impairment of fertility. No carcinogenic or mutagenic studies have been performed using doxapram. Doxapram did not adversely affect the breeding performance of rats.
Pregnancy Category B. Reproduction studies have been performed in rats at doses up to 1.6 times the human dose and have revealed no evidence of impaired fertility or harm to the fetus due to doxapram. There are, however, no adequate and well-controlled studies in pregnant women. Since the animals in the reproduction studies were dosed by the IM and oral routes and animal reproduction studies, in general, are not always predictive of human response, this drug should be used during pregnancy only if clearly needed.
Nursing mothers. It is not known whether this drug is excreted in human milk. Because many drugs are excreted in human milk, caution should be exercised when doxapram hydrochloride is administered to a nursing mother.
Pediatric use. The use of the preservative benzyl alcohol in the newborn has been associated with metabolic, CNS, respiratory, circulatory, and renal dysfunction. Safety and effectiveness in children below the age of 12 years have not been established.

ADVERSE REACTIONS

The following adverse reactions have been reported:
1. *Central and autonomic nervous systems.*
   Pyrexia, flushing, sweating; pruritus and paresthesia, such as a feeling of warmth, burning, or hot sensation, especially in the area of genitalia and perineum; apprehension, disorientation, pupillary dilatation, headache, dizziness, hyperactivity, involuntary movements, muscle spasticity, increased deep tendon reflexes, clonus, bilateral Babinski, and convulsions.
2. *Respiratory.*
   Dyspnea, cough, tachypnea, laryngospasm, bronchospasm, hiccough, and rebound hypoventilation.
3. *Cardiovascular.*
   Phlebitis, variations in heart rate, lowered T-waves, arrhythmias, chest pain, tightness in chest. A mild to moderate increase in blood pressure is commonly noted and may be of concern in patients with severe cardiovascular diseases.

Table I. Dopram Injectable Dosage for postanesthetic use — I.V.

I.V. Administration	Recommended dosage mg/kg	mg/lb	Maximum dose per single injection mg/kg	mg/lb	Maximum total dose mg/kg	mg/lb
Single Injection	0.5–1.0	0.25–0.5	1.5	0.70	1.5	0.70
Repeat Injections (5 min. intervals)	0.5–1.0	0.25–0.5	1.5	0.70	2.0	1.0
Infusion	0.5–1.0	0.25–0.5	—	—	4.0	2.0

4. *Gastrointestinal.*
Nausea, vomiting, diarrhea, desire to defecate.
5. *Genitourinary.*
Stimulation of urinary bladder with spontaneous voiding; urinary retention.
6. *Laboratory determinations.*
A decrease in hemoglobin, hematocrit, or red blood cell count has been observed in postoperative patients. In the presence of pre-existing leukopenia, a further decrease in WBC has been observed following anesthesia and treatment with doxapram hydrochloride. Elevation of BUN and albuminuria have also been observed. As some of the patients cited above had received multiple drugs concomitantly, a cause and effect relationship could not be determined.

OVERDOSAGE

Signs and Symptoms. Symptoms of overdosage are extensions of the pharmacologic effects of the drug. Excessive pressor effect, tachycardia, skeletal muscle hyperactivity, and enhanced deep tendon reflexes may be early signs of overdosage. Therefore, the blood pressure, pulse rate and deep tendon reflexes should be evaluated periodically and the dosage or infusion rate adjusted accordingly.
Convulsive seizures are unlikely at recommended dosages. In unanesthetized animals, the convulsant dose is 70 times greater than the respiratory stimulant dose. Intravenous LD_{50} values in the mouse and rat were approximately 75 mg/kg and in the cat and dog were 40–80 mg/kg.
Except for management of chronic obstructive pulmonary disease associated with acute hypercapnia, the maximum recommended dosage is 3 GRAMS/24 HOURS. (See Dosage and Administration.)
Management. There is no specific antidote for doxapram. Management should be symptomatic. Short-acting intravenous barbiturates, oxygen and resuscitative equipment should be used as needed for supportive treatment.
There is no evidence that doxapram is dialyzable; further, the half-life of doxapram makes it unlikely that dialysis would be appropriate in managing overdose with this drug.

DOSAGE AND ADMINISTRATION

1. Doxapram hydrochloride is compatible with 5% and 10% dextrose in water or normal saline. ADMIXTURE OF DOXAPRAM WITH ALKALINE SOLUTIONS SUCH AS 2.5% THIOPENTAL SODIUM, BICARBONATE, OR AMINOPHYLLINE WILL RESULT IN PRECIPITATION OR GAS FORMATION.
2. *In postanesthetic use.*
   a. By i.v. injection (see Table I. Dosage for postanesthetic use—I.V.) Slow administration of the drug and careful observation of the patient during administration and for some time subsequently are advisable.
   b. By infusion. The solution is prepared by adding 250 mg of doxapram (12.5 mL) to 250 mL of dextrose or saline solution. The infusion is initiated at a rate of approximately 5 mg/minute until a satisfactory respiratory response is observed, and maintained at a rate of 1–3 mg/minute. The rate of infusion should be adjusted to sustain the desired level of respiratory stimulation with a minimum of side effects. The recommended total dosage by infusion is 4 mg/kg (2.0 mg/lb), or approximately 300 mg for the average adult.

3. *In the management of drug-induced CNS depression.* (See Table II. Dosage for drug-induced CNS depression.)
METHOD ONE
Using Single and/or Repeat Single I.V. *Injections.*
   a. Give priming dose of 1.0 mg/lb (2.0 mg/kg) body weight and repeat in 5 minutes.
   b. Repeat same dose q1–2h until patient wakens. Watch for relapse into unconsciousness or development of respiratory depression, since Dopram does not affect the metabolism of CNS-depressant drugs.
   c. If relapse occurs, resume injections q1–2h until arousal is sustained, or total maximum daily dose (3 grams) is given. Allow patients to sleep until 24 hours have elapsed from first injection of Dopram, using assisted or automatic respiration if necessary.
   d. Repeat procedure the following day until patient breathes spontaneously and sustains desired level of consciousness, or until maximum dosage (3 grams) is given.
   e. Repetitive doses should be administered only to patients who have shown response to the initial dose.
   f. Failure to respond appropriately indicates the need for neurologic evaluation for a possible central nervous system source of sustained coma.

METHOD TWO
By Intermittent I.V. *Infusion.*
   a. Give priming dose as in Method One.
   b. If patient wakens, watch for relapse; if no response, continue general supportive treatment for 1–2 hours and repeat Dopram. If some respiratory stimulation occurs, prepare I.V. infusion by adding 250 mg of Dopram (12.5 mL) to 250 mL of saline or dextrose solution. Deliver at rate of 1–3 mg/min (60–180 mL/hr) according to size of patient and depth of coma. Discontinue Dopram if patient begins to waken or at end of 2 hours.
   c. Continue supportive treatment for $\frac{1}{2}$ to 2 hours and repeat Step b.
   d. Do not exceed 3 grams/day.
4. *Chronic obstructive pulmonary disease associated with acute hypercapnia.*
   a. One vial of doxapram (400 mg) should be mixed with 180 mL of dextrose or saline solution (concentration of 2.0 mg/mL). The infusion should be started at 1–2 mg/minute ($\frac{1}{2}$–1 mL/minute); if indicated, increase to a maximum of 3 mg/minute. Arterial blood gases should be determined prior to the onset of doxapram's administration and at least every half hour during the two hours of infusion to insure against the insidious development of CO_2-RETENTION AND ACIDOSIS. Alteration of oxygen concentration or flow rate may necessitate adjustment in the rate of doxapram infusion.
   b. Predictable blood gas patterns are more readily established with a continuous infusion of doxapram. If the blood gases show evidence of deterioration, the infusion of doxapram should be discontinued.
   c. ADDITIONAL INFUSIONS BEYOND THE SINGLE MAXIMUM TWO HOUR ADMINISTRATION PERIOD ARE NOT RECOMMENDED.
Parenteral drug products should be inspected visually for particulate matter and discoloration prior to administration, whenever solution and container permit.

HOW SUPPLIED

Dopram Injectable (doxapram hydrochloride injection) is available in 20 mL multiple dose vials containing 20 mg of doxapram hydrochloride per mL. with benzyl alcohol 0.9% as the preservative (NDC 0031-4849-83).
Store at Controlled Room Temperature, Between 15°C and 30°C (59°F and 86°F).
Manufactured for A. H. Robins Company, Richmond, Virginia 23220 by Elkins-Sinn, Inc., Cherry Hill, New Jersey 08003-4099.
Shown in Product Identification Section, page 425

ENTOZYME®   R
[ĕn′to-zīm]
Pancreatic Enzyme Replacement

DESCRIPTION

Entozyme tablets are available for oral administration. Each tablet contains:
Pancreatin, USP equivalent .... 300 mg
which provides not less than the following enzymatic activity—
Lipase .... 600 USP Units
Protease ....7,500 USP Units
Amylase ....7,500 USP Units
Natural Digestive Enzymes
Inactive Ingredients: Acacia, Acetylated Monoglycerides, Calcium Carbonate, Calcium Sulfate, Carnauba Wax, Cellulose Acetate Phthalate, Corn Starch, Diethyl Phthalate, Edible Ink, FD&C Blue 2 Aluminum Lake, Gelatin, Microcrystalline Cellulose, Polysorbates, Shellac, Stearic Acid, Sucrose, Titanium Dioxide, White Wax. May contain FD&C Red 40 and Yellow 6 Aluminum Lakes.

CLINICAL PHARMACOLOGY

Entozyme enhances proteolysis by its peptic and tryptic activity, carbohydrate digestion by amylolytic activity, and fat emulsification and transport by lipolytic activity.

INDICATIONS AND USAGE

Entozyme is indicated for the treatment of exocrine pancreatic insufficiency.

CONTRAINDICATIONS

Entozyme is contraindicated in patients with known hypersensitivity to the drug.

WARNINGS

Do not take this product if you are allergic to pork.
Do not take this product unless directed by a physician.
Do not exceed the labeled dose unless directed by a physician.
Do not chew tablets.
Swallow tablets quickly to lessen potential for mouth irritation.

PRECAUTIONS

Carcinogenesis, mutagenesis. Long-term studies in animals have not been performed to evaluate carcinogenic potential.
Pregnancy Category C. Animal reproduction studies have not been conducted with Entozyme. It is not known whether Entozyme can cause fetal harm when administered to a pregnant woman or can affect reproduction capacity. Entozyme should be given to a pregnant woman only if clearly needed.
Nursing mothers. It is not known whether this drug is excreted in human milk. Because many drugs are excreted in human milk, caution should be exercised when Entozyme is administered to a nursing woman.
Pediatric Use. Safety and effectiveness in children have not been established.

ADVERSE REACTIONS

Skin rash is the most frequently reported adverse reaction to Entozyme, and appears to be associated with hypersensitivity to pork protein in the pancreatin. At high doses, a laxative effect may occur.

OVERDOSAGE

Excessive dosage may produce a laxative effect. Systemic toxicity does not occur.

DOSAGE AND ADMINISTRATION

Two tablets with each meal and 2 tablets taken with food eaten between meals or as directed by a physician. Entozyme tablets should be swallowed whole and not crushed or chewed.

Continued on next page

Table II. Dopram Injectable Dosage for drug-induced CNS depression.

Level of Depression	METHOD ONE Priming dose single/repeat i.v. injection mg/kg	mg/lb	METHOD TWO Rate of intermittent i.v. infusion mg/kg/hr	mg/lb/hr
Mild*	1.0	0.5	1.0–2.0	0.5–1.0
Moderate†	2.0	1.0	2.0–3.0	1.0–1.5

*Mild Depression
Class 0: Asleep, but can be aroused and can answer questions.
Class 1: Comatose, will withdraw from painful stimuli, reflexes intact.

†Moderate Depression
Class 2: Comatose, will not withdraw from painful stimuli, reflexes intact.
Class 3: Comatose, reflexes absent, no depression of circulation or respiration.

A. H. Robins—Cont.

HOW SUPPLIED

White, coated tablets, monogrammed AHR and 5050 in bottles of 100 (NDC 0031-5050-63).
Store at controlled room temperature, between 15°C and 30°C (59°F and 86°F). Dispense in tight container.

Shown in Product Identification Section, page 425

EXNA® Tablets   ℞
[ĕks'nă]
brand of Benzthiazide Tablets, USP

DESCRIPTION

Exna (benzthiazide) is a diuretic available in round, yellow, scored tablets engraved AHR and 5449 for oral administration. Each tablet contains 50 mg benzthiazide.
Inactive Ingredients: Corn Starch, Dibasic Calcium Phosphate, FD&C Yellow 5, Lactose, Magnesium Stearate, Polyethylene Glycol , Sodium Lauryl Sulfate.
Benzthiazide is a white, crystalline powder with a characteristic odor, freely soluble in alkaline solution.
The chemical name is 6-chloro-3-[[(phenylmethyl) thio]methyl] -2H-1,2,4-benzothiadiazine-7-sulfonamide 1,1-dioxide.

CLINICAL PHARMACOLOGY

Exna is a diuretic and antihypertensive. It affects the renal tubular mechanism of electrolyte reabsorption. At maximal therapeutic dosage, all thiazides are approximately equal in their diuretic potency. The mechanism whereby thiazides function in the control of hypertension is unknown. Exna increases excretion of sodium and chloride in approximately equivalent amounts. Natriuresis may be accompanied by some loss of potassium and bicarbonate.
In humans, benzthiazide is excreted in the urine almost entirely unchanged. Following a single oral dose of Exna Tablets or benzthiazide solution, 1% and 4.3% of the respective doses were recovered in the urine in 24 hr. The relative bioavailability of Exna Tablets was determined to be about 25% in reference to benzthiazide solution.

INDICATIONS

Exna (benzthiazide) is indicated as adjunctive therapy in edema associated with congestive heart failure, hepatic cirrhosis and corticosteroid and estrogen therapy.
Exna has also been found useful in edema due to various forms of renal dysfunction as: nephrotic syndrome; acute glomerulonephritis; and chronic renal failure.
Exna is indicated in the management of hypertension either as the sole therapeutic agent or to enhance the effectiveness of other antihypertensive drugs in the more severe forms of hypertension.
Use in Pregnancy. The routine use of diuretics in an otherwise healthy woman is inappropriate and exposes mother and fetus to unnecessary hazard. Diuretics do not prevent development of toxemia of pregnancy, and there is no satisfactory evidence that they are useful in the treatment of developed toxemia.
Edema during pregnancy may arise from pathological causes or from the physiologic and mechanical consequences of pregnancy. Thiazides are indicated in pregnancy when edema is due to pathologic causes, just as they are in the absence of pregnancy (however, see Warnings, below). Dependent edema in pregnancy, resulting from restriction of venous return by the expanded uterus, is properly treated through elevation of the lower extremities and use of support hose; use of diuretics to lower intravascular volume in this case is illogical and unnecessary. There is hypervolemia during normal pregnancy which is harmful to neither the fetus nor the mother (in the absence of cardiovascular disease), but which is associated with edema, including generalized edema, in the majority of pregnant women. If this edema produces discomfort, increased recumbency will often provide relief. In rare instances, this edema may cause extreme discomfort which is not relieved by rest. In these cases, a short course of diuretics may provide relief and may be appropriate.

CONTRAINDICATIONS

Anuria. Hypersensitivity to this or other sulfonamide-derived drugs.

WARNINGS

Thiazides should be used with caution in severe renal disease. In patients with renal disease, thiazides may precipitate azotemia. Cumulative effects of the drug may develop in patients with impaired renal function.
Thiazides should be used with caution in patients with impaired hepatic function or progressive liver disease, since minor alterations of fluid and electrolyte balance may precipitate hepatic coma.
Sensitivity reactions may occur in patients with a history of allergy or bronchial asthma.

The possibility of exacerbation or activation of systemic lupus erythematosus has been reported.
Latent diabetes mellitus may become manifest during thiazide administration; hyperuricemia or frank gout may also be precipitated in certain patients. The antihypertensive effect of the drug may be enhanced in the postsympathectomy patient.

PRECAUTIONS

General: All patients receiving thiazide therapy should be observed for clinical signs of fluid or electrolyte imbalance; namely, hyponatremia, hypochloremic alkalosis, and hypokalemia.
Dilutional hyponatremia may occur in edematous patients in hot weather; appropriate therapy is water restriction, rather than administration of salt except in rare instances when hyponatremia is life threatening.
In actual salt depletion, appropriate replacement is the therapy of choice. Any chloride deficit is generally mild and usually does not require specific treatment except under extraordinary circumstances (as in liver disease or renal disease).
Hypokalemia may develop with thiazides as with any other potent diuretic especially with brisk diuresis. Inadequate oral electrolyte intake will also contribute to hypokalemia. This product contains FD&C Yellow No. 5 (tartrazine) which may cause allergic-type reactions (including bronchial asthma) in certain susceptible individuals. Although the overall incidence of FD&C Yellow No. 5 (tartrazine) sensitivity in the general population is low, it is frequently seen in patients who have aspirin hypersensitivity.
Information for patients: Warning signs of electrolyte imbalance are: dryness of mouth, thirst, weakness, lethargy, drowsiness, restlessness, muscle pains or cramps. muscular fatigue, hypotension, oliguria, tachycardia, and gastrointestinal disturbances such as nausea and vomiting.
Laboratory tests: Periodic determination of serum electrolytes to detect possible electrolyte imbalance should be performed at appropriate intervals. When the patient is vomiting excessively or receiving parenteral fluids, serum and urine electrolyte determinations are particularly important. In patients with renal impairment, nonprotein nitrogen or blood urea nitrogen level should be tested periodically; rising values would indicate progressive renal impairment and careful reappraisal of therapy is necessary with consideration given to withholding or discontinuing diuretic therapy.
Drug interaction: Thiazides may add to or potentiate the action of other hypotensive drugs. Potentiation occurs with ganglionic or peripheral adrenergic-blocking drugs.
Thiazides may increase the responsiveness to tubocurarine.
Thiazides may decrease arterial responsiveness to norepinephrine. This diminution is not sufficient to preclude effectiveness of the pressor agent for therapeutic use.
Insulin requirement in diabetic patients may be increased, decreased, or unchanged.
Medication such as digitalis may also influence serum electrolytes. Digitalis therapy may exaggerate metabolic effects of hypokalemia especially with reference to myocardial activity.
Drug/Laboratory Test Interactions: Thiazides may decrease serum PBI levels without signs of thyroid disturbance.
Carcinogenesis, mutagenesis, impairment of fertility: No animal carcinogenicity or mutagenesis studies on benzthiazide are known.
Pregnancy-teratogenic effects: Pregnancy Category C. Benzthiazide has an embryocidal effect in rats when given in doses several hundred times the human dose. Exna (benzthiazide) can cause fetal harm when administered to a pregnant woman. Fetal or neonatal jaundice has been reported. Thrombocytopenia and possibly other adverse reactions have occurred in the adult. If this drug is used during pregnancy, or if patient becomes pregnant while taking this drug, the patient should be apprised of the potential hazard to the fetus.
Thiazides cross the placental barrier and appear in cord blood.
Nursing mothers: It is not known whether this drug is excreted in human milk. Because many drugs are excreted in human milk, caution should be exercised when Exna is administered to a nursing mother.
Pediatric use: Safety and effectiveness in children have not been established.

ADVERSE REACTIONS

The following adverse reactions have been observed, but there is not enough systematic collection of data to support an estimate of their frequency.
Gastrointestinal System: jaundice (intrahepatic cholestatic jaundice); pancreatitis; gastric irritation; vomiting; cramping; nausea; anorexia; diarrhea; constipation.
Central Nervous System: dizziness; restlessness; paresthesia; headache; xanthopsia.
Hematologic: aplastic anemia; thrombocytopenia; agranulocytosis; leukopenia.

Dermatologic-Hypersensitivity: necrotizing angiitis (vasculitis) (cutaneous vasculitis); purpura; urticaria; rash; photosensitivity.
Cardiovascular: Orthostatic hypotension may occur and may be aggravated by alcohol, barbiturates or narcotics.
Other: hyperglycemia; glycosuria; hyperuricemia; weakness; muscle spasm.
Whenever adverse reactions are moderate or severe, thiazide dosage should be reduced or therapy withdrawn.

OVERDOSAGE

Symptoms of overdosage include electrolyte imbalance and signs of potassium deficiency such as confusion, dizziness, muscular weakness, and gastrointestinal disturbances. General supportive measures including replacement of fluids and electrolytes may be indicated in treatment of overdosage.

DOSAGE AND ADMINISTRATION

Therapy should be individualized according to patient response. This therapy should be titrated to gain maximal therapeutic response as well as the minimal dose possible to maintain that therapeutic response.

	Diuretic	Antihypertensive
Benzthiazide	50 to 200 mg	50 to 200 mg

Edema: *Initiation of diuresis:* 50 to 200 mg daily should be used for several days, or until dry weight is attained. With 100 mg or more daily, it is generally preferable to administer benzthiazide in two doses, following morning and evening meals.
Maintenance of diuresis: 50 to 150 mg daily depending upon the patient's response. To maintain effectiveness, reduction to minimal effective dosage should be gradual.
Hypertension: *Initiation of antihypertensive therapy:* 50 to 100 mg daily is the average dose. It may be given in two doses of 25 mg or 50 mg each after breakfast and after lunch. This dosage may be continued until a therapeutic drop in blood pressure occurs.
Maintenance of antihypertensive therapy: Dosage should be adjusted according to the patient response, either upward to as much as 50 mg q.i.d. or downward to the minimal effective dosage level.

HOW SUPPLIED

Exna (benzthiazide) is supplied in 50 mg round, yellow, scored tablets engraved AHR and 5449, packaged in bottles of 100 (NDC 0031-5449-63).
Store at controlled room temperature, between 15°C and 30°C (59°F and 86°F).
Dispense in tight container.

Shown in Product Identification Section, page 425

MICRO–K EXTENCAPS®   ℞
[mi'cro" K ĕks"tĕn'caps]
MICRO–K 10 EXTENCAPS®   ℞
(Potassium Chloride Extended-Release Capsules, USP)

DESCRIPTION

Micro-K Extencaps are pale orange, hard gelatin capsules, each containing 600 mg of dispersible, small crystalline particles of potassium chloride (equivalent to 8 mEq K), monogrammed Micro-K and AHR/5720.
Micro-K 10 Extencaps are pale orange and opaque white, hard gelatin capsules, each containing 750 mg of dispersible, small crystalline particles of potassium chloride (equivalent to 10 mEq K) monogrammed Micro-K 10 and AHR/5730. Each particle of potassium chloride (KCl) is microencapsulated with a polymeric coating which allows for the controlled release of potassium and chloride ions over an eight-to ten-hour period. The dispersibility of the microcapsules and the controlled release of ions are intended to minimize the likelihood of high localized concentrations of potassium chloride and resultant mucosal ulceration within the gastrointestinal tract.
The polymeric coating forming the microcapsules functions as a water-permeable membrane. Fluids pass through the membrane and gradually dissolve the potassium chloride within the microcapsules. The resulting potassium chloride solution slowly diffuses outward through the membrane.
Inactive Ingredients: Edible Ink, Ethylcellulose, FD&C Blue 2 Aluminum Lake, FD&C Yellow 6, Gelatin, Magnesium Stearate, Sodium Lauryl Sulfate, Titanium Dioxide. May contain FD&C Red 40 and Yellow 6 Aluminum Lakes.

ACTIONS

Potassium ion is the principal intracellular cation of most body tissues. Potassium ions participate in a number of essential physiological processes, including the maintenance of intracellular tonicity, the transmission of nerve impulses, the contraction of cardiac, skeletal, and smooth muscle and the maintenance of normal renal function.

Potassium depletion may occur whenever the rate of potassium loss through renal excretion and/or loss from the gastrointestinal tract exceeds the rate of potassium intake. Such depletion usually develops slowly as a consequence of prolonged therapy with oral diuretics, primary or secondary hyperaldosteronism, diabetic ketoacidosis, severe diarrhea, or inadequate replacement of potassium in patients on prolonged parenteral nutrition. Potassium depletion due to these causes is usually accompanied by a concomitant deficiency of chloride and is manifested by hypokalemia and metabolic alkalosis. Potassium depletion may produce weakness, fatigue, disturbances of cardiac rhythm (primarily ectopic beats), prominent U-waves in the electrocardiogram, and in advanced cases, flaccid paralysis and/or impaired ability to concentrate urine.

Potassium depletion associated with metabolic alkalosis is managed by correcting the fundamental causes of the deficiency whenever possible and administering supplemental potassium chloride, in the form of high potassium food or potassium chloride solution, capsules or tablets. In rare circumstances (e.g., patients with renal tubular acidosis) potassium depletion may be associated with metabolic acidosis and hyperchloremia. In such patients potassium replacement should be accomplished with potassium salts other than the chloride, such as potassium bicarbonate, potassium citrate, or potassium acetate.

INDICATIONS

BECAUSE OF REPORTS OF INTESTINAL AND GASTRIC ULCERATION AND BLEEDING WITH SLOW-RELEASE POTASSIUM CHLORIDE PREPARATIONS, THESE DRUGS SHOULD BE RESERVED FOR THOSE PATIENTS WHO CANNOT TOLERATE OR REFUSE TO TAKE LIQUID OR EFFERVESCENT POTASSIUM PREPARATIONS OR FOR PATIENTS IN WHOM THERE IS A PROBLEM OF COMPLIANCE WITH THESE PREPARATIONS.

1. For therapeutic use in patients with hypokalemia with or without metabolic alkalosis; in digitalis intoxication and in patients with hypokalemic familial periodic paralysis.
2. For prevention of potassium depletion when the dietary intake of potassium is inadequate in the following conditions: patients receiving digitalis and diuretics for congestive heart failure; hepatic cirrhosis with ascites; states of aldosterone excess with normal renal function; potassium-losing nephropathy, and certain diarrheal states.
3. The use of potassium salts in patients receiving diuretics for uncomplicated essential hypertension is often unnecessary when such patients have a normal dietary pattern. Serum potassium should be checked periodically, however, and, if hypokalemia occurs, dietary supplementation with potassium-containing foods may be adequate to control milder cases. In more severe cases, supplementation with potassium salts may be indicated.

CONTRAINDICATIONS

Potassium supplements are contraindicated in patients with hyperkalemia since a further increase in serum potassium concentration in such patients can produce cardiac arrest. Hyperkalemia may complicate any of the following conditions: chronic renal failure, systemic acidosis such as diabetic acidosis, acute dehydration, extensive tissue breakdown as in severe burns, adrenal insufficiency, or the administration of a potassium-sparing diuretic (e.g., spironolactone, triamterene, amiloride) (see OVERDOSAGE).

Controlled release formulations of potassium chloride have produced esophageal ulceration in certain cardiac patients with esophageal compression due to an enlarged left atrium. Potassium supplementation, when indicated in such patients, should be given as a liquid preparation.

All solid oral dosage forms of potassium chloride are contraindicated in any patient in whom there is structural, pathological (e.g., diabetic gastroparesis) or pharmacologic (use of anticholinergic agents or other agents with anticholinergic properties at sufficient doses to exert anticholinergic effects) cause for arrest or delay in capsule passage through the gastrointestinal tract.

WARNINGS

Hyperkalemia. In patients with impaired mechanisms for excreting potassium, the administration of potassium salts can produce hyperkalemia and cardiac arrest. This occurs most commonly in patients given potassium by the intravenous route but may also occur in patients given potassium orally. Potentially fatal hyperkalemia can develop rapidly and be asymptomatic.

The use of potassium salts in patients with chronic renal disease, or any other condition which impairs potassium excretion, requires particularly careful monitoring of the serum potassium concentration and appropriate dosage adjustments.

Interaction with Potassium-Sparing Diuretics. Hypokalemia should not be treated by the concomitant administration of potassium salts and a potassium-sparing diuretic (e.g., spironolactone or triamterene), since the simultaneous administration of these agents can produce severe hyperkalemia.

Interaction with Angiotensin Converting Enzyme Inhibitors. Angiotensin converting enzyme (ACE) inhibitors (e.g., captopril, enalapril) will produce some potassium retention by inhibiting aldosterone production. Potassium supplements should be given to patients receiving ACE inhibitors only with close monitoring.

Gastrointestinal lesions. Potassium chloride tablets have produced stenotic and/or ulcerative lesions of the small bowel and deaths, in addition to upper gastrointestinal bleeding. These lesions are caused by a high localized concentration of potassium ion in the region of a rapidly dissolving tablet which injures the bowel wall and thereby produces obstruction, hemorrhage, or perforation.

Micro-K Extencaps contain microcapsules which disperse upon dissolution of the hard gelatin capsule. The microcapsules are formulated to provide a controlled release of potassium chloride. The dispersibility of the microcapsules and the controlled release of ions from the microcapsules are intended to minimize the possibility of a high local concentration near the gastrointestinal mucosa and the ability of the KCl to cause stenosis or ulceration. Other means of accomplishing this (e.g., incorporation of KCl into a wax matrix) have reduced the frequency of such lesions to less than one per 100,000 patient years (compared to 40–50 per 100,000 patient years with enteric-coated KCl), but have not eliminated them. The frequency of GI lesions with Micro-K Extencaps is, at present, unknown. Micro-K Extencaps should be discontinued immediately and the possibility of bowel obstruction or perforation considered if severe vomiting, abdominal pain, distention, or gastrointestinal bleeding occurs.

Metabolic Acidosis. Hypokalemia in patients with metabolic *acidosis* should be treated with an alkalinizing potassium salt such as potassium bicarbonate, potassium citrate, or potassium acetate.

PRECAUTIONS

General: The diagnosis of potassium depletion is ordinarily made by demonstrating hypokalemia in a patient with a clinical history suggesting some cause for potassium depletion. In interpreting the serum potassium level, the physician should bear in mind that acute alkalosis per se can produce hypokalemia in the absence of a deficit in total body potassium, while acute acidosis per se can increase the serum potassium concentration into the normal range even in the presence of a reduced total body potassium. The treatment of potassium depletion, particularly in the presence of cardiac disease, renal disease, or acidosis, requires careful attention to acid-base balance and appropriate monitoring of serum electrolytes, the electrocardiogram, and the clinical status of the patient.

Information for Patients:
Physicians should consider reminding the patient of the following:
To take each dose with meals and with water or other suitable liquid.
To take this medicine following the frequency and amount prescribed by the physician. This is especially important if the patient is also taking diuretics and/or digitalis preparations.
To check with the physician if there is trouble swallowing capsules or if the capsules seem to stick in the throat.
To check with the physician at once if tarry stools or other evidence of gastrointestinal bleeding is noticed.
To take each dose without crushing, chewing, or sucking the capsule.

Laboratory Tests:
Regular serum potassium determinations are recommended, especially in patients with renal insufficiency or diabetic nephropathy.
When blood is drawn for analysis of plasma potassium it is important to recognize that artifactual elevations can occur after improper venipuncture technique or as a result of *in vitro* hemolysis of the sample.

Drug Interactions:
Potassium-sparing diuretic, angiotensin converting enzyme inhibitors: see WARNINGS.

Carcinogenesis, Mutagenesis, Impairment of Fertility: Carcinogenicity, mutagenicity and fertility studies in animals have not been performed. Potassium is a normal dietary constituent.

Pregnancy Category C:
Animal reproduction studies have not been conducted with Micro-K. It is unlikely that potassium supplementation that does not lead to hyperkalemia would have an adverse effect on the fetus or would affect reproductive capacity.

Nursing Mothers:
The normal potassium ion content of human milk is about 13 mEq per liter. Since oral potassium becomes part of the body potassium pool, so long as body potassium is not excessive, the contribution of potassium chloride supplementation should have little or no effect on the level in human milk.

Pediatric Use:
Safety and effectiveness in children have not been established.

ADVERSE REACTIONS

One of the most severe adverse effects is hyperkalemia (see CONTRAINDICATIONS, WARNINGS, AND OVERDOSAGE).

Gastrointestinal bleeding and ulceration have been reported in patients treated with Micro-K Extencaps (see WARNINGS).

In addition to gastrointestinal bleeding and ulceration, perforation and obstruction have been reported in patients treated with other solid KCl dosage forms, and may occur with Micro-K Extencaps.

The most common adverse reactions to the oral potassium salts are nausea, vomiting, abdominal pain/discomfort, and diarrhea. These symptoms are due to irritation of the gastrointestinal tract and are best managed by taking the dose with meals, or reducing the amount taken at one time.

OVERDOSAGE

The administration of oral potassium salts to persons with normal excretory mechanisms for potassium rarely causes serious hyperkalemia. However, if excretory mechanisms are impaired or if potassium is administered too rapidly intravenously, potentially fatal hyperkalemia can result (see Contraindications and Warnings). It is important to recognize that hyperkalemia is usually asymptomatic and may be manifested only by an increased serum potassium concentration and characteristic electrocardiogram changes (peaking of T-waves, loss of P-wave, depression of S-T segment, and prolongation of the QT interval). Late manifestations include muscle paralysis and cardiovascular collapse from cardiac arrest.

Treatment measures for hyperkalemia include the following: (1) elimination of foods and medications containing potassium and of potassium-sparing diuretics; (2) intravenous administration of 300 to 500 ml/hr of 10% dextrose solution containing 10–20 units of insulin per 1,000 ml; (3) correction of acidosis, if present, with intravenous sodium bicarbonate; (4) use of exchange resins, hemodialysis, or peritoneal dialysis.

In treating hyperkalemia, it should be recalled that in patients who have been stabilized on digitalis, too rapid a lowering of the serum potassium concentration can produce digitalis toxicity.

DOSAGE AND ADMINISTRATION

The usual dietary intake of potassium by the average adult is 40 to 80 mEq per day. Potassium depletion sufficient to cause hypokalemia usually requires the loss of 200 or more mEq of potassium from the total body store.

Dosage must be adjusted to the individual needs of each patient, but typically is around 20 mEq per day for the prevention of hypokalemia and 40 to 100 mEq per day for the treatment of potassium depletion.

	For Prevention	For Treatment
Micro-K Extencaps (8 mEq K)	2 or 3 Extencaps/day (16–24 mEq K)	5 to 12 Extencaps/day (40–96 mEq K)
Micro-K 10 Extencaps (10 mEq K)	2 Extencaps/day (20 mEq K)	4 to 10 Extencaps/day (40–100 mEq K)

If more than 2 Extencaps are prescribed per day, the total daily dosage should be divided into two or more separate doses. Those patients having difficulty swallowing the capsules may be advised to sprinkle the contents onto a spoonful of soft food to facilitate ingestion.

HOW SUPPLIED

Micro-K Extencaps® are pale orange capsules monogrammed Micro-K and AHR/5720, each containing 600 mg microencapsulated potassium chloride (equivalent to 8 mEq K) in bottles of 100 (NDC 0031-5720-63), 500 (NDC 0031-5720-70) and Dis-Co® unit dose packs of 100 (NDC 0031-5720-64).

Micro-K 10 Extencaps® are pale orange and opaque white capsules monogrammed Micro-K 10 and AHR/5730, each containing 750 mg microencapsulated potassium chloride (equivalent to 10 mEq K) in bottles of 100 (NDC 0031-5730-63), 100 Unit-of-Use (NDC 0031-5730-68), bottles of 500 (NDC 0031-5730-70), and Dis-Co® unit dose packs of 100 (NDC 0031-5730-64).

Store at controlled room temperature, between 15°C and 30°C (59°F and 86°F). Dispense in tight container.

CAUTION: Federal law prohibits dispensing without a prescription.

Animal Toxicology: The ulcerogenic potential of microencapsulated KCl was studied in anesthetized cats by direct applications on exteriorized gastric mucosa. The microcapsules of KCl were found to be non-ulcerogenic and signifi-

Continued on next page

Prescribing information on A. H. Robins products listed here is based on official labeling in effect June 1, 1992, with Indications, Contraindications, Warnings, Precautions, Adverse Reactions, and Dosage stated in full.

A. H. Robins—Cont.

cantly less irritating than wax-matrix tablets and 20% solution of KCl.

In groups of monkeys (up to 8 monkeys per group) receiving different formulations of potassium chloride at equivalent daily dosage (2400 mg KCl) for four and one-half days, Micro-K Extencaps showed no tendency to cause intestinal ulceration (similar to liquid KCl and a wax-matrix preparation but in contrast to an enteric-coated KCl tablet) and minimal gastric irritation (less than a wax-matrix preparation).

Shown in Product Identification Section, page 425

MICRO–K® LS   ℞

[*mi'cro"k*]
brand of Potassium Chloride
Extended-Release Formulation
for Liquid Suspension

DESCRIPTION

Micro-K LS is an oral dosage form of microencapsulated potassium chloride. Each packet contains 1.5 g of potassium chloride, USP equivalent to 20 mEq of potassium. Micro-K LS is comprised of specially formulated granules. After reconstitution with 2–6 fl oz of water and 1 minute of stirring, the suspension is odorless and tasteless.

Each crystal of potassium chloride (KCl) is microencapsulated with an insoluble polymeric coating which functions as a semipermeable membrane; it allows for the controlled release of potassium and chloride ions over an eight–ten hour period. The controlled release of K^+ ions by the microcapsular membrane is intended to reduce the likelihood of a high localized concentration of potassium chloride at any point on the mucosa of the gastrointestinal tract. Fluids pass through the membrane and gradually dissolve the potassium chloride within the microcapsules. The resulting potassium chloride solution slowly diffuses outward through the membrane.

Micro-K LS is an electrolyte replenisher. The chemical name of the active ingredient is potassium chloride and the structural formula is KCl. Potassium Chloride, USP occurs as a white, granular powder or as colorless crystals. It is odorless and has a saline taste. Its solutions are neutral to litmus. It is freely soluble in water and insoluble in alcohol.

Inactive Ingredients: Docusate Sodium, Ethylcellulose, Povidone, Silicon Dioxide, Sucrose, and another ingredient.

CLINICAL PHARMACOLOGY

The potassium ion is the principal intracellular cation of most body tissues. Potassium ions participate in a number of essential physiological processes including the maintenance of intracellular tonicity, the transmission of nerve impulses, the contraction of cardiac, skeletal, and smooth muscle, and the maintenance of normal renal function.

The intracellular concentration of potassium is approximately 150 to 160 mEq per liter. The normal adult plasma concentration is 3.5 to 5 mEq per liter. An active ion transport system maintains this gradient across the plasma membrane.

Potassium is a normal dietary constituent and under steady-state conditions the amount of potassium absorbed from the gastrointestinal tract is equal to the amount excreted in the urine. The usual dietary intake of potassium is 50 to 100 mEq per day.

Potassium depletion will occur whenever the rate of potassium loss through renal excretion and/or loss from the gastrointestinal tract exceeds the rate of potassium intake. Such depletion usually develops as a consequence of therapy with diuretics, primary or secondary hyperaldosteronism, diabetic ketoacidosis, or inadequate replacement of potassium in patients on prolonged parenteral nutrition. Depletion can develop rapidly with severe diarrhea, especially if associated with vomiting. Potassium depletion due to these causes is usually accompanied by a concomitant loss of chloride and is manifested by hypokalemia and metabolic alkalosis. Potassium depletion may produce weakness, fatigue, disturbances of cardiac rhythm (primarily ectopic beats), prominent U-waves in the electrocardiogram, and, in advanced cases, flaccid paralysis and/or impaired ability to concentrate urine.

If potassium depletion associated with metabolic alkalosis cannot be managed by correcting the fundamental cause of the deficiency, e.g., where the patient requires long-term diuretic therapy, supplemental potassium in the form of high potassium food or potassium chloride may be able to restore normal potassium levels.

In rare circumstances (e.g., patients with renal tubular acidosis) potassium depletion may be associated with metabolic acidosis and hyperchloremia. In such patients potassium replacement should be accomplished with potassium salts other than the chloride, such as potassium bicarbonate, potassium citrate, potassium acetate, or potassium gluconate.

INDICATIONS AND USAGE

BECAUSE OF REPORTS OF INTESTINAL AND GASTRIC ULCERATION AND BLEEDING WITH CONTROLLED RELEASE POTASSIUM CHLORIDE PREPARATIONS, THESE DRUGS SHOULD BE RESERVED FOR THOSE PATIENTS WHO CANNOT TOLERATE OR REFUSE TO TAKE IMMEDIATE RELEASE LIQUIDS/EFFERVESCENT POTASSIUM PREPARATIONS OR FOR PATIENTS IN WHOM THERE IS A PROBLEM OF COMPLIANCE WITH THESE PREPARATIONS.

1. For the treatment of patients with hypokalemia, with or without metabolic alkalosis; in digitalis intoxication; and in patients with hypokalemic familial periodic paralysis. If hypokalemia is the result of diuretic therapy, consideration should be given to the use of a lower dose of diuretic, which may be sufficient without leading to hypokalemia.

2. For the prevention of hypokalemia in patients who would be at particular risk if hypokalemia were to develop, e.g., digitalized patients or patients with significant cardiac arrhythmias, hepatic cirrhosis with ascites, states of aldosterone excess with normal renal function, potassium losing nephropathy, and certain diarrheal states.

The use of potassium salts in patients receiving diuretics for uncomplicated essential hypertension is often unnecessary when such patients have a normal dietary pattern and when low doses of the diuretic are used. Serum potassium should be checked periodically, however, and if hypokalemia occurs, dietary supplementation with potassium-containing foods may be adequate to control milder cases. In more severe cases, and if dose adjustment of the diuretic is ineffective or unwarranted, supplementation with potassium salts may be indicated.

CONTRAINDICATIONS

Potassium supplements are contraindicated in patients with hyperkalemia since a further increase in serum potassium concentration in such patients can produce cardiac arrest. Hyperkalemia may complicate any of the following conditions: chronic renal failure, systemic acidosis such as diabetic acidosis, acute dehydration, extensive tissue breakdown as in severe burns, adrenal insufficiency, or the administration of a potassium-sparing diuretic (e.g., spironolactone, triamterene, amiloride) (see OVERDOSAGE).

Controlled release formulations of potassium chloride have produced esophageal ulceration in certain cardiac patients with esophageal compression due to an enlarged left atrium. Potassium supplementation, when indicated in such patients, should be given as an immediate release liquid preparation.

All solid oral dosage forms of potassium chloride are contraindicated in any patient in whom there is structural, pathological (e.g., diabetic gastroparesis) or pharmacologic (use of anticholinergic agents or other agents with anticholinergic properties at sufficient doses to exert anticholinergic effects) cause for arrest or delay in tablet or capsule-passage through the gastrointestinal tract.

WARNINGS

Hyperkalemia (see OVERDOSAGE). In patients with impaired mechanisms for excreting potassium, the administration of potassium salts can produce hyperkalemia and cardiac arrest. This occurs most commonly in patients given potassium by the intravenous route but may also occur in patients given potassium orally. Potentially fatal hyperkalemia can develop rapidly and be asymptomatic. The use of potassium salts in patients with chronic renal disease, or any other condition which impairs potassium excretion, requires particularly careful monitoring of the serum potassium concentration and appropriate dosage adjustment.

Interaction with Potassium-Sparing Diuretics. Hypokalemia should not be treated by the concomitant administration of potassium salts and a potassium-sparing diuretic (e.g., spironolactone, triamterene or amiloride) since the simultaneous administration of these agents can produce severe hyperkalemia.

Interaction with Angiotensin Converting Enzyme Inhibitors. Angiotensin converting enzyme (ACE) inhibitors (e.g., captopril, enalapril) will produce some potassium retention by inhibiting aldosterone production. Potassium supplements should be given to patients receiving ACE inhibitors only with close monitoring.

Gastrointestinal Lesions. Solid oral dosage forms of potassium chloride can produce ulcerative and/or stenotic lesions of the gastrointestinal tract. Based on spontaneous adverse reaction reports, enteric coated preparations of potassium chloride are associated with an increased frequency of small bowel lesions (40–50 per 100,000 patient years) compared to sustained release wax matrix formulations (less than one per 100,000 patient years). Because of the lack of extensive marketing experience with microencapsulated products, a comparison between such products and wax matrix or enteric coated products is not available. Micro-K LS is administered as a liquid suspension of microencapsulated potassium chloride formulated to provide a controlled rate of release of potassium chloride and thus to minimize the possibility of a

high local concentration of potassium near the gastrointestinal wall.

Prospective trials have been conducted in normal human volunteers in which the upper gastrointestinal tract was evaluated by endoscopic inspection before and after one week of solid oral potassium chloride therapy. The ability of this model to predict events occurring in usual clinical practice is unknown. Trials which approximated usual clinical practice did not reveal any clear differences between the wax matrix and microencapsulated dosage forms. In contrast, there was a higher incidence of gastric and duodenal lesions in subjects receiving a high dose of a wax matrix controlled release formulation under conditions which did not resemble usual or recommended clinical practice (i.e., 96 mEq per day in divided doses of potassium chloride administered to fasted patients, in the presence of an anticholinergic drug to delay gastric emptying). The upper gastrointestinal lesions observed by endoscopy were asymptomatic and were not accompanied by evidence of bleeding (hemoccult testing). The relevance of these findings to the usual conditions (i.e., nonfasting, no anticholinergic agent, smaller doses) under which controlled release potassium chloride products are used is uncertain; epidemiologic studies have not identified an elevated risk, compared to microencapsulated products, for upper gastrointestinal lesions in patients receiving wax matrix formulations. Micro-K LS should be discontinued immediately and the possibility of ulceration, obstruction or perforation considered if severe vomiting, abdominal pain, distention, or gastrointestinal bleeding occurs.

Diarrhea or Dehydration. Micro-K LS contains, as a dispersing agent, docusate sodium, which also increases stool water and is used as a stool softener. Clinical studies with Micro-K LS indicate that minor changes in stool consistency may be common, although usually are well-tolerated. However, rarely patients may experience diarrhea or cramping abdominal pain. Patients with severe or chronic diarrhea or who are dehydrated ordinarily should not be prescribed Micro-K LS.

Metabolic Acidosis. Hypokalemia in patients with metabolic acidosis should be treated with an alkalinizing potassium salt such as potassium bicarbonate, potassium citrate, potassium acetate, or potassium gluconate.

PRECAUTIONS

General: The diagnosis of potassium depletion is ordinarily made by demonstrating hypokalemia in a patient with a clinical history suggesting some cause for potassium depletion. In interpreting the serum potassium level, the physician should bear in mind that acute alkalosis *per se* can produce hypokalemia in the absence of a deficit in total body potassium while acute acidosis *per se* can increase the serum potassium concentration into the normal range even in the presence of a reduced total body potassium. The treatment of potassium depletion, particularly in the presence of cardiac disease, renal disease, or acidosis requires careful attention to acid-base balance and appropriate monitoring of serum electrolytes, the electrocardiogram, and the clinical status of the patient.

Information for Patients: Physicians should consider reminding the patient of the following:

To take each dose with meals mixed in water or other suitable liquid.

To take this medicine following the frequency and amount prescribed by the physician. This is especially important if the patient is also taking diuretics and/or digitalis preparations.

To inform patients that this product contains as a dispersing agent the stool softener, docusate sodium, which may change stool consistency, or rarely produce diarrhea or cramps.

To check with the physician at once if tarry stools or other evidence of gastrointestinal bleeding is noticed.

Laboratory Tests: Regular serum potassium determinations are recommended, especially in patients with renal insufficiency or diabetic nephropathy.

When blood is drawn for analysis of plasma potassium, it is important to recognize that artifactual elevations can occur after improper venipuncture technique or as a result of *in vitro* hemolysis of the sample.

Drug Interactions: Potassium-sparing diuretics, angiotensin converting enzyme inhibitors: see WARNINGS.

Carcinogenesis, Mutagenesis, Impairment of Fertility: Carcinogenicity, mutagenicity, and fertility studies in animals have not been performed. Potassium is a normal dietary constituent.

Pregnancy Category C. Animal reproduction studies have not been conducted with Micro-K LS. It is unlikely that potassium supplementation that does not lead to hyperkalemia would have an adverse effect on the fetus or would affect reproductive capacity.

Nursing Mothers: The normal potassium ion content of human milk is about 13 mEq per liter. Since oral potassium becomes part of the body potassium pool, so long as body potassium is not excessive, the contribution of potassium chloride supplementation should have little or no effect on the level in human milk.

Pediatric Use: Safety and effectiveness in children have not been established.

ADVERSE REACTIONS

One of the most severe adverse effects is hyperkalemia (see CONTRAINDICATIONS, WARNINGS, AND OVERDOSAGE).

Gastrointestinal bleeding and ulceration have been reported in patients treated with microencapsulated KCl (see WARNINGS).

In addition to bleeding and ulceration, perforation and obstruction have been reported in patients treated with solid KCl dosage forms, and may occur with Micro-K LS.

The most common adverse reactions to the oral potassium salts are nausea, vomiting, flatulence, abdominal pain/discomfort, and diarrhea. These symptoms are due to irritation of the gastrointestinal tract and are best managed by taking the dose with meals, or reducing the amount taken at one time.

Skin rash has been reported rarely with potassium preparations.

In a controlled clinical study Micro-K LS was associated with an increased frequency of gastrointestinal intolerance (e.g., diarrhea, loose stools, abdominal pain, etc.) compared to equal doses (100 mEq/day) of Micro-K Extencaps (see WARNINGS, Diarrhea or Dehydration). This finding was attributed to an inactive ingredient used in the Micro-K LS formulation that is not present in the Micro-K Extencaps formulation.

OVERDOSAGE

The administration of oral potassium salts to persons with normal excretory mechanisms for potassium rarely causes serious hyperkalemia. However, if excretory mechanisms are impaired, or if potassium is administered too rapidly intravenously, potentially fatal hyperkalemia can result (see CONTRAINDICATIONS and WARNINGS). It is important to recognize that hyperkalemia is usually asymptomatic and may be manifested only by an increased serum potassium concentration (6.5–8.0 mEq/L) and characteristic electrocardiographic changes (peaking of T-waves, loss of P-wave, depression of S-T segment, and prolongation of the QT interval). Late manifestations include muscle paralysis and cardiovascular collapse from cardiac arrest (9–12 mEq/L).

Treatment measures for hyperkalemia include the following:

1. Elimination of foods and medications containing potassium and of any agents with potassium-sparing properties;
2. Intravenous administration of 300 to 500 mL/hr of 10% dextrose solution containing 10–20 units of crystalline insulin per 1,000 mL;
3. Correction of acidosis, if present, with intravenous sodium bicarbonate;
4. Use of exchange resins, hemodialysis, or peritoneal dialysis.

In treating hyperkalemia, it should be recalled that in patients who have been stabilized on digitalis, too rapid a lowering of the serum potassium concentration can produce digitalis toxicity.

DOSAGE AND ADMINISTRATION

The usual dietary potassium intake by the average adult is 50 to 100 mEq per day. Potassium depletion sufficient to cause hypokalemia usually requires the loss of 200 or more mEq of potassium from the total body store.

Dosage must be adjusted to the individual needs of each patient. The dose for the prevention of hypokalemia is typically in the range of 20 mEq per day. Doses of 40–100 mEq per day or more are used for the treatment of potassium depletion. Dosage should be divided if more than 20 mEq per day are given such that no more than 20 mEq is given in a single dose.

Usual Adult dose—One Micro-K LS 20 mEq packet 1 to 5 times daily, depending on the requirements of the patient. This product must be suspended in a liquid, preferably water, or sprinkled on food prior to ingestion.

Suspension in Water: Pour contents of packet slowly into approximately 2–6 fluid ounces (1/4–3/4 glassful) of water. Stir thoroughly for approximately 1 minute until slightly thickened, then drink. The entire contents of the packet must be used immediately and not stored for future use. Any microcapsule/water mixture should be used immediately and not stored for future use.

Suspension in Liquids other than Water: Studies conducted using orange juice, tomato juice, apple juice and milk as the suspending liquid have shown that the quantity of fluid used to suspend one Micro-K LS packet MUST be limited to ***2 fluid ounces (1/4 glassful)***. The use of volumes greater than 2 fluid ounces substantially reduces the dose of potassium chloride delivered. If a liquid other than water is used to suspend Micro-K LS then the contents of the packet should be slowly poured into ***2 fluid ounces (1/4 glassful)*** of liquid. Stir thoroughly for approximately 1 minute, then drink. The entire contents of the packet must be used immediately and not stored for future use. Any microcapsule/liquid mixture should be used immediately and not stored for future use.

Sprinkling Contents on Food: Micro-K LS may be given on soft food that may be swallowed easily without chewing, such as applesauce or pudding. After sprinkling the contents of the packet on the food, it should be swallowed immediately without chewing and followed with a glass of cool water, milk, or juice to ensure complete swallowing of all the microcapsules. Do not store microcapsule/food mixture for future use.

HOW SUPPLIED

Micro-K LS containing 1.5 g microencapsulated potassium chloride (equivalent to 20 mEq K) per packet in cartons of 30 (NDC 0031-5760-56) and 100 packets (NDC 0031-5760-63).

Store at controlled room temprature, between 15°C and 30°C (59°F and 86°F).

CAUTION: Federal law prohibits dispensing without prescription.

PHENAPHEN® WITH CODEINE NO. 2 ℞ Ⓒ III
PHENAPHEN® WITH CODEINE NO. 3 ℞ Ⓒ III
PHENAPHEN® WITH CODEINE NO. 4 ℞ Ⓒ III

[fen 'ah-fen"]

(Acetaminophen and Codeine Phosphate Capsules)

DESCRIPTION

Each Phenaphen® with Codeine No. 2 capsule contains:

Acetaminophen, USP .... 325 mg
Codeine Phosphate, USP .... 15 mg
(Warning: May be habit forming)

Inactive Ingredients: Corn Starch, D&C Yellow 10, Edible Ink, FD&C Blue 1, FD&C Red 40, FD&C Yellow 6, Gelatin, Magnesium Stearate, Sodium Starch Glycolate, Stearic Acid.

Each Phenaphen® with Codeine No. 3 capsule contains:

Acetaminophen, USP .... 325 mg
Codeine Phosphate, USP .... 30 mg
(Warning: May be habit forming)

Inactive Ingredients: D&C Yellow 10, Edible Ink, FD&C Blue 1, (FD&C Green 3 *and* Red 40), FD&C Yellow 6, Gelatin, Magnesium Stearate, Sodium Starch Glycolate, Stearic Acid.

Each Phenaphen® with Codeine No. 4 capsule contains:

Acetaminophen, USP .... 325 mg
Codeine Phosphate, USP .... 60 mg
(Warning: May be habit forming)

Inactive Ingredients: Corn Starch, D&C Yellow 10, Edible Ink, FD&C Green 3 or Blue 1, FD&C Yellow 6, Gelatin, Lactose, Magnesium Stearate, Sodium Starch Glycolate, Stearic Acid.

Acetaminophen, 4′-hydroxyacetanilide, is a non-opiate, non-salicylate analgesic and antipyretic which occurs as a white, odorless, crystalline powder, possessing a slightly bitter taste.

Codeine is an alkaloid, obtained from opium or prepared from morphine by methylation. Codeine phosphate occurs as fine, white, needle-shaped crystals, or white, crystalline powder. It is affected by light. Its chemical name is: 7,8-didehydro-4, 5α-epoxy-3-methoxy-17-methylmorphinan-6α-ol phosphate (1:1) (salt) hemihydrate.

CLINICAL PHARMACOLOGY

Phenaphen with Codeine capsules combine the analgesic effects of a centrally acting analgesic, codeine, with a peripherally acting analgesic, acetaminophen. Both ingredients are well absorbed orally. The plasma elimination half-life ranges from 1 to 4 hours for acetaminophen, and from 2.5 to 3 hours for codeine.

Codeine retains at least one-half of its analgesic activity when administered orally. A reduced first-pass metabolism of codeine by the liver accounts for the greater oral efficacy of codeine when compared to most other morphine-like narcotics. Following absorption, codeine is metabolized by the liver and metabolic products are excreted in the urine.

Approximately 10 percent of the administered codeine is demethylated to morphine, which may account for its analgesic activity.

Acetaminophen is distributed throughout most fluids of the body and is metabolized primarily in the liver. Little unchanged drug is excreted in the urine, but most metabolic products appear in the urine within 24 hours.

INDICATIONS AND USAGE

Phenaphen with Codeine capsules are indicated for the relief of mild to moderately severe pain.

CONTRAINDICATIONS

Acetaminophen and codeine phosphate should not be administered to patients who have previously exhibited hypersensitivity to codeine or acetaminophen.

PRECAUTIONS

General

Head Injury and Increased Intracranial Pressure: The respiratory depressant effects of narcotics and their capacity to elevate cerebrospinal fluid pressure may be markedly exaggerated in the presence of head injury, other intracranial lesions or a pre-existing increase in intracranial pressure. Furthermore, narcotics produce adverse reactions which may obscure the clinical course of patients with head injuries.

Acute Abdominal Conditions: The administration of this product or other narcotics may obscure the diagnosis or clinical course of patients with acute abdominal conditions.

Special risk patients: This drug should be given with caution to certain patients such as the elderly or debilitated, and those with severe impairment of hepatic or renal function, hypothyroidism, Addison's disease, and prostatic hypertrophy or urethral structure.

Information for Patients: Codeine may impair the mental and/or physical abilities required for the performance of potentially hazardous tasks such as driving a car or operating machinery. The patient using this drug should be cautioned accordingly.

The patient should understand the single-dose and 24-hour dose limits and the time interval between doses.

Drug Interactions: Patients receiving other narcotic analgesics, antipsychotics, antianxiety agents, or other CNS depressants (including alcohol) concomitantly with this drug may exhibit an additive CNS depression. When such combined therapy is contemplated, the dose of one or both agents should be reduced.

The concurrent use of anticholinergics with codeine may produce paralytic ileus.

Carcinogenesis, Mutagenesis, Impairment of Fertility: No long-term studies in animals have been performed with acetaminophen or codeine to determine carcinogenic potential or effects on fertility.

Acetaminophen and codeine have been found to have no mutagenic potential using the Ames Salmonella-Microsomal Activation test, the Basc test on Drosophila germ cells, and the Micronucleus test on mouse bone marrow.

Pregnancy:

Teratogenic Effects: Pregnancy Category C.

Codeine: A study in rats and rabbits reported no teratogenic effect of codeine administered during the period of organogenesis in doses ranging from 5 to 120 mg/kg. In the rat, doses at the 120 mg/kg level, in the toxic range for the adult animal, were associated with an increase in embryo resorption at the time of implantation. In another study a single 100 mg/kg dose of codeine administered in pregnant mice reportedly resulted in delayed ossification in the offspring.

There are no studies in humans, and the significance of these findings to humans, if any, is not known.

Acetaminophen and codeine phosphate should be used during pregnancy only if the potential benefit justifies the potential risk to the fetus.

Nonteratogenic Effects: Dependence has been reported in newborns whose mothers took opiates regularly during pregnancy. Withdrawal signs include irritability, excessive crying, tremors, hyperreflexia, fever, vomiting, and diarrhea. These signs usually appear during the first few days of life.

Labor and Delivery: Narcotic analgesics cross the placental barrier. The closer to delivery and the larger the dose used, the greater the possibility of respiratory depression in the newborn. Narcotic analgesics should be avoided during labor if delivery of a premature infant is anticipated. If the mother has received narcotic analgesics during labor, newborn infants should be observed closely for signs of respiratory depression. Resuscitation may be required (see "Overdosage"). The effect of codeine, if any, on the later growth, development, and functional maturation of the child is unknown.

Nursing Mothers: Some studies, but not others, have reported detectable amounts of codeine in breast milk. The levels are probably not clinically significant after usual therapeutic dosage. The possibility of clinically important amounts being excreted in breast milk in individuals abusing codeine should be considered.

ADVERSE REACTIONS

The most frequently observed adverse reactions include lightheadedness, dizziness, sedation, shortness of breath, nausea and vomiting. These effects seem to be more prominent in ambulatory than in non-ambulatory patients, and some of these adverse reactions may be alleviated if the patient lies down. Other adverse reactions include allergic re-

Continued on next page

Prescribing information on A. H. Robins products listed here is based on official labeling in effect June 1, 1992, with Indications, Contraindications, Warnings, Precautions, Adverse Reactions, and Dosage stated in full.

A. H. Robins—Cont.

actions, euphoria, dysphoria, constipation, abdominal pain and pruritus.
At higher doses, codeine has most of the disadvantages of morphine including respiratory depression.

DRUG ABUSE AND DEPENDENCE
Acetaminophen and codeine phosphate capsules are a Schedule III controlled substance.
Codeine can produce drug dependence of the morphine type and, therefore, has the potential for being abused. Psychic dependence, physical dependence and tolerance may develop upon repeated administration of this drug, and it should be prescribed and administered with the same degree of caution appropriate to the use of other oral narcotic-containing medications.

OVERDOSAGE
Acetaminophen:
Signs and Symptoms: In acute acetaminophen overdosage, dose-dependent, potentially fatal hepatic necrosis is the most serious adverse effect. Renal tubular necrosis, hypoglycemic coma and thrombocytopenia may also occur.
In adults, hepatic toxicity has rarely been reported with acute overdoses of less than 10 grams and fatalities with less than 15 grams. Importantly, young children seem to be more resistant than adults to the hepatotoxic effect of an acetaminophen overdose. Despite this, the measures outlined below should be initiated in any adult or child suspected of having ingested an acetaminophen overdose.
Early symptoms following a potentially hepatotoxic overdose may include: nausea, vomiting, diaphoresis and general malaise. Clinical and laboratory evidence of hepatic toxicity may not be apparent until 48 to 72 hours post-ingestion.
Treatment: The stomach should be emptied promptly by lavage or by induction of emesis with syrup of ipecac. Patients' estimates of the quantity of a drug ingested are notoriously unreliable. Therefore, if an acetaminophen overdose is suspected, a serum acetaminophen assay should be obtained as early as possible, but no sooner than four hours following ingestion. Liver function studies should be obtained initially and repeated at 24-hour intervals.
The antidote, N-acetylcysteine, should be administered as early as possible, preferably within 16 hours of the overdose ingestion for optimal results, but in any case, within 24 hours. Following recovery, there are no residual, structural or functional hepatic abnormalities.
Codeine:
Signs and Symptoms: Serious overdose with codeine is characterized by respiratory depression (a decrease in respiratory rate and/or tidal volume, Cheyne-Stokes respiration, cyanosis), extreme somnolence progressing to stupor or coma, skeletal muscle flaccidity, cold and clammy skin, and sometimes bradycardia and hypotension. In severe overdosage, apnea, circulatory collapse, cardiac arrest and death may occur.
Treatment: Primary attention should be given to the reestablishment of adequate respiratory exchange through provision of a patent airway and the institution of assisted or controlled ventilation. The narcotic antagonist naloxone is a specific antidote against respiratory depression which may result from overdosage or unusual sensitivity to narcotics, including codeine. Therefore, an appropriate dose of naloxone hydrochloride (see package insert) should be administered, preferably by the intravenous route, and simultaneously with efforts at respiratory resuscitation. Since the duration of action of codeine may exceed that of the antagonist, the patient should be kept under continued surveillance and repeated doses of the antagonist should be administered as needed to maintain adequate respiration.
An antagonist should not be administered in the absence of clinically significant respiratory or cardiovascular depression. Oxygen, intravenous fluids, vasopressors and other supportive measures should be employed as indicated.
Gastric emptying may be useful in removing unabsorbed drug.

DOSAGE AND ADMINISTRATION
Dosage should be adjusted according to severity of pain and response of the patient.
The usual adult dosage is:

	Single Doses (Range)	Maximum 24 Hour Dose
Codeine Phosphate	15 mg–60 mg	360 mg
Acetaminophen	300 mg–1000 mg	4000 mg

Doses may be repeated up to every 4 hours.
The prescriber must determine the number of capsules per dose, and the maximum number of capsules per 24 hours, based upon the above dosage guidance. This information should be conveyed in the prescription.
For children, the single dose of codeine phosphate is 0.5 mg/kg.
This dose may be repeated up to every four hours.
It should be kept in mind, however, that tolerance to codeine can develop with continued use and that the incidence of untoward effects is dose related. Adult doses of codeine higher than 60 mg fail to give commensurate relief of pain but merely prolong analgesia and are associated with an appreciably increased incidence of undesirable side effects. Equivalently high doses in children would have similar effects.

HOW SUPPLIED
Phenaphen with Codeine No. 2, black and yellow capsules in bottles of 100 (NDC 0031-6242-63).
Phenaphen with Codeine No. 3, black and green capsules in bottles of 100 (NDC 0031-6257-63) and 500 (NDC 0031-6257-70) and Dis-Co® Unit Dose Packs (4×25's) (NDC 0031-6257-61).
Phenaphen with Codeine No. 4, green and white capsules in bottles of 100 (NDC 0031-6274-63) and 500 (NDC 0031-6274-70).
Store at controlled room temperature, between 15°C and 30°C (59°F and 86°F).
Dispense capsules in tight, light-resistant container.
Shown in Product Identification Section, page 425

PHENAPHEN®-650 WITH CODEINE TABLETS ℞ Ⓒ
[fen 'ah-fen"]
(Acetaminophen and Codeine Phosphate Tablets)

DESCRIPTION
Each Phenaphen®-650 with Codeine tablet contains:
Acetaminophen, USP .... 650 mg
Codeine Phosphate, USP .... 30 mg
(Warning: May be habit forming)
Inactive Ingredients: Calcium Sulfate, Corn Starch, Microcrystalline Cellulose, Polyethylene Glycol, Povidone, Colloidal Silicon Dioxide, Sodium Starch Glycolate, Stearic Acid.
Acetaminophen, 4'-hydroxyacetanilide, is a non-opiate, non-salicylate analgesic and antipyretic which occurs as a white, odorless, crystalline powder, possessing a slightly bitter taste.
Codeine is an alkaloid, obtained from opium or prepared from morphine by methylation. Codeine phosphate occurs as fine, white, needle-shaped crystals, or white, crystalline powder. It is affected by light. Its chemical name is: 7,8-didehydro-4, 5α-epoxy-3-methoxy-17-methylmorphinan-6α-ol phosphate (1:1) (salt) hemihydrate.
Clinical Pharmacology
Phenaphen-650 with Codeine combines the analgesic effects of a centrally acting analgesic, codeine, with a peripherally acting analgesic, acetaminophen. Both ingredients are well absorbed orally. The plasma elimination half-life ranges from 1 to 4 hours for acetaminophen, and from 2.5 to 3 hours for codeine.
Codeine retains at least one-half of its analgesic activity when administered orally. A reduced first-pass metabolism of codeine by the liver accounts for the greater oral efficacy of codeine when compared to most other morphine-like narcotics. Following absorption, codeine is metabolized by the liver and metabolic products are excreted in the urine. Approximately 10 percent of the administered codeine is demethylated to morphine, which may account for its analgesic activity.
Acetaminophen is distributed throughout most fluids of the body and is metabolized primarily in the liver. Little unchanged drug is excreted in the urine, but most metabolic products appear in the urine within 24 hours.

INDICATIONS AND USAGE
Phenaphen-650 with Codeine Tablets are indicated for the relief of mild to moderately severe pain.

CONTRAINDICATIONS
Acetaminophen and codeine phosphate should not be administered to patients who have previously exhibited hypersensitivity to codeine or acetaminophen.

PRECAUTIONS
General:
Head Injury and Increased Intracranial Pressure. The respiratory depressant effects of narcotics and their capacity to elevate cerebrospinal fluid pressure may be markedly exaggerated in the presence of head injury, other intracranial lesions or a pre-existing increase in intracranial pressure. Furthermore, narcotics produce adverse reactions which may obscure the clinical course of patients with head injuries.
Acute Abdominal Conditions. The administration of this product or other narcotics may obscure the diagnosis or clinical course in patients with acute abdominal conditions.
Special Risk Patients. This drug should be given with caution to certain patients such as the elderly or debilitated, and those with severe impairment of hepatic or renal function, hypothyroidism, Addison's disease, and prostatic hypertrophy or, urethral stricture.
Information for Patients. Codeine may impair the mental and/or physical abilities required for the performance of potentially hazardous tasks such as driving a car or operating machinery. The patient using this drug should be cautioned accordingly.
The patient should understand the single-dose and 24 hour dose limits and the time interval between doses.
Drug Interactions. Patients receiving other narcotic analgesics, antipsychotics, antianxiety agents, or other CNS depressants (including alcohol) concomitantly with this drug may exhibit additive CNS depression. When such combined therapy is contemplated, the dose of one or both agents should be reduced.
The concurrent use of anticholinergics with codeine may produce paralytic ileus.
Carcinogenesis, Mutagenesis, Impairment of Fertility: No long-term studies in animals have been performed with acetaminophen or codeine to determine carcinogenic potential or effects on fertility.
Acetaminophen and codeine have been found to have no mutagenic potential using the Ames Salmonella-Microsomal Activation test, the Basc test on Drosophila germ cells, and the Micronucleus test on mouse bone marrow.
Pregnancy:
Teratogenic Effects: Pregnancy Category C.
Codeine: A study in rats and rabbits reported no teratogenic effect of codeine administered during the period of organogenesis in doses ranging from 5 to 120 mg/kg. In the rat, doses at the 120 mg/kg level, in the toxic range for the adult animal, were associated with an increase in embryo resorption at the time of implantation. In another study a single 100 mg/kg dose of codeine administered to pregnant mice reportedly resulted in delayed ossification in the offspring.
There are no studies in humans, and the significance of these findings to humans, if any, is not known.
Acetaminophen and codeine phosphate should be used during pregnancy only if the potential benefit justifies the potential risk to the fetus.
Nonteratogenic Effects: Dependence has been reported in newborns whose mothers took opiates regularly during pregnancy. Withdrawal signs include irritability, excessive crying, tremors, hyperreflexia, fever, vomiting, and diarrhea. These signs usually appear during the first days of life.
Labor and Delivery: Narcotic analgesics cross the placental barrier. The closer to delivery and the larger the dose used, the greater the possibility of respiratory depression in the newborn. Narcotic analgesics should be avoided during labor if delivery of a premature infant is anticipated. If the mother has received narcotic analgesics during labor, newborn infants should be observed closely for signs of respiratory depression. Resuscitation may be required (see "Overdosage"). The effect of codeine, if any, on the later growth, development, and functional maturation of the child is unknown.
Nursing Mothers: Some studies, but not others, have reported detectable amounts of codeine in breast milk. The levels are probably not clinically significant after usual therapeutic dosage. The possibility of clinically important amounts being excreted in breast milk in individuals abusing codeine should be considered.

ADVERSE REACTIONS
The most frequently observed adverse reactions include lightheadedness, dizziness, sedation, shortness of breath, nausea and vomiting. These effects seem to be more prominent in ambulatory than non-ambulatory patients, and some of these adverse reactions may be alleviated if the patient lies down. Other adverse reactions include allergic reactions, euphoria, dysphoria, constipation, abdominal pain and pruritus.
At higher doses, codeine has most of the disadvantages of morphine including respiratory depression.
Drug Abuse and Dependence
Acetaminophen and codeine phosphate tablets are a Schedule III controlled substance.
Codeine can produce drug dependence of the morphine type and, therefore, has the potential for being abused. Psychic dependence, physical dependence and tolerance may develop upon repeated administration of this drug, and it should be prescribed and administered with the same degree of caution appropriate to the use of other oral narcotic-containing medications.

OVERDOSAGE
Acetaminophen:
Signs and Symptoms: In acute acetaminophen overdosage, dose-dependent, potentially fatal hepatic necrosis is the most serious adverse effect. Renal tubular necrosis, hypoglycemic coma and thrombocytopenia may also occur.
In adults, hepatic toxicity has rarely been reported with acute overdoses of less than 10 grams and fatalities with less than 15 grams. Importantly, young children seem to be more resistant than adults to the hepatotoxic effect of an acetaminophen overdose. Despite this, the measures outlined below

should be initiated in any adult or child suspected of having ingested an acetaminophen overdose.

Early symptoms following a potentially hepatotoxic overdose may include: nausea, vomiting, diaphoresis and general malaise. Clinical and laboratory evidence of hepatic toxicity may not be apparent until 48 to 72 hours post-ingestion.

Treatment: The stomach should be emptied promptly by lavage or by induction of emesis with syrup of ipecac. Patients' estimates of the quantity of a drug ingested are notoriously unreliable. Therefore, if an acetaminophen overdose is suspected, a serum acetaminophen assay should be obtained as early as possible, but no sooner than four hours following ingestion. Liver function studies should be obtained initially and repeated at 24-hour intervals.

The antidote, N-acetylcysteine, should be administered as early as possible, preferably within 16 hours of the overdose ingestion for optimal results, but in any case, within 24 hours. Following recovery, there are no residual, structural or functional hepatic abnormalities.

Codeine:

Signs and Symptoms: Serious overdose with codeine is characterized by respiratory depression (a decrease in respiratory rate and/or tidal volume, Cheyne-Stokes respiration, cyanosis), extreme somnolence progressing to stupor or coma, skeletal muscle flaccidity, cold and clammy skin, and sometimes bradycardia and hypotension. In severe overdosage, apnea, circulatory collapse, cardiac arrest and death may occur.

Treatment: Primary attention should be given to the reestablishment of adequate respiratory exchange through provision of a patent airway and the institution of assisted or controlled ventilation. The narcotic antagonist naloxone is a specific antidote against respiratory depression which may result from overdosage or unusual sensitivity to narcotics, including codeine. Therefore, an appropriate dose of naloxone hydrochloride (see package insert) should be administered, preferably by the intravenous route, and simultaneously with efforts at respiratory resuscitation. Since the duration of action of codeine may exceed that of the antagonist, the patient should be kept under continued surveillance and repeated doses of the antagonist should be administered as needed to maintain adequate respiration.

An antagonist should not be administered in the absence of clinically significant respiratory or cardiovascular depression. Oxygen, intravenous fluids, vasopressors and other supportive measures should be employed as indicated.

Gastric emptying may be useful in removing unabsorbed drug.

DOSAGE AND ADMINISTRATION

Dosage should be adjusted according to severity of pain and response of the patient.

The usual adult dosage is:

	Single Doses (Range)	Maximum 24 Hour Dose
Codeine Phosphate	15 mg–60 mg	360 mg
Acetaminophen	300 mg–1000 mg	4000 mg

Doses may be repeated up to every 4 hours.

The prescriber must determine the number of tablets per dose, and the maximum number of tablets per 24 hours, based upon the above dosage guidance. This information should be conveyed in the prescription.

For children, the single dose of codeine phosphate is 0.5 mg/kg.

This dose may be repeated up to every four hours.

It should be kept in mind, however, that tolerance to codeine can develop with continued use and that the incidence of untoward effects is dose related. Adult doses of codeine higher than 60 mg fail to give commensurate relief of pain but merely prolong analgesia and are associated with an appreciably increased incidence of undesirable side effects. Equivalently high doses in children would have similar effects.

HOW SUPPLIED

Phenaphen-650 with Codeine is available as a scored, white, capsule-shaped compressed tablet, engraved AHR and 6251 containing 650 mg acetaminophen and 30 mg of codeine phosphate in bottles of 50 (NDC 0031-6251-60).

Store at controlled room temperature, between 15°C and 30°C (59°F and 86°F).

Dispense tablets in tight, light-resistant container.

Shown in Product Identification Section, page 425

PONDIMIN® TABLETS   ℞ ℂⅣ

[pŏn´dĭ-min]

brand of Fenfluramine Hydrochloride

Tablets—20 mg

DESCRIPTION

Pondimin (fenfluramine hydrochloride) is an anorectic drug for oral administration. Immediate release tablets containing 20 mg fenfluramine hydrochloride are orange, scored, compressed tablets engraved AHR and 6447.

Inactive Ingredients: Corn Starch, FD&C Yellow 6, Magnesium Stearate, Microcrystalline Cellulose, Silicon Dioxide, Sodium Lauryl Sulfate.

Pondimin has the chemical name, N-ethyl-α-methyl-3-(trifluoromethyl) benzeneethanamine hydrochloride.

CLINICAL PHARMACOLOGY

Fenfluramine is a sympathomimetic amine, the pharmacologic activity of which differs somewhat from that of the prototype drugs of this class used in obesity, the amphetamines, in appearing to produce more central nervous system depression than stimulation.

The mechanism of action of Pondimin is unclear but may be related to brain levels (or turnover rates) of serotonin or to increased glucose utilization. The antiappetite effects of Pondimin are suppressed by serotonin-blocking drugs and by drugs that lower brain levels of the amine. Furthermore, decreased serotonin levels produced by selective brain lesions suppress the action of Pondimin.

In a study of 20 normal males, fenfluramine increased glucose utilization, resulting in decreased blood glucose levels. Experimental work in animals suggested that increased glucose utilization activated the satiety center and decreased the activity of the feeding center. Perhaps by this mechanism Pondimin inhibits appetite. The relationship between glucose utilization and serotonin has not been clarified.

Fenfluramine is well-absorbed from the gastrointestinal tract, and a maximal anorectic effect is generally seen after 2 to 4 hours. In man, fenfluramine is de-ethylated to norfenfluramine which is subsequently oxidized to m-trifluoromethyl benzoic acid and excreted as the glycine conjugate, m-trifluoromethylhippuric acid. Other compounds found in the urine include unchanged fenfluramine and norfenfluramine.

The rate of excretion of fenfluramine is pH dependent, with much smaller amounts appearing in an alkaline than in an acid urine.

The half-life of fenfluramine is said to be about 20 hours, compared with 5 hours for amphetamines; however, if urinary excretion is rapid and the pH maintained in the acidic range (below pH 5), half-life can be reduced to 11 hours. Fenfluramine and norfenfluramine reach steady state concentrations in plasma within 3 to 4 days following chronic dosage.

The greatest weight loss is seen in those patients who maintain the highest levels of Pondimin. A 2-to-3-kg weight loss over 6 weeks is associated with a plasma level of 0.1 mcg/mL (or 10 mcg/100 mL).

Fenfluramine is widely distributed in almost all body tissues. It is soluble in lipids and crosses the blood-brain barrier. Fenfluramine crosses the placenta readily in monkeys.

INDICATIONS AND USAGE

Pondimin is indicated in the management of exogenous obesity as a short-term (a few weeks) adjunct in a regimen of weight reduction based on caloric restriction.

Drugs of this class used in obesity are commonly known as "anorectics" or "anorexigenics." It has not been established, however, that the action of such drugs in treating obesity is primarily one of appetite suppression. Other central nervous system actions or metabolic effects may be involved.

Adult obese subjects instructed in dietary management and treated with "anorectic" drugs, lose more weight on the average than those treated with placebo and diet, as determined in relatively short-term trials.

The average magnitude of increased weight loss of drug-treated patients over placebo-treated is only a fraction of a pound a week. The rate of weight loss is greatest in the first weeks of therapy for both drug and placebo subjects and tends to decrease in succeeding weeks. The possible origins of the increased weight loss due to the various drug effects are not established. The average amount of weight loss associated with the use of an "anorectic" drug varies from trial to trial, and the increased weight loss appears to be related in part to variables other than the drug prescribed such as the physician-investigator, the population treated and the diet prescribed. Studies do not permit conclusions as to the relative importance of the drug and non-drug factors on weight loss.

The natural history of obesity is measured in years, whereas the studies cited are restricted to a few weeks duration; thus, the total impact of drug-induced weight loss over that of diet alone must be considered clinically limited.

CONTRAINDICATIONS

Fenfluramine is contraindicated in patients with glaucoma or with hypersensitivity to fenfluramine or other sympathomimetic amines. Do not administer fenfluramine during or within 14 days following the administration of monoamine oxidase inhibitors, since hypertensive crises may result. Patients with a history of drug abuse should not receive the drug.

Do not administer fenfluramine to patients with alcoholism since psychiatric symptoms (paranoia, depression, psychosis) have been reported in a few such patients who had been administered this drug.

Fenfluramine should also generally be avoided in patients with psychotic illness. There have been reports of schizophrenic patients who have become agitated, delusional, and assaultive.

A fatal cardiac arrest has been reported shortly after the induction of anesthesia in a patient who had been taking fenfluramine prior to surgery. Fenfluramine may have a catecholamine-depleting effect when administered for prolonged periods of time; therefore, potent anesthetic agents should be administered with caution to patients taking fenfluramine. If general anesthesia cannot be avoided, full cardiac monitoring and facilities for instant resuscitative measures are a minimum necessity.

WARNINGS

When tolerance to the "anorectic" effect develops, the maximum recommended dose should not be exceeded in an attempt to increase the effect; rather, the drug should be discontinued.

PRECAUTIONS

General. Fenfluramine differs in its pharmacological profile from other "anorectic" drugs with which the prescribing practitioner may be familiar. Correspondingly, there are possible adverse effects not associated with other "anorectics"; such effects include those of diarrhea, sedation, and depression. The possibility of these effects should be weighed against the possible advantage of decreased central nervous system stimulation and/or abuse potential.

There have been four cases of pulmonary hypertension reported in association with fenfluramine use. Two cases were apparently reversible after discontinuation of fenfluramine, but evidence of pulmonary hypertension recurred in one of these patients upon rechallenge with fenfluramine. A third patient was initially improved with nifedipine treatment, but was noted to have increased pulmonary arterial pressure again at a four month follow up visit. Finally, an irreversible and fatal case of pulmonary hypertension has been reported in a patient who had seven 1-month courses of fenfluramine in the twelve years prior to death. Patients taking fenfluramine should be advised to report immediately any deterioration in exercise tolerance.

Use only with caution in hypertension, with monitoring of blood pressure, since evidence is insufficient to rule out a possible adverse effect on blood pressure in some hypertensive patients. The drug is not recommended in severely hypertensive patients. The drug is not recommended for patients with symptomatic cardiovascular disease including arrhythmias.

Caution should be exercised in prescribing fenfluramine for patients with a history of mental depression. Further depression of mood may become evident while the patient is on fenfluramine or following withdrawal of fenfluramine. Symptoms of depression occurring immediately following abrupt withdrawal can be readily controlled by reinstituting Pondimin, followed by a gradual tapering off of the daily dose.

Information for Patients. Fenfluramine may impair the ability of the patient to engage in potentially hazardous activities such as operating machinery or driving a motor vehicle (see "Adverse Reactions"); the patient should be cautioned accordingly. Patient should also be advised to avoid alcoholic beverages while taking Pondimin.

Drug Interactions. Fenfluramine may increase slightly the effect of antihypertensive drugs, e.g., guanethidine, methyldopa, reserpine.

Other CNS depressant drugs should be used with caution in patients taking fenfluramine, since the effects may be additive.

Carcinogenesis, Mutagenesis. No carcinogenic studies or mutagenic studies have been undertaken with this drug.

Pregnancy Category C. Pondimin was shown to produce a questionable embryotoxic effect in rats and a reduced conception rate when given in a dose of 20 times the human dose. However, additional reproduction studies in rats, rabbits, mice, and monkeys at doses up to, respectively, 5 times, 20 times, 1 time, and 5 times the human dose yielded negative results.

There are no adequate and well-controlled studies in pregnant women. Pondimin should be used during pregnancy only if the potential benefit justifies the potential risk to the fetus.

Labor and Delivery. The effect of fenfluramine during labor or delivery on the mother and the fetus is unknown. The effect on later growth, development, and functional maturation of the child is unknown.

Nursing Mothers. It is not known whether this drug is excreted in human milk. Because many drugs are excreted in

Continued on next page

Prescribing information on A. H. Robins products listed here is based on official labeling in effect June 1, 1992, with Indications, Contraindications, Warnings, Precautions, Adverse Reactions, and Dosage stated in full.

A. H. Robins—Cont.

human milk, caution should be exercised when fenfluramine is administered to a nursing mother.

Pediatric Use. Safety and effectiveness in children below the age of 12 years have not been established.

ADVERSE REACTIONS

The most common adverse reactions of fenfluramine are drowsiness, diarrhea, and dry mouth. Less frequent adverse reactions reported in association with fenfluramine are:

Central nervous system. Dizziness; confusion; incoordination; headache; elevated mood; depression; anxiety, nervousness, or tension; insomnia; weakness or fatigue; increased or decreased libido; agitation, dysarthria.

Gastrointestinal. Constipation; abdominal pain; nausea.

Autonomic. Sweating; chills; blurred vision.

Genitourinary. Dysuria; urinary frequency.

Cardiovascular. Palpitation; hypotension; hypertension; fainting; pulmonary hypertension.

Skin. Rash; urticaria; burning sensation.

Miscellaneous. Eye irritation; myalgia; fever; chest pain; bad taste.

DRUG ABUSE AND DEPENDENCE

Pondimin (fenfluramine hydrochloride) is a controlled substance in Schedule IV. Fenfluramine is related chemically to the amphetamines, although it differs somewhat pharmacologically. The amphetamines and related stimulant drugs have been extensively abused and can produce tolerance and severe psychological dependence, as well as other adverse organic and mental changes. In this regard, there has been a report of abuse of fenfluramine by subjects with a history of abuse of other drugs. Abuse of 80 to 400 milligrams of the drug has been reported to be associated with euphoria, derealization, and perceptual changes. Fenfluramine did not produce signs of dependence in animals and appears to produce sedation more often than CNS stimulation at therapeutic doses. Its abuse potential appears qualitatively different from that of amphetamines. The possibility that fenfluramine may induce dependence should be kept in mind when evaluating the desirability of including the drug in the weight reduction programs of individual patients.

OVERDOSAGE

Signs and Symptoms: Only limited data have been reported concerning clinical effects and management of overdosage of fenfluramine.

Agitation and drowsiness, confusion, flushing, tremor (or shivering), fever, sweating, abdominal pain, hyperventilation, and dilated non-reactive pupils seem frequent in fenfluramine overdosage. Reflexes may be either exaggerated or depressed and some patients may have rotary nystagmus. Tachycardia may be present, but blood pressure may be normal or only slightly elevated. Convulsions, coma, and ventricular extrasystoles, culminating in ventricular fibrillation, and cardiac arrest, may occur at higher dosages.

Human Toxicity. Less than 5 mg/kg are toxic to humans. Five-ten mg/kg may produce coma and convulsions. Reported single overdoses have ranged from 300 to 2000 mg; the lowest reported fatal dose was a few hundred mg in a small child, and the highest reported nonfatal dose was 1800 mg in an adult. Most deaths were apparently due to respiratory failure and cardiac arrest.

Toxic effects will appear within 30 to 60 minutes and may progress rapidly to potentially fatal complications in 90 to 240 minutes. Symptoms may persist for extended periods depending upon the dose ingested.

Management. After overdosage, only a small percentage of the drug is excreted in the urine. Forced acid diuresis has been recommended only in extreme cases in which the patient survives the early hours of intoxication but fails to show decisive improvement from other measures. Hemodialysis and peritoneal dialysis are of theoretical advantage but have not been used clinically.

Reportedly the treatment of fenfluramine intoxication should include:

- *Gastric lavage* (but not drug-induced emesis because the patient may become unconscious at a very early stage.)
- In the event that gastric lavage is not feasible due to trismus, consult an anesthesiologist for endotracheal intubation after administration of muscle relaxants; only then gastric evacuation should be tried.
- Administration of activated charcoal after emesis or lavage may reduce absorption of drug.
- *Monitoring of vital functions.* If necessary, mechanical respiration, defibrillation, or "cardioversion" should be instituted.
- *Drug therapy.* Diazepam or phenobarbital for convulsions or muscular hyperactivity. In the presence of extreme tachycardia; propranolol; in the presence of ventricular extrasystoles; lidocaine; in the presence of hyperpyrexia; chlorpromazine.

Since fenfluramine has been shown to have a slight lowering effect on blood sugar in some patients, the theoretical possi-

bility of hypoglycemia should be borne in mind although this effect has not been reported in cases of clinical overdosage.

DOSAGE AND ADMINISTRATION

The usual dose is one 20 mg tablet three times daily before meals. Depending on the degree of effectiveness and side effects, the dosage may be increased at weekly intervals by one tablet (20 mg) daily until a maximum dosage of two tablets three times daily is attained. Total dosage of fenfluramine should not exceed 120 mg per day.

HOW SUPPLIED

Pondimin is available in 20 mg orange, scored, compressed tablets monogrammed AHR and 6447, in bottles of 100 (NDC 0031-6447-63) and 500 (NDC 0031-6447-70).

Store at controlled room temperature, between 15°C and 30°C (59°F and 86°F).

Dispense in well-closed container.

Shown in Product Identification Section, page 425

QUINIDEX EXTENTABS®   ℞
[kwĭn 'ĭ "dĕks ĕks "tĕn 'tabs]
brand of Quinidine Sulfate Extended-release Tablets, USP

DESCRIPTION

Quinidex Extentabs (quinidine sulfate extended-release tablets) are constructed to release one-third of their alkaloidal salt, quinidine sulfate (100 mg), on reaching the stomach, to begin absorption in the upper intestinal tract. The remaining two-thirds of the active drug (200 mg) is evenly distributed throughout a homogeneous core which slowly dissolves as it moves along the intestinal tract, releasing the quinidine sulfate for continuous absorption over an 8–12 hour period. Each Quinidex Extentabs tablet contains 300 mg of quinidine sulfate, the equivalent of 248.6 mg of the anhydrous quinidine alkaloid.

Chemically, quinidine sulfate is cinchonan-9-ol,6'-methoxy-, (9s)-sulfate(2:1) (salt) dihydrate.

Inactive Ingredients: Acacia, Acetylated Monoglycerides, Calcium Sulfate, Carnauba Wax, Edible Ink, FD&C Blue 2, Gelatin, Guar Gum, Magnesium Oxide, Magnesium Stearate, Polysorbates, Shellac, Sucrose, Titanium Dioxide, White Wax and other ingredients, one of which is a corn derivative. May contain FD&C Red 40 and FD&C Yellow 6 Aluminum Lakes.

ACTION

The action of quinidine in preventing aberrant cardiac rhythms of atrial and ventricular origin resides in its ability to (a) depress excitability of cardiac muscle, (b) slow the rate of spontaneous rhythm, (c) decrease vagal tone, and (d) prolong conduction and effective refractory period.

INDICATIONS AND USAGE

Quinidex Extentabs are indicated for the treatment of:
- Premature atrial and ventricular contractions.
- Paroxysmal atrial tachycardia.
- Paroxysmal A-V junctional rhythm.
- Atrial flutter.
- Paroxysmal atrial fibrillation.
- Established atrial fibrillation when therapy is appropriate.
- Paroxysmal ventricular tachycardia when not associated with complete heartblock.
- Maintenance therapy after electrical conversion of atrial fibrillation and/or flutter.

CONTRAINDICATIONS

Intraventricular conduction defects. Complete A-V block. A-V conduction disorders caused by digitalis intoxication. Aberrant impulses and abnormal rhythms due to escape mechanisms. Idiosyncrasy or hypersensitivity to quinidine or related cinchona derivatives. Myasthenia gravis.

WARNINGS

In the treatment of atrial flutter, reversion to sinus rhythm may be preceded by a progressive reduction in the degree of A-V block to a 1:1 ratio, resulting in an extremely rapid ventricular rate. This possible hazard may be reduced by digitalization prior to administration of quinidine.

Reports in the literature indicate that serum concentrations of digoxin may increase and may even double when quinidine is administered concurrently. Patients on concomitant therapy should be carefully monitored for digitalis toxicity. Reduction of digoxin dosage may have to be considered. Manifestations of quinidine cardiotoxicity such as excessive prolongation of the QT interval, widening of the QRS complex and ventricular tachyarrhythmias mandate immediate discontinuation of the drug and/or close clinical and electrocardiographic monitoring.

In susceptible individuals, such as those with marginally compensated cardiovascular disease, quinidine may produce clinically important depression of cardiac function manifested by hypotension, bradycardia, or heartblock. Quinidine therapy should be carefully monitored in such individuals.

Quinidine should be used with extreme caution in patients with incomplete AV block since complete AV block and asystole may be produced. Quinidine may cause abnormalities of cardiac rhythm in digitalized patients and therefore should be used with caution in the presence of digitalis intoxication. Quinidine should be used with caution in patients exhibiting renal, cardiac or hepatic insufficiency because of potential accumulation of quinidine in serum, leading to toxicity.

Patients taking quinidine occasionally have syncopal episodes which usually result from ventricular tachycardia or fibrillation. This syndrome has not been shown to be related to dose or serum levels. Syncopal episodes frequently terminate spontaneously or in response to treatment, but sometimes are fatal.

Cases of hepatotoxicity, including granulomatous hepatitis, due to quinidine hypersensitivity have been reported. Unexplained fever and/or elevation of hepatic enzymes, particularly in the early stages of therapy, warrant consideration of possible hepatotoxicity. Monitoring liver function during the first 4–8 weeks should be considered. Cessation of quinidine in these cases usually results in the disappearance of toxicity.

PRECAUTIONS

General—All the precautions applying to regular quinidine therapy apply to this product. Hypersensitivity or anaphylactoid reactions to quinidine, although rare, should be considered, especially during the first weeks of therapy. Hospitalization for close clinical observation, electrocardiographic monitoring, and determination of serum quinidine levels are indicated when large doses of quinidine are used or with patients who present an increased risk.

Information for Patients—As with all solid dosage medications, Quinidex Extentabs should be taken with an adequate amount of fluid, preferably with the patient in an upright position to facilitate swallowing. They should be swallowed whole in order to preserve the controlled-release mechanism.

Laboratory Tests—Periodic blood counts and liver and kidney function tests should be performed during long-term therapy; the drug should be discontinued if blood dyscrasias or evidence of hepatic or renal dysfunction occurs.

Drug Interactions

Drug	Effect
Quinidine with anticholinergic drugs	Additive vagolytic effect
Quinidine with cholinergic drugs	Antagonism of cholinergic effects
Quinidine with carbonic anhydrase inhibitors, sodium bicarbonate, thiazide diuretics	Alkalinization of urine resulting in decreased excretion of quinidine
Quinidine with coumarin anticoagulants	Reduction of clotting factor concentrations
Quinidine with tubocurare, succinylcholine and decamethonium	Potentiation of neuro-muscular blockade
Quinidine with phenothiazines and reserpine	Additive cardiac depressive effects
Quinidine with hepatic enzyme-inducing drugs (phenobarbital, phenytoin, rifampin)	Decreased plasma half-life of quinidine
Quinidine with digoxin	Increased serum concentration of digoxin (See Warnings)
Quinidine with amiodarone	Increased serum concentration of quinidine
Quinidine with cimetidine	Prolonged quinidine half-life and an increase in serum quinidine level
Quinidine with ranitidine	Premature ventricular contractions and/or bigeminy
Quinidine with verapamil	Increased quinidine half-life and an increase in serum quinidine level; potential hypotensive reactions
Quinidine with nifedipine	Decreased serum concentrations of quinidine

Carcinogenesis: Studies in animals have not been performed to evaluate the carcinogenic potential of quinidine.

Pregnancy, Teratogenic Effects: Pregnancy Category C. Animal reproduction studies have not been conducted with quinidine. There are no adequate and well-controlled studies in pregnant women. Quinidex Extentabs should be administered to a pregnant woman only if clearly indicated.

Nonteratogenic Effects: Like quinine, quinidine has been reported to have oxytocic properties. The significance of this property in the clinical setting has not been established.

Labor and Delivery—There is no known use for Quinidex Extentabs in labor and delivery. However, quinidine has

been reported to have oxytocic properties. The significance of this property in the clinical setting has not been established.

Nursing Mothers—Because of passage of the drug into breast milk, caution should be exercised when Quinidex Extentabs are administered to a nursing woman.

Pediatric Use—There are no adequate and well-controlled studies establishing the safety and effectiveness of Quinidex Extentabs in children.

ADVERSE REACTIONS

Symptoms of cinchonism, such as ringing in the ears, loss of hearing, dizziness, lightheadedness, headache, nausea, and/or disturbed vision may appear in sensitive patients after a single dose of the drug. The most frequently encountered side effects to quinidine are gastrointestinal.

Gastrointestinal—Nausea, vomiting, abdominal pain, diarrhea, anorexia, granulomatous hepatitis (which may be preceded by fever), esophagitis.

Cardiovascular—Ventricular extrasystoles occurring at a rate of one or more every 6 normal beats; widening of the QRS complex and prolonged QT interval; complete A-V block; ventricular tachycardia and fibrillation; ventricular flutter; torsade de pointes; arterial embolism; hypotension; syncope.

Central Nervous System—Headache, vertigo, apprehension, excitement, confusion, delirium, dementia, ataxia, depression.

Ophthalmologic and Otologic—Disturbed hearing (tinnitus, decreased auditory acuity), disturbed vision (mydriasis, blurred vision, disturbed color perception, photophobia, diplopia, night blindness, scotomata), optic neuritis, reduced visual field.

Dermatologic—Cutaneous flushing with intense pruritus, photosensitivity, urticaria, rash, eczema, exfoliative eruptions, psoriasis, abnormalities of pigmentation.

Hypersensitivity—Angioedema, acute asthmatic episode, vascular collapse, respiratory arrest, hepatotoxicity, granulomatous hepatitis (See Warnings), purpura, vasculitis.

Hematologic—Thrombocytopenia, thrombocytopenic purpura, agranulocytosis, acute hemolytic anemia, hypoprothrombinemia, leukocytosis, shift to left in WBC differential, neutropenia.

Immunologic—Systemic lupus erythematosus, lupus nephritis.

Miscellaneous—Fever, increase in serum skeletal muscle creatine phosphokinase, arthralgia, myalgia.

OVERDOSAGE

Symptoms—Overdosage of quinidine can lead to accelerated idioventricular rhythm, morphologic appearance of QRS complexes, prolonged QT intervals, intermittent sinus capture beats, paroxysms of tachycardia, ventricular arrhythmias, hypotension, oliguria, respiratory depression, pulmonary edema, acidosis, seizures, and coma.

Treatment—Early treatment to empty the stomach using syrup of ipecac and/or gastric lavage is recommended. Since Quinidex Extentabs cannot be removed through a nasogastric tube, gastric lavage should be followed by saline cathartics. Administration of activated charcoal may reduce absorption. Other general supportive measures should be employed as indicated by patient response. In severe cases, circulation should be stabilized and measurements of pulmonary capillary wedge pressure should be performed to assure adequate left ventricular filling pressure. Electrolyte and blood gas abnormalities should be corrected. In quinidine-induced vasodilation, catecholamines and other alpha-adrenergic agonists may be tried. Arrhythmias may be treated with lidocaine, pacing, and cardioversion. Administration of sodium lactate reportedly reduces the cardiotoxicity of quinidine; however, sodium lactate is contraindicated in the presence of alkalosis as increased urinary pH can lead to an increase in the renal tubular absorption of quinidine. Acidification of the urine may enhance the urinary excretion of quinidine.

DOSAGE AND ADMINISTRATION

One or two Quinidex Extentabs tablets every 8 to 12 hours as may be required to achieve the desired therapeutic effect.

HOW SUPPLIED

White, sugar-coated Extentabs tablets, monogrammed Quinidex and AHR in bottles of 100 (NDC 0031-6649-63), 250 (NDC 0031-6649-67), and Dis-Co® Unit Dose packs of 100 (NDC 0031-6649-64).

Store at controlled room temperature, between 15°C and 30°C (59°F and 86°F).

Dispense in well-closed, light-resistant container.

Shown in Product Identification Section, page 425

REGLAN® ℞

[*rĕg'lan*]

(Metoclopramide Hydrochloride)
Tablets, Syrup and Injectable

DESCRIPTION

For oral administration, **Reglan Tablets** (metoclopramide hydrochloride) **10 mg** are white. scored, capsule-shaped tablets engraved Reglan on one side and AHR 10 on the opposite side.

Each tablet contains:

Metoclopramide base 10 mg
(as the monohydrochloride monohydrate)

Inactive Ingredients: Magnesium Stearate, Mannitol, Microcrystalline Cellulose, Stearic Acid.

Reglan Tablets (metoclopramide hydrochloride) **5 mg** are green, elliptical-shaped tablets engraved Reglan 5 on one side and AHR on the opposite side.

Each tablet contains:

Metoclopramide base 5 mg
(as the monohydrochloride monohydrate)

Inactive Ingredients: Corn Starch, D&C Yellow 10 Lake, FD&C Blue 1 Aluminum Lake, Lactose, Microcrystalline Cellulose, Silicon Dioxide, Stearic Acid.

Reglan Syrup (metoclopramide hydrochloride) is an orange-colored, palatable, aromatic, sugar-free liquid.

Each 5 mL (1 teaspoonful) contains:

Metoclopramide base 5 mg
(as the monohydrochloride monohydrate)

Inactive Ingredients: Citric Acid, FD&C Yellow 6, Flavors, Glycerin, Methylparaben, Propylparaben, Sorbitol, Water.

For parenteral administration, **Reglan Injectable** (metoclopramide hydrochloride) is a clear, colorless, sterile solution with a pH of 4.5–6.5 for intravenous or intramuscular administration.

CONTAIN NO PRESERVATIVE.

2 mL and 10 mL **single dose** vials/ampuls; 30 mL **single dose** vial

Each **1** mL contains:

Metoclopramide base 5 mg
(as the monohydrochloride monohydrate)

Sodium Chloride, USP 8.5 mg, Water for Injection, USP q.s. pH adjusted, when necessary, with hydrochloric acid and/or sodium hydroxide.

Metoclopramide hydrochloride is a white crystalline, odorless substance, freely soluble in water. Chemically, it is 4-amino-5-chloro-N-[2-(diethylamino)ethyl]-2-methoxy benzamide monohydrochloride monohydrate. Molecular weight: 354.3.

CLINICAL PHARMACOLOGY

Metoclopramide stimulates motility of the upper gastrointestinal tract without stimulating gastric, biliary, or pancreatic secretions. Its mode of action is unclear. It seems to sensitize tissues to the action of acetylcholine. The effect of metoclopramide on motility is not dependent on intact vagal innervation, but it can be abolished by anticholinergic drugs.

Metoclopramide increases the tone and amplitude of gastric (especially antral) contractions, relaxes the pyloric sphincter and the duodenal bulb, and increases peristalsis of the duodenum and jejunum resulting in accelerated gastric emptying and intestinal transit. It increases the resting tone of the lower esophageal sphincter. It has little, if any effect on the motility of the colon or gallbladder.

In patients with gastroesophageal reflux and low LESP (lower esophageal sphincter pressure), single oral doses of metoclopramide produce dose-related increases in LESP. Effects begin at about 5 mg and increase through 20 mg (the largest dose tested). The increase in LESP from a 5 mg dose lasts about 45 minutes and that of 20 mg lasts between 2 and 3 hours. Increased rate of stomach emptying has been observed with single oral doses of 10 mg.

The antiemetic properties of metoclopramide appear to be a result of its antagonism of central and peripheral dopamine receptors. Dopamine produces nausea and vomiting by stimulation of the medullary chemoreceptor trigger zone (CTZ), and metoclopramide blocks stimulation of the CTZ by agents like l-dopa or apomorphine which are known to increase dopamine levels or to possess dopamine-like effects. Metoclopramide also abolishes the slowing of gastric emptying caused by apomorphine.

Like the phenothiazines and related drugs, which are also dopamine antagonists, metoclopramide produces sedation and may produce extrapyramidal reactions, although these are comparatively rare (See Warnings). Metoclopramide inhibits the central and peripheral effects of apomorphine, induces release of prolactin and causes a transient increase in circulating aldosterone levels, which may be associated with transient fluid retention.

The onset of pharmacological action of metoclopramide is 1 to 3 minutes following an intravenous dose, 10 to 15 minutes following intramuscular administration, and 30 to 60 minutes following an oral dose; pharmacological effects persist for 1 to 2 hours.

Pharmacokinetics: Metoclopramide is rapidly and well absorbed. Relative to an intravenous dose of 20 mg, the absolute oral bioavailability of metoclopramide is 80% ± 15.5% as demonstrated in a crossover study of 18 subjects. Peak plasma concentrations occur at about 1–2 hr after a single oral dose. Similar time to peak is observed after individual doses at steady state.

In a single dose study of 12 subjects the area under the drug concentration-time curve increases linearly with doses from 20 to 100 mg. Peak concentrations increase linearly with dose; time to peak concentrations remains the same; whole body clearance is unchanged; and the elimination rate remains the same. The average elimination half-life in individuals with normal renal function is 5–6 hr. Linear kinetic processes adequately describe the absorption and elimination of metoclopramide.

Approximately 85% of the radioactivity of an orally administered dose appears in the urine within 72 hr. Of the 85% eliminated in the urine, about half is present as free or conjugated metoclopramide.

The drug is not extensively bound to plasma proteins (about 30%). The whole body volume of distribution is high (about 3.5 L/kg) which suggests extensive distribution of drug to the tissues.

Renal impairment affects the clearance of metoclopramide. In a study with patients with varying degrees of renal impairment, a reduction in creatinine clearance was correlated with a reduction in plasma clearance, renal clearance, non-renal clearance, and increase in elimination half-life. The kinetics of metoclopramide in the presence of renal impairment remained linear however. The reduction in clearance as a result of renal impairment suggests that adjustment downward of maintenance dosage should be done to avoid drug cumulation.

INDICATIONS AND USAGE

Symptomatic gastroesophageal reflux: Reglan Tablets and Syrup are indicated as short-term (4 to 12 weeks) therapy for adults with symptomatic, documented gastroesophageal reflux who fail to respond to conventional therapy.

The principal effect of metoclopramide is on symptoms of postprandial and daytime heartburn with less observed effect on nocturnal symptoms. If symptoms are confined to particular situations, such as following the evening meal, use of metoclopramide as single doses prior to the provocative situation should be considered, rather than using the drug throughout the day. Healing of esophageal ulcers and erosions has been endoscopically demonstrated at the end of a 12-week trial using doses of 15 mg q.i.d. As there is no documented correlation between symptoms and healing of esophageal lesions, patients with documented lesions should be monitored endoscopically.

Diabetic gastroparesis (diabetic gastric stasis). Reglan (metoclopramide hydrochloride) is indicated for the relief of symptoms associated with acute and recurrent diabetic gastric stasis. The usual manifestations of delayed gastric emptying (e.g., nausea, vomiting, heartburn, persistent fullness after meals and anorexia) appear to respond to Reglan within different time intervals. Significant relief of nausea occurs early and continues to improve over a three-week period. Relief of vomiting and anorexia may precede the relief of abdominal fullness by one week or more.

The prevention of nausea and vomiting associated with emetogenic cancer chemotherapy. Reglan Injectable is indicated for the prophylaxis of vomiting associated with emetogenic cancer chemotherapy.

The prevention of postoperative nausea and vomiting. Reglan Injectable is indicated for the prophylaxis of postoperative nausea and vomiting in those circumstances where nasogastric suction is undesirable.

Small bowel intubation. Reglan Injectable may be used to facilitate small bowel intubation in adults and children in whom the tube does not pass the pylorus with conventional maneuvers.

Radiological examination. Reglan Injectable may be used to stimulate gastric emptying and intestinal transit of barium in cases where delayed emptying interferes with radiological examination of the stomach and/or small intestine.

CONTRAINDICATIONS

Metoclopramide should not be used whenever stimulation of gastrointestinal motility might be dangerous, e.g., in the presence of gastrointestinal hemorrhage, mechanical obstruction, or perforation.

Metoclopramide is contraindicated in patients with pheochromocytoma because the drug may cause a hypertensive crisis, probably due to release of catecholamines from the

Continued on next page

Prescribing information on A. H. Robins products listed here is based on official labeling in effect June 1, 1992, with Indications, Contraindications, Warnings, Precautions, Adverse Reactions, and Dosage stated in full.

A. H. Robins—Cont.

tumor. Such hypertensive crises may be controlled by phentolamine.

Metoclopramide is contraindicated in patients with known sensitivity or intolerance to the drug.

Metoclopramide should not be used in epileptics or patients receiving other drugs which are likely to cause extrapyramidal reactions, since the frequency and severity of seizures or extrapyramidal reactions may be increased.

WARNINGS

Mental depression has occurred in patients with and without prior history of depression. Symptoms have ranged from mild to severe and have included suicidal ideation and suicide. Metoclopramide should be given to patients with a prior history of depression only if the expected benefits outweigh the potential risks.

Extrapyramidal symptoms, manifested primarily as acute dystonic reactions, occur in approximately 1 in 500 patients treated with the usual adult dosages of 30–40 mg/day of metoclopramide. These usually are seen during the first 24–48 hours of treatment with metoclopramide, occur more frequently in children and young adults, and are even more frequent at the higher doses used in prophylaxis of vomiting due to cancer chemotherapy. These symptoms may include involuntary movements of limbs and facial grimacing, torticollis, oculogyric crisis, rhythmic protrusion of tongue, bulbar type of speech, trismus, or dystonic reactions resembling tetanus. Rarely, dystonic reactions may present as stridor and dyspnea, possibly due to laryngospasm. If these symptoms should occur, inject 50 mg Benadryl® (diphenhydramine hydrochloride) intramuscularly, and they usually will subside. Cogentin® (benztropine mesylate), 1 to 2 mg intramuscularly, may also be used to reverse these reactions.

Parkinsonian-like symptoms have occurred, more commonly within the first 6 months after beginning treatment with metoclopramide, but occasionally after longer periods. These symptoms generally subside within 2–3 months following discontinuance of metoclopramide. Patients with preexisting Parkinson's disease should be given metoclopramide cautiously, if at all, since such patients may experience exacerbation of parkinsonian symptoms when taking metoclopramide.

Tardive Dyskinesia: Tardive dyskinesia, a syndrome consisting of potentially irreversible, involuntary, dyskinetic movements may develop in patients treated with metoclopramide. Although the prevalence of the syndrome appears to be highest among the elderly, especially elderly women, it is impossible to predict which patients are likely to develop the syndrome. Both the risk of developing the syndrome and the likelihood that it will become irreversible are believed to increase with the duration of treatment and the total cumulative dose.

Less commonly, the syndrome can develop after relatively brief treatment periods at low doses; in these cases, symptoms appear more likely to be reversible.

There is no known treatment for established cases of tardive dyskinesia although the syndrome may remit, partially or completely, within several weeks-to-months after metoclopramide is withdrawn. Metoclopramide itself, however, may suppress (or partially suppress) the signs of tardive dyskinesia, thereby masking the underlying disease process. The effect of this symptomatic suppression upon the long-term course of the syndrome is unknown. Therefore, the use of metoclopramide for the symptomatic control of tardive dyskenesia is not recommended.

PRECAUTIONS

General. In one study in hypertensive patients, intravenously administered metoclopramide was shown to release catecholamines; hence, caution should be exercised when metoclopramide is used in patients with hypertension.

Intravenous injections of undiluted metoclopramide should be made slowly allowing 1 to 2 minutes for 10 mg since a transient but intense feeling of anxiety and restlessness, followed by drowsiness, may occur with rapid administration.

Intravenous administration of Reglan Injectable diluted in a parenteral solution should be made slowly over a period of not less than 15 minutes.

Giving a promotility drug such as metoclopramide theoretically could put increased pressure on suture lines following a gut anastomosis or closure. Although adverse events related to this possibility have not been reported to date, the possibility should be considered and weighed when deciding whether to use metoclopramide or nasogastric suction in the prevention of postoperative nausea and vomiting.

Information for patients: Metoclopramide may impair the mental and/or physical abilities required for the performance of hazardous tasks such as operating machinery or driving a motor vehicle. The ambulatory patient should be cautioned accordingly.

Drug Interactions. The effects of metoclopramide on gastrointestinal motility are antagonized by anticholinergic drugs

and narcotic analgesics. Additive sedative effects can occur when metoclopramide is given with alcohol, sedatives, hypnotics, narcotics or tranquilizers.

The finding that metoclopramide releases catecholamines in patients with essential hypertension suggests that it should be used cautiously, if at all, in patients receiving monoamine oxidase inhibitors.

Absorption of drugs from the stomach may be diminished (e.g., digoxin) by metoclopramide, whereas absorption of drugs from the small bowel may be accelerated (e.g., acetaminophen, tetracycline, levodopa, ethanol).

Gastroparesis (gastric stasis) may be responsible for poor diabetic control in some patients. Exogenously administered insulin may begin to act before food has left the stomach and lead to hypoglycemia. Because the action of metoclopramide will influence the delivery of food to the intestines and thus the rate of absorption, insulin dosage or timing of dosage may require adjustment.

Carcinogenesis, Mutagenesis, Impairment of Fertility: A 77-week study was conducted in rats with oral doses up to about 40 times the maximum recommended human daily dose. Metoclopramide elevates prolactin levels and the elevation persists during chronic administration. Tissue culture experiments indicate that approximately one-third of human breast cancers are prolactin-dependent *in vitro*, a factor of potential importance if the prescription of metoclopramide is contemplated in a patient with previously detected breast cancer. Although disturbances such as galactorrhea, amenorrhea, gynecomastia, and impotence have been reported with prolactin-elevating drugs, the clinical significance of elevated serum prolactin levels is unknown for most patients. An increase in mammary neoplasms has been found in rodents after chronic administration of prolactin-stimulating neuroleptic drugs and metoclopramide. Neither clinical studies nor epidemiologic studies conducted to date, however, have shown an association between chronic administration of these drugs and mammary tumorigenesis; the available evidence is too limited to be conclusive at this time.

An Ames mutagenicity test performed on metoclopramide was negative.

Pregnancy Category B. Reproduction studies performed in rats, mice, and rabbits by the i.v., i.m., s.c. and oral routes at maximum levels ranging from 12 to 250 times the human dose have demonstrated no impairment of fertility or significant harm to the fetus due to metoclopramide. There are, however, no adequate and well-controlled studies in pregnant women. Because animal reproduction studies are not always predictive of human response, this drug should be used during pregnancy only if clearly needed.

Nursing Mothers. Metoclopramide is excreted in human milk. Caution should be exercised when metoclopramide is administered to a nursing mother.

ADVERSE REACTIONS

In general, the incidence of adverse reactions correlates with the dose and duration of metoclopramide administration. The following reactions have been reported, although in most instances, data do not permit an estimate of frequency.

CNS Effects. Restlessness, drowsiness, fatigue and lassitude occur in approximately 10% of patients receiving the most commonly prescribed dosage of 10 mg q.i.d. (see Precautions). Insomnia, headache, confusion, dizziness or mental depression with suicidal ideation (see Warnings) occur less frequently. In cancer chemotherapy patients being treated with 1–2 mg/kg per dose, incidence of drowsiness is about 70%. There are isolated reports of convulsive seizures without clearcut relationship to metoclopramide. Rarely, hallucinations have been reported.

Extrapyramidal Reactions (EPS). Acute dystonic reactions, the most common type of EPS associated with metoclopramide, occur in approximately 0.2% of patients (1 in 500) treated with 30 to 40 mg of metoclopramide per day. In cancer chemotherapy patients receiving 1–2 mg/kg per dose, the incidence is 2% in patients over the ages of 30–35, and 25% or higher in children and young adults who have not had prophylactic administration of diphenhydramine. Symptoms include involuntary movements of limbs, facial grimacing, torticollis, oculogyric crisis, rhythmic protrusion of tongue, bulbar type of speech, trismus, opisthotonus (tetanus-like reactions) and rarely, stridor and dyspnea, possibly due to laryngospasm; ordinarily these symptoms are readily reversed by diphenhydramine (see Warnings).

Parkinsonian-like symptoms may include bradykinesia, tremor, cogwheel rigidity, mask-like facies (see Warnings). Tardive dyskinesia most frequently is characterized by involuntary movements of the tongue, face, mouth or jaw, and sometimes by involuntary movements of the trunk and/or extremities; movements may be choreoathetotic in appearance (see Warnings).

Motor restlessness (akathisia) may consist of feelings of anxiety, agitation, jitteriness, and insomnia, as well as inability to sit still, pacing, foot-tapping. These symptoms may disappear spontaneously or respond to a reduction in dosage.

Endocrine Disturbances. Galactorrhea, amenorrhea, gynecomastia, impotence secondary to hyperprolactinemia (see

Precautions). Fluid retention secondary to transient elevation of aldosterone (see Clinical Pharmacology).

Cardiovascular. Hypotension, hypertension supraventricular tachycardia, and bradycardia (see Contraindications, Precautions).

Gastrointestinal. Nausea and bowel disturbances, primarily diarrhea.

Hepatic. Rarely, cases of hepatotoxicity, characterized by such findings as jaundice and altered liver function tests, when metoclopramide was administered with other drugs with known hepatotoxic potential.

Renal. Urinary frequency and incontinence.

Hematologic. A few cases of neutropenia, leukopenia, or agranulocytosis, generally without clearcut relationship to metoclopramide. Methemoglobinemia, especially with overdosage in neonates (see Overdosage).

Allergic Reactions. A few cases of rash, urticaria, or bronchospasm, especially in patients with a history of asthma. Rarely, angioneurotic edema, including glossal or laryngeal edema.

Miscellaneous. Visual disturbances. Porphyria. Rare occurrences of neuroleptic malignant syndrome (NMS) have been reported. This potentially fatal syndrome is comprised of the symptom complex of hyperthermia, altered consciousness, muscular rigidity and autonomic dysfunction.

Transient flushing of the face and upper body, without alterations in vital signs, following high doses intravenously.

OVERDOSAGE

Symptoms of overdosage may include drowsiness, disorientation and extrapyramidal reactions. Anticholinergic or antiparkinson drugs or antihistamines with anticholinergic properties may be helpful in controlling the extrapyramidal reactions. Symptoms are self-limiting and usually disappear within 24 hours.

Hemodialysis removes relatively little metoclopramide, probably because of the small amount of the drug in blood relative to tissues. Similarly, continuous ambulatory peritoneal dialysis does not remove significant amounts of drug. It is unlikely that dosage would need to be adjusted to compensate for losses through dialysis. Dialysis is not likely to be an effective method of drug removal in overdose situations.

Methemoglobinemia has occurred in premature and full-term neonates who were given overdoses of metoclopramide (1–4 mg/kg/day orally, intramuscularly or intravenously for 1–3 or more days). Methemoglobinemia has not been reported in neonates treated with 0.5 mg/kg/day in divided doses. Methemoglobinemia can be reversed by the intravenous administration of methylene blue.

DOSAGE AND ADMINISTRATION

For the relief of symptomatic gastroesophageal reflux: Administer from 10 mg to 15 mg Reglan (Metoclopramide Hydrochloride) orally up to q.i.d. 30 minutes before each meal and at bedtime, depending upon symptoms being treated and clinical response (see Clinical Pharmacology and Indications). If symptoms occur only intermittently or at specific times of the day, use of metoclopramide in single doses up to 20 mg prior to the provoking situation may be preferred rather than continuous treatment. Occasionally, patients (such as elderly patients) who are more sensitive to the therapeutic or adverse effects of metoclopramide will require only 5 mg per dose.

Experience with esophageal erosions and ulcerations is limited, but healing has thus far been documented in one controlled trial using q.i.d. therapy at 15 mg/dose, and this regimen should be used when lesions are present, so long as it is tolerated (see Adverse Reactions). Because of the poor correlation between symptoms and endoscopic appearance of the esophagus, therapy directed at esophageal lesions is best guided by endoscopic evaluation.

Therapy longer than 12 weeks has not been evaluated and cannot be recommended.

For the relief of symptoms associated with diabetic gastroparesis (diabetic gastric stasis): Administer 10 mg of metoclopramide 30 minutes before each meal and at bedtime for two to eight weeks, depending upon response and the likelihood of continued well-being upon drug discontinuation.

The initial route of administration should be determined by the severity of the presenting symptoms. If only the earliest manifestations of diabetic gastric stasis are present, oral administration of Reglan may be initiated. However, if severe symptoms are present, therapy should begin with Reglan Injectable (I.M. or I.V.). Doses of 10 mg may be administered slowly by the intravenous route over a 1- to 2-minute period.

Administration of Reglan Injectable up to 10 days may be required before symptoms subside, at which time oral administration may be instituted. Since diabetic gastric stasis is frequently recurrent, Reglan therapy should be reinstituted at the earliest manifestation.

For the prevention of nausea and vomiting associated with emetogenic cancer chemotherapy: For doses in excess of 10 mg, Reglan Injectable should be diluted in 50 mL of a parenteral solution.

The preferred parenteral solution is Sodium Chloride Injection (normal saline), which when combined with Reglan Injectable, can be stored frozen for up to 4 weeks. Reglan Injectable is degraded when admixed and frozen with Dextrose-5% in Water. Reglan Injectable diluted in Sodium Chloride Injection, Dextrose-5% in Water, Dextrose-5% in 0.45% Sodium Chloride, Ringer's Injection or Lactated Ringer's Injection may be stored up to 48 hours (without freezing) after preparation if protected from light. All dilutions may be stored unprotected from light under normal light conditions up to 24 hours after preparation.

Intravenous infusions should be made slowly over a period of not less than 15 minutes, 30 minutes before beginning cancer chemotherapy and repeated every 2 hours for two doses, then every 3 hours for three doses.

The initial two doses should be 2 mg/kg if highly emetogenic drugs such as cisplatin or dacarbazine are used alone or in combination. For less emetogenic regimens, 1 mg/kg per dose may be adequate.

If extrapyramidal symptoms should occur, inject 50 mg Benadryl® (diphenhydramine hydrochloride) intramuscularly, and EPS usually will subside.

For the prevention of postoperative nausea and vomiting: Reglan Injectable should be given intramuscularly near the end of surgery. The usual adult dose is 10 mg; however, doses of 20 mg may be used.

To facilitate small bowel intubation: If the tube has not passed the pylorus with conventional maneuvers in 10 minutes, a single dose (undiluted) may be administered slowly by the intravenous route over a 1- to 2-minute period.

The recommended single dose is: Adults—10 mg metoclopramide base. Children (6–14 years of age)—2.5 to 5 mg metoclopramide base; (under 6 years of age)—0.1 mg/kg metoclopramide base.

To aid in radiological examinations: In patients where delayed gastric emptying interferes with radiological examination of the stomach and/or small intestine, a single dose may be administered slowly by the intravenous route over a 1- to 2-minute period.

For dosage, see intubation, above.

Use in Patients with Renal or Hepatic Impairment: Since metoclopramide is excreted principally through the kidneys, in those patients whose creatinine clearance is below 40 mL/min, therapy should be initiated at approximately one-half the recommended dosage. Depending upon clinical efficacy and safety considerations, the dosage may be increased or decreased as appropriate.

See Overdosage section for information regarding dialysis. Metoclopramide undergoes minimal hepatic metabolism, except for simple conjugation. Its safe use has been described in patients with advanced liver disease whose renal function was normal.

NOTE: Parenteral drug products should be inspected visually for particulate matter and discoloration prior to administration, whenever solution and container permit.

Admixture Compatibilities. Reglan (metoclopramide hydrochloride) Injectable is compatible for mixing and injection with the following dosage forms to the extent indicated below:

Physically and Chemically Compatible up to 48 hours. Cimetidine Hydrochloride (SK&F), Mannitol, USP (Abbott), Potassium Acetate, USP (Invenex), Potassium Chloride, USP (ESI), Potassium Phosphate, USP (Invenex).

Physically Compatible up to 48 hours. Ascorbic Acid, USP (Abbott), Benztropine Mesylate, USP (MS&D), Cytarabine, USP (Upjohn), Dexamethasone Sodium Phosphate, USP (ESI, MS&D), Diphenhydramine Hydrochloride, USP (Parke-Davis), Doxorubicin Hydrochloride, USP (Adria), Heparin Sodium, USP (ESI), Hydrocortisone Sodium Phosphate (MS&D), Lidocaine Hydrochloride, USP (ESI), Magnesium Sulfate, USP (ESI), Multi-Vitamin Infusion (must be refrigerated-USV), Vitamin B Complex with Ascorbic Acid (Roche).

Physically Compatible up to 24 hours (Do not use if precipitation occurs). Aminophylline, USP (ESI), Clindamycin Phosphate, USP (Upjohn), Cyclophosphamide, USP (Mead-Johnson), Insulin, USP (Lilly), Methylprednisolone Sodium Succinate, USP (ESI).

Conditionally Compatible (Use within one hour after mixing or may be infused directly into the same running IV line). Ampicillin Sodium, USP (Bristol), Calcium Gluconate, USP (ESI), Cisplatin (Bristol), Erythromycin Lactobionate, USP (Abbott), Methotrexate Sodium, USP (Lederle), Penicillin G Potassium, USP (Squibb), Tetracycline Hydrochloride, USP (Lederle).

Incompatible (Do Not Mix). Cephalothin Sodium, USP (Lilly), Chloramphenicol Sodium, USP (Parke-Davis), Sodium Bicarbonate, USP (Abbott).

HOW SUPPLIED

Each white, capsule-shaped, scored Reglan® Tablet contains 10 mg metoclopramide base (as the monohydrochloride monohydrate). Available in bottles of 100 (NDC 0031-6701-63), and 500 tablets (NDC 0031-6701-70) and Dis-Co® Unit Dose Packs of 100 tablets (NDC 0031-6701-64).

Container	Total Contents #	Concentration #	Administration
2 mL single dose vial/ampul	10 mg	5 mg/mL	FOR IV or IM ADMINISTRATION
10 mL single dose vial/ampul	50 mg	5 mg/mL	FOR IV INFUSION ONLY; DILUTE BEFORE USING
30 mL single dose vial	150 mg	5 mg/mL	FOR IV INFUSION ONLY; DILUTE BEFORE USING

\# Metoclopramide base (as the monohydrochloride monohydrate)

Each green, elliptical-shaped Reglan® Tablet contains 5 mg metoclopramide base (as the monohydrochloride monohydrate). Available in bottles of 100 (NDC 0031-6705-63) and Dis-Co® Unit Dose Packs of 100 tablets (NDC 0031-6705-64). Dispense in tight, light-resistant container.

Reglan® Syrup, 5 mg metoclopramide base (as the monohydrochloride monohydrate) per 5 mL, available in pints (NDC 0031-6706-25) and 10 mL Dis-Co® Unit Dose Packs (10 × 10s) (NDC 0031-6706-26). Dispense syrup in tight, light-resistant container.

Preservative-free:
Reglan® Injectable, **5 mg** metoclopramide base (as the monohydrochloride monohydrate) **per mL**; available in 2 mL single dose vials in cartons of 25 (NDC 0031-6709-72), 10 mL single dose vials in cartons of 25 (NDC 0031-6709-78); 30 mL single dose vials in cartons of 6 (NDC 0031-6709-85) and in cartons of 25 (NDC 0031-6709-24); 2 mL ampuls in cartons of 5 (NDC 0031-6709-90) and 25 (NDC 0031-6709-95); 10 mL ampuls in cartons of 25 (NDC 0031-6709-94).

[See table above.]

Store vials and ampuls in carton until used. Do not store open single dose vials or ampuls for later use, as they contain no preservative.

Dilutions may be stored unprotected from light under normal light conditions up to 24 hours after preparation.

TABLETS, SYRUP AND INJECTABLE SHOULD BE STORED AT CONTROLLED ROOM TEMPERATURE BETWEEN 15°C and 30°C (59°F and 86°F).

Reglan Injectable is manufactured for Pharmaceutical Division, A. H. Robins Company, Richmond, Virginia 23220 by Elkins-Sinn, Inc., Cherry Hill, NJ 08003.

Tablets Shown in Product Identification Section, page 425

ROBAXIN® INJECTABLE   ℞
[ro"baks'in]
brand of Methocarbamol Injection, USP

DESCRIPTION

Methocarbamol has the following chemical name: 3-(2-methoxyphenoxy)-1,2-propanediol 1-carbamate.

Robaxin Injectable is a parenteral dosage form.

Each mL contains:

Methocarbamol, USP **100 mg**; Polyethylene Glycol 300, NF 0.5 mL; Water for Injection, USP q.s. pH adjusted, when necessary, with hydrochloric acid and/or sodium hydroxide.

AFTER MIXING WITH I.V. INFUSION FLUIDS, **DO NOT REFRIGERATE.**

ACTIONS

The mechanism of action of methocarbamol in humans has not been established, but may be due to general central nervous system depression. It has no direct action on the contractile mechanism of striated muscle, the motor end plate or the nerve fiber.

INDICATIONS

The injectable form of methocarbamol is indicated as an adjunct to rest, physical therapy, and other measures for the relief of discomfort associated with acute, painful musculoskeletal conditions. The mode of action of this drug has not been clearly identified, but may be related to its sedative properties. Methocarbamol does not directly relax tense skeletal muscles in man.

CONTRAINDICATIONS

Robaxin Injectable should not be administered to patients with known or suspected renal pathology. This caution is necessary because of the presence of polyethylene glycol 300 in the vehicle.

A much larger amount of polyethylene glycol 300 than is present in recommended doses of Robaxin Injectable is known to have increased pre-existing acidosis and urea retention in patients with renal impairment. Although the amount present in this preparation is well within the limits of safety, caution dictates this contraindication.

Robaxin Injectable is contraindicated in patients hypersensitive to any of the ingredients.

WARNINGS

Since methocarbamol may possess a general central nervous system depressant effect, patients receiving Robaxin Inject-

able (methocarbamol injection) should be cautioned about combined effects with alcohol and other CNS depressants.

Safe use of Robaxin Injectable has not been established with regard to possible adverse effects upon fetal development. Therefore, Robaxin Injectable should not be used in women who are or may become pregnant and particularly during early pregnancy unless in the judgment of the physician the potential benefits outweigh the possible hazards.

PRECAUTIONS

As with other agents administered either intravenously or intramuscularly, careful supervision of dose and rate of injection should be observed. Rate of injection should not exceed 3 mL per minute—i.e., one 10 mL vial in approximately three minutes. Since Robaxin Injectable is hypertonic, vascular extravasation must be avoided. A recumbent position will reduce the likelihood of side reactions.

Blood aspirated into the syringe does not mix with the hypertonic solution. This phenomenon occurs with many other intravenous preparations. The blood may be safely injected with the methocarbamol, or the injection may be stopped when the plunger reaches the blood, whichever the physician prefers.

The total dosage should not exceed 30 mL (three vials) a day for more than three consecutive days except in the treatment of tetanus.

Caution should be observed in using the injectable form in suspected or known epileptic patients.

Safety and effectiveness in children below the age of 12 years have not been established except in tetanus. See special directions for use in tetanus.

It is not known whether this drug is secreted in human milk. As a general rule, nursing should not be undertaken while a patient is on a drug since many drugs are excreted in human milk.

Methocarbamol may cause a color interference in certain screening tests for 5-hydroxyindoleacetic acid (5-HIAA) and vanillylmandelic acid (VMA).

ADVERSE REACTIONS

Dizziness, lightheadedness, drowsiness, vertigo, fainting, syncope, hypotension, gastrointestinal upset, metallic taste, thrombophlebitis, sloughing at the site of injection, pain at the site of injection, anaphylactic reaction, urticaria, pruritus, rash, conjunctivitis with nasal congestion, flushing, nystagmus, diplopia, mild muscular incoordination, bradycardia, blurred vision, headache, fever. In most cases of syncope there was spontaneous recovery. In others, epinephrine, injectable steroids and/or injectable antihistamines were employed to hasten recovery. Certain of these complaints may have been due to any overly rapid rate of intravenous injection.

The onset of convulsive seizures during intravenous administration has been reported, including instances in known epileptics. The psychic trauma of the procedure may have been a contributing factor. Although several observers have reported success in terminating epileptiform seizures with Robaxin Injectable, its administration to patients with epilepsy is not recommended.

DOSAGE AND ADMINISTRATION

For Intravenous and Intramuscular Use Only. Total adult dosage should not exceed 30 mL (3 vials) a day for more than 3 consecutive days except in the treatment of tetanus. A like course may be repeated after a lapse of 48 hours if the condition persists. Dosage and frequency of injection should be based on the severity of the condition being treated and therapeutic response noted.

For the relief of symptoms of moderate degree, 10 mL (one vial) may be adequate. Ordinarily this injection need not be repeated, as the administration of the oral form will usually sustain the relief initiated by the injection. For the severest cases or in postoperative conditions in which oral administration is not feasible, 20 to 30 mL (two to three vials) may be required.

Continued on next page

Prescribing information on A. H. Robins products listed here is based on official labeling in effect June 1, 1992, with Indications, Contraindications, Warnings, Precautions, Adverse Reactions, and Dosage stated in full.

A. H. Robins—Cont.

Directions for Intravenous Use. Robaxin Injectable may be administered undiluted directly into the vein at a *maximum rate of three mL per minute*. It may also be added to an intravenous drip of Sodium Chloride Injection (Sterile Isotonic Sodium Chloride Solution for Parenteral Use) or five per cent Dextrose Injection (Sterile 5 per cent Dextrose Solution); one vial given as a single dose should not be diluted to more than 250 mL for I. V. infusion. Care should be exercised to avoid vascular extravasation of this hypertonic solution which may result in thrombophlebitis. It is preferable that the patient be in a recumbent position during and for at least 10 to 15 minutes following the injection.

Directions for Intramuscular Use. When the intramuscular route is indicated, not more than five mL (one-half vial) should be injected into each gluteal region. The injections may be repeated at eight hour intervals, if necessary. When satisfactory relief of symptoms is achieved, it can usually be maintained with tablets.

Not Recommended for Subcutaneous Administration.

Special Directions for Use in Tetanus: There is clinical evidence which suggests that methocarbamol may have a beneficial effect in the control of the neuromuscular manifestations of tetanus. It does not, however, replace the usual procedure of debridement, tetanus antitoxin, penicillin, tracheotomy, attention to fluid balance, and supportive care. Robaxin Injectable should be added to the regimen as soon as possible.

For adults: Inject one or two vials directly into the tubing of a previously inserted indwelling needle. An additional 10 mL or 20 mL may be added to the infusion bottle so that a total of up to 30 mL (three vials) is given as the initial dose (note Precautions). This procedure should be repeated every six hours until conditions allow for the insertion of a nasogastric tube. Crushed Robaxin (methocarbamol) tablets suspended in water or saline may then be given through this tube. Total daily oral doses up to 24 grams may be required as judged by patient response.

For children: A minimum initial dose of 15 mg/kg is recommended. This dosage may be repeated every six hours as indicated. The maintenance dosage may be given by injection into the tubing or by I.V. infusion with an appropriate quantity of fluid. See directions for I.V. use.

HOW SUPPLIED

Robaxin Injectable—10 mL single dose vials in packages of 5 (NDC 0031-7409-87) and 25 (NDC 0031-7409-94).
Manufactured for A. H. ROBINS CO., by ELKINS-SINN, INC.

Shown in Product Identification Section, page 425

ROBAXIN®   ℞
[ro"baks'ĭn]
brand of Methocarbamol Tablets, USP
500 mg per tablet
ROBAXIN®-750   ℞
brand of Methocarbamol Tablets, USP
750 mg per tablet

DESCRIPTION

Inactive Ingredients: ROBAXIN—Corn Starch, FD&C Yellow 6 Aluminum Lake, Hydroxypropyl Cellulose, Hydroxypropyl Methylcellulose, Magnesium Stearate, Polysorbate 20, Povidone, Propylene Glycol, Saccharin Sodium, Sodium Lauryl Sulfate, Sodium Starch Glycolate, Stearic Acid, Titanium Dioxide.
ROBAXIN-750—Corn Starch, D&C Yellow 10 Aluminum Lake, FD&C Yellow 6 Aluminum Lake, Hydroxypropyl Cellulose, Hydroxypropyl Methylcellulose, Magnesium Stearate, Polysorbate 20, Povidone, Propylene Glycol, Saccharin Sodium, Sodium Lauryl Sulfate, Sodium Starch Glycolate, Stearic Acid, Titanium Dioxide.
Methocarbamol has the following chemical name: 3-(2-methoxyphenoxy)-1,2-propanediol 1-carbamate.

ACTIONS

The mechanism of action of methocarbamol in humans has not been established, but may be due to general central nervous system depression. It has no direct action on the contractile mechanism of striated muscle, the motor end plate or the nerve fiber.

INDICATIONS

Robaxin (methocarbamol) is indicated as an adjunct to rest, physical therapy, and other measures for the relief of discomforts associated with acute, painful musculoskeletal conditions. The mode of action of this drug has not been clearly identified, but may be related to its sedative properties. Methocarbamol does not directly relax tense skeletal muscles in man.

CONTRAINDICATIONS

Robaxin is contraindicated in patients hypersensitive to any of the ingredients.

WARNINGS

Since methocarbamol may possess a general central nervous system depressant effect, patients receiving Robaxin/Robaxin-750 (methocarbamol tablets) should be cautioned about combined effects with alcohol and other CNS depressants.

Safe use of methocarbamol has not been established with regard to possible adverse effects upon fetal development. Therefore, methocarbamol tablets should not be used in women who are or may become pregnant and particularly during early pregnancy unless in the judgment of the physician the potential benefits outweigh the possible hazards.

PRECAUTIONS

Safety and effectiveness in children below the age of 12 years have not been established.
It is not known whether this drug is secreted in human milk. As a general rule, nursing should not be undertaken while a patient is on a drug since many drugs are excreted in human milk.
Methocarbamol may cause a color interference in certain screening tests for 5-hydroxyindoleacetic acid (5-HIAA) and vanilmandelic acid (VMA).

ADVERSE REACTIONS

Lightheadedness, dizziness, drowsiness, nausea, allergic manifestations such as urticaria, pruritus, rash, conjunctivitis with nasal congestion, blurred vision, headache, fever.

DOSAGE AND ADMINISTRATION

Robaxin (methocarbamol), 500 mg—Adults: initial dosage, 3 tablets q.i.d.; maintenance dosage, 2 tablets q.i.d.
Robaxin-750 (methocarbamol), 750 mg — Adults: initial dosage, 2 tablets q.i.d.; maintenance dosage, 1 tablet q.4h. or 2 tablets t.i.d.
Six grams a day are recommended for the first 48 to 72 hours of treatment. (For severe conditions 8 grams a day may be administered.) Thereafter, the dosage can usually be reduced to approximately 4 grams a day.

HOW SUPPLIED

Robaxin—light orange, round, film-coated tablets monogrammed Robaxin and AHR in bottles of 100 (NDC 0031-7429-63), 500 (NDC 0031-7429-70) and Dis-Co® unit dose packs of 100 (NDC 0031-7429-64).
Robaxin-750—orange, capsule-shaped, film-coated tablets monogrammed Robaxin-750 and AHR in bottles of 100 (NDC 0031-7449-63), 500 (NDC 0031-7449-70), and Dis-Co® unit dose packs of 100 (NDC 0031-7449-64).
Store at Controlled Room Temperature, between 15°C and 30°C (59°F and 86°F).
Dispense in tight container.
Also available in the injectable form, 1 g methocarbamol in each 10 ml vial (NDC 0031-7409).

Shown in Product Identification Section, page 425

ROBAXISAL® TABLETS   ℞
[ro"baks'ĭ-sal"]

DESCRIPTION

For oral administration, Robaxisal is available as a pink and white laminated tablet containing:
Methocarbamol, USP ....400 mg
Aspirin, USP ....325 mg
Inactive Ingredients: Corn Starch, FD&C Red 3, Magnesium Stearate, Povidone, Sodium Lauryl Sulfate, Sodium Starch Glycolate, Stearic Acid.
Methocarbamol has the following chemical name: 3-(2-Methoxyphenoxy)-1,2-propanediol 1-Carbamate.

ACTIONS

Robaxisal provides a double approach to the management of discomforts associated with musculoskeletal disorders.
Methocarbamol. The mechanism of action of methocarbamol in humans has not been established, but may be due to general central nervous system depression. It has no direct action on the contractile mechanism of striated muscle, the motor end plate or the nerve fiber.
Aspirin. Aspirin is a mild analgesic with anti-inflammatory and antipyretic activity.

INDICATIONS

Robaxisal is indicated as an adjunct to rest, physical therapy, and other measures for the relief of discomfort associated with acute, painful musculoskeletal conditions. The mode of action of methocarbamol has not been clearly identified but may be related to its sedative properties. Methocarbamol does not directly relax tense skeletal muscles in man.

CONTRAINDICATIONS

Hypersensitivity to methocarbamol or aspirin.

WARNINGS

Salicylates have been reported to be associated with the development of Reye syndrome in children and teenagers with chicken pox, influenza, and influenza-like infections. Since methocarbamol may possess a general central nervous system depressant effect, patients receiving Robaxisal should be cautioned about combined effects with alcohol and other CNS depressants.

PRECAUTIONS

Products containing aspirin should be administered with caution to patients with gastritis or peptic ulceration, or those receiving hypoprothrombinemic anticoagulants.
Methocarbamol may cause a color interference in certain screening tests for 5-hydroxyindoleacetic acid (5-HIAA) and vanilmandelic acid (VMA).
Pregnancy. Safe use of Robaxisal has not been established with regard to possible adverse effects upon fetal development. Therefore, Robaxisal should not be used in women who are or may become pregnant and particularly during early pregnancy unless in the judgment of the physician the potential benefits outweigh the possible hazards.
Nursing Mothers. It is not known whether methocarbamol is secreted in human milk; however, aspirin does appear in human milk in moderate amounts. It can produce a bleeding tendency either by interfering with the function of the infant's platelets or by decreasing the amount of prothrombin in the blood. The risk is minimal if the mother takes the aspirin just after nursing and if the infant has an adequate store of vitamin K. As a general rule, nursing should not be undertaken while a patient is on a drug.
Pediatric Use. Safety and effectiveness in children 12 years of age and below have not been established.
Use in Activities Requiring Mental Alertness. Robaxisal may rarely cause drowsiness. Until the patient's response has been determined, he should be cautioned against the operation of motor vehicles or dangerous machinery.

ADVERSE REACTIONS

The most frequent adverse reaction to methocarbamol is dizziness or lightheadedness and nausea. This occurs in about one in 20–25 patients. Less frequent reactions are drowsiness, blurred vision, headache, fever, allergic manifestations such as urticaria, pruritus, and rash.
Adverse reactions that have been associated with the use of aspirin include: nausea and other gastrointestinal discomfort, gastritis, gastric erosion, vomiting, constipation, diarrhea, angio-edema, asthma, rash, pruritus, urticaria. Gastrointestinal discomfort may be minimized by taking Robaxisal with food.

DOSAGE AND ADMINISTRATION

Adults and children over 12 years of age: Two tablets four times daily. Three tablets four times daily may be used in severe conditions for one to three days in patients who are able to tolerate salicylates. These dosage recommendations provide respectively 3.2 and 4.8 grams of methocarbamol per day. For Chicken Pox or Flu, see Warnings.

OVERDOSAGE

Toxicity due to overdosage of methocarbamol is unlikely; however, acute overdosage of aspirin may cause symptoms of salicylate intoxication.
Treatment of Overdosage. Supportive therapy for 24 hours, as methocarbamol is excreted within that time. If salicylate intoxication occurs, especially in children, the hyperpnea may be controlled with sodium bicarbonate. Judicious use of 5% CO_2 with 95% O_2 may be of benefit. Abnormal electrolyte patterns should be corrected with appropriate fluid therapy.

HOW SUPPLIED

Robaxisal® is supplied as pink and white laminated, compressed tablets in bottles of 100 (NDC 0031-7469-63), 500 (NDC 0031-7469-70) and Dis-Co® Unit Dose Packs of 100 (NDC 0031-7469-64).
Store at controlled room temperature, between 15°C and 30°C (59°F and 86°F).
Dispense in well-closed container.
Shown in Product Identification Section, page 425

ROBINUL® TABLETS   ℞
[ro'bĭ-nul]
ROBINUL® FORTE TABLETS   ℞
brand of Glycopyrrolate Tablets, USP

DESCRIPTION

Robinul and Robinul Forte tablets contain the synthetic anticholinergic, glycopyrrolate. Glycopyrrolate is a quaternary ammonium compound with the following chemical name: 3-[(cyclopentylhydroxyphenylacetyl)oxy]-1,1-dimethylpyrrolidinium bromide.

Robinul tablets are scored, compressed white tablets engraved AHR. Each tablet contains:
Glycopyrrolate, USP .... 1 mg
Robinul Forte tablets are scored, compressed white tablets engraved AHR/2.
Each tablet contains:
Glycopyrrolate, USP .... 2 mg
Inactive Ingredients: Dibasic Calcium Phosphate, Lactose, Magnesium Stearate, Povidone, Sodium Starch Glycolate.

ACTIONS

Glycopyrrolate, like other anticholinergic (antimuscarinic) agents, inhibits the action of acetylcholine on structures innervated by postganglionic cholinergic nerves and on smooth muscles that respond to acetylcholine but lack cholinergic innervation. These peripheral cholinergic receptors are present in the autonomic effector cells of smooth muscle, cardiac muscle, the sino-atrial node, the atrioventricular node, exocrine glands, and, to a limited degree, in the autonomic ganglia. Thus, it diminishes the volume and free acidity of gastric secretions and controls excessive pharyngeal, tracheal, and bronchial secretions.
Glycopyrrolate antagonizes muscarinic symptoms (e.g., bronchorrhea, bronchospasm, bradycardia, and intestinal hypermotility) induced by cholinergic drugs such as the anticholinesterases.
The highly polar quaternary ammonium group of glycopyrrolate limits its passage across lipid membranes, such as the blood-brain barrier, in contrast to atropine sulfate and scopolamine hydrobromide, which are non-polar tertiary amines which penetrate lipid barriers easily.

INDICATIONS

For use as adjunctive therapy in the treatment of peptic ulcer.

CONTRAINDICATIONS

Glaucoma; obstructive uropathy (for example, bladder neck obstruction due to prostatic hypertrophy); obstructive disease of the gastrointestinal tract (as in achalasia, pyloroduodenal stenosis, etc.); paralytic ileus; intestinal atony of the elderly or debilitated patient; unstable cardiovascular status in acute hemorrhage; severe ulcerative colitis; toxic megacolon complicating ulcerative colitis; myasthenia gravis. Robinul (glycopyrrolate) tablets are contraindicated in those patients with a hypersensitivity to glycopyrrolate.

WARNINGS

In the presence of a high environmental temperature, heat prostration (fever and heat stroke due to decreased sweating) can occur with use of Robinul.
Diarrhea may be an early symptom of incomplete intestinal obstruction, especially in patients with ileostomy or colostomy. In this instance treatment with this drug would be inappropriate and possibly harmful.
Robinul (glycopyrrolate) may produce drowsiness or blurred vision. In this event, the patient should be warned not to engage in activities requiring mental alertness such as operating a motor vehicle or other machinery, or performing hazardous work while taking this drug.
Theoretically, with overdosage, a curare-like action may occur, i.e., neuromuscular blockade leading to muscular weakness and possible paralysis.
Pregnancy. The safety of this drug during pregnancy has not been established. The use of any drug during pregnancy requires that the potential benefits of the drug be weighed against possible hazards to mother and child. Reproduction studies in rats revealed no teratogenic effects from glycopyrrolate; however, the potent anticholinergic action of this agent resulted in diminished rates of conception and of survival at weaning, in a dose-related manner. Other studies in dogs suggest that this may be due to diminished seminal secretion which is evident at high doses of glycopyrrolate. Information on possible adverse effects in the pregnant female is limited to uncontrolled data derived from marketing experience. Such experience has revealed no reports of teratogenic or other fetus-damaging potential. No controlled studies to establish the safety of the drug in pregnancy have been performed.
Nursing mothers. It is not known whether this drug is secreted in human milk. As a general rule, nursing should not be undertaken while a patient is on a drug since many drugs are excreted in human milk.
Pediatric Use. Since there is no adequate experience in children who have received this drug, safety and efficacy in children have not been established.

PRECAUTIONS

Use Robinul with caution in the elderly and in all patients with:
- Autonomic neuropathy.
- Hepatic or renal disease.
- Ulcerative colitis—large doses may suppress intestinal motility to the point of producing a paralytic ileus and for this reason may precipitate or aggravate "toxic megacolon," a serious complication of the disease.
- Hyperthyroidism, coronary heart disease, congestive heart failure, cardiac tachyarrhythmias, tachycardia, hypertension and prostatic hypertrophy.
- Hiatal hernia associated with reflux esophagitis, since anticholinergic drugs may aggravate this condition.

ADVERSE REACTIONS

Anticholinergics produce certain effects, most of which are extensions of their fundamental pharmacological actions. Adverse reactions to anticholinergics in general may include xerostomia; decreased sweating; urinary hesitancy and retention; blurred vision; tachycardia; palpitations; dilatation of the pupil; cycloplegia; increased ocular tension; loss of taste; headaches; nervousness; mental confusion; drowsiness; weakness; dizziness; insomnia; nausea; vomiting; constipation; bloated feeling; impotence; suppression of lactation; severe allergic reaction or drug idiosyncrasies including anaphylaxis, urticaria and other dermal manifestations.
Robinul (glycopyrrolate) is chemically a quaternary ammonium compound; hence, its passage across lipid membranes, such as the blood-brain barrier, is limited in contrast to atropine sulfate and scopolamine hydrobromide. For this reason the occurrence of CNS related side effects is lower, in comparison to their incidence following administration of anticholinergics which are chemically tertiary amines that can cross this barrier readily.

OVERDOSAGE

The symptoms of overdosage of glycopyrrolate are peripheral in nature rather than central.
1. To guard against further absorption of the drug—use gastric lavage, cathartics and/or enemas.
2. To combat peripheral anticholinergic effects (residual mydriasis, dry mouth, etc.)—utilize a quaternary ammonium anticholinesterase, such as neostigmine methylsulfate.
3. To combat hypotension—use pressor amines (norepinephrine, metaraminol) i.v.; and supportive care.
4. To combat respiratory depression—administer oxygen; utilize a respiratory stimulant such as Dopram® i.v.; artificial respiration.

DOSAGE AND ADMINISTRATION

The dosage of Robinul or Robinul Forte should be adjusted to the needs of the individual patient to assure symptomatic control with a minimum of adverse reactions. The presently recommended maximum daily dosage of glycopyrrolate is 8 mg.
Robinul (glycopyrrolate, 1 mg) tablets. The recommended initial dosage of Robinul for adults is one tablet three times daily (in the morning, early afternoon, and at bedtime). Some patients may require two tablets at bedtime to assure overnight control of symptoms. For maintenance, a dosage of one tablet twice a day is frequently adequate.
Robinul Forte (glycopyrrolate, 2 mg) tablets. The recommended dosage of Robinul Forte for adults is one tablet two or three times daily at equally spaced intervals.
Robinul tablets are not recommended for use in children under the age of 12 years.

DRUG INTERACTIONS

There are no known drug interactions.

HOW SUPPLIED

Robinul (glycopyrrolate, 1 mg) tablets in bottles of 100 (NDC 0031-7824-63) and 500 (NDC 0031-7824-70).
Robinul Forte (glycopyrrolate, 2 mg) tablets in bottles of 100 (NDC 0031-7840-63).

Shown in Product Identification Section, page 425

ROBINUL® INJECTABLE ℞

[ro'bĭ-nul]
brand of Glycopyrrolate Injection, USP

DESCRIPTION

Robinul (glycopyrrolate) is a synthetic anticholinergic agent.
Each 1 mL contains:
Glycopyrrolate, USP .... 0.2 mg
Water for Injection, USP .... q.s.
Benzyl Alcohol, NF (preservative) 0.9%
pH adjusted, when necessary, with hydrochloric acid and/or sodium hydroxide.
For Intramuscular or Intravenous administration.
Glycopyrrolate is a quaternary ammonium compound with the following chemical name:
3[(cyclopentylhydroxyphenylacetyl)oxy]-1,1-dimethylpyrrolidinium bromide.
Unlike atropine, glycopyrrolate is completely ionized at physiological pH values.
Robinul Injectable is a clear, colorless, sterile liquid; pH 2.0–3.0.

CLINICAL PHARMACOLOGY

Glycopyrrolate, like other anticholinergic (antimuscarinic) agents, inhibits the action of acetylcholine on structures innervated by postganglionic cholinergic nerves and on smooth muscles that respond to acetylcholine but lack cholinergic innervation. These peripheral cholinergic receptors are present in the autonomic effector cells of smooth muscle, cardiac muscle, the sinoatrial node, the atrioventricular node, exocrine glands, and, to a limited degree, in the autonomic ganglia. Thus, it diminishes the volume and free acidity of gastric secretions and controls excessive pharyngeal, tracheal, and bronchial secretions.
Glycopyrrolate antagonizes muscarinic symptoms (e.g., bronchorrhea, bronchospasm, bradycardia, and intestinal hypermotility) induced by cholinergic drugs such as the anticholinesterases.
The highly polar quaternary ammonium group of glycopyrrolate limits its passage across lipid membranes, such as the blood-brain barrier, in contrast to atropine sulfate and scopolamine hydrobromide, which are non-polar tertiary amines which penetrate lipid barriers easily.
Peak effects occur approximately 30 to 45 minutes after intramuscular administration. The vagal blocking effects persist for 2 to 3 hours and the antisialagogue effects persist up to 7 hours, periods longer than for atropine. With intravenous injection, the onset of action is generally evident within one minute.

INDICATIONS AND USAGE

In Anesthesia: Robinul (glycopyrrolate) Injectable is indicated for use as a preoperative antimuscarinic to reduce salivary, tracheobronchial, and pharyngeal secretions; to reduce the volume and free acidity of gastric secretions; and, to block cardiac vagal inhibitory reflexes during induction of anesthesia and intubation. When indicated, Robinul Injectable may be used intraoperatively to counteract drug-induced or vagal traction reflexes with the associated arrhythmias. Glycopyrrolate protects against the peripheral muscarinic effects (e.g., bradycardia and excessive secretions) of cholinergic agents such as neostigmine and pyridostigmine given to reverse the neuromuscular blockade due to non-depolarizing muscle relaxants.
In Peptic Ulcer: For use in adults as adjunctive therapy for the treatment of peptic ulcer when rapid anticholinergic effect is desired or when oral medication is not tolerated.

CONTRAINDICATIONS

Known hypersensitivity to glycopyrrolate.
Due to its benzyl alcohol content, Robinul Injectable should not be used in newborns (children less than 1 month of age).
In addition, in the management of ***peptic ulcer*** patients, because of the longer duration of therapy, Robinul Injectable may be contraindicated in patients with concurrent glaucoma; obstructive uropathy (for example, bladder neck obstruction due to prostatic hypertrophy); obstructive disease of the gastrointestinal tract (as in achalasia, pyloroduodenal stenosis, etc.); paralytic ileus, intestinal atony of the elderly or debilitated patient; unstable cardiovascular status in acute hemorrhage; severe ulcerative colitis; toxic megacolon complicating ulcerative colitis; myasthenia gravis.

WARNINGS

This drug should be used with great caution, if at all, in patients with glaucoma or asthma.
In the ambulatory patient. Robinul (glycopyrrolate) may produce drowsiness or blurred vision. The patient should be cautioned regarding activities requiring mental alertness such as operating a motor vehicle or other machinery or performing hazardous work while taking this drug.
In addition, in the presence of a high environmental temperature, heat prostration (fever and heat stroke due to decreased sweating) can occur with use of Robinul (glycopyrrolate).
Diarrhea may be an early symptom of incomplete intestinal obstruction, especially in patients with ileostomy or colostomy. In this instance treatment with Robinul (glycopyrrolate) would be inappropriate and possibly harmful.

PRECAUTIONS

General.
Investigate any tachycardia before giving glycopyrrolate since an increase in the heart rate may occur.
Use with caution in patients with: coronary artery disease; congestive heart failure; cardiac arrhythmias; hypertension; hyperthyroidism.
In managing ulcer patients, use Robinul with caution in the elderly and in all patients with autonomic neuropathy, hepatic or renal disease, ulcerative colitis or hiatal hernia, since anticholinergic drugs may aggravate these conditions.
With overdosage, a curare-like action may occur.
Drug Interactions. The intravenous administration of any anticholinergic in the presence of cyclopropane anesthesia can result in ventricular arrhythmias; therefore, caution should be observed if Robinul (glycopyrrolate) Injectable is

Continued on next page

Prescribing information on A. H. Robins products listed here is based on official labeling in effect June 1, 1992, with Indications, Contraindications, Warnings, Precautions, Adverse Reactions, and Dosage stated in full.

A. H. Robins—Cont.

used during cyclopropane anesthesia. If the drug is given in small incremental doses of 0.1 mg or less, the likelihood of producing ventricular arrhythmias is reduced.
Carcinogenesis, mutagenesis, impairment of fertility. Long-term studies in animals have not been performed to evaluate carcinogenic potential. In the teratology studies, diminished rates of conception and of survival at weaning were observed in rats, in a dose-related manner. Studies in dogs suggest that this may be due to diminished seminal secretion which is evident at high doses of glycopyrrolate.
Pregnancy Category B. Reproduction studies have been performed in rats and rabbits up to 1000 times the human dose and have revealed no teratogenic effects from glycopyrrolate. There are, however, no adequate and well-controlled studies in pregnant women. Because animal reproduction studies are not always predictive of human response, this drug should be used during pregnancy only if clearly needed.
Nursing Mothers. It is not known whether this drug is excreted in human milk. Because many drugs are excreted in human milk, caution should be exercised when Robinul is administered to a nursing woman.
Pediatric Use. Safety and effectiveness in children below the age of 12 years have not been established for the management of peptic ulcer.

ADVERSE REACTIONS

Anticholinergics produce certain effects, most of which are extensions of their pharmacologic actions. Adverse reactions to anticholinergics in general may include dry mouth; urinary hesitancy and retention; blurred vision due to mydriasis; increased ocular tension; tachycardia; palpitation; decreased sweating; loss of taste; headache; nervousness; drowsiness; weakness; dizziness; insomnia; nausea; vomiting; impotence; suppression of lactation; constipation; bloated feeling; severe allergic reaction or drug idiosyncrasies including anaphylaxis; urticaria and other dermal manifestations; some degree of mental confusion and/or excitement, especially in elderly persons.
Robinul is chemically a quaternary ammonium compound; hence, its passage across lipid membranes, such as the blood-brain barrier is limited in contrast to atropine sulfate and scopolamine hydrobromide. For this reason the occurrence of CNS related side effects is lower, in comparison to their incidence following administration of anticholinergics which are chemically tertiary amines that can cross this barrier readily.

OVERDOSAGE

To combat peripheral anticholinergic effects, a quaternary ammonium anticholinesterase such as neostigmine methylsulfate (which does not cross the blood-brain barrier) may be given intravenously in increments of 0.25 mg in adults. This dosage may be repeated every five to ten minutes until anticholinergic over-activity is reversed or up to a maximum of 2.5 mg. Proportionately smaller doses should be used in children. Indication for repetitive doses of neostigmine should be based on close monitoring of the decrease in heart rate and the return of bowel sounds.
In the unlikely event that CNS symptoms (excitement, restlessness, convulsions, psychotic behavior) occur, physostigmine (which does cross the blood-brain barrier) should be used. Physostigmine 0.5 to 2 mg should be slowly administered intravenously and repeated as necessary up to a total of 5 mg in adults. Proportionately smaller doses should be used in children.
Fever should be treated symptomatically. In the event of a curare-like effect on respiratory muscles, artificial respiration should be instituted and maintained until effective respiratory action returns.

DOSAGE AND ADMINISTRATION

Robinul (glycopyrrolate) Injectable may be administered intramuscularly, or intravenously, without dilution, in the following indications:
Adults: *Preanesthetic Medication.* The recommended dose of Robinul (glycopyrrolate) Injectable is 0.002 mg (0.01 mL) per pound of body weight by intramuscular injection, given 30 to 60 minutes prior to the anticipated time of induction of anesthesia or at the time the preanesthetic narcotic and/or sedative are administered.
Intraoperative Medication. Robinul (glycopyrrolate) Injectable may be used during surgery to counteract drug induced or vagal traction reflexes with the associated arrhythmias (e.g., bradycardia). It should be administered intravenously as single doses of 0.1 mg (0.5 mL) and repeated, as needed, at intervals of 2–3 minutes. The usual attempts should be made to determine the etiology of the arrhythmia, and the surgical or anesthetic manipulations necessary to correct parasympathetic imbalance should be performed.
Reversal of Neuromuscular Blockade. The recommended dose of Robinul (glycopyrrolate) Injectable is 0.2 mg (1.0 mL) for each 1.0 mg of neostigmine or 5.0 mg of pyridostigmine. In order to minimize the appearance of cardiac side effects, the drugs may be administered simultaneously by intravenous injection and may be mixed in the same syringe.
Children: (Read Contraindications) *Preanesthetic Medication.* The recommended dose of Robinul (glycopyrrolate) Injectable in children 1 month to 12 years of age is 0.002 mg (0.01 mL) per pound of body weight intramuscularly, given 30 to 60 minutes prior to the anticipated time of induction of anesthesia or at the time the preanesthetic narcotic and/or sedative are administered.
Children 1 month to 2 years of age may require up to 0.004 mg (0.02 mL) per pound of body weight.
Intraoperative Medication. Because of the long duration of action of Robinul (glycopyrrolate) if used as preanesthetic medication, additional Robinul (glycopyrrolate) Injectable for anticholinergic effect intraoperatively is rarely needed; in the event it is required the recommended pediatric dose is 0.002 mg (0.01 mL) per pound of body weight intravenously, not to exceed 0.1 mg (0.5 mL) in a single dose which may be repeated, as needed, at intervals of 2–3 minutes. The usual attempts should be made to determine the etiology of the arrhythmia, and the surgical or anesthetic manipulations necessary to correct parasympathetic imbalance should be performed.
Reversal of Neuromuscular Blockade. The recommended pediatric dose of Robinul (glycopyrrolate) Injectable is 0.2 mg (1.0 mL) for each 1.0 mg of neostigmine or 5.0 mg of pyridostigmine. In order to minimize the appearance of cardiac side effects, the drugs may be administered simultaneously by intravenous injection and may be mixed in the same syringe.
Adults: *Peptic Ulcer.* The usual recommended dose of Robinul Injectable is 0.1 mg (0.5 mL) administered at 4-hour intervals, 3 or 4 times daily intravenously or intramuscularly. Where more profound effect is required, 0.2 mg (1.0 mL) may be given. Some patients may need only a single dose, and frequency of administration should be dictated by patient response up to a maximum of four times daily.
Robinul Injectable is not recommended for peptic ulcers in children under 12 years of age. (See Precautions.)
NOTE: Parenteral drug products should be inspected visually for particulate matter and discoloration prior to administration whenever solution and container permit.
Admixture Compatibilities. Robinul (glycopyrrolate) Injectable is compatible for mixing and injection with the following injectable dosage forms: 5% and 10% glucose in water or saline; atropine sulfate, USP; Antilirium® (physostigmine salicylate); Benadryl® (diphenhydramine HCl); codeine phosphate, USP; Emete-Con® (benzquinamide HCl); hydromorphone HCl, USP; Inapsine® (droperidol); Innovar® (droperidol and fentanyl citrate); Largon® (propiomazine HCl); Levo-Dromoran® (levorphanol tartrate); lidocaine, USP; Mepergan® (meperidine and promethazine HCls); meperidine HCl, USP; Mestinon® /Regonol® (pyridostigmine bromide); morphine sulfate, USP; Nisentil® (alphaprodine HCl); Nubain® (nalbuphine HCl); Numorphan® (oxymorphone HCl); Pantopon® (opium alkaloids HCls); procaine HCl, USP; promethazine HCl, USP; Prostigmin® (neostigmine methylsulfate, USP); scopolamine HBr, USP; Sparine® (promazine HCl); Stadol® (butorphanol tartrate); Sublimaze® (fentanyl citrate); Talwin® (pentazocine lactate); Tigan® (trimethobenzamide HCl); Vesprin® (triflupromazine HCl); and Vistaril® (hydroxyzine HCl).
Robinul Injectable may be administered via the tubing of a running infusion of physiological saline or lactated Ringer's solution.
Since the stability of glycopyrrolate is questionable above a pH of 6.0, do *not* combine Robinul Injectable in the same syringe with Brevital® (methohexital Na); Chloromycetin® (chloramphenicol Na succinate); Dramamine® (dimenhydrinate); Nembutal® (pentobarbital Na); Pentothal® (thiopental Na); Seconal® (secobarbital Na); sodium bicarbonate (Abbott); or Valium® (diazepam). A gas will evolve or a precipitate may form. Mixing with Decadron® (dexamethasone Na phosphate) or a buffered solution of lactated Ringer's solution will result in a pH higher than 6.0.
Mixing chlorpromazine HCl, USP, or Compazine® (prochlorperazine) with other agents in a syringe is not recommended by the manufacturer, although the mixture with Robinul Injectable is physically compatible.

HOW SUPPLIED

Robinul (glycopyrrolate) Injectable, 0.2 mg/mL, is available in 1 mL single dose vials packaged in 5's (NDC 0031-7890-87), and 25's (NDC 0031-7890-11), 2 mL single dose vials packaged in 25's (NDC 0031-7890-95), 5 mL multiple dose vials packaged individually (NDC 0031-7890-93) and in 25's (NDC 0031-7890-06), and 20 mL (NDC 0031-7890-83) multiple dose vials.
Store at controlled room temperature, between 15°C and 30°C (59°F and 86°F).
Manufactured for A. H. Robins Company, by Elkins-Sinn, Inc.

Shown in Product Identification Section, page 425

ROBITUSSIN A–C® Ⓒ

[*ro"bĭ-tuss'ĭn*]
Expectorant
Cough Suppressant
Sugar-Free

Robitussin and Codeine
Each 5 mL (1 teaspoonful) contains:
Guaifenesin, USP .... 100 mg
Codeine Phosphate, USP .... 10 mg
(Warning: May be habit forming)
Alcohol 3.5 percent
In a palatable, aromatic syrup
Inactive Ingredients: Caramel, Citric Acid, FD&C Red 40, Flavors, Glycerin, Saccharin Sodium, Sodium Benzoate, Sorbitol, Water.

ACTIONS

Robitussin A-C combines the expectorant, guaifenesin, with the cough suppressant, codeine. Guaifenesin enhances the output of lower respiratory tract fluid. The enhanced flow of less viscid secretions promotes and facilitates the removal of mucus. Codeine is a centrally acting agent which elevates the threshold for cough.
As a result, dry, unproductive coughs become more productive and less frequent.
Under Federal law, Robitussin A-C is available without a prescription. Certain state laws may differ. The container label contains the following indications, warnings and drug interaction precaution statements and directions:

INDICATIONS

Temporarily controls cough due to minor throat and bronchial irritation as may occur with the common cold or inhaled irritants. Helps loosen phlegm (mucus) and thin bronchial secretions to make coughs more productive.

WARNINGS

A persistent cough may be a sign of a serious condition. If cough persists for more than 1 week, tends to recur, or is accompanied by fever, rash, or persistent headache, consult a doctor. Do not take this product for persistent or chronic cough such as occurs with smoking, asthma, chronic bronchitis, emphysema, or if cough is accompanied by excessive phlegm (mucus) unless directed by a doctor. Adults and children who have a chronic pulmonary disease or shortness of breath, or children who are taking other drugs, should not take this product unless directed by a doctor. May cause or aggravate constipation. As with any drug, if you are pregnant or nursing a baby, seek the advice of a health professional before using this product.
PROFESSIONAL NOTE: Guaifenesin has been shown to produce a color interference with certain clinical laboratory determinations of 5-hydroxyindoleacetic acid (5-HIAA) and vanillylmandelic acid (VMA).

DRUG INTERACTION PRECAUTION

Caution should be used when taking this product with sedatives, tranquilizers and drugs used for depression, especially monoamine oxidase inhibitors (MAOIs). These combinations may cause greater sedation (drowsiness) than is caused by the products used alone.

DIRECTIONS

Take orally as stated below or use as directed by a doctor.
Adults and children 12 years of age and over: 2 teaspoonfuls every 4 hours, not to exceed 12 teaspoonfuls in a 24-hour period; children 6 to under 12 years: 1 teaspoonful every 4 hours, not to exceed 6 teaspoonfuls in a 24-hour period; children under 6 years: consult a doctor. A special measuring device should be used to give an accurate dose of this product to children under 6 years of age. Giving a higher dose than recommended by a doctor could result in serious side effects for a child. Use of codeine-containing preparations is not recommended for children under 2 years of age. Do not exceed recommended dosage.

HOW SUPPLIED

Bottles of 2 fl. oz. (NDC 0031-8674-05), 4 fl. oz. (NDC 0031-8674-12), pints (NDC 0031-8674-25), and gallons (NDC 0031-8674-29).

ROBITUSSIN® -DAC Ⓒ

[*ro"bĭ-tuss'ĭn*]
Expectorant
Nasal Decongestant
Cough-Suppressant
Sugar-Free

Each 5 mL (1 teaspoonful) contains:
Guaifenesin, USP .... 100 mg
Pseudoephedrine
Hydrochloride, USP .... 30 mg
Codeine Phosphate, USP .... 10 mg
(Warning: May be habit forming)
In a palatable, aromatic syrup
Alcohol 1.9 percent

Mean Decrease in Seated and Standing Blood Pressure (BP) by Guanfacine Dosage Group					
Vital Sign n =	Placebo 63	0.5 mg 63	1 mg 64	2 mg 58	3 mg 59
Change in Systolic (seated) BP	–5	–5	–14	–12	–16
Change in Diastolic (seated) BP	–7	–6	–13	–13	–13
Change in Systolic (standing) BP	–3	–5	–11	– 9	–15
Change in Diastolic (standing) BP	–5	–4	– 9	–10	–12

Inactive Ingredients: Caramel, Citric Acid, FD&C Red 40, Flavors, Glycerin, Saccharin Sodium, Sodium Benzoate, Sorbitol, Water.

ACTIONS

Robitussin-DAC combines the expectorant, guaifenesin, the nasal decongestant, pseudoephedrine, and the cough suppressant, codeine. Guaifenesin enhances the output of lower respiratory tract fluid. The enhanced flow of less viscid secretions promotes and facilitates the removal of mucus. Codeine is a centrally acting agent which elevates the threshold for cough. As a result, dry, unproductive coughs become more productive and less frequent. The nasal decongestant, pseudoephedrine, reduces the swelling of nasal passages.

Under Federal law, Robitussin-DAC is available without a prescription. Certain state laws may differ, The container label contains the following indications, warnings and drug interaction precaution statements and directions:

INDICATIONS

Temporarily relieves nasal congestion and controls cough due to minor throat and bronchial irritation as may occur with the common cold or inhaled irritants. Temporarily restores freer breathing through the nose. Helps loosen phlegm (mucus) and thin bronchial secretions to make coughs more productive.

WARNINGS

A persistent cough may be a sign of a serious condition. If cough persists for more than 1 week, tends to recur, or is accompanied by fever, rash, or persistent headache, consult a doctor. Do not take this product for persistent or chronic cough such as occurs with smoking, asthma, chronic bronchitis, emphysema, or if cough is accompanied by excessive phlegm (mucus) unless directed by a doctor. Adults and children who have a chronic pulmonary disease or shortness of breath, or children who are taking other drugs, should not take this product unless directed by a doctor. Do not take this product if you have high blood pressure, heart disease, diabetes or thyroid disease, except under the advice and supervision of a doctor. Do not exceed recommended dosage because at higher doses nervousness, dizziness or sleeplessness may occur. May cause or aggravate constipation. As with any drug, if you are pregnant or nursing a baby, seek the advice of a health professional before using this product.

PROFESSIONAL NOTE: Guaifenesin has been shown to produce a color interference with certain clinical laboratory determinations of 5-hydroxyindoleacetic acid (5-HIAA) and vanillylmandelic acid (VMA).

DRUG INTERACTION PRECAUTION

Do not take this product if you are presently taking a prescription drug for high blood pressure or depression, especially monoamine oxidase inhibitors (MAOIs), without first consulting your doctor.

DIRECTIONS

Take orally as stated below or use as directed by a doctor. Adults and children 12 years of age and over: 2 teaspoonfuls every 4 hours, not to exceed 8 teaspoonfuls in a 24-hour period; children 6 to under 12 years: 1 teaspoonful every 4 hours, not to exceed 4 teaspoonfuls in a 24-hour period; children under 6 years: consult a doctor. A special measuring device should be used to give an accurate dose of this product to children under 6 years of age. Giving a higher dose than recommended by a doctor could result in serious side effects for a child. Use of codeine-containing preparations is not recommended for children under 2 years of age. Do not exceed recommended dosage.

HOW SUPPLIED

Bottles of 4 fl. oz. (NDC 0031-8680-12) and one pint (NDC 0031-8680-25).

TENEX® Tablets ℞
[ten 'ex]
(Guanfacine Hydrochloride)
1 mg
2 mg

DESCRIPTION

Tenex (guanfacine hydrochloride) is a centrally acting antihypertensive with α_2-adrenoceptor agonist properties in tablet form for oral administration.

The chemical name of Tenex (guanfacine hydrochloride) is N-amidino-2-(2,6-dichlorophenyl) acetamide hydrochloride and its molecular weight is 282.56.

Guanfacine hydrochloride is a white to off-white powder; sparingly soluble in water and alcohol and slightly soluble in acetone. The tablets contain the following inactive ingredients:

1 mg—FD&C Red 40 aluminum lake, Lactose, Microcrystalline cellulose, Povidone, Stearic Acid.

2 mg—D&C Yellow 10 aluminum lake, Lactose, Microcrystalline cellulose, Povidone, Stearic Acid.

CLINICAL PHARMACOLOGY

Tenex (guanfacine hydrochloride) is an orally active antihypertensive agent whose principal mechanism of action appears to be stimulation of central α_2-adrenergic receptors. By stimulating these receptors, guanfacine reduces sympathetic nerve impulses from the vasomotor center to the heart and blood vessels. This results in a decrease in peripheral vascular resistance and a reduction in heart rate.

Controlled clinical trials in patients with mild to moderate hypertension who were receiving a thiazide-type diuretic have defined the dose-response relationship for blood pressure response and adverse reactions of guanfacine given at bedtime and have shown that the blood pressure response to guanfacine can persist for 24 hours after a single dose. In the dose-response study, patients were randomized to placebo or to doses of 0.5, 1, 2, and 3 mg of guanfacine, each given at bedtime. The observed mean changes from baseline, tabulated below, indicate the similarity of response for placebo and the 0.5 mg dose. Doses of 1, 2, and 3 mg resulted in decreased blood pressure in the sitting position with no real differences among the three doses. In the standing position there was some increase in response with dose.

[See table above.]

While most of the effectiveness of guanfacine was present at 1 mg, adverse reactions at this dose were not clearly distinguishable from those associated with placebo. Adverse reactions were clearly present at 2 and 3 mg (see Adverse Reactions).

In a placebo-controlled study of Tenex (guanfacine hydrochloride) a significant decrease in blood pressure was maintained for a full 24 hours after dosing. While there was no significant difference between the 12 and 24 hour blood pressure readings, the fall in blood pressure at 24 hours was numerically smaller, suggesting possible escape of blood pressure in some patients and the need for individualization of therapy.

In a double-blind, randomized trial, either guanfacine or clonidine was given at recommended doses with 25 mg chlorthalidone for 24 weeks and then abruptly discontinued. Results showed equal degrees of blood pressure reduction with the two drugs and there was no tendency for blood pressures to increase despite maintenance of the same daily dose of the two drugs. Signs and symptoms of rebound phenomena were infrequent upon discontinuation of either drug. Abrupt withdrawal of clonidine produced a rapid return of diastolic and especially, systolic blood pressure to approximately pretreatment levels, with occasional values significantly greater than baseline, whereas guanfacine withdrawal produced a more gradual increase to pre-treatment levels, but also with occasional values significantly greater than baseline.

Pharmacodynamics: Hemodynamic studies in man showed that the decrease in blood pressure observed after single-dose or long-term oral treatment with guanfacine was accompanied by a significant decrease in peripheral resistance and a slight reduction in heart rate (5 beats/min). Cardiac output under conditions of rest or exercise was not altered by guanfacine.

Tenex (guanfacine hydrochloride) lowered elevated plasma renin activity and plasma catecholamine levels in hypertensive patients, but this does not correlate with individual blood-pressure responses.

Growth hormone secretion was stimulated with single oral doses of 2 and 4 mg of guanfacine. Long-term use of Tenex had no effect on growth hormone levels.

Guanfacine had no effect on plasma aldosterone. A slight but insignificant decrease in plasma volume occurred after one month of guanfacine therapy. There were no changes in mean body weight or electrolytes.

Pharmacokinetics: Relative to an intravenous dose of 3 mg, the absolute oral bioavailability of guanfacine is about 80%. Peak plasma concentrations occur from 1 to 4 hours with an average of 2.6 hours after single oral doses or at steady state. The area under the concentration-time curve (AUC) increases linearly with the dose.

In individuals with normal renal function, the average elimination half-life is approximately 17 hr (range 10–30 hr). Younger patients tend to have shorter elimination half-lives (13–14 hr) while older patients tend to have half-lives at the upper end of the range. Steady state blood levels were attained within 4 days in most subjects.

In individuals with normal renal function, guanfacine and its metabolites are excreted primarily in the urine. Approximately 50% (40–75%) of the dose is eliminated in the urine as unchanged drug; the remainder is eliminated mostly as conjugates of metabolites produced by oxidative metabolism of the aromatic ring.

The guanfacine-to-creatinine clearance ratio is greater than 1.0, which would suggest that tubular secretion of drug occurs.

The drug is approximately 70% bound to plasma proteins, independent of drug concentration.

The whole body volume of distribution is high (a mean of 6.3 L/kg), which suggests a high distribution of drug to the tissues.

The clearance of guanfacine in patients with varying degrees of renal insufficiency is reduced, but plasma levels of drug are only slightly increased compared to patients with normal renal function. When prescribing for patients with renal impairment, the low end of the dosing range should be used. Patients on dialysis also can be given usual doses of guanfacine hydrochloride as the drug is poorly dialyzed.

INDICATIONS AND USAGE

Tenex (guanfacine hydrochloride) is indicated in the management of hypertension. Since dosing information (see Dosage and Administration) has been established in the presence of a thiazide-type diuretic; Tenex should, therefore, be used in patients who are already receiving a thiazide-type diuretic.

CONTRAINDICATIONS

Tenex is contraindicated in patients with known hypersensitivity to guanfacine hydrochloride.

PRECAUTIONS

General. Like other antihypertensive agents, Tenex (guanfacine hydrochloride) should be used with caution in patients with severe coronary insufficiency, recent myocardial infarction, cerebrovascular disease or chronic renal or hepatic failure.

Sedation. Tenex, like other orally active central alpha-2-adrenergic agonists, causes sedation or drowsiness, especially when beginning therapy. These symptoms are dose-related (see Adverse Reactions). When Tenex is used with other centrally active depressants (such as phenothiazines, barbiturates, or benzodiazepines), the potential for additive sedative effects should be considered.

Rebound. Abrupt cessation of therapy with orally active central alpha-2 adrenergic agonists may be associated with increases (from depressed on-therapy levels) in plasma and urinary catecholamines, symptoms of "nervousness and anxiety" and, less commonly, increases in blood pressure to levels significantly greater than those prior to therapy.

Information for Patients. Patients who receive Tenex should be advised to exercise caution when operating dangerous machinery or driving motor vehicles until it is determined that they do not become drowsy or dizzy from the medication. Patients should be warned that their tolerance for alcohol and other CNS depressants may be diminished. Patients should be advised not to discontinue therapy abruptly.

Laboratory Tests. In clinical trials, no clinically relevant laboratory test abnormalities were identified as causally related to drug during short-term treatment with Tenex (guanfacine hydrochloride).

Drug Interactions. The potential for increased sedation when Tenex is given with other CNS-depressant drugs should be appreciated.

The administration of guanfacine concomitantly with a known microsomal enzyme inducer (phenobarbital or phenytoin) to two patients with renal impairment reportedly resulted in significant reductions in elimination half-life and plasma concentration. In such cases, therefore, more frequent dosing may be required to achieve or maintain the desired hypotensive response. Further, if guanfacine is to be discontinued in such patients, careful tapering of the dosage may be necessary in order to avoid rebound phenomena (see *Rebound* above).

Continued on next page

Prescribing information on A. H. Robins products listed here is based on official labeling in effect June 1, 1992, with Indications, Contraindications, Warnings, Precautions, Adverse Reactions, and Dosage stated in full.

A. H. Robins—Cont.

Anticoagulants. Ten patients who were stabilized on oral anticoagulants were given guanfacine, 1–2 mg/day, for 4 weeks. No changes were observed in the degree of anticoagulation.

In several well-controlled studies, guanfacine was administered together with diuretics with no drug interactions reported. In the long-term safety studies, Tenex was given concomitantly with many drugs without evidence of any interactions. The principal drugs given (number of patients in parentheses) were: cardiac glycosides (115), sedatives and hypnotics (103), coronary vasodilators (52), oral hypoglycemics (45), cough and cold preparations (45), NSAIDs (38), antihyperlipidemics (29), antigout drugs (24), oral contraceptives (18), bronchodilators (13), insulin (10), and beta blockers (10).

Drug/Laboratory Test Interactions. No laboratory test abnormalities related to the use of Tenex (guanfacine hydrochloride) have been identified.

Carcinogenesis, Mutagenesis, Impairment of Fertility. No carcinogenic effect was observed in studies of 78 weeks in mice at doses more than 150 times the maximum recommended human dose and 102 weeks in rats at doses more than 100 times the maximum recommended human dose. In a variety of test models guanfacine was not mutagenic.

No adverse effects were observed in fertility studies in male and female rats.

Pregnancy Category B. Administration of guanfacine to rats at 70 times the maximum recommended human dose and rabbits at 20 times the maximum recommended human dose resulted in no evidence of impaired fertility or harm to the fetus. Higher doses (100 and 200 times the maximum recommended human dose in rabbits and rats respectively) were associated with reduced fetal survival and maternal toxicity. Rat experiments have shown that guanfacine crosses the placenta.

There are, however, no adequate and well-controlled studies in pregnant women. Because animal reproduction studies are not always predictive of human response, this drug should be used during pregnancy only if clearly needed.

Labor and Delivery. Tenex (guanfacine hydrochloride) is not recommended in the treatment of acute hypertension associated with toxemia of pregnancy. There is no information available on the effects of guanfacine on the course of labor and delivery.

Nursing Mothers. It is not known whether Tenex (guanfacine hydrochloride) is excreted in human milk. Because many drugs are excreted in human milk, caution should be exercised when Tenex is administered to a nursing woman. Experiments with rats have shown that guanfacine is excreted in the milk.

Pediatric Use. Safety and effectiveness in children under 12 years of age have not been demonstrated. Therefore, the use of Tenex in this age group is not recommended.

ADVERSE REACTIONS

Adverse reactions noted with Tenex (guanfacine hydrochloride) are similar to those of other drugs of the central α-2 adrenoreceptor agonist class: dry mouth, sedation (somnolence), weakness (asthenia), dizziness, constipation, and impotence. While the reactions are common, most are mild and tend to disappear on continued dosing.

Skin rash with exfoliation has been reported in a few cases; although clear cause and effect relationships to Tenex could not be established, should a rash occur, Tenex should be discontinued and the patient monitored appropriately.

In a 12-week placebo-controlled, dose-response study the frequency of the most commonly observed adverse reactions showed a clear dose relationship from 0.5 to 3 mg, as follows: [See table at bottom of page.]

There were 41 premature terminations because of adverse reactions in this study. The percent of patients who terminated and the dose at which they terminated were as follows:

Dose:	Placebo	0.5 mg	1 mg	2 mg	3 mg
Terminated:	6.9%	4.2%	3.2%	6.9%	8.3%

Reasons for dropouts among patients who received guanfacine were: somnolence, headache, weakness, dry mouth, dizziness, impotence, insomnia, constipation, syncope, urinary incontinence, conjunctivitis, paresthesia, and dermatitis.

In a second placebo-controlled study in which the dose could be adjusted upward to 3 mg per day in 1-mg increments at 3-week intervals, i.e., a setting more similar to ordinary clinical use, the most commonly recorded reactions were: dry mouth 47%, constipation 16%, fatigue 12%, somnolence 10%, asthenia 6%, dizziness 6%, headache 4%, and insomnia 4%.

Reasons for dropouts among patients who received guanfacine were: somnolence, dry mouth, dizziness, impotence, constipation, confusion, depression, and palpitations.

In the clonidine/guanfacine comparison described in Clinical Pharmacology, the most common adverse reactions noted were:

	Guanfacine (n = 279)	Clonidine (n = 278)
Dry mouth	30%	37%
Somnolence	21%	35%
Dizziness	11%	8%
Constipation	10%	5%
Fatigue	9%	8%
Headache	4%	4%
Insomnia	4%	3%

Adverse reactions occurring in 3% or less of patients in the three controlled trials were:

Cardiovascular—	bradycardia, palpitations, substernal pain
Gastrointestinal—	abdominal pain, diarrhea, dyspepsia, dysphagia, nausea
CNS—	amnesia, confusion, depression, insomnia, libido decrease
ENT disorders—	rhinitis, taste perversion, tinnitus
Eye disorders—	conjunctivitis, iritis, vision disturbance
Musculoskeletal—	leg cramps, hypokinesia
Respiratory—	dyspnea
Dermatologic—	dermatitis, pruritus, purpura, sweating
Urogenital—	testicular disorder, urinary incontinence
Other—	malaise, paresthesia, paresis

Adverse reaction reports tend to decrease over time. In an open-label trial of one year's duration, 580 hypertensive subjects were given guanfacine, titrated to achieve goal blood pressure, alone (51%), with diuretic (38%), with beta blocker (3%), with diuretic plus beta blocker (6%), or with diuretic plus vasodilator (2%). The mean daily dose of guanfacine reached was 4.7 mg.

Adverse Reactions	Incidence of adverse reactions at any time during the study	Incidence of adverse reactions at the end of one year
	N=580	N=580
Dry mouth	60%	15%
Drowsiness	33%	6%
Dizziness	15%	1%
Constipation	14%	3%
Weakness	5%	1%
Headache	4%	0.2%
Insomnia	5%	0%

There were 52 (8.9%) dropouts due to adverse effects in this 1-year trial. The causes were: dry mouth (n = 20), weakness (n = 12), constipation (n = 7), somnolence (n = 3), nausea (n = 3), orthostatic hypotension (n = 2), insomnia (n = 1), rash (n = 1), nightmares (n = 1), headache (n = 1), and depression (n = 1).

Postmarketing Experience. An open-label postmarketing study involving 21,718 patients was conducted to assess the safety of Tenex (guanfacine hydrochloride) 1 mg/day given at bedtime for 28 days. Tenex was administered with or without other antihypertensive agents. Adverse events reported in the postmarketing study at an incidence greater than 1% included dry mouth, dizziness, somnolence, fatigue, headache and nausea. The most commonly reported adverse events in this study were the same as those observed in controlled clinical trials.

Less frequent, possibly Tenex-related events observed in the postmarketing study and/or reported spontaneously include:

BODY AS A WHOLE: asthenia, chest pain, edema, malaise, tremor

CARDIOVASCULAR: bradycardia, palpitations, syncope, tachycardia

CENTRAL NERVOUS SYSTEM: paresthesias, vertigo

EYE DISORDERS; blurred vision

GASTROINTESTINAL SYSTEM: abdominal pain, constipation, diarrhea, dyspepsia

LIVER AND BILIARY SYSTEM: abnormal liver function tests

MUSCULO-SKELETAL SYSTEM: arthralgia, leg cramps, leg pain, myalgia

PSYCHIATRIC: agitation, anxiety, confusion, depression, insomnia, nervousness

REPRODUCTIVE SYSTEM, MALE: impotence

RESPIRATORY SYSTEM: dyspnea

SKIN AND APPENDAGES: alopecia, dermatitis, exfoliative dermatitis, pruritus, rash

SPECIAL SENSES: alterations in taste

URINARY SYSTEM: nocturia, urinary frequency

Rare, serious disorders with no definitive cause and effect relationship to Tenex have been reported spontaneously and/or in the postmarketing study. These events include acute renal failure, cardiac fibrillation, cerebrovascular accident, congestive heart failure, heart block, and myocardial infarction.

Drug Abuse and Dependence: No reported abuse or dependence has been associated with the administration of Tenex (guanfacine hydrochloride).

OVERDOSAGE

Signs and Symptoms. Drowsiness, lethargy, bradycardia and hypotension have been observed following overdose with guanfacine.

A 25-year-old female intentionally ingested 60 mg. She presented with severe drowsiness and bradycardia of 45 beats/minute. Gastric lavage was performed and an infusion of isoproterenol (0.8 mg in 12 hours) was administered. She recovered quickly and without sequelae.

A 28-year-old female who ingested 30–40 mg developed only lethargy, was treated with activated charcoal and a cathartic, was monitored for 24 hours, and was discharged in good health.

A 2-year-old male weighing 12 kg, who ingested up to 4 mg of guanfacine, developed lethargy. Gastric lavage (followed by activated charcoal and sorbitol slurry via NG tube) removed some tablet fragments within 2 hours after ingestion, and vital signs were normal. During 24-hour observation in ICU, systolic pressure was 58 and heart rate 70 at 16 hours post-ingestion. No intervention was required, and child was discharged fully recovered the next day.

Treatment of Overdosage. Gastric lavage and infusion of isoproterenol, as appropriate.

Guanfacine is not dialyzable in clinically significant amounts (2.4%).

DOSAGE AND ADMINISTRATION

The recommended dose of Tenex (guanfacine hydrochloride) is 1 mg daily given at bedtime to minimize somnolence. Patients should already be receiving a thiazide type diuretic.

If after 3 to 4 weeks of therapy, 1 mg does not give a satisfactory result, doses of 2 and then subsequently 3 mg may be given, although most of the effect of Tenex is seen at 1 mg (see Clinical Pharmacology). Some patients may show a rise in pressure toward the end of the dosing interval; in this event a divided dose may be utilized.

Higher daily doses (rarely up to 40 mg/day, in divided doses) have been used, but adverse reactions increase significantly with doses above 3 mg/day and there is no evidence of increased efficacy. No studies have established an appropriate dose or dosing interval when Tenex (guanfacine hydrochloride) is given as the sole antihypertensive agent.

The frequency of rebound hypertension is low, but rebound can occur. When rebound occurs, it does so after 2–4 days, which is delayed compared with clonidine hydrochloride. This is consistent with the longer half-life of guanfacine. In most cases, after abrupt withdrawal of guanfacine, blood pressure returns to pretreatment levels slowly (within 2–4 days) without ill effects.

HOW SUPPLIED

Tenex is available in 2 tablet strengths of guanfacine (as the hydrochloride salt) as follows:

1 mg—light pink, diamond-shaped tablet embossed with a 1 and engraved AHR on one side and engraved TENEX on the other side in bottles of 100 (NDC 0031-8901-63) and 500 (NDC 0031-8901-70) and Dis-Co® Unit Dose Packs of 100 (NDC 0031-8901-64).

2 mg—yellow, diamond-shaped tablet, one side engraved TENEX, other side engraved 2 with AHR below it in bottles of 100 (NDC 0031-8903-63).

Adverse Reaction	Assigned Treatment Group				
	Placebo	0.5 mg	1.0 mg	2.0 mg	3.0 mg
n=	73	72	72	72	72
Dry Mouth	5 (7%)	4 (5%)	6 (8%)	8 (11%)	20 (28%)
Somnolence	1 (1%)	3 (4%)	0 (0%)	1 (1%)	10 (14%)
Asthenia	0 (0%)	2 (3%)	0 (0%)	2 (2%)	7 (10%)
Dizziness	2 (2%)	1 (1%)	3 (4%)	6 (8%)	3 (4%)
Headache	3 (4%)	4 (3%)	3 (4%)	1 (1%)	2 (2%)
Impotence	1 (1%)	1 (0%)	0 (0%)	1 (1%)	3 (4%)
Constipation	0 (0%)	0 (0%)	0 (0%)	1 (1%)	1 (1%)
Fatigue	3 (3%)	2 (3%)	2 (3%)	5 (6%)	3 (4%)

Store at controlled room temperature, between 15°C and 30°C (59°F and 86°F). Dispense in tight, light-resistant container.
Shown in Product Identification Section, page 425

VIOKASE®   ℞
[*vi 'o-kās*]
(Pancrelipase, USP)
Tablets
Powder

DESCRIPTION
Viokase (Pancrelipase, USP) is a pancreatic enzyme concentrate of porcine origin containing standardized lipase, protease, and amylase as well as other pancreatic enzymes. Viokase is available in tablet and powder dosage form for oral administration.
The enzyme potencies of the tablets and powder are:

	Each Tablet	Each 0.7g powder ($\frac{1}{4}$ teaspoonful)
Lipase, USP Units	8,000	16,800
Protease, USP Units	30,000	70,000
Amylase, USP Units	30,000	70,000

Inactive Ingredients:
TABLETS—Lactose, Magnesium Stearate, Sodium Chloride, Stearic Acid.
POWDER—Lactose, Sodium Chloride

CLINICAL PHARMACOLOGY
The natural digestive enzymes in Viokase hydrolyze fats into fatty acids and glycerol, split protein into amino acids, and convert carbohydrates to dextrins and short chain sugars. Under conditions of the USP test method (in vitro) Viokase has the following total digestive capacity:

	Each Tablet	Each 0.7g powder
Dietary Fat, grams	28	59
Dietary Protein, grams	30	70
Dietary Starch, grams	30	70

Viokase Tablets are not enteric coated.
The digestive capacity of a pancreatic enzyme concentrate depends on the amount that passes through the stomach unchanged and is available at the site of action in the small intestine.

INDICATIONS
Viokase (Pancrelipase, USP) is indicated as a digestive aid in the treatment of exocrine pancreatic insufficiency as associated with but not limited to cystic fibrosis, chronic pancreatitis, pancreatectomy, or obstruction of the pancreas ducts.

CONTRAINDICATIONS
Do not use in patients hypersensitive to pork protein.

PRECAUTIONS
General: Individuals previously sensitized to trypsin, pancreatin or pancrelipase may have allergic manifestations.
Information for patients: Viokase should not be held in the mouth as the proteolytic action may cause irritation of the mucosa.
Avoid inhalation of the powder when administering Viokase.
Carcinogenesis, Mutagenesis, Impairment of Fertility: Long-term studies in animals have not been performed to evaluate carcinogenic potential.
Pregnancy Category C. Animal reproduction studies have not been conducted with Viokase. It is also not known whether Viokase can cause fetal harm when administered to a pregnant woman or can affect reproduction capacity. Viokase should be given to a pregnant woman only if clearly needed.
Nursing Mothers: It is not known whether this drug is excreted in human milk. Because many drugs are excreted in human milk, caution should be exercised when Viokase is administered to a nursing mother.

ADVERSE REACTIONS
The dust or finely powdered pancreatic enzyme concentrate is irritating to the nasal mucosa and the respiratory tract. It has been documented that inhalation of the airborne powder can precipitate an asthma attack. The literature also contains several references to asthma due to inhalation in patients sensitized to pancreatic enzyme concentrates. Extremely high doses of exogenous pancreatic enzymes have been associated with hyperuricemia and hyperuricosuria. Overdosage of pancreatic enzyme concentrate may cause diarrhea or transient intestinal upset.

OVERDOSAGE
Acute toxicity determinations in animals have not been possible since the maximum dose that could be given orally produced no toxic reaction. In chronic feeding tests, rats developed swollen salivary glands. This is believed due to the proteolytic activity and the mucosal irritation caused by tissue digestion.
No acute toxic reactions have been reported.

DOSAGE AND ADMINISTRATION
Powder: Dosage for patients with cystic fibrosis—$\frac{1}{4}$ teaspoonful (0.7 grams) with meals.
Tablets: Dosage for patients with cystic fibrosis or chronic pancreatitis—1 to 3 tablets with meals or as directed by physician. As a digestive aid in patients with pancreatectomy or obstruction of pancreatic ducts—1 to 2 tablets taken at 2-hour intervals or as directed by physician.

HOW SUPPLIED
Tablets—Tan, round, compressed tablets engraved Viokase/AHR on one side and 9111 on the other side in bottles of 100 (NDC 0031-9111-63) and 500 (NDC 0031-9111-70).
Powder—Tan powder in bottles of 4 oz. (113.5 grams) (NDC 0031-9115-12) and 8 oz. (227 grams) (NDC 0031-9115-25).
Store in tightly closed container in a dry place at a temperature not exceeding 25°C (77°F).
Dispense tablets and powder in tight container, preferably with a desiccant.

CLINICAL STUDIES
The effectiveness of Viokase as a digestive aid in the treatment of patients with exocrine pancreatic insufficiency has been documented in the literature as follows:
1. Regan, PT, Malagelada J-R, DiMagno EP, Glanzman SL, Go VLW: Comparative effects of antacids, cimetidine and enteric coating on the therapeutic response to oral enzymes in severe pancreatic insufficiency. N. Engl. J. Med. 297:854-8, 1977.
2. Graham DY: Enzyme replacement therapy of exocrine pancreatic insufficiency in man. N. Engl. J. Med. 296:1314-7, 1977.
Shown in Product Identification Section, page 425

A.H. Robins Consumer Products Division
1405 CUMMINGS DRIVE
RICHMOND, VA 23230

ALLBEE® WITH C CAPLETS   OTC
[*all-be'*]

(See PDR For Nonprescription Drugs.)

ALLBEE® C–800 TABLETS   OTC
ALLBEE® C–800 plus IRON TABLETS
[*all-be'*]

(See PDR For Nonprescription Drugs.)

DIMACOL® CAPLETS   OTC
[*di 'mă-col*]

(See PDR For Nonprescription Drugs.)

DIMETANE EXTENTABS®   OTC
[*di 'mĕ-tāne eks "tĕn 'tabs*]
brand of Brompheniramine Maleate, USP
8 mg and 12 mg

(See PDR For Nonprescription Drugs.)

DIMETANE®   OTC
[*di 'mĕ-tāne*]
brand of Brompheniramine Maleate, USP
Tablets—4 mg
Elixir—2 mg/5 ml
  Alcohol, 3%

(See PDR For Nonprescription Drugs.)

DIMETANE® DECONGESTANT ELIXIR   OTC
[*di 'mĕ-tāne*]
DIMETANE® DECONGESTANT CAPLETS

(See PDR For Nonprescription Drugs.)

DIMETAPP® Cold and Flu   OTC
[*di ' mĕ-tap*]

(See PDR For Nonprescription Drugs.)

DIMETAPP® ELIXIR   OTC
[*di 'mĕ-tap*]

(See PDR For Nonprescription Drugs.)

DIMETAPP® DM ELIXIR   OTC
[*di 'mĕ-tap*]

(See PDR For Nonprescription Drugs.)

ROBITUSSIN®   OTC
[*ro "bĭ-tuss 'ĭn*]
ROBITUSSIN® CF
ROBITUSSIN® DM
ROBITUSSIN® PE

(See PDR For Nonprescription Drugs.)

12-HOUR EXTENTABS   OTC
(formerly Dimetapp® 12-Hour Extentabs)
[*twelv au 'ər eks "tĕn 'tabs*]

(See PDR For Nonprescription Drugs.)

Z–BEC®   OTC
[*zē 'bĕk*]

(See PDR For Nonprescription Drugs.)

E. C. Robins Company, Inc.
E. C. Robins/William P. Poythress
3911 DEEP ROCK ROAD
P. O. BOX 71600
RICHMOND, VA 23255

E.C. Robins Co. is not affiliated with A.H. Robins or American Home Products.

NDC 0095	Product	
—0040	**Antrocol Tablets and**	℞
—0042	**Antrocol Elixir**	℞
	Each tablet and teaspoon (5 ml) of elixir Contains: Atropine Sulfate 0.195 mg; Phenobarbital, 16 mg (Elixir, 20% Alcohol)	
—0015	**Bensulfoid Tablets**	℞
	(Bensulfoid, 130 mg [33% Collodial Sulfur])	
—0016	**Bensulfoid Cream**	OTC
	Sulfur, 8%; Resorcinol 2%; Alcohol, 10%)	
—6006	**Lodrane LD**	℞
	(Brompheniramine Maleate, 6 mg; Pseudoephedrine HCl, 60 mg—Sustained Release, Dye Free)	
—0050	**Mudrane Tablets**	℞
	Potassium Iodide, 195 mg; Aminophylline, 130 mg; Ephedrine HCl, 16 mg; Phenobarbital, 8 mg)	
—0032	**Mudrane-2 Tablets**	℞
	(Potassium Iodide, 195 mg; Aminophylline, 130 mg)	
—0051	**Mudrane GG Tablets**	℞
	(Aminophylline, 130 mg; Guaifenesin, 100 mg; Ephedrine HCl, 16 mg; Phenobarbital, 8 mg)	
—0053	**Mudrane GG Elixir**	℞
	(Each 5 ml/ Guaifenesin, 26 mg; Theophylline, 20 mg; Phenobarbital, 2.5 mg; Ephedrine HCl, 4 mg; Alcohol, 20%)	
—0033	**Mudrane GG-2 Tablets**	℞
	(Guaifenesin, 100 mg; Aminophylline, 130 mg)	
—0141	**Panacet 5/500 Tablets**	℞ ⓒ
	(Hydrocodone Bitartrate 5 mg; Acetaminophen 500 mg)	
—0131	**Panasal 5/500 Tablets**	℞ ⓒ
	(Hydrocodone Bitartrate 5 mg; Aspirin 500 mg)	
—0021	**Panalgesic Gold Cream**	OTC
	(Methyl Salicylate, 35%; Menthol, 4%)	
—0120	**Panalgesic Gold Liniment**	OTC
	(Methyl Salicylate, 55%; Camphor, 3.1%; Menthol, 1.25%)	

Continued on next page

E. C. Robins—Cont.

—0065 Pneumotussin HC ℞ C-III
(Guaifenesin, 100 mg; Hydrocodone Bitartrate, 5 mg)

—0600 Pneumomist ℞
(Guaifenesin, 600 mg—Sustained Release, Dye Free)

—0023 Solfoton Tablets and ℞ C-IV
—0025 Solfoton Capsules ℞ C-IV
(Phenobarbital, 16 mg)

—0031 Uro-Phosphate Tablets ℞
(Methenamine, 300 mg; Sodium Biphosphate, 500 mg)

Roche Dermatologics

a division of Hoffmann-La Roche Inc.
NUTLEY, NJ 07110

ACCUTANE® ℞

[acc 'u-tane]
(isotretinoin/Roche)
CAPSULES

The following text is complete prescribing information based on official labeling in effect June 1, 1992.

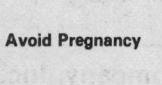

Avoid Pregnancy

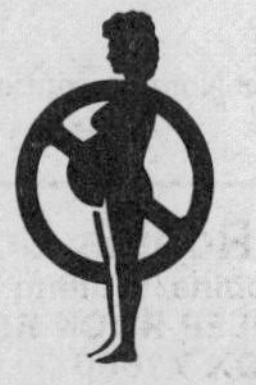

CONTRAINDICATION AND WARNING

Accutane must not be used by females who are pregnant or who may become pregnant while undergoing treatment. There is an extremely high risk that a deformed infant will result if pregnancy occurs while taking Accutane in any amount even for short periods. Potentially all exposed fetuses can be affected.

Accutane is contraindicated in women of childbearing potential unless the patient meets all of the following conditions:

- **has severe disfiguring cystic acne that is recalcitrant to standard therapies**
- **is reliable in understanding and carrying out instructions**
- **is capable of complying with the mandatory contraceptive measures**
- **has received both oral and written warnings of the hazards of taking Accutane during pregnancy and the risk of possible contraception failure and has acknowledged her understanding of these warnings in writing**
- **has had a negative serum pregnancy test within two weeks prior to beginning therapy (It is also recommended that pregnancy testing and contraception counseling be repeated on a monthly basis. To encourage compliance with this recommendation, the physician should prescribe no more than a one month supply of the drug.)**
- **will begin therapy only on the second or third day of the next normal menstrual period**

Major human fetal abnormalities related to Accutane administration have been documented: CNS abnormalities (including cerebral abnormalities, cerebellar malformation, hydrocephalus, microcephaly, cranial nerve deficit); skull abnormality; external ear abnormalities (including anotia, micropinna, small or absent external auditory canals); eye abnormalities (including microphthalmia); cardiovascular abnormalities; facial dysmorphia; thymus gland abnormality; parathyroid hormone deficiency. In some cases death has occurred with certain of the abnormalities previously noted. Cases of IQ scores less than 85 with or without obvious CNS abnormalities have also been reported. There is an increased risk of spontaneous abortion. In addition, premature births have been reported.

Effective contraception must be used for at least one month before beginning Accutane therapy, during therapy and for one month following discontinuation of therapy even where there has been a history of infertility, unless due to hysterectomy. It is recommended that two reliable forms of contraception be used simultaneously unless abstinence is the chosen method.

If pregnancy does occur during treatment, the physician and patient should discuss the desirability of continuing the pregnancy.

Accutane should be prescribed only by physicians who have special competence in the diagnosis and treatment of severe recalcitrant cystic acne, are experienced in the use of systemic retinoids and understand the risk of teratogenicity if Accutane is used during pregnancy.

DESCRIPTION

Accutane (isotretinoin/Roche), a retinoid which inhibits sebaceous gland function and keratinization, is available in 10-mg, 20-mg and 40-mg soft gelatin capsules for oral administration. Each capsule also contains beeswax, butylated hydroxyanisole, edetate disodium, hydrogenated soybean oil flakes, hydrogenated vegetable oil and soybean oil. Gelatin capsules contain glycerin and parabens (methyl and propyl), with the following dye systems: 10 mg—iron oxide (red) and titanium dioxide; 20 mg—FD&C Red No. 3, FD&C Blue No. 1 and titanium dioxide; 40 mg—FD&C Yellow No. 6, D&C Yellow No. 10 and titanium dioxide.

Chemically, isotretinoin is 13-*cis* -retinoic acid and is related to both retinoic acid and retinol (vitamin A). It is a yellow-orange to orange crystalline powder with a molecular weight of 300.44.

CLINICAL PHARMACOLOGY

The exact mechanism of action of Accutane is unknown.

Cystic Acne: Clinical improvement in cystic acne patients occurs in association with a reduction in sebum secretion. The decrease in sebum secretion is temporary and is related to the dose and duration of treatment with Accutane, and reflects a reduction in sebaceous gland size and an inhibition of sebaceous gland differentiation.[1]

Clinical Pharmacokinetics: The pharmacokinetic profile of isotretinoin is predictable and can be described using linear pharmacokinetic theory.

After oral administration of 80 mg (two 40-mg capsules), peak blood concentrations ranged from 167 to 459 ng/mL (mean 256 ng/mL) and mean time to peak was 3.2 hours in normal volunteers, while in acne patients peak concentrations ranged from 98 to 535 ng/mL (mean 262 ng/mL) with a mean time to peak of 2.9 hours. The drug is 99.9% bound in human plasma almost exclusively to albumin. The terminal elimination half-life of isotretinoin ranged from 10 to 20 hours in volunteers and patients. Following an 80-mg liquid suspension oral dose of ^{14}C-isotretinoin, ^{14}C-activity in blood declined with a half-life of 90 hours. Relatively equal amounts of radioactivity were recovered in the urine and feces with 65% to 83% of the dose recovered.

The major identified metabolite in blood is 4-*oxo* -isotretinoin. The mean elimination half-life of this metabolite is 25 hours (range 17–50 hours). Tretinoin and 4-*oxo* -tretinoin were also observed. After two 40-mg capsules of isotretinoin, maximum concentrations of the metabolite of 87 to 399 ng/mL occurred at 6 to 20 hours. The blood concentration of the major metabolite generally exceeded that of isotretinoin after six hours.

When taken with food or milk, the oral absorption of isotretinoin is increased.

The mean $\pm$ SD minimum steady-state blood concentration of isotretinoin was 160 $\pm$ 19 ng/mL in ten patients receiving 40-mg *b.i.d.* doses. After single and multiple doses, the mean ratio of areas under the blood concentration:time curves of 4-*oxo* -isotretinoin to isotretinoin was 3 to 3.5.

Tissue Distribution in Animals: Tissue distribution of ^{14}C-isotretinoin in rats after oral dosing revealed high concentrations of radioactivity in many tissues after 15 minutes, with a maximum in one hour, and declining to nondetectable levels by 24 hours in most tissues. After seven days, however, low levels of radioactivity were detected in the liver, ureter, adrenal, ovary and lacrimal gland.

INDICATIONS AND USAGE

Cystic Acne: Accutane is indicated for the treatment of severe recalcitrant cystic acne, and a single course of therapy has been shown to result in complete and prolonged remission of disease in many patients.[1–3] If a second course of therapy is needed, it should not be initiated until at least eight weeks after completion of the first course, since experience has shown that patients may continue to improve while off drug.

Because of significant adverse effects associated with its use, Accutane should be reserved for patients with severe cystic acne who are unresponsive to conventional therapy, including systemic antibiotics.

CONTRAINDICATIONS

Pregnancy: Category X. See boxed CONTRAINDICATION and WARNING.

Accutane should not be given to patients who are sensitive to parabens, which are used as preservatives in the gelatin capsule.

WARNINGS

***Pseudotumor cerebri:* Accutane use has been associated with a number of cases of pseudotumor cerebri (benign intracranial hypertension). Early signs and symptoms of pseudotumor cerebri include papilledema, headache, nausea and vomiting, and visual disturbances. Patients with these symptoms should be screened for papilledema and, if present, they should be told to discontinue Accutane immediately and be referred to a neurologist for further diagnosis and care.**

Decreased Night Vision: A number of cases of decreased night vision have occurred during Accutane therapy. Because the onset in some patients was sudden, patients should be advised of this potential problem and warned to be cautious when driving or operating any vehicle at night. Visual problems should be carefully monitored.

Corneal opacities: Corneal opacities have occurred in patients receiving Accutane for acne and more frequently when higher drug dosages were used in patients with disorders of keratinization. All Accutane patients experiencing visual difficulties should discontinue the drug and have an ophthalmological examination. The corneal opacities that have been observed in patients treated with Accutane have either completely resolved or were resolving at follow-up six to seven weeks after discontinuation of the drug. See ADVERSE REACTIONS.

Inflammatory Bowel Disease: Accutane has been temporally associated with inflammatory bowel disease (including regional ileitis) in patients without a prior history of intestinal disorders. Patients experiencing abdominal pain, rectal bleeding or severe diarrhea should discontinue Accutane immediately.

Lipids: Blood lipid determinations should be performed before Accutane is given and then at intervals until the lipid response to Accutane is established, which usually occurs within four weeks. See PRECAUTIONS.

Approximately 25% of patients receiving Accutane experienced an elevation in plasma triglycerides. Approximately 15% developed a decrease in high density lipoproteins and about 7% showed an increase in cholesterol levels. These effects on triglycerides, HDL and cholesterol were reversible upon cessation of Accutane therapy.

Patients with increased tendency to develop hypertriglyceridemia include those with diabetes mellitus, obesity, increased alcohol intake and familial history.

The cardiovascular consequences of hypertriglyceridemia are not well understood, but may increase the patient's risk status. In addition, elevation of serum triglycerides in excess of 800 mg/dL has been associated with acute pancreatitis. Therefore, every attempt should be made to control significant triglyceride elevation.

Some patients have been able to reverse triglyceride elevation by reduction in weight, restriction of dietary fat and alcohol, and reduction in dose while continuing Accutane.[4] An obese male patient with Darier's disease developed elevated triglycerides and subsequent eruptive xanthomas.[5]

Hyperostosis: In clinical trials of disorders of keratinization with a mean dose of 2.24 mg/kg/day, a high prevalence of skeletal hyperostosis was noted. Two children showed x-ray findings suggestive of premature closure of the epiphysis. Additionally, skeletal hyperostosis was noted in six of eight patients in a prospective study of disorders of keratinization.[6] Minimal skeletal hyperostosis has also been observed by x-rays in prospective studies of cystic acne patients treated with a single course of therapy at recommended doses.

Hepatotoxicity: Several cases of clinical hepatitis have been noted which are considered to be possibly or probably related to Accutane therapy. Additionally, mild to moderate elevations of liver enzymes have been observed in approximately 15% of individuals treated during clinical trials, some of which normalized with dosage reduction or continued administration of the drug. If normalization does not readily occur or if hepatitis is suspected during treatment with Accutane, the drug should be discontinued and the etiology further investigated.

Animal Studies: In rats given 32 or 8 mg/kg/day of isotretinoin for 18 months or longer, the incidences of focal calcification, fibrosis and inflammation of the myocardium, calcification of coronary, pulmonary and mesenteric arteries and metastatic calcification of the gastric mucosa were greater than in control rats of similar age. Focal endocardial and myocardial calcifications associated with calcification of the coronary arteries were observed in two dogs after approximately six to seven months of treatment with isotretinoin at a dosage of 60 to 120 mg/kg/day.

In dogs given isotretinoin chronically at a dosage of 60 mg/kg/day, corneal ulcers and corneal opacities were encountered at a higher incidence than in control dogs. In general, these ocular changes tended to revert toward normal when treatment with isotretinoin was stopped, but did not completely clear during the observation period.

In rats given isotretinoin at a dosage of 32 mg/kg/day for approximately 15 weeks, long bone fracture has been observed.

PRECAUTIONS

Information for Patients: **Women of childbearing potential should be instructed that they must not be pregnant when Accutane therapy is initiated, and that they should use effective contraception while taking Accutane and for one month after Accutane has been stopped. They should also sign a consent form prior to beginning Accutane therapy. See boxed CONTRAINDICATION AND WARNING.**

Because of the relationship of Accutane to vitamin A, patients should be advised against taking vitamin supplements containing vitamin A to avoid additive toxic effects.

Patients should be informed that transient exacerbation of acne has been seen, generally during the initial period of therapy.

Patients should be informed that they may experience decreased tolerance to contact lenses during and after therapy.

It is recommended that patients not donate blood during therapy and for at least one month following discontinuance of the drug.

Laboratory Tests: The incidence of hypertriglyceridemia is 1 patient in 4 on Accutane therapy. Pretreatment and follow-up blood lipids should be obtained under fasting conditions. After consumption of alcohol at least 36 hours should elapse before these determinations are made. It is recommended that these tests be performed at weekly or biweekly intervals until the lipid response to Accutane is established.

Since elevations of liver enzymes have been observed during clinical trials, pretreatment and follow-up liver function tests should be performed at weekly or biweekly intervals until the response to Accutane has been established.

Certain patients receiving Accutane have experienced problems in the control of their blood sugar. In addition, new cases of diabetes have been diagnosed during Accutane therapy, although no causal relationship has been established.

Some patients undergoing vigorous physical activity while on Accutane therapy have experienced elevated CPK levels; however, the clinical significance is unknown.

Carcinogenesis, Mutagenesis, Impairment of Fertility: In Fischer 344 rats given isotretinoin at dosages of 32 or 8 mg/kg/day for greater than 18 months, there was an increased incidence of pheochromocytoma. The incidence of adrenal medullary hyperplasia was also increased at the higher dosage. The relatively high level of spontaneous pheochromocytomas occurring in the Fischer 344 rat makes it a poor model for study of this tumor, since the increase in adrenal medullary proliferative lesions following chronic treatment with relatively high dosages of isotretinoin may be an accentuation of a genetic predisposition in the Fischer 344 rat, and its relevance to the human population is not clear. In addition, a decreased incidence of liver adenomas, liver angiomas and leukemia was noted at the dose levels of 8 and 32 mg/kg/day.

The Ames test was conducted in two laboratories. The results of the tests in one laboratory were negative while in the second laboratory a weakly-positive response (less than 1.6 × background) was noted in S. typhimurium TA100 when the assay was conducted with metabolic activation. No dose-response effect was seen and all other strains were negative. Additionally, other tests designed to assess genotoxicity (Chinese hamster cell assay, mouse micronucleus test, S. cerevisiae D7 assay, *in vitro* clastogenesis assay in human-derived lymphocytes and unscheduled DNA synthesis assay) were all negative.

No adverse effects on gonadal function, fertility, conception rate, gestation or parturition were observed at dose levels of 2, 8 or 32 mg/kg/day in male and female rats.

In dogs, testicular atrophy was noted after treatment with isotretinoin for approximately 30 weeks at dosages of 60 or 20 mg/kg/day. In general, there was microscopic evidence for appreciable depression of spermatogenesis but some sperm were observed in all testes examined and in no instance were completely atrophic tubules seen. In studies in 66 human males, 30 of whom were patients with cystic acne, no significant changes were noted in the count or motility of spermatozoa in the ejaculate. In a study of 50 men (ages 17–32 years) receiving Accutane therapy for cystic acne, no significant effects were seen on ejaculate volume, sperm count, total sperm motility, morphology or seminal plasma fructose.

Pregnancy: **Category X. See boxed CONTRAINDICATION AND WARNING.**

Nursing Mothers: It is not known whether this drug is excreted in human milk. Because of the potential for adverse effects, nursing mothers should not receive Accutane.

ADVERSE REACTIONS

Clinical: Many of the side effects and adverse reactions seen or expected in patients receiving Accutane are similar to those described in patients taking high doses of vitamin A. The percentages of adverse reactions listed below reflect the total experience in Accutane studies, including investigational studies of disorders of keratinization, with the exception of those pertaining to dry skin and mucous membranes. These latter reflect the experience only in patients with cystic acne because reactions relating to dryness are more commonly recognized as adverse reactions in this disease. Included in this category are dry skin, skin fragility, pruritus, epistaxis, dry nose and dry mouth, which may be seen in up to 80% of cystic acne patients.

The most frequent adverse reaction to Accutane is cheilitis, which occurs in over 90% of patients. A less frequent reaction was conjunctivitis (about two patients in five).

Skeletal hyperostosis has been observed on x-rays of patients treated with Accutane. See WARNINGS. Other types of bone abnormalities have also been reported; however, no causal relatioinship has been established.

Approximately 16% of patients treated with Accutane developed musculoskeletal symptoms (including arthralgia) during treatment. In general, these were mild to moderate and have occasionally required discontinuation of drug. Less frequently, transient pain in the chest has also been reported. These symptoms generally cleared rapidly after discontinuation of Accutane but in rare cases have persisted.

In less than one patient in ten—rash (including erythema, seborrhea and eczema); thinning of hair, which in rare cases has persisted.

In approximately one patient in twenty—peeling of palms and soles, skin infections, nonspecific urogenital findings, nonspecific gastrointestinal symptoms, fatigue, headache and increased susceptibility to sunburn.

Accutane has been associated with a number of cases of pseudotumor cerebri, some of which involved concomitant use of tetracyclines. See WARNINGS.

The following CNS reactions have been reported and may bear no relationship to therapy—seizures, emotional instability, dizziness, nervousness, drowsiness, malaise, weakness, insomnia, lethargy and paresthesias.

Depression has been reported in some patients on Accutane therapy. In some of these patients, this has subsided with discontinuation of therapy and recurred with reinstitution of therapy.

The following reactions have been reported in less than 1% of patients and may bear no relationship to therapy—changes in skin pigment (hypo- and hyperpigmentation), flushing, urticaria, bruising, disseminated herpes simplex, edema, hair problems (other than thinning), hirsutism, respiratory infections, weight loss, erythema nodosum, paronychia, nail dystrophy, bleeding and inflammation of the gums, abnormal menses, optic neuritis, photophobia, eye lid inflammation, arthritis, anemia, palpitation, tachycardia, lymphadenopathy, sweating, tinnitus and voice alteration.

A few isolated reports of vasculitis, including Wegener's granulomatosis, have been received, but no causal relationship to Accutane therapy has been established.

In Accutane studies to date, of 72 patients who had normal pretreatment ophthalmological examinations, five developed corneal opacities while on Accutane (all five patients had a disorder of keratinization). Corneal opacities have also been reported in cystic acne patients treated with Accutane. See WARNINGS. Dry eyes and decrease in night vision have been reported and in rare instances have persisted. See WARNINGS. Cataracts and visual disturbances have also been reported.

Accutane has been temporally associated with inflammatory bowel disease. See WARNINGS.

As may be seen with healing cystic acne lesions, an occasional exaggerated healing response, manifested by exuberant granulation tissue with crusting, has also been reported in patients receiving therapy with Accutane. Pyogenic granuloma has also been diagnosed in a number of cases.

Laboratory: Accutane therapy induces change in serum lipids in a significant number of treated subjects. Approximately 25% of patients had elevation of plasma triglycerides. Five out of 135 patients treated for cystic acne and 32 out of 298 total subjects treated for all diagnoses showed an elevation of triglycerides above 500 mg percent. About 16% of patients showed a mild to moderate decrease in serum high density lipoprotein (HDL) levels while receiving treatment with Accutane and about 7% of patients experienced minimal elevations of serum cholesterol during treatment. Abnormalities of serum triglycerides, HDL and cholesterol were reversible upon cessation of Accutane therapy.

Approximately 40% of patients receiving Accutane developed elevated sedimentation rates, often from elevated baseline values.

From one in ten to one in five patients showed decreases in red blood cell parameters and white blood cell counts, elevated platelet counts, white cells in the urine, increased alkaline phosphatase, SGOT, SGPT, GGTP or LDH. See WARNINGS: Hepatotoxicity.

Less than one in ten patients showed proteinuria, microscopic or gross hematuria, elevated fasting blood sugar, elevated CPK, hyperuricemia or thrombocytopenia.

Dose Relationship and Duration: Cheilitis and hypertriglyceridemia are usually dose-related.

Most adverse reactions were reversible when therapy was discontinued; however, some have persisted after cessation of therapy. (See WARNINGS and ADVERSE REACTIONS.)

Overdosage: The oral LD_{50} of isotretinoin is greater than 4000 mg/kg in rats and mice and is approximately 1960 mg/kg in rabbits. Overdose has been associated with transient headache, vomiting, facial flushing, cheilosis, abdominal pain, headache, dizziness and ataxia. All symptoms quickly resolved without apparent residual effects.

DOSAGE AND ADMINISTRATION

The recommended dosage range for Accutane is 0.5 to 2 mg/kg given in two divided doses daily for 15 to 20 weeks. In studies comparing 0.1, 0.5 and 1 mg/kg/day,[7] it was found that all doses provided initial clearing of disease but there was a greater need for retreatment with the lower dose(s).

It is recommended that for most patients the initial dose of Accutane be 0.5 to 1 mg/kg/day. Patients whose disease is very severe or is primarily manifest on the body may require up to the maximum recommended dose, 2 mg/kg/day. During treatment, the dose may be adjusted according to response of the disease and/or the appearance of clinical side effects—some of which may be dose-related.

If the total cyst count has been reduced by more than 70 percent prior to completing 15 to 20 weeks of treatment, the drug may be discontinued. After a period of two months or more off therapy, and if warranted by persistent or recurring severe cystic acne, a second course of therapy may be initiated. Contraceptive measures must be followed for any subsequent course of therapy.

Accutane should be administered with food.

ACCUTANE DOSING BY BODY WEIGHT

Body Weight		Total Mg/Day		
kilograms	pounds	0.5 mg/kg	1 mg/kg	2 mg/kg
40	88	20	40	80
50	110	25	50	100
60	132	30	60	120
70	154	35	70	140
80	176	40	80	160
90	198	45	90	180
100	220	50	100	200

HOW SUPPLIED

Soft gelatin capsules, 10 mg (light pink), imprinted ACCUTANE 10 ROCHE. Boxes of 100 containing 10 Prescription Paks of 10 capsules (NDC 0004-0155-49).

Soft gelatin capsules, 20 mg (maroon), imprinted ACCUTANE 20 ROCHE. Boxes of 100 containing 10 Prescription Paks of 10 capsules (NDC 0004-0169-49).

Soft gelatin capsules, 40 mg (yellow), imprinted ACCUTANE 40 ROCHE. Boxes of 100 containing 10 Prescription Paks of 10 capsules (NDC 0004-0156-49).

Store at 59° to 86°F; 15°to 30°C. Protect from light.

REFERENCES

1. Peck GL, Olsen TG, Yoder FW, Strauss JS, Downing DT, Pandya M, Butkus D, Arnaud-Battandier J: Prolonged remissions of cystic and conglobate acne with 13-*cis*-retinoic acid. *N Engl J Med 300*:329–333, 1979. 2. Farrell LN, Strauss JS, Stranieri AM: The treatment of severe cystic acne with 13-*cis*-retinoic acid. Evaluation of sebum production and the clinical response in a multiple-dose trial. *J Am Acad Dermatol 3*:602–611, 1980. 3. Jones H, Blanc D, Cunliffe WJ: 13-*cis*-retinoic acid and acne. *Lancet 2*:1048–1049, 1980. 4. Katz RA, Jorgensen H, Nigra TP: Elevation of serum triglyceride levels from oral isotretinoin in disorders of keratinization. *Arch Dermatol 116*:1369–1372, 1980. 5. Dicken CH, Connolly SM: Eruptive xanthomas associated with isotretinoin (13-*cis*-retinoic acid). *Arch Dermatol 116*:951–952, 1980. 6. Ellis CN, Madison KC, Pennes DR, Martel W, Voorhees JJ: Isotretinoin therapy is associated with early skeletal radiographic changes. *J Am Acad Dermatol 10*:1024–1029, 1984. 7. Strauss JS, Rapini RP, Shalita AR, Konecky E, Pochi PE, Comite H, Exner JH: Isotretinoin therapy for acne: Results of a multicenter dose-response study. *J Am Acad Dermatol 10*:490–496, 1984.

PATIENT INFORMATION/CONSENT

Accutane must not be used by females who are pregnant or who may become pregnant while undergoing treatment.

IMPORTANT INFORMATION AND WARNING: Accutane can cause severe birth defects if it is taken when a woman is pregnant. There is an extremely high risk that you will have a severely deformed baby if:

- you are pregnant when you start taking Accutane,
- you become pregnant while you are taking Accutane,
- you do not wait at least one month after you stop taking Accutane before becoming pregnant.

It is recommended that you and your doctor schedule an appointment every month to repeat the pregnancy test and check your body's response to Accutane. For your health and well-being, be sure to keep your appointments as scheduled.

Continued on next page

Roche Dermatologics—Cont.

THE CONSENT

My treatment with Accutane has been personally explained to me by Dr. ______________.

The following points of information, among others, have been specifically discussed and made clear:

1. I, ______________________________,
(Patient's Name)
understand that Accutane is a very powerful medicine used to treat severe cystic acne that did not get better with other treatments including oral antibiotics.
INITIALS: ________
2. I understand that I must not take Accutane if I am or may become pregnant during treatment.
INITIALS: ________
3. I understand that severe birth defects have occurred in babies of women who took Accutane during pregnancy. I have been warned by my doctor that there is an extremely high risk of severe damage to my unborn baby if I am or become pregnant while taking Accutane.
INITIALS: ________
4. I have been told by my doctor that effective birth control (contraception) must be used for at least one month before starting Accutane, all during Accutane therapy and for at least one month after Accutane treatment has stopped. My doctor has recommended that I either abstain from sexual intercourse or use two reliable kinds of birth control at the same time. I have also been told that any method of birth control can fail.
INITIALS: ________
5. I know that I must have a blood test that shows I am not pregnant within two weeks before starting Accutane, and I understand that I must wait until the second or third day of my next normal menstrual period before starting Accutane. INITIALS: ________
6. My doctor has told me that I can participate in the "Patient Referral" program for an initial free pregnancy test and birth control counseling session by a consulting physician.
INITIALS: ________
7. I also know that I must immediately stop taking Accutane if I become pregnant while taking the drug and immediately contact my doctor to discuss the desirability of continuing the pregnancy. INITIALS: ________
8. I have carefully read the Accutane patient brochure, "Important information concerning your treatment with Accutane," given to me by my doctor. I understand all of its contents and have talked over any questions I have with my doctor. INITIALS: ________
9. I am not now pregnant, nor do I plan to become pregnant for at least 30 days after I have completely finished taking Accutane. INITIALS: ________
10. My doctor has told me that I can participate in a survey concerning Accutane use in women by completing an additional form. INITIALS: ________

I now authorize Dr. ______________ to begin my treatment with Accutane.

____
Patient, Parent or Guardian Date

Address
____
____

Telephone Number

I have fully explained to the patient, ______________, the nature and purpose of the treatment described above and the risks to women of childbearing potential. I have asked the patient if she has any questions regarding her treatment with Accutane and have answered those questions to the best of my ability.

____
Physician Date

Revised: May 1990

Shown in Product Identification Section, page 425

EFUDEX® ℞
[ef'u-dex]
(fluorouracil/Roche)

The following text is complete prescribing information based on official labeling in effect June 1, 1992.

DESCRIPTION

Efudex solutions and cream are topical preparations containing the fluorinated pyrimidine 5-fluorouracil, an antineoplastic antimetabolite.

Efudex Solution consists of 2% or 5% fluorouracil/Roche on a weight/weight basis, compounded with propylene glycol, tris(hydroxymethyl) aminomethane, hydroxypropyl cellulose, parabens (methyl and propyl) and disodium edetate.

Efudex Cream contains 5% fluorouracil/Roche in a vanishing cream base consisting of white petrolatum, stearyl alcohol, propylene glycol, polysorbate 60 and parabens (methyl and propyl).

ACTIONS

There is evidence that the metabolism of fluorouracil in the anabolic pathway blocks the methylation reaction of deoxyuridylic acid to thymidylic acid. In this fashion fluorouracil interferes with the synthesis of deoxyribonucleic acid (DNA) and to a lesser extent inhibits the formation of ribonucleic acid (RNA). Since DNA and RNA are essential for cell division and growth, the effect of fluorouracil may be to create a thymine deficiency which provokes unbalanced growth and death of the cell. The effects of DNA and RNA deprivation are most marked on those cells which grow more rapidly and which take up fluorouracil at a more rapid pace. The catabolic metabolism of fluorouracil results in degradative products (e.g., CO_2, urea, α-fluoro-β-alanine) which are inactive. Studies in man with topical application of ^{14}C-labeled Efudex demonstrated insignificant absorption as measured by ^{14}C content of plasma, urine and respiratory CO_2.

INDICATIONS

Efudex is recommended for the topical treatment of multiple actinic or solar keratoses. In the 5% strength it is also useful in the treatment of superficial basal cell carcinomas, when conventional methods are impractical, such as with multiple lesions or difficult treatment sites. The diagnosis should be established prior to treatment, since this new method has not been proven effective in other types of basal cell carcinomas. With isolated, easily accessible lesions, conventional techniques are preferred since success with such lesions is almost 100% with these methods. The success rate with Efudex cream and solution is approximately 93%. This 93% success rate is based on 113 lesions in 54 patients. Twenty-five lesions treated with the solution produced one failure and 88 lesions treated with the cream produced 7 failures.

CONTRAINDICATIONS

Efudex is contraindicated in patients with known hypersensitivity to any of its components.

WARNINGS

If an occlusive dressing is used, there may be an increase in the incidence of inflammatory reactions in the adjacent normal skin. A porous gauze dressing may be applied for cosmetic reasons without increase in reaction.

Prolonged exposure to ultraviolet rays should be avoided while under treatment with Efudex because the intensity of the reaction may be increased.

Usage in Pregnancy: Safety for use in pregnancy has not been established.

PRECAUTIONS

If Efudex is applied with the fingers, the hands should be washed immediately afterward. Efudex should be applied with care near the eyes, nose and mouth. Solar keratoses which do not respond should be biopsied to confirm the diagnosis. Patients should be forewarned that the reaction in the treated areas may be unsightly during therapy, and, in some cases, for several weeks following cessation of therapy. Follow-up biopsies should be performed as indicated in the management of superficial basal cell carcinoma.

ADVERSE REACTIONS

The most frequently encountered local reactions are pain, pruritus, hyperpigmentation and burning at the site of application. Other local reactions include allergic contact dermatitis, scarring, soreness, tenderness, suppuration, scaling and swelling.

Also reported are alopecia, insomnia, stomatitis, irritability, medicinal taste, photosensitivity, lacrimation, telangiectasia and urticaria, although a causal relationship is remote.

Laboratory abnormalities reported are leukocytosis, thrombocytopenia, toxic granulation and eosinophilia.

DOSAGE AND ADMINISTRATION

When Efudex is applied to a lesion, a response occurs with the following sequence: erythema, usually followed by vesiculation, erosion, ulceration, necrosis and epithelization.

Actinic or solar keratosis: Apply cream or solution twice daily in an amount sufficient to cover the lesions. Medication should be continued until the inflammatory response reaches the erosion, necrosis and ulceration stage, at which time use of the drug should be terminated. The usual duration of therapy is from two to four weeks. Complete healing of the lesions may not be evident for one to two months following cessation of Efudex therapy.

Superficial basal cell carcinomas: **Only the 5% strength is recommended.** Apply cream or solution twice daily in an amount sufficient to cover the lesions. Treatment should be continued for at least three to six weeks. Therapy may be required for as long as 10 to 12 weeks before the lesions are obliterated. As in any neoplastic condition, the patient should be followed for a reasonable period of time to determine if a cure has been obtained.

HOW SUPPLIED

Efudex Solution, 10-ml drop dispensers—containing 2% or 5% fluorouracil/Roche on a weight/weight basis, compounded with propylene glycol, tris(hydroxymethyl)-aminomethane, hydroxypropyl cellulose, parabens (methyl and propyl) and disodium edetate.

Efudex Cream, 25-Gm tubes—containing 5% fluorouracil/Roche in a vanishing cream base consisting of white petrolatum, stearyl alcohol, propylene glycol, polysorbate 60 and parabens (methyl and propyl).

Revised: November 1981

SOLATENE® ℞
[sol 'a-teen]
(beta-carotene/Roche)
capsules

The following text is complete prescribing information based on official labeling in effect June 1, 1992.

DESCRIPTION

Solatene (beta-carotene) is available in capsules for oral administration. Each capsule is composed of beadlets containing 30 mg beta-carotene, ascorbyl palmitate, corn starch, dl-α-tocopherol, gelatin, peanut oil and sucrose. Gelatin capsule shells may contain parabens (methyl and propyl), potassium sorbate, FD&C Blue No. 1, D&C Yellow No. 10, FD&C Red No. 3, FD&C Green No. 3 and titanium dioxide.

Beta-carotene, precursor of vitamin A, is a carotenoid pigment occurring naturally in green and yellow vegetables. Chemically, beta-carotene has the empirical formula $C_{40}H_{56}$ and a calculated molecular weight of 536.85. Trans-beta-carotene is a red, crystalline compound which is insoluble in water.

CLINICAL PHARMACOLOGY

Beta-carotene, a provitamin A, belongs to the class of carotenoid pigments. In terms of its vitamin activity, 6 μg of dietary beta-carotene is considered equivalent to 1 μg of vitamin A (retinol). Bioavailability of beta-carotene depends on the presence of fat in the diet to act as a carrier, and bile in the intestinal tract for its absorption. Beta-carotene is metabolized, primarily in the intestine, to vitamin A at a rate of approximately 50% to 60% of normal dietary intake and falls off rapidly as intake goes up. In humans, an appreciable amount of unchanged beta-carotene is absorbed and stored in various tissues, especially the depot fat. Small amounts may be converted to vitamin A in the liver. The vitamin A derived from beta-carotene follows the same metabolic pathway as that from dietary sources. The major route of elimination is fecal excretion. Excessive ingestion of carotenes is not harmful, but it may cause yellow coloration of the skin, which disappears upon reduction or cessation of intake.

INDICATIONS AND USAGE

Solatene is used to reduce the severity of photosensitivity reactions in patients with erythropoietic protoporphyria (EPP).

CONTRAINDICATIONS

Solatene is contraindicated in patients with known hypersensitivity to the drug.

WARNINGS

Solatene has not been shown to be effective as a sunscreen.

PRECAUTIONS

General: Solatene should be used with caution in patients with impaired renal or hepatic function because safe use in the presence of these conditions has not been established.

Information for Patients: Patients receiving Solatene should be advised against taking supplementary vitamin A since Solatene administration will fulfill normal vitamin A requirements. They should be cautioned to continue sun protection, and forewarned that their skin may appear slightly yellow while receiving Solatene.

Carcinogenesis, Mutagenesis, Impairment of Fertility: Long-term studies in animals to determine carcinogenesis have not been completed. *In vitro* and *in vivo* studies to evaluate mutagenic potential were negative. No effects on fertility in male rats were observed at doses as high as 500 mg/kg/day (100 times the recommended human dose).

Pregnancy: Teratogenic Effects: Pregnancy Category C. Beta-carotene has been shown to be fetotoxic (*i.e.,* cause an increase in resorption rate), but not teratogenic when given to rats at doses 300 to 400 times the maximum recommended human dose. No such fetotoxicity was observed at 75 times the maximum recommended human dose or less. A three-generation reproduction study in rats receiving beta-carotene at a dietary concentration of 0.1% (1000 ppm) has revealed no evidence of impaired fertility or effect on the fetus. There are no adequate and well-controlled studies in pregnant women. Solatene should be used during pregnancy only if the potential benefit justifies the potential risk to the fetus.

Nursing Mothers: It is not known whether this drug is excreted in human milk. Because many drugs are excreted in human milk, caution should be exercised when Solatene is administered to a nursing mother.

ADVERSE REACTIONS

Some patients may have occasional loose stools while taking Solatene. This reaction is sporadic and may not require discontinuance of medication. Other reactions which have been reported rarely are ecchymoses and arthralgia.

OVERDOSAGE

There are no reported cases of overdosage. The oral LD_{50} of beta-carotene (suspended in 5% gum acacia solution) in mice and rats is greater than 20,000 mg/kg. No lethality was observed in mice following administration of 30-mg beadlet capsules (ground and suspended in 5% gum acacia) at a dose of 1200 mg/kg beta-carotene.

DOSAGE AND ADMINISTRATION

Solatene may be administered either as a single daily dose or in divided doses, preferably with meals.

Usage in Children: The usual dosage for children under 14 is 30 to 150 mg (1 to 5 capsules) per day. Capsules may be opened and the contents mixed in orange juice or tomato juice to aid administration.

Usage in Adults: The usual adult dosage is 30 to 300 mg (1 to 10 capsules) per day.

Dosage should be adjusted depending on the severity of the symptoms and the response of the patient. Several weeks of therapy are necessary to accumulate enough Solatene in the skin to exert its effect. Patients should be instructed not to increase exposure to sunlight until they appear carotenemic (first seen as yellowness of palms and soles). This usually occurs after two to six weeks of therapy. Exposure to the sun may then be increased gradually. The protective effect is not total and each patient should establish his or her own limits of exposure.

HOW SUPPLIED

Solatene is available in blue and green capsules, each containing 30 mg of beta-carotene—bottles of 100 (NDC 0004-0115-01). Imprint on capsules: SOLATENE ROCHE.
Revised: April 1989

Shown in Product Identification Section, page 426

TEGISON®   ℞
[*teg'is-on*]
etretinate/Roche
CAPSULES

The following text is complete prescribing information based on official labeling in effect June 1, 1992.

CONTRAINDICATION

Tegison must not be used by females who are pregnant, who intend to become pregnant, or who are unreliable or may not use reliable contraception while undergoing treatment. The period of time during which pregnancy must be avoided after treatment is concluded has not been determined. Tegison blood levels of 0.5 to 12 ng/mL have been reported in 5 of 47 patients in the range of 2.1 to 2.9 years after treatment was concluded. The length of time necessary to wait after discontinuation of treatment to assure that no drug will be detectable in the blood has not been determined. The significance of undetectable blood levels relative to the risk of teratogenicity is unknown.

Major human fetal abnormalities related to Tegison administration have been reported, including meningomyelocoele, meningoencephalocoele, multiple synostoses, facial dysmorphia, syndactylies, absence of terminal phalanges, malformations of hip, ankle and forearm, low set ears, high palate, decreased cranial volume, and alterations of the skull and cervical vertebrae on x-ray.

Women of childbearing potential must not be given Tegison until pregnancy is excluded. It is strongly recommended that a pregnancy test be performed within two weeks prior to initiating Tegison therapy. Tegison therapy should start on the second or third day of the next normal menstrual period. An effective form of contraception must be used for at least one month before Tegison therapy, during therapy and following discontinuation of Tegison therapy for an indefinite period of time.

Females should be fully counseled on the serious risks to the fetus should they become pregnant while undergoing treatment or after discontinuation of therapy. If pregnancy does occur, the physician and patient should discuss the desirability of continuing the pregnancy.

TABLE I
ADVERSE EVENTS FREQUENTLY REPORTED DURING CLINICAL TRIALS
PERCENT OF PATIENTS REPORTING

BODY SYSTEM	>75%	50–75%	25–50%	10–25%
Mucocutaneous	Dry nose Chapped lips	Excessive thirst Sore mouth	Nosebleed	Cheilitis Sore tongue
Dermatologic	Loss of hair Palm/sole/ fingertip peeling	Dry skin Itching Rash Red scaly face Skin fragility	Bruising Sunburn	Nail disorder Skin peeling
Musculoskeletal	Hyperostosis*	Bone/joint pain	Muscle cramps	
Central Nervous		Fatigue	Headache	Fever
Special Senses		Irritation of eyes	Eyeball pain Eyelid abnormalities	Abnormalities of: —conjunctiva —cornea —lens —retina Conjunctivitis Decrease in visual acuity Double vision
Gastrointestinal			Abdominal pain Changes in appetite	Nausea

*In a retrospective study of 45 patients, 38 of whom received long-term etretinate therapy, 32 (84%) had radiographic evidence of hyperotosis. See WARNINGS.

DESCRIPTION

Tegison (brand of etretinate/Roche), a retinoid, is available in 10-mg and 25-mg gelatin capsules for oral administration. Each capsule also contains corn starch, lactose and talc. Gelatin capsule shells contain parabens (methyl and propyl) and potassium sorbate, with the following dye systems: 10 mg—iron oxide (yellow, black and red). FD&C Blue No. 2 and titanium dioxide (yellow, black and red) and titanium dioxide.

Chemically, etretinate is ethyl (*all-E*)-9-(4-methoxy-2,3,6-trimethylphenyl)-3,7-dimethyl-2,4,6,8-nonate traenoate and is related to both retinoic acid and retinol (vitamin A). It is a greenish-yellow to yellow powder with a calculated molecular weight of 354.5.

CLINICAL PHARMACOLOGY

The mechanism of action of Tegison is unknown.

Clinical: Improvement in psoriatic patients occurs in association with a decrease in scale, erythema and thickness of lesions, as well as histological evidence of normalization of epidermal differentiation, decreased stratum corneum thickness and decreased inflammation in the epidermis and dermis.

Pharmacokinetics: The pharmacokinetic profile of etretinate is predictable and is linear following single and multiple doses. Etretinate is extensively metabolized following oral dosing, with significant first-pass metabolism to the acid form, which also has the all-*trans* structure and is pharmacologically active. Subsequent metabolism results in the 13-*cis* acid form, chain-shortened breakdown products and conjugates that are ultimately excreted in the bile and urine.

After a six-month course of therapy with doses ranging from 25 mg once daily to 25 mg four times daily, Cmax values ranged from 102 to 389 ng/mL and occurred at Tmax values of two to six hours. In one study the apparent terminal half-life after six months of therapy was approximately 120 days. In another study of 47 patients treated chronically with etretinate, 5 had detectable serum drug levels (in the range of 0.5 to 12 ng/mL) 2.1 to 2.9 years after therapy was discontinued. The long half-life appears to be due to storage of etretinate in adipose tissue.

Etretinate is more than 99% bound to plasma proteins, predominantly lipoproteins, whereas its active metabolite, the all-*trans* acid form, is predominantly bound to albumin. Concentrations of etretinate in blister fluid after six weeks of dosing were approximately one-tenth of those observed in plasma. Concentrations of etretinate and its all-*trans* acid metabolite in epidermal specimens obtained after 1 to 36 months of therapy were a function of location; subcutis > > serum > epidermis > dermis. Similarly, liver concentrations of etretinate in patients receiving therapy for six months were generally higher than concomitant plasma concentrations and tended to be higher in livers with a higher degree of fatty infiltration.

Studies in normal volunteers indicated that, when compared with the fasting state, the absorption of etretinate was increased by whole milk or a high-lipid diet.

INDICATIONS AND USAGE

Tegison is indicated for the treatment of severe recalcitrant psoriasis, including the erythrodermic and generalized pustular types. Because of significant adverse effects associated with its use, Tegison should be prescribed only by physicians knowledgeable in the systemic use of retinoids and reserved for patients with severe recalcitrant psoriasis who are unresponsive to or intolerant of standard therapies; topical tar plus UVB light; psoralens plus UVA light; systemic corticosteroids; and methotrexate.

The use of Tegison resulted in clinical improvement in the majority of patients treated. Complete clearing of the disease was observed after four to nine months of therapy in 13% of all patients treated for severe psoriasis. This included complete clearing in 16% of patients with erythrodermic psoriasis and 37% of patients with generalized pustular psoriasis.

After discontinuation of Tegison the majority of patients experience some degree of relapse by the end of two months. After relapse, subsequent four- to nine-month courses of Tegison therapy resulted in approximately the same clinical response as experienced during the initial course of therapy.

CONTRAINDICATIONS

Pregnancy: Category X. See boxed CONTRAINDICATION.

WARNINGS

Pseudotumor cerebri: Tegison and other retinoids have been associated with cases of pseudotumor cerebri (benign intracranial hypertension). Early signs and symptoms of pseudotumor cerebri include papilledema, headache, nausea and vomiting, and visual disturbances. Patients with these symptoms should be examined for papilledema and, if present, they should discontinue Tegison immediately and be referred for neurologic diagnosis and care.

Hepatoxicity: Of the 652 patients treated in U.S. clinical trials, ten had clinical or histologic hepatitis considered possibly or probably related to Tegison treatment. Liver function tests returned to normal in eight of these patients after Tegison was discontinued; one patient had histologic changes resembling chronic active hepatitis six months off therapy, and one patient had no follow-up available. There have been four reports of hepatitis-related deaths worldwide; two of these patients had received etretinate for a month or less before presenting with hepatic symptoms. Elevations of AST (SGOT), ALT (SGPT) or LDH have occurred in 18%, 23% and 15%, respectively, of individuals treated with Tegison. Cases with pathology findings of hepatic fibrosis, necrosis and/or cirrhosis which may be related to Tegison therapy have been reported. If hepatoxicity is suspected during treatment with Tegison, the drug should be discontinued and the etiology further investigated.

Ophthalmic effects: Corneal erosion, abrasion, irregularity and punctate staining have occurred in patients treated with Tegison, although these effects were absent or improved after therapy was stopped in those patients who had follow-up examinations. Corneal opacities have occurred in patients receiving isotretinoin; they had either completely re-

Continued on next page

Roche Dermatologics—Cont.

solved or were resolving at follow-up six to seven weeks after discontinuation of the drug. Other ophthalmic effects that have occurred in Tegison patients include decreased visual acuity and blurring of vision, minimal posterior subcapsular cataract, iritis, blot retinal hemorrhage, scotoma and photophobia. A number of cases of decreased night vision have occurred during Tegison therapy. Because the onset in some patients was sudden, patients should be advised of this potential problem and warned to be cautious when driving or operating any vehicle at night. Any Tegison patient experiencing visual difficulties should discontinue the drug and have an ophthalmological examination.

Hyperostosis: There is a very high likelihood of the development of hyperostosis with Tegison therapy. In one clinical trial, 45 patients with a mean age of 40 years were retrospectively evaluated for evidence of hyperostosis. They had received etretinate at a mean dose of 0.8 mg/kg for a mean duration of 33 months at the time of x-ray. Eleven patients had psoriasis, while 34 patients had a disorder of keratinization. Of these, 38 patients who continued to receive etretinate at an average dose of 0.8 mg/kg/day for an average duration of 60 months, 32 (84%) had radiographic evidence of extraspinal tendon and ligament calcification. The most common sites of involvement were the ankles (76%), pelvis (53%) and knees (42%); spinal changes were uncommon. Involvement tended to be bilateral and multifocal. There were no bone or joint symptoms at the sites of radiographic abnormalities in 47% of the affected patients.

Lipids: Blood lipid determinations should be performed before Tegison is administered and then at intervals of one or two weeks until the lipid response to Tegison is established; this usually occurs within four to eight weeks.

Approximately 45% of patients receiving Tegison during clinical trials experienced an elevation of plasma triglycerides. Approximately 37% developed a decrease in high density lipoproteins and about 16% showed an increase in cholesterol levels. These effects on triglycerides, HDL and cholesterol were reversible after cessation of Tegison therapy. Patients with an increased tendency to develop hypertriglyceridemia include those with diabetes mellitus, obesity, increased alcohol intake or a familial history of these conditions.

Hypertriglyceridemia, hypercholesterolemia and lowered HDL may increase a patient's cardiovascular risk status. In addition, elevation of serum triglycerides in excess of 800 mg/dL has been associated with acute pancreatitis. Therefore, every attempt should be made to control significant elevations of triglycerides or cholesterol or significant decreases in HDL. Some patients have been able to reverse triglyceride and cholesterol elevations or HDL decrease by reduction in weight or restriction of dietary fat and alcohol while continuing Tegison therapy.

Cardiovascular effects: During clinical trials of 652 patients, 21 significant cardiovascular adverse incidents were reported, all in patients who had a strong history of cardiovascular risk. These incidents were not considered related to Tegison therapy except for two cases of myocardial infarction: one which was considered possibly related to Tegison therapy and one for which a relationship was not specified.

Animal studies: In general, the signs of etretinate toxicity in rats, mice and dogs are dose-related with respect to incidence, onset and severity. In rodents, the most striking manifestations of this toxicity are bone fractures; no evidence of fractures was observed in a one-year dog study. Other dose-related changes in some animals treated with etretinate in subchronic or chronic toxicity studies include alopecia, erythema, reductions in body weight and food consumption, stiffness, altered gait, hematologic changes, elevations in serum alkaline phosphatase and testicular atrophy with microscopic evidence of reduced spermatogenesis.

PRECAUTIONS

Information for Patients: Women of childbearing potential should be advised that they must not be pregnant when Tegison therapy is initiated, and that they should use an effective form of contraception for one month prior to Tegison therapy, while taking Tegison and after Tegison has been discontinued. Tegison has been found in the blood of some patients two to three years after the drug was discontinued. See boxed CONTRAINDICATION.

Because of the relationship of Tegison to vitamin A, patients should be advised against taking vitamin A supplements to avoid possible additive toxic effects.

Patients should be advised that transient exacerbation of psoriasis is commonly seen during the initial period of therapy.

Patients should be informed that they may experience decreased tolerance to contact lenses during and after therapy.

Laboratory Tests: See WARNINGS section. In clinical studies, the incidence of hypertriglyceridemia was one patient in two, that of hypercholesterolemia one patient in six, and that of decreased HDL one patient in three during Tegison

therapy. Pretreatment and follow-up blood lipids should be obtained under fasting conditions. If alcohol has been consumed, at least 36 hours should elapse before these determinations are made. It is recommended that these tests be performed at weekly or biweekly intervals until the lipid response to Tegison is established.

Elevations of AST (SGOT), ALT (SGPT) or LDH have occurred in 18%, 23% and 15%, respectively, of individuals treated with Tegison. It is recommended that these tests be performed prior to initiation of Tegison therapy, at one to two week intervals for the first one to two months of therapy and thereafter at intervals of one to three months, depending on the response to Tegison administration.

Drug Interactions: Little information is available on drug interactions with Tegison; however, concomitant consump-

tion of milk increases the absorption of etretinate. See *Pharmacokinetics* and DOSAGE AND ADMINISTRATION sections.

Carcinogenesis, Mutagenesis, Impairment of Fertility:
Carcinogenesis: In a two-year study, male or female Sprague-Dawley rats given etretinate by dietary admixture at doses up to 3 mg/kg/day (two times the maximum recommended human therapeutic dose) had no increase in tumor incidence. In an 80-week study, Crl:CD-1 (ICR) BR mice were given etretinate by dietary admixture at doses of 1 to 5 mg/kg/day. An increased incidence of blood vessel tumors (hemangiomas and hemangiosarcomas in several different tissue sites) was noted in the high-dose male group (4 to 5 mg/kg/day) but not in the female group.

TABLE II
LESS FREQUENT ADVERSE EVENTS REPORTED DURING CLINICAL TRIALS
(SOME OF WHICH MAY BEAR NO RELATIONSHIP TO THERAPY)
PERCENT OF PATIENTS REPORTING

BODY SYSTEM	1–10%	<1%
Mucocutaneous	Dry eyes Mucous membrane abnormalities Dry mouth Gingival bleeding/inflammation	Decreased mucous secretion Rhinorrhea
Dermatologic	Hair abnormalities Bullous eruption Cold/clammy skin Onycholysis Paronychia Pyogenic granuloma Changes in perspiration	Abnormal skin odor Granulation tissue Healing impairment Herpes simplex Hirsutism Increased pore size Sensory skin changes Skin atrophy Skin fissures Skin infection Skin nodule Skin ulceration Urticaria
Musculoskeletal	Myalgia	Gout Hyperkinesia Hypertonia
Central Nervous System	Dizziness Lethargy Changes in sensation Pain Rigors	Abnormal thinking Amnesia Anxiety Depression Pseudotumor cerebri Emotional lability Faint feeling Flu-like symptoms
Special Senses	Abnormal lacrimation Abnormal vision Abnormalities of: —Extraocular musculature —Ocular tension —Pupil —Vitreous Earache Otitis externa	Change in equilibrium Ear drainage Ear infection Hearing change Night vision decrease Photophobia Visual change Scotoma
Gastrointestinal	Hepatitis	Constipation Diarrhea Melena Flatulence Weight loss Oral ulcers Taste perversion Tooth caries
Cardiovascular	Cardiovascular thrombotic or obstructive events Edema	Atrial fibrillation Chest pain Coagulation disorder Phlebitis Postural hypotension Syncope
Respiratory	Dyspnea	Coughing Increased sputum Dysphonia Pharyngitis
Renal		Kidney stones
Urogenital		Abnormal menses Atrophic vaginitis Dysuria Polyuria Urinary retention
Other	Malignant neoplasms	

TABLE III
LABORATORY ABNORMALITIES REPORTED DURING CLINICAL TRIALS
PERCENT OF PATIENTS REPORTING

BODY SYSTEM	25–50%	10–25%	1–10%
Hematologic	Increased: —MCHC (60%) —MCH —Reticulocytes —PTT —ESR	Decreased: —Hemoglobin/HCT —RBC —MCV Increased platelets Increased or decreased: —WBC and components —Prothrombin time	Decreased: —Platelets —MCH —MCHC —PTT Increased: —Hemoglobin/HCT —RBC
Urinary		WBC in urine	Proteinuria Glycosuria Microscopic hematuria Casts in urine Acetonuria Hemoglobinuria
Hepatic	Increased triglycerides	Increased: —AST (SGOT) —ALT (SGPT) —Alkaline phosphatase —GGTP —Globulin —Cholesterol	Increased bilirubin Increased or decreased: —Total protein —Albumin
Renal			Increased: —BUN —Creatinine
Electrolytes	Increased or decreased potassium	Increased or decreased: —Venous CO_2 —Sodium —Chloride	
Miscellaneous	Increased or decreased: —Calcium —Phosphorus	Increased or decreased FBS	Increased CPK

Mutagenesis: Etretinate was evaluated by the Ames test in a host-mediated assay, in the micronucleus test, and in a "treat and plate" test using the diploid yeast strain S. cerevisiae D7. Except for a weakly positive response in the Ames test using the tester strain TA 100, there was no evidence of genotoxicity. No differences in the rate of sister chromatid exchange (SCE) were noted in lymphocytes of patients before and after four weeks of treatment with therapeutic doses of etretinate.

Impairment of Fertility: In a study of fertility and general reproductive performance in rats, no etretinate-related effects were observed at doses up to 2.5 mg/kg/day. At a dose of 5 mg/kg/day (approximately three times the maximum recommended human therapeutic dose) the readiness of the treated animals to copulate was reduced but the pregnancy rate was unaffected. The number of viable young at birth and their postnatal weight gain and survival were adversely affected at the high dose. The pregnancy rate of the untreated first generation animals and postnatal weight gain of the untreated second generation animals were also reduced. No adverse effects on sperm production were noted in 12 psoriatic patients given 75 mg/day of etretinate for one month and 50 mg/day for an additional two months. However, testicular atrophy was noted in subchronic and chronic rat studies and in a chronic dog study, in some cases at doses approaching those recommended for use in humans. Decreased sperm counts were reported in a 13-week dog study at doses as low as 3 mg/kg/day (approximately twice the maximum recommended human dose). Spermatogenic arrest also was reported with chronic administration of the all-trans metabolite to dogs.

Pregnancy: Category X. See boxed CONTRAINDICATION.
The following limited preliminary data must not be read or understood to diminish the serious risk of teratogenicity set forth in the boxed pregnancy CONTRAINDICATION.
Thirty women worldwide have been reported as having taken one or more doses of Tegison during pregnancy. In 29 cases in which information was available, there were a total of ten congenital abnormalities. The occurrence of congenital abnormalities was four of 20 among delivered infants, two of two among spontaneously aborted fetuses, and four of seven among induced abortions.
A further 38 women were reported to have become pregnant within 24 months after discontinuing Tegison therapy. Because congenital abnormalities have been reported in these pregnancies, it cannot be stated that there is a "safe" time to become pregnant after Tegison therapy. In 37 cases in which information was available, there were a total of three con-

genital abnormalities. The occurrence of congential abnormalities was two of 29 among delivered infants, zero of one among spontaneously aborted fetuses, and one of five among induced abortions. Two stillbirths with no apparent congenital abnormalities were attributed to other causes.
Nonteratogenic Effects: No adverse effects on various parameters of late gestation and lactation were observed in rats at doses of etretinate up to 4 mg/kg/day (approximately three times the maximum human recommended dose). At doses of 8 mg/kg/day (approximately five times the maximum human recommended dose) of etretinate, the rate of stillbirths was increased and neonatal weight gain and survival rate were markedly reduced.
Nursing Mothers: Studies have shown that etretinate is excreted in the milk of lactating rats; however, it is not known whether this drug is excreted in human milk. Because of the potential for adverse effects, nursing mothers should not receive Tegison.
Pediatric Use: No clinical studies have been conducted in the U. S. using Tegison in children. Ossification of interosseous ligaments and tendons of the extremities has been reported. Two children showed x-ray changes suggestive of premature epiphyseal closure during treatment with Tegison. Skeletal hyperostosis has also been reported after treatment with isotretinoin. It is not known if any of these effects occur more commonly in children, but concern should be greater because of the growth process. Pretreatment x-rays for bone age including x-rays of the knees, followed by yearly monitoring, are advised. In addition, pain or limitation of motion should be evaluated with appropriate radiological examination. Because of the lack of data on the use of etretinate in children and the possibility of their being more sensitive to effects of the drug, this product should be used only when all alternative therapies have been exhausted.

ADVERSE EVENTS
Clinical: Hepatitis was observed in about 1.5% of patients treated with Tegison in clinical trials. Pathology findings of hepatic fibrosis, necrosis and/or cirrhosis have been reported. See WARNINGS section.
Tegison has been associated with pseudotumor cerebri. See WARNINGS section.
Hypervitaminosis A produces a wide spectrum of signs and symptoms of primarily the mucocutaneous, musculoskeletal, hepatic and central nervous systems. Nearly all of the clinical adverse events reported to date with Tegison administration resemble those of the hypervitaminosis A syndrome.

Table I lists the adverse events frequently reported during clinical trials in which 652 patients were treated either for psoriasis (591 patients) or a disorder of keratinization (61 patients). Table II lists less frequently reported adverse events in these same patients. However the number of patients evaluated for each adverse event was not 652 in every case.
[See Table I on page 1963.]
[See Table II on preceding page.]
Laboratory: Tegison therapy induces change in serum lipids in a significant number of treated patients. Approximately 45% of patients experienced elevation in serum triglycerides, 37% a decrease in high density lipoproteins and 16% an increase in cholesterol levels.
Approximately 46% of patients has elevations of triglycerides above 250 mg/dL, 54% had decreases of HDL below 36 mg%, and 19% had elevations of cholesterrol above 300 mg%. One case of eruptive xanthomas associated with triglyceride levels greater than 1000 mg% has been reported. Elevations of AST (SGOT), ALT (SGPT) or LDH were experienced by 18%, 23% and 15%, respectively, of individuals treated with Tegison. In most of the patients, the elevations were slight to moderate and became normal either during therapy or after cessation of treatment. See WARNINGS section.
Table III list the laboratory abnormalities reported during clinical trials. Data for patients who received intermittent courses of therapy for periods up to five years are included. Any instance of two consecutive values outside the range of normal, or an abnormal value with no follow-up during therapy, was considered to be possibly related to Tegison.

OVERDOSAGE
There has been no experience with acute overdosage in humans.
The acute oral and intraperitoneal toxicities (LD_{50}) of etretinate capsules in mice and rats were greater than 4000 mg/kg. The acute oral toxicity (LD_{50}) of etretinate substance in 4% solution was 2300 mg/kg in mice and 1300 mg/kg in rats.

DOSAGE AND ADMINISTRATION
There is intersubject variation in the absorption and the rate of metabolism of Tegison. Individualization of dosage is required to achieve the maximal therapeutic response with a tolerable degree of side effects. Therapy with Tegison should generally be initiated at a dosage of 0.75 to 1 mg/kg of body weight/day taken in divided doses. A maximum dose of 1.5 mg/kg/day should not be exceeded. Erythrodermic psoriasis may respond to lower initial doses of 0.25 mg/kg/day increased by 0.25 mg/kg/day each week until optimal initial response is attained.
Maintenance doses of 0.5 to 0.75 mg/kg/day may be initiated after initial response, generally after 8 to 16 weeks of therapy. In general, therapy should be terminated in patients whose lesions have sufficiently resolved. Relapses may be treated as outlined for initial therapy.
Tegison should be administered with food.

HOW SUPPLIED
Brown and green capsules, 10 mg, imprinted TEGISON 10 ROCHE; Prescription Paks of 30 (NDC 0004-0177-57).
Brown and caramel capsules, 25 mg, imprinted TEGISON 25 ROCHE; Prescription Paks of 30 (NDC 0004-0179-57).
STORE AT 59° TO 86°F; 15° TO 30°C. PROTECT FROM LIGHT.
Revised: December 1986
Shown in Product Identification Section, page 426

Roche Laboratories
a division of Hoffmann-La Roche Inc.
NUTLEY, NJ 07110

ALURATE® ELIXIR
[al 'u-rate]
(aprobarbital/Roche)

The following text is complete prescribing information based on official labeling in effect June 1, 1992.
The following sections contain information specifically applicable to Alurate as well as information pertinent to other barbiturates. The information pertinent to other barbiturates should be considered when administering Alurate.

DESCRIPTION
Alurate (aprobarbital/Roche) is an intermediate-acting barbiturate which is used as a sedative-hypnotic. As with other barbiturates, it acts as a CNS depressant. Alurate is available for oral administration as a red elixir providing 40 mg of aprobarbital per teaspoonful (5 ml) in a vehicle containing 20 percent alcohol, dextrose, saccharin, sorbitol, sucrose, FD&C Yellow No. 6, FD&C Red No. 40, flavors and water. Chemically, aprobarbital is 5-allyl-5-isopropylbarbituric acid. It is a

Continued on next page

Roche Laboratories—Cont.

bitter, white crystalline powder with an empirical formula of $C_{10}H_{14}N_2O_3$ and a molecular weight of 210.23.

CLINICAL PHARMACOLOGY

Barbiturates are capable of producing all levels of CNS mood alteration from excitation to mild sedation, hypnosis and deep coma. Overdosage can produce death. In high enough therapeutic doses, barbiturates induce anesthesia.

Barbiturates depress the sensory cortex, decrease motor activity, alter cerebellar function and produce drowsiness, sedation and hypnosis.

Barbiturate-induced sleep differs from physiological sleep. Sleep laboratory studies have demonstrated that barbiturates reduce the amount of time spent in the rapid eye movement (REM) phase of sleep or dreaming stage. Also, Stages III and IV sleep are decreased. Patients may experience markedly increased dreaming, nightmares and/or insomnia if barbiturates are prescribed for a period of time and then abruptly withdrawn. It is recommended that dosage be reduced gradually over a period of 5 or 6 days to lessen REM rebound and disturbed sleep (for example, decrease the dose from 3 to 2 doses a day for 1 week).

In studies, secobarbital sodium and pentobarbital sodium have been found to lose most of their effectiveness for both inducing and maintaining sleep by the end of 2 weeks of continued drug administration, even with the use of multiple doses. Other barbiturates might also be expected to lose their effectiveness for inducing and maintaining sleep after about 2 weeks. Therefore, as sleep medications, the barbiturates are of limited value beyond short-term use.

Barbiturates have little analgesic action at subanesthetic doses. Rather, they may increase the reaction to painful stimuli. All barbiturates exhibit anticonvulsant activity in anesthetic doses; however, only phenobarbital, mephobarbital and metharbital are effective as oral anticonvulsants in subhypnotic doses.

Barbiturates are respiratory depressants; the degree of depression is dose-dependent. With hypnotic doses, respiratory depression produced by barbiturates is similar to that which occurs during physiologic sleep. Hypnotic doses also cause a slight decrease in blood pressure and heart rate.

Studies in laboratory animals have shown that barbiturates cause reduction in the tone and contractility of the uterus, ureters and urinary bladder. However, concentrations of the drugs required to produce this effect in humans are not reached with sedative-hypnotic doses.

Barbiturates do not impair normal hepatic function, but have been shown to induce liver microsomal enzymes, thus altering the metabolism of certain other drugs. (See Precautions — Drug Interactions section.)

Pharmacokinetics: Barbiturates are absorbed in varying degrees following oral administration. The onset of action for oral barbiturate administration varies from 20 to 60 minutes. Duration of action, which is related to the rate at which the barbiturates are redistributed throughout the body, varies among persons and in the same person from time to time. Aprobarbital, which is an intermediate-acting barbiturate, has a duration of action ranging from 6 to 8 hours.

Barbiturates are weak acids that are absorbed and rapidly distributed to all tissues and fluids, with high concentrations in the brain, liver and kidneys. Lipid solubility of the barbiturates is the dominant factor in their distribution throughout the body. Barbiturates are bound to plasma and tissue proteins to a varying degree, with the degree of binding increasing directly as a function of lipid solubility. Aprobarbital is approximately 20 percent plasma protein-bound. The half-life of aprobarbital ranges from 14 to 34 hours with a mean half-life of 24 hours.

Barbiturates are metabolized primarily by the hepatic microsomal enzyme system; the metabolic products are excreted in the urine and, less commonly, in the feces. Approximately 13 to 24 percent of aprobarbital is eliminated unchanged in the urine. The inactive metabolites of the barbiturates are excreted as conjugates of glucuronic acid.

INDICATIONS AND USAGE

Alurate is indicated for sedation and induction of sleep, on a short-term basis, in conditions requiring a sedative-hypnotic.

CONTRAINDICATIONS

Barbiturates are contraindicated in patients with known barbiturate sensitivity. Barbiturates are also contraindicated in patients with a history of manifest or latent porphyria.

WARNINGS

Habit forming: Barbiturates may be habit forming. Tolerance and psychological and physical dependence may occur with continued use. (See Drug Abuse and Dependence section.) Patients who have a psychological dependence on barbiturates may increase the dosage or decrease the dosage interval without consulting a physician and may subsequently develop a physical dependence. To minimize the possibility of overdosage or the development of dependence, the quantity of sedative-hypnotic barbiturates prescribed or

dispensed should be limited to the amount required between appointments. Abrupt cessation after prolonged use may result in withdrawal symptoms, including delirium, convulsions and possibly death.

Barbiturates should be withdrawn gradually from any patient known to be taking excessive doses over long periods of time.

Acute or chronic pain: Caution should be exercised when barbiturates are administered to patients with acute or chronic pain, because paradoxical excitement may be induced or important symptoms may be masked.

Use in pregnancy: Barbiturates can cause fetal damage when administered to a pregnant woman. Retrospective case-controlled studies have suggested a connection between maternal consumption of barbiturates and a higher than expected incidence of fetal abnormalities. Following oral administration, barbiturates readily cross the placental barrier and are distributed throughout the placenta and fetal tissues, with highest concentrations found in the liver and brain.

Withdrawal symptoms occur in infants born to mothers who receive barbiturates throughout the last trimester of pregnancy. (See Drug Abuse and Dependence section.) If this drug is used during pregnancy, or if the patient becomes pregnant while taking this drug, the patient should be apprised of the potential hazard to the fetus.

Synergistic effects: The concomitant use of alcohol or other CNS depressants may produce additive CNS-depressant effects.

PRECAUTIONS

General: Barbiturates may be habit forming. Tolerance and psychological and physical dependence may occur with continued use. (See Drug Abuse and Dependence section.) Barbiturates should be administered with caution, if at all, to patients who are mentally depressed, have suicidal tendencies, or a history of drug abuse. Elderly or debilitated patients may react to barbiturates with marked excitement, depression and confusion. In some persons, barbiturates repeatedly produce excitement rather than depression. In patients with hepatic damage, barbiturates should be administered with caution, and initially in reduced doses. Barbiturates should not be administered to patients showing the premonitory signs of hepatic coma.

Information for Patients: The use of barbiturates carries with it an associated risk of psychological and/or physical dependence. The patient should be warned against increasing the dose of the drug without consulting a physician.

Barbiturates may impair mental and/or physical abilities required for the performance of potentially hazardous tasks, such as driving a car or operating machinery.

Alcohol should not be consumed while taking barbiturates. Concurrent use of barbiturates with other CNS depressants (*e.g.,* alcohol, narcotics, tranquilizers, antihistamines) may result in additional CNS depressant effects.

Laboratory Tests: Prolonged therapy with barbiturates should be accompanied by periodic laboratory evaluation of organ systems, including hematopoietic, renal and hepatic systems.

Drug Interactions: Most reports of clinically significant drug interactions occurring with the barbiturates have involved phenobarbital. However, the application of these data to other barbiturates appears valid and warrants serial blood level determinations of the relevant drugs when there are multiple therapies.

1. *Anticoagulants.* Phenobarbital lowers the plasma levels of dicumarol (name previously used: bishydroxycoumarin) and causes a decrease in anticoagulant activity as measured by the prothrombin time. Barbiturates can induce hepatic microsomal enzymes resulting in increased metabolism of and decreased anticoagulant response to oral anticoagulants (*e.g.,* warfarin, acenocoumarol, dicumarol and phenprocoumon). Patients stabilized on anticoagulant therapy may require dosage adjustments if barbiturates are added to or withdrawn from their dosage regimen.

2. *Corticosteroids.* Barbiturates appear to enhance the metabolism of exogenous corticosteroids, probably through the induction of hepatic microsomal enzymes. Patients stabilized on corticosteroid therapy may require dosage adjustments if barbiturates are added to or withdrawn from their dosage regimen.

3. *Griseofulvin.* Phenobarbital appears to interfere with the absorption of orally administered griseofulvin, thus decreasing its blood level. This effect on therapeutic response has not been established; however, it would be preferable to avoid concomitant administration of these drugs.

4. *Doxycycline.* Phenobarbital has been shown to shorten the half-life of doxycycline for as long as two weeks after discontinuance of the barbiturate therapy. This action is probably the result of induction of hepatic microsomal enzymes that metabolize the antibiotic. If phenobarbital and doxycycline are administered concurrently, the clinical response to doxycycline should be monitored closely.

5. *Phenytoin, sodium valproate, valproic acid.* The effect of barbiturates on the metabolism of phenytoin appears to be

variable. Some investigators report an accelerating effect, while others report no effect. Because the effect is not predictable, phenytoin and barbiturate blood levels should be monitored more frequently if these drugs are given concurrently. Sodium valproate and valproic acid appear to decrease barbiturate metabolism; therefore, barbiturate blood levels should be monitored and appropriate dosage adjustments made.

6. *Central nervous system depressants.* The concomitant use of other central nervous system depressants, including other sedatives or hypnotics, antihistamines, tranquilizers or alcohol, may produce additive effects.

7. *Monoamine oxidase inhibitors (MAOI).* MAOI prolong the effects of barbiturates, probably because metabolism of the barbiturates is inhibited.

8. *Estradiol, estrone, progesterone and other steroidal hormones.* Pretreatment with or concurrent administration of phenobarbital may decrease the effect of estradiol by increasing its metabolism. There have been reports of patients treated with antiepileptic drugs (*e.g.,* phenobarbital) who became pregnant while taking oral contraceptives. An alternate contraceptive method might be suggested to women taking phenobarbital.

Carcinogenesis: 1. Animal data. Phenobarbital sodium is carcinogenic in mice and rats after lifetime administration. In mice, it produced benign and malignant liver cell tumors. In rats, benign liver cell tumors were observed very late in life.

2. Human data. In a 29-year epidemiological study of 9136 patients who were treated on an anticonvulsant protocol which included phenobarbital sodium, results indicated a higher than normal incidence of hepatic carcinoma. Previously, some of these patients were treated with Thorotrast, a drug which is known to produce hepatic carcinomas. Thus, this study did not provide sufficient evidence that phenobarbital sodium is carcinogenic in humans.

A retrospective study of 84 children with brain tumors matched to 73 normal controls and 78 cancer controls (malignant disease other than brain tumors) suggested an association between exposure to barbiturates prenatally and an increased incidence of brain tumors.

Pregnancy: 1. Teratogenic Effects. Pregnancy Category D. See Warnings section.

2. Nonteratogenic Effects. Reports of infants suffering from long-term barbiturate exposure *in utero* include the acute withdrawal syndrome of seizures and hyperirritability from birth. A delayed onset of the symptoms may be seen for up to 14 days. (See Drug Abuse and Dependence section.)

Labor and Delivery: Hypnotic doses of barbiturates do not appear to significantly impair uterine activity during labor. Full anesthetic doses of barbiturates decrease the force and frequency of uterine contractions. Administration of sedative-hypnotic barbiturates to the mother during labor may result in respiratory depression in the newborn.

Premature infants are particularly susceptible to the depressant effects of barbiturates. If barbiturates are used during labor and delivery, resuscitation equipment should be available.

Data are not currently available to evaluate the effect of these barbiturates when forceps delivery or other intervention is necessary. Also, data are not available to determine the effect of these barbiturates on the later growth, development and functional maturation of the child.

Nursing mothers: Small amounts of barbiturates are excreted in the human milk. Because of the potential for serious adverse reactions in nursing infants from barbiturates, a decision should be made whether to discontinue nursing or to discontinue the drug, taking into account the importance of the drug to the mother.

Pediatric use: Safety and effectiveness in children have not been established.

ADVERSE REACTIONS

The following adverse reactions have been reported following the use of Alurate in an incidence of less than 1 in 100 patients.

Nervous system: Dizziness, nervousness.

Digestive system: Nausea and vomiting.

Other reported reactions: Headache, hypersensitivity reactions (skin rashes) and purpura.

Although the following adverse reactions have not been reported with Alurate, they have been compiled from surveillance of thousands of hospitalized patients receiving barbiturates and should be considered when administering Alurate:

More than 1 in 100 patients. The most common adverse reaction estimated to occur at a rate of 1 to 3 patients per 100 is:

Nervous system: Somnolence.

Less than 1 in 100 patients. Adverse reactions estimated to occur at a rate of less than 1 in 100 patients are listed below, grouped by organ system and by decreasing order of occurrence:

Nervous system: Agitation, confusion, hyperkinesia, ataxia, CNS depression, nightmares, psychiatric disturbances, hallucinations, insomnia, anxiety, thinking abnormality.

Concentration of Barbiturate in the Blood Versus Degree of CNS Depression

Barbiturate	Onset/ duration	Degree of depression in nontolerant persons*				
		1	2	3	4	5
		Barbiturate blood levels in ppm (mcg/ml)				
Pentobarbital	Fast/short	≤ 2	0.5 to 3	10 to 15	12 to 25	15 to 40
Secobarbital	Fast/short	≤ 2	0.5 to 5	10 to 15	15 to 25	15 to 40
Amobarbital	Intermediate/ intermediate	≤ 3	2 to 10	30 to 40	30 to 60	40 to 80
Butabarbital	Intermediate/ intermediate	≤ 5	3 to 25	40 to 60	50 to 80	60 to 100
Phenobarbital	Slow/long	≤ 10	5 to 40	50 to 80	70 to 120	100 to 200

*Categories of degree of depression in nontolerant persons:
1. Under the influence and appreciably impaired for purposes of driving a motor vehicle or performing tasks requiring alertness and unimpaired judgment and reaction time.
2. Sedated, therapeutic range, calm, relaxed, and easily aroused.
3. Comatose, difficult to arouse, significant depression of respiration.
4. Compatible with death in aged or ill persons or in presence of obstructed airway, other toxic agents, or exposure to cold.
5. Usual lethal level, the upper end of the range includes those who received some supportive treatment.

Respiratory system: Hypoventilation, apnea.
Cardiovascular system: Bradycardia, hypotension, syncope.
Digestive system: Constipation.
Other reported reactions: Hypersensitivity reactions (angioedema, exfoliative dermatitis), fever, liver damage, megaloblastic anemia following chronic phenobarbital use.

DRUG ABUSE AND DEPENDENCE

Alurate is subject to Class III control under the Federal Controlled Substances Act.

Barbiturates may be habit forming. Tolerance, psychological dependence and physical dependence may occur especially following prolonged use of high doses of barbiturates. Daily administration in excess of 400 mg of pentobarbital or secobarbital for approximately 90 days is likely to produce some degree of physical dependence. A dosage of from 600 to 800 mg taken for at least 35 days is sufficient to produce withdrawal seizures. The average daily dose for the barbiturate addict is usually about 1.5 grams. As tolerance to barbiturates develops, the amount needed to maintain the same level of intoxication increases; tolerance to fatal dosage, however, does not increase more than twofold. As this occurs, the margin between an intoxicating dosage and fatal dosage becomes smaller.

Symptoms of acute intoxication with barbiturates include unsteady gait, slurred speech and sustained nystagmus. Mental signs of chronic intoxication include confusion, poor judgment, irritability, insomnia and somatic complaints. Symptoms of barbiturate dependence are similar to those of chronic alcoholism. If an individual appears to be intoxicated with alcohol to a degree that is radically disproportionate to the amount of alcohol in his or her blood, the use of barbiturates should be suspected. The lethal dose of a barbiturate is far less if alcohol is also ingested.

The symptoms of barbiturate withdrawal can be severe and may cause death. Minor withdrawal symptoms may appear 8 to 12 hours after the last dose of a barbiturate. These symptoms usually appear in the following order: anxiety, muscle twitching, tremor of hands or fingers, progressive weakness, dizziness, distortion in visual perception, nausea, vomiting, insomnia and orthostatic hypotension. Major withdrawal symptoms (convulsions and delirium) may occur within 16 hours and last up to 5 days after abrupt cessation of these drugs. Intensity of withdrawal symptoms gradually declines over a period of approximately 15 days. Individuals susceptible to barbiturate abuse and dependence include alcoholics and opiate abusers, as well as other sedative-hypnotic and amphetamine abusers.

Drug dependence to barbiturates arises from repeated administration of a barbiturate or an agent with barbiturate-like effect on a continuous basis, generally in amounts exceeding therapeutic dosage levels. The characteristics of drug dependence to barbiturates include: (a) a strong desire or need to continue taking the drug; (b) a tendency to increase the dose; (c) a psychic dependence on the effects of the drug related to subjective and individual appreciation of those effects; and (d) a physical dependence on the effects of the drug requiring its presence for maintenance of homeostasis and resulting in a definite, characteristic and self-limited abstinence syndrome when the drug is withdrawn.

Treatment of barbiturate dependence consists of cautious and gradual withdrawal of the drug. Barbiturate-dependent patients can be withdrawn by using a number of different withdrawal regimens. In all cases withdrawal takes an extended period of time. One method involves substituting 30 mg of phenobarbital for each 100 mg of the short-acting barbiturate which the patient has been taking. The total daily amount of phenobarbital is then administered in 4 divided doses, not to exceed 600 mg daily. Should signs of withdrawal occur on the first day of treatment, a loading dose of 200 mg of phenobarbital may be administered IM, and the daily oral dosage increased. After stabilization with phenobarbital is achieved, the total daily dose of phenobarbital is decreased by 30 mg a day as long as withdrawal is proceeding smoothly. An alternative method of treatment is to decrease the daily dosage of the barbiturate which the patient has been taking by 10 percent/day, if tolerated by the patient.

Infants physically dependent on barbiturates may be given phenobarbital 3 to 10 mg/kg/day. After withdrawal symptoms (hyperactivity, disturbed sleep, tremors, hyperreflexia) are relieved, the dosage of phenobarbital should be gradually decreased and completely withdrawn over a 2-week period.

OVERDOSAGE

The toxic dose of barbiturates varies considerably. In general, an oral dose of 1 gram of most barbiturates produces serious poisoning in an adult. Death commonly occurs after ingestion of 2 to 10 grams of barbiturate. Barbiturate intoxication may be confused with alcoholism, bromide intoxication and with various neurological disorders.

Acute overdosage with barbiturates is manifested by CNS and respiratory depression which may progress to Cheyne-Stokes respiration, areflexia, constriction of the pupils to a slight degree (though in severe poisoning they may show paralytic dilation), oliguria, tachycardia, hypotension, lowered body temperature and coma. Typical shock syndrome (apnea, circulatory collapse, respiratory arrest and death) may occur.

In extreme overdose, all electrical activity in the brain may cease, in which case the EEG may be "flat," which does not necessarily indicate clinical death. This effect is fully reversible unless hypoxic damage occurs. Consideration should be given to the possibility of barbiturate intoxication even in situations that appear to involve trauma.

Complications such as pneumonia, pulmonary edema, cardiac arrhythmias, congestive heart failure and renal failure may occur. Uremia may increase CNS sensitivity to barbiturates if renal function is impaired. Differential diagnosis should include hypoglycemia, head trauma, cerebrovascular accidents, convulsive states and diabetic coma. Blood levels from acute overdosage for some barbiturates are listed in the accompanying table. [See table above.]

Treatment of overdosage is mainly supportive and consists of the following:

1. Maintenance of an adequate airway, with assisted respiration and oxygen administration as necessary.

2. Monitoring of vital signs and fluid balance.

3. If the patient is conscious and has not lost the gag reflex, emesis may be induced with ipecac. Care should be taken to prevent pulmonary aspiration of vomitus. After completion of vomiting, 30 grams activated charcoal, in a glass of water, may be administered.

4. If emesis is contraindicated, gastric lavage may be performed with a cuffed endotracheal tube in place with the patient in the face down position. Activated charcoal may be left in the emptied stomach and a saline cathartic administered.

5. Fluid therapy and other standard treatment for shock, if needed.

6. If renal function is normal, forced diuresis may aid in the elimination of the barbiturate. *Alkalinization of the urine increases renal excretion of some barbiturates, especially* phenobarbital, *aprobarbital* and mephobarbital (which is metabolized to phenobarbital).

7. Although not recommended as a routine procedure, hemodialysis may be used in severe barbiturate intoxication or if the patient is anuric or in shock.

8. Patient should be rolled from side to side every 30 minutes.

9. Antibiotics should be given if pneumonia is suspected.

10. Appropriate nursing care to prevent hypostatic pneumonia, decubiti, aspiration and other complications in patients with altered states of consciousness.

DOSAGE AND ADMINISTRATION

Usual Adult Dosage: As a sedative, one 5-ml teaspoonful (40 mg) three times daily; for mild insomnia, one to two 5-ml teaspoonfuls before retiring; for pronounced insomnia, two to four 5-ml teaspoonfuls before retiring.

Special Patient Population: Dosage should be reduced in the elderly or debilitated because these patients may be more sensitive to barbiturates. Dosage should be reduced for patients with impaired renal function or hepatic disease.

HOW SUPPLIED

Elixir (red) providing 40 mg of aprobarbital/Roche per 5 ml in a vehicle containing 20 percent alcohol — bottles of 16 oz (1 pint) (NDC 0004-1000-28).
Revised: March 1985

ANCOBON®   ℞

[an 'co-bon]
(flucytosine/Roche)

The following text is complete prescribing information based on official labeling in effect June 1, 1992.

> **WARNING**
>
> Use with extreme caution in patients with impaired renal function. Close monitoring of hematologic, renal and hepatic status of all patients is essential. These instructions should be thoroughly reviewed before administration of Ancobon.

DESCRIPTION

Ancobon (flucytosine/Roche), an antifungal agent, is available as 250-mg and 500-mg capsules for oral administration. Each capsule also contains corn starch, lactose and talc. Gelatin capsule shells contain parabens (butyl, methyl, propyl) and sodium propionate, with the following dye systems: 250-mg capsules—black iron oxide, FD&C Blue No. 1, FD&C Yellow No. 6, D&C Yellow No. 10 and titanium dioxide; 500-mg capsules—black iron oxide and titanium dioxide. Chemically, flucytosine is 5-fluorocytosine, a fluorinated pyrimidine which is related to fluorouracil and floxuridine. It is a white to off-white crystalline powder with a molecular weight of 129.09.

CLINICAL PHARMACOLOGY

Flucytosine is rapidly and virtually completely absorbed following oral administration. Bioavailability estimated by comparing the area under the curve of serum concentrations after oral and intravenous administration showed 78% to 89% absorption of the oral dose. Peak blood concentrations of 30 to 40 mcg/mL were reached within two hours of administration of a 2-Gm oral dose to normal subjects. The mean blood concentrations were approximately 70 to 80 mcg/mL one to two hours after a dose in patients with normal renal function who received a six-week regimen of flucytosine (150 mg/kg/day given in divided doses every 6 hours) in combination with amphotericin B. The half-life in the majority of normal subjects ranged between 2.4 and 4.8 hours. Flucytosine is excreted via the kidneys by means of glomerular filtration without significant tubular reabsorption. More than 90% of the total radioactivity after oral administration was recovered in the urine as intact drug. Approximately 1% of the dose is present in the urine as the α-fluoro-β-ureido-propionic acid metabolite. A small portion of the dose is excreted in the feces.

The half-life of flucytosine is prolonged in patients with renal insufficiency; the average half-life in nephrectomized or anuric patients was 85 hours (range: 29.9 to 250 hours). A linear correlation was found between the elimination rate constant of flucytosine and creatinine clearance.

In vitro studies have shown that 2.9% to 4% of flucytosine is protein-bound over the range of therapeutic concentrations found in the blood. Flucytosine readily penetrates the blood-brain barrier, achieving clinically significant concentrations in cerebrospinal fluid. Studies in pregnant rats have shown that flucytosine injected intraperitoneally crosses the placental barrier (see PRECAUTIONS).

MICROBIOLOGY

Flucytosine has *in vitro* and *in vivo* activity against Candida and Cryptococcus. Although the exact mode of action is unknown, it has been proposed that flucytosine acts directly on fungal organisms by competitive inhibition of purine and

Continued on next page

Roche Laboratories—Cont.

pyrimidine uptake and indirectly by intracellular metabolism to 5-fluorouracil. Flucytosine enters the fungal cell via cytosine permease; thus, flucytosine is metabolized to 5-fluorouracil within in fungal organisms. The 5-fluorouracil is extensively incorporated into fungal RNA and inhibits synthesis of both DNA and RNA. The result is unbalanced growth and death of the fungal organism. Antifungal synergism between Ancobon and polyene antibiotics, particularly amphotericin B, has been reported.

ACTIONS

Flucytosine has *in vitro* and *in vivo* activity against Candida and Cryptococcus. The exact mode of action against these fungi is not known. Ancobon is not metabolized significantly when given orally to man.

SUSCEPTIBILITY

Cryptococcus: Most strains initially isolated from clinical material have shown flucytosine minimal inhibitory concentrations (MIC's) ranging from .46 to 7.8 mcg/mL. Any isolate with an MIC greater than 12.5 mcg/mL is considered resistant. *In vitro* resistance has developed in originally susceptible strains during therapy. It is recommended that clinical cultures for susceptibility testing be taken initially and at weekly intervals during therapy. The initial culture should be reserved as a reference in susceptibilty testing of subsequent isolates.

Candida: As high as 40 to 50 percent of the pretreatment clinical isolates of Candida have been reported to be resistant to flucytosine. It is recommended that susceptibility studies be performed as early as possible and be repeated during therapy. An MIC value greater than 100 mcg/mL is considered resistant.

Interference with *in vitro* activity of flucytosine occurs in complex or semisynthetic media. In order to rely upon the recommended *in vitro* interpretations of susceptibility, it is essential that the broth medium and the testing procedure used be that described by Shadomy.[1]

INDICATIONS AND USAGE

Ancobon is indicated only in the treatment of serious infections caused by susceptible strains of Candida and/or Cryptococcus. *Candida:* Septicemia, endocarditis and urinary system infections have been effectively treated with flucytosine. Limited trials in pulmonary infections justify the use of flucytosine. *Cryptococcus:* Meningitis and pulmonary infections have been treated effectively. Studies in septicemias and urinary tract infections are limited, but good responses have been reported.

CONTRAINDICATIONS

Ancobon should not be used in patients with a known hypersensitivity to the drug.

WARNINGS

Ancobon must be given with extreme caution to patients with impaired renal function. Since Ancobon is excreted primarily by the kidneys, renal impairment may lead to accumulation of the drug. Ancobon blood concentrations should be monitored to determine the adequacy of renal excretion in such patients.[1] Dosage adjustments should be made in patients with renal insufficiency to prevent progressive accumulation of active drug.

Ancobon must be given with extreme caution to patients with bone marrow depression. Patients may be more prone to depression of bone marrow function if they: 1) have a hematologic disease, 2) are being treated with radiation or drugs which depress bone marrow, or 3) have a history of treatment with such drugs or radiation. Frequent monitoring of hepatic function and of the hematopoietic system is indicated during therapy.

PRECAUTIONS

General: Before therapy with Ancobon is instituted, electrolytes (because of hypokalemia) and the hematologic and renal status of the patient should be determined (see WARNINGS). Close monitoring of the patient during therapy is essential.

Laboratory tests: Since renal impairment can cause progressive accumulation of the drug, blood concentrations and kidney function should be monitored during therapy. Hematologic status (leucocyte and thrombocyte count) and liver function (alkaline phosphatase, SGOT and SGPT) should be determined at frequent intervals during treatment as indicated.

Drug interactions: Cytosine arabinoside, a cytostatic agent, has been reported to inactivate the antifungal activity of Ancobon by competitive inhibition. Drugs which impair glomerular filtration may prolong the biological half-life of flucytosine. Antifungal synergism between Ancobon and polyene antibiotics, particularly amphotericin B, has been reported.

Drug/laboratory test interactions: Measurement of serum creatinine levels should be determined by the Jaffe method, since Ancobon does not interfere with the determination of creatinine values by this method, as it does when the dry-slide enzymatic method with the Kodak Ektachem analyzer is used.

Carcinogenesis, mutagenesis, impairment of fertility: Ancobon has not undergone adequate animal testing to evaluate carcinogenic potential. The mutagenic potential of Ancobon was evaluated in Ames-type studies with five different mutants of *S. typhimurium* and no mutagenicity was detected in the presence or absence of activating enzymes. Ancobon was nonmutagenic in three different repair assay systems.

There have been no adequate trials in animals on the effects of Ancobon on fertility or reproductive performance. The fertility and reproductive performance of the offspring (F_1 generation) of mice treated with 100, 200 or 400 mg/kg/day of flucytosine on days 7 to 13 of gestation was studied; the *in utero* treatment had no adverse effect on the fertility or reproductive performance of the offspring.

Pregnancy: Teratogenic effects. Pregnancy Category C. Ancobon has been shown to be teratogenic in the rat and mouse at doses of 40 mg/kg/day (*i.e.,* 0.27 times the maximum recommended human dose). There are no adequate and well-controlled studies in pregnant women. Ancobon should be used during pregnancy only if the potential benefit justifies the potential risk to the fetus.

The teratogenicity of Ancobon is apparently species-related. Although there is confirmation of rat teratogenicity in the published literature, three studies in the mouse and studies in the rabbit and monkey have failed to reveal a teratogenic liability.

Nursing mothers: It is not known whether this drug is excreted in human milk. Because many drugs are excreted in human milk and because of the potential for serious adverse reactions in nursing infants from Ancobon, a decision should be made whether to discontinue nursing or to discontinue the drug, taking into account the importance of the drug to the mother.

Pediatric use: Safety and effectiveness in children have not been established.

ADVERSE REACTIONS

The adverse reactions which have occurred during treatment with Ancobon are grouped according to organ system affected.

Cardiovascular: Cardiac arrest.

Respiratory: Respiratory arrest, chest pain, dyspnea.

Dermatologic: Rash, pruritus, urticaria, photosensitivity.

Gastrointestinal: Nausea, emesis, abdominal pain, diarrhea, anorexia, dry mouth, duodenal ulcer, gastrointestinal hemorrhage, hepatic dysfunction, jaundice, ulcerative colitis, bilirubin elevation.

Genitourinary: Azotemia, creatinine and BUN elevation, crystalluria, renal failure.

Hematologic: Anemia, agranulocytosis, aplastic anemia, eosinophilia, leukopenia, pancytopenia, thrombocytopenia.

Neurologic: Ataxia, hearing loss, headache, paresthesia, parkinsonism, peripheral neuropathy, pyrexia, vertigo, sedation.

Psychiatric: Confusion, hallucinations, psychosis.

Miscellaneous: Fatigue, hypoglycemia, hypokalemia, weakness.

OVERDOSAGE

There is no experience with intentional overdosage. It is reasonable to expect that overdosage may produce pronounced manifestations of the known clinical adverse reactions. Prolonged serum concentrations in excess of 100 mcg/mL may be associated with an increased incidence of toxicity, especially gastrointestinal (diarrhea, nausea, vomiting), hematologic (leukopenia, thrombocytopenia) and hepatic (hepatitis).

In the management of overdosage, prompt gastric lavage or the use of an emetic is recommended. Adequate fluid intake should be maintained, by the intravenous route if necessary, since Ancobon is excreted unchanged via the renal tract. The hematologic parameters should be monitored frequently; liver and kidney function should be carefully monitored. Should any abnormalities appear in any of these parameters, appropriate therapeutic measures should be instituted. Since hemodialysis has been shown to rapidly reduce serum concentrations in anuric patients, this method may be considered in the management of overdosage.

DOSAGE AND ADMINISTRATION

The usual dosage of Ancobon is 50 to 150 mg/kg/day administered in divided doses at 6-hour intervals. Nausea or vomiting may be reduced or avoided if the capsules are given a few at a time over a 15-minute period. If the BUN or the serum creatinine is elevated, or if there are other signs of renal impairment, the initial dose should be at the lower level (see WARNINGS).

HOW SUPPLIED

Capsules, 250 mg (gray and green), imprinted ANCOBON® 250 ROCHE; bottles of 100 (NDC 0004-0077-01). *Capsules,* 500 mg (gray and white), imprinted ANCOBON® 500 ROCHE, bottles of 100 (NDC 0004-0079-01).

REFERENCE

1. Shadomy S: *Appl Microbiol 17:* 871–877, June 1969.

Revised: November 1987

Shown in Product Identification Section, page 425

ARFONAD® ℞

[ar'fo-nad]

(trimethaphan camsylate/Roche)

Ampuls

The following text is complete prescribing information based on official labeling in effect June 1, 1992.

DESCRIPTION

Arfonad (trimethaphan camsylate/Roche) Injection, a vasodepressor agent, is available as a sterile solution to be used only for intravenous infusion. Each 10-mL ampul contains 500 mg trimethaphan camsylate compounded with 0.013% sodium acetate and hydrochloric acid to adjust pH to approximately 5.2.

Trimethaphan camsylate is a sulfonium derivative. The chemical name is (+)-1,3-dibenzyldecahydro-2-oxoimidazo[4,5-*c*]thieno[1,2-*a*]-thiolium 2-oxo-10-bornanesulfonate (1:1). It occurs as white crystals or a white, crystalline powder which is freely soluble in water and alcohol. It has a molecular weight of 596.80.

CLINICAL PHARMACOLOGY

Trimethaphan camsylate is primarily a ganglionic blocking agent. It blocks transmission in autonomic ganglia without producing any preceding or concomitant change in the membrane potentials of the ganglion cells. It does not modify the conduction of impulses in the preganglionic or postganglionic neurons and does not prevent the release of acetylcholine by preganglionic impulses. Trimethaphan camsylate produces ganglionic blockade by occupying receptor sites on the ganglion cells and by stabilizing the postsynaptic membranes against the action of acetylcholine liberated from the presynaptic nerve endings.

In addition to ganglionic blocking, trimethaphan camsylate may also exert a direct peripheral vasodilator effect. By inducing vasodilation, it causes pooling of blood in the dependent periphery and the splanchnic system. The vasodilation results in a lowering of the blood pressure. Trimethaphan camsylate liberates histamine.

Trimethaphan crosses the placenta. Other pharmacokinetic data are unavailable because there is no acceptable assay procedure for the determination of trimethaphan in biological specimens.

INDICATIONS AND USAGE

Arfonad is indicated for the production of controlled hypotension during surgery; for the short term (acute) control of blood pressure in hypertensive emergencies; and in the emergency treatment of pulmonary edema in patients with pulmonary hypertension associated with systemic hypertension.

CONTRAINDICATIONS

Arfonad is contraindicated in those conditions where hypotension may subject the patient to undue risk, *e.g.,* uncorrected anemia, hypovolemia, shock (both incipient and frank), asphyxia or uncorrected respiratory insufficiency. Inadequate availability of fluids and inability to replace blood for technical reasons may also constitute contraindications.

WARNINGS

Arfonad is a powerful hypotensive drug and should always be diluted before use.

It is recommended that the use of Arfonad to produce hypotension in surgical or medical indications be limited to physicians with proper training in this technique. Adequate facilities, equipment and personnel should be available for vigilant monitoring of the circulation since Arfonad is an extremely potent hypotensive agent. Adequate oxygenation must be assured throughout the treatment period, especially in regard to coronary and cerebral circulation.

Arfonad should be used with extreme caution in patients with arteriosclerosis, cardiac disease, hepatic or renal disease, degenerative disease of the central nervous system, Addison's disease or diabetes, and in patients who are under treatment with steroids.

Usage in Pregnancy: **Arfonad can cause fetal harm when administered to a pregnant woman. Trimethaphan camsylate crosses the placenta, decreasing fetal gastrointestinal motility and resulting in meconium ileus. In addition, Arfonad-induced hypotension may have other serious adverse effects on the fetus. If Arfonad is used during pregnancy, or if the patient becomes pregnant while taking Arfonad, the patient should be apprised of the potential hazard to the fetus.**

PRECAUTIONS

General: Arfonad should be used with extreme caution in the elderly or debilitated. Because Arfonad liberates hista-

mine, it should be used with caution in patients with a history of allergies.

Respiratory depression and arrest have occurred during Arfonad administration, although a causal relationship has not been firmly established. The patient's respiratory status must be monitored closely, particularly if large doses of Arfonad are used.

Occasionally, patients may fail to show an adequate hypotensive response to Arfonad admnistration. When this is observed, administration should be discontinued and other methods to control hypertension instituted. Tachyphylaxis has also been reported.

NOTE: Because Arfonad causes mydriasis, pupillary dilation does not necessarily indicate anoxia or the depth of anesthesia.

Drug interactions: Arfonad should be used with care in patients who have been receiving antihypertensive drugs, since an additive hypotensive effect may occur. Arfonad may also have an additive hypotensive effect when administered with anesthetic agents, especially spinal anesthetics. Procainamide also has an additive hypotensive effect with Arfonad. Diuretic agents may markedly enhance the responses evoked by ganglionic-blocking drugs. Arfonad may also prolong the effects of neuromuscular blocking agents such as tubocurarine chloride or succinylcholine chloride, especially when large doses of Arfonad are administered.

Concomitant therapy with other drugs can considerably modify the dose of Arfonad necessary to achieve the desired response. In general, the deeper the plane of anesthesia, the smaller the dose of Arfonad that is required to produce hypotension; conversely, less anesthetic is required after hypotension has been induced by Arfonad.

Carcinogenesis, mutagenesis and impairment of fertility: Arfonad has not undergone adequate animal testing to evaluate its carcinogenic potential. The mutagenicity of Arfonad has not been studied nor has the drug been evaluated for effects on fertility.

Pregnancy: Teratogenic effects—Pregnancy Category D. See WARNINGS section.

Nonteratogenic effects—See WARNINGS section.

Nursing mothers: It is not known whether Arfonad is excreted in human milk. Because of the potential for serious adverse reactions from Arfonad in nursing infants, mothers who require Arfonad should be advised not to nurse.

Pediatric use: Safety and effectiveness in children have not been established.

ADVERSE REACTIONS

The adverse reactions produced by Arfonad are primarily due to its nonselective blockade of the autonomic nervous system. The following adverse reactions have been observed, but there is not enough systematic collection of data to support an estimate of their frequency.

Cardiovascular: Tachycardia, precipitation of angina, syncope which may occur without warning. *Respiratory:* Respiratory depression and arrest have occurred during Arfonad administration, although a causal relationship has not been firmly established. *Gastrointestinal:* Paralytic ileus, dry mouth, constipation, occasional diarrhea, abdominal discomfort, anorexia, heartburn, nausea, vomiting, eructation. *Genitourinary:* Urinary hesitancy, decreased potentia. *Ophthalmic:* Cycloplegia, mydriasis, difficulty in accommodation, conjunctival suffusion. *Miscellaneous:* Subjective chilliness, weakness, restlessness, urticaria, itching. Arfonad prevents surgically-induced elevation of blood glucose and decreases serum potassium slightly.

Generally, side effects are decreased when dosage is reduced or the drug is temporarily discontinued.

OVERDOSAGE

Vasopressor agents may be used to correct excessive hypotension during surgery or to effect a more rapid return to normotensive levels. Phenylephrine HCl or mephentermine sulfate should be tried initially and norepinephrine should be reserved for refractory cases.

The acute intravenous toxicity of trimethaphan camsylate is as follows:

Species	LD$_{50}$ mg/kg
mouse	21
rat	21
rabbit	23
dog	0.75
guinea pig	13
monkey	>8

DOSAGE AND ADMINISTRATION

Arfonad must always be diluted and administered by intravenous infusion. Solutions should be freshly prepared and any unused portions discarded. For this purpose a 0.1 percent (1 mg/mL) concentration of Arfonad in 5% Dextrose Injection USP, normal saline solution, or Ringer's Injection USP should be employed. Arfonad is stable in these diluents for at least 24 hours at room temperature. Use of other diluents is not recommended, since experience with them has not been reported.

Arfonad is physically incompatible with thiopental, gallamine triethiodide, tubocurarine chloride, iodides, bromides and strongly alkaline solutions. **Therefore, the infusion fluid used for administration of Arfonad should not be employed as a vehicle for the simultaneous administration of any other drugs.**

One (1) ampul of Arfonad—10 mL, 50 mg/mL—should be diluted to 500 mL. Since individual response varies, the rate of administration must be adjusted to the requirements of each patient.

When Arfonad is given, the patient should be positioned so as to avoid cerebral anoxia. During surgery, adequate anesthesia should be established. Intravenous drip with Arfonad is started at an average rate of 3 mL to 4 mL (3 mg to 4 mg) per minute (see chart below). The rate of administration is then adjusted to maintain the desired level of hypotension. Since there is a marked variation of individual response, **frequent blood pressure determinations are essential to maintain proper control.** Rates from as low as 0.3 mL (0.3 mg) per minute to rates exceeding 6 mL (6 mg) per minute have been found necessary, based upon clinical experience.

0.1% (1 mg/mL) CONCENTRATION OF ARFONAD

Delivery System Drops/mL	Drops/Min to Obtain 3–4 mL (3–4 mg) Arfonad
10	30–40
15	45–60
60	180–240

During surgery, administration of Arfonad should be stopped prior to wound closure in order to permit blood pressure to return to normal. A systolic pressure of 100 mm will usually be attained within 10 minutes after stopping Arfonad.

Parenteral drug products should be inspected visually for particulate matter and discoloration prior to administration, whenever solution and container permit.

HOW SUPPLIED

10 mL Ampuls (500 mg trimethaphan camsylate/10 mL)—boxes of 10 (NDC 0004-1900-06).

Arfonad is stable under refrigeration (36° to 46°F or 2° to 8°C). Arfonad should not be frozen as ampul breakage may result from ice formation.

Revised: February 1988

AZO GANTANOL®   ℞
[a "zo gan 'tan-ol]

The following text is complete prescribing information based on official labeling in effect June 1, 1992.

DESCRIPTION

Azo Gantanol combines the antibacterial effectiveness of sulfamethoxazole (Gantanol®) with the local urinary analgesic activity of phenazopyridine hydrochloride. Each tablet contains 0.5 Gm sulfamethoxazole/Roche and 100 mg phenazopyridine hydrochloride. Each tablet also contains carnauba wax, castor oil, corn starch, docusate sodium, magnesium stearate, polyvinyl acetate, polyvinyl alcohol, pregelatinized starch, shellac and FD&C Red No. 3, and may contain red and brown synthetic iron oxides.

Gantanol (sulfamethoxazole/Roche) is an intermediate-dosage sulfonamide. Sulfamethoxazole is an almost white, odorless, tasteless compound. Chemically, it is N^1-(5-methyl-3-isoxazolyl) sulfanilamide.

Phenazopyridine hydrochloride is a urinary analgesic. Chemically, it is 3-phenylazo-2,6-diaminopyridine hydrochloride.

Sulfonamides exist in the blood as free, conjugated (acetylated and possibly other forms) and protein-bound forms. The "free" form is considered to be the therapeutically active form. It has been shown that approximately 70 per cent of Gantanol is protein bound in the blood;[1] of the unbound portion 80 to 90 per cent is in the nonacetylated form.[2,3] Excretion of sulfonamides is chiefly by the kidneys with glomerular filtration as the primary mechanism.

ACTIONS

The systemic sulfonamides are bacteriostatic agents. The spectrum of activity is similar for all. Sulfonamides competitively inhibit bacterial synthesis of folic acid (pteroylglutamic acid) from para-aminobenzoic acid. Resistant strains are capable of utilizing folic acid precursors or preformed folic acid.

Phenazopyridine hydrochloride has a specific analgesic effect in the urinary tract, promptly relieving pain and burning.

INDICATIONS

For the initial treatment of uncomplicated urinary tract infections caused by susceptible strains of the following microorganisms: *Escherichia coli, Klebsiella* species, *Enterobacter* species, *Proteus mirabilis, Proteus vulgaris* and *Staphylococcus aureus* when relief of symptoms of pain, burning or urgency is needed during the first 2 days of therapy. Treat-

ment with Azo Gantanol should not exceed 2 days. There is a lack of evidence that the combination of sulfamethoxazole and phenazopyridine hydrochloride provides greater benefit than sulfamethoxazole alone after 2 days. Treatment beyond 2 days should only be continued with Gantanol (sulfamethoxazole/Roche). (See DOSAGE AND ADMINISTRATION section.)

Important note. In vitro sulfonamide sensitivity tests are not always reliable. The test must be carefully coordinated with bacteriologic and clinical response. When the patient is already taking sulfonamides, follow-up cultures should have aminobenzoic acid added to the culture media.

Currently, the increasing frequency of resistant organisms is a limitation of the usefulness of antibacterial agents including the sulfonamides.

Wide variation in blood levels may result with identical doses. Blood levels should be measured in patients receiving sulfonamides for serious infections. Free sulfonamide blood levels of 5 to 15 mg per 100 ml may be considered therapeutically effective for most infections, with blood levels of 12 to 15 mg per 100 ml optimal for serious infections; 20 mg per 100 ml should be the maximum total sulfonamide level, as adverse reactions occur more frequently above this level.

CONTRAINDICATIONS

Children below age 12. Hypersensitivity to sulfonamides. Pregnancy at term and during the nursing period, because sulfonamides pass the placenta and are excreted in the milk and may cause kernicterus.

Because Azo Gantanol contains phenazopyridine hydrochloride it is contraindicated in glomerulonephritis, severe hepatitis, uremia, and pyelonephritis of pregnancy with gastrointestinal disturbances.

WARNINGS

Usage in Pregnancy: The safe use of sulfonamides in pregnancy has not been established. The teratogenicity potential of most sulfonamides has not been thoroughly investigated in either animals or humans. However, a significant increase in the incidence of cleft palate and other bony abnormalities of offspring has been observed when certain sulfonamides of the short, intermediate and long-acting types were given to pregnant rats and mice at high oral doses (7 to 25 times the human therapeutic dose).

Deaths associated with the administration of sulfonamides have been reported from hypersensitivity reactions, hepatocellular necrosis, agranulocytosis, aplastic anemia and other blood dyscrasias.

The presence of clinical signs such as sore throat, fever, arthralgia, cough, shortness of breath, pallor, purpura or jaundice may be early indications of serious reactions, including serious blood disorders. Complete blood counts should be done frequently in patients receiving sulfonamides.

The frequency of renal complications is considerably lower in patients receiving the more soluble sulfonamides. Urinalysis with careful microscopic examination should be obtained frequently in patients receiving sulfonamides.

PRECAUTIONS

Sulfonamides should be given with caution to patients with impaired renal or hepatic function and to those with severe allergy or bronchial asthma. In glucose-6-phosphate dehydrogenase-deficient individuals, hemolysis may occur. This reaction is frequently dose-related. Adequate fluid intake must be maintained in order to prevent crystalluria and stone formation.

Carcinogenesis: Azo Gantanol has not undergone adequate trials relating to carcinogenicity; each component, however, has been evaluated separately. Rats appear to be especially susceptible to the goitrogenic effects of sulfonamides, and long-term administration of sulfonamides has resulted in thyroid malignancies in this species. Long-term administration of phenazopyridine hydrochloride has induced neoplasia in rats (large intestine) and mice (liver). Although no association between phenazopyridine hydrochloride and human neoplasia has been reported, adequate epidemiological studies have not been conducted.

ADVERSE REACTIONS

Blood dyscrasias: Agranulocytosis, aplastic anemia, thrombocytopenia, leukopenia, hemolytic anemia, purpura, hypoprothrombinemia, methemoglobinemia, and eosinophilia.

Allergic reactions: Erythema multiforme (Stevens-Johnson syndrome), generalized skin eruptions, epidermal necrolysis, urticaria, serum sickness, pruritus, exfoliative dermatitis, anaphylactoid reactions, periorbital edema, conjunctival and scleral injection, photosensitization, arthralgia and allergic myocarditis.

Gastrointestinal reactions: Nausea, emesis, abdominal pains, hepatitis, hepatocellular necrosis, diarrhea, anorexia, pancreatitis and stomatitis.

C.N.S. reactions: Headache, peripheral neuritis, mental depression, convulsions, ataxia, hallucinations, tinnitus, vertigo and insomnia.

Continued on next page

Roche Laboratories—Cont.

Miscellaneous reactions: Drug fever, chills, and toxic nephrosis with oliguria and anuria. Polyarteritis nodosa and L.E. phenomenon have occurred.

Respiratory reactions: Pulmonary infiltrates.

The sulfonamides bear certain chemical similarities to some goitrogens, diuretics (acetazolamide and the thiazides) and oral hypoglycemic agents. Goiter production, diuresis and hypoglycemia have occurred rarely in patients receiving sulfonamides. Cross-sensitivity may exist with these agents.

DOSAGE AND ADMINISTRATION

Azo Gantanol is intended for the acute, painful phase of urinary tract infections. The usual dosage in adults is 4 tablets initially followed by 2 tablets morning and evening for up to 2 days. Treatment with Azo Gantanol should not exceed 2 days. Treatment beyond 2 days should only be continued with Gantanol (sulfamethoxazole/Roche).

NOTE: Patients should be told that the orange-red dye (phenazopyridine HCl) will color the urine soon after ingestion of the medication.

HOW SUPPLIED

Tablets, red, film-coated, each containing 0.5 Gm sulfamethoxazole/Roche and 100 mg phenazopyridine HCl—bottles of 100.

REFERENCES

1. Struller, T.: *Antibiot. Chemother.,* 14: 179, 1968.
2. Boger, W. P., and Gavin, J. J.: *Antibiotics and Chemother.,* 10:572, 1960.
3. Brandman, O., and Engelberg, R.: *Curr. Therap. Res.,* 2:364, 1960.

Revised: July 1988

Shown in Product Identification Section, page 425

AZO GANTRISIN®   ℞
[a "zo gan 'tris-in]

The following text is complete prescribing information based on official labeling in effect June 1, 1992.

DESCRIPTION

Azo Gantrisin is a combination drug containing 500 mg of the antibacterial sulfisoxazole and 50 mg of the urinary analgesic phenazopyridine hydrochloride per tablet for oral administration. Each tablet also contains carnauba wax, castor oil, docusate sodium, hydrogenated cottonseed oil, magnesium stearate, pregelatinized starch, shellac, FD&C Red No. 3 and D&C Red No. 28.

Sulfisoxazole, an antibacterial sulfonamide, is N^1-(3,4-dimethyl-5-isoxazoyl) sulfanilamide. It is a white to slightly yellowish, odorless, slightly bitter, crystalline powder which is soluble in alcohol and very slightly soluble in water. Sulfisoxazole has an empirical formula of $C_{11}H_{13}N_3O_3S$, a molecular weight of 267.30.

Phenazopyridine hydrochloride, a local urinary analgesic, is 2,6-diamino-3-(phenylazo) pyridine monohydrochloride. It is a light or dark red to dark violet, odorless, slightly bitter, crystalline powder with an empirical formula of $C_{11}H_{11}N_5 \cdot HCl$, a molecular weight of 249.70.

CLINICAL PHARMACOLOGY

Following oral administration, sulfisoxazole is rapidly and completely absorbed; the small intestine is the major site of absorption, but some of the drug is absorbed from the stomach. Sulfonamides are present in the blood as free, conjugated (acetylated and possibly other forms) and protein-bound forms. The amount present as "free" drug is considered to be the therapeutically active form. Approximately 85% of a dose of sulfisoxazole is bound to plasma proteins, primarily to albumin; 65% to 72% of the unbound portion is in the nonacetylated form.

Maximum plasma concentrations of intact sulfisoxazole following a single 2-Gm oral dose of sulfisoxazole to healthy adult volunteers ranged from 127 to 211 mcg/mL (mean 169 mcg/mL), and the time of peak plasma concentration ranged from 1 to 4 hours (mean 2.5 hours). The elimination half-life of sulfisoxazole ranged from 4.6 to 7.8 hours after oral administration. The elimination of sulfisoxazole has been shown to be slower in elderly subjects (63 to 75 years) with diminished renal function (creatinine clearance 37 to 68 mL/min).[1] After multiple-dose oral administration of 500 mg q.i.d. to healthy volunteers, the average steady-state plasma concentrations of intact sulfisoxazole ranged from 49.9 to 88.8 mcg/mL (mean 63.4 mcg/mL).[2]

Wide variation in blood levels may result following identical doses of a sulfonamide. Blood levels should be measured in patients receiving sulfonamides at the higher recommended doses or being treated for serious infections. Free sulfonamide blood levels of 50 to 150 mcg/mL may be considered therapeutically effective for most infections, with blood levels of 120 to 150 mcg/mL being optimal for serious infections. The maximum sulfonamide level should not exceed 200 mcg/mL, since adverse reactions occur more frequently above this concentration.

Sulfisoxazole and its acetylated metabolites are excreted primarily by the kidneys through glomerular filtration. Concentrations of sulfisoxazole are considerbly higher in the urine than in the blood. The mean urinary recovery following oral administration of sulfisoxazole is 97% within 48 hours; 52% of this is intact drug, and the remaining is the N^4-acetylated metabolite.

Sulfisoxazole is distributed only in extracellular body fluid. It is excreted in human milk. It readily crosses the placental barrier and enters into fetal circulation and also crosses the blood-brain barrier. In healthy subjects, cerebrospinal fluid concentrations of sulfisoxazole vary; in patients with meningitis, however, concentrations of free drug in cerebrospinal fluid as high as 94 mcg/mL have been reported.

Phenazopyridine hydrochloride has a specific local analgesic effect in the urinary tract, promptly relieving pain and burning. In six healthy subjects, 90% of a 600 mg oral dose of phenazopyridine hydrochloride was eliminated in the urine in 24 hours, 41% as unchanged drug and 49% as metabolites. No additional pharmacokinetic data are available on this drug.

Microbiology: The sulfonamides are bacteriostatic agents and the spectrum of activity is similar for all. Sulfonamides inhibit bacterial synthesis of dihydrofolic acid by preventing the condensation of the pteridine with aminobenzoic acid through competitive inhibition of the enzyme dihydropteroate synthetase. Resistant strains have altered dihydropteroate synthetase with reduced affinity for sulfonamides or produce increased quantities of aminobenzoic acid.

INDICATIONS AND USAGE

Azo Gantrisin is indicated for the initial treatment of uncomplicated urinary tract infections caused by susceptible strains of the following microorganisms: *Escherichia coli, Klebiella* species, *Enterobacter* species, *Proteus mirabilis, Proteus vulgaris* and *Staphylococcus aureus* when relief of symptoms of pain, burning or urgency is needed during the first 2 days of therapy. There is a lack of evidence that the combination of sulfisoxazole and phenazopyridine hydrochloride provides greater benefit than sulfisoxazole alone after 2 days. Therefore, treatment with Azo Gantrisin should not exceed 2 days, and the remaining therapeutic course should be completed with sulfisoxazole alone. (See DOSAGE AND ADMINISTRATION section.)

The frequency of resistant organisms limits the usefulness of sulfonamides as sole therapy in the treatment of urinary tract infections.

Important Note: In vitro susceptibility tests for sulfonamides are not always reliable. When the patient is already taking sulfonamides, follow-up cultures should have aminobenzoic acid added to the culture media.

CONTRAINDICATIONS

Azo Gantrisin is contraindicated in the following patient populations:

Patients with a known sensitivity to either of its components;

Children younger than 2 months;

Pregnant women *at term*; and

Mothers nursing infants less than 2 months of age.

Use in pregnant women at term, in children less than 2 months of age and in mothers nursing infants less than 2 months of age is contraindicated because sulfonamides may promote kernicterus in the newborn by displacing bilirubin from plasma proteins.

Because Azo Gantrisin contains phenazopyridine hydrochloride, it is also contraindicated in patients with glomerulonephritis, severe hepatitis, uremia, and pyelonephritis of pregnancy with gastrointestinal disturbances.

WARNINGS: FATALITIES ASSOCIATED WITH THE ADMINISTRATION OF SULFONAMIDES, ALTHOUGH RARE, HAVE OCCURRED DUE TO SEVERE REACTIONS, INCLUDING STEVENS-JOHNSON SYNDROME, TOXIC EPIDERMAL NECROLYSIS, FULMINANT HEPATIC NECROSIS, AGRANULOCYTOSIS, APLASTIC ANEMIA AND OTHER BLOOD DYSCRASIAS.

SULFONAMIDES, INCLUDING AZO GANTRISIN, SHOULD BE DISCONTINUED AT THE FIRST APPEARANCE OF SKIN RASH OR ANY SIGN OF ADVERSE REACTION. In rare instances a skin rash may be followed by a more severe reaction, such as Stevens-Johnson syndrome, toxic epidermal necrolysis, hepatic necrosis and serious blood disorders. (See PRECAUTIONS.)

Clinical signs such as rash, sore throat, fever, arthralgia, pallor, purpura or jaundice may be early indications of serious reactions.

Cough, shortness of breath and pulmonary infiltrates are hypersensitivity reactions of the respiratory tract that have been reported in association with sulfonamide treatment.

The sulfonamides should not be used for the treatment of group A beta-hemolytic streptococcal infections. In the established infection, they will not eradicate the streptococcus and, therefore, will not prevent sequelae such as rheumatic fever.

Pseudomembranous coilitis has been reported with nearly all antibacterial agents, including sulfisoxazole, and may range in severity from mild to life-threatening. Therefore, it is important to consider this diagnosis in patients who present with diarrhea subsequent to the administration of antibacterial agents.

Treatment with antibacterial agents alters the normal flora of the colon and may permit overgrowth of clostridia. Studies indicate that a toxin product by *Clostridium difficile* is one primary cause of "antibiotic-associated colitis."

After the diagnosis of pseudomembranous colitis has been established, therapeutic measures should be initiated. Mild cases of pseudomembranous colitis usually respond to drug discontinuation alone. In moderate to severe cases, consideration should be given to management with fluids and electrolytes, protein supplementation, and treatment with an oral antibacterial drug effective against *C. difficile.*

PRECAUTIONS

General: Sulfonamides should be given with caution to patients with impaired renal or hepatic function and to those with severe allergy or bronchial asthma. In glucose-6-phosphate dehydrogenase-deficient individuals, hemolysis may occur; this reaction is frequently dose-related.

The frequency of resistant organisms limits the usefulness of sulfonamides as sole therapy in the treatment of urinary tract infections. Since sulfonamides are bacteriostatic and not bacteriocidal, a complete course is needed to prevent immediate regrowth and the development of resistant uropathogens.

Information for Patients: Patients should maintain an adequate fluid intake to prevent crystalluria and stone formation. Patients should also be told that soon after ingestion of this medication, the phenazopyridine HCl component will produce a reddish-orange discoloration of the urine.

Laboratory Tests: Complete blood counts should be done frequently in patients receiving sulfonamides. If a significant reduction in the count of any formed blood element is noted, sulfonamide therapy should be discontinued. Urinalysis with careful microscopic examination and renal function tests should be performed during therapy, particularly for those patients with impaired renal function. Blood levels should be measured in patients receiving a sulfonamide for serious infections. (See INDICATIONS AND USAGE.)

Drug Interactions: It has been reported that sulfisoxazole may prolong the prothrombin time in patients who are receiving anticoagulants, including warfarin. This interaction should be kept in mind when Azo Gantrisin is given to patients already on anticoagulant therapy, and the coagulation time should be reassessed.

It has been proposed that sulfisoxazole competes with thiopental for plasma protein binding. In one study involving 48 patients, intravenous sulfisoxazole resulted in a decrease in the amount of thiopental required for anesthesia and in a shortening of the awakening time. It is not known whether chronic oral doses of sulfisoxazole have a similar effect. Until more is known about this interaction, physicians should be aware that patients receiving sulfisoxazole might require less thiopental for anesthesia.

Sulfonamides can displace methotrexate from plasma protein-binding sites, thus increasing free methotrexate concentrations. Studies in man have shown sulfisoxazole infusions to decrease plasma protein-bound methotrexate by one-fourth.

Sulfisoxazole can also potentiate the blood sugar-lowering activity of sulfonylureas.

Carcinogenesis, Mutagenesis, Impairment of Fertility:

Carcinogenesis: Azo Gantrisin has not undergone adequate trials relating to carcinogenicity; each component, however, has been evaluated separately. Sulfisoxazole was not carcinogenic in either sex when administered to mice by gavage for 103 weeks at dosages up to approximately 36 times the recommended human dose or to rats at 7 times the human dose. Rats appear to be especially susceptible to the goitrogenic effects of sulfonamides, and long-term administration of sulfonamides has resulted in thyroid malignancies in this species. Long-term administration of phenazopyridine hydrochloride has induced neoplasia in rats (large intestine) and mice (liver). Although no association between phenazopyridine hydrochloride and human neoplasia has been reported, adequate epidemiological studies have not been conducted.

Mutagenesis: There are no studies available that adequately evaluate the mutagenic potential of Azo Gantrisin or either of its components. However, sulfisoxazole was not observed to be mutagenic in *E. coli* Sd-4-73 when tested in the absence of a metabolic activating system.

Impairment of Fertility: Azo Gantrisin has not undergone adequate trials relating to impairment of fertility. In a reproduction study in rats given 14 times the human dose per day of sulfisoxazole, no effects were observed regarding mating behavior, conception rate or fertility index (percent pregnant). In a single 2-litter reproductive study of rats given 10 times the recommended human dose, phenazopyridine demonstrated no adverse effect on fertility.

Pregnancy:
Teratogenic Effects: Pregnancy Category C. At dosages 14 times the human daily dose, sulfisoxazole was not teratogenic in either rats or rabbits. However, in two other teratogenicity studies, cleft palates developed in both rats and mice after administration of 9 to 18 times the human therapeutic dose of sulfisoxazole. Phenazopyridine has not been adequately tested in animals for teratogenicity; however, data from a single study demonstrated no congenital malformations in rats given 10 times the human daily dose.
There are no adequate or well-controlled studies of Azo Gantrisin in either laboratory animals or in pregnant women. It is not known whether Azo Gantrisin can cause fetal harm when administered to a pregnant woman prior to term or can affect reproduction capacity. Azo Gantrisin should be used during pregnancy only if the potential benefit justifies the potential risk to the fetus.
Nonteratogenic Effects: Kernicterus may occur in the newborn as a result of treatment of a pregnant woman *at term* with sulfonamides. (See CONTRAINDICATIONS.)
Nursing Mothers: Azo Gantrisin is excreted in human milk. Because of the potential for the development of kernicterus in neonates due to the displacement of bilirubin from plasma proteins by sulfisoxazole, a decision should be made whether to discontinue nursing or discontinue the drug taking into account the importance of the drug to the mother. (See CONTRAINDICATIONS.)
Pediatric Use: Safety and effectiveness in children have not been established. Not for use in children under 2 months of age. (See CONTRAINDICATIONS.)

ADVERSE REACTIONS

Included in the listing that follows are adverse reactions that have been reported with other sulfonamide products; pharmacologic similarities require that each of the reactions be considered with Azo Gantrisin administration.
Allergic/Dermatologic: Anaphylaxis, erythema multiforme (Stevens-Johnson syndrome), toxic epidermal necrolysis, exfoliative dermatitis, angioedema, arteritis and vasculitis, allergic myocarditis, serum sickness, rash, urticaria, pruritus, photosensitivity, and conjuctival and scleral injection. In addition, periarteritis nodosa and systemic lupus erythematosus have been reported. (See WARNINGS.)
Cardiovascular: Tachycardia, palpitations, syncope and cyanosis.
Endocrine: The sulfonamides bear certain chemical similarities to some goitrogens, diuretics (acetazolamide and the thiazides) and oral hypoglycemic agents. Cross-sensitivity may exist with these agents. Development of goiter, diuresis and hypoglycemia have occurred rarely in patients receiving sulfonamides.
Gastrointestinal: Hepatitis, hepatocellular necrosis, jaundice, pseudomembranous colitis, nausea, emesis, anorexia, abdominal pain, diarrhea, gastrointestinal hemorrhage, melena, flatulence, glossitis, stomatitis, salivary gland enlargement and pancreatitis.
Onset of pseudomembranous colitis symptoms may occur during or after treatment with sulfisoxazole, a component of Azo Gantrisin. (See WARNINGS.)
Both components of Azo Gantrisin have been reported to cause increased elevation of liver-associated enzymes in patients with hepatitis.
Genitourinary: Crystalluria, hematuria, BUN and creatinine elevations, nephritis and toxic nephrosis with oliguria and anuria. Acute renal failure and urinary retention have also been reported. The frequency of renal complications, commonly associated with some sulfonamides, is lower in patients receiving the more soluble sulfonamides such as sulfisoxazole.
Hematologic: Leukopenia, agranulocytosis, aplastic anemia, thrombocytopenia, purpura, hemolytic anemia, anemia, eosinophilia, clotting disorders including hypoprothrombinemia and hypofibrinogenemia, sulfhemoglobinemia and methemoglobinemia.
Musculoskeletal: Arthralgia and myalgia.
Neurologic: Headache, dizziness, peripheral neuritis, paresthesia, convulsions, tinnitus, vertigo, ataxia and intracranial hypertension.
Psychiatric: Psychosis, hallucinations, disorentation, depression and anxiety.
Respiratory: Cough, shortness of breath and pulmonary infiltrates. (See WARNINGS.)
Vascular: Angioedema, arteritis and vasculitis.
Miscellaneous: Edema (including periorbital), pyrexia, drowsiness, weakness, fatigue, lassitude, rigors, flushing, hearing loss, insomnia and pneumonitis.

OVERDOSAGE

The amount of a single dose that is associated with symptoms of overdosage or is likely to be life-threatening has not been reported. Signs and symptoms of overdosage with Azo Gantrisin include anorexia, colic, nausea, vomiting, headache, dizziness, drowsiness, and unconsciousness. Pyrexia, hematuria and crystalluria may be noted. Blood dyscrasias and jaundice are potential late manifestations of overdosage.
General principles of treatment include the immediate discontinuation of the drug, instituting gastric lavage or emesis, forcing oral fluids, and administering intravenous fluids if urine output is low and renal function is normal. The patient should be monitored with blood counts and appropriate blood chemistries, including electrolytes. If the patient becomes cyanotic, the possibility of methemoglobinemia should be considered and, if present, the condition should be treated appropriately with intravenous 1% methylene blue. If a significant blood dyscrasia or jaundice occurs, specific therapy should be instituted for these complications.
Peritoneal dialysis is not effective, and hemodialysis is only moderately effective in removing sulfonamides.

DOSAGE AND ADMINISTRATION

The recommended dosage in adults is 4 tablets initially, followed by 2 tablets four times daily for up to two days. **Treatment with Azo Gantrisin should not exceed 2 days.** A full course of therapy for an uncomplicated urinary tract infection should be completed with sulfisoxazole alone.

HOW SUPPLIED

Each red, film-coated tablet contains 500 mg sulfisoxazole/Roche and 50 mg phenazopyridine HCl. Azo Gantrisin is available in bottles of 100 tablets (NDC-0004-0012-01) and 500 tablets (NDC-0004-0012-14). Imprint on tablets; AZO GANTRISIN® ROCHE.

REFERENCES

1. Boivert A, Barbeau G, Belanger PM: Pharmacokinetics of sulfisoxazole in young and elderly subjects. *Gerontology 30:* 125–131, 1984.
2. Oie S, Gambertoglio JG, Fleckenstein L: Comparison of the disposition of total and unbound sulfisoxazole after single and multiple dosing. *J Pharmacokinet Biopharm 10:* 157–172, 1982.

Revised: September 1990

Shown in Product Identification Section, page 425

BACTRIM™ I.V. INFUSION ℞

[bac'trim]
(trimethoprim and sulfamethoxazole/Roche)

The following text is complete prescribing information based on official labeling in effect June 1, 1992.

DESCRIPTION

Bactrim (trimethoprim and sulfamethoxazole) I.V. Infusion, a sterile solution for intravenous infusion only, is a synthetic antibacterial combination product. Each 5 mL contains 80 mg trimethoprim (16 mg/mL) and 400 mg sulfamethoxazole (80 mg/mL) compounded with 40% propylene glycol, 10% ethyl alcohol and 0.3% diethanolamine; 1% benzyl alcohol and 0.1% sodium metabisulfite added as preservatives, water for injection, and pH adjusted to approximately 10 with sodium hydroxide.
Trimethoprim is 2,4-diamino-5-(3,4,5-trimethoxybenzyl) pyrimidine. It is a white to light yellow, odorless, bitter compound with a molecular weight of 290.3.
Sulfamethoxazole is N^1-(5-methyl-3-isoxazolyl)sulfanilamide. It is an almost white, odorless, tasteless compound with a molecular weight of 253.28.

CLINICAL PHARMACOLOGY

Following a one-hour intravenous infusion of a single dose of 160 mg trimethoprim and 800 mg sulfamethoxazole to 11 patients whose weight ranged from 105 lbs to 165 lbs (mean, 143 lbs), the peak plasma concentrations of trimethoprim and sulfamethoxazole were 3.4 ± 0.3 μg/mL and 46.3 ± 2.7 μg/mL, respectively. Following repeated intravenous administration of the same dose at eight-hour intervals, the mean plasma concentrations just prior to and immediately after each infusion at steady state were 5.6 ± 0.6 μg/mL and 8.8 ± 0.9 μg/mL for trimethoprim and 70.6 ± 7.3 μg/mL and 105.6 ± 10.9 μg/mL for sulfamethoxazole. The mean plasma half-life was 11.3 ± 0.7 hours for trimethoprim and 12.8 ± 1.8 hours for sulfamethoxazole. All of these 11 patients had normal renal function, and their ages ranged from 17 to 78 years (median, 60 years).[1]
Pharmacokinetic studies in children and adults suggest an age-dependent half-life of trimethoprim, as indicated in the following table.[2]

Age (years)	No. of Patients	Mean TMP Half-life (hours)
<1	2	7.67
1–10	9	5.49
10–20	5	8.19
20–63	6	12.82

Patients with severely impaired renal function exhibit an increase in the half-lives of both components, requiring dosage regimen adjustment (See DOSAGE AND ADMINISTRATION section).
Both trimethoprim and sulfamethoxazole exist in the blood as unbound, protein-bound and metabolized forms; sulfamethaxazole also exists as the conjugated form. The metabolism of sulfamethoxazole occurs predominately by N_4-acetylation, although the glucuronide conjugate has been identified. The principal metabolites of trimethoprim are the 1- and 3-oxides and the 3'- and 4'-hydroxy derivatives. The free forms of trimethoprim and sulfamethoxazole are considered to be the therapeutically active forms. Approximately 44% of trimethoprim and 70% of sulfamethoxazole are bound to plasma proteins. The presence of 10 mg percent sulfamethoxazole in plasma decreases the protein binding of trimethoprim by an insignificant degree; trimethoprim does not influence the protein binding of sulfamethoxazole.
Excretion of trimethoprim and sulfamethoxazole is primarily by the kidneys through both glomerular filtration and tubular secretion. Urine concentrations of both trimethoprim and sulfamethoxazole are considerably higher than are the concentrations in the blood. The percent of dose excreted in urine over a 12-hour period following the intravenous administration of the first dose of 240 mg of trimethoprim and 1200 mg of sulfamethoxazole on day 1 ranged from 17% to 42.4% as free trimethoprim; 7% to 12.7% as free sulfamethoxazole; and 36.7% to 56% as total (free plus the N_4-acetylated metabolite) sulfamethoxazole. When administered together as Bactrim, neither trimethoprim nor sulfamethoxazole affects the urinary excretion pattern of the other. Both trimethoprim and sulfamethoxazole distribute to sputum and vaginal fluid; trimethoprim also distributes to bronchial secretions, and both pass the placental barrier and are excreted in breast milk.
Microbiology: Sulfamethoxazole inhibits bacterial synthesis of dihydrofolic acid by competing with *para*-aminobenzoic acid (PABA). Trimethoprim blocks the production of tetrahydrofolic acid from dihydrofolic acid by binding to and reversibly inhibiting the required enzyme, dihydrofolate reductase. Thus, Bactrim blocks two consecutive steps in the biosynthesis of nucleic acids and proteins essential to many bacteria.
In vitro studies have shown that bacterial resistance develops more slowly with Bactrim than with either trimethoprim or sulfamethoxazole alone.
In vitro serial dilution tests have shown that the spectrum of antibacterial activity of Bactrim includes common bacterial pathogens with the exception of *Pseudomonas aeruginosa.* The following organisms are usually susceptible: *Escherichia coli, Klebsiella* species, *Enterobacter* species, *Morganella morganii, Proteus mirabilis,* indole-positive *Proteus* species including *Proteus vulgaris, Haemophilus influenzae* (including ampicillin-resistant strains), *Streptococcus pneumoniae, Shigella flexneri* and *Shigella sonnei.* It should be noted, however, that there are little clinical data on the use of Bactrim I.V. Infusion in serious systemic infections due to *Haemophilus influenzae* and *Streptococcus pneumoniae.*
[See table on next page.]
The recommended quantitative disc susceptibility method may be used for estimating the susceptibility of bacteria to Bactrim.[3,4] With this procedure, a report from the laboratory of "Susceptible to trimethoprim and sulfamethoxazole" indicates that the infection is likely to respond to therapy with Bactrim. If the infection is confined to the urine, a report of "Intermediate susceptibility to trimethoprim and sulfamethoxazole" also indicates that the infection is likely to respond. A report of "Resistant to trimethoprim and sulfamethoxazole" indicates that the infection is unlikely to respond to therapy with Bactrim.

INDICATIONS AND USAGE

PNEUMOCYSTIS CARINII PNEUMONIA: Bactrim I.V. Infusion is indicated in the treatment of *Pneumocystis carinii* pneumonia in children and adults.
SHIGELLOSIS: Bactrim I.V. Infusion is indicated in the treatment of enteritis caused by susceptible strains of *Shigella flexneri* and *Shigella sonnei* in children and adults.
URINARY TRACT INFECTIONS: Bactrim I.V. Infusion is indicated in the treatment of severe or complicated urinary tract infections due to susceptible strains of *Escherichia coli, Klebsiella* species, *Enterobacter* species, *Morganella morganii* and *Proteus* species when oral administration of Bactrim is not feasible and when the organism is not susceptible to single-agent antibacterials effective in the urinary tract.
Although appropriate culture and susceptibility studies should be performed, therapy may be started while awaiting the results of these studies.

CONTRAINDICATIONS

Hypersensitivity to trimethoprim or sulfonamides. Patients with documented megaloblastic anemia due to folate deficiency. Pregnancy at term and during the nursing period, because sulfonamides pass the placenta and are excreted in the milk and may cause kernicterus. Infants less than two months of age.

WARNINGS

FATALITIES ASSOCIATED WITH THE ADMINISTRATION OF SULFONAMIDES, ALTHOUGH RARE, HAVE OCCURRED DUE TO SEVERE REACTIONS, INCLUDING STEVENS-JOHNSON SYNDROME, TOXIC EPIDERMAL NE-

Continued on next page

Roche Laboratories—Cont.

CROLYSIS, FULMINANT HEPATIC NECROSIS, AGRANULOCYTOSIS, APLASTIC ANEMIA AND OTHER BLOOD DYCRASIAS.

BACTRIM SHOULD BE DISCONTINUED AT THE FIRST APPEARANCE OF SKIN RASH OR ANY SIGN OF ADVERSE REACTION. Clinical signs, such as rash, sore throat, fever, arthralgia, cough, shortness of breath, pallor, purpura or jaundice may be early indications of serious reactions. In rare instances a skin rash may be followed by more severe reactions, such as Stevens-Johnson syndrome, toxic epidermal necrolysis, hepatic necrosis or serious blood disorder. Complete blood counts should be done frequently in patients receiving sulfonamides.

BACTRIM SHOULD NOT BE USED IN THE TREATMENT OF STREPTOCOCCAL PHARYNGITIS. Clinical studies have documented that patients with group A β-hemolytic streptococcal tonsillopharyngitis have a greater incidence of bacteriologic failure when treated with Bactrim than do those patients treated with penicillin, as evidenced by failure to eradicate this organism from the tonsillopharyngeal area.

Bactrim I.V. Infusion contains sodium metabisulfite, a sulfite that may cause allergic-type reactions, including anaphylactic symptoms and life-threatening or less severe asthmatic episodes in certain susceptible people. The overall prevalence of sulfite sensitivity in the general population is unknown and probably low. Sulfite sensitivity is seen more frequently in asthmatic than in nonasthmatic people.

PRECAUTIONS

General: Bactrim should be given with caution to patients with impaired renal or hepatic function, to those with possible folate deficiency (*e.g.,* the elderly, chronic alcoholics, patients receiving anticonvulsant therapy, patients with malabsorption syndrome, and patients in malnutrition states) and to those with severe allergies or bronchial asthma. In glucose-6-phosphate dehydrogenase deficient individuals, hemolysis may occur. This reaction is frequently dose-related.

Local irritation and inflammation due to extravascular infiltration of the infusion have been observed with Bactrim I.V. Infusion. If these occur the infusion should be discontinued and restarted at another site.

Use in the Elderly: There may be an increased risk of severe adverse reactions in elderly patients, particularly when complicating conditions exist, *e.g.,* impaired kidney and/or liver function, or concomitant use of other drugs. Severe skin reactions, generalized bone marrow suppression (see WARNINGS and ADVERSE REACTIONS sections) or a specific decrease in platelets (with or without purpura) are the most frequently reported severe adverse reactions in elderly patients. In those concurrently receiving certain diuretics, primarily thiazides, an increased incidence of thrombocytopenia with purpura has been reported. Appropriate dosage adjustments should be made for patients with impaired kidney function (see DOSAGE AND ADMINISTRATION section).

Use in the Treatment of Pneumocystis Carinii Pneumonia in Patients with Acquired Immunodeficiency Syndrome (AIDS): AIDS patients may not tolerate or respond to Bactrim in the same manner as non-AIDS patients. The incidence of side effects, particularly rash, fever, leukopenia, and elevated aminotransferase (transaminase) values, with Bactrim therapy in AIDS patients who are being treated for *Pneumocystis carinii* pneumonia has been reported to be greatly increased compared with the incidence normally associated with the use of Bactrim in non-AIDS patients.

Laboratory Tests: Appropriate culture and susceptibility studies should be performed before and throughout treatment. Complete blood counts should be done frequently in patients receiving Bactrim; if a significant reduction in the count of any formed blood element is noted, Bactrim should be discontinued. Urinalyses with careful microscopic examination and renal function tests should be performed during therapy, particularly for those patients with impaired renal function.

Drug Interactions: In elderly patients concurrently receiving certain diuretics, primarily thiazides, an increased incidence of thrombocytopenia with purpura has been reported.

It has been reported that Bactrim may prolong the prothrombin time in patients who are receiving the anticoagulant warfarin. This interaction should be kept in mind when Bactrim is given to patients already on anticoagulant therapy, and the coagulation time should be reassessed.

Bactrim may inhibit the hepatic metabolism of phenytoin. Bactrim, given at a common clinical dosage, increased the phenytoin half-life by 39% and decreased the phenytoin metabolic clearance rate by 27%. When administering these drugs concurrently, one should be alert for possible excessive phenytoin effect.

Sulfonamides can also displace methotrexate from plasma protein binding sites, thus increasing free methotrexate concentrations.

Drug/Laboratory Test Interactions: Bactrim, specifically the trimethoprim component, can interfere with a serum methotrexate assay as determined by the competitive binding protein technique (CBPA) when a bacterial dihydrofolate reductase is used as the binding protein. No interference occurs, however, if methotrexate is measured by a radioimmunoassay (RIA).

The presence of trimethoprim and sulfamethoxazole may also interfere with the Jaffé alkaline picrate reaction assay for creatinine, resulting in overestimations of about 10% in the range of normal values.

Carcinogenesis, Mutagenesis, Impairment of Fertility:

Carcinogenesis: Long-term studies in animals to evaluate carcinogenic potential have not been conducted with Bactrim I.V. Infusion.

Mutagenesis: Bacterial mutagenic studies have not been performed with sulfamethoxazole and trimethoprim in combination. Trimethoprim was demonstrated to be nonmutagenic in the Ames assay. No chromosomal damage was observed in human leukocytes cultured *in vitro* with sulfamethoxazole and trimethoprim alone or in combination; the concentrations used exceeded blood levels of these compounds following therapy with Bactrim. Observations of leukocytes obtained from patients treated with Bactrim revealed no chromosomal abnormalities.

Impairment of Fertility: Bactrim I.V. Infusion has not been studied in animals for evidence of impairment of fertility. However, studies in rats at oral dosages as high as 70 mg/kg trimethoprim plus 350 mg/kg sulfamethoxazole daily showed no adverse effects on fertility or general reproductive performance.

Pregnancy: Teratogenic Effects: Pregnancy Category C. In rats, oral doses of 533 mg/kg sulfamethoxazole or 200 mg/kg trimethoprim produced teratological effects manifested mainly as cleft palates.

The highest dose which did not cause cleft palates in rats was 512 mg/kg sulfamethoxazole or 192 mg/kg trimethoprim when administered separately. In two studies in rats, no teratology was observed when 512 mg/kg of sulfamethoxazole was used in combination with 128 mg/kg of trimethoprim. In one study, however, cleft palates were observed in one litter out of 9 when 355 mg/kg of sulfamethoxazole was used in combination with 88 mg/kg of trimethoprim.

In some rabbit studies, an overall increase in fetal loss (dead and resorbed and malformed conceptuses) was associated with doses of trimethoprim 6 times the human therapeutic dose.

While there are no large, well-controlled studies on the use of trimethoprim and sulfamethoxazole in pregnant women, Brumfitt and Pursell,[5] in a retrospective study, reported the outcome of 186 pregnancies during which the mother received either placebo or oral trimethoprim and sulfamethoxazole. The incidence of congenital abnormalities was 4.5% (3 of 66) in those who received placebo and 3.3% (4 of 120) in those receiving trimethoprim and sulfamethoxazole. There were no abnormalities in the 10 children whose mothers received the drug during the first trimester. In a separate survey, Brumfitt and Pursell also found no congenital abnormalities in 35 children whose mothers had received oral trimethoprim and sulfamethoxazole at the time of conception or shortly thereafter.

Because trimethoprim and sulfamethoxazole may interfere with folic acid metabolism, Bactrim I.V. Infusion should be used during pregnancy only if the potential benefit justifies the potential risk to the fetus.

Nonteratogenic Effects: See CONTRAINDICATIONS section.

Nursing Mothers: See CONTRAINDICATIONS section.

Pediatric Use: Bactrim I.V. Infusion is not recommended for infants younger than two months of age (see CONTRAINDICATIONS section).

ADVERSE REACTIONS

The most common adverse effects are gastrointestinal disturbances (nausea, vomiting, anorexia) and allergic skin reactions (such as rash and urticaria). **FATALITIES ASSOCIATED WITH THE ADMINISTRATION OF SULFONAMIDES, ALTHOUGH RARE, HAVE OCCURRED DUE TO SEVERE REACTIONS, INCLUDING STEVENS-JOHNSON SYNDROME, TOXIC EPIDERMAL NECROLYSIS, FULMINANT HEPATIC NECROSIS, AGRANULOCYTOSIS, APLASTIC ANEMIA AND OTHER BLOOD DYSCRASIAS (SEE WARNINGS SECTION).** Local reaction, pain and slight irritation on I.V. administration are infrequent. Thrombophlebitis has rarely been observed.

Hematologic: Agranulocytosis, aplastic anemia, thrombocytopenia, leukopenia, neutropenia, hemolytic anemia, megaloblastic anemia, hypoprothrombinemia, methemoglobinemia, eosinophilia.

Allergic Reactions: Stevens-Johnson syndrome, toxic epidermal necrolysis, anaphylaxis, allergic myocarditis, erythema multiforme, exfoliative dermatitis, angioedema, drug fever, chills, Henoch-Schoenlein purpura, serum sickness-like syndrome, generalized allergic reactions, generalized skin eruptions, conjunctival and scleral injection, photosensitivity, pruritus, urticaria and rash. In addition, periarteritis nodosa and systemic lupus erythematosus have been reported.

Gastrointestinal: Hepatitis (including cholestatic jaundice and hepatic necrosis), elevation of serum transaminase and bilirubin, pseudomembraneous enterocolitis, pancreatitis, stomatitis, glossitis, nausea, emesis, abdominal pain, diarrhea, anorexia.

Genitourinary: Renal failure, interstitial nephritis, BUN and serum creatinine elevation, toxic nephrosis with oliguria and anuria, and crystalluria.

Neurologic: Aseptic meningitis, convulsions, peripheral neuritis, ataxia, vertigo, tinnitus, headache.

Psychiatric: Hallucinations, depression, apathy, nervousness.

Endocrine: The sulfonamides bear certain chemical similarities to some goitrogens, diuretics (acetazolamide and the thiazides) and oral hypoglycemic agents. Cross-sensitivity may exist with these agents. Diuresis and hypoglycemia have occurred rarely in patients receiving sulfonamides.

Musculoskeletal: Arthralgia and myalgia.

Respiratory: Pulmonary infiltrates.

Miscellaneous: Weakness, fatigue, insomnia.

OVERDOSAGE

Acute: Since there has been no extensive experience in humans with single doses of Bactrim I.V. Infusion in excess of 25 mL (400 mg trimethoprim and 2000 mg sulfamethoxazole), the maximum tolerated dose in humans is unknown. Signs and symptoms of overdosage reported with sulfonamides include anorexia, colic, nausea, vomiting, dizziness, headache, drowsiness and unconsciousness. Pyrexia, hematuria and crystalluria may be noted. Blood dyscrasias and jaundice are potential late manifestations of overdosage.

Signs of acute overdosage with trimethoprim include nausea, vomiting, dizziness, headache, mental depression, confusion and bone marrow depression.

General principles of treatment include the administration of intraveneous fluids if urine output is low and renal function is normal. Acidification of the urine will increase renal elimination of trimethoprim. The patient should be monitored with blood counts and appropriate blood chemistries, including electrolytes. If a significant blood dyscrasia or jaundice occurs, specific therapy should be instituted for these complications. Peritoneal dialysis is not effective and hemodialysis is only moderately effective in eliminating trimethoprim and sulfamethoxazole.

Chronic: Use of Bactrim I.V. Infusion at high doses and/or for extended periods of time may cause bone marrow depression manifested as thrombocytopenia, leukopenia and/or megaloblastic anemia. If signs of bone marrow depression occur, the patient should be given leucovorin 5 to 15 mg daily until normal hematopoiesis is restored.

Animal Toxicity: The LD_{50} of Bactrim I.V. Infusion in mice is 700 mg/kg or 7.3 mL/kg; in rats and rabbits the LD_{50} is

REPRESENTATIVE MINIMUM INHIBITORY CONCENTRATION VALUES FOR BACTRIM-SUSCEPTIBLE ORGANISMS (MIC—μg/mL)

Bacteria	TMP alone	SMX alone	TMP/SMX (1:20) TMP	TMP/SMX (1:20) SMX
Escherichia coli	0.05–1.5	1.0–245	0.05–0.5	0.95–9.5
Proteus species (indole positive)	0.5–5.0	7.35–300	0.05–1.5	0.95–28.5
Morganella morganii	0.5–5.0	7.35–300	0.05–1.5	0.95–28.5
Proteus mirabilis	0.5–1.5	7.35–30	0.05–0.15	0.95–2.85
Klebsiella species	0.15–5.0	2.45–245	0.05–1.5	0.95–28.5
Enterobacter species	0.15–5.0	2.45–245	0.05–1.5	0.95–28.5
Haemophilus influenzae	0.15–1.5	2.85–95	0.015–0.15	0.285–2.85
Streptococcus pneumoniae	0.15–1.5	7.35–24.5	0.05–0.15	0.95–2.85
*Shigella flexneri**	<0.01–0.04	<0.16–>320	<0.002–0.03	0.04–0.625
*Shigella sonnei**	0.02–0.08	0.625–>320	0.004–0.06	0.08–1.25

TMP = trimethoprim SMX = sulfamethoxazole

*Rudoy RC, Nelson JD, Haltalin KC: *Antimicrob Agents Chemother* 5:439–443, May 1974.

> 500 mg/kg or > 5.2 mL/kg. The vehicle produced the same LD_{50} in each of these species as the active drug.
The signs and symptoms noted in mice, rats and rabbits with Bactrim I.V. Infusion or its vehicle at the high I.V. doses used in acute toxicity studies included ataxia, decreased motor activity, loss of righting reflex, tremors or convulsions, and/or respiratory depression.

DOSAGE AND ADMINISTRATION

CONTRAINDICATED IN INFANTS LESS THAN TWO MONTHS OF AGE. CAUTION—BACTRIM I.V. INFUSION MUST BE DILUTED IN 5% DEXTROSE IN WATER SOLUTION PRIOR TO ADMINISTRATION. DO NOT MIX BACTRIM I.V. INFUSION WITH OTHER DRUGS OR SOLUTIONS. RAPID INFUSION OR BOLUS INJECTION MUST BE AVOIDED.
DOSAGE:
Children and Adults:
PNEUMOCYSTIS CARINII PNEUMONIA: Total daily dose is 15 to 20 mg/kg (based on the trimethoprim component) given in three or four equally divided doses every 6 to 8 hours for up to 14 days. One investigator noted that a total daily dose of 10 to 15 mg/kg was sufficient in ten adult patients with normal renal function.[6]
SEVERE URINARY TRACT INFECTIONS AND SHIGELLOSIS: Total daily dose is 8 to 10 mg/kg (based on the trimethoprim component) given in two to four equally divided doses every 6, 8 or 12 hours for up to 14 days for severe urinary tract infections and 5 days for shigellosis. The maximum recommended daily dose is 60 mL per day.
For Patients with Impaired Renal Function: When renal function is impaired, a reduced dosage should be employed using the following table:

Creatinine Clearance (mL/min)	Recommended Dosage Regimen
Above 30	Usual standard regimen
15–30	½ the usual regimen
Below 15	Use not recommended

Method of Preparation: Bactrim I.V. Infusion must be diluted. EACH 5 ML SHOULD BE ADDED TO 125 ML OF 5% DEXTROSE IN WATER. After diluting with 5% dextrose in water the solution should not be refrigerated and should be used within 6 hours. If a dilution of 5 mL per 100 mL of 5% dextrose in water is desired, it should be used within 4 hours. If upon visual inspection there is cloudiness or evidence of crystallization after mixing, the solution should be discarded and a fresh solution prepared.
Multidose Vials: After initial entry into the vial, the remaining contents must be used within 48 hours.
The following infusion systems have been tested and found satisfactory: unit-dose glass containers; unit-dose polyvinyl chloride and polyolefin containers. No other systems have been tested and therefore no others can be recommended.
Dilution: EACH 5 ML OF BACTRIM I.V. INFUSION SHOULD BE ADDED TO 125 ML OF 5% DEXTROSE IN WATER.
NOTE: *In those instances where fluid restriction is desirable,* each 5 mL may be added to 75 mL of 5% dextrose in water. Under these circumstances the solution should be mixed just prior to use and should be administered within two (2) hours. If upon visual inspection there is cloudiness or evidence of crystallization after mixing, the solution should be discarded and a fresh solution prepared.
DO NOT MIX BACTRIM I.V. INFUSION–5% DEXTROSE IN WATER WITH DRUGS OR SOLUTIONS IN THE SAME CONTAINER.
ADMINISTRATION: The solution should be given by intravenous infusion over a period of 60 to 90 minutes. Rapid infusion or bolus injection must be avoided. Bactrim I.V. Infusion should not be given intramuscularly.

HOW SUPPLIED

5-mL *ampuls,* containing 80 mg trimethoprim (16 mg/mL) and 400 mg sulfamethoxazole (80 mg/mL) for infusion with 5% dextrose in water. Boxes of 10 (NDC 0004-1943-06).
5-mL *vials,* containing 80 mg trimethoprim (16 mg/mL) and 400 mg sulfamethoxazole (80 mg/mL) for infusion with 5% dextrose in water. Boxes of 10 (NDC 0004-1956-01).
10-mL *vials,* containing 160 mg trimethoprim (16 mg/mL) and 800 mg sulfamethoxazole (80 mg/mL) for infusion with 5% dextrose in water. Boxes of 10 (NDC 0004-1955-01).
30-mL *multidose vials,* each 5 mL containing 80 mg trimethoprim (16 mg/mL) and 400 mg sulfamethoxazole (80 mg/mL) for infusion with 5% dextrose in water. Boxes of 1 (NDC 0004-1958-01).
STORE AT ROOM TEMPERATURE (15°–30°C or 59°–86°F). DO NOT REFRIGERATE.
Bactrim is also available as *DS (double strength) Tablets* (white, notched, capsule shaped), containing 160 mg trimethoprim and 800 mg sulfamethoxazole—bottles of 100 (NDC 0004-0117-01), 250 (NDC 0004-0117-04) and 500 (NDC 0004-0117-14); Tel-E-Dose® packages of 100 (NDC 0004-0117-49); Prescription Paks of 20 (NDC 0004-0117-54). Imprint on tablets: (front) BACTRIM-DS; (back) ROCHE.
Tablets (light green, scored, capsule shaped), containing 80 mg trimethoprim and 400 mg sulfamethoxazole—bottles of 100 (NDC 0004-0050-01); Tel-E-Dose® packages of 100 (NDC 0004-0050-49); Prescription Paks of 40 (NDC 0004-0050-34). Imprint on tablets: (front) BACTRIM; (back) ROCHE.
Pediatric Suspension (pink, cherry flavored), containing 40 mg trimethoprim and 200 mg sulfamethoxazole per teaspoonful (5 mL)—bottles of 100 mL (NDC 0004-1033-01) and 16 oz (1 pint) (NDC 0004-1033-28).
Suspension (pink, fruit-licorice flavored), containing 40 mg trimethoprim and 200 mg sulfamethoxazole per teaspoonful (5 mL)—bottles of 16 oz (1 pint) (NDC 0004-1015-28).

REFERENCES

1. Grose WE, Bodey GP, Loo TL: Clinical Pharmacology of Intravenously Administered Trimethoprim-Sulfamethoxazole. *Antimicrob Agents Chemother 15*:447-451, Mar 1979. 2. Siber GR, Gorham C, Durbin W, Lesko L, Levin MJ: Pharmacology of Intravenous Trimethoprim-Sulfamethoxazole in Children and Adults. *Current Chemotherapy and Infectious Diseases,* American Society for Microbiology, Washington, D.C., 1980, Vol. 1, pp. 691-692. 3. Bauer AW, Kirby WMM, Sherris JC, Turck M: Antibiotic Susceptibility Testing by a Standardized Single Disk Method. *Am J Clin Pathol 45*:493-496, Apr 1966. 4. Approved Standard ASM-2 Performance Standards for Antimicrobial Disc Susceptibility Test: National Committee for Clinical Laboratory Standards, 771 East Lancaster Avenue, Villanova, Pennsylvania 19085. 5. Brumfitt W, Pursell R: Trimethoprim/Sulfamethoxazole in the Treatment of Bacteriuria in Women. *J Infect Dis 128* (Suppl): S657-S663, Nov 1973. 6. Winston DJ, Lau WK, Gale RP, Young LS: Trimethoprim-Sulfamethoxazole for the Treatment of *Pneumocystis carinii* pneumonia. *Ann Intern Med 92*:762-769, June 1980.
Revised: June 1992

BACTRIM™ ℞

[*bac 'trim*]
(trimethoprim and sulfamethoxazole/Roche)
DS (double strength) Tablets
Tablets
Suspension
and
Pediatric Suspension

The following text is complete prescribing information based on official labeling in effect June 1, 1992.

DESCRIPTION

Bactrim (trimethoprim and sulfamethoxazole) is a synthetic antibacterial combination product available in DS (double strength) tablets, tablets, pediatric suspension and suspension for oral administration. Each DS tablet contains 160 mg trimethoprim and 800 mg sulfamethoxazole plus magnesium stearate, pregelatinized starch and sodium starch glycolate. Each tablet contains 80 mg trimethoprim and 400 mg sulfamethoxazole plus magnesium stearate, pregelatinized starch, sodium starch glycolate, FD&C Blue No. 1 lake, FD&C Yellow No. 6 lake and D&C Yellow No. 10 lake. Each teaspoonful (5 mL) of the pediatric suspension or suspension contains 40 mg trimethoprim and 200 mg sulfamethoxazole in a vehicle containing 0.3 percent alcohol, edetate disodium, glycerin, microcrystalline cellulose, parabens (methyl and propyl), polysorbate 80, saccharin sodium, simethicone, sorbitol, sucrose, FD&C Yellow No. 6, FD&C Red No. 40, flavors and water.
Trimethoprim is 2,4-diamino-5-(3,4,5-trimethoxybenzyl) pyrimidine. It is a white to light yellow, odorless, bitter compound with a molecular weight of 290.3.
Sulfamethoxazole is N^1-(5-methyl-3-isoxazolyl) sulfanilamide. It is an almost white, odorless, tasteless compound with a molecular weight of 253.28.

CLINICAL PHARMACOLOGY

Bactrim is rapidly absorbed following oral administration. Both sulfamethoxazole and trimethoprim exist in the blood as unbound, protein-bound and metabolized forms; sulfamethoxazole also exists as the conjugated form. The metabolism of sulfamethoxazole occurs predominately by N_4-acetylation, although the glucuronide conjugate has been identified. The principal metabolites of trimethoprim are the 1- and 3-oxides and the 3'- and 4'-hydroxy derivatives. The free forms of sulfamethoxazole and trimethoprim are considered to be the therapeutically active forms. Approximately 44% of trimethoprim and 70% of sulfamethoxazole are bound to plasma proteins. The presence of 10 mg percent sulfamethoxazole in plasma decreases the protein binding of trimethoprim by an insignificant degree; trimethoprim does not influence the protein binding of sulfamethoxazole.
Peak blood levels for the individual components occur 1 to 4 hours after oral administration. The mean serum half-lives of sulfamethoxazole and trimethoprim are 10 and 8 to 10 hours, respectively. However, patients with severely impaired renal function exhibit an increase in the half-lives of both components, requiring dosage regimen adjustment (see DOSAGE AND ADMINISTRATION section). Detectable amounts of trimethoprim and sulfamethoxazole are present in the blood 24 hours after drug administration. During administration of 160 mg trimethoprim and 800 mg sulfamethoxazole *b.i.d.,* the mean steady-state plasma concentration of trimethoprim was 1.72 μg/mL. The steady-state mean plasma levels of free and total sulfamethoxazole were 57.4 μg/mL and 68.0 μg/mL, respectively. These steady-state levels were achieved after three days of drug administration.[1]
Excretion of sulfamethoxazole and trimethoprim is primarily by the kidneys through both glomerular filtration and tubular secretion. Urine concentrations of both sulfamethoxazole and trimethoprim are considerably higher than are the concentrations in the blood. The average percentage of the dose recovered in urine from 0 to 72 hours after a single oral dose of Bactrim is 84.5% for total sulfonamide and 66.8% for free trimethoprim. Thirty percent of the total sulfonamide is excreted as free sulfamethoxazole, with the remaining as N_4-acetylated metabolite.[2] When administered together as Bactrim, neither sulfamethoxazole nor trimethoprim affects the urinary excretion pattern of the other.
Both trimethoprim and sulfamethoxazole distribute to sputum, vaginal fluid and middle ear fluid; trimethoprim also distributes to bronchial secretion, and both pass the placental barrier and are excreted in breast milk.
Microbiology: Sulfamethoxazole inhibits bacterial synthesis of dihydrofolic acid by competing with *para*-aminobenzoic acid (PABA). Trimethoprim blocks the production of tetrahydrofolic acid from dihydrofolic acid by binding to and reversibly inhibiting the required enzyme, dihydrofolate reductase. Thus, Bactrim blocks two consecutive steps in the biosynthesis of nucleic acids and proteins essential to many bacteria.
In vitro studies have shown that bacterial resistance develops more slowly with Bactrim than with either trimethoprim or sulfamethoxazole alone.
In vitro serial dilution tests have shown that the spectrum of antibacterial activity of Bactrim includes the common urinary tract pathogens with the exception of *Pseudomonas aeruginosa.* The following organisms are usually susceptible: *Escherichia coli, Klebsiella* species, *Enterobacter* species, *Morganella morganii, Proteus mirabilis,* and indole-positive *Proteus* species including *Proteus vulgaris.* The usual spectrum of antimicrobial activity of Bactrim includes the following bacterial pathogens isolated from middle ear exudate and from bronchial secretions: *Haemophilus influenzae,* including ampicillin-resistant strains, and *Streptococcus pneumoniae. Shigella flexneri* and *Shigella sonnei* are usually susceptible. The usual spectrum also includes enterotoxigenic strains of *Escherichia coli* (ETEC) causing bacterial gastroenteritis.
[See table on next page.]
The recommended quantitative disc susceptibility method may be used for estimating the susceptibility of bacteria to Bactrim.[3,4] With this procedure, a report from the laboratory of "Susceptible to trimethoprim and sulfamethoxazole" indicates that the infection is likely to respond to therapy with Bactrim. If the infection is confined to the urine, a report of "Intermediate susceptibility to trimethoprim and sulfamethoxazole" also indicates that the infection is likely to respond. A report of "Resistant to trimethoprim and sulfamethoxazole" indicates that the infection is unlikely to respond to therapy with Bactrim.

INDICATIONS AND USAGE

URINARY TRACT INFECTIONS: For the treatment of urinary tract infections due to susceptible strains of the following organisms: *Escherichia coli, Klebsiella* species, *Enterobacter* species, *Morganella morganii, Proteus mirabilis* and *Proteus vulgaris.* It is recommended that initial episodes of uncomplicated urinary tract infections be treated with a single effective antibacterial agent rather than the combination.
ACUTE OTITIS MEDIA: For the treatment of acute otitis media in children due to susceptible strains of *Streptococcus pneumoniae* or *Haemophilus influenzae* when in the judgment of the physician Bactrim offers some advantage over the use of other antimicrobial agents. To date, there are limited data on the safety of repeated use of Bactrim in children under two years of age. Bactrim is not indicated for prophylactic or prolonged administration in otitis media at any age.
ACUTE EXACERBATIONS OF CHRONIC BRONCHITIS IN ADULTS: For the treatment of acute exacerbations of chronic bronchitis due to susceptible strains of *Streptococcus pneumoniae* or *Haemophilus influenzae* when in the judgment of the physician Bactrim offers some advantage over the use of a single antimicrobial agent.
SHIGELLOSIS: For the treatment of enteritis caused by susceptible strains of *Shigella flexneri* and *Shigella sonnei* when antibacterial therapy is indicated.

Continued on next page

Roche Laboratories—Cont.

PNEUMOCYSTIS CARINII PNEUMONIA: For the treatment of documented *Pneumocystis carinii* pneumonia.
TRAVELERS' DIARRHEA IN ADULTS: For the treatment of travelers' diarrhea due to susceptible strains of enterotoxigenic *E. coli.*

CONTRAINDICATIONS

Hypersensitivity to trimethoprim or sulfonamides. Patients with documented megaloblastic anemia due to folate deficiency. Pregnancy at term and during the nursing period, because sulfonamides pass the placenta and are excreted in the milk and may cause kernicterus. Infants less than two months of age.

WARNINGS

FATALITIES ASSOCIATED WITH THE ADMINISTRATION OF SULFONAMIDES, ALTHOUGH RARE, HAVE OCCURRED DUE TO SEVERE REACTIONS, INCLUDING STEVENS-JOHNSON SYNDROME, TOXIC EPIDERMAL NECROLYSIS, FULMINANT HEPATIC NECROSIS, AGRANULOCYTOSIS, APLASTIC ANEMIA AND OTHER BLOOD DYSCRASIAS.

BACTRIM SHOULD BE DISCONTINUED AT THE FIRST APPEARANCE OF SKIN RASH OR ANY SIGN OF ADVERSE REACTION. Clinical signs, such as rash, sore throat, fever, arthralgia, cough, shortness of breath, pallor, purpura or jaundice may be early indications of serious reactions. In rare instances a skin rash may be followed by more severe reactions, such as Stevens-Johnson syndrome, toxic epidermal necrolysis, hepatic necrosis or serious blood disorder. Complete blood counts should be done frequently in patients receiving sulfonamides.

BACTRIM SHOULD NOT BE USED IN THE TREATMENT OF STREPTOCOCCAL PHARYNGITIS. Clinical studies have documented that patients with group A β-hemolytic streptococcal tonsillopharyngitis have a greater incidence of bacteriologic failure when treated with Bactrim than do those patients treated with penicillin, as evidenced by failure to eradicate this organism from the tonsillopharyngeal area.

PRECAUTIONS

General: Bactrim should be given with caution to patients with impaired renal or hepatic function, to those with possible folate deficiency (*e.g.,* the elderly, chronic alcoholics, patients receiving anticonvulsant therapy, patients with malabsorption syndrome, and patients in malnutrition states) and to those with severe allergies or bronchial asthma. In glucose-6-phosphate dehydrogenase deficient individuals, hemolysis may occur. This reaction is frequently dose-related.

Use in the Elderly: There may be an increased risk of severe adverse reactions in elderly patients, particularly when complicating conditions exist, *e.g.,* impaired kidney and/or liver function, or concomitant use of other drugs. Severe skin reactions, generalized bone marrow suppression (see WARNINGS and ADVERSE REACTIONS sections) or a specific decrease in platelets (with or without purpura) are the most frequently reported severe adverse reactions in elderly patients. In those concurrently receiving certain diuretics, primarily thiazides, an increased incidence of thrombocytopenia with purpura has been reported. Appropriate dosage adjustments should be made for patients with impaired kidney function (see DOSAGE AND ADMINISTRATION section).

Use in the Treatment of Pneumocystis Carinii Pneumonia in Patients with Acquired Immunodeficiency Syndrome (AIDS): AIDS patients may not tolerate or respond to Bactrim in the same manner as non-AIDS patients. The incidence of side effects, particularly rash, fever, leukopenia and elevated aminotransferase (transaminase) values, with Bactrim therapy in AIDS patients who are being treated for *Pneumocystis carinii* pneumonia has been reported to be greatly increased compared with the incidence normally associated with the use of Bactrim in non-AIDS patients.

Information for Patients: Patients should be instructed to maintain an adequate fluid intake in order to prevent crystalluria and stone formation.

Laboratory Tests: Complete blood counts should be done frequently in patients receiving Bactrim; if a significant reduction in the count of any formed blood element is noted, Bactrim should be discontinued. Urinalyses with careful microscopic examination and renal function tests should be performed during therapy, particularly for those patients with impaired renal function.

Drug Interactions: In elderly patients concurrently receiving certain diuretics, primarily thiazides, an increased incidence of thrombocytopenia with purpura has been reported. It has been reported that Bactrim may prolong the prothrombin time in patients who are receiving the anticoagulant warfarin. This interaction should be kept in mind when Bactrim is given to patients already on anticoagulant therapy, and the coagulation time should be reassessed.

Bactrim may inhibit the hepatic metabolism of phenytoin. Bactrim, given at a common clinical dosage, increased the phenytoin half-life by 39% and decreased the phenytoin metabolic clearance rate by 27%. When administering these drugs concurrently, one should be alert for possible excessive phenytoin effect.

Sulfonamides can also displace methotrexate from plasma protein binding sites, thus increasing free methotrexate concentrations.

Drug/Laboratory Test Interactions: Bactrim, specifically the trimethoprim component, can interfere with a serum methotrexate assay as determined by the competitive binding protein technique (CBPA) when a bacterial dihydrofolate reductase is used as the binding protein. No interference occurs, however, if methotrexate is measured by a radioimmunoassay (RIA).

The presence of trimethoprim and sulfamethoxazole may also interfere with the Jaffé alkaline picrate reaction assay for creatinine, resulting in overestimations of about 10% in the range of normal values.

Carcinogenesis, Mutagenesis, Impairment of Fertility:
Carcinogenesis: Long-term studies in animals to evaluate carcinogenic potential have not been conducted with Bactrim.

Mutagenesis: Bacterial mutagenic studies have not been performed with sulfamethoxazole and trimethoprim in combination. Trimethoprim was demonstrated to be nonmutagenic in the Ames assay. No chromosomal damage was observed in human leukocytes *in vitro* with sulfamethoxazole and trimethoprim alone or in combination; the concentrations used exceeded blood levels of these compounds following therapy with Bactrim. Observations of leukocytes obtained from patients treated with Bactrim revealed no chromosomal abnormalities.

Impairment of Fertility: No adverse effects on fertility or general reproductive performance were observed in rats given oral dosages as high as 70 mg/kg/day trimethoprim plus 350 mg/kg/day sulfamethoxazole.

Pregnancy: Teratogenic Effects: Pregnancy Category C. In rats, oral doses of 533 mg/kg sulfamethoxazole or 200 mg/kg trimethoprim produced teratologic effects manifested mainly as cleft palates.

The highest dose which did not cause cleft palates in rats was 512 mg/kg sulfamethoxazole or 192 mg/kg trimethoprim when administered separately. In two studies in rats, no teratology was observed when 512 mg/kg of sulfamethoxazole was used in combination with 128 mg/kg of trimethoprim. In one study, however, cleft palates were observed in one litter out of 9 when 355 mg/kg of sulfamethoxazole was used in combination with 88 mg/kg of trimethoprim.

In some rabbit studies, an overall increase in fetal loss (dead and resorbed and malformed conceptuses) was associated with doses of trimethoprim 6 times the human therapeutic dose.

While there are no large, well-controlled studies on the use of trimethoprim and sulfamethoxazole in pregnant women, Brumfitt and Pursell,[5] in a retrospective study, reported the outcome of 186 pregnancies during which the mother received either placebo or trimethoprim and sulfamethoxazole. The incidence of congenital abnormalities was 4.5% (3 of 66) in those who received placebo and 3.3% (4 of 120) in those receiving trimethoprim and sulfamethoxazole. There were no abnormalities in the 10 children whose mothers received the drug during the first trimester. In a separate survey, Brumfitt and Pursell also found no congenital abnormalities in 35 children whose mothers had received oral trimethoprim and sulfamethoxazole at the time of conception or shortly thereafter.

Because trimethoprim and sulfamethoxazole may interfere with folic acid metabolism, Bactrim should be used during pregnancy only if the potential benefit justifies the potential risk to the fetus.

Nonteratogenic Effects: See CONTRAINDICATIONS section.

Nursing Mothers: See CONTRAINDICATIONS section.

Pediatric Use: Bactrim is not recommended for infants younger than two months of age (see INDICATIONS and CONTRAINDICATIONS sections).

ADVERSE REACTIONS

The most common adverse effects are gastrointestinal disturbances (nausea, vomiting, anorexia) and allergic skin reactions (such as rash and urticaria). **FATALITIES ASSOCIATED WITH THE ADMINISTRATION OF SULFONAMIDES, ALTHOUGH RARE, HAVE OCCURRED DUE TO SEVERE REACTIONS, INCLUDING STEVENS-JOHNSON SYNDROME, TOXIC EPIDERMAL NECROLYSIS, FULMINANT HEPATIC NECROSIS, AGRANULOCYTOSIS, APLASTIC ANEMIA AND OTHER BLOOD DYSCRASIAS (SEE WARNINGS SECTION).**

Hematologic: Agranulocytosis, aplastic anemia, thrombocytopenia, leukopenia, neutropenia, hemolytic anemia, megaloblastic anemia, hypoprothrombinemia, methemoglobinemia, eosinophilia.

Allergic Reactions: Stevens-Johnson syndrome, toxic epidermal necrolysis, anaphylaxis, allergic myocarditis, erythema multiforme, exfoliative dermatitis, angioedema, drug fever, chills, Henoch-Schoenlein purpura, serum sickness-like syndrome, generalized allergic reactions, generalized skin eruptions, photosensitivity, conjunctival and scleral injection, pruritus, urticaria and rash. In addition, periarteritis nodosa and systemic lupus erythematosus have been reported.

Gastrointestinal: Hepatitis (including cholestatic jaundice and hepatic necrosis), elevation of serum transaminase and bilirubin, pseudomembranous enterocolitis, pancreatitis, stomatitis, glossitis, nausea, emesis, abdominal pain, diarrhea, anorexia.

Genitourinary: Renal failure, interstitial nephritis, BUN and serum creatinine elevation, toxic nephrosis with oliguria and anuria, and crystalluria.

Neurologic: Aseptic meningitis, convulsions, peripheral neuritis, ataxia, vertigo, tinnitus, headache.

Psychiatric: Hallucinations, depression, apathy, nervousness.

Endocrine: The sulfonamides bear certain chemical similarities to some goitrogens, diuretics (acetazolamide and the thiazides) and oral hypoglycemic agents. Cross-sensitivity may exist with these agents. Diuresis and hypoglycemia have occurred rarely in patients receiving sulfonamides.

Musculoskeletal: Arthralgia and myalgia.

Respiratory: Pulmonary infiltrates.

Miscellaneous: Weakness, fatigue, insomnia.

OVERDOSAGE

Acute: The amount of a single dose of Bactrim that is either associated with symptoms of overdosage or is likely to be life-threatening has not been reported. Signs and symptoms of overdosage reported with sulfonamides include anorexia, colic, nausea, vomiting, dizziness, headache, drowsiness and unconsciousness. Pyrexia, hematuria and crystalluria may be noted. Blood dyscrasias and jaundice are potential late manifestations of overdosage.

Signs of acute overdosage with trimethoprim include nausea, vomiting, dizziness, headache, mental depression, confusion and bone marrow depression.

General principles of treatment include the institution of gastric lavage or emesis, forcing oral fluids, and the administration of intravenous fluids if urine output is low and renal function is normal. Acidification of the urine will increase renal elimination of trimethoprim. The patient should be monitored with blood counts and appropriate blood chemistries, including electrolytes. If a significant blood dyscrasia or jaundice occurs, specific therapy should be instituted for

REPRESENTATIVE MINIMUM INHIBITORY CONCENTRATION VALUES FOR BACTRIM-SUSCEPTIBLE ORGANISMS
(MIC—μg/mL)

Bacteria	TMP alone	SMX alone	TMP/SMX (1:20) TMP	SMX
Escherichia coli	0.05–1.5	1.0–245	0.05–0.5	0.95–9.5
Escherichia coli (enterotoxigenic strains)	0.015–0.15	0.285–>950	0.005–0.15	0.095–2.85
Proteus species (indole positive)	0.5–5.0	7.35–300	0.05–1.5	0.95–28.5
Morganella morganii	0.5–5.0	7.35–300	0.05–1.5	0.95–28.5
Proteus mirabilis	0.5–1.5	7.35–30	0.05–0.15	0.95–2.85
Klebsiella species	0.15–5.0	2.45–245	0.05–1.5	0.95–28.5
Enterobacter species	0.15–5.0	2.45–245	0.05–1.5	0.95–28.5
Haemophilus influenzae	0.15–1.5	2.85–95	0.015–0.15	0.285–2.85
Streptococcus pneumoniae	0.15–1.5	7.35–24.5	0.05–0.15	0.95–2.85
*Shigella flexneri**	<0.01–0.04	<0.16–>320	<0.002–0.03	0.04–0.625
*Shigella sonnei**	0.02–0.08	0.625–>320	0.004–0.06	0.08–1.25

TMP = trimethoprim SMX = sulfamethoxazole
*Rudoy RC, Nelson JD, Haltalin KC: *Antimicrob Agents Chemother 5:* 439–443, May 1974.

these complications. Peritoneal dialysis is not effective and hemodialysis is only moderately effective in eliminating trimethoprim and sulfamethoxazole.

Chronic: Use of Bactrim at high doses and/or for extended periods of time may cause bone marrow depression manifested as thrombocytopenia, leukopenia and/or megaloblastic anemia. If signs of bone marrow depression occur, the patient should be given leucovorin 5 to 15 mg daily until normal hematopoiesis is restored.

DOSAGE AND ADMINISTRATION

Not recommended for use in infants less than two months of age.

URINARY TRACT INFECTIONS AND SHIGELLOSIS IN ADULTS AND CHILDREN, AND ACUTE OTITIS MEDIA IN CHILDREN:

Adults: The usual adult dosage in the treatment of urinary tract infections is one Bactrim DS (double strength) tablet, two Bactrim tablets or four teaspoonfuls (20 mL) of Bactrim Pediatric Suspension or Bactrim Suspension every 12 hours for 10 to 14 days. An identical daily dosage is used for 5 days in the treatment of shigellosis.

Children: The recommended dose for children with urinary tract infections or acute otitis media is 8 mg/kg trimethoprim and 40 mg/kg sulfamethoxazole per 24 hours, given in two divided doses every 12 hours for 10 days. An identical daily dosage is used for 5 days in the treatment of shigellosis. The following table is a guideline for the attainment of this dosage:

Children two months of age or older:

Weight		Dose—every 12 hours	
lb	kg	Teaspoonfuls	Tablets
22	10	1 teasp. (5 mL)	—
44	20	2 teasp. (10 mL)	1 tablet
66	30	3 teasp. (15 mL)	1½ tablets
88	40	4 teasp. (20 mL)	2 tablets or 1 DS tablet

For Patients with Impaired Renal Function: When renal function is impaired, a reduced dosage should be employed using the following table:

Creatinine Clearance (mL/min)	Recommended Dosage Regimen
Above 30	Usual standard regimen
15–30	½ the usual regimen
Below 15	Use not recommended

ACUTE EXACERBATIONS OF CHRONIC BRONCHITIS IN ADULTS:

The usual adult dosage in the treatment of acute exacerbations of chronic bronchitis is one Bactrim DS (double strength) tablet, two Bactrim tablets or four teaspoonfuls (20 mL) of Bactrim Pediatric Suspension or Bactrim Suspension every 12 hours for 14 days.

PNEUMOCYSTIS CARINII PNEUMONIA:

The recommended dosage for patients with documented *Pneumocystis carinii* pneumonia is 20 mg/kg trimethoprim and 100 mg/kg sulfamethoxazole per 24 hours given in equally divided doses every 6 hours for 14 days. The following table is a guideline for the attainment of this dosage in children:

Weight		Dose—every six hours	
lb	kg	Teaspoonfuls	Tablets
18	8	1 teasp. (5 mL)	—
35	16	2 teasp. (10 mL)	1 tablet
53	24	3 teasp. (15 mL)	1½ tablets
70	32	4 teasp. (20 mL)	2 tablets or 1 DS tablet

TRAVELERS' DIARRHEA IN ADULTS:

For the treatment of travelers' diarrhea, the usual adult dosage is one Bactrim DS (double strength) tablet; two Bactrim tablets or four teaspoonfuls (20 mL) of Bactrim Suspension or Pediatric Suspension every 12 hours for 5 days.

HOW SUPPLIED

DS (double strength) Tablets (white, notched, capsule shaped), containing 160 mg trimethoprim and 800 mg sulfamethoxazole—bottles of 100 (NDC 0004-0117-01), 250 (NDC 0004-0117-04), and 500 (NDC 0004-0117-14); Tel-E-Dose® packages of 100 (NDC 0004-0117-49); Prescription Paks of 20 (NDC 0004-0117-54). Imprint on tablets: (front) BACTRIM-DS; (back) ROCHE.

Tablets (light green, scored, capsule shaped), containing 80 mg trimethoprim and 400 mg sulfamethoxazole—bottles of 100 (NDC 0004-0050-01); Tel-E-Dose® packages of 100 (NDC

0004-0050-49); Prescription Paks of 40 (NDC 0004-0050-34). Imprint on tablets: (front) BACTRIM; (back) ROCHE.

Pediatric Suspension (pink, cherry flavored), containing 40 mg trimethoprim and 200 mg sulfamethoxazole per teaspoonful (5 mL)—bottles of 100 mL (NDC 0004-1033-01) and 16 oz (1 pint) (NDC 0004-1033-28).

Suspension (pink, fruit-licorice flavored), containing 40 mg trimethoprim and 200 mg sulfamethoxazole per teaspoonful (5 mL)—bottles of 16 oz (1 pint) (NDC 0004-1015-28).

TABLETS SHOULD BE STORED AT 15°–30°C (59°–86°F) IN A DRY PLACE AND PROTECTED FROM LIGHT.

SUSPENSIONS SHOULD BE STORED AT 15°–30°C (59°–86°F) AND PROTECTED FROM LIGHT.

REFERENCES

1. Kremers P, Duvivier J, Heusghem C: Pharmacokinetic Studies of Co-Trimoxazole in Man after Single and Repeated Doses. *J Clin Pharmacol 14:* 112–117, Feb-Mar 1974. 2. Kaplan SA, *et al:* Pharmacokinetic Profile of Trimethoprim-Sulfamethoxazole in Man. *J Infect Dis 128* (Suppl): S547–S555, Nov 1973. 3. *Federal Register 37:* 20527–20529, 1972. 4. Bauer AW, Kirby WMM, Sherris JC, Turck M: Antibiotic Susceptibility Testing by a Standardized Single Disk Method. *Am J Clin Path 45:* 493–496, Apr 1966. 5. Brumfitt W, Pursell R: Trimethoprim/Sulfamethoxazole in the Treatment of Bacteriuria in Women. *J Infect Dis 128* (Suppl): S657–S663, Nov 1973.

Revised: June 1990

Shown in Product Identification Section, page 425

BEROCCA® TABLETS   ℞

[ber-o'ka]

The following text is complete prescribing information based on official labeling in effect June 1, 1992.
(See accompanying table [below].)

Each tablet also contains acacia, calcium sulfate, carnauba wax, hydrogenated vegetable oil, magnesium oxide, magnesium stearate, povidone, shellac, sodium benzoate, sugar and talc with the following dyes: FD&C Blue No. 1, FD&C Yellow No. 6, D&C Yellow No. 10 and titanium dioxide.

DESCRIPTION

Berocca is a prescription-only oral multivitamin tablet specially formulated for prophylactic or therapeutic nutritional supplementation in conditions requiring water-soluble vitamins.

Berocca tablets supply *therapeutic* levels of ascorbic acid, vitamins B_1, B_2, B_6, niacin and pantothenic acid and a *supplemental* level of vitamin B_{12}. Berocca tablets also supply a supplemental level of folic acid for pregnant or lactating women and a therapeutic level for adults and children four or more years of age.

CLINICAL PHARMACOLOGY

Vitamins are essential for normal metabolic functions including hematopoiesis. The B-complex vitamins are necessary for the conversion of carbohydrate, protein and fat into tissue and energy.

Ascorbic acid (C) is involved in collagen formation and tissue repair.

The water-soluble vitamins (B-complex and C) are not significantly stored by the body; excess quantities are excreted in the urine. They must be replenished regularly through diet or other means to maintain essential tissue levels. Thus, these vitamins are rapidly depleted in conditions interfering with their intake or absorption.

INDICATIONS AND USAGE

Berocca is indicated for supportive nutritional supplementation in conditions in which water-soluble vitamins are required prophylactically or therapeutically. These include:

Conditions causing depletion, or reduced absorption or bioavailability of water-soluble vitamins—

Gastrointestinal disorders, chronic alcoholism, febrile illnesses, prolonged or wasting diseases, hyperthyroidism or poorly controlled diabetes.

Conditions resulting in increased needs for water-soluble vitamins—

Pregnancy, severe burns, recovery from surgery.

CONTRAINDICATIONS

Berocca is contraindicated in patients known to be hypersensitive to any of its components.

WARNINGS

Berocca is not intended for treatment of pernicious anemia or other megaloblastic anemias where vitamin B_{12} is deficient. Neurologic involvement may develop or progress, despite temporary remission of anemia, in patients with vitamin B_{12} deficiency who receive supplemental folic acid and who are inadequately treated with B_{12}.

PRECAUTIONS

General: Certain conditions listed above may require additional nutritional supplementation. During pregnancy, for instance, supplementation with fat-soluble vitamins and minerals may be required according to the dietary habits of the individual. Berocca is not intended for treatment of severe specific deficiencies.

Information for the Patient: Because toxic reactions have been reported with injudicious use of certain vitamins, urge patients to follow your specific instructions regarding dosage regimen. As with any medication, advise patients to keep Berocca out of reach of children.

Drug and Treatment Interactions: As little as 5 mg pyridoxine daily can decrease the efficacy of levodopa in the treatment of parkinsonism. Therefore, Berocca is not recommended for patients undergoing such therapy.

ADVERSE REACTIONS

Adverse reactions have been reported with specific vitamins, but generally at levels substantially higher than those in Berocca. However, allergic and idiosyncratic reactions are possible at lower levels.

DOSAGE AND ADMINISTRATION

Usual adult dosage: one tablet daily.
Berocca is available on prescription only.

HOW SUPPLIED

Light green, capsule-shaped tablets—bottles of 100 (NDC 0004-0020-01) and 500 (NDC 0004-0020-14).
Imprint on tablets: BEROCCA®
                    ROCHE

Revised: November 1985
Shown in Product Identification Section, page 425

BEROCCA® PLUS TABLETS   ℞

[ber-o'ka]

The following text is complete prescribing information based on official labeling in effect June 1, 1992.
(See accompanying table [on next page].)

DESCRIPTION

Berocca Plus is a prescription-only oral multivitamin/mineral tablet specially formulated for prophylactic or therapeutic nutritional supplementation in physiologically stressful conditions.

Berocca Plus supplies: *therapeutic* levels of water-soluble vitamins (ascorbic acid and all B-complex vitamins except biotin; *supplemental* levels of biotin, fat-soluble vitamins (A and E) and minerals (iron, chromium, manganese, copper and zinc); plus magnesium.

CLINICAL PHARMACOLOGY

Vitamins and minerals are essential for normal metabolic functions including hematopoiesis. The B-complex vitamins are necessary for the conversion of carbohydrate, protein and fat into tissue and energy. Ascorbic acid is involved in tissue repair and collagen formation. Vitamin A is necessary for proper functioning of the retina; it appears to be essential to the integrity of epithelial cells. Vitamin E is an antioxidant which preserves essential cellular constituents. Magnesium is a structural component of body tissues; iron, chromium, manganese, copper and zinc serve as catalysts in enzyme systems which perform vital cellular functions.

Each Berocca® tablet contains:	Quantity	U.S. RDA—Adults and children 4 or more years of age	U.S. RDA—Pregnant or lactating women
Vitamin C (ascorbic acid)	500 mg	60 mg	60 mg
Vitamin B_1 (as thiamine mononitrate)	15 mg	1.5 mg	1.7 mg
Vitamin B_2 (riboflavin)	15 mg	1.7 mg	2 mg
Niacin (as niacinamide)	100 mg	20 mg	20 mg
Vitamin B_6 (as pyridoxine HCl)	4 mg	2 mg	2.5 mg
Pantothenic acid (as calcium *d*-pantothenate)	18 mg	10 mg	10 mg
Folic acid	0.5 mg	0.4 mg	0.8 mg
Vitamin B_{12} (cyanocobalamin)	5 mcg	6 mcg	8 mcg

Continued on next page

Roche Laboratories—Cont.

Each Berocca® Plus tablet contains:	Quantity	U.S. RDA—Adults and children 4 or more years of age	U.S. RDA—Pregnant or lactating women
Fat-Soluble Vitamins			
Vitamin A (as vitamin A acetate)	5000 IU	5000 IU	8000 IU
Vitamin E	30 IU	30 IU	30 IU
(as *dl*-alpha tocopheryl acetate)			
Water-Soluble Vitamins			
Vitamin C (ascorbic acid)	500 mg	60 mg	60 mg
Vitamin B_1 (as thiamine mononitrate)	20 mg	1.5 mg	1.7 mg
Vitamin B_2 (riboflavin)	20 mg	1.7 mg	2 mg
Niacin (as niacinamide)	100 mg	20 mg	20 mg
Vitamin B_6 (as pyridoxine HCl)	25 mg	2 mg	2.5 mg
Biotin	0.15 mg	0.30 mg	0.30 mg
Pantothenic acid	25 mg	10 mg	10 mg
(as calcium pantothenate)			
Folic acid	0.8 mg	0.4 mg	0.8 mg
Vitamin B_{12} (cyanocobalamin)	50 mcg	6 mcg	8 mcg
Minerals			
Iron (as ferrous fumarate)	27 mg	18 mg	18 mg
Chromium (as chromium nitrate)	0.1 mg	0.05–0.2 mg*	
Magnesium (as magnesium oxide)	50 mg	400 mg	450 mg
Manganese (as manganese dioxide)	5 mg	2.5–5 mg*	
Copper (as cupric oxide)	3 mg	2 mg	2 mg
Zinc (as zinc oxide)	22.5 mg	15 mg	15 mg

Each tablet also contains carnauba wax, ethylcellulose, ethyl vanillin, hydroxypropyl methylcellulose, magnesium stearate, povidone, silicon dioxide, stearic acid, triacetin and flavor with the following dyes: yellow iron oxide and titanium dioxide.
*Not established. Estimated by NAS/NRC as safe and adequate daily dietary intake for adults.

Water-soluble vitamins (B-complex and C) are not significantly stored by the body and must be replaced continually to maintain essential tissue levels; excess quantities are excreted in urine. These vitamins are rapidly depleted in conditions interfering with their intake or absorption. Berocca Plus supplies therapeutic levels of vitamin C and all B-complex vitamins (except biotin).

Fat-soluble vitamins and several trace minerals, however, can accumulate in the body and do not need replacement as frequently. Therefore, Berocca Plus supplies more conservative levels of vitamins A and E and various essential minerals.

Specifically, Berocca Plus contains an adequate level of vitamin B_6 (25 mg) to normalize the tryptophan metabolism disturbance which has been associated with the use of estrogenic oral contraceptives or other estrogen therapy. It provides zinc (22.5 mg) which facilitates wound healing, the level of folic acid (0.8 mg) recommended during pregnancy, and ascorbic acid (500 mg) which has been demonstrated to improve the absorption of inorganic iron.

INDICATIONS

Berocca Plus is indicated for prophylactic or therapeutic nutritional supplementation in physiologically stressful conditions. These include:

Conditions causing depletion, or reduced absorption or bioavailability of essential vitamins and minerals—

Inadequate intake due to highly restricted or unbalanced diets such as those frequently associated with anorexic conditions and other states of severe malnutrition.

Gastrointestinal disorders, chronic alcoholism, chronic or acute infections (especially those involving febrile illness), prolonged or wasting disease, congestive heart failure, hyperthyroidism, poorly controlled diabetes or other physiologic stress.

Also, patients on estrogenic oral contraceptives or other estrogen therapy, antibacterials which affect intestinal microflora, or other interfering drugs.

Certain conditions resulting from severe B-vitamin or ascorbic acid deficiency—

Cheilosis, gingivitis, stomatitis and certain other classic water-soluble vitamin deficiency syndromes.

Conditions resulting in increased needs for essential vitamins and minerals—

Recovery from surgery or trauma involving severe burns, fractures or other extensive tissue damage.

Also, pregnant women and those with heavy menstrual bleeding.

CONTRAINDICATIONS

Berocca Plus is contraindicated in patients hypersensitive to any of its components.

WARNINGS

Not intended for treatment of pernicious anemia or other megaloblastic anemias where vitamin B_{12} is deficient. Neurologic involvement may develop or progress, despite temporary remission of anemia, in patients with vitamin B_{12} deficiency who receive supplemental folic acid and who are inadequately treated with B_{12}.

PRECAUTIONS

General: Certain conditions listed above may require additional nutritional supplementation. During pregnancy, for instance, supplementation with vitamin D and calcium may be required according to the dietary habits of the individual. Berocca Plus is not intended for treatment of severe specific deficiencies.

Information for the Patient: Because toxic reactions have been reported with injudicious use of certain vitamins and minerals, urge patients to follow your specific instructions regarding dosage regimen. Advise patients to keep Berocca Plus out of reach of children.

Drug and Treatment Interactions: As litte as 5 mg pyridoxine daily can decrease the efficacy of levodopa in the treatment of parkinsonism. Therefore, Berocca Plus is not recommended for patients undergoing such therapy.

ADVERSE REACTIONS

Adverse reactions have been reported with specific vitamins and minerals, but generally at levels substantially higher than those in Berocca Plus. However, allergic and idiosyncratic reactions are possible at lower levels. Iron, even at the usual recommended levels, has been associated with gastrointestinal intolerance in some patients.

DOSAGE AND ADMINISTRATION

Usual adult dosage: one tablet daily. Not recommended for children. *Berocca Plus is available on prescription only.*

HOW SUPPLIED

Golden yellow, capsule-shaped tablets—bottles of 100. Imprint on tablets: (front) BEROCCA PLUS; (back) ROCHE. Revised: November 1985

Shown in Product Identification Section, page 426

BUMEX®   ℞
[*bu 'mex*]
(bumetanide/Roche)
TABLETS
INJECTION

The following text is complete prescribing information based on official labeling in effect June 1, 1992.

> **WARNING**
>
> Bumex (bumetanide/Roche) is a potent diuretic which, if given in excessive amounts, can lead to a profound diuresis with water and electrolyte depletion. Therefore, careful medical supervision is required, and dose and dosage schedule have to be adjusted to the individual patient's needs. (See DOSAGE AND ADMINISTRATION.)

DESCRIPTION

Bumex® (bumetanide/Roche) is a loop diuretic, available as scored tablets, 0.5 mg (light green), 1 mg (yellow) and 2 mg (peach) for oral administration; each tablet also contains lactose, magnesium stearate, microcrystalline cellulose, corn starch and talc, with the following dye systems: 0.5 mg—D&C Yellow No. 10 and FD&C Blue No. 1; 1 mg—D&C Yellow No. 10; 2 mg—red iron oxide. Also as 2-mL ampuls, 2-mL vials, 4-mL vials and 10-mL vials (0.25 mg/mL) for intravenous or intramuscular injection as a sterile solution, each 2 mL of which contains 0.5 mg (0.25 mg/mL) bumetanide compounded with 0.85% sodium chloride and 0.4% ammonium acetate as buffers; 0.01% edetate disodium; 1% benzyl alcohol as preservative, and pH adjusted to approximately 7 with sodium hydroxide.

Chemically, bumetanide is 3-(butylamino)-4-phenoxy-5-sulfamoylbenzoic acid. It is a practically white powder having a calculated molecular weight of 364.41.

CLINICAL PHARMACOLOGY

Bumex is a loop diuretic with a rapid onset and short duration of action. Pharmacological and clinical studies have shown that 1 mg Bumex has a diuretic potency equivalent to approximately 40 mg furosemide. The major site of Bumex action is the ascending limb of the loop of Henle.

The mode of action has been determined through various clearance studies in both humans and experimental animals. Bumex inhibits sodium reabsorption in the ascending limb of the loop of Henle, as shown by marked reduction of free-water clearance (^CH_2O) during hydration and tubular free-water reabsorption (T^CH_2O) during hydropenia. Reabsorption of chloride in the ascending limb is also blocked by Bumex, and Bumex is somewhat more chloruretic than natriuretic.

Potassium excretion is also increased by Bumex, in a dose-related fashion.

Bumex may have an additional action in the proximal tubule. Since phosphate reabsorption takes place largely in the proximal tubule, phosphaturia during Bumex-induced diuresis is indicative of this additional action. This is further supported by the reduction in the renal clearance of Bumex by probenecid, associated with diminution in the natriuretic response. This proximal tubular activity does not seem to be related to an inhibition of carbonic anhydrase. Bumex does not appear to have a noticeable action on the distal tubule. Bumex decreases uric acid excretion and increases serum uric acid. Following oral administration of Bumex the onset of diuresis occurs in 30 to 60 minutes. Peak activity is reached between 1 and 2 hours. At usual doses (1 to 2 mg) diuresis is largely complete within 4 hours; with higher doses, the diuretic action lasts for 4 to 6 hours. Diuresis starts within minutes following an intravenous injection and reaches maximum values within 15 to 30 minutes.

Several pharmacokinetic studies have shown that Bumex, administered orally or parenterally, is eliminated rapidly in humans, with a half-life of between 1 and $1\frac{1}{2}$ hours. Plasma protein-binding is in the range of 94% to 96%.

Oral administration of carbon-14 labeled Bumex to human volunteers revealed that 81% of the administered radioactivity was excreted in the urine, 45% of it as unchanged drug. Urinary and biliary metabolites identified in this study were formed by oxidation of the N-butyl side chain. Biliary excretion of Bumex amounted to only 2% of the administered dose.

INDICATIONS AND USAGE

Bumex is indicated for the treatment of edema associated with congestive heart failure, hepatic and renal disease, including the nephrotic syndrome.

Almost equal diuretic response occurs after oral and parenteral administration of Bumex. Therefore, if impaired gastrointestinal absorption is suspected or oral administration is not practical, Bumex should be given by the intramuscular or intravenous route.

Successful treatment with Bumex following instances of allergic reactions to furosemide suggests a lack of cross-sensitivity.

CONTRAINDICATIONS

Bumex is contraindicated in anuria. Although Bumex can be used to induce diuresis in renal insufficiency, any marked increase in blood urea nitrogen or creatinine, or the development of oliguria during therapy of patients with progressive renal disease, is an indication for discontinuation of treatment with Bumex. Bumex is also contraindicated in patients in hepatic coma or in states of severe electrolyte depletion until the condition is improved or corrected. Bumex is contraindicated in patients hypersensitive to this drug.

WARNINGS

1. Volume and electrolyte depletion. The dose of Bumex should be adjusted to the patient's need. Excessive doses or too frequent administration can lead to profound water loss, electrolyte depletion, dehydration, reduction in blood volume and circulatory collapse with the possibility of vascular thrombosis and embolism, particularly in elderly patients.
2. Hypokalemia. Hypokalemia can occur as a consequence of Bumex administration. Prevention of hypokalemia requires particular attention in the following conditions: patients receiving digitalis and diuretics for congestive heart failure, hepatic cirrhosis and ascites, states of aldosterone excess with normal renal function, potassium-losing nephropathy, certain diarrheal states, or other states where hypokalemia is thought to represent particular added risks to the patient, *i.e.*, history of ventricular arrhythmias.

In patients with hepatic cirrhosis and ascites, sudden alterations of electrolyte balance may precipitate hepatic encephalopathy and coma. Treatment in such patients is best initiated in the hospital with small doses and careful monitoring of the patient's clinical status and electrolyte balance. Supplemental potassium and/or spironolactone may prevent hypokalemia and metabolic alkalosis in these patients.

3. Ototoxicity. In cats, dogs and guinea pigs, Bumex has been shown to produce ototoxicity. In these test animals Bumex was 5 to 6 times more potent than furosemide and, since the diuretic potency of Bumex is about 40 to 60 times furosemide, it is anticipated that blood levels necessary to produce ototoxicity will rarely be achieved. The potential exists, however, and must be considered a risk of intravenous therapy, especially at high doses, repeated frequently in the face of renal excretory function impairment. Potentiation of aminoglycoside ototoxicity has not been tested for Bumex. Like other members of this class of diuretics, Bumex probably shares this risk.

4. Allergy to sulfonamides. Patients allergic to sulfonamides may show hypersensitivity to Bumex.

5. Thrombocytopenia. Since there have been rare spontaneous reports of thrombocytopenia from postmarketing experience, patients should be observed regularly for possible occurrence of thrombocytopenia.

PRECAUTIONS

General: Serum potassium should be measured periodically and potassium supplements or potassium-sparing diuretics added if necessary. Periodic determinations of other electrolytes are advised in patients treated with high doses or for prolonged periods, particularly in those on low salt diets. Hyperuricemia may occur; it has been asymptomatic in cases reported to date. Reversible elevations of the BUN and creatinine may also occur, especially in association with dehydration and particularly in patients with renal insufficiency. Bumex may increase urinary calcium excretion with resultant hypocalcemia.

Laboratory Tests: Studies in normal subjects receiving Bumex revealed no adverse effects on glucose tolerance, plasma insulin, glucagon and growth hormone levels, but the possibility of an effect on glucose metabolism exists. Periodic determinations of blood sugar should be done, particularly in patients with diabetes or suspected latent diabetes.

Patients under treatment should be observed regularly for possible occurrence of blood dyscrasias, liver damage or idiosyncratic reactions, which have been reported occasionally in foreign marketing experience. The relationship of these occurrences to Bumex use is not certain.

Drug Interactions:

1. Drugs with ototoxic potential (see WARNINGS): Especially in the presence of impaired renal function, the use of parenterally administered Bumex in patients to whom aminoglycoside antibiotics are also being given should be avoided, except in life-threatening conditions.

2. Drugs with nephrotoxic potential: There has been no experience on the concurrent use of Bumex with drugs known to have a nephrotoxic potential. Therefore, the simultaneous administration of these drugs should be avoided.

3. Lithium: Lithium should generally not be given with diuretics (such as Bumex) because they reduce its renal clearance and add a high risk of lithium toxicity.

4. Probenecid: Pretreatment with probenecid reduces both the natriuresis and hyperreninemia produced by Bumex. This antagonistic effect of probenecid on Bumex natriuresis is not due to a direct action on sodium excretion but is probably secondary to its inhibitory effect on renal tubular secretion of bumetanide. Thus, probenecid should not be administered concurrently with Bumex.

5. Indomethacin: Indomethacin blunts the increases in urine volume and sodium excretion seen during Bumex treatment and inhibits the bumetanide-induced increase in plasma renin activity. Concurrent therapy with Bumex is thus not recommended.

6. Antihypertensives: Bumex may potentiate the effect of various antihypertensive drugs, necessitating a reduction in the dosage of these drugs.

7. Digoxin: Interaction studies in humans have shown no effect on digoxin blood levels.

8. Anticoagulants: Interaction studies in humans have shown Bumex to have no effect on warfarin metabolism or on plasma prothrombin activity.

Carcinogenesis, Mutagenesis, Impairment of Fertility: Bumex was devoid of mutagenic activity in various strains of *Salmonella typhimurium* when tested in the presence or absence of an *in vitro* metabolic activation system. An 18-month study showed an increase in mammary adenomas of questionable significance in female rats receiving oral doses of 60 mg/kg/day (2000 times a 2-mg human dose). A repeat study at the same doses failed to duplicate this finding.

Reproduction studies were performed to evaluate general reproductive performance and fertility in rats at oral dose levels of 10, 30, 60 or 100 mg/kg/day. The pregnancy rate was slightly decreased in the treated animals; however, the differences were small and not statistically significant.

Pregnancy: Teratogenic Effects: Pregnancy Category C. Bumex is neither teratogenic nor embryocidal in mice when given in doses up to 3400 times the maximum human therapeutic dose.

Bumex has been shown to be nonteratogenic, but it has a slight embryocidal effect in rats when given in doses of 3400 times the maximum human therapeutic dose and in rabbits at doses of 3.4 times the maximum human therapeutic dose. In one study, moderate growth retardation and increased incidence of delayed ossification of sternebrae were observed in rats at oral doses of 100 mg/kg/day, 3400 times the maximum human therapeutic dose. These effects were associated with maternal weight reductions noted during dosing. No such adverse effects were observed at 30 mg/kg/day (1000 times the maximum human therapeutic dose). No fetotoxicity was observed at 1000 to 2000 times the human therapeutic dose.

In rabbits, a dose-related decrease in litter size and an increase in resorption rate were noted at oral doses of 0.1 and 0.3 mg/kg/day (3.4 and 10 times the maximum human therapeutic dose). A slightly increased incidence of delayed ossification of sternebrae occurred at 0.3 mg/kg/day; however, no such adverse effects were observed at the dose of 0.03 mg/kg/day. The sensitivity of the rabbit to Bumex parallels the marked pharmacologic and toxicologic effects of the drug in this species.

Bumex was not teratogenic in the hamster at an oral dose of 0.5 mg/kg/day (17 times the maximum human therapeutic dose). Bumex was not teratogenic when given intravenously to mice and rats at doses up to 140 times the maximum human therapeutic dose.

There are no adequate and well-controlled studies in pregnant women. A small investigational experience in the United States and marketing experience in other countries to date have not indicated any evidence of adverse effects on the fetus, but these data do not rule out the possibility of harmful effects. Bumex should be given to a pregnant woman only if the potential benefit justifies the potential risk to the fetus.

Nursing Mothers: It is not known whether this drug is excreted in human milk. As a general rule, nursing should not be undertaken while the patient is on Bumex since it may be excreted in human milk.

Pediatric Use: Safety and effectiveness in children below the age of 18 have not been established.

ADVERSE REACTIONS

The most frequent clinical adverse reactions considered probably or possibly related to Bumex are muscle cramps (seen in 1.1% of treated patients), dizziness (1.1%), hypotension (0.8%), headache (0.6%), nausea (0.6%), and encephalopathy (in patients with preexisting liver disease) (0.6%). One or more of these adverse reactions have been reported in approximately 4.1% of Bumex-treated patients.

Less frequent clinical adverse reactions to Bumex are impaired hearing (0.5%), pruritus (0.4%), electrocardiogram changes (0.4%), weakness (0.2%), hives (0.2%), abdominal pain (0.2%), arthritic pain (0.2%), musculoskeletal pain (0.2%), rash (0.2%) and vomiting (0.2%). One or more of these adverse reactions have been reported in approximately 2.9% of Bumex-treated patients.

Other clinical adverse reactions, which have each occurred in approximately 0.1% of patients, are vertigo, chest pain, ear discomfort, fatigue, dehydration, sweating, hyperventilation, dry mouth, upset stomach, renal failure, asterixis, itching, nipple tenderness, diarrhea, premature ejaculation and difficulty maintaining an erection.

Laboratory abnormalities reported have included hyperuricemia (in 18.4% of patients tested), hypochloremia (14.9%), hypokalemia (14.7%), azotemia (10.6%), hyponatremia (9.2%), increased serum creatinine (7.4%), hyperglycemia (6.6%), and variations in phosphorus (4.5%), CO_2 content (4.3%), bicarbonate (3.1%) and calcium (2.4%). Although manifestations of the pharmacologic action of Bumex, these conditions may become more pronounced by intensive therapy.

Also reported have been thrombocytopenia (0.2%) and deviations in hemoglobin (0.8%), prothrombin time (0.8%), hematocrit (0.6%), WBC (0.3%) and differential counts (0.1%). There have been rare spontaneous reports of thrombocytopenia from postmarketing experience.

Diuresis induced by Bumex may also rarely be accompanied by changes in LDH (1.0%), total serum bilirubin (0.8%), serum proteins (0.7%), SGOT (0.6%), SGPT (0.5%), alkaline phosphatase (0.4%), cholesterol (0.4%) and creatinine clearance (0.3%). Increases in urinary glucose (0.7%) and urinary protein (0.3%) have also been seen.

OVERDOSAGE

Overdosage can lead to acute profound water loss, volume and electrolyte depletion, dehydration, reduction of blood volume and circulatory collapse with a possibility of vascular thrombosis and embolism. Electrolyte depletion may be manifested by weakness, dizziness, mental confusion, anorexia, lethargy, vomiting and cramps. Treatment consists of replacement of fluid and electrolyte losses by careful moni-

toring of the urine and electrolyte output and serum electrolyte levels.

DOSAGE AND ADMINISTRATION

Dosage should be individualized with careful monitoring of patient response.

Oral Administration: The usual total daily dosage of Bumex is 0.5 to 2.0 mg and in most patients is given as a single dose.

If the diuretic response to an initial dose of Bumex is not adequate, in view of its rapid onset and short duration of action, a second or third dose may be given at 4- to 5-hour intervals up to a maximum daily dose of 10 mg. An intermittent dose schedule, whereby Bumex is given on alternate days or for 3 to 4 days with rest periods of 1 to 2 days in between, is recommended as the safest and most effective method for the continued control of edema. In patients with hepatic failure, the dosage should be kept to a minimum, and if necessary, dosage increased very carefully.

Because cross-sensitivity with furosemide has rarely been observed, Bumex can be substituted at approximately a 1:40 ratio of Bumex to furosemide in patients allergic to furosemide.

Parenteral Administration: Bumex may be administered parenterally (IV or IM) to patients in whom gastrointestinal absorption may be impaired or in whom oral administration is not practical.

Parenteral treatment should be terminated and oral treatment instituted as soon as possible.

The usual initial dose is 0.5 to 1.0 mg intravenously or intramuscularly. Intravenous administration should be given over a period of 1 to 2 minutes. If the response to an initial dose is deemed insufficient, a second or third dose may be given at intervals of 2 to 3 hours, but should not exceed a daily dosage of 10 mg.

Miscibility and Parenteral Solutions: The compatibility tests of Bumex injection (0.25 mg/mL, 2-mL ampuls) with 5% dextrose in water, 0.9% sodium chloride, and lactated Ringer's solution in both glass and plasticized PVC (Viaflex) containers have shown no significant absorption effect with either containers, nor a measurable loss of potency due to degradation of the drug. However, solutions should be freshly prepared and used within 24 hours.

Parenteral drug products should be inspected visually for particulate matter and discoloration prior to administration whenever solution and container permit.

HOW SUPPLIED

Tablets 0.5 mg (light green), bottles of 100 (NDC 0004-0125-01) and 500 (NDC 0004-0125-14); Tel-E-Dose® packages of 100 (NDC 0004-0125-49). 1 mg (yellow), bottles of 100 (NDC 0004-0121-01) and 500 (NDC 0004-0121-14); Tel-E-Dose® packages of 100 (NDC 0004-0121-49). 2 mg (peach), bottles of 100 (NDC 0004-0162-01); Tel-E-Dose® packages of 100 (NDC 0004-0162-07).

Imprint on tablets: 0.5 mg—ROCHE BUMEX 0.5; 1 mg—ROCHE BUMEX 1; 2 mg—ROCHE BUMEX 2.

Ampuls (0.25 mg/mL), 2 mL, boxes of 10 (NDC 0004-1944-06).

Vials (0.25 mg/mL), 2 mL, boxes of 10 (NDC 0004-1968-01); 4 mL, boxes of 10 (NDC 0004-1969-01); 10 mL, boxes of 10 (NDC 0004-1970-01).

Store all tablets, vials and ampuls at 59° to 86° F.

Revised: February 1991

Shown in Product Identification Section, page 426

FANSIDAR®   ℞

[*fan 'sid-ar*]

(sulfadoxine and pyrimethamine/Roche)

TABLETS

The following text is complete prescribing information based on official labeling in effect June 1, 1992.

> **WARNING: FATALITIES ASSOCIATED WITH THE ADMINISTRATION OF FANSIDAR HAVE OCCURRED DUE TO SEVERE REACTIONS, INCLUDING STEVENS-JOHNSON SYNDROME AND TOXIC EPIDERMAL NECROLYSIS. FANSIDAR PROPHYLAXIS SHOULD BE DISCONTINUED AT THE FIRST APPEARANCE OF SKIN RASH, IF A SIGNIFICANT REDUCTION IN THE COUNT OF ANY FORMED BLOOD ELEMENTS IS NOTED, OR UPON THE OCCURRENCE OF ACTIVE BACTERIAL OR FUNGAL INFECTIONS.**

DESCRIPTION

Fansidar is an antimalarial agent, each tablet containing 500 mg N^1-(5,6-dimethoxy-4-pyrimidinyl) sulfanilamide (sulfadoxine) and 25 mg 2,4-diamino-5-(p-chlorophenyl)-6-ethylpyrimidine (pyrimethamine). Each tablet also contains corn starch, gelatin, lactose, magnesium stearate and talc.

Continued on next page

Roche Laboratories—Cont.

CLINICAL PHARMACOLOGY

Fansidar is an antimalarial agent which acts by reciprocal potentiation of its two components, achieved by a sequential blockade of two enzymes involved in the biosynthesis of folinic acid within the parasites. Fansidar is effective against certain strains of *Plasmodium falciparum* that are resistant to chloroquine.

Both the sulfadoxine and the pyrimethamine of Fansidar are absorbed orally and are excreted mainly by the kidney. Following a single tablet administration, sulfadoxine peak plasma concentrations of 51 to 76 mcg/ml were achieved in 2.5 to 6 hours and the pyrimethamine peak plasma concentrations of 0.13 to 0.4 mcg/ml were achieved in 1.5 to 8 hours. The apparent half-life of elimination of sulfadoxine ranged from 100 to 231 hours with a mean of 169 hours, whereas pyrimethamine half-lives ranged from 54 to 148 hours with a mean of 111 hours. Both drugs appear in breast milk of nursing mothers.

INDICATIONS AND USAGE

Fansidar is indicated for the treatment of *P. falciparum* malaria for those patients in whom chloroquine resistance is suspected. Malaria prophylaxis with Fansidar is indicated for travelers to areas where chloroquine-resistant *P. falciparum* malaria is endemic. However, strains of *P. falciparum* may be encountered which have developed resistance to Fansidar.

CONTRAINDICATIONS

Prophylactic (repeated) use of Fansidar is contraindicated in patients with severe renal insufficiency, marked liver parenchymal damage or blood dyscrasias. Hypersensitivity to pyrimethamine or sulfonamides. Patients with documented megaloblastic anemia due to folate deficiency. Infants less than two months of age. Pregnancy at term and during the nursing period because sulfonamides pass the placenta and are excreted in the milk and may cause kernicterus.

WARNINGS

FATALITIES ASSOCIATED WITH THE ADMINISTRATION OF FANSIDAR HAVE OCCURRED DUE TO SEVERE REACTIONS, INCLUDING STEVENS-JOHNSON SYNDROME AND TOXIC EPIDERMAL NECROLYSIS. FANSIDAR PROPHYLAXIS SHOULD BE DISCONTINUED AT THE FIRST APPEARANCE OF SKIN RASH, IF A SIGNIFICANT REDUCTION IN THE COUNT OF ANY FORMED BLOOD ELEMENTS IS NOTED, OR UPON THE OCCURRENCE OF ACTIVE BACTERIAL OR FUNGAL INFECTIONS.

Fatalities associated with the administration of sulfonamides, although rare, have occurred due to severe reactions, including fulminant hepatic necrosis, agranulocytosis, aplastic anemia and other blood dyscrasias. Fansidar prophylactic regimen has been reported to cause leukopenia during a treatment of two months or longer. This leukopenia is generally mild and reversible.

PRECAUTIONS

1. *General:* Fansidar should be given with caution to patients with impaired renal or hepatic function, to those with possible folate deficiency and to those with severe allergy or bronchial asthma. As with some sulfonamide drugs, in glucose-6-phosphate dehydrogenase-deficient individuals, hemolysis may occur. Urinalysis with microscopic examination and renal function tests should be performed during therapy of those patients who have impaired renal function.

2. *Information for the patient:* Patients should be warned that at the first appearance of a skin rash, they should stop use of Fansidar and seek medical attention immediately. Adequate fluid intake must be maintained in order to prevent crystalluria and stone formation.

Patients should also be warned that the appearance of sore throat, fever, arthralgia, cough, shortness of breath, pallor, purpura, jaundice or glossitis may be early indications of serious disorders which require prophylactic treatment to be stopped and medical treatment to be sought.

Females should be cautioned against becoming pregnant and should not breast feed their infants during Fansidar therapy or prophylactic treatment.

Patients should be warned to keep Fansidar out of reach of children.

3. *Laboratory tests:* Periodic blood counts and analysis of urine for crystalluria are desirable during prolonged prophylaxis.

4. *Drug interactions:* There have been reports which may indicate an increase in incidence and severity of adverse reactions when chloroquine is used with Fansidar as compared to the use of Fansidar alone. Fansidar is compatible with quinine and with antibiotics. However, antifolic drugs such as sulfonamides or trimethoprim-sulfamethoxazole combinations should not be used while the patient is receiving Fansidar for antimalarial prophylaxis. Fansidar has not been reported to interfere with antidiabetic agents.

If signs of folic acid deficiency develop, Fansidar should be discontinued. Folinic acid (leucovorin) may be administered in doses of 5 mg to 15 mg intramuscularly daily, for 3 days or longer, for depressed platelet or white blood cell counts in patients with drug-induced folic acid deficiency when recovery is too slow.

5. *Carcinogenesis, mutagenesis, impairment of fertility:* Pyrimethamine was not found carcinogenic in female mice or in male and female rats. The carcinogenic potential of pyrimethamine in male mice could not be assessed from the study because of markedly reduced life-span. Pyrimethamine was found to be mutagenic in laboratory animals and also in human bone marrow following 3 or 4 consecutive daily doses totaling 200 mg to 300 mg. Pyrimethamine was not found mutagenic in the Ames test. Testicular changes have been observed in rats treated with 105 mg/kg/day of Fansidar and with 15 mg/kg/day of pyrimethamine alone. Fertility of male rats and the ability of male or female rats to mate were not adversely affected at dosages of up to 210 mg/kg/day of Fansidar. The pregnancy rate of female rats was not affected following their treatment with 10.5 mg/kg/day, but was significantly reduced at dosages of 31.5 mg/kg/day or higher, a dosage approximately 30 times the weekly human prophylactic dose or higher.

6. *Pregnancy:* Teratogenic effects: Pregnancy Category C. Fansidar has been shown to be teratogenic in rats when given in weekly doses approximately 12 times the weekly human prophylactic dose. Teratology studies with pyrimethamine plus sulfadoxine (1:20) in rats showed the minimum oral teratogenic dose to be approximately 0.9 mg/kg pyrimethamine plus 18 mg/kg sulfadoxine. In rabbits, no teratogenic effects were noted at oral doses as high as 20 mg/kg pyrimethamine plus 400 mg/kg sulfadoxine.

There are no adequate and well-controlled studies in pregnant women. However, due to the teratogenic effect shown in animals and because pyrimethamine plus sulfadoxine may interfere with folic acid metabolism, Fansidar therapy should be used during pregnancy only if the potential benefit justifies the potential risk to the fetus. Women of childbearing potential who are traveling to areas where malaria is endemic should be warned against becoming pregnant.

Nonteratogenic effects: See "CONTRAINDICATIONS" section.

7. *Nursing mothers:* See "CONTRAINDICATIONS" section.

8. *Pediatric use:* Fansidar should not be given to infants less than two months of age because of inadequate development of the glucuronide-forming enzyme system.

ADVERSE REACTIONS

For completeness, all major reactions to sulfonamides and to pyrimethamine are included below, even though they may not have been reported with Fansidar. See "WARNINGS" and "PRECAUTIONS" (Information for the Patient) sections.

Blood dyscrasias: Agranulocytosis, aplastic anemia, megaloblastic anemia, thrombopenia, leukopenia, hemolytic anemia, purpura, hypoprothrombinemia, methemoglobinemia and eosinophilia.

Allergic reactions: Erythema multiforme, Stevens-Johnson syndrome, generalized skin eruptions, toxic epidermal necrolysis, urticaria, serum sickness, pruritus, exfoliative dermatitis, anaphylactoid reactions, periorbital edema, conjunctival and scleral injection, photosensitization, arthralgia and allergic myocarditis.

Gastrointestinal reactions: Glossitis, stomatitis, nausea, emesis, abdominal pains, hepatitis, hepatocellular necrosis, diarrhea and pancreatitis.

C.N.S. reactions: Headache, peripheral neuritis, mental depression, convulsions, ataxia, hallucinations, tinnitus, vertigo, insomnia, apathy, fatigue, muscle weakness and nervousness.

Respiratory reactions: Pulmonary infiltrates.

Miscellaneous reactions: Drug fever, chills, and toxic nephrosis with oliguria and anuria. Periarteritis nodosa and L. E. phenomenon have occurred.

The sulfonamides bear certain chemical similarities to some goitrogens, diuretics (acetazolamide and the thiazides) and oral hypoglycemic agents. Diuresis and hypoglycemia have occurred rarely in patients receiving sulfonamides. Cross-sensitivity may exist with these agents. Rats appear to be especially susceptible to the goitrogenic effects of sulfonamides, and long-term administration has produced thyroid malignancies in the species.

OVERDOSAGE

Acute intoxication may be manifested by anorexia, vomiting and central nervous system stimulation (including convulsions), followed by megaloblastic anemia, leukopenia, thrombocytopenia, glossitis and crystalluria. In acute intoxication, emesis and gastric lavage followed by purges may be of benefit. The patient should be adequately hydrated to prevent renal damage. The renal and hematopoietic systems should be monitored for at least one month after an overdosage. If the patient is having convulsions, the use of a parenteral barbiturate is indicated. For depressed platelet or white blood cell counts, folinic acid (leucovorin) should be administered in a dosage of 5 mg to 15 mg intramuscularly daily for 3 days or longer.

DOSAGE AND ADMINISTRATION

(See Indications and Usage Section):

(a) *Treatment of acute attack of malaria*

A single dose of the following number of Fansidar Tablets is used in sequence with quinine or alone:

Adults	2 to 3 tablets
9 to 14 years	2 tablets
4 to 8 years	1 tablet
Under 4 years	½ tablet

(b) *Malaria prophylaxis*

The first dose of Fansidar should be taken one or two days before departure to an endemic area; administration should be continued during the stay and for four to six weeks after return.

	Once Weekly	Once Every Two Weeks
Adults	1 tablet	2 tablets
9 to 14 years	¾ tablet	1½ tablets
4 to 8 years	½ tablet	1 tablet
Under 4 years	¼ tablet	½ tablet

HOW SUPPLIED

Scored tablets, containing 500 mg sulfadoxine and 25 mg pyrimethamine—boxes of 25 (NDC-0004-0161-03).

Revised: May 1987

Shown in Product Identification Section, page 426

FLUOROURACIL ℞
[flu "ro-u 'ra-sil]
INJECTION

The following text is complete prescribing information based on official labeling in effect June 1, 1992.

WARNING

It is recommended that FLUOROURACIL be given only by or under the supervision of a qualified physician who is experienced in cancer chemotherapy and who is well versed in the use of potent antimetabolites. Because of the possibility of severe toxic reactions, it is recommended that patients be hospitalized at least during the initial course of therapy.

DESCRIPTION

FLUOROURACIL INJECTION/Roche, an antineoplastic antimetabolite, is a sterile, nonpyrogenic injectable solution for intravenous administration. Each 10-mL contains 500 mg fluorouracil; pH is adjusted to approximately 9.2 with sodium hydroxide.

Chemically, fluorouracil, a fluorinated pyrimidine, is 5-fluoro-2,4 (*1H,3H*)-pyrimidinedione. It is a white to practically white crystalline powder which is sparingly soluble in water. The molecular weight of fluorouracil is 130.08.

CLINICAL PHARMACOLOGY

There is evidence that the metabolism of fluorouracil in the anabolic pathway blocks the methylation reaction of deoxyuridylic acid to thymidylic acid. In this manner, fluorouracil interferes with the synthesis of deoxyribonucleic acid (DNA) and to a lesser extent inhibits the formation of ribonucleic acid (RNA). Since DNA and RNA are essential for cell division and growth, the effect of fluorouracil may be to create a thymine deficiency which provokes unbalanced growth and death of the cell. The effects of DNA and RNA deprivation are most marked on those cells which grow more rapidly and which take up fluorouracil at a more rapid rate.

Following intravenous injection, fluorouracil distributes into tumors, intestinal mucosa, bone marrow, liver and other tissues throughout the body. In spite of its limited lipid solubility, fluorouracil diffuses readily across the blood-brain barrier and distributes into cerebrospinal fluid and brain tissue.

Seven to twenty percent of the parent drug is excreted unchanged in the urine in six hours; of this over 90% is excreted in the first hour. The remaining percentage of the administered dose is metabolized, primarily in the liver. The catabolic metabolism of fluorouracil results in degradation products (*e.g.,* CO_2, urea and α-fluoro-β-alanine) which are inactive. The inactive metabolites are excreted in the urine over the next 3 to 4 hours. When fluorouracil is labeled in the six carbon position, thus preventing the ^{14}C metabolism to CO_2, approximately 90% of the total radioactivity is excreted in the urine. When fluorouracil is labeled in the two carbon position approximately 90% of the total radioactivity is excreted in expired CO_2. Ninety percent of the dose is accounted for during the first 24 hours following intravenous administration.

Following intravenous administration of fluorouracil, the mean half-life of elimination from plasma is approximately 16 minutes, with a range of 8 to 20 minutes, and is dose dependent. No intact drug can be detected in the plasma three hours after an intravenous injection.

INDICATIONS AND USAGE

Fluorouracil is effective in the palliative management of carcinoma of the colon, rectum, breast, stomach and pancreas.

CONTRAINDICATIONS

Fluorouracil therapy is contraindicated for patients in a poor nutritional state, those with depressed bone marrow function, those with potentially serious infections or those with a known hypersensitivity to Fluorouracil.

WARNINGS

THE DAILY DOSE OF FLUOROURACIL IS NOT TO EXCEED 800 MG. IT IS RECOMMENDED THAT PATIENTS BE HOSPITALIZED DURING THEIR FIRST COURSE OF TREATMENT.

Fluorouracil should be used with extreme caution in poor risk patients with a history of high-dose pelvic irradiation or previous use of alkylating agents, those who have a widespread involvement of bone marrow by metastatic tumors or those with impaired hepatic or renal function.

Pregnancy: Teratogenic effects: Pregnancy category D. Fluorouracil may cause fetal harm when administered to a pregnant woman. Fluorouracil has been shown to be teratogenic in laboratory animals. Fluorouracil exhibited maximum teratogenicity when given to mice as single intraperitoneal injections of 10 to 40 mg/kg on day 10 or 12 of gestation. Similarly, intraperitoneal doses of 12 to 37 mg/kg given to rats between days 9 and 12 of gestation and intramuscular doses of 3 to 9 mg given to hamsters between days 8 and 11 of gestation were teratogenic. Malformations included cleft palates, skeletal defects and deformed appendages, paws and tails. The dosages which were teratogenic in animals are 1 to 3 times the maximum recommended human therapeutic dose. In monkeys, divided doses of 40 mg/kg given between days 20 and 24 of gestation were not teratogenic.

There are no adequate and well-controlled studies with Fluorouracil in pregnant women. While there is no evidence of teratogenicity in humans due to Fluorouracil, it should be kept in mind that other drugs which inhibit DNA synthesis (*e.g.,* methotrexate and aminopterin) have been reported to be teratogenic in humans. Women of childbearing potential should be advised to avoid becoming pregnant. If the drug is used during pregnancy, or if the patient becomes pregnant while taking the drug, the patient should be told of the potential hazard to the fetus. Fluorouracil should be used during pregnancy only if the potential benefit justifies the potential risk to the fetus.

Combination Therapy: Any form of therapy which adds to the stress of the patient, interferes with nutrition or depresses bone marrow function will increase the toxicity of Fluorouracil.

PRECAUTIONS

General: Fluorouracil is a highly toxic drug with a narrow margin of safety. Therefore, patients should be carefully supervised, since therapeutic response is unlikely to occur without some evidence of toxicity. Severe hematological toxicity, gastrointestinal hemorrhage and even death may result from the use of Fluorouracil despite meticulous selection of patients and careful adjustment of dosage. Although severe toxicity is more likely in poor risk patients, fatalities may be encountered occasionally even in patients in relatively good condition.

Therapy is to be discontinued promptly whenever one of the following signs of toxicity appears:

Stomatitis or esophagopharyngitis, at the first visible sign.
Leukopenia (WBC under 3500) or a rapidly falling white blood count.
Vomiting, intractable.
Diarrhea, frequent bowel movements or watery stools.
Gastrointestinal ulceration and bleeding.
Thrombocytopenia (platelets under 100,000).
Hemorrhage from an site.

The administration of 5-fluorouracil has been associated with the occurrence of palmar-plantar erythrodysesthesia syndrome, also known as hand-foot syndrome. This syndrome has been characterized as a tingling sensation of hands and feet which may progress over the next few days to pain when holding objects or walking. The palms and soles become symmetrically swollen and erythematous with tenderness of the distal phalanges, possibly accompanied by desquamation. Interruption of therapy is followed by gradual resolution over 5 to 7 days. Although pyridoxine has been reported to ameliorate the palmar-plantar erythrodysesthesia syndrome, its safety and effectiveness have not been established.

Information for Patients: Patients should be informed of expected toxic effects, particularly oral manifestations. Patients should be alerted to the possibility of alopecia as a result of therapy and should be informed that it is usually a transient effect.

Laboratory Tests: White blood counts with differential are recommended before each dose.

Drug Interactions: Leucovorin calcium may enhance the toxicity of fluorouracil.

Also see WARNINGS section.

Carcinogenesis, Mutagenesis, Impairment of Fertility: Carcinogenesis: Long-term studies in animals to evaluate the carcinogenic potential of fluorouracil have not been conducted. However, there was no evidence of carcinogenicity in small groups of rats given fluorouracil orally at doses of 0.01, 0.3, 1 or 3 mg per rat 5 days per week for 52 weeks, followed by a six-month observation period. Also, in other studies, 33 mg/kg of fluorouracil was administered intravenously to male rats once a week for 52 weeks followed by observation for the remainder of their lifetimes with no evidence of carcinogenicity. Female mice were given 1 mg of fluorouracil intravenously once a week for 16 weeks with no effect on the incidence of lung adenomas. On the basis of the available data, no evaluation can be made of the carcinogenic risk of fluorouracil to humans.

Mutagenesis: Oncogenic transformation of fibroblasts from mouse embryo has been induced *in vitro* by fluorouracil, but the relationship between oncogenicity and mutagenicity is not clear. Fluorouracil has been shown to be mutagenic to several strain of *Salmonella typhimurium*, including TA 1535, TA 1537 and TA 1538, and to *Saccharomyces cerevisiae*, although no evidence of mutagenicity was found with *Salmonella typhimurium* strains TA 92, TA 98 and TA 100. In addition, a positive effect was observed in the micronucleus test on bone marrow cells of the mouse, and fluorouracil at very high concentrations produced chromosomal breaks in hamster fibroblasts *in vitro*.

Impairment of fertility: Fluorouracil has not been adequately studied in animals to permit an evaluation of its effects on fertility and general reproductive performance. However, doses of 125 or 250 mg/kg, administered intraperitoneally, have been shown to induce chromosomal aberrations and changes in chromosomal organization of spermatogonia in rats. Spermatogonial differentiation was also inhibited by fluorouracil, resulting in transient infertility. However, in studies with a strain of mouse which is sensitive to the induction of sperm head abnormalities after exposure to a range of chemical mutagens and carcinogens, fluorouracil did not produce any abnormalities at oral doses of up to 80 mg/kg/day. In female rats, fluorouracil, administered intraperitoneally at weekly doses of 25 or 50 mg/kg for three weeks during the pre-ovulatory phases of oogenesis, significantly reduced the incidence of fertile matings, delayed the development of pre- and postimplantation embryos, increased the incidence of pre-implantation lethality and induced chromosomal anomalies in these embryos. In a limited study in rabbits, a single 25 mg/kg dose of fluorouracil or 5 daily doses of 5 mg/kg had no effect on ovulation, appeared not to affect implantation and had only a limited effect in producing zygote destruction. Compounds such as fluorouracil, which interfere with DNA, RNA and protein synthesis, might be expected to have adverse effects on gametogenesis.

Pregnancy: Pregnancy Category D. See WARNINGS section.

Nonteratogenic effects: Fluorouracil has not been studied in animals for its effects on peri- and postnatal development. However, fluorouracil has been shown to cross the placenta and enter into fetal circulation in the rat. Administration of fluorouracil has resulted in increased resorptions and embryolethality in rats. In monkeys, maternal doses higher than 40 mg/kg resulted in abortion of all embryos exposed to fluorouracil. Compounds which inhibit DNA, RNA and protein synthesis might be expected to have adverse effects on peri- and postnatal development.

Nursing Mothers: It is not known whether fluorouracil is excreted in human milk. Because fluorouracil inhibits DNA, RNA and protein synthesis, mothers should not nurse while receiving this drug.

Pediatric Use: Safety and effectiveness in children have not been established.

ADVERSE REACTIONS

Stomatitis and esophagopharyngitis (which made lead to sloughing and ulceration), diarrhea, anorexia, nausea and emesis are commonly seen during therapy.

Leukopenia usually follows every course of adequate therapy with Fluorouracil. The lowest white blood cell counts are commonly observed between the 9th and 14th days after the first course of treatment, although uncommonly the maximal depression may be delayed for as long as 20 days. By the 30th day the count has usually returned to the normal range.

Alopecia and dermatitis may be seen in a substantial number of cases. The dermatitis most often seen is a pruritic maculopapular rash usually appearing on the extremities and less frequently on the trunk. It is generally reversible and usually responsive to symptomatic treatment.

Other adverse reactions are:

Hematologic: pancytopenia, thrombocytopenia, agranulocytosis, anemia.

Cardiovascular: myocardial ischemia, angina.

Gastrointestinal: gastrointestinal ulceration and bleeding.

Allergic reactions: anaphylaxis and generalized allergic reactions.

Neurologic: acute cerebellar syndrome (which may pesist following discontinuance of treatment), nystagmus, headache.

Dermatologic: dry skin; fissuring; photosensitivity, as manifested by erythema or increased pigmentation of the skin; vein pigmentation, palmar-plantar erythrodysesthesia syndrome, as manifested by tingling of the hands and feet followed by pain, erythema and swelling.

Ophthalmic: lacrimal duct stenosis, visual changes, lacrimation, photophobia.

Psychiatric: disorientation, confusion, euphoria.

Miscellaneous: thrombophlebitis, epistaxis, nail changes (including loss of nails).

OVERDOSAGE

The possibility of overdosage with Fluorouracil is unlikely in view of the mode of administration. Nevertheless, the anticipated manifestations would be nausea, vomiting, diarrhea, gastrointestinal ulceration and bleeding, bone marrow depression (including thrombocytopenia, leukopenia and agranulocytosis). No specific antidotal therapy exists. Patients who have been exposed to an overdose of Fluorouracil should be monitored hematologically for at least four weeks. Should abnormalities appear, appropriate therapy should be utilized.

The acute intravenous toxicity of fluorouracil is as follows:

Species	LD_{50} (mg/kg±S.E.)
Mouse	340±17
Rat	165±26
Rabbit	27±5.1
Dog	31.5±3.8

DOSAGE AND ADMINISTRATION

General Instructions: Fluorouracil Injection should be administered only intravenously, using care to avoid extravasation. No dilution is required.

All dosages are based on the patient's actual weight. However, the estimated lean body mass (dry weight) is used if the patient is obese or if there has been a spurious weight gain due to edema, ascites or other forms of abnormal fluid retention.

It is recommended that prior to treatment each patient be carefully evaluated in order to estimate as accurately as possible the optimum initial dosage of Fluorouracil.

Dosage: Twelve mg/kg are given intravenously once daily for four successive days. The daily dose should not exceed 800 mg. *If no toxicity is observed,* 6 mg/kg are given on the 6th, 8th, 10th and 12th days *unless toxicity occurs.* No therapy is given on the 5th, 7th, 9th or 11th days. *Therapy is to be discontinued at the end of the 12th day, even if no toxicity has become apparent.* (See WARNINGS and PRECAUTIONS sections.)

Poor risk patients or those who are not in an adequate nutritional state (see CONTRAINDICATIONS and WARNINGS sections) should receive 6 mg/kg/day for three days. *If no toxicity is observed,* 3 mg/kg may be given on the 5th, 7th and 9th days *unless toxicity occurs.* No therapy is given on the 4th, 6th or 8th days. The daily dose should not exceed 400 mg.

A sequence of injections on either schedule constitutes a "course of therapy."

Maintenance Therapy: In instances where toxicity has not been a problem, it is recommended that therapy be continued using either of the following schedules:

1. Repeat dosage of first course every 30 days after the last day of the previous course of treatment.
2. When toxic signs resulting from the initial course of therapy have subsided, administer a maintenance dosage of 10 to 15 mg/kg/week as a single dose. Do not exceed 1 Gm per week.

The patient's reaction to the previous course of therapy should be taken into account in determining the amount of the drug to be used, and the dosage should be adjusted accordingly. Some patients have received from 9 to 45 courses of treatment during periods which ranged from 12 to 60 months.

Procedures for proper handling and disposal of anticancer drugs should be considered. Several guidelines on this subject have been published.[1–6] There is no general agreement that all of the procedures recommended in the guidelines are necessary or appropriate.

Note: Parenteral drug products should be inspected visually for particulate matter and discoloration prior to administration, whenever solution and container permit. Although the Fluorouracil solution may discolor slightly during storage, the potency and safety are not adversely affected. If a precipitate occurs due to exposure to low temperatures, resolubilize by heating to 140°F and shaking vigorously; allow to cool to body temperature before using.

Continued on next page

Roche Laboratories—Cont.

HOW SUPPLIED

For intravenous use—10-mL single-use vials, boxes of 10 (NDC 0004-1977-01). Each 10 mL contains 500 mg fluorouracil in a colorless to faint yellow aqueous solution, with pH adjusted to approximately 9.2 with sodium hydroxide.
Store at room temperature (59° to 86°F; 15° to 30°C). Protect from light.

REFERENCES

1. Recommendations for the safe handling of parenteral antineoplastic drugs. Washington, DC, U.S. Government Printing Office (NIH Publication No. 83-2621).
2. AMA Council Report. Guidelines for handling parenteral antineoplastics. *JAMA 253:* 1590–1592, Mar 15, 1985.
3. National Study Commission on Cytotoxic Exposure: Recommendations for handling cytotoxic agents. Available from Louis P. Jeffrey, ScD, Director of Pharmacy Services, Rhode Island Hospital, 593 Eddy Street, Providence, Rhode Island 02902.
4. Clinical Oncological Society of Australia: Guidelines and recommendations for safe handling of antineoplastic agents. *Med J Aust 1:* 426–428, Apr 30, 1983.
5. Jones RB, Frank R, Mass T: Safe handling of chemotherapeutic agents: a report from the Mount Sinai Medical Center. *CA 33:* 258–263, Sept–Oct 1983.
6. ASHP technical assistance bulletin on handling cytotoxic drugs in hospitals. *Am J Hosp Pharm 42:* 131–137, Jan 1985.

Revised: June 1991

STERILE ℞
FUDR
[ef-u-dee-are]
(floxuridine/Roche)

FOR INTRA-ARTERIAL INFUSION ONLY
The following text is complete prescribing information based on official labeling in effect June 1, 1992.

WARNING
It is recommended that FUDR be given only by or under the supervision of a qualified physician who is experienced in cancer chemotherapy and intra-arterial drug therapy and is well versed in the use of potent antimetabolites.
Because of the possibility of severe toxic reactions, all patients should be hospitalized for initiation of the first course of therapy.

DESCRIPTION

Sterile FUDR (floxuridine/Roche), an antineoplastic antimetabolite, is available as a sterile, nonpyrogenic, lyophilized powder for reconstitution. Each vial contains 500 mg of floxuridine which is to be reconstituted with 5 mL of sterile water for injection. An appropriate amount of reconstituted solution is then diluted with a parenteral solution for intra-arterial infusion (see DOSAGE AND ADMINISTRATION section).
Floxuridine is a fluorinated pyrimidine. Chemically, floxuridine is 2′-deoxy-5-fluorouridine with an empirical formula of $C_9H_{11}FN_2O_5$. It is a white to off-white odorless solid which is freely soluble in water.
The 2% aqueous solution has a pH of between 4.0 to 5.5. The molecular weight of floxuridine is 246.19.

CLINICAL PHARMACOLOGY

When FUDR is given by rapid intra-arterial injection it is apparently rapidly catabolized to 5-fluorouracil. Thus, rapid injection of FUDR produces the same toxic and antimetabolic effects as does 5-fluorouracil. The primary effect is to interfere with the synthesis of deoxyribonucleic acid (DNA) and to a lesser extent inhibit the formation of ribonucleic acid (RNA). However, when FUDR is given by continuous intra-arterial infusion its direct anabolism to FUDR-monophosphate is enhanced, thus increasing the inhibition of DNA.
Floxuridine is metabolized in the liver. The drug is excreted intact and as urea, fluorouracil, α-fluoro-β-ureidopropionic acid, dihydrofluorouracil, α-fluoro-β-guanidopropionic acid and α-fluoro-β-alanine in the urine; it is also expired as respiratory carbon dioxide. Pharmacokinetic data on intra-arterial infusion of FUDR are not available.

INDICATIONS AND USAGE

FUDR is effective in the palliative management of gastrointestinal adenocarcinoma metastatic to the liver, when given by continuous regional intra-arterial infusion in carefully selected patients who are considered incurable by surgery or other means. Patients with known disease extending beyond an area capable of infusion via a single artery should, except in unusual circumstances, be considered for systemic therapy with other chemotherapeutic agents.

CONTRAINDICATIONS

FUDR therapy is contraindicated for patients in a poor nutritional state, those with depressed bone marrow function or those with potentially serious infections.

WARNINGS

BECAUSE OF THE POSSIBILITY OF SEVERE TOXIC REACTIONS, ALL PATIENTS SHOULD BE HOSPITALIZED FOR THE FIRST COURSE OF THERAPY.
FUDR should be used with extreme caution in poor risk patients with impaired hepatic or renal function or a history of high-dose pelvic irradiation or previous use of alkylating agents. The drug is not intended as an adjuvant to surgery.
FUDR may cause fetal harm when administered to a pregnant woman. It has been shown to be teratogenic in the chick embryo, mouse (at doses of 2.5 to 100 mg/kg) and rat (at doses of 75 to 150 mg/kg). Malformations included cleft palates; skeletal defects; and deformed appendages, paws and tails. The dosages which were teratogenic in animals are 4.2 to 125 times the recommended human therapeutic dose.
There are no adequate and well-controlled studies with FUDR in pregnant women. If this drug is used during pregnancy or if the patient becomes pregnant while taking (receiving) this drug, the patient should be apprised of the potential hazard to the fetus. Women of childbearing potential should be advised to avoid becoming pregnant.
Combination therapy: Any form of therapy which adds to the stress of the patient, interferes with nutrition or depresses bone marrow function will increase the toxicity of FUDR.

PRECAUTIONS

General: Sterile FUDR is a highly toxic drug with a narrow margin of safety. Therefore, patients should be carefully supervised since therapeutic response is unlikely to occur without some evidence of toxicity. Severe hematological toxicity, gastrointestinal hemorrhage and even death may result from the use of FUDR despite meticulous selection of patients and careful adjustment of dosage. Although severe toxicity is more likely in poor risk patients, fatalities may be encountered occasionally even in patients in relatively good condition.
Therapy is to be discontinued promptly whenever one of the following signs of toxicity appears:
Myocardial ischemia
Stomatitis or esophagopharyngitis, at the first visible sign
Leukopenia (WBC under 3500) or a rapidly falling white blood count
Vomiting, intractable
Diarrhea, frequent bowel movements or watery stools
Gastrointestinal ulceration and bleeding
Thrombocytopenia (platelets under 100,000)
Hemorrhage from any site
Information for patients: Patients should be informed of expected toxic effects, particularly oral manifestations. Patients should be alerted to the possibility of alopecia as a result of therapy and should be informed that it is usually a transient effect.
Laboratory tests: Careful monitoring of the white blood count and platelet count is recommended.
Drug interactions: See WARNINGS section.
Carcinogenesis, mutagenesis, impairment of fertility:
Carcinogenesis: Long-term studies in animals to evaluate the carcinogenic potential of floxuridine have not been conducted. On the basis of the available data, no evaluation can be made of the carcinogenic risk of FUDR to humans.
Mutagenesis: Oncogenic transformation of fibroblasts from mouse embryo has been induced *in vitro* by FUDR, but the relationship between oncogenicity and mutagenicity is not clear. Floxuridine has also been shown to be mutagenic in human leukocytes *in vitro* and in the *Drosophila* test system. In addition, 5-fluorouracil, to which floxuridine is catabolized when given by intra-arterial injection, has been shown to be mutagenic in *in vitro* tests.
Impairment of fertility: The effects of floxuridine on fertility and general reproductive performance have not been studied in animals. However, because floxuridine is catabolized to 5-fluorouracil, it should be noted that 5-fluorouracil has been shown to induce chromosomal aberrations and changes in chromosome organization of spermatogonia in rats at doses of 125 or 250 mg/kg, administered intraperitoneally.
Spermatogonial differentiation was also inhibited by fluorouracil, resulting in transient infertility. In female rats, fluorouracil, administered intraperitoneally at doses of 25 or 50 mg/kg during the preovulatory phase of oogenesis, significantly reduced the incidence of fertile matings, delayed the development of pre- and post-implantation embryos, increased the incidence of preimplantation lethality and induced chromosomal anomalies in these embryos. Compounds such as FUDR, which interfere with DNA, RNA and protein synthesis, might be expected to have adverse effects on gametogenesis.
Pregnancy: Teratogenic effects: Pregnancy category D. See WARNINGS section. Floxuridine has been shown to be teratogenic in the chick embryo, mouse (at doses of 2.5 to 100 mg/kg) and rat (at doses of 75 to 150 mg/kg). Malformations included cleft palates, skeletal defects and deformed appendages, paws and tails. The dosages which were teratogenic in animals are 4.2 to 125 times the recommended human therapeutic dose.
There are no adequate and well-controlled studies with FUDR in pregnant women. While there is no evidence of teratogenicity in humans due to FUDR, it should be kept in mind that other drugs which inhibit DNA synthesis (*e.g.,* methotrexate and aminopterin) have been reported to be teratogenic in humans. FUDR should be used during pregnancy only if the potential benefit justifies the potential risk to the fetus.
Nonteratogenic effects: Floxuridine has not been studied in animals for its effects on peri- and postnatal development. However, compounds which inhibit DNA, RNA and protein synthesis might be expected to have adverse effects on peri- and postnatal development.
Nursing mothers: It is not known whether FUDR is excreted in human milk. Because FUDR inhibits DNA and RNA synthesis, mothers should not nurse while receiving this drug.
Pediatric use: Safety and effectiveness in children have not been established.

ADVERSE REACTIONS

Adverse reactions to the arterial infusion of FUDR are generally related to the procedural complications of regional arterial infusion.
The more common adverse reactions to the drug are nausea, vomiting, diarrhea, enteritis, stomatitis and localized erythema. The more common laboratory abnormalities are anemia, leukopenia, thrombocytopenia and elevations of alkaline phosphatase, serum transaminase, serum bilirubin and lactic dehydrogenase.
Other adverse reactions are:
Gastrointestinal: duodenal ulcer, duodenitis, gastritis, bleeding, gastroenteritis, glossitis, pharyngitis, anorexia, cramps, abdominal pain; possible intra- and extrahepatic biliary sclerosis, as well as acalculous cholecystitis.
Dermatologic: alopecia, dermatitis, nonspecific skin toxicity, rash.
Cardiovascular: myocardial ischemia.
Miscellaneous clinical reactions: fever, lethargy, malaise, weakness.
Laboratory abnormalities: BSP, prothrombin, total proteins, sedimentation rate and thrombopenia.
Procedural complications of regional arterial infusion: arterial aneurysm; arterial ischemia; arterial thrombosis; embolism; fibromyositis; thrombophlebitis; hepatic necrosis; abscesses; infection at catheter site; bleeding at catheter site; catheter blocked, displaced or leaking.
The following adverse reactions have not been reported with FUDR but have been noted following the administration of 5-fluorouracil. While the possibility of these occurring following FUDR therapy is remote because of its regional administration, one should be alert for these reactions following the administration of FUDR because of the pharmacological similarity of these two drugs: pancytopenia, agranulocytosis, myocardial ischemia, angina, anaphylaxis, generalized allergic reactions, acute cerebellar syndrome, nystagmus, headache, dry skin, fissuring, photosensitivity, pruritic maculopapular rash, increased pigmentation of the skin, vein pigmentation, lacrimal duct stenosis, visual changes, lacrimation, photophobia, disorientation, confusion, euphoria, epistaxis and nail changes, including loss of nails.

OVERDOSAGE

The possibility of overdosage with FUDR is unlikely in view of the mode of administration. Nevertheless, the anticipated manifestations would be nausea, vomiting, diarrhea, gastrointestinal ulceration and bleeding, bone marrow depression (including thrombocytopenia, leukopenia and agranulocytosis).
No specific antidotal therapy exists. Patients who have been exposed to an overdosage of FUDR should be monitored hematologically for at least four weeks. Should abnormalities appear, appropriate therapy should be utilized.
The acute intravenous toxicity of floxuridine is as follows:

Species	LD_{50} (mg/kg ± S.E.)
Mouse	880 ± 51
Rat	670 ± 73
Rabbit	94 ± 19.6
Dog	157 ± 46

DOSAGE AND ADMINISTRATION

Each vial must be reconstituted with 5 mL of sterile water for injection to yield a solution containing approximately 100 mg of floxuridine/mL. The calculated daily dose(s) of the drug is then diluted with 5% dextrose or 0.9% sodium chloride injection to a volume appropriate for the infusion apparatus to be used. The administration of FUDR is best achieved with the use of an appropriate pump to overcome pressure in large arteries and to ensure a uniform rate of infusion.

Parenteral drug products should be inspected visually for particulate matter and discoloration prior to administration whenever solution and container permit.

The recommended therapeutic dosage schedule of FUDR by continuous arterial infusion is 0.1 to 0.6 mg/kg/day. The higher dosage ranges (0.4 to 0.6 mg) are usually employed for hepatic artery infusion because the liver metabolizes the drug, thus reducing the potential for systemic toxicity. Therapy can be given until adverse reactions appear. (See PRECAUTIONS section.) When these side effects have subsided, therapy may be resumed. The patient should be maintained on therapy as long as response to FUDR continues.

Procedures for proper handling and disposal of anticancer drugs should be considered. Several guidelines on this subject have been published.[1–6] There is no general agreement that all of the procedures recommended in the guidelines are necessary or appropriate.

HOW SUPPLIED

500 mg Sterile FUDR (floxuridine) powder in a 5-mL vial (NDC 0004-1935-08). This is to be reconstituted with 5 mL sterile water for injection.

The sterile powder should be stored at 59° to 86°F (15° to 30°C). Reconstituted vials should be stored under refrigeration (36° to 46°F, 2° to 8°C) for not more than two weeks.

REFERENCES

1. Recommendations for the safe handling of parenteral antineoplastic drugs. Washington, DC, U.S. Government Printing Office (NIH Publication No. 83-2621).
2. AMA Council Report. Guidelines for handling parenteral antineoplastics. *JAMA 253:* 1590–1592, Mar 15, 1985.
3. National Study Commission on Cytotoxic Exposure: Recommendations for handling cytotoxic agents. Available from Louis P. Jeffrey, ScD, Director of Pharmacy Services, Rhode Island Hospital, 593 Eddy Street, Providence, Rhode Island 02902.
4. Clinical Oncological Society of Australia: Guidelines and recommendations for safe handling of antineoplastic agents. *Med J Aust 1:* 426–428, Apr 30, 1983.
5. Jones RB, Frank R, Mass T: Safe handling of chemotherapeutic agents: a report from the Mount Sinai Medical Center. *CA 33:* 258–263, Sept–Oct 1983.
6. ASHP technical assistance bulletin on handling cytotoxic drugs in hospitals. *Am J Hosp Pharm 42:* 131–137, Jan 1985.

Revised: October 1989

GANTANOL® ℞

[*gan 'tan-ol*]
sulfamethoxazole/Roche
TABLETS • SUSPENSION

The following text is complete prescribing information based on official labeling in effect June 1, 1992.

DESCRIPTION

Gantanol® (brand of sulfamethoxazole/Roche) is an intermediate-dosage antibacterial sulfonamide available in tablets and suspension. Each tablet contains 0.5 Gm sulfamethoxazole plus corn starch, polyvinyl acetate, polyvinyl alcohol, magnesium stearate, FD&C Blue No. 1 Lake, FD&C Yellow No. 6 Lake and D&C Yellow No. 10 Lake. Each teaspoonful (5 mL) of the suspension contains 0.5 Gm sulfamethoxazole in a vehicle containing carboxyvinyl polymer, citric acid, edetate disodium, methylcellulose, saccharin, saccharin sodium, simethicone, sodium benzoate, sodium citrate, sodium hydroxide, sodium lauryl sulfate, sorbitol, sucrose, FD&C Red. No. 40, flavors and water.

Sulfamethoxazole is *N*[1]-(5-methyl-3-isoxazolyl) sulfanilamide. It is an almost white, odorless, tasteless compound with a molecular weight of 253.28.

CLINICAL PHARMACOLOGY

Sulfamethoxazole is rapidly absorbed following oral administration. It exists in the blood as unbound, protein-bound, metabolized and conjugated forms. The metabolism of sulfamethoxazole occurs predominately by N_4-acetylation, although the glucuronide conjugate has been identified. The free form is considered to be the therapeutically active form. Approximately 70% of sulfamethoxazole is bound to plasma proteins; of the unbound portion, 80% to 90% is in the nonacetylated form.

Following a single 1-Gm oral dose in 12 volunteer male subjects, the mean peak plasma concentration of 38 mcg/mL of intact sulfamethoxazole was achieved by 2 hours. The mean half-life of sulfamethoxazole is approximately 10 hours. However, patients with severely impaired renal function, as shown by a creatinine clearance of less than 30 mL/minute, exhibit an increase of the half-life of sulfamethoxazole, requiring dosage regimen adjustment.

Sulfamethoxazole is excreted primarily by the kidneys chiefly through glomerular filtration but also through tubular secretion. Urine concentrations of sulfamethoxazole are considerably higher than are the concentrations in blood. Eighty percent to 100 percent of the dose is excreted in the urine as total sulfamethoxazole, of which 30% is intact drug with the remaining as the N_4-acetylated metabolite.

Sulfamethoxazole diffuses into cerebrospinal fluid, with peak concentrations occurring at 8 hours and reaching approximately 14% of simultaneous plasma concentrations. The drug has also been shown to distribute to aqueous humor, vaginal fluid and middle ear fluid; it also passes the placental barrier and is excreted in breast milk.

Microbiology: The systemic sulfonamides are bacteriostatic agents and the spectrum of activity is similar for all. Sulfonamides inhibit bacterial synthesis of dihydrofolic acid by competing with *para*-aminobenzoic acid (PABA). Resistant strains are capable of utilizing folic acid precursors or preformed folic acid.

INDICATIONS AND USAGE

Acute, recurrent or chronic urinary tract infections (primarily pyelonephritis, pyelitis and cystitis) due to susceptible organisms (usually *E. coli, Klebsiella-Enterbacter,* staphylococcus, *Proteus mirabilis* and, less frequently, *Proteus vulgaris*) in the absence of obstructive uropathy or foreign bodies.

Meningococcal meningitis prophylaxis when sulfonamide-sensitive group A strains are known to prevail in family groups or larger closed populations. (The prophylactic usefulness of sulfonamides when group B or C infections are prevalent has not been proven and in closed population groups may be harmful.)

Acute otitis media due to *Haemophilus influenzae* when used concomitantly with adequate doses of penicillin.

Trachoma, Inclusion conjunctivitis, Nocardiosis, Chancroid.

Toxoplasmosis as adjunctive therapy with pyrimethamine.

Malaria due to chloroquine-resistant strains of *Plasmodium falciparum,* when used as adjunctive therapy.

Important note: In vitro sulfonamide susceptibility tests are not always reliable. The test must be carefully coordinated with bacteriologic and clinical response. When the patient is already taking sulfonamides, follow-up cultures should have aminobenzoic acid added to the culture media.

Currently, the increasing frequency of resistant organisms is a limitation of the usefulness of antibacterial agents including the sulfonamides, especially in the treatment of chronic and recurrent urinary tract infections.

Wide variation in blood concentrations may result with identical doses. Blood concentrations should be measured in patients receiving sulfonamides for serious infections. Free sulfonamide blood concentrations of 5 to 15 mg/100 mL may be considered therapeutically effective for most infections, with blood concentrations of 12 to 15 mg/100 mL optimal for serious infections; 20 mg/100 mL should be the maximum total sulfonamide concentration, since adverse reactions occur more frequently above this concentration.

CONTRAINDICATIONS

Hypersensitivity to sulfonamides. Infants less than 2 months of age (except in the treatment of congenital toxoplasmosis as adjunctive therapy with pyrimethamine). Pregnancy at term and during the nursing period because sulfonamides pass the placenta and are excreted in the milk and may cause kernicterus.

WARNINGS

The sulfonamides should not be used for the treatment of group A beta-hemolytic streptococcal infections. In an established infection, they will not eradicate the streptococcus, and therefore will not prevent sequelae such as rheumatic fever and glomerulonephritis.

Deaths associated with the administration of sulfonamides have been reported from hypersensitivity reactions, hepatocellular necrosis, agranulocytosis, aplastic anemia and other blood dyscrasias.

The presence of clinical signs such as sore throat, fever, arthralgia, cough, shortness of breath, pallor, purpura or jaundice may be early indications of serious reactions, including serious blood disorders.

PRECAUTIONS

General: Sulfonamides should be given with caution to patients with impaired renal or hepatic function and to those with severe allergy or bronchial asthma. In glucose-6-phosphate dehydrogenase-deficient individuals, hemolysis may occur. This reaction is frequently dose-related.

Information for patients: Patients should be instructed to maintain an adequate fluid intake in order to prevent crystalluria and stone formation.

Laboratory tests: Complete blood counts should be done frequently in patients receiving sulfonamides. If a significant reduction in the count of any formed blood element is noted, Gantanol should be discontinued. Urinalyses with careful microscopic examination and renal function tests should be performed during therapy, particularly for those patients with impaired renal function.

Drug interactions: In elderly patients concurrently receiving certain diuretics, primarily thiazides, an increased incidence of thrombopenia with purpura has been reported.

It has been reported that sulfamethoxazole may prolong the prothrombin time in patients who are receiving the anticoagulant warfarin. This interaction should be kept in mind when Gantanol is given to patients already on anticoagulant therapy, and the coagulation time should be reassessed.

Sulfamethoxazole may inhibit the hepatic metabolism of phenytoin. At a 1.6 Gm dose, sulfamethoxazole produced a slight but significant increase in the half-life of phenytoin but did not produce a corresponding decrease in the metabolic clearance rate. When administering these drugs concurrently, one should be alert for possible excessive phenytoin effect.

Sulfonamides can also displace methotrexate from plasma protein-binding sites, thus increasing free methotrexate concentrations.

The presence of sulfamethoxazole may interfere with the Jaffé alkaline picrate reaction assay for creatinine, resulting in overestimations of about 10% in the range of normal values.

Carcinogenesis, mutagenesis, impairment of fertility: Carcinogenesis: Sulfamethoxazole has not been adequately tested in animals to permit an evaluation of its carcinogenic potential.

Mutagenesis: Bacterial mutagenic studies have not been performed with sulfamethoxazole. No chromosomal damage was observed in human leukocytes cultured *in vitro* with sulfamethoxazole; the concentrations used exceeded blood levels of sulfamethoxazole following therapy with Gantanol.

Impairment of fertility: No adverse effects on fertility or general reproductive performance were observed in rats given sulfamethoxazole in oral dosages as high as 350 mg/kg/day.

Pregnancy: Teratogenic Effects: Pregnancy Category C. In rats, oral doses of 533 mg/kg of sulfamethoxazole produced teratologic effects manifested mainly as cleft palates. The highest dose which did not cause cleft palates in rats was 512 mg/kg of sulfamethoxazole. In rabbits, 150 to 350 mg/kg/day increased maternal mortality but had no deleterious effects on fetal development.

There are no adequate and well-controlled studies of Gantanol in pregnant women. Gantanol should be used during pregnancy only if the potential benefit justifies the potential risk to the fetus.

Nonteratogenic effects: See CONTRAINDICATIONS section.

Nursing mothers: See CONTRAINDICATIONS section.

Pediatric Use: Gantanol is not recommended in infants under 2 months of age, except in the treatment of congenital toxoplasmosis as adjunctive therapy with pyrimethamine. (See CONTRAINDICATIONS section.) At the present time there are insufficient clinical data on prolonged or recurrent therapy in chronic renal diseases of children under 6 years of age.

ADVERSE REACTIONS

Included in the listing that follows are adverse reactions that have not been reported with this specific drug; however, the pharmacologic similarities among the sulfonamides require that each of the reactions be considered with Gantanol administration.

Hematologic: Agranulocytosis, aplastic anemia, thrombocytopenia, leukopenia, hemolytic anemia, purpura, hypoprothrombinemia, methemoglobinemia, neutropenia, eosinophilia.

Allergic Reactions: Anaphylaxis, allergic myocarditis, serum sickness, conjunctival and scleral injection, generalized allergic reactions. In addition, periarteritis nodosa and systemic lupus erythematosus have been reported.

Dermatologic: Stevens-Johnson syndrome, epidermal necrolysis, erythema multiforme, exfoliative dermatitis, photosensitivity, pruritus, urticaria, rash, generalized skin eruptions.

Gastrointestinal: Hepatitis, hepatocellular necrosis, pseudomembranous enterocolitis, pancreatitis, stomatitis, glossitis, nausea, emesis, abdominal pain, diarrhea, anorexia.

Genitourinary: Creatinine elevation, toxic nephrosis with oliguria and anuria. The frequency of renal complications is considerably lower in patients receiving the more soluble sulfonamides.

Neurologic: Convulsions, peripheral neuritis, ataxia, vertigo, tinnitus, headache.

Psychiatric: Hallucinations, depression, apathy.

Endocrine: The sulfonamides bear certain chemical similarities to some goitrogens, diuretics (acetazolamide and the thiazides) and oral hypoglycemic agents. Cross-sensitivity may exist with these agents. Diuresis and hypoglycemia have occurred rarely in patients receiving sulfonamides.

Musculoskeletal: Arthralgia, myalgia.

Respiratory: Pulmonary infiltrates.

Miscellaneous: Edema (including periorbital), pyrexia, chills, weakness, fatigue, insomnia.

OVERDOSAGE

Acute: The amount of a single dose of sulfamethoxazole that is either associated with symptoms of overdosage or is likely to be life-threatening has not been reported. Signs and symptoms of overdosage reported with sulfonamides include

Continued on next page

Roche Laboratories—Cont.

anorexia, colic, nausea, vomiting, dizziness, headache, drowsiness and unconsciousness. Pyrexia, hematuria and crystalluria may be noted. Blood dyscrasias and jaundice are potential late manifestations of overdosage.

General principles of treatment include the institution of gastric lavage or emesis; forcing oral fluids; and the administration of intravenous fluids if urine output is low and renal function is normal. The patient should be monitored with blood counts and appropriate blood chemistries, including electrolytes. If a significant blood dyscrasia or jaundice occurs, specific therapy should be instituted for these complications. Peritoneal dialysis is not effective and hemodialysis is only moderately effective in eliminating sulfamethoxazole.

Chronic: Use of sulfamethoxazole at high doses and/or for extended periods of time may cause bone marrow depression manifested as thrombocytopenia, leukopenia and/or megaloblastic anemia. If signs of bone marrow depression occur, the patient should be given leucovorin 3 to 6 mg intramuscularly daily for three days, or as required to restore normal hematopoiesis.

Animal Toxicity: The oral LD_{50} of sulfamethoxazole is 2300 mg/kg in mice, 3000 mg/kg in rats and > 2000 mg/kg in rabbits.

DOSAGE AND ADMINISTRATION

Systemic sulfonamides are contraindicated in infants under 2 months of age, except in the treatment of congenital toxoplasmosis as adjunctive therapy with pyrimethamine.

The usual dosage schedules are as follows:

Children

Infants (2 Months or Older) and Children	Initial Dose (50–60 mg/kg)	Dose Morning and Evening Daily Thereafter (25–30 mg/kg)
20 lbs	1 tablet or 1 teasp. (0.5 Gm)	½ tablet or ½ teasp. (0.25 Gm)
40 lbs	2 tablets or 2 teasp. (1 Gm)	1 tablet or 1 teasp. (0.5 Gm)
60 lbs	3 tablets or 3 teasp. (1.5 Gm)	1½ tablets or 1½ teasp. (0.75 Gm)
80 lbs	4 tablets or 4 teasp. (2 Gm)	2 tablets or 2 teasp. (1 Gm)

The maximum dose for children should not exceed 75 mg/kg/24 hours.

Adults		
Mild to Moderate Infections	4 tablets or 4 teasp. (2 Gm)	2 tablets or 2 teasp. (1 Gm)

Note: One teaspoonful equals 5 ml.

Severe Infections: 4 tablets or 4 teaspoonfuls (2 Gm) initially, followed by 2 tablets or 2 teaspoonfuls (1 Gm) three times daily thereafter.

Patients with impaired renal function (creatinine clearance below 20 to 30 mL/min) require decreased dosage adjustment.

HOW SUPPLIED

Tablets (pale green, scored), containing 0.5 Gm sulfamethoxazole—bottles of 100 (NDC 0004-0010-01); Tel-E-Dose® packages of 100 (NDC 0004-0010-49). Imprint on tablets: GANTANOL® ROCHE.

Suspension, 10%, containing 0.5 Gm sulfamethoxazole per teaspoonful (5 mL); cherry-flavored—bottles of 1 pint (473 mL) (NDC 0004-1002-28).

Revised: July 1988

Shown in Product Identification Section, page 426

GANTRISIN®   ℞
[*gan 'tris-in*]
(sulfisoxazole diolamine/Roche)
OPHTHALMIC SOLUTION
OPHTHALMIC OINTMENT

The following text is complete prescribing information based on official labeling in effect June 1, 1992.

DESCRIPTION

Gantrisin (sulfisoxazole diolamine/Roche) Ophthalmic Solution and Ointment are antibacterial sulfonamide preparations specifically intended for topical ophthalmic use. The solution is a sterile, isotonic preparation containing 4% (40 mg/ml) sulfisoxazole in the form of the diolamine salt, and phenylmercuric nitrate 1:100,000 as a preservative. The solution has a physiologic pH, and does not cause significant stinging or burning on application. The ointment is a sterile preparation containing 4% sulfisoxazole in the form of the

diolamine salt, compounded with white petrolatum, mineral oil and phenylmercuric nitrate 1:50,000 as a preservative. Chemically, sulfisoxazole diolamine is N^1-(3,4-dimethyl-5-isoxazolyl)sulfanilamide compound with 2,2'-iminodiethanol (1:1). It is a white to off-white, odorless, crystalline powder that is freely soluble in water and soluble in alcohol. Sulfisoxazole diolamine has a molecular weight of 372.44.

CLINICAL PHARMACOLOGY

Sulfonamides do not appear to be appreciably absorbed from mucous membranes.

Microbiology: Sulfonamides exert a bacteriostatic effect against a wide range of gram-positive and gram-negative microorganisms. Sulfonamides inhibit bacterial synthesis of dihydrofolic acid by competing with *para*-aminobenzoic acid (PABA). Resistant strains are capable of utilizing folic acid precursors or preformed folic acid. Currently, the increasing frequency of resistant organisms is a limitation of the usefulness of antibacterial agents, including the sulfonamides.

INDICATIONS

For the treatment of conjunctivitis, corneal ulcers and other superficial ocular infections due to susceptible microorganisms, and as an adjunct in systemic sulfonamide therapy of trachoma.

CONTRAINDICATIONS

Hypersensitivity to sulfonamides or to other ingredients in the formulation. Infants less than 2 months of age. Pregnancy at term and during the nursing period because sulfonamides pass the placenta and are excreted in the milk and may cause kernicterus.

PRECAUTIONS

General: Ophthalmic ointments may retard corneal healing. Nonsusceptible organisms, including fungi, may proliferate with the use of these preparations. Sulfonamides are inactivated by the *para*-aminobenzoic acid present in purulent exudates. Should undesirable reactions occur, discontinue Gantrisin immediately.

Information for patients: Patients using Gantrisin Ophthalmic Solution should be instructed not to touch the dropper tip to any surface, since contamination of the solution may result.

Drug Interactions: Gantrisin Ophthalmic Solution and Ointment are incompatible with preparations containing silver. *In vitro* antagonism with sulfisoxazole diolamine and gentamicin sulfate (Garamycin) has been reported.

Carcinogenesis, mutagenesis, impairment of fertility: Carcinogenesis: Carcinogenic studies have not been performed with ophthalmic preparations of sulfisoxazole. Sulfisoxazole was not carcinogenic in either sex when administered by gavage for 103 weeks at dosages up to 2000 mg/kg/day in mice or 400 mg/kg/day in rats. Mutagenesis: Bacterial mutagenic studies have not been performed with sulfisoxazole. However, Gantrisin was not observed to be mutagenic in *E. coli* Sd-4-73 when tested in the absence of a metabolic activating system. Impairment of fertility: Fertility studies have not been performed with ophthalmic preparations of sulfisoxazole. No effects on mating behavior, conception rate or fertility index (percent pregnant) were observed in a reproduction study in rats given oral dosages of 800 mg/kg/day sulfisoxazole.

Pregnancy: Teratogenic effects: Pregnancy Category C. Teratogenic studies of ophthalmic preparations of sulfisoxazole have not been performed in laboratory animals. Sulfisoxazole was not teratogenic in either rats or rabbits at oral dosages of 800 mg/kg/day. However, in another teratogenicity study, cleft palates developed in both rats and mice after oral administration of 1000 mg/kg/day sulfisoxazole; skeletal defects were also observed in rats. This dose is 9 to 18 times the usual adult dosage for oral Gantrisin.

There are no adequate and well-controlled studies of Gantrisin in pregnant women. Gantrisin Ophthalmic Solution and Ointment should be used during pregnancy only if the potential benefit justifies the potential risk to the fetus.

Nursing mothers: See CONTRAINDICATIONS section.

Pediatric use: Gantrisin Ophthalmic Solution is not recommended for use in infants younger than 2 months of age.

ADVERSE REACTIONS

Topical application of the sulfonamides may produce sensitization and preclude later systemic use of these drugs. In addition, patients who have been sensitized by systemic sulfonamide administration may exhibit hypersensitivity reactions following topical application of the drugs.

Ophthalmic: Ocular irritation, chemosis, itching.

Included in the listing that follows are adverse reactions that have not been reported with these dosage forms but have been reported for the systemically absorbed sulfonamides.

Hematologic: Agranulocytosis, aplastic anemia, thrombocytopenia, leukopenia, hemolytic anemia, purpura, hypoprothrombinemia and methemoglobinemia.

Allergic reactions: Erythema multiforme (Stevens-Johnson syndrome), generalized skin eruptions, epidermal necrolysis, urticaria, serum sickness, pruritus, exfoliative dermatitis, anaphylactoid reactions, periorbital edema, conjunctival

and scleral injection, photosensitization, arthralgia and allergic myocarditis.

Gastrointestinal reactions: Nausea, emesis, abdominal pains, hepatitis, hepatocellular necrosis, diarrhea, anorexia, pancreatitis and stomatitis.

C.N.S. reactions: Headache, peripheral neuritis, mental depression, convulsions, ataxia, hallucinations, tinnitus, vertigo and insomnia.

Miscellaneous reactions: Drug fever, chills, and toxic nephrosis with oliguria and anuria. Periarteritis, nodosa and L.E. phenomenon have occurred.

Endocrine: The sulfonamides bear certain chemical similarities to some goitrogens, diuretics (acetazolamide and the thiazides) and oral hypoglycemic agents. Goiter production, diuresis and hypoglycemia have occurred rarely in patients receiving sulfonamides. Cross sensitivity may exist with these agents.

DOSAGE AND ADMINISTRATION

Solution: Instill two or three drops in the eye three or more times daily. Care should be taken not to touch dropper tip to any surface, since contamination of the solution may result.

Ointment: Instill small amount in the lower conjunctival sac one to three times daily and at bedtime.

HOW SUPPLIED

Gantrisin Ophthalmic Solution, containing 4% (40 mg/ml) sulfisoxazole in the form of the diolamine salt—½ oz bottles with dropper (NDC 0004-1702-39).

Gantrisin Ophthalmic Ointment, containing 4% sulfisoxazole in the form of the diolamine salt—⅛ oz tubes (NDC 0004-1501-41).

Both dosage forms are stable at room temperature and do not require refrigeration.

Revised: August 1985

GANTRISIN®   ℞
[*gan 'tris-in*]
sulfisoxazole/Roche Tablets
GANTRISIN®   ℞
acetyl sulfisoxazole/Roche
Pediatric Suspension and Syrup

The following text is complete prescribing information based on official labeling in effect June 1, 1992.

DESCRIPTION

Gantrisin (brand of sulfisoxazole/Roche) is an antibacterial sulfonamide available in tablets, pediatric suspension and syrup for oral administration. Each tablet contains 0.5 Gm sulfisoxazole with corn starch, gelatin, lactose and magnesium stearate. Each teaspoonful (5 mL) of the pediatric suspension contains the equivalent of approximately 0.5 Gm sulfisoxazole in the form of acetyl sulfisoxazole in a vehicle containing 0.3 percent alcohol, carboxymethylcellulose (sodium), citric acid, methylcellulose, parabens (methyl and propyl), partial invert sugar, sodium citrate, sorbitan monolaurate, sucrose, flavors and water. Each teaspoonful (5 mL) of the syrup contains the equivalent of approximately 0.5 Gm sulfisoxazole in the form of acetyl sulfisoxazole in a vehicle containing 0.9 percent alcohol, benzoic acid, carrageenan, citric acid, cocoa, sodium citrate, sorbitan monolaurate, sucrose, flavors and water.

Sulfisoxazole is N^1-(3,4-dimethyl-5-isoxazolyl)sulfanilamide. It is a white to slightly yellowish, odorless, slightly bitter, crystalline powder that is soluble in alcohol and very slightly soluble in water. Sulfisoxazole has a molecular weight of 267.30.

Acetyl sulfisoxazole, the tasteless form of sulfisoxazole, is N^1-acetyl sulfisoxazole and must be distinguished from N^4-acetyl sulfisoxazole, which is a metabolite of sulfisoxazole. Acetyl sulfisoxazole is a white or slightly yellow, crystalline powder that is slightly soluble in alcohol and practically insoluble in water. Acetyl sulfisoxazole has a molecular weight of 309.34.

CLINICAL PHARMACOLOGY

Following oral administration, sulfisoxazole is rapidly and completely absorbed; the small intestine is the major site of absorption, but some of the drug is absorbed from the stomach. Sulfisoxazole exists in the blood as unbound, proteinbound and conjugated forms. Sulfisoxazole is metabolized primarily by acetylation and oxidation in the liver. The free form is considered to be the therapeutically active form. Approximately 85% of sulfisoxazole is bound to plasma proteins, primarily to albumin; of the unbound portion, 65% to 72% is in the nonacetylated form.

Maximum plasma concentrations of intact sulfisoxazole following a single 2-Gm oral dose of sulfisoxazole to healthy adult volunteers ranged from 127 to 211 mcg/mL (mean, 169 mcg/mL) and the time of peak plasma concentration ranged from 1 to 4 hours (mean, 2.5 hours). The half-life of elimination of sulfisoxazole ranged from 4.6 to 7.8 hours after oral administration. The elimination of sulfisoxazole has been shown to be slower in elderly subjects (63 to 75 years) with diminished renal function (creatinine clearance, 37 to

68 mL/min).[1] After multiple dose oral administration of 500 mg Q.I.D. to healthy volunteers, the average steady-state plasma concentrations of intact sulfisoxazole ranged from 49.9 to 88.8 mcg/mL (mean, 63.4 mcg/mL).[2]

N^1-acetyl sulfisoxazole is metabolized to sulfisoxazole by digestive enzymes in the gastrointestinal tract and is absorbed as sulfisoxazole. This enzymatic splitting is presumed to be responsible for slower absorption and lower peak blood concentrations than are attained following administration of an equal oral dose of sulfisoxazole. With continued administration of acetyl sulfisoxazole, blood concentrations approximate those of sulfisoxazole. Following a single 4-Gm dose of acetyl sulfisoxazole to healthy volunteers, maximum plasma concentrations of sulfisoxazole ranged from 122 to 282 mcg/mL (mean, 181 mcg/mL) for the pediatric suspension and from 101 to 202 mcg/mL (mean, 144 mcg/mL) for the syrup, and occurred between 2 and 6 hours postadministration. The half-lives of elimination from plasma ranged from 5.4 to 7.4 and from 5.9 to 8.5 hours, respectively.

Sulfisoxazole and acetylated metabolites are excreted primarily by the kidneys through glomerular filtration. Urine concentrations of sulfisoxazole are considerably higher than are the concentrations in blood. The mean urinary excretion recovery following oral administration of sulfisoxazole is 97% within 48 hours, of which 52% is intact drug, with the remaining as the N^4-acetylated metabolite. Following administration of acetyl sulfisoxazole syrup or suspension, approximately 58% is excreted in the urine as total drug within 72 hours.

Sulfisoxazole is distributed only in extracellular body water. It readily crosses the placental barrier and enters into fetal circulation; it is also secreted in breast milk. It also crosses the blood-brain barrier. In healthy subjects, cerebrospinal fluid concentrations of sulfisoxazole vary; in patients with meningitis, however, concentrations of free drug as high as 94 mcg/mL have been reported.

Microbiology: The systemic sulfonamides are bacteriostatic agents. The spectrum of activity is similar for all. Sulfonamides inhibit bacterial synthesis of dihydrofolic acid by competing with *para*-aminobenzoic acid (PABA). Resistant strains are capable of utilizing folic acid precursors or preformed folic acid.

INDICATIONS AND USAGE

Acute, recurrent or chronic urinary tract infections (primarily pyelonephritis, pyelitis and cystitis) due to susceptible organisms (usually *Escherichia coli, Klebsiella-Enterobacter,* staphylococcus, *Proteus mirabilis* and, less frequently, *Proteus vulgaris*) in the absence of obstructive uropathy or foreign bodies.

Meningococcal meningitis where the organism has been demonstrated to be susceptible. *Haemophilus influenzae* meningitis as adjunctive therapy with parenteral streptomycin.

Meningococcal meningitis prophylaxis when sulfonamide-sensitive group A strains are known to prevail in family groups or larger closed populations. (The prophylactic usefulness of sulfonamides when group B or C infections are prevalent has not been proven and in closed population groups may be harmful.)

Acute otitis media due to *Haemophilus influenzae* when used concomitantly with adequate doses of penicillin or erythromycin (see appropriate labeling for prescribing information).

Trachoma. Inclusion conjunctivitis. Nocardiosis. Chancroid.

Toxoplasmosis as adjunctive therapy with pyrimethamine.

Malaria due to chloroquine-resistant strains of *Plasmodium falciparum,* when used as adjunctive therapy.

Important Note: In vitro sulfonamide susceptibility tests are not always reliable. The test must be carefully coordinated with bacteriologic and clinical response. When the patient is already taking sulfonamides, follow-up cultures should have aminobenzoic acid added to the culture media.

Currently, the increasing frequency of resistant organisms is a limitation of the usefulness of antibacterial agents including the sulfonamides, especially in the treatment of chronic and recurrent urinary tract infections.

Wide variation in blood concentrations may result with identical doses. Blood concentrations should be measured in patients receiving sulfonamides for serious infections. Free sulfonamide blood concentrations of 5 to 15 mg/100 mL may be considered therapeutically effective for most infections, with blood concentrations of 12 to 15 mg/100 mL optimal for serious infections; 20 mg/100 mL should be the maximum total sulfonamide concentration, since adverse reactions occur more frequently above this concentration.

CONTRAINDICATIONS

Hypersensitivity to sulfonamides. Infants less than 2 months of age (except in the treatment of congenital toxoplasmosis as adjunctive therapy with pyrimethamine). Pregnancy at term and during the nursing period, because sulfonamides pass the placenta and are excreted in the milk and may cause kernicterus.

WARNINGS

The sulfonamides should not be used for the treatment of group A beta-hemolytic streptococcal infections. In an established infection, they will not eradicate the streptococcus, and therefore will not prevent sequelae such as rheumatic fever and glomerulonephritis.

Deaths associated with the administration of sulfonamides have been reported from hypersensitivity reactions, hepatocellular necrosis, agranulocytosis, aplastic anemia and other blood dyscrasias.

The presence of clinical signs such as sore throat, fever, arthralgia, cough, shortness of breath, pallor, purpura or jaundice may be early indications of serious reactions, including serious blood disorders.

PRECAUTIONS

General: Sulfonamides should be given with caution to patients with impaired renal or hepatic function and to those with severe allergy or bronchial asthma. In glucose-6-phosphate dehydrogenase-deficient individuals, hemolysis may occur. This reaction is frequently dose-related. Patients should be instructed to maintain an adequate fluid intake in order to prevent crystalluria and stone formation.

Laboratory tests: Complete blood counts should be done frequently in patients receiving sulfonamides. If a significant reduction in the count of any formed blood element is noted, Gantrisin should be discontinued. Urinalyses with careful microscopic examination and renal function tests should be performed during therapy, particularly for those patients with impaired renal function.

Drug interactions: It has been reported that sulfisoxazole may prolong the prothrombin time in patients who are receiving the anticoagulant warfarin. This interaction should be kept in mind when Gantrisin is given to patients already on anticoagulant therapy, and the coagulation time should be reassessed.

It has been proposed that sulfisoxazole competes with thiopental for plasma protein binding. In one study involving 48 patients, intravenous sulfisoxazole reduced the amount of thiopental required for anesthesia and shortened the awakening time. It is not known whether chronic oral doses of sulfisoxazole would have a similar effect. Until more is known about this interaction, physicians should be aware that patients receiving sulfisoxazole might require less thiopental for anesthesia.

Sulfonamides can displace methotrexate from plasma protein-binding sites, thus increasing free methotrexate concentrations. Studies in man have shown sulfisoxazole infusions to decrease plasma protein-bound methotrexate by one-fourth.

Sulfisoxazole can also potentiate the blood sugar lowering activity of sulfonylureas.

Carcinogenesis, mutagenesis, impairment of fertility: Carcinogenesis: Sulfisoxazole was not carcinogenic in either sex when administered by gavage for 103 weeks at dosages up to 2000 mg/kg/day to mice or 400 mg/kg/day to rats.

Mutagenesis: Bacterial mutagenic studies have not been performed with sulfisoxazole. However, Gantrisin was not observed to be mutagenic in *E. coli* Sd-4-73 when tested in the absence of a metabolic activating system.

Impairment of fertility: No effects on mating behavior, conception rate or fertility index (percent pregnant) were observed in a reproduction study in rats given 800 mg/kg/day sulfisoxazole.

Pregnancy: Teratogenic effects: Pregnancy Category C. Sulfisoxazole was not teratogenic in either rats or rabbits at dosages of 800 mg/kg/day. However, in another teratogenicity study, cleft palates developed in both rats and mice after administration of 1000 mg/kg/day sulfisoxazole; skeletal defects were also observed in rats. This dose is 9 to 18 times the usual adult dosage for Gantrisin.

There are no adequate and well-controlled studies of Gantrisin in pregnant women. Gantrisin should be used during pregnancy only if the potential benefit justifies the potential risk to the fetus.

Nonteratogenic effects: See CONTRAINDICATIONS section.

Nursing mothers: See CONTRAINDICATIONS section.

Pediatric use: Gantrisin is not recommended for use in infants younger than 2 months of age except in the treatment of congenital toxoplasmosis as adjunctive therapy with pyrimethamine. (See CONTRAINDICATIONS section.)

ADVERSE REACTIONS

Included in the listing that follows are adverse reactions that have not been reported with this specific drug; however, the pharmacologic similarities among the sulfonamides require that each of the reactions be considered with the administration of any of the Gantrisin dosage forms.

Hematologic: Agranulocytosis, aplastic anemia, thrombocytopenia, leukopenia, hemolytic anemia, purpura, hypoprothrombinemia, methemoglobinemia, eosinophilia.

Allergic reactions: Anaphylaxis, allergic myocarditis, serum sickness, conjunctival and scleral injection, generalized allergic reactions. In addition, periarteritis nodosa and systemic lupus erythematosus have been reported.

Dermatologic: Stevens-Johnson syndrome, epidermal necrolysis, erythema multiforme, exfoliative dermatitis, photosensitivity, pruritus, urticaria, rash, generalized skin eruptions.

Gastrointestinal: Hepatitis, hepatocellular necrosis, pseudomembranous enterocolitis, pancreatitis, stomatitis, glossitis, nausea, emesis, abdominal pain, diarrhea, anorexia.

Genitourinary: Creatinine elevation, toxic nephrosis with oliguria and anuria. The frequency of renal complications is considerably lower in patients receiving the more soluble sulfonamides.

Neurologic: Convulsions, peripheral neuritis, ataxia, vertigo, tinnitus, headache.

Psychiatric: Hallucinations, depression, apathy.

Endocrine: The sulfonamides bear certain chemical similarities to some goitrogens, diuretics (acetazolamide and the thiazides) and oral hypoglycemic agents. Cross-sensitivity may exist with these agents. Diuresis and hypoglycemia have occurred rarely in patients receiving sulfonamides.

Musculoskeletal: Arthralgia, myalgia.

Respiratory: Pulmonary infiltrates.

Miscellaneous: Edema (including periorbital), pyrexia, chills, weakness, fatigue, insomnia.

OVERDOSAGE

The amount of a single dose of sulfisoxazole that is either associated with symptoms of overdosage or is likely to be life-threatening has not been reported. Signs and symptoms of overdosage reported with sulfonamides include anorexia, colic, nausea, vomiting, dizziness, headache, drowsiness and unconsciousness. Pyrexia, hematuria and crystalluria may be noted. Blood dyscrasias and jaundice are potential late manifestations of overdosage.

General principles of treatment include the immediate discontinuation of the drug; institution of gastric lavage or emesis; forcing oral fluids; and the administration of intravenous fluids if urine output is low and renal function is normal. The patient should be monitored with blood counts and appropriate blood chemistries, including electrolytes. If a significant blood dyscrasia or jaundice occurs, specific therapy should be instituted for these complications. Peritoneal dialysis is not effective and hemodialysis is only moderately effective in eliminating sulfonamides.

The acute toxicity of sulfisoxazole in animals is as follows:

Species	LD_{50} ± S.E. (mg/kg)
mouse	5700 ± 235
rats	> 10,000
rabbits	> 2,000

DOSAGE AND ADMINISTRATION

Systemic sulfonamides are contraindicated in infants under 2 months of age, except in the treatment of congenital toxoplasmosis as adjunctive therapy with pyrimethamine.

Usual dose for infants over 2 months of age and children: Initial dose: One-half of the 24-hour dose. Maintenance dose: 150 mg/kg/24 hours or 4 Gm/M^2/24 hours—dose to be divided into 4 to 6 doses/24 hours. The maximum dose should not exceed 6 Gm/24 hours.

Usual adult dose: Initial dose: 2 to 4 Gm. Maintenance dose: 4 to 8 Gm/24 hours, divided in 4 to 6 doses/24 hours.

HOW SUPPLIED

Tablets (white, scored), containing 0.5 Gm sulfisoxazole—bottles of 100 (NDC 0004-0009-01) and 500 (NDC 0004-0009-14); Tel-E-Dose® packages of 100 (NDC 0004-0009-49). Imprint on tablets: ROCHE GANTRISIN®.

Pediatric Suspension (raspberry flavored), containing acetyl sulfisoxazole equivalent to approximately 0.5 Gm sulfisoxazole per teaspoonful (5 mL)—bottles of 4 oz (NDC 0004-1003-30) and 16 oz (1 pint) (NDC 0004-1003-28).

Syrup (chocolate flavored), containing acetyl sulfisoxazole equivalent to approximately 0.5 Gm sulfisoxazole per teaspoonful (5 mL)—bottles of 16 oz (1 pint) (NDC 0004-1004-28).

REFERENCES

1. Boisvert A, Barbeau G, Belanger PM: Pharmacokinetics of sulfisoxazole in young and elderly subjects. *Gerontology 30:* 125–131, 1984
2. Oie S, Gambertoglio JG, Fleckenstein L: Comparison of the disposition of total and unbound sulfisoxazole after single and multiple dosing. *J Pharmacokinet Biopharm 10:* 157–172, 1982

Revised: July 1988

Shown in Product Identification Section, page 426

HIVID® ℞

[hiv'id]

(zalcitabine)

TABLETS

The following text is complete prescribing information based on official labeling in effect June 1, 1992.

Continued on next page

Roche Laboratories—Cont.

WARNING:
HIVID® (ZALCITABINE) IN COMBINATION WITH ZIDOVUDINE (ZDV) IS INDICATED FOR THE TREATMENT OF ADULT PATIENTS WITH ADVANCED HIV INFECTION (CD4 CELL COUNT ≤300 CELLS/mm^3) WHO HAVE DEMONSTRATED SIGNIFICANT CLINICAL OR IMMUNOLOGIC DETERIORATION. THIS INDICATION IS BASED ON LIMITED DATA FROM TWO SMALL STUDIES IN WHICH ZIDOVUDINE-NAIVE PATIENTS WITH A CD4 CELL COUNT ≤300 CELLS/mm^3 WHO WERE TREATED WITH HIVID PLUS ZIDOVUDINE HAD A GREATER CD4 RESPONSE THAN PATIENTS TREATED WITH ZIDOVUDINE ALONE (SEE DESCRIPTION OF STUDIES). NEITHER STUDY INCLUDED A CONCURRENT CONTROL GROUP TAKING THE CURRENTLY RECOMMENDED ZIDOVUDINE DOSE OF 100 mg q4h, AND THESE STUDIES WERE NOT DESIGNED TO MEASURE THE CLINICAL EFFICACY OF THE COMBINATION. AT PRESENT NO DATA ARE AVAILABLE ON THE COMBINED USE OF HIVID AND ZIDOVUDINE IN PATIENTS WHO HAVE PREVIOUSLY RECEIVED ZIDOVUDINE MONOTHERAPY, ALTHOUGH CONTROLLED STUDIES ARE ONGOING. RESULTS ARE ALSO CURRENTLY UNAVAILABLE FROM CONTROLLED STUDIES EVALUATING THE EFFECT OF COMBINED USE OF HIVID AND ZIDOVUDINE ON THE CLINICAL PROGRESSION OF HIV INFECTION (SUCH AS SURVIVAL OR THE INCIDENCE OF OPPORTUNISTIC INFECTIONS).
BECAUSE ZIDOVUDINE HAS BEEN SHOWN TO PROLONG SURVIVAL AND DECREASE THE INCIDENCE OF OPPORTUNISTIC INFECTIONS IN PATIENTS WITH ADVANCED HIV DISEASE, ZIDOVUDINE MONOTHERAPY SHOULD BE CONSIDERED AS INITIAL THERAPY FOR ADULT PATIENTS WITH HIV INFECTION WHO HAVE EVIDENCE OF IMPAIRED IMMUNITY (CD4 CELL COUNTS OF ≤500 CELLS/mm^3).
THE MAJOR CLINICAL TOXICITIES OF HIVID ARE PERIPHERAL NEUROPATHY AND, MUCH LESS FREQUENTLY, PANCREATITIS. MODERATE OR SEVERE PERIPHERAL NEUROPATHY, WHICH FOR SOME PATIENTS WAS CLINICALLY DISABLING, OCCURRED IN 17% TO 31% OF PATIENTS TREATED WITH HIVID MONOTHERAPY DEPENDING ON SEVERITY AND PRESUMED RELATIONSHIP TO DRUG. IT IS UNKNOWN AT THIS TIME WHETHER THE RISK OF PERIPHERAL NEUROPATHY IS INCREASED WITH THE USE OF COMBINATION THERAPY OVER THAT OBSERVED WITH HIVID MONOTHERAPY. THERE ARE NO DATA REGARDING THE USE OF HIVID IN PATIENTS WITH PREEXISTING PERIPHERAL NEUROPATHY SINCE THESE PATIENTS WERE EXCLUDED FROM CLINICAL TRIALS; THEREFORE, HIVID SHOULD BE USED WITH EXTREME CAUTION IN THESE PATIENTS. THE OCCURRENCE OF PERIPHERAL NEUROPATHY IN PATIENTS TREATED WITH HIVID WAS GREATER IN PATIENTS WITH MORE ADVANCED HIV DISEASE (SEE WARNINGS).
DOCUMENTED FATAL PANCREATITIS HAS BEEN OBSERVED WITH THE ADMINISTRATION OF HIVID ALONE OR IN COMBINATION WITH ZIDOVUDINE. THE USE OF BOTH HIVID AND ZIDOVUDINE SHOULD BE SUSPENDED IMMEDIATELY IN PATIENTS WHO DEVELOP ANY SYMPTOMS SUGGESTIVE OF PANCREATITIS UNTIL THIS DIAGNOSIS IS EXCLUDED (SEE WARNINGS). OVERALL, PANCREATITIS IS AN UNCOMMON COMPLICATION OF HIVID MONOTHERAPY, OCCURRING IN <1% OF PATIENTS.
TOXICITIES PREVIOUSLY ASSOCIATED WITH ZIDOVUDINE MONOTHERAPY ARE LIKELY TO OCCUR IN PATIENTS TREATED WITH COMBINED HIVID AND ZIDOVUDINE THERAPY. IT IS HIGHLY RECOMMENDED THAT PHYSICIANS REFER TO THE WARNINGS AND PRECAUTIONS DESCRIBED IN THE ZIDOVUDINE COMPLETE PRODUCT INFORMATION BEFORE PRESCRIBING COMBINATION THERAPY WITH HIVID AND ZIDOVUDINE.
IT IS RECOMMENDED THAT THE DECISION TO USE HIVID SHOULD BE MADE IN CONSULTATION WITH A PHYSICIAN EXPERIENCED IN THE CARE OF PATIENTS WITH HIV INFECTION.

DESCRIPTION

HIVID is the Hoffmann-La Roche brand of zalcitabine [formerly called dideoxycytidine (ddC)], a synthetic pyrimidine nucleoside analogue active against the human immunodeficiency virus (HIV). HIVID is available as film-coated tablets for oral administration in strengths of 0.375 mg and 0.750 mg. Each tablet also contains the inactive ingredients lactose, microcrystalline cellulose, croscarmellose sodium, magnesium stearate, hydroxypropyl methylcellulose, polyethylene glycol and polysorbate 80 along with the following colorant system: 0.375 mg tablet—synthetic brown, black, red and yellow iron oxide, and titanium dioxide; 0.750 mg tablet—synthetic black iron oxide titanium dioxide. The chemical name for zalcitabine is 4-amino-1-beta-D-2′,3′-dideoxyribofuranosyl-2-(1H)-pyrimidone or 2′,3′-dideoxycytidine with the molecular formula $C_9H_{13}N_3O_3$ and a molecular weight of 211.22.
Zalcitabine is a white to off-white crystalline powder with an aqueous solubility of 76.4 mg/mL at 25°C.

CLINICAL PHARMACOLOGY

Mechanism of Action: Zalcitabine is a synthetic nucleoside analogue of the naturally occurring nucleoside 2′-deoxycytidine in which the 3′-hydroxyl group is replaced by hydrogen. Within cells, zalcitabine is converted to the active metabolite, dideoxycytidine 5′-triphosphate (ddCTP), by cellular enzymes. ddCTP serves as an alternative substrate to deoxycytidine triphosphate (dCTP) for HIV-reverse transcriptase and inhibits the in vitro replication of HIV-1 by inhibition of viral DNA synthesis. This inhibition has been demonstrated in vitro in human primary cell cultures and in established cell lines. In DNA biosynthesis, DNA chain extension occurs through the formation of a phosphodiester bridge between the 3′-hydroxyl group of the growing end of a DNA chain and the 5′-phosphate group of the incoming deoxynucleotide. Because ddCTP lacks the 3′-hydroxyl group required for chain elongation, its incorporation into a growing DNA chain leads to premature chain termination. ddCTP serves as a competitive inhibitor of the natural substrate, dCTP, for the active site of the viral reverse transcriptase and thus further inhibits viral DNA synthesis.
The active metabolite, ddCTP, also has a high affinity for cellular mitochondrial DNA polymerase gamma and has been reported to be incorporated into the DNA of cells in culture. However, DNA chain termination with cellular DNA polymerases has not been demonstrated.
The half-life of ddCTP in established cell lines and in human peripheral blood mononuclear cells in culture has been determined to be in the range of 2.6 to 10 hours.
Microbiology: The anti-HIV activity of zalcitabine was determined in a variety of human T-cell lines infected with different strains of HIV. The in vitro anti-HIV activity of zalcitabine varied greatly depending upon the time between virus infection and zalcitabine treatment of cell cultures, the ratio of the number of infectious virus particles to the number of cells, the kind of assay and the cell type used. When established cell lines were infected with a large excess of virus per cell and drug added soon after infection, the concentration of zalcitabine required to inhibit HIV-1 replication by 50% (ID_{50}) was generally in the range of 30 nM to 500 nM (1 nM = 0.21 ng/mL). In these cell lines, >95% inhibition of viral replication was achieved with 100 nM to 1000 nM zalcitabine. Zalcitabine blocked virus-induced cytopathic effects in cell lines in culture at a concentration of 30 nM to 300 nM. In assays measuring the inhibition of p24 viral antigen, the ID_{50} of zalcitabine was in the range of 1 nM to 500 nM, and the 90% inhibitory concentration (ID_{90}) was in the range of 500 nM to 1000 nM. In peripheral blood mononuclear cell cultures infected with HIV-1 (LAV strain) at a low ratio of virus to cells and assayed for HIV-reverse transcriptase, ID_{50} and ID_{90} values for zalcitabine were determined to be 11 nM and 100 nM, respectively. In monocyte/macrophage cultures infected with HIV (Ba-L strain) and treated with zalcitabine, the ID_{90} value was <10 nM when assayed for viral p24 antigen. However, viral replication in monocyte/macrophage cultures infected with a lymphotropic isolate of HIV (LAV-1 strain) was not inhibited at 100,000 nM. Comparative studies of the antiviral activity of zalcitabine against HIV-1 and HIV-2 in vitro revealed no significant difference in sensitivity between the two viruses when activity was determined by measuring viral cytopathic effect. The relationship of the in vitro inhibition of HIV by zalcitabine to the inhibition of HIV replication in infected people, or the clinical response to therapy, has not been established.
The results of cytotoxicity studies in various cell lines demonstrated that the concentration of the drug necessary to inhibit the cell growth by 50% (EC_{50}) was in the range of 5000 nM to >100,000 nM. In vitro combination studies have demonstrated that zalcitabine and zidovudine have an additive or synergistic antiviral effect, depending on the cell line used, without increased cytotoxicity over that observed for either agent alone.
The potential for development of clinically significant zalcitabine-resistant virus in patients with HIV infection who received HIVID has not been adequately studied to date. Zalcitabine-resistant virus has not been isolated directly from patients who received this drug. However, reduced zalcitabine sensitivity in vitro was reported in hybrid virus constructs made with portions of the HIV genome obtained from a patient who received intermittent HIVID therapy for over 18 months. Combination therapy of HIVID plus zidovudine does not appear to prevent the emergence of zidovudine-resistant isolates. However, studies with zidovudine-resistant virus isolates indicate zidovudine-resistant strains remain sensitive to zalcitabine.
Pharmacokinetics: The pharmacokinetics of zalcitabine has been evaluated in studies in HIV-infected patients following 0.01 mg/kg, 0.03 mg/kg and 1.5 mg oral doses, and a 1.5 mg intravenous dose administered as a 1-hour infusion.
Absorption and Bioavailability in Adults: Following oral administration to HIV-infected patients, the mean absolute bioavailability of zalcitabine was >80% (30% CV, range 23% to 124%, n=19). The absorption rate of a 1.5 mg oral dose of zalcitabine (n=20) was reduced when administered with food. This resulted in a 39% decrease in mean maximum plasma concentrations (C_{max}) from 25.2 ng/mL (35% CV, range 11.6 to 37.5 ng/mL) to 15.5 ng/mL) (24% CV, range 9.1 to 23.7 ng/mL), and a twofold increase in time to achieve maximum plasma concentrations from a mean of 0.8 hours under fasting conditions to 1.6 hours when the drug was given with food. The extent of absorption (as reflected by AUC) was decreased by 14%, from 72 ng·hr/mL (28% CV, range 43 to 119 ng·hr/mL) to 62 ng·hr/mL (23% CV, range 42 to 91 ng·hr/mL). The clinical relevance of these decreases is unknown.
Distribution in Adults: The steady-state volume of distribution following IV administration of a 1.5 mg dose of zalcitabine averaged 0.534 (±0.127) L/kg (24% CV, range 0.304 to 0.734 L/kg, n=20). Cerebrospinal fluid obtained from 9 patients at 2 to 3.5 hours following 0.06 mg/kg or 0.09 mg/kg IV infusion showed measurable concentrations of zalcitabine. The CSF:plasma concentration ratio ranged from 9% to 37% (mean 20%), demonstrating penetration of the drug through the blood-brain barrier. The clinical relevance of these ratios has not been evaluated.
Metabolism and Elimination in Adults: Zalcitabine is phosphorylated intracellularly to zalcitabine triphosphate, the active substrate for HIV-reverse transcriptase. Concentrations of zalcitabine triphosphate are too low for quantitation following administration of therapeutic doses to humans.

Zalcitabine metabolism in humans has not been fully evaluated. Zalcitabine does not appear to undergo a significant degree of metabolism by the liver. Renal excretion appears to be the primary route of elimination, and accounted for approximately 70% of an orally-administered, radiolabeled dose (i.e., total radioactivity) within 24 hours after dosing (n=6). The mean elimination half-life is 2 hours and generally ranges from 1 to 3 hours in individual patients. Total body clearance following an intravenous dose averages 285 mL/min (29% CV, range 165 to 447 mL/min). Less than 10% of a radiolabeled dose of zalcitabine appears in the feces.
In patients with impaired kidney function, prolonged elimination of zalcitabine may be expected. Results from 7 patients with renal impairment (estimated CrCl <55 mL/min) indicate that the half-life was prolonged (up to 8.5 hours) in these patients compared to those with normal renal function. Maximum plasma concentrations were higher in some patients after a single dose.
In patients with normal renal function, the pharmacokinetics of zalcitabine was not altered during three times daily multiple dosing (n=9). Accumulation of drug in plasma during this regimen was negligible. The drug was <4% bound to plasma proteins, indicating that drug interactions involving binding-site displacement are unlikely (see *Drug Interactions*).
Pharmacokinetics in Children: Limited pharmacokinetic data have been reported for five HIV-positive children using doses of 0.03 and 0.04 mg/kg HIVID administered orally every 6 hours.[1] The mean bioavailability of zalcitabine in this study was 54% and mean apparent systemic clearance was 150 mL/min/m^2. Due to the small number of subjects and different analytical techniques, it is difficult to make comparisons between pediatric and adult data.

INDICATIONS AND USAGE

Combination Therapy with Zidovudine in Advanced HIV Infection: HIVID (zalcitabine) in combination with zidovudine is indicated for the treatment of adult patients with advanced HIV infection (CD4 cell count ≤300 cells/mm^3) who have demonstrated significant clinical or immunologic deterioration. This indication is based on limited data from two small studies in which zidovudine-naive patients with a CD4 cell count ≤300 cells/mm^3 who were treated with HIVID plus zidovudine had a greater CD4 response than patients treated with zidovudine alone (see *Description of Studies*). Neither study included a concurrent control group taking the current recommended zidovudine dose of 100 mg q4h, and these studies were not designed to measure the clinical efficacy of the combination. No data are currently available on the combined use of HIVID and zidovudine in patients who have previously received zidovudine monotherapy, although controlled studies are ongoing. At present there are no data available from controlled or uncontrolled studies addressing whether an effect on CD4 cell count would be observed by the addition of HIVID to patients who are currently receiving zidovudine or who had previously been exposed to antiretroviral therapy. Because zidovudine has been shown to prolong survival and decrease the incidence of

opportunistic infections in patients with advanced HIV disease, zidovudine monotherapy should be considered as initial therapy for adult patients with HIV infection who have evidence of impaired immunity (CD4 cell counts of ≤500 cells/mm^3).

Description of Studies: *Combination Trials:* The combined use of HIVID and zidovudine is based on limited data from two small studies. The first was a Phase 1/2, open-label, dose-ranging study (N3447/ACTG 106) that evaluated several dose combinations of HIVID and zidovudine. The second study was a randomized Phase 2 study (BW 34,225-02) designed to evaluate the virologic and immunologic effects of the combined administration of two nucleoside analogues (zidovudine combined with either HIVID or didanosine). Both studies used an experimental regimen of zidovudine administered three times daily, and neither was designed to assess the clinical efficacy of the combination.

Data from a study of HIVID alternating with zidovudine at doses of HIVID higher than currently recommended (ACTG 047) have shown results comparable to those observed in N3447/ACTG 106 in zidovudine-naive patients. A parallel study in patients who were previously hematologically intolerant to zidovudine monotherapy but then changed to an alternating HIVID and zidovudine regimen (ACTG 050) showed greater toxicity and less CD4 response. The applicability of the results from the two studies using alternating regimens to the recommended combination regimen is uncertain.

HIVID GIVEN IN COMBINATION WITH ZIDOVUDINE IN ADULT ZIDOVUDINE-NAIVE PATIENTS WITH ADVANCED HIV INFECTION (CD4 CELL COUNT ≤200 CELLS/mm^3 [N3447/ACTG 106]): This Phase 1/2 study of therapy with concomitant HIVID and zidovudine is an ongoing, six-arm, open-label, dose-escalating study with randomization within blocks of two arms. Doses being studied are HIVID 0.005 and 0.01 mg/kg q8h administered concomitantly with zidovudine 100 or 200 mg q8h, as well as zidovudine 50 mg q8h alone or combined with HIVID 0.005 mg/kg q8h. No control arm of zidovudine monotherapy at the currently approved regimen was included in this study. A total of 56 zidovudine-naive patients with advanced HIV infection (CD4 cell count ≤200 cells/mm^3) were entered. Patients have now been treated for a median duration varying across groups from 36 to 72 weeks; median CD4 cell counts at entry were 75 cells/mm^3. An earlier analysis of this study has been published.[2]

[See Table 1 above.]

Table 1. Baseline Characteristics

Study	BW 34,225-02 Combination HIVID + ZDV	BW 34,225-02 ZDV	N3300/ACTG 114 ZDV (No Prior ZDV)	N3447/ACTG 106 (Four Pooled Combination Arms)
n	45	47	262	36
Accrual Date	5/91–11/91	5/91–11/91	8/89–9/90	7/89–5/90
Baseline Median CD4 (cells/mm^3)	125	153	85	70
CD4 Range (cells/mm^3)	1–301	11–288	5–289	3–188
% Male	89%	92%	93%	97%
% Caucasian	60%	66%	79%	89%
% Homosexual	51%	55%	77%	69%
% AIDS	22%	15%	26%	44%

Treatment regimens with 150 mg/day of zidovudine showed less activity than those with ≥300 mg/day of zidovudine; therefore, the four treatment regimens that included ≥300 mg/day zidovudine were pooled for CD4 and weight analyses (see Table 1 for baseline characteristics). For safety analyses, data from all five combination arms were pooled. Although the clinical outcomes were monitored while subjects were on therapy, the study was not designed to evaluate clinical outcome as an efficacy parameter.

There were eight deaths during the study. Twenty of the 56 patients who entered developed an AIDS-defining opportunistic infection, neoplasm or condition. These AIDS-defining events were equally distributed among the six treatment arms.

A total of 37 patients prematurely withdrew from the study. Nine patients discontinued therapy because of adverse events. Of these 9 patients, 2 were discontinued for peripheral neuropathy, 5 for hematologic abnormalities, 1 for nausea and vomiting, 1 for myositis.

The effect of study therapy on CD4 cell counts is presented later in this section. A mean peak increase in weight of 4.5 kg for the pool of the four combination regimens was observed. Body weight was maintained above baseline for >1 year for patients who remained on study.

HIVID GIVEN IN COMBINATION WITH ZIDOVUDINE IN PATIENTS WITH HIV INFECTION, ≤4 WEEKS PRIOR ZIDOVUDINE AND CD4 CELL COUNTS ≤300 CELLS/mm^3 (BW 34,225-02): An unscheduled analysis of CD4 changes for patients administered either combined HIVID and zidovudine therapy, or zidovudine monotherapy, was obtained from this ongoing, double-blind, randomized, Phase 2 controlled trial. The trial was designed to compare the antiviral and immunologic effects of zidovudine monotherapy administered three times daily to that of combination therapy with either HIVID and zidovudine or didanosine and zidovudine. Subjects were HIV-infected patients with CD4 cell counts at entry ≤300 cells/mm^3 who had received <4 weeks of zidovudine.

The unscheduled analysis of CD4 cell count changes in this study included only the group receiving zidovudine alone (200 mg q8h, a currently experimental regimen) and the HIVID plus zidovudine group. At the time of this analysis, 45 patients were randomized to the combination of HIVID and zidovudine and 47 patients to the zidovudine-monotherapy arm. Median duration of treatment was 13 weeks for the zidovudine-monotherapy group and 14 weeks for the group receiving HIVID and zidovudine; median CD4 cell counts at entry were 153 cells/mm^3 and 125 cells/mm^3, respectively.

The primary end point of this study is emergence of viral resistance. Data on viral resistance, clinical outcome (survival, incidence of opportunistic infection) or the incidence of adverse events are not currently available. Change in CD4 cell count was the only outcome variable analyzed from this study.

ANALYSIS OF CD4 CELL COUNTS IN COMBINATION TRIALS: The activity of combination HIVID and zidovudine was assessed using CD4 cell counts as a marker of biologic activity. In controlled trials, zidovudine monotherapy has been associated with clinical benefit (improved survival and decreased incidence of opportunistic infection) and transient increases in CD4 cell counts. Evidence of efficacy of HIVID in combination with zidovudine is based only on improvements in CD4 cell counts.

Definitions of outcome were applied to data from patients receiving HIVID in combination with zidovudine. Analyses included the following:

1. Mean change from baseline in CD4 cell counts at various time points during therapy;
2. Longitudinal changes during study: time weighted average of serial CD4 cell counts adjusted (normalized) for baseline CD4 cell counts (NAUC). (NAUC = Cumulative AUC of CD4 cell count up to time t/baseline CD4 count × t.) NAUCs that exceed a value of 1 indicate that the average CD4 level during therapy is increased over the baseline CD4 cell count;
3. Presence of a "response" where response was defined as one of the following: a) the greater of either a 75-cell or 75% increase over baseline CD4 cell count maintained for a minimum of two consecutive visits at least 21 days apart (75:75 response), or b) the greater of either a 50-cell or 50% increase over baseline CD4 cell count maintained for a minimum of two consecutive visits at least 21 days apart (50:50 response).

Definitions of outcome measures 2 and 3 were not specified in the two study protocols but were applied post hoc and have not been previously correlated with clinical outcome. In the discussion below, the outcomes for the control group referred to as N3300/ACTG 114 are results for subjects in the zidovudine arm of a large, prospective study comparing zidovudine to HIVID monotherapy. The figures cited are for those patients with no previous zidovudine exposure. Comparisons across clinical studies must be interpreted cautiously due to possible differences in study population, selection bias between studies, and different methodologies for measuring CD4 cells counts.

Figure 1 displays the CD4 cell response for those patients receiving HIVID in combination with zidovudine in BW 34,225-02 and in N3447/ACTG 106 (pooled response for the combination regimens of HIVID with ≥300 mg/day of zidovudine). It also depicts the CD4 cell response for zidovudine-monotherapy arm from BW34,225-02 and for those zidovudine patients in N3300/ACTG 114 who were zidovudine-naive at entry. Table 1 describes the baseline characteristics of those populations whose CD4 data were analyzed as presented in Figure 1 and Table 2. Table 2 lists the NAUC response at weeks 12 and 24 for BW 34,225-02, N3447/ACTG 106 and N3300/ACTG 114.

Results of the CD4 analyses are as follows:

1. *Mean Change from Baseline:* Results for changes in CD4 cell count from baseline are displayed in Figure 1 for BW 34,225-02, N3447/ACTG 106 and N3300/ACTG 114 (ZDV-monotherapy arm).
2. *Longitudinal Changes during Study:* In BW 34,225-02, 84% of patients receiving combination HIVID and zidovudine had an NAUC >1 at week 12 (89% at week 24) compared to 72% of patients receiving zidovudine monotherapy (200 mg q8h) at week 12 (68% at week 24). In a contemporary zidovudine-treated control group (N3300/ACTG 114), 87% of the zidovudine-treated patients had an NAUC >1 at week 12 (81% at week 24). In the open-label study N3447/ACTG106, 97% of patients administered HIVID in combination with ≥300 mg/day of zidovudine had an NAUC>1 at weeks 12 and 24.
3. *Response:* In BW 34,225-02, 38% of patients receiving combination HIVID and zidovudine had a 50:50 response at week 24 compared to 21% of patients in the zidovudine-monotherapy group. In the zidovudine-contemporary control group (N3300/ACTG 114), 34% of patients had a 50:50 response at week 24. In N3447/ACTG 106, 70% of patients receiving HIVID combined with zidovudine (≥300 mg/day) had a 50:50 response at week 24.

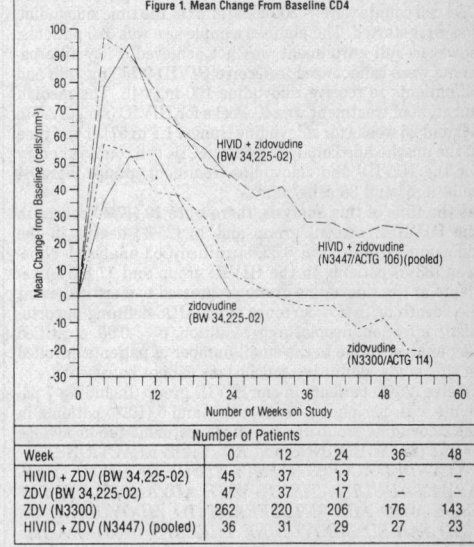

Figure 1. Mean Change From Baseline CD4

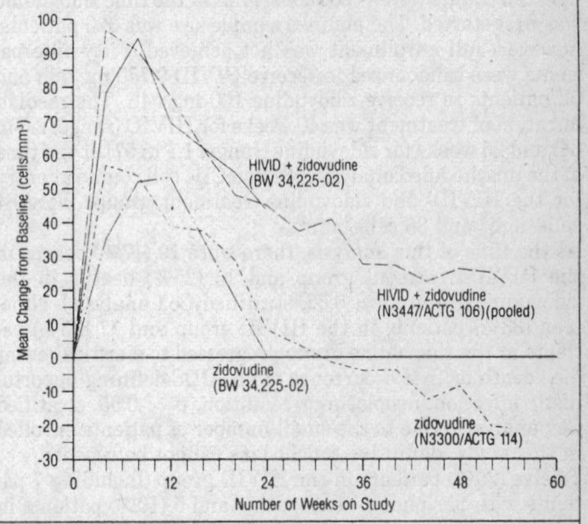

Number of Patients					
Week	0	12	24	36	48
HIVID + ZDV (BW 34,225-02)	45	37	13	–	–
ZDV (BW 34,225-02)	47	37	17	–	–
ZDV (N3300)	262	220	206	176	143
HIVID + ZDV (N3447) (pooled)	36	31	29	27	23

[See Table 2 on next page.]

Additional Monotherapy and Combination Studies of HIVID: *Monotherapy Trials:* HIVID was studied in two controlled comparative trials (N3300/ACTG 114 and N3492/ACTG 119) of patients with AIDS or advanced ARC (CD4 cell count ≤200 cells/mm^3), and in a randomized, dose-comparison, expanded-access safety study (N3544) of HIVID in patients with advanced HIV disease who were intolerant to zidovudine or who showed evidence of clinical progression while on zidovudine therapy. Information from these monotherapy studies is included to describe the safety profile of HIVID (see ADVERSE REACTIONS).

The parameters of efficacy evaluated in the controlled comparative studies of HIVID included the clinical end points of survival and opportunistic infection. The expanded-access safety program (N3544) was designed primarily as a dose-comparison safety study.

HIVID MONOTHERAPY IN ADULT PATIENTS WITH AIDS OR ADVANCED ARC AND ≤3 MONTHS OF PRIOR ZIDOVUDINE THERAPY (N3300/ACTG 114): This study was a randomized, double-blind, parallel, controlled trial of HIVID at 26 medical centers in patients with AIDS or advanced ARC (CD4 cell count ≤200 cells/mm^3) who previously received ≤3 months of zidovudine. Patients received either HIVID 0.750 mg q8h or zidovudine 200 mg q4h, later reduced to 100 mg g4h. Three hundred and twenty patients were randomized to receive HIVID and 315 patients randomized to receive zidovudine with a median duration of treatment of 44 weeks (range: 1.1 to 96) and 53 weeks (range: 0.3 to 96), respectively. Median CD4 cell count at entry was 90 cells/mm^3 and 87 cells/mm^3 for the HIVID- and zidovudine-treatment groups, respectively.

This study was terminated on the basis of 1-year survival results that showed a signficant difference in survival favoring the zidovudine group, with 59 deaths in the HIVID group versus 33 deaths in the zidovudine group (p = .007, stratified Cox analysis). One hundred and thirty patients (41%) in the HIVID group and 95 patients (30%) in the zidovudine group progressed to a critical event at the time of the 1-year analysis (i.e., death or fist occurrence of an AIDS-defining opportunistic infection, neoplasm or condition, p=0.02).

Toxicities requiring discontinuation were primarily peripheral neuropathy in the HIVID group and hematologic toxicity in the zidovudine group. Overall; 60 (20%) patients receiving HIVID developed moderate or severe neuropathy

Continued on next page

Roche Laboratories—Cont.

considered by the investigator to be possibly or probably drug related; 33 (10%) of patients were reported to have prematurely discontinued study therapy because of peripheral neuropathy. Of 315 zidovudine patients, 22 (7%) were discontinued due to hematologic toxicity. At the time of the 1-year interim analysis, 187 (58%) of HIVID-treated patients discontinued for any reason and 59 (18%) discontinued treatment due to an adverse event. By comparison, 142 (45%) patients treated with zidovudine discontinued for any reason and 33 (11%) discontinued for adverse events (see WARNINGS and ADVERSE REACTIONS).

HIVID MONOTHERAPY IN ADULTS WITH AIDS OR ADVANCED ARC AND ≤48 WEEKS OF PRIOR ZIDOVUDINE THERAPY (N3492/ACTG 119): This is a nine center, randomized, open-label, parallel, controlled trial of HIVID in patients with AIDS or advance ARC who previously received ≥48 weeks of zidovudine. This trial enrolled patients whose CD4 cell counts were ≤200 cells/mm^3 at the time zidovudine was first started. The planned sample size was 320 patients; however, full enrollment was not achieved. Fifty-nine patients were randomized to receive HIVID 0.750 mg q8h and 52 patients to receive zidovudine 100 mg q4h. The median duration of treatment was 40 weeks for HIVID (range: 2.3 to 64) and 25 weeks for zidovudine (range: 1.1 to 57) at the time of the unscheduled analysis. Median CD4 cell counts at entry for the HIVID- and zidovudine-treatment groups were 84 cells/mm^3 and 88 cells/mm^3.

At the time of this analysis, there were 10 (17%) deaths in the HIVID-treatment group and 13 (25%) deaths in the zidovudine group ($p = 0.52$, stratified Cox analysis). Nineteen (33%) patients in the HIVID group and 17 (33%) patients in the zidovudine group progressed to a critical event (i.e., death or first occurrence of an AIDS-defining opportunistic infection, neoplasm or condition, $p = 0.95$, stratified Cox analysis). Due to the small number of patients enrolled in this study, definitive conclusions cannot be reached.

Twelve (20%) patients in the HIVID group (including 7 patients with peripheral neuropathy) and 5 (10%) patients in the zidovudine group discontinued treatment due to adverse events (see WARNINGS and ADVERSE REACTIONS).

EXPANDED-ACCESS SAFETY STUDY OF HIVID THERAPY IN ADULT PATIENTS WITH ADVANCED HIV DISEASE WHO ARE INTOLERANT TO ZIDOVUDINE OR HAD FAILED ZIDOVUDINE THERAPY (N3544): A randomized, open-label, dose-comparison safety study was initiated in patients with advanced HIV disease (CD4 cell count ≤200 cells/mm^3) who were intolerant to zidovudine, for whom zidovudine was contraindicated, or who were clinically deteriorating despite zidovudine therapy. An interim analysis was performed for 3479 patients, 1757 in the HIVID 0.375 mg q8h and 1722 in the HIVID 0.750 mg q8h groups, with a median duration of treatment of 16 weeks (range: 0.1 to 61). Mean CD4 cell counts at entry were similar for the 0.375 mg (83 cells/mm^3) and 0.750 mg (79 cells/mm^3) HIVID groups.

Two hundred seventy-nine patients discontinued for an adverse event, including 164 (5%) with peripheral neuropathy (97 in the high-dose group and 67 in the low-dose group) and 11 (0.3%) with pancreatitis (7 in the high-dose group and 4 in the low dose-group) (see ADVERSE REACTIONS).

No statistically significant difference in survival was found for the deaths reported at the interim analysis. Subsequently, to better define survival in the two dose groups, survival data on 3920 patients with follow-up information as of February 1, 1992, were validated by telephone survey. There was a total of 556 deaths, 296 in the low-dose group and 260 in the high-dose group ($p = 0.59$, Cox regression analysis).

Alternating Trials: Alternating regimens of HIVID and zidovudine were studied in two open-label, controlled, multiarm, dose-ranging trials (ACTG 047 and ACTG 050). ACTG 047 evaluated regimens of HIVID and zidovudine alternating weekly and alternating monthly. Regimens were also included with HIVID alternating weekly with no therapy, zidovudine alternating weekly with no therapy and continuous zidovudine therapy. All patients were zidovudine-naive. Median CD4 cell counts at entry for patients in various arms of ACTG 047 ranged from 59 to 161 cells/mm^3. ACTG 050 evaluated the same dose schedules of HIVID and zidovudine as ACTG 047 in patients who demonstrated previous hematologic intolerance to zidovudine. ACTG 050 did not include a continuous zidovudine group. Median CD4 cells counts at entry for patients in the various arms of ACTG 050 ranged from 22 to 45 cells/mm^3. Doses of HIVID evaluated in both trials were 0.01 mg/kg and 0.03 mg/kg q4h. These doses were higher than those used in the previously discussed monotherapy or combination trials. In ACTG 047, 3 of the 4 alternating regimens had improvements in CD4 cell counts that were higher and sustained above baseline longer than the continuous zidovudine-monotherapy control arm. The occurrence of toxicity in some of the alternating arms was higher than that seen in the monotherapy studies of HIVID or in N3447/ACTG 106. Overall, 24% of patients had to discontinue therapy for adverse events. Patients in ACTG 050 did not tolerate alternating HIVID and zidovudine regimens as well as zidovudine-naive patients in ACTG 047 (see WARNINGS).

CONTRAINDICATIONS

HIVID is contraindicated in patients with clinically significant hypersensitivity to zalcitabine or to any of the excipients contained in the tablets.

WARNINGS

1. *PERIPHERAL NEUROPATHY:*

THE MAJOR CLINICAL TOXICITY OF HIVID IS PERIPHERAL NEUROPATHY, WHICH OCCURRED IN 17% TO 31% OF SUBJECTS TREATED IN PHASE 2/3 MONOTHERAPY STUDIES DEPENDING ON SEVERITY AND PRESUMED RELATIONSHIP TO DRUG. BY COMPARISON, NEUROPATHY OCCURRED IN 0% TO 12% OF ZIDOVUDINE-TREATED PATIENTS. THESE DATA ARE SUMMARIZED IN TABLE 3. DATA ARE VERY LIMITED ON THE OCCURRENCE OF PERIPHERAL NEUROPATHY WITH THE COMBINED USE OF HIVID AND ZIDOVUDINE.

HIVID-related peripheral neuropathy is a sensorimotor neuropathy characterized initially by numbness and burning dysesthesia involving the distal extremities. These symptoms may be followed by sharp shooting pains or severe continuous burning pain if the drug is not withdrawn. The neuropathy may progress to severe pain requiring narcotic analgesics and is potentially irreversible, especially if HIVID is not stopped promptly. In some patients, symptoms of neuropathy may initially progress despite discontinuation of HIVID. With prompt discontinuation of HIVID, the neuropathy is usually slowly reversible.

There are no data regarding the use of HIVID in patients with preexisting peripheral neuropathy since these patients were excluded from clinical trials; therefore, HIVID should be used with extreme caution in these patients. HIVID should also be used with particular caution in patients with low CD4 cell counts (CD4 <50 cells/mm^3) for whom the risk of developing peripheral neuropathy while on HIVID therapy is greater. Careful monitoring is strongly recommended for these individuals. Individuals with moderate or severe peripheral neuropathy, as evidenced by symptoms accompanied by objective findings, are advised to avoid HIVID.

HIVID should be stopped promptly when moderate discomfort from numbness, tingling, burning or pain of the extremities progresses, or any related symptoms occur that are accompanied by an objective finding. In a large ongoing clinical trial, peripheral neuropathy requiring HIVID interruption is defined as moderate discomfort of the lower extremities (requiring non-narcotic analgesics) that is bilateral and persists for ≥3 days, or mild symptoms accompanied by the loss of a previously present Achilles reflex. If symptoms resolve to mild intensity, rechallenge with half-dosage is permitted. Peripheral neuropathy requiring permanent discontinuation of HIVID has been defined in clinical trials as any severe discomfort of the extremities requiring narcotic analgesics or moderate discomfort progressing for ≥1 week. (These definitions are based on the cumulative experience with HIVID and do not correspond to the definitions used in Table 3, for which symptoms could be more severe.)

2. *PANCREATITIS:*

DOCUMENTED FATAL PANCREATITIS HAS BEEN OBSERVED WITH THE ADMINISTRATION OF HIVID ALONE OR THE COMBINATION OF HIVID WITH ZIDOVUDINE. Pancreatitis is an uncommon complication of HIVID monotherapy, occurring in <1% of patients. The occurrence of asymptomatic elevated serum amylase of any etiology while on HIVID monotherapy was also <1%. Of 633 patients treated with HIVID in the expanded-access safety study (N3544) who had a history of prior pancreatitis or increased amylase, 10 (1.6%) developed pancreatitis and an additional 10 (1.6%) developed asymptomatic elevated serum amylase. There was no apparent difference in the occurrence of pancreatitis between the two doses of HIVID in the expanded-access trial (N3544).

Caution should be exercised when administering HIVID to any patient with a history of pancreatitis or known risk factor for the development of pancreatitis. To date, in an ongoing, blinded, combination study, one patient has died of fulminant pancreatitis possibly related to HIVID and/or zidovudine. Another patient who received concomitant intravenous pentamidine and HIVID died of fulminant pancreatitis possibly related to the concomitant use of HIVID and intravenous pentamidine.

Patients with a history of pancreatitis or a history of elevated serum amylase should be followed more closely while on HIVID therapy. The signficance of an asymptomatic increase in serum amylase levels in HIV-infected patients prior to starting HIVID or while on HIVID is inclear. Treatment with HIVID should be interrupted in the setting of a rising serum amylase level associated with dysglycemia, rising triglyceride level, decreasing serum calcium or other parameters or symptoms suggestive of impending pancreatitis, until a clinical diagnosis is reached. Treatment with HIVID should also be interrupted if treatment with another durg known to cause pancreatitis (e.g., intravenous pentamidine) is required (see *Drug Interactions*).

Treatment with HIVID and zidovudine should be stopped immediately if nausea, vomiting, abdominal pain or other symptoms suggestive of pancreatitis develop, until a definitive diagnosis can be established. HIVID should be restarted only after pancreatitis has been ruled out. If clinical pancreatitis develops during HIVID administration, it is recommended that HIVID be permanently discontinued.

3. *OTHER SERIOUS TOXICITIES:*

a. *Esophageal Ulcers:* Infrequent cases of esophageal ulcers have been attributed to HIVID therapy. Interruption of HIVID should be considered in patients who develop esophageal ulcers that do not respond to specific treatment for opportunistic pathogens in order to assess a possible relationship to HIVID.

b. *Cardiomyopathy/Congestive Heart Failure:* Cardiomyopathy and congestive heart failure in patients with AIDS have been associated with the use of nucleoside antiretroviral agents. Infrequent cases have been reported in patients receiving HIVID. In one case, the investigator considered that the exacerbation of preexising cardiomyopathy was possibly related to HIVID. Treatment with HIVID in patients with baseline cardiomyopathy or history of congestive heart failure should be approached with caution.

c. *Anaphylactoid Reaction:* There has been one report of anaphylactoid reaction occurring in a patient receiving both HIVID and zidovudine in an alternating regimen. In addition, there have been several reports of urticaria without other signs of anaphylaxis.

BECAUSE SEVERE ADVERSE EFFECTS MAY BE ATTRIBUTABLE TO EITHER THE HIVID OR THE ZIDOVUDINE COMPONENTS OF COMBINATION THERAPY, OR TO THEIR COMBINATION, THE COMPLETE PRODUCT

Table 2. CD4 Response Analyses

Study	BW 34,225-02		N3300/ACTG 114 No Prior ZDV	N3447/ACTG 106 HIVID + ZDV
Dose	0.750 mg+200 mg q8h HIVID+ZDV	200 mg q8h ZDV[a]	200 mg q4h ZDV[b]	Four Pooled Combination Arms[c]
Mean Peak Increase in CD4	+94 cells/mm^3 (week 8)	+53 cells/mm^3 (week 12)	+57 cells/mm^3 (week 4)	+97 cells/mm^3 (week 4)
Week 12				
NAUC >1	84%	72%	87%	97%
Median NAUC	1.4	1.2	1.50	2.37
25–25	—	—	47%	82%
50–50	—	—	29%	70%
75–75	—	—	13%	46%
Week 24				
NAUC >1	89%	68%	81%	97%
Median NAUC	1.5	1.3	1.39	2.10
25–25	51%	43%	54%	85%
50–50	38%	21%	34%	70%
75–75	31%	9%	18%	49%

[a] Dosage of ZDV used was not the currently approved dose and interval of ZDV 200 mg q4h for 4 weeks, followed by 100 mg q4h.

[b] Reduced to 100 mg q4h ZDV when dose was approved.

[c] The pooled concomitant regimens of HIVID + ZDV included:

A = HIVID 0.005 mg/kg q8h + ZDV 100 mg q8h

B = HIVID 0.005 mg/kg q8h + ZDV 200 mg q8h

D = HIVID 0.01 mg/kg q8h + ZDV 100 mg q8h

E = HIVID 0.01 mg/kg q8h + ZDV 200 mg q8h

Table 3. Percentage of Patients with Moderate or Severe Peripheral Neuropathy[a]

Study[b]	N3300/ACTG 114		N3492/ACTG 119		N3447/ACTG 106
Investigator's Assessment of Relationship	HIVID 0.750 mg q8h n=320	ZDV[c] 200 mg q4h n=318[d]	HIVID 0.750 mg q8h n=59	ZDV 100 mg q4h n=52	HIVID + ZDV Pooled Concomitant Regimens n=47[e]
All Relationships[f]	31	12	24	10	21
Possible/Probable	20	6	17	0	4

[a] All adverse events related to peripheral neuropathy were pooled to include all potentially related signs and symptoms of neuopathy (i.e., tingling, numbness, weakness, or pain of the hands/arms or feet/legs).

[b] Median duration of treatment for N3300 wasa 44 weeks for HIVID, 53 weeks for ZDV; for N3492, 39 weeks for HIVID, 25 weeks for ZDV and for N3447 treatment ranged from 22 to 92 weeks among the arms.

[c] Reduced to 100 mg q4h ZDV when dose was approved.

[d] 315 patients randomized to ZDV arm. 3 patients randomized to HIVID inadvertently received ZDV for short periods; they did not develop any symptoms of neuropathy. For safety analyses, the 3 patients were included in the denominators of both HIVID and ZDV arms.

[e] Excluded are 9 patients who received ZDV alone for the greater part of the study. Only 8 patients were treated with the recommended combination regimen; all other patients were treated at lower doses of HIVID and/or ZDV.

[f] Unrelated, remotely, possibly or probably related to drug therapy.

INFORMATION FOR ZIDOVUDINE SHOULD BE CONSULTED BEFORE INITIATION OF COMBINATION THERAPY OR REINSTITUTION OF MONOTHERAPY WITH ZIDOVUDINE FOLLOWING AN ADVERSE REACTION.

PRECAUTIONS

General: Information regarding the safety of combined HIVID and zidovudine therapy is limited; the safety profile of HIVID has been characterized primarily in monotherapy trials. The safety profile of HIVID in children younger than 13 years of age and in asymptomatic HIV-infected individuals has not been established.

Patients receiving HIVID or any other antiretroviral therapy may continue to develop opportunistic infections and other complications of HIV infection, and therefore, should remain under close clinical observation by physicians experienced in the treatment of patients with HIV-associated diseases.

1. *Renal Impairment:* Patients with renal impairment (estimated creatinine clearance <55 mL/min) may be at a greater risk of toxicity from HIVID due to decreased drug clearance. HIVID dosage reduction for patients with more impaired renal function should be considered as follows: estimated creatinine clearance 10 to 40 mL/min—reduce the HIVID dose to 0.750 mg q12h; estimated creatinine clearance <10 mL/min—reduce the HIVID dose to 0.750 mg q24h.

2. *Hepatic Impairment:* The use of HIVID may be associated with exacerbation of hepatic dysfunction, especially in individuals with preexisting liver disease or with a history of ethanol abuse. Of 85 patients in the expanded-access safety study (N3544) with a prior history of liver function test (LFT) elevation before starting HIVID, 10 (12%) developed increases in LFTs >5 times the upper limit of normal while on HIVID. Such patients should be closely monitored by their physician, and dose reduction or interruption of drug therapy should be considered if necessary. Zidovudine use has also been associated with increases in liver function tests.

Information for Patients: Patients should be informed that HIVID is not a cure for HIV infection, that they may continue to develop illnesses associated with advanced HIV infection including opportunistic infections, and that HIVID has not been shown to reduce the incidence or frequency of such illnesses. Since it is frequently difficult to determine whether symptoms are a result of drug effect or underlying disease manifestation, patients should be encouraged to report all changes in their condition to their physician. Patients should be informed that the use of HIVID or other antiretroviral drugs do not preclude the ongoing need to maintain practices designed to prevent transmission of HIV. Patients should be instructed that the major toxicity of HIVID is peripheral neuropathy. Pancreatitis is another serious and potentially life-threatening toxicity that has been reported in <1% of patients treated with HIVID monotherapy. Patients should be advised of the early symptoms of both of these conditions and instructed to promptly report them to their physician. Since the development of peripheral neuropathy appears to be dose-related to HIVID,

patients should be advised to follow their physicians' instructions regarding the prescribed dose. Patients should be informed that the long-term effects of HIVID in combination with zidovudine are presently unknown.

Women of childbearing age should use effective contraception while using HIVID.

Laboratory Tests: Complete blood counts and clinical chemistry tests should be performed prior to initiating combination therapy with HIVID and zidovudine and at appropriate intervals thereafter. Baseline testing of serum amylase and triglyceride levels should be performed in individuals with a prior history of pancreatitis, increased amylase, those on parenteral nutrition or with a history of ethanol abuse.

Drug Interactions: The concomitant use of HIVID with drugs that have the potential to cause peripheral neuropathy should be avoided where possible. Drugs which have been associated with peripheral neuropathy include chloramphenicol, cisplatin, dapsone, disulfiram, ethionamide, glutethimide, gold, hydralazine, iodoquinol, isoniazid, metronidazole, nitrofurantoin, phenytoin, ribavirin and vincristine. Concomitant use of HIVID with didanosine is not recommended.

Drugs such as amphotercin, foscarnet and aminoglycosides may increase the risk of developing peripheral neuropathy or other HIVID-associated toxicities by interfering with the renal clearance of zalcitabine (and thereby raising systemic exposure). Patients who require the use of one of these drugs with HIVID and zidovudine should have frequent clinical and laboratory monitoring with dosage adjustment for any significant change in renal function.

Treatment with HIVID should be interrupted when the use of a drug that has the potential to cause pancreatitis is required. One death due to fulminant pancreatitis possibly related to HIVID and intravenous pentamidine was reported. If intravenous pentamidine is required to treat *Pneumocystis carinii* pneumonia, treatment with HIVID should be interrupted (see WARNINGS).

Possible interactions of HIVID with other concomitant medications have not been formally investigated.

Carcinogenesis, Mutagenesis and Impairment of Fertility: Carcinogenesis: Carcinogenicity studies in animals have not yet been performed.

Mutagenesis: Ames tests using seven different tester strains, with and without metabolic activation, were performed with no evidence of mutagenicity. Chinese hamster lung cell tests, with and without metabolic activation, and mouse lymphoma cell tests were performed and there was no evidence of mutagenicity. An unscheduled DNA synthesis assay was performed in rat hepatocytes with no increases in DNA repair. Human peripheral blood lymphocytes were exposed to zalcitabine, with and without metabolic activation, and at 1.5 mcg/mL and higher, dose-related increases in chromosomal aberration were seen. Oral doses of zalcitabine at 2500 and 4500 mg/kg were clastogenic in the mouse micronucleus assay.

Impairment of Fertility: Fertility and reproductive performance were assessed in rats at plasma concentrations up to 2142 times those achieved with the maximum recommended human dose (MRHD) based on AUC measurements. No adverse effects on rate of conception or general reproductive performance were observed. The highest dose was associated with embryolethality and evidence of teratogenicity. The next lower dose studied (plasma concentrations equivalent to 485 times the MRHD) was associated with a lower frequency of embryotoxicity but no teratogenicity.

Pregnancy: Teratogenic Effects: Pregnancy Category C. Zalcitabine has been shown to be teratogenic in mice at calculated exposure levels of 1365 and 2730 times that at the MRHD (based on AUC measurements). In rats, zalcitabine was teratogenic at a calculated exposure level of 2142 times the MRHD but not at an exposure level of 485 times the MRHD. There are no adequate and well-controlled studies of zalcitabine in pregnant women. HIVID should be used during prenancy only if the potential benefit justifies the potential risk to the fetus. Fertile women should not receive HIVID unless they are using effective contraception during therapy.

Nonteratogenic Effects: Increased embryolethality was observed in pregnant mice at doses 2730 times the MRHD and in rats above 485 times the MRHD (based on AUC measurements). Average fetal body weight was significantly decreased in mice at doses of 1365 times the MRHD and in rats at 2142 times the MRHD.

Nursing Mothers: It is not known whether zalcitabine is excreted in human milk. Because many drugs are excreted in human milk and the potential exists for serious adverse reactions from HIVID in nursing infants, a decision should be made whether to discontinue nursing or to discontinue the drug, taking into account the importance of the drug to the mother. It is currently recommended practice in the United States that HIV-infected women do not breastfeed infants regardless of the use of antiretroviral agents.

Table 4. Percentage of Patients with Clinical Adverse Experiences Considered Possibly or Probably Related to Study Drug Occurring in >3% of Patients Treated in HIVID-Monotherapy Trials

Body System/ Adverse Event	N3300/ACTG 114[a] ≤3 Months Prior ZDV				N3492/ACTG 119[a] ≥12 Months Prior ZDV			
	HIVID 0.750 mg q8h n=320		ZDV[b] 200 mg q4h n=318[c]		HIVID 0.750 mg q8h n=59		ZDV[b] 100 mg q4h N=52	
	mild/ mod/ sev	mod/ sev	mild/ mod/ sev	mod/ sev	mild/ mod/ sev	mod/ sev	mild/ mod/ sev	mod/ sev
Peripheral Neuopathy	S	E	E	T	A	B	L E 3	
Gastrointestinal								
Oral Ulcers	13.4	7.8	6.3	3.1	16.9	15.3	1.9	1.9
Nausea	7.2	2.8	19.5	8.2	3.4	1.7	0.0	0.0
Dysphagia	3.4	3.1	0.0	0.0	1.7	1.7	0.0	0.0
Anorexia	3.1	1.9	6.0	2.5	0.0	0.0	0.0	0.0
Abdominal Pain	2.8	0.9	2.5	1.6	5.1	3.4	0.0	0.0
Vomiting	2.2	0.9	5.0	3.5	1.7	1.7	0.0	0.0
Skin and Appendages								
Rash	7.8	4.1	5.3	3.1	0.0	0.0	0.0	0.0
Pruritus	4.7	2.8	5.3	2.2	0.0	0.0	0.0	0.0
Central and Periph NS								
Headache	8.8	5.0	12.6	6.6	0.0	0.0	0.0	0.0
Dizziness	3.1	1.3	2.8	1.3	0.0	0.0	0.0	0.0
Musculoskeletal								
Myalgia	5.3	2.2	6.3	3.1	1.7	1.7	1.9	1.9
Body as a Whole								
Fatigue	7.8	3.8	12.3	8.5	3.4	1.7	3.8	3.8
Respiratory								
Pharyngitis	2.2	1.9	0.0	0.0	5.1	3.4	0.0	0.0

[a] Median duration of treatment for N3300 was 44 weeks for HIVID, 53 weeks for ZDV; for N3492, treatment was 39 weeks for HIVID, 25 weeks for ZDV.

[b] Reduced to 100 mg q4h ZDV when dose was approved.

[c] 315 patients randomized to ZDV arm. 3 patients on HIVID inadvertently received ZDV. For safety analyses, the 3 patients were included in the denominators of both HIVID and ZDV arms.

Continued on next page

Roche Laboratories—Cont.

Pediatric Use: Safety and effectiveness of HIVID in combination with zidovudine or as monotherapy in HIV-infected children younger than 13 years of age has not been established.

ADVERSE REACTIONS
(SEE WARNINGS). ONLY LIMITED SAFETY DATA ARE AVAILABLE ON THE COMBINED USE OF HIVID WITH ZIDOVUDINE. The following data on adverse reactions are based primarily on the administration of HIVID at the recommended dose, as a single agent, to patients with AIDS or advanced ARC (CD4 cell count ≤ 200 cells/mm[3]). Table 3 summarizes the occurrence of moderate or severe peripheral neuropathy. Table 4 summarizes clinical adverse events or symptoms at least possibly related to HIVID therapy that occurred in at least 3% of all HIVID-treated patients with advanced HIV disease who were enrolled in the two comparative monotherapy trials (N3300/ACTG 114, N3492/ACTG 119) of HIVID versus zidovudine. Clinical adverse events in the combination HIVID and zidovudine Protocol N3447/ACTG 106 are included in Table 5.
[See Table 3 and Table 4 on preceding page.]

Table 5. Number and Percentage of Patients with Clinical Adverse Experiences Considered Possibly or Probably Related to Study Drug Occurring in > 3% of Patients

Body System/ Adverse Event	HIVID + ZDV Combination Trial Pooled Concomitant Regimens[a] mild/mod/sev		N3447/ACTG 106[b] No Prior ZDV mod/sev	
	n = 47 (%)			
Peripheral Neuropathy	S E E	T A B L E	3	
Gastrointestinal				
Nausea	17	(36.2)	4	(8.5)
Oral Ulcers	13	(27.7)	2	(4.3)
Abdominal Pain	10	(21.3)	4	(8.5)
Diarrhea	7	(14.9)	5	(10.6)
Vomiting	7	(14.9)	1	(2.1)
Anorexia	6	(12.8)	3	(6.4)
Constipation	3	(6.4)	1	(2.1)
Skin and Appendages				
Pruritus	7	(14.9)	2	(4.3)
Rash	7	(14.9)	1	(2.1)
Erythematous Rash	3	(6.4)	1	(2.1)
Night Sweats	3	(6.4)	1	(2.1)
Maculopapular Rash	2	(4.3)	1	(2.1)
Follicular Rash	2	(4.3)	0	(0.0)
Central and Periph NS				
Headache	18	(38.3)	4	(8.5)
Musculoskeletal				
Myalgia	7	(14.9)	1	(2.1)
Arthralgia	4	(8.5)	1	(2.1)
Body as a Whole				
Fatigue	16	(34.0)	4	(8.5)
Fever	7	(14.9)	1	(2.1)
Rigors	4	(8.5)	1	(2.1)
Chest Pain	3	(6.4)	1	(2.1)
Weight Decrease	3	(6.4)	2	(4.3)
Respiratory				
Pharyngitis	4	(8.5)	1	(2.1)

[a] Excluded are 9 patients who received ZDV alone for the greater part of the study. Only 8 patients were treated with the recommended combination regimen; all other patients were treated at lower doses of HIVID and/or ZDV.
[b] Median duration of treatment ranged from 22 to 92 weeks among the arms.

Monotherapy Trials: Clinical adverse events of all intensities classified as at least possibly related to HIVID that occurred in <3% of HIVID-treated patients in N3300/ACTG 114 are listed below. Events are listed in decreasing order of frequency within each body system.
Body as a Whole: weight decrease (1.9%); chest pain (1.6%); fever, asthenia, pain, substernal chest pain (<1%).
Cardiovascular: heart racing (1%).
Gastrointestinal: abdominal pain (<2.8%); diarrhea (2.5%); vomiting (2.2%); dry mouth (1.6%); esophageal ulcers (1.6%); dyspepsia (1.3%); glossitis (1.3%); constipation, esophageal pain, rectal hemorrhage, hemorrhoids, rectal ulcers, flatulence, tongue ulceration, enlarged abdomen, gum disorder (<1%).
Hepatic: hepatocellular damage, hepatitis (<1%).
Musculoskeletal: arthralgia (1.9%); shoulder pain, leg cramps, foot pain (<1%).

Table 6. Percentage of Patients with Laboratory Abnormalities[a]

	Monotherapy				Combination Therapy
	N3300/ACTG 114		N3492/ACTG 119		N3447/ACTG 106
	≤ 3 Months Prior ZDV		≥ 12 Months Prior ZDV		No Prior ZDV
	n=635		n=111		n=47
	HIVID 0.750 mg q8h n=320	ZDV[b] 200 mg q4h n=315	HIVID 0.750 mg q8h n=59	ZDV 100 mg q4h n=52	Pooled Concomitant Regimens n=47[c]
Laboratory Abnormality					
Anemia (< 7.5 g/dL)	5.0	14.3	5.1	7.7	8.5
Leukopenia (< 1500 cells/mm[3])	9.4	12.1	11.9	15.4	2.1
Neutropenia (< 750 cells/mm[3])	8.8	19.7	5.1	11.5	8.5
Eosinophilia (> 1000 or 25%)	5.8	2.3	5.2	0.0	4.3
Thrombocytopenia (< 50,000 cells/mm[3])	4.4	2.9	0.0	5.8	4.3
SGPT (> 250 U/L)	10.0	8.6	8.5	7.7	8.5
SGOT (> 250 U/L)	5.6	5.1	6.8	5.8	4.3
Alkaline Phosphatase (> 625 U/L)	3.1	3.2	0.0	9.6	2.1

[a] All percentages based on number of patients tested, not on number of patients in study. Median duration of treatment for N3300 was 44 weeks for HIVID, 53 weeks for ZDV; for N3492, 39 weeks for HIVID, 25 weeks for ZDV and for N3447 treatment ranged from 22 to 92 weeks among the arms.
[b] Reduced to 100 mg q4h ZDV when dose was approved.
[c] Excluded are 9 patients who received ZDV alone for the greater part of the study. Only 8 patients were treated with the recommended combination regimen; all other patients were treated at lower doses of HIVID and/or ZDV.

Table 7. Percentage of Patients with Clinical Adverse Experiences Considered Possibly or Probably Related to Study Drug Occurring in > 1% of Patients Treated in the HIVID Expanded-Access Program

	N3544[a] ZDV Intolerant or Failure			
	HIVID 0.375 mg q8h n=1757		HIVID 0.750 mg q8h n=1722	
Body System/ Adverse Event	mild/mod/sev	mod/sev	mild/mod/sev	mod/sev
Peripheral Neuropathy	10.8	5.9	14.9	7.8
Gastrointestinal				
Nausea	1.5	0.8	1.5	0.9
Ulcerative Stomatitis	1.4	0.6	2.6	1.7
Abdominal Pain	1.3	0.9	1.2	0.6
Aphthous Stomatitis	1.1	0.6	2.2	1.3
Diarrhea	0.9	0.4	1.0	0.6
Skin and Appendages				
Rash	1.2	0.6	1.4	0.6
Central and Periph NS				
Headache	0.7	0.2	1.2	0.7
Musculoskeletal				
Pain, Feet	0.9	0.3	2.1	1.2

[a] Median duration of treatment was 16 weeks.

Nervous: hypertonia, tremor, hand tremor, twitching (<1%).
Psychiatric: confusion (1.3%); impaired concentration (1.3%); amnesia, insomnia, somnolence, depression (<1%).
Respiratory: pharyngitis (2.2%); coughing, dyspnea, cyanosis (<1%).
Skin: dermatitis (1.3%); maculopapular rash, night sweats, alopecia, urticaria, erythematous papules (<1%).
Special Senses and Vision: taste perversion, xerophthalmia, abnormal vision, eye pain, tinnitus (<1%).
Urinary System: micturition frequency, abnormal renal function, acute renal failure, renal cyst (<1%).
Table 6 summarizes protocol grades 3-4 laboratory abnormalities occurring in HIVID monotherapy Protocols N3300/ACTG 114, N3492/ACTG 119 and combination HIVID and zidovudine Protocol N3447/ACTG 106.
Clinical adverse events and protocol grades 3-4 laboratory abnormalities that occurred in >1% of patients in the expanded-access safety study (N3544) are listed in Tables 7 and 8. The median duration of treatment was 16 weeks.
[See Table 8 on next page.]

Clinical adverse events at least possibly related to HIVID occurring in <1% of patients treated with either 0.375 mg or 0.750 mg q8h HIVID in the expanded-access safety study (N3544) are listed below by body system:
Body as a Whole: fatigue, fever, pain, malaise, asthenia, chest pain, generalized edema, weight decrease.
Cardiovascular: hypertension, palpitation, syncope, atrial fibrillation, tachycardia.
Gastrointestinal: vomiting, increased amylase, flatulence, anorexia, dyspepsia, esophageal ulcers, stomatitis, tongue ulceration, constipation, dry mouth, dysphagia, eructation, gastritis, gastrointestinal hemorrhage, pancreatitis, glossitis, left quadrant pain, salivary gland enlargement, jaundice, esophageal pain, esophagitis, rectal ulcers.
Endocrine: diabetes mellitus, hyperglycemia, hypocalcemia, impotence, hot flushes.
Hematologic: epistaxis.
Hepatic: abnormal hepatic function, hepatitis, jaundice.
Musculoskeletal: myalgia, arm pain, arthralgia, arthritis, arthropathy, cold feet, leg cramps, myositis, shoulder pain, wrist pain, cold extremities.
Nervous: seizures, ataxia, abnormal coordination, Bell's palsy, dizziness, dysphonia, hyperkinesia, hypokinesia, migraine, neuralgia, neuritis, stupor, tremor, vertigo.
Psychiatric: insomnia, agitation, depersonalization, hallucination, emotional lability, nervousness, confusion, anxiety, depression, euphoria, manic reaction, dementia, amnesia, somnolence, abnormal thinking, impaired concentration, abnormal crying.
Respiratory: pharyngitis, coughing, dyspnea, flu-like symptoms.
Skin: maculopapular rash, pruritus, dermatitis, skin lesions, acne, alopecia, bullous eruptions, follicular rash, flushing, increased sweating, urticaria.
Special Senses and Vision: abnormal vision, ear blockage, parosmia, loss of taste, taste perversion, burning eyes, eye itching, eye abnormality, deafness.
Urinary System: gout, toxic nephropathy, polyuria, renal calculus, acute renal failure, hyperuricemia.
Combination Trials: Only limited safety data are available on the combined use of HIVID with zidovudine. One patient with advanced HIV disease in study N3447/ACTG 106 died of refractory acidosis, mild pancreatitis, hepatomegaly with

Table 8. Percentage of Patients with Laboratory Abnormalities[a]

	Expanded Access (N3544)[b]	
	Dose Comparison Randomized ZDV Intolerant, ZDV Failure	
	n=3479	
	HIVID 0.375 mg q8h n=1757	HIVID 0.750 mg q8h n=1722
Laboratory Abnormality		
Anemia (<7.6 gm/dL)	3.5	4.1
Leukopenia (<1500 cells/mm^3)	8.8	10.2
Neutropenia (<750 cells/mm^3)	9.3	9.5
Eosinophilia (>1000 or 25%)	2.0	2.8
Thrombocytopenia (<50,000 cells/mm^3)	3.2	2.3
SGPT (>250 U/L)	2.7	3.3
SGOT (>250 U/L)	2.4	2.6
Alkaline Phosphatase (>650 U/L)	2.8	2.3

[a] All percentages based on number of patients tested, not on number of patients in study.
[b] Median duration of treatment was 16 weeks.

steatosis, and an unexplained neurological syndrome. The investigator assessed this event as remotely related to zidovudine and/or the combination of HIVID and zidovudine. Adverse events observed in this study are listed in Table 5. Only eight patients were treated with the recommended combination regimen; all other patients were treated with lower doses of HIVID and/or zidovudine. The occurrence of clinical adverse events at each dosage combination of HIVID and zidovudine did not vary significantly. There are no safety data currently available from the BW 34,225-02 study.

OVERDOSAGE

Acute Overdosage: There is little experience with acute HIVID overdosage and the sequelae are unknown. There is no known antidote for HIVID overdosage. It is not known whether zalcitabine is dialyzable by peritoneal dialysis or hemodialysis.

Chronic Overdosage: In an initial dose-finding study in which zalcitabine was administered at doses 25 times (0.25 mg/kg q8h) the currently recommended dose, one patient discontinued HIVID after one and one-half weeks of treatment subsequent to the development of a rash and fever. In the early Phase 1 studies, all patients receiving zalcitabine at approximately six times the current total daily recommended dose experienced peripheral neuropathy by week 10. Eighty percent of patients who received approximately two times the current total daily recommended dose experienced peripheral neuropathy by week 12.

DOSAGE AND ADMINISTRATION

The recommended combination regimen is one 0.750 mg tablet of HIVID orally, administered concomitantly with 200 mg of zidovudine every 8 hours (2.25 mg HIVID total daily dose and 600 mg zidovudine total daily dose). Based on pharmacokinetic weight-ranging data, there is no need to dose-reduce for weight down to 30 kg.

Monitoring of Patients: Periodic complete blood counts and clinical chemistry tests should be performed. Serum amylase levels should be monitored in those individuals who have a history of elevated amylase, pancreatitis, ethanol abuse, who are on parenteral nutrition or who are otherwise at high risk of pancreatitis. Careful monitoring for signs or symptoms suggestive of peripheral neuropathy is recommended, particularly in individuals with a low CD4 cell count or who are at a greater risk of developing peripheral neuropathy while on therapy (see WARNINGS).

Dose Adjustment for Combination Therapy with HIVID and Zidovudine: For recipients of combination therapy with HIVID and zidovudine, dose adjustments for either drug should be based on the known toxicity profile of the individual drugs. For toxicities more likely to be associated with HIVID (e.g., peripheral neuropathy, severe oral ulcers). HIVID should be interrupted or dose-reduced (see WARNINGS and PRECAUTIONS). For patients experiencing toxicities more likely to be associated with zidovudine (e.g., anemia, granulocytopenia), zidovudine should be interrupted or dose-reduced first. For any interruption of HIVID, and especially if HIVID is permanently discontinued, the zidovudine dosage schedule should be adjusted from 200 mg q8h to 100 mg q4h as recommended in the complete product information for zidovudine. FOR SEVERE TOXICITIES OR TOXICITIES IN WHICH THE CAUSATIVE DRUG IS UNCLEAR OR THOSE PERSISTING AFTER DOSE INTERRUPTION OR REDUCTION OF ONE DRUG, THE OTHER DRUG SHOULD ALSO BE INTERRUPTED OR DOSE-REDUCED. PHYSICIANS SHOULD REFER TO THE COMPLETE PRODUCT INFORMATION FOR ZIDOVUDINE FOR A DESCRIPTION OF KNOWN ZIDOVUDINE-ASSOCIATED ADVERSE REACTIONS. Since HIVID is not indicated for use as monotherapy, alternative antiretroviral therapy should be considered for patients who are unable to tolerate zidovudine as part of a combination regimen with HIVID.

Patients developing moderate discomfort with signs or symptoms of peripheral neuropathy (e.g., numbness, tingling, hypesthesias, burning or shooting pains of the lower or upper extremities, or loss of vibratory sense or ankle reflex). should stop HIVID, especially when these symptoms are bilateral and progress for >72 hours. HIVID-associated peripheral neuropathy may continue to worsen despite interruption of HIVID. HIVID should be reintroduced at 50% dose—0.375 mg q8h only if all findings related to peripheral neuropathy have improved to mild symptoms. HIVID should be permanently discontinued when patients experience severe discomfort related to peripheral neuropathy or moderate discomfort progressing for ≥1 week. If other moderate to severe clinical adverse reactions or laboratory abnormalities (such as increased liver function tests) occur, then both HIVID and zidovudine should be interrupted until the adverse reaction abates. Either zidovudine monotherapy or HIVID and zidovudine therapy should then be carefully reintroduced at lower doses if appropriate. If adverse reactions recur at the reduced dose, therapy should be discontinued. The minimum effective dose of HIVID in combination with zidovudine for the treatment of adult patients with advanced HIV infection has not been established.

In patients with poor bone marrow reserve, particularly those patients with advanced symptomatic HIV disease, frequent monitoring of hematologic indices is recommended to detect serious anemia or granulocytopenia (see WARNINGS). Significant toxicities, such as anemia (hemoglobin of <7.5 g/dL or reduction of >25% of baseline) and/or granulocytopenia (granulocyte count of <750 cells/mm^3 or reduction of >50% from baseline), may require treatment interruption of HIVID and zidovudine until evidence of marrow recovery is observed (see WARNINGS). For less severe anemia or granulocytopenia, a reduction in daily dose of zidovudine may be adequate. In patients who experience hematologic toxicity, reduction in hemoglobin may occur as early as 2 to 4 weeks after initiation of therapy, and granulocytopenia usually occurs after 6 to 8 weeks of therapy. In patients who develop significant anemia, dose modification does not necessarily eliminate the need for transfusion. If marrow recovery occurs following dose modification, gradual increases in dose may be appropriate depending on hematologic indices and patient tolerance. For more details, refer to the complete product information for zidovudine.

HOW SUPPLIED

HIVID 0.375 mg tablets are oval, beige, film-coated tablets with "HIVID 0.375" imprinted on one side and "ROCHE" on the other side—bottles of 100 (NDC 0004-0220-01). HIVID 0.750 mg tablets are oval, gray, film-coated tablets with "HIVID 0.750" imprinted on one side and "ROCHE" on the other side—bottles of 100 (NDC 0004-0221-01).

The tablets should be stored in tightly closed bottles at 59° to 87°F (15° to 30°C).

REFERENCES

1. Pizzo PA, Butler K, Balis, F, et al. Dideoxycytidine alone and in an alternating schedule with zid,vudine in children with symptomatic human immunodeficiency virus infection. *J Pediatr.* 1990;117(5):799–808. 2. Meng TC, Fischl MA, Boota AH, et al. Combination therapy with zidovudine and dideoxycytidine in patients with advanced human immunodeficiency virus infection. *Ann Intern Med.* 1992;116:13–20.

June 1992

Shown in Product Identification Section, page 426

KLONOPIN®

[*klon 'o-pin*]
(clonazepam/Roche)
(formerly known as Clonopin®)

The following text is complete prescribing information based on official labeling in effect June 1, 1992.

DESCRIPTION

Klonopin is available as scored tablets containing 0.5 mg, 1 mg or 2 mg clonazepam/Roche. Each tablet also contains lactose, magnesium stearate, microcrystalline cellulose and corn starch, with the following dye systems: 0.5 mg—FD&C Yellow No. 6; 1 mg—FD&C Blue No. 1 and FD&C Blue No. 2.

Chemically, clonazepam is 5-(2-chlorophenyl)-1,3-dihydro-7-nitro-2H-1,4-benzodiazepin-2-one. It is a light yellow crystalline powder. It has a molecular weight of 315.7.

ACTIONS

In laboratory animals, Klonopin exhibits several pharmacologic properties which are characteristic of the benzodiazepine class of drugs. Convulsions produced in rodents by pentylenetetrazol or electrical stimulation are antagonized, as are convulsions produced by photic stimulation in susceptible baboons. A taming effect in aggressive primates, muscle weakness and hypnosis are likewise produced by Klonopin. In humans it is capable of suppressing the spike and wave discharge in absence seizures (petit mal) and decreasing the frequency, amplitude, duration and spread of discharge in minor motor seizures.

Single oral dose administration of Klonopin to humans gave maximum blood levels of drug, in most cases, within one to two hours. The half-life of the parent compound varied from approximately 18 to 50 hours, and the major route of excretion was in the urine. In humans, five metabolites have been identified. In general, the biotransformation of clonazepam followed two pathways: oxidative hydroxylation at the C-3 position and reduction of the 7-nitro function to form 7-amino and/or 7-acetyl-amino derivatives.

INDICATIONS

Klonopin is useful alone or as an adjunct in the treatment of the Lennox-Gastaut syndrome (petit mal variant), akinetic and myoclonic seizures. In patients with absence seizures (petit mal) who have failed to respond to succinimides, Klonopin may be useful.

In some studies, up to 30% of patients have shown a loss of anticonvulsant activity, often within three months of administration. In some cases, dosage adjustment may reestablish efficacy.

CONTRAINDICATIONS

Klonopin should not be used in patients with a history of sensitivity to benzodiazepines, nor in patients with clinical or biochemical evidence of significant liver disease. It may be used in patients with open angle glaucoma who are receiving appropriate therapy, but is contraindicated in acute narrow angle glaucoma.

WARNINGS

Since Klonopin produces CNS depression, patients receiving this drug should be cautioned against engaging in hazardous occupations requiring mental alertness, such as operating machinery or driving a motor vehicle. They should also be warned about the concomitant use of alcohol or other CNS-depressant drugs during Klonopin therapy (see Drug Interactions).

Usage in Pregnancy: The effects of Klonopin in human pregnancy and nursing infants are unknown.

Recent reports suggest an association between the use of anticonvulsant drugs by women with epilepsy and an elevated incidence of birth defects in children born to these women. Data are more extensive with respect to diphenylhydantoin and phenobarbital, but these are also the most commonly prescribed anticonvulsants; less systematic or anecdotal reports suggest a possible similar association with the use of all known anticonvulsant drugs.

The reports suggesting an elevated incidence of birth defects in children of drug-treated epileptic women cannot be regarded as adequate to prove a definite cause and effect relationship. There are intrinsic methodologic problems in obtaining adequate data on drug teratogenicity in humans; the possibility also exists that other factors, *e.g.*, genetic factors or the epileptic condition itself, may be more important than drug therapy in leading to birth defects. The great majority of mothers on anticonvulsant medication deliver normal infants. It is important to note that anticonvulsant drugs should not be discontinued in patients in whom the drug is administered to prevent seizures because of the strong possibility of precipitating status epilepticus with attendant hypoxia and threat to life. In individual cases where the severity and frequency of the seizure disorder are such that the removal of medication does not pose a serious threat to the patient, discontinuation of the drug may be considered prior to and during pregnancy, although it cannot be said with any confidence that even mild seizures do not pose some hazards to the developing embryo or fetus.

These considerations should be weighed in treating or counseling epileptic women of childbearing potential.

Use of Klonopin in women of childbearing potential should be considered only when the clinical situation warrants the risk. Mothers receiving Klonopin should not breast feed their infants.

In a two-generation reproduction study with Klonopin given orally to rats at 10 or 100 mg/kg/day, there was a decrease in the number of pregnancies and a decrease in the number of offspring surviving until weaning. When Klonopin was administered orally to pregnant rabbits at 0.2, 1.0, 5.0 or 10.0 mg/kg/day, a nondose-related incidence of cleft palates,

Continued on next page

Roche Laboratories—Cont.

open eyelids, fused sternebrae and limb defects was observed at the 0.2 and 5.0 mg/kg/day levels. Nearly all of the malformations were seen from one dam in each of the affected dosages.

Usage in Children: Because of the possibility that adverse effects on physical or mental development could become apparent only after many years, a benefit-risk consideration of the long-term use of Klonopin is important in pediatric patients.

Withdrawal symptoms of the barbiturate type have occurred after the discontinuation of benzodiazepines. (See DRUG ABUSE AND DEPENDENCE section.)

PRECAUTIONS

When used in patients in whom several different types of seizure disorders coexist, Klonopin may increase the incidence or precipitate the onset of generalized tonic-clonic seizures (grand mal). This may require the addition of appropriate anticonvulsants or an increase in their dosages. The concomitant use of valproic acid and clonazepam may produce absence status.

Periodic blood counts and liver function tests are advisable during long-term therapy with Klonopin.

The abrupt withdrawal of Klonopin, particularly in those patients on long-term, high-dose therapy, may precipitate status epilepticus. Therefore, when discontinuing Klonopin, gradual withdrawal is essential. While Klonopin is being gradually withdrawn, the simultaneous substitution of another anticonvulsant may be indicated. Metabolites of Klonopin are excreted by the kidneys; to avoid their excess accumulation, caution should be exercised in the administration of the drug to patients with impaired renal function.

Klonopin may produce an increase in salivation. This should be considered before giving the drug to patients who have difficulty handling secretions. Because of this and the possibility of respiratory depression, Klonopin should be used with caution in patients with chronic respiratory diseases.

Information for patients: To assure the safe and effective use of benzodiazepines, patients should be informed that, since benzodiazepines may produce psychological and physical dependence, it is advisable that they consult with their physician before either increasing the dose or abruptly discontinuing this drug.

ADVERSE REACTIONS

The most frequently occurring side effects of Klonopin are referable to CNS depression. Experience to date has shown that drowsiness has occurred in approximately 50% of patients and ataxia in approximately 30%. In some cases, these may diminish with time; behavior problems have been noted in approximately 25% of patients. Others, listed by system, are:

Neurologic: Abnormal eye movements, aphonia, choreiform movements, coma, diplopia, dysarthria, dysdiadochokinesis, "glassy-eyed" appearance, headache, hemiparesis, hypotonia, nystagmus, respiratory depression, slurred speech, tremor, vertigo.

Psychiatric: Confusion, depression, amnesia, hallucinations, hysteria, increased libido, insomnia, psychosis, suicidal attempt (the behavior effects are more likely to occur in patients with a history of psychiatric disturbances).

Respiratory: Chest congestion, rhinorrhea, shortness of breath, hypersecretion in upper respiratory passages.

Cardiovascular: Palpitations.

Dermatologic: Hair loss, hirsutism, skin rash, ankle and facial edema.

Gastrointestinal: Anorexia, coated tongue, constipation, diarrhea, dry mouth, encopresis, gastritis, hepatomegaly, increased appetite, nausea, sore gums.

Genitourinary: Dysuria, enuresis, nocturia, urinary retention.

Musculoskeletal: Muscle weakness, pains.

Miscellaneous: Dehydration, general deterioration, fever, lymphadenopathy, weight loss or gain.

Hematopoietic: Anemia, leukopenia, thrombocytopenia, eosinophilia.

Hepatic: Transient elevations of serum transaminases and alkaline phosphatase.

DRUG ABUSE AND DEPENDENCE

Withdrawal symptoms, similar in character to those noted with barbiturates and alcohol (*e.g.,* convulsions, psychosis, hallucinations, behavioral disorder, tremor, abdominal and muscle cramps) have occurred following abrupt discontinuance of clonazepam. The more severe withdrawal symptoms have usually been limited to those patients who received excessive doses over an extended period of time. Generally milder withdrawal symptoms (*e.g.,* dysphoria and insomnia) have been reported following abrupt discontinuance of benzodiazepines taken continuously at therapeutic levels for several months. Consequently, after extended therapy, abrupt discontinuation should generally be avoided and a gradual dosage tapering schedule followed. Addiction-prone individuals (such as drug addicts or alcoholics) should be under careful surveillance when receiving clonazepam or other psychotropic agents because of the predisposition of such patients to habituation and dependence.

DRUG INTERACTIONS

The CNS-depressant action of the benzodiazepine class of drugs may be potentiated by alcohol, narcotics, barbiturates, nonbarbiturate hypnotics, antianxiety agents, the phenothiazines, thioxanthene and butyrophenone classes of antipsychotic agents, monoamine oxidase inhibitors and the tricyclic antidepressants, and by other anticonvulsant drugs.

OVERDOSAGE

Symptoms of Klonopin overdosage, like those produced by other CNS depressants, include somnolence, confusion, coma and diminished reflexes. Treatment includes monitoring of respiration, pulse and blood pressure, general supportive measures and immediate gastric lavage. Intravenous fluids should be administered and an adequate airway maintained. Hypotension may be combated by the use of levarterenol or metaraminol. Methylphenidate or caffeine and sodium benzoate may be given to combat CNS depression. Dialysis is of no known value.

DOSAGE AND ADMINISTRATION

Infants and Children: Klonopin is administered orally. In order to minimize drowsiness, the initial dose for infants and children (up to 10 years of age or 30 kg of body weight) should be between 0.01 and 0.03 mg/kg/day but not to exceed 0.05 mg/kg/day given in two or three divided doses. Dosage should be increased by no more than 0.25 to 0.5 mg every third day until a daily maintenance dose of 0.1 to 0.2 mg/kg of body weight has been reached unless seizures are controlled or side effects preclude further increase. Whenever possible, the daily dose should be divided into three equal doses. If doses are not equally divided, the largest dose should be given before retiring.

Adults: The initial dose for adults should not exceed 1.5 mg/day divided into three doses. Dosage may be increased in increments of 0.5 to 1 mg every three days until seizures are adequately controlled or until side effects preclude any further increase. Maintenance dosage must be individualized for each patient depending upon response. Maximum recommended daily dose is 20 mg.

The use of multiple anticonvulsants may result in an increase of depressant adverse effects. This should be considered before adding Klonopin to an existing anticonvulsant regimen.

HOW SUPPLIED

Scored tablets—0.5 mg, orange; 1 mg, blue; 2 mg, white—bottles of 100; Tel-E-Dose® packages of 100, available in boxes of four reverse-numbered cards of 25.

Revised: July 1991

Shown in Product Identification Section, page 426

KONAKION® ℞

[ko-nak 'e-on]

(phytonadione/Roche)

INJECTION

The following text is complete prescribing information based on official labeling in effect June 1, 1992.

DESCRIPTION

Konakion (phytonadione/Roche) Injection, a prothrombogenic vitamin, is an essentially clear, light yellow, sterile, aqueous dispersion of vitamin K_1. It is intended for intramuscular administration only. Konakion Injection is available in the following concentrations:

0.5-mL Ampuls —each 0.5 mL contains 1 mg phytonadione (vitamin K_1) compounded with 10 mg polysorbate 80, 0.45% phenol as preservative, 10.4 mg propylene glycol, 0.17 mg sodium acetate and 0.00002 mL glacial acetic acid.

1-mL Ampuls —each mL contains 10 mg phytonadione (vitamine K_1) compounded with 40 mg polysorbate 80, 20.7 mg propylene glycol, 0.8 mg sodium acetate and 0.00006 mL glacial acetic acid.

Phytonadione is a fat-soluble naphthoquinone derivative which is identical to naturally occurring vitamin K_1. Chemically, phytonadione is 1,4-naphthalenedione, 2-methyl-3-(3,7,11,15-tetramethyl-2-hexadecenyl)-[R-[R*, R*-(E)]]. It is a clear, yellow to amber, very viscous liquid and is insoluble in water and slightly soluble in alcohol. It has a molecular weight of 450.70.

CLINICAL PHARMACOLOGY

Phytonadione possesses the same type and degree of activity as does naturally occurring vitamin K, which is necessary for the synthesis in the liver of blood coagulation factors prothrombin (factor II), proconvertin (factor VII), plasma thromboplastin component (factor IX) and Stuart factor (factor X). The prothrombin test is sensitive to the concentrations of factors II, VII and X. The mechanism by which vitamin K_1 promotes formation of these clotting factors involves the hepatic post-translational carboxylation of specific glutamate residues to gamma-carboxylglutamate residues in proteins involved in coagulation, thus leading to their activation.

Following intramuscular injection, phytonadione is readily absorbed, almost entirely by way of the lymph. After absorption, phytonadione is initially concentrated in the liver, but the concentration declines rapidly. Very little vitamin K accumulates in tissues. There is considerable evidence that the synthesis of prothrombin and the related vitamin K-dependent blood clotting factors are linked to a metabolic cycle in which vitamin K_1 is oxidized and reduced to its inactive 2,3 epoxide metabolite. This vitamin K epoxide cycle is mediated by at least two enzymes which have been partially characterized as phytonadione epoxidase and phytonadione epoxide reductase. Phytonadione is known to cross the placenta.

Following intravenous administration of tritiated vitamin K_1, the half-life of elimination of phytonadione ranged from two to four hours. The lipid-soluble radioactivity in the plasma, which is assumed to represent the injected phytonadione, was rapidly cleared and resembles the clearance of orally administered phytonadione.

The action of the aqueous dispersion when administered parenterally is generally detectable within an hour or two, and hemorrhage is usually controlled within three to six hours. A normal prothrombin level may often be obtained in 12 to 14 hours.

INDICATIONS AND USAGE

Konakion is indicated for:

- anticoagulant-induced prothrombin deficiency;
- prophylaxis and therapy of hemorrhagic disease of the newborn;
- hypoprothrombinemia due to oral antibacterial therapy;
- hypoprothrombinemia secondary to factors limiting absorption or synthesis of vitamin K, *e.g.,* obstructive jaundice, biliary fistula, sprue, ulcerative colitis, celiac disease, intestinal resection, cystic fibrosis of the pancreas and regional enteritis;
- other drug-induced hypoprothrombinemia (such as that due to salicylates) when it is definitely shown that the result is due to interference with vitamin K metabolism.

In the prophylaxis and treatment of hemorrhagic disease of the newborn, Konakion has demonstrated a greater margin of safety than that of the water-soluble vitamin K analogs.

CONTRAINDICATIONS

Konakion is contraindicated in patients with known hypersensitivity to the drug.

WARNINGS

Konakion does not directly counteract the effects of oral anticoagulants, but it promotes the synthesis of prothrombin by the liver, usually within two hours. Fresh plasma or blood transfusions may be required for severe blood loss or lack of response to vitamin K. Phytonadione will not counteract the anticoagulant action of heparin.

When vitamin K_1 is used to correct excessive anticoagulant-induced hypoprothrombinemia but anticoagulant therapy is still indicated, the patient is again faced with the clotting hazards existing prior to starting the anticoagulant therapy. Phytonadione is not a clotting agent, but overzealous therapy with vitamin K may restore conditions which originally permitted thromboembolic phenomena. Dosage, therefore, should be kept as low as possible, and prothrombin time should be checked regularly as clinical conditions indicate.

PRECAUTIONS

General: Temporary resistance to prothrombin-depressing anticoagulants may result, especially when larger doses of phytonadione are used. If relatively large doses have been employed, it may be necessary when reinstituting anticoagulant therapy to use somewhat larger doses of the prothrombin-depressing anticoagulant or one which has a different mode of action, such as heparin.

Since the liver is the site of metabolic synthesis of prothrombin, hypoprothrombinemia resulting from hepatocellular damage is not corrected by administration of vitamin K. Repeated large doses of vitamin K are not warranted in liver disease if the response to initial use of the vitamin is unsatisfactory (Koller test).

Failure to respond to vitamin K may indicate that a coagulation defect is present or that the condition being treated is unresponsive to vitamin K.

Laboratory tests: The dose and frequency of administration and duration of treatment depend on the severity of the prothrombin deficiency and should be regulated by repeated determinations of prothrombin time.

Drug interactions: Because vitamin K_1 is a pharmacologic antagonist to coumarin and indanedione derivatives, patients being treated with these anticoagulants should not receive Konakion except for the treatment of excessive hypoprothrombinemia.

Carcinogenesis, mutagenesis, impairment of fertility: Konakion has not undergone adequate animal testing to evaluate carcinogenic or mutagenic potential, or impairment of fertility.

Pregnancy: Teratogenic effects: Pregnancy Category C. Animal reproduction studies have not been conducted with

phytonadione. When menaquinone (vitamin K_2), which is structurally similar to phytonadione, was administered to mice and rats on gestation days 7 through 14 at maximum doses of 1000 mg/kg/day (p.o.) and 100 mg/kg/day (i.p.), no teratogenicity was observed. It is not known whether Konakion can cause fetal harm when administered to pregnant women or can affect reproductive capacity. Konakion should be given to pregnant women only if clearly needed.

Nonteratogenic effects: Retardation of skeletal ossification has been reported in mice with vitamin K_2 (menaquinone).

Nursing mothers: A study has shown that vitamin K is excreted in human milk. This should be considered if it is necessary to administer Konakion to a nursing mother.

Pediatric use: Hemolysis and jaundice in newborns, particularly in premature infants, may be related to the dose of Konakion. Therefore, the recommended dose should not be exceeded (see ADVERSE REACTIONS and DOSAGE AND ADMINISTRATION sections).

ADVERSE REACTIONS

Allergic reactions: The possibility of allergic reactions, including an anaphylactoid reaction, should be kept in mind.

Miscellaneous: Pain, swelling and tenderness at the injection site have occurred rarely.

Although Konakion has a greater margin of safety than the water-soluble vitamin K analogs, hyperbilirubinemia has been reported in the newborn, particularly in prematures when used at 5 to 10 times the recommended dosage. This effect, with the possibility of attendant kernicterus, should be considered if such dosages are deemed necessary.

In patients with severe hepatic disease, large doses of phytonadione may further depress liver function. Paradoxically, the administration of excessive doses of vitamin K or its analogs in an attempt to correct the hypoprothrombinemia associated with severe hepatitis or cirrhosis may actually result in a further depression of the concentration of prothrombin (also see PRECAUTIONS: *General* section).

OVERDOSAGE

There are no data available on overdosage of Konakion in man. Phytonadione is nontoxic to animals, even when given in huge amounts. The acute toxicity of vitamin K_1 is as follows:

Species	Route	LD_{50}
Mouse	p.o.	> 25 Gm/kg
Mouse	i.p.	> 25 Gm/kg
Mouse*	i.v.	57 (48–112) mg/kg

*Konakion formulation used

If anticoagulation is needed following overdosage of phytonadione, heparin may be used.

DOSAGE AND ADMINISTRATION

The U.S. Recommended Daily Allowances for vitamin K in humans have not been established officially. The adequate daily dietary intake of vitamin K for adults has been estimated to be 70 to 140 mcg; for infants 10 to 20 mcg; for children and adolescents 15 to 100 mcg. The dietary abundance of vitamin K normally satisfies the requirements except for the neonatal period of 5 to 8 days.

Prevention and Therapy of Neonatal Hemorrhage Due to Vitamin K Deficiency: Vitamin K_1 0.5 to 1.0 mg should be administered intramuscularly to the infant immediately after delivery. This may be repeated after two to three weeks if the mother has received anticoagulant, anticonvulsant, antituberculous or recent antibiotic therapy during her pregnancy. These mothers may be given 1.0 to 5.0 mg of vitamin K_1 intramuscularly 12 to 24 hours before delivery. Due to inefficient placental transport, however, this should not be considered a substitute for the prophylactic administration of vitamin K_1 to the infant immediately after delivery.

For the treatment of severe, life-threatening hemorrhage, administration of blood or blood products such as fresh frozen plasma, in addition to parenteral vitamin K_1, may be needed (see WARNINGS).

When the expected clinical response is not observed, additional coagulation studies should be carried out to more clearly define the cause of the bleeding.

Because of the possibility that breast-fed infants who develop diarrhea may have decreased bacterial synthesis, as well as insufficient dietary intake of vitamin K_1, the American Academy of Pediatrics recommends that breast-fed infants who develop diarrhea that persists for longer than a few days should be given an additional injection of vitamin K_1 (1.0 mg).

Therapy of Hypoprothrombinemia Induced by Anticoagulant Therapy (except Heparin) in Adults: Vitamin K_1 should be administered intramuscularly at the dose of 5 to 10 mg initially; up to 20 mg if necessary.

In the presence of severe or active bleeding, transfusion of blood or fresh frozen plasma may be required (see WARNINGS).

Therapy of Hypoprothrombinemia Due to Other Causes in Adults:

Antibacterial therapy:	5 to 20 mg intramuscularly.
Other drugs (e.g. salicylates):	2 to 20 mg intramuscularly.
Factors limiting synthesis or absorption of vitamin K:	2 to 20 mg intramuscularly.

In older children and adults, injection of Konakion should be in the upper outer quadrant of the buttocks. In infants and young children, the anterolateral aspect of the thighs or the deltoid region is preferred so that danger of sciatic nerve injury is avoided.

It is recommended that Konakion be injected by itself, since phytonadione injection has been reported to be incompatible with many drugs in admixtures.

Parenteral drug products should be inspected visually for particulate matter and discoloration prior to administration, whenever solution and container permit. Slight opalescence may occur with Konakion ampuls, but this does not affect the safety or potency of the product.

Konakion is stable in the air, but it is photosensitive, decomposing with loss of potency on exposure to light. Therefore, it should be stored in a dark place and protected from light at all times. Konakion need not be refrigerated.

HOW SUPPLIED

0.5-mL Ampuls (1 mg phytonadione/0.5 mL)—boxes of 10 (NDC 0004-1907-06).

1-mL Ampuls (10 mg phytonadione/mL)—boxes of 10 (NDC 0004-1908-06).

STORE AT ROOM TEMPERATURE (15° to 30°C; 59° to 86°F). DO NOT FREEZE. PROTECT FROM LIGHT AT ALL TIMES.

Revised: August 1991

LARIAM® ℞

[*lar-é-um*]

(mefloquine hydrochloride)
TABLETS

The following text is complete prescribing information based on official labeling in effect June 1, 1992.

DESCRIPTION

Lariam (mefloquine hydrochloride) is an antimalarial agent available as 250-mg tablets of mefloquine hydrochloride (equivalent to 228.0 mg of the free base) for oral administration.

Mefloquine hydrochloride is a 4-quinolinemethanol derivative with the specific chemical name of (R*, S*)-(±)-α-2-piperidinyl-2,8-bis (trifluoromethyl)-4-quinolinemethanol hydrochloride. It is a 2-aryl substituted chemical structural analog of quinine. The drug is a white to almost white crystalline compound, slightly soluble in water.

Mefloquine hydrochloride has a calculated molecular weight of 414.78.

The inactive ingredients are ammonium-calcium alginate, corn starch, crospovidone, lactose, magnesium stearate, microcrystalline cellulose, poloxamer #331 and talc.

CLINICAL PHARMACOLOGY

Mefloquine is an antimalarial agent which acts as a blood schizonticide. Its exact mechanism of action is not known.

Pharmacokinetic studies of mefloquine in healthy male subjects showed that a significant lagtime occurred after drug administration, and the terminal elimination half-life varied widely (13 to 24 days) with a mean of about three weeks. Mefloquine is a mixture of enantiomeric molecules whose rates of release, absorption, transport, action, degradation and elimination may differ. A valid pharmacokinetic model may not exist in such a case.

Additional studies in European subjects showed slightly greater concentrations of drug for longer periods of time. The absorption half-life was 0.36 to 2.0 hours, and the terminal elimination half-life was 15 to 33 days. The primary metabolite was identified and its concentrations were found to surpass the concentrations of mefloquine.

Multiple-dose kinetic studies confirmed the long elimination half-lives previously observed. The mean metabolite to mefloquine ratio measured at steady-state was found to range between 2.3 and 8.6.

The total clearance of the drug, which is essentially all hepatic, is approximately 30 mL/min. The volume of distribution, approximately 20 L/kg, indicates extensive distribution. The drug is highly bound (98%) to plasma proteins and concentrated in blood erythrocytes, the target cells in malaria, at a relatively constant erythrocyte-to-plasma concentration ratio of about 2.

The pharmacokinetics of mefloquine in patients with compromised renal function and compromised hepatic function have not been studied.

In vitro and *in vivo* studies showed no hemolysis associated with glucose-6-phosphate dehydrogenase deficiency. (See ANIMAL TOXICOLOGY for additional information.)

INDICATIONS AND USAGE

Treatment of Acute Malaria Infections: Lariam is indicated for the treatment of mild to moderate acute malaria caused by mefloquine-susceptible strains of *Plasmodium falciparum* (both chloroquine-susceptible and resistant strains) or by *Plasmodium vivax.* There are insufficient clinical data to document the effect of mefloquine in malaria caused by *P. ovale* or *P. malariae.*

Note: Patients with acute *P. vivax* malaria, treated with Lariam, are at high risk of relapse because Lariam does not eliminate exoerythrocytic (hepatic phase) parasites. To avoid relapse, after initial treatment of the acute infection with Lariam, patients should subsequently be treated with an 8-aminoquinoline (*e.g.,* primaquine).

Prevention of Malaria: Lariam is indicated for the prophylaxis of *P. falciparum* and *P. vivax* malaria infections, including prophylaxis of chloroquine-resistant strains of *P. falciparum.*

CONTRAINDICATIONS

Use of this drug is contraindicated in patients with a known hypersensitivity to mefloquine or related compounds.

WARNINGS

In case of life-threatening, serious or overwhelming malaria infections due to *P. falciparum,* patients should be treated with an intravenous antimalarial drug. Following completion of intravenous treatment, Lariam may be given orally to complete the course of therapy.

Concomitant administration of Lariam and quinine, quinidine or drugs producing beta-adrenergic blockade may produce electrocardiographic abnormalities or cardiac arrest. Concomitant administration of Lariam and quinine or chloroquine may increase the risk of convulsions. (See PRECAUTIONS: Drug Interactions.)

PRECAUTIONS

General: Caution should be exercised with regard to driving, piloting airplanes and operating machines, as dizziness, a disturbed sense of balance or neuropsychiatric reactions have been reported during the use of Lariam. During prophylactic use, if signs of unexplained anxiety, depression, restlessness or confusion are noticed, these may be considered prodromal to a more serious event. In these cases, the drug must be discontinued.

This drug has not been administered for longer than one year. If the drug is to be administered for a prolonged period, periodic evaluations including liver function tests should be performed. Although retinal abnormalities seen in humans with long-term chloroquine use have not been observed with mefloquine use, long-term feeding of mefloquine to rats resulted in dose-related ocular lesions (retinal degeneration, retinal edema and lenticular opacity at 12.5 mg/kg/day and higher). (See ANIMAL TOXICOLOGY.) Therefore, periodic ophthalmic examinations are recommended.

Laboratory Tests: Periodic evaluation of hepatic function should be performed during prolonged prophylaxis.

Drug Interactions: Drug-drug interactions with Lariam have not been explored in detail. There is one report of cardiopulmonary arrest, with full recovery, in a patient who was taking a beta blocker (propranolol). Although no cardiovascular action of mefloquine hydrochloride, a myocardial depressant, has been observed during clinical trials, parenteral studies in animals show that it possesses 20% of the antifibrillatory action of quinidine and produces 50% of the increase in the PR interval reported with quinine. The effect of mefloquine hydrochloride on the compromised cardiovascular system has not been evaluated. The benefits of Lariam therapy should be weighed against the possibility of adverse effects in patients with cardiac disease.

Lariam should not be used concurrently with quinine or quinidine. If these drugs are to be used in the initial treatment of severe malaria, Lariam administration should be delayed at least twelve hours after the last dose.

Patients taking Lariam while taking valproic acid had loss of seizure control and lower than expected valproic acid blood levels. Therefore, patients concurrently taking antiseizure medication and Lariam should have the blood level of their antiseizure medication monitored and the dosage adjusted appropriately.

In clinical trials the concomitant administration of sulfadoxine and pyrimethamine did not alter the adverse reaction profile.

Carcinogenesis, Mutagenesis, Impairment of Fertility:

Carcinogenesis: The carcinogenic potential of mefloquine was studied in rats and mice in two-year feeding studies at doses up to 30 mg/kg/day. No treatment-related increases in tumor of any type were noted.

Mutagenesis: The mutagenic potential of mefloquine was studied in a variety of assay systems including: Ames test, a host-mediated assay in mice, fluctuation tests and a mouse micronucleus assay. Several of these assays were performed with and without prior metabolic activation. In no instance was evidence obtained for the mutagenicity of mefloquine.

Impairment of Fertility: Fertility studies in rats at doses of 5, 20 and 50 mg/kg/day of mefloquine have demonstrated adverse effects on fertility in the male at the high dose of 50 mg/kg/day, and in the female at doses of 20 and

Continued on next page

Roche Laboratories—Cont.

50 mg/kg/day. Histopathological lesions were noted in the epididymides from male rats at doses of 20 and 50 mg/kg/day. Administration of 250 mg/week of mefloquine (base) in adult males for 22 weeks failed to reveal any deleterious effects on human spermatozoa.

Pregnancy: Teratogenic Effects. Pregnancy Category C. Mefloquine has been demonstrated to be teratogenic in rats and mice at a dose of 100 mg/kg/day. In rabbits, a high dose of 160 mg/kg/day was embryotoxic and teratogenic, and a dose of 80 mg/kg/day was teratogenic but not embryotoxic. There are no adequate and well-controlled studies in pregnant women. Mefloquine should be used during pregnancy only if the potential benefit justifies the potential risk to the fetus. Women of childbearing potential who are traveling to areas where malaria is endemic should be warned against becoming pregnant.

Nursing Mothers: Based on a study in a few subjects, low concentrations (3 to 4%) of mefloquine were excreted in human milk following a dose equivalent to 250 mg of the free base. Caution should be exercised when mefloquine is administered to a nursing woman.

Pediatric Use: Safety and effectiveness in children have not been established. Two studies of mefloquine in children living in endemic areas for *P. falciparum* were conducted. All children in these studies had at least a low level of parasitemia and 18 to 40% had significant parasitemia with or without mild malaria symptoms. When given 20 to 30 mg/kg of mefloquine as a single dose, all children with fever became afebrile, and 92% of those with significant parasitemia had a satisfactory response to treatment. While incomplete follow-up was obtained in these studies, nausea and vomiting occurred in approximately 10 and 20%, respectively, and dizziness was seen in approximately 40% of children.

ADVERSE REACTIONS

Clinical: At the doses used for treatment of acute malaria infections, the symptoms possibly attributable to drug administration cannot be distinguished from those symptoms usually attributable to the disease itself.

Among subjects who received mefloquine for prophylaxis of malaria, the most frequently observed adverse experience was vomiting (3%). Dizziness, syncope, extrasystoles and other complaints affecting less than 1% were also reported. Among subjects who received mefloquine for treatment, the most frequently observed adverse experiences included: dizziness, myalgia, nausea, fever, headache, vomiting, chills, diarrhea, skin rash, abdominal pain, fatigue, loss of appetite and tinnitus. Those side effects occurring in less than 1% included bradycardia, hair loss, emotional problems, pruritus, asthenia, transient emotional disturbances and telogen effluvium (loss of resting hair). Seizures have also been reported.

Two serious adverse reactions were cardiopulmonary arrest in one patient shortly after ingesting a single prophylactic dose of mefloquine while concomitantly using propranolol (see WARNINGS and PRECAUTIONS), and encephalopathy of unknown etiology during prophylactic mefloquine administration. The relationship of encephalopathy to drug administration could not be clearly established.

The following additional adverse reactions have been reported during post-marketing surveillance: vertigo, visual disturbances and central nervous system disturbances (*e.g.* psychotic manifestations, hallucinations, confusion, anxiety and depression).

Laboratory: The most frequently observed laboratory alterations which could be possibly attributable to drug administration were decreased hematocrit, transient elevation of transaminases, leukopenia and thrombocytopenia. These alterations were observed in patients with acute malaria who received treatment doses of the drug and were attributed to the disease itself.

During prophylactic administration of mefloquine to indigenous populations in malaria-endemic areas, the following occasional alterations in laboratory values were observed: transient elevation of transaminases, leukocytosis or thrombocytopenia.

OVERDOSAGE

Induce vomiting and see a physician immediately because of the potential cardiotoxic effect. Treat vomiting or diarrhea with standard fluid therapy.

DOSAGE AND ADMINISTRATION (See INDICATIONS AND USAGE section):

(a) Treatment of mild to moderate malaria in adults caused by *P. vivax* or mefloquine-susceptible strains of *P. falciparum*—five tablets (1250 mg) mefloquine hydrochloride to be given as a single oral dose. The drug should not be taken on an empty stomach and should be administered with at least 8 oz (240 mL) of water.

Note: Patients with acute *P. vivax* malaria, treated with Lariam, are at high risk of relapse because Lariam does not eliminate exoerythrocytic (hepatic phase) parasites. To avoid relapse after initial treatment of the acute infection with Lariam, patients should subsequently be treated with an 8-aminoquinoline (*e.g.*, primaquine).

(b) Malaria prophylaxis—one tablet (250 mg) mefloquine hydrochloride once weekly for four weeks, then one tablet every other week.

Prophylactic drug administration should be initiated one week prior to departure to an endemic area. It is suggested that the same day of the week be used each time the drug is administered. To avoid development of malaria after return from an endemic area, prophylaxis should be continued for four additional weeks. For prolonged stays in an endemic area this may be achieved by continuing the recommended dosage schedule, once weekly for four weeks, then once every other week, until the traveler has taken three doses following return to a malaria-free area. Tablets should not be taken on an empty stomach and should be administered with at least 8 oz (240 mL) of water.

HOW SUPPLIED

Lariam is available as scored, white, round tablets, containing 250 mg of mefloquine hydrochloride in unit-dose foil strips in cartons containing 25 (NDC 0004-0172-02). Imprint on tablets: LARIAM 250 ROCHE.

Tablets should be stored at 15°–30°C (59°–86°F).

ANIMAL TOXICOLOGY

Ocular lesions were observed in rats fed mefloquine daily for two years. All surviving rats given 30 mg/kg/day had ocular lesions in both eyes characterized by retinal degeneration, opacity of the lens and retinal edema. Similar but less severe lesions were observed in 80% of female and 22% of male rats fed 12.5 mg/kg/day for two years. At doses of 5 mg/kg/day, only corneal lesions were observed. They occurred in 9% of rats studied.

Revised: February 1990

Manufactured by
F. HOFFMANN-LA ROCHE & CO., LTD.
Basle, Switzerland
Distributed by
ROCHE LABORATORIES
a division of Hoffmann-La Roche Inc.
340 Kingsland Street
Nutley, New Jersey 07110-1199

Shown in Product Identification Section, page 426

LAROBEC® TABLETS   ℞
[*lar 'o-bek*]

The following text is complete prescribing information based on official labeling in effect June 1, 1992.

Each Larobec® tablet contains:	Quantity	U.S. RDA— Adults and children 4 or more years of age
Water-Soluble Vitamins		
Vitamin C (ascorbic acid)	500 mg	60 mg
Vitamin B₁ (as thiamine mononitrate)	15 mg	1.5 mg
Vitamin B₂ (riboflavin)	15 mg	1.7 mg
Niacin (as niacinamide)	100 mg	20 mg
Pantothenic acid (as calcium *d*-pantothenate)	18 mg	10 mg
Folic acid	0.5 mg	0.4 mg
Vitamin B₁₂ (cyanocobalamin)	5 mcg	6 mcg

Each tablet also contains acacia, calcium sulfate, carnauba wax, hydrogenated vegetable oil, magnesium oxide, magnesium stearate, povidone, shellac, sodium benzoate, sugar and talc with the following dyes: FD&C Yellow No. 6, D&C Yellow No. 10 and titanium dioxide.

DESCRIPTION

Larobec is a prescription-only oral multivitamin tablet specially formulated for patients who require prophylactic or therapeutic nutritional supplementation of water-soluble vitamins and are receiving levodopa therapy for Parkinson's disease and syndrome. Larobec provides *therapeutic* levels of ascorbic acid, vitamins B₁, B₂, niacin, pantothenic acid and folic acid and a *supplemental* level of vitamin B₁₂ *without* pyridoxine (vitamin B₆), which has been reported to reduce the clinical benefits of levodopa therapy.

CLINICAL PHARMACOLOGY

Vitamins are essential for maintenance of normal metabolic functions including hematopoiesis. The water-soluble vitamins play vital roles in the conversion of carbohydrate, protein and fat into tissue and energy. *Thiamine (B₁)* acts as a coenzyme in carbohydrate metabolism. *Riboflavin (B₂)* functions as a coenzyme in the electron transport system associated with conversion of tissue oxidations into usable energy. *Niacin* serves as a coenzyme in oxidation-reduction reactions in tissue respiration. *Pantothenic acid* functions as a coenzyme in various metabolic acetylation reactions. *Folic acid* and *cyanocobalamin (B₁₂)* are metabolically interrelated. They are essential to nucleic acid synthesis and normal maturation of red blood cells. *Ascorbic acid (C)* performs a vital function in the process of cellular respiration, and is involved in both carbohydrate and amino acid metabolism. It is essential for collagen formation and tissue repair.

The water-soluble vitamins (B-complex and C) are not significantly stored by the body; excess quantities are excreted in the urine. They must be replenished regularly through diet or other means to maintain essential tissue levels. Thus these vitamins are rapidly depleted in conditions interfering with their intake or absorption.

INDICATIONS AND USAGE

Larobec is indicated for supportive nutritional supplementation when a water-soluble vitamin formulation (without pyridoxine) is required prophylactically or therapeutically in patients who are undergoing treatment with levodopa.

CONTRAINDICATIONS

Larobec is contraindicated in patients known to be hypersensitive to any of its components.

WARNINGS

Administration of vitamin B₆ may be required if signs of pyridoxine deficiency develop. Folic acid in doses above 0.1 mg daily may obscure pernicious anemia. Larobec is not intended for treatment of pernicious anemia or other megaloblastic anemias where vitamin B₁₂ is deficient. Neurologic involvement may develop or progress, despite temporary remission of anemia, in patients with vitamin B₁₂ deficiency who receive supplemental folic acid and who are inadequately treated with B₁₂.

PRECAUTIONS

General: Certain patients may require additional nutritional supplementation with fat-soluble vitamins and minerals according to the dietary habits of the individual. Larobec is not intended for treatment of severe specific vitamin deficiencies.

Information for the Patient: Because toxic reactions have been reported with injudicious use of certain vitamins, urge patients to follow your specific instructions regarding dosage regimen. As with any medication, advise patients to keep Larobec out of reach of children.

ADVERSE REACTIONS

Adverse reactions have been reported with specific vitamins, but generally at levels substantially higher than those in Larobec. However, allergic and idiosyncratic reactions are possible at lower levels.

DOSAGE AND ADMINISTRATION

Usual adult dosage: one tablet daily.
Larobec is available on prescription only.

HOW SUPPLIED

Orange-colored, capsule-shaped tablets—bottles of 100 (NDC 0004-0073-01).
Imprint on tablets: LAROBEC® ROCHE
Revised: November 1985

Shown in Product Identification Section, page 426

LARODOPA®   ℞
[*lar "o-do 'pa*]
(levodopa/Roche)

The following text is complete prescribing information based on official labeling in effect June 1, 1992.

> In order to reduce the high incidence of adverse reactions, it is necessary to individualize the therapy and to gradually increase the dosage to the desired therapeutic level.

DESCRIPTION

Larodopa is available as tablets containing 0.1 Gm, 0.25 Gm or 0.5 Gm levodopa. Each tablet also contains corn starch, magnesium stearate, microcrystalline cellulose, povidone, talc and D&C Red No. 7 lake dye.

Chemically, levodopa is (−)-3-(3,4-dihydroxyphenyl)-*L*-alanine. It is a colorless, crystalline compound, slightly soluble in water and insoluble in alcohol, with a molecular weight of 197.2.

ACTIONS

Evidence indicates that the symptoms of Parkinson's disease are related to depletion of striatal dopamine. Since dopamine apparently does not cross the blood-brain barrier, its administration is ineffective in the treatment of Parkinson's disease. However, levodopa, the levo-rotatory isomer of dihydroxyphenylalanine (dopa) which is the metabolic precursor of dopamine, does cross the blood-brain barrier. Presumably it is converted into dopamine in the basal ganglia. This is generally thought to be the mechanism whereby oral

levodopa acts in relieving the symptoms of Parkinson's disease.

The major urinary metabolites of levodopa in man appear to be dopamine and homovanillic acid (HVA). In 24-hour urine samples, HVA accounts for 13 to 42 percent of the ingested dose of levodopa.

INDICATIONS

Larodopa is indicated in the treatment of idiopathic Parkinson's disease (Paralysis Agitans), postencephalitic parkinsonism, symptomatic parkinsonism which may follow injury to the nervous system by carbon monoxide intoxication, and manganese intoxication. It is indicated in those elderly patients believed to develop parkinsonism in association with cerebral arteriosclerosis.

CONTRAINDICATIONS

Monoamine oxidase (MAO) inhibitors and Larodopa should not be given concomitantly and these inhibitors must be discontinued two weeks prior to initiating therapy with Larodopa. Larodopa is contraindicated in patients with known hypersensitivity to the drug and in narrow angle glaucoma.

Because levodopa may activate a malignant melanoma, it should not be used in patients with suspicious, undiagnosed skin lesions or a history of melanoma.

WARNINGS

Larodopa should be administered cautiously to patients with severe cardiovascular or pulmonary disease, bronchial asthma, renal, hepatic or endocrine disease.

Care should be exercised in administering Larodopa to patients with a history of myocardial infarction who have residual atrial, nodal or ventricular arrhythmias. If Larodopa is necessary in this type of patient, it should be used in a facility with a coronary care unit or an intensive care unit.

One must be on the alert for the possibility of upper gastrointestinal hemorrhage in those patients with a past history of active peptic ulcer disease.

All patients should be carefully observed for the development of depression with concomitant suicidal tendencies. Psychotic patients should be treated with caution.

Pyridoxine hydrochloride (vitamin B_6) in oral doses of 10 to 25 mg rapidly reverses the toxic and therapeutic effects of Larodopa. This should be considered before recommending vitamin preparations containing pyridoxine hydrochloride (vitamin B_6).

Usage in Pregnancy: The safety of Larodopa in women who are or who may become pregnant has not been established; hence it should be given only when the potential benefits have been weighed against possible hazards to mother and child. Studies in rodents have shown that levodopa at dosages in excess of 200 mg/kg/day has an adverse effect on fetal and postnatal growth and viability.

Larodopa should not be used in nursing mothers.

Usage in Children: The safety of Larodopa under the age of 12 has not been established.

PRECAUTIONS

Periodic evaluations of hepatic, hematopoietic, cardiovascular and renal function are recommended during extended therapy in all patients.

Patients with chronic wide angle glaucoma may be treated cautiously with Larodopa, provided the intraocular pressure is well controlled and the patient monitored carefully for changes in intraocular pressure during therapy.

Postural hypotensive episodes have been reported as adverse reactions. Therefore, Larodopa should be administered to patients on antihypertensive drug cautiously (for patients receiving pargyline, see note on MAO inhibitors contraindications), and it may be necessary to adjust the dosage of the antihypertensive drugs.

ADVERSE REACTIONS

The most serious adverse reactions associated with the administration of Larodopa having frequent occurrences are: adventitious movements such as choreiform and/or dystonic movements. Other serious adverse reactions with a lower incidence are: cardiac irregularities and/or palpitations, orthostatic hypotensive episodes, bradykinetic episodes (the "on-off" phenomena), mental changes including paranoid ideation and psychotic episodes, depression with or without the development of suicidal tendencies, dementia, and urinary retention.

Rarely, gastrointestinal bleeding, development of duodenal ulcer, hypertension, phlebitis, hemolytic anemia, agranulocytosis, and convulsions have been observed. (The causal relationship between convulsions and Larodopa has not been established.)

Adverse reactions of a less serious nature having a relatively frequent occurrence are the following: anorexia, nausea and vomiting with or without abdominal pain and distress, dry mouth, dysphagia, sialorrhea, ataxia, increased hand tremor, headache, dizziness, numbness, weakness and faintness, bruxism, confusion, insomnia, nightmares, hallucinations and delusions, agitation and anxiety, malaise, fatigue and euphoria. Occurring with a lesser order of frequency are the following: muscle twitching and blepharospasm (which

may be taken as an early sign of overdosage; consideration of dosage reduction may be made at this time), trismus, burning sensation of the tongue, bitter taste, diarrhea, constipation, flatulence, flushing, skin rash, increased sweating, bizarre breathing patterns, urinary incontinence, diplopia, blurred vision, dilated pupils, hot flashes, weight gain or loss, dark sweat and/or urine.

Rarely, oculogyric crises, sense of stimulation, hiccups, development of edema, loss of hair, hoarseness, priapism and activation of latent Horner's syndrome have been observed. Elevations of blood urea nitrogen, SGOT, SGPT, LDH, bilirubin, alkaline phosphatase or protein-bound iodine have been reported; and the significance of this is not known. Occasional reductions in WBC, hemoglobin, and hematocrit have been noted.

Leukopenia has occurred and requires cessation, at least temporarily, of Larodopa administration. The Coombs test has occasionally become positive during extended therapy. Elevations of uric acid have been noted when colorimetric method was used but not when uricase method was used.

OVERDOSAGE

For acute overdosage general supportive measures should be employed, along with immediate gastric lavage. Intravenous fluids should be administered judiciously and an adequate airway maintained.

Electrocardiographic monitoring should be instituted and the patient carefully observed for the possible development of arrhythmias; if required, appropriate antiarrhythmic therapy should be given. Consideration should be given to the possibility of multiple drug ingestion by the patient. To date, no experience has been reported with dialysis; hence its value in Larodopa overdosage is not known. Although pyridoxine hydrochloride (vitamin B_6) has been reported to reverse the antiparkinson effects of Larodopa, its usefulness in the management of acute overdosage has not been established.

DOSAGE AND ADMINISTRATION

The optimal daily dose of Larodopa, *i.e.*, the dose producing maximal improvement with tolerated side effects, must be determined and *carefully titrated for each individual patient.* The usual initial dosage is 0.5 to 1 Gm daily, divided in two or more doses with food.

The total daily dosage is then increased gradually in increments not more than 0.75 Gm every three to seven days as tolerated. The usual optimal therapeutic *dosage should not exceed 8 Gm.* The exceptional patient may carefully be given more than 8 Gms as required. In some patients, a significant therapeutic response may not be obtained until six months of treatment.

In the event general anesthesia is required, Larodopa therapy may be continued as long as the patient is able to take fluids and medication by mouth. If therapy is temporarily interrupted, the usual daily dosage may be administered as soon as the patient is able to take oral medication. Whenever therapy has been interrupted for longer periods, dosage should again be adjusted gradually; however, in many cases the patient can be rapidly titrated to his previous therapeutic dosage.

HOW SUPPLIED

Tablets, pink, scored, each containing levodopa/Roche 0.1 Gm (NDC 0004-0072-01), 0.25 Gm (NDC 0004-0057-01) or 0.5 Gm (NDC 0004-0056-01)—bottles of 100.

Revised: May 1991

Shown in Product Identification Section, page 426

LEVO-DROMORAN®　　Ⓒ

[lee "vo dro 'mo-ran]
(levorphanol tartrate/Roche)
Ampuls ● Vials ● Tablets

The following text is complete prescribing information based on official labeling in effect June 1, 1992.

DESCRIPTION

Levo-Dromoran is available as 1-ml ampuls containing 2 mg levorphanol tartrate compounded with 0.2% parabens (methyl and propyl) as preservatives and sodium hydroxide to adjust pH to approximately 4.3; as 10-ml vials containing 2 mg levorphanol tartrate per ml, compounded with 0.45% phenol as preservative and sodium hydroxide to adjust pH to approximately 4.3; and as scored tablets, each containing 2 mg levorphanol tartrate plus lactose, corn starch, stearic acid and talc.

Levo-Dromoran is a highly potent synthetic analgesic with properties and actions similar to those of morphine. It produces a degree of analgesia at least equal to that of morphine and greater than that of meperidine at far smaller doses than either. It is longer acting than either; from 6 to 8 hours of pain relief can be expected with Levo-Dromoran whether given orally or by injection. It is almost as effective orally as it is parenterally. Its safety margin is about equal to that of morphine, but it is less likely to produce nausea, vomiting and constipation.

INDICATIONS

Levo-Dromoran is recommended whenever a narcotic-analgesic is required. It is recommended for the relief of pain whether moderate or severe. For example, it may be used in alleviating pain due to biliary and renal colic, myocardial infarction, and severe trauma; intractable pain due to cancer and other tumors; and for postoperative pain relief. Used preoperatively, it allays apprehension, provides prolonged analgesia, reduces thiopental requirements and shortens recovery-room time. Levo-Dromoran is compatible with a wide range of anesthetic agents. It is a useful supplement to nitrous oxide-oxygen anesthesia. It has been given by slow intravenous injection for special indications.

CONTRAINDICATIONS

As with the use of morphine, Levo-Dromoran is contraindicated in acute alcoholism, bronchial asthma, increased intracranial pressure, respiratory depression and anoxia.

WARNING

May be habit forming. Levo-Dromoran is a narcotic with an addiction liability similar to that of morphine, and for this reason the same precautions should be taken in administering the drug as with morphine. As with all narcotics, Levo-Dromoran should be used in early pregnancy only when expected benefits outweigh risks.

PRECAUTIONS

To counteract narcotic-induced respiratory depression, a narcotic antagonist, such as Narcan (naloxone hydrochloride), is recommended and should be readily available whenever Levo-Dromoran is used by parenteral administration.

ADVERSE REACTIONS

As is true with the use of any narcotic-analgesic, nausea, emesis and dizziness are not uncommon in the ambulatory patient. Respiratory depression, hypotension, urinary retention and various cardiac arrhythmias have been infrequently reported following the use of Levo-Dromoran, primarily in surgical patients. Occasional allergic reactions in the form of skin rash or urticaria have been reported. Pruritus or sweating are rarely observed.

DOSAGE AND ADMINISTRATION

Good medical practice dictates that the dose of any narcotic-analgesic be appropriate to the degree of pain to be relieved. This is especially important during the postoperative period because (a) residual CNS-depressant effects of anesthetic agents may still be present, and (b) later, gradual lessening of pain may not warrant full narcotizing doses. The average adult dose is 2 mg orally or subcutaneously. The dosage may be increased to 3 mg, if necessary.

ANTIDOTE FOR OVERDOSAGE

In the event of overdosage of Levo-Dromoran, an appropriate dose of a narcotic antagonist, such as Narcan (naloxone HCl), should be administered; consult the prescribing information of the specific narcotic antagonist for details about use.

HOW SUPPLIED

Ampuls, 1 ml (boxes of 10). Each ml of solution contains 2 mg levorphanol tartrate/Roche (WARNING: May be habit forming).

Multiple Dose Vials, 10 ml, 2 mg/ml (boxes of 1). Each ml of solution contains 2 mg levorphanol tartrate/Roche (WARNING: May be habit forming).

Oral Tablets, 2 mg, scored (bottles of 100). Each tablet contains 2 mg levorphanol tartrate/Roche (WARNING: May be habit forming).

Narcotic order required.

Revised: September 1985

Shown in Product Identification Section, page 426

MARPLAN® TABLETS　　℞

[mar 'plan]
(isocarboxazid/Roche)

The following text is complete prescribing information based on official labeling in effect June 1, 1992.

DESCRIPTION

Marplan (isocarboxazid/Roche), an amine-oxidase inhibitor, is available for oral administration in 10-mg tablets. Each tablet also contains gelatin, lactose, magnesium stearate, corn starch, talc, FD&C Red No. 3 and FD&C Yellow No. 6. Chemically, isocarboxazid is 5-methyl-3-isoxazolecarboxylic acid 2-benzylhydrazide.

Isocarboxazid is a colorless, crystalline substance with very little taste.

ACTIONS

Isocarboxazid, a potent inhibitor of amine-oxidase, exhibits antidepressant activity. *In vivo* and *in vitro* studies demonstrated inhibition of amine-oxidase in the brain, heart and liver.

Continued on next page

Roche Laboratories—Cont.

The oral LD_{50} in mice was 171 mg/kg and in rats, 270 mg/kg. In rats administered 120 mg/kg daily for 6 weeks, isocarboxazid produced a reduction of growth rate and appetite. In chronic tolerance studies of 24 weeks duration, hyperexcitability and depression of growth rate occurred in male rats given oral doses of 5 mg/kg/day and in both sexes of this species given 10 mg/kg/day orally. The relevance of these findings to the clinical use of Marplan is not known. No hematologic changes were observed.
Dogs given 15 mg/kg/day for 2 weeks showed emetic effects and a slight lowering of hemoglobin and hematocrit. No adverse effects were noted, however, at doses of 10 mg/kg/day for 6 weeks. Given as successively increasing daily oral doses to a dog, isocarboxazid was tolerated up to 40 mg/kg.
Monkeys given 20 mg/kg/day orally for 2 weeks tolerated the drug with no apparent adverse effects.
Reproduction studies were carried out in rats given 0.5 and 5 mg/kg/day of isocarboxazid as a dietary mixture for 10 weeks prior to mating and continuing through two mating cycles to the weaning of the second litter. The parent animals remained in good condition throughout the test period. Litters of the treated groups compared favorably with those of the controls. No evidence of teratogenic effects was seen in any of the young.

INDICATIONS: Based on a review of this drug by the National Academy of Sciences—National Research Council and/or other information, FDA has classified the indications as follows:
"Probably" effective for the treatment of depressed patients who are refractory to tricyclic antidepressants or electroconvulsive therapy and depressed patients in whom tricyclic antidepressants are contraindicated.
Final classification of the less-than-effective indications requires further investigation.

Careful selection of candidates for Marplan—with due regard to the symptomatology of the patient and to the properties of the compound—will result in more effective therapy. Complete review of the package insert is advised before initiating treatment.

CONTRAINDICATIONS

Marplan is contraindicated in patients with known hypersensitivity to the drug, severe impairment of liver or renal function, congestive heart failure or pheochromocytoma.
The potentiation of sympathomimetic substances by MAO inhibitors may result in *hypertensive crisis;* therefore, patients taking Marplan should not be given *sympathomimetic drugs* (including amphetamines, methyldopa, levodopa, dopamine, and tryptophan as well as epinephrine and norepinephrine) nor *foods with a high concentration of tryptophan* (broad beans) or *tyramine* (cheese, beers, wines, alcohol-free and reduced-alcohol beer and wine products, pickled herring, chicken livers, yeast extract). Excessive amounts of caffeine can also cause hypertensive reactions.
These hypertensive crises can be fatal, due to circulatory collapse or intracranial bleeding. Hypertensive crises are characterized by some or all of the following symptoms: occipital headache which may radiate frontally, neck stiffness or soreness, nausea, vomiting, photophobia, dilated pupils, sweating (sometimes with fever and sometimes with cold, clammy skin) and palpitations. Either tachycardia or bradycardia may be present, and can be associated with constricting chest pain. These crises usually occur within several hours after the ingestion of a contraindicated substance. Marplan should be discontinued immediately upon the occurrence of palpitations or frequent headaches.
Recommended treatment in hypertensive crisis: Marplan should be discontinued and therapy to lower blood pressure should be started immediately. A successful method of treatment is with an alpha-adrenergic blocking agent such as phentolamine, 5 mg, I.V., or pentolinium, 3 mg, subcutaneously. These drugs should be administered slowly to avoid excessive hypotension. Fever should be managed by external cooling.
Marplan should not be administered together with or immediately following other MAO inhibitors or dibenzazepines. Such combinations can produce hypertensive crisis, fever, marked sweating, excitation, delirium, tremor, twitching, convulsions, coma, and circulatory collapse. Marplan should also not be used in combination with buspirone, since several cases of elevated blood pressure have been reported in patients taking MAO inhibitors who were then given buspirone. At least 10 days should elapse between the discontinuation of Marplan and the institution of another antidepressant or buspirone, or the discontinuation of another MAO inhibitor and the institution of Marplan.
Some other amine-oxidase inhibitors commonly used in this country include pargyline HCl, phenelzine sulfate and tranylcypromine.
Some dibenzazepine-related compounds are antidepressants commonly used in this country, including amitriptyline HCl, amoxapine, desipramine HCl, doxepin HCl, imipramine HCl, maprotiline HCl, nortriptyline HCl, protriptyline HCl, and trimipramine maleate. Carbamazepine and cyclobenzaprine HCl are also dibenzazepines.
MAO inhibitors, including Marplan, are contraindicated in patients receiving clomipramine hydrochloride (Anafranil®).
Patients taking Marplan should not undergo elective surgery requiring general anesthesia. Should spinal anesthesia be essential, consideration should be given to possible combined hypotensive effects of Marplan and the blocking agent. Also, they should not be given cocaine or local anesthetic solutions containing sympathomimetic vasoconstrictors. Marplan should be discontinued at least 10 days prior to elective surgery.
Marplan should not be used in combination with CNS depressants such as narcotics and ethanol (see PRECAUTIONS for barbiturates). Circulatory collapse and death have been reported from the combination of amine-oxidase inhibitors and a single dose of meperidine. In addition, serious hyperpyrexia can occur following administration of this combination. It is thought that this latter reaction may be mediated by release of 5-hydroxytryptamine, as it does not occur in experimental animals pretreated with inhibitors of 5-HT synthesis.
The combination of MAO inhibitors and dextromethorphan has been reported to cause brief episodes of psychosis or bizarre behavior.
The combination of MAO inhibitors and tryptophan has been reported to cause behavioral and neurologic syndromes, including disorientation, confusion, amnesia, delirium, agitation, hypomanic signs, ataxia, myoclonus, hyperreflexia, shivering, ocular oscillations and Babinski signs.
There have been reports of serious reactions (including hyperthermia, rigidity, myoclonus, hypertension and mental changes, particularly confusion and hypomania) in patients receiving fluoxetine in combination with an MAO inhibitor, or even in patients who have very recently dicontinued from fluoxetine and are then started on an MAO inhibitor. Therefore, Marplan should not be used in combination with fluoxetine, or even shortly after stopping fluoxetine. Fluoxetine and its major metabolite have very long elimination half-lives and at least 5 weeks should be allowed after stopping fluoxetine and starting Marplan. In addition, there should be an interval of at least 10 days between discontinuation of Marplan and initiation of fluoxetine.

WARNINGS

Because the most serious reactions to Marplan relate to effects on blood pressure, it is not advisable to use this drug in elderly or debilitated patients or in the presence of hypertension, cardiovascular or cerebrovascular disease. Patients with severe or frequent headaches should not be considered as candidates for therapy with Marplan because headaches during therapy may be the first symptom of a hypertensive reaction to the drug.
Marplan should be used with caution in combination with antihypertensive drugs including thiazide diuretics since hypotension may result.
In patients who may be suicidal risks, no single form of treatment, such as Marplan, electroshock or other therapy, should be relied on as a sole therapeutic measure. The strictest supervision, and preferably hospitalization, are advised.
Warning to patient: All patients taking Marplan should be warned against self-medication with proprietary cold, hay fever or reducing preparations, since most of these contain sympathomimetic agents. They should be warned against eating the foods previously mentioned that contain high concentrations of tyramine or tryptophan. Beverages containing caffeine should be used in moderation. Patients should be instructed to report promptly the occurrence of headache or other unusual symptoms.
Use in Children: Marplan is not recommended for use in patients under 16 years of age since there are no controlled studies of safety or efficacy in this group.
Use in Pregnancy: Safe use of Marplan during pregnancy or lactation has not yet been established. Before prescribing Marplan in pregnancy, lactation, or in women of childbearing age, the potential benefit of the drug should be weighed against its possible hazard to mother and child. (See ACTIONS.)

PRECAUTIONS

Concomitant use of Marplan and other psychotropic agents is not recommended because of possible potentiating effects and decreased margin of safety. This is especially true in patients who may subject themselves to an overdosage of drugs. If combination therapy is indicated, careful consideration should be given to the pharmacology of all agents to be employed. The effects of Marplan may persist for a substantial period after discontinuation of the drug, and this should be borne in mind when another drug is prescribed following Marplan. To avoid potentiation, the physician wishing to terminate treatment with Marplan and begin therapy with another agent should allow for an interval of 10 days.
Marplan should be used cautiously in hyperactive or agitated patients, as well as schizophrenic patients, because it may cause excessive stimulation. Characteristically, in manic-depressive states there may be a tendency for patients to swing from a depressive to a manic phase. If such a swing should occur during Marplan therapy, brief discontinuation of the drug, followed by resumption of therapy at a reduced dosage, is advised.
Clinical evidence indicates only a low incidence of altered liver function or jaundice in patients treated with Marplan. It is difficult to differentiate most cases of drug-induced hepatocellular jaundice from viral hepatitis since they are histopathologically and biochemically indistinguishable. Moreover, many of the clinical signs and symptoms are identical. While some of the few cases of jaundice reported during Marplan therapy may have been drug-induced, the reaction is rare. Nevertheless, Marplan is an amine-oxidase inhibitor and, as with the use of all these agents, it is advisable to watch for hepatic complications. It is suggested that periodic liver function tests, such as bilirubins, alkaline phosphatase or transaminases, be performed during Marplan therapy; use of the drug should be discontinued at the first sign of hepatic dysfunction or jaundice. In patients with impaired renal function, Marplan should be used cautiously to prevent accumulation.
Marplan appears to have varying effects in epileptic patients; while some have a decrease in frequency of seizures, others have more seizures. Appropriate consideration must be given to the latter possibility if Marplan is prescribed for such patients.
All patients taking Marplan should be watched for symptoms of postural hypotension. If such hypotension occurs, the dose should be reduced or the drug discontinued.
Since the MAO inhibitors, including Marplan, potentiate hexobarbital hypnosis in animals, the dose of barbiturates if given concomitantly should be reduced.
Since the MAO inhibitors inhibit the destruction of serotonin, which is believed to be released from tissue stores by rauwolfia alkaloids, caution should be exercised when these drugs are used together.
There is conflicting evidence as to whether MAO inhibitors affect glucose metabolism or potentiate hypoglycemic agents. This should be considered if Marplan is used in diabetics.

ADVERSE REACTIONS

Marplan is a potent therapeutic agent with a relatively low incidence of adverse reactions. Since Marplan affects many enzyme systems of the body, a variety of side effects may be anticipated. The most frequently noted have been orthostatic hypotension, associated in some patients with falling, disturbances in cardiac rate and rhythm, complaints of dizziness and vertigo, constipation, headache, overactivity, hyperreflexia, tremors and muscle twitching, mania, hypomania, jitteriness, confusion and memory impairment, insomnia, peripheral edema, weakness, fatigue, dryness of the mouth, blurred vision, hyperhidrosis, anorexia and body weight changes, gastrointestinal disturbances, and minor sensitivity reactions such as skin rashes. Isolated cases of akathisia, ataxia, black tongue, coma, dysuria, euphoria, hematologic changes, incontinence, neuritis, photosensitivity, sexual disturbances, spider telangiectases and urinary retention have been reported. These side effects sometimes necessitate discontinuation of therapy. In rare instances, hallucinations have been reported with high dosages, but they have disappeared upon reduction of dosage or discontinuation of therapy. Toxic amblyopia was reported in one psychiatric patient who had received isocarboxazid for about a year; no causal relationship to isocarboxazid was established. Impaired water excretion compatible with the syndrome of inappropriate secretion of antidiuretic hormone (SIADH) has been reported.

DOSAGE AND ADMINISTRATION

As with other potent drugs, for maximum therapeutic effect the dosage of Marplan must be individually adjusted on the basis of careful observation of the patient. The usual starting dose is 30 mg daily, to be given in single or divided doses. Marplan has a cumulative effect; therefore, as soon as clinical improvement is observed, the dosage should be reduced to a maintenance level of 10 to 20 mg daily (or less). Since daily doses larger than 30 mg may cause an increase in the incidence or severity of side effects, it is recommended that this dosage generally not be exceeded. Many patients may show a favorable response to Marplan therapy within a week or less; however, since Marplan acts by directly affecting enzyme metabolism, a beneficial effect may not be seen in some patients for three or four weeks. If no response is obtained by then, continued administration is unlikely to help.

MANAGEMENT OF OVERDOSAGE

The lethal dose of Marplan in man is not known. There has been one report of a fatality in a patient who ingested 400 mg of Marplan together with an unspecified amount of another drug. Major overdosage may be evidenced by symptoms such

as tachycardia, hypotension, coma, convulsions, respiratory depression, sluggish reflexes, pyrexia and diaphoresis; these signs may persist for 8 to 14 days. General supportive measures should be employed, along with immediate gastric lavage or emetics. If the latter are given, the danger of aspiration must be borne in mind. An adequate airway should be maintained, with supplemental oxygen if necessary. The mechanism by which amine-oxidase inhibitors produce hypotension is not fully understood, but there is evidence that these agents block the vascular bed response. Thus it is suggested that plasma may be of value in the management of this hypotension. Administration of pressor amines such as Levophed® (levarterenol bitartrate) may be of limited value (note that their effects may be potentiated by Marplan). Continue treatment for several days until homeostasis is restored. Liver function studies are recommended during the 4 to 6 weeks after recovery, as well as at the time of overdosage. As with the management of intentional overdosage with any drug, it should be borne in mind that multiple agents may have been ingested.

HOW SUPPLIED

Tablets, 10 mg isocarboxazid/Roche each, peach-colored, scored—bottles of 100 (NDC 0004-0032-01).

Revised: September 1990

Shown in Product Identification Section, page 426

MATULANE® ℞

[*mat'u-lane*]

procarbazine hydrochloride/Roche

CAPSULES

The following text is complete prescribing information based on official labeling in effect June 1, 1992.

> **WARNING**
> **It is recommended that MATULANE be given only by or under the supervision of a physician experienced in the use of potent antineoplastic drugs. Adequate clinical and laboratory facilities should be available to patients for proper monitoring of treatment.**

DESCRIPTION

Matulane (procarbazine hydrochloride/Roche), a hydrazine derivative antineoplastic agent, is available as capsules containing the equivalent of 50 mg procarbazine as the hydrochloride. Each capsule also contains corn starch, mannitol and talc. Gelatin capsule shells contain parabens (methyl and propyl), potassium sorbate, titanium tioxide, FD&C Yellow No. 6 and D&C Yellow No. 10.

Chemically, procarbazine hydrochloride is *N*-isopropyl-α-(2-methylhydrazino)-*p*-toluamide monohydrochloride. It is a white to pale yellow crystalline powder which is soluble but unstable in water or aqueous solutions. The molecular weight of procarbazine hydrochloride is 257.76.

CLINICAL PHARMACOLOGY

The precise mode of cytotoxic action of procarbazine has not been clearly defined. There is evidence that the drug may act by inhibition of protein, RNA and DNA synthesis. Studies have suggested that procarbazine may inhibit transmethylation of methyl groups of methionine into t-RNA. The absence of functional t-RNA could cause the cessation of protein synthesis and consequently DNA and RNA synthesis. In addition, procarbazine may directly damage DNA. Hydrogen peroxide, formed during the auto-oxidation of the drug, may attack protein sulfhydryl groups contained in residual protein which is tightly bound to DNA.

Procarbazine is metabolized primarily in the liver and kidneys. The drug appears to be auto-oxidized to the azo derivative with the release of hydrogen peroxide. The azo derivative isomerizes to the hydrazone, and following hydrolysis splits into a benzyladehyde derivative and methylhydrazine. The methylhydrazine is further degraded to CO_2 and CH_4 and possibly hydrazine, whereas the aldehyde is oxidized to *N*-isopropylterephthalamic acid, which is excreted in the urine.

Procarbazine is rapidly and completely absorbed. Following oral administration of 30 mg of ^{14}C-labeled procarbazine, maximum peak plasma radioactive concentrations were reached within 60 minutes.

After intravenous injection, the plasma half-life of procarbazine is approximately 10 minutes. Approximately 70% of the radioactivity is excreted in the urine as *N*-isopropylterephthalamic acid within 24 hours following both oral and intravenous administration of ^{14}C-labeled procarbazine.

Procarbazine crosses the blood-brain barrier and rapidly equilibrates between plasma and cerebrospinal fluid after oral administration.

INDICATIONS AND USAGE

Matulane is indicated for use in combination with other anticancer drugs for the treatment of Stage III and IV Hodgkin's disease. Matulane is used as part of the MOPP (nitrogen mustard, vincristine, procarbazine, prednisone) regimen.

CONTRAINDICATIONS

Matulane is contraindicated in patients with known hypersensitivity to the drug or inadequate marrow reserve as demonstrated by bone marrow aspiration. Due consideration of this possible state should be given to each patient who has leukopenia, thrombocytopenia or anemia.

WARNINGS

To minimize CNS depression and possible potentiation, barbiturates, antihistamines, narcotics, hypotensive agents or phenothiazines should be used with caution. Ethyl alcohol should not be used since there may be an Antabuse (disulfiram)-like reaction. Because Matulane exhibits some monoamine oxidase inhibitory activity, sympathomimetic drugs, tricyclic antidepressant drugs (*e.g.*, amitriptyline HCl, imipramine HCl) and other drugs and foods with known high tyramine content, such as wine, yogurt, ripe cheese and bananas, should be avoided. A further phenomenon of toxicity common to many hydrazine derivatives is hemolysis and the appearance of Heinz-Ehrlich inclusion bodies in erythrocytes.

Pregnancy: Teratogenic effects: Pregnancy Category D. Procarbazine hydrochloride can cause fetal harm when administered to a pregnant woman. While there are no adequate and well-controlled studies with procarbazine hydrochloride in pregnant women, there are case reports of malformations in the offspring of women who were exposed to procarbazine hydrochloride in combination with other antineoplastic agents during pregnancy. Matulane should be used during pregnancy only if the potential benefit justifies the potential risk to the fetus. If this drug is used during pregnancy, or if the patient becomes pregnant while taking this drug, the patient should be apprised of the potential hazard to the fetus. Women of childbearing potential should be advised to avoid becoming pregnant. Procarbazine hydrochloride is teratogenic in the rat when given at doses approximately 4 to 13 times the maximum recommended human therapeutic dose of 6 mg/kg/day.

Nonteratogenic effects: Procarbazine hydrochloride has not been adequately studied in animals for its effects on peri- and postnatal development. However, neurogenic tumors were noted in the offspring of rats given intravenous injections of 125 mg/kg of procarbazine hydrochloride on day 22 of gestation. Compounds which inhibit DNA, RNA and protein synthesis might be expected to have adverse effects on peri- and postnatal development.

Carcinogenesis, mutagenesis and impairment of fertility: Carcinogenesis: The carcinogenicity of procarbazine hydrochloride in mice, rats and monkeys has been reported in a considerable number of studies. Instances of a second nonlymphoid malignancy, including acute myelocytic leukemia, have been reported in patients with Hodgkin's disease treated with procarbazine in combination with other chemotherapy and/or radiation. The International Agency for Research on Cancer (IARC) considers that there is "sufficient evidence" for the human carcinogenicity of procarbazine hydrochloride when it is given in intensive regimens which include other antineoplastic agents but that there is inadequate evidence of carcinogenicity in humans given procarbazine hydrochloride alone.

Mutagenesis: Procarbazine hydrochloride has been shown to be mutagenic in a variety of bacterial and mammalian test systems.

Impairment of fertility: Azoospermia and antifertility effects associated with procarbazine hydrochloride administration in combination with other chemotherapeutic agents for treating Hodgkin's disease have been reported in human clinical studies. Since these patients received multicombination therapy, it is difficult to determine to what extent procarbazine hydrochloride alone was involved in the male germ-cell damage. The usual Segment 1 fertility/reproduction studies in laboratory animals have not been carried out with procarbazine hydrochloride. However, compounds which inhibit DNA, RNA and/or protein synthesis might be expected to have adverse effects on gametogenesis. Unscheduled DNA synthesis in the testis of rabbits and decreased fertility in male mice treated with procarbazine hydrochloride have been reported.

PRECAUTIONS

General: Undue toxicity may occur if Matulane is used in patients with impairment of renal and/or hepatic function. When appropriate, hospitalization for the initial course of treatment should be considered.

If radiation or a chemotherapeutic agent known to have marrow-depressant activity has been used, an interval of one month or longer without such therapy is recommended before starting treatment with Matulane. The length of this interval may also be determined by evidence of bone marrow recovery based on successive bone marrow studies.

Prompt cessation of therapy is recommended if any one of the following occurs:

- Central nervous system signs or symptoms such as paresthesias, neuropathies or confusion.
- Leukopenia (white blood count under 4000).
- Thrombocytopenia (platelets under 100,000).
- Hypersensitivity reaction.
- Stomatitis—The first small ulceration or persistent spot soreness around the oral cavity is a signal for cessation of therapy.
- Diarrhea—Frequent bowel movements or watery stools.
- Hemorrhage or bleeding tendencies.

Bone marrow depression often occurs 2 to 8 weeks after the start of treatment. If leukopenia occurs, hospitalization of the patient may be needed for appropriate treatment to prevent systemic infection.

Information for patients: Patients should be warned not to drink alcoholic beverages while on Matulane therapy since there may be an Antabuse (disulfiram)-like reaction. They should also be cautioned to avoid foods with known high tyramine content such as wine, yogurt, ripe cheese and bananas. Over-the-counter drug preparations which contain antihistamines or sympathomimetic drugs should also be avoided. Patients taking Matulane should also be warned against the use of prescription drugs without the knowledge and consent of their physician.

Laboratory tests: Baseline laboratory data should be obtained prior to initiation of therapy. The hematologic status as indicated by hemoglobin, hematocrit, white blood count (WBC), differential, reticulocytes and platelets should be monitored closely—at least every 3 or 4 days.

Hepatic and renal evaluation are indicated prior to beginning therapy. Urinalysis, transaminase, alkaline phosphatase and blood urea nitrogen tests should be repeated at least weekly.

Drug interactions: See WARNINGS section.

No cross-resistance with other chemotherapeutic agents, radiotherapy or steroids has been demonstrated.

Carcinogenesis, mutagenesis and impairment of fertility: See WARNINGS section.

Pregnancy: Pregnancy Category D. See WARNINGS section.

Nursing mothers: It is not known whether Matulane is excreted in human milk. Because of the potential for tumorigenicity shown for procarbazine hydrochloride in animal studies, mothers should not nurse while receiving this drug.

ADVERSE REACTIONS

Leukopenia, anemia and thrombopenia occur frequently. Nausea and vomiting are the most commonly reported side effects.

Other adverse reactions are:

Hematologic: Pancytopenia; eosinophilia; hemolytic anemia; bleeding tendencies such as petechiae, purpura, epistaxis and hemoptysis.

Gastrointestinal: Hepatic dysfunction, jaundice, stomatitis, hematemesis, melena, diarrhea, dysphagia, anorexia, abdominal pain, constipation, dry mouth.

Neurologic: Coma, convulsions, neuropathy, ataxia, paresthesia, nystagmus, diminished reflexes, falling, foot drop, headache, dizziness, unsteadiness.

Cardiovascular: Hypotension, tachycardia, syncope.

Ophthalmic: Retinal hemorrhage, papilledema, photophobia, diplopia, inability to focus.

Respiratory: Pneumonitis, pleural effusion, cough.

Dermatologic: Herpes, dermatitis, pruritus, alopecia, hyperpigmentation, rash, urticaria, flushing.

Allergic: Generalized allergic reactions.

Genitourinary: Hematuria, urinary frequency, nocturia.

Musculoskeletal: Pain, including myalgia and arthralgia; tremors.

Psychiatric: Hallucinations, depression, apprehension, nervousness, confusion, nightmares.

Endocrine: Gynecomastia in prepubertal and early pubertal boys.

Miscellaneous: Intercurrent infections, hearing loss, pyrexia, diaphoresis, lethargy, weakness, fatigue, edema, chills, insomnia, slurred speech, hoarseness, drowsiness.

Second nonlymphoid malignancies, including acute myelocytic leukemia and malignant myelosclerosis, and azoospermia have been reported in patients with Hodgkin's disease treated with procarbazine in combination with other chemotherapy and/or radiation.

OVERDOSAGE

The major manifestations of overdosage with Matulane would be anticipated to be nausea, vomiting, enteritis, diarrhea, hypotension, tremors, convulsions and coma. Treatment should consist of either the administration of an emetic or gastric lavage. General supportive measures such as intravenous fluids are advised. Since the major toxicity of procarbazine hydrochloride is hematologic and hepatic, patients should have frequent complete blood counts and liver function tests throughout their period of recovery and for a minimum of two weeks thereafter. Should abnormalities appear in any of these determinations, appropriate measures for correction and stabilization should be immediately undertaken.

Continued on next page

Roche Laboratories—Cont.

The estimated mean lethal dose of procarbazine hydrochloride in laboratory animals varied from approximately 150 mg/kg in rabbits to 1300 mg/kg in mice.

DOSAGE AND ADMINISTRATION

The following doses are for administration of the drug as a single agent. When used in combination with other anticancer drugs, the Matulane dose should be appropriately reduced, *e.g.,* in the MOPP regimen, the Matulane dose is 100 mg/m^2 daily for 14 days. All dosages are based on the patient's actual weight. However, the estimated lean body mass (dry weight) is used if the patient is obese or if there has been a spurious weight gain due to edema, ascites or other forms of abnormal fluid retention.

Adults—To minimize the nausea and vomiting experienced by a high percentage of patients beginning Matulane therapy, single or divided doses of 2 to 4 mg/kg/day for the first week are recommended. Daily dosage should then be maintained at 4 to 6 mg/kg/day until maximum response is obtained or until the white blood count falls below 4000/cmm or the platelets fall below 100,000/cmm. When maximum response is obtained, the dose may be maintained at 1 to 2 mg/kg/day. Upon evience of hematologic or other toxicity (see PRECAUTIONS section), the drug should be discontinued until there has been satisfactory recovery. After toxic side effects have subsided, therapy may then be resumed at the discretion of the physician, based on clinical evaluation and appropriate laboratory studies, at a dosage of 1 to 2 mg/kg/day.

Children—Very close clinical monitoring is mandatory. Undue toxicity, evidenced by tremors, coma and convulsions, has occurred in a few cases. Dosage, therefore, should be individualized. The following dosage schedule is provided as a guideline only.

Fifty (50) mg per square meter of body surface per day is recommended for the first week. Dosage should then be maintained at 100 mg per square meter of body surface per day until maximum response is obtained or until leukopenia or thrombocytopenia occurs. When maximum response is attained, the dose may be maintained at 50 mg per square meter of body surface per day. Upon evidence of hematologic or other toxicity (see PRECAUTIONS section), the drug should be discontinued until there has been satisfactory recovery, based on clinical evaluation and appropriate laboratory tests. After toxic side effects have subsided, therapy may then be resumed.

Procedures for proper handling and disposal of anticancer drugs should be considered. Several guidelines on this subject have been published.[1–6] There is no general agreement that all of the procedures recommended in the guidelines are necessary or appropriate.

HOW SUPPLIED

Capsules, ivory, containing the equivalent of 50 mg procarbazine as the hydrochloride; bottles of 100 (NDC 0004-0053-01). Imprint on capsules; MATULANE® ROCHE.

REFERENCES

1. Recommendations for the safe handling of parenteral antineoplastic drugs. Washington, DC, U.S. Government Printing Office (NIH Publication No. 83-2621).
2. AMA Council Report. Guidelines for handling parenteral antineoplastics. *JAMA 253*:1590–1592, Mar 15, 1985.
3. National Study Commission on Cytotoxic Exposure: Recommendations for handling cytotoxic agents. Available from Louis P. Jeffrey, ScD, Director of Pharmacy Services, Rhode Island Hospital, 593 Eddy Street, Providence, Rhode Island 02902.
4. Clinical Oncological Society of Australia: Guidelines and recommendations for safe handling of antineoplastic agents. *Med. J. Aust 1*:426–428, Apr 30, 1983.
5. Jones RB, Frank R. Mass T: Safe handling of chemotherapeutic agents: a report from the Mount Sinai Medical Center. *CA 33*:258–263, Sept–Oct 1983.
6. ASHP technical assistance bulletin on handling cytotoxic drugs in hospitals. *Am J Hosp Pharm 42*:131–137, Jan 1985.

Revised: January 1987

Shown in Product Identification Section, page 426

MAZICON™ ℞

[*măs'ĕ-kŏn"*]
(flumazenil/Roche)
Injection

The following text is complete prescribing information based on official labeling in effect June 1, 1992.

DESCRIPTION

MAZICON™ (flumazenil/Roche) is a benzodiazepine receptor antagonist. Chemically, flumazenil is ethyl 8-fluoro-5,6-dihydro-5-methyl-6-oxo-4H-imidazo[1,5-a](1,4) benzodiazepine-3-carboxylate. Flumazenil has an imidazobenzodiazepine structure, a calculated molecular weight of 303.3.

Flumazenil is a white to off-white crystalline compound with an octanol:buffer partition coefficient of 14 to 1 at pH 7.4. It is insoluble in water but slightly soluble in acidic aqueous solutions. MAZICON is available as a sterile parenteral dosage form for intravenous administration. Each mL contains 0.1 mg of flumazenil compounded with 1.8 mg of methylparaben, 0.2 mg of propylparaben, 0.9% sodium chloride, 0.01% edetate disodium, and 0.01% acetic acid; the pH is adjusted to approximately 4 with hydrochloric acid and/or, if necessary, sodium hydroxide.

CLINICAL PHARMACOLOGY

Flumazenil, an imidazobenzodiazepine derivative, antagonizes the actions of benzodiazepines on the central nervous system. Flumazenil competitively inhibits the activity at the benzodiazepine recognition site on the GABA/benzodiazepine receptor complex. Flumazenil is a weak partial agonist in some animal models of activity, but has little or no agonist activity in man.

Flumazenil does not antagonize the central nervous system effects of drugs affecting GABA-ergic neurons by means other than the benzodiazepine receptor (including ethanol, barbiturates, or general anesthetics) and does not reverse the effects of opioids.

PHARMACODYNAMICS: Intravenous MAZICON has been shown to antagonize sedation, impairment of recall and psychomotor impairment produced by benzodiazepines in healthy human volunteers.

The duration and degree of reversal of benzodiazepine effects are related to the dose and plasma concentrations of flumazenil as shown in the following data from a study in normal volunteers.

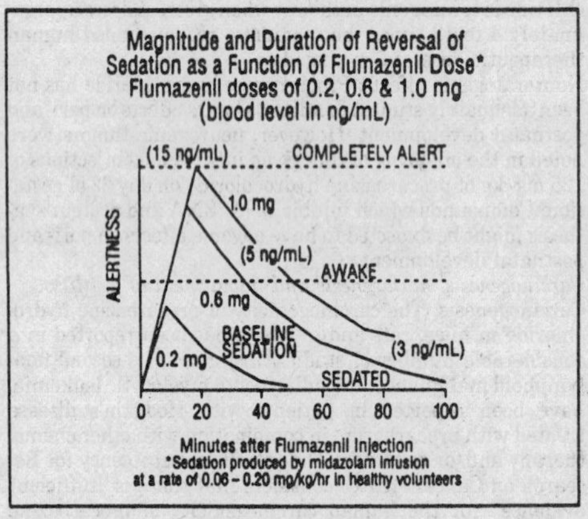

Generally, doses of approximately 0.1 to 0.2 mg (corresponding to peak plasma levels of 3 to 6 ng/mL) produce partial antagonism, whereas higher doses of 0.4 to 1.0 mg (peak plasma levels of 12 to 28 ng/mL) usually produce complete antagonism in patients who have received the usual sedating doses of benzodiazepines. The onset of reversal is usually evident within 1 to 2 minutes after the injection is completed. Eighty percent response will be reached within 3 minutes, with the peak effect occurring at 6 to 10 minutes. The duration and degree of reversal are related to the plasma concentration of the sedating benzodiazepine as well as the dose of MAZICON given.

In healthy volunteers, MAZICON did not alter intraocular pressure when given alone and reversed the decrease in intraocular pressure seen after admininstration of midazolam.

PHARMACOKINETICS: After IV administration, plasma concentrations of flumazenil follow a two compartment open pharmacokinetic model with an initial distribution half-life of 7 to 15 minutes and a terminal half-life of 41 to 79 minutes. Peak concentrations of flumazenil are proportional to dose, with an apparent initial volume of distribution of 0.5 L/kg. After redistribution the apparent volume of distribution (V_{ss}) ranges from 0.77 to 1.60L/kg. Protein binding is approximately 50% and the drug shows no preferential partitioning into red blood cells.

Flumazenil is a highly extracted drug. Clearance of flumazenil occurs primarily by hepatic metabolism and is dependent on hepatic blood flow. In pharmacokinetic studies of normal volunteers, total clearance ranges from 0.7 to 1.3 L/hr/kg, with less than 1% of the administered dose eliminated unchanged in the urine. The major metabolites of flumazenil identified in urine are the de-ethylated free acid and its glucuronide conjugate. In preclinical studies there was no evidence of pharmacologic activity exhibited by the de-ethylated free acid. Elimination of radiolabelled drug is essentially complete within 72 hours, with 90% to 95% of the radioactivity appearing in urine and 5% to 10% in the feces.

Pharmacokinetic Parameters Following a 5-minute infusion of a total of 1.0 mg of MAZICON Mean (Coefficient of variation, Range)

C_{max} (ng/mL)	24 (38%, 11–43)
AUC (ng* hr/mL)	15 (22%, 10–22)
V_{SS} (L/kg)	1 (24%, 0.8–1.6)
Cl (L/hr/kg)	1 (20%, 0.7–1.4)
Half-life (min)	54 (21%, 41–79)

The pharmacokinetics of flumazenil are not significantly affected by gender, age, renal failure (creatinine clearance < 10 mL/min), or hemodialysis beginning 1 hour after drug administration. Mean total clearance is decreased to 40% to 60% of normal in patients with moderate liver dysfunction and to 25% of normal in patients with severe liver dysfunction compared with age-matched healthy subjects. This results in a prolongation of the half-life from 0.8 hours in healthy subjects to 1.3 hours in patients with moderate hepatic impairment and 2.4 hours in severely impaired patients. Ingestion of food during an intravenous infusion of the drug results in a 50% increase in clearance, most likely due to the increased hepatic blood flow that accompanies a meal. The pharmacokinetic profile of flumazenil is unaltered in the presence of benzodiazepine agonists and the kinetic profiles of those benzodiazepines are unaltered by flumazenil.

CLINICAL TRIALS

MAZICON has been administered to reverse the effects of benzodiazepines in conscious sedation, general anesthesia, and the management of suspected benzodiazepine overdose.

CONSCIOUS SEDATION: MAZICON was studied in four trials in 970 patients who received an average of 30 mg diazepam or 10 mg midazolam for sedation (with or without a narcotic) in conjunction with both inpatient and outpatient diagnostic or surgical procedures. MAZICON was effective in reversing the sedating and psychomotor effects of the benzodiazepine, however, amnesia was less completely and less consistently reversed. In these studies, MAZICON was administered as an initial dose of 0.4 mg I.V. (two doses of 0.2 mg) with additional 0.2 mg doses as needed to achieve complete awakening, up to a maximum total dose of 1.0 mg.

Seventy-eight percent of patients receiving flumazenil responded by becoming completely alert. Of those patients, approximately half responded to doses of 0.4 to 0.6 mg, while the other half responded to doses of 0.8 to 1.0 mg. Adverse effects were infrequent in patients who received 1 mg of MAZICON or less, although injection site pain, agitation and anxiety did occur. Reversal of sedation was not associated with any increase in the frequency of inadequate analgesia or increase in narcotic demand in these studies. While most patients remained alert throughout the 3 hour post-procedure observation period, resedation was observed to occur in 3% to 9% of the patients, and was most common in patients who had received high doses of benzodiazepine. (See PRECAUTIONS.)

GENERAL ANESTHESIA: MAZICON was studied in four trials in 644 patients who received midazolam as an induction and/or maintenance agent in both balanced and inhalational anesthesia. Midazolam was generally administered in doses ranging from 5 to 80 mg, alone and/or in conjunction with muscle relaxants, nitrous oxide, regional or local anesthetics, narcotics and/or inhalational anesthetics. Flumazenil was given as an initial dose of 0.2 mg IV, with additional 0.2 mg doses as needed to reach a complete response, up to a maximum total dose of 1.0 mg. These doses were effective in reversing sedation and restoring psychomotor function, but did not completely restore memory as tested by picture recall. MAZICON was not as effective in the reversal of sedation in patients who had received multiple anesthetic agents in addition to benzodiazepines.

Eighty-one percent of patients sedated with midazolam responded to flumazenil by becoming completely alert or just slightly drowsy. Of those patients, 36% responded to doses of 0.4 to 0.6 mg, while 64% responded to doses of 0.8 to 1.0 mg.

Resedation in patients who responded to MAZICON occurred in 10% to 15% of patients studied and was more common with larger doses of midazolam (> 20 mg), long procedures (> 60 minutes) and use of neuromuscular blocking agents. (See PRECAUTIONS.)

MANAGEMENT OF SUSPECTED BENZODIAZEPINE OVERDOSE: MAZICON was studied in two trials in 497 patients who were presumed to have taken an overdose of a benzodiazepine, either alone or in combination with a variety of other agents. In these trials, 299 patients were proven to have taken a benzodiazepine as part of the overdose, and 80% of the 148 who received MAZICON responded by an improvement in level of consciousness. Of the patients who responded to flumazenil, 75% responded to a total dose of 1.0 to 3.0 mg.

Reversal of sedation was associated with an increased frequency of symptoms of CNS excitation. Of the patients treated with flumazenil, 1% to 3% were treated for agitation or anxiety. Serious side effects were uncommon, but six seizures were observed in 446 patients treated with flumazenil in these studies. Four of these 6 patients had ingested a large

dose of cyclic antidepressants, which increased the risk of seizures. (See WARNINGS.)

INDIVIDUALIZATION OF DOSAGE

GENERAL PRINCIPLES: The serious adverse effects of MAZICON are related to the reversal of benzodiazepine effects. Using more than the minimally effective dose of MAZICON is tolerated by most patients but may complicate the management of patients who are physically dependent on benzodiazepines or patients who are depending on benzodiazepines for therapeutic effect (such as suppression of seizures in cyclic antidepressant overdose).

In high-risk patients, it is important to administer the smallest amount of MAZICON that is effective. The 1-minute wait between individual doses in the dose-titration recommended for general clinical populations may be too short for high risk patients. This is because it takes 6 to 10 minutes for any single dose of flumazenil to reach full effects. Practitioners should slow the rate of administration of MAZICON administered to high risk patients as recommended below.

ANESTHESIA AND CONSCIOUS SEDATION: MAZICON is well tolerated at the recommended doses in individuals who have no tolerance to (or dependence on) benzodiazepines. The recommended dosages and titration rates in anesthesia and conscious sedation (0.2 to 1.0 mg given at 0.2 mg/min) are well tolerated in patients receiving the drug for reversal of a single benzodiazepine exposure in most clinical settings (see Adverse Events). The major risk will be resedation because the duration of effect of a long-acting (or large dose of a short-acting) benzodiazepine may exceed that of MAZICON. Resedation may be treated by giving a repeat dose at no less than 20-minute intervals. For repeat treatment, no more than 1.0 mg (at 0.2 mg/min doses) should be given at any one time and no more than 3.0 mg should be given in any one hour.

OVERDOSE PATIENTS: The risk of confusion, agitation, emotional lability and perceptual distortion with the doses recommended in patients with benzodiazepine overdose (3 to 5 mg administered as 0.5 mg/min) may be greater than that expected with lower doses and slower administration. The recommended doses represent a compromise between a desirable slow awakening and the need for prompt response and a persistent effect in the overdose situation. If circumstances permit, the physician may elect to use the 0.2 mg/minute titration rate to slowly awaken the patient over 5 to 10 minutes, which may help to reduce signs and symptoms on emergence.

MAZICON has no effect in cases where benzodiazepines are not responsible for sedation. Once doses of 3 to 5 mg have been reached without clinical response, additional MAZICON is likely to have no effect.

PATIENTS TOLERANT TO BENZODIAZEPINES: MAZICON may cause benzodiazepine withdrawal symptoms in individuals who have been taking benzodiazepines long enough to have some degree of tolerance. Patients who had been taking benzodiazepines prior to entry into the MAZICON trials who were given flumazenil in doses over 1 mg experienced withdrawal-like events 2 to 5 times more frequently than patients who received less than 1 mg.

In patients who may have tolerance to benzodiazepines, as indicated by clinical history or by the need for larger than usual doses of benzodiazepine, slower titration rates of 0.1 mg/min and lower total doses may help reduce the frequency of emergent confusion and agitation. In such cases special care must be taken to monitor the patients for resedation because of the lower doses of MAZICON used.

PATIENTS PHYSICALLY DEPENDENT ON BENZODIAZEPINES: MAZICON is known to precipitate withdrawal seizures in patients who are physically dependent on benzodiazepines, even if such dependence was established in a relatively few days of high dose sedation in Intensive Care Unit environments. The risk of either seizures or resedation in such cases is high and patients have experienced seizures before regaining consciousness. MAZICON should be used in such settings with extreme caution, since the use of flumazenil in this situation has not been studied and no information as to dose and rate of titration is available. MAZICON should be used in such patients only if the potential benefits of using the drug outweigh the risks of precipitated seizures. Physicians are directed to the scientific literature for the most current information in this area.

INDICATIONS AND USAGE

MAZICON is indicated for the complete or partial reversal of the sedative effects of benzodiazepines in cases where general anesthesia has been induced and/or maintained with benzodiazepines, where sedation has been produced with benzodiazepines for diagnostic and therapeutic procedures, and for the management of benzodiazepine overdose.

CONTRAINDICATIONS

MAZICON is contraindicated:

- in patients with a known hypersensitivity to flumazenil or to benzodiazepines.
- in patients who have been given a benzodiazepine for control of a potentially life-threatening condition (*e.g.* control of intracranial pressure or status epilepticus).
- in patients who are showing signs of serious cyclic antidepressant overdose. (See WARNINGS.)

WARNINGS

THE USE OF MAZICON HAS BEEN ASSOCIATED WITH THE OCCURRENCE OF SEIZURES.
THESE ARE MOST FREQUENT IN PATIENTS WHO HAVE BEEN ON BENZODIAZEPINES FOR LONG-TERM SEDATION OR IN OVERDOSE CASES WHERE PATIENTS ARE SHOWING SIGNS OF SERIOUS CYCLIC ANTIDEPRESSANT OVERDOSE.
PRACTITIONERS SHOULD INDIVIDUALIZE THE DOSAGE OF MAZICON AND BE PREPARED TO MANAGE SEIZURES.

Risk of Seizures: The reversal of benzodiazepine effects may be associated with the onset of seizures in certain high-risk populations. Possible risk factors for seizures include: concurrent major sedative-hypnotic drug withdrawal, recent therapy with repeated doses of parenteral benzodiazepines, myoclonic jerking or seizure activity prior to flumazenil administration in overdose cases, or concurrent cyclic antidepressant poisoning.

MAZICON is not recommended in cases of serious cyclic antidepressant poisoning, as manifested by motor abnormalities (twitching, rigidity, focal seizure), dysrhythmia (wide QRS, ventricular dysrhythmia, heart block), anticholinergic signs (mydriasis, dry mucosa, hypo-peristalsis), and cardiovascular collapse at presentation. In such cases MAZICON should be withheld and the patient should be allowed to remain sedated (with ventilatory and circulatory support as needed) until the signs of antidepressant toxicity have subsided. Treatment with MAZICON has no known benefit to the seriously ill mixed-overdose patient other than reversing sedation and should not be used in cases where seizures (from any cause) are likely.

Most convulsions associated with flumazenil administration require treatment and have been successfully managed with benzodiazepines, phenytoin or barbiturates. Because of the presence of flumazenil, higher than usual doses of benzodiazepines may be required.

HYPOVENTILATION: Patients who have received MAZICON for the reversal of benzodiazepine effects (after conscious sedation or general anesthesia) should be monitored for resedation, respiratory depression, or other residual benzodiazepine effects for an appropriate period (up to 120 minutes) based on the dose and duration of effect of the benzodiazepine employed.

This is because MAZICON has not been established as an effective treatment for hypoventilation due to benzodiazepine administration. The availability of flumazenil does not diminish the need for prompt detection of hypoventilation and the ability to effectively intervene by establishing an airway and assisting ventilation.

MAZICON may not fully reverse postoperative airway problems or ventilatory insufficiency induced by benzodazepines. In addition, even if MAZICON is initially effective, such problems may recur because the effects of MAZICON wear off before the effects of many benzodiazepines.

Overdose cases should always be monitored for resedation until the patients are stable and resedation is unlikely.

PRECAUTIONS

RETURN OF SEDATION: MAZICON may be expected to improve the alertness of patients recovering from a procedure involving sedation or anesthesia with benzodiazepines, but should not be substituted for an adequate period of postprocedure monitoring. The availability of MAZICON does not reduce the risks associated with the use of large doses of benzodiazepines for sedation.

Patients should be monitored for resedation, respiratory depression (See WARNINGS), or other persistent or recurrent agonist effects for an adequate period of time after administration of MAZICON.

Resedation is least likely in cases where MAZICON is administered to reverse a low dose of a short-acting benzodiazepine (< 10 mg midazolam). It is most likely in cases where a large single or cumulative dose of a benzodiazepine has been given in the course of a long procedure along with neuromuscular blocking agents and multiple anesthetic agents.

Profound resedation was observed in 1% to 3% of patients in the clinical studies. In clinical situations where resedation must be prevented, physicians may wish to repeat the initial dose (up to 1 mg of MAZICON given at 0.2 mg/min) at 30 minutes and possibly again at 60 minutes. This dosage schedule, although not studied in clinical trials, was effective in preventing resedation in a pharmacologic study in normal volunteers.

USE IN THE ICU: MAZICON should be used with caution in the Intensive Care Unit because of the increased risk of unrecognized benzodiazepine dependence in such settings. MAZICON may produce convulsions in patients physically dependent on benzodiazepines (See INDIVIDUALIZATION OF DOSAGE AND WARNINGS).

Administration of MAZICON to diagnose benzodiazepine-induced sedation in the Intensive Care Unit is not recommended due to the risk of adverse events as described above. In addition, the prognostic significance of a patient's failure to respond to flumazenil in cases confounded by metabolic disorder, traumatic injury, drugs other than benzodiazepines, or any other reasons not associated with benzodiazepine receptor occupancy is not known.

USE IN OVERDOSE: MAZICON is intended as an adjunct to, not as a substitute for, proper management of airway, assisted breathing, circulatory access and support, internal decontamination by lavage and charcoal, and adequate clinical evaluation.

Necessary measures should be instituted to secure airway, ventilation and intravenous access prior to administering flumazenil. Upon arousal patients may attempt to withdraw endotracheal tubes and/or intravenous lines as the result of confusion and agitation following awakening.

HEAD INJURY: MAZICON should be used with caution in patients with head injury as it may be capable of precipitating convulsions or altering cerebral blood flow in patients receiving benzodiazepines. It should be used only by practitioners prepared to manage such complications should they occur.

USE WITH NEUROMUSCULAR BLOCKING AGENTS: MAZICON should not be used until the effects of neuromuscular blockade have been fully reversed.

USE IN PSYCHIATRIC PATIENTS: MAZICON has been reported to provoke panic attacks in patients with a history of panic disorder.

PAIN ON INJECTION: To minimize the likelihood of pain or inflammation at the injection site, MAZICON should be administered through a freely flowing intravenous infusion into a large vein. Local irritation may occur following extravasation into perivascular tissues.

USE IN RESPIRATORY DISEASE: The primary treatment of patients with serious lung disease who experience serious respiratory depression due to benzodiazepines should be appropriate ventilatory support (See PRECAUTIONS) rather than the administration of MAZICON. Flumazenil is capable of partially reversing benzodiazepine-induced alterations in ventilatory drive in healthy volunteers, but has not been shown to be clinically effective.

USE IN CARDIOVASCULAR DISEASE: MAZICON did not increase the work of the heart when used to reverse benzodiazepines in cardiac patients when given at a rate of 0.1 mg/min in total doses of less than 0.5 mg in studies reported in the clinical literature. Flumazenil alone had no significant effects of cardiovascular parameters when administered to patients with stable ischemic heart disease.

USE IN LIVER DISEASE: The clearance of MAZICON is reduced to 40% to 60% of normal in patients with mild to moderate hepatic disease and to 25% of normal in patients with severe hepatic dysfunction (See PHARMACOKINETICS). While the dose of flumazenil used for initial reversal of benzodiazepine effects is not affected, repeat doses of the drug in liver disease should be reduced in size or frequency.

USE IN DRUG AND ALCOHOL DEPENDENT PATIENTS: MAZICON should be used with caution in patients with alcoholism and other drug dependencies due to the increased frequency of benzodiazepine tolerance and dependence observed in these patient populations.

MAZICON is not recommended either as a treatment for benaodiazepine dependence or for the management of protracted benzodiazepine abstinence syndromes, as such use has not been studied.

The administration of flumazenil can precipitate benzodiazepine withdrawal in animals and man. This has been seen in healthy volunteers treated with therapeutic doses of oral lorazepam for up to 2 weeks who exhibited effects such as hot flushes, agitation and tremor when treated with cumulative doses of up to 3 mg doses of flumazenil.

Similar adverse experiences suggestive of flumazenil precipitation of benzodiazepine withdrawal have occurred in some patients in clinical trials. Such patients had a short-lived syndrome characterized by dizziness, mild confusion, emotional lability, agitation (with signs and symptoms of anxiety), and mild sensory distortions. This response was dose-related, most common at doses above 1 mg, rarely required treatment other than reassurance and was usually short lived. When required (5 to 10 cases), these patients were successfully treated with usual doses of a barbiturate, a benzodiazepine, or other sedative drug.

Practitioners should assume that flumazenil administration may trigger dose-dependent withdrawal syndromes in patients with established physical dependence on benzodiazepines and may complicate the management of withdrawal syndromes for alcohol, barbiturates and cross-tolerant sedatives.

DRUG INTERACTIONS

Interaction with central nervous system depressants other than benzodiazepines has not been specifically studied; however, no deleterious interactions were seen when MAZICON was administered after narcotics, inhalational anesthetics, muscle relaxants and muscle relaxant antagonists administered in conjunction with sedation or anesthesia.

Continued on next page

Roche Laboratories—Cont.

Particular caution is necessary when using MAZICON in cases of mixed drug overdosage since the toxic effects (such as convulsions and cardiac dysrhythmias) of other drugs taken in overdose (especially cyclic antidepressants) may emerge with the reversal of the benzodiazepine effect by flumazenil. (See WARNINGS).

The pharmacokinetics of benzodiazepines are unaltered in the presence of flumazenil.

USE IN AMBULATORY PATIENTS: The effects of MAZICON may wear off before a long-acting benzodiazepine is completely cleared from the body. In general, if a patient shows no signs of sedation within 2 hours after a 1.0 mg dose of flumazenil, serious resedation at a later time is unlikely. An adequate period of observation must be provided for any patient in whom either long-acting benzodiazepines (such as diazepam) or large doses of short-acting benzodiazepines (such as > 10 mg of midazolam) have been used. (See INDI-VIDUALIZATION OF DOSAGE.)

Because of the increased risk of adverse reactions in patients who have been taking benzodiazepines on a regular basis, it is particularly important that physicians query carefully about benzodiazepine, alcohol and sedative use as part of the history prior to any procedure in which the use of MAZICON is planned. (See DRUG AND ALCOHOL DEPENDENT PATIENTS.)

INFORMATION FOR PATIENTS: MAZICON does not consistently reverse amnesia. Patients cannot be expected to remember information told to them in the post-procedure period and instructions given to patients should be reinforced in writing or given to a responsible family member. Physicians are advised to discuss with their patients, both before surgery and at discharge, that although the patient may feel alert at the time of discharge, the effects of the benzodiazepine may recur. As a result, the patient should be instructed, preferably in writing, that their memory and judgement may be impaired and specifically advised:

1. Not to engage in any activities requiring complete alertness, and not to operate hazardous machinery or a motor vehicle until at least 18 to 24 hours after discharge, and it is certain no residual sedative effects of the benzodiazepine remain.
2. Not to take any alcohol or non-prescription drugs for 18 to 24 hours after flumazenil administration or if the effects of the benzodiazepine persist.

LABORATORY TESTS: No specific laboratory tests are recommended to follow the patient's response or to identify possible adverse reactions.

DRUG/LABORATORY TEST INTERACTIONS: The possible interaction of flumazenil with commonly used laboratory tests has not been evaluated.

CARCINOGENESIS, MUTAGENESIS, IMPAIRMENT OF FERTILITY: Carcinogenesis: No studies in animals to evaluate the carcinogenic potential of flumazenil have been conducted.

Mutagenesis: No evidence for mutagenicity was noted in the Ames test using five different tester strains. Assays for mutagenic potential in *S. cerevisiae* D7 and in Chinese hamster cells were considered to be negative as were blastogenesis assays *in vitro* in peripheral human lymphocytes and *in vivo* in a mouse micronucleus assay. Flumazenil caused a slight increase in unscheduled DNA synthesis in rat hepatocyte culture at concentrations which were also cytotoxic; no increase in DNA repair was observed in male mouse germ cells in an *in vivo* DNA repair assay.

Impairment of fertility: A reproduction study in male and female rats did not show any impairment of fertility at oral dosages of 125 mg/kg/day. From the available data on the area under the curve (AUC) in animals and man the dose represented 120 × the human exposure from a maximum recommended intravenous dose of 5 mg.

PREGNANCY: CATEGORY C. There are no adequate and well-controlled studies of the use of flumazenil in pregnant women. Flumazenil should be used during pregnancy only if the potential benefit justifies the potential risk to the fetus. Teratogenic Effects: Flumazenil has been studied for teratogenicity in rats and rabbits following oral treatments of up to 150 mg/kg/day. The treatments during the major organogenesis were on days 6 to 15 of gestation in the rat and days 6 to 18 of gestation in the rabbit. No teratogenic effects were observed in rats or rabbits at 150 mg/kg; the dose, based on the available data on the area under the plasma concentration-time curve (AUC) represented 120 × 600 × the human exposure from a maximum recommended intravenous dose of 5 mg in humans. In rabbits, embryocidal effects (as evidenced by increased pre-implantation and post-implantation losses) were observed at 50 mg/kg or 200 × the human exposure from a maximum recommended intravenous dose of 5 mg. The no-effect dose of 15 mg/kg in rabbits represents 60 × the human exposure.

Nonteratogenic Effects: An animal reproduction study was conducted in rats at oral dosages of 5, 25 and 125 mg/kg/day of flumazenil. Pup survival was decreased during the lactat-

ing period, pup liver weight at weaning was increased for the high-dose group (125 mg/kg/day) and incisor eruption and ear opening in the offspring were delayed; the delay in ear opening was associated with a delay in the appearance of the auditory startle response. No treatment-related adverse effects were noted for the other dose groups. Based on the available data from AUC, the effect level (125 mg/kg), represents 120 × the human exposure from 5 mg, the maximum recommended intravenous dose in humans. The no-effect level represents 24 × the human exposure from an intravenous dose of 5 mg.

LABOR AND DELIVERY: The use of MAZICON to reverse the effects of benzodiazepines used during labor and delivery is not recommended because the effects of the drug in the newborn are unknown.

NURSING MOTHERS: Caution should be exercised when deciding to administer MAZICON to a nursing woman because it is not known whether flumazenil is excreted in human milk.

PEDIATRIC USE: MAZICON is not recommended for use in children (either for the reversal of sedation, the management of overdose or the resuscitation of the newborn), as no clinical studies have been performed to determine the risks, benefits and dosages to be used.

GERATRIC USE: The pharmacokinetics of flumazenil have been studied in the elderly and are not significantly different from younger patients. Several studies of MAZICON in patients over the age of 65 and one study in patients over the age of 80 suggest that while the doses of benzodiazepine used to induce sedation should be reduced, ordinary doses of MAZICON may be used for reversal.

ADVERSE REACTIONS

SERIOUS ADVERSE REACTIONS: Deaths have occurred in patients who received MAZICON in a variety of clinical settings. The majority of deaths occurred in patients with serious underlying disease or in patients who had ingested large amounts of non-benzodiazepine drugs, (usually cyclic antidepressants) as part of an overdose.

Serious adverse events have occurred in all clinical settings, and convulsions are the most common serious adverse event reported. MAZICON administration has been associated with the onset of convulsions in patients who are relying on benzodiazepine effects to control seizures, are physically dependent on benzodiazepines, or who have ingested large doses of other drugs. (See WARNINGS.)

Two of the 446 patients who received MAZICON in controlled clinical trials for the management of a benzodiazepine overdosage had cardiac dysrhythmias (1 ventricular tachycardia, 1 junctional tachycardia).

ADVERSE EVENTS IN CLINICAL STUDIES: The following adverse reactions were considered to be related to MAZICON administration (both alone and for the reversal of benzodiazepine effects) and were reported in studies involving 1875 individuals who received flumazenil in controlled trials. Adverse events most frequently associated with flumazenil alone were limited to dizziness, injection site pain, increased sweating, headache and abnormal or blurred vision (3% to 9%).

BODY AS A WHOLE: Fatigue (asthenia, malaise), Headache, Injection Site Pain*, Injection Site Reaction (thrombophlebitis, skin abnormality, rash)

CARDIOVASCULAR SYSTEM: Cutaneous vasodilation (sweating, flushing, hot flushes)

DIGESTIVE SYSTEM: Nausea and Vomiting (11%)

NERVOUS SYSTEM: Agitation (anxiety, nervousness, dry mouth, tremor, palpitations, insomnia, dyspnea, hyperventilation)*, Dizziness (vertigo, ataxia) (10%), Emotional lability (crying abnormal, depersonalization, euphoria, increased tears, depression, dysphoria, paranoia)

SPECIAL SENSES: Abnormal Vision (visual field defect, diplopia), Paresthesia (sensation abnormal, hypoesthesia)

All adverse reactions occurred in 1% to 3% of cases unless otherwise marked.

Observed percentage reported if greater than 9%.

The following adverse events were observed infrequently (less than 1%) in the clinical studies, but were judged as probably related to MAZICON administration and/or reversal of benzodiazepine effects:

NERVOUS SYSTEM: Confusion (difficulty concentrating, delirium), Convulsions (See WARNINGS), Somnolence (stupor)

SPECIAL SENSES: Abnormal Hearing (transient hearing impairment, hyperacusis, tinnitus).

The following adverse events occurred with frequencies less than 1% in the clinical trials. Their relationship to MAZICON administration is unknown, but they are included as alerting information for the physician.

BODY AS A WHOLE: Rigors, shivering.

CARDIOVASCULAR: Arrythmia (atrial, nodal, ventricular extrasystoles), bradycardia, tachycardia, hypertension, chest pain.

DIGESTIVE SYSTEM: Hiccup.

NERVOUS SYSTEM: Speech disorder (dysphonia, thick tongue).

* indicates reaction in 3% to 9% of cases.

Not included in this list is operative site pain that occurred with the same frequency in patients receiving placebo as in patients receiving flumazenil for reversal of sedation following a surgical procedure.

DRUG ABUSE AND DEPENDENCE

MAZICON acts as a benzodiazepine antagonist, blocks the effects of benzodiazepines in animals and man, antagonizes benzodiazepine reinforcement in animal models, produces dysphoria in normal subjects, and has had no reported abuse in foreign marketing.

Although MAZICON has a benzodiazepine-like structure it does not act as a benzodiazepine agonist in man and is not a controlled substance.

OVERDOSAGE

Large intravenous doses of MAZICON, when administered to healthy normal volunteers in the absence of a benzodiazepine agonist, produced no serious adverse reactions, severe signs or symptoms, or clinically significant laboratory test abnormalities. In clinical studies, most adverse reactions to flumazenil were an extension of the pharmacologic effects of the drug in reversing benzodiazepine effects.

Reversal with an excessively high dose of MAZICON may produce anxiety, agitation, increased muscle tone, hyperesthesia and possibly convulsions. Convulsions have been treated with barbiturates, benzodiazepines and phenytoin, generally with prompt resolution of the seizures. (See WARNINGS.)

DOSE AND ADMINISTRATION

MAZICON is recommended for intravenous use only. It is compatible with 5% dextrose in water, lactated Ringer's and normal saline solutions. If MAZICON is drawn into a syringe or mixed with any of these solutions, it should be discarded after 24 hours. For optimum sterility, MAZICON should remain in the vial until just before use. As with all parenteral drug products, MAZICON should be inspected visually for particulate matter and discoloration prior to administration, whenever solution and container permit.

To minimize the likelihood of pain at the injection site, MAZICON should be administered through a freely running intravenous infusion into a large vein.

REVERSAL OF CONSCIOUS SEDATION OR IN GENERAL ANESTHESIA: For the reversal of the sedative effects of benzodiazepines administered for conscious sedation or general anesthesia, the recommended initial dose of MAZICON is 0.2 mg (2 mL) administered intravenously over 15 seconds. If the desired level of consciousness is not obtained after waiting an additional 45 seconds, a further dose of 0.2 mg (2 mL) can be injected and repeated at 60-second intervals where necessary (up to a maximum of 4 additional times) to a maximum total dose of 1 mg (10 mL). The dose should be individualized based on the patient's response, with most patients responding to doses of 0.6 to 1 mg. (See INDIVIDUALIZATION OF DOSAGE.)

In the event of resedation, repeated doses may be administered at 20 minute intervals as needed. For repeat treatment, no more than 1 mg (given as 0.2 mg/min) should be administered at any one time, and no more than 3 mg should be given in any one hour.

It is recommended that MAZICON be administered as the series of small injections described (not as a single bolus injection) to allow the practitioner to control the reversal of sedation to the approximate endpoint desired and to minimize the possibility of adverse effects. (See INDIVIDUALIZATION OF DOSAGE.)

MANAGEMENT OF SUSPECTED BENZODIAZEPINE OVERDOSE: For initial management of a known or suspected benzodiazepine overdose, the recommended initial dose of MAZICON is 0.2 mg (2 mL) administered intravenously over 30 seconds. If the desired level of consciousness is not obtained after waiting 30 seconds, a further dose of 0.3 mg (3 mL) can be administered over another 30 seconds. Further doses of 0.5 mg (5 mL) can be administered over 30 seconds at 1-minute intervals up to a cumulative dose of 3 mg. Do not rush the administration of MAZICON. Patients should have a secure airway and intravenous access before administration of the drug and be awakened gradually. (See PRECAUTIONS.)

Most patients with benzodiazepine overdose will respond to a cumulative dose of 1 to 3 mg of MAZICON, and doses beyond 3 mg do not reliably produce additional effects. On rare occasions, patients with a partial response at 3 mg may require additional titration up to a total dose of 5 mg (administered slowly in the same manner).

If a patient has not responded 5 minutes after receiving a cumulative dose of 5 mg MAZICON, the major cause of sedation is likely not to be due to benzodiazepines, and additional MAZICON is likely to have no effect.

In the event of resedation, repeated doses may be given at 20-minute intervals if needed. For repeat treatment, no more than 1 mg (given as 0.5 mg/min) should be given at any one time and no more than 3 mg should be given in any one hour.

SAFETY AND HANDLING: MAZICON is supplied in sealed dosage forms and poses no known risk to the health care provider. Routine care should be taken to avoid aerosol genera-

tion when preparing syringes for injection, and spilled medication should be rinsed from the skin with cool water.

HOW SUPPLIED

5 mL multiple-use vials containing 0.1 mg/mL flumazenil: Boxes of 1 (NDC 0004-6904-09); boxes of 10 (NDC 0004-6904-14).

10 mL multiple-use vials containing 0.1 mg/mL flumazenil: Boxes of 1 (NDC 0004-6905-09); boxes of 10 (NDC 0004-6905-14).

Store at 59° to 86°F (15° to 30°C).

Revised April 1992

NIPRIDE®   ℞

[ny'pryde]
(sodium nitroprusside/Roche)

The following text is complete prescribing information based on official labeling in effect June 1, 1992.

> After reconstitution, Nipride (sodium nitroprusside/Roche) is not suitable for direct injection. **The reconstituted solution must be further diluted in sterile 5% dextrose injection before infusion (see Dosage and Administration).**
>
> Nipride can cause **precipitous decreases in blood pressure (see Dosage and Administration).** In patients not properly monitored, these decreases can lead to **irreversible ischemic injuries or death.** Nipride should be used only when available equipment and personnel allow blood pressure to be continuously monitored.
>
> Except when used briefly or at low (< 2 μg/kg/min) infusion rates, sodium nitroprusside injection gives rise to important quantities of cyanide ion, which can reach **toxic, potentially lethal levels (see Warnings).** The usual dose rate is 0.5 to 10 μg/kg/min, but **infusion at the maximum dose rate should never last more than 10 minutes.** If blood pressure has not been adequately controlled after 10 minutes of infusion at the maximum rate, administration of Nipride should be terminated immediately.
>
> Although acid-base balance and venous oxygen concentration should be monitored and may indicate cyanide toxicity, these laboratory tests provide imperfect guidance.
>
> This package insert should be thoroughly reviewed before administration of Nipride infusion.

DESCRIPTION

Sodium nitroprusside is disodium pentacyanonitrosylferrate(2-)dihydrate, an inorganic hypotensive agent whose molecular formula is $Na_2[Fe(CN)_5 \ NO] \cdot 2H_2O$, and whose molecular weight is 297.95. Dry sodium nitroprusside is a reddish-brown powder, soluble in water. In an aqueous solution infused intravenously, sodium nitroprusside is a rapid-acting vasodilator, active on both arteries and veins.

Sodium nitroprusside solution is rapidly degraded by trace contaminants, often with resulting color changes (see **Dosage and Administration**). The solution is also sensitive to certain wavelengths of light, and it must be protected from light in clinical use.

Each 5-mL vial contains the equivalent of 50 mg sodium nitroprusside dihydrate.

CLINICAL PHARMACOLOGY

The principal pharmacological action of sodium nitroprusside is relaxation of vascular smooth muscle and consequent dilatation of peripheral arteries and veins. Other smooth muscle (*e.g.*, uterus, duodenum) is not affected. Sodium nitroprusside is more active on veins than on arteries, but this selectivity is much less marked than that of nitroglycerin.

Dilatation of the veins promotes peripheral pooling of blood and decreases venous return to the heart, thereby reducing left ventricular end-diastolic pressure and pulmonary capillary wedge pressure (preload). Arteriolar relaxation reduces systemic vascular resistance, systolic arterial pressure and mean arterial pressure (afterload). Dilatation of the coronary arteries also occurs.

In association with the decrease in blood pressure, sodium nitroprusside administered intravenously to hypertensive and normotensive patients produces slight increases in heart rate and a variable effect on cardiac output. In hypertensive patients, moderate doses induce renal vasodilatation roughly proportional to the decrease in systemic blood pressure, so there is no appreciable change in renal blood flow or glomerular filtration rate.

In normotensive subjects, acute reduction of mean arterial pressure to 60 to 75 mm Hg by infusion of sodium nitroprusside caused a significant increase in renin activity. In the same study, ten renovascular-hypertensive patients given sodium nitroprusside had significant increases in renin release from the involved kidney at mean arterial pressures of 90 to 137 mm Hg.

The hypotensive effect of sodium nitroprusside is seen within a minute or two after the start of an adequate infusion, and it dissipates almost as rapidly after an infusion is discontinued. The effect is augmented by ganglionic blocking agents and inhaled anesthetics.

Pharmacokinetics and Metabolism: Infused sodium nitroprusside is rapidly distributed to a volume that is approximately coextensive with the extracellular space. The drug is cleared from this volume by intraerythrocytic reaction with hemoglobin (Hgb), and sodium nitroprusside's resulting circulatory half-life is about 2 minutes.

The products of the nitroprusside/hemoglobin reaction are cyanmethemoglobin (cyanmetHgb) and cyanide ion (CN^-). Safe use of sodium nitroprusside injection must be guided by knowledge of the further metabolism of these products. As shown in the diagram below, the essential features of nitroprusside metabolism are:

- one molecule of sodium nitroprusside is metabolized by combination with hemoglobin to produce one molecule of cyanmethemoglobin, and four CN^- ions;
- methemoglobin, obtained from hemoglobin, can sequester cyanide as cyanmethemoglobin;
- thiosulfate reacts with cyanide to produce thiocyanate;
- thiocyanate is eliminated in the urine;
- cyanide not otherwise removed binds to cytochromes; and
- cyanide is much more toxic than methemoglobin or thiocyanate.

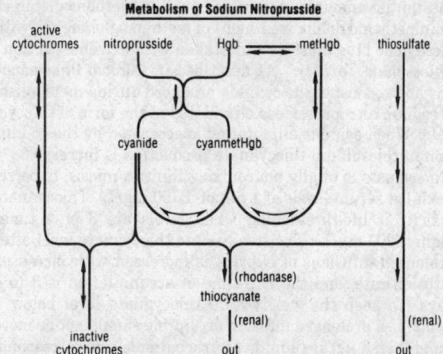

Metabolism of Sodium Nitroprusside

Cyanide ion is normally found in serum; it is derived from dietary substrates and from tobacco smoke. Cyanide binds avidly (but reversibly) to ferric ion (Fe^{+++}), most body stores of which are found in erythrocyte methemoglobin (metHgb) and in mitochondrial cytochromes. When CN^- is infused or generated within the bloodstream, essentially all of it is bound to methemoglobin until intraerythrocytic methemoglobin has been saturated.

When the Fe^{+++} of cytochromes is bound to cyanide, the cytochromes are unable to participate in oxidative metabolism. In this situation, cells may be able to provide for their energy needs by utilizing anaerobic pathways, but they thereby generate an increasing body burden of lactic acid. Other cells may be unable to utilize these alternate pathways, and they may die hypoxic deaths.

CN^- levels in packed erythrocytes are typically less than 1 μmol/L (less than 25 μg/L); levels are roughly doubled in heavy smokers.

At healthy steady-state, most people have less than 1% of their hemoglobin in the form of methemoglobin. Nitroprusside metabolism can lead to methemoglobin formation (a) through dissociation of cyanmethemoglobin formed in the original reaction of sodium nitroprusside with Hgb and (b) by direct oxidation of Hgb by the released nitroso group. Relatively large quantities of sodium nitroprusside, however, are required to produce significant methemoglobinemia.

At physiologic methemoglobin levels, the CN^- binding capacity of packed red cells is a little less than 200 μmol/L (5 mg/L). Cytochrome toxicity is seen at levels only slightly higher, and death has been reported at levels from 300 to 3000 μmol/L (8 to 80 mg/L). Put another way, a patient with a normal red-cell mass (35 mL/kg) and normal methemoglobin levels can buffer about 175 μg/kg of CN^-, corresponding to a little less than 500 μg/kg of infused sodium nitroprusside. Some cyanide is eliminated from the body as expired hydrogen cyanide, but most is enzymatically converted to thiocyanate (SCN^-) by thiosulfate-cyanide sulfur transferase (rhodanase, EC 2.8.1.1), a mitochondrial enzyme. The enzyme is normally present in great excess, so the reaction is rate-limited by the availability of sulfur donors, especially thiosulfate, cystine and cysteine.

Thiosulfate is a normal constituent of serum, produced from cysteine by way of β-mercaptopyruvate. Physiological levels of thiosulfate are typically about 0.1 mmol/L (11 mg/L), but they are approximately twice this level in children and in adults who are not eating. Infused thiosulfate is cleared from the body (primarily by the kidneys) with a $t_{1/2}$ of about 20 minutes.

When thiosulfate is being supplied only by normal physiologic mechanisms, conversion of CN^- to SCN^- generally proceeds at about 1 μg/kg/min. This rate of CN^- clearance corresponds to steady-state processing of a sodium nitroprusside infusion of slightly more than 2 μg/kg/min. CN^- begins to accumulate when sodium nitroprusside infusions exceed this rate.

Thiocyanate (SCN^-) is also a normal physiological constituent of serum, with normal levels typically in the range of 50 to 250 μmol/L (3 to 15 mg/L). Clearance of SCN^- is primarily renal, with a $t_{1/2}$ of about 3 days. In renal failure, the $t_{1/2}$ can be doubled or tripled.

Clinical Trials: Baseline-controlled clinical trials have uniformly shown that sodium nitroprusside has a prompt hypotensive effect, at least initially, in all populations. With increasing rates of infusion, sodium nitroprusside has been able to lower blood pressure without an observed limit of effect.

Clinical trials have also shown that the hypotensive effect of sodium nitroprusside is associated with reduced blood loss in a variety of major surgical procedures.

Many trials have verified the clinical significance of the metabolic pathways described above. In patients receiving unopposed infusions of sodium nitroprusside, cyanide and thiocyanate levels have increased with increasing rates of sodium nitroprusside infusion. Mild to moderate metabolic acidosis has usually accompanied higher cyanide levels, but peak base deficits have lagged behind the peak cyanide levels by an hour or more.

Progressive tachyphylaxis to the hypotensive effects of sodium nitroprusside has been reported in several trials and numerous case reports. This tachyphylaxis has frequently been attributed to concomitant cyanide toxicity, but the only evidence adduced for this assertion has been the observation that in patients treated with sodium nitroprusside and found to be resistant to its hypotensive effects, cyanide levels are often found to be elevated. In the only reported *comparisons* of cyanide levels in resistant and nonresistant patients, cyanide levels did *not* correlate with tachyphylaxis. The mechanism of tachyphylaxis to sodium nitroprusside remains unknown.

INDICATIONS AND USAGE

Nipride is indicated for the immediate reduction of blood pressure of patients in hypertensive crises. Concomitant longer-acting antihypertensive medication should be administered so that the duration of treatment with Nipride can be minimized.

Nipride is also indicated for producing controlled hypotension in order to reduce bleeding during surgery.

CONTRAINDICATIONS

Nipride should not be used in the treatment of compensatory hypertension, where the primary hemodynamic lesion is aortic coarctation or arteriovenous shunting.

Nipride should not be used to produce hypotension during surgery in patients with known inadequate cerebral circulation or in moribund patients (A.S.A. Class 5E) coming to emergency surgery.

Patients with congenital (Leber's) optic atrophy or with tobacco amblyopia have unusually high cyanide/thiocyanate ratios. These rare conditions are probably associated with defective or absent rhodanase, and Nipride use should be avoided in these patients.

WARNINGS

(See also the boxed warning at the beginning of this insert.)

The principal hazards of Nipride administration are excessive hypotension and excessive accumulation of cyanide (**see also Overdosage and Dosage and Administration**).

Excessive Hypotension: Small transient excesses in the infusion rate of Nipride can result in excessive hypotension, sometimes to levels so low as to compromise the perfusion of vital organs. These hemodynamic changes may lead to a variety of associated symptoms: see Adverse Reactions. Nitroprusside-induced hypotension will be self-limited within 1 to 10 minutes after discontinuation of the nitroprusside infusion; during these few minutes, it may be helpful to put the patient into a head-down (Trendelenburg) position to maximize venous return. **If hypotension persists more than a few minutes after discontinuation of the infusion of Nipride, Nipride is not the cause, and the true cause must be sought.**

Cyanide Toxicity: As described in **Clinical Pharmacology** above, sodium nitroprusside infusions at rates above 2 μg/kg/min generate cyanide ion (CN^-) faster than the body can normally dispose of it. (When sodium thiosulfate is given, as described under **Dosage and Administration,** the body's capacity for CN^- elimination is greatly increased.) Methemoglobin normally present in the body can buffer a certain amount of CN^-, but the capacity of this system is exhausted by the CN^- produced from about 500 μg/kg of sodium nitroprusside. This amount of sodium nitroprusside is administered in less than an hour when the drug is administered at 10 μg/kg/min (the maximum recommended rate). Thereaf-

Continued on next page

Roche Laboratories—Cont.

ter, the toxic effects of CN^- may be rapid, serious and even lethal.

The true rates of clinically important cyanide toxicity cannot be assessed from spontaneous reports or published data. Most patients reported to have experienced such toxicity have received relatively prolonged infusions, and the only patients whose deaths have been unequivocally attributed to nitroprusside-induced cyanide toxicity have been patients who had received nitroprusside infusions at rates (30 to 120 μg/kg/min) much greater than those now recommended. Elevated cyanide levels, metabolic acidosis, and marked clinical deterioration; however, have occasionally been reported in patients who received infusions at recommended rates for only a few hours and even, in one case, for only 35 minutes. In some of these cases, infusion of sodium thiosulfate caused dramatic clinical improvement, supporting the diagnosis of cyanide toxicity.

Cyanide toxicity may manifest itself as venous hyperoxemia with bright red venous blood, as cells become unable to extract the oxygen delivered to them; metabolic (lactic) acidosis; air hunger; confusion; and death. Cyanide toxicity due to causes other than nitroprusside has been associated with angina pectoris and myocardial infarction; ataxia, seizures and stroke; and other diffuse ischemic damage.

Hypertensive patients, and patients concomitantly receiving other antihypertensive medications, may be more sensitive to the effects of sodium nitroprusside than normal subjects.

PRECAUTIONS

General: Like other vasodilators, sodium nitroprusside can cause increases in intracranial pressure. In patients whose intracranial pressure is already elevated, Nipride should be used only with extreme caution.

Hepatic: Use caution when administering Nipride to patients with hepatic insufficency.

Use in Anesthesia: When Nipride (or any other vasodilator) is used for controlled hypotension during anesthesia, the patient's capacity to compensate for anemia and hypovolemia may be diminished. If possible, pre-existing anemia and hypovolemia should be corrected prior to administration of Nipride.

Hypotensive anesthetic techniques may also cause abnormalities of the pulmonary ventilation/perfusion ratio. Patients intolerant of these abnormalities may require a higher fraction of inspired oxygen.

Extreme caution should be exercised in patients who are especially poor surgical risks (A.S.A. Classes 4 and 4E).

Laboratory Tests: The cyanide-level assay is technically difficult, and cyanide levels in body fluids other than packed red blood cells are difficult to interpret. Cyanide toxicity will lead to lactic acidosis and venous hyperoxemia, but these findings may not be present until an hour or more after the cyanide capacity of the body's red-cell mass has been exhausted.

Drug Interactions: The hypotensive effect of sodium nitroprusside is augmented by that of most other hypotensive drugs, including ganglionic blocking agents, negative inotropic agents and inhaled anesthetics.

Carcinogenesis, mutagenesis, impairment of fertility: Nipride has not undergone adequate carcinogenicity testing in animals. The mutagenic potential of Nipride has not been assessed. Nipride has not been tested for effects on fertility.

Pregnancy: Teratogenic effects: Pregnancy Category C. There are no adequate or well-controlled studies of Nipride in either laboratory animals or pregnant women. It is not known whether Nipride can cause fetal harm when administered to a pregnant woman or can affect reproductive capacity. Nipride should be given to a pregnant woman only if clearly needed.

Nonteratogenic effects: In three studies in pregnant ewes, nitroprusside was shown to cross the placental barrier. Fetal cyanide levels were shown to be dose-related to maternal levels of nitroprusside. The metabolic transformation of sodium nitroprusside given to pregnant ewes led to fatal levels of cyanide in the fetuses. The infusion of 25 μg/kg/min of sodium nitroprusside for one hour in pregnant ewes resulted in the death of all fetuses. Pregnant ewes infused with 1 μg/kg/min of sodium nitroprusside for one hour delivered normal lambs.

The effects of administering sodium thiosulfate in pregnancy, either by itself or as a co-infusion with sodium nitroprusside, are completely unknown.

Nursing Mothers: It is not known whether sodium nitroprusside and its metabolites are excreted in human milk. Because many drugs are excreted in human milk and because of the potential for serious adverse reactions in nursing infants from Nipride, a decision should be made whether to discontinue nursing or to discontinue the drug, taking into account the importance of the drug to the mother.

Pediatric Use: **See Dosage and Administration.**

ADVERSE REACTIONS

The most important adverse reactions to sodium nitroprusside are the avoidable ones of excessive hypotension and cyanide toxicity, described above under **Warnings.** The adverse reactions described in this section develop less rapidly and, as it happens, less commonly.

Methemoglobinemia: As described in **Clinical Pharmacology** above, sodium nitroprusside infusions can cause sequestration of hemoglobin as methemoglobin. The back-conversion process is normally rapid, and clinically significant methemoglobinemia (> 10%) is seen only rarely in patients receiving Nipride. Even patients congenitally incapable of back-converting methemoglobin should demonstrate 10% methemoglobinemia only after they have received about 10 mg/kg of Nipride, and a patient receiving Nipride at the maximum recommended rate (10 μg/kg/min) would take over 16 hours to reach this total accumulated dose.

Methemoglobin levels can be measured by most clinical laboratories. The diagnosis should be suspected in patients who have received > 10 mg/kg of sodium nitroprusside and who exhibit signs of impaired oxygen delivery despite adequate cardiac output and adequate arterial pO_2. Classically, methemoglobinemic blood is described as chocolate brown, without color change on exposure to air.

When methemoglobinemia is diagnosed, the treatment of choice is 1 to 2 mg/kg of methylene blue, administered intravenously over several minutes. In patients likely to have substantial amounts of cyanide bound to methemoglobin as cyanmethemoglobin, treatment of methemoglobinemia with methylene blue must be undertaken with extreme caution.

Thiocyanate Toxicity: As described in **Clinical Pharmacology** above, most of the cyanide produced during metabolism of sodium nitroprusside is eliminated in the form of thiocyanate. When cyanide elimination is accerated by the co-infusion of thiosulfate, thiocyanate production is increased.

Thiocyanate is mildly neurotoxic (tinnitus, miosis, hyperreflexia) at serum levels of 1 mmol/L (60 mg/L). Thiocyanate toxicity is life-threatening when levels are 3 or 4 times higher (200 mg/L). The steady-state thiocyanate level after prolonged infusions of Nipride is increased with increased infusion rate, and the half-time of accumulation is 3 to 4 days. To keep the steady-state thiocyanate level below 1 mmol/L, a prolonged infusion of Nipride should not be more rapid than 3 μg/kg/min; in anuric patients, the corresponding limit is just 1 μg/kg/min. When prolonged infusions are more rapid than these, thiocyanate levels should be measured daily.

Physiologic maneuvers (*e.g.,* those that alter the pH of the urine) are not known to increase the elimination of thiocyanate. Thiocyanate clearance rates during dialysis, on the other hand, can approach the blood flow rate of the dialyzer.

Thiocyanate interferes with iodine uptake by the thyroid.

Abdominal pain, apprehension, diaphoresis, "dizziness," headache, muscle twitching, nausea, palpitations, restlessness, retching, and retrosternal discomfort have been noted when the blood pressure was too rapidly reduced. These symptoms quickly disappeared when the infusion was slowed or discontinued, and they did not reappear with a continued (or resumed) slower infusion.

Other adverse reactions reported are:

Cardiovascular: Bradycardia, electrocardiographic changes, tachycardia.

Dermatologic: Rash.

Endocrine: Hypothyrodism.

Gastrointestinal: Ileus.

Hematologic: Decreased platelet aggregation, methemoglobinemia.

Neurologic: Increased intracranial pressure.

Miscellaneous: Flushing, venous streaking, irritation at the infusion site.

OVERDOSAGE

Overdosage of nitroprusside can be manifested as excessive hypotension or cyanide toxicity (**see Warnings**) or as thiocyanate toxicity (**see Adverse Reactions**).

The acute intravenous mean lethal doses (LD_{50}) of nitroprusside in rabbits, dogs, mice and rats are 2.8, 5.0, 8.4 and 11.2 mg/kg, respectively.

Treatment of cyanide toxicity: Cyanide levels can be measured by many laboratories, and blood-gas studies that can detect venous hyperoxemia or acidosis are widely available. **Acidosis may not appear until more than an hour after the appearance of dangerous cyanide levels, and laboratory tests should not be awaited. Reasonable suspicion of cyanide toxicity is adequate grounds for initiation of treatment.**

Treatment of cyanide toxicity consists of:

- discontinuing the administration of Nipride.
- providing a buffer for cyanide by using sodium nitrite to convert as much hemoglobin into methemoglobin as the patient can safely tolerate; and then
- infusing sodium thiosulfate in sufficent quantity to convert the cyanide into thiocyanate.

The necessary medications for this treatment are contained in commercially available Cyanide Antidote Kits. Alternatively, discrete stocks of medications can be used.

Hemodialysis is ineffective in removal of cyanide, but it will eliminate most thiocyanate.

Cyanide Antidote Kits contain both amyl nitrite and sodium nitrite for induction of methemoglobinemia. The amyl nitrite is supplied in the form of inhalant ampuls, for administration in environments where intravenous administration of sodium nitrite may be delayed. In a patient who already has a patent intravenous line, use of amyl nitrite confers no benefit that is not provided by infusion of sodium nitrite.

Sodium nitrite is available in a 3% solution, and 4 to 6 mg/kg (about 0.2 mL/kg) should be injected over 2 to 4 minutes. This dose can be expected to convert about 10% of the patient's hemoglobin into methemoglobin; this level of methemoglobinemia is not associated with any important hazard of its own. The nitrite infusion may cause transient vasodilatation and hypotension, and this hypotension must, if it occurs, be routinely managed.

Immediately after infusion of the sodium nitrite, sodium thiosulfate should be infused. This agent is available in 10% and 25% solutions, and the recommended dose is 150 to 200 mg/kg; a typical adult dose is 50 mL of the 25% solution. Thiosulfate treatment of an acutely cyanide-toxic patient will raise thiocyanate levels, but not to a dangerous degree. The nitrite/thiosulfate regimen may be repeated, at half the original doses, after two hours.

DOSAGE AND ADMINISTRATION

Solution of the powder: The contents of a 50-mg Nipride vial should be dissolved in 2 to 3 mL of dextrose in water. No other diluent should be used.

Dilution to proper strength for infusion: Depending on the desired concentration, the initially reconstituted solution containing 50 mg of sodium nitroprusside must be further diluted in 250 to 1000 mL of sterile 5% dextrose injection. The diluted solution should be protected from light by promptly wrapping with aluminum foil or other opaque material. It is not necessary to cover the infusion drip chamber or the tubing.

Verification of the chemical integrity of the product: Sodium nitroprusside solution can be inactivated by reactions with trace contaminants. The products of these reactions are often blue, green or red, much brighter than the faint brownish color of unreacted sodium nitroprusside. Discolored solutions, or solutions in which particulate matter is visible, should not be used. If properly protected from light, the freshly reconstituted and diluted solution is stable for 24 hours.

No other drugs should be administered in the same solution with Nipride.

Avoidance of excessive hypotension: While the average effective rate in adults and children is about 3 μg/kg/min, some patients will become dangerously hypotensive when they receive Nipride at this rate. Infusion of Nipride should therefore be started at a very low rate (0.3 μg/kg/min), with gradual upward titration every few minutes until the desired effect is achieved or the maximum recommended infusion rate (10 μg/kg/min) has been reached.

Because sodium nitroprusside's hypotensive effect is very rapid in onset and in dissipation, small variations in infusion rate can lead to wide, undesirable variations in blood pressure. **Nipride should not be infused through ordinary IV apparatus regulated only by gravity and mechanical clamps. Only an infusion pump, preferably a volumetric pump, should be used.**

Because sodium nitroprusside can induce essentially unlimited blood-pressure reduction, **the blood pressure of a patient receiving this drug must be continuously monitored,** using either a continually reinflated sphygmomanometer or (preferably) an intra-arterial pressure sensor. Special caution should be used in elderly patients, since they may be more sensitive to the hypotensive effects of the drug.

The table below shows the infusion rates for adults and children of various weights corresponding to the recommended initial and maximal doses (0.3 μg/kg/min and 10 μg/kg/min, respectively). Some of the listed infusion rates are so slow or so rapid as to be impractical, and these practicalities must be considered when the concentration to be used is selected. Note that when the concentration used in a given patient is changed, the tubing is still filled with a solution at the previous concentration.

Avoidance of cyanide toxicity: As described in **Clinical Pharmacology** above, when more than 500 μg/kg of sodium nitroprusside is administered faster than 2 μg/kg/min, cyanide is generated faster than the unaided patient can eliminate it. Administration of sodium thiosulfate has been shown to increase the rate of cyanide processing, reducing the hazard of cyanide toxicity. Although toxic reactions to sodium thiosulfate have not been reported, the co-infusion regimen has not been extensively studied and it cannot be recommended without reservation. In one study, sodium thiosulfate appeared to potentiate the hypotensive effects of sodium nitroprusside.

Infusion Rates (mL/hour) to Achieve Initial (0.3 μg/kg/min) and Maximal (10 μg/kg/min) Dosing of Nipride

Volume		250 mL		500 mL		1000 mL	
Nipride		50 mg		50 mg		50 mg	
concentration		200 μg/mL		100 μg/mL		50 μg/mL	
pt weight							
kg	lbs	init	max	init	max	init	max
10	22	1	30	2	60	4	120
20	44	2	60	4	120	7	240
30	66	3	90	5	180	11	360
40	88	4	120	7	240	14	480
50	110	5	150	9	300	18	600
60	132	5	180	11	360	22	720
70	154	6	210	13	420	25	840
80	176	7	240	14	480	29	960
90	198	8	270	16	540	32	1080
100	220	9	300	18	600	36	1200

Co-infusions of sodium thiosulfate have been administered at rates of 5 to 10 times that of sodium nitroprusside. Care must be taken to avoid the indiscriminate use of prolonged or high doses of sodium nitroprusside with sodium thiosulfate as this may result in thiocyanate toxicity and hypovolemia. Incautious administration of Nipride must still be avoided, and all of the precautions concerning Nipride administration must still be observed.

Consideration of methemoglobinemia and thiocyanate toxicity: Rare patients receiving more than 10 mg/kg of sodium nitroprusside will develop methemoglobinemia; other patients, especially those with impaired renal function, will predictably develop thiocyanate toxicity after prolonged, rapid infusions. In accordance with the descriptions in **Adverse Reactions** above, patients with suggestive findings should be tested for these toxicities.

HOW SUPPLIED

Nipride is supplied in 5-mL amber-colored vials containing the equivalent of 50 mg sodium nitroprusside dihydrate for reconstitution with dextrose in water—boxes of 1 (NDC 0004-1938-08). Store the 5 mL amber-colored vials at 59° to 86°F.

Revised: November 1990

PROVOCHOLINE® ℞

[*pro "vo-kol 'leen*]
(methacholine Cl/Roche)

The following text is complete prescribing information based on official labeling in effect June 1, 1992.

PROVOCHOLINE IS A BRONCHOCONSTRICTOR AGENT FOR DIAGNOSTIC PURPOSES ONLY AND SHOULD NOT BE USED AS A THERAPEUTIC AGENT. PROVOCHOLINE INHALATION CHALLENGE SHOULD BE PERFORMED ONLY UNDER THE SUPERVISION OF A PHYSICIAN TRAINED IN AND THOROUGHLY FAMILIAR WITH ALL ASPECTS OF THE TECHNIQUE OF METHACHOLINE CHALLENGE, ALL CONTRAINDICATIONS, WARNINGS AND PRECAUTIONS, AND THE MANAGEMENT OF RESPIRATORY DISTRESS.
EMERGENCY EQUIPMENT AND MEDICATION SHOULD BE IMMEDIATELY AVAILABLE TO TREAT ACUTE RESPIRATORY DISTRESS.
PROVOCHOLINE SHOULD BE ADMINISTERED ONLY BY INHALATION. SEVERE BRONCHOCONSTRICTION AND REDUCTION IN RESPIRATORY FUNCTION CAN RESULT FROM THE ADMINISTRATION OF PROVOCHOLINE. PATIENTS WITH SEVERE HYPERREACTIVITY OF THE AIRWAYS CAN EXPERIENCE BROCHOCONSTRICTION AT A DOSAGE AS LOW AS 0.025 MG/ML (0.125 CUMULATIVE UNITS). IF SEVERE BRONCHOCONSTRICTION OCCURS, IT SHOULD BE REVERSED IMMEDIATELY BY THE ADMINISTRATION OF A RAPID-ACTING INHALED BRONCHODILATOR AGENT (BETA AGONIST). BECAUSE OF THE POTENTIAL FOR SEVERE BRONCHOCONSTRICTION, PROVOCHOLINE CHALLENGE SHOULD NOT BE PERFORMED IN ANY PATIENT WITH CLINICALLY APPARENT ASTHMA, WHEEZING, OR VERY LOW BASELINE PULMONARY FUNCTION TESTS (*E.G.*, FEV_1 LESS THAN 1 TO 1.5 LITER OR LESS THAN 70% OF THE PREDICTED VALUES). PLEASE CONSULT STANDARD NOMOGRAMS FOR PREDICTED VALUES.[1]

DESCRIPTION

Provocholine (brand of methacholine chloride/Roche) is a parasympathomimetic (cholinergic) bronchoconstrictor agent to be adminsitered in solution only, by inhalation, for diagnostic purposes. Each 5-mL vial contains 100 mg of methacholine Cl powder which is to be reconstituted with 0.9% sodium chloride injection containing 0.4% phenol (pH 7.0). See DOSAGE AND ADMINISTRATION for dilution procedures, concentrations and schedule of administration. Chemically, methacholine Cl (the active ingredient) is 1-propanaminium, 2-(acetyloxy)-*N,N,N*, -trimethyl,-chloride. It is a white to practically white deliquescent compound, soluble in water. Methacholine Cl has an empirical formula of $C_8H_{18}ClNO_2$ and a calculated molecular weight of 195.69.

CLINICAL PHARMACOLOGY

Methacholine Cl is the β-methyl homolog of acetylcholine and differs from the latter primarily in its greater duration and selectivity of action. Bronchial smooth muscle contains significant parasympathetic (cholinergic) innervation. Bronchoconstriction occurs when the vagus nerve is stimulated and acetylcholine is released from the nerve endings. Muscle constriction is essentially confined to the local site of release because acetylcholine is rapidly inactivated by acetylcholinesterase.

Compared with acetylcholine, methacholine Cl is more slowly hydrolyzed by acetylcholinesterase and is almost totally resistant to inactivation by nonspecific cholinesterase or pseudocholinesterase.

When a sodium chloride solution containing methacholine Cl is inhaled, subjects with asthma are markedly more sensitive to methacholine-induced bronchoconstriction than are healthy subjects. This difference in response is the pharmacologic basis for the Provocholine inhalation diagnostic challenge. However, it should be recognized that methacholine challenge may occasionally be positive after influenza, upper respiratory infections or immunizations, in very young or very old patients, or in patients with chronic lung disease (cystic fibrosis, sarcoidosis, tuberculosis, chronic obstructive pulmonary disease). The challenge may also be positive in patients with allergic rhinitis without asthma, in smokers, in patients after exposure to air pollutants, or in patients who have had or will in the future develop asthma.

There are no metabolic and pharmacokinetic data available on methacholine Cl.

INDICATIONS AND USAGE

Provocholine is indicated for the diagnosis of bronchial airway hyperreactivity in subjects who do not have clinically apparent asthma.

CONTRAINDICATIONS

Provocholine is contraindicated in patients with known hypersensitivity to this drug or to other parasympathomimetic agents.

Repeated administration of Provocholine by inhalation other than on the day that a patient undergoes challenge with increasing doses is contraindicated.

Inhalation challenge should not be performed in patients receiving any beta-adrenergic blocking agent because in such patients responses to methacholine Cl can be exaggerated or prolonged, and may not respond as readily to accepted modalities of treatment (see WARNINGS box).

PRECAUTIONS

General: Administration of Provocholine to patients with epilepsy, cardiovascular disease accompanied by bradycardia, vagotonia, peptic ulcer disease, thyroid disease, urinary tract obstruction or other condition that could be adversely affected by a cholinergic agent should be undertaken only if the physician feels benefit to the individual outweighs the potential risks.

Information for Patients: To assure the safe and effective use of Provocholine inhalation challenge, the following instructions and information should be given to patients:

1. Patients should be instructed regarding symptoms that may occur as a result of the test and how such symptoms can be managed.
2. A female patient should inform her physician if she is pregnant, or the date of her last onset of menses, or the date and result of her last pregnancy test. (See PRECAUTIONS: *Pregnancy.*)

Carcinogenesis, Mutagenesis, Impairment of Fertility: There have been no studies with methacholine Cl that would permit an evaluation of its carcinogenic or mutagenic potential or of its effect on fertility.

Pregnancy: Teratogenic Effects: Pregnancy Category C. Animal reproduction studies have not been conducted with methacholine Cl. It is not known whether methacholine Cl can cause fetal harm when administered to a pregnant patient or affect reproductive capacity. Methacholine Cl should be given to a pregnant woman only if clearly needed.

IN FEMALES OF CHILDBEARING POTENTIAL, PROVOCHOLINE INHALATION CHALLENGE SHOULD BE PERFORMED EITHER WITHIN TEN DAYS FOLLOWING THE ONSET OF MENSES OR WITHIN TWO WEEKS OF A NEGATIVE PREGNANCY TEST.

Nursing Mothers: Provocholine inhalation challenge should not be administered to a nursing mother since it is not known whether methacholine Cl when inhaled is excreted in breast milk.

Pediatric Use: The safety and efficacy of Provocholine inhalation challenge have not been established in children below the age of 5 years.

ADVERSE REACTIONS

Adverse reactions associated with 153 inhaled methacholine Cl challenges include one occurrence each of headache, throat irritation, lightheadedness and itching.

Provocholine is to be administered only by inhalation. When administered orally or by injection, methacholine Cl is reported to be associated with nausea and vomiting, substernal pain or pressure, hypotension, fainting and transient complete heart block. (See OVERDOSAGE.)

OVERDOSAGE

Provocholine is to be administered only by inhalation. When administered orally or by injection, overdosage with methacholine Cl can result in a syncopal reaction, with cardiac arrest and loss of consciousness. Serious toxic reactions should be treated with 0.5 mg to 1 mg of atropine sulfate, administered IM or IV.

The acute (24-hour) oral LD_{50} of methacholine Cl and related compounds is 1100 mg/kg in the mouse and 750 mg/kg in the rat.

Cynomolgus monkeys were exposed to a 2% (20 mg/mL) aerosol of methacholine Cl in acute (10-minute) and subchronic (7-day) inhalation toxicity studies. In the former study, animals exposed to the aerosol for up to 10 minutes demonstrated an increase in respiratory rate and decrease in tidal volume after 30 seconds. These changes peaked at 2 minutes and were followed by a rise in pulmonary resistance and a decrease in compliance. Pulmonary function returned to normal 20 to 25 minutes after exposure ended. In the 7-day study, monkeys were given daily inhalations equivalent to the maximum and roughly five times the maximum standard human dose. Although the typical pulmonary response/recovery sequence was observed, distinct changes in airway resistance were noted at the end of the study. These changes were not rapidly reversed in the maximum equivalent standard-dose group, which was observed for 9 weeks.

DOSAGE AND ADMINISTRATION

Before Provocholine inhalation challenge is begun, baseline pulmonary function tests must be performed. A subject to be challenged must have an FEV_1 of at least 70% of the predicted value.

The target level for a positive challenge is a 20% reduction in the FEV_1 compared with the baseline value after inhalation of the control sodium chloride solution. This target value should be calculated and recorded before Provocholine challenge is started.

Dilutions: (Note: Do not inhale powder. Do not handle this material if you have asthma or hay fever.) All dilutions should be made with 0.9% sodium chloride injection containing 0.4% phenol (pH 7.0). After adding the sodium chloride solution, shake each vial to obtain a clear solution.

Vial A. Add 4 mL of 0.9% sodium chloride injection containing 0.4% phenol (pH 7.0) to the 5-ML vial containing 100 mg of Provocholine. This is *vial A*, which contains a concentration of 25 mg/mL.

Vial B. Remove 3 mL from vial A (25 mg/mL), transfer to another vial and add 4.5 mL of 0.9% sodium chloride injection containing 0.4% phenol (pH 7.0). This is *vial B*, which contains a concentration of 10 mg/mL. An alternative method of preparing vial B is to remove 1 mL from vial A and add 1.5 mL of 0.9% sodium chloride injection containing 0.4% phenol (pH 7.0).

Vial C. Remove 1 mL from vial A (25 mg/mL), transfer to another vial and add 9 mL of 0.9% sodium chloride injection containing 0.4% phenol (pH 7.0). This is *vial C*, which contains a concentration of 2.5 mg/mL. (This step depletes the contents of vial A if the first dilution method under Vial B directions is used.)

Vial D. Remove 1 mL from vial C (2.5 mg/mL), transfer to another vial and add 9 mL of 0.9% sodium chloride injection containing 0.4% phenol (pH 7.0). This is *vial D*, which contains a concentration of 0.25 mg/mL.

Vial E. Remove 1 mL from vial D (0.25 mg/mL), transfer to another vial and add 9 mL of 0.9% sodium chloride injection containing 0.4% phenol (pH 7.0). This is *vial E*, which contains a concentration of 0.025 mg/mL.

Dilutions A through D should be stored at 36° to 46°F in a refrigerator and can be stored for up to two weeks. (The unreconstituted powder should be stored at 59° to 86°F.) After this time, discard the vials and prepare new dilutions. Freezing does not affect the stability of dilutions A through D. Vial E must be prepared on the day of challenge. A bacterial-retentive filter (porosity 0.22μ) should be used when transferring a solution from each vial to a nebulizer.

Procedure: A standardized procedure for inhalation has been developed.

Continued on next page

Roche Laboratories—Cont.

Serial Concentration	Number of Breaths	Cumulative Units per Concentration	Total Cumulative Units
0.025 mg/mL	5	0.125	0.125
0.25 mg/mL	5	1.25	1.375
2.5 mg/mL	5	12.5	13.88
10.0 mg/mL	5	50.0	63.88
25.0 mg/mL	5	125.0	188.88

The challenge is performed by giving a subject ascending serial concentrations of Provocholine. At each concentration, five breaths are administered by a nebulizer that permits intermittent delivery time of 0.6 seconds by either a Y-tube or a breath-actuated timing device (dosimeter).
At each of five inhalations of a serial concentration, the subject begins at functional residual capacity (FRC) and slowly and completely inhales the dose delivered. Within five minutes, FEV_1 values are determined. The procedure ends either when there is a 20% or greater reduction in the FEV_1 compared with the baseline sodium chloride solution value (*i.e.,* a positive response) or if 188.88 total cumulative units has been administered (see table below) and the FEV_1 has been reduced by 14% or less (*i.e.,* a negative response). If there is a reduction of 15% to 19% in the FEV_1 compared with baseline, either the challenge may be repeated at that concentration or a higher concentration may be given as long as the dosage administered does not result in total cumulative units exceeding 188.88.
The following is a suggested schedule for the administration of Provocholine challenge. Cumulative units are calculated by multiplying the number of breaths by the concentration administered.
Total cumulative units is the sum of cumulative units for each concentration administered. [See table above.]
An inhaled beta-agonist may be administered after Provocholine challenge to expedite the return of the FEV_1 to baseline and to relieve the discomfort of the subject. Most patients revert to normal pulmonary function within 5 minutes following bronchodilators or within 30 to 45 minutes without any bronchodilator.

HOW SUPPLIED

5-mL vials containing 100 mg of methacholine chloride powder which is to be reconstituted with 0.9% sodium chloride injection containing 0.4% phenol (pH 7.0)—boxes of 1 (NDC 0004-6102-01). Store the powder at 59° to 86°F. Refrigerate the reconstituted solutions at 36° to 46°F.

REFERENCE

1. Morris JF, Koski WA, Johnson LC: Spirometric standards for healthy nonsmoking adults. *Am Rev Resp Dis 103*:57–67, Jan 1971.

Revised: February 1988

ROCALTROL® ℞

[ro-cal'trol]
(calcitriol/Roche)
CAPSULES

The following text is complete prescribing information based on official labeling in effect June 1, 1992.

DESCRIPTION

Rocaltrol (calcitriol/Roche) is a synthetic vitamin D analog which is active in the regulation of the absorption of calcium from the gastrointestinal tract and its utilization in the body. It is available in capsules containing 0.25 mcg or 0.5 mcg calcitriol/Roche. Each capsule also contains butylated hydroxyanisole (BHA), butylated hydroxytoluene (BHT) and fractionated triglyceride of coconut oil. Gelatin capsule shells contain glycerin, parabens (methyl and propyl) and sorbitol, with the following dye systems: 0.25 mcg—FD&C Yellow No. 6 and titanium dioxide; 0.5 mcg—FD&C Red No. 3, FD&C Yellow No. 6 and titanium dioxide.
Calcitriol is a colorless, crystalline compound which occurs naturally in humans. It has a calculated molecular weight of 416.65 and is soluble in organic solvents but relatively insoluble in water. Chemically, calcitriol is 9,10-seco(5Z,7E)-5,7,10(19)-cholestatriene-1α, 3β, 25-triol.
The other names frequently used for calcitriol are 1α,25-dihydroxycholecalciferol, 1,25-dihydroxyvitamin D_3, 1,25-DHCC, $1,25(OH)_2D_3$ and 1,25-diOHC.

CLINICAL PHARMACOLOGY

Man's natural supply of vitamin D depends mainly on exposure to the ultraviolet rays of the sun for conversion of 7-dehydrocholesterol in the skin to vitamin D_3 (cholecalciferol). Vitamin D_3 must be metabolically activated in the liver and the kidney before it is fully active as a regulator of calcium and phosphorus metabolism at target tissues. The initial transformation of vitamin D_3 is catalyzed by a vitamin D_3-25-hydroxylase enzyme (25-OHase) present in the liver, and the product of this reaction is 25-hydroxyvitamin D_3 [25-$(OH)D_3$]. Hydroxylation of 25-$(OH)D_3$ occurs in the mitochondria of kidney tissue, activated by the renal 25-hydroxyvitamin D_3-1 alpha-hydroxylase (alpha-OHase), to produce 1,25-$(OH)_2D_3$ (calcitriol), the active form of vitamin D_3. Several metabolites of calcitriol have been identified which include:

1α, 25, $(OH)_2$-24-oxo-D_3
1α, 23,25$(OH)_3$-24-oxo-D_3
1α, 24R,25$(OH)_3D_3$
1α, 25R$(OH)_2$-26-23S-lactone D_3
1α, 25S,26$(OH)_3D_3$
1α, 25$(OH)_2$-23-oxo-D_3
1α, 25R,26$(OH)_3$-23-oxo-D_3
1α, (OH)24,25,26,27-tetranor-COOH-D_3

The two known sites of action of calcitriol are intestine and bone. A calcitriol receptor-binding protein appears to exist in the mucosa of human intestine. Additional evidence suggests that calcitriol may also act on the kidney and the parathyroid glands. Calcitriol is the most active known form of vitamin D_3 in stimulating intestinal calcium transport. In acutely uremic rats calcitriol has been shown to stimulate intestinal calcium absorption. The kidneys of uremic patients cannot adequately synthesize calcitriol, the active hormone formed from precursor vitamin D. Resultant hypocalcemia and secondary hyperparathyroidism are a major cause of the metabolic bone disease of renal failure. However, other bone-toxic substances which accumulate in uremia (*e.g.,* aluminum) may also contribute.
The beneficial effect of Rocaltrol in renal osteodystrophy appears to result from correction of hypocalcemia and secondary hyperparathyroidism. It is uncertain whether Rocaltrol produces other independent beneficial effects.
Calcitriol is rapidly absorbed from the intestine. Peak serum concentrations (above basal values) were reached within 3 to 6 hours following oral administration of single doses of 0.25 to 1.0 mcg of Rocaltrol. The half-life of calcitriol elimination from serum was found to range from 3 to 6 hours. Following a single oral dose of 0.5 mcg, mean serum concentrations of calcitriol rose from a baseline value of 40.0 ± 4.4 (S.D.) pg/ml to 60.0 ± 4.4 pg/ml at 2 hours, and declined to 53.0 ± 6.9 at 4 hours, 50 ± 7.0 at 8 hours, 44 ± 4.6 at 12 hours and 41.5 ± 5.1 at 24 hours. The duration of pharmacologic activity of a single dose of calcitriol is about 3 to 5 days.
Calcitriol and other vitamin D metabolites are transported in blood, bound to specific plasma proteins. Enterohepatic recycling and biliary excretion of calcitriol occurs. Following intravenous administration of radiolabeled calcitriol in normal subjects, approximately 27% and 7% of the radioactivity appeared in the feces and urine, respectively, within 24 hours. When a 1-mcg oral dose of radiolabeled calcitriol was administered to normals, approximately 10% of the total radioactivity appeared in urine within 24 hours. Cumulative excretion of radioactivity on the sixth day following intravenous administration of radiolabeled calcitriol averaged 16% in urine and 49% in feces.
There is evidence that maternal calcitriol may enter the fetal circulation. Calcitriol may be excreted in human milk.

INDICATIONS AND USAGE

Rocaltrol is indicated in the management of hypocalcemia and the resultant metabolic bone disease in patients undergoing chronic renal dialysis. In these patients, Rocaltrol administration enhances calcium absorption, reduces serum alkaline phosphatase levels and may reduce elevated parathyroid hormone levels and the histological manifestations of osteitis fibrosa cystica and defective mineralization.
Rocaltrol is also indicated in the management of hypocalcemia and its clinical manifestations in patients with postsurgical hypoparathyroidism, idiopathic hypoparathyroidism, and pseudohypoparathyroidism.

CONTRAINDICATIONS

Rocaltrol should not be given to patients with hypercalcemia or evidence of vitamin D toxicity.

WARNINGS

Since Rocaltrol is the most potent metabolite of vitamin D available, pharmacologic doses of vitamin D and its derivatives should be withheld during Rocaltrol treatment to avoid possible additive effects and hypercalcemia.
Both appropriate oral phosphate-binders and a low phosphate diet should be used to control serum phosphate levels in patients undergoing dialysis.
Magnesium-containing antacids and Rocaltrol should not be used concomitantly in patients on chronic renal dialysis because such use may lead to the development of hypermagnesemia.
Overdosage of any form of vitamin D is dangerous (see also OVERDOSAGE). Progressive hypercalcemia due to overdosage of vitamin D and its metabolites may be so severe as to require emergency attention. Chronic hypercalcemia can lead to generalized vascular calcification, nephrocalcinosis and other soft-tissue calcification. **The serum calcium times phospate (Ca × P) product should not be allowed to exceed 70.** Radiographic evaluation of suspect anatomical regions may be useful in the early detection of this condition.
Studies in dogs and rats given calcitriol for up to 26 weeks have shown that small increases of calcitriol above endogenous levels can lead to abnormalities of calcium metabolism with the potential for calcification of many tissues in the body.

PRECAUTIONS

General: Excessive dosage of Rocaltrol induces hypercalcemia and in some instances hypercalciuria; therefore, early in treatment during dosage adjustment, serum calcium should be determined twice weekly. In dialysis patients, a fall in serum alkaline phosphatase levels usually antedates the appearance of hypercalcemia and may be an indication of impending hypercalcemia. Should hypercalcemia develop, the drug should be discontinued immediately. Rocaltrol should be given cautiously to patients on digitalis, because hypercalcemia in such patients may precipitate cardiac arrhythmias.
In patients with normal renal function, chronic hypercalcemia may be associated with an increase in serum creatinine. While this is usually reversible, it is important in such patients to pay careful attention to those factors which may lead to hypercalcemia. Rocaltrol therapy should always be started at the lowest possible dose and should not be increased without careful monitoring of the serum calcium. An estimate of daily dietary calcium intake should be made and the intake adjusted when indicated.
Patients with normal renal function taking Rocaltrol should avoid dehydration. Adequate fluid intake should be maintained.
Information for the patient: The patient and his or her parents or spouse should be informed about compliance with dosage instructions, adherence to instructions about diet and calcium supplementation and avoidance of the use of unapproved nonprescription drugs. Patients should also be carefully informed about the symptoms of hypercalcemia (see ADVERSE REACTIONS section).
Laboratory tests: For dialysis patients, serum calcium, phosphorus, magnesium and alkaline phosphatase should be determined periodically. For hypoparathyroid patients, serum calcium, phosphorus and 24-hour urinary calcium should be determined periodically.
Drug interactions: Cholestyramine has been reported to reduce intestinal absorption of fat-soluble vitamins; as such it may impair intestinal absorption of Rocaltrol. (Also see WARNINGS and PRECAUTIONS [General] sections.)
Carcinogenesis, mutagenesis, impairment of fertility: Long-term studies in animals have not been conducted to evaluate the carcinogenic potential of Rocaltrol. There was no evidence of mutagenicity as studied by the Ames method. No significant effects of Rocaltrol on fertility and/or general reproductive performances were reported.
Pregnancy: Teratogenic effects: Pregnancy Category C. Rocaltrol has been found to be teratogenic in rabbits when given in doses 4 and 15 times the dose recommended for human use. All 15 fetuses in 3 litters at these doses showed external and skeletal abnormalities. However, none of the other 23 litters (156 fetuses) showed significant abnormalities compared with controls. Teratogenicity studies in rats showed no evidence of teratogenic potential. There are no adequate and well-controlled studies in pregnant women. Rocaltrol should be used during pregnancy only if the potential benefit justifies the potential risk to the fetus.
Nonteratogenic effects: In the rabbit, dosages of 0.3 mcg/kg/day administered on days 7 to 18 of gestation resulted in 19% maternal mortality, a decrease in mean fetal body weight and a reduced number of newborn surviving to 24 hours. A study of peri- and postnatal development in rats resulted in hypercalcemia in the offspring of dams given Rocaltrol at doses of 0.08 or 0.3 mcg/ kg/day, hypercalcemia and hypophosphatemia in dams at doses of 0.08 or 0.3 mcg/kg/day, and increased serum urea nitrogen in dams given Rocaltrol at a dose of 0.3 mcg/kg/day. In another study in rats, maternal weight gain was slightly reduced at a dose of 0.3 mcg/kg/day administered on days 7 to 15 of gestation.
The offspring of a woman administered 17 to 36 mcg/day of Rocaltrol (17 to 144 times the recommended dose) during pregnancy manifested mild hypercalcemia in the first two days of life which returned to normal at day 3.
Nursing mothers: Calcitriol may be excreted in human milk. Because many drugs are excreted in human milk and because of the potential for serious adverse reactions from Rocaltrol in nursing infants, a mother should not nurse while taking this drug.

Pediatric use: Safety and efficacy of Rocaltrol in children undergoing dialysis have not been established.

ADVERSE REACTIONS

Since Rocaltrol is believed to be the active hormone which exerts vitamin D activity in the body, adverse effects are, in general, similar to those encountered with excessive vitamin D intake. The early and late signs and symptoms of vitamin D intoxication associated with hypercalcemia include:

Early: Weakness, headache, somnolence, nausea, vomiting, dry mouth, constipation, muscle pain, bone pain and metallic taste.

Late: Polyuria, polydipsia, anorexia, weight loss, nocturia, conjunctivitis (calcific), pancreatitis, photophobia, rhinorrhea, pruritus, hyperthermia, decreased libido, elevated BUN, albuminuria, hypercholesterolemia, elevated SGOT and SGPT, ectopic calcification, nephrocalcinosis, hypertension, cardiac arrhythmias and, rarely, overt psychosis.

In clinical studies on hypoparathyroidism and pseudohypoparathyroidism, hypercalcemia was noted on at least one occasion in about 1 in 3 patients and hypercalciuria in about 1 in 7. Elevated serum creatinine levels were observed in about 1 in 6 patients (approximately one half of whom had normal levels at baseline).

One case of erythema multiforme was confirmed by rechallenge.

OVERDOSAGE

Administration of Rocaltrol to patients in excess of their daily requirements can cause hypercalcemia, hypercalciuria and hyperphosphatemia. High intake of calcium and phosphate concomitant with Rocaltrol may lead to similar abnormalities. High levels of calcium in the dialysate bath may contribute to the hypercalcemia.

Treatment of Hypercalcemia and Overdosage: General treatment of hypercalcemia (greater than 1 mg/dl above the upper limit of the normal range) consists of immediate discontinuation of Rocaltrol therapy, institution of a low calcium diet and withdrawal of calcium supplements. Serum calcium levels should be determined daily until normocalcemia ensues. Hypercalcemia frequently resolves in two to seven days. When serum calcium levels have returned to within normal limits, Rocaltrol therapy may be reinstituted at a dose of 0.25 mcg/day less than prior therapy. Serum calcium levels should be obtained at least twice weekly after all dosage changes and subsequent dosage titration. In dialysis patients, persistent or markedly elevated serum calcium levels may be corrected by dialysis against a calcium-free dialysate.

Treatment of Accidental Overdosage of Rocaltrol: The treatment of acute accidental overdosage of Rocaltrol should consist of general supportive measures. If drug ingestion is discovered within a relatively short time, induction of emesis or gastric lavage may be of benefit in preventing further absorption. If the drug has passed through the stomach, the administration of mineral oil may promote its fecal elimination. Serial serum electrolyte determinations (especially calcium), rate of urinary calcium excretion and assessment of electrocardiographic abnormalities due to hypercalcemia should be obtained. Such monitoring is critical in patients receiving digitalis. Discontinuation of supplemental calcium and a low calcium diet are also indicated in accidental overdosage. Due to the relatively short duration of the pharmacological action of calcitriol, further measures are probably unnecessary. Should, however, persistent and markedly elevated serum calcium levels occur, there are a variety of therapeutic alternatives which may be considered, depending on the patient's underlying condition. These include the use of drugs such as phosphates and corticosteroids as well as measures to induce an appropriate forced diuresis. The use of peritoneal dialysis against a calcium-free dialysate has also been reported.

DOSAGE AND ADMINISTRATION

The optimal daily dose of Rocaltrol must be carefully determined for each patient.

The effectiveness of Rocaltrol therapy is predicated on the assumption that each patient is receiving an adequate daily intake of calcium. The U.S. RDA for calcium in adults is 800 to 1200 mg. To ensure that each patient receives an adequate daily intake of calcium, the physician should either prescribe a calcium supplement or instruct the patient in proper dietary measures.

Dialysis patients: The recommended initial dose of Rocaltrol is 0.25 mcg/day. If a satisfactory response in the biochemical parameters and clinical manifestations of the disease state is not observed, dosage may be increased by 0.25 mcg/day at four- to eight-week intervals. During this titration period, serum calcium levels should be obtained at least twice weekly, and if hypercalcemia is noted, the drug should be immediately discontinued until normocalcemia ensues.

Patients with normal or only slightly reduced serum calcium levels may respond to Rocaltrol doses of 0.25 mcg every other day. Most patients undergoing hemodialysis respond to doses between 0.5 and 1 mcg/day.

Oral Rocaltrol may normalize plasma ionized calcium in some uremic patients, yet fail to suppress parathyroid hyperfunction. In these individuals with autonomous parathyroid hyperfunction, oral Rocaltrol may be useful to maintain normocalcemia, but has not been shown to be adequate treatment for hyperparathyroidism.

Hypoparathyroidism: The recommended initial dose of Rocaltrol is 0.25 mcg/day given in the morning. If a satisfactory response in the biochemical parameters and clinical manifestations of the disease is not observed, the dose may be increased at two- to four-week intervals. During the dosage titration period, serum calcium levels should be obtained at least twice weekly and, if hypercalcemia is noted, Rocaltrol should be immediately discontinued until normocalcemia ensues. Careful consideration should also be given to lowering the dietary calcium intake.

Most adult patients and pediatric patients age 6 years and older have responded to dosages in the range of 0.5 to 2 mcg daily. Pediatric patients in the 1–5 year age group with hypoparathyroidism have usually been given 0.25 to 0.75 mcg daily. The number of treated patients with pseudohypoparathyroidism less than 6 years of age is too small to make dosage recommendations.

HOW SUPPLIED

0.25 mcg calcitriol/Roche in soft gelatin, light orange, oval capsules, imprinted ROCALTROL 0.25 ROCHE; bottles of 30 (NDC 0004-0143-23), and bottles of 100, (NDC 0004-0143-01).

0.5 mcg calcitriol/Roche in soft gelatin, dark orange, oblong capsules, imprinted ROCALTROL 0.5 ROCHE; bottles of 100, (NDC 0004-0144-01).

Rocaltrol should be protected from heat and light.

Revised: June 1990

Shown in Product Identification Section, page 426

ROCEPHIN®   ℞

[ro-sef'in]

(ceftriaxone sodium/Roche)

The following text is complete prescribing information based on official labeling in effect June 1, 1992.

DESCRIPTION

Rocephin® (ceftriaxone sodium/Roche) is a sterile, semisynthetic, broad-spectrum cephalosporin antibiotic for intravenous or intramuscular administration. Ceftriaxone sodium is 5-Thia-1-azabicyclo[4.2.0]oct-2-ene-2-carboxylic acid, 7-[[(2-amino-4-thiazolyl)(methoxyimino) acetyl]-amino]-8-oxo-3-[[(1, 2, 5, 6-tetrahydro-2-methyl-5, 6-dioxo-1, 2, 4-triazin-3-yl)thio]methyl]-, disodium salt, [6R-[6α,7β(Z)]]-.

The chemical formula of ceftriaxone sodium is $C_{18}H_{16}N_8Na_2O_7S_3 \cdot 3.5H_2O$. It has a calculated molecular weight of 661.59.

Rocephin is a white to yellowish-orange crystalline powder which is readily soluble in water, sparingly soluble in methanol and very slightly soluble in ethanol. The pH of a 1% aqueous solution is approximately 6.7. The color of Rocephin solutions ranges from light yellow to amber, depending on the length of storage, concentration and diluent used.

Rocephin contains approximately 83 mg (3.6 mEq) of sodium per gram of ceftriaxone activity.

CLINICAL PHARMACOLOGY

Average plasma concentrations of ceftriaxone following a single 30-minute intravenous (I.V.) infusion of a 0.5, 1 or 2 gm dose and intramuscular (I.M.) administration of a single 0.5 or 1 gm dose in healthy subjects are presented in Table 1.

Ceftriaxone was completely absorbed following I.M. administration with mean maximum plasma concentrations occurring between two and three hours postdosing. Multiple I.V. or I.M. doses ranging from 0.5 to 2 gm at 12- to 24-hour intervals resulted in 15 to 36% accumulation of ceftriaxone above single dose values.

Ceftriaxone concentrations in urine are high, as shown in Table 2.

Thirty-three to 67% of a ceftriaxone dose was excreted in the urine as unchanged drug and the remainder was secreted in the bile and ultimately found in the feces as microbiologically inactive compounds. After a 1 gm I.V. dose, average concentrations of ceftriaxone, determined from one to three hours after dosing, were 581 mcg/mL in the gallbladder bile, 788 mcg/mL in the common duct bile, 898 mcg/mL in the cystic duct bile, 78.2 mcg/gm in the gallbladder wall and 62.1 mcg/mL in the concurrent plasma.

Over a 0.15 to 3 gm dose range in healthy adult subjects, the values of elimination half-life ranged from 5.8 to 8.7 hours; apparent volume of distribution from 5.78 to 13.5 L; plasma clearance from 0.58 to 1.45 L/hour; and renal clearance from 0.32 to 0.73 L/hour. Ceftriaxone is reversibly bound to human plasma proteins, and the binding decreased from a value of 95% bound at plasma concentrations of <25 mcg/mL to a value of 85% bound at 300 mcg/mL.

The average values of maximum plasma concentration, elimination half-life, plasma clearance and volume of distribution after a 50 mg/kg I.V. dose and after a 75 mg/kg I.V. dose in pediatric patients suffering from bacterial meningitis are shown in Table 3. Ceftriaxone penetrated the inflamed meninges of infants and children; CSF concentrations after a 50 mg/kg I.V. dose and after a 75 mg/kg I.V. dose are also shown in Table 3.

TABLE 1
Ceftriaxone Plasma Concentrations After Single Dose Administration

Dose/Route	Average Plasma Concentrations (mcg/mL)								
	0.5 hr	1 hr	2 hr	4 hr	6 hr	8 hr	12 hr	16 hr	24 hr
0.5 gm I.V.*	82	59	48	37	29	23	15	10	5
0.5 gm I.M.	30	41	43	39	31	25	16	ND†	ND
1 gm I.V.*	151	111	88	67	53	43	28	18	9
1 gm I.M.	40	68	76	68	56	44	29	ND	ND
2 gm I.V.*	257	192	154	117	89	74	46	31	15

* I.V. doses were infused at a constant rate over 30 minutes.

† ND = Not determined.

TABLE 2
Urinary Concentrations of Ceftriaxone After Single Dose Administration

Dose/Route	Average Urinary Concentrations (mcg/mL)					
	0–2 hr	2–4 hr	4–8 hr	8–12 hr	12–24 hr	24–48 hr
0.5 gm I.V.	526	366	142	87	70	15
0.5 gm I.M.	115	425	308	127	96	28
1 gm I.V.	995	855	293	147	132	32
1 gm I.M.	504	628	418	237	ND*	ND
2 gm I.V.	2692	1976	757	274	198	40

* ND = Not determined.

TABLE 3
Average Pharmacokinetic Parameters of Ceftriaxone in Pediatric Patients with Meningitis

	50 mg/kg I.V.	75 mg/kg I.V.
Maximum Plasma Concentrations (mcg/mL)	216	275
Elimination Half-life (hr)	4.6	4.3
Plasma Clearance (mL/hr/kg)	49	60
Volume of Distribution (mL/kg)	338	373
CSF Concentration—inflamed meninges (mcg/mL)	5.6	6.4
Range (mcg/mL)	1.3–18.5	1.3–44
Time after dose (hr)	3.7 (± 1.6)	3.3 (± 1.4)

Continued on next page

Roche Laboratories—Cont.

Compared to that in healthy adult subjects, the pharmacokinetics of ceftriaxone were only minimally altered in elderly subjects and in patients with renal impairment or hepatic dysfunction (Table 4); therefore, dosage adjustments are not necessary for these patients with ceftriaxone dosages up to 2 gm per day. Ceftriaxone was not removed to any significant extent from the plasma by hemodialysis. In 6 of 26 dialysis patients, the elimination rate of ceftriaxone was markedly reduced, suggesting that plasma concentrations of ceftriaxone should be monitored in these patients to determine if dosage adjustments are necessary.

TABLE 4
Average Pharmacokinetic Parameters of Ceftriaxone in Humans

Subject Group	Elimination Half-Life (hr)	Plasma Clearance (L/hr)	Volume of Distribution (L)
Healthy Subjects	5.8–8.7	0.58–1.45	5.8–13.5
Elderly Subjects (mean age, 70.5 yr)	8.9	0.83	10.7
Patients with renal impairment			
Hemodialysis patients (0–5 mL/min)*	14.7	0.65	13.7
Severe (5–15 mL/min)	15.7	0.56	12.5
Moderate (16–30 mL/min)	11.4	0.72	11.8
Mild (31–60 mL/min)	12.4	0.70	13.3
Patients with liver disease	8.8	1.1	13.6

*Creatinine clearance.

MICROBIOLOGY: The bactericidal activity of ceftriaxone results from inhibition of cell wall synthesis. Ceftriaxone has a high degree of stability in the presence of beta-lactamases, both penicillinases and cephalosporinases, of gram-negative and gram-positive bacteria. Ceftriaxone is usually active against the following microorganisms *in vitro* and in clinical infections (see INDICATIONS AND USAGE):

GRAM-NEGATIVE AEROBES:
Acinetobacter calcoaceticus
Enterobacter aerogenes
Enterobacter cloacae
Escherichia coli
Haemophilus influenzae (including ampicillin-resistant strains)
Haemophilus parainfluenzae
Klebsiella oxytoca
Klebsiella pneumoniae
Morganella morganii
Neisseria gonorrhoeae (including penicillinase- and nonpenicillinase-producing strains)
Neisseria meningitidis
Proteus mirabilis
Proteus vulgaris
Serratia marcescens

Ceftriaxone is also active against many strains of *Pseudomonas aeruginosa.*

Note: Many strains of the above organisms that are multiply resistant to other antibiotics, *e.g.,* penicillins, cephalosporins and aminoglycosides, are susceptible to ceftriaxone.

GRAM-POSITIVE AEROBES
Staphylococcus aureus (including penicillinase-producing strains)
Staphylococcus epidermidis
Streptococcus pneumoniae
Streptococcus pyogenes
Viridans group streptococci

Note: Methicillin-resistant streptococci are resistant to cephalosporins, including ceftriaxone. Most strains of Group D streptococci and enterococci, *e.g., Enterococcus (Streptococcus) faecalis,* are resistant.

ANAEROBES:
Bacteroides fragilis
Clostridium species
Peptostreptococcus species

Note: Most strains of *C. difficile* are resistant.

Ceftriaxone also demonstrates *in vitro* activity against most strains of the following microorganisms, although the clinical significance is unknown:

GRAM-NEGATIVE AEROBES
Citrobacter diversus
Citrobacter freundii
Providencia species (including *Providencia rettgeri*)
Salmonella species (including *S. typhi*)
Shigella species

GRAM-POSITIVE AEROBES:
Streptococcus agalactiae

ANAEROBES
Bacteroides bivius
Bacteroides melaninogenicus

SUSCEPTIBILITY TEST: Diffusion Techniques: Quantitative methods that require measurement of zone diameters give the most precise estimate of the susceptibility of bacteria to antimicrobial agents. One such procedure[1] which has been recommended for use with disks to test susceptibility of organisms to ceftriaxone uses a 30-mcg ceftriaxone disk. Interpretation involves the correlation of the diameters obtained in the disk test with the minimum inhibitory concentration (MIC) for ceftriaxone.

Reports from the laboratory giving results of the standardized single disk susceptibility test using a 30-mcg ceftriaxone disk should be interpreted for ceftriaxone according to the following criteria:

Zone Diameter (mm)	Interpretation
≥18	(S) Susceptible
14–17	(MS) Moderately Susceptible
≤13	(R) Resistant

A report of "Susceptible" indicates that the pathogen is likely to be inhibited by generally achievable levels. A report of "Moderately Susceptible" suggests that the organism would be susceptible if high dosage (not to exceed 4 gm per day) is used or if the infection is confined to tissues and fluids in which high antimicrobial levels are attained. A report of "Resistant" indicates that achievable concentrations are unlikely to be inhibitory, and other therapy should be selected.

Standardized procedures require the use of laboratory control organisms. The 30-mcg cefuroxime disk should give the following zone diameters:

Organism	Zone Diameter (mm)
Staphylococcus aureus ATCC® 25923	22–28
Escherichia coli ATCC® 25922	29–35
Pseudomonas aeruginosa ATCC® 27853	17–23

Dilution Techniques:
Use a standardized dilution method[2] (broth, agar, microdilution) or equivalent with ceftriaxone powder. The MIC values obtained should be interpreted according to the following criteria:

MIC (mcg/mL)	Interpretation
≤16	Susceptible
>16–<64	Moderately Susceptible
≥64	Resistant

As with standard diffusion techniques, dilution methods require the use of laboratory control organisms. Standard ceftriaxone powder should provide the following MIC values:

Organism	MIC (mcg/mL)
Staphylococcus aureus ATCC® 29213	1–8
Escherichia coli ATCC® 25922	0.03–0.12
Pseudomonas aeruginosa ATCC® 27853	8–32

INDICATIONS AND USAGE

Rocephin is indicated for the treatment of the following infections when caused by susceptible organisms:

LOWER RESPIRATORY TRACT INFECTIONS caused by *Streptococcus pneumoniae, Staphylococcus aureus, Haemophilus influenzae, Haemophilus parainfluenzae, Klebsiella pneumoniae, Escherichia coli, Enterobacter aerogenes, Proteus mirabilis* or *Serratia marcescens.*

SKIN AND SKIN STRUCTURE INFECTIONS caused by *Staphylococcus aureus, Staphylococcus epidermidis, Streptococcus pyogenes, Viridans* group streptococci, *Escherichia coli, Enterobacter cloacae, Klebsiella oxytoca, Klebsiella pneumoniae, Proteus mirabilis, Morganella morganii*, Pseudomonas aeruginosa, Serratia marcescens, Acinetobacter calcoaceticus, Bacteroides fragilis** or *Peptostreptococcus* species.

URINARY TRACT INFECTIONS (complicated and uncomplicated) caused by *Escherichia coli, Proteus mirabilis, Proteus vulgaris, Morganella morganii* or *Klebsiella pneumoniae.*

UNCOMPLICATED GONORRHEA (cervical/urethral and rectal) caused by *Neisseria gonorrhoeae,* including both penicillinase- and nonpenicillinase-producing strains, and pharyngeal gonorrhea caused by nonpenicillinase-producing strains of *Neisseria gonorrhoeae.*

PELVIC INFLAMMATORY DISEASE caused by *Neisseria gonorrhoeae.*

BACTERIAL SEPTICEMIA caused by *Staphylococcus aureus, Streptococcus pneumoniae, Escherichia coli, Haemophilus influenzae* or *Klebsiella pneumoniae.*

BONE AND JOINT INFECTIONS caused by *Staphylococcus aureus, Streptococcus pneumoniae, Escherichia coli, Proteus mirabilis, Klebsiella pneumoniae* or *Enterobacter* species.

INTRA-ABDOMINAL INFECTIONS caused by *Escherichia coli, Klebsiella pneumoniae, Bacteroides fragilis, Clostridium* species (Note: most strains of *C. difficile* are resistant) or *Peptostreptococcus* species.

MENINGITIS caused by *Haemophilus influenzae, Neisseria meningitidis* or *Streptococcus pneumoniae.* Rocephin has also been used successfully in a limited number of cases of meningitis and shunt infection caused by *Staphylococcus epidermidis** and *Escherichia coli.**

SURGICAL PROPHYLAXIS: The preoperative administration of a single 1 gm dose of Rocephin may reduce the incidence of postoperative infections in patients undergoing surgical procedures classified as contaminated or potentially contaminated (*e.g.,* vaginal or abdominal hysterectomy) and in surgical patients for whom infection at the operative site would present serious risk (*e.g.,* during coronary artery bypass surgery). Although Rocephin has been shown to have been as effective as cefazolin in the prevention of infection following coronary artery bypass surgery, no placebo-controlled trials have been conducted to evaluate any cephalosporin antibiotic in the prevention of infection following coronary artery bypass surgery.

*Efficacy for this organism in this organ system was studied in fewer than ten infections.

When administered prior to surgical procedures for which it is indicated, a single 1 gm dose of Rocephin provides protection from most infections due to susceptible organisms throughout the course of the procedure.

Before instituting treatment with Rocephin, appropriate specimens should be obtained for isolation of the causative organism and for determination of its susceptibility to the drug. Therapy may be instituted prior to obtaining results of susceptibility testing.

Note: Most strains of enterococci are resistant to ceftriaxone.

CONTRAINDICATIONS

Rocephin is contraindicated in patients with known allergy to the cephalosporin class of antibiotics.

WARNINGS

BEFORE THERAPY WITH ROCEPHIN IS INSTITUTED, CAREFUL INQUIRY SHOULD BE MADE TO DETERMINE WHETHER THE PATIENT HAS HAD PREVIOUS HYPERSENSITIVITY REACTIONS TO CEPHALOSPORINS, PENICILLINS OR OTHER DRUGS. THIS PRODUCT SHOULD BE GIVEN CAUTIOUSLY TO PENICILLIN-SENSITIVE PATIENTS. ANTIBIOTICS SHOULD BE ADMINISTERED WITH CAUTION TO ANY PATIENT WHO HAS DEMONSTRATED SOME FORM OF ALLERGY, PARTICULARLY TO DRUGS. SERIOUS ACUTE HYPERSENSITIVITY REACTIONS MAY REQUIRE THE USE OF SUBCUTANEOUS EPINEPHRINE AND OTHER EMERGENCY MEASURES.

Pseudomembranous colitis has been reported with nearly all antibacterial agents, including ceftriaxone, and may range in severity from mild to life-threatening. Therefore, it is important to consider this diagnosis in patients who present with diarrhea subsequent to the administration of antibacterial agents.

Treatment with antibacterial agents alters the normal flora of the colon and may permit overgrowth of clostridia. Studies indicate that a toxin produced by *Clostridium difficile* is one primary cause of "antibiotic-associated colitis."

After the diagnosis of pseudomembranous colitis has been established, therapeutic measures should be initiated. Mild cases of pseudomembranous colitis usually respond to drug discontinuance alone. In moderate to severe cases, consideration should be given to management with fluids and electrolytes, protein supplementation and treatment with an oral antibacterial drug effective against *C. difficile.*

PRECAUTIONS

GENERAL: Although transient elevations of BUN and serum creatinine have been observed, at the recommended dosages, the nephrotoxic potential of Rocephin is similar to that of other cephalosporins.

Ceftriaxone is excreted via both biliary and renal excretion (see CLINICAL PHARMACOLOGY). Therefore, patients with renal failure normally require no adjustment in dosage when usual doses of Rocephin are administered, but concentrations of drug in the serum should be monitored periodically. If evidence of accumulation exists, dosage should be decreased accordingly.

Dosage adjustments should not be necessary in patients with hepatic dysfunction; however, in patients with both hepatic dysfunction and significant renal disease, Rocephin dosage should not exceed 2 gm daily without close monitoring of serum concentrations.

Alterations in prothrombin times have occurred rarely in patients treated with Rocephin. Patients with impaired vitamin K synthesis or low vitamin K stores (*e.g.,* chronic hepatic disease and malnutrition) may require monitoring of prothrombin time during Rocephin treatment. Vitamin K ad-

Diluent	Concentration mg/mL	Storage Room Temp. (25°C)	Refrigerated (4°C)
Sterile Water for	100	3 days	10 days
Injection	250	24 hours	3 days
0.9% Sodium	100	3 days	10 days
Chloride Solution	250	24 hours	3 days
5% Dextrose	100	3 days	10 days
Solution	250	24 hours	3 days
Bacteriostatic Water +	100	24 hours	10 days
0.9% Benzyl Alcohol	250	24 hours	3 days
1% Lidocaine Solution	100	24 hours	10 days
(without epinephrine)	250	24 hours	3 days

ministration (10 mg weekly) may be necessary if the prothrombin time is prolonged before or during therapy.

Prolonged use of Rocephin may result in overgrowth of nonsusceptible organisms. Careful observation of the patient is essential. If superinfection occurs during therapy, appropriate measures should be taken.

Rocephin should be prescribed with caution in individuals with a history of gastrointestinal disease, especially colitis.

Rare cases have been reported in which sonographic abnormalities are seen in the gallbladder of patients treated with Rocephin; these patients may also have symptoms of gallbladder disease. These abnormalities are variously described as sludge, precipitations, echoes with shadows, and may be misinterpreted as concretions. The chemical nature of the sonographically-detected material has not been determined. The condition appears to be transient and reversible when Rocephin is discontinued and conservative management employed. Therefore, Rocephin should be discontinued in patients who develop signs and symptoms suggestive of gallbladder disease and/or the sonographic findings described above.

CARCINOGENESIS, MUTAGENESIS, IMPAIRMENT OF FERTILITY:

Carcinogenesis: Considering the maximum duration of treatment and the class of the compound, carcinogenicity studies with ceftriaxone in animals have not been performed. The maximum duration of animal toxicity studies was six months.

Mutagenesis: Genetic toxicology tests included the Ames test, a micronucleus test and a test for chromosomal aberrations in human lymphocytes cultured *in vitro* with ceftriaxone. Ceftriaxone showed no potential for mutagenic activity in these studies.

Impairment of Fertility: Ceftriaxone produced no impairment of fertility when given intravenously to rats at daily doses up to 586 mg/kg/day, approximately 20 times the recommended clinical dose of 2 gm/day.

PREGNANCY: Teratogenic Effects: Pregnancy Category B. Reproductive studies have been performed in mice and rats at doses up to 20 times the usual human dose and have no evidence of embryotoxicity, fetotoxicity or teratogenicity. In primates, no embryotoxicity or teratogenicity was demonstrated at a dose approximately three times the human dose. There are, however, no adequate and well-controlled studies in pregnant women. Because animal reproductive studies are not always predictive of human response, this drug should be used during pregnancy only if clearly needed.

Nonteratogenic Effects: In rats, in the Segment I (fertility and general reproduction) and Segment III (perinatal and postnatal) studies with intravenously administered ceftriaxone, no adverse effects were noted on various reproductive parameters during gestation and lactation, including postnatal growth, functional behavior and reproductive ability of the offspring, at doses of 586 mg/kg/day or less.

NURSING MOTHERS: Low concentrations of ceftriaxone are excreted in human milk. Caution should be exercised when Rocephin is administered to a nursing woman.

PEDIATRIC USE: Safety and effectiveness of Rocephin in neonates, infants and children have been established for the dosages described in the DOSAGE AND ADMINISTRATION section. *In vitro* studies have shown that ceftriaxone, like some other cephalosporins, can displace bilirubin from serum albumin. Rocephin should not be administered to hyperbilirubinemic neonates, especially prematures.

ADVERSE REACTIONS

Rocephin is generally well tolerated. In clinical trials, the following adverse reactions, which were considered to be related to Rocephin therapy or of uncertain etiology, were observed:

LOCAL REACTIONS—pain, induration or tenderness at the site of injection (1%). Less frequently reported (less than 1%) was phlebitis after I.V. administration.

HYPERSENSITIVITY—rash (1.7%). Less frequently reported (less than 1%) were pruritus, fever or chills.

HEMATOLOGIC—eosinophilia (6%), thrombocytosis (5.1%) and leukopenia (2.1%). Less frequently reported (less than 1%) were anemia, hemolytic anemia, neutropenia, lymphopenia, thrombocytopenia and prolongation of the prothrombin time.

GASTROINTESTINAL—diarrhea (2.7%). Less frequently reported (less than 1%) were nausea or vomiting, and dysgeusia. Onset of pseudomembranous colitis symptoms may occur during or after antibiotic treatment (see WARNINGS).

HEPATIC—elevations of SGOT (3.1%) or SGPT (3.3%). Less frequently reported (less than 1%) were elevations of alkaline phosphatase and bilirubin.

RENAL—elevations of the BUN (1.2%). Less frequently reported (less than 1%) were elevations of creatinine and the presence of casts in the urine.

CENTRAL NERVOUS SYSTEM—headache or dizziness were reported occasionally (less than 1%).

GENITOURINARY—moniliasis or vaginitis were reported occasionally (less than 1%).

MISCELLANEOUS—diaphoresis and flushing were reported occasionally (less than 1%).

Other rarely observed adverse reactions (less than 0.1%) include leukocytosis, lymphocytosis, monocytosis, basophilia, a decrease in the prothrombin time, jaundice, gallbladder sludge, glycosuria, hematuria, anaphylaxis, bronchospasm, serum sickness, abdominal pain, colitis, flatulence, dyspepsia, palpitations and epistaxis.

DOSAGE AND ADMINISTRATION

Rocephin may be administered intravenously or intramuscularly.

ADULTS: The usual adult daily dose is 1 to 2 grams given once a day (or in equally divided doses twice a day) depending on the type and severity of infection. The total daily dose should not exceed 4 grams.

For the treatment of uncomplicated gonococcal infections, a single intramuscular dose of 250 mg is recommended.

For preoperative use (surgical prophylaxis), a single dose of 1 gram administered ½ to 2 hours before surgery is recommended.

CHILDREN: For the treatment of skin and skin structure infections, the recommended total daily dose is 50 to 75 mg/kg given once a day (or in equally divided doses twice a day). The total daily dose should not exceed 2 grams.

For the treatment of serious miscellaneous infections other than meningitis, the recommended total daily dose is 50 to 75 mg/kg, given in divided doses every 12 hours. The total daily dose should not exceed 2 grams.

In the treatment of meningitis, a daily dose of 100 mg/kg (not to exceed 4 grams), given in divided doses every 12 hours, should be administered with or without a loading dose of 75 mg/kg.

Generally, Rocephin therapy should be continued for at least two days after the signs and symptoms of infection have disappeared. The usual duration is 4 to 14 days; in complicated infections, longer therapy may be required.

When treating infections caused by *Streptococcus pyogenes*, therapy should be continued for at least ten days.

No dosage adjustment is necessary for patients with impairment of renal or hepatic function; however, blood levels should be monitored in patients with severe renal impairment (*e.g.*, dialysis patients) and in patients with both renal and hepatic dysfunctions.

DIRECTIONS FOR USE: Intramuscular Administration: Reconstitute Rocephin powder with the appropriate diluent (see COMPATIBILITY-STABILITY section).

Vial Dosage Size	Amount of Diluent to be Added
250 mg	0.9 mL
500 mg	1.8 mL
1 gm	3.6 mL
2 gm	7.2 mL

After reconstitution, each 1 mL of solution contains approximately 250 mg equivalent of ceftriaxone. If required, more dilute solutions could be utilized. As with all intramuscular preparations, Rocephin should be injected well within the body of a relatively large muscle; aspiration helps to avoid unintentional injection into a blood vessel.

Intravenous Administration: Rocephin should be administered intravenously by infusion over a period of 30 minutes. Concentrations between 10 mg/mL and 40 mg/mL are recommended; however, lower concentrations may be used if desired. Reconstitute vials or "piggyback" bottles with an appropriate I.V. diluent (see COMPATIBILITY-STABILITY section).

Vial Dosage Size	Amount of Diluent to be Added
250 mg	2.4 mL
500 mg	4.8 mL
1 gm	9.6 mL
2 gm	19.2 mL

After reconstitution, each 1 mL of solution contains approximately 100 mg equivalent of ceftriaxone. Withdraw entire contents and dilute to the desired concentration with the appropriate I.V. diluent.

Piggyback Bottle Dosage Size	Amount of Diluent to be Added
1 gm	10 mL
2 gm	20 mL

After reconstitution, further dilute to 50 mL or 100 mL volumes with the appropriate I.V. diluent.

10 gm Bulk Pharmacy Container: This dosage size is *NOT FOR DIRECT ADMINISTRATION.* Reconstitute powder with 95 mL of an appropriate I.V. diluent. Before parenteral administration, withdraw the required amount, then further dilute to the desired concentration.

COMPATIBILITY AND STABILITY: Rocephin sterile powder should be stored at room temperature—77°F (25°C)—or below and protected from light. After reconstitution, protection from normal light is not necessary. The color of solutions ranges from light yellow to amber, depending on the length of storage, concentration and diluent used.

Rocephin *intramuscular* solutions remain stable (loss of potency less than 10%) for the following time periods:

[See table above.]

Rocephin *intravenous* solutions, at concentrations of 10, 20 and 40 mg/mL, remain stable (loss of potency less than 10%) for the following time periods stored in glass or PVC containers: [See table below.]

Similarly, Rocephin *intravenous* solutions, at concentrations of 100 mg/mL, remain stable in the I.V. piggyback glass containers for the above specified time periods.

The following *intravenous* Rocephin solutions are stable at room temperature (25°C) for 24 hours, at concentrations between 10 mg/mL and 40 mg/mL: Sodium Lactate (PVC container), 10% Invert Sugar (glass container), 5% Sodium Bicarbonate (glass container), Freamine III (glass container), Normosol-M in 5% Dextrose (glass and PVC containers), Ionosol-B in 5% Dextrose (glass container), 5% Mannitol (glass container), 10% Mannitol (glass container).

After the indicated stability time periods, unused portions of solutions should be discarded.

Rocephin reconstituted with 5% Dextrose or 0.9% Sodium Chloride solution at concentrations between 10 mg/mL and 40 mg/mL, and then stored in frozen state (−20°C) in PVC (Viaflex) or polyolefin containers, remains stable for 26 weeks.

Frozen solutions should be thawed at room temperature before use. After thawing, unused portions should be discarded. **DO NOT REFREEZE.**

Rocephin solutions should *not* be physically mixed with or piggybacked into solutions containing other antimicrobial drugs or into diluent solutions other than those listed above, due to possible incompatibility.

Diluent	Storage Room Temp. (25°C)	Refrigerated (4°C)
Sterile Water	3 days	10 days
0.9% Sodium Chloride Solution	3 days	10 days
5% Dextrose Solution	3 days	10 days
10% Dextrose Solution	3 days	10 days
5% Dextrose + 0.9% Sodium Chloride Solution*	3 days	Incompatible
5% Dextrose + 0.45% Sodium Chloride Solution	3 days	Incompatible

*Data available for 10–40 mg/mL concentrations in this diluent in PVC containers only.

ANIMAL PHARMACOLOGY

Concretions consisting of the precipitated calcium salt of ceftriaxone have been found in the gallbladder bile of dogs and baboons treated with ceftriaxone.

These appeared as a gritty sediment in dogs that received 100 mg/kg/day for four weeks. A similar phenomenon has been observed in baboons but only after a protracted dosing period (6 months) at higher dose levels (335 mg/kg/day or

Continued on next page

Roche Laboratories—Cont.

more). The likelihood of this occurrence in humans is considered to be low, since ceftriaxone has a greater plasma half-life in humans, the calcium salt of ceftriaxone is more soluble in human gallbladder bile and the calcium content of human gallbladder bile is relatively low.

HOW SUPPLIED

Rocephin (ceftriaxone sodium/Roche) is supplied as a sterile crystalline powder in glass vials and piggyback bottles. The following packages are available:

Vials containing 250 mg equivalent of ceftriaxone. Boxes of 1 (NDC 0004-1962-02) and boxes of 10 (NDC 0004-1962-01).
Vials containing 500 mg equivalent of ceftriaxone. Boxes of 1 (NDC 0004-1963-02) and boxes of 10 (NDC 0004-1963-01).
Vials containing 1 gm equivalent of ceftriaxone. Boxes of 1 (NDC 0004-1964-04) and boxes of 10 (NDC 0004-1964-01).
Piggyback bottles containing 1 gm equivalent of ceftriaxone. Boxes of 10 (NDC 0004-1964-03).
Vials containing 2 gm equivalent of ceftriaxone. Boxes of 10 (NDC 0004-1965-01).
Piggyback bottles containing 2 gm equivalent of ceftriaxone. Boxes of 10 (NDC 0004-1965-03).
Bulk pharmacy containers, containing 10 gm equivalent of ceftriaxone. Boxes of 1 (NDC 0004-1971-01). NOT FOR DIRECT ADMINISTRATION.
Rocephin (ceftriaxone sodium/Roche) is also supplied as a sterile crystalline powder in ADD-Vantage®* Vials as follows:
ADD-Vantage Vials containing 1 gm equivalent of ceftriaxone. Boxes of 10 (NDC 0004-1964-05).
ADD-Vantage Vials containing 2 gm equivalent of ceftriaxone. Boxes of 10 (NDC 0004-1965-05).
Rocephin (ceftriaxone sodium/Roche) injection is also supplied premixed as a frozen, iso-osmotic, sterile, nonpyrogenic solution of ceftriaxone sodium in 50 mL single dose Galaxy®† containers (PL 2040 plastic). The following strengths are available:
1 gm equivalent of ceftriaxone, iso-osmotic with approximately 1.9 gm Dextrose Hydrous, USP, added (NDC 0004-2002-78).
2 gm equivalent of ceftriaxone, iso-osmotic with approximately 1.2 gm Dextrose Hydrous, USP, added (NDC 0004-2003-78).
NOTE: Store Rocephin in the frozen state at or below −20°C/−4°F.
Rocephin, supplied as a frozen, iso-osmotic, sterile, nonpyrogenic solution in Galaxy® containers (PL 2040 plastic), is manufactured for Roche Laboratories, a division of Hoffmann-La Roche Inc., by Baxter Healthcare Corporation, Deerfield, Illinois 60015.

REFERENCES

1. National Committee for Clinical Standards, *Performance Standards for Antimicrobial Disk Susceptibility Tests* —Fourth Edition. Approved Standard NCCLS Document M2-A4, Vol. 10, No. 7, NCCLS, Villanova, PA, 1990.
2. National Committee for Clinical Laboratory Standards, *Methods for Dilution Antimicrobial Susceptibility Tests for Bacteria That Grow Aerobically*—Second Edition. Approved Standard NCCLS Document M7-A2, Vol. 10, No. 8, NCCLS, Villanova, PA, 1990.
Revised: January 1992

* Registered trademark of Abbott Laboratories, Inc.
† Registered trademark of Baxter International Inc.

ROFERON®–A　　　℞
[ro-fear'on]
(Interferon alfa-2a, recombinant/Roche)

The following text is complete prescribing information based on official labeling in effect June 1, 1992.

DESCRIPTION

Roferon®–A (Interferon alfa-2a, recombinant/Roche) is a sterile protein product for use by injection. Roferon-A is manufactured by recombinant DNA technology that employs a genetically engineered *E. coli* bacterium containing DNA that codes for the human protein. Interferon alfa-2a, recombinant/Roche is a highly purified protein containing 165 amino acids, and it has an approximate molecular weight of 19,000 daltons. The purification procedure includes affinity chromatography using a murine monoclonal antibody. Fermentation is carried out in a defined nutrient medium containing the antibiotic tetracycline hydrochloride, 5 mg/L. However, the presence of the antibiotic is not detectable in the final product. Roferon-A is supplied as an injectable solution or as a sterile powder for injection with its accompanying diluent.

Injectable Solution:
3 million IU Roferon-A per vial —The solution is colorless and each mL contains 3 million IU of Interferon alfa-2a, recombinant/Roche, 9 mg sodium chloride, 5 mg Albumin (Human) and 3 mg phenol as a preservative.
18 million IU Roferon-A per vial —The solution is colorless and each mL contains 6 million IU of Interferon alfa-2a, recombinant/Roche, 9 mg sodium chloride, 5 mg Albumin (Human) and 3 mg phenol as a preservative. Each 0.5 mL contains 3 million IU of Interferon alfa-2a, recombinant/Roche.
36 million IU Roferon-A per vial —The solution is colorless and each mL contains 36 million IU of Interferon alfa-2a, recombinant/Roche, 9 mg sodium chloride, 5 mg Albumin (Human) and 3 mg phenol as a preservative.

Sterile Powder for Injection:
18 million IU Roferon-A per vial —The powder is white to beige and when reconstituted with Diluent for Sterile Powder for Injection each 1 mL of reconstituted solution contains 6 million IU of Interferon alfa-2a, recombinant/Roche, 9 mg sodium chloride, 5 mg Albumin (Human) and 3 mg phenol as a preservative. Each 0.5 mL contains 3 million IU of Interferon alfa-2a, recombinant/Roche.
Diluent for Sterile Powder for Injection:
3 mL per vial —Each mL contains 6 mg sodium chloride, 3.3 mg Albumin (Human) and 3 mg phenol as a preservative.
The specific activity of Interferon alfa-2a, recombinant/Roche is 2×10^8 IU/mg protein. The route of administration is subcutaneous or intramuscular.

CLINICAL PHARMACOLOGY

The mechanism by which Interferon alfa-2a, recombinant/Roche, or any other interferon, exerts antitumor activity is not clearly understood. However, it is believed that direct antiproliferative action against tumor cells and modulation of the host immune response play important roles in the antitumor activity.
The biological activities of Interferon alfa-2a, recombinant/Roche are species-restricted, *i.e.*, they are expressed in a very limited number of species other than humans. As a consequence, preclinical evaluation of Interferon alfa-2a, recombinant/Roche has involved *in vitro* experiments with human cells and some *in vivo* experiments. [1] Using human cells in culture, Interferon alfa-2a, recombinant/Roche has been shown to have antiproliferative and immunomodulatory activities that are very similar to those of the mixture of interferon alfa subtypes produced by human leukocytes. *In vivo*, Interferon alfa-2a, recombinant/Roche has been shown to inhibit the growth of several human tumors growing in immunocompromised (nude) mice. Because of its species-restricted activity, it has not been possible to demonstrate antitumor activity in immunologically intact syngeneic tumor model systems, where effects on the host immune system would be observable. However, such antitumor activity has been repeatedly demonstrated with, for example, mouse interferon-alfa in transplantable mouse tumor systems. The clinical significance of these findings is unknown.
The metabolism of Interferon alfa-2a, recombinant/Roche is consistent with that of alfa interferons in general. Alfa interferons are totally filtered through the glomeruli and undergo rapid proteolytic degradation during tubular reabsorption, rendering a negligible reappearance of intact alfa interferon in the systemic circulation. Small amounts of radiolabeled Interferon alfa-2a, recombinant/Roche appear in the urine of isolated rat kidneys, suggesting near complete reabsorption of Interferon alfa-2a, recombinant/Roche catabolites. Liver metabolism and subsequent biliary excretion are considered minor pathways of elimination for alfa interferons.
The serum concentrations of Interferon alfa-2a, recombinant/Roche reflected a large intersubject variation in both healthy volunteers and patients with disseminated cancer.

In healthy people, Interferon alfa-2a, recombinant/Roche exhibited an elimination half-life of 3.7 to 8.5 hours (mean 5.1 hours), volume of distribution at steady-state of 0.223 to 0.748 L/kg (mean 0.400 L/kg) and a total body clearance of 2.14 to 3.62 mL/min/kg (mean 2.79 mL/min/kg) after a 36 million IU (2.2×10^8 pg) intravenous infusion. After intramuscular and subcutaneous administrations of 36 million IU, peak serum concentrations ranged from 1500 to 2580 pg/mL (mean 2020 pg/mL) at a mean time to peak of 3.8 hours and from 1250 to 2320 pg/mL (mean 1730 pg/mL) at a mean time to peak of 7.3 hours, respectively. The apparent fraction of the dose absorbed after intramuscular injection was greater than 80%.
The pharmacokinetics of Interferon alfa-2a, recombinant/Roche after single intramuscular doses to patients with disseminated cancer were similar to those found in healthy volunteers. Dose proportional increases in serum concentrations were observed after single doses up to 198 million IU. There were no changes in the distribution or elimination of Interferon alfa-2a, recombinant/Roche during twice daily (0.5 to 36 million IU), once daily (1 to 54 million IU), or three times weekly (1 to 136 million IU) dosing regimens up to 28 days of dosing. Multiple intramuscular doses of Interferon alfa-2a, recombinant/Roche resulted in an accumulation of 2 to 4 times the single dose serum concentrations. Pharmacokinetic information in patients with hairy cell leukemia or AIDS-related Kaposi's sarcoma is presently unknown.
Serum neutralizing activity, determined by a highly sensitive enzyme immunoassay and a neutralization bioassay, was detected in approximately 25% of all patients who received Roferon-A.[2] Antibodies to human leukocyte interferon may occur spontaneously in certain clinical conditions (cancer, systemic lupus erythematosus, herpes zoster) in patients who have never received exogenous interferon.[3] The significance of the appearance of serum neutralizing activity is not known.
The acute parenteral toxicity of Interferon alfa-2a, recombinant/Roche has been studied in mice, rats, rabbits and ferrets at doses up to 30 million IU/kg intravenously, and 500 million IU/kg intramuscularly. No treatment-related mortality was noted in any species given Interferon alfa-2a, recombinant/Roche by any of the routes of administration.
EFFECTS ON HAIRY CELL LEUKEMIA: During the first one to two months of treatment of patients with hairy cell leukemia, significant depression of hematopoiesis was likely to occur. Subsequently, there was improvement in circulating blood cell counts.
Of the 75 patients who were evaluable for efficacy following at least 16 weeks of therapy, 46 (61%) achieved complete or partial response. Twenty-one patients (28%) had a minor remission, eight (11%) remained stable, and none had worsening of disease. All patients who achieved either a complete or partial response had complete or partial normalization of all peripheral blood elements including hemoglobin level, white blood cell, neutrophil, monocyte and platelet counts with a concomitant decrease in peripheral blood and bone marrow hairy cells. Responding patients also exhibited a marked reduction in red blood cell and platelet transfusion requirements, a decrease in infectious episodes and improvement in performance status. The probability of survival for two years in patients receiving Roferon-A (94%) was statistically increased compared to a historical control group (75%).
EFFECTS ON AIDS-RELATED KAPOSI'S SARCOMA: In six studies with Roferon-A, doses of 3 to 54 million IU daily were evaluated for the treatment of AIDS-related Kaposi's sarcoma in more than 350 patients. Four dosage regimens of Roferon-A were evaluated for initial induction. Thirty-nine patients received 3 million IU daily; 99 patients received an escalating regimen of 3 million, 9 million and 18 million IU each daily for 3 days, followed by 36 million IU daily; 119 patients received 36 million IU daily; and 16 patients received doses greater than 36 million IU to a maximum of 54 million IU daily. An additional 91 patients received Roferon-A in combination with vinblastine. The best response rate associated with acceptable toxicity was observed when Roferon-A was administered as a single agent at a dose of 36 million IU daily. The escalating regimen of 3 to 36 million IU daily provided equivalent therapeutic benefit with some amelioration of acute toxicity in some patients. In AIDS-related Kaposi's sarcoma, lower doses were less effective in inducing tumor regression and doses higher than 36 million IU daily were associated with unacceptable toxicity.
As summarized in Table 1, the likelihood of response to Roferon-A varied with the clinical manifestations of human immunodeficiency virus (HIV) infection. Patients with prior opportunistic infection or B symptoms are unlikely to respond to treatment with Roferon-A. [See table below.]
In the 28 patients evaluated who had prior opportunistic infection or B symptoms, the response rate was 3.6%.
Patients who were otherwise asymptomatic, with no prior opportunistic infection and near-normal levels of CD_4 lymphocytes, experienced higher response rates. Responding patients with a baseline CD_4 lymphocyte count greater than 200 cells/mm³ had a distinct survival advantage over both responding patients with a baseline CD_4 lymphocyte count of 200 cells/mm³ or less and nonresponding patients regardless

Table 1

Likelihood of Response to Roferon-A in Patients with
AIDS-Related Kaposi's Sarcoma

No. Pts.*	CD₄(T₄) Lymphocyte Count (cells/mm³)	Objective Response Rate (%)		
		CR	PR	Total
83	0–200	3.6	3.6	7.2
51	>200–400	15.7	11.8	27.5
33	>400	24.2	21.2	45.4

* Patients had no prior opportunistic infection or B symptoms. B symptoms include night sweats, weight loss of greater than 10% of body weight or 15 lbs., or fever greater than 100°F without an identifiable source of infection.

of their baseline CD_4 lymphocyte count. Median survival for responding patients with CD_4 lymphocyte counts of greater than 200 to 400 cells/mm^3 had not been reached but was greater than 32.7 months from the initiation of therapy. For responding patients with CD_4 lymphocyte counts of greater than 400 cells/mm^3, the median survival had not been reached but was greater than 29.5 months.

A classification system for staging AIDS-related Kaposi's sarcoma has been described based on location and extent of disease. In studies of Roferon-A, no difference was noted in response rates for patients with different stages of Kaposi's sarcoma. Likelihood of response was related to manifestations of HIV Infection (baseline CD_4 lymphocyte count, prior opportunistic infection or B symptons) and not to extent of tumor involvement. The median time to response was 2.7 months. The median duration of response for patients achieving a partial or complete response was 6.3 and 20.7 months, respectively. Complete and partial responses lasting in excess of three years have been observed. Therapy was discontinued because of progression of Kaposi's sarcoma, development of severe opportunistic infection or severe adverse effects. The median time to discontinuation of treatment was 12.5 months for responding patients and 2.3 months for patients who did not respond.

INDICATIONS AND USAGE

Roferon-A is indicated for use in the treatment of hairy cell leukemia and AIDS-related Kaposi's sarcoma in select patients 18 years of age or older. Studies have shown that Roferon-A can produce clinically meaningful tumor regression or disease stabilization in patients with hairy cell leukemia or in patients with AIDS-related Kaposi's sarcoma.[4–6]

FOR PATIENTS WITH HAIRY CELL LEUKEMIA: Prior to initiation of therapy, tests should be performed to quantitate peripheral blood hemoglobin, platelets, granulocytes and hairy cells and bone marrow hairy cells. These parameters should be monitored periodically (*e.g.,* monthly) during treatment to determine whether response to treatment has occurred. If a patient does not respond within six months, treatment should be discontinued. If a response to treatment does occur, treatment should be continued until no further improvement is observed and these laboratory parameters have been stable for about three months. It is not known whether continued treatment after that time is beneficial. Studies are in progress to evaluate this question.

FOR PATIENTS WITH AIDS-RELATED KAPOSI'S SARCOMA: Roferon-A is useful for the treatment of AIDS-related Kaposi's sarcoma in a select group of patients. In determining whether a patient should be treated, the physician should assess the likelihood of response based on the clinical manifestations of HIV infection and the manifestations of Kaposi's sarcoma requiring treatment. See CLINICAL PHARMACOLOGY.

Indicator lesion measurements and total lesion count should be performed before initiation of therapy. These parameters should be monitored periodically (*e.g.,* monthly) during treatment to determine whether response to treatment or disease stabilization has occurred. When disease stabilization or a response to treatment occurs, treatment should continue until there is no further evidence of tumor or until discontinuation is required because of a severe opportunistic infection or adverse effects.

CONTRAINDICATIONS

Roferon-A is contraindicated in patients with known hypersensitivity to alfa interferon, mouse immunoglobulin or any component of the product.

WARNINGS

Roferon-A should be administered under the guidance of a qualified physician. (See DOSAGE AND ADMINISTRATION.) Appropriate management of the therapy and its complications is possible only when adequate diagnostic and treatment facilities are readily available.

Roferon-A should not be used for the treatment of visceral AIDS-related Kaposi's sarcoma associated with rapidly progressive or life-threatening disease.

Roferon-A should be used with caution in patients with severe preexisting cardiac disease, severe renal or hepatic disease, seizure disorders and/or compromised central nervous system function.

Because of the possibility of severe or even fatal adverse reactions, patients should be informed not only of the benefits of therapy but also of the risks involved.

Roferon-A should be administered with caution to patients with cardiac disease or with any history of cardiac illness. No direct cardiotoxic effect has been demonstrated, but it is likely that acute, self-limited toxicities (*i.e.,* fever, chills) frequently associated with Roferon-A administration may exacerbate preexisting cardiac conditions. Rarely, myocardial infarction has occurred in patients receiving Roferon-A. Cases of cardiomyopathy have been observed on rare occasions in patients treated with alfa-interferons.

Caution should be exercised when administering Roferon-A to patients with myelosuppression or when Roferon-A is used in combination with other agents that are known to cause myelosuppression. Syngeristic toxicity has been observed when Roferon-A is administered in combination with zidovudine (AZT).[7] The effects of Roferon-A when combined with other drugs used in the treatment of AIDS-related disease are not known.

Central nervous system adverse reactions have been reported in a number of patients. These reactions included decreased mental status, exaggerated central nervous system function, and dizziness. More severe obtundation and coma have been rarely observed. Most of these abnormalities were mild and reversible within a few days to three weeks upon dose reduction or discontinuation of Roferon-A therapy. Careful periodic neuropsychiatric monitoring of all patients is recommended.

Leukopenia and elevation of hepatic enzymes occurred frequently but were rarely dose-limiting. Thrombocytopenia occurred less frequently. Proteinuria and increased cells in urinary sediment were also seen infrequently. Rarely, significant hepatic, renal and myelosuppressive toxicities were noted.

PRECAUTIONS

General: In all instances where the use of Roferon-A is considered for chemotherapy, the physician must evaluate the need and usefulness of the drug against the risk of adverse reactions. Most adverse reactions are reversible if detected early. If severe reactions occur, the drug should be reduced in dosage or discontinued and appropriate corrective measures should be taken according to the clinical judgment of the physician. Reinstitution of Roferon-A therapy should be carried out with caution and with adequate consideration of the further need for the drug and alertness as to possible recurrence of toxicity.

The minimum effective doses of Roferon-A for treatment of hairy cell leukemia and AIDS-related Kaposi's sarcoma have not been established. Variations in dosage and adverse reactions exist among different brands of Interferon. Therefore, do not use different brands of Interferon in a single treatment regimen.

Information for Patient: Patients should be cautioned not to change brands of Interferon without medical consultation, as a change in dosage may result. Patients should be informed regarding the potential benefits and risks attendant to the use of Roferon-A. If home use is determined to be desirable by the physician, instructions on appropriate use should be given, including review of the contents of the enclosed Patient Information Sheet. Patients should be well hydrated, especially during the initial stages of treatment.

Patients should be thoroughly instructed in the importance of proper disposal procedures and cautioned against reusing syringes and needles. If home use is prescribed, a puncture resistant container for the disposal of used syringes and needles should be supplied to the patient. The full container should be disposed of according to directions provided by the physician.

Patients receiving high dose alfa-interferon should be cautioned against performing tasks that require complete mental alertness such as operating machinery or driving a motor vehicle.

Laboratory Tests: Complete blood counts and clinical chemistry tests should be performed before initiation of Roferon-A therapy and at appropriate periods during therapy. Since responses of hairy cell leukemia and AIDS-related Kaposi's sarcoma are not generally observed for one to three months after initiation of treatment, very careful monitoring for severe depression of blood cell counts is warranted during the initial phase of treatment.

Those patients who have preexisting cardiac abnormalities and/or are in advanced stages of cancer should have electrocardiograms taken before and during the course of treatment.

Carcinogenesis, Mutagenesis and Impairment of Fertility:

Carcinogenesis: Roferon-A has not been tested for its carcinogenic potential.

Mutagenesis: A. Internal studies—Ames tests using six different tester strains, with and without metabolic activation, were performed with Roferon-A up to a concentration of 1920 µg/plate. There was no evidence of mutagenicity.

Human lymphocyte cultures were treated *in vitro* with Roferon-A at noncytotoxic concentrations. No increase in the incidence of chromosomal damage was noted.

B. Published studies—There are no published studies on the mutagenic potential of Roferon-A. However, a number of studies on the genotoxicity of human leukocyte interferon have been reported.

A chromosomal defect following the addition of human leukocyte interferon to lymphocyte cultures from a patient suffering from a lymphoproliferative disorder has been reported.

In contrast, other studies have failed to detect chromosomal abnormalities following treatment of lymphocyte cultures from healthy volunteers with human leukocyte interferon.

It has also been shown that human leukocyte interferon protects primary chick embryo fibroblasts from chromosomal aberrations produced by gamma rays.

Impairment of Fertility: Roferon-A has been studied for its effect on fertility in Macaca mulatta (rhesus monkeys). Nonpregnant rhesus females treated with Roferon-A at doses of 5 and 25 milion IU/kg/day have shown menstrual cycle irregularities, including prolonged or shortened menstrual periods and erratic bleeding; these cycles were considered to be anovulatory on the basis that reduced progesterone levels were noted and that expected increases in preovulatory estrogen and luteinizing hormones were not observed. These monkeys returned to a normal menstrual rhythm following discontinuation of treatment.

Drug Interactions: Roferon-A, apparently through an unknown effect on certain microsomal enzyme systems, has been reported to reduce the clearance of theophylline.[8,9] The clinical relevance of this interaction is presently unknown. Interactions between Roferon-A and other drugs have not been fully evaluated. Caution should be exercised when administering Roferon-A in combination with other potentially myelosuppressive agents. See WARNINGS.

PREGNANCY

Teratogenic Effects: Pregnancy Category C. Roferon-A has been shown to demonstrate a statistically significant increase in abortifacient activity in rhesus monkeys when given at approximately 20 to 500 times the human dose. A study in pregnant rhesus monkeys treated with 1, 5 or 25 million IU/kg/day of Roferon-A in their early to midfetal period (days 22 to 70 of gestation) has failed to demonstrate teratogenic activity for Roferon-A.

There are no adequate and well-controlled studies in pregnant women.

Nonteratogenic Effects: Dose-related abortifacient activity was observed in pregnant rhesus monkeys treated with 1, 5 or 25 million IU/kg/day of Roferon-A in their early to midfetal period (days 22 to 70 of gestation). A late-fetal period study (days 79 to 100 of gestation) is in progress and as yet there have been no reports of any increased rate of abortion.

Usage in Pregnancy: Safe use in human pregnancy has not been established. Therefore, Roferon-A should be used during pregnancy only if the potential benefit justifies the potential risk to the fetus. Information from primate studies showed dose-related menstrual irregularities and an increased incidence of spontaneous abortions. Decreases in serum estradiol and progesterone concentrations have been reported in women treated with human leukocyte interferon.[10] Therefore, fertile women should not receive Roferon-A unless they are using effective contraception during the therapy period.

Male fertility and teratologic evaluations have yielded no significant adverse effects to date.

Nursing Mothers: It is not known whether this drug is excreted in human milk. Because many drugs are excreted in human milk and because of the potential for serious adverse reactions in nursing infants from Roferon-A, a decision should be made whether to discontinue nursing or to discontinue the drug, taking into account the importance of the drug to the mother.

Pediatric Use: Safety and effectiveness in children under 18 years of age have not been established.

ADVERSE REACTIONS

The following data on adverse reactions are based on the subcutaneous or intramuscular administration of Roferon-A as a single agent. Most of the adverse reactions reported were mild to moderate and diminished in severity and number with continued therapy. More severe adverse reactions were observed at higher doses and may require dose reduction.

FOR PATIENTS WITH HAIRY CELL LEUKEMIA:

Flu-like Symptoms—Fever (98%), fatigue (89%), myalgia (73%), headache (71%), chills (64%) and arthralgia (5%).

Gastrointestinal—Anorexia (46%), nausea (32%), diarrhea (29%) and emesis (10%).

Central and Peripheral Nervous System—Dizziness (21%), paresthesia (6%), numbness (6%) and transient impotence (6%).

Skin—Rash (18%), dry skin or pruritus (13%) and partial alopecia (8%).

Other—Dryness or inflammation of the oropharynx (16%), weight loss (14%), change in taste (13%), diaphoresis (8%) and reactivation of herpes liabialis (8%).

Rarely (< 3%), central nervous system effects including decreased mental status, depression, visual disturbances, sleep disturbances and nervousness, as well as cardiac adverse events, including hypertension, chest pain, arrhythmias and palpitations, were reported. Adverse experiences that occurred rarely, and may have been related to underlying disease, included epistaxis, bleeding gums, ecchymosis and petechiae. Miscellaneous adverse events, such as night sweats, urticaria, conjunctivitis and inflammation at the site of injection, were also rarely observed.

FOR PATIENTS WITH AIDS-RELATED KAPOSI'S SARCOMA:

Flu-like Symptoms—Fatigue (95%), fever (74%), myalgia (69%), headache (66%), chills (41%) and arthralgia (24%).

Continued on next page

Roche Laboratories—Cont.

Gastrointestinal—Anorexia (65%), nausea (51%), diarrhea (42%), emesis (17%) and abdominal pain (15%).
Central and Peripheral Nervous System—Dizziness (40%), decreased mental status (17%), depression (16%), paresthesia (8%), confusion (8%), diaphoresis (7%), visual disturbances (5%), sleep disturbances (5%) and numbness (3%).
Pulmonary and Cardiovascular—Coughing (27%), dyspnea (11%), edema (9%), chest pain (4%) and hypotension (4%).
Skin—Partial alopecia (22%), rash (11%) and dry skin or pruritus (5%).
Other—Weight loss (25%), change in taste (25%), dryness or inflammation of the oropharynx (14%), night sweats (8%) and rhinorrhea (4%).
Occasionally (<3%) nervous system effects including anxiety, nervousness, emotional lability, vertigo and forgetfulness, as well as cardiac adverse events, including palpitations and arrhythmia, were reported. Other adverse experiences that occurred occasionally (<3%) and may have been related to underlying disease, included sinusitis, constipation, chest congestion, urticaria, and flatulence. Adverse experiences which occurred rarely (<1%) included ataxia, seizures, cyanosis, gastric distress, bronchospasm, pain at injection site, earache, eye irritation and rhinitis. Miscellaneous adverse experiences such as poor coordination, lethargy, muscle contractions, neuropathy, tremor, involuntary movement, syncope, aphasia, aphonia, dysarthria, amnesia, weakness, and flushing of skin were observed in less than 0.5% of patients. Cases of cardiomyopathy have been observed on rare occasions in patients treated with alfa-interferons.
In other investigational studies of Roferon-A, in addition to the adverse experiences noted above, other adverse experiences that occurred included: abdominal fullness, hypermotility, hepatitis, gait disturbance, hallucinations, encephalopathy. psychomotor retardation, coma, stroke, transient ischemic attacks, dysphasia, sedation, apathy, irritability, hyperactivity, claustrophobia, loss of libido, congestive heart failure, myocardial infarction, Raynaud's phenomenon, hot flashes, tachypnea, and excessive salivation. These adverse experiences occurred rarely (<1%).
ABNORMAL LABORATORY TEST VALUES: The percentage of patients with hairy cell leukemia or AIDS-related Kaposi's sarcoma who experienced a significant abnormal laboratory test value (NCI grades III or IV) at least once during their treatment with Roferon-A is shown in the following table:

ABNORMAL LABORATORY TEST VALUES

	Hairy Cell Leukemia (n=63)	AIDS-Related Kaposi's Sarcoma (n=241)
Leukopenia	NA*	49%
Neutropenia	NA	52%
Thrombocytopenia	NA	35%
Decreased Hemoglobin	NA	27%
SGOT	42%	46%
Alkaline Phosphatase	8%	11%
LDH	13%	10%
Bilirubin	2%	<1%
BUN	4%	0%
Serum Creatinine	2%	<1%
Proteinuria	0%	<1%

*Not Applicable—Patient's initial hematologic laboratory test values were abnormal due to their underlying disease.

Increases in fasting serum glucose, serum phosphorus and serum uric acid levels and decreases in serum calcium levels were also observed in less than 5% of patients.

DOSAGE AND ADMINISTRATION

The recommended dosages of Roferon-A differ for hairy cell leukemia and AIDS-related Kaposi's sarcoma. See indication-specific dosages below.
HAIRY CELL LEUKEMIA—The induction dose of Roferon-A is 3 million IU daily for 16 to 24 weeks, administered as a subcutaneous or intramuscular injection. Subcutaneous administration is particularly suggested for, but not limited to, thrombocytopenia patients (platelet count <50,000) or for patients at risk for bleeding. The recommended maintenance dose is 3 million IU, three times per week. Dose reduction by one-half or withholding of individual doses may be needed when severe adverse reactions occur. The use of doses higher than 3 million IU is not recommended in hairy cell leukemia. The 36 million IU dosage form should not be used for the treatment of hairy cell leukemia.
Patients should be treated for approximately six months before the physician determines whether to continue therapy in patients who respond or discontinue therapy in patients who did not respond. Patients with hairy cell leukemia have been treated for up to 24 consecutive months. The optimal duration of treatment for this disease has not been determined.
AIDS-RELATED KAPOSI'S SARCOMA—The recommended induction dose of Roferon-A is 36 million IU daily for 10 to 12 weeks, administered as an intramuscular or subcutaneous injection. Subcutaneous administration is particularly suggested for, but not limited to, patients who are thrombocytopenic (platelet count <50,000) or who are at risk for bleeding. The recommended maintenance dose is 36 million IU, three times per week. Dose reductions by one-half or withholding of individual doses may be required when severe adverse reactions occur. An escalating schedule of 3 million IU, 9 million IU and 18 million IU each daily for 3 days followed by 36 million IU daily for the remainder of the 10 to 12 week induction period has also produced equivalent therapeutic benefit with some amelioration of the acute toxicity in some patients.
When disease stabilization or a response to treatment occurs, treatment should continue until there is no further evidence of tumor or until discontinuation is required because of a severe opportunistic infection or adverse effects. The optimal duration of treatment for this disease has not been determined.
If severe reactions occur, the dose should be modified (50% reduction) or therapy should be temporarily discontinued until the adverse reactions abate. The need for dose reduction should take into account the effects of prior X-ray therapy or chemotherapy that may have compromised bone marrow reserve. The minimum effective doses of Roferon-A for the treatment of hairy cell leukemia and AIDS-related Kaposi's sarcoma have not been established.
Parenteral drug products should be inspected visually for particulate matter and discoloration before administration, whenever solution and container permit.

HOW SUPPLIED

Injectable Solution:
3 million IU Roferon-A per vial—Each 1 mL contains 3 million IU of Interferon alfa-2a, recombinant/Roche, 9 mg sodium chloride, 5 mg Albumin (Human) and 3 mg phenol as a preservative. Boxes of 1 (NDC 0004-1987-09).
18 million IU Roferon-A per vial—Each 1 mL contains 6 million IU of Interferon alfa-2a, recombinant/Roche, 9 mg sodium chloride, 5 mg Albumin (Human) and 3 mg phenol as a preservative. Each 0.5 mL contains 3 million IU of Interferon alfa-2a, recombinant/Roche. Boxes of 1 (NDC 0004-1988-09).
36 million IU Roferon-A per vial—Each 1 mL contains 36 million IU of Interferon alfa-2a, recombinant/Roche, 9 mg sodium chloride, 5 mg Albumin (Human) and 3 mg phenol as a preservative. This dosage form should not be used for the treatment of hairy cell leukemia. Boxes of 1 (NDC 0004-2005-09).
Sterile Powder for Injection:
18 million IU Roferon-A per vial—Reconstitute with 3 mL diluent and swirl gently to dissolve. When reconstituted with accompanying Diluent for Roferon-A, each 1 mL of reconstituted solution contains 6 million IU Interferon alfa-2a, recombinant/Roche, 9 mg sodium chloride, 5 mg Albumin (Human) and 3 mg phenol as a preservative. Each 0.5 mL contains 3 million IU of Interferon alfa-2a, recombinant/Roche. Once the powder is reconstituted, it must be used within 30 days. Boxes of 1 (NDC 0004-1993-09).

STORAGE

The sterile powder and its accompanying diluent, the reconstituted solution and the injectable solution should be stored in the refrigerator at 36° to 46°F (2° to 8°C). Do *not* freeze or shake.

REFERENCES

1. Trown PW *et al: Cancer 57* (Suppl.): 1648–1656, 1986. 2. Itri LM *et al: Cancer 59*:668–674, 1987. 3. Jones GJ, Itri LM: *Cancer 57* (Suppl.): 1709–1715, 1986. 4. Foon KA *et al: Blood 64* (Suppl. 1): 164a, 1984. 5. Quesada JR *et al: Cancer 57* (Suppl.): 1678–1680, 1986. 6. Krown SE *et al: N Eng. J Med 308:* 1071–1076, 1983. 7. Krown SE *et al: Proc Am Soc Clin Oncol 7:* 1, 1988. 8. Williams SJ *et al: Lancet 2:* 939–941, 1987. 9. Jonkman JHG *et al: Br J Clin Pharmacol 2(27)* 795–802, 1989. 10. Kauppila A *et al: Int J Cancer 29:* 291–294, 1982.
Revised: November 1990

SYNKAYVITE® ℞
(menadiol sodium diphosphate/Roche)
INJECTION

The following text is complete product information based on official labeling in effect June 1, 1992.

DESCRIPTION

Synkayvite (menadiol sodium diphosphate/Roche) Injection, a synthetic water-soluble derivative of menadione (vitamin K_3), is a sterile aqueous solution intended for intramuscular, intravenous or subcutaneous administration. Synkayvite Injection is available in the following concentrations:
1-ml Ampuls, 5 mg/ml—each ml contains 5 mg menadiol sodium diphosphate compounded with 2.5 mg sodium metabisulfite, 0.45% phenol as preservative, 0.4% sodium chloride for isotonicity and sodium hydroxide to adjust pH to approximately 8.0.
1-ml Ampuls, 10 mg/ml—each ml contains 10 mg menadiol sodium diphosphate compounded with 2.5 mg sodium metabisulfite, 0.45% phenol as preservative, 0.4% sodium chloride for isotonicity and sodium hydroxide to adjust pH to approximately 8.0.
2-ml Ampuls, 75 mg/2 ml—each 2 ml contains 75 mg menadiol sodium diphosphate compounded with 5 mg sodium metabisulfite, 0.45% phenol as preservative, 0.4% sodium chloride for isotonicity and sodium hydroxide to adjust pH to approximately 8.0.
Chemically, menadiol sodium diphosphate is 2-methyl-1,4-naphthalenediol bis (dihydrogen phosphate) tetrasodium salt, hexahydrate. It is a white to pink hygroscopic powder with a characteristic odor and is very soluble in water and insoluble in alcohol. It has a molecular weight of 530.18.

CLINICAL PHARMACOLOGY

Synkayvite is converted *in vivo* to menadione (vitamin K_3). Its potency is approximately one-half that of menadione. Synkayvite is similar in activity to naturally occurring vitamin K, which is necessary for the synthesis in the liver of blood coagulation factors prothrombin (factor II), proconvertin (factor VII), thromboplastin (factor IX) and Stuart factor (factor X). The prothrombin test is sensitive to the concentrations of factors II, VII and X. The mechanism by which vitamin K_1 promotes formation of these clotting factors is not known, but animal data suggest that it acts as an enzyme or catalyst upon a substrate within the liver or combines with an apoenzyme (AE) to form an active enzyme (AE-K) which then is involved in prothrombin synthesis.
Pharmacokinetic data are unavailable because there is no acceptable assay procedure for the determination of menadiol in biological specimens. The physiochemical properties of menadiol sodium diphosphate indicate a negligible potential for absorption problems. The action of menadiol sodium diphosphate is generally detectable within one to two hours following parenteral administration; the prothrombin time often returns to normal in 8 to 24 hours. Vitamin K appears to pass through the placenta.

INDICATIONS AND USAGE

Synkayvite Injection is indicated for the treatment of hypoprothrombinemia secondary to factors limiting absorption or synthesis of vitamin K, *e.g.,* obstructive jaundice, biliary fistula, sprue, ulcerative colitis, celiac disease, intestinal resection, cystic fibrosis of the pancreas, regional enteritis and antibacterial therapy.
It is also indicated in hypoprothrombinemia secondary to administration of salicylates.
Synkayvite Injection may also be used as a liver function test, although newer methods are available.

CONTRAINDICATIONS

Vitamin K, or any of its synthetic analogs, should not be administered to the mother during the *last few weeks of pregnancy* as a prophylactic measure against physiologic hypoprothrombinemia or hemorrhagic disease of the newborn.
Synkayvite is contraindicated in patients with known hypersensitivity to the drug.

WARNINGS

Synkayvite Injection should not be used in the prophylaxis and treatment of hemorrhagic disease of the newborn, because phytonadione/Roche (Konakion®) is safer than the water-soluble vitamin K analogs.
Synkayvite and other water-soluble vitamin K analogs are ineffective in the treatment of oral anticoagulant-induced hypoprothrombinemia and, therefore, should not be used in its treatment. Synkayvite will not counteract the anticoagulant action of heparin.
Synkayvite Injection contains sodium metabisulfite, a sulfite that may cause allergic-type reactions, including anaphylactic symptoms and life-threatening or less severe asthmatic episodes in certain susceptible people. The overall prevalence of sulfite sensitivity in the general population is unknown and probably low. Sulfite sensitivity is seen more frequently in asthmatic than in nonasthmatic people.

PRECAUTIONS

General: Temporary resistance to prothrombin-depressing anticoagulants may result, especially when larger doses of Synkayvite are used. If relatively large doses have been employed, it may be necessary when reinstituting anticoagulant therapy to use somewhat larger doses of prothrombin-depressing anticoagulant or one which has a different mode of action, such as heparin.
Since the liver is the site of metabolic synthesis of prothrombin, hypoprothrombinemia resulting from hepatocellular damage is not corrected by administration of vitamin K. Repeated large doses of vitamin K are not warranted in liver disease if the response to initial use of the vitamin is unsatisfactory (Koller test).
Failure to respond to vitamin K may indicate that a coagulation defect is present or that the condition being treated is unresponsive to vitamin K.
Laboratory Tests: The dose, route and frequency of administration and duration of treatment depend on the severity of

the prothrombin deficiency and should be regulated by repeated determinations of prothrombin time.

Drug Interactions: Patients being treated with coumarin and indandione derivative anticoagulants are extremely sensitive to changes in available vitamin K. Therefore, large doses of menadione or menadiol sodium diphosphate may decrease patient sensitivity to oral anticoagulants, although these vitamin K analogs are ineffective in treating anticoagulant overdosage.

Drug/Laboratory Test Interactions: Menadione has been reported to interfere with the modified Reedy, Jenkins, Thorn procedure for determining urinary 17-hydroxycorticosteroids, producing falsely elevated levels.

Carcinogenesis, Mutagenesis and Impairment of Fertility: Synkayvite has not undergone adequate animal testing to evaluate carcinogenic potential. The mutagenicity of Synkayvite has not been evaluated in the Ames test. Synkayvite has not been evaluated for effects on fertility.

Pregnancy: Teratogenic Effects: Pregnancy Category C. Segment II reproduction studies have not been conducted with menadiol. However, menadione (vitamin K_3) was nonteratogenic in rats at doses of 15 and 150 mg/day. The 150 mg/day dose in rats is approximately 872 times the maximum human therapeutic dose of 30 mg daily for the treatment of hypoprothrombinemia and 350 times the human dose of 75 mg for the liver function test. It is not known whether Synkayvite can cause fetal harm when administered to a pregnant woman or can affect reproductive capacity. Synkayvite should be given to a pregnant woman only if clearly needed.

Nonteratogenic effects: Retardation of skeletal ossification and an increase in fetal resorptions have been reported in rats with menadione (vitamin K_3).

Menadione and its derivatives have been implicated in producing hemolytic anemia, hyperbilirubinemia and kernicterus in the newborn, especially in premature infants, when administered to the mother prior to delivery or to the newborn. A marked hyperbilirubinemia has been reported in premature infants of mothers given menadione 2 to 112 hours prior to delivery. Synkayvite given parenterally during labor caused an elevation in prothrombin levels in 16 of 22 infants. (Also see **Contraindications** section.)

Nursing Mothers: A study has shown that vitamin K is excreted in human milk. This should be considered if it is necessary to administer Synkayvite to a nursing mother.

Pediatric Use: See **Warnings** section.

ADVERSE REACTIONS

In adults, bromsulfalein retention and prolongation of prothrombin time have been reported after maximum doses of vitamin K analogs. In infants (particularly premature babies), excessive doses of vitamin K analogs may cause increased bilirubinemia in the first few days of life. This, in turn, may result in kernicterus, which may lead to brain damage or even death. Immaturity is apparently an important factor in the appearance of toxic reactions to vitamin K analogs as full-term and larger premature infants demonstrate greater tolerance than smaller premature infants. (Also see **Warnings** section.)

Menadione can induce erythrocyte hemolysis in persons having a genetic deficiency of glucose-6-phosphate dehydrogenase in their red blood cells.

In patients with severe hepatic disease, large doses of menadione may further depress liver function. Paradoxically, the administration of excessive doses of vitamin K or its analogs in an attempt to correct the hypoprothrombinemia associated with severe hepatitis or cirrhosis may actually result in a further depression of the concentration of prothrombin. (Also see **Precautions,** *General,* section.)

Occasional allergic reactions, such as skin rash and urticaria, have been reported.

OVERDOSAGE

There are no data available on overdosage of Synkayvite in man. The administration of large doses of menadione and its derivatives to animals has resulted in the production of anemia, polycythemia, splenomegaly, renal and hepatic damage and death.

The acute intravenous toxicity of Synkayvite is as follows:

	$LD_{50} \pm S.D.$
Mouse	500 ± 55 mg/kg
Rat	400 ± 65 mg/kg

DOSAGE AND ADMINISTRATION

The U.S. Recommended Daily Allowances for vitamin K in humans have not been established officially. The adequate daily dietary intake of vitamin K for adults has been estimated to be 70 to 140 mcg; for infants 10 to 20 mcg; for children and adolescents 15 to 100 mcg. The dietary abundance of vitamin K normally satisfies the requirements except for the neonatal period of 5 to 8 days.

Synkayvite may be injected subcutaneously, intramuscularly or intravenously. The response after intravenous administration may be more prompt, but more sustained action follows intramuscular or subcutaneous use.

Duration of treatment and frequency of dosage should be governed by blood prothrombin-time determination. In the absence of impaired liver function, a single dose usually corrects hypoprothrombinemia in 8 to 24 hours. Injections should be repeated in 12 hours if tests at this time show no evidence of improvement.

Following are the usual recommended dosages:

	ADULTS	CHILDREN
For treatment of hypoprothrombinemia	5 to 15 mg once or twice daily	5 to 10 mg once or twice daily
For liver function test	75 mg intravenously	

Parenteral drug products should be inspected visually for particulate matter and discoloration prior to administration, whenever solution and container permit. Synkayvite Injection is incompatible with protein hydrolysate.

HOW SUPPLIED

1-ml Ampuls (5 mg menadiol sodium diphosphate/ml) —boxes of 10 (NDC 0004-1923-06).
1-ml Ampuls (10 mg menadiol sodium diphosphate/ml) —boxes of 10 (NDC 0004-1924-06).
2-ml Ampuls (75 mg menadiol sodium diphosphate/2 ml) —boxes of 10 (NDC 0004-1925-06).
Store at room temperature (15° to 30°C or 59° to 86°F). Synkayvite need not be refrigerated.
Revised: February 1987

SYNKAYVITE®   ℞
(menadiol sodium diphosphate/Roche)
TABLETS

The following text is complete product information based on official labeling in effect June 1, 1992.

DESCRIPTION

Synkayvite (menadiol sodium diphosphate/Roche), a synthetic, water-soluble derivative of menadione (vitamin K_3), is available for oral administration in 5-mg tablets. Each tablet also contains gelatin, lactose, magnesium stearate, corn starch and talc. Chemically, menadiol sodium diphosphate is 2-methyl-1,4-naphthalenediol bis (dihydrogen phosphate) tetrasodium salt, hexahydrate. It is a white to pink hygroscopic powder with a characteristic odor and is very soluble in water and insoluble in alcohol. It has a molecular weight of 530.18.

CLINICAL PHARMACOLOGY

Synkayvite is converted *in vivo* to menadione (vitamin K_3). Its potency is approximately one-half that of menadione. Synkayvite is similar in activity to naturally occurring vitamin K, which is necessary for the synthesis in the liver of blood coagulation factors prothrombin (factor II), proconvertin (factor VII), thromboplastin (factor IX) and Stuart factor (factor X). The prothrombin test is sensitive to the concentrations of factors II, VII and X. The mechanism by which vitamin K_1 promotes formation of these clotting factors is not known, but animal data suggest that it acts as an enzyme or catalyst upon a substrate within the liver or combines with an apoenzyme (AE) to form an active enzyme (AE-K) which then is involved in prothrombin synthesis.

Pharmacokinetic data are unavailable because there is no acceptable assay procedure for the determination of menadiol in biological specimens. The physiochemical properties of menadiol sodium diphosphate indicate a negligible potential for absorption problems. The onset and duration of action following oral administration are not known. Vitamin K appears to pass through the placenta.

INDICATIONS AND USAGE

Synkayvite Tablets are indicated for:
—vitamin K deficiency secondary to the administration of antibacterial therapy;
—hypoprothrombinemia secondary to obstructive jaundice and biliary fistulas;
—hypoprothrombinemia secondary to administration of salicylates.

CONTRAINDICATIONS

Vitamin K, or any of its synthetic analogs, should not be administered to the mother *during the last few weeks of pregnancy* as a prophylactic measure against physiologic hypoprothrombinemia or hemorrhagic disease of the newborn. Synkayvite is contraindicated in patients with known hypersensitivity to the drug.

WARNINGS

Synkayvite and other water-soluble vitamin K analogs are ineffective in the treatment of oral anticoagulant-induced hypoprothrombinemia and should, therefore, not be used in its treatment. Synkayvite will not counteract the anticoagulant action of heparin.

PRECAUTIONS

General: Temporary resistance to prothrombin-depressing anticoagulants may result, especially when larger doses of Synkayvite are used. If relatively large doses have been employed, it may be necessary when reinstituting anticoagulant therapy to use somewhat larger doses of the prothrom-

bin-depressing anticoagulant or one which has a different mode of action, such as heparin.

Since the liver is the site of metabolic synthesis of prothrombin, hypoprothrombinemia resulting from hepatocellular damage is not corrected by administration of vitamin K. Repeated large doses of vitamin K are not warranted in liver disease if the response to initial use of the vitamin is unsatisfactory (Koller test).

Failure to respond to vitamin K may indicate that a coagulation defect is present or that the condition being treated is unresponsive to vitamin K.

Information for Patients: To assure safe and effective use of this drug, the following information and instructions should be given to the patient:

1. Take this medication exactly as directed by your doctor. Do not increase or decrease the prescribed dosage, or take it more often, or take it for a longer period of time than instructed.

2. If you miss a dose, take it as soon as possible, and then continue with your normal dosing schedule. Do not take the missed dose if it is almost time for your next dose; continue on your normal schedule and inform your doctor about any doses that you miss. If you have any questions about this, ask your doctor or pharmacist.

3. Inform all doctors and pharmacists that you are taking this medication; other medicines may affect the way this medicine works.

4. Before starting or stopping any other medications, including nonprescription drugs such as aspirin, check with your doctor or pharmacist.

5. A blood test should be performed at regular intervals to determine how this medicine is working. This will help your doctor decide the best dosing schedule for you.

6. Inform your doctor if you are pregnant or become pregnant while using this drug, even though vitamin K has not been shown to cause birth defects or other problems. Also inform your doctor if you are nursing.

Laboratory Tests: The dose, route and frequency of administration and duration of treatment depend on the severity of the prothrombin deficiency and should be regulated by repeated determinations of prothrombin time.

Drug Interactions: Patients being treated with coumarin and indandione derviative anticoagulants are extremely sensitive to changes in available vitamin K. Therefore, large doses of menadione or menadiol sodium diphosphate may decrease patient sensitivity to oral anticoagulants, although these vitamin K analogs are ineffective in treating anticoagulant overdosage.

Drug/Laboratory Test Interactions: Menadione has been reported to interfere with the modified Reddy, Jenkins, Thorn procedure for determining urinary 17-hydroxycorticosteroids, producing falsely elevated levels.

Carcinogenesis, Mutagenesis and Impairment of Fertility: Synkayvite has not undergone adequate animal testing to evaluate carcinogenic potential. The mutagenicity of Synkayvite has not been evaluated in the Ames test. Synkayvite has not been evaluated for effects on fertility.

Pregnancy: Teratogenic Effects: Pregnancy Category C. Segment II reproduction studies have not been conducted with menadiol. However, menadione (vitamin K_3) was nonteratogenic in rats at doses of 15 and 150 mg/day. The 150 mg/day dose in rats is approximately 2640 times the maximum human therapeutic dose of 10 mg daily. It is not known whether Synkayvite can cause fetal harm when administered to a pregnant woman or can affect reproductive capacity. Synkayvite should be given to a pregnant woman only if clearly needed.

Nonteratogenic Effects: Retardation of skeletal ossification and an increase in fetal resorptions have been reported in rats with menadione (vitamin K_3).

Menadione and its derivatives have been implicated in producing hemolytic anemia, hyperbilirubinemia and kernicterus in the newborn, especially in premature infants, when administered to the mother prior to delivery or to the newborn. A marked hyperbilirubinemia has been reported in premature infants of mothers given menadione 2 to 112 hours prior to delivery. Synkayvite given parenterally during labor caused an elevation in prothrombin levels in 16 of 22 infants. (Also see **Contraindications** section.)

Nursing Mothers: A study has shown that vitamin K is excreted in human milk. This should be considered if it is necessary to administer Synkayvite to a nursing mother.

ADVERSE REACTIONS

Bromsulfalein retention and prolongation of prothrombin time have been reported after maximum doses of vitamin K analogs.

Menadione can induce erythrocyte hemolysis in persons having a genetic deficiency of glucose-6-phosphate dehydrogenase in their red blood cells.

In patients with severe hepatic disease, large doses of menadione may further depress liver function. Paradoxically, the administration of excessive doses of vitamin K or its analogs in an attempt to correct the hypoprothrombinemia associ-

Continued on next page

Roche Laboratories—Cont.

ated with severe hepatitis or cirrhosis may actually result in a further depression of the concentration of prothrombin. (Also see **Precautions,** *General,* section.)
Occasional allergic reactions, such as skin rash and urticaria, have been reported. There have also been minor instances of gastric disturbance.

OVERDOSAGE

There are no data on overdosage of Synkayvite in man. The administration of large doses of menadione and its derivatives to animals has resulted in the production of anemia, polycythemia, splenomegaly, renal and hepatic damage and death.
The acute oral toxicity of Synkayvite is as follows:

	$LD_{50} \pm$ S.D.
Mouse	6172 ± 966 mg/kg
Rat	5250 ± 740 mg/kg

DOSAGE AND ADMINISTRATION

The U.S. Recommended Daily Allowances for vitamin K in humans have not been established officially. The adequate daily dietary intake of vitamin K for adults has been estimated to be 70 to 140 mcg. The dietary abundance of vitamin K normally satisfies these requirements.
Following are the usual recommended dosages:

For hypoprothrombinemia secondary to obstructive jaundice and biliary fistulas	5 mg daily
For hypoprothrombinemia secondary to the administration of antibacterials or salicylates	5 to 10 mg daily

HOW SUPPLIED

White tablets containing 5 mg menadiol sodium diphosphate—bottls of 100 (NDC 0004-0037-01). Imprint on tablets: (front) SYNKAYVITE 5; (back) ROCHE.
Note: Slight pink discoloration of tablets does not affect the safety and efficacy of Synkayvite.
Store at room temperature (15° to 30° C or 59° to 86° F).
Revised: March 1985

Shown in Product Identification Section, page 426

TARACTAN® ℞
[tar-ac 'tan]
(chlorprothixene/Roche)
TABLETS

TARACTAN® ℞
(chlorprothixene lactate and HCl/Roche)
CONCENTRATE

TARACTAN® ℞
(chlorprothixene HCl/Roche)
AMPULS

The following text is complete prescribing information based on official labeling in effect June 1, 1992.

DESCRIPTION

Tablets—each containing 10 mg, 25 mg, 50 mg or 100 mg chlorprothixene; each tablet also contains acacia, corn starch, dibasic calcium phosphate, gelatin, magnesium stearate, shellac, sugar, talc, hydrogenated vegetable oil, wax (beeswax and carnauba) and other ingredients, with the following dye systems: 10-mg, 25-mg and 50-mg tablets—FD&C Blue No. 2, FD&C Yellow No. 5 and FD&C Yellow No. 6; 100-mg tablets—FD&C Blue No. 2, FD&C Red No. 3 and FD&C Yellow No. 5. Concentrate—100 mg/5 mL as the lactate and hydrochloride, fruit flavored; also contains benzoic acid, edetate disodium, glycerin, hydrochloric acid, lactic acid, magnesium aluminum silicate, parabens (methyl and propyl), polyoxyethylene (8) stearate, silicone emulsion, sodium hydroxide, sorbitol, sucrose, FD&C Red No. 40, FD&C Blue No. 1, FD&C Yellow No. 6, flavors and water. Ampuls—25 mg/2 mL as the hydrochloride, with 0.2% parabens (methyl and propyl) added as preservatives and pH adjusted to approximately 3.4 with HCl.
Taractan (chlorprothixene/Roche) is a thioxanthene derivative. Chemically, it is the alpha isomer of 2-chloro-*N, N*-dimethylthioxanthene-Δ^9, γ-propylamine. In chemical structure chlorprothixene resembles the phenothiazines; however, in place of the nitrogen (N) in the phenothiazine ring, chlorprothixene carries a carbon atom with a double bond to a side chain.

ACTIONS

EEG changes following the injection of Taractan into cats suggest that it acts on the brain stem. Effects demonstrated were the synchronization of the EEG tracings during rest, a shortening of cortical activation obtained by stimulation of the reticular formation, and modifications of elicited potentials.

INDICATIONS

Taractan is indicated for the management of manifestations of psychotic disorders. Taractan has not been shown effective in the management of behavioral complications in patients with mental retardation.

CONTRAINDICATIONS

Circulatory collapse, comatose states due to central depressant drugs (alcohol, hypnotics, opiates, etc.) and known sensitivity to the drug are contraindications.

WARNINGS

Tardive Dyskinesia: Tardive dyskinesia, a syndrome consisting of potentially irreversible, involuntary, dyskinetic movements, may develop in patients treated with neuroleptic (antipsychotic) drugs. Although the prevalence of the syndrome appears to be highest among the elderly, especially elderly women, it is impossible to rely upon prevalence estimates to predict, at the inception of neuroleptic treatment, which patients are likely to develop the syndrome. Whether neuroleptic drug products differ in their potential to cause tardive dyskinesia is unknown.
Both the risk of developing the syndrome and the likelihood that it will become irreversible are believed to increase as the duration of treatment and the total cumulative dose of neuroleptic drugs increase. However, the syndrome can develop, although much less commonly, after relatively brief treatment periods at low doses.
There is no known treatment for established cases of tardive dyskinesia, although the syndrome may remit, partially or completely, if neuroleptic treatment is withdrawn. Neuroleptic treatment itself, however, may suppress (or partially suppress) the signs and symptoms of the syndrome and thereby may possibly mask the underlying disease process. The effect that symptomatic suppression has upon the long-term course of the syndrome is unknown.
Given these considerations, neuroleptics should be prescribed in a manner that is most likely to minimize the occurrence of tardive dyskinesia. Chronic neuroleptic treatment should generally be reserved for patients who suffer from a chronic illness that 1) is known to respond to neuroleptic drugs, and 2) for whom alternative, equally effective, but potentially less harmful treatments are not available or appropriate. In patients who do require chronic treatment, the smallest dose and the shortest duration of treatment producing a satisfactory clinical response should be sought. The need for continued treatment should be reassessed periodically.
If signs and symptoms of tardive dyskinesia appear in a patient on neuroleptics, drug discontinuation should be considered. However, some patients may require treatment despite the presence of the syndrome.
(For further information about the description of tardive dyskinesia and its clinical detection, please refer to the sections on Information for Patients and Adverse Reactions.)
Neuroleptic Malignant Syndrome: A potentially fatal symptom complex sometimes referred to as neuroleptic malignant syndrome (NMS) has been reported in association with antipsychotic drugs. Clinical manifestations of NMS are hyperpyrexia, muscle rigidity, altered mental status and evidence of autonomic instability (irregular pulse or blood pressure, tachycardia, diaphoresis and cardiac dysrhythmias).
The diagnostic evaluation of patients with this syndrome is complicated. In arriving at a diagnosis, it is important to identify cases where the clinical presentation includes both serious medical illness (*e.g.,* pneumonia, systemic infection, etc.) and untreated or inadequately treated extrapyramidal signs and symptoms (EPS). Other important considerations in the differential diagnosis include central anticholinergic toxicity, heat stroke, drug fever and primary central nervous system (CNS) pathology.
The management of NMS should include 1) immediate discontinuation of antipsychotic drugs and other drugs not essential to concurrent therapy, 2) intensive symptomatic treatment and medical monitoring, and 3) treatment of any concomitant serious medical problems for which specific treatments are available. There is no general agreement about specific pharmacological treatment regimens for uncomplicated NMS.
If a patient requires antipsychotic drug treatment after recovery from NMS, the potential reintroduction of drug therapy should be carefully considered. The patient should be carefully monitored, since recurrences of NMS have been reported.
Usage in Pregnancy: The safety of Taractan during pregnancy or lactation in humans has not been established. Therefore, use of Taractan in women who may become pregnant requires weighing the drug's potential benefits against its possible hazards to mother and child. For the results of reproductive and teratogenic studies in rats and rabbits see **Animal Pharmacology and Toxicology.**
This drug may impair the mental and/or physical abilities required for the performance of hazardous tasks such as operating machinery or driving a motor vehicle; therefore, the patient should be cautioned accordingly.
As in the case of other CNS-acting drugs, patients receiving Taractan should be cautioned about possible combined effects with alcohol.
The safety and efficacy of Taractan have not been established for oral administration in children under age 6 or for parenteral use in those under age 12.

PRECAUTIONS

Because of its structural similarity to the phenothiazines, all of the precautions associated with phenothiazine therapy should be considered when patients receive Taractan. Therefore, Taractan should be used with caution in patients who:
—are receiving barbiturates or narcotics, because of additive effects of central nervous system depressants. The dosage of the narcotic or barbiturate should be reduced when given concomitantly with Taractan.
—are receiving atropine or related drugs, because of additive anticholinergic effects.
—have a history of epilepsy. When necessary, Taractan may be used concomitantly with anticonvulsant drugs. However, use of Taractan may lower the convulsive threshold; therefore, an adequate dosage of the anticonvulsant should be maintained.
—are exposed to extreme heat or phosphorous insecticides.
—have cardiovascular disease.
—have respiratory impairment due to acute pulmonary infections or chronic respiratory disorders such as severe asthma or emphysema.
The concurrent use of Taractan and electroshock treatment should be reserved for those patients for whom it is essential, but the hazards may be increased.
Taractan may augment or interfere with the absorption, metabolism or therapeutic activity of other psychotropic drugs and vice versa.
The appearance of signs of blood dyscrasias requires immediate discontinuance of the drug and the institution of appropriate therapy.
The possibility of liver damage, variations in thyroid function, pigmentary retinopathy, lenticular or corneal deposits and development of irreversible dyskinesias should be kept in mind when patients are on prolonged therapy.
When used in the treatment of agitated states accompanying depression, the usual precautions indicated with such patients are necessary, particularly the recognition that a suicidal tendency may be present and protective measures necessary.
Taractan has been demonstrated to have a prominent uricosuric effect when used at usual therapeutic doses. Consequently clinicians should be alert to the possible occurrence of acute renal insufficiency after voluntary overdose of chlorprothixene or during the first days of treatment, especially in dehydrated patients.
Taractan tablets contain FD&C Yellow No. 5 (tartrazine) which may cause allergic-type reactions (including bronchial asthma) in certain susceptible individuals. Although the overall incidence of FD&C Yellow No. 5 (tartrazine) sensitivity in the general population is low, it is frequently seen in patients who also have aspirin hypersensitivity.
Information for Patients: Given the likelihood that some patients exposed chronically to neuroleptics will develop tardive dyskinesia, it is advised that all patients in whom chronic use is contemplated be given, if possible, full information about this risk. The decision to inform patients and/or their guardians must obviously take into account the clinical circumstances and the competency of the patient to understand the information provided.
Abrupt Withdrawal: Taractan is not known to produce physical dependence. However, gastritis, nausea and vomiting, dizziness and tremulousness have been reported following abrupt cessation of high-dose therapy.
Neuroleptic drugs elevate prolactin levels; the elevation persists during chronic administration. Tissue culture experiments indicate that approximately one-third of human breast cancers are prolactin-dependent *in vitro,* a factor of potential importance if the prescription of these drugs is contemplated in a patient with a previously detected breast cancer. Although disturbances such as galactorrhea, amenorrhea, gynecomastia and impotence have been reported, the clinical significance of elevated serum prolactin levels is unknown for most patients. An increase in mammary neoplasms has been found in rodents after chronic administration of neuroleptic drugs. Neither clinical studies nor epidemiologic studies conducted to date, however, have shown an association between chronic administration of these drugs and mammary tumorigenesis; the available evidence is considered too limited to be conclusive at this time.

ADVERSE REACTIONS

General Introduction: Untoward events reported in association with a drug's use can be classified into three general categories: 1) those which are more or less predictable extensions of the pharmacological activity of the drug; 2) those which are caused by the drug, but in an unpredictable and/or idiosyncratic manner (*e.g.,* jaundice, agranulocytosis, etc.); and 3) those which have occurred in circumstances where evidence of a causal link to the drug's use is inconclusive.

The first section describes the neurological events that are commonly seen in association with the use of neuroleptics, regardless of mechanism. The second and third sections present events that have been reported in association with the use of Taractan and of phenothiazine derivatives, respectively.

Common Reactions Linked to the Use of Neuroleptics: Untoward Neurological Events: The following section details events that have been reported to occur in association with the use of neuroleptics or drugs which share the ability to block CNS dopamine receptors.

The common acute neurological untoward effects of neuroleptics consist of dystonia, akathisia and pseudoparkinsonism.

Chronic use of neuroleptics, including Taractan, may be associated with the development of tardive dyskinesia. The salient features of this syndrome are described below and in the WARNINGS section. Additional details about the common acute neurological impairments also follow.

Tardive Dyskinesia: Clinical picture and detection. The syndrome is characterized by involuntary choreoathetoid movements which variously involve the tongue, face, mouth, lips or jaw (*e.g.,* protrusion of the tongue, puffing of the cheeks, puckering of the mouth, chewing movements), trunk and extremities. The severity of the syndrome and the degree of impairment produced vary widely.

The syndrome may become clinically recognizable either during treatment, upon dosage reduction, or upon withdrawal of treatment. Movements may decrease in intensity and may disappear altogether if further treatment with neuroleptics is withheld. It is generally believed that reversibility is more likely after short- rather than long-term neuroleptic exposure. Consequently, early detection of tardive dyskinesia is important. To increase the likelihood of detecting the syndrome at the earliest possible time, the dosage of neuroleptic drug should be reduced periodically (if clinically possible) and the patient observed for signs of the disorder. This maneuver is critical, for neuroleptic drugs may mask the signs of the syndrome.

Neuroleptic Malignant Syndrome: See **Warnings**.

Acute Neurological Effects:

1. Dystonia. This may present as acute, reversible torticollis, opisthotonos, carpopedal spasm, trismus, dysphagia, respiratory difficulty, oculogyric crisis, and protrusion of the tongue. Treatment consists of the parenteral administration of either an anticholinergic antiparkinsonism agent or diphenhydramine.
2. Akathisia. Akathisia presents as constant motor restlessness. It is often confused with agitation and the differential diagnosis can be difficult. One feature that may permit a distinction is that the patient with akathisia often complains, *when asked,* about his or her inability to stop moving. The importance of the differential diagnosis is that akathisia should *not* be treated with an increased dose of neuroleptic. In the treatment of akathisia, the dose of antipsychotic may be lowered until the motor restlessness has subsided. The efficacy of anticholinergic treatment of this side effect is unestablished.
3. Pseudoparkinsonism. Pseudoparkinsonism refers to a drug-induced state similar to the classic syndrome. Its features include a generalized increase in muscle tone, often accompanied by "cogwheeling," tremor, and other signs and symptoms of the spontaneously occurring syndrome (*i.e.,* bradyphrenia, bradykinesia, masked facies, drooling, difficulty initiating movements, lack of associated movements, micrographia, etc.). Generally, anticholinergic antiparkinsonism agents (*i.e.,* benztropine, biperiden, procyclidine, or trihexyphenidyl) and amantadine are helpful in alleviating symptoms that cannot be managed by neuroleptic dose reduction. The value of prophylactic antiparkinsonism drug therapy has not been established. The need for continued use of antiparkinsonism medication should be reevaluated periodically.

Adverse Reactions Associated with Taractan: See **Warnings** and **Adverse Reactions:** *Common Reactions Linked to the Use of Neuroleptics: Untoward Neurological Events.*

Note: Sudden death has occasionally been reported in patients who have received phenothiazines. In some cases death was apparently due to cardiac arrest; in others the cause appeared to be asphyxia due to failure of the cough reflex. In some patients the cause could not be determined nor could it be established that death was due to the phenothiazine.

Taractan commonly causes sedation and hypotension.

The following adverse reactions have been reported with Taractan:

Central Nervous System: The most frequently occurring effect is initial drowsiness which usually disappears with or without dose adjustments. Hyperactivity or stimulation can occur, sometimes requiring discontinuation of the medication. Convulsions, particularly in patients with a history of EEG abnormalities, have been reported. Ataxia.

Autonomic Nervous System: Dry mouth, nasal stuffiness, visual changes and constipation have been occasionally reported. Headache. Gastric upset.

Cardiovascular System: Postural hypotension, tachycardia (especially with sudden marked increase in dosage) and dizziness have been reported. In the event that a vasoconstrictor is required, Levophed® (levarterenol) or Aramine (metaraminol) are the most suitable. Other pressor agents, including epinephrine, should not be used, as a paradoxical further lowering of the blood pressure may ensue.

EKG changes—particularly nonspecific, usually reversible Q and T wave distortions—have been observed in some patients receiving phenothiazine tranquilizers. Their relationship to myocardial damage has not been confirmed.

Skin: Dermatitis and urticarial type skin reactions have been observed infrequently. Photosensitivity is rare but undue exposure to the sun should be avoided.

Hepatotoxicity: Jaundice has been reported occasionally.

Hematological Disorders: Agranulocytosis, eosinophilia, leukopenia, hemolytic anemia, thrombocytopenic purpura and pancytopenia have been reported very rarely.

Endocrine Disorders: Galactorrhea and increased libido have been reported in isolated cases.

Other: Excessive weight gain and excessive thirst have occasionally been reported. Hyperpyrexia, paradoxical exacerbation of psychotic symptoms and ocular changes may also occur. Insomnia. Weakness.

Adverse Reactions Associated with Phenothiazine Derivatives: See **Warnings** and **Adverse Reactions:** *Common Reactions Linked to the Use of Neuroleptics: Untoward Neurological Events.*

Adverse Reactions Associated with Phenothiazine Derivatives: The following adverse reactions have not been reported specifically for Taractan nor have they been observed with every phenothiazine derivative; however, because of pharmacological similarities of Taractan to the various phenothiazine derivatives, they should be considered when administering drugs of this class.

Central Nervous System: Extrapyramidal symptoms (opisthotonos, oculogyric crisis, hyperreflexia); grand mal convulsions; altered cerebrospinal fluid proteins; cerebral edema; intensification and prolongation of the action of central nervous system depressants (opiates, analgesics, antihistamines, barbiturates, alcohol), atropine, exposure to extreme heat or organophosphorus insecticides.

Autonomic Nervous System: Obstipation; adynamic ileus; inhibition of ejaculation.

Cardiovascular System: Cardiac arrest; bradycardia; faintness.

Hepatotoxicity: Biliary stasis.

Endocrine Disorders: Lactation; gynecomastia; menstrual irregularities; moderate breast engorgement; hyperglycemia, hypoglycemia, glycosuria.

Allergic Reactions: Itching; erythema; eczema up to exfoliative dermatitis; asthma; laryngeal edema; angioneurotic edema; anaphylactoid reactions.

Other: Enlargement of the parotid gland; catatonic-like states; peripheral edema, reversed epinephrine effect; systemic lupus erythematosus-like syndrome; pigmentary retinopathy; with prolonged administration of substantial doses—skin pigmentation, epithelial keratopathy, and lenticular and corneal deposits.

DOSAGE AND ADMINISTRATION

Dosage should be individually adjusted according to diagnosis and severity of the condition. In general, small doses should be used initially, and increased to the optimal effective level as rapidly as possible based on therapeutic response. When higher dosage is required, greater sedation may be encountered; therefore, patients should be closely supervised. Lethargy and drowsiness are readily controlled by dosage reduction. Initially, lower doses (10 to 25 mg three or four times daily) should be used for elderly or debilitated patients.

For convenience in prescribing and dispensing, all recommended dosages are expressed as strengths of the active moiety, chlorprothixene.

Taractan may be administered orally as tablets or concentrate. The concentrate, containing 100 mg of the drug per 5 mL teaspoonful, is pleasantly flavored and may be administered alone or in milk, water, fruit juices, coffee and carbonated beverages.

ORAL	AVERAGE DAILY DOSE
Adults:	Initially, 25 to 50 mg three or four times daily; to be increased as needed. Dosages exceeding 600 mg daily are rarely required.
Children (over 6 years of age):	10 to 25 mg three or four times daily.
PARENTERAL Not to be used in children under the age of 12.	25 to 50 mg I.M. up to three or four times daily.

Pain or induration at the site of injection is minimal. Since postural hypotension may occur in some patients, injection should be given with the patient seated or recumbent. If hypotension does occur, recovery is usually spontaneous; however, the patient should be observed until symptoms of weakness or dizziness pass.

As soon as the acutely agitated patient is brought under control, oral medication should be instituted. The changeover should be made gradually, with oral and parenteral doses being given alternately on the same day, then oral doses only, adjusted to the required maintenance level.

OVERDOSAGE

Taractan can be fatal in overdosage in the range of 2.5 to 4 Gm or above. Manifestations of overdosage are drowsiness, coma, respiratory depression, hypotension (which may appear after a delay of several hours and may persist for two to three days), tachycardia, pyrexia and constricted pupils. Convulsions, hyperactivity and hematuria may be seen in the recovery period.

Treatment is essentially symptomatic. Early gastric lavage is recommended, along with supportive measures such as I.V. fluids and the maintenance of an adequate airway. Severe hypotension usually responds to the use of levarterenol or metaraminol. Should coma be prolonged, caffeine and sodium benzoate, or ethamivan may be used, but the possibility must be borne in mind that these may lead to a convulsive episode. Should convulsions occur, the judicious use of sodium amytal is recommended. **Epinephrine must not be used in these patients.**

HOW SUPPLIED

Tablets — 10 mg, 25 mg, 50 mg or 100 mg chlorprothixene/Roche—bottles of 100.

Concentrate—containing, in each teaspoonful, chlorprothixene/Roche 100 mg base (as the lactate and hydrochloride)—bottles of 16 fluid ounces (1 pint).

Ampuls—containing chlorprothixene/Roche 25 mg/2 mL as the hydrochloride—boxes of 10.

ANIMAL PHARMACOLOGY AND TOXICOLOGY

In mice, the oral LD_{50} of the two oral dosage forms of chlorprothixene were 350 $\pm$ 27 mg/kg (as the 2 per cent concentrate) and 220 $\pm$ 24 mg/kg (as the tablet form ground and suspended in 5 per cent gum acacia). For the injectable form the intramuscular LD_{50} in mice was greater than 125 mg/kg.

Reproduction Studies: Reproductive and teratological studies in rats and rabbits were performed at levels of 12 and 24 mg/kg. In the rats, a decreased conception rate and an increased incidence of stillborns was noted at both levels. An increased number of resorptions was noted only at the high dose level. There was a decrease in the number of implantation sites at both doses. The number of live fetuses per litter and the mean fetal body weights were reduced slightly at 12 mg/kg and more so at 24 mg/kg. No teratological effects were observed. No deleterious effects on reproduction were seen in rabbits nor were any teratological findings noted.

Revised: July 1991

TEL-E-DOSE®

Tel-E-Dose is a unit package designed by Roche for convenience in dispensing medications in the hospital and nursing home. Each unit, sealed against contamination and moisture, is clearly identified by product name and strength and carries the control number and expiration date.

Currently available in this package form are the following products: Bactrim™ (80 mg trimethoprim and 400 mg sulfamethoxazole) tablets; Bactrim™ DS (160 mg trimethoprim and 800 mg sulfamethoxazole) tablets; Bumex® (bumetanide HCl) tablets, 0.5 mg, 1 mg, 2 mg; Fansidar® (500 mg sulfadoxine and 25 mg pryrimethamine) tablets; Gantanol® (sulfamethoxazole) tablets, 0.5 Gm; Gantrisin® (sulfisoxazole) tablets, 0.5 Gm; Klonopin® (clonazepam) tablets, 0.5 mg, 1 mg, 2 mg; Trimpex® (trimethoprim) tablets, 100 mg.

Shown in Product Identification Section, page 425

TRIMPEX® ℞

[trim 'pex]
(trimethoprim/Roche)
TABLETS

The following text is complete prescribing information based on official labeling in effect June 1, 1992.

DESCRIPTION

Trimpex (trimethoprim/Roche) is a synthetic antibacterial available as 100-mg tablets for oral administration. Each tablet also contains lactose, magnesium stearate, sodium starch glycolate and pregelatinized starch.

Trimethoprim is 2,4-diamino-5-(3,4,5-trimethoxybenzyl)-pyrimidine. It is a white to light yellow, odorless, bitter compound with a molecular weight of 290.3.

CLINICAL PHARMACOLOGY

Trimethoprim is rapidly absorbed following oral administration. It exists in the blood as unbound, protein-bound and

Continued on next page

Roche Laboratories—Cont.

metabolized forms. Ten to twenty percent of trimethoprim is metabolized, primarily in the liver; the remainder is excreted unchanged in the urine. The principal metabolites of trimethoprim are the 1- and 3-oxides and the 3'- and 4'-hydroxy derivatives. The free form is considered to be the therapeutically active form. Approximately 44% of trimethoprim is bound to plasma proteins.

Mean peak plasma concentrations of approximately 1.0 mcg/ml occur 1 to 4 hours after oral administration of a single 100-mg dose. A single 200-mg dose will result in plasma concentrations approximately twice as high. The half-life of trimethoprim ranges from 8 to 10 hours. However, patients with severely impaired renal function exhibit an increase in the half-life of trimethoprim, which requires either dosage regimen adjustment or not using the drug in such patients (see DOSAGE AND ADMINISTRATION section). During a 13-week study of trimethoprim administered at a dosage of 50 mg *q.i.d.*, the mean minimum steady-state concentration of the drug was 1.1 mcg/ml. Steady-state concentrations were achieved within 2 to 3 days of chronic administration and were maintained throughout the experimental period.

Excretion of trimethoprim is primarily by the kidneys through glomerular filtration and tubular secretion. Urine concentrations of trimethoprim are considerably higher than are the concentrations in the blood. After a single oral dose of 100 mg, urine concentrations of trimethoprim ranged from 30 to 160 mcg/ml during the 0- to 4-hour period and declined to approximately 18 to 91 mcg/ml during the 8- to 24-hour period. A 200-mg single oral dose will result in trimethoprim urine concentrations approximately twice as high. After oral administration, 50% to 60% of trimethoprim is excreted in urine within 24 hours, approximately 80% of this being unmetabolized trimethoprim.

Since normal vaginal and fecal flora are the source of most pathogens causing urinary tract infections, it is relevant to consider the distribution of trimethoprim into these sites. Concentrations of trimethoprim in vaginal secretions are consistently greater than those found simultaneously in the serum, being typically 1.6 times the concentrations of simultaneously obtained serum samples. Sufficient trimethoprim is excreted in the feces to markedly reduce or eliminate trimethoprim-susceptible organisms from the fecal flora. The dominant non-*Enterobacteriaceae* fecal organisms, *Bacteroides* spp. and *Lactobacillus* spp., are not susceptible to trimethoprim concentrations obtained with the recommended dosage.

Trimethoprim also passes the placental barrier and is excreted in breast milk.

Microbiology: Trimpex blocks the production of tetrahydrofolic acid from dihydrofolic acid by binding to and reversibly inhibiting the required enzyme, dihydrofolate reductase. This binding is very much stronger for the bacterial enzyme than for the corresponding mammalian enzyme. Thus, Trimpex selectively interferes with bacterial biosynthesis of nucleic acids and proteins.

In vitro serial dilution tests have shown that the spectrum of antibacterial activity of Trimpex includes the common urinary tract pathogens with the exception of *Pseudomonas aeruginosa.*

Representative Minimum Inhibitory Concentrations for Trimethoprim-Susceptible Organisms

Bacteria	Trimethoprim MIC—mcg/ml (Range)
Escherichia coli	0.05—1.5
Proteus mirabilis	0.5—1.5
Klebsiella pneumoniae	0.5—5.0
Enterobacter species	0.5—5.0
Staphylococcus species (coagulase-negative)	0.15—5.0

The recommended quantitative disc susceptibility method[1,2] may be used for estimating the susceptibility of bacteria to Trimpex. With this procedure, reports from the laboratory giving results using the 5-mcg trimethoprim disc should be interpreted according to the following criteria: Organisms producing zones of 16 mm or greater are classified as susceptible, whereas those producing zones of 11 to 15 mm are classified as having intermediate susceptibility. A report from the laboratory of "Susceptible to trimethoprim" or "Intermediate susceptibility to trimethoprim" indicates that the infection is likely to respond when, as in uncomplicated urinary tract infections, effective therapy is dependent upon the urine concentration of trimethoprim. Organisms producing zones of 10 mm or less are reported as resistant, indicating that other therapy should be selected.

Dilution methods for determining susceptibility are also used, and results are reported as the minimum drug concentration inhibiting microbial growth (MIC).[3] If the MIC is 8 mcg per ml or less, the microorganism is considered "susceptible." If the MIC is 16 mcg per ml or greater, the microorganism is considered "resistant."

INDICATIONS AND USAGE

For the treatment of initial episodes of uncomplicated urinary tract infections due to susceptible strains of the following organisms: *Escherichia coli, Proteus mirabilis, Klebsiella pneumoniae, Enterobacter* species and coagulase-negative *Staphylococcus* species, including *S. saprophyticus*.

Cultures and susceptibility tests should be performed to determine the susceptibility of the bacteria to trimethoprim. Therapy may be initiated prior to obtaining the results of these tests.

CONTRAINDICATIONS

Trimpex is contraindicated in individuals hypersensitive to trimethoprim and in those with documented megaloblastic anemia due to folate deficiency.

WARNINGS

Serious hypersensitivity reactions have been reported rarely in patients on trimethoprim therapy. Trimethoprim has been reported rarely to interfere with hematopoiesis, especially when administered in large doses and/or for prolonged periods.

The presence of clinical signs such as sore throat, fever, pallor or purpura may be early indications of serious blood disorders.

PRECAUTIONS

General: Trimethoprim should be given with caution to patients with possible folate deficiency. Folates may be administered concomitantly without interfering with the antibacterial action of trimethoprim. Trimethoprim should also be given with caution to patients with impaired renal or hepatic function. If any clinical signs of a blood disorder are noted in a patient receiving trimethoprim, a complete blood count should be obtained and the drug discontinued if a significant reduction in the count of any formed blood element is found.

Drug interactions: Trimpex may inhibit the hepatic metabolism of phenytoin. Trimethoprim, given at a common clinical dosage, increased the phenytoin half-life by 51% and decreased the phenytoin metabolic clearance rate by 30%. When administering these drugs concurrently, one should be alert for possible excessive phenytoin effect.

Drug/laboratory test interactions: Trimethoprim can interfere with a serum methotrexate assay as determined by the competitive binding protein technique (CBPA) when a bacterial dihydrofolate reductase is used as the binding protein. No interference occurs, however, if methotrexate is measured by a radioimmunoassay (RIA).

The presence of trimethoprim may also interfere with the Jaffé alkaline picrate reaction assay for creatinine resulting in overestimations of about 10% in the range of normal values.

Carcinogenesis, mutagenesis, impairment of fertility:

Carcinogenesis: Long-term studies in animals to evaluate carcinogenic potential have not been conducted with trimethoprim.

Mutagenesis: Trimethoprim was demonstrated to be nonmutagenic in the Ames assay. No chromosomal damage was observed in human leukocytes cultured *in vitro* with trimethoprim; the concentration used exceeded blood levels following therapy with Trimpex.

Impairment of fertility: No adverse effects on fertility or general reproductive performance were observed in rats given trimethoprim in oral dosages as high as 70 mg/kg/day for males and 14 mg/kg/day for females.

Pregnancy: Teratogenic effects: Pregnancy Category C. Trimethoprim has been shown to be teratogenic in the rat when given in doses 40 times the human dose. In some rabbit studies, the overall increase in fetal loss (dead and resorbed and malformed conceptuses) was associated with doses 6 times the human therapeutic dose.

While there are no large well-controlled studies on the use of trimethoprim in pregnant women, Brumfitt and Pursell,[4] in a retrospective study, reported the outcome of 186 pregnancies during which the mother received either placebo or trimethoprim in combination wih sulfamethoxazole. The incidence of congenital abnormalities was 4.5% (3 of 66) in those who received placebo and 3.3% (4 of 120) in those receiving trimethoprim plus sulfamethoxazole. There were no abnormalities in the 10 children whose mothers received the drug during the first trimester. In a separate survey, Brumfitt and Pursell also found no congenital abnormalities in 35 children whose mothers had received trimethoprim plus sulfamethoxazole at the time of conception or shortly thereafter.

Because trimethoprim may interfere with folic acid metabolism, Trimpex should be used during pregnancy only if the potential benefit justifies the potential risk to the fetus.

Nonteratogenic effects: The oral administration of trimethoprim to rats at a dose of 70 mg/kg/day commencing with the last third of gestation and continuing through parturition and lactation caused no deleterious effects on gestation or pup growth and survival.

Nursing mothers: Trimethoprim is excreted in human milk. Because trimethoprim may interfere with folic acid metabolism, caution should be exercised when Trimpex is administered to a nursing woman.

Pediatric use: The safety of trimethoprim in infants under two months of age has not been demonstrated. The effectiveness of trimethoprim has not been established in children under 12 years of age.

ADVERSE REACTIONS

The adverse effects encountered most often with trimethoprim were rash and pruritus. Other adverse effects reported involved the gastrointestinal and hematopoietic systems.

Dermatologic: Rash, pruritus and phototoxic skin eruptions. At the recommended dosage regimens of 100 mg *b.i.d.* or 200 mg *q.d.*, each for 10 days, the incidence of rash is 2.9% to 6.7%. In clinical studies which employed high doses of Trimpex, an elevated incidence of rash was noted. These rashes were maculopapular, morbilliform, pruritic and generally mild to moderate, appearing 7 to 14 days after the initiation of therapy.

Hypersensitivity: There have been rare reports of exfoliative dermatitis, erytherma multiforme, Stevens-Johnson syndrome, Lyell syndrome, anaphylaxis and aseptic meningitis.

Gastrointestinal: Epigastric distress, nausea, vomiting and glossitis. Elevation of serum transaminase and bilirubin.

Hematologic: Thrombocytopenia, leukopenia, neutropenia, megaloblastic anemia and methemoglobinemia.

Miscellaneous: Fever, increases in BUN and serum creatinine levels.

OVERDOSAGE

Acute: Signs of acute overdosage with trimethoprim may appear following ingestion of 1 gram or more of the drug and include nausea, vomiting, dizziness, headaches, mental depression, confusion and bone marrow depression (see CHRONIC OVERDOSAGE).

Treatment consists of gastric lavage and general supportive measures. Acidification of the urine will increase renal elimination of trimethoprim. Peritoneal dialysis is not effective and hemodialysis only moderately effective in eliminating the drug.

Chronic: Use of trimethoprim at high doses and/or for extended periods of time may cause bone marrow depression manifested as thrombocytopenia, leukopenia and/or megaloblastic anemia. If signs of bone marrow depression occur, trimethoprim should be discontinued and the patient should be given leucovorin, 3 to 6 mg intramuscularly daily for three days, or as required to restore normal hematopoiesis.

DOSAGE AND ADMINISTRATION

The usual oral adult dosage is 100 mg (one tablet) every 12 hours or 200 mg (two tablets) every 24 hours, each for 10 days. The use of trimethoprim in patients with a creatinine clearance of less than 15 ml/min is not recommended. For patients with a creatinine clearance of 15 to 30 ml/min, the dose should be 50 mg every 12 hours.

The effectiveness of trimethoprim has not been established in children under 12 years of age.

HOW SUPPLIED

100-mg tablets (white, elliptical, scored)—bottles of 100 (NDC 0004-0127-01); Tel-E-Dose® packages of 100 (NDC 0004-0127-49). Imprint on tablets: TRIMPEX 100 ROCHE.

REFERENCES

1. Bauer AW, Kirby WMM, Sherris JC, Turck M: Antibiotic Susceptibility Testing by Standardized Single Disk Method, *Am J Clin Pathol 45*:493–496, 1966.
2. Approved Standard ASM-2 Performance Standards for Antimicrobial Disc Susceptibility Test; National Committee for Clinical Laboratory Standards, 771 East Lancaster Avenue, Villanova, Pennsylvania 19085.
3. Ericsson HM, Sherris JC: Antibiotic Sensitivity Testing. Report of an International Collaborative Study. *Acta Pathol Microbiol Scand* [B] (Suppl 217): 1–90, 1971.
4. Brumfitt W, Pursell R: Trimethoprim/Sulfamethoxazole in the Treatment of Bacteriuria in Women, *J Infect Dis 128* (Suppl): S657–S663, 1973.

Revised: September 1988

Shown in Product Identification Section, page 426

VALRELEASE® ℭ

[*val 're-lease*]
(diazepam/Roche)
CAPSULES
A slow-release dosage form of Valium® (diazepam/Roche)

The following text is complete prescribing information based on official labeling in effect June 1, 1992.

DESCRIPTION

Diazepam is a benzodiazepine derivative developed through original Roche research. Chemically, diazepam is 7-chloro-1,3-dihydro-1-methyl-5-phenyl-2*H*-1,4-benzodiazepin-2-one.

It is a colorless crystalline compound, insoluble in water and has a molecular weight of 284.74.

Valrelease capsules provide the actions of Valium® (diazepam/Roche) in a slow-release dosage form.

Valrelease capsule shells contain the following dye system: FD&C Blue No. 1, FD&C Yellow No. 6 and D&C Yellow No. 10.

PHARMACOLOGY

In animals, diazepam appears to act on parts of the limbic system, the thalamus and hypothalamus, and induces calming effects. Diazepam, unlike chlorpromazine and reserpine, has no demonstrable peripheral autonomic blocking action, nor does it produce extrapyramidal side effects; however, animals treated with diazepam do have a transient ataxia at higher doses. Diazepam was found to have transient cardiovascular depressor effects in dogs. Long-term experiments in rats revealed no disturbances of endocrine function.

Oral LD_{50} of diazepam is 720 mg/kg in mice and 1240 mg/kg in rats. Intraperitoneal administration of 400 mg/kg to a monkey resulted in death on the sixth day.

Reproduction Studies: A series of rat reproduction studies was performed with diazepam in oral doses of 1, 10, 80 and 100 mg/kg. At 100 mg/kg there was a decrease in the number of pregnancies and surviving offspring in these rats. Neonatal survival of rats at doses lower than 100 mg/kg was within normal limits. Several neonates in these rat reproduction studies showed skeletal or other defects. Further studies in rats at doses up to and including 80 mg/kg/day did not reveal teratological effects on the offspring.

In humans, measurable blood levels of diazepam were obtained in maternal and cord blood, indicating placental transfer of the drug.

The administration of one 15-mg Valrelease capsule results in blood levels of diazepam over a 24-hour period which are comparable to those of 5-mg Valium tablets given three times daily.

The mean time to maximum plasma diazepam concentrations after administration of 15-mg Valrelease capsules to eleven fasted subjects was 5.3 hours. The harmonic mean half-life of diazepam was 36 hours. The range of average minimum steady-state plasma diazepam concentrations during once daily administration of 15-mg Valrelease capsules to eleven normal subjects was 196 to 341 ng/ml.

INDICATIONS

Valrelease is indicated for the management of anxiety disorders or for the short-term relief of the symptoms of anxiety. Anxiety or tension associated with the stress of everyday life usually does not require treatment with an anxiolytic.

Valrelease is a useful adjunct for the relief of skeletal muscle spasm due to reflex spasm to local pathology (such as inflammation of the muscles or joints, or secondary to trauma); spasticity caused by upper motor neuron disorders (such as cerebral palsy and paraplegia); athetosis; and stiff-man syndrome.

The effectiveness of diazepam in long-term use, that is, more than 4 months, has not been assessed by systematic clinical studies. The physician should periodically reassess the usefulness of the drug for the individual patient.

CONTRAINDICATIONS

Valrelease is contraindicated in patients with a known hypersensitivity to this drug and, because of lack of sufficient clinical experience, in children under 6 months of age. It may be used in patients with open angle glaucoma who are receiving appropriate therapy, but is contraindicated in acute narrow angle glaucoma.

WARNINGS

Valrelease is not of value in the treatment of psychotic patients and should not be employed in lieu of appropriate treatment. As is true of most preparations containing CNS-acting drugs, patients receiving Valrelease should be cautioned against engaging in hazardous occupations requiring complete mental alertness such as operating machinery or driving a motor vehicle.

If the use of Valrelease in patients with seizure disorders results in an increase in the frequency and/or severity of grand mal seizures, there may be a need to increase the dosage of standard anticonvulsant medication.

Abrupt withdrawal of Valrelease in patients with a history of seizures may also be associated with a temporary increase in the frequency and/or severity of seizures.

Since Valrelease has a central nervous system depressant effect, patients should be advised against the simultaneous ingestion of alcohol and other CNS-depressant drugs during Valrelease therapy.

Usage in Pregnancy: **An increased risk of congenital malformations associated with the use of minor tranquilizers (diazepam, meprobamate and chlordiazepoxide) during the first trimester of pregnancy has been suggested in several studies. Because use of these drugs is rarely a matter of urgency, their use during this period should almost always be avoided. The possibility that a woman of childbearing potential may be pregnant at the time of institution of therapy should be considered. Patients should be advised that if they become pregnant during therapy or intend to become pregnant they should communicate with their physicians about the desirability of discontinuing the drug.**

Management of Overdosage: Manifestations of diazepam overdosage include somnolence, confusion, coma and diminished reflexes. Respiration, pulse and blood pressure should be monitored, as in all cases of drug overdosage, although, in general, these effects have been minimal following overdosage. General supportive measures should be employed, along with immediate gastric lavage. Intravenous fluids should be administered and an adequate airway maintained. Hypotension may be combated by the use of Levophed® (levarterenol) or Aramine (metaraminol). Dialysis is of limited value. As with the management of intentional overdosage with any drug, it should be borne in mind that multiple agents may have been ingested.

Withdrawal symptoms of the barbiturate type have occurred after the discontinuation of benzodiazepines. (See DRUG ABUSE AND DEPENDENCE section.)

PRECAUTIONS

If Valrelease is to be combined with other psychotropic agents or anticonvulsant drugs, careful consideration should be given to the pharmacology of the agents to be employed—particularly with known compounds which may potentiate the action of diazepam, such as phenothiazines, narcotics, barbiturates, MAO inhibitors and other antidepressants. The usual precautions are indicated for severely depressed patients or those in whom there is any evidence of latent depression; particularly the recognition that suicidal tendencies may be present and protective measures may be necessary. The usual precautions in treating patients with impaired renal or hepatic function should be observed.

In elderly and debilitated patients, it is recommended that the dosage be limited to the smallest effective amount to preclude the development of ataxia or oversedation (2 mg to 2½ mg once or twice daily, initially, to be increased gradually as needed and tolerated).

NOTE: If 2 or 2½ mg is the desired dose, scored Valium® (diazepam/Roche) tablets should be used.

The clearance of Valium and certain other benzodiazepines can be delayed in association with Tagamet (cimetidine) administration. The clinical significance of this is unclear.

Information for Patients: To assure the safe and effective use of benzodiazepines, patients should be informed that, since benzodiazepines may produce psychological and physical dependence, it is advisable that they consult with their physician before either increasing the dose or abruptly discontinuing this drug.

ADVERSE REACTIONS

Side effects most commonly reported were drowsiness, fatigue and ataxia. Infrequently encountered were confusion, constipation, depression, diplopia, dysarthria, headache, hypotension, incontinence, jaundice, changes in libido, nausea, changes in salivation, skin rash, slurred speech, tremor, urinary retention, vertigo and blurred vision. Paradoxical reactions such as acute hyperexcited states, anxiety, hallucinations, increased muscle spasticity, insomnia, rage, sleep disturbances and stimulation have been reported; should these occur, use of the drug should be discontinued.

Because of isolated reports of neutropenia and jaundice, periodic blood counts and liver function tests are advisable during long-term therapy. Minor changes in EEG patterns, usually low-voltage fast activity, have been observed in patients during and after diazepam therapy and are of no known significance.

DRUG ABUSE AND DEPENDENCE

Withdrawal symptoms, similar in character to those noted with barbiturates and alcohol (convulsions, tremor, abdominal and muscle cramps, vomiting and sweating), have occurred following abrupt discontinuance of diazepam. The more severe withdrawal symptoms have usually been limited to those patients who had received excessive doses over an extended period of time. Generally milder withdrawal symptoms (*e.g.*, dysphoria and insomnia) have been reported following abrupt discontinuance of benzodiazepines taken continuously at therapeutic levels for several months. Consequently, after extended therapy, abrupt discontinuation should generally be avoided and a gradual dosage tapering schedule followed. Addiction-prone individuals (such as drug addicts or alcoholics) should be under careful surveillance when receiving diazepam or other psychotropic agents because of the predisposition of such patients to habituation and dependence.

DOSAGE AND ADMINISTRATION

Dosage should be individualized for maximum beneficial effect. While the usual daily dosages given below will meet the needs of most patients, there will be some who may require higher doses. In such cases dosage should be increased cautiously to avoid adverse effects.

Whenever oral Valium® (diazepam/Roche), 5 mg t.i.d., would be considered the appropriate dosage, one 15-mg Valrelease capsule daily may be used.

Note: If 1 mg or 2½ mg is the desired dose, scored Valium (diazepam/Roche) tablets should be used.

Valrelease 15-mg capsules are recommended for elderly or debilitated patients and children only when it has been determined that 5 mg oral Valium t.i.d. is the optimal daily dose. Oral Valium is not recommended for children under 6 months of age.

Adults:	USUAL DAILY DOSE
Management of Anxiety Disorders and Relief of Symptoms of Anxiety.	Depending upon severity of symptoms—1 or 2 (15 to 30 mg) capsules once daily
Adjunctively for Relief of Skeletal Muscle Spasm.	1 or 2 capsules (15 to 30 mg) once daily

HOW SUPPLIED

For oral administration, Valrelease (diazepam/Roche) capsules—15 mg (yellow and blue)—bottles of 100; Prescription Paks of 30.

Revised: February 1988

Shown in Product Identification Section, page 426

VERSED® ℞

[*ver-sed'*]

midazolam HCl/Roche

INJECTION

The following text is complete prescribing information based on official labeling in effect June 1, 1992.

> Intravenous VERSED has been associated with respiratory depression and respiratory arrest, especially when used for conscious sedation. In some cases, where this was not recognized promptly and treated effectively, death or hypoxic encephalopathy has resulted. Intravenous VERSED should be used only in hospital or ambulatory care settings, including physicians' offices, that provide for continuous monitoring of respiratory and cardiac function. Immediate availability of resuscitative drugs and equipment and personnel trained in their use should be assured. (See WARNINGS.)
>
> The initial intravenous dose for conscious sedation may be as little as 1 mg, but should not exceed 2.5 mg in a normal healthy adult. Lower doses are necessary for older (over 60 years) or debilitated patients and in patients receiving concomitant narcotics or other CNS depressants. The initial dose and all subsequent doses should never be given as a bolus; administer over at least 2 minutes and allow an additional 2 or more minutes to fully evaluate the sedative effect. The use of the 1 mg/mL formulation or dilution of the 1 mg/mL or 5 mg/mL formulation is recommended to facilitate slower injection. See DOSAGE AND ADMINISTRATION for complete dosing information.

DESCRIPTION

VERSED (brand of midazolam hydrochloride/Roche) is a water-soluble benzodiazepine available as a sterile, nonpyrogenic parenteral dosage form for intravenous or intramuscular injection. Each mL contains midazolam hydrochloride equivalent to 1 mg or 5 mg midazolam compounded with 0.8% sodium chloride and 0.01% disodium edetate, with 1% benzyl alcohol as preservative; the pH is adjusted to approximately 3 with hydrochloric acid and, if necessary, sodium hydroxide.

Midazolam is a white to light yellow crystalline compound, insoluble in water. The hydrochloride salt of midazolam, which is formed *in situ*, is soluble in aqueous solutions. Chemically, midazolam HCl is 8-chloro-6-(2-fluorophenyl)-1-methyl-4*H*-imidazo[1,5-a][1,4] benzodiazepine hydrochloride. Midazolam hydrochloride has the empirical formula $C_{18}H_{13}ClFN_3 \cdot HCl$, a calculated molecular weight of 362.25.

CLINICAL PHARMACOLOGY

VERSED is a short-acting benzodiazepine central nervous system depressant.

The effects of VERSED on the CNS are dependent on the dose administered, the route of administration, and the presence or absence of other premedications. Onset time of sedative effects after IM administration was 15 minutes, with peak sedation occurring 30 to 60 minutes following injection. In one study, when tested the following day, 73% of the patients who received VERSED intramuscularly had no recall of memory cards shown 30 minutes following drug administration; 40% had no recall of the memory cards shown 60 minutes following drug administration.

Sedation after IV injection was achieved within 3 to 5 minutes; the time of onset is affected by total dose administered and the concurrent administration of narcotic premedication. Seventy-one percent of the patients in the endoscopy

Continued on next page

Roche Laboratories—Cont.

studies had no recall of introduction of the endoscope; 82% of the patients had no recall of withdrawal of the endoscope. When VERSED is given intravenously as an anesthetic induction agent, induction of anesthesia occurs in approximately 1.5 minutes when narcotic premedication has been administered and in 2 to 2.5 minutes without narcotic premedication or with sedative premedication. Some impairment in a test of memory was noted in 90% of the patients studied.

VERSED, used as directed, does not delay awakening from general anesthesia. Gross tests of recovery after awakening (orientation, ability to stand and walk, suitability for discharge from the recovery room, return to baseline Trieger competency) usually indicate recovery within 2 hours but recovery may take up to 6 hours in some cases. When compared with patients who received thiopental, patients who received midazolam generally recovered at a slightly slower rate.

In patients without intracranial lesions, induction with VERSED is associated with a moderate decrease in cerebrospinal fluid pressure (lumbar puncture measurements), similar to that seen following use of thiopental. Preliminary data in intracranial surgical patients with normal intracranial pressure but decreased compliance (subarachnoid screw measurements) show comparable elevations of intracranial pressure with VERSED and with thiopental during intubation.

Usual intramuscular premedicating doses of VERSED do not depress the ventilatory response to carbon dioxide stimulation to a clinically significant extent. Induction doses of VERSED depress the ventilatory response to carbon dioxide stimulation for 15 minutes or more beyond the duration of ventilatory depression following administration of thiopental. Impairment of ventilatory response to carbon dioxide is more marked in patients with chronic obstructive pulmonary disease (COPD). Sedation with intravenous VERSED does not adversely affect the mechanics of respiration (resistance, static recoil, most lung volume measurements); total lung capacity and peak expiratory flow decrease significantly but static compliance and maximum expiratory flow at 50% of awake total lung capacity (Vmax) increase.

In cardiac hemodynamic studies, induction with VERSED was associated with a slight to moderate decrease in mean arterial pressure, cardiac output, stroke volume and systemic vascular resistance. Slow heart rates (less than 65/minute), particularly in patients taking propranolol for angina, tended to rise slightly; faster heart rates (e.g., 85/minute) tended to slow slightly.

The following preliminary pharmacokinetic data for midazolam have been reported. In normal subjects and healthy patients intravenous midazolam exhibited an elimination half-life of 1.2 to 12.3 hours, a large volume of distribution (0.95 to 6.6 L/kg) and a plasma clearance of 0.15 to 0.77 L/hr/kg. Clinical effects of VERSED do not directly correlate with the blood concentrations of midazolam. Following intravenous administration, less than 0.03% of the dose is excreted in the urine as intact midazolam. Midazolam is rapidly metabolized to 1-hydroxymethyl midazolam, which is conjugated, with subsequent excretion in the urine. Approximately 45% to 57% of the dose is excreted in the urine as the conjugate of 1-hydroxymethyl midazolam, the major metabolite of midazolam. The half-life of elimination of 1-hydroxymethyl midazolam is similar to the parent compound. The concentration of midazolam is 10- to 30-fold greater than that of 1-hydroxymethyl midazolam after single IV administration.

In a small group of patients (n=11) with congestive heart failure, there appeared to be a 2- to 3-fold increase in the elimination half-life and volume of distribution of midazolam; however, the total body clearance of midazolam appeared to remain unchanged at a single 5-mg intravenous dose. There was no apparent change in the pharmacokinetic profile following the intravenous administration of 5 mg of midazolam to a small group of patients (n=12) with hepatic dysfunction. There was a 1.5- to 2-fold increase in elimination half-life, total body clearance and volume of distribution in a small group of patients (n=15) with chronic renal failure.

In a small group (n=12) of surgical patients, aged 49 to 60 years old, given 0.2 mg/kg midazolam intravenously, there appeared to be a small increase in the volume of distribution and elimination half-life with little change in total body clearance compared to an equal number of younger surgical patients (aged 18 to 30).

The mean absolute bioavailability of midazolam following intramuscular administration is greater than 90%. The mean time of maximum midazolam plasma concentrations following intramuscular dosing occurs within 45 minutes postadministration. Peak concentrations of midazolam as well as 1-hydroxymethyl midazolam after intramuscular administration are about one-half of those achieved after equivalent intravenous doses. The pharmacokinetic profile

of elimination after intramuscularly administered midazolam is comparable to that observed following intravenous administration of the drug. Dose-linearity relationships have not been adequately defined.

Midazolam is approximately 97% plasma protein-bound in normal subjects and patients with renal failure. In animals, midazolam has been shown to cross the blood-brain barrier. In animals and in humans, midazolam has been shown to cross the placenta and enter into fetal circulation. Midazolam is excreted in human milk. (See PRECAUTIONS: Nursing mothers).

INDICATIONS

Injectable VERSED is indicated—

- intramuscularly for preoperative sedation (induction of sleepiness or drowsiness and relief of apprehension) and to impair memory of perioperative events;
- intravenously as an agent for conscious sedation prior to short diagnostic or endoscopic procedures, such as bronchoscopy, gastroscopy, cystoscopy, coronary angiography and cardiac catheterization, either alone or with a narcotic;
- intravenously for induction of general anesthesia, before administration of other anesthetic agents. With the use of narcotic premedication, induction of anesthesia can be attained within a relatively narrow dose range and in a short period of time. Intravenous VERSED can also be used as a component of intravenous supplementation of nitrous oxide and oxygen (balanced anesthesia) *for short surgical procedures;* longer procedures have not been studied.

When used intravenously, VERSED is associated with a high incidence of partial or complete impairment of recall for the next several hours. (See CLINICAL PHARMACOLOGY.)

CONTRAINDICATIONS

Injectable VERSED is contraindicated in patients with a known hypersensitivity to the drug. Benzodiazepines are contraindicated in patients with acute narrow angle glaucoma. Benzodiazepines may be used in patients with open angle glaucoma only if they are receiving appropriate therapy. Measurements of intraocular pressure in patients without eye disease show a moderate lowering following induction with VERSED; patients with glaucoma have not been studied.

VERSED is not intended for intrathecal or epidural administration due to the presence of the preservative benzyl alcohol in dosage form.

WARNINGS

VERSED must never be used without individualization of dosage. Prior to the intravenous administration of VERSED in any dose, the immediate availability of oxygen, resuscitative equipment and skilled personnel for the maintenance of a patent airway and support of ventilation should be ensured. Patients should be continuously monitored for early signs of underventilation or apnea, which can lead to hypoxia/cardiac arrest unless effective countermeasures are taken immediately. Vital signs should continue to be monitored during the recovery period. Because intravenous VERSED depresses respiration (see CLINICAL PHARMACOLOGY) and because opioid agonists and other sedatives can add to this depression, VERSED should be administered as an induction agent only by a person trained in general anesthesia and should be used for conscious sedation only in the presence of personnel skilled in early detection of underventilation, maintaining a patent airway and supporting ventilation. **When used for conscious sedation, VERSED should not be administered by rapid or single bolus intravenous administration.**

Serious cardiorespiratory adverse events have occurred. These have included respiratory depression, apnea, respiratory arrest and/or cardiac arrest, sometimes resulting in death. There have also been rare reports of hypotensive episodes requiring treatment during or after diagnostic or surgical manipulations in patients who have received VERSED. Hypotension occurred more frequently in the conscious sedation studies in patients premedicated with a narcotic.

Reactions such as agitation, involuntary movements (including tonic/clonic movements and muscle tremor), hyperactivity and combativeness have been reported. These reactions may be due to inadequate or excessive dosing or improper administration of VERSED; however, consideration should be given to the possibility of cerebral hypoxia or true paradoxical reactions. Should such reactions occur, the response to each dose of VERSED and all other drugs, including local anesthetics, should be evaluated before proceeding.

Concomitant use of barbiturates, alcohol or other central nervous system depressants may increase the risk of underventilation or apnea and may contribute to profound and/or prolonged drug effect. Narcotic premedication also depresses the ventilatory response to carbon dioxide stimulation.

Higher risk surgical patients, elderly patients and debilitated patients require lower dosages, whether premedicated or not. Patients with chronic obstructive pulmonary disease are unusually sensitive to the respiratory depressant effect of VERSED. Patients with chronic renal failure and patients

with congestive heart failure eliminate midazolam more slowly. (See CLINICAL PHARMACOLOGY.) Because elderly patients frequently have inefficient function of one or more organ systems, and because dosage requirements have been shown to decrease with age, reduced initial dosage of VERSED is recommended and the possibility of profound and/or prolonged effect should be considered.

Injectable VERSED should not be administered to patients in shock or coma, or in acute alcohol intoxication with depression of vital signs. Particular care should be exercised in the use of intravenous VERSED in patients with uncompensated acute illnesses, such as severe fluid or electrolyte disturbances.

The hazards of intra-arterial injection of VERSED solutions in humans are unknown; therefore, precautions against unintended intra-arterial injection should be taken. Extravasation should also be avoided.

The safety and efficacy of VERSED following non-intravenous and non-intramuscular routes of administration have not been established. VERSED should only be administered intramuscularly or intravenously.

The decision as to when patients who have received injectable VERSED, particularly on an outpatient basis, may again engage in activities requiring complete mental alertness, operate hazardous machinery or drive a motor vehicle must be individualized. Gross tests of recovery from the effects of VERSED (see CLINICAL PHARMACOLOGY) cannot be relied upon alone to predict reaction time under stress. This drug is never used alone during anesthesia and the contribution of other perioperative drugs and events can vary. It is recommended that no patient operate hazardous machinery or a motor vehicle until the effects of the drug, such as drowsiness, have subsided or until the day after anesthesia and surgery, whichever is longer.

Usage in Pregnancy: An increased risk of congenital malformations associated with the use of benzodiazepine drugs (diazepam and chlordiazepoxide) has been suggested in several studies. If this drug is used during pregnancy, the patient should be apprised of the potential hazard to the fetus.

PRECAUTIONS

General: Intravenous doses of VERSED should be decreased for elderly and for debilitated patients. (See WARNINGS and DOSAGE AND ADMINISTRATION.) These patients will also probably take longer to recover completely after VERSED administration for the induction of anesthesia.

VERSED does not protect against the increase in intracranial pressure or against the heart rate rise and/or blood pressure rise associated with endotracheal intubation under light general anesthesia.

Information for patients: To assure safe and effective use of benzodiazepines, the following information and instructions should be communicated to the patient when appropriate:

1. Inform your physician about any alcohol consumption and medicine you are now taking, including drugs you buy without a prescription. Alcohol has an increased effect when consumed with benzodiazepines; therefore, caution should be exercised regarding simultaneous ingestion of alcohol during benzodiazepine treatment.
2. Inform your physician if you are pregnant or are planning to become pregnant.
3. Inform your physician if you are nursing.

Drug interactions: The sedative effect of intravenous VERSED is accentuated by premedication, particularly narcotics (e.g., morphine, meperidine and fentanyl) and also secobarbital and Innovar (fentanyl and droperidol). Consequently, the dosage of VERSED should be adjusted according to the type and amount of premedication administered. (See DOSAGE AND ADMINISTRATION.)

A moderate reduction in induction dosage requirements of thiopental (about 15%) has been noted following use of intramuscular VERSED for premedication.

The intravenous administration of VERSED decreases the minimum alveolar concentration (MAC) of halothane required for general anesthesia. This decrease correlates with the dose of VERSED administered.

Although the possibility of minor interactive effects has not been fully studied, VERSED and pancuronium have been used together in patients without noting clinically significant changes in dosage, onset or duration. VERSED does not protect against the characteristic circulatory changes noted after administration of succinylcholine or pancuronium and does not protect against the increased intracranial pressure noted following administration of succinylcholine. VERSED does not cause a clinically significant change in dosage, onset or duration of a single intubating dose of succinylcholine.

No significant adverse interactions with commonly used premedications or drugs used during anesthesia and surgery (including atropine, scopolamine, glycopyrrolate, diazepam, hydroxyzine, d-tubocurarine, succinylcholine and nondepolarizing muscle relaxants) or topical local anesthetics (including lidocaine, dyclonine HCl and Cetacaine) have been observed.

The clearance of midazolam and certain other benzodiazepines may be delayed with the concomitant administration

of cimetidine (but not ranitidine). The clinical significance of this interaction is unclear.

Drug/laboratory test interactions: Midazolam has not been shown to interfere with results obtained in clinical laboratory tests.

Carcinogenesis, mutagenesis, impairment of fertility:

Carcinogenesis: Midazolam maleate was administered with diet in mice and rats for two years at dosages of 1, 9 and 80 mg/kg/day. In female mice in the highest dose group there was a marked increase in the incidence of hepatic tumors. In high dose male rats there was a small but statistically significant increase in benign thyroid follicular cell tumors. Dosages of 9 mg/kg/day of midazolam maleate (25 times a human dose of 0.35 mg/kg) do not increase the incidence of tumors. The pathogenesis of induction of these tumors is not known. These tumors were found after chronic administration, whereas human use will ordinarily be of single or several doses.

Mutagenesis: Midazolam did not have mutagenic activity in *Salmonella typhimurium* (5 bacterial strains), Chinese hamster lung cells (V79), human lymphocytes, or in the micronucleus test in mice.

Impairment of fertility: A reproduction study in male and female rats did not show any impairment of fertility at dosages up to ten times the human IV dose of 0.35 mg/kg.

Pregnancy: Teratogenic effects: Pregnancy Category D. See WARNINGS section.

Segment II teratology studies, performed with midazolam maleate injectable in rabbits and rats at 5 and 10 times the human dose of 0.35 mg/kg, did not show evidence of teratogenicity.

Nonteratogenic effects: Studies in rats showed no adverse effects on reproductive parameters during gestation and lactation. Dosages tested were approximately 10 times the human dose of 0.35 mg/kg.

Labor and delivery: In humans, measurable levels of midazolam were found in maternal venous serum, umbilical venous and arterial serum and amniotic fluid, indicating placental transfer of the drug. Following intramuscular administration of 0.05 mg/kg of midazolam, both the venous and the umbilical arterial serum concentrations were lower than maternal concentrations.

The use of injectable VERSED in obstetrics has not been evaluated in clinical studies. Because midazolam is transferred transplacentally and because other benzodiazepines given in the last weeks of pregnancy have resulted in neonatal CNS depression, VERSED is not recommended for obstetrical use.

Nursing mothers: Midazolam is excreted in human milk. VERSED is not recommended for use in nursing mothers.

Pediatric use: Safety and effectiveness of VERSED in children below the age of 18 years have not been established.

ADVERSE REACTIONS

See WARNINGS concerning serious cardiorespiratory events and possible paradoxical reactions. Fluctuations in vital signs were the most frequently seen findings following parenteral administration of VERSED and included decreased tidal volume and/or respiratory rate decrease (23.3% of patients following IV and 10.8% of patients following IM administration) and apnea (15.4% of patients following IV administration), as well as variations in blood pressure and pulse rate.

The following additional adverse reactions were reported after intramuscular administration:

headache (1.3%)	*Local effects at IM injection site*
	pain (3.7%)
	induration (0.5%)
	redness (0.5%)
	muscle stiffness (0.3%)

Administration of IM VERSED to elderly and/or higher risk surgical patients has been associated with rare reports of death under circumstances compatible with cardiorespiratory depression. In most of these cases, the patients also received other central nervous system depressants capable of depressing respiration, especially narcotics (see DOSAGE AND ADMINISTRATION).

The following additional adverse reactions were reported subsequent to intravenous administration:

hiccoughs (3.9%)	*Local effects at the IV site*
nausea (2.8%)	tenderness (5.6%)
vomiting (2.6%)	pain during injection (5.0%)
coughing (1.3%)	redness (2.6%)
"oversedation" (1.6%)	induration (1.7%)
headache (1.5%)	phlebitis (0.4%)
drowsiness (1.2%)	

Other adverse experiences, observed mainly following IV injection and occurring at an incidence of less than 1.0%, are as follows:

Respiratory: Laryngospasm, bronchospasm, dyspnea, hyperventilation, wheezing, shallow respirations, airway obstruction, tachypnea.

Cardiovascular: Bigeminy, premature ventricular contractions, vasovagal episode, bradycardia, tachycardia, nodal rhythm.

Gastrointestinal: Acid taste, excessive salivation, retching.

CNS/Neuromuscular: Retrograde amnesia, euphoria, hallucination, confusion, argumentativeness, nervousness, anxiety, grogginess, restlessness, emergence delirium or agitation, prolonged emergence from anesthesia, dreaming during emergence, sleep disturbance, insomnia, nightmares, athetoid movements, seizure-like activity, ataxia, dizziness, dysphoria, slurred speech, dysphonia, paresthesia.

Special sense: Blurred vision, diplopia, nystagmus, pinpoint pupils, cyclic movements of eyelids, visual disturbance, difficulty focusing eyes, ears blocked, loss of balance, light-headedness.

Integumentary: Hive-like elevation at injection site, swelling or feeling of burning, warmth or coldness at injection site.

Hypersensitivity: Allergic reactions including anaphylactoid reactions, hives, rash, pruritus.

Miscellaneous: Yawning, lethargy, chills, weakness, toothache, faint feeling, hematoma.

DRUG ABUSE AND DEPENDENCE

Midazolam is subject to Schedule IV control under the Controlled Substances Act of 1970.

Midazolam was actively self-administered in primate models used to assess the positive reinforcing effects of psychoactive drugs.

Midazolam produced physical dependence of a mild to moderate intensity in cynomolgus monkeys after 5 to 10 weeks of administration. Available data concerning the drug abuse and dependence potential of midazolam suggest that its abuse potential is at least equivalent to that of diazepam.

OVERDOSAGE

While there is insufficient human data on overdosage with VERSED, the manifestations of VERSED overdosage are expected to be similar to those observed with other benzodiazepines and include sedation, somnolence, confusion, impaired coordination, diminished reflexes, coma and untoward effects on vital signs. No evidence of specific organ toxicity from VERSED overdosage would be expected.

Treatment of overdosage: Treatment of injectable VERSED overdosage is the same as that followed for overdosage with other benzodiazepines. Respiration, pulse rate and blood pressure should be monitored and general supportive measures should be employed. Attention should be given to the maintenance of a patent airway and support of ventilation. An intravenous infusion should be started. Should hypotension develop, treatment may include intravenous fluid therapy, repositioning, judicious use of vasopressors appropriate to the clinical situation, if indicated, and other appropriate countermeasures. There is no information as to whether peritoneal dialysis, forced diuresis or hemodialysis are of any value in the treatment of midazolam overdosage.

DOSAGE AND ADMINISTRATION

VERSED is a potent sedative agent which requires slow administration and individualization of dosage. Clinical experience has shown VERSED to be 3 to 4 times as potent per mg as diazepam. BECAUSE SERIOUS AND LIFE-THREATENING CARDIORESPIRATORY ADVERSE EVENTS HAVE BEEN REPORTED, PROVISION FOR MONITORING, DETECTION AND CORRECTION OF THESE REACTIONS MUST BE MADE FOR EVERY PATIENT TO WHOM VERSED INJECTION IS ADMINISTERED, REGARDLESS OF AGE OR HEALTH STATUS. Excess doses or rapid or single bolus intravenous administration may result in respiratory depression and/or arrest. (See WARNINGS.)

Reactions such as agitation, involuntary movements, hyperactivity and combativeness have been reported. Should such reactions occur, caution should be exercised before continuing administration of VERSED. (See WARNINGS.)

VERSED should only be administered IM or IV (See WARNINGS.)

Care should be taken to avoid intra-arterial injection or extravasation. (See WARNINGS.)

VERSED Injection may be mixed in the same syringe with the following frequently used premedications: morphine sulfate, meperidine, atropine sulfate or scopolamine. VERSED, at a concentration of 0.5 mg/mL, is compatible with 5% dextrose in water and 0.9% sodium chloride for up to 24 hours and with lactated Ringer's solution for up to 4 hours. Both the 1 mg/mL and 5 mg/mL formulations of VERSED may be diluted with 0.9% sodium chloride or 5% dextrose in water.

INTRAMUSCULARLY	USUAL ADULT DOSE
For preoperative sedation (induction of sleepiness or drowsiness and relief of apprehension) and to impair memory of perioperative events. For intramuscular use, VERSED should be injected deep in a large muscle mass.	The recommended premedication dose of VERSED for good risk (ASA Physical Status I & II) adult patients below the age of 60 years is 0.07 to 0.08 mg/kg IM (approximately 5 mg IM) administered approximately one hour before surgery. The dose must be individualized and reduced when IM VERSED is administered to patients with chronic obstructive pulmonary disease, other higher risk surgical patients, patients 60 or more years of age, and patients who have received concomitant narcotics or other CNS depressants (see ADVERSE REACTIONS). In a study of patients 60 years or older, who did not receive concomitant administration of narcotics, 2 to 3 mg (0.02 to 0.05 mg/kg) of VERSED produced adequate sedation during the preoperative period. The dose of 1 mg IM VERSED may suffice for some older patients if the anticipated intensity and duration of sedation is less critical. As with any potential respiratory depressant, these patients require observation for signs of cardiorespiratory depression after receiving IM VERSED. Onset is within 15 minutes, peaking at 30 to 60 minutes. It can be administered concomitantly with atropine sulfate or scopolamine hydrochloride and reduced doses of narcotics.
INTRAVENOUSLY *Conscious Sedation* (See INDICATIONS): Narcotic premedication results in less variability in patient response and a reduction in dosage of VERSED. For peroral procedures, the use of an appropriate topical anesthetic is recommended. For bronchoscopic procedures, the use of narcotic premedication is recommended. **VERSED 1 mg/mL formulation is recommended for conscious sedation, to facilitate slower injection. Both the 1 mg/mL and the 5 mg/mL formulations may be diluted with 0.9% sodium chloride or 5% dextrose in water.**	**When used for conscious sedation, dosage must be individualized and titrated. VERSED should not be administered by rapid or single bolus intravenous administration. Individual response will vary with age, physical status and concomitant medications, but may also vary independent of these factors. (See WARNINGS concerning cardiac/respiratory arrest.)** 1. *Healthy adults* below the age of 60:* Titrate *slowly* to the desired effect, *e.g.*, the initiation of slurred speech. Some patients may respond to as little as 1 mg. No more than 2.5 mg should be given over a period of at least 2 minutes. Wait an additional 2 or more minutes to fully evaluate the sedative effect. If further titration is necessary, continue to titrate, using small increments, to the appropriate level of sedation. Wait an additional 2 or more minutes after each increment to fully evaluate the sedative effect. A total dose greater than 5 mg is not usually necessary to reach the desired endpoint. If narcotic premedication or other CNS depressants are used, patients will require approximately 30% less VERSED than unpremedicated patients. 2. *Patients age 60 or older, and debilitated or chronically ill patients:* Because the danger of underventilation or apnea is greater in elderly patients and those with chronic disease states or decreased pulmonary reserve, and because the peak effect may take longer in these patients, increments should be

Continued on next page

Roche Laboratories—Cont.

smaller and the rate of injection slower.

Titrate *slowly* to the desired effect, *e.g.*, the initiation of slurred speech. Some patients may respond to as little as 1 mg. No more than 1.5 mg should be given over a period of no less than 2 minutes. Wait an additional 2 or more minutes to fully evaluate the sedative effect. If additional titration is necessary, it should be given at a rate of no more than 1 mg over a period of 2 minutes, waiting an additional 2 or more minutes each time to fully evaluate the sedative effect. Total doses greater than 3.5 mg are not usually necessary.

If concomitant CNS depressant premedications are used in these patients, they will require at least 50% less VERSED than healthy young unpremedicated patients.

3. *Maintenance dose:*
Additional doses to maintain the desired level of sedation may be given in increments of 25% of the dose used to first reach the sedative endpoint, but again only by slow titration, especially in the elderly and chronically ill or debilitated patient. These additional doses should be given *only* after a thorough clinical evaluation clearly indicates the need for additional sedation.

Induction of Anesthesia:
For induction of general anesthesia, before administration of other anesthetic agents.

Individual response to the drug is variable, particularly when a narcotic premedication is not used. The dosage should be titrated to the desired effect according to the patient's age and clinical status.

When VERSED is used before other intravenous agents for induction of anesthesia, the initial dose of each agent may be significantly reduced, at times to as low as 25% of the usual initial dose of the individual agents.

Unpremedicated Patients:
In the absence of premedication, an average adult under the age of 55 years will usually require an initial dose of 0.3 to 0.35 mg/kg for induction, administered over 20 to 30 seconds and allowing 2 minutes for effect. If needed to complete induction, increments of approximately 25% of the patient's initial dose may be used; induction may instead be completed with volatile liquid inhalational anesthetics. In resistant cases, up to 0.6 mg/kg total dose may be used for induction, but such larger doses may prolong recovery.

Unpremedicated patients over the age of 55 years usually require less VERSED for induction; an initial dose of 0.3 mg/kg is recommended. Unpremedicated patients with severe systemic disease or other debilitation usually require less VERSED for induction. An initial dose of 0.2 to 0.25 mg/kg will usually suffice; in some cases, as little as 0.15 mg/kg may suffice.

Premedicated Patients:
When the patient has received sedative or narcotic premedication, particularly narcotic premedication, the range of recommended doses is 0.15 to 0.35 mg/kg.

In average adults below the age of 55 years, a dose of 0.25 mg/kg, administered over 20 to 30 seconds and allowing 2 minutes for effect, will usually suffice.

The initial dose of 0.2 mg/kg is recommended for good risk (ASA I & II) surgical patients over the age of 55 years.

In some patients with severe systemic disease or debilitation, as little as 0.15 mg/kg may suffice.

Narcotic premedication frequently used during clinical trials included fentanyl (1.5 to 2 μg/kg IV, administered five minutes before induction), morphine (dosage individualized, up to 0.15 mg/kg IM), meperidine (dosage individualized, up to 1 mg/kg IM) and Innovar (0.02 mL/kg IM). Sedative premedications were hydroxyzine pamoate (100 mg orally) and sodium secobarbital (200 mg orally). Except for intravenous fentanyl, administered five minutes before induction, all other premedications should be administered approximately one hour prior to the time anticipated for VERSED induction.

Incremental injections of approximately 25% of the induction dose should be given in response to signs of lightening of anesthesia and repeated as necessary.

Injectable VERSED can also be used during maintenance of anesthesia, *for short surgical procedures,* as a component of balanced anesthesia. Effective narcotic premedication is especially recommended in such cases. Long surgical procedures have not been studied.

Note: Parenteral drug products should be inspected visually for particulate matter and discoloration prior to administration, whenever solution and container permit.

HOW SUPPLIED

Package configurations containing midazolam hydrochloride equivalent to **5 mg** midazolam/mL:
1-mL vials (5 mg)—boxes of 10 (NDC 0004-1974-01);
2-mL vials (10 mg)—boxes of 10 (NDC 0004-1973-01);
5-mL vials (25 mg)—boxes of 10 (NDC 0004-1975-01);
10-mL vials (50 mg)—boxes of 10 (NDC 0004-1946-01);
2-mL Tel-E-Ject® disposable syringes (10 mg)—boxes of 10 (NDC 0004-1947-01).
Package configurations containing midazolam hydrochloride equivalent to **1 mg** midazolam/mL:
2-mL vials (2 mg)—boxes of 10 (NDC 0004-1998-06);
5-mL vials (5 mg)—boxes of 10 (NDC 0004-1999-01);
10-mL vials (10 mg)—boxes of 10 (NDC 0004-2000-06).
Store at 59° to 86°F (15° to 30°C).

Revised: June 1991

EDUCATIONAL MATERIAL

Please contact your Roche representative concerning availability of educational programs and material.

Products are cross-indexed by
generic and chemical names
in the
YELLOW SECTION.

Roche Products Inc.
MANATI, PUERTO RICO 00674

DALMANE®   ℞
[dal'mane]
(flurazepam hydrochloride/Roche)
Capsules

The following text is complete prescribing information based on official labeling in effect June 1, 1992.

DESCRIPTION

Dalmane is available as capsules containing 15 mg or 30 mg flurazepam hydrochloride/Roche. Each 15-mg capsule also contains corn starch, lactose, magnesium stearate and talc; gelatin capsule shells may contain methyl and propyl parabens and potassium sorbate, with the following dye systems: FD&C Red No. 3, FD&C Yellow No. 6 and D&C Yellow No. 10. Each 30-mg capsule also contains corn starch, lactose and magnesium stearate; gelatin capsule shells may contain methyl and propyl parabens and potassium sorbate, with the following dye systems: FD&C Blue No. 1, FD&C Yellow No. 6, D&C Yellow No. 10 and either FD&C Red No. 3 or FD&C Red No. 40.

Flurazepam hydrochloride is chemically 7-chloro-1-[2-(diethylamino) ethyl]-5-(*o* -fluorophenyl) -1, 3-dihydro-2*H* -1, 4-benzodiazepin-2-one dihydrochloride. It is a pale yellow, crystalline compound, freely soluble in U.S.P. alcohol and very soluble in water. It has a molecular weight of 460.826.

CLINICAL PHARMACOLOGY

Flurazepam hydrochloride is rapidly absorbed from the G.I. tract. Flurazepam is rapidly metabolized and is excreted primarily in the urine. Following a single oral dose, peak flurazepam plasma concentrations ranging from 0.5 to 4.0 ng/ml occur at 30 to 60 minutes post-dosing. The harmonic mean apparent half-life of flurazepam is 2.3 hours. The blood level profile of flurazepam and its major metabolites was determined in man following the oral administration of 30 mg daily for 2 weeks. The N_1-hydroxyethyl-flurazepam was measurable only during the early hours after a 30-mg dose and was not detectable after 24 hours. The major metabolite in blood was N_1-desalkyl-flurazepam, which reached steady-state (plateau) levels after 7 to 10 days of dosing, at levels approximately five- to sixfold greater than the 24-hour levels observed on Day 1. The half-life of elimination of N_1-desalkyl-flurazepam ranged from 47 to 100 hours. The major urinary metabolite is conjugated N_1-hydroxyethyl-flurazepam which accounts for 22 to 55 percent of the dose. Less than 1% of the dose is excreted in the urine as N_1-desalkyl-flurazepam.

This pharmacokinetic profile may be responsible for the clinical observation that flurazepam is increasingly effective on the second or third night of consecutive use and that for one or two nights after the drug is discontinued both sleep latency and total wake time may still be decreased.

INDICATIONS

Dalmane is a hypnotic agent useful for the treatment of insomnia characterized by difficulty in falling asleep, frequent nocturnal awakenings, and/or early morning awakening. Dalmane can be used effectively in patients with recurring insomnia or poor sleeping habits, and in acute or chronic medical situations requiring restful sleep. Sleep laboratory studies have objectively determined that Dalmane is effective for at least 28 consecutive nights of drug administration. Since insomnia is often transient and intermittent, short-term use is usually sufficient. Prolonged use of hypnotics is usually not indicated and should only be undertaken concomitantly with appropriate evaluation of the patient.

CONTRAINDICATIONS

Dalmane is contraindicated in patients with known hypersensitivity to the drug.

Usage in Pregnancy: Benzodiazepines may cause fetal damage when administered during pregnancy. An increased risk of congenital malformations associated with the use of diazepam and chlordiazepoxide during the first trimester of pregnancy has been suggested in several studies.

Dalmane is contraindicated in pregnant women. Symptoms of neonatal depression have been reported; a neonate whose mother received 30 mg of Dalmane nightly for insomnia during the 10 days prior to delivery appeared hypotonic and inactive during the first four days of life. Serum levels of N_1-desalkyl-flurazepam in the infant indicated transplacental circulation and implicate this long-acting metabolite in this case. If there is a likelihood of the patient becoming pregnant while receiving flurazepam, she should be warned of the potential risks to the fetus. Patients should be instructed to discontinue the drug prior to becoming pregnant. The possibility that a woman of child-bearing potential may be pregnant at the time of institution of therapy should be considered.

WARNINGS

Patients receiving Dalmane should be cautioned about possible combined effects with alcohol and other CNS depres-

sants. Also, caution patients that an additive effect may occur if alcoholic beverages are consumed during the day following the use of Dalmane for nighttime sedation. The potential for this interaction continues for several days following discontinuance of flurazepam, until serum levels of psychoactive metabolites have declined.

Patients should also be cautioned about engaging in hazardous occupations requiring complete mental alertness such as operating machinery or driving a motor vehicle after ingesting the drug, including potential impairment of the performance of such activities which may occur the day following ingestion of Dalmane.

Usage in Children: Clinical investigations of Dalmane have not been carried out in children. Therefore, the drug is not currently recommended for use in persons under 15 years of age.

Withdrawal symptoms of the barbiturate type have occurred after the discontinuation of benzodiazepines. (See DRUG ABUSE AND DEPENDENCE section.)

PRECAUTIONS

Since the risk of the development of oversedation, dizziness, confusion and/or ataxia increases substantially with larger doses in elderly and debilitated patients, it is recommended that in such patients the dosage be limited to 15 mg. If Dalmane is to be combined with other drugs having known hypnotic properties or CNS-depressant effects, due consideration should be given to potential additive effects.

The usual precautions are indicated for severely depressed patients or those in whom there is any evidence of latent depression; particularly the recognition that suicidal tendencies may be present and protective measures may be necessary.

The usual precautions should be observed in patients with impaired renal or hepatic function and chronic pulmonary insufficiency.

Information for Patients: To assure the safe and effective use of benzodiazepines, patients should be informed that since benzodiazepines may produce psychological and physical dependence, it is advisable that they consult with their physician before either increasing the dose or abruptly discontinuing this drug.

ADVERSE REACTIONS

Dizziness, drowsiness, light-headedness, staggering, ataxia and falling have occurred, particularly in elderly or debilitated persons. Severe sedation, lethargy, disorientation and coma, probably indicative of drug intolerance or overdosage, have been reported.

Also reported were headache, heartburn, upset stomach, nausea, vomiting, diarrhea, constipation, gastrointestinal pain, nervousness, talkativeness, apprehension, irritability, weakness, palpitations, chest pains, body and joint pains and genitourinary complaints. There have also been rare occurrences of leukopenia, granulocytopenia, sweating, flushes, difficulty in focusing, blurred vision, burning eyes, faintness, hypotension, shortness of breath, pruritus, skin rash, dry mouth, bitter taste, excessive salivation, anorexia, euphoria, depression, slurred speech, confusion, restlessness, hallucinations, and elevated SGOT, SGPT, total and direct bilirubins, and alkaline phosphatase. Paradoxical reactions, *e.g.*, excitement, stimulation and hyperactivity, have also been reported in rare instances.

DRUG ABUSE AND DEPENDENCE

Withdrawal symptoms, similar in character to those noted with barbiturates and alcohol (convulsions, tremor, abdominal and muscle cramps, vomiting and sweating), have occurred following abrupt discontinuance of benzodiazepines. The more severe withdrawal symptoms have usually been limited to those patients who had received excessive doses over an extended period of time. Generally milder withdrawal symptoms (*e.g.*, dysphoria and insomnia) have been reported following abrupt discontinuance of benzodiazepines taken continuously at therapeutic levels for several months. Consequently, after extended therapy, abrupt discontinuation should generally be avoided and a gradual dosage tapering schedule followed. Addiction-prone individuals (such as drug addicts or alcoholics) should be under careful surveillance when receiving flurazepam or other psychotropic agents because of the predisposition of such patients to habituation and dependence.

DOSAGE AND ADMINISTRATION

Dosage should be individualized for maximal beneficial effects. The usual adult dosage is 30 mg before retiring. In some patients, 15 mg may suffice. In elderly and /or debilitated patients, 15 mg is usually sufficient for a therapeutic response and it is therefore recommended that therapy be initiated with this dosage.

OVERDOSAGE

Manifestations of Dalmane overdosage include somnolence, confusion and coma. Respiration, pulse and blood pressure should be monitored as in all cases of drug overdosage. General supportive measures should be employed, along with immediate gastric lavage. Intravenous fluids should be administered and an adequate airway maintained. Hypotension and CNS depression may be combated by judicious use of appropriate therapeutic agents. The value of dialysis has not been determined. If excitation occurs in patients following Dalmane overdosage, barbiturates should not be used. As with the management of intentional overdosage with any drug, it should be borne in mind that multiple agents may have been ingested.

HOW SUPPLIED

Dalmane (flurazepam hydrochloride/Roche) capsules—15 mg, orange and ivory; 30 mg, red and ivory—bottles of 100 and 500.

Revised: August 1991

Shown in Product Identification Section, page 426

ENDEP® ℞

[en 'dep]

(amitriptyline HCl/Roche)

TABLETS

The following text is complete prescribing information based on official labeling in effect June 1, 1992.

DESCRIPTION

Endep (amitriptyline HCl/Roche), a tricyclic antidepressant, is available as 10-mg, 25-mg, 50-mg, 75-mg, 100-mg and 150-mg tablets for oral administration. Each tablet also contains corn starch, ethylcellulose, hydroxypropyl methylcellulose, lactose, magnesium stearate, microcrystalline cellulose, povidone, talc and triacetin, with the following dye systems: 10 mg, 25 mg, 50 mg and 75 mg—FD&C Yellow No. 6 and D&C Yellow No. 10; 100 mg and 150 mg—D&C Red No. 30 and FD&C Yellow No. 6.

Amitriptyline HCl, a dibenzocycloheptadiene derivative, is a white or practically white crystalline compound that is freely soluble in water. It is designated chemically as 10,11-dihydro-*N,N*-dimethyl-5 *H*-dibenzo[*a,d*]cycloheptene-$\Delta^{5,\gamma}$-propylamine hydrochloride. The molecular weight is 313.87. The empirical formula is $C_{20}H_{23}N \cdot HCl$.

CLINICAL PHARMACOLOGY

Endep is an antidepressant with sedative effects. Its mechanism of action in man is not known. It is not a monoamine oxidase inhibitor, and it does not act primarily by stimulation of the central nervous system.

Amitriptyline inhibits the membrane pump mechanism responsible for uptake of norepinephrine and serotonin in adrenergic and serotonergic neurons. Pharmacologically this action may potentiate or prolong neuronal activity, since reuptake of these biogenic amines is important physiologically in terminating its transmitting activity. This interference with reuptake of norepinephrine and/or serotonin is believed by some to underlie the antidepressant activity of amitriptyline.

Amitriptyline undergoes extensive metabolism primarily through N-demethylation to nortriptyline, an active metabolite, followed by extensive hydroxylation to their respective 10-hydroxy metabolites which are eliminated as glucuronide conjugates.

Following a single oral dose of 75 mg of amitriptyline HCl, the mean maximum plasma concentrations of 39.4 ng/ml of amitriptyline and 16.1 ng/ml of nortriptyline were reached in approximately 4 and 10 hours, respectively. The average minimum steady-state plasma concentrations in patients receiving 50 mg of amitriptyline HCl, three times a day for an average of 32 days, were 81 ng/ml for amitriptyline, 71 ng/ml for nortriptyline, 12 ng/ml for 10-hydroxyamitriptyline, 91 ng/ml for conjugated 10-hydroxyamitriptyline, 82 ng/ml for 10-hydroxynortriptyline and 176 ng/ml for conjugated 10-hydroxynortriptyline. Steady-state plasma concentrations are usually reached by day 14. The mean apparent half-life of elimination of amitriptyline is 22.4 hours and the apparent half-life of elimination of nortriptyline is 26.0 hours. Amitriptyline is approximately 96% bound to plasma proteins.

Amitriptyline has been shown to cross the blood-brain barrier in cats, mice and rats. It has also been shown to pass the placental barrier and to enter fetal circulation in mice after intramuscular and intravenous administration. Amitriptyline is excreted in human breast milk.

INDICATIONS AND USAGE

Endep is indicated for the relief of symptoms of depression. Endogenous depression is more likely to be alleviated than are other depressive states.

CONTRAINDICATIONS

Endep is contraindicated in patients who have shown prior hypersensitivity to this agent; cross-sensitivity to other tricyclic antidepressants can occur.

Endep should not be given concomitantly with a monoamine oxidase inhibitor. Hyperpyretic crises, severe convulsions and deaths have occurred in patients receiving tricyclic antidepressant and monoamine oxidase inhibiting drugs simultaneously. When it is desired to replace a monoamine oxidase inhibitor with Endep, a minimum of 14 days should be allowed to elapse after the former is discontinued. Endep should then be initiated cautiously with gradual increase in dosage until optimum response is achieved.

Endep is not recommended for use during the acute recovery phase following myocardial infarction.

WARNINGS

Endep may block the antihypertensive action of guanethidine or similarly acting compounds.

Endep should be used with caution in patients with a history of seizures and, because of its atropine-like action, in patients with a history of urinary retention, angle-closure glaucoma or increased intraocular pressure. In patients with angle-closure glaucoma, even average doses may precipitate an attack.

Patients with cardiovascular disorders should be watched closely. Tricyclic antidepressant drugs, including Endep, particularly when given in high doses, have been reported to produce arrhythmias, sinus tachycardia and prolongation of the conduction time. Myocardial infarction and stroke have been reported with drugs of this class.

Close supervision is required when Endep is given to hyperthyroid patients or those receiving thyroid medication.

Amitriptyline HCl may enhance the response to alcohol and the effects of barbiturates and other CNS depressants. In patients who may use alcohol excessively, it should be borne in mind that the potentiation may increase the danger inherent in any suicide attempt or overdosage. Delirium has been reported with concurrent administration of amitriptyline HCl and disulfiram.

PRECAUTIONS

General: Schizophrenic patients may develop increased symptoms of psychosis; patients with paranoid symptomatology may have an exaggeration of such symptoms. Depressed patients, particularly those with known manic-depressive illness, may experience a shift to mania or hypomania. In these circumstances, the dose of Endep may be reduced or a major tranquilizer such as perphenazine may be administered concurrently.

The possibility of suicide in depressed patients remains during treatment and until significant remission occurs. Potentially suicidal patients should not have access to large quantities of this drug. Prescriptions should be written for the smallest amount feasible.

Concurrent administration of Endep and electroshock therapy may increase the hazards associated with such therapy. Such treatment should be limited to patients for whom it is essential.

Amitriptyline HCl should be used with caution in patients with impaired liver function.

Both elevation and lowering of blood sugar levels have been reported.

The drug should be discontinued several days before elective surgery, if possible.

Information for Patients: When being treated with amitriptyline HCl, patients should be advised as to the possible impairment of mental and/or physical abilities required for performance of hazardous tasks, such as operating machinery or driving a motor vehicle.

Patients receiving amitriptyline HCl should also be cautioned about the possible combined effects with alcohol, barbiturates and other CNS depressants.

Drug Interactions: MAO inhibitors—see CONTRAINDICATIONS section. Thyroid medications; alcohol, barbiturates and other CNS depressants; and guanethidine or similarly acting compounds—see WARNINGS section.

When Endep is given with anticholinergic agents or sympathomimetic drugs, including epinephrine combined with local anesthetics, close supervision and careful adjustment of dosages are required.

Paralytic ileus may occur in patients taking tricyclic antidepressants in combination with anticholinergic-type drugs.

Cimetidine is reported to reduce hepatic metabolism of certain tricyclic antidepressants, thereby delaying elimination and increasing steady-state concentrations of these drugs. Clinically significant effects have been reported with the tricyclic antidepressants when used concomitantly with cimetidine (Tagamet). Increases in plasma levels of tricyclic antidepressants, and in the frequency and severity of side effects, particularly anticholinergic, have been reported when cimetidine was added to the drug regimen. Discontinuation of cimetidine in well-controlled patients receiving tricyclic antidepressants and cimetidine may decrease the plasma levels and efficacy of the antidepressants.

Caution is advised if patients receive large doses of ethchlorvynol concurrently. Transient delirium has been reported in patients who were treated with one gram of ethchlorvynol and 75 to 150 mg of amitriptyline HCl.

Carcinogenesis, Mutagenesis, Impairment of Fertility: Carcinogenesis: Amitriptyline HCl has not been adequately studied in animals to permit an evaluation of its carcinogenic potential. However, in a study during which relatively small numbers of rats received amitriptyline HCl as a

Continued on next page

Roche Products—Cont.

dietary admixture at dosages up to 100 mg/kg/day for 78 weeks, no increase in the incidence of any tumor was reported.

Mutagenesis: Amitriptyline HCl was tested in a bacterial mutagenesis assay (Ames test) in the presence and absence of activating enzymes. No evidence for mutagenicity was found using *Salmonella* tester strains TA 1535, TA 100, TA 98 and TA 1537 at concentrations up to 5000 mcg/plate.

Impairment of Fertility: Amitriptyline HCl was studied in a Segment I fertility and general reproduction study in rats at dosages up to 20 mg/kg/day. There were no adverse effects on fertility, fetal growth and development, litter size, pup survival or pup growth. Similarly, no adverse effects were reported in a rat litter test in which amitriptyline HCl was administered at dosages up to 20 mg/kg/day.

Pregnancy: Teratogenic Effects: Pregnancy Category C. Animal reproduction studies have been inconclusive, and clinical experience has been limited. Amitriptyline HCl was tested in rats and in rabbits for teratogenic potential at dosages up to 20 mg/kg/day. Although stunting and increased neonatal mortality were observed in rabbits, there was no evidence for teratogenicity in either rats or rabbits. In a brief report, amitriptyline HCl was shown to be teratogenic in the hamster at dosages up to 100 mg/kg administered intraperitoneally on day 8 of gestation. In a more detailed study, amitriptyline HCl was shown to produce malformations in the rabbit at dosages of 15 to 60 mg/kg/day and in the mouse at dosages of 14 to 56 mg/kg/day. In another study, amitriptyline HCl was shown to be teratogenic in JBT/Jd and JBT/Ju strains of mice at dosages of 60 to 65 mg/kg, respectively; these dosages are near the litter LD_{50}. The dosages which were teratogenic in animals ranged from 10.5 to 70 times the maximum recommended adult maintenance dosage of 100 mg/day of Endep and from 3.5 to 23 times the maximum recommended initial dosage for hospitalized patients (300 mg/day).

There are no adequate or well-controlled studies of Endep in pregnant women. Endep should be used during pregnancy only if the potential benefit justifies the potential risk to the fetus.

Nonteratogenic Effects: Amitriptyline HCl was tested in rats in a Segment II study at dosages up to 20 mg/kg/day. No significant adverse effects were observed in the peri- or postnatal development and growth of pups.

Nursing Mothers: Amitriptyline and its metabolite, nortriptyline, are excreted in breast milk. Because of the potential for serious adverse reactions from Endep in nursing infants, a decision should be made whether to discontinue nursing or to discontinue the drug, taking into account the importance of the drug to the mother.

Pediatric Use: Safety and effectiveness in children below the age of 12 have not been established.

ADVERSE REACTIONS

Note: Included in this listing which follows are a few adverse reactions which have not been reported with this specific drug. However, pharmacological similarities among the tricyclic antidepressant drugs require that each of the reactions be considered when Endep is administered.

Cardiovascular: Hypotension, particularly orthostatic hypotension, hypertension, tachycardia, palpitation, myocardial infarction, arrhythmias, heart block, stroke.

CNS and Neuromuscular: Confusional states; disturbed concentration; disorientation; delusions; hallucinations; excitement; anxiety; restlessness; insomnia; nightmares; numbness; tingling and paresthesias of the extremities; peripheral neuropathy; incoordination; ataxia; tremors; seizures; alteration in EEG patterns; extrapyramidal symptoms; tinnitus.

Anticholinergic: Dry mouth, blurred vision, disturbance of accommodation, increased intraocular pressure, constipation, paralytic ileus, urinary retention, dilatation of urinary tract.

Allergic: Skin rash, urticaria, photosensitization, edema of face and tongue.

Hematologic: Bone marrow depression including agranulocytosis, leukopenia, eosinophilia, purpura, thrombocytopenia.

Gastrointestinal: Nausea, epigastric distress, vomiting, anorexia, stomatitis, peculiar taste, diarrhea, parotid swelling, black tongue. Rarely, hepatitis (including altered liver function and jaundice).

Endocrine: Testicular swelling and gynecomastia in the male, breast enlargement and galactorrhea in the female, increased or decreased libido, elevation and lowering of blood sugar levels, syndrome of inappropriate ADH (antidiuretic hormone) secretion.

Other: Dizziness, weakness, fatigue, headache, weight gain or loss, edema, increased perspiration, urinary frequency, mydriasis, drowsiness, alopecia.

Withdrawal Symptoms: Abrupt cessation of treatment after prolonged administration may produce nausea, headache and malaise. Gradual dosage reduction has been reported to produce, within two weeks, transient symptoms including irritability, restlessness, and dream and sleep disturbance. These symptoms are not indicative of addiction. Rare instances have been reported of mania or hypomania occurring within 2 to 7 days following cessation of chronic therapy with tricyclic antidepressants.

OVERDOSAGE

Manifestations: High doses may cause temporary confusion, disturbed concentration or transient visual hallucinations. Overdosage may cause drowsiness; hypothermia; tachycardia and other arrhythmic abnormalities, such as bundle branch block; ECG evidence of impaired conduction; congestive heart failure; dilated pupils; disorders of ocular motility; convulsions; severe hypotension; stupor and coma. Other symptoms may be agitation, hyperactive reflexes, muscle rigidity, vomiting, hyperpyrexia or any of those listed in the ADVERSE REACTIONS section.

Treatment: **All patients suspected of having taken an overdosage should be admitted to a hospital as soon as possible.** Treatment is symptomatic and supportive. Empty the stomach as quickly as possible by emesis followed by gastric lavage upon arrival at the hospital. Following gastric lavage, activated charcoal may be administered. Twenty to 30 Gm of activated charcoal may be given every four to six hours during the first 24 to 48 hours after ingestion. An ECG should be taken and close monitoring of cardiac function instituted if there is any sign of abnormality. Maintain an open airway and adequate fluid intake; regulate body temperature.

The intravenous administration of 1 to 3 mg of physostigmine salicylate has been reported to reverse the symptoms of tricyclic antidepressant poisoning. Because physostigmine is rapidly metabolized, the dosage of physostigmine should be repeated as required, particularly if life-threatening signs such as arrhythmias, convulsions and deep coma recur or persist after the initial dosage of physostigmine. Because physostigmine itself may be toxic, it is not recommended for routine use.

Standard measures should be used to manage circulatory shock and metabolic acidosis. Cardiac arrhythmias may be treated with neostigmine, pyridostigmine or propranolol. Should cardiac failure occur, the use of digitalis should be considered. Close monitoring of cardiac function for not less than five days is advisable. Anticonvulsants may be given to control convulsions. Amitriptyline increases the CNS depressant action but not the anticonvulsant action of barbiturates; therefore, an inhalation anesthetic, diazepam or paraldehyde is recommended for control of convulsions.

Dialysis is of no value because of low plasma concentrations of the drug.

Since overdosage is often deliberate, patients may attempt suicide by other means during the recovery phase.

Deaths by deliberate or accidental overdosage have occurred with this class of drugs.

The acute oral toxicity of amitriptyline HCl is as follows:

Species	$LD_{50} \pm$ S.E. (mg/kg)
Mouse	260 ± 16
Rat	617 ± 50
Rabbit	446 ± 32
Dog	~ 290

DOSAGE AND ADMINISTRATION

Oral Dosage: Dosage should be initiated at a low level and increased gradually, noting carefully the clinical response and any evidence of intolerance.

Initial Dosage for Adults: Twenty-five mg 3 times a day usually is satisfactory for outpatients. If necessary, this may be increased to a total of 150 mg a day. Increases are made preferably in the late afternoon and/or bedtime doses. A sedative effect may be apparent before the antidepressant effect is noted, but an adequate therapeutic effect may take as long as 30 days to develop.

An alternative method of initiating therapy in outpatients is to begin with 50 to 100 mg amitriptyline HCl at bedtime. This may be increased by 25 to 50 mg as necessary in the bedtime dose to a total of 150 mg per day.

Hospitalized patients may require 100 mg a day initially. This can be increased gradually to 200 mg a day if necessary. A small number of hospitalized patients may need as much as 300 mg a day.

Adolescent and Elderly Patients: In general, lower dosages are recommended for these patients. Ten mg 3 times a day with 20 mg at bedtime may be satisfactory in adolescent and elderly patients who do not tolerate higher dosages.

Maintenance: The usual maintenance dosage of amitriptyline HCl is 50 to 100 mg per day. In some patients 40 mg per day is sufficient. For maintenance therapy the total daily dosage may be given in a single dose preferably at bedtime. When satisfactory improvement has been reached, dosage should be reduced to the lowest amount that will maintain relief of symptoms. It is appropriate to continue maintenance therapy 3 months or longer to lessen the possibility of relapse.

Usage in Children: In view of the lack of experience in children, this drug is not recommended at the present time for patients under 12 years of age.

Plasma Levels: Because of the wide variation in the absorption and distribution of tricyclic antidepressants in body fluids, it is difficult to directly correlate plasma levels and therapeutic effect. However, determination of plasma levels may be useful in identifying patients who appear to have toxic effects and may have excessively high levels, or those in whom lack of absorption or noncompliance is suspected. Adjustments in dosage should be made according to the patient's clinical response and not on the basis of plasma levels.

HOW SUPPLIED

10-mg tablets, orange, round, film-coated, scored—bottles of 100 (NDC 0140-0106-01). Imprint on tablets: ENDEP 10 ROCHE.

25-mg tablets, orange, round, film-coated, scored—bottles of 100 (NDC 0140-0107-01). Imprint on tablets: ENDEP 25 ROCHE.

50-mg tablets, orange, round, film-coated, scored—bottles of 100 (NDC 0140-0109-01). Imprint on tablets: ENDEP 50 ROCHE.

75-mg tablets, yellow, round, film-coated, scored—bottles of 100 (NDC 0140-0114-01). Imprint on tablets: ENDEP 75 ROCHE.

100-mg tablets, peach, round, film-coated, scored—bottles of 100 (NDC 0140-0116-01). Imprint on tablets: ENDEP 100 ROCHE.

150-mg tablets, salmon, round, film-coated, scored—bottles of 100 (NDC 0140-0124-01). Imprint on tablets: ENDEP 150 ROCHE.

Revised: July 1988

Shown in Product Identification Section, page 426

LIBRAX® ℞
[lib'rax]

The following text is complete prescribing information based on official labeling in effect June 1, 1992.

COMPOSITION

Each capsule contains 5 mg chlordiazepoxide hydrochloride (Librium®) and 2.5 mg clidinium bromide (Quarzan®).

DESCRIPTION

Librax combines in a single capsule formulation the antianxiety action of Librium (chlordiazepoxide hydrochloride/Roche) and the anticholinergic/spasmolytic effects of Quarzan (clidinium bromide/Roche), both exclusive developments of Roche research.

Each Librax capsule contains 5 mg chlordiazepoxide hydrochloride and 2.5 mg clidinium bromide. Each capsule also contains corn starch, lactose and talc. Gelatin capsule shells may contain methyl and propyl parabens and potassium sorbate, with the following dye systems: D&C Yellow No. 10 and either FD&C Blue No. 1 or FD&C Green No. 3.

Librium (chlordiazepoxide hydrochloride/Roche) is a versatile therapeutic agent of proven value for the relief of anxiety and tension. It is indicated when anxiety, tension or apprehension are significant components of the clinical profile. It is among the safer of the effective psychopharmacologic compounds.

Chlordiazepoxide hydrochloride is 7-chloro-2-methylamino-5-phenyl-3H-1, 4-benzodiazepine 4-oxide hydrochloride. A colorless, crystalline substance, it is soluble in water. It is unstable in solution and the powder must be protected from light. The molecular weight is 336.22.

Quarzan (clidinium bromide/Roche) is a synthetic anticholinergic agent which has been shown in experimental and clinical studies to have a pronounced antispasmodic and antisecretory effect on the gastrointestinal tract.

ANIMAL PHARMACOLOGY

Chlordiazepoxide hydrochloride has been studied extensively in many species of animals and these studies are suggestive of action on the limbic system of the brain,[1,2,3] which recent evidence indicates is involved in emotional responses.[4,5]

Hostile monkeys were made tame by oral drug doses which did not cause sedation. Chlordiazepoxide hydrochloride revealed a "taming" action with the elimination of fear and aggression.[6] The taming effect of chlordiazepoxide hydrochloride was further demonstrated in rats made vicious by lesions in the septal area of the brain. The drug dosage which effectively blocked the vicious reaction was well below the dose which caused sedation in these animals.[6]

The oral LD_{50} of single doses of chlordiazepoxide hydrochloride, calculated according to the method of Miller and Tainter,[7] is 720 ± 51 mg/kg as determined in mice observed over a period of five days following dosage.

Clidinium bromide is an effective anticholinergic agent with activity approximating that of atropine sulfate against acetylcholine-induced spasms in isolated intestinal strips. On oral administration in mice it proved an effective antisialagogue in preventing pilocarpine-induced salivation. Sponta-

neous intestinal motility in both rats and dogs is reduced following oral dosing with 0.1 to 0.25 mg/kg. Potent cholinergic ganglionic blocking effects (vagal) are produced with intravenous usage in anesthetized dogs.

Oral doses of 2.5 mg/kg to dogs produced signs of nasal dryness and slight pupillary dilation. In two other species, monkeys and rabbits, doses of 5 mg/kg, p.o., given three times daily for 5 days did not produce apparent secretory or visual changes.

The oral LD_{50} of single doses of clidinium bromide is 860 ± 57 mg/kg as determined in mice observed over a period of 5 days following dosage; the calculations were made according to the method of Miller and Tainter.[7]

Effects on Reproduction: Reproduction studies in rats fed chlordiazepoxide hydrochloride, 10, 20 and 80 mg/kg daily, and bred through one or two matings showed no congenital anomalies, nor were there adverse effects on lactation of the dams or growth of the newborn. However, in another study at 100 mg/kg daily there was noted a significant decrease in the fertilization rate and a marked decrease in the viability and body weight of offspring which may be attributable to sedative activity, thus resulting in lack of interest in mating and lessened maternal nursing and care of the young.[8,9] One neonate in each of the first and second matings in the rat reproduction study at the 100 mg/kg dose exhibited major skeletal defects. Further studies are in progress to determine the significance of these findings.

Two series of reproduction experiments with clidinium bromide were carried out in rats, employing dosages of 2.5 and 10 mg/kg daily in each experiment. In the first experiment clidinium bromide was administered for a 9-week interval prior to mating; no untoward effect on fertilization or gestation was noted. The offspring were taken by caesarean section and did not show a significant incidence of congenital anomalies when compared to control animals. In the second experiment adult animals were given clidinium bromide for ten days prior to and through two mating cycles. No significant effects were observed on fertility, gestation, viability of offspring or lactation, as compared to control animals, nor was there a significant incidence of congenital anomalies in the offspring derived from these experiments.

A reproduction study of Librax was carried out in rats through two successive matings. Oral daily doses were administered in two concentrations: 2.5 mg/kg chlordiazepoxide hydrochloride with 1.25 mg/kg clidinium bromide, or 25 mg/kg chlordiazepoxide hydrochloride with 12.5 mg/kg clidinium bromide. In the first mating no significant differences were noted between the control or the treated groups, with the exception of a slight decrease in the number of animals surviving during lactation among those receiving the highest dosage. As with all anticholinergic drugs, an inhibiting effect on lactation may occur. In the second mating similar results were obtained except for a slight decrease in the number of pregnant females and in the percentage of offspring surviving until weaning. No congenital anomalies were observed in both matings in either the control or treated groups. Additional animal reproduction studies are in progress.

INDICATIONS

Based on a review of this drug by the National Academy of Sciences—National Research Council and/or other information, FDA has classified the indications as follows:

"Possibly" effective: as adjunctive therapy in the treatment of peptic ulcer and in the treatment of the irritable bowel syndrome (irritable colon, spastic colon, mucous colitis) and acute enterocolitis.

Final classification of the less-than-effective indications requires further investigation.

CONTRAINDICATIONS

Librax is contraindicated in the presence of glaucoma (since the anticholinergic component may produce some degree of mydriasis) and in patients with prostatic hypertrophy and benign bladder neck obstruction. It is contraindicated in patients with known hypersensitivity to chlordiazepoxide hydrochloride and/or clidinium bromide.

WARNINGS

As in the case of other preparations containing CNS-acting drugs, patients receiving Librax should be cautioned about possible combined effects with alcohol and other CNS depressants. For the same reason, they should be cautioned against hazardous occupations requiring complete mental alertness such as operating machinery or driving a motor vehicle.

Usage in Pregnancy: **An increased risk of congenital malformations associated with the use of minor tranquilizers (chlordiazepoxide, diazepam and meprobamate) during the first trimester of pregnancy has been suggested in several studies. Because use of these drugs is rarely a matter of urgency, their use during this period should almost always be avoided. The possibility that a woman of childbearing potential may be pregnant at the time of institution of therapy should be considered. Patients should be advised that if they become pregnant during therapy or intend to become pregnant they should communicate with their physicians about the desirability of discontinuing the drug.**

As with all anticholinergic drugs, an inhibiting effect on lactation may occur. (See Animal Pharmacology.)

Management of Overdosage: Manifestations of Librium (chlordiazepoxide hydrochloride/Roche) overdosage include somnolence, confusion, coma and diminished reflexes. Respiration, pulse and blood pressure should be monitored, as in all cases of drug overdosage, although, in general, these effects have been minimal following Librium overdosage.

While the signs and symptoms of Librax overdosage may be produced by either of its components, usually such symptoms will be overshadowed by the anticholinergic actions of Quarzan (clidinium bromide/Roche). The symptoms of overdosage of Quarzan are excessive dryness of mouth, blurring of vision, urinary hesitancy and constipation.

General supportive measures should be employed, along with immediate gastric lavage. Administer physostigmine (Antilirium) 0.5 to 2 mg at a rate of no more than 1 mg per minute. This may be repeated in 1 to 4 mg doses if arrhythmias, convulsions or deep coma recur. Intravenous fluids should be administered and an adequate airway maintained. Hypotension may be combated by the use of Levophed® (levarterenol) or Aramine (metaraminol). Ritalin (methylphenidate) or caffeine and sodium benzoate may be given to combat CNS-depressive effects. Dialysis is of limited value. Should excitation occur, barbiturates should not be used. As with the management of intentional overdosage with any drug, it should be borne in mind that multiple agents may have been ingested.

Withdrawal symptoms of the barbiturate type have occurred after the discontinuation of benzodiazepines. (See DRUG ABUSE AND DEPENDENCE section.)

PRECAUTIONS

In elderly and debilitated patients, it is recommended that the dosage be limited to the smallest effective amount to preclude the development of ataxia, oversedation, or confusion (not more than two Librax capsules per day initially, to be increased gradually as needed and tolerated). In general, the concomitant administration of Librax and other psychotropic agents is not recommended. If such combination therapy seems indicated, careful consideration should be given to the pharmacology of the agents to be employed—particularly when the known potentiating compounds such as the MAO inhibitors and phenothiazines are to be used. The usual precautions in treating patients with impaired renal or hepatic function should be observed.

Paradoxical reactions to chlordiazepoxide hydrochloride, *e.g.*, excitement, stimulation and acute rage, have been reported in psychiatric patients and should be watched for during Librax therapy. The usual precautions are indicated when chlordiazepoxide hydrochloride is used in the treatment of anxiety states where there is any evidence of impending depression; it should be borne in mind that suicidal tendencies may be present and protective measures may be necessary. Although clinical studies have not established a cause and effect relationship, physicians should be aware that variable effects on blood coagulation have been reported very rarely in patients receiving oral anticoagulants and Librium (chlordiazepoxide hydrochloride).

Information for Patients: To assure the safe and effective use of benzodiazepines, patients should be informed that, since benzodiazepines may produce psychological and physical dependence, it is advisable that they consult with their physician before either increasing the dose or abruptly discontinuing this drug.

ADVERSE REACTIONS[10]

No side effects or manifestations not seen with either compound alone have been reported with the administration of Librax. However, since Librax contains chlordiazepoxide hydrochloride and clidinium bromide, the possibility of untoward effects which may be seen with either of these two compounds cannot be excluded.

When chlordiazepoxide hydrochloride has been used alone the necessity of discontinuing therapy because of undesirable effects has been rare.[11] Drowsiness,[12] ataxia[13] and confusion[9] have been reported in some patients—particularly the elderly and debilitated.[9] While these effects can be avoided in almost all instances by proper dosage adjustment, they have occasionally been observed at the lower dosage ranges. In a few instances syncope has been reported.[14]

Other adverse reactions reported during therapy with Librium (chlordiazepoxide hydrochloride/Roche) include isolated instances of skin eruptions,[12] edema,[15] minor menstrual irregularities,[12] nausea and constipation,[16] extrapyramidal symptoms,[9] as well as increased and decreased libido. Such side effects have been infrequent and are generally controlled with reduction of dosage. Changes in EEG patterns (low-voltage fast activity) have been observed in patients during and after Librium treatment.[17]

Blood dyscrasias,[10] including agranulocytosis,[18] jaundice and hepatic dysfunction[19] have occasionally been reported during therapy with Librium. When Librium treatment is protracted, periodic blood counts and liver function tests are advisable.

Adverse effects reported with use of *Librax* are those typical of anticholinergic agents, *i.e.*, dryness of the mouth, blurring of vision, urinary hesitancy and constipation. Constipation has occurred most often when Librax therapy has been combined with other spasmolytic agents and/or a low residue diet.

DRUG ABUSE AND DEPENDENCE

Withdrawal symptoms, similar in character to those noted with barbiturates and alcohol (convulsions, tremor, abdominal and muscle cramps, vomiting and sweating), have occurred following abrupt discontinuance of chlordiazepoxide. The more severe withdrawal symptoms have usually been limited to those patients who had received excessive doses over an extended period of time. Generally milder withdrawal symptoms (*e.g.*, dysphoria and insomnia) have been reported following abrupt discontinuance of benzodiazepines taken continuously at therapeutic levels for several months. Consequently, after extended therapy, abrupt discontinuation should generally be avoided and a gradual dosage tapering schedule followed. Addiction-prone individuals (such as drug addicts or alcoholics) should be under careful surveillance when receiving chlordiazepoxide or other psychotropic agents because of the predisposition of such patients to habituation and dependence.

DOSAGE

Because of the varied individual responses to tranquilizers and anticholinergics, the optimum dosage of Librax varies with the diagnosis and response of the individual patient. The dosage, therefore, should be individualized for maximum beneficial effects. The usual maintenance dose is 1 or 2 capsules, 3 or 4 times a day administered before meals and at bedtime.

HOW SUPPLIED

Librax is available in green capsules, each containing 5 mg chlordiazepoxide hydrochloride (Librium®) and 2.5 mg clidinium bromide (Quarzan®)—bottles of 100 (NDC 0140-0007-01) and 500 (NDC 0140-0007-14); Tel-E-Dose® packages of 100 (NDC 0140-0007-49).

REFERENCES

1. Schallek, W., *et al:* Arch. Int. Pharmacodyn. *149*:467-483, 1964.
2. Himwich, H. E., *et al:* J. Neuropsych. *3* (Suppl. 1):S15-S26, August 1962.
3. Morillo, A., *et al:* Psychopharmacologia *3* (No. 5):386-394, 1962.
4. MacLean, P. D.: Psychosomatic Med. *17:* 355-366, September 1955.
5. Morgan, C. T.: Physiological Psychology, 3rd Ed.; New York, McGraw-Hill, 1965.
6. Randall, L. O. *et al:* J. Pharm. Exper. Therap. *129*:163-171, June 1960.
7. Miller, L. C. and Tainter, M. C.: Proc. Soc. Exp. Biol. & Med. 57:261, 1944.
8. Zbinden, G., *et al:* Toxicology and Applied Pharmacology *3*:619-637, November 1961.
9. Data on file, Hoffmann-La Roche Inc., Nutley, New Jersey.
10. Bibliography and References available on request from Roche Laboratories.
11. Rickels, K. *et al:* Med. Times *93*:238-245, March 1965.
12. Tobin, J. M. *et al:* J. Amer. Med. Assoc. *174:* 1242-1249, November 1960.
13. Jenner, F. A., *et al:* J. Ment. Sci. *107*:575-582, May 1961.
14. Robinson, R. C. V.: Dis. Nerv. System *21*:43-45, March 1960.
15. Rose, J. T.: Amer. J. Psychiat. *120*:899-900, March 1964.
16. Hines, L. R.: Curr. Therap. Res. *2*:227-236, June 1960.
17. Gibbs, F. A. and Gibbs, E. L.: J. Neuropsych., 3 (Suppl. 1):S73-S78, August 1962.
18. Kaelbling, R., *et al:* J. Amer. Med. Assoc. *174*:1863-1865, December 1960.
19. Cacioppo, J., *et al:* Amer. J. Psychiat. *117*:1040-1041, May 1961.

Revised: February 1988

Shown in Product Identification Section, page 426

LIBRITABS® ℂ

[lib'rit-abs]

(chlordiazepoxide/Roche)

The following text is complete prescribing information based on official labeling in effect June 1, 1992.

Continued on next page

Roche Products—Cont.

DESCRIPTION

Libritabs, the original chlordiazepoxide and prototype for the benzodiazepine compounds, was synthesized and developed at Hoffmann-LaRoche Inc. It is a versatile therapeutic agent of proven value for the relief of anxiety. Libritabs is among the safer of the effective psychopharmacologic compounds available, as demonstrated by extensive clinical evidence.

Libritabs is available as tablets containing 5 mg, 10 mg or 25 mg chlordiazepoxide. Each tablet also contains corn starch, ethylcellulose, hydroxypropyl methylcellulose, lactose, magnesium stearate, microcrystalline cellulose and triacetin; with FD&C Blue No. 1, D&C Yellow No. 10 and FD&C Yellow No. 6 dyes.

Chlordiazepoxide is 7-chloro-2-(methylamino)-5-phenyl-3H-1,4-benzodiazepine 4-oxide. A yellow crystalline substance, it is insoluble in water. The powder must be protected from light. The molecular weight is 299.76.

ACTIONS

Libritabs (chlordiazepoxide/Roche) has antianxiety, sedative, appetite-stimulating and weak analgesic actions. The precise mechanism of action is not known. The drug blocks EEG arousal from stimulation of the brain stem reticular formation. It takes several hours for peak blood levels to be reached and the half-life of the drug is between 24 and 48 hours. After the drug is discontinued plasma levels decline slowly over a period of several days. Chlordiazepoxide is excreted in the urine, with 1 to 2% unchanged and 3 to 6% as a conjugate.

Animal Pharmacology: The drug has been studied extensively in many species of animals and these studies are suggestive of action on the limbic system of the brain, which recent evidence indicates is involved in emotional response. Hostile monkeys were made tame by oral doses which did not cause sedation. Chlordiazepoxide HCl revealed a "taming" action with the elimination of fear and aggression. The taming effect of chlordiazepoxide HCl was further demonstrated in rats made vicious by lesions in the septal area of the brain. The drug dosage which effectively blocked the vicious reaction was well below the dose which caused sedation in these animals.

The LD_{50} of parenterally administered chlordiazepoxide HCl was determined in mice (72 hours) and rats (5 days), and calculated according to the method of Miller and Tainter, with the following results: mice, I.V., 123 $\pm$12 mg/kg; mice, I.M., 366 $\pm$7 mg/kg; rats, I.V., 120 $\pm$7 mg/kg; rats, I.M., >160 mg/kg.

Effects on Reproduction: Reproduction studies in rats fed 10, 20 and 80 mg/kg daily and bred through one or two matings showed no congenital anomalies, nor were there adverse effects on lactation of the dams or growth of the newborn. However, in another study at 100 mg/kg daily there was noted a significant decrease in the fertilization rate and a marked decrease in the viability and body weight of offspring which may be attributable to sedative activity, thus resulting in lack of interest in mating and lessened maternal nursing and care of the young. One neonate in each of the first and second matings in the rat reproduction study at the 100 mg/kg dose exhibited major skeletal defects. Further studies are in progress to determine the significance of these findings.

INDICATIONS

Libritabs is indicated for the management of anxiety disorders or for the short-term relief of symptoms of anxiety, withdrawal symptoms of acute alcoholism, and preoperative apprehension and anxiety. Anxiety or tension associated with the stress of everyday life usually does not require treatment with an anxiolytic.

The effectiveness of Libritabs in long-term use, that is, more than 4 months, has not been assessed by systematic clinical studies. The physician should periodically reassess the usefulness of the drug for the individual patient.

CONTRAINDICATIONS

Libritabs is contraindicated in patients with known hypersensitivity to the drug.

WARNINGS

Chlordiazepoxide may impair the mental and/or physical abilities required for the performance of potentially hazardous tasks such as driving a vehicle or operating machinery. Similarly, it may impair mental alertness in children. The concomitant use of alcohol or other central nervous system depressants may have an additive effect. PATIENTS SHOULD BE WARNED ACCORDINGLY.

Usage in Pregnancy: An increased risk of congenital malformations associated with the use of minor tranquilizers (chlordiazepoxide, diazepam and meprobamate) during the first trimester of pregnancy has been suggested in several studies. Because use of these drugs is rarely a matter of urgency, their use during this period should almost always be avoided. The possibility that a woman of childbearing potential may be pregnant at the time of institution of therapy should be considered. Patients should be advised that if they become pregnant during therapy or intend to become pregnant they should communicate with their physicians about the desirability of discontinuing the drug.

Withdrawal symptoms of the barbiturate type have occurred after the discontinuation of benzodiazepines. (See DRUG ABUSE AND DEPENDENCE section.)

PRECAUTIONS

In elderly and debilitated patients, it is recommended that the dosage be limited to the smallest effective amount to preclude the development of ataxia or oversedation (10 mg or less per day initially, to be increased gradually as needed and tolerated). In general, the concomitant administration of Libritabs and other psychotropic agents is not recommended. If such combination therapy seems indicated, careful consideration should be given to the pharmacology of the agents to be employed — particularly when the known potentiating compounds such as the MAO inhibitors and phenothiazines are to be used. The usual precautions in treating patients with impaired renal or hepatic function should be observed.

Paradoxical reactions, *e.g.*, excitement, stimulation and acute rage, have been reported in psychiatric patients and in hyperactive aggressive children, and should be watched for during Libritabs therapy. The usual precautions are indicated when Libritabs is used in the treatment of anxiety states where there is any evidence of impending depression; it should be borne in mind that suicidal tendencies may be present and protective measures may be necessary. Although clinical studies have not established a cause and effect relationship, physicians should be aware that variable effects on blood coagulation have been reported very rarely in patients receiving oral anticoagulants and Libritabs. In view of isolated reports associating chlordiazepoxide with exacerbation of porphyria, caution should be exercised in prescribing chlordiazepoxide to patients suffering from this disease.

Information for Patients: To assure the safe and effective use of benzodiazepines, patients should be informed that, since benzodiazepines may produce psychological and physical dependence it is advisable that they consult with their physician before either increasing the dose or abruptly discontinuing this drug.

ADVERSE REACTIONS

The necessity of discontinuing therapy because of undesirable effects has been rare. Drowsiness, ataxia and confusion have been reported in some patients — particularly the elderly and debilitated. While these effects can be avoided in almost all instances by proper dosage adjustment, they have occasionally been observed at the lower dosage ranges. In a few instances syncope has been reported.

Other adverse reactions reported during therapy include isolated instances of skin eruptions, edema, minor menstrual irregularities, nausea and constipation, extrapyramidal symptoms, as well as increased and decreased libido. Such side effects have been infrequent and are generally controlled with reduction of dosage. Changes in EEG patterns (low-voltage fast activity) have been observed in patients during and after Libritabs treatment.

Blood dyscrasias (including agranulocytosis), jaundice and hepatic dysfunction have occasionally been reported during therapy. When Libritabs treatment is protracted, periodic blood counts and liver function tests are advisable.

DRUG ABUSE AND DEPENDENCE

Chlordiazepoxide tablets are classified by the Drug Enforcement Administration as a Schedule IV controlled substance. Withdrawal symptoms, similar in character to those noted with barbiturates and alcohol (convulsions, tremor, abdominal and muscle cramps, vomiting and sweating), have occurred following abrupt discontinuance of chlordiazepoxide. The more severe withdrawal symptoms have usually been limited to those patients who had received excessive doses over an extended period of time. Generally milder withdrawal symptoms (*e.g.*, dysphoria and insomnia) have been reported following abrupt discontinuance of benzodiazepines taken continuously at therapeutic levels for several months. Consequently, after extended therapy, abrupt discontinuation should generally be avoided and a gradual dosage tapering schedule followed. Addiction-prone individuals (such as drug addicts or alcoholics) should be under careful surveillance when receiving chlordiazepoxide or other psychotropic agents because of the predisposition of such patients to habituation and dependence.

OVERDOSAGE

Manifestations of Libritabs overdosage include somnolence, confusion, coma and diminished reflexes. Respiration, pulse and blood pressure should be monitored, as in all cases of drug overdosage, although, in general, these effects have been minimal following Libritabs overdosage. General supportive measures should be employed, along with immediate gastric lavage. Intravenous fluids should be administered and an adequate airway maintained. Hypotension may be combated by the use of Levophed® (norepinephrine) or Aramine (metaraminol). Dialysis is of limited value. There have been occasional reports of excitation in patients following chlordiazepoxide overdosage; if this occurs barbiturates should not be used. As with the management of intentional overdosage with any drug, it should be borne in mind that multiple agents may have been ingested.

DOSAGE AND ADMINISTRATION

Because of the wide range of clinical indications for Libritabs, the optimum dosage varies with the diagnosis and response of the individual patient. The dosage, therefore, should be individualized for maximum beneficial effects.

ADULTS	Usual Daily Dose
Relief of mild and moderate anxiety disorders and symptoms of anxiety	5 mg or 10 mg, 3 or 4 times daily
Relief of severe anxiety disorders and symptoms of anxiety	20 mg or 25 mg, 3 or 4 times daily
Geriatric patients, or in the presence of debilitating disease	5 mg, 2 to 4 times daily

Preoperative apprehension and anxiety:
On days preceding surgery, 5 to 10 mg orally, 3 or 4 times daily. If used as preoperative medication, 50 to 100 mg I.M.* one hour prior to surgery.

CHILDREN	Usual Daily Dose
Because of the varied response of children to CNS-acting drugs, therapy should be initiated with the lowest dose and increased as required. Since clinical experience in children under 6 years of age is limited, the use of the drug in this age group is not recommended.	5 mg, 2 to 4 times daily (may be increased in some children to 10 mg, 2 or 3 times daily)

For the relief of withdrawal symptoms of acute alcoholism, the parenteral form* is usually used initially. If the drug is administered orally, the suggested initial dose is 50 to 100 mg, to be followed by repeated doses as needed until agitation is controlled — up to 300 mg per day. Dosage should then be reduced to maintenance levels.

* See package insert for injectable Librium (chlordiazepoxide HCl/Roche).

HOW SUPPLIED

5-mg tablets, green, round, film-coated, scored—bottles of 100. Imprint on tablets: (front) LIBRITABS® 5, (back) ROCHE.

10-mg tablets, green, round, film-coated, scored—bottles of 100. Imprint on tablets: (front) LIBRITABS® 10, (back) ROCHE.

25-mg tablets, green, round, film-coated, scored—bottles of 100. Imprint on tablets: (front) LIBRITABS® 25, (back) ROCHE.

Revised: August 1988

Shown in Product Identification Section, page 426

LIBRIUM® CAPSULES   ℞

[*lib 'ree-um*]
(chlordiazepoxide HCl/Roche)

The following text is complete prescribing information based on official labeling in effect June 1, 1992.

DESCRIPTION

Librium, the original chlordiazepoxide HCl and prototype for the benzodiazepine compounds, was synthesized and developed at Hoffmann-La Roche Inc. It is a versatile therapeutic agent of proven value for the relief of anxiety. Librium is among the safer of the effective psychopharmacologic compounds available, as demonstrated by extensive clinical evidence.

Librium is available as capsules containing 5 mg, 10 mg or 25 mg chlordiazepoxide HCl. Each capsule also contains corn starch, lactose and talc. Gelatin capsule shells may contain methyl and propyl parabens and potassium sorbate, with the following dye systems: 5-mg capsules—FD&C Yellow No. 6 plus D&C Yellow No. 10 and either FD&C Blue No. 1 or FD&C Green No. 3. 10-mg capsules—FD&C Yellow No. 6 plus D&C Yellow No. 10 and either FD&C Blue No. 1 plus FD&C Red No. 3 or FD&C Green No. 3 plus FD&C Red No. 40. 25-mg capsules—D&C Yellow No. 10 and either FD&C Green No. 3 or FD&C Blue No. 1.

Chlordiazepoxide hydrochloride is 7-chloro-2-(methylamino)-5-phenyl-3H-1,4-benzodiazepine 4-oxide hydrochloride. A white to practically white crystalline substance, it is soluble

in water. It is unstable in solution and the powder must be protected from light. The molecular weight is 336.22.

ACTIONS

Librium (chlordiazepoxide HCl/Roche) has antianxiety, sedative, appetite-stimulating and weak analgesic actions. The precise mechanism of action is not known. The drug blocks EEG arousal from stimulation of the brain stem reticular formation. It takes several hours for peak blood levels to be reached and the half-life of the drug is between 24 and 48 hours. After the drug is discontinued plasma levels decline slowly over a period of several days. Chlordiazepoxide is excreted in the urine, with 1 to 2% unchanged and 3 to 6% as a conjugate.

Animal Pharmacology: The drug has been studied extensively in many species of animals and these studies are suggestive of action on the limbic system of the brain, which recent evidence indicates is involved in emotional responses.

Hostile monkeys were made tame by oral drug doses which did not cause sedation. Chlordiazepoxide HCl revealed a "taming" action with the elimination of fear and aggression. The taming effect of chlordiazepoxide HCl was further demonstrated in rats made vicious by lesions in the septal area of the brain. The drug dosage which effectively blocked the vicious reaction was well below the dose which caused sedation in these animals.

The LD_{50} of parenterally administered chlordiazepoxide HCl was determined in mice (72 hours) and rats (5 days), and calculated according to the method of Miller and Tainter, with the following results: mice, I.V., 123 $\pm$12 mg/kg; mice, I.M., 366 $\pm$7 mg/kg; rats, I.V., 120 $\pm$7 mg/kg; rats, I.M., >160 mg/kg.

Effects on Reproduction: Reproduction studies in rats fed 10, 20 and 80 mg/kg daily and bred through one or two matings showed no congenital anomalies, nor were there adverse effects on lactation of the dams or growth of the newborn. However, in another study at 100 mg/kg daily there was noted a significant decrease in the fertilization rate and a marked decrease in the viability and body weight of offspring which may be attributable to sedative activity, thus resulting in lack of interest in mating and lessened maternal nursing and care of the young. One neonate in each of the first and second matings in the rat reproduction study at the 100 mg/kg dose exhibited major skeletal defects. Further studies are in progress to determine the significations of these findings.

INDICATIONS

Librium is indicated for the management of anxiety disorders or for the short-term relief of symptoms of anxiety, withdrawal symptoms of acute alcoholism, and preoperative apprehension and anxiety. Anxiety or tension associated with the stress of everyday life usually does not require treatment with an anxiolytic.

The effectiveness of Librium in long-term use, that is, more than 4 months, has not been assessed by systematic clinical studies. The physician should periodically reassess the usefulness of the drug for the individual patient.

CONTRAINDICATIONS

Librium is contraindicated in patients with known hypersensitivity to the drug.

WARNINGS

Chlordiazepoxide HCl may impair the mental and/or physical abilities required for the performance of potentially hazardous tasks such as driving a vehicle or operating machinery. Similarly, it may impair mental alertness in children. The concomitant use of alcohol or other central nervous system depressants may have an additive effect. PATIENTS SHOULD BE WARNED ACCORDINGLY.

Usage in Pregnancy: An increased risk of congenital malformations associated with the use of minor tranquilizers (chlordiazepoxide, diazepam and meprobamate) during the first trimester of pregnancy has been suggested in several studies. Because use of these drugs is rarely a matter of urgency, their use during this period should almost always be avoided. The possibility that a woman of childbearing potential may be pregnant at the time of institution of therapy should be considered. Patients should be advised that if they become pregnant during therapy or intend to become pregnant they should communicate with their physicians about the desirability of discontinuing the drug.

Withdrawal symptoms of the barbiturate type have occurred after the discontinuation of benzodiazepines. (See DRUG ABUSE AND DEPENDENCE section.)

PRECAUTIONS

In elderly and debilitated patients, it is recommended that the dosage be limited to the smallest effective amount to preclude the development of ataxia or oversedation (10 mg or less per day initially, to be increased gradually as needed and tolerated). In general, the concomitant administration of Librium and other psychotropic agents is not recommended. If such combination therapy seems indicated, careful consideration should be given to the pharmacology of the agents to be employed — particularly when the known potentiating compounds such as the MAO inhibitors and phenothiazines are to be used. The usual precautions in treating patients with impaired renal or hepatic function should be observed.

Paradoxical reactions, *e.g.,* excitement, stimulation and acute rage, have been reported in psychiatric patients and in hyperactive aggressive children, and should be watched for during Librium therapy. The usual precautions are indicated when Librium is used in the treatment of anxiety states where there is any evidence of impending depression; it should be borne in mind that suicidal tendencies may be present and protective measures may be necessary. Although clinical studies have not established a cause and effect relationship, physicians should be aware that variable effects on blood coagulation have been reported very rarely in patients receiving oral anticoagulants and Librium. In view of isolated reports associating chlordiazepoxide with exacerbation of porphyria, caution should be exercised in prescribing chlordiazepoxide to patients suffering from this disease.

Information for Patients: To assure the safe and effective use of benzodiazepines, patients should be informed that, since benzodiazepines may produce psychological and physical dependence it is advisable that they consult with their physician before either increasing the dose or abruptly discontinuing this drug.

ADVERSE REACTIONS

The necessity of discontinuing therapy because of undesirable effects has been rare. Drowsiness, ataxia and confusion have been reported in some patients — particularly the elderly and debilitated. While these effects can be avoided in almost all instances by proper dosage adjustment, they have occasionally been observed at the lower dosage ranges. In a few instances syncope has been reported.

Other adverse reactions reported during therapy include isolated instances of skin eruptions, edema, minor menstrual irregularities, nausea and constipation, extrapyramidal symptoms, as well as increased and decreased libido. Such side effects have been infrequent and are generally controlled with reduction of dosage. Changes in EEG patterns (low-voltage fast activity) have been observed in patients during and after Librium treatment.

Blood dyscrasias (including agranulocytosis), jaundice and hepatic dysfunction have occasionally been reported during therapy. When Librium treatment is protracted, periodic blood counts and liver function tests are advisable.

DRUG ABUSE AND DEPENDENCE

Chlordiazepoxide hydrochloride capsules are classified by the Drug Enforcement Administration as a Schedule IV controlled substance.

Withdrawal symptoms, similar in character to those noted with barbiturates and alcohol (convulsions, tremor, abdominal and muscle cramps, vomiting and sweating), have occurred following abrupt discontinuance of chlordiazepoxide. The more severe withdrawal symptoms have usually been limited to those patients who had received excessive doses over an extended period of time. Generally milder withdrawal symptoms (*e.g.,* dysphoria and insomnia) have been reported following abrupt discontinuance of benzodiazepines taken continuously at therapeutic levels for several months. Consequently, after extended therapy, abrupt discontinuation should generally be avoided and a gradual dosage tapering schedule followed. Addiction-prone individuals (such as drug addicts or alcoholics) should be under careful surveillance when receiving chlordiazepoxide or other psychotropic agents because of the predisposition of such patients to habituation and dependence.

OVERDOSAGE

Manifestations of Librium overdosage include somnolence, confusion, coma and diminished reflexes. Respiration, pulse and blood pressure should be monitored, as in all cases of drug overdosage, although, in general, these effects have been minimal following Librium overdosage. General supportive measures should be employed, along with immediate gastric lavage. Intravenous fluids should be administered and an adequate airway maintained. Hypotension may be combated by the use of Levophed® (norepinephrine) or Aramine (metaraminol). Dialysis is of limited value. There have been occasional reports of excitation in patients following chlordiazepoxide HCl overdosage; if this occurs barbiturates should not be used. As with the management of intentional overdosage with any drug, it should be borne in mind that multiple agents may have been ingested.

DOSAGE AND ADMINISTRATION

Because of the wide range of clinical indications for Librium, the optimum dosage varies with the diagnosis and response of the individual patient. The dosage, therefore, should be individualized for maximum beneficial effects.

HOW SUPPLIED

Librium (chlordiazepoxide HCl/Roche) capsules—5 mg, green and yellow; 10 mg, green and black; 25 mg, green and white—bottles of 100 and 500; Tel-E-Dose® packages of 100, available in boxes of 4 reverse-numbered cards of 25, and in boxes containing 10 strips of 10.

ADULTS	Usual Daily Dose
Relief of mild and moderate anxiety disorders and symptoms of anxiety	5 mg or 10 mg, 3 or 4 times daily
Relief of severe anxiety disorders and symptoms of anxiety	20 mg or 25 mg, 3 or 4 times daily
Geriatric patients, or in the presence of debilitating disease	5 mg, 2 to 4 times daily

Preoperative apprehension and anxiety: On days preceding surgery, 5 to 10 mg orally, 3 or 4 times daily. If used as preoperative medication, 50 to 100 mg I.M.* one hour prior to surgery.

CHILDREN	Usual Daily Dose
Because of the varied response of children to CNS-acting drugs, therapy should be initiated with the lowest dose and increased as required. Since clinical experience in children under 6 years of age is limited, the use of the drug in this age group is not recommended.	5 mg, 2 to 4 times daily (may be increased in some children to 10 mg, 2 or 3 times daily)

For the relief of withdrawal symptoms of acute alcoholism, the parenteral form* is usually used initially. If the drug is administered orally, the suggested initial dose is 50 to 100 mg, to be followed by repeated doses as needed until agitation is controlled — up to 300 mg per day. Dosage should then be reduced to maintenance levels.

* See package insert for injectable Librium (chlordiazepoxide HCl/Roche).

Revised: July 1988

Shown in Product Identification Section, page 426

LIBRIUM® INJECTABLE Ⓒ
[lib'ree-um]
(chlordiazepoxide HCl/Roche)

Librium Injectable is manufactured by Hoffmann-La Roche Inc., Nutley, N.J. 07110 and distributed by Roche Products Inc., Manati, P.R. 00674.

The following text is complete prescribing information based on official labeling in effect June 1, 1992.

DESCRIPTION

Librium is a versatile therapeutic agent of proven value for the relief of anxiety and tension.

Librum is the first of a new class, unrelated chemically and pharmacologically to other types of tranquilizers. Librium promptly relieves anxiety and is among the safer of the effective psychopharmacologic compounds available.

Chlordiazepoxide HCl is 7-chloro-2-methylamino-5-phenyl-3H-1,4-benzodiazepine 4-oxide hydrochloride. A colorless, crystalline substance, it is soluble in water. It is unstable in solution and the powder must be protected from light. The molecular weight is 336.22.

ANIMAL PHARMACOLOGY

The drug has been studied extensively in many species of animals and these studies are suggestive of action on the limbic system of the brain, which recent evidence indicates is involved in emotional responses.

Hostile monkeys were made tame by oral drug doses which did not cause sedation. Librium revealed a "taming" action with the elimination of fear and aggression. The taming effect of Librium was further demonstrated in rats made vicious by lesions in the septal area of the brain. The drug dosage which effectively blocked the vicious reaction was well below the dose which caused sedation in these animals.

The LD_{50} of parenterally administered chlordiazepoxide HCl was determined in mice (72 hours) and rats (5 days), and calculated according to the method of Miller and Tainter, with the following results: mice, I.V., 123 $\pm$ 12 mg/kg; mice, I.M., 366 $\pm$ 7 mg/kg; rats, I.V., 120 $\pm$ 7 mg/kg; rats, I.M., >160 mg/kg.

Effects on Reproduction: Reproduction studies in rats fed 10, 20 and 80 mg/kg daily and bred through one or two matings showed no congenital anomalies, nor were there adverse effects on lactation of the dams or growth of the newborn. However, in another study at 100 mg/kg daily there was noted a significant decrease in the fertilization rate and a marked decrease in the viability and body weight of offspring which may be attributable to sedative activity, thus resulting in lack of interest in mating and lessened maternal nursing and care of the young. One neonate in each of the first and second matings in the rat reproduction study at the 100

Continued on next page

Roche Products—Cont.

mg/kg dose exhibited major skeletal defects. Further studies are in progress to determine the significance of these findings.

INDICATIONS

Injectable Librium is indicated for the management of anxiety disorders or for the short-term relief of symptoms of anxiety, withdrawal symptoms of acute alcoholism, and preoperative apprehension and anxiety. Anxiety or tension associated with the stress of everyday life usually does not require treatment with an anxiolytic.

CONTRAINDICATIONS

Librium is contraindicated in patients with known hypersensitivity to the drug.

WARNINGS

As in the case of other CNS-acting drugs, patients receiving Librium should be cautioned about possible combined effects with alcohol and other CNS depressants.

As is true of all preparations containing CNS-acting drugs, patients receiving Librium should be cautioned against hazardous occupations requiring complete mental alertness such as operating machinery or driving a motor vehicle.

Usage in Pregnancy: **An increased risk of congenital malformations associated with the use of minor tranquilizers (chlordiazepoxide, diazepam and meprobamate) during the first trimester of pregnancy has been suggested in several studies. Because use of these drugs is rarely a matter of urgency, their use during this period should almost always be avoided. The possibility that a woman of childbearing potential may be pregnant at the time of institution of therapy should be considered. Patients should be advised that if they become pregnant during therapy or intend to become pregnant they should communicate with their physicians about the desirability of discontinuing the drug.**

Management of Overdosage: Manifestations of Librium overdosage include somnolence, confusion, coma and diminished reflexes. Respiration, pulse and blood pressure should be monitored, as in all cases of drug overdosage, although, in general, these effects have been minimal following Librium overdosage. General supportive measures should be employed, along with immediate gastric lavage.

Intravenous fluids should be administered and an adequate airway maintained. Hypotension may be combated by the use of Levophed® (levarterenol) or Aramine (metaraminol). Dialysis is of limited value. There have been occasional reports of excitation in patients following Librium overdosage; if this occurs barbiturates should not be used. As with the management of intentional overdosage with any drug, it should be borne in mind that multiple agents may have been ingested.

Withdrawal symptoms of the barbiturate type have occurred after the discontinuation of benzodiazepines. (See DRUG ABUSE AND DEPENDENCE section.)

PRECAUTIONS

Injectable Librium (intramuscular or intravenous) is indicated primarily in acute states, and patients receiving this form of therapy should be kept under observation, preferably in bed, for a period of up to three hours. Ambulatory patients should not be permitted to operate a vehicle following an injection. Injectable Librium should not be given to patients in shock or comatose states. Reduced dosage (usually 25 to 50 mg) should be used for elderly or debilitated patients, and for children age twelve or older. In general, the concomitant administration of Librium and other psychotropic agents is not recommended. If such combination therapy seems indicated, careful consideration should be given to the pharmacology of the agents to be employed—particularly when the known potentiating compounds such as the MAO inhibitors and phenothiazines are to be used. The usual precautions in treating patients with impaired renal or hepatic function should be observed.

Paradoxical reactions, *e.g.,* excitement, stimulation and acute rage, have been reported in psychiatric patients and in hyperactive aggressive children, and should be watched for during Librium therapy. The usual precautions are indicated when Librium is used in the treatment of anxiety states where there is any evidence of impending depression; it should be borne in mind that suicidal tendencies may be present and protective measures may be necessary. Although clinical studies have not established a cause and effect relationship, physicians should be aware that variable effects on blood coagulation have been reported very rarely in patients receiving oral anticoagulants and Librium. In view of isolated reports associating chlordiazepoxide with exacerbation of porphyria, caution should be exercised in prescribing chlordiazepoxide to patients suffering from this disease.

ADVERSE REACTIONS

The necessity of discontinuing therapy because of undesirable effects has been rare. Drowsiness, ataxia and confusion are more commonly seen in the elderly and debilitated.

Other adverse reactions reported during therapy include isolated instances of syncope, hypotension, tachycardia, skin eruptions, edema, minor menstrual irregularities, nausea and constipation, extrapyramidal symptoms, blurred vision, as well as increased and decreased libido. Such side effects have been infrequent and are generally controlled with reduction of dosage. Similarly, hypotension associated with spinal anesthesia has occurred. Pain following intramuscular injection has been reported. Changes in EEG patterns (low-voltage fast activity) have been observed in patients during and after Librium treatment.

Blood dyscrasias (including agranulocytosis), jaundice and hepatic dysfunction, have occasionally been reported during therapy. When Librium treatment is protracted, periodic blood counts and liver function tests are advisable.

DRUG ABUSE AND DEPENDENCE

Withdrawal symptoms, similar in character to those noted with barbiturates and alcohol (convulsions, tremor, abdominal and muscle cramps, vomiting and sweating), have occurred following abrupt discontinuance of chlordiazepoxide. The more severe withdrawal symptoms have usually been limited to those patients who had received excessive doses over an extended period of time. Generally milder withdrawal symptoms (*e.g.,* dysphoria and insomnia) have been reported following abrupt discontinuance of benzodiazepines taken continuously at therapeutic levels for several months. Consequently, after extended therapy, abrupt discontinuation should generally be avoided and a gradual dosage tapering schedule followed. Addiction-prone individuals (such as drug addicts or alcoholics) should be under careful surveillance when receiving chlordiazepoxide or other psychotropic agents because of the predisposition of such patients to habituation and dependence.

PREPARATION AND ADMINISTRATION OF SOLUTIONS

Solutions of Librium for intramuscular or intravenous use should be prepared aseptically. Sterilization by heating should not be attempted.

Intramuscular: Add 2 ml of *Special Intramuscular Diluent* to contents of 5-ml dry-filled amber ampul of Librium Sterile Powder (100 mg). Avoid excessive pressure in injecting this special diluent into the ampul containing the powder since bubbles will form on the surface of the solution. Agitate gently until completely dissolved. Solution should be prepared immediately before administration. Any unused solution should be discarded. Deep intramuscular injection should be given *slowly* into the upper outer quadrant of the gluteus muscle.

Caution: Librium solution made with the Special Intramuscular Diluent should not be given intravenously because of the air bubbles which form when the intramuscular diluent is added to the Librium powder. Do not use diluent solution if it is opalescent or hazy.

Intravenous: In most cases, intramuscular injection is the preferred route of administration of Injectable Librium since beneficial effects are usually seen within 15 to 30 minutes. When, in the judgment of the physician, even more rapid action is mandatory, Injectable Librium may be administered intravenously. A suitable solution for intravenous administration may be prepared as follows: Add 5 ml of *sterile physiological saline* or *sterile water for injection* to contents of 5-ml dry-filled amber ampul of Librium Sterile Powder (100 mg). Agitate gently until thoroughly dissolved. Solution should be prepared immediately before administration. Any unused portion should be discarded. *Intravenous injection should be given slowly over a one-minute period.*

Caution: Librium solution made with physiological saline or sterile water for injection should not be given intramuscularly because of pain on injection.

DOSAGE

Dosage should be individualized according to the diagnosis and the response of the patient. While 300 mg may be given during a 6-hour period, this dose should not be exceeded in any 24-hour period. [See table at top of next column.]

In most cases, acute symptoms may be rapidly controlled by parenteral administration so that subsequent treatment, if necessary, may be given orally. (See package insert for Oral Librium.)

HOW SUPPLIED

For Parenteral Administration: Ampuls—Duplex package consisting of a 5-ml dry-filled ampul containing 100 mg chlordiazepoxide HCl in dry crystalline form, and a 2-ml ampul of Special Intramuscular Diluent (for intramuscular administration) compounded with 1.5% benzyl alcohol, 4% polysorbate 80, 20% propylene glycol, 1.6% maleic acid and

INDICATION	ADULT DOSAGE*
Withdrawal Symptoms of Acute Alcoholism	50 to 100 mg I.M. or I.V. initially; repeat in 2 to 4 hours, if necessary
Acute or Severe Anxiety Disorders or Symptoms of Anxiety	50 to 100 mg I.M. or I.V. initially; then 25 to 50 mg 3 or 4 times daily, if necessary
Preoperative Apprehension and Anxiety	50 to 100 mg I.M. one hour prior to surgery

* Lower doses (usually 25 to 50 mg) should be used for elderly or debilitated patients, and for older children. Since clinical experience in children under 12 years of age is limited, the use of the drug in this age group is not recommended.

sodium hydroxide to adjust pH to approximately 3.0. Boxes of 10.

CAUTION

Before preparing solution for intramuscular or intravenous administration, please read instructions for PREPARATION AND ADMINISTRATION OF SOLUTIONS.

Revised: February 1988

LIMBITROL® Ⓒ

[*lim 'bit-roll*]
(chlordiazepoxide and amitriptyline HCl/Roche)
DS (double strength) Tablets
Tablets

The following text is complete prescribing information based on official labeling in effect June 1, 1992.

DESCRIPTION

Limbitrol combines for oral administration, chlordiazepoxide, an agent for the relief of anxiety and tension, and amitriptyline, an antidepressant. It is available in DS (double strength) white, film-coated tablets, each containing 10 mg chlordiazepoxide and 25 mg amitriptyline (as the hydrochloride salt); and in blue, film-coated tablets, each containing 5 mg chlordiazepoxide and 12.5 mg amitriptyline (as the hydrochloride salt). Each tablet also contains corn starch, ethylcellulose, hydroxypropyl methylcellulose, lactose, magnesium stearate, povidone and triacetin; Limbitrol tablets contain the following dye: FD&C Blue No. 1; Limbitrol DS tablets contain no dye.

Chlordiazepoxide is a benzodiazepine with the formula 7-chloro-2-(methylamino)-5-phenyl-3*H* -1,4-benzodiazepine 4-oxide. It is a slightly yellow crystalline material and is insoluble in water. The molecular weight is 299.76.

Amitriptyline is a dibenzocycloheptadiene derivative. The formula is 10,11-dihydro-*N,N*-dimethyl-5H -dibenzo[a,d]- cycloheptene-$\Delta^{5,\gamma}$ -propylamine hydrochloride. It is a white or practically white crystalline compound that is freely soluble in water. The molecular weight is 313.87.

ACTIONS

Both components of Limbitrol exert their action in the central nervous system. Extensive studies with chlordiazepoxide in many animal species suggest action in the limbic system. Recent evidence indicates that the limbic system is involved in emotional response. Taming action was observed in some species. The mechanism of action of amitriptyline in man is not known, but the drug appears to interfere with the reuptake of norepinephrine into adrenergic nerve endings. This action may prolong the sympathetic activity of biogenic amines.

INDICATIONS

Limbitrol is indicated for the treatment of patients with moderate to severe depression associated with moderate to severe anxiety.

The therapeutic response to Limbitrol occurs earlier and with fewer treatment failures than when either amitriptyline or chlordiazepoxide is used alone.

Symptoms likely to respond in the first week of treatment include: insomnia, feelings of guilt or worthlessness, agitation, psychic and somatic anxiety, suicidal ideation and anorexia.

CONTRAINDICATIONS

Limbitrol is contraindicated in patients with hypersensitivity to either benzodiazepines or tricyclic antidepressants. It should not be given concomitantly with a monoamine oxidase inhibitor. Hyperpyretic crises, severe convulsions and deaths have occurred in patients receiving a tricyclic antidepressant and a monoamine oxidase inhibitor simultaneously. When it is desired to replace a monoamine oxidase inhibitor with Limbitrol, a minimum of 14 days should be allowed to elapse after the former is discontinued. Limbitrol should then be initiated cautiously with gradual increase in dosage until optimum response is achieved.

This drug is contraindicated during the acute recovery phase following myocardial infarction.

WARNINGS

Because of the atropine-like action of the amitriptyline component, great care should be used in treating patients with a history of urinary retention or angle-closure glaucoma. In patients with glaucoma, even average doses may precipitate an attack. Severe constipation may occur in patients taking tricyclic antidepressants in combination with anticholinergic-type drugs.

Patients with cardiovascular disorders should be watched closely. Tricyclic antidepressant drugs, particularly when given in high doses, have been reported to produce arrhythmias, sinus tachycardia and prolongation of conduction time. Myocardial infarction and stroke have been reported in patients receiving drugs of this class.

Because of the sedative effects of Limbitrol, patients should be cautioned about combined effects with alcohol or other CNS depressants. The additive effects may produce a harmful level of sedation and CNS depression.

Patients receiving Limbitrol should be cautioned against engaging in hazardous occupations requiring complete mental alertness, such as operating machinery or driving a motor vehicle.

Usage in Pregnancy: Safe use of Limbitrol during pregnancy and lactation has not been established. Because of the chlordiazepoxide component, please note the following:

An increased risk of congenital malformations associated with the use of minor tranquilizers (chlordiazepoxide, diazepam and meprobamate) during the first trimester of pregnancy has been suggested in several studies. Because use of these drugs is rarely a matter of urgency, their use during this period should almost always be avoided. The possibility that a woman of childbearing potential may be pregnant at the time of institution of therapy should be considered. Patients should be advised that if they become pregnant during therapy or intend to become pregnant they should communicate with their physicians about the desirability of discontinuing the drug.

Withdrawal symptoms of the barbiturate type have occurred after the discontinuation of benzodiazepines. (See DRUG ABUSE AND DEPENDENCE section.)

PRECAUTIONS

General: Use with caution in patients with a history of seizures.

Close supervision is required when Limbitrol is given to hyperthyroid patients or those on thyroid medication.

The usual precautions should be observed when treating patients with impaired renal or hepatic function.

Patients with suicidal ideation should not have easy access to large quantities of the drug. The possibility of suicide in depressed patients remains until significant remission occurs.

Essential Laboratory Tests: Patients on prolonged treatment should have periodic liver function tests and blood counts.

Drug and Treatment Interactions: Because of its amitriptyline component, Limbitrol may block the antihypertensive action of guanethidine or compounds with a similar mechanism of action.

The effects of concomitant administration of Limbitrol and other psychotropic drugs have not been evaluated. Sedative effects may be additive.

Cimetidine is reported to reduce hepatic metabolism of certain tricyclic antidepressants and benzodiazepines, thereby delaying elimination and increasing steady state concentrations of these drugs. Clinically significant effects have been reported with the tricyclic antidepressants when used concomitantly with cimetidine (Tagamet).

The drug should be discontinued several days before elective surgery.

Concurrent administration of ECT and Limbitrol should be limited to those patients for whom it is essential.

Pregnancy: See WARNINGS section.

Nursing Mothers: It is not known whether this drug is excreted in human milk. As a general rule, nursing should not be undertaken while a patient is on a drug, since many drugs are excreted in human milk.

Pediatric Use: Safety and effectiveness in children below the age of 12 years have not been established.

Elderly Patients: In elderly and debilitated patients it is recommended that dosage be limited to the smallest effective amount to preclude the development of ataxia, oversedation, confusion or anticholinergic effects.

Information for Patients: To assure the safe and effective use of benzodiazepines, patients should be informed that, since benzodiazepines may produce psychological and physical dependence, it is advisable that they consult with their physician before either increasing the dose or abruptly discontinuing this drug.

ADVERSE REACTIONS

Adverse reactions to Limbitrol are those associated with the use of either component alone. Most frequently reported were drowsiness, dry mouth, constipation, blurred vision, dizziness and bloating. Other side effects occurring less commonly included vivid dreams, impotence, tremor, confusion

and nasal congestion. Many symptoms common to the depressive state, such as anorexia, fatigue, weakness, restlessness and lethargy, have been reported as side effects of treatment with both Limbitrol and amitriptyline.

Granulocytopenia, jaundice and hepatic dysfunction of uncertain etiology have also been observed rarely with Limbitrol. When treatment with Limbitrol is prolonged, periodic blood counts and liver function tests are advisable.

Note: Included in the listing which follows are adverse reactions which have not been reported with Limbitrol. However, they are included because they have been reported during therapy with one or both of the components or closely related drugs.

Cardiovascular: Hypotension, hypertension, tachycardia, palpitations, myocardial infarction, arrhythmias, heart block, stroke.

Psychiatric: Euphoria, apprehension, poor concentration, delusions, hallucinations, hypomania and increased or decreased libido.

Neurologic: Incoordination, ataxia, numbness, tingling and paresthesias of the extremities, extrapyramidal symptoms, syncope, changes in EEG patterns.

Anticholinergic: Disturbance of accommodation, paralytic ileus, urinary retention, dilatation of urinary tract.

Allergic: Skin rash, urticaria, photosensitization, edema of face and tongue, pruritus.

Hematologic: Bone marrow depression including agranulocytosis, eosinophilia, purpura, thrombocytopenia.

Gastrointestinal: Nausea, epigastric distress, vomiting, anorexia, stomatitis, peculiar taste, diarrhea, black tongue.

Endocrine: Testicular swelling and gynecomastia in the male, breast enlargement, galactorrhea and minor menstrual irregularities in the female, elevation and lowering of blood sugar levels, and syndrome of inappropriate ADH (antidiuretic hormone) secretion.

Other: Headache, weight gain or loss, increased perspiration, urinary frequency, mydriasis, jaundice, alopecia, parotid swelling.

DRUG ABUSE AND DEPENDENCE

Withdrawal symptoms, similar in character to those noted with barbiturates and alcohol (convulsions, tremor, abdominal and muscle cramps, vomiting and sweating), have occurred following abrupt discontinuance of chlordiazepoxide. The more severe withdrawal symptoms have usually been limited to those patients who had received excessive doses over an extended period of time. Generally milder withdrawal symptoms (*e.g.*, dysphoria and insomnia) have been reported following abrupt discontinuance of benzodiazepines taken continuously at therapeutic levels for several months. Withdrawal symptoms (*e.g.*, nausea, headache and malaise) have also been reported in association with abrupt amitriptyline discontinuation. Consequently, after extended therapy, abrupt discontinuation should generally be avoided and a gradual dosage tapering schedule followed. Addiction-prone individuals (such as drug addicts or alcoholics) should be under careful surveillance when receiving chlordiazepoxide or other psychotropic agents because of the predisposition of such patients to habituation and dependence.

OVERDOSAGE

There has been limited experience with Limbitrol overdosage *per se;* the manifestations of overdosage and recommendations for treatment are based on clinical experience with its components. Primary concern should be with the dangers associated with amitriptyline overdosage. Deaths by deliberate or accidental overdosage have occurred with this class of drugs.

All patients suspected of having an overdosage of Limbitrol should be admitted to a hospital as soon as possible.

Manifestations: High doses may cause drowsiness, temporary confusion, disturbed concentration or transient visual hallucinations. Overdosage may cause hypothermia, tachycardia and other arrhythmias, ECG evidence of impaired conduction (such as bundle branch block), congestive heart failure, dilated pupils, convulsions, severe hypotension, stupor and coma. Other symptoms may be agitation, hyperactive reflexes, muscle rigidity, vomiting, hyperpyrexia or any of those listed under Adverse Reactions.

Treatment: Empty the stomach as quickly as possible by emesis or lavage. In the comatose patient a cuff endotracheal tube should be placed in position prior to either of these measures. The instillation of activated charcoal into the stomach also should be considered. If the patient is stuporous but responds to stimuli, only close observation and nursing care may be required. It is essential to maintain an adequate airway and fluid intake. Body temperature should be watched closely and appropriate measures taken should deviations occur.

The intramuscular or slow intravenous administration of 1 to 3 mg in adults (or 0.5 mg in children) of physostigmine salicylate (Antilirium)[1-3] has been reported to reverse the manifestations of amitriptyline overdosage. Because of its relatively short half-life, additional doses may be needed at intervals of 30 minutes to 2 hours.

Convulsions may be treated by the use of an inhalation anesthetic rather than the use of barbiturates. Cardiac monitoring is advisable, and the cautious use of digitalis or other antiarrhythmic agents should be considered if serious cardiovascular abnormalities occur. Serum potassium levels should be monitored and kept within normal limits by the use of appropriate I.V. fluids. Standard measures including oxygen, I.V. fluids, plasma expanders and corticosteroids may be used to control circulatory shock.

Dialysis is unlikely to be of value, as it has not proven useful in overdosages of either amitriptyline or chlordiazepoxide. Since many suicidal attempts involve multiple drugs including barbiturates, the possibility of dialysis being beneficial for removal of other drugs should not be overlooked.

Treatment should be continued for at least 48 hours, along with cardiac monitoring in patients who do not respond to therapy promptly. Since relapses are frequent, patients should be hospitalized until their conditions remain stable without physostigmine for at least 24 hours.

Since overdosage is often deliberate, patients may attempt suicide by other means during the recovery phase.

References:

1. Granacher RP, Baldessarini RJ: Physostigmine: Its use in acute anticholinergic syndrome with antidepressant and antiparkinson drugs. *Arch Gen Psychiatry* 32:375–380, March 1975.

2. Burks JS, Walker JE, Rumack BH, Ott JE: Tricyclic antidepressant poisoning: Reversal of coma, choreoathetosis, and myoclonus by physostigmine. *JAMA* 230:1405–1407, Dec. 9, 1974.

3. Snyder BD, Blonde L, McWhirter WR: Reversal of amitriptyline intoxication by physostigmine. *JAMA* 230:1433–1434, Dec. 9, 1974.

DOSAGE AND ADMINISTRATION

Optimum dosage varies with the severity of the symptoms and the response of the individual patient. When a satisfactory response is obtained, dosage should be reduced to the smallest amount needed to maintain the remission. The larger portion of the total daily dose may be taken at bedtime. In some patients, a single dose at bedtime may be sufficient. In general, lower dosages are recommended for elderly patients.

Limbitrol DS (double strength) Tablets are recommended in an initial dosage of three or four tablets daily in divided doses; this may be increased to six tablets daily as required. Some patients respond to smaller doses and can be maintained on two tablets daily.

Limbitrol Tablets in an initial dosage of three or four tablets daily in divided doses may be satisfactory in patients who do not tolerate higher doses.

HOW SUPPLIED

DS (double strength) Tablets, containing 10 mg chlordiazepoxide and 25 mg amitriptyline (as the hydrochloride salt)—bottles of 100 and 500; Tel-E-Dose® packages of 100.

Tablets, containing 5 mg chlordiazepoxide and 12.5 mg amitriptyline (as the hydrochloride salt)—bottles of 100 and 500; Tel-E-Dose® packages of 100.

Revised: May 1991

Shown in Product Identification Section, page 426

MENRIUM® 5-2   ℞

[men 'ree-um]
Each tablet contains 5 mg chlordiazepoxide and 0.2 mg water-soluble esterified estrogens.

MENRIUM® 5-4   ℞

Each tablet contains 5 mg chlordiazepoxide and 0.4 mg water-soluble esterified estrogens.

MENRIUM® 10-4   ℞

Each tablet contains 10 mg chlordiazepoxide and 0.4 mg water-soluble esterified estrogens.

Menrium tablets are manufactured by Hoffmann-La Roche Inc., Nutley, N.J. 07110 and distributed by Roche Products Inc., Manati, P.R. 00674.

The following text is complete prescribing information based on official labeling in effect June 1, 1992.

Since estrogens are a component of Menrium, please note:

1. ESTROGENS HAVE BEEN REPORTED TO INCREASE THE RISK OF ENDOMETRIAL CARCINOMA.

Three independent case control studies have shown an increased risk of endometrial cancer in postmenopausal women exposed to exogenous estrogens for prolonged periods.[1-3] This risk was independent of the other known risk factors for endometrial cancer. These studies are further supported by the finding that incidence rates of endometrial cancer have increased sharply since 1969 in eight different areas of the United States

Continued on next page

Roche Products—Cont.

with population-based cancer reporting systems, an increase which may be related to the rapidly expanding use of estrogens during the last decade.[4] The three case control studies reported that the risk of endometrial cancer in estrogen users was about 4.5 to 13.9 times greater than in nonusers. The risk appears to depend on both duration of treatment[1] and on estrogen dose.[3] In view of these findings, when estrogens are used for the treatment of menopausal symptoms, the lowest dose that will control symptoms should be utilized and medication should be discontinued as soon as possible. When prolonged treatment is medically indicated, the patient should be reassessed on at least a semiannual basis to determine the need for continued therapy. Although the evidence must be considered preliminary, one study suggests that cyclic administration of low doses of estrogen may carry less risk than continuous administration;[3] it therefore appears prudent to utilize such a regimen.

Close clinical surveillance of all women taking estrogens is important. In all cases of undiagnosed persistent or recurring abnormal vaginal bleeding, adequate diagnostic measures should be undertaken to rule out malignancy.

There is no evidence at present that "natural" estrogens are more or less hazardous than "synthetic" estrogens at equiestrogenic doses.

2. ESTROGENS SHOULD NOT BE USED DURING PREGNANCY

The use of female sex hormones, both estrogens and progestogens, during early pregnancy may seriously damage the offspring. It has been shown that females exposed in utero to diethylstilbestrol, a nonsteroidal estrogen, have an increased risk of developing, in later life, a form of vaginal or cervical cancer that is ordinarily extremely rare.[5,6] This risk has been estimated as not greater than 4 per 1000 exposures.[7] Furthermore, a high percentage of such exposed women (from 30 to 90 percent) have been found to have vaginal adenosis,[8-12] epithelial changes of the vagina and cervix. Although these changes are histologically benign, it is not known whether they are precursors of malignancy. Although similar data are not available with the use of other estrogens, it cannot be presumed they would not induce similar changes.

Several reports suggest an association between intrauterine exposure to female sex hormones and congenital anomalies, including congenital heart defects and limb reduction defects.[13-16] One case control study[16] estimated a 4.7-fold increased risk of limb reduction defects in infants exposed in utero to sex hormones (oral contraceptives, hormone withdrawal tests for pregnancy, or attempted treatment for threatened abortion). Some of these exposures were very short and involved only a few days of treatment. The data suggest that the risk of limb reduction defects in exposed fetuses is somewhat less than 1 per 1,000. In the past, female sex hormones have been used during pregnancy in an attempt to treat threatened or habitual abortion. There is considerable evidence that estrogens are ineffective for these indications, and there is no evidence from well-controlled studies that progestogens are effective for these uses.

If Menrium is used during pregnancy, or if the patient becomes pregnant while taking this drug, she should be apprised of the potential risks to the fetus, and the advisability of pregnancy continuation.

DESCRIPTION

Menrium tablets are available in three strengths: Menrium 5-2, containing 5 mg chlordiazepoxide and 0.2 mg water-soluble esterified estrogens; Menrium 5-4, containing 5 mg chlordiazepoxide and 0.4 mg water-soluble esterified estrogens; and Menrium 10-4, containing 10 mg chlordiazepoxide and 0.4 mg water-soluble esterified estrogens. Each tablet also contains acacia, calcium stearate, calcium sulfate, carnauba wax, corn starch, lactose, pregelatinized starch, sodium bicarbonate, sucrose and flavor, with the following dye systems: Menrium 5-2 and Menrium 5-4—FD&C Blue 1, FD&C Yellow No. 6 and D&C Yellow No. 10; Menrium 10-4—FD&C Blue No. 1 and FD&C Red No. 3.

Menrium affords in a single formulation the psychotropic action of Librium® (chlordiazepoxide/Roche) and hormonal replacement in the form of water-soluble esterified estrogens (expressed in terms of sodium estrone sulfate) to provide comprehensive management of the menopausal syndrome or the climacteric.

Librium (chlordiazepoxide/Roche) is a versatile therapeutic agent of proven value for the relief of anxiety and tension. It is indicated when anxiety, tension or apprehension are sig-

nificant components of the clinical profile. It is among the safer of the effective psychopharmacologic compounds. Chlordiazepoxide is 7-chloro-2-methylamino-5-phenyl-3H-1, 4-benzodiazepine 4-oxide. It is a slightly yellow, crystalline material and is insoluble in water. The molecular weight is 299.75.

Water-soluble esterified estrogens provide hormonal replacement in the menopausal patient, the need for which is widely recognized and accepted. Esterified estrogens is a mixture of the sodium salts of the sulfate esters of the estrogenic substances, principally estrone, that are of the type excreted by pregnant mares. It is a white to buff-colored, amorphous powder, odorless or having a slight, characteristic odor.

CLINICAL PHARMACOLOGY

The estrogenic component of Menrium is water-soluble esterified estrogens—steroidal compounds—which occur naturally. The action of this substance is substantially equal to the action of both conjugated estrogens, also naturally occurring, and synthetic estrogenic substances.

Menopausal changes, such as atrophic changes of the genital tract and breasts due to a slow decline in estrogen secretion, may be reversed by substitution therapy with estrogenic substances.

Estrogens are, in general, completely absorbed following oral administration. Estrogens are detoxified by the liver, and excretion occurs by way of the urine and the feces.

Librium (chlordiazepoxide HCl/Roche) has antianxiety and sedative actions. The drug has been studied extensively in many species of animals and these studies are suggestive of action on the limbic system of the brain, which recent evidence indicates is involved in emotional responses. However, the precise mechanism of action in man is not known. The drug blocks EEG arousal from stimulation of the brain stem reticular formation. The mean ±S.E. plasma peak time is 1.4 (±0.3) hours, and the half-life ranges between 7.1 and 19.8 hours with a mean ±S.E. half-life of 12.0 (±0.7) hours. After the drug is discontinued, plasma levels are usually at the lowest quantitatively detectable amounts by 48 to 72 hours. Chlordiazepoxide HCl is excreted in urine with 1% or less unchanged and 12 to 34% recoverable as conjugates.

INDICATIONS

Menrium is indicated in the management of the manifestations generally associated with the menopausal syndrome—anxiety and tension, vasomotor complaints and hormonal deficiency states.

MENRIUM HAS NOT BEEN SHOWN TO BE EFFECTIVE FOR ANY PURPOSE DURING PREGNANCY AND ITS USE MAY CAUSE SEVERE HARM TO THE FETUS (SEE BOXED WARNING).

CONTRAINDICATIONS

Menrium is contraindicated in patients with known hypersensitivity to chlordiazepoxide and/or esterified estrogens. Estrogens should not be used in women (or men) with any of the following conditions:

1. Known or suspected cancer of the breast except in appropriately selected patients being treated for metastatic disease.
2. Known or suspected estrogen-dependent neoplasia.
3. Known or suspected pregnancy. (See Boxed Warning.)
4. Undiagnosed abnormal genital bleeding.
5. Active thrombophlebitis or thromboembolic disorders.
6. A past history of thrombophlebitis, thrombosis, or thromboembolic disorders associated with previous estrogen use.

WARNINGS

1. *Induction of malignant neoplasms.* Long term continuous administration of natural and synthetic estrogens in certain animal species increases the frequency of carcinomas of the breast, cervix, vagina, and liver. There is now evidence that estrogens increase the risk of carcinoma of the endometrium in humans. (See Boxed Warning.)

At the present time there is no satisfactory evidence that estrogens given to postmenopausal women increase the risk of cancer of the breast,[17] although a recent long-term followup of a single physician's practice has raised this possibility.[18] Because of the animal data, there is a need for caution in prescribing estrogens for women with a strong family history of breast cancer or who have breast nodules, fibrocystic disease, or abnormal mammograms.

2. *Gall bladder disease.* A recent study has reported a 2- to 3-fold increase in the risk of surgically confirmed gall bladder disease in women receiving postmenopausal estrogens,[17] similar to the 2-fold increase previously noted in users of oral contraceptives.[19,24] In the case of oral contraceptives the increased risk appeared after two years of use.[24]

3. *Effects similar to those caused by estrogen-progestogen oral contraceptives.* There are several serious adverse effects of oral contraceptives, most of which have not, up to now, been documented as consequences of postmenopausal estrogen therapy. This may reflect the comparatively low doses of estrogen used in postmenopausal women. It would be expected that the larger doses of estrogen used to treat pros-

tatic or breast cancer or postpartum breast engorgement are more likely to result in these adverse effects, and, in fact, it has been shown that there is an increased risk of thrombosis in men receiving estrogens for prostatic cancer and women for postpartum breast engorgement.[20-23]

a. *Thromboembolic disease.* It is now well established that users of oral contraceptives have an increased risk of various thromboembolic and thrombotic vascular diseases, such as thrombophlebitis, pulmonary embolism, stroke, and myocardial infarction.[24-31] Cases of retinal thrombosis, mesenteric thrombosis, and optic neuritis have been reported in oral contraceptive users. There is evidence that the risk of several of these adverse reactions is related to the dose of the drug.[32,33] An increased risk of postsurgery thromboembolic complications has also been reported in users of oral contraceptives.[34,35] If feasible, estrogen should be discontinued at least 4 weeks before surgery of the type associated with an increased risk of thromboembolism, or during periods of prolonged immobilization.

While an increased rate of thromboembolic and thrombotic disease in postmenopausal users of estrogens has not been found,[17,36] this does not rule out the possibility that such an increase may be present or that subgroups of women who have underlying risk factors or who are receiving relatively large doses of estrogens may have increased risk. Therefore, estrogens should not be used in persons with active thrombophlebitis or thromboembolic disorders, and they should not be used in persons with a history of such disorders in association with estrogen use. They should be used with caution in patients with cerebral vascular or coronary artery disease and only for those in whom estrogens are clearly needed. Large doses of estrogen (5 mg conjugated estrogens per day), comparable to those used to treat cancer of the prostate and breast, have been shown in a large prospective clinical trial in men[37] to increase the risk of nonfatal myocardial infarction, pulmonary embolism and thrombophlebitis. When estrogen doses of this size are used, any of the thromboembolic and thrombotic adverse effects associated with oral contraceptive use should be considered a clear risk.

b. *Hepatic adenoma.* Benign hepatic adenomas appear to be associated with the use of oral contraceptives.[38-40] Although benign, and rare, these may rupture and may cause death through intra-abdominal hemorrhage. Such lesions have not yet been reported in association with other estrogen or progestogen preparations but should be considered in estrogen users having abdominal pain and tenderness, abdominal mass, or hypovolemic shock. Hepatocellular carcinoma has also been reported in women taking estrogen-containing oral contraceptives.[39] The relationship of this malignancy to these drugs is not known at this time.

c. *Elevated blood pressure.* Increased blood pressure is not uncommon in women using oral contraceptives. There is now a report that this may occur with the use of estrogens in the menopause[41] and blood pressure should be monitored with estrogen use, especially if high doses are used.

d. *Glucose tolerance.* A worsening of glucose tolerance has been observed in a significant percentage of patients on estrogen-containing oral contraceptives. For this reason, diabetic patients should be carefully observed while receiving estrogen.

4. *Hypercalcemia.* Administration of estrogens may lead to severe hypercalcemia in patients with breast cancer and bone metastases. If this occurs, the drug should be stopped and appropriate measures taken to reduce the serum calcium level.

As in the case of other preparations containing CNS-acting drugs, patients receiving Menrium should be cautioned about possible combined effects with alcohol and other CNS depressants. Other causes of manifestations of the menopausal syndrome, such as pregnancy, should be excluded. As is true of all preparations containing CNS-acting drugs, patients receiving Menrium should be cautioned against hazardous occupations requiring complete mental alertness such as operating machinery or driving a motor vehicle.

Physical and Psychological Dependence: Withdrawal symptoms have not been observed in more than 1300 subjects during clinical trials with Menrium. Physical and psychological dependence have rarely been reported in persons taking recommended doses of Librium (chlordiazepoxide/ Roche). However, caution must be exercised in administering Librium to individuals known to be addiction-prone or those whose history suggests they may increase the dosage on their own initiative. Withdrawal symptoms following discontinuation of chlordiazepoxide hydrochloride have been reported. These symptoms (including convulsions) are similar to those seen with barbiturates.

PRECAUTIONS

A. General Precautions.

1. A complete medical and family history should be taken prior to the initiation of any estrogen therapy. The pretreatment and periodic physical examinations should include special reference to blood pressure, breasts, abdomen, and pelvic organs, and should include a Papanicolaou smear. As a general rule, estrogen should not be prescribed for longer

than one year without another physical examination being performed.

2. Fluid retention—Because estrogens may cause some degree of fluid retention, conditions which might be influenced by this factor, such as epilepsy, migraine, and cardiac or renal dysfunction, require careful observation.

3. Certain patients may develop undesirable manifestations of excessive estrogenic stimulation, such as abnormal or excessive uterine bleeding, mastodynia, etc.

4. Oral contraceptives appear to be associated with an increased incidence of mental depression.[24] Although it is not clear whether this is due to the estrogenic or progestogenic component of the contraceptive, patients with a history of depression should be carefully observed.

5. Preexisting uterine leiomyomata may increase in size during estrogen use.

6. The lowest effective dose appropriate for the specific indication should be utilized. Studies of the addition of a progestin for seven or more days of a cycle of estrogen administration have reported a lowered incidence of endometrial hyperplasia. Morphological and biochemical studies of endometrium suggest that 10 to 13 days of progestin are needed to provide maximal maturation of the endometrium and to eliminate any hyperplastic changes. Whether this will provide protection from endometrial carcinoma has not been clearly established. There are possible additional risks which may be associated with the inclusion of progestin in estrogen replacement regimens. The potential risks include adverse effects on carbohydrate and lipid metabolism. The choice of progestin and dosage may be important in minimizing these adverse effects.

7. The pathologist should be advised of estrogen therapy when relevant specimens are submitted.

8. Patients with a past history of jaundice during pregnancy have an increased risk of recurrence of jaundice while receiving estrogen-containing oral contraceptive therapy. If jaundice develops in any patient receiving estrogen, the medication should be discontinued while the cause is investigated.

9. Estrogens may be poorly metabolized in patients with impaired liver function and they should be administered with caution in such patients.

10. Because estrogens influence the metabolism of calcium and phosphorus, they should be used with caution in patients with metabolic bone diseases that are associated with hypercalcemia or in patients with renal insufficiency.

11. Because of the effects of estrogens on epiphyseal closure, they should be used judiciously in young patients in whom bone growth is not complete.

12. Certain endocrine and liver function tests may be affected by estrogen-containing oral contraceptives. The following similar changes may be expected with larger doses of estrogen:

a. Increased sulfobromophthalein retention.

b. Increased prothrombin and factors VII, VIII, IX, and X; decreased antithrombin 3; increased norepinephrine-induced platelet aggregability.

c. Increased thyroid binding globulin (TBG) leading to increased circulating total thyroid hormone, as measured by PBI, T4 by column, or T4 by radioimmunoassay. Free T3 resin uptake is decreased, reflecting the elevated TBG; free T4 concentration is unaltered.

d. Impaired glucose tolerance.

e. Decreased pregnanediol excretion.

f. Reduced response to metyrapone test.

g. Reduced serum folate concentration.

h. Increased serum triglyceride and phospholipid concentration.

B. Information for the Patient.
See Text of Patient Package Insert which follows below.

WHAT YOU SHOULD KNOW ABOUT ESTROGENS

Estrogens are female hormones produced by the ovaries. The ovaries make several different kinds of estrogens. In addition, scientists have been able to make a variety of synthetic estrogens. As far as we know, all these estrogens have similar properties and therefore much the same usefulness, side effects, and risks. This leaflet is intended to help you understand what estrogens are used for, the risks involved in their use, and how to use them as safely as possible.

This leaflet includes the most important information about estrogens, but not all the information. If you want to know more, you can ask your doctor or pharmacist to let you read the package insert prepared for the doctor.

USES OF ESTROGEN

Estrogens are prescribed by doctors for a number of purposes, including:

1. To provide estrogen during a period of adjustment when a woman's ovaries no longer produce it, in order to prevent certain uncomfortable symptoms of estrogen deficiency. (All women normally stop producing estrogens, generally between the ages of 45 and 55; this is called the menopause.)

2. To prevent symptoms of estrogen deficiency when a woman's ovaries have been removed surgically before the natural menopause.

3. To prevent pregnancy. (Estrogens are given along with a progestogen, another female hormone; these combinations are called oral contraceptives or birth control pills. Patient labeling is available to women taking oral contraceptives and they will not be discussed in this leaflet.)

4. To treat certain cancers in women and men.

5. To prevent painful swelling of the breasts after pregnancy in women who choose not to nurse their babies.

THERE IS NO PROPER USE OF ESTROGENS IN A PREGNANT WOMAN.

ESTROGENS IN THE MENOPAUSE

In the natural course of their lives, all women eventually experience a decrease in estrogen production. This usually occurs between ages 45 and 55 but may occur earlier or later. Sometimes the ovaries may need to be removed before natural menopause by an operation, producing a "surgical menopause."

When the amount of estrogen in the blood begins to decrease, many women may develop typical symptoms: Feelings of warmth in the face, neck, and chest or sudden intense episodes of heat and sweating throughout the body (called "hot flashes" or "hot flushes"). These symptoms are sometimes very uncomfortable. A few women eventually develop changes in the vagina (called "atrophic vaginitis") which cause discomfort, especially during and after intercourse. Estrogens can be prescribed to treat these symptoms of the menopause. It is estimated that considerably more than half of all women undergoing the menopause have only mild symptoms or no symptoms at all and therefore do not need estrogens. Other woman may need estrogens for a few months, while their bodies adjust to lower estrogen levels. Sometimes the need will be for periods longer than six months. In an attempt to avoid overstimulation of the uterus (womb), estrogens are usually given cyclically during each month of use, that is three weeks of pills followed by one week without pills.

Sometimes women experience nervous symptoms or depression during menopause. There is no evidence that estrogens are effective for such symptoms and they should not be used to treat them, although other treatment may be needed.

You may have heard that taking estrogens for long periods (years) after the menopause will keep your skin soft and supple and keep you feeling young. There is no evidence that this is so, however, and such long-term treatment carries important risks.

Estrogens to Prevent Swelling of the Breasts After Pregnancy: If you do not breast feed your baby after delivery, your breasts may fill up with milk and become painful and engorged. This usually begins about 3 to 4 days after delivery and may last for a few days to up to a week or more. Sometimes the discomfort is severe, but usually it is not and can be controlled by pain relieving drugs such as aspirin and by binding the breasts up tightly. Estrogens can be used to try to prevent the breasts from filling up. While this treatment is sometimes successful, in many cases the breasts fill up to some degree in spite of treatment. The dose of estrogens needed to prevent pain and swelling of the breasts is much larger than the dose needed to treat symptoms of the menopause and this may increase your chances of developing blood clots in the legs or lungs (see below). Therefore, it is important that you discuss the benefits and the risks of estrogen use with your doctor if you have decided not to breast feed your baby.

The Dangers of Estrogens:

1. *Cancer of the uterus.* If estrogens are used in the postmenopausal period for more than a year, there is an increased risk of *endometrial cancer* (cancer of the uterus). Women taking estrogens have roughly 5 to 10 times as great a chance of getting this cancer as women who take no estrogens. To put this another way, while a postmenopausal woman not taking estrogens has 1 chance in 1,000 each year of getting cancer of the uterus, a woman taking estrogens has 5 to 10 chances in 1,000 each year. For this reason *it is important to take estrogens only when you really need them.*

The risk of this cancer is greater the longer estrogens are used and also seems to be greater when larger doses are taken. For this reason *it is important to take the lowest dose of estrogen that will control symptoms and to take it only as long as it is needed.* If estrogens are needed for longer periods of time, your doctor will want to reevaluate your need for estrogens at least every six months.

Women using estrogens should report any irregular vaginal bleeding to their doctors; such bleeding may be of no importance, but it can be an early warning of cancer of the uterus. If you have undiagnosed vaginal bleeding, you should not use estrogens until a diagnosis is made and you are certain there is no cancer of the uterus.

If you have had your uterus completely removed (total hysterectomy), there is no danger of developing cancer of the uterus.

2. *Other possible cancers.* Estrogens can cause development of other tumors in animals, such as tumors of the breast, cervix, vagina, or liver, when given for a long time. At present there is no good evidence that women using estrogen in the menopause have an increased risk of such tumors, but

there is no way yet to be sure they do not; and one study raises the possibility that use of estrogens in the menopause may increase the risk of breast cancer many years later. This is a further reason to use estrogens only when clearly needed. While you are taking estrogens, it is important that you go to your doctor at least once a year for a physical examination. Also, if members of your family have had breast cancer or if you have breast nodules or abnormal mammograms (breast x-rays), your doctor may wish to carry out more frequent examinations of your breasts.

3. *Gall bladder disease.* Women who use estrogens after menopause are more likely to develop gall bladder disease needing surgery as women who do not use estrogens. Birth control pills have a similar effect.

4. *Abnormal blood clotting.* Oral contraceptives increase the risk of blood clotting in various parts of the body. This can result in a stroke (if the clot is in the brain), a heart attack (clot in a blood vessel of the heart), or a pulmonary embolus (a clot which forms in the legs or pelvis, then breaks off and travels to the lungs). Any of these can be fatal.

At this time use of estrogens in the menopause is not known to cause such blood clotting, but this has not been fully studied and there could still prove to be such a risk. It is recommended that if you have had clotting in the legs or lungs or a heart attack or stroke while you were using estrogens or birth control pills, you should not use estrogens (unless they are being used to treat cancer of the breast or prostate). If you have had a stroke or heart attack or if you have angina pectoris, estrogens should be used with great caution and only if clearly needed (for example, if you have severe symptoms of the menopause).

The larger doses of estrogen used to prevent swelling of the breasts after pregnancy have been reported to cause clotting in the legs and lungs.

Special Warning About Pregnancy: You should not receive estrogen if you are pregnant. If this should occur, there is a greater than usual chance that the developing child will be born with a birth defect, although the possibility remains fairly small. A female child may have an increased risk of developing cancer of the vagina or cervix later in life (in the teens or twenties). Every possible effort should be made to avoid exposure to estrogens during pregnancy. If exposure occurs, see your doctor.

Other Effects of Estrogens: In addition to the serious known risks of estrogens described above, estrogens have the following side effects and potential risks:

1. *Nausea and vomiting.* The most common side effect of estrogen therapy is nausea. Vomiting is less common.

2. *Effects on breasts.* Estrogens may cause breast tenderness or enlargement and may cause the breasts to secrete a liquid. These effects are not dangerous.

3. *Effects on the uterus.* Estrogens may cause benign fibroid tumors of the uterus to get larger.

Some women will have menstrual bleeding when estrogens are stopped. But if the bleeding occurs on days you are still taking estrogens you should report this to your doctor.

4. *Effects on liver.* Women taking oral contraceptives develop on rare occasions a tumor of the liver which can rupture and bleed into the abdomen. So far, these tumors have not been reported in women using estrogens in the menopause, but you should report any swelling or unusual pain or tenderness in the abdomen to your doctor immediately. Women with a past history of jaundice (yellowing of the skin and white parts of the eyes) may get jaundice again during estrogen use. If this occurs, stop taking estrogens and see your doctor.

5. *Other effects.* Estrogens may cause excess fluid to be retained in the body. This may make some conditions worse, such as epilepsy, migraine, heart disease, or kidney disease.

SUMMARY

Estrogens have important uses, but they have serious risks as well. You must decide, with your doctor, whether the risks are acceptable to you in view of the benefits of treatment. Except where your doctor has prescribed estrogens for use in special cases of cancer of the breast or prostate, you should not use estrogens if you have cancer of the breast or uterus, are pregnant, have undiagnosed abnormal vaginal bleeding, clotting in the legs or lungs, or have had a stroke, heart attack or angina, or clotting in the legs or lungs in the past while you were taking estrogens.

You can use estrogens as safely as possible by understanding that your doctor will require regular physical examinations while you are taking them and will try to discontinue the drug as soon as possible and use the smallest dose possible. Be alert for signs of trouble including:

1. Abnormal bleeding from the vagina.

2. Pains in the calves or chest or sudden shortness of breath, or coughing blood (indicating possible clots in the legs, heart, or lungs).

3. Severe headache, dizziness, faintness, or changes in vision (indicating possible developing clots in the brain or eye).

4. Breast lumps (you should ask your doctor how to examine your own breasts).

Continued on next page

Roche Products—Cont.

5. Jaundice (yellowing of the skin).
6. Mental depression.

Based on his or her assessment of your medical needs, your doctor has prescribed this drug for you. Do not give the drug to anyone else.

C. **Pregnancy:** See Contraindications and Box Warning.
D. **Nursing Mothers:** As a general principle, the administration of any drug to nursing mothers should be done only when clearly necessary since many drugs are excreted in human milk.

In elderly and debilitated patients, it is recommended that the dosage be limited to the smallest effective amount to preclude the development of ataxia or oversedation (10 mg chlordiazepoxide or less per day initially, to be increased gradually as needed and tolerated). In general, the concomitant administration of Menrium and other psychotropic agents is not recommended. If such combination therapy seems indicated, careful consideration should be given to the pharmacology of the agents to be employed—particularly when the known potentiating compounds such as the MAO inhibitors and phenothiazines are to be used. The usual precautions in treating patients with impaired renal or hepatic function should be observed.

Paradoxical reactions to chlordiazepoxide, e.g., excitement, stimulation and acute rage, have been reported in psychiatric patients and should be watched for during Menrium therapy. The usual precautions are indicated when chlordiazepoxide is used in the treatment of anxiety states where there is any evidence of impending depression; it should be borne in mind that suicidal tendencies may be present and protective measures may be necessary. Although clinical studies have not established a cause and effect relationship, physicians should be aware that variable effects on blood coagulation have been reported very rarely in patients receiving oral anticoagulants and Librium (chlordiazepoxide/Roche).

ADVERSE REACTIONS

No side effects or manifestations not seen with either compound alone have been reported with the administration of Menrium. However, since Menrium contains chlordiazepoxide and water-soluble esterified estrogens, the possibility of untoward effects which may be seen with either of these two compounds cannot be excluded.

(See Warnings regarding induction of neoplasia, adverse effects on the fetus, increased incidence of gall bladder disease, and adverse effects similar to those of oral contraceptives, including thromboembolism.) The following additional adverse reactions have been reported with estrogenic therapy, including oral contraceptives:

1. *Genitourinary system.*
Breakthrough bleeding, spotting, change in menstrual flow.
Dysmenorrhea.
Premenstrual-like syndrome.
Amenorrhea during and after treatment.
Increase in size of uterine fibromyomata.
Vaginal candidiasis.
Change in cervical eversion and in degree of cervical secretion.
Cystitis-like syndrome.
2. *Breasts.*
Tenderness, enlargement, secretion.
3. *Gastrointestinal.*
Nausea, vomiting.
Abdominal cramps, bloating.
Cholestatic jaundice.
4. *Skin.*
Chloasma or melasma which may persist when drug is discontinued.
Erythema multiforme.
Erythema nodosum.
Hemorrhagic eruption.
Loss of scalp hair.
Hirsutism.
5. *Eyes.*
Steepening of corneal curvature.
Intolerance to contact lenses.
6. *CNS.*
Headache, migraine, dizziness.
Mental depression.
Chorea.
7. *Miscellaneous.*
Increase or decrease in weight.
Reduced carbohydrate tolerance.
Aggravation of porphyria.
Edema.
Changes in libido.
When chlordiazepoxide has been used alone the necessity of discontinuing therapy because of undesirable effects has been rare. Drowsiness, ataxia and confusion have been reported in some patients—particularly the elderly and debilitated. While these effects can be avoided in almost all instances by proper dosage adjustment, they have occasionally

been observed at the lower dosage ranges. In a few instances syncope has been reported.

Other adverse reactions reported during therapy include isolated instances of skin eruptions, edema, minor menstrual irregularities, nausea and constipation, extrapyramidal symptoms, as well as increased and decreased libido. Such side effects have been infrequent and are generally controlled with reduction of dosage. Changes in EEG patterns (low-voltage fast activity) have been observed in patients during and after Librium (chlordiazepoxide/Roche) treatment.

Blood dyscrasias, including agranulocytosis, jaundice and hepatic dysfunction have occasionally been reported during therapy. When Librium treatment is protracted, periodic blood counts and liver function tests are advisable.

Management of Overdosage: Numerous reports of ingestion of large doses of estrogen-containing oral contraceptives by young children indicate that serious ill effects do not occur. Overdosage of estrogen may cause nausea, and withdrawal bleeding may occur in females. Manifestations of Librium (chlordiazepoxide/Roche) overdosage include somnolence, confusion, coma and diminished reflexes. Respiration, pulse and blood pressure should be monitored, as in all cases of drug overdosage, although, in general, these effects have been minimal following Librium overdosage. General supportive measures should be employed, along with immediate gastric lavage. Intravenous fluids should be administered and an adequate airway maintained. Hypotension may be combated by the use of Levophed® (levarterenol) or Aramine (metaraminol). Dialysis is of limited value. There have been occasional reports of excitation in patients following chlordiazepoxide overdosage; if this occurs barbiturates should not be used. As with the management of intentional overdosage with any drug, it should be borne in mind that multiple agents may have been ingested.

DOSAGE

The lowest dose that will control symptoms should be chosen and medication should be discontinued as promptly as possible.

MENRIUM 5-2—for the majority of patients with the menopausal syndrome or the climacteric having anxiety and tension and hormonal deficiency states requiring estrogen replacement—One tablet, t.i.d.

MENRIUM 5-4—for patients with the menopausal syndrome or the climacteric with anxiety and tension and more severe vasomotor manifestations —One tablet, t.i.d.

MENRIUM 10-4—for patients with the menopausal syndrome or the climacteric with pronounced anxiety and tension and marked vasomotor complaints—One tablet, t.i.d. Therapy should be continued for 21-day courses, followed by one-week rest periods. While these dosage schedules will prove generally satisfactory, individual adjustment of dosage is desirable, since some patients may obtain satisfactory relief with as little as one tablet daily of Menrium 5-2.

Treated patients with an intact uterus should be monitored closely for signs of endometrial cancer and appropriate diagnostic measures should be taken to rule out malignancy in the event of persistent or recurring abnormal vaginal bleeding.

HOW SUPPLIED

Menrium 5-2, light green tablets; Menrium 5-4, dark green tablets; and Menrium 10-4, purple tablets—bottles of 100.

PHYSICIAN REFERENCES

1. Ziel HK, Finkel WD: *N Engl J Med 293* :1167–1170, 1975
2. Smith DC, et al: *N Engl J Med 293* :1164–1167, 1975
3. Mack TM, et al: *N Engl J Med 294* :1262–1267, 1976
4. Weiss NS, Szekely DR, Austin DF: *N Engl J Med 294* :1259–1262, 1976
5. Herbst AL, Ulfelder H, Poskanzer DC: *N Engl J Med 284* :878–881, 1971
6. Greenwald P, et al: *N Engl J Med 285* :390–392, 1971
7. Lanier A, et al: *Mayo Clin Proc 48* :793–799, 1973
8. Herbst A, Kurman R, Scully R: *Obstet Gynecol 40* :287–298, 1972
9. Herbst A, et al: *Am J Obstet Gynecol 118* :607–615, 1974
10. Herbst, A, et al: *N Engl J Med 292* :334–339, 1975
11. Stafl A, et al: *Obstet Gynecol 43* :118–128, 1974
12. Sherman AI, et al: *Obstet Gynecol 44* :531–545, 1974
13. Gal I, Kirman B, Stern J: *Nature 216* :83, 1967
14. Levy EP, Cohen A, Fraser FC: *Lancet 1* :611, 1973
15. Nora J, Nora A: *Lancet 1* :941–942, 1973
16. Janerich DT, Piper JM, Glebatis DM: *N Engl J Med 291* :697–700, 1974
17. Boston Collaborative Drug Surveillance Program: *N Engl J Med 290* :15–19, 1974
18. Hoover R, et al: *N Engl J Med 295* :401–405, 1976
19. Boston Collaborative Drug Surveillance Program: *Lancet 1* :1399–1404, 1973
20. Daniel DG, Campbell H, Turnbull AC: *Lancet 2* :287–289, 1967
21. The Veterans Administration Cooperative Urological Research Group: *J Urol 98* :516–522, 1967
22. Bailar JC: *Lancet 2* :560, 1967
23. Blackard C, et al: *Cancer 26* :249–256, 1970
24. Royal College of General Practitioners: *J Coll Gen Pract 13* :267–279, 1967
25. Inman WHW, Vessey MP: *Br Med J 2* :193–199, 1968
26. Vessey MP, Doll R: *Br Med J 2* :651–657, 1969
27. Sartwell PE, et al: *Am J Epidemiol 90* :365–380, 1969
28. Collaborative Group for the Study of Stroke in Young Women: *N Engl J Med 288* :871–878, 1973
29. Collaborative Group for the Study of Stroke in Young Women: *JAMA 231* :718–722, 1975
30. Mann JI, Inman WHW: *Br Med J 2* :245–248, 1975
31. Mann JI, et al: *Br Med J 2* :241–245, 1975
32. Inman WHW, et al: *Br Med J 2* :203–209, 1970
33. Stolley PD, et al: *Am J Epidemiol 102* :197–208, 1975
34. Vessey MP, et al: *Br Med J 3* :123–126, 1970
35. Greene GR, Sartwell PE: *Am J Public Health 62* :680–685, 1972
36. Rosenberg L, Armstrong MB, Jick H: *N Engl J Med 294* :1256–1259, 1976
37. Coronary Drug Project Research Group: *JAMA 214* :1303–1313, 1970
38. Baum J, et al: *Lancet 2* :926–928, 1973
39. Mays ET, et al: *JAMA 235* :730–732, 1976
40. Edmondson HA, Henderson B, Benton B: *N Engl J Med 294* :470–472, 1976
41. Pfeffer RI, Van Den Noort S: *Am J Epidemiol 103* :445–456, 1976
Revised: July 1987

Shown in Product Identification Section, page 426

QUARZAN®   ℞
[kwar'zan]
(clidinium bromide/Roche)
CAPSULES

The following text is complete prescribing information based on official labeling in effect June 1, 1992.

DESCRIPTION

Clidinium bromide is 3-hydroxy-1-methylquinuclidinium bromide benzilate. A white or nearly white crystalline compound, it is soluble in water and has a calculated molecular weight of 432.36.

Clidinium bromide is a quaternary ammonium compound with anticholinergic and antispasmodic activity. Quarzan is available as green and red opaque capsules each containing 2.5 mg clidinium bromide, and green and grey opaque capsules each containing 5 mg clidinium bromide. Each capsule also contains corn starch, lactose and talc. Gelatin capsule shells contain methyl and propyl parabens and potassium sorbate, with the following dye systems: 2.5-mg capsules—FD&C Blue No. 1, FD&C Green No. 3, FD&C Red No. 3, D&C Red No. 33 and D&C Yellow No. 10. 5-mg capsules—FD&C Green No. 3, D&C Red No. 33, FD&C Yellow No. 6 and D&C Yellow No. 10.

ACTIONS

Quarzan inhibits gastrointestinal motility and diminishes gastric acid secretion. Its anticholinergic activity approximates that of atropine sulfate and propantheline bromide.

INDICATIONS

Quarzan is effective as adjunctive therapy in peptic ulcer disease. **Quarzan has not been shown to be effective in contributing to the healing of peptic ulcer, decreasing the rate of recurrence or preventing complications.**

CONTRAINDICATIONS

Known hypersensitivity to clidinium bromide or to other anticholinergic drugs, glaucoma, obstructive uropathy (for example, bladder neck obstruction due to prostatic hypertrophy), obstructive disease of the gastrointestinal tract (for example, pyloroduodenal stenosis), paralytic ileus, intestinal atony of the elderly or debilitated patient, unstable cardiovascular status in acute hemorrhage, severe ulcerative colitis, toxic megacolon complicating ulcerative colitis, myasthenia gravis.

WARNINGS

Quarzan may produce drowsiness or blurred vision. The patient should be cautioned regarding activities requiring mental alertness such as operating a motor vehicle or other machinery or performing hazardous work while taking this drug. In the presence of high environmental temperature, heat prostration (fever and heat stroke) may occur with the use of anticholinergics due to decreased sweating. Diarrhea may be an early symptom of incomplete intestinal obstruction, especially in patients with ileostomy or colostomy. Use of anticholinergics in patients with suspected intestinal obstruction would be inappropriate and possibly harmful. With overdosage, a curare-like action may occur, *i.e.*, neuromuscular blockade leading to muscular weakness and possible paralysis.

Usage in Pregnancy: No controlled studies in humans have been performed to establish the safety of the drug in preg-

nancy. Uncontrolled data derived from clinical usage have failed to show abnormalities attributable to its use. Reproduction studies in rats have failed to show any impaired fertility or abnormality in the fetuses that might be associated with the use of Quarzan. Use of any drug in pregnancy or in women of childbearing potential requires that the potential benefit of the drug be weighed against the possible hazards to mother and fetus.

Nursing Mothers: As with all anticholinergic drugs, Quarzan may be secreted in human milk and may inhibit lactation. As a general rule, nursing should not be undertaken while a patient is on Quarzan, or the drug should not be used by nursing mothers.

Pediatric Use: Since there is no adequate experience in children who have received this drug, safety and efficacy in children have not been established.

PRECAUTIONS

Use Quarzan with caution in the elderly and in all patients with autonomic neuropathy, hepatic or renal disease, ulcerative colitis— large doses may suppress intestinal motility to the point of producing a paralytic ileus and for this reason precipitate or aggravate "toxic megacolon," a serious complication of the disease; hyperthyroidism; coronary heart disease; congestive heart failure; cardiac tachy-arrhythmias; tachycardia; hypertension; prostatic hypertrophy; hiatal hernia associated with reflux esophagitis, since anticholinergic drugs may aggravate this condition.

ADVERSE REACTIONS

As with other anticholinergic drugs, the most frequently reported adverse effects are dryness of mouth, blurring of vision, urinary hesitancy and constipation. Other adverse effects reported with the use of anticholinergic drugs include decreased sweating, urinary retention, tachycardia, palpitations, dilatation of the pupils, cycloplegia, increased ocular tension, loss of taste, headaches, nervousness, mental confusion, drowsiness, weakness, dizziness, insomnia, nausea, vomiting, bloated feeling, impotence, suppression of lactation and severe allergic reactions or drug idiosyncrasies including anaphylaxis, urticaria and other dermal manifestations.

OVERDOSAGE

The symptoms of overdosage with Quarzan progress from an intensification of the usual side effects to CNS disturbances (from restlessness and excitement to psychotic behavior), circulatory changes (flushing, tachycardia, fall in blood pressure, circulatory failure), respiratory failure, paralysis and coma.

Treatment should consist of: *General measures* —(1) gastric lavage, (2) maintenance of adequate airway, using artificial respiration if needed, (3) administration of i.v. fluids, and (4) for fever: alcohol sponging or ice packs.

Specific measures—(1) Antidotes: physostigmine (Antilirium) 0.5 to 2 mg, i.v., repeated as needed up to a total of 5 mg; or pilocarpine, 5 mg, s.c. at intervals until mouth is moist; neostigmine may also be useful. (2) Against excitement: sodium pentothal 2% may be given i.v. or chloral hydrate (100 to 200 ml, 2% solution) *rectally.* (3) Against hypotension and circulatory collapse: levarterenol (Levophed®) or metaraminol (Aramine) infusions. (4) Against CNS depression: caffeine and sodium benzoate.

The usefulness of dialysis is not known.

DOSAGE AND ADMINISTRATION

For maximum efficacy, dosage should be individualized according to severity of symptoms and occurrence of side effects. The usual dosage is 2.5 to 5 mg three or four times daily before meals and at bedtime. Dosage in excess of 20 mg daily is usually not required to obtain maximum effectiveness. For the aged or debilitated, one 2.5-mg capsule three times daily before meals is recommended. The desired pharmacological effect of the drug is unlikely to be attained without occasional side effects.

DRUG INTERACTIONS

No specific drug interactions are known.

HOW SUPPLIED

Opaque capsules, 2.5 mg, green and red—bottles of 100 (NDC 0140-0119-01); 5 mg, green and grey—bottles of 100 (NDC 0140-0120-01).

Revised: January 1986

Shown in Product Identification Section, page 426

TEL-E-DOSE®

Tel-E-Dose is a unit package designed by Roche for convenience in dispensing medications in the hospital and nursing home. Each unit, sealed against contamination and moisture, is clearly identified by product name and strength and carries the control number and expiration date.

Currently available in this package form are the following products: Librax® (5 mg chlordiazepoxide HCl and 2.5 mg clidinium Br) capsules; Librium® (chlordiazepoxide HCl) capsules, 5 mg, 10 mg, 25 mg; Limbitrol® (5 mg chlordiazepoxide and 12.5 mg amitriptyline HCl) tablets; Limbitrol® DS (10 mg chlordiazepoxide and 25 mg amitriptyline HCl) tablets; Valium® (diazepam) tablets, 2 mg, 5 mg, 10 mg.

Shown in Product Identification Section, page 426

VALIUM® Injectable Ⓒ

[*val'ee-um*]

(diazepam/Roche)

Valium Injectable is manufactured by Hoffmann-La Roche Inc., Nutley, N.J. 07110 and distributed by Roche Products Inc., Manati, P.R. 00674.

The following text is complete prescribing information based on official labeling in effect June 1, 1992.

DESCRIPTION

Each ml contains 5 mg diazepam/Roche compounded with 40% propylene glycol, 10% ethyl alcohol, 5% sodium benzoate and benzoic acid as buffers, and 1.5% benzyl alcohol as preservative.

Diazepam is a benzodiazepine derivative developed through original Roche research. Chemically, diazepam is 7-chloro-1, 3-dihydro-1-methyl-5-phenyl-2H-1,4-benzodiazepin-2-one. It is a colorless crystalline compound, insoluble in water and has a molecular weight of 284.74.

ACTIONS

In animals, diazepam appears to act on parts of the limbic system, the thalamus and hypothalamus, and induces calming effects. Diazepam, unlike chlorpromazine and reserpine, has no demonstrable peripheral autonomic blocking action, nor does it produce extrapyramidal side effects; however, animals treated with diazepam do have a transient ataxia at higher doses. Diazepam was found to have transient cardiovascular depressor effects in dogs. Long-term experiments in rats revealed no disturbances of endocrine function. Injections into animals have produced localized irritation of tissue surrounding injection sites and some thickening of veins after intravenous use.

INDICATIONS

Valium is indicated for the management of anxiety disorders or for the short-term relief of the symptoms of anxiety. Anxiety or tension associated with the stress of everyday life usually does not require treatment with an anxiolytic.

In acute alcohol withdrawal, Valium may be useful in the symptomatic relief of acute agitation, tremor, impending or acute delirium tremens and hallucinosis.

As an adjunct prior to endoscopic procedures if apprehension, anxiety or acute stress reactions are present, and to diminish the patient's recall of the procedures. (See WARNINGS.)

Valium is a useful adjunct for the relief of skeletal muscle spasm due to reflex spasm to local pathology (such as inflammation of the muscles or joints, or secondary to trauma); spasticity caused by upper motor neuron disorders (such as cerebral palsy and paraplegia); athetosis; stiff-man syndrome; and tetanus.

Injectable Valium is a useful adjunct in status epilepticus and severe recurrent convulsive seizures.

Valium is a useful premedication (the I.M. route is preferred) for relief of anxiety and tension in patients who are to undergo surgical procedures. Intravenously, prior to cardioversion for the relief of anxiety and tension and to diminish the patient's recall of the procedure.

CONTRAINDICATIONS

Injectable Valium is contraindicated in patients with a known hypersensitivity to this drug; acute narrow angle glaucoma; and open angle glaucoma unless patients are receiving appropriate therapy.

WARNINGS

When used intravenously, the following procedures should be undertaken to reduce the possibility of venous thrombosis, phlebitis, local irritation, swelling, and, rarely, vascular impairment: the solution should be injected slowly, taking at least one minute for each 5 mg (1 ml) given; do not use small veins, such as those on the dorsum of the hand or wrist; extreme care should be taken to avoid intra-arterial administration or extravasation.

Do not mix or dilute Valium with other solutions or drugs in syringe or infusion flask. If it is not feasible to administer Valium directly I.V., it may be injected slowly through the infusion tubing as close as possible to the vein insertion.

Extreme care must be used in administering Injectable Valium, particularly by the I.V. route, to the elderly, to very ill patients and to those with limited pulmonary reserve because of the possibility that apnea and/or cardiac arrest may occur. Concomitant use of barbiturates, alcohol, or other central nervous system depressants increases depression with increased risk of apnea. Resuscitative equipment including that necessary to support respiration should be readily available.

When Valium is used with a narcotic analgesic, the dosage of the narcotic should be reduced by at least one-third and administered in small increments. In some cases the use of a narcotic may not be necessary.

Injectable Valium should not be administered to patients in shock, coma, or in acute alcoholic intoxication with depression of vital signs. As is true of most CNS-acting drugs, patients receiving Valium should be cautioned against engaging in hazardous occupations requiring complete mental alertness, such as operating machinery or driving a motor vehicle.

Tonic status epilepticus has been precipitated in patients treated with I.V. Valium for petit mal status or petit mal variant status.

***Usage in Pregnancy:* An increased risk of congenital malformations associated with the use of minor tranquilizers (diazepam, meprobamate and chlordiazepoxide) during the first trimester of pregnancy has been suggested in several studies. Because use of these drugs is rarely a matter of urgency, their use during this period should almost always be avoided. The possibility that a woman of childbearing potential may be pregnant at the time of institution of therapy should be considered. Patients should be advised that if they become pregnant during therapy or intend to become pregnant they should communicate with their physicians about the desirability of discontinuing the drug.**

In humans, measurable amounts of diazepam were found in maternal and cord blood, indicating placental transfer of the drug. Until additional information is available, Valium Injectable is not recommended for obstetrical use.

Use in Children: Efficacy and safety of parenteral Valium has not been established in the neonate (30 days or less of age).

Prolonged central nervous system depression has been observed in neonates, apparently due to inability to biotransform Valium into inactive metabolites.

In pediatric use, in order to obtain maximal clinical effect with the minimum amount of drug and thus to reduce the risk of hazardous side effects, such as apnea or prolonged periods of somnolence, it is recommended that the drug be given slowly over a three-minute period in a dosage not to exceed 0.25 mg/kg. After an interval of 15 to 30 minutes the initial dosage can be safely repeated. If, however, relief of symptoms is not obtained after a third administration, adjunctive therapy appropriate to the condition being treated is recommended.

Withdrawal symptoms of the barbiturate type have occurred after the discontinuation of benzodiazepines. (See DRUG ABUSE AND DEPENDENCE section.)

PRECAUTIONS

Although seizures may be brought under control promptly, a significant proportion of patients experience a return to seizure activity, presumably due to the short-lived effect of Valium after I.V. administration. The physician should be prepared to re-administer the drug. However, Valium is not recommended for maintenance, and once seizures are brought under control, consideration should be given to the administration of agents useful in longer term control of seizures.

If Valium is to be combined with other psychotropic agents or anticonvulsant drugs, careful consideration should be given to the pharmacology of the agents to be employed—particularly with known compounds which may potentiate the action of Valium, such as phenothiazines, narcotics, barbiturates, MAO inhibitors and other antidepressants. In highly anxious patients with evidence of accompanying depression, particularly those who may have suicidal tendencies, protective measures may be necessary. The usual precautions in treating patients with impaired hepatic function should be observed. Metabolites of Valium are excreted by the kidney; to avoid their excess accumulation, caution should be exercised in the administration to patients with compromised kidney function.

Since an increase in cough reflex and laryngospasm may occur with peroral endoscopic procedures, the use of a topical anesthetic agent and the availability of necessary countermeasures are recommended.

Until additional information is available, injectable diazepam is not recommended for obstetrical use.

Injectable Valium has produced hypotension or muscular weakness in some patients particularly when used with narcotics, barbiturates or alcohol.

Lower doses (usually 2 mg to 5 mg) should be used for elderly and debilitated patients.

The clearance of Valium and certain other benzodiazepines can be delayed in association with Tagamet (cimetidine) administration. The clinical significance of this is unclear.

ADVERSE REACTIONS

Side effects most commonly reported were drowsiness, fatigue and ataxia; venous thrombosis and phlebitis at the site of injection. Other adverse reactions less frequently reported

Continued on next page

Roche Products—Cont.

include: *CNS:* confusion, depression, dysarthria, headache, hypoactivity, slurred speech, syncope, tremor, vertigo. *G.I.:* constipation, nausea. *G.U.:* incontinence, changes in libido, urinary retention. *Cardiovascular:* bradycardia, cardiovascular collapse, hypotension. *EENT:* blurred vision, diplopia, nystagmus. *Skin:* urticaria, skin rash. *Other:* hiccups, changes in salivation, neutropenia, jaundice. Paradoxical reactions such as acute hyperexcited states, anxiety, hallucinations, increased muscle spasticity, insomnia, rage, sleep disturbances and stimulation have been reported; should these occur, use of the drug should be discontinued. Minor changes in EEG patterns, usually low-voltage fast activity, have been observed in patients during and after Valium therapy and are of no known significance.

In peroral endoscopic procedures, coughing, depressed respiration, dyspnea, hyperventilation, laryngospasm and pain in throat or chest have been reported.

Because of isolated reports of neutropenia and jaundice, periodic blood counts and liver function tests are advisable during long-term therapy.

DRUG ABUSE AND DEPENDENCE

Withdrawal symptoms, similar in character to those noted with barbiturates and alcohol (convulsions, tremor, abdominal and muscle cramps, vomiting and sweating), have occurred following abrupt discontinuance of diazepam. The more severe withdrawal symptoms have usually been limited to those patients who had received excessive doses over an extended period of time. Generally milder withdrawal symptoms (*e.g.*, dysphoria and insomnia) have been reported following abrupt discontinuance of benzodiazepines taken continuously at therapeutic levels for several months. Consequently, after extended therapy, abrupt discontinuation should generally be avoided and a gradual dosage tapering schedule followed. Addiction-prone individuals (such as drug addicts or alcoholics) should be under careful surveillance when receiving diazepam or other psychotropic agents because of the predisposition of such patients to habituation and dependence.

DOSAGE AND ADMINISTRATION

Dosage should be individualized for maximum beneficial effect. The usual recommended dose in older children and adults ranges from 2 mg to 20 mg I.M. or I.V., depending on the indication and its severity. In some conditions, *e.g.*, tetanus, larger doses may be required. (See dosage for specific indications.) In acute conditions the injection may be re-

Status Epilepticus and Severe Recurrent Convulsive Seizures: In the convulsing patient, the I.V. route is by far preferred. This injection should be administered slowly. However, if I.V. administration is impossible, the I.M. route may be used.

Preoperative Medication: To relieve anxiety and tension. (If atropine, scopolamine or other premedications are desired, they must be administered in separate syringes.)

Cardioversion: To relieve anxiety and tension and to reduce recall of procedure.

5 mg to 10 mg initially (I.V. preferred). This injection may be repeated if necessary at 10 to 15 minute intervals up to a maximum dose of 30 mg.
If necessary, therapy with Valium may be repeated in 2 to 4 hours; however, residual active metabolites may persist, and readministration should be made with this consideration. Extreme caution must be exercised with individuals with chronic lung disease or unstable cardiovascular status.

10 mg, I.M. (preferred route), before surgery.

5 mg to 15 mg, I.V., within 5 to 10 minutes prior to the procedure.

Infants over 30 days of age and children under 5 years, 0.2 mg to 0.5 mg slowly every 2 to 5 minutes up to a maximum of 5 mg (I.V. preferred). Children 5 years or older, 1 mg every 2 to 5 minutes up to a maximum of 10 mg (slow I.V. administration preferred). Repeat in 2 to 4 hours if necessary. EEG monitoring of the seizure may be helpful.

peated within one hour although an interval of 3 to 4 hours is usually satisfactory. Lower doses (usually 2 mg to 5 mg) and slow increase in dosage should be used for elderly or debilitated patients and when other sedative drugs are administered. (See WARNINGS and ADVERSE REACTIONS.)

For dosage in infants above the age of 30 days and children, see the specific indications below. When intravenous use is indicated, facilities for respiratory assistance should be readily available.

Intramuscular: Injectable Valium should be injected deeply into the muscle.

Intravenous use: (See WARNINGS, particularly for use in children.) The solution should be injected slowly, taking at least one minute for each 5 mg (1 ml) given. Do not use small veins, such as those on the dorsum of the hand or wrist. Extreme care should be taken to avoid intra-arterial administration or extravasation.

Do not mix or dilute Valium with other solutions or drugs in syringe or infusion flask. If it is not feasible to administer Valium directly I.V., it may be injected slowly through the infusion tubing as close as possible to the vein insertion. [See table below.]

Once the acute symptomatology has been properly controlled with Injectable Valium, the patient may be placed on oral therapy with Valium if further treatment is required.

Management of Overdosage:

Manifestations of Valium overdosage include somnolence, confusion, coma, and diminished reflexes. Respiration, pulse and blood pressure should be monitored, as in all cases of drug overdosage, although, in general, these effects have been minimal. General supportive measures should be employed, along with intravenous fluids, and an adequate airway maintained. Hypotension may be combated by the use of Levophed® (levarterenol) or Aramine (metaraminol). Dialysis is of limited value.

HOW SUPPLIED

Ampuls, 2 ml, boxes of 10; Vials, 10 ml, boxes of 1; Tel-E-Ject® (disposable syringes), 2 ml, boxes of 10.

ANIMAL PHARMACOLOGY

Oral LD$_{50}$ of diazepam is 720 mg/kg in mice and 1240 mg/kg in rats. Intraperitoneal administration of 400 mg/kg to a monkey resulted in death on the sixth day. [See table above.]

Reproduction Studies: A series of rat reproduction studies was performed with diazepam in oral doses of 1, 10, 80 and 100 mg/kg given for periods ranging from 60–228 days prior to mating. At 100 mg/kg there was a decrease in the number of pregnancies and surviving offspring in these rats. These effects may be attributable to prolonged sedative activity, resulting in lack of interest in mating and lessened maternal nursing and care of the young. Neonatal survival of rats at doses lower than 100 mg/kg was within normal limits. Several neonates, both controls and experimentals, in these rat reproduction studies showed skeletal or other defects. Further studies in rats at doses up to and including 80 mg/kg/day did not reveal significant teratological effects on the offspring. Rabbits were maintained on doses of 1, 2, 5 and 8 mg/kg from day 6 through day 18 of gestation. No adverse effects on reproduction and no teratological changes were noted.

Revised: February 1988

Shown in Product Identification Section, page 426

RECOMMENDED DOSAGE FOR *INJECTABLE VALIUM®* (diazepam/Roche)

	USUAL ADULT DOSAGE	DOSAGE RANGE IN CHILDREN (I.V. administration should be made slowly)
Moderate Anxiety Disorders and Symptoms of Anxiety	2 mg to 5 mg, I.M. or I.V. Repeat in 3 to 4 hours, if necessary.	
Severe Anxiety Disorders and Symptoms of Anxiety	5 mg to 10 mg, I.M. or I.V. Repeat in 3 to 4 hours, if necessary.	
Acute Alcohol Withdrawal: As an aid in symptomatic relief of acute agitation, tremor, impending or acute delirium tremens and hallucinosis.	10 mg, I.M. or I.V. initially, then 5 mg to 10 mg in 3 to 4 hours, if necessary.	
Endoscopic Procedures: Adjunctively, if apprehension, anxiety or acute stress reactions are present prior to endoscopic procedures. Dosage of narcotics should be reduced by at least a third and in some cases may be omitted. See *Precautions* for peroral procedures.	Titrate I.V. dosage to desired sedative response, such as slurring of speech, with slow administration immediately prior to the procedure. Generally 10 mg or less is adequate, but up to 20 mg I.V. may be given, particularly when concomitant narcotics are omitted. If I.V. cannot be used, 5 mg to 10 mg I.M. approximately 30 minutes prior to the procedure.	
Muscle Spasm: Associated with local pathology, cerebral palsy, athetosis, stiff-man syndrome or tetanus.	5 mg to 10 mg, I.M. or I.V. initially, then 5 mg to 10 mg in 3 to 4 hours, if necessary. For tetanus, larger doses may be required.	For tetanus in infants over 30 days of age, 1 mg to 2 mg I.M. or I.V., slowly, repeated every 3 to 4 hours as necessary. In children 5 years or older, 5 mg to 10 mg repeated every 3 to 4 hours may be required to control tetanus spasms. Respiratory assistance should be available.

VALIUM® TABLETS ℞
[*val 'ee-um*]
(diazepam/Roche)

The following text is complete prescribing information based on official labeling in effect June 1, 1992.

DESCRIPTION

Valium (brand of diazepam/Roche) is a benzodiazepine derivative developed through original Roche research. Chemically, diazepam is 7- chloro - 1,3 - dihydro - 1 - methyl - 5 - phenyl - 2H-1,4-benzodiazepin-2-one. It is a colorless crystalline compound, insoluble in water and has a molecular weight of 284.74.

Valium 5-mg tablets contain FD&C Yellow No. 6 and D&C Yellow No. 10 dyes. Valium 10-mg tablets contain FD&C Blue No. 1 dye. Valium 2-mg tablets contain no dye.

PHARMACOLOGY

In animals Valium appears to act on parts of the limbic system, the thalamus and hypothalamus, and induces calming effects. Valium, unlike chlorpromazine and reserpine, has no demonstrable peripheral autonomic blocking action, nor does it produce extrapyramidal side effects; however, animals treated with Valium do have a transient ataxia at higher doses. Valium was found to have transient cardiovascular depressor effects in dogs. Long-term experiments in rats revealed no disturbances of endocrine function.

Oral LD_{50} of diazepam is 720 mg/kg in mice and 1240 mg/kg in rats. Intraperitoneal administration of 400 mg/kg to a monkey resulted in death on the sixth day.

Reproduction Studies: A series of rat reproduction studies was performed with diazepam in oral doses of 1, 10, 80 and 100 mg/kg. At 100 mg/kg there was a decrease in the number of pregnancies and surviving offspring in these rats. Neonatal survival of rats at doses lower than 100 mg/kg was within normal limits. Several neonates in these rat reproduction studies showed skeletal or other defects. Further studies in rats at doses up to and including 80 mg/kg/day did not reveal teratological effects on the offspring.

In humans, measurable blood levels of Valium were obtained in maternal and cord blood, indicating placental transfer of the drug.

INDICATIONS

Valium is indicated for the management of anxiety disorders or for the short-term relief of the symptoms of anxiety. Anxiety or tension associated with the stress of everyday life usually does not require treatment with an anxiolytic.

In acute alcohol withdrawal, Valium may be useful in the symptomatic relief of acute agitation, tremor, impending or acute delirium tremens and hallucinosis.

Valium is a useful adjunct for the relief of skeletal muscle spasm due to reflex spasm to local pathology (such as inflammation of the muscles or joints, or secondary to trauma); spasticity caused by upper motor neuron disorders (such as cerebral palsy and paraplegia); athetosis; and stiff-man syndrome.

Oral Valium may be used adjunctively in convulsive disorders, although it has not proved useful as the sole therapy.

The effectiveness of Valium in long-term use, that is, more than 4 months, has not been assessed by systematic clinical studies. The physician should periodically reassess the usefulness of the drug for the individual patient.

CONTRAINDICATIONS

Valium is contraindicated in patients with a known hypersensitivity to this drug and, because of lack of sufficient clinical experience, in children under 6 months of age. It may be used in patients with open angle glaucoma who are receiving appropriate therapy, but is contraindicated in acute narrow angle glaucoma.

WARNINGS

Valium is not of value in the treatment of psychotic patients and should not be employed in lieu of appropriate treatment.

As is true of most preparations containing CNS-acting drugs, patients receiving Valium should be cautioned against engaging in hazardous occupations requiring complete mental alertness such as operating machinery or driving a motor vehicle.

As with other agents which have anticonvulsant activity, when Valium is used as an adjunct in treating convulsive disorders, the possibility of an increase in the frequency and/or severity of grand mal seizures may require an increase in the dosage of standard anticonvulsant medication. Abrupt withdrawal of Valium in such cases may also be associated with a temporary increase in the frequency and/or severity of seizures.

Since Valium has a central nervous system depressant effect, patients should be advised against the simultaneous ingestion of alcohol and other CNS-depressant drugs during Valium therapy.

Usage in Pregnancy: **An increased risk of congenital malformations associated with the use of minor tranquilizers (diazepam, meprobamate and chlordiazepoxide) during the first trimester of pregnancy has been suggested in several studies. Because use of these drugs is rarely a matter of urgency, their use during this period should almost always be avoided. The possibility that a woman of childbearing potential may be pregnant at the time of institution of therapy should be considered. Patients should be advised that if they become pregnant during therapy or intend to become pregnant they should communicate with their physicians about the desirability of discontinuing the drug.**

Management of Overdosage: Manifestations of Valium overdosage include somnolence, confusion, coma and diminished reflexes. Respiration, pulse and blood pressure should be monitored, as in all cases of drug overdosage, although, in general, these effects have been minimal following overdosage. General supportive measures should be employed, along with immediate gastric lavage. Intravenous fluids should be administered and an adequate airway maintained. Hypotension may be combated by the use of Levophed® (levarterenol) or Aramine (metaraminol). Dialysis is of limited value. As with the management of intentional overdosage with any drug, it should be borne in mind that multiple agents may have been ingested.

Withdrawal symptoms of the barbiturate type have occurred after the discontinuation of benzodiazepines. (See DRUG ABUSE AND DEPENDENCE section.)

PRECAUTIONS

If Valium is to be combined with other psychotropic agents or anticonvulsant drugs, careful consideration should be given to the pharmacology of the agents to be employed—particularly with known compounds which may potentiate the action of Valium, such as phenothiazines, narcotics, barbiturates, MAO inhibitors and other antidepressants. The usual precautions are indicated for severely depressed patients or those in whom there is any evidence of latent depression; particularly the recognition that suicidal tendencies may be present and protective measures may be necessary. The usual precautions in treating patients with impaired renal or hepatic function should be observed.

In elderly and debilitated patients, it is recommended that the dosage be limited to the smallest effective amount to preclude the development of ataxia or oversedation (2 mg to 2½ mg once or twice daily, initially, to be increased gradually as needed and tolerated).

The clearance of Valium and certain other benzodiazepines can be delayed in association with Tagamet (cimetidine) administration. The clinical significance of this is unclear.

Information for Patients: To assure the safe and effective use of benzodiazepines, patients should be informed that, since benzodiazepines may produce psychological and physical dependence, it is advisable that they consult with their physician before either increasing the dose or abruptly discontinuing this drug.

ADVERSE REACTIONS

Side effects most commonly reported were drowsiness, fatigue and ataxia. Infrequently encountered were confusion, constipation, depression, diplopia, dysarthria, headache, hypotension, incontinence, jaundice, changes in libido, nausea, changes in salivation, skin rash, slurred speech, tremor, urinary retention, vertigo and blurred vision. Paradoxical reactions such as acute hyperexcited states, anxiety, hallucinations, increased muscle spasticity, insomnia, rage, sleep disturbances and stimulation have been reported; should these occur, use of the drug should be discontinued.

Because of isolated reports of neutropenia and jaundice, periodic blood counts and liver function tests are advisable during long-term therapy. Minor changes in EEG patterns, usually low-voltage fast activity, have been observed in patients during and after Valium therapy and are of no known significance.

DRUG ABUSE AND DEPENDENCE

Withdrawal symptoms, similar in character to those noted with barbiturates and alcohol (convulsions, tremor, abdominal and muscle cramps, vomiting and sweating), have occurred following abrupt discontinuance of diazepam. The more severe withdrawal symptoms have usually been limited to those patients who had received excessive doses over an extended period of time. Generally milder withdrawal symptoms (*e.g.,* dysphoria and insomnia) have been reported following abrupt discontinuation of benzodiazepines taken continuously at therapeutic levels for several months. Consequently, after extended therapy, abrupt discontinuation should generally be avoided and a gradual dosage tapering schedule followed. Addiction-prone individuals (such as drug addicts or alcoholics) should be under careful surveillance when receiving diazepam or other psychotropic agents because of the predisposition of such patients to habituation and dependence.

DOSAGE AND ADMINISTRATION

Dosage should be individualized for maximum beneficial effect. While the usual daily dosages given above will meet the needs of most patients, there will be some who may require higher doses. In such cases dosage should be increased cautiously to avoid adverse effects. [See table above.]

HOW SUPPLIED

For oral administration, round, scored tablets with a cut out "V" design—2 mg, white; 5 mg, yellow; 10 mg, blue—bottles of 100 and 500. Tel-E-Dose® packages of 100, available in boxes of 4 reverse-numbered cards of 25, and in boxes containing 10 strips of 10.

Imprint on tablets:

2 mg:
2 VALIUM® (front)
ROCHE (scored side)

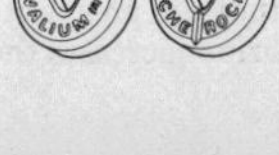

	USUAL DAILY DOSE
Adults:	
Management of Anxiety Disorders and Relief of Symptoms of Anxiety	Depending upon severity of symptoms—2 mg to 10 mg, 2 to 4 times daily
Symptomatic Relief in Acute Alcohol Withdrawal.	10 mg, 3 or 4 times during the first 24 hours, reducing to 5 mg, 3 or 4 times daily as needed
Adjunctively for Relief of Skeletal Muscle Spasm.	2 mg to 10 mg, 3 or 4 times daily
Adjunctively in Convulsive Disorders.	2 mg to 10 mg, 2 to 4 times daily
Geriatric Patients, or in the presence of debilitating disease.	2 mg to 2½ mg, 1 or 2 times daily initially; increase gradually as needed and tolerated
Children:	
Because of varied responses to CNS-acting drugs, initiate therapy with lowest dose and increase as required. Not for use in children under 6 months.	1 mg to 2½ mg, 3 or 4 times daily initially; increase gradually as needed and tolerated

5 mg:
5 VALIUM® (front)
ROCHE (scored side)

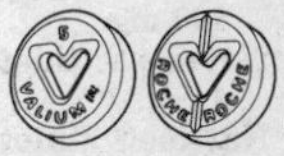

10 mg:
10 VALIUM® (front)
ROCHE (scored side)

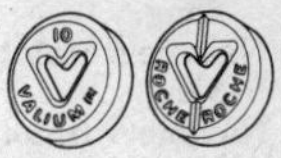

Revised: July 1988

Shown in Product Identification Section, page 426

Roerig Division

Pfizer Incorporated
235 EAST 42nd STREET
NEW YORK, NY 10017

Product Identification Codes

To provide quick and positive identification of Roerig Division products, we have imprinted the product identification number of the National Drug Code on most tablets and capsules.

In order that you may quickly identify a product by its code number, we have compiled below a numerical list of code numbers with their corresponding product names. We are also listing the code numbers by alphabetical order of products.

Numerical Listing

Product Ident. Number	Product
035	**Spectrobid® (bacampicillin HCl) Tablets, 400 mg., equivalent to 280 mg. ampicillin**
092	**Urobiotic®-250 (oxytetracycline HCl 250 mg. with sulfamethizole 250 mg. and phenazopyridine 50 mg.) Capsules**
143	**Geocillin® (carbenicillin indanyl sodium) Tablets, equivalent to 382 mg. carbenicillin**
159	**TAO® (troleandomycin) Capsules, 250 mg.**
210	**Antivert® (meclizine HCl) Tablets, 12.5 mg.**
211	**Antivert® /25 (meclizine HCl) Tablets, 25 mg.**
214	**Antivert® /50 (meclizine HCl) Tablets, 50 mg.**
254	**Marax® (ephedrine sulfate, 25 mg; theophylline, 130 mg; and Atarax® [hydroxyzine HCl], 10 mg) Tablets**
275	**Cardura® (doxazosin mesylate) Tablets, 1 mg.**
276	**Cardura® (doxazosin mesylate) Tablets, 2 mg.**
277	**Cardura® (doxazosin mesylate) Tablets, 4 mg.**
278	**Cardura® (doxazosin mesylate) Tablets, 8 mg.**

Continued on next page

Roerig—Cont.

341	Diflucan® (fluconazole) Tablets, 50 mg.
342	Diflucan® (fluconazole) Tablets, 100 mg.
343	Diflucan® (fluconazole) Tablets, 200 mg.
490	Zoloft™ (sertraline HCl) Tablets, 50 mg.
491	Zoloft™ (sertraline HCl) Tablets, 100 mg.
534	Sinequan® (doxepin HCl) Capsules 10 mg.
535	Sinequan® (doxepin HCl) Capsules 25 mg.
536	Sinequan® (doxepin HCl) Capsules 50 mg.
537	Sinequan® (doxepin HCl) Capsules 150 mg.
538	Sinequan® (doxepin HCl) Capsules 100 mg.
539	Sinequan® (doxepin HCl) Capsules 75 mg.
560	Atarax® (hydroxyzine HCl) Tablets, 10 mg.
561	Atarax® (hydroxyzine HCl) Tablets, 25 mg.
562	Atarax® (hydroxyzine HCl) Tablets, 50 mg.
563	Atarax® (hydroxyzine HCl) Tablets, 100 mg.
571	Navane® (thiothixene) Capsules, 1 mg.
572	Navane® (thiothixene) Capsules, 2 mg.
573	Navane® (thiothixene) Capsules, 5 mg.
574	Navane® (thiothixene) Capsules, 10 mg.
577	Navane® (thiothixene) Capsules, 20 mg.

Alphabetical Listing

Prod. Ident.

Number	Product
210	Antivert® (meclizine HCl) Tablets, 12.5 mg.
211	Antivert® /25 (meclizine HCl) Tablets, 25 mg.
214	Antivert® /50 (meclizine HCl) Tablets, 50 mg.
560	Atarax® (hydroxyzine HCl) Tablets, 10 mg.
561	Atarax® (hydroxyzine HCl) Tablets, 25 mg.
562	Atarax® (hydroxyzine HCl) Tablets, 50 mg.
563	Atarax® (hydroxyzine HCl) Tablets, 100 mg.
275	Cardura® (doxazosin mesylate) Tablets, 1 mg.
276	Cardura® (doxazosin mesylate) Tablets, 2 mg.
277	Cardura® (doxazosin mesylate) Tablets, 4 mg.
278	Cardura® (doxazosin mesylate) Tablets, 8 mg.
341	Diflucan® fluconazole) Tablets 50 mg.
342	Diflucan® (fluconazole) Tablets 100 mg.
343	Diflucan® (fluconazole) Tablets 200 mg.
143	Geocillin® (carbenicillin indanyl sodium) Tablets equivalent to 382 mg. carbenicillin
254	Marax® (ephedrine sulfate, 25 mg; theophylline, 130 mg; and Atarax® [hydroxyzine HCl], 10 mg) Tablets
571	Navane® (thiothixene) Capsules, 1 mg.
572	Navane® (thiothixene) Capsules, 2 mg.
573	Navane® (thiothixene) Capsules, 5 mg.
574	Navane® (thiothixene) Capsules, 10 mg.
577	Navane® (thiothixene) Capsules, 20 mg.
534	Sinequan® (doxepin HCl) Capsules 10 mg.
535	Sinequan® (doxepin HCl) Capsules 25 mg.
536	Sinequan® (doxepin HCl) Capsules 50 mg.
539	Sinequan® (doxepin HCl) Capsules 75 mg.
538	Sinequan® (doxepin HCl) Capsules 100 mg.
537	Sinequan® (doxepin HCl) Capsules 150 mg.
035	Spectrobid® (bacampicillin HCl) Tablets, 400 mg., equivalent to 280 mg. ampicillin
159	TAO® (troleandomycin) Capsules, 250 mg.
092	Urobiotic®-250 (oxytetracycline HCl 250 mg. with sulfamethizole 250 mg. and phenazopyridine 50 mg.) Capsules
490	Zoloft™ (sertraline HCl) Tablets, 50 mg.
491	Zoloft™ (sertraline HCl) Tablets, 100 mg.

ANTIVERT® TABLETS   ℞
[ăn 'tĭ-vert "]
(12.5 mg. meclizine HCl)
ANTIVERT®/25 TABLETS   ℞
(25 mg. meclizine HCl)
ANTIVERT®/50 TABLETS   ℞
(50 mg. meclizine HCl)

DESCRIPTION
Chemically, Antivert (meclizine HCl) is 1-(p-chloro-α-phenyl-benzyl) -4- (m -methylbenzyl)piperazine dihydrochloride monohydrate.

Inert ingredients for the tablets are: dibasic calcium phosphate; magnesium stearate; polyethylene glycol; starch; sucrose. The 12.5 mg tablets also contain: Blue 1. The 25 mg tablets also contain: Yellow 6 Lake; Yellow 10 Lake. The 50 mg tablets also contain: Blue 1 Lake; Yellow 10 Lake.
Inert ingredients for the chewable tablets are: lactose, magnesium stearate; raspberry flavor; Red 40; saccharin sodium; siliceous earth; starch; talc.

ACTIONS
Antivert is an antihistamine which shows marked protective activity against nebulized histamine and lethal doses of intravenously injected histamine in guinea pigs. It has a marked effect in blocking the vasodepressor response to histamine, but only a slight blocking action against acetylcholine. Its activity is relatively weak in inhibiting the spasmogenic action of histamine on isolated guinea pig ileum.

INDICATIONS
Based on a review of this drug by the National Academy of Sciences-National Research Council and/or other information, FDA has classified the indications as follows:
Effective: Management of nausea and vomiting, and dizziness associated with motion sickness.
Possibly Effective: Management of vertigo associated with diseases affecting the vestibular system.
Final classification of the less than effective indications requires further investigation.

CONTRAINDICATIONS
Meclizine HCl is contraindicated in individuals who have shown a previous hypersensitivity to it.

WARNINGS
Since drowsiness may, on occasion, occur with use of this drug, patients should be warned of this possibility and cautioned against driving a car or operating dangerous machinery.
Patients should avoid alcoholic beverages while taking the drug. Due to its potential anticholinergic action, this drug should be used with caution in patients with asthma, glaucoma, or enlargement of the prostate gland.
USAGE IN CHILDREN:
Clinical studies establishing safety and effectiveness in children have not been done; therefore, usage is not recommended in children under 12 years of age.
USAGE IN PREGNANCY:
Pregnancy Category B. Reproduction studies in rats have shown cleft palates at 25–50 times the human dose. Epidemiological studies in pregnant women, however, do not indicate that meclizine increases the risk of abnormalities when administered during pregnancy. Despite the animal findings, it would appear that the possibility of fetal harm is remote. Nevertheless, meclizine, or any other medication, should be used during pregnancy only if clearly necessary.

ADVERSE REACTIONS
Drowsiness, dry mouth and, on rare occasions, blurred vision have been reported.

DOSAGE AND ADMINISTRATION
Vertigo:
For the control of vertigo associated with diseases affecting the vestibular system, the recommended dose is 25 to 100 mg. daily, in divided dosage, depending upon clinical response.
Motion Sickness:
The initial dose of 25 to 50 mg. of Antivert should be taken one hour prior to embarkation for protection against motion sickness. Thereafter, the dose may be repeated every 24 hours for the duration of the journey.

HOW SUPPLIED
Antivert—12.5 mg tablets: bottles of 100 (NDC 0662-2100-66), 1000 (NDC 0662-2100-82).
Antivert/25—25 mg tablets: bottles of 100 (NDC 0662-2110-66), 1000 (NDC 0662-2110-82).
Antivert/50—50 mg tablets: bottles of 100 (NDC 0662-2140-66).

69-2148-37-7
Shown in Product Identification Section, page 426

ATARAX®   ℞
[ăt 'ā-raks "]
(hydroxyzine hydrochloride)
TABLETS AND SYRUP

DESCRIPTION
Hydroxyzine hydrochloride is designated chemically as 1-(p-chlorobenzhydryl) 4-[2-(2-hydroxyethoxy)-ethyl] piperazine dihydrochloride.
Inert ingredients for the tablets are: acacia; carnauba wax; dibasic calcium phosphate; gelatin; lactose; magnesium stearate; precipitated calcium carbonate; shellac; sucrose; talc; white wax. The 10 mg tablets also contain: sodium hydroxide; starch; titanium dioxide; Yellow 6 Lake. The 25 mg tablets also contain: starch; velo dark green. The 50 mg tablets also contain: starch; velo yellow. The 100 mg tablets also contain: alginic acid; Blue 1; polyethylene glycol; Red 3.
Inert ingredients for the syrup are: alcohol; menthol; peppermint oil; sodium benzoate; spearmint oil; sucrose; water.

CLINICAL PHARMACOLOGY
Atarax is unrelated chemically to the phenothiazines, reserpine, meprobamate, or the benzodiazepines.
Atarax is not a cortical depressant, but its action may be due to a suppression of activity in certain key regions of the subcortical area of the central nervous system. Primary skeletal muscle relaxation has been demonstrated experimentally. Bronchodilator activity, and antihistaminic and analgesic effects have been demonstrated experimentally and confirmed clinically. An antiemetic effect, both by the apomorphine test and the veriloid test, has been demonstrated. Pharmacological and clinical studies indicate that hydroxyzine in therapeutic dosage does not increase gastric secretion or acidity and in most cases has mild antisecretory activity. Hydroxyzine is rapidly absorbed from the gastrointestinal tract and Atarax's clinical effects are usually noted within 15 to 30 minutes after oral administration.

INDICATIONS
For symptomatic relief of anxiety and tension associated with psychoneurosis and as an adjunct in organic disease states in which anxiety is manifested.
Useful in the management of pruritus due to allergic conditions such as chronic urticaria and atopic and contact dermatoses, and in histamine-mediated pruritus.
As a sedative when used as premedication and following general anesthesia, **Hydroxyzine may potentiate meperidine (Demerol®) and barbiturates,** so their use in pre-anesthetic adjunctive therapy should be modified on an individual basis. Atropine and other belladonna alkaloids are not affected by the drug. Hydroxyzine is not known to interfere with the action of digitalis in any way and it may be used concurrently with this agent.
The effectiveness of hydroxyzine as an antianxiety agent for long term use, that is more than 4 months, has not been assessed by systematic clinical studies. The physician should reassess periodically the usefulness of the drug for the individual patient.

CONTRAINDICATIONS
Hydroxyzine, when administered to the pregnant mouse, rat, and rabbit, induced fetal abnormalities in the rat and mouse at doses substantially above the human therapeutic range. Clinical data in human beings are inadequate to establish safety in early pregnancy. Until such data are available, hydroxyzine is contraindicated in early pregnancy.

Hydroxyzine is contraindicated for patients who have shown a previous hypersensitivity to it.

WARNINGS

Nursing Mothers: It is not known whether this drug is excreted in human milk. Since many drugs are so excreted, hydroxyzine should not be given to nursing mothers.

PRECAUTIONS

THE POTENTIATING ACTION OF HYDROXYZINE MUST BE CONSIDERED WHEN THE DRUG IS USED IN CONJUNCTION WITH CENTRAL NERVOUS SYSTEM DEPRESSANTS SUCH AS NARCOTICS, NON-NARCOTIC ANALGESICS AND BARBITURATES. Therefore when central nervous system depressants are administered concomitantly with hydroxyzine their dosage should be reduced. Since drowsiness may occur with use of this drug, patients should be warned of this possibility and cautioned against driving a car or operating dangerous machinery while taking Atarax. Patients should be advised against the simultaneous use of other CNS depressant drugs, and cautioned that the effect of alcohol may be increased.

ADVERSE REACTIONS

Side effects reported with the administration of Atarax (hydroxyzine hydrochloride) are usually mild and transitory in nature.

Anticholinergic: Dry mouth.

Central Nervous System: Drowsiness is usually transitory and may disappear in a few days of continued therapy or upon reduction of the dose. Involuntary motor activity including rare instances of tremor and convulsions have been reported, usually with doses considerably higher than those recommended. Clinically significant respiratory depression has not been reported at recommended doses.

OVERDOSAGE

The most common manifestation of Atarax overdosage is hypersedation. As in the management of overdosage with any drug, it should be borne in mind that multiple agents may have been taken.

If vomiting has not occurred spontaneously, it should be induced. Immediate gastric lavage is also recommended. General supportive care, including frequent monitoring of the vital signs and close observation of the patient, is indicated. Hypotension, though unlikely, may be controlled with intravenous fluids and Levophed® (levarterenol), or Aramine® (metaraminol). Do not use epinephrine as Atarax counteracts its pressor action.

There is no specific antidote. It is doubtful that hemodialysis would be of any value in the treatment of overdosage with hydroxyzine. However, if other agents such as barbiturates have been ingested concomitantly, hemodialysis may be indicated. There is no practical method to quantitate hydroxyzine in body fluids or tissue after its ingestion or administration.

DOSAGE

For symptomatic relief of anxiety and tension associated with psychoneurosis and as an adjunct in organic disease states in which anxiety is manifested: in adults, 50–100 mg q.i.d.: children under 6 years, 50 mg daily in divided doses and over 6 years, 50–100 mg daily in divided doses.

For use in the management of pruritus due to allergic conditions such as chronic urticaria and atopic and contact dermatoses, and in histamine-mediated pruritus: in adults, 25 mg t.i.d. or q.i.d.; children under 6 years, 50 mg daily in divided doses and over 6 years, 50–100 mg daily in divided doses.

As a sedative when used as a premedication and following general anesthesia: 50–100 mg in adults, and 0.6 mg/kg in children.

When treatment is initiated by the intramuscular route of administration, subsequent doses may be administered orally.

As with all medications, the dosage should be adjusted according to the patient's response to therapy.

SUPPLY

Atarax Tablets

10 mg: 100's (NDC 0049-5600-66), 500's (NDC 0049-5600-73), Unit Dose 10 × 10's (NDC 0049-5600-41), and Unit of Use 40's (NDC 0049-5600-43)—orange tablets

25 mg: 100's (NDC 0049-5610-66), 500's (NDC 0049-5610-73), Unit Dose 10 × 10's (NDC 0049-5610-41)

50 mg: 100's (NDC 0049-5620-66), 500's (NDC 0049-5620-73)—yellow tablets

Atarax 100 Tablets

100 mg: 100's (NDC 0049-5630-66)—red tablets

Atarax Syrup

10 mg per teaspoon (5 ml): 1 pint bottles (NDC 0049-5590-93)

Alcohol Content—Ethyl Alcohol—0.5% v/v

BIBLIOGRAPHY

Available on request.

77-0618-00-4

Shown in Product Identification Section, page 426

CARDURA® ℞

(doxazosin mesylate)
Tablets

DESCRIPTION

CARDURA (doxazosin mesylate) is a quinazoline compound that is a selective inhibitor of the alpha$_1$ subtype of alpha adrenergic receptors. The chemical name of doxazosin mesylate is 1-(4-amino-6,7-dimethoxy-2-quinazolinyl)-4-(1,4-benzodioxan-2-ylcarbonyl) piperazine methanesulfonate. The empirical formula for doxazosin mesylate is $C_{23}H_{25}N_5O_5 \cdot CH_4O_3S$ and the molecular weight is 547.6. It has the following structure:

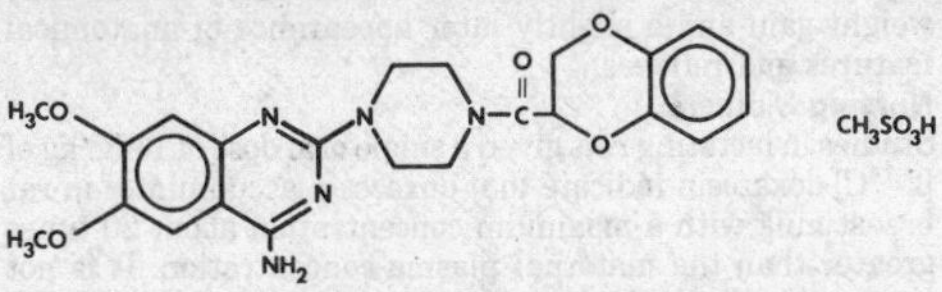

CARDURA (doxazosin mesylate) is freely soluble in dimethylsulfoxide, soluble in dimethylformamide, slightly soluble in methanol, ethanol, and water (0.8% at 25°C), and very slightly soluble in acetone and methylene chloride. CARDURA is available as colored tablets for oral use and contains 1 mg (white), 2 mg (yellow), 4 mg (orange) and 8 mg (green) of doxazosin as the free base.

The inactive ingredients for all tablets are: microcrystalline cellulose, lactose, sodium starch glycolate, magnesium stearate and sodium lauryl sulfate. The 2 mg tablet contains D & C yellow 10, FD & C yellow 6; the 4 mg tablet contains FD & C yellow 6; the 8 mg tablet contains FD & C blue 10 and D & C yellow 10.

CLINICAL PHARMACOLOGY

Mechanism of Action

The mechanism of action of CARDURA (doxazosin mesylate) is selective blockade of the alpha$_1$ (postjunctional) subtype of alpha adrenergic receptors. Studies in normal human subjects have shown that doxazosin competitively antagonized the pressor effects of phenylephrine (an alpha$_1$ agonist) and the systolic pressor effect of norepinephrine. Doxazosin and prazosin have similar abilities to antagonize phenylephrine. The antihypertensive effect of CARDURA results from a decrease in systemic vascular resistance. The parent compound, doxazosin, is primarily responsible for the antihypertensive activity. The low plasma concentrations of known active and inactive metabolites of doxazosin (2-piperazinyl, 6'- and 7'-hydroxy and 6- and 7-O-desmethyl compounds) compared to parent drug indicate that the contribution of even the most potent compound (6'-hydroxy) to the antihypertensive effect of doxazosin in man is probably small.

Pharmacokinetics

After oral administration of therapeutic doses, peak plasma levels of CARDURA (doxazosin mesylate) occur at about 2–3 hours. Bioavailability is approximately 65%, reflecting first pass metabolism of doxazosin by the liver. The effect of food on the bioavailability of doxazosin has not been determined. CARDURA is extensively metabolized in the liver, mainly by O-demethylation of the quinazoline nucleus or hydroxylation of the benzodioxan moiety. In a study of two subjects administered radiolabelled doxazosin 2 mg orally and 1 mg intravenous on two separate occasions, approximately 63% of the dose was eliminated in the feces and 9% of the dose was found in the urine. On average only 4.8% of the dose was excreted as unchanged drug in the feces and only a trace of the total radioactivity in the urine was attributed to unchanged drug. At the plasma concentrations achieved by therapeutic doses approximately 98% of the circulating drug is bound to plasma proteins.

Plasma elimination of doxazosin is biphasic, with a terminal elimination half life of about 22 hours. Steady-state studies in hypertensive patients given doxazosin doses of 2–16 mg once daily showed linear kinetics and dose proportionality. In two studies, following the administration of 2 mg orally once daily, the mean accumulation ratios (steady state AUC vs first dose AUC) were 1.2 and 1.7. Enterohepatic recycling is suggested by secondary peaking of plasma doxazosin concentrations.

Although several active metabolites of doxazosin have been identified, the pharmacokinetics of these metabolites have not been characterized.

Pharmacokinetic studies in elderly patients and patients with renal impairment have shown no significant alterations compared to younger patients with normal renal function. There have, however, been no studies of patients with liver impairment, nor studies of the effects of drugs known to influence hepatic metabolism (e.g. cimetidine). Use of doxazosin in patients with altered liver function should be undertaken with particular caution, if at all, as excretion is almost wholly hepatic.

Pharmacodynamics

Administration of CARDURA (doxazosin mesylate) results in a reduction in systemic vascular resistance. In patients with hypertension there is little change in cardiac output. Maximum reductions in blood pressure usually occur 2–6 hours after dosing and are associated with a small increase in standing heart rate. Like other alpha$_1$-adrenergic blocking agents, doxazosin has a greater effect on blood pressure and heart rate in the standing position.

In a pooled analysis of placebo controlled studies with about 300 patients per treatment group, doxazosin, at doses of 1–16 mg given once daily, lowered blood pressure at 24 hours by about 10/8 mmHg compared to placebo in the standing position and about 9/5 mmHg in the supine position. Peak blood pressure effects (1–6 hours) were larger by about 50–75% (i.e., trough values were about 55–70% of peak effect), with the larger peak-trough differences seen in systolic pressures. There was no apparent difference in the blood pressure response of Caucasians and blacks or of patients above and below age 65. In these predominantly normocholesterolemic patients doxazosin produced small reductions in total serum cholesterol (2–3%), LDL cholesterol (4%), and a similarly small increase in HDL/total cholesterol ratio (4%). The clinical significance of these findings is uncertain. In the same patient population, patients receiving CARDURA gained a mean of 0.6 kg compared to a mean loss of 0.1 kg for placebo patients.

INDICATIONS AND USAGE

CARDURA (doxazosin mesylate) is indicated for the treatment of hypertension. CARDURA may be used alone or in combination with diuretics or beta-adrenergic blocking agents. There is limited experience with CARDURA in combination with angiotensin converting enzyme inhibitors or calcium channel blockers.

CONTRAINDICATIONS

CARDURA is contraindicated in patients with a known sensitivity to quinazolines (e.g. prazosin, terazosin).

WARNINGS

Syncope and "First-dose" Effect:

Doxazosin, like other alpha-adrenergic blocking agents, can cause marked hypotension, especially in the upright position, with syncope and other postural symptoms such as dizziness. Marked orthostatic effects are most common with the first dose but can also occur when there is a dosage increase, or if therapy is interrupted for more than a few days. To decrease the likelihood of excessive hypotension and syncope, it is essential that treatment be initiated with the 1 mg dose. The 2, 4, and 8 mg tablets are not for initial therapy. Dosage should then be adjusted slowly (see DOSAGE AND ADMINISTRATION section) with increases in dose every two weeks. Additional antihypertensive agents should be added with caution.

Patients being titrated with doxazosin should be cautioned to avoid situations where injury could result should syncope occur.

In an early investigational study of the safety and tolerance of increasing daily doses of doxazosin in normotensives beginning at 1 mg/day, only 2 of 6 subjects could tolerate more than 2 mg/day without experiencing symptomatic postural hypotension. In another study of 24 healthy normotensive male subjects receiving initial doses of 2 mg/day of doxazosin, seven (29%) of the subjects experienced symptomatic postural hypotension between 0.5 and 6 hours after the first dose necessitating termination of the study. In this study 2 of the normotensive subjects experienced syncope. Subsequent trials in hypertensive patients always began doxazosin dosing at 1 mg/day resulting in a 4% incidence of postural side effects at 1 mg/day with no cases of syncope.

In multiple dose clinical trials involving over 1500 patients with dose titration every one to two weeks, syncope was reported in 0.7% of patients. None of these events occurred at the starting dose of 1 mg and 1.2% (8/664) occurred at 16 mg/day.

If syncope occurs, the patient should be placed in a recumbent position and treated supportively as necessary.

PRECAUTIONS

General

1. Orthostatic Hypotension:

While syncope is the most severe orthostatic effect of CARDURA, other symptoms of lowered blood pressure, such as dizziness, lightheadedness, or vertigo, can occur, especially at initiation of therapy or at the time of dose increases. These were common in clinical trials, occurring in up to 23% of all patients treated and causing discontinuation of therapy in about 2%.

In placebo controlled titration trials orthostatic effects were minimized by beginning therapy at 1 mg per day and titrating every two weeks to 2.4 or 8 mg per day. There was an increased frequency of orthostatic effects in patients given 8 mg or more, 10%, compared to 5% at 1–4 mg and 3% in the placebo group.

Patients in occupations in which orthostatic hypotension could be dangerous should be treated with particular caution.

Continued on next page

Roerig—Cont.

If hypotension occurs, the patient should be placed in the supine position and, if this measure is inadequate, volume expansion with intravenous fluids or vasopressor therapy may be used. A transient hypotensive response is not a contraindication to further doses of CARDURA.

2. Impaired liver function:
CARDURA should be administered with caution to patients with evidence of impaired hepatic function or to patients receiving drugs known to influence hepatic metabolism (see CLINICAL PHARMACOLOGY). There is no controlled clinical experience with CARDURA in patients with these conditions.

3. Leukopenia/Neutropenia:
Analysis of hematologic data from patients receiving CARDURA in controlled clinical trials showed that the mean WBC (N = 474) and mean neutrophil counts (N = 419) were decreased by 2.4% and 1.0% respectively, compared to placebo, a phenomenon seen with other alpha blocking drugs. A search through a data base of 2400 patients revealed 4 in which drug-related neutropenia could not be ruled out. Two had a single low value on the last day of treatment. Two had stable, non-progressive neutrophil counts in the 1000/mm^3 range over periods of 20 and 40 weeks. In cases where follow-up was available the WBCs and neutrophil counts returned to normal after discontinuation of CARDURA. No patients became symptomatic as a result of the low WBC or neutrophil counts.

Information for Patients:
Patients should be made aware of the possibility of syncopal and orthostatic symptoms, especially at the initation of therapy, and urged to avoid driving or hazardous tasks for 24 hours after the first dose, after a dosage increase, and after interruption of therapy when treatment is resumed. They should be cautioned to avoid situations where injury could result should syncope occur during initiation of doxazosin therapy. They should also be advised of the need to sit or lie down when symptoms of lowered blood pressure occur, although these symptoms are not always orthostatic, and to be careful when rising from a sitting or lying position. If dizziness, lightheadedness, or palpitations are bothersome they should be reported to the physician, so that dose adjustment can be considered. Patients should also be told that drowsiness or somnolence can occur with doxazosin, requiring caution in people who must drive or operate heavy machinery.

Drug Interactions:
Most (98%) of plasma doxazosin is protein bound. *In vitro* data in human plasma indicate that CARDURA has no effect on protein binding of digoxin, warfarin, phenytoin or indomethacin. There is no information on the effect of other highly plasma protein bound drugs on doxazosin binding. CARDURA has been administered without any evidence of an adverse drug interaction to patients receiving thiazide diuretics, beta blocking agents, and nonsteroidal anti-inflammatory drugs.

Drug/Laboratory test interactions:
None known.

Cardiac Toxicity in Animals:
An increased incidence of myocardial necrosis or fibrosis was displayed by Sprague-Dawley rats after 6 months of dietary administration at concentrations calculated to provide 80 mg doxazosin/kg/day and after 12 months of dietary administration at concentrations calculated to provide 40 mg doxazosin/kg/day (150 times the maximum recommended human dose assuming a patient weight of 60 kg). Myocardial fibrosis was observed in both rats and mice treated in the same manner with 40 mg doxazosin/kg/day for 18 months. No cardiotoxicity was observed at lower doses (up to 10 or 20 mg/kg/day, depending on the study) in either species. These lesions were not observed after 12 months of oral dosing in dogs and Wistar rats at maximum doses of 20 mg/kg/day and 100 mg/kg/day, respectively. There is no evidence that similar lesions occur in humans.

Carcinogenesis, Mutagenesis and Impairment of Fertility:
Chronic dietary administration (up to 24 months) of doxazosin mesylate at maximally tolerated concentrations (highest dose 40 mg/kg: about 150 times the maximum recommended human dose of 16 mg/60 kg) revealed no evidence of carcinogenicity in rats. There was also no evidence of carcinogenicity in a similarly conducted study (up to 18 months of dietary administration) in mice. The mouse study, however, was compromised by the failure to use a maximally tolerated dose of doxazosin.
Mutagenicity studies revealed no drug- or metabolite-related effects at either chromosomal or subchromosomal levels.
Studies in rats showed reduced fertility in males treated with doxazosin at oral doses of 20 (but not 5 or 10) mg/kg/day, about 75 times the maximum recommended human dose. This effect was reversible within two weeks of drug withdrawal.

Pregnancy
Teratogenic Effects, Pregnancy Category B. Studies in rabbits and rats at daily oral doses of up to 40 and 20 mg/kg, respectively (150 and 75 times the maximum recommended daily dose of 16 mg, assuming a patient weight of 60 kg), have revealed no evidence of harm to the fetus. The rabbit study, however, was compromised by the failure to use a maximally tolerated dose of doxazosin. There are no adequate and well-controlled studies in pregnant women. Because animal reproduction studies are not always predictive of human response, CARDURA should be used during pregnancy only if clearly needed.
Radioactivity was found to cross the placenta following oral administration of labelled doxazosin to pregnant rats.
Nonteratogenic Effects. In peri-postnatal studies in rats, postnatal development at maternal doses of 40 or 50 mg/kg/day of doxazosin was delayed as evidenced by slower body weight gain and a slightly later appearance of anatomical features and reflexes.

Nursing Mothers
Studies in lactating rats given a single oral dose of 1 mg/kg of [2-^{14}C]-doxazosin indicate that doxazosin accumulates in rat breast milk with a maximum concentration about 20 times greater than the maternal plasma concentration. It is not known whether this drug is excreted in human milk. Because many drugs are excreted in human milk, caution should be exercised when CARDURA is administered to a nursing mother.

Pediatric Use
Safety and effectiveness in children have not been established.

ADVERSE REACTIONS

CARDURA has been administered to approximately 4000 patients, of whom 1679 were included in the clinical development program. In that program, minor adverse effects were frequent, but led to discontinuation of treatment in only 7% of patients. In placebo-controlled studies adverse effect occurred in 49% and 40% of patients in the doxazosin and placebo groups, respectively, and led to discontinuation in 2% of patients in each group. The major reasons for discontinuation were postural effects (2%), edema, malaise/fatigue, and some heart rate disturbance, each about 0.7%.
In controlled clinical trials directly comparing CARDURA to placebo there was no significant difference in the incidence of side effects, except for dizziness (including postural), weight gain, somnolence and fatigue/malaise. Postural effects and edema appeared to be dose related.
The prevalence rates presented below are based on combined data from placebo-controlled studies involving once daily administration of doxazosin at doses ranging from 1–16 mg. Table 1 summarizes those adverse experiences (possibly/probably related) reported for patients in these studies where the prevalence rate in the doxazosin group was at least 0.5% or where the reaction is of particular interest.
Additional adverse reactions have been reported, but these are, in general, not distinguishable from symptoms that might have occurred in the absence of exposure to doxazosin. The following adverse reactions occurred with a frequency of between 0.5% and 1%: syncope, hypoesthesia, increased sweating, agitation, increased weight. The following additional adverse reactions were reported by <0.5% of 3960 patients who received doxazosin in controlled or open, short- or long-term clinical studies, including international studies. *Cardiovascular System:* angina pectoris, myocardial infarction, cerebrovascular accident; *Autonomic Nervous System:* pallor; *Metabolic:* thirst, gout, hypokalemia; *Hematopoietic:* lymphadenopathy, purpura; *Reproductive System:* breast pain; *Skin Disorders:* alopecia, dry skin, eczema; *Central Nervous System:* paresis, tremor, twitching, confusion, migraine, impaired concentration; *Psychiatric:* paroniria, amnesia, emotional lability, abnormal thinking, depersonalization; *Special Senses:* parosmia, earache, taste perversion, photophobia, abnormal lacrimation; *Gastrointestinal System:* increased appetite, anorexia, fecal incontinence, gastroenteritis; *Respiratory System:* bronchospasm, sinusitis, coughing, pharyngitis; *Urinary System:* renal calculus; *General Body System:* hot flushes, back pain, infection, fever/rigors, decreased weight, influenza-like symptoms.
CARDURA has not been associated with any clinically significant changes in routine biochemical tests. No clinically relevant adverse effects were noted on serum potassium, serum glucose, uric acid, blood urea nitrogen, creatinine or liver function tests. CARDURA has been associated with decreases in white blood cell counts (See Precautions).

OVERDOSAGE

No data are available in regard to overdosage in humans. The oral LD_{50} of doxazosin is greater than 1000 mg/kg in mice and rats. The most likely manifestation of overdosage would be hypotension, for which the usual treatment would be intravenous infusion of fluid. As doxazosin is highly protein bound, dialysis would not be indicated.

DOSAGE AND ADMINISTRATION

DOSAGE MUST BE INDIVIDUALIZED. The initial dosage of CARDURA in hypertensive patients is 1 mg given once daily. This starting dose is intended to minimize the frequency of postural hypotension and first dose syncope associated with CARDURA. Postural effects are most likely to occur between 2 and 6 hours after a dose. Therefore blood pressure measurements should be taken during this time period after the first dose and with each increase in dose. Depending on the individual patient's standing blood pressure response (based on measurements taken at 2–6 hours postdose and 24 hours postdose), dosage may then be increased to 2 mg and thereafter if necessary to 4 mg, 8 mg and 16 mg to achieve the desired reduction in blood pressure. **Increases in dose beyond 4 mg increase the likelihood of excessive postural effects including syncope, postural dizziness/vertigo, postural hypotension. At a titrated dose of 16 mg once daily the frequency of postural effects is about 12% compared to 3% for placebo.**

TABLE 1
ADVERSE REACTIONS DURING
PLACEBO CONTROLLED STUDIES

	Doxazosin (N=339)	Placebo (N=336)
Cardiovascular		
Dizziness	19%	9%
Vertigo	2%	1%
Postural Hypotension	0.3%	0%
Edema	4%	3%
Palpitation	2%	3%
Arrhythmia	1%	0%
Hypotension	1%	0%
Tachycardia	0.3%	1%
Peripheral Ischemia	0.3%	0%
Skin Appendages		
Rash	1%	1%
Pruritus	1%	1%
Musculoskeletal		
Arthralgia/Arthritis	1%	0%
Muscle Weakness	1%	0%
Myalgia	1%	0%
Central & Peripheral N.S.		
Headache	14%	16%
Paresthesia	1%	1%
Kinetic Disorders	1%	0%
Ataxia	1%	0%
Hypertonia	1%	0%
Muscle Cramps	1%	0%
Autonomic		
Mouth Dry	2%	2%
Flushing	1%	0%
Special Senses		
Vision Abnormal	2%	1%
Conjunctivitis/Eye Pain	1%	1%
Tinnitus	1%	0.3%
Psychiatric		
Somnolence	5%	1%
Nervousness	2%	2%
Depression	1%	1%
Insomnia	1%	1%
Sexual Dysfunction	2%	1%
Gastrointestinal		
Nausea	3%	4%
Diarrhea	2%	3%
Constipation	1%	1%
Dyspepsia	1%	1%
Flatulence	1%	1%
Abdominal Pain	0%	2%
Vomiting	0%	1%
Respiratory		
Rhinitis	3%	1%
Dyspnea	1%	1%
Epistaxis	1%	0%
Urinary		
Polyuria	2%	0%
Urinary Incontinence	1%	0%
Micturation Frequency	0%	2%
General		
Fatigue/Malaise	12%	6%
Chest Pain	2%	2%
Asthenia	1%	1%
Face Edema	1%	0%
Pain	2%	2%

HOW SUPPLIED

CARDURA (doxazosin mesylate) is available as colored tablets for oral administration. Each tablet contains doxazosin mesylate equivalent to 1 mg (white), 2 mg (yellow), 4 mg (orange) or 8 mg (green) of the active constituent, doxazosin.

CARDURA® TABLETS are available as 1 mg (white), 2 mg (yellow), 4 mg (orange) and 8 mg (green) scored tablets.

Bottles of 100: 1 mg (NDC 0049-2750-66)
2 mg (NDC 0049-2760-66)
4 mg (NDC 0049-2770-66)
8 mg (NDC 0049-2780-66)

Recommended Storage: Store below 86°F(30°C).

CAUTION: Federal law prohibits dispensing without prescription.

Roerig
A Division of Pfizer Inc, N.Y., N.Y. 10017
65-4538-00-0 Issued Nov. 1990
Shown in Product Identification Section, page 427

CEFOBID® ℞

[sĕf'ō-bĭd]
(cefoperazone sodium)
and cefoperazone sodium injection
For Intravenous or Intramuscular Use

DESCRIPTION

CEFOBID (cefoperazone sodium) is a sterile, semisynthetic, broad-spectrum, parenteral cephalosporin antibiotic for intravenous or intramuscular administration. It is the sodium salt of 7-[D(-)-α-(4-ethyl-2,3-dioxo-1-piperazinecarboxamido)- α-(4-hydroxyphenyl)acetamido]-3-[(l-methyl-1H-tetrazol-5-yl)thiomethyl]-3-cephem-4-carboxylic acid. Its chemical formula is $C_{25}H_{26}N_9NaO_8S_2$ with a molecular weight of 667.65. The structural formula is given below:

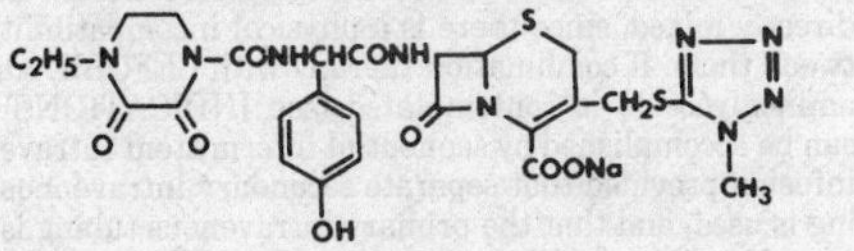

CEFOBID contains 34 mg sodium (1.5 mEq) per gram. CEFOBID is a white powder which is freely soluble in water. The pH of a 25% (w/v) freshly reconstituted solution varies between 4.5–6.5 and the solution ranges from colorless to straw yellow depending on the concentration.

CEFOBID in crystalline form is supplied in vials equivalent to 1 g or 2 g of cefoperazone and in Piggyback Units for intravenous administration equivalent to 1 g or 2 g cefoperazone. CEFOBID is also supplied premixed as a frozen, sterile, nonpyrogenic, iso-osmotic solution equivalent to 1 g or 2 g cefoperazone in plastic containers. After thawing, the solution is intended for intravenous use.

The plastic container is fabricated from specially formulated polyvinyl chloride. Solutions in contact with the plastic container can leach out certain of its chemical components in very small amounts within the expiration period, e.g., di-2-ethylhexyl phthalate (DEHP), up to 5 parts per million. However, the safety of the plastic has been confirmed in tests in animals according to the USP biological tests for plastic containers, as well as by tissue culture toxicity studies.

CLINICAL PHARMACOLOGY

High serum and bile levels of CEFOBID are attained after a single dose of the drug. Table 1 demonstrates the serum concentrations of CEFOBID in normal volunteers following either a single 15-minute constant rate intravenous infusion of 1, 2, 3 or 4 grams of the drug, or a single intramuscular injection of 1 or 2 grams of the drug.

[See table above.]

The mean serum half-life of CEFOBID is approximately 2.0 hours, independent of the route of administration.

In vitro studies with human serum indicate that the degree of CEFOBID reversible protein binding varies with the serum concentration from 93% at 25 mcg/ml of CEFOBID to 90% at 250 mcg/ml and 82% at 500 mcg/ml.

CEFOBID achieves therapeutic concentrations in the following body tissues and fluids:

Tissue or Fluid	Dose	Concentration
Ascitic Fluid	2 g	64 mcg/ml
Cerebrospinal Fluid (in patients with inflamed meninges)	50 mg/kg	1.8 mcg/ml to 8.0 mcg/ml
Urine	2 g	3,286 mcg/ml
Sputum	3 g	6.0 mcg/ml
Endometrium	2 g	74 mcg/g
Myometrium	2 g	54 mcg/g
Palatine Tonsil	1 g	8 mcg/g
Sinus Mucous Membrane	1 g	8 mcg/g
Umbilical Cord Blood	1 g	25 mcg/ml
Amniotic Fluid	1 g	4.8 mcg/ml
Lung	1 g	28 mcg/g
Bone	2 g	40 mcg/g

CEFOBID is excreted mainly in the bile. Maximum bile concentrations are generally obtained between one and three hours following drug administration and exceed concurrent

TABLE 1. Cefoperazone Serum Concentrations

Dose/Route	Mean Serum Concentrations (mcg/ml) 0*	0.5 hr	1 hr	2 hr	4 hr	8 hr	12 hr
1 g IV	153	114	73	38	16	4	0.5
2 g IV	252	153	114	70	32	8	2
3 g IV	340	210	142	89	41	9	2
4 g IV	506	325	251	161	71	19	6
1 g IM	32**	52	65	57	33	7	1
2 g IM	40**	69	93	97	58	14	4

*Hours post-administration, with 0 time being the end of the infusion.
**Values obtained 15 minutes post-injection.

serum concentrations by up to 100 times. Reported biliary concentrations of CEFOBID range from 66 mcg/ml at 30 minutes to as high as 6000 mcg/ml at 3 hours after an intravenous bolus injection of 2 grams.

Following a single intramuscular or intravenous dose, the urinary recovery of CEFOBID over a 12-hour period averages 20–30%. No significant quantity of metabolites has been found in the urine. Urinary concentrations greater than 2200 mcg/ml have been obtained following a 15-minute infusion of a 2 g dose. After an IM injection of 2 g, peak urine concentrations of almost 1000 mcg/ml have been obtained, and therapeutic levels are maintained for 12 hours.

Repeated administration of CEFOBID at 12-hour intervals does not result in accumulation of the drug in normal subjects. Peak serum concentrations, areas under the curve (AUC's), and serum half-lives in patients with severe renal insufficiency are not significantly different from those in normal volunteers. In patients with hepatic dysfunction, the serum half-life is prolonged and urinary excretion is increased. In patients with combined renal and hepatic insufficiencies, CEFOBID may accumulate in the serum.

CEFOBID has been used in pediatrics, but the safety and effectiveness in children have not been established. The half-life of CEFOBID in serum is 6–10 hours in low birth-weight neonates.

Microbiology

CEFOBID is active *in vitro* against a wide range of aerobic and anaerobic, gram-positive and gram-negative pathogens. The bactericidal action of CEFOBID results from the inhibition of bacterial cell wall synthesis. CEFOBID has a high degree of stability in the presence of beta-lactamases produced by most gram-negative pathogens. CEFOBID is usually active against organisms which are resistant to other beta-lactam antibiotics because of beta-lactamase production. CEFOBID is usually active against the following organisms *in vitro* and in clinical infections:

Gram-Positive Aerobes:
Staphylococcus aureus, penicillinase and non-penicillinase-producing strains
Staphylococcus epidermidis
Streptococcus pneumoniae (formerly *Diplococcus pneumoniae*)
Streptococcus pyogenes (Group A beta-hemolytic streptococci)
Streptococcus agalactiae (Group B beta-hemolytic streptococci)
Enterococcus (*Streptococcus faecalis, S. faecium* and *S. durans*)

Gram-Negative Aerobes:
Escherichia coli
Klebsiella species (including *K. pneumoniae*)
Enterobacter species
Citrobacter species
Haemophilus influenzae
Proteus mirabilis
Proteus vulgaris
Morganella morganii (formerly *Proteus morganii*)
Providencia stuartii
Providencia rettgeri (formerly *Proteus rettgeri*)
Serratia marcescens
Pseudomonas aeruginosa
Pseudomonas species
Some strains of *Acinetobacter calcoaceticus*
Neisseria gonorrhoeae

Anaerobic Organisms:
Gram-positive cocci (including *Peptococcus* and *Peptostreptococcus*)
Clostridium species
Bacteroides fragilis
Other *Bacteroides* species

CEFOBID is also active *in vitro* against a wide variety of other pathogens although the clinical significance is unknown. These organisms include: *Salmonella* and *Shigella* species, *Serratia liquefaciens, N. meningitidis, Bordetella pertussis, Yersinia enterocolitica, Clostridium difficile, Fusobacterium* species, *Eubacterium* species and beta-lactamase producing strains of *H. influenzae* and *N. gonorrhoeae.*

Susceptibility Testing:

Diffusion Technique. For the disk diffusion method of susceptibility testing, a 75 mcg CEFOBID diffusion disk should be used. Organisms should be tested with the CEFOBID 75 mcg disk since CEFOBID has been shown *in vitro* to be active against organisms which are found to be resistant to other beta-lactam antibiotics.

Tests should be interpreted by the following criteria:

Zone Diameter	Interpretation
Greater than or equal to 21 mm	Susceptible
16–20 mm	Moderately Susceptible
Less than or equal to 15 mm	Resistant

Quantitative procedures that require measurement of zone diameters give the most precise estimate of susceptibility. One such method which has been recommended for use with the CEFOBID 75 mcg disk is the NCCLS approved standard. (Performance Standards for Antimicrobic Disk Susceptibility Tests. Second Information Supplement Vol. 2 No. 2 pp. 49–69. Publisher—National Committee for Clinical Laboratory Standards, Villanova, Pennsylvania.)

A report of "susceptible" indicates that the infecting organism is likely to respond to CEFOBID therapy and a report of "resistant" indicates that the infecting organism is not likely to respond to therapy. A "moderately susceptible" report suggests that the infecting organism will be susceptible to CEFOBID if a higher than usual dosage is used or if the infection is confined to tissues and fluids (e.g., urine or bile) in which high antibiotic levels are attained.

Dilution Techniques. Broth or agar dilution methods may be used to determine the minimal inhibitory concentration (MIC) of CEFOBID. Serial twofold dilutions of CEFOBID should be prepared in either broth or agar. Broth should be inoculated to contain 5×10^5 organisms/ml and agar "spotted" with 10^4 organisms.

MIC test results should be interpreted in light of serum, tissue, and body fluid concentrations of CEFOBID. Organisms inhibited by CEFOBID at 16 mcg/ml or less are considered susceptible, while organisms with MIC's of 17–63 mcg/ml are moderately susceptible. Organisms inhibited at CEFOBID concentrations of greater than or equal to 64 mcg/ml are considered resistant, although clinical cures have been obtained in some patients infected by such organisms.

INDICATIONS AND USAGE

CEFOBID is indicated for the treatment of the following infections when caused by susceptible organisms:

Respiratory Tract Infections caused by *S. pneumoniae, H. influenzae, S. aureus* (penicillinase and non-penicillinase producing strains), *S. pyogenes** (Group A beta-hemolytic streptococci), *P. aeruginosa, Klebsiella pneumoniae, E. coli, Proteus mirabilis*, and *Enterobacter* species.

Peritonitis and Other Intra-abdominal Infections caused by *E. coli, P. aeruginosa,** and anaerobic gram-negative bacilli (including *Bacteroides fragilis*).

Bacterial Septicemia caused by *S. pneumoniae, S. agalactiae*, S. aureus, Pseudomonas aeruginosa*, E. coli, Klebsiella* spp.,* Klebsiella pneumoniae* , Proteus species* (indole-positive and indole-negative), *Clostridium* spp.* and anaerobic gram-positive cocci.*

Infections of the Skin and Skin Structures caused by *S. aureus* (penicillinase and non-penicillinase producing strains), *S. pyogenes**, and *P. aeruginosa.*

Pelvic Inflammatory Disease, Endometritis, and Other Infections of the Female Genital Tract caused by *N. gonorrhoeae, S. epidermidis*, S. agalactiae, E. coli, Clostridium* spp.,* *Bacteroides* species (including *Bacteroides fragilis*) and anaerobic gram-positive cocci.

Urinary Tract Infections caused by *Escherichia coli* and *Pseudomonas aeruginosa.*

Enterococcal Infections: Although cefoperazone has been shown to be clinically effective in the treatment of infections caused by enterococci in cases of **peritonitis and other intra-abdominal infections, infections of the skin and skin structures, pelvic inflammatory disease, endometritis and other infections of the female genital tract, and urinary tract infection,*** the majority of clinical isolates of enterococci tested

*Efficacy of this organism in this organ system was studied in fewer than 10 infections.

Continued on next page

Roerig—Cont.

are not susceptible to cefoperazone but fall just at or in the intermediate zone of susceptibilty, and are moderately resistant to cefoperazone. However, *in vitro* susceptibility testing may not correlate directly with *in vivo* results. Despite this, cefoperazone therapy has resulted in clinical cures of enterococcal infections, chiefly in polymicrobial infections. Cefoperazone should be used in enterococcal infections with care and at doses that achieve satisfactory serum levels of cefoperazone.

Susceptibility Testing

Before instituting treatment with CEFOBID, appropriate specimens should be obtained for isolation of the causative organism and for determination of its susceptibility to the drug. Treatment may be started before results of susceptibility testing are available.

Combination Therapy

Synergy between CEFOBID and aminoglycosides has been demonstrated with many gram-negative bacilli. However, such enhanced activity of these combinations is not predictable. If such therapy is considered, *in vitro* susceptibility tests should be performed to determine the activity of the drugs in combination, and renal function should be monitored carefully. (See PRECAUTIONS, and DOSAGE AND ADMINISTRATION sections).

CONTRAINDICATIONS

CEFOBID is contraindicated in patients with known allergy to the cephalosporin-class of antibiotics.

WARNINGS

BEFORE THERAPY WITH CEFOBID IS INSTITUTED, CAREFUL INQUIRY SHOULD BE MADE TO DETERMINE WHETHER THE PATIENT HAS HAD PREVIOUS HYPERSENSITIVITY REACTIONS TO CEPHALOSPORINS, PENICILLINS OR OTHER DRUGS. THIS PRODUCT SHOULD BE GIVEN CAUTIOUSLY TO PENICILLIN-SENSITIVE PATIENTS. ANTIBIOTICS SHOULD BE ADMINISTERED WITH CAUTION TO ANY PATIENT WHO HAS DEMONSTRATED SOME FORM OF ALLERGY, PARTICULARLY TO DRUGS. SERIOUS ACUTE HYPERSENSITIVITY REACTIONS MAY REQUIRE THE USE OF SUBCUTANEOUS EPINEPHRINE AND OTHER EMERGENCY MEASURES.

PSEUDOMEMBRANOUS COLITIS HAS BEEN REPORTED WITH THE USE OF CEPHALOSPORINS (AND OTHER BROAD-SPECTRUM ANTIBIOTICS); THEREFORE, IT IS IMPORTANT TO CONSIDER ITS DIAGNOSIS IN PATIENTS WHO DEVELOP DIARRHEA IN ASSOCIATION WITH ANTIBIOTIC USE.

Treatment with broad-spectrum antibiotics alters normal flora of the colon and may permit overgrowth of clostridia. Studies indicate a toxin produced by *Clostridium difficile* is one primary cause of antibiotic-associated colitis. Cholestyramine and colestipol resins have been shown to bind the toxin *in vitro*.

Mild cases of colitis may respond to drug discontinuance alone.

Moderate to severe cases should be managed with fluid, electrolyte, and protein supplementation as indicated.

When the colitis is not relieved by drug discontinuance or when it is severe, oral vancomycin is the treatment of choice for antibiotic-associated pseudomembranous colitis produced by *C. difficile*. Other causes of colitis should also be considered.

PRECAUTIONS

Although transient elevations of the BUN and serum creatinine have been observed, CEFOBID alone does not appear to cause significant nephrotoxicity. However, concomitant administration of aminoglycosides and other cephalosporins has caused nephrotoxicity.

CEFOBID is extensively excreted in bile. The serum half-life of CEFOBID is increased 2–4 fold in patients with hepatic disease and/or biliary obstruction. In general, total daily dosage above 4 g should not be necessary in such patients. If higher dosages are used, serum concentrations should be monitored.

Because renal excretion is not the main route of elimination of CEFOBID (see CLINICAL PHARMACOLOGY), patients with renal failure require no adjustment in dosage when usual doses are administered. When high doses of CEFOBID are used, concentrations of drug in the serum should be monitored periodically. If evidence of accumulation exists, dosage should be decreased accordingly.

The half-life of CEFOBID is reduced slightly during hemodialysis. Thus, dosing should be scheduled to follow a dialysis period. In patients with both hepatic dysfunction and significant renal disease, CEFOBID dosage should not exceed 1–2 g daily without close monitoring of serum concentrations.

As with other antibiotics, vitamin K deficiency has occurred rarely in patients treated with CEFOBID. The mechanism is most probably related to the suppression of gut flora which normally synthesize this vitamin. Those at risk include patients with a poor nutritional status, malabsorption states (e.g., cystic fibrosis), alcoholism, and patients on prolonged hyper-alimentation regimens (administered either intravenously or via a naso-gastric tube). Prothrombin time should be monitored in these patients and exogenous vitamin K administered as indicated.

A disulfiram-like reaction characterized by flushing, sweating, headache, and tachycardia has been reported when alcohol (beer, wine) was ingested within 72 hours after CEFOBID administration. Patients should be cautioned about the ingestion of alcoholic beverages following the administration of CEFOBID. A similar reaction has been reported with other cephalosporins.

Prolonged use of CEFOBID may result in the overgrowth of nonsusceptible organisms. Careful observation of the patient is essential. If superinfection occurs during therapy, appropriate measures should be taken.

CEFOBID should be prescribed with caution in individuals with a history of gastrointestinal disease, particularly colitis.

Drug Laboratory Test Interactions

A false-positive reaction for glucose in the urine may occur with Benedict's or Fehling's solution.

Carcinogenesis, Mutagenesis, Impairment of Fertility

Long term studies in animals have not been performed to evaluate carcinogenic potential. The maximum duration of CEFOBID animal toxicity studies is six months. In none of the *in vivo* or *in vitro* genetic toxicology studies did CEFOBID show any mutagenic potential at either the chromosomal or subchromosomal level. CEFOBID produced no impairment of fertility and had no effects on general reproductive performance or fetal development when administered subcutaneously at daily doses up to 500 to 1000 mg/kg prior to and during mating, and to pregnant female rats during gestation. These doses are 10 to 20 times the estimated usual single clinical dose. CEFOBID had adverse effects on the testes of prepubertal rats at all doses tested. Subcutaneous administration of 1000 mg/kg per day (approximately 16 times the average adult human dose) resulted in reduced testicular weight, arrested spermatogenesis, reduced germinal cell population and vacuolation of Sertoli cell cytoplasm. The severity of lesions was dose dependent in the 100 to 1000 mg/kg per day range; the low dose caused a minor decrease in spermatocytes. This effect has not been observed in adult rats. Histologically the lesions were reversible at all but the highest dosage levels. However, these studies did not evaluate subsequent development of reproductive function in the rats. The relationship of these findings to humans is unknown.

Usage in Pregnancy

Pregnancy Category B: Reproduction studies have been performed in mice, rats, and monkeys at doses up to 10 times the human dose and have revealed no evidence of impaired fertility or harm to the fetus due to CEFOBID. There are, however, no adequate and well controlled studies in pregnant women. Because animal reproduction studies are not always predictive of human response, this drug should be used during pregnancy only if clearly needed.

Usage in Nursing Mothers

Only low concentrations of CEFOBID are excreted in human milk. Although CEFOBID passes poorly into breast milk of nursing mothers, caution should be exercised when CEFOBID is administered to a nursing woman.

Pediatric Use

Safety and effectiveness in children have not been established. For information concerning testicular changes in prepubertal rats (see Carcinogenesis, Mutagenesis, Impairment of Fertility).

ADVERSE REACTIONS

In clinical studies the following adverse effects were observed and were considered to be related to CEFOBID therapy or of uncertain etiology:

Hypersensitivity: As with all cephalosporins, hypersensitivity manifested by skin reactions (1 patient in 45), drug fever (1 in 260), or a change in Coombs' test (1 in 60) has been reported. These reactions are more likely to occur in patients with a history of allergies, particularly to penicillin.

Hematology: As with other beta-lactam antibiotics, reversible neutropenia may occur with prolonged administration. Slight decreases in neutrophil count (1 patient in 50) have been reported. Decreased hemoglobins (1 in 20) or hematocrits (1 in 20) have been reported, which is consistent with published literature on other cephalosporins. Transient eosinophilia has occurred in 1 patient in 10.

Hepatic: Of 1285 patients treated with cefoperazone in clinical trials, one patient with a history of liver disease developed significantly elevated liver function enzymes during CEFOBID therapy. Clinical signs and symptoms of nonspecific hepatitis accompanied these increases. After CEFOBID therapy was discontinued, the patient's enzymes returned to pre-treatment levels and the symptomatology resolved. As with other antibiotics that achieve high bile levels, mild transient elevations of liver function enzymes have been observed in 5–10% of the patients receiving CEFOBID therapy. The relevance of these findings, which were not accompanied by overt signs or symptoms of hepatic dysfunction, has not been established.

Gastrointestinal: Diarrhea or loose stools has been reported in 1 in 30 patients. Most of these experiences have been mild or moderate in severity and self-limiting in nature. In all cases, these symptoms responded to symptomatic therapy or ceased when cefoperazone therapy was stopped. Nausea and vomiting have been reported rarely.

Symptoms of pseudomembranous colitis can appear during or for several weeks subsequent to antibiotic therapy (see WARNINGS).

Renal Function Tests: Transient elevations of the BUN (1 in 16) and serum creatinine (1 in 48) have been noted.

Local Reactions: CEFOBID is well tolerated following intramuscular administration. Occasionally, transient pain (1 in 140) may follow administration by this route. When CEFOBID is administered by intravenous infusion some patients may develop phlebitis (1 in 120) at the infusion site.

DOSAGE AND ADMINISTRATION

The usual adult daily dose of CEFOBID is 2 to 4 grams per day administered in divided doses every 12 hours.

In severe infections or infections caused by less sensitive organisms, the total daily dose and/or frequency may be increased. Patients have been successfully treated with a total daily dosage of 6–12 grams divided into 2, 3 or 4 administrations ranging from 1.5 to 4 grams per dose.

In a pharmacokinetic study, a total daily dose of 16 grams was administered to severely immunocompromised patients by constant infusion without complications. Steady state serum concentrations were approximately 150 mcg/ml in these patients.

When treating infections caused by *Streptococcus pyogenes*, therapy should be continued for at least 10 days.

Solutions of CEFOBID and aminoglycoside should not be directly mixed, since there is a physical incompatibility between them. If combination therapy with CEFOBID and an aminoglycoside is contemplated (see INDICATIONS) this can be accomplished by sequential intermittent intravenous infusion provided that separate secondary intravenous tubing is used, and that the primary intravenous tubing is adequately irrigated with an approved diluent between doses. It is also suggested that CEFOBID be administered prior to the aminoglycoside. *In vitro* testing of the effectiveness of drug combination(s) is recommended.

RECONSTITUTION

The following solutions may be used for the initial reconstitution of CEFOBID sterile powder:

Table 1. Solutions for Initial Reconstitution.

- 5% Dextrose Injection (USP)
- 5% Dextrose and 0.9% Sodium Chloride Injection (USP)
- 5% Dextrose and 0.2% Sodium Chloride Injection (USP)
- 10% Dextrose Injection (USP)
- Bacteriostatic Water for Injection [Benzyl Alcohol or Parabens] (USP)*†
- 0.9% Sodium Chloride Injection (USP)
- Normosol® M and 5% Dextrose Injection
- Normosol® R
- Sterile Water for Injection*

* Not to be used as a vehicle for intravenous infusion

† Preparations containing Benzyl Alcohol should not be used in neonates.

General Reconstitution Procedures

CEFOBID sterile powder for intravenous or intramuscular use may be initially reconstituted with any compatible solution mentioned above in Table 1. Solutions should be allowed to stand after reconstitution to allow any foaming to dissipate to permit visual inspection for complete solubilization. Vigorous and prolonged agitation may be necessary to solubilize CEFOBID in higher concentrations (above 333 mg cefoperazone/ml). The maximum solubility of CEFOBID sterile powder is approximately 475 mg cefoperazone/ml of compatible diluent.

Preparation For Intravenous Use

General. CEFOBID concentrations between 2 mg/ml and 50 mg/ml are recommended for intravenous administration.

Preparation of Vials. Vials of CEFOBID sterile powder may be initially reconstituted with a minimum of 2.8 ml per gram of cefoperazone of any compatible reconstituting solution appropriate for intravenous administration listed above in Table 1. For ease of reconstitution the use of 5 ml of compatible solution per gram of CEFOBID is recommended. The entire quantity of the resulting solution should then be withdrawn for further dilution and administration using any of the following vehicles for intravenous infusion:

Table 2. Vehicles for Intravenous Infusion.

- 5% Dextrose Injection (USP)
- 5% Dextrose and Lactated Ringer's Injection
- 5% Dextrose and 0.9% Sodium Chloride Injection (USP)
- 5% Dextrose and 0.2% Sodium Chloride Injection (USP)
- 10% Dextrose Injection (USP)
- Lactated Ringer's Injection (USP)
- 0.9% Sodium Chloride Injection (USP)
- Normosol® M and 5% Dextrose Injection
- Normosol® R

	Final Cefoperazone Concentration	Step 1 Volume of Sterile Water	Step 2 Volume of 2% Lidocaine	Withdrawable Volume*†
1 g vial	333 mg/ml	2.0 ml	0.6 ml	3 ml
	250 mg/ml	2.8 ml	1.0 ml	4 ml
2 g vial	333 mg/ml	3.8 ml	1.2 ml	6 ml
	250 mg/ml	5.4 ml	1.8 ml	8 ml

When a diluent other than Lidocaine HCl Injection (USP) is used reconstitute as follows:

	Cefoperazone Concentration	Volume of Diluent to be Added	Withdrawable Volume*
1 g vial	333 mg/ml	2.6 ml	3 ml
	250 mg/ml	3.8 ml	4 ml
2 g vial	333 mg/ml	5.0 ml	6 ml
	250 mg/ml	7.2 ml	8 ml

* There is sufficient excess present to allow for withdrawal of the stated volume.
† Final lidocaine concentration will approximate that obtained if a 0.5% Lidocaine Hydrochloride Solution is used as diluent.

Preparation of Piggy Back Units. CEFOBID sterile powder in Piggy Back Units for intravenous use may be prepared by adding between 20 ml and 40 ml of any appropriate diluent listed in Table 2 per gram of cefoperazone. If 5% Dextrose and Lactated Ringer's Injection or Lactated Ringer's Injection (USP) is the chosen vehicle for administration the CEFOBID sterile powder should initially be reconstituted using 2.8–5 ml per gram of any compatible reconstituting solution listed in Table 1 prior to the final dilution.
The resulting intravenous solution should be administered in one of the following manners:
Intermittent Infusion: Solutions of CEFOBID should be administered over a 15–30 minute time period.
Continuous Infusion: CEFOBID can be used for continuous infusion after dilution to a final concentration of between 2 and 25 mg cefoperazone per ml.

Preparation For Intramuscular Injection
Any suitable solution listed above may be used to prepare CEFOBID sterile powder for intramuscular injection. When concentrations of 250 mg/ml or more are to be administered, a lidocaine solution should be used. These solutions should be prepared using a combination of Sterile Water for Injection and 2% Lidocaine Hydrochloride Injection (USP) that approximates a 0.5% Lidocaine Hydrochloride Solution. A two-step dilution process as follows is recommended: First, add the required amount of Sterile Water for Injection and agitate until CEFOBID powder is completely dissolved. Second, add the required amount of 2% lidocaine and mix. [See table above.]

DIRECTIONS FOR USE OF CEFOBID (cefoperazone sodium) INJECTION IN PLASTIC CONTAINERS
CEFOBID supplied premixed as a frozen, sterile, iso-osmotic solution in plastic containers is to be administered either as continuous or intermittent infusion.

Thaw container at room temperature. After thawing, check for minute leaks by squeezing bag firmly. If leaks are found, discard solution as sterility may be impaired. Additives should not be introduced into this solution. Do not use if the solution is cloudy or precipitated or if the seal is not intact. After thawing, the solution is stable for 10 days if stored under refrigeration (5°C) and for 48 hours at room temperature. DO NOT REFREEZE. Use sterile equipment.
CAUTION: Do not use plastic container in series connections. Such use could result in air embolism due to residual air being drawn from the primary container before administration of the fluid from the secondary container is complete.
Preparation for administration
1. Suspend container from eyelet support.
2. Remove plastic protector from outlet port at bottom of container.
3. Attach administration set. Refer to complete directions accompanying set.
Storage and Stability: CEFOBID sterile powder is to be stored at or below 25°C (77°F) and protected from light prior to reconstitution. After reconstitution, protection from light is not necessary.
The following parenteral diluents and approximate concentrations of CEFOBID provide stable solutions under the following conditions for the indicated time periods. (After the indicated time periods, unused portions of solutions should be discarded.) [See table below.]

HOW SUPPLIED
CEFOBID sterile powder is available in vials containing cefoperazone sodium equivalent to 1 gram cefoperazone × 10 (NDC 0049-1201-83), and 2 gram cefoperazone × 10 (NDC 0049-1202-83) for intramuscular and intravenous administration.
CEFOBID sterile powder is available in Piggyback Units containing cefoperazone sodium equivalent to 1 gram cefo-

Controlled Room Temperature (15°–25°C/59°–77°F) 24 Hours	Approximate Concentrations
Bacteriostatic Water for Injection [Benzyl Alcohol or Parabens] (USP)	300 mg/ml
5% Dextrose Injection (USP)	2 mg to 50 mg/ml
5% Dextrose and Lactated Ringer's Injection	2 mg to 50 mg/ml
5% Dextrose and 0.9% Sodium Chloride Injection (USP)	2 mg to 50 mg/ml
5% Dextrose and 0.2% Sodium Chloride Injection (USP)	2 mg to 50 mg/ml
10% Dextrose Injection (USP)	2 mg to 50 mg/ml
Lactated Ringer's Injection (USP)	2 mg/ml
0.5% Lidocaine Hydrochloride Injection (USP)	300 mg/ml
0.9% Sodium Chloride Injection (USP)	2 mg to 300 mg/ml
Normosol® M and 5% Dextrose Injection	2 mg to 50 mg/ml
Normosol® R	2 mg to 50 mg/ml
Sterile Water for Injection	300 mg/ml

Reconstituted CEFOBID solutions may be stored in glass or plastic syringes, or in glass or flexible plastic parenteral solution containers.

Refrigerator Temperature (2°–8°C/36°–46°F) 5 Days	Approximate Concentrations
Bacteriostatic Water for Injection [Benzyl Alcohol or Parabens] (USP)	300 mg/ml
5% Dextrose Injection (USP)	2 mg to 50 mg/ml
5% Dextrose and 0.9% Sodium Chloride Injection (USP)	2 mg to 50 mg/ml
5% Dextrose and 0.2% Sodium Chloride Injection (USP)	2 mg to 50 mg/ml
Lactated Ringer's Injection (USP)	2 mg/ml
0.5% Lidocaine Hydrochloride Injection (USP)	300 mg/ml
0.9% Sodium Chloride Injection (USP)	2 mg to 300 mg/ml
Normosol® M and 5% Dextrose Injection	2 mg to 50 mg/ml
Normosol® R	2 mg to 50 mg/ml
Sterile Water for Injection	300 mg/ml

Reconstituted CEFOBID solutions may be stored in glass or plastic syringes, or in glass or flexible plastic parenteral solution containers.

Freezer Temperature (−20° to −10°C/−4° to 14°F) 3 Weeks	Approximate Concentrations
5% Dextrose Injection (USP)	50 mg/ml
5% Dextrose and 0.9% Sodium Chloride Injection (USP)	2 mg/ml
5% Dextrose and 0.2% Sodium Chloride Injection (USP)	2 mg/ml

5 Weeks	
0.9% Sodium Chloride Injection (USP)	300 mg/ml
Sterile Water for Injection	300 mg/ml

Reconstituted CEFOBID solutions may be stored in plastic syringes, or in flexible plastic parenteral solution containers. Frozen samples should be thawed at room temperature before use. After thawing, unused portions should be discarded. Do not refreeze.

perazone × 10 (NDC 0049-1211-83), and 2 gram cefoperazone × 10 (NDC 0049-1212-83) for intravenous administration. CEFOBID (cefoperazone sodium) injection is supplied premixed as a frozen, sterile, nonpyrogenic, iso-osmotic solution in plastic containers. Each 50 mL unit contains cefoperazone sodium equivalent to 1 g cefoperazone with approximately 2.3 g dextrose hydrous USP added (NDC 0049-1216-18) or 2 g cefoperazone with approximately 1.8 g dextrose hydrous USP added (NDC 0049-1215-18). The solution is iso-osmotic (approximately 300 mOsmol/L), and solution pH may have been adjusted with sodium hydroxide and/or hydrochloric acid. Do not store above −20°C.
CEFOBID supplied as a frozen, sterile, nonpyrogenic, iso-osmotic solution in 50 ml plastic containers is manufactured for Roerig Division of Pfizer Pharmaceuticals by Baxter Healthcare Corporation, Deerfield, IL 60015.

70-4169-00-4

CEFOBID®   ℞
[sĕf'ō-bĭd]
Sterile Cefoperazone Sodium, USP
PHARMACY BULK PACKAGE
NOT FOR DIRECT INFUSION

DESCRIPTION
CEFOBID (cefoperazone sodium) is a sterile, semisynthetic, broad-spectrum, parenteral cephalosporin antibiotic for intravenous or intramuscular administration. It is the sodium salt of 7-[(R)-2-(4-ethyl-2,3-dioxo-1-piperazine-carboxamido)-2-(p-hydroxyphenyl)acetamido-3-[[(l-methyl-H-tetrazol-5-yl)thio]methyl]-8-oxo-5-thia-1-azabicyclo[4.2.0] oct-2-ene-2-carboxylate. Its chemical formula is $C_{25}H_{26}N_9NaO_8S_2$ with a molecular weight of 667.65. The structural formula is given below:

CEFOBID contains 34 mg sodium (1.5 mEq) per gram. CEFOBID is a white powder which is freely soluble in water. The pH of a 25% (w/v) freshly reconstituted solution varies between 4.5–6.5 and the solution ranges from colorless to straw yellow depending on the concentration. CEFOBID in crystalline form is supplied in vials equivalent to 1 g or 2 g of cefoperazone and in Piggyback Units for intravenous administration equivalent to 1 g or 2 g cefoperazone. CEFOBID is also supplied premixed as a frozen, sterile, nonpyrogenic, iso-osmotic solution equivalent to 1 g or 2 g cefoperazone in plastic containers. After thawing, the solution is intended for intravenous use.
The plastic container is fabricated from specially formulated polyvinyl chloride. Solutions in contact with the plastic container can leach out certain of its chemical components in very small amounts within the expiration period, e.g., di 2-ethylhexyl phthalate (DEHP), up to 5 parts per million. However, the safety of the plastic has been confirmed in tests in animals according to the USP biological tests for plastic containers, as well as by tissue culture toxicity studies.
A pharmacy bulk package is a container of a sterile preparation for parenteral use that contains many single doses. This Pharmacy Bulk Package is for use in a pharmacy admixture service; it provides many single doses of cefoperazone for addition to suitable parenteral fluids in the preparation of admixtures for intravenous infusion. (See DOSAGE AND ADMINISTRATION, and DIRECTIONS FOR PROPER USE OF PHARMACY BULK PACKAGE).

CLINICAL PHARMACOLOGY
High serum and bile levels of CEFOBID are attained after a single dose of the drug. Table 1 demonstrates the serum concentrations of CEFOBID in normal volunteers following either a single 15-minute constant rate intravenous infusion of 1, 2, 3 or 4 grams of the drug, or a single intramuscular injection of 1 or 2 grams of the drug. [See next page.]
The mean serum half-life of CEFOBID is approximately 2.0 hours, independent of the route of administration.
In vitro studies with human serum indicate that the degree of CEFOBID reversible protein binding varies with the serum concentration from 93% at 25 mcg/ml of CEFOBID to 90% at 250 mcg/ml and 82% at 500 mcg/ml.
CEFOBID achieves therapeutic concentrations in the following body tissues and fluids: [See second table next page.]
CEFOBID is excreted mainly in the bile. Maximum bile concentrations are generally obtained between one and three hours following drug administration and exceed concurrent serum concentrations by up to 100 times. Reported biliary concentrations of CEFOBID range from 66 mcg/ml at 30

Continued on next page

Roerig—Cont.

TABLE 1. Cefoperazone Serum Concentrations

Dose/Route	Mean Serum Concentrations (mcg/ml)						
	0*	0.5 hr	1 hr	2 hr	4 hr	8 hr	12 hr
1 g IV	153	114	73	38	16	4	0.5
2 g IV	252	153	114	70	32	8	2
3 g IV	340	210	142	89	41	9	2
4 g IV	506	325	251	161	71	19	6
1 g IM	32**	52	65	57	33	7	1
2 g IM	40**	69	93	97	58	14	4

*Hours post-administration, with 0 time being the end of the infusion.
**Values obtained 15 minutes post-injection.

Tissue or Fluid	Dose	Concentration
Ascitic Fluid	2 g	64 mcg/ml
Cerebrospinal Fluid (in patients with inflamed meninges)	50 mg/kg	1.8 mcg/ml to 8.0 mcg/ml
Urine	2 g	3,286 mcg/ml
Sputum	3 g	6.0 mcg/ml
Endometrium	2 g	74 mcg/g
Myometrium	2 g	54 mcg/g
Palatine Tonsil	1 g	8 mcg/g
Sinus Mucous Membrane	1 g	8 mcg/g
Umbilical Cord Blood	1 g	25 mcg/ml
Amniotic Fluid	1 g	4.8 mcg/ml
Lung	1 g	28 mcg/g
Bone	2 g	40 mcg/g

minutes to as high as 6000 mcg/ml at 3 hours after an intravenous bolus injection of 2 grams.

Following a single intramuscular or intravenous dose, the urinary recovery of CEFOBID over a 12-hour period averages 20–30%. No significant quantity of metabolites has been found in the urine. Urinary concentrations greater than 2200 mcg/ml have been obtained following a 15-minute infusion of a 2 g dose. After an IM injection of 2 g, peak urine concentrations of almost 1000 mcg/ml have been obtained, and therapeutic levels are maintained for 12 hours.

Repeated administration of CEFOBID at 12-hour intervals does not result in accumulation of the drug in normal subjects. Peak serum concentrations, areas under the curve (AUC's), and serum half-lives in patients with severe renal insufficiency are not significantly different from those in normal volunteers. In patients with hepatic dysfunction, the serum half-life is prolonged and urinary excretion is increased. In patients with combined renal and hepatic insufficiencies, CEFOBID may accumulate in the serum.

CEFOBID has been used in pediatrics, but the safety and effectiveness in children have not been established. The half-life of CEFOBID in serum is 6–10 hours in low birth-weight neonates.

Microbiology

CEFOBID is active *in vitro* against a wide range of aerobic and anaerobic, gram-positive and gram-negative pathogens. The bactericidal action of CEFOBID results from the inhibition of bacterial cell wall synthesis. CEFOBID has a high degree of stability in the presence of beta-lactamases produced by most gram-negative pathogens. CEFOBID is usually active against organisms which are resistant to other beta-lactam antibiotics because of beta-lactamase production. CEFOBID is usually active against the following organisms *in vitro* and in clinical infections:

Gram-Positive Aerobes:

Staphylococcus aureus, penicillinase and non-penicillinase-producing strains
Staphylococcus epidermidis
Streptococcus pneumoniae (formerly *Diplococcus pneumoniae*)
Streptococcus pyogenes (Group A beta-hemolytic streptococci)
Streptococcus agalactiae (Group B beta-hemolytic streptococci)
Enterococcus (*Streptococcus faecalis*, *S. faecium* and *S. durans*)

Gram-Negative Aerobes:

Escherichia coli
Klebsiella species (including *K. pneumoniae*)
Enterobacter species
Citrobacter species
Haemophilus influenzae
Proteus mirabilis
Proteus vulgaris
Morganella morganii (formerly *Proteus morganii*)
Providencia stuartii
Providencia rettgeri (formerly *Proteus rettgeri*)
Serratia marcescens
Pseudomonas aeruginosa
Pseudomonas species
Some strains of *Acinetobacter calcoaceticus*
Neisseria gonorrhoeae

Anaerobic Organisms:

Gram-positive cocci (including *Peptococcus* and *Peptostreptococcus*)
Clostridium species
Bacteroides fragilis
Other *Bacteroides* species

CEFOBID is also active *in vitro* against a wide variety of other pathogens although the clinical significance is unknown. These organisms include: *Salmonella* and *Shigella* species, *Serratia liquefaciens*, *N. meningitidis*, *Bordetella pertussis*, *Yersinia enterocolitica*, *Clostridium difficile*, *Fusobacterium* species, *Eubacterium* species and beta-lactamase producing strains of *H. influenzae* and *N. gonorrhoeae.*

SUSCEPTIBILITY TESTING

Diffusion Technique. For the disk diffusion method of susceptibility testing, a 75 mcg CEFOBID diffusion disk should be used. Organisms should be tested with the CEFOBID 75 mcg disk since CEFOBID has been shown *in vitro* to be active against organisms which are found to be resistant to other beta-lactam antibiotics.

Tests should be interpreted by the following criteria:

Zone Diameter	Interpretation
Greater than or equal to 21 mm	Susceptible
16–20 mm	Moderately Susceptible
Less than or equal to 15 mm	Resistant

Quantitative procedures that require measurement of zone diameters give the most precise estimate of susceptibility. One such method which has been recommended for use with the CEFOBID 75 mcg disk is the NCCLS approved standard. (Performance Standards for Antimicrobic Disk Susceptibility Tests. Second Information Supplement Vol. 2 No. 2 pp. 49–69. Publisher—National Committee for Clinical Laboratory Standards, Villanova, Pennsylvania.)

A report of "susceptible" indicates that the infecting organism is likely to respond to CEFOBID therapy and a report of "resistant" indicates that the infecting organism is not likely to respond to therapy. A "moderately susceptible" report suggests that the infecting organism will be susceptible to CEFOBID if a higher than usual dosage is used or if the infection is confined to tissues and fluids (e.g., urine or bile) in which high antibiotic levels are attained.

Dilution Techniques. Broth or agar dilution methods may be used to determine the minimal inhibitory concentration (MIC) of CEFOBID. Serial twofold dilutions of CEFOBID should be prepared in either broth or agar. Broth should be inoculated to contain 5×10^5 organisms/ml and agar "spotted" with 10^4 organisms.

MIC test results should be interpreted in light of serum, tissue, and body fluid concentrations of CEFOBID. Organisms inhibited by CEFOBID at 16 mcg/ml or less are considered susceptible, while organisms with MIC's of 17–63 mcg/ml are moderately susceptible. Organisms inhibited at CEFOBID concentrations of greater than or equal to 64 mcg/ml are considered resistant, although clinical cures have been obtained in some patients infected by such organisms.

INDICATIONS AND USAGE

CEFOBID is indicated for the treatment of the following infections when caused by susceptible organisms:

Respiratory Tract Infections caused by *S. pneumoniae*, *H. influenzae*, *S. aureus* (penicillinase and non-penicillinase producing strains), *S. pyogenes** (Group A beta-hemolytic streptococci), *P. aeruginosa*, *Klebsiella pneumoniae*, *E. coli*, *Proteus mirabilis*, and *Enterobacter* species.

Peritonitis and Other Intra-abdominal Infections caused by *E. coli*, *P. aeruginosa*,* anaerobic and gram-negative bacilli (including *Bacteroides fragilis*).

Bacterial Septicemia caused by *S. pneumoniae*, *S. agalactiae**, *S. aureus*, *Pseudomonas aeruginosa**, *E. coli*, *Klebsiella* spp.,* *Klebsiella pneumoniae**, *Proteus* species* (indole-positive and indole-negative), *Clostridium* spp.* and anaerobic gram-positive cocci.*

Infections of the Skin and Skin Structures caused by *S. aureus* (penicillinase and non-penicillinase producing strains), *S. pyogenes**, and *P. aeruginosa.*

Pelvic Inflammatory Disease, Endometritis, and Other Infections of the Female Genital Tract caused by *N. gonorrhoeae*, *S. epidermidis**, *S. agalactiae*, *E. coli*, *Clostridium* spp.,* *Bacteroides* species (including *Bacteroides fragilis*) and anaerobic gram-positive cocci.

Urinary Tract Infections caused by *Escherichia coli*, and *Pseudomonas aeruginosa.*

Enterococcal Infections: Although cefoperazone has been shown to be clinically effective in the treatment of infections caused by enterococci in cases of **peritonitis and other intra-abdominal infections, infections of the skin and skin structures, pelvic inflammatory disease, endometritis and other infections of the female genital tract, and urinary tract infection,*** the majority of clinical isolates of enterococci tested are not susceptible to cefoperazone but fall just at or in the intermediate zone of susceptibilty, and are moderately resistant to cefoperazone. However, *in vitro* susceptibility testing may not correlate directly with *in vivo* results. Despite this, cefoperazone therapy has resulted in clinical cures of enterococcal infections, chiefly in polymicrobial infections. Cefoperazone should be used in enterococcal infections with care and at doses that achieve satisfactory serum levels of cefoperazone.

Susceptibility Testing

Before instituting treatment with CEFOBID, appropriate specimens should be obtained for isolation of the causative organism and for determination of its susceptibility to the drug. Treatment may be started before results of susceptibility testing are available.

Combination Therapy

Synergy between CEFOBID and aminoglycosides has been demonstrated with many gram-negative bacilli. However, such enhanced activity of these combinations is not predictable. If such therapy is considered, *in vitro* susceptibility tests should be performed to determine the activity of the drugs in combination, and renal function should be monitored carefully. (See PRECAUTIONS, and DOSAGE AND ADMINISTRATION sections).

CONTRAINDICATIONS

CEFOBID is contraindicated in patients with known allergy to the cephalosporin-class of antibiotics.

WARNINGS

BEFORE THERAPY WITH CEFOBID IS INSTITUTED, CAREFUL INQUIRY SHOULD BE MADE TO DETERMINE WHETHER THE PATIENT HAS HAD PREVIOUS HYPERSENSITIVITY REACTIONS TO CEPHALOSPORINS, PENICILLINS OR OTHER DRUGS. THIS PRODUCT SHOULD BE GIVEN CAUTIOUSLY TO PENICILLIN-SENSITIVE PATIENTS. ANTIBIOTICS SHOULD BE ADMINISTERED WITH CAUTION TO ANY PATIENT WHO HAS DEMONSTRATED SOME FORM OF ALLERGY, PARTICULARLY TO DRUGS. SERIOUS ACUTE HYPERSENSITIVITY REACTIONS MAY REQUIRE THE USE OF SUBCUTANEOUS EPINEPHRINE AND OTHER EMERGENCY MEASURES.

PSEUDOMEMBRANOUS COLITIS HAS BEEN REPORTED WITH THE USE OF CEPHALOSPORINS (AND OTHER BROAD-SPECTRUM ANTIBIOTICS); THEREFORE, IT IS IMPORTANT TO CONSIDER ITS DIAGNOSIS IN PATIENTS WHO DEVELOP DIARRHEA IN ASSOCIATION WITH ANTIBIOTIC USE.

Treatment with broad-spectrum antibiotics alters normal flora of the colon and may permit overgrowth of clostridia. Studies indicate a toxin produced by *Clostridium difficile* is one primary cause of antibiotic-associated colitis. Cholestyramine and colestipol resins have been shown to bind the toxin *in vitro.*

Mild cases of colitis may respond to drug discontinuance alone.

Moderate to severe cases should be managed with fluid, electrolyte, and protein supplementation as indicated.

When the colitis is not relieved by drug discontinuance or when it is severe, oral vancomycin is the treatment of choice for antibiotic-associated pseudomembranous colitis produced by *C. difficile.* Other causes of colitis should also be considered.

PRECAUTIONS

Although transient elevations of the BUN and serum creatinine have been observed, CEFOBID alone does not appear to cause significant nephrotoxicity. However, concomitant administration of aminoglycosides and other cephalosporins has caused nephrotoxicity.

CEFOBID is extensively excreted in bile. The serum half-life of CEFOBID is increased 2–4 fold in patients with hepatic disease and/or biliary obstruction. In general, total daily dosage above 4 g should not be necessary in such patients. If higher dosages are used, serum concentrations should be monitored.

Because renal excretion is not the main route of elimination of CEFOBID (see CLINICAL PHARMACOLOGY), patients with renal failure require no adjustment in dosage when usual doses are administered. When high doses of CEFOBID

*Efficacy of this organism in this organ system was studied in fewer than 10 infections.

are used, concentrations of drug in the serum should be monitored periodically. If evidence of accumulation exists, dosage should be decreased accordingly.

The half-life of CEFOBID is reduced slightly during hemodialysis. Thus, dosing should be scheduled to follow a dialysis period. In patients with both hepatic dysfunction and significant renal disease, CEFOBID dosage should not exceed 1–2 g daily without close monitoring of serum concentrations.

As with other antibiotics, vitamin K deficiency has occurred rarely in patients treated with CEFOBID. The mechanism is most probably related to the suppression of gut flora which normally synthesize this vitamin. Those at risk include patients with a poor nutritional status, malabsorption states (e.g., cystic fibrosis), alcoholism, and patients on prolonged hyper-alimentation regimens (administered either intravenously or via a naso-gastric tube). Prothrombin time should be monitored in these patients and exogenous vitamin K administered as indicated.

A disulfiram-like reaction characterized by flushing, sweating, headache, and tachycardia has been reported when alcohol (beer, wine) was ingested within 72 hours after CEFOBID administration. Patients should be cautioned about the ingestion of alcoholic beverages following the administration of CEFOBID. A similar reaction has been reported with other cephalosporins.

Prolonged use of CEFOBID may result in the overgrowth of nonsusceptible organisms. Careful observation of the patient is essential. If superinfection occurs during therapy, appropriate measures should be taken.

CEFOBID should be prescribed with caution in individuals with a history of gastrointestinal disease, particularly colitis.

Drug Laboratory Test Interactions

A false-positive reaction for glucose in the urine may occur with Benedict's or Fehling's solution.

Carcinogenesis, Mutagenesis, Impairment of Fertility

Long term studies in animals have not been performed to evaluate carcinogenic potential. The maximum duration of CEFOBID animal toxicity studies is six months. In none of the *in vivo* or *in vitro* genetic toxicology studies did CEFOBID show any mutagenic potential at either the chromosomal or subchromosomal level. CEFOBID produced no impairment of fertility and had no effects on general reproductive performance or fetal development when administered subcutaneously at daily doses up to 500 to 1000 mg/kg prior to and during mating, and to pregnant female rats during gestation. These doses are 10 to 20 times the estimated usual single clinical dose. CEFOBID had adverse effects on the testes of prepubertal rats at all doses tested. Subcutaneous administration of 1000 mg/kg per day (approximately 16 times the average adult human dose) resulted in reduced testicular weight, arrested spermatogenesis, reduced germinal cell population and vacuolation of Sertoli cell cytoplasm. The severity of lesions was dose dependent in the 100 to 1000 mg/kg per day range; the low dose caused a minor decrease in spermatocytes. This effect has not been observed in adult rats. Histologically the lesions were reversible at all but the highest dosage levels. However, these studies did not evaluate subsequent development of reproductive function in the rats. The relationship of these findings to humans is unknown.

Usage in Pregnancy

Pregnancy Category B: Reproduction studies have been performed in mice, rats, and monkeys at doses up to 10 times the human dose and have revealed no evidence of impaired fertility or harm to the fetus due to CEFOBID. There are, however, no adequate and well controlled studies in pregnant women. Because animal reproduction studies are not always predictive of human response, this drug should be used during pregnancy only if clearly needed.

Usage in Nursing Mothers

Only low concentrations of CEFOBID are excreted in human milk. Although CEFOBID passes poorly into breast milk of nursing mothers, caution should be exercised when CEFOBID is administered to a nursing woman.

Pediatric Use

Safety and effectiveness in children have not been established. For information concerning testicular changes in prepubertal rats (see Carcinogenesis, Mutagenesis, Impairment of Fertility).

ADVERSE REACTIONS

In clinical studies the following adverse effects were observed and were considered to be related to CEFOBID therapy or of uncertain etiology:

Hypersensitivity: As with all cephalosporins, hypersensitivity manifested by skin reactions (1 patient in 45), drug fever (1 in 260), or a change in Coombs' test (1 in 60) has been reported. These reactions are more likely to occur in patients with a history of allergies, particularly to penicillin.

Hematology: As with other beta-lactam antibiotics, reversible neutropenia may occur with prolonged administration. Slight decreases in neutrophil count (1 patient in 50) have been reported. Decreased hemoglobins (1 in 20) or hematocrits (1 in 20) have been reported, which is consistent with published literature on other cephalosporins. Transient eosinophilia has occurred in 1 patient in 10.

Controlled Room Temperature (15°–25°C/59°–77°F) 24 Hours	Approximate Concentrations
Bacteriostatic Water for Injection [Benzyl Alcohol or Parabens] (USP)	300 mg/ml
5% Dextrose Injection (USP)	2 mg to 50 mg/ml
5% Dextrose and Lactated Ringer's Injection	2 mg to 50 mg/ml
5% Dextrose and 0.9% Sodium Chloride Injection (USP)	2 mg to 50 mg/ml
5% Dextrose and 0.2% Sodium Chloride Injection (USP)	2 mg to 50 mg/ml
10% Dextrose Injection (USP)	2 mg to 50 mg/ml
Lactated Ringer's Injection (USP)	2 mg/ml
0.5% Lidocaine Hydrochloride Injection (USP)	300 mg/ml
0.9% Sodium Chloride Injection (USP)	2 mg to 300 mg/ml
Normosol® M and 5% Dextrose Injection	2 mg to 50 mg/ml
Normosol® R	2 mg to 50 mg/ml
Sterile Water for Injection	100 mg to 300 mg/ml

Reconstituted CEFOBID solutions may be stored in glass or plastic syringes, or in glass or flexible plastic parenteral solution containers.

Refrigerator Temperature (2°–8°C/36°–46°F) 5 Days	Approximate Concentrations
Bacteriostatic Water for Injection [Benzyl Alcohol or Parabens] (USP)	300 mg/ml
5% Dextrose Injection (USP)	2 mg to 50 mg/ml
5% Dextrose and 0.9% Sodium Chloride Injection (USP)	2 mg to 50 mg/ml
5% Dextrose and 0.2% Sodium Chloride Injection (USP)	2 mg to 50 mg/ml
Lactated Ringer's Injection (USP)	2 mg/ml
0.5% Lidocaine Hydrochloride Injection (USP)	300 mg/ml
0.9% Sodium Chloride Injection (USP)	2 mg to 300 mg/ml
Normosol® M and 5% Dextrose Injection	2 mg to 50 mg/ml
Normosol® R	2 mg to 50 mg/ml
Sterile Water for Injection	100 mg to 300 mg/ml

Reconstituted CEFOBID solutions may be stored in glass or plastic syringes, or in glass or flexible plastic parenteral solution containers.

Freezer Temperature (−20° to −10°C/−4° to 14°F)	Approximate Concentrations
3 Weeks	
5% Dextrose Injection (USP)	50 mg/ml
5% Dextrose and 0.9% Sodium Chloride Injection (USP)	2 mg/ml
5% Dextrose and 0.2% Sodium Chloride Injection (USP)	2 mg/ml
5 Weeks	
0.9% Sodium Chloride Injection (USP)	300 mg/ml
Sterile Water for Injection	300 mg/ml

Reconstituted CEFOBID solutions may be stored in plastic syringes, or in flexible plastic parenteral solution containers. Frozen samples should be thawed at room temperature before use. After thawing, unused portions should be discarded. Do not refreeze.

Hepatic: Of 1285 patients treated with cefoperazone in clinical trials, one patient with a history of liver disease developed significantly elevated liver function enzymes during CEFOBID therapy. Clinical signs and symptoms of nonspecific hepatitis accompanied these increases. After CEFOBID therapy was discontinued, the patient's enzymes returned to pre-treatment levels and the symptomatology resolved. As with other antibiotics that achieve high bile levels, mild transient elevations of liver function enzymes have been observed in 5–10% of the patients receiving CEFOBID therapy. The relevance of these findings, which were not accompanied by overt signs or symptoms of hepatic dysfunction, has not been established.

Gastrointestinal: Diarrhea or loose stools has been reported in 1 in 30 patients. Most of these experiences have been mild or moderate in severity and self-limiting in nature. In all cases, these symptoms responded to symptomatic therapy or ceased when cefoperazone therapy was stopped. Nausea and vomiting have been reported rarely.

Symptoms of pseudomembranous colitis can appear during or for several weeks subsequent to antibiotic therapy (see WARNINGS).

Renal Function Tests: Transient elevations of the BUN (1 in 16) and serum creatinine (1 in 48) have been noted.

Local Reactions: CEFOBID is well tolerated following intramuscular administration. Occasionally, transient pain (1 in 140) may follow administration by this route. When CEFOBID is administered by intravenous infusion some patients may develop phlebitis (1 in 120) at the infusion site.

DOSAGE AND ADMINISTRATION

Sterile cefoperazone sodium can be administered by IM or IV injection (following dilution). However, the intent of this pharmacy bulk package is for the preparation of solutions for IV infusion only.

The usual adult daily dose of CEFOBID is 2 to 4 grams per day administered in equally divided doses every 12 hours.

In severe infections or infections caused by less sensitive organisms, the total daily dose and/or frequency may be increased. Patients have been successfully treated with a total daily dosage of 6–12 grams divided into 2, 3 or 4 administrations ranging from 1.5 to 4 grams per dose.

In a pharmacokinetic study, a total daily dose of 16 grams was administered to severely immunocompromised patients by constant infusion without complications. Steady state serum concentrations were approximately 150 mcg/ml in these patients.

When treating infections caused by *Streptococcus pyogenes*, therapy should be continued for at least 10 days.

Solutions of CEFOBID and aminoglycoside should not be directly mixed, since there is a physical incompatibility between them. If combination therapy with CEFOBID and an aminoglycoside is contemplated (see INDICATIONS) this can be accomplished by sequential intermittent intravenous infusion provided that separate secondary intravenous tubing is used, and that the primary intravenous tubing is adequately irrigated with an approved diluent between doses. It is also suggested that CEFOBID be administered prior to the aminoglycoside. *In vitro* testing of the effectiveness of drug combination(s) is recommended.

RECONSTITUTION

The following solutions may be used for the initial reconstitution of CEFOBID sterile powder:

Table 1. Solutions for Initial Reconstitution

5% Dextrose Injection (USP)
5% Dextrose and 0.9% Sodium Chloride Injection (USP)
5% Dextrose and 0.2% Sodium Chloride Injection (USP)
10% Dextrose Injection (USP)
Bacteriostatic Water for Injection [Benzyl Alcohol or Parabens] (USP)*†
0.9% Sodium Chloride Injection (USP)
Normosol® M and 5% Dextrose Injection
Normosol® R
Sterile Water for Injection*

* Not to be used as a vehicle for intravenous infusion

† Preparations containing Benzyl Alcohol should not be used in neonates.

General Reconstitution Procedures

CEFOBID sterile powder for intravenous or intramuscular use may be initially reconstituted with any compatible solution mentioned above in Table 1. Solutions should be allowed to stand after reconstitution to allow any foaming to dissipate to permit visual inspection for complete solubilization. Vigorous and prolonged agitation may be necessary to solubilize CEFOBID in higher concentrations (above 333 mg cefoperazone/ml). The maximum solubility of CEFOBID sterile powder is approximately 475 mg cefoperazone/ml of compatible diluent.

Preparation For Intravenous Use

General. CEFOBID concentrations between 2 mg/ml and 50 mg/ml are recommended for intravenous administration.

Table 2. Vehicles for Intravenous Infusion

5% Dextrose Injection (USP)
5% Dextrose and Lactated Ringer's Injection
5% Dextrose and 0.9% Sodium Chloride Injection (USP)
5% Dextrose and 0.2% Sodium Chloride Injection(USP)
10% Dextrose Injection (USP)
Lactated Ringer's Injection (USP)
0.9% Sodium Chloride Injection (USP)
Normosol® M and 5% Dextrose Injection
Normosol® R

DIRECTIONS FOR PROPER USE OF PHARMACY BULK PACKAGE

The 10 gram vial should be reconstituted with 95 ml of sterile water for injection in two separate aliquots in a suitable

Continued on next page

Roerig—Cont.

work area such as a laminar flow hood. Add 45 ml of solution, shake to dissolve and add 50 ml, shake for final solution. The resulting solution will contain 100 mg/ml of cefoperazone. This closure may be penetrated only one time after reconstitution, if needed, using a suitable sterile transfer device or dispensing set which allows measured dispensing of the contents.
Discard unused solution within 24 hours of initial entry.

Reconstituted Bulk Solutions Should Not Be Used For Direct Infusion.

Although after reconstitution of the Pharmacy Bulk Package, no significant loss of potency occurs for 24 hours at room temperature and for 5 days if refrigerated, transfer individual dose to appropriate intravenous infusion solutions as soon as possible following reconstitution of the bulk package. Discard unused portions of solution held longer than these recommended periods at room temperature or under refrigeration. The stability of the solution which has been transferred into a container varies according to diluent and concentration. (See STORAGE AND STABILITY.)
The 10 gram vials may be further diluted with the parenteral diluents listed under **Table 2. Vehicles for Intravenous Infusion.** The parenteral diluents and approximate concentrations of CEFOBID that provide stable solutions are presented under STORAGE AND STABILITY.
Parenteral drug products should be inspected visually for particulate matter and discoloration prior to administration, whenever solution and container permit.

DIRECTIONS FOR USE OF CEFOBID (cefoperazone sodium) INJECTION IN PLASTIC CONTAINERS

CEFOBID supplied premixed as a frozen, sterile, iso-osmotic solution in plastic containers is to be administered either as continuous or intermittent infusion.
Thaw container at room temperature. After thawing, check for minute leaks by squeezing bag firmly. If leaks are found, discard solution as sterility may be impaired. Additives should not be introduced into this solution. Do not use if the solution is cloudy or precipitated or if the seal is not intact. After thawing, the solution is stable for 10 days if stored under refrigeration (5°C) and for 48 hours at room temperature. DO NOT REFREEZE. Use sterile equipment.
CAUTION: Do not use plastic container in series connections. Such use could result in air embolism due to residual air being drawn from the primary container before administration of the fluid from the secondary container is complete.

Preparation for Administration

1. Suspend container from eyelet support.
2. Remove plastic protector from outlet port at bottom of container.
3. Attach administration set. Refer to complete directions accompanying set.

STORAGE AND STABILITY

CEFOBID sterile powder is to be stored at or below 25°C (77°F) and protected from light prior to reconstitution. After reconstitution, protection from light is not necessary.
The following parenteral diluents and approximate concentrations of CEFOBID provide stable solutions under the following conditions for the indicated time periods. (After the indicated time periods, unused portions of solutions should be discarded.) [See table on preceding page.]

HOW SUPPLIED

CEFOBID sterile powder is available in Pharmacy Bulk Package containing cefoperazone sodium equivalent to 10 g cefoperazone × 1 (NDC 0049-1219-28).

OTHER SIZE PACKAGES AVAILABLE

CEFOBID sterile powder is available in vials containing cefoperazone sodium equivalent to 1 g cefoperazone × 10 (NDC 0049-1201-83) and 2 g cefoperazone × 10 (NDC 0049-1202-83) for intramuscular and intravenous administration.
CEFOBID sterile powder is available in Piggyback Units containing cefoperazone sodium equivalent to 1 gram cefoperazone × 10 (NDC 0049-1211-83), and 2 g cefoperazone × 10 (NDC 0049-1212-83).
CEFOBID (cefoperazone sodium) injection is supplied premixed as a frozen, sterile, nonpyrogenic, iso-osmotic solution in plastic containers. Each 50 mL unit contains cefoperazone sodium equivalent to 1 g cefoperazone with approximately 2.3 g dextrose hydrous USP added (NDC 0049-1216-18) or 2 g cefoperazone with approximately 1.8 g dextrose hydrous USP added (NDC 0049-1215-18). The solution is iso-osmotic (approximately 300 mOsmol/L), and solution pH may have been adjusted with sodium hydroxide and/or hydrochloric acid. Do not store above −20°C.
CEFOBID supplied as a frozen, sterile, nonpyrogenic, iso-osmotic solution in 50 ml plastic containers is manufactured for Roerig Division of Pfizer Pharmaceuticals by Baxter Healthcare Corporation, Deerfield, IL 60015.

70-4482-00-2 Issued April 1990

DIFLUCAN® ℞
(fluconazole)
Tablets
Injections (for intravenous infusion only)

DESCRIPTION

DIFLUCAN (fluconazole), the first of a new class of synthetic broad-spectrum bis-triazole antifungal agents, is available as tablets for oral administration and as a sterile solution for intravenous use in glass and in Viaflex® Plus plastic containers.
Fluconazole is designated chemically as 2,4-difluoro-α,α¹-bis(1H-1,2,4-triazol-1-ylmethyl)benzyl alcohol with an empirical formula of $C_{13}H_{12}F_2N_6O$ and molecular weight 306.3. The structural formula is:

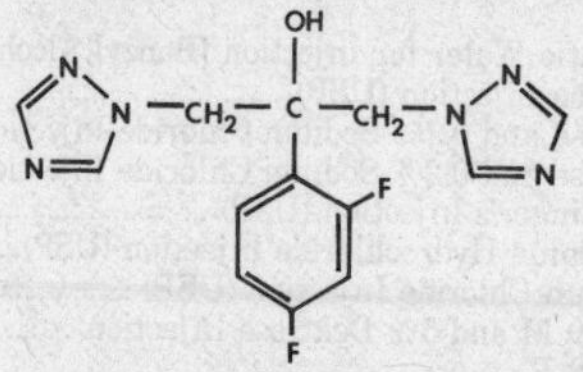

Fluconazole is a white crystalline solid which is slightly soluble in water and saline.
DIFLUCAN tablets contain 50, 100, or 200 mg of fluconazole and the following inactive ingredients: microcrystalline cellulose, dibasic calcium phosphate anhydrous, povidone, croscarmellose sodium, FD&C Red No. 40 aluminum lake dye, and magnesium stearate.
DIFLUCAN for injection is an iso-osmotic, sterile, nonpyrogenic solution of fluconazole in a sodium chloride diluent. Each mL contains 2 mg of fluconazole and 9 mg of sodium chloride. The pH ranges from 4.0 to 8.0. Injection volumes of 100 mL and 200 mL are packaged in glass and in Viaflex® Plus plastic containers.
The Viaflex® Plus plastic container is fabricated from a specially formulated polyvinyl chloride (PL 146® Plastic) (Viaflex and PL 146 are registered trademarks of Baxter International Inc.). The amount of water that can permeate from inside the container into the overwrap is insufficient to affect the solution significantly. Solutions in contact with the plastic container can leach out certain of its chemical components in very small amounts within the expiration period, e.g. di-2-ethylhexylphthalate (DEHP), up to 5 parts per million. However, the suitability of the plastic has been confirmed in tests in animals according to USP biological tests for plastic containers as well as by tissue culture toxicity studies.

CLINICAL PHARMACOLOGY

Mode of Action

Fluconazole is a highly selective inhibitor of fungal cytochrome P-450 sterol C-14 alpha-demethylation. Mammalian cell demethylation is much less sensitive to fluconazole inhibition. The subsequent loss of normal sterols correlates with the accumulation of 14 alpha-methyl sterols in fungi and may be responsible for the fungistatic activity of fluconazole.

Pharmacokinetics and Metabolism

The pharmacokinetic properties of fluconazole are similar following administration by the intravenous or oral routes. In normal volunteers, the bioavailability of orally administered fluconazole is over 90% compared with intravenous administration.
Peak plasma concentrations (Cmax) in fasted normal volunteers occur between 1 and 2 hours with a terminal plasma elimination half-life of approximately 30 hours (range 20–50 hours) after oral administration.
In fasted normal volunteers, administration of a single oral 400 mg dose of DIFLUCAN (fluconazole) leads to a mean Cmax of 6.72 μg/mL (range: 4.12 to 8.08 μg/mL) and after single oral doses of 50–400 mg, fluconazole plasma concentrations and AUC (area under the plasma concentration-time curve) are dose proportional.
Steady-state concentrations are reached within 5–10 days following oral doses of 50–400 mg given once daily. Administration of a loading dose (on Day 1) of twice the usual daily dose results in plasma concentrations close to steady state by the second day. The apparent volume of distribution of fluconazole approximates that of total body water. Plasma protein binding is low (11–12%). Following either single- or multiple-oral doses for up to 14 days, fluconazole penetrates into all body fluids studied (see table below). In normal volunteers, saliva concentrations of fluconazole were equal to or slightly greater than plasma concentrations regardless of dose, route, or duration of dosing. In patients with bronchiectasis, sputum concentrations of fluconazole following a single 150 mg oral dose were equal to plasma concentrations at both 4 and 24 hours post dose. In patients with fungal meningitis, fluconazole concentrations in the CSF are approximately 80% of the corresponding plasma concentrations.

Tissue or Fluid	Ratio of Fluconazole Tissue (Fluid)/Plasma Concentration*
Cerebrospinal fluid†	.5–.9
Saliva	1
Sputum	1
Blister fluid	1
Urine	10
Normal skin	10
Nails	1
Blister skin	2

* Relative to concurrent concentrations in plasma in subjects with normal renal function.
† Independent of degree of meningeal inflammation.

In normal volunteers, fluconazole is cleared primarily by renal excretion, with approximately 80% of the administered dose appearing in the urine as unchanged drug. About 11% of the dose is excreted in the urine as metabolites.
The pharmacokinetics of fluconazole are markedly affected by reduction in renal function. There is an inverse relationship between the elimination half-life and creatinine clearance. The dose of DIFLUCAN may need to be reduced in patients with impaired renal function (see Dosage and Administration). A 3-hour hemodialysis session decreases plasma concentrations by approximately 50%.
In normal volunteers, DIFLUCAN administration (doses ranging from 200 mg to 400 mg once daily for up to 14 days) was associated with small and inconsistent effects on testosterone concentrations, endogenous corticosteroid concentrations, and the ACTH-stimulated cortisol response.

Drug Interaction Studies

Oral Contraceptives: Single and multiple 50 mg oral doses of DIFLUCAN were administered to healthy women taking oral contraceptives. The AUC for ethinyl estradiol was decreased by 16%, but no changes were observed in levonorgestrel pharmacokinetics.
Gastrointestinal Drugs: In fasted normal volunteers, absorption of orally administered DIFLUCAN does not appear to be affected by agents that increase gastric pH. Single dose administration of DIFLUCAN (100 mg) with cimetidine (400 mg) resulted in a 13% reduction in AUC (range 4% to 32%) and 21% reduction in Cmax (range 20% to 40%) of fluconazole. Administration of MAALOX® (20 mL) immediately prior to a single dose of DIFLUCAN (100 mg) had no effect on the absorption or elimination of fluconazole.
Hydrochlorothiazide: Concomitant oral administration of 100 mg DIFLUCAN and 50 mg hydrochlorothiazide for 10 days in normal volunteers resulted in an increase of 41% in Cmax and an increase of 43% in AUC of fluconazole, compared to DIFLUCAN given alone. Overall, the plasma concentrations of fluconazole were approximately 1–2 μg/mL higher with concomitant diuretic. These changes are attributable to a mean net reduction of approximately 20% in the renal clearance of fluconazole.
Rifampin: Administration of a single oral 200 mg dose of DIFLUCAN after chronic rifampin administration resulted in a 25% decrease in AUC and a 20% shorter half-life of fluconazole in normal volunteers. (See Precautions.)
Warfarin: A single dose of warfarin (15 mg) given to normal volunteers, following 14 days of orally administered DIFLUCAN (200 mg) resulted in a 12% increase in the prothrombin time response (area under the prothrombin time-time curve). One of 13 subjects experienced a 2-fold increase in his prothrombin time response. (See Precautions.)
Oral Hypoglycemic Agents: The effects of fluconazole on the pharmacokinetics of the sulfonylurea oral hypoglycemic agents tolbutamide, glipizide and glyburide were examined in three placebo-controlled crossover studies in normal volunteers. All subjects received the sulfonylurea alone and following treatment with 100 mg of DIFLUCAN as a single daily oral dose for 7 days. DIFLUCAN administration resulted in significant increases in Cmax and AUC of the sulfonylurea. Several subjects in these three studies experienced symptoms consistent with hypoglycemia. In the glyburide study, several volunteers required oral glucose treatment. (See Precautions.)
Phenytoin: Concomitant administration of oral DIFLUCAN (200 mg) at steady state with phenytoin at steady state resulted in an average increase of 75% of phenytoin AUC values in normal volunteers. (See Precautions.)
Cyclosporine: Stable bone marrow transplant patients receiving twice daily doses of cyclosporine, who were administered DIFLUCAN (100 mg) as a single oral dose for 14 days, demonstrated slight increases in cyclosporine Cmax, Cmin (minimum plasma concentration) and AUC values which did not achieve statistical significance. There have been several literature reports associating concomitant administration of high doses of DIFLUCAN with an increase in cyclosporine plasma concentrations in renal transplant patients with or without impaired renal function. (See Precautions.)

Zidovudine and Pentamidine: Formal interaction studies have not been completed for DIFLUCAN and concomitant zidovudine and aerosolized pentamidine isethionate.

Microbiology

Fluconazole exhibits *in vitro* activity against *Cryptococcus neoformans* and *Candida spp.* Fungistatic activity has also been demonstrated in normal and immunocompromised animal models for systemic and intracranial fungal infections due to *Cryptococcus neoformans* and for systemic infections due to *Candida albicans.* Development of resistance to fluconazole has not been studied.

In common with other azole antifungal agents, most fungi show a higher apparent sensitivity to fluconazole *in vivo* than *in vitro.* Fluconazole administered orally and/or intravenously was active in a variety of animal models of fungal infection using standard laboratory strains of fungi. Activity has been demonstrated against fungal infections caused by *Aspergillus flavus* and *Aspergillus fumigatus* in normal mice. Fluconazole has also been shown to be active in animal models of endemic mycoses, including one model of *Blastomyces dermatitidis* pulmonary infections in normal mice; one model of *Coccidioides immitis* intracranial infections in normal mice; and several models of *Histoplasma capsulatum* pulmonary infection in normal and immunosuppressed mice. The clinical significance of results obtained in these studies is unknown.

Concurrent administration of fluconazole and amphotericin B in infected normal and immunosuppressed mice showed the following results: a small additive antifungal effect in systemic infection with *C. albicans,* no interaction in intracranial infection with *Cr. neoformans,* and antagonism of the two drugs in systemic infection with *Asp. fumigatus.* The clinical significance of results obtained in these studies is unknown.

INDICATIONS AND USAGE

DIFLUCAN (fluconazole) is indicated for the treatment of:
1. Oropharyngeal and esophageal candidiasis. DIFLUCAN is also effective for the treatment of serious systemic candidal infections, including urinary tract infection, peritonitis, and pneumonia.
2. Cryptococcal meningitis.

Specimens for fungal culture and other relevant laboratory studies (serology, histopathology) should be obtained prior to therapy to isolate and identify causative organisms. Therapy may be instituted before the results of the cultures and other laboratory studies are known; however, once these results become available, anti-infective therapy should be adjusted accordingly.

CONTRAINDICATIONS

DIFLUCAN (fluconazole) is contraindicated in patients who have shown hypersensitivity to fluconazole or to any of its excipients. There is no information regarding cross hypersensitivity between fluconazole and other azole antifungal agents. Caution should be used in prescribing DIFLUCAN to patients with hypersensitivity to other azoles.

WARNINGS

In rare cases, anaphylaxis has been reported.

Patients who develop abnormal liver function tests during DIFLUCAN therapy should be monitored for the development of more severe hepatic injury. Although serious hepatic reactions have been rare and the causal association with DIFLUCAN uncertain, if clinical signs and symptoms consistent with liver disease develop that may be attributable to fluconazole, DIFLUCAN should be discontinued. (See Adverse Reactions.)

Immunocompromised patients who develop rashes during treatment with DIFLUCAN should be monitored closely and the drug discontinued if lesions progress. (See Adverse Reactions.)

PRECAUTIONS

Drug Interactions (See Clinical Pharmacology)

DIFLUCAN (fluconazole) increased the prothrombin time after warfarin administration. Careful monitoring of prothrombin time in patients receiving DIFLUCAN and coumarin-type anticoagulants is recommended.

DIFLUCAN increased the plasma concentrations of phenytoin. Careful monitoring of phenytoin concentrations in patients receiving DIFLUCAN and phenytoin is recommended.

DIFLUCAN has been infrequently associated with an increase in cyclosporine concentrations in renal transplant patients with or without impaired renal function. Careful monitoring of cyclosporine concentrations in patients receiving DIFLUCAN and cyclosporine is recommended.

DIFLUCAN increased the plasma concentrations and reduced the metabolism of tolbutamide, glyburide and glipizide. When DIFLUCAN is used concomitantly with these or other sulfonylurea oral hypoglycemic agents, blood glucose concentrations should be carefully monitored, and the dose of the sulfonylurea should be adjusted as necessary.

Rifampin enhances the metabolism of concurrently administered DIFLUCAN. Depending on clinical circumstances, consideration should be given to increasing the dose of DIFLUCAN when it is administered with rifampin.

Physicians should be aware that drug-drug interaction studies with other medications have not been conducted, but such interactions may occur.

Carcinogenesis, Mutagenesis and Impairment of Fertility

Fluconazole showed no evidence of carcinogenic potential in mice and rats treated orally for 24 months at doses of 2.5, 5 or 10 mg/kg/day (approximately 2–7× the recommended human dose). Male rats treated with 5 and 10 mg/kg/day had an increased incidence of hepatocellular adenomas.

Fluconazole, with or without metabolic activation, was negative in tests for mutagenicity in 4 strains of *S. typhimurium,* and in the mouse lymphoma L5178Y system. Cytogenetic studies *in vivo* (murine bone marrow cells, following oral administration of fluconazole) and *in vitro* (human lymphocytes exposed to fluconazole at 1000 μg/mL) showed no evidence of chromosomal mutations.

Fluconazole did not affect the fertility of male or female rats treated orally with daily doses of 5, 10 or 20 mg/kg or with parenteral doses of 5, 25 or 75 mg/kg, although the onset of parturition was slightly delayed at 20 mg/kg p.o. In an intravenous perinatal study in rats at 5, 20 and 40 mg/kg, dystocia and prolongation of parturition were observed in a few dams at 20 mg/kg (approximately 5–15× the recommended human dose) and 40 mg/kg, but not at 5 mg/kg. The disturbances in parturition were reflected by a slight increase in the number of still-born pups and decrease of neonatal survival at these dose levels. The effects on parturition in rats are consistent with the species specific estrogen-lowering property produced by high doses of fluconazole. Such a hormone change has not been observed in women treated with fluconazole. (See Clinical Pharmacology.)

Pregnancy

Teratogenic Effects. Pregnancy Category C: Fluconazole was administered orally to pregnant rabbits during organogenesis in two studies, at 5, 10 and 20 mg/kg and at 5, 25, and 75 mg/kg respectively. Maternal weight gain was impaired at all dose levels, and abortions occurred at 75 mg/kg (approximately 20–60× the recommended human dose); no adverse fetal effects were detected. In several studies in which pregnant rats were treated orally with fluconazole during organogenesis, maternal weight gain was impaired and placental weights were increased at 25 mg/kg. There were no fetal effects at 5 or 10 mg/kg; increases in fetal anatomical variants (supernumerary ribs, renal pelvis dilation) and delays in ossification were observed at 25 and 50 mg/kg and higher doses. At doses ranging from 80 mg/kg (approximately 20–60× the recommended human dose) to 320 mg/kg, embryolethality in rats was increased and fetal abnormalities included wavy ribs, cleft palate and abnormal cranio-facial ossification. These effects are consistent with the inhibition of estrogen synthesis in rats and may be a result of known effects of lowered estrogen on pregnancy, organogenesis and parturition.

There are no adequate and well controlled studies in pregnant women. DIFLUCAN should be used in pregnancy only if the potential benefit justifies the possible risk to the fetus.

Nursing Mothers

Fluconazole is secreted in human milk at concentrations similar to plasma. Therefore, the use of DIFLUCAN in nursing mothers is not recommended.

Pediatric Use

Efficacy of DIFLUCAN has not been established in children. A small number of patients from age 3 to 13 years have been treated safely with DIFLUCAN using doses of 3–6 mg/kg daily.

ADVERSE REACTIONS

Sixteen percent of over 4000 patients treated with DIFLUCAN (fluconazole) in clinical trials of 7 days or more experienced adverse events. Treatment was discontinued in 1.5% of patients due to adverse clinical events and in 1.3% of patients due to laboratory test abnormalities.

In combined clinical trials and foreign marketing experience prior to U.S. marketing, patients with serious underlying disease (predominantly AIDS or malignancy) rarely have developed serious hepatic reactions or exfoliative skin disorders during treatment with DIFLUCAN (See Warnings). Two of these hepatic reactions and one exfoliative skin disorder (Stevens-Johnson syndrome) were associated with a fatal outcome. Because most of these patients were receiving multiple concomitant medications, including many known to be hepatotoxic or associated with exfoliative skin disorders, the causal association of these reactions with DIFLUCAN therapy is uncertain.

Clinical adverse events were reported more frequently in HIV infected patients (21%) than in non-HIV infected patients (13%); however, the patterns in HIV infected and non-HIV infected patients were similar. The proportions of patients discontinuing therapy due to clinical adverse events were similar in the two groups (1.5%).

The following treatment-related clinical adverse events occurred at an incidence of 1% or greater in 4048 patients receiving DIFLUCAN for 7 or more days in clinical trials: nausea 3.7%, headache 1.9%, skin rash 1.8%, vomiting 1.7%, abdominal pain 1.7%, and diarrhea 1.5%.

In two comparative trials evaluating the efficacy of DIFLUCAN for the suppression of relapse of cryptococcal meningitis, a statistically significant increase was observed in median AST (SGOT) levels from a baseline value of 30 IU/L to 41 IU/L in one trial and 34 IU/L to 66 IU/L in the other. The overall rate of serum transaminase elevations of more than 8 times the upper limit of normal was approximately 1% in fluconazole-treated patients in clinical trials. These elevations occurred in patients with severe underlying disease, predominantly AIDS or malignancies, most of whom were receiving multiple concomitant medications, including many known to be hepatotoxic. The incidence of abnormally elevated serum transaminases was greater in patients taking DIFLUCAN concomitantly with one or more of the following medications: rifampin, phenytoin, isoniazid, valproic acid, or oral sulfonylurea hypoglycemic agents.

In rare cases, anaphylaxis has been reported.

The following adverse experiences occurred under conditions (e.g. open trials, marketing experience) where a causal association is uncertain.

Central Nervous System: seizures

Hematopoietic and Lymphatic: leukopenia, thrombocytopenia.

DOSAGE AND ADMINISTRATION

SINCE ORAL ABSORPTION IS RAPID AND ALMOST COMPLETE, THE DAILY DOSE OF DIFLUCAN (FLUCONAZOLE) IS THE SAME FOR ORAL AND INTRAVENOUS ADMINISTRATION.

The daily dose of DIFLUCAN should be based on the infecting organism and the patient's response to therapy. Treatment should be continued until clinical parameters or laboratory tests indicate that active fungal infection has subsided. An inadequate period of treatment may lead to recurrence of active infection. Patients with AIDS and cryptococcal meningitis or recurrent oropharyngeal candidiasis usually require maintenance therapy to prevent relapse.

The recommended dosage of DIFLUCAN for oropharyngeal candidiasis is 200 mg on the first day, followed by 100 mg once daily. Clinical evidence of oropharyngeal candidiasis generally resolves within several days, but treatment should be continued for at least 2 weeks to decrease the likelihood of relapse.

The recommended dosage of DIFLUCAN for esophageal candidiasis is 200 mg on the first day, followed by 100 mg once daily. Doses up to 400 mg/day may be used, based on medical judgment of the patient's response to therapy. Patients with esophageal candidiasis should be treated for a minimum of three weeks and for at least two weeks following resolution of symptoms.

For systemic candidiasis, the recommended dosage of DIFLUCAN is 400 mg on the first day, followed by 200 mg once daily. These patients should be treated for a minimum of 4 weeks and for at least 2 weeks following resolution of symptoms.

For cryptococcal meningitis, the recommended dosage of DIFLUCAN is 400 mg on the first day, followed by 200 mg once daily. A dosage of 400 mg once daily may be used, based on medical judgment of the patient's response to therapy. The recommended duration of treatment for initial therapy of cryptococcal meningitis is 10–12 weeks after the cerebrospinal fluid becomes culture negative. The recommended dosage of DIFLUCAN for suppression of relapse of cryptococcal meningitis in patients with AIDS is 200 mg once daily.

Dosage In Patients With Impaired Renal Function

Fluconazole is cleared primarily by renal excretion as unchanged drug. In patients with impaired renal function, an initial loading dose of 50 to 400 mg should be given. After the loading dose, the daily dose (according to indication) should be based on the following table:

DIFLUCAN

Creatinine Clearance (mL/min)	Percent of Recommended Dose
>50	100%
21–50	50%
11–20	25%
Patients receiving regular hemodialysis	one recommended dose after each dialysis

These are suggested dose adjustments based on pharmacokinetics following administration of single doses. Further adjustment may be needed depending upon clinical condition.

When serum creatinine is the only measure of renal function available, the following formula (based on sex, weight, and age of the patient) should be used to estimate the creatinine clearance.

Males:	$\dfrac{\text{Weight (kg)} \times (140 - \text{age})}{72 \times \text{serum creatinine (mg/100mL)}}$
Females:	$0.85 \times \text{above value}$

DIFLUCAN may be administered either orally or by intravenous infusion. DIFLUCAN injection has been used safely for up to fourteen days of intravenous therapy. The intravenous

Continued on next page

Roerig—Cont.

infusion of DIFLUCAN should be administered at a maximum rate of approximately 200 mg/hour, given as a continuous infusion.
DIFLUCAN injections in glass and Viaflex® Plus plastic containers are intended only for intravenous administration using sterile equipment.
Parenteral drug products should be inspected visually for particulate matter and discoloration prior to administration whenever solution and container permit.
Do not use if the solution is cloudy or precipitated or if the seal is not intact.

DIRECTIONS FOR IV USE OF DIFLUCAN In Viaflex® Plus Plastic Containers

Do not remove unit from overwrap until ready for use. The overwrap is a moisture barrier. The inner bag maintains the sterility of the product.
WARNING: Do not use plastic containers in series connections. Such use could result in air embolism due to residual air being drawn from the primary container before administration of the fluid from the secondary container is completed.

To Open

Tear overwrap down side at slit and remove solution container. Some opacity of the plastic due to moisture absorption during the sterilization process may be observed. This is normal and does not affect the solution quality or safety. The opacity will diminish gradually. After removing overwrap, check for minute leaks by squeezing inner bag firmly. If leaks are found discard solution as sterility may be impaired. DO NOT ADD SUPPLEMENTARY MEDICATION.

Preparation for Administration

1. Suspend container from eyelet support.
2. Remove plastic protector from outlet port at bottom of container.
3. Attach administration set. Refer to complete directions accompanying set.

OVERDOSAGE

There has been one reported case of overdosage with DIFLUCAN. A 42-year old patient infected with human immunodeficiency virus developed hallucinations and exhibited paranoid behavior after reportedly ingesting 8,200 mg of DIFLUCAN. The patient was admitted to the hospital, and his condition resolved within 48 hours.
In the event of overdose, symptomatic treatment (with supportive measures and gastric lavage if clinically indicated) should be instituted.
Fluconazole is largely excreted in urine. A three hour hemodialysis session decreases plasma levels by approximately 50%.
In mice and rats receiving very high doses of fluconazole, clinical effects, in both species, included decreased motility and respiration, ptosis, lacrimation, salivation, urinary incontinence, loss of righting reflex and cyanosis; death was sometimes preceded by clonic convulsions.

HOW SUPPLIED

DIFLUCAN Tablets: Pink trapezoidal tablets containing 50, 100 or 200 mg of fluconazole are packaged in bottles or unit dose blisters.
DIFLUCAN Tablets are supplied as follows:
DIFLUCAN 50 mg Tablets: Engraved with DIFLUCAN and 50 on the front and ROERIG on the back.
NDC 0049-3410-30 Bottles of 30
DIFLUCAN 100 mg Tablets: Engraved with DIFLUCAN and 100 on the front and ROERIG on the back.
NDC 0049-3420-30 Bottles of 30
NDC 0049-3420-41 Unit dose package of 100
DIFLUCAN 200 mg Tablets: Engraved with DIFLUCAN and 200 on the front and ROERIG on the back.
NDC 0049-3430-30 Bottles of 30
NDC 0049-3430-41 Unit dose package of 100
Storage: Store tablets below 86°F (30°C).
DIFLUCAN Injections: DIFLUCAN injections for intravenous infusion administration are formulated as sterile iso-osmotic solutions containing 2 mg/mL of fluconazole. They are supplied in glass bottles or in Viaflex® Plus plastic containers containing volumes of 100 mL or 200 mL affording doses of 200 mg and 400 mg of fluconazole, respectively.
DIFLUCAN Injections in Glass Bottles:
NDC 0049-3371-26 Fluconazole 200 mg/100 mL×6
NDC 0049-3372-26 Fluconazole 400 mg/200 mL×6
Storage: Store between 86°F (30°C) and 41°F (5°C). Protect from freezing.
DIFLUCAN Injections in Viaflex® Plus Plastic Containers:
NDC 0049-3435-26 Fluconazole 200 mg/100 mL×6
NDC 0049-3436-26 Fluconazole 400 mg/200 mL×6
Storage: Store between 77°F (25°C) and 41°F (5°C). Brief exposure up to 104°F (40°C) does not adversely affect the product. Protect from freezing.
70-4526-00-5

Shown in Product Identification Section, page 427

EMETE-CON® ℞

[ă-mĕt ′ă-kŏn ″]
(benzquinamide hydrochloride)
For Intramuscular and Intravenous Use

DESCRIPTION

Benzquinamide is a non-amine-depleting benzoquinolizine derivative, chemically unrelated to the phenothiazines and to other antiemetics.
Chemically, Emete-con (benzquinamide hydrochloride) is N,N-diethyl-1,3,4,6,7,11b-hexahydro-2-hydroxy-9,10-dimethoxy- 2H-benzo-[a]quinolizine-3-carboxamide acetate hydrochloride. The empirical formula is $C_{22}H_{32}N_2O_5 \cdot HCl$ and the molecular weight is 441.

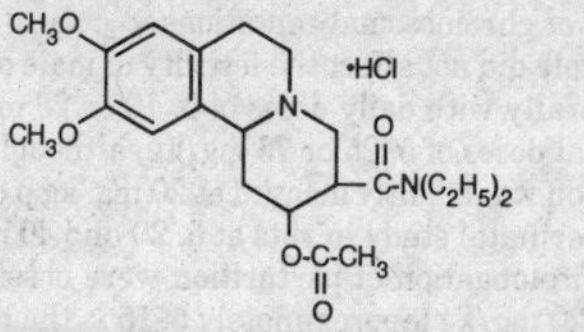

Emete-con for injection contains benzquinamide hydrochloride equivalent to 50 mg/vial of benzquinamide. When reconstituted with 2.2 ml of proper diluent, each vial yields 2 ml of a solution containing benzquinamide hydrochloride equivalent to 25 mg/ml of benzquinamide. When reconstituted this product maintains its potency for 14 days at room temperature.

ACTIONS

Benzquinamide HCl exhibited antiemetic, antihistaminic, mild anticholinergic and sedative action in animals. Studies conducted in dogs and human volunteers have demonstrated suppression of apomorphine-induced vomiting; however, relevance to clinical efficacy has not been established. The mechanism of action in humans is unknown. The onset of antiemetic activity in humans usually occurs within 15 minutes.
Benzquinamide metabolism has been studied in animals and in man. In both species, 5-10% of an administered dose is excreted unchanged in the urine. The remaining drug undergoes metabolic transformation in the liver by at least three pathways to a spectrum of metabolites which are excreted in the urine and in the bile, from which the more polar metabolites are not reabsorbed but are excreted in the feces. The half-life in plasma of Emete-con is about 40 minutes. More than 95% of an administered dose was excreted within 72 hours in animal studies using C14-labeled benzquinamide. In blood, benzquinamide is about 58% bound to plasma protein.

INDICATIONS

Emete-con is indicated for the prevention and treatment of nausea and vomiting associated with anesthesia and surgery.
Since the incidence of postoperative and postanesthetic vomiting has decreased with the adoption of modern techniques and agents, the prophylactic use of Emete-con should be restricted to those patients in whom emesis would endanger the results of surgery or result in harm to the patient.

CONTRAINDICATIONS

Emete-con is contraindicated in individuals who have demonstrated hypersensitivity to the drug.

WARNINGS

Use in Pregnancy
No teratogenic effects of benzquinamide were demonstrated in reproduction studies in chick embryos, mice, rats and rabbits. The relevance of these data to the human is not known. However, safe use of this drug in pregnancy has not been established and its use in pregnancy is not recommended.
Use in Children
As the data available at present are insufficient to establish proper dosage in children, the use of Emete-con in children is not recommended.
Intravenous use
Sudden increase in blood pressure and transient arrhythmias (premature ventricular and auricular contractions) have been reported following intravenous administration of benzquinamide. Until a more predictable pattern of the effect of intravenous benzquinamide has been established, the intramuscular route of administration is considered preferable. The intravenous route of administration should be restricted to patients without cardiovascular disease and receiving no preanesthetic and/or concomitant cardiovascular drugs.
If patients receiving pressor agents or epinephrine-like drugs are also given benzquinamide, the latter should be given in fractions of the normal dose. Blood pressure should be monitored. Safeguards against hypertensive reactions are particularly important in hypertensive patients.

PRECAUTIONS

Benzquinamide, like other antiemetics, may mask signs of overdosage of toxic drugs or may obscure diagnosis of such conditions as intestinal obstruction and brain tumor.

ADVERSE REACTIONS

The following adverse reactions have been reported in subjects who have received benzquinamide. However, drowsiness appears to be the most common reaction. One case of pronounced allergic reaction has been encountered, characterized by pyrexia and urticaria.
System Affected
Autonomic Nervous System: Dry mouth, shivering, sweating, hiccoughs, flushing, salivation, blurred vision.
Cardiovascular System: Hypertension, hypotension, dizziness, atrial fibrillation, premature auricular and ventricular contractions.
Hypertensive episodes have occurred after IM and IV administration.
Central Nervous System: Drowsiness, insomnia, restlessness, headache, excitement, nervousness.
Gastrointestinal System: Anorexia, nausea.
Musculoskeletal System: Twitching, shaking/tremors, weakness.
Skin: Hives/rash.
Other Systems: Fatigue, shaking chills, increased temperature.

DOSAGE AND ADMINISTRATION

Intramuscular: 50 mg (0.5 mg/kg–1.0 mg/kg)
First dose may be repeated in one hour with subsequent doses every 3-4 hours, as necessary. The precautions applicable to all intramuscular injections should be observed. Emete-con should be injected well within the mass of a larger muscle. The deltoid area should be used only if well developed. Injections should not be made into the lower and mid-thirds of the upper arm. Aspiration of the syringe should be carried out to avoid inadvertent intravascular injection. Therapeutic blood levels and demonstrable antiemetic activity appear within fifteen minutes of intramuscular administration. When the objective of therapy is the prevention of nausea and vomiting, intramuscular administration is recommended at least fifteen minutes prior to emergence from anesthesia.
Intravenous: 25 mg (0.2 mg/kg–0.4 mg/kg as a single dose) administered slowly (1 ml per 0.5 to 1 minute). Subsequent doses should be given intramuscularly.
The intravenous route of administration should be restricted to patients without cardiovascular disease (See WARNINGS). If it is necessary to use Emete-con intravenously in elderly or debilitated patients, benzquinamide should be administered cautiously and the lower dose range is recommended.
This preparation must be initially reconstituted with 2.2 ml of Sterile Water for Injection, Bacteriostatic Water for Injection with benzyl alcohol or with methylparaben and propylparaben. This procedure yields 2 ml of a solution equivalent to 25 mg benzquinamide/ml, which maintains its potency for 14 days at room temperature.

OVERDOSAGE

Manifestations: On the basis of acute animal toxicology studies, gross Emete-con overdosage in humans might be expected to manifest itself as a combination of Central Nervous System stimulant and depressant effects. This speculation is derived from experimental studies in which intravenous doses of benzquinamide, at least 150 times the human therapeutic dose, were administered to dogs.
Treatment: There is no specific antidote for Emete-con overdosage. General supportive measures should be instituted, as indicated. Atropine may be helpful. Although there has been no direct experience with dialysis, it is not likely to be of value, since benzquinamide is extensively bound to plasma protein.

HOW SUPPLIED

Emete-con for IM/IV use is available in a vial containing benzquinamide HCl equivalent to 50 mg of benzquinamide in packages of 10 vials.

CAUTION

Federal law prohibits dispensing without prescription.
60-1787-00-4

GEOCILLIN® ℞

[gē′ō-sil-ĭn]
(carbenicillin indanyl sodium)
TABLETS
For Oral Use

DESCRIPTION

Geocillin, a semisynthetic penicillin, is the sodium salt of the indanyl ester of Geopen® (carbenicillin disodium). The chemical name is:

1-(5-Indanyl)-N-(2-carboxy-3,3-dimethyl-7-oxo-4-thia-1-azabicyclo[3.2.0] hept-6-yl)-2-phenylmalonamate monosodium salt.

The structural formula is:

The empirical formula is: $C_{26}H_{25}N_2NaO_6S$ and mol. wt. is 516.55.

Geocillin tablets are yellow, capsule-shaped and film-coated, made of a white crystalline solid. Carbenicillin is freely soluble in water. Each Geocillin tablet contains 382 mg of carbenicillin, 118 mg of indanyl sodium ester. Each Geocillin tablet contains 23 mg of sodium.

Inert ingredients are: glycine; magnesium stearate and sodium lauryl sulfate. May also include the following: hydroxypropyl cellulose; hydroxypropyl methylcellulose; opaspray (which may include Blue 2 Lake, Yellow 6 Lake, Yellow 10 Lake, and other inert ingredients); opadry light yellow (which may contain D&C Yellow 10 Lake, FD&C Yellow 6 Lake and other inert ingredients); opadry clear (which may contain other inert ingredients).

CLINICAL PHARMACOLOGY

Free carbenicillin is the predominant pharmacologically active fraction of Geocillin. Carbenicillin exerts its antibacterial activity by interference with final cell wall synthesis of susceptible bacteria.

Geocillin is acid stable, and rapidly absorbed from the small intestine following oral administration. It provides relatively low plasma concentrations of antibiotic and is primarily excreted in the urine. After absorption, Geocillin is rapidly converted to carbenicillin by hydrolysis of the ester linkage. Following ingestion of a single 500 mg tablet of Geocillin, a peak carbenicillin plasma concentration of approximately 6.5 mcg/ml is reached in 1 hour. About 30% of this dose is excreted in the urine unchanged within 12 hours, with another 6% excreted over the next 12 hours.

In a multiple dose study utilizing volunteers with normal renal function, the following mean urine and serum levels of carbenicillin were achieved:

[See table above.]

Microbiology

The antibacterial activity of Geocillin is due to its rapid conversion to carbenicillin by hydrolysis after absorption. Though Geocillin provides substantial *in vitro* activity against a variety of both gram-positive and gram-negative microorganisms, the most important aspect of its profile is in its antipseudomonal and antiproteal activity. Because of the high urine levels obtained following administration, Geocillin has demonstrated clinical efficacy in urinary infections due to susceptible strains of:

Escherichia coli
Proteus mirabilis
Proteus vulgaris
Morganella morganii (formerly *Proteus morganii*)
Pseudomonas species
Providencia rettgeri (formerly *Proteus rettgeri*)
Enterobacter species
Enterococci (*S. faecalis*)

In addition, *in vitro* data, not substantiated by clinical studies, indicate the following pathogens to be usually susceptible to Geocillin:

Staphylococcus species (nonpenicillinase producing)
Streptococcus species

Resistance

Most *Klebsiella* species are usually resistant to the action of Geocillin. Some strains of *Pseudomonas* species have developed resistance to carbenicillin.

Susceptibility Testing

Geopen (carbenicillin disodium) Susceptibility Powder or 100 ug. Geopen Susceptibility Discs may be used to determine microbial susceptibility to Geocillin using one of the following standard methods recommended by the National Committee for Clinical Laboratory Standards:

M2-A3, "Performance Standards for Antimicrobial Disk Susceptibility Tests"
M7-A, "Methods for Dilution Antimicrobial Susceptibility Tests for Bacteria that Grow Aerobically"
M11-A, "Reference Agar Dilution Procedure for Antimicrobial Susceptibility Testing of Anaerobic Bacteria"
M17-P, "Alternative Methods for Antimicrobial Susceptibility Testing of Anaerobic Bacteria"

Tests should be interpreted by the following criteria:

	Disk Diffusion Zone diameter (mm)		
Organisms	Suscept.	Intermed.	Resist.
Enterobacter	≥ 23	18–22	≤ 17
Pseudomonas sp.	≥ 17	14–16	≤ 13

	Dilution MIC (μ/ml)		
		Moderately	
Organisms	Suscept.	Suscept.	Resist.
Enterobacter	≤ 16	32	≥ 64
Pseudomonas sp.	≤ 128	—	≥ 156

Interpretations of susceptible, intermediate, and resistant correlate zone size diameters with MIC values. A laboratory report of "susceptible" indicates that the suspected causative microorganism most likely will respond to therapy with carbenicillin. A laboratory report of "resistant" indicates that the infecting microorganism most likely will not respond to therapy. A laboratory report of "moderately susceptible" indicates that the microorganism is most likely susceptible if a high dosage of carbenicillin is used, or if the infection is such that high levels of carbenicillin may be attained as in urine. A report of "intermediate" using the disk diffusion method may be considered an equivocal result, and dilution tests may be indicated.

INDICATIONS AND USAGE

Geocillin (carbenicillin indanyl sodium) is indicated in the treatment of acute and chronic infections of the upper and lower urinary tract and in asymptomatic bacteriuria due to susceptible strains of the following organisms:

Escherichia coli
Proteus mirabilis
Morganella morganii
   (formerly *Proteus morganii*)
Providencia rettgeri
   (formerly *Proteus rettgeri*)
Proteus vulgaris
Pseudomonas
Enterobacter
Enterococci

Geocillin is also indicated in the treatment of prostatitis due to susceptible strains of the following organisms:

Escherichia coli
   Enterococcus (*S. faecalis*)
Proteus mirabilis
Enterobacter sp.

WHEN HIGH AND RAPID BLOOD AND URINE LEVELS OF ANTIBIOTIC ARE INDICATED, THERAPY WITH GEOPEN (CARBENICILLIN DISODIUM) SHOULD BE INITIATED BY PARENTERAL ADMINISTRATION FOLLOWED, AT THE PHYSICIAN'S DISCRETION, BY ORAL THERAPY.

NOTE: Susceptibility testing should be performed prior to and during the course of therapy to detect the possible emergence of resistant organisms which may develop.

CONTRAINDICATIONS

Geocillin is ordinarily contraindicated in patients who have a known penicillin allergy.

WARNINGS

Serious and occasionally fatal hypersensitivity (anaphylactic) reactions have been reported in patients on oral penicillin therapy. Although anaphylaxis is more frequent following parenteral therapy, it has occurred in patients on oral penicillins. These reactions are more apt to occur in individuals with a history of penicillin hypersensitivity and/or a history of sensitivity to multiple allergens.

There have been reports of individuals with a history of penicillin hypersensitivity who have experienced severe hypersensitivity reactions when treated with a cephalosporin, and vice versa. Before initiating therapy with a penicillin, careful inquiry should be made concerning previous hypersensitivity reactions to penicillins, cephalosporins, or other allergens. If an allergic reaction occurs, the drug should be discontinued and the appropriate therapy instituted.

SERIOUS ANAPHYLACTOID REACTIONS REQUIRE IMMEDIATE EMERGENCY TREATMENT WITH EPINEPHRINE. OXYGEN, INTRAVENOUS STEROIDS AND AIRWAY MANAGEMENT, INCLUDING INTUBATION, SHOULD ALSO BE ADMINISTERED AS INDICATED.

PRECAUTIONS

General: As with any penicillin preparation, an allergic response, including anaphylaxis, may occur particularly in a hypersensitive individual.

Long term use of Geocillin may result in the overgrowth of nonsusceptible organisms. If superinfection occurs during therapy, appropriate measures should be taken.

Since carbenicillin is primarily excreted by the kidney, patients with severe renal impairment (creatinine clearance of less than 10 ml/min) will not achieve therapeutic urine levels of carbenicillin.

In patients with creatinine clearance of 10–20 ml/min it may be necessary to adjust dosage to prevent accumulation of drug.

Laboratory Tests: As with other penicillins, periodic assessment of organ system function including renal, hepatic, and hematopoietic systems is recommended during prolonged therapy.

Drug Interactions: Geocillin (carbenicillin indanyl sodium) blood levels may be increased and prolonged by concurrent administration of probenecid.

Carcinogenesis, Mutagenesis, Impairment of Fertility: There are no long-term animal or human studies to evaluate carcinogenic potential. Rats fed 250–1000 mg/kg/day for 18 months developed mild liver pathology (e.g., bile duct hyperplasia) at all dose levels, but there was no evidence of drug-related neoplasia. Geocillin administered at daily doses ranging to 1000 mg/kg had no apparent effect on the fertility or reproductive performance of rats.

Pregnancy Category B: Reproduction studies have been performed at dose levels of 1000 or 500 mg/kg in rats, 200 mg/kg in mice, and at 500 mg/kg in monkeys with no harm to fetus due to Geocillin. There are, however, no adequate and well controlled studies in pregnant women. Because animal reproduction studies are not always predictive of human response, this drug should be used during pregnancy only if clearly needed.

Labor and Delivery: It is not known whether the use of Geocillin in humans during labor or delivery has immediate or delayed adverse effects on the fetus, prolongs the duration of labor, or increases the likelihood that forceps delivery or other obstetrical intervention or resuscitation of the newborn will be necessary.

Nursing Mothers: Carbenicillin class antibiotics are excreted in milk although the amounts excreted are unknown; therefore, caution should be exercised if administered to a nursing woman.

Pediatric Use: Since only limited clinical data is available to date in children, the safety of Geocillin administration in this age group has not yet been established.

ADVERSE REACTIONS

The following adverse reactions have been reported as possibly related to Geocillin administration in controlled studies which include 344 patients receiving Geocillin.

Gastrointestinal: The most frequent adverse reactions associated with Geocillin therapy are related to the gastrointestinal tract. Nausea, bad taste, diarrhea, vomiting, flatulence, and glossitis were reported. Abdominal cramps, dry mouth, furry tongue, rectal bleeding, anorexia, and unspecified epigastric distress were rarely reported.

Dermatologic: Hypersensitivity reactions such as skin rash, urticaria, and less frequently pruritus.

Hematologic: As with other penicillins, anemia, thrombocytopenia, leukopenia, neutropenia, and eosinophilia have infrequently been observed. The clinical significance of these abnormalities is not known.

Miscellaneous: Other reactions rarely reported were hyperthermia, headache, itchy eyes, vaginitis, and loose stools.

Abnormalities of Hepatic Function Tests: Mild SGOT elevations have been observed following Geocillin administration.

Continued on next page

DRUG	DOSE	Mean Urine Concentration of Carbenicillin mcg/ml Hours After Initial Dose		
		0–3	3–6	6–24
Geocillin	1 tablet q.6 hr	1130	352	292
Geocillin	2 tablets q.6 hr	1428	789	809

Mean serum concentrations of carbenicillin in this study for these dosages are:

DRUG	DOSE	Mean Serum Concentration mcg/ml Hours After Initial Dose								
		½	1	2	4	6	24	25	26	28
Geocillin	1 tablet q.6 hr	5.1	6.5	3.2	1.9	0.0	0.4	8.8	5.4	0.4
Geocillin	2 tablets q.6 hr	6.1	9.6	7.9	2.6	0.4	0.8	13.2	12.8	3.8

Roerig—Cont.

OVERDOSAGE

Geocillin is generally nontoxic. Geocillin when taken in excessive amounts may produce mild gastrointestinal irritation. The drug is rapidly excreted in the urine and symptoms are transitory. The usual symptoms of anaphylaxis may occur in hypersensitive individuals.

Carbenicillin blood levels achievable with Geocillin are very low, and toxic reactions as a function of overdosage should not occur systematically. The oral LD_{50} in mice is 3,600 mg/kg, in rats 2,000 mg/kg, and in dogs is in excess of 500 mg/kg. The lethal human dose is not known.

Although never reported, the possibility of accumulation of indanyl should be considered when large amounts of Geocillin are ingested. Free indole, which is a phenol derivative, may be potentially toxic. In general 8–15 grams of phenol, and presumably a similar amount of indole, are required orally before toxicity (peripheral vascular collapse) may occur. The metabolic by-products of indole are nontoxic. In patients with hepatic failure it may be possible for unmetabolized indole to accumulate.

The metabolic by-products of Geocillin, indanyl sulfate and glucuronide, as well as free carbenicillin, are dialyzable.

DOSAGE AND ADMINISTRATION

Geocillin is available as a coated tablet to be administered orally.

Usual Adult Dose

URINARY TRACT INFECTIONS	
Escherichia coli, Proteus species, and *Enterobacter*	1–2 tablets 4 times daily
Pseudomonas and *Enterococcus*	2 tablets 4 times daily
PROSTATITIS	
Escherichia coli, Proteus mirabilis, Enterobacter and *Enterococcus*	2 tablets 4 times daily

HOW SUPPLIED

Geocillin is available as film-coated tablets in bottles of 100's (NDC 0049-1430-66), and unit-dose packages of 100 (10 × 10's) (NDC 0049-1430-41). Each tablet contains carbenicillin indanyl sodium equivalent to 382 mg of carbenicillin.

69-1970-00-2

Shown in Product Identification Section, page 427

MARAX® ℞

[*mā'rax*]

(ephedrine sulfate, theophylline, hydroxyzine HCl)

TABLETS AND DF SYRUP

CONTENTS

	Each Tablet Contains:	Each Teaspoon (5 ml.) Syrup Contains:
Ephedrine Sulfate	25 mg.	6.25 mg.
Theophylline	130 mg.	32.50 mg.
Atarax® (hydroxyzine HCl)	10 mg.	2.5 mg.
Alcohol (Ethyl Alcohol)		5% v/v.

Inert ingredients for tablets are: alginic acid; magnesium stearate; precipitated calcium carbonate; sodium lauryl sulfate.

Inert ingredients for syrup are: alcohol; cherry flavor; hydrochloric acid; sodium benzoate; special flavor compound; sucrose; water.

ACTIONS

The action of ephedrine as a vasoconstrictor is well known. It is therefore of significant benefit in symptomatic relief of the congestion occurring in bronchial asthma. As a bronchodilator, it has a slower onset but longer duration of action than does epinephrine, which, in contrast to ephedrine, is not effective upon oral administration.

The diverse actions of theophylline—bronchospasmolytic, cardiovascular, and diuretic—are well established, and make it a particularly useful drug in the treatment of bronchial asthma, both in the acute attack and in the prophylactic therapy of the disease.

Atarax (hydroxyzine HCl) modifies the central stimulatory action of ephedrine preventing excessive excitation in patients on Marax therapy.

In animal studies Atarax has demonstrated antiserotonin activity and antispasmodic potency of a nonspecific nature.

Marax-DF Syrup produces an expectorant action wherein the tenacity of the sputum is decreased and the ease of expectoration is increased.

INDICATIONS

Based on a review of this drug by the National Academy of Sciences-National Research Council and/or other information, FDA has classified the indications as follows:

"Possibly" Effective: For controlling bronchospastic disorders.

Final classification of the less than effective indication requires further investigation.

CONTRAINDICATIONS

Because of the ephedrine, Marax is contraindicated in cardiovascular disease, hyperthyroidism, and hypertension. This drug is contraindicated in individuals who have shown hypersensitivity to the drug or its components.

Hydroxyzine, when administered to the pregnant mouse, rat, and rabbit induced fetal abnormalities in the rat at doses substantially above the human therapeutic range. Clinical data in human beings are inadequate to establish safety in early pregnancy. Until such data are available, hydroxyzine is contraindicated in early pregnancy.

PRECAUTIONS

Because of the ephedrine component this drug should be used with caution in elderly males or those with known prostatic hypertrophy.

The potentiating action of hydroxyzine, although mild, must be taken into consideration when the drug is used in conjunction with central nervous system depressants; and when other central nervous system depressants are administered concomitantly with hydroxyzine their dosage should be reduced. Patients should be cautioned that hydroxyzine can increase the effect of alcohol.

Patients should be warned—because of the hydroxyzine component—of the possibility of drowsiness occurring and cautioned against driving a car or operating dangerous machinery while taking this drug.

ADVERSE REACTIONS

With large doses of ephedrine, excitation, tremulousness, insomnia, nervousness, palpitation, tachycardia, precordial pain, cardiac arrhythmias, vertigo, dryness of the nose and throat, headache, sweating, and warmth may occur. Because ephedrine is a sympathomimetic agent some patients may develop vesical sphincter spasm and resultant urinary hesitation, and occasionally acute urinary retention. This should be borne in mind when administering preparations containing ephedrine to elderly males or those with known prostatic hypertrophy. At the recommended dose for Marax, a side effect occasionally reported is palpitation, and this can be controlled with dosage adjustment, additional amounts of concurrently administered Atarax (hydroxyzine HCl), or discontinuation of the medication. When ephedrine is given three or more times daily patients may develop tolerance after several weeks of therapy.

Theophylline when given on an empty stomach frequently causes gastric irritation accompanied by upper abdominal discomfort, nausea, and vomiting. Administration of the medication after meals will serve to minimize this side effect. Theophylline may cause diuresis and cardiac stimulation.

The amount of Atarax present in Marax has not resulted in disturbing side effects. When used alone specifically as a tranquilizer in the normal dosage range (25 to 50 mg. three or four times a day), side effects are infrequent; even at these higher doses, no serious side effects have been reported and confirmed to date. Those which do occasionally occur when Atarax is used alone are drowsiness, xerostomia and, at extremely high doses, involuntary motor activity, unsteadiness of gait, neuromuscular weakness, all of which may be controlled by reduction of the dosage or discontinuation of the medication.

With the relatively low dose of Atarax in Marax, these effects are not likely to occur. In addition, the ataractic action of Atarax may modify the cardiac stimulatory action of ephedrine, and concurrently, increasing the amount of Atarax may control or abolish this undesirable effect of ephedrine.

DOSAGE AND ADMINISTRATION

The dosage of Marax should be adjusted according to the severity of complaints, and the patient's individual toleration.

Tablets: In general, an adult dose of 1 tablet, 2 to 4 times daily, should be sufficient. Some patients are controlled adequately with ½ to 1 tablet at bedtime. The time interval between doses should not be shorter than four hours. The dosage for children over 5 years of age and for adults who are sensitive to ephedrine, is one-half the usual adult dose. Clinical experience to date has been confined to ages above 5 years.

Syrup: The dose for children over 5 years of age is 1 teaspoon (5 ml.), 3 to 4 times daily. Dosage for children 2 to 5 years of age is ½ to 1 teaspoon (2.5-5 ml.), 3 to 4 times daily. Not recommended for children under 2 years of age.

HOW SUPPLIED

Marax Tablets are available as scored, dye free, m-shaped tablets in bottles of 100 (NDC 0049-2540-66) and 500 (NDC 0049-2540-73).

Marax-DF Syrup is available in pints (NDC 0049-2550-93) and gallons (NDC 0049-2550-54) as a colorless syrup, free of all coal tar dyes, and should be dispensed in tight, light-resistant containers (USP).

69-0928-00-7
66-2265-00-4

Shown in Product Identification Section, page 427

NAVANE® ℞

[*nah'vān*]

(thiothixene) CAPSULES

NAVANE® ℞

(thiothixene hydrochloride) CONCENTRATE

DESCRIPTION

Navane (thiothixene) is a thioxanthene derivative. Specifically, it is the *cis* isomer of N,N-dimethyl-9-[3-(4-methyl-1-piperazinyl)-propylidene] thioxanthene-2-sulfonamide.

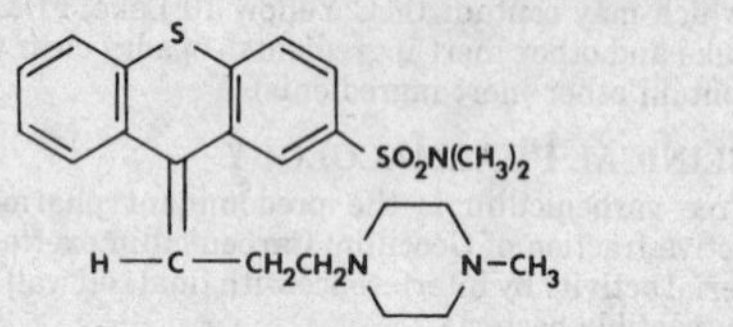

The thioxanthenes differ from the phenothiazines by the replacement of nitrogen in the central ring with a carbon-linked side chain fixed in space in a rigid structural configuration. An N,N-dimethyl sulfonamide functional group is bonded to the thioxanthene nucleus.

Inert ingredients for the capsule formulations are: hard gelatin capsules (which contain gelatin and titanium dioxide; may contain Yellow 10, Yellow 6, Blue 1, Green 3, Red 3, and other inert ingredients); lactose; magnesium stearate; sodium lauryl sulfate; starch.

Inert ingredients for the oral concentrate formulation are: alcohol; cherry flavor; dextrose; passion fruit flavor; sorbitol solution; water.

ACTIONS

Navane is a psychotropic agent of the thioxanthene series. Navane possesses certain chemical and pharmacological similarities to the piperazine phenothiazines and differences from the aliphatic group of phenothiazines.

INDICATIONS

Navane is effective in the management of manifestations of psychotic disorders. Navane has not been evaluated in the management of behavioral complications in patients with mental retardation.

CONTRAINDICATIONS

Navane is contraindicated in patients with circulatory collapse, comatose states, central nervous system depression due to any cause, and blood dyscrasias. Navane is contraindicated in individuals who have shown hypersensitivity to the drug. It is not known whether there is a cross sensitivity between the thioxanthenes and the phenothiazine derivatives, but this possibility should be considered.

WARNINGS

Tardive Dyskinesia—Tardive dyskinesia, a syndrome consisting of potentially irreversible, involuntary, dyskinetic movements may develop in patients treated with neuroleptic (antipsychotic) drugs. Although the prevalence of the syndrome appears to be highest among the elderly, especially elderly women, it is impossible to rely upon prevalence estimates to predict, at the inception of neuroleptic treatment, which patients are likely to develop the syndrome. Whether neuroleptic drug products differ in their potential to cause tardive dyskinesia is unknown.

Both the risk of developing the syndrome and the likelihood that it will become irreversible are believed to increase as the duration of treatment and the total cumulative dose of neuroleptic drugs administered to the patient increase. However, the syndrome can develop, although much less commonly, after relatively brief treatment periods at low doses.

There is no known treatment for established cases of tardive dyskinesia, although the syndrome may remit, partially or completely, if neuroleptic treatment is withdrawn. Neuroleptic treatment, itself, however, may suppress (or partially suppress) the signs and symptoms of the syndrome and thereby may possibly mask the underlying disease process. The effect that symptomatic suppression has upon the long-term course of the syndrome is unknown.

Given these considerations, neuroleptics should be prescribed in a manner that is most likely to minimize the occur-

rence of tardive dyskinesia. Chronic neuroleptic treatment should generally be reserved for patients who suffer from a chronic illness that, 1) is known to respond to neuroleptic drugs, and 2) for whom alternative, equally effective, but potentially less harmful treatments are *not* available or appropriate. In patients who do require chronic treatment, the smallest dose and the shortest duration of treatment producing a satisfactory clinical response should be sought. The need for continued treatment should be reassessed periodically.

If signs and symptoms of tardive dyskinesia appear in a patient on neuroleptics, drug discontinuation should be considered. However, some patients may require treatment despite the presence of the syndrome.

(For further information about the description of tardive dyskinesia and its clinical detection, please refer to "Information for Patients" in the PRECAUTIONS section, and to the ADVERSE REACTIONS section.)

Neuroleptic Malignant Syndrome (NMS)—A potentially fatal symptom complex sometimes referred to as Neuroleptic Malignant Syndrome (NMS) has been reported in association with antipsychotic drugs. Clinical manifestations of NMS are hyperpyrexia, muscle rigidity, altered mental status and evidence of autonomic instability (irregular pulse or blood pressure, tachycardia, diaphoresis, and cardiac dysrhythmias).

The diagnostic evaluation of patients with this syndrome is complicated. In arriving at a diagnosis, it is important to identify cases where the clinical presentation includes both serious medical illness (e.g., pneumonia, systemic infection, etc.) and untreated or inadequately treated extrapyramidal signs and symptoms (EPS). Other important considerations in the differential diagnosis include central anticholinergic toxicity, heat stroke, drug fever and primary central nervous system (CNS) pathology.

The management of NMS should include 1) immediate discontinuation of antipsychotic drugs and other drugs not essential to concurrent therapy, 2) intensive symptomatic treatment and medical monitoring, and 3) treatment of any concomitant serious medical problems for which specific treatments are available. There is no general agreement about specific pharmacological treatment regimens for uncomplicated NMS.

If a patient requires antipsychotic drug treatment after recovery from NMS, the potential reintroduction of drug therapy should be carefully considered. The patient should be carefully monitored, since recurrences of NMS have been reported.

Usage in Pregnancy—Safe use of Navane during pregnancy has not been established. Therefore, this drug should be given to pregnant patients only when, in the judgment of the physician, the expected benefits from the treatment exceed the possible risks to mother and fetus. Animal reproduction studies and clinical experience to date have not demonstrated any teratogenic effects.

In the animal reproduction studies with Navane, there was some decrease in conception rate and litter size, and an increase in resorption rate in rats and rabbits. Similar findings have been reported with other psychotropic agents. After repeated oral administration of Navane to rats (5 to 15 mg/kg/day), rabbits (3 to 50 mg/kg/day), and monkeys (1 to 3 mg/kg/day) before and during gestation, no teratogenic effects were seen.

Usage in Children—The use of Navane in children under 12 years of age is not recommended because safe conditions for its use have not been established.

As is true with many CNS drugs, Navane may impair the mental and/or physical abilities required for the performance of potentially hazardous tasks such as driving a car or operating machinery, especially during the first few days of therapy. Therefore, the patient should be cautioned accordingly.

As in the case of other CNS-acting drugs, patients receiving Navane (thiothixene) should be cautioned about the possible additive effects (which may include hypotension) with CNS depressants and with alcohol.

PRECAUTIONS

General: An antiemetic effect was observed in animal studies with Navane; since this effect may also occur in man, it is possible that Navane may mask signs of overdosage of toxic drugs and may obscure conditions such as intestinal obstruction and brain tumor.

In consideration of the known capability of Navane and certain other psychotropic drugs to precipitate convulsions, extreme caution should be used in patients with a history of convulsive disorders or those in a state of alcohol withdrawal, since it may lower the convulsive threshold. Although Navane potentiates the actions of the barbiturates, the dosage of the anticonvulsant therapy should not be reduced when Navane is administered concurrently.

Though exhibiting rather weak anticholinergic properties, Navane should be used with caution in patients who might be exposed to extreme heat or who are receiving atropine or related drugs.

Use with caution in patients with cardiovascular disease. Caution as well as careful adjustment of the dosages is indicated when Navane is used in conjunction with other CNS depressants.

Also, careful observation should be made for pigmentary retinopathy, and lenticular pigmentation (fine lenticular pigmentation has been noted in a small number of patients treated with Navane for prolonged periods). Blood dyscrasias (agranulocytosis, pancytopenia, thrombocytopenic purpura), and liver damage (jaundice, biliary stasis), have been reported with related drugs.

Neuroleptic drugs elevate prolactin levels; the elevation persists during chronic administration. Tissue culture experiments indicate that approximately one-third of human breast cancers are prolactin dependent *in vitro*, a factor of potential importance if the prescription of these drugs is contemplated in a patient with a previously detected breast cancer. Although disturbances such as galactorrhea, amenorrhea, gynecomastia, and impotence have been reported, the clinical significance of elevated serum prolactin levels is unknown for most patients. An increase in mammary neoplasms has been found in rodents after chronic administration of neuroleptic drugs. Neither clinical studies nor epidemiologic studies conducted to date, however, have shown an association between chronic administration of these drugs and mammary tumorigenesis; the available evidence is considered too limited to be conclusive at this time.

Information for Patients: Given the likelihood that some patients exposed chronically to neuroleptics will develop tardive dyskinesia, it is advised that all patients in whom chronic use is contemplated be given, if possible, full information about this risk. The decision to inform patients and/or their guardians must obviously take into account the clinical circumstances and the competency of the patient to understand the information provided.

ADVERSE REACTIONS

NOTE: Not all of the following adverse reactions have been reported with Navane. However, since Navane has certain chemical and pharmacologic similarities to the phenothiazines, all of the known side effects and toxicity associated with phenothiazine therapy should be borne in mind when Navane is used.

Cardiovascular Effects: Tachycardia, hypotension, lightheadedness, and syncope. In the event hypotension occurs, epinephrine should not be used as a pressor agent since a paradoxical further lowering of blood pressure may result. Nonspecific EKG changes have been observed in some patients receiving Navane. These changes are usually reversible and frequently disappear on continued Navane therapy. The incidence of these changes is lower than that observed with some phenothiazines. The clinical significance of these changes is not known.

CNS Effects: Drowsiness, usually mild, may occur although it usually subsides with continuation of Navane therapy. The incidence of sedation appears similar to that of the piperazine group of phenothiazines but less than that of certain aliphatic phenothiazines. Restlessness, agitation and insomnia have been noted with Navane. Seizures and paradoxical exacerbation of psychotic symptoms have occurred with Navane infrequently.

Hyperreflexia has been reported in infants delivered from mothers having received structurally related drugs.

In addition, phenothiazine derivatives have been associated with cerebral edema and cerebrospinal fluid abnormalities. Extrapyramidal symptoms, such as pseudo-parkinsonism, akathisia and dystonia have been reported. Management of these extra-pyramidal symptoms depends upon the type and severity. Rapid relief of acute symptoms may require the use of an injectable antiparkinson agent. More slowly emerging symptoms may be managed by reducing the dosage of Navane and/or administering an oral antiparkinson agent.

Persistent Tardive Dyskinesia: As with all antipsychotic agents tardive dyskinesia may appear in some patients on long term therapy or may occur after drug therapy has been discontinued. The syndrome is characterized by rhythmical involuntary movements of the tongue, face, mouth or jaw (e.g., protrusion of tongue, puffing of cheeks, puckering of mouth, chewing movements). Sometimes these may be accompanied by involuntary movements of extremities.

Since early detection of tardive dyskinesia is important, patients should be monitored on an ongoing basis. It has been reported that fine vermicular movement of the tongue may be an early sign of the syndrome. If this or any other presentation of the syndrome is observed, the clinician should consider possible discontinuation of neuroleptic medication. (See Warnings section.)

Hepatic Effects: Elevations of serum transaminase and alkaline phosphatase, usually transient, have been infrequently observed in some patients. No clinically confirmed cases of jaundice attributable to Navane have been reported.

Hematologic Effects: As is true with certain other psychotropic drugs, leukopenia and leucocytosis, which are usually transient, can occur occasionally with Navane. Other anti-

psychotic drugs have been associated with agranulocytosis, eosinophilia, hemolytic anemia, thrombocytopenia and pancytopenia.

Allergic Reactions: Rash, pruritus, urticaria, photosensitivity and rare cases of anaphylaxis have been reported with Navane. Undue exposure to sunlight should be avoided. Although not experienced with Navane, exfoliative dermatitis and contact dermatitis (in nursing personnel), have been reported with certain phenothiazines.

Endocrine Disorders: Lactation, moderate breast enlargement and amenorrhea have occurred in a small percentage of females receiving Navane. If persistent, this may necessitate a reduction in dosage or the discontinuation of therapy. Phenothiazines have been associated with false positive pregnancy tests, gynecomastia, hypoglycemia, hyperglycemia and glycosuria.

Autonomic Effects: Dry mouth, blurred vision, nasal congestion, constipation, increased sweating, increased salivation and impotence have occurred infrequently with Navane therapy. Phenothiazines have been associated with miosis, mydriasis, and adynamic ileus.

Other Adverse Reactions: Hyperpyrexia, anorexia, nausea, vomiting, diarrhea, increase in appetite and weight, weakness or fatigue, polydipsia, and peripheral edema.

Although not reported with Navane, evidence indicates there is a relationship between phenothiazine therapy and the occurrence of a systemic lupus erythematosus-like syndrome.

Neuroleptic Malignant Syndrome (NMS): Please refer to the text regarding NMS in the WARNINGS section.

NOTE: Sudden deaths have occasionally been reported in patients who have received certain phenothiazine derivatives. In some cases the cause of death was apparently cardiac arrest or asphyxia due to failure of the cough reflex. In others, the cause could not be determined nor could it be established that death was due to phenothiazine administration.

DOSAGE AND ADMINISTRATION

Dosage of Navane should be individually adjusted depending on the chronicity and severity of the condition. In general, small doses should be used initially and gradually increased to the optimal effective level, based on patient response. Some patients have been successfully maintained on once-a-day Navane therapy.

The use of Navane in children under 12 years of age is not recommended because safe conditions for its use have not been established.

In milder conditions, an initial dose of 2 mg. three times daily. If indicated, a subsequent increase to 15 mg./day total daily dose is often effective.

In more severe conditions, an initial dose of 5 mg. twice daily. The usual optimal dose is 20 to 30 mg. daily. If indicated, an increase to 60 mg./day total daily dose is often effective. Exceeding a total daily dose of 60 mg. rarely increases the beneficial response.

OVERDOSAGE

Manifestations include muscular twitching, drowsiness and dizziness. Symptoms of gross overdosage may include CNS depression, rigidity, weakness, torticollis, tremor, salivation, dysphagia, hypotension, disturbances of gait, or coma.

Treatment: Essentially symptomatic and supportive. Early gastric lavage is helpful. Keep patient under careful observation and maintain an open airway, since involvement of the extrapyramidal system may produce dysphagia and respiratory difficulty in severe overdosage. If hypotension occurs, the standard measures for managing circulatory shock should be used (I.V. fluids and/or vasoconstrictors).

If a vasoconstrictor is needed, levarterenol and phenylephrine are the most suitable drugs. Other pressor agents, including epinephrine, are not recommended, since phenothiazine derivatives may reverse the usual pressor action of these agents and cause further lowering of blood pressure.

If CNS depression is marked, symptomatic treatment is indicated. Extrapyramidal symptoms may be treated with antiparkinson drugs.

There are no data on the use of peritoneal or hemodialysis, but they are known to be of little value in phenothiazine intoxication.

HOW SUPPLIED

Navane (thiothixene) Capsules
Bottles of 100's: 1 mg (NDC 0049-5710-66); 2 mg (NDC 0049-5720-66); 5 mg (NDC 0049-5730-66); 10 mg (NDC 0049-5740-66); 20 mg (NDC 0049-5770-66). 1000's: 2 mg (NDC 0049-5720-82); 5 mg (NDC 0049-5730-82); 10 mg (NDC 0049-5740-82). 500's: 20 mg (NDC 0049-5770-73).
Unit Doses of: 1 mg (NDC 0049-5710-41); 2 mg (NDC 0049-5720-41); 5 mg (NDC 0049-5730-41); 10 mg (NDC 0049-5740-41); and 20 mg (NDC 0049-5770-41).
Navane (thiothixene hydrochloride) Concentrate is available in 120 ml (4 oz.) bottles (NDC 0049-5750-47) with an accompanying dropper calibrated at 2 mg, 3 mg, 4 mg, 5 mg, 6 mg, 8 mg, and 10 mg; in 30 ml (1 oz.) bottles (NDC 0049-5750-51) with an accompanying dropper calibrated at 2 mg, 3 mg, 4

Continued on next page

Roerig—Cont.

mg, and 5 mg. Each ml. contains thiothixene hydrochloride equivalent to 5 mg. of thiothixene. Contains alcohol, U.S.P. 7.0% v/v. (small loss unavoidable).

77-1655-00-7

Shown in Product Identification Section, page 427

NAVANE® ℞
[nah 'vān]
(thiothixene hydrochloride)
Intramuscular
2 mg./ml. 5 mg./ml.

DESCRIPTION

Navane (thiothixene hydrochloride) is a thioxanthene derivative. Specifically, thiothixene is the *cis* isomer of N,N-dimethyl-9-[3-(4-methyl-1-piperazinyl)-propylidene]thioxanthene-2-sulfonamide.

The thioxanthenes differ from the phenothiazines by the replacement of nitrogen in the central ring with a carbon-linked side chain fixed in space in a rigid structural configuration. An N,N-dimethyl sulfonamide functional group is bonded to the thioxanthene nucleus.

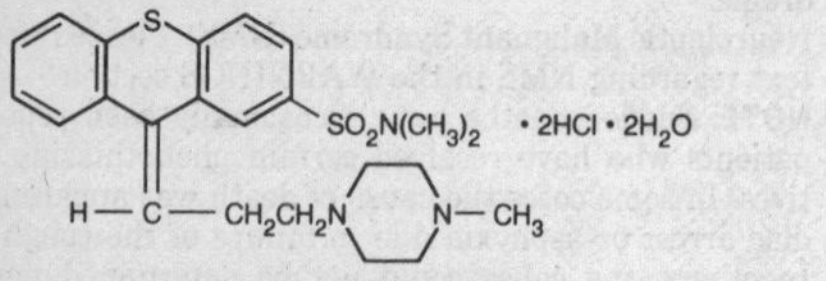

thiothixene hydrochloride

Inert ingredients for the intramuscular solution formulation are: dextrose; benzyl alcohol; propyl gallate.

Inert ingredient for the intramuscular for injection formulation is: mannitol.

ACTIONS

Navane is a psychotropic agent of the thioxanthene series. Navane possesses certain chemical and pharmacological similarities to the piperazine phenothiazines and differences from the aliphatic group of phenothiazines. Navane's mode of action has not been clearly established.

INDICATIONS

Navane is effective in the management of manifestations of psychotic disorders. Navane has not been evaluated in the management of behavioral complications in patients with mental retardation.

CONTRAINDICATIONS

Navane is contraindicated in patients with circulatory collapse, comatose states, central nervous system depression due to any cause, and blood dyscrasias. Navane is contraindicated in individuals who have shown hypersensitivity to the drug. It is not known whether there is a cross sensitivity between the thioxanthenes and the phenothiazine derivatives, but this possibility should be considered.

WARNINGS

Tardive Dyskinesia—Tardive dyskinesia, a syndrome consisting of potentially irreversible, involuntary, dyskinetic movements may develop in patients treated with neuroleptic (antipsychotic) drugs. Although the prevalence of the syndrome appears to be highest among the elderly, especially elderly women, it is impossible to rely upon prevalence estimates to predict, at the inception of neuroleptic treatment, which patients are likely to develop the syndrome. Whether neuroleptic drug products differ in their potential to cause tardive dyskinesia is unknown.

Both the risk of developing the syndrome and the likelihood that it will become irreversible are believed to increase as the duration of treatment and the total cumulative dose of neuroleptic drugs administered to the patient increase. However, the syndrome can develop, although much less commonly, after relatively brief treatment periods at low doses.

There is no known treatment for established cases of tardive dyskinesia, although the syndrome may remit, partially or completely, if neuroleptic treatment is withdrawn. Neuroleptic treatment, itself, however, may suppress (or partially suppress) the signs and symptoms of the syndrome and thereby may possibly mask the underlying disease process. The effect that symptomatic suppression has upon the long-term course of the syndrome is unknown.

Given these considerations, neuroleptics should be prescribed in a manner that is most likely to minimize the occurrence of tardive dyskinesia. Chronic neuroleptic treatment should generally be reserved for patients who suffer from a chronic illness that, 1) is known to respond to neuroleptic drugs, and, 2) for whom alternative, equally effective, but potentially less harmful treatments are *not* available or appropriate. In patients who do require chronic treatment, the smallest dose and the shortest duration of treatment producing a satisfactory clinical response should be sought. The need for continued treatment should be reassessed periodically.

If signs and symptoms of tardive dyskinesia appear in a patient on neuroleptics, drug discontinuation should be considered. However, some patients may require treatment despite the presence of the syndrome.

(For further information about the description of tardive dyskinesia and its clinical detection, please refer to "Information for Patients" in the PRECAUTIONS section, and to the ADVERSE REACTIONS section.)

Neuroleptic Malignant Syndrome (NMS)—A potentially fatal symptom complex sometimes referred to as Neuroleptic Malignant Syndrome (NMS) has been reported in association with antipsychotic drugs. Clinical manifestations of NMS are hyperpyrexia, muscle rigidity, altered mental status and evidence of autonomic instability (irregular pulse or blood pressure, tachycardia, diaphoresis, and cardiac dysrhythmias).

The diagnostic evaluation of patients with this syndrome is complicated. In arriving at a diagnosis, it is important to identify cases where the clinical presentation includes both serious medical illness (e.g., pneumonia, systemic infection, etc.) and untreated or inadequately treated extrapyramidal signs and symptoms (EPS). Oher important considerations in the differential diagnosis include central anticholinergic toxicity, heat stroke, drug fever and primary central nervous system (CNS) pathology.

The management of NMS should include 1) immediate discontinuation of antipsychotic drugs and other drugs not essential to concurrent therapy, 2) intensive symptomatic treatment and medical monitoring, and 3) treatment of any concomitant serious medical problems for which specific treatments are available. There is no general agreement about specific pharmacological treatment regimens for uncomplicated NMS.

If a patient requires antipsychotic drug treatment after recovery from NMS, the potential reintroduction of drug therapy should be carefully considered. The patient should be carefully monitored, since recurrences of NMS have been reported.

Usage in Pregnancy—Safe use of Navane during pregnancy has not been established. Therefore, this drug should be given to pregnant patients only when, in the judgment of the physician, the expected benefits from treatment exceed the possible risks to mother and fetus. Animal reproductive studies and clinical experience to date have not demonstrated any teratogenic effects.

In the animal reproduction studies with Navane, there was some decrease in conception rate and litter size, and an increase in resorption rate in rats and rabbits, changes which have been similarly reported with other psychotropic agents. After repeated oral administration of Navane to rats (5 to 15 mg./kg./day), rabbits (3 to 50 mg./kg./day), and monkeys (1 to 3 mg./kg./day) before and during gestation, no teratogenic effects were seen. (See Precautions).

Usage in Children—The use of Navane in children under 12 years of age is not recommended because safety and efficacy in the pediatric age group have not been established.

As is true with many CNS drugs, Navane may impair the mental and/or physical abilities required for the performance of potentially hazardous tasks such as driving a car or operating machinery, especially during the first few days of therapy. Therefore, the patient should be cautioned accordingly.

As in the case of other CNS-acting drugs, patients receiving Navane should be cautioned about the possible additive effects (which may include hypotension) with CNS depressants and with alcohol.

PRECAUTIONS

General: An antiemetic effect was observed in animal studies with Navane (thiothixene hydrochloride); since this effect may also occur in man, it is possible that Navane may mask signs of overdosage of toxic drugs and may obscure conditions such as intestinal obstruction and brain tumor.

In consideration of the known capability of Navane and certain other psychotropic drugs to precipitate convulsions, extreme caution should be used in patients with a history of convulsive disorders, or those in a state of alcohol withdrawal since it may lower the convulsive threshold. Although Navane potentiates the actions of the barbiturates, the dosage of the anticonvulsant therapy should not be reduced when Navane is administered concurrently.

Caution as well as careful adjustment of the dosage is indicated when Navane is used in conjunction with other CNS depressants other than anticonvulsant drugs.

Though exhibiting rather weak anticholinergic properties, Navane should be used with caution in patients who are known or suspected to have glaucoma, or who might be exposed to extreme heat, or who are receiving atropine or related drugs.

Use with caution in patients with cardiovascular disease.

Also, careful observation should be made for pigmentary retinopathy, and lenticular pigmentation (fine lenticular pigmentation has been noted in a small number of patients treated with Navane for prolonged periods). Blood dyscrasias (agranulocytosis, pancytopenia, thrombocytopenic purpura), and liver damage (jaundice, biliary stasis), have been reported with related drugs.

Undue exposure to sunlight should be avoided. Photosensitive reactions have been reported in patients on Navane.

As with all intramuscular preparations, Navane Intramuscular should be injected well within the body of a relatively large muscle. The preferred sites are the upper outer quadrant of the buttock (i.e., gluteus maximus) and the mid-lateral thigh.

The deltoid area should be used only if well developed such as in certain adults and older children, and then only with caution to avoid radial nerve injury. Intramuscular injections should not be made into the lower and mid-thirds of the upper arm. As with all intramuscular injections, aspiration is necessary to help avoid inadvertent injection into a blood vessel.

Neuroleptic drugs elevate prolactin levels; the elevation persists during chronic administration. Tissue culture experiments indicate that approximately one-third of human breast cancers are prolactin dependent *in vitro*, a factor of potential importance if the prescription of these drugs is contemplated in a patient with a previously detected breast cancer. Although disturbances such as galactorrhea, amenorrhea, gynecomastia, and impotence have been reported, the clinical significance of elevated serum prolactin levels is unknown for most patients. An increase in mammary neoplasms has been found in rodents after chronic administration of neuroleptic drugs. Neither clinical studies nor epidemiologic studies conducted to date, however, have shown an association between chronic administration of these drugs and mammary tumorigenesis; the available evidence is considered too limited to be conclusive at this time.

Information for Patients: Given the likelihood that some patients exposed chronically to neuroleptics will develop tardive dyskinesia, it is advised that all patients in whom chronic use is contemplated be given, if possible, full information about this risk. The decision to inform patients and/or their guardians must obviously take into account the clinical circumstances and the competency of the patient to understand the information provided.

ADVERSE REACTIONS

NOTE: Not all of the following adverse reactions have been reported with Navane. However, since Navane has certain chemical and pharmacologic similarities to the phenothiazines, all of the known side effects and toxicity associated with phenothiazine therapy should be borne in mind when Navane is used.

Cardiovascular Effects: Tachycardia, hypotension, lightheadedness, and syncope. In the event hypotension occurs, epinephrine should not be used as a pressor agent since a paradoxical further lowering of blood pressure may result. Nonspecific EKG changes have been observed in some patients receiving Navane. These changes are usually reversible and frequently disappear on continued Navane therapy. The clinical significance of these changes is not known.

CNS Effects: Drowsiness, usually mild, may occur although it usually subsides with continuation of Navane therapy. The incidence of sedation appears similar to that of the piperazine group of phenothiazines, but less than that of certain aliphatic phenothiazines. Restlessness, agitation and insomnia have been noted with Navane. Seizures and paradoxical exacerbation of psychotic symptoms have occurred with Navane infrequently.

Hyperreflexia has been reported in infants delivered from mothers having received structurally related drugs.

In addition, phenothiazine derivatives have been associated with cerebral edema and cerebrospinal fluid abnormalities.

Extrapyramidal symptoms, such as pseudo-parkinsonism, akathisia, and dystonia have been reported. Management of these extrapyramidal symptoms depends upon the type and severity. Rapid relief of acute symptoms may require the use of an injectable antiparkinson agent. More slowly emerging symptoms may be managed by reducing the dosage of Navane and/or administering an oral antiparkinson agent.

Persistent Tardive Dyskinesia: As with all antipsychotic agents tardive dyskinesia may appear in some patients on long term therapy or may occur after drug therapy has been discontinued. The syndrome is characterized by rhythmical involuntary movements of the tongue, face, mouth or jaw (e.g., protrusion of tongue, puffing of cheeks, puckering of mouth, chewing movements). Sometimes these may be accompanied by involuntary movements of extremities.

Since early detection of tardive dyskinesia is important, patients should be monitored on an ongoing basis. It has been reported that fine vermicular movement of the tongue may be an early sign of the syndrome. If this or any other presentation of the syndrome is observed, the clinician should consider possible discontinuation of neuroleptic medication. (See Warnings section.)

Hepatic Effects: Elevations of serum transaminase and alkaline phosphatase, usually transient, have been infrequently observed in some patients. No clinically confirmed cases of jaundice attributable to Navane (thiothixene hydrochloride) have been reported.

Hematologic Effects: As is true with certain other psychotropic drugs, leukopenia and leucocytosis, which are usually transient, can occur occasionally with Navane. Other antipsychotic drugs have been associated with agranulocytosis, eosinophilia, hemolytic anemia, thrombocytopenia and pancytopenia.

Allergic Reactions: Rash, pruritus, urticaria, and rare cases of anaphylaxis have been reported with Navane. Undue exposure to sunlight should be avoided. Although not experienced with Navane, exfoliative dermatitis, contact dermatitis (in nursing personnel), have been reported with certain phenothiazines.

Endocrine Disorders: Lactation, moderate breast enlargement and amenorrhea have occurred in a small percentage of females receiving Navane. If persistent, this may necessitate a reduction in dosage or the discontinuation of therapy. Phenothiazines have been associated with false positive pregnancy tests, gynecomastia, hypoglycemia, hyperglycemia, and glycosuria.

Autonomic Effects: Dry mouth, blurred vision, nasal congestion, constipation, increased sweating, increased salivation, and impotence have occurred infrequently with Navane therapy. Phenothiazines have been associated with miosis, mydriasis, and adynamic ileus.

Other Adverse Reactions: Hyperpyrexia, anorexia, nausea, vomiting, diarrhea, increase in appetite and weight, weakness or fatigue, polydipsia and peripheral edema.

Although not reported with Navane, evidence indicates there is a relationship between phenothiazine therapy and the occurrence of a systemic lupus erythematosus-like syndrome.

Neuroleptic Malignant Syndrome (NMS): Please refer to the text regarding NMS in the WARNINGS section.

NOTE: Sudden deaths have occasionally been reported in patients who have received certain phenothiazine derivatives. In some cases the cause of death was apparently cardiac arrest or asphyxia due to failure of the cough reflex. In others, the cause could not be determined nor could it be established that death was due to phenothiazine administration.

DOSAGE AND ADMINISTRATION

Preparation

Navane (thiothixene hydrochloride) Intramuscular Solution is ready for use as supplied.

Navane (thiothixene hydrochloride) Intramuscular For Injection must be reconstituted with 2.2 ml of Sterile Water for Injection.

For Intramuscular Use Only

Dosage of Navane should be individually adjusted depending on the chronicity and severity of the condition. In general, small doses should be used initially and gradually increased to the optimal effective level, based on patient response.

Usage in children under 12 years of age is not recommended.

Where more rapid control and treatment of acute behavior is desirable, the intramuscular form of Navane may be indicated. It is also of benefit where the very nature of the patient's symptomatology, whether acute or chronic, renders oral administration impractical or even impossible.

For treatment of acute symptomatology or in patients unable or unwilling to take oral medication, the usual dose is 4 mg. of Navane Intramuscular administered 2 to 4 times daily. Dosage may be increased or decreased depending on response. Most patients are controlled on a total daily dosage of 16 to 20 mg. The maximum recommended dosage is 30 mg./day. An oral form should supplant the injectable form as soon as possible. It may be necessary to adjust the dosage when changing from the intramuscular to oral dosage forms. Dosage recommendations for Navane Capsules and Concentrate can be found in the Navane oral package insert.

OVERDOSAGE

Manifestations include muscular twitching, drowsiness, and dizziness. Symptoms of gross overdosage may include CNS depression, rigidity, weakness, torticollis, tremor, salivation, dysphagia, hypotension, disturbances of gait, or coma.

Treatment: Essentially symptomatic and supportive. Keep patient under careful observation and maintain an open airway, since involvement of the extrapyramidal system may produce dysphagia and respiratory difficulty in severe overdosage. If hypotension occurs, the standard measures for managing circulatory shock should be used (I.V. fluids and/or vasoconstrictors).

If a vasoconstrictor is needed, levarterenol and phenylephrine are the most suitable drugs. Other pressor agents, including epinephrine, are not recommended, since phenothiazine derivatives may reverse the usual pressor elevating action of these agents and cause further lowering of blood pressure.

If CNS depression is marked, symptomatic treatment is indicated. Extrapyramidal symptoms may be treated with antiparkinson drugs.

There are no data on the use of peritoneal or hemodialysis, but they are known to be of little value in phenothiazine intoxication.

HOW SUPPLIED

Navane (thiothixene hydrochloride) Intramuscular Solution is available in a 2 ml. amber glass vial in packages of 10 vials (NDC 0049-5760-83). Each ml. contains thiothixene hydrochloride equivalent to 2 mg. of thiothixene, dextrose 5% w/v, benzyl alcohol 0.9% w/v, and propyl gallate 0.02% w/v.

Navane (thiothixene hydrochloride) Intramuscular For Injection is available in amber glass vials in packages of 10 vials (NDC 0049-5765-83). When reconstituted with 2.2 ml of STERILE WATER FOR INJECTION, each ml contains thiothixene hydrochloride equivalent to 5 mg of thiothixene, and 59.6 mg of mannitol. The reconstituted solution of Navane Intramuscular For Injection may be stored for 48 hours at room temperature before discarding.

70-1865-00-3
70-4177-00-4

Buffered
PFIZERPEN® ℞
(penicillin G potassium)
for Injection

DESCRIPTION

Buffered Pfizerpen (penicillin G potassium) for Injection is a sterile, pyrogen-free powder for reconstitution. Buffered Pfizerpen for Injection is an antibacterial agent for intramuscular, continuous intravenous drip, intrapleural or other local infusion, and intrathecal administration.

Each million units contains approximately 6.8 milligrams of sodium (0.3 mEq) and 65.6 milligrams of potassium (1.68 mEq).

Chemically, Pfizerpen is monopotassium 3,3-dimethyl-7oxo-6-(2-phenylacetamido)-4-thia-1-azabicyclo (3.2.0) heptane-2-carboxylate. It has a molecular weight of 372.48 and the following chemical structure.

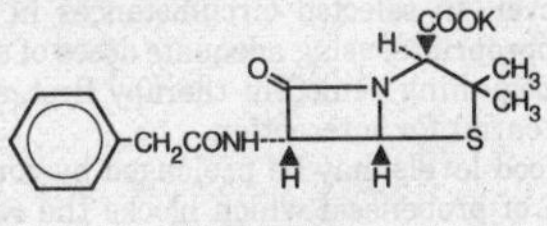

Formula
$C_{16}H_{17}KN_2O_4S$

Penicillin G potassium is a colorless or white crystal, or a white crystalline powder which is odorless, or practically so, and moderately hygroscopic. Penicillin G potassium is very soluble in water. The pH of the reconstituted product is between 6.0–8.5.

CLINICAL PHARMACOLOGY

Aqueous penicillin G is rapidly absorbed following both intramuscular and subcutaneous injection. Initial blood levels following parenteral administration are high but transient. Penicillins bind to serum proteins, mainly albumin. Therapeutic levels of the penicillins are easily achieved under normal circumstances in extracellular fluid and most other body tissues. Penicillins are distributed in varying degrees into pleural, pericardial, peritoneal, ascitic, synovial, and interstitial fluids. Penicillins are excreted in breast milk. Penetration into the cerebrospinal fluid, eyes, and prostate is poor. Penicillins are rapidly excreted in the urine by glomerular filtration and active tubular secretion, primarily as unchanged drug. Approximately 60 percent of the total dose of 300,000 units is excreted in the urine within this 5 hour period. For this reason high and frequent doses are required to maintain the elevated serum levels desirable in treating certain severe infections in individuals with normal kidney function. In neonates and young infants, and in individuals with impaired kidney function, excretion is considerably delayed.

Microbiology

Penicillin G exerts a bactericidal action against penicillin-susceptible microorganisms during the stage of active multiplication. It acts through the inhibition of biosynthesis of cell wall mucopeptide rendering the cell wall osmotically unstable. It is not active against the penicillinase-producing bacteria, which include many strains of staphylococci. While *in vitro* studies have demonstrated the susceptibility of most strains of the following organisms, clinical efficacy for infections other than those included in the INDICATIONS AND USAGE section has not been documented. Penicillin G exerts high *in vitro* activity against staphylococci (except penicillinase-producing strains), streptococci (groups A, C, G, H, L, and M), and pneumococci. Other organisms susceptible to penicillin G are *N. gonorrhoeae, Corynebacterium diphtheriae, Bacillus anthracis,* Clostridia, *Actinomyces bovis, Streptobacillus moniliformis, Listeria monocytogenes* and Leptospira. *Treponema pallidum* is extremely sensitive to the bactericidal action of penicillin G. Some species of gram-negative bacilli are sensitive to moderate to high concentrations of the drug obtained with intravenous administration. These include most strains of *Escherichia coli;* all strains of *Proteus mirabilis,* Salmonella and Shigella; and some strains of *Aerobacter aerogenes* and *Alcaligenes faecalis.*

Penicillin acts synergistically with gentamicin or tobramycin against many strains of enterococci.

Susceptibility Testing: Penicillin G Susceptibility Powder or 10 units Penicillin G Susceptibility Discs may be used to determine microbial susceptibility to penicillin G using one of the following standard methods recommended by the National Committee for Laboratory Standards:

M2-A3, "Performance Standards for Antimicrobial Disk Susceptibility Tests"

M7-A, "Methods for Dilution Antimicrobial Susceptibility Tests for Bacteria that Grow Aerobically"

M11-A, "Reference Agar Dilution Procedure for Antimicrobial Susceptibility Testing of Anaerobic Bacteria"

M17-P, "Alternative Methods for Antimicrobial Susceptibility Testing of Anaerobic Bacteria"

Tests should be interpreted by the following criteria:

	Zone Diameter, nearest whole mm		
	Susceptible	Moderately Susceptible	Resistant
Staphylococci	≥29	—	≤28
N. gonorrhoeae	≥20	—	≤19
Enterococci	—	≥15	≤14
Non-enterococcal streptococci and *L. monocytogenes*	≥28	20–27	≤19

	Approximate MIC Correlates	
	Susceptible	Resistant
Staphylococci	≤0.1 μg/mL	β-lactamase
N. gonorrhoeae	≤0.1 μg/mL	β-lactamase
Enterococci	—	≥16 μg/mL
Non-enterococcal streptococci and *L. monocytogenes*	≤0.12 μg/mL	≥4 μg/mL

Interpretations of susceptible, intermediate, and resistant correlate zone size diameters with MIC values. A laboratory report of "susceptible" indicates that the suspected causative microorganism most likely will respond to therapy with penicillin G. A laboratory report of "resistant" indicates that the infecting microorganism most likely will not respond to therapy. A laboratory report of "moderately susceptible" indicates that the microorganism is most likely susceptible if a high dosage of penicillin G is used, or if the infection is such that high levels of penicillin G may be attained, as in urine. A report of "intermediate" using the disk diffusion method may be considered an equivocal result, and dilution tests may be indicated.

Control organisms are recommended for susceptibility testing. Each time the test is performed the following organisms should be included. The range for zones of inhibition is shown below;

Control Organism	Zone of Inhibition Range
Staphylococcus aureus (ATCC 25923)	27–35

INDICATIONS AND USAGE

Aqueous penicillin G (parenteral) is indicated in the therapy of severe infections caused by penicillin G-susceptible microorganisms when rapid and high penicillin levels are required in the conditions listed below. Therapy should be guided by bacteriological studies (including susceptibility tests) and by clinical response.

The following infections will usually respond to adequate dosage of aqueous penicillin G (parenteral):

Streptococcal infections.

NOTE: Streptococci in groups A, C, H, G, L, and M are very sensitive to penicillin G. Some group D organisms are sensitive to the high serum levels obtained with aqueous penicillin G.

Aqueous penicillin (parenteral) is the penicillin dosage form of choice for bacteremia, empyema, severe pneumonia, pericarditis, endocarditis, meningitis, and other severe infections caused by sensitive strains of the gram-positive species listed above.

Pneumococcal infections.
Staphylococcal infections —penicillin G sensitive.
Other infections:
Anthrax.
Actinomycosis.
Clostridial infections (including tetanus).
Diphtheria (to prevent carrier state).
Erysipeloid (*Erysipelothrix insidiosa*) endocarditis.
Fusospirochetal infections—severe infections of the oropharynx (Vincent's), lower respiratory tract and genital area due to *Fusobacterium fusiformisans* spirochetes.

Continued on next page

Roerig—Cont.

Gram-negative bacillary infections (bateremias)—(*E. coli, A. aerogenes, A. faecalis,* Salmonella, Shigella and *P. mirabilis*).
Listeria infections (*Listeria monocytogenes*).
Meningitis and endocarditis.
Pasteurella infections (*Pasteurella multocida*).
Bacteremia and meningitis.
Rat-bite fever (*Spirillum minus* or *Streptobacillus moniliformis*).
Gonorrheal endocarditis and arthritis (*N. gonorrhoeae*).
Syphilis (*T. pallidum*) including congenital syphilis.
Meningococcic meningitis.

Although no controlled clinical efficacy studies have been conducted, aqueous crystalline penicillin G for injection and penicillin G procaine suspension have been suggested by the American Heart Association and the American Dental Association for use as part of a combined parenteral-oral regimen for prophylaxis against bacterial endocarditis in patients with congenital heart disease or rheumatic, or other acquired valvular heart disease when they undergo dental procedures and surgical procedures of the upper respiratory tract.[1] Since it may happen that *alpha* hemolytic streptococci relatively resistant to penicillin may be found when patients are receiving continuous oral penicillin for secondary prevention of rheumatic fever, prophylactic agents other than penicillin may be chosen for these patients and prescribed in addition to their continuous rheumatic fever prophylactic regimen.

NOTE: When selecting antibiotics for the prevention of bacterial endocarditis the physician or dentist should read the full joint statement of the American Heart Association and the American Dental Association.[1]

CONTRAINDICATIONS

A history of a previous hypersensitivity reaction to any penicillin is a contraindication.

WARNINGS

Serious and occasionally fatal hypersensitivity (anaphylactoid) reactions have been reported in patients on penicillin therapy. These reactions are more likely to occur in individuals with a history of penicillin hypersensitivity and/or a history of sensitivity to multiple allergens. There have been reports of individuals with a history of penicillin hypersensitivity who have experienced severe reactions when treated with cephalosporins. Before initiating therapy with any penicillin, careful inquiry should be made concerning previous hypersensitivity reactions to penicillin, cephalosporins, or other allergens. If an allergic reaction occurs, the drug should be discontinued and the appropriate therapy instituted. Serious anaphylactoid reactions require immediate emergency treatment with epinephrine. Oxygen, intravenous steroids, and airway management including incubation, should also be administered as indicated.

PRECAUTIONS

General: Penicillin should be used with caution in individuals with histories of significant allergies and/or asthma.

Intramuscular Therapy: Care should be taken to avoid intravenous or accidental intraarterial administration, or injection into or near major peripheral nerves or blood vessels, since such injections may produce neurovascular damage. Particular care should be taken with IV administration because of the possibility of thrombophlebitis.

In streptococcal infections, therapy must be sufficient to eliminate the organism (10 days minimum) otherwise the sequelae of streptococcal disease may occur. Cultures should be taken following the completion of treatment to determine whether streptococci have been eradicated.

The use of antibiotics may result in overgrowth of nonsusceptible organisms. Constant observation of the patient is essential. If new infections due to bacteria or fungi appear during therapy, the drug should be discontinued and appropriate measures taken. Whenever allergic reactions occur, penicillin should be withdrawn unless, in the opinion of the physician, the condition being treated is life threatening and amenable only to penicillin therapy.

Aqueous penicillin G by the intravenous route in high doses (above 10 million units), should be administered slowly because of the adverse effects of electrolyte imbalance from either the potassium or sodium content of the penicillin. Potassium penicillin G contains 1.7 mEq potassium and 0.3 mEq sodium per million units. The patient's renal, cardiac, and vascular status should be evaluated and if impairment of function is suspected or known to exist a reduction in the total dosage should be considered. Frequent evaluation of electrolyte balance, renal and hematopoietic function is recommended during therapy when high doses of intravenous aqueous penicillin G are used.

Laboratory Tests: In prolonged therapy with penicillin, periodic evaluation of the renal, hepatic, and hematopoietic systems is recommended for organ system dysfunction. This is particularly important in prematures, neonates and other infants, and when high doses are used.

Positive Coomb's tests have been reported after large intravenous doses.

Monitor serum potassium and implement corrective measures when necessary.

When treating gonococcal infections in which primary and secondary syphilis are suspected, proper diagnostic procedures, including dark field examinations, should be done before receiving penicillin and monthly serological tests made for at least four months. All cases of penicillin treated syphilis should receive clinical and serological examinations every six months for two to three years.

In suspected staphylococcal infections, proper laboratory studies, including susceptibility tests, should be performed.

In streptococcal infections, cultures should be taken following completion of treatment to determine whether streptococci have been eradicated. Therapy must be sufficient to eliminate the organism (a minimum of 10 days), otherwise the sequelae of streptococcal disease (e.g., endocarditis, rheumatic fever) may occur.

Drug Interactions: Concurrent administration of bacteriostatic antibiotics (e.g., erythromycin, tetracycline) may diminish the bactericidal effects of penicillins by slowing the rate of bacterial growth. Bactericidal agents work most effectively against the immature cell wall of rapidly proliferating microorganisms. This has been demonstrated *in vitro:* however, the clinical significance of this interaction is not well documented. There are few clinical situations in which the concurrent use of "static" and "cidal" antibiotics are indicated. However, in selected circumstances in which such therapy is appropriate, using adequate doses of antibacterial agents and beginning penicillin therapy first, should minimize the potential for interaction.

Penicillin blood levels may be prolonged by concurrent administration of probenecid which blocks the renal tubular secretion of penicillins.

Displacement of penicillin from plasma protein binding sites will elevate the level of free penicillin in the serum.

Carcinogenesis, Mutagenesis, Impairment of Fertility: No information on long-term studies are available on the carcinogenesis, mutagenesis, or the impairment of fertility with the use of penicillins.

Pregnancy Category B—*Teratogenic Effects:* Reproduction studies performed in the mouse, rat, and rabbit have revealed no evidence of impaired fertility or harm to the fetus due to penicillin G. Human experience with the penicillins during pregnancy has not shown any positive evidence of adverse effects on the fetus. There are, however, no adequate and well controlled studies in pregnant women showing conclusively that harmful effects of these drugs on the fetus can be excluded. Because animal reproduction studies are not always predictive of human response, this drug should be used during pregnancy only if clearly needed.

Nursing Mothers: Penicillins are excreted in human milk. Caution should be exercised when penicillin G is administered to a nursing woman.

Pediatric Use: Penicillins are excreted largely unchanged by the kidney. Because of incompletely developed renal function in infants, the rate of elimination will be slow. Use caution in administering to newborns and evaluate organ system function frequently.

ADVERSE REACTIONS

Penicillin is a substance of low toxicity but does have a significant index of sensitization. The following hypersensitivity reactions have been reported: skin rashes ranging from maculopapular eruptions to exfoliative dermatitis; urticaria; and reactions resembling serum sickness, including chills, fever, edema, arthralgia and prostration. Severe and occasionally fatal anaphylaxis has occurred (see "WARNINGS").

Hemolytic anemia, leucopenia, thrombocytopenia, nephropathy, and neuropathy are rarely observed adverse reactions and are usually associated with high intravenous dosage. Patients given continuous intravenous therapy with penicillin G potassium in high dosage (10 million to 100 million units daily) may suffer severe or even fatal potassium poisoning, particularly if renal insufficiency is present. Hyperreflexia, convulsions and coma may be indicative of this syndrome.

Cardiac arrhythmias and cardiac arrest may also occur. (High dosage of penicillin G sodium may result in congestive heart failure due to high sodium intake.)

The Jarisch-Herxheimer reaction has been reported in patients treated for syphilis.

OVERDOSAGE

Neurological adverse reactions, including convulsions, may occur with the attainment of high CSF levels of beta-lactams. In case of overdosage, discontinue medication, treat symptomatically, and institute supportive measures as required. Penicillin G potassium is hemodialyzable.

DOSAGE AND ADMINISTRATION

Severe infections due to Susceptible Strains of Streptococci, Pneumococci and Staphylococci—bacteremia, pneumonia, endocarditis, pericarditis, empyema, meningitis and other severe infections—a minimum of 5 million units daily.

Syphilis—Aqueous penicillin G may be used in the treatment of acquired and congenital syphilis, but because of the necessity of frequent dosage, hospitalization is recommended. Dosage and duration of therapy will be determined by age of patient and stage of the disease.

Gonorrheal endocarditis—a minimum of 5 million units daily.

Meningococcic meningitis—1–2 million units intramuscularly every 2 hours, or continuous IV drip of 20–30 million units/day.

Actinomycosis—1–6 million units/day for cervicofacial cases; 10–20 million units/day for thoracic and abdominal disease.

Clostridial infections—20 million units/day; penicillin is adjunctive therapy to antitoxin.

Fusospirochetal infections—severe infections of oropharynx, lower respiratory tract and genital area—5–10 million units/day.

Rat-bite fever (*Spirillum minus* or *Streptobacillus moniliformis*)—12–15 million units/day for 3–4 weeks.

Listeria infections (*Listeria monocytogenes*).
Neonates—500,000 to 1 million units/day.
Adults with meningitis—15–20 million units/day for 2 weeks.
Adults with endocarditis—15–20 million units/day for 4 weeks.

Pasteurella infections (*Pasteurella multocida*).
Bacteremia and meningitis—4–6 million units/day for 2 weeks.

Erysipeloid (*Erysipelothrix insidiosa*).
Endocarditis—2–20 million units/day for 4–6 weeks.

Gram-negative bacillary infections (*E. coli, Enterobacter aerogenes, A. faecalis,* Salmonella, Shigella and *Proteus mirabilis*).
Bacteremia—20–80 million units/day.

Diphtheria (carrier state): 300,000–400,000 units of penicillin/day in divided doses for 10–12 days.

Anthrax—A minimum of 5 million units of penicillin/day in divided doses until cure is effected.

For prophylaxis against bacterial endocarditis[1] in patients with congenital heart disease or rheumatic, or other acquired valvular heart disease when undergoing dental procedures or surgical procedures of the upper respiratory tract, use a combined parenteral-oral regimen. One million units of aqueous crystalline penicillin G (30,000 units/kg in children) intramuscularly mixed with 600,000 units procaine penicillin G (600,000 units for children) should be given one-half to one hour before the procedure. Oral penicillin V (phenoxymethyl penicillin), 500 mg for adults or 250 mg for children less than 60 lb, should be given every 6 hours for 8 doses. Doses for children should not exceed recommendations for adults for a single dose or for a 24 hour period.

Reconstitution

The following table shows the amount of solvent required for solution of various concentrations.
[See table below.]

Approx. Desired Concentration (units/ml)	Approx. Volume (ml) 1,000,000 units	Solvent for Vial of 5,000,000 units	Infusion Only 20,000,000 units
50,000	20.0	—	—
100,000	10.0	—	—
250,000	4.0	18.2	75.0
500,000	1.8	8.2	33.0
750,000	—	4.8	—
1,000,000	—	3.2	11.5

When the required volume of solvent is greater than the capacity of the vial, the penicillin can be dissolved by first injecting only a portion of the solvent into the vial, then withdrawing the resultant solution and combining it with the remainder of the solvent in a larger sterile container.

Buffered Pfizerpen (penicillin G potassium) for Injection is highly water soluble. It may be dissolved in small amounts of Water for Injection, or Sterile Isotonic Sodium Chloride Solution for Parenteral Use. All solutions should be stored in a refrigerator. When refrigerated, penicillin solutions may be stored for seven days without significant loss of potency.

Buffered Pfizerpen for Injection may be given intramuscularly or by continuous intravenous drip for dosages of 500,000, 1,000,000, or 5,000,000 units. It is also suitable for intrapleural, intraarticular, and other local instillations.

THE 20,000,000 UNIT DOSAGE MAY BE ADMINISTERED BY INTRAVENOUS INFUSION ONLY.

(1) Intramuscular Injection: Keep total volume of injection small. The intramuscular route is the preferred route of ad-

ministration. Solutions containing up to 100,000 units of penicillin per ml of diluent may be used with a minimum of discomfort. Greater concentration of penicillin G per ml is physically possible and may be employed where therapy demands. When large dosages are required, it may be advisable to administer aqueous solutions of penicillin by means of continuous intravenous drip.

(2) Continuous Intravenous Drip: Determine the volume of fluid and rate of its administration required by the patient in a 24-hour period in the usual manner for fluid therapy, and add the appropriate daily dosage of penicillin to this fluid. For example, if an adult patient requires 2 liters of fluid in 24 hours and a daily dosage of 10 million units of penicillin, add 5 million units to 1 liter and adjust the rate of flow so that the liter will be infused in 12 hours.

(3) Intrapleural or Other Local Infusion: If fluid is aspirated, give infusion in a volume equal to $\frac{1}{4}$ or $\frac{1}{2}$ the amount of fluid aspirated, otherwise, prepare as for intramuscular injection.

(4) Intrathecal Use: The intrathecal use of penicillin in meningitis must be highly individualized. It should be employed only with full consideration of the possible irritating effects of penicillin when used by this route. The preferred route of therapy in bacterial meningitides is intravenous, supplemented by intramuscular injection.

Parenteral drug products should be inspected visually for particulate matter and discoloration prior to administration, whenever solution and container permit.

Sterile solution may be left in refrigerator for one week without significant loss of potency.

HOW SUPPLIED

Buffered Pfizerpen (penicillin G potassium) for Injection is available in vials containing respectively 5,000,000 units × 10's (NDC 0049-0520-83), 5,000,000 units × 100's (NDC 0049-0520-95), 20,000,000 units × 1's (NDC 0049-0530-28), and a bulk pharmacy package of 20,000,000 units × 10's (NDC 0049-0530-83) of dry powder for reconstitution; buffered with sodium citrate and citric acid to an optimum pH.

Each million units contains approximately 6.8 milligrams of sodium (0.3 mEq) and 65.6 milligrams of potassium (1.68 mEq).

Store the dry powder below 86°F (30°C).

REFERENCE

1. American Heart Association. 1977. Prevention of bacterial endocarditis. Circulation. 56:139A–143A.

70-4209-00-5

PFIZERPEN®–AS ℞
(penicillin G procaine)
in Aqueous Suspension
For Intramuscular Use Only

DESCRIPTION

Pfizerpen-AS (penicillin G procaine) is a highly potent antibacterial agent effective against a wide variety of pathogenic organisms. It is an equimolecular compound of procaine and penicillin G in aqueous suspension for intramuscular administration.

Pfizerpen-AS is supplied in 10 ml vials (3,000,000 units).

Chemically, Pfizerpen-AS is: 3,3-Dimethyl-7-oxo-6-(2-phenylacetamido)-4-thia-1-azabicyclo [3.2.0] heptane-2-carboxylic acid compound with 2-(diethylamino) ethyl-p-aminobenzoate (1:1) monohydrate.

It has a molecular weight of 588.72 and the following chemical structure:

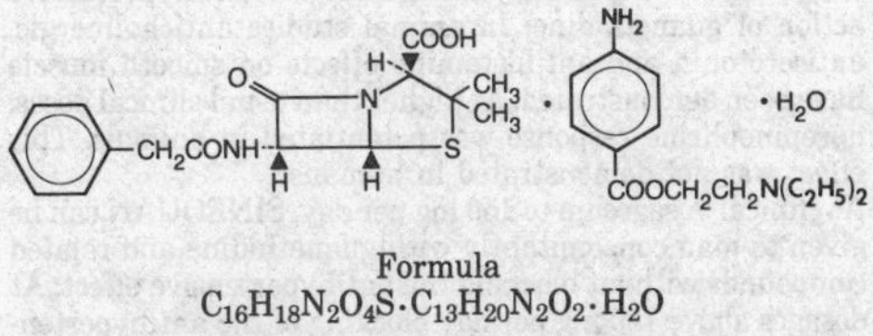

Formula
$C_{16}H_{18}N_2O_4S \cdot C_{13}H_{20}N_2O_2 \cdot H_2O$

Penicillin G procaine is a white, fine crystal, or a white, very fine microcrystalline powder. Penicillin G procaine is odorless or practically so and 1 gram is soluble in 250 ml water. The pH of the aqueous suspension is between 5.0–7.5.

CLINICAL PHARMACOLOGY

Penicillin G procaine is an equimolecular compound of procaine and penicillin G administered intramuscularly as a suspension. It dissolves slowly at the site of injection, giving a plateau type of blood level at about 4 hours, which falls slowly over a period of the next 15–20 hours.

Approximately 60% of penicillin G is bound to serum protein. The drug is distributed throughout the body tissues in widely varying amounts. Highest levels are found in the kidneys with lesser amounts in the liver, skin, and intestines. Penicillin G penetrates into all other tissues to a lesser degree with a very small level found in the cerobrospinal fluid. With normal kidney function the drug is excreted rapidly by tubular excretion. In neonates and young infants, and in individuals with impaired kidney function, excretion is considerably delayed. Approximately 60%–90% of a dose of parenteral penicillin G is excreted in the urine within 24–36 hours. Penicillin G crosses the placental barrier and is found in the amniotic fluid and cord serum.

Microbiology

Penicillin G exerts a bactericidal action against penicillin-susceptible microorganisms during the stage of active multiplication. It acts through the inhibition of biosynthesis of cell wall mucopeptide. It is not active against the penicillinase-producing bacteria, which include many strains of staphylococci. While *in vitro* studies have demonstrated the susceptibility of most strains of the following organisms, clinical efficacy for infections other than those included in the INDICATIONS AND USAGE section has not been documented.

Penicillin G exerts high *in vitro* activity against staphylococci (except penicillinase-producing strains), streptococci (groups A, C, G, H, L, and M), and pneumococci. Other organisms sensitive to penicillin G are *N. gonorrhoeae. Corynebacterium diphtheriae, Bacillus anthracis,* Clostridia, *Actinomyces bovis. Streptobacillus moniliformis, Listeria monocytogenes,* and Leptospira. *Treponema pallidum* is extremely sensitive to the bactericidal action of penicillin G.

Penicillin acts synergistically with gentamicin or tobramycin against many strains of enterococci.

Susceptibility Testing: Penicillin G Susceptibility Powder or 10 units Penicillin G Susceptibility Discs may be used to determine microbial susceptibility to penicillin G using one of the following standard methods recommended by the National Committee for Laboratory Standards:

M2-A3, "Performance Standards for Antimicrobial Disk Susceptibility Tests"

M7-A, "Methods for Dilution Antimicrobial Susceptibility Tests for Bacteria that Grow Aerobically"

M11-A, "Reference Agar Dilution Procedure for Antimicrobial Susceptibility Testing of Anaerobic Bacteria"

M17-P, "Alternative Methods for Antimicrobial Susceptibility Testing of Anaerobic Bacteria"

Tests should be interpreted by the following criteria:

	Zone Diameter, nearest whole mm		
	Susceptible	Moderately Susceptible	Resistant
Staphylococci	≥29	—	≤28
N. gonorrhoeae	≥20	—	≤19
Enterococci	—	≥15	≤14
Non-enterococcal streptococci and *L. monocytogenes*	≥28	20–27	≤19

	Approximate MIC Correlates	
	Susceptible	Resistant
Staphylococci	≤0.1 μg/mL	β-lactamase
N. gonorrhoeae	≤0.1 μg/mL	β-lactamase
Enterococci	—	≥16 μg/mL
Non-enterococcal streptococci and *L. monocytogenes*	≤0.12 μg/mL	≥4 μg/mL

Interpretations of susceptible, intermediate, and resistant correlate zone size diameters with MIC values. A laboratory report of "susceptible" indicates that the suspected causative microorganism most likely will respond to therapy with penicillin G. A laboratory report of "resistant" indicates that the infecting microorganism most likely will not respond to therapy. A laboratory report of "moderately susceptible" indicates that the microorganism is most likely susceptible if a high dosage of penicillin G is used, or if the infection is such that high levels of penicillin G may be attained as in urine. A report of "intermediate" using the disk diffusion method may be considered an equivocal result, and dilution tests may be indicated.

Control organisms are recommended for susceptibility testing. Each time the test is performed the following organisms should be included. The range for zones of inhibition is shown below:

Control Organism	Zone of Inhibition Range
Staphylococcus aureus (ATCC 25923)	27–35

INDICATIONS AND USAGE

Penicillin G procaine is indicated in the treatment of moderately severe infections in both adults and children due to penicillin G-susceptible microorganisms that are susceptible to the low and persistent serum levels common to this particular dosage form in the indications listed below. Therapy should be guided by bacteriological studies (including susceptibility tests) and by clinical response.

NOTE: When high sustained serum levels are required, aqueous penicillin G either IM or IV should be used.

The following infections will usually respond to adequate dosages of intramuscular penicillin G procaine.

Streptococcal infections Group A (without bacteremia). Moderately severe to severe infections of the upper respiratory tract (including middle ear infections-otitis media), skin and soft tissue infections, scarlet fever, and erysipelas.

NOTE: Streptococci in groups A, C, H, G, L, and M are very sensitive to penicillin G. Other groups, including group D (enterococcus) are resistant. Aqueous penicillin is recommended for streptococcal infections with bacteremia.

Pneumococcal infections: Moderately severe infections of the respiratory tract (including middle ear infections-otitis media).

NOTE: Severe pneumonia, empyema, bacteremia, pericarditis, meningitis, peritonitis, and purulent or septic arthritis of pneumoccal etiology are better treated with aqueous penicillin G during the acute stage.

Staphylococcal infections: penicillin G-sensitive. Moderately severe infections of the skin and soft tissues.

NOTE: Reports indicate an increasing number of strains of staphylococci resistant to penicillin G emphasizing the need for culture and sensitivity studies in treating suspected staphylococcal infections.

Indicated surgical procedures should be performed.

Fusospirochetosis (Vincent's gingivitis and pharyngitis). Moderately severe infections of the oropharynx respond to therapy with penicillin G procaine.

NOTE: Necessary dental care should be accomplished in infections involving the gum tissue.

Treponema pallidum (syphilis): all stages.

N. gonorrhoeae: acute and chronic (without bacteremia).

Yaws, Bejel, Pinta.

C. diphtheriae —penicillin G procaine as an adjunct to antitoxin for prevention of the carrier stage.

Anthrax.

Streptobacillus moniliformis and *Spirillum minus* infections (rat bite fever).

Erysipeloid.

Subacute bacterial endocarditis (group A streptococcus) only in extremely sensitive infections.

Prophylaxis Against Bacterial Endocarditis —Although no controlled clinical efficacy studies have been conducted, aqueous crystalline penicillin G for injection and penicillin G procaine suspension have been suggested by the American Heart Association and the American Dental Association for use as part of a combined parenteral-oral regimen for prophylaxis against bacterial endocarditis in patients with congenital heart disease or rheumatic, or other acquired valvular heart disease when they undergo dental procedures and surgical procedures of the upper respiratory tract.[1] Since it may happen that *alpha* hemolytic streptococci relatively resistant to penicillin may be found when patients are receiving continuous oral penicillin for secondary prevention of rheumatic fever, prophylactic agents other than penicillin may be chosen for these patients and prescribed in addition to their continuous rheumatic fever prophylactic regimen.

NOTE: When selecting antibiotics for the prevention of bacterial endocarditis the physician or dentist should read the full joint statement of the American Heart Association and the American Dental Association.[1]

CONTRAINDICATIONS

A previous hypersensitivity reaction to any penicillin or procaine is a contraindication.

WARNINGS

Serious and occasionally fatal hypersensitivity (anaphylactoid) reactions have been reported in patients on penicillin therapy. These reactions are more likely to occur in individuals with a history of penicillin hypersensitivity and/or a history of sensitivity to multiple allergens. There have been reports of individuals with a history of penicillin hypersensitivity who have experienced severe reactions when treated with cephalosporins. Before initiating therapy with any penicillin, careful inquiry should be made concerning previous hypersensitivity reactions to penicillin, cephalosporins, or other allergens. If an allergic reaction occurs, the drug should be discontinued and the appropriate therapy instituted. Serious anaphylactoid reactions require immediate emergency treatment with epinephrine. Oxygen, intravenous steroids, and airway management—including intubation, should be administered as indicated.

Immediate toxic reactions to procaine may occur in some individuals, particularly when a large single dose is administered in the treatment of gonorrhea (4.8 million units). These reactions may be manifested by mental disturbances including anxiety, confusion, agitation, depression, weakness, seizures, hallucinations, combativeness, and expressed "fear of impending death." The reactions noted in carefully controlled studies occurred in approximately one in 500 patients treated for gonorrhea. Reactions are transient, lasting from 15–30 minutes.

Continued on next page

Roerig—Cont.

PRECAUTIONS

General: Penicillin should be used with caution in individuals with histories of significant allergies and/or asthma.

Intramuscular Therapy: Care should be taken to avoid intravenous or accidental intraarterial administration, or injection into or near major peripheral nerves or blood vessels, since such injections may produce neurovascular damage.

As with all intramuscular preparations, Pfizerpen-AS (penicillin G procaine) should be injected well within the body of a relatively large muscle, ADULTS: The preferred site is the upper quadrant of the buttock (i.e., gluteus maximus), or the mid-lateral thigh. CHILDREN: It is recommended that intramuscular injections be given preferably in the mid-lateral muscles of the thigh. In infants and small children the periphery of the upper outer quadrant of the gluteal region should only be used when necessary, such as in burn patients, in order to minimize the possibility of damage to the sciatic nerve.

The deltoid area should be used only if well developed, such as in certain adults and older children, and then only with caution to avoid radial nerve injury. Intramuscular injections should not be made into the lower and mid-third of the upper arm. As with all intramuscular injections, aspiration is necessary to help avoid inadvertent injection into a blood vessel.

In streptococcal infections, therapy must be sufficient to eliminate the organism (10 days minimum), otherwise the sequelae of streptococcal disease may occur. Cultures should be taken following completion of treatment to determine whether streptococci have been eradicated.

The use of antibiotics may result in overgrowth of nonsusceptible organisms. Constant observation of the patient is essential. If new infections due to bacteria or fungi appear during therapy, the drug should be discontinued and appropriate measures taken. Whenever allergic reactions occur, penicillin should be withdrawn unless, in the opinion of the physician, the condition being treated is life threatening and amenable only to penicillin therapy.

A small percentage of patients are sensitive to procaine. If there is a history of sensitivity make the usual test: Inject intradermally 0.1 ml of a 1 to 2 percent solution. Development of an erythema, wheal, flare, or eruption indicates procaine sensitivity. Sensitivity should be treated by the usual methods, including barbiturates, and penicillin G procaine preparations should not be used. Antihistamines appear beneficial in treatment of procaine reactions.

Laboratory Tests: In prolonged therapy with penicillin, periodic evaluation of the renal, hepatic, and hematopoietic systems is recommended. This is particularly important in prematures, neonates and other infants, and when high doses are used.

When treating gonococcal infections in which primary or secondary syphilis may be suspected, proper diagnostic procedures, including dark field examinations, should be done. In all cases in which concomitant syphilis is suspected, monthly serological tests should be made for at least four months. All cases of penicillin treated syphilis should receive clinical and serological examinations every six months for two to three years.

In suspected staphylococcal infections, proper laboratory studies, including susceptibility tests, should be performed.

In streptococcal infections, cultures should be taken following completion of treatment to determine whether streptoccci have been eradicated.

Drug Interactions: Concurrent administration of bacteriostatic antibiotics (e.g., erythromycin, tetracycline) may diminish the bactericidal effects of penicillins by slowing the rate of bacterial growth. Bactericidal agents work most effectively against the immature cell wall of rapidly proliferating microorganisms. This has been demonstrated *in vitro*; however, the clinical significance of this interaction is not well documented. There are few clinical situations in which the concurrent use of "static" and "cidal" antibiotics are indicated. However, in selected circumstances in which such therapy is appropriate, using adequate doses of antibacterial agents and beginning penicillin therapy first, should minimize the potential for interaction.

Penicillin blood levels may be prolonged by concurrent administration of probenecid which blocks the renal tubular secretion of penicillins.

Displacement of penicillins from plasma protein binding sites will elevate the level of free penicillin in the serum.

Carcinogenesis, Mutagenesis, Impairment of Fertility: No information or long-term studies are available on the carcinogenesis, mutagenesis, or the impairment of fertility with the use of penicillin.

Pregnancy Category B. *Teratogenic Effects:* Reproduction studies performed in the mouse, rat, and rabbit have revealed no evidence of impaired fertility or harm to the fetus due to penicillin G. Human experience with the penicillins during pregnancy has not shown any positive evidence of adverse effects on the fetus. There are, however, no adequate and well controlled studies in pregnant women showing conclusively that harmful effects of these drugs on the fetus can be excluded. Because animal reproduction studies are not always predictive of human response, this drug should be used during pregnancy only if clearly needed.

Nursing Mothers: Penicillin G procaine has been reported in milk. Caution should be exercised when penicillin G is administered to a nursing woman.

Pediatric Use: Penicillins are excreted largely unchanged by the kidney. Because of incompletely developed renal function in infants, the rate of elimination will be slow. Use caution in administering to newborns and evaluate organ system function frequently.

ADVERSE REACTIONS

Penicillin is a substance of low toxicity, but does possess a significant index of sensitization. The following hypersensitivity reactions associated with use of penicillin have been reported: skin rashes, ranging from maculopapular eruptions to exfoliative dermatitis; urticaria, serum sickness-like reactions, including chills, fever, edema, arthralgia, and prostration. Severe and often fatal anaphylaxis has been reported (see WARNINGS). As with other treatments for syphilis, the Jarisch-Herxheimer reaction has been reported. Procaine toxicity manifestations have been reported (see WARNINGS). Procaine hypersensitivity reactions have not been reported with this drug.

OVERDOSAGE

In case of overdosage, discontinue medication, treat symptomatically, and institute supportive measures as required. Convulsions have been reported in individuals receiving 4.8 million units.

Penicillin is hemodialyzable.

DOSAGE AND ADMINISTRATION

Pediatric Dosage Schedule: In children under 3 months of age, the absorption of aqueous penicillin G produces such high and sustained levels that penicillin G procaine dosage forms offer no advantages and are usually unnecessary.

In children under 12 years of age, dosage should be adjusted in accordance with the age and weight of the child, and the severity of the infection.

Under 2 years of age, the dose may be divided between the two buttocks if necessary.

Penicillin G procaine (aqueous) is for intramuscular injection only.

Recommended Dosage for Penicillin G Procaine Aqueous

Pneumonia (pneumococcal), moderately severe (uncomplicated): 600,000–1,000,000 units daily.

Streptococcal infections (group A), moderately severe to severe tonsillitis, erysipelas, scarlet fever, upper respiratory tract, skin and soft tissue: 600,000–1,000,000 units daily for a minimum of 10 days.

Staphylococcal infections, moderately severe to severe: 600,000–1,000,000 units daily.

Bacterial endocarditis (group A streptococci), only in extremely sensitive infections: 600,000–1,000,000 units daily.

For prophylaxis against bacterial endocarditis[1] in patients with congenital heart disease or rheumatic or other acquired valvular heart disease, when undergoing dental procedures or surgical procedures of the upper respiratory tract, use a combined parenteral-oral regimen. One million units of aqueous crystalline penicillin G (30,000 units/kg in children) intramuscularly, mixed with 600,000 units penicillin G (600,000 units for children) should be given one-half to one hour before the procedure. Oral penicillin V (phenoxymethyl penicillin), 500 mg for adults or 250 mg for children less than 60 lb. should be given every six hours for 8 doses. Doses for children should not exceed recommendations for adults for a single dose or for a 24 hour period.

Syphilis: Primary, secondary and latent with a negative spinal fluid in adults and children over 12 years of age: 600,000 units daily for 8 days, total 4,800,000 units.

Late (tertiary neurosyphilis and latent syphilis with positive spinal fluid examination or no spinal fluid examination): 600,000 units daily for 10–15 days, total 6–9 million units.

Congenital syphilis (early and late): 50,000 units/kg per day for a minimum of 10 days.

Yaws, Bejel, and *Pinta:* Treatment as syphilis in corresponding stage of disease.

Gonorrheal infections (uncomplicated): Men or women–4.8 million units intramuscularly divided into at least two doses and injected at different sites at one visit, together with 1 gram of oral probenecid, preferably given at least 30 minutes prior to the injection.

NOTE: Gonorrheal endocarditis should be treated intensively with aqueous penicillin G.

Diphtheria —adjunctive therapy with antitoxin: 300,000–600,000 units daily.

Diphtheria —carrier state: 300,000 units daily for 10 days.

Anthrax —cutaneous: 600,000–1,000,000 units/day.

Vincent's infection (fusospirochetosis): 600,000–1,000,000 units/day.

Erysipeloid: 600,000–1,000,000 units/day.

Streptobacillus moniliformis and *Spirillum minus* (rat bite fever): 600,000–1,000,000 units/day.

Parenteral drug products should be inspected visually for particulate matter and discoloration prior to administration, whenever solution and container permit.

HOW SUPPLIED

Pfizerpen-AS (penicillin G procaine) in Aqueous Suspension is supplied in 10 ml vials (3,000,000 units)—packages of 10 (NDC 0049-0540-95), packages of 100 (NDC 0049-0540-95). Each ml contains 300,000 units penicillin G as penicillin G procaine, and as w/v 0.8% sodium citrate, 0.15% sodium carboxymethylcellulose, 25% of sorbitol solution U.S.P., 0.6% polyvinylpyrrolidone, and 0.6% lecithin.

Preservatives: 0.103% methylparaben, 0.011% propylparaben.

The product should be stored between 2°–8°C (36°–46°F).

REFERENCE

1. American Heart Association, 1977. Prevention of Bacterial Endocarditis. Circulation 56:139A-143A.

70-0033-00-0

SINEQUAN® ℞

[*sin 'a-kwon*]
(doxepin HCl)
Capsules
Oral Concentrate

DESCRIPTION

SINEQUAN (doxepin hydrochloride) is one of a class of psychotherapeutic agents known as dibenzoxepin tricyclic compounds. The molecular formula of the compound is $C_{19}H_{21}NO \cdot HCl$ having a molecular weight of 316. It is a white crystalline solid readily soluble in water, lower alcohols and chloroform.

Inert ingredients for the capsule formulations are: hard gelatin capsules (which may contain Blue 1, Red 3, Red 40, Yellow 10, and other inert ingredients); magnesium stearate; sodium lauryl sulfate; starch.

Inert ingredients for the oral concentrate formulation are: glycerin; methylparaben; peppermint oil; propylparaben; water.

CHEMISTRY

SINEQUAN (doxepin HCl) is a dibenzoxepin derivative and is the first of a family of tricyclic psychotherapeutic agents. Specifically, it is an isomeric mixture of: 1-Propanamine, 3-dibenz [*b,e*] oxepin-11(6*H*)ylidene-*N,N*,-dimethyl-, hydrochloride.

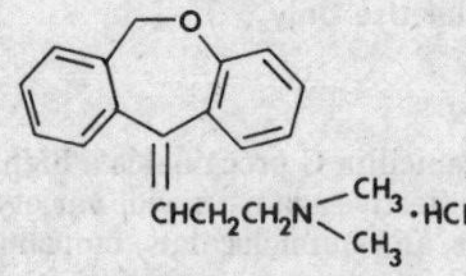

SINEQUAN (doxepin HCl)

ACTIONS

The mechanism of action of SINEQUAN (doxepin HCl) is not definitely known. It is not a central nervous system stimulant nor a monoamine oxidase inhibitor. The current hypothesis is that the clinical effects are due, at least in part, to influences on the adrenergic activity at the synapses so that deactivation of norepinephrine by reuptake into the nerve terminals is prevented. Animal studies suggest that doxepin HCl does not appreciably antagonize the antihypertensive action of guanethidine. In animal studies anticholinergic, antiserotonin and antihistamine effects on smooth muscle have been demonstrated. At higher than usual clinical doses, norepinephrine response was potentiated in animals. This effect was not demonstrated in humans.

At clinical dosages up to 150 mg per day, SINEQUAN can be given to man concomitantly with guanethidine and related compounds without blocking the antihypertensive effect. At dosages above 150 mg per day blocking of the antihypertensive effect of these compounds has been reported.

SINEQUAN is virtually devoid of euphoria as a side effect. Characteristic of this type of compound, SINEQUAN has not been demonstrated to produce the physical tolerance or psychological dependence associated with addictive compounds.

INDICATIONS

SINEQUAN is recommended for the treatment of:

1. Psychoneurotic patients with depression and/or anxiety.
2. Depression and/or anxiety associated with alcoholism (not to be taken concomitantly with alcohol).
3. Depression and/or anxiety associated with organic disease (the possibility of drug interaction should be considered if the patient is receiving other drugs concomitantly).

4. Psychotic depressive disorders with associated anxiety including involutional depression and manic-depressive disorders.

The target symptoms of psychoneurosis that respond particularly well to SINEQUAN include anxiety, tension, depression, somatic symptoms and concerns, sleep disturbances, guilt, lack of energy, fear, apprehension and worry.

Clinical experience has shown that SINEQUAN is safe and well-tolerated even in the elderly patient. Owing to lack of clinical experience in the pediatric population, SINEQUAN is not recommended for use in children under 12 years of age.

CONTRAINDICATIONS

SINEQUAN is contraindicated in individuals who have shown hypersensitivity to the drug. Possibility of cross sensitivity with other dibenzoxepines should be kept in mind.

SINEQUAN is contraindicated in patients with glaucoma or a tendency to urinary retention. These disorders should be ruled out, particularly in older patients.

WARNINGS

The once-a-day dosage regimen of SINEQUAN in patients with intercurrent illness or patients taking other medications should be carefully adjusted. This is especially important in patients receiving other medications with anticholinergic effects.

Usage in Geriatrics

The use of SINEQUAN on a once-a-day dosage regimen in geriatric patients should be adjusted carefully based on the patient's condition.

Usage in Pregnancy

Reproduction studies have been performed in rats, rabbits, monkeys and dogs and there was no evidence of harm to the animal fetus. The relevance to humans is not known. Since there is no experience in pregnant women who have received this drug, safety in pregnancy has not been established. There has been a report of apnea and drowsiness occurring in a nursing infant whose mother was taking SINEQUAN.

Usage in Children

The use of SINEQUAN in children under 12 years of age is not recommended because safe conditions for its use have not been established.

DRUG INTERACTIONS

MAO Inhibitors

Serious side effects and even death have been reported following the concomitant use of certain drugs with MAO inhibitors. Therefore, MAO inhibitors should be discontinued at least two weeks prior to the cautious initiation of therapy with SINEQUAN. The exact length of time may vary and is dependent upon the particular MAO inhibitor being used, the length of time it has been administered, and the dosage involved.

Cimetidine

Cimetidine has been reported to produce clinically significant fluctuations in steady-state serum concentrations of various tricyclic antidepressants. Serious anticholinergic symptoms (i.e., severe dry mouth, urinary retention and blurred vision) have been associated with elevations in the serum levels of tricyclic antidepressant when cimetidine therapy is initiated. Additionally, higher than expected tricyclic antidepressant levels have been observed when they are begun in patients already taking cimetidine. In patients who have been reported to be well controlled on tricyclic antidepressants receiving concurrent cimetidine therapy, discontinuation of cimetidine has been reported to decrease established steady-state serum tricyclic antidepressant levels and compromise their therapeutic effects.

Alcohol

It should be borne in mind that alcohol ingestion may increase the danger inherent in any intentional or unintentional SINEQUAN overdosage. This is especially important in patients who may use alcohol excessively.

Tolazamide

A case of severe hypoglycemia has been reported in a type II diabetic patient maintained on tolazamide (1 gm/day) 11 days after the addition of doxepin (75 mg/day).

PRECAUTIONS

Since drowsiness may occur with the use of this drug, patients should be warned of the possibility and cautioned against driving a car or operating dangerous machinery while taking the drug. Patients should also be cautioned that their response to alcohol may be potentiated.

Since suicide is an inherent risk in any depressed patient and may remain so until significant improvement has occurred, patients should be closely supervised during the early course of therapy. Prescriptions should be written for the smallest feasible amount.

Should increased symptoms of psychosis or shift to manic symptomatology occur, it may be necessary to reduce dosage or add a major tranquilizer to the dosage regimen.

ADVERSE REACTIONS

NOTE: Some of the adverse reactions noted below have not been specifically reported with SINEQUAN use. However, due to the close pharmacological similarities among the tricyclics, the reactions should be considered when prescribing SINEQUAN (doxepin HCl).

Anticholinergic Effects: Dry mouth, blurred vision, constipation, and urinary retention have been reported. If they do not subside with continued therapy, or become severe, it may be necessary to reduce the dosage.

Central Nervous System Effects: Drowsiness is the most commonly noticed side effect. This tends to disappear as therapy is continued. Other infrequently reported CNS side effects are confusion, disorientation, hallucinations, numbness, paresthesias, ataxia, extrapyramidal symptoms, seizures, tardive dyskinesia, and tremor.

Cardiovascular: Cardiovascular effects including hypotension, hypertension, and tachycardia have been reported occasionally.

Allergic: Skin rash, edema, photosensitization, and pruritus have occasionally occurred.

Hematologic: Eosinophilia has been reported in a few patients. There have been occasional reports of bone marrow depression manifesting as agranulocytosis, leukopenia, thrombocytopenia, and purpura.

Gastrointestinal: Nausea, vomiting, indigestion, taste disturbances, diarrhea, anorexia, and aphthous stomatitis have been reported. (See anticholinergic effects.)

Endocrine: Raised or lowered libido, testicular swelling, gynecomastia in males, enlargement of breasts and galactorrhea in the female, raising or lowering of blood sugar levels, and syndrome of inappropriate antidiuretic hormone secretion have been reported with tricyclic administration.

Other: Dizziness, tinnitus, weight gain, sweating, chills, fatigue, weakness, flushing, jaundice, alopecia, headache, exacerbation of asthma, and hyperpyrexia (in association with chlorpromazine) have been occasionally observed as adverse effects.

Withdrawal Symptoms: The possibility of development of withdrawal symptoms upon abrupt cessation of treatment after prolonged SINEQUAN administration should be borne in mind. These are not indicative of addiction and gradual withdrawal of medication should not cause these symptoms.

DOSAGE AND ADMINISTRATION

For most patients with illness of mild to moderate severity, a starting daily dose of 75 mg is recommended. Dosage may subsequently be increased or decreased at appropriate intervals and according to individual response. The usual optimum dose range is 75 mg/day to 150 mg/day.

In more severely ill patients higher doses may be required with subsequent gradual increase to 300 mg/day if necessary. Additional therapeutic effect is rarely to be obtained by exceeding a dose of 300 mg/day.

In patients with very mild symptomatology or emotional symptoms accompanying organic disease, lower doses may suffice. Some of these patients have been controlled on doses as low as 25-50 mg/day.

The total daily dosage of SINEQUAN may be given on a divided or once-a-day dosage schedule. If the once-a-day schedule is employed the maximum recommended dose is 150 mg/day. This dose may be given at bedtime. **The 150 mg capsule strength is intended for maintenance therapy only and is not recommended for initiation of treatment.**

Anti-anxiety effect is apparent before the antidepressant effect. Optimal antidepressant effect may not be evident for two to three weeks.

OVERDOSAGE

A. Signs and Symptoms
   1. Mild: Drowsiness, stupor, blurred vision, excessive dryness of mouth.
   2. Severe: Respiratory depression, hypotension, coma, convulsions, cardiac arrhythmias and tachycardias.

   Also: urinary retention (bladder atony), decreased gastrointestinal motility (paralytic ileus), hyperthermia (or hypothermia), hypertension, dilated pupils, hyperactive reflexes.

B. Management and Treatment
   1. Mild: Observation and supportive therapy is all that is usually necessary.
   2. Severe: Medical management of severe SINEQUAN overdosage consists of aggressive supportive therapy. If the patient is conscious, gastric lavage, with appropriate precautions to prevent pulmonary aspiration, should be performed even though SINEQUAN is rapidly absorbed. The use of activated charcoal has been recommended, as has been continuous gastric lavage with saline for 24 hours or more. An adequate airway should be established in comatose patients and assisted ventilation used if necessary. EKG monitoring may be required for several days, since relapse after apparent recovery has been reported. Arrhythmias should be treated with the appropriate antiarrhythmic agent. It has been reported that many of the cardiovascular and CNS symptoms of tricyclic antidepressant poisoning in adults may be reversed by the slow intravenous administration of 1 mg to 3 mg of physostigmine salicylate. Because physostigmine is rapidly metabolized, the dosage should be repeated as required. Convulsions may respond to standard anticonvulsant therapy, however, barbiturates may potentiate any respiratory depression. Dialysis and forced diuresis generally are not of value in the management of overdosage due to high tissue and protein binding of SINEQUAN.

SUPPLY

SINEQUAN is available as capsules containing doxepin HCl equivalent to:

10 mg—100's (NDC 0662-5340-66), 1000's (NDC 0662-5340-82).

25 mg—100's (NDC 0662-5350-66), (NDC 0049-5350-66); 1000's (NDC 0662-5350-82), 5000's (NDC 0662-5350-94), Unit Dose 10×10's (NDC 0662-5350-41).

50 mg—100's (NDC 0662-5360-66), (NDC 0049-5360-66); 1000's (NDC 0662-5360-82), 5000's (NDC 0662-5360-94).

75 mg—100's (NDC 0662-5390-66), 1000's (NDC 0662-5390-82).

100 mg—100's (NDC 0662-5380-66), 1000's (NDC 0662-5380-82).

150 mg—50's (NDC 0662-5370-50), 500's (NDC 0662-5370-73).

SINEQUAN Oral Concentrate is available in 120 ml bottles (NDC 0662-5100-47) with an accompanying dropper calibrated at 5 mg, 10 mg, 15 mg, 20 mg, and 25 mg. Each ml contains doxepin HCl equivalent to 10 mg doxepin. Just prior to administration, SINEQUAN Oral Concentrate should be diluted with approximately 120 ml of water, whole or skimmed milk, or orange, grapefruit, tomato, prune or pineapple juice. SINEQUAN Oral Concentrate is not physically compatible with a number of carbonated beverages. For those patients requiring antidepressant therapy who are on methadone maintenance, SINEQUAN Oral Concentrate and methadone syrup can be mixed together with Gatorade®, lemonade, orange juice, sugar water, Tang®, or water; but not with grape juice. Preparation and storage of bulk dilutions is not recommended.

65-2135-37-7

Shown in Product Identification Section, page 427

SPECTROBID® ℞

[spek 'trō-bid]

(bacampicillin HCl)

TABLETS and POWDER for ORAL SUSPENSION

DESCRIPTION

SPECTROBID (bacampicillin HCl) is a member of the ampicillin class of semi-synthetic penicillins derived from the basic penicillin nucleus: 6-aminopenicillanic acid. SPECTROBID, as well as ampicillin and other ampicillin analogues, is acid resistant and suitable for oral administration.

SPECTROBID is the hydrochloride salt of 1-ethoxycarbonyloxyethyl ester of ampicillin, available either as tablets or as a microencapsulated oral suspension. During the process of absorption from the gastrointestinal tract, SPECTROBID is hydrolyzed rapidly to ampicillin, a well characterized and effective antibacterial agent. Each 400 mg tablet of SPECTROBID is chemically equivalent to 280 mg of ampicillin, and 125 mg/5 ml of the oral suspension is chemically equivalent to 87.5 mg of ampicillin.

Chemically, SPECTROBID is 1′-ethoxycarbonyloxyethyl -6 - (D-α aminophenylacetamide) - penicillinate hydrochloride.

It has a molecular weight of 501.96 and the following structural formula:

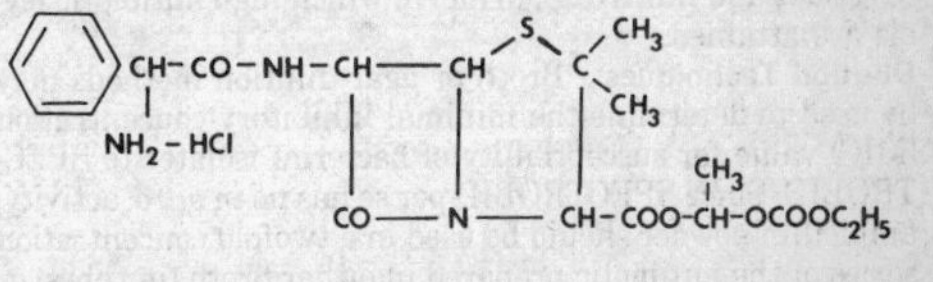

Inert ingredients for the tablets are: hydroxypropyl methylcellulose; lactose; magnesium stearate; microcrystalline cellulose; opaspray.

Inert ingredients for the oral suspension are: carboxymethylcellulose sodium; cherry flavor; compressible sugar; ethylcellulose; hydroxypropyl cellulose; mannitol; saccharin sodium; sodium bicarbonate; titanium dioxide; xanthan gum.

ACTIONS

Clinical Pharmacology

SPECTROBID is characterized by its more complete and more rapid absorption from the GI tract than ampicillin. SPECTROBID tablets of 400 mg, 800 mg, and 1600 mg have provided ampicillin peak serum concentrations of 7.9, 12.9, and 20.1 mcg/ml. These peak levels are approximately three times the levels obtained with administration of equivalent amounts of ampicillin. The areas-under-the-serum-concentration curves obtained during the first 6 hours were 24.8 and 12.9 mcg/ml/hr., when bacampicillin HCl 800 mg and

Continued on next page

Roerig—Cont.

ampicillin 500 mg were administered to adults. (See Graph 1.) Graph 2 shows the serum ampicillin curves following a 28 mg/kg dose of bacampicillin HCl and a 25 mg/kg dose of ampicillin in infants and young children. The areas-under-the-serum-concentration curves were 28.2 and 13.1 respectively. The absorption of the SPECTROBID oral suspension was shown to be equivalent to that of the 400 mg tablet in fasting adult volunteers. A 400 mg dose of suspension gave a peak serum ampicillin concentration of 7.6 mcg/ml and the tablet gave a peak of 7.2 mcg/ml. In fasting pediatric patients a 12.5 mg/kg dose provided a peak of 8.4 mcg/ml.
After oral administration of SPECTROBID tablet or suspension, ampicillin activity in serum peaks at 0.7–0.9 hours (compared to 1.5–2.0 hours after administration of ampicillin). Serum ampicillin half-life is 1.1 hours after either SPECTROBID or ampicillin administration.
Peak tissue and body fluid ampicillin concentrations also are higher after administration of SPECTROBID. Utilizing a special skin window technique to determine ampicillin levels, therapeutic levels in the interstitial fluid were higher and more prolonged after SPECTROBID than after ampicillin administration. SPECTROBID is stable in the presence of gastric acid. SPECTROBID oral suspension absorption is affected by food. Food does not retard absorption of SPECTROBID tablets which may be given without regard to meals. SPECTROBID has been shown to be rapidly and well absorbed after oral administration, with about 75% of a given dose being recoverable in the urine as active ampicillin within 8 hours of administration. Urinary excretion can be delayed by concurrent administration of probenecid. The active moiety of SPECTROBID (i.e., ampicillin) diffuses readily into most body tissues and fluids. In serum, ampicillin is only 20% protein-bound, compared to 60–90% for other penicillins.

Microbiology

SPECTROBID per se has no *in vitro* antibacterial activity and owes its *in vivo* bactericidal activity to the parent compound, ampicillin. The ampicillin class of penicillins (including SPECTROBID) has a broad spectrum of activity against many gram-negative and gram-positive bacteria. Like other penicillins, the ampicillin class of penicillins inhibits the synthesis of cell wall mucopeptide.
Ampicillin class antibiotics are inactivated by β-lactamases produced by certain strains of *Enterobacter, Citrobacter, Haemophilus influenzae,* and *Escherichia coli,* and by most strains of staphylococci and indole-positive *Proteus* spp. Ampicillin class antibiotics are not active against *Pseudomonas, Klebsiella,* or *Serratia* spp.

Susceptibility Testing:

Elution Technique: For the automated method of susceptibility testing (i.e., Autobac™), gram-negative organisms should be tested with the 4.5 mcg ampicillin elution disk, while gram-positive organisms should be tested with the 0.22 mcg disk.

Diffusion Technique: For the Kirby-Bauer method of susceptibility testing, a 10 mcg ampicillin diffusion disk should be used. With this procedure, a laboratory report of "susceptible" indicates that the infecting organism is likely to respond to SPECTROBID therapy, and a report of "resistant" indicates that the infecting organism is not likely to respond to therapy. An "intermediate susceptibility" report suggests that the infecting organism would be susceptible to SPECTROBID if a high dosage is used or if the infection is confined to tissues and fluids (e.g., urine) in which high antibiotic levels are attained.

Dilution Techniques: Broth or agar dilution methods may be used to determine the minimal inhibitory concentration (MIC) value for susceptibility of bacterial isolates to SPECTROBID. Since SPECTROBID per se has no *in vitro* activity, ampicillin powder should be used in a twofold concentration series of the antibiotic prepared in either broth (in tubes) or agar (in petri plates). Tubes should be inoculated to contain 10^4 to 10^5 organisms/ml or plates "spotted" with 10^3 to 10^4 organisms.

INDICATIONS AND USAGE

SPECTROBID is indicated for the treatment of the following infections when caused by ampicillin-susceptible organisms:

1. Upper and Lower Respiratory Tract Infections (including acute exacerbations of chronic bronchitis) due to streptococci (β-hemolytic streptococci, *Streptococcus pyogenes*), pneumococci (*Streptococcus pneumoniae*), nonpenicillinase-producing staphylococci and *H. influenzae;*
2. Urinary Tract Infections due to *E. coli, Proteus mirabilis,* and *Streptococcus faecalis* (enterococci);
3. Skin and Skin Structure Infections due to streptococci and susceptible staphylococci;
4. Gonorrhea (acute uncomplicated urogenital infections) due to *Neisseria gonorrhoeae.*

Bacteriological studies to determine the causative organisms and their susceptibility to SPECTROBID (i.e., ampicillin) should be performed. Therapy may be instituted prior to obtaining results of susceptibility testing. Indicated surgical procedures should be performed.

GRAPH 1.
Comparison of Bacampicillin HCl 800 mg, Ampicillin 500 mg, and Amoxicillin 500 mg

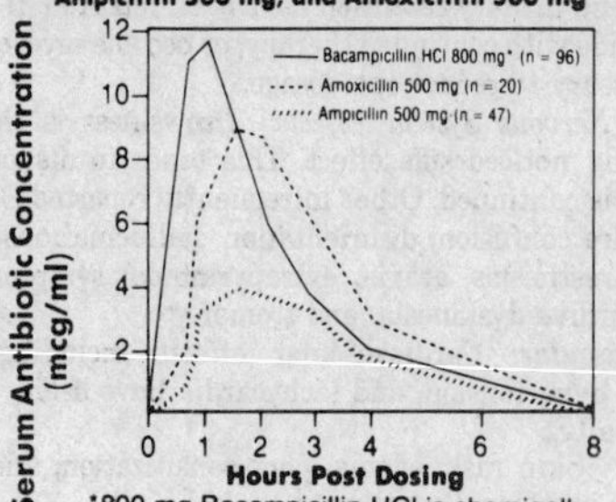

*800 mg Bacampicillin HCl is chemically equivalent to 560 mg of Ampicillin

GRAPH 2.
Crossover Comparison of Bacampicillin HCl Oral Suspension (28 mg/kg)* with Ampicillin Oral Suspension (25 mg/kg) in Fasted Infants and Children (n = 7).

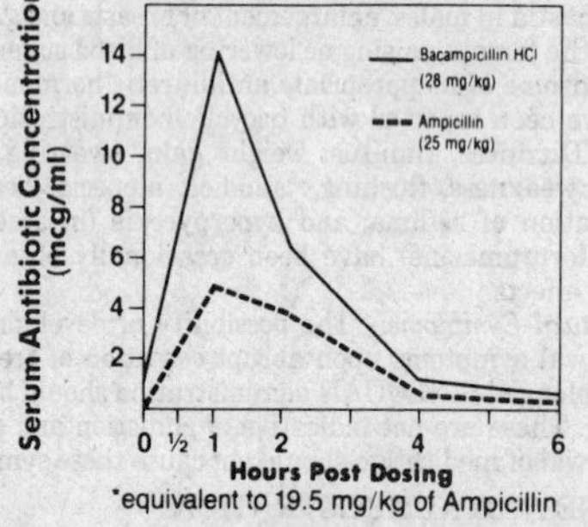

*equivalent to 19.5 mg/kg of Ampicillin

CONTRAINDICATIONS

The use of ampicillin class antibiotics is contraindicated in individuals with a history of an allergic reaction to any of the penicillin antibiotics and/or cephalosporins.

WARNINGS

Serious and occasional fatal hypersensitivity (anaphylactic) reactions have been reported in patients on penicillin therapy. Although anaphylaxis is more frequent following parenteral therapy, it has occurred in patients on oral penicillins. These reactions are more apt to occur in individuals with a history of penicillin hypersensitivity and/or hypersensitivity to multiple allergens.
There have been reports of individuals with a history of penicillin hypersensitivity who have experienced severe reactions when treated with cephalosporins. Before therapy with a penicillin, careful inquiry should be made concerning previous hypersensitivity reactions to penicillins, cephalosporins, and other allergens.
IF AN ALLERGIC REACTION OCCURS, THE DRUG SHOULD BE DISCONTINUED AND THE APPROPRIATE THERAPY INSTITUTED. SERIOUS ANAPHYLACTOID REACTIONS REQUIRE IMMEDIATE EMERGENCY TREATMENT WITH EPINEPHRINE. OXYGEN, INTRAVENOUS STEROIDS, AND AIRWAY MANAGEMENT, INCLUDING INTUBATION, SHOULD ALSO BE ADMINISTERED AS INDICATED.

PRECAUTIONS

1. General: The possibility of superinfections with mycotic or bacterial pathogens should be kept in mind during therapy. If superinfections occur (usually involving *Aerobacter, Pseudomonas,* or *Candida*), the drug should be discontinued and appropriate therapy instituted.
As with any potent agent, it is advisable to check periodically for organ system dysfunction during prolonged therapy. This includes renal, hepatic, and hematopoietic systems and is particularly important in prematures, neonates, and patients with liver or renal impairments.
A high percentage of patients with mononucleosis who receive ampicillin develop a skin rash. Thus, ampicillin class antibiotics should not be administered to patients with mononucleosis.

2. Clinically Significant Drug Interactions: The concurrent administration of allopurinol and ampicillin increases substantially the incidence of rashes in patients receiving both drugs as compared to patients receiving ampicillin alone. It is not known whether this potentiation of ampicillin rashes is due to allopurinol or the hyperuricemia present in these patients. There are no data available on the incidence of rash in patients treated concurrently with SPECTROBID (bacampicillin HCl) and allopurinol. SPECTROBID should not be co-administered with Antabuse (disulfiram).

3. Drug and Laboratory Test Interactions: When testing for the presence of glucose in urine using Clinitest™, Benedict's Solution, or Fehling's Solution, high urine concentrations of ampicillin may result in false-positive reactions. Therefore, it is recommended that glucose tests based on enzymatic glucose oxidase reactions (such as Clinistix™ or Testape™) be used.
Following administration of ampicillin to pregnant women a transient decrease in plasma concentration of total conjugated estriol, estriol-glucuronide, conjugated estrone and estradiol, has been noted.

4. Pregnancy Category B: Reproduction studies have been performed in mice and rats at SPECTROBID doses of up to 750 mg/kg (more than 25 times the human dose) and have revealed no evidence of impaired fertility or harm to the fetus due to SPECTROBID.
There are, however, no adequate and well controlled studies in pregnant women. Because animal reproduction studies are not always predictive of human response, this drug should be used during pregnancy only if clearly needed.

5. Carcinogenesis, Mutagenesis, Impairment of Fertility: No carcinogenicity or mutagenicity studies were conducted. No impairment of fertility and no significant effect on general reproductive performance was observed in rats administered oral doses of up to 750 mg/kg of bacampicillin HCl per day prior to and during mating and gestation. In addition, bacampicillin HCl caused no drug-related effects on the reproductive organs of rats or dogs receiving daily oral doses of up to 800 and 650 mg/kg respectively for 6 months.

6. Labor and Delivery: Oral ampicillin class antibiotics are generally poorly absorbed during labor. Studies in guinea pigs showed that intravenous administration of ampicillin decreased the uterine tone, frequency of contractions, height of contractions, and duration of contractions. However, it is not known whether use of SPECTROBID in humans during labor or delivery has immediate or delayed adverse effects on the fetus, prolongs the duration of labor, or increases the likelihood that forceps delivery or other obstetrical intervention or resuscitation of the newborn will be necessary.

7. Nursing Mothers: Ampicillin class antibiotics are excreted in milk; therefore, caution should be exercised when ampicillin class antibiotics are administered to a nursing woman.

8. Pediatric Use: SPECTROBID tablets are indicated for children weighing 25 kg or more. The SPECTROBID oral suspension is indicated for children and infants weighing less than 25 kg or in those children not able to swallow a tablet.

ADVERSE REACTIONS

As with other penicillins, it may be expected that untoward reactions will be essentially limited to sensitivity phenomena. They are more likely to occur in individuals who have previously demonstrated hypersensitivity to penicillins and in those with a history of allergy, asthma, hay fever, or urticaria.
In well controlled clinical trials conducted in the U.S. the most frequent adverse reactions to SPECTROBID were epigastric upset (2%) and diarrhea (2%). Increased dosage may result in an increased incidence of diarrhea. In the same clinical trials the most frequent adverse effects for amoxicillin were diarrhea (4%) and nausea (2%).
The following adverse reactions have been reported for ampicillin.

Gastrointestinal: diarrhea, gastritis, stomatitis, nausea, vomiting, glossitis, black "hairy" tongue, enterocolitis, and pseudomembranous colitis.

Hypersensitivity Reactions: skin rashes, urticaria, erythema multiforme, and an occasional case of exfoliative dermatitis. These reactions may be controlled with antihistamines and, if necessary, systemic corticosteroids. Whenever such reactions occur, the drug should be discontinued, unless the opinion of the physician dictates otherwise.
Serious and occasional fatal hypersensitivity (anaphylactic) reactions can occur with oral penicillins. (See WARNINGS).

Liver: A moderate rise in serum glutamic oxaloacetic transaminase (SGOT) has been noted in some ampicillin treated patients, but the significance of this finding is unknown. In well controlled clinical trials no difference was noted between ampicillin and SPECTROBID with regard to the incidence of liver function test abnormalities.

Hemic and Lymphatic Systems: Anemia, thrombocytopenia, thrombocytopenic purpura, eosinophilia, leukopenia, and agranulocytosis have been reported during therapy with penicillins. These reactions are usually reversible on discontinuation of therapy and are believed to be hypersensitivity phenomena.

DOSAGE AND ADMINISTRATION

SPECTROBID tablets may be given without regard to meals. SPECTROBID oral suspension should be administered to fasting patients.

UPPER RESPIRATORY TRACT INFECTIONS (including otitis media) due to streptococci, pneumococci, nonpenicillinase-producing staphylococci and *H. influenzae;*
URINARY TRACT INFECTIONS due to *E. coli, Proteus mirabilis,* and *Streptococcus faecalis;*
SKIN AND SKIN STRUCTURES INFECTIONS due to streptococci and susceptible staphylococci:
Usual Dosage
Adults: 1 × 400 mg tablet every 12 hours (for patients weighing 25 kg or more).
Children: 25 mg/kg per day in 2 equally divided doses at 12 hour intervals.
IN SEVERE INFECTIONS OR THOSE CAUSED BY LESS SUSCEPTIBLE ORGANISMS:
Usual Dosage
Adults: 2 × 400 mg tablets every 12 hours (for patients weighing 25 kg or more).
Children: 50 mg/kg per day in 2 equally divided doses at 12 hour intervals.
LOWER RESPIRATORY TRACT INFECTIONS due to streptococci, pneumococci, nonpenicillinase-producing staphylococci, and *H. influenzae:*
Usual Dosage
Adults: 2 × 400 mg tablets every 12 hours (for patients weighing 25 kg or more).
Children: 50 mg/kg per day in 2 equally divided doses at 12 hour intervals.
GONORRHEA—acute uncomplicated urogenital infections due to *N. gonorrhoeae* (males and females):
1.6 grams (4 × 400 mg tablet plus 1 gram probenecid) as a single oral dose.
No pediatric dosage has been established.
Cases of gonorrhea with a suspected lesion of syphilis should have dark field examination before receiving SPECTROBID and monthly serological tests for a minimum of four months.
Larger doses may be required for stubborn or severe infections.
It should be recognized that in the treatment of chronic urinary tract infections, frequent bacteriological and clinical appraisals are necessary. Smaller doses than those recommended above should not be used. In stubborn infections, therapy may be required for several weeks. It may be necessary to continue clinical and/or bacteriological follow-up for several months after cessation of therapy. Except for gonorrhea, treatment should be continued for a minimum of 48 to 72 hours beyond the time that the patient becomes asymptomatic or evidence of bacterial eradication has been obtained.
IT IS RECOMMENDED THAT THERE BE AT LEAST 10 DAYS' TREATMENT FOR ANY INFECTION CAUSED BY HEMOLYTIC STREPTOCOCCI TO PREVENT THE OCCURRENCE OF ACUTE RHEUMATIC FEVER OR GLOMERULONEPHRITIS.
Directions for Mixing Oral Suspension:
Prepare suspension at the time of dispensing as follows:
Prior to reconstitution, tap bottle to thoroughly loosen powder. Add the required amount (see table below) of water to the contents of the bottle in approximately two equally divided portions and SHAKE WELL after each addition. Let stand at least 30 minutes and SHAKE WELL just prior to administering each dose. Each level teaspoon (5 ml) will contain 125 mg of bacampicillin HCl.

Final Volume after reconstitution	Amount of Water Required for reconstitution
70 ml	53 ml
100 ml	75 ml

Reconstituted suspension *must be stored under refrigeration and discarded after 10 days.*

HOW SUPPLIED
SPECTROBID (bacampicillin HCl) Tablets
400 mg (NDC 0049-0350-66): white, film-coated, oblong, unscored are available in bottles of 100.
SPECTROBID (bacampicillin HCl) Powder for Oral Suspension.
Each 5 ml of reconstituted suspension contains 125 mg of bacampicillin HCl.
Bottles containing the following volumes are available: 70 ml (NDC 0049-0357-37), 100 ml (NDC 0049-0357-44).

69-4092-00-5

Shown in Product Identification Section, page 427

TAO® ℞
[tā′ō]
(troleandomycin)
Capsules

DESCRIPTION
TAO (troleandomycin) is a synthetically derived acetylated ester of oleandomycin, an antibiotic elaborated by a species of *Streptomyces antibioticus.* It is a white crystalline compound, insoluble in water, but readily soluble and stable in the presence of gastric juice. The compound has a molecular weight of 814 and corresponds to the empirical formula $C_{41}H_{67}NO_{15}$.
Inert ingredients in the formulation are: hard gelatin capsules (which may contain inert ingredients); lactose; magnesium stearate; sodium lauryl sulfate; starch.

ACTIONS
TAO is an antibiotic shown to be active *in vitro* against the following gram-positive organisms:
Streptococcus pyogenes
Diplococcus pneumoniae
Susceptibility plate testing: If the Kirby-Bauer method of disc sensitivity is used, a 15 mcg. oleandomycin disc should give a zone of over 18 mm when tested against a troleandomycin sensitive bacterial strain.

INDICATIONS
Diplococcus pneumoniae
Pneumococcal pneumonia due to susceptible strains.
Streptococcus pyogenes
Group A beta-hemolytic streptococcal infections of the upper respiratory tract.
Injectable benzathine penicillin G is considered by the American Heart Association to be the drug of choice in the treatment and prevention of streptococcal pharyngitis and in long term prophylaxis of rheumatic fever.
Troleandomycin is generally effective in the eradication of streptococci from the nasopharynx. However, substantial data establishing the efficacy of TAO in the subsequent prevention of rheumatic fever are not available at present.

CONTRAINDICATIONS
Troleandomycin is contraindicated in patients with known hypersensitivity to this antibiotic.

WARNINGS
Usage in Pregnancy: Safety for use in pregnancy has not been established.
The administration of troleandomycin has been associated with an allergic type of cholestatic hepatitis. Some patients receiving troleandomycin for more than two weeks or in repeated courses have shown jaundice accompanied by right upper quadrant pain, fever, nausea, vomiting, eosinophilia, and leukocytosis. These changes have been reversible on discontinuance of the drug. Liver function tests should be monitored in patients on such dosage, and the drug discontinued if abnormalities develop. Reports in the literature have suggested that the concurrent use of ergotamine-containing drugs and troleandomycin may induce ischemic reactions. Therefore, the concurrent use of ergotamine-containing drugs and troleandomycin should be avoided. Troleandomycin should be administered with caution to patients concurrently receiving estrogen containing oral contraceptives.
Studies in chronic asthmatic patients have suggested that the concurrent use of theophylline and troleandomycin may result in elevated serum concentrations of theophylline. Therefore, it is recommended that patients receiving such concurrent therapy be observed for signs of theophylline toxicity, and that therapy be appropriately modified if such signs develop.

PRECAUTIONS
Troleandomycin is principally excreted by the liver.
Caution should be exercised in administering the antibiotic to patients with impaired hepatic function.

ADVERSE REACTIONS
The most frequent side effects of troleandomycin preparations are gastrointestinal, such as abdominal cramping and discomfort, and are dose related. Nausea, vomiting, and diarrhea occur infrequently with usual oral doses.
During prolonged or repeated therapy, there is a possibility of overgrowth of nonsusceptible bacteria or fungi. If such infections occur, the drug should be discontinued and appropriate therapy instituted.
Mild allergic reactions such as urticaria and other skin rashes have occurred. Serious allergic reactions, including anaphylaxis, have been reported.

DOSAGE AND ADMINISTRATION
Clinical judgment based on the type of infection and its severity should determine dosage within the below listed ranges.
Adults: 250 to 500 mg 4 times a day
Children: 125 to 250 mg (3-5 mg/lb or 6.6 to 11 mg/kg) every 6 hours
When used in streptococcal infection, therapy should be continued for ten days.

HOW SUPPLIED
TAO is supplied as:
Capsules 250 mg: Each capsule contains troleandomycin equivalent to 250 mg of oleandomycin; bottle of 100 (NDC 0049-1590-66).

69-1800-00-7

Shown in Product Identification Section, page 427

TERRA-CORTRIL® ℞
Terramycin ® (oxytetracycline HCl)
—Cortril® (hydrocortisone acetate)
OPHTHALMIC SUSPENSION

DESCRIPTION
Terra-Cortril suspension combines the antibiotic, oxytetracycline HCl ($C_{22}H_{24}N_2O_9 \cdot HCl$) and the adrenocorticoid, hydrocortisone acetate ($C_{23}H_{32}O_6$). **Each ml of Terra-Cortril contains Terramycin (oxytetracycline HCl) equivalent to 5 mg of oxytetracycline, and 15 mg of Cortril (hydrocortisone acetate) incorporated in mineral oil with aluminum tristearate.**

For Ophthalmic Use Only.

CLINICAL PHARMACOLOGY
Corticosteroids suppress the inflammatory response to a variety of agents and they probably delay or slow healing. Since corticoids may inhibit the body's defense mechanism against infection, a concomitant antimicrobial drug may be used when this inhibition is considered to be clinically significant in a particular case.
The anti-infective component in the combination is included to provide action against specific organisms susceptible to it.
Terramycin is considered active against the following microorganisms:
Rickettsiae (Rocky Mountain spotted fever, typhus fever and the typhus group, Q fever, rickettsialpox and tick fevers),
Mycoplasma pneumoniae (PPLO, Eaton Agent),
Agents of psittacosis and ornithosis,
Agents of lymphogranuloma venereum and granuloma inguinale,
The spirochetal agent of relapsing fever (*Borrelia recurrentis*).
The following gram-negative microorganisms:
Haemophilus ducreyi (chancroid),
Pasteurella pestis and *Pasteurella tularensis,*
Bartonella bacilliformis,
Bacteroides species,
Vibrio comma and *Vibrio fetus,*
Brucella species (in conjunction with streptomycin).
Because many strains of the following groups of microorganisms have been shown to be resistant to tetracyclines, culture and susceptibility testing are recommended.
Oxytetracycline is indicated for treatment of infections caused by the following gram-negative microorganisms, when bacteriologic testing indicates appropriate susceptibility to the drug:
Escherichia coli,
Enterobacter aerogenes (formerly *Aerobacter aerogenes*),
Shigella species,
Mima species and *Herellea* species,
Haemophilus influenzae (respiratory infections),
Klebsiella species (respiratory and urinary infections).
Oxytetracycline is indicated for treatment of infections caused by the following gram-positive microorganisms when bacteriologic testing indicates appropriate susceptibility to the drug:
Streptococcus species:
Up to 44 percent of strains of *Streptococcus pyogenes* and 74 percent of *Streptococcus faecalis* have been found to be resistant to tetracycline drugs. Therefore, tetracyclines should not be used for streptococcal disease unless the organism has been demonstrated to be sensitive.
For upper respiratory infections due to Group A beta-hemolytic streptococci, pencillin is the usual drug of choice, including prophylaxis of rheumatic fever.
Diplococcus pneumoniae,
Staphylococcus aureus, skin and soft tissue infections. Oxytetracycline is not the drug of choice in the treatment of any type of staphylococcus infections.
When penicillin is contraindicated, tetracyclines are alternative drugs in the treatment of infections due to:
Neisseria gonorrhoeae,
Treponema pallidum and *Treponema pertenue* (syphilis and yaws),
Listeria monocytogenes,
Clostridium species,
Bacillus anthracis,
Fusobacterium fusiforme (Vincent's infection),
Actinomyces species.
Tetracyclines are indicated in the treatment of trachoma, although the infectious agent is not always eliminated, as judged by immunofluorescence.
Inclusion conjunctivitis may be treated with oral tetracyclines or with a combination of oral and topical agents.
When a decision to administer both a corticoid and an antimicrobial is made, the administration of such drugs in combination has the advantage of greater patient compliance and convenience, with the added assurance that the appropriate dosage of both drugs is administered, plus assured compatibility of ingredients when both types of drug are in

Continued on next page

Roerig—Cont.

the same formulation and, particularly, that the correct volume of drug is delivered and retained.

The relative potency of corticosteroids depends on the molecular structure, concentration, and release from the vehicle.

INDICATIONS AND USAGE

For steroid-responsive inflammatory ocular conditions for which a corticosteroid is indicated and where bacterial infection or risk of bacterial ocular infection exists.

Ocular steroids are indicated in inflammatory conditions of the palpebral and bulbar conjunctiva, cornea, and anterior segment of the globe where the inherent risk of steroid use in certain infective conjunctivitides is accepted to obtain a diminution in edema and inflammation. They are also indicated in chronic anterior uveitis and corneal injury from chemical radiation, thermal burns, or penetration of foreign bodies. The use of a combination drug with an anti-infective component is indicated where the risk of infection is high or where there is an expectation that potentially dangerous numbers of bacteria will be present in the eye.

The particular anti-infective drug in this product is active against the following common bacterial eye pathogens:

Staphylococcus aureus
Streptococci, including *Streptococcus pneumoniae*
Escherichia coli
Neisseria species

The product does not provide adequate coverage against:

Haemophilus influenzae
Klebsiella/Enterobacter species
Pseudomonas aeruginosa
Serratia marcescens

CONTRAINDICATIONS

Epithelial herpes simplex keratitis (dendritic keratitis), vaccinia, varicella, and many other viral diseases of the cornea and conjunctiva. Mycobacterial infection of the eye. Fungal diseases of ocular structures. Hypersensitivity to a component of the medication. (Hypersensitivity to the antibiotic component occurs at a higher rate than for other components.)

The use of these combinations is always contraindicated after uncomplicated removal of a corneal foreign body.

WARNINGS

Prolonged use may result in glaucoma, with damage to the optic nerve, defects in visual acuity and fields of vision, and posterior subcapsular cataract formation. Prolonged use may suppress the host response and thus increase the hazard of secondary ocular infections. In those diseases causing thinning of the cornea or sclera, perforations have been known to occur with the use of topical steroids. In acute purulent conditions of the eye, steroids may mask infection or enhance existing infection. If these products are used for 10 days or longer, intraocular pressure should be routinely monitored even though it may be difficult in children and uncooperative patients.

Employment of steroid medication in the treatment of herpes simplex requires great caution.

PRECAUTIONS

The initial prescription and renewal of the medication order beyond 20 milliliters should be made by a physician only after examination of the patient with the aid of magnification, such as slit lamp biomicroscopy and, where appropriate, fluorescein staining.

The possibility of persistent fungal infections of the cornea should be considered after prolonged steroid dosing.

ADVERSE REACTIONS

Adverse reactions have occurred with steroid/anti-infective combination drugs which can be attributed to the steroid component, the anti-infective component, or the combination. Exact incidence figures are not available since no denominator of treated patients is available.

Reactions occurring most often from the presence of the anti-infective ingredient are allergic sensitizations. The reactions due to the steroid component in decreasing order of frequency are: elevation of intraocular pressure (IOP) with possible development of glaucoma, and infrequent optic nerve damage; posterior subcapsular cataract formation; and delayed wound healing.

Secondary Infection: The development of secondary infection has occurred after use of combinations containing steroids and antimicrobials. Fungal infections of the cornea are particularly prone to develop coincidentally with long-term applications of steroid. The possibility of fungal invasion must be considered in any persistent corneal ulceration where steroid treatment has been used.

Secondary bacterial ocular infection following suppression of host responses also occurs.

DOSAGE AND ADMINISTRATION

Instill 1 or 2 drops of Terra-Cortril Ophthalmic Suspension into the affected eye three times daily.

Not more than 20 milliliters should be prescribed initially and the prescription should not be refilled without further evaluation as outlined in "Precautions" above.

HOW SUPPLIED

Terra-Cortril Ophthalmic Suspension (NDC 0049-0670-48) is supplied in 5 ml vials with separate sterile dropper.

60-2323-00-3

TERRAMYCIN®   ℞
(oxytetracycline)
INTRAMUSCULAR SOLUTION*
FOR INTRAMUSCULAR USE ONLY
contains 2% lidocaine

DESCRIPTION

Oxytetracycline is a product of the metabolism of *Streptomyces rimosus* and is one of the family of tetracycline antibiotics.

Oxytetracycline diffuses readily through the placenta into the fetal circulation, into the pleural fluid and, under some circumstances, into the cerebrospinal fluid. It appears to be concentrated in the hepatic system and excreted in the bile, so that it appears in the feces, as well as in the urine, in a biologically active form.

COMPOSITION

[See table below.]

ACTIONS

Oxytetracycline is primarily bacteriostatic and is thought to exert its antimicrobial effect by the inhibition of protein synthesis. Oxytetracycline is active against a wide range of gram-negative and gram-positive organisms.

The drugs in the tetracycline class have closely similar antimicrobial spectra, and cross resistance among them is common. Microorganisms may be considered susceptible if the M.I.C. (minimum inhibitory concentration) is not more than 4.0 mcg/ml and intermediate if the M.I.C. is 4.0 to 12.5 mcg/ml.

Susceptibility plate testing: A tetracycline disc may be used to determine microbial susceptibility to drugs in the tetracycline class. If the Kirby-Bauer method of disc susceptibility testing is used, a 30 mcg tetracycline disc should give a zone of at least 19 mm when tested against an oxytetracycline-susceptible bacterial strain.

Tetracyclines are readily absorbed and are bound to plasma proteins in varying degree. They are concentrated by the liver in the bile and excreted in the urine and feces at high concentrations and in a biologically active form.

INDICATIONS

Oxytetracycline is indicated in infections caused by the following microorganisms:

Rickettsiae (Rocky Mountain spotted fever, typhus fever and the typhus group, Q fever, rickettsialpox and tick fevers).

Mycoplasma pneumoniae (PPLO, Eaton Agent),

Agents of psittacosis and ornithosis,

Agents of lymphogranuloma venereum and granuloma inguinale,

The spirochetal agent of relapsing fever *(Borrelia recurrentis).*

The following gram-negative microorganisms:

Haemophilus ducreyi (chancroid),

Pasteurella pestis, and *Pasteurella tularensis,*

Bartonella bacilliformis,

Bacteroides species,

Vibrio comma and *Vibrio fetus,*

Brucella species (in conjunction with streptomycin).

Because many strains of the following groups of microorganisms have been shown to be resistant to tetracyclines, culture and susceptibility testing are recommended.

Oxytetracycline is indicated for treatment of infections caused by the following gram-negative microorganisms,

*U.S. Pat. Nos. 3,017,323 and 3,026,248

when bacteriologic testing indicates appropriate susceptibility to the drug:

Escherichia coli,
Enterobacter aerogenes (formerly *Aerobacter aerogenes),*
Shigella species,
Mima species and *Herellea* species,
Haemophilus influenzae (respiratory infections),
Klebsiella species (respiratory and urinary infections).

Oxytetracycline is indicated for treatment of infections caused by the following gram-positive microorganisms when bacteriologic testing indicates appropriate susceptibility to the drug:

Streptococcus species;

Up to 44 percent of strains of *Streptococcus pyogenes* and 74 percent of *Streptococcus faecalis* have been found to be resistant to tetracycline drugs. Therefore, tetracyclines should not be used for streptococcal disease unless the organism has been demonstrated to be sensitive.

For upper respiratory infections due to Group A beta-hemolytic streptococci, penicillin is the usual drug of choice, including prophylaxis of rheumatic fever.

Diplococcus pneumoniae,
Staphylococcus aureus, skin and soft tissue infections. Oxytetracycline is not the drug of choice in the treatment of any type of staphylococcal infections.

When penicillin is contraindicated, tetracyclines are alternative drugs in the treatment of infections due to:

Neisseria gonorrhoeae,
Treponema pallidum and *Treponema pertenue* (syphilis and yaws),
Listeria monocytogenes,
Clostridium species,
Bacillus anthracis,
Fusobacterium fusiforme (Vincent's infection),
Actinomyces species.

In acute intestinal amebiasis, the tetracyclines may be a useful adjunct to amebicides.

Tetracyclines are indicated in the treatment of trachoma, although the infectious agent is not always eliminated, as judged by immunofluorescence.

Inclusion conjunctivitis may be treated with oral tetracyclines or with a combination of oral and topical agents.

CONTRAINDICATIONS

This drug is contraindicated in persons who have shown hypersensitivity to any of the tetracyclines.

WARNINGS

THE USE OF TETRACYCLINES DURING TOOTH DEVELOPMENT (LAST HALF OF PREGNANCY, INFANCY, AND CHILDHOOD TO THE AGE OF 8 YEARS) MAY CAUSE PERMANENT DISCOLORATION OF THE TEETH (YELLOW-GRAY-BROWN). This adverse reaction is more common during long term use of the drugs but has been observed following repeated short term courses. Enamel hypoplasia has also been reported. *TETRACYCLINES, THEREFORE, SHOULD NOT BE USED IN THIS AGE GROUP UNLESS OTHER DRUGS ARE NOT LIKELY TO BE EFFECTIVE OR ARE CONTRAINDICATED.*

If renal impairment exists, even usual oral or parenteral doses may lead to excessive systemic accumulation of the drug and possible liver toxicity. Under such conditions, lower than usual total doses are indicated and, if therapy is prolonged, serum level determinations of the drug may be advisable. This hazard is of particular importance in the parenteral administration of tetracyclines to pregnant or postpartum patients with pyelonephritis. When used under these circumstances, the blood level should not exceed 15 mcg/ml and liver function tests should be made at frequent intervals. Other potentially hepatotoxic drugs should not be prescribed concomitantly.

(In the presence of renal dysfunction, particularly in pregnancy, intravenous tetracycline therapy in daily doses exceeding 2 grams has been associated with deaths due to liver failure.)

Photosensitivity manifested by an exaggerated sunburn reaction has been observed in some individuals taking tetracyclines. Patients apt to be exposed to direct sunlight or ul-

---

Terramycin Intramuscular
contents per ml (w/v)

Ingredient	2 ml Single Dose Ampules		10 ml/Vial Multidose
	100 mg/2 ml	250 mg/2 ml	50 mg/ml 10 ml (5 × 2 ml Doses)
oxytetracycline	50 mg	125 mg	50 mg
lidocaine	2.0%	2.0%	2.0%
magnesium chloride hexahydrate	2.5%	6.0%	2.5%
sodium formaldehyde sulfoxylate	0.5%	0.5%	0.3%
α-monothioglycerol	—	—	1.0%
monoethanolamine	approx. 1.7%	approx. 4.2%	approx. 2.6%
citric acid	—	—	1.0%
propyl gallate	—	—	0.02%
propylene glycol	75.2%	67.0%	74.1%
water	18.8%	16.8%	18.5%

traviolet light should be advised that this reaction can occur with tetracycline drugs, and treatment should be discontinued at the first evidence of skin erythema.

The antianabolic action of the tetracyclines may cause an increase in BUN. While this is not a problem in those with normal renal function, in patients with significantly impaired function, higher serum levels of this drug may lead to azotemia, hyperphosphatemia, and acidosis.

The product contains sodium formaldehyde sulfoxylate which serves as an antioxidant. Upon oxidation, this compound can form a potential sulfiting agent. Sulfiting agents may cause allergic-type reactions including anaphylactic symptoms and life-threatening or less severe asthmatic episodes in certain susceptible people. The over-all prevalence of sulfite sensitivity in the general population is unknown and probably low. Sulfite sensitivity is seen more frequently in asthmatic than in nonasthmatic people.

Usage in pregnancy. (See above "Warnings" about use during tooth development.)

Results of animal studies indicate that tetracyclines cross the placenta, are found in fetal tissues and can have toxic effects on the developing fetus (often related to retardation of skeletal development). Evidence of embryotoxicity has also been noted in animals treated early in pregnancy.

Usage in newborns, infants, and children. (See above "Warnings" about use during tooth development).

All tetracyclines form a stable calcium complex in any bone-forming tissue. A decrease in the fibula growth rate has been observed in prematures given oral tetracycline in doses of 25 mg/kg every 6 hours. This reaction was shown to be reversible when the drug was discontinued.

Tetracyclines are present in the milk of lactating women who are taking a drug in this class.

PRECAUTIONS

As with all intramuscular preparations, Terramycin (oxytetracycline) Intramuscular Solution should be injected well within the body of a relatively large muscle. ADULTS: The preferred sites are the upper outer quadrant of the buttock, (i.e., gluteus maximus), and the mid-lateral thigh. CHILDREN: It is recommended that intramuscular injections be given preferably in the mid-lateral muscles of the thigh. In infants and small children the periphery of the upper outer quadrant of the gluteal region should be used only when necessary, such as in burn patients, in order to minimize the possibility of damage to the sciatic nerve.

The deltoid area should be used only if well developed such as in certain adults and older children, and then only with caution to avoid radial nerve injury. Intramuscular injections should not be made into the lower and mid-thirds of the upper arm. As with all intramuscular injections, aspiration is necessary to help avoid inadvertent injection into a blood vessel.

As with other antibiotic preparations, use of this drug may result in overgrowth of nonsusceptible organisms, including fungi. If superinfection occurs, the antibiotic should be discontinued and appropriate therapy instituted.

In venereal diseases when coexistent syphilis is suspected, a dark field examination should be done before treatment is started and the blood serology repeated monthly for at least 4 months.

Because tetracyclines have been shown to depress plasma prothrombin activity, patients who are on anticoagulant therapy may require downward adjustment of their anticoagulant dosage.

In long term therapy, periodic laboratory evaluation of organ systems, including hematopoietic, renal and hepatic studies should be performed.

All infections due to Group A beta-hemolytic streptococci should be treated for at least 10 days.

Since bacteriostatic drugs may interfere with the bactericidal action of penicillin, it is advisable to avoid giving tetracycline in conjunction with penicillin.

ADVERSE REACTIONS

Local irritation may be present after intramuscular injection. The injection should be deep, with care taken not to injure the sciatic nerve nor inject intravascularly.

Gastrointestinal: anorexia, nausea, vomiting, diarrhea, glossitis, dysphagia, enterocolitis, and inflammatory lesions (with monilial overgrowth) in the anogenital region. These reactions have been caused by both the oral and parenteral administration of tetracyclines.

Skin: maculopapular and erythematous rashes. Exfoliative dermatitis has been reported but is uncommon. Photosensitivity is discussed above. (See "Warnings").

Renal toxicity: Rise in BUN has been reported and is apparently dose related. (See "Warnings").

Hypersensitivity reactions: Urticaria, angioneurotic edema, anaphylaxis, anaphylactoid purpura, pericarditis, and exacerbation of systemic lupus erythematosus.

Bulging fontanels in infants and benign intracranial hypertension in adults have been reported in individuals receiving full therapeutic dosages. These conditions disappeared rapidly when the drug was discontinued.

Blood: Hemolytic anemia, thrombocytopenia, neutropenia, and eosinophilia have been reported.

When given over prolonged periods, tetracyclines have been reported to produce brown-black microscopic discoloration of thyroid glands. No abnormalities of thyroid function studies are known to occur.

DOSAGE AND ADMINISTRATION

Intramuscular Administration:

Adults: The usual daily dose is 250 mg administered once every 24 hours or 300 mg given in divided doses at 8 to 12 hour intervals.

For children above eight years of age: 15–25 mg/kg body weight up to a maximum of 250 mg per single daily injection. Dosage may be divided and given at 8 to 12 hour intervals.

Intramuscular therapy should be reserved for situations in which oral therapy is not feasible.

The intramuscular administration of oxytetracycline produces lower blood levels than oral administration in the recommended dosages. Patients placed on intramuscular oxytetracycline should be changed to the oral dosage form as soon as possible. If rapid, high blood levels are needed, oxytetracycline should be administered intravenously.

In patients with renal impairment: (See "Warnings") Total dosage should be decreased by reduction of recommended individual doses and/or by extending time intervals between doses.

HOW SUPPLIED

Terramycin (oxytetracycline) Intramuscular Solution is available as follows:

250 mg/2 ml—in 2 ml pre-scored glass ampules, packages of 5 (NDC 0049-0770-09).

100 mg/2 ml—in 2 ml pre-scored glass ampules, packages of 5 (NDC 0049-0760-09).

50 mg/ml—in 10 ml multiple dose vials, packages of 5 (NDC 0049-0750-77).

70-1051-00-2

TERRAMYCIN® ℞

(oxytetracycline HCl with polymyxin B sulfate)
OPHTHALMIC OINTMENT
STERILE

DESCRIPTION

Each gram of sterile ointment contains oxytetracycline HCl equivalent to 5 mg oxytetracycline, 10,000 units of polymyxin B sulfate, white petrolatum, and liquid petrolatum.

ACTIONS

Terramycin® is a widely used antibiotic with clinically proved activity against gram-positive and gram-negative bacteria, rickettsiae, spirochetes, large viruses, and certain protozoa.

Polymyxin B Sulfate, one of a group of related antibiotics derived from *Bacillus polymyxa*, is rapidly bactericidal. This action is exclusively against gram-negative organisms. It is particularly effective against *Pseudomonas aeruginosa (B. pyocyaneus)* and Koch-Weeks bacillus, frequently found in local infections of the eye.

There is thus made available a particularly effective antimicrobial combination of the broad-spectrum antibiotic Terramycin as well as polymyxin B sulfate against primarily causative or secondarily infecting organisms.

INDICATIONS

The sterile preparation, Terramycin with Polymyxin B Sulfate Ophthalmic Ointment, is indicated for the treatment of superficial ocular infections involving the conjunctiva and/or cornea caused by Terramycin with Polymyxin B Sulfate-susceptible organisms.

It may be administered topically alone, or as an adjunct to systemic therapy.

It is effective in infections caused by susceptible strains of staphylococci, streptococci, pneumococci, *Hemophilus influenzae, Pseudomonas aeruginosa*, Koch-Weeks bacillus, and *Proteus*.

CONTRAINDICATIONS

This drug is contraindicated in individuals who have shown hypersensitivity to any of its components.

PRECAUTIONS

As with all antibiotic preparations, use of this drug may result in overgrowth of nonsusceptible organisms, including fungi. If superinfection occurs, the antibiotic should be discontinued and appropriate specific therapy should be instituted.

ADVERSE REACTIONS

Terramycin with Polymyxin B Sulfate Ophthalmic Ointment is well tolerated by the epithelial membranes and other tissues of the eye. Allergic or inflammatory reactions due to individual hypersensitivity are rare.

DOSAGE AND ADMINISTRATION

Approximately ½ inch of the ointment is squeezed from the tube onto the lower lid of the affected eye two to four times daily.

The patient should be instructed to avoid contamination of the tip of the tube when applying the ointment.

HOW SUPPLIED

Terramycin with Polymyxin B Sulfate Ophthalmic Ointment is supplied in ⅛ oz., (3.5 g) tubes (NDC 0049-0801-08).

60-2324-00-1

UNASYN® ℞

(ampicillin sodium/sulbactam sodium)

DESCRIPTION

UNASYN is an injectable antibacterial combination consisting of the semisynthetic antibiotic ampicillin sodium and the beta-lactamase inhibitor sulbactam sodium for intravenous and intramuscular administration.

Ampicillin sodium is derived from the penicillin nucleus, 6-aminopenicillanic acid. Chemically, it is monosodium (2S, 5R, 6R)-6-[(R)-2-amino-2-phenylacetamido]-3,3-dimethyl-7-oxo-4-thia-1-azabicyclo[3.2.0]heptane-2-carboxylate and has a molecular weight of 371.39. Its chemical formula is $C_{16}H_{18}N_3NaO_4S$. The structural formula is:

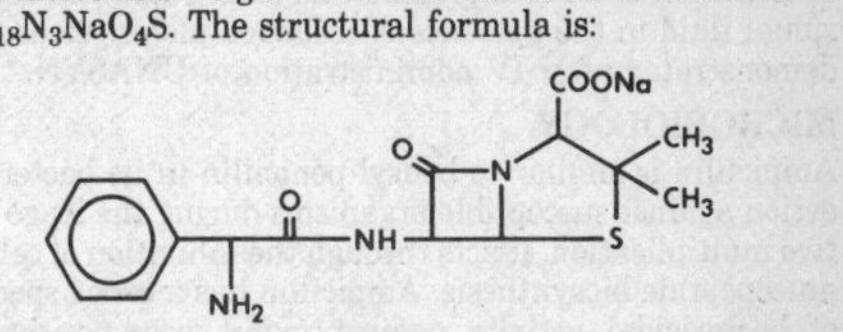

Sulbactam sodium is a derivative of the basic penicillin nucleus. Chemically, sulbactam sodium is sodium penicillinate sulfone; sodium (2S, 5R)-3,3-dimethyl-7-oxo-4-thia-1-azabicyclo[3.2.0]heptane-2-carboxylate 4,4-dioxide. Its chemical formula is $C_8H_{10}NNaO_5S$ with a molecular weight of 255.22. The structural formula is:

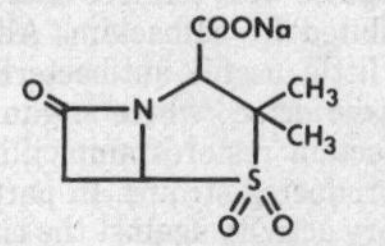

UNASYN, ampicillin sodium/sulbactam sodium parenteral combination, is available as a white to off-white dry powder for reconstitution. UNASYN dry powder is freely soluble in aqueous diluents to yield pale yellow to yellow solutions containing ampicillin sodium and sulbactam sodium equivalent to 250 mg ampicillin per mL and 125 mg sulbactam per mL. The pH of the solutions is between 8.0 and 10.0.

Dilute solutions (up to 30 mg ampicillin and 15 mg sulbactam per mL) are essentially colorless to pale yellow. The pH of dilute solutions remains the same.

1.5 g of UNASYN (1 g ampicillin as the sodium salt plus 0.5 g sulbactam as the sodium salt) parenteral contains approximately 115 mg (5 mEq) of sodium.

3 g of UNASYN (2 g ampicillin as the sodium salt plus 1 g sulbactam as the sodium salt) parenteral contains approximately 230 mg (10 mEq) sodium.

CLINICAL PHARMACOLOGY

General: Immediately after completion of a 15-minute intravenous infusion of UNASYN, peak serum concentrations of ampicillin and sulbactam are attained. Ampicillin serum levels are similar to those produced by the administration of equivalent amounts of ampicillin alone. Peak ampicillin serum levels ranging from 109 to 150 mcg/mL are attained after administration of 2000 mg of ampicillin plus 1000 mg sulbactam and 40 to 71 mcg/mL after administration of 1000 mg ampicillin plus 500 mg sulbactam. The corresponding mean peak serum levels for sulbactam range from 48 to 88 mcg/mL and 21 to 40 mcg/mL, respectively. After an intramuscular injection of 1000 mg ampicillin plus 500 mg sulbactam, peak ampicillin serum levels ranging from 8 to 37 mcg/mL and peak sulbactam serum levels ranging from 6 to 24 mcg/mL are attained.

The mean serum half-life of both drugs is approximately 1 hour in healthy volunteers.

Approximately 75 to 85% of both ampicillin and sulbactam are excreted unchanged in the urine during the first 8 hours after administration of UNASYN to individuals with normal renal function. Somewhat higher and more prolonged serum levels of ampicillin and sulbactam can be achieved with the concurrent administration of probenecid.

In patients with impaired renal function the elimination kinetics of ampicillin and sulbactam are similarly affected, hence the ratio of one to the other will remain constant

Continued on next page

Roerig—Cont.

whatever the renal function. The dose of UNASYN in such patients should be administered less frequently in accordance with the usual practice for ampicillin (see Dosage and Administration).
Ampicillin has been found to be approximately 28% reversibly bound to human serum protein and sulbactam approximately 38% reversibly bound.
The following average levels of ampicillin and sulbactam were measured in the tissues and fluids listed:

TABLE A
Concentration of UNASYN in Various Body Tissues and Fluids

Fluid or Tissue	Dose (grams) Ampicillin/ Sulbactam	Concentration (mcg/mL or mcg/g) Ampicillin/ Sulbactam
Peritoneal Fluid	0.5/0.5 IV	7/14
Blister Fluid (Cantharides)	0.5/0.5 IV	8/20
Tissue Fluid	1/0.5 IV	8/4
Intestinal Mucosa	0.5/0.5 IV	11/18
Appendix	2/1 IV	3/40

Penetration of both ampicillin and sulbactam into cerebrospinal fluid in the presence of inflamed meninges has been demonstrated after IV administration of UNASYN.

MICROBIOLOGY

Ampicillin is similar to benzyl penicillin in its bactericidal action against susceptible organisms during the stage of active multiplication. It acts through the inhibition of cell wall mucopeptide biosynthesis. Ampicillin has a broad spectrum of bactericidal activity against many gram-positive and gram-negative aerobic and anaerobic bacteria. (Ampicillin is, however, degraded by beta-lactamases and therefore the spectrum of activity does not normally include organisms which produce these enzymes.)
A wide range of beta-lactamases found in microorganisms resistant to penicillins and cephalosporins have been shown in biochemical studies with cell free bacterial systems to be irreversibly inhibited by sulbactam. Although sulbactam alone possesses little useful antibacterial activity except against the *Neisseriaciae*, whole organism studies have shown that sulbactam restores ampicillin activity against beta-lactamase producing strains. In particular, sulbactam has good inhibitory activity against the clinically important plasmid mediated beta-lactamases most frequently responsible for transferred drug resistance. Sulbactam has no effect on the activity of ampicillin against ampicillin susceptible strains.
The presence of sulbactam in the UNASYN formulation effectively extends the antibiotic spectrum of ampicillin to include many bacteria normally resistant to it and to other beta-lactam antibiotics. Thus, UNASYN possesses the properties of a broad-spectrum antibiotic and a beta-lactamase inhibitor.
While *in vitro* studies have demonstrated the susceptibility of most strains of the following organisms, clinical efficacy for infections other than those included in the indications section has not been documented.
Gram-Positive Bacteria: *Staphylococcus aureus* (beta-lactamase and non-beta-lactamase producing), *Staphylococcus epidermidis* (beta-lactamase and non-beta-lactamase producing), *Staphylococcus saprophyticus* (beta-lactamase and non-beta-lactamase producing), *Streptococcus faecalis*† (Enterococcus), *Streptococcus pneumoniae*† (formerly *D. pneumoniae*), *Streptococcus pyogenes*†, *Streptococcus viridans*†.
Gram-Negative Bacteria: *Hemophilus influenzae* (beta-lactamase and non-beta-lactamase producing). *Moraxella (Branhamella) catarrhalis* (beta-lactamase and non-beta-lactamase producing). *Escherichia coli* (beta-lactamase and non-beta-lactamase producing). *Klebsiella* species (all known strains are beta-lactamase procuding). *Proteus mirabilis* (beta-lactamase and non-beta-lactamase producing). *Proteus vulgaris, Providencia rettgeri, Providencia stuartii, Morganella morganii,* and *Neisseria gonorrhoeae* (beta-lactamase and non-beta-lactamase producing).
Anaerobes: *Clostridium* species†, *Peptococcus* species†, *Peptostreptococcus* species, *Bacteroides* species, including *B. fragilis.*

Susceptibility Testing
Diffusion Technique: For the Kirby-Bauer method of susceptibility testing, a 20 mcg (10 mcg ampicillin + 10 mcg sulbactam) diffusion disk should be used. The method is one outlined in the NCCLS publication M 2-A4.[1] With this procedure, a report from the laboratory of "Susceptible" indicates that the infecting organism is likely to respond to UNASYN therapy and a report of "Resistant" indicates that the infecting organism is not likely to respond to therapy. An "Intermediate" susceptibility report suggests that the infecting organism would be susceptible to UNASYN if a higher dosage is used or if the infection is confined to tissues or fluids (e.g., urine) in which high antibiotic levels are attained.

†These are not beta-lactamase producing strains and, therefore, are susceptible to ampicillin alone.

Recommended ampicillin/sulbactam, Susceptibility Ranges[1,2,3]

	Resistant	Intermediate	Susceptible
Gram(-) and Staphylococcus			
Bauer/Kirby Zone Sizes	≤11 mm	12–13 mm	≥14 mm
MIC (mcg of ampicillin/mL)	≥32	16	≤8
Hemophilus influenzae			
Bauer/Kirby Zone Sizes	≤19	—	≥20
MIC (mcg of ampicillin/mL)	≥4	—	≤2

[1]The non-beta-lactamase producing organisms which are normally susceptible to ampicillin, such as *Streptococci*, will have similar zone sizes as for ampicillin disks.
[2]*Staphylococci* resistant to methicillin, oxacillin, or nafcillin must be considered resistant to UNASYN.
[3]The quality control cultures should have the following assigned daily ranges for ampicillin/sulbactam:

		Disks	Mode MIC (mcg/mL ampicillin/mcg/mL sulbactam)
E. coli	(ATCC 25922)	20–24 mm	2/1
S. aureus	(ATCC 25923)	29–37 mm	0.12/0.06
E. coli	(ATCC 35218)	13–19 mm	8/4

Dilution Techniques: Broth or agar dilution methods may be used to determine the minimal inhibitory concentration (MIC) value for susceptibility of bacterial isolates to ampicillin/sulbactam. The method used is one outlined in the NCCLS publication M 7-A2.[2] Tubes should be inoculated to contain 10^5 to 10^6 organisms/mL or plates "spotted" with 10^4 organisms.
The recommended dilution method employs a constant ampicillin/sulbactam ratio of 2:1 in all tubes with increasing concentrations of ampicillin. MIC's are reported in terms of ampicillin concentration in the presence of sulbactam at a constant 2 parts ampicillin to 1 part sulbactam.
[See table above.]

INDICATIONS AND USAGE

UNASYN is indicated for the treatment of infections due to susceptible strains of the designated microorganisms in the conditions listed below.
Skin and Skin Structure Infections caused by beta-lactamase producing strains of *Staphylococcus aureus, Escherichia coli*, Klebsiella* spp.* (including *K. pneumoniae*), Proteus mirabilis*, Bacteroides fragilis*, Enterobacter* spp.*, and *Acinetobacter calcoaceticus**.
Intra-Abdominal Infections caused by beta-lactamase producing strains of *Escherichia coli, Klebsiella* spp. (including *K. pneumoniae*), Bacteroides* spp. (including *B. fragilis*), and *Enterobacter* spp*.
Gynecological Infections caused by beta-lactamase producing strains of *Escherichia coli**, and *Bacteroides* spp.* (including *B. fragilis*)*.
While UNASYN is indicated only for the conditions listed above, infections caused by ampicillin-susceptible organisms are also amenable to treatment with UNASYN due to its ampicillin content. Therefore, mixed infections caused by ampicillin-susceptible organisms and beta-lactamase producing organisms susceptible to UNASYN should not require the addition of another antibiotic.
Appropriate culture and susceptibility tests should be performed before treatment in order to isolate and identify the organisms causing infection and to determine their susceptibility to UNASYN.
Therapy may be instituted prior to obtaining the results from bacteriological and susceptibility studies, when there is reason to believe the infection may involve any of the beta-lactamase producing organisms listed above in the indicated organ systems. Once the results are known, therapy should be adjusted if appropriate.

CONTRAINDICATIONS

The use of UNASYN is contraindicated in individuals with a history of hypersensitivity reactions to any of the penicillins.

WARNINGS

SERIOUS AND OCCASIONALLY FATAL HYPERSENSITIVITY (ANAPHYLACTIC) REACTIONS HAVE BEEN REPORTED IN PATIENTS ON PENICILLIN THERAPY. THESE REACTIONS ARE MORE APT TO OCCUR IN INDIVIDUALS WITH A HISTORY OF PENICILLIN HYPERSENSITIVITY AND/OR HYPERSENSITIVITY REACTIONS TO MULTIPLE ALLERGENS. THERE HAVE BEEN REPORTS OF INDIVIDUALS WITH A HISTORY OF PENICILLIN HYPERSENSITIVITY WHO HAVE EXPERIENCED SEVERE REACTIONS WHEN TREATED WITH CEPHALOSPORINS. BEFORE THERAPY WITH A PENICILLIN, CAREFUL INQUIRY SHOULD BE MADE CONCERNING PREVIOUS HYPERSENSITIVITY REACTIONS TO PENICILLINS, CEPHALOSPORINS, AND OTHER ALLERGENS. IF AN ALLERGIC REACTION OCCURS, UNASYN SHOULD BE DISCONTINUED AND THE APPROPRIATE THERAPY INSTITUTED.
SERIOUS ANAPHYLACTOID REACTIONS REQUIRE IMMEDIATE EMERGENCY TREATMENT WITH EPINEPHRINE. OXYGEN, INTRAVENOUS STEROIDS, AND AIRWAY MANAGEMENT, INCLUDING INTUBATION, SHOULD ALSO BE ADMINISTERED AS INDICATED.
Pseudomembranous colitis has been reported with nearly all antibacterial agents, including UNASYN, and has ranged in severity from mild to life-threatening. Therefore, it is important to consider this diagnosis in patients who present with diarrhea subsequent to the administration of antibacterial agents.
Treatment with antibacterial agents alters the normal flora of the colon and may permit overgrowth of clostridia. Studies indicate that toxin produced by *Clostridium difficile* is one primary cause of "antibiotic-associated colitis."
Mild cases of pseudomembranous colitis usually respond to drug discontinuation alone. In moderate to severe cases, consideration should be given to management with fluids and electrolytes, protein supplementation and treatment with an antibacterial drug clinically effective against *C. difficile* colitis.

PRECAUTIONS

General: A high percentage of patients with mononucleosis who receive ampicillin develop a skin rash. Thus, ampicillin class antibiotics should not be administered to patients with mononucleosis. In patients treated with UNASYN the possibility of superinfections with mycotic or bacterial pathogens should be kept in mind during therapy. If superinfections occur (usually involving *Pseudomonas* or *Candida*), the drug should be discontinued and/or appropriate therapy instituted.
Drug Interactions: Probenecid decreases the renal tubular secretion of ampicillin and sulbactam. Concurrent use of probenecid with UNASYN may result in increased and prolonged blood levels of ampicillin and sulbactam. The concurrent administration of allopurinol and ampicillin increases substantially the incidence of rashes in patients receiving both drugs as compared to patients receiving ampicillin alone. It is not known whether this potentiation of ampicillin rashes is due to allopurinol or the hyperuricemia present in these patients. There are no data with UNASYN and allopurinol administered concurrently. UNASYN and aminoglycosides should not be reconstituted together due to the *in vitro* inactivation of aminoglycosides by the ampicillin component of UNASYN.
Drug/Laboratory Test Interactions: Administration of UNASYN will result in high urine concentration of ampicillin. High urine concentrations of ampicillin may result in false positive reactions when testing for the presence of glucose in urine using Clinitest™, Benedict's Solution or Fehling's Solution. It is recommended that glucose tests based on enzymatic glucose oxidase reactions (such as Clinistix™ or Testape™) be used. Following administration of ampicillin to pregnant women, a transient decrease in plasma concentration of total conjugated estriol, estriol-glucuronide, conjugated estrone and estradiol has been noted. This effect may also occur with UNASYN.
Carcinogenesis, Mutagenesis, Impairment of Fertility: Long-term studies in animals have not been performed to evaluate carcinogenic or mutagenic potential.
Pregnancy
Pregnancy Category B: Reproduction studies have been performed in mice, rats, and rabbits at doses up to ten (10) times the human dose and have revealed no evidence of impaired fertility or harm to the fetus due to UNASYN. There are, however, no adequate and well controlled studies in pregnant women. Because animal reproduction studies are not always predictive of human response, this drug should be used during pregnancy only if clearly needed. (See—Drug/Laboratory Test Interactions.)

*Efficacy for this organism in this organ system was studied in fewer than 10 infections.

Labor and Delivery: Studies in guinea pigs have shown that intravenous administration of ampicillin decreased the uterine tone, frequency of contractions, height of contractions, and duration of contractions. However, it is not known whether the use of UNASYN in humans during labor or delivery has immediate or delayed adverse effects on the fetus, prolongs the duration of labor, or increases the likelihood that forceps delivery or other obstetrical intervention or resuscitation of the newborn will be necessary.

Nursing Mothers: Low concentrations of ampicillin and sulbactam are excreted in the milk; therefore, caution should be exercised when UNASYN is administered to a nursing woman.

Pediatric Use: The efficacy and safety of UNASYN have not been established in infants and children under the age of 12.

ADVERSE REACTIONS

UNASYN is generally well tolerated. The following adverse reactions have been reported.

Local Adverse Reactions

Pain at IM injection site—16%
Pain at IV injection site—3%
Thrombophlebitis—3%

Systemic Adverse Reactions

The most frequently reported adverse reactions were diarrhea in 3% of the patients and rash in less than 2% of the patients.

Additional systemic reactions reported in less than 1% of the patients were: itching, nausea, vomiting, candidiasis, fatigue, malaise, headache, chest pain, flatulence, abdominal distension, glossitis, urine retention, dysuria, edema, facial swelling, erythema, chills, tightness in throat, substernal pain, epistaxis and mucosal bleeding.

Adverse Laboratory Changes

Adverse laboratory changes without regard to drug relationship that were reported during clinical trials were:

Hepatic: Increased AST (SGOT), ALT (SGPT), alkaline phosphatase, and LDH.

Hematologic: Decreased hemoglobin, hematocrit, RBC, WBC, neutrophils, lymphocytes, platelets and increased lymphocytes, monocytes, basophils, eosinophils, and platelets.

Blood Chemistry: Decreased serum albumin and total proteins.

Renal: Increased BUN and creatinine.

Urinalysis: Presence of RBC's and hyaline casts in urine.

The following adverse reactions have been reported with ampicillin-class antibiotics and can also occur with UNASYN.

Gastrointestinal: Gastritis, stomatitis, black "hairy" tongue, and enterocolitis. Onset of pseudomembranous colitis symptoms may occur during or after antibiotic treatment (see WARNINGS).

Hypersensitivity Reactions: Urticaria, erythema multiforme, and an occasional case of exfoliative dermatitis have been reported. These reactions may be controlled with antihistamines and, if necessary, systemic corticosteroids. Whenever such reactions occur, the drug should be discontinued, unless the opinion of the physician dictates otherwise. Serious and occasional fatal hypersensitivity (anaphylactic) reactions can occur with a penicillin (see **WARNINGS**).

Hematologic: In addition to the adverse laboratory changes listed above for UNASYN, agranulocytosis has been reported during therapy with penicillins. All of these reactions are usually reversible on discontinuation of therapy and are believed to be hypersensitivity phenomena.

OVERDOSAGE

Neurological adverse reactions, including convulsions, may occur with the attainment of high CSF levels of beta-lactams. Ampicillin may be removed from circulation by hemodialysis. The molecular weight, degree of protein binding and pharmacokinetics profile of sulbactam suggest that this compound may also be removed by hemodialysis.

DOSAGE AND ADMINISTRATION

UNASYN may be administered by either the IV or the IM routes.

For IV administration, the dose can be given by slow intravenous injection over at least 10–15 minutes or can also be delivered, in greater dilutions with 50–100 mL of a compatible diluent as an intravenous infusion over 15–30 minutes.

UNASYN may be administered by deep intramuscular injection. (See Preparation for Intramuscular Injection.)

The recommended adult dosage of UNASYN is 1.5 g (1 g ampicillin as the sodium salt plus 0.5 g sulbactam as the sodium salt) to 3 g (2 g ampicillin as the sodium salt plus 1 g sulbactam as the sodium salt) every six hours. This 1.5 to 3 g range represents the total of ampicillin content plus the sulbactam content of UNASYN, and corresponds to a range of 1 g ampicillin/0.5 g sulbactam to 2 g ampicillin/1 g sulbactam. The total dose of sulbactam should not exceed 4 grams per day.

Impaired Renal Function

In patients with impairment of renal function the elimination kinetics of ampicillin and sulbactam are similarly affected, hence the ratio of one to the other will remain constant whatever the renal function. The dose of UNASYN in such patients should be administered less frequently in accordance with the usual practice for ampicillin and according to the following recommendations:

UNASYN Dosage Guide For Patients With Renal Impairment

Creatinine Clearance (mL/min/1.73m²)	Ampicillin/ Sulbactam Half-Life (Hours)	Recommended UNASYN Dosage
≥30	1	1.5–3.0 g q 6h–q 8h
15–29	5	1.5–3.0 g q 12h
5–14	9	1.5–3.0 g q 24h

When only serum creatinine is available, the following formula (based on sex, weight, and age of the patient) may be used to convert this value into creatinine clearance. The serum creatinine should represent a steady state of renal function.

Males $\frac{\text{weight (kg)} \times (140-\text{age})}{72 \times \text{serum creatinine}}$

Females $0.85 \times \text{above value}$

COMPATABILITY, RECONSTITUTION AND STABILITY

UNASYN sterile powder is to be stored at or below 30°C (86°F) prior to reconstitution.

When concomitant therapy with aminoglycosides is indicated, UNASYN and aminoglycosides should be reconstituted and administered separately, due to the *in vitro* inactivation of aminoglycosides by any of the aminopenicillins.

DIRECTIONS FOR USE

General Dissolution Procedures: UNASYN sterile powder for intravenous and intramuscular use may be reconstituted with any of the compatible diluents described in this insert. Solutions should be allowed to stand after dissolution to allow any foaming to dissipate in order to permit visual inspection for complete solubilization.

Preparation for Intravenous Use

1.5 g and 3.0 g Bottles: UNASYN sterile powder in piggyback units may be reconstituted directly to the desired concentrations using any of the following parenteral diluents. Reconstitution of UNASYN, at the specified concentrations, with these diluents provide stable solutions for the time periods indicated in the following table: (After the indicated time periods, any unused portions of solutions should be discarded.) [See table above.]

Diluent	Maximum Concentration (mg/mL) UNASYN (Ampicillin/Sulbactam)	Use Periods
Sterile Water for Injection	45 (30/15)	8 hrs @ 25°C
	45 (30/15)	48 hrs @ 4°C
	30 (20/10)	72 hrs @ 4°C
0.9% Sodium Chloride Injection	45 (30/15)	8 hrs @ 25°C
	45 (30/15)	48 hrs @ 4°C
	30 (20/10)	72 hrs @ 4°C
5% Dextrose Injection	30 (20/10)	2 hrs @ 25°C
	30 (20/10)	4 hrs @ 4°C
	3 (2/1)	4 hrs @ 25°C
Lactated Ringer's Injection	45 (30/15)	8 hrs @ 25°C
	45 (30/15)	24 hrs @ 4°C
M/6 Sodium Lactate Injection	45 (30/15)	8 hrs @ 25°C
	45 (30/15)	8 hrs @ 4°C
5% Dextrose in 0.45% Saline	3 (2/1)	4 hrs @ 25°C
	15 (10/5)	4 hrs @ 4°C
10% Invert Sugar	3 (2/1)	4 hrs @ 25°C
	30 (20/10)	3 hrs @ 4°C

If piggyback bottles are unavailable, standard vials of UNASYN sterile powder may be used. Initially, the vials may be reconstituted with Sterile Water for Injection to yield solutions containing 375 mg UNASYN per mL (250 mg ampicillin/125 mg sulbactam per mL). An appropriate volume should then be immediately diluted with a suitable parenteral diluent to yield solutions containing 3 to 45 mg UNASYN per mL (2 to 30 mg ampicillin/1 to 15 mg sulbactam per mL).

1.5 g ADD-Vantage® Vials: UNASYN in the ADD-Vantage® system is intended as a single dose for intravenous administration after dilution with the ADD-Vantage® Flexible Diluent Container containing 50 mL, 100 mL or 250 mL of 0.9% Sodium Chloride Injection, USP.

3 g ADD-Vantage® Vials: UNASYN in the ADD-Vantage® system is intended as a single dose for intravenous administration after dilution with the ADD-Vantage® Flexible Diluent Container containing 100 mL or 250 mL of 0.9% Sodium Chloride Injection. USP. UNASYN in the ADD-Vantage® system is to be reconstituted with 0.9% Sodium Chloride Injection, USP only. See INSTRUCTIONS FOR USE OF THE ADD-Vantage® VIAL. Reconstitution of UNASYN, at the specified concentration, with 0.9% Sodium Chloride Injection, USP provides stable solutions for the time period indicated below:

Diluent	Maximum Concentration (mg/mL) UNASYN (Ampicillin/Sulbactam)	Use Period
0.9% Sodium Chloride Injection	30 (20/10)	8 hrs @ 25°C

In 0.9% Sodium Chloride Injection, USP

The final diluted solution of UNASYN should be completely administered *within 8 hours* in order to assure proper potency.

Preparation for Intramuscular Injection

1.5 g and 3.0 g Standard Vials: Vials for intramuscular use may be reconstituted with Sterile Water for Injection USP, 0.5% Lidocaine Hydrochloride Injection USP or 2% Lidocaine Hydrochloride Injection USP. Consult the following table for recommended volumes to be added to obtain solutions containing 375 mg UNASYN per mL (250 mg ampicillin/125 mg sulbactam per mL). Note: *Use only freshly prepared solutions and administer within one hour after preparation.*

UNASYN Vial Size	Volume of Diluent to be Added	Withdrawal Volume*
1.5 g	3.2 mL	4.0 mL
3.0 g	6.4 mL	8.0 mL

*There is sufficient excess present to allow withdrawal and administration of the stated volumes.

Animal Pharmacology: While reversible glycogenosis was observed in laboratory animals, this phenomenon was dose- and time-dependent and is not expected to develop at the therapeutic doses and corresponding plasma levels attained during the relatively short periods of combined ampicillin/sulbactam therapy in man.

HOW SUPPLIED

UNASYN (ampicillin sodium/sulbactam sodium) is supplied as a sterile off-white dry powder in glass vials and piggyback bottles. The following packages are available:

Vials containing 1.5 g (NDC 0049-0013-83) equivalent of UNASYN (1 g ampicillin as the sodium salt plus 0.5 g sulbactam as the sodium salt)

Vials containing 3 g (NDC 0049-0014-83) equivalent of UNASYN (2 g ampicillin as the sodium salt plus 1 g sulbactam as the sodium salt)

Bottles containing 1.5 g (NDC 0049-0022-83) equivalent of UNASYN (1 g ampicillin as the sodium salt plus 0.5 g sulbactam as the sodium salt)

Bottles containing 3 g (NDC 0049-0023-83) equivalent of UNASYN (2 g ampicillin as the sodium salt plus 1 g sulbactam as the sodium salt)

ADD-Vantage® vials containing 1.5 g (NDC 0049-0031-83) equivalent of UNASYN (1 g ampicillin as the sodium salt plus 0.5 g sulbactam as the sodium salt) are distributed by Pfizer Inc.

ADD-Vantage® vials containing 3 g (NDC 0049-0032-83) equivalent of UNASYN (2 g ampicillin as the sodium salt plus 1 g sulbactum as the sodium salt) are distributed by Pfizer Inc.

The 1.5 g UNASYN ADD-Vantage® vials are only to be used with Abbott Laboratories' ADD-Vantage® Flexible Diluent Container containing 0.9% Sodium Chloride Injection, USP, 50 mL, 100 mL, or 250 mL sizes.

The 3 g UNASYN ADD-Vantage® vials are only to be used with Abbott Laboratories' ADD-Vantage® Flexible Diluent Container containing 0.9% Sodium Chloride Injection. USP, 100 mL or 250 mL sizes.

INSTRUCTIONS FOR USE OF THE ADD-Vantage® VIAL

To Open Diluent Container: Peel overwrap from the corner and remove container. Some opacity of the plastic due to moisture absorption during the sterilization process may be observed. This is normal and does not affect the solution quality or safety. The opacity will diminish gradually.

To Assemble Vial and Flexible Diluent Container: (Use Aseptic Technique)

1. Remove the protective covers from the top of the vial and the vial port on the diluent container as follows:

Continued on next page

Roerig—Cont.

a. To remove the breakaway vial cap, swing the pull ring over the top of the vial and pull down far enough to start the opening (see Figure 1), pull the ring approximately half way around the cap and then pull straight up to remove the cap (see Figure 2).

NOTE: Do not access vial with syringe.

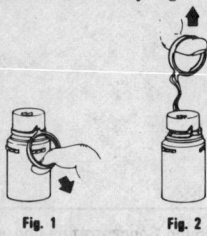

Fig. 1   Fig. 2

b. To remove the vial port cover, grasp the tab on the pull ring, pull up to break the three tie strings, then pull back to remove the cover. (See Figure 3.)
2. Screw the vial into the vial port until it will go no further. THE VIAL MUST BE SCREWED IN TIGHTLY TO ASSURE A SEAL. This occurs approximately ½ turn (180°) after the first audible click. (See Figure 4.) The clicking sound does not assure a seal, the vial must be turned as far as it will go.
NOTE: Once vial is sealed, do not attempt to remove. (See Figure 4.)
3. Recheck the vial to assure that it is tight by trying to turn it further in the direction of assembly.
4. Label appropriately.

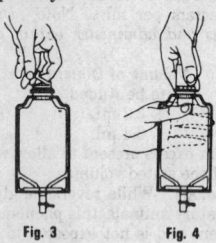

Fig. 3   Fig. 4

To Prepare Admixture
1. Squeeze the bottom of the diluent container gently to inflate the portion of the container surrounding the end of the drug vial.
2. With the other hand, push the drug vial down into the container telescoping the walls of the container. Grasp the inner cap of the vial through the walls of the container. (See Figure 5.)
3. Pull the inner cap from the drug vial. (See Figure 6.) Verify that the rubber stopper has been pulled out, allowing the drug and diluent to mix.
4. Mix container contents thoroughly and use within the specified time.

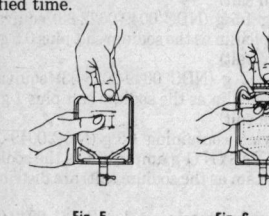

Fig. 5   Fig. 6

70-4361-00-9

REFERENCES
1. National Committee for Clinical Laboratory Standards, *Performance Standards for Antimicrobial Disk Susceptibility Tests*—Fourth Edition. Approved Standard NCCLS Document M2-A4, Vol. 10, No. 7 NCCLS. Villanova, PA. April 1990.
2. National Committee for Clinical Laboratory Standards, *Methods for Dilution Antimicrobial Susceptibility Tests for Bacteria that Grow Aerobically.* Second Edition. Approved Standard NCCLS Document M7-A2. Vol. 10, No 8 NCCLS. Villanova, PA. April 1990.

UROBIOTIC®-250
[u "rō-bī-ot 'ik]
Each capsule contains
Oxytetracycline hydrochloride equivalent to 250 mg. oxytetracycline
Sulfamethizole .... 250 mg.
Phenazopyridine hydrochloride .... 50 mg.

Inert ingredients in the formulation are: hard gelatin capsules (which may contain Green 3, Yellow 6, Yellow 10 and other inert ingredients); magnesium stearate; sodium lauryl sulfate; starch.

ACTIONS
Urobiotic-250 is a product designed for use specifically in urinary tract infections. Terramycin (oxytetracycline HCl) is a widely used antibiotic with clinically proved activity against gram-positive and gram-negative bacteria, rickettsiae, spirochetes, large viruses, and certain protozoa. Terramycin is well tolerated and well absorbed after oral administration. It diffuses readily through the placenta and is present in the fetal circulation. It diffuses into the pleural fluid, and under some circumstances, into the cerebrospinal fluid. Oxytetracycline HCl appears to be concentrated in the hepatic system and is excreted in the bile. It is excreted in the urine and in the feces, in high concentrations, in a biologically active form.
Sulfamethizole is a chemotherapeutic agent active against a number of important gram-positive and gram-negative bacteria. This sulfonamide is well absorbed, has a low degree of acetylation, and is extremely soluble. Because of these features and its rapid renal excretion, sulfamethizole has a low order of toxicity and provides prompt and high concentrations of the active drug in the urinary tract.
Phenazopyridine is an orally absorbed agent which produces prompt and effective local analgesia and relief of urinary symptoms by virtue of its rapid excretion in the urinary tract. These effects are confined to the genitourinary system and are not accompanied by generalized sedation or narcosis.

INDICATIONS
Based on a review of this drug by the National Academy of Sciences-National Research Council and/or other information, FDA has classified the indications as follows:
"Lacking substantial evidence of effectiveness as a fixed combination":
Urobiotic-250 is indicated in the therapy of a number of genitourinary infections caused by susceptible organisms. These infections include the following: pyelonephritis, pyelitis, ureteritis, cystitis, prostatitis, and urethritis.
Since both Terramycin and sulfamethizole provide effective levels in blood, tissue, and urine, Urobiotic-250 provides a multiple antimicrobial approach at the site of infection. Both antibacterial components are active against the most common urinary pathogens, including *Escherichia coli, Pseudomonas aeruginosa, Aerobacter aerogenes, Streptococcus faecalis, Streptococcus hemolyticus, and Micrococcus pyogenes.* Urobiotic-250 is particularly useful in the treatment of infections caused by bacteria more sensitive to the combination than to either component alone. The combination is also of value in those cases with mixed infections, and in those instances where the causative organism is unknown pending laboratory isolation.
Final classification of the less than effective indications require further investigation. Clinical studies to substantiate the efficacy of Urobiotic-250 are ongoing. Completion of these ongoing studies will provide data for final classification of these indications.

CONTRAINDICATIONS
This drug is contraindicated in individuals who have shown hypersensitivity to any of its components.
This drug, because of the sulfonamide component, should not be used in patients with a history of sulfonamide sensitivities, and in pregnant females at term.

WARNINGS
If renal impairment exists, even usual oral or parenteral doses may lead to excessive systemic accumulation of the drug and possible liver toxicity. Under such conditions, lower than usual doses are indicated and if therapy is prolonged, tetracycline serum level determinations may be advisable.
Oxytetracycline HCl, which is one of the ingredients of Urobiotic-250, may form a stable calcium complex in any bone-forming tissue with no serious harmful effects reported thus far in humans. However, use of oxytetracycline during tooth development (last trimester of pregnancy, neonatal period and early childhood) may cause discoloration of the teeth (yellow-grey-brownish). This effect occurs mostly during long term use of the drug but it also has been observed in usual short treatment courses.
Because of its sulfonamide content, this drug should be used only after critical appraisal in patients with liver damage, renal damage, urinary obstruction, or blood dyscrasias. Deaths have been reported from hypersensitivity reactions, agranulocytosis, aplastic anemia, and other blood dyscrasias associated with sulfonamide administration. When used

intermittently, or for a prolonged period, blood counts and liver and kidney function tests should be performed.
Certain hypersensitive individuals may develop a photodynamic reaction precipitated by exposure to direct sunlight during the use of this drug. This reaction is usually of the photoallergic type which may also be produced by other tetracycline derivatives. Individuals with a history of photosensitivity reactions should be instructed to avoid exposure to direct sunlight while under treatment with this or other tetracycline drugs, and treatment should be discontinued at first evidence of skin discomfort.
NOTE: Reactions of a photoallergic nature are exceedingly rare with Terramycin (oxytetracycline HCl). Phototoxic reactions are not believed to occur with Terramycin.

PRECAUTIONS
As with all antibiotic preparations, use of this drug may result in overgrowth of nonsusceptible organisms, including fungi. If superinfection occurs, the antibiotic should be discontinued and appropriate specific therapy should be instituted. This drug should be used with caution in persons having histories of significant allergies and/or asthma.

ADVERSE REACTIONS
Glossitis, stomatitis, proctitis, nausea, diarrhea, vaginitis, and dermatitis, as well as reactions of an allergic nature, may occur during oxytetracycline HCl therapy, but are rare. If adverse reactions, individual idiosyncrasy, or allergy occur, discontinue medication. Rare instances of esophagitis and esophageal ulcerations have been reported in patients receiving capsule forms of drugs in the tetracycline class. Most of these patients took medications immediately before going to bed. (See Dosage and Administration.)
With oxytetracycline therapy bulging fontanels in infants and benign intracranial hypertension in adults have been reported in individuals receiving full therapeutic dosages. These conditions disappeared rapidly when the drug was discontinued.
As in all sulfonamide therapy, the following reactions may occur: nausea, vomiting, diarrhea, hepatitis, pancreatitis, blood dyscrasias, neuropathy, drug fever, skin rash, infection of the conjunctiva and sclera, petechiae, purpura, hematuria and crystalluria. The dosage should be decreased or the drug withdrawn, depending upon the severity of the reaction.

DOSAGE AND ADMINISTRATION
Urobiotic-250 is recommended in adults only. A dose of 1 capsule four times daily is suggested. In refractory cases 2 capsules four times a day may be used.
Therapy should be continued for a minimum of seven days or until bacteriologic cure in acute urinary tract infections. Administration of adequate amounts of fluid along with capsule forms of drugs in the tetracycline class is recommended to wash down the drugs and reduce the risk of esophageal irritation and ulceration. (See Adverse Reactions.)
To aid absorption of the drug, it should be given at least one hour before or two hours after eating. Aluminum hydroxide gel given with antibiotics has been shown to decrease their absorption and is contraindicated.

SUPPLY
Urobiotic-250 capsules: bottles of 50 (NDC 0049-0920-50).

LITERATURE AVAILABLE
Yes.

70-1636-00-9
Shown in Product Identification Section, page 427

VIBRAMYCIN® Hyclate   ℞
[vī "bra-mī 'sin]
(doxycycline hyclate for injection)
INTRAVENOUS
For Intravenous Use Only

DESCRIPTION
Vibramycin (doxycycline hyclate for injection) Intravenous is a broad–spectrum antibiotic synthetically derived from oxytetracycline, and is available as Vibramycin Hyclate (doxycycline hydrochloride hemiethanolate hemihydrate). The chemical designation of this light-yellow crystalline powder is alpha-6-deoxy-5-oxytetracycline. Doxycycline has a high degree of lipoid solubility and a low affinity for calcium binding. It is highly stable in normal human serum.

ACTIONS
Doxycycline is primarily bacteriostatic and thought to exert its antimicrobial effect by the inhibition of protein synthesis. Doxycycline is active against a wide range of gram-positive and gram-negative organisms.
The drugs in the tetracycline class have closely similar antimicrobial spectra and cross resistance among them is common. Microorganisms may be considered susceptible to doxycycline (likely to respond to doxycycline therapy) if the minimum inhibitory concentration (M.I.C.) is not more than 4.0 mcg/ml. Microorganisms may be considered intermediate (harboring partial resistance) if the M.I.C. is 4.0 to 12.5 mcg/

ml and resistant (not likely to respond to therapy) if the M.I.C. is greater than 12.5 mcg/ml.

Susceptibility plate testing: If the Kirby-Bauer method of disc susceptibility testing is used, a 30 mcg doxycycline disc should give a zone of at least 16 mm when tested against a doxycycline-susceptible bacterial strain. A tetracycline disc may be used to determine microbial susceptibility. If the Kirby-Bauer method of disc susceptibility testing is used, a 30 mcg tetracycline disc should give a zone of at least 19 mm when tested against a tetracycline-susceptible bacterial strain.

Tetracyclines are readily absorbed and are bound to plasma proteins in varying degree. They are concentrated by the liver in the bile, and excreted in the urine and feces at high concentrations and in a biologically active form.

Following a single 100 mg dose administered in a concentration of 0.4 mg/ml in a one-hour infusion, normal adult volunteers average a peak of 2.5 mcg/ml, while 200 mg of a concentration of 0.4 mg/ml administered over two hours averaged a peak of 3.6 mcg/ml.

Excretion of doxycycline by the kidney is about 40 percent/72 hours in individuals with normal function (creatinine clearance about 75 ml/min.). This percentage excretion may fall as low as 1-5 percent/72 hours in individuals with severe renal insufficiency (creatinine clearance below 10 ml/min.). Studies have shown no significant difference in serum half-life of doxycycline (range 18-22 hours) in individuals with normal and severely impaired renal function.

Hemodialysis does not alter this serum half-life of doxycycline.

INDICATIONS

Doxycycline is indicated in infections caused by the following microorganisms:

Rickettsiae (Rocky Mountain spotted fever, typhus fever, and the typhus group, Q fever, rickettsialpox and tick fevers).

Mycoplasma pneumoniae (PPLO, Eaton Agent).

Agents of psittacosis and ornithosis.

Agents of lymphogranuloma venereum and granuloma inguinale.

The spirochetal agent of relapsing fever *(Borrelia recurrentis).*

The following gram-negative microorganisms:

Haemophilus ducreyi (chancroid),

Pasteurella pestis and *Pasteurella tularensis,*

Bartonella bacilliformis,

Bacteroides species,

Vibrio comma and *Vibrio fetus,*

Brucella species (in conjunction with streptomycin).

Because many strains of the following groups of microorganisms have been shown to be resistant to tetracyclines, culture and susceptibility testing are recommended. Doxycycline is indicated for treatment of infections caused by the following gram-negative microorganisms when bacteriologic testing indicates appropriate susceptibility to the drug:

Escherichia coli,

Enterobacter aerogenes (formerly *Aerobacter aerogenes),*

Shigella species,

Mima species and *Herellea* species,

Haemophilus influenzae (respiratory infections),

Klebsiella species (respiratory and urinary infections).

Doxycycline is indicated for treatment of infections caused by the following gram-positive microorganisms when bacteriologic testing indicates appropriate susceptibility to the drug:

Streptococcus species:

Up to 44 percent of strains of *Streptococcus pyogenes* and 74 percent of *Streptococcus faecalis* have been found to be resistant to tetracycline drugs. Therefore, tetracyclines should not be used for streptococcal disease unless the organism has been demonstrated to be sensitive.

For upper respiratory infections due to group A beta-hemolytic streptococci, penicillin is the usual drug of choice, including prophylaxis of rheumatic fever.

Diplococcus pneumoniae,

Staphylococcus aureus, respiratory, skin and soft tissue infections. Tetracyclines are not the drugs of choice in the treatment of any type of staphylococcal infections.

When penicillin is contraindicated, doxycycline is an alternative drug in the treatment of infections due to:

Neisseria gonorrhoeae and *N. meningitidis,*

Treponema pallidum and *Treponema pertenue* (syphilis and yaws),

Listeria monocytogenes,

Clostridium species,

Bacillus anthracis,

Fusobacterium fusiforme (Vincent's infection),

Actinomyces species.

In acute intestinal amebiasis, doxycycline may be a useful adjunct to amebicides.

Doxycycline is indicated in the treatment of trachoma, although the infectious agent is not always eliminated, as judged by immunofluorescence.

CONTRAINDICATIONS

This drug is contraindicated in persons who have shown hypersensitivity to any of the tetracyclines.

WARNINGS

THE USE OF DRUGS OF THE TETRACYCLINE CLASS DURING TOOTH DEVELOPMENT (LAST HALF OF PREGNANCY, INFANCY AND CHILDHOOD TO THE AGE OF 8 YEARS) MAY CAUSE PERMANENT DISCOLORATION OF THE TEETH (YELLOW-GRAY-BROWN). This adverse reaction is more common during long-term use of the drugs but has been observed following repeated short-term courses. Enamel hypoplasia has also been reported. *TETRACYCLINE DRUGS, THEREFORE, SHOULD NOT BE USED IN THIS AGE GROUP UNLESS OTHER DRUGS ARE NOT LIKELY TO BE EFFECTIVE OR ARE CONTRAINDICATED.*

Photosensitivity manifested by an exaggerated sunburn reaction has been observed in some individuals taking tetracyclines. Patients apt to be exposed to direct sunlight or ultraviolet light should be advised that this reaction can occur with tetracycline drugs, and treatment should be discontinued at the first evidence of skin erythema.

The antianabolic action of the tetracyclines may cause an increase in BUN. Studies to date indicate that this does not occur with the use of doxycycline in patients with impaired renal function.

Usage in Pregnancy

(See above WARNINGS about use during tooth development.)

Vibramycin Intravenous has not been studied in pregnant patients. It should not be used in pregnant women unless, in the judgment of the physician, it is essential for the welfare of the patient.

Results of animal studies indicate that tetracyclines cross the placenta, are found in fetal tissues and can have toxic effects on the developing fetus (often related to retardation of skeletal development). Evidence of embryotoxicity has also been noted in animals treated early in pregnancy.

Usage in Children

The use of Vibramycin Intravenous in children under 8 years is not recommended because safe conditions for its use have not been established.

(See above WARNINGS about use during tooth development.)

As with other tetracyclines, doxycycline forms a stable calcium complex in any bone-forming tissue. A decrease in the fibula growth rate has been observed in prematures given oral tetracycline in doses of 25 mg/kg every 6 hours. This reaction was shown to be reversible when the drug was discontinued.

Tetracyclines are present in the milk of lactating women who are taking a drug in this class.

PRECAUTIONS

As with other antibiotic preparations, use of this drug may result in overgrowth of nonsusceptible organisms, including fungi. If superinfection occurs, the antibiotic should be discontinued and appropriate therapy instituted.

In venereal diseases when coexistent syphilis is suspected, a dark field examination should be done before treatment is started and the blood serology repeated monthly for at least 4 months.

Because tetracyclines have been shown to depress plasma prothrombin activity, patients who are on anticoagulant therapy may require downward adjustment of their anticoagulant dosage.

In long-term therapy, periodic laboratory evaluation of organ systems, including hematopoietic, renal, and hepatic studies should be performed.

All infections due to group A beta-hemolytic streptococci should be treated for at least 10 days.

Since bacteriostatic drugs may interfere with the bactericidal action of penicillin, it is advisable to avoid giving tetracycline in conjunction with penicillin.

ADVERSE REACTIONS

Gastrointestinal: anorexia, nausea, vomiting, diarrhea, glossitis, dysphagia, enterocolitis, and inflammatory lesions (with monilial overgrowth) in the anogenital region. Hepatotoxicity has been reported rarely. These reactions have been caused by both the oral and parenteral administration of tetracyclines.

Skin: maculopapular and erythematous rashes. Exfoliative dermatitis has been reported but is uncommon. Photosensitivity is discussed above. (See WARNINGS.)

Renal toxicity: Rise in BUN has been reported and is apparently dose related. (See WARNINGS.)

Hypersensitivity reactions: urticaria, angioneurotic edema, anaphylaxis, anaphylactoid purpura, pericarditis and exacerbation of systemic lupus erythematosus.

Bulging fontanels in infants and benign intracranial hypertension in adults have been reported in individuals receiving full therapeutic dosages. These conditions disappeared rapidly when the drug was discontinued.

Blood: Hemolytic anemia, thrombocytopenia, neutropenia and eosinophilia have been reported.

When given over prolonged periods, tetracyclines have been reported to produce brown-black microscopic discoloration of thyroid glands. No abnormalities of thyroid function studies are known to occur.

DOSAGE AND ADMINISTRATION

Note: Rapid administration is to be avoided. Parenteral therapy is indicated only when oral therapy is not indicated. Oral therapy should be instituted as soon as possible. If intravenous therapy is given over prolonged periods of time, thrombophlebitis may result.

THE USUAL DOSAGE AND FREQUENCY OF ADMINISTRATION OF VIBRAMYCIN I.V. (100-200 MG/DAY) DIFFERS FROM THAT OF THE OTHER TETRACYCLINES (1-2 G/DAY). EXCEEDING THE RECOMMENDED DOSAGE MAY RESULT IN AN INCREASED INCIDENCE OF SIDE EFFECTS.

Studies to date have indicated that Vibramycin at the usual recommended doses does not lead to excessive accumulation of the antibiotic in patients with renal impairment.

Adults: The usual dosage of Vibramycin I.V. is 200 mg on the first day of treatment administered in one or two infusions. Subsequent daily dosage is 100 to 200 mg depending upon the severity of infection, with 200 mg administered in one or two infusions.

In the treatment of primary and secondary syphilis, the recommended dosage is 300 mg daily for at least 10 days.

For children above eight years of age: The recommended dosage schedule for children weighing 100 pounds or less is 2 mg/lb. of body weight on the first day of treatment, administered in one or two infusions. Subsequent daily dosage is 1 to 2 mg/lb. of body weight given as one or two infusions, depending on the severity of the infection. For children over 100 pounds the usual adult dose should be used. (See WARNINGS Section for Usage in Children.)

General: The duration of infusion may vary with the dose (100 to 200 mg per day), but is usually one to four hours. A recommended minimum infusion time for 100 mg of a 0.5 mg/ml solution is one hour. Therapy should be continued for at least 24-48 hours after symptoms and fever have subsided. The therapeutic antibacterial serum activity will usually persist for 24 hours following recommended dosage.

Intravenous solutions should not be injected intramuscularly or subcutaneously. Caution should be taken to avoid the inadvertent introduction of the intravenous solution into the adjacent soft tissue.

PREPARATION OF SOLUTION

To prepare a solution containing 10 mg/ml, the contents of the vial should be reconstituted with 10 ml (for the 100 mg/vial container) or 20 ml (for the 200 mg/vial container) of Sterile Water for Injection or any of the ten intravenous infusion solutions listed below. Each 100 mg of Vibramycin (i.e., withdraw entire solution from the 100 mg vial) is further diluted with 100 ml to 1000 ml of the intravenous solutions listed below. Each 200 mg of Vibramycin (i.e., withdraw entire solution from the 200 mg vial) is further diluted with 200 ml to 2000 ml of the following intravenous solutions:

1. Sodium Chloride Injection, USP
2. 5% Dextrose Injection, USP
3. Ringer's Injection, USP
4. Invert Sugar, 10% in Water
5. Lactated Ringer's Injection, USP
6. Dextrose 5% in Lactated Ringer's
7. Normosol-M® in D5-W (Abbott)
8. Normosol-R® in D5-W (Abbott)
9. Plasma-Lyte® 56 in 5% Dextrose (Travenol)
10. Plasma-Lyte® 148 in 5% Dextrose (Travenol)

This will result in desired concentrations of 0.1 to 1.0 mg/ml. Concentrations lower than 0.1 mg/ml or higher than 1.0 mg/ml are not recommended.

Stability:

Vibramycin IV is stable for 48 hours in solution when diluted with Sodium Chloride Injection, USP, or 5% Dextrose Injection, USP, to concentrations between 1.0 mg/ml and 0.1 mg/ml and stored at 25°C. Vibramycin IV in these solutions is stable under fluorescent light for 48 hours, but must be protected from direct sunlight during storage and infusion. Reconstituted solutions (1.0 to 0.1 mg/ml) may be stored up to 72 hours prior to start of infusion if refrigerated and protected from sunlight and artificial light. Infusion must then be completed within 12 hours. Solutions must be used within these time periods or discarded.

Vibramycin IV, when diluted with Ringer's Injection, USP, or Invert Sugar, 10% in Water, or Normosol-M® in D5-W (Abbott), or Normosol-R® in D5-W (Abbott), or Plasma-Lyte® 56 in 5% Dextrose (Travenol), or Plasma-Lyte® 148 in 5% Dextrose (Travenol) to a concentration between 1.0 mg/ml and 0.1 mg/ml, must be completely infused within 12

Continued on next page

Roerig—Cont.

hours after reconstitution to ensure adequate stability. During infusion, the solution must be protected from direct sunlight. Reconstituted solutions (1.0 to 0.1 mg/ml) may be stored up to 72 hours prior to start of infusion if refrigerated and protected from sunlight and artifical light. Infusion must then be completed within 12 hours. Solutions must be used within these time periods or discarded.
When diluted with Lactated Ringer's Injection, USP, or Dextrose 5% in Lactated Ringer's, infusion of the solution (ca. 1.0 mg/ml) or lower concentrations (not less than 0.1 mg/ml) must be completed within six hours after reconstitution to ensure adequate stability. During infusion, the solution must be protected from direct sunlight. Solutions must be used within this time period or discarded.
Solutions of Vibramycin (doxycycline hyclate for injection) at a concentration of 10 mg/ml in Sterile Water for Injection, when frozen immediately after reconstitution are stable for 8 weeks when stored at −20°C. If the product is warmed, care should be taken to avoid heating it after the thawing is complete. Once thawed the solution should not be refrozen.

HOW SUPPLIED

Vibramycin (doxycycline hyclate for injection) Intravenous is available as a sterile powder in a vial containing doxycycline hyclate equivalent to 100 mg of doxycycline with 480 mg of ascorbic acid, packages of 5 (NDC 0049-0960-77), and in individually packaged vials containing doxycycline hyclate equivalent to 200 mg of doxycycline with 960 mg of ascorbic acid (NDC 0049-0980-81).

65-1940-00-2

LITERATURE AVAILABLE

Yes.

VISTARIL® ℞

(hydroxyzine hydrochloride)
Intramuscular Solution
For Intramuscular Use Only

CHEMISTRY

Hydroxyzine hydrochloride is designated chemically as 1-(p-chlorobenzhydryl) 4-[2-(2-hydroxyethoxy) ethyl] piperazine dihydrochloride.

ACTIONS

VISTARIL (hydroxyzine hydrochloride) is unrelated chemically to phenothiazine, reserpine, and meprobamate. Hydroxyzine has demonstrated its clinical effectiveness in the chemotherapeutic aspect of the total management of neuroses and emotional disturbances manifested by anxiety, tension, agitation, apprehension or confusion.
Hydroxyzine has been shown clinically to be a rapid-acting true ataraxic with a wide margin of safety. It induces a calming effect in anxious, tense, psychoneurotic adults and also in anxious, hyperkinetic children without impairing mental alertness. It is not a cortical depressant, but its action may be due to a suppression of activity in certain key regions of the subcortical area of the central nervous system.
Primary skeletal muscle relaxation has been demonstrated experimentally.
Hydroxyzine has been shown experimentally to have antispasmodic properties, apparently mediated through interference with the mechanism that reponds to spasmogenic agents such as serotonin, acetylcholine, and histamine.
Antihistaminic effects have been demonstrated experimentally and confirmed clinically.
An antiemetic effect, both by the apomorphine test and the veriloid test, has been demonstrated. Pharmacological and clinical studies indicate that hydroxyzine in therapeutic dosage does not increase gastric secretion or acidity and in most cases provides mild antisecretory benefits.

INDICATIONS

The total management of anxiety, tension, and psychomotor agitation in conditions of emotional stress requires in most instances a combined approach of psychotherapy and chemotherapy. Hydroxyzine has been found to be particularly useful for this latter phase of therapy in its ability to render the disturbed patient more amenable to psychotherapy in long term treatment of the psychoneurotic and psychotic, although it should not be used as the sole treatment of psychosis or of clearly demonstrated cases of depression.
Hydroxyzine is also useful in alleviating the manifestations of anxiety and tension as in the preparation for dental procedures and in acute emotional problems. It has also been recommended for the management of anxiety associated with organic disturbances and as adjunctive therapy in alcoholism and allergic conditions with strong emotional overlay, such as in asthma, chronic urticaria, and pruritus.
VISTARIL (hydroxyzine hydrochloride) Intramuscular Solution is useful in treating the following types of patients when intramuscular administration is indicated:

1. The acutely disturbed or hysterical patient.
2. The acute or chronic alcoholic with anxiety withdrawal symptoms or delirium tremens.
3. As pre- and postoperative and pre- and postpartum adjunctive medication to permit reduction in narcotic dosage, allay anxiety and control emesis.

VISTARIL (hydroxyzine hydrochloride) has also demonstrated effectiveness in controlling nausea and vomiting, excluding nausea and vomiting of pregnancy. (See Contraindications.)
In prepartum states, the reduction in narcotic requirement effected by hydroxyzine is of particular benefit to both mother and neonate.
Hydroxyzine benefits the cardiac patient by its ability to allay the associated anxiety and apprehension attendant to certain types of heart disease. Hydroxyzine is not known to interfere with the action of digitalis in any way and may be used concurrently with this agent.
The effectiveness of hydroxyzine in long term use, that is, more than 4 months, has not been assessed by systematic clinical studies. The physician should reassess periodically the usefulness of the drug for the individual patient.

CONTRAINDICATIONS

Hydroxyzine hydrochloride intramuscular solution is intended only for intramuscular administration and should not, under any circumstances, be injected subcutaneously, intra-arterially, or intravenously.
This drug is contraindicated for patients who have shown a previous hypersensitivity to it.
Hydroxyzine, when administered to the pregnant mouse, rat, and rabbit, induced fetal abnormalities in the rat at doses substantially above the human therapeutic range. Clinical data in human beings are inadequate to establish safety in early pregnancy. Until such data are available, hydroxyzine is contraindicated in early pregnancy.

PRECAUTIONS

THE POTENTIATING ACTION OF HYDROXYZINE MUST BE CONSIDERED WHEN THE DRUG IS USED IN CONJUNCTION WITH CENTRAL NERVOUS SYSTEM DEPRESSANTS SUCH AS NARCOTICS, BARBITURATES, AND ALCOHOL. Rarely, cardiac arrests and death have been reported in association with the combined use of hydroxyzine hydrochloride IM and other CNS depressants. Therefore when central nervous system depressants are administered concomitantly with hydroxyzine their dosage should be reduced up to 50 per cent. The efficacy of hydroxyzine as adjunctive pre- and postoperative sedative medication has also been well established, especially as regards its ability to allay anxiety, control emesis, and reduce the amount of narcotic required.
HYDROXYZINE MAY POTENTIATE NARCOTICS AND BARBITURATES, so their use in preanesthetic adjunctive therapy should be modified on an individual basis. Atropine and other belladonna alkaloids are not affected by the drug. When hydroxyzine is used preoperatively or prepartum, narcotic requirements may be reduced as much as 50 per cent. Thus, when 50 mg of VISTARIL (hydroxyzine hydrochloride) Intramuscular Solution is employed, meperidine dosage may be reduced from 100 mg to 50 mg. The administration of meperidine may result in severe hypotension in the postoperative patient or any individual whose ability to maintain blood pressure has been compromised by a depleted blood volume. Meperidine should be used with great caution and in reduced dosage in patients who are receiving other pre- and/or postoperative medications and in whom there is a risk of respiratory depression, hypotension, and profound sedation or coma occurring. Before using any medications concomitant with hydroxyzine, the manufacturer's prescribing information should be read carefully.
Since drowsiness may occur with the use of this drug, patients should be warned of this possibility and cautioned against driving a car or operating dangerous machinery while taking this drug.
As with all intramuscular preparations, VISTARIL Intramuscular Solution should be injected well within the body of a relatively large muscle. Inadvertent subcutaneous injection may result in significant tissue damage.
ADULTS: The preferred site is the upper outer quadrant of the buttock, (i.e., gluteus maximus), or the mid-lateral thigh.
CHILDREN: It is recommended that intramuscular injections be given preferably in the mid-lateral muscles of the thigh. In infants and small children the periphery of the upper outer quadrant of the gluteal region should be used only when necessary, such as in burn patients, in order to minimize the possibility of damage to the sciatic nerve.
The deltoid area should be used only if well developed such as in certain adults and older children, and then only with caution to avoid radial nerve injury. Intramuscular injections should not be made into the lower and mid-third of the upper arm. As with all intramuscular injections, aspiration is necessary to help avoid inadvertent injection into a blood vessel.

ADVERSE REACTIONS

Therapeutic doses of hydroxyzine seldom produce impairment of mental alertness. However, drowsiness may occur; if so, it is usually transitory and may disappear in a few days of continued therapy or upon reduction of the dose. Dryness of the mouth may be encountered at higher doses. Extensive clinical use has substantiated the absence of toxic effects on the liver or bone marrow when administered in the recommended doses for over four years of uninterrupted therapy. The absence of adverse effects has been further demonstrated in experimental studies in which excessively high doses were administered.
Involuntary motor activity, including rare instances of tremor and convulsions, has been reported, usually with doses considerably higher than those recommended. Continuous therapy with over one gram per day has been employed in some patients without these effects having been encountered.

DOSAGE AND ADMINISTRATION

The recommended dosages for VISTARIL (hydroxyzine hydrochloride) Intramuscular Solution are:

For adult psychiatric and emotional emergencies, including acute alcoholism.	I.M.: 50–100 mg stat., and q. 4–6h., p.r.n.
Nausea and vomiting excluding nausea and vomiting of pregnancy.	Adults: 25–100 mg I.M. Children: 0.5 mg/lb. body weight I.M.
Pre- and postoperative adjunctive medication.	Adults: 25–100 mg I.M. Children: 0.5 mg/lb. body weight I.M.
Pre- and postpartum adjunctive therapy.	25–100 mg I.M.

As with all potent medications, the dosage should be adjusted according to the patient's response to therapy.
FOR ADDITIONAL INFORMATION ON THE ADMINISTRATION AND SITE OF SELECTION SEE PRECAUTIONS SECTION. NOTE: VISTARIL (hydroxyzine hydrochloride) Intramuscular Solution may be administered without further dilution.
Patients may be started on intramuscular therapy when indicated. They should be maintained on oral therapy whenever this route is practicable.

SUPPLY

VISTARIL (hydroxyzine hydrochloride) Intramuscular Solution
Multi-Dose Vials
25 mg/ml; 10 ml vials (NDC 0049-5450-74)
50 mg/ml; 10 ml vials (NDC 0049-5460-74)
Unit Dose Vials
50 mg/ml–1 ml fill; packages of 25 vials (NDC 0049-5462-76)
100 mg/2 ml–2 ml fill; packages of 25 vials (NDC 0049-5460-76)

FORMULA

Dosage Strength	25 mg/1 ml	50 mg/1 ml 100 mg/2 ml
Hydroxyzine hydrochloride	25 mg/ml	50 mg/ml
Benzyl Alcohol	0.9%	0.9%
Sodium hydroxide	to adjust to optimum pH	

BIBLIOGRAPHY

Available upon request.

70-0843-00-4

ZOLOFT™ ℞

(sertraline hydrochloride)
Tablets

DESCRIPTION

ZOLOFT™ (sertraline hydrochloride) is an antidepressant for oral administration. It is chemically unrelated to tricylic, tetracyclic, or other available antidepressant agents. It has a molecular weight of 342.7. Sertraline hydrochloride has the following chemical name: (1S-cis)-4-(3-4-dichlorophenyl)-1,2,3,4-tetrahydro-N-methyl-1-naphthalenamine hydrochloride. The empirical formula $C_{17}H_{17}NCl_2 \cdot HCl$ is represented by the following structural formula:

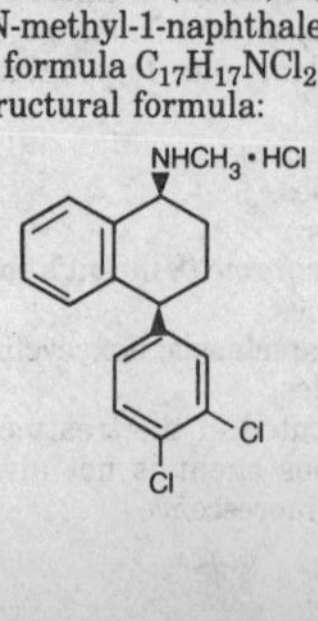

Sertraline hydrochloride is a white crystalline powder that is slightly soluble in water and isopropyl alcohol, and sparingly soluble in ethanol.

ZOLOFT is supplied for oral administration as scored tablets containing sertraline hydrochloride equivalent to 50 and 100 mg of sertraline and the following inactive ingredients: dibasic calcium phosphate dihydrate, FD&C Blue #2 aluminum lake (in 50 mg tablet), hydroxypropyl cellulose, hydroxypropyl methylcellulose, magnesium stearate, microcrystalline cellulose, polyethylene glycol, polysorbate 80, sodium starch glycolate, synthetic yellow iron oxide (in 100 mg tablet), and titanium dioxide.

CLINICAL PHARMACOLOGY

Pharmacodynamics

The mechanism of action of sertraline is presumed to be linked to its inhibition of CNS neuronal uptake of serotonin (5HT). Studies at clinically relevant doses in man have demonstrated that sertraline blocks the uptake of serotonin into human platelets. *In vitro* studies in animals also suggest that sertraline is a potent and selective inhibitor of neuronal serotonin reuptake and has only very weak effects on norepinephrine and dopamine neuronal reuptake. *In vitro* studies have shown that sertraline has no significant affinity for adrenergic (alpha$_1$, alpha$_2$, beta), cholinergic, GABA, dopaminergic, histaminergic, serotonergic (5HT$_{1A}$, 5HT$_{1B}$, 5HT$_2$), or benzodiazepine receptors; antagonism of such receptors has been hypothesized to be associated with various anticholinergic, sedative, and cardiovascular effects for other psychotropic drugs. The chronic administration of sertraline was found in animals to downregulate brain norepinephrine receptors, as has been observed with other clinically effective antidepressants. Sertraline does not inhibit monoamine oxidase.

Pharmacokinetics

Systemic Bioavailability—In man, following oral once-daily dosing over the range of 50 to 200 mg for 14 days, mean peak plasma concentrations (Cmax) of sertraline occurred between 4.5 to 8.4 hours postdosing. The average terminal elimination half-life of plasma sertraline is about 26 hours. Based on this pharmacokinetic parameter, steady-state sertraline plasma levels should be achieved after approximately one week of once-daily dosing. Linear dose-proportional pharmacokinetics were demonstrated in a single dose study in which the Cmax and area under the plasma concentration time curve (AUC) of sertraline were proportional to dose over a range of 50 to 200 mg. Consistent with the terminal elimination half-life, there is an approximately two-fold accumulation, compared to a single dose, of sertraline with repeated dosing over a 50 to 200 mg dose range. The single-dose bioavailability of sertraline tablets is approximately equal to an equivalent dose of solution.

The effects of food on the bioavailability of sertraline were studied in subjects administered a single-dose with and without food. AUC was slightly increased when drug was administered with food but the Cmax was 25% greater, while the time to reach peak plasma concentration decreased from 8 hours post-dosing to 5.5 hours.

Metabolism—Sertraline undergoes extensive first pass metabolism. The principal initial pathway of metabolism for sertraline is N-demethylation. N-desmethylsertraline has a plasma terminal elimination half-life of 62 to 104 hours. Both *in vitro* biochemical and *in vivo* pharmacological testing have shown N-desmethylsertraline to be substantially less active than sertraline. Both sertraline and N-desmethylsertraline undergo oxidative deamination and subsequent reduction, hydroxylation, and glucuronide conjugation. In a study of radiolabeled sertraline involving two healthy male subjects, sertraline accounted for less than 5% of the plasma radioactivity. About 40–45% of the administered radioactivity was recovered in urine in 9 days. Unchanged sertraline was not detectable in the urine. For the same period, about 40–45% of the administered radioactivity was accounted for in feces, including 12–14% unchanged sertraline.

Desmethylsertraline exhibits time-related, dose dependent increases in AUC (0–24 hour), Cmax and Cmin, with about a 5–9 fold increase in these pharmacokinetic parameters between day 1 and day 14.

Protein Binding—*In vitro* protein binding studies performed with radiolabeled ^{3}H-sertraline showed that sertraline is highly bound to serum proteins (98%) in the range of 20 to 500 ng/mL. However, at up to 300 and 200 ng/mL concentrations, respectively, sertraline and N-desmethylsertraline did not alter the plasma protein binding of two other highly protein bound drugs, viz., warfarin and propranolol (see Precautions).

Age—Sertraline plasma clearance in a group of 16 (8 male, 8 female) elderly patients treated for 14 days at dose of 100 mg/day was approximately 40% lower than in a similarly studied group of younger (25 to 32 y.o.) individuals. Steady state, therefore, should be achieved after 2 to 3 weeks in older patients. The same study showed a decreased clearance of desmethylsertraline in older males, but not in older females.

Liver Disease and Renal Disease—The pharmacokinetics of sertraline in patients with significant hepatic or renal dysfunction have not been determined.

INDICATIONS AND USAGE

ZOLOFT (sertraline hydrochloride) is indicated for the treatment of depression. The efficacy of ZOLOFT in the treatment of a major depressive episode was established in six to eight week controlled trials of outpatients whose diagnoses corresponded most closely to the DSM-III category of major depressive disorder.

A major depressive episode implies a prominent and relatively persistent depressed or dysphoric mood that usually interferes with daily functioning (nearly every day for at least 2 weeks); it should include at least 4 of the following 8 symptoms: change in appetite, change in sleep, psychomotor agitation or retardation, loss of interest in usual activities or decrease in sexual drive, increased fatigue, feelings of guilt or worthlessness, slowed thinking or impaired concentration, and a suicide attempt or suicidal ideation.

The antidepressant action of ZOLOFT in hospitalized depressed patients has not been adequately studied.

A study of depressed outpatients who had responded to ZOLOFT during an initial eight-week open treatment phase and were then randomized to continuation on ZOLOFT or placebo demonstrated a significantly lower relapse rate over the next eight weeks for patients taking ZOLOFT compared to those on placebo. However, the effectiveness of ZOLOFT in long-term use, that is, for more than 16 weeks, has not been systematically evaluated in controlled trials. Therefore, the physician who elects to use ZOLOFT for extended periods should periodically reevaluate the long-term usefulness of the drug for the individual patient.

CONTRAINDICATIONS

None known.

WARNINGS

In patients receiving another serotonin reuptake inhibitor drug in combination with a monoamine oxidase inhibitor (MAOI), there have been reports of serious, sometimes fatal, reactions including hyperthermia, rigidity, myoclonus, autonomic instability with possible rapid fluctuations of vital signs, and mental status changes that include extreme agitation progressing to delirium and coma. These reactions have also been reported in patients who have recently discontinued that drug and have been started on an MAOI. Some cases presented with features resembling neuroleptic malignant syndrome. Therefore, it is recommended that ZOLOFT (sertraline hydrochloride) not be used in combination with an MAOI, or within 14 days of discontinuing treatment with an MAOI. Similarly, at least 14 days should be allowed after stopping ZOLOFT before starting an MAOI.

PRECAUTIONS

General

Activation of Mania/Hypomania—During premarketing testing, hypomania or mania occurred in approximately 0.4% of ZOLOFT (sertraline hydrochloride) treated patients. Activation of mania/hypomania has also been reported in a small proportion of patients with Major Affective Disorder treated with other marketed antidepressants.

Weight Loss—Significant weight loss may be an undesirable result of treatment with sertraline for some patients, but on average, patients in controlled trials had minimal, 1 to 2 pound weight loss, versus smaller changes on placebo. Only rarely have sertraline patients been discontinued for weight loss.

Seizure—ZOLOFT has not been evaluated in patients with a seizure disorder. These patients were excluded from clinical studies during the product's premarket testing. Accordingly, like other antidepressants, ZOLOFT should be introduced with care in epileptic patients.

Suicide—The possibility of a suicide attempt is inherent in depression and may persist until significant remission occurs. Close supervision of high risk patients should accompany initial drug therapy. Prescriptions for ZOLOFT should be written for the smallest quantity of tablets consistent with good patient management, in order to reduce the risk of overdose.

Weak Uricosuric Effect—ZOLOFT is associated with a mean decrease in serum uric acid of approximately 7%. The clinical significance of this weak uricosuric effect is unknown, and there have been no reports of acute renal failure with ZOLOFT.

Use in Patients with Concomitant Illness—Clinical experience with ZOLOFT in patients with certain concomitant systemic illness is limited. Caution is advisable in using ZOLOFT in patients with diseases or conditions that could affect metabolism or hemodynamic responses.

ZOLOFT has not been evaluated or used to any appreciable extent in patients with a recent history of myocardial infarction or unstable heart disease. Patients with these diagnoses were excluded from clinical studies during the product's premarket testing. However, the electrocardiograms of 774 patients who received ZOLOFT in double-blind trials were evaluated and the data indicate that ZOLOFT is not associ-

ated with the development of significant ECG abnormalities. ZOLOFT is extensively metabolized by the liver. The pharmacokinetics of ZOLOFT have not been studied in patients with significant hepatic dysfunction nor have patients with significant hepatic dysfunction been evaluated during treatment with ZOLOFT. Accordingly, ZOLOFT should be used with caution in such patients.

Since ZOLOFT is extensively metabolized, excretion of unchanged drug in urine is a minor route of elimination. However, until the pharmacokinetics of ZOLOFT have been studied in patients with renal impairment and until adequate numbers of patients with severe renal impairment have been evaluated during chronic treatment with ZOLOFT, it should be used with caution in such patients.

Interference with Cognitive and Motor Performance—In controlled studies, ZOLOFT did not cause sedation and did not interfere with psychomotor performance.

Information for Patients

Physicians are advised to discuss the following issues with patients for whom they prescribe ZOLOFT:

Patients should be told that although ZOLOFT has not been shown to impair the ability of normal subjects to perform tasks requiring complex motor and mental skills in laboratory experiments, drugs that act upon the central nervous system may affect some individuals adversely.

Patients should be told that although ZOLOFT has not been shown in experiments with normal subjects to increase the mental and motor skill impairments caused by alcohol, the concomitant use of ZOLOFT and alcohol in depressed patients is not advised.

Patients should be told that while no adverse interaction of ZOLOFT with over-the-counter (OTC) drug products is known to occur, the potential for interaction exists. Thus, the use of any OTC product should be initiated cautiously according to the directions of use given for the OTC product. Patients should be advised to notify their physician if they become pregnant or intent to become pregnant during therapy.

Patients should be advised to notify their physician if they are breast feeding an infant.

Laboratory Tests

None.

Drug Interactions

Potential Effects of Coadministration of Drugs Highly Bound to Plasma Proteins—Because sertraline is tightly bound to plasma protein, the administration of ZOLOFT (sertraline hydrochloride) to a patient taking another drug which is tightly bound to protein, (e.g., warfarin, digitoxin) may cause a shift in plasma concentrations potentially resulting in an adverse effect. Conversely, adverse effects may result from displacement of protein bound ZOLOFT by other tightly bound drugs.

In a study comparing prothrombin time AUC (0–120 hr) following dosing with warfarin (0.75 mg/kg) before and after 21 days of dosing with either ZOLOFT (50–200 mg/day) or placebo, there was a mean increase in prothrombin time of 8% relative to baseline for ZOLOFT compared to a 1% decrease for placebo (p < 0.02). The normalization of prothrombin time for the ZOLOFT group was delayed compared to the placebo group. The clinical significance of this change is unknown. Accordingly, prothrombin time should be carefully monitored when ZOLOFT therapy is initiated or stopped.

CNS Active Drugs—In a study comparing the disposition of intravenously administered diazepam before and after 21 days of dosing with either ZOLOFT (50 to 200 mg/day escalating dose) or placebo, there was a 32% decrease relative to baseline in diazepam clearance for the ZOLOFT group compared to a 19% decrease relative to baseline for the placebo group (p < 0.03). There was a 23% increase in Tmax for desmethyldiazepam in the ZOLOFT group compared to a 20% decrease in the placebo group (p < 0.03). The clinical significance of these changes is unknown.

In a placebo-controlled trial in normal volunteers, the administration of two doses of ZOLOFT did not significantly alter steady-state lithium levels or the renal clearance of lithium.

Nonetheless, at this time, it is recommended that plasma lithium levels be monitored following initiation of ZOLOFT therapy with appropriate adjustments to the lithium dose. The risk of using ZOLOFT in combination with other CNS active drugs has not been systematically evaluated. Consequently, caution is advised if the concomitant administration of ZOLOFT and such drugs is required.

Hypoglycemic Drugs—In a placebo-controlled trial in normal volunteers, administration of ZOLOFT for 22 days (including 200 mg/day for the final 13 days) caused a statistically significant 16% decrease from baseline in the clearance of tolbutamide following an intravenous 1000 mg dose. ZOLOFT administration did not noticeably change either the plasma protein binding or the apparent volume of distribution of tolbutamide, suggesting that the decreased clearance was due to a change in the metabolism of the drug. The clini-

Continued on next page

Roerig—Cont.

cal significance of this decrease in tolbutamide clearance is unknown.

Atenolol—ZOLOFT (100 mg) when administered to 10 healthy male subjects had no effect on the beta-adrenergic blocking ability of atenolol.

Microsomal Enzyme Induction—Preclinical studies have shown ZOLOFT to induce hepatic microsomal enzymes. In clinical studies, ZOLOFT was shown to induce hepatic enzymes minimally as determined by a small (5%) but statistically significant decrease in antipyrine half-life following administration of 200 mg/day for 21 days. This small change in antipyrine half-life reflects a clinically insignificant change in hepatic metabolism.

Electroconvulsive Therapy—There are no clinical studies establishing the risks or benefits of the combined use of electroconvulsive therapy (ECT) and ZOLOFT.

Alcohol—Although ZOLOFT did not potentiate the cognitive and psychomotor effects of alcohol in experiments with normal subjects, the concomitant use of ZOLOFT and alcohol in depressed patients is not recommended.

Carcinogenesis, Mutagenesis, Impairment of Fertility
Lifetime carcinogenicity studies were carried out in CD-1 mice and Long-Evans rats at doses up to 40 mg/kg in mice (10 times, on a mg/kg basis, and the same, on a mg/m² basis, as the maximum recommended human dose) and at doses up to 40 mg/kg in rats (10 times, on a mg/kg basis, and 2 times, on a mg/m² basis, the maximum recommended human dose). There was a dose-related increase in the incidence of liver adenomas in male mice receiving sertraline at 10–40 mg/kg. No increase was seen in female mice or in rats of either sex receiving the same treatments, nor was there an increase in hepatocellular carcinomas. Liver adenomas have a variable rate of spontaneous occurrence in the CD-1 mouse and are of unknown significance to humans. There was an increase in follicular adenomas of the thyroid in female rats receiving sertraline at 40 mg/kg; this was not accompanied by thyroid hyperplasia. While there was an increase in uterine adenocarcinomas in rats receiving sertraline at 10–40 mg/kg compared to placebo controls, this effect was not clearly drug related.

Sertraline had no genotoxic effects, with or without metabolic activation, based on the following assays: bacterial mutation assay; mouse lymphoma mutation assay; and tests for cytogenetic aberrations *in vivo* in mouse bone marrow and *in vitro* in human lymphocytes.

A decrease in fertility was seen in one of two rat studies at a dose of 80 mg/kg (20 times the maximum human dose on a mg/kg basis and 4 times on a mg/m² basis).

Pregnancy-Pregnancy Category B
Teratogenic Effects—Reproduction studies have been performed in rats and rabbits at doses up to approximately 20 times and 10 times the maximum daily human mg/kg dose (4 to 4.5 times the mg/m² dose), respectively.

There was no evidence of teratogenicity at any dose level. At doses approximately 2.5–10 times the maximum daily human mg/kg dose, sertraline was associated with delayed ossification in fetuses, probably secondary to effects on the dams.

There are no adequate and well-controlled studies in pregnant women. Because animal reproduction studies are not always predictive of human response, this drug should be used during pregnancy only if clearly needed.

Non-teratogenic Effects—There was also decreased neonatal survival following maternal administration of sertraline at doses as low as approximately 5 times the maximum human mg/kg dose. The decrease in pup survival was shown to be most probably due to *in utero* exposure to sertraline. The clinical significance of these effects is unknown.

Labor and Delivery—The effect of ZOLOFT on labor and delivery in humans is unknown.

Nursing Mothers—It is not known whether, and if so in what amount, sertraline or its metabolites are excreted in human milk. Because many drugs are excreted in human milk, caution should be exercised when ZOLOFT is administered to a nursing woman.

Pediatric Use—Safety and effectivenesss in children have not been established.

Geriatric Use—Several hundred elderly patients have participated in clinical studies with ZOLOFT. The pattern of adverse reactions in the elderly was similar to that in younger patients.

ADVERSE REACTIONS

Commonly Observed—The most commonly observed adverse events associated with the use of ZOLOFT (sertraline hydrochloride) and not seen at an equivalent incidence among placebo treated patients were: gastrointestinal complaints, including nausea, diarrhea/loose stools and dyspepsia; tremor; dizziness; insomnia; somnolence; increased sweating; dry mouth; and male sexual dysfunction (primarily ejaculatory delay).

Associated with Discontinuation of Treatment—Fifteen percent of 2710 subjects who received ZOLOFT in premar-

keting multiple dose clinical trials discontinued treatment due to an adverse event. The more common events (reported by at least 1% of subjects) associated with discontinuation included agitation, insomnia, male sexual dysfunction (primarily ejaculatory delay), somnolence, dizziness, headache, tremor, anorexia, diarrhea/loose stools, nausea, and fatigue.
Incidence in Controlled Clinical Trials—The table that follows enumerates adverse events that occurred at a frequency of 1% or more among ZOLOFT patients who participated in controlled trials comparing titrated ZOLOFT with placebo. Most patients received doses of 50 to 200 mg per day. The prescriber should be aware that these figures cannot be used to predict the incidence of side effects in the course of usual medical practice where patient characteristics and other factors differ from those which prevailed in the clinical trials. Similarly, the cited frequencies cannot be compared with figures obtained from other clinical investigations involving different treatments, uses, and investigators. The cited figures, however, do provide the prescribing physician with some basis for estimating the relative contribution of drug and non-drug factors to the side effect incidence rate in the population studied.

Treatment-Emergent Adverse Experience Incidence in Placebo-Controlled Clinical Trials*

Adverse Experience	(Percent of Patients Reporting)	
	Zoloft (N=861)	Placebo (N=853)
Autonomic Nervous System Disorders		
Mouth Dry	16.3	9.3
Sweating Increased	8.4	2.9
Cardiovascular		
Palpitations	3.5	1.6
Chest Pain	1.0	1.6
Centr. & Periph. Nerv. System Disorders		
Headache	20.3	19.0
Dizziness	11.7	6.7
Tremor	10.7	2.7
Paresthesia	2.0	1.8
Hypoesthesia	1.7	0.6
Twitching	1.4	0.1
Hypertonia	1.3	0.4
Disorders of Skin and Appendages		
Rash	2.1	1.5
Gastrointestinal Disorders		
Nausea	26.1	11.8
Diarrhea/Loose Stools	17.7	9.3
Constipation	8.4	6.3
Dyspepsia	6.0	2.8
Vomiting	3.8	1.8
Flatulence	3.3	2.5
Anorexia	2.8	1.6
Abdominal Pain	2.4	2.2
Appetite Increased	1.3	0.9
General		
Fatigue	10.6	8.1
Hot Flushes	2.2	0.5
Fever	1.6	0.6
Back Pain	1.5	0.9
Metabolic and Nutritional Disorders		
Thirst	1.4	0.9
Musculoskeletal System Disorders		
Myalgia	1.7	1.5
Psychiatric Disorders		
Insomnia	16.4	8.8
Sexual Dysfunction-Male (1)	15.5	2.2
Somnolence	13.4	5.9
Agitation	5.6	4.0
Nervousness	3.4	1.9
Anxiety	2.6	1.3
Yawning	1.9	0.2
Sexual Dysfunction-Female (2)	1.7	0.2
Concentration Impaired	1.3	0.5
Reproductive		
Menstrual Disorder (2)	1.0	0.5
Respiratory System Disorders		
Rhinitis	2.0	1.5
Pharyngitis	1.2	0.9
Special Senses		
Vision Abnormal	4.2	2.1
Tinnitus	1.4	1.1
Taste Perversion	1.2	0.7
Urinary System Disorders		
Micturition Frequency	2.0	1.2
Micturition Disorder	1.4	0.5

*Events reported by at least 1% of patients treated with ZOLOFT are included.
(1)—% based on male patients only: 271 ZOLOFT (primarily ejaculatory delay) and 271 placebo patients.
(2)—% based on female patients only: 590 ZOLOFT and 582 placebo patients.

Other Events Observed During the Premarketing Evaluation of ZOLOFT (sertraline hydrochloride): During its premarketing assessment, multiple doses of ZOLOFT were administered to approximately 2700 subjects. The conditions and

duration of exposure to ZOLOFT varied greatly, and included (in overlapping categories) clinical pharmacology studies, open and double-blind studies, uncontrolled and controlled studies, inpatient and outpatient studies, fixed-dose and titration studies, and studies for indications other than depression. Untoward events associated with this exposure were recorded by clinical investigators using terminology of their own choosing. Consequently, it is not possible to provide a meaningful estimate of the proportion of individuals experiencing adverse events without first grouping similar types of untoward events into a smaller number of standardized event categories.

In the tabulations that follow, a World Health Organization dictionary of terminology has been used to classify reported adverse events. The frequencies presented, therefore, represent the proportion of the approximately 2700 individuals exposed to multiple doses of ZOLOFT who experienced an event of the type cited on at least one occasion while receiving ZOLOFT. All events are included except those already listed in the previous table and those reported in terms so general as to be uninformative. It is important to emphasize that although the events reported occurred during treatment with ZOLOFT, they were not necessarily caused by it. Events are further categorized by body system and listed in order of decreasing frequency according to the following definitions: frequent adverse events are those occurring on one or more occasions in at least 1/100 patients (only those not already listed in the tabulated results from placebo controlled trials appear in this listing); infrequent adverse events are those occurring in 1/100 to 1/1000 patients; rare events are those occurring in fewer than 1/1000 patients. Events of major clinical importance are also described in the PRECAUTIONS section.

Autonomic Nervous System Disorders—*Infrequent:* flushing, mydriasis, increased saliva, cold clammy skin; *Rare:* pallor.

Cardiovascular—*Infrequent:* postural dizziness, hypertension, hypotension, postural hypotension, edema, dependent edema, periorbital edema, peripheral edema, peripheral ischemia, syncope, tachycardia: *Rare:* percordial chest pain, substernal chest pain, aggravated hypertension, myocardial infarction, varicose veins.

Central and Peripheral Nervous System Disorders—*Frequent:* confusion; *Infrequent:* ataxia, abnormal coordination, abnormal gait, hyperesthesia, hyperkinesia, hypokinesia, migraine, nystagmus, vertigo; *Rare:* local anesthesia, coma, convulsions, dyskinesia, dysphonia, hyporeflexia, hypotonia, ptosis.

Disorders of Skin and Appendages—*Infrequent:* acne, alopecia, pruritus, erythematous rash, maculopapular rash, dry skin; *Rare:* bullous eruption, dermatitis, erythema multiforme, abnormal hair texture, hypertrichosis, photosensitivity reaction, follicular rash, skin discoloration, abnormal skin odor, urticaria.

Endocrine Disorders—*Rare:* exophthalmos, gynecomastia.

Gastrointestinal Disorders—*Infrequent:* dysphagia, eructation; *Rare:* diverticulitis, fecal incontinence, gastritis, gastroenteritis, glossitis, gum hyperplasia, hemorrhoids, hiccup, melena, hemorrhagic peptic ulcer, proctitis, stomatitis, ulcerative stomatitis, tenesmus, tongue edema, tongue ulceration.

General—*Frequent:* asthenia; *Infrequent:* malaise, generalized edema, rigors, weight decrease, weight increase; *Rare:* enlarged abdomen, halitosis, otitis media, aphthous stomatitis.

Hematopoietic and Lymphatic—*Infrequent:* lymphadenopathy, purpura; *Rare:* anemia, anterior chamber eye hemorrhage.

Metabolic and Nutritional Disorders—*Rare:* dehydration, hypercholesterolemia, hypoglycemia.

Musculoskeletal System Disorders—*Infrequent:* arthralgia, arthrosis, dystonia, muscle cramps, muscle weakness; *Rare:* hernia.

Psychiatric Disorders—*Infrequent:* abnormal dreams, aggressive reaction, amnesia, apathy, delusion, depersonalization, depression, aggravated depression, emotional lability, euphoria, hallucination, neurosis, paranoid reaction, suicide ideation and attempt, teeth-grinding, abnormal thinking; *Rare:* hysteria, somnambulism, withdrawal syndrome.

Reproductive—*Infrequent:* dysmenorrhea (2), intermenstrual bleeding (2); *Rare:* amenorrhea (2), balanoposthitis (1), breast enlargement (2), female breast pain (2), leukorrhea (2), menorrhagia (2), atrophic vaginitis (2).
(1)—% based on male subjects only: 1005.
(2)—% based on female subjects only: 1705.

Respiratory System Disorders—*Infrequent:* bronchospasm, coughing, dyspnea, epistaxis; *Rare:* bradypnea, hyperventilation, sinusitis, stridor.

Special Senses—*Infrequent:* abnormal accommodation, conjunctivitis, diplopia, earache, eye pain, xerophthalmia; *Rare:* abnormal lacrimation, photophobia, visual field defect.

Urinary System Disorders—*Infrequent:* dysuria, face edema, nocturia, polyuria, urinary incontinence; *Rare:* oliguria, renal pain, urinary retention.

Laboratory Tests—In man, asymptomatic elevations in serum transaminases (SGOT [or AST] and SGPT [or ALT])

have been reported infrequently (approximately 0.8%) in association with ZOLOFT administration. These hepatic enzyme elevations usually occurred within the first 1 to 9 weeks of drug treatment and promptly diminished upon drug discontinuation.

ZOLOFT therapy was associated with small mean increases in total cholesterol (approximately 3%) and triglycerides (approximately 5%), and a small mean decrease in serum uric acid (approximately 7%) of no apparent clinical importance.

DRUG ABUSE AND DEPENDENCE

Controlled Substance Class—ZOLOFT (sertraline hydrochloride) is not a controlled substance.

Physical and Psychological Dependence—ZOLOFT has not been systematically studied, in animals or humans, for its potential for abuse, tolerance, or physical dependence. However, the premarketing clinical experience with ZOLOFT did not reveal any tendency for a withdrawal syndrome or any drug-seeking behavior. As with any new CNS active drug, physicians should carefully evaluate patients for history of drug abuse and follow such patients closely, observing them for signs of ZOLOFT misuse or abuse (e.g., development of tolerance, incrementation of dose, drug-seeking behavior).

OVERDOSAGE

Human Experience—There have been 3 cases of ZOLOFT (sertraline hydrochloride) overdosage (approximately 750-2,100 mg). No specific therapy was required for any of the 3 patients, all of whom recovered completely.

Management of Overdoses—Establish and maintain an airway, insure adequate oxygenation and ventilation. Activated charcoal, which may be used with sorbitol, may be as or more effective than emesis or lavage, and should be considered in treating overdose.

Cardiac and vital signs monitoring is recommended along with general symptomatic and supportive measures.

There are no specific antidotes for ZOLOFT.

Due to the large volume of distribution of ZOLOFT, forced diuresis, dialysis, hemoperfusion, and exchange transfusion are unlikely to be of benefit.

In managing overdosage, consider the possibility of multiple drug involvement. The physician should consider contacting a poison control center on the treatment of any overdose.

DOSE AND ADMINISTRATION

Initial Treatment—ZOLOFT (sertraline hydrochloride) treatment should be initiated with a dose of 50 mg once daily. While a relationship between dose and antidepressant effect has not been established, patients were dosed in a range of 50–200 mg/day in the clinical trials demonstrating the antidepressant effectiveness of ZOLOFT. Consequently, patients not responding to a 50 mg dose may benefit from dose increases up to a maximum of 200 mg/day. Given the 24 hour elimination half-life of ZOLOFT, dose changes should not occur at intervals of less than 1 week.

ZOLOFT should be administered once daily, either in the morning or evening.

As indicated under Precautions, particular care should be used in patients with hepatic and/or renal impairment.

Maintenance/Continuation/Extended Treatment—There is evidence to suggest that depressed patients responding during an initial 8 week treatment phase will continue to benefit during an additional 8 weeks of treatment. While there are insufficient data regarding any benefits from treatment beyond 16 weeks, it is generally agreed among expert psychopharmacologists that acute episodes of depression require several months or longer of sustained pharmacological therapy. Whether the dose of antidepressant needed to induce remission is identical to the dose needed to maintain and/or sustain euthymia is unknown.

HOW SUPPLIED

ZOLOFT™ capsular-shaped scored tablets, containing sertraline hydrochloride equivalent to 50 and 100 mg of sertraline, are packaged in bottles.

ZOLOFT™ 50 mg Tablets: light blue film coated tablets engraved on the front with ZOLOFT and on the back scored and engraved with 50 mg.
NDC 0049-4900-50   Bottles of 50
ZOLOFT™ 100 mg Tablets: light yellow film coated tablets engraved on the front with ZOLOFT and on the back scored and engraved with 100 mg.
NDC 0049-4910-50   Bottles of 50
Store at controlled room temperature of 59°F to 86°F (15° to 30°C).

Roerig
Pfizer

Division of Pfizer Inc, N.Y., N.Y. 10017
65-4721-00-0   Issued Jan. 1992
Shown in Product Identification Section, page 427

EDUCATIONAL MATERIAL

Printed Material

1. *Zoloft Product Monograph*—A comprehensive review of Zoloft including its chemistry, pharmacology, pharmacokinetics and pharmacodynamics, clinical effectiveness, safety and tolerability profile, and indications for clinical use. Available from Roerig and Pratt Pharmaceutical representatives.
2. *Dealing with Depression: Taking Steps in the Right Direction*—A brochure for depressed patients offers information on depression and its treatment as well as advice for effectively communicating with physicians about the disease. Available from Roerig and Pratt Pharmaceutical representatives.
3. *Unmasking Depression: Seeing Things in a Different Light*—A brochure for the undiagnosed depressed patient features a self-assessment multiple-choice examination, information on depression and its treatment, and advice for effectively communicating with physicians about the disease. Available from Roerig and Pratt Pharmaceutical representatives.

Films/Videos

1. "Controlling Hypertension at its Source: Cardura and the New Era of Vasculoaction". This 8 minute film explains the success of doxazosin in reducing total peripheral resistance by selectively blocking the peripheral alpha-1 receptor. Drs. Dzau and Pool discuss the benefits of vasculoaction in managing blood pressures. Available from Roerig Representative.
2. "Say Goodbye to High Blood Pressure"—A one hour patient education video. An informative look at the causes, effects, and treatments plus a daily exercise and relaxation program.
3. "Sexual Function: Impotence and the Hypertensive Male"—This film examines the mechanism of erectile functioning and factors that inhibit this action. Two prominent physicians, Dr. Culley Carson and Dr. Steven Schwab from Duke University, narrate this film, which focuses on the antihypertensive medications that cause sexual dysfunction and products such as Cardura that do not. The new data from the Treatment of Mild Hypertension Study (TOMHS) is incorporated into this film to show physicians that Cardura does not adversely affect sexual functioning.
4. *Zoloft in the Management of Depressive Illness*—presents the clinical efficacy, safety, and pharmacologic profiles of Zoloft. Available for showing by Roerig and Pratt Pharmaceutical representatives.
5. *The Role of Serotonin in Mood and Behavior*—clearly demonstrates the current understanding of the role of serotonin in depressive illness. A comparative perspective of the presumed mechanisms of action of antidepressants as well as a representation of receptor blockade and its effect on side effects are vividly depicted via computer animation. Available for showing by Roerig and Pratt Pharmaceutical representatives.
6. *Taking Control of Depression: Mending the Mind*—leading experts in depression speak directly to patients in a reassuring and hopeful tone that can support your efforts. Available for your lending library by Roerig and Pratt Pharmaceutical representatives.

Computer Programs (IBM Compatible)

"Coronary Heart Disease Risk Factor Modification"—Allows calculation of a 10-year CHD risk estimate from the Framingham data base utilizing age, sex, smoking status, left ventricular hypertrophy, diabetes, blood pressure (diastolic or systolic), total cholesterol, and HDL cholesterol. Available from Roerig Representative.

Samples

Cardura (doxazosin mesylate) Tablets—1 mg
Diflucan (fluconazole) Tablets—100 mg
Navane (thiothixene) Capsules—2 mg, 5 mg
Sinequan (doxepin HCl) Capsules—25 mg, 50 mg
Unasyn (ampicillin sodium/sulbactam sodium) vials—1.5 mg
Zoloft (sertraline HCl) Tablets—50 mg
TOLL FREE NUMBER FOR CARDURA
1-800-4LOWER BP (1-800-456-9372)

Products are
listed alphabetically
in the
PINK SECTION.

Ross Laboratories
COLUMBUS, OH 43216

ALIMENTUM®
[al "ah-men 'tum]
Protein Hydrolysate Formula
With Iron
● **Ready To Feed**

For most current information, refer to product labels.

ALITRAQ™
[al 'ah-trak ']
Specialized Elemental Nutrition
With Glutamine

USAGE

A complete, elemental feeding designed for metabolically stressed patients with impaired GI function. AlitraQ helps maintain nutritional status and provides supplemental glutamine to nourish the GI tract and restore glutamine depleted during catabolic dysfunction.
Not for parenteral use.

AVAILABILITY

Powder:
2.68 oz (76 g) packets; 24 packets per case; No. 50630.

COMPOSITION

INGREDIENTS

Hydrolyzed cornstarch, soy hydrolysate, sucrose, L-glutamine, fructose, medium-chain triglycerides (fractionated coconut oil), safflower oil, whey protein concentrate, lactalbumin hydrolysate, magnesium sulfate, L-arginine, calcium phosphate tribasic, L-leucine, L-valine, L-lysine, potassium phosphate dibasic, potassium citrate, L-phenylalanine, sodium citrate, L-isoleucine, L-threonine, L-tyrosine, L-methionine, sodium chloride, ascorbic acid, L-histidine, choline chloride, L-tryptophan, natural and artificial flavors, taurine, carnitine, carrageenan, niacinamide, calcium pantothenate, zinc sulfate, ferrous sulfate, vitamin A palmitate, alpha-tocopheryl acetate, thiamine chloride hydrochloride, pyridoxine hydrochloride, riboflavin, manganese sulfate, cupric sulfate, folic acid, biotin, potassium iodide, sodium molybdate, phylloquinone, chromium chloride, sodium selenite, cyanocobalamin and vitamin D_3.

Nutrients (grams)	Per 300 Calories* (1 packet)
Protein	15.8
Fat	4.65
Carbohydrate	49.5

*In standard dilution (76 g of Alitraq powder mixed in 250 mL of water)
(FAN 790-01)

CLEAR EYES®   OTC
[klēr īz]
Lubricating Eye Redness Reliever Drops

(See PDR For Nonprescription Drugs or PDR For Ophthalmology.)

CLEAR EYES® ACR   OTC
[klēr īz]
Astringent/Lubricating Eye Redness Reliever Drops

(See PDR For Nonprescription Drugs or PDR For Ophthalmology.)

EAR DROPS BY MURINE   OTC
See Murine Ear Wax Removal
System/Murine Ear Drops

(See PDR For Nonprescription Drugs.)

ENSURE®
[en-shur ']
Liquid Nutrition

USAGE

For complete, balanced nutrition. Ensure can be used as a sole source of nutrition or as a dietary supplement. As a low-

Continued on next page

Ross Laboratories—Cont.

residue feeding, Ensure can be used for patients on low residue diagnostic test diets. Ensure can be used on sodium-restricted, low-cholesterol, lactose-restricted or gluten-free diets. Ensure may be fed orally or by tube. Ensure is useful whenever the patient's medical, surgical or psychological state causes inadequate dietary intake. Two quarts (2000 Calories) of Ensure meet or surpass 100% of the U.S. RDA for vitamins and minerals for adults and children 4 or more years of age.

Not for parenteral use.

AVAILABILITY

Ready To Use:
8-fl-oz bottles; 24 per case; Vanilla, No. 708.
8-fl-oz cans; 24 per case; Chocolate, No. 701 (retail), Chocolate, No. 50462 (institution); Black Walnut, No. 703; Coffee, No. 704; Strawberry, No. 705 (retail), Strawberry, No. 50648 (institution); Eggnog, No. 710; Vanilla, No. 711 (retail), Vanilla, No. 50460 (institution).
32-fl-oz cans; 6 per case; Vanilla, No. 733; Chocolate, No. 799.
Powder:
14-oz (400 g) cans; 6 per case; Vanilla, No. 750.

COMPOSITION

Ready To Use Vanilla (Other flavors and Vanilla Powder at standard dilution have similar composition and nutrient values. For specific information, see product labels.)

INGREDIENTS

Ⓓ-D Water, corn syrup, sucrose, corn oil, sodium and calcium caseinates, soy protein isolate, potassium citrate, magnesium chloride, soy lecithin, calcium phosphate tribasic, sodium citrate, natural and artificial flavor, potassium chloride, ascorbic acid, choline chloride, carrageenan, zinc sulfate, ferrous sulfate, alpha-tocopheryl acetate, niacinamide, calcium pantothenate, manganese sulfate, thiamine chloride hydrochloride, pyridoxine hydrochloride, riboflavin, cupric sulfate, vitamin A palmitate, folic acid, biotin, sodium molybdate, chromium chloride, potassium iodide, sodium selenite, phylloquinone, cyanocobalamin and vitamin D_3.
Nutrients per 8 fl oz: Calories, 250; Protein, 8.8 g; Carbohydrate, 34.3 g; Fat, 8.8 g; Cholesterol, < 5 mg; Sodium, 200 mg; Potassium, 370 mg.
(FAN 793-04)

ENSURE PLUS®

[en-shur']
High Calorie Liquid Nutrition

USAGE

As a high-calorie liquid food providing complete, balanced nutrition. Caloric density is 1500 Calories per liter, 50% more than that of most other liquid feedings. Ensure Plus is intended for use when extra calories and correspondingly higher concentrations of protein and most other nutrients are needed to achieve a required calorie intake in a limited volume. When used to provide total nutrition, Ensure Plus can deliver the high-calorie intakes required by patients who are nutritionally depleted, and who may not be able to tolerate large-volume intakes. As a dietary supplement, Ensure Plus can supply extra calories and protein for those patients unable to consume adequate nutrition.

Not for parenteral use.

AVAILABILITY

Ready To Use:
8-fl-oz bottles; 24 per case; Vanilla, No. 741.
8-fl-oz cans; 24 per case; Chocolate, No. 702 (retail), Chocolate, No. 50466 (institution); Vanilla, No. 707 (retail), Vanilla, No. 50464 (institution); Eggnog, No. 716; Coffee, No. 717; Strawberry, No. 718 (retail), Strawberry, No. 50646 (institution).
32-fl-oz cans; 6 per case; Vanilla, No. 688; Chocolate, No. 698; Strawberry, No. 51172.
1-liter Ross Ready-To-Hang® Enteral Feeding Containers; 8 per case; No. 50340.

COMPOSITION

Ready To Use Vanilla (Other flavors and Ready-To-Hang have similar composition. For specific information, see product labels.)

INGREDIENTS

Ⓓ-D Water, corn syrup, corn oil, sodium and calcium caseinates, sucrose, soy protein isolate, magnesium chloride, potassium citrate, calcium phosphate tribasic, soy lecithin, natural and artificial flavor, sodium citrate, potassium chloride, choline chloride, ascorbic acid, zinc sulfate, ferrous sulfate, alpha-tocopheryl acetate, carrageenan, niacinamide, calcium pantothenate, manganese sulfate, thiamine chloride hydrochloride, pyridoxine hydrochloride, riboflavin, cupric sulfate, vitamin A palmitate, folic acid, biotin, sodium

molybdate, chromium chloride, potassium iodide, sodium selenite, phylloquinone, cyanocobalamin and vitamin D_3.
Nutrients per 8 fl oz: Calories, 355; Protein, 13.0 g; Carbohydrate, 47.3 g; Fat, 12.6 g; Cholesterol, < 5 mg; Sodium, 250 mg; Potassium, 460 mg.
(FAN 793-04)

ENSURE® WITH FIBER

[en-shur']
Complete, Balanced Liquid Nutrition

USAGE

As a fiber-containing, nutritionally complete liquid food, Ensure With Fiber is useful for persons who can benefit from increased dietary fiber and supplemental nutrition. The fiber level in Ensure With Fiber helps maintain normal bowel function and is useful for those who need to increase the dietary fiber content of their diet. Ensure With Fiber is suitable for persons who do not require a low-residue diet. Although intended primarily as an oral feeding, Ensure With Fiber may be fed by tube.

Not for parenteral use.

AVAILABILITY

Ready To Use:
8-fl-oz cans; 24 per case; Vanilla, No. 759 (retail), Vanilla, No. 50650 (institution); Chocolate, No. 756.
32-fl-oz cans; 6 per case; Vanilla, No. 706.

COMPOSITION

Vanilla (Chocolate flavor has similar composition. For specific information, see product label.)

INGREDIENTS

Ⓓ-D Water, hydrolyzed cornstarch, sucrose, corn oil, sodium and calcium caseinates, soy fiber (a source of dietary fiber), soy protein isolate, natural and artificial flavor, potassium citrate, magnesium chloride, soy lecithin, calcium phosphate tribasic, sodium citrate, potassium chloride, choline chloride, ascorbic acid, zinc sulfate, ferrous sulfate, alpha-tocopheryl acetate, niacinamide, calcium pantothenate, manganese sulfate, thiamine chloride hydrochloride, pyridoxine hydrochloride, cupric sulfate, riboflavin, vitamin A palmitate, folic acid, biotin, sodium molybdate, chromium chloride, potassium iodide, sodium selenite, phylloquinone, cyanocobalamin and vitamin D_3.
Nutrients per 8 fl oz: Calories, 260; Protein, 9.4 g; Carbohydrate, 38.3 g*; Fat, 8.8 g; Cholesterol, < 5 mg; Sodium, 200 mg; Potassium, 400 mg.

*Includes 5 g soy fiber (a source of dietary fiber that provides 10 Calories and 3.4 g total dietary fiber).
(FAN 857-04)

GLUCERNA®

[glu-ser'nah]
**Specialized Nutrition with Fiber
for Patients with Abnormal Glucose
Tolerance**

USAGE

As a high-fiber, low-carbohydrate, enteral formula providing complete nutrition for patients with abnormal glucose tolerance. Glucerna has a unique formulation designed to maintain or improve nutritional status, yet enhance blood glucose control. Glucerna can be used as a tube feeding or oral supplement in persons with type I or type II diabetes mellitus or stress-induced hyperglycemia.

Not for parenteral use.

AVAILABILITY

Ready To Use:
8-fl-oz cans; 24 per case; Vanilla, No. 50240. 1-liter Ross Ready-To-Hang® Enteral Feeding Containers; 8 per case; No. 51206.

INGREDIENTS

Ⓓ-D Water, hydrolyzed cornstarch, hi-oleic safflower oil, sodium and calcium caseinate, soy fiber, fructose, soy oil, soy lecithin, magnesium chloride, calcium phosphate tribasic, sodium citrate, natural and artificial flavors, potassium chloride, m-inositol, potassium citrate, choline chloride, potassium phosphate dibasic, ascorbic acid, L-carnitine, taurine, zinc sulfate, ferrous sulfate, alpha-tocopheryl acetate, niacinamide, calcium pantothenate, manganese sulfate, thiamine chloride hydrochloride, pyridoxine hydrochloride, cupric sulfate, riboflavin, vitamin A palmitate, folic acid, biotin, sodium molybdate, chromium chloride, potassium iodide, sodium selenite, phylloquinone, cyanocobalamin and vitamin D_3.

Nutrients (Grams/8 fl oz): Protein, 9.9; Fat, 13.2; Carbohydrate, 22.2*; L-carnitine, 0.034; Taurine, 0.025; m-Inositol, 0.20; Water, 207. Calories per mL, 1.0; Calories per fl oz, 29.6.

*Includes soy fiber (a source of dietary fiber that provides 10 Calories and 3.4 g total dietary fiber).
(FAN 689-02)

ISOMIL®

[ī'sō-mil]
Soy Protein Formula With Iron
● **Powder**
● **Concentrated Liquid**
● **Ready To Feed**

For most current information, refer to product labels.

ISOMIL® SF

[ī'sō-mil]
Sucrose-Free Soy Protein Formula With Iron
● **Concentrated Liquid**

For most current information, refer to product labels.

JEVITY®

[jev'ə-tē"]
Isotonic Liquid Nutrition with Fiber

USAGE

As a fiber-containing, isotonic, high-nitrogen, nutritionally complete liquid food for tube feeding, Jevity helps patients maintain normal bowel function. The fiber source, soy polysaccharide, helps control diarrhea and constipation associated with tube feeding. The high-nitrogen and concentrated vitamin/mineral content of Jevity makes it ideal for patients with increased nutrient needs and/or reduced caloric requirements. Because it is fortified with selenium, chromium, molybdenum, carnitine and taurine, Jevity can be used as the sole source of nutrition for extended periods of time.

Not for parenteral use.

AVAILABILITY

Ready To Use:
8-fl-oz cans; 24 per case; No. 143.
32-fl-oz cans; 6 per case; No. 50330.
1-liter Ross Ready-To-Hang® Enteral Feeding Containers; 8 per case; No. 682.

COMPOSITION

INGREDIENTS

Ⓓ-D Water, hydrolyzed cornstarch, sodium and calcium caseinates, soy fiber (a source of dietary fiber), medium-chain triglycerides (fractionated coconut oil), corn oil, soy oil, calcium phosphate tribasic, potassium citrate, magnesium chloride, soy lecithin, sodium citrate, potassium chloride, magnesium sulfate, choline chloride, ascorbic acid, taurine, L-carnitine, zinc sulfate, ferrous sulfate, alpha-tocopheryl acetate, niacinamide, calcium pantothenate, manganese sulfate, cupric sulfate, thiamine chloride hydrochloride, pyridoxine hydrochloride, riboflavin, vitamin A palmitate, folic acid, biotin, sodium molybdate, chromium chloride, potassium iodide, sodium selenite, phylloquinone, cyanocobalamin and vitamin D_3.
Nutrients (Grams/8 fl oz): Protein, 10.5; Fat, 8.7; Carbohydrate, 35.9*; L-carnitine, 0.027; Taurine, 0.027; Water, 197. Calories per mL, 1.06; Calories per fl oz, 31.3.

*Includes soy fiber (a source of dietary fiber that provides 10 Calories and 3.4 g total dietary fiber).
(FAN 725-03)

MURINE®   OTC

[mur'ēn]
Lubricating Eye Drops

(See PDR For Nonprescription Drugs or PDR For Ophthalmology.)

MURINE® PLUS   OTC

[mur'ēn]
Lubricating Redness Reliever Eye Drops

(See PDR For Nonprescription Drugs or PDR For Ophthalmology.)

MURINE® EAR WAX REMOVAL SYSTEM/MURINE® EAR DROPS   OTC
[mur'ēn]
Carbamide Peroxide Ear Wax Removal Aid

(See PDR For Nonprescription Drugs.)

NEPRO™
[nep'rō]
Specialized Liquid Nutrition

USAGE

As a moderate-protein, low-electrolyte, low-fluid, high-calorie formula, Nepro is designed to provide balanced nutrition for dialyzed patients with chronic or acute renal failure. Nepro may be fed orally or by tube. It can be used as a primary or supplemental source of nutrition for dialyzed renal patients.
Not for parenteral use.

AVAILABILITY
Ready To Use
8-fl-oz cans; 24 per case; Vanilla, No. 50632.

COMPOSITION

INGREDIENTS

Ⓓ-D Water, hydrolyzed cornstarch, high-oleic safflower oil, calcium, magnesium and sodium caseinates, sucrose, soy oil, soy lecithin, natural and artificial flavors, calcium carbonate, potassium citrate, sodium chloride, sodium citrate, choline chloride, magnesium hydroxide, calcium hydroxide, ascorbic acid, L-carnitine, taurine, zinc sulfate, alpha-tocopheryl acetate, ferrous sulfate, niacinamide, calcium pantothenate, manganese sulfate, pyridoxine hydrochloride, cupric sulfate, thiamine chloride hydrochloride, riboflavin, folic acid, vitamin A palmitate, biotin, potassium iodide, sodium selenite, phylloquinone, cyanocobalamin and vitamin D_3.
Nutrients (Grams/8 fl oz): Protein, 16.6; Fat, 22.7; Carbohydrate, 51.1; L-carnitine, 0.062; Taurine, 0.038; Water, 167. Calories per mL, 2.0; Calories per fl oz, 59.4.
(FAN 823-02)

OSMOLITE®
[oz'mō-līt]
Isotonic Liquid Nutrition

USAGE

As an isotonic liquid food providing complete, balanced nutrition. Osmolite is isotonic so it is useful for patients sensitive to hyperosmotic feedings. Osmolite may be used as a tube feeding (nasogastric, nasoduodenal or jejunal) or as an oral feeding. Two quarts (2000 Calories) of Osmolite meet or surpass 100% of the U.S. RDA for vitamins and minerals for adults and children 4 or more years of age.
Not for parenteral use.

AVAILABILITY
Ready To Use:
8-fl-oz bottles; 24 per case; No. 715.
8-fl-oz cans; 24 per case; No. 709.
32-fl-oz cans; 6 per case; No. 738.
1-liter Ross Ready-To-Hang® Enteral Feeding Containers; 8 per case; No. 50350.

COMPOSITION
Ready To Use (Ready-To-Hang has similar composition. For specific information, see product label.)

INGREDIENTS

Ⓓ-D Water, hydrolyzed cornstarch, casein, medium-chain triglycerides (fractionated coconut oil), corn oil, soy protein isolate, soy oil, potassium citrate, soy lecithin, calcium phosphate tribasic, magnesium chloride, carrageenan, choline chloride, ascorbic acid, magnesium sulfate, taurine, L-carnitine, sodium citrate, zinc sulfate, ferrous sulfate, alpha-tocopheryl acetate, niacinamide, calcium pantothenate, manganese sulfate, thiamine chloride hydrochloride, pyridoxine hydrochloride, riboflavin, cupric sulfate, vitamin A palmitate, folic acid, biotin, sodium molybdate, chromium chloride, potassium iodide, sodium selenite, phylloquinone, cyanocobalamin and vitamin D_3.
Nutrients (Grams/8 fl oz): Protein, 8.8; Fat, 9.1; Carbohydrate, 34.3; L-Carnitine, 0.019; Taurine, 0.019; Water, 199. Calories per mL, 1.06; Calories per fl oz, 31.3.
(FAN 689-05)

OSMOLITE® HN
[oz'mō-līt]
High Nitrogen Isotonic Liquid Nutrition

USAGE

As a high-nitrogen, isotonic liquid food providing complete, balanced nutrition. Osmolite HN was designed to meet the needs of tube-fed patients with decreased energy requirements or increased protein needs, with intolerance to hyperosmolar feedings or with fat maldigestion/malabsorption. Osmolite HN helps tube-fed patients get the vitamins, minerals and protein they need when their volume intake is low. Osmolite HN may be used as a tube feeding (nasogastric, nasoduodenal or jejunal).
Not for parenteral use.

AVAILABILITY
Ready To Use:
8-fl-oz bottles; 24 per case; No. 736.
8-fl-oz cans; 24 per case; No. 735.
32-fl-oz cans; 6 per case; No. 739.
1-liter Ross Ready-To-Hang® Enteral Feeding Containers; 8 per case; No. 668.

COMPOSITION
Ready To Use (Ready-To-Hang has similar composition. For specific information, see product label.)

INGREDIENTS

Ⓓ-D Water, hydrolyzed cornstarch, casein, medium-chain triglycerides (fractionated coconut oil), corn oil, soy protein isolate, soy oil, magnesium chloride, potassium citrate, calcium phosphate tribasic, soy lecithin, sodium citrate, potassium chloride, choline chloride, ascorbic acid, carrageenan, potassium phosphate dibasic, taurine, L-carnitine, zinc sulfate, ferrous sulfate, alpha-tocopheryl acetate, niacinamide, calcium pantothenate, manganese sulfate, thiamine chloride hydrochloride, pyridoxine hydrochloride, cupric sulfate, riboflavin, vitamin A palmitate, folic acid, biotin, sodium molybdate, chromium chloride, potassium iodide, sodium selenite, phylloquinone, cyanocobalamin and vitamin D_3.
Nutrients (Grams/8 fl oz): Protein, 10.5; Fat, 8.7; Carbohydrate, 33.4; L-Carnitine, 0.027; Taurine, 0.027; Water, 199. Calories per mL, 1.06; Calories per fl oz, 31.3.
(FAN 725-06)

PEDIAFLOR® Drops   ℞
[pē'dē-a-flor"]
Sodium Fluoride Oral Solution, USP

DESCRIPTION
One dropperful (1.0 mL) provides:
Fluoride .... 0.5 mg
  (as sodium fluoride .... 1.1 mg)

Inactive Ingredients: Alcohol less than 0.5%, citric acid, methylparaben, propylparaben, sorbitol, water, artificial flavoring and other ingredients.

INDICATIONS AND USAGE
As an aid in the prevention of dental caries in infants and children.

CONTRAINDICATIONS
Should be used only where the fluoride content of the drinking water supply is known to be 0.7 parts per million or less.

PRECAUTIONS
The recommended dosage should not be exceeded since chronic overdosage of fluoride may result in mottling of tooth enamel and osseous changes.

OVERDOSAGE
In children, acute ingestion of 10 to 20 mg of sodium fluoride may cause excessive salivation and gastrointestinal disturbances; 500 mg may be fatal. Oral and/or intravenous fluids containing calcium may be indicated.

DOSAGE AND ADMINISTRATION
Daily dosage —under 2 years of age, one-half dropperful or less; 2 years of age, one dropperful; 3 years of age or older, two dropperfuls or less as directed by physician or dentist.

AVAILABILITY
50-mL bottles, calibrated dropper enclosed; ℞; **NDC** 0074-0101-50.

PEDIALYTE®
[pē'dē-ah-līt"]
Oral Electrolyte Maintenance Solution

USAGE
To restore fluid and minerals lost in diarrhea and vomiting; for maintenance of water and electrolytes following corrective parenteral therapy for severe diarrhea.

Features:
- Ready To Use—no mixing or dilution necessary.
- Balanced electrolytes to replace stool losses and provide maintenance requirements.
- Provides glucose to promote sodium and water absorption.
- Unflavored form available for young infants; fruit-flavored form available to enhance compliance in older infants and children.
- Plastic liter bottles are resealable and easy to pour.
- No coloring added.
- Widely available in grocery, drug and convenience stores.

Pedialyte, Rehydralyte Administration Guide

For Infants and Young Children

Age	2 Weeks	3	6 Months	9	1	1½	2	2½ Years	3	3½	4
Approximate Weight[2]											
(lb)	7	13	17	20	23	25	28	30	32	35	38
(kg)	3.2	6.0	7.8	9.2	10.2	11.4	12.6	13.6	14.6	16.0	17.0
PEDIALYTE UNFLAVORED or FRUIT-FLAVORED fl oz/day for maintenance*	13 to 16	28 to 32	34 to 40	38 to 44	41 to 46	45 to 50	48 to 53	51 to 56	54 to 58	56 to 60	57 to 62
REHYDRALYTE fl oz/day for Replacement for 5% Dehydration (including maintenance)*	18 to 21	38 to 42	47 to 53	53 to 59	58 to 63	64 to 69	69 to 74	74 to 79	78 to 82	83 to 87	85 to 90
REHYDRALYTE fl oz/day for Replacement for 10% Dehydration (including maintenance)*	23 to 26	48 to 52	60 to 66	68 to 74	75 to 80	83 to 88	90 to 95	97 to 102	102 to 106	110 to 114	113 to 118

Administration Guide does not apply to infants less than 1 week of age. For children over 4 years, maintenance intakes may exceed 2 liters daily.

1. Extrapolated from Barness L: Nutrition and nutritional disorders, in Behrman RE, Vaughan VC III: *Nelson Textbook of Pediatrics,* ed 12. Philadelphia, WB Saunders Co, 1983, pp 136-138.
2. Weight based on the 50th percentile of weight for age of the National Center for Health Statistics (NCHS) reference data. Hamill PVV, Drizd TA, Johnson CL, et al: Physical growth: National Center for Health Statistics percentiles. *Am J Clin Nutr* 1979; 32:607-629.
* Fluid intakes do not take into account ongoing stool losses. Fluid loss in the stool should be replaced by consumption of an extra amount of Pedialyte or Rehydralyte equal to stool losses in addition to the amounts given in this Administration Guide.

Ross Laboratories—Cont.

AVAILABILITY

1 liter (33.8-fl-oz) plastic bottles; 8 per case; Unflavored, No. 336—NDC 0074-6470-32; Fruit-flavored, No. 365—NDC 0074-6471-32.

8-fl-oz bottles; 4 six-packs per case; Unflavored, No. 160—NDC 0074-6470-08. For hospital use, Pedialyte is available in the Ross Hospital Formula System.

DOSAGE

Administration Guide to restore fluid and minerals lost in diarrhea and vomiting (Pedialyte Unflavored or Fruit-Flavored) and management of mild to moderate dehydration secondary to moderate to severe diarrhea (Rehydralyte® Oral Electrolyte Rehydration Solution).

Pedialyte (Unflavored or Fruit-Flavored) or Rehydralyte should be offered frequently in amounts tolerated. Total daily intake should be adjusted to meet individual needs, based on thirst and response to therapy. The suggested intakes for maintenance are based on water requirements for ordinary energy expenditure.[1] The suggested intakes for replacement are based on fluid losses of 5% or 10% of body weight, including maintenance requirement.
[See table on preceding page.]

COMPOSITION

Unflavored Pedialyte (Fruit-Flavored Pedialyte has similar composition and nutrient value. For specific information, see product label.)

INGREDIENTS

(Pareve, ⓤ) Water, dextrose, potassium citrate, sodium chloride and sodium citrate.

Provides:	Per 8 Fl Oz	Per Liter	Per 32 Fl Oz
Sodium (mEq)	10.6	45	42.4
Potassium (mEq)	4.7	20	18.8
Chloride (mEq)	8.3	35	33.2
Citrate (mEq)	7.1	30	28.4
Dextrose (g)	5.9	25	23.6
Calories	24	100	96

(FAN 806-01)

PEDIASURE®
[pē'dē-ah-shur"]
Liquid Nutrition for Children

USAGE

As a nutritionally complete, balanced, isotonic enteral formula especially designed for tube or oral feeding of children 1 to 6 years of age. May be used as the sole source of nutrition or as a supplement. PediaSure meets or exceeds 100% of the NAS-NRC RDAs for protein, vitamins and minerals for children 1 to 6 years of age in 1000 mL. Calcium/phosphorus ratio of 1.2:1 meets recommendations by the American Academy of Pediatrics Committee on Nutrition (AAP-CON) for growing children. Fortified with biotin, choline, inositol, taurine and L-carnitine.

Not for parenteral use.

Not intended for infants under 1 year of age unless specified by a physician.

AVAILABILITY

Ready To Use:
8-fl-oz cans; 24 per case; Vanilla, No. 373.

INGREDIENTS

ⓤ-D Water, hydrolyzed cornstarch, sucrose, sodium caseinate, high oleic safflower oil, soy oil, fractionated coconut oil (medium-chain triglycerides), whey protein concentrate, calcium phosphate tribasic, natural and artificial flavor, magnesium chloride, potassium citrate, potassium phosphate dibasic, potassium chloride, soy lecithin, mono- and diglycerides, choline chloride, carrageenan, ascorbic acid, m-inositol, taurine, ferrous sulfate, zinc sulfate, niacinamide, alpha-tocopheryl acetate, L-carnitine, calcium pantothenate, manganese sulfate, thiamine chloride hydrochloride, pyridoxine hydrochloride, riboflavin, cupric sulfate, vitamin A palmitate, folic acid, biotin, vitamin D₃, potassium iodide, sodium selenite, sodium molybdate, phylloquinone and cyanocobalamin.

Nutrients (Grams/8 fl oz): Protein, 7.1; Fat, 11.8; Carbohydrate, 26; L-Carnitine, 0.004; Taurine, 0.017; Water, 200. Calories per mL, 1.0; Calories per fl oz, 29.6.
(FAN 688-02)

PEDIAZOLE®   ℞
[pē'dē-e-zōl"]
**erythromycin ethylsuccinate
and sulfisoxazole acetyl for oral suspension**

DESCRIPTION

Pediazole is a combination of erythromycin ethylsuccinate, USP and sulfisoxazole acetyl, USP. When reconstituted with water as directed on the label, the granules form a white, strawberry-banana flavor suspension which provides 200 mg erythromycin activity and the equivalent of 600 mg of sulfisoxazole per teaspoonful (5 mL).

Erythromycin is produced by a strain of *Streptomyces erythraeus* and belongs to the macrolide group of antibiotics. It is basic and readily forms salts and esters. Erythromycin ethylsuccinate is an ester of erythromycin.

Sulfisoxazole acetyl or N[1]-acetyl sulfisoxazole is an ester of sulfisoxazole. Chemically, sulfisoxazole is N[1]-(3,4-dimethyl-5-isoxazolyl) sulfanilamide.

Inactive Ingredients: Citric acid, magnesium aluminum silicate, poloxamer, sodium carboxymethylcellulose, sodium citrate, sucrose, artificial flavoring and other ingredients.

ACTIONS

Clinical Pharmacology: Orally administered erythromycin ethylsuccinate suspension is reliably and readily absorbed and serum levels are comparable when administered to patients in either the fasting or non-fasting state. After absorption, erythromycin diffuses readily into most body fluids. In the presence of normal hepatic function, erythromycin is concentrated in the liver and excreted in the bile; the effect of hepatic dysfunction on excretion of erythromycin by the liver into the bile is not known. After oral administration, less than 5 percent of the activity of the administered dose can be recovered in the urine.

Erythromycin crosses the placental barrier but fetal plasma levels are generally low.

Sulfisoxazole acetyl is deacetylated by enzymatic hydrolysis in the gastrointestinal tract from which it is readily absorbed as sulfisoxazole. Sulfisoxazole exists in the blood primarily bound to serum proteins as well as conjugated and in the active or free form. Metabolic pathways include N[4]-acetylation and oxidation with approximately 80 percent of an administered dose being excreted by the kidney within 24 hours.

Serum half-life for total erythromycin and free sulfisoxazole is about 1.5 and 6 hours, respectively.

Microbiology: Pediazole has been formulated to contain sulfisoxazole for concomitant use with erythromycin. The mode of action of erythromycin is by inhibition of protein synthesis without affecting nucleic acid synthesis. Sulfonamides, including sulfisoxazole, possess bacteriostatic activity. This bacteriostatic agent acts by means of competitively inhibiting bacterial synthesis of folic acid (pteroylglutamic acid) from para-amino-benzoic acid. Resistance to erythromycin blood levels ordinarily achieved has been demonstrated by some strains of *Hemophilus influenzae*. Pediazole is usually active against *Hemophilus influenzae in vitro*, including ampicillin-resistant strains.

Quantitative methods that require measurements of zone diameters give the most precise estimates of antibiotic susceptibility. One such standardized procedure, the ASM-2 method published by the National Committee for Clinical Laboratory Standards (NCCLS), has been recommended for use with discs to test susceptibility to erythromycin and sulfisoxazole. Interpretation involves correlation of the diameters obtained in the disc test with Minimal Inhibitory Concentrations (MIC) values for erythromycin and sulfisoxazole. If the standardized ASM-2 procedure of disc susceptibility is used, a 15 mcg erythromycin disc should give a zone diameter of at least 18 mm when tested against an erythromycin-susceptible bacterial strain and a 250-300 mcg sulfisoxazole disc should give a zone diameter of at least 17 mm when tested against a sulfisoxazole-susceptible bacterial strain.

In vitro sulfonamide sensitivity tests are not always reliable because media containing excessive amounts of thymidine are capable of reversing the inhibitory effect of sulfonamides which may result in false resistant reports. The tests must be carefully coordinated with bacteriological and clinical responses. When the patient is already taking sulfonamides follow-up cultures should have aminobenzoic acid added to the isolation media but not to subsequent susceptibility test media.

INDICATION

For treatment of ACUTE OTITIS MEDIA in children that is caused by susceptible strains of *Hemophilus influenzae.*

CONTRAINDICATIONS

Known hypersensitivity to either erythromycin or sulfonamides.

Infants less than 2 months of age.

Pregnancy at term and during the nursing period, because sulfonamides pass into the placental circulation and are excreted in human breast milk and may cause kernicterus in the infant.

WARNINGS

FATALITIES ASSOCIATED WITH THE ADMINISTRATION OF SULFONAMIDES, ALTHOUGH RARE, HAVE OCCURRED DUE TO SEVERE REACTIONS INCLUDING STEVENS-JOHNSON SYNDROME, TOXIC EPIDERMAL NECROLYSIS, FULMINANT HEPATIC NECROSIS, AGRANULOCYTOSIS, APLASTIC ANEMIA, AND OTHER BLOOD DYSCRASIAS.

Clinical signs such as sore throat, fever, pallor, rash, purpura, or jaundice may be early indications of serious reactions.

PEDIAZOLE SHOULD BE DISCONTINUED AT THE FIRST APPEARANCE OF SKIN RASH OR ANY SIGN OF ADVERSE REACTION. In some instances a skin rash may be followed by a more severe reaction, such as Stevens-Johnson syndrome, toxic epidermal necrolysis, hepatic necrosis and serious blood disorders.

COMPLETE BLOOD COUNT SHOULD BE DONE FREQUENTLY IN PATIENTS RECEIVING SULFONAMIDES.

Usage in Pregnancy (SEE ALSO: CONTRAINDICATIONS): The safe use of erythromycin or sulfonamides in pregnancy has not been established. The teratogenic potential of most sulfonamides has not been thoroughly investigated in either animals or humans. However, a significant increase in the incidence of cleft palate and other bony abnormalities of offspring has been observed when certain sulfonamides of the short, intermediate and long-acting types were given to pregnant rats and mice at high oral doses (7 to 25 times the human therapeutic dose).

The frequency of renal complications is considerably lower in patients receiving the most soluble sulfonamides such as sulfisoxazole. Urinalysis with careful microscopic examination should be obtained frequently in patients receiving sulfonamides.

PRECAUTIONS

Erythromycin is principally excreted by the liver. Caution should be exercised in administering the antibiotic to patients with impaired hepatic function. There have been reports of hepatic dysfunction, with or without jaundice occurring in patients receiving oral erythromycin products.

Recent data from studies of erythromycin reveal that its use in patients who are receiving high doses of theophylline may be associated with an increase of serum theophylline levels and potential theophylline toxicity. In case of theophylline toxicity and/or elevated serum theophylline levels, the dose of theophylline should be reduced while the patient is receiving concomitant erythromycin therapy.

Surgical procedures should be performed when indicated.

Sulfonamide therapy should be given with caution to patients with impaired renal or hepatic function and in those patients with a history of severe allergy or bronchial asthma. In the presence of a deficiency in the enzyme glucose-6-phosphate dehydrogenase, hemolysis may occur. This reaction is frequently dose-related. Adequate fluid intake must be maintained in order to prevent crystalluria and renal stone formation.

ADVERSE REACTIONS

The most frequent side effects of oral erythromycin preparations are gastrointestinal, such as abdominal cramping and discomfort, and are dose-related. Nausea, vomiting and diarrhea occur infrequently with usual oral doses. During prolonged or repeated therapy, there is a possibility of overgrowth of nonsusceptible bacteria or fungi. If such infections occur, the drug should be discontinued and appropriate therapy instituted. The overall incidence of these latter side effects reported for the combined administration of erythromycin and a sulfonamide is comparable to those observed in patients given erythromycin alone. Mild allergic reactions such as urticaria and other skin rashes have occurred. Serious allergic reactions, including anaphylaxis, have been reported with erythromycin.

There have been isolated reports of reversible hearing loss occurring chiefly in patients with renal insufficiency and in patients receiving high doses of erythromycin.

The following untoward effects have been associated with the use of sulfonamides:

Blood Dyscrasias: Agranulocytosis, aplastic anemia, thrombocytopenia, leukopenia, hemolytic anemia, purpura, hypoprothrombinemia and methemoglobinemia.

Allergic Reactions: Erythema multiforme (Stevens-Johnson syndrome), generalized skin eruptions, epidermal necrolysis, urticaria, serum sickness, pruritus, exfoliative dermatitis, anaphylactoid reactions, periorbital edema, conjunctival and scleral injection, photosensitization, arthralgia and allergic myocarditis.

Gastrointestinal Reactions: Nausea, emesis, abdominal pains, hepatitis, diarrhea, anorexia, pancreatitis and stomatitis.

CNS Reactions: Headache, peripheral neuritis, mental depression, convulsions, ataxia, hallucinations, tinnitus, vertigo and insomnia.

Miscellaneous Reactions: Drug fever, chills and toxic nephrosis with oliguria or anuria. Periarteritis nodosa and LE phenomenon have occurred.

The sulfonamides bear certain chemical similarities to some goitrogens, diuretics (acetazolamide and the thiazides) and oral hypoglycemic agents. Goiter production, diuresis and hypoglycemia have occurred rarely in patients receiving sulfonamides. Cross-sensitivity may exist with these agents. Rats appear to be especially susceptible to the goitrogenic effects of sulfonamides, and long-term administration has produced thyroid malignancies in the species.

DOSAGE AND ADMINISTRATION

PEDIAZOLE SHOULD NOT BE ADMINISTERED TO INFANTS UNDER 2 MONTHS OF AGE BECAUSE OF CONTRAINDICATIONS OF SYSTEMIC SULFONAMIDES IN THIS AGE GROUP.

For Acute Otitis Media in Children: The dose of Pediazole can be calculated based on the erythromycin component (50 mg/kg/day) or the sulfisoxazole component (150 mg/kg/day to a maximum of 6 g/day). Pediazole should be administered in equally divided doses four times a day for 10 days. Pediazole may be administered without regard to meals. The following approximate dosage schedule is recommended for using Pediazole:

Children: Two months of age or older

Weight	Dose—every 6 hours
Less than 8 kg (18 lb)	Adjust dosage by body weight
8 kg (18 lb)	½ teaspoonful (2.5 mL)
16 kg (35 lb)	1 teaspoonful (5 mL)
24 kg (53 lb)	1½ teaspoonfuls (7.5 mL)
Over 45 kg (over 100 lb)	2 teaspoonfuls (10 mL)

HOW SUPPLIED

Pediazole Suspension is available for teaspoon dosage in 100-mL (**NDC** 0074-8030-13), 150-mL (**NDC** 0074-8030-43), 200-mL (**NDC** 0074-8030-53) and 250 mL (**NDC** 0074-8030-73) bottles, in the form of granules to be reconstituted with water. The suspension provides erythromycin ethylsuccinate equivalent to 200 mg erythromycin activity and sulfisoxazole acetyl equivalent to 600 mg sulfisoxazole per teaspoonful (5 mL).
(.9830)

PERATIVE™

[*per'ah-tiv*]
Specialized Liquid Nutrition

USAGE

As complete, balanced nutrition for use in the nutritional management of metabolically stressed patients with injuries such as multiple fractures, wounds, burns, surgery and the associated conditions of hypermetabolism, catabolism and susceptibility to sepsis.
Not for parenteral use.

AVAILABILITY

Ready To Use:
8-fl-oz cans; 24 cans per case; No. 50628.

COMPOSITION

INGREDIENTS

Ⓤ-D Water, hydrolyzed cornstarch, partially hydrolyzed sodium caseinate, lactalbumin hydrolysate, canola oil, medium-chain triglycerides (fractionated coconut oil), L-arginine, corn oil, magnesium chloride, potassium citrate, calcium phosphate tribasic, citric acid, soy lecithin, ascorbic acid, potassium phosphate dibasic, choline chloride, carrageenan, potassium chloride, taurine, L-carnitine, zinc sulfate, ferrous sulfate, alpha-tocopheryl acetate, niacinamide, calcium pantothenate, manganese sulfate, beta-carotene, cupric sulfate, thiamine chloride hydrochloride, pyridoxine hydrochloride, riboflavin, vitamin A palmitate, folic acid, biotin, sodium molybdate, chromium chloride, potassium iodide, sodium selenite, phylloquinone, cyanocobalamin and vitamin D₃.

Nutrients (Grams/8 fl oz): Protein, 15.8; Fat, 8.8; Carbohydrate, 42.0; L-carnitine, 0.031; Taurine, 0.031; Water, 187. Calories per fl oz, 38.5.
(FAN 851-01)

POLYCOSE®

[*pol'ē-kōs*]
Glucose Polymers

USAGE

As a source of calories (derived solely from carbohydrate) for persons with increased caloric needs or those unable to meet their caloric needs with their normal diet. Polycose is particularly useful in supplying carbohydrate calories for protein-, electrolyte- and fat-restricted diets. Polycose is minimally sweet and mixes readily with most foods and beverages.

PRECAUTIONS

NOT FOR PARENTERAL USE.
Polycose is nutritionally incomplete and should not be used as the sole source of nutrition. Polycose is for enteral use only and should be used as directed by a health care professional.
FOR INFANT USE: Not to be fed undiluted. USE ONLY AS SPECIFICALLY DIRECTED BY A PHYSICIAN.

AVAILABILITY

Powder: 12.3 oz (350g) cans; 6 per case; No. 746.
Liquid: (43% solution): 4.2-fl-oz bottles; 48 per case; No. 431.

COMPOSITION

Powder: (Pareve, Ⓤ) Glucose polymers derived from controlled hydrolysis of cornstarch.
Nutrients (per 100 grams):

Carbohydrate		94 g
Water		6 g
Calcium	Does not exceed	30 mg (1.5 mEq)
Sodium	Does not exceed	110 mg (4.8 mEq)
Potassium	Does not exceed	10 mg (0.3 mEq)
Chloride	Does not exceed	223 mg (6.3 mEq)
Phosphorus	Does not exceed	5 mg
Calories		380

Approximate Caloric Equivalents:
1 level teaspoonful (2 g) = 8 Calories; 1 level tablespoonful (6 g) = 23 Calories; ¼ cup (25 g) = 95 Calories; ⅓ cup (33 g) = 125 Calories; ½ cup (50 g) = 190 Calories; 1 cup (100 g) = 380 Calories.
(FAN 366-01)

COMPOSITION

Liquid: (Pareve, Ⓤ) Water and glucose polymers derived from controlled hydrolysis of cornstarch.
Nutrients (per 100 mL):

Carbohydrate		50 g
Water		70 g
Calcium	Does not exceed	20 mg (1.0 mEq)
Sodium	Does not exceed	70 mg (3.0 mEq)
Potassium	Does not exceed	6 mg (0.15 mEq)
Chloride	Does not exceed	140 mg (3.9 mEq)
Phosphorus	Does not exceed	3 mg
Calories		200

Approximate Caloric Equivalents:
1 mL = 2 Calories; 1 fl oz = 60 Calories; 100 mL = 200 Calories.
(FAN 483-01)

PRAMET® FA   ℞

[*pram'et*]
**Vitamin/Mineral Prescription
for Expectant and
New Mothers**

DESCRIPTION

Each Pramet FA Filmtab® Film-Sealed oral tablet provides:
Vitamins

Vitamin A (as acetate, may contain palmitate) 1.2 mg	4000	I.U.
Vitamin D (cholecalciferol, 10 mcg)	400	I.U.
Vitamin C (ascorbic acid)	100	mg
Folic Acid	1	mg
Vitamin B₁ (thiamine mononitrate)	3	mg
Vitamin B₂ (riboflavin)	2	mg
Niacinamide	10	mg
Vitamin B₆ (pyridoxine hydrochloride)	5	mg
Vitamin B₁₂ (cyanocobalamin)	3	mcg
Pantothenic Acid (as calcium pantothenate)	0.92	mg
Minerals		
Calcium (as calcium carbonate)	250	mg
Iodine (as calcium iodate)	100	mcg
Elemental Iron* (300 mg ferrous sulfate USP)	60	mg
Copper (as cupric chloride)	0.15	mg

* In controlled-release form—Gradumet®

Inactive Ingredients: Cellulosic polymers, corn starch, DC Yellow No. 10, FDC Blue No. 1, magnesium stearate, methyl acrylate-methyl methacrylate copolymer, microcrystalline cellulose, polyethylene glycols, povidone, propylene glycol, talc, titanium dioxide and vanillin.

INDICATIONS AND USAGE

To help prevent vitamin and mineral deficiencies during and after pregnancy and for treatment of megaloblastic anemias. 1 mg of folic acid has been found to be effective therapy for megaloblastic anemias of pregnancy and lactation.

WARNING

Folic acid alone is improper therapy in the treatment of pernicious anemia and other megaloblastic anemias where vitamin B₁₂ is deficient.

PRECAUTION

Folic acid may mask the presence of pernicious anemia in that hematologic remission may occur while neurologic manifestations remain progressive.

ADVERSE REACTION

Allergic sensitization has been reported following both oral and parenteral administration of folic acid.

OVERDOSAGE

Acute overdosage of iron may cause nausea and vomiting and, in severe cases, cardiovascular collapse and death. The estimated lethal dose of orally ingested elemental iron is 300 mg per kg body weight. Serum iron and total iron-binding capacity may be used as guides for use of chelating agents such as deferoxamine.
Store below 77°F (25°C).

DOSAGE AND ADMINISTRATION

One tablet daily, or as directed by physician.

HOW SUPPLIED

100-tablet bottles; ℞; **NDC** 0074-0147-01.
(.1901)

PRAMILET® FA   ℞

[*pram'e-let"*]
**Prenatal Vitamin/Mineral Preparation
with Folic Acid**

DESCRIPTION

Each Pramilet FA Filmtab® Film-Sealed oral tablet provides:
Vitamins

Vitamin A (as acetate, may contain palmitate) 1.2 mg	4000	I.U.
Vitamin D (cholecalciferol, 10 mcg)	400	I.U.
Vitamin C (as sodium ascorbate)	60	mg
Folic Acid	1	mg
Vitamin B₁ (thiamine mononitrate)	3	mg
Vitamin B₂ (riboflavin)	2	mg
Niacinamide	10	mg
Vitamin B₆ (pyridoxine hydrochloride)	3	mg
Vitamin B₁₂ (cyanocobalamin)	3	mcg
Calcium Pantothenate	1	mg
Minerals		
Calcium (as calcium carbonate)	250	mg
Iodine (as calcium iodate)	100	mcg
Elemental Iron (as ferrous fumarate)	40	mg
Magnesium (as magnesium oxide)	10	mg
Copper (as cupric chloride)	0.15	mg
Zinc (as zinc oxide)	0.085	mg

Inactive Ingredients: Cellulosic polymers, cornstarch, crospovidone, D&C Red No. 33, FDC Blue No. 1, propylene glycol, magnesium stearate, povidone, sorbic acid, sorbitan monooleate, titanium dioxide and vanillin.

INDICATIONS AND USAGE

To help prevent vitamin and mineral deficiencies during and after pregnancy and for treatment of megaloblastic anemias. 1 mg of folic acid has been found to be effective therapy for megaloblastic anemias of pregnancy and lactation.

WARNING

Folic acid alone is improper therapy in the treatment of pernicious anemia and other megaloblastic anemias where vitamin B₁₂ is deficient.

PRECAUTION

Folic acid may mask the presence of pernicious anemia in that hematologic remission may occur while neurologic manifestations remain progressive.

ADVERSE REACTION

Allergic sensitization has been reported following both oral and parenteral administration of folic acid.

OVERDOSAGE

Acute overdosage of iron may cause nausea and vomiting and, in severe cases, cardiovascular collapse and death. The estimated lethal dose of orally ingested elemental iron is 300 mg per kg body weight. Serum iron and total iron-binding capacity may be used as guides for use of chelating agents such as deferoxamine.
Store below 77°F (25°C).

DOSAGE AND ADMINISTRATION

One tablet daily, or as directed by physician.

HOW SUPPLIED

100-tablet bottles; ℞; **NDC** 0074-0121-01.
(.1901)

Continued on next page

Ross Laboratories—Cont.

PROMOTE™
[pruh-mōt]
High Protein Liquid Nutrition

USAGE
As a high-protein, nutritionally complete liquid food, Promote is designed for patients who may benefit from an increased protein intake. It has a low nutrient base and permits nonambulatory patients, with energy requirements as low as 1250 Calories, to meet 100% of the highest age/sex-specific NAS-NRC RDAs for protein, vitamins and minerals. Promote has a mild vanilla flavor, making it useful as a high-protein oral supplement.
Not for parenteral use.

AVAILABILITY
Ready To Use:
8-fl-oz cans; 24 cans per case; No. 50774.

COMPOSITION

INGREDIENTS
Ⓤ-D Water, Hydrolyzed Cornstarch, Sodium and Calcium Caseinates, Sucrose, High-Oleic Safflower Oil, Canola Oil, Medium-Chain Triglycerides (Fractionated Coconut Oil), Soy Protein Isolate, Natural and Artificial Flavors, Magnesium Phosphate, Potassium Citrate, Potassium Chloride, Sodium Citrate, Calcium Citrate, Soy Lecithin, Calcium Carbonate, Choline Chloride, Potassium Phosphate Dibasic, Ascorbic Acid, Calcium Phosphate Dibasic, Carrageenan, Taurine, L-Carnitine, Zinc Sulfate, Ferrous Sulfate, Alpha-Tocopheryl Acetate, Niacinamide, Calcium Pantothenate, Manganese Sulfate, Cupric Sulfate, Thiamine Chloride Hydrochloride, Pyridoxine Hydrochloride, Riboflavin, Vitamin A Palmitate, Folic Acid, Biotin, Sodium Molybdate, Chromium Chloride, Potassium Iodide, Sodium Selenite, Phylloquinone, Cyanocobalamin and Vitamin D_3.
Nutrients (Grams/8 fl oz): Protein, 14.8; Fat, 6.2; Carbohydrate, 30.8; L-carnitine, 0.029; Taurine, 0.029; Water, 199. Calories per mL, 1.0; Calories per fl oz, 29.6.
FAN 805-01

PULMOCARE®
[pul'mō-kār]
**Specialized Nutrition
for Pulmonary Patients**

USAGE
For the dietary management of respiratory insufficiency, the high-fat and low-carbohydrate content of Pulmocare is designed to reduce carbon dioxide production and respiratory quotient, thus diminishing ventilatory requirements. Pulmocare can be used for enteral tube feeding or oral supplementation and is appropriate for ambulatory or ventilator-dependent patients.
Not for parenteral use.

AVAILABILITY
8-fl-oz cans; 24 per case; Vanilla, No. 699; Strawberry, No. 50180.
1-liter Ross Ready-To-Hang® Enteral Feeding Containers; 8 per case; No. 51204.

COMPOSITION
Vanilla (Strawberry flavor has similar composition. For specific information, see product label.)

INGREDIENTS
Ⓤ-D Water, corn oil, sodium and calcium caseinates, sucrose, hydrolyzed cornstarch, magnesium chloride, soy lecithin, calcium phosphate tribasic, potassium citrate, sodium citrate, natural and artificial flavor, potassium phosphate dibasic, choline chloride, ascorbic acid, sodium chloride, zinc sulfate, ferrous sulfate, alpha-tocopheryl acetate, niacinamide, carrageenan, calcium pantothenate, manganese sulfate, cupric sulfate, thiamine chloride hydrochloride, pyridoxine hydrochloride, riboflavin, vitamin A palmitate, folic acid, biotin, sodium molybdate, chromium chloride, potassium iodide, sodium selenite, phylloquinone, cyanocobalamin and vitamin D_3.
Nutrients (Grams/8 fl oz): Protein, 14.8; Fat, 21.8; Carbohydrate, 25.0; Water, 186. Calories per mL, 1.5; Calories per fl oz, 44.4.
(FAN 689-04)

REHYDRALYTE®
[rē-hī'drə-līt″]
Oral Electrolyte Rehydration Solution

USAGE
For replacement of water and electrolytes lost during moderate to severe diarrhea.
Features:
● Ready To Use—no mixing or dilution necessary.
● Safe, economical alternative to IV therapy.
● 75 mEq of sodium per liter for effective replacement of fluid deficits.
● 2½% glucose solution to promote sodium and water absorption and provide energy.
● Available in pharmacies.

AVAILABILITY
8-fl-oz bottles; 4 six-packs per case; No. 162; NDC 0074-0162-01.

DOSAGE
(See Administration Guide under Pedialyte)

INGREDIENTS
(Pareve, Ⓤ) Water, dextrose, sodium chloride, potassium citrate and sodium citrate.

Provides:	Per 8 Fl Oz	Per Liter
Sodium (mEq)	17.7	75
Potassium (mEq)	4.7	20
Chloride (mEq)	15.4	65
Citrate (mEq)	7.1	30
Dextrose (g)	5.9	25
Calories	24	100

(FAN 564-01)

RONDEC® Oral Drops   ℞
[ron'dek]
RONDEC® Syrup
RONDEC® Tablet   ℞
RONDEC–TR® Tablet   ℞

DESCRIPTION
Antihistamine/Decongestant for oral use
For infants
RONDEC® Oral Drops
Each dropperful (1 mL) contains carbinoxamine maleate, 2 mg; pseudoephedrine hydrochloride, 25 mg.
Inactive Ingredients: Citric acid, DC Red No. 33, FDC Yellow No. 6, glycerin, methylparaben, propylparaben, purified water, sodium benzoate, sodium citrate, sorbitol and artificial flavoring.
For young children
RONDEC® Syrup
Each teaspoonful (5 mL) contains carbinoxamine maleate, 4 mg; pseudoephedrine hydrochloride, 60 mg.
Inactive Ingredients: Citric acid, DC Red No. 33, FDC Yellow No. 6, glycerin, methylparaben, propylparaben, purified water, sodium benzoate, sodium citrate, sorbitol and artificial flavoring.
For adults and children 6 years and over
RONDEC® Tablet
Each Filmtab® tablet contains carbinoxamine maleate, 4 mg; pseudoephedrine hydrochloride, 60 mg.
Inactive Ingredients: Cellulosic polymers, FDC Yellow No. 6, hydrogenated vegetable oil wax, lactose, magnesium stearate, microcrystalline cellulose, polyethylene glycol, povidone, propylene glycol, silicon dioxide, sodium starch glycolate, sorbitan monooleate, titanium dioxide and vanillin.
For adults and children 12 years and over
RONDEC-TR® Tablet
Each timed-release Filmtab tablet contains carbinoxamine maleate, 8 mg; pseudoephedrine hydrochloride, 120 mg.
Inactive Ingredients: Castor oil, cellulosic polymers, confectioner's sugar, corn starch, FDC Blue No. 1, lactose, magnesium stearate, methyl acrylate-methyl methacrylate copolymer, microcrystalline cellulose, povidone, propylene glycol, sorbitan monooleate and titanium dioxide.
Carbinoxamine maleate (2-[p-Chloro-α-[2-(dimethylamino) ethoxy] benzyl] pyridine maleate) is one of the ethanolamine class of H_1 antihistamines.
Pseudoephedrine hydrochloride (Benzenemethanol, α-[1-(methylamino) ethyl]-, [S-(R*, R*)]-, hydrochloride) is the hydrochloride of pseudoephedrine, a naturally occurring dextrorotatory stereoisomer of ephedrine.

CLINICAL PHARMACOLOGY
Antihistaminic and decongestant actions.
Carbinoxamine maleate possesses H_1 antihistaminic activity and mild anticholinergic and sedative effects. Serum half-life for carbinoxamine is estimated to be 10 to 20 hours. Virtually no intact drug is excreted in the urine.
Pseudoephedrine hydrochloride is an oral sympathomimetic amine that acts as a decongestant to respiratory tract mucous membranes. While its vasoconstrictor action is similar to that of ephedrine, pseudoephedrine has less pressor effect

in normotensive adults. Serum half-life for pseudoephedrine is 6 to 8 hours. Acidic urine is associated with faster elimination of the drug. About one half of the administered dose is excreted in the urine.

INDICATIONS AND USAGE
For symptomatic relief of seasonal and perennial allergic rhinitis and vasomotor rhinitis.
Rondec Oral Drops, Rondec Syrup and Rondec Tablet are immediate-release dosage forms allowing titration of dose up to four times a day.
Rondec-TR Tablet utilizes a gradual-release mechanism providing approximately a 12-hour therapeutic effect, thus allowing twice-daily dosage.

CONTRAINDICATIONS
Patients with hypersensitivity or idiosyncrasy to any ingredients, patients taking monoamine oxidase (MAO) inhibitors, patients with narrow-angle glaucoma, urinary retention, peptic ulcer, severe hypertension or coronary artery disease, or patients undergoing an asthmatic attack.

WARNINGS
Use in Pregnancy: Safety for use during pregnancy has not been established.
Nursing Mothers: Use with caution in nursing mothers.
Special Risk Patients: Use with caution in patients with hypertension or ischemic heart disease, and persons older than 60 years.

PRECAUTIONS
Use with caution in patients with hypertension, heart disease, asthma, hyperthyroidism, increased intraocular pressure, diabetes mellitus and prostatic hypertrophy.
Information for Patients: Avoid alcohol and other CNS depressants while taking these products. Patients sensitive to antihistamines may experience moderate to severe drowsiness. Patients sensitive to sympathomimetic amines may note mild CNS stimulation. While taking these products, exercise care in driving or operating appliances, machinery, etc.
Drug Interactions: Antihistamines may enhance the effects of tricyclic antidepressants, barbiturates, alcohol, and other CNS depressants. MAO inhibitors prolong and intensify the anticholinergic effects of antihistamines. Sympathomimetic amines may reduce the antihypertensive effects of reserpine, veratrum alkaloids, methyldopa and mecamylamine. Effects of sympathomimetics are increased with MAO inhibitors and beta-adrenergic blockers.

Pregnancy Category C.: Animal reproduction studies have not been conducted with these products. It is also not known whether these products can cause fetal harm when administered to a pregnant woman or affect reproduction capacity. Give to pregnant women only if clearly needed.

ADVERSE REACTIONS
Antihistamines: Sedation, dizziness, diplopia, vomiting, diarrhea, dry mouth, headache, nervousness, nausea, anorexia, heartburn, weakness, polyuria and dysuria and, rarely, excitability in children.
Sympathomimetic Amines: Convulsions, CNS stimulation, cardiac arrhythmias, respiratory difficulty, increased heart rate or blood pressure, hallucinations, tremors, nervousness, insomnia, weakness, pallor and dysuria.

OVERDOSAGE
No information is available as to specific results of an overdose of these products. The signs, symptoms and treatment described below are those of H_1 antihistamines and ephedrine overdose.
Symptoms: Should antihistamine effects predominate, central action constitutes the greatest danger. In the small child, symptoms include excitation, hallucination, ataxia, incoordination, tremors, flushed face and fever. Convulsions, fixed and dilated pupils, coma and death may occur in severe cases. In the adult, fever and flushing are uncommon; excitement leading to convulsions and postictal depression is often preceded by drowsiness and coma. Respiration is usually not seriously depressed; blood pressure is usually stable.
Should sympathomimetic symptoms predominate, central effects include restlessness, dizziness, tremor, hyperactive reflexes, talkativeness, irritability and insomnia. Cardiovascular and renal effects include difficulty in micturition, headache, flushing, palpitation, cardiac arrhythmias, hypertension with subsequent hypotension and circulatory collapse. Gastrointestinal effects include dry mouth, metallic taste, anorexia, nausea, vomiting, diarrhea and abdominal cramps.
Treatment: a) Evacuate stomach as condition warrants. Activated charcoal may be useful. *b)* Maintain a non-stimulating environment. *c)* Monitor cardiovascular status. *d)* Do not give stimulants. *e)* Reduce fever with cool sponging. *f)* Support respiration. *g)* Use sedatives or anticonvulsants to control CNS excitation and convulsions. *h)* Physostigmine may reverse anticholinergic symptoms. *i)* Ammonium chloride may acidify the urine to increase excretion of

pseudoephedrine. *j*) Further care is symptomatic and supportive.

DOSAGE AND ADMINISTRATION

Age	Dose*	Frequency*
Rondec Oral Drops		
for oral use only		
1–3 months	¼ dropperful (¼ mL)	q.i.d.
3–6 months	½ dropperful (½ mL)	q.i.d.
6–9 months	¾ dropperful (¾ mL)	q.i.d.
9–18 months	1 dropperful (1 mL)	q.i.d.
Rondec Syrup and		
Rondec Tablet		
18 months–		
6 years	½ teaspoonful (2.5 mL)	q.i.d.
adults and		
children	1 teaspoonful (5 mL)	q.i.d.
6 years and	or	
over	1 tablet	
Rondec-TR Tablet		
adults and children		
12 years and over	1 tablet	b.i.d.

*In mild cases or in particularly sensitive patients, less frequent or reduced doses may be adequate.

HOW SUPPLIED

Rondec Oral Drops, berry-flavored, in 30-mL bottles for dropper dosage, **NDC** 0074-5783-30. Calibrated shatterproof dropper enclosed in each carton. Container meets safety closure requirements.
Rondec Syrup, berry-flavored, in 16-fl-oz (1-pint) bottles, **NDC** 0074-5782-16; and 4-fl-oz bottles, **NDC** 0074-5782-04. Dispense in USP tight glass container.
Rondec Tablet, Filmtab tablets, in bottles of 100, **NDC** 0074-5726-13; and bottles of 500, **NDC** 0074-5726-53. Each orange-colored tablet marked with Ross "R" and the number 5726 for professional identification. Dispense in USP tight container.
Rondec-TR Tablet, Filmtab tablets, in bottles of 100, **NDC** 0074-6240-13. Each blue-colored tablet marked with Ross "R" and the number 6240 for professional identification. Dispense in USP tight container.
Recommended storage: Store below 86°F (30°C).
(.1901)

RONDEC®–DM Syrup ℞
[ron 'dek]
RONDEC®–DM Oral Drops ℞

DESCRIPTION

Antihistamine/Decongestant/Antitussive for oral use
For adults and children
Rondec®-DM Syrup
Each teaspoonful (5 mL) contains carbinoxamine maleate, 4 mg; pseudoephedrine hydrochloride, 60 mg; dextromethorphan hydrobromide, 15 mg.
Inactive Ingredients: Citric acid, DC Red No. 33, FDC Blue No. 1, glycerin, menthol, purified water, sodium benzoate, sodium citrate, sorbitol, natural and artificial flavoring and other ingredients.
For infants
Rondec®-DM Oral Drops
Each dropperful (1 mL) contains carbinoxamine maleate, 2 mg; pseudoephedrine hydrochloride, 25 mg; dextromethorphan hydrobromide, 4 mg.
Inactive Ingredients: Citric acid, DC Red No. 33, FDC Blue No. 1, glycerin, menthol, purified water, sodium benzoate, sodium citrate, sorbitol, natural and artificial flavoring and other ingredients.
Carbinoxamine maleate (2-[p-Chloro-α-[2-(dimethylamino) ethoxy]benzyl]pyridine maleate) is one of the ethanolamine class of H_1 antihistamines.
Pseudoephedrine hydrochloride (Benzenemethanol, α-[1-(methylamino) ethyl]-, [S-(R*, R*)]-, hydrochloride) is the hydrochloride of pseudoephedrine, a naturally occurring dextrorotatory stereoisomer of ephedrine.
Dextromethorphan hydrobromide (Morphinan, 3-methoxy-17-methyl-, (9α, 13α, 14α) -, hydrobromide, monohydrate) is the hydrobromide of d-form racemethorphan.

CLINICAL PHARMACOLOGY

Antihistaminic, decongestant and antitussive actions.
Carbinoxamine maleate possesses H_1 antihistaminic activity and mild anticholinergic and sedative effects. Serum half-life for carbinoxamine is estimated to be 10 to 20 hours. Virtually no intact drug is excreted in the urine.
Pseudoephedrine hydrochloride is an oral sympathomimetic amine that acts as a decongestant to respiratory tract mucous membranes. While its vasoconstrictor action is similar to that of ephedrine, pseudoephedrine has less pressor effect in normotensive adults. Serum half-life for pseudoephedrine is 6 to 8 hours. Acidic urine is associated with faster elimination of the drug. About one half of the administered dose is excreted in the urine.

Dextromethorphan hydrobromide is a nonnarcotic antitussive with effectiveness equal to codeine. It acts in the medulla oblongata to elevate the cough threshold. Dextromethorphan does not produce analgesia or induce tolerance, and has no potential for addiction. At usual doses, it will not depress respiration or inhibit ciliary activity. Dextromethorphan is rapidly metabolized, with trace amounts of the parent compound in blood and urine. About one half of the administered dose is excreted in the urine as conjugated metabolites.

INDICATIONS AND USAGE

For relief of coughs and upper respiratory symptoms, including nasal congestion, associated with allergy or the common cold.

CONTRAINDICATIONS

Patients with hypersensitivity or idiosyncrasy to any ingredients, patients taking monoamine oxidase (MAO) inhibitors, patients with narrow-angle glaucoma, urinary retention, peptic ulcer, severe hypertension or coronary artery disease, or patients undergoing an asthmatic attack.

WARNINGS

Use in Pregnancy: Safety for use during pregnancy has not been established.
Nursing Mothers: Use with caution in nursing mothers.
Special Risk Patients: Use with caution in patients with hypertension or ischemic heart disease, and persons older than 60 years.

PRECAUTIONS

Before prescribing medication to suppress or modify cough, identify and provide therapy for the underlying cause of cough.
Use with caution in patients with hypertension, heart disease, asthma, hyperthyroidism, increased intraocular pressure, diabetes mellitus and prostatic hypertrophy.
Information for Patients: Avoid alcohol and other CNS depressants while taking these products. Patients sensitive to antihistamines may experience moderate to severe drowsiness. Patients sensitive to sympathomimetic amines may note mild CNS stimulation. While taking these products, exercise care in driving or operating appliances, machinery, etc.
Drug Interactions: Antihistamines may enhance the effects of tricyclic antidepressants, barbiturates, alcohol, and other CNS depressants. MAO inhibitors prolong and intensify the anticholinergic effects of antihistamines. Sympathomimetic amines may reduce the antihypertensive effects of reserpine, veratrum alkaloids, methyldopa and mecamylamine. Effects of sympathomimetics are increased with MAO inhibitors and beta-adrenergic blockers. The cough-suppressant action of dextromethorphan and narcotic antitussives are additive.
Pregnancy Category C.: Animal reproduction studies have not been conducted with Rondec-DM. It is also not known whether these products can cause fetal harm when administered to a pregnant woman or affect reproduction capacity. Give to pregnant women only if clearly needed.

ADVERSE REACTIONS

Antihistamines: Sedation, dizziness, diplopia, vomiting, diarrhea, dry mouth, headache, nervousness, nausea, anorexia, heartburn, weakness, polyuria and dysuria and, rarely, excitability in children.
Sympathomimetic Amines: Convulsions, CNS stimulation, cardiac arrhythmias, respiratory difficulty, increased heart rate or blood pressure, hallucinations, tremors, nervousness, insomnia, weakness, pallor and dysuria.
Dextromethorphan: Drowsiness and GI disturbance.

OVERDOSAGE

No information is available as to specific results of an overdose of these products. The signs, symptoms and treatment described below are those of H_1 antihistamine, ephedrine and dextromethorphan overdose.
Symptoms: Should antihistamine effects predominate, central action constitutes the greatest danger. In the small child, predominant symptoms are excitation, hallucination, ataxia, incoordination, tremors, flushed face and fever. Convulsions, fixed and dilated pupils, coma and death may occur in severe cases. In the adult, fever and flushing are uncommon; excitement leading to convulsions and postictal depression is often preceded by drowsiness and coma. Respiration is usually not seriously depressed; blood pressure is usually stable.
Should sympathomimetic symptoms predominate, central effects include restlessness, dizziness, tremor, hyperactive reflexes, talkativeness, irritability and insomnia. Cardiovascular and renal effects include difficulty in micturition, headache, flushing, palpitation, cardiac arrhythmias, hypertension with subsequent hypotension and circulatory collapse. Gastrointestinal effects include dry mouth, metallic taste, anorexia, nausea, vomiting, diarrhea and abdominal cramps.
Dextromethorphan may cause respiratory depression with a large overdose.

Treatment: *a*) Evacuate stomach as condition warrants. Activated charcoal may be useful. *b*) Maintain a nonstimulating environment. *c*) Monitor cardiovascular status. *d*) Do not give stimulants. *e*) Reduce fever with cool sponging. *f*) Treat respiratory depression with naloxone if dextromethorphan toxicity is suspected. *g*) Use sedatives or anticonvulsants to control CNS excitation and convulsions. *h*) Physostigmine may reverse anticholinergic symptoms. *i*) Ammonium chloride may acidify the urine to increase urinary excretion of pseudoephedrine. *j*) Further care is symptomatic and supportive.

DOSAGE AND ADMINISTRATION

Age	Dose*	Frequency*
Rondec-DM Syrup		
18 months–	½ teaspoonful	
6 years	(2.5 mL)	q.i.d.
adults and	1 teaspoonful	
children 6	(5 mL)	q.i.d.
years and over		
Rondec-DM Oral Drops		
for oral use only		
1–3 months	¼ dropperful (¼ mL)	q.i.d.
3–6 months	½ dropperful (½ mL)	q.i.d.
6–9 months	¾ dropperful (¾ mL)	q.i.d.
9–18 months	1 dropperful (1 mL)	q.i.d.

*In mild cases or in particularly sensitive patients, less frequent or reduced doses may be adequate.

HOW SUPPLIED

Rondec-DM Syrup, grape-flavored, in 16-fl-oz (1-pint) bottles, **NDC** 0074-5640-16; and 4-fl-oz bottles, **NDC** 0074-5640-04. Dispense in USP tight, light-resistant, glass container. Avoid exposure to excessive heat.
Rondec-DM Oral Drops, grape-flavored, in 30-mL bottles for dropper dosage. Calibrated, shatterproof dropper enclosed in each carton. Container meets safety closure requirements. **NDC** 0074-5639-30. Avoid exposure to excessive heat.
(.7890)

ROSS HOSPITAL FORMULA SYSTEM
Products for hospital nursery use

ALIMENTUM®
Protein Hydrolysate Formula With Iron
  Availability: Ready To Feed
  8-fl-oz glass bottles; 24 per case; No. 862.

ISOMIL® 20 (20 Cal/fl oz)
Soy Protein Formula With Iron
  Availability: Ready To Feed
  4-fl-oz glass bottles; 48 per case; No. 406.
  4-fl-oz plastic bottles; 48 per case; No. 50568.
  8-fl-oz glass bottles; 24 per case; No. 871.

PEDIALYTE®
Oral Electrolyte Maintenance Solution
  Availability: Ready To Use
  8-fl-oz glass bottles; 24 per case; No. 806.

SIMILAC® 13 (13 Cal/fl oz)
Low-Iron Infant Formula
  Availability: Ready To Feed
  4-fl-oz glass bottles; 48 per case; No. 408.

SIMILAC® 20 (20 Cal/fl oz)
Low-Iron Infant Formula
  Availability: Ready To Feed
  4-fl-oz glass bottles; 48 per case; No. 415.
  4-fl-oz plastic bottles; 48 per case; No. 50558.
  8-fl-oz glass bottles; 24 per case; No. 841.

SIMILAC® WITH IRON 20
Infant Formula
  Availability: Ready To Feed
  4-fl-oz glass bottles; 48 per case; No. 426.
  4-fl-oz plastic bottles; 48 per case; No. 50564.
  8-fl-oz glass bottles; 24 per case; No. 858.

SIMILAC® 24 (24 Cal/fl oz)
Low-Iron Infant Formula
  Availability: Ready To Feed
  4-fl-oz glass bottles; 48 per case; No. 404.
  4-fl-oz plastic bottles; 48 per case; No. 50560.

SIMILAC® WITH IRON 24
Infant Formula
  Availability: Ready To Feed
  4-fl-oz glass bottles; 48 per case; No. 403.
  4-fl-oz plastic bottles; 48 per case; No. 50566.

SIMILAC® 27 (27 Cal/fl oz)
Low-Iron Infant Formula
  Availability: Ready To Feed
  4-fl-oz glass bottles; 48 per case; No. 427.

Continued on next page

Ross Laboratories—Cont.

SIMILAC NATURAL CARE®
Low-Iron Human Milk Fortifier
Availability: Ready To Use
4-fl-oz glass bottles; 48 per case; No. 443.

SIMILAC® PM 60/40
Low-Iron Infant Formula
Availability: Ready To Feed
4-fl-oz glass bottles; 48 per case; No. 424.

SIMILAC® SPECIAL CARE® 20 (20 Cal/fl oz)
Low-Iron Premature Infant Formula
Availability: Ready To Feed
4-fl-oz glass bottles; 48 per case; No. 439.
4-fl-oz plastic bottles; 48 per case; No. 50570.

SIMILAC® SPECIAL CARE® 24 (24 Cal/fl oz)
Low-Iron Premature Infant Formula
Availability: Ready To Feed
4-fl-oz glass bottles; 48 per case; No. 433.
4-fl-oz plastic bottles; 48 per case; No. 50572.

SIMILAC® SPECIAL CARE® WITH IRON 24
Premature Infant Formula
Availability: Ready To Feed
4-fl-oz glass bottles; 48 per case; No. 478.
4-fl-oz plastic bottles; 48 per case; No. 50574.

STERILIZED WATER
Availability: Ready To Feed
4-fl-oz glass bottles; 48 per case; No. 432.
4-fl-oz plastic bottles; 48 per case; No. 50550.
8-fl-oz glass bottles; 24 per case; No. 879.

5% GLUCOSE WATER
Availability: Ready To Feed
4-fl-oz glass bottles; 48 per case; No. 405.
4-fl-oz plastic bottles; 48 per case; No. 50552.

10% GLUCOSE WATER
Availability: Ready To Feed
4-fl-oz glass bottles; 48 per case; No. 410.
4-fl-oz plastic bottles; 48 per case; No. 50554.

ROSS METABOLIC FORMULA SYSTEM

CALCILO XD®
Low-Calcium/Vitamin D-Free
Infant Formula With Iron
Powder: 14.1-oz cans, measuring scoop enclosed; 6 per case; No. 378.

PROVIMIN®
Protein-Vitamin-Mineral
Formula Component With Iron
Powder: 5.3-oz (150 g) cans, 6 per case; No. 50260.

RCF®
Ross Carbohydrate Free
Low-Iron Soy Protein Formula Base
Concentrated Liquid: 13-fl-oz cans; 12 per case; No. 108.

SIMILAC® PM 60/40
[sim 'e-lak]
Low-Iron Infant Formula
Powder: 1-lb cans, measuring scoop enclosed; 6 per case; No. 00850.
For hospital use, Ready To Feed Similac PM 60/40 in disposable nursing bottles is available in the Ross Hospital Formula System. (Ready To Feed has similar composition and nutrient values as Powder. For specific information see bottle tray.)

SELSUN® ℞
[sel 'sun]
(2.5% selenium sulfide lotion, USP)

DESCRIPTION
A liquid antiseborrheic, antifungal preparation for topical application. Contains: Selenium sulfide 2 ½% w/v in aqueous suspension; also contains: bentonite, lauric diethanolamide, ethylene glycol monostearate, titanium dioxide, amphoteric-2, sodium lauryl sulfate, sodium phosphate (monobasic), glyceryl monoricinoleate, citric acid, captan and perfume.

CLINICAL PHARMACOLOGY
Selenium sulfide appears to have a cytostatic effect on cells of the epidermis and follicular epithelium, reducing corneocyte production.

INDICATIONS AND USAGE
Treatment of tinea versicolor, seborrheic dermatitis of scalp and treatment of dandruff.

CONTRAINDICATIONS
Not to be used by patients allergic to ingredients.

PRECAUTIONS
General: Not to be used when inflammation or exudation is present as increased absorption may occur.
Information for Patients: See Warnings and Precautions section under Application Instructions.
Carcinogenesis: Dermal application of 25% and 50% solutions of 2.5% selenium sulfide lotion on mice over an 88 week period, indicated no carcinogenic effects.
Pregnancy: WHEN USED FOR THE TREATMENT OF TINEA VERSICOLOR, SELSUN IS CLASSIFIED AS PREGNANCY CATEGORY C. Animal reproduction studies have not been conducted with SELSUN. It is also not known whether SELSUN can cause fetal harm when applied to body surfaces of a pregnant woman or can affect reproduction capacity. Under ordinary circumstances SELSUN should not be used for the treatment of tinea versicolor in pregnant women.
Pediatric Use: Safety and effectiveness in infants have not been established.

ADVERSE REACTIONS
In decreasing order of severity: skin irritation; occasional reports of increase in normal hair loss; discoloration of hair (can be avoided or minimized by thorough rinsing of hair after treatment). As with other shampoos, oiliness or dryness of hair and scalp may occur.

OVERDOSAGE
Accidental Oral Ingestion:
No documented reports of serious toxicity in humans resulting from acute ingestion of SELSUN, however, acute toxicity studies in animals suggest that ingestion of large amounts could result in potential human toxicity. Evacuation of the stomach contents should be considered in cases of acute oral ingestion.

DOSAGE AND ADMINISTRATION
See application instructions.
Treatment of tinea versicolor: Apply to affected areas and lather with a small amount of water. Allow product to remain on skin for 10 minutes, then rinse thoroughly. Repeat procedure once a day for 7 days.
Treatment of seborrheic dermatitis and dandruff: Usually two applications each week for two weeks will afford control. After this, may be used at less frequent intervals —weekly, every two weeks, or every 3 or 4 weeks in some cases. Should not be applied more frequently than required to maintain control.
APPLICATION INSTRUCTIONS: Keep tightly capped.
Shake well before using. Product may damage jewelry; remove jewelry before use.
For treatment of tinea versicolor:
1. Apply to affected areas and lather with a small amount of water.
2. Allow to remain on skin for 10 minutes.
3. Rinse body thoroughly.
4. Repeat this procedure once a day for 7 days.
For treatment of dandruff and seborrheic dermatitis of the scalp:
1. Massage about 1 or 2 teaspoonfuls of shampoo into wet scalp.
2. Allow to remain on scalp for 2 to 3 minutes.
3. Rinse scalp thoroughly.
4. Repeat application and rinse thoroughly.
5. After treatment, wash hands well.
6. Repeat treatments as directed by physician.
WARNINGS AND PRECAUTIONS:
For External Use Only. Do not use on broken skin or inflamed areas. If allergic reactions occur, discontinue use. Avoid getting shampoo in eyes or in contact with genital area and skin folds as it may cause irritation and burning. These areas should be thoroughly rinsed after application. Keep this and all medicines out of reach of children.
Store below 86°F (30°C).

HOW SUPPLIED
4-fl-oz bottles (NDC 0074-2660-04).
(.1921)

SELSUN BLUE®   OTC
[sel 'sun]
Dandruff Shampoo
(selenium sulfide lotion, 1%)

Selsun Blue is a non-prescription anti-dandruff shampoo containing the active ingredient selenium sulfide, 1%, in a freshly scented, pH balanced formula to leave hair clean and manageable. Available in Dry, Oily, Regular, Extra Conditioning and Extra Medicated formulas (contains 0.5% menthol).

INACTIVE INGREDIENTS
Dry formula—Acetylated lanolin alcohol, ammonium laureth sulfate, ammonium lauryl sulfate, cetyl acetate, citric acid, cocamide DEA, cocamidopropyl betaine, DMDM hydantoin, FD&C blue No. 1, fragrance, hydroxypropyl methylcellulose, magnesium aluminum silicate, polysorbate 80, sodium chloride, titanium dioxide, water and other ingredients.
Regular formula—Ammonium laureth sulfate, ammonium lauryl sulfate, citric acid, cocamide DEA, cocamidopropyl betaine, DMDM hydantoin, FD&C blue No. 1, fragrance, hydroxypropyl methylcellulose, magnesium aluminum silicate, sodium chloride, titanium dioxide, water and other ingredients.
Oily formula—Ammonium laureth sulfate, ammonium lauryl sulfate, citric acid, cocamide DEA, cocamidopropyl betaine, DMDM hydantoin, FD&C blue No. 1, fragrance, hydroxypropyl methylcellulose, magnesium aluminum silicate, sodium chloride, titanium dioxide, water and other ingredients.
Extra Conditioning formula—Acetylated lanolin alcohol, aloe, ammonium laureth sulfate, ammonium lauryl sulfate, cetyl acetate, citric acid, cocamide DEA, cocamidopropyl betaine, DMDM hydantoin, FD&C blue No. 1, fragrance, glycol disterate, hydroxypropyl methylcellulose, magnesium aluminum silicate, polysorbate 80, propylene glycol, sodium chloride, TEA-lauryl sulfate, titanium dioxide, water and other ingredients.
Extra Medicated formula—Ammonium laureth sulfate, ammonium lauryl sulfate, citric acid, cocamide DEA, cocamidopropyl betaine, DMDM hydantoin, D&C red No. 33, FD&C blue No. 1, fragrance, hydroxypropyl methylcellulose, magnesium aluminum silicate, sodium chloride, TEA-lauryl sulfate, water and other ingredients.

Clinical testing has shown Selsun Blue to be as safe and effective as other leading shampoos in helping control dandruff symptoms with regular use.

DIRECTIONS
Shake well. Lather, rinse, repeat. For best results, use regularly.

WARNINGS
For external use only. Avoid contact with eyes. If this happens, rinse thoroughly with water. If condition worsens or does not improve, consult doctor. Keep out of reach of children. **CAUTION** If used on bleached, tinted, or permanent waved hair, rinse for 5 minutes.

HOW SUPPLIED
4-, 7- and 11-fl-oz plastic bottles.
(FAN 2301-02)

SELSUN GOLD FOR WOMEN™   OTC
[sel 'sun]
Dandruff Shampoo
(selenium sulfide lotion, 1%)

Selsun Gold for Women allows you to shampoo, condition and control dandruff flaking and itching with one shampoo. This formula contains patented ingredients to leave hair soft, shiny and manageable. You won't need a separate conditioner to have beautiful hair. May be used on color-treated or permed hair, if used as directed.

INACTIVE INGREDIENTS
Ammonium lauryl sulfate, ammonium laureth sulfate, citric acid, cocamide DEA, DI (hydrogenated) tallow phthalic acid amide, dimethicone, DMDM hydantoin, hydroxypropyl methylcellulose, purified water, sodium citrate and fragrance.

DIRECTIONS
Shake well. Shampoo and rinse thoroughly. For best results, use regularly, at least twice a week or as directed by a doctor.

WARNINGS
For external use only. Avoid contact with the eyes. If contact occurs, rinse eyes thoroughly with water. If condition worsens or does not improve after regular use of this product as directed, consult a doctor. Keep this and all drugs out of the reach of children.

HOW SUPPLIED
4-, 7- and 11-fl-oz plastic bottles.
(FAN 2336-01)

SIMILAC®
[sim 'e-lak]
Low-Iron Infant Formula
● **Powder**
● **Concentrated Liquid**
● **Ready To Feed**

For most current information, refer to product labels.

SIMILAC® SPECIAL CARE®
WITH IRON 24
Premature Infant Formula
● Ready To Feed

For most current information, refer to product labels.

SIMILAC® WITH IRON
[sim'e-lak]
Infant Formula
● Powder
● Concentrated Liquid
● Ready To Feed

For most current information, refer to product labels.

SUPLENA™
[suh-plĕn'ah]
Specialized Liquid Nutrition

USAGE
For patients requiring protein, electrolyte and fluid restrictions. Suplena is a high-calorie, low-nitrogen, low-electrolyte liquid food. In the dietary management of patients prone to uremia, Suplena helps maintain nutritional status while minimizing accumulation of nitrogenous wastes, fluid and electrolytes. It can be used as a supplement to the prescribed diet or as the sole source of nutrition under medical supervision.
Not for parenteral use.

AVAILABILITY
Ready To Feed
8-fl-oz cans; 24 per case; Vanilla, No. 50164.

INGREDIENTS
ⓊD Water, hydrolyzed cornstarch, high-oleic safflower oil, sodium and calcium caseinates, sucrose, soy oil, soy lecithin, natural and artificial flavors, calcium carbonate, potassium citrate, magnesium phosphate dibasic, calcium phosphate tribasic, choline chloride, sodium chloride, ascorbic acid, taurine, carrageenan, L-carnitine, potassium chloride, zinc sulfate, alpha-tocopheryl acetate, ferrous sulfate, niacinamide, calcium pantothenate, manganese sulfate, pyridoxine hydrochloride, cupric sulfate, thiamine chloride hydrochloride, riboflavin, folic acid, vitamin A palmitate, biotin, potassium iodide, sodium selenite, phylloquinone, cyanocobalamin and vitamin D_3.
Nutrients (Grams/8 fl oz): Protein, 7.1; Fat, 22.7; Carbohydrate, 60.6; L-carnitine, 0.038; Taurine, 0.038; Water, 169. Calories per mL, 2.0; Calories per fl oz, 59.4.
(FAN 798-03)

SURVANTA®   ℞
beractant
intratracheal suspension

Sterile Suspension
For Intratracheal Use Only

DESCRIPTION
SURVANTA® (beractant) Intratracheal Suspension is a sterile, non-pyrogenic pulmonary surfactant intended for intratracheal use only. It is a natural bovine lung extract containing phospholipids, neutral lipids, fatty acids, and surfactant-associated proteins to which colfosceril palmitate (dipalmitoylphosphatidylcholine), palmitic acid, and tripalmitin are added to standardize the composition and to mimic surface-tension lowering properties of natural lung surfactant. The resulting composition provides 25 mg/mL phospholipids (including 11.0-15.5 mg/mL disaturated phosphatidylcholine), 0.5-1.75 mg/mL triglycerides, 1.4-3.5 mg/mL free fatty acids, and less than 1.0 mg/mL protein. It is suspended in 0.9% sodium chloride solution, and heat-sterilized. SURVANTA contains no preservatives. Its protein content consists of two hydrophobic, low molecular weight, surfactant-associated proteins commonly known as SP-B and SP-C. It does not contain the hydrophilic, large molecular weight surfactant-associated protein known as SP-A.
Each mL of SURVANTA contains 25 mg of phospholipids. It is an off-white to light brown liquid supplied in single-use glass vials containing 8 mL (200 mg phospholipids).

CLINICAL PHARMACOLOGY
Endogenous pulmonary surfactant lowers surface tension on alveolar surfaces during respiration and stabilizes the alveoli against collapse at resting transpulmonary pressures. Deficiency of pulmonary surfactant causes Respiratory Distress Syndrome (RDS) in premature infants. SURVANTA replenishes surfactant and restores surface activity to the lungs of these infants.

Activity
In vitro, SURVANTA reproducibly lowers minimum surface tension to less than 8 dynes/cm as measured by the pulsating bubble surfactometer and Wilhelmy Surface Balance. *In situ*, SURVANTA restores pulmonary compliance to excised rat lungs artificially made surfactant-deficient. *In vivo*, single SURVANTA doses improve lung pressure-volume measurements, lung compliance, and oxygenation in premature rabbits and sheep.

Animal Metabolism
SURVANTA is administered directly to the target organ, the lungs, where biophysical effects occur at the alveolar surface. In surfactant-deficient premature rabbits and lambs, alveolar clearance of radio-labelled lipid components of SURVANTA is rapid. Most of the dose becomes lung-associated within hours of administration, and the lipids enter endogenous surfactant pathways of reutilization and recycling. In surfactant-sufficient adult animals, SURVANTA clearance is more rapid than in premature and young animals. There is less reutilization and recycling of surfactant in adult animals.
Limited animal experiments have not found effects of SURVANTA on endogenous surfactant metabolism. Precursor incorporation and subsequent secretion of saturated phosphatidylcholine in premature sheep are not changed by SURVANTA treatments.
No information is available about the metabolic fate of the surfactant-associated proteins in SURVANTA. The metabolic disposition in humans has not been studied.

Clinical Studies
Clinical effects of SURVANTA were demonstrated in six single-dose and four multiple-dose randomized, multicenter, controlled clinical trials involving approximately 1700 infants. Three open trials, including a Treatment IND, involved more than 4800 infants. Each dose of SURVANTA in all studies was 100 mg phospholipids/kg birth weight and was based on published experience with Surfactant TA, a lyophilized powder dosage form of SURVANTA having the same composition.

Prevention Studies
Infants of 600-1250 g birth weight and 23 to 29 weeks estimated gestational age were enrolled in two *multiple-dose* studies. A dose of SURVANTA was given within 15 minutes of birth to prevent the development of RDS. Up to three additional doses in the first 48 hours, as often as every 6 hours, were given if RDS subsequently developed and infants required mechanical ventilation with an $FiO_2 \geq 0.30$. Results of the studies at 28 days of age are shown in Table 1.

TABLE 1

Study 1

	SURVANTA	Control	P-Value
Number infants studied	119	124	
Incidence of RDS (%)	27.6	63.5	< 0.001
Death due to RDS (%)	2.5	19.5	< 0.001
Death or BPD due to RDS (%)	48.7	52.8	0.536
Death due to any cause (%)	7.6	22.8	0.001
Air Leaks[a] (%)	5.9	21.7	0.001
Pulmonary interstitial emphysema (%)	20.8	40.0	0.001

Study 2[b]

	SURVANTA	Control	P-Value
Number infants studied	91	96	
Incidence of RDS (%)	28.6	48.3	0.007
Death due to RDS (%)	1.1	10.5	0.006
Death or BPD due to RDS (%)	27.5	44.2	0.018
Death due to any cause[c] (%)	16.5	13.7	0.633
Air Leaks[a] (%)	14.5	19.6	0.374
Pulmonary interstitial emphysema (%)	26.5	33.2	0.298

[a] Pneumothorax or pneumopericardium
[b] Study discontinued when Treatment IND initiated
[c] No cause of death in the SURVANTA group was significantly increased; the higher number of deaths in this group was due to the sum of all causes.

Rescue Studies
Infants of 600-1750 g birth weight with RDS requiring mechanical ventilation and an $FiO_2 \geq 0.40$ were enrolled in two *multiple-dose* rescue studies. The initial dose of SURVANTA was given after RDS developed and before 8 hours of age. Infants could receive up to three additional doses in the first 48 hours, as often as every 6 hours, if they required mechanical ventilation and an $FiO_2 \geq 0.30$. Results of the studies at 28 days of age are shown in Table 2.
[See table at top of next column.]

TABLE 2

Study 3[a]

	SURVANTA	Control	P-Value
Number infants studied	198	193	
Death due to RDS (%)	11.6	18.1	0.071
Death or BPD due to RDS (%)	59.1	66.8	0.102
Death due to any cause (%)	21.7	26.4	0.285
Air Leaks[b] (%)	11.8	29.5	< 0.001
Pulmonary interstitial emphysema (%)	16.3	34.0	< 0.001

Study 4

	SURVANTA	Control	P-Value
Number infants studied	204	203	
Death due to RDS (%)	6.4	22.3	< 0.001
Death or BPD due to RDS (%)	43.6	63.4	< 0.001
Death due to any cause (%)	15.2	28.2	0.001
Air Leaks[b] (%)	11.2	22.2	0.005
Pulmonary interstitial emphysema (%)	20.8	44.4	< 0.001

[a] Study discontinued when Treatment IND initiated
[b] Pneumothorax or pneumopericardium

Acute Clinical Effects
Marked improvements in oxygenation may occur within minutes of administration of SURVANTA.
All controlled clinical studies with SURVANTA provided information regarding the acute effects of SURVANTA on the arterial-alveolar oxygen ratio (a/APO₂), FiO₂, and mean airway pressure (MAP) during the first 48 to 72 hours of life. Significant improvements in these variables were sustained for 48-72 hours in SURVANTA-treated infants in four single-dose and two multiple-dose rescue studies and in two multiple-dose prevention studies. In the single-dose prevention studies, FiO₂ improved significantly.

INDICATIONS AND USAGE
SURVANTA is indicated for prevention and treatment ("rescue") of Respiratory Distress Syndrome (RDS) (hyaline membrane disease) in premature infants. SURVANTA significantly reduces the incidence of RDS, mortality due to RDS and air leak complications.
Prevention
In premature infants less than 1250 g birth weight or with evidence of surfactant deficiency, give SURVANTA as soon as possible, preferably within 15 minutes of birth.
Rescue
To treat infants with RDS confirmed by x-ray and requiring mechanical ventilation, give SURVANTA as soon as possible, preferably by 8 hours of age.

CONTRAINDICATIONS
None known.

WARNINGS
SURVANTA is intended for intratracheal use only.
SURVANTA CAN RAPIDLY AFFECT OXYGENATION AND LUNG COMPLIANCE. Therefore, its use should be restricted to a highly supervised clinical setting with immediate availability of clinicians experienced with intubation, ventilator management, and general care of premature infants. Infants receiving SURVANTA should be frequently monitored with arterial or transcutaneous measurement of systemic oxygen and carbon dioxide.
DURING THE DOSING PROCEDURE, TRANSIENT EPISODES OF BRADYCARDIA AND DECREASED OXYGEN SATURATION HAVE BEEN REPORTED. If these occur, stop the dosing procedure and initiate appropriate measures to alleviate the condition. After stabilization, resume the dosing procedure.

PRECAUTIONS
General
Rales and moist breath sounds can occur transiently after administration. Endotracheal suctioning or other remedial action is not necessary unless clear-cut signs of airway obstruction are present.
Increased probability of post-treatment nosocomial sepsis in SURVANTA-treated infants was observed in the controlled clinical trials (Table 3). The increased risk for sepsis among SURVANTA-treated infants was not associated with increased mortality among these infants. The causative organisms were similar in treated and control infants. There was no significant difference between groups in the rate of post-treatment infections other than sepsis.
Use of SURVANTA in infants less than 600 g birth weight or greater than 1750 g birth weight has not been evaluated in controlled trials. There is no controlled experience with use of SURVANTA in conjunction with experimental therapies

Continued on next page

Ross Laboratories—Cont.

for RDS (eg, high-frequency ventilation or extracorporeal membrane oxygenation).

No information is available on the effects of doses other than 100 mg phospholipids/kg, more than four doses, dosing more frequently than every 6 hours, or administration after 48 hours of age.

Carcinogenesis, Mutagenesis, Impairment of Fertility
Reproduction studies in animals have not been completed. Mutagenicity studies were negative. Carcinogenicity studies have not been performed with SURVANTA.

ADVERSE REACTIONS
The most commonly reported adverse experiences were associated with the dosing procedure. In the multiple-dose controlled clinical trials, transient bradycardia occurred with 11.9% of doses. Oxygen desaturation occurred with 9.8% of doses.

Other reactions during the dosing procedure occurred with fewer than 1% of doses and included endotracheal tube reflux, pallor, vasoconstriction, hypotension, endotracheal tube blockage, hypertension, hypocarbia, hypercarbia, and apnea. No deaths occurred during the dosing procedure, and all reactions resolved with symptomatic treatment.

The occurrence of concurrent illnesses common in premature infants was evaluated in the controlled trials. The rates in all controlled studies are in Table 3.

TABLE 3

| | All Controlled Studies | | |
| | SURVANTA | Control | |
Concurrent Event	(%)	(%)	P-Value[a]
Patent ductus arteriosus	46.9	47.1	0.814
Intracranial hemorrhage	48.1	45.2	0.241
Severe intracranial hemorrhage	24.1	23.3	0.693
Pulmonary air leaks	10.9	24.7	<0.001
Pulmonary interstitial emphysema	20.2	38.4	<0.001
Necrotizing enterocolitis	6.1	5.3	0.427
Apnea	65.4	59.6	0.283
Severe apnea	46.1	42.5	0.114
Post-treatment sepsis	20.7	16.1	0.019
Post-treatment infection	10.2	9.1	0.345
Pulmonary hemorrhage	7.2	5.3	0.166

[a] P-value comparing groups in controlled studies

When all controlled studies were pooled, there was no difference in intracranial hemorrhage. However, in one of the single-dose rescue studies and one of the multiple-dose prevention studies, the rate of intracranial hemorrhage was significantly higher in SURVANTA patients than control patients (63.3% v 30.8%, P=0.001; and 48.8% v 34.2%, P=0.047, respectively). The rate in a Treatment IND involving approximately 4400 infants was lower than in the controlled trials.

In the controlled clinical trials, there was no effect of SURVANTA on results of common laboratory tests: white blood cell count and serum sodium, potassium, bilirubin, creatinine.

More than 3700 pretreatment and post-treatment serum samples were tested by Western Blot immunoassay for antibodies to surfactant-associated proteins SP-B and SP-C. No IgG or IgM antibodies were detected.

Several other complications are known to occur in premature infants. The following conditions were reported in the controlled clinical studies. The rates of the complications were not different in treated and control infants, and none of the complications were attributed to SURVANTA.

Respiratory: lung consolidation, blood from the endotracheal tube, deterioration after weaning, respiratory decompensation, subglottic stenosis, paralyzed diaphragm, respiratory failure.

Cardiovascular: hypotension, hypertension, tachycardia, ventricular tachycardia, aortic thrombosis, cardiac failure, cardio-respiratory arrest, increased apical pulse, persistent fetal circulation, air embolism, total anomalous pulmonary venous return.

Gastrointestinal: abdominal distention, hemorrhage, intestinal perforations, volvulus, bowel infarct, feeding intolerance, hepatic failure, stress ulcer.

Renal: renal failure, hematuria.

Hematologic: coagulopathy, thrombocytopenia, disseminated intravascular coagulation.

Central Nervous System: seizures.

Endocrine/Metabolic: adrenal hemorrhage, inappropriate ADH secretion, hyperphosphatemia.

Musculoskeletal: inguinal hernia.

Systemic: fever, deterioration.

Follow-Up Evaluations
To date, no long-term complications or sequelae of SURVANTA therapy have been found.

Single-Dose Studies
Six-month adjusted-age follow-up evaluations of 232 infants (115 treated) demonstrated no clinically important differences between treatment groups in pulmonary and neurologic sequelae, incidence or severity of retinopathy of prematurity, rehospitalizations, growth, or allergic manifestations.

Multiple-Dose Studies
Six-month adjusted age follow-up evaluations have not been completed. Preliminarily, in 605 (333 treated) of 916 surviving infants, there are trends for decreased cerebral palsy and need for supplemental oxygen in SURVANTA infants. Wheezing at the time of examination tended to be more frequent among SURVANTA infants, although there was no difference in bronchodilator therapy.

Twelve-month follow-up data from the multiple-dose studies have been completed in 328 (171 treated) of 909 surviving infants. To date no significant differences between treatments have been found, although there is a trend toward less wheezing in SURVANTA infants in contrast to the six month results.

OVERDOSAGE
Overdosage with SURVANTA has not been reported. Based on animal data, overdosage might result in acute airway obstruction. Treatment should be symptomatic and supportive.

Rales and moist breath sounds can transiently occur after SURVANTA is given, and do not indicate overdosage. Endotracheal suctioning or other remedial action is not required unless clear-cut signs of airway obstruction are present.

DOSAGE AND ADMINISTRATION
FOR INTRATRACHEAL ADMINISTRATION ONLY.
SURVANTA should be administered by or under the supervision of clinicians experienced in intubation, ventilator management, and general care of premature infants.

Marked improvements in oxygenation may occur within minutes of administration of SURVANTA. Therefore, frequent and careful clinical observation and monitoring of systemic oxygenation are essential to avoid hyperoxia.

Review of audiovisual instructional materials describing dosage and administration procedures is recommended before using SURVANTA. Materials are available upon request from Ross Laboratories.

Dosage
Each dose of SURVANTA is 100 mg of phospholipids/kg birth weight (4 mL/kg). The SURVANTA DOSING CHART shows the total dosage for a range of birth weights.

SURVANTA DOSING CHART

WEIGHT (grams)	TOTAL DOSE (mL)	WEIGHT (grams)	TOTAL DOSE (mL)
600- 650	2.6	1301-1350	5.4
651- 700	2.8	1351-1400	5.6
701- 750	3.0	1401-1450	5.8
751- 800	3.2	1451-1500	6.0
801- 850	3.4	1501-1550	6.2
851- 900	3.6	1551-1600	6.4
901- 950	3.8	1601-1650	6.6
951-1000	4.0	1651-1700	6.8
1001-1050	4.2	1701-1750	7.0
1051-1100	4.4	1751-1800	7.2
1101-1150	4.6	1801-1850	7.4
1151-1200	4.8	1851-1900	7.6
1201-1250	5.0	1901-1950	7.8
1251-1300	5.2	1951-2000	8.0

Four doses of SURVANTA can be administered in the first 48 hours of life. Doses should be given no more frequently than every 6 hours.

Directions for Use
SURVANTA should be inspected visually for discoloration prior to administration. The color of SURVANTA is off-white to light brown. If settling occurs during storage, swirl the vial gently (DO NOT SHAKE) to redisperse. Some foaming at the surface may occur during handling and is inherent in the nature of the product.

SURVANTA is stored refrigerated (2-8°C). Before administration, SURVANTA should be warmed by standing at room temperature for at least 20 minutes or warmed in the hand for at least 8 minutes. ARTIFICIAL WARMING METHODS SHOULD NOT BE USED. If a prevention dose is to be given, preparation of SURVANTA should begin before the infant's birth.

Unopened, unused vials of SURVANTA that have been warmed to room temperature may be returned to the refrigerator within 8 hours of warming, and stored for future use. Drug should not be warmed and returned to the refrigerator more than once. Each single-use vial of SURVANTA should

be entered only once. Used vials with residual drug should be discarded.
SURVANTA DOES NOT REQUIRE RECONSTITUTION OR SONICATION BEFORE USE.

Dosing Procedures
General
SURVANTA is administered intratracheally by instillation through a 5 French end-hole catheter inserted into the infant's endotracheal tube with the tip of the catheter protruding just beyond the end of the endotracheal tube above the infant's carina. Before inserting the catheter through the endotracheal tube, the length of the catheter should be shortened. SURVANTA should not be instilled into a mainstem bronchus.

It is important to ensure homogenous distribution of SURVANTA throughout the lungs. In the controlled clinical trials, each dose was divided into four quarter-doses. Each quarter-dose was administered with the infant in a different position. The sequence of positions was:
• Head and body inclined slightly down, head turned to the right
• Head and body inclined slightly down, head turned to the left
• Head and body inclined slightly up, head turned to the right
• Head and body inclined slightly up, head turned to the left
See illustrations below for recommended positioning of infants.

ILLUSTRATIONS

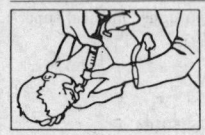
1. Infant's head and body inclined down, head turned to the right.

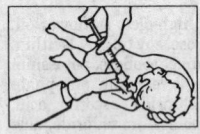
2. Head and body inclined down, head turned to the left.

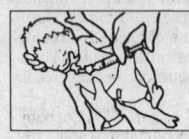
3. Head and body inclined up, head turned to the right.

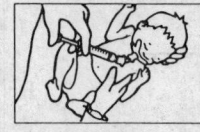
4. Head and body inclined up, head turned to the left.

The dosing procedure is facilitated if one person administers the dose while another person positions and monitors the infant.

First Dose
Determine the total dose of SURVANTA from the SURVANTA DOSING CHART based on the infant's birth weight. Slowly withdraw the entire contents of the vial into a plastic syringe through a large-gauge needle (eg, at least 20 gauge). DO NOT FILTER SURVANTA AND AVOID SHAKING.

Attach the premeasured 5 French end-hole catheter to the syringe. Fill the catheter with SURVANTA. Discard excess SURVANTA through the catheter so that only the total dose to be given remains in the syringe.

BEFORE ADMINISTERING SURVANTA, assure proper placement and patency of the endotracheal tube. At the discretion of the clinician, the endotracheal tube may be suctioned before administering SURVANTA. The infant should be allowed to stabilize before proceeding with dosing.

In the prevention strategy, weigh, intubate and stabilize the infant. Administer the dose as soon as possible after birth, preferably within 15 minutes. Position the infant appropriately and gently inject the first quarter-dose through the catheter over 2-3 seconds.

After administration of the first quarter-dose, remove the catheter from the endotracheal tube. Manually ventilate with a hand-bag with sufficient oxygen to prevent cyanosis, at a rate of 60 breaths/minute, and sufficient positive pressure to provide adequate air exchange and chest wall excursion.

In the rescue strategy, the first dose should be given as soon as possible after the infant is placed on a ventilator for management of RDS. In the clinical trials, immediately before instilling the first quarter-dose, the infant's ventilator set-

tings were changed to rate 60/minute, inspiratory time 0.5 second, and FiO₂ 1.0.

Position the infant appropriately and gently inject the first quarter-dose through the catheter over 2–3 seconds. After administration of the first quarter-dose, remove the catheter from the endotracheal tube. Return the infant to the mechanical ventilator.

In both strategies, ventilate the infant for at least 30 seconds or until stable. Reposition the infant for instillation of the next quarter-dose.

Instill the remaining quarter-doses using the same procedures. After instillation of each quarter-dose, remove the catheter and ventilate for at least 30 seconds or until the infant is stabilized. After instillation of the final quarter-dose, remove the catheter without flushing it. Do not suction the infant for 1 hour after dosing unless signs of significant airway obstruction occur.

AFTER COMPLETION OF THE DOSING PROCEDURE, RESUME USUAL VENTILATOR MANAGEMENT AND CLINICAL CARE.

Repeat Doses

The dosage of SURVANTA for repeat doses is also 100 mg phospholipids/kg and is based on the infant's birth weight. The infant should not be reweighed for determination of the SURVANTA dosage. Use the SURVANTA DOSING CHART to determine the total dosage.

The need for additional doses of SURVANTA is determined by evidence of continuing respiratory distress. Using the following criteria for redosing, significant reductions in mortality due to RDS were observed in the multiple-dose clinical trials with SURVANTA.

> Dose no sooner than 6 hours after the preceding dose if the infant remains intubated and requires at least 30% inspired oxygen to maintain a PaO₂ less than or equal to 80 torr.
>
> Radiographic confirmation of RDS should be obtained before administering additional doses to those who received a prevention dose.

Prepare SURVANTA and position the infant for administration of each quarter-dose as previously described. After instillation of each quarter-dose, remove the dosing catheter from the endotracheal tube and ventilate the infant for at least 30 seconds or until stable.

In the clinical studies, ventilator settings used to administer repeat doses were different than those used for the first dose. For repeat doses, the FiO₂ was increased by 0.20 or an amount sufficient to prevent cyanosis. The ventilator delivered a rate of 30/minute with an inspiratory time less than 1.0 second. If the infant's pretreatment rate was 30 or greater, it was left unchanged during SURVANTA instillation.

Manual hand-bag ventilation should not be used to administer repeat doses. DURING THE DOSING PROCEDURE, VENTILATOR SETTINGS MAY BE ADJUSTED AT THE DISCRETION OF THE CLINICIAN TO MAINTAIN APPROPRIATE OXYGENATION AND VENTILATION.

AFTER COMPLETION OF THE DOSING PROCEDURE, RESUME USUAL VENTILATOR MANAGEMENT AND CLINICAL CARE.

Dosing Precautions

If an infant experiences bradycardia or oxygen desaturation during the dosing procedure, stop the dosing procedure and initiate appropriate measures to alleviate the condition. After the infant has stabilized, resume the dosing procedure. Rales and moist breath sounds can occur transiently after administration of SURVANTA. Endotracheal suctioning or other remedial action is unnecessary unless clear-cut signs of airway obstruction are present.

HOW SUPPLIED

SURVANTA (beractant) Intratracheal Suspension is supplied in single-use glass vials containing 8 mL of SURVANTA (NDC 0074-1040-08). Each milliliter contains 25 mg of phospholipids (200 mg phospholipids/8 mL) suspended in 0.9% sodium chloride solution. The color is off-white to light brown.

Store unopened vials at refrigeration temperature (2-8°C). Protect from light. Store vials in carton until ready for use. Vials are for single use only. Upon opening, discard unused drug.

June, 1991

TRONOLANE®   OTC
[tron 'e-lān]
Anesthetic Cream for Hemorrhoids
Hemorrhoidal Suppositories

(See PDR For Nonprescription Drugs.)

VI-DAYLIN® ADC VITAMINS Drops   OTC
[vī "dā 'lin]
Dietary Supplement of
Vitamins A, D and C

DESCRIPTION

One dropperful (1.0 mL) provides:

Vitamins		% U.S. RDA*	% U.S. RDA**
Vitamin A	1500 I.U.	100	60
Vitamin D	400 I.U.	100	100
Vitamin C	35 mg	100	87

INGREDIENTS

Propylene glycol, polysorbate 80, ascorbic acid, methylparaben (preservative), vitamin A palmitate, propylparaben (preservative), and ergocalciferol in corn oil, in a glycerin-water vehicle with added artificial pineapple-fruit flavoring and caramel coloring. Contains only a trace (less than ½%) of alcohol.

Contains no sugar.

*% U.S. Recommended Daily Allowance for infants.

**% U.S. Recommended Daily Allowance for children under 4 years of age.

INDICATIONS AND USAGE

Dietary supplement of vitamins A, D and C for infants and children under 4 years of age.

DOSAGE AND ADMINISTRATION

One dropperful daily, or as directed by physician.

HOW SUPPLIED

50-mL Spil-gard® bottles, calibrated dropper enclosed; OTC; List No. 0105-04.
Store below 77°F (25°C).
.1901

VI-DAYLIN® ADC VITAMINS + IRON   OTC
Drops
[vī "dā 'lin]
Dietary Supplement of Vitamins A, D and C
with Iron

DESCRIPTION

One dropperful (1.0 mL) provides:

Vitamins		% U.S. RDA*	% U.S. RDA**
Vitamin A	1500 I.U.	100	60
Vitamin D	400 I.U.	100	100
Vitamin C	35 mg	100	87
Minerals			
Iron	10 mg	66	100

INGREDIENTS

Polysorbate 80, ferrous sulfate, ascorbic acid, vitamin A palmitate, benzoic acid (preservative), methylparaben (preservative), and ergocalciferol in corn oil, in a glycerin-water vehicle with added artificial flavoring and coloring.

Contains no sugar.

*% U.S. Recommended Daily Allowance for infants.

**% U.S. Recommended Daily Allowance for children under 4 years of age.

INDICATIONS AND USAGE

Dietary supplement of vitamins A, D and C with iron for infants and children under 4 years of age.

DOSAGE AND ADMINISTRATION

One dropperful daily, or as directed by physician.

HOW SUPPLIED

50-mL Spil-gard® bottles; calibrated dropper enclosed; OTC; List No. 0117-01.
Store below 77°F (25°C).
.1901

VI-DAYLIN® MULTIVITAMIN Drops   OTC
[vī "dā 'lin]
Multivitamin Supplement

DESCRIPTION

One dropperful (1.0 mL) provides:

Vitamins			% U.S. RDA*	% U.S. RDA**
Vitamin A	1500	I.U.	100	60
Vitamin D	400	I.U.	100	100
Vitamin E	5	I.U.	100	50
Vitamin C	35	mg	100	87
Thiamine (Vitamin B₁)	0.5	mg	100	71
Riboflavin (Vitamin B₂)	0.6	mg	100	75
Niacin	8	mg	100	88
Vitamin B₆	0.4	mg	100	57
Vitamin B₁₂	1.5	mcg	75	50

INGREDIENTS

Ascorbic acid, d-alpha-tocopheryl acid succinate, niacinamide, benzoic acid (preservative), ferric ammonium citrate (stabilizer), riboflavin-5'-phosphate sodium, methylparaben (preservative), thiamine hydrochloride, pyridoxine hydrochloride, ergocalciferol in corn oil, disodium edetate (stabilizer) and cyanocobalamin in a glycerin-water vehicle with added artificial flavoring. Contains only a trace (less than ½%) of alcohol.

Contains no sugar.

*% U.S. Recommended Daily Allowance for infants.

**% U.S. Recommended Daily Allowance for children under 4 years of age.

INDICATIONS AND USAGE

Multivitamin supplement for infants and children under 4 years of age.

DOSAGE AND ADMINISTRATION

One dropperful daily, or as directed by physician.

HOW SUPPLIED

50-mL Spil-gard® bottles, calibrated dropper enclosed; OTC; List No. 0103-04.
Store below 77°F (25°C).
.1901

VI-DAYLIN® MULTIVITAMIN + IRON   OTC
Drops
[vī "dā 'lin]
Multivitamin/Iron Supplement

DESCRIPTION

One dropperful (1.0 mL) provides:

Vitamins			% U.S. RDA*	% U.S. RDA**
Vitamin A	1500	I.U.	100	60
Vitamin D	400	I.U.	100	100
Vitamin E	5	I.U.	100	50
Vitamin C	35	mg	100	87
Thiamine (Vitamin B₁)	0.5	mg	100	71
Riboflavin (Vitamin B₂)	0.6	mg	100	75
Niacin	8	mg	100	88
Vitamin B₆	0.4	mg	100	57
Minerals				
Iron	10	mg	66	100

INGREDIENTS

Ferrous sulfate, ascorbic acid, d-alpha-tocopheryl acid succinate, niacinamide, vitamin A palmitate, benzoic acid (preservative), riboflavin-5'-phosphate sodium, thiamine hydrochloride, methylparaben (preservative), pyridoxine hydrochloride and ergocalciferol in corn oil, in a glycerin-water vehicle with added artificial coloring and flavoring. Contains only a trace (less than ½%) of alcohol.

Contains no sugar.

*% U.S. Recommended Daily Allowance for infants.

**% U.S. Recommended Daily Allowance for children under 4 years of age.

INDICATIONS AND USAGE

Multivitamin supplement with iron for infants and children under 4 years of age.

ADMINISTRATION AND DOSAGE

One dropperful daily, or as directed by physician.

HOW SUPPLIED

50-mL Spil-gard® bottles, calibrated dropper enclosed; OTC; List No. 0116-01.
Store below 77°F (25°C).
.1901

VI-DAYLIN®/F ADC VITAMINS   ℞
Drops With Fluoride
[vī "dā 'lin]
ADC Vitamins/Fluoride

DESCRIPTION

One dropperful (1.0 mL) provides:
Fluoride   0.25 mg

Vitamins			% U.S. RDA*	% U.S. RDA**
Vitamin A	1500	I.U.	100	60
Vitamin D	400	I.U.	100	100
Vitamin C	35	mg	100	87

Continued on next page

Ross Laboratories—Cont.

Active Ingredients: Ascorbic acid, vitamin A palmitate, sodium fluoride and ergocalciferol.
Inactive Ingredients: Alcohol approximately 0.3%, caramel coloring, corn oil, glycerin, methylparaben, polysorbate 80, propylene glycol, propylparaben, water, artificial and natural flavoring, and other ingredients.
Contains no sugar.
  *%U.S. Recommended Daily Allowance for infants.
 **% U.S. Recommended Daily Allowance for children under 4 years of age.

INDICATIONS AND USAGE
As an aid in the prevention of dental caries in infants and children, and in the prophylaxis of vitamin A, D and C deficiencies.

CONTRAINDICATIONS
Should be used only where the fluoride content of the drinking water supply is known to be 0.7 parts per million or less.

PRECAUTIONS
The recommended dosage should not be exceeded since chronic overdosage of fluoride may result in mottling of tooth enamel and osseous changes.

OVERDOSAGE
In children, acute ingestion of 10 to 20 mg of sodium fluoride may cause excessive salivation and gastrointestinal disturbances; 500 mg may be fatal. Oral and/or intravenous fluids containing calcium may be indicated.

DOSAGE AND ADMINISTRATION
One dropperful daily, or as directed by physician or dentist.

HOW SUPPLIED
50-mL Spil-gard® bottles, calibrated dropper enclosed; ℞;
NDC 0074-1106-50.
Store below 77°F (25°C).
.5880

VI-DAYLIN®/F ADC VITAMINS + IRON   ℞
Drops With Fluoride
[vī″dā′lin]
ADC Vitamins/Fluoride/Iron Supplement

DESCRIPTION
One dropperful (1.0 mL) provides:
Fluoride   0.25 mg

Vitamins			% U.S. RDA*	% U.S. RDA**
Vitamin A	1500 I.U.		100	60
Vitamin D	400 I.U.		100	100
Vitamin C	35 mg		100	87
Minerals				
Iron	10 mg		66	100

Active Ingredients: Ascorbic acid, ferrous sulfate, vitamin A palmitate, sodium fluoride and ergocalciferol.
Inactive Ingredients: Benzoic acid, caramel coloring, glycerin, methylparaben, polysorbate 80, water, artificial flavoring and other ingredients.
Contains no sugar.
  *%U.S. Recommended Daily Allowance for infants.
 **%U.S. Recommended Daily Allowance for children under 4 years of age.

INDICATIONS AND USAGE
As an aid in the prevention of dental caries in infants and children, and in the prophylaxis of iron and vitamin A, D and C deficiencies.

CONTRAINDICATIONS
Should be used only where the fluoride content of the drinking water supply is known to be 0.7 parts per million or less.

PRECAUTIONS
The recommended dosage should not be exceeded since chronic overdosage of fluoride may result in mottling of tooth enamel and osseous changes. In infants, oral iron-containing preparations may cause temporary darkening of the membrane covering the teeth.

OVERDOSAGE
In children, acute ingestion of 10 to 20 mg of sodium fluoride may cause excessive salivation and gastrointestinal disturbances; 500 mg may be fatal. Oral and/or intravenous fluids containing calcium may be indicated.
Acute overdosage of iron may cause nausea and vomiting and, in severe cases, cardiovascular collapse and death. The estimated lethal dose of orally ingested elemental iron is 300 mg per kg body weight. Serum iron and total iron-binding capacity may be used as guides for use of chelating agents such as deferoxamine.

DOSAGE AND ADMINISTRATION
One dropperful daily, or as directed by physician or dentist.

HOW SUPPLIED
50-mL Spil-gard® bottles, calibrated dropper enclosed; ℞;
NDC 0074-8929-50.
Store below 77°F (25°C).
.5880

VI-DAYLIN®/F MULTIVITAMIN   ℞
Drops With Fluoride
[vī″dā′lin]
Multivitamins/Fluoride

DESCRIPTION
One dropperful (1.0 mL) provides:
Fluoride   0.25 mg

Vitamins			% U.S. RDA*	% U.S. RDA**
Vitamin A	1500	I.U.	100	60
Vitamin D	400	I.U.	100	100
Vitamin E	5	I.U.	100	50
Vitamin C	35	mg	100	87
Thiamine (Vitamin B₁)	0.5	mg	100	71
Riboflavin (Vitamin B₂)	0.6	mg	100	75
Niacin	8	mg	100	88
Vitamin B₆	0.4	mg	100	57

Active Ingredients: Ascorbic acid, niacinamide, d-alpha tocopheryl acid succinate, riboflavin-5′-phosphate sodium, sodium fluoride, vitamin A palmitate, thiamine hydrochloride, pyridoxine hydrochloride and ergocalciferol.
Inactive Ingredients: Alcohol less than 0.1%, benzoic acid, caramel coloring, corn oil, glycerin, methylparaben, water, natural flavoring and other ingredients. No artificial sweeteners.
Contains no sugar.
  *%U.S. Recommended Daily Allowance for infants.
 **%U.S. Recommended Daily Allowance for children under 4 years of age.

INDICATIONS AND USAGE
As an aid in the prevention of dental caries in infants and children, and in the prophylaxis of appropriate vitamin deficiencies.

CONTRAINDICATIONS
Should be used only where the fluoride content of the drinking water supply is known to be 0.7 parts per million or less.

PRECAUTIONS
The recommended dosage should not be exceeded since chronic overdosage of fluoride may result in mottling of tooth enamel and osseous changes.

OVERDOSAGE
In children, acute ingestion of 10 to 20 mg of sodium fluoride may cause excessive salivation and gastrointestinal disturbances; 500 mg may be fatal. Oral and/or intravenous fluids containing calcium may be indicated.

DOSAGE AND ADMINISTRATION
One dropperful daily, or as directed by physician or dentist.

HOW SUPPLIED
50-mL Spil-gard® bottles, calibrated dropper enclosed; ℞;
NDC 0074-1104-50.
Store below 77°F (25°C).
.6880

VI-DAYLIN®/F MULTIVITAMIN + IRON   ℞
Drops With Fluoride
[vī″dā′lin]
Multivitamins/Fluoride/Iron Supplement

DESCRIPTION
One dropperful (1.0 mL) provides:
Fluoride   0.25 mg

Vitamins			% U.S. RDA*	% U.S. RDA**
Vitamin A	1500	I.U.	100	60
Vitamin D	400	I.U.	100	100
Vitamin E	5	I.U.	100	50
Vitamin C	35	mg	100	87
Thiamine (Vitamin B₁)	0.5	mg	100	71
Riboflavin (Vitamin B₂)	0.6	mg	100	75
Niacin	8	mg	100	88
Vitamin B₆	0.4	mg	100	57
Minerals				
Iron	10	mg	66	100

Active Ingredients: Ascorbic acid, ferrous sulfate, niacinamide, d-alpha tocopheryl acid succinate, vitamin A palmitate, riboflavin-5′-phosphate sodium, thiamine hydrochloride, sodium fluoride, pyridoxine hydrochloride and ergocalciferol.
Inactive Ingredients: Alcohol less than 0.1%, benzoic acid, caramel coloring, corn oil, glycerin, methylparaben, water, natural flavoring and other ingredients.
Contains no sugar.
  *%U.S. Recommended Daily Allowance for infants.
 **%U.S. Recommended Daily Allowance for children under 4 years of age.

INDICATIONS AND USAGE
As an aid in the prevention of dental caries in infants and children and in the prophylaxis of iron and appropriate vitamin deficiencies.

CONTRAINDICATIONS
Should be used only where the fluoride content of the drinking water supply is known to be 0.7 parts per million or less.

PRECAUTIONS
The recommended dosage should not be exceeded since chronic overdosage of fluoride may result in mottling of tooth enamel and osseous changes. In infants, oral iron-containing preparations may cause temporary darkening of the membrane covering the teeth.

OVERDOSAGE
In children, acute ingestion of 10 to 20 mg of sodium fluoride may cause excessive salivation and gastrointestinal disturbances; 500 mg may be fatal. Oral and/or intravenous fluids containing calcium may be indicated.
Acute overdosage of iron may cause nausea and vomiting and, in severe cases, cardiovascular collapse and death. The estimated lethal dose of orally ingested elemental iron is 300 mg per kg body weight. Serum iron and total iron-binding capacity may be used as guides for use of chelating agents such as deferoxamine.

DOSAGE AND ADMINISTRATION
One dropperful daily, or as directed by physician or dentist.

HOW SUPPLIED
50-mL Spil-gard® bottles, calibrated dropper enclosed; ℞;
NDC 0074-8928-50.
Store below 77°F (25°C).
.5880

VI-DAYLIN® MULTIVITAMIN   OTC
Chewable Tablets
[vī″dā′lin]
Multivitamin Supplement

DESCRIPTION
Each chewable tablet provides:

Vitamins			%U.S. RDA*	%U.S. RDA**
Vitamin A	2500	I.U.	100	50
Vitamin D	400	I.U.	100	100
Vitamin E	15	I.U.	150	50
Vitamin C	60	mg	150	100
Folic Acid	0.3	mg	150	75
Thiamine (Vitamin B₁)	1.05	mg	150	70
Riboflavin (Vitamin B₂)	1.2	mg	150	70
Niacin	13.5	mg	150	67
Vitamin B₆	1.05	mg	150	52
Vitamin B₁₂	4.5	mcg	150	75

INGREDIENTS
Sucrose and dextrins, sodium ascorbate, niacinamide, dl-alpha tocopheryl acetate, ascorbic acid, vitamin A palmitate, riboflavin, pyridoxine hydrochloride, thiamine mononitrate, cholecalciferol, folic acid and cyanocobalamin. Made with natural sweeteners, artificial flavoring and artificially colored with natural ingredients.
  *% U.S. Recommended Daily Allowance for children under 4 years of age.
 **% U.S. Recommended Daily Allowance for adults and children 4 or more years of age.

INDICATIONS AND USAGE
Multivitamin supplement for children and adults.

DOSAGE AND ADMINISTRATION
One chewable tablet daily, or as directed by physician.

HOW SUPPLIED
100-tablet bottles; OTC; List No. 4519-13.
Store below 77°F (25°C).
.1901

VI-DAYLIN® MULTIVITAMIN + IRON   OTC
Chewable Tablets
[vī"dā'lin]
Multivitamin/Iron Supplement

DESCRIPTION
Each chewable tablet provides:

Vitamins			% U.S. RDA*	% U.S. RDA**
Vitamin A	2500	I.U.	100	50
Vitamin D	400	I.U.	100	100
Vitamin E	15	I.U.	150	50
Vitamin C	60	mg	150	100
Folic Acid	0.3	mg	150	75
Thiamine (Vitamin B₁)	1.05	mg	150	70
Riboflavin (Vitamin B₂)	1.2	mg	150	70
Niacin	13.5	mg	150	67
Vitamin B₆	1.05	mg	150	52
Vitamin B₁₂	4.5	mcg	150	75
Minerals				
Iron	12	mg	120	66

INGREDIENTS
Sucrose and dextrins, mannitol, sodium ascorbate, niacinamide, ferrous fumarate, dl-alpha tocopheryl acetate, ascorbic acid, artificial flavors, vitamin A palmitate, riboflavin, pyridoxine hydrochloride, thiamine mononitrate, FD&C yellow #6, cholecalciferol, folic acid and cyanocobalamin.

*%U.S. Recommended Daily Allowance for children under 4 years of age.

**%U.S. Recommended Daily Allowance for adults and children 4 or more years of age.

INDICATIONS AND USAGE
Multivitamin supplement with iron for children and adults.

DOSAGE AND ADMINISTRATION
One tablet daily, or as directed by physician.

HOW SUPPLIED
100-tablet bottles; OTC; List No. 4520-13.
Store below 77°F (25°C).
.1901

VI-DAYLIN®/F MULTIVITAMIN   ℞
Chewable Tablets With Fluoride
[vī"dā'lin]
Multivitamins/Fluoride

DESCRIPTION
Each chewable tablet provides:
Fluoride (as sodium fluoride) 1 mg

Vitamins			%U.S. RDA*	%U.S. RDA**
Vitamin A (as palmitate, 0.75 mg)	2500	I.U.	100	50
Vitamin D (as cholecalciferol, 10 mcg)	400	I.U.	100	100
Vitamin E (as dl-alpha tocopheryl acetate)	15	I.U.	150	50
Vitamin C (as sodium ascorbate, 40 mg; ascorbic acid, 20 mg)	60	mg	150	100
Folic Acid	0.3	mg	150	75
Vitamin B₁ (as thiamine mononitrate)	1.05	mg	150	70
Vitamin B₂ (as riboflavin)	1.2	mg	150	70
Niacin (as niacinamide)	13.5	mg	150	67
Vitamin B₆ (as pyridoxine hydrochloride)	1.05	mg	150	52
Vitamin B₁₂ (as cyanocobalamin)	4.5	mcg	150	75

*%U.S. Recommended Daily Allowance for children under 4 years of age.

**%U.S. Recommended Daily Allowance for adults and children 4 or more years of age.

INACTIVE INGREDIENTS
Cellulosic polymers, citric acid, corn starch, DC Yellow No. 10, dextrin, FDC Yellow No. 6, magnesium stearate, sucrose, artificial flavoring and other ingredients.

INDICATIONS AND USAGE
As an aid in the prevention of dental caries in children, and in the prophylaxis of appropriate vitamin deficiencies.

CONTRAINDICATIONS
Should be used only where the fluoride content of the drinking water supply is known to be 0.7 parts per million or less.

PRECAUTIONS
The recommended dosage should not be exceeded since chronic overdosage of fluoride may result in mottling of tooth enamel and osseous changes.

OVERDOSAGE
In children, acute ingestion of 10 to 20 mg of sodium fluoride may cause excessive salivation and gastrointestinal disturbances: 500 mg may be fatal. Oral and/or intravenous fluids containing calcium may be indicated.

DOSAGE AND ADMINISTRATION
Children 3 years of age or older, 1 chewable tablet daily; age 2 to 3 years, ½ chewable tablet daily; or as directed by physician or dentist.

HOW SUPPLIED
100-tablet bottles; ℞; NDC 0074-7626-13.
Store below 77°F (25°C).
.1901

VI-DAYLIN®/F MULTIVITAMIN + IRON   ℞
Chewable Tablets With Fluoride
[vī"dā'lin]
Multivitamins/Fluoride/Iron

DESCRIPTION
Each chewable tablet provides:
Fluoride (as sodium fluoride) 1 mg

Vitamins			% U.S. RDA*	% U.S. RDA**
Vitamin A (as palmitate, 0.75 mg)	2500	I.U.	100	50
Vitamin D (as cholecalciferol, 10 mcg)	400	I.U.	100	100
Vitamin E (as dl-alpha tocopheryl acetate)	15	I.U.	150	50
Vitamin C (as sodium ascorbate, 40 mg; ascorbic acid, 20 mg)	60	mg	150	100
Folic Acid	0.3	mg	150	75
Vitamin B₁ (as thiamine mononitrate)	1.05	mg	150	70
Vitamin B₂ (as riboflavin)	1.2	mg	150	70
Niacin (as niacinamide)	13.5	mg	150	67
Vitamin B₆ (as pyridoxine hydrochloride)	1.05	mg	150	52
Vitamin B₁₂ (as cyanocobalamin)	4.5	mcg	150	75
Minerals				
Iron (as ferrous fumarate)	12	mg	120	66

*%U.S. Recommended Daily Allowance for children under 4 years of age.

**%U.S. Recommended Daily Allowance for adults and children 4 or more years of age.

INACTIVE INGREDIENTS
Carmine No. 40, cellulosic polymers, citric acid, corn starch, dextrin, FDC Yellow No. 6, magnesium stearate, mannitol, sodium chloride, sucrose, tricalcium phosphate, artificial flavoring and other ingredients.

INDICATIONS AND USAGE
As an aid in the prevention of dental caries in children, and in the prophylaxis of iron and appropriate vitamin deficiencies.

CONTRAINDICATIONS
Should be used only where the fluoride content of the drinking water supply is known to be 0.7 parts per million or less.

PRECAUTIONS
The recommended dosage should not be exceeded since chronic overdosage of fluoride may result in mottling of tooth enamel and osseous changes.

OVERDOSAGE
In children, acute ingestion of 10 to 20 mg of sodium fluoride may cause excessive salivation and gastrointestinal disturbances; 500 mg may be fatal. Oral and/or intravenous fluids containing calcium may be indicated.
Acute overdosage of iron may cause nausea and vomiting and, in severe cases, cardiovascular collapse and death. The estimated lethal dose of orally ingested elemental iron is 300 mg per kg body weight. Serum iron and total iron-binding capacity may be used as guides for use of chelating agents such as deferoxamine.

DOSAGE AND ADMINISTRATION
Children 3 years of age or older, one chewable tablet daily; age 2-3 years, ½ chewable tablet daily; or as directed by physician or dentist.

HOW SUPPLIED
100-tablet bottles; ℞; NDC 0074-7621-13.
Store below 77°F (25°C).
.1901

VI-DAYLIN® MULTIVITAMIN Liquid   OTC
[vī"dā'lin]
Multivitamin Supplement

DESCRIPTION
One teaspoonful (5.0 mL) provides:

Vitamins			% U.S. RDA*	% U.S. RDA**
Vitamin A	2500	I.U.	100	50
Vitamin D	400	I.U.	100	100
Vitamin E	15	I.U.	150	50
Vitamin C	60	mg	150	100
Thiamine (Vitamin B₁)	1.05	mg	150	70
Riboflavin (Vitamin B₂)	1.2	mg	150	70
Niacin	13.5	mg	150	67
Vitamin B₆	1.05	mg	150	52
Vitamin B₁₂	4.5	mcg	150	75

*%U.S. Recommended Daily Allowance for children under 4 years of age.

**%U.S. Recommended Daily Allowance for adults and children 4 or more years of age.

INGREDIENTS
Glucose, sucrose, ascorbic acid, polysorbate 80, d-alpha tocopheryl acetate, niacinamide, acacia, cysteine hydrochloride (stabilizer), benzoic acid (preservative), vitamin A palmitate, methylparaben (preservative), pyridoxine hydrochloride, riboflavin, thiamine hydrochloride, ergocalciferol in corn oil, and cyanocobalamin in an aqueous vehicle with added natural citrus flavor and artificial color. Contains only a trace of alcohol (not more than ½%).

INDICATIONS AND USAGE
Multivitamin supplement for children and adults.

DOSAGE AND ADMINISTRATION
One teaspoonful daily, or as directed by physician.

HOW SUPPLIED
16-fl-oz (pint) bottles; OTC; List No. 3606-03.
8-fl-oz bottles; OTC; List No. 3606-02.
Store below 77°F (25°C).
.1901

VI-DAYLIN® MULTIVITAMIN + IRON   OTC
Liquid
[vī"dā'lin]
Multivitamin/Iron Supplement

DESCRIPTION
One teaspoonful (5.0 mL) provides:

Vitamins			% U.S. RDA*	% U.S. RDA**
Vitamin A	2500	I.U.	100	50
Vitamin D	400	I.U.	100	100
Vitamin E	15	I.U.	150	50
Vitamin C	60	mg	150	100
Thiamine (Vitamin B₁)	1.05	mg	150	70
Riboflavin (Vitamin B₂)	1.2	mg	150	70
Niacin	13.5	mg	150	67
Vitamin B₆	1.05	mg	150	52
Vitamin B₁₂	4.5	mcg	150	75
Minerals				
Iron	10	mg	100	55

*%U.S. Recommended Daily Allowance for children under 4 years of age.

**%U.S. Recommended Daily Allowance for adults and children 4 or more years of age.

INGREDIENTS
Glucose, sucrose, ascorbic acid, ferrous gluconate, polysorbate 80, d-alpha tocopheryl acetate, citric acid, niacinamide, acacia, cysteine hydrochloride (stabilizer), benzoic acid (preservative), methylparaben (preservative), vitamin A palmitate, riboflavin-5'-phosphate sodium, pyridoxine hydrochloride, thiamine hydrochloride, propylparaben (preservative), ergocalciferol in corn oil, and cyanocobalamin in an aqueous vehicle with added natural citrus flavor and artificial color. Contains only a trace of alcohol (not more than ½%).

Continued on next page

Ross Laboratories—Cont.

INDICATIONS AND USAGE
Multivitamin supplement with iron for children and adults.

DOSAGE AND ADMINISTRATION
One teaspoonful daily, or as directed by physician.

HOW SUPPLIED
16-fl-oz (pint) bottles; OTC; List No. 6992-03.
8-fl-oz bottles; OTC; List No. 6992-02.
Store below 77°F (25°C).
.1901

VITAL® HIGH NITROGEN
[vī′tel]
Nutritionally Complete
Partially Hydrolyzed Diet

USAGE
As a source of total or supplemental nutrition for patients with impaired gastrointestinal function (limited digestion/absorption). VITAL HIGH NITROGEN may be used as a tube feeding (nasogastric, nasoduodenal or jejunal) or as an oral feeding. Five servings (1500 Calories) meet or exceed 100% of the daily U.S. RDA for vitamins and minerals for adults and children 4 or more years of age.
Not for parenteral use.

AVAILABILITY
Powder: 2.79 oz (79 g) packets; 24 packets per case; Vanilla, No. 766.

COMPOSITION

INGREDIENTS
Hydrolyzed cornstarch, protein components (partially hydrolyzed whey, meat and soy), sucrose, safflower oil, medium-chain triglycerides (fractionated coconut oil), artificial and natural flavor, magnesium sulfate, calcium phosphate tribasic, potassium phosphate dibasic, L-tyrosine, magnesium chloride, L-leucine, L-valine, sodium chloride, L-isoleucine, L-phenylalanine, L-histidine, choline chloride, ascorbic acid, L-methionine, L-threonine, soy lecithin, mono- and diglycerides, L-tryptophan, zinc sulfate, ferrous sulfate, niacinamide, alpha-tocopheryl acetate, calcium pantothenate, manganese sulfate, thiamine chloride hydrochloride, cupric sulfate, pyridoxine hydrochloride, riboflavin, vitamin A palmitate, potassium citrate, folic acid, biotin, sodium molybdate, chromium chloride, potassium iodide, sodium selenite, phylloquinone, cyanocobalamin and vitamin D_3.

Nutrients: (grams)	Per 300 Calories* (1 packet)	Per 1500 Calories* (5 packets)
Protein	12.5	62.5
Fat	3.25	16.25
Carbohydrate	55.4	277
Water (Max)	5.2	26.0

*In standard dilution (79 g of Vital High Nitrogen Powder mixed in 255 mL of water).
(FAN 768-04)

Roxane Laboratories, Inc.
P.O. 16532
COLUMBUS, OH 43216-6532

HOSPITAL UNIT DOSE

Hospital Unit Dose—Roxane, was developed to aid in improved drug distribution and administration. With Hospital Unit Dose, each single unit of medication moves from our quality controlled production lines to the patient's bedside in tamper resistant containers, labeled for positive identification, thus protecting dosage integrity to the point of administration.

The following products are currently available in Hospital Unit Dose:

Acetaminophen Oral Solution USP (lime) 325mg/10.15mL, 650mg/20.3mL
Acetaminophen Oral Solution USP (cherry) 160mg/5mL, 325mg/10.15mL, 650mg/20.3mL
Acetaminophen Suppositories USP 120mg, 650mg
Acetaminophen Tablets USP 325mg, 500mg, 650mg
Acetaminophen 120mg and Codeine Phosphate 12mg Elixir USP
Acetaminophen 300mg and Codeine Phosphate 30mg Tablets USP
Aluminum Hydroxide Gel USP (Flavored) 2700mg/30mL
Aluminum Hydroxide, Concentrate, 2700mg/20mL, 4050mg/30mL
Aluminum Hydroxide Tablets 500mg
Alumina and Magnesia Oral Suspension USP 30 mL
Alumina, Magnesia, and Simethicone Oral Suspension USP I 15mL, 30mL
Alumina, Magnesia, and Simethicone Oral Suspension USP II 15mL, 30mL
Aminophylline Tablets USP 100mg, 200mg
Aminophylline Oral Solution USP 210mg/10mL, 315mg/15mL
Amitriptyline Hydrochloride Tablets USP 10mg, 25mg, 50mg, 75mg, 100mg
Aromatic Cascara Fluidextract USP 5mL
Aromatic Castor Oil USP 30mL, 60mL
Ascorbic Acid Tablets USP 500mg
Bisacodyl Suppositories USP 10mg
Calcium Carbonate Tablets USP 1250mg
Calcium Carbonate Oral Suspension 1250mg/5mL
Calcium Gluconate Tablets USP 500mg
Castor Oil USP 30mL, 60mL
Chloral Hydrate Syrup USP 500mg/10mL, 1g/10mL
Chloral Hydrate Capsules USP 500mg
Chlorpheniramine Maleate Tablets USP 4mg
Cocaine Hydrochloride Topical Solution 4%/4mL, 10%/4mL
Cocaine Hydrochloride Viscous Topical Solution 4%/4mL, 10%/4mL
Codeine Phosphate Oral Solution 15mg/5mL
Codeine Sulfate Tablets USP 15mg, 30mg, 60mg
Dexamethasone Oral Solution 0.5mg/5mL, 2mg/20mL
Dexamethasone Tablets USP 0.5mg, 0.75mg, 1mg, 1.5mg, 2mg, 4mg, 6mg
Diazepam Oral Solution 5 mg/5 mL, 10 mg/10 mL
Diazepam Tablets USP 2mg, 5mg, 10mg
Digoxin Elixir USP 0.125mg/2.5mL, 0.25mg/5mL
DHT (Dihydrotachysterol) Tablets USP 0.125mg, 0.2mg
Diluent (Flavored) for Oral Use 15mL
Diphenhydramine Hydrochloride Elixir USP 25mg/10mL
Diphenoxylate Hydrochloride 2.5mg and Atropine Sulfate 0.025mg Tablets USP
Diphenoxylate Hydrochloride and Atropine Sulfate Oral Solution USP 5mL, 10mL
Docusate Sodium Capsules USP 50mg, 100mg, 250mg
Docusate Sodium Syrup USP 50mg/15mL, 100mg/30mL
Docusate Sodium 100mg with Casanthranol 30mg Capsules
Ferrous Sulfate Oral Solution USP 300mg/5mL
Ferrous Sulfate Tablets USP 300mg
Furosemide Oral Solution 40mg/5mL, 80mg/10mL
Furosemide Tablets USP 20mg, 40mg, 80mg
Guaifenesin Syrup USP 100mg/5mL, 200mg/10mL, 300mg/15mL
Haloperidol Tablets USP 0.5 mg, 1 mg, 2 mg, 5 mg, 10 mg and 20 mg
Hydromorphone Hydrochloride Tablets USP 2mg, 4mg
Imipramine Hydrochloride Tablets USP 10mg, 25mg, 50mg
Iodinated Glycerol and Codeine Phosphate Oral Solution 5mL, 10mL (each 5mL contains 30mg Iodinated Glycerol and 10mg Codeine Phosphate)
Iodinated Glycerol and Dextromethorphan Oral Solution 5mL, 10mL (each 5mL contains 30mg Iodinated Glycerol and 10mg Dextromethorphan Hydrobromide)
Iodinated Glycerol Elixir 60mg/5mL
Ipecac Syrup USP 15mL, 30mL
Isoetharine Inhalation Solution USP 0.1%, 2.5mL
Isoetharine Inhalation Solution USP 0.125%, 4mL
Isoetharine Inhalation Solution USP 0.167%, 3mL
Isoetharine Inhalation Solution USP 0.2%, 2.5mL

Isoetharine Inhalation Solution USP 0.25%, 2mL
Kaolin-Pectin Suspension 30mL
Lactulose Syrup USP 10mg/15mL
Levorphanol Tartrate Tablets USP 2 mg
Lidocaine Viscous 2% 20mL
Lithium Carbonate Capsules USP 150mg, 300mg, 600mg
Lithium Carbonate Tablets USP 300mg
Lithium Citrate Syrup USP 8mEq per 5mL, 16mEq per 10mL
Loperamide Hydrochloride Capsules USP 2mg
Loperamide Hydrochloride Oral Solution 1mg/5mL, 2mg/10mL, 4mg/20mL
Methadone Hydrochloride Tablets USP 5mg, 10mg
Metoclopramide Syrup 10mg/10mL
Milk of Magnesia USP 15mL, 30mL
Milk of Magnesia Concentrated Flavored 10mL, 15mL, 20mL
Milk of Magnesia—Cascara Suspension Concentrated 15mL
Milk of Magnesia—Mineral Oil Emulsion 30mL
Milk of Magnesia—Mineral Oil Emulsion (Flavored) 30mL
Mineral Oil, Topical Light, USP 10mL, 30mL
Mineral Oil USP 30mL
Morphine Sulfate Tablets 15mg, 30mg
Morphine Sulfate Oral Solution 10mg/5mL, 20mg/10mL
Neomycin Sulfate Tablets USP 500mg
Nystatin Oral Suspension USP 100,000 USP units per mL
Paregoric USP 5mL
Oramoprh SR Tablets (Morphine sulfate sustained release tablets) 30mg, 60mg, 100mg
Phenobarbital Elixir USP 20mg/5mL, 30mg/7.5mL
Phenobarbital Tablets USP 15mg, 30mg, 60mg, 100mg
Potassium Chloride Oral Solution USP 10% (15mEq/11.25mL), (20mEq/15mL), (30mEq/22.5mL), (40mEq/30mL)
Prednisolone Tablets USP 5mg
Prednisone Oral Solution 5mg/5mL
Prednisone Tablets USP 1mg, 2.5mg, 5mg, 10mg, 20mg, 50mg
Propantheline Bromide Tablets USP 15mg
Propoxyphene Hydrochloride Capsules USP 65mg
Propranolol Hydrochloride Tablets USP 10mg, 20mg, 40mg, 60mg, 80mg
Propranolol Hydrochloride Oral Solution 20 mg/5 mL and 40 mg/5 mL
Pseudoephedrine Hydrochloride Tablets USP 30mg, 60mg
Quinidine Sulfate Tablets USP 200mg, 300mg
Roxanol UD (morphine sulfate concentrated oral solution) 10mg/2.5 mL, 20mg/5mL, 30mg/1.5 mL
Rescudose 10mg/2.5mL
Roxanol Suppositories 5mg, 10mg, 20mg, 30mg
Roxicet Oral Solution (Oxycodone Hydrochloride 5mg and Acetaminophen 325mg/5mL)
Roxicet Tablets (Oxycodone and Acetaminophen Tablets USP 5mg/325mg)
Roxicet 5/500 Caplets (Oxycodone and Acetaminophen Tablets USP, 5mg/500mg)
Roxicodone Oral Solution (Oxycodone Hydrochloride Oral Solution USP 5mg/5mL)
Roxicodone Tablets (Oxycodone Tablets USP 5mg)
Roxiprin Tablets (Oxycodone Hydrochloride 4.5mg, Oxycodone Terephthalate 0.38mg, and Aspirin 325mg Tablets USP)
Saliva Substitute
Sodium Chloride Inhalation Solution USP (Normal Saline) Sterile 0.9% 3mL, 5mL
Sodium Phosphates Oral Solution USP 30mL
Sodium Polystyrene Sulfonate Suspension 60mL, and 120mL Enema Package, 200 mL Enema Package
Sulfamethoxazole and Trimethoprim Tablets USP (Regular Strength) 400mg Sulfamethoxazole and 80mg Trimethoprim, (Double Strength) 800mg Sulfamethoxazole and 160 mg Trimethoprim
Theophylline Oral Solution 80mg/15mL, 100mg/18.75mL, 160mg/30mL
Torecan Suppositories (thiethylperazine maleate Suppositories USP) 10mg
Torecan Tablets (thiethylperazine maleate tablets USP) 10mg

As research continues, new Roxane Laboratories' products will be available in Hospital Unit Dose packages.

DHT™   ℞
Dihydrotachysterol
Tablets USP and Intensol

DESCRIPTION
Each tablet contains:
Dihydrotachysterol .... 0.125 mg, 0.2 mg, or 0.4 mg
Each mL of Intensol contains:
Dihydrotachysterol .... 0.2 mg
Dihydrotachysterol is a synthetic reduction product of tachysterol, a close isomer of vitamin D. Chemically Dihydrotachysterol is *9,10- Secoergosta-5,7,22-tri-en-3β- ol.*
Dihydrotachysterol acts as a blood calcium regulator.

CLINICAL PHARMACOLOGY

Dihydrotachysterol is hydroxylated in the liver to 25-hydroxydihydrotachysterol, which is the major circulating active form of the drug. It does not undergo further hydroxylation by the kidney and therefore is the analogue of 1,25-dihydroxyvitamin D. Dihydrotachysterol is effective in the elevation of serum calcium by stimulating intestinal calcium absorption and mobilizing bone calcium in the absence of parathyroid hormone and of functioning renal tissue. Dihydrotachysterol also increases renal phosphate excretion. In contrast to parathyroid extract, Dihydrotachysterol is active when taken orally, exerts a slow but persistent effect, and may be used for long periods without increasing the dosage or causing tolerance. Dihydrotachysterol is faster-acting than pharmacologic doses of vitamin D and is less persistent after cessation of treatment, thus decreasing the risk of accumulation and of hypercalcemia.

INDICATIONS AND USAGE

Dihydrotachysterol is indicated for the treatment of acute, chronic, and latent forms of postoperative tetany, idiopathic tetany, and hypoparathyroidism.

CONTRAINDICATIONS

Contraindicated in patients with hypercalcemia, abnormal sensitivity to the effects of vitamin D, and hypervitaminosis D.

PRECAUTIONS

General: The difference between therapeutic dose and intoxicating dose may be small in any patient and therefore dosage must be individualized and periodically reevaluated. In patients with renal osteodystrophy accompanied by hyperphosphatemia, maintenance of a normal serum phosphorus level by dietary phosphate restriction and/or administration of aluminum gels as intestinal phosphate binders is essential to prevent metastatic calcification.

Because of its effect on serum calcium, Dihydrotachysterol should be administered to pregnant patients or to patients with renal stones only when, in the judgment of the physician, the potential benefits outweigh the possible hazards.

Laboratory tests: **To prevent hypercalcemia, treatment should always be controlled by regular determinations of blood calcium level, which should be maintained within the normal range.**

Drug interactions: Administration of thiazide diuretics to hypoparathyroid patients who are concurrently being treated with Dihydrotachysterol may cause hypercalcemia.

Pregnancy: Teratogenic effects —Pregnancy Category C: Animal reproduction studies have shown fetal abnormalities in several species associated with hypervitaminosis D. These are similar to the supravalvular aortic stenosis syndrome described in infants by Black in England (1963). This syndrome was characterized by supravalvular aortic stenosis, elfin facies, and mental retardation.

There are no adequate and well-controlled studies in pregnant women. Dihydrotachysterol should be used during pregnancy only if the potential benefit justifies the potential risk to the fetus.

Nursing mothers: It is not known whether this drug is excreted in human milk. Because many drugs are excreted in human milk, caution should be exercised when Dihydrotachysterol is administered to a nursing woman.

OVERDOSAGE

The effects of Dihydrotachysterol can persist for up to one month after cessation of treatment.

Manifestations: Toxicity associated with Dihydrotachysterol is similar to that seen with large doses of vitamin D. Overdosage is manifested by symptoms of hypercalcemia, i.e., weakness, headache, anorexia, nausea, vomiting, abdominal cramps, diarrhea, constipation, vertigo, tinnitus, ataxia, hypotonia, lethargy, depression, amnesia, disorientation, hallucinations, syncope, and coma. Impairment of renal function may result in polyuria, polydipsia, and albuminuria. Widespread calcification of soft tissues, including heart, blood vessels, kidneys, and lungs, can occur. Death can result from cardiovascular or renal failure.

Treatment: Treatment of overdosage consists of withdrawal of Dihydrotachysterol, bed rest, liberal intake of fluids, a low-calcium diet, and administration of a laxative. Hypercalcemic crisis with dehydration, stupor, coma, and azotemia requires more vigorous treatment. The first step should be hydration of the patient. Intravenous saline may quickly and significantly increase urinary calcium excretion. A loop diuretic (furosemide or ethacrynic acid) may be given with the saline infusion to further increase renal calcium excretion. Other reported therapeutic measures include dialysis or the administration of citrates, sulfates, phosphates, corticosteroids, EDTA (ethylenediaminetetraacetic acids), and mithramycin via appropriate regimens.

DOSAGE AND ADMINISTRATION

The dosage depends on the nature and seriousness of the disorder and should be adapted to each individual patient.

Serum calcium levels should be maintained between 9 to 10 mg per 100 mL.

The following dosage schedule will serve as a guide:

Initial dose: 0.8 mg to 2.4 mg daily for several days.

Maintenance dose: 0.2 mg to 1.0 mg daily as required for normal serum calcium levels. The average maintenance dose is 0.6 mg daily. This dose may be supplemented with 10 to 15 grams of calcium lactate or gluconate by mouth daily.

HOW SUPPLIED

0.125 mg white tablets.

NDC 0054-8172-25: Unit dose, 10 tablets per strip, 10 strips per shelf pack, 10 shelf packs per shipper.

NDC 0054-4190-19: Bottles of 50 tablets.

0.2 mg pink tablets.

NDC 0054-8182-25: Unit dose, 10 tablets per strip, 10 strips per shelf pack, 10 shelf packs per shipper.

NDC 0054-4189-25: Bottles of 100 tablets.

0.4 mg white tablets.

NDC 0054-4191-19: Bottles of 50 tablets.

Intensol 0.2 mg/mL

NDC 0054-3170-44: Bottles of 30 mL with calibrated dropper (graduated 0.25 mL to 1.0 mL)

LITHIUM CARBONATE   ℞
CAPSULES USP 150 mg, 300 mg, and 600 mg
TABLETS USP 300 mg

> **WARNING**
>
> Lithium toxicity is closely related to serum lithium levels, and can occur at doses close to therapeutic levels. Facilities for prompt and accurate serum lithium determinations should be available before initiating therapy.

DESCRIPTION

Each tablet for oral administration contains:

Lithium Carbonate .... 300 mg

Each capsule for oral administration contains:

Lithium Carbonate .... 150 mg, 300 mg, or 600 mg

Inactive Ingredients:

The capsules contain talc, gelatin, FD&C Red No. 40, titanium dioxide, and the imprinting ink contains FD&C Blue No. 2, FD&C Yellow No. 6, FD&C Red No. 40, synthetic black iron oxide, and pharmaceutical glaze. The tablets contain calcium stearate, microcrystalline cellulose, povidone, sodium lauryl sulfate, and sodium starch glycolate.

Lithium Carbonate is a white, light alkaline powder with molecular formula Li_2CO_3 and molecular weight 73.89. Lithium is an element of the alkali-metal group with atomic number 3, atomic weight 6.94 and an emission line at 671 nm on the flame photometer. Lithium acts as an antimanic.

CLINICAL PHARMACOLOGY

Preclinical studies have shown that lithium alters sodium transport in nerve and muscle cells and effects a shift toward intraneuronal metabolism of catecholamines, but the specific biochemical mechanism of lithium action in mania is unknown.

INDICATIONS AND USAGE

Lithium carbonate is indicated in the treatment of manic episodes of Bipolar Disorder. Bipolar Disorder, Manic (DSM-III) is equivalent to Manic Depressive illness, Manic, in the older DSM-II terminology.

Lithium is also indicated as a maintenance treatment for individuals with a diagnosis of Bipolar Disorder. Maintenance therapy reduces the frequency of manic episodes and diminishes the intensity of those episodes which may occur. Typical symptoms of mania include pressure of speech, motor hyperactivity, reduced need for sleep, flight of ideas, grandiosity, or poor judgment, aggressiveness, and possibly hostility. When given to a patient experiencing a manic episode, lithium may produce a normalization of symptomatology within 1 to 3 weeks.

CONTRAINDICATIONS

Lithium should generally not be given to patients with significant renal or cardiovascular disease, severe debilitation or dehydration, or sodium depletion, and to patients receiving diuretics, since the risk of lithium toxicity is very high in such patients. If the psychiatric indication is life-threatening, and if such a patient fails to respond to other measures, lithium treatment may be undertaken with extreme caution, including daily serum lithium determinations and adjustment to the usually low doses ordinarily tolerated by these individuals. In such instances, hospitalization is a necessity.

WARNINGS

Lithium may cause fetal harm when administered to a pregnant woman. There have been reports of lithium having adverse effects on nidation in rats, embryo viability in mice, and metabolism in-vitro of rat testis and human spermatozoa have been attributed to lithium, as have teratogenicity in submammalian species and cleft palates in mice. Studies in rats, rabbits and monkeys have shown no evidence of lith-

ium-induced teratology. Data from lithium birth registries suggest an increase in cardiac and other anomalies, especially Ebstein's anomaly. If the patient becomes pregnant while taking lithium, she should be apprised of the potential risk to the fetus. If possible, lithium should be withdrawn for at least the first trimester unless it is determined that this would seriously endanger the mother.

Chronic lithium therapy may be associated with diminution of renal concentrating ability, occasionally presenting as nephrogenic diabetes insipidus, with polyuria and polydipsia. Such patients should be carefully managed to avoid dehydration with resulting lithium retention and toxicity. This condition is usually reversible when lithium is discontinued. Morphologic changes with glomerular and interstitial fibrosis and nephron-atrophy have been reported in patients on chronic lithium therapy. Morphologic changes have been seen in bipolar patients never exposed to lithium. The relationship between renal functional and morphologic changes and their association with lithium therapy has not been established. To date, lithium in therapeutic doses has not been reported to cause end-stage renal disease.

When kidney function is assessed, for baseline data prior to starting lithium therapy or thereafter, routine urinalysis and other tests may be used to evaluate tubular function (e.g., urine specific gravity or osmolality following a period of water deprivation, or 24-hour urine volume) and glomerular function (e.g., serum creatinine or creatinine clearance). During lithium therapy, progressive or sudden changes in renal function, even within the normal range, indicate the need for reevaluation of treatment.

Lithium toxicity is closely related to serum lithium levels, and can occur at doses close to therapeutic levels (see DOSAGE AND ADMINISTRATION).

PRECAUTIONS

General: The ability to tolerate lithium is greater during the acute manic phase and decreases when manic symptoms subside (See DOSAGE AND ADMINISTRATION).

The distribution space of lithium approximates that of total body water. Lithium is primarily excreted in urine with insignificant excretion in feces. Renal excretion of lithium is proportional to its plasma concentration. The half-life of elimination of lithium is approximately 24 hours. Lithium decreases sodium reabsorption by the renal tubules which could lead to sodium depletion. Therefore, it is essential for the patient to maintain a normal diet, including salt, and an adequate fluid intake (2500-3000 mL) at least during the initial stabilization period. Decreased tolerance to lithium has been reported to ensue from protracted sweating or diarrhea and, if such occur, supplemental fluid and salt should be administered.

In addition to sweating and diarrhea, concomitant infection with elevated temperatures may also necessitate a temporary reduction or cessation of medication.

Previously existing underlying thyroid disorders do not necessarily constitute a contraindication to lithium treatment; where hypothyroidism exists, careful monitoring of thyroid function during lithium stabilization and maintenance allows for correction of changing thyroid parameters, if any. Where hypothyroidism occurs during lithium stabilization and maintenance, supplemental thyroid treatment may be used.

Information for the patients: Outpatients and their families should be warned that the patient must discontinue lithium therapy and contact his physician if such clinical signs of lithium toxicity as diarrhea, vomiting, tremor, mild ataxia, drowsiness, or muscular weakness occur.

Lithium may impair mental and/or physical abilities. Caution patients about activities requiring alertness (e.g., operating vehicles or machinery).

Drug interactions: *Combined use of haloperidol and lithium:* An encephalopathic syndrome (characterized by weakness, lethargy, fever, tremulousness and confusion, extrapyramidal symptoms, leucocytosis, elevated serum enzymes, BUN and FBS) followed by irreversible brain damage has occurred in a few patients treated with lithium plus haloperidol. A causal relationship between these events and the concomitant administration of lithium and haloperidol has not been established; however, patients receiving such combined therapy should be monitored closely for early evidence of neurological toxicity and treatment discontinued promptly if such signs appear.

The possibility of similar adverse interactions with other antipsychotic medication exists.

Lithium may prolong the effects of neuromuscular blocking agents. Therefore, neuromuscular blocking agents should be given with caution to patients receiving lithium.

Indomethacin and piroxicam have been reported to increase significantly steady state plasma lithium levels. In some cases lithium toxicity has resulted from such interactions. There is also evidence that other non-steroidal, anti-inflammatory agents may have a similar effect. When such combi-

Continued on next page

Roxane Laboratories—Cont.

nations are used, increased plasma lithium level monitoring is recommended.
Caution should be used when lithium and diuretics or angiotensin converting enzyme (ACE) inhibitors are used concomitantly because sodium loss may reduce the renal clearance of lithium and increase serum lithium levels with risk of lithium toxicity. When such combinations are used, the lithium dosage may need to be decreased, and more frequent monitoring of lithium plasma levels is recommended.
Pregnancy: Teratogenic effects—Pregnancy Category D, See "Warnings" section.
Nursing mothers: Lithium is excreted in human milk. Nursing should not be undertaken during lithium therapy except in rare and unusual circumstances where, in the view of the physician, the potential benefits to the mother outweigh possible hazards to the child.
Usage in Children: Since information regarding the safety and effectiveness of lithium in children under 12 years of age is not available, its use in such patients is not recommended at this time. There has been a report of a transient syndrome of acute dystonia and hyperreflexia occurring in a 15 kg child who ingested 300 mg lithium carbonate.

ADVERSE REACTIONS

Lithium toxicity: The likelihood of toxicity increases with increasing serum lithium levels. Serum lithium levels greater than 1.5 mEq/l carry a greater risk than lower levels. However, patients sensitive to lithium may exhibit toxic signs at serum levels below 1.5 mEq/l.
Diarrhea, vomiting, drowsiness, muscular weakness and lack of coordination may be early signs of lithium toxicity, and can occur at lithium levels below 2.0 mEq/l. At higher levels, giddiness, ataxia, blurred vision, tinnitus and a large output of dilute urine may be seen. Serum lithium levels above 3.0 mEq/l may produce a complex clinical picture involving multiple organs and organ systems. Serum lithium levels should not be permitted to exceed 2.0 mEq/l during the acute treatment phase.
Fine hand tremor, polyuria and mild thirst may occur during initial therapy for the acute manic phase, and may persist throughout treatment. Transient and mild nausea and general discomfort may also appear during the first few days of lithium administration.
These side effects are an inconvenience rather than a disabling condition, and usually subside with continued treatment or a temporary reduction or cessation of dosage. If persistent, a cessation of dosage is indicated.
The following adverse reactions have been reported and do not appear to be directly related to serum lithium levels.
Neuromuscular: tremor, muscle hyperirritability (fasciculations, twitching, clonic movements of whole limbs), ataxia, choreo-athetotic movements, hyperactive deep tendon reflexes.
Central Nervous System: Blackout spells, epileptiform seizures, slurred speech, dizziness, vertigo, incontinence of urine or feces, somnolence, psychomotor retardation, restlessness, confusion, stupor, coma, acute dystonia, downbeat nystagmus.
Cardiovascular: cardiac arrhythmia, hypotension, peripheral circulatory collapse.
Neurological: Cases of pseudotumor cerebri (increased intracranial pressure and papilledema) have been reported with lithium use. If undetected, this condition may result in enlargement of the blind spot, constriction of visual fields and eventual blindness due to optic atrophy. Lithium should be discontinued, if clinically possible, if this syndrome occurs.
Gastrointestinal: anorexia, nausea, vomiting, diarrhea.
Genitourinary: albuminuria, oliguria, polyuria, glycosuria.
Dermatologic: drying and thinning of hair, anesthesia of skin, chronic folliculitis, xerosis cutis, alopecia and exacerbation of psoriasis.
Autonomic Nervous System: blurred vision, dry mouth.
Thyroid Abnormalities: euthyroid goiter and/ or hypothyroidism (including myxedema) accompanied by lower T_3 and T_4. Iodine 131 uptake may be elevated. (See PRECAUTIONS). Paradoxically, rare cases of hyperthyroidism have been reported.
EEG Changes: diffuse slowing, widening of frequency spectrum, potentiation and disorganization of background rhythm.
EKG Changes: reversible flattening, isoelectricity or inversion of T-waves.
Miscellaneous: fatigue, lethargy, transient scotomata, dehydration, weight loss, tendency to sleep.
Miscellaneous reactions unrelated to dosage are: transient electroencephalographic and electrocardiographic changes, leucocytosis, headache, diffuse nontoxic goiter with or without hypothyroidism, transient hyperglycemia, generalized pruritis with or without rash, cutaneous ulcers, albuminuria, worsening of organic brain syndromes, excessive weight gain, edematous swelling of ankles or wrists, and thirst or polyuria, sometimes resembling diabetes insipidus, and metallic taste.
A single report has been received of the development of painful discoloration of fingers and toes and coldness of the extremities within one day of the starting of treatment of lithium. The mechanism through which these symptoms (resembling Raynaud's Syndrome) developed is not known. Recovery followed discontinuance.

OVERDOSAGE

The toxic levels for lithium are close to the therapeutic levels. It is therefore important that patients and their families be cautioned to watch for early symptoms and to discontinue the drug and inform the physician should they occur. Toxic symptoms are listed in detail under ADVERSE REACTIONS.
Treatment: No specific antidote for lithium poisoning is known. Early symptoms of lithium toxicity can usually be treated by reduction or cessation of dosage of the drug and resumption of the treatment at a lower dose after 24 to 48 hours. In severe cases of lithium poisoning, the first and foremost goal of treatment consists of elimination of this ion from the patient.
Treatment is essentially the same as that used in barbiturate poisoning: 1) gastric lavage, 2) correction of fluid and electrolyte imbalance and 3) regulation of kidney functioning. Urea, mannitol, and aminophylline all produce significant increases in lithium excretion. Hemodialysis is an effective and rapid means of removing the ion from the severely toxic patient. Infection prophylaxis, regular chest X-rays, and preservation of adequate respiration are essential.

DOSAGE AND ADMINISTRATION

Acute Mania: Optimal patient response to Lithium Carbonate usually can be established and maintained with 600 mg t.i.d. Such doses will normally produce an effective serum lithium level ranging between 1.0 and 1.5 mEq/l. Dosage must be individualized according to serum levels and clinical response. Regular monitoring of the patient's clinical state and of serum lithium levels is necessary. Serum levels should be determined twice per week during the acute phase, and until the serum level and clinical condition of the patient have been stabilized.
Long-term Control: The desirable serum lithium levels are 0.6 to 1.2 mEq/l. Dosage will vary from one individual to another, but usually 300 mg t.i.d. or q.i.d. will maintain this level. Serum lithium levels in uncomplicated cases receiving maintenance therapy during remission should be monitored at least every two months.
Patients abnormally sensitive to lithium may exhibit toxic signs at serum levels of 1.0 to 1.5 mEq/l. Elderly patients often respond to reduced dosage, and may exhibit signs of toxicity at serum levels ordinarily tolerated by other patients.
N.B.: Blood samples for serum lithium determination should be drawn immediately prior to the next dose when lithium concentrations are relatively stable (i.e., 8–12 hours after the previous dose.) Total reliance must not be placed on serum levels alone. Accurate patient evaluation requires both clinical and laboratory analysis.

HOW SUPPLIED

Lithium Carbonate Tablets USP
300 mg white, scored tablets (Identified 54 452)
NDC 0054-8528-25: Unit dose, 10 tablets per strip, 10 strips per shelf pack, 10 shelf packs per shipper.
(For Institutional Use Only).
NDC 0054-4527-25: Bottles of 100 tablets.
NDC 0054-4527-31: Bottles of 1000 tablets.
Lithium Carbonate Capsules USP
150 mg white opaque colored capsules (size 4) (Identified 54 213).
NDC 0054-8526-25: Unit dose, 10 capsules per strip, 10 strips per shelf pack, 10 shelf packs per shipper.
(For Institutional Use Only).
NDC 0054-2526-25: Bottles of 100 capsules.
NDC 0054-2526-31: Bottles of 1000 capsules.
300 mg flesh-colored capsules (size 2) (Identified 54 463).
NDC 0054-8527-25: Unit dose, 10 capsules per strip, 10 strips per shelf pack, 10 shelf packs per shipper.
(For Institutional Use Only).
NDC 0054-2527-25: Bottles of 100 capsules.
NDC 0054-2527-31: Bottles of 1000 capsules.
600 mg white opaque/flesh colored capsules (size 0) (Identified 54 702).
NDC 0054-8531-25: Unit dose, 10 capsules per strip, 10 strips per shelf pack, 10 shelf packs per shipper.
(For Institutional Use Only.)
NDC 0054-2531-25: Bottles of 100 capsules.
NDC 0054-2531-31: Bottles of 1000 capsules.
Caution: Federal law prohibits dispensing without prescription.
4055500 Revised June 1989
069

LITHIUM CITRATE SYRUP USP ℞

8 mEq of Lithium per 5 mL, 16mEq of Lithium per 10 mL
SUGAR FREE
FOR ORAL ADMINISTRATION ONLY

DESCRIPTION

Lithium Citrate Syrup is a palatable oral dosage form of lithium ion. Lithium citrate is prepared in solution from lithium hydroxide and citric acid in a ratio approximating di-lithium citrate:
Each 5 mL of Lithium Citrate Syrup contains 8 mEq of lithium ion (Li+), equivalent to the amount of lithium in 300 mg of lithium carbonate and alcohol 0.3% v/v.
Inactive ingredients:
The syrup contains alcohol, sorbitol, flavoring, water, and other ingredients.
Lithium is an element of the alkali-metal group with atomic number 3, atomic weight 6.94, and an emission line at 671 nm on the flame photometer.

HOW SUPPLIED

Lithium Citrate Syrup, 8 mEq per 5 mL
NDC 0054-8529-04: Unit dose Patient Cup™ filled to deliver 5 mL, ten 5 mL Patient Cups™ per shelf pack, ten shelf packs per shipper. (For Institutional Use Only).
NDC 0054-3527-63: Bottles of 500 mL.
Lithium Citrate Syrup, 16 mEq per 10 mL
NDC 0054-8530-04: Unit dose Patient Cup™ filled to deliver 10 mL, ten 10 mL Patient Cups™ per shelf pack, ten shelf packs per shipper. (For Institutional Use Only).
Refer to Lithium Carbonate Capsules and Tablets heading for complete text.

MARINOL® Ⓒ ℞

(Dronabinol)

(WARNING: May be habit forming)

DESCRIPTION

Each capsule for oral administration contains:
Dronabinol .... 2.5 mg, 5 mg, or 10 mg
(Warning: May be habit forming)
MARINOL brand of dronabinol (delta-9-tetrahydrocannabinol, THC), [(6a*R-trans*)-6a,7,8,10a-tetrahydro-6,6,9-trimethyl-3-pentyl-6*H*-dibenzo[*b,d*]pyran-1-ol] is the principal psychoactive substance present in *Cannabis sativa L.* (marijuana). It has the empirical formula $C_{21}H_{30}O_2$ with the molecular weight of 314.45. It has the following structural formula:

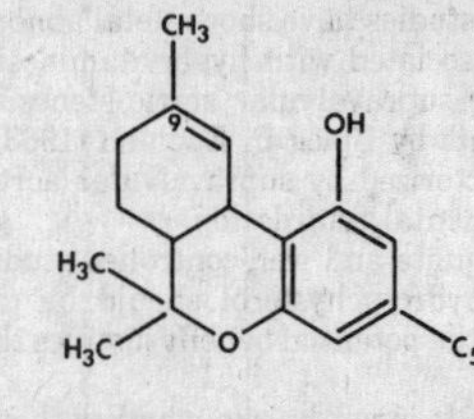

MARINOL is chemically synthesized and formulated in sesame oil and encapsulated in round soft gelatin capsules for oral administration.

CLINICAL PHARMACOLOGY

Non-therapeutic Effects
Dronabinol, commonly known as delta-9-THC, is one of the major active substances in marijuana. For practical purposes, the non-therapeutic effects of dronabinol may be considered essentially identical to those of marijuana and other centrally active cannabinoids. MARINOL is highly abusable and can produce both physical and psychological dependence.
Dronabinol has complex effects upon the central nervous system. Subjects using cannabis may experience changes in mood (euphoria, detachment, depression, anxiety, panic, paranoia, etc.), decrements in cognitive performance and memory, a decreased ability to control drives and impulses, and alterations in the experience of reality (e.g., distortions in the perception of objects and the sense of time, hallucinations, etc.). These latter phenomena appear to be more common when larger doses of dronabinol are administered; however, a full blown picture of psychosis (psychotic organic brain syndrome) may occur in patients receiving doses within the lower portion of the therapeutic range.
Reliable information on the behavioral effects of chronic dronabinol use is not available; however, it has been reported that chronic use of cannabis may be associated with decrements in motivation, cognition, judgment, etc. (Whether these impairments reflect the underlying character of individuals chronically abusing cannabis or are a result of the use of cannabis is not known.)
Dronabinol, used within or slightly above the recommended dose range, has several systemic effects of interest. It characteristically causes an increase in heart rate and conjunctival

injection. Its effects on blood pressure are inconsistent, but occasional subjects have experienced orthostatic hypotension and/or fainting upon standing. In one study, a slight, but consistent, decrease in oral temperature was recorded. The potential of dronabinol to cause tolerance and physical dependence was examined in a 30 day rising dose tolerance study. Following thirty days of use, tolerance developed to the cardiovascular and subjective effects of dronabinol administered at doses up to 210 mg/day. An initial tachycardia induced by dronabinol was replaced successively by normal sinus rhythm and then bradycardia. A fall in supine blood pressure, made worse by standing, was also observed initially. Within days, however, these effects disappeared, indicating the development of tolerance.

A withdrawal syndrome, consisting of irritability, insomnia, and restlessness, was observed in some subjects within 12 hours following abrupt withdrawal of dronabinol. The syndrome reached its peak intensity at 24 hours when subjects exhibited "hot flashes", sweating, rhinorrhea, loose stools, hiccoughs and anorexia. The syndrome was essentially complete within 96 hours.

Electroencephalographic changes recorded following dronabinol discontinuation were consistent with a withdrawal syndrome. While on drug, dronabinol produced a decrease in REM sleep. Following discontinuation, a marked rebound of REM sleep occurred. Several subjects reported impressions of disturbed sleep for several weeks after discontinuing high dose dronabinol. Dronabinol is not an opioid, and does not cause opioid-like effects upon respiration or pupil size.

Metabolism and Pharmacokinetics

Reliable information on the pharmacokinetics of MARINOL is not yet available. The following summary highlights important aspects of the literature concerning the absorption, distribution, metabolism and elimination of dronabinol; however, differences in the preparation, formulation and method of administration make it difficult to extrapolate this information directly to the drug product, MARINOL. Following oral administration, dronabinol has a systemic availability of 10 to 20% relative to an I.V. dose, indicating that the drug undergoes extensive first pass metabolism. Numerous metabolites have been identified, including 11-hydroxy-tetrahydrocannabinol, which is psychoactive. Dronabinol has a volume of distribution about 100 times as large as the plasma volume.

The maximum plasma concentrations of dronabinol, the 11-hydroxy metabolite, and several other metabolites occur approximately 2 to 3 hours after oral dosing. Biliary excretion is the major route of elimination. Within 72 hours following oral administration, approximately 50% of the dose is recovered in feces; another ten to fifteen percent appears in the urine either unchanged or as a metabolite. Renal clearance in normals is approximately one-tenth of the glomerular filtration rate.

The elimination phase of dronabinol exhibits biphasic kinetics with an alpha half-life of about 4 hours and a terminal half-life of 25 to 36 hours. The principal active metabolite, 11-OH-delta-9-THC, appears in the plasma in roughly the same mg quantities as its parent. The terminal plasma half-life for the 11-OH-delta-9-THC is approximately 15–18 hours. Thus, extended use of MARINOL at the doses recommended in this labeling may cause the accumulation of toxic amounts of dronabinol and its metabolites.

INDICATIONS AND USAGE

MARINOL is indicated for the treatment of the nausea and vomiting associated with cancer chemotherapy in patients who have failed to respond adequately to conventional antiemetic treatments. This restriction is required because a substantial proportion of patients treated with MARINOL can be expected to experience disturbing psychotomimetic reactions not observed with other antiemetic agents.

Because of its potential to alter the mental state, MARINOL is intended for use under circumstances that permit close supervision of the patient by a responsible individual. MARINOL is highly abusable and controlled under Schedule II of the Controlled Substances Act. Prescriptions of MARINOL should be limited to the amount necessary for a single cycle of chemotherapy (i.e., a few days).

Evidence supporting the efficacy of MARINOL in the treatment of nausea and vomiting induced by cancer chemotherapy was obtained from a variety of sources. The most persuasive evidence was obtained in subjects being treated with MOPP for Hodgkin's and non-Hodgkin's lymphomas. Other evidence supports the conclusion that MARINOL is effective against nausea and vomiting induced by other cancer chemotherapy regimens employed in the treatment of a wide variety of tumor types.

CONTRAINDICATIONS

MARINOL is contraindicated in patients whose nausea and vomiting arises from any cause other than cancer chemotherapy.

MARINOL is contraindicated in any patient known to be hypersensitive to either dronabinol or sesame oil.

WARNINGS

Because of its profound effects on the mental status, patients should be warned not to drive, operate complex machinery, or engage in any activity requiring sound judgment and unimpaired coordination while receiving treatment with MARINOL. The effects of MARINOL may persist for a variable and unpredictable period of time following its oral administration. Dronabinol is highly lipid soluble and its metabolites may persist in tissues, including plasma, for days. Because of individual variation in response and tolerance to the effects of MARINOL, the physician should determine on clinical grounds the period of patient supervision required. Patients receiving MARINOL should be closely observed, if possible within an inpatient setting. This is especially important during the treatment of naive patients. However, even patients experienced with MARINOL (or cannabis) may have serious untoward responses not predicted by prior uneventful exposures. Because a psychotic patient is a potential danger to him/herself and/or others, any patient who has a psychotic experience with MARINOL should be closely observed in an appropriate setting until his/her mental state returns to normal. The patient should not be given additional doses of MARINOL until he/she has been examined, and the circumstances evaluated, by a physician. If the clinical situation warrants it, a lower dose of MARINOL may be administered under very close supervision. The patient should be counseled about the experience and should share in the decision about further use of MARINOL.

MARINOL should not be taken with alcohol, sedatives, hypnotics, or other psychotomimetic substances.

PRECAUTIONS

General: Because it may cause a general increase in central sympathomimetic activity, MARINOL should be used with caution in persons with hypertension or heart disease. MARINOL should be used cautiously in manic, depressive, or schizophrenic patients as the symptoms of these disease states may be unmasked by the use of cannabinoids. MARINOL should be used with caution in individuals receiving other psychoactive drugs.

Information for Patients: Persons taking MARINOL should be alerted to the additive central nervous system depression resulting from simultaneous use of MARINOL and alcohol or barbiturates. This combination should be avoided. Operation of machinery or a motor vehicle should be avoided during MARINOL therapy. Patients using MARINOL should be made aware of possible changes in mood and other adverse behavioral effects of the drug so as to avoid panic in the event of such manifestations. Patients should remain under supervision of a responsible adult while using MARINOL.

Drug Interactions: The effects of MARINOL on blood ethanol levels are complex. During sub-chronic MARINOL administration (60 mg/day) for ten days, absorption of ethanol was delayed, resulting in lower and delayed peak blood alcohol levels. Metabolism of ethanol was increased in some subjects and decreased in others. The overall rate of ethanol disappearance was decreased by about ten percent.

Carcinogenesis, Mutagenesis, and Impairment of Fertility: Carcinogenicity studies have not been performed with MARINOL. Reproductive studies in mice (approximately 32–400 times the human dose) and rats (approximately 8–32 times the human dose) demonstrate that MARINOL causes a decrease in pregnancy rate. In a long-term rat study (77 days), oral administration of MARINOL at doses 3–17 times the human dose reduced ventral prostate, seminal vesicle and epididymal weights and caused a decrease in seminal fluid volume. Decreases in spermatogenesis, number of developing germ cells, and number of Leydig cells in the testis were also observed. However, sperm count, mating success and testosterone levels were not affected. The significance of these animal findings in humans is not known.

Pregnancy: Pregnancy Category B. Reproduction studies have been performed in mice, rats and rabbits at doses up to 400 times, 32 times, and 10 times the human dose, respectively, and have revealed no evidence of teratogenicity due to MARINOL. At these dose levels in mice and rats, which produced substantial reductions in maternal weight gain, MARINOL caused a decrease in the number of viable pups, an increase in fetal mortality and an increase in early resorptions. Such effects were dose dependent and less apparent at lower doses which produced less maternal toxicity. There are, however, no adequate and well-controlled studies in pregnant women. Because animal reproduction studies are not always predictive of human response, this drug should be used during pregnancy only if clearly needed.

Nursing Mothers: MARINOL is concentrated and secreted in human milk and is absorbed by the nursing baby. Because the effects on the infant of chronic exposure to MARINOL and its metabolites are unknown, nursing mothers should not use MARINOL.

ADVERSE REACTIONS

In controlled clinical trials, the most frequently reported adverse reactions involved the central nervous system. In decreasing order of frequency these events were drowsiness, dizziness, muddled thinking and brief impairment of coordi-

nation, sensory and perceptual functions. Easy laughing, elation and heightened awareness, often termed a "high", was observed in 24% of MARINOL patients.

The incidences listed in the following table are derived from comparative double-blind, crossover or parallel design trials in which patients received MARINOL, an active control drug (usually prochlorperazine) or placebo.

The figures cited cannot be used to predict precisely the incidence of untoward events in the course of usual medical practice where patient characteristics and other factors often differ from those obtained in the clinical trials. Furthermore, these figures should not be compared with those obtained in other clinical studies involving related drug products and placebo, as each group of drug trials are conducted under a different set of conditions.

FREQUENCY OF ADVERSE EFFECTS FROM CONTROLLED STUDIES

Body System/ Adverse Reaction	MARINOL (n=317) %	Control (n=263) %	Placebo (n=68) %
CENTRAL NERVOUS SYSTEM:			
Drowsiness	48	33	49
Dizziness	21	5	1
Anxiety	16	3	24
Muddled Thinking	12	1	1
Perceptual Difficulties	11	1	0
Coordination Impairment	9	2	10
Irritability/Weird Feeling	7	3	0
Depression	7	3	15
Weak, Sluggish	6	3	1
Headache	6	4	4
Hallucinations	5	0	0
Memory Lapse	5	1	0
Unsteadiness, Ataxia	4	1	0
Paranoia	2	0	0
Depersonalization	2	0	0
Disorientation, Confusion	1	0	2
AUTONOMIC NERVOUS SYSTEM:			
Dry Mouth	3	1	1
Paresthesia	3	0	1
Visual Distortions	3	0	0
CARDIOVASCULAR:			
Tachycardia	1	1	0
Postural Hypotension	1	0	0

In addition to the events enumerated above, the following have been reported at a frequency below one percent: CENTRAL NERVOUS SYSTEM: tinnitus, nightmares; AUTONOMIC NERVOUS SYSTEM: speech difficulty, facial flushing, perspiring; CARDIOVASCULAR: syncope; GASTROINTESTINAL: diarrhea, fecal incontinence; MUSCULOSKELETAL: muscular pains.

DRUG ABUSE AND DEPENDENCE

MARINOL is highly abusable and controlled as delta-9-tetrahydrocannabinol under Schedule II of the Controlled Substances Act. Prescriptions of MARINOL should be limited to the amount necessary for a single cycle of chemotherapy (i.e., a few days).

It is not known what proportion of individuals exposed chronically to MARINOL or other cannabinoids will develop either psychological or physical dependence. Long-term use of these compounds has been associated with disorders of motivation, judgment, and cognition. It is not clear, though, if this is a manifestation of the underlying personalities of chronic users of this class of drugs, or if cannabinoids are directly responsible for these effects. An abstinence syndrome has been reported following discontinuation of high doses of delta-9-THC (210 mg per day). The acute phase was characterized by psychic distress, insomnia, and signs of autonomic hyperactivity (sweating, rhinorrhea, loose stools, hiccoughs). A protracted abstinence phase may have occurred as subjects reported sleep disturbances for several weeks after delta-9-THC discontinuation.

OVERDOSAGE

Signs and symptoms of overdosage are an extension of the psychotomimetic and physiologic effects of MARINOL, and, therefore, the clinical picture of overdosage may vary widely from patient to patient. Overdosages may be considered to be of two types: those at therapeutic doses, and those at higher, non-therapeutic doses.

Overdosage at Prescribed Dosages

Overdosage may be considered to have occurred even at prescribed dosages if disturbing psychiatric symptoms have occurred. In these cases, the patient should be observed in a quiet environment and supportive measures, including reassurance, should be used. Subsequent doses should be held until the patient has returned to baseline; routine dosing may then be resumed if clinically indicated, though this should be at a lower dosage. In controlled clinical trials, all such disturbing reactions spontaneously disappeared within 24 hours without specific medical therapy.

Continued on next page

Roxane Laboratories—Cont.

Particular attention should be paid to the vital signs in these patients, as tachycardia and both hyper- and hypotension are common adverse reactions. These signs should be monitored and treated, if necessary, in the usual manner according to the judgment of the physician.

Overdosage at Multiples of Prescribed Dosages

No cases of overdosage in multiples of prescribed dosages were reported in the controlled clinical studies. Few deaths have been reported from the use of dronabinol in any of its many forms (e.g., hashish, marijuana, etc.). Two incidents of death following the ingestion of large overdoses of Indian Hemp have been reported, while one death resulting from smoking cannabis herb and/or resin has appeared. No estimate of actual dosages was provided in either case. However, from a case of severe coma due to cannabis in a young French soldier, who recovered with conventional supportive therapy (intubation, I.V. fluids), it has been estimated that the acute lethal intravenous dose of dronabinol would be on the order of 1000–2000 mg total dose. Although this is a crude extrapolation at best, it represents a five to ten-fold multiple of the maximum oral dose recommended for MARINOL in a twenty-four hour period.

DOSAGE AND ADMINISTRATION

MARINOL is best administered at an initial dose of 5 mg/M^2, given 1–3 hours prior to the administration of chemotherapy, then every 2–4 hours after chemotherapy is given, for a total of 4–6 doses/day. Should the 5 mg/M^2 dose prove to be ineffective, and in the absence of significant side effects, the dose may be escalated by 2.5 mg/M^2 increments to a maximum of 15 mg/M^2 per dose. Caution should be exercised, however, as the incidence of disturbing psychiatric symptoms increases significantly at this maximum dose.

HOW SUPPLIED

MARINOL CAPSULES (Dronabinol solution in soft gelatin capsules).

2.5 mg white capsules (Identified RL).

NDC 0054-2601-11: Bottles of 25 capsules.

5 mg dark brown capsules (Identifed RL)

NDC 0054-2602-11: Bottles of 25 capsules.

10 mg orange capsules (Identifed RL)

NDC 0054-2603-11: Bottles of 25 capsules.

MARINOL capsules should be preserved in a well sealed container, and stored in a cool place

MARINOL® is a registered trademark of and is marketed under license from Unimed, Inc.

DEA ORDER FORM REQUIRED.

Shown in Product Identification Section, page 427

METHADONE HYDROCHLORIDE ℂ ℞
ORAL SOLUTION USP
TABLETS USP

(WARNING: May be habit forming)

CONDITIONS FOR DISTRIBUTION AND USE OF METHADONE PRODUCTS:
Code of Federal Regulations,
Title 21, Sec. 291.505

METHADONE PRODUCTS, WHEN USED FOR TREATMENT OF NARCOTIC ADDICTION IN DETOXIFICATION OR MAINTENANCE PROGRAMS, SHALL BE DISPENSED ONLY BY APPROVED HOSPITAL PHARMACIES, APPROVED COMMUNITY PHARMACIES, AND MAINTENANCE PROGRAMS APPROVED BY THE FOOD AND DRUG ADMINISTRATION AND THE DESIGNATED STATE AUTHORITY.

APPROVED MAINTENANCE PROGRAMS SHALL DISPENSE AND USE METHADONE IN ORAL FORM ONLY AND ACCORDING TO THE TREATMENT REQUIREMENTS STIPULATED IN THE FEDERAL METHADONE REGULATIONS (21 CFR 291.505).

FAILURE TO ABIDE BY THE REQUIREMENTS IN THESE REGULATIONS MAY RESULT IN CRIMINAL PROSECUTION, SEIZURE OF THE DRUG SUPPLY, REVOCATION OF THE PROGRAM APPROVAL, AND INJUNCTION PRECLUDING OPERATION OF THE PROGRAM.

A METHADONE PRODUCT, WHEN USED AS AN ANALGESIC, MAY BE DISPENSED IN ANY LICENSED PHARMACY.

DESCRIPTION

Each 5 mL of Methadone Hydrochloride Oral Solution contains:

Methadone Hydrochloride .... 5 mg or 10 mg

(**Warning:** May be habit forming)

Alcohol 8%

Each tablet for oral administration contains:

Methadone Hydrochloride .... 5 mg or 10 mg

(**Warning:** May be habit forming)

Inactive Ingredients:

The oral solution contains alcohol, FD&C Red No. 40, FD&C Yellow No. 6, flavoring, glycol, sorbitol, water, and other ingredients.

The tablets contain magnesium steareate, microcrystalline cellulose, and starch (corn).

Chemically, Methadone Hydrochloride is 3-Heptanone, 6-(dimethylamino)-4,4-diphenyl-, hydrochloride.

Methadone Hydrochloride acts as a narcotic analgesic.

CLINICAL PHARMACOLOGY

Methadone Hydrochloride is a synthetic narcotic analgesic with multiple actions quantitatively similar to those of morphine, the most prominent of which involve the central nervous system and organs composed of smooth muscle. The principal actions of therapeutic value are analgesia and sedation and detoxification or temporary maintenance in narcotic addiction. The methadone abstinence syndrome, although qualitatively similar to that of morphine, differs in that the onset is slower, the course is more prolonged, and the symptoms are less severe.

When administered orally, methadone is approximately one-half as potent as when given parenterally. Oral administration results in a delay of the onset, a lowering of the peak, and an increase in the duration of analgesic effect.

INDICATIONS AND USAGE

Methadone Hydrochloride is indicated for relief of severe pain, for detoxification treatment of narcotic addiction, and for temporary maintenance treatment of narcotic addiction.

Note

If methadone is administered for treatment of heroin dependence for more than three weeks, the procedure passes from treatment of the acute withdrawal syndrome (detoxification) to maintenance therapy. Maintenance treatment is permitted to be undertaken only by approved methadone programs. This does not preclude the maintenance treatment of an addict who is hospitalized for medical conditions other than addiction and who requires temporary maintenance during the critical period of his stay or whose enrollment has been verified in a program which has approval for maintenance treatment with methadone.

CONTRAINDICATIONS

Hypersensitivity to methadone.

WARNINGS

Methadone Hydrochloride Tablets are for oral administration only and *must not* be used for injection. It is recommended that Methadone Hydrochloride Tablets, if dispensed, be packaged in child-resistant containers and kept out of the reach of children to prevent accidental ingestion.

Methadone Hydrochloride, a narcotic, is a Schedule II controlled substance under the Federal Controlled Substances Act. Appropriate security measures should be taken to safeguard stocks of methadone against diversion.

DRUG DEPENDENCE — METHADONE CAN PRODUCE DRUG DEPENDENCE OF THE MORPHINE TYPE AND, THEREFORE, HAS THE POTENTIAL FOR BEING ABUSED. PSYCHIC DEPENDENCE, PHYSICAL DEPENDENCE, AND TOLERANCE MAY DEVELOP UPON REPEATED ADMINISTRATION OF METHADONE, AND IT SHOULD BE PRESCRIBED AND ADMINISTERED WITH THE SAME DEGREE OF CAUTION APPROPRIATE TO THE USE OF MORPHINE.

Interaction with Other Central-Nervous-System Depressants —Methadone should be used with caution and in reduced dosage in patients who are concurrently receiving other narcotic analgesics, general anesthetics, phenothiazines, other tranquilizers, sedative-hypnotics, tricyclic antidepressants, and other C.N.S. depressants (including alcohol). Respiratory depression, hypotension, and profound sedation or coma may result.

Anxiety —Since methadone, as used by tolerant subjects at a constant maintenance dosage, is not a tranquilizer, patients who are maintainedon this drug will react to life problems and stresses with the same symptoms of anxiety as do other individuals. The physician should not confuse such symptoms with those of narcotic abstinence and should not attempt to treat anxiety by increasing the dosage of methadone. The action of methadone in maintenance treatment is limited to the control of narcotic symptoms and is ineffective for relief of general anxiety.

Head Injury and Increased Intracranial Pressure —The respiratory depressant effects of methadone and its capacity to elevate cerebrospinal-fluid pressure may be markedly exaggerated in the presence of increased intracranial pressure. Furthermore, narcotics produce side effects that may obscure the clinical course of patients with head injuries. In such patients, methadone must be used with caution and only if it is deemed essential.

Asthma and Other Respiratory Conditions— Methadone should be used with caution in patients having an acute asthmatic attack, in those with chronic obstructive pulmonary disease or cor pulmonale, and in individuals with a substantially decreased respiratory reserve, preexisting respiratory depression, hypoxia, or hypercapnia. In such patients, even usual therapeutic doses of narcotics may decrease respiratory drive while simultaneously increasing airway resistance to the point of apnea.

Hypotensive Effect —The administration of methadone may result in severe hypotension in an individual whose ability to maintain his blood pressure has already been compromised by a depleted blood volume or concurrent administration of such drugs as the phenothiazines or certain anesthetics.

Use in Ambulatory Patients —Methadone may impair the mental and/or physical abilities required for the performance of potentially hazardous tasks, such as driving a car or operating machinery. The patient should be cautioned accordingly.

Methadone, like other narcotics, may produce orthostatic hypotension in ambulatory patients.

Use in Pregnancy —Safe use in pregnancy has not been established in relation to possible adverse effects on fetal development. Therefore, methadone should not be used in pregnant women unless, in the judgment of the physician, the potential benefits outweigh the possible hazards.

Methadone is not recommended for obstetric analgesia because its long duration of action increases the probability of respiratory depression in the newborn.

Use in Children —Methadone is not recommended for use as an analgesic in children, since documented clinical experience has been insufficient to establish a suitable dosage regimen for the pediatric age group.

PRECAUTIONS

Interaction with Pentazocine **—Patients who are addicted to heroin or who are on the methadone maintenance program may experience withdrawal symptoms when given pentazocine.**

Interaction with Rifampin —The concurrent administration of rifampin may possibly reduce the blood concentration of methadone. The mechanism by which rifampin may decrease blood concentrations of methadone is not fully understood, although enhanced microsomal drug-metabolized enzymes may influence drug disposition.

Acute Abdominal Conditions —The administration of methadone or other narcotics may obscure the diagnosis or clinical course in patients with acute abdominal conditions.

Interaction with Monoamine Oxidase (MAO) Inhibitors— Therapeutic doses of meperidine have precipitated severe reactions in patients concurrently receiving monoamine oxidase inhibitors or those who have received such agents within 14 days. Similar reactions thus far have not been reported with methadone; but if the use of methadone is necessary in such patients, a sensitivity test should be performed in which repeated small incremental doses are administered over the course of several hours while the patient's condition and vital signs are under careful observation.

Special-Risk Patients —Methadone should be given with caution and the initial dose should be reduced in certain patients, such as the elderly or debilitated and those with severe impairment of hepatic or renal function, hypothyroidism, Addison's disease, prostatic hypertrophy, or urethral stricture.

ADVERSE REACTIONS

THE MAJOR HAZARDS OF METHADONE, AS OF OTHER NARCOTIC ANALGESICS, ARE RESPIRATORY DEPRESSION AND, TO A LESSER DEGREE, CIRCULATORY DEPRESSION. RESPIRATORY ARREST, SHOCK, AND CARDIAC ARREST HAVE OCCURRED.

The most frequently observed adverse reactions include lightheadedness, dizziness, sedation, nausea, vomiting, and sweating. These effects seem to be more prominent in ambulatory patients and in those who are not suffering severe chronic pain. In such individuals, lower doses are advisable. Some adverse reactions may be alleviated in the ambulatory patient if he lies down.

Other adverse reactions include the following:

Central Nervous System —Euphoria, dysphoria, weakness, headache, insomnia, agitation, disorientation, and visual disturbances.

Gastrointestinal —Dry mouth, anorexia, constipation, and biliary tract spasm.

Cardiovascular —Flushing of the face, bradycardia, palpitation, faintness, and syncope.

Genitourinary —Urinary retention or hesitancy, antidiuretic effect, and reduced libido and/or potency.

Allergic —Pruritus, urticaria, other skin rashes, edema, and, rarely, hemorrhagic urticaria.

ADMINISTRATION AND DOSAGE

For relief of Severe Pain —Dosage should be adjusted according to the severity of the pain and the response of the patient.

Occasionally it may be necessary to exceed the usual dosage recommended in cases of exceptionally severe chronic pain or in those patients who have become tolerant to the analgesic effect of narcotics.

For severe acute pain, the usual adult dose is 2.5 mg to 10 mg every three to four hours as necessary.

For Detoxification Treatment—THE DRUG SHALL BE ADMINISTERED DAILY UNDER CLOSE SUPERVISION AS FOLLOWS:

A detoxification treatment course shall not exceed 21 days and may not be repeated earlier than four weeks after completion of the preceding course.

The oral form of administration is preferred. However, if the patient is unable to ingest oral medication, he may be started on the parenteral form initially.

In detoxification, the patient may receive methadone when there are significant symptoms of withdrawal. The dosage schedules indicated below are recommended but could be varied in accordance with clinical judgment. Initially, a single dose of 15 to 20 mg of methadone will often be sufficient to suppress withdrawal symptoms. Additional methadone may be provided if withdrawal symptoms are not suppressed or if symptoms reappear. When patients are physically dependent on high doses, it may be necessary to exceed these levels. Forty mg per day in single or divided doses will usually constitute an adequate stabilizing dosage level. Stabilization can be continued for two to three days, and then the amount of methadone normally will be gradually decreased. The rate at which methadone is decreased will be determined separately for each patient. The dose of methadone can be decreased on a daily basis or at two-day intervals, but the amount of intake shall always be sufficient to keep withdrawal symptoms at a tolerable level. In hospitalized patients, a daily reduction of 20 percent of the total dose may be tolerated and may cause little discomfort. In ambulatory patients, a somewhat slower schedule may be needed. If methadone is administered for more than three weeks, the procedure is considered to have progressed from detoxification or treatment of the acute withdrawal syndrome to maintenance treatment, even though the goal and intent may be eventual total withdrawal.

OVERDOSAGE

Symptoms—Serious overdosage of methadone is characterized by respiratory depression (a decrease in respiratory rate and/or tidal volume, Cheyne-Stokes respiration, cyanosis), extreme somnolence progressing to stupor or coma, maximally constricted pupils, skeletal-muscle flaccidity, cold and clammy skin, and sometimes, bradycardia and hypotension. In severe overdosage, particularly by the intravenous route, apnea, circulatory collapse, cardiac arrest, and death may occur.

Treatment—Primary attention should be given to the reestablishment of adequate respiratory exchange through provision of a patent airway and institution of assisted or controlled ventilation. If a nontolerant person, especially a child, takes a large dose of methadone, effective narcotic antagonists are available to counteract the potentially lethal respiratory depression. **The physician must remember, however, that methadone is a long-acting depressant (36 to 48 hours), whereas the antagonists act for much shorter periods (one to three hours).** The patient must, therefore, be monitored continuously for recurrence of respiratory depression and treated repeatedly with the narcotic antagonist as needed. If the diagnosis is correct and respiratory depression is due only to overdosage of methadone, the use of other respiratory stimulants is not indicated.

An antagonist should not be administered in the absence of clinically significant respiratory or cardiovascular depression. Intravenously administered narcotic antagonists (naloxone and nalorphine) are the drugs of choice to reverse signs of intoxication. These agents should be given repeatedly until the patient's status remains satisfactory. The hazard that the narcotic agent will further depress respiration is less likely with the use of naloxone.

Oxygen, intravenous fluids, vasopressors, and other supportive measures should be employed as indicated.

Note
IN AN INDIVIDUAL PHYSICALLY DEPENDENT ON NARCOTICS, THE ADMINISTRATION OF THE USUAL DOSE OF A NARCOTIC ANTAGONIST WILL PRECIPITATE AN ACUTE WITHDRAWAL SYNDROME. THE SEVERITY OF THIS SYNDROME WILL DEPEND ON THE DEGREE OF PHYSICAL DEPENDENCE AND THE DOSE OF THE ANTAGONIST ADMINISTERED. THE USE OF A NARCOTIC ANTAGONIST IN SUCH A PERSON SHOULD BE AVOIDED IF POSSIBLE. IF IT MUST BE USED TO TREAT SERIOUS RESPIRATORY DEPRESSION IN THE PHYSICALLY DEPENDENT PATIENT, THE ANTAGONIST SHOULD BE ADMINISTERED WITH EXTREME CARE AND BY TITRATION WITH SMALLER THAN USUAL DOSES OF THE ANTAGONIST.

HOW SUPPLIED
Methadone Hydrochloride Oral Solution USP
5 mg per 5 mL
NDC 0054-3555-63: Bottles of 500 mL
10 mg per 5 mL
NDC 0054-3556-63: Bottles of 500 mL
Methadone Hydrochloride Tablets USP
5 mg white, scored identified (54 210) tablets.
NDC 0054-4570-25: Bottle of 100 tablets.
NDC 0054-8553-24: Unit dose, 25 tablets per card (reverse numbered), 4 cards per shipper.
10 mg white, scored identified (54 142) tablets.
NDC 0054-4571-25: Bottle of 100 tablets.
NDC 0054-8554-24: Unit dose, 25 tablets per card (reverse numbered), 4 cards per shipper.

Caution: Federal law prohibits dispensing without prescription.
4056400
099   Revised September 1989

MORPHINE SULFATE IMMEDIATE RELEASE Ⓒ ℞ ORAL SOLUTION
(WARNING: May be habit forming.)
MORPHINE SULFATE IMMEDIATE RELEASE Ⓒ ℞ TABLETS
(WARNING: May be habit forming.)

DESCRIPTION
Each 5 mL of Morphine Sulfate Oral Solution contains:
Morphine Sulfate .... 10 or 20 mg
(WARNING: May be habit forming.)
Each tablet for oral administration contains:
Morphine Sulfate .... 15 or 30 mg
(WARNING: May be habit forming.)

HOW SUPPLIED
Morphine Sulfate Oral Solution
(Unflavored).
10 mg per 5 mL.
NDC 0054-8585-16: Unit dose Patient Cup™ filled to deliver 5 mL (10 mg Morphine Sulfate), ten 5 mL Patient Cups™ per shelf pack, four shelf packs per shipper.
NDC 0054-8586-16: Unit dose Patient Cup™ filled to deliver 10 mL (20 mg Morphine Sulfate), ten 10 mL Patient Cups™ per shelf pack, four shelf packs per shipper.
NDC 0054-3785-49: 100 mL "Unit of use" calibrated bottle.
NDC 0054-3785-63: Bottles of 500 mL.
20 mg per 5 mL.
NDC 0054-3786-49: 100 mL "Unit of Use" calibrated bottle.
NDC 0054-3786-63: Bottles of 500 mL.
Tablets
15 mg white scored, identified (54/733) tablets.
NDC 0054-8582-24: Unit dose, 25 tablets per card (reverse numbered), 4 cards per shipper.
NDC 0054-4582-25: Bottles of 100 tablets.
30 mg white scored, identified (54/262) tablets.
NDC 0054-8583-24: Unit dose, 25 tablets per card (reverse numbered), 4 cards per shipper.
NDC 0054-4583-25: Bottles of 100 Tablets.
DEA Order Form Required

ORAMORPH SR™ Ⓒ ℞
(MORPHINE SULFATE)
SUSTAINED RELEASE TABLETS
30 mg, 60 mg, 100 mg
(WARNING: May be habit forming.)

NOTE
THIS IS A SUSTAINED RELEASE DOSAGE FORM. PATIENT SHOULD BE INSTRUCTED TO SWALLOW THE TABLET AS A WHOLE; THE TABLE SHOULD NOT BE BROKEN IN HALF, NOR SHOULD IT BE CRUSHED OR CHEWED.
THE SUSTAINED RELEASE OF MORPHINE FROM ORAMORPH SR SHOULD BE TAKEN INTO CONSIDERATION IN EVENT OF ADVERSE REACTIONS OR OVERDOSAGE.

DESCRIPTION
Each tablet for oral administration contains:
Morphine sulfate ....30 mg, 60 mg, or 100 mg
(**WARNING:** May be habit forming)
in a tablet that provides for sustained release of the medication.

Morphine sulfate occurs as white, feathery, silky crystals, cubical masses of crystals, or white crystalline powder; it is soluble in water and slightly soluble in alcohol. Morphine has a pKa of 7.9, with an octanol/water partition coefficient of 1.42 at pH 7.4. At this pH, the tertiary amino group is mostly ionized, making the molecule water-soluble. Morphine is significantly more water-soluble than any other opioid in clinical use.

Chemically, morphine sulfate is 7,8-didehydro-4,5α-epoxy-17-methyl-morphinian-3,6α-diol sulfate (2:1)(salt) pentahydrate, and has the following structural formula:

Each ORAMORPH SR Tablet contains 30 mg, 60 mg, or 100 mg Morphine Sulfate USP. Inactive ingredients: Lactose, Hydroxypropyl Methylcellulose, Colloidal Silicon Dioxide, and Stearic Acid.

CLINICAL PHARMACOLOGY
Morphine is the prototype of many narcotic drugs that interact predeominantly with the opioid μ-receptor. These μ-binding sites are discretely distributed in the human brain, with high densities in the posterior amygdala, hypothalamus, thalamus, nucleus caudatus, putamen, and certain cortical areas. They are also found on the terminal axons of primary afferents with laminae I and II (substantia gelatinosa) of the spinal cord and in the spinal nucleus of the trigeminal nerve.

In clinical settings, morphine exerts its principal pharmacological effect on the central nervous system and gastrointestinal tract. Its primary actions of therapeutic value are analgesia and sedation. Morphine appears to increase the patient's tolerance for pain and to decrease discomfort, although the presence of the pain itself may still be recognized. In addition to analgesia, alterations in mood, euphoria and dysphoria, and drowsiness commonly occur.

Morphine depresses various respiratory centers, depresses the cough reflex, and constricts the pupils. Analgesically effective blood levels of morphine may cause nausea and vomiting directly by stimulating the chemoreceptor trigger zone, but nausea and vomiting are significantly more common in ambulatory than in recumbent patients, as is postural syncope.

Morphine increases the tone and decreases the propulsive contractions of the smooth muscle of the gastrointestinal tract. The resultant prolongation in gastrointestinal transit time is responsible for the constipating effect of morphine. Because morphine may increase biliary-tract pressure, some patients with biliary colic may experience worsening rather than relief of pain.

While morphine generally increases the tone of urinary-tract smooth muscle, the net effect tends to be variable, in some cases producing urinary urgency, in others, difficulty in urination.

In therapeutic doses, morphine does not usually exert major effects on the cardiovascular system. Some patients, however, exhibit a propensity to develop orthostatic hypotension and fainting. Rapid intravenous injection is more likely to precipitate a fall in blood pressure than oral dosing.

Morphine can cause histamine release, which appears to be responsible for dilation of cutaneous blood vessels, with resulting flushing of the face and neck, pruritus, and sweating.

PHARMACOKINETICS
ORAMORPH SR Tablets are a sustained release oral dosage form of morphine sulfate. Only about 40% of the administered dose reaches the central compartment because of first-pass effect (i.e., metabolism in the gut wall and liver). Once absorbed, morphine is distributed to skeletal muscle, kidneys, liver, intestinal tract, lungs, spleen and brain. Morphine also crosses the placental membrane and has been found in breast milk.

For all practical purposes, virtually all morphine is converted to glucuronide metabolites; only a small fraction (less than 5%) of absorbed morphine is demethylated. Among these glucuronide metabolites, morphine-3-glucuronide is present in the highest plasma concentration following oral administration; a smaller fraction is converted to morphine-6-glucuronide, which has the greater analgesic activity of these two metabolites.

Continued on next page

Roxane Laboratories—Cont.

The glucuronide system has a high capacity and is not easily saturated, even in disease. Therefore, the rate of delivery of morphine to the gut and liver does not influence the total and/or the relative quantities of the various metabolites formed.

The pharmacokinetic parameters following oral administration of ORAMORPH SR, presented in the table below, show considerable inter-subject variation, but are representative of average values reported in the literature. The volume of distribution (Vd) for morphine is 4 liters per kilogram (L/kg), and the terminal elimination half-life is approximately 2 to 4 hours.

[See table below.]

Following the administration of conventional, immediate-release, oral morphine products, approximately 50% of the morphine that will ever reach the central compartment, reaches it within 30 minutes. Following the administration of an equal amount of ORAMORPH SR to normal volunteers, however, 50% of absorption occurs, on average, after 1.5 hours.

The possible effect of food upon the systemic bioavailability of ORAMORPH SR has not been evaluated.

Although variation in the physico-mechanical properties of a formulation of an oral morphine drug product can affect both its absolute bioavailability and its absorption rate constant (k_a), morphine distribution and clearance are unchanged, as they are fundamental properties of morphine in the organism. However, in chronic use, the possibility of shifts in metabolite-to-parent drug ratios cannot be excluded.

When immediate-release oral morphine or ORAMORPH SR is given on a fixed dosing regimen, steady-state is achieved in about one day.

For a given dose and dosing interval, the Area-Under-the-Curve (AUC) and average blood concentration of morphine at steady-state (C_{SS}) will be independent of the type of oral formulation administered, as long as the formulations have the same absolute bioavailability. The absorption rate of a formulation will, however, affect the maximum (C_{max}) and minimum (C_{min}) plasma concentrations and the time between administration and their occurrence. For any fixed dose and dosing interval, ORAMORPH SR will have, at steady-state, a lower C_{max} and a higher C_{min} than conventional immediate-release morphine, which might be a therapeutic advantage in chronic pain control (see also PHARMACODYNAMICS).

The clearance of morphine occurs primarily as renal excretion of morphine-3-glucuronide. A small amount of the glucuronide conjugate is excreted in the bile, and there is some minor enterohepatic recycling; about 10% of the glucuronide conjugate is excreted in the feces. Because morphine is essentially metabolized in the liver, the effects of renal disease on morphine's clearance are not likely to be pronounced. As with any drug, however, caution should be taken to guard against unanticipated accumulation if renal and/or hepatic function is seriously impaired.

PHARMACODYNAMICS

In clinical settings, morphine's primary actions of therapeutic value are analgesia and sedation. Opiate analgesia involves at least three anatomical areas of the central nervous system: the periaqueductal -periventricular gray matter, the ventromedial medulla, and the spinal cord. Morphine appears to increase the patient's tolerance for pain, and to decrease the discomfort, although the presence of pain itself may still be recognized.

While there is considerable variability in the relationship between morphine blood concentration and analgesic response, effective analgesia probably will not occur below some minimum blood level in a given patient. The minimum effective blood level for analgesia will vary among patients, especially among patients who have been previously treated with potent μ-agonist opioids. Similarly, there is a considerable variability in the relationship between morphine plasma concentration and untoward clinical responses, but higher concentrations are more likely to be toxic.

In contrast to immediate-release morphine, after dosing with ORAMORPH SR, the morphine blood levels show reduced fluctuation between peak and trough plasma levels; that means that they are more centered within the theoretical 'therapeutic window'. On the other hand, the reduced fluctuation in morphine plasma concentration might conceivably affect other phenomena, as for example, the rate of tolerance induction.

ORAMORPH SR is an analgesic intended for patients who require chronic morphine analgesia and who will have, in consequence, markedly different degrees of pharmacodynamic tolerance for opioid drugs. Morphine and similar opioids induce tolerance to their effects, so that a shortening of the duration of satisfactory analgesia may be the first sign of an increase in tolerance.

Once patients are started on morphine, the dose required for satisfactory analgesia will rise, with the rate of development of tolerance varying, depending on the patient's prior narcotic use, level of pain, degree of anxiety, use of other CNS-active drugs, circulatory status, total daily dose, and the dosing interval.

INDICATIONS AND USAGE

ORAMORPH SR is indicated for the relief of pain in patients who require opioid analgesics for more than a few days.

CONTRAINDICATIONS

ORAMORPH SR is contraindicated in patients with respiratory depression in the absence of resuscitative equipment, in patients with acute or severe bronchial asthma and in patients with known hypersensitivity to morphine.

ORAMORPH SR is contraindicated in any patient who has or is suspected of having a paralytic ileus.

WARNINGS

IMPAIRED RESPIRATION:

Respiratory depression is the chief hazard of all morphine preparations. Respiratory depression occurs more frequently in the elderly and debilitated patients, as well as in those suffering from conditions accompanied by hypoxia or hypercapnia when even moderate therapeutic doses may dangerously decrease pulmonary ventiliation.

Morphine should be used with extreme caution in patients who have a decreased respiratory reserve (e.g., emphysema, severe obesity, kyphoscoliosis, or paralysis of the phrenic nerve). ORAMORPH SR should not be given in cases of chronic asthma, upper airway obstruction, or in any other chronic pulmonary disorder without due consideration of the known risk of acute respiratory failure following morphine administration in such patients.

DRUG ABUSE AND DEPENDENCE CONTROLLED SUBSTANCE:

Morphine sulfate is a Schedule II narcotic under the United States Controlled Substance Act (21 U.S.C. 801–886).

Morphine is the most commonly cited prototype for narcotic substances that possess an addiction-forming or addiction-sustaining liability. A patient may be at risk for developing a dependence to morphine if used improperly or for overly long periods of time. As with all potent opioids which are μ-agonists, tolerance as well as psychological and physical dependence to morphine may develop irrespective of the route of administration (oral, intravenous, intramuscular, intrathecal, epidural). Individuals with a prior history of opioid or other substance abuse or dependence, being more apt to respond to eurphorogenic and reinforcing properties of morphine, would be considered to be at greater risk.

Care must be taken to avert withdrawal symptoms when morphine is discontinued abruptly or upon administration of a narcotic antagonist.

PRECAUTIONS

General Precautions:

Selection of patients for treatment with ORAMORPH SR should be governed by the same principles that apply to the use of morphine or other potent opioid analgesics. Narcotic analgesics are drugs that have a narrow therapeutic index in the old, the sick, and the infirm, i.e., the very population in which their use is indicated. Physicians should individualize treatment with ORAMORPH SR in every case, weighing the need for analgesia against the risk of serious or fatal reactions to the drug.

Use in Patients with Increased Intracranial Pressure or with Head Injury:

ORAMORPH SR should be used with extreme caution in patients with increased intracranial pressure or with head injury. The respiratory depressant effects of morphine (increased pCO_2) may result in elevation of cerebrospinal fluid pressure and may thus be markedly exaggerated in the presence of head injury, other intracranial lesions, or a pre-existing increased intracranial pressure. Morphine produces effects which may obscure neurologic signs of further increases in pressure in patients with head injuries. Pupillary changes (miosis), associated with morphine, may conceal the existence, extent, and course of intracranial pathology.

Use in Hepatic or Renal Disease:

The clearance of morphine may be reduced in patients with hepatic dysfunction, while the clearance of its metabolites may be decreased in renal dysfunction. This will be manifested by both, a prolonged elimination half-life and the accumulation of levels of either morphine or its metabolites in excess of those produced in normals, with the potential for an increase of adverse effects (see WARNINGS and ADVERSE REACTIONS). These changes in morphine pharmacodynamics, in patients with hepatic or renal dysfunctions, should be considered when adjusting the dose and dosage intervals, taking also into account the slow-release character of ORAMORPH SR.

Drug Interactions:

Use with Other Central Nervous System Depressants:

The depressant effects of morphine are potentiated by the presence of other CNS depressants such as alcohol, sedatives, antihistaminics, or psychotropic drugs. Use of neuroleptics in conjunction with oral morphine may increase the risk of respiratory depression, hypotension and profound sedation or coma.

Interaction with Mixed Agonist/Antagonist Opioid Analgesics:

Agonist/antagonist analgesics (i.e., pentazocine, nalbuphine, butorphanol, or buprenorphine) should NOT be administered to patients who have received or are receiving a course of therapy with a pure opioid agonist analgesic. In these patients, the mixed agonist/antagonist may alter the analgesic effect or may precipitate withdrawal symptoms.

Carcinogenesis, Mutagenesis, Impairment of Fertility:

Studies of morphine sulfate in animals to evaluate the drug's carcinogenic and mutagenic potential or the effect on fertility have not been conducted.

Pregnancy:

Teratogenic Effects—Category C: There are no well-controlled studies in women, but marketing experience does not include any evidence of adverse effects on the fetus following routine (short-term) clinical use of morphine sulfate products. Although there is no clearly defined risk, such experience cannot exclude the possibility of infrequent or subtle damage to the human fetus.

ORAMORPH SR should be used in pregnant women only when clearly needed. (See also: PRECAUTIONS: Labor and Delivery, and DRUG ABUSE AND DEPENDENCE CONTROLLED SUBSTANCE.)

Nonteratogenic Effects:

Infants born from mothers who have been taking morphine chronically may exhibit withdrawal symptoms.

Labor and Delivery:

ORAMORPH SR is not recommended for use in women during and immediately prior to labor. Occasionally, opioid analgesics may prolong labor through actions which temporarily reduce the strength, duration and frequency of uterine contractions.

Neonates, whose mothers received opioid analgesics during labor, should be observed closely for signs of respiratory depression. A specific narcotic antagonist, naloxone, should be available for reversal of narcotic-induced respiratory depression in the neonate.

Nursing Mothers:

ORAMORPH SR should not be given to nursing mothers because morphine is excreted in maternal milk. Effects on

TABLE OF APPROXIMATE[1] AVERAGE PHARMACOKINETIC PARAMETERS FOLLOWING ORAL DOSING OF ORAMORPH SR ™

Pharmacokinetic Parameter (scientific notation) (unit)		Dose of ORAMORPH SR 30 mg	60 mg	100 mg
Bioavailability (oral compared to injectable)		approximately 40%		
Time-to-peak plasma concentration {T_{max}}(h)	mean (range)	3.8 (1–7)	3.8 (2–7)	3.6 (1.5–12)
Peak plasma concentration {C_{max}} (ng/mL) [single dose]	mean (range)	9.9 (5.0–18.6)	16.1 (10.0–25.3)	27.4 14.1–46.1)
Volume of distribution (calculated from mean clearance and terminal half-life) {Vd(β)} (L/kg)	mean		4 L/kg	

Dose metabolized = approximately 90%

Morphine metabolites (%) = morphine-3-glucuronide (55–75%), morphine-6-glucuronide (1–5%)

[1]Derived from pharmacokinetic studies in 24 normal volunteers

the nursing infant are not known, but withdrawal symptoms can occur in breast-fed infants when maternal administration of morphine sulfate is stopped.

Pediatric Use:
ORAMORPH SR has not been evaluated in children. Its use in the pediatric population is, therefore, not recommended.

Use in the Aged:
The pharmacodynamic effects of morphine in the aged are more variable than in the younger population. Patients will vary widely in the effective initial dose, rate of development of tolerance, and the frequency and magnitude of associated adverse effects as the dose is increased. Individualization of doses must receive careful attention in elderly patients.

Information for Patients:
If clinically advisable, patients receiving ORAMORPH SR brand or morphine sulfate sustained release tablets, should be given the following instructions by the physician:

1. Morphine may produce psychological and/or physical dependence. For this reason, the dose of the drug should not be increased without consulting a physician.
2. Morphine may impair mental and/or physical ability required for the performance of potentially hazardous tasks (e.g., driving, operating machinery).
3. Morphine should not be taken with alcohol or other CNS depressants (sleep aids, tranquilizers) because additive effects, including CNS depression, may occur. A physician should be consulted if other prescription and/or over-the-counter medications are currently being used or are prescribed for future use.
4. For women of childbearing potential, who become or are planning to become pregnant, a physician should be consulted regarding analgesics and other drug use.

ADVERSE REACTIONS

> NOTE: THE SUSTAINED RELEASE OF MORPHINE FROM ORAMORPH SR SHOULD BE TAKEN INTO CONSIDERATION IN THE EVENT OF OCCURRING ADVERSE REACTIONS.

Adverse reactions caused by morphine are essentially those observed with other opioid analgesics. They include the following *major hazards:* **respiratory depression,** and less frequently, **circulatory depression, apnea, shock** and **cardiac arrest** secondary to respiratory and/or circulatory depression.

Most Frequently Observed Reactions:
Constipation, nausea, vomiting, lightheadedness, dizziness, sedation, dysphoria, euphoria, and sweating. Some of these effects seem to be more prominent in ambulatory patients and in those not experiencing severe pain. Some adverse reactions in ambulatory patients may be alleviated if the patient is in a supine position.

Less Frequently Observed Reactions:
Body as a Whole: Edema, antidiuretic effect, chills, muscle tremor, muscle rigidity.
Cardiovascular: Flushing of the face, tachycardia, bradycardia, palpitation, faintness, syncope, hypotension, hypertension.
Gastrointestinal: Dry mouth, biliary tract spasm, laryngospasm, anorexia, diarrhea, cramps, taste alterations.
Genitourinary: Urine retention or hesitance, reduced libido and/or potency.
Nervous System: Weakness, headache, agitation, tremor, uncoordinated muscle movements, seizure, paresthesia, alterations of mood (nervousness, apprehension, depression, floating feelings), dreams, transient hallucination and disorientation, visual disturbances, insomnia, increased intracranial pressure.
Skin: Pruritus, urticaria and other skin rashes.
Special Senses: Blurred vision, nystagmus, diplopia, miosis.

DRUG ABUSE AND DEPENDENCE

Opioid analgesics may cause psychological and physical dependence (see WARNINGS). Physical dependence results in withdrawal symptoms in patients who abruptly discontinue the drug, or these symptoms may be precipitated through the administration of drugs with antagonistic activity, e.g., naloxone or mixed agonist/antagonist analgesics (pentazocine, etc.; see also OVERDOSAGE). Physical dependence usually does not occur, to a clinically significant degree, until several weeks of continued opioid usage. Tolerance, in which increasingly larger doses are required to produce the same degree of analgesia, is initially manifested by a shortened duration of a analgesic effect and, subsequently, by decreases in the intensity of analgesia. In patients with chronic pain, as well as in opioid-tolerant cancer patients, the administration of ORAMORPH SR (morphine sulfate) should be guided by the degree of tolerance manifested. Physical dependence, *per se*, is not ordinarily a concern when one is dealing with opioid-tolerant patients whose pain and suffering is associated with an irreversible illness.

If ORAMORPH SR is abruptly discontinued, an abstinence syndrome may occur. Withdrawal symptoms, in patients dependent on morphine, begin shortly before the time of the next scheduled dose, reaching a peak at 36 to 72 hours after the last dose, and then slowly subside over a period of 7 to 10 days. Symptoms include yawning, sweating, lacrimation, rhinorrhea, restless sleep, dilated pupils, gooseflesh, irritability, tremor, nausea, vomiting, and diarrhea.

Treatment of the abstinence syndrome is primarily symptomatic and supportive, including maintenance of proper fluid and electrolyte balance. If withdrawal has inadvertently been precipitated in a patient who requires narcotics for pain management, the withdrawal syndrome can be terminated rapidly by the administration of an appropriate dose of a pure agonist opioid, such as morphine. The degree of physical dependence of a patient on ORAMORPH SR can be intentionally reduced by a gradual reduction of dosage and symptomatic treatment of withdrawal symptomatology.

OVERDOSAGE

> NOTE: THE SUSTAINED RELEASE OF MORPHINE FROM ORAMORPH SR SHOULD BE TAKEN INTO CONSIDERATION IN THE EVENT OF AN OVERDOSAGE.

Overdosage of morphine is characterized by respiratory depression, with or without concomitant CNS depression. Since respiratory arrest may result either through direct depression of the respiratory center, or as the result of hypoxia, primary attention should be given to the establishment of adequate respiratory exchange through provision of a patent airway and institution of assisted, or controlled, ventilation. The narcotic antagonist, naloxone, is a specific antidote. An initial dose of 0.4 to 2 mg of naloxone should be administered intravenously, simultaneously with respiratory resuscitation. If the desired degree of counteraction and improvement in respiratory function is not obtained, naloxone may be repeated at 2 to 3 minute intervals. If no response is observed after 10 mg of naloxone has been administered, the diagnosis of narcotic-induced, or partial narcotic-induced, toxicity should be questioned. Intramuscular or subcutaneous administration may be used if the intravenous route is not available.

As the duration of effect of naloxone is considerably shorter than that of ORAMORPH SR, repeated administration may be necessary. Patients should be closely observed for evidence of renarcotization.

> NOTE: In a individual physically dependent on opioids, administration of the usual dose of the antagonist will precipitate an acute withdrawal syndrome. The severity of the withdrawal syndrome produced will depend on the degree of physical dependence and the dose of the antagonist administered. Use of a narcotic antagonist in such a person should be avoided. If necessary to treat serious respiratory depression in a physically dependent patient, the antagonist should be administered with extreme care and by titration with smaller than usual dose of the antagonist.

When indicated, gut decontamination should be performed via emesis and/or activated charcoal (60 to 100 g in adults, 1 to 2 g/kg in children) with cathartic. Since ORAMORPH SR is a sustained release product, absorption may be expected to continue for many hours, particularly following an overdose, combined with decreased peristaltic activity of the gastrointestinal tract.

Supportive measures (including oxygen, vasopressors) should be employed in the management of circulatory shock and pulmonary edema accompanying overdose as indicated. Cardiac arrest or arrhythmias may require cardiac massage or defibrillation.

DOSAGE AND ADMINISTRATION

(See also: CLINICAL PHARMACOLOGY, WARNINGS and PRECAUTIONS sections.)

ORAMORPH SR is intended for use in patients who require more than several days of continuous treatment with a potent opioid analgesic. The sustained release nature of the formulation allows it to be administered on a more convenient schedule than conventional immediate-release oral morphine products (see CLINICAL PHARMACOLOGY—PHARMACOKINETICS). However, ORAMORPH SR does not release morphine continuously over the course of a dosing interval. The administration of single doses of ORAMORPH SR on a q12h dosing schedule will result in peak and trough plasma levels similar to those following an identical daily dose of morphine administered using conventional oral formulations on a q4h regimen. If pain is not controlled for a full 12 hours, then the dosing interval should be shortened, but to no less than 8 hours.

As with any potent opioid, it is critical to adjust the dosing regimen for each patient individually, taking into account the patient's prior analgesic treatment experience. Although it is not possible to enumerate every condition that is important to the selection of the initial dose and dosing interval of ORAMORPH SR, attention should be given to (1) the daily dose, potency and characteristics of a pure agonist, or mixed agonist-antagonist, the patient has been taking previously, (2) the reliability of the relative potentcy estimate to calculate the dose of morphine needed [N.B.: potency estimates may vary with the route of administration], (3) the fact that roughly only 40% of the morphine sulfate in ORAMORPH SR becomes available after pre-systemic metabolization in the intestinal wall and liver, (4) the degree of opioid tolerance, and (5) the general condition and medical status of the patient.

The following dosing recommendation for ORAMORPH SR therefore, can only be considered suggested approaches to the series of clinical decisions in the management of pain of an individual patient.

Conversion from Conventional Immediate-Release Oral Morphine to ORAMORPH SR:
A patient's daily morphine requirement is established by using the Daily Oral Morphine Requirement of the immediate-release formulation which gives the Daily Oral Morphine Requirement for ORAMORPH SR. Since ORAMORPH SR is given on an 'every 12 hour' schedule, the single dose of ORAMORPH SR is half of the Daily Oral Morphine Requirement. Dose and dosing interval is adjusted as needed (see discussion below). For initial conversion, the 30 mg tablet strength is recommended for patients with a daily morphine requirement of 120 mg or less.

Conversion from Parental Morphine or Other Opioid Analgesics (parental or oral) to ORAMORPH SR:
Because of uncertainty about relative estimates of opioid potency and cross tolerance, as well as intersubject variation, initial dosing regimens should be conservative, i.e., an underestimation of the 24-hour oral morphine requirement is preferred to an overestimate. To this end, initial individual doses of ORAMORPH SR should be estimated conservatively. In patients whose daily morphine requirements are expected to be less than or equal to 120 mg per day, the 30 mg tablet strength is recommended for the initial titration period. Once a stable dose regimen is reached, the patient can be converted to the 60 mg or 100 mg tablet strength, as appropriate.

Estimates of the relative potency of opioids are only approximate, and are influenced by route of administration, individual patient differences, and possibly, by the patient's medical condition. Consequently, it is difficult to recommend any precise rule for converting a patient to ORAMORPH SR directly. However, the following general points should be considered:

1. *Parenteral to oral morphine ratio:* Estimates of the oral-to-parenteral potency of morphine vary. Some authorities suggest that a dose of morphine only 3 times the daily parenteral morphine requirement may be sufficient in chronic use settings. (3 times the Daily Parenteral Morphine Requirement = the Daily Oral Morphine Requirement)
2. *Oral parenteral or oral opioids to oral morphine:* Because of a lack of reliable relative potency assays, specific recommendations are not possible. In general, it is safer to underestimate the Total Daily Dose of ORAMORPH SR required and rely upon *ad hoc* supplementation to deal with inadequate analgesia (see discussion which follows).

Use of ORAMORPH SR as the First Opioid Analgesic:
There has been no systematic evaluation of ORAMORPH SR as an initial opioid analgesic in the management of pain. Because it may be more difficult to titrate a patient using a sustained release morphine, it is ordinarily advisable to begin treatment using an immediate release formulation, such as Roxanol Solution.

Considerations in the Adjustment of Dosing Regimens.
Whatever the approach, if signs of excessive opioid effects are observed early in a dosing interval, the next dose should be reduced. If this adjustment leads to inadequate analgesia, i.e., 'breakthrough' pain occurs late in the dosing interval, the dosing interval may be shortened. Alternatively, a supplemental dose of a short-acting analgesic may be given.

As experience is gained, adjustments can be made to obtain an appropriate balance between pain relief, opioid side effects and the convenience of the dosing schedule.

In adjusting dose requirements, it is recommended that the dosing interval never be extended beyond 12 hours, because the administration of very large single doses of ORAMORPH SR may lead to acute overdosage.

For patients with low daily morphine requirements, precise titration may be difficult, because the smallest available dosage form of ORAMORPH SR contains 30 mg of morphine. In this regard, adjustment in dose should NOT be attempted by breaking or crushing the tablets. ORAMORPH SR tablets are intended to be swallowed whole.

Conversion from ORAMORPH SR to Parenteral Opioids:
When converting a patient from ORAMORPH SR to parenteral opioids, it is best to assume that the parenteral to oral potency relationship is high. NOTE THAT THIS IS THE CONVERSE OF THE STRATEGY USED WHEN THE DIRECTION OF CONVERSION IS FROM THE PARENTERAL TO ORAL FORMULATIONS. IN BOTH CASES,

Continued on next page

Roxane Laboratories—Cont.

HOWEVER, THE AIM IS TO ESTIMATE THE NEW DOSE CONSERVATIVELY. For example, to estimate the required 24-hour dose of morphine for IM use, one could employ a conversion of 1 mg of morphine IM for every 6 mg of morphine as ORAMORPH SR. Of course, the IM 24-hour dose would have to be divided by six and administered on a q4h regimen. This approach is recommended because it is least likely to cause overdosage.

NOTE: ORAMORPH SR TABLET MUST BE SWALLOWED WHOLE. DO NOT BREAK THE TABLET IN HALF. DO NOT CRUSH OR CHEW.

HOW SUPPLIED

ORAMORPH SR™ (Morphine Sulfate)
Sustained Release Tablets
30 mg white tablets (Identified 54 090)
[Embossed with 30]
NDC 0054-8805-24: Unit dose, 25 tablets per card (reverse numbered), 4 cards per shipper.
NDC 0054-4805-19: Bottles of 50 tablets.
NDC 0054-4805-25: Bottles of 100 tablets.
NDC 0054-4805-27: Bottles of 250 tablets.
60 mg white tablets (Identified 54 933)
[Embossed with 60]
NDC 0054-8792-11: Unit dose, 25 tablets per card (reverse numbered), 1 card per shipper.
NDC 0054-4792-25: Bottles of 100 tablets.
100 mg white tablets (Identified 54 862)
[Embossed with 100]
NDC 0054-8793-11: Unit dose, 25 tablets per card (reverse numbered), 1 card per shipper.
NDC 0054-4793-25: Bottles of 100 tablets.
      DEA Order Form Required.
Dispense in a tight, light-resistant container.
Storage: ORAMORPH SR Tablets should be stored in unopened containers at or below room temperature.
Caution: Federal law prohibits dispensing without prescription. Federal law prohibits the transfer of this drug to any person other than the patient for whom it was prescribed.
Safety and Handling Instructions:
ORAMORPH SR is supplied as tablets that pose little risk of direct exposure to health care personnel and should be handled and disposed of in accordance with hospital policy. Patients and their families should be instructed to dispose of ORAMORPH SR tablets, that are no longer needed, down the toilet.
4073301   Issued October 1991
Roxane
Laboratories, Inc.
Columbus, Ohio 43216
   Shown in Product Identification Section, page 427

PREDNISONE TABLETS USP   ℞
1 mg, 2.5 mg, 5 mg, 10 mg, 20 mg, or 50 mg

HOW SUPPLIED

1 mg white, scored tablets, gluten-free (Identified 54 092).
NDC 0054-8739-25: Unit dose, 10 tablets per strip, 10 strips per shelf pack, 10 shelf packs per shipper.
NDC 0054-4741-25: Bottles of 100 tablets.
2.5 mg white, scored tablets, gluten-free (Identified 54 339).
NDC 0054-8740-25: Unit dose, 10 tablets per strip, 10 strips per shelf pack, 10 shelf packs per shipper.
NDC 0054-4742-25: Bottles of 100 tablets.
5 mg white, scored tablets, gluten-free (Identified 54 612).
NDC 0054-8724-25: Unit dose, 10 tablets per strip, 10 strips per shelf pack, 10 shelf packs per shipper.
NDC 0054-4728-25: Bottles of 100 tablets.
NDC 0054-4728-31: Bottles of 1000 tablets.
10 mg white, scored tablets, gluten-free (Identified 54 899).
NDC 0054-8725-25: Unit dose, 10 tablets per strip, 10 strips per shelf pack, 10 shelf packs per shipper.
NDC 0054-4730-25: Bottles of 100 tablets.
NDC 0054-4730-29: Bottles of 500 tablets.
20 mg white, scored tablets, gluten-free (Identified 54 760).
NDC 0054-8726-25: Unit dose, 10 tablets per strip, 10 strips per shelf pack, 10 shelf packs per shipper.
NDC 0054-4729-25: Bottles of 100 tablets.
NDC 0054-4729-29: Bottles of 500 tablets.
50 mg white, scored tablets, gluten-free (Identified 54 343).
NDC 0054-8729-25: Unit dose, 10 tablets per strip, 10 strips per shelf pack, 10 shelf packs per shipper.
NDC 0054-4733-25: Bottles of 100 tablets.

ROXANOL™   ⒸⅡ ℞
[rox'-ĕ-nŭl]
Morphine Sulfate Immediate Release, Concentrated Oral Solution
20 mg per mL
      (WARNING: May be habit forming.)

ROXANOL 100™
Morphine Sulfate Immediate Release, Concentrated Oral Solution
100 mg per 5 mL
      (WARNING: May be habit forming.)

ROXANOL™UD
Morphine Sulfate Immediate Release, Concentrated Oral Solution
30 mg/1.5 mL
      (WARNING: May be habit forming.)

ROXANOL™UD
Morphine Sulfate (Immediate Release) Oral Solution
10 mg/2.5 mL, 20 mg/5 mL
      (WARNING: May be habit forming.)

RESCUDOSE™
Morphine Sulfate Immediate Release Oral Solution
10 mg per 2.5 mL
      (WARNING: May be habit forming.)

DESCRIPTION
Each mL of Roxanol™ contains:
Morphine Sulfate .... 20 mg
      (Warning: May be habit forming.)
Each 5 mL of Roxanol 100™ contains:
Morphine Sulfate .... 100 mg
      (Warning: May be habit forming.)
Each 2.5 mL of Rescudose™ contains:
Morphine Sulfate .... 10 mg
      (Warning: May be habit forming.)
Chemically, Morphine Sulfate is, Morphinan-3,6-diol, 7,8-didehydro-4,5-epoxy-17-methyl-, (5α,6α)-, sulfate (2:1) (salt), pentahydrate.
Morphine Sulfate acts as a narcotic analgesic.

CLINICAL PHARMACOLOGY
The major effects of morphine are on the central nervous system and the bowel. Opioids act as agonists, interacting with stereospecific and saturable binding sites or receptors in the brain and other tissues.
Morphine is about two-thirds absorbed from the gastrointestinal tract with the maximum analgesic effect occurring 60 minutes post administration.

INDICATIONS AND USAGE
Morphine is indicated for the relief of severe acute and severe chronic pain.

CONTRAINDICATIONS
Hypersensitivity to morphine; respiratory insufficiency or depression; severe CNS depression; attack of bronchial asthma; heart failure secondary to chronic lung disease; cardiac arrhythmias; increased intracranial or cerebrospinal pressure; head injuries; brain tumor; acute alcoholism; delirium tremens; convulsive disorders; after biliary tract surgery; suspected surgical abdomen; surgical anastomosis; concomitantly with MAO inhibitors or within 14 days of such treatment.

WARNINGS
Morphine can cause tolerance, psychological and physical dependence. Withdrawal will occur on abrupt discontinuation or administration of a narcotic antagonist.
Interaction with Other Central-Nervous-System Depressants—Morphine should be used with caution and in reduced dosage in patients who are concurrently receiving other narcotic analgesics, general anesthetics, phenothiazines, other tranquilizers, sedative-hypnotics, tricyclic antidepressants, and other CNS depressants (including alcohol). Respiratory depression, hypotension, and profound sedation or coma may result.

PRECAUTIONS
General:
Head Injury and Increased Intracranial Pressure —The respiratory depressant effects of morphine and its capacity to elevate cerebrospinal-fluid pressure may be markedly exaggerated in the presence of increased intracranial pressure. Furthermore, narcotics produce side effects that may obscure the clinical course of patients with head injuries. In such patients, morphine must be used with caution and only if it is deemed essential.
Asthma and Other Respiratory Conditions —Morphine should be used with caution in patients having an acute asthmatic attack, in those with chronic obstructive pulmonary disease or cor pulmonale, and in individuals with a substantially decreased respiratory reserve, preexisting respiratory depression, hypoxia, or hypercapnia. In such patients, even usual therapeutic doses of narcotics may decrease respira-

tory drive while simultaneously increasing airway resistance to the point of apnea.
Hypotensive Effect —The administration of morphine may result in severe hypotension in an individual whose ability to maintain his blood pressure has already been compromised by a depleted blood volume or concurrent administration of such drugs as the phenothiazines or certain anesthetics.
Special-Risk Patients —Morphine should be given with caution and the initial dose should be reduced in certain patients, such as the elderly or debilitated and those with severe impairment of hepatic or renal function, hypothyroidism, Addison's disease, prostatic hypertrophy, or urethral stricture.
Acute Abdominal Conditions —The administration of morphine or other narcotics may obscure the diagnosis or clinical course in patients with acute abdominal conditions.
Information for patients:
Use in Ambulatory Patients —Morphine may impair the mental and/or physical abilities required for the performance of potentially hazardous tasks, such as driving a car or operating machinery. The patient should be cautioned accordingly.
Morphine, like other narcotics, may produce orthostatic hypotension in ambulatory patients.
Patients should be cautioned about the combined effects of alcohol or other central nervous system depressants with morphine.
Drug interactions:
Generally, effects of morphine may be potentiated by alkalizing agents and antagonized by acidifying agents. Analgesic effect of morphine is potentiated by chlorpromazine and methocarbamol. CNS depressants such as anaesthetics, hypnotics, barbiturates, phenothiazines, chloral hydrate, glutethimide, sedatives, MAO inhibitors (including procarbazine hydrochloride), antihistamines, β-blockers (propranolol), alcohol, furazolidone and other narcotics may enhance the depressant effects of morphine.
Morphine may increase anticoagulant activity of coumarin and other anticoagulants.
Carcinogenicity/Mutagenicity:
Long-term studies to determine the carcinogenic and mutagenic potential of morphine are not available.
Pregnancy:
Teratogenic Effects —Pregnancy Category C: Animal production studies have not been conducted with morphine. It is also not known whether morphine can cause fetal harm when administered to a pregnant woman or can affect reproduction capacity. Morphine should be given to a pregnant woman only if clearly needed.
Labor and Delivery:
Morphine readily crosses the placental barrier and, if administered during labor, may lead to respiratory depression in the neonate.
Nursing Mothers:
Morphine has been detected in human milk. For this reason, caution should be exercised when morphine is administered to a nursing woman.
Pediatric Usage:
Safety and effectiveness in children have not been established.

ADVERSE REACTIONS
THE MAJOR HAZARDS OF MORPHINE AS OF OTHER NARCOTIC ANALGESICS, ARE RESPIRATORY DEPRESSION AND, TO A LESSER DEGREE, CIRCULATORY DEPRESSION, RESPIRATORY ARREST, SHOCK, AND CARDIAC ARREST HAVE OCCURRED.
The most frequently observed adverse reactions include lightheadedness, dizziness, sedation, nausea, vomiting, and sweating. These effects seem to be more prominent in ambulatory patients and in those who are not suffering severe pain. In such individuals, lower doses are advisable. Some adverse reactions may be alleviated in the ambulatory patient if he lies down.
Other adverse reactions include the following:
Central Nervous System —Euphoria, dysphoria, weakness, headache, insomnia, agitation, disorientation, and visual disturbances.
Gastrointestinal —Dry mouth, anorexia, constipation, and biliary tract spasm.
Cardiovascular —Flushing of the face, bradycardia, palpitation, faintness, and syncope.
Genitourinary —Urinary retention or hesitancy, anti-diuretic effect, and reduced libido and/or potency.
Allergic —Pruritus, urticaria, other skin rashes, edema, and, rarely hemorrhagic urticaria.
Treatment of the most frequent adverse reactions:
Constipation —Ample intake of water or other liquids should be encouraged. Concomitant administration of a stool softener and a peristaltic stimulant with the narcotic analgesic can be an effective preventive measure for those patients in need of therapeutics. If elimination does not occur for two days, an enema should be administered to prevent impaction.

In the event diarrhea occurs, seepage around a fecal impaction is a possible cause to consider before antidiarrheal measures are employed.

Nausea and Vomiting—Phenothiazines and antihistamines can be effective treatments for nausea of the medullary and vestibular sources respectively. However, these drugs may potentiate the side effects of the narcotics or the antinauseant.

Drowsiness (sedation)—Once pain control is achieved, undesirable sedation can be minimized by titrating the dosage to a level that just maintains a tolerable pain or pain free state.

DRUG ABUSE AND DEPENDENCE

Morphine Sulfate, narcotic, is a Schedule II controlled substance under the Federal Controlled Substance Act. As with other narcotics, some patients may develop a physical and psychological dependence on morphine. They may increase dosage without consulting a physician and subsequently may develop a physical dependence on the drug. In such cases, abrupt discontinuance may precipitate typical withdrawal symptoms, including convulsions. Therefore the drug should be withdrawn gradually from any patient known to be taking excessive dosages over a long period of time.

In treating the terminally ill patient the benefit of pain relief may outweigh the possibility of drug dependence. *The chance of drug dependence is substantially reduced when the patient is placed on scheduled narcotic programs instead of a "pain to relief-of-pain" cycle typical of a PRN regimen.*

OVERDOSAGE

Signs and Symptoms: Serious overdose with morphine is characterized by respiratory depression (a decrease in respiratory rate and/or tidal volume, Cheyne-Stokes respiration, cyanosis), extreme somnolence progressing to stupor or coma, skeletal muscle flaccidity, cold or clammy skin, and sometimes bradycardia and hypotension. In severe overdosage, apnea, circulatory collapse, cardiac arrest and death may occur.

Treatment: Primary attention should be given to the re-establishment of adequate respiratory exchange through provision of a patent airway and the institution of assisted or controlled ventilation. The narcotic antagonist naloxone is a specific antidote against respiratory depression which may result from overdosage or unusual sensitivity to narcotics, including morphine. Therefore, an appropriate dose of naloxone (usual initial adult dose: 0.4 mg) should be administered, preferably by the intravenous route and simultaneously with efforts at respiratory resuscitation. Since the duration of action of morphine may exceed that of the antagonist, the patient should be kept under continued surveillance and repeated doses of the antagonist should be administered as needed to maintain adequate respiration.

An antagonist should not be administered in the absence of clinically significant respiratory or cardiovascular depression.

Oxygen, intravenous fluids, vasopressors and other supportive measures should be employed as indicated.

Gastric emptying may be useful in removing unabsorbed drug.

DOSAGE AND ADMINISTRATION

ROXANOL™ and ROXANOL 100™—Usual Adult Oral Dose: 10 to 30 mg every 4 hours or as directed by physician. Dosage is a patient dependent variable, therefore increased dosage may be required to achieve adequate analgesia.

For control of chronic, agonizing pain in patients with certain terminal disease, this drug should be administered on a regularly scheduled basis, every 4 hours, at the lowest dosage level that will achieve adequate analgesia.

Note: Medication may suppress respiration in the elderly, the very ill, and those patients with respiratory problems, therefore lower doses may be required.

Morphine Dosage Reduction: During the first two to three days of effective pain relief, the patient may sleep for many hours. This can be misinterpreted as the effect of excessive analgesic dosing rather than the first sign of relief in a pain exhausted patient. The dose, therefore, should be maintained for at least three days before reduction, if respiratory activity and other vital signs are adequate.

Following successful relief of severe pain, periodic attempts to reduce the narcotic dose should be made. Smaller doses or complete discontinuation of the narcotic analgesic may become feasible due to a physiologic change or the improved mental state of the patient.

HOW SUPPLIED

Roxanol™
Morphine Sulfate (Immediate Release)
Concentrated Oral Solution
20 mg per mL
NDC 0054-3751-44: Bottles of 30 mL with calibrated dropper.
NDC 0054-3751-50: Bottles of 120 mL with calibrated dropper.

Roxanol 100™
Morphine Sulfate (Immediate Release)
Concentrated Oral Solution
100 mg per 5 mL
NDC 0054-3751-58: Bottles of 240 mL with calibrated patient spoon.

Roxanol™ UD
Morphine Sulfate (Immediate Release)
Oral Solution
10 mg per 2.5 mL
NDC 0054-8781-11: Unit dose vial of 2.5 mL (10 mg Morphine Sulfate), 25 reverse number vials per carton.
20 mg per 5 mL
NDC 0054-8785-11: Unit dose vial of 5 mL (20 mg Morphine Sulfate), 25 reverse number vials per carton.

Morphine Sulfate (Immediate Release)
Concentrated Oral Solution
30 mg per 1.5 mL
NDC 0054-8788-11: Unit dose vial of 1.5 mL (30 mg Morphine Sulfate), 25 reverse number vials per carton.

Rescudose™
Morphine Sulfate (Immediate Release)
Oral Solution
10 mg per 2.5 mL
NDC 0054-8789-11: Unit dose vial of 2.5 mL (10 mg Morphine Sulfate), 25 vials per container.
DEA Order Form Required
Shown in Product Identification Section, page 427

ROXICET™ Tablets   ℂ ℞
[*rox-ē-cĕt*]
Oxycodone and Acetaminophen Tablets USP
(Oxycodone Hydrochloride 5 mg and Acetaminophen 325 mg)
(WARNING: May be habit forming)

ROXICET™ Oral Solution   ℂ ℞
Oxycodone and Acetaminophen Oral Solution
(Oxycodone Hydrochloride 5 mg and Acetaminophen 325 mg Oral Solution per 5 mL)
(WARNING: May be habit forming)

ROXICET 5/500™ Caplet   ℂ ℞
Oxycodone and Acetaminophen Tablets USP
(Oxycodone Hydrochloride 5 mg and Acetaminophen 500 mg)
(WARNING: May be habit forming)

DESCRIPTION

Each tablet contains:
Oxycodone Hydrochloride+ .... 5 mg
          (**Warning:** May Be Habit Forming)
Acetaminophen.. 325 mg
Each 5 mL contains:
Oxycodone Hydrochloride+ .... 5 mg
          (**Warning:** May Be Habit Forming)
Acetaminophen.. 325 mg
Alcohol... 0.4%
Each caplet contains:
Oxycodone Hydrochloride+ .... 5 mg
          Warning: May be Habit Forming)
Acetaminophen.. 500 mg
(+5 mg Oxycodone HCl is equivalent to 4.4815 mg Oxycodone.)

HOW SUPPLIED

ROXICET™ Tablets, Oxycodone and Acetaminophen Tablets USP (Oxycodone Hydrochloride 5 mg and Acetaminophen 325 mg) white scored tablets (Identified 54 543).
NDC 0054-8650-24: Unit dose, 25 tablets per card (reverse numbered), 4 cards per shipper.
NDC 0054-4650-25: Bottles of 100 tablets.
NDC 0054-4650-29: Bottles of 500 tablets.
ROXICET™ Oral Solution,
Oxycodone and Acetaminophen Oral Solution (Oxycodone Hydrochloride 5 mg and Acetaminophen 325 mg Oral Solution per 5 mL)
NDC 0054-8648-16: Unit dose Patient Cups™ filled to deliver 5 mL (Oxycodone Hydrochloride 5 mg, Acetaminophen 325 mg), ten 5 mL Patient Cups™ per shelf pack, 4 shelf packs per shipper.
NDC 0054-3686-63: Bottles of 500 mL.
ROXICET 5/500™ Caplets,
Oxycodone and Acetaminophen Tablets USP (Oxycodone Hydrochloride 5 mg and Acetaminophen 500 mg), white scored capsule-shaped tablets (Identified 54 730).
NDC 0054-8784-24: Unit dose, 25 caplets per card (reverse numbered), 4 cards per shipper.
NDC 0054-4784-25: Bottles of 100 caplets.
Store at Controlled Room Temperature (15°–30°C (59°–86°F).
DEA Order Form Required.
Caution: Federal law prohibits dispensing without prescription.

ROXICODONE™   ℂ ℞
[*rox-ē-cō-dōne*]
(oxycodone hydrochloride)
Tablets USP, Oral Solution USP, and Intensol™

DESCRIPTION

Each tablet contains:
Oxycodone Hydrochloride .... 5 mg
          (**WARNING: May be habit forming**)
Each 5 mL Oral Solution contains:
Oxycodone Hydrochloride .... 5 mg
          (**WARNING: May be habit forming**)
Each mL Intensol™ contains:
Oxycodone Hydrochloride .... 20 mg
          (**WARNING: May be habit forming**)
Inactive Ingredients:
The tablets contain microcrystalline cellulose and stearic acid.
The oral solution contains alcohol, FD&C Red No. 40, flavoring, glycol, sorbitol, water, and other ingredients.
The Intensol™ contains citric acid, sodium benzoate, and water.
Oxycodone is 14-hydroxydihydrocodeinone, a white odorless crystalline powder which is derived from the opium alkaloid, thebaine.

ACTIONS

The analgesic ingredient, oxycodone, is a semisynthetic narcotic with multiple actions qualitatively similar to those of morphine; the most prominent of these involve the central nervous system and organs composed of smooth muscle. The principal actions of therapeutic value of oxycodone are analgesia and sedation.

Oxycodone is similar to codeine and methadone in that it retains at least one half of its analgesic activity when administered orally.

INDICATIONS

For the relief of moderate to moderately severe pain.

CONTRAINDICATIONS

Hypersensitivity to oxycodone.

WARNINGS

Drug Dependence: Oxycodone can produce drug dependence of the morphine type, and therefore, has the potential for being abused. Psychic dependence, physical dependence and tolerance may develop upon repeated administration of this drug, and it should be prescribed and administered with the same degree of caution appropriate to the use of other oral narcotic-containing medications. Like other narcotic-containing medications, this drug is subject to the Federal Controlled Substances Act.

Usage in Ambulatory Patients: Oxycodone may impair the mental and/or physical abilities required for the performance of potentially hazardous tasks such as driving a car or operating machinery. The patient using this drug should be cautioned accordingly.

Interaction with Other Central Nervous System Depressants: Patients receiving other narcotic analgesics, general anesthetics, phenothiazines, other tranquilizers, sedative-hypnotics or other CNS depressants (including alcohol) concomitantly with oxycodone hydrochloride may exhibit an additive CNS depression. When such combined therapy is contemplated, the dose of one or both agents should be reduced.

Usage In Pregnancy: Safe use in pregnancy has not been established relative to possible adverse effects on fetal development. Therefore, this drug should not be used in pregnant women unless, in the judgment of the physician, the potential benefits outweigh the possible hazards.

Usage In Children: This drug should not be administered to children.

PRECAUTIONS

Head Injury and Increased Intracranial Pressure: The respiratory depressant effects of narcotics and their capacity to elevate cerebrospinal fluid pressure may be markedly exaggerated in the presence of head injury, other intracranial lesions or a pre-existing increase in intracranial pressure. Furthermore, narcotics produce adverse reactions which may obscure the clinical course of patients with head injuries.

Acute Abdominal Conditions: The administration of this drug or other narcotics may obscure the diagnosis or clinical course in patients with acute abdominal conditions.

Special Risk Patients: This drug should be given with caution to certain patients such as the elderly, or debilitated, and those with severe impairment of hepatic or renal function, hypothyroidism, Addison's disease and prostatic hypertrophy or urethral stricture.

ADVERSE REACTIONS

The most frequently observed adverse reactions include light headedness, dizziness, sedation, nausea and vomiting. These

Continued on next page

Roxane Laboratories—Cont.

effects seem to be more prominent in ambulatory than in nonambulatory patients, and some of these adverse reactions may be alleviated if the patient lies down.
Other adverse reactions include euphoria, dysphoria, constipation, skin rash and pruritus.

DOSAGE AND ADMINISTRATION
Dosage should be adjusted to the severity of the pain and the response of the patient. It may occasionally be necessary to exceed the usual dosage recommended below in cases of more severe pain or in those patients who have become tolerant to the analgesic effects of narcotics. This drug is given orally. The usual adult dose is one 5 mg tablet or 5 mL every 6 hours as needed for pain.

DRUG INTERACTIONS
The CNS depressant effects of oxycodone hydrochloride may be additive with that of other CNS depressants. See WARNINGS.

MANAGEMENT OF OVERDOSAGE
Signs and Symptoms: Serious overdose of oxycodone hydrochloride is characterized by respiratory depression (a decrease in respiratory rate and/or tidal volume, Cheyne-Stokes respiration, cyanosis), extreme somnolence progessing to stupor or coma, skeletal muscle flaccidity, cold and clammy skin, and sometimes bradycardia and hypotension. In severe overdosage, apnea, circulatory collapse, cardiac arrest and death may occur.
Treatment: Primary attention should be given to the reestablishment of adequate respiratory exchange through provision of a patent airway and the institution of assisted or controlled ventilation. The narcotic antagonist naloxone is a specific antidote against respiratory depression which may result from overdosage or unusual sensitivity to narcotics, including oxycodone. Therefore, an appropriate dose of naloxone (usual initial adult dose: 0.4 mg) should be administered, preferably by the intravenous route, simultaneously with efforts at respiratory resuscitation. Since the duration of action of oxycodone may exceed that of the antagonist, the patient should be kept under continued surveillance and repeated doses of the antagonist should be administered as needed to maintain adequate respiration.
An antagonist should not be administered in the absence of clinically significant respiratory or cardiovascular depression.
Oxygen, intravenous fluids, vasopressors and other supportive measures should be employed as indicated.
Gastric emptying may be useful in removing unabsorbed drug.

HOW SUPPLIED
5 mg white scored tablets. (Identified 54 582).
NDC 0054-8657-24: Unit dose, 25 tablets per card (reverse numbered), 4 cards per shipper.
NDC 0054-4657-25: Bottles of 100 tablets.
5 mg per 5 mL Oral Solution.
NDC 0054-8545-16: Unit dose Patient Cups™ filled to deliver 5 mL (oxycodone hydrochloride 5 mg), ten 5 mL Patient Cups™ per shelf pack, 4 shelf packs per shipper.
NDC 0054-3682-63: Bottles of 500 mL.
20 mg per mL Intensol™
(Concentrated Oral Solution)
NDC 0054-3683-44: Bottles of 30 mL with calibrated dropper [graduations of 0.25 mL (5 mg), 0.5 mL (10 mg), 0.75 mL (15 mg), and 1 mL (20 mg) on the dropper].
DEA Order Form Required
091 Revised September 1991

SODIUM POLYSTRENE
SULFONATE SUSPENSION USP ℞

CATION-EXCHANGE RESIN

DESCRIPTION
Sodium Polystyrene Sulfonate Suspension USP can be administered orally or in an enema and contains the following per 60 mL:

Sodium Polystyrene Sulfonate USP	15 g
Sorbitol USP	14.1 g
Alcohol	0.1%

The suspension is carmel-cherry-flavored and also contains Propylene Glycol USP, Microcrystalline Cellulose and Carboxymethylcellulose Sodium, Methylparaben NF, Propylparaben NF, Saccharin Sodium USP, Flavors and Purified Water USP.
Sodium Polystyrene Sulfonate is a benzene, diethenyl-, polymer with ethenylbenzene, sulfonated, sodium salt.
The sodium content of the suspension is 1500 mg (65 mEq) per 60 mL. It is a brown, slightly viscous suspension with an *in-vitro* exchange capacity of approximately 3.1 mEq (*in-vivo* approximately 1 mEq) of potassium per 4 mL (1 gram) of suspension.

CLINICAL PHARMACOLOGY
As the resin passes along the intestine or is retained in the colon after administration by enema, the sodium ions are partially released and are replaced by potassium ions. For the most part, this action occurs in the large intestine, which excretes potassium ions to a greater degree than does the small intestine. The efficiency of this process is limited and unpredictably variable. It commonly approximates the order of 33%, but the range is so large that definite indices of electrolyte balance must be clearly monitored. Metabolic data are unavailable.

INDICATIONS AND USAGE
Sodium Polystyrene Sulfonate suspension is indicated to treatment of hyperkalemia.

CONTRAINDICATIONS
Sodium Polystyrene Sulfonate suspension is contraindicated in patients with hypokalema or those patients who are hypersensitive to it.

WARNINGS
Alternative Therapy in Severe Hyperkalemia:
Since the effective lowering of serum potassium with Sodium Polystyrene Sulfonate may take hours to days, treatment with this drug alone may be insufficient to rapidly correct severe hyperkalemia associated with states of rapid tissue breakdown (e.g., burns and renal failure) or hyperkalemia so marked as to constitute a medical emergency. Therefore, other definite measures, including dialysis, should always be considered and may be imperative.
Hypokalemia:
Serious potassium deficiency can occur from Sodium Polystyrene Sulfonate therapy. The effect must be carefully controlled by frequent serum potassium determination within each 24 hour period. Since intracellular potassium deficiency is not always reflected by serum potassium levels, the level at which treatment with Sodium Polystyrene Sulfonate should be discontinued must be determined individually for each patient. Important aids in making this determination are the patient's clinical condition and electrocardiogram. Early clinical signs of severe hypokalemia include a pattern of irritable confusion and delayed thought processes. Electocardiographically, severe hypokalemia is often associated with a lengthened Q-T interval, widening, flattening, or inversion of the T wave, and prominent U waves. Also, cardiac arrhythmias may occur, such as premature atrial, nodal, and ventricular contractions, and supraventricular and ventricular tachycardias. The toxic effects of digitalis are likely to be exaggerated. Marked hypokalemia can also be manifested by severe muscle weakness, at times extending into frank paralysis.
Electrolyte Disturbances:
Like all cation-exchange resins, Sodium Polystyrene Sulfonate is not totally selective (for potassium) in its actions, and small amounts of other cations such as magnesium and calcium can also be lost during treatment. Accordingly, patients receiving Sodium Polystyrene Sulfonate should be monitored for all applicable electrolyte disturbances.
Systemic Alkalosis:
Systemic alkalosis has been reported after cation-exchange resins were administered orally in combination with nonabsorbable cation-donating antacids and laxatives such as magnesium hydroxide and aluminum carbonate. Magnesium hydroxide should not be administered with Sodium Polystyrene Sulfonate. One case of grand mal seizure has been reported in a patient with chronic hypocalcemia of renal failure who was given Sodium Polystyrene Sulfonate with magnesium hydroxide as a laxative. (See PRECAUTIONS, Drug Interactions).

PRECAUTIONS
Caution is advised when Sodium Polystyrene Sulfonate is administered to patients who cannot tolerate even a small increase in sodium loads (i.e., severe congestive heart failure, severe hypotension, or marked edema). In such instances compensatory restriction of sodium intake from other sources may be indicated.
If constipation occurs, patients should be treated with sorbitol (from 10 to 20 mL of 70% syrup every 2 hours or as needed to produce 1 to 2 watery stools daily) a measure which also reduces any tendency to fecal impaction.
Drug Interactions:
Antacids: The simultaneous oral administration of Sodium Polystyrene Sulfonate suspension with nonabsorbable cation-donating antacids and laxatives may reduce the resin's potassium exchange capability.
Systemic alkalosis has been reported after cation-exchange resins were administered orally in combination wth nonabsorbable cation-donating antacids and laxatives such as magnesium hydroxide and aluminum carbonate. Magnesium hydroxide should not be administered with Sodium Polystyrene Sulfonate suspension. One case of grand mal seizure has been reported in a patient with chronic hypocalcemia of renal failure who was given Sodium Polystyrene Sulfonate with magnesium hydroxide as a laxative. Intestinal obstruction due to concretions of aluminum hydroxide when used in combination with Sodium Polystyrene Sulfonate has been reported.
Digitalis: The toxic effects of digitalis on the heart, especially various ventricular arrhythmias and A-V nodal dissociation, are likely to be exaggerated by hypokalemia, even in the face of serum digoxin concentrations in the "normal range". (See WARNINGS.)
Carcinogenesis, Mutagenesis, Impairment of Fertility:
Studies have not been performed.
Pregnancy Category C: Animal reproduction studies have not been conducted with Sodium Polystyrene Sulfonate. It is also not known whether Sodium Polystyrene Sulfonate can cause fetal harm when administered to a pregnant woman or can affect reproduction capacity. Sodium Polystyrene Sulfonate should be given to a pregnant woman only if clearly needed.
Nursing Mothers: It is not known whether this drug is excreted in human milk. Because many drugs are excreted in human milk, caution should be exercised when Sodium Polystyrene Sulfonate is administered to a nursing woman.

ADVERSE REACTIONS
Sodium Polystyrene Sulfonate may cause some degree of gastric irritation. Anorexia, nausea, vomiting, and constipation may occur especially if high doses are given. Also, hypokalemia, hypocalcemia, and significant sodium retention may occur. Occasionally diarrhea develops. Large doses in elderly individuals may cause fecal impaction (see PRECAUTIONS). This effect may be obviated through usage of the resin in enemas as described under DOSAGE AND ADMINISTRATION. Rare instances of colonic necrosis have been reported. Intestinal obstruction due to concretions of aluminum hydroxide, when used in combination with Sodium Polystyrene Sulfonate, has been reported.

DOSAGE AND ADMINISTRATION
Oral Administration
The average daily adult dose is 15 g (60 mL) to 60 g (240 mL) of suspension. This is best provided by administering 15 g (60 mL) of Sodium Polystyrene Sulfonate suspension one to four times daily. Each 60 mL of Sodium Polystyrene Sulfonate suspension contains 1500 mg (65 mEq) of sodium. Since the *in-vivo* efficiency of sodium-potassium exchange resins is approximately 33%, about one-third of the resin's actual sodium content is being delivered to the body.
In smaller children and infants, lower doses should be employed by using as a guide a rate of 1 mEq of potassium per gram of resin as the basis of calculation.
The suspension may be introduced into the stomach through a plastic tube and, if desired, mixed with a diet appropriate for a patient in renal failure.
Rectal Administration:
The suspension may also be given, although with less effective results, as a retention enema for adults of 30 g (120 mL) to 50 g (200 mL) every six hours. The enema should be retained as long as possible and followed by a cleansing enema.
After an initial cleansing enema, a soft, large size (French 28) rubber tube is inserted into the rectum for a distance of 20 cm, with the tip well into the sigmoid colon and taped in place. The suspension is introduced at body temperature by gravity. The suspension is flushed with 50 or 100 mL of fluid, following which the tube is clamped and left in place. If back leakage occurs, the hips are elevated on pillows or a knee-chest position is taken temporarily. The suspension is kept in the sigmoid colon for several hours, if possible. Then the colon is irrigated with a nonsodium-containing solution at body temperature in order to remove the resin. Two quarts of flushing solution may be necessary. The returns are drained constantly through a Y tube connection. Particular attention should be paid to this cleansing enema when sorbitol has been used.
The intensity and duration of therapy depend upon the severity and resistance of hyperkalemia.

HOW SUPPLIED
Sodium Polystyrene Sulfonate Suspension USP, 15 g per 60 mL (an amber-colored, cherry/caramel-flavored suspension)
NDC 0054-8816-11: Unit dose bottle filled to deliver 60 mL, 10 bottles per shipper.
NDC 0054-8815-01: Unit dose enema bottle filled to contain 120 mL (for use in delivering the suspension rectally through appropriate tubing).
NDC 0054-8817-55: Unit dose enema bottle filled to contain 200 mL (for use in delivering the suspension rectally through appropriate tubing).
NDC 0054-3805-63: Bottle of 500 mL.
Note: Sodium Polystyrene Sulfonate suspension should not be heated for to do so may alter the exchange properties of the resin.

SHAKE WELL BEFORE USING
Dispense in a tight container as defined in the USP/NF.
Store at Controlled Room Temperature 15°–30°C (59°–86°F).

Caution: Federal law prohibits dispensing without prescription.

4073700   Revised May 1992
052
Roxane
Laboratories, Inc.
Columbus, Ohio 43216

TORECAN®   ℞
(thiethylperazine maleate
tablets USP)
(thiethylperazine malate
injection USP)
(for intramuscular use only)
(thiethylperazine maleate
suppositories USP)

Caution: Federal law prohibits dispensing without prescription.

DESCRIPTION
Torecan® (thiethylperazine) is a phenothiazine. Thiethylperazine is characterized by a substituted thioethyl group at position 2 in the phenothiazine nucleus, and a piperazine moiety in the side chain. The chemical designation is: 2-ethyl-mercapto-10-[3'(1''-methyl-piperazinyl-4'')-propyl-1']phenothiazine. Thiethylperazine has the following structural formula:

Tablet, 10 mg, for oral administration
ACTIVE INGREDIENT: thiethylperazine maleate USP, 10 mg. *INACTIVE INGREDIENTS*: acacia, carnauba wax, FD&C Yellow No. 5 aluminum lake (tartrazine), FD& C Yellow No. 6 aluminum lake, gelatin, lactose, magnesium stearate, povidone, sodium benzoate, sorbitol, starch, stearic acid, sucrose, talc, titanium dioxide.
Ampul, 2 ml, for intramuscular administration
ACTIVE INGREDIENT: thiethylperazine malate USP, 10 mg per 2 ml. *INACTIVE INGREDIENTS*: sodium metabisulfite NF, 0.5 mg; ascorbic acid USP, 2.0 mg; sorbitol NF, 40 mg; carbon dioxide gas q.s.; water for injection USP, q.s. to 2 ml.
Suppository, 10 mg, for rectal administration
ACTIVE INGREDIENT: thiethylperazine maleate USP, 10 mg. *INACTIVE INGREDIENT*: cocoa butter NF.

ACTIONS
The pharmacodynamic action of Torecan® (thiethylperazine) in humans is unknown. However, a direct action of Torecan on both the CTZ and the vomiting center may be concluded from induced vomiting experiments in animals.

INDICATIONS
Torecan® (thiethylperazine) is indicated for the relief of nausea and vomiting.

CONTRAINDICATIONS
Severe central nervous system (CNS) depression and comatose states.
In patients who have demonstrated a hypersensitivity reaction (e.g., blood dyscrasias, jaundice) to phenothiazines.
Because severe hypotension has been reported after the intravenous administration of phenothiazines, this route of administration is contraindicated.
Usage in Pregnancy: Torecan® (thiethylperazine) is contraindicated in pregnancy.

WARNINGS
Torecan® (thiethylperazine) injection contains sodium metabisulfite, a sulfite that may cause allergic-type reactions including anaphylactic symptoms and life-threatening or less severe asthmatic episodes in certain susceptible people. The overall prevalence of sulfite sensitivity in the general population is unknown and probably low. Sulfite sensitivity is seen more frequently in asthmatic than in nonasthmatic people.
Phenothiazines are capable of potentiating CNS depressants (e.g., anesthetics, opiates, alcohol, etc.) as well as atropine and phosphorus insecticides.
Since Torecan® (thiethylperazine) may impair mental and/or physical ability required in the performance of potentially hazardous tasks such as driving a car or operating machinery, it is recommended that patients be warned accordingly.
Postoperative Nausea and Vomiting: With the use of this drug to control postoperative nausea and vomiting occurring in patients undergoing elective surgical procedures, restlessness and postoperative CNS depression during anesthesia

recovery may occur. Possible postoperative complications of a severe degree of any of the known reactions of this class of drug must be considered. Postural hypotension may occur after an initial injection, rarely with the tablet or suppository.
The administration of epinephrine should be avoided in the treatment of drug-induced hypotension in view of the fact that phenothiazines may induce a reversed epinephrine effect on occasion.
Should a vasoconstrictive agent be required, the most suitable are norepinephrine bitartrate and phenylephrine.
The use of this drug has not been studied following intracardiac and intracranial surgery.
Usage in Pediatrics: The safety and efficacy of Torecan in children under 12 years of age has not been established.
Nursing Mothers: Information is not available concerning the secretion of Torecan in the milk of nursing mothers. As a general rule, nursing should not be undertaken while a patient is on a drug, since many drugs are secreted in human milk.

PRECAUTIONS
Abnormal movements such as extrapyramidal symptoms (E.P.S.) (e.g., dystonia, torticollis, dysphasia, oculogyric crises, akathisia) have occurred. Convulsions have also been reported. The varied symptom complex is more likely to occur in young adults and children. Extrapyramidal effects must be treated by reduction of dosage or cessation of medication.
Torecan® (thiethylperazine) tablets contain FD&C Yellow No. 5 (tartrazine) which may cause allergic-type reactions (including bronchial asthma) in certain susceptible individuals. Although the overall incidence of FD&C Yellow No. 5 (tartrazine) sensitivity in the general population is low, it is frequently seen in patients who also have aspirin hypersensitivity.
Postoperative Nausea and Vomiting: When used in the treatment of the nausea and/or vomiting associated with anesthesia and surgery, it is recommended that Torecan® (thiethylperazine) should be administered by deep intramuscular injection at or shortly before the termination of anesthesia.

ADVERSE REACTIONS
Central Nervous System: Serious: Convulsions have been reported. Extrapyramidal symptoms (E.P.S.) may occur, such as dystonia, torticollis, oculogyric crises, akathisia and gait disturbances. Others: Occasional cases of dizziness, headache, fever and restlessness have been reported.
Drowsiness may occur on occasion, following an initial injection. Generally this effect tends to subside with continued therapy or is usually alleviated by a reduction in dosage.
Autonomic Nervous System: Dryness of the mouth and nose, blurred vision, tinnitus. An occasional case of sialorrhea together with altered gustatory sensation has been observed.
Endocrine System: Peripheral edema of the arms, hands and face.
Hepatotoxicity: An occasional case of cholestatic jaundice has been observed.
Other: An occasional case of cerebral vascular spasm and trigeminal neuralgia has been reported.
Phenothiazine Derivatives: The physician should be aware that the following have occurred with one or more phenothiazines and should be considered whenever one of these drugs is used:
Blood Dyscrasias Serious—Agranulocytosis, leukopenia, thrombocytopenia, aplastic anemia, pancytopenia. Other—Eosinophilia, leukocytosis.
Autonomic Reactions Miosis, obstipation, anorexia, paralytic ileus.
Cutaneous Reactions Serious—Erythema, exfoliative dermatitis, contact dermatitis.
Hepatotoxicity Serious—Jaundice, biliary stasis.
Cardiovascular Effects Serious—Hypotension, rarely leading to cardiac arrest; electrocardiographic (ECG) changes.
Extrapyramidal Symptoms Serious—Akathisia, agitation, motor restlessness, dystonic reactions, trismus, torticollis, opisthotonos, oculogyric crises, tremor, muscular rigidity, akinesia—some of which have persisted for several months or years especially in patients of advanced age with brain damage.
Endocrine Disturbances Menstrual irregularities, altered libido, gynecomastia, weight gain. False positive pregnancy tests have been reported.
Urinary Disturbances Retention, incontinence.
Allergic Reactions Serious—Fever, laryngeal edema, angioneurotic edema, asthma.
Others: Hyperpyrexia, Behavioral effects suggestive of a paradoxical reaction have been reported. These include excitement, bizarre dreams, aggravation of psychoses and toxic confusional states. While there is no evidence at present that ECG changes observed in patients receiving phenothiazines are in any way precursors of any significant disturbance of cardiac rhythm, it should be noted that sudden and unexpected deaths apparently due to cardiac arrest have been

reported in a few instances in hospitalized psychotic patients previously showing characteristic ECG changes. A peculiar skin-eye syndrome has also been recognized as a side effect following long-term treatment with certain phenothiazines. This reaction is marked by progressive pigmentation of areas of the skin or conjunctiva and/or accompanied by discoloration of the exposed sclera and cornea. Opacities of the anterior lens and cornea described as irregular or stellate in shape have also been reported.
Drug Interactions: Phenothiazines are capable of potentiating CNS depressants (e.g., anesthetics, opiates, alcohol, etc.) as well as atropine and phosphorus insecticides.
Phenothiazines may induce a reversed epinephrine effect on occasion.

DOSAGE AND ADMINISTRATION
Adult: Usual daily dose range is 10 mg to 30 mg. *ORAL*: One tablet one to three times daily. *INTRAMUSCULAR*: 2 ml IM, one to three times daily. (See PRECAUTIONS.) *SUPPOSITORY*: Insert one suppository, one to three times daily.
Children: Appropriate dosage of Torecan® (thiethylperazine) has not been determined in children.

HOW SUPPLIED
Tablets Each tablet contains 10 mg thiethylperazine maleate, USP.
NDC 0054-8748-25: Unit dose tablets, 10 tablets per strip, 10 strips per shelf pack.
NDC 0054-4748-25: Bottles of 100 tablets.
Ampuls: Each 2 ml ampul contains in aqueous solution 10 mg thiethylperazine malate, USP. Boxes of 20 and 100.
Storage: Below 86°F; protect from light.
Administer only if clear and colorless.
Suppositories: Each containing 10 mg thiethylperazine maleate, USP. Packages of 12.
Storage: Below 77°F; tight container (sealed foil).
Manufactured by
Sandoz Pharmaceuticals Corporation
East Hanover, NJ 07936
Distributed by
Roxane Laboratories Inc.
Columbus OH 43216

Rystan Company, Inc.
47 CENTER AVENUE
P.O. BOX 214
LITTLE FALLS, NJ 07424-0214

CHLORESIUM®   OTC
[*klor-eez'ium*]
Ointment and Solution
Healing and Deodorizing Agent

COMPOSITION
Ointment: 0.5% Chlorophyllin Copper Complex in a hydrophilic base. Solution: 0.2% Chlorophyllin Copper Complex in isotonic saline solution.

ACTIONS AND USES
To promote healing and to relieve itching and discomfort of minor wounds, burns, surface ulcers, cuts, abrasions and skin irritations. To reduce malodors in wounds and surface ulcers.

ADMINISTRATION AND DOSAGE
Ointment: Apply generously and cover with an appropriate dressing, or as directed by physician. Dressings preferably changed no more often than every 48 to 72 hours. Solution: Apply full strength as continuous wet dressing, or as directed by physician.

SIDE EFFECTS
CHLORESIUM Ointment and Solution are soothing and nontoxic. Sensitivity reactions are extremely rare, and only

Continued on next page

Rystan—Cont.

a few instances of slight itching or irritation have been reported.

HOW SUPPLIED

Ointment: 1 oz and 4 oz tubes, 1 lb. jars (NDC 0263-5155-01 and -04, -16). Solution: 8 fl oz and 32 fl oz bottles (NDC 0263-5158-08 and -32).

DERIFIL® Tablets   OTC
[der'ah-fil]
Internal Deodorant

COMPOSITION

100 mg chlorophyllin copper complex per tablet.

INDICATIONS

Oral deodorant for internal use: 1. An aid to reduce fecal odor due to incontinence, 2. An aid to reduce odor from a colostomy or ileostomy.

DIRECTIONS

Adults and children 12 years of age and over: Oral dosage is one to two tablets daily in divided doses as required. If odor is not controlled, take up to an additional tablet daily in divided doses as required. The smallest effective dose should be used. Do not exceed 3 tablets daily. Children under 12 years of age: consult a doctor. In ostomies, tablets may be either taken by mouth or placed in the appliance.

SIDE EFFECTS

When used as directed, no toxic effects have been reported. As with any drug, do not exceed the recommended dosage. A temporary mild laxative effect may be noted, and the fecal discharge is commonly stained dark green.

WARNING

If cramps or diarrhea occurs, reduce the dosage. If symptoms persist, consult your doctor.

HOW SUPPLIED

Dark green, round, film-coated tablet with "R" on one side and score on other. Each tablet contains 100 mg Chlorophyllin Copper Complex. Bottles of 30 (NDC 0263-5001-03), 100 (NDC 0263-5001-10), and 1000 tablets (NDC 0263-5001-11).

PANAFIL® Ointment   ℞
[pan'ah-fil]
PANAFIL®—WHITE Ointment   ℞

CAUTION

Federal law prohibits dispensing without prescription.

DESCRIPTION

PANAFIL® Ointment is an enzymatic debriding-healing ointment which contains standardized papain 10%, urea USP 10% and chlorophyllin copper complex 0.5% in a hydrophilic base. Inactive ingredients are: White Petrolatum, USP; Propylene Glycol, USP; Stearyl Alcohol, NF; Sorbitan Monostearate, NF; Polyoxyl 40 Stearate, NF; Boric Acid, NF; Sodium Borate, NF; Chlorobutanol (Anhydrous), NF as a preservative. PANAFIL-WHITE is identical except that the chlorophyllin copper complex is omitted.

CLINICAL PHARMACOLOGY

Papain, the proteolytic enzyme derived from the fruit of carica papaya, is a potent digestant of nonviable protein matter, but is harmless to viable tissue. It has the unique advantage of being active over a wide pH range, 3 to 12. Despite its recognized value as a digestive agent, papain is relatively ineffective when used alone as a debriding agent, primarily because it requires the presence of activators to exert its digestive function.

Urea is combined with papain to provide two supplementary chemical actions: 1) to expose by solvent action the activators of papain (sulfhydryl groups) which are always present, but not necessarily accessible, in the nonviable tissue or debris of lesions, and 2) to denature the nonviable protein matter in lesions and thereby render it more susceptible to enzymatic digestion. In pharmacologic studies involving digestion of beef powder, Miller[1] showed that the combination of papain and urea produced twice as much digestion as papain alone. Chlorophyllin copper complex adds healing action to the cleansing action of the proteolytic papain-urea combination. The basic wound-healing properties of chlorophyllin copper complex are promotion of healthy granulations, control of local inflammation and reduction of wound odors.[2] Specifically, chlorophyllin copper complex inhibits the hemagglutinating and inflammatory properties of protein degradation products in the wound, including the products of enzymatic digestion, thus providing an additional protective factor.[1,3] The incorporation of chlorophyllin copper complex in PANAFIL® Ointment permits its continuous use for as long

as desired to help produce and then maintain a clean wound base and to promote healing.

INDICATIONS AND USES

Ointment is suggested for treatment of acute and chronic lesions such as varicose, diabetic and decubitus ulcers, burns, postoperative wounds, pilonidal cyst wounds, carbuncles and miscellaneous traumatic or infected wounds.

Ointment is applied continuously throughout treatment of these conditions (1) for enzymatic debridement of necrotic tissue and liquefaction of fibrinous, purulent debris, (2) to **keep** the wound clean, and simultaneously (3) to promote normal healing.

CONTRAINDICATIONS

None known.

PRECAUTIONS

See Dosage and Administration.
Not to be used in eyes.

ADVERSE REACTIONS

Ointment is generally well tolerated and nonirritating. A small percentage of patients may experience a transient "burning" sensation on application of the ointment. Occasionally, the profuse exudate resulting from enzymatic digestion may cause irritation. In such cases, more frequent changes of dressings until exudate diminishes will alleviate discomfort.

DOSAGE AND ADMINISTRATION

Apply Ointment directly to lesion and cover with appropriate dressing. When practicable, daily or twice daily changes of dressings are preferred. Longer intervals between redressings (two or three days) have proved satisfactory, and Ointment may be applied under pressure dressings. At each redressing, the lesion should be irrigated with isotonic saline solution or other mild cleansing solution (except hydrogen peroxide solution, which may inactivate the papain) to remove any accumulation of liquefied necrotic material.

NOTE

Papain may also be inactivated by the salts of heavy metals (lead, silver, mercury, etc.) Contact with medications containing these metals should be avoided.

HOW SUPPLIED

PANAFIL—1 oz. tubes, (NDC 0263-5145-01).
1 lb. jars, (NDC 0263-5145-16).
PANAFIL-WHITE—1 oz. tubes, (NDC-0263-5148-01)

REFERENCES

1–3 Data on file.

PROPHYLLIN®   OTC
[pro-fil'in]
Wet Dressing Powder and Ointment

COMPOSITION

Powder: Each packet contains 2.3 grams Sodium Propionate. One packet (or one level teaspoonful of bulk powder) in 8 fluid ounces of water makes a solution containing approximately 1% Sodium Propionate. Chlorophyllin Copper Complex present for its deodorizing effect.

Ointment: 5% Sodium Propionate and 0.0125% Chlorophyllin Copper Complex in an emollient ointment base.

HOW SUPPLIED

Powder: Cartons of 12 packets and in 4 oz. jars (NDC 0263-5182-12 and 04). Ointment: 1 oz. tubes (NDC 0263-5185-01).

Sandoz Nutrition Corporation
Clinical Products Division
MINNEAPOLIS, MN 55416

TOLEREX®
Maintenance Elemental Diet

**Nutritional Information
And Use Instructions**
The **Tolerex®** diet is a nutritionally complete elemental diet formulated for the nutritional management of patients with impaired digestion and or malabsorption.

COMPOSITION

The **Tolerex** diet is a chemically defined diet composed of all essential nutrients in simple, readily absorbable form: free amino acids, predigested carbohydrates, safflower oil, vitamins, minerals, electrolytes and trace elements. One 80-gram packet provides 300 Calories and 0.98 grams of available nitrogen with a caloric density of 1 Calorie per ml when diluted with 255 ml water to a total standard dilution volume of 300 ml:

	Amount per 80 g	Amount per 1000 ml (Standard dilution)	Energy Distribution
Total energy (Calories)	300	1000	
Amino acids (free base equivalent)	6.18 g	20.6 g	8.2%
Carbohydrate (dry basis)	67.9 g	226.3 g	90.5%
Fat	0.435 g	1.45 g	1.3%
Linoleic acid	0.348 g	1.16 g	1.0%

Six 80-g packets of the **Tolerex** diet supply 5.88 grams of available nitrogen, 2.61 grams fat, 408 grams carbohydrate, and the following vitamins, minerals, electrolytes and amino acid profile:

Vitamins Minerals and Trace Elements	Per 1000 m (Standard dilution)	Per 6 Packets (480 Grams)	% U.S. RDA Per 6 Packets
Vitamin A	2778 IU	5000 IU	100
Vitamin D₃	222 IU	400 IU	100
Vitamin E	16.7 IU	30 IU	100
Vitamin C	33.3 mg	60 mg	100
Folic Acid	0.22 mg	0.4 mg	100
Thiamine	0.83 mg	1.5 mg	100
Riboflavin	0.94 mg	1.7 mg	100
Niacin	11.1 mg	20 mg	100
Vitamin B₆	1.11 mg	2 mg	100
Vitamin B₁₂	3.33 mcg	6 mcg	100
Biotin	0.17 mg	0.3 mg	100
Pantothenic Acid	5.55 mg	10 mg	100
Vitamin K₁	37.2 mcg	67 mcg	*
Choline	40.9 mg	73.7 mg	*
Calcium	0.55 g	1 g	100
Phosphorus	0.55 g	1 g	100
Iodine	83.3 mcg	150 mcg	100
Iron	10 mg	18 mg	100
Magnesium	222 mg	400 mg	100
Copper	1.11 mg	2 mg	100
Zinc	8.33 mg	15 mg	100
Manganese	1.56 mg	2.81 mg	*
Selenium†	83.3 mcg	150 mcg	*
Molybdenum†	83.3 mcg	150 mcg	*
Chromium†	27.8 mcg	50 mcg	*

* No U.S. RDA established.
† Represents amounts of these elements added.

Electrolytes	mEq per 1000 ml (Standard dilution)	Wt per 1000 ml (Standard dilution)
CATIONS		
Sodium	20.4	468 mg
Potassium	30.0	1172 mg
Calcium	27.7	556 mg
Magnesium	18.3	222 mg
Manganese	0.057	1.56 mg
Iron	0.358	10 mg
Copper	0.035	1.11 mg
Zinc	0.255	8.33 mg
Selenium†	0.002*	83.3 mcg
Molybdenum†	0.002**	83.3 mcg
Chromium†	0.002	27.8 mcg
ANIONS		
Chloride	26.8	950 mg
Phosphorus	54.0‡	556 mg
Acetate	18.7	1106 mg
Iodide	0.0007	83.3 mcg

†Represents amounts of these elements added.
*Calculated as Selenite SeO_3^{-2}
**Calculated as Molybdate MoO_4^{-2}
‡Calculated as Phosphate PO_4^{-3}

Amino Acid Profile	% Total Amino Acids
ESSENTIAL	
L-Isoleucine	4.55
L-Leucine	7.20
L-Valine	5.02
L-Lysine	5.41
L-Methionine	4.66
L-Phenylalanine	5.18
L-Threonine	4.55
L-Tryptophan	1.41
Total essential amino acids	37.98

Day	Strength	Approx Rate (ml/hour)	Diet (No of Packets)	Total Water (ml)	Volume (ml)	Calories (Cal)	Nitrogen (g)
1	½	75	3	1,665	1,800	900	3
2	⅔	75	4	1,620	1,800	1,200	4
3	Full	75	6	1,530	1,800	1,800	6

NON-ESSENTIAL

L-Alanine	4.85
L-Arginine	8.87
L-Aspartic Acid	10.35
L-Glutamine	17.07
Glycine	7.91
L-Histidine	2.21
L-Proline	6.48
L-Serine	3.34
L-Tyrosine	0.94
Total non-essential amino acids	62.02

In the standard solution of 1 Calorie/ml, the Tolerex diet has a pH of approximately 5.5 and an average osmolality of 550 mOsm/kg.

ACTIONS AND USES

The Tolerex diet is a nutritionally complete, elemental diet that is rapidly utilized, since absorption can take place without the aid of peptidases. The Tolerex diet is absorbed within the first 100 cm of functional small intestine. It is essentially a no-residue diet. There is minimal stimulation of biliary, pancreatic, and intestinal secretions, because of its free L-amino acid nitrogen (protein) source, glucose oligo-saccharide primary energy source, and low fat content. The low fat content also permits rapid gastric emptying and minimizes gastric residuals, thus reducing the possibility of aspiration. The balanced amino acid profile of the Tolerex diet allows optimum utilization and retention of its readily absorbed, elemental nitrogen source.

The Tolerex diet is useful as a maintenance diet in the dietary management of patients suffering from intractable diarrhea, impaired digestion and absorption which are secondary to a variety of diseases and disorders such as gastrointestinal disease, e.g., Crohns disease, irradiated bowel, intestinal atresia; and conditions leading to partial function of the gastrointestinal tract, e.g., immediate postoperative malnutrition, pancreatitis, fistula, partial obstruction, short-bowel syndrome. The Tolerex diet is also useful as an aid in preparing the bowel for diagnostic and surgical procedures, and as a transitional diet between parenteral and normal oral feeding. It is well tolerated by patients with known food sensitivities because it contains crystalline pure amino acids rather than whole protein or protein derivatives. The Tolerex diet has been proven useful as an elimination diet for patients undergoing diagnosis of specific food allergens.

One packet diluted with 255 ml (8½ oz) of water makes a single serving. Six packets of the Tolerex diet mixed thoroughly with 1530 ml of water provide a full day's supply for the average adult with 1800 Calories, 5.88 grams available nitrogen, 2.61 grams fat, and 408 grams carbohydrate. The Tolerex diet is a perishable liquid food when in solution. A full day's supply may be prepared at one time and stored in the refrigerator for up to 24 hours; shake the liquid briefly before serving. Do not leave at room temperature for more than 8 hours.

The Tolerex diet may be administered via a nasogastric, esophagostomy, gastrostomy, or jejunostomy feeding tube. Because of the diet's homogeneity and low viscosity, small bore feeding tubes (16 gauge catheter or #5 French feeding tube) may be used to optimize patient tolerance. It is suggested that the diet be given at room temperature by continuous drip technique using a suitable infusion pump. At the 1 Calorie per ml dilution, the Tolerex diet supplies most of the daily fluid requirements. Additional fluids should be given when necessary to maintain adequate urine output.

During the first two days of use, the Tolerex diet may need to be overdiluted for the osmotically sensitive patient, gradually concentrating up to full strength. The following administration schedule will facilitate GI adaptation, in most patients, within three days.

[See table above.]

If diarrhea is encountered, provide an antidiarrheal agent, which will often allow uninterrupted titration of the diet. Regress the rate and/or strength of the diet if needed. Then continue with progressive schedule until desired caloric/nitrogen intake is achieved.

The Tolerex diet also may be given orally, but should be flavored and served chilled over ice. The Vivonex™ Flavor Packets were specifically developed for this purpose, although other flavoring agents may be used if their contribution to the elemental and nutritional qualities of the diet are kept in mind. The Tolerex diet should be sipped slowly, preferably with a straw, when served as a beverage. Initiate oral feeding with a dilute solution, e.g., one packet diluted with 555 ml (18½ oz) water, and gradually increase volume and concentration.

PRECAUTIONS

Tolerex Diet:
DO NOT ADMINISTER THE TOLEREX DIET PARENTERALLY.
For use only under medical supervision.

Nausea, vomiting, abdominal cramps and distention, and diarrhea have been reported. Nausea is usually due to a high feeding rate, while diarrhea may be caused by a high diet concentration, low serum albumin, and concomitant medication. If intolerance is encountered, consider: 1) reverting one step in the above administration schedule, and then continuing slowly with a progressive schedule until desired caloric and nitrogen intake is achieved, 2) giving the Tolerex diet at room temperature, 3) repleting the patient's serum albumin level within normal range, 4) using a continuous drip technique, and 5) monitoring the patient's medication for potential GI side effects. Local water conditions also have been implicated in instances of diarrhea. Using sterile water in diet preparation has been reported to be effective in this circumstance.

Aspiration is an uncommon complication with the Tolerex diet because of its low fat content. However, the likelihood of aspiration may be reduced by radiologically confirming the anatomic position of the feeding tube, elevating the head of the bed 30° while the patient is receiving diet intragastrically, and limiting the administration rate to 150 ml/hour or less, depending upon patient tolerance. Jejunal administration should also be considered.

Diabetics receiving this diet should be closely monitored. Use in children may require adjusting the daily consumption to meet the Recommended Daily Allowance for the age group involved.

Vivonex Flavor Packets:
Vivonex Flavor Packets, except vanilla, contain citric acid. Patients with renal insufficiency should not use citric acid-containing flavor packets concurrently with aluminum based gels used as phosphate binders.

Additional professional and technical information is available through your local Sandoz Nutrition representative.

SUPPLY INFORMATION: The Tolerex diet (NDC 0212-4580-72) is available in cartons of six 80-g sealed packets for individual servings. Each packet provides 300 Calories in a total volume of 300 ml when mixed with 255 ml water.

The Vivonex Flavor Packets are available in Vanilla (NDC 0212-7190-74), Raspberry (NDC 0212-7200-74), Orange-Pineapple (NDC 0212-7160-74), Lemon-Lime (NDC 0212-7170-74), and Cherry-Vanilla (NDC 0212-7180-74) flavors.

CLINICAL PRODUCTS DIVISION
SANDOZ
NUTRITION
CORPORATION
MINNEAPOLIS, MN 55416 U.S.A.
© 1992 CLINICAL PRODUCTS DIVISION,   824600
SANDOZ NUTRITION CORP, MPLS., MN 55416   82

VIVONEX® T•E•N
Total Enteral Nutrition
An effective substitute for total parenteral nutrition (TPN)

The Vivonex® T.E.N. diet is a high nitrogen, elemental (100% free amino acids) diet for total enteral nutrition. The Vivonex diet is an effective substitute for intravenous feeding (TPN), except in patients where enteral feeding may be contraindicated (i.e., less than 60 cm of functioning small intestine). Its high essential to nonessential amino acid ratio (52:48), enhanced branched-chain amino acid content (33% of total amino acids), and optimal quantity of protein-sparing carbohydrate in a 175:1 Calorie to nitrogen ratio, make it especially useful in stressed, catabolic patients. The Vivonex diet will further benefit those patients with gastrointestinal impairment requiring a low residue feeding that permits maximal absorption with minimal digestion.

INDICATIONS
The Vivonex diet is recommended in the dietary management of the following conditions:
- Early postoperative feeding
  —immediate postoperative malnutrition
  —select multiple trauma/major surgery
- Impaired digestion and absorption
  —Crohns disease
  —irradiated bowel
  —intestinal atresia
  —pancreatitis
  —fistula
  —partial obstruction
  —short-bowel syndrome
  —acquired immunodeficiency syndrome with GI involvement
- Bowel preparation prior to diagnostic and surgical procedures
- Transitional diet between parenteral and normal oral feeding
- Food sensitivities

COMPOSITION: The Vivonex diet is a chemically defined diet composed of all essential nutrients in simple, readily absorbable form: free amino acids, predigested carbohydrates, safflower oil, vitamins, minerals, electrolytes, and trace elements. One 80.4-gram packet provides 300 Calories and 1.71 grams of available nitrogen with a caloric density of 1 Calorie per ml when diluted with 250 ml water to a total standard dilution volume of 300 ml:

	Amount per 80.4g	Amount per 1000 ml (standard dilution)	Energy Distribution
Total energy (Calories)	300	1000	
Amino acids (free base equivalent)	11.46g	38.20g	15.3%
Carbohydrate (dry basis)	61.67g	205.57g	82.2%
Fat	0.83g	2.77g	2.5%
Linoleic acid	0.65g	2.17g	2.0%

Ten 80.4-gram packets of the Vivonex diet meet or exceed the quantity of nutrients and energy required daily by the average catabolic adult: 17.1 grams of available nitrogen, 115 grams amino acids, 8.33 grams fat, 617 grams carbohydrate, and the following vitamins, minerals, electrolytes, and amino acid profile:

Vitamins, Minerals and Trace Elements	Per 1000 ml (standard dilution)	Per 10 Packets (804 Grams)	% U.S. RDA Per 10 Packets
Vitamin A	2500 IU	7500 IU	150
Vitamin D₃	200 IU	600 IU	150
Vitamin E	15 IU	45 IU	150
Vitamin C	60 mg	180 mg	300
Folic Acid	0.4 mg	1.2 mg	300
Thiamine	1.5 mg	4.5 mg	300
Riboflavin	1.7 mg	5.1 mg	300
Niacin	20 mg	60 mg	300
Vitamin B₆	2 mg	6 mg	300
Vitamin B₁₂	6 mcg	18 mcg	300
Biotin	0.3 mg	0.9 mg	300
Pantothenic Acid	10 mg	30 mg	300
Vitamin K₁	22.3 mcg	67 mcg	*
Choline	73.7 mg	221 mg	*
Calcium	0.5 g	1.5 g	150
Phosphorus	0.5 g	1.5 g	150
Iodine	75 mcg	225 mcg	150
Iron	9 mg	27 mg	150
Magnesium	200 mg	600 mg	150
Copper	1 mg	3 mg	150
Zinc	10 mg	30 mg	200
Manganese	0.94 mg	2.81 mg	*
Selenium†	50 mcg	150 mcg	*
Molybdenum†	50 mcg	150 mcg	*
Chromium†	16.67 mcg	50 mcg	*

* No U.S. RDA established.

† Represents amounts of these elements added.

Electrolytes	mEq per 1000 ml (standard dilution)	Wt. Per 1000 ml (standard dilution)
Cations		
Sodium	20	460 mg
Potassium	20	782 mg
Calcium	25	500 mg
Magnesium	16.5	200 mg
Manganese	0.034	937 mcg
Iron	0.322	9 mg
Copper	0.032	1 mg
Zinc	0.306	10 mg
Selenium†	0.001*	50 mcg
Molybdenum†	0.001**	50 mcg
Chromium†	0.001	17 mcg
Anions		
Chloride	23.1	819 mg
Phosphorus	48.5‡	500 mg
Acetate	31.0	1830 mg
Iodide	0.0006	75 mcg

†Represents amounts of these elements added
*Calculated as Selenite, SeO_3^{-2}
**Calculated as Molybdate, MoO_4^{-2}
‡Calculated as Phosphate, PO_4^{-3}

Continued on next page

Sandoz Nutrition—Cont.

Day	Strength	Approx. Rate (ml/hour)	Vivonex Diet (no. of packets)	+	Water (ml)	=	Total Volume (ml)	Calories (Cal.)	Nitrogen (g)
1	½	50	2	+	1100	=	1200	600	3.42
2	½	100	4	+	2200	=	2400	1200	6.84
3	¾	100	6	+	2100	=	2400	1800	10.26
4	Full	100	8	+	2000	=	2400	2400	13.68

Amino Acid Profile	% Total Amino Acids
Essential	
L-Isoleucine	8.27
L-Leucine	16.56
L-Valine	8.27
L-Lysine	5.10
L-Methionine	3.66
L-Phenylalanine	5.16
L-Threonine	4.00
L-Tryptophan	1.28
Total essential amino acids	52.30
Non-essential	
L-Alanine	5.18
L-Arginine	7.64
L-Aspartic Acid	7.01
L-Glutamine	12.85
Glycine	4.01
L-Histidine	2.36
L-Proline	4.88
L-Serine	2.93
L-Tyrosine	0.84
Total non-essential amino acids	47.70
Branched-chain amino acids (Isoleucine, Leucine, Valine)	33.10
Aromatic amino acids (Phenylalanine, Tyrosine)	6.00
Branched-chain: Aromatic amino acid molar ratio	7.4:1

In the standard dilution of 1 Calorie/ml, the Vivonex diet has a pH of approximately 5.0 and an average osmolality of 630 mOsm/kg.

MIXING AND STORAGE

To prepare 300 ml full strength diet (1 packet):
1. Add 1 packet of diet to 250 ml of warm water in a 1 pint container.
2. Cover and shake for 20 seconds.
Any remaining undissolved particles will dissolve spontaneously after standing 5–10 minutes.
NOTE: For larger quantities the container should be no more than ¾ full after diet is added to water, and more time may be required to shake product into solution. The Vivonex diet can also be blenderized if desired. The Vivonex diet is a perishable liquid food when in solution. A full day's supply may be prepared at one time and stored in the refrigerator for up to 48 hours; shake the liquid briefly before serving. Do not leave at room temperature for more than 8 hours.

FEEDING TUBE ADMINISTRATION

The Vivonex diet may be administered via a nasogastric, nasointestinal, esophagostomy, gastrostomy, or jejunostomy feeding tube. Because of its homogeneity and low viscosity, small bore feeding tubes (16 gauge catheter or #5 French tube) may be used to optimize patient tolerance. The diet should be given at room temperature by continuous drip technique, or using a suitable infusion pump. At the 1 Calorie per ml dilution, the Vivonex diet supplies most of the daily fluid requirements. Additional fluids should be given when necessary to maintain hydration and adequate urine output.

Generally, patient tolerance is optimized with any enteral diet by beginning with a dilute solution, titrating up to the desired calorie and nitrogen input. Although a more aggressive administration schedule may be considered, especially for gastric feeding or patients with a serum albumin level greater than 3.5 g/dl, the following schedule has been found to facilitate adaptation in most patients:
[See table above.]

Once the Vivonex diet is being administered full strength, nutrient intake can be increased by raising the continuous flow rate in 25 ml increments and/or raising the concentration, e.g., one packet + 150 ml water = 200 ml of 1.5 Cal/ml diet.

Diarrhea is the most common side effect with any liquid diet. Concomitant use of an antidiarrheal will often allow uninterrupted titration of the diet. However, in some instances, it may be necessary to revert one step to a more dilute solution, maintaining the patient at the last tolerated rate until free of symptoms for eight hours. Then continue with progressive schedule until desired calorie and nitrogen intake is achieved.

ORAL ADMINISTRATION

For oral use, the Vivonex diet should be flavored and served chilled over ice. Vivonex™ Flavor Packets were specifically developed for this purpose, although other flavoring agents may be used if their contribution to the elemental and nutritional qualities of the diet are kept in mind. The Vivonex diet should be sipped slowly, preferably through a straw, when served as a beverage. Initiate oral feeding with dilute solution, e.g., one packet diluted with 550 ml (18⅓ oz.), and gradually increase volume and concentration.

PRECAUTIONS

Vivonex Diet:
DO NOT ADMINISTER THE VIVONEX DIET PARENTERALLY. For use only under medical supervision. Nausea, vomiting, abdominal cramps, distention, and diarrhea are possible. Nausea and diarrhea are usually due to feeding rate or diet concentration. Local water conditions may be implicated in instances of diarrhea. Preparing diet with deionized or distilled water may be effective in this circumstance.
Aspiration is an uncommon complication with the Vivonex diet because of its low fat content. However, radiologically confirm the anatomic position of the feeding tube, elevate the head of the bed 30° while the patient is receiving diet intragastrically, and control the administration to 150 ml/hour or less, depending upon patient tolerance. Jejunal administration should also be considered.
Diabetics and patients with renal insufficiency receiving this diet should be closely monitored. Use in children may require adjusting the daily consumption to meet the Recommended Daily Allowance for the age group involved.
Vivonex Flavor Packets:
Vivonex Flavor Packets, except vanilla, contain citric acid. Patients with renal insufficiency should not use citric acid-containing flavor packets concurrently with aluminum based gels used as phosphate binders.

SUPPLY INFORMATION

The Vivonex T.E.N. diet (NDC 0212-7278-73) is available in cartons of ten 80.4-gram sealed packets, each providing 300 Calories.
Vivonex Flavor Packets are available in Vanilla (NDC 0212-7190-74), Raspberry (NDC 0212-7200-74), Orange-Pineapple (NDC 0212-7160-74), Lemon-Lime (NDC 0212-7170-74) and Cherry-Vanilla (NDC 0212-7180-74) flavors.
Additional professional and technical information on all Vivonex products is available through local Sandoz Nutrition representatives.

<u>CLINICAL PRODUCTS DIVISION</u>
SANDOZ
NUTRITION
CORPORATION
MINNEAPOLIS, MN 55416 U.S.A.
© 1992 CLINICAL PRODUCTS DIVISION,   824500
SANDOZ NUTRITION CORP, MPLS. MN 55416   82

Sandoz Pharmaceuticals/ Consumer Division
Division of Sandoz Pharmaceuticals Corp.
59 RT. 10
EAST HANOVER, NJ 07936

ACID MANTLE® CREME   OTC
[ă'sĭd-mănt'l]
Topical Creme

(See PDR For Nonprescription Drugs.)

CAMA® ARTHRITIS PAIN RELIEVER   OTC
[kă'măh]

(See PDR For Nonprescription Drugs.)

DORCOL® CHILDREN'S COUGH SYRUP   OTC
[door'call]

(See PDR For Nonprescription Drugs.)

DORCOL® CHILDREN'S DECONGESTANT LIQUID   OTC
[door'call]

(See PDR For Nonprescription Drugs.)

DORCOL® CHILDREN'S LIQUID COLD FORMULA   OTC
[door'call]

(See PDR For Nonprescription Drugs.)

GAS-X® CHEWABLE TABLETS and EXTRA STRENGTH GAS-X® CHEWABLE TABLETS   OTC
Simethicone - Anti-Gas

(See PDR For Nonprescription Drugs.)

THERAFLU®   OTC
Flu and Cold Medicine
Flu, Cold & Cough Medicine
Maximum Strength Nighttime Flu, Cold & Cough Medicine

(See PDR For Nonprescription Drugs.)

TRIAMINIC® ALLERGY MEDICINE   OTC
[trī"ah-mĭn'ĭc]

(See PDR For Nonprescription Drugs.)

TRIAMINIC® CHEWABLE TABLETS   OTC
For Children
[trī"ah-mĭn'ĭc]

(See PDR For Nonprescription Drugs.)

TRIAMINIC® COLD MEDICINE   OTC
[trī"ah-mĭn'ĭc]

(See PDR For Nonprescription Drugs.)

TRIAMINIC® EXPECTORANT   OTC
[trī"ah-mĭn'ĭc]
The Congestion Medicine

(See PDR For Nonprescription Drugs.)

TRIAMINIC® EXPECTORANT DH   ©
[trī"ah-mĭn'ĭc]

DESCRIPTION

Each teaspoonful (5 ml) of TRIAMINIC Expectorant DH contains: hydrocodone bitartrate 1.67 mg (Warning: May be habit forming), phenylpropanolamine hydrochloride 12.5 mg, pheniramine maleate 6.25 mg, pyrilamine maleate 6.25 mg, and guaifenesin 100 mg. Other ingredients: alcohol (5%), benzoic acid, Blue 1, flavors, purified water, saccharin sodium, sorbitol, sucrose, Yellow 10, Yellow 6.
Phenylpropanolamine hydrochloride, a sympathomimetic drug, is structurally related to ephedrine and amphetamine. Pheniramine maleate is an antihistamine of the alkylamine class while pyrilamine maleate belongs to the ethylenediamine class.
The expectorant component is guaifenesin (3-(o-methoxyphenoxy)-1,2- propanediol) which helps loosen and thus clear the bronchial passageways of bothersome, thickened mucus. The antitussive component, hydrocodone, is 7,8 dihydrocodeinone, a derivative of codeine.

CLINICAL PHARMACOLOGY

Phenylpropanolamine presumably acts on α-adrenergic receptors in the mucosa of the respiratory tract producing vasoconstriction which results in shrinkage of swollen mucous membranes, reduction of tissue hyperemia, edema and

nasal congestion, and an increase in nasal airway patency. Antihistamines competitively act as H_1 receptor antagonists of histamine. They exhibit anticholinergic (drying) and sedative side effects. There are several classes of antihistamines which vary with respect to potency, dosage and the relative incidence of side effects. Antihistamines inhibit the effects of histamine on capillary permeability and on vascular, bronchial and many other types of smooth muscle.

By increasing respiratory tract fluid, guaifenesin reduces the viscosity of tenacious secretions and acts as an expectorant. The drug is effective in productive as well as nonproductive cough, but is of particular value in dry, nonproductive cough which tends to injure the mucous membranes of the air passages.

Hydrocodone is a centrally acting narcotic antitussive providing cough relief for up to 6 hours.

INDICATIONS

For relief of troublesome cough, nasal congestion and postnasal drip associated with colds, nasal allergies, sinusitis, and rhinitis. Also effective for relief of severe, prolonged or refractory cough associated with other respiratory disorders. For the relief of symptoms associated with allergic rhinitis such as sneezing, rhinorrhea, pruritus and lacrimation.

CONTRAINDICATIONS

TRIAMINIC Expectorant DH is contraindicated in patients exhibiting hypersensitivity to any of the ingredients. Antihistamines are contraindicated in patients receiving monoamine oxidase inhibitors since these agents may prolong and intensify the anticholinergic effects of antihistamines (see Drug Interactions). Antihistamines *should not* be used to treat lower respiratory tract symptoms or be given to premature or newborn infants. Sympathomimetic agents such as phenylpropanolamine are contraindicated in patients with severe hypertension, severe coronary artery disease and in those taking monoamine oxidase inhibitors. Narcotic analgesics are contraindicated in patients with acute respiratory depression. Continuous dosage over an extended period is generally contraindicated since hydrocodone can cause addiction.

Nursing Mothers: Because of the higher risk of antihistamines for premature and newborn infants, antihistamine therapy is contraindicated in nursing mothers.

WARNINGS

TRIAMINIC Expectorant DH can produce drug dependence, and therefore has the potential for abuse.

Sympathomimetic agents should be used with caution in patients with hypertension, hyperthyroidism, diabetes mellitus and cardiovascular disease. Antihistamines should be used with caution in patients with narrow angle glaucoma, stenosing peptic ulcer, pyloroduodenal obstruction, symptomatic prostatic hypertrophy, bladder neck obstruction or chronic pulmonary disease. Narcotic analgesics should be used with caution in patients with chronic respiratory impairment, cardiac arrhythmias, history of convulsions, history of drug dependence, gallbladder disease or impaired renal or hepatic function.

Use in the Elderly (Approximately 60 Years or Older): Antihistamines are more likely to cause dizziness, sedation and hypotension in elderly patients. Overdosage of sympathomimetic agents in this age group may cause hallucinations, convulsions, CNS depression or death. Geriatric patients may be more susceptible to the effects of hydrocodone, especially the respiratory depressant effects.

PRECAUTIONS

General: Use with caution in patients with hypertension, hyperthyroidism, diabetes mellitus, cardiovascular disease, bronchial asthma, increased intraocular pressure (see WARNINGS). Before prescribing medication to suppress or modify cough, it is important to ascertain that the underlying cause of cough is identified, that modification of cough does not increase the risk of clinical complications, and that appropriate therapy for the primary disease is provided.

Information for Patients: Patients should be informed of the potential for sedation or drowsiness and cautioned about engaging in activities requiring mental alertness such as driving or operating machinery. The concomitant consumption of alcoholic beverages or other sedative drugs should be avoided.

Drug Interactions:

(1) Monoamine oxidase inhibitors: MAO inhibitors may prolong and intensify the anticholinergic effects of antihistamines and potentiate the pressor effects of sympathomimetics.

(2) Alcohol and CNS depressants: These agents potentiate the sedative effects of antihistamines and hydrocodone. The CNS and respiratory depressant effects of some opioids may be exaggerated and prolonged by phenothiazines, alcohol, CNS depressants, MAO inhibitors, and tricyclic antidepressants; the mechanism of this supra-additive effect is not fully understood, but may involve alterations in the rate of metabolic transformation of the opioid or alterations in neurotransmitters involved in opioid actions.

(3) Certain antihypertensives: Sympathomimetics may reduce the antihypertensive effects of methyldopa, mecamylamine, reserpine and veratrum alkaloids.

Drug/Laboratory Test Interactions: Guaifenesin or its metabolites may cause color interference with the VMA test for catechols. It may also falsely elevate the level of urinary 5HIAA in certain serotonin metabolite chemical tests because of color interference.

Carcinogenesis, Mutagenesis, Impairment of Fertility: No data are available on the long-term potential for carcinogenicity, mutagenicity or impairment of fertility in animals or humans.

Pregnancy: *Pregnancy Category C*— Animal reproduction studies have not been conducted. Safe use in pregnancy has not been established relative to possible adverse effects on fetal development. Therefore, this product should not be used in pregnant patients unless, in the judgement of the physician, the potential benefits outweigh possible hazards.

Nursing Mothers: See CONTRAINDICATIONS.

Pediatric Use: TRIAMINIC Expectorant DH is intended for administration to children 1 to 12 years of age (see DOSAGE AND ADMINISTRATION). It is important to note the variability of response infants and small children exhibit to antihistamines and sympathomimetics. As in adults, the combination of an antihistamine and sympathomimetic can elicit either mild stimulation or mild sedation in children. In the young child, mild stimulation is the response most frequently seen. In infants and children, overdosage of antihistamines may cause hallucinations, convulsions or death. Pediatric patients may be more susceptible to the effects of hydrocodone, especially the respiratory depressant effects.

ADVERSE REACTIONS

The most frequent adverse reactions are underlined.

(1) General: urticaria, drug rash, anaphylactic shock, photosensitivity, excessive perspiration, chills, dryness of mouth, nose and throat.

(2) Cardiovascular System: hypotension, headache, palpitations, tachycardia, extrasystoles.

(3) Hematologic System: hemolytic anemia, thrombocytopenia, agranulocytosis.

(4) Nervous System: <u>sedation, sleepiness, dizziness, disturbed coordination,</u> fatigue, confusion, restlessness, excitation, nervousness, tremor, irritability, insomnia, euphoria, paresthesias, blurred vision, diplopia, vertigo, tinnitus, acute labyrinthitis, hysteria, neuritis, convulsions, CNS depression, hallucinations.

(5) GI System: <u>epigastric distress,</u> anorexia, nausea, vomiting, diarrhea, <u>constipation.</u>

(6) GU System: urinary frequency, difficult urination, urinary retention, early menses.

(7) Respiratory System: thickening of bronchial secretions, tightness of chest and wheezing, nasal stuffiness.

DRUG ABUSE AND DEPENDENCE: Tolerance and physical dependence may occur following prolonged administration of hydrocodone.

OVERDOSAGE

Symptoms: The triad of coma, pinpoint pupils, and depressed respiration strongly suggest hydrocodone poisoning. Serious overdose with TRIAMINIC Expectorant DH may be characterized by respiratory depression, extreme somnolence progressing to stupor or coma, convulsions, skeletal muscle flaccidity, cold and clammy skin, and sometimes bradycardia and hypotension. In severe overdosage, apnea, circulatory collapse, cardiac arrest and death may occur. In the presence of fever and dehydration excitation may occur in children.

Treatment of Overdosage: Primary attention should be given to the reestablishment of adequate respiratory exchange through provision of patent airway and the institution of assisted or controlled ventilation. The narcotic antagonists naloxone and levallorphan are specific antidotes against respiratory depression which may result from overdosage or unusual sensitivity to narcotics, including hydrocodone. An appropriate dose of one of these antagonists should be administered, preferably by the intravenous route, simultaneously with efforts at respiratory resuscitation. The fact that an opioid antagonist may precipitate withdrawal symptoms in patients who are physically dependent on hydrocodone must be kept in mind and dosage titrated accordingly. Since the duration of action of hydrocodone may exceed that of the antagonist, the patient should be kept under continued surveillance and repeated doses of the antagonist should be administered as needed to maintain adequate respiration. Oxygen, intravenous fluids, vasopressors and other supportive measures should be employed as indicated, including treatment for anticholinergic drug intoxication. Gastric emptying may be useful in removing unabsorbed drug. Activated charcoal may be of benefit.

DOSAGE AND ADMINISTRATION

Adults—2 teaspoonfuls every 4 hours; children 6 to 12—1 teaspoonful every 4 hours; children 1 to 6—1/2 teaspoonful every 4 hours.

HOW SUPPLIED

TRIAMINIC Expectorant DH (green), in pint bottles. Store at room temperature. TRIAMINIC Expectorant DH is a Schedule III controlled substance.

TRIAMINIC® EXPECTORANT WITH CODEINE Ⓒ

[*trī″ah-mĭn′ĭc*]

DESCRIPTION

Each teaspoonful (5 ml) of TRIAMINIC Expectorant with Codeine contains: codeine phosphate 10 mg (Warning: May be habit forming), phenylpropanolamine hydrochloride 12.5 mg, guaifenesin 100 mg. Other ingredients: alcohol (5%), benzoic acid, Blue 1, flavors, purified water, sorbitol, sucrose. Yellow 10.

INDICATIONS

For prompt, temporary relief of coughs and nasal congestion due to the common cold. Helps loosen bronchial secretions to drain bronchial tubes.

WARNINGS

A persistent cough may be a sign of a serious condition. If cough persists for more than 1 week, tends to recur, or is accompanied by fever, rash, or persistent headache, consult a physician. Do not take this product for more than 7 days. If symptoms do not improve or are accompanied by fever consult a physician. Do not take this product for persistent or chronic cough such as occurs with smoking, asthma, chronic bronchitis, or emphysema, or where cough is accompanied by excessive phlegm (sputum) unless directed by a physician. Adults and children who have a chronic pulmonary disease or shortness of breath, or children who are taking other drugs, should not take this product unless directed by a physician. This product may cause or aggravate constipation. Do not take this product if you have heart disease, high blood pressure, thyroid disease, diabetes, or difficulty in urination due to enlargement of the prostate gland unless directed by a physician. As with any drug if you are pregnant or nursing a baby, seek the advice of a health professional before using this product. Keep this and all drugs out of the reach of children. In case of accidental overdose, seek professional assistance or contact a Poison Control Center immediately.

DRUG INTERACTION PRECAUTION

Do not take this product if you are presently taking a prescription drug for high blood pressure or depression, without first consulting a physician.

DOSAGE

Adults and children 12 years of age and over: 2 teaspoonfuls every 4 hours. Children 6 to under 12 years of age: 1 teaspoonful every 4 hours. Unless directed by a physician, do not exceed 6 doses in 24 hours. Children under 6 years of age: Consult a physician.

A dispensing device (such as a dropper calibrated for age or weight) should be dispensed along with the product when it is intended for use in children 2 to under 6 years of age to prevent possible overdose due to improper measuring of the dose.

Parents should be instructed to obtain and use a calibrated measuring device for administering the drug to the child, to use extreme care in measuring the dosage, and not to exceed the recommended daily dosage.

Codeine is not recommended for use in children under 2 years of age. Children under 2 years may be more susceptible to the respiratory depressant effects of codeine, including respiratory arrest, coma, and death.

HOW SUPPLIED

TRIAMINIC Expectorant with Codeine (green), in pint bottles. TRIAMINIC Expectorant with Codeine is a Schedule V controlled substance.

TRIAMINIC® NITE LIGHT® OTC

Nighttime Cough and Cold Medicine for Children

[*trī″ah-min′ic*]

(See PDR For Nonprescription Drugs.)

TRIAMINIC® ORAL INFANT DROPS ℞

[*trī″ah-mĭn′ĭc*]

DESCRIPTION

Each ml of TRIAMINIC Oral Infant Drops contains: phenylpropanolamine hydrochloride 20 mg, pheniramine maleate 10 mg, and pyrilamine maleate 10 mg. Other ingredients: benzoic acid, flavor, glycerin, purified water, Red 33, saccharin sodium, sorbitol, sucrose, Yellow 6.

Continued on next page

Sandoz Consumer—Cont.

This product combines the nasal decongestant properties of phenylpropanolamine hydrochloride with the antihistaminic activities of pheniramine maleate and pyrilamine maleate.

Phenylpropanolamine hydrochloride, a sympathomimetic drug, is structurally related to ephedrine and amphetamine. Pheniramine maleate is an antihistamine of the alkylamine class while pyrilamine maleate belongs to the ethylenediamine class.

CLINICAL PHARMACOLOGY

Phenylpropanolamine presumably acts on α-adrenergic receptors in the mucosa of the respiratory tract producing vasoconstriction which results in shrinkage of swollen mucous membranes, reduction of tissue hyperemia, edema and nasal congestion, and an increase in nasal airway patency. Antihistamines competitively act as H_1 receptor antagonists of histamine. They exhibit anticholinergic (drying) and sedative side effects. There are several classes of antihistamines which vary with respect to potency, dosage and the relative incidence of side effects. Antihistamines inhibit the effects of histamine on capillary permeability and on vascular, bronchial and many other types of smooth muscle.

INDICATIONS AND USAGE

For relief from such symptoms as nasal congestion and post-nasal drip associated with colds, allergies, sinusitis and rhinitis. Also for relief of symptoms associated with allergic rhinitis such as sneezing, rhinorrhea, pruritus and lacrimation.

CONTRAINDICATIONS

TRIAMINIC Oral Infant Drops are contraindicated in patients exhibiting hypersensitivity to any of the ingredients. Antihistamines are contraindicated in patients receiving monoamine oxidase inhibitors since these agents may prolong and intensify the anticholinergic and CNS depressant effects of antihistamines (see Drug Interactions). Antihistamines should not be used to treat lower respiratory tract symptoms or be given to premature or newborn infants. Sympathomimetic agents such as phenylpropanolamine are contraindicated in patients with severe hypertension, severe coronary artery disease and in those taking monoamine oxidase inhibitors.

WARNINGS

Sympathomimetic agents should be used with caution in patients with hypertension, hyperthyroidism, diabetes mellitus and cardiovascular disease. Antihistamines should be used with caution in patients with narrow angle glaucoma, stenosing peptic ulcer, pyloroduodenal obstruction, symptomatic prostatic hypertrophy, bladder neck obstruction or chronic pulmonary disease.

PRECAUTIONS

General: see WARNINGS.
Information For Patients: Antihistamines have additive effects with other CNS depressants (hypnotics, sedatives, tranquilizers, alcohol, etc.) Mothers should be informed of the potential for sedation or drowsiness when prescribing antihistamine preparations. Patients should be cautioned against mechanical activity requiring alertness.
Drug Interactions:
(1) Monoamine oxidase inhibitors: MAO inhibitors prolong and intensify the anticholinergic effects of antihistamines and potentiate the pressor effects of sympathomimetics.
(2) Alcohol and CNS depressants: These agents potentiate the sedative effects of antihistamines.
(3) Certain antihypertensives: Sympathomimetics may reduce the antihypertensive effects of methyldopa, mecamylamine, reserpine and veratrum alkaloids.
Carcinogenesis, Mutagenesis, Impairment Of Fertility: No data are available on the long-term potential for carcinogenicity, mutagenicity or impairment of fertility in animals or humans.
Pediatric Use: TRIAMINIC Oral Infant Drops have been formulated to provide safe and effective symptomatic relief for infants and small children. Precise dosage (on a body weight basis) is facilitated through the use of the plastic squeeze bottle with attached dropper tip (see DOSAGE AND ADMINISTRATION). It is important to note the variability of response infants and small children exhibit to antihistamines and sympathomimetics. As in adults, the combination of an antihistamine and sympathomimetic can elicit either mild stimulation or mild sedation in children. In the young child, mild stimulation is the response most frequently seen. In infants and children, overdosage of antihistamines may cause hallucinations, convulsions or death.

ADVERSE REACTIONS

The most frequent adverse reactions are underlined.
(1) *General:* urticaria, drug rash, anaphylactic shock, photosensitivity, excessive perspiration, chills, dryness of mouth, nose, and throat.

(2) *Cardiovascular System:* hypotension, headache, palpitations, tachycardia, extrasystoles.
(3) *Hematologic System:* hemolytic anemia, thrombocytopenia, agranulocytosis.
(4) *Nervous System:* sedation, sleepiness, dizziness, disturbed coordination, fatigue, confusion, restlessness, excitation, nervousness, tremor, irritability, insomnia, euphoria, paresthesias, blurred vision, diplopia, vertigo, tinnitus, acute labyrinthitis, hysteria, neuritis, convulsions, CNS depression, hallucinations.
(5) *GI System:* epigastric distress, anorexia, nausea, vomiting, diarrhea, constipation.
(6) *GU System:* urinary frequency, difficult urination, urinary retention.
(7) *Respiratory System:* thickening of bronchial secretions, tightness of chest and wheezing, nasal stuffiness.

OVERDOSAGE

TRIAMINIC product overdosage reactions may vary from central nervous system depression to stimulation. Stimulation is particularly likely in children. Atropine-like signs and symptoms—dry mouth; fixed, dilated pupils; flushing—and gastrointestinal symptoms may also occur.
If vomiting has not occurred spontaneously, the conscious patient should be induced to vomit. This is best done by having the patient drink a glass of water or milk after which they should be made to gag. Precautions against aspiration must be taken, especially in infants and children.
If vomiting is unsuccessful, gastric lavage is indicated within 3 hours after ingestion, and even later if large amounts of milk or cream were given beforehand. Isotonic and ½ isotonic saline is the lavage solution of choice.
Saline cathartics, such as milk of magnesia, draw water by osmosis into the bowel and therefore are valuable for their action in rapid dilution of bowel content.
Stimulants should *not* be used. Vasopressors may be used to treat hypotension.

DOSAGE AND ADMINISTRATION

1 drop per 2 pounds of body weight administered orally 4 times daily. The prescribed number of drops may be put directly into child's mouth or on a spoon for administration.

HOW SUPPLIED

TRIAMINIC Oral Infant Drops, in 15 ml plastic squeeze bottles which deliver approximately 24 drops per ml. Store TRIAMINIC Oral Infant Drops at room temperature.

TRIAMINIC® SYRUP   OTC
[trī"ah-mĭn'ĭc]
For Colds and Allergies

(See PDR For Nonprescription Drugs.)

TRIAMINIC–DM® SYRUP   OTC
[trī"ah-mĭn'ĭc]
Cough Relief Without Alcohol

(See PDR For Nonprescription Drugs.)

TRIAMINIC-12® MAXIMUM STRENGTH   OTC
12 HOUR RELIEF
[trī"ah-mĭn'ĭc]
Cold and Allergy Tablets

(See PDR For Nonprescription Drugs.)

TRIAMINICIN® COLD, ALLERGY,   OTC
SINUS MEDICINE
[trī"ah-mĭn'ĭ-sĭn]
Multisymptom Tablets

(See PDR For Nonprescription Drugs.)

TRIAMINICOL® MULTI-SYMPTOM   OTC
COLD AND COUGH MEDICINE
[trī"ah-mĭn'ĭ-call]

(See PDR For Nonprescription Drugs.)

TRIAMINICOL® MULTI-SYMPTOM   OTC
RELIEF
[trī"ah-mĭn'ĭ-call]
When the Cold Comes With a Cough

(See PDR For Nonprescription Drugs.)

Sandoz Pharmaceuticals Corp.
Dorsey Division
Sandoz Division
ROUTE 10
EAST HANOVER, NJ 07936

ASBRON G® Elixir and   ℞
[az'bron]
ASBRON G® Inlay-Tabs®   ℞

The following prescribing information is based on official labeling in effect on August 1, 1992.

DESCRIPTION

Each ASBRON G® Inlay-Tab® and tablespoonful (15 ml) of ASBRON G® Elixir contains: theophylline sodium glycinate 300 mg (equivalent to 150 mg theophylline), guaifenesin 100 mg. The elixir supplies the active ingredients in a solution containing 15% alcohol by volume. ASBRON G® contains a bronchodilator and an expectorant.

Theophylline sodium glycinate, a methylxanthine, is a white crystalline powder that is freely soluble in water, has a slight ammoniacal odor and a bitter taste. It is an equimolar mixture of theophylline sodium and glycine buffered by an additional mole of the essential amino acid, glycine.

The expectorant component is guaifenesin (formerly called glyceryl guaiacolate) which helps loosen and thus clear the bronchial passageways of bothersome, thickened mucus. Guaifenesin, 3-(o-methoxyphenoxy)-1,2-propanediol, occurs as a fine, white powder having a bitter, aromatic taste and a slight odor of guaiacol. The powder tends to become lumpy on storage. It is freely soluble in alcohol and soluble in water.

Asbron G® Elixir
Active Ingredients: Guaifenesin USP and Theophylline Sodium Glycinate USP.
Inactive Ingredients: Alcohol, Benzoic Acid, Blue 1, Citric Acid, Natural and Artificial Flavorings, Purified Water, Saccharin, Saccharin Sodium, Sodium Chloride, Sorbitol, Sucrose and Yellow 10.

Asbron G® Inlay Tabs®
Active Ingredients: Guaifenesin USP and Theophylline Sodium Glycinate USP.
Inactive Ingredients: Blue 1, Calcium Stearate, Calcium Sulfate, Colloidal Silicon Dioxide, Sodium Starch Glycolate, Starch, Stearic Acid, Sucrose and Yellow 10.

CLINICAL PHARMACOLOGY

Theophylline sodium glycinate is more stable in the presence of hydrochloric acid due to the buffering action of glycine with subsequent reduction of the chance of theophylline precipitation in the stomach. This and the high solubility of the product are suggested as the reasons why this product has better gastric tolerance than aminophylline.

Theophylline, the active ingredient of theophylline sodium glycinate, accounts for 50% of the weight of this compound. Theophylline sodium glycinate is highly effective in relaxing the smooth muscle of the bronchioles and the pulmonary blood vessels, thus acting primarily as a bronchodilator, pulmonary vasodilator and smooth muscle relaxant. Like other xanthines, theophylline sodium glycinate is a coronary vasodilator, a diuretic, a cerebral, cardiac and skeletal muscle stimulant.

Theophylline acts by inhibiting phosphodiesterase which causes an increase in intracellular cyclic AMP. This action produces smooth muscle relaxation and inhibits the release of histamine and other bronchoconstricting mediators from mast cells.

In vitro, using human white blood cells, theophylline has been shown to react synergistically with beta agonists to increase intracellular cyclic AMP. More data is required to clearly establish if theophylline and the beta agonists are synergistic or additive in vivo.

Even after prolonged therapy, it has not been possible to demonstrate the development of tolerance to theophylline sodium glycinate.

The half-life of theophylline varies from individual to individual. Since effective bronchodilatation depends upon maintaining serum theophylline levels between 10-20 mg/dl (10-20 mcg/ml), the determination of serum theophylline can be of value.

The half-life of theophylline is prolonged in alcoholism, in patients with reduced hepatic or renal function, congestive heart failure and in patients receiving antibiotics such as triacetyloleandomycin, erythromycin, clindamycin and lincomycin. Fever can also prolong theophylline half-life.

Cigarette smoking (1-2 packs per day) enhances theophylline elimination. The half-life of theophylline is shortened with cigarette smoking. This effect is probably related to the induction of enzymes and requires between three months and two years to normalize after stopping tobacco usage.

By increasing respiratory tract fluid, guaifenesin reduces the viscosity of tenacious secretions and acts as an expectorant. The drug is effective in productive as well as nonproductive cough, but is of particular value in dry, nonproduc-

THEOPHYLLINE ELIMINATION CHARACTERISTICS

Group	Theophylline Renal Clearance Rates	Half-Life Average
1. Children	1.4 ml/kg/min	3.5 hours
2. Adults with uncomplicated asthma	1.2 ml/kg/min	7 hours
3. Older Adults with chronic obstructive pulmonary disease	0.6 ml/kg/min	up to 24 hours
4. Adults with chronic obstructive pulmonary disease and cor pulmonale or other causes of heart failure and liver pathology	0.6 ml/kg/min and less	may exceed 24 hours
5. Young smokers	Not available	4.3 hours

Drug	Effect
Aminophylline with Lithium Carbonate	Increased excretion of Lithium Carbonate
Aminophylline with Propranolol	Antagonism of Propranolol effect
Theophylline with Furosemide	Increased Diuresis
Theophylline with Hexamethonium	Decreased Hexamethonium-induced chronotropic effect
Theophylline with Reserpine	Reserpine-induced Tachycardia
Theophylline with Cimetidine	Increased theophylline blood levels
Theophylline with clindamycin, troleandomycin, erythromycin, lincomycin	Increased theophylline blood levels

tive cough which tends to injure the mucous membranes of the air passages.
[See top table.]

INDICATIONS AND USAGE
For relief of acute bronchial asthma and for reversible bronchospasm associated with chronic bronchitis and emphysema.

CONTRAINDICATIONS
Asbron G® Inlay-Tabs® and Asbron G® Elixir are contraindicated in individuals who have shown hypersensitivity to any of the components.

WARNINGS
There is an excellent correlation between high theophylline blood levels and the clinical manifestations of toxicity in (1) patients with lowered body plasma clearances (due to transient cardiac decomposition), (2) chronic obstructive lung disease or patients with liver dysfunction, (3) patients who are older than 55 years of age, particularly males.
There are often no early signs of theophylline toxicity such as nausea and restlessness which may appear in up to 50% of patients. Convulsions or ventricular arrhythmias may be the first signs of toxicity.
Excessive doses of theophylline sodium glycinate may be expected to be toxic and serum theophylline levels are recommended to monitor therapy. The incidence of toxicity increases significantly at levels greater than 20 mcg/ml. Many patients who have higher theophylline serum levels exhibit tachycardia. Theophylline products often worsen preexisting arrhythmias.
Asbron G® Inlay-Tabs®, Asbron G® Elixir and other oral theophylline compounds should never be used to treat status asthma.

PRECAUTIONS
General: Theophylline should be used with caution in patients with severe cardiovascular disease, severe hypoxemia, hypertension, hyperthyroidism, acute myocardial injury, obstructive lung disease, liver disease, in the elderly and in neonates.
Great caution should be used in giving theophylline to patients in congestive heart failure. Such patients have markedly prolonged theophylline blood levels which have persisted for long periods after discontinuation of the drug. Smokers have a shorter mean half-life of theophylline than nonsmokers and may require larger doses of theophylline.

Theophylline sodium glycinate should not be administered concurrently with other theophylline containing products. Theophylline should be given with caution to patients with a history of peptic ulcer. Theophylline may act as a local irritant in the gastrointestinal tract.
Information for Patients: The importance of adherence to the prescribed dosage regimen should be stressed. Patients should be informed of symptoms associated with theophylline toxicity such as nausea and restlessness.
Laboratory Tests: There is great patient-to-patient variation in the serum half-life of theophylline. Therefore, when possible, serum theophylline levels should be measured to assist in titration of dosage.
Drug Interactions: The use of theophylline sodium glycinate with ephedrine and other sympathomimetic bronchodilators may result in a significant increase in side effects. [See second table above.]

Drug/Laboratory Test Interactions
Theophylline has been shown to increase the urinary excretion of catecholamines. The VMA test for catechols may be falsely elevated by guaifenesin. Theophylline may increase the apparent serum uric acid in certain manual or automated chemical procedures by being treated as if it were uric acid. Guaifenesin may increase renal clearance for urate and thereby lower the serum uric acid. It may also falsely elevate the level of urinary 5HIAA in certain serotonin metabolite chemical tests.

Carcinogenesis, Mutagenesis, Impairment of Fertility: No data are available on the long-term potential for carcinogenicity, mutagenicity or impairment of fertility in animals or humans.

Pregnancy: *Pregnancy Category C*—Animal reproduction studies have not been conducted with ASBRON G®. Safe use in pregnancy has not been established relative to possible adverse effects in fetal development.
Therefore, theophylline should not be used in pregnant patients unless, in the judgment of the physician, the potential benefits outweigh possible hazards.

Nursing Mothers: It is not known whether this drug is excreted in human milk. Because many drugs are excreted in human milk, caution should be observed when Asbron G® Inlay-Tabs® or Asbron G® Elixir is administered to a nursing mother.
Pediatric Use: See Dosage and Administration Section for mg/kg dosage in pediatric patients.

ADVERSE REACTIONS
Included in this listing which follows are adverse reactions, some of which may have been reported with theophylline sodium glycinate. However, pharmacological similarities among the xanthine drugs require that each of the reactions be considered when theophylline is administered. The most consistent adverse reactions are usually due to overdosage of theophylline sodium glycinate and are:

1. Gastrointestinal: nausea, vomiting, epigastric pain, hematemesis, diarrhea.
2. Central Nervous System: headaches, irritability, restlessness, insomnia, reflex hyperexcitability, muscle twitching, clonic and tonic generalized convulsions.
3. Cardiovascular: palpitation, tachycardia, extrasystoles, flushing hypotension, circulatory failure, life-threatening ventricular arrhythmias.
4. Respiratory: tachypnea.
5. Renal: albuminuria, increased excretion of renal tubular cells and red blood cells: potentiation of diuresis.
6. Others: hyperglycemia and inappropriate ADH syndrome.

OVERDOSAGE (Management)
A. If potential oral overdose is established and seizure has not occurred: (1) induce vomiting and resort to gastric lavage if the patient fails to vomit within 20-30 minutes; (2) administer a cathartic (this is particularly important if sustained-release preparations have been taken) and activated charcoal after successful vomiting has been induced or adequate gastric lavage performed.
B. If patient is having a seizure: (1) establish an airway; (2) administer O_2; (3) treat the seizure with intravenous diazepam 0.1 to 0.3 mg/kg up to 10 mg; (4) monitor vital signs, maintain blood pressure and provide adequate hydration.
C. Post-Seizure Coma: (1) maintain airway and oxygenation; (2) if a result of oral medication, follow above recommendations to prevent absorption of drug, but tracheal intubation and lavage will have to be performed instead of inducing emesis, and the cathartic and charcoal will need to be introduced via a large bore gastric lavage tube; (3) continue to provide full supportive care and adequate hydration while waiting for drug to be metabolized. In general, the drug is metabolized sufficiently rapidly so as to not warrant consideration of dialysis.

DOSAGE AND ADMINISTRATION
Therapeutic serum levels associated with optimal likelihood for benefit and minimal risk of toxicity are between 10-20 mcg/ml. There is great variation from patient to patient in the dosage of theophylline needed to achieve a therapeutic blood level because of variable rates of elimination. Because of this and because of the relatively narrow therapeutic blood level range associated with optimal results, the monitoring of serum theophylline levels is highly recommended. (See Laboratory Tests)
Usual Dosage: Adults—1 or 2 tablets or tablespoonfuls (15-30 ml), 3 or 4 times daily. Children 6 to 12—2 or 3 teaspoonfuls (10-15 ml), 3 or 4 times daily. Children 3 to 6—1 to 1½ teaspoonfuls (5-7.5 ml), 3 or 4 times daily. Children 1 to 3—½ to 1 teaspoonful (2.5-5 ml), 3 or 4 times daily.

Dosage Titration: [See table below.]

A. **FOR PATIENTS NOT CURRENTLY RECEIVING THEOPHYLLINE PRODUCTS:**

B. **FOR PATIENTS CURRENTLY RECEIVING THEOPHYLLINE PRODUCTS:** Determine, where possible, the time, amount, route of administration and form of the patient's last dose of theophylline.

The loading dose for theophylline will be based on the principle that each 0.5 mg/kg of theophylline administered as a loading dose will result in a 1 mcg/ml increase in serum theophylline concentration. Ideally, then, the loading dose should be deferred if a serum theophylline concentration can be rapidly obtained. If this is not possible, the clinician must exercise his judgment in selecting a dose based on the potential for benefit and risk. When there is sufficient respiratory distress to warrant a small risk, 2.5 mg/kg of theophylline is likely to increase the serum concentration when administered as a loading dose in rapidly absorbed form by only about 5 mcg/ml. If the patient is not already experiencing theophylline toxicity, this is unlikely to result in dangerous adverse effects.
Measurement of serum theophylline concentration during chronic therapy: Blood for peak theophylline determinations should be obtained 1-2 hours after a dose of theophylline sodium glycinate. When determining theophylline serum concentrations in patients who have received chronic therapy, it is essential to establish that no doses were omitted in the 48 hours prior to the determination. Missed doses

	Oral Loading Dose (Theophylline Sodium Glycinate)	Maintenance Dose For Next 12 Hours (Theophylline Sodium Glycinate)	Maintenance Dose Beyond 12 Hours (Theophylline Sodium Glycinate)
1. Infants	8 mg/kg *(4 mg/kg)	3-8 mg/kg q6h *(1.5-4.0 mg/kg q6h)	4-6 mg/kg q6h *(2-3 mg/kg q6h)**
2. Children 6 months to 9 years	12 mg/kg *(6 mg/kg)	8 mg/kg q4h *(4 mg/kg q4h)	8 mg/kg q6h *(4 mg/kg q6h)
3. Children age 9-16 and young adult smokers	12 mg/kg *(6 mg/kg)	6 mg/kg q4h *(3 mg/kg q4h)	6 mg/kg q6h *(3 mg/kg q6h)
4. Otherwise healthy nonsmoking adults	12 mg/kg *(6 mg/kg)	6 mg/kg q6h *(3 mg/kg q6h)	6 mg/kg q8h *(3 mg/kg q8h)
5. Older patients and patients with Cor pulmonale	12 mg/kg *(6 mg/kg)	4 mg/kg q6h *(2 mg/kg q6h)	4 mg/kg q8h *(2 mg/kg q8h)
6. Patients with congestive heart failure, liver failure	12 mg/kg *(6 mg/kg)	4 mg/kg q8h *(2 mg/kg q8h)	2-4 mg/kg q12h *(1-2 mg/kg q12h)

Equivalent theophylline dosage indicated in parenthesis and marked with an (*).
** PEDIATRICS, Vol. 55, No. 5, May, 1975.

Continued on next page

Sandoz—Cont.

Age	Theophylline Sodium Glycinate	Equivalent Theophylline
Under 9 years	48 mg/kg/day	24 mg/kg/day
9-12 years	40 mg/kg/day	20 mg/kg/day
12-16 years	36 mg/kg/day	18/mg/kg/day
Over 16 years	26 mg/kg/day or 1800 mg/day (WHICHEVER IS LESS)	13 mg/kg/day or 900 mg/day (WHICHEVER IS LESS)

could result in recommendations of future doses that would cause serious toxicity due to overdosage.

DOSAGE ADJUSTMENT BASED ON SERUM THEOPHYLLINE MEASUREMENTS WHEN THESE INSTRUCTIONS HAVE NOT BEEN FOLLOWED MAY RESULT IN RECOMMENDATIONS THAT PRESENT RISK OF TOXICITY TO THE PATIENT.

PATIENTS SHOULD NEVER BE MAINTAINED ON A DOSAGE OF THEOPHYLLINE THAT IS NOT WELL TOLERATED. Patients experiencing toxic side effects should be instructed to skip the next regular dose and to resume theophylline therapy at a lower dosage when all side effects have disappeared.

Maximum Dose Without Measurement of Serum Concentration: Not to exceed the following: (WARNING: DO NOT ATTEMPT TO MAINTAIN ANY DOSAGE THAT IS NOT WELL TOLERATED.)

[See table above.]

Use ideal (lean) body weight for obese patients in computing dosage.

Dosage should always be calculated on the basis of ideal (lean) body weight when mg/kg doses are stated. Theophylline does not distribute into fatty tissues. NEVER ATTEMPT TO MAINTAIN A DOSAGE THAT IS NOT WELL TOLERATED BY THE PATIENT.

HOW SUPPLIED

Asbron G® Inlay-Tabs®, green, round, compressed tablet with white inlay, imprinted "Asbron G" on one side, "78-202" on the other. In bottles of 100. Asbron G® Elixir, green, in pint bottles.

CAUTION: Federal law prohibits dispensing without prescription.

[ASB-Z3 Issued June 22, 1987]

BELLERGAL-S® ℞
[bel'er-gal]
TABLETS

CAUTION: Federal law prohibits dispensing without prescription.

The following prescribing information is based on official labeling in effect on August 1, 1992.

AUTONOMIC STABILIZER

DESCRIPTION

Each Bellergal-S® tablet contains: phenobarbital, USP, (Warning: may be habit forming), 40 mg; ergotamine tartrate, USP, 0.6 mg; Bellafoline® (levorotatory alkaloids of belladonna) 0.2 mg.

Inactive Ingredients: colloidal silicon dioxide, color additives including FD&C Blue #1, FD&C Red #40, FD&C Yellow #5, FD&C Yellow #6(Sunset Yellow), gelatin, lactose, magnesium stearate, malic acid, polyvinyl acetate resins, stearic acid, sucrose and tartaric acid.

CLINICAL PHARMACOLOGY

Based on the concept that functional disorders frequently involve hyperactivity of both the sympathetic and parasympathetic nervous systems, the ingredients in Bellergal-S are combined to provide a balanced preparation designed to correct imbalance of the autonomic nervous system. The integrated action of Bellergal-S is effected through the combined administration of ergotamine and the levorotatory alkaloids of belladonna, specific inhibitors of the sympathetic and parasympathetic respectively, reinforced by the synergistic action of phenobarbital in dampening the cortical centers. It should be noted that on a weight basis the levorotatory alkaloids of belladonna have approximately twice the pharmacological effects as do the usual racemic mixtures.

INDICATIONS AND USAGE

Bellergal-S is employed in the management of disorders characterized by nervous tension and exaggerated autonomic response: *Menopausal disorders* with hot flushes, sweats, restlessness and insomnia; *cardiovascular disorders* with palpitation, tachycardia, chest oppression and vasomotor disturbances; *gastrointestinal disorders* with hypermotility, hypersecretion, "nervous stomach," and alternately diarrhea and constipation; interval treatment of *recurrent, throbbing headache.*

CONTRAINDICATIONS

Peripheral vascular disease, coronary heart disease, hypertension, impaired hepatic or renal function, sepsis, pregnancy, nursing mothers and glaucoma. The concomitant administration of ergotamine and dopamine should be avoided, due to the increased potential for ischemic vasoconstriction. Phenobarbital is contraindicated in patients with a history of manifest or latent porphyria. Phenobarbital is contraindicated in those patients in whom the drug produces restlessness and/or excitement. Bellergal-S is contraindicated in patients with a demonstrated hypersensitivity to any of the components.

WARNINGS

Total weekly dosage of ergotamine tartrate should not exceed 10 mg. (This dosage corresponds to 16 Bellergal-S tablets.) Due to the presence of a barbiturate, may be habit forming.

PRECAUTIONS

Even though the ergotamine tartrate content of this product is low and untoward effects have been rare and of minor significance, caution should be exercised if large or prolonged dosage is contemplated, and physicians should be alert to possible peripheral vascular complications in patients sensitive to ergot. Due to the presence of the anticholinergic agent, special caution should be exercised in the use of this drug in patients with bronchial asthma or obstructive uropathy.

Bellergal-S contains FD&C Yellow #5 (tartrazine) which may cause allergic-type reactions (including bronchial asthma) in certain susceptible individuals. Although the overall incidence of FD&C Yellow #5 (tartrazine) sensitivity in the general population is low, it is frequently seen in patients who also have aspirin hypersensitivity.

Information for Patients

Patients on large or prolonged dosage should be asked to report numbness or tingling of extremities, claudication or other symptoms of peripheral vasoconstriction.

Drug Interaction

1. *Oral Anticoagulants:* Phenobarbital may lower the plasma levels of dicumarol (name previously used: bishydroxycoumarin) and may cause a decrease in anticoagulant activity as measured by the prothrombin time. More frequent monitoring of prothrombin time responses is indicated whenever phenobarbital is initiated or discontinued, and the dosage of anticoagulants should be adjusted accordingly.

2. *CNS Depressants:* Combined administration of phenobarbital and CNS depressants such as alcohol, tricyclic antidepressants, phenothiazines and narcotic analgesics may result in a potentiation of the depressant action.

3. *Beta Adrenergic Blocking Agents:* Although proof is lacking, several reports in the literature suggest a possible interaction between ergot alkaloids and beta adrenergic blocking agents. This interaction may result in excessive vasoconstriction. Although many patients can apparently take propranolol and ergot alkaloids without ill effects, there is enough evidence of an interaction to dictate closer surveillance of patients so treated.

4. *Hepatic Metabolism:* Through the mechanism of enzyme induction caused by phenobarbital, a number of substances have been shown to be metabolized at an increased rate. In these cases, clinical responses should be closely monitored and appropriate dosage adjustments made. Included are such substances as griseofulvin, quinidine, doxycycline and estrogen. Although the meaning of published reports regarding the effects of phenobarbital on estrogen metabolism are unclear at this time, if avoidance of pregnancy is critical, consideration should be given to alternative methods of contraception.

5. *Phenytoin, Sodium Valproate, Valproic Acid:* The effect of barbiturates on the metabolism of phenytoin appears to be variable. Some investigators report an accelerating effect, while others report no effect. Because the effect of barbiturates on the metabolism of phenytoin is not predictable, phenytoin and barbiturate blood levels should be monitored more frequently if these drugs are given concurrently. Sodium valproate and valproic acid appear to decrease barbiturate metabolism; therefore, barbiturate blood levels should be monitored and appropriate dosage adjustments made as indicated.

6. *Tricyclic Antidepressants:* Due to the presence of levorotatory alkaloids of belladonna, concomitant administration of tricyclic antidepressants may result in additive anticholinergic effects.

Carcinogenesis

No data are available on the long-term potential for carcinogenicity in animals or humans.

Pregnancy

Pregnancy Category X—due to the potential uterotonic effects of the ergot alkaloids, the use of Bellergal-S® during pregnancy is contraindicated. See "Contraindications" section.

Nursing Mothers

A number of ergot alkaloids inhibit the secretion of prolactin. Therefore, Bellergal-S is contraindicated in nursing mothers. See "Contraindications" section.

Pediatric Use

Safety and effectiveness in children have not been established.

ADVERSE REACTIONS

Tingling and other paresthesias of the extremities, blurred vision, palpitations, dry mouth, decreased sweating, decreased gastrointestinal motility, urinary retention, tachycardia, flushing, and drowsiness occur rarely.

DRUG ABUSE AND DEPENDENCE

Barbiturates may be habit-forming. Tolerance, psychological dependence, and physical dependence may occur especially following prolonged use of high doses. Daily administration in excess of 400 mg of pentobarbital or secobarbital for approximately 90 days is likely to produce some degree of physical dependence. By way of comparison, the phenobarbital component of Bellergal-S at the highest recommended daily dosage amounts to 80 mg.

OVERDOSAGE

Management of Overdosage: While severe symptoms of overdosage with Bellergal-S have not been reported, theoretically they could occur. It is imperative to note that overdosage symptoms with Bellergal-S may be attributable to any one or more of the three active ingredients. Which toxic manifestation might predominate in any individual case would be impossible to predict but one should be alert to the various possibilities. When anticholinergic/antispasmodic drugs are taken in sufficient overdose to produce such severe symptoms, prompt treatment should be instituted. Gastric lavage and other measures to limit intestinal absorption should be initiated without delay.

Cholinesterase inhibitors administered parenterally may be necessary for treatment of the serious manifestations of anticholinergic overdosage. Additionally, symptomatic therapy, including oxygen, sedatives and control of hyperthermia may be necessary.

Acute barbiturate overdosage symptoms with Bellergal-S, while possible, have not been reported. While the usual procedures for handling barbiturate poisoning should be employed, keep in mind the possibility of anticholinergic overdosing effects.

Acute ergot overdosage symptoms with Bellergal-S, while possible, have not been reported. The usual procedures for handling ergot overdosage include the administration of a peripheral vasodilator to counteract the vasospasm.

DOSAGE AND ADMINISTRATION

One tablet in the morning and one tablet in the evening.

HOW SUPPLIED

Compressed tablets of tri-colored pattern: dark green, orange and light lemon yellow, scored on one side, embossed "78-31" on other side, in bottles of 100. (NDC #0078-0031-05)

[BEG-Z15 Issued May 1, 1987]

Shown in Product Identification Section, page 427

CAFERGOT® ℞
[kaf'er-got]
(ergotamine tartrate and caffeine) TABLETS, USP
(ergotamine tartrate and caffeine) SUPPOSITORIES, USP

CAUTION: Federal law prohibits dispensing without prescription.

The following prescribing information is based on official labeling in effect on August 1, 1992.

DESCRIPTION

CAFERGOT®

(ergotamine tartrate and caffeine) Tablet

ergotamine tartrate USP	1 mg
caffeine USP	100 mg

Inactive Ingredients: acacia, carnauba wax, lactose, methylparaben, povidone, propylparaben, sodium benzoate, sorbitol, starch, stearic acid, sucrose, synthetic black ferric oxide, synthetic red ferric oxide, synthetic yellow ferric oxide, talc, tartaric acid, and titanium dioxide.

CAFERGOT®
(ergotamine tartrate and caffeine) Suppository

ergotamine tartrate USP	2 mg
caffeine USP	100 mg

Inactive Ingredients: cocoa butter NF and tartaric acid NF.
CAFERGOT® (ergotamine tartrate and caffeine) suppositories are *sealed* in foil to afford protection from cocoa butter leakage. If an unavoidable period of exposure to heat softens the suppository, it should be chilled in ice-cold water to solidify it before removing the foil.

CLINICAL PHARMACOLOGY

Ergotamine is an alpha adrenergic blocking agent with a direct stimulating effect on the smooth muscle of peripheral and cranial blood vessels and produces depression of central vasomotor centers. The compound also has the properties of serotonin antagonism. In comparison to hydrogenated ergotamine, the adrenergic blocking actions are less pronounced and vasoconstrictive actions are greater.
Caffeine, also a cranial vasoconstrictor, is added to further enhance the vasoconstrictive effect without the necessity of increasing ergotamine dosage.
Many migraine patients experience excessive nausea and vomiting during attacks, making it impossible for them to retain any oral medication. In such cases, therefore, the only practical means of medication is through the rectal route where medication may reach the cranial vessels directly, evading the splanchnic vasculature and the liver.

INDICATIONS AND USAGE

Cafergot® (ergotamine tartrate and caffeine)
Indicated as therapy to abort or prevent vascular headache, e.g., migraine, migraine variants or so-called "histaminic cephalalgia".

CONTRAINDICATIONS

CAFERGOT® (ergotamine tartrate and caffeine) may cause fetal harm when administered to pregnant women. CAFERGOT® (ergotamine tartrate and caffeine) is contraindicated in women who are or may become pregnant. If this drug is used during pregnancy or if the patient becomes pregnant while taking this product, the patient should be apprised of the potential hazard to the fetus.
Peripheral vascular disease, coronary heart disease, hypertension, impaired hepatic or renal function and sepsis.
Hypersensitivity to any of the components.

PRECAUTIONS

General
Although signs and symptoms of ergotism rarely develop even after long term intermittent use of the orally or rectally administered drugs, care should be exercised to remain within the limits of recommended dosage.
Ergotism is manifested by intense arterial vasoconstriction, producing signs and symptoms of peripheral vascular ischemia. Ergotamine induces vasoconstriction by a direct action on vascular smooth muscle. In chronic intoxication with ergot derivatives, headache, intermittent claudication, muscle pains, numbness, coldness and pallor of the digits may occur. If the condition is allowed to progress untreated, gangrene can result.
While most cases of ergotism associated with ergotamine treatment result from frank overdosage, some cases have involved apparent hypersensitivity. There are few reports of ergotism among patients taking doses within the recommended limits or for brief periods of time. In rare instances, patients, particularly those who have used the medication indiscriminately over long periods of time, may display withdrawal symptoms consisting of rebound headache upon discontinuation of the drug.
Rare cases of a solitary rectal or anal ulcer have occurred from abuse of ergotamine suppositories usually in higher than recommended doses or with continual use at the recommended dose for many years. Spontaneous healing occurs within usually 4-8 weeks after drug withdrawal.
Information for Patients
Patients should be advised that two tablets or one suppository of CAFERGOT® (ergotamine tartrate and caffeine) should be taken at the first sign of a migraine headache. No more than 6 tablets or 2 suppositories should be taken for any single migraine attack. No more than 10 tablets or 5 suppositories should be taken during any 7-day period. CAFERGOT® (ergotamine tartrate and caffeine) should be used only for migraine headaches. It is not effective for other types of headaches and it lacks analgesic properties. Patients should be advised to report to the physician immediately any of the following: numbness or tingling in the fingers and toes, muscle pain in the arms and legs, weakness in the legs, pain in the chest or temporary speeding or slowing of the heart rate, swelling or itching.
Drug Interactions
CAFERGOT® (ergotamine tartrate and caffeine) should not be administered with other vasoconstrictors. Use with sympathomimetics (pressor agents) may cause extreme elevation of blood pressure. The beta-blocker Inderal (propranolol) has been reported to potentiate the vasoconstrictive action of CAFERGOT® (ergotamine tartrate and caffeine) by blocking the vasodilating property of epinephrine. Nicotine may provoke vasoconstriction in some patients, predisposing to a greater ischemic response to ergot therapy.
The blood levels of ergotamine-containing drugs are reported to be elevated by the concomitant administration of macrolide antibiotics and vasospastic reactions have been reported with therapeutic doses of the ergotamine-containing drugs when coadministered with these antibiotics.
Pregnancy
Teratogenic Effects
Pregnancy Category X: There are no studies on the placental transfer or teratogenicity of the combined products of CAFERGOT® (ergotamine tartrate and caffeine). Caffeine is known to cross the placenta and has been shown to be teratogenic in animals. Ergotamine crosses the placenta in small amounts, although it does not appear to be embryotoxic in this quantity. However, prolonged vasoconstriction of the uterine vessels and/or increased myometrial tone leading to reduced myometrial and placental blood flow may have contributed to fetal growth retardation observed in animals. (*See CONTRAINDICATIONS*)
Nonteratogenic Effects
CAFERGOT® (ergotamine tartrate and caffeine) is contraindicated in pregnancy due to the oxytocic effects of ergotamine. (*See CONTRAINDICATIONS*)
Labor and Delivery
CAFERGOT® (ergotamine tartrate and caffeine) is contraindicated in labor and delivery due to its oxytocic effect which is maximal in the third trimester. (*See CONTRAINDICATIONS*)
Nursing Mothers
Ergot drugs are known to inhibit prolactin but there are no reports of decreased lactation with CAFERGOT® (ergotamine tartrate and caffeine). Ergotamine is excreted in breast milk and may cause symptoms of vomiting, diarrhea, weak pulse and unstable blood pressure in nursing infants. Because of the potential for serious adverse reactions in nursing infants from CAFERGOT® (ergotamine tartrate and caffeine), a decision should be made whether to discontinue nursing or discontinue the drug, taking into account the importance of the drug to the mother.
Pediatric Use
Safety and effectiveness in children have not been established.

ADVERSE REACTIONS

Cardiovascular: Vasoconstrictive complications of a serious nature may occur at times. These include ischemia, cyanosis, absence of pulse, cold extremities, gangrene, precordial distress and pain, EKG changes and muscle pains. Although these effects occur most commonly with long-term therapy at relatively high doses, they have also been reported with short-term or normal doses. Other cardiovascular adverse effects include transient tachycardia or bradycardia and hypertension.
Gastrointestinal: Nausea and vomiting; rectal or anal ulcer (from overuse of suppositories).
Neurological: paresthesias, numbness, weakness, and vertigo.
Allergic: Localized edema and itching.
Miscellaneous: There have been a few reports of patients on CAFERGOT® (ergotamine tartrate and caffeine) therapy developing retroperitoneal and/or pleuropulmonary fibroses.

DRUG ABUSE AND DEPENDENCE

There have been reports of drug abuse and psychological dependence in patients on CAFERGOT® (ergotamine tartrate and caffeine) therapy. Due to the chronicity of vascular headaches, it is imperative that patients be advised not to exceed recommended dosages with long-term use to avoid ergotism. (*See PRECAUTIONS*)

OVERDOSAGE

The toxic effects of an acute overdosage of CAFERGOT® (ergotamine tartrate and caffeine) are due primarily to the ergotamine component. The amount of caffeine is such that its toxic effects will be overshadowed by those of ergotamine. Symptoms include vomiting, numbness, tingling, pain and cyanosis of the extremities associated with diminished or absent peripheral pulses; hypertension or hypotension; drowsiness, stupor, coma, convulsions and shock. A case has been reported of reversible bilateral papillitis with ring scotomata in a patient who received five times the recommended daily adult dose over a period of 14 days.
Treatment consists of removal of the offending drug by induction of emesis, gastric lavage, and catharsis. Maintenance of adequate pulmonary ventilation, correction of hypotension, and control of convulsions and blood pressure are important considerations. Treatment of peripheral vasospasm should consist of warmth, but not heat, and protection of the ischemic limbs. Vasodilators may be beneficial but caution must be exercised to avoid aggravating an already existent hypotension.

DOSAGE AND ADMINISTRATION

Procedure
For the best results, dosage should start at the first sign of an attack.

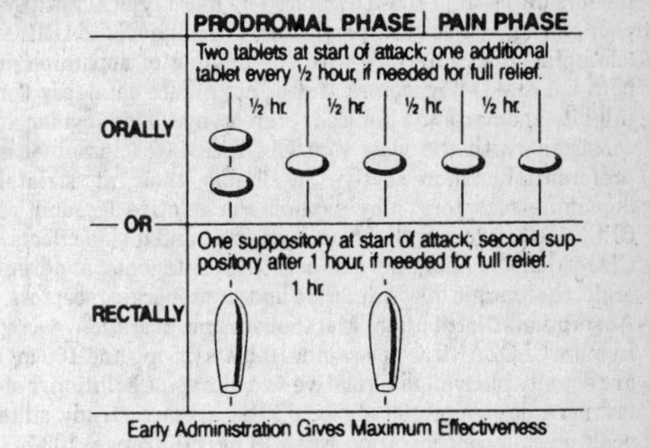
PRODROMAL PHASE | PAIN PHASE
Two tablets at start of attack; one additional tablet every ½ hour, if needed for full relief.
½ hr. ½ hr. ½ hr. ½ hr.
ORALLY
OR
One suppository at start of attack; second suppository after 1 hour, if needed for full relief.
1 hr.
RECTALLY
Early Administration Gives Maximum Effectiveness

MAXIMUM ADULT DOSAGE

Orally
Total dose for any one attack should not exceed 6 tablets.
Rectally
Two suppositories is the maximum dose for an individual attack.
Total weekly dosage should not exceed 10 tablets or 5 suppositories.
In carefully selected patients, with due consideration of maximum dosage recommendations, administration of the drug at bedtime may be an appropriate short-term preventive measure.

HOW SUPPLIED

CAFERGOT®
(ergotamine tartrate and caffeine) Tablets
Shell pink colored, sugar coated, imprinted "CAFERGOT" on one side, "S" on other side.
Bottles of 250 (NDC 0078-0034-28).
Cartons of three SigPak® (dispensing unit) packages, each containing 30 tablets in individual blisters (NDC 0078-0034-42).
Store and Dispense
Below 77°F (25°C); tight, light-resistant container.
CAFERGOT®
(ergotamine tartrate and caffeine) Suppositories
Sealed in fuchsia-colored aluminum foil, imprinted "S CAFERGOT® SUPPOSITORY 78-33 SANDOZ".
Boxes of 12 (NDC 0078-0033-02).
Store and Dispense
Below 77°F (25°C); tight container (sealed foil).
[CAF-Z27 Issued January 15, 1992]
Shown in Product Identification Section, page 427

CLOZARIL® ℞
[*klō 'ză-ril*]
(clozapine) TABLETS

CAUTION: Federal law prohibits dispensing without a prescription.
The following prescribing information is based on official labeling in effect on August 10, 1992.

DESCRIPTION

CLOZARIL® (clozapine), an atypical antipsychotic drug, is a tricyclic dibenzodiazepine derivative, 8-chloro-11-(4-methyl-1-piperazinyl)-5*H*-dibenzo [*b,e*] [1,4] diazepine.
The structural formula is:

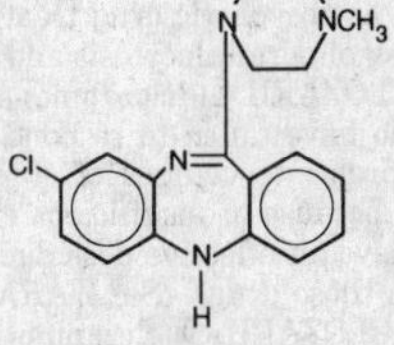
N
NCH3
Cl
N
N
H

$C_{18}H_{19}ClN_4$ Mol. wt. 326.83

CLOZARIL® (clozapine) is available in pale yellow tablets of 25 mg and 100 mg for oral administration.
25 mg and 100 mg Tablets
Active Ingredient: clozapine is a yellow, crystalline powder, very slightly soluble in water.
Inactive Ingredients: colloidal silicon dioxide, lactose, magnesium stearate, mineral oil, povidone, starch and talc.

CLINICAL PHARMACOLOGY

Pharmacodynamics
CLOZARIL® (clozapine) is classified as an 'atypical' antipsychotic drug because its profile of binding to dopamine

Continued on next page

Sandoz—Cont.

receptors and its effects on various dopamine mediated behaviors differ from those exhibited by more typical antipsychotic drug products. In particular, although CLOZARIL® (clozapine) does interfere with the binding of dopamine at both D-1 and D-2 receptors, it does not induce catalepsy nor inhibit apomorphine-induced stereotypy. This evidence, consistent with the view that CLOZARIL® (clozapine) is preferentially more active at limbic than at striatal dopamine receptors, may explain the relative freedom of CLOZARIL® (clozapine) from extrapyramidal side effects.
CLOZARIL® (clozapine) also acts as an antagonist at adrenergic, cholinergic, histaminergic and serotonergic receptors.

Absorption, Distribution, Metabolism and Excretion

In man, CLOZARIL® (clozapine) tablets (25 mg and 100 mg) are equally bioavailable relative to a clozapine solution. Following a dosage of 100 mg b.i.d., the average steady state peak plasma concentration was 319 ng/mL (range: 102-771 ng/mL), occurring at the average of 2.5 hours (range: 1-6 hours) after dosing. The average minimum concentration at steady state was 122 ng/mL (range: 41-343 ng/mL), after 100 mg b.i.d. dosing. Food does not appear to affect the systemic bioavailability of CLOZARIL® (clozapine). Thus, CLOZARIL® (clozapine) may be administered with or without food.

Clozapine is approximately 95% bound to serum proteins. The interaction between CLOZARIL® (clozapine) and other highly protein-bound drugs has not been fully evaluated but may be important. *(See PRECAUTIONS)*

Clozapine is almost completely metabolized prior to excretion and only trace amounts of unchanged drug are detected in the urine and feces. Approximately 50% of the administered dose is excreted in the urine and 30% in the feces. The demethylated, hydroxylated and N-oxide derivatives are components in both urine and feces. Pharmacological testing has shown the desmethyl metabolite to have only limited activity, while the hydroxylated and N-oxide derivatives were inactive.

The mean elimination half-life of clozapine after a single 75 mg dose was 8 hours (range: 4-12 hours), compared to a mean elimination half-life, after achieving steady state with 100 mg b.i.d. dosing, of 12 hours (range: 4-66 hours). A comparison of single-dose and multiple-dose administration of clozapine showed that the elimination half-life increased significantly after multiple dosing relative to that after single-dose administration, suggesting the possibility of concentration dependent pharmacokinetics. However, at steady state, linearly dose-proportional changes with respect to AUC (area under the curve), peak and minimum clozapine plasma concentrations were observed after administration of 37.5 mg, 75 mg, and 150 mg b.i.d.

Human Pharmacology

In contrast to more typical antipsychotic drugs, CLOZARIL® (clozapine) therapy produces little or no prolactin elevation.

As is true of more typical antipsychotic drugs, clinical EEG studies have shown that CLOZARIL® (clozapine) increases delta and theta activity and slows dominant alpha frequencies. Enhanced synchronization occurs, and sharp wave activity and spike and wave complexes may also develop. Patients on rare occasions may report an intensification of dream activity during CLOZARIL® (clozapine) therapy. REM sleep was found to be increased to 85% of the total sleep time. In these patients, the onset of REM sleep occurred almost immediately after falling asleep.

INDICATIONS AND USAGE

CLOZARIL® (clozapine) is indicated for the management of severely ill schizophrenic patients who fail to respond adequately to standard antipsychotic drug treatment. Because of the significant risk of agranulocytosis and seizure associated with its use, CLOZARIL® (clozapine) should be used only in patients who have failed to respond adequately to treatment with appropriate courses of standard antipsychotic drugs, either because of insufficient effectiveness or the inability to achieve an effective dose due to intolerable adverse effects from those drugs. *(See WARNINGS)*

The effectiveness of CLOZARIL® (clozapine) in a treatment resistant schizophrenic population was demonstrated in a 6-week study comparing CLOZARIL® (clozapine) and chlorpromazine. Patients meeting DSM-III criteria for schizophrenia and having a mean BPRS total score of 61 were demonstrated to be treatment resistant by history and by open, prospective treatment with haloperidol before entering into the double-blind phase of the study. The superiority of CLOZARIL® (clozapine) to chlorpromazine was documented in statistical analyses employing both categorical and continuous measures of treatment effect.

Because of the significant risk of agranulocytosis and seizure, events which both present a continuing risk over time, the extended treatment of patients failing to show an acceptable level of clinical response should ordinarily be avoided. In addition, the need for continuing treatment in patients exhibiting beneficial clinical responses should be periodically re-evaluated.

CONTRAINDICATIONS

CLOZARIL® (clozapine) is contraindicated in patients with myeloproliferative disorders, or a history of CLOZARIL® (clozapine)-induced agranulocytosis or severe granulocytopenia. CLOZARIL® (clozapine) should not be used simultaneously with other agents having a well-known potential to suppress bone marrow function. As with more typical antipsychotic drugs, CLOZARIL® (clozapine) is contraindicated in severe central nervous system depression or comatose states from any cause.

WARNINGS

General

BECAUSE OF THE SIGNIFICANT RISK OF AGRANULOCYTOSIS, A POTENTIALLY LIFE-THREATENING ADVERSE EVENT *(SEE FOLLOWING)*, CLOZARIL® (clozapine) SHOULD BE RESERVED FOR USE IN THE TREATMENT OF SEVERELY ILL SCHIZOPHRENIC PATIENTS WHO FAIL TO SHOW AN ACCEPTABLE RESPONSE TO ADEQUATE COURSES OF STANDARD ANTIPSYCHOTIC DRUG TREATMENT, EITHER BECAUSE OF INSUFFICIENT EFFECTIVENESS OR THE INABILITY TO ACHIEVE AN EFFECTIVE DOSE DUE TO INTOLERABLE ADVERSE EFFECTS FROM THOSE DRUGS. CONSEQUENTLY, BEFORE INITIATING TREATMENT WITH CLOZARIL® (clozapine), IT IS STRONGLY RECOMMENDED THAT A PATIENT BE GIVEN AT LEAST 2 TRIALS, EACH WITH A DIFFERENT STANDARD ANTIPSYCHOTIC DRUG PRODUCT, AT AN ADEQUATE DOSE, AND FOR AN ADEQUATE DURATION.

PATIENTS WHO ARE BEING TREATED WITH CLOZARIL® (clozapine) MUST HAVE A BASELINE WHITE BLOOD CELL (WBC) AND DIFFERENTIAL COUNT BEFORE INITIATION OF TREATMENT, AND A WBC COUNT EVERY WEEK THROUGHOUT TREATMENT, AND FOR 4 WEEKS AFTER THE DISCONTINUATION OF CLOZARIL® (clozapine).

CLOZARIL® (clozapine) IS AVAILABLE ONLY THROUGH A DISTRIBUTION SYSTEM THAT ENSURES WEEKLY WBC TESTING PRIOR TO DELIVERY OF THE NEXT WEEK'S SUPPLY OF MEDICATION.

Agranulocytosis

Agranulocytosis, defined as a granulocyte count (polys + bands) of less than 500/mm^3, has been estimated to occur in association with CLOZARIL® (clozapine) use at a cumulative incidence at 1 year of approximately 1.3%, based on the occurrence of 15 US cases out of 1743 patients exposed to CLOZARIL® (clozapine) during its clinical testing prior to domestic marketing. All of these cases occurred at a time when the need for close monitoring of WBC counts was already recognized. This reaction could prove fatal if not detected early and therapy interrupted. Of the 149 cases of agranulocytosis reported worldwide in association with CLOZARIL® (clozapine) use as of December 31, 1989, 32% were fatal. However, few of these deaths occurred since 1977, at which time the knowledge of CLOZARIL® (clozapine)-induced agranulocytosis became more widespread, and close monitoring of WBC counts more widely practiced. Nevertheless, it is unknown at present what the case fatality rate will be for CLOZARIL® (clozapine)-induced agranulocytosis, despite strict adherence to the recommendation for weekly monitoring of WBC counts. In the US, under a weekly WBC monitoring system in premarketing studies and in postmarketing experience with CLOZARIL® (clozapine), there have been 68 cases of agranulocytosis and one associated fatality as of January 1, 1991.

Because of the substantial risk of agranulocytosis in association with CLOZARIL® (clozapine) use, which may persist over an extended period of time, patients must have a blood sample drawn for a WBC count before initiation of treatment with CLOZARIL® (clozapine), and must have subsequent WBC counts done at least weekly for the duration of therapy, as well as for 4 weeks thereafter. The distribution of CLOZARIL® (clozapine) is contingent upon performance of the required blood tests.

Treatment should not be initiated if the WBC count is less than 3500/mm^3, or if the patient has a history of a myeloproliferative disorder, or previous CLOZARIL® (clozapine)-induced agranulocytosis or granulocytopenia. Patients should be advised to report immediately the appearance of lethargy, weakness, fever, sore throat or any other signs of infection. If, after the initiation of treatment, the total WBC count has dropped below 3500/mm^3 or it has dropped by a substantial amount from baseline, even if the count is above 3500/mm^3, or if immature forms are present, a repeat WBC count and a differential count should be done. If subsequent WBC counts and the differential count reveal a total WBC count between 3000 and 3500/mm^3 and a granulocyte count above 1500/mm^3, twice weekly WBC counts and differential counts should be performed.

If the total WBC count falls below 3000/mm^3 or the granulocyte count below 1500/mm^3, CLOZARIL® (clozapine) therapy should be interrupted, WBC count and differential should be performed daily, and patients should be carefully monitored for flu-like symptoms or other symptoms suggestive of infection. CLOZARIL® (clozapine) therapy may be resumed if no symptoms of infection develop, and if the total WBC count returns to levels above 3000/mm^3 and the granulocyte count returns to levels above 1500/mm^3. However, in this event, twice-weekly WBC counts and differential counts should continue until total WBC counts return to levels above 3500/mm^3.

If the total WBC count falls below 2000/mm^3 or the granulocyte count falls below 1000/mm^3, bone marrow aspiration should be considered to ascertain granulopoietic status. Protective isolation with close observation may be indicated if granulopoiesis is determined to be deficient. Should evidence of infection develop, the patient should have appropriate cultures performed and an appropriate antibiotic regimen instituted.

Patients whose total WBC counts fall below 2000/mm^3, or granulocyte counts below 1000/mm^3 during CLOZARIL® (clozapine) therapy should have daily WBC count and differential. These patients should not be re-challenged with CLOZARIL® (clozapine). Patients discontinued from CLOZARIL® (clozapine) therapy due to significant WBC suppression have been found to develop agranulocytosis upon re-challenge, often with a shorter latency on re-exposure. To reduce the chances of re-challenge occurring in patients who have experienced significant bone marrow suppression during CLOZARIL® (clozapine) therapy, a single, national master file will be maintained confidentially.

Except for evidence of significant bone marrow suppression during initial CLOZARIL® (clozapine) therapy, there are no established risk factors, based on worldwide experience, for the development of agranulocytosis in association with CLOZARIL® (clozapine) use. However, a disproportionate number of the US cases of agranulocytosis occurred in patients of Jewish background compared to the overall proportion of such patients exposed during domestic development of CLOZARIL® (clozapine). Most of the US cases occurred within 4-10 weeks of exposure, but neither dose nor duration is a reliable predictor of this problem. No patient characteristics have been clearly linked to the development of agranulocytosis in association with CLOZARIL® (clozapine) use, but agranulocytosis associated with other antipsychotic drugs has been reported to occur with a greater frequency in women, the elderly and in patients who are cachectic or have serious underlying medical illness; such patients may also be at particular risk with CLOZARIL® (clozapine).

To reduce the risk of agranulocytosis developing undetected, CLOZARIL® (clozapine) is available only through a distribution system that ensures weekly WBC testing prior to delivery of the next week's supply of medication.

Seizures

Seizure has been estimated to occur in association with CLOZARIL® (clozapine) use at a cumulative incidence at one year of approximately 5%, based on the occurrence of one or more seizures in 61 of 1743 patients exposed to CLOZARIL® (clozapine) during its clinical testing prior to domestic marketing (i.e., a crude rate of 3.5%). Dose appears to be an important predictor of seizure, with a greater likelihood of seizure at the higher CLOZARIL® (clozapine) doses used.

Caution should be used in administering CLOZARIL® (clozapine) to patients having a history of seizures or other predisposing factors. Because of the substantial risk of seizure associated with CLOZARIL® (clozapine) use, patients should be advised not to engage in any activity where sudden loss of consciousness could cause serious risk to themselves or others, e.g., the operation of complex machinery, driving an automobile, swimming, climbing, etc.

Adverse Cardiovascular and Respiratory Effects

Orthostatic hypotension with or without syncope can occur with CLOZARIL® (clozapine) treatment and may represent a continuing risk in some patients. Rarely (approximately 1 case per 3,000 patients), collapse can be profound and be accompanied by respiratory and/or cardiac arrest. Orthostatic hypotension is more likely to occur during initial titration in association with rapid dose escalation and may even occur on first dose. In one

report, initial doses as low as 12.5 mg were associated with collapse and respiratory arrest. When restarting patients who have had even a brief interval off CLOZARIL® (clozapine), i.e., 2 days or more since the last dose, it is recommended that treatment be reinitiated with one-half of a 25 mg tablet (12.5 mg) once or twice daily (see DOSAGE AND ADMINISTRATION). Some of the cases of collapse/respiratory arrest/cardiac arrest during initial treatment occurred in patients who were being administered benzodiazepines; similar events have been reported in patients taking other psychotropic drugs or even CLOZARIL® (clozapine) by itself. Although it has not been established that there is an interaction between CLOZARIL® (clozapine) and benzodiazepines or other psychotropics, caution is advised when clozapine is initiated in patients taking a benzodiazepine or any other psychotropic drug.

Tachycardia, which may be sustained, has also been observed in approximately 25% of patients taking CLOZARIL® (clozapine), with patients having an average increase in pulse rate of 10-15 bpm. The sustained tachycardia is not simply a reflex response to hypotension, and is present in all positions monitored. Either tachycardia or hypotension may pose a serious risk for an individual with compromised cardiovascular function.

A minority of CLOZARIL® (clozapine) treated patients experience ECG repolarization changes similar to those seen with other antipsychotic drugs, including S-T segment depression and flattening or inversion of T waves, which all normalize after discontinuation of CLOZARIL® (clozapine). The clinical significance of these changes is unclear. However, in clinical trials with CLOZARIL® (clozapine), several patients experienced significant cardiac events, including ischemic changes, myocardial infarction, nonfatal arrhythmias and sudden unexplained death. In addition there have been postmarketing reports of congestive heart failure and myocarditis in association with CLOZARIL® (clozapine) use. Causality assessment was difficult in many of these cases because of serious preexisting cardiac disease and plausible alternative causes. Rare instances of sudden, unexplained death have been reported in psychiatric patients, with or without associated antipsychotic drug treatment, and the relationship of these events to antipsychotic drug use is unknown.

CLOZARIL® (clozapine) should be used with caution in patients with known cardiovascular and/or pulmonary disease, and the recommendation for gradual titration of dose should be carefully observed.

Neuroleptic Malignant Syndrome (NMS)
A potentially fatal symptom complex sometimes referred to as Neuroleptic Malignant Syndrome (NMS) has been reported in association with antipsychotic drugs. Clinical manifestations of NMS are hyperpyrexia, muscle rigidity, altered mental status and evidence of autonomic instability (irregular pulse or blood pressure, tachycardia, diaphoresis, and cardiac dysrhythmias).

The diagnostic evaluation of patients with this syndrome is complicated. In arriving at a diagnosis, it is important to identify cases where the clinical presentation includes both serious medical illness (e.g., pneumonia, systemic infection, etc.) and untreated or inadequately treated extrapyramidal signs and symptoms (EPS). Other important considerations in the differential diagnosis include central anticholinergic toxicity, heat stroke, drug fever and primary central nervous system (CNS) pathology.

The management of NMS should include 1) immediate discontinuation of antipsychotic drugs and other drugs not essential to concurrent therapy, 2) intensive symptomatic treatment and medical monitoring, and 3) treatment of any concomitant serious medical problems for which specific treatments are available. There is no general agreement about specific pharmacological treatment regimens for uncomplicated NMS.

If a patient requires antipsychotic drug treatment after recovery from NMS, the potential reintroduction of drug therapy should be carefully considered. The patient should be carefully monitored, since recurrences of NMS have been reported.

There have been several reported cases of NMS in patients receiving CLOZARIL® (clozapine), usually in combination with lithium or other CNS-active agents.

Tardive Dyskinesia
A syndrome consisting of potentially irreversible, involuntary, dyskinetic movements may develop in patients treated with antipsychotic drugs. Although the prevalence of the syndrome appears to be highest among the elderly, especially elderly women, it is impossible to rely upon prevalence estimates to predict, at the inception of treatment, which patients are likely to develop the syndrome.

There are several reasons for predicting that CLOZARIL® (clozapine) may be different from other antipsychotic drugs in its potential for inducing tardive dyskinesia, including the preclinical finding that it has a relatively weak dopamine blocking effect and the clinical finding of a virtual absence of

certain acute extrapyramidal symptoms, e.g., dystonia. A few cases of tardive dyskinesia have been reported in patients on CLOZARIL® (clozapine) who had been previously treated with other antipsychotic agents, so that a causal relationship cannot be established. There have been no reports of tardive dyskinesia directly attributable to CLOZARIL® (clozapine) alone. Nevertheless, it cannot be concluded, without more extended experience, that CLOZARIL® (clozapine) is incapable of inducing this syndrome.

Both the risk of developing the syndrome and the likelihood that it will become irreversible are believed to increase as the duration of treatment and the total cumulative dose of antipsychotic drugs administered to the patient increase. However, the syndrome can develop, although much less commonly, after relatively brief treatment periods at low doses. There is no known treatment for established cases of tardive dyskinesia, although the syndrome may remit, partially or completely, if antipsychotic drug treatment is withdrawn. Antipsychotic drug treatment, itself, however, may suppress (or partially suppress) the signs and symptoms of the syndrome and thereby may possibly mask the underlying process. The effect that symptom suppression has upon the long-term course of the syndrome is unknown.

Given these considerations, CLOZARIL® (clozapine) should be prescribed in a manner that is most likely to minimize the occurrence of tardive dyskinesia. As with any antipsychotic drug, chronic CLOZARIL® (clozapine) use should be reserved for patients who appear to be obtaining substantial benefit from the drug. In such patients, the smallest dose and the shortest duration of treatment should be sought. The need for continued treatment should be reassessed periodically.

If signs and symptoms of tardive dyskinesia appear in a patient on CLOZARIL® (clozapine), drug discontinuation should be considered. However, some patients may require treatment with CLOZARIL® (clozapine) despite the presence of the syndrome.

PRECAUTIONS
General
Because of the significant risk of agranulocytosis and seizure, both of which present a continuing risk over time, the extended treatment of patients failing to show an acceptable level of clinical response should ordinarily be avoided. In addition, the need for continuing treatment in patients exhibiting beneficial clinical responses should be periodically re-evaluated.

The mechanism of CLOZARIL® (clozapine)-induced agranulocytosis is unknown; nonetheless, the possibility that causative factors may interact synergistically to increase the risk and/or severity of bone marrow suppression warrants consideration. Therefore, CLOZARIL® (clozapine) should not be used with other agents having a well-known potential to suppress bone marrow function.

Fever
During CLOZARIL® (clozapine) therapy, patients may experience transient temperature elevations above 100.4°F (38°C), with the peak incidence within the first 3 weeks of treatment. While this fever is generally benign and self limiting, it may necessitate discontinuing patients from treatment. On occasion, there may be an associated increase or decrease in WBC count. Patients with fever should be carefully evaluated to rule out the possibility of an underlying infectious process or the development of agranulocytosis. In the presence of high fever, the possibility of Neuroleptic Malignant Syndrome (NMS) must be considered. There have been several reports of NMS in patients receiving CLOZARIL® (clozapine), usually in combination with lithium or other CNS-active drugs. [See Neuroleptic Malignant Syndrome (NMS), under WARNINGS]

Anticholinergic Toxicity
CLOZARIL® (clozapine) has very potent anticholinergic effects and great care should be exercised in using this drug in the presence of prostatic enlargement or narrow angle glaucoma.

Interference with Cognitive and Motor Performance
Because of initial sedation, CLOZARIL® (clozapine) may impair mental and/or physical abilities, especially during the first few days of therapy. The recommendations for gradual dose escalation should be carefully adhered to, and patients cautioned about activities requiring alertness.

Use in Patients with Concomitant Illness
Clinical experience with CLOZARIL® (clozapine) in patients with concomitant systemic diseases is limited. Nevertheless, caution is advisable in using CLOZARIL® (clozapine) in patients with hepatic, renal or cardiac disease.

Information for Patients
Physicians are advised to discuss the following issues with patients for whom they prescribe CLOZARIL® (clozapine):
—Patients who are to receive CLOZARIL® (clozapine) should be warned about the significant risk of developing agranulocytosis. They should be informed that weekly blood tests are required to monitor for the occurrence of agranulocytosis, and that CLOZARIL® (clozapine) tablets will be made available only through a special program designed to ensure the required blood monitoring. Pa-

tients should be advised to report immediately the appearance of lethargy, weakness, fever, sore throat, malaise, mucous membrane ulceration or other possible signs of infection. Particular attention should be paid to any flu-like complaints or other symptoms that might suggest infection.
—Patients should be informed of the significant risk of seizure during CLOZARIL® (clozapine) treatment, and they should be advised to avoid driving and any other potentially hazardous activity while taking CLOZARIL® (clozapine).
—Patients should be advised of the risk of orthostatic hypotension, especially during the period of initial dose titration.
—Patients should be informed that if they stop taking CLOZARIL® (clozapine) for more than 2 days, they should not restart their medication at the same dosage, but should contact their physician for dosing instructions.
—Patients should notify their physician if they are taking, or plan to take, any prescription or over-the-counter drugs or alcohol.
—Patients should notify their physician if they become pregnant or intend to become pregnant during therapy.
—Patients should not breast feed an infant if they are taking CLOZARIL® (clozapine).

Drug Interactions
The risks of using CLOZARIL® (clozapine) in combination with other drugs have not been systematically evaluated. The mechanism of CLOZARIL® (clozapine)-induced agranulocytosis is unknown; nonetheless, the possibility that causative factors may interact synergistically to increase the risk and/or severity of bone marrow suppression warrants consideration. Therefore, CLOZARIL® (clozapine) should not be used with other agents having a well-known potential to suppress bone marrow function.

Given the primary CNS effects of CLOZARIL® (clozapine), caution is advised in using it concomitantly with other CNS-active drugs.

Orthostatic hypotension in patients taking clozapine can, in rare cases (approximately 1 case per 3,000 patients), be accompanied by profound collapse and respiratory and/or cardiac arrest. Some of the cases of collapse/respiratory arrest/cardiac arrest during initial treatment occurred in patients who were being administered benzodiazepines; similar events have been reported in patients taking other psychotropic drugs or even CLOZARIL® (clozapine) by itself. Although it has not been established that there is an interaction between CLOZARIL® (clozapine) and benzodiazepines or other psychotropics, caution is advised when clozapine is initiated in patients taking a benzodiazepine or any other psychotropic drug.

Because CLOZARIL® (clozapine) is highly bound to serum protein, the administration of CLOZARIL® (clozapine) to a patient taking another drug which is highly bound to protein (e.g., warfarin, digitoxin) may cause an increase in plasma concentrations of these drugs, potentially resulting in adverse effects. Conversely, adverse effects may result from displacement of protein-bound CLOZARIL® (clozapine) by other highly bound drugs.

Cimetidine may increase plasma levels of CLOZARIL® (clozapine), potentially resulting in adverse effects. Phenytoin may decrease CLOZARIL® (clozapine) plasma levels, resulting in a decrease in effectiveness of a previously effective CLOZARIL® (clozapine) dose.

CLOZARIL® (clozapine) may also potentiate the hypotensive effects of antihypertensive drugs and the anticholinergic effects of atropine-type drugs. The administration of epinephrine should be avoided in the treatment of drug-induced hypotension because of a possible reverse epinephrine effect.

Carcinogenesis, Mutagenesis, Impairment of Fertility
No carcinogenic potential was demonstrated in long-term studies in mice and rats at doses approximately 7 times the typical human dose on a mg/kg basis. Fertility in male and female rats was not adversely affected by clozapine. Clozapine did not produce genotoxic or mutagenic effects when assayed in appropriate bacterial and mammalian tests.

Pregnancy Category B
Reproduction studies have been performed in rats and rabbits at doses of approximately 2-4 times the human dose and have revealed no evidence of impaired fertility or harm to the fetus due to clozapine. There are, however, no adequate and well-controlled studies in pregnant women. Because animal reproduction studies are not always predictive of human response, and in view of the desirability of keeping the administration of all drugs to a minimum during pregnancy, this drug should be used only if clearly needed.

Nursing Mothers
Animal studies suggest that clozapine may be excreted in breast milk and have an effect on the nursing infant. Therefore, women receiving CLOZARIL® (clozapine) should not breast feed.

Continued on next page

Sandoz—Cont.

Pediatric Use
Safety and effectiveness in children below age 16 have not been established.

ADVERSE REACTIONS
Associated with Discontinuation of Treatment
Sixteen percent of 1080 patients who received CLOZARIL® (clozapine) in premarketing clinical trials discontinued treatment due to an adverse event, including both those that could be reasonably attributed to CLOZARIL® (clozapine) treatment and those that might more appropriately be considered intercurrent illness. The more common events considered to be causes of discontinuation included: CNS, primarily drowsiness/sedation, seizures, dizziness/syncope; cardiovascular, primarily tachycardia, hypotension and ECG changes; gastrointestinal, primarily nausea/vomiting; hematologic, primarily leukopenia/granulocytopenia/agranulocytosis; and fever. None of the events enumerated accounts for more than 1.7% of all discontinuations attributed to adverse clinical events.

Commonly Observed
Adverse events observed in association with the use of CLOZARIL® (clozapine) in clinical trials at an incidence of greater than 5% were: central nervous system complaints, including drowsiness/sedation, dizziness/vertigo, headache and tremor; autonomic nervous system complaints, including salivation, sweating, dry mouth and visual disturbances; cardiovascular findings, including tachycardia, hypotension and syncope; and gastrointestinal complaints, including constipation and nausea; and fever. Complaints of drowsiness/sedation tend to subside with continued therapy or dose reduction. Salivation may be profuse, especially during sleep, but may be diminished with dose reduction.

Incidence in Clinical Trials
The table at right enumerates adverse events that occurred at a frequency of 1% or greater among CLOZARIL® (clozapine) patients who participated in clinical trials. These rates are not adjusted for duration of exposure.

Other Events Observed During the Premarketing Evaluation of CLOZARIL® (clozapine)
This section reports additional, less frequent adverse events which occurred among the patients taking CLOZARIL® (clozapine) in clinical trials. Various adverse events were reported as part of the total experience in these clinical studies; a causal relationship to CLOZARIL® (clozapine) treatment cannot be determined in the absence of appropriate controls in some of the studies. The table above enumerates adverse events that occurred at a frequency of at least 1% of patients treated with CLOZARIL® (clozapine). The list below includes all additional adverse experiences reported as being temporally associated with the use of the drug which occurred at a frequency less than 1%, enumerated by organ system.

Central Nervous System—loss of speech, amentia, tics, poor coordination, delusions/hallucinations, involuntary movement, stuttering, dysarthria, amnesia/memory loss, histrionic movements, libido increase or decrease, paranoia, shakiness, Parkinsonism, and irritability.

Cardiovascular System—edema, palpitations, phlebitis/thrombophlebitis, cyanosis, premature ventricular contraction, bradycardia, and nose bleed.

Gastrointestinal System—abdominal distention, gastroenteritis, rectal bleeding, nervous stomach, abnormal stools, hematemesis, gastric ulcer, bitter taste, and eructation.

Urogenital System—dysmenorrhea, impotence, breast pain/discomfort, and vaginal itch/infection.

Autonomic Nervous System—numbness, polydypsia, hot flashes, dry throat, and mydriasis.

Integumentary (Skin)—pruritus, pallor, eczema, erythema, bruise, dermatitis, petechiae, and urticaria.

Musculoskeletal System—twitching and joint pain.

Respiratory System—coughing, pneumonia/pneumonia-like symptoms, rhinorrhea, hyperventilation, wheezing, bronchitis, laryngitis, and sneezing.

Hemic and Lymphatic System—anemia and leukocytosis.

Miscellaneous—chills/chills with fever, malaise, appetite increase, ear disorder, hypothermia, eyelid disorder, bloodshot eyes, and nystagmus.

Postmarketing Clinical Experience
Postmarketing experience has shown an adverse experience profile similar to that presented above. Reports of adverse events temporally associated with CLOZARIL® (clozapine) that may have no causal relationship to the drug include the following: salivary gland swelling, periorbital edema, paralytic ileus, atrial fibrillation, hyperuricemia, hyperglycemia, priapism, pleural effusion, myasthenic syndrome, cholestasis, and possible mild cataplexy.

DRUG ABUSE AND DEPENDENCE
Physical and psychological dependence have not been reported or observed in patients taking CLOZARIL® (clozapine).

Treatment-Emergent Adverse Experience Incidence Among Patients Taking CLOZARIL® (clozapine) in Clinical Trials (N = 842) (Percentage of Patients Reporting)

Body System Adverse Event[a]	Percent
Central Nervous System	
Drowsiness/Sedation	39
Dizziness/Vertigo	19
Headache	7
Tremor	6
Syncope	6
Disturbed sleep/Nightmares	4
Restlessness	4
Hypokinesia/Akinesia	4
Agitation	4
Seizures (convulsions)	3[b]
Rigidity	3
Akathisia	3
Confusion	3
Fatigue	2
Insomnia	2
Hyperkinesia	1
Weakness	1
Lethargy	1
Ataxia	1
Slurred speech	1
Depression	1
Epileptiform movements/Myoclonic jerks	1
Anxiety	1
Cardiovascular	
Tachycardia	25[b]
Hypotension	9
Hypertension	4
Chest pain/Angina	1
ECG change/Cardiac abnormality	1
Gastrointestinal	
Constipation	14
Nausea	5
Abdominal discomfort/Heartburn	4
Nausea/Vomiting	3
Vomiting	3
Diarrhea	2
Liver test abnormality	1
Anorexia	1
Urogenital	
Urinary abnormalities	2
Incontinence	1
Abnormal ejaculation	1
Urinary urgency/frequency	1
Urinary retention	1
Autonomic Nervous System	
Salivation	31
Sweating	6
Dry mouth	6
Visual disturbances	5
Integumentary (Skin)	
Rash	2
Musculoskeletal	
Muscle weakness	1
Pain (back, neck, legs)	1
Muscle spasm	1
Muscle pain, ache	1
Respiratory	
Throat discomfort	1
Dyspnea, shortness of breath	1
Nasal congestion	1
Hemic/Lymphatic	
Leukopenia/Decreased WBC/Neutropenia	3
Agranulocytosis	1[b]
Eosinophilia	1
Miscellaneous	
Fever	5
Weight gain	4
Tongue numb/sore	1

[a] Events reported by at least 1% of CLOZARIL® (clozapine) patients are included.
[b] Rate based on population of approximately 1700 exposed during premarket clinical evaluation of CLOZARIL® (clozapine).

OVERDOSAGE
Human Experience
The most commonly reported signs and symptoms associated with CLOZARIL® (clozapine) overdose are: altered states of consciousness, including drowsiness, delirium and coma; tachycardia; hypotension; respiratory depression or failure; hypersalivation. Seizures have occurred in a minority of reported cases. Fatal overdoses have been reported with CLOZARIL® (clozapine), generally at doses above 2500 mgs. There have also been reports of patients recovering from overdoses well in excess of 4 gms.

Management of Overdose
Establish and maintain an airway; ensure adequate oxygenation and ventilation. Activated charcoal, which may be used with sorbitol, may be as or more effective than emesis or lavage, and should be considered in treating overdosage. Cardiac and vital signs monitoring is recommended along with general symptomatic and supportive measures. Additional surveillance should be continued for several days because of the risk of delayed effects. Avoid epinephrine and derivatives when treating hypotension, and quinidine and procainamide when treating cardiac arrhythmia.

There are no specific antidotes for CLOZARIL® (clozapine). Forced diuresis, dialysis, hemoperfusion and exchange transfusion are unlikely to be of benefit.

In managing overdosage, the physician should consider the possibility of multiple drug involvement.

Up-to-date information about the treatment of overdose can often be obtained from a certified Regional Poison Control Center. Telephone numbers of certified Poison Control Centers are listed in the Physicians' Desk Reference (PDR).

DOSAGE AND ADMINISTRATION
In order to minimize the risk of agranulocytosis, CLOZARIL® (clozapine) is available only through a distribution system that ensures weekly WBC testing prior to delivery of the next week's supply of medication. Upon initiation of CLOZARIL® (clozapine) therapy, up to a 1 week supply of additional CLOZARIL® (clozapine) tablets may be provided to the patient to be held for emergencies (e.g., weather, holidays).

Initial Treatment
It is recommended that treatment with CLOZARIL® (clozapine) begin with one-half of a 25 mg tablet (12.5 mg) once or twice daily and then be continued with daily dosage increments of 25-50 mg/day, if well-tolerated, to achieve a target dose of 300-450 mg/day by the end of 2 weeks. Subsequent dosage increments should be made no more than once or twice-weekly, in increments not to exceed 100 mg. Cautious titration and a divided dosage schedule are necessary to minimize the risks of hypotension, seizure, and sedation.

In the multicenter study that provides primary support for the effectiveness of CLOZARIL® (clozapine) in patients resistant to standard antipsychotic drug treatment, patients were titrated during the first 2 weeks up to a maximum dose of 500 mg/day, on a t.i.d. basis, and were then dosed in a total daily dose range of 100-900 mg/day, on a t.i.d. basis thereafter, with clinical response and adverse effects as guides to correct dosing.

Therapeutic Dose Adjustment
Daily dosing should continue on a divided basis as an effective and tolerable dose level is sought. While many patients may respond adequately at doses between 300-600 mg/day, it may be necessary to raise the dose to the 600-900 mg/day range to obtain an acceptable response. [Note: In the multicenter study providing the primary support for the superiority of CLOZARIL® (clozapine) in treatment resistant patients, the mean and median CLOZARIL® (clozapine) doses were both approximately 600 mg/day.]

Because of the possibility of increased adverse reactions at higher doses, particularly seizures, patients should ordinarily be given adequate time to respond to a given dose level before escalation to a higher dose is contemplated.

Dosing should not exceed 900 mg/day.

Because of the significant risk of agranulocytosis and seizure, events which both present a continuing risk over time, the extended treatment of patients failing to show an acceptable level of clinical response should ordinarily be avoided.

Maintenance Treatment
While the maintenance effectiveness of CLOZARIL® (clozapine) in schizophrenia is still under study, the effectiveness of maintenance treatment is well established for many other antipsychotic drugs. It is recommended that responding patients be continued on CLOZARIL® (clozapine), but at the lowest level needed to maintain remission. Because of the significant risk associated with the use of CLOZARIL® (clozapine), patients should be periodically reassessed to determine the need for maintenance treatment.

Discontinuation of Treatment
In the event of planned termination of CLOZARIL® (clozapine) therapy, gradual reduction in dose is recommended over a 1-2 week period. However, should a patient's medical condition require abrupt discontinuation (e.g., leukopenia), the patient should be carefully observed for the recurrence of psychotic symptoms.

Re-initiation of Treatment in Patients Previously Discontinued

When restarting patients who have had even a brief interval off CLOZARIL® (clozapine), i.e., 2 days or more since the last dose, it is recommended that treatment be reinitiated with one-half of a 25 mg tablet (12.5 mg) once or twice daily *(see WARNINGS).* If that dose is well tolerated, it may be feasible to titrate patients back to a therapeutic dose more quickly than is recommended for initial treatment. However, any patient who has previously experienced respiratory or cardiac arrest with initial dosing, but was then able to be successfully titrated to a therapeutic dose, should be re-titrated with extreme caution after even 24 hours of discontinuation.

Certain additional precautions seem prudent when re-initiating treatment. The mechanisms underlying CLOZARIL® (clozapine)-induced adverse reactions are unknown. It is conceivable, however, that re-exposure of a patient might enhance the risk of an untoward event's occurrence and increase its severity. Such phenomena, for example, occur when immune mediated mechanisms are responsible. Consequently, during the re-initiation of treatment, additional caution is advised. Patients discontinued for WBC counts below 2000/mm^3 or a granulocyte count below 1000/mm^3 must *not* be restarted on CLOZARIL® (clozapine). *(See WARNINGS)*

HOW SUPPLIED

CLOZARIL® (clozapine) is available only through a distribution system that ensures weekly WBC testing prior to delivery of the next week's supply of medication.

CLOZARIL® (clozapine) is available as 25 mg and 100 mg round, pale yellow compressed tablets, engraved "CLOZARIL" on one side, and dosage strength (25 or 100) on the other side.

25 mg

Bottle of 100 (NDC 0078-0126-05).

SandoPak® unit-dose packages of 100: 2 × 5 strips, 10 blisters per strip (NDC 0078-0126-06).

100 mg

Bottle of 100 (NDC 0078-0127-05).

SandoPak® unit-dose packages of 100: 2 × 5 strips, 10 blisters per strip (NDC 0078-0127-06).

Store and Dispense

Storage temperature should not exceed 86°F (30°C). Drug dispensing should not ordinarily exceed a weekly supply. Dispensing should be contingent upon the results of a WBC count.

[CLO-Z7 Issued June 1, 1992]

Shown in Product Identification Section, page 427

D.H.E. 45®* ℞

(dihydroergotamine mesylate) injection, USP

CAUTION: Federal law prohibits dispensing without prescription.

The following prescribing information is based on official labeling in effect on August 1, 1992.

DESCRIPTION

D.H.E. 45® is hydrogenated ergotamine as the mesylate. It is a clear, colorless, stable ampul solution containing per mL:

dihydroergotamine mesylate, USP	1mg
methanesulfonic acid/ sodium hydroxide	qs to pH 3.6±0.4
alcohol, USP	6.1% by vol.
glycerin, USP	15% by wt.
water for injection, USP, qs to	1 mL

ACTIONS

Dihydroergotamine is an alpha adrenergic blocking agent with a direct stimulating effect on the smooth muscle of peripheral and cranial blood vessels, and produces depression of central vasomotor centers. The compound also has the properties of serotonin antagonism. In comparison to ergotamine, the adrenergic blocking actions are more pronounced, the vasoconstrictive actions somewhat less pronounced, and there is reduced incidence and degree of nausea and vomiting.

Onset of action occurs in 15 to 30 minutes following intramuscular administration and persists for 3-4 hours.

Repeated dosage at 1 hour intervals up to 3 hours may be required to obtain maximal effect.

INDICATIONS

As therapy to abort or prevent vascular headache, e.g., migraine, migraine variants, or so-called "histaminic cephalalgia" when rapid control is desired or when other routes of administration are not feasible.

CONTRAINDICATIONS

Peripheral vascular disease, coronary heart disease, hypertension, impaired hepatic or renal function, sepsis and pregnancy. Hypersensitivity.

*Also known as Dyhydergot®

ADVERSE REACTIONS

Numbness and tingling of fingers and toes, muscle pains in the extremities, weakness in the legs, precordial distress and pain, transient tachycardia or bradycardia, nausea, vomiting, localized edema and itching.

There have been reports of pleural and retroperitoneal fibrosis in patients following prolonged use of dihydroergotamine.

DOSAGE AND ADMINISTRATION

For vascular headache, 1 mL intramuscularly at first warning sign of headache, repeated at 1 hour intervals to a total of 3 mL. Optimal results are obtained by titrating the dose for several headaches to find the minimal effective dose for each patient and this dose should then be employed at onset of subsequent attacks. Where more rapid effect is desired, the intravenous route may be employed to a maximum of 2 mL. Total weekly dosage should not exceed 6 mL.

OVERDOSAGE

Failure to observe the upper limits of repeated parenteral dosage may result in eventual onset of the peripheral toxic signs and symptoms of ergotism. Treatment includes discontinuance of the drug, warmth, vasodilators, and good nursing care to prevent tissue damage.

HOW SUPPLIED

As a clear, colorless and stable solution in ampuls containing:

dihydroergotamine mesylate, USP	1 mg
methanesulfonic acid/ sodium hydroxide	qs to pH 3.6±0.4
alcohol, USP	6.1% by vol.
glycerin, USP	15% by wt.
water for injection, USP, qs to	1 mL

Ampuls, 1 mL size—boxes of 20.

Store and Dispense

Store below 77°F (25°C). To assure constant potency, protect the ampuls from light. In the event the ampul solution becomes discolored, it should not be used.

[DHE-Z21 Issued January 15, 1992.]

DIAPID® ℞

[dī'a-pid"]

(lypressin nasal solution, USP) NASAL SPRAY

CAUTION: Federal law prohibits dispensing without prescription.

The following prescribing information is based on official labeling in effect on August 1, 1992.

DESCRIPTION

Diapid® (lypressin nasal solution, USP) Nasal Spray contains synthetic lysine-8-vasopressin with an activity of 50 USP Posterior Pituitary (Pressor) Units per mL (0.185 mg/mL).

The molecular formula of lysine-8-vasopressin is $C_{46}H_{65}N_{13}O_{12}S_2$; its structural formula may be represented as follows:

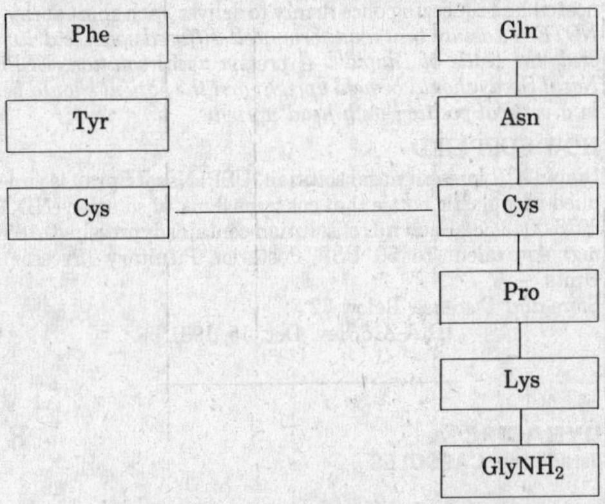

It is an antidiuretic with vasoconstrictor activity.

Diapid® (lypressin nasal solution, USP) Nasal Spray is provided for intra-nasal administration as a solution containing per 1 mL, 50 USP Posterior Pituitary (Pressor) Units of synthetic lysine-8-vasopressin and the following inactive ingredients: acetic acid, NF, chlorobutanol, NF, (max. 0.1%), citric acid, USP, disodium phosphate, USP, glycerin, USP, methylparaben, NF, propylparaben, NF, purified water, USP, sodium acetate, USP, sodium chloride, USP, sorbitol solution, USP.

CLINICAL PHARMACOLOGY

Lysine-8-vasopressin is a polypeptide and is one of the two known naturally occurring molecular forms of mammalian posterior pituitary antidiuretic hormone. It is identical to the vasopressin produced naturally in swine pituitaries. This synthetic vasopressin differs from that produced in humans in that it contains lysine instead of arginine in its structure. It is present as a protein-free substance in Diapid® (lypressin nasal solution, USP) Nasal Spray. Unlike preparations of posterior pituitary antidiuretic hormone of animal origin, Diapid® (lypressin nasal solution, USP) Nasal Spray is completely free of oxytocin and foreign proteins.

The principal pharmacologic action of lysine-8-vasopressin, the active ingredient of Diapid® (lypressin nasal solution, USP) Nasal Spray, is similar to that of arginine-8-vasopressin, the posterior pituitary antidiuretic hormone occurring in man. Diapid® (lypressin nasal solution, USP) Nasal Spray increases the rate of reabsorption of solute free water from the distal renal tubules, without significantly modifying the rate of glomerular filtration, producing a fall in free water clearance and an increase in urinary osmolality. The rates of solute and creatinine excretion noted with therapeutic doses of Diapid® (lypressin nasal solution, USP) Nasal Spray suggest that sodium clearance and glomerular filtration rates are essentially unaltered by this hormone. Diapid® (lypressin nasal solution, USP) Nasal Spray is relatively free of oxytocic activity when used within the recommended therapeutic dose levels.

It possesses little pressor activity, the ratio of pressor to antidiuretic activity being in the range of 1:1000.

The antidiuretic effect produced by Diapid® (lypressin nasal solution, USP) Nasal Spray begins rapidly and usually reaches a peak within 30–120 minutes. Its usual duration of action is 3–8 hours.

INDICATIONS

Diapid® (lypressin nasal solution, USP) Nasal Spray is indicated for the control or prevention of the symptoms and complications of diabetes insipidus due to deficiency of endogenous posterior pituitary antidiuretic hormone in both children and adults. These symptoms and complications include polydipsia, polyuria, and dehydration. It is particularly useful in patients with diabetes insipidus who have become unresponsive to other forms of therapy or who experience various types of local and/or systemic reactions, allergic reactions, or other undesirable effects (e.g., excessive fluid retention) from preparations of posterior pituitary antidiuretic hormone of animal origin.

CONTRAINDICATIONS

Hypersensitivity. (See PRECAUTIONS)

WARNINGS

Cardiovascular pressor effects with Diapid® (lypressin nasal solution, USP) Nasal Spray are minimal or absent when it is administered as a nasal spray in therapeutic doses. Nevertheless, it should be used with caution in patients for whom such effects would not be desirable because mild blood pressure elevation has been noted in unanesthetized subjects who received lypressin intravenously. Large doses intranasally may cause coronary artery constriction and caution should be observed in treating patients with coronary artery disease. There have been reports of acute myocardial infarction in patients taking Diapid® (lypressin nasal solution, USP) Nasal Spray.[1]

[1]Adverse reaction file, Sandoz Pharmaceuticals

PRECAUTIONS

General

The effectiveness of Diapid® (lypressin nasal solution, USP) Nasal Spray may be lessened in patients with nasal congestion, allergic rhinitis, and upper respiratory infections because these conditions may interfere with absorption of the drug by the nasal mucosa. In this event, larger doses of Diapid® (lypressin nasal solution, USP) Nasal Spray, or adjunctive therapy, may be needed.

Patients with a known sensitivity to antidiuretic hormone should be tested for sensitivity to Diapid® (lypressin nasal solution, USP) Nasal Spray. *(See CONTRAINDICATIONS)*

Information For Patients

Diapid® (lypressin nasal solution, USP) Nasal Spray is indicated for the treatment of diabetes insipidus, a disorder in which the lack of a specific hormone, vasopressin, prevents the kidneys from conserving water. As a result, excess urine is produced which can lead to dehydration. The symptoms of this disorder are mainly excessive urination and thirst. Diapid® (lypressin nasal solution, USP) Nasal Spray provides the body with a synthetic form of vasopressin and thus prevents these symptoms.

Patients should be instructed on how to regulate their daily dosage according to their degree of excessive urination and thirst. Once established, daily requirements should remain stable for a long period of time. In case of nasal congestion due to allergic conditions or upper respiratory tract infections which interferes with the absorption of the drug by the nasal mucosa, patients may require larger doses of Diapid® (lypressin nasal solution, USP) Nasal Spray or an alternate form of therapy. Patients should be advised to consult their physician if this circumstance arises.

Continued on next page

Sandoz—Cont.

To assure a uniform delivery of spray with Diapid® (lypressin nasal solution, USP) Nasal Spray, the bottle should be held upright and the patient should be sitting or standing with the head upright.

Diapid® (lypressin nasal solution, USP) Nasal Spray is indicated for use in the treatment of diabetes insipidus *only.* It should not be used in the therapy of other disorders or conditions.

Carcinogenesis, Mutagenesis, Impairment of Fertility

No long-term studies in animals have been performed to evaluate carcinogenic potential. Reproductive studies have not been conducted in animals or humans to test whether lypressin constitutes a potential problem in relation to mutagenesis or impairment of fertility in either females or males. However, as a posterior pituitary antidiuretic hormone it is unlikely to evoke detrimental reproductive effects. Commercially available since September, 1970, lypressin has not been reported to have been related to any instance of fetal abnormality, infertility or impotence.

Pregnancy Category C

Animal reproduction studies have not been conducted with Diapid® (lypressin nasal solution, USP) Nasal Spray. It is not known whether Diapid® (lypressin nasal solution, USP) Nasal Spray can cause fetal harm when administered to a pregnant woman or can affect reproduction capacity. Diapid® (lypressin nasal solution, USP) Nasal Spray should be given to a pregnant woman only if clearly needed.

Nursing Mothers

It is not known whether this drug is excreted in human milk. Because many drugs are excreted in human milk, a decision should be made whether to discontinue nursing or to discontinue the drug, taking into account the importance of the drug to the mother.

Pediatric Use

The usual dosage in children is the same as for adults (*See DOSAGE AND ADMINISTRATION*). Safety and efficacy have not been demonstrated in children less than six weeks of age.

ADVERSE REACTIONS

Cardiovascular pressor effects with Diapid® (lypressin nasal solution, USP) Nasal Spray are minimal when it is administered as a nasal spray in therapeutic doses. (*See WARNINGS*)

With clinical use of Diapid® (lypressin nasal solution, USP) Nasal Spray, adverse reactions, in general, have been infrequent and mild. Such reactions have included rhinorrhea, nasal congestion, irritation and pruritus of the nasal passages, nasal ulceration, headache, conjunctivitis, heartburn secondary to excessive nasal administration with drippage into the pharynx, abdominal and muscle cramps and increased bowel movements. Periorbital edema, with itching, has been reported. Inadvertent inhalation of Diapid® (lypressin nasal solution, USP) Nasal Spray has resulted in substernal tightness, coughing, and transient dyspnea. Tolerance or tachyphylaxis to Diapid® (lypressin nasal solution, USP) Nasal Spray has not been reported to date.

Hypersensitivity manifested by positive skin test has been reported.

DRUG ABUSE AND DEPENDENCE

There have been no reports of drug abuse or dependence with Diapid® (lypressin nasal solution, USP) Nasal Spray.

OVERDOSAGE

The lethal dose of Diapid® (lypressin nasal solution, USP) Nasal Spray has not been established. The I.V. LD_{50} of Diapid® (lypressin nasal solution, USP) in rats is 7266 mg/kg. The oral or intraperitoneal administration of Diapid® (lypressin nasal solution, USP) Nasal Spray to rats in doses up to 20mL (1000 I.U.)/100 gm resulted in no deaths.

Diapid® (lypressin nasal solution, USP) Nasal Spray is a polypeptide and is therefore subject to inactivation by the proteolytic enzymes of the alimentary tract. Hence, Diapid® (lypressin nasal solution, USP) Nasal Spray is NOT ABSORBED from the gastrointestinal tract, and, for this reason, ingestion of this drug is not likely to have toxic effects. The only reasonable route of significant acute overdosage with Diapid® (lypressin nasal solution, USP) Nasal Spray is by excessive use of the nasal spray.

Inadvertent or intentional excessive use of Diapid® (lypressin nasal solution, USP) Nasal Spray may result in significant water retention, and if the overdosage is high enough and associated with a very high fluid intake, the possibility of water intoxication does arise. The symptoms of water intoxication include headache, anorexia, nausea, vomiting, abdominal pain, lethargy, drowsiness, unconsciousness and grand mal-type seizures. The dilution factor associated with marked water retention lowers the electrolyte concentration in the blood.

A patient being treated with Diapid® (lypressin nasal solution, USP) Nasal Spray for diabetes insipidus misunderstood the therapeutic recommendations and used the spray vigorously according to thirst. As a result, marked water retention with related hyponatremia developed. These conditions were relieved by decreasing the frequency of use of the nasal spray.

The treatment of Diapid® (lypressin nasal solution, USP) Nasal Spray overdose should include the following:

1. Discontinue the drug and restrict fluid intake. As the duration of action of Diapid® (lypressin nasal solution, USP) Nasal Spray is from 3–8 hours, these measures alone usually suffice for simple water retention.
2. Correction of electrolyte imbalance as indicated in water intoxication with the I.V. administration of 200-300 mL of 5% saline solution over several hours sufficient to raise the serum sodium to a level at which the symptoms will improve.
3. When there is the possibility of congestive heart failure due to the fluid overload, the simultaneous administration of furosemide with the hypertonic saline usually causes a diuresis sufficient to reduce cardiac overload. Potassium and other electrolyte levels must be monitored with the use of furosemide.
4. If I.V. fluid administration is considered necessary when the serum sodium has been raised to normal, the slow infusion of isotonic saline is advised to maintain normal serum sodium levels.

DOSAGE AND ADMINISTRATION

Patients should be instructed to administer 1 or 2 sprays of Diapid® (lypressin nasal solution, USP) Nasal Spray to one or both nostrils whenever frequency of urination becomes increased or significant thirst develops. (One spray provides approximately 2 USP Posterior Pituitary [Pressor] Units.)

The usual dosage for adults and children six weeks and older is 1 or 2 sprays in each nostril four times daily. An additional dose at bedtime is often helpful to eliminate nocturia, if it is not controlled with the regular daily dosage. For patients requiring more than 2 sprays per nostril every 4–6 hours, it is recommended that the time interval between doses be reduced rather than increasing the number of sprays at each dose. (More than 2 or 3 sprays in each nostril usually results in wastage because the unabsorbed excess will drain posteriorly, by way of the nasopharynx, into the digestive tract where it will be inactivated.)

Diapid® (lypressin nasal solution, USP) Nasal Spray permits individualization of dosage necessary to control the symptoms of diabetes insipidus. Patients quickly learn to regulate their dosage in accordance with their degree of polyuria and thirst, and once determined, daily requirements remain fairly stable for months and years. Although most patients require 1 or 2 sprays of Diapid® (lypressin nasal solution, USP) Nasal Spray in each nostril four times daily, dosage has ranged from 1 spray per day at bedtime to 10 sprays in each nostril every 3-4 hours. Requirements of the larger doses may represent greater severity of disease or other phenomena, such as poor nasal absorption. A seeming requirement for larger doses of lypressin may be due to the presence of mixed hypothalamichypophyseal and nephrogenic diabetes insipidus, the latter condition being unresponsive to administration of antidiuretic hormone.

Diapid® (lypressin nasal solution, USP) Nasal Spray is conveniently administered, from a compact and portable, plastic squeeze bottle, by inserting the nozzle of the bottle into the nostril and squeezing once firmly to deliver each short spray.

NOTE: To assure that a uniform, well-diffused spray is delivered, the bottle of Diapid® (lypressin nasal solution, USP) Nasal Spray should be held upright and the patient should be in a vertical position with head upright.

HOW SUPPLIED

Diapid® (lypressin nasal solution, USP) Nasal Spray is supplied in a plastic bottle that contains 8 mL of solution (NDC 0078-0042-38). Each mL of solution contains lypressin (0.185 mg) equivalent to 50 USP Posterior Pituitary (Pressor) Units.

Store and Dispense: Below 72°F.

[DIA-Z16 Rev. Dec. 15, 1991.]

DYNACIRC®
(isradipine) CAPSULES ℞

CAUTION: Federal law prohibits dispensing without prescription.

The following prescribing information is based on official labeling in effect on August 1, 1992.

DESCRIPTION

DynaCirc® (isradipine) is a calcium antagonist available for oral administration in capsules containing 2.5 mg or 5 mg. The structural formula of isradipine is given above.

[See chemical structure at top of next column.]

Chemically, isradipine is 3,5-Pyridinedicarboxylic acid, 4-(4-benzofurazanyl)-1,4-dihydro-2,6-dimethyl-, methyl 1-methylethyl ester. It has a molecular weight of 371.39. Isradipine is a yellow, fine crystalline powder which is odorless or has a faint characteristic odor. Isradipine is practically insoluble in water (<10 mg/L at 37°C), but is soluble in ethanol and

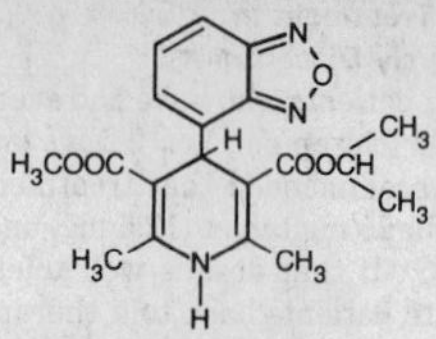

freely soluble in acetone, chloroform, and methylene chloride.

Active Ingredient: isradipine

Inactive Ingredients: colloidal silicon dioxide, D&C Red No. 7 Calcium Lake, FD&C Red No. 40 (5 mg capsule only), FD&C Yellow No. 6 Aluminum Lake, gelatin, lactose, starch, titanium dioxide and other ingredients.

The 2.5 mg and 5 mg capsules may also contain: benzyl alcohol, butylparaben, edetate calcium disodium, methylparaben, propylparaben, sodium propionate.

CLINICAL PHARMACOLOGY

Mechanism of Action

Isradipine is a dihydropyridine calcium channel blocker. It binds to calcium channels with high affinity and specificity and inhibits calcium flux into cardiac and smooth muscle. The effects observed in mechanistic experiments *in vitro* and studied in intact animals and man are compatible with this mechanism of action and are typical of the class.

Except for diuretic activity, the mechanism of which is not clearly understood, the pharmacodynamic effects of isradipine observed in whole animals can also be explained by calcium channel blocking activity, especially dilating effects in arterioles which reduce systemic resistance and lower blood pressure, with a small increase in resting heart rate. Although like other dihydropyridine calcium channel blockers, isradipine has negative inotropic effects *in vitro,* studies conducted in intact anesthetized animals have shown that the vasodilating effect occurs at doses lower than those which affect contractility. In patients with normal ventricular function, isradipine's afterload reducing properties lead to some increase in cardiac output.

Effects in patients with impaired ventricular function have not been fully studied.

Clinical Effects

Dose-related reductions in supine and standing blood pressure are achieved within 2-3 hours following single oral doses of 2.5 mg, 5 mg, 10 mg, and 20 mg DynaCirc® (isradipine), with a duration of action (at least 50% of peak response) of more than 12 hours following administration of the highest dose.

DynaCirc® (isradipine) has been shown in controlled, double-blind clinical trials to be an effective antihypertensive agent when used as monotherapy, or when added to therapy with thiazide-type diuretics. During chronic administration, divided doses (b.i.d.) in the range of 5 mg–20 mg daily have been shown to be effective, with response at trough (prior to next dose) over 50% of the peak blood pressure effect. The response is dose-related between 5-10 mg daily. DynaCirc® (isradipine) is equally effective in reducing supine, sitting, and standing blood pressure.

On chronic administration, increases in resting pulse rate averaged about 3-5 beats/min. These increases were not dose-related.

Hemodynamics

In man, peripheral vasodilation produced by DynaCirc® (isradipine) is reflected by decreased systemic vascular resistance and increased cardiac output. Hemodynamic studies conducted in patients with normal left ventricular function produced, following intravenous isradipine administration, increases in cardiac index, stroke volume index, coronary sinus blood flow, heart rate, and peak positive left ventricular dP/dt. Systemic, coronary, and pulmonary vascular resistance were decreased. These studies were conducted with doses of isradipine which produced clinically significant decreases in blood pressure. The clinical consequences of these hemodynamic effects, if any, have not been evaluated.

Effects on heart rate are variable, dependent upon rate of administration and presence of underlying cardiac condition. While increases in both peak positive dP/dt and LV ejection fraction are seen when intravenous isradipine is given, it is impossible to conclude that these represent a positive inotropic effect due to simultaneous changes in preload and afterload. In patients with coronary artery disease undergoing atrial pacing during cardiac catheterization, intravenous isradipine diminished abnormalities of systolic performance. In patients with moderate left ventricular dysfunction, oral and intravenous isradipine in doses which reduce blood pressure by 12-30%, resulted in improvement in cardiac index without increase in heart rate, and with no change or reduction in pulmonary capillary wedge pressure. Combination of isradipine and propranolol did not significantly affect left ventricular dP/dt max. The clinical consequences of these effects have not been evaluated.

Electrophysiologic Effects

In general, no detrimental effects on the cardiac conduction system were seen with the use of DynaCirc® (isradipine).

		DynaCirc® (isradipine)				
	All Doses	2.5 mg b.i.d.	5 mg b.i.d.†	10 mg b.i.d.††	Placebo	Active Controls*
N=	934	199	150	59	297	414
Adverse Experience	%	%	%	%	%	%
Headache	13.7	12.6	10.7	22.0	14.1	9.4
Dizziness	7.3	8.0	5.3	3.4	4.4	8.2
Edema	7.2	3.5	8.7	8.5	3.0	2.9
Palpitations	4.0	1.0	4.7	5.1	1.4	1.5
Fatigue	3.9	2.5	2.0	8.5	0.3	6.3
Flushing	2.6	3.0	2.0	5.1	0.0	1.2
Chest Pain	2.4	2.5	2.7	1.7	2.4	2.9
Nausea	1.8	1.0	2.7	5.1	1.7	3.1
Dyspnea	1.8	0.5	2.7	3.4	1.0	2.2
Abdominal Discomfort	1.7	0.0	3.3	1.7	1.7	3.9
Tachycardia	1.5	1.0	1.3	3.4	0.3	0.5
Rash	1.5	1.5	2.0	1.7	0.3	0.7
Pollakiuria	1.5	2.0	1.3	3.4	0.0	<1.0
Weakness	1.2	0.0	0.7	0.0	0.0	1.2
Vomiting	1.1	1.0	1.3	0.0	0.3	0.2
Diarrhea	1.1	0.0	2.7	3.4	2.0	1.9

† Initial dose of 2.5 mg b.i.d. followed by maintenance dose of 5.0 mg b.i.d.
†† Initial dose of 2.5 mg b.i.d. followed by sequential titration to 5.0 mg b.i.d., 7.5 mg b.i.d., and maintenance dose of 10.0 mg b.i.d.
* Propranolol, prazosin, hydrochlorothiazide, enalapril, captopril.

Electrophysiologic studies were conducted on patients with normal sinus and atrioventricular node function. Intravenous isradipine in doses which reduce systolic blood pressure did not affect PR, QRS, AH* or HV* intervals.

No changes were seen in Wenckebach cycle length, atrial, and ventricular refractory periods. Slight prolongation of QTc interval of 3% was seen in one study. Effects on sinus node recovery time (CSNRT) were mild or not seen.

In patients with sick sinus syndrome, at doses which significantly reduced blood pressure, intravenous isradipine resulted in no depressant effect on sinus and atrioventricular node function.

Pharmacokinetics and Metabolism

Isradipine is 90-95% absorbed and is subject to extensive first-pass metabolism, resulting in a bioavailability of about 15-24%. Isradipine is detectable in plasma within 20 minutes after administration of single oral doses of 2.5-20 mg, and peak concentrations of approximately 1 ng/mL/mg dosed occur about 1.5 hours after drug administration. Administration of DynaCirc® (isradipine) with food significantly increases the time to peak by about an hour, but has no effect on the total bioavailability (area under the curve) of the drug. Isradipine is 95% bound to plasma proteins. Both peak plasma concentration and AUC exhibit a linear relationship to dose over the 0-20 mg dose range. The elimination of isradipine is biphasic with an early half-life of 1½-2 hours, and a terminal half-life of about 8 hours. The total body clearance of isradipine is 1.4 L/min and the apparent volume of distribution is 3 L/kg.

Isradipine is completely metabolized prior to excretion, and no unchanged drug is detected in the urine. Six metabolites have been characterized in blood and urine, with the mono acids of the pyridine derivative and a cyclic lactone product accounting for >75% of the material identified. Approximately 60-65% of an administered dose is excreted in the urine and 25-30% in the feces. Mild renal impairment (creatinine clearance 30-80 mL/min) increases the bioavailability (AUC) of isradipine by 45%. Progressive deterioration reverses this trend, and patients with severe renal failure (creatinine clearance <10 mL/min) who have been on hemodialysis show a 20-50% lower AUC than healthy volunteers. No pharmacokinetic information is available on drug therapy during hemodialysis. In elderly patients, C_{max} and AUC are increased by 13% and 40%, respectively; in patients with hepatic impairment, C_{max} and AUC are increased by 32% and 52%, respectively *(see DOSAGE AND ADMINISTRATION).*

INDICATIONS AND USAGE

Hypertension

DynaCirc® (isradipine) is indicated in the management of hypertension. It may be used alone or concurrently with thiazide-type diuretics.

CONTRAINDICATIONS

DynaCirc® (isradipine) is contraindicated in individuals who have shown hypersensitivity to any of the ingredients in the formulation.

WARNINGS

None.

PRECAUTIONS

General

Blood Pressure: Because DynaCirc® (isradipine) decreases peripheral resistance, like other calcium blockers DynaCirc® (isradipine) may occasionally produce symptomatic hypotension. However, symptoms like syncope and severe dizziness have rarely been reported in hypertensive patients administered DynaCirc® (isradipine), particularly at the initial recommended doses *(see DOSAGE AND ADMINISTRATION).*

Use in Patients with Congestive Heart Failure: Although acute hemodynamic studies in patients with congestive heart failure have shown that DynaCirc® (isradipine) reduced afterload without impairing myocardial contractility, it has a negative inotropic effect at high doses *in vitro,* and possibly in some patients. Caution should be exercised when using the drug in congestive heart failure patients, particularly in combination with a beta-blocker.

Drug Interactions

Nitroglycerin: DynaCirc® (isradipine) has been safely coadministered with nitroglycerin.

Hydrochlorothiazide: A study in normal healthy volunteers has shown that concomitant administration of DynaCirc® (isradipine) and hydrochlorothiazide does not result in altered pharmacokinetics of either drug. In a study in hypertensive patients, addition of isradipine to existing hydrochlorothiazide therapy did not result in any unexpected adverse effects, and isradipine had an additional antihypertensive effect.

Propranolol: In a single dose study in normal volunteers, coadministration of propranolol had a small effect on the rate but no effect on the extent of isradipine bioavailability. Coadministration of DynaCirc® (isradipine) resulted in significant increases in AUC (27%) and C_{max} (58%) and decreases in t_{max} (23%) of propranolol.

Digoxin: The concomitant administration of DynaCirc® (isradipine) and digoxin in a single-dose pharmacokinetic study did not affect renal, non-renal, and total body clearance of digoxin.

Fentanyl Anesthesia: Severe hypotension has been reported during fentanyl anesthesia with concomitant use of a beta blocker and a calcium channel blocker. Even though such interactions have not been seen in clinical studies with DynaCirc® (isradipine), an increased volume of circulating fluids might be required if such an interaction were to occur.

Carcinogenesis, Mutagenesis, Impairment of Fertility

Treatment of male rats for 2 years with 2.5, 12.5, or 62.5 mg/kg/day isradipine admixed with the diet (approximately 6, 31, and 156 times the maximum recommended daily dose based on a 50 kg man) resulted in dose dependent increases in the incidence of benign Leydig cell tumors and testicular hyperplasia relative to untreated control animals. These findings, which were replicated in a subsequent experiment, may have been indirectly related to an effect of isradipine on circulating gonadotropin levels in the rats; a comparable endocrine effect was not evident in male patients receiving therapeutic doses of the drug on a chronic basis. Treatment of mice for two years with 2.5, 15, or 80 mg/kg/day isradipine in the diet (approximately 6, 38, and 200 times the maximum recommended daily dose based on a 50 kg man) showed no evidence of oncogenicity. There was no evidence of mutagenic potential based on the results of a battery of mutagenicity tests. No effect on fertility was observed in male and female rats treated with up to 60 mg/kg/day isradipine.

Pregnancy

Pregnancy Category C: Isradipine was administered orally to rats and rabbits during organogenesis. Treatment of pregnant rats with doses of 6, 20, or 60 mg/kg/day produced a significant reduction in maternal weight gain during treatment with the highest dose (150 times the maximum recommended human daily dose) but with no lasting effects on the mother or the offspring. Treatment of pregnant rabbits with doses of 1, 3, or 10 mg/kg/day (2.5, 7.5, and 25 times the maximum recommended human daily dose) produced decrements in maternal body weight gain and increased fetal resorptions at the two higher doses. There was no evidence of embryotoxicity at doses which were not maternotoxic and no evidence of teratogenicity at any dose tested. In a peri/postnatal administration study in rats, reduced maternal body weight gain during late pregnancy at oral doses of 20 and 60 mg/kg/day isradipine was associated with reduced birth weights and decreased peri and postnatal pup survival.

Nursing Mothers

It is not known whether DynaCirc® (isradipine) is excreted in human milk. Because many drugs are excreted in human milk, and because of the potential for adverse effects of DynaCirc® (isradipine) on nursing infants, a decision should be made as to whether to discontinue nursing or discontinue the drug, taking into account the importance of the drug to the mother.

Pediatric Use

Safety and effectiveness have not been established in children.

*AH = conduction time from low right atrium to His bundle deflection, or AV nodal conduction time; HV = conduction time through the His bundle and the bundle branch-Purkinje system.

ADVERSE REACTIONS

In multiple dose U.S. studies in hypertension, 1228 patients received DynaCirc® (isradipine) alone or in combination with other agents, principally a thiazide diuretic, 934 of them in controlled comparisons with placebo or active agents. An additional 652 patients (which includes 374 normal volunteers) received DynaCirc® (isradipine) in U.S. studies of conditions other than hypertension, and 1321 patients received DynaCirc® (isradipine) in non-U.S. studies. About 500 patients received DynaCirc® (isradipine) in long-term hypertension studies, 410 of them for at least 6 months. The adverse reaction rates given below are principally based on controlled hypertension studies, but rarer serious events are derived from all exposures to DynaCirc® (isradipine), including foreign marketing experience.

Most adverse reactions were mild and related to the vasodilatory effects of DynaCirc® (dizziness, edema, palpitations, flushing, tachycardia), and many were transient. About 5% of isradipine patients left studies prematurely because of adverse reactions (vs. 3% of placebo patients and 6% of active control patients), principally due to headache, edema, dizziness, palpitations, and gastrointestinal disturbances.

The table above shows the most common adverse reactions, volunteered or elicited, considered by the investigator to be at least possibly drug related. The results for the DynaCirc® (isradipine) treated patients are presented for all doses pooled together (reported by 1% or greater of patients receiving any dose of isradipine), and also for the two treatment regimens most applicable to the treatment of hypertension with DynaCirc® (isradipine): (1) initial and maintenance dose of 2.5 mg b.i.d., and (2) initial dose of 2.5 mg b.i.d. followed by maintenance dose of 5.0 mg b.i.d.

Except for headache, which is not clearly drug-related (see table above), the more frequent adverse reactions listed above show little change, or increase slightly, in frequency over time, as shown in the following table:

[See table on next page.]

Edema, palpitations, fatigue, and flushing appear to be dose-related, especially at the higher doses of 15-20 mg/day.

In open-label, long-term studies of up to two years in duration, the adverse events reported were generally the same as those reported in the short-term controlled trials. The overall frequencies of these adverse events were slightly higher in the long-term than in the controlled studies, but as in the controlled trials most adverse reactions were mild and transient.

The following adverse events were reported in 0.5-1.0% of the isradipine-treated patients in hypertension studies, or are rare. More serious events from this and other data sources, including postmarketing exposure, are shown in italics. The relationship of these adverse events to isradipine administration is uncertain.

Skin

Pruritus, *urticaria*

Musculoskeletal

Cramps of legs/feet

Respiratory

Cough

Continued on next page

Sandoz—Cont.

Incidence Rates for DynaCirc® (isradipine) (All Doses) by Week (%)

Week	1	2	3	4	5	6
N	694	906	649	847	432	494
Adverse Reaction						
Headache	6.5	6.1	5.2	5.2	5.8	4.5
Dizziness	1.6	1.9	1.7	2.2	2.3	2.0
Edema	1.2	2.5	3.2	3.2	5.3	5.5
Palpitations	1.2	1.3	1.4	1.9	2.1	1.4
Fatigue	0.4	1.0	1.4	1.2	1.2	1.6
Flushing	1.2	1.3	2.0	1.4	2.1	1.4

Week	7	8	9	10	11	12
N	153	377	261	362	107	105
Adverse Reaction						
Headache	2.0	2.7	1.9	2.8	2.8	3.8
Dizziness	2.0	1.9	2.3	3.9	4.7	3.8
Edema	5.9	5.0	4.6	4.7	3.8	3.8
Palpitations	1.3	0.8	0.8	1.7	1.9	2.9
Fatigue	2.0	2.7	1.5	1.4	0.9	1.9
Flushing	3.3	1.3	1.1	0.8	0.0	0.0

Cardiovascular
Shortness of breath, hypotension, *atrial fibrillation, ventricular fibrillation, myocardial infarction, heart failure.*
Gastrointestinal
Abdominal discomfort, constipation, diarrhea.
Urogenital
Nocturia
Nervous System
Drowsiness, insomnia, lethargy, nervousness, impotence, decreased libido, depression, *syncope, paresthesia* (which includes numbness and tingling), *transient ischemic attack, stroke.*
Autonomic
Hyperhidrosis, visual disturbance, dry mouth, numbness.
Miscellaneous
Throat discomfort, *leukopenia, elevated liver function tests.*

OVERDOSAGE

Although there is no well documented experience with DynaCirc® (isradipine) overdosage, available data suggest that, as with other dihydropyridines, gross overdosage would result in excessive peripheral vasodilation with subsequent marked and probably prolonged systemic hypotension. Clinically significant hypotension overdosage calls for active cardiovascular support including monitoring of cardiac and respiratory function, elevation of lower extremities, and attention to circulating fluid volume and urine output. A vasoconstrictor (such as epinephrine, norepinephrine, or levarterenol) may be helpful in restoring vascular tone and blood pressure, provided that there is no contraindication to its use. Since isradipine is highly protein-bound, dialysis is not likely to be of benefit.
Significant lethality was observed in mice given oral doses of over 200 mg/kg and rabbits given about 50 mg/kg of isradipine. Rats tolerated doses of over 2000 mg/kg without effects on survival.

DOSAGE AND ADMINISTRATION

The dosage of DynaCirc® (isradipine) should be individualized. The recommended initial dose of DynaCirc® (isradipine) is 2.5 mg b.i.d. alone or in combination with a thiazide diuretic. An antihypertensive response usually occurs within 2-3 hours. Maximal response may require 2-4 weeks. If a satisfactory reduction in blood pressure does not occur after this period, the dose may be adjusted in increments of 5 mg/day at 2-4 week intervals up to a maximum of 20 mg/day. Most patients, however, show no additional response to doses above 10 mg/day, and adverse effects are increased in frequency above 10 mg/day.
The bioavailability of DynaCirc® (increased AUC) is increased in elderly patients (above 65 years of age), patients with hepatic functional impairment, and patients with mild renal impairment. Ordinarily, the starting dose should still be 2.5 mg b.i.d. in these patients.

HOW SUPPLIED

DynaCirc® (isradipine) Capsules:
2.5 mg, white, imprinted twice with the DynaCirc® (isradipine) logo and "DynaCirc" on one end, and "2.5" and " ⑧ " on the other. Bottles of 100 capsules (NDC 0078-0226-05); bottles of 60 capsules (NDC 0078-0226-44); and SandoPak® (unit-dose) packages of 100, 10 strips, 10 blisters (2×5) per strip (NDC 0078-0226-06).

5 mg, light pink, imprinted twice with the DynaCirc® (isradipine) logo and "DynaCirc" on one end, and "5" and " ⑧ " on the other. Bottles of 100 capsules (NDC 0078-0227-05); bottles of 60 capsules (NDC 0078-0227-44); and San-

doPak® (unit-dose) packages of 100, 10 strips, 10 blisters (2×5) per strip (NDC 0078-0227-06).
Store and Dispense: Below 86°F (30°C) in a tight container. Protect from light.
[DYN-Z2 Issued December 31, 1990]
Shown in Product Identification Section, page 427

ELDEPRYL®   ℞
(selegiline hydrochloride)
Tablets

This product is marketed by Sandoz Pharmaceuticals Corporation. Please refer to Somerset Pharmaceuticals, Inc., for complete prescribing information, page 2351.
Shown in Product Identification Section, page 432

FIORICET®   ℞
[fē "or '-set]
(Butalbital, Acetaminophen, and Caffeine Tablets, USP)

CAUTION: Federal law prohibits dispensing without prescription.
The following prescribing information is based on official labeling in effect on August 1, 1992.

DESCRIPTION

Each Fioricet® (Butalbital, Acetaminophen, and Caffeine Tablets, USP) for oral administration contains:
butalbital*, USP .... 50 mg
*WARNING: May be habit forming.
acetaminophen, USP .... 325 mg
caffeine, USP .... 40 mg
Active Ingredients: butalbital, USP, acetaminophen, USP, and caffeine, USP.
Inactive Ingredients: crospovidone, FD&C Blue #1, magnesium stearate, microcrystalline cellulose, povidone, pregelatinized starch, and stearic acid.
Butalbital, 5-allyl-5-isobutylbarbituric acid, a white, odorless, crystalline powder having a slightly bitter taste, is a short to intermediate-acting barbiturate. Its structure is as follows:

$$CH_2{=}CHCH_2$$
$$(CH_3)_2CHCH_2$$

$C_{11}H_{16}N_2O_3$ Mol. wt. 224.26

Acetaminophen, 4'-hydroxyacetanilide, is a non-opiate, non-salicylate analgesic, and antipyretic which occurs as a white, odorless, crystalline powder possessing a slightly bitter taste. Its structure is as follows:

$$HO{-}\bigcirc{-}NHCOCH_3$$

$C_8H_9NO_2$ Mol. wt. 151.16

Caffeine, 1,3,7-trimethylxanthine, is a central nervous system stimulant which occurs as a white powder or white glis-

tening needles. It also has a bitter taste. Its structure is as follows:

$C_8H_{10}N_4O_2$ Mol. wt. 194.19

CLINICAL PHARMACOLOGY

Pharmacologically, Fioricet® (Butalbital, Acetaminophen, and Caffeine Tablets) combines the analgesic properties of acetaminophen-caffeine with the anxiolytic and muscle relaxant properties of butalbital.

INDICATIONS AND USAGE

Fioricet® (Butalbital, Acetaminophen, and Caffeine Tablets) is indicated for the relief of the symptom complex of tension (or muscle contraction) headache.

CONTRAINDICATIONS

Hypersensitivity to acetaminophen, caffeine or barbiturates. Patients with porphyria.

PRECAUTIONS

General
Barbiturates should be administered with caution, if at all, to patients who are mentally depressed, have suicidal tendencies, or a history of drug abuse.
Elderly or debilitated patients may react to barbiturates with marked excitement, depression, and confusion. In some persons, barbiturates repeatedly produce excitement rather than depression.
Information for Patients
Practitioners should give the following information and instructions to patients receiving barbiturates:
A. The use of barbiturates carries with it an associated risk of psychological and/or physical dependence. The patient should be warned against increasing the dose of the drug without consulting a physician.
B. Barbiturates may impair mental and/or physical abilities required for the performance of potentially hazardous tasks (*e.g.,* driving, operating machinery, etc.).
C. Alcohol should not be consumed while taking barbiturates. Concurrent use of the barbiturates with other CNS depressants (e.g., alcohol, narcotics, tranquilizers, and antihistamines) may result in additional CNS depressant effects.
Drug Interactions
Patients receiving narcotic analgesics, antipsychotics, antianxiety agents, or other CNS depressants (including alcohol) concomitantly with Fioricet® (Butalbital, Acetaminophen, and Caffeine Tablets) may exhibit additive CNS depressant effects.

Drugs	Effect
Butalbital w/coumarin anticoagulants	Decreased effect of anticoagulant because of increased metabolism resulting from enzyme induction.
Butalbital w/tricyclic antidepressants	Decreased blood levels of the antidepressant.

Usage in Pregnancy
Adequate studies have not been performed in animals to determine whether this drug affects fertility in males or females, has teratogenic potential or has other adverse effects on the fetus. There are no well-controlled studies in pregnant women. Although there is no clearly defined risk, one cannot exclude the possibility of infrequent or subtle damage to the human fetus. Fioricet® (Butalbital, Acetaminophen, and Caffeine Tablets) should be used in pregnant women only when clearly needed.
Nursing Mothers
The effects of Fioricet® (Butalbital, Acetaminophen, and Caffeine Tablets) on infants of nursing mothers are not known. Barbiturates are excreted in the breast milk of nursing mothers. The serum levels in infants are believed to be insignificant with therapeutic doses.
Pediatric Use
Safety and effectiveness in children below the age of 12 have not been established.

ADVERSE REACTIONS

The most frequent adverse reactions are drowsiness and dizziness. Less frequent adverse reactions are lightheadedness and gastrointestinal disturbances including nausea, vomiting, and flatulence. Mental confusion or depression can occur due to intolerance or overdosage of butalbital.

Several cases of dermatological reactions including toxic epidermal necrolysis and erythema multiforme have been reported.

DRUG ABUSE AND DEPENDENCE

Prolonged use of barbiturates can produce drug dependence, characterized by psychic dependence and tolerance. The abuse liability of Fioricet® (Butalbital, Acetaminophen, and Caffeine Tablets) is similar to that of other barbiturate-containing drug combinations. Caution should be exercised when prescribing medication for patients with a known propensity for taking excessive quantities of drugs, which is not uncommon in patients with chronic tension headache.

OVERDOSAGE

The toxic effects of acute overdosage of Fioricet® (Butalbital, Acetaminophen, and Caffeine Tablets) are attributable mainly to its barbiturate component, and, to a lesser extent, acetaminophen. Because toxic effects of caffeine occur in very high dosages only, the possibility of significant caffeine toxicity from Fioricet® (Butalbital, Acetaminophen, and Caffeine Tablets) overdosage is unlikely.

Barbiturate

Signs and Symptoms

Drowsiness, confusion, coma; respiratory depression; hypotension; shock.

Treatment

1. Maintenance of an adequate airway, with assisted respiration and oxygen administration as necessary.
2. Monitoring of vital signs and fluid balance.
3. If the patient is conscious and has not lost the gag reflex, emesis may be induced with ipecac. Care should be taken to prevent pulmonary aspiration of vomitus. After completion of vomiting, 30 grams of activated charcoal in a glass of water may be administered.
4. If emesis is contraindicated, gastric lavage may be performed with a cuffed endotracheal tube in place with the patient in the facedown position. Activated charcoal may be left in the emptied stomach and a saline cathartic administered.
5. Fluid therapy and other standard treatment of shock, if needed.
6. If renal function is normal, forced diuresis may aid in the elimination of the barbiturate. Alkalinization of the urine increases renal excretion of some barbiturates, especially phenobarbital.
7. Although not recommended as a routine procedure, hemodialysis may be used in severe barbiturate intoxication or if the patient is anuric or in shock.

Acetaminophen

Signs and Symptoms

In acute acetaminophen overdosage, dose-dependent, potentially fatal hepatic necrosis is the most serious adverse effect. Renal tubular necrosis, hypoglycemic coma, and thrombocytopenia may also occur.

In adults, hepatic toxicity has rarely been reported with acute overdoses of less than 10 grams and fatalities with less than 15 grams. Importantly, young children seem to be more resistant than adults to the hepatotoxic effect of an acetaminophen overdose.

Early symptoms following a potentially hepatotoxic overdosage may include: nausea, vomiting, diaphoresis, and general malaise. Clinical and laboratory evidence of hepatic toxicity may not be apparent until 48–72 hours post-ingestion.

Treatment

The stomach should be emptied promptly by lavage or by induction of emesis with syrup of ipecac. Patients' estimates of the quantity of a drug ingested are notoriously unreliable. Therefore, if an acetaminophen overdose is suspected, a serum acetaminophen assay should be obtained as early as possible, but no sooner than four hours following ingestion. Liver function studies should be obtained initially and repeated at 24-hour intervals.

The antidote, N-acetylcysteine, should be administered as early as possible, preferably within 16 hours of the overdose ingestion for optimal results, but in any case, within 24 hours. Following recovery, there are no residual, structural or functional hepatic abnormalities.

DOSAGE AND ADMINISTRATION

One or 2 tablets every 4 hours as needed. Do not exceed 6 tablets per day.

HOW SUPPLIED

Fioricet® (Butalbital, Acetaminophen, and Caffeine Tablets, USP), containing 50 mg butalbital, 325 mg acetaminophen, and 40 mg caffeine, is available as light-blue, round compressed tablets, engraved "FIORICET" and "⚠" on one side, three-head profile "S" on other side. Bottles of 100 (NDC 0078-0084-05) and 500 (NDC 0078-0084-08).

SandoPak® (unit-dose) packages of 100, 10 blister strips of 10 tablets (NDC 0078-0084-06).

Store and Dispense

Store below 86°F (30°C); dispense in a tight container.

[FCT-Z12 Issued January 15, 1992]

Shown in Product Identification Section, page 427

FIORICET® with CODEINE ©III ℞

[fē″or′-set]

(butalbital, acetaminophen, caffeine, and codeine phosphate)

CAPSULES

CAUTION: Federal law prohibits dispensing without prescription.

The following prescribing information is based on official labeling in effect on August 1, 1992.

DESCRIPTION

Fioricet® with Codeine (butalbital, acetaminophen, caffeine, and codeine phosphate) is supplied in capsule form for oral administration.

Each capsule contains:

codeine phosphate, USP	30 mg (½ gr)
Warning: May be habit-forming.	
butalbital, USP	50 mg
Warning: May be habit-forming.	
caffeine, USP	40 mg
acetaminophen, USP	325 mg

Codeine phosphate [morphine-3-methyl ether phosphate (1:1) (salt) hemihydrate, $C_{18}H_{24}NO_7P$, anhydrous mw 397.37], a white crystalline powder, is a narcotic analgesic and antitussive.

Butalbital (5-allyl-5-isobutylbarbituric acid, $C_{11}H_{16}N_2O_3$, mw 224.26), a slightly bitter, white crystalline powder, is a short-to intermediate-acting barbiturate.

Caffeine (1,3,7-trimethylxanthine, $C_8H_{10}N_4O_2$, mw 194.19), a bitter, white crystalline powder, is a central nervous system stimulant.

Acetaminophen (4′-hydroxyacetanilide, $C_8H_9NO_2$, mw 151.16), a slightly bitter white crystalline powder, is a non-opiate, non-salicylate analgesic and antipyretic.

Active Ingredients: codeine phosphate, USP, butalbital, USP, caffeine, USP, and acetaminophen, USP.

Inactive Ingredients: black iron oxide, colloidal silicon dioxide, D&C Red #7 (calcium lake), D&C Red #33, FD&C Blue #1, FD&C Blue #1 (aluminum lake), gelatin, magnesium stearate, pregelatinized starch, red iron oxide, sodium lauryl sulfate, and titanium dioxide.

May also include: benzyl alcohol, butylparaben, carboxymethylcellulose sodium, edetate calcium disodium, methylparaben, propylparaben, silicon dioxide, and sodium propionate.

CLINICAL PHARMACOLOGY

Fioricet® with Codeine is a combination drug product intended as a treatment for tension headache.

Fioricet® consists of a fixed combination of butalbital 50 mg, acetaminophen 325 mg and caffeine 40 mg. The role each component plays in the relief of the complex of symptoms known as tension headache is incompletely understood.

Pharmacokinetics

The behavior of the individual components is described below.

Codeine

Codeine is readily absorbed from the gastrointestinal tract. It is rapidly distributed from the intravascular spaces to the various body tissues, with preferential uptake by parenchymatous organs such as the liver, spleen and kidney. Codeine crosses the blood-brain barrier, and is found in fetal tissue and breast milk. The plasma concentration does not correlate with brain concentration or relief of pain; however, codeine is not bound to plasma proteins and does not accumulate in body tissues.

The plasma half-life is about 2.9 hours. The elimination of codeine is primarily via the kidneys, and about 90% of an oral dose is excreted by the kidneys within 24 hours of dosing. The urinary secretion products consist of free and glucuronide conjugated codeine (about 70%), free and conjugated norcodeine (about 10%), free and conjugated morphine (about 10%), normorphine (4%), and hydrocodone (1%). The remainder of the dose is excreted in the feces.

At therapeutic doses, the analgesic effect reaches a peak within 2 hours and persists between 4 and 6 hours.

See **OVERDOSAGE** for toxicity information.

Butalbital

Butalbital is well absorbed from the gastrointestinal tract and is expected to distribute to most tissues in the body. Barbiturates in general may appear in breast milk and readily cross the placental barrier. They are bound to plasma and tissue proteins to a varying degree and binding increases directly as a function of lipid solubility.

Elimination of butalbital is primarily via the kidney (59%–88% of the dose) as unchanged drug or metabolites. The plasma half-life is about 35 hours. Urinary excretion products include parent drug (about 3.6% of the dose), 5-isobutyl-5-(2,3-dihydroxypropyl) barbituric acid (about 24% of the dose), 5-allyl-5(3-hydroxy-2-methyl-1-propyl) barbituric acid (about 4.8% of the dose), products with the barbituric acid ring hydrolyzed with excretion of urea (about 14% of the dose), as well as unidentified materials. Of the material excreted in the urine, 32% is conjugated.

See **OVERDOSAGE** for toxicity information.

Caffeine

Like most xanthines, caffeine is rapidly absorbed and distributed in all body tissues and fluids, including the CNS, fetal tissues, and breast milk.

Caffeine is cleared through metabolism and excretion in the urine. The plasma half-life is about 3 hours. Hepatic biotransformation prior to excretion results in about equal amounts of 1-methyl-xanthine and 1-methyluric acid. Of the 70% of the dose that is recovered in the urine, only 3% is unchanged drug.

See **OVERDOSAGE** for toxicity information.

Acetaminophen

Acetaminophen is rapidly absorbed from the gastrointestinal tract and is distributed throughout most body tissues. The plasma half-life is 1.25–3 hours, but may be increased by liver damage and following overdosage. Elimination of acetaminophen is principally by liver metabolism (conjugation) and subsequent renal excretion of metabolites. Approximately 85% of an oral dose appears in the urine within 24 hours of administration, most as the glucuronide conjugate, with small amounts of other conjugates and unchanged drug.

See **OVERDOSAGE** for toxicity information.

INDICATIONS

Fioricet® with Codeine is indicated for the relief of the symptom complex of tension (or muscle contraction) headache.

Evidence supporting the efficacy and safety of Fioricet® with Codeine in the treatment of multiple recurrent headaches is unavailable. Caution in this regard is required because codeine and butalbital are habit-forming and potentially abusable.

CONTRAINDICATIONS

Fioricet® with Codeine is contraindicated under the following conditions:

—Hypersensitivity or intolerance to acetaminophen, caffeine, butalbital, or codeine.

—Patients with porphyria.

WARNINGS

In the presence of head injury or other intracranial lesions, the respiratory depressant effects of codeine and other narcotics may be markedly enhanced, as well as their capacity for elevating cerebrospinal fluid pressure. Narcotics also produce other CNS depressant effects, such as drowsiness, that may further obscure the clinical course of the patients with head injuries.

Codeine or other narcotics may obscure signs on which to judge the diagnosis or clinical course of patients with acute abdominal conditions.

Butalbital and codeine are both habit-forming and potentially abusable. Consequently, the extended use of Fioricet® with Codeine is not recommended.

PRECAUTIONS

General

Fioricet® with Codeine should be prescribed with caution in certain special-risk patients such as the elderly or debilitated, and those with severe impairment of renal or hepatic function, head injuries, elevated intracranial pressure, acute abdominal conditions, hypothyroidism, urethral stricture, Addison's disease, or prostatic hypertrophy.

Information for patients

Fioricet® with Codeine may impair mental and/or physical abilities required for the performance of potentially hazardous tasks such as driving a car or operating machinery. Such tasks should be avoided while taking Fioricet® with Codeine.

Alcohol and other CNS depressants may produce an additive CNS depression, when taken with Fioricet® with Codeine, and should be avoided.

Codeine and butalbital may be habit-forming. Patients should take the drug only for as long as it is prescribed, in the amounts prescribed, and no more frequently than prescribed.

Laboratory tests

In patients with severe hepatic or renal disease, effects of therapy should be monitored with serial liver and/or renal function tests.

Drug interactions

The CNS effects of butalbital may be enhanced by monoamine oxidase (MAO) inhibitors.

Fioricet® with Codeine may enhance the effects of:

—Other narcotic analgesics, alcohol, general anesthetics, tranquilizers such as chlordiazepoxide, sedative-hypnotics, or other CNS depressants, causing increased CNS depression.

Continued on next page

Sandoz—Cont.

Drug/laboratory test interactions

Codeine

Codeine may increase serum amylase levels.

Acetaminophen

Acetaminophen may produce false-positive test results for urinary 5-hydroxyindoleacetic acid.

Carcinogenesis, mutagenesis, impairment of fertility

No adequate studies have been conducted in animals to determine whether acetaminophen, codeine and butalbital have a potential for carcinogenesis or mutagenesis. No adequate studies have been conducted in animals to determine whether acetaminophen and butalbital have a potential for impairment of fertility.

Pregnancy

Teratogenic effects

Pregnancy category C: Animal reproduction studies have not been conducted with Fioricet® with Codeine. It is also not known whether Fioricet® with Codeine can cause fetal harm when administered to a pregnant woman or can affect reproduction capacity. Fioricet® with Codeine should be given to a pregnant woman only when clearly needed.

Nonteratogenic effects

Withdrawal seizures were reported in a two-day-old male infant whose mother had taken a butalbital-containing drug during the last 2 months of pregnancy. Butalbital was found in the infant's serum. The infant was given phenobarbital 5 mg/kg, which was tapered without further seizure or other withdrawal symptoms.

Labor and delivery

Use of codeine during labor may lead to respiratory depression in the neonate.

Nursing mothers

Caffeine, barbiturates, acetaminophen and codeine are excreted in breast milk in small amounts, but the significance of their effects on nursing infants is not known. Because of potential for serious adverse reactions in nursing infants from Fioricet® with Codeine (butalbital, acetaminophen, caffeine, and codeine phosphate), a decision should be made whether to discontinue nursing or to discontinue the drug, taking into account the importance of the drug to the mother.

Pediatric use

Safety and effectiveness in children below the age of 12 have not been established.

ADVERSE REACTIONS

Frequently observed

The most frequently reported adverse reactions are drowsiness, lightheadedness, dizziness, sedation, shortness of breath, nausea, vomiting, abdominal pain, and intoxicated feeling.

Infrequently observed

All adverse events tabulated below are classified as infrequent.

Central nervous: headache, shaky feeling, tingling, agitation, fainting, fatigue, heavy eyelids, high energy, hot spells, numbness, sluggishness, seizure. Mental confusion, excitement or depression can also occur due to intolerance, particularly in elderly or debilitated patients, or due to overdosage of butalbital.

Autonomic nervous: dry mouth, hyperhidrosis.

Gastrointestinal: difficulty swallowing, heartburn, flatulence, constipation.

Cardiovascular: tachycardia.

Musculoskeletal: leg pain, muscle fatigue.

Genitourinary: diuresis.

Miscellaneous: pruritus, fever, earache, nasal congestion, tinnitus, euphoria, allergic reactions.

The following adverse reactions have been voluntarily reported as temporally associated with Fiorinal® with Codeine, a related product containing aspirin, butalbital, caffeine, and codeine.

Central nervous: abuse, addiction, anxiety, disorientation, hallucination, hyperactivity, insomnia, libido decrease, nervousness, neuropathy, psychosis, sexual activity increase, slurred speech, twitching, unconsciousness, vertigo.

Autonomic nervous: epistaxis, flushing, miosis, salivation.

Gastrointestinal: anorexia, appetite increased, diarrhea, esophagitis, gastroenteritis, gastrointestinal spasms, hiccup, mouth burning, pyloric ulcer.

Cardiovascular: chest pain, hypotensive reaction, palpitations, syncope.

Skin: erythema, erythema multiforme, exfoliative dermatitis, hives, rash, toxic epidermal necrolysis.

Urinary: kidney impairment, urinary difficulty.

Miscellaneous: allergic reaction, anaphylactic shock, cholangiocarcinoma, drug interaction with erythromycin (stomach upset), edema.

The following adverse drug events may be borne in mind as potential effects of the components of Fioricet® with Codeine. Potential effects of high dosage are listed in the OVERDOSAGE section.

Acetaminophen: allergic reactions, rash, thrombocytopenia, agranulocytosis.

Caffeine: cardiac stimulation, irritability, tremor, dependence, nephrotoxicity, hyperglycemia.

Codeine: nausea, vomiting, drowsiness, lightheadedness, constipation, pruritus.

Several cases of dermatological reactions, including toxic epidermal necrolysis and erythema multiforme, have been reported for Fioricet® (Butalbital, Acetaminophen, and Caffeine Tablets, USP).

DRUG ABUSE AND DEPENDENCE

Controlled substance

Fioricet® with Codeine is controlled by the Drug Enforcement Administration and is classified under Schedule III.

Abuse and dependence

Codeine

Codeine can produce drug dependence of the morphine type and, therefore, has the potential for being abused. Psychological dependence, physical dependence, and tolerance may develop upon repeated administration and it should be prescribed and administered with the same degree of caution appropriate for the use of other oral narcotic medications.

Butalbital

Barbiturates may be habit-forming: Tolerance, psychological dependence, and physical dependence may occur especially following prolonged use of high doses of barbiturates. The average daily dose for the barbiturate addict is usually about 1,500 mg. As tolerance to barbiturates develops, the amount needed to maintain the same level of intoxication increases; tolerance to a fatal dosage, however, does not increase more than two-fold. As this occurs, the margin between an intoxication dosage and fatal dosage becomes smaller. The lethal dose of a barbiturate is far less if alcohol is also ingested. Major withdrawal symptoms (convulsions and delirium) may occur within 16 hours and last up to 5 days after abrupt cessation of these drugs. Intensity of withdrawal symptoms gradually declines over a period of approximately 15 days. Treatment of barbiturate dependence consists of cautious and gradual withdrawal of the drug. Barbiturate-dependent patients can be withdrawn by using a number of different withdrawal regimens. One method involves initiating treatment at the patient's regular dosage level and gradually decreasing the daily dosage as tolerated by the patient.

OVERDOSAGE

Following an acute overdosage of Fioricet® with Codeine, toxicity may result from the barbiturate, the codeine, or the acetaminophen. Toxicity due to the caffeine is less likely, due to the relatively small amounts in this formulation.

Signs and symptoms

Toxicity from ***barbiturate*** poisoning include drowsiness, confusion, and coma; respiratory depression; hypotension; and hypovolemic shock. Toxicity from ***codeine*** poisoning includes the opioid triad of: pinpoint pupils, depression of respiration, and loss of consciousness. Convulsions may occur. In ***acetaminophen*** overdosage: dose-dependent, potentially fatal hepatic necrosis is the most serious adverse effect. Renal tubular necroses, hypoglycemic coma, and thrombocytopenia may also occur. Early symptoms following a potentially hepatotoxic overdose may include: nausea, vomiting, diaphoresis, and general malaise. Clinical and laboratory evidence of hepatic toxicity may not be apparent until 48–72 hours post-ingestion. In adults hepatic toxicity has rarely been reported with acute overdoses of less than 10 grams, or fatalities with less than 15 grams. Acute ***caffeine*** poisoning may cause insomnia, restlessness, tremor, and delirium, tachycardia, and extrasystoles.

Treatment

A single or multiple overdose with Fioricet® with Codeine is a potentially lethal polydrug overdose, and consultation with a regional poison control center is recommended. Immediate treatment includes support of cardiorespiratory function and measures to reduce drug absorption. Vomiting should be induced mechanically, or with syrup of ipecac, if the patient is alert (adequate pharyngeal and laryngeal reflexes). Oral activated charcoal (1 g/kg) should follow gastric emptying. The first dose should be accompanied by an appropriate cathartic. If repeated doses are used, the cathartic might be included with alternate doses as required. Hypotension is usually hypovolemic and should respond to fluids. Pressors should be avoided. A cuffed endotracheal tube should be inserted before gastric lavage of the unconscious patient and, when necessary, to provide assisted respiration. If renal function is normal, forced diuresis may aid in the elimination of the barbiturate. Alkalinization of the urine increases renal excretion of some barbiturates, especially phenobarbital.

Meticulous attention should be given to maintaining adequate pulmonary ventilation. In severe cases of intoxication, peritoneal dialysis, or preferably hemodialysis may be considered. If hypoprothrombinemia occurs due to acetaminophen overdose, vitamin K should be administered intravenously.

Naloxone, a narcotic antagonist, can reverse respiratory depression and coma associated with opioid overdose. Naloxone 0.4–2 mg is given parenterally. Since the duration of action of codeine may exceed that of the naloxone, the patient should be kept under continuous surveillance and repeated doses of the antagonist should be administered as needed to maintain adequate respiration. A narcotic antagonist should not be administered in the absence of clinically significant respiratory or cardiovascular depression.

If the dose of acetaminophen may have exceeded 140 mg/kg, N-acetyl-cysteine should be administered as early as possible. Serum acetaminophen levels should be obtained, since levels 4 or more hours following ingestion help predict acetaminophen toxicity. Do not await acetaminophen assay results before initiating treatment. Hepatic enzymes should be obtained initially, and repeated at 24-hour intervals.

Methemoglobinemia over 30% should be treated with methylene blue by slow intravenous administration.

Toxic doses (for adults)

Butalbital: toxic dose 1.0 g
(20 capsules of Fioricet® with Codeine)

Acetaminophen: toxic dose 10 g
(30 capsules of Fioricet® with Codeine)

Caffeine: toxic dose 1.0 g
(25 capsules of Fioricet® with Codeine)

Codeine: toxic dose 240 mg
(8 capsules of Fioricet® with Codeine)

DOSAGE AND ADMINISTRATION

One or 2 capsules every 4 hours. Total daily dosage should not exceed 6 capsules.

Extended and repeated use of this product is not recommended because of the potential for physical dependence.

HOW SUPPLIED

Fioricet® with Codeine Capsules

Dark blue, opaque cap with a grey, opaque body. Cap is imprinted twice in light-blue with "FIORICET" and "CODEINE". Body is imprinted twice with four-head profile "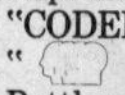" in red.

Bottle of 100 (NDC 0078-0243-05)

ControlPak® unit-dose package of 25; continuous reverse-numbered roll of sealed blisters (NDC 0078-0243-13).

Store and dispense

Below 86°F (30°C); tight container.

[FCD-Z1 Issued July, 1992]

FIORINAL® Ⓒⅲ ℞

[fē-ōr 'i-nol]

TABLETS/CAPSULES

CAUTION: Federal law prohibits dispensing without prescription.

The following prescribing information is based on official labeling in effect on August 1, 1992.

DESCRIPTION

Each Fiorinal® Tablet or Capsule for oral administration contains: butalbital, USP, 50 mg (Warning: May be habit forming); aspirin, USP, 325 mg; caffeine, USP, 40 mg.

Butalbital, 5-allyl-5-isobutyl-barbituric acid, a white odorless crystalline powder; is a short- to intermediate-acting barbiturate.

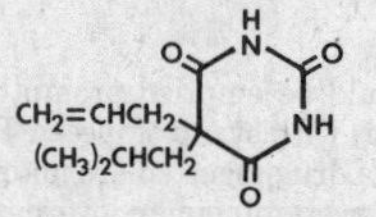

Tablets

Active Ingredients: aspirin, USP, butalbital, USP, and caffeine, USP.

Inactive Ingredients: alginic acid, lactose, microcrystalline cellulose, povidone, stearic acid, and another ingredient.

Capsules

Active Ingredients: aspirin, USP, butalbital, USP, and caffeine, USP.

Inactive Ingredients: D&C Yellow #10, gelatin, microcrystalline cellulose, sodium lauryl sulfate, starch, and talc.

May Also Include: benzyl alcohol, butylparaben, color additives including FD&C Blue #1, FD&C Green #3, FD&C Yellow #6, edetate calcium disodium, methylparaben, propylparaben, silicon dioxide, sodium propionate.

ACTIONS

Pharmacologically, Fiorinal® combines the analgesic properties of aspirin with the anxiolytic and muscle relaxant properties of butalbital.

The clinical effectiveness of Fiorinal® in tension headache has been established in double-blind, placebo-controlled, multi-clinic trials. A factorial design study compared Fiorinal® with each of its major components. This study demonstrated that each component contributes to the efficacy of Fiorinal® in the treatment of the target symptoms of tension headache (headache pain, psychic tension, and mus-

cle contraction in the head, neck, and shoulder region). For each symptom and the symptom complex as a whole, Fiorinal® was shown to have significantly superior clinical effects to either component alone.

INDICATIONS

Fiorinal® is indicated for the relief of the symptom complex of tension (or muscle contraction) headache.

CONTRAINDICATIONS

Hypersensitivity to aspirin, caffeine, or barbiturates. Patients with porphyria.

WARNINGS

Drug Dependency

Prolonged use of barbiturates can produce drug dependence, characterized by psychic dependence, and less frequently, physical dependence and tolerance. The abuse liability of Fiorinal® is similar to that of other barbiturate-containing drug combinations. Caution should be exercised when prescribing medication for patients with a known propensity for taking excessive quantities of drugs, which is not uncommon in patients with chronic tension headache.

Use in Ambulatory Patients

Fiorinal® may impair the mental and/or physical abilities required for the performance of potentially hazardous tasks, such as driving a car or operating machinery. The patient should be cautioned accordingly. Central Nervous System depressant effects of butalbital may be additive with those of other CNS depressants. Concurrent use with other sedative-hypnotics or alcohol should be avoided. When such combined therapy is necessary, the dose of one or more agents may need to be reduced.

Use in Pregnancy

Adequate studies have not been performed in animals to determine whether this drug affects fertility in males or females, has teratogenic potential, or has other adverse effects on the fetus. While there are no well-controlled studies in pregnant women, over twenty years of marketing and clinical experience does not include any positive evidence of adverse effects on the fetus. Although there is no clearly defined risk, such experience cannot exclude the possibility of infrequent or subtle damage to the human fetus. Fiorinal® should be used in pregnant women only when clearly needed.

Nursing Mothers

The effects of Fiorinal® on infants of nursing mothers are not known. Salicylates and barbiturates are excreted in the breast milk of nursing mothers. The serum levels in infants are believed to be insignificant with therapeutic doses.

PRECAUTIONS

Salicylates should be used with extreme caution in the presence of peptic ulcer or coagulation abnormalities.

Pediatric Use

Safety and effectiveness in children below the age of 12 have not been established.

ADVERSE REACTIONS

The most frequent adverse reactions are drowsiness and dizziness. Less frequent adverse reactions are lightheadedness and gastrointestinal disturbances including nausea, vomiting, and flatulence. A single incidence of bone marrow suppression has been reported with the use of Fiorinal®. Several cases of dermatological reactions including toxic epidermal necrolysis and erythema multiforme have been reported.

OVERDOSAGE

The toxic effects of acute overdosage of Fiorinal® are attributable mainly to its barbiturate component, and, to a lesser extent, aspirin. Because toxic effects of caffeine occur in very high dosages only, the possibility of significant caffeine toxicity from Fiorinal® overdosage is unlikely. Symptoms attributable to *acute barbiturate poisoning* include drowsiness, confusion, and coma; respiratory depression; hypotension; shock. Symptoms attributable to *acute aspirin poisoning* include hyperpnea; acid-base disturbances with development of metabolic acidosis; vomiting and abdominal pain; tinnitus; hyperthermia; hypoprothrombinemia; restlessness; delirium; convulsions. *Acute caffeine poisoning* may cause insomnia, restlessness, tremor, and delirium; tachycardia and extrasystoles. *Treatment* consists primarily of management of barbiturate intoxication and the correction of the acid-base imbalance due to salicylism. Vomiting should be induced mechanically or with emetics in the conscious patient. Gastric lavage may be used if the pharyngeal and laryngeal reflexes are present and if less than 4 hours have elapsed since ingestion. A cuffed endotracheal tube should be inserted before gastric lavage of the unconscious patient and when necessary to provide assisted respiration. Diuresis, alkalinization of the urine, and correction of electrolyte disturbances should be accomplished through administration of intravenous fluids such as 1% sodium bicarbonate in 5% dextrose in water. Meticulous attention should be given to maintaining adequate pulmonary ventilation. Correction of hypotension may require the administration of levarterenol bitartrate or phenylephrine hydrochloride by intravenous infusion. In severe cases of intoxication, peritoneal dialysis, hemodialysis, or exchange transfusion may be lifesaving. Hypoprothrombinemia should be treated with Vitamin K, intravenously.

DOSAGE AND ADMINISTRATION

One or 2 tablets or capsules every 4 hours. Total daily dose should not exceed 6 tablets or capsules.

HOW SUPPLIED

Fiorinal® Capsules

Color is bright Kelly green and lime green, imprinted "FIORINAL 78-103" on each half of capsule. Packages of 100 (NDC 0078-0103-05) and 500 (NDC 0078-0103-08). Also available in ControlPak® package, 25 capsules (continuous reverse-numbered roll of sealed blisters) (NDC 0078-0103-13).

Fiorinal® Tablets

White, compressed tablet, engraved "FIORINAL" on one side, "SANDOZ" on other side. Packages of 100 (NDC 0078-0104-05) and 1000 (NDC 0078-0104-09). Also available in SandoPak® (unit-dose) package of 100 tablets individually blister-sealed (NDC 0078-0104-06).

Store and Dispense

Below 77°F (25°C), tight container.

[FIO-ZZ30 Issued November 15, 1990.]

Shown in Product Identification Section, page 427

FIORINAL® with CODEINE Ⓒ ℞

[fē-or´ĭ-nol]

(butalbital, aspirin, caffeine, and codeine phosphate) CAPSULES

CAUTION: Federal law prohibits dispensing without prescription.

The following prescribing information is based on official labeling in effect on August 1, 1992.

DESCRIPTION

Fiorinal® with Codeine (butalbital, aspirin, caffeine, and codeine phosphate) is supplied in capsule form for oral administration. Each capsule contains:

codeine phosphate, USP .... 30 mg (1/2 gr)
Warning: May be habit forming.
butalbital, USP .... 50 mg
Warning: May be habit forming.
caffeine, USP .... 40 mg
aspirin, USP .... 325 mg

Codeine phosphate occurs as fine, white, needle-shaped crystals, or white, crystalline powder. It is affected by light. Its chemical name is 7,8-didehydro-4,5α-epoxy-3-methoxy-17-methylmorphinan-6α-ol phosphate (1:1) (salt) hemihydrate.

Butalbital, 5-allyl-5-isobutyl-barbituric acid, a white odorless crystalline powder, is a short- to intermediate-acting barbiturate. Its molecular weight is 224.26 and its empirical formula is $C_{11}H_{16}N_2O_3$.

Caffeine, 1,3,7-trimethylxanthine, is a central nervous stimulant which occurs as a white powder or white glistening needles.

Aspirin is benzoic acid, 2-(acetyloxy)-, with an empirical formula of $C_9H_8O_4$.

Inactive Ingredients: D&C Yellow #10, FD&C Blue #1, FD&C Red #3, FD&C Yellow #6, gelatin, microcrystalline cellulose, sodium lauryl sulfate, starch, talc, titanium dioxide.

May Also Include: benzyl alcohol, butylparaben, edetate calcium disodium, glycerin, methylparaben, propylparaben, silicon dioxide, sodium propionate.

CLINICAL PHARMACOLOGY

Fiorinal® with Codeine is a combination drug product intended as a treatment for tension headache.

Fiorinal® consists of a fixed combination of caffeine 40 mg, butalbital 50 mg, and aspirin 325 mg. The role each component plays in the relief of the complex of symptoms known as tension headache is incompletely understood.

Pharmacokinetics

Bioavailability: The bioavailability of the components of the fixed combination of Fiorinal® with Codeine is identical to their bioavailability when Fiorinal® and Codeine are administered separately in equivalent molar doses.

The behavior of the individual components is described below.

Aspirin

The systemic availability of aspirin after an oral dose is highly dependent on the dosage form, the presence of food, the gastric emptying time, gastric pH, antacids, buffering agents, and particle size. These factors affect not necessarily the extent of absorption of total salicylates but more the stability of aspirin prior to absorption.

During the absorption process and after absorption, aspirin is mainly hydrolyzed to salicylic acid and distributed to all body tissues and fluids, including fetal tissues, breast milk, and the central nervous system (CNS). Highest concentrations are found in plasma, liver, renal cortex, heart, and lung. In plasma, about 50%-80% of the salicylic acid and its metabolites are loosely bound to plasma proteins.

The clearance of total salicylates is subject to saturable kinetics; however, first-order elimination kinetics are still a good approximation for doses up to 650 mg. The plasma half-life for aspirin is about 12 minutes and for salicylic acid and/or total salicylates is about 3.0 hours.

The elimination of therapeutic doses is through the kidneys either as salicylic acid or other biotransformation products. The renal clearance is greatly augmented by an alkaline urine as is produced by concurrent administration of sodium bicarbonate or potassium citrate.

The biotransformation of aspirin occurs primarily in the hepatocytes. The major metabolites are salicyluric acid (75%), the phenolic and acyl glucuronides of salicylate (15%), and gentisic and gentisuric acid (1%). The bioavailability of the aspirin component of Fiorinal® with Codeine capsules is equivalent to that of a solution except for a slower rate of absorption. A peak concentration of 8.80 μg/mL was obtained at 40 minutes after a 650 mg dose.

See *OVERDOSAGE* for toxicity information.

Codeine

Codeine is readily absorbed from the gastrointestinal tract. It is rapidly distributed from the intravascular spaces to the various body tissues, with preferential uptake by parenchymatous organs such as the liver, spleen, and kidney. Codeine crosses the blood-brain barrier, and is found in fetal tissue and breast milk. Codeine is not bound to plasma proteins and does not accumulate in body tissues.

The plasma half-life is about 2.9 hours. The elimination of codeine is primarily via the kidneys, and about 90% of an oral dose is excreted by the kidneys within 24 hours of dosing. The urinary secretion products consist of free and glucuronide-conjugated codeine (about 70%), free and conjugated norcodeine (about 10%), free and conjugated morphine (about 10%), normorphine (4%), and hydrocodone (1%). The remainder of the dose is excreted in the feces.

At therapeutic doses, the analgesic effect reaches a peak within 2 hours and persists between 4 and 6 hours.

The bioavailability of the codeine component of Fiorinal® with Codeine capsules is equivalent to that of a solution. Peak concentrations of 198 ng/mL were obtained at 1 hour after a 60 mg dose.

See *OVERDOSAGE* for toxicity information.

Butalbital

Butalbital is well absorbed from the gastrointestinal tract and is expected to distribute to most of the tissues in the body. Barbiturates, in general, may appear in milk and readily cross the placental barrier. They are bound to plasma and tissue proteins to a varying degree and binding increases directly as a function of lipid solubility.

Elimination of butalbital is primarily via the kidney (59%-88% of the dose) as unchanged drug or metabolites. The plasma half-life is about 35 hours. Urinary excretion products included parent drug (about 3.6% of the dose), 5-isobutyl-5-(2,3-dihydroxypropyl) barbituric acid (about 24% of the dose), 5-allyl-5(3-hydroxy-2-methyl-1-propyl) barbituric acid (about 4.8% of the dose), products with the barbituric acid ring hydrolyzed with excretion of urea (about 14% of the dose), as well as unidentified materials. Of the material excreted in the urine, 32% was conjugated.

The bioavailability of the butalbital component of Fiorinal® with Codeine capsules is equivalent to that of a solution except for a decrease in the rate of absorption. A peak concentration of 2020 ng/mL is obtained at about 1.5 hours after a 100 mg dose.

See *OVERDOSAGE* for toxicity information.

Caffeine

Like most xanthines, caffeine is rapidly absorbed and distributed in all body tissues and fluids, including the CNS, fetal tissues, and breast milk.

Caffeine is cleared rapidly through metabolism and excretion in the urine. The plasma half-life is about 3 hours. Hepatic biotransformation prior to excretion results in about equal amounts of 1-methyl-xanthine and 1-methyluric acid. Of the 70% of the dose that has been recovered in the urine, only 3% was unchanged drug.

The bioavailability of the caffeine component for Fiorinal® with Codeine capsules is equivalent to that of a solution except for a slightly longer time to peak. A peak concentration of 1660 ng/mL was obtained in less than an hour for an 80 mg dose.

See *OVERDOSAGE* for toxicity information.

INDICATIONS

Fiorinal® with Codeine is indicated for the relief of the symptom complex of tension (or muscle contraction) headache.

Evidence supporting the efficacy of Fiorinal® with Codeine is derived from 2 multi-clinic trials that compared patients with tension headache randomly assigned to 4 parallel treatments: Fiorinal® with Codeine, codeine, Fiorinal®, and placebo. Response was assessed over the course of the first 4 hours of each of 2 distinct headaches, separated by at least 24 hours. Fiorinal® with Codeine proved statistically signifi-

Continued on next page

Sandoz—Cont.

cantly superior to each of its components (Fiorinal®, codeine) and to placebo on measures of pain relief.

Evidence supporting the efficacy and safety of Fiorinal® with Codeine in the treatment of multiple recurrent headaches is unavailable. Caution in this regard is required because codeine and butalbital are habit-forming and potentially abusable.

CONTRAINDICATIONS

Fiorinal® with Codeine is contraindicated under the following conditions:

1. Hypersensitivity or intolerance to aspirin, caffeine, butalbital or codeine.
2. Patients with a hemorrhagic diathesis (e.g., hemophilia, hypoprothrombinemia, von Willebrand's disease, the thrombocytopenias, thrombasthenia and other ill-defined hereditary platelet dysfunctions, severe vitamin K deficiency and severe liver damage.)
3. Patients with the syndrome of nasal polyps, angioedema and bronchospastic reactivity to aspirin or other nonsteroidal anti-inflammatory drugs. Anaphylactoid reactions have occurred in such patients.
4. Peptic ulcer or other serious gastrointestinal lesions.
5. Patients with porphyria.

WARNINGS

Therapeutic doses of aspirin can cause anaphylactic shock and other severe allergic reactions. It should be ascertained if the patient is allergic to aspirin, although a specific history of allergy may be lacking.

Significant bleeding can result from aspirin therapy in patients with peptic ulcer or other gastrointestinal lesions, and in patients with bleeding disorders.

Aspirin administered pre-operatively may prolong the bleeding time.

In the presence of head injury or other intracranial lesions, the respiratory depressant effects of codeine and other narcotics may be markedly enhanced, as well as their capacity for elevating cerebrospinal fluid pressure. Narcotics also produce other CNS depressant effects, such as drowsiness, that may further obscure the clinical course of patients with head injuries.

Codeine or other narcotics may obscure signs on which to judge the diagnosis or clinical course of patients with acute abdominal conditions.

Butalbital and codeine are both habit-forming and potentially abusable. Consequently, the extended use of Fiorinal® with Codeine is not recommended.

Results from epidemiologic studies indicate an association between aspirin and Reye Syndrome. Caution should be used in administering this product to children, including teenagers, with chicken pox or flu.

PRECAUTIONS

General

Fiorinal® with Codeine should be prescribed with caution for certain special-risk patients such as the elderly or debilitated, and those with severe impairment of renal or hepatic function, coagulation disorders, or head injuries.

Aspirin should be used with caution in patients on anticoagulant therapy and in patients with underlying hemostatic defects.

Precautions should be taken when administering salicylates to persons with known allergies. Hypersensitivity to aspirin is particularly likely in patients with nasal polyps, and relatively common in those with asthma.

Information for Patients

Patients should be informed that Fiorinal® with Codeine contains aspirin and should not be taken by patients with an aspirin allergy.

Fiorinal® with Codeine may impair the mental and/or physical abilities required for performance of potentially hazardous tasks such as driving a car or operating machinery. Such tasks should be avoided while taking Fiorinal® with Codeine.

Alcohol and other CNS depressants may produce an additive CNS depression when taken with Fiorinal® with Codeine, and should be avoided.

Codeine and butalbital may be habit-forming. Patients should take the drug only for as long as it is prescribed, in the amounts prescribed, and no more frequently than prescribed.

Laboratory Tests

In patients with severe hepatic or renal disease, effects of therapy should be monitored with serial liver and/or renal function tests.

Drug Interactions

The CNS effects of butalbital may be enhanced by monoamine oxidase (MAO) inhibitors.

In patients receiving concomitant corticosteroids and chronic use of aspirin, withdrawal of corticosteroids may result in salicylism because corticosteroids enhance renal clearance of salicylates and their withdrawal is followed by return to normal rates of renal clearance.

Fiorinal® with Codeine may enhance the effects of:

1. Oral anticoagulants, causing bleeding by inhibiting prothrombin formation in the liver and displacing anticoagulants from plasma protein binding sites.
2. Oral antidiabetic agents and insulin, causing hypoglycemia by contributing an additive effect, if dosage of Fiorinal® with Codeine exceeds maximum recommended daily dosage.
3. 6-mercaptopurine and methotrexate, causing bone marrow toxicity and blood dyscrasias by displacing these drugs from secondary binding sites, and, in the case of methotrexate, also reducing its excretion.
4. Non-steroidal anti-inflammatory agents, increasing the risk of peptic ulceration and bleeding by contributing additive effects.
5. Other narcotic analgesics, alcohol, general anesthetics, tranquilizers such as chlordiazepoxide, sedative-hypnotics, or other CNS depressants, causing increased CNS depression.

Fiorinal® with Codeine may diminish the effects of:

Uricosuric agents such as probenecid and sulfinpyrazone, reducing their effectiveness in the treatment of gout. Aspirin competes with these agents for protein binding sites.

Drug/Laboratory Test Interactions

Aspirin: Aspirin may interfere with the following laboratory determinations in blood: serum amylase, fasting blood glucose, cholesterol, protein, serum glutamic-oxalacetic transaminase (SGOT), uric acid, prothrombin time and bleeding time. Aspirin may interfere with the following laboratory determinations in urine: glucose, 5-hydroxyindoleacetic acid, Gerhardt ketone, vanillylmandelic acid (VMA), uric acid, diacetic acid, and spectrophotometric detection of barbiturates.

Codeine: Codeine may increase serum amylase levels.

Carcinogenesis, Mutagenesis, Impairment of Fertility

Adequate long-term studies have been conducted in mice and rats with aspirin, alone or in combination with other drugs, in which no evidence of carcinogenesis was seen. No adequate studies have been conducted in animals to determine whether aspirin has a potential for mutagenesis or impairment of fertility. No adequate studies have been conducted in animals to determine whether butalbital has a potential for carcinogenesis, mutagenesis, or impairment of fertility.

Usage in Pregnancy

Teratogenic Effects:

Pregnancy Category C. Animal reproduction studies have not been conducted with Fiorinal® with Codeine. It is also not known whether Fiorinal® with Codeine can cause fetal harm when administered to a pregnant woman or can affect reproduction capacity. Fiorinal® with Codeine should be given to a pregnant woman only when clearly needed.

Nonteratogenic Effects:

Although Fiorinal® with Codeine was not implicated in the birth defect, a female infant was born with lissencephaly, pachygyria and heterotopic gray matter. The infant was born 8 weeks prematurely to a woman who had taken an average of 90 Fiorinal® with Codeine capsules each month from the first few days of pregnancy. The child's development was mildly delayed and from one year of age she had partial simple motor seizures.

Withdrawal seizures were reported in a two-day-old male infant whose mother had taken a butalbital-containing drug during the last 2 months of pregnancy. Butalbital was found in the infant's serum. The infant was given phenobarbital 5mg/kg, which was tapered without further seizure or other withdrawal symptoms.

Studies of aspirin use in pregnant women have not shown that aspirin increases the risk of abnormalities when administered during the first trimester of pregnancy. In controlled studies involving 41,337 pregnant women and their offspring, there was no evidence that aspirin taken during pregnancy caused stillbirth, neonatal death or reduced birth weight. In controlled studies of 50,282 pregnant women and their offspring, aspirin administration in moderate and heavy doses during the first four lunar months of pregnancy showed no teratogenic effect.

Reproduction studies have been performed in rabbits and rats at doses up to 150 times the human dose and have revealed no evidence of impaired fertility or harm to the fetus due to codeine.

Therapeutic doses of aspirin in pregnant women close to term may cause bleeding in mother, fetus, or neonate. During the last 6 months of pregnancy, regular use of aspirin in high doses may prolong pregnancy and delivery.

Labor and Delivery

Ingestion of aspirin prior to delivery may prolong delivery or lead to bleeding in the mother or neonate. Use of codeine during labor may lead to respiratory depression in the neonate.

Nursing Mothers

Aspirin, caffeine, barbiturates and codeine are excreted in breast milk in small amounts, but the significance of their effects on nursing infants is not known. Because of potential for serious adverse reactions in nursing infants from Fiorinal® with Codeine, a decision should be made whether to discontinue nursing or to discontinue the drug, taking into account the importance of the drug to the mother.

Pediatric Use

Safety and effectiveness in children below the age of 12 have not been established.

ADVERSE REACTIONS

Commonly Observed

The most commonly reported adverse events associated with the use of Fiorinal® with Codeine and not reported at an equivalent incidence by placebo-treated patients were nausea and/or abdominal pain, drowsiness, and dizziness.

Associated with Treatment Discontinuation

Of the 382 patients treated with Fiorinal® with Codeine in controlled clinical trials, three (0.8%) discontinued treatment with Fiorinal® with Codeine because of adverse events. One patient each discontinued treatment for the following reasons: gastrointestinal upset; lightheadedness and heavy eyelids; and drowsiness and generalized tingling.

Incidence in Controlled Clinical Trials

The following table summarizes the incidence rates of the adverse events reported by at least 1% of the Fiorinal® with Codeine treated patients in controlled clinical trials comparing Fiorinal® with Codeine to placebo, and provides a comparison to the incidence rates reported by the placebo-treated patients.

The prescriber should be aware that these figures cannot be used to predict the incidence of side effects in the course of usual medical practice where patient characteristics and other factors differ from those that prevailed in the clinical trials. Similarly, the cited frequencies cannot be compared with figures obtained from other clinical investigations involving different treatments, uses, and investigators.

Adverse Events Reported by at Least 1% of Fiorinal® with Codeine Treated Patients During Placebo Controlled Clinical Trials

Body System/ Adverse Event	Incidence Rate of Adverse Events	
	Fiorinal®/Codeine (N=382)	Placebo (N=377)
Central Nervous		
Drowsiness	2.4%	0.5%
Dizziness/		
Lightheadedness	2.6%	0.5%
Intoxicated Feeling	1.0%	0%
Gastrointestinal		
Nausea/		
Abdominal Pain	3.7%	0.8%

Other Adverse Events Reported During Controlled Clinical Trials

The listing that follows represents the proportion of the 382 patients exposed to Fiorinal® with Codeine while participating in the controlled clinical trials who reported, on at least one occasion, an adverse event of the type cited. All reported adverse events, except those already presented in the previous table, are included. It is important to emphasize that, although the adverse events reported did occur while the patient was receiving Fiorinal® with Codeine, the adverse events were not necessarily caused by Fiorinal® with Codeine.

Adverse events are classified by body system and frequency. "Frequent" is defined as an adverse event which occurred in at least 1/100 (1%) of the patients; all adverse events listed in the previous table are frequent. "Infrequent" is defined as an adverse event that occurred in less than 1/100 patients but at least 1/1000 patients. All adverse events tabulated below are classified as infrequent.

Central Nervous: headache, shaky feeling, tingling, agitation, fainting, fatigue, heavy eyelids, high energy, hot spells, numbness, and sluggishness.

Autonomic Nervous: dry mouth and hyperhidrosis.

Gastrointestinal: vomiting, difficulty swallowing, and heartburn.

Cardiovascular: tachycardia.

Musculoskeletal: leg pain and muscle fatigue.

Genitourinary: diuresis.

Miscellaneous: pruritus, fever, earache, nasal congestion, and tinnitus.

Voluntary reports of adverse drug events, temporally associated with Fiorinal® with Codeine, that have been received since market introduction and that were not reported in clinical trials by the patients treated with Fiorinal® with Codeine, are listed below. Many or most of these events may have no causal relationship with the drug and are listed according to body system.

Central Nervous: Abuse, addiction, anxiety, depression, disorientation, hallucination, hyperactivity, insomnia, libido decrease, nervousness, neuropathy, psychosis, sedation, sexual activity increase, slurred speech, twitching, unconsciousness, vertigo.

Autonomic Nervous: epistaxis, flushing, miosis, salivation.
Gastrointestinal: anorexia, appetite increased, constipation, diarrhea, esophagitis, gastroenteritis, gastrointestinal spasm, hiccup, mouth burning, pyloric ulcer.
Cardiovascular: chest pain, hypotensive reaction, palpitations, syncope.
Skin: erythema, erythema multiforme, exfoliative dermatitis, hives, rash, toxic epidermal necrolysis.
Urinary: kidney impairment, urinary difficulty.
Miscellaneous: allergic reaction, anaphylactic shock, cholangiocarcinoma, drug interaction with erythromycin (stomach upset), edema.
The following adverse drug events may be borne in mind as potential effects of the components of Fiorinal® with Codeine. Potential effects of high dosage are listed in the *OVERDOSAGE* section of this insert.
Aspirin: occult blood loss, hemolytic anemia, iron deficiency anemia, gastric distress, heartburn, nausea, peptic ulcer, prolonged bleeding time, acute airway obstruction, renal toxicity when taken in high doses for prolonged periods, impaired urate excretion, hepatitis.
Caffeine: cardiac stimulation, irritability, tremor, dependence, nephrotoxicity, hyperglycemia.
Codeine: nausea, vomiting, drowsiness, lightheadedness, constipation, pruritus.

DRUG ABUSE AND DEPENDENCE

Fiorinal® with Codeine is controlled by the Drug Enforcement Administration and is classified under Schedule III.

Codeine

Codeine can produce drug dependence of the morphine type and, therefore, has the potential for being abused. Psychological dependence, physical dependence, and tolerance may develop upon repeated administration and it should be prescribed and administered with the same degree of caution appropriate to the use of other oral narcotic medications.

Butalbital

Barbiturates may be habit forming: Tolerance, psychological dependence, and physical dependence may occur especially following prolonged use of high doses of barbiturates. The average daily dose for the barbiturate addict is usually about 1,500 mg. As tolerance to barbiturates develops, the amount needed to maintain the same level of intoxication increases; tolerance to a fatal dosage, however, does not increase more than two-fold. As this occurs, the margin between an intoxication dosage and fatal dosage becomes smaller. The lethal dose of a barbiturate is far less if alcohol is also ingested. Major withdrawal symptoms (convulsions and delirium) may occur within 16 hours and last up to 5 days after abrupt cessation of these drugs. Intensity of withdrawal symptoms gradually declines over a period of approximately 15 days. Treatment of barbiturate dependence consists of cautious and gradual withdrawal of the drug. Barbiturate-dependent patients can be withdrawn by using a number of different withdrawal regimens. One method involves initiating treatment at the patient's regular dosage level and gradually decreasing the daily dosage as tolerated by the patient.

OVERDOSAGE

The toxic effects of acute overdosage of Fiorinal® with Codeine capsules are attributable mainly to the barbiturate and codeine components, and, to a lesser extent, aspirin. Because toxic effects of caffeine occur in very high dosages only, the possibility of significant caffeine toxicity from Fiorinal® with Codeine overdosage is unlikely.

Signs and Symptoms

Symptoms attributable to *acute barbiturate poisoning* include drowsiness, confusion, and coma; respiratory depression; hypotension; shock. Symptoms attributable to *acute aspirin poisoning* include hyperpnea; acid-base disturbances with development of metabolic acidosis; vomiting and abdominal pain; tinnitus, hyperthermia; hypoprothrombinemia; restlessness; delirium; convulsions. *Acute caffeine poisoning* may cause insomnia, restlessness, tremor, and delirium; tachycardia and extrasystoles. Symptoms of *acute codeine poisoning* include the triad of: pinpoint pupils, marked depression of respiration, and loss of consciousness. Convulsions may occur.

Treatment

The following paragraphs describe one approach to the treatment of overdose with Fiorinal® with Codeine. However, because strategies for the management of an overdose continually evolve, consultation with a regional poison control center is strongly encouraged.
Treatment consists primarily of management of barbiturate intoxication, reversal of the effects of codeine, and the correction of the acid-base imbalance due to salicylism. Vomiting should be induced mechanically or with emetics in the conscious patient. Gastric lavage may be used if the pharyngeal and laryngeal reflexes are present and if less than 4 hours have elapsed since ingestion. A cuffed endotracheal tube should be inserted before gastric lavage of the unconscious patient and when necessary to provide assisted respiration. Diuresis, alkalinization of the urine, and correction of electrolyte disturbances should be accomplished through administration of intravenous fluids such as 1% sodium bicarbonate and 5% dextrose in water.
Meticulous attention should be given to maintaining adequate pulmonary ventilation. Correction of hypotension may require the administration of levarterenol bitartrate or phenylephrine hydrochloride by intravenous infusion. In severe cases of intoxication, peritoneal dialysis, hemodialysis, or exchange transfusion may be lifesaving. Hypoprothrombinemia should be treated with vitamin K, intravenously.
Methemoglobinemia over 30% should be treated with methylene blue by slow intravenous administration.
Naloxone, a narcotic antagonist, can reverse respiratory depression and coma associated with opioid overdose. Typically, a dose of 0.4 mg to 2 mg is given parenterally and may be repeated if an adequate response is not achieved. Since the duration of action of codeine may exceed that of the antagonist, the patient should be kept under continued surveillance and repeated doses of the antagonist should be administered as needed to maintain adequate respiration. A narcotic antagonist should not be administered in the absence of clinically significant respiratory or cardiovascular depression.

Toxic and Lethal Doses

Butalbital:	toxic dose 1.0 g (adult); lethal dose 2.0–5.0 g
Aspirin:	toxic blood level greater than 30 mg/100 mL; lethal dose 10–30 g (adult)
Caffeine:	toxic dose greater than 1.0 g; lethal dose unknown
Codeine:	lethal dose 0.5–1.0 g (adult)

DOSAGE AND ADMINISTRATION

One or 2 capsules every 4 hours. Total daily dosage should not exceed 6 capsules.
Extended and repeated use of this product is not recommended because of the potential for physical dependence.

HOW SUPPLIED

Fiorinal® with Codeine Capsules, imprinted "⚠ F-C" on one half, "SANDOZ 78-107" other half, color is blue and yellow, in bottles of 100 capsules and in ControlPak® package, 25 capsules (continuous reverse-numbered roll of sealed blisters).

[FWC-Z26 issued November 1, 1990]
Shown in Product Identification Section, page 427

HYDERGINE® ℞
[*hī'der-jēn*]
(ergoloid mesylates) tablets, USP (ORAL)
(ergoloid mesylates) tablets, USP (SUBLINGUAL)
(ergoloid mesylates) liquid

HYDERGINE® LC ℞
(ergoloid mesylates) liquid capsules

CAUTION: Federal law prohibits dispensing without prescription.
The following prescribing information is based on official labeling in effect on August 1, 1992.

DESCRIPTION AND TYPE

Hydergine® tablet 1 mg, Hydergine® sublingual tablet 1 mg and Hydergine® LC (liquid capsule) 1 mg, each contains ergoloid mesylates USP as follows: dihydroergocornine mesylate 0.333 mg, dihydroergocristine mesylate 0.333 mg, and dihydroergocryptine (dihydro-alpha-ergocryptine and dihydro-beta-ergocryptine in the proportion of 2:1) mesylate 0.333 mg, representing a total of 1 mg.
Inactive Ingredients:
1 mg, Oral Tablets: lactose, povidone, starch, stearic acid, and talc
1 mg, Sublingual Tablets: gelatin, mannitol, starch, stearic acid, and sucrose
Liquid Capsules: ascorbic acid, gelatin, glycerin, methylparaben, polyethylene glycol, propylparaben, propylene glycol, sorbitol, and titanium dioxide
Hydergine® sublingual tablet 0.5 mg, each contains ergoloid mesylates USP as follows: dihydroergocornine mesylate 0.167 mg, dihydroergocristine mesylate 0.167 mg, and dihydroergocryptine (dihydro-alpha-ergocryptine and dihydro-beta-ergocryptine in the proportion of 2:1) mesylate 0.167 mg, representing a total of 0.5 mg.
Inactive Ingredients: gelatin, mannitol, starch, stearic acid, and sucrose
Hydergine® liquid 1 mg/mL, each mL contains ergoloid mesylates USP as follows: dihydroergocornine mesylate 0.333 mg, dihydroergocristine mesylate 0.333 mg, and dihydroergocryptine (dihydro-alpha-ergocryptine and dihydro-beta-ergocryptine in the proportion of 2:1) mesylate 0.333 mg, representing a total of 1 mg; alcohol, 28.5% by volume.
Inactive Ingredients: alcohol, glycerin, propylene glycol, and purified water

Pharmacokinetic Properties

Pharmacokinetic studies have been performed in normal volunteers with the help of radiolabelled drug as well as employing a specific radioimmunoassay technique. From the urinary excretion quotient of orally and intravenously administered tritium-labelled Hydergine® (ergoloid mesylates) the absorption of ergoloid was calculated to be 25%. Following oral administration, peak levels of 0.5 ng Eq/mL/mg were achieved within 1.5–3 hr. Bioavailability studies with the specific radioimmunoassay confirm that ergoloid is rapidly absorbed from the gastrointestinal tract, with mean peak levels of 0.05–0.13 ng/mL/mg (with extremes of 0.03 and 0.18 ng/mL/mg) achieved within 0.6–1.3 hr. (with extremes of 0.4 and 2.8 hr.). The finding of lower peak levels of ergoloid compared to the total drug-metabolite composite is consistent with a considerable first pass liver metabolism, with less than 50% of the therapeutic moiety reaching the systemic circulation. The elimination of radioactivity, representing ergoloid plus metabolites bearing the radiolabel, was biphasic with half-lives of 4 and 13 hr. The mean half-life of unchanged ergoloid in plasma is about 2.6–5.1 hr; after 3 half-lives ergoloid plasma levels are less than 10% of radioactivity levels, and by 24 hr no ergoloid is detectable.
Bioequivalence studies were performed comparing Hydergine® oral tablets (administered orally) with Hydergine® sublingual tablets (administered sublingually), Hydergine® oral tablets with Hydergine® liquid and Hydergine® oral tablets with Hydergine® LC (liquid capsules). The oral tablet, sublingual tablet and liquid capsule oral forms were shown to be bioequivalent. Within the bioequivalence limits, the liquid capsule showed a statistically significant (12%) greater bioavailability than the oral tablet. In the study comparing the oral tablet and liquid forms, both forms tested showed an equivalent rate of absorption and an equivalent peak plasma concentration (C_{max}).

ACTIONS

There is no specific evidence which clearly establishes the mechanism by which Hydergine® (ergoloid mesylates) preparations produce mental effects, nor is there conclusive evidence that the drug particularly affects cerebral arteriosclerosis or cerebrovascular insufficiency.

INDICATIONS

A proportion of individuals over sixty who manifest signs and symptoms of an idiopathic decline in mental capacity (i.e., cognitive and interpersonal skills, mood, self-care, apparent motivation) can experience some symptomatic relief upon treatment with Hydergine® (ergoloid mesylates) preparations. The identity of the specific trait(s) or condition(s), if any, which would usefully predict a response to Hydergine® (ergoloid mesylates) therapy is not known. It appears, however, that those individuals who do respond come from groups of patients who would be considered clinically to suffer from some ill-defined process related to aging or to have some underlying dementing condition (i.e., primary progressive dementia, Alzheimer's dementia, senile onset, multi-infarct dementia).
Before prescribing Hydergine® (ergoloid mesylates), the physician should exclude the possibility that the patient's signs and symptoms arise from a potentially reversible and treatable condition. Particular care should be taken to exclude delirium and dementiform illness secondary to systemic disease, primary neurological disease, or primary disturbance of mood. Hydergine® (ergoloid mesylates) preparations are not indicated in the treatment of acute or chronic psychosis, regardless of etiology (see **CONTRAINDICATIONS** section).
The decision to use Hydergine® (ergoloid mesylates) in the treatment of an individual with a symptomatic decline in mental capacity of unknown etiology should be continually reviewed since the presenting clinical picture may subsequently evolve sufficiently to allow a specific diagnosis and a specific alternative treatment. In addition, continued clinical evaluation is required to determine whether any initial benefit conferred by Hydergine® (ergoloid mesylates) therapy persists with time.
The efficacy of Hydergine® (ergoloid mesylates) was evaluated using a special rating scale known as the SCAG (Sandoz Clinical Assessment-Geriatric). The specific items on this scale on which modest but statistically significant changes were observed at the end of twelve weeks include: mental alertness, confusion, recent memory, orientation, emotional lability, self-care, depression, anxiety/fears, cooperation, sociability, appetite, dizziness, fatigue, bothersome(ness), and an overall impression of clinical status.

CONTRAINDICATIONS

Hydergine® (ergoloid mesylates) preparations are contraindicated in individuals who have previously shown hypersensitivity to the drug. Hydergine® (ergoloid mesylates) preparations are also contraindicated in patients who have psychosis, acute or chronic, regardless of etiology.

Continued on next page

Sandoz—Cont.

PRECAUTIONS

Practitioners are advised that because the target symptoms are of unknown etiology, careful diagnosis should be attempted before prescribing Hydergine® (ergoloid mesylates) preparations.

ADVERSE REACTIONS

Hydergine® (ergoloid mesylates) preparations have not been found to produce serious side effects. Some sublingual irritation with the sublingual tablets, transient nausea, and gastric disturbances have been reported. Hydergine® (ergoloid mesylates) preparations do not possess the vasoconstrictor properties of the natural ergot alkaloids.

DOSAGE AND ADMINISTRATION

1 mg three times daily.
Alleviation of symptoms is usually gradual and results may not be observed for 3–4 weeks.

HOW SUPPLIED

Hydergine® tablets (for oral use)
1 mg
Round, white, engraved "HYDERGINE® 1" on one side, " Ⓢ " other side.
NDC 0078-0070-05: bottles of 100
NDC 0078-0070-06: SandoPak® unit-dose packages of 100
NDC 0078-0070-08: bottles of 500
NDC 0078-0070-18: SandoPak® unit-dose packages of 500
Hydergine® sublingual tablets
1 mg
Oval, white, engraved "HYDERGINE®" on one side, "78-77" other side.
NDC 0078-0077-05: bottles of 100
NDC 0078-0077-09: bottles of 1000
0.5 mg
Round, white, engraved "HYDERGINE®0.5" on one side, " Ⓢ " other side.
NDC 0078-0051-05: bottles of 100
Hydergine® liquid
1 mg/mL
Supplied with an accompanying dropper graduated to deliver 1 mg.
NDC 0078-0100-36: bottles of 100 mL
Hydergine® LC (liquid capsules)
1 mg
Oblong, off-white, branded "HYDERGINE® LC 1 mg" on one side, " Ⓢ " other side.
NDC 0078-0101-05: bottles of 100
NDC 0078-0101-06: SandoPak® unit-dose packages of 100
NDC 0078-0101-08: bottles of 500
NDC 0078-0101-18: SandoPak® unit-dose packages of 500
(Encapsulated by R. P. Scherer, N.A.
Clearwater, Florida 33518)
[HYD-ZZ28 Issued June 30, 1991]
Shown in Product Identification Section, page 427

KLORVESS® EFFERVESCENT GRANULES, and ℞
[klor'ves"]
KLORVESS® (potassium chloride) ℞
10% LIQUID

The following prescribing information is based on official labeling in effect on August 1, 1992.

DESCRIPTION

KLORVESS® EFFERVESCENT GRANULES: Each packet (2.8 g) contains 20 mEq each of potassium and chloride supplied by potassium chloride 1.125 g, potassium bicarbonate 0.5 g, lysine hydrochloride 0.913 g in a sodium-, sugar- and carbohydrate-free effervescent formulation. Dissolution of the packet contents in water provides the potassium and chloride available for oral ingestion as potassium chloride, potassium bicarbonate, potassium citrate and lysine hydrochloride.
Active Ingredients: lysine hydrochloride USP, potassium bicarbonate USP and potassium chloride USP
Inactive Ingredients: citric acid, flavorings, polyethylene glycol and saccharin
KLORVESS® (potassium chloride) 10% LIQUID: Each tablespoonful (15 ml) contains 20 mEq of potassium chloride (provided by potassium chloride 1.5 g), in a palatable, cherry and pit flavored vehicle, alcohol 0.75%.
Active Ingredient: potassium chloride USP
Inactive Ingredients: alcohol, malic acid, natural flavor, purified water, saccharin sodium, sodium benzoate and sucrose

INDICATIONS

For the prevention and treatment of potassium depletion and hypokalemic-hypochloremic alkalosis. Deficits of body potassium and chloride can occur as a consequence of therapy with potent diuretic agents and adrenal corticosteroids.

CONTRAINDICATIONS

Severe renal impairment characterized by azotemia or oliguria, untreated Addison's disease, Familial Periodic Paralysis, acute dehydration, heat cramps, patients receiving aldosterone-inhibiting or potassium-sparing diuretic agents or hyperkalemia from any cause.

PRECAUTIONS

In response to a rise in the concentration of body potassium, renal excretion of the ion is increased. In the presence of normal renal function and hydration, it is difficult to produce potassium intoxication by oral potassium salt supplements.
Since the extent of potassium deficiency cannot be accurately determined, it is prudent to proceed cautiously in undertaking potassium replacement. Periodic evaluations of the patient's clinical status, serum electrolytes and the EKG should be carried out when replacement therapy is undertaken. This is particularly important in patients with cardiac disease and those patients receiving digitalis.
High serum concentrations of potassium may cause death through cardiac depression, arrhythmia or cardiac arrest.
To minimize gastrointestinal irritation associated with potassium chloride preparations, patients should dissolve the packet contents of KLORVESS® EFFERVESCENT GRANULES in 3 to 4 ounces of cold water, fruit juice or other liquid, or dilute each tablespoonful of KLORVESS® (potassium chloride) 10% LIQUID in 3 to 4 ounces of cold water. Both of these solutions should be ingested slowly with or immediately after meals.

ADVERSE REACTIONS

Abdominal discomfort, diarrhea, nausea and vomiting may occur with the use of potassium salts.
The symptoms and signs of potassium intoxication include paresthesias, heaviness, muscle weakness and flaccid paralysis of the extremities. Potassium intoxication can produce listlessness, mental confusion, a fall in blood pressure, shock, cardiac arrhythmias, heart block and cardiac arrest.
The EKG picture of hyperkalemia is characterized by the early appearance of tall, peaked T waves. The R wave is decreased in amplitude and the S wave deepens; the QRS complex widens progressively. The P wave widens and decreases in amplitude until it disappears. Occasionally, an apparent elevation of the RS-T junction and a cove plane RS-T segment and T wave will be noted in AVL.

DOSAGE AND ADMINISTRATION

KLORVESS® EFFERVESCENT GRANULES:
Adults—One packet (20 mEq each of potassium and chloride) completely dissolved in 3 to 4 ounces of cold water, fruit juice or other liquid 2 to 4 times daily depending upon the requirements of the patient.
KLORVESS® (potassium chloride) 10% LIQUID:
Adults —One tablespoonful (15 ml) of Klorvess Liquid (20 mEq of potassium chloride) completely diluted in 3 to 4 ounces of cold water 2 to 4 times daily depending upon the requirements of the patient.
Both of these solutions should be ingested slowly with meals or immediately after eating. Deviations from these recommended dosages may be indicated in certain cases of hypokalemia based upon the patient's status. The average total daily dosage must be governed by the patient's response as determined by frequent evaluation of serum electrolytes, EKG and clinical status.

OVERDOSAGE

Potassium intoxication may result from overdosage of potassium or from therapeutic dosage in conditions stated under "Contraindications." Hyperkalemia, when detected, must be treated immediately because lethal levels can be reached in a few hours.

TREATMENT OF HYPERKALEMIA:

1. Dextrose solution, 10 to 25% containing 10 units of crystalline insulin per 20 g dextrose, given IV in a dose of 300 to 500 ml in an hour.
2. Adsorption and exchange of potassium using sodium or ammonium cycle cation exchange resins, orally and as a retention enema. (Caution: Ammonium compounds should not be used in patients with hepatic cirrhosis.)
3. Hemodialysis and peritoneal dialysis.
4. The use of potassium-containing foods or medicaments must be eliminated.
In digitalized patients too rapid a lowering of plasma potassium concentration can cause digitalis toxicity.

HOW SUPPLIED

KLORVESS® EFFERVESCENT GRANULES—packages of 30 packets (2.8 g each). KLORVESS® (potassium chloride) 10% LIQUID (dark red) – as a cherry and pit flavored liquid in pint bottles.
NOTE: Occasionally, Klorvess Granules packets may appear to be slightly swollen due to a small amount of moisture that may have been included during packaging. The quality of the product is not affected.
[KLO-Z4 Issued February 20, 1986]

KLORVESS® ℞
[klor'ves"]
EFFERVESCENT TABLETS

CAUTION: Federal law prohibits dispensing without prescription.
The following prescribing information is based on official labeling in effect on August 1, 1992.

DESCRIPTION

Each dry, sodium- and sugar-free effervescent tablet contains 20 mEq each of potassium and chloride supplied by potassium chloride 1.125 g, potassium bicarbonate 0.5 g, lysine hydrochloride 0.913 g. Dissolution of the tablet in water provides the potassium and chloride available for oral ingestion as potassium chloride, potassium bicarbonate, potassium citrate and lysine hydrochloride.
Active Ingredients: lysine hydrochloride USP, potassium bicarbonate USP and potassium chloride USP
Inactive Ingredients: citric acid, flavorings, polyethylene glycol and saccharin

INDICATIONS

For the prevention and treatment of potassium depletion and hypokalemic-hypochloremic alkalosis. Deficits of body potassium and chloride can occur as a consequence of therapy with potent diuretic agents and adrenal corticosteroids.

CONTRAINDICATIONS

Severe renal impairment characterized by azotemia or oliguria, untreated Addison's disease, Familial Periodic Paralysis, acute dehydration, heat cramps, patients receiving aldosterone-inhibiting or potassium-sparing diuretic agents or hyperkalemia from any cause.

PRECAUTIONS

In response to a rise in the concentration of body potassium, renal excretion of the ion is increased. In the presence of normal renal function and hydration, it is difficult to produce potassium intoxication by oral potassium salt supplements.
Since the extent of potassium deficiency cannot be accurately determined, it is prudent to proceed cautiously in undertaking potassium replacement. Periodic evaluations of the patient's clinical status, serum electrolytes and the EKG should be carried out when replacement therapy is undertaken. This is particularly important in patients with cardiac disease and those patients receiving digitalis.
High serum concentrations of potassium may cause death through cardiac depression, arrhythmia or cardiac arrest.
To minimize gastrointestinal irritation associated with potassium chloride preparations, patients should dissolve each Klorvess® Effervescent Tablet in 3 or 4 ounces of cold water or fruit juice. This solution should be ingested slowly with or immediately after meals.

ADVERSE REACTIONS

Abdominal discomfort, diarrhea, nausea and vomiting may occur with the use of potassium salts.
The symptoms and signs of potassium intoxication include paresthesias, heaviness, muscle weakness and flaccid paralysis of the extremities. Potassium intoxication can produce listlessness, mental confusion, a fall in blood pressure, shock, cardiac arrhythmias, heart block and cardiac arrest.
The EKG picture of hyperkalemia is characterized by the early appearance of tall, peaked T waves. The R wave is decreased in amplitude and the S wave deepens; the QRS complex widens progressively. The P wave widens and decreases in amplitude until it disappears. Occasionally, an apparent elevation of the RS-T junction and a cove plane RS-T segment and T wave will be noted in AVL.

DOSAGE AND ADMINISTRATION

Adults—One Klorvess® Effervescent Tablet (20 mEq each of potassium and chloride) completely dissolved in 3 to 4 ounces of cold water or fruit juice 2 to 4 times daily depending upon the requirements of the patient.
The solution should be ingested slowly with meals or immediately after eating. Deviations from these recommended dosages may be indicated in certain cases of hypokalemia based upon the patient's status. The average total daily dosage must be governed by the patient's response as determined by frequent evaluation of serum electrolytes, EKG and clinical status.

OVERDOSAGE

Potassium intoxication may result from overdosage of potassium or from therapeutic dosage in conditions stated under "Contraindications." Hyperkalemia, when detected, must be treated immediately because lethal levels can be reached in a few hours.

TREATMENT OF HYPERKALEMIA:

1. Dextrose solution, 10 or 25% containing 10 units of crystalline insulin per 20 g dextrose, given IV in a dose of 300 to 500 ml in an hour.
2. Adsorption and exchange of potassium using sodium or ammonium cycle cation exchange resins, orally and as a retention enema. (Caution: Ammonium compounds should not be used in patients with hepatic cirrhosis.)

3. Hemodialysis and peritoneal dialysis.
4. The use of potassium-containing foods or medicaments must be eliminated.

In digitalized patients too rapid a lowering of plasma potassium concentration can cause digitalis toxicity.

HOW SUPPLIED

Klorvess® Effervescent Tablets (white)—60 and 1000 tablets. Each tablet is individually foil wrapped.
Store and dispense: Below 86°F (30°C).
U.S. Patent No. 3,970,750
[KLO-ZZ3 Issued February 20, 1986]

MELLARIL®* ℞

[*mel'ah-ril"*]
(thioridazine HCl) TABLETS, USP
(thioridazine HCl) ORAL SOLUTION, USP

MELLARIL-S® ℞

(thioridazine) ORAL SUSPENSION, USP

FOR ORAL ADMINISTRATION

CAUTION: Federal law prohibits dispensing without prescription.

The following prescribing information is based on official labeling in effect on August 1, 1992.

DESCRIPTION

Mellaril® (thioridazine) is 2-methylmercapto-10-[2-(N-methyl-2-piperidyl) ethyl] phenothiazine.

The presence of a thiomethyl radical ($S\text{-}CH_3$) in position 2, conventionally occupied by a halogen, is unique and could account for the greater toleration obtained with recommended doses of thioridazine as well as a greater specificity of psychotherapeutic action.

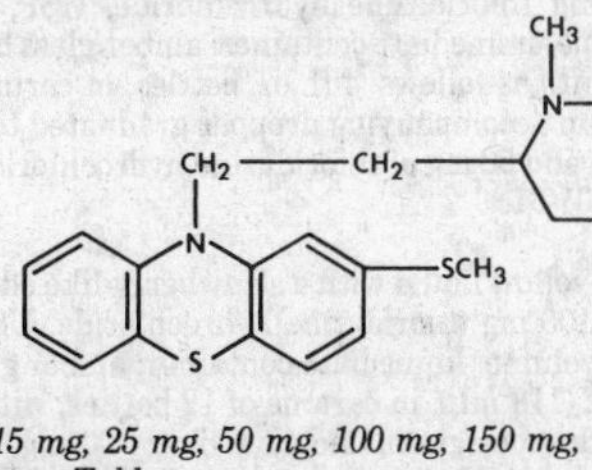

10 mg, 15 mg, 25 mg, 50 mg, 100 mg, 150 mg, and 200 mg Tablets
Active Ingredient: thioridazine HCl, USP
10 mg Tablets
Inactive Ingredients: acacia, calcium sulfate dihydrate, carnauba wax, D&C Yellow #10, FD&C Blue #1, FD&C Yellow #6, gelatin, lactose, methylparaben, povidone, propylparaben, sodium benzoate, starch, stearic acid, sucrose, synthetic black iron oxide, talc, titanium dioxide, and other ingredients.
15 mg Tablets
Inactive Ingredients: acacia, calcium sulfate dihydrate, carnauba wax, D&C Red #7, gelatin, lactose, methylparaben, povidone, propylparaben, starch, stearic acid, sucrose, synthetic black iron oxide, talc, titanium dioxide, and other ingredients.
25 mg Tablets
Inactive Ingredients: acacia, calcium sulfate dihydrate, carnauba wax, gelatin, lactose, methylparaben, povidone, propylparaben, sodium benzoate, starch, stearic acid, sucrose, synthetic black iron oxide, synthetic iron oxide, talc, titanium dioxide, and other ingredients.
50 mg Tablets
Inactive Ingredients: acacia, calcium sulfate dihydrate, carnauba wax, gelatin, lactose, sodium benzoate, starch, stearic acid, sucrose, synthetic black iron oxide, talc, titanium dioxide, and other ingredients.
100 mg Tablets
Inactive Ingredients: acacia, calcium sulfate dihydrate, carnauba wax, D&C Yellow #10, FD&C Blue #1, FD&C Blue #2, FD&C Yellow #6, lactose, povidone, sodium benzoate, sorbitol, starch, stearic acid, sucrose, synthetic black iron oxide, talc, titanium dioxide, and other ingredients.
150 mg Tablets
Inactive Ingredients: acacia, calcium sulfate dihydrate, carnauba wax, D&C Yellow #10, FD&C Green #3, FD&C Yellow #6, lactose, methylparaben, povidone, propylparaben, sodium benzoate, starch, stearic acid, sucrose, synthetic black iron oxide, talc, titanium dioxide, and other ingredients.
200 mg Tablets
Inactive Ingredients: acacia, calcium sulfate dihydrate, carnauba wax, D&C Red #7, gelatin, lactose, magnesium stearate, methylparaben, povidone, propylparaben, starch, stearic acid, sucrose, synthetic black iron oxide, talc, titanium dioxide, and other ingredients.

*Also known as Mellerettes and Mallorol.

30 mg and 100 mg Concentrate
Active Ingredient: thioridazine HCl, USP
30 mg Concentrate
Inactive Ingredients: alcohol, 3.0%, flavor, methylparaben, propylparaben, purified water, and sorbitol solution. May contain sodium hydroxide or hydrochloric acid to adjust the pH.
100 mg Concentrate
Inactive Ingredients: alcohol, 4.2%, flavor, glycerin, methylparaben, propylparaben, purified water, sorbitol solution, and sucrose. May contain sodium hydroxide or hydrochloric acid to adjust pH.
25 mg and 100 mg Oral Suspension
Active Ingredient: each 5 mL contains thioridazine, USP, equivalent to 25 mg and 100 mg thioridazine HCl, USP respectively.
25 mg Oral Suspension
Inactive Ingredients: carbomer 934, flavor, polysorbate 80, purified water, sodium hydroxide, and sucrose.
100 mg Oral Suspension
Inactive Ingredients: carbomer 934, D&C Yellow #10, FD&C Yellow #6, flavor, polysorbate 80, purified water, sodium hydroxide, and sucrose.

CLINICAL PHARMACOLOGY

Mellaril® (thioridazine) is effective in reducing excitement, hypermotility, abnormal initiative, affective tension, and agitation through its inhibitory effect on psychomotor functions. Successful modification of such symptoms is the prerequisite for, and often the beginning of, the process of recovery in patients exhibiting mental and emotional disturbances.

Thioridazine's basic pharmacological activity is similar to that of other phenothiazines, but certain specific qualities have come to light which support the observation that the clinical spectrum of this drug shows significant differences from those of the other agents of this class. Minimal antiemetic activity and minimal extrapyramidal stimulation, notably pseudoparkinsonism, are distinctive features of this drug.

INDICATIONS

For the management of manifestations of psychotic disorders.

For the short-term treatment of moderate to marked depression with variable degrees of anxiety in adult patients and for the treatment of multiple symptoms such as agitation, anxiety, depressed mood, tension, sleep disturbances, and fears in geriatric patients.

For the treatment of severe behavioral problems in children marked by combativeness and/or explosive hyperexcitable behavior (out of proportion to immediate provocations), and in the short-term treatment of hyperactive children who show excessive motor activity with accompanying conduct disorders consisting of some or all of the following symptoms: impulsivity, difficulty sustaining attention, aggressivity, mood lability, and poor frustration tolerance.

CONTRAINDICATIONS

In common with other phenothiazines, Mellaril® (thioridazine) is contraindicated in severe central nervous system depression or comatose states from any cause. It should also be noted that hypertensive or hypotensive heart disease of extreme degree is a contraindication of phenothiazine administration.

WARNINGS

Tardive Dyskinesia

Tardive dyskinesia, a syndrome consisting of potentially irreversible, involuntary, dyskinetic movements may develop in patients treated with neuroleptic (antipsychotic) drugs. Although the prevalence of the syndrome appears to be highest among the elderly, especially elderly women, it is impossible to rely upon prevalence estimates to predict, at the inception of neuroleptic treatment, which patients are likely to develop the syndrome. Whether neuroleptic drug products differ in their potential to cause tardive dyskinesia is unknown.

Both the risk of developing the syndrome and the likelihood that it will become irreversible are believed to increase as the duration of treatment and the total cumulative dose of neuroleptic drugs administered to the patient increase. However, the syndrome can develop, although much less commonly, after relatively brief treatment periods at low doses.

There is no known treatment for established cases of tardive dyskinesia, although the syndrome may remit, partially or completely, if neuroleptic treatment is withdrawn. Neuroleptic treatment itself, however, may suppress (or partially suppress) the signs and symptoms of the syndrome and thereby may possibly mask the underlying disease process. The effect that symptomatic suppression has upon the long-term course of the syndrome is unknown.

Given these considerations, neuroleptics should be prescribed in a manner that is most likely to minimize the occurrence of tardive dyskinesia. Chronic neuroleptic treatment should generally be reserved for patients who suffer from a chronic illness that, 1) is known to respond to neuroleptic drugs, and, 2) for whom alternative, equally effective, but potentially less harmful treatments are *not* available or appropriate. In patients who do require chronic treatment, the smallest dose and the shortest duration of treatment producing a satisfactory clinical response should be sought. The need for continued treatment should be reassessed periodically.

If signs and symptoms of tardive dyskinesia appear in a patient on neuroleptics, drug discontinuation should be considered. However, some patients may require treatment despite the presence of the syndrome.

(For further information about the description of tardive dyskinesia and its clinical detection, please refer to the sections on *Information for Patients* and *ADVERSE REACTIONS.)*

It has been suggested in regard to phenothiazines in general, that people who have demonstrated a hypersensitivity reaction (e.g. blood dyscrasias, jaundice) to one may be more prone to demonstrate a reaction to others. Attention should be paid to the fact that phenothiazines are capable of potentiating central nervous system depressants (e.g. anesthetics, opiates, alcohol, etc.) as well as atropine and phosphorus insecticides. Physicians should carefully consider benefit versus risk when treating less severe disorders.

Reproductive studies in animals and clinical experience to date have failed to show a teratogenic effect with Mellaril® (thioridazine). However, in view of the desirability of keeping the administration of all drugs to a minimum during pregnancy, Mellaril® (thioridazine) should be given only when the benefits derived from treatment exceed the possible risks to mother and fetus.

Neuroleptic Malignant Syndrome (NMS)

A potentially fatal symptom complex sometimes referred to as Neuroleptic Malignant Syndrome (NMS) has been reported in association with antipsychotic drugs. Clinical manifestations of NMS are hyperpyrexia, muscle rigidity, altered mental status, and evidence of autonomic instability (irregular pulse or blood pressure, tachycardia, diaphoresis, and cardiac dysrhythmias).

The diagnostic evaluation of patients with this syndrome is complicated. In arriving at a diagnosis, it is important to identify cases where the clinical presentation includes both serious medical illness (e.g. pneumonia, systemic infection, etc.) and untreated or inadequately treated extrapyramidal signs and symptoms (EPS). Other important considerations in the differential diagnosis include central anticholinergic toxicity, heat stroke, drug fever, and primary central nervous system (CNS) pathology.

The management of NMS should include, 1) immediate discontinuation of antipsychotic drugs and other drugs not essential to concurrent therapy, 2) intensive symptomatic treatment and medical monitoring, and 3) treatment of any concomitant serious medical problems for which specific treatments are available. There is no general agreement about specific pharmacological treatment regimens for uncomplicated NMS.

If a patient requires antipsychotic drug treatment after recovery from NMS, the potential reintroduction of drug therapy should be carefully considered. The patient should be carefully monitored, since recurrences of NMS have been reported.

PRECAUTIONS

Leukopenia and/or agranulocytosis and convulsive seizures have been reported but are infrequent. Mellaril® (thioridazine) has been shown to be helpful in the treatment of behavioral disorders in epileptic patients, but anticonvulsant medication should also be maintained. Pigmentary retinopathy, which has been observed primarily in patients taking larger than recommended doses, is characterized by diminution of visual acuity, brownish coloring of vision, and impairment of night vision; examination of the fundus discloses deposits of pigment. The possibility of this complication may be reduced by remaining within the recommended limits of dosage.

Where patients are participating in activities requiring complete mental alertness (e.g. driving) it is advisable to administer the phenothiazines cautiously and to increase the dosage gradually. Female patients appear to have a greater tendency to orthostatic hypotension than male patients. The administration of epinephrine should be avoided in the treatment of drug-induced hypotension in view of the fact that phenothiazines may induce a reversed epinephrine effect on occasion. Should a vasoconstrictor be required, the most suitable are levarterenol and phenylephrine.

Neuroleptic drugs elevate prolactin levels; the elevation persists during chronic administration. Tissue culture experiments indicate that approximately one-third of human breast cancers are prolactin dependent in vitro, a factor of potential importance if the prescription of these drugs is contemplated in a patient with a previously detected breast cancer. Although disturbances such as galactorrhea, amenorrhea, gynecomastia, and impotence have been reported, the clinical significance of elevated serum prolactin levels is unknown for most patients. An increase in mammary neo-

Continued on next page

Sandoz—Cont.

plasms has been found in rodents after chronic administration of neuroleptic drugs. Neither clinical studies nor epidemiologic studies conducted to date, however, have shown an association between chronic administration of these drugs and mammary tumorigenesis; the available evidence is considered too limited to be conclusive at this time.
Concurrent administration of propranolol (100-800 mg daily) has been reported to produce increases in plasma levels of thioridazine (approximately 50%-400%) and its metabolites (approximately 80%-300%).
Pindolol: Concurrent administration of pindolol and thioridazine have resulted in moderate, dose-related increases in the serum levels of thioridazine and two of its metabolites, as well as higher than expected serum pindolol levels.
It is recommended that a daily dose in excess of 300 mg be reserved for use only in severe neuropsychiatric conditions.
Information for Patients: Given the likelihood that some patients exposed chronically to neuroleptics will develop tardive dyskinesia, it is advised that all patients in whom chronic use is contemplated be given, if possible, full information about this risk. The decision to inform patients and/or their guardians must obviously take into account the clinical circumstances and the competency of the patient to understand the information provided.

ADVERSE REACTIONS

In the recommended dosage ranges with Mellaril® (thioridazine) most side effects are mild and transient.
Central Nervous System: Drowsiness may be encountered on occasion, especially where large doses are given early in treatment. Generally, this effect tends to subside with continued therapy or a reduction in dosage. Pseudoparkinsonism and other extrapyramidal symptoms may occur but are infrequent. Nocturnal confusion, hyperactivity, lethargy, psychotic reactions, restlessness, and headache have been reported but are extremely rare.
Autonomic Nervous System: Dryness of mouth, blurred vision, constipation, nausea, vomiting, diarrhea, nasal stuffiness, and pallor have been seen.
Endocrine System: Galactorrhea, breast engorgement, amenorrhea, inhibition of ejaculation, and peripheral edema have been described.
Skin: Dermatitis and skin eruptions of the urticarial type have been observed infrequently. Photosensitivity is extremely rare.
Cardiovascular System: ECG changes have been reported. (See *Phenothiazine Derivatives: Cardiovascular Effects*)
Other: Rare cases described as parotid swelling have been reported following administration of Mellaril® (thioridazine).

Post Introduction Reports

These are voluntary reports of adverse events temporally associated with Mellaril® (thioridazine) that were received since marketing, and there may be no causal relationship between Mellaril® (thioridazine) use and these events: priapism.

Phenothiazine Derivatives

It should be noted that efficacy, indications, and untoward effects have varied with the different phenothiazines. It has been reported that old age lowers the tolerance for phenothiazines. The most common neurological side effects in these patients are parkinsonism and akathisia. There appears to be an increased risk of agranulocytosis and leukopenia in the geriatric population. The physician should be aware that the following have occurred with one or more phenothiazines and should be considered whenever one of these drugs is used:
Autonomic Reactions: Miosis, obstipation, anorexia, paralytic ileus.
Cutaneous Reactions: Erythema, exfoliative dermatitis, contact dermatitis.
Blood Dyscrasias: Agranulocytosis, leukopenia, eosinophilia, thrombocytopenia, anemia, aplastic anemia, pancytopenia.
Allergic Reactions: Fever, laryngeal edema, angioneurotic edema, asthma.
Hepatotoxicity: Jaundice, biliary stasis.
Cardiovascular Effects: Changes in the terminal portion of the electrocardiogram, including prolongation of the Q-T interval, lowering and inversion of the T-wave, and appearance of a wave tentatively identified as a bifid T or a U wave have been observed in some patients receiving the phenothiazine tranquilizers, including Mellaril® (thioridazine). To date, these appear to be due to altered repolarization and not related to myocardial damage. They appear to be reversible. While there is no evidence at present that these changes are in any way precursors of any significant disturbance of cardiac rhythm, it should be noted that several sudden and unexpected deaths apparently due to cardiac arrest have occurred in patients previously showing characteristic electrocardiographic changes while taking the drug. The use of periodic electrocardiograms has been proposed but would appear to be of questionable value as a predictive device.
Hypotension, rarely resulting in cardiac arrest.
Extrapyramidal Symptoms: Akathisia, agitation, motor restlessness, dystonic reactions, trismus, torticollis, opisthotonus, oculogyric crises, tremor, muscular rigidity, akinesia.
Tardive Dyskinesia: Chronic use of neuroleptics may be associated with the development of tardive dyskinesia. The salient features of this syndrome are described in the *WARNINGS* section and subsequently.
The syndrome is characterized by involuntary choreoathetoid movements which variously involve the tongue, face, mouth, lips, or jaw (e.g. protrusion of the tongue, puffing of cheeks, puckering of the mouth, chewing movements), trunk, and extremities. The severity of the syndrome and the degree of impairment produced vary widely.
The syndrome may become clinically recognizable either during treatment, upon dosage reduction, or upon withdrawal of treatment. Movements may decrease in intensity and may disappear altogether if further treatment with neuroleptics is withheld. It is generally believed that reversibility is more likely after short rather than long-term neuroleptic exposure. Consequently, early detection of tardive dyskinesia is important. To increase the likelihood of detecting the syndrome at the earliest possible time, the dosage of neuroleptic drug should be reduced periodically (if clinically possible) and the patient observed for signs of the disorder. This maneuver is critical, for neuroleptic drugs may mask the signs of the syndrome.
Neuroleptic Malignant Syndrome (NMS): Chronic use of neuroleptics may be associated with the development of Neuroleptic Malignant Syndrome. The salient features of this syndrome are described in the *WARNINGS* section and subsequently. Clinical manifestations of NMS are hyperpyrexia, muscle rigidity, altered mental status, and evidence of autonomic instability (irregular pulse or blood pressure, tachycardia, diaphoresis, and cardiac dysrhythmias).
Endocrine Disturbances: Menstrual irregularities, altered libido, gynecomastia, lactation, weight gain, edema. False positive pregnancy tests have been reported.
Urinary Disturbances: Retention, incontinence.
Others: Hyperpyrexia. Behavioral effects suggestive of a paradoxical reaction have been reported. These include excitement, bizarre dreams, aggravation of psychoses, and toxic confusional states. More recently, a peculiar skin-eye syndrome has been recognized as a side effect following long-term treatment with phenothiazines. This reaction is marked by progressive pigmentation of areas of the skin or conjunctiva and/or accompanied by discoloration of the exposed sclera and cornea. Opacities of the anterior lens and cornea described as irregular or stellate in shape have also been reported. Systemic lupus erythematosus-like syndrome.

DOSAGE

Dosage must be individualized according to the degree of mental and emotional disturbance. In all cases, the smallest effective dosage should be determined for each patient.

Adults

Psychotic manifestations: The usual starting dose is 50-100 mg three times a day, with a gradual increment to a maximum of 800 mg daily if necessary. Once effective control of symptoms has been achieved, the dosage may be reduced gradually to determine the minimum maintenance dose. The total daily dosage ranges from 200-800 mg, divided into two to four doses.
For the short-term treatment of moderate to marked depression with variable degrees of anxiety in adult patients and for the treatment of multiple symptoms such as agitation, anxiety, depressed mood, tension, sleep disturbances, and fears in geriatric patients: The usual starting dose is 25 mg three times a day. Dosage ranges from 10 mg two to four times a day in milder cases to 50 mg three or four times a day for more severely disturbed patients. The total daily dosage range is from 20 mg to a maximum of 200 mg.

Children

Mellaril® (thioridazine) is not intended for children under 2 years of age. For children aged 2-12 the dosage of thioridazine hydrochloride ranges from 0.5 mg to a maximum of 3.0 mg/Kg/day. For children with moderate disorders, 10 mg two or three times a day is the usual starting dose. For hospitalized, severely disturbed, or psychotic children, 25 mg two or three times daily is the usual starting dose. Dosage may be increased gradually until optimum therapeutic effect is obtained or the maximum has been reached.

HOW SUPPLIED

Mellaril® (thioridazine HCl) Tablets

Bottles of 100 and 1000 tablets for all strengths and SandoPak® (unit-dose) package of 100 tablets for all strengths except the 150 mg strength.
10 mg
Bright chartreuse, coated tablets; " △ " imprinted on one side, "78-2" imprinted on the other side, in black. Bottle of 100, NDC 0078-0002-05, bottle of 1000, NDC 0078-0002-09, SandoPak® package, NDC 0078-0002-06.
15 mg
Pink, coated tablets; " △ " imprinted on one side, "78-8" imprinted on the other side, in black. Bottle of 100, NDC 0078-0008-05, bottle of 1000, NDC 0078-0008-09, SandoPak® package, NDC 0078-0008-06.
25 mg
Light tan, coated tablets; " △ " imprinted on one side, "MELLARIL 25" imprinted on the other side, in black. Bottle of 100, NDC 0078-0003-05, bottle of 1000, NDC 0078-0003-09, SandoPak® package, NDC 0078-0003-06.
50 mg
White, coated tablets; " △ " imprinted on one side, "MELLARIL 50" imprinted on the other side, in black. Bottle of 100, NDC 0078-0004-05, bottle of 1000, NDC 0078-0004-09, SandoPak® package, NDC 0078-0004-06.
100 mg
Light green, coated tablets; " △ " imprinted on one side, "MELLARIL 100" imprinted on the other side, in black. Bottle of 100, NDC 0078-0005-05, bottle of 1000, NDC 0078-0005-09, SandoPak® package, NDC 0078-0005-06.
150 mg
Yellow, coated tablets; " △ " imprinted on one side, "MELLARIL 150" imprinted on the other side, in black. Bottle of 100, NDC 0078-0006-05, bottle of 1000, NDC 0078-0006-09.
200 mg
Pink, coated tablets; " △ " imprinted on one side, "MELLARIL 200" imprinted on the other side, in black. Bottle of 100, NDC 0078-0007-05, bottle of 1000, NDC 0078-0007-09, SandoPak® package, NDC 0078-0007-06.
Store and Dispense
Below 86°F (30°C); tight container.

Mellaril® (thioridazine HCl) Concentrate

30 mg/mL
A clear, straw-yellow liquid with a cherry-like odor. Each mL contains 30 mg thioridazine hydrochloride, USP, alcohol, 3.0% by volume. Immediate container: amber glass bottles of 4 fl. oz. (118 mL) as follows: 4 fl. oz. bottles, in cartons of 12 bottles, with an accompanying dropper graduated to deliver 10 mg, 25 mg, and 50 mg of thioridazine hydrochloride, USP, NDC 0078-0001-31.
100 mg/mL
A clear, light-yellow liquid with a strawberry-like odor. Each mL contains 100 mg thioridazine hydrochloride, USP, alcohol, 4.2% by volume. Immediate container: amber glass bottles of 4 fl. oz. (118 mL), in cartons of 12 bottles, with an accompanying dropper graduated to deliver 100 mg, 150 mg, and 200 mg of thioridazine hydrochloride, USP, NDC 0078-0009-31.
Store and Dispense
Below 86°F (30°C); tight, amber glass bottle.
The concentrate may be diluted with distilled water, acidified tap water, or suitable juices. Each dose should be so diluted just prior to administration—preparation and storage of bulk dilutions is not recommended.

Mellaril-S® (thioridazine) Oral Suspension

25 mg/5 mL
An off-white suspension with a buttermint taste and a peppermint odor. Each 5 mL contains thioridazine, USP, equivalent to 25 mg thioridazine hydrochloride, USP. Buttermint-flavored in pint bottles, NDC 0078-0068-33.
100 mg/5 mL
A yellow suspension with a buttermint taste and a peppermint odor. Each 5 mL contains thioridazine, USP, equivalent to 100 mg thioridazine hydrochloride, USP. Buttermint-flavored in pint bottles, NDC 0078-0069-33.
Store and Dispense
Below 77°F (25°C); tight, amber glass bottle.
Additional information available to physicians.

[MEL-Z48 Issued February 15, 1991]

Shown in Product Identification Section, page 427

MESANTOIN® ℞

*[meh-san 'toyn]**
(mephenytoin) tablets, USP

CAUTION: Federal law prohibits dispensing without prescription.
The following prescribing information is based on official labeling in effect on August 1, 1992.

DESCRIPTION

Mesantoin® (mephenytoin) is 3-methyl 5,5-phenyl-ethyl-hydantoin. It may be considered to be the hydantoin homolog of the barbiturate mephobarbital. Mesantoin (mephenytoin) has the following structure:

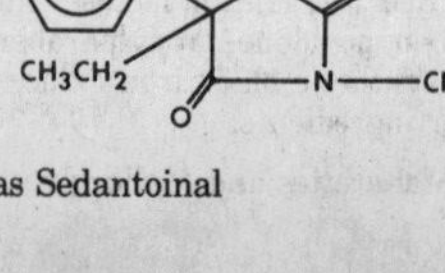

*Also known as Sedantoinal

Active Ingredient: mephenytoin, USP
Inactive Ingredients: FD&C Red #3, gelatin, lactose, starch, stearic acid, and sucrose

ACTIONS

Mephenytoin exhibits pharmacologic effects similar to both diphenylhydantoin and the barbiturates in antagonizing experimental seizures in laboratory animals. Mephenytoin produces behavioral and electroencephalographic effects in man which are similar to those produced by barbiturates.

INDICATIONS

For the control of grand mal, focal, Jacksonian, and psychomotor seizures in those patients who have been refractory to less toxic anticonvulsants.

CONTRAINDICATIONS

Hypersensitivity to hydantoin products.

WARNINGS

Mephenytoin should be used only after safer anticonvulsants have been given an adequate trial and have failed.
As with all anticonvulsants, dose reduction must be gradual so as to minimize the risk of precipitating seizures.
Patients should be cautioned about possible additive effects of alcohol and other CNS depressants. Acute alcohol intoxication may increase the anticonvulsant effect due to decreased metabolic breakdown. Chronic alcohol abuse may result in decreased anticonvulsant effect due to enzyme induction.
Usage in Pregnancy: The effects of mephenytoin in human pregnancy and nursing infants are unknown.
Recent reports suggest an association between the use of anticonvulsant drugs by women with epilepsy and an elevated incidence of birth defects in children born to these women. Data are more extensive with respect to diphenylhydantoin and phenobarbital, but these are also the most commonly prescribed anticonvulsants; less systematic or anecdotal reports suggest a possible similar association with the use of all known anticonvulsant drugs.
The reports suggesting an elevated incidence of birth defects in children of drug-treated epileptic women cannot be regarded as adequate to prove a definite cause and effect relationship. There are intrinsic methodologic problems in obtaining adequate data on drug teratogenicity in humans; the possibility also exists that other factors, e.g., genetic factors or the epileptic condition itself, may be more important than drug therapy in leading to birth defects. The great majority of mothers on anticonvulsant medication deliver normal infants. It is important to note that anticonvulsant drugs should not be discontinued in patients in whom the drug is administered to prevent major seizures because of the strong possibility of precipitating status epilepticus with attendant hypoxia and threat to life. In individual cases where the severity and frequency of the seizure disorder are such that the removal of medication does not pose a serious threat to the patient, discontinuation of the drug may be considered prior to and during pregnancy, although it cannot be said with any confidence that even minor seizures do not pose some hazards to the developing embryo or fetus.
The prescribing physician will wish to weigh these considerations in treating or counseling epileptic women of childbearing potential.

PRECAUTIONS

The patient taking Mesantoin (mephenytoin) must be kept under close medical supervision at all times since serious adverse reactions may emerge.
Because the primary site of degradation is the liver, it is recommended that screening tests of liver function precede introduction of the drug.
Some patients may show side reactions as the result of individual sensitivity. These reactions can be broken down into three types respectively according to severity: 1) blood dyscrasias; 2) skin and mucous membrane manifestations; and 3) central effects. The blood, skin and mucous membrane manifestations are the more important since they can be more serious in nature. Since mephenytoin has been reported to produce blood dyscrasia in certain instances, the patient must be instructed that in the event any unusual symptoms develop (e.g. sore throat, fever, mucous membrane bleeding, glandular swelling, cutaneous reaction), he must discontinue the drug and report for examination immediately. It is recommended that blood examinations be made (total white cell count and differential count) during the initial phase of administration. Such tests are best made: a) before starting medication; b) after 2 weeks on a low dosage; c) again after 2 weeks when full dosage is reached; d) thereafter, monthly for a year; e) from then on, every 3 months. If the neutrophils drop to between 2500 and 1600/cu.mm., counts are made every 2 weeks. Stop medication if the count drops to 1600.

ADVERSE REACTIONS

A number of side effects and toxic reactions have been reported with Mesantoin® (mephenytoin) as well as with other hydantoin compounds. Many of these appear to be dose related while others seem to be a manifestation of a hypersensitivity reaction to these drugs.

Blood Dyscrasias
Leukopenia, neutropenia, agranulocytosis, thrombocytopenia and pancytopenia have occurred. Eosinophilia, monocytosis, and leukocytosis have been described. Simple anemia, hemolytic anemia, megaloblastic anemia and aplastic anemia have occurred but are uncommon.

Skin and Mucous Membrane Manifestations
Maculopapular, morbilliform, scarlatiniform, urticarial, purpuric (associated with thrombocytopenia) and non-specific skin rashes have been reported. Exfoliative dermatitis, erythema multiforme (Stevens-Johnson Syndrome), toxic epidermal necrolysis and fatal dermatitides have been described on rare occasions. Skin pigmentation and rashes associated with a lupus erythematosus syndrome have also been reported.

Central Effects
Drowsiness is dose-related and may be reduced by a reduction in dose. Ataxia, diplopia, nystagmus, dysarthria, fatigue, irritability, choreiform movements, depression and tremor have been encountered.
Nervousness, nausea, vomiting, sleeplessness and dizziness may occur during the initial stages of therapy. Generally, these symptoms are transient, often disappearing with continued treatment.
Mental confusion and psychotic disturbances and increased seizures have been reported, but a definite causal relationship with the drug is uncertain.

Miscellaneous
Hepatitis, jaundice and nephrosis have been reported but a definite cause and effect relationship between the drug and these effects has not been established.
Alopecia, weight gain, edema, photophobia, conjunctivitis and gum hyperplasia have been encountered.
Polyarthropathy, pulmonary fibrosis, lupus erythematosus syndrome and lymphadenopathy which simulates Hodgkin's Disease have also been observed.

DOSAGE AND ADMINISTRATION

Dosage of antiepileptic therapy should be adjusted to the needs of the individual patient. Maintenance dosage is that smallest amount of antiepileptic necessary to suppress seizures completely or reduce their frequency. Optimum dosage is attained by starting with ½ or 1 tablet of Mesantoin (mephenytoin) per day during the first week and thereafter increasing the daily dose by ½ or 1 tablet at weekly intervals. No dose should be increased until it has been taken for at least one week.
The average dose of Mesantoin (mephenytoin) for adults ranges from 2 to 6 tablets (0.2 to 0.6 Gm.) daily. In some instances it may be necessary to administer as much as 8 tablets or more daily in order to obtain full seizure control. Children usually require from 1 to 4 tablets (0.1 Gm. to 0.4 Gm.) according to nature of seizures and age.
When the physician wishes to replace the anticonvulsant now being employed with Mesantoin (mephenytoin), he should give ½ to 1 tablet of Mesantoin (mephenytoin) daily during the first week and gradually increase the daily dose at weekly intervals while gradually reducing that of the drug being discontinued. The transition can be made smoothly over a period of three to six weeks. If seizures are not completely controlled with the dose so attained, the daily dose should then be increased by a one-tablet increment at weekly intervals to the point of maximum effect. If the patient had also been receiving phenobarbital, it is well to continue it until the transition is completed, at which time gradual withdrawal of the phenobarbital may be tried.

HOW SUPPLIED

Each tablet contains 100 mg mephenytoin and is scored to permit half-tablet dosage. Packages of 100 tablets. Tablets embossed "78/52" and scored on one side, " " other side.

[MES-Z16 Issued July 27, 1987]

METAPREL® ℞

(metaproterenol sulfate USP)
INHALATION AEROSOL BRONCHODILATOR

CAUTION: Federal law prohibits dispensing without prescription.
The following prescribing information is based on official labeling in effect on August 1, 1992.

PRESCRIBING INFORMATION

DESCRIPTION

Metaprel® (metaproterenol sulfate USP) Inhalation Aerosol is a bronchodilator administered by oral inhalation. Each Metaprel® (metaproterenol sulfate USP) Inhalation Aerosol contains 150 mg of metaproterenol sulfate as a micronized powder. This is sufficient medication for 200 inhalations. Each metered dose delivers through the mouthpiece 0.65 mg of metaproterenol sulfate (each mL contains 15 mg). The inert ingredients are dichlorodifluoromethane, dichlorotetrafluoroethane, and trichloromonofluoromethane as propellants, and sorbitan trioleate.
Metaprel® (metaproterenol sulfate USP), 1-(3,5-dihydroxyphenyl)-2-isopropylaminoethanol sulfate, is a white, crystalline, racemic mixture of 2 optically active isomers. It has the following chemical structure:

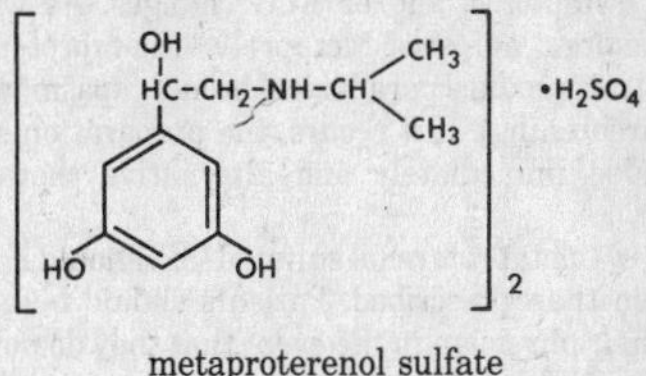

metaproterenol sulfate
(Metaprel®)

$(C_{11}H_{17}NO_3)_2 \cdot H_2SO_4$ Mol. wt. 520.59

CLINICAL PHARMACOLOGY

In vitro studies and *in vivo* pharmacologic studies have demonstrated that Metaprel® (metaproterenol sulfate USP) has a preferential effect on beta-2 adrenergic receptors compared with isoproterenol. While it is recognized that beta-2 adrenergic receptors are the predominant receptors in bronchial smooth muscle, recent data indicate that there is a population of beta-2 receptors in the human heart existing in a concentration between 10%-50%. The precise function of these, however, is not yet established. *(See WARNINGS)*
The pharmacologic effects of beta adrenergic agonist drugs, including Metaprel® (metaproterenol sulfate USP), are at least in part attributable to stimulation through beta adrenergic receptors of intracellular adenyl cyclase, the enzyme which catalyzes the conversion of adenosine triphosphate (ATP) to cyclic-3′, 5′-adenosine monophosphate (c-AMP). Increased c-AMP levels are associated with relaxation of bronchial smooth muscle and inhibition of release of mediators of immediate hypersensitivity from cells, especially from mast cells.

Pharmacokinetics
Absorption, biotransformation, and excretion studies in humans following administration by inhalation have shown that approximately 3% of the actuated dose is absorbed intact through the lungs. The major metabolite, metaproterenol-3-O-sulfate, is produced in the gastrointestinal tract. Metaprel® (metaproterenol sulfate USP) is not metabolized by catechol-O-methyltransferase nor have glucuronide conjugates been isolated to date.
Pulmonary function tests performed concomitantly usually show improvement following aerosol Metaprel® (metaproterenol sulfate USP) administration, e.g., an increase in the 1-second forced expiratory volume (FEV_1), maximum expiratory flow rate, forced vital capacity, and/or a decrease in airway resistance. The resultant decrease in airway obstruction may relieve the dyspnea associated with bronchospasm.
Controlled single- and multiple-dose studies have been performed with pulmonary function monitoring. The duration of effect of a *single dose* of 2-3 inhalations of Metaprel® (metaproterenol sulfate USP) (that is, the period of time during which there is a 20% or greater increase in FEV_1) has varied from 1-5 hours.
In repetitive-dosing studies (up to q.i.d.), the duration of effect for a similar dose of Metaprel® (metaproterenol sulfate USP) has ranged from about 1-2.5 hours. Present studies are inadequate to explain the divergence in duration of the FEV_1 effect between single- and repetitive-dosing studies, respectively.
Recent studies in laboratory animals (minipigs, rodents, and dogs) recorded the occurrence of cardiac arrhythmias and sudden death (with histologic evidence of myocardial necrosis) when beta agonists and methylxanthines were administered concurrently. The significance of these findings when applied to humans is currently unknown.

INDICATIONS AND USAGE

Metaprel® (metaproterenol sulfate USP) is indicated as a bronchodilator for bronchial asthma and for reversible bronchospasm which may occur in association with bronchitis and emphysema.

CONTRAINDICATIONS

Use in patients with cardiac arrhythmias associated with tachycardia is contraindicated.
Although rare, immediate hypersensitivity reactions can occur. Therefore, Metaprel® (metaproterenol sulfate USP) Inhalation Aerosol is contraindicated in patients with a history of hypersensitivity to any of its components.

WARNINGS

Fatalities have been reported following excessive use of Metaprel® (metaproterenol sulfate USP) as with other sympathomimetic inhalation preparations, and the exact cause is unknown. Cardiac arrest was noted in several cases.

Continued on next page

Sandoz—Cont.

Metaprel® (metaproterenol sulfate USP), like other beta adrenergic agonists, can produce a significant cardiovascular effect in some patients, as measured by pulse rate, blood pressure, symptoms, and/or ECG changes. As with other beta adrenergic aerosols, Metaprel® (metaproterenol sulfate USP) can produce paradoxical bronchospasm (which can be life threatening). If it occurs, the preparation should be discontinued immediately and alternative therapy instituted.
Metaprel® (metaproterenol sulfate USP) should not be used more often than prescribed. Patients should be advised to contact their physician in the event that they do not respond to their usual dose of a sympathomimetic amine aerosol.

PRECAUTIONS

General
Extreme care must be exercised with respect to the administration of additional sympathomimetic agents.
Since metaproterenol is a sympathomimetic amine, it should be used with caution in patients with cardiovascular disorders, including ischemic heart disease, hypertension or cardiac arrhythmias, in patients with hyperthyroidism or diabetes mellitus, and in patients who are unusually responsive to sympathomimetic amines or who have convulsive disorders. Significant changes in systolic and diastolic blood pressure could be expected to occur in some patients after use of any beta adrenergic bronchodilator.

Information for Patients
Appropriate care should be exercised when considering the administration of additional sympathomimetic agents. A sufficient interval of time should elapse prior to administration of another sympathomimetic agent.

Drug Interactions
Other beta adrenergic aerosol bronchodilators should not be used concomitantly with Metaprel® (metaproterenol sulfate USP) because they may have additive effects. Beta adrenergic agonists should be administered with caution to patients being treated with monoamine oxidase inhibitors or tricyclic antidepressants, since the action of beta adrenergic agonists on the vascular system may be potentiated.

Carcinogenesis/Mutagenesis/Impairment of Fertility
In an 18-month study in mice, Metaprel® (metaproterenol sulfate USP) produced an increase in benign ovarian tumors in females at doses corresponding to 320 and 640 times the maximum recommended dose (based on a 50 kg individual). In a 2-year study in rats, a non-significant incidence of benign leiomyomata of the mesovarium was noted at 640 times the maximum recommended dose. The relevance of these findings to man is not known. Mutagenic studies with Metaprel® (metaproterenol sulfate USP) have not been conducted. Reproduction studies in rats revealed no evidence of impaired fertility.

Pregnancy: Teratogenic Effects
Pregnancy Category C. Metaprel® (metaproterenol sulfate USP) has been shown to be teratogenic and embryotoxic in rabbits when given in doses corresponding to 640 times the maximum recommended dose. These effects included skeletal abnormalities, hydrocephalus, and skull bone separation. Results of other studies in rabbits, rats, or mice have not revealed any teratogenic, embryocidal, or fetotoxic effects. There are no adequate and well-controlled studies in pregnant women. Metaprel® (metaproterenol sulfate USP) should be used during pregnancy only if the potential benefit justifies the potential risk to the fetus.

Nursing Mothers
It is not known whether Metaprel® (metaproterenol sulfate USP) is excreted in human milk; therefore, Metaprel® (metaproterenol sulfate USP) should be used during nursing only if the potential benefit justifies the possible risk to the newborn.

Pediatric Use
Safety and effectiveness in children below the age of 12 have not been established. Studies are currently under way in this age group.

ADVERSE REACTIONS

Adverse reactions are similar to those noted with other sympathomimetic agents.
The most frequent adverse reaction to Metaprel® (metaproterenol sulfate USP) administered by metered-dose inhaler among 251 patients in 90-day controlled clinical trials was nervousness. This was reported in 6.8% of patients. Less frequent adverse experiences, occurring in 1%-4% of patients were headache, dizziness, palpitations, gastrointestinal distress, tremor, throat irritation, nausea, vomiting, cough, and asthma exacerbation. Tachycardia occurred in less than 1% of patients.

OVERDOSAGE

The expected symptoms with overdosage are those of excessive beta-stimulation and/or any of the symptoms listed under adverse reactions, e.g. angina, hypertension or hypotension, arrhythmias, nervousness, headache, tremor, dry mouth, palpitation, nausea, dizziness, fatigue, malaise, and insomnia.
Treatment consists of discontinuation of metaproterenol together with appropriate symptomatic therapy.

DOSAGE AND ADMINISTRATION

The usual single dose is 2-3 inhalations. With repetitive dosing, inhalation should usually not be repeated more often than about every 3-4 hours. Total dosage per day should not exceed 12 inhalations.
Metaprel® (metaproterenol sulfate USP) Inhalation Aerosol is not recommended for children under 12 years of age. It is recommended that the physician titrate dosage according to each individual patient's response to therapy.

HOW SUPPLIED

Each Metaprel® (metaproterenol sulfate USP) Inhalation Aerosol contains 150 mg of metaproterenol sulfate as a micronized powder in inert propellants. This is sufficient medication for 200 inhalations. Each metered dose delivers through the mouthpiece 0.65 mg metaproterenol sulfate (each mL contains 15 mg). Metaprel® (metaproterenol sulfate USP) Inhalation Aerosol with Mouthpiece (NDC 0078-0209-57), net contents 14 g (10 mL). The mouthpiece is white with a clear, colorless sleeve and a purple protective cap. Metaprel® (metaproterenol sulfate USP) Inhalation Aerosol Refill (NDC 0078-0209-53), net contents 14 g (10 mL).

Storage
Store between 59°F (15°C) and 77°F (25°C). Avoid excessive humidity.

INSTRUCTIONS FOR USE

1. Insert metal canister into clear end of mouthpiece.
2. Remove protective cap, invert canister and shake well before each use.

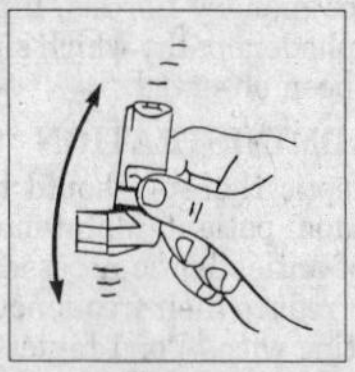

3. Enclose mouthpiece with the lips. The base of the canister should be held vertically.

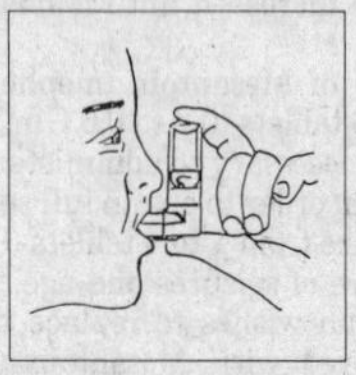

4. Exhale deeply, then inhale slowly through the mouth and at the same time firmly press once on the upended canister base; continue to inhale deeply. Hold your breath for a few seconds and then remove the mouthpiece from the mouth and exhale slowly.
5. One inhalation is often enough to obtain relief. The inhalation can be repeated once or twice, if necessary, or as your physician directs. Wait at least 2 minutes before repeating the inhalation. In most cases, the dose should not be repeated more often than every 3-4 hours. No more than 12 inhalations should be taken in 1 day.
6. Replace protective cap after use.

WARNING: Do not exceed the dose prescribed by your physician. If difficulty in breathing persists, contact your physician immediately.

Note: When full, the container holds enough medication for at least 200 inhalations. Check regularly, by shaking the cylinder or container, to determine whether it contains any medication. When it first seems empty, there are still about 10 doses left. Refill containers for the plastic mouthpiece are available when prescribed by your physician.

Keep the mouthpiece clean. Wash with hot water. If soap is used, rinse thoroughly with plain water.

Never open the container holding the medication. Opening it is dangerous and renders the contents useless.

Caution: Contents under pressure. Do not puncture or incinerate container. Do not expose to heat or store at temperatures above 120°F. Keep out of reach of small children.

Manufactured by:
3M Health Care Specialties Division
Bldg. 225-1N, 3M Center
St. Paul, MN 55144-1000
Distributed by:
SANDOZ
PHARMACEUTICALS
CORPORATION
EAST HANOVER, N.J. 07936
Licensed from Boehringer Ingelheim Pharmaceuticals, Inc.
[MTP-ZZ(200)6 Issued September 30, 1991]

METAPREL® ℞

(metaproterenol sulfate USP)
SYRUP
10 mg/5 mL
TABLETS
10 mg; 20 mg

CAUTION: Federal law prohibits dispensing without prescription.
The following prescribing information is based on official labeling in effect on August 1, 1992.

DESCRIPTION

Syrup: Each 5 mL of Metaprel® (metaproterenol sulfate USP) syrup contains metaproterenol sulfate USP 10 mg. Inactive Ingredients: edetate disodium, flavor, hydroxyethyl cellulose, methylparaben, propylparaben, purified water, Red 40, saccharin, and sorbitol.
Tablets: Each Metaprel® (metaproterenol sulfate USP) tablet, 10 mg and 20 mg, contains metaproterenol sulfate USP 10 mg and 20 mg respectively.
Other Ingredients: colloidal silicon dioxide, dibasic calcium phosphate, lactose, magnesium stearate, and starch.
Chemically, Metaprel® (metaproterenol sulfate USP) is 1-(3, 5-dihydroxyphenyl)-2-isopropylaminoethanol sulfate, a white crystalline, racemic mixture of two optically active isomers.
Its chemical structure is:

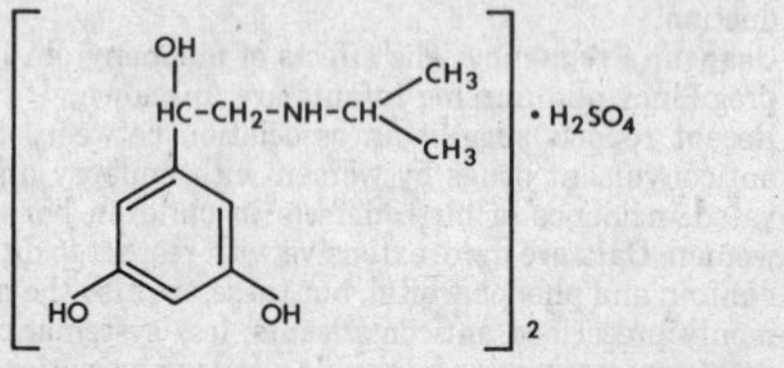

$(C_{11}H_{17}NO_3)_2 \cdot H_2SO_4$ Mol wt 520.59

ACTIONS

Metaprel® (metaproterenol sulfate USP) is a potent beta-adrenergic stimulator. It is postulated that beta-adrenergic stimulants produce many of their pharmacological effects by activation of adenyl cyclase, the enzyme which catalyzes the conversion of adenosine triphosphate to cyclic adenosine monophosphate.
Absorption, biotransformation and excretion studies in humans following oral administration, have indicated that an average of 40% of the drug is absorbed; it is not metabolized by catechol-O-methyltransferase or sulfatase enzymes in the gut but is excreted primarily as glucuronic acid conjugates.
Syrup: When administered orally, Metaprel® (metaproterenol sulfate USP) decreases reversible bronchospasm. Pulmonary function tests performed after the administration of Metaprel® (metaproterenol sulfate USP) usually show improvement, e.g., an increase in the one-second forced expiratory volume (FEV_1), an increase in maximum expiratory flow rate, an increase in peak expiratory flow rate, an increase in forced vital capacity, and/or a decrease in airway resistance. The decrease in airway obstruction may relieve the dyspnea associated with bronchospasm. Pulmonary function has been monitored in controlled single- and multiple-dose studies. The duration of effect of a single dose of Metaprel® (metaproterenol sulfate USP) Syrup (that is, the period of time during which there is a 15% or greater increase in mean FEV_1) was up to 4 hours.
Tablets: When administered orally, Metaprel® (metaproterenol sulfate USP) decreases reversible bronchospasm. Pulmonary function tests performed concomitantly usually show improvement following Metaprel® (metaproterenol sulfate USP) administration, e.g., an increase in the one-second forced expiratory volume (FEV_1), an increase in maximum expiratory flow rate, an increase in forced vital capacity, and/or a decrease in airway resistance. The resultant decrease in airway obstruction may relieve the dyspnea associated with bronchospasm.
Controlled single- and multiple-dose studies have been performed with pulmonary function monitoring. The mean duration of effect of a single dose of 20 mg of Metaprel® (metaproterenol sulfate USP) (that is, the period of time during which there is a 15% or greater increase in FEV_1) was up to 4 hours. Four controlled multiple-dose 60-day studies, comparing the effectiveness of metaproterenol sulfate tablets with ephedrine tablets, have been performed. Because of difficulties in study design, only one study was available which could be analyzed in depth. This study showed a loss of efficacy with time for both metaproterenol sulfate and ephedrine. Therefore, the physician should take this phenomenon into account in evaluating the individual patient's overall management. Further studies are in progress to adequately explain these results.
Recent studies in laboratory animals (minipigs, rodents and dogs) recorded the occurrence of cardiac arrhythmias and sudden death (with histologic evidence of myocardial necrosis) when beta agonists and methylxanthines were adminis-

tered concurrently. The significance of these findings when applied to humans is currently unknown.

INDICATIONS

Metaprel® (metaproterenol sulfate USP) is indicated as a bronchodilator for bronchial asthma, and for reversible bronchospasm which may occur in association with bronchitis and emphysema.

CONTRAINDICATIONS

Use in patients with cardiac arrhythmias associated with tachycardia is contraindicated.

Although rare, immediate hypersensitivity reactions can occur. Therefore, Metaprel® (metaproterenol sulfate USP) is contraindicated in patients with a history of hypersensitivity to any of its components.

PRECAUTIONS

Extreme care must be exercised with respect to the administration of additional sympathomimetic agents. A sufficient interval of time should elapse prior to administration of another sympathomimetic agent.

Because metaproterenol sulfate is a sympathomimetic drug, it should be used with great caution in patients with hypertension, coronary artery disease, congestive heart failure, hyperthyroidism and diabetes, or when there is sensitivity to sympathomimetic amines.

Usage in Pregnancy

Safety in pregnancy has not been established. Metaproterenol should not be used except with caution during pregnancy, weighing the drug's benefit to the patient against potential risk to the fetus. Studies of metaproterenol in mice, rats and rabbits have revealed no significant teratogenic effects at oral doses up to 50 mg/kg (31 times the recommended daily human oral dose). In rabbits, fetal loss and teratogenic effects have been observed at and above oral doses of 50 and 100 mg/kg, respectively.

ADVERSE REACTIONS

Adverse reactions such as tachycardia, hypertension, palpitations, nervousness, tremor, nausea and vomiting have been reported. These reactions are similar to those noted with other sympathomimetic agents.

DOSAGE AND ADMINISTRATION

Syrup: Children aged 6-9 years or weight under 60 lbs—1 teaspoonful 3 or 4 times a day. Children over 9 years or weight over 60 lbs—2 teaspoonfuls 3 or 4 times a day. Experience in children under the age of 6 is limited to 78 children. Of this number, 40 were treated with metaproterenol sulfate for at least 1 month. In this group, daily doses of approximately 1.3-2.6 mg/kg were well tolerated. Adults—2 teaspoonfuls 3 or 4 times a day.

Tablets: The usual adult dose is 20 mg 3 or 4 times a day. Children aged 6-9 years or weight under 60 lbs—10 mg 3 or 4 times a day. Over 9 years or weight over 60 lbs—20 mg 3 or 4 times a day. Metaprel® (metaproterenol sulfate USP) tablets are not recommended for use in children under 6 years at this time. *(Please refer to the ACTIONS section for further information on clinical experience with this product.)*

If Metaprel® (metaproterenol sulfate USP) is administered before or after other sympathomimetic bronchodilators, caution should be exercised with respect to possible potentiation of adrenergic effects.

OVERDOSAGE

The symptoms of overdosage are those of excessive beta-adrenergic stimulation listed under *ADVERSE REACTIONS.*

HOW SUPPLIED

Metaprel® (metaproterenol sulfate USP) Syrup

Available as a cherry-flavored syrup, 10 mg per teaspoonful (5 mL), in pint bottles, NDC 0078-0211-33.

Store and Dispense

Controlled room temperature 15°-30°C (59°-86°F); tight, light-resistant container.

Metaprel® (metaproterenol sulfate USP) Tablets

10 mg Tablets

White, scored, round, imprinted "78-212" on one side, "10" on the other side. Bottle of 100 tablets, NDC 0078-0212-05.

20 mg Tablets

White, scored, round, imprinted "78-213" on one side, "20" on the other side. Bottle of 100 tablets, NDC 0078-0213-05.

Store and Dispense

Controlled room temperature 15°-30°C (59°-86°F); tight, light-resistant container.

Under license from
Boehringer Ingelheim Pharmaceuticals, Inc.
[MTP-Z3 Issued June 1, 1990]

METAPREL®   ℞

(metaproterenol sulfate USP)

INHALATION SOLUTION 5%, Bronchodilator

CAUTION: Federal law prohibits dispensing without prescription.

The following prescribing information is based on official labeling in effect on August 1, 1992.

PRESCRIBING INFORMATION

DESCRIPTION

Metaprel® (metaproterenol sulfate USP) Inhalation Solution is a bronchodilator administered by oral inhalation with the aid of a hand bulb nebulizer or an intermittent positive pressure breathing apparatus (IPPB). It contains Metaprel® (metaproterenol sulfate USP) 5% in a pH-adjusted aqueous solution containing benzalkonium chloride and edetate disodium as preservatives.

Chemically, Metaprel® (metaproterenol sulfate USP) is 1-(3,5 dihydroxyphenyl)-2-isopropylaminoethanol sulfate, a white crystalline, racemic mixture of two optically active isomers.

Its chemical structure is:

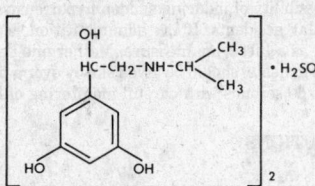

Metaproterenol Sulfate USP
(Metaprel®)

$(C_{11}H_{17}NO_3)_2 \cdot H_2SO_4$ Mol. wt. 520.59

CLINICAL PHARMACOLOGY

Metaprel® (metaproterenol sulfate USP) is a potent beta-adrenergic stimulator with a rapid onset of action. It is postulated that beta-adrenergic stimulants produce many of their pharmacological effects by activation of adenyl cyclase, the enzyme which catalyzes the conversion of adenosine triphosphate to cyclic adenosine monophosphate.

Absorption, biotransformation and excretion studies following administration by inhalation have not been performed. Following oral administration in humans, an average of 40% of the drug is absorbed; it is not metabolized by catechol-O-methyltransferase but is excreted primarily as glucuronic acid conjugates.

Recent studies in laboratory animals (minipigs, rodents and dogs) recorded the occurrence of cardiac arrhythmias and sudden death (with histologic evidence of myocardial necrosis) when beta agonists and methylxanthines were administered concurrently. The significance of these findings when applied to humans is currently unknown.

INDICATIONS AND USAGE

Metaprel® (metaproterenol sulfate USP) Inhalation Solution is indicated as a bronchodilator for bronchial asthma and for reversible bronchospasm which may occur in association with bronchitis and emphysema.

Following controlled single-dose studies by an intermittent positive pressure breathing apparatus (IPPB) and by hand bulb nebulizers, significant improvement (15% or greater increase in FEV_1) occurred within 5-30 minutes and persisted for periods varying from 2-6 hours.

In these studies, the longer duration of effect occurred in the studies in which the drug was administered by IPPB, i.e. 6 hours versus 2-3 hours when administered by hand bulb nebulizer. In these studies, the doses used were 0.3 mL by IPPB and 10 inhalations by hand bulb nebulizer.

In controlled repetitive-dosing studies by IPPB and by hand bulb nebulizer, the onset of effect occurred within 5-30 minutes and the duration ranged from 4-6 hours. In these studies, the doses used were 0.3 mL b.i.d. or t.i.d. when given by IPPB, and 10 inhalations q.i.d. (no more often than q4h) when given by hand bulb nebulizer. As in the single-dose studies, effectiveness was measured as a sustained increase in FEV_1 of 15% or greater. In these repetitive-dosing studies, there was no apparent difference in duration between the two methods of delivery.

Clinical studies were conducted in which the effectiveness of Metaprel® (metaproterenol sulfate USP) Inhalation Solution was evaluated by comparison with that of isoproterenol hydrochloride over periods of 2-3 months. Both drugs continued to produce significant improvement in pulmonary function throughout this period of treatment.

CONTRAINDICATIONS

Use in patients with cardiac arrhythmias associated with tachycardia is contraindicated.

Although rare, immediate hypersensitivity reactions can occur. Therefore, Metaprel® (metaproterenol sulfate USP) is contraindicated in patients with a history of hypersensitivity to any of its components.

WARNINGS

Excessive use of adrenergic aerosols is potentially dangerous. Fatalities have been reported following excessive use of Metaprel® (metaproterenol sulfate USP) as with other sympathomimetic inhalation preparations, and the exact cause is unknown. Cardiac arrest was noted in several cases. Paradoxical bronchoconstriction with repeated excessive administration has been reported with sympathomimetic agents. Patients should be advised to contact their physician in the event that they do not respond to their *usual dose* of sympathomimetic amine aerosol.

PRECAUTIONS

Because Metaprel® (metaproterenol sulfate USP) Inhalation Solution is a sympathomimetic drug, it should be used with great caution in patients with hypertension, coronary artery disease, congestive heart failure, hyperthyroidism or diabetes, or when there is sensitivity to sympathomimetic amines.

Information for Patients

Extreme care must be exercised with respect to the administration of additional sympathomimetic agents. A sufficient interval of time should elapse prior to administration of another sympathomimetic agent.

Carcinogenesis

Long-term studies in mice and rats to evaluate the oral carcinogenic potential of metaproterenol sulfate have not been completed.

Pregnancy

Teratogenic Effects: Pregnancy Category C. Metaprel® (metaproterenol sulfate USP) has been shown to be teratogenic and embryocidal in rabbits when given orally in doses 620 times the human inhalation dose; the teratogenic effects included skeletal abnormalities and hydrocephalus with bone separation. Oral reproduction studies in mice, rats and rabbits showed no teratogenic or embryocidal effect at 50 mg/kg, or 310 times the human inhalation dose. There are no adequate and well-controlled studies in pregnant women. Metaprel® (metaproterenol sulfate USP) Inhalation Solution should be used during pregnancy only if the potential benefit justifies the potential risk to the fetus.

Nursing Mothers

It is not known whether this drug is excreted in human milk. Because many drugs are excreted in human milk, caution should be exercised when Metaprel® (metaproterenol sulfate USP) is administered to a nursing woman.

Pediatric Use

Safety and effectiveness in children below the age of 12 have not been established.

ADVERSE REACTIONS

Adverse reactions are similar to those noted with other sympathomimetic agents.

The most frequent adverse reactions to Metaprel® (metaproterenol sulfate USP) are nervousness and tachycardia which occur in about 1 in 7 patients, tremor which occurs in about 1 in 20 patients and nausea which occurs in about 1 in 50 patients. Less frequent adverse reactions are hypertension, palpitations, vomiting and bad taste which occur in approximately 1 in 300 patients.

OVERDOSAGE

The symptoms of overdosage are those of excessive beta-adrenergic stimulation listed under *ADVERSE REACTIONS.* These reactions usually do not require treatment other than reduction of dosage and/or frequency of administration.

DOSAGE AND ADMINISTRATION

Metaprel® (metaproterenol sulfate USP) Inhalation Solution is administered by oral inhalation with the aid of a hand bulb nebulizer or an intermittent positive pressure breathing apparatus (IPPB).

Usually, treatment need not be repeated more often than every 4 hours to relieve acute attacks of bronchospasm. As part of a total treatment program in chronic bronchospastic pulmonary diseases, Metaprel® (metaproterenol sulfate USP) Inhalation Solution may be administered 3-4 times a day.

As with all medications, the physician should begin therapy with the lowest effective dose and then titrate the dosage according to the individual patient's requirement.

[See table below.]

Method of Administration	Usual Single dose	Range	Dilution
Hand nebulizer	10 inhalations	5–15 inhalations	No dilution
IPPB	0.3 mL	0.2–0.3 mL	Diluted in approx. 2.5 mL of saline solution or other diluent

Continued on next page

Sandoz—Cont.

Metaprel® (metaproterenol sulfate USP) Inhalation Solution is not recommended for use in children under 12 years of age.

HOW SUPPLIED

Metaprel® (metaproterenol sulfate USP) Inhalation Solution is supplied as a 5% solution in bottles of 10 mL with accompanying calibrated dropper, NDC 0078-0210-26.

Store and Dispense

Do not store above 77°F (25°C). Protect from light.

Do not use the solution if its color is pinkish or darker than slightly yellow or if it contains a precipitate.

Under license from Boehringer Ingelheim Pharmaceuticals, Inc.

SANDOZ
PHARMACEUTICALS
CORPORATION
EAST HANOVER, NJ 07936
[MTP-SZ4 issued June 1, 1991]
2270-42

METHERGINE®   ℞

[meth 'er-gin]

(methylergonovine maleate) TABLETS, USP
(methylergonovine maleate) INJECTION, USP

CAUTION: Federal law prohibits dispensing without prescription.

The following prescribing information is based on official labeling in effect on August 1, 1992.

DESCRIPTION

Methergine® (methylergonovine maleate) is a semi-synthetic ergot alkaloid used for the prevention and control of postpartum hemorrhage.

Methergine® (methylergonovine maleate) is available in sterile ampuls of 1 mL, containing 0.2 mg methylergonovine maleate for intramuscular or intravenous injection and in tablets for oral ingestion containing 0.2 mg methylergonovine maleate.

Tablets

Active Ingredient: methylergonovine maleate USP, 0.2 mg

Inactive Ingredients: acacia, carnauba wax, D&C Red #7, FD&C Blue #1, lactose, mixed parabens, povidone, sodium benzoate, starch, stearic acid, sucrose, talc, tartaric acid, and titanium dioxide.

Ampuls, 1 mL, clear, colorless solution

Active Ingredient: methylergonovine maleate USP, 0.2 mg

Inactive Ingredients: sodium chloride USP 3 mg, tartaric acid NF 0.25 mg, water for injection USP qs to 1 mL.

Chemically, methylergonovine maleate is designated as ergoline-8-carboxamide, 9,10-didehydro-N-[1-(hydroxymethyl)propyl]-6-methyl-, [8β(S)]-, (Z)-2-butenedioate (1:1) (salt).

Its structural formula is:

$C_{20}H_{25}N_3O_2 \cdot C_4H_4O_4$ Mol. wt.—455.51

CLINICAL PHARMACOLOGY

Methergine® (methylergonovine maleate) acts directly on the smooth muscle of the uterus and increases the tone, rate, and amplitude of rhythmic contractions. Thus, it induces a rapid and sustained tetanic uterotonic effect which shortens the third stage of labor and reduces blood loss. The onset of action after i.v. administration is immediate; after i.m. administration, 2-5 minutes, and after oral administration, 5-10 minutes.

Pharmacokinetic studies have utilized radioimmunoassay techniques. After i.v. injection of 0.2 mg, Methergine® (methylergonovine maleate) is rapidly distributed from plasma to peripheral tissues within an alpha-phase half-life of 2-3 minutes or less. The beta-phase elimination half-life is 20-30 minutes or more, but clinical effects continue for about 3 hours.[1,2]

Intramuscular injection of 0.2 mg afforded peak plasma concentrations of over 3 ng/mL at t_{max} of 0.5 hours. After 2 hours, total plasma clearance was 120-240 mL/minute.

After oral administration, bioavailability was reported as

60% with no cumulation after repeated doses. During delivery, with parenteral injection, bioavailability increased to 78%.

Excretion is rapid and appears to be partially renal and partially hepatic. Whether the drug is able to penetrate the blood/brain barrier has not been determined.

INDICATIONS AND USAGE

For routine management after delivery of the placenta; postpartum atony and hemorrhage; subinvolution. Under full obstetric supervision, it may be given in the second stage of labor following delivery of the anterior shoulder.

CONTRAINDICATIONS

Hypertension; toxemia; pregnancy; and hypersensitivity.

WARNINGS

This drug should not be administered i.v. routinely because of the possibility of inducing sudden hypertensive and cerebrovascular accidents. If i.v. administration is considered essential as a lifesaving measure, Methergine® (methylergonovine maleate) should be given slowly over a period of no less than 60 seconds with careful monitoring of blood pressure.

PRECAUTIONS

General

Caution should be exercised in the presence of sepsis, obliterative vascular disease, hepatic or renal involvement. Also use with caution during the second stage of labor. The necessity for manual removal of a retained placenta should occur only rarely with proper technique and adequate allowance of time for its spontaneous separation.

Drug Interactions

Caution should be exercised when Methergine® (methylergonovine maleate) is used concurrently with other vasoconstrictors or ergot alkaloids.

Carcinogenesis, mutagenesis, impairment of fertility

No long-term studies have been performed in animals to evaluate carcinogenic potential. The effect of the drug on fertility has not been determined.

Pregnancy

Category C. Animal reproductive studies have not been conducted with Methergine® (methylergonovine maleate). It is also not known whether methylergonovine maleate can cause fetal harm or can affect reproductive capacity. Use of Methergine® (methylergonovine maleate) is contraindicated during pregnancy. (See INDICATIONS AND USAGE)

Labor and Delivery

The uterotonic effect of Methergine® (methylergonovine maleate) is utilized after delivery to assist involution and decrease hemorrhage, shortening the third stage of labor.

Nursing Mothers

Methergine® (methylergonovine maleate) may be administered orally for a maximum of 1 week postpartum to control uterine bleeding. Recommended dosage is 1 tablet (0.2 mg) 3 or 4 times daily. At this dosage level a small quantity of drug appears in mothers' milk.

Adverse effects have not been described, but caution should be exercised when Methergine® (methylergonovine maleate) is administered to a nursing woman.

ADVERSE REACTIONS

The most common adverse reaction is hypertension associated in several cases with seizure and/or headache. Hypotension has also been reported. Nausea and vomiting have occurred occasionally. Rarely observed reactions have included, in order of severity: transient chest pains, dyspnea, hematuria, thrombophlebitis, water intoxication, hallucinations, leg cramps, dizziness, tinnitus, nasal congestion, diarrhea, diaphoresis, palpitation, and foul taste.[3]

DRUG ABUSE AND DEPENDENCE

Methergine® (methylergonovine maleate) has not been associated with drug abuse or dependence of either a physical or psychological nature.

OVERDOSE

Symptoms of acute overdose may include: nausea, vomiting, abdominal pain, numbness, tingling of the extremities, rise in blood pressure, in severe cases followed by hypotension, respiratory depression, hypothermia, convulsions, and coma. Because reports of overdosage with Methergine® (methylergonovine maleate) are infrequent, the lethal dose in humans has not been established. The oral LD_{50} (in mg/kg) for the mouse is 187, the rat 93, and the rabbit 4.5.[4] Several cases of accidental Methergine® (methylergonovine maleate) injection in newborn infants have been reported, and in such cases 0.2 mg represents an overdose of great magnitude. However, recovery occurred in all but one case following a period of respiratory depression, hypothermia, hypertonicity with jerking movements, and, in one case, a single convulsion.

Also, several children 1-3 years of age have accidentally ingested up to 10 tablets (2 mg) with no apparent ill effects. A postpartum patient took 4 tablets at one time in error and reported paresthesias and clamminess as her only symptoms.

Treatment of acute overdosage is symptomatic and includes the usual procedures of:

1. removal of offending drug by inducing emesis, gastric lavage, catharsis, and supportive diuresis.
2. maintenance of adequate pulmonary ventilation, especially if convulsions or coma develop.
3. correction of hypotension with pressor drugs as needed.
4. control of convulsions with standard anticonvulsant agents.
5. control of peripheral vasospasm with warmth to the extremities if needed.[5]

DOSAGE AND ADMINISTRATION

Parenteral drug products should be inspected visually for particulate matter and discoloration prior to administration.

Intramuscularly

1 mL, 0.2 mg, after delivery of the anterior shoulder, after delivery of the placenta, or during the puerperium. May be repeated as required, at intervals of 2-4 hours.

Intravenously

Dosage same as intramuscular. (See WARNINGS)

Orally

One tablet, 0.2 mg, 3 or 4 times daily in the puerperium for a maximum of 1 week.

HOW SUPPLIED

Tablets

0.2 mg round, coated, orchid, branded "78-54" one side, "SANDOZ" other side. Bottles of 100 (NDC 0078-0054-05) and 1000 (NDC 0078-0054-09). SandoPak® (unit dose) packages of 100, 10 blister strips of 10 tablets (NDC 0078-0054-06).

Ampuls

1 mL size, boxes of 20 (NDC 0078-0053-03) and 50 (NDC 0078-0053-04).

Store and dispense

Tablets: Below 77°F; tight, light-resistant container.

Ampuls: Below 77°F; protect from light—administer only if solution is clear and colorless.

References

1. Mantyla, R. and Kants, J.: Clinical Pharmacokinetics of Methylergometrine (Methylergonovine). Int. J. Clin. Pharmacol. Ther. Toxicol. 19(9): 386-391, 1981
2. Iwamura, S. and Kambegawa, A.: Determination of Methylergometrine and Dihydroergotoxine in Biological Fluids. J. Pharm. Dyn. 4: 275-281, 1981
3. Information on Adverse Reactions supplied by Medical Services Dept., Sandoz Pharmaceuticals, E. Hanover, N.J., based on computerized clinical reports.
4. Berde, B. and Schild, H.O.: *Ergot Alkaloids and Related Compounds*, Springer-Verlag, New York, 1978, p. 810
5. Treatment of Acute Overdosage. Sandoz Dorsey Rx Products. Sandoz Inc., Medical Services Department.
[MET-Z21 Issued April 1, 1991]

MIACALCIN®   ℞

[mī"ă-kal'sin]

(calcitonin-salmon) INJECTION, SYNTHETIC

CAUTION: Federal law prohibits dispensing without prescription.

The following prescribing information is based on official labeling in effect on August 1, 1992.

DESCRIPTION

Calcitonin is a polypeptide hormone secreted by the parafollicular cells of the thyroid gland in mammals and by the ultimobranchial gland of birds and fish.

Miacalcin® (calcitonin-salmon) Injection, Synthetic is a synthetic polypeptide of 32 amino acids in the same linear sequence that is found in calcitonin of salmon origin. This is shown by the following graphic formula:

It is provided in sterile solution for subcutaneous or intramuscular injection. Each milliliter contains: calcitonin-salmon 200 I.U.; acetic acid, USP, 2.25 mg; phenol, USP, 5.0 mg; sodium acetate trihydrate, USP, 2.0 mg; sodium chloride, USP, 7.5 mg; water for injection, USP, qs to 1.0 mL. The activity of Miacalcin® (calcitonin-salmon) is stated in International Units based on bioassay in comparison with the International Reference Preparation of calcitonin-salmon for Bioassay, distributed by the National Institute for Biological Standards and Control, Holly Hill, London.

CLINICAL PHARMACOLOGY

Calcitonin acts primarily on bone, but direct renal effects and actions on the gastrointestinal tract are also recognized. Calcitonin-salmon appears to have actions essentially identi-

cal to calcitonins of mammalian origin, but its potency per mg is greater and it has a longer duration of action. The actions of calcitonin on bone and its role in normal human bone physiology are still incompletely understood.

Bone—Single injections of calcitonin cause a marked transient inhibition of the ongoing bone resorptive process. With prolonged use, there is a persistent, smaller decrease in the rate of bone resorption. Histologically, this is associated with a decreased number of osteoclasts and an apparent decrease in their resorptive activity. Decreased osteocytic resorption may also be involved. There is some evidence that initially bone formation may be augmented by calcitonin through increased osteoblastic activity. However, calcitonin will probably not induce a long-term increase in bone formation. Animal studies indicate that endogenous calcitonin, primarily through its action on bone, participates with parathyroid hormone in the homeostatic regulation of blood calcium. Thus, high blood calcium levels cause increased secretion of calcitonin which, in turn, inhibits bone resorption. This reduces the transfer of calcium from bone to blood and tends to return blood calcium to the normal level. The importance of this process in humans has not been determined. In normal adults, who have a relatively low rate of bone resorption, the administration of exogenous calcitonin results in only a slight decrease in serum calcium. In normal children and in patients with generalized Paget's disease, bone resorption is more rapid and decreases in serum calcium are more pronounced in response to calcitonin.

Paget's Disease of Bone (osteitis deformans)—Paget's disease is a disorder of uncertain etiology characterized by abnormal and accelerated bone formation and resorption in one or more bones. In most patients only small areas of bone are involved and the disease is not symptomatic. In a small fraction of patients, however, the abnormal bone may lead to bone pain and bone deformity, cranial and spinal nerve entrapment, or spinal cord compression. The increased vascularity of the abnormal bone may lead to high output congestive heart failure.

Active Paget's disease involving a large mass of bone may increase the urinary hydroxyproline excretion (reflecting breakdown of collagen-containing bone matrix) and serum alkaline phosphatase (reflecting increased bone formation). Calcitonin-salmon, presumably by an initial blocking effect on bone resorption, causes a decreased rate of bone turnover with a resultant fall in the serum alkaline phosphatase and urinary hydroxyproline excretion in approximately 2/3 of patients treated. These biochemical changes appear to correspond to changes toward more normal bone, as evidenced by a small number of documented examples of: 1) radiologic regression of Pagetic lesions, 2) improvement of impaired auditory nerve and other neurologic function, 3) decreases (measured) in abnormally elevated cardiac output. These improvements occur extremely rarely, if ever, spontaneously (elevated cardiac output may disappear over a period of years when the disease slowly enters a sclerotic phase; in the cases treated with calcitonin, however, the decreases were seen in less than one year.)

Some patients with Paget's disease who have good biochemical and/or symptomatic responses initially, later relapse. Suggested explanations have included the formation of neutralizing antibodies and the development of secondary hyperparathyroidism, but neither suggestion appears to explain adequately the majority of relapses.

Although the parathyroid hormone levels do appear to rise transiently during each hypocalcemic response to calcitonin, most investigators have been unable to demonstrate persistent hypersecretion of parathyroid hormone in patients treated chronically with calcitonin-salmon.

Circulating antibodies to calcitonin after 2-18 months' treatment have been reported in about half of the patients with Paget's disease in whom antibody studies were done, but calcitonin treatment remained effective in many of these cases. Occasionally, patients with high antibody titers are found. These patients usually will have suffered a biochemical relapse of Paget's disease and are unresponsive to the acute hypocalcemic effects of calcitonin.

Hypercalcemia—In clinical trials, calcitonin-salmon has been shown to lower the elevated serum calcium of patients with carcinoma (with or without demonstrated metastases), multiple myeloma or primary hyperparathyroidism (lesser response). Patients with higher values for serum calcium tend to show greater reduction during calcitonin therapy. The decrease in calcium occurs about 2 hours after the first injection and lasts for about 6-8 hours. Calcitonin-salmon given every 12 hours maintained a calcium lowering effect for about 5-8 days, the time period evaluated for most patients during the clinical studies. The average reduction of 8-hour post-injection serum calcium during this period was about 9 percent.

Kidney—Calcitonin increases the excretion of filtered phosphate, calcium, and sodium by decreasing their tubular reabsorption. In some patients, the inhibition of bone resorption by calcitonin is of such magnitude that the consequent reduction of filtered calcium load more than compensates for the decrease in tubular reabsorption of calcium. The result

in these patients is a decrease rather than an increase in urinary calcium.

Transient increases in sodium and water excretion may occur after the initial injection of calcitonin. In most patients, these changes return to pretreatment levels with continued therapy.

Gastrointestinal Tract—Increasing evidence indicates that calcitonin has significant actions on the gastrointestinal tract. Short-term administration results in marked transient decreases in the volume and acidity of gastric juice and in the volume and the trypsin and amylase content of pancreatic juice. Whether these effects continue to be elicited after each injection of calcitonin during chronic therapy has not been investigated.

Metabolism—The metabolism of calcitonin-salmon has not yet been studied clinically. Information from animal studies with calcitonin-salmon and from clinical studies with calcitonins of porcine and human origin suggest that calcitonin-salmon is rapidly metabolized by conversion to smaller inactive fragments, primarily in the kidneys, but also in the blood and peripheral tissues. A small amount of unchanged hormone and its inactive metabolites are excreted in the urine.

It appears that calcitonin-salmon cannot cross the placental barrier and its passage to the cerebrospinal fluid or to breast milk has not been determined.

INDICATIONS AND USAGE

Miacalcin® (calcitonin-salmon) Injection, Synthetic is indicated for the treatment of symptomatic Paget's disease of bone, for the treatment of hypercalcemia, and for the treatment of postmenopausal osteoporosis.

Paget's Disease—At the present time, effectiveness has been demonstrated principally in patients with moderate to severe disease characterized by polyostotic involvement with elevated serum alkaline phosphatase and urinary hydroxyproline excretion.

In these patients, the biochemical abnormalities were substantially improved (more than 30% reduction) in about 2/3 of patients studied, and bone pain was improved in a similar fraction. A small number of documented instances of reversal of neurologic deficits has occurred, including improvement in the basilar compression syndrome, and improvement of spinal cord and spinal nerve lesions. At present, there is too little experience to predict the likelihood of improvement of any given neurologic lesion. Hearing loss, the most common neurologic lesion of Paget's disease, is improved infrequently (4 of 29 patients studied audiometrically).

Patients with increased cardiac output due to extensive Paget's disease have had measured decreases in cardiac output while receiving calcitonin. The number of treated patients in this category is still too small to predict how likely such a result will be.

The large majority of patients with localized, especially monostotic disease do not develop symptoms and most patients with mild symptoms can be managed with analgesics. There is no evidence that the prophylactic use of calcitonin is beneficial in asymptomatic patients, although treatment may be considered in exceptional circumstances in which there is extensive involvement of the skull or spinal cord with the possibility of irreversible neurologic damage. In these instances, treatment would be based on the demonstrated effect of calcitonin on Pagetic bone, rather than on clinical studies in the patient population in question.

Hypercalcemia—Miacalcin® (calcitonin-salmon) Injection, Synthetic is indicated for early treatment of hypercalcemic emergencies, along with other appropriate agents, when a rapid decrease in serum calcium is required, until more specific treatment of the underlying disease can be accomplished. It may also be added to existing therapeutic regimens for hypercalcemia such as intravenous fluids and furosemide, oral phosphate or corticosteroids, or other agents.

Postmenopausal Osteoporosis—Miacalcin® (calcitonin-salmon) Injection, Synthetic is indicated for the treatment of postmenopausal osteoporosis in conjunction with an adequate calcium and vitamin D intake to prevent the progressive loss of bone mass. The evidence of efficacy was based on an increase in total body calcium. No significant differences were observed in bone density measurements of the distal radius, and the clinical studies were not designed to detect differences in fracture rates.

CONTRAINDICATIONS

Clinical allergy to synthetic calcitonin-salmon.

WARNINGS

Allergic Reactions

Because calcitonin is protein in nature, the possibility of a systemic allergic reaction exists. **Administration of calcitonin-salmon has been reported in a few cases to cause serious allergic-type reactions (e.g. bronchospasm, swelling of the tongue or throat, and anaphylactic shock), and in one case, death attributed to anaphylaxis.** The usual provisions should be made for the emergency treatment of such a reaction should it occur. Allergic reactions should be differentiated from generalized flushing and hypotension.

Skin testing should be considered prior to treatment with calcitonin, particularly for patients with suspected sensitivity to calcitonin. The following procedure is suggested: Prepare a dilution of 10 I.U. per mL by withdrawing 1/20 mL (0.05 mL) in a tuberculin syringe and filling it to 1.0 mL with Sodium Chloride Injection, USP. Mix well, discard 0.9 mL and inject, intracutaneously 0.1 mL (approximately 1 I.U.) on the inner aspect of the forearm. Observe the injection site 15 minutes after injection. The appearance of more than mild erythema or wheal constitutes a positive response.

The incidence of osteogenic sarcoma is known to be increased in Paget's disease. Pagetic lesions, with or without therapy, may appear by X-ray to progress markedly, possibly with some loss of definition of periosteal margins. Such lesions should be evaluated carefully to differentiate these from osteogenic sarcoma.

PRECAUTIONS

1. General

The administration of calcitonin possibly could lead to hypocalcemic tetany under special circumstances although no cases have yet been reported. Provisions for parenteral calcium administration should be available during the first several administrations of calcitonin.

2. Laboratory Tests

Periodic examinations of urine sediment of patients on chronic therapy are recommended.

Coarse granular casts and casts containing renal tubular epithelial cells were reported in young adult volunteers at bed rest who were given calcitonin-salmon to study the effect of immobilization on osteoporosis. There was no other evidence of renal abnormality and the urine sediment became normal after calcitonin was stopped. Urine sediment abnormalities have not been reported by other investigators.

3. Instructions for the Patient

Careful instruction in sterile injection technique should be given to the patient, and to other persons who may administer Miacalcin® (calcitonin-salmon) Injection, Synthetic.

4. Carcinogenesis, Mutagenesis, and Impairment of Fertility

An increased incidence of pituitary adenomas has been observed in one-year toxicity studies in Sprague-Dawley rats administered calcitonin-salmon at dosages of 20 and 80 I.U./kg/day and in Fisher 344 rats given 80 I.U./kg/day. The relevance of these findings to humans is unknown. Calcitonin-Salmon was not mutagenic in tests using *Salmonella typhimurium, Escherichia coli,* and Chinese Hamster V79 cells.

5. Pregnancy: Teratogenic Effects

Category C

Calcitonin-salmon has been shown to cause a decrease in fetal birth weights in rabbits when given in doses 14-56 times the dose recommended for human use. Since calcitonin does not cross the placental barrier, this finding may be due to metabolic effects on the pregnant animal. There are no adequate and well-controlled studies in pregnant women. Miacalcin® (calcitonin-salmon) Injection, Synthetic should be used during pregnancy only if the potential benefit justifies the potential risk to the fetus.

6. Nursing Mothers

It is not known whether this drug is excreted in human milk. As a general rule, nursing should not be undertaken while a patient is on this drug since many drugs are excreted in human milk. Calcitonin has been shown to inhibit lactation in animals.

7. Pediatric Use

Disorders of bone in children referred to as juvenile Paget's disease have been reported rarely. The relationship of these disorders to adult Paget's disease has not been established and experience with the use of calcitonin in these disorders is very limited. There are no adequate data to support the use of Miacalcin® (calcitonin-salmon) Injection, Synthetic in children.

ADVERSE REACTIONS

Gastrointestinal System

Nausea with or without vomiting has been noted in about 10% of patients treated with calcitonin. It is most evident when treatment is first initiated and tends to decrease or disappear with continued administration.

Dermatologic/Hypersensitivity

Local inflammatory reactions at the site of subcutaneous or intramuscular injection have been reported in about 10% of patients. Flushing of face or hands occurred in about 2-5% of patients. Skin rashes, nocturia, pruritus of the ear lobes, feverish sensation, pain in the eyes, poor appetite, abdominal pain, edema of feet, and salty taste have been reported in patients treated with calcitonin-salmon. Administration of calcitonin-salmon has been reported in a few cases to cause serious allergic-type reactions (e.g. bronchospasm, swelling of the tongue or throat, and anaphylactic shock), and in one case, death attributed to anaphylaxis [see *Warnings*].

OVERDOSAGE

A dose of 1000 I.U. subcutaneously may produce nausea and vomiting as the only adverse effects. Doses of 32 units per kg per day for 1-2 days demonstrate no other adverse effects.

Continued on next page

Sandoz—Cont.

Data on chronic high dose administration are insufficient to judge toxicity.

DOSAGE AND ADMINISTRATION

Paget's Disease —The recommended starting dose of calcitonin-salmon in Paget's disease is 100 I.U. (0.5 mL) per day administered subcutaneously (preferred for outpatient self-administration) or intramuscularly. Drug effect should be monitored by periodic measurement of serum alkaline phosphatase and 24-hour urinary hydroxyproline (if available) and evaluations of symptoms. A decrease toward normal of the biochemical abnormalities is usually seen, if it is going to occur, within the first few months. Bone pain may also decrease during that time. Improvement of neurologic lesions, when it occurs, requires a longer period of treatment, often more than one year.

In many patients, doses of 50 I.U. (0.25 mL) per day or every other day are sufficient to maintain biochemical and clinical improvement. At the present time, however, there are insufficient data to determine whether this reduced dose will have the same effect as the higher dose on forming more normal bone structure. It appears preferable, therefore, to maintain the higher dose in any patient with serious deformity or neurological involvement.

In any patient with a good response initially who later relapses, either clinically or biochemically, the possibility of antibody formation should be explored. The patient may be tested for antibodies by an appropriate specialized test or evaluated for the possibility of antibody formation by critical clinical evaluation.

Patient compliance should also be assessed in the event of relapse.

In patients who relapse, whether because of antibodies or for unexplained reasons, a dosage increase beyond 100 I.U. per day does not usually appear to elicit an improved response.

Hypercalcemia —The recommended starting dose of Miacalcin® (calcitonin-salmon) Injection, Synthetic in hypercalcemia is 4 I.U./kg body weight every 12 hours by subcutaneous or intramuscular injection. If the response to this dose is not satisfactory after one or two days, the dose may be increased to 8 I.U./kg every 12 hours. If the response remains unsatisfactory after two more days, the dose may be further increased to a maximum of 8 I.U./kg every 6 hours.

Postmenopausal Osteoporosis —The recommended dose of calcitonin is 100 I.U. per day administered subcutaneously or intramuscularly. Patients should also receive supplemental calcium such as calcium carbonate 1.5 g daily and an adequate vitamin D intake (400 units daily). An adequate diet is also essential.

If the volume of Miacalcin® (calcitonin-salmon) Injection, Synthetic to be injected exceeds 2 mL, intramuscular injection is preferable and multiple sites of injection should be used.

Parenteral drug products should be inspected visually for particulate matter and discoloration prior to administration whenever solution and container permit.

HOW SUPPLIED

Miacalcin® (calcitonin-salmon) Injection, Synthetic is available as a sterile solution in individual 2 mL vials containing 200 I.U. per mL (NDC 0078-0149-23).

Store in Refrigerator—Between 2°-8°C (36°-46°F).

Manufactured by
Schering-Plough Products, Inc.
Manati, Puerto Rico
for Sandoz Pharmaceuticals Corporation
East Hanover, NJ 07936
[MIA-Z5(PR) Issued April 1, 1992]
Shown in Product Identification Section, page 427

NEO–CALGLUCON® (calcium glubionate)
Syrup, USP
[nē'ō cal"glū'kon]
Palatable and Readily Absorbable Calcium Supplement.

The following prescribing information is based on official labeling in effect on August 1, 1992.

DESCRIPTION

Each teaspoonful (5 mL) of NEO-CALGLUCON® (calcium glubionate) Syrup, USP contains: glubionate calcium 1.8 g, (calcium content 115 mg—providing the same amount as 1.2 g calcium gluconate). Other ingredients: benzoic acid, caramel, citric acid, flavors, purified water, saccharin sodium, sorbitol, sucrose.

Adequate calcium intake is particularly important during periods of bone growth in childhood and adolescence, during pregnancy and lactation. An adequate supply of calcium is considered important in adults, especially those over 40, to prevent a negative calcium balance which may contribute to the development of osteoporosis. The following are the US

NEO-CALGLUCON® (calcium glubionate) Syrup, USP

		Grams of Supplemental Calcium Provided Daily	Percentage of US Recommended Daily Allowance (US RDA)
I.	As a Dietary Supplement: Adults and children 4 or more years of age—1 tablespoonful 3 times daily.	1.0 g	104
	Pregnant or lactating women— 1 tablespoonful 4 times daily.	1.4 g	106
	Children under 4 years of age— 2 teaspoonfuls 3 times daily.	0.7 g	86
	Infants—1 teaspoonful 5 times daily (may be taken undiluted, mixed with infant's formula or fruit juice).	0.6 g	96
	(Part of need is supplied by diet)		

NEO-CALGLUCON® (calcium glubionate) Syrup, USP

		Grams of Supplemental Ca Provided Daily
II.	In the treatment of Calcium Deficiency States:	

Tetany of the Newborn (Tetany of the newborn appears to be a transient physiologic hypoparathyroidism related to the maturation of the parathyroid glands. Adequate parathyroid gland function usually occurs within one week after birth.)

Serum calcium should be determined before therapy is instituted. Hypocalcemia is defined as a serum calcium below 8 mg/100 mL or 4 mEq/liter. It is advisable to lower the solute and phosphorus loads in the feeding as well as to provide extra calcium. Intravenous administration of calcium solutions may be necessary for prompt relief of symptoms.

Dose: Infants with confirmed hypocalcemia may be benefited by the oral administration of calcium salts so as to provide ELEMENTAL CALCIUM in a dosage of 50 to 150 mg/kg/day divided into three or more doses. (NEO-CALGLUCON® calcium glubionate) Syrup, USP contains 115 mg ELEMENTAL CALCIUM per 5 mL teaspoon.)

The lower dosage range should be employed if calcium is also being provided by the parenteral route. Whole milk formulas which are high in phosphorus should be eliminated in order to increase the calcium/phosphorus ratio. Supplemental oral calcium should be gradually reduced over a period of two or three weeks after the condition has completely stabilized.

See left-hand column

Hypoparathyroidism
Acute
    Intravenous administration of calcium solutions may be necessary for prompt correction of hypocalcemia. Supplementary calcium should be given orally as soon as possible.

Dose: 1–3 tablespoonfuls 3 times daily	1.0–3.1
Chronic	
Dose: 1–3 tablespoonfuls daily	0.3–1.0
Pseudohypoparathyroidism	
Dose: 1–3 tablespoonfuls daily	0.3–1.0
Osteoporosis, postmenopausal and senile	
Dose: 1–2 tablespoonfuls 3 times daily	1.0–2.1

Rickets and Osteomalacia
Treatment of these disorders consists of the administration of Vitamin D orally. The addition of calcium to the therapeutic regimen may be desirable to provide calcium needed for remineralization and to avoid hypocalcemia which occurs not infrequently in the early days of treatment. Dosages should be those recommended above under Dietary Supplement.

Government Recommended Daily Allowances (US RDA) of calcium.

Age Period	Calcium Requirements
Infants	0.6 g
Children under 4 years	0.8 g
Adults and children over 4	1.0 g
Pregnant and lactating women	1.3 g

Eight ounces of whole milk provide approximately 267 mg of calcium. One tablespoonful (15 mL) of NEO-CALGLUCON® (calcium glubionate) Syrup, USP contains 345 mg of calcium.

INDICATIONS

1. As a *dietary supplement* where calcium intake may be inadequate:
   a. childhood and adolescence
   b. pregnancy
   c. lactation
   d. postmenopausal females and in the aged
2. In the *treatment* of calcium deficiency states which may occur in diseases such as:

    a. tetany of the newborn*
    b. hypoparathyroidism, acute* and chronic
    c. pseudohypoparathyroidism
    d. postmenopausal and senile osteoporosis
    e. rickets and osteomalacia
*As a supplement to parenterally administered calcium.

CONTRAINDICATIONS

Patients with renal calculi.

WARNINGS

Certain dietary substances interfere with the absorption of calcium. These include oxalic acid (found in large quantities in rhubarb and spinach), phytic acid (bran and whole cereals) and phosphorus (milk and other dairy products). Administration of corticosteroids may interfere with calcium absorption.

PRECAUTIONS

When calcium is administered in therapeutic amounts for prolonged periods, hypercalcemia and hypercalciuria may result. This is most likely to occur in patients with hypoparathyroidism who are receiving high doses of Vitamin D. It can be avoided by frequent checks of plasma and urine calcium levels. Urine calcium levels may rise before plasma calcium

levels. The former may be checked by determining 24-hour calcium excretion or by the Sulkowitch test.

ADVERSE REACTIONS

NEO-CALGLUCON® (calcium glubionate) Syrup, USP is exceptionally well tolerated. Gastrointestinal disturbances are exceedingly rare. A fatal case of hypercalcemia associated with an overdose of NEO-CALGLUCON® (calcium glubionate) Syrup, USP has been reported in a two pound neonate. Symptoms of hypercalcemia include anorexia, nausea, vomiting, constipation, abdominal pain, dryness of the mouth, thirst and polyuria.

DOSAGE AND ADMINISTRATION

NEO-CALGLUCON® (calcium glubionate) Syrup, USP should be administered before meals to enhance absorption.

[See table on preceding page.]

HOW SUPPLIED

NEO-CALGLUCON® (calcium glubionate) Syrup, USP (straw yellow) in pint bottles.

Store and Dispense: Below 86° F (30°C); glass bottle.

PAMELOR® ℞

[pam 'ah-lar"]

(nortriptyline HCl) CAPSULES, USP

(nortriptyline HCl) ORAL SOLUTION, USP

CAUTION: Federal law prohibits dispensing without prescription.

The following prescribing information is based on official labeling in effect on August 1, 1992.

DESCRIPTION

Pamelor® (nortriptyline HCl) is 1-Propanamine, 3-(10,11-dihydro-5*H*-dibenzo[*a,d*]cyclohepten-5-ylidene)-*N*-methyl-, hydrochloride.

The structural formula is as follows:

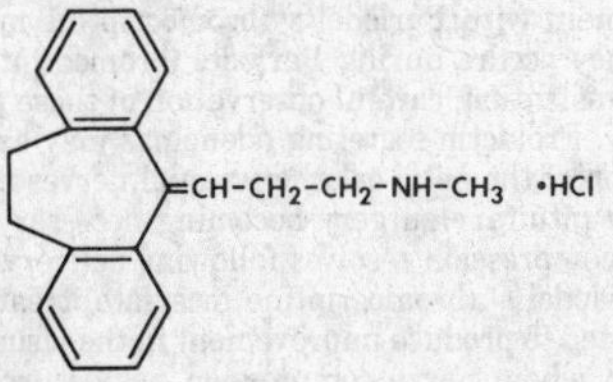

$C_{19}H_{21}N \cdot HCl$ Mol. wt. 299.8

10 mg, 25 mg, 50 mg, and 75 mg Capsules

Active Ingredient: nortriptyline HCl, USP

10 mg, 25 mg, and 75 mg Capsules

Inactive Ingredients: D&C Yellow #10, FD&C Yellow #6, gelatin, silicone fluid, sodium lauryl sulfate, starch, and titanium dioxide.

May Also Include: benzyl alcohol, butylparaben, edetate calcium disodium, methylparaben, propylparaben, silicon dioxide, and sodium propionate.

50 mg Capsules

Inactive Ingredients: gelatin, silicone fluid, sodium lauryl sulfate, starch, and titanium dioxide.

May Also Include: benzyl alcohol, butylparaben, edetate calcium disodium, methylparaben, propylparaben, silicon dioxide, sodium bisulfite (capsule shell only), and sodium propionate.

Solution

Active Ingredient: nortriptyline HCl, USP

Inactive Ingredients: alcohol, benzoic acid, flavoring, purified water, and sorbitol.

ACTIONS

The mechanism of mood elevation by tricyclic antidepressants is at present unknown. Pamelor® (nortriptyline HCl) is not a monoamine oxidase inhibitor. It inhibits the activity of such diverse agents as histamine, 5-hydroxytryptamine, and acetylcholine. It increases the pressor effect of norepinephrine but blocks the pressor response of phenethylamine. Studies suggest that Pamelor® (nortriptyline HCl) interferes with the transport, release, and storage of catecholamines. Operant conditioning techniques in rats and pigeons suggest that Pamelor® (nortriptyline HCl) has a combination of stimulant and depressant properties.

INDICATIONS

Pamelor® (nortriptyline HCl) is indicated for the relief of symptoms of depression. Endogenous depressions are more likely to be alleviated than are other depressive states.

CONTRAINDICATIONS

The use of Pamelor® (nortriptyline HCl) or other tricyclic antidepressants concurrently with a monoamine oxidase (MAO) inhibitor is contraindicated. Hyperpyretic crises, severe convulsions, and fatalities have occurred when similar tricyclic antidepressants were used in such combinations. It is advisable to have discontinued the MAO inhibitor for at least two weeks before treatment with Pamelor® (nortriptyline HCl) is started. Patients hypersensitive to Pamelor® (nortriptyline HCl) should not be given the drug.

Cross-sensitivity between Pamelor® (nortriptyline HCl) and other dibenzazepines is a possibility.

Pamelor® (nortriptyline HCl) is contraindicated during the acute recovery period after myocardial infarction.

WARNINGS

Patients with cardiovascular disease should be given Pamelor® (nortriptyline HCl) only under close supervision because of the tendency of the drug to produce sinus tachycardia and to prolong the conduction time. Myocardial infarction, arrhythmia, and strokes have occurred. The antihypertensive action of guanethidine and similar agents may be blocked. Because of its anticholinergic activity, Pamelor® (nortriptyline HCl) should be used with great caution in patients who have glaucoma or a history of urinary retention. Patients with a history of seizures should be followed closely when Pamelor® (nortriptyline HCl) is administered, inasmuch as this drug is known to lower the convulsive threshold. Great care is required if Pamelor® (nortriptyline HCl) is given to hyperthyroid patients or to those receiving thyroid medication, since cardiac arrhythmias may develop.

Pamelor® (nortriptyline HCl) may impair the mental and/or physical abilities required for the performance of hazardous tasks, such as operating machinery or driving a car; therefore, the patient should be warned accordingly.

Excessive consumption of alcohol in combination with nortriptyline therapy may have a potentiating effect, which may lead to the danger of increased suicidal attempts or overdosage, especially in patients with histories of emotional disturbances or suicidal ideation.

The concomitant administration of quinidine and nortriptyline may result in a significantly longer plasma half-life, higher AUC, and lower clearance of nortriptyline.

Use in Pregnancy—Safe use of Pamelor® (nortriptyline HCl) during pregnancy and lactation has not been established; therefore, when the drug is administered to pregnant patients, nursing mothers, or women of childbearing potential, the potential benefits must be weighed against the possible hazards. Animal reproduction studies have yielded inconclusive results.

Use in Children—This drug is not recommended for use in children, since safety and effectiveness in the pediatric age group have not been established.

PRECAUTIONS

The use of Pamelor® (nortriptyline HCl) in schizophrenic patients may result in an exacerbation of the psychosis or may activate latent schizophrenic symptoms. If the drug is given to overactive or agitated patients, increased anxiety and agitation may occur. In manic-depressive patients, Pamelor® (nortriptyline HCl) may cause symptoms of the manic phase to emerge.

Administration of reserpine during therapy with a tricyclic antidepressant has been shown to produce a "stimulating" effect in some depressed patients.

Troublesome patient hostility may be aroused by the use of Pamelor® (nortriptyline HCl). Epileptiform seizures may accompany its administration, as is true of other drugs of its class.

Close supervision and careful adjustment of the dosage are required when Pamelor® (nortriptyline HCl) is used with other anticholinergic drugs and sympathomimetic drugs.

Concurrent administration of cimetidine and tricyclic antidepressants can produce clinically significant increases in the plasma concentrations of the tricyclic antidepressant.

The patient should be informed that the response to alcohol may be exaggerated.

When it is essential, the drug may be administered with electroconvulsive therapy, although the hazards may be increased. Discontinue the drug for several days, if possible, prior to elective surgery.

The possibility of a suicidal attempt by a depressed patient remains after the initiation of treatment; in this regard, it is important that the least possible quantity of drug be dispensed at any given time.

Both elevation and lowering of blood sugar levels have been reported.

A case of significant hypoglycemia has been reported in a type II diabetic patient maintained on chlorpropamide (250 mg/day), after the addition of nortriptyline (125 mg/day).

ADVERSE REACTIONS

Note: Included in the following list are a few adverse reactions that have not been reported with this specific drug. However, the pharmacologic similarities among the tricyclic antidepressant drugs require that each of the reactions be considered when nortriptyline is administered.

Cardiovascular—Hypotension, hypertension, tachycardia, palpitation, myocardial infarction, arrhythmias, heart block, stroke.

Psychiatric—Confusional states (especially in the elderly) with hallucinations, disorientation, delusions; anxiety, restlessness, agitation; insomnia, panic, nightmares; hypomania; exacerbation of psychosis.

Neurologic—Numbness, tingling, paresthesias of extremities; incoordination, ataxia, tremors; peripheral neuropathy; extrapyramidal symptoms; seizures, alteration in EEG patterns; tinnitus.

Anticholinergic—Dry mouth and, rarely, associated sublingual adenitis; blurred vision, disturbance of accommodation, mydriasis; constipation, paralytic ileus; urinary retention, delayed micturition, dilation of the urinary tract.

Allergic—Skin rash, petechiae, urticaria, itching, photosensitization (avoid excessive exposure to sunlight); edema (general or of face and tongue), drug fever, cross-sensitivity with other tricyclic drugs.

Hematologic—Bone marrow depression, including agranulocytosis; eosinophilia; purpura; thrombocytopenia.

Gastrointestinal—Nausea and vomiting, anorexia, epigastric distress, diarrhea, peculiar taste, stomatitis, abdominal cramps, black-tongue.

Endocrine—Gynecomastia in the male, breast enlargement and galactorrhea in the female; increased or decreased libido, impotence; testicular swelling; elevation or depression of blood sugar levels; syndrome of inappropriate ADH (antidiuretic hormone) secretion.

Other—Jaundice (simulating obstructive), altered liver function; weight gain or loss; perspiration; flushing; urinary frequency, nocturia; drowsiness, dizziness, weakness, fatigue; headache; parotid swelling; alopecia.

Withdrawal Symptoms—Though these are not indicative of addiction, abrupt cessation of treatment after prolonged therapy may produce nausea, headache, and malaise.

DOSAGE AND ADMINISTRATION

Pamelor® (nortriptyline HCl) is not recommended for children.

Pamelor® (nortriptyline HCl) is administered orally in the form of capsules or liquid. Lower than usual dosages are recommended for elderly patients and adolescents. Lower dosages are also recommended for outpatients than for hospitalized patients who will be under close supervision. The physician should initiate dosage at a low level and increase it gradually, noting carefully the clinical response and any evidence of intolerance. Following remission, maintenance medication may be required for a longer period of time at the lowest dose that will maintain remission.

If a patient develops minor side effects, the dosage should be reduced. The drug should be discontinued promptly if adverse effects of a serious nature or allergic manifestations occur.

Usual Adult Dose—25 mg three or four times daily; dosage should begin at a low level and be increased as required. As an alternate regimen, the total daily dosage may be given once a day. When doses above 100 mg daily are administered, plasma levels of nortriptyline should be monitored and maintained in the optimum range of 50-150 ng/mL. Doses above 150 mg/day are not recommended.

Elderly and Adolescent Patients—30-50 mg/day, in divided doses, or the total daily dosage may be given once a day.

OVERDOSAGE

Toxic overdosage may result in confusion, restlessness, agitation, vomiting, hyperpyrexia, muscle rigidity, hyperactive reflexes, tachycardia, ECG evidence of impaired conduction, shock, congestive heart failure, stupor, coma, and CNS stimulation with convulsions followed by respiratory depression. Deaths have occurred following overdosage with drugs of this class.

No specific antidote is known. General supportive measures are indicated, with gastric lavage. Respiratory assistance is apparently the most effective measure when indicated. The use of CNS depressants may worsen the prognosis.

The administration of barbiturates for control of convulsions alleviates an increase in the cardiac work load but should be undertaken with caution to avoid potentiation of respiratory depression.

Intramuscular paraldehyde or diazepam provides anticonvulsant activity with less respiratory depression than do the barbiturates; diazepam seems to be preferred.

The use of digitalis and/or physostigmine may be considered in case of serious cardiovascular abnormalities or cardiac failure.

The value of dialysis has not been established.

HOW SUPPLIED

Capsules: Pamelor® (nortriptyline HCl) Capsules, USP, equivalent to 10 mg, 25 mg, 50 mg, and 75 mg base, are available in bottles of 100 (10 mg: NDC 0078-0086-05; 25 mg: NDC 0078-0087-05; 50 mg: NDC 0078-0078-05; 75 mg: NDC 0078-0079-05). 10 mg, 25 mg, and 50 mg are available in SandoPak® (unit-dose) box of 100 individually labeled blisters, each containing 1 capsule (10 mg: NDC 0078-0086-06; 25 mg: NDC 0078-0087-06; 50 mg: NDC 0078-0078-06). Pamelor® (nortriptyline HCl) Capsules, USP 25 mg are also available in bottles of 500 (NDC 0078-0087-08).

Continued on next page

Sandoz—Cont.

10 mg capsules branded "SANDOZ" on one half, "PAMELOR 10 mg" other half; 25 mg capsules branded "SANDOZ" on one half, "PAMELOR 25 mg" other half; 50 mg capsules branded "SANDOZ" on one half, "PAMELOR 50 mg" other half; and 75 mg capsules branded "SANDOZ" on one half, "PAMELOR 75 mg" other half.
Store and Dispense: Below 86°F (30°C); tight container.
Solution: Pamelor® (nortriptyline HCl) Solution, USP, equivalent to 10 mg base per 5 mL, is supplied in 16-fluid-ounce bottles (NDC 0078-0016-33). Alcohol content 4%.
Store and Dispense: Below 86°F (30°C); tight, light-resistant container.

[PAM-Z21 Issued July 1, 1990]
Shown in Product Identification Section, page 427

PARLODEL® ℞

[*par'lō-del"*]
SnapTabs® (bromocriptine mesylate) TABLETS, USP
(bromocriptine mesylate) CAPSULES

CAUTION: Federal law prohibits dispensing without prescription.
The following prescribing information is based on official labeling in effect on August 1, 1992.

DESCRIPTION

Parlodel® (bromocriptine mesylate) is an ergot derivative with potent dopamine receptor agonist activity. Each Parlodel® (bromocriptine mesylate) SnapTabs® tablet for oral administration contains 2½ mg and each capsule contains 5 mg bromocriptine (as the mesylate). Parlodel® (bromocriptine mesylate) is chemically designated as (1) Ergotaman-3′, 6′, 18-trione, 2-bromo-12′-hydroxy-2′-(1-methylethyl)-5′-(2-methylpropyl)-, (5′α) monomethanesulfonate (salt); (2) 2-bromoergocryptine monomethanesulfonate (salt).*

Structural Formula

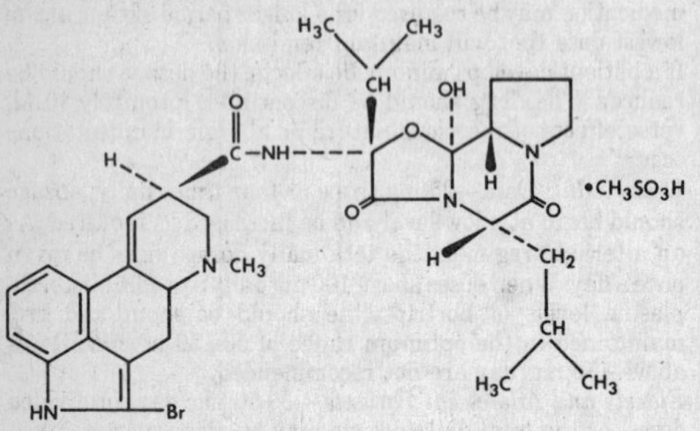

2.5 mg SnapTabs®
Active Ingredient: bromocriptine mesylate, USP
Inactive Ingredients: colloidal silicon dioxide, lactose, magnesium stearate, povidone, starch, and another ingredient
5 mg Capsules
Active Ingredient: bromocriptine mesylate, USP
Inactive Ingredients: colloidal silicon dioxide, gelatin, lactose, magnesium stearate, red iron oxide, silicon dioxide, sodium bisulfite, sodium lauryl sulfate, starch, titanium dioxide, yellow iron oxide, and another ingredient

CLINICAL PHARMACOLOGY

Parlodel® (bromocriptine mesylate) is a dopamine receptor agonist, which activates post-synaptic dopamine receptors. The dopaminergic neurons in the tuberoinfundibular process modulate the secretion of prolactin from the anterior pituitary by secreting a prolactin inhibitory factor (thought to be dopamine); in the corpus striatum the dopaminergic neurons are involved in the control of motor function. Clinically, Parlodel® (bromocriptine mesylate) significantly reduces plasma levels of prolactin in patients with physiologically elevated prolactin as well as in patients with hyperprolactinemia. The inhibition of physiological lactation as well as galactorrhea in pathological hyperprolactinemic states is obtained at dose levels that do not affect secretion of other tropic hormones from the anterior pituitary. Experiments have demonstrated that bromocriptine induces long lasting stereotyped behavior in rodents and turning behavior in rats having unilateral lesions in the substantia nigra. These actions, characteristic of those produced by dopamine, are inhibited by dopamine antagonists and suggest a direct action of bromocriptine on striatal dopamine receptors.
Parlodel® (bromocriptine mesylate) is a nonhormonal, nonestrogenic agent that inhibits the secretion of prolactin in humans, with little or no effect on other pituitary hormones, except in patients with acromegaly, where it lowers elevated blood levels of growth hormone in the majority of patients.
In about 75% of cases of amenorrhea and galactorrhea, Parlodel® (bromocriptine mesylate) therapy suppresses the galactorrhea completely, or almost completely, and reinitiates normal ovulatory menstrual cycles.
Menses are usually reinitiated prior to complete suppression of galactorrhea; the time for this on average is 6-8 weeks. However, some patients respond within a few days, and others may take up to 8 months.
Galactorrhea may take longer to control depending on the degree of stimulation of the mammary tissue prior to therapy. At least a 75% reduction in secretion is usually observed after 8-12 weeks. Some patients may fail to respond even after 12 months of therapy.
Parlodel® (bromocriptine mesylate), by virtue of its ability to inhibit prolactin secretion, acts to prevent physiological lactation in women when therapy is started after delivery and continued for two to three weeks. There is no evidence that Parlodel® (bromocriptine mesylate) acts on the mammary tissues to prevent lactation, as is the case with estrogen-containing preparations.
In many acromegalic patients, Parlodel® (bromocriptine mesylate) produces a prompt and sustained reduction in circulating levels of serum growth hormone.
Parlodel® (bromocriptine mesylate) produces its therapeutic effect in the treatment of Parkinson's disease, a clinical condition characterized by a progressive deficiency in dopamine synthesis in the substantia nigra, by directly stimulating the dopamine receptors in the corpus striatum. In contrast, levodopa exerts its therapeutic effect only after conversion to dopamine by the neurons of the substantia nigra, which are known to be numerically diminished in this patient population.

PHARMACOKINETICS

The pharmacokinetics and metabolism of bromocriptine in human subjects were studied with the help of radioactively labeled drug. Twenty-eight percent of an oral dose was absorbed from the gastrointestinal tract. The blood levels following a 2½ mg dose were in the range of 2-3 ng equivalents/ml. Plasma levels were in the range of 4-6 ng equivalents/ml indicating that the red blood cells did not contain appreciable amounts of drug and/or metabolites. *In vitro* experiments showed that the drug was 90-96% bound to serum albumin.
Bromocriptine was completely metabolized prior to excretion. The major route of excretion of absorbed drug was via the bile. Only 2.5-5.5% of the dose was excreted in the urine. Almost all (84.6%) of the administered dose was excreted in the feces in 120 hours.

INDICATIONS AND USAGE

Hyperprolactinemia-associated Dysfunctions
Parlodel® (bromocriptine mesylate) is indicated for the treatment of dysfunctions associated with **hyperprolactinemia** including **amenorrhea** with or without **galactorrhea, infertility or hypogonadism.** Parlodel® (bromocriptine mesylate) treatment is indicated in patients with **prolactin-secreting adenomas,** which may be the basic underlying endocrinopathy contributing to the above clinical presentations. **Reduction in tumor size** has been demonstrated in both male and female patients with macroadenomas. In cases where adenectomy is elected, a course of Parlodel® (bromocriptine mesylate) therapy may be used to reduce the tumor mass prior to surgery.
Prevention of Physiological Lactation
Parlodel® (bromocriptine mesylate) SnapTabs® are indicated for the prevention of physiological lactation (secretion, congestion, and engorgement) occurring:

1. After parturition when the mother elects not to breast feed the infant, or when breast feeding is contraindicated.
2. After stillbirth or abortion.

The physician should keep in mind that the incidence of significant painful engorgement is low and usually responsive to appropriate supportive therapy. In contrast with supportive therapy, Parlodel® (bromocriptine mesylate) prevents the secretion of prolactin, thus inhibiting lactogenesis and the subsequent development of secretion, congestion and engorgement.
Once Parlodel® (bromocriptine mesylate) therapy is stopped, 18% to 40% of patients experience rebound of breast secretion, congestion or engorgement, which is usually mild to moderate in severity.
Acromegaly
Parlodel® (bromocriptine mesylate) therapy is indicated in the treatment of acromegaly. Parlodel® (bromocriptine mesylate) therapy, alone or as adjunctive therapy with pituitary irradiation or surgery, reduces serum growth hormone by 50% or more in approximately one-half of patients treated, although not usually to normal levels.
Since the effects of external pituitary radiation may not become maximal for several years, adjunctive therapy with Parlodel® (bromocriptine mesylate) offers potential benefit before the effects of irradiation are manifested.
Parkinson's Disease
Parlodel® (bromocriptine mesylate) SnapTabs® or capsules are indicated in the treatment of the signs and symptoms of idiopathic or postencephalitic Parkinson's disease. As adjunctive treatment to levodopa (alone or with a peripheral decarboxylase inhibitor), Parlodel® (bromocriptine mesylate) therapy may provide additional therapeutic benefits in those patients who are currently maintained on optimal dosages of levodopa, those who are beginning to deteriorate (develop tolerance) to levodopa therapy, and those who are experiencing "end of dose failure" on levodopa therapy. Parlodel® (bromocriptine mesylate) therapy may permit a reduction of the maintenance dose of levodopa and, thus may ameliorate the occurrence and/or severity of adverse reactions associated with long-term levodopa therapy such as abnormal involuntary movements (e.g., dyskinesias) and the marked swings in motor function ("on-off" phenomenon). Continued efficacy of Parlodel® (bromocriptine mesylate) therapy during treatment of more than two years has not been established.
Data are insufficient to evaluate potential benefit from treating newly diagnosed Parkinson's disease with Parlodel® (bromocriptine mesylate). Studies have shown, however, significantly more adverse reactions (notably nausea, hallucinations, confusion and hypotension) in Parlodel® (bromocriptine mesylate) treated patients than in levodopa/carbidopa treated patients. Patients unresponsive to levodopa are poor candidates for Parlodel® (bromocriptine mesylate) therapy.

CONTRAINDICATIONS

Uncontrolled hypertension, toxemia of pregnancy, sensitivity to any ergot alkaloids.

WARNINGS

Since hyperprolactinemia with amenorrhea/galactorrhea and infertility has been found in patients with pituitary tumors, a complete evaluation of the pituitary is indicated before treatment with Parlodel® (bromocriptine mesylate).
If pregnancy occurs during Parlodel (bromocriptine mesylate) administration, careful observation of these patients is mandatory. Prolactin-secreting adenomas may expand and compression of the optic or other cranial nerves may occur, emergency pituitary surgery becoming necessary. In most cases, the compression resolves following delivery. Reinitiation of Parlodel® (bromocriptine mesylate) treatment has been reported to produce improvement in the visual fields of patients in whom nerve compression has occurred during pregnancy. The safety of Parlodel® (bromocriptine mesylate) treatment during pregnancy to the mother and fetus has not been established.
Symptomatic hypotension can occur in patients treated with Parlodel® (bromocriptine mesylate) for any indication.
In postpartum studies with Parlodel® (bromocriptine mesylate), decreases in supine systolic and diastolic pressures of greater than 20 mm and 10 mm Hg, respectively, have been observed in almost 30% of patients receiving Parlodel® (bromocriptine mesylate). On occasion, the drop in supine systolic pressure was as much as 50-59 mm of Hg. Since decreases in blood pressure are frequently noted during the puerperium independent of drug therapy, it is likely that many of these decreases in blood pressure observed with Parlodel® (bromocriptine mesylate) therapy were not drug induced. **While hypotension during the start of therapy with Parlodel® (bromocriptine mesylate) occurs in some patients, 50 cases of hypertension have been reported, sometimes at the initiation of therapy, but often developing in the second week of therapy. Seizures have been reported in 38 cases (including 4 cases of status epilepticus), both with and without the prior development of hypertension occurring mostly in postpartum patients up to 14 days after initiation of treatment. Fifteen cases of stroke during Parlodel® (bromocriptine mesylate) therapy have been reported mostly in postpartum patients whose prenatal and obstetric courses had been uncomplicated. Many of these patients experiencing seizures and/or strokes reported developing a constant and often progressively severe headache hours to days prior to the acute event. Some cases of strokes and seizures during therapy with Parlodel® (bromocriptine mesylate) were also preceded by visual disturbances (blurred vision, and transient cortical blindness). Four cases of acute myocardial infarction have been reported, including 3 cases receiving Parlodel® (bromocriptine mesylate) for the prevention of physiological lactation. The relationship of these adverse reactions to Parlodel® (bromocriptine mesylate) administration is not certain. The use of Parlodel® (bromocriptine mesylate) is not recommended for patients with uncontrolled hypertension or toxemia of pregnancy. Although there is no conclusive evidence which demonstrates the interaction between Parlodel® (bromocriptine mesylate) and other ergot alkaloids, the concomitant use of these medications is not recommended. Particular attention should be paid to patients who have recently received other drugs that can alter the blood pressure. Parlodel® (bromocriptine mesylate) therapy for the prevention of postpartum lactation should not be initiated until the vital signs have been stabilized and**

---
*U.S. Pat. Nos. 3.752.814 and 3.752.888

no sooner than four hours after delivery. Periodic monitoring of the blood pressure, particularly during the first weeks of therapy and especially during the postpartum period, is prudent. If hypertension, severe, progressive, or unremitting headache (with or without visual disturbance), or evidence of CNS toxicity develops, drug therapy should be discontinued and the patient should be evaluated promptly.

Long-term treatment (6-36 months) with Parlodel® (bromocriptine mesylate) in doses ranging from 20-100 mg/day has been associated with pulmonary infiltrates, pleural effusion and thickening of the pleura in a few patients. In those instances in which Parlodel® (bromocriptine mesylate) treatment was terminated, the changes slowly reverted towards normal.

PRECAUTIONS

General

Safety and efficacy of Parlodel® (bromocriptine mesylate) have not been established in patients with renal or hepatic disease. Care should be exercised when administering Parlodel® (bromocriptine mesylate) therapy concomitantly with other medications known to lower blood pressure.

Hyperprolactinemic States

The relative efficacy of Parlodel® (bromocriptine mesylate) versus surgery in preserving visual fields is not known. Patients with rapidly progressive visual field loss should be evaluated by a neurosurgeon to help decide on the most appropriate therapy. Since pregnancy is often the therapeutic objective in many hyperprolactinemic patients presenting with amenorrhea/galactorrhea and hypogonadism (infertility), a careful assessment of the pituitary is essential to detect the presence of a prolactin-secreting adenoma. Patients not seeking pregnancy, or those harboring large adenomas, should be advised to use contraceptive measures, other than oral contraceptives, during treatment with Parlodel® (bromocriptine mesylate). Since pregnancy may occur prior to reinitiation of menses, a pregnancy test is recommended at least every four weeks during the amenorrheic period, and, once menses are reinitiated, every time a patient misses a menstrual period. Treatment with Parlodel® (bromocriptine mesylate) SnapTabs® or capsules should be discontinued as soon as pregnancy has been established. Patients must be monitored closely throughout pregnancy for signs and symptoms that may signal the enlargement of a previously undetected or existing prolactin-secreting tumor. Discontinuation of Parlodel® (bromocriptine mesylate) treatment in patients with known macroadenomas has been associated with rapid regrowth of tumor and increase in serum prolactin in most cases.

Use in Pregnancy

In human studies with Parlodel® (bromocriptine mesylate) there have been 1276 reported pregnancies, which have yielded 1109 live and 4 stillborn infants from women who took Parlodel® (bromocriptine mesylate) during pregnancy. The majority of these patients received Parlodel® (bromocriptine mesylate) therapy during the first two to three weeks of pregnancy and several received the drug for up to three months and five were treated for the entire period of gestation. Several studies in the literature reported on the use of Parlodel® (bromocriptine mesylate) during the final weeks of pregnancy to reduce plasma levels of prolactin in cases where possible pituitary tumor expansion occurred. Among the 1113 infants, 37 cases of congenital anomalies have been reported. There were 9 major malformations which included 3 limb reduction defects and 28 minor malformations which include 8 hip dislocations. The total incidence of malformations (3.3%) and the incidence of spontaneous abortions (11%) in this group of pregnancies does not exceed that generally reported for the population at large. There were three hydatidiform moles, two of which occurred in the same patient.

Physiological Lactation

Decreases in the blood pressure are common during the puerperium and, since Parlodel® (bromocriptine mesylate) therapy is known to produce hypotension and, rarely, hypertension in some patients, the drug should not be administered until the vital signs have been stabilized. Because the development of hypertension may be delayed, it is prudent to monitor the blood pressure periodically during the first weeks of therapy. If hypertension, severe, progressive, or unremitting headache (with or without visual disturbance), or evidence of CNS toxicity develops, drug therapy should be discontinued and the patient should be evaluated promptly.

Acromegaly

Cold sensitive digital vasospasm has been observed in some acromegalic patients treated with Parlodel® (bromocriptine mesylate). The response, should it occur, can be reversed by reducing the dose of Parlodel® (bromocriptine mesylate) and may be prevented by keeping the fingers warm. Cases of severe gastrointestinal bleeding from peptic ulcers have been reported, some fatal. Although there is no evidence that Parlodel® (bromocriptine mesylate) increases the incidence of peptic ulcers in acromegalic patients, symptoms suggestive of peptic ulcer should be investigated thoroughly and treated appropriately.

Possible tumor expansion while receiving Parlodel® (bromocriptine mesylate) therapy has been reported in a few patients. Since the natural history of growth hormone secreting tumors is unknown, all patients should be carefully monitored and, if evidence of tumor expansion develops, discontinuation of treatment and alternative procedures considered.

Parkinson's Disease

Safety during long-term use for more than two years at the doses required for parkinsonism has not been established.

As with any chronic therapy, periodic evaluation of hepatic, hematopoietic, cardiovascular, and renal function is recommended. Symptomatic hypotension can occur and, therefore, caution should be exercised when treating patients receiving antihypertensive drugs.

High doses of Parlodel® (bromocriptine mesylate) may be associated with confusion and mental disturbances. Since parkinsonian patients may manifest mild degrees of dementia, caution should be used when treating such patients.

Parlodel® (bromocriptine mesylate) administered alone or concomitantly with levodopa may cause hallucinations (visual or auditory). Hallucinations usually resolve with dosage reduction; occasionally, discontinuation of Parlodel® (bromocriptine mesylate) is required. Rarely, after high doses, hallucinations have persisted for several weeks following discontinuation of Parlodel® (bromocriptine mesylate).

As with levodopa, caution should be exercised when administering Parlodel® (bromocriptine mesylate) to patients with a history of myocardial infarction who have a residual atrial, nodal, or ventricular arrhythmia.

Retroperitoneal fibrosis has been reported in a few patients receiving long-term therapy (2-10 years) with Parlodel® (bromocriptine mesylate) in doses ranging from 30 to 140 mg daily.

Nursing Mothers

Since it prevents lactation, Parlodel® (bromocriptine mesylate) should not be administered to mothers who elect to breast feed infants.

Pediatric Use

Safety and efficacy of Parlodel® (bromocriptine mesylate) have not been established in children under the age of 15.

INFORMATION FOR PATIENTS

When initiating therapy, all patients receiving Parlodel® (bromocriptine mesylate) should be cautioned with regard to engaging in activities requiring rapid and precise responses, such as driving an automobile or operating machinery since dizziness (8-16%), drowsiness (8%), faintness, fainting (8%), and syncope (less than 1%) have been reported early in the course of therapy. Patients receiving Parlodel® (bromocriptine mesylate) for hyperprolactinemic states associated with macroadenoma or those who have had previous transsphenoidal surgery, should be told to report any persistent watery nasal discharge to their physician. Patients receiving Parlodel® (bromocriptine mesylate) for treatment of a macroadenoma should be told that discontinuation of drug may be associated with rapid regrowth of the tumor and recurrence of their original symptoms. Patients receiving Parlodel® (bromocriptine mesylate) for the prevention of physiological lactation should be advised to stop the drug and seek prompt medical attention including blood pressure evaluation should severe, progressive, or unremitting headache develop during therapy.

DRUG INTERACTIONS

Lack or decrease in efficacy may occur in patients receiving Parlodel® (bromocriptine mesylate) when they are treated concurrently with drugs which have dopamine antagonist activity, e.g. phenothiazines, butyrophenones. This may be a problem particularly for patients treated with Parlodel® (bromocriptine mesylate) for macroadenomas. Although there is no conclusive evidence demonstrating interactions between Parlodel® (bromocriptine mesylate) and other ergot derivatives, the concomitant use of these medications is not recommended.

ADVERSE REACTIONS

Hyperprolactinemic Indications

The incidence of adverse effects is quite high (69%) but these are generally mild to moderate in degree. Therapy was discontinued in approximately 5% of patients because of adverse effects. These in decreasing order of frequency are: nausea (49%), headache (19%), dizziness (17%), fatigue (7%), lightheadedness (5%), vomiting (5%), abdominal cramps (4%), nasal congestion (3%), constipation (3%), diarrhea (3%) and drowsiness (3%).

A slight hypotensive effect may accompany Parlodel® (bromocriptine mesylate) treatment. The occurrence of adverse reactions may be lessened by temporarily reducing dosage to one-half SnapTabs® tablet two or three times daily. A few cases of cerebrospinal fluid rhinorrhea have been reported in patients receiving Parlodel® (bromocriptine mesylate) for treatment of large prolactinomas. This has occurred rarely, usually only in patients who have received previous transsphenoidal surgery, pituitary radiation, or both, and who were receiving Parlodel® (bromocriptine mesylate) for tumor recurrence. It may also occur in previously untreated patients whose tumor extends into the sphenoid sinus.

Physiological Lactation

Twenty-three percent of patients treated within the recommended dosage range for the prevention of physiological lactation had at least one side effect, but they were generally mild to moderate in degree. Therapy was discontinued in approximately 3% of patients. The most frequently occurring adverse reactions were: headache (10%), dizziness (8%), nausea (7%), vomiting (3%), fatigue (1.0%), syncope (0.7%), diarrhea (0.4%) and cramps (0.4%). Decreases in blood pressure (≥20 mm Hg systolic and ≥10 mm Hg diastolic) occurred in 28% of patients at least once during the first three postpartum days; these were usually of a transient nature. Reports of fainting in the puerperium may possibly be related to this effect. Serious adverse reactions reported include 38 cases of seizures (including 4 cases of status epilepticus), 15 cases of stroke, and 3 cases of myocardial infarction among postpartum patients. Seizure cases were not necessarily accompanied by the development of hypertension. An unremitting and often progressively severe headache, sometimes accompanied by visual disturbance, often preceded by hours to days many cases of seizure and/or stroke. Most patients had shown no evidence of toxemia during the pregnancy. One stroke case was associated with sagittal sinus thrombosis, and another was associated with cerebral and cerebellar vasculitis. One case of myocardial infarction was associated with unexplained disseminated intravascular coagulation and a second occurred in conjunction with use of another ergot alkaloid. The relationship of these adverse reactions to Parlodel® (bromocriptine mesylate) administration has not been established.

Acromegaly

The most frequent adverse reactions encountered in acromegalic patients treated with Parlodel® (bromocriptine mesylate) were: nausea (18%), constipation (14%), postural/orthostatic hypotension (6%), anorexia (4%), dry mouth/nasal stuffiness (4%), indigestion/dyspepsia (4%), digital vasospasm (3%), drowsiness/tiredness (3%) and vomiting (2%). Less frequent adverse reactions (less than 2%) were: gastrointestinal bleeding, dizziness, exacerbation of Raynaud's Syndrome, headache and syncope. Rarely (less than 1%) hair loss, alcohol potentiation, faintness, lightheadedness, arrhythmia, ventricular tachycardia, decreased sleep requirement, visual hallucinations, lassitude, shortness of breath, bradycardia, vertigo, paresthesia, sluggishness, vasovagal attack, delusional psychosis, paranoia, insomnia, heavy headedness, reduced tolerance to cold, tingling of ears, facial pallor and muscle cramps have been reported.

Parkinson's Disease

In clinical trials in which bromocriptine was administered with concomitant reduction in the dose of levodopa/carbidopa, the most common newly appearing adverse reactions were: nausea, abnormal involuntary movements, hallucinations, confusion, "on-off" phenomenon, dizziness, drowsiness, faintness/fainting, vomiting, asthenia, abdominal discomfort, visual disturbance, ataxia, insomnia, depression, hypotension, shortness of breath, constipation, and vertigo.

Less common adverse reactions which may be encountered include: anorexia, anxiety, blepharospasm, dry mouth, dysphagia, edema of the feet and ankles, erythromelalgia, epileptiform seizure, fatigue, headache, lethargy, mottling of skin, nasal stuffiness, nervousness, nightmares, paresthesia, skin rash, urinary frequency, urinary incontinence, urinary retention, and rarely, signs and symptoms of ergotism such as tingling of fingers, cold feet, numbness, muscle cramps of feet and legs or exacerbation of Raynaud's Syndrome.

Abnormalities in laboratory tests may include elevations in blood urea nitrogen, SGOT, SGPT, GGPT, CPK, alkaline phosphatase and uric acid, which are usually transient and not of clinical significance.

DOSAGE AND ADMINISTRATION

General

It is recommended that Parlodel® (bromocriptine mesylate) be taken with food. Patients should be evaluated frequently during dose escalation to determine the lowest dosage that produces a therapeutic response.

Hyperprolactinemic Indications

The initial dosage of Parlodel® (bromocriptine mesylate) is ½ to one 2½ mg SnapTabs® tablet daily. An additional 2½ mg SnapTabs® tablet may be added to the treatment regimen as tolerated every 3-7 days until an optimal therapeutic response is achieved. The therapeutic dosage usually is 5-7.5 mg and ranges from 2.5-15 mg/day.

In order to reduce the likelihood of prolonged exposure to Parlodel® (bromocriptine mesylate) should an unsuspected pregnancy occur, a mechanical contraceptive should be used in conjunction with Parlodel® (bromocriptine mesylate) therapy until normal ovulatory menstrual cycles have been restored. Contraception may then be discontinued in patients desiring pregnancy.

Continued on next page

Sandoz—Cont.

Thereafter, if menstruation does not occur within 3 days of the expected date, Parlodel® (bromocriptine mesylate) therapy should be discontinued and a pregnancy test performed.

Prevention of Physiological Lactation

Therapy should be started only after the patient's vital signs have been stabilized and no sooner than four hours after delivery. The recommended therapeutic dosage is one 2½ mg SnapTabs® tablet of Parlodel® (bromocriptine mesylate) twice daily. The usual dosage range is 2.5-7.5 mg daily. Parlodel® (bromocriptine mesylate) therapy should be continued for 14 days; however, therapy may be given up to 21 days if necessary.

Acromegaly

Virtually all acromegalic patients receiving therapeutic benefit from Parlodel® (bromocriptine mesylate) also have reductions in circulating levels of growth hormone. Therefore, periodic assessment of circulating levels of growth hormone will, in most cases, serve as a guide in determining the therapeutic potential of Parlodel® (bromocriptine mesylate). If, after a brief trial with Parlodel® (bromocriptine mesylate) therapy, no significant reduction in growth hormone levels has taken place, careful assessment of the clinical features of the disease should be made, and if no change has occurred, dosage adjustment or discontinuation of therapy should be considered.

The initial recommended dosage is ½ to one 2½ mg Parlodel® (bromocriptine mesylate) SnapTabs® tablet on retiring (with food) for 3 days. An additional ½ to 1 SnapTabs® tablet should be added to the treatment regimen as tolerated every 3-7 days until the patient obtains optimal therapeutic benefit. Patients should be reevaluated monthly and the dosage adjusted based on reductions of growth hormone or clinical response. The usual optimal therapeutic dosage range of Parlodel® (bromocriptine mesylate) varies from 20 to 30 mg per day in most patients. The maximal dosage should not exceed 100 mg per day.

Patients treated with pituitary irradiation should be withdrawn from Parlodel® (bromocriptine mesylate) therapy on a yearly basis to assess both the clinical effects of radiation on the disease process as well as the effects of Parlodel® (bromocriptine mesylate) therapy. Usually a four to eight week withdrawal period is adequate for this purpose. Recurrence of the signs/symptoms or increases in growth hormone indicate the disease process is still active and further courses of Parlodel® (bromocriptine mesylate) should be considered.

Parkinson's Disease

The basic principle of Parlodel® (bromocriptine mesylate) therapy is to initiate treatment at a low dosage and, on an individual basis, increase the daily dosage slowly until a maximum therapeutic response is achieved. The dosage of levodopa during this introductory period should be maintained, if possible. The initial dose of Parlodel® (bromocriptine mesylate) is ½ of a 2½ mg SnapTabs® tablet twice daily with meals. Assessments are advised at two week intervals during dosage titration to ensure that the lowest dosage producing an optimal therapeutic response is not exceeded. If necessary, the dosage may be increased every 14 to 28 days by 2½ mg per day with meals. Should it be advisable to reduce the dosage of levodopa because of adverse reactions, the daily dosage of Parlodel® (bromocriptine mesylate), if increased, should be accomplished gradually in small (2½ mg) increments.

The safety of Parlodel® (bromocriptine mesylate) has not been demonstrated in dosages exceeding 100 mg per day.

HOW SUPPLIED

SnapTabs®, 2½ mg

Round, white, scored SnapTabs® each containing 2½ mg bromocriptine (as the mesylate) in packages of 30 (NDC 0078-0017-15) and 100 (NDC 0078-0017-05). Engraved "PARLODEL 2½" on one side and scored on reverse side.

Capsules, 5 mg

Caramel and white capsules, each containing 5 mg bromocriptine (as the mesylate) in packages of 30 (NDC 0078-0102-15) and 100 (NDC 0078-0102-05). Imprinted "PARLODEL 5 mg" on one half and " " on other half.

Store and Dispense

Below 77°F (25°C); tight, light-resistant container.

[PAR-Z21 Issued April 15, 1991]

Shown in Product Identification Section, page 427

RESTORIL® CIV ℞

[res'tah-ril"]

(temazepam) CAPSULES

CAUTION: Federal law prohibits dispensing without prescription.

The following prescribing information is based on official labeling in effect on August 1, 1992.

DESCRIPTION

Restoril® (temazepam) is a benzodiazepine hypnotic agent. The chemical name is 7-chloro-1,3-dihydro-3-hydroxy-1-methyl-5-phenyl- *2H* -1,4-benzodiazepin-2-one, and the structural formula is:

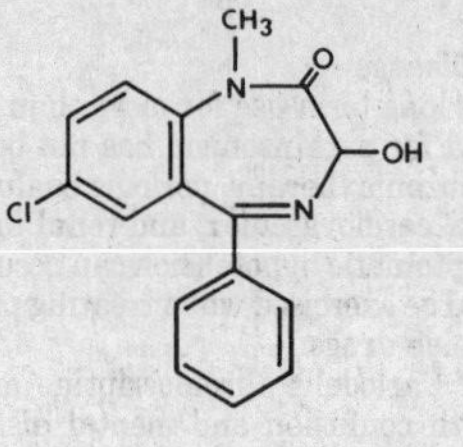

$C_{16}H_{13}ClN_2O_2$ Mol. wt. 300.74

Temazepam is a white, crystalline substance, very slightly soluble in water and sparingly soluble in alcohol USP.

Restoril® (temazepam) capsules, 15 mg and 30 mg, are for oral administration.

15 mg and 30 mg Capsules

Active Ingredient: temazepam

15 mg Capsules

Inactive Ingredients: FD&C Blue #1, FD&C Red #3, gelatin, lactose, magnesium stearate, sodium lauryl sulfate, synthetic red ferric oxide, and titanium dioxide.

May also include: benzyl alcohol, butylparaben, edetate calcium disodium, methylparaben, propylparaben, silicon dioxide, sodium propionate, and another ingredient.

30 mg Capsules

Inactive Ingredients: FD&C Blue #1, FD&C Red #3, gelatin, lactose, magnesium stearate, sodium lauryl sulfate, and titanium dioxide.

May also include: benzyl alcohol, butylparaben, edetate calcium disodium, methylparaben, propylparaben, silicon dioxide, sodium propionate, and another ingredient.

CLINICAL PHARMACOLOGY

Restoril® (temazepam) improved sleep parameters in clinical studies. Residual medication effects ("hangover") were essentially absent. Early morning awakening, a particular problem in the geriatric patient, was significantly reduced.

In sleep laboratory studies, Restoril® (temazepam) significantly improved sleep maintenance parameters [e.g., wake time after sleep onset, total sleep time, and the number of nocturnal awakenings]. There was no significant reduction in sleep latency. REM sleep was essentially unchanged, slow wave sleep was decreased, and no rebound effects occurred in these sleep stages. Transient sleep disturbance, mainly during the first night, occurred after withdrawal of the drug. In these studies, there was no evidence of tolerance when patients were given Restoril® (temazepam) nightly for approximately one month.

A single and a multiple dose absorption, distribution, metabolism, and excretion (ADME) study using ^3H-labeled drug, as well as a bioavailability study, were carried out in normal volunteers. Absorption was complete and detectable blood levels were achieved at 20-40 minutes; peak concentration was reached at 2-3 hours. There was minimal (approximately 8%) first pass metabolism.

The only significant metabolite present in blood was the O-conjugate. The unchanged drug was 96% bound to plasma proteins. The blood level decline of the parent drug was biphasic with the short half-life ranging from 0.4-0.6 hours and the terminal half-life from 9.5-12.4 hours (mean: 10 hours), depending on the study population and method of determination. Metabolites were formed with a half-life of 10 hours and excreted with a half-life of approximately 2 hours. Thus, formation of the major metabolite is the rate limiting step in the biodisposition of temazepam. There is no accumulation of metabolites. The area under the blood concentration/time curve was directly proportional to the dose in the 0-45 mg range.

Temazepam was completely metabolized prior to excretion; 80%-90% of the dose appeared in the urine. The major metabolite was the O-conjugate of temazepam (90%); the O-conjugate of N-demethyl temazepam was a minor metabolite (7%). There were no active metabolites.

At a dose of 30 mg once a day for 8 weeks, no evidence of enzyme induction was found in man.

The steady state plasma concentration measured under therapeutic sleep laboratory conditions was 382 ± 192 ng/mL, 2.5 hours after a 30 mg dose, and 26 ng/mL at 24 hours. On a once-a-day regimen, steady state was attained on the third day.

INDICATIONS AND USAGE

Restoril® (temazepam) is indicated for the relief of insomnia associated with the complaints of difficulty in falling asleep, frequent nocturnal awakenings, and/or early morning awakenings. In clinical trials there is a perception by patients that Restoril® (temazepam) decreases sleep latency, but sleep laboratory studies have not confirmed such an effect when the drug was administered within 30 minutes of retiring.

Since insomnia is often transient and intermittent, the prolonged administration of Restoril® (temazepam) is generally not necessary or recommended. Restoril® (temazepam) has been employed for sleep maintenance for up to 35 consecutive nights of drug administration in sleep laboratory studies.

Since insomnia may be a symptom of several other disorders, the possibility that the complaint may be related to a condition for which there is more specific treatment should be considered.

CONTRAINDICATIONS

Benzodiazepines may cause fetal damage when administered during pregnancy. An increased risk of congenital malformations associated with the use of diazepam and chlordiazepoxide during the first trimester of pregnancy has been suggested in several studies. Transplacental distribution has resulted in neonatal CNS depression following the ingestion of therapeutic doses of a benzodiazepine hypnotic during the last weeks of pregnancy.

Reproduction studies in animals with temazepam were performed in rats and rabbits. In a perinatal-postnatal study in rats, oral doses of 60 mg/kg/day resulted in increasing nursling mortality. Teratology studies in rats demonstrated increased fetal resorptions at doses of 30 and 120 mg/kg in one study and increased occurrence of rudimentary ribs, which are considered skeletal variants, in a second study at doses of 240 mg/kg or higher. In rabbits, occasional abnormalities such as exencephaly and fusion or asymmetry of ribs were reported without dose relationship. Although these abnormalities were not found in the concurrent control group, they have been reported to occur randomly in historical controls. At doses of 40 mg/kg or higher, there was an increased incidence of the 13th rib variant when compared to the incidence in concurrent and historical controls.

Restoril® (temazepam) is contraindicated in pregnant women. If there is a likelihood of the patient becoming pregnant while receiving temazepam, she should be warned of the potential risk to the fetus. Patients should be instructed to discontinue the drug prior to becoming pregnant. The possibility that a woman of childbearing potential may be pregnant at the time of institution of therapy should be considered.

WARNINGS

Patients receiving Restoril® (temazepam) should be cautioned about possible combined effects with alcohol and other CNS depressants.

Withdrawal symptoms (of the barbiturate type) have occurred after the abrupt discontinuation of benzodiazepines. *(See DRUG ABUSE AND DEPENDENCE)*

PRECAUTIONS

General

Since the risk of the development of oversedation, dizziness, confusion, and/or ataxia increases substantially with larger doses of benzodiazepines in elderly and debilitated patients, 15 mg of Restoril® (temazepam) is recommended as the initial dosage for such patients.

Restoril® (temazepam) should be administered with caution in severely depressed patients or those in whom there is any evidence of latent depression; it should be recognized that suicidal tendencies may be present and protective measures may be necessary.

The usual precautions should be observed in patients with impaired renal or hepatic function and in patients with chronic pulmonary insufficiency.

If Restoril® (temazepam) is to be combined with other drugs having known hypnotic properties or CNS-depressant effects, consideration should be given to potential additive effects.

The possibility of a synergistic effect exists with the co-administration of Restoril® (temazepam) and diphenhydramine. One case of stillbirth at term has been reported 8 hours after a pregnant patient received Restoril® (temazepam) and diphenhydramine. A cause and effect relationship has not yet been determined. (*See CONTRAINDICATIONS*)

Information for Patients

Patients receiving Restoril® (temazepam) should be cautioned about possible combined effects with alcohol and other CNS depressants. Patients should be cautioned not to operate machinery or drive a motor vehicle after ingesting the drug.

Patients should also be advised that, because benzodiazepines may produce psychological and physical dependence, they should consult with their physician before increasing the dose. In addition, they should be cautioned that a temporary disturbance of nocturnal sleep and other symptoms may result from discontinuation of the drug. Patients taking 30 mg or more for more than a few nights should be advised not to abruptly discontinue this drug without first consulting with their physician.

Laboratory Tests

The usual precautions should be observed in patients with impaired renal or hepatic function and in patients with

chronic pulmonary insufficiency. Abnormal liver function tests as well as blood dyscrasias have been reported with benzodiazepines.

Carcinogenesis, Impairment of Fertility

No carcinogenic potential was demonstrated in long-term studies in mice and rats. Fertility in male and female rats was not adversely affected by Restoril® (temazepam).

Pregnancy

Pregnancy Category X. (*See CONTRAINDICATIONS*)

Nursing Mothers

It is not known whether this drug is excreted in human milk. Because many drugs are excreted in human milk, caution should be exercised when Restoril® (temazepam) is administered to a nursing woman.

Pediatric Use

Safety and effectiveness in children below the age of 18 years have not been established.

ADVERSE REACTIONS

During clinical studies in which 795 patients received Restoril® (temazepam), the drug was well tolerated. Side effects were usually mild and transient. These 795 patients included 175 subjects who received Restoril® (temazepam) during daytime waking hours, sometimes in excess of recommended therapeutic dosage, in studies to evaluate dosage levels for safety and pharmacokinetic profiles.

The most common adverse reactions were drowsiness (17%), dizziness (7%), and lethargy (5%).

Other side effects include confusion, euphoria, and relaxed feeling (2%–3%). Less commonly reported were weakness, anorexia, and diarrhea (1%–2%). Rarely reported were tremor, ataxia, lack of concentration, loss of equilibrium, falling, and palpitations (less than 1%).

Hallucinations, horizontal nystagmus, and paradoxical reactions, including excitement, stimulation, and hyperactivity were rare (less than 0.5%).

DRUG ABUSE AND DEPENDENCE

Controlled Substance

Restoril® (temazepam) is a controlled substance in Schedule IV.

Abuse and Dependence

Withdrawal symptoms, similar in character to those noted with barbiturates and alcohol (convulsions, tremor, abdominal, and muscle cramps, vomiting, and sweating), have occurred following abrupt discontinuance of benzodiazepines. The more severe withdrawal symptoms have usually been limited to those patients who received excessive doses over an extended period of time. Generally milder withdrawal symptoms (e.g., dysphoria and insomnia) have been reported following abrupt discontinuance of benzodiazepines taken continuously at therapeutic levels for several months. Consequently, after extended therapy at doses higher than 15 mg, abrupt discontinuation should generally be avoided and a gradual dosage tapering schedule followed. As with any hypnotic, caution must be exercised in administering Restoril® (temazepam) to individuals known to be addiction-prone or to those whose history suggests they may increase the dosage on their own initiative. It is desirable to limit repeated prescriptions without adequate medical supervision.

OVERDOSAGE

Manifestations of acute overdosage of Restoril® (temazepam) can be expected to reflect the CNS effects of the drug and include somnolence, confusion, and coma, with reduced or absent reflexes, respiratory depression, and hypotension. If the patient is conscious, vomiting should be induced mechanically or with emetics. Gastric lavage should be employed utilizing concurrently a cuffed endotracheal tube if the patient is unconscious to prevent aspiration and pulmonary complications. Maintenance of adequate pulmonary ventilation is essential. The use of pressor agents intravenously may be necessary to combat hypotension. Fluids should be administered intravenously to encourage diuresis. The value of dialysis has not been determined. If excitation occurs, barbiturates should not be used. It should be borne in mind that multiple agents may have been ingested.

The oral LD_{50} was 1963 mg/kg in mice, 1833 mg/kg in rats, and >2400 mg/kg in rabbits.

DOSAGE AND ADMINISTRATION

The recommended usual adult dose is 30 mg before retiring. In some patients, 15 mg may be sufficient. As with all medications, dosage should be individualized for maximal beneficial effects. In elderly and/or debilitated patients it is recommended that therapy be initiated with 15 mg until individual responses are determined.

HOW SUPPLIED

Restoril® (temazepam) Capsules

15 mg, maroon and pink, imprinted "RESTORIL 15 mg" and "FOR SLEEP" twice on each capsule; 30 mg, maroon and blue, imprinted "RESTORIL 30 mg" and "FOR SLEEP" twice on each capsule. Supplied in bottles of 100, 15 mg (NDC 0078-0098-05) and 30 mg (NDC 0078-0099-05) and bottles of 500, 15 mg (NDC 0078-0098-08) and 30 mg (NDC 0078-0099-08). ControlPak® (continuous reverse-numbered roll of sealed blisters) packages of 25 capsules, 15 mg (NDC 0078-0098-13) and 30 mg (NDC 0078-0099-13). SandoPak® (unit-dose) packages of 100 individually labeled blisters, each containing one capsule, 15 mg (NDC 0078-0098-06) and 30 mg (NDC 0078-0099-06).

[RES-Z12 Issued July 10, 1989]

Shown in Product Identification Section, page 427

SANDIMMUNE® ℞

[san 'di-mewn]

(cyclosporine, USP) SOFT GELATIN CAPSULES

SANDIMMUNE® ℞

(cyclosporine) ORAL SOLUTION, USP

SANDIMMUNE® ℞

(cyclosporine concentrate for injection) AMPULS, USP FOR INFUSION ONLY

CAUTION: Federal law prohibits dispensing without prescription.

The following prescribing information is based on official labeling in effect on August 1, 1992.

WARNING

Only physicians experienced in immunosuppressive therapy and management of organ transplant patients should prescribe Sandimmune® (cyclosporine, USP). Patients receiving the drug should be managed in facilities equipped and staffed with adequate laboratory and supportive medical resources. The physician responsible for maintenance therapy should have complete information requisite for the follow-up of the patient.

Sandimmune® (cyclosporine, USP) should be administered with adrenal corticosteroids but not with other immunosuppressive agents. Increased susceptibility to infection and the possible development of lymphoma may result from immunosuppression.

The absorption of cyclosporine during chronic administration of Sandimmune® soft gelatin capsules and oral solution was found to be erratic. It is recommended that patients taking the soft gelatin capsules or oral solution over a period of time be monitored at repeated intervals for cyclosporine blood levels and subsequent dose adjustments be made in order to avoid toxicity due to high levels and possible organ rejection due to low absorption of cyclosporine. This is of special importance in liver transplants. Numerous assays are being developed to measure blood levels of cyclosporine. Comparison of levels in published literature to patient levels using current assays must be done with detailed knowledge of the assay methods employed. *(See Blood Level Monitoring under DOSAGE AND ADMINISTRATION)*

DESCRIPTION

Cyclosporine, the active principle in Sandimmune® (cyclosporine, USP) is a cyclic polypeptide immunosuppressant agent consisting of 11 amino acids. It is produced as a metabolite by the fungus species Tolypocladium inflatum Gams.

Chemically, cyclosporine is designated as [*R*-[*R**,*R**-(*E*)]]-cyclic(L-alanyl-D-alanyl-*N*-methyl-L-leucyl-*N*-methyl-L-leucyl-*N*-methyl -L- valyl -3- hydroxy- *N*, 4-dimethyl-L-2-amino-6-octenoyl-L -α- amino-butyryl-*N*-methylglycyl-*N*-methyl-L-leucyl-L-valyl-*N*-methyl-L-leucyl).

Sandimmune® (cyclosporine, USP) soft gelatin capsules are available in 25 mg and 100 mg strengths.

Each 25 mg capsule contains:

cyclosporine, USP ....25 mg

alcohol, USP dehydrated ....max 12.7% by volume

Each 100 mg capsule contains:

cyclosporine, USP ....100 mg

alcohol, USP dehydrated ....max 12.7% by volume

Inactive Ingredients: corn oil, gelatin, glycerol, Labrafil M 2125 CS (polyoxyethylated glycolysed glycerides), red iron oxide, sorbitol, titanium dioxide, and other ingredients.

Sandimmune® (cyclosporine) oral solution, USP, is available in 50 mL bottles.

Each mL contains:

cyclosporine, USP ....100 mg

alcohol, Ph. Helv. ....12.5% by volume

dissolved in an olive oil, Ph. Helv./Labrafil M 1944 CS (polyoxyethylated oleic glycerides) vehicle which must be further diluted with milk, chocolate milk or orange juice before oral administration.

Sandimmune® (cyclosporine concentrate for injection) ampuls, USP, are available in a 5 mL sterile ampul for I.V. administration.

Each mL contains:

cyclosporine, USP ....50 mg

*Cremophor EL

(polyoxyethylated castor oil) ....650 mg

alcohol, Ph. Helv. ....32.9% by volume

nitrogen ....qs

which must be diluted further with 0.9% Sodium Chloride Injection or 5% Dextrose Injection before use.

The chemical structure of cyclosporine (also known as cyclosporin A) is:

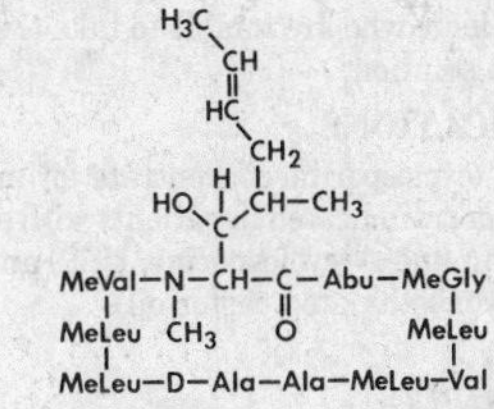

$C_{62}H_{111}N_{11}O_{12}$ Mol. Wt. 1202.63

CLINICAL PHARMACOLOGY

Sandimmune® (cyclosporine, USP) is a potent immunosuppressive agent which in animals prolongs survival of allogeneic transplants involving skin, heart, kidney, pancreas, bone marrow, small intestine, and lung. Sandimmune® (cyclosporine, USP) has been demonstrated to suppress some humoral immunity and to a greater extent, cell-mediated reactions such as allograft rejection, delayed hypersensitivity, experimental allergic encephalomyelitis, Freund's adjuvant arthritis, and graft vs. host disease in many animal species for a variety of organs.

Successful kidney, liver, and heart allogeneic transplants have been performed in man using Sandimmune® (cyclosporine, USP).

The exact mechanism of action of Sandimmune® (cyclosporine, USP) is not known. Experimental evidence suggests that the effectiveness of cyclosporine is due to specific and reversible inhibition of immunocompetent lymphocytes in the G_0 or G_1-phase of the cell cycle. T-lymphocytes are preferentially inhibited. The T-helper cell is the main target, although the T-suppressor cell may also be suppressed. Sandimmune® (cyclosporine, USP) also inhibits lymphokine production and release including interleukin-2 or T-cell growth factor (TCGF).

No functional effects on phagocytic (changes in enzyme secretions not altered, chemotactic migration of granulocytes, macrophage migration, carbon clearance *in vivo*) or tumor cells (growth rate, metastasis) can be detected in animals. Sandimmune® (cyclosporine, USP) does not cause bone marrow suppression in animal models or man.

The absorption of cyclosporine from the gastrointestinal tract is incomplete and variable. Peak concentrations (C_{max}) in blood and plasma are achieved at about 3.5 hours. C_{max} and area under the plasma or blood concentration/time curve (AUC) increase with the administered dose; for blood the relationship is curvilinear (parabolic) between 0 and 1400 mg. As determined by a specific assay, C_{max} is approximately 1.0 ng/mL/mg of dose for plasma and 2.7–1.4 ng/mL/mg of dose for blood (for low to high doses). Compared to an intravenous infusion, the absolute bioavailability of the oral solution is approximately 30% based upon the results in 2 patients. The bioavailability of Sandimmune® (cyclosporine, USP) soft gelatin capsules is equivalent to Sandimmune® (cyclosporine) oral solution, USP.

Cyclosporine is distributed largely outside the blood volume. In blood the distribution is concentration dependent. Approximately 33%–47% is in plasma, 4%–9% in lymphocytes, 5%–12% in granulocytes, and 41%–58% in erythrocytes. At high concentrations, the uptake by leukocytes and erythrocytes becomes saturated. In plasma, approximately 90% is bound to proteins, primarily lipoproteins.

The disposition of cyclosporine from blood is biphasic with a terminal half-life of approximately 19 hours (range: 10-27 hours). Elimination is primarily biliary with only 6% of the dose excreted in the urine.

Cyclosporine is extensively metabolized but there is no major metabolic pathway. Only 0.1% of the dose is excreted in the urine as unchanged drug. Of 15 metabolites characterized in human urine, 9 have been assigned structures. The major pathways consist of hydroxylation of the Cγ-carbon of 2 of the leucine residues, Cη -carbon hydroxylation, and cyclic ether formation (with oxidation of the double bond) in the side chain of the amino acid 3-hydroxyl-*N*,4-dimethyl-L-2-amino-6-octenoic acid and *N*-demethylation of *N*-methyl leucine residues. Hydrolysis of the cyclic peptide chain or conjugation of the aforementioned metabolites do not appear to be important biotransformation pathways.

INDICATIONS AND USAGE

Sandimmune® (cyclosporine, USP) is indicated for the prophylaxis of organ rejection in kidney, liver, heart allogeneic transplants. It is always to be used with adrenal corticoste-

*Cremophor is the registered trademark of BASF Aktiengesellschaft.

Continued on next page

Sandoz—Cont.

roids. The drug may also be used in the treatment of chronic rejection in patients previously treated with other immunosuppressive agents.

Because of the risk of anaphylaxis, Sandimmune® (cyclosporine concentrate for injection) ampuls, USP, should be reserved for patients who are unable to take the soft gelatin capsules or oral solution.

CONTRAINDICATIONS

Sandimmune® (cyclosporine concentrate for injection) ampuls, USP, are contraindicated in patients with a hypersensitivity to Sandimmune® (cyclosporine, USP) and/or Cremophor® EL (polyoxyethylated castor oil).

WARNINGS

(See boxed WARNINGs)

Sandimmune® (cyclosporine, USP), when used in high doses, can cause hepatotoxicity and nephrotoxicity.

It is not unusual for serum creatinine and BUN levels to be elevated during Sandimmune® (cyclosporine, USP) therapy. These elevations in renal transplant patients do not necessarily indicate rejection, and each patient must be fully evaluated before dosage adjustment is initiated.

Nephrotoxicity has been noted in 25% of cases of renal transplantation, 38% of cases of cardiac transplantation, and 37% of cases of liver transplantation. Mild nephrotoxicity was generally noted 2–3 months after transplant and consisted of an arrest in the fall of the pre-operative elevations of BUN and creatinine at a range of 35–45 mg/dl and 2.0–2.5 mg/dl respectively. These elevations were often responsive to dosage reduction.

More overt nephrotoxicity was seen early after transplantation and was characterized by a rapidly rising BUN and creatinine. Since these events are similar to rejection episodes care must be taken to differentiate between them. This form of nephrotoxicity is usually responsive to Sandimmune® (cyclosporine, USP) dosage reduction.

Although specific diagnostic criteria which reliably differentiate renal graft rejection from drug toxicity have not been found, a number of parameters have been significantly associated to one or the other. It should be noted however, that up to 20% of patients may have simultaneous nephrotoxicity and rejection.

[See table below.]

A form of chronic progressive cyclosporine-associated nephrotoxicity is characterized by serial deterioration in renal function and morphologic changes in the kidneys. From 5%–15% of transplant recipients will fail to show a reduction in a rising serum creatinine despite a decrease or discontinuation of cyclosporine therapy. Renal biopsies from these patients will demonstrate an interstitial fibrosis with tubular atrophy. In addition, toxic tubulopathy, peritubular capillary congestion, arteriolopathy, and a striped form of interstitial fibrosis with tubular atrophy may be present. Though none of these morphologic changes is entirely specific, a histologic diagnosis of chronic progressive cyclosporine-associated nephrotoxicity requires evidence of these. When considering the development of chronic nephrotoxicity it is noteworthy that several authors have reported an association between the appearance of interstitial fibrosis and higher cumulative doses or persistently high circulating trough levels of cyclosporine. This is particularly true during the first 6 posttransplant months when the dosage tends to be highest and when, in kidney recipients, the organ appears to be most vulnerable to the toxic effects of cyclosporine. Among other contributing factors to the development of interstitial fibrosis in these patients must be included, prolonged perfusion time, warm ischemia time, as well as episodes of acute toxicity, and acute and chronic rejection. The reversibility of interstitial fibrosis and its correlation to renal function have not yet been determined.

Impaired renal function at any time requires close monitoring, and frequent dosage adjustment may be indicated. In patients with persistent high elevations of BUN and creatinine who are unresponsive to dosage adjustments, consideration should be given to switching to other immunosuppressive therapy. In the event of severe and unremitting rejection, it is preferable to allow the kidney transplant to be rejected and removed rather than increase the Sandimmune®

(cyclosporine, USP) dosage to a very high level in an attempt to reverse the rejection.

Occasionally patients have developed a syndrome of thrombocytopenia and microangiopathic hemolytic anemia which may result in graft failure. The vasculopathy can occur in the absence of rejection and is accompanied by avid platelet consumption within the graft as demonstrated by Indium[111] labeled platelet studies. Neither the pathogenesis nor the management of this syndrome is clear. Though resolution has occurred after reduction or discontinuation of Sandimmune® (cyclosporine, USP) and 1) administration of streptokinase and heparin or 2) plasmapheresis, this appears to depend upon early detection with Indium[111] labeled platelet scans. *(See ADVERSE REACTIONS)*

Significant hyperkalemia (sometimes associated with hyperchloremic metabolic acidosis) and hyperuricemia have been seen occasionally in individual patients.

Hepatotoxicity has been noted in 4% of cases of renal transplantation, 7% of cases of cardiac transplantation, and 4% of cases of liver transplantation. This was usually noted during the first month of therapy when high doses of Sandimmune® (cyclosporine, USP) were used and consisted of elevations of hepatic enzymes and bilirubin. The chemistry elevations usually decreased with a reduction in dosage. As in patients receiving other immunosuppressants, those patients receiving Sandimmune® (cyclosporine, USP) are at increased risk for development of lymphomas and other malignancies, particularly those of the skin. The increased risk appears related to the intensity and duration of immunosuppression rather than to the use of specific agents. Because of the danger of oversuppression of the immune system, which can also increase susceptibility to infection, Sandimmune® (cyclosporine, USP) should not be administered with other immunosuppressive agents except adrenal corticosteroids. The efficacy and safety of cyclosporine in combination with other immunosuppressive agents has not been determined. There have been reports of convulsions in adult and pediatric patients receiving cyclosporine, particularly in combination with high dose methylprednisolone.

Rarely (approximately 1 in 1000), patients receiving Sandimmune® (cyclosporine concentrate for injection) ampuls, USP, have experienced anaphylactic reactions. Although the exact cause of these reactions is unknown, it is believed to be due to the Cremophor® EL (polyoxyethylated castor oil) used as the vehicle for the I.V. formulation. These reactions have consisted of flushing of the face and upper thorax, acute respiratory distress with dyspnea and wheezing, blood pressure changes, and tachycardia. One patient died after respiratory arrest and aspiration pneumonia. In some cases, the reaction subsided after the infusion was stopped.

Patients receiving Sandimmune® (cyclosporine concentrate for injection) ampuls, USP, should be under continuous observation for at least the first 30 minutes following start of the infusion and at frequent intervals thereafter. If anaphylaxis occurs, the infusion should be stopped. An aqueous solution of epinephrine 1:1000 should be available at the bedside as well as a source of oxygen.

Anaphylactic reactions have not been reported with the soft gelatin capsules or oral solution which lack Cremophor® EL (polyoxyethylated castor oil). In fact, patients experiencing anaphylactic reactions have been treated subsequently with the soft gelatin capsules or oral solution without incident. Care should be taken in using Sandimmune® (cyclosporine, USP) with nephrotoxic drugs. *(See PRECAUTIONS)*

PRECAUTIONS

General

Patients with malabsorption may have difficulty in achieving therapeutic levels with Sandimmune® soft gelatin capsules or oral solution.

Hypertension is a common side effect of Sandimmune® (cyclosporine, USP) therapy. *(See ADVERSE REACTIONS)* Mild or moderate hypertension is more frequently encountered than severe hypertension and the incidence decreases over time. Antihypertensive therapy may be required. Control of blood pressure can be accomplished with any of the common antihypertensive agents. However, since cyclosporine may cause hyperkalemia, potassium-sparing diuretics should not be used. While calcium antagonists can be effective agents in treating cyclosporine-associated hypertension, care should be taken since interference with cyclosporine metabolism may require a dosage adjustment. *(See Drug Interactions)*

During treatment with Sandimmune® (cyclosporine, USP), vaccination may be less effective; and the use of live attenuated vaccines should be avoided.

Information for Patients

Patients should be informed of the necessity of repeated laboratory tests while they are receiving the drug. They should be given careful dosage instructions, advised of the potential risks during pregnancy, and informed of the increased risk of neoplasia.

Nephrotoxicity vs Rejection

Parameter	Nephrotoxicity	Rejection
History	Donor > 50 years old or hypotensive Prolonged kidney preservation Prolonged anastamosis time Concomitant nephrotoxic drugs	Antidonor immune response Retransplant patient
Clinical	Often > 6 weeks postop[b] Prolonged initial nonfunction (acute tubular necrosis)	Often < 4 weeks postop[b] Fever > 37.5° C Weight gain > 0.5 Kg Graft swelling and tenderness Decrease in daily urine volume > 500 mL (or 50%)
Laboratory	CyA serum trough level > 200 ng/mL Gradual rise in Cr (<0.15 mg/dl/day)[a] Cr plateau < 25% above baseline BUN/Cr ≥ 20	CyA serum trough level < 150 ng/mL Rapid rise in Cr (> 0.3 mg/dl/day)[a] Cr > 25% above baseline BUN/Cr < 20
Biopsy	Arteriolopathy (medial hypertrophy[a], hyalinosis, nodular deposits, intimal thickening, endothelial vacuolization, progressive scarring) Tubular atrophy, isometric vacuolization, isolated calcifications Minimal edema Mild focal infiltrates[c] Diffuse interstitial fibrosis, often striped form	Endovasculitis[c] (proliferation[a], intimal arteritis[b], necrosis, sclerosis) Tubulitis with RBC[b] and WBC[b] casts, some irregular vacuolization Interstitial edema[c] and hemorrhage[b] Diffuse moderate to severe mononuclear infiltrates[d] Glomerulitis (Mononuclear Cells)[c]
Aspiration Cytology	CyA deposits in tubular and endothelial cells Fine isometric vacuolization of tubular cells	Inflammatory infiltrate with mononuclear phagocytes, macrophages, lymphoblastoid cells, and activated T-cells These strongly express HLA-DR antigens
Urine Cytology	Tubular cells with vacuolization and granularization	Degenerative tubular cells, plasma cells, and lymphocyturia > 20% of sediment
Manometry	Intracapsular pressure < 40 mm Hg[b]	Intracapsular pressure > 40 mm Hg[b]
Ultrasonography	Unchanged graft cross sectional area	Increase in graft cross sectional area A-P diameter ≥ Transverse diameter
Magnetic Resonance Imagery	Normal appearance	Loss of distinct corticomedullary junction, swelling, image intensity of parachyma approaching that of psoas, loss of hilar fat
Radionuclide Scan	Normal or generally decreased perfusion Decrease in tubular function (^{131}I-hippuran) > decrease in perfusion (^{99m}Tc DTPA)	Patchy arterial flow Decrease in perfusion > decrease in tubular function Increased uptake of Indium 111 labeled platelets or Tc-99m in colloid
Therapy	Responds to decreased Sandimmune® (cyclosporine, USP)	Responds to increased steroids or antilymphocyte globulin

[a] $p < 0.05$, [b] $p < 0.01$, [c] $p < 0.001$, [d] $p < 0.0001$

Laboratory Tests

Renal and liver functions should be assessed repeatedly by measurement of BUN, serum creatinine, serum bilirubin, and liver enzymes.

Drug Interactions

All of the individual drugs cited below are well substantiated to interact with Sandimmune® (cyclosporine, USP).

Drugs That Exhibit Nephrotoxic Synergy

gentamicin	amphotericin B
tobramycin	ketoconazole
vancomycin	melphalan
cimetidine	trimethoprim with
ranitidine	sulfamethoxazole
diclofenac	azapropazon

Careful monitoring of renal function should be practiced when Sandimmune® (cyclosporine, USP) is used with nephrotoxic drugs.

Drugs That Alter Cyclosporine Levels

Cyclosporine is extensively metabolized by the liver. Therefore, circulating cyclosporine levels may be influenced by drugs that affect hepatic microsomal enzymes, particularly the cytochrome P-450 system. Substances known to inhibit these enzymes will decrease hepatic metabolism and increase cyclosporine levels. Substances that are inducers of cytochrome P-450 activity will increase hepatic metabolism and decrease cyclosporine levels. Monitoring of circulating cyclosporine levels and appropriate Sandimmune® (cyclosporine, USP) dosage adjustment are essential when these drugs are used concomitantly (*see Blood Level Monitoring*).

Drugs That Increase Cyclosporine Levels

diltiazem	ketoconazole
nicardipine	fluconazole
verapamil	itraconazole
danazol	erythromycin
bromocriptine	methylprednisolone
metoclopramide	

Drugs That Decrease Cyclosporine Levels

rifampin	phenytoin
phenobarbital	carbamazepine

Other Drug Interactions

Reduced clearance of prednisolone, digoxin and lovastatin have been observed when these drugs are administered with Sandimmune® (cyclosporine, USP). In addition, a decrease in the apparent volume of distribution of digoxin has been reported after Sandimmune® (cyclosporine, USP) administration. Severe digitalis toxicity has been seen within days of starting cyclosporine in several patients taking digoxin. Sandimmune® (cyclosporine, USP) should not be used with potassium-sparing diuretics because hyperkalemia can occur. During treatment with Sandimmune® (cyclosporine, USP), vaccination may be less effective; and the use of live vaccines should be avoided. Myositis has occurred with concomitant lovastatin, frequent gingival hyperplasia with nifedipine, and convulsions with high dose methylprednisolone. Further information on drugs that have been reported to interact with Sandimmune® (cyclosporine, USP) is available from Sandoz Pharmaceuticals Corporation.

Carcinogenesis, Mutagenesis, and Impairment of Fertility

Cyclosporine gave no evidence of mutagenic or teratogenic effects in appropriate test systems. Only at dose levels toxic to dams, were adverse effects seen in reproduction studies in rats. *(See Pregnancy)*

Carcinogenicity studies were carried out in male and female rats and mice. In the 78-week mouse study, at doses of 1, 4, and 16 mg/kg/day, evidence of a statistically significant trend was found for lymphocytic lymphomas in females, and the incidence of hepatocellular carcinomas in mid-dose males significantly exceeded the control value. In the 24-month rat study, conducted at 0.5, 2, and 8 mg/kg/day, pancreatic islet cell adenomas significantly exceeded the control rate in the low dose level. The hepatocellular carcinomas and pancreatic islet cell adenomas were not dose related. No impairment in fertility was demonstrated in studies in male and female rats.

Cyclosporine has not been found mutagenic/genotoxic in the Ames Test, the V79-HGPRT Test, the micronucleus test in mice and Chinese hamsters, the chromosome-aberration tests in Chinese hamster bone-marrow, the mouse dominant lethal assay, and the DNA-repair test in sperm from treated mice. A recent study analyzing sister chromatid exchange (SCE) induction by cyclosporine using human lymphocytes *in vitro* gave indication of a positive effect (i.e., induction of SCE), at high concentrations in this system.

An increased incidence of malignancy is a recognized complication of immunosuppression in recipients of organ transplants. The most common forms of neoplasms are non-Hodgkin's lymphoma and carcinomas of the skin. The risk of malignancies in cyclosporine recipients is higher than in the normal, healthy population but similar to that in patients receiving other immunosuppressive therapies. It has been reported that reduction or discontinuance of immunosuppression may cause the lesions to regress.

Body System/ Adverse Reactions	Randomized Kidney Patients		All Sandimmune® Patients		
	Sandimmune® (N=227) %	Azathioprine (N=228) %	Kidney (N=705) %	Heart (N=112) %	Liver (N=75) %
Genitourinary					
Renal Dysfunction	32	6	25	38	37
Cardiovascular					
Hypertension	26	18	13	53	27
Cramps	4	<1	2	<1	0
Skin					
Hirsutism	21	<1	21	28	45
Acne	6	8	2	2	1
Central Nervous System					
Tremor	12	0	21	31	55
Convulsions	3	1	1	4	5
Headache	2	<1	2	15	4
Gastrointestinal					
Gum Hyperplasia	4	0	9	5	16
Diarrhea	3	<1	3	4	8
Nausea/Vomiting	2	<1	4	10	4
Hepatotoxicity	<1	<1	4	7	4
Abdominal Discomfort	<1	0	<1	7	0
Autonomic Nervous System					
Paresthesia	3	0	1	2	1
Flushing	<1	0	4	0	4
Hematopoietic					
Leukopenia	2	19	<1	6	0
Lymphoma	<1	0	1	6	1
Respiratory					
Sinusitis	<1	0	4	3	7
Miscellaneous					
Gynecomastia	<1	0	<1	4	3

Pregnancy

Pregnancy Category C. Sandimmune® (cyclosporine) oral solution, USP, has been shown to be embryo- and fetotoxic in rats and rabbits when given in doses 2–5 times the human dose. At toxic doses (rats at 30 mg/kg/day and rabbits at 100 mg/kg/day), Sandimmune® (cyclosporine) oral solution, USP, was embryo- and fetotoxic as indicated by increased pre- and postnatal mortality and reduced fetal weight together with related skeletal retardations. In the well-tolerated dose range (rats at up to 17 mg/kg/day and rabbits at up to 30 mg/kg/day), Sandimmune® (cyclosporine) oral solution, USP, proved to be without any embryolethal or teratogenic effects.

There are no adequate and well-controlled studies in pregnant women. Sandimmune® (cyclosporine, USP) should be used during pregnancy only if the potential benefit justifies the potential risk to the fetus.

The following data represent the reported outcomes of 116 pregnancies in women receiving Sandimmune® (cyclosporine, USP) during pregnancy, 90% of whom were transplant patients, and most of whom received Sandimmune® (cyclosporine, USP) throughout the entire gestational period. Since most of the patients were not prospectively identified, the results are likely to be biased toward negative outcomes. The only consistent patterns of abnormality were premature birth (gestational period of 28 to 36 weeks) and low birth weight for gestational age. It is not possible to separate the effects of Sandimmune® (cyclosporine, USP) on these pregnancies from the effects of the other immunosuppressants, the underlying maternal disorders, or other aspects of the transplantation milieu. Sixteen fetal losses occurred. Most of the pregnancies (85 of 100) were complicated by disorders; including, pre-eclampsia, eclampsia, premature labor, abruptio placentae, oligohydramnios, Rh incompatibility and fetoplacental dysfunction. Preterm delivery occurred in 47%. Seven malformations were reported in 5 viable infants and in 2 cases of fetal loss. Twenty-eight percent of the infants were small for gestational age. Neonatal complications occurred in 27%. In a report of 23 children followed up to 4 years, postnatal development was said to be normal. More information on cyclosporine use in pregnancy is available from Sandoz Pharmaceuticals Corporation.

Nursing Mothers

Since Sandimmune® (cyclosporine, USP) is excreted in human milk, nursing should be avoided.

Pediatric Use

Although no adequate and well controlled studies have been conducted in children, patients as young as 6 months of age have received the drug with no unusual adverse effects.

ADVERSE REACTIONS

The principal adverse reactions of Sandimmune® (cyclosporine, USP) therapy are renal dysfunction, tremor, hirsutism, hypertension, and gum hyperplasia.

Hypertension, which is usually mild to moderate, may occur in approximately 50% of patients following renal transplantation and in most cardiac transplant patients.

Glomerular capillary thrombosis has been found in patients treated with cyclosporine and may progress to graft failure. The pathologic changes resemble those seen in the hemolytic-uremic syndrome and include thrombosis of the renal microvasculature, with platelet-fibrin thrombi occluding glomerular capillaries and afferent arterioles, microangiopathic hemolytic anemia, thrombocytopenia, and decreased renal function. Similar findings have been observed when other immunosuppressives have been employed posttransplantation.

Hypomagnesemia has been reported in some, but not all, patients exhibiting convulsions while on cyclosporine therapy. Although magnesium-depletion studies in normal subjects suggest that hypomagnesemia is associated with neurologic disorders, multiple factors, including hypertension, high dose methylprednisolone, hypocholesterolemia, and nephrotoxicity associated with high plasma concentrations of cyclosporine appear to be related to the neurological manifestations of cyclosporine toxicity.

The following reactions occurred in 3% or greater of 892 patients involved in clinical trials of kidney, heart, and liver transplants: [See table above.]

The following reactions occurred in 2% or less of patients: allergic reactions, anemia, anorexia, confusion, conjunctivitis, edema, fever, brittle fingernails, gastritis, hearing loss, hiccups, hyperglycemia, muscle pain, peptic ulcer, thrombocytopenia, tinnitus.

The following reactions occurred rarely: anxiety, chest pain, constipation, depression, hair breaking, hematuria, joint pain, lethargy, mouth sores, myocardial infarction, night sweats, pancreatitis, pruritus, swallowing difficulty, tingling, upper GI bleeding, visual disturbance, weakness, weight loss.

[See tables on next page.]

Cremophor® EL (polyoxyethylated castor oil) is known to cause hyperlipemia and electrophoretic abnormalities of lipoproteins. These effects are reversible upon discontinuation of treatment but are usually not a reason to stop treatment.

OVERDOSAGE

There is a minimal experience with overdosage. Because of the slow absorption of Sandimmune® soft gelatin capsules or oral solution, forced emesis would be of value up to 2 hours after administration. Transient hepatotoxicity and nephrotoxicity may occur which should resolve following drug withdrawal. General supportive measures and symptomatic treatment should be followed in all cases of overdosage. Sandimmune® (cyclosporine, USP) is not dialyzable to any great extent, nor is it cleared well by charcoal hemoperfusion. The oral LD_{50} is 2329 mg/kg in mice, 1480 mg/kg in rats, and >1000 mg/kg in rabbits. The I.V. LD_{50} is 148 mg/kg in mice, 104 mg/kg in rats, and 46 mg/kg in rabbits.

DOSAGE AND ADMINISTRATION

Sandimmune® (cyclosporine, USP) Soft Gelatin Capsules and Sandimmune® (cyclosporine) Oral Solution, USP

The initial oral dose of Sandimmune® (cyclosporine, USP) should be given 4-12 hours prior to transplantation as a single dose of 15 mg/kg. Although a daily single dose of 14–18 mg/kg was used in most clinical trials, few centers continue to use the highest dose, most favoring the lower end of the scale. There is a trend towards use of even lower initial doses for renal transplantation in the ranges of 10–14 mg/kg/day.

Continued on next page

Sandoz—Cont.

The initial single daily dose is continued postoperatively for 1–2 weeks and then tapered by 5% per week to a maintenance dose of 5–10 mg/kg/day. Some centers have successfully tapered the maintenance dose to as low as 3 mg/kg/day in selected *renal* transplant patients without an apparent rise in rejection rate.

(See Blood Level Monitoring below)

In pediatric usage, the same dose and dosing regimen may be used as in adults although in several studies children have required and tolerated higher doses than those used in adults.

Adjunct therapy with adrenal corticosteroids is recommended. Different tapering dosage schedules of prednisone appear to achieve similar results. A dosage schedule based on the patient's weight started with 2.0 mg/kg/day for the first 4 days tapered to 1.0 mg/kg/day by 1 week, 0.6 mg/kg/day by 2 weeks, 0.3 mg/kg/day by 1 month, and 0.15 mg/kg/day by 2 months and thereafter as a maintenance dose. Another center started with an initial dose of 200 mg tapered by 40 mg/day until reaching 20 mg/day. After 2 months at this dose, a further reduction to 10 mg/day was made. Adjustments in dosage of prednisone must be made according to the clinical situation.

To make Sandimmune® (cyclosporine) oral solution, USP, more palatable, the oral solution may be diluted with milk, chocolate milk, or orange juice preferably at room temperature. Patients should avoid switching diluents frequently. Sandimmune® soft gelatin capsules and oral solution should be administered on a consistent schedule with regard to time of day and relation to meals.

Take the prescribed amount of Sandimmune® (cyclosporine, USP) from the container using the pipette supplied, after removal from the protective cover, and transfer the solution to a glass of milk, chocolate milk, or orange juice. Stir well and drink at once. Do not allow to stand before drinking. It is best to use a glass container and rinse it with more diluent to ensure that the total dose is taken. After use, dry the outside of the pipette with a clean towel and replace it in the protective cover. To avoid cloudiness, do not rinse the pipette with water or other cleaning agents. If the pipette requires cleaning, it must be completely dry before resuming use.

Sandimmune® (cyclosporine concentrate for injection) ampuls, USP
FOR INFUSION ONLY

Note: Anaphylactic reactions have occurred with Sandimmune® (cyclosporine concentrate for injection) ampuls, USP. (*See WARNINGS*)

Patients unable to take Sandimmune® soft gelatin capsules or oral solution pre- or postoperatively may be treated with the I.V. concentrate. **Sandimmune® (cyclosporine concentrate for injection) ampuls, USP, are administered at ⅓ the oral dose.** The initial dose of Sandimmune® (cyclosporine concentrate for injection) ampuls, USP, should be given 4–12 hours prior to transplantation as a single I.V. dose of 5–6 mg/kg/day. This daily single dose is continued postoperatively until the patient can tolerate the soft gelatin capsules or oral solution. Patients should be switched to Sandimmune® soft gelatin capsules or oral solution as soon as possible after surgery. In pediatric usage, the same dose and dosing regimen may be used, although higher doses may be required.

Adjunct steroid therapy is to be used. (*See aforementioned*)

Immediately before use, the I.V. concentrate should be diluted 1 mL Sandimmune® (cyclosporine concentrate for injection) ampuls, USP in 20 mL to 100 mL 0.9% Sodium Chloride Injection or 5% Dextrose Injection and given in a slow intravenous infusion over approximately 2–6 hours. Diluted infusion solutions should be discarded after 24 hours.

The Cremophor® EL (polyoxyethylated castor oil) contained in the concentrate for intravenous infusion can cause phthalate stripping from PVC.

Parenteral drug products should be inspected visually for particulate matter and discoloration prior to administration, whenever solution and container permit.

Blood Level Monitoring

Several study centers have found blood level monitoring of cyclosporine useful in patient management. While no fixed relationships have yet been established, in one series of 375 consecutive cadaveric renal transplant recipients, dosage was adjusted to achieve specific whole blood 24-hour trough levels of 100–200 ng/mL as determined by high-pressure liquid chromatography (HPLC).

Of major importance to blood level analysis is the type of assay used. The above levels are specific to the parent cyclosporine molecule and correlate directly to the new monoclonal specific radioimmunoassays (mRIA-sp). Nonspecific assays are also available which detect the parent compound molecule and various of its metabolites. Older studies often

Renal Transplant Patients in Whom Therapy was Discontinued

Reason for Discontinuation	Randomized Patients Sandimmune® (N=227) %	Azathioprine (N=228) %	All Sandimmune® Patients (N=705) %
Renal Toxicity	5.7	0	5.4
Infection	0	0.4	0.9
Lack of Efficacy	2.6	0.9	1.4
Acute Tubular Necrosis	2.6	0	1.0
Lymphoma/ Lymphoproliferative Disease	0.4	0	0.3
Hypertension	0	0	0.3
Hematological Abnormalities	0	0.4	0
Other	0	0	0.7

Sandimmune® (cyclosporine, USP) was discontinued on a temporary basis and then restarted in 18 additional patients.

Infectious Complications in the Randomized Renal Transplant Patients

Complication	Sandimmune® Treatment (N=227) % of Complications	Standard Treatment* (N=228) % of Complications
Septicemia	5.3	4.8
Abscesses	4.4	5.3
Systemic Fungal Infection	2.2	3.9
Local Fungal Infection	7.5	9.6
Cytomegalovirus	4.8	12.3
Other Viral Infections	15.9	18.4
Urinary Tract Infections	21.1	20.2
Wound and Skin Infections	7.0	10.1
Pneumonia	6.2	9.2

* Some patients also received ALG.

cited levels using a nonspecific assay which were roughly twice those of specific assays. Assay results are not interchangeable and their use should be guided by their approved labeling. If plasma specimens are employed, levels will vary with the temperature at the time of separation from whole blood. Plasma levels may range from ½–⅕ of whole blood levels. Refer to individual assay labeling for complete instructions. In addition, *Transplantation Proceedings* (June 1990) contains position papers and a broad consensus generated at the Cyclosporine-Therapeutic Drug Monitoring conference that year. Blood level monitoring is not a replacement for renal function monitoring or tissue biopsies.

HOW SUPPLIED

Sandimmune® (cyclosporine) Soft Gelatin Capsules
25 mg
Oblong, pink, branded " ⑤ 78/240". SandoPak® unit-dose packages of 30 capsules, 3 blister cards of 10 capsules (NDC 0078-0240-15)
100 mg
Oblong, dusty rose, branded " ⑤ 78/241". SandoPak® unit-dose packages of 30 capsules, 3 blister cards of 10 capsules (NDC 0078-0241-15)
Store and Dispense
In the original unit-dose container at temperatures below 77°F (25°C).

Sandimmune® (cyclosporine) Oral Solution, USP, is supplied in 50 mL bottles containing 100 mg of cyclosporine per mL (NDC 0078-0110-22). A graduated pipette for dispensing is provided.
Store and Dispense
In the original container at temperatures below 86°F (30°C). Do not store in the refrigerator. Once opened, the contents must be used within 2 months.

Sandimmune® (cyclosporine concentrate for injection) ampuls, USP, for intravenous infusion are supplied in a 5 mL sterile ampul containing 50 mg of cyclosporine per mL, in boxes of 10 ampuls (NDC 0078-0109-01).
Store and Dispense
At temperatures below 86°F (30°C) and protected from light. Protect from freezing.

Sandimmune® (cyclosporine, USP) Soft Gelatin Capsules
Manufactured by
R.P. Scherer GmbH
EBERBACH/BADEN, WEST GERMANY
Manufactured for
Sandoz Pharmaceuticals Corporation
East Hanover, NJ 07936
Sandimmune® (cyclosporine) oral solution, USP and Sandimmune® (cyclosporine concentrate for injection) ampuls, USP
FOR INFUSION ONLY
Manufactured by
SANDOZ PHARMA LTD., Basle, Switzerland
Manufactured for
Sandoz Pharmaceuticals Corporation
East Hanover, NJ 07936
[SDI-Z12(A4) Issued July 15, 1991]
Shown in Product Identification Section, page 427

IMMUNE GLOBULIN INTRAVENOUS (HUMAN) SANDOGLOBULIN® ℞
Lyophilized Preparation

CAUTION: US Federal law prohibits dispensing without prescription.
The following prescribing information is based on official labeling in effect on August 1, 1992.

DESCRIPTION

Immune Globulin Intravenous (Human)* Sandoglobulin® is a sterile, highly purified polyvalent antibody product containing in concentrated form all the IgG antibodies which regularly occur in the donor population (1). This immunoglobulin preparation is produced by cold alcohol fractionation from the plasma of over 16,000 volunteer US donors. Part of the fractionation may be performed by another US-licensed manufacturer. Sandoglobulin® (IGIV) is made suitable for intravenous use by treatment at acid pH in the presence of trace amounts of pepsin (2,3). The preparation contains at least 96% of IgG and with a neutral unbuffered diluent has a pH of 6.6 ± 0.2. Most of the immunoglobulins are monomeric (7 S) IgG; the remainder consists of dimeric IgG and a small amount of polymeric IgG, traces of IgA and IgM and immunoglobulin fragments (4). The distribution of the IgG subclasses corresponds to that of normal serum (5,6,7,8). Final container lyophilized units are prepared so as to contain 1, 3 or 6 g protein with 1.67 g sucrose and less than 20 mg NaCl per gram of protein. The lyophilized preparation is devoid of any preservatives and may be reconstituted with sterile water, 5% dextrose or 0.9% saline to a solution with protein concentrations ranging from 3%-12%. The patient's fluid, electrolyte and caloric requirements should be considered in selecting an appropriate diluent and concentration.

Table 1
Calculated Sandoglobulin® (IGIV) Osmolality (mOsm/kg)

| Diluent | Concentration | | | |
	3%	6%	9%	12%
0.9% NaCl	498	690	882	1074
5% Dextrose	444	636	828	1020
Sterile Water	192	384	576	768

CLINICAL PHARMACOLOGY

This product contains a broad spectrum of antibody specificities against bacterial, viral, parasitic, and mycoplasma

*Hereinafter referred to as IGIV.

antigens, that are capable of both opsonization and neutralization of microbes and toxins. The 3 week half-life of Immune Globulin Intravenous (Human) Sandoglobulin® corresponds to that of Immune Globulin (Human) for intramuscular use, although individual variations in half-life have been observed (9,10). Appropriate doses of Sandoglobulin® (IGIV) restore abnormally low immunoglobulin G levels to the normal range. One hundred percent of the infused dose is available in the recipient's circulation immediately after infusion. After approximately 6 days an equilibrium is reached between the intra- and extravascular compartments. This is distributed approximately 50% intravascular and 50% extravascular. In comparison, after the intramuscular injection of an intramuscular immune globulin, the IgG requires 2-5 days to reach its maximum concentration in the intravascular compartment. This concentration corresponds to about 40% of the injected dose (10).

While Sandoglobulin® (IGIV) has been shown to be effective in some cases of idiopathic thrombocytopenic purpura (ITP) (*see INDICATIONS AND USAGE*), the mechanism of action in ITP has not been fully elucidated.

Toxicity from overdose has not been observed on regimens of 0.4 g/kg body weight each day for 5 days (11,12,13). Sucrose is added to Sandoglobulin® (IGIV) for reasons of stability, solubility, and safety.

The intravenous administration of the sucrose used for stabilizing Immune Globulin Intravenous (Human) Sandoglobulin® is considered to be innocuous (14). Because sucrose is excreted unchanged in the urine when given intravenously, Sandoglobulin® (IGIV) may be given to diabetics, without compensatory changes in insulin dosage regimen.

INDICATIONS AND USAGE
Immunodeficiency
Sandoglobulin® (IGIV) is indicated for the maintenance treatment of patients with primary immunodeficiencies, e.g., in common variable immunodeficiency, severe combined immunodeficiency, and primary immunoglobulin deficiency syndromes such as X-linked agammaglobulinemia (12,15,16,17). Sandoglobulin® (IGIV) is preferable to intramuscular Immune Globulin (Human) preparations in treating patients who require an immediate and high increase in the intravascular immunoglobulin level (10), in patients with limited muscle mass, and in patients with bleeding tendencies for whom intramuscular injections are contraindicated. The infusions must be repeated at regular intervals.

Idiopathic Thrombocytopenic Purpura (ITP)
Acute
A controlled study was performed in children in which Sandoglobulin® (IGIV) was compared with steroids for the treatment of acute (defined as less than 6 months duration) ITP. In this study sequential platelet levels of 30,000, 100,000, and 150,000/μl were all achieved faster with Sandoglobulin® (IGIV) than steroids and without any of the side effects associated with steroids (11,18). However, it should be noted that many cases of acute ITP in childhood resolve spontaneously within weeks to months. Immune Globulin Intravenous (Human) Sandoglobulin® has been used with good results in the treatment of acute ITP in adult patients (19,20,21). In a study involving 10 adults with ITP of less than 16 weeks duration, Sandoglobulin® (IGIV) therapy raised the platelet count to the normal range after a 5 day course. This effect lasted a mean of over 173 days (22).
Chronic
Children and adults with chronic (defined as greater than 6 months duration) ITP have also shown an increase (sometimes temporary) in platelet counts upon administration of Sandoglobulin® (IGIV) (18,22,23,24,25,26). Therefore, in situations that require a rapid rise in platelet count, for example prior to surgery or in control of excessive bleeding, use of Sandoglobulin® (IGIV) should be considered. In children with chronic ITP, Sandoglobulin® (IGIV) therapy resulted in a mean rise in platelet count of 312,000/μl with a duration of increase ranging from 2-6 months (23,26). Sandoglobulin® (IGIV) therapy may be considered as a means to defer or avoid splenectomy (25,26,27). In adults, Sandoglobulin® (IGIV) therapy has been shown to be effective in maintaining the platelet count in an acceptable range with or without periodic booster therapy. The mean rise in platelet count was 93,000/μl and the average duration of the increase was 20-24 days (22,23). However, it should be noted that not all patients will respond. Even in those patients who do respond, this treatment should not be considered to be curative.

CONTRAINDICATIONS
As with all blood products containing IgA, Sandoglobulin® (IGIV) is contraindicated in patients with selective IgA deficiency, who possess antibody to IgA. It may also be contraindicated in patients who have had severe systemic reactions to the intravenous or intramuscular administration of human immune globulin.

WARNINGS
Patients with agamma- or extreme hypogammaglobulinemia who have never before received immunoglobulin substitution treatment or whose time from last treatment is

greater than 8 weeks, may be at risk of developing inflammatory reactions on rapid infusion of Immune Globulin Intravenous (Human) Sandoglobulin® (over 20 drops [1 mL] per minute). These reactions are manifested by a rise in temperature, chills, nausea, and vomiting. The patient's vital signs should be monitored continuously and he should be carefully observed throughout the infusion, since these reactions on rare occasions may lead to shock. Epinephrine should be available for treatment of an acute anaphylactic reaction. Particular care should be exercised when Sandoglobulin® (IGIV) is administered to patients with paraproteins (17).

PRECAUTIONS
It is generally advisable not to dilute plasma derivatives with other infusable drugs. Sandoglobulin® (IGIV) should be given by a separate infusion line. No other medications or fluids should be mixed with the Sandoglobulin® (IGIV) preparation.
Pregnancy
Pregnancy Category C: Animal reproduction studies have not been conducted with Sandoglobulin® (IGIV). It is also not known whether Sandoglobulin® (IGIV) can cause fetal harm when administered to a pregnant woman or can affect reproduction capacity. Sandoglobulin® (IGIV) should be given to a pregnant woman only if clearly needed (21).
Intact immune globulins such as those contained in Sandoglobulin® (IGIV) cross the placenta from maternal circulation increasingly after 30 weeks gestation (28,29). In cases of maternal ITP where Sandoglobulin® (IGIV) was administered to the mother prior to delivery, the platelet response and clinical effect were similar in the mother and neonate (21,29-38).
Pediatric Use
High dose administration of Immune Globulin Intravenous (Human) Sandoglobulin® in children with acute or chronic idiopathic thrombocytopenic purpura did not reveal any pediatric-specific hazard (11).
Antibodies in Immune Globulin Intravenous (Human) may interfere with the response to live viral vaccines such as measles, mumps, and rubella. Immunizing physicians should be informed of recent therapy with Immune Globulin Intravenous (Human) so that appropriate precautions may be taken.

ADVERSE REACTIONS
Adverse reactions to Sandoglobulin® (IGIV) are rare and occur in less than 1% of patients who are not immunodeficient. Agammaglobulinemic and hypogammaglobulinemic patients who have never received immunoglobulin substitution therapy before or whose time from last treatment is greater than 8 weeks may show adverse reactions if the initial infusion flow rate exceeds 20 drops (1 mL) per minute. This occurs in approximately 10% of such cases.
These reactions, which generally become apparent only 30 minutes to 1 hour after the beginning of the infusion, are as follows: flushing of the face, feelings of tightness in the chest, chills, fever, dizziness, nausea, diaphoresis, and hypotension. In such cases the infusion should be temporarily stopped until the symptoms have subsided. Immediate anaphylactoid and hypersensitivity reactions due to previous sensitization of the recipient to certain antigens, most commonly IgA, may be observed in exceptional cases, described under *CONTRAINDICATIONS* (12,13,39).
In patients with ITP, who receive higher doses (0.4 g/kg/day or greater) 2.9% of infusions may result in adverse reactions (18). Headache, generally mild, is the most common symptom noted, occurring during or following 2% of infusions.

DOSAGE AND ADMINISTRATION
Adult and Child Substitution Therapy
The usual dose of Sandoglobulin® (IGIV) in immunodeficiency syndromes is 0.2 g/kg of body weight administered once a month by intravenous infusion. If the clinical response is inadequate, the dose may be increased to 0.3 g/kg of body weight or the infusion may be repeated more frequently than once a month (12,15,16,17).
The first infusion of Immune Globulin Intravenous (Human) Sandoglobulin® in previously untreated agammaglobulinemic or hypogammaglobulinemic patients must be given as a 3% immunoglobulin solution (use the total volume of fluid provided, or see *Table 2*, to reconstitute the lyophilized product). Start with a flow rate of 10-20 drops (0.5-1.0 mL) per minute. After 15-30 minutes the rate of infusion may be further increased to 30-50 drops (1.5-2.5 mL) per minute. After the first bottle of 3% solution is infused and the patient shows good tolerance, subsequent infusions may be administered at a higher rate or concentration. Such increases should be made gradually allowing 15-30 minutes before each increment.
Recent investigations confirm that Sandoglobulin® (IGIV) is well tolerated and not likely to produce side effects when infused at higher rates (13). However, the first infusion of Sandoglobulin® (IGIV) in previously untreated agammaglobulinemic and hypogammaglobulinemic patients may lead to systemic side effects. Some of the effects may occur as a result of the reaction between the antibodies administered and free antigens in the blood and tissues of the immunodefi-

cient recipient (13, 39). When free antigen is no longer present, further administration of Sandoglobulin® (IGIV) to immunodeficient patients as well as to normal individuals usually does not cause further untoward side effects.
Therapy of Idiopathic
Thrombocytopenic Purpura (ITP)
Induction
0.4 g/kg of body weight on 2-5 consecutive days.
Acute ITP-Childhood
In acute ITP of childhood, if an initial platelet count response to the first two doses is adequate (30-50,000/μl), therapy may be discontinued after the second day of the 5 day course (18).
Maintenance-Chronic ITP
In adults and children, if after induction therapy the platelet count falls to less than 30,000/μl and/or the patient manifests clinically significant bleeding, 0.4 g/kg of body weight may be given as a single infusion. If an adequate response does not result, the dose can be increased to 0.8-1.0 g/kg of body weight given as a single infusion (19, 40).
Reconstitution
For a 3% solution from the Sandoglobulin® (IGIV) kit
1. Tear off the protective caps from the bottle containing the solvent and the Immune Globulin Intravenous (Human) Sandoglobulin®. Disinfect both rubber stoppers with alcohol.
2. Remove the protective cover from one end of the transfer set and insert the needle through the rubber stopper into the bottle containing the solvent.
3. Remove the cover from the other needle and plunge the inverted Sandoglobulin® (IGIV) bottle onto it, as shown in 3.
4. Invert the two bottles so that the solvent flows into the Sandoglobulin® (IGIV) bottle.
5. Discard the empty solvent bottle and the transfer set.

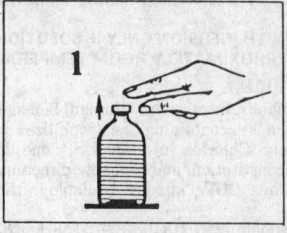

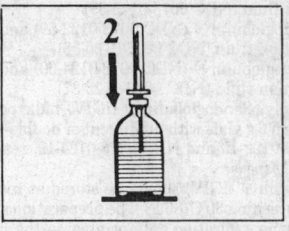

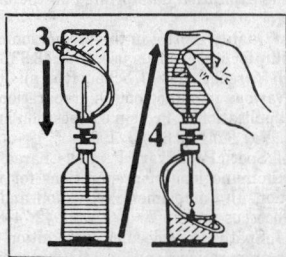

For a 6% solution from the Sandoglobulin® (IGIV) kit
1. Follow steps 1-3 aforementioned.
2. Invert the two bottles so that the solvent flows into the Immune Globulin Intravenous (Human) Sandoglobulin® bottle. Use half the solvent by removing the solvent bottle with transfer needle as soon as the fluid reaches the 6% mark printed on the Sandoglobulin® (IGIV) label.
3. Discard any unused solvent and the transfer set.
To reconstitute Sandoglobulin® (IGIV) from the multivial bulk pack, or when using other diluents or higher concentrations, *Table 2* indicates the volume of sterile diluent required. Observing aseptic technique, this volume should be drawn into a sterile hypodermic syringe and needle. The diluent is then injected into the corresponding Sandoglobulin® (IGIV) vial size. [See table 2 on next page.]
If large doses of Sandoglobulin® (IGIV) are to be administered, several reconstituted vials of identical concentration and diluent may be pooled in an empty sterile glass or plastic i.v. infusion container using aseptic technique.
Sandoglobulin® (IGIV) normally dissolves within a few min-

Continued on next page

Sandoz—Cont.

Table 2
Required Diluent Volume

Concentration	1 g Vial	3 g Vial	6 g Vial
3%	33.0 cc	100 cc	200 cc
6%	16.5 cc	50 cc	100 cc
9%	11.0 cc	33 cc	66 cc
12%	8.3 cc	25 cc	50 cc

utes, though in exceptional cases it may take up to 20 minutes.

DO NOT SHAKE! Excessive shaking will cause foaming.

Any undissolved particles should respond to careful rotation of the bottle. Avoid foaming. Parenteral drug products should be inspected visually for particulate matter and discoloration prior to administration, whenever solution and container permit.

Filtering of Sandoglobulin® (IGIV) is acceptable but not required. Pore sizes of 15 microns or larger will be less likely to slow infusion, especially with higher Sandoglobulin® (IGIV) concentrations. Antibacterial filters (0.2 microns) may be used.

When reconstitution of Sandoglobulin® (IGIV) occurs outside of sterile laminar air flow conditions, administration must begin promptly with partially used vials discarded. When reconstitution is carried out in a sterile laminar flow hood using aseptic technique, administration may begin within 24 hours provided the solution has been refrigerated during that time. Do not freeze Sandoglobulin® (IGIV) solution.

PROCEED WITH INFUSION ONLY IF SOLUTION IS CLEAR AND AT APPROXIMATELY ROOM TEMPERATURE!

HOW SUPPLIED

Immune Globulin Intravenous (Human) Sandoglobulin® is supplied as a kit containing the lyophilized preparation, sterile Sodium Chloride Injection USP, one double-ended spike for reconstitution, and complete directions for use.

Sandoglobulin® (IGIV) kits are available in three package sizes:

- 1 g Sandoglobulin® (NDC 0078-0120-58) and 33 mL reconstitution fluid (NDC 0078-0125-39)
- 3 g Sandoglobulin® (NDC 0078-0122-59) and 100 mL reconstitution fluid (NDC 0078-0125-36)
- 6 g Sandoglobulin® (NDC 0078-0124-60) and 200 mL reconstitution fluid (NDC 0078-0125-37)

Alternatively, Sandoglobulin® (IGIV) bulk packs contain ten 3 g or ten 6 g vials without diluent or double-ended spikes (NDC 0078-0122-19 and NDC 0078-0124-19, respectively).

Store and Dispense

Sandoglobulin® (IGIV) should be stored at room temperature not exceeding 30°C (86°F). The preparation should not be used after the expiration date printed on the label.

References

1. Gardi A: Quality control in the production of an immunoglobulin for intravenous use. *Blut* **48**:337–344, 1984.
2. Römer J, Morgenthaler JJ, Scherz R, et al: Characterization of various immunoglobulin-preparations for intravenous application. I. Protein composition and antibody content. *Vox Sang* **42**:62–73, 1982.
3. Römer J, Späth PJ, Skvaril F, et al: Characterization of various immunoglobulin preparations for intravenous application. II. Complement activation and binding to Staphylococcus protein A. *Vox Sang* **42**:74–80, 1982.
4. Römer J, Späth PJ: Molecular composition of immunoglobulin preparations and its relation to complement activation, in Nydegger UE (ed): *Immunohemotherapy: A Guide to Immunoglobulin Prophylaxis and Therapy.* London, Academic Press, 1981, p 123.
5. Skvaril F, Roth-Wicky B, and Barandun S: IgG subclasses in human-γ-globulin preparations for intravenous use and their reactivity with Staphylococcus protein A. *Vox Sang* **38**:147, 1980.
6. Skvaril F: Qualitative and quantitative aspects of IgG subclasses in i.v. immunoglobulin preparations, in Nydegger UE (ed): *Immunohemotherapy: A Guide to Immunoglobulin Prophylaxis and Therapy.* London, Academic Press, 1981, p 113.
7. Skvaril F, and Barandun S: In vitro characterization of immunoglobulins for intravenous use, in Alving BM, Finlayson JS (eds): *Immunoglobulins: Characteristics and Uses of Intravenous Preparations,* DHHS Publication No. (FDA)-80-9005. US Government Printing Office, 1980, pp 201–206.
8. Burckhardt JJ, Gardi A, Oxelius V, et al: Immunoglobulin G subclass distribution in three human intravenous immunoglobulin preparations. *Vox Sang* **57**:10–14, 1989.
9. Morell A, and Skvaril F: Struktur und biologische Eigenschaften von Immunoglobulinen und γ-Globulin-Präparaten. II. Eigenschaften von γ-Globulin-Präparaten. *Schweiz Med Wochenschr* **110**:80, 1980.
10. Morell A, Schürch B, Ryser D, et al: In vivo behavior of gamma globulin preparations. *Vox Sang* **38**:272, 1980.
11. Imbach P, Barandun S, d'Apuzzo V, et al: High-dose intravenous gamma globulin for idiopathic thrombocytopenic purpura in childhood. *Lancet* **1**:1228, 1981.
12. Barandun S, Morell A, Skvaril F: Clinical experiences with immunoglobulin for intravenous use, in Alving BM, Finlayson JS (eds): *Immunoglobulins: Characteristics and Uses of Intravenous Preparations.* DHHS Publication No. (FDA)-80-9005. US Government Printing Office, 1980, pp 31–35.
13. Barandun S, Morell A: Adverse reactions to immunoglobulin preparations, in Nydegger UE (ed): *Immunohemotherapy: A Guide to Immunoglobulin Prophylaxis and Therapy.* London, Academic Press, 1981, p 223.
14. Wade A (ed): *Martindale: The Extra Pharmacopoeia,* ed 27. London, The Pharmaceutical Press, 1979, p 65.
15. Joller PW, Barandun S, Hitzig WH: Neue Möglichkeiten der Immunoglobulin-Ersatztherapie bei Antikörpermangel. Syndrom. *Schweiz Med Wochenschr* **110**:1451, 1980.
16. Barandun S, Imbach P, Morell A, et al: Clinical indications for immunoglobulin infusion, in Nydegger UE (ed): *Immunohemotherapy: A Guide to Immunoglobulin Prophylaxis and Therapy.* London, Academic Press, 1981, p 275.
17. Cunningham-Rundles C, Smithwick EM, Siegal FP, et al: Treatment of primary humoral immunodeficiency disease with intravenous (pH 4.0 treated) gamma globulin, in Nydegger UE (ed): *Immunohemotherapy: A Guide to Immunoglobulin Prophylaxis and Therapy.* London, Academic Press, 1981, p 283.
18. Imbach P, Wagner HP, Berchtold W, et al: Intravenous immunoglobulin versus oral corticosteroids in acute immune thrombocytopenic purpura in childhood. *Lancet* **2**:464, 1985.
19. Fehr J, Hofmann V, Kappeler U: Transient reversal of thrombocytopenia in idiopathic thrombocytopenic purpura by high-dose intravenous gamma globulin. *N Engl J Med* **306**:1254, 1982.
20. Müeller-Eckhardt C, Küenzlen E, Thilo-Körner D, et al: High-dose intravenous immunoglobulin for posttransfusion purpura. *N Engl J Med* **308**:287, 1983.
21. Wenske G, Gaedicke G, Küenzlen E, et al: Treatment of idiopathic thrombocytopenic purpura in pregnancy by high-dose intravenous immunoglobulin. *Blut* **46**:347–353, 1983.
22. Newland AC, Treleaven JG, Minchinton B, et al: High-dose intravenous IgG in adults with autoimmune thrombocytopenia. *Lancet* **1**:84–87, 1983.
23. Bussel JB, Kimberly RP, Inman RD, et al: Intravenous gammaglobulin for chronic idiopathic thrombocytopenic purpura. *Blood* **62**:480–486, 1983.
24. Abe T, Matsuda J, Kawasugi K, et al: Clinical effect of intravenous immunoglobulin in chronic idiopathic thrombocytopenic purpura. *Blut* **47**:69–75, 1983.
25. Bussel JB, Schulman I, Hilgartner MW, et al: Intravenous use of gamma globulin in the treatment of chronic immune thrombocytopenic purpura as a means to defer splenectomy. *J Pediatr* **103**:651–654, 1983.
26. Imholz B, et al: Intravenous immunoglobulin (i.v. IgG) for previously treated acute or for chronic idiopathic thrombocytopenic purpura (ITP) in childhood: A prospective multicenter study. *Blut* **56**:63-68, 1988.
27. Lusher JM, and Warrier I: Use of intravenous gamma globulin in children with idiopathic thrombocytopenic purpura and other immune thrombocytopenias. *Am J Med* **83(suppl 4A)**:10–16, 1987.
28. Hammarstrom L, and Smith CI: Placental transfer of intravenous immunoglobulin. *Lancet* **1**:681, 1986.
29. Sidiropoulos D, et al: Transplacental passage of intravenous immunoglobulin in the last trimester of pregnancy. *J Pediatr* **109**:505–508, 1986.
30. Wenske G, et al: Idiopathic thrombocytopenic purpura in pregnancy and neonatal period. *Blut* **48**:377–382, 1984.
31. Fabris P, et al: Successful treatment of a steroid-resistant form of idiopathic thrombocytopenic purpura in pregnancy with high doses of intravenous immunoglobulins. *Acta Haemat* **77**:107–110, 1987.
32. Coller BS, et al: Management of severe ITP during pregnancy with intravenous immunoglobulin (IVIgG). *Clin Res* **33**:545A, 1985.
33. Tchernia G, et al: Management of immune thrombocytopenia in pregnancy: Response to infusions of immunoglobulins. *Am J Obstet Gynecol* **148**:225–226, 1984.
34. Newland AC, et al: Intravenous IgG for autoimmune thrombocytopenia in pregnancy. *N Engl J Med* **310**:261–262, 1984.
35. Morgenstern GR, et al: Autoimmune thrombocytopenia in pregnancy: New approach to management. *Br Med J* **287**:584, 1983.
36. Ciccimarra F, et al: Treatment of neonatal passive immune thrombocytopenia. *J Pediat* **105**:677-678, 1984.
37. Rose VL, and Gordon LI: Idiopathic thrombocytopenic purpura in pregnancy. Successful management with immunoglobulin infusion. *JAMA* **254**:2626–2628, 1985.
38. Gounder MP, et al: Intravenous gammaglobulin therapy in the management of a patient with idiopathic thrombocytopenic purpura and a warm autoimmune erythrocyte panagglutinin during pregnancy. *Obstet Gynecol* **67**:741–746, 1986.
39. Cunningham-Rundles C, Day NK, Wahn V, et al: Reactions to intravenous gamma globulin infusions and immune complex formation, in Nydegger UE (ed): *Immunohemotherapy: A Guide to Immunoglobulin Prophylaxis and Therapy.* London, Academic Press, 1981, p 447.
40. Bussel JB, Pham LC, Hilgartner MW, et al: Long-term maintenance of adults with ITP using intravenous gamma globulin. Abstract, *American Society of Hematology.* New Orleans, December, 1985.

Manufactured by:
CENTRAL LABORATORY
BLOOD TRANSFUSION SERVICE
SWISS RED CROSS
Wankdorfstrasse 10, 3000 Berne 22
Switzerland
US License No. 647
Distributed by:
SANDOZ PHARMACEUTICALS CORPORATION
East Hanover, NJ 07936
[SGL-Z12 Issued August 15, 1991]

Shown in Product Identification Section, page 427

SANDOSTATIN® ℞
octreotide acetate
INJECTION

CAUTION: Federal law prohibits dispensing without a prescription.

The following prescribing information is based on official labeling in effect on August 1, 1992.

DESCRIPTION

Sandostatin® (octreotide acetate) Injection, a cyclic octapeptide prepared as a clear sterile solution of octreotide, acetate salt, in buffered sodium chloride for administration by deep subcutaneous (intrafat) injection. Octreotide acetate, known chemically as L-Cysteinamide, D-phenylalanyl-L-cysteinyl-L-phenylalanyl-D-tryptophyl-L-lysyl-L-threonyl-N-[2-hydroxy-1-(hydroxymethyl)propyl]-, cyclic (2→7) disulfide; [R-(R*, R*)] acetate salt, is a long-acting octapeptide with pharmacologic actions mimicking those of the natural hormone somatostatin.

Sandostatin® (octreotide acetate) Injection is available as: sterile 1 mL ampuls in 3 strengths, containing 50, 100, or 500 mcg octreotide (as acetate), and sterile 5 mL multi-dose vials in 2 strengths, containing 200 and 1000 mcg/mL of octreotide (as acetate).

Each ampul also contains:

acetic acid, glacial, USP	2.0 mg
sodium acetate trihydrate, USP	2.0 mg
sodium chloride, USP	7.0 mg
water for injection, qs to	1.0 mL

Each mL of the multi-dose vials also contains:

acetic acid, glacial, USP	2.0 mg
sodium acetate trihydrate, USP	2.0 mg
sodium chloride, USP	7.0 mg
phenol, USP	5.0 mg
water for injection, qs to	1.0 mL

Acetic acid and sodium acetate trihydrate are added to provide a buffered solution, pH 4.2 $\pm$ 0.3.

The molecular weight of octreotide acetate is 1019.3 (free peptide, $C_{49}H_{66}N_{10}O_{10}S_2$) and its amino acid sequence is:

H-D-Phe-Cys-Phe-D-Trp-Lys-Thr-Cys-Thr-ol,
x CH_3COOH where x = 1.4 to 2.5

CLINICAL PHARMACOLOGY

Sandostatin® (octreotide acetate) exerts pharmacological actions similar to the natural hormone somatostatin. In normal subjects, it has the ability to suppress secretion of serotonin and the gastroenteropancreatic peptides: gastrin, vasoactive intestinal peptide, insulin, glucagon, secretin, motilin, and pancreatic polypeptide. In addition, Sandostatin® (octreotide acetate) suppresses growth hormone (under both basal and stimulated conditions). It also suppresses the LH response to GnRH. In animals, Sandostatin® (octreotide acetate) is a more potent inhibitor of growth hormone, glucagon, and insulin release than natural somatostatin with greater selectivity for growth hormone and glucagon suppression. Sandostatin® (octreotide acetate), like somatostatin, decreases splanchnic blood flow.

By virtue of these pharmacological actions, Sandostatin® (octreotide acetate) has been used to treat the symptoms associated with metastatic carcinoid tumors (flushing and diarrhea), and Vasoactive Intestinal Peptide (VIP) secreting adenomas (watery diarrhea).

Pharmacokinetics
After subcutaneous injection, octreotide is absorbed rapidly and completely from the injection site. Peak concentrations of 5.2 ng/mL (100 mcg dose) were reached 0.4 hours after dosing. Using a specific radioimmunoassay, intravenous and subcutaneous doses were found to be bioequivalent. Peak concentrations and area under the curve values were dose proportional both after s.c. or i.v. single doses up to 400 mcg and with multiple doses of 200 mcg t.i.d. (600 mcg/day). Clearance was reduced by about 66% suggesting non-linear kinetics of the drug at daily doses of 600 mcg/day as compared to 150 mcg/day. The relative decrease in clearance with doses above 600 mcg/day is not defined.
The distribution of octreotide from plasma was rapid ($t\alpha 1/2 = 0.2$ h) and the volume of distribution was estimated to be 13.6 L. In blood, the distribution into the erythrocytes was found to be negligible and about 65% was bound in the plasma in a concentration-independent manner. Binding was mainly to lipoprotein and, to a lesser extent, to albumin.
The elimination of octreotide from plasma had an apparent half-life of 1.7 hours compared with 1–3 minutes with the natural hormone. The duration of action of Sandostatin® (octreotide acetate) is variable but extends up to 12 hours depending upon the type of tumor. About 32% of the dose is excreted unchanged into the urine. In an elderly population, dose adjustments may be necessary due to a significant increase in the half-life (46%) and a significant decrease in the clearance (26%) of the drug.
In patients with severe renal failure requiring dialysis, clearance was reduced to about half that found in normal subjects (from approximately 10 L/h to 4.5 L/h). The effect of hepatic diseases on the disposition of octreotide is unknown.

INDICATIONS AND USAGE

General
Sandostatin® (octreotide acetate) therapy is indicated for control of symptoms in patients with metastatic carcinoid and vasoactive intestinal peptide-secreting tumors (VIPomas).
Data are insufficient to determine whether Sandostatin® (octreotide acetate) decreases the size, rate of growth, or development of metastases in patients with these tumors.
Sandostatin® (octreotide acetate) has been used in patients ranging in age from 1 month to 83 years without any drug limiting toxicity.

Carcinoid Tumors
Sandostatin® (octreotide acetate) is indicated for the symptomatic treatment of patients with metastatic carcinoid tumors where it suppresses or inhibits the severe diarrhea and flushing episodes associated with the disease.

Vasoactive Intestinal Peptide Tumors (VIPomas)
Sandostatin® (octreotide acetate) is indicated for the treatment of the profuse watery diarrhea associated with VIP-secreting tumors. Significant improvement has been noted in the overall condition of these otherwise therapeutically unresponsive patients. Therapy with Sandostatin® (octreotide acetate) results in improvement in electrolyte abnormalities, e.g., hypokalemia, often enabling reduction of fluid and electrolyte support.

CONTRAINDICATIONS

Sensitivity to this drug or any of its components.

WARNINGS

Sandostatin® (octreotide acetate) therapy, like the natural hormone, somatostatin, may be associated with cholelithiasis, presumably by altering fat absorption and possibly by decreasing the motility of the gallbladder. Preliminary data from controlled studies of patients being treated with Sandostatin® (octreotide acetate) for psoriasis or acromegaly suggest a 15%–20% incidence of the development of gallstones or sludge. Therefore, patients being treated with Sandostatin® (octreotide acetate) should be monitored periodically for gallbladder disease using ultrasound evaluations of the gallbladder and bile ducts. Surgical intervention has been required in a few patients who developed severe abdominal pain associated with cholelithiasis while on Sandostatin® (octreotide acetate) therapy.

PRECAUTIONS

General
In the treatment of patients with carcinoid syndrome or VIPomas, dosage adjustment may be required to maintain symptomatic control.
Sandostatin® (octreotide acetate) therapy is occasionally associated with mild transient hypo- or hyperglycemia due to alterations in the balance between the counterregulatory hormones; insulin, glucagon, and growth hormone. Patients should be closely observed on introduction of Sandostatin® (octreotide acetate) therapy and at each change of dosage for symptomatic evidence of hyper- or hypoglycemia.
Data on the effect of chronic therapy with Sandostatin® (octreotide acetate) on hypothalamic/pituitary function has not been obtained. A progressive drop in T_4 levels has been reported, culminating in clinical and biochemical hypothyroidism after 19 months of therapy in 1 clinical trial patient (carcinoid) receiving 1500 mcg of Sandostatin® (octreotide acetate) daily. Therefore, baseline and periodic thyroid function tests using total and free T_4 are advised to monitor patients.
In insulin-dependent diabetics, reduction of insulin requirements may result following initiation of Sandostatin® (octreotide acetate) therapy.
There is evidence that Sandostatin® (octreotide acetate) therapy may alter absorption of dietary fats in some patients. It is suggested that periodic quantitative 72-hour fecal fat and serum carotene determinations be performed to aid in the assessment of possible drug-induced aggravation of fat malabsorption.
In patients with severe renal failure requiring dialysis, the half-life of the drug may be increased, necessitating adjustment of the maintenance dosage.
Because decreased gallbladder contractility and bile stasis may result from treatment with Sandostatin® (octreotide acetate), baseline and periodic ultrasonography may be useful to assess the presence of gallstones *(see WARNINGS)*.

Information for Patients
Careful instruction in sterile subcutaneous injection technique should be given to the patients and to other persons who may administer Sandostatin® (octreotide acetate) Injection.

Laboratory Tests
Laboratory tests that may be helpful as biochemical markers in determining and following patient response depend on the specific tumor. Based on diagnosis, measurement of the following substances may be useful in monitoring the progress of therapy:

Carcinoid: 5-HIAA (urinary 5-hydroxyindole acetic acid), plasma serotonin, plasma Substance P
VIPoma: VIP (plasma vasoactive intestinal peptide)

Baseline and periodic total and/or free T_4 measurements should be performed during chronic therapy *(see PRECAUTIONS—General)*.

Drug Interactions
Many patients with carcinoid syndrome or VIPomas being treated with Sandostatin® (octreotide acetate) have also been, or are being, treated with many other drugs to control the symptomatology or progression of the disease, generally without serious drug interaction. Included are chemotherapeutic agents, H_2 antagonists, antimotility agents, drugs affecting glycemic states, solutions for electrolyte and fluid support or hyperalimentation, antihypertensive diuretics, and antidiarrheal agents.
Where symptoms are severe and Sandostatin® (octreotide acetate) therapy is added to other therapies used to control glycemic states such as sulfonylureas, insulin, diazoxide and to beta blockers or agents for the control of fluid and electrolyte balance, patients must be monitored closely and adjustment made in the other therapies as the symptoms of the disease are controlled. Imbalances in fluid and electrolytes or glycemic state may be secondary to correction of pre-existing abnormalities and not necessarily to a direct metabolic action of Sandostatin® (octreotide acetate) Injection. Adjustment of the dosage of drugs, such as insulin, affecting glucose metabolism may be required following initiation of Sandostatin® (octreotide acetate) therapy in patients with diabetes.
Since Sandostatin® (octreotide acetate) has been associated with alterations in nutrient absorption, its effect on absorption of any orally administered drugs should be carefully considered. A single case of transplant rejection episode (renal/whole pancreas) in a patient immunosuppressed with cyclosporine has been reported. Sandostatin® (octreotide acetate) treatment to reduce exocrine secretion and close a fistula in this patient resulted in decreases in blood levels of cyclosporine and may have contributed to the rejection episode.

Drug Laboratory Test Interactions
No known interference exists with clinical laboratory tests, including amine or peptide determinations.

Carcinogenesis/Mutagenesis/Impairment of Fertility
Studies in laboratory animals have demonstrated no mutagenic potential of Sandostatin® (octreotide acetate). No long-term studies in animals to assess carcinogenicity have been completed. Sandostatin® (octreotide acetate) did not impair fertility in rats at doses up to 1 mg/kg/day.

Pregnancy Category B
Reproduction studies have been performed in rats and rabbits at doses up to 30 times the highest human dose and have revealed no evidence of impaired fertility or harm to the fetus due to Sandostatin® (octreotide acetate). There are, however, no adequate and well-controlled studies in pregnant women. Because animal reproduction studies are not always predictive of human response, this drug should be used during pregnancy only if clearly needed.

Nursing Mothers
It is not known whether this drug is excreted in human milk. Because many drugs are excreted in milk, caution should be exercised when Sandostatin® (octreotide acetate) is administered to a nursing woman.

Pediatric Use
Experience with Sandostatin® (octreotide acetate) in the pediatric population is limited. The youngest patient to receive the drug was 1 month old. Doses of 1-10 mcg/kg body weight were well tolerated in the young patients. A single case of an infant (nesidioblastosis) was complicated by a seizure thought to be independent of Sandostatin® (octreotide acetate) therapy.

ADVERSE REACTIONS

Preliminary data from controlled psoriasis and acromegaly studies suggest a 15%–20% incidence in the development of gallstones or sludge in patients being treated with Sandostatin® (octreotide acetate) Injection. Additional adverse reactions by patient group and in the total cohort (N = 491) of patients for which final data is available follow. These adverse reactions were largely of mild to moderate severity and of short duration.
[See tables above.]

Adverse Reactions Occurring in 3%–10% of Patients

Reaction	Number Reporting: Carcinoid and VIPoma Patients N = 211 (%)	Other Patients N = 280 (%)	Total N = 491 (%)
Nausea	16 (7.6)	31 (11.1)	47 (9.6)
Injection Site Pain	16 (7.6)	21 (7.5)	37 (7.5)
Diarrhea	10 (4.7)	24 (8.6)	34 (6.9)
Abdominal Pain/Discomfort	6 (2.8)	27 (9.6)	33 (6.7)
Loose Stools	3 (1.4)	18 (6.4)	21 (4.3)
Vomiting	4 (1.9)	15 (5.4)	19 (3.9)

Adverse Reactions Occurring in 1%–3% of Patients

Reaction	Number Reporting: Carcinoid and VIPoma Patients N = 211 (%)	Other Patients N = 280 (%)	Total N = 491 (%)
Headache	3 (1.4)	7 (2.5)	10 (2.0)
Fat Malabsorption	5 (2.4)	3 (1.1)	8 (1.6)
Dizziness/Light-headedness	3 (1.4)	5 (1.8)	8 (1.6)
Hyperglycemia	3 (1.4)	5 (1.8)	8 (1.6)
Fatigue	2 (0.9)	5 (1.8)	7 (1.4)
Flushing	3 (1.4)	4 (1.4)	7 (1.4)
Hypoglycemia	1 (0.5)	5 (1.8)	6 (1.2)
Edema	2 (0.9)	3 (1.1)	5 (1.0)
Asthenia/Weakness	4 (1.9)	1 (0.4)	5 (1.0)
Injection Site/Wheal/Erythema	4 (1.9)	1 (0.4)	5 (1.0)

In addition, the following infrequent reactions were reported (fewer than 1% of patients):

Gastrointestinal
Constipation, flatulence, hepatitis, jaundice, slight increase in liver enzymes, rectal disorder (spasm), GI bleeding, stomach swollen, heartburn, fluttering sensation, abnormal stools, and cholelithiasis.

Continued on next page

Sandoz—Cont.

Integumentary
Hair loss, thinning of skin, skin flaking, bruising, bleeding from a superficial wound, pruritus, and rash.
Musculoskeletal
Backache pain, muscle pain, muscle cramping, joint pain, shoulder and leg pain, leg cramps, and chest pain.
Cardiovascular
Shortness of breath, hypertensive reaction, thrombophlebitis, ischemia, congestive heart failure, hypertension, palpitations, orthostatic BP decrease, and chest pain.
CNS
Anxiety, anorexia, convulsions, depression, drowsiness, vertigo, hyperesthesia, pounding in head, insomnia, irritability, libido decrease/frigidity, forgetfulness, malaise, nervousness, shakiness, syncope, tremor, and Bell's Palsy.
Respiratory
Rhinorrhea
Endocrine
Galactorrhea
Clinical hypothyroidism requiring thyroid hormone replacement was observed after 19 months of therapy with 1500 mcg daily of Sandostatin® (octreotide acetate) in a clinical trial patient. A progressive fall to low total and free T_4 values was observed, without an elevated TSH, indicative of hypothalamic-pituitary dysfunction, probably related to Sandostatin® (octreotide acetate) therapy.
Urogenital
Oliguria, pollakiuria, prostatitis, and urine hyperosmolarity.
Autonomic
Burning sensation, dry mouth, numbness, hyperhidrosis, hyperdipsia, warm feeling, and visual disturbance.
Miscellaneous
Chills, fever, throat discomfort, increased CPK, arm pain, and eyes burning.
Evaluation of 20 patients treated for at least 6 months has failed to demonstrate titers of antibodies exceeding background levels.

OVERDOSAGE
Specific information on Sandostatin® (octreotide acetate) overdosage is not available as no frank overdosage has occurred in any patient to date. Bolus i.v. injections of 1 mg (1000 mcg) given to healthy volunteers have been tolerated without serious complication. In research studies single intravenous dosages of up to 30 mg (30,000 mcg) over 20 minutes or 120 mg (120,000 mcg) over 8 hours have been given without serious ill effect.
Based on the pharmacological properties of Sandostatin® (octreotide acetate), acute overdosage may be expected to produce hyper- or hypoglycemia, depending on the endocrine status of the patient and type of peptide-secreting tumor involved. Hyper- and hypoglycemia may be manifested by neurologic and mental disturbances such as loss of sensory or motor function, incoordination, visual blurring, dizziness, drowsiness, and disturbed consciousness. These conditions should resolve with temporary withdrawal of the drug and symptomatic treatment.
The i.v. LD_{50} is 72 mg/kg in mice and 18 mg/kg in rats.

DOSAGE AND ADMINISTRATION
Sandostatin® (octreotide acetate) may be administered subcutaneously or intravenously. Subcutaneous injection is the usual route of administration of Sandostatin® (octreotide acetate) for control of symptoms. Pain with subcutaneous administration may be reduced by using the smallest volume that will deliver the desired dose. Multiple subcutaneous injections at the same site within short periods of time should be avoided. Sites should be rotated in a systematic manner.
Parenteral drug products should be inspected visually for particulate matter and discoloration prior to administration. **Do not use if particulates and/or discoloration are observed.** Proper sterile technique should be used in the preparation of parenteral admixtures to minimize the possibility of microbial contamination. **Sandostatin® (octreotide acetate) is not compatible in Total Parenteral Nutrition (TPN) solutions because of the formation of a glycosyl octreotide conjugate which may decrease the efficacy of the product.**
Sandostatin® (octreotide acetate) is stable in sterile isotonic saline solutions or sterile solutions of dextrose 5% in water for 24 hours. It may be diluted in volumes of 50–200 mL and infused intravenously over 15–30 minutes or administered by IV push over 3 minutes. In emergency situations (e.g.: carcinoid crisis) it may be given by rapid bolus.
The initial dosage is 50 mcg, administered subcutaneously, once or twice daily. Thereafter, the number of injections and dosage may be increased gradually based on patient tolerability and response. Dosage information for patients with specific tumors follows. The drug is usually given in a b.i.d. or t.i.d. schedule.
Carcinoid Tumors
The suggested daily dosage of Sandostatin® (octreotide acetate) during the first 2 weeks of therapy ranges from 100–600 mcg/day in 2–4 divided doses (mean daily dosage is 300 mcg). In the clinical studies, the **median** daily maintenance dosage was approximately 450 mcg, but clinical and biochemical benefits were obtained in some patients with as little as 50 mcg, while others required doses up to 1500 mcg/day. However, experience with doses above 750 mcg/day is limited.
VIPomas
Daily dosages of 200–300 mcg in 2–4 divided doses are recommended during the initial 2 weeks of therapy (range 150–750 mcg) to control symptoms of the disease. On an individual basis, dosage may be adjusted to achieve a therapeutic response, but usually doses above 450 mcg/day are not required.

HOW SUPPLIED
Sandostatin® (octreotide acetate) Injection is available in 1 mL ampuls and 5 mL multi-dose vials as follows:
Ampuls
50 mcg/mL octreotide (as acetate)
Package of 20 ampuls (NDC 0078-0180-03)
Package of 50 ampuls (NDC 0078-0180-04)
100 mcg/mL octreotide (as acetate)
Package of 20 ampuls (NDC 0078-0181-03)
Package of 50 ampuls (NDC 0078-0181-04)
500 mcg/mL octreotide (as acetate)
Package of 20 ampuls (NDC 0078-0182-03)
Package of 50 ampuls (NDC 0078-0182-04)
Multi-Dose Vials
200 mcg/mL octreotide (as acetate)
Box of one (NDC 0078-0183-25)
1000 mcg/mL octreotide (as acetate)
Box of one (NDC 0078-0184-25)
Storage
For prolonged storage, Sandostatin® (octreotide acetate) ampuls and multi-dose vials should be stored in the refrigerator at 2°–8°C (36°–46°F). Ampuls can **only** be stored at room temperature (20°–30°C or 70°–86°F) for the day they will be used.
The ampuls are manufactured by
SANDOZ PHARMA LTD.,
Basle, Switzerland
for
SANDOZ PHARMACEUTICALS CORPORATION
East Hanover, New Jersey 07936
The multi-dose vials are manufactured by
SCHERING-PLOUGH PRODUCTS, INC.
Manati, Puerto Rico
for
SANDOZ PHARMACEUTICALS CORPORATION
East Hanover, New Jersey 07936
[SDS-ZZ7 Issued August, 1992]
Shown in Product Identification Section, page 428

SANOREX® CIV ℞
[san 'ō-rex ″]
(mazindol) tablets, USP

CAUTION: Federal law prohibits dispensing without prescription.
The following prescribing information is based on official labeling in effect on August 1, 1992.

DESCRIPTION
SANOREX® (mazindol) is an imidazoisoindole anorectic agent. It is chemically designated as 5-(4-chlorophenyl)-2,5-dihydro-3*H*-imidazo[2,1-*a*]isoindol-5-ol), a tautomeric form of 2-[2′-(p-chlorobenzoyl) phenyl]-2-imidazoline, and has the following structure:

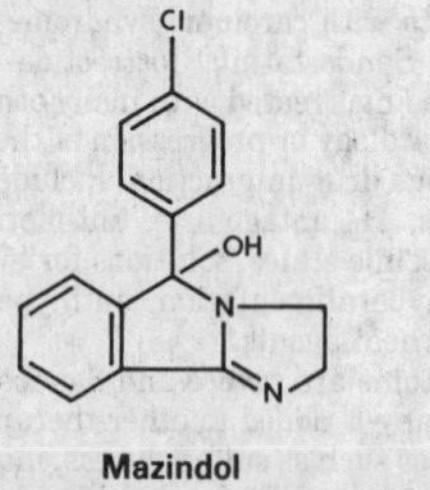

Mazindol

$C_{16}H_{13}ClN_2O$ Mol. wt. 284.74

1 mg and 2 mg Tablets
Active Ingredient: mazindol, USP.
Inactive Ingredients: calcium sulfate dihydrate, NF; lactose, NF; magnesium stearate, NF; povidone, USP; starch, NF; and talc, USP.

ACTIONS
SANOREX® (mazindol), although an isoindole, has pharmacologic activity similar in many ways to the prototype drugs used in obesity, the amphetamines. Actions include central nervous system stimulation in humans and animals, as well as such amphetamine-like effects in animals as the production of stereotyped behavior. Animal experiments also suggest certain differences from phenethylamine anorectic drugs, e.g., amphetamine, with respect to site and mechanism of action; for example, mazindol appears to exert its primary effects on the limbic system. The significance of these differences for humans is uncertain. It does not cause brain norepinephrine depletion in animals; on the other hand, it does appear to inhibit storage site uptake of norepinephrine as is suggested by its marked potentiation of the effect of exogenous norepinephrine on blood pressure in dogs *(see WARNINGS)* and on smooth muscle contraction *in vitro*.
Tolerance has been demonstrated with all drugs of this class in which this phenomenon has been studied.
Drugs used in obesity are commonly known as "anorectics" or "anorexigenics." It has not been established, however, that the action of such drugs in treating obesity is exclusively one of appetite suppression. Other central nervous system actions, or metabolic effects may be involved as well.
Adult obese subjects instructed in dietary management and treated with anorectic drugs, lose more weight on the average than those treated with placebo and diet, as determined in relatively short-term clinical trials.
The average magnitude of increased weight loss of drug-treated patients over placebo-treated patients in studies of anorectics in general is ordinarily only a fraction of a pound a week. The rate of weight loss is greatest in the first weeks of therapy for both drug and placebo subjects and tends to decrease in succeeding weeks.
The amount of weight loss associated with the use of SANOREX® (mazindol), as with other anorectic drugs, varies from trial to trial, and the increased weight loss appears to be related in part to variables other than the drugs prescribed, such as the interaction between physician-investigator and the patient, the population treated, and the diet prescribed. The importance of non-drug factors in such weight loss has not been elucidated.
The natural history of obesity is measured in years, whereas, most studies cited are restricted to a few weeks' duration; thus, the total impact of drug-induced weight loss over that of diet alone must be considered clinically limited.

INDICATION
SANOREX® (mazindol) is indicated in the management of exogenous obesity as a short-term (a few weeks) adjunct in a regimen of weight reduction based on caloric restriction. The limited usefulness of agents of this class *(see ACTIONS)* should be measured against possible risk factors inherent in their use, such as those described below.

CONTRAINDICATIONS
Glaucoma; hypersensitivity or idiosyncrasy to SANOREX® (mazindol).
Agitated states.
Patients with a history of drug abuse.
During or within 14 days following the administration of monoamine oxidase inhibitors, (hypertensive crises may result).

WARNINGS
Tolerance to the effect of many anorectic drugs may develop within a few weeks; if this occurs, the recommended dose should not be exceeded in an attempt to increase the effect; rather, the drug should be discontinued.
SANOREX® (mazindol) may impair the ability of the patient to engage in potentially hazardous activities such as operating machinery or driving a motor vehicle; the patient should therefore be cautioned accordingly.
Drug Interactions
SANOREX® (mazindol) may decrease the hypotensive effect of guanethidine; patients should be monitored accordingly.
SANOREX® (mazindol) may markedly potentiate the pressor effect of exogenous catecholamines. If it should be necessary to give a pressor amine agent (e.g., levarterenol or isoproterenol) to a patient in shock (e.g., from a myocardial infarction) who has recently been taking SANOREX® (mazindol), extreme care should be taken in monitoring blood pressure at frequent intervals and initiating pressor therapy with a low initial dose and careful titration.
Drug Dependence
SANOREX® (mazindol) shares important pharmacologic properties with amphetamines. Amphetamines and related stimulant drugs have been extensively abused and can produce tolerance and severe psychologic dependence. In this regard, the manifestations of chronic overdosage or withdrawal of SANOREX® (mazindol) have not been determined in humans. Abstinence effects have been observed in dogs after abrupt cessation for prolonged periods. There was some self-administration of the drug in monkeys. EEG studies and "liking" scores in human subjects yielded equivocal results. While the abuse potential of SANOREX® (mazindol) has not been further defined, the possibility of dependence should be kept in mind when evaluating the desirability of including SANOREX® (mazindol) as part of a weight reduction program.

Usage in Pregnancy
SANOREX® (mazindol) was studied in reproduction experiments in rats and rabbits and an increase in neonatal mortality and a possible increased incidence of rib anomalies in rats were observed at relatively high doses.
Although these studies have not indicated important adverse effects, use of mazindol by women who are or may become pregnant requires that the potential benefit be weighed against the possible hazard to mother and infant.
Usage in Children
SANOREX® (mazindol) is not recommended for use in children under 12 years of age.

PRECAUTIONS

Insulin requirements in diabetes mellitus may be altered in association with the use of mazindol and the concomitant dietary regimen.
The least amount feasible should be prescribed or dispensed at one time in order to minimize the possibility of overdosage.
Use only with caution in hypertension with monitoring of blood pressure, since evidence is insufficient to rule out a possible adverse effect on blood pressure in some hypertensive patients. The drug is not recommended in severely hypertensive patients. The drug is not recommended for patients with symptomatic cardiovascular disease including arrhythmias.

ADVERSE REACTIONS

The most common adverse effects of SANOREX® (mazindol) are dry mouth, tachycardia, constipation, nervousness and insomnia.
Cardiovascular: Palpitation, tachycardia.
Central Nervous System: Overstimulation, restlessness, dizziness, insomnia, dysphoria, tremor, headache, depression, drowsiness, weakness.
Gastrointestinal: Dryness of the mouth, unpleasant taste, diarrhea, constipation, nausea, other gastrointestinal disturbances.
Skin: Rash, excessive sweating, clamminess.
Endocrine: Impotence, changes in libido have rarely been observed with SANOREX® (mazindol).
Eye: Treatment of dogs with high doses of SANOREX® (mazindol) for long periods resulted in some corneal opacities, reversible on cessation of medication. No such effect has been observed in humans.

DOSAGE AND ADMINISTRATION

Usual dosage is 1 mg three times daily, one hour before meals; or 2 mg once daily, one hour before lunch. The lowest effective dose should be used. To determine the lowest effective dose, therapy with SANOREX® (mazindol) may be initiated at 1 mg once a day, and adjusted to the need and response of the patient. Should G.I. discomfort occur, SANOREX® (mazindol) may be taken with meals.

OVERDOSAGE

There are no data as yet on acute overdosage with SANOREX® (mazindol) in humans.
Manifestations of acute overdosage with amphetamines and related substances include restlessness, tremor, rapid respiration, dizziness. Fatigue and depression may follow the stimulatory phase of overdosage. Cardiovascular effects include tachycardia, hypertension and circulatory collapse. Gastrointestinal symptoms include nausea, vomiting and abdominal cramps. While similar manifestations of overdosage may be seen with SANOREX® (mazindol), their exact nature has yet to be determined. The management of acute intoxication is largely symptomatic. Data are not available on the treatment of acute intoxication with SANOREX® (mazindol) by hemodialysis or peritoneal dialysis, but the substance is poorly soluble except at very acid pH.

HOW SUPPLIED

SANOREX® (mazindol) Tablets, USP
SANOREX® (mazindol) is available in 1 mg elliptical, white tablets, engraved "SANOREX" one side, "78-71" other side; and in 2 mg round, white scored tablets, engraved "78/66" one side, "SANDOZ" other side, in packages of 100 (NDC 0078-0071-05 and NDC 0078-0066-05, respectively).
Store and dispense
Below 77°F (25°C); tight container.
[SNX-Z14 Issued January 1, 1991]

SANSERT® ℞

[san 'surt]
(methysergide maleate) TABLETS, USP

CAUTION: Federal law prohibits dispensing without prescription.
The following prescribing information is based on official labeling in effect on August 1, 1992.

> **WARNING**
> **Retroperitoneal Fibrosis, Pleuropulmonary Fibrosis and Fibrotic Thickening of Cardiac Valves May Occur in Patients Receiving Long-term Methysergide Maleate Therapy. Therefore, This Preparation Must be Reserved for Prophylaxis in Patients Whose Vascular Headaches are Frequent and/or Severe and Uncontrollable and Who Are Under Close Medical Supervision.**
> ***(See also WARNINGS section)***

DESCRIPTION

Sansert® (methysergide maleate) is a partially synthetic compound structurally related to lysergic acid butanolamide, well-known as methylergonovine in obstetrical practice as an oxytocic agent.
Chemically, methysergide maleate is designated as ergoline-8-carboxamide,9,10-didehydro-*N*-[1-(hydroxymethyl)propyl]-1,6-dimethyl-, (8β)-, (*Z*)-2-butenedioate (1:1) (salt).
Its structural formula is:

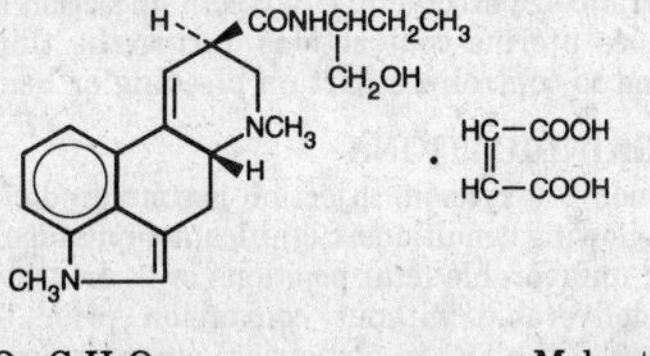

$C_{21}H_{27}N_3O_2 \cdot C_4H_4O_4$ Mol. wt. 469.54

Methylation in the number 1 position of the ring structure enormously enhances the antagonism to serotonin which is present to a much lesser degree in the partially methylated compound (methylergonovine maleate) as well as profoundly altering other pharmacologic properties.
Active Ingredient: methysergide maleate, USP.
Inactive Ingredients: acacia, carnauba wax, colloidal silicon dioxide, FD&C Blue #1, FD&C Yellow #5, gelatin, lactose, malic acid, povidone, sodium benzoate, starch, stearic acid, sucrose, synthetic black iron oxide, talc, and titanium dioxide.

ACTIONS

Sansert® (methysergide maleate) has been shown, *in vitro* and *in vivo*, to inhibit or block the effects of serotonin, a substance which may be involved in the mechanism of vascular headaches. Serotonin has been variously described as a central neurohumoral agent or chemical mediator, as a "headache substance" acting directly or indirectly to lower pain threshold (others in this category include tyramine; polypeptides, such as bradykinin; histamine; and acetylcholine), as an intrinsic "motor hormone" of the gastrointestinal tract, and as a "hormone" involved in connective tissue reparative processes. Suggestions have been made by investigators as to the mechanism whereby methysergide produces its clinical effects, but this has not been finally established.

INDICATIONS

For the prevention or reduction of intensity and frequency of vascular headaches in the following kinds of patients:

1. Patients suffering from one or more severe vascular headaches per week.
2. Patients suffering from vascular headaches that are uncontrollable or so severe that preventive therapy is indicated regardless of the frequency of the attack.

CONTRAINDICATIONS

Pregnancy, peripheral vascular disease, severe arteriosclerosis, severe hypertension, coronary artery disease, phlebitis or cellulitis of the lower limbs, pulmonary disease, collagen diseases or fibrotic processes, impaired liver or renal function, valvular heart disease, debilitated states and serious infections.

WARNINGS

With long-term, uninterrupted administration, retroperitoneal fibrosis or related conditions—pleuropulmonary fibrosis and cardiovascular disorders with murmurs or vascular bruits have been reported. Patients must be warned to report immediately the following symptoms: cold, numb, and painful hands and feet; leg cramps on walking; any type of girdle, flank, or chest pain, or any associated symptomatology. Should any of these symptoms develop, methysergide should be discontinued. Continuous administration should not exceed 6 months. There must be a drug-free interval of 3-4 weeks after each 6-month course of treatment. The dosage should be reduced gradually during the last 2-3 weeks of each treatment course to avoid "headache rebound."
The drug is not recommended for use in children.

PRECAUTIONS

All patients receiving Sansert® (methysergide maleate) should remain under constant supervision of the physician and be examined regularly for the development of fibrotic or vascular complications. *(See ADVERSE REACTIONS)*
The manifestations of retroperitoneal fibrosis, pleuropulmonary fibrosis, and vascular shutdown have shown a high incidence of regression once Sansert® (methysergide maleate) is withdrawn. These facts should be borne in mind to avoid unnecessary surgical intervention. Cardiac murmurs, which may indicate endocardial fibrosis, have shown varying degrees of regression, with complete disappearance in some and persistence in others.
Sansert® (methysergide maleate) has been specifically designed for the prophylaxis of vascular headache and has no place in the management of the acute attack.
Sansert® (methysergide maleate) tablets contain FD&C Yellow No. 5 (tartrazine) which may cause allergic-type reactions (including bronchial asthma) in certain susceptible individuals. Although the overall incidence of FD&C Yellow No. 5 (tartrazine) sensitivity in the general population is low, it is frequently seen in patients who also have aspirin hypersensitivity.

ADVERSE REACTIONS

Within the recommended dose levels, the following side effects have been reported:
1) Fibrotic Complications
Fibrotic changes have been observed in the retroperitoneal, pleuropulmonary, cardiac, and other tissues, either singly or, very rarely, in combination.
Retroperitoneal Fibrosis
This nonspecific fibrotic process is usually confined to the retroperitoneal connective tissue above the pelvic brim and may present clinically with one or more symptoms such as general malaise, fatigue, weight loss, backache, low grade fever (elevated sedimentation rate), urinary obstruction (girdle or flank pain, dysuria, polyuria, oliguria, elevated BUN), vascular insufficiency of the lower limbs (leg pain, Leriche syndrome, edema of legs, thrombophlebitis). The single most useful diagnostic procedure in suspected cases of retroperitoneal fibrosis is intravenous pyelography. Typical deviation and obstruction of one or both ureters may be observed.
Pleuropulmonary Complications
A similar nonspecific fibrotic process, limited to the pleural and immediately subjacent pulmonary tissues, usually presents clinically with dyspnea, tightness and pain in the chest, pleural friction rubs, and pleural effusion. These findings may be confirmed by chest X-ray.
Cardiac Complications
Nonrheumatic fibrotic thickenings of the aortic root and of the aortic and mitral valves usually present clinically with cardiac murmurs and dyspnea.
Other Fibrotic Complications
Several cases of fibrotic plaques, simulating Peyronie's Disease have been described.
2) Cardiovascular Complications
Encroachment of retroperitoneal fibrosis on the aorta, inferior vena cava and their common iliac branches may result in vascular insufficiency of the lower limbs, the presenting features of which are mentioned under *Retroperitoneal Fibrosis.*
Intrinsic vasoconstriction of large and small arteries, involving one or more vessels or merely a segment of a vessel, may occur at any stage of therapy. Depending on the vessel involved, this complication may present with chest pain, abdominal pain, or cold, numb, painful extremities with or without paresthesias and diminished or absent pulses. Progression to ischemic tissue damage has rarely been reported. Prompt withdrawal of the drug at the first signs of impaired circulation is recommended (see *WARNINGS*) to obviate such effects.
Postural hypotension and tachycardia have also been observed.
3) Gastrointestinal Symptoms
Nausea, vomiting, diarrhea, heartburn, abdominal pain. These effects tend to appear early and can frequently be obviated by gradual introduction of the medication and by administration of the drug with meals. Constipation and elevation of gastric HCl have also been reported.
4) CNS Symptoms
Insomnia, drowsiness, mild euphoria, dizziness, ataxia, lightheadedness, hyperesthesia, unworldly feelings (described variously as "dissociation", "hallucinatory experiences", etc.). Some of these symptoms may be associated with vascular headaches, per se, and may, therefore, be unrelated to the drug.
5) Dermatological Manifestations
Facial flush, telangiectasia, and nonspecific rashes have rarely been reported. Increased hair loss may occur, but in many instances the tendency has abated despite continued therapy.
6) Edema
Peripheral edema, and, more rarely, localized brawny edema may occur.
Dependent edema has responded to lowered doses, salt restriction, or diuretics.

Continued on next page

Sandoz—Cont.

7) Weight Gain
Weight gain may be a reason to caution patients regarding their caloric intake.
8) Hematological Manifestations
Neutropenia, eosinophilia.
9) Miscellaneous
Weakness, arthralgia, myalgia.

DOSAGE AND ADMINISTRATION

Usual adult dose 4-8 mg daily. Tablets to be given with meals.
Note: There must be a medication-free interval of 3-4 weeks after every 6-month course of treatment. (See WARNINGS)
No pediatric dosage has been established.
If, after a 3-week trial period, efficacy has not been demonstrated, longer administration of Sansert® (methysergide maleate) is unlikely to be of benefit.

HOW SUPPLIED

Sansert® (methysergide maleate) Tablets, USP
Bottles of 100 tablets, each tablet containing 2 mg of methysergide maleate, USP. Imprinted "78-58" on one side, "SANDOZ" other side.
[SAN-Z23 Issued June 1, 1991]

SYNTOCINON® ℞

[sin "tō 'si-non]
(oxytocin injection, USP)
Injection

CAUTION: Federal law prohibits dispensing without prescription.
The following prescribing information is based on official labeling in effect on August 1, 1992.

DESCRIPTION

Syntocinon® (oxytocin) injection is a synthetic nonapeptide. For intravenous or intramuscular administration.
Each 1 mL of Syntocinon® solution contains 10 USP or International Units of oxytocin and the following inactive ingredients:

sodium acetate, USP	1 mg
sodium chloride, USP	0.017 mg
chlorobutanol, NF	0.5%
alcohol, USP	0.61% by vol.
acetic acid, NF, qs to	pH 4 ± .3
water for injection, USP, qs to	1 ml

The Syntocinon® solution in each ampul is sterile.
Syntocinon® (oxytocin) is a cyclic (1–6) nonapeptide with the following chemical name.
Glycinamide, L-cysteinyl-L-tyrosyl-L-isoleucyl-L-glutaminyl-L-asparaginyl-L-cysteinyl-L-prolyl-L-leucyl-, cyclic (1–6)-disulfide
Its Chemical Abstract Registry number is: 50-56-6; and its chemical formula is shown below:

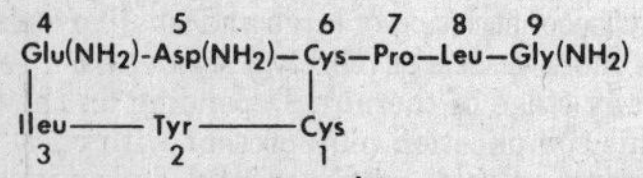
4 5 6 7 8 9
Glu(NH2)-Asp(NH2)—Cys—Pro—Leu—Gly(NH2)
Ileu—Tyr—Cys
3 2 1

oxytocin

CLINICAL PHARMACOLOGY

The pharmacologic and clinical properties of Syntocinon® (oxytocin) are identical with the naturally occurring oxytocic principle of the posterior lobe of the pituitary. Syntocinon® (oxytocin) injection does not contain the amino acids characteristic of vasopressin, and therefore has fewer and less severe cardiovascular effects. Syntocinon® (oxytocin) exerts a selective action on the smooth musculature of the uterus, particularly toward the end of pregnancy, during labor and immediately following delivery. Oxytocin stimulates rhythmic contractions of the uterus, increases the frequency of existing contractions, and raises the tone of the uterine musculature.
Syntocinon® (oxytocin), when given in appropriate doses during pregnancy, is capable of eliciting graded increases in uterine motility from a moderate increase in the rate and force of spontaneous motor activity to sustained tetanic contraction.
Syntocinon® (oxytocin) is promptly effective after parenteral administration. Following intramuscular injection, the myotonic effect on the uterus appears in 3–7 minutes, and persists for 30–60 minutes. With intravenous injection, the uterine effect appears within one minute and is of more brief duration.

INDICATIONS AND USAGE

IMPORTANT NOTICE
Syntocinon® (oxytocin) injection is indicated for the medical rather than the elective induction of labor. Available data and information are inadequate to define the benefits to risk considerations in the use of the drug product for elective induction. Elective induction of labor is defined as the initiation of labor for convenience in an individual with a term pregnancy who is free of medical indications.

Antepartum: Syntocinon® (oxytocin) is indicated for the initiation or improvement of uterine contractions, where this is desirable and considered suitable, in order to achieve early vaginal delivery for fetal or maternal reasons. It is indicated for (1) induction of labor in patients with a medical indication for the initiation of labor, such as Rh problems, maternal diabetes, pre-eclampsia at or near term, when delivery is in the best interest of mother and fetus or when membranes are prematurely ruptured and delivery is indicated; (2) stimulation or reinforcement of labor, as in selected cases of uterine inertia; (3) as adjunctive therapy in the management of incomplete or inevitable abortion. In the first trimester, curettage is generally considered primary therapy. In the second trimester abortion, oxytocin infusion will often be successful in emptying the uterus. Other means of therapy, however, may be required in such cases.
Postpartum: Syntocinon® (oxytocin) injection is indicated to produce uterine contractions during the third stage of labor and to control postpartum bleeding or hemorrhage.

CONTRAINDICATIONS

Syntocinon® (oxytocin) injection is contraindicated in any of the following conditions: Significant cephalopelvic disproportion; unfavorable fetal positions or presentations which are undeliverable without conversion prior to delivery (transverse lies); i.e., in obstetrical emergencies where the benefit-to-risk ratio for either the fetus or the mother favors surgical intervention; in cases of fetal distress where delivery is not imminent; prolonged use in uterine inertia or severe toxemia; hypertonic uterine patterns; patients with hypersensitivity to the drug; induction or augmentation of labor in those cases where vaginal delivery is contraindicated, such as cord presentation or prolapse, total placental previa, and vasa previa.

WARNINGS

Syntocinon® (oxytocin), when given for induction or stimulation of labor, must be administered only by the intravenous route and with adequate medical supervision in a hospital.

PRECAUTIONS

General: **All patients receiving intravenous oxytocin must be under continuous observation by trained personnel with a thorough knowledge of the drug and qualified to identify complications. A physician qualified to manage any complications should be immediately available.**
When properly administered, oxytocin should stimulate uterine contractions similar to those seen in normal labor. Overstimulation of the uterus by improper administration can be hazardous to both mother and fetus. Even with proper administration and adequate supervision, hypertonic contractions can occur in patients whose uteri are hypersensitive to oxytocin.
Except in unusual circumstances, oxytocin should not be administered in the following conditions: prematurity, borderline cephalopelvic disproportion, previous major surgery on the cervix or uterus including cesarean section, over-distention of the uterus, grand multiparity, or invasive cervical carcinoma. Because of the variability of the combinations of factors which may be present in the conditions listed above, the definition of "unusual circumstances" must be left to the judgment of the physician. The decision can only be made by carefully weighing the potential benefits which oxytocin can provide in a given case against rare but definite potential for the drug to produce hypertonicity or tetanic spasm.
Maternal deaths due to hypertensive episodes, subarachnoid hemorrhage, rupture of the uterus, and fetal deaths due to various causes have been reported associated with the use of parenteral oxytocic drugs for induction of labor or for augmentation in the first and second stages of labor.
Oxytocin has been shown to have an intrinsic antidiuretic effect, acting to increase water reabsorption from the glomerular filtrate. Consideration should, therefore, be given to the possibility of water intoxication, particularly when oxytocin is administered continuously by infusion and the patient is receiving fluids by mouth.
Drug Interactions: Severe hypertension has been reported when oxytocin was given three to four hours following prophylactic administration of a vasoconstrictor in conjunction with caudal block anesthesia. Cyclopropane anesthesia may modify oxytocin's cardiovascular effects, so as to produce unexpected results such as hypotension. Maternal sinus bradycardia with abnormal atrioventricular rhythms has also been noted when oxytocin was used concomitantly with cyclopropane anesthesia.
Carcinogenesis, Mutagenesis, Impairment of Fertility: There are no animal or human studies on the carcinogenicity and mutagenicity of this drug, nor is there any information on its effect on fertility.
Pregnancy: Teratogenic Effects. Animal reproduction studies have not been conducted with oxytocin. There are no known indications for use in the first trimester of pregnancy other than in relation to spontaneous or induced abortion. Based on the wide experience with this drug and its chemical structure and pharmacological properties, it would not be expected to present a risk of fetal abnormalities when used as indicated.
Nonteratogenic Effects. See **ADVERSE REACTIONS** in the fetus or infant.
Labor and Delivery: See **INDICATIONS AND USAGE.**
Nursing Mothers: Syntocinon® (oxytocin) may be found in small quantities in mother's milk. If a patient requires the drug postpartum to control severe bleeding, she should not commence nursing until the day after Syntocinon® has been discontinued.
Pediatric Use: Syntocinon® (oxytocin) is not intended for use in children.

ADVERSE REACTIONS

The following adverse reactions have been reported in the mother: Anaphylactic reaction, Postpartum hemorrhage, Cardiac arrhythmia, Fatal afibrinogenemia, Nausea, Vomiting, Premature ventricular contractions and Pelvic hematoma.
Excessive dosage or hypersensitivity to the drug may result in uterine hypertonicity, spasm, tetanic contraction, or rupture of the uterus.
The possibility of increased blood loss and afibrinogenemia should be kept in mind when administering the drug.
Severe water intoxication with convulsions and coma has occurred, associated with a slow oxytocin infusion over a 24-hour period. Maternal death due to oxytocin-induced water intoxication has been reported.
The following adverse reactions have been reported in the fetus or infant:
Due to induced uterine motility: Bradycardia, Premature ventricular contractions and other arrhythmias, Permanent CNS or brain damage and Fetal death.
Due to use of oxytocin in the mother: Low Apgar scores at 5 minutes, Neonatal jaundice and Neonatal retinal hemorrhage.

DRUG ABUSE AND DEPENDENCE

There is no evidence that Syntocinon® (oxytocin) has been abused or has provoked drug dependence.

OVERDOSAGE

Overdosage with oxytocin depends essentially on uterine hyperactivity, whether or not due to hypersensitivity to this agent. Hyperstimulation with strong (hypertonic) or prolonged (tetanic) contractions, or a resting tone of 15 to 20 mm H_2O or more between contractions can lead to tumultuous labor, uterine rupture, cervical and vaginal lacerations, postpartum hemorrhage, uteroplacental hypoperfusion, and variable deceleration of fetal heart, fetal hypoxia, hypercapnia or death. Water intoxication with convulsions, which is caused by the inherent antidiuretic effect of oxytocin, is a serious complication that may occur if large doses (40 to 50 mL/minute) are infused for long periods. Treatment of water intoxication consists of discontinuation of oxytocin, restriction of fluid intake, diuresis, IV hypertonic saline solution, correction of electrolyte imbalance, control of convulsions with judicious use of a barbiturate and special nursing care for the comatose patient.

DOSAGE AND ADMINISTRATION

Dosage of oxytocin is determined by uterine response. The following dosage information is based upon the various regimens and indications in general use. Parenteral drug products should be inspected visually for particulate matter and discoloration prior to administration, wherever solution and container permit.
A. Induction or Stimulation of Labor
Intravenous infusion (drip method) is the only acceptable method of administration for the induction or stimulation of labor.
Accurate control of the rate of infusion flow is essential. An infusion pump or other such device and frequent monitoring of strength of contractions and fetal heart rate are necessary for the safe administration of oxytocin for the induction or stimulation of labor. If uterine contractions become too powerful, the infusion can be abruptly stopped, and oxytocin stimulation of the uterine musculature will soon wane.
1. An intravenous infusion of non-oxytocin containing solution should be started. Physiologic electrolyte solution should be used except under unusual circumstances.
2. To prepare the usual solution for infusion, the contents of one 1-mL ampul are combined aseptically with 1,000 mL of nonhydrating dilutent. The combined solution, rotated in the infusion bottle to insure thorough mixing contains 10 mU/mL. Add the container with dilute oxytocin solution to the system through use of a constant infusion pump or other such device, to control accurately the rate of infusion.
3. The initial dose should be no more than 1–2 mU/minute. The dose may be gradually increased in increments of no more than 1–2 mU/minute, until a contraction pattern has been established, which is similar to normal labor.

4. The fetal heart rate, resting uterine tone, and the frequency, duration, and force of contractions should be monitored.
5. The oxytocin infusion should be discontinued immediately in the event of uterine hyperactivity or fetal distress. Oxygen should be administered to the mother. The mother and the fetus must be evaluated by the responsible physician.

B. Control of Postpartum Uterine Bleeding
1. *Intravenous Infusion (Drip Method):* To control postpartum bleeding, 10–40 units of oxytocin may be added to 1,000 mL of a non-hydrating dilutent and run at a rate necessary to control uterine atony.
2. *Intramuscular Administration:* 1 mL (10 units) of oxytocin can be given after delivery of the placenta.

C. Treatment of Incomplete or Inevitable Abortion
Intravenous infusion with physiologic saline solution, 500 mL, or 5% dextrose in physiologic saline solution to which 10 units of Syntocinon® (oxytocin) have been added should be infused at a rate of 20–40 drops/minute.

HOW SUPPLIED

Ampuls: 1 mL (10 USP units) size, boxes of 20 (NDC 0078-0060-03), 50 (NDC 0078-0060-04) and 100 (NDC 0078-0060-05).
Store and dispense: Below 77°F; DO NOT FREEZE.
[SYT-Z20 (BB) Issued July 15, 1986]

SYNTOCINON® ℞
[sin"tō'si-non]
(oxytocin nasal solution, USP)
NASAL SPRAY

CAUTION: Federal law prohibits dispensing without prescription.
The following prescribing information is based on official labeling in effect on August 1, 1992.

DESCRIPTION

Each mL contains 40 USP Units (International Units) Syntocinon® (oxytocin) and the following: chlorobutanol, NF max. 0.05%; citric acid, USP; dried sodium phosphate, USP; glycerin, USP; methylparaben, NF; propylparaben, NF; purified water, USP; sodium chloride, USP; sorbitol solution, USP.
Oxytocin is one of the polypeptide hormones of the posterior lobe of the pituitary gland. The pharmacologic and clinical properties of Syntocinon® (oxytocin nasal solution, USP) Nasal Spray are identical with the oxytocic and the galactokinetic principle of the natural hormone.
Synthetic oxytocin has the formula $C_{43}H_{66}N_{12}O_{12}S_2$, with a molecular weight of 1007.19. It is represented structurally[1] as:

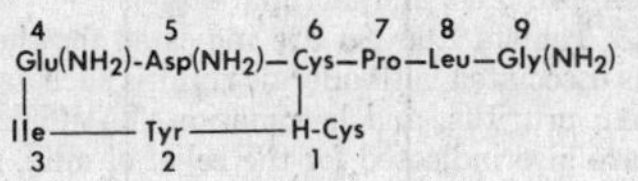
4 5 6 7 8 9
Glu(NH2)-Asp(NH2)-Cys-Pro-Leu-Gly(NH2)
Ile Tyr H-Cys
3 2 1
Oxytocin

Since oxytocin, a polypeptide, is subject to inactivation by the proteolytic enzymes of the alimentary tract, it is **not absorbed from the gastrointestinal tract.**

CLINICAL PHARMACOLOGY

Syntocinon® (oxytocin nasal solution, USP) Nasal Spray acts specifically on the myoepithelial elements surrounding the alveoli of the breast, and making up the walls of the lactiferous ducts, causing their smooth muscle fibers to contract and thus force milk into the large ducts or sinuses where it is more readily available to the baby. Oxytocin does not possess galactopoietic properties and its use is intended only for the purpose of milk ejection.

Pharmacokinetics
Syntocinon® (oxytocin nasal solution, USP) Nasal Spray is promptly absorbed by the nasal mucosa to enter the systemic circulation. Intranasal application of the spray preparation, however, is a practical and effective method of administration. Half-life is extremely short—less than 10 minutes—and oxytocin is then rapidly removed from plasma by the kidney, liver, and lactating mammary gland. The enzyme oxytocinase is believed to be elaborated by placental and uterine tissues. This enzyme inactivates the hormone by cleavage of the cysteine-tyrosine peptide bond. Excretion is mainly urinary following inactivation of metabolites.[2]

INDICATIONS AND USAGE

Syntocinon® (oxytocin nasal solution, USP) Nasal Spray is indicated to assist initial postpartum milk ejection from the breasts once milk formation has commenced.

CONTRAINDICATIONS

Pregnancy and hypersensitivity are the only known contraindications.

PRECAUTIONS

General
No particular information regarding any special care to be exercised by the practitioner for safe and effective use of the drug is known at this time.

Information for Patients
The squeeze bottle should be held in an upright position when administering the drug to the nose and the patient should be in a sitting position rather than lying down. If preferred, the solution can be instilled in drop form by inverting the squeeze bottle and exerting very gentle pressure on its walls.

Carcinogenesis, Mutagenesis, Impairment of Fertility
There are no animal or human studies on the carcinogenicity and mutagenicity of this drug, nor is there any information on its effect on fertility.

Pregnancy
Category X. (*See CONTRAINDICATIONS*) Syntocinon® (oxytocin nasal solution, USP) Nasal Spray is contraindicated during pregnancy since it may provoke a uterotonic effect to precipitate contractions and abortion. Its proper use is during the first week postpartum, as needed.

Nursing Mothers
While harmful effects on the newborn have not been reported, it should be noted that Syntocinon® (oxytocin nasal solution, USP) Nasal Spray is intended to be used only for **initial** milk propulsion and ejection during the first week postpartum, and not for continued use. Caution shall be exercised when Syntocinon® (oxytocin nasal solution, USP) Nasal Spray is administered to a nursing mother since oxytocin is known to be excreted in human milk.

ADVERSE REACTIONS

Lack of efficacy has been the most frequent adverse effect (seven cases), followed by nasal irritation and/or rhinorrhea, uterine bleeding, excessive uterine contractions, and lacrimation.
One case each of seizure and "psychotic state" are the most severe reactions reported. No other reactions have been described.[3]

DRUG ABUSE AND DEPENDENCE

These problems have not been encountered with Syntocinon® (oxytocin nasal solution, USP) Nasal Spray. This may be due to the fact that synthetic oxytocin acts like the natural posterior pituitary hormone. Also, its clinical use is limited to the first week following delivery, to assist in initial milk letdown.

OVERDOSAGE

No case of overdosage with Syntocinon® (oxytocin nasal solution, USP) Nasal Spray has been reported since the preparation became commercially available in 1961. It is theoretically possible for very large doses to be self-administered depending on the topical tolerance of the nasal mucosa. With such massive use, painful uterine contractions could be induced, although these effects persist for only about 15 minutes.[4] Also, an antidiuretic effect could occur resulting in water intoxication. Should this ensue, diuresis should be forced with appropriate agents such as furosemide.[5]

DOSAGE AND ADMINISTRATION

One spray into one or both nostrils two to three minutes before nursing or pumping of breasts.

HOW SUPPLIED

Syntocinon® (oxytocin nasal solution, USP) Nasal Spray in squeeze bottles containing: 2 mL oxytocin solution, NDC 0078-0061-23 or 5 mL oxytocin solution, NDC 0078-0061-25.
Store and dispense: Below 77°F; DO NOT FREEZE.

References

1. U.S.P. XXI, p. 777.
2. Goodman and Gilman: The Pharmacological Basis of Therapeutics. Sixth Ed., 937–8.
3. Data collected by the Medical Services Department, Sandoz Pharmaceuticals Corporation.
4. Borglin, N.E.: The use of intranasal oxytocin for the induction of labor. Zbl. Gynak. **85**: 193–199 (Feb. 9) 1963.
5. Sandoz Overdosage Manual, 1984, Syntocinon® Injection.

[SYT-ZZ13 Issued July 15, 1988]

TAVIST® ℞
(clemastine) SYRUP 0.5 mg-5 ml
(present as clemastine fumarate 0.67 mg/5 ml)

CAUTION: Federal law prohibits dispensing without prescription.
The following prescribing information is based on official labeling in effect on August 1, 1992.

DESCRIPTION

Each teaspoonful (5 ml) of Tavist® (clemastine fumarate) Syrup for oral administration contains clemastine 0.5 mg (present as clemastine fumarate 0.67 mg). Other ingredients: alcohol 5.5%, flavors, methylparaben, propylene glycol, propylparaben, purified water, saccharin sodium, sorbitol in a buffered solution. Tavist® (clemastine fumarate) belongs to the benzhydryl ether group of antihistaminic compounds. The chemical name is (+)-(2R)-2-[2-[[(R)-p-Chloro-α-methyl-α-phenylbenzyl]-oxy]ethyl]-1-methylpyrrolidine fumarate* and has the following structural formula:

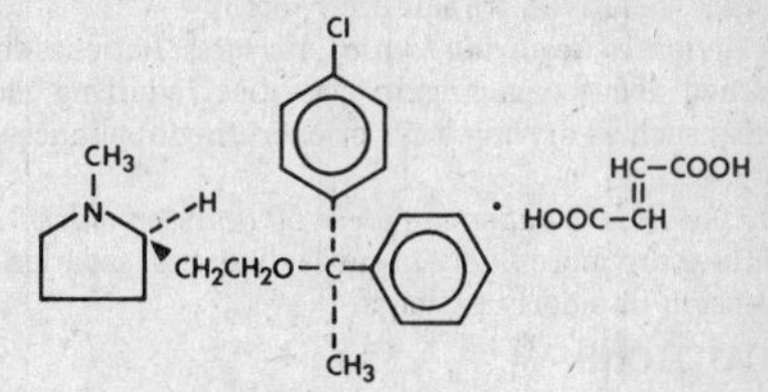
Cl
CH3
N
H
CH2CH2O-C
CH3
HC-COOH
HOOC-CH

AHFS Classification 4:00
CAS Registration Number 14976-57-9

Clemastine fumarate occurs as a colorless to faintly yellow, practically odorless, crystalline powder. Tavist® (clemastine fumarate) Syrup has an approximate pH of 6.2.

CLINICAL PHARMACOLOGY

Tavist® (clemastine fumarate) is an antihistamine with anticholinergic (drying) and sedative side effects. Antihistamines competitively antagonize various physiological effects of histamine including increased capillary permeability and dilatation, the formation of edema, the "flare" and "itch" response, and gastrointestinal and respiratory smooth muscle constriction. Within the vascular tree, H_1-receptor antagonists inhibit both the vasoconstrictor and vasodilator effects of histamine. Depending on the dose, H_1-receptor antagonists can produce CNS stimulation or depression. Most antihistamines exhibit central and/or peripheral anticholinergic activity. Antihistamines act by competitively blocking H_1-receptor sites. Antihistamines do not pharmacologically antagonize or chemically inactivate histamine, nor do they prevent the release of histamine.

PHARMACOKINETICS

Antihistamines are well-absorbed following oral administration. Chlorpheniramine maleate, clemastine fumarate, and diphenhydramine hydrochloride achieve peak blood levels within 2-5 hours following oral administration. The absorption of antihistamines is often partially delayed by the use of controlled release dosage forms. In these instances, plasma concentrations from identical doses of the immediate and controlled release dosage forms will not be similar.
Tissue distribution of the antihistamines in humans has not been established.
Antihistamines appear to be metabolized in the liver chiefly via mono- and didemethylation and glucuronide conjugation. Antihistamine metabolites and small amounts of unchanged drug are excreted in the urine. Small amounts of the drugs may also be excreted in breast milk.
In normal human subjects who received histamine injections over a 24-hour period, the antihistaminic activity of Tavist® (clemastine fumarate) reached a peak at 5-7 hours, persisted for 10-12 hours and, in some cases, for as long as 24 hours. Pharmacokinetic studies in man utilizing ^3H and ^{14}C labeled compound demonstrates that: Tavist® (clemastine fumarate) is rapidly absorbed from the gastrointestinal tract, peak plasma concentrations are attained in 2-4 hours, and urinary excretion is the major mode of elimination.

INDICATIONS AND USAGE

Tavist® (clemastine fumarate) Syrup is indicated for the relief of symptoms associated with allergic rhinitis such as sneezing, rhinorrhea, pruritus and lacrimation. Tavist® (clemastine fumarate) Syrup is indicated for use in pediatric populations (age 6 years through 12) and adults (see *DOSAGE AND ADMINISTRATION*).
It should be noted that Tavist® (clemastine fumarate) is indicated for the relief of mild uncomplicated allergic skin manifestations of urticaria and angioedema at the 2 mg dosage level only.

CONTRAINDICATIONS

Antihistamines are contraindicated in patients hypersensitive to the drug or to other antihistamines of similar chemical structure (see *PRECAUTIONS—Drug Interactions*).
Antihistamines *should not* be used *in newborn or premature infants.* Because of the higher risk of antihistamines for infants generally and for newborns and prematures in particular, antihistamine therapy is contraindicated *in nursing mothers* (see *PRECAUTIONS—Nursing Mothers*).

WARNINGS

Antihistamines should be used with considerable caution in patients with: narrow angle glaucoma, stenosing peptic ulcer, pyloroduodenal obstruction, symptomatic prostatic hypertrophy, and bladder neck obstruction.

*U.S. Patent No. 3,097,212.

Continued on next page

Sandoz—Cont.

Use with CNS Depressants: Tavist® (clemastine fumarate) has additive effects with alcohol and other CNS depressants (hypnotics, sedatives, tranquilizers, etc.)
Use in Activities Requiring Mental Alertness: Patients should be warned about engaging in activities requiring mental alertness such as driving a car or operating appliances, machinery, etc.
Use in the Elderly (approximately 60 years or older): Antihistamines are more likely to cause dizziness, sedation, and hypotension in elderly patients.

PRECAUTIONS

General: Tavist® (clemastine fumarate) should be used with caution in patients with: history of bronchial asthma, increased intraocular pressure, hyperthyroidism, cardiovascular disease, and hypertension.
Information for Patients:
Patients taking antihistamines should receive the following information and instructions:
1. Antihistamines are prescribed to reduce allergic symptoms.
2. Patients should be questioned regarding a history of glaucoma, peptic ulcer, urinary retention, or pregnancy before starting antihistamine therapy.
3. Patients should be told not to take alcohol, sleeping pills, sedatives, or tranquilizers while taking antihistamines.
4. Antihistamines may cause drowsiness, dizziness, dry mouth, blurred vision, weakness, nausea, headache, or nervousness in some patients.
5. Patients should avoid driving a car or working with hazardous machinery until they assess the effects of this medicine.
6. Patients should be told to store this medicine in a tightly closed container in a dry, cool place away from heat or direct sunlight and out of the reach of children.

Drug Interactions:
Additive CNS depression may occur when antihistamines are administered concomitantly with other CNS depressants including barbiturates, tranquilizers, and alcohol. Patients receiving antihistamines should be advised against the concurrent use of other CNS depressant drugs.
Monoamine oxidase (MAO) inhibitors prolong and intensify the anticholinergic effects of antihistamines.
Carcinogenesis, Mutagenesis, Impairment of Fertility:
Carcinogenesis and Mutagenesis: In a 2-year oral study in the rat at a dose of 84 mg/kg (about 500 times the adult human dose) and an 85-week oral study in the mouse at 206 mg/kg (about 1300 times the adult human dose), clemastine fumarate showed no evidence of carcinogenesis. No mutagenic studies have been conducted with clemastine fumarate.
Impairment of Fertility: Oral doses of clemastine fumarate in the rat produced a decrease in mating ability of the male at 312 times the adult human dose. This effect was not found at 156 times the adult human dose.
Pregnancy:
Pregnancy Category B: Oral reproduction studies performed with clemastine fumarate in rats and rabbits at doses up to 312 and 188 times the adult human doses respectively, have revealed no evidence of teratogenic effects.
There are no adequate and well-controlled studies of Tavist® (clemastine fumarate) Syrup in pregnant women. Because animal reproduction studies are not always predictive of human response, this drug should be used in pregnancy only if clearly needed.
Nursing Mothers:
Although quantitative determinations of antihistaminic drugs in breast milk have not been reported, qualitative tests have documented the excretion of diphenhydramine, pyrilamine, and tripelennamine in human milk.
Because of the potential for adverse reactions in nursing infants from antihistamines, a decision should be made whether to discontinue nursing or to discontinue the drug.
Pediatric Use:
The safety and efficacy of Tavist® (clemastine fumarate) Syrup has been confirmed in the pediatric population (age 6 years through 12). Safety and dose tolerance studies have confirmed children 6 through 11 years tolerated dosage ranges of 0.75 to 2.25 mg clemastine. In infants and children particularly, antihistamines in overdosage may produce hallucinations, convulsions, and death. Symptoms of antihistamine toxicity in children may include fixed dilated pupils, flushed face, dry mouth, fever, excitation, hallucinations, ataxia, incoordination, athetosis, tonic-clonic convulsions, and postictal depression (see *OVERDOSAGE*).

ADVERSE REACTIONS

The most frequent adverse reactions are underlined:
Nervous System: Sedation, sleepiness, dizziness, disturbed coordination, fatigue, confusion, restlessness, excitation, nervousness, tremor, irritability, insomnia, euphoria, paresthesia, blurred vision, diplopia, vertigo, tinnitus, acute labyrinthitis, hysteria, neuritis, convulsions.
Gastrointestinal System: Epigastric distress, anorexia, nausea, vomiting, diarrhea, constipation.
Respiratory System: Thickening of bronchial secretions, tightness of chest and wheezing, nasal stuffiness.
Cardiovascular System: Hypotension, headache, palpitations, tachycardia, extrasystoles.
Hematologic System: Hemolytic anemia, thrombocytopenia, agranulocytosis.
Genitourinary System: Urinary frequency, difficult urination, urinary retention, early menses.
General: Urticaria, drug rash, anaphylactic shock, photosensitivity, excessive perspiration, chills, dryness of mouth, nose and throat.

OVERDOSAGE

Antihistamine overdosage reactions may vary from central nervous system depression to stimulation. In children, stimulation predominates initially in a syndrome which may include excitement, hallucinations, ataxia, incoordination, muscle twitching, athetosis, hyperthermia, cyanosis convulsions, tremors, and hyperreflexia followed by postictal depression and cardio-respiratory arrest. Convulsions in children may be preceded by mild depression. Dry mouth, fixed dilated pupils, flushing of the face, and fever are common. In adults, CNS depression, ranging from drowsiness to coma, is more common. The convulsant dose of antihistamines lies near the lethal dose. Convulsions indicate a poor prognosis. In both children and adults, coma and cardiovascular collapse may occur. Deaths are reported especially in infants and children.
There is no specific therapy for acute overdosage with antihistamines. The latent period from ingestion to appearance of toxic effects is characteristically short (½-2 hours). General symptomatic and supportive measures should be instituted promptly and maintained for as long as necessary.
Since overdoses of other classes of drugs (i.e., tricyclic antidepressants) may also present anticholinergic symptomatology, appropriate toxicological analysis should be performed as soon as possible to identify the causative agent.
In the conscious patient, vomiting should be induced even though it may have occurred spontaneously. If vomiting cannot be induced, gastric lavage is indicated. Adequate precautions must be taken to protect against aspiration, especially in infants and children. Charcoal slurry or other suitable agents should be instilled into the stomach after vomiting or lavage. Saline cathartics or milk of magnesia may be of additional benefit.
In the unconscious patient, the airway should be secured with a cuffed endotracheal tube before attempting to evacuate the gastric contents. Intensive supportive and nursing care is indicated, as for any comatose patient.
If breathing is significantly impaired, maintenance of an adequate airway and mechanical support of respiration is the most effective means of providing adequate oxygenation.
Hypotension is an early sign of impending cardiovascular collapse and should be treated vigorously. Although general supportive measures are important, specific treatment with intravenous infusion of a vasopressor titrated to maintain adequate blood pressure may be necessary.
Do not use with CNS stimulants.
Convulsions should be controlled by careful administration of diazepam or a short-acting barbiturate, repeated as necessary. Physostigmine may also be considered for use in controlling centrally mediated convulsions.
Ice packs and cooling sponge baths, not alcohol, can aid in reducing the fever commonly seen in children. A more detailed review of antihistamine toxicology and overdose management is available in Gosselin, R.E., et al., "Clinical Toxicology of Commercial Products."

DOSAGE AND ADMINISTRATION

DOSAGE SHOULD BE INDIVIDUALIZED ACCORDING TO THE NEEDS AND RESPONSE OF THE PATIENT.
Pediatric: Children aged 6 to 12 years:
For Symptoms of Allergic Rhinitis—The starting dose is 1 teaspoonful (0.5 mg clemastine) twice daily. Since single doses of up to 2.25 mg clemastine were well tolerated by this age group, dosage may be increased as required, but not to exceed 6 teaspoonsful daily (3 mg clemastine).
For Urticaria and Angioedema—The starting dose is 2 teaspoonsful (1 mg clemastine) twice daily, not to exceed 6 teaspoonsful daily (3 mg clemastine).
Adults and Children 12 Years and Over:
For Symptoms of Allergic Rhinitis—The starting dose is 2 teaspoonsful (1.0 mg clemastine) twice daily. Dosage may be increased as required, but not to exceed 12 teaspoonsful daily (6 mg clemastine).
For Urticaria and Angioedema—The starting dose is 4 teaspoonsful (2 mg clemastine) twice daily, not to exceed 12 teaspoonsful daily (6 mg clemastine).

HOW SUPPLIED

Tavist® (clemastine fumarate) Syrup: clemastine 0.5 mg/5 ml (present as clemastine fumarate 0.67mg/5 ml). A clear, colorless liquid with a citrus flavor, in 4 fl. oz. bottle (NDC 0078-0222-31).
Store and dispense: Below 77°F (25°C) tight, amber glass bottle. Store in an upright position.
[TAS-Z3 Issued April 1, 1986]

TAVIST 1® ℞
CLEMASTINE FUMARATE TABLETS, USP, 1.34 MG
TAVIST® ℞
CLEMASTINE FUMARATE TABLETS, USP, 2.68 MG

CAUTION: Federal law prohibits dispensing without prescription.
The following prescribing information is based on official labeling in effect on August 1, 1992.

DESCRIPTION

TAVIST® (clemastine fumarate, USP) belongs to the benzhydryl ether group of antihistaminic compounds. The chemical name is (+)-2-[2-[(p-chloro-α-methyl-α-phenylbenzyl) oxy]ethyl]-1-methyl-pyrrolidine* hydrogen fumarate.

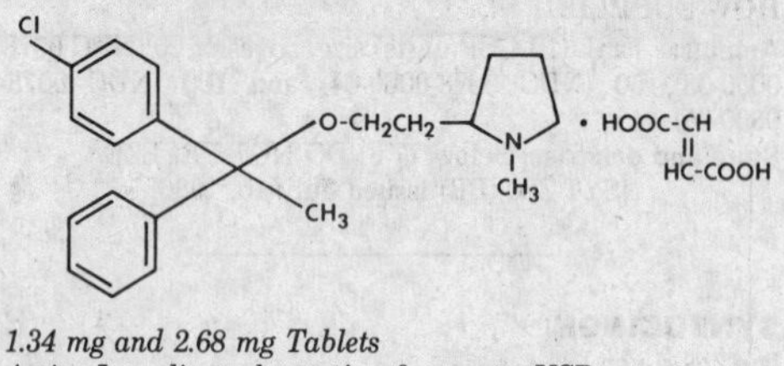

1.34 mg and 2.68 mg Tablets
Active Ingredient: clemastine fumarate, USP
Inactive Ingredients: lactose, povidone, starch, stearic acid, and talc

ACTIONS

TAVIST® is an antihistamine with anticholinergic (drying) and sedative side effects. Antihistamines appear to compete with histamine for cell receptor sites on effector cells. The inherently long duration of antihistaminic effects of TAVIST® has been demonstrated in wheal and flare studies. In normal human subjects who received histamine injections over a 24-hour period, the antihistaminic activity of TAVIST® reached a peak at 5-7 hours, persisted for 10-12 hours and, in some cases, for as long as 24 hours. Pharmacokinetic studies in man utilizing ^{3}H and ^{14}C labeled compound demonstrates that: TAVIST® (clemastine fumarate, USP) is rapidly and nearly completely absorbed from the gastrointestinal tract, peak plasma concentrations are attained in 2-4 hours, and urinary excretion is the major mode of elimination.

INDICATIONS

TAVIST-1® Tablets, 1.34 mg are indicated for the relief of symptoms associated with allergic rhinitis such as sneezing, rhinorrhea, pruritus, and lacrimation.
TAVIST® Tablets 2.68 mg are indicated for the relief of symptoms associated with allergic rhinitis such as sneezing, rhinorrhea, pruritus, and lacrimation. TAVIST® Tablets 2.68 mg are also indicated for the relief of mild, uncomplicated allergic skin manifestations of urticaria and angioedema.
It should be noted that TAVIST® (clemastine fumarate, USP) is indicated for the dermatologic indications at the 2.68 mg dosage level only.

CONTRAINDICATIONS

Use in Nursing Mothers
Because of the higher risk of antihistamines for infants generally and for newborns and prematures in particular, antihistamine therapy is contraindicated in nursing mothers.
Use in Lower Respiratory Disease
Antihistamines *should not* be used to treat lower respiratory tract symptoms including asthma.
Antihistamines are also contraindicated in the following conditions:
Hypersensitivity to TAVIST® (clemastine fumarate, USP) or other antihistamines of similar chemical structure.
Monamine oxidase inhibitor therapy. *(See Drug Interaction Section)*

WARNINGS

Antihistamines should be used with considerable caution in patients with: narrow angle glaucoma, stenosing peptic ulcer, pyloroduodenal obstruction, symptomatic prostatic hypertrophy, and bladder neck obstruction.
Use in Children
Safety and efficacy of TAVIST® have not been established in children under the age of 12.
Use in Pregnancy
Experience with this drug in pregnant women is inadequate to determine whether there exists a potential for harm to the developing fetus.

*U.S. Patent No. 3,097,212

Use with CNS Depressants

TAVIST® has additive effects with alcohol and other CNS depressants (hypnotics, sedatives, tranquilizers, etc.).

Use in Activities Requiring Mental Alertness

Patients should be warned about engaging in activities requiring mental alertness such as driving a car or operating appliances, machinery, etc.

Use in the Elderly (approximately 60 years or older)

Antihistamines are more likely to cause dizziness, sedation, and hypotension in elderly patients.

PRECAUTIONS

TAVIST® (clemastine fumarate, USP) should be used with caution in patients with: history of bronchial asthma, increased intraocular pressure, hyperthyroidism, cardiovascular disease, and hypertension.

Drug Interactions

MAO inhibitors prolong and intensify the anticholinergic (drying) effects of antihistamines.

ADVERSE REACTIONS

Transient drowsiness, the most common adverse reaction associated with TAVIST® (clemastine fumarate, USP), occurs relatively frequently and may require discontinuation of therapy in some instances.

Antihistaminic Compounds

It should be noted that the following reactions have occurred with one or more antihistamines and, therefore, should be kept in mind when prescribing drugs belonging to this class, including TAVIST®. The most frequent adverse reactions are underlined.

1. *General:* Urticaria, drug rash, anaphylactic shock, photosensitivity, excessive perspiration, chills, dryness of mouth, nose, and throat.
2. *Cardiovascular System:* Hypotension, headache, palpitations, tachycardia, extrasystoles.
3. *Hematologic System:* Hemolytic anemia, thrombocytopenia, agranulocytosis.
4. *Nervous System:* Sedation, sleepiness, dizziness, disturbed coordination, fatigue, confusion, restlessness, excitation, nervousness, tremor, irritability, insomnia, euphoria, parasthesias, blurred vision, diplopia, vertigo, tinnitus, acute labyrinthitis, hysteria, neuritis, convulsions.
5. *GI System:* Epigastric distress, anorexia, nausea, vomiting, diarrhea, constipation.
6. *GU System:* Urinary frequency, difficult urination, urinary retention, early menses.
7. *Respiratory System:* Thickening of bronchial secretions, tightness of chest and wheezing, nasal stuffiness.

OVERDOSAGE

Antihistamine overdosage reactions may vary from central nervous system depression to stimulation. Stimulation is particularly likely in children. Atropine-like signs and symptoms: dry mouth; fixed, dilated pupils; flushing; and gastrointestinal symptoms may also occur.

If vomiting has not occurred spontaneously the conscious patient should be induced to vomit. This is best done by having him drink a glass of water or milk after which he should be made to gag. Precautions against aspiration must be taken, especially in infants and children.

If vomiting is unsuccessful gastric lavage is indicated within 3 hours after ingestion and even later if large amounts of milk or cream were given beforehand. Isotonic and ½ isotonic saline is the lavage solution of choice.

Saline cathartics, such as milk of magnesia, by osmosis draw water into the bowel and therefore, are valuable for their action in rapid dilution of bowel content.

Stimulants should *not* be used.

Vasopressors may be used to treat hypotension.

DOSAGE AND ADMINISTRATION

DOSAGE SHOULD BE INDIVIDUALIZED ACCORDING TO THE NEEDS AND RESPONSE OF THE PATIENT.

TAVIST-1® Tablets 1.34 mg

The recommended starting dose is one tablet twice daily. Dosage may be increased as required, but not to exceed six tablets daily.

TAVIST® Tablets 2.68 mg

The maximum recommended dosage is one tablet three times daily. Many patients respond favorably to a single dose which may be repeated as required, but not to exceed three tablets daily.

HOW SUPPLIED

TAVIST-1® Tablets 1.34 mg clemastine fumarate

White, oval, compressed, scored tablet, engraved "TAVIST 1" on both sides. Packages of 100.

TAVIST® Tablets 2.68 mg clemastine fumarate

White, round, compressed tablet, engraved "78/72" and scored on one side, "TAVIST" on other. Packages of 100.

Store and Dispense

Controlled room temperature, between 15°–30°C (59°–86°F); tight, light-resistant container.

[TAV-Z5 Issued September 1, 1991]

Shown in Product Identification Section, page 428

TAVIST D® ℞

(clemastine fumarate and phenylpropanolamine HCl extended-release tablets)
TABLETS

CAUTION: Federal law prohibits dispensing without prescription.

The following prescribing information is based on official labeling in effect on August 1, 1992.

DESCRIPTION

Each Tavist D® (clemastine fumarate and phenylpropanolamine HCl extended-release) tablet for oral administration contains 1.34 mg clemastine fumarate, USP (equivalent to 1 mg of the free base) and 75 mg phenylpropanolamine hydrochloride, USP. The clemastine fumarate is in the outer shell of the tablet and is immediately released upon dissolution. The tablet's core is a sustained-release matrix which releases the phenylpropanolamine hydrochloride over a 12-hour period at a rate that produces blood levels bioequivalent to those obtained by the administration of 25 mg standard release tablets of phenylpropanolamine hydrochloride every four hours for three doses. Clemastine fumarate belongs to the benzhydryl ether group of antihistaminic compounds. The chemical name is (+)-(2*R*)-2-[2-[[(*R*)-*p*-Chloro-α-methyl-α-phenylbenzyl]oxy]ethyl]-1-methylpyrrolidine fumarate (1:1) and the structural formula is:

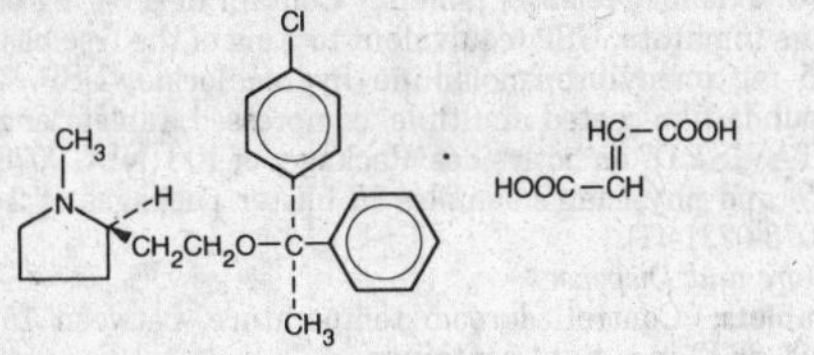

$C_{21}H_{26}ClNO.C_4H_4O_4$ Mol. wt. 459.97

Phenylpropanolamine hydrochloride is a sympathomimetic, orally effective nasal decongestant. Sympathomimetic compounds, whether catecholamines or non-catecholamines, can be regarded as compounds produced by substitution on the phenylethylamine nucleus common to all these sympathomimetic products, whether their action is on the Alpha receptors of the sympathetic nervous system or on Beta-1 or Beta-2 receptors. The chemical name for phenylpropanolamine hydrochloride is benzenemethanol, α-(1-aminoethyl)-, hydrochloride, (R^*,S^*)-, (±) and the structural formula is:

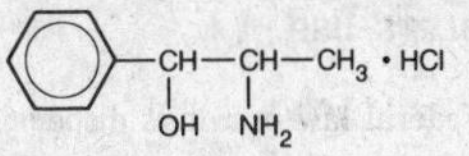

$C_9H_{13}NO.HCl$ Mol. wt. 187.67

Active Ingredients: clemastine fumarate, USP, and phenylpropanolamine HCl, USP.

Inactive Ingredients: colloidal silicon dioxide, NF; D&C Yellow #10; dibasic calcium phosphate dihydrate, USP; lactose, NF; magnesium stearate, NF; methylcellulose, USP; polyethylene glycol, NF; povidone, USP; starch, NF; synthetic polymers; and titanium dioxide, USP.

CLINICAL PHARMACOLOGY

Clemastine fumarate is an antihistamine with anticholinergic (drying) and sedative side effects. Antihistamines appear to compete with histamine for cell receptor sites on effector cells. The inherently long duration of antihistaminic effects of clemastine fumarate has been demonstrated in wheal and flare studies. In normal human subjects who received intradermal histamine injections over a 24-hour period, the antihistaminic activity of clemastine fumarate, as demonstrated by inhibition of the wheal and flare reaction, reached a peak at 5–7 hours, persisted for 10–12 hours and, in some cases, for as long as 24 hours. Pharmacokinetic studies in man utilizing ^3H and ^{14}C labeled compound demonstrate that clemastine fumarate is rapidly and nearly completely absorbed from the gastrointestinal tract, peak plasma concentrations are attained in 2–4 hours, and urinary excretion is the major mode of elimination.

Phenylpropanolamine hydrochloride is an Alpha adrenergic stimulator producing nasal decongestion by constriction of arterioles and precapillary arterioles in the nasal mucosa. Phenylpropanolamine hydrochloride is one of the most widely used oral nasal decongestants; it is similar in action to ephedrine, but produces less central nervous system stimulation.

In adult subjects who were given one Tavist D® (clemastine fumarate and phenylpropanolamine HCl extended-release) tablet, the average peak plasma concentration of phenylpropanolamine was 85.4 ng/mL ± 13.1 (S.D.) which occurred at about 4.3 hours. In this crossover study these same subjects were given a 25 mg phenylpropanolamine hydrochloride tablet every 4 hours for 3 consecutive doses plus a single dose of a TAVIST 1® clemastine fumarate tablet, USP, 1.34 mg. The average peak concentration of phenylpropanolamine was found to be 67.6 ng/mL ± 11.6 (S.D.) which occurred at about 8.2 hours.

In another study, adult subjects received Tavist D® (clemastine fumarate and phenylpropanolamine HCl extended-release) tablets every 12 hours for 4 consecutive days. The average peak concentration of phenylpropanolamine was found to be 117.29 ng/mL ± 14.52 (S.D.) which occurred at about 6.2 hours after the morning dose. In this crossover study these same subjects received a 25 mg phenylpropanolamine hydrochloride tablet every 4 hours for 4 consecutive days. In addition they received a TAVIST 1® clemastine fumarate tablet, USP, 1.34 mg, every 12 hours for 4 consecutive days. The average peak concentration of phenylpropanolamine was found to be 107.92 ng/mL ± 15.97 (S.D.) which occurred at about 4.8 hours after the first dose in the morning.

INDICATIONS AND USAGE

Tavist D® (clemastine fumarate and phenylpropanolamine HCl extended-release) tablets are indicated for the relief of symptoms associated with allergic rhinitis such as sneezing, rhinorrhea, pruritus of the eyes, nose or throat, lacrimation, and nasal congestion.

CONTRAINDICATIONS

Tavist D® (clemastine fumarate and phenylpropanolamine HCl extended-release) tablets are contraindicated in patients hypersensitive to any of the components or to other antihistamines of similar chemical structure. Antihistamines should not be used in newborn or premature infants or in nursing mothers. Antihistamines should not be used to treat lower respiratory tract symptoms including asthma.

Tavist D® (clemastine fumarate and phenylpropanolamine HCl extended-release) tablets are contraindicated in patients receiving monoamine oxidase inhibitors (See *PRECAUTIONS — Drug Interactions*) and in patients with severe hypertension or severe coronary artery disease.

WARNINGS

Antihistamines such as clemastine fumarate should be used with considerable caution in patients with: narrow angle glaucoma, stenosing peptic ulcer, pyloroduodenal obstruction, symptomatic prostatic hypertrophy, and bladder neck obstruction. Sympathomimetic drugs such as phenylpropanolamine hydrochloride should be used with caution in hypertension, cardiovascular disease, diabetes mellitus, and uncontrolled hyperthyroidism.

Use with CNS Depressants: Antihistamines have additive effects with alcohol and other CNS depressants (hypnotics, sedatives, tranquilizers, etc.).

Use in Activities Requiring Mental Alertness: Patients should be warned about engaging in activities requiring mental alertness such as driving a car or operating appliances, machinery, etc.

Use in the Elderly (approximately 60 years or older): Antihistamines are more likely to cause dizziness, sedation, and hypotension in elderly patients. Overdosages of sympathomimetics in this age group may cause hallucinations, convulsions, CNS depression, and death in elderly patients.

Use in Children: Safety and effectiveness of Tavist D® (clemastine fumarate and phenylpropanolamine HCl extended-release) tablets have not been established in children under the age of 12. In infants and children, especially, antihistamines in *overdosage* may cause hallucinations, convulsions, or death. As in adults, antihistamines may diminish mental alertness, but they may also produce excitation, particularly in young children.

PRECAUTIONS

General: Tavist D® (clemastine fumarate and phenylpropanolamine HCl extended-release) tablets should be used with caution in patients with: History of bronchial asthma, increased intraocular pressure, hyperthyroidism, cardiovascular disease, hypertension, diabetes mellitus, and prostate disease. (See *WARNINGS*)

Information for Patients: Patients should be informed of the potential for sedation or drowsiness and warned about driving or operating machinery. The concomitant consumption of alcoholic beverages or other sedative drugs should be avoided.

Due to the inherently long-acting nature of clemastine fumarate and due to the sustained-release of phenylpropanolamine hydrochloride from the tablet's core, Tavist D® (clemastine fumarate and phenylpropanolamine HCl extended-release) tablets provide prolonged symptomatic relief (10–14 hours).

Drug Interactions

1. Monoamine oxidase inhibitors: MAO inhibitors prolong and intensify the anticholinergic effects of antihistamines and potentiate the pressor effects of sympathomimetics.
2. Alcohol and CNS depressants: These agents potentiate the sedative effects of antihistamines.

Continued on next page

Sandoz—Cont.

3. Certain antihypertensives: Sympathomimetics may reduce the antihypertensive effects of methyldopa, mecamylamine, reserpine, and veratrum alkaloids.

Carcinogenesis and Mutagenesis: Carcinogenic studies have not been conducted on the drug combination of clemastine fumarate/phenylpropanolamine hydrochloride. In a two-year oral study in the rat at a dose of 84 mg/kg (about 1500 times the human dose) and an 85-week oral study in the mouse at 206 mg/kg (about 3800 times the human dose), clemastine fumarate showed no evidence of carcinogenesis. No mutagenic studies have been conducted with clemastine fumarate, phenylpropanolamine hydrochloride or the drug combination.

Impairment of Fertility: Oral doses of clemastine fumarate alone in the rat produced a decrease in mating ability of the male at 933 times the human dose. This effect was not found at 466 times the human dose.

Pregnancy: *Category B*—Oral reproduction studies performed with clemastine fumarate alone in rats and rabbits at doses up to 933 and 560 times the human dose, respectively, have revealed no evidence of teratogenic effects. Reproduction studies have not been conducted with phenylpropanolamine hydrochloride alone.

Oral reproduction studies on the drug combination in a ratio of 1 part of clemastine fumarate to 49 parts of phenylpropanolamine hydrochloride in rats and rabbits at doses up to 100 and 67 times the human dose, respectively, have revealed no evidence of teratogenic effects. Adverse reactions attributed to the pharmacological effects of phenylpropanolamine were as follows:

Rats—Impaired weight gain and deaths in dams at 33 times the human dose and a slight increase in pre-implantation loss and prenatal deaths, and reduced fetal weights at 100 times the human dose.

Rabbits—Increased maternal deaths at 20 times the human dose, and increased maternal deaths and weight loss plus a slight increase in prenatal deaths (within normal limits) at 67 times the human dose.

There are no adequate and well controlled studies of Tavist D® (clemastine fumarate and phenylpropanolamine HCl extended-release) tablets in pregnant women. Because animal reproductive studies are not always predictive of human response, this drug should be used in pregnancy only if clearly needed.

Nursing Mothers: (See *CONTRAINDICATIONS*).

ADVERSE REACTIONS

Antihistaminic Compounds: It should be noted that the following reactions have occurred with one or more antihistamines and, therefore, should be kept in mind when prescribing drugs belonging to this class, including clemastine fumarate. The most frequent adverse reactions reported with clemastine fumarate are underlined.

1. *General:* Urticaria, drug rash, anaphylactic shock, photosensitivity, excessive perspiration, chills, dryness of mouth, nose, and throat.
2. *Cardiovascular System:* Hypotension, headache, palpitations, tachycardia, extrasystoles.
3. *Hematologic System:* Hemolytic anemia, thrombocytopenia, agranulocytosis.
4. *Nervous System:* <u>Sedation,</u> <u>sleepiness,</u> <u>dizziness,</u> <u>disturbed coordination,</u> fatigue, confusion, restlessness, excitation, nervousness, tremor, irritability, insomnia, euphoria, paresthesias, blurred vision, diplopia, vertigo, tinnitus, acute labyrinthitis, hysteria, neuritis, convulsions.
5. *Gastrointestinal System:* <u>Epigastric</u> <u>distress,</u> anorexia, nausea, vomiting, diarrhea, constipation.
6. *Genitourinary System:* Urinary frequency, difficult urination, urinary retention, early menses.
7. *Respiratory System:* <u>Thickening</u> <u>of</u> <u>bronchial</u> <u>secretions,</u> tightness of chest and wheezing, nasal stuffiness.

Sympathomimetic Compounds: *Nervous System*—At higher doses may cause drowsiness, dizziness, nervousness, or sleeplessness, and especially in children may cause excitability. Phenylpropanolamine hydrochloride may cause elevated blood pressure and tachyarrhythmias, especially in hyperthyroid patients.

OVERDOSAGE

Antihistamine overdosage reactions may vary from central nervous system depression to stimulation. Stimulation is particularly likely in children. Atropine-like signs and symptoms: dry mouth; fixed, dilated pupils; flushing; and gastrointestinal symptoms may also occur.

Overdosage of the phenylpropanolamine hydrochloride may produce tachycardia, pupillary dilation, excitation, and arrhythmias.

If vomiting has not occurred spontaneously, the conscious patient should be induced to vomit. This is best done by having the patient drink a glass of water or milk along with an appropriate amount of Syrup of Ipecac. Precautions against aspiration must be taken, especially in infants and children.

If vomiting is unsuccessful within 20 minutes, gastric lavage is indicated within 3 hours after ingestion and even later if large amounts of milk or cream were given beforehand. Isotonic and 1/2 isotonic saline is the lavage solution of choice. *Saline cathartics,* such as milk of magnesia, by osmosis draw water into the bowel and therefore are valuable for their action in rapid dilution of bowel content.

Stimulants should *not* be used.

Activated charcoal has been demonstrated to interfere with phenylpropanolamine absorption.

The value of dialysis has not been established.

The concentration of phenylpropanolamine hydrochloride or clemastine fumarate in biological fluids associated with toxicity is not known.

The amount of Tavist D® (clemastine fumarate and phenylpropanolamine HCl extended-release) tablets in single doses associated with significant signs of overdose or death is not known.

The oral LD_{50} for a mixture containing 50 mg phenylpropanolamine hydrochloride and 1.34 mg clemastine fumarate is 1277 mg/kg in mice, 602 mg/kg in rats, and 634 mg/kg in rabbits.

DOSAGE AND ADMINISTRATION

Adults and children twelve years and over: One tablet swallowed whole every twelve hours.

HOW SUPPLIED

Tavist D® (clemastine fumarate and phenylpropanolamine HCl extended-release) tablets: Containing 1.34 mg clemastine fumarate, USP (equivalent to 1 mg of the free base) and 75 mg phenylpropanolamine hydrochloride, USP. White, round, film-coated multiple compressed tablet, engraved "TAVIST D" on both sides. Packages of 100 (NDC 0078-0221-05) and physician's samples in blister packages of 2 (NDC 0078-0221-41).

Store and Dispense

Tablets: Controlled room temperature, between 15°–30°C (59°–86°F) in a tight container.

Blister Packages: Dry place at controlled room temperature, between 15°–30°C (59°–86°F).

SANDOZ
PHARMACEUTICALS
CORPORATION
EAST HANOVER, NJ 07936

[TAD-Z7 Issued April 1, 1992]

Shown in Product Identification Section, page 428

VISKEN® ℞

[vis 'kin]

(pindolol) TABLETS, USP

CAUTION: Federal law prohibits dispensing without prescription.

The following prescribing information is based on official labeling in effect on August 1, 1992.

DESCRIPTION

Visken® (pindolol), a synthetic beta-adrenergic receptor blocking agent with intrinsic sympathomimetic activity is 4-(2-hydroxy-3-isopropylamino-propoxy)-indole.

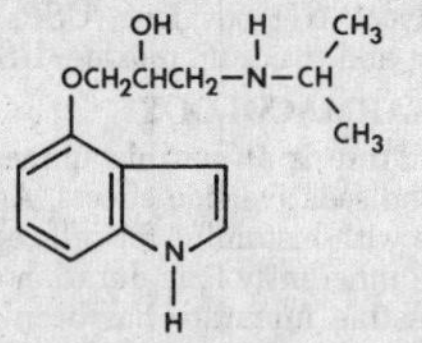

Mol. wt. 248.3

Pindolol is a white to off-white odorless powder soluble in organic solvents and aqueous acids.

5 mg and 10 mg Tablets

Active Ingredient: pindolol

Inactive Ingredients: colloidal silicon dioxide, magnesium stearate, microcrystalline cellulose, and pregelatinized starch.

CLINICAL PHARMACOLOGY

Visken® (pindolol) is a non-selective beta-adrenergic antagonist (beta-blocker) which possesses intrinsic sympathomimetic activity (ISA) in therapeutic dosage ranges but does not possess quinidine-like membrane stabilizing activity.

PHARMACODYNAMICS

In standard pharmacologic tests in man and animals, Visken® (pindolol) attenuates increases in heart rate, systolic blood pressure, and cardiac output resulting from exercise and isoproterenol administration, thus confirming its beta-blocking properties. The ISA or partial agonist activity of Visken® (pindolol) is mediated directly at the adrenergic receptor sites and may be blocked by other beta-blockers. In catecholamine depleted animal experiments, ISA is manifested as an increase in the inotropic and chronotropic activity of the myocardium. In man, ISA is manifested by a smaller reduction in the resting heart rate (4-8 beats/min) than is seen with drugs lacking ISA. There is also a smaller reduction in resting cardiac output. The clinical significance of this observation has not been evaluated and there is no evidence, or reason to believe, that exercise cardiac output is less affected by Visken® (pindolol).

Visken® (pindolol) has been shown in controlled, double-blind clinical studies to be an effective antihypertensive agent when used as monotherapy, or when added to therapy with thiazide-type diuretics. Divided dosages in the range of 10-60 mg daily have been shown to be effective. As monotherapy, Visken® (pindolol) is as effective as propranolol, α-methyldopa, hydrochlorothiazide, and chlorthalidone in reducing systolic and diastolic blood pressure. The effect on blood pressure is not orthostatic, i.e. Visken® (pindolol) was equally effective in reducing the supine and standing blood pressure.

In open, long-term studies up to 4 years, no evidence of diminution of the blood pressure lowering response was observed. An average 3-pound increase in body weight has been noted in patients treated with Visken® (pindolol) alone, a larger increase than was observed with propranolol or placebo. The weight gain appeared unrelated to blood pressure response and was not associated with an increased risk of heart failure, although edema was more common than in control patients. Visken® (pindolol) does not have a consistent effect on plasma renin activity.

The mechanism of the antihypertensive effects of beta-blocking agents has not been established, but several mechanisms have been postulated: 1) an effect on the central nervous system resulting in a reduced sympathetic outflow to the periphery, 2) competitive antagonism of catecholamines at peripheral (especially cardiac) adrenergic receptor sites, leading to decreased cardiac output, 3) an inhibition of renin release. These mechanisms appear less likely for pindolol than other beta-blockers in view of the modest effect on resting cardiac output and renin.

Beta-blockade therapy is useful when it is necessary to suppress the effects of beta-adrenergic agonists in order to achieve therapeutic goals. However, in certain clinical situations, (e.g., cardiac failure, heart block, bronchospasm), the preservation of an adequate sympathetic tone may be necessary to maintain vital functions. Although a beta-antagonist with ISA such as Visken® (pindolol) does not eliminate sympathetic tone entirely, there is no controlled evidence that it is safer than other beta-blockers in such conditions as heart failure, heart block, or bronchospasm or is less likely to cause those conditions. In single dose studies of the effects of beta-blockers on FEV_1, Visken® (pindolol) was indistinguishable from other non-cardioselective agents in its reduction of FEV_1, and its reduction in the effectiveness of an exogenous beta agonist.

Exacerbation of angina and, in some cases, myocardial infarction and ventricular dysrhythmias have been reported after abrupt discontinuation of therapy with beta-adrenergic blocking agents in patients with coronary artery disease. Abrupt withdrawal of these agents in patients without coronary artery disease has resulted in transient symptoms, including tremulousness, sweating, palpitation, headache, and malaise. Several mechanisms have been proposed to explain these phenomena, among them increased sensitivity to catecholamines because of increased numbers of beta receptors.

PHARMACOKINETICS AND METABOLISM

Visken® (pindolol) is rapidly and reproducibly absorbed (greater than 95%), achieving peak plasma concentrations within 1 hour of drug administration. Visken® (pindolol) has no significant first-pass effect. The blood concentrations are proportional in a linear manner to the administered dose in the range of 5-20 mg. Upon repeated administration to the same subject, variation is minimal. After a single dose, intersubject variation for peak plasma concentrations was about 4 fold (e.g., 45-167 ng/mL for a 20 mg dose). Upon multiple dosing, intersubject variation decreased to 2-2.5 fold. Visken® (pindolol) is only 40% bound to plasma proteins and is evenly distributed between plasma and red cells. The volume of distribution in healthy subjects is about 2 L/kg.

Visken® (pindolol) undergoes extensive metabolism in animals and man. In man, 35%-40% is excreted unchanged in the urine and 60%-65% is metabolized primarily to hydroxy-metabolites which are excreted as glucuronides and ethereal sulfates. The polar metabolites are excreted with a half-life of approximately 8 hours and thus multiple dosing therapy (q.8H) results in a less than 50% accumulation in plasma. About 6%-9% of an administered intravenous dose is excreted by the bile into the feces.

The disposition of Visken® (pindolol) after oral administration is monophasic with a half-life in healthy subjects or hypertensive patients with normal renal function of approximately 3-4 hours. Following t.i.d. administration (q.8H), no significant accumulation of Visken® (pindolol) is observed.

In elderly hypertensive patients with normal renal function, the half-life of Visken® (pindolol) is more variable, averaging about 7 hours, but with values as high as 15 hours.

In hypertensive patients with renal diseases, the half-life is within the range expected for healthy subjects. However, a significant decrease (50%) in volume of distribution (V_D) is

observed in uremic patients and V_D appears to be directly correlated to creatinine clearance. Therefore, renal drug clearance is significantly reduced in uremic patients, resulting in a significant decrease in urinary excretion of unchanged drug. Uremic patients with a creatinine clearance of less than 20 mL/min generally excreted less than 15% of the administered dose unchanged in the urine.
In patients with histologically diagnosed cirrhosis of the liver, the elimination of Visken® (pindolol) was more variable in rate and generally significantly slower than in healthy subjects. The total body clearance of Visken® (pindolol) in cirrhotic patients ranged from about 50-300 mL/min and was directly correlated to antipyrine clearance. The half-life ranges from 2.5 hours to greater than 30 hours. These findings strongly suggest that caution should be exercised in dosage adjustments of Visken® (pindolol) in such patients.
The bioavailability of Visken® (pindolol) is not significantly affected by co-administration of food, hydralazine, hydrochlorothiazide or aspirin. Visken® (pindolol) has no effect on warfarin activity or the clinical effectiveness of digoxin, although small transient decreases in plasma digoxin concentrations were noted.

INDICATIONS AND USAGE

Visken® (pindolol) is indicated in the management of hypertension. It may be used alone or concomitantly with other antihypertensive agents, particularly with a thiazide-type diuretic.

CONTRAINDICATIONS

Visken® (pindolol) is contraindicated in: 1) bronchial asthma; 2) overt cardiac failure; 3) cardiogenic shock; 4) second and third degree heart block; 5) severe bradycardia. *(See WARNINGS)*

WARNINGS

Cardiac Failure: Sympathetic stimulation may be a vital component supporting circulatory function in patients with congestive heart failure, and its inhibition by beta-blockade may precipitate more severe failure. Although beta-blockers should be avoided in overt congestive heart failure, if necessary, Visken® (pindolol) can be used with caution in patients with a history of failure who are well-compensated, usually with digitalis and diuretics. Beta-adrenergic blocking agents do not abolish the inotropic action of digitalis on heart muscle.

In Patients Without History of Cardiac Failure: In patients with latent cardiac insufficiency, continued depression of the myocardium with beta-blocking agents over a period of time can in some cases lead to cardiac failure. At the first sign or symptom of impending cardiac failure, patients should be fully digitalized and/or be given a diuretic, and the response observed closely. If cardiac failure continues, despite adequate digitalization and diuretic, Visken® (pindolol) therapy should be withdrawn (gradually if possible).

Exacerbation of Ischemic Heart Disease Following Abrupt Withdrawal: Hypersensitivity to catecholamines has been observed in patients withdrawn from beta-blocker therapy; exacerbation of angina and, in some cases, myocardial infarction have occurred after *abrupt* discontinuation of such therapy. When discontinuing chronically administered Visken® (pindolol), particularly in patients with ischemic heart disease, the dosage should be gradually reduced over a period of 1-2 weeks and the patient should be carefully monitored. If angina markedly worsens or acute coronary insufficiency develops, Visken® (pindolol) administration should be reinstituted promptly, at least temporarily, and other measures appropriate for the management of unstable angina should be taken. Patients should be warned against interruption or discontinuation of therapy without the physician's advice. Because coronary artery disease is common and may be unrecognized, it may be prudent not to discontinue Visken® (pindolol) therapy abruptly even in patients treated only for hypertension.

Nonallergic Bronchospasm (e.g., chronic bronchitis, emphysema)—Patients with Bronchospastic Diseases Should in General Not Receive Beta-Blockers: Visken® (pindolol) should be administered with caution since it may block bronchodilation produced by endogenous or exogenous catecholamine stimulation of $beta_2$ receptors.

Major Surgery: Because beta blockade impairs the ability of the heart to respond to reflex stimuli and may increase the risks of general anesthesia and surgical procedures, resulting in protracted hypotension or low cardiac output, it has generally been suggested that such therapy should be withdrawn several days prior to surgery. Recognition of the increased sensitivity to catecholamines of patients recently withdrawn from beta-blocker therapy, however, has made this recommendation controversial. If possible, beta-blockers should be withdrawn well before surgery takes place. In the event of emergency surgery, the anesthesiologist should be informed that the patient is on beta-blocker therapy.
The effects of Visken® (pindolol) can be reversed by administration of beta-receptor agonists such as isoproterenol, dopamine, dobutamine, or levarterenol. Difficulty in restarting and maintaining the heart beat has also been reported with beta-adrenergic receptor blocking agents.

Diabetes and Hypoglycemia: Beta-adrenergic blockade may prevent the appearance of premonitory signs and symptoms (e.g., tachycardia and blood pressure changes) of acute hypoglycemia. This is especially important with labile diabetics. Beta-blockade also reduces the release of insulin in response to hyperglycemia; therefore, it may be necessary to adjust the dose of antidiabetic drugs.

Thyrotoxicosis: Beta-adrenergic blockade may mask certain clinical signs (e.g., tachycardia) of hyperthyroidism. Patients suspected of developing thyrotoxicosis should be managed carefully to avoid abrupt withdrawal of beta-blockade which might precipitate a thyroid crisis.

PRECAUTIONS

Impaired Renal or Hepatic Function: Beta-blocking agents should be used with caution in patients with impaired hepatic or renal function. Poor renal function has only minor effects on Visken® (pindolol) clearance, but poor hepatic function may cause blood levels of Visken® (pindolol) to increase substantially.

Information for Patients: Patients, especially those with evidence of coronary artery insufficiency, should be warned against interruption or discontinuation of Visken® (pindolol) therapy without the physician's advice. Although cardiac failure rarely occurs in properly selected patients, patients being treated with beta-adrenergic blocking agents should be advised to consult the physician at the first sign or symptom of impending failure.

Drug Interactions: Catecholamine-depleting drugs (e.g., reserpine) may have an additive effect when given with beta-blocking agents. Patients receiving Visken® (pindolol) plus a catecholamine-depleting agent should, therefore, be closely observed for evidence of hypotension and/or marked bradycardia which may produce vertigo, syncope, or postural hypotension.
Visken® (pindolol) has been used with a variety of antihypertensive agents, including hydrochlorothiazide, hydralazine, and guanethidine without unexpected adverse interactions.
Visken® (pindolol) has been shown to increase serum thioridazine levels when both drugs are co-administered. Visken® (pindolol) levels may also be increased with this combination.

Carcinogenesis, Mutagenesis, Impairment of Fertility: In chronic oral toxicologic studies (1-2 years) in mice, rats, and dogs, Visken® (pindolol) did not produce any significant toxic effects. In 2-year oral carcinogenicity studies in rats and mice in doses as high as 59 mg/kg/day and 124 mg/kg/day (50 and 100 times the maximum recommended human dose), respectively, Visken® (pindolol) did not produce any neoplastic, preneoplastic, or nonneoplastic pathologic lesions. In fertility and general reproductive performance studies in rats, Visken® (pindolol) caused no adverse effects at a dose of 10 mg/kg.
In the male fertility and general reproductive performance test in rats, definite toxicity characterized by mortality and decreased weight gain was observed in the group given 100 mg/kg/day. At 30 mg/kg/day, decreased mating was associated with testicular atrophy and/or decreased spermatogenesis. This response is not clearly drug related, however, as there was no dose response relationship within this experiment and no similar effect on testes of rats administered Visken® (pindolol) as a dietary admixture for 104 weeks. There appeared to be an increase in prenatal mortality in males given 100 mg/kg but development of offspring was not impaired.
In females administered Visken® (pindolol) prior to mating through day 21 of lactation, mating behavior was decreased at 100 mg/kg and 30 mg/kg. At these dosages there also was increased mortality of offspring. Prenatal mortality was increased at 10 mg/kg but there was not a clear dose response relationship in this experiment. There was an increased resorption rate at 100 mg/kg observed in females necropsied on the 15th day of gestation.

Pregnancy—Category B: Studies in rats and rabbits exceeding 100 times the maximum recommended human doses, revealed no embryotoxicity or teratogenicity. Since there are no adequate and well-controlled studies in pregnant women, and since animal reproduction studies are not always predictive of human response, Visken® (pindolol), as with any drug, should be employed during pregnancy only if the potential benefit justifies the potential risk to the fetus.

Nursing Mothers: Since Visken® (pindolol) is secreted in human milk, nursing should not be undertaken by mothers receiving the drug.

Pediatric Use: Safety and effectiveness in children have not been established.

CLINICAL LABORATORY

Minor persistent elevations in serum transaminases (SGOT, SGPT) have been noted in 7% of patients during Visken® (pindolol) administration, but progressive elevations were not observed and liver injury has not been reported in the medical literature over a 10-year period of marketing. Alkaline phosphatase, lactic acid dehydrogenase (LDH), and uric acid are also elevated on rare occasions. The significance of these findings is unknown.

ADVERSE REACTIONS

Most adverse reactions have been mild. The incidences listed in the following table are derived from 12-week comparative double-blind, parallel design trials in hypertensive patients given Visken® (pindolol) as monotherapy, given various active control drugs as monotherapy, or given placebo. Data for Visken® (pindolol) and the positive controls were pooled from several trials because no striking differences were seen in the individual studies, with 1 exception. When considering all adverse reactions reported, the frequency of edema was noticeably higher in positive control trials [16% Visken® (pindolol) vs. 9% positive control] than in placebo controlled trials [6% Visken® (pindolol) vs. 3% placebo]. The table includes adverse reactions either volunteered or elicited, and at least possibly drug related, which were reported in greater than 2% of Visken® (pindolol) patients and other selected important reactions.
[See table above.]

Adverse Reactions which were Volunteered or Elicited (and at least possibly drug related)

Body System/Adverse Reactions	Visken® (pindolol) (N = 322) %	Active Controls* (N = 188) %	Placebo (N = 78) %
Central Nervous System			
Bizarre or Many Dreams	5	0	6
Dizziness	9	11	1
Fatigue	8	4	4
Hallucinations	<1	0	0
Insomnia	10	3	10
Nervousness	7	3	5
Weakness	4	2	1
Autonomic Nervous System			
Paresthesia	3	1	6
Cardiovascular			
Dyspnea	5	4	6
Edema	6	3	1
Heart Failure	<1	<1	0
Palpitations	<1	1	0
Musculoskeletal			
Chest Pain	3	1	3
Joint Pain	7	4	4
Muscle Cramps	3	1	0
Muscle Pain	10	9	8
Gastrointestinal			
Abdominal Discomfort	4	4	5
Nausea	5	2	1
Skin			
Pruritus	1	<1	0
Rash	<1	<1	1

*Active Controls: Patients received either propranolol, α-methyldopa or a diuretic (hydrochlorothiazide or chlorthalidone).

The following selected (potentially important) adverse reactions were seen in 2% or fewer patients and their relation-

Continued on next page

Sandoz—Cont.

ship to Visken® (pindolol) is uncertain. CENTRAL NERVOUS SYSTEM: anxiety, lethargy; AUTONOMIC NERVOUS SYSTEM: visual disturbances, hyperhidrosis; CARDIOVASCULAR: bradycardia, claudication, cold extremities, heart block, hypotension, syncope, tachycardia, weight gain; GASTROINTESTINAL: diarrhea, vomiting; RESPIRATORY: wheezing; UROGENITAL: impotence, pollakiuria; MISCELLANEOUS: eye discomfort or burning eyes.

POTENTIAL ADVERSE EFFECTS

In addition, other adverse effects not aforementioned have been reported with other beta-adrenergic blocking agents and should be considered potential adverse effects of Visken® (pindolol).
Central Nervous System: Reversible mental depression progressing to catatonia; an acute reversible syndrome characterized by disorientation for time and place, short-term memory loss, emotional lability, slightly clouded sensorium, and decreased performance on neuropsychometrics.
Cardiovascular: Intensification of AV block. *(See CONTRAINDICATIONS)*
Allergic: Erythematous rash; fever combined with aching and sore throat; laryngospasm; respiratory distress.
Hematologic: Agranulocytosis; thrombocytopenic and non-thrombocytopenic purpura.
Gastrointestinal: Mesenteric arterial thrombosis; ischemic colitis.
Miscellaneous: Reversible alopecia; Peyronie's disease.
The oculomucocutaneous syndrome associated with the beta-blocker practolol has not been reported with Visken® (pindolol) during investigational use and extensive foreign experience amounting to over 4 million patient-years.

OVERDOSAGE

No specific information on emergency treatment of overdosage is available. Therefore, on the basis of the pharmacologic actions of Visken® (pindolol), the following general measures should be employed as appropriate in addition to gastric lavage:
Excessive Bradycardia: administer atropine; if there is no response to vagal blockade, administer isoproterenol cautiously.
Cardiac Failure: digitalize the patient and/or administer diuretic. It has been reported that glucagon may be useful in this situation.
Hypotension: administer vasopressors, e.g., epinephrine or levarterenol, with serial monitoring of blood pressure. (There is evidence that epinephrine may be the drug of choice.)
Bronchospasm: administer a beta$_2$ stimulating agent such as isoproterenol and/or a theophylline derivative.
A case of an acute overdosage has been reported with an intake of 500 mg of Visken® (pindolol) by a hypertensive patient. Blood pressure increased and heart rate was ≥80 beats/min. Recovery was uneventful. In another case, 250 mg of Visken® (pindolol) was taken with 150 mg diazepam and 50 mg nitrazepam, producing coma and hypotension. The patient recovered in 24 hours.

DOSAGE AND ADMINISTRATION

The dosage of Visken® (pindolol) should be individualized. The recommended initial dose of Visken® (pindolol) is 5 mg b.i.d. alone or in combination with other antihypertensive agents. An antihypertensive response usually occurs within the first week of treatment. Maximal response, however, may take as long as or occasionally longer than 2 weeks. If a satisfactory reduction in blood pressure does not occur within 3-4 weeks, the dose may be adjusted in increments of 10 mg/day at these intervals up to a maximum of 60 mg/day.

HOW SUPPLIED

White, uncoated, heart-shaped tablets; 5 mg and 10 mg, packages of 100. 5 mg tablets engraved "VISKEN 5" on one side, and embossed "V" on other side (NDC 0078-0111-05). 10 mg tablets engraved "VISKEN 10" on one side, and embossed "V" on other side (NDC 0078-0073-05).
Store and Dispense: Below 86°F (30°C); tight, light-resistant container.

[VIS-Z12 Issued March 15, 1990]
Shown in Product Identification Section, page 428

Products are cross-indexed
by product classifications
in the
BLUE SECTION.

Sanofi Winthrop Pharmaceuticals
**90 PARK AVENUE
NEW YORK, NY 10016**

Winthrop Pharmaceuticals' products are now distributed by Sanofi Winthrop Pharmaceuticals.

ARALEN® Hydrochloride   ℞
**brand of chloroquine hydrochloride
injection, USP**

> For Malaria and
> Extraintestinal Amebiasis

> WARNING: PHYSICIANS SHOULD COMPLETELY FAMILIARIZE THEMSELVES WITH THE COMPLETE CONTENTS OF THIS LEAFLET BEFORE PRESCRIBING ARALEN.

DESCRIPTION

Parenteral solution, each mL containing 50 mg of the dihydrochloride salt equivalent to 40 mg of chloroquine base. ARALEN hydrochloride, a 4-aminoquinoline compound, is chemically 7- (Chloro - 4 - [[4 - diethylamino) - 1 - methylbutyl] amino]-quinoline dihydrochloride, a white, crystalline substance, freely soluble in water.

ACTIONS

The compound is a highly active antimalarial and amebicidal agent.
ARALEN hydrochloride has been found to be highly active against the erythrocytic forms of *Plasmodium vivax* and *malariae* and most strains of *Plasmodium falciparum* (but not the gametocytes of *P. falciparum*). The precise mechanism of action of the drug is not known.
ARALEN hydrochloride does not prevent relapses in patients with vivax or malariae malaria because it is not effective against exoerythrocytic forms of the parasite, nor will it prevent vivax or malariae infection when administered as a prophylactic. It is highly effective as a suppressive agent in patients with vivax or malariae malaria, in terminating acute attacks, and significantly lengthening the interval between treatment and relapse. In patients with falciparum malaria it abolishes the acute attack and effects complete cure of the infection, unless due to a resistant strain of *P. falciparum.*

INDICATIONS

ARALEN hydrochloride is indicated for the treatment of extraintestinal amebiasis and for treatment of acute attacks of malaria due to *P. vivax, P. malariae, P. ovale,* and susceptible strains of *P. falciparum* when oral therapy is not feasible.

CONTRAINDICATIONS

Use of this drug is contraindicated in the presence of retinal or visual field changes either attributable to 4- aminoquinoline compounds or to any other etiology, and in patients with known hypersensitivity to 4-aminoquinoline compounds. However, in the treatment of acute attacks of malaria caused by susceptible strains of plasmodia, the physician may elect to use this drug after carefully weighing the possible benefits and risks to the patient.

WARNINGS

Children and infants are extremely susceptible to adverse effects from an overdose of parenteral ARALEN and sudden deaths have been recorded after such administration. In no instance should the single dose of parenteral ARALEN administered to infants or children exceed 5 mg base per kg.
In recent years it has been found that certain strains of *P. falciparum* have become resistant to 4-aminoquinoline compounds (including chloroquine and hydroxychloroquine) as shown by the fact that normally adequate doses have failed to prevent or cure clinical malaria or parasitemia. Treatment with quinine or other specific forms of therapy is therefore advised for patients infected with a resistant strain of parasites.
Use of ARALEN should be avoided in patients with psoriasis, for it may precipitate a severe attack of psoriasis. Some authors consider the use of 4-aminoquinoline compounds contraindicated in patients with porphyria since the condition may be exacerbated.
Irreversible retinal damage has been observed in some patients who had received long-term or high-dosage 4-aminoquinoline therapy. Retinopathy has been reported to be dose related.
If there is any indication (past or present) of abnormality in the visual acuity, visual field, or retinal macular areas (such

as pigmentary changes, loss of foveal reflex), or any visual symptoms (such as light flashes and streaks) which are not fully explainable by difficulties of accommodation or corneal opacities, the drug should be discontinued immediately and the patient closely observed for possible progression. Retinal changes (and visual disturbances) may progress even after cessation of therapy.
Usage in Pregnancy. Usage of this drug during pregnancy should be avoided except in the suppression or treatment of malaria when in the judgment of the physician the benefit outweighs the possible hazard. It should be noted that radioactively tagged chloroquine administered intravenously to pregnant pigmented CBA mice passed rapidly across the placenta, accumulated selectively in the melanin structures of the fetal eyes and was retained in the ocular tissues for five months after the drug had been eliminated from the rest of the body.[1]

PRECAUTIONS

Since the drug is known to concentrate in the liver, it should be used with caution in patients with hepatic disease or alcoholism or in conjunction with known hepatotoxic drugs.
The drug should be administered with caution to patients having G-6-PD (glucose-6-phosphate dehydrogenase) deficiency.

ADVERSE REACTIONS

Respiratory depression, cardiovascular collapse, shock, convulsions, and death have been reported with overdoses of ARALEN hydrochloride, brand of chloroquine hydrochloride injection, especially in infants and children.
Any of the adverse reactions associated with short-term oral administration of chloroquine phosphate must be considered a possibility with chloroquine hydrochloride. Cardiovascular effects, such as hypotension and electrocardiographic changes (particularly inversion or depression of the T-wave, widening of the QRS complex), have rarely been noted in patients receiving usual antimalarial doses of the drug. Mild and transient headache, pruritus, psychic stimulation, visual disturbances (blurring of vision and difficulty of focusing or accommodation), pleomorphic skin eruptions, and gastrointestinal complaints (anorexia, nausea, vomiting, diarrhea, abdominal cramps) have been observed.
Instances of convulsive seizures associated with oral chloroquine therapy in patients with extraintestinal amebiasis have been reported.
A few cases of a nerve type of deafness have been reported after prolonged therapy, usually in high doses. Tinnitus and reduced hearing have been reported, in a patient with preexistent auditory damage, after administration of only 500 mg once a week for a few months. Since neuromyopathy, blood dyscrasias, lichen planus-like eruptions, and skin and mucosal pigmentary changes have been noted during prolonged oral therapy, their occurrence with this dosage form is possible.
Patients with retinal changes may be asymptomatic, especially in early cases, or may complain of nyctalopia and scotomatous vision with field defects of paracentral, pericentral ring types, and typically temporal scotomas, eg, difficulty in reading with words tending to disappear, seeing only half an object, misty vision, and fog before the eyes. Rarely scotomatous vision may occur without observable retinal changes.

DOSAGE AND ADMINISTRATION

Malaria —**Adult Dose.** An initial dose of 4 mL or 5 mL (160 mg to 200 mg chloroquine base) may be injected intramuscularly and repeated in 6 hours if necessary. The total parenteral dosage in the first 24 hours should not exceed 800 mg chloroquine base. Treatment by mouth should be started as soon as practicable and continued until a course of approximately 1.5 g of base in 3 days is completed.
Pediatric Dose. Infants and children are extremely susceptible to overdosage of parenteral ARALEN. Severe reactions and deaths have occurred. In the pediatric age range, parenteral ARALEN dosage should be calculated in proportion to the adult dose based upon body weight. The recommended single dose in infants and children is 5 mg base per kg. This dose may be repeated in 6 hours; however, the total dose in any 24 hour period should not exceed 10 mg base per kg of body weight. Parenteral administration should be terminated and oral therapy instituted as soon as possible.
Extraintestinal Amebiasis —In adult patients not able to tolerate oral therapy, from 4 mL to 5 mL (160 mg to 200 mg chloroquine base) may be injected daily for 10 to 12 days. Oral administration should be substituted or resumed as soon as possible.

OVERDOSAGE

Inadvertent toxic doses may produce respiratory depression or shock with hypotension. Respiratory depression is treated by artificial respiration and administration of oxygen. In shock with hypotension, a potent vasopressor, such as NEO-SYNEPHRINE® hydrochloride, brand of phenylephrine hydrochloride, USP, should be given intramuscularly in doses of 2 mg to 5 mg.

HOW SUPPLIED
Ampuls of 5 mL, box of 5 (NDC 0024-0074-01)

REFERENCE
Ullberg S, Lindquist N G, Sjostrand S E: Accumulation of chorio-retinotoxic drugs in the foetal eye. *Nature* 1970; 227:1257.

AW-100-H

ARALEN® Phosphate ℞
brand of chloroquine phosphate tablets, USP

For Malaria and Extraintestinal Amebiasis

WARNING
PHYSICIANS SHOULD COMPLETELY FAMILIARIZE THEMSELVES WITH THE COMPLETE CONTENTS OF THIS LEAFLET BEFORE PRESCRIBING ARALEN.

DESCRIPTION
ARALEN phosphate, brand of chloroquine phosphate, USP, is a 4-aminoquinoline compound for oral administration. It is a white, odorless, bitter tasting, crystalline substance, freely soluble in water.
ARALEN phosphate is an antimalarial and amebicidal drug. Chemically, it is 7-chloro- 4-[[4- (diethylamino) -1-methylbutyl]amino] quinoline phosphate (1:2).
Inactive Ingredients: Acacia, Carnauba Wax, D&C Red #7, Dibasic Calcium Phosphate, Gelatin, Kaolin, Liquid Glucose, Magnesium Stearate, Parabens, Pharmaceutical Glaze, Povidone, Sodium Benzoate, Starch, Sucrose, Talc, Titanium Dioxide, Yellow Wax.

CLINICAL PHARMACOLOGY
ARALEN phosphate has been found to be highly active against the erythrocytic forms of *Plasmodium vivax* and *Plasmodium malariae* and most strains of *Plasmodium falciparum* (but not the gametocytes of *P. falciparum*).
The mechanism of plasmodicidal action of chloroquine is not completely certain. While the drug can inhibit certain enzymes, its effect is believed to result, at least in part, from its interaction with DNA.
Chloroquine is rapidly and almost completely absorbed from the gastrointestinal tract, and only a small proportion of the administered dose is found in the stools. Approximately 55% of the drug in the plasma is bound to nondiffusible plasma constituents. Excretion of chloroquine is quite slow, but is increased by acidification of the urine. Chloroquine is deposited in the tissues in considerable amounts. In animals, from 200 to 700 times the plasma concentration may be found in the liver, spleen, kidney, and lung; leukocytes also concentrate the drug. The brain and spinal cord, in contrast, contain only 10 to 30 times the amount present in plasma.
Chloroquine undergoes appreciable degradation in the body. The main metabolite is desethylchloroquine, which accounts for one fourth of the total material appearing in the urine; bisdesethylchloroquine, a carboxylic acid derivative, and other metabolic products as yet uncharacterized are found in small amounts. Slightly more than half of the urinary drug products can be accounted for as unchanged chloroquine.

Microbiology
ARALEN phosphate has been found to be highly active against the erythrocytic forms of *Plasmodium vivax* and *malariae* and most strains of *Plasmodium falciparum* (but not the gametocytes of *P. falciparum*). The precise mechanism of action of the drug is not known.
In vitro studies with trophozoites of *Entamoeba histolytica* have demonstrated that ARALEN phosphate also possesses amebicidal activity comparable to that of emetine.

INDICATIONS AND USAGE
ARALEN phosphate, brand of chloroquine phosphate, is indicated for the suppressive treatment and for acute attacks of malaria due to *P. vivax, P. malariae, P. ovale,* and susceptible strains of *P. falciparum.* The drug is also indicated for the treatment of extraintestinal amebiasis.
ARALEN phosphate does not prevent relapses in patients with vivax or malariae malaria because it is not effective against exoerythrocytic forms of the parasite, nor will it prevent vivax or malariae infection when administered as a prophylactic. It is highly effective as a suppressive agent in patients with vivax or malariae malaria, in terminating acute attacks, and significantly lengthening the interval between treatment and relapse. In patients with falciparum malaria it abolishes the acute attack and effects complete cure of the infection, unless due to a resistant strain of *P. falciparum.*

CONTRAINDICATIONS
Use of this drug is contraindicated in the presence of retinal or visual field changes either attributable to 4-aminoquinoline compounds or to any other etiology, and in patients with known hypersensitivity to 4-aminoquinoline compounds. However, in the treatment of acute attacks of malaria caused by susceptible strains of plasmodia, the physician may elect to use this drug after carefully weighing the possible benefits and risks to the patient.

WARNINGS
In recent years it has been found that certain strains of *P. falciparum* have become resistant to 4-aminoquinoline compounds (including chloroquine and hydroxychloroquine) as shown by the fact that normally adequate doses have failed to prevent or cure clinical malaria or parasitemia. Treatment with quinine or other specific forms of therapy is therefore advised for patients infected with a resistant strain of parasites.
Irreversible retinal damage has been observed in some patients who had received long-term or high-dosage 4-aminoquinoline therapy. Retinopathy has been reported to be dose related.
When prolonged therapy with any antimalarial compound is contemplated, initial (base line) and periodic ophthalmologic examinations (including visual acuity, expert slit-lamp, funduscopic, and visual field tests) should be performed.
If there is any indication (past or present) of abnormality in the visual acuity, visual field, or retinal macular areas (such as pigmentary changes, loss of foveal reflex), or any visual symptoms (such as light flashes and streaks) which are not fully explainable by difficulties of accommodation or corneal opacities, the drug should be discontinued immediately and the patient closely observed for possible progression. Retinal changes (and visual disturbances) may progress even after cessation of therapy.
All patients on long-term therapy with this preparation should be questioned and examined periodically, including testing knee and ankle reflexes, to detect any evidence of muscular weakness. If weakness occurs, discontinue the drug.
A number of fatalities have been reported following the accidental ingestion of chloroquine, sometimes in relatively small doses (0.75 g or 1 g chloroquine phosphate in one 3-year-old child). Patients should be strongly warned to keep this drug out of the reach of children because they are especially sensitive to the 4-aminoquinoline compounds.
Use of ARALEN phosphate, brand of chloroquine phosphate tablets, in patients with psoriasis may precipitate a severe attack of psoriasis. When used in patients with porphyria the condition may be exacerbated. The drug should not be used in these conditions unless in the judgment of the physician the benefit to the patient outweighs the possible hazard.

PRECAUTIONS

General
If any severe blood disorder appears which is not attributable to the disease under treatment, discontinuance of the drug should be considered.
Since this drug is known to concentrate in the liver, it should be used with caution in patients with hepatic disease or alcoholism or in conjunction with known hepatotoxic drugs.
The drug should be administered with caution to patients having G-6-PD (glucose-6-phosphate dehydrogenase) deficiency.

Laboratory Tests
Complete blood cell counts should be made periodically if patients are given prolonged therapy.

Nursing Mothers
Because of the potential for serious adverse reactions in nursing infants from chloroquine, a decision should be made whether to discontinue nursing or to discontinue the drug, taking into account the importance of the drug to the mother.

Pediatric Use
See WARNINGS and DOSAGE AND ADMINISTRATION.

ADVERSE REACTIONS
Ocular reactions: Irreversible retinal damage in patients receiving long-term or high-dosage 4-aminoquinoline therapy; visual disturbances (blurring of vision and difficulty of focusing or accommodation); nyctalopia; scotomatous vision with field defects of paracentral, pericentral ring types, and typically temporal scotomas, eg, difficulty in reading with words tending to disappear, seeing half an object, misty vision, and fog before the eyes.
Neuromuscular reactions: Convulsive seizures.
Auditory reactions: Nerve type deafness; tinnitus, reduced hearing in patients with preexisting auditory damage.
Gastrointestinal reactions: Anorexia, nausea, vomiting, diarrhea, abdominal cramps.
Dermatologic reactions: Pleomorphic skin eruptions, skin and mucosal pigmentary changes; lichen planus-like eruptions, pruritus, and hair loss.
CNS reactions: Mild and transient headache, psychic stimulation.
Cardiovascular reactions: Rarely, hypotension, electrocardiographic change.

OVERDOSAGE
Symptoms: Chloroquine is very rapidly and completely absorbed after ingestion. Toxic doses of chloroquine can be fatal. As little as 1 g may be fatal in children. Toxic symptoms can occur within minutes. These consist of headache, drowsiness, visual disturbances, nausea and vomiting, cardiovascular collapse, and convulsions followed by sudden and early respiratory and cardiac arrest. The electrocardiogram may reveal atrial standstill, nodal rhythm, prolonged intraventricular conduction time, and progressive bradycardia leading to ventricular fibrillation and/or arrest.
Treatment: Treatment is symptomatic and must be prompt with immediate evacuation of the stomach by emesis (at home, before transportation to the hospital) or gastric lavage until the stomach is completely emptied. If finely powdered, activated charcoal is introduced by stomach tube, after lavage, and within 30 minutes after ingestion of the antimalarial, it may inhibit further intestinal absorption of the drug. To be effective, the dose of activated charcoal should be at least five times the estimated dose of chloroquine ingested.
Convulsions, if present, should be controlled before attempting gastric lavage. If due to cerebral stimulation, cautious administration of an ultra short-acting barbiturate may be tried but, if due to anoxia, it should be corrected by oxygen administration and artificial respiration. In shock with hypotension, a potent vasopressor should be administered. Because of the importance of supporting respiration, tracheal intubation or tracheostomy, followed by gastric lavage, may also be necessary. Peritoneal dialysis and exchange transfusions have also been suggested to reduce the level of the drug in the blood.
A patient who survives the acute phase and is asymptomatic should be closely observed for at least six hours. Fluids may be forced, and sufficient ammonium chloride (8 g daily in divided doses for adults) may be administered for a few days to acidify the urine to help promote urinary excretion in cases of both overdosage or sensitivity.

DOSAGE AND ADMINISTRATION
The dosage of chloroquine phosphate is often expressed or calculated as the base. Each 500 mg tablet of ARALEN phosphate, brand of chloroquine phosphate, is equivalent to 300 mg base. In infants and children the dosage is preferably calculated on the body weight.
Malaria: Suppression—**Adult Dose:** 500 mg (= 300 mg base) on exactly the same day of each week.
Pediatric Dose: The weekly suppressive dosage is 5 mg calculated as base, per kg of body weight, but should not exceed the adult dose regardless of weight.
If circumstances permit, suppressive therapy should begin two weeks prior to exposure. However, failing this in adults, an initial double (loading) dose of 1 g (= 600 mg base), or in children 10 mg base/kg may be taken in two divided doses, six hours apart. The suppressive therapy should be continued for eight weeks after leaving the endemic area.

For Treatment of Acute Attack
Adults: An initial dose of 1 g (= 600 mg base) followed by an additional 500 mg (= 300 mg base) after six to eight hours and a single dose of 500 mg (= 300 mg base) on each of two consecutive days. This represents a total dose of 2.5 g chloroquine phosphate or 1.5 g base in three days.
The dosage for adults may also be calculated on the basis of body weight; this method is preferred for infants and children. A total dose representing 25 mg of base per kg of body weight is administered in three days, as follows:
First dose: 10 mg base per kg (but not exceeding a single dose of 600 mg base).
Second dose: 5 mg base per kg (but not exceeding a single dose of 300 mg base) 6 hours after first dose.
Third dose: 5 mg base per kg 18 hours after second dose.
Fourth dose: 5 mg base per kg 24 hours after third dose.
For radical cure of *vivax* and *malariae* malaria concomitant therapy with an 8-aminoquinoline compound is necessary.
Extraintestinal Amebiasis: Adults, 1 g (600 mg base) daily for two days, followed by 500 mg (300 mg base) daily for at least two to three weeks. Treatment is usually combined with an effective intestinal amebicide.

HOW SUPPLIED
Tablets of 500 mg (= 300 mg base), bottles of 25 (NDC 0024-0077-01).
Pink, sugar-coated convex tablets, ½ inch in diameter with an uncoated core, containing 500 mg chloroquine phosphate, equivalent to 300 mg of chloroquine base.

AW-123-M

Shown in Product Identification Section, page 428

Continued on next page

This product information was prepared in August 1992. On these and other products of Sanofi Winthrop Pharmaceuticals, detailed information may be obtained on a current basis by direct inquiry to Product Information Services, 90 Park Avenue, New York, NY 10016 (toll free 1-800-446-6267).

Sanofi Winthrop—Cont.

ATABRINE® Hydrochloride   ℞
brand of quinacrine hydrochloride tablets, USP

> For Chemotherapy of Giardiasis, Tapeworm, and Malaria

> WARNING: PHYSICIANS SHOULD COMPLETELY FAMILIARIZE THEMSELVES WITH THE COMPLETE CONTENTS OF THIS LEAFLET BEFORE PRESCRIBING ATABRINE.

DESCRIPTION
Each tablet contains 100 mg of quinacrine hydrochloride, a bright yellow, odorless, bitter crystalline powder that is water soluble (1:35).
Inactive Ingredients: Pharmaceutical Glaze, Starch, Stearic Acid, Talc.

ACTIONS
ATABRINE eradicates certain intestinal cestodes, for example, beef tapeworm (*Taenia saginata*), pork tapeworm (*Taenia solium*), dwarf tapeworm (*Hymenolepis nana*) and probably fish tapeworm (*Diphyllobothrium latum*), and eliminates *Giardia lamblia* from the intestinal tract. It exerts both suppressive and therapeutic action in malaria. It destroys erythrocytic asexual forms (trophozoites) of vivax, falciparum, and quartan malaria, and sexual forms (gametocytes) of vivax and quartan malaria; however, it is ineffective against falciparum gametocytes and against sporozoites of all forms of malaria.

INDICATIONS
ATABRINE is indicated for the treatment of giardiasis and cestodiasis. It is also occasionally used for the treatment and suppression of malaria.

CONTRAINDICATIONS
Treatment of pregnant women with cestodiasis or giardiasis should be postponed until after delivery because quinacrine crosses the placenta and these conditions generally are not life-threatening.
Since ATABRINE increases the toxicity of the antimalarial agent, primaquine, ATABRINE is contraindicated for concomitant use with this drug.

WARNINGS
Patients should be strongly warned to keep this drug out of the reach of children. Quinacrine occasionally causes a transitory psychosis and therefore should be used with special caution in patients over 60 years of age or in those with a history of psychosis.
In recent years it has been found that certain strains of *Plasmodium falciparum* have become resistant to synthetic antimalarial compounds (including quinacrine) as shown by the fact that normally adequate doses have failed to prevent or cure clinical malaria or parasitemia. Treatment with quinine or other specific forms of therapy is therefore advised for patients infected with a resistant strain of parasites.
Use of ATABRINE in patients with psoriasis may precipitate a severe attack of psoriasis. When used in patients with porphyria the condition may be exacerbated. The drug should not be used in these conditions unless in the judgment of the physician the benefit to the patient outweighs the possible hazard.
Usage in Pregnancy. Usage of this drug in the suppression or treatment of malaria during pregnancy should be avoided except when in the judgment of the physician the benefit outweighs the possible hazard.

PRECAUTIONS
Since the drug is known to concentrate in the liver, it should be used with caution in patients with hepatic disease or alcoholism or in conjunction with known hepatotoxic drugs.
Complete blood cell counts should be made periodically if patients are given prolonged therapy. If any severe blood disorder appears which is not attributable to the disease under treatment, discontinuance of the drug should be considered. The drug should be administered with caution to patients having G-6-PD (glucose-6-phosphate dehydrogenase) deficiency.
Patients receiving prolonged ATABRINE, brand of quinacrine hydrochloride, therapy should be instructed to promptly report any visual disturbances and to receive periodic complete ophthalmologic examinations (see ADVERSE REACTIONS).

ADVERSE REACTIONS
The drug temporarily imparts a yellow color to the urine and skin (but does not cause jaundice).
Following administration in doses adequate for the treatment of an acute malarial attack, mild and transient headache, dizziness, and gastrointestinal complaints (diarrhea, anorexia, nausea, abdominal cramps and, on rare occasions, vomiting) may occur. Other infrequent but reversible side effects include pleomorphic skin eruptions, neuropsychiatric disturbances (nervousness, vertigo, irritability, emotional change, nightmares, and transient psychosis). Rarely, episodes of convulsions and transient toxic psychosis have been observed after ATABRINE doses of only 50 mg to 100 mg three times a day for a few days. Aplastic anemia, hepatitis, and lichen planus-like eruptions have been described, especially after long periods of malaria suppressive therapy with quinacrine. Exfoliative dermatitis can develop as a primary reaction to the drug or as a secondary response to other types of quinacrine-induced symptoms. Contact dermatitis can also occur. Epileptiform convulsions have been reported following the administration of massive doses.
Cases of reversible corneal edema or deposits, manifested by visual halos, focusing difficulty and blurred vision, have been reported in patients taking ATABRINE as long-term suppressive therapy for malaria.
Retinopathy has been reported rarely in patients who received relatively high doses of ATABRINE for prolonged periods in the treatment of certain chronic diseases. Retinopathy has not been reported as a result of ATABRINE use in malaria suppression or in the short-term treatment of parasitic diseases. (See PRECAUTIONS.)
Single large doses used for the treatment of tapeworm (0.6 g) may produce severe headache, nausea and vomiting, abdominal cramps, and slight diarrhea.

DOSAGE AND ADMINISTRATION
Treatment of Malaria—*Adults and children over 8 years,* 200 mg orally with 1 g of sodium bicarbonate every six hours for 5 doses, then 100 mg three times daily for six days (total dosage 2.8 g in seven days). *Children from 4 to 8 years,* 200 mg three times the first day, then 100 mg two times daily for six days. *Children from 1 to 4 years,* 100 mg three times the first day, then 100 mg once daily for six days. Medication should be taken after meals, with a full glass of water, tea, or fruit juice.
Suppression of Malaria—*Adults,* 100 mg orally once daily. *Children,* 50 mg daily. Medication should be maintained for one to three months.
Giardiasis—*Adults,* 100 mg three times daily for five to seven days. *Children,* 7 mg/kg/day given in three divided doses (maximum 300 mg/day) after meals for five days will eradicate the infestation in over 90 percent of children. The stool may be examined two weeks later and a repeat course given if indicated. The bitter taste of the pulverized tablets may be disguised by administration in jam or honey.
Tapeworm (Beef, Pork, and Fish)—(1) Preliminary bland, semisolid, nonfat diet, or milk diet on the day before medication, with fasting following the evening meal. A saline purge or purge and cleansing enema before treatment if desired. (2) *Adults,* four doses of 200 mg ten minutes apart (total dose, 800 mg). Sodium bicarbonate 600 mg with each dose in order to reduce the tendency to nausea and vomiting. *Children from 5 to 10 years,* a total dose of 400 mg. *Children from 11 to 14 years,* a total dose of 600 mg, divided into three or four doses administered ten minutes apart. Sodium bicarbonate 300 mg with each dose if desired. (3) Saline purge one to two hours later. The expelled worm is stained yellow, facilitating identification of scolex.
Dwarf Tapeworm—(1) *Adults,* the night before medication 1 tablespoon of sodium sulfate. *Children,* half adult dose. (2) *Adults,* on first day, 900 mg of the antimalarial compound orally, on an empty stomach, in three portions twenty minutes apart, with sodium sulfate purge one and one-half hours later. On the following three days, 100 mg three times daily. *Children from 4 to 8 years,* initial dose of 200 mg, followed by 100 mg after breakfast for three days. *Children from 8 to 10 years,* initial dose of 300 mg, followed by 100 mg twice daily for three days. *Children from 11 to 14 years,* initial dose of 400 mg, followed by 100 mg three times daily for three days.

OVERDOSAGE
Manifestations: Although extremely large doses of quinacrine may prove fatal (eg, 6.8 g intraduodenally, by error in a case of tapeworm infestation), some adults in suicidal attempts have taken enormous doses orally (eg, 7.5 g, 18 g, 25 g with unknown amount expelled by vomiting) and have survived. Toxic effects of large doses include excitation of the central nervous system with restlessness, insomnia, psychic stimulation, and convulsions, gastrointestinal disorders (nausea, vomiting, abdominal cramps, diarrhea), vascular collapse with hypotension, shock, cardiac arrhythmias or arrest, and yellow pigmentation of the skin.
Treatment: Treatment is symptomatic with evacuation of the stomach by emesis or gastric lavage. Convulsions, if present, should be controlled before attempting gastric lavage. If due to cerebral stimulation, an ultrashort-acting barbiturate

may be administered cautiously. If due to anoxia, it should be corrected by administration of oxygen, artificial respiration or, in shock with hypotension, by vasopressor therapy. In vascular collapse, vasopressors should be administered. Because of the importance of supporting respiration, tracheal intubation or tracheostomy may be advisable.
A patient who survives the acute phase and is asymptomatic should be closely observed for at least six hours. Fluids may be forced, and ammonium chloride (8 g daily in divided doses for adults) may be administered to acidify the urine to help promote urinary excretion in cases of both overdosage or sensitivity.

HOW SUPPLIED
Tablets of 100 mg, bottle of 100 (NDC 0024-0082-04)

            AW-91-K

BRONKEPHRINE®   ℞
brand of ethylnorepinephrine hydrochloride injection, USP
IN AQUEOUS SOLUTION

DESCRIPTION
BRONKEPHRINE is ethylnorepinephrine hydrochloride injection, USP. Each mL contains 2 mg ethylnorepinephrine HCl in a sterile isotonic solution of 0.7% sodium chloride with acetone sodium bisulfite 0.2% as preservative. The pH is adjusted to 2.9 to 4.5 with NaOH or HCl. BRONKEPHRINE is a synthetic sympathomimetic amine intended for subcutaneous or intramuscular injection. The chemical name is 1,2-Benzenediol,4-(2-amino-1-hydroxybutyl)-, hydrochloride.

CLINICAL PHARMACOLOGY
BRONKEPHRINE is primarily a beta-adrenergic agonist. Its actions are similar to those of isoproterenol, although it is less potent. Its bronchodilating properties closely simulate those of epinephrine but without significant pressor effects. It thus may be safer than epinephrine for hypertensive patients and severely ill patients in whom such effects are undesirable. It is particularly adapted for use in children because of its relative lack of adverse effects, especially central nervous system excitation. It also may be of value in diabetic asthmatics due to its lack of glycogenolytic activity.
Metabolic and pharmacokinetic data are unavailable.

INDICATIONS AND USAGE
BRONKEPHRINE is indicated for use as a bronchodilator for bronchial asthma and for reversible bronchospasm that may occur in association with bronchitis and emphysema.

CONTRAINDICATIONS
BRONKEPHRINE is contraindicated in patients who are hypersensitive to any of its ingredients or with idiosyncrasy to sympathomimetic drugs.

WARNINGS
BRONKEPHRINE should not be administered along with epinephrine or other sympathomimetic amines because these drugs are direct cardiac stimulants and may cause excessive tachycardia.
Contains acetone sodium bisulfite, a sulfite that may cause allergic-type reactions including anaphylactic symptoms and life-threatening or less severe asthmatic episodes in certain susceptible people. The overall prevalence of sulfite sensitivity in the general population is unknown and probably low. Sulfite sensitivity is seen more frequently in asthmatic than in nonasthmatic people.

PRECAUTIONS
BRONKEPHRINE should be used with caution in persons with cardiovascular disease, a history of stroke or coronary artery disease. It is a potent drug and may cause toxic symptoms through idiosyncratic response or overdosage.
Care should be taken in anatomical selection of injection sites to avoid inadvertent intraneural or intravascular injection.
Carcinogenesis, Mutagenesis, Impairment of Fertility: Long-term animal studies of BRONKEPHRINE to evaluate carcinogenic potential and reproduction studies in animals have not been performed. There is no evidence from human data that BRONKEPHRINE may be carcinogenic or mutagenic or that it impairs fertility.
Pregnancy Category C: Animal reproduction studies have not been conducted with BRONKEPHRINE. It is not known whether BRONKEPHRINE can cause fetal harm when administered to a pregnant woman or can affect reproduction capacity. BRONKEPHRINE should be given to a pregnant woman only if clearly needed and the potential benefits outweigh the risk.
Nursing Mothers: It is not known whether BRONKEPHRINE is excreted in human milk; however, because many drugs are excreted in human milk, caution should be exercised when BRONKEPHRINE is administered to a nursing woman.

ADVERSE REACTIONS

BRONKEPHRINE, brand of ethylnorepinephrine hydrochloride injection, is generally well tolerated. It may, however, produce changes in blood pressure (elevation or depression) or pulse rate (elevation), palpitation, headache, dizziness or nausea; as with other sympathomimetic amines.

OVERDOSAGE

The signs and symptoms of overdosage with BRONKEPHRINE are those typical of any sympathomimetic amine. Treatment should be symptomatic.

DOSAGE AND ADMINISTRATION

The usual adult dose by subcutaneous or intramuscular injection is 0.5 mL to 1 mL. Depending on severity of the asthmatic attack, smaller doses (0.3 mL to 0.5 mL) may suffice. Dosage in children varies according to age and weight; usually 0.1 mL to 0.5 mL is sufficient.

HOW SUPPLIED

Uni-Nest™—Sterile single-dose ampuls of 1 mL, box of 25. (NDC 0024-1001-25)
PROTECT AMPULS FROM LIGHT.

BW-96 B

BRONKODYL®   ℞
brand of theophylline capsules, USP
100 mg and 200 mg

DESCRIPTION

Theophylline is a bronchodilator structurally classified as a xanthine derivative. It occurs as a white, odorless, crystalline powder having a bitter taste. Theophylline anhydrous has the chemical name 1H-Purine-2, 6-dione, 3, 7-dihydro-1, 3-dimethyl-.
BRONKODYL is available as 100 mg, brown and white capsules and 200 mg, green and white capsules intended for oral administration, containing 100 mg of theophylline anhydrous and 200 mg of theophylline anhydrous respectively.
Inactive Ingredients: Benzyl Alcohol, Gelatin, Lactose, Magnesium Stearate, Methyl Propylparaben and Butylparaben, Colloidal Silicon Dioxide. Sodium Propionate, Sodium Starch Glycolate. Capsule **100 mg** contains FD&C Blue #1, Red #3, Yellow #6. Capsule **200 mg** contains D&C Yellow #10, FD&C Blue #1, Yellow #6.

HOW SUPPLIED

100 mg, brown and white, hard gelatin capsules, bottles of 100 **NDC** 0024-1036-10
200 mg, green and white, hard gelatin capsules, bottles of 100 **NDC** 0024-1037-10
Mfd. by KV Pharmaceutical Co., St. Louis, Missouri 63144
For complete prescribing information, see package insert or contact Product Information Services.

BW-98E

BRONKOLIXIR®   OTC

(See PDR For Nonprescription Drugs.)

BRONKOSOL®   ℞
brand of isoetharine inhalation solution, USP, 1%
BRONCHODILATOR SOLUTION FOR ORAL INHALATION

DESCRIPTION

Isoetharine hydrochloride, USP, 1% also contains: Acetone Sodium Bisulfite, Glycerin, Parabens, Purified Water, Sodium Chloride, and Sodium Citrate.

BRONKOMETER®   ℞
brand of isoetharine mesylate inhalation aerosol, USP

DESCRIPTION

BRONKOMETER is a complete pocket nebulizer containing isoetharine mesylate 0.61% (w/w). BRONKOMETER also contains: alcohol 30% (w/w), ascorbic acid 0.1% (w/w) as a preservative, dichlorodifluoromethane and dichlorotetrafluoroethane as propellants, menthol, and saccharin.
Isoetharine mesylate is 1,2-Benzenediol, 4-[1-hydroxy-2-[(1-methylethyl)amino]-butyl]-, methanesulfonate (salt). The BRONKOMETER unit delivers approximately 20 metered doses per mL of solution. Each average 56 mg delivery contains 340 µg isoetharine.

CLINICAL PHARMACOLOGY

Isoetharine is a sympathomimetic amine with preferential affinity for Beta$_2$ adrenergic receptor sites of bronchial and certain arteriolar musculature, and a lower order of affinity for Beta$_1$ adrenergic receptors. Its activity in symptomatic relief of bronchospasm is rapid and of relatively long duration. By relieving bronchospasm, BRONKOSOL and

---

BRONKOMETER help give prompt relief and significantly increase vital capacity.

INDICATIONS AND USAGE

BRONKOSOL and BRONKOMETER are indicated for use as bronchodilators for bronchial asthma and for reversible bronchospasm that may occur in association with bronchitis and emphysema.

CONTRAINDICATION

BRONKOSOL and BRONKOMETER should not be administered to patients who are hypersensitive to any of their ingredients.

WARNINGS

BRONKOSOL contains acetone sodium bisulfite, a sulfite that may cause allergic-type reactions including anaphylactic symptoms and life-threatening or less severe asthmatic episodes in certain susceptible people. The overall prevalence of sulfite sensitivity in the general population is unknown and probably low. Sulfite sensitivity is seen more frequently in asthmatic than in nonasthmatic people.
Excessive use of an adrenergic aerosol should be discouraged as it may lose its effectiveness. Occasional patients have been reported to develop severe paradoxical airway resistance with repeated excessive use of an aerosol adrenergic inhalation preparation. The cause of this refractory state is unknown. It is advisable that in such instances the use of the aerosol adrenergic be discontinued immediately and alternative therapy instituted, since in the reported cases the patients did not respond to other forms of therapy until the drug was withdrawn. Cardiac arrest has been noted in several instances.
BRONKOSOL and BRONKOMETER should not be administered along with epinephrine or other sympathomimetic amines, since these drugs are direct cardiac stimulants and may cause excessive tachycardia. They may, however, be alternated if desired.
Usage in Pregnancy: Although there has been no evidence of teratogenic effects with this drug, use of any drug in pregnancy, lactation, or in women of childbearing potential requires that the potential benefit of the drug be weighed against its possible hazard to the mother or child.

PRECAUTIONS

Dosage must be carefully adjusted in patients with hyperthyroidism, hypertension, acute coronary disease, cardiac asthma, limited cardiac reserve, and in individuals sensitive to sympathomimetic amines, since overdosage may result in tachycardia, palpitation, nausea, headache, or epinephrine-like side effects.

ADVERSE REACTIONS

Although BRONKOSOL and BRONKOMETER are relatively free of toxic side effects, too frequent use may cause tachycardia, palpitation, nausea, headache, changes in blood pressure, anxiety, tension, restlessness, insomnia, tremor, weakness, dizziness, and excitement, as is the case with other sympathomimetic amines.

DOSAGE AND ADMINISTRATION

BRONKOSOL can be administered by hand nebulizer, oxygen aerosolization, or intermittent positive pressure breathing (IPPB). Usually treatment need not be repeated more often than every four hours, although in severe cases more frequent administration may be necessary.

Method of Administration	Usual Dose	Range	Usual Dilution
Hand nebulizer	4 inhalations	3-7 inhalations	undiluted
Oxygen aerosolization*	½ mL	¼-½ mL	1:3 with saline or other diluent
IPPB†	½ mL	¼-1 mL	1:3 with saline or other diluent

* Administered with oxygen flow adjusted to 4 to 6 liters/minute over a period of 15 to 20 minutes.
† Usually an inspiratory flow rate of 15 liters/minute at a cycling pressure of 15 cm H$_2$O is recommended. It may be necessary, according to patient and type of IPPB apparatus, to adjust flow rate to 6 to 30 liters per minute, cycling pressure to 10 to 15 cm H$_2$0, and further dilution according to needs of patient.

BRONKOMETER®

DOSAGE AND ADMINISTRATION

The average adult dose is one or two inhalations. Occasionally, more may be required. It is important, however, to wait one full minute after the initial one or two inhalations in order to be certain whether another is necessary. In most cases, inhalations need not be repeated more often than every four hours, although more frequent administration may be necessary in severe cases.

HOW SUPPLIED

BRONKOMETER, brand of isoetharine mesylate inhalation aerosol
Vial of 10 mL, with oral nebulizer (NDC 0024-1040-01)
Refill only, 10 mL (NDC 0024-1041-01)
Vial of 15 mL, with oral nebulizer (NDC 0024-1040-03)
Refill only, 15 mL (NDC 0024-1041-03)
The bronchodilator isoetharine is also available in a convenient solution for use with conventional nebulizers, by oxygen aerosolization, and in IPPB machines as BRONKOSOL, brand of isoetharine inhalation solution, 1%. It is supplied as follows:
Bottle of 10 mL (NDC 0024-1071-10)
Bottle of 30 mL (NDC 0024-1071-30)

    Manufactured by Sterling Pharmaceuticals Inc.
        Barceloneta, Puerto Rico 00617

BRONKOTABS®   OTC

(See PDR For Nonprescription Drugs.)

CARBOCAINE® HYDROCHLORIDE   ℞
brand of mepivacaine hydrochloride
injection, USP

THESE SOLUTIONS ARE NOT INTENDED FOR SPINAL ANESTHESIA OR DENTAL USE

DESCRIPTION

Mepivacaine hydrochloride is 2-Piperidinecarboxamide, *N*-(2,6-dimethylphenyl)-1-methyl-, monohydrochloride.
It is a white crystalline odorless powder, soluble in water, but very resistant to both acid and alkaline hydrolysis.
CARBOCAINE hydrochloride is a local anesthetic available as sterile isotonic solutions in concentrations of 1%, 1.5%, and 2% for injection via local infiltration, peripheral nerve block, and caudal and lumbar epidural blocks.
Mepivacaine hydrochloride is related chemically and pharmacologically to the amide-type local anesthetics. It contains an amide linkage between the aromatic nucleus and the amino group. [See table on next page.]
The pH of the solutions is adjusted between 4.5 and 6.8 with sodium hydroxide or hydrochloric acid.

CLINICAL PHARMACOLOGY

Local anesthetics block the generation and the conduction of nerve impulses, presumably by increasing the threshold for electrical excitation in the nerve, by slowing the propagation of the nerve impulse, and by reducing the rate of rise of the action potential. In general, the progression of anesthesia is related to the diameter, myelination, and conduction velocity of affected nerve fibers. Clinically, the order of loss of nerve function is as follows: pain, temperature, touch, proprioception, and skeletal muscle tone.
Systemic absorption of local anesthetics produces effects on the cardiovascular and central nervous systems. At blood concentrations achieved with normal therapeutic doses, changes in cardiac conduction, excitability, refractoriness, contractility, and peripheral vascular resistance are minimal. However, toxic blood concentrations depress cardiac conduction and excitability, which may lead to atrioventricular block and ultimately to cardiac arrest. In addition, myocardial contractility is depressed and peripheral vasodilation occurs, leading to decreased cardiac output and arterial blood pressure.
Following systemic absorption, local anesthetics can produce central nervous system stimulation, depression, or both. Apparent central stimulation is manifested as restlessness, tremors, and shivering, progressing to convulsions, followed by depression and coma progressing ultimately to respiratory arrest. However, the local anesthetics have a primary depressant effect on the medulla and on higher centers. The depressed stage may occur without a prior excited stage.
Pharmacokinetics
The rate of systemic absorption of local anesthetics is dependent upon the total dose and concentration of drug administered, the route of administration, the vascularity of the administration site, and the presence or absence of epinephrine in the anesthetic solution. A dilute concentration of epinephrine (1:200,000 or 5 µg/mL) usually reduces the rate of absorption and plasma concentration of CARBOCAINE, how-

Continued on next page

This product information was prepared in August 1992. On these and other products of Sanofi Winthrop Pharmaceuticals, detailed information may be obtained on a current basis by direct inquiry to Product Information Services, 90 Park Avenue, New York, NY 10016 (toll free 1-800-446-6267).

Sanofi Winthrop—Cont.

ever, it has been reported that vasoconstrictors do not significantly prolong anesthesia with CARBOCAINE.

Onset of anesthesia with CARBOCAINE is rapid, the time of onset for sensory block ranging from about 3 to 20 minutes depending upon such factors as the anesthetic technique, the type of block, the concentration of the solution, and the individual patient. The degree of motor blockade produced is dependent on the concentration of the solution. A 0.5% solution will be effective in small superficial nerve blocks while the 1% concentration will block sensory and sympathetic conduction without loss of motor function. The 1.5% solution will provide extensive and often complete motor block and the 2% concentration of CARBOCAINE will produce complete sensory and motor block of any nerve group.

The duration of anesthesia also varies depending upon the technique and type of block, the concentration, and the individual. Mepivacaine will normally provide anesthesia which is adequate for 2 to 2½ hours of surgery.

Local anesthetics are bound to plasma proteins in varying degrees. Generally, the lower the plasma concentration of drug, the higher the percentage of drug bound to plasma. Local anesthetics appear to cross the placenta by passive diffusion. The rate and degree of diffusion is governed by the degree of plasma protein binding, the degree of ionization, and the degree of lipid solubility. Fetal/maternal ratios of local anesthetics appear to be inversely related to the degree of plasma protein binding, because only the free, unbound drug is available for placental transfer. CARBOCAINE is approximately 75% bound to plasma proteins. The extent of placental transfer is also determined by the degree of ionization and lipid solubility of the drug. Lipid soluble, nonionized drugs readily enter the fetal blood from the maternal circulation.

Depending upon the route of administration, local anesthetics are distributed to some extent to all body tissues, with high concentrations found in highly perfused organs such as the liver, lungs, heart, and brain.

Various pharmacokinetic parameters of the local anesthetics can be significantly altered by the presence of hepatic or renal disease, addition of epinephrine, factors affecting urinary pH, renal blood flow, the route of drug administration, and the age of the patient. The half-life of CARBOCAINE in adults is 1.9 to 3.2 hours and in neonates 8.7 to 9 hours. Mepivacaine, because of its amide structure, is not detoxified by the circulating plasma esterases. It is rapidly metabolized, with only a small percentage of the anesthetic (5 percent to 10 percent) being excreted unchanged in the urine. The liver is the principal site of metabolism, with over 50% of the administered dose being excreted into the bile as metabolites. Most of the metabolized mepivacaine is probably resorbed in the intestine and then excreted into the urine since only a small percentage is found in the feces. The principal route of excretion is via the kidney. Most of the anesthetic and its metabolites are eliminated within 30 hours. It has been shown that hydroxylation and N-demethylation, which are detoxification reactions, play important roles in the metabolism of the anesthetic. Three metabolites of mepivacaine have been identified from human adults: two phenols, which are excreted almost exclusively as their glucuronide conjugates, and the N-demethylated compound (2', 6'-pipecoloxylidide).

Mepivacaine does not ordinarily produce irritation or tissue damage, and does not cause methemoglobinemia when administered in recommended doses and concentrations.

INDICATIONS AND USAGE

CARBOCAINE, brand of mepivacaine hydrochloride, is indicated for production of local or regional analgesia and anesthesia by local infiltration, peripheral nerve block techniques, and central neural techniques including epidural and caudal blocks.

The routes of administration and indicated concentrations for CARBOCAINE are:

local infiltration	0.5% (via dilution) or 1%
peripheral nerve blocks	1% and 2%
epidural block	1%, 1.5%, 2%
caudal block	1%, 1.5%, 2%

See DOSAGE AND ADMINISTRATION for additional information. Standard textbooks should be consulted to determine the accepted procedures and techniques for the administration of CARBOCAINE.

CONTRAINDICATIONS

CARBOCAINE is contraindicated in patients with a known hypersensitivity to it or to any local anesthetic agent of the amide-type or to other components of solutions of CARBOCAINE.

Composition of Available Solutions*

	1% Single-Dose 30 mL Vial mg/mL	1% Multiple-Dose 50 mL Vial mg/mL	1.5% Single-Dose 30 mL Vial mg/mL	2% Single-Dose 20 mL Vial mg/mL	2% Multiple-Dose 50 mL Vial mg/mL
Mepivacaine hydrochloride	10	10	15	20	20
Sodium chloride	6.6	7	5.6	4.6	5
Potassium chloride	0.3		0.3	0.3	
Calcium chloride	0.33		0.33	0.33	
Methylparaben		1			1

*In Water for Injection

WARNINGS

LOCAL ANESTHETICS SHOULD ONLY BE EMPLOYED BY CLINICIANS WHO ARE WELL VERSED IN DIAGNOSIS AND MANAGEMENT OF DOSE-RELATED TOXICITY AND OTHER ACUTE EMERGENCIES WHICH MIGHT ARISE FROM THE BLOCK TO BE EMPLOYED, AND THEN ONLY AFTER INSURING THE <u>IMMEDIATE</u> AVAILABILITY OF OXYGEN, OTHER RESUSCITATIVE DRUGS, CARDIOPULMONARY RESUSCITATIVE EQUIPMENT, AND THE PERSONNEL RESOURCES NEEDED FOR PROPER MANAGEMENT OF TOXIC REACTIONS AND RELATED EMERGENCIES. (See also ADVERSE REACTIONS and PRECAUTIONS.) DELAY IN PROPER MANAGEMENT OF DOSE-RELATED TOXICITY, UNDERVENTILATION FROM ANY CAUSE, AND/OR ALTERED SENSITIVITY MAY LEAD TO THE DEVELOPMENT OF ACIDOSIS, CARDIAC ARREST AND, POSSIBLY, DEATH.

Local anesthetic solutions containing antimicrobial preservatives (ie, those supplied in multiple-dose vials) should not be used for epidural or caudal anesthesia because safety has <u>not</u> been established with regard to intrathecal injection, either intentionally or inadvertently, of such preservatives. It is essential that aspiration for blood or cerebrospinal fluid (where applicable) be done prior to injecting any local anesthetic, both the original dose and all subsequent doses, to avoid intravascular or subarachnoid injection. However, a negative aspiration does not ensure against an intravascular or subarachnoid injection.

Reactions resulting in fatality have occurred on rare occasions with the use of local anesthetics.

CARBOCAINE with epinephrine or other vasopressors should not be used concomitantly with ergot-type oxytocic drugs, because a severe persistent hypertension may occur. Likewise, solutions of CARBOCAINE containing a vasoconstrictor, such as epinephrine, should be used with extreme caution in patients receiving monoamine oxidase inhibitors (MAOI) or antidepressants of the triptyline or imipramine types, because severe prolonged hypertension may result.

Local anesthetic procedures should be used with caution when there is inflammation and/or sepsis in the region of the proposed injection.

Mixing or the prior or intercurrent use of any local anesthetic with CARBOCAINE cannot be recommended because of insufficient data on the clinical use of such mixtures.

PRECAUTIONS

General

The safety and effectiveness of local anesthetics depend on proper dosage, correct technique, adequate precautions, and readiness for emergencies. Resuscitative equipment, oxygen, and other resuscitative drugs should be available for immediate use. (See WARNINGS and ADVERSE REACTIONS.) During major regional nerve blocks, the patient should have IV fluids running via an indwelling catheter to assure a functioning intravenous pathway. The lowest dosage of local anesthetic that results in effective anesthesia should be used to avoid high plasma levels and serious adverse effects. Injections should be made slowly, with frequent aspirations before and during the injection to avoid intravascular injection. Current opinion favors fractional administration with constant attention to the patient, rather than rapid bolus injection. Syringe aspirations should also be performed before and during each supplemental injection in continuous (intermittent) catheter techniques. An intravascular injection is still possible even if aspirations for blood are negative. During the administration of epidural anesthesia, it is recommended that a test dose be administered initially and the effects monitored before the full dose is given. When using a "continuous" catheter technique, test doses should be given prior to both the original and all reinforcing doses, because plastic tubing in the epidural space can migrate into a blood vessel or through the dura. When clinical conditions permit, an effective test dose should contain epinephrine (10 µg to 15 µg have been suggested) to serve as a warning of unintended intravascular injection. If injected into a blood vessel, this amount of epinephrine is likely to produce an "epinephrine response" within 45 seconds, consisting of an increase of pulse and blood pressure, circumoral pallor, palpitations, and nervousness in the unsedated patient. The sedated patient may exhibit only a pulse rate increase of 20 or more beats per minute for 15 or more seconds. Therefore, following the test dose, the heart rate should be monitored

for a heart rate increase. The test dose should also contain 45 mg to 50 mg of CARBOCAINE to detect an unintended intrathecal administration. This will be evidenced within a few minutes by signs of spinal block (eg, decreased sensation of the buttocks, paresis of the legs, or, in the sedated patient, absent knee jerk).

Injection of repeated doses of local anesthetics may cause significant increases in plasma levels with each repeated dose due to slow accumulation of the drug or its metabolites or to slow metabolic degradation. Tolerance to elevated blood levels varies with the status of the patient. Debilitated, elderly patients, and acutely ill patients should be given reduced doses commensurate with their age and physical status. Local anesthetics should also be used with caution in patients with severe disturbances of cardiac rhythm, shock, heart block, or hypotension.

Careful and constant monitoring of cardiovascular and respiratory (adequacy of ventilation) vital signs, and the patient's state of consciousness should be performed after each local anesthetic injection. It should be kept in mind at such times that restlessness, anxiety, incoherent speech, lightheadedness, numbness and tingling of the mouth and lips, metallic taste, tinnitus, dizziness, blurred vision, tremors, twitching, depression, or drowsiness may be early warning signs of central nervous system toxicity.

Local anesthetic solutions containing a vasoconstrictor should be used cautiously and in carefully restricted quantities in areas of the body supplied by end arteries or having otherwise compromised blood supply such as digits, nose, external ear, penis. Patients with hypertensive vascular disease may exhibit exaggerated vasoconstrictor response. Ischemic injury or necrosis may result.

Mepivacaine should be used with caution in patients with known allergies and sensitivities.

Because amide-type local anesthetics such as CARBOCAINE, brand of mepivacaine hydrochloride, are metabolized by the liver and excreted by the kidneys, these drugs, especially repeat doses, should be used cautiously in patients with hepatic and renal disease. Patients with severe hepatic disease, because of their inability to metabolize local anesthetics normally, are at a greater risk of developing toxic plasma concentrations. Local anesthetics should also be used with caution in patients with impaired cardiovascular function because they may be less able to compensate for functional changes associated with the prolongation of AV conduction produced by these drugs.

Serious dose-related cardiac arrhythmias may occur if preparations containing a vasoconstrictor such as epinephrine are employed in patients during or following the administration of potent inhalation anesthetics. In deciding whether to use these products concurrently in the same patient, the combined action of both agents upon the myocardium, the concentration and volume of vasoconstrictor used, and the time since injection, when applicable, should be taken into account.

Many drugs used during the conduct of anesthesia are considered potential triggering agents for familial malignant hyperthermia. Because it is not known whether amide-type local anesthetics may trigger this reaction and because the need for supplemental general anesthesia cannot be predicted in advance, it is suggested that a standard protocol for management should be available. Early unexplained signs of tachycardia, tachypnea, labile blood pressure, and metabolic acidosis may precede temperature elevation. Successful outcome is dependent on early diagnosis, prompt discontinuance of the suspect triggering agent(s), and institution of treatment, including oxygen therapy, indicated supportive measures, and dantrolene. (Consult dantrolene sodium intravenous package insert before using.)

Use in Head and Neck Area

Small doses of local anesthetics injected into the head and neck area may produce adverse reactions similar to systemic toxicity seen with unintentional intravascular injections of larger doses. The injection procedures require the utmost care.

Confusion, convulsions, respiratory depression, and/or respiratory arrest, and cardiovascular stimulation or depression have been reported. These reactions may be due to intra-arterial injection of the local anesthetic with retrograde flow to the cerebral circulation. Patients receiving these blocks should have their circulation and respiration monitored and

be constantly observed. Resuscitative equipment and personnel for treating adverse reactions should be immediately available. Dosage recommendations should not be exceeded.

Information for Patients
When appropriate, patients should be informed in advance that they may experience temporary loss of sensation and motor activity, usually in the lower half of the body, following proper administration of caudal or epidural anesthesia. Also, when appropriate, the physician should discuss other information including adverse reactions listed in the package insert on CARBOCAINE, brand of mepivacaine hydrochloride.

Clinically Significant Drug Interactions
The administration of local anesthetic solutions containing epinephrine or norepinephrine to patients receiving monoamine oxidase inhibitors or tricyclic antidepressants may produce severe, prolonged hypertension. Concurrent use of these agents should generally be avoided. In situations when concurrent therapy is necessary, careful patient monitoring is essential.

Concurrent administration of vasopressor drugs and of ergot-type oxytocic drugs may cause severe, persistent hypertension or cerebrovascular accidents.

Phenothiazines and butyrophenones may reduce or reverse the pressor effect of epinephrine.

Carcinogenesis, Mutagenesis, and Impairment of Fertility
Long-term studies in animals of most local anesthetics including mepivacaine to evaluate the carcinogenic potential have not been conducted. Mutagenic potential or the effect on fertility has not been determined. There is no evidence from human data that CARBOCAINE may be carcinogenic or mutagenic or that it impairs fertility.

Pregnancy Category C
Animal reproduction studies have not been conducted with mepivacaine. There are no adequate and well-controlled studies in pregnant women of the effect of mepivacaine on the developing fetus. Mepivacaine hydrochloride should be used during pregnancy only if the potential benefit justifies the potential risk to the fetus. This does not preclude the use of CARBOCAINE at term for obstetrical anesthesia or analgesia. (See *Labor and Delivery*.)

CARBOCAINE has been used for obstetrical analgesia by the epidural, caudal, and paracervical routes without evidence of adverse effects on the fetus when no more than the maximum safe dosages are used and strict adherence to technique is followed.

Labor and Delivery
Local anesthetics rapidly cross the placenta, and when used for epidural, paracervical, caudal, or pudendal block anesthesia, can cause varying degrees of maternal, fetal, and neonatal toxicity. (See *Pharmacokinetics*—CLINICAL PHARMACOLOGY.) The incidence and degree of toxicity depend upon the procedure performed, the type and amount of drug used, and the technique of drug administration. Adverse reactions in the parturient, fetus, and neonate involve alterations of the central nervous system, peripheral vascular tone, and cardiac function.

Maternal hypotension has resulted from regional anesthesia. Local anesthetics produce vasodilation by blocking sympathetic nerves. Elevating the patient's legs and positioning her on her left side will help prevent decreases in blood pressure. The fetal heart rate also should be monitored continuously and electronic fetal monitoring is highly advisable.

Epidural, paracervical, caudal, or pudendal anesthesia may alter the forces of parturition through changes in uterine contractility or maternal expulsive efforts. In one study, paracervical block anesthesia was associated with a decrease in the mean duration of first stage labor and facilitation of cervical dilation. Epidural anesthesia has been reported to prolong the second stage of labor by removing the parturient's reflex urge to bear down or by interfering with motor function. The use of obstetrical anesthesia may increase the need for forceps assistance.

The use of some local anesthetic drug products during labor and delivery may be followed by diminished muscle strength and tone for the first day or two of life. The long-term significance of these observations is unknown.

Fetal bradycardia may occur in 20 to 30 percent of patients receiving paracervical block anesthesia with the amide-type local anesthetics and may be associated with fetal acidosis. Fetal heart rate should always be monitored during paracervical anesthesia. Added risk appears to be present in prematurity, postmaturity, toxemia of pregnancy, and fetal distress. The physician should weigh the possible advantages against dangers when considering paracervical block in these conditions. Careful adherence to recommended dosage is of the utmost importance in obstetrical paracervical block. Failure to achieve adequate analgesia with recommended doses should arouse suspicion of intravascular or fetal intracranial injection.

Cases compatible with unintended fetal intracranial injection of local anesthetic solution have been reported following intended paracervical or pudendal block or both. Babies so affected present with unexplained neonatal depression at birth which correlates with high local anesthetic serum levels and usually manifest seizures within six hours. Prompt

Recommended Concentrations and Doses of CARBOCAINE

Procedure	Concentration	Total Dose mL	Total Dose mg	Comments
Cervical, brachial, intercostal, pudendal nerve block	1%	5–40	50–400	Pudendal block: one half of total dose injected each side.
	2%	5–20	100–400	
Transvaginal block (paracervical plus pudendal)	1%	up to 30 (both sides)	up to 300 (both sides)	One half of total dose injected each side. See PRECAUTIONS.
Paracervical block	1%	up to 20 (both sides)	up to 200 (both sides)	One half of total dose injected each side. This is maximum recommended dose per 90-minute period in obstetrical and non-obstetrical patients. Inject slowly, 5 minutes between sides. See PRECAUTIONS.
Caudal and Epidural block	1%	15–30	150–300	Use only single-dose vials which do not contain a preservative.
	1.5%	10–25	150–375	
	2%	10–20	200–400	
Infiltration	1%	up to 40	up to 400	An equivalent amount of a 0.5% solution (prepared by diluting the 1% solution with Sodium Chloride Injection, USP) may be used for large areas.
Therapeutic block (pain management)	1%	1–5	10–50	
	2%	1–5	20–100	

Unused portions of solutions not containing preservatives should be discarded.

use of supportive measures combined with forced urinary excretion of the local anesthetic has been used successfully to manage this complication.

Case reports of maternal convulsions and cardiovascular collapse following use of some local anesthetics for paracervical block in early pregnancy (as anesthesia for elective abortion) suggest that systemic absorption under these circumstances may be rapid. The recommended maximum dose of the local anesthetic should not be exceeded. Injection should be made slowly and with frequent aspiration. Allow a five-minute interval between sides.

It is extremely important to avoid aortocaval compression by the gravid uterus during administration of regional block to parturients. To do this, the patient must be maintained in the left lateral decubitus position or a blanket roll or sandbag may be placed beneath the right hip and the gravid uterus displaced to the left.

Nursing Mothers
It is not known whether local anesthetic drugs are excreted in human milk. Because many drugs are excreted in human milk, caution should be exercised when local anesthetics are administered to a nursing woman.

Pediatric Use
Guidelines for the administration of mepivacaine to children are presented in DOSAGE AND ADMINISTRATION.

ADVERSE REACTIONS
Reactions to CARBOCAINE, brand of mepivacaine hydrochloride, are characteristic of those associated with other amide-type local anesthetics. A major cause of adverse reactions to this group of drugs is excessive plasma levels, which may be due to overdosage, inadvertent intravascular injection, or slow metabolic degradation.

Systemic
The most commonly encountered acute adverse experiences which demand immediate countermeasures are related to the central nervous system and the cardiovascular system. These adverse experiences are generally dose related and due to high plasma levels which may result from overdosage, rapid absorption from the injection site, diminished tolerance, or from unintentional intravascular injection of the local anesthetic solution. In addition to systemic dose-related toxicity, unintentional subarachnoid injection of drug during the intended performance of caudal or lumbar epidural block or nerve blocks near the vertebral column (especially in the head and neck region) may result in underventilation or apnea ("Total or High Spinal"). Also, hypotension due to loss of sympathetic tone and respiratory paralysis or underventilation due to cephalad extension of the motor level of anesthesia may occur. This may lead to secondary cardiac arrest if untreated. Factors influencing plasma protein binding, such as acidosis, systemic diseases which alter protein production, or competition of other drugs for protein binding sites, may diminish individual tolerance.

Central Nervous System Reactions
These are characterized by excitation and/or depression. Restlessness, anxiety, dizziness, tinnitus, blurred vision, or tremors may occur, possibly proceeding to convulsions. However, excitement may be transient or absent, with depression being the first manifestation of an adverse reaction. This may quickly be followed by drowsiness merging into unconsciousness and respiratory arrest. Other central nervous system effects may be nausea, vomiting, chills, and constriction of the pupils.

The incidence of convulsions associated with the use of local anesthetics varies with the procedure used and the total dose administered. In a survey of studies of epidural anesthesia, overt toxicity progressing to convulsions occurred in approximately 0.1% of local anesthetic administrations.

Cardiovascular Reactions
High doses or, inadvertent intravascular injection, may lead to high plasma levels and related depression of the myocardium, decreased cardiac output, heart block, hypotension (or sometimes hypertension), bradycardia, ventricular arrhythmias, and possibly cardiac arrest). (See WARNINGS, PRECAUTIONS, and OVERDOSAGE sections.)

Allergic
Allergic-type reactions are rare and may occur as a result of sensitivity to the local anesthetic or to other formulation ingredients, such as the antimicrobial preservative methylparaben, contained in multiple-dose vials. These reactions are characterized by signs such as urticaria, pruritus, erythema, angioneurotic edema (including laryngeal edema), tachycardia, sneezing, nausea, vomiting, dizziness, syncope, excessive sweating, elevated temperature, and possibly, anaphylactoid-like symptomatology (including severe hypotension). Cross sensitivity among members of the amide-type local anesthetic group has been reported. The usefulness of screening for sensitivity has not been definitely established.

Neurologic
The incidences of adverse neurologic reactions associated with the use of local anesthetics may be related to the total dose of local anesthetic administered and are also dependent upon the particular drug used, the route of administration,

Continued on next page

This product information was prepared in August 1992. On these and other products of Sanofi Winthrop Pharmaceuticals, detailed information may be obtained on a current basis by direct inquiry to Product Information Services, 90 Park Avenue, New York, NY 10016 (toll free 1-800-446-6267).

Sanofi Winthrop—Cont.

and the physical status of the patient. Many of these effects may be related to local anesthetic techniques, with or without a contribution from the drug.

In the practice of caudal or lumbar epidural block, occasional unintentional penetration of the subarachnoid space by the catheter or needle may occur. Subsequent adverse effects may depend partially on the amount of drug administered intrathecally and the physiological and physical effects of a dural puncture. A high spinal is characterized by paralysis of the legs, loss of consciousness, respiratory paralysis, and bradycardia.

Neurologic effects following epidural or caudal anesthesia may include spinal block of varying magnitude (including high or total spinal block); hypotension secondary to spinal block; urinary retention; fecal and urinary incontinence; loss of perineal sensation and sexual function; persistent anesthesia, paresthesia, weakness, paralysis of the lower extremities, and loss of sphincter control all of which may have slow, incomplete, or no recovery; headache; backache; septic meningitis; meningismus; slowing of labor; increased incidence of forceps delivery; cranial nerve palsies due to traction on nerves from loss of cerebrospinal fluid.

Neurologic effects following other procedures or routes of administration may include persistent anesthesia, paresthesia, weakness, paralysis, all of which may have slow, incomplete, or no recovery.

OVERDOSAGE

Acute emergencies from local anesthetics are generally related to high plasma levels encountered during therapeutic use of local anesthetics or to unintended subarachnoid injection of local anesthetic solution. (See ADVERSE REACTIONS, WARNINGS, and PRECAUTIONS.)

Management of Local Anesthetic Emergencies

The first consideration is prevention, best accomplished by careful and constant monitoring of cardiovascular and respiratory vital signs and the patient's state of consciousness after each local anesthetic injection. At the first sign of change, oxygen should be administered.

The first step in the management of systemic toxic reactions, as well as underventilation or apnea due to unintentional subarachnoid injection of drug solution, consists of immediate attention to the establishment and maintenance of a patent airway and effective assisted or controlled ventilation with 100% oxygen with a delivery system capable of permitting immediate positive airway pressure by mask. This may prevent convulsions if they have not already occurred.

If necessary, use drugs to control the convulsions. A 50 mg to 100 mg bolus IV injection of succinylcholine will paralyze the patient without depressing the central nervous or cardiovascular systems and facilitate ventilation. A bolus IV dose of 5 mg to 10 mg of diazepam or 50 mg to 100 mg of thiopental will permit ventilation and counteract central nervous system stimulation, but these drugs also depress central nervous system, respiratory, and cardiac function, add to postictal depression and may result in apnea. Intravenous barbiturates, anticonvulsant agents, or muscle relaxants should only be administered by those familiar with their use. Immediately after the institution of these ventilatory measures, the adequacy of the circulation should be evaluated. Supportive treatment of circulatory depression may require administration of intravenous fluids, and when appropriate, a vasopressor dictated by the clinical situation (such as ephedrine or epinephrine to enhance myocardial contractile force).

Endotracheal intubation, employing drugs and techniques familiar to the clinician may be indicated after initial administration of oxygen by mask, if difficulty is encountered in the maintenance of a patent airway or if prolonged ventilatory support (assisted or controlled) is indicated.

Recent clinical data from patients experiencing local anesthetic induced convulsions demonstrated rapid development of hypoxia, hypercarbia, and acidosis within a minute of the onset of convulsions. These observations suggest that oxygen consumption and carbon dioxide production are greatly increased during local anesthetic convulsions and emphasize the importance of immediate and effective ventilation with oxygen which may avoid cardiac arrest.

If not treated immediately, convulsions with simultaneous hypoxia, hypercarbia, and acidosis, plus myocardial depression from the direct effects of the local anesthetic may result in cardiac arrhythmias, bradycardia, asystole, ventricular fibrillation, or cardiac arrest. Respiratory abnormalities, including apnea, may occur. Underventilation or apnea due to unintentional subarachnoid injection of local anesthetic solution may produce these same signs and also lead to cardiac arrest if ventilatory support is not instituted. If cardiac arrest should occur, standard cardiopulmonary resuscitative measures should be instituted and maintained for a prolonged period if necessary. Recovery has been reported after prolonged resuscitative efforts.

The supine position is dangerous in pregnant women at term because of aortocaval compression by the gravid uterus. Therefore during treatment of systemic toxicity, maternal hypotension, or fetal bradycardia following regional block, the parturient should be maintained in the left lateral decubitus position if possible, or manual displacement of the uterus off the great vessels be accomplished.

The mean seizure dosage of mepivacaine in rhesus monkeys was found to be 18.8 mg/kg with mean arterial plasma concentration of 24.4 µg/mL. The intravenous and subcutaneous LD_{50} in mice is 23 mg/kg to 35 mg/kg and 280 mg/kg respectively.

DOSAGE AND ADMINISTRATION

The dose of any local anesthetic administered varies with the anesthetic procedure, the area to be anesthetized, the vascularity of the tissues, the number of neuronal segments to be blocked, the depth of anesthesia and degree of muscle relaxation required, the duration of anesthesia desired, individual tolerance and the physical condition of the patient. The smallest dose and concentration required to produce the desired result should be administered. Dosages of CARBOCAINE should be reduced for elderly and debilitated patients and patients with cardiac and/or liver disease. The rapid injection of a large volume of local anesthetic solution should be avoided and fractional doses should be used when feasible.

For specific techniques and procedures, refer to standard textbooks.

The recommended single adult dose (or the total of a series of doses given in one procedure) of CARBOCAINE, brand of mepivacaine hydrochloride, for unsedated, healthy, normal-sized individuals should not usually exceed 400 mg. The recommended dosage is based on requirements for the average adult and should be reduced for elderly or debilitated patients.

While maximum doses of 7 mg/kg (550 mg) have been administered without adverse effect, these are not recommended, except in exceptional circumstances and under no circumstances should the administration be repeated at intervals of less than 1½ hours. The total dose for any 24-hour period should not exceed 1000 mg because of a slow accumulation of the anesthetic or its derivatives or slower than normal metabolic degradation or detoxification with repeat administration (see CLINICAL PHARMACOLOGY and PRECAUTIONS).

Children tolerate the local anesthetic as well as adults. However, the pediatric dose should be ***carefully measured*** as a percentage of the total adult dose ***based on weight***, and should not exceed 5 mg/kg to 6 mg/kg (2.5 mg/lb to 3 mg/lb) in children, especially those weighing less than 30 lb. In children ***under 3 years of age or weighing less than 30 lb*** concentrations less than 2% (eg, 0.5% to 1.5%) should be employed.

Unused portions of solutions not containing preservatives, ie, those supplied in single-dose vials, should be discarded following initial use.

This product should be inspected visually for particulate matter and discoloration prior to administration whenever solution and container permit. Solutions which are discolored or which contain particulate matter should not be administered.

[See table at top of preceding page.]

HOW SUPPLIED

Single-dose vials and multiple-dose vials of CARBOCAINE may be sterilized by autoclaving at 15 pound pressure, 121°C (250°F) for 15 minutes. Solutions of CARBOCAINE may be reautoclaved when necessary. Do not administer solutions which are discolored or which contain particulate matter.

THESE SOLUTIONS ARE NOT INTENDED FOR SPINAL ANESTHESIA OR DENTAL USE.

1% Single-dose vials of 30 mL (NDC 0024-0231-01)
1% Multiple-dose vials of 50 mL (NDC 0024-0232-01)
1.5% Single-dose vials of 30 mL (NDC 0024-0234-01)
2% Single-dose vials of 20 mL (NDC 0024-0236-01)
2% Multiple-dose vials of 50 mL (NDC 0024-0237-01)

Store at controlled room temperature between 15°C to 30°C (59°F to 86°F); brief exposure up to 40°C (104°F) does not adversely affect the product.

For full prescribing information on the dental use of CARBOCAINE see Eastman Kodak Company product listing in this publication.

CW-60-U

CARPUJECT® Sterile Cartridge-Needle Unit ℞

Sanofi Winthrop Pharmaceuticals offers a broad line of injectable drug products in unit of use pre-filled cartridges. Each cartridge is clearly labelled by medication name and dosage calibrations. In addition each individual cartridge label and outer package is specially color-coded allowing for ease of identification, making the system easily adaptable to any hospital setting.

The cartridges are packaged in a unique DETECTO-SEAL® tamper detection package specially designed to discourage narcotic diversion and allow for easy inventory analysis. This package contains a sturdy aluminum shield to prevent plunger end diversion.

Prior to injection the pre-filled cartridges are placed in a unique sturdy plastic holder. This full-length holder provides secure, stable injections and is lightweight, durable, and reusable in design.

In addition, the holder utilized for CARPUJECT has an open-ended barrel allowing for release of used needles into most any disposal bin. This holder is designed with nursing personnel in mind to eliminate the need for recapping needles and minimize the potential for needle stick injuries.

The following products are currently available in CARPUJECT Sterile Cartridge-Needle Unit.

Product	Units/Package
atropine and DEMEROL® Injection atropine sulfate and meperidine HCl, USP (C-II)	
0.4 mg and 50 mg (22 G × 1¼") 0024-0021-01	10 (1 mL fill in 2 mL)
0.4 mg and 75 mg (22 G × 1¼") 0024-0022-02	10 (1 mL fill in 2 mL)
CODEINE Phosphate Injection, USP (C-II)	
30 mg (22 G × 1¼") 0024-0272-02	10 (2 mL)
60 mg (22 G × 1¼") 0024-0274-02	10 (2 mL)
DEMEROL® Hydrochloride brand of meperidine HCl injection, USP (C-II)	
25 mg (22 G × 1¼") 0024-0324-02	10 (1 mL fill in 2 mL)
50 mg (22 G × 1¼") 0024-0325-02	10 (1 mL fill in 2 mL)
75 mg (22 G × 1¼") 0024-0326-02	10 (1 mL fill in 2 mL)
100 mg (22 G × 1¼") 0024-0328-02	10 (1 mL fill in 2 mL)
DIAZEPAM Injection, USP (C-IV)	
10 mg/2 mL (22 G × 1¼") 0024-0376-02	10 (2 mL)
FENTANYL Citrate Injection, USP (C-II)	
100 µg/2 mL (22 G × 1¼") 0024-0682-02	10 (2 mL)
250 µg/5 mL (22 G × 1¼") 0024-0682-05	10 (5 mL)
FUROSEMIDE Injection, USP	
10 mg/mL (22 G × 1¼") 0024-0611-03	10 (2 mL)
10 mg/mL (22 G × 1¼") 0024-0611-50	50 (2 mL)
10 mg/mL (22 G × 1¼") 0024-0609-40	10 (4mL fill in 5 mL)
10 mg/mL (22 G × 1¼") 0024-0609-25	25 (4 mL fill in 5 mL)
HEPARIN LOCK FLUSH Solution, USP	
10 USP heparin U/mL (25 G × ⅝") 0024-0721-12	50 (1 mL fill in 2 mL)
100 USP heparin U/mL (25 G × ⅝") 0024-0722-12	50 (1 mL fill in 2 mL)
HEPARIN LOCK FLUSH Solution, USP	
10 USP heparin U/mL (25 G × ⅝") 0024-0721-13	50 (2 mL fill in 2 mL)
100 USP heparin U/mL (25 G × ⅝") 0024-0722-13	50 (2 mL fill in 2 mL)
HEPARIN LOCK FLUSH Solution, USP With InterLink™ System Cannula:	
10 USP heparin U/mL 0024-0721-16	50 (1 mL fill in 2 mL)
10 USP heparin U/mL 0024-0721-17	50 (2 mL)
100 USP heparin U/mL 0024-0722-16	50 (1 mL fill in 2 mL)
100 USP heparin U/mL 0024-0722-17	50 (2 mL)
HEP-PAK® Convenience Package[1]	
10 USP heparin U/mL (25 G × ⅝") 0024-0725-03	50 × 3
100 USP heparin U/mL (25 G × ⅝") 0024-0736-03	50 × 3

HEP-PAK® 2 Convenience Package[2]
10 USP heparin U/mL   50 × 2
(25 G × 5/8") 0024-0741-12
100 USP heparin U/mL   50 × 2
(25 G × 5/8") 0024-0742-12

HEP-PAK® CVC Convenience Package[3]
10 USP heparin U/2 mL   30 × 3
(25 G × 5/8") 0024-0725-02
100 USP heparin U/2 mL   30 × 3
(25 G × 5/8") 0024-0736-02

HEPARIN Sodium Injection, USP
5000 USP heparin U/mL   10 (1 mL fill in 2 mL)
(25 G × 5/8") 0024-0793-02
5000 USP heparin U/mL   50 (1 mL fill in 2 mL)
(25 G × 5/8") 0024-0793-12

HEPARIN Sodium Injection, USP
Preservative-Free
5000 USP heparin U/0.5 mL 10 (0.5 mL fill in 2 mL)
(25 G × 5/8") 0024-0733-05
5000 USP heparin U/0.5 mL 50 (0.5 mL fill in 2 mL)
(25 G × 5/8") 0024-0733-15

HEPARIN Sodium Injection, USP
Preservative-Free
10 000 USP heparin U/mL   10 (1 mL fill in 2 mL)
(25 G × 5/8") 0024-0733-02
10 000 USP heparin U/mL   50 (1 mL fill in 2 mL)
(25 G × 5/8") 0024-0733-12

HYDROMORPHONE Hydrochloride   Ⓒ(II)
Injection, USP
1 mg (22 G ×1¼")   10 (1 mL fill in 2 mL)
0024-0726-02
2 mg (22 G × 1¼")   10 (1 mL fill in 2 mL)
0024-0728-02
4 mg (22 G × 1¼")   10 (1 mL fill in 2 mL)
0024-0727-02

HYDROXYZINE Hydrochloride Injection, USP
25 mg (22 G × 1¼")   10 (1 mL fill in 2 mL)
0024-0711-02
50 mg (22 G × 1¼")   10 (1 mL fill in 2 mL)
0024-0712-02
100 mg (22 G × 1¼")   10 (2 mL)
0024-0713-02

MORPHINE Sulfate Injection, USP   Ⓒ(II)
2 mg (25 G × 5/8")   10 (1 mL fill in 2 mL)
0024-1257-02
4 mg (25 G × 5/8")   10 (1 mL fill in 2 mL)
0024-1258-02
8 mg (22 G × 1¼")   10 (1 mL fill in 2 mL)
0024-1259-02
8 mg (25 G × 5/8")   10 (1 mL fill in 2 mL)
0024-1260-02
10 mg (22 G × 1¼")   10 (1 mL fill in 2 mL)
0024-1261-02
10 mg (25 G × 5/8")   10 (1 mL fill in 2 mL)
0024-1263-02
15 mg (22 G × 1¼")   10 (1 mL fill in 2 mL)
0024-1262-02
15 mg (25 G × 5/8")   10 (1 mL fill in 2 mL)
0024-1264-02

NEO-SYNEPHRINE® Hydrochloride
brand of phenylephrine HCl injection, USP
10 mg (22 G × 1¼")   50 (1 mL fill in 2 mL)
0024-1340-02

PHENYTOIN Sodium Injection, USP
100 mg/2 mL (22 G × 1¼")   10 (2 mL)
0024-1549-01
250 mg/5 mL (22 G × 1¼")   10 (5 mL)
0024-1549-05

PROCAINAMIDE Hydrochloride, USP
500 mg   10 (2 mL)
(22 G × 1¼")
0024-1526-02

PROCHLORPERAZINE Edisylate Injection, USP
10 mg/2 mL (22 G × 1¼")   10 (2 mL)
0024-1598-01

SODIUM Chloride Injection, USP, 0.9%
(22 G × 1¼")   50 (2 mL)
0024-1811-02
(22 G × 1¼")   25 (3 mL fill in 5 mL)
0024-1811-03
(22 G × 1¼")   25 (5 mL)
0024-1811-05
(25 G × 5/8")   50 (2 mL)
0024-1815-02

(25 G × 5/8")   25 (3 mL fill in 5 mL)
0024-1815-03
(25 G × 5/8")   25 (5 mL)
0024-1815-05

SAL-PAK™ 2 Convenience Package[4]
(22 G × 1¼")   50 (2 mL)
0024-1811-20
(25 G × 1¼")   50 (2 mL)
0024-1815-20

TALWIN® Injection   Ⓒ(IV)
brand of pentazocine lactate injection, USP
30 mg (22 G × 1¼")   10 (1 mL fill in 2 mL)
0024-1917-02
45 mg (22 G × 1¼")   10 (1.5 mL fill in 2 mL)
0024-1918-02
60 mg (22 G × 1¼")   10 (2 mL)
0024-1919-02

TRIMETHOBENZAMIDE
Hydrochloride Injection, USP
200 mg (22 G × 1¼")   10 (2 mL)
0024-1955-03

VERAPAMIL Hydrochloride
5 mg (22 G × 1¼")   10 (2 mL)
0024-2110-03

EMPTY STERILE CARPUJECT
(22 G × 1¼")   10 (2 mL)
(25 G × 5/8")   10 (2 mL)

[1] Each HEP-PAK® contains one cartridge of Heparin Lock Flush Solution, USP (10 U/mL or 100 U/mL) with two cartridges of Sodium Chloride Injection, USP, 0.9% (2 mL).
[2] Each HEP-PAK® 2 contains one cartridge of Heparin Lock Flush Solution (10 U/mL or 100 U/mL) with one cartridge of Sodium Chloride Injection, USP, 0.9% (2 mL).
[3] Each HEP-PAK® CVC Convenience Package contains one cartridge of Heparin Lock Flush Solution 2 mL fill (20 or 200 U/2 mL) with two cartridges of Sodium Chloride Injection, USP, 0.9% (2 mL).
[4] Each SAL-PAK™ contains 2 cartridges of Sodium Chloride Injection, USP, 0.9%, (2 mL fill in 2 mL cartridge).
[5] InterLink is a trademark of Baxter Healthcare Corp. U.S. Pat. No. D321, 250; Pat. Pending.

DANOCRINE®   ℞
brand of danazol capsules, USP

DESCRIPTION
DANOCRINE, brand of danazol, is a synthetic steroid derived from ethisterone. Chemically, danazol is 17α-Pregna-2,4-dien-20-yno[2,3-d]-isoxazol-17-ol.
Inactive Ingredients: Benzyl Alcohol, Gelatin, Lactose, Magnesium Stearate, Parabens, Sodium Propionate, Starch, Talc. CAPSULES 50 mg and 200 mg contain D&C Yellow #10, FD&C Red #3. CAPSULE 100 mg contains D&C Yellow #10, FD&C Yellow #6.

CLINICAL PHARMACOLOGY
DANOCRINE suppresses the pituitary-ovarian axis. This suppression is probably a combination of depressed hypothalamic-pituitary response to lowered estrogen production, the alteration of sex steroid metabolism, and interaction of danazol with sex hormone receptors. The only other demonstrable hormonal effect is weak androgenic activity. DANOCRINE depresses the output of both follicle-stimulating hormone (FSH) and luteinizing hormone (LH).
Recent evidence suggests a direct inhibitory effect at gonadal sites and a binding of DANOCRINE to receptors of gonadal steroids at target organs.
Bioavailability studies indicate that blood levels do not increase proportionally with increases in the administered dose. When the dose of DANOCRINE is doubled, the increase in plasma levels is only about 35% to 40%.
In the treatment of endometriosis, DANOCRINE alters the normal and ectopic endometrial tissue so that it becomes inactive and atrophic. Complete resolution of endometrial lesions occurs in the majority of cases.
Changes in vaginal cytology and cervical mucus reflect the suppressive effect of DANOCRINE on the pituitary-ovarian axis.
In the treatment of fibrocystic breast disease, DANOCRINE usually produces partial to complete disappearance of nodularity and complete relief of pain and tenderness. Changes in the menstrual pattern may occur.
Generally, the pituitary-suppressive action of DANOCRINE is reversible. Ovulation and cyclic bleeding usually return within 60 to 90 days when therapy with DANOCRINE is discontinued.
In the treatment of hereditary angioedema, DANOCRINE at effective doses prevents attacks of the disease characterized by episodic edema of the abdominal viscera, extremities,

face, and airway which may be disabling and, if the airway is involved, fatal. In addition, DANOCRINE corrects partially or completely the primary biochemical abnormality of hereditary angioedema by increasing the levels of the deficient C1 esterase inhibitor (C1EI). As a result of this action the serum levels of the C4 component of the complement system are also increased.

INDICATIONS AND USAGE
Endometriosis. DANOCRINE is indicated for the treatment of endometriosis amenable to hormonal management.
Fibrocystic Breast Disease. Most cases of symptomatic fibrocystic breast disease may be treated by simple measures (eg, padded brassieres and analgesics).
In infrequent patients, symptoms of pain and tenderness may be severe enough to warrant treatment by suppression of ovarian function. DANOCRINE is usually effective in decreasing nodularity, pain, and tenderness. It should be stressed to the patient that this treatment is not innocuous in that it involves considerable alterations of hormone levels and that recurrence of symptoms is very common after cessation of therapy.
Hereditary Angioedema. DANOCRINE is indicated for the prevention of attacks of angioedema of all types (cutaneous, abdominal, laryngeal) in males and females.

CONTRAINDICATIONS
DANOCRINE should not be administered to patients with:
1. Undiagnosed abnormal genital bleeding.
2. Markedly impaired hepatic, renal, or cardiac function.
3. Pregnancy. (See WARNINGS.)
4. Breast feeding.
5. Porphyria—DANOCRINE can induce ALA synthetase activity and hence porphyrin metabolism.

WARNINGS

> **Use of danazol in pregnancy is contraindicated. A sensitive test (eg, beta subunit test if available) capable of determining early pregnancy is recommended immediately prior to start of therapy. Additionally a nonhormonal method of contraception should be used during therapy. If a patient becomes pregnant while taking danazol, administration of the drug should be discontinued and the patient should be apprised of the potential risk to the fetus. Exposure to danazol in utero may result in androgenic effects on the female fetus; reports of clitoral hypertrophy, labial fusion, urogenital sinus defect, vaginal atresia, and ambiguous genitalia have been received. (See PRECAUTIONS: Pregnancy, Teratogenic Effects.)**

Thromboembolism, thrombotic and thrombophlebitic events including sagittal sinus thrombosis and life-threatening or fatal strokes have been reported.
Experience with long-term therapy with danazol is limited. Peliosis hepatis and benign hepatic adenoma have been observed with long-term use. Peliosis hepatis and hepatic adenoma may be silent until complicated by acute, potentially life-threatening intra-abdominal hemorrhage. The physician therefore should be alert to this possibility. Attempts should be made to determine the lowest dose that will provide adequate protection. If the drug was begun at a time of exacerbation of hereditary angioneurotic edema due to trauma, stress or other cause, periodic attempts to decrease or withdraw therapy should be considered.
Danazol has been associated with several cases of benign intracranial hypertension also known as pseudotumor cerebri. Early signs and symptoms of benign intracranial hypertension include papilledema, headache, nausea and vomiting, and visual disturbances. Patients with these symptoms should be screened for papilledema and, if present, the patients should be advised to discontinue danazol immediately and be referred to a neurologist for further diagnosis and care.

A temporary alteration of lipoproteins in the form of decreased high density lipoproteins and possibly increased low density lipoproteins has been reported during danazol therapy. These alterations may be marked, and prescribers should consider the potential impact on the risk of atherosclerosis and coronary artery disease in accordance with the potential benefit of the therapy to the patient.
Before initiating therapy of fibrocystic breast disease with DANOCRINE, carcinoma of the breast should be excluded. However, nodularity, pain, tenderness due to fibrocystic

Continued on next page

This product information was prepared in August 1992. On these and other products of Sanofi Winthrop Pharmaceuticals, detailed information may be obtained on a current basis by direct inquiry to Product Information Services, 90 Park Avenue, New York, NY 10016 (toll free 1-800-446-6267).

Sanofi Winthrop—Cont.

breast disease may prevent recognition of underlying carcinoma before treatment is begun. Therefore, if any nodule persists or enlarges during treatment, carcinoma should be considered and ruled out.

Patients should be watched closely for signs of androgenic effects some of which may not be reversible even when drug administration is stopped.

PRECAUTIONS

Because DANOCRINE, brand of danazol capsules, may cause some degree of fluid retention, conditions that might be influenced by this factor, such as epilepsy, migraine, or cardiac or renal dysfunction, require careful observation.

Since hepatic dysfunction manifested by modest increases in serum transaminase levels has been reported in patients treated with DANOCRINE, periodic liver function tests should be performed (see WARNINGS and ADVERSE REACTIONS).

Administration of danazol has been reported to cause exacerbation of the manifestations of acute intermittent porphyria. (See CONTRAINDICATIONS.)

Drug Interactions: Prolongation of prothrombin time occurs in patients stabilized on warfarin. Therapy with danazol may cause an increase in carbamazepine levels in patients taking both drugs.

Laboratory Tests: Danazol treatment may interfere with laboratory determinations of testosterone, androstenedione, and dehydroepiandrosterone.

Carcinogenesis, Mutagenesis, Impairment of Fertility: No valid studies have been performed to assess the carcinogenicity of DANOCRINE.

Pregnancy, Teratogenic Effects: (See CONTRAINDICATIONS.) Pregnancy Category X. DANOCRINE administered orally to pregnant rats from the 6th through the 15th day of gestation at doses up to 250 mg/kg/day (7–15 times the human dose) did not result in drug-induced embryotoxicity or teratogenicity, nor difference in litter size, viability or weight of offspring compared to controls. In rabbits, the administration of DANOCRINE on days 6–18 of gestation at doses of 60 mg/kg/day and above (2–4 times the human dose) resulted in inhibition of fetal development.

Nursing Mothers: (See CONTRAINDICATIONS.)

Pediatric Use: Safety and effectiveness in children have not been established.

ADVERSE REACTIONS

The following events have been reported in association with the use of DANOCRINE:

Andogren-like effects include weight gain, acne, and seborrhea. Mild hirsutism, edema, hair loss, voice change, which may take the form of hoarseness, sore throat, or of instability or deepening of pitch, may occur and may persist after cessation of therapy. Hypertrophy of the clitoris is rare.

Other possible endocrine effects include menstrual disturbances in the form of spotting, alteration of the timing of the cycle and amenorrhea. Although cyclical bleeding and ovulation usually return within 60 to 90 days after discontinuation of therapy with DANOCRINE, persistent amenorrhea has occasionally been reported.

Flushing, sweating, vaginal dryness and irritation, and reduction in breast size may reflect lowering of estrogen. Nervousness and emotional liability have been reported. In the male a modest reduction in spermatogenesis may be evident during treatment. Abnormalities in semen volume, viscosity, sperm count, and motility may occur in patients receiving long-term therapy.

Hepatic dysfunction, as evidenced by reversible elevated serum enzymes and/or jaundice, has been reported in patients receiving a daily dosage of DANOCRINE of 400 mg or more. It is recommended that patients receiving DANOCRINE be monitored for hepatic dysfunction by laboratory tests and clinical observation. Serious hepatic toxicity including cholestatic jaundice, peliosis hepatis, and hepatic adenoma have been reported. (See WARNINGS and PRECAUTIONS.)

Abnormalities in laboratory tests may occur during therapy with DANOCRINE including CPK, glucose tolerance, glucagon, thyroid binding globulin, sex hormone binding globulin, other plasma proteins, lipids and lipoproteins.

The following reactions have been reported, a causal relationship to the administration of DANOCRINE has neither been confirmed nor refuted; *allergic:* urticaria, pruritus and rarely, nasal congestion; *CNS effects:* headache, nervousness and emotional lability, dizziness and fainting, depression, fatigue, sleep disorders, tremor, paresthesias, weakness, visual disturbances, and rarely, benign intracranial hypertension, anxiety, changes in appetite, chills, and rarely Guillain-Barré syndrome; *gastrointestinal:* gastroenteritis, nausea, vomiting, constipation, and rarely, pancreatitis; *musculoskeletal:* muscle cramps or spasms, or pains, joint pain, joint lockup, joint swelling, pain in back, neck, or extremities, and rarely, carpal tunnel syndrome which may be secondary to fluid retention; *genitourinary:* hematuria, prolonged posttherapy amenorrhea; *hematologic:* an increase in red cell and platelet count. Reversible erythrocytosis, leukocytosis or polycythemia may be provoked. Eosinophilia, leukopenia and thrombocytopenia have also been noted. *Skin:* rashes (maculopapular, vesicular, papular, purpuric, petechial), and rarely, sun sensitivity, Stevens-Johnson syndrome; *other:* increased insulin requirements in diabetic patients, changes in libido, elevation in blood pressure, and rarely, cataracts, bleeding gums, fever, pelvic pain, nipple discharge.

DOSAGE AND ADMINISTRATION

Endometriosis. In moderate to severe disease, or in patients infertile due to endometriosis, a starting dose of 800 mg given in two divided doses is recommended. Amenorrhea and rapid response to painful symptoms is best achieved at this dosage level. Gradual downward titration to a dose sufficient to maintain amenorrhea may be considered depending upon patient response. For mild cases, an initial daily dose of 200 mg to 400 mg given in two divided doses is recommended and may be adjusted depending on patient response. **Therapy should begin during menstruation. Otherwise, appropriate tests should be performed to ensure that the patient is not pregnant while on therapy with DANOCRINE. (See CONTRAINDICATIONS and WARNINGS.) It is essential that therapy continue uninterrupted for 3 to 6 months but may be extended to 9 months if necessary.** After termination of therapy, if symptoms recur, treatment can be reinstituted.

Fibrocystic Breast Disease. The total daily dosage of DANOCRINE, brand of danazol capsules, for fibrocystic breast disease ranges from 100 mg to 400 mg given in two divided doses depending upon patient response. **Therapy should begin during menstruation. Otherwise, appropriate tests should be performed to ensure that the patient is not pregnant while on therapy with DANOCRINE.** A nonhormonal method of contraception is recommended when DANOCRINE is administered at this dose, since ovulation may not be suppressed.

In most instances, breast pain and tenderness are significantly relieved by the first month and eliminated in 2 to 3 months. Usually elimination of nodularity requires 4 to 6 months of uninterrupted therapy. Regular menstrual patterns, irregular menstrual patterns, and amenorrhea each occur in approximately one-third of patients treated with 100 mg of DANOCRINE. Irregular menstrual patterns and amenorrhea are observed more frequently with higher doses. Clinical studies have demonstrated that 50% of patients may show evidence of recurrence of symptoms within one year. In this event, treatment may be reinstated.

Hereditary Angioedema. The dosage requirements for continuous treatment of hereditary angioedema with DANOCRINE, brand of danazol capsules, should be individualized on the basis of the clinical response of the patient. It is recommended that the patient be started on 200 mg, two or three times a day. After a favorable initial response is obtained in terms of prevention of episodes of edematous attacks, the proper continuing dosage should be determined by decreasing the dosage by 50% or less at intervals of one to three months or longer if frequency of attacks prior to treatment dictates. If an attack occurs, the daily dosage may be increased by up to 200 mg. During the dose adjusting phase, close monitoring of the patient's response is indicated, particularly if the patient has a history of airway involvement.

HOW SUPPLIED

Capsules of 200 mg (orange), bottles of 60 (NDC 0024-0305-60).

Capsules of 200 mg (orange), bottles of 100 (NDC 0024-0305-06).

Capsules of 100 mg (yellow), bottles of 100 (NDC 0024-0304-06).

Capsules of 50 mg (orange and white), bottles of 100 (NDC 0024-0303-06).

Manufactured by Sterling Pharmaceuticals Inc.
Barceloneta, Puerto Rico 00617

DW-254-W(0)

Shown in Product Identification Section, page 428

DEMEROL® Hydrochloride Ⓒ℞
brand of meperidine hydrochloride, USP

DESCRIPTION

Meperidine hydrochloride is ethyl 1-methyl-4-phenylisonipecotate hydrochloride, a white crystalline substance with a melting point of 186°C to 189°C. It is readily soluble in water and has a neutral reaction and a slightly bitter taste. The solution is not decomposed by a short period of boiling.

The syrup is a pleasant-tasting, nonalcoholic, banana-flavored solution containing 50 mg of DEMEROL hydrochloride, brand of meperidine hydrochloride, per 5 mL teaspoon (25 drops contain 13 mg of DEMEROL hydrochloride). The tablets contain 50 mg or 100 mg of the analgesic.

DEMEROL hydrochloride injectable is supplied in Carpuject® Sterile Cartridge-Needle Unit of 2.5% (25 mg/1 mL), 5% (50 mg/1 mL), 7.5% (75 mg/ 1 mL), and 10% (100 mg/1 mL). Uni-Amp® Unit Dose Pak—ampuls of 5% solution (25 mg/0.5 mL), (50 mg/1 mL), (75 mg/1.5 mL), 100 mg/2 mL), and 10% solution (100 mg/1 mL). Uni-Nest™ Pak—ampuls of 5% solution (25 mg/0.5 mL), (50 mg/1 mL), (75 mg/1.5 mL), (100 mg/2 mL), and 10% solution (100 mg/1 mL). Multiple-dose vials of 5% and 10% solutions contain metacresol 0.1% as preservative.

The pH of DEMEROL solution is adjusted between 3.5 and 6 with sodium hydroxide or hydrochloric acid.

DEMEROL hydrochloride, brand of meperidine hydrochloride, 5 percent solution has a specific gravity of 1.0086 at 20°C and 10 percent solution, a specific gravity of 1.0165 at 20°C.

Inactive Ingredients—TABLETS: Calcium Sulfate, Dibasic Calcium Phosphate, Starch, Stearic Acid, Talc.

SYRUP: Benzoic Acid, Flavor, Liquid Glucose, Purified Water, Saccharin Sodium.

CLINICAL PHARMACOLOGY

Meperidine hydrochloride is a narcotic analgesic with multiple actions qualitatively similar to those of morphine; the most prominent of these involve the central nervous system and organs composed of smooth muscle. The principal actions of therapeutic value are analgesia and sedation.

There is some evidence which suggests that meperidine may produce less smooth muscle spasm, constipation, and depression of the cough reflex than equianalgesic doses of morphine. Meperidine, in 60 mg to 80 mg parenteral doses, is approximately equivalent in analgesic effect to 10 mg of morphine. The onset of action is slightly more rapid than with morphine, and the duration of action is slightly shorter. Meperidine is significantly less effective by the oral than by the parenteral route, but the exact ratio of oral to parenteral effectiveness is unknown.

INDICATIONS AND USAGE

For the relief of moderate to severe pain (parenteral and oral forms)

For preoperative medication (parenteral form only)

For support of anesthesia (parenteral form only)

For obstetrical analgesia (parenteral form only)

CONTRAINDICATIONS

Hypersensitivity to meperidine.

Meperidine is contraindicated in patients who are receiving monoamine oxidase (MAO) inhibitors or those who have recently received such agents. Therapeutic doses of meperidine have occasionally precipitated unpredictable, severe, and occasionally fatal reactions in patients who have received such agents within 14 days. The mechanism of these reactions is unclear, but may be related to a preexisting hyperphenylalaninemia. Some have been characterized by coma, severe respiratory depression, cyanosis, and hypotension, and have resembled the syndrome of acute narcotic overdose. In other reactions the predominant manifestations have been hyperexcitability, convulsions, tachycardia, hyperpyrexia, and hypertension. Although it is not known that other narcotics are free of the risk of such reactions, virtually all of the reported reactions have occurred with meperidine. If a narcotic is needed in such patients, a sensitivity test should be performed in which repeated, small, incremental doses of morphine are administered over the course of several hours while the patient's condition and vital signs are under careful observation. (Intravenous hydrocortisone or prednisolone have been used to treat severe reactions, with the addition of intravenous chlorpromazine in those cases exhibiting hypertension and hyperpyrexia. The usefulness and safety of narcotic antagonists in the treatment of these reactions is unknown.)

Solutions of DEMEROL and barbiturates are chemically incompatible.

WARNINGS

Drug Dependence. Meperidine can produce drug dependence of the morphine type and therefore has the potential for being abused. Psychic dependence, physical dependence, and tolerance may develop upon repeated administration of meperidine, and it should be prescribed and administered with the same degree of caution appropriate to the use of morphine. Like other narcotics, meperidine is subject to the provisions of the Federal narcotic laws.

Interaction with Other Central Nervous System Depressants. MEPERIDINE SHOULD BE USED WITH GREAT CAUTION AND IN REDUCED DOSAGE IN PATIENTS WHO ARE CONCURRENTLY RECEIVING OTHER NARCOTIC ANALGESICS, GENERAL ANESTHETICS, PHENOTHIAZINES, OTHER TRANQUILIZERS (SEE DOSAGE AND ADMINISTRATION), SEDATIVE-HYPNOTICS (INCLUDING BARBITURATES), TRICYCLIC ANTIDEPRESSANTS, AND OTHER CNS DEPRESSANTS (INCLUDING ALCOHOL). RESPIRATORY DEPRESSION, HYPOTENSION, AND PROFOUND SEDATION OR COMA MAY RESULT.

Head Injury and Increased Intracranial Pressure. The respiratory depressant effects of meperidine and its capacity to elevate cerebrospinal fluid pressure may be markedly exaggerated in the presence of head injury, other intracranial

lesions, or a preexisting increase in intracranial pressure. Furthermore, narcotics produce adverse reactions which may obscure the clinical course of patients with head injuries. In such patients, meperidine must be used with extreme caution and only if its use is deemed essential.

Intravenous Use. If necessary, meperidine may be given intravenously, but the injection should be given very slowly, preferably in the form of a diluted solution. Rapid intravenous injection of narcotic analgesics, including meperidine, increases the incidence of adverse reactions; severe respiratory depression, apnea, hypotension, peripheral circulatory collapse, and cardiac arrest have occurred. Meperidine should not be administered intravenously unless a narcotic antagonist and the facilities for assisted or controlled respiration are immediately available. When meperidine is given parenterally, especially intravenously, the patient should be lying down.

Asthma and Other Respiratory Conditions. Meperidine should be used with extreme caution in patients having an acute asthmatic attack, patients with chronic obstructive pulmonary disease or cor pulmonale, patients having a substantially decreased respiratory reserve, and patients with preexisting respiratory depression, hypoxia, or hypercapnia. In such patients, even usual therapeutic doses of narcotics may decrease respiratory drive while simultaneously increasing airway resistance to the point of apnea.

Hypotensive Effect. The administration of meperidine may result in severe hypotension in the postoperative patient or any individual whose ability to maintain blood pressure has been compromised by a depleted blood volume or the administration of drugs such as the phenothiazines or certain anesthetics.

Usage in Ambulatory Patients. Meperidine may impair the mental and/or physical abilities required for the performance of potentially hazardous tasks such as driving a car or operating machinery. The patient should be cautioned accordingly.

Meperidine, like other narcotics, may produce orthostatic hypotension in ambulatory patients.

Usage in Pregnancy and Lactation. Meperidine should not be used in pregnant women prior to the labor period, unless in the judgment of the physician the potential benefits outweigh the possible hazards, because safe use in pregnancy prior to labor has not been established relative to possible adverse effects on fetal development.

When used as an obstetrical analgesic, meperidine crosses the placental barrier and can produce depression of respiration and psychophysiologic functions in the newborn. Resuscitation may be required (see section on **OVERDOSAGE**). Meperidine appears in the milk of nursing mothers receiving the drug.

PRECAUTIONS

As with all intramuscular preparations DEMEROL intramuscular injection should be injected well within the body of a large muscle.

Supraventricular Tachycardias. Meperidine should be used with caution in patients with atrial flutter and other supraventricular tachycardias because of a possible vagolytic action which may produce a significant increase in the ventricular response rate.

Convulsions. Meperidine may aggravate preexisting convulsions in patients with convulsive disorders. If dosage is escalated substantially above recommended levels because of tolerance development, convulsions may occur in individuals without a history of convulsive disorders.

Acute Abdominal Conditions. The administration of meperidine or other narcotics may obscure the diagnosis or clinical course in patients with acute abdominal conditions.

Special Risk Patients. Meperidine should be given with caution and the initial dose should be reduced in certain patients such as the elderly or debilitated, and those with severe impairment of hepatic or renal function, hypothyroidism, Addison's disease, and prostatic hypertrophy or urethral stricture.

ADVERSE REACTIONS

The major hazards of meperidine, as with other narcotic analgesics, are respiratory depression and, to a lesser degree, circulatory depression; respiratory arrest, shock, and cardiac arrest have occurred.

The most frequently observed adverse reactions include lightheadedness, dizziness, sedation, nausea, vomiting, and sweating. These effects seem to be more prominent in ambulatory patients and in those who are not experiencing severe pain. In such individuals, lower doses are advisable. Some adverse reactions in ambulatory patients may be alleviated if the patient lies down.

Other adverse reactions include:

Nervous System. Euphoria, dysphoria, weakness, headache, agitation, tremor, uncoordinated muscle movements, severe convulsions, transient hallucinations and disorientation, visual disturbances. Inadvertent injection about a nerve trunk may result in sensory-motor paralysis which is usually, though not always, transitory.

Gastrointestinal. Dry mouth, constipation, biliary tract spasm.

Cardiovascular. Flushing of the face, tachycardia, bradycardia, palpitation, hypotension (see Warnings), syncope, phlebitis following intravenous injection.

Genitourinary. Urinary retention.

Allergic. Pruritus, urticaria, other skin rashes, wheal and flare over the vein with intravenous injection.

Other. Pain at injection site; local tissue irritation and induration following subcutaneous injection, particularly when repeated; antidiuretic effect.

DOSAGE AND ADMINISTRATION

For Relief of Pain

Dosage should be adjusted according to the severity of the pain and the response of the patient. While subcutaneous administration is suitable for occasional use, intramuscular administration is preferred when repeated doses are required. If intravenous administration is required, dosage should be decreased and the injection made very slowly, preferably utilizing a diluted solution. Meperidine is less effective orally than on parenteral administration. The dose of DEMEROL should be proportionately reduced (usually by 25 to 50 percent) when administered concomitantly with phenothiazines and many other tranquilizers since they potentiate the action of DEMEROL, brand of meperidine.

Adults. The usual dosage is 50 mg to 150 mg intramuscularly, subcutaneously, or orally, every 3 or 4 hours as necessary.

Children. The usual dosage is 0.5 mg/lb to 0.8 mg/lb intramuscularly, subcutaneously, or orally up to the adult dose, every 3 or 4 hours as necessary.

Each dose of the syrup sho[illegible]n one-half glass of water, since if taken u[illegible]ert a slight topical anesthetic effect on mu[illegible]es.

For Preoperative Medication

Adults. The usual dosage is 50 mg to 100 mg intramuscularly or subcutaneously, 30 to 90 minutes before the beginning of anesthesia.

Children. The usual dosage is 0.5 mg/lb to 1 mg/lb intramuscularly or subcutaneously up to the adult dose, 30 to 90 minutes before the beginning of anesthesia.

For Support of Anesthesia

Repeated slow intravenous injections of fractional doses (eg, 10 mg/mL) or continuous intravenous infusion of a more dilute solution (eg, 1 mg/mL) should be used. The dose should be titrated to the needs of the patient and will depend on the premedication and type of anesthesia being employed, the characteristics of the particular patient, and the nature and duration of the operative procedure.

For Obstetrical Analgesia

The usual dosage is 50 mg to 100 mg intramuscularly or subcutaneously when pain becomes regular, and may be repeated at 1- to 3-hour intervals.

OVERDOSAGE

Symptoms. Serious overdosage with meperidine is characterized by respiratory depression (a decrease in respiratory rate and/or tidal volume, Cheyne-Stokes respiration, cyanosis), extreme somnolence progressing to stupor or coma, skeletal muscle flaccidity, cold and clammy skin, and sometimes bradycardia and hypotension. In severe overdosage, particularly by the intravenous route, apnea, circulatory collapse, cardiac arrest, and death may occur.

Treatment. Primary attention should be given to the reestablishment of adequate respiratory exchange through provision of a patent airway and institution of assisted or controlled ventilation. The narcotic antagonist, naloxone hydrochloride, is a specific antidote against respiratory depression which may result from overdosage or unusual sensitivity to narcotics, including meperidine. Therefore, an appropriate dose of this antagonist should be administered, preferably by the intravenous route, simultaneously with efforts at respiratory resuscitation.

An antagonist should not be administered in the absence of clinically significant respiratory or cardiovascular depression.

Oxygen, intravenous fluids, vasopressors, and other supportive measures should be employed as indicated.

In cases of overdosage with DEMEROL, brand of meperidine, tablets, the stomach should be evacuated by emesis or gastric lavage.

NOTE: In an individual physically dependent on narcotics, the administration of the usual dose of a narcotic antagonist will precipitate an acute withdrawal syndrome. The severity of this syndrome will depend on the degree of physical dependence and the dose of antagonist administered. The use of narcotic antagonists in such individuals should be avoided if possible. If a narcotic antagonist must be used to treat serious respiratory depression in the physically dependent patient, the antagonist should be administered with extreme care and only one-fifth to one-tenth the usual initial dose administered.

HOW SUPPLIED

For Parenteral Use

Detecto-Seal ® — *Carpuject* ® **Sterile Cartridge-Needle Unit**—*2.5 percent* (25 mg per 1 mL) **NDC** 0024-0324-02, *5 percent* (50 mg per 1 mL) **NDC** 0024-0325-02, *7.5 percent* (75 mg per 1 mL) **NDC** 0024-0326-02; and *10 percent* (100 mg per 1 mL) **NDC** 0024-0328-02 all in boxes of 10.

Each cartridge is only partially-filled based upon product volume to permit mixture with other sterile materials in accordance with the best judgment of the physician.

Uni-Amp ®—*5 percent solution;* ampuls of 0.5 mL (25 mg) **NDC** 0024-0361-04, 1 mL (50 mg) **NDC** 0024-0362-04, 1½ mL (75 mg) **NDC** 0024-0363-04, and 2 mL (100 mg) **NDC** 0024-0364-04 all in boxes of 25; and *10 percent solution,* ampuls of 1 mL (100 mg) **NDC** 0024-0365-04 in boxes of 25.

Uni-Nest ™—*5 percent solution;* ampuls of 0.5 mL (25 mg) **NDC** 0024-0371-04, 1 mL (50 mg) **NDC** 0024-0372-04, 1½ mL (75 mg) **NDC** 0024-0373-04, and 2 mL (100 mg) **NDC** 0024-0374-04 all in boxes of 25; and *10 percent solution,* ampuls of 1 mL (100 mg) **NDC** 0024-0375-04 in boxes of 25.

Vials—*5 percent* multiple-dose vials of 30 mL **NDC** 0024-0329-01, and *10 percent* multiple-dose vials of 20 mL **NDC** 0024-0331-01 all in boxes of 1.

Note: The pH of DEMEROL solutions is adjusted between 3.5 and 6 with sodium hydroxide or hydrochloric acid. Multiple-dose vials contain metacresol 0.1 percent as preservative. No preservatives are added to the ampuls or CARPUJECT Sterile Cartridge-Needle Units.

For Oral Use

Tablets of 50 mg, bottles of 100 (**NDC** 0024-0335-04) and 500 (**NDC** 0024-0335-06); Hospital Blister Pak of 25 (**NDC** 0024-0335-02); 100 mg, bottles of 100 (**NDC** 0024-0337-04) and 500 (**NDC** 0024-0337-06); Hospital Blister Pak of 25 (**NDC** 0024-0337-02).

Syrup, nonalcoholic, banana-flavored 50 mg per 5 mL teaspoon, bottles of 16 fl oz (**NDC** 0024-0332-06).

DW-55-HH

Shown in Product Identification Section, page 428

INOCOR® LACTATE INJECTION ℞

brand of amrinone lactate
Sterile Intravenous Solution

DESCRIPTION

INOCOR lactate injection, brand of amrinone lactate, represents a new class of cardiac inotropic agents distinct from digitalis glycosides or catecholamines. Amrinone lactate is designated chemically as 5-Amino[3,4′-bipyridin]-6(1*H*)-one 2-hydroxypropanate.

Amrinone is a pale yellow crystalline compound with a molecular weight of 187.2 and an empirical formula of $C_{10}H_9N_3O$. Each mole of lactic acid has a molecular weight of 90.08 and an empirical formula of $C_3H_6O_3$. The solubilities of amrinone at pH's 4.1, 6.0, and 8.0 are 25, 0.9, and 0.7 mg/mL, respectively.

INOCOR lactate injection is available as a sterile solution in 20 mL ampuls for intravenous administration. Each mL contains INOCOR lactate equivalent to 5 mg of base and 0.25 mg of sodium metabisulfite added as a preservative in Water for Injection. All dosages expressed in the package insert are expressed in terms of the base, amrinone. The pH is adjusted to between 3.2 to 4.0 with lactic acid or sodium hydroxide. The total concentration of lactic acid can vary between 5.0 mg/mL and 7.5 mg/mL.

CLINICAL PHARMACOLOGY

INOCOR lactate injection is a positive inotropic agent with vasodilator activity, different in structure and mode of action from either digitalis glycosides or catecholamines.

The mechanism of its inotropic and vasodilator effects has not been fully elucidated.

With respect to its inotropic effect, experimental evidence indicates that it is not a beta-adrenergic agonist. It inhibits myocardial cyclic adenosine monophosphate (c-AMP) phosphodiesterase activity and increases cellular levels of c-AMP. Unlike digitalis, it does not inhibit sodium-potassium adenosine triphosphatase activity.

With respect to its vasodilatory activity, INOCOR reduces afterload and preload by its direct relaxant effect on vascular smooth muscle.

Pharmacokinetics

Following intravenous bolus (1 to 2 minutes) injection of 0.68 mg/kg to 1.2 mg/kg to normal volunteers, INOCOR had a

Continued on next page

This product information was prepared in August 1992. On these and other products of Sanofi Winthrop Pharmaceuticals, detailed information may be obtained on a current basis by direct inquiry to Product Information Services, 90 Park Avenue, New York, NY 10016 (toll free 1-800-446-6267).

Sanofi Winthrop—Cont.

volume of distribution of 1.2 liters/kg, and following a distributive phase half-life of about 4.6 minutes in plasma, had a mean apparent first-order terminal elimination half-life of about 3.6 hours. In patients with congestive heart failure receiving infusions of INOCOR the mean apparent first-order terminal elimination half-life was about 5.8 hours.

Amrinone has been shown in one study to be 10% to 22% bound to human plasma protein by ultrafiltration in vitro, and in another study 35% to 49% bound by either ultrafiltration or equilibrium dialysis.

The primary route of excretion in man is *via* the urine as both amrinone and several metabolites (N-glycolyl, N-acetate, O-glucuronide and N-glucuronide). In normal volunteers, approximately 63% of an oral dose of ^{14}C-labelled amrinone was excreted in the urine over a 96-hour period. In the first 8 hours, 51% of the radioactivity in the urine was amrinone with 5% as the N-acetate, 8% as the N-glycolate, and less than 5% for each glucuronide. Approximately 18% of the administered dose was excreted in the feces in 72 hours.

In a 24-hour nonradioactive intravenous study, 10% to 40% of the dose was excreted in urine as unchanged amrinone with the N-acetyl metabolite representing less than 2% of the dose.

In congestive heart failure patients, after a loading bolus dose, steady-state plasma levels of about 2.4 µg/mL were able to be maintained by an infusion of 5 µg/kg/min to 10 µg/kg/min. In some congestive heart failure patients, with associated compromised renal and hepatic perfusion, it is possible that plasma levels of amrinone may rise during the infusion period; therefore, in these patients, it may be necessary to monitor the hemodynamic response and/or drug level. The principal measures of patient response include cardiac index, pulmonary capillary wedge pressure, central venous pressure, and their relationship to plasma concentrations. Additionally, measurements of blood pressure, urine output, and body weight may prove useful, as may such clinical symptoms as orthopnea, dyspnea, and fatigue.

Pharmacodynamics

In patients with depressed myocardial function, INOCOR lactate injection produces a prompt increase in cardiac output due to its inotropic and vasodilator actions.

Following a single intravenous bolus dose of INOCOR of 0.75 mg/kg to 3 mg/kg in patients with congestive heart failure, dose-related maximum increases in cardiac output occur (of about 28% at 0.75 mg/kg to about 61% at 3 mg/kg). The peak effect occurs within 10 minutes at all doses. The duration of effect depends upon dose, lasting about ½ hour at 0.75 mg/kg and approximately 2 hours at 3 mg/kg.

Over the same range of doses, pulmonary capillary wedge pressure and total peripheral resistance show dose-related decreases (mean maximum decreases of 29% in pulmonary capillary wedge pressure and 29% in systemic vascular resistance). At doses up to 3.0 mg/kg dose-related decreases in diastolic pressure (up to 13%) have been observed. Mean arterial pressure decreases (9.7%) at a dose of 3.0 mg/kg. The heart rate is generally unchanged.

The changes in hemodynamic parameters are maintained during continuous intravenous infusion and for several hours thereafter.

INOCOR lactate injection, brand of amrinone lactate, is effective in fully digitalized patients without causing signs of cardiac glycoside toxicity. Its inotropic effects are additive to those of digitalis. In cases of atrial flutter/fibrillation, it is possible that INOCOR may increase ventricular response rate because of its slight enhancement of A/V conduction. In these cases, prior treatment with digitalis is recommended.

Improvement in left ventricular function and relief of congestive heart failure in patients with ischemic heart disease have been observed. The improvement has occurred without inducing symptoms or electrocardiographic signs of myocardial ischemia.

At constant heart rate and blood pressure, increases in cardiac output occur without measurable increases in myocardial oxygen consumption or changes in arteriovenous oxygen difference.

Inotropic activity is maintained following repeated intravenous doses of INOCOR. Administration of INOCOR produces hemodynamic and symptomatic benefits to patients not satisfactorily controlled by conventional therapy with diuretics and cardiac glycosides.

INDICATIONS AND USAGE

INOCOR lactate injection is indicated for the short-term management of congestive heart failure. Because of limited experience and potential for serious adverse effects (see ADVERSE REACTIONS), INOCOR should be used only in patients who can be closely monitored and who have not responded adequately to digitalis, diuretics, and/or vasodilators. Although most patients have been studied hemodynamically for periods only up to 24 hours, some patients were studied for longer periods and demonstrated consistent hemodynamic and clinical effects. The duration of therapy should depend on patient responsiveness.

CONTRAINDICATIONS

INOCOR lactate injection is contraindicated in patients who are hypersensitive to it.

It is also contraindicated in those patients known to be hypersensitive to bisulfites.

WARNING

Contains sodium metabisulfite, a sulfite that may cause allergic-type reactions including anaphylactic symptoms and life-threatening or less severe asthmatic episodes in certain susceptible people. The overall prevalence of sulfite sensitivity in the general population is unknown and probably low. Sulfite sensitivity is seen more frequently in asthmatic than in nonasthmatic people.

PRECAUTIONS

General

INOCOR lactate injection should not be used in patients with severe aortic or pulmonic valvular disease in lieu of surgical relief of the obstruction. Like other inotropic agents, it may aggravate outflow tract obstruction in hypertrophic subaortic stenosis.

During intravenous therapy with INOCOR lactate injection, blood pressure and heart rate should be monitored and the rate of infusion slowed or stopped in patients showing excessive decreases in blood pressure.

Patients who have received vigorous diuretic therapy may have insufficient cardiac filling pressure to respond adequately to INOCOR lactate injection, in which case cautious liberalization of fluid and electrolyte intake may be indicated.

Supraventricular and ventricular arrhythmias have been observed in the v[illegible]h-risk population treated. While amrinone per se h[illegible]wn to be arrhythmogenic, the potential for a[illegible]t in congestive heart failure itself, may be [illegible]ny drug or combination of drugs.

Thrombocytopenia and hepatotoxicity have been noted (see ADVERSE REACTIONS).

USE IN ACUTE MYOCARDIAL INFARCTION

No clinical trials have been carried out in patients in the acute phase of postmyocardial infarction. Therefore, INOCOR lactate injection, brand of amrinone lactate, is not recommended in these cases.

Laboratory Tests

Fluid and Electrolytes: Fluid and electrolyte changes and renal function should be carefully monitored during amrinone lactate therapy. Improvement in cardiac output with resultant diuresis may necessitate a reduction in the dose of diuretic. Potassium loss due to excessive diuresis may predispose digitalized patients to arrhythmias. Therefore, hypokalemia should be corrected by potassium supplementation in advance of or during amrinone use.

Drug Interactions

In a relatively limited experience, no untoward clinical manifestations have been observed in patients in which INOCOR lactate injection was used concurrently with the following drugs: digitalis glycosides; lidocaine, quinidine; metoprolol, propranolol; hydralazine, prazosin; isosorbide dinitrate, nitroglycerine; chlorthalidone, ethacrynic acid, furosemide, hydrochlorothiazide, spironolactone; captopril; heparin, warfarin; potassium supplements; insulin; diazepam.

One case report of excessive hypotension has been reported when amrinone was used concurrently with disopyramide. Until additional experience is available, concurrent administration with NORPACE® (disopyramide) should be undertaken with caution.

Chemical Interactions

A chemical interaction occurs slowly over a 24-hour period when the intravenous solution of INOCOR lactate injection is mixed directly with dextrose(glucose)-containing solutions. **THEREFORE, INOCOR LACTATE INJECTION SHOULD NOT BE DILUTED WITH SOLUTIONS THAT CONTAIN DEXTROSE (GLUCOSE) PRIOR TO INJECTION.**

A chemical interaction occurs immediately, which is evidenced by the formation of a precipitate when furosemide is injected into an intravenous line of an infusion of amrinone. Therefore, furosemide should not be administered in intravenous lines containing amrinone.

Carcinogenesis, Mutagenesis, Impairment of Fertility

There was no suggestion of a carcinogenic potential with amrinone when administered orally for up to two years to rats and mice at dose levels up to the maximally tolerated dose of 80 mg/kg/day.

The mouse micronucleus test (at 7.5 to 10 times the maximum human dose) and the Chinese hamster ovary chromosome aberration assay were positive indicating both clastogenic potential and suppression of the number of polychromatic erythrocytes. However, the Ames Salmonella assay, mouse lymphoma study, and cultured human lymphocyte metaphase analysis were all negative. The clastogenic effects are in contrast to negative results obtained in the rat male and female fertility studies, and a three-generation study in rats, both with oral dosing.

Slight prolongation of the rat gestation period was seen in these studies at dose levels of 50 mg/kg/day and 100 mg/kg/day. Dystocia occurred in dams receiving 100 mg/kg/day resulting in increased numbers of stillbirths, decreased litter size, and poor pup survival.

Pregnancy Category C

In New Zealand white rabbits, amrinone has been shown to produce fetal skeletal and gross external malformations at oral doses of 16 mg/kg and 50 mg/kg which were toxic for the rabbit. Studies in French Hy/Cr rabbits using oral doses up to 32 mg/kg/day did not confirm this finding. No malformations were seen in rats receiving amrinone intravenously at the maximum dose used, 15 mg/kg/day (approximately the recommended daily intravenous dose for patients with congestive heart failure). There are no adequate and well-controlled studies in pregnant women. Amrinone should be used during pregnancy only if the potential benefit justifies the potential risk to the fetus.

Nursing Mothers

Caution should be exercised when amrinone is administered to nursing women, since it is not known whether it is excreted in human milk.

Pediatric Use

Safety and effectiveness in children have not been established.

ADVERSE REACTIONS

Thrombocytopenia: Intravenous INOCOR lactate injection, brand of amrinone lactate, resulted in platelet count reductions to below 100,000/mm^3 or normal limits in 2.4 percent of the patients.

It is more common in patients receiving prolonged therapy. To date, in closely-monitored clinical trials, in patients whose platelet counts were not allowed to remain depressed, no bleeding phenomena have been observed.

Platelet reduction is dose dependent and appears due to a decrease in platelet survival time. Several patients who developed thrombocytopenia while receiving amrinone had bone marrow examinations which were normal. There is no evidence relating platelet reduction to immune response or to a platelet activating factor.

Gastrointestinal Effects: Gastrointestinal adverse reactions reported with INOCOR lactate injection during clinical use included nausea (1.7%), vomiting (0.9%), abdominal pain (0.4%), and anorexia (0.4%).

Cardiovascular Effects: Cardiovascular adverse reactions reported with INOCOR lactate injection include arrhythmia (3%) and hypotension (1.3%).

Hepatic Toxicity: In dogs, at IV doses between 9 mg/kg/day and 32 mg/kg/day, amrinone showed dose-related hepatotoxicity manifested either as enzyme elevation or hepatic cell necrosis or both. Hepatotoxicity has been observed in man following long-term oral dosing and has been observed, in a limited experience (0.2%), following intravenous administration of amrinone. There have also been rare reports of enzyme and bilirubin elevation and jaundice.

Hypersensitivity: There have been reports of several apparent hypersensitivity reactions in patients treated with oral amrinone for about two weeks. Signs and symptoms were variable but included pericarditis, pleuritis and ascites (1 case), myositis with interstitial shadowing on chest x-ray and elevated sedimentation rate (1 case) and vasculitis with nodular pulmonary densities, hypoxemia, and jaundice (1 case). The first patient died, not necessarily of the possible reaction, while the last two resolved with discontinuation of therapy. None of the cases were rechallenged so that attribution to amrinone is not certain, but possible hypersensitivity reactions should be considered in any patient maintained for a prolonged period on amrinone.

General: Additional adverse reactions observed in intravenous amrinone clinical studies include fever (0.9%), chest pain (0.2%), and burning at the site of injection (0.2%).

Management of Adverse Reactions

Platelet Count Reductions: Asymptomatic platelet count reduction (to $<150{,}000/mm^3$) may be reversed within one week of a decrease in drug dosage. Further, with no change in drug dosage, the count may stabilize at lower than predrug levels without any clinical sequelae. Pre-drug platelet counts and frequent platelet counts during therapy are recommended to assist in decisions regarding dosage modifications.

Should a platelet count less than 150,000/mm^3 occur, the following actions may be considered:

- Maintain total daily dose unchanged, since in some cases counts have either stabilized or returned to pretreatment levels.
- Decrease total daily dose.
- Discontinue amrinone if, in the clinical judgment of the physician, risk exceeds the potential benefit.

Gastrointestinal Side Effects: While gastrointestinal side effects were seen infrequently with intravenous therapy, should severe or debilitating ones occur, the physician may wish to reduce dosage or discontinue the drug based on the usual benefit-to-risk considerations.

Hepatic Toxicity: In clinical experience to date with intravenous administration, hepatotoxicity has been observed

LOADING DOSE DETERMINATION
0.75 mg/kg (undiluted)

Patient Weight in kg	30	40	50	60	70	80	90	100	110	120
mL of undiluted INOCOR Inj	4.5	6.0	7.5	9.0	10.5	12.0	13.5	15.0	16.5	18.0

rarely. If acute marked alterations in liver enzymes occur together with clinical symptoms suggesting an idiosyncratic hypersensitivity reaction, amrinone therapy should be promptly discontinued.

If less than marked enzyme alterations occur without clinical symptoms, these nonspecific changes should be evaluated on an individual basis. The clinician may wish to continue amrinone, reduce dosage, or discontinue the drug based on the usual benefit/risk considerations.

OVERDOSAGE

A death has been reported with a massive accidental overdose (840 mg over three hours by initial bolus and infusion) of amrinone, although causal relation is uncertain. Diligence should be exercised during product preparation and administration.

Doses of INOCOR lactate injection may produce hypotension because of its vasodilator effect. If this occurs, amrinone administration should be reduced or discontinued. No specific antidote is known, but general measures for circulatory support should be taken.

In rats, the LD_{50} of amrinone, as the lactate salt, was 102 mg/kg or 130 mg/kg intravenously in two different studies and 132 mg/kg orally (intragastrically); as a suspension in aqueous gum tragacanth the oral LD_{50} was 239 mg/kg.

DOSAGE AND ADMINISTRATION

Loading doses of INOCOR lactate injection should be administered as supplied (undiluted). Infusions of INOCOR lactate injection may be administered in normal, or half normal saline solution to a concentration of 1 mg/mL to 3 mg/mL. Diluted solutions should be used within 24 hours.

INOCOR lactate injection, brand of amrinone lactate, may be injected into running dextrose (glucose) infusions through a Y-Connector or directly into the tubing where preferable.

Chemical Interactions

A chemical interaction occurs slowly over a 24-hour period when the intravenous solution of INOCOR lactate injection is mixed directly with dextrose (glucose)-containing solutions. **THEREFORE, INOCOR LACTATE INJECTION SHOULD NOT BE DILUTED WITH SOLUTIONS THAT CONTAIN DEXTROSE (GLUCOSE) PRIOR TO INJECTION.**

A chemical interaction occurs immediately, which is evidenced by the formation of a precipitate when furosemide is injected into an intravenous line of an infusion of amrinone. Therefore, furosemide should not be administered in intravenous lines containing amrinone.

The following procedure is recommended for the administration of INOCOR lactate injection:

1. Initiate therapy with a 0.75 mg/kg loading dose given slowly over 2 to 3 minutes. [See table above.]
2. Continue therapy with a maintenance infusion between 5 μg/kg/min and 10 μg/kg/min.
3. Based on clinical response, an additional loading dose of 0.75 mg/kg may be given 30 minutes after the initiation of therapy.
4. The rate of infusion usually ranges from 5 μg/kg/min to 10 μg/kg/min such that the recommended total daily dose (including loading doses) does not exceed 10 mg/kg. A limited number of patients studied at higher doses support a dosage regimen up to 18 mg/kg/day for shortened durations of therapy.

The following infusion rate chart may be used to assure that the calculations are made correctly.

To utilize the chart, the concentration of amrinone infusion solution used must be 2.5 mg/mL (2500 μg/mL). This concentration is prepared by mixing the amrinone solution with an equal volume of diluent (normal or half normal saline). [See table below.]

INOCOR I.V. (amrinone) INFUSION RATE (mL/hr) CHART
Using 2.5 mg/mL Infusion Concentration*

Patient Weight in kg	30	40	50	60	70	80	90	100	110	120
Dosage: 5.0 μg/kg/min	4	5	6	7	8	10	11	12	13	14
7.5 μg/kg/min	5	7	9	11	13	14	16	18	20	22
10.0 μg/kg/min	7	10	12	14	17	19	22	24	26	29

Example: A 70 kg patient would require a loading dose of 10.5 mL of undiluted INOCOR. If the physician selects a dose of 7.5 μg/kg/min for the infusion, the flow rate would be 13 mL/hr at the 2.5 mg/mL concentration of INOCOR.

*Dilution: To prepare the 2.5 mg/mL concentration recommended for infusion mix INOCOR with an equal volume of diluent. For example, mix three 20 mL ampuls of INOCOR (3×20 mL=60 mL) with 60 mL of diluent for a total volume of 120 mL of the final 2.5 mg/mL solution of INOCOR.

5. The rate of administration and the duration of therapy should be adjusted according to the response of the patient. The physician may wish to reduce or titrate the infusion downward based on clinical responsiveness or untoward effects.

The above dosing regimens can be expected to place most patients' plasma concentration of amrinone at approximately 3 μg/mL. Increases in cardiac index show a linear relationship to plasma concentration of a range of 0.5 μg/mL to 7 μg/mL. No observations have been made at greater plasma concentrations.

Patient improvement may be reflected by increases in cardiac output, reduction in pulmonary capillary wedge pressure, and such clinical responses as a lessening of dyspnea and an improvement in other symptoms of heart failure, such as orthopnea and fatigue.

Monitoring central venous pressure (CVP) may be valuable in the assessment of hypotension and fluid balance management. Prior correction or adjustment of fluid/electrolytes is essential to obtain satisfactory response with amrinone.

Parenteral drug products should be inspected visually and should not be used if particulate matter or discoloration is observed.

HOW SUPPLIED

Ampuls of 20 mL sterile, clear yellow solution containing INOCOR 5 mg/mL, box of 5 (NDC 0024-0888-20). Each 1 mL contains INOCOR lactate equivalent to 5 mg base and 0.25 mg sodium metabisulfite in Water for Injection. The pH of INOCOR lactate injection, brand of amrinone lactate, is adjusted to a range of 3.2 to 4.0 with lactic acid or sodium hydroxide.

Protect INOCOR lactate ampuls from light. Ampul packaging is light resistant for protection during storage.
Store at room temperature.

NORPACE, trademark, G. D. Searle & Co.

Manufactured by Sterling Pharmaceuticals Inc.
Barceloneta, Puerto Rico 00617

IW-161-Z

FOR MEDICAL INFORMATION ON INOCOR CALL TOLL FREE 1-800-446-6267.

ISUPREL® ℞

brand of isoproterenol hydrochloride injection, USP
Sterile Injection 1:5000

DESCRIPTION

Isoproterenol hydrochloride is 3,4-Dihydroxy-α-[(isopropylamino)methyl] benzyl alcohol hydrochloride, a synthetic sympathomimetic amine that is structurally related to epinephrine but acts almost exclusively on beta receptors.

Each milliliter of the sterile 1:5000 solution contains ISUPREL, brand of isoproterenol hydrochloride injection, USP, 0.2 mg, lactic acid 0.12 mg, sodium chloride 7.0 mg, sodium lactate 1.8 mg, sodium metabisulfite (as preservative) 1.0 mg, and Water for Injection qs ad 1.0 mL.

The pH is adjusted between 3.5 and 4.5 with hydrochloric acid. The air in the ampuls has been displaced by nitrogen gas.

The sterile 1:5000 solution can be administered by the intravenous, intramuscular, subcutaneous, or intracardiac routes.

CLINICAL PHARMACOLOGY

Isoproterenol hydrochloride injection acts primarily on the heart and on smooth muscle of bronchi, skeletal muscle vasculature, and alimentary tract. The positive inotropic and chronotropic actions of the drug result in an increase in minute blood flow. There is an increase in heart rate, an approximately unchanged stroke volume, and an increase in ejection velocity. The rate of discharge of cardiac pacemakers is increased with isoproterenol hydrochloride injection. Venous return to the heart is increased through a decreased compliance of the venous bed. Systemic resistance and pulmonary vascular resistance are decreased, and there is an increase in coronary and renal blood flow. Systolic blood pressure may increase and diastolic blood pressure may decrease. Mean arterial blood pressure is usually unchanged or reduced. The peripheral and coronary vasodilating effects of the drug may aid tissue perfusion.

Isoproterenol hydrochloride injection relaxes most smooth muscle, the most pronounced effect being on bronchial and gastrointestinal smooth muscle. It produces marked relaxation in the smaller bronchi and may even dilate the trachea and main bronchi past the resting diameter.

Isoproterenol hydrochloride injection is metabolized primarily in the liver by COMT. The duration of action of isoproterenol hydrochloride injection may be longer than epinephrine, but it is still brief.

INDICATIONS AND USAGE

Isoproterenol hydrochloride injection is indicated:

- For mild or transient episodes of heart block that do not require electric shock or pacemaker therapy.
- For serious episodes of heart block and Adams-Stokes attacks (except when caused by ventricular tachycardia or fibrillation). (See CONTRAINDICATIONS.)
- For use in cardiac arrest until electric shock or pacemaker therapy, the treatments of choice, is available. (See CONTRAINDICATIONS.)
- For bronchospasm occurring during anesthesia.
- As an adjunct to fluid and electrolyte replacement therapy and the use of other drugs and procedures in the treatment of hypovolemic and septic shock, low cardiac output (hypoperfusion) states, congestive heart failure, and cardiogenic shock. (See WARNINGS.)

CONTRAINDICATIONS

Use of isoproterenol hydrochloride injection is contraindicated in patients with tachyarrhythmias; tachycardia or heartblock caused by digitalis intoxication; ventricular arrhythmias which require inotropic therapy; and angina pectoris.

WARNINGS

Isoproterenol hydrochloride injection, by increasing myocardial oxygen requirements while decreasing effective coronary perfusion, may have a deleterious effect on the injured or failing heart. Most experts discourage its use as the initial agent in treating cardiogenic shock following myocardial infarction. However, when a low arterial pressure has been elevated by other means, isoproterenol hydrochloride injection may produce beneficial hemodynamic and metabolic effects.

In a few patients, presumably with organic disease of the AV node and its branches, isoproterenol hydrochloride injection has paradoxically been reported to worsen heart block or to precipitate Adams-Stokes attacks during normal sinus rhythm or transient heart block.

Contains sodium metabisulfite, a sulfite that may cause allergic-type reactions including anaphylactic symptoms and life-threatening or less severe asthmatic episodes in certain susceptible people. The overall prevalence of sulfite sensitivity in the general population is unknown and probably low. Sulfite sensitivity is seen more frequently in asthmatic than in nonasthmatic people.

PRECAUTIONS

General

Isoproterenol hydrochloride injection should generally be started at the lowest recommended dose. This may be gradually increased, if necessary, while carefully monitoring the patient. Doses sufficient to increase the heart rate to more than 130 beats per minute may increase the likelihood of inducing ventricular arrhythmias. Such increases in heart rate will also tend to increase cardiac work and oxygen requirements which may adversely affect the failing heart or the heart with a significant degree of arteriosclerosis.

Particular caution is necessary in administering isoproterenol hydrochloride injection to patients with coronary artery

Continued on next page

This product information was prepared in August 1992. On these and other products of Sanofi Winthrop Pharmaceuticals, detailed information may be obtained on a current basis by direct inquiry to Product Information Services, 90 Park Avenue, New York, NY 10016 (toll free 1-800-446-6267).

Sanofi Winthrop—Cont.

disease, coronary insufficiency, diabetes, hyperthyroidism, and sensitivity to sympathomimetic amines.

Adequate filling of the intravascular compartment by suitable volume expanders is of primary importance in most cases of shock, and should precede the administration of vasoactive drugs. In patients with normal cardiac function, determination of central venous pressure is a reliable guide during volume replacement. If evidence of hypoperfusion persists after adequate volume replacement, isoproterenol hydrochloride injection may be given.

In addition to the routine monitoring of systemic blood pressure, heart rate, urine flow, and the electrocardiograph, the response to therapy should also be monitored by frequent determination of the central venous pressure and blood gases. Patients in shock should be closely observed during isoproterenol hydrochloride injection administration. If the heart rate exceeds 110 beats per minute, it may be advisable to decrease the infusion rate or temporarily discontinue the infusion. Determinations of cardiac output and circulation time may also be helpful. Appropriate measures should be taken to ensure adequate ventilation. Careful attention should be paid to acid-base balance and to the correction of electrolyte disturbances. In cases of shock associated with bacteremia, suitable antimicrobial therapy is, of course, imperative.

Drug Interactions
Isoproterenol hydrochloride injection and epinephrine should not be administered simultaneously because both drugs are direct cardiac stimulants and their combined effects may induce serious arrhythmias. The drugs may, however, be administered alternately provided a proper interval has elapsed between doses.

ISUPREL, brand of isoproterenol, should be used with caution, if at all, when potent inhalational anesthetics such as halothane are employed because of potential to sensitize the myocardium to effects of sympathomimetic amines.

Carcinogenesis, Mutagenesis, Impairment of Fertility
Long-term studies in animals to evaluate the carcinogenic potential of isoproterenol hydrochloride have not been done. Mutagenic potential and effect on fertility have not been determined. There is no evidence from human experience that isoproterenol hydrochloride injection may be carcinogenic or mutagenic or that it impairs fertility.

Pregnancy Category C
Animal reproduction studies have not been conducted with isoproterenol hydrochloride. It is also not known whether isoproterenol hydrochloride can cause fetal harm when administered to a pregnant woman or can affect reproduction capacity. Isoproterenol hydrochloride should be given to a pregnant woman only if clearly needed.

Nursing Mothers
It is not known whether this drug is excreted in human milk. Because many drugs are excreted in human milk, caution should be exercised when isoproterenol hydrochloride injection is administered to a nursing woman.

ADVERSE REACTIONS

The following reactions to isoproterenol hydrochloride injection have been reported:

CNS: Nervousness, headache, dizziness.
Cardiovascular: Tachycardia, palpitations, angina, Adams-Stokes attacks, pulmonary edema, hypertension, hypotension, ventricular arrhythmias, tachyarrhythmias.

In a few patients, presumably with organic disease of the AV node and its branches, isoproterenol hydrochloride injection has been reported to precipitate Adams-Stokes seizures during normal sinus rhythm or transient heart block.

Other: Flushing of the skin, sweating, mild tremors, weakness.

OVERDOSAGE

The acute toxicity of isoproterenol hydrochloride in animals is much less than that of epinephrine. Excessive doses in animals or man can cause a striking drop in blood pressure, and repeated large doses in animals may result in cardiac enlargement and focal myocarditis.

In case of accidental overdosage as evidenced mainly by tachycardia or other arrhythmias, palpitations, angina, hypotension, or hypertension, reduce rate of administration or discontinue isoproterenol hydrochloride injection until patient's condition stabilizes. Blood pressure, pulse, respiration, and EKG should be monitored.

It is not known whether isoproterenol hydrochloride is dialyzable.

The oral LD_{50} of isoproterenol hydrochloride in mice is $3,850$ mg/kg $\pm$ $1,190$ mg/kg of pure drug in solution.

DOSAGE AND ADMINISTRATION

ISUPREL injection 1:5000 should generally be started at the lowest recommended dose and the rate of administration gradually increased if necessary while carefully monitoring the patient. The usual route of administration is by intravenous infusion or bolus intravenous injection. In dire emergencies, the drug may be administered by intracardiac injection. If time is not of the utmost importance, initial therapy by intramuscular or subcutaneous injection is preferred. [See first table below.]

There are no well-controlled studies in children to establish appropriate dosing; however, the American Heart Association recommends an initial infusion rate of 0.1μg/kg/min, with the usual range being 0.1μg/kg/min to 1.0μg/kg/min. [See table at bottom of page.]

Parenteral drug products should be inspected visually for particulate matter and discoloration prior to administration, whenever solution and container permit. Such solution should not be used.

HOW SUPPLIED

Ampuls of 1 mL (0.2 mg) UNI-NEST™ PAK of 25 (NDC 0024-0866-25)
Ampuls of 5 mL (1 mg) box of 10 (NDC 0024-0866-02)
Protect from light. Keep in opaque container until used.
Store in a cool place between 8°C to 15°C (46° F to 59° F). Do not use if the injection is pinkish to brownish in color or contains a precipitate.

IW-33-X

ISUPREL®   ℞
brand of isoproterenol hydrochloride inhalation aerosol, USP
MISTOMETER®

Potent Bronchodilator

DESCRIPTION

ISUPREL MISTOMETER is a beta agonist sympathomimetic bronchodilator. It is a complete nebulizing unit consisting of a plastic-coated vial of aerosol solution, detachable plastic mouthpiece with built-in nebulizer, and protective cap. The vial contains isoproterenol hydrochloride 0.25% (w/w) with inert ingredients of alcohol 33% (w/w) and ascorbic acid 0.1% (w/w) and, as propellants, dichlorodifluoromethane and dichlorotetrafluoroethane.

Chemically, isoproterenol hydrochloride is 3,4-Dihydroxy-α-[(isopropylamino)methyl]benzyl alcohol hydrochloride.

The contents permit the delivery of not less than 200 actuations from the 11.2 g (10 mL) vial and not less than 300 actuations from the 16.8 g (15 mL) vial. The MISTOMETER delivers a measured dose of 131 μg of the bronchodilator in a fine, even mist for inhalation.

CLINICAL PHARMACOLOGY

ISUPREL relaxes bronchial spasm and facilitates expectoration of pulmonary secretions by acting almost exclusively on beta receptors. It is frequently effective when epinephrine and other drugs fail, and it has a wide margin of safety.

ISUPREL is readily absorbed when given as an aerosol. It is metabolized primarily in the liver and other tissues by catechol-O-methyltransferase (COMT).

Recent studies in laboratory animals (minipigs, rodents, and dogs) recorded the occurrence of cardiac arrhythmias and sudden death (with histologic evidence of myocardial necrosis) when beta agonists and methylxanthines were concomitantly administered. The significance of these findings when applied to human usage is currently unknown.

INDICATIONS AND USAGE

ISUPREL is indicated for the relief of bronchospasm associated with acute and chronic asthma and reversible bronchospasm which may be associated with chronic bronchitis or emphysema.

CONTRAINDICATIONS

Use of isoproterenol in patients with preexisting cardiac arrhythmias associated with tachycardia is generally considered contraindicated because the cardiac stimulant effect of the drug may aggravate such disorders. The use of this medication is contraindicated in those patients who have a known hypersensitivity to isoproterenol or to any of the other components of this drug.

WARNINGS

Excessive use of an adrenergic aerosol should be discouraged as it may lose its effectiveness.

In patients with status asthmaticus and abnormal blood gas tensions, improvement in vital capacity and in blood gas tensions may not accompany apparent relief of bronchospasm. Facilities for administering oxygen mixtures and ventilatory assistance are necessary for such patients.

Occasional patients have been reported to develop severe paradoxical airway resistance with repeated, excessive use of isoproterenol inhalation preparations. The cause of this

---

Recommended dosage for adults with heart block, Adams-Stokes attacks, and cardiac arrest:

Route of Administration	Preparation of Dilution	Initial Dose	Subsequent Dose Range*
Bolus intravenous injection	Dilute 1 mL (0.2 mg) to 10 mL with Sodium Chloride Injection, USP, or 5% Dextrose Injection, USP	0.02 mg to 0.06 mg (1 mL to 3 mL of diluted solution)	0.01 mg to 0.2 mg (0.5 mL to 10 mL of diluted solution)
Intravenous infusion	Dilute 10 mL (2 mg) in 500 mL of 5% Dextrose Injection, USP	5 μg/min. (1.25 mL of diluted solution per minute)	
Intramuscular	Use Solution 1:5000 undiluted	0.2 mg (1 mL)	0.02 mg to 1 mg (0.1 mL to 5 mL)
Subcutaneous	Use Solution 1:5000 undiluted	0.2 mg (1 mL)	0.15 mg to 0.2 mg (0.75 mL to 1 mL)
Intracardiac	Use Solution 1:5000 undiluted	0.02 mg (0.1 mL)	

*Subsequent dosage and method of administration depend on the ventricular rate and the rapidity with which the cardiac pacemaker can take over when the drug is gradually withdrawn.

Recommended dosage for adults with shock and hypoperfusion states:

Route of Administration	Preparation of Dilution†	Infusion Rate††
Intravenous infusion	Dilute 5 mL (1 mg) in 500 mL of 5% Dextrose Injection, USP	0.5 μg to 5 μg per minute (0.25 mL to 2.5 mL of diluted solution)

† Concentrations up to 10 times greater have been used when limitation of volume is essential.
†† Rates over 30 μg per minute have been used in advanced stages of shock. The rate of infusion should be adjusted on the basis of heart rate, central venous pressure, systemic blood pressure, and urine flow. If the heart rate exceeds 110 beats per minute, it may be advisable to decrease or temporarily discontinue the infusion.

Recommended dosage for adults with bronchospasm occurring during anesthesia:

Route of Administration	Preparation of Dilution	Initial Dose	Subsequent Dose
Bolus intravenous injection	Dilute 1 mL (0.2 mg) to 10 mL with Sodium Chloride Injection, USP, or 5% Dextrose Injection, USP	0.01 mg to 0.02 mg (0.5 mL to 1 mL of diluted solution)	The initial dose may be repeated when necessary

refractory state is unknown. It is advisable that in such instances the use of this preparation be discontinued immediately and alternative therapy instituted, since in the reported cases the patients did not respond to other forms of therapy until the drug was withdrawn.
Deaths have been reported following excessive use of isoproterenol inhalation preparations and the exact cause is unknown. Cardiac arrest was noted in several instances.

PRECAUTIONS

General
Isoproterenol should be used with caution in patients with cardiovascular disorders including coronary insufficiency, diabetes, or hyperthyroidism, and in persons sensitive to sympathomimetic amines.
A single treatment with the ISUPREL MISTOMETER is usually sufficient for controlling isolated attacks of asthma. Any patient who requires more than three aerosol treatments within a 24-hour period should be under the close supervision of a physician. Further therapy with the bronchodilator aerosol alone is inadvisable when three to five treatments within six to twelve hours produce minimal or no relief.

Information for Patients
Do not inhale more often than directed by your physician. Read enclosed instructions before using (see attachment to insert). Do not exceed the dose prescribed by your physician. If difficulty in breathing persists, contact your physician immediately. Avoid spraying in eyes. Contents under pressure. Do not break or incinerate. Do not store at temperatures above 120°F. Keep out of reach of children.

Drug Interactions
Epinephrine should not be administered concomitantly with ISUPREL, as both drugs are direct cardiac stimulants and their combined effects may induce serious arrhythmia. If desired they may, however, be alternated, provided an interval of at least four hours has elapsed.

Carcinogenesis, Mutagenesis, Impairment of Fertility
Long-term chronic toxicity studies in animals have not been done to evaluate isoproterenol in these areas.

Pregnancy Category C
Animal reproduction studies have not been conducted with isoproterenol hydrochloride. It is also not known whether isoproterenol hydrochloride can cause fetal harm when administered to a pregnant woman or can affect reproduction capacity. Isoproterenol hydrochloride should be given to a pregnant woman only if clearly needed.

Nursing Mothers
It is not known whether this drug is excreted in human milk. Because many drugs are excreted in human milk, caution should be exercised when isoproterenol hydrochloride is administered to a nursing woman.

Pediatric Use
In general, the technique of ISUPREL MISTOMETER in administration to children is similar to that of adults, since children's smaller ventilatory exchange capacity automatically provides proportionally smaller aerosol intake.

ADVERSE REACTIONS

The mist from the ISUPREL MISTOMETER contains alcohol but is generally very well tolerated. An occasional patient may experience some transient throat irritation which has been attributed to the alcohol content.
Serious reactions to ISUPREL, brand of isoproterenol hydrochloride inhalation aerosol, are infrequent. The following reactions, however, have been reported:
CNS: Nervousness, headache, dizziness, weakness.
Gastrointestinal: Nausea, vomiting.
Cardiovascular: Tachycardia, palpitations, precordial distress, anginal-type pain.
Other: Flushing of the skin, tremor, and sweating.
The inhalation route is usually accompanied by a minimum of side effects. These untoward reactions disappear quickly and do not, as a rule, inconvenience the patient to the extent that the drug must be discontinued. No cumulative effects have been reported.

OVERDOSAGE

Overdosage of ISUPREL may produce signs and symptoms typical of excessive sympathomimetic effects, including tachycardia, palpitations, nervousness, nausea, and vomiting. Excessive use of adrenergic aerosols may result in loss of effectiveness or severe paradoxical airway resistance. Cardiac arrest has been noted in several instances. In all cases of overdose or excessive use of ISUPREL, the drug should be discontinued immediately and vital functions supported until the patient is stabilized. It is not known whether isoproterenol hydrochloride is dialyzable.
The acute oral LD_{50} in mice is 3,850 mg/kg $\pm$ 1,190 mg/kg of pure drug in solution (isoproterenol hydrochloride). In dogs, the toxic dose is 1,000 times the therapeutic dose. Converted to the amount used clinically in man, this would be about 2,500 times the therapeutic dose.

DOSAGE AND ADMINISTRATION

This drug may not be dispensed without a prescription.
Acute Bronchial Asthma: Hold the MISTOMETER in an inverted position. Close lips and teeth around open end of mouthpiece. Breathe out, expelling as much air from the lungs as possible; then inhale deeply while pressing down on the bottle to activate spray mechanism. Try to hold breath for a few seconds before exhaling. Wait one full minute in order to determine the effect before considering a second inhalation. A treatment may be repeated up to 5 times daily if necessary. (See PRECAUTIONS.) If carefully instructed, children quickly learn to keep the stream of mist clear of the teeth and tongue, thereby assuring inhalation into the lungs. Occlusion of the nares of very young children may be advisable to make inhalation certain.
Warm water should be run through the mouthpiece once daily to wash it and prevent clogging.
The mouthpiece may also be sanitized by immersion in alcohol.
Bronchospasm in Chronic Obstructive Lung Disease: The MISTOMETER provides a convenient aerosol method for delivering ISUPREL, brand of isoproterenol hydrochloride inhalation aerosol. The treatment described above for Acute Bronchial Asthma may be repeated at not less than 3 to 4 hour intervals as part of a programmed regimen of treatment of obstructive lung disease complicated by a reversible bronchospastic component. One application from the MISTOMETER may be regarded as equivalent in effectiveness to 5 to 7 operations of a hand-bulb nebulizer using a 1:100 solution.

Children's Dosage
In general, the technique of ISUPREL MISTOMETER in administration to children is similar tc that of adults, since children's smaller ventilatory exchange capacity automatically provides proportionally smaller aerosol intake.

HOW SUPPLIED

ISUPREL MISTOMETER is supplied as a metered dose aerosol providing 131 μg of isoproterenol hydrochloride per actuation.
Vial of 11.2 g (10 mL) with oral nebulizer
(NDC 0024-0878-05)
Vial of 16.8 g (15 mL) with oral nebulizer
(NDC 0024-0878-01)
Refill only, 16.8 g (15 mL)
(NDC 0024-0879-01)
Store at controlled room temperature 15°C to 30°C (59°F to 86°F).

Manufactured by Sterling Pharmaceuticals Inc.
Barceloneta, Puerto Rico 00617

IW-67-DD

ISUPREL® Hydrochloride ℞
brand of isoproterenol
inhalation solution, USP
SOLUTION 1:200
SOLUTION 1:100

Potent Bronchodilator

DESCRIPTION

ISUPREL hydrochloride, brand of isoproterenol inhalation solution, is a beta agonist sympathomimetic bronchodilator.
Solution 1:200 contains isoproterenol hydrochloride 5 mg/mL.
Inactive Ingredients: Chlorobutanol 0.5 percent and Sodium Metabisulfite 0.3 percent as preservatives, Citric Acid, Glycerin, Purified Water, and Sodium Chloride.
Solution 1:100 contains isoproterenol hydrochloride 10 mg/mL.
Inactive Ingredients: Chlorobutanol 0.5 percent and Sodium Metabisulfite 0.3 percent as preservatives, Citric Acid, Purified Water, Saccharin Sodium, Sodium Chloride, and Sodium Citrate.
Isoproterenol hydrochloride is soluble in water (1 g isoproterenol hydrochloride dissolves in 3 mL H_2O). The solutions have a pH range of 3 to 4.5.
Chemically, isoproterenol hydrochloride is 3,4-Dihydroxy-α-[(isopropylamino)methyl]benzyl alcohol hydrochloride.
The air in the bottles has been displaced by nitrogen gas.

CLINICAL PHARMACOLOGY

ISUPREL relaxes bronchial spasm and facilitates expectoration of pulmonary secretions by acting almost exclusively on beta receptors. It is frequently effective when epinephrine and other drugs fail, and it has a wide margin of safety.
ISUPREL is readily absorbed when given as an aerosol. It is metabolized primarily in the liver and other tissues by catechol-0 methyltransferase (COMT).
Recent studies in laboratory animals (minipigs, rodents, and dogs) recorded the occurrence of cardiac arrhythmias and sudden death (with histologic evidence of myocardial necrosis) when beta agonists and methylxanthines were concomitantly administered. The significance of these findings when applied to human usage is currently unknown.

INDICATIONS AND USAGE

ISUPREL is indicated for the relief of bronchospasm associated with acute and chronic asthma and reversible bronchospasm which may be associated with chronic bronchitis or emphysema.

CONTRAINDICATION

Use of isoproterenol in patients with preexisting cardiac arrhythmias associated with tachycardia is generally considered contraindicated because the cardiac stimulant effect of the drug may aggravate such disorders.

WARNINGS

Excessive use of an adrenergic aerosol should be discouraged as it may lose its effectiveness.
In patients with status asthmaticus and abnormal blood gas tensions, improvement in vital capacity and in blood gas tensions may not accompany apparent relief of bronchospasm. Facilities for administering oxygen mixtures and ventilatory assistance are necessary for such patients.
Occasional patients have been reported to develop severe paradoxical airway resistance with repeated, excessive use of isoproterenol inhalation preparations. The cause of this refractory state is unknown. It is advisable that in such instances the use of this preparation be discontinued immediately and alternative therapy instituted, since in the reported cases the patients did not respond to other forms of therapy until the drug was withdrawn.
Deaths have been reported following excessive use of isoproterenol inhalation preparations and the exact cause is unknown. Cardiac arrest was noted in several instances.
Contains sodium metabisulfite, a sulfite that may cause allergic-type reactions including anaphylactic symptoms and life-threatening or less severe asthmatic episodes in certain susceptible people. The overall prevalence of sulfite sensitivity in the general population is unknown and probably low. Sulfite sensitivity is seen more frequently in asthmatic than in nonasthmatic people.

PRECAUTIONS

General: Isoproterenol should be used with caution in patients with cardiovascular disorders including coronary insufficiency, diabetes, or hyperthyroidism, and in persons sensitive to sympathomimetic amines.
Any patient who requires more than three aerosol treatments within a 24-hour period should be under the close supervision of his physician. Further therapy with the bronchodilator aerosol alone is inadvisable when three to five treatments within six to twelve hours produce minimal or no relief.
When compressed oxygen is employed as the aerosol propellant, the percentage of oxygen used should be determined by the patient's individual requirements to avoid depression of respiratory drive.
Drug Interactions: Epinephrine should not be administered concomitantly with ISUPREL, as both drugs are direct cardiac stimulants and their combined effects may induce serious arrhythmia. If desired they may, however, be alternated, provided an interval of at least four hours has elapsed.
Carcinogenesis, Mutagenesis, Impairment of Fertility: Long-term chronic toxicity studies in animals have not been done to evaluate isoproterenol in these areas.
Pregnancy Category C: Animal reproduction studies have not been conducted with isoproterenol hydrochloride. It is also not known whether isoproterenol hydrochloride can cause fetal harm when administered to a pregnant woman or can affect reproduction capacity. Isoproterenol hydrochloride should be given to a pregnant woman only if clearly needed.
Nursing Mothers: It is not known whether this drug is excreted in human milk. Because many drugs are excreted in human milk, caution should be exercised when isoproterenol hydrochloride is administered to a nursing woman.
Pediatric Use: In general, the technique of isoproterenol hydrochloride solution in administration to children is similar to that of adults, since children's smaller ventilatory exchange capacity automatically provides proportionally smaller aerosol intake. However, it is generally recommended that the 1:200 solution (rather than the 1:100) be used for an acute attack of bronchospasm, and no more than 0.25 mL of the 1:200 solution should be used for each 10 to 15 minute programmed treatment in chronic bronchospastic disease.

ADVERSE REACTIONS

Serious reactions to ISUPREL are infrequent. The following reactions, however, have been reported:

Continued on next page

This product information was prepared in August 1992. On these and other products of Sanofi Winthrop Pharmaceuticals, detailed information may be obtained on a current basis by direct inquiry to Product Information Services, 90 Park Avenue, New York, NY 10016 (toll free 1-800-446-6267).

Sanofi Winthrop—Cont.

CNS: Nervousness, headache, dizziness, weakness.
Gastrointestinal: Nausea, vomiting.
Cardiovascular: Tachycardia, palpitations, precordial distress, anginal-type pain.
Other: Flushing of the skin, tremor, and sweating.
The inhalation route is usually accompanied by a minimum of side effects. These untoward reactions disappear quickly and do not as a rule, inconvenience the patient to the extent that the drug must be discontinued. No cumulative effects have been reported.

OVERDOSAGE

Overdosage of ISUPREL may produce signs and symptoms typical of excessive sympathomimetic effects, including tachycardia, palpitations, nervousness, nausea, and vomiting. Excessive use of adrenergic aerosols may result in loss of effectiveness or severe paradoxical airway resistance. Cardiac arrest has been noted in several instances. In all cases of overdose or excessive use of ISUPREL, the drug should be discontinued immediately and vital functions supported until the patient is stabilized. It is not known whether isoproterenol hydrochloride is dialyzable.
The acute oral LD_{50} in mice is 3,850 mg/kg $\pm$ 1,190 mg/kg of pure drug in solution (isoproterenol hydrochloride). In dogs, the toxic dose is 1,000 times the therapeutic dose. Converted to the amount used clinically in man, this would be about 2,500 times the therapeutic dose.

DOSAGE AND ADMINISTRATION

ISUPREL hydrochloride solutions can be administered as an aerosol mist by hand-bulb nebulizer, compressed air or oxygen operated nebulizer, or by intermittent positive pressure breathing (IPPB) devices. The method of delivery, and the treatment regimen employed in the management of the reversible bronchospastic element accompanying bronchial asthma, chronic bronchitis, and chronic obstructive lung diseases, will depend on such factors as the severity of the bronchospasm, patient age, tolerance to the medication, complicating cardiopulmonary conditions, and whether therapy is for an intermittent acute attack of bronchospasm or is part of a programmed treatment regimen for constant bronchospasm.
Acute Bronchial Asthma. *Hand-Bulb Nebulizer*—Depending on the frequency of treatment and the type of nebulizer used, a volume of solution of ISUPREL, sufficient for not more than one day's treatment, should be placed in the nebulizer using the dropper provided. In time, the patient can learn to adjust the volume required. For adults and children, the 1:200 solution is administered by hand-bulb nebulization in a dosage of 5 to 15 deep inhalations (using an all glass or plastic nebulizer). In adults, the 1:100 solution may be used if a stronger solution seems to be indicated. The dose is 3 to 7 deep inhalations. If after about 5 to 10 minutes inadequate relief is observed, these doses may be repeated one more time. If the acute attack recurs, treatments may be repeated up to 5 times daily if necessary. (See PRECAUTIONS.)
Bronchospasm in Chronic Obstructive Lung Disease. *Hand-Bulb Nebulizer*—A solution of 1:200 or 1:100 of ISUPREL may be administered daily at not less than 3 to 4 hour intervals for subacute bronchospastic attacks or as part of a programmed treatment regimen in patients with chronic obstructive lung disease with a reversible bronchospastic component. An adequate dose is usually 5 to 15 deep inhalations, using the 1:200 solution. Some patients with severe attacks of bronchospasm may require 3 to 7 deep inhalations using the 1:100 solution of ISUPREL.
Nebulization by Compressed Air or Oxygen—A method often used in patients with severe chronic obstructive lung disease is to deliver the isoproterenol mist *in more dilute form over a longer period of time.* The purpose is, not so much to increase the dose supplied, as to achieve progressively deeper bronchodilatation and thus insure that the mist achieves maximum penetration of the finer bronchioles. In this method, 0.5 mL of a 1:200 solution of ISUPREL is diluted to 2 mL to 2.5 mL with water or isotonic saline to achieve a use concentration of 1:800 to 1:1000. If desired, 0.25 mL of the 1:100 solution may be similarly diluted to achieve the same use concentration. The diluted solution is placed in a nebulizer (eg, DeVilbiss #640 unit) connected to either a source of compressed air or oxygen. The flow rate is regulated to suit the particular nebulizer so that the diluted solution of ISUPREL will be delivered over approximately 10 to 20 minutes. A treatment may be repeated up to 5 times daily if necessary. Although the total delivered dose of ISUPREL is somewhat higher than with the treatment regimen employing the hand-bulb nebulizer, patients usually tolerate it well because of the greater dilution and longer application-time factors.
Intermittent Positive Pressure Breathing (IPPB)—Diluted solutions of 1:200 or 1:100 of ISUPREL are used in a programmed regimen for the treatment of reversible bronchospasm in patients with chronic obstructive lung disease who require intermittent positive pressure breathing therapy.

These devices generally have a small nebulizer, usually of 3 mL to 5 mL capacity, on a patient-operated side arm. The effectiveness of IPPB therapy is greatly enhanced by the simultaneous use of aerosolized bronchodilators. As with compressed air or oxygen operated nebulizers, the usual regimen is to place 0.5 mL of 1:200 solution of ISUPREL diluted to 2 mL to 2.5 mL with water or isotonic saline in the nebulizer cup and follow the IPPB manufacturer's operating instructions. IPPB-bronchodilator treatments are usually administered over 15 to 20 minutes, up to 5 times daily if necessary.
Children's Dosage: In general, the technique of isoproterenol hydrochloride solution in administration to children is similar to that of adults, since children's smaller ventilatory exchange capacity automatically provides proportionally smaller aerosol intake. However, it is generally recommended that the 1:200 solution (rather than the 1:100) be used for an acute attack of bronchospasm, and no more than 0.25 mL of the 1:200 solution should be used for each 10 to 15 minute programmed treatment in chronic bronchospastic disease.

HOW SUPPLIED

Solution 1:100 contains isoproterenol hydrochloride 1% (10 mg/mL).
Solution 1:200 contains isoproterenol hydrochloride 0.5% (5 mg/mL).
Solution 1:100
  bottle of 10 mL   **NDC** 0024-0873-01
Solution 1:200
  bottle of 10 mL   **NDC** 0024-0871-01
  bottle of 60 mL   **NDC** 0024-0871-03
Protect from light. Do not use the solutions if they are pinkish to brownish in color or contain a precipitate. Although solutions of ISUPREL left in nebulizers will remain clear and potent for many days, for sanitary reasons it is recommended that they be changed daily.
Store at controlled room temperature 15°C to 30°C (59°F to 86°F).

Manufactured by Sterling Pharmaceuticals Inc.
Barceloneta, Puerto Rico 00617

IW-154-F

ISUPREL® Hydrochloride   ℞
brand of isoproterenol hydrochloride tablets, USP
GLOSSETS®

DESCRIPTION

Each tablet contains 10 mg or 15 mg isoproterenol hydrochloride in a rapidly disintegrating base consisting of lactose, saccharin sodium, sodium metabisulfite 2 mg per tablet as antioxidant, starch, and talc.

HOW SUPPLIED

ISUPREL GLOSSETS 10 mg, bottle of 50
(NDC 0024-0875-02)
For complete prescribing information, see package insert or contact Product Information Services.

KAYEXALATE®   ℞
brand of sodium polystyrene sulfonate, USP

> **Cation-Exchange Resin**

DESCRIPTION

KAYEXALATE, brand of sodium polystyrene sulfonate, is a benzene, diethenyl-, polymer with ethenylbenzene, sulfonated, sodium salt.
The drug is a light brown to brown, finely ground, powdered form of sodium polystyrene sulfonate, a cation-exchange resin prepared in the sodium phase with an in vitro exchange capacity of approximately 3.1 mEq (in vivo approximately 1 mEq) of potassium per gram. The sodium content is approximately 100 mg (4.1 mEq) per gram of the drug. It can be administered orally or in an enema.

CLINICAL PHARMACOLOGY

As the resin passes along the intestine or is retained in the colon after administration by enema, the sodium ions are partially released and are replaced by potassium ions. For the most part, this action occurs in the large intestine, which excretes potassium ions to a greater degree than does the small intestine. The efficiency of this process is limited and unpredictably variable. It commonly approximates the order of 33 percent but the range is so large that definitive indices of electrolyte balance must be clearly monitored.
Metabolic data are unavailable.

INDICATION AND USAGE

KAYEXALATE is indicated for the treatment of hyperkalemia.

CONTRAINDICATIONS

KAYEXALATE is contraindicated in patients with hypokalemia or those patients who are hypersensitive to it.

WARNINGS

Alternative Therapy in Severe Hyperkalemia:
Since effective lowering of serum potassium with KAYEXALATE may take hours to days, treatment with this drug alone may be insufficient to rapidly correct severe hyperkalemia associated with states of rapid tissue breakdown (eg, burns and renal failure) or hyperkalemia so marked as to constitute a medical emergency. Therefore, other definitive measures, including dialysis, should always be considered and may be imperative.
Hypokalemia: Serious potassium deficiency can occur from therapy with KAYEXALATE. The effect must be carefully controlled by frequent serum potassium determinations within each 24-hour period. Since intracellular potassium deficiency is not always reflected by serum potassium levels, the level at which treatment with KAYEXALATE should be discontinued must be determined individually for each patient. Important aids in making this determination are the patient's clinical condition and electrocardiogram. Early clinical signs of severe hypokalemia include a pattern of irritable confusion and delayed thought processes. Electrocardiographically, severe hypokalemia is often associated with a lengthened Q-T interval, widening, flattening, or inversion of the T wave, and prominent U waves. Also, cardiac arrhythmias may occur, such as premature atrial, nodal, and ventricular contractions, and supraventricular and ventricular tachycardias. The toxic effects of digitalis are likely to be exaggerated. Marked hypokalemia can also be manifested by severe muscle weakness, at times extending into frank paralysis.
Electrolyte Disturbances: Like all cation-exchange resins, KAYEXALATE is not totally selective (for potassium) in its actions, and small amounts of other cations such as magnesium and calcium can also be lost during treatment. Accordingly, patients receiving KAYEXALATE should be monitored for all applicable electrolyte disturbances.
Systemic Alkalosis: Systemic alkalosis has been reported after cation-exchange resins were administered orally in combination with nonabsorbable cation-donating antacids and laxatives such as magnesium hydroxide and aluminum carbonate. Magnesium hydroxide should not be administered with KAYEXALATE. One case of grand mal seizure has been reported in a patient with chronic hypocalcemia of renal failure who was given KAYEXALATE with magnesium hydroxide as laxative. (See PRECAUTIONS, Drug Interactions.)

PRECAUTIONS

Caution is advised when KAYEXALATE is administered to patients who cannot tolerate even a small increase in sodium loads (ie, severe congestive heart failure, severe hypertension, or marked edema). In such instances compensatory restriction of sodium intake from other sources may be indicated.
If constipation occurs, patients should be treated with sorbitol (from 10 mL to 20 mL of 70 percent syrup every two hours or as needed to produce one or two watery stools daily), a measure which also reduces any tendency to fecal impaction.
Drug Interactions
Antacids: The simultaneous oral administration of KAYEXALATE with nonabsorbable cation-donating antacids and laxatives may reduce the resin's potassium exchange capability.
Systemic alkalosis has been reported after cation-exchange resins were administered orally in combination with nonabsorbable cation-donating antacids and laxatives such as magnesium hydroxide and aluminum carbonate. Magnesium hydroxide should not be administered with KAYEXALATE. One case of grand mal seizure has been reported in a patient with chronic hypocalcemia of renal failure who was given KAYEXALATE with magnesium hydroxide as a laxative. Intestinal obstruction due to concretions of aluminum hydroxide when used in combination with KAYEXALATE has been reported.
Digitalis: The toxic effects of digitalis on the heart, especially various ventricular arrhythmias and A-V nodal dissociation, are likely to be exaggerated by hypokalemia, even in the face of serum digoxin concentrations in the "normal range". (See WARNINGS.)
Carcinogenesis, Mutagenesis, Impairment of Fertility
Studies have not been performed.
Pregnancy Category C
Animal reproduction studies have not been conducted with KAYEXALATE. It is also not known whether KAYEXALATE can cause fetal harm when administered to a pregnant woman or can affect reproduction capacity. KAYEXALATE should be given to a pregnant woman only if clearly needed.
Nursing Mothers
It is not known whether this drug is excreted in human milk. Because many drugs are excreted in human milk, caution

should be exercised when KAYEXALATE is administered to a nursing woman.

ADVERSE REACTIONS

KAYEXALATE may cause some degree of gastric irritation. Anorexia, nausea, vomiting, and constipation may occur especially if high doses are given. Also, hypokalemia, hypocalcemia, and significant sodium retention may occur. Occasionally diarrhea develops. Large doses in elderly individuals may cause fecal impaction (see PRECAUTIONS). This effect may be obviated through usage of the resin in enemas as described under DOSAGE AND ADMINISTRATION. Rare instances of colonic necrosis have been reported. Intestinal obstruction due to concretions of aluminum hydroxide, when used in combination with KAYEXALATE, has been reported.

DOSAGE AND ADMINISTRATION

Suspension of this drug should be freshly prepared and not stored beyond 24 hours.

The average daily adult dose of the resin is 15 g to 60 g. This is best provided by administering 15 g (approximately 4 *level* teaspoons) of KAYEXALATE one to four times daily. One gram of KAYEXALATE contains 4.1 mEq of sodium; one level teaspoon contains approximately 3.5 g of KAYEXALATE and 15 mEq of sodium. (A heaping teaspoon may contain as much as 10 g to 12 g of KAYEXALATE, brand of sodium polystyrene sulfonate.) Since the in vivo efficiency of sodium-potassium exchange resins is approximately 33 percent, about one third of the resin's actual sodium content is being delivered to the body.

In smaller children and infants, lower doses should be employed by using as a guide a rate of 1 mEq of potassium per gram of resin as the basis for calculation.

Each dose should be given as a suspension in a small quantity of water or, for greater palatability, in syrup. The amount of fluid usually ranges from 20 mL to 100 mL, depending on the dose, or may be simply determined by allowing 3 mL to 4 mL per gram of resin. Sorbitol may be administered in order to combat constipation.

The resin may be introduced into the stomach through a plastic tube and, if desired, mixed with a diet appropriate for a patient in renal failure.

The resin may also be given, although with less effective results, in an enema consisting (for adults) of 30 g to 50 g every six hours. Each dose is administered as a warm emulsion (at body temperature) in 100 mL of aqueous vehicle, such as sorbitol. The emulsion should be agitated gently during administration. The enema should be retained as long as possible and followed by a cleansing enema.

After an initial cleansing enema, a soft, large size (French 28) rubber tube is inserted into the rectum for a distance of about 20 cm, with the tip well into the sigmoid colon, and taped in place. The resin is then suspended in the appropriate amount of aqueous vehicle at body temperature and introduced by gravity, while the particles are kept in suspension by stirring. The suspension is flushed with 50 mL or 100 mL of fluid, following which the tube is clamped and left in place. If back leakage occurs, the hips are elevated on pillows or a knee-chest position is taken temporarily. A somewhat thicker suspension may be used, but care should be taken that no paste is formed, because the latter has a greatly reduced exchange surface and will be particularly ineffective if deposited in the rectal ampulla. The suspension is kept in the sigmoid colon for several hours, if possible. Then, the colon is irrigated with nonsodium containing solution at body temperature in order to remove the resin. Two quarts of flushing solution may be necessary. The returns are drained constantly through a Y tube connection. Particular attention should be paid to this cleansing enema when sorbitol has been used.

The intensity and duration of therapy depend upon the severity and resistance of hyperkalemia.

HOW SUPPLIED

Store at room temperature.

KAYEXALATE should not be heated for to do so may alter the exchange properties of the resin.

Caution: Federal law prohibits dispensing without prescription.

KAYEXALATE is available as a powder in jars of 1 pound (453.6 g), **NDC 0024-1075-01.**

KW 2-P

LEVOPHED® Bitartrate ℞

brand of norepinephrine bitartrate injection, USP

DESCRIPTION

Norepinephrine (sometimes referred to as *l-arterenol/Levarterenol* or *l-norepinephrine*) is a sympathomimetic amine which differs from epinephrine by the absence of a methyl group on the nitrogen atom.

Norepinephrine Bitartrate is (-)-α-(aminomethyl)-3,4-dihydroxybenzyl alcohol tartrate (1:1) (salt) monohydrate.

LEVOPHED is supplied in sterile aqueous solution in the form of the bitartrate salt to be administered by intravenous infusion following dilution. Norepinephrine is sparingly soluble in water, very slightly soluble in alcohol and ether, and readily soluble in acids. Each mL of LEVOPHED bitartrate injection contains the equivalent of 1 mg base of LEVOPHED, sodium chloride for isotonicity, and not more than 2 mg of sodium metabisulfite as an antioxidant. It has a pH of 3 to 4.5. The air in the ampuls has been displaced by nitrogen gas.

CLINICAL PHARMACOLOGY

LEVOPHED functions as a peripheral vasoconstrictor (alpha-adrenergic action) and as an inotropic stimulator of the heart and dilator of coronary arteries (beta-adrenergic action).

INDICATIONS AND USAGE

For blood pressure control in certain acute hypotensive states (eg, pheochromocytomectomy, sympathectomy, poliomyelitis, spinal anesthesia, myocardial infarction, septicemia, blood transfusion, and drug reactions).

As an adjunct in the treatment of cardiac arrest and profound hypotension.

CONTRAINDICATIONS

LEVOPHED should not be given to patients who are hypotensive from blood volume deficits except as an emergency measure to maintain coronary and cerebral artery perfusion until blood volume replacement therapy can be completed. If LEVOPHED is continuously administered to maintain blood pressure in the absence of blood volume replacement, the following may occur: severe peripheral and visceral vasoconstriction, decreased renal perfusion and urine output, poor systemic blood flow despite "normal" blood pressure, tissue hypoxia, and lactate acidosis.

LEVOPHED should also not be given to patients with mesenteric or peripheral vascular thrombosis (because of the risk of increasing ischemia and extending the area of infarction) unless, in the opinion of the attending physician, the administration of LEVOPHED is necessary as a life-saving procedure.

Cyclopropane and halothane anesthetics increase cardiac autonomic irritability and therefore seem to sensitize the myocardium to the action of intravenously administered epinephrine or norepinephrine. Hence, the use of LEVOPHED during cyclopropane and halothane anesthesia is generally considered contraindicated because of the risk of producing ventricular tachycardia or fibrillation.

The same type of cardiac arrhythmias may result from the use of LEVOPHED in patients with profound hypoxia or hypercarbia.

WARNINGS

LEVOPHED should be used with extreme caution in patients receiving monoamine oxidase inhibitors (MAOI) or antidepressants of the triptyline or imipramine types, because severe, prolonged hypertension may result.

LEVOPHED Bitartrate Injection contains sodium metabisulfite, a sulfite that may cause allergic-type reactions including anaphylactic symptoms and life-threatening or less severe asthmatic episodes in certain susceptible people. The overall prevalence of sulfite sensitivity in the general population is unknown. Sulfite sensitivity is seen more frequently in asthmatic than in nonasthmatic people.

PRECAUTIONS

General

Avoid Hypertension: Because of the potency of LEVOPHED and because of varying response to pressor substances, the possibility always exists that dangerously high blood pressure may be produced with overdoses of this pressor agent. It is desirable, therefore, to record the blood pressure every two minutes from the time administration is started until the desired blood pressure is obtained, then every five minutes if administration is to be continued.

The rate of flow must be watched constantly, and the patient should never be left unattended while receiving LEVOPHED. Headache may be a symptom of hypertension due to overdosage.

Site of Infusion: Whenever possible, infusions of LEVOPHED should be given into a large vein, particularly an antecubital vein because, when administered into this vein, the risk of necrosis of the overlying skin from prolonged vasoconstriction is apparently very slight. Some authors have indicated that the femoral vein is also an acceptable route of administration. A catheter tie-in technique should be avoided, if possible, since the obstruction to blood flow around the tubing may cause stasis and increased local concentration of the drug. Occlusive vascular diseases (for example, atherosclerosis, arteriosclerosis, diabetic endarteritis, Buerger's disease) are more likely to occur in the lower than in the upper extremity. Therefore, one should avoid the veins of the leg in elderly patients or in those suffering from such disorders. Gangrene has been reported in a lower extremity when infusions of LEVOPHED were given in an ankle vein.

Extravasation: The infusion site should be checked frequently for free flow. Care should be taken to avoid extravasation of LEVOPHED (norepinephrine) into the tissues, as local necrosis might ensue due to the vasoconstrictive action of the drug. Blanching along the course of the infused vein, sometimes without obvious extravasation, has been attributed to vasa vasorum constriction with increased permeability of the vein wall, permitting some leakage.

This also may progress on rare occasions to superficial slough, particularly during infusion into leg veins in elderly patients or in those suffering from obliterative vascular disease. Hence, if blanching occurs, consideration should be given to the advisability of changing the infusion site at intervals to allow the effects of local vasoconstriction to subside.

> **IMPORTANT—Antidote for Extravasation Ischemia:** To prevent sloughing and necrosis in areas in which extravasation has taken place, the area should be infiltrated as soon as possible with 10 mL to 15 mL of saline solution containing from 5 mg to 10 mg of **Regitine® (brand of phentolamine),** an adrenergic blocking agent. A syringe with a fine hypodermic needle should be used, with the solution being infiltrated liberally throughout the area, which is easily identified by its cold, hard, and pallid appearance. Sympathetic blockade with phentolamine causes immediate and conspicuous local hyperemic changes if the area is infiltrated within 12 hours. Therefore, phentolamine should be given as soon as possible after the extravasation is noted.

Drug Interactions: Cyclopropane and halothane anesthetics increase cardiac automatic irritability and therefore seem to sensitize the myocardium to the action of intravenously administered epinephrine or norepinephrine. Hence, the use of LEVOPHED, brand of norepinephrine bitartrate injection, during cyclopropane and halothane anesthesia is generally considered contraindicated because of the risk of producing ventricular tachycardia or fibrillation. The same type of cardiac arrhythmias may result from the use of LEVOPHED in patients with profound hypoxia or hypercarbia.

LEVOPHED should be used with extreme caution in patients receiving monoamine oxidase inhibitors (MAOI) or antidepressants of the triptyline or imipramine types, because severe, prolonged hypertension may result.

Carcinogenesis, Mutagenesis, Impairment of Fertility: Studies have not been performed.

Pregnancy Category C: Animal reproduction studies have not been conducted with LEVOPHED. It is also not known whether LEVOPHED can cause fetal harm when administered to a pregnant woman or can affect reproduction capacity. LEVOPHED should be given to a pregnant woman only if clearly needed.

Nursing Mothers: It is not known whether this drug is excreted in human milk. Because many drugs are excreted in human milk, caution should be exercised when LEVOPHED is administered to a nursing woman.

Pediatric Use: Safety and effectiveness in children have not been established.

ADVERSE REACTIONS

The following reactions can occur:

Body As A Whole: Ischemic injury due to potent vasoconstrictor action and tissue hypoxia.

Cardiovascular System: Bradycardia, probably as a reflex result of a rise in blood pressure, arrhythmias.

Nervous System: Anxiety, transient headache.

Respiratory System: Respiratory difficulty.

Skin and Appendages: Extravasation necrosis at injection site.

Prolonged administration of any potent vasopressor may result in plasma volume depletion which should be continuously corrected by appropriate fluid and electrolyte replacement therapy. If plasma volumes are not corrected, hypotension may recur when LEVOPHED is discontinued, or blood pressure may be maintained at the risk of severe peripheral and visceral vasoconstriction (eg, decreased renal perfusion) with diminution in blood flow and tissue perfusion with subsequent tissue hypoxia and lactic acidosis and possible ischemic injury. Gangrene of extremities has been rarely reported.

Regitine, trademark, CIBA Pharmaceutical Company

Continued on next page

This product information was prepared in August 1992. On these and other products of Sanofi Winthrop Pharmaceuticals, detailed information may be obtained on a current basis by direct inquiry to Product Information Services, 90 Park Avenue, New York, NY 10016 (toll free 1-800-446-6267).

Sanofi Winthrop—Cont.

Overdoses or conventional doses in hypersensitive persons (eg, hyperthyroid patients) cause severe hypertension with violent headache, photophobia, stabbing retrosternal pain, pallor, intense sweating, and vomiting.

OVERDOSAGE

Overdosage with LEVOPHED may result in headache, severe hypertension, reflex bradycardia, marked increase in peripheral resistance, and decreased cardiac output. In case of accidental overdosage, as evidenced by excessive blood pressure elevation, discontinue LEVOPHED until the condition of the patient stabilizes.

DOSAGE AND ADMINISTRATION

Norepinephrine Bitartrate Injection is a concentrated, potent drug which must be diluted in dextrose containing solutions prior to infusion. An infusion of LEVOPHED should be given into a large vein (see PRECAUTIONS).

Restoration of Blood Pressure In Acute Hypotensive States

Blood volume depletion should always be corrected as fully as possible before any vasopressor is administered. When, as an emergency measure, intra-aortic pressures must be maintained to prevent cerebral or coronary artery ischemia, LEVOPHED bitartrate, brand of norepinephrine bitartrate injection, can be administered before and concurrently with blood volume replacement.

Diluent: LEVOPHED should be diluted in 5 percent dextrose injection or 5 percent dextrose and sodium chloride injections. These dextrose containing fluids are protection against significant loss of potency due to oxidation. **Administration in saline solution alone is not recommended.** Whole blood or plasma, if indicated to increase blood volume, should be administered separately (for example, by use of a Y-tube and individual containers if given simultaneously).

Average Dosage: Add a 4 mL ampul (4 mg) of LEVOPHED to 1000 mL of a 5 percent dextrose containing solution. Each 1 mL of this dilution contains 4 μg of the base of LEVOPHED. Give this solution by intravenous infusion. Insert a plastic intravenous catheter through a suitable bore needle well advanced centrally into the vein and securely fixed with adhesive tape, avoiding, if possible, a catheter tie-in technique as this promotes stasis. An IV drip chamber or other suitable metering device is essential to permit an accurate estimation of the rate of flow in drops per minute. After observing the response to an initial dose of 2 mL to 3 mL (from 8 μg to 12 μg of base) per minute, adjust the rate of flow to establish and maintain a low normal blood pressure (usually 80 mm Hg to 100 mm Hg systolic) sufficient to maintain the circulation to vital organs. In previously hypertensive patients, it is recommended that the blood pressure should be raised no higher than 40 mm Hg below the preexisting systolic pressure. The average maintenance dose ranges from 0.5 mL to 1 mL per minute (from 2 μg to 4 μg of base).

High Dosage: Great individual variation occurs in the dose required to attain and maintain an adequate blood pressure. In all cases, dosage of LEVOPHED should be titrated according to the response of the patient. Occasionally much larger or even enormous daily doses (as high as 68 mg base or 17 ampuls) may be necessary if the patient remains hypotensive, but occult blood volume depletion should always be suspected and corrected when present. Central venous pressure monitoring is usually helpful in detecting and treating this situation.

Fluid Intake: The degree of dilution depends on clinical fluid volume requirements. If large volumes of fluid (dextrose) are needed at a flow rate that would involve an excessive dose of the pressor agent per unit of time, a solution more dilute than 4 μg per mL should be used. On the other hand, when large volumes of fluid are clinically undesirable, a concentration greater than 4 μg per mL may be necessary.

Duration of Therapy: The infusion should be continued until adequate blood pressure and tissue perfusion are maintained without therapy. Infusions of LEVOPHED should be reduced gradually, avoiding abrupt withdrawal. In some of the reported cases of vascular collapse due to acute myocardial infarction, treatment was required for up to six days.

Adjunctive Treatment in Cardiac Arrest

Infusions of LEVOPHED are usually administered intravenously during cardiac resuscitation to restore and maintain an adequate blood pressure after an effective heartbeat and ventilation have been established by other means. [The powerful beta-adrenergic stimulating action of LEVOPHED is also thought to increase the strength and effectiveness of systolic contractions once they occur.]

Average Dosage: To maintain systemic blood pressure during the management of cardiac arrest, LEVOPHED bitartrate, brand of norepinephrine bitartrate injection, is used in the same manner as described under Restoration of Blood Pressure in Acute Hypotensive States.

Parenteral drug products should be inspected visually for particulate matter and discoloration prior to use, whenever solution and container permit.

HOW SUPPLIED

LEVOPHED Bitartrate, brand of norepinephrine bitartrate injection, contains the equivalent of 4 mg base of LEVOPHED per each 4 mL ampul.

Do not use the solution if its color is pinkish or darker than slightly yellow or if it contains a precipitate.

Avoid contact with iron salts, alkalis, or oxidizing agents.

Supplied as:

Ampuls of 4 mL in boxes of 10, NDC 0024-1123-02.

Store at room temperature. Protect from light.

Caution: Federal law prohibits dispensing without prescription.

LW-34-X

MARCAINE® HYDROCHLORIDE ℞

brand of bupivacaine hydrochloride injection, USP

MARCAINE® HYDROCHLORIDE ℞

WITH EPINEPHRINE 1:200,000 (AS BITARTRATE)

brand of bupivacaine and epinephrine injection, USP

DESCRIPTION

Bupivacaine hydrochloride is 2-Piperidinecarboxamide, 1-butyl-*N*-(2,6-dimethylphenyl)-, monohydrochloride, monohydrate, a white crystalline powder that is freely soluble in 95 percent ethanol, soluble in water, and slightly soluble in chloroform or acetone.

Epinephrine is (-)-3, 4-Dihydroxy-α-[(methylamino)methyl] benzyl alcohol.

MARCAINE hydrochloride is available in sterile isotonic solutions with and without epinephrine (as bitartrate) 1:200,000 for injection via local infiltration, peripheral nerve block, and caudal and lumbar epidural blocks. Solutions of MARCAINE may be autoclaved if they do not contain epinephrine.

Bupivacaine is related chemically and pharmacologically to the aminoacyl local anesthetics. It is a homologue of mepivacaine and is chemically related to lidocaine. All three of these anesthetics contain an amide linkage between the aromatic nucleus and the amino, or piperidine group. They differ in this respect from the procaine-type local anesthetics, which have an ester linkage.

MARCAINE hydrochloride—Sterile isotonic solutions containing sodium chloride. In multiple-dose vials, each 1 mL also contains 1 mg methylparaben as antiseptic preservative. The pH of these solutions is adjusted to between 4 and 6.5 with sodium hydroxide or hydrochloric acid.

MARCAINE hydrochloride with epinephrine 1:200,000 (as bitartrate)—Sterile isotonic solutions containing sodium chloride. Each 1 mL contains bupivacaine hydrochloride and 0.0091 mg epinephrine bitartrate, with 0.5 mg sodium metabisulfite, 0.001 mL monothioglycerol, and 2 mg ascorbic acid as antioxidants, 0.0017 mL 60% sodium lactate buffer, and 0.1 mg edetate calcium disodium as stabilizer. In multiple-dose vials, each 1 mL also contains 1 mg methylparaben as antiseptic preservative. The pH of these solutions is adjusted to between 3.4 and 4.5 with sodium hydroxide or hydrochloric acid. The specific gravity of MARCAINE 0.5% with epinephrine 1:200,000 (as bitartrate) at 25°C is 1.008 and at 37°C is 1.008.

CLINICAL PHARMACOLOGY

Local anesthetics block the generation and the conduction of nerve impulses, presumably by increasing the threshold for electrical excitation in the nerve, by slowing the propagation of the nerve impulse, and by reducing the rate of rise of the action potential. In general, the progression of anesthesia is related to the diameter, myelination, and conduction velocity of affected nerve fibers. Clinically, the order of loss of nerve function is as follows: (1) pain, (2) temperature, (3) touch, (4) proprioception, and (5) skeletal muscle tone.

Systemic absorption of local anesthetics produces effects on the cardiovascular and central nervous systems (CNS). At blood concentrations achieved with normal therapeutic doses, changes in cardiac conduction, excitability, refractoriness, contractility, and peripheral vascular resistance are minimal. However, toxic blood concentrations depress cardiac conduction and excitability, which may lead to atrioventricular block, ventricular arrhythmias, and cardiac arrest, sometimes resulting in fatalities. In addition, myocardial contractility is depressed and peripheral vasodilation occurs, leading to decreased cardiac output and arterial blood pressure. Recent clinical reports and animal research suggest that these cardiovascular changes are more likely to occur after unintended intravascular injection of bupivacaine. Therefore, incremental dosing is necessary.

Following systemic absorption, local anesthetics can produce central nervous system stimulation, depression, or both. Apparent central stimulation is manifested as restlessness, tremors and shivering progressing to convulsions, followed by depression and coma progressing ultimately to respiratory arrest. However, the local anesthetics have a primary depressant effect on the medulla and on higher centers. The depressed stage may occur without a prior excited state.

Pharmacokinetics: The rate of systemic absorption of local anesthetics is dependent upon the total dose and concentration of drug administered, the route of administration, the vascularity of the administration site, and the presence or absence of epinephrine in the anesthetic solution. A dilute concentration of epinephrine (1:200,000 or 5 μg/mL) usually reduces the rate of absorption and peak plasma concentration of MARCAINE, permitting the use of moderately larger total doses and sometimes prolonging the duration of action.

The onset of action with MARCAINE is rapid and anesthesia is long lasting. The duration of anesthesia is significantly longer with MARCAINE than with any other commonly used local anesthetic. It has also been noted that there is a period of analgesia that persists after the return of sensation, during which time the need for strong analgesics is reduced.

The onset of action following dental injections is usually 2 to 10 minutes and anesthesia may last two or three times longer than lidocaine and mepivacaine for dental use, in many patients up to 7 hours. The duration of anesthetic effect is prolonged by the addition of epinephrine 1:200,000.

Local anesthetics are bound to plasma proteins in varying degrees. Generally, the lower the plasma concentration of drug the higher the percentage of drug bound to plasma proteins.

Local anesthetics appear to cross the placenta by passive diffusion. The rate and degree of diffusion is governed by (1) the degree of plasma protein binding, (2) the degree of ionization, and (3) the degree of lipid solubility. Fetal/maternal ratios of local anesthetics appear to be inversely related to the degree of plasma protein binding, because only the free, unbound drug is available for placental transfer. MARCAINE with a high protein binding capacity (95%) has a low fetal/maternal ratio (0.2 to 0.4). The extent of placental transfer is also determined by the degree of ionization and lipid solubility of the drug. Lipid soluble, nonionized drugs readily enter the fetal blood from the maternal circulation.

Depending upon the route of administration, local anesthetics are distributed to some extent to all body tissues, with high concentrations found in highly perfused organs such as the liver, lungs, heart, and brain.

Pharmacokinetic studies on the plasma profile of MARCAINE after direct intravenous injection suggest a three-compartment open model. The first compartment is represented by the rapid intravascular distribution of the drug. The second compartment represents the equilibration of the drug throughout the highly perfused organs such as the brain, myocardium, lungs, kidneys, and liver. The third compartment represents an equilibration of the drug with poorly perfused tissues, such as muscle and fat. The elimination of drug from tissue distribution depends largely upon the ability of binding sites in the circulation to carry it to the liver where it is metabolized.

After injection of MARCAINE for caudal, epidural, or peripheral nerve block in man, peak levels of bupivacaine in the blood are reached in 30 to 45 minutes, followed by a decline to insignificant levels during the next three to six hours.

Various pharmacokinetic parameters of the local anesthetics can be significantly altered by the presence of hepatic or renal disease, addition of epinephrine, factors affecting urinary pH, renal blood flow, the route of drug administration, and the age of the patient. The half-life of MARCAINE (bupivacaine) in adults is 2.7 hours and in neonates 8.1 hours.

Amide-type local anesthetics such as MARCAINE are metabolized primarily in the liver via conjugation with glucuronic acid. Patients with hepatic disease, especially those with severe hepatic disease, may be more susceptible to the potential toxicities of the amide-type local anesthetics. Pipecoloxylidine is the major metabolite of MARCAINE.

The kidney is the main excretory organ for most local anesthetics and their metabolites. Urinary excretion is affected by urinary perfusion and factors affecting urinary pH. Only 6% of bupivacaine is excreted unchanged in the urine.

When administered in recommended doses and concentrations, MARCAINE does not ordinarily produce irritation or tissue damage and does not cause methemoglobinemia.

INDICATIONS AND USAGE

MARCAINE is indicated for the production of local or regional anesthesia or analgesia for surgery, dental and oral surgery procedures, diagnostic and therapeutic procedures, and for obstetrical procedures. Only the 0.25% and 0.5% concentrations are indicated for obstetrical anesthesia. (See WARNINGS.)

Experience with nonobstetrical surgical procedures in pregnant patients is not sufficient to recommend use of 0.75% concentration of MARCAINE in these patients.

MARCAINE is not recommended for intravenous regional anesthesia (Bier Block). See WARNINGS.

The routes of administration and indicated MARCAINE concentrations are:

Sanofi Winthrop—Cont.

temporary loss of sensation and motor activity, usually in the lower half of the body, following proper administration of caudal or epidural anesthesia. Also, when appropriate, the physician should discuss other information including adverse reactions in the package insert of MARCAINE.

Patients receiving dental injections of MARCAINE (bupivacaine) should be cautioned not to chew solid foods or test the anesthetized area by biting or probing until anesthesia has worn off (up to 7 hours).

Clinically Significant Drug Interactions: The administration of local anesthetic solutions containing epinephrine or norepinephrine to patients receiving monoamine oxidase inhibitors or tricyclic antidepressants may produce severe, prolonged hypertension. Concurrent use of these agents should generally be avoided. In situations when concurrent therapy is necessary, careful patient monitoring is essential.

Concurrent administration of vasopressor drugs and of ergot-type oxytocic drugs may cause severe, persistent hypertension or cerebrovascular accidents.

Phenothiazines and butyrophenones may reduce or reverse the pressor effect of epinephrine.

Carcinogenesis, Mutagenesis, Impairment of Fertility: Long-term studies in animals of most local anesthetics including bupivacaine to evaluate the carcinogenic potential have not been conducted. Mutagenic potential or the effect on fertility has not been determined. There is no evidence from human data that MARCAINE may be carcinogenic or mutagenic or that it impairs fertility.

Pregnancy Category C: Decreased pup survival in rats and an embryocidal effect in rabbits have been observed when bupivacaine hydrochloride was administered to these species in doses comparable to nine and five times respectively the maximum recommended daily human dose (400 mg). There are no adequate and well-controlled studies in pregnant women of the effect of bupivacaine on the developing fetus. Bupivacaine hydrochloride should be used during pregnancy only if the potential benefit justifies the potential risk to the fetus. This does not exclude the use of MARCAINE at term for obstetrical anesthesia or analgesia. (See ***Labor and Delivery.***)

Labor and Delivery: SEE BOXED WARNING REGARDING OBSTETRICAL USE OF 0.75% MARCAINE.

MARCAINE is contraindicated for obstetrical paracervical block anesthesia.

Local anesthetics rapidly cross the placenta, and when used for epidural, caudal, or pudendal block anesthesia, can cause varying degrees of maternal, fetal, and neonatal toxicity. (See ***Pharmacokinetics*** in **CLINICAL PHARMACOLOGY.**) The incidence and degree of toxicity depend upon the procedure performed, the type, and amount of drug used, and the technique of drug administration. Adverse reactions in the parturient, fetus, and neonate involve alterations of the central nervous system, peripheral vascular tone, and cardiac function.

Maternal hypotension has resulted from regional anesthesia. Local anesthetics produce vasodilation by blocking sympathetic nerves. Elevating the patient's legs and positioning her on her left side will help prevent decreases in blood pressure. The fetal heart rate also should be monitored continuously and electronic fetal monitoring is highly advisable.

Epidural, caudal, or pudendal anesthesia may alter the forces of parturition through changes in uterine contractility or maternal expulsive efforts. Epidural anesthesia has been reported to prolong the second stage of labor by removing the parturient's reflex urge to bear down or by interfering with motor function. The use of obstetrical anesthesia may increase the need for forceps assistance.

The use of some local anesthetic drug products during labor and delivery may be followed by diminished muscle strength and tone for the first day or two of life. This has not been reported with bupivacaine.

It is extremely important to avoid aortocaval compression by the gravid uterus during administration of regional block to parturients. To do this, the patient must be maintained in the left lateral decubitus position or a blanket roll or sandbag may be placed beneath the right hip and gravid uterus displaced to the left.

Nursing Mothers: It is not known whether local anesthetic drugs are excreted in human milk. Because many drugs are excreted in human milk, caution should be exercised when local anesthetics are administered to a nursing woman.

Pediatric Use: Until further experience is gained in children younger than 12 years, administration of MARCAINE in this age group is not recommended.

ADVERSE REACTIONS

Reactions to MARCAINE (bupivacaine) are characteristic of those associated with other amide-type local anesthetics. A major cause of adverse reactions to this group of drugs is excessive plasma levels, which may be due to overdosage, unintentional intravascular injection, or slow metabolic degradation.

The most commonly encountered acute adverse experiences which demand immediate countermeasures are related to the central nervous system and the cardiovascular system. These adverse experiences are generally dose related and due to high plasma levels which may result from overdosage, rapid absorption from the injection site, diminished tolerance, or from unintentional intravascular injection of the local anesthetic solution. In addition to systemic dose-related toxicity, unintentional subarachnoid injection of drug during the intended performance of caudal or lumbar epidural block or nerve blocks near the vertebral column (especially in the head and neck region) may result in underventilation or apnea ("Total or High Spinal"). Also, hypotension due to loss of sympathetic tone and respiratory paralysis or underventilation due to cephalad extension of the motor level of anesthesia may occur. This may lead to secondary cardiac arrest if untreated. Factors influencing plasma protein binding, such as acidosis, systemic diseases which alter protein production, or competition of other drugs for protein binding sites, may diminish individual tolerance.

Central Nervous System Reactions: These are characterized by excitation and/or depression. Restlessness, anxiety, dizziness, tinnitus, blurred vision, or tremors may occur, possibly proceeding to convulsions. However, excitement may be transient or absent, with depression being the first manifestation of an adverse reaction. This may quickly be followed by drowsiness merging into unconsciousness and respiratory arrest. Other central nervous system effects may be nausea, vomiting, chills, and constriction of the pupils.

The incidence of convulsions associated with the use of local anesthetics varies with the procedure used and the total dose administered. In a survey of studies of epidural anesthesia, overt toxicity progressing to convulsions occurred in approximately 0.1% of local anesthetic administrations.

Cardiovascular System Reactions: High doses or unintentional intravascular injection may lead to high plasma levels and related depression of the myocardium, decreased cardiac output, heartblock, hypotension, bradycardia, ventricular arrhythmias, including ventricular tachycardia and ventricular fibrillation, and cardiac arrest. (See **WARNINGS, PRECAUTIONS,** and **OVERDOSAGE** sections.)

Allergic: Allergic-type reactions are rare and may occur as a result of sensitivity to the local anesthetic or to other formulation ingredients, such as the antimicrobial preservative methylparaben contained in multiple-dose vials or sulfites in epinephrine-containing solutions. These reactions are characterized by signs such as urticaria, pruritus, erythema, angioneurotic edema (including laryngeal edema), tachycardia, sneezing, nausea, vomiting, dizziness, syncope, excessive sweating, elevated temperature, and, possibly, anaphylactoid-like symptomatology (including severe hypotension). Cross sensitivity among members of the amide-type local anesthetic group has been reported. The usefulness of screening for sensitivity has not been definitely established.

Neurologic: The incidences of adverse neurologic reactions associated with the use of local anesthetics may be related to the total dose of local anesthetic administered and are also dependent upon the particular drug used, the route of administration, and the physical status of the patient. Many of these effects may be related to local anesthetic techniques, with or without a contribution from the drug.

In the practice of caudal or lumbar epidural block, occasional unintentional penetration of the subarachnoid space by the catheter or needle may occur. Subsequent adverse effects may depend partially on the amount of drug administered intrathecally and the physiological and physical effects of a dural puncture. A high spinal is characterized by paralysis of the legs, loss of consciousness, respiratory paralysis, and bradycardia.

Neurologic effects following epidural or caudal anesthesia may include spinal block of varying magnitude (including high or total spinal block); hypotension secondary to spinal block; urinary retention; fecal and urinary incontinence; loss of perineal sensation and sexual function; persistent anesthesia, paresthesia, weakness, paralysis of the lower extremities and loss of sphincter control all of which may have slow, incomplete, or no recovery; headache; backache; septic meningitis; meningismus; slowing of labor; increased incidence of forceps delivery; and cranial nerve palsies due to traction on nerves from loss of cerebrospinal fluid.

Neurologic effects following other procedures or routes of administration may include persistent anesthesia, paresthesia, weakness, paralysis, all of which may have slow, incomplete, or no recovery.

OVERDOSAGE

Acute emergencies from local anesthetics are generally related to high plasma levels encountered during therapeutic use of local anesthetics or to unintended subarachnoid injection of local anesthetic solution. (See **ADVERSE REACTIONS, WARNINGS,** and **PRECAUTIONS.**)

Management of Local Anesthetic Emergencies: The first consideration is prevention, best accomplished by careful and constant monitoring of cardiovascular and respiratory vital signs and the patient's state of consciousness after each local anesthetic injection. At the first sign of change, oxygen should be administered.

The first step in the management of systemic toxic reactions, as well as underventilation or apnea due to unintentional subarachnoid injection of drug solution, consists of immediate attention to the establishment and maintenance of a patent airway and effective assisted or controlled ventilation with 100% oxygen with a delivery system capable of permitting immediate positive airway pressure by mask. This may prevent convulsions if they have not already occurred.

If necessary, use drugs to control the convulsions. A 50 mg to 100 mg bolus IV injection of succinylcholine will paralyze the patient without depressing the central nervous or cardiovascular systems and facilitate ventilation. A bolus IV dose of 5 mg to 10 mg of diazepam or 50 mg to 100 mg of thiopental will permit ventilation and counteract central nervous system stimulation, but these drugs also depress central nervous system, respiratory, and cardiac function, add to postictal depression and may result in apnea. Intravenous barbiturates, anticonvulsant agents, or muscle relaxants should only be administered by those familiar with their use. Immediately after the institution of these ventilatory measures, the adequacy of the circulation should be evaluated. Supportive treatment of circulatory depression may require administration of intravenous fluids, and when appropriate, a vasopressor dictated by the clinical situation (such as ephedrine or epinephrine to enhance myocardial contractile force).

Endotracheal intubation, employing drugs and techniques familiar to the clinician, may be indicated after initial administration of oxygen by mask if difficulty is encountered in the maintenance of a patent airway, or if prolonged ventilatory support (assisted or controlled) is indicated.

Recent clinical data from patients experiencing local anesthetic-induced convulsions demonstrated rapid development of hypoxia, hypercarbia, and acidosis with bupivacaine within a minute of the onset of convulsions. These observations suggest that oxygen consumption and carbon dioxide production are greatly increased during local anesthetic convulsions and emphasize the importance of immediate and effective ventilation with oxygen which may avoid cardiac arrest.

If not treated immediately, convulsions with simultaneous hypoxia, hypercarbia, and acidosis plus myocardial depression from the direct effects of the local anesthetic may result in cardiac arrhythmias, bradycardia, asystole, ventricular fibrillation, or cardiac arrest. Respiratory abnormalities, including apnea, may occur. Underventilation or apnea due to unintentional subarachnoid injection of local anesthetic solution may produce these same signs and also lead to cardiac arrest if ventilatory support is not instituted. *If cardiac arrest should occur, successful outcome may require prolonged resuscitative efforts.*

The supine position is dangerous in pregnant women at term because of aortocaval compression by the gravid uterus. Therefore during treatment of systemic toxicity, maternal hypotension or fetal bradycardia following regional block, the parturient should be maintained in the left lateral decubitus position if possible, or manual displacement of the uterus off the great vessels be accomplished.

The mean seizure dosage of bupivacaine in rhesus monkeys was found to be 4.4 mg/kg with mean arterial plasma concentration of 4.5 µg/mL. The intravenous and subcutaneous LD_{50} in mice is 6 mg/kg to 8 mg/kg and 38 mg/kg to 54 mg/kg respectively.

DOSAGE AND ADMINISTRATION

The dose of any local anesthetic administered varies with the anesthetic procedure, the area to be anesthetized, the vascularity of the tissues, the number of neuronal segments to be blocked, the depth of anesthesia and degree of muscle relaxation required, the duration of anesthesia desired, individual tolerance, and the physical condition of the patient. The smallest dose and concentration required to produce the desired result should be administered. Dosages of MARCAINE should be reduced for elderly and debilitated patients and patients with cardiac and/or liver disease. The rapid injection of a large volume of local anesthetic solution should be avoided and fractional (incremental) doses should be used when feasible.

For specific techniques and procedures, refer to standard textbooks.

In recommended doses, MARCAINE (bupivacaine) produces complete sensory block, but the effect on motor function differs among the three concentrations.

0.25%—when used for caudal, epidural, or peripheral nerve block, produces incomplete motor block. Should be used for operations in which muscle relaxation is not important, or when another means of providing muscle relaxation is used concurrently. Onset of action may be slower than with the 0.5% or 0.75% solutions.

0.5%—provides motor blockade for caudal, epidural, or nerve block, but muscle relaxation may be inadequate for operations in which complete muscle relaxation is essential.

- local infiltration — 0.25%
- peripheral nerve block — 0.25% and 0.5%
- retrobulbar block — 0.75%
- sympathetic block — 0.25%
- lumbar epidural — 0.25%, 0.5%, and 0.75% (0.75% not for obstetrical anesthesia)
- caudal — 0.25% and 0.5%
- epidural test dose — 0.5% with epinephrine 1:200,000
- dental blocks — 0.5% with epinephrine 1:200,000

(See **DOSAGE AND ADMINISTRATION** for additional information.)

Standard textbooks should be consulted to determine the accepted procedures and techniques for the administration of MARCAINE.

CONTRAINDICATIONS

MARCAINE is contraindicated in obstetrical paracervical block anesthesia. Its use in this technique has resulted in fetal bradycardia and death.

MARCAINE (bupivacaine) is contraindicated in patients with a known hypersensitivity to it or to any local anesthetic agent of the amide-type or to other components of MARCAINE solutions.

WARNINGS

THE 0.75% CONCENTRATION OF MARCAINE IS NOT RECOMMENDED FOR OBSTETRICAL ANESTHESIA. THERE HAVE BEEN REPORTS OF CARDIAC ARREST WITH DIFFICULT RESUSCITATION OR DEATH DURING USE OF MARCAINE FOR EPIDURAL ANESTHESIA IN OBSTETRICAL PATIENTS. IN MOST CASES, THIS HAS FOLLOWED USE OF THE 0.75% CONCENTRATION. RESUSCITATION HAS BEEN DIFFICULT OR IMPOSSIBLE DESPITE APPARENTLY ADEQUATE PREPARATION AND APPROPRIATE MANAGEMENT. CARDIAC ARREST HAS OCCURRED AFTER CONVULSIONS RESULTING FROM SYSTEMIC TOXICITY, PRESUMABLY FOLLOWING UNINTENTIONAL INTRAVASCULAR INJECTION. THE 0.75% CONCENTRATION SHOULD BE RESERVED FOR SURGICAL PROCEDURES WHERE A HIGH DEGREE OF MUSCLE RELAXATION AND PROLONGED EFFECT ARE NECESSARY.

LOCAL ANESTHETICS SHOULD ONLY BE EMPLOYED BY CLINICIANS WHO ARE WELL VERSED IN DIAGNOSIS AND MANAGEMENT OF DOSE-RELATED TOXICITY AND OTHER ACUTE EMERGENCIES WHICH MIGHT ARISE FROM THE BLOCK TO BE EMPLOYED, AND THEN ONLY AFTER INSURING THE *IMMEDIATE* AVAILABILITY OF OXYGEN, OTHER RESUSCITATIVE DRUGS, CARDIOPULMONARY RESUSCITATIVE EQUIPMENT, AND THE PERSONNEL RESOURCES NEEDED FOR PROPER MANAGEMENT OF TOXIC REACTIONS AND RELATED EMERGENCIES. (See also ADVERSE REACTIONS, PRECAUTIONS, and OVERDOSAGE.) DELAY IN PROPER MANAGEMENT OF DOSE-RELATED TOXICITY, UNDERVENTILATION FROM ANY CAUSE, AND/OR ALTERED SENSITIVITY MAY LEAD TO THE DEVELOPMENT OF ACIDOSIS, CARDIAC ARREST AND, POSSIBLY, DEATH.

Local anesthetic solutions containing antimicrobial preservatives, ie, those supplied in multiple-dose vials, should not be used for epidural or caudal anesthesia because safety has not been established with regard to intrathecal injection, either intentionally or unintentionally, of such preservatives.

It is essential that aspiration for blood or cerebrospinal fluid (where applicable) be done prior to injecting any local anesthetic, both the original dose and all subsequent doses, to avoid intravascular or subarachnoid injection. However, a negative aspiration does *not* ensure against an intravascular or subarachnoid injection.

MARCAINE with epinephrine 1:200,000 or other vasopressors should not be used concomitantly with ergot-type oxytocic drugs, because a severe persistent hypertension may occur. Likewise, solutions of MARCAINE containing a vasoconstrictor, such as epinephrine, should be used with extreme caution in patients receiving monoamine oxidase inhibitors (MAOI) or antidepressants of the triptyline or imipramine types, because severe prolonged hypertension may result.

Until further experience is gained in children younger than 12 years, administration of MARCAINE in this age group is not recommended.

Mixing or the prior or intercurrent use of any other local anesthetic with MARCAINE cannot be recommended because of insufficient data on the clinical use of such mixtures.

There have been reports of cardiac arrest and death during the use of MARCAINE for intravenous regional anesthesia (Bier Block). Information on safe dosages and techniques of administration of MARCAINE in this procedure is lacking.

Therefore, MARCAINE is not recommended for use in this technique.

MARCAINE hydrochloride with epinephrine 1:200,000 contains sodium metabisulfite, a sulfite that may cause allergic-type reactions including anaphylactic symptoms and life-threatening or less severe asthmatic episodes in certain susceptible people. The overall prevalence of sulfite sensitivity in the general population is unknown and probably low. Sulfite sensitivity is seen more frequently in asthmatic than in nonasthmatic people. Single-dose ampuls and single-dose vials of *MARCAINE hydrochloride* without epinephrine do not contain sodium metabisulfite.

PRECAUTIONS

General: The safety and effectiveness of local anesthetics depend on proper dosage, correct technique, adequate precautions, and readiness for emergencies. Resuscitative equipment, oxygen, and other resuscitative drugs should be available for immediate use. (See WARNINGS, ADVERSE REACTIONS, and OVERDOSAGE.) During major regional nerve blocks, the patient should have IV fluids running via an indwelling catheter to assure a functioning intravenous pathway. The lowest dosage of local anesthetic that results in effective anesthesia should be used to avoid high plasma levels and serious adverse effects. The rapid injection of a large volume of local anesthetic solution should be avoided and fractional (incremental) doses should be used when feasible.

Epidural Anesthesia: During epidural administration of MARCAINE, 0.5% and 0.75% solutions should be administered in incremental doses of 3 mL to 5 mL with sufficient time between doses to detect toxic manifestations of unintentional intravascular or intrathecal injection. Injections should be made slowly, with frequent aspirations before and during the injection to avoid intravascular injection. Syringe aspirations should also be performed before and during each supplemental injection in continuous (intermittent) catheter techniques. An intravascular injection is still possible even if aspirations for blood are negative.

During the administration of epidural anesthesia, it is recommended that a test dose be administered initially and the effects monitored before the full dose is given. When using a "continuous" catheter technique, test doses should be given prior to both the original and all reinforcing doses, because plastic tubing in the epidural space can migrate into a blood vessel or through the dura. When clinical conditions permit, the test dose should contain epinephrine (10 μg to 15 μg has been suggested) to serve as a warning of unintended intravascular injection. If injected into a blood vessel, this amount of epinephrine is likely to produce a transient "epinephrine response" within 45 seconds, consisting of an increase in heart rate and/or systolic blood pressure, circumoral pallor, palpitations, and nervousness in the unsedated patient. The sedated patient may exhibit only a pulse rate increase of 20 or more beats per minute for 15 or more seconds. Therefore, following the test dose, the heart rate should be monitored for a heart rate increase. Patients on beta-blockers may not manifest changes in heart rate, but blood pressure monitoring can detect a transient rise in systolic blood pressure. The test dose should also contain 10 mg to 15 mg of MARCAINE or an equivalent amount of another local anesthetic to detect an unintended intrathecal administration. This will be evidenced within a few minutes by signs of spinal block (eg, decreased sensation of the buttocks, paresis of the legs, or, in the sedated patient, absent knee jerk). The Test Dose formulation of MARCAINE contains 15 mg of bupivacaine and 15 μg of epinephrine in a volume of 3 mL. An intravascular or subarachnoid injection is still possible even if results of the test dose are negative. The test dose itself may produce a systemic toxic reaction, high spinal or epinephrine-induced cardiovascular effects.

Injection of repeated doses of local anesthetics may cause significant increases in plasma levels with each repeated dose due to slow accumulation of the drug or its metabolites, or to slow metabolic degradation. Tolerance to elevated blood levels varies with the status of the patient. Debilitated, elderly patients and acutely ill patients should be given reduced doses commensurate with their age and physical status. Local anesthetics should also be used with caution in patients with hypotension or heartblock.

Careful and constant monitoring of cardiovascular and respiratory (adequacy of ventilation) vital signs and the patient's state of consciousness should be performed after each local anesthetic injection. It should be kept in mind at such times that restlessness, anxiety, incoherent speech, lightheadedness, numbness and tingling of the mouth and lips, metallic taste, tinnitus, dizziness, blurred vision, tremors, twitching, depression, or drowsiness may be early warning signs of central nervous system toxicity.

Local anesthetic solutions containing a vasoconstrictor should be used cautiously and in carefully restricted quantities in areas of the body supplied by end arteries or having otherwise compromised blood supply such as digits, nose, external ear, or penis. Patients with hypertensive vascular disease may exhibit exaggerated vasoconstrictor response. Ischemic injury or necrosis may result.

Because amide-type local anesthetics such as MARCAINE (bupivacaine) are metabolized by the liver, these drugs, especially repeat doses, should be used cautiously in patients with hepatic disease. Patients with severe hepatic disease, because of their inability to metabolize local anesthetics normally, are at a greater risk of developing toxic plasma concentrations. Local anesthetics should also be used with caution in patients with impaired cardiovascular function because they may be less able to compensate for functional changes associated with the prolongation of AV conduction produced by these drugs.

Serious dose-related cardiac arrhythmias may occur if preparations containing a vasoconstrictor such as epinephrine are employed in patients during or following the administration of potent inhalation anesthetics. In deciding whether to use these products concurrently in the same patient, the combined action of both agents upon the myocardium, the concentration and volume of vasoconstrictor used, and the time since injection, when applicable, should be taken into account.

Many drugs used during the conduct of anesthesia are considered potential triggering agents for familial malignant hyperthermia. Because it is not known whether amide-type local anesthetics may trigger this reaction and because the need for supplemental general anesthesia cannot be predicted in advance, it is suggested that a standard protocol for management should be available. Early unexplained signs of tachycardia, tachypnea, labile blood pressure, and metabolic acidosis may precede temperature elevation. Successful outcome is dependent on early diagnosis, prompt discontinuance of the suspect triggering agent(s) and prompt institution of treatment, including oxygen therapy, indicated supportive measures and dantrolene. (Consult dantrolene sodium intravenous package insert before using.)

Use in Head and Neck Area: Small doses of local anesthetics injected into the head and neck area, including retrobulbar, dental and stellate ganglion blocks, may produce adverse reactions similar to systemic toxicity seen with unintentional intravascular injections of larger doses. The injection procedures require the utmost care. Confusion, convulsions, respiratory depression, and/or respiratory arrest, and cardiovascular stimulation or depression have been reported. These reactions may be due to intra-arterial injection of the local anesthetic with retrograde flow to the cerebral circulation. They may also be due to puncture of the dural sheath of the optic nerve during retrobulbar block with diffusion of any local anesthetic along the subdural space to the midbrain. Patients receiving these blocks should have their circulation and respiration monitored and be constantly observed. Resuscitative equipment and personnel for treating adverse reactions should be immediately available. Dosage recommendations should not be exceeded. (See DOSAGE AND ADMINISTRATION.)

Use in Ophthalmic Surgery: Clinicians who perform retrobulbar blocks should be aware that there have been reports of respiratory arrest following local anesthetic injection. Prior to retrobulbar block, as with all other regional procedures, the immediate availability of equipment, drugs, and personnel to manage respiratory arrest or depression, convulsions, and cardiac stimulation or depression should be assured (see also WARNINGS and *Use in Head and Neck Area*, above). As with other anesthetic procedures, patients should be constantly monitored following ophthalmic blocks for signs of these adverse reactions, which may occur following relatively low total doses. A concentration of 0.75% bupivacaine is indicated for retrobulbar block; however, this concentration is not indicated for any other peripheral nerve block, including the facial nerve, and not indicated for local infiltration, including the conjunctiva (see INDICATIONS and PRECAUTIONS, *General*). Mixing MARCAINE with other local anesthetics is not recommended because of insufficient data on the clinical use of such mixtures.

When MARCAINE 0.75% is used for retrobulbar block, complete corneal anesthesia usually precedes onset of clinically acceptable external ocular muscle akinesia. Therefore, presence of akinesia rather than anesthesia alone should determine readiness of the patient for surgery.

Use in Dentistry: Because of the long duration of anesthesia, when MARCAINE 0.5% with epinephrine is used for dental injections, patients should be cautioned about the possibility of inadvertent trauma to tongue, lips, and buccal mucosa and advised not to chew solid foods or test the anesthetized area by biting or probing.

Information for Patients: When appropriate, patients should be informed in advance that they may experience

Continued on next page

This product information was prepared in August 1992. On these and other products of Sanofi Winthrop Pharmaceuticals, detailed information may be obtained on a current basis by direct inquiry to Product Information Services, 90 Park Avenue, New York, NY 10016 (toll free 1-800-446-6267).

0.75%—produces complete motor block. Most useful for epidural block in abdominal operations requiring complete muscle relaxation, and for retrobulbar anesthesia. Not for obstetrical anesthesia.

The duration of anesthesia with MARCAINE is such that for most indications, a single dose is sufficient.

Maximum dosage limit must be individualized in each case after evaluating the size and physical status of the patient, as well as the usual rate of systemic absorption from a particular injection site. Most experience to date is with single doses of MARCAINE up to 225 mg with epinephrine 1:200,000 and 175 mg without epinephrine; more or less drug may be used depending on individualization of each case. These doses may be repeated up to once every three hours. In clinical studies to date, total daily doses have been up to 400 mg. Until further experience is gained, this dose should not be exceeded in 24 hours. The duration of anesthetic effect may be prolonged by the addition of epinephrine.

The dosages in Table 1 have generally proved satisfactory and are recommended as a guide for use in the average adult. These dosages should be reduced for elderly or debilitated patients. Until further experience is gained, MARCAINE (bupivacaine) is not recommended for children younger than 12 years. MARCAINE is contraindicated for obstetrical paracervical blocks, and is not recommended for intravenous regional anesthesia (Bier Block).

Use in Epidural Anesthesia: During epidural administration of MARCAINE, 0.5% and 0.75% solutions should be administered in incremental doses of 3 mL to 5 mL with sufficient time between doses to detect toxic manifestatons of unintentional intravascular or intrathecal injection. In obstetrics, only the 0.5% and 0.25% concentrations should be used; incremental doses of 3 mL to 5 mL of the 0.5% solution not exceeding 50 mg to 100 mg at any dosing interval are recommended. Repeat doses should be preceded by a test dose containing epinephrine if not contraindicated. Use only the single-dose ampuls and single-dose vials for caudal or epidural anesthesia; the multiple-dose vials contain a preservative and therefore should not be used for these procedures.

Test Dose for Caudal and Lumbar Epidural Blocks: The Test Dose of MARCAINE (0.5% bupivacaine with 1:200,000 epinephrine in a 3 mL ampul) is recommended for use as a test dose when clinical conditions permit prior to caudal and lumbar epidural blocks. This may serve as a warning of unintended intravascular or subarachnoid injection. (See **PRECAUTIONS**.) The pulse rate and other signs should be monitored carefully immediately following each test dose administration to detect possible intravascular injection, and adequate time for onset of spinal block should be allotted to detect possible intrathecal injection. An intravascular or subarachnoid injection is still possible even if results of the test dose are negative. The test dose itself may produce a systemic toxic reaction, high spinal or cardiovascular effects from the epinephrine. (See **WARNINGS** and **OVERDOSAGE**.)

Use in Dentistry: The 0.5% concentration with epinephrine is recommended for infiltration and block injection in the maxillary and mandibular area when a longer duration of local anesthetic action is desired, such as for oral surgical procedures generally associated with significant postoperative pain. The average dose of 1.8 mL (9 mg) per injection site will usually suffice; an occasional second dose of 1.8 mL (9 mg) may be used if necessary to produce adequate anesthesia after making allowance for 2 to 10 minutes onset time. (See **CLINICAL PHARMACOLOGY**.) The lowest effective dose should be employed and time should be allowed between injections; it is recommended that the total dose for all injection sites, *spread out* over a single dental sitting, should not ordinarily exceed 90 mg for a healthy adult patient (ten 1.8 mL injections of 0.5% MARCAINE with epinephrine, bupivacaine and epinephrine). Injections should be made slowly and with frequent aspirations. Until further experience is gained, MARCAINE in dentistry is not recommended for children younger than 12 years.

Unused portions of solution not containing preservatives, ie, those supplied in single-dose ampuls and single-dose vials, should be discarded following initial use.

This product should be inspected visually for particulate matter and discoloration prior to administration whenever solution and container permit. Solutions which are discolored or which contain particulate matter should not be administered. [See table above.]

HOW SUPPLIED

These solutions are not for spinal anesthesia.
Store at controlled room temperature, between 15°C and 30°C (59°F and 86°F).
MARCAINE hydrochloride — Solutions of MARCAINE (bupivacaine) that do not contain epinephrine may be autoclaved. Autoclave at 15-pound pressure, 121°C (250°F) for 15 minutes.
0.25%—Contains 2.5 mg bupivacaine hydrochloride per mL.
Single-dose ampuls of 50 mL, box of 5
                        NDC 0024-1212-02
Single-dose vials of 10 mL, box of 10
                        NDC 0024-1212-10

Table 1. Recommended Concentrations and Doses of MARCAINE

Type of Block	Conc.	Each Dose (mL)	Each Dose (mg)	Motor Block[1]
Local infiltration	0.25%[4]	up to max.	up to max.	—
Epidural	0.75%[2,4]	10–20	75–150	complete
	0.5%[4]	10–20	50–100	moderate to complete
	0.25%[4]	10–20	25–50	partial to moderate
Caudal	0.5%[4]	15–30	75–150	moderate to complete
	0.25%[4]	15–30	37.5–75	moderate
Peripheral nerves	0.5%[4]	5 to max.	25 to max.	moderate to complete
	0.25%[4]	5 to max.	12.5 to max.	moderate to complete
Retrobulbar[3]	0.75%[4]	2–4	15–30	complete
Sympathetic	0.25%	20–50	50–125	—
Dental[3]	0.5% w/epi	1.8–3.6 per site	9–18 per site	—
Epidural[3] Test Dose	0.5% w/epi	2–3	10–15 (10–15 micrograms epinephrine)	—

[1]With continuous (intermittent) techniques, repeat doses increase the degree of motor block. The first repeat dose of 0.5% may produce complete motor block. Intercostal nerve block with 0.25% may also produce complete motor block for intra-abdominal surgery.
[2]For single-dose use, not for intermittent (catheter) epidural technique. Not for obstetrical anesthesia.
[3]See PRECAUTIONS.
[4]Solutions with or without epinephrine.

Single-dose vials of 30 mL, box of 10
                        NDC 0024-1212-30
Multiple-dose vials of 50 mL, box of 1
                        NDC 0024-1217-01
0.5%—Contains 5 mg bupivacaine hydrochloride per mL.
Single-dose ampuls of 30 mL, box of 5
                        NDC 0024-1213-02
Single-dose vials of 10 mL, box of 10
                        NDC 0024-1213-10
Single-dose vials of 30 mL, box of 10
                        NDC 0024-1213-30
Multiple-dose vials of 50 mL, box of 1
                        NDC 0024-1218-01
0.75%—Contains 7.5 mg bupivacaine hydrochloride per mL.
Single-dose ampuls of 30 mL, box of 5
                        NDC 0024-1214-02
Single-dose vials of 10 mL, box of 10
                        NDC 0024-1214-10
Single-dose vials of 30 mL, box of 10
                        NDC 0024-1214-30

MARCAINE hydrochloride with epinephrine 1:200,000 (as bitartrate)—Solutions of MARCAINE that contain epinephrine should not be autoclaved and should be protected from light. Do not use the solution if its color is pinkish or darker than slightly yellow or if it contains a precipitate.
0.25%—with epinephrine 1:200,000
Contains 2.5 mg bupivacaine hydrochloride per mL.
Single-dose ampuls of 50 mL, box of 5
                        NDC 0024-1222-02
Single-dose vials of 10 mL, box of 10
                        NDC 0024-1222-10
Single-dose vials of 30 mL, box of 10
                        NDC 0024-1222-30
Multiple-dose vials of 50 mL, box of 1
                        NDC 0024-1227-01
0.5%—with epinephrine 1:200,000
Contains 5 mg bupivacaine hydrochloride per mL.
Single-dose ampuls of 3 mL, box of 10
                        NDC 0024-1223-03
Single-dose ampuls of 30 mL, box of 5
                        NDC 0024-1223-02
Single-dose vials of 10 mL, box of 10
                        NDC 0024-1223-10
Single-dose vials of 30 mL, box of 10
                        NDC 0024-1223-30
Multiple-dose vials of 50 mL, box of 1
                        NDC 0024-1228-01
0.75%—with epinephrine 1:200,000
Contains 7.5 mg bupivacaine hydrochloride per mL.
Single-dose ampuls of 30 mL, box of 5
                    NDC 0024-1224-02
                    MW-126-N

For full prescribing information on the dental use of MARCAINE see Eastman Kodak Company product listing in this publication.

MARCAINE® Spinal
brand of bupivacaine in dextrose injection, USP   ℞

STERILE HYPERBARIC SOLUTION FOR SPINAL ANESTHESIA

DESCRIPTION

Bupivacaine hydrochloride is 2-Piperidinecarboxamide, 1-butyl-N-(2,6-dimethylphenyl)-, monohydrochloride, monohydrate, a white crystalline powder that is freely soluble in 95 percent ethanol, soluble in water, and slightly soluble in chloroform or acetone.
Dextrose is D-glucopyranose monohydrate.
MARCAINE Spinal is available in sterile hyperbaric solution for subarachnoid injection (spinal block).
Bupivacaine hydrochloride is related chemically and pharmacologically to the aminoacyl local anesthetics. It is a homologue of mepivacaine and is chemically related to lidocaine. All three of these anesthetics contain an amide linkage between the aromatic nucleus and the amino or piperidine group. They differ in this respect from the procaine-type local anesthetics, which have an ester linkage.
Each 1 mL of MARCAINE Spinal contains 7.5 mg bupivacaine hydrochloride and 82.5 mg dextrose. The pH of this solution is adjusted to between 4.0 and 6.5 with sodium hydroxide or hydrochloric acid.
The specific gravity of MARCAINE Spinal is between 1.030 and 1.035 at 25° C and 1.03 at 37° C.
MARCAINE Spinal does not contain any preservatives.

CLINICAL PHARMACOLOGY

Local anesthetics block the generation and the conduction of nerve impulses, presumably by increasing the threshold for electrical excitation in the nerve, by slowing the propagation of the nerve impulse, and by reducing the rate of rise of the action potential. In general, the progression of anesthesia is related to the diameter, myelination, and conduction velocity of affected nerve fibers. Clinically, the order of loss of nerve function is as follows: (1) pain, (2) temperature, (3) touch, (4) proprioception, and (5) skeletal muscle tone.
Systemic absorption of local anesthetics produces effects on the cardiovascular and central nervous systems (CNS). At blood concentrations achieved with normal therapeutic doses, changes in cardiac conduction, excitability, refractoriness, contractility, and peripheral vascular resistance are minimal. However, toxic blood concentrations depress cardiac conduction and excitability, which may lead to atrioventricular block, ventricular arrhythmias, and cardiac arrest, sometimes resulting in fatalities. In addition, myocardial contractility is depressed and peripheral vasodilation occurs, leading to decreased cardiac output and arterial blood pres-

Continued on next page

This product information was prepared in August 1992. On these and other products of Sanofi Winthrop Pharmaceuticals, detailed information may be obtained on a current basis by direct inquiry to Product Information Services, 90 Park Avenue, New York, NY 10016 (toll free 1-800-446-6267).

Sanofi Winthrop—Cont.

sure. Recent clinical reports and animal research suggest that these cardiovascular changes are more likely to occur after unintended direct intravascular injection of bupivacaine. Therefore, when epidural anesthesia with bupivacaine is considered, incremental dosing is necessary.

Following systemic absorption, local anesthetics can produce central nervous system stimulation, depression, or both. Apparent central stimulation is manifested as restlessness, tremors and shivering, progressing to convulsions, followed by depression and coma progressing ultimately to respiratory arrest. However, the local anesthetics have a primary depressant effect on the medulla and on higher centers. The depressed stage may occur without a prior excited stage.

Pharmacokinetics: The rate of systemic absorption of local anesthetics is dependent upon the total dose and concentration of drug administered, the route of administration, the vascularity of the administraton site, and the presence or absence of epinephrine in the anesthetic solution. A dilute concentration of epinephrine (1:200,000 or 5 μg/mL) usually reduces the rate of absorption and peak plasma concentration of MARCAINE, permitting the use of moderately larger total doses and sometimes prolonging the duration of action.

The onset of action with MARCAINE is rapid and anesthesia is long lasting. The duration of anesthesia is significantly longer with MARCAINE than with any other commonly used local anesthetic. It has also been noted that there is a period of analgesia that persists after the return of sensation, during which time the need for strong analgesics is reduced.

The onset of sensory blockade following spinal block with MARCAINE Spinal is very rapid (within one minute); maximum motor blockade and maximum dermatome level are achieved within 15 minutes in most cases. Duration of sensory blockade (time to return of complete sensation in the operative site or regression of two dermatomes) following a 12 mg dose averages 2 hours with or without 0.2 mg epinephrine. The time to return of complete motor ability with 12 mg MARCAINE Spinal averages 3½ hours without the addition of epinephrine and 4½ hours if 0.2 mg epinephrine is added. When compared to equal milligram doses of hyperbaric tetracaine, the duration of sensory blockade was the same but the time to complete motor recovery was significantly longer for tetracaine. Addition of 0.2 mg epinephrine significantly prolongs the motor blockade and time to first postoperative narcotic with MARCAINE Spinal.

Local anesthetics appear to cross the placenta by passive diffusion. The rate and degree of diffusion is governed by (1) the degree of plasma protein binding, (2) the degree of ionization, and (3) the degree of lipid solubility. Fetal/maternal ratios of local anesthetics appear to be inversely related to the degree of plasma protein binding, because only the free, unbound drug is available for placental transfer. MARCAINE with a high protein binding capacity (95%) has a low fetal/maternal ratio (0.2 to 0.4). The extent of placental transfer is also determined by the degree of ionization and lipid solubility of the drug. Lipid soluble, nonionized drugs readily enter the fetal blood from the maternal circulation.

Depending upon the route of administration, local anesthetics are distributed to some extent to all body tissues, with high concentrations found in highly perfused organs such as the liver, lungs, heart, and brain.

Pharmacokinetic studies on the plasma profiles of MARCAINE after direct intravenous injection suggest a three-compartment open model. The first compartment is represented by the rapid intravascular distribution of the drug. The second compartment represents the equilibration of the drug throughout the highly perfused organs such as the brain, myocardium, lungs, kidneys, and liver. The third compartment represents an equilibration of the drug with poorly perfused tissues, such as muscle and fat. The elimination of drug from tissue distribution depends largely upon the ability of binding sites in the circulation to carry it to the liver where it is metabolized.

Various pharmacokinetic parameters of the local anesthetics can be significantly altered by the presence of hepatic or renal disease, addition of epinephrine, factors affecting urinary pH, renal blood flow, the route of drug administration, and the age of the patient. The half-life of MARCAINE in adults is 2.7 hours and in neonates 8.1 hours.

Amide-type local anesthetics such as MARCAINE are metabolized primarily in the liver via conjugation with glucuronic acid. Patients with hepatic disease, especially those with severe hepatic disease, may be more susceptible to the potential toxicities of the amide-type local anesthetics. Pipecolylxylidine is the major metabolite of MARCAINE.

The kidney is the main excretory organ for most local anesthetics and their metabolites. Urinary excretion is affected by urinary perfusion and factors affecting urinary pH. Only 6% of bupivacaine is excreted unchanged in the urine.

When administered in recommended doses and concentrations, MARCAINE does not ordinarily produce irritation or tissue damage and does not cause methemoglobinemia.

INDICATIONS AND USAGE

MARCAINE Spinal, brand of bupivacaine in dextrose injection, is indicated for the production of subarachnoid block (spinal anesthesia).

Standard textbooks should be consulted to determine the accepted procedures and techniques for the administration of spinal anesthesia.

CONTRAINDICATIONS

MARCAINE Spinal is contraindicated in patients with a known hypersensitivity to it or to any local anesthetic agent of the amide-type.

The following conditions preclude the use of spinal anesthesia:

1. Severe hemorrhage, severe hypotension or shock and arrhythmias, such as complete heart block, which severely restrict cardiac output.
2. Local infection at the site of proposed lumbar puncture.
3. Septicemia.

WARNINGS

LOCAL ANESTHETICS SHOULD ONLY BE EMPLOYED BY CLINICIANS WHO ARE WELL VERSED IN DIAGNOSIS AND MANAGEMENT OF DOSE-RELATED TOXICITY AND OTHER ACUTE EMERGENCIES WHICH MIGHT ARISE FROM THE BLOCK TO BE EMPLOYED, AND THEN ONLY AFTER INSURING THE **IMMEDIATE** AVAILABILITY OF OXYGEN, OTHER RESUSCITATIVE DRUGS, CARDIOPULMONARY RESUSCITATIVE EQUIPMENT, AND THE PERSONNEL RESOURCES NEEDED FOR PROPER MANAGEMENT OF TOXIC REACTIONS AND RELATED EMERGENCIES. (See also ADVERSE REACTIONS and PRECAUTIONS.) DELAY IN PROPER MANAGEMENT OF DOSE-RELATED TOXICITY, UNDERVENTILATION FROM ANY CAUSE AND/OR ALTERED SENSITIVITY MAY LEAD TO THE DEVELOPMENT OF ACIDOSIS, CARDIAC ARREST, AND, POSSIBLY, DEATH.

Spinal anesthetics should not be injected during uterine contractions, because spinal fluid current may carry the drug further cephalad than desired.

A free flow of cerebrospinal fluid during the performance of spinal anesthesia is indicative of entry into the subarachnoid space. However, aspiration should be performed before the anesthetic solution is injected to confirm entry into the subarachnoid space and to avoid intravascular injection.

MARCAINE solutions containing epinephrine or other vasopressors should not be used concomitantly with ergot-type oxytocic drugs, because a severe persistent hypertension may occur. Likewise, solutions of MARCAINE containing a vasoconstrictor, such as epinephrine, should be used with extreme caution in patients receiving monoamine oxidase inhibitors (MAOI) or antidepressants of the triptyline or imipramine types, because severe prolonged hypertension may result.

Until further experience is gained in patients younger than 18 years, administration of MARCAINE in this age group is not recommended.

Mixing or the prior or intercurrent use of any other local anesthetic with MARCAINE cannot be recommended because of insufficient data on the clinical use of such mixtures.

PRECAUTIONS

General: The safety and effectiveness of spinal anesthetics depend on proper dosage, correct technique, adequate precautions, and readiness for emergencies. Resuscitative equipment, oxygen, and other resuscitative drugs should be available for immediate use. (See WARNINGS and ADVERSE REACTONS.) The patient should have IV fluids running via an indwelling catheter to assure a functioning intravenous pathway. The lowest dosage of local anesthetic that results in effective anesthesia should be used. Aspiration for blood should be performed before injection and injection should be made slowly. Tolerance varies with the status of the patient. Elderly patients and acutely ill patients may require reduced doses. Reduced doses may also be indicated in patients with increased intra-abdominal pressure (including obstetrical patients), if otherwise suitable for spinal anesthesia.

There should be careful and constant monitoring of cardiovascular and respiratory (adequacy of ventilation) vital signs and the patient's state of consciousness after local anesthetic injection. Restlessness, anxiety, incoherent speech, lightheadedness, numbness and tingling of the mouth and lips, metallic taste, tinnitus, dizziness, blurred vision, tremors, depression, or drowsiness may be early warning signs of central nervous system toxicity.

Spinal anesthetics should be used with caution in patients with severe disturbances of cardiac rhythm, shock, or heart block.

Sympathetic blockade occurring during spinal anesthesia may result in peripheral vasodilation and hypotension, the extent depending on the number of dermatomes blocked. Blood pressure should, therefore, be carefully monitored especially in the early phases of anesthesia. Hypotension may be controlled by vasoconstrictors in dosages depending on the severity of hypotension and response of treatment. The level of anesthesia should be carefully monitored because it is not always controllable in spinal techniques.

Because amide-type local anesthetics such as MARCAINE are metabolized by the liver, these drugs, especially repeat doses, should be used cautiously in patients with hepatic disease. Patients with severe hepatic disease, because of their inability to metabolize local anesthetics normally, are at a greater risk of developing toxic plasma concentrations.

Local anesthetics should also be used with caution in patients with impaired cardiovascular function because they may be less able to compensate for functional changes associated with the prolongation of AV conduction produced by these drugs. However, dosage recommendations for spinal anesthesia are much lower than dosage recommendations for other major blocks and most experience regarding hepatic and cardiovascular disease dose-related toxicity is derived from these other major blocks.

Serious dose-related cardiac arrhythmias may occur if preparations containing a vasoconstrictor such as epinephrine are employed in patients during or following the administration of potent inhalation agents. In deciding whether to use these products concurrently in the same patient, the combined action of both agents upon the myocardium, the concentration and volume of vasoconstrictor used, and the time since injection, when applicable, should be taken into account.

Many drugs used during the conduct of anesthesia are considered potential triggering agents for familial malignant hyperthermia. Because it is not known whether amide-type local anesthetics may trigger this reaction and because the need for supplemental general anesthesia cannot be predicted in advance, it is suggested that a standard protocol for management should be available. Early unexplained signs of tachycardia, tachypnea, labile blood pressure, and metabolic acidosis may precede temperature elevation. Successful outcome is dependent on early diagnosis, prompt discontinuance of the suspect triggering agent(s) and institution of treatment, including oxygen therapy, indicated supportive measures, and dantrolene. (Consult dantrolene sodium intravenous package insert before using.)

The following conditions may preclude the use of spinal anesthesia, depending upon the physician's evaluation of the situation and ability to deal with the complications or complaints which may occur:

- Preexisting diseases of the central nervous system, such as those attributable to pernicious anemia, poliomyelitis, syphilis, or tumor.
- Hematological disorders predisposing to coagulopathies or patients on anticoagulant therapy. Trauma to a blood vessel during the conduct of spinal anesthesia may, in some instances, result in uncontrollable central nervous system hemorrhage or soft tissue hemorrhage.
- Chronic backache and preoperative headache.
- Hypotension and hypertension.
- Technical problems (persistent paresthesias, persistent bloody tap).
- Arthritis or spinal deformity.
- Extremes of age.
- Psychosis or other causes of poor cooperation by the patient.

Information for Patients: When appropriate, patients should be informed in advance that they may experience temporary loss of sensation and motor activity, usually in the lower half of the body, following proper administration of spinal anesthesia. Also, when appropriate, the physician should discuss other information including adverse reactions in the MARCAINE Spinal package insert.

Clinically Significant Drug Interactions: The administration of local anesthetic solutions containing epinephrine or norepinephrine to patients receiving monoamine oxidase inhibitors or tricyclic antidepressants may produce severe, prolonged hypertension. Concurrent use of these agents should generally be avoided. In situations when concurrent therapy is necessary, careful patient monitoring is essential. Concurrent administration of vasopressor drugs and of ergot-type oxytocic drugs may cause severe persistent hypertension or cerebrovascular accidents.

Phenothiazines and butyrophenones may reduce or reverse the pressor effect of epinephrine.

Carcinogenesis, Mutagenesis, and Impairment of Fertility: Long-term studies in animals of most local anesthetics including bupivacaine to evaluate the carcinogenic potential have not been conducted. Mutagenic potential or the effect on fertility have not been determined. There is no evidence from human data that MARCAINE Spinal, brand of bupivacaine in dextrose injection, may be carcinogenic or mutagenic or that it impairs fertility.

Pregnancy Category C: Decreased pup survival in rats and an embryocidal effect in rabbits have been observed when bupivacaine hydrochloride was administered to these species in doses comparable to 230 and 130 times respectively the

maximum recommended human spinal dose. There are no adequate and well-controlled studies in pregnant women of the effect of bupivacaine on the developing fetus. Bupivacaine hydrochloride should be used during pregnancy only if the potential benefit justifies the potential risk to the fetus. This does not exclude the use of MARCAINE Spinal at term for obstetrical anesthesia. (See ***Labor and Delivery.***)

Labor and Delivery: Spinal anesthesia has a recognized use during labor and delivery. Bupivacaine hydrochloride, when administered properly, via the epidural route in doses 10 to 12 times the amount used in spinal anesthesia has been used for obstetrical analgesia and anesthesia without evidence of adverse effects on the fetus.

Maternal hypotension has resulted from regional anesthesia. Local anesthetics produce vasodilation by blocking sympathetic nerves. Elevating the patient's legs and positioning her on her left side will help prevent decreases in blood pressure. The fetal heart rate also should be monitored continuously and electronic fetal monitoring is highly advisable.

It is extremely important to avoid aortocaval compression by the gravid uterus during administrations of regional block to parturients. To do this, the patient must be maintained in the left lateral decubitus position or a blanket roll or sandbag may be placed beneath the right hip and the gravid uterus displaced to the left.

Spinal anesthesia may alter the forces of parturition through changes in uterine contractility or maternal expulsive efforts. Spinal anesthesia has also been reported to prolong the second stage of labor by removing the parturient's reflex urge to bear down or by interfering with motor function. The use of obstetrical anesthesia may increase the need for forceps assistance.

The use of some local anesthetic drug products during labor and delivery may be followed by diminished muscle strength and tone for the first day or two of life. This has not been reported with bupivacaine.

There have been reports of cardiac arrest during use of MARCAINE 0.75% solution for epidural anesthesia in obstetrical patients. The package insert for MARCAINE hydrochloride for epidural, nerve block, etc, has a more complete discussion of preparation for, and management of, this problem. These cases are compatible with systemic toxicity following unintended intravascular injection of the much larger doses recommended for epidural anesthesia and have not occurred within the dose range of bupivacaine hydrochloride 0.75% recommended for spinal anesthesia in obstetrics. The 0.75% concentration of MARCAINE is therefore not recommended for obstetrical epidural anesthesia. MARCAINE Spinal, brand of bupivacaine in dextrose injection, is recommended for spinal anesthesia in obstetrics.

Nursing Mothers: It is not known whether local anesthetic drugs are excreted in human milk. Because many drugs are excreted in human milk, caution should be exercised when local anesthetics are administered to a nursing woman.

Pediatric Use: Until further experience is gained in patients younger than 18 years, administration of MARCAINE Spinal in this age group is not recommended.

ADVERSE REACTIONS

Reactions to bupivacaine are characteristic of those associated with other amide-type local anesthetics.

The most commonly encountered acute adverse experiences which demand immediate countermeasures following the administration of spinal anesthesia are hypotension due to loss of sympathetic tone and respiratory paralysis or underventilation due to cephalad extension of the motor level of anesthesia. These may lead to cardiac arrest if untreated. In addition, dose-related convulsions and cardiovascular collapse may result from diminished tolerance, rapid absorption from the injection site, or from unintentional intravascular injection of a local anesthetic solution. Factors influencing plasma protein binding, such as acidosis, systemic diseases which alter protein production, or competition of other drugs for protein binding sites, may diminish individual tolerance.

Respiratory System: Respiratory paralysis or underventilation may be noted as a result of upward extension of the level of spinal anesthesia and may lead to secondary hypoxic cardiac arrest if untreated. Preanesthetic medication, intraoperative analgesics and sedatives, as well as surgical manipulation, may contribute to underventilation. This will usually be noted within minutes of the injection of spinal anesthetic solution, but because of differing maximal onset times, differing intercurrent drug usage and differing surgical manipulation, it may occur at any time during surgery or the immediate recovery period.

Cardiovascular System: Hypotension due to loss of sympathetic tone is a commonly encountered extension of the clinical pharmacology of spinal anesthesia. This is more commonly observed in patients with shrunken blood volume, shrunken interstitial fluid volume, cephalad spread of the local anesthetic, and/or mechanical obstruction of venous return. Nausea and vomiting are frequently associated with hypotensive episodes following the administration of spinal anesthesia. High doses, or inadvertent intravascular injection, may lead to high plasma levels and related depression of the myocardium, decreased cardiac output, bradycardia, heart block, ventricular arrhythmias, and, possibly, cardiac arrest. (See **WARNINGS, PRECAUTIONS,** and **OVERDOSAGE** sections.)

Central Nervous System: Respiratory paralysis or underventilation secondary to cephalad spread of the level of spinal anesthesia (see *Respiratory System*) and hypotension for the same reason (see *Cardiovascular System*) are the two most commonly encountered central nervous system-related adverse observations which demand immediate countermeasures.

High doses or inadvertent intravascular injection may lead to high plasma levels and related central nervous system toxicity characterized by excitement and/or depression. Restlessness, anxiety, dizziness, tinnitus, blurred vision, or tremors may occur, possibly proceeding to convulsions. However, excitement may be transient or absent, with depression being the first manifestation of an adverse reaction. This may quickly be followed by drowsiness merging into unconsciousness and respiratory arrest.

Neurologic: The incidences of adverse neurologic reactions associated with the use of local anesthetics may be related to the total dose of local anesthetic administered and are also dependent upon the particular drug used, the route of administration, and the physical status of the patient. Many of these effects may be related to local anesthetic techniques, with or without a contribution from the drug.

Neurologic effects following spinal anesthesia may include loss of perineal sensation and sexual function; persistent anesthesia, paresthesia, weakness and paralysis of the lower extremities, and loss of sphincter control all of which may have slow, incomplete, or no recovery; hypotension; high or total spinal block; urinary retention; headache; backache; septic meningitis; meningismus; arachnoiditis; slowing of labor; increased incidence of forceps delivery; shivering; cranial nerve palsies due to traction on nerves from loss of cerebrospinal fluid; and fecal and urinary incontinence.

Allergic: Allergic-type reactions are rare and may occur as a result of sensitivity to the local anesthetic. These reactions are characterized by signs such as urticaria, pruritus, erythema, angioneurotic edema (including laryngeal edema), tachycardia, sneezing, nausea, vomiting, dizziness, syncope, excessive sweating, elevated temperature, and, possibly, anaphylactoid-like symptomatology (including severe hypotension). Cross sensitivity among members of the amide-type local anesthetic group has been reported. The usefulness of screening for sensitivity has not been definitely established.

Other: Nausea and vomiting may occur during spinal anesthesia.

OVERDOSAGE

Acute emergencies from local anesthetics are generally related to high plasma levels encountered during therapeutic use or to underventilation (and perhaps apnea) secondary to upward extension of spinal anesthesia. Hypotension is commonly encountered during the conduct of spinal anesthesia due to relaxation of sympathetic tone, and sometimes, contributory mechanical obstruction of venous return.

Management of Local Anesthetic Emergencies: The first consideration is prevention, best accomplished by careful and constant monitoring of cardiovascular and respiratory vital signs and the patient's state of consciousness after each local anesthetic injection. At the first sign of change, oxygen should be administered.

The first step in the management of systemic toxic reactions, as well as underventilation or apnea due to a high or total spinal, consists of ***immediate*** *attention to the establishment and maintenance of a patent airway and effective assisted or controlled ventilation with 100% oxygen with a delivery system capable of permitting immediate positive airway pressure by mask.* This may prevent convulsions if they have not already occurred.

If necessary, use drugs to control the convulsions. A 50 mg to 100 mg bolus IV injection of succinylcholine will paralyze the patient without depressing the central nervous or cardiovascular systems and facilitate ventilation. A bolus IV dose of 5 mg to 10 mg of diazepam or 50 mg to 100 mg of thiopental will permit ventilation and counteract central nervous system stimulation, but these drugs also depress central nervous system, respiratory and cardiac function, add to postictal depression and may result in apnea. Intravenous barbiturates, anticonvulsant agents, or muscle relaxants should only be administered by those familiar with their use. Immediately after the institution of these ventilatory measures, the adequacy of the circulation should be evaluated. Supportive treatment of circulatory depression may require administration of intravenous fluids, and, when appropriate, a vasopressor dictated by the clinical situation (such as ephedrine or epinephrine to enhance myocardial contractile force).

Hypotension due to sympathetic relaxation may be managed by giving intravenous fluids (such as isotonic saline or lactated Ringer's solution), in an attempt to relieve mechanical obstruction of venous return, or by using vasopressors (such as ephedrine which increases the force of myocardial contractions) and, if indicated, by giving plasma expanders or whole blood.

Endotracheal intubation, employing drugs and techniques familiar to the clinician, may be indicated after initial administration of oxygen by mask if difficulty is encountered in the maintenance of a patent airway, or if prolonged ventilatory support (assisted or controlled) is indicated.

Recent clinical data from patients experiencing local anesthetic-induced convulsions demonstrated rapid development of hypoxia, hypercarbia, and acidosis with bupivacaine within a minute of the onset of convulsions. These observations suggest that oxygen consumption and carbon dioxide production are greatly increased during local anesthetic convulsions and emphasize the importance of immediate and effective ventilation with oxygen which may avoid cardiac arrest.

If not treated immediately, convulsions with simultaneous hypoxia, hypercarbia, and acidosis plus myocardial depression from the direct effects of the local anesthetic may result in cardiac arrhythmias, bradycardia, asystole, ventricular fibrillation, or cardiac arrest. Respiratory abnormalities, including apnea, may occur. Underventilation or apnea due to a high or total spinal may produce these same signs and also lead to cardiac arrest if ventilatory support is not instituted. If cardiac arrest should occur, standard cardiopulmonary resuscitative measures should be instituted and maintained for a prolonged period if necessary. Recovery has been reported after prolonged resuscitative efforts.

The supine position is dangerous in pregnant women at term because of aortocaval compression by the gravid uterus. Therefore during treatment of systemic toxicity, maternal hypotension, or fetal bradycardia following regional block, the parturient should be maintained in the left lateral decubitus position if possible, or manual displacement of the uterus off the great vessels be accomplished.

The mean seizure dosage of bupivacaine in rhesus monkeys was found to be 4.4 mg/kg with mean arterial plasma concentration of 4.5 μg/mL. The intravenous and subcutaneous LD_{50} in mice is 6 mg/kg to 8 mg/kg and 38 mg/kg to 54 mg/kg respectively.

DOSAGE AND ADMINISTRATION

The dose of any local anesthetic administered varies with the anesthetic procedure, the area to be anesthetized, the vascularity of the tissues, the number of neuronal segments to be blocked, the depth of anesthesia and degree of muscle relaxation required, the duration of anesthesia desired, individual tolerance, and the physical condition of the patient. The smallest dose and concentration required to produce the desired result should be administered. Dosages of MARCAINE Spinal, brand of bupivacaine in dextrose injection, should be reduced for elderly and debilitated patients and patients with cardiac and/or liver disease.

For specific techniques and procedures, refer to standard textbooks.

The extent and degree of spinal anesthesia depend upon several factors including dosage, specific gravity of the anesthetic solution, volume of solution used, force of injection, level of puncture, and position of the patient during and immediately after injection.

Seven and one-half mg (7.5 mg or 1.0 mL) MARCAINE Spinal has generally proven satisfactory for spinal anesthesia for lower extremity and perineal procedures including TURP and vaginal hysterectomy. Twelve mg (12.0 mg or 1.6 mL) has been used for lower abdominal procedures such as abdominal hysterectomy, tubal ligation, and appendectomy. These doses are recommended as a guide for use in the average adult and may be reduced for the elderly or debilitated patients. Because experience with MARCAINE Spinal is limited in patients below the age of 18 years, dosage recommendations in this age group cannot be made.

Obstetrical Use: Doses as low as 6 mg bupivacaine hydrochloride have been used for vaginal delivery under spinal anesthesia. The dose range of 7.5 mg to 10.5 mg (1 mL to 1.4 mL) bupivacaine hydrochloride has been used for Cesarean section under spinal anesthesia.

In recommended doses, MARCAINE Spinal produces complete motor and sensory block.

Unused portions of solutions should be discarded following initial use.

MARCAINE Spinal should be inspected visually for discoloration and particulate matter prior to administration; solutions which are discolored or which contain particulate matter should not be administered.

Continued on next page

This product information was prepared in August 1992. On these and other products of Sanofi Winthrop Pharmaceuticals, detailed information may be obtained on a current basis by direct inquiry to Product Information Services, 90 Park Avenue, New York, NY 10016 (toll free 1-800-446-6267).

Sanofi Winthrop—Cont.

HOW SUPPLIED

Single-dose ampuls of 2 mL (15 mg bupivacaine hydrochloride with 165 mg dextrose), in Uni-Nest™ Unit Dose Pak of 10 (NDC 0024-1229-10)

Store at controlled room temperature, between 15° C and 30° C (59° F and 86° F).

MARCAINE Spinal solution may be autoclaved once at 15 pound pressure, 121° C (250° F) for 15 minutes. Do not administer any solution which is discolored or contains particulate matter.

MW-246-B

MEBARAL® Ⓒ℞

brand of mephobarbital tablets, USP

DESCRIPTION

Mephobarbital, 5-Ethyl-1-methyl-5-phenylbarbituric acid, is a barbiturate with sedative, hypnotic, and anticonvulsant properties. It occurs as a white, nearly odorless, tasteless powder and is slightly soluble in water and in alcohol. MEBARAL is available as tablets for oral administration.
Inactive Ingredients: Lactose, Starch, Stearic Acid, Talc.

CLINICAL PHARMACOLOGY

Barbiturates are capable of producing all levels of CNS mood alteration from excitation to mild sedation, to hypnosis, and deep coma. Overdosage can produce death. In high enough therapeutic doses, barbiturates induce anesthesia.

Barbiturates depress the sensory cortex, decrease motor activity, alter cerebellar function, and produce drowsiness, sedation, and hypnosis.

Barbiturates are respiratory depressants. The degree of respiratory depression is dependent upon dose. With hypnotic doses, respiratory depression produced by barbiturates is similar to that which occurs during physiologic sleep with slight decrease in blood pressure and heart rate.

Studies in laboratory animals have shown that barbiturates cause reduction in the tone and contractility of the uterus, ureters, and urinary bladder. However, concentrations of the drugs required to produce this effect in humans are not reached with sedative-hypnotic doses.

Barbiturates do not impair normal hepatic function, but have been shown to induce liver microsomal enzymes, thus increasing and/or altering the metabolism of barbiturates and other drugs. (See PRECAUTIONS—Drug Interactions.)

MEBARAL exerts a strong sedative and anticonvulsant action but has a relatively mild hypnotic effect. It reduces the incidence of epileptic seizures in grand mal and petit mal. MEBARAL usually causes little or no drowsiness or lassitude. Hence, when it is used as a sedative or anticonvulsant, patients usually become more calm, more cheerful, and better adjusted to their surroundings without clouding of mental faculties. MEBARAL is reported to produce less sedation than does phenobarbital.

Barbiturates are weak acids that are absorbed and rapidly distributed to all tissues and fluids with high concentrations in the brain, liver, and kidneys. Lipid solubility of the barbiturates is the dominant factor in their distribution within the body. Barbiturates are bound to plasma and tissue proteins to a varying degree with the degree of binding increasing directly as a function of lipid solubility.

Approximately 50% of an oral dose of mephobarbital is absorbed from the gastrointestinal tract. Therapeutic plasma concentrations for mephobarbital have not been established nor has the half-life been determined. Following oral administration, the onset of action of the drug is 30 to 60 minutes and the duration of action is 10 to 16 hours. The primary route of mephobarbital metabolism is N-demethylation by the microsomal enzymes of the liver to form phenobarbital. Phenobarbital may be excreted in the urine unchanged or further metabolized to *p*-hydroxyphenobarbital and excreted in the urine as glucuronide or sulfate conjugates. About 75% of a single oral dose of mephobarbital is converted to phenobarbital in 24 hours.

Therefore, chronic administration of mephobarbital may lead to an accumulation of phenobarbital (not mephobarbital) in plasma. It has not been determined whether mephobarbital or phenobarbital is the active agent during long-time mephobarbital therapy.

INDICATIONS AND USAGE

MEBARAL is indicated for use as a sedative for the relief of anxiety, tension, and apprehension, and as an anticonvulsant for the treatment of grand mal and petit mal epilepsy.

CONTRAINDICATIONS

Hypersensitivity to any barbiturate. Manifest or latent porphyria.

WARNINGS

Habit Forming

Barbiturates may be habit forming. Tolerance, psychological, and physical dependence may occur with continued use. (See DRUG ABUSE AND DEPENDENCE and CLINICAL PHARMACOLOGY.) Patients who have psychological dependence on barbiturates may increase the dosage or decrease the dosage interval without consulting a physician and may subsequently develop a physical dependence on barbiturates. To minimize the possibility of overdosage or the development of dependence, the prescribing and dispensing of sedative-hypnotic barbiturates should be limited to the amount required for the interval until the next appointment. Abrupt cessation after prolonged use in the dependent person may result in withdrawal symptoms, including delirium, convulsions, and possibly death. Barbiturates should be withdrawn gradually from any patient known to be taking excessive dosage over long periods of time. (See DRUG ABUSE AND DEPENDENCE.)

Acute or Chronic Pain

Caution should be exercised when barbiturates are administered to patients with acute or chronic pain, because paradoxical excitement could be induced or important symptoms could be masked. However, the use of barbiturates as sedatives in the postoperative surgical period and as adjuncts to cancer chemotherapy is well established.

Use in Pregnancy

Barbiturates can cause fetal damage when administered to a pregnant woman. Retrospective, case-controlled studies have suggested a connection between the maternal consumption of barbiturates and a higher than expected incidence of fetal abnormalities. Following oral or parenteral administration, barbiturates readily cross the placental barrier and are distributed throughout fetal tissues with highest concentrations found in the placenta, fetal liver, and brain. Fetal blood levels approach maternal blood levels following parenteral administration.

Withdrawal symptoms occur in infants born to mothers who receive barbiturates throughout the last trimester of pregnancy. (See DRUG ABUSE AND DEPENDENCE.) If this drug is used during pregnancy, or if the patient becomes pregnant while taking this drug, the patient should be apprised of the potential hazard to the fetus.

Synergistic Effects

The concomitant use of alcohol or other CNS depressants may produce additive CNS depressant effects.

PRECAUTIONS

General

Barbiturates may be habit forming. Tolerance and psychological and physical dependence may occur with continuing use. (See DRUG ABUSE AND DEPENDENCE.) Barbiturates should be administered with caution, if at all, to patients who are mentally depressed, have suicidal tendencies, or a history of drug abuse.

Elderly or debilitated patients may react to barbiturates with marked excitement, depression, and confusion. In some persons, barbiturates repeatedly produce excitement rather than depression.

In patients with hepatic damage, barbiturates should be administered with caution and initially in reduced doses. Barbiturates should not be administered to patients showing the premonitory signs of hepatic coma.

Status epilepticus may result from the abrupt discontinuation of MEBARAL, even when administered in small daily doses in the treatment of epilepsy.

Caution and careful adjustment of dosage are required when MEBARAL, brand of mephobarbital tablets, is used in patients with impaired renal, cardiac, or respiratory function and in patients with myasthenia gravis and myxedema. The least quantity feasible should be prescribed or dispensed at any one time in order to minimize the possibility of acute or chronic overdosage.

Vitamin D Deficiency: MEBARAL may increase vitamin D requirements, possibly by increasing vitamin D metabolism via enzyme induction. Rarely, rickets and osteomalacia have been reported following prolonged use of barbiturates.

Vitamin K: Bleeding in the early neonatal period due to coagulation defects may follow exposure to anticonvulsant drugs *in utero;* therefore, vitamin K should be given to the mother before delivery or to the child at birth.

Information for the Patient

Practitioners should give the following information and instructions to patients receiving barbiturates.

1. The use of barbiturates carries with it an associated risk of psychological and/or physical dependence. The patient should be warned against increasing the dose of the drug without consulting a physician.
2. Barbiturates may impair mental and/or physical abilities required for the performance of potentially hazardous tasks (eg, driving, operating machinery, etc).
3. Alcohol should not be consumed while taking barbiturates. Concurrent use of the barbiturates with other CNS depressants (eg, alcohol, narcotics, tranquilizers, and antihistamines) may result in additional CNS depressant effects.

Laboratory Tests

Prolonged therapy with barbiturates should be accompanied by periodic laboratory evaluation of organ systems, including hematopoietic, renal, and hepatic systems. (See PRECAUTIONS [General] and ADVERSE REACTIONS.)

Drug Interactions

Most reports of clinically significant drug interactions occurring with the barbiturates have involved phenobarbital. However, the application of these data to other barbiturates appears valid and warrants serial blood level determinations of the relevant drugs when there are multiple therapies.

1. *Anticoagulants.* Phenobarbital lowers the plasma levels of dicumarol (name previously used: bishydroxycoumarin) and causes a decrease in anticoagulant activity as measured by the prothrombin time. Barbiturates can induce hepatic microsomal enzymes resulting in increased metabolism and decreased anticoagulant response of oral anticoagulants (eg, warfarin, acenocoumarol, dicumarol, and phenprocoumon). Patients stabilized on anticoagulant therapy may require dosage adjustments if barbiturates are added to or withdrawn from their dosage regimen.
2. *Corticosteroids.* Barbiturates appear to enhance the metabolism of exogenous corticosteroids probably through the induction of hepatic microsomal enzymes. Patients stabilized on corticosteroid therapy may require dosage adjustments if barbiturates are added to or withdrawn from their dosage regimen.
3. *Griseofulvin.* Phenobarbital appears to interfere with the absorption of orally administered griseofulvin, thus decreasing its blood level. The effect of the resultant decreased blood levels of griseofulvin on therapeutic response has not been established. However, it would be preferable to avoid concomitant administration of these drugs.
4. *Doxycycline.* Phenobarbital has been shown to shorten the half-life of doxycycline for as long as 2 weeks after barbiturate therapy is discontinued.

This mechanism is probably through the induction of hepatic microsomal enzymes that metabolize the antibiotic. If phenobarbital and doxycycline are administered concurrently, the clinical response to doxycycline should be monitored closely.

5. *Phenytoin, Sodium Valproate, Valproic Acid.* The effect of barbiturates on the metabolism of phenytoin appears to be variable. Some investigators report an accelerating effect, while others report no effect. Because the effect of barbiturates on the metabolism of phenytoin is not predictable, phenytoin and barbiturate blood levels should be monitored more frequently if these drugs are given concurrently. Sodium valproate and valproic acid appear to decrease barbiturate metabolism; therefore, barbiturate blood levels should be monitored and appropriate dosage adjustments made as indicated.
6. *Central Nervous System Depressants.* The concomitant use of other central nervous system depressants, including other sedatives or hypnotics, antihistamines, tranquilizers, or alcohol, may produce additive depressant effects.
7. *Monoamine Oxidase Inhibitors (MAOI).* MAOI prolong the effects of barbiturates probably because metabolism of the barbiturate is inhibited.
8. *Estradiol, Estone, Progesterone, and other Steroidal Hormones.* Pretreatment with or concurrent administration of phenobarbital may decrease the effect of estradiol by increasing its metabolism. There have been reports of patients treated with antiepileptic drugs (eg, phenobarbital) who become pregnant while taking oral contraceptives. An alternant contraceptive method might be suggested to women taking phenobarbital.

Carcinogenesis

Animal Data. Phenobarbital sodium is carcinogenic in mice and rats after lifetime administration. In mice, it produced benign and malignant liver cell tumors. In rats, benign liver cell tumors were observed very late in life. Phenobarbital is the major metabolite of MEBARAL.

Human Data. In a 29-year epidemiological study of 9,136 patients who were treated on an anticonvulsant protocol which included phenobarbital, results indicated a higher than normal incidence of hepatic carcinoma. Previously, some of these patients were treated with thorotrast, a drug which is known to produce hepatic carcinomas. Thus, this study did not provide sufficient evidence that phenobarbital sodium is carcinogenic in humans. Phenobarbital is the major metabolite of MEBARAL, brand of mephobarbital tablets.

A retrospective study of 84 children with brain tumors matched to 73 normal controls and 78 cancer controls (malignant disease other than brain tumors) suggested an association between exposure to barbiturates prenatally and an increased incidence of brain tumors.

Pregnancy

Teratogenic Effects. Pregnancy Category D—See WARNINGS—Use in Pregnancy.

Nonteratogenic Effects. Reports of infants suffering from long-term barbiturate exposure *in utero* included the acute withdrawal syndrome of seizures and hyperirritability from

birth to a delayed onset of up to 14 days. (See DRUG ABUSE AND DEPENDENCE.)

Labor and Delivery.

Hypnotic doses of these barbiturates do not appear to significantly impair uterine activity during labor. Full anesthetic doses of barbiturates decrease the force and frequency of uterine contractions. Administration of sedative-hypnotic barbiturates to the mother during labor may result in respiratory depression in the newborn. Premature infants are particularly susceptible to the depressant effects of barbiturates. If barbiturates are used during labor and delivery, resuscitation equipment should be available.

Data are currently not available to evaluate the effect of these barbiturates when forceps delivery or other intervention is necessary. Also, data are not available to determine the effect of these barbiturates on the later growth, development, and functional maturation of the child.

Nursing Mothers.

Caution should be exercised when a barbiturate is administered to a nursing woman since small amounts of barbiturates are excreted in the milk.

ADVERSE REACTIONS

The following adverse reactions and their incidence were compiled from surveillance of thousands of hospitalized patients. Because such patients may be less aware of certain of the milder adverse effects of barbiturates, the incidence of these reactions may be somewhat higher in fully ambulatory patients.

More than 1 in 100 Patients. The most common adverse reaction estimated to occur at a rate of 1 to 3 patients per 100 is:

Nervous System: Somnolence.

Less than 1 in 100 Patients. Adverse reactions estimated to occur at a rate of less than 1 in 100 patients listed below, grouped by organ system, and by decreasing order of occurrence are:

Nervous System: Agitation, confusion, hyperkinesia, ataxia, CNS depression, nightmares, nervousness, psychiatric disturbance, hallucinations, insomnia, anxiety, dizziness, thinking abnormality.

Respiratory System: Hypoventilation, apnea.

Cardiovascular System: Bradycardia, hypotension, syncope.

Digestive System: Nausea, vomiting, constipation.

Other Reported Reactions: Headache, hypersensitivity reactions (angioedema, skin rashes, exfoliative dermatitis), fever, liver damage, megaloblastic anemia following chronic phenobarbital use.

DRUG ABUSE AND DEPENDENCE

Mephobarbital is a controlled substance in Narcotic Schedule IV. Barbiturates may be habit forming. Tolerance, psychological dependence, and physical dependence may occur especially following prolonged use of high doses of barbiturates. As tolerance to barbiturates develops, the amount needed to maintain the same level of intoxication increases; tolerance to a fatal dosage, however, does not increase more than two-fold. As this occurs, the margin between an intoxicating dosage and fatal dosage becomes smaller.

Symptoms of acute intoxication with barbiturates include unsteady gait, slurred speech, and sustained nystagmus. Mental signs of chronic intoxication include confusion, poor judgment, irritability, insomnia, and somatic complaints. Symptoms of barbiturate dependence are similar to those of chronic alcoholism. If an individual appears to be intoxicated with alcohol to a degree that is radically disproportionate to the amount of alcohol in his or her blood the use of barbiturates should be suspected. The lethal dose of a barbiturate is far less if alcohol is also ingested.

The symptoms of barbiturate withdrawal can be severe and may cause death. Minor withdrawal symptoms may appear 8 to 12 hours after the last dose of a barbiturate. These symptoms usually appear in the following order: anxiety, muscle twitching, tremor of hands and fingers, progressive weakness, dizziness, distortion in visual perception, nausea, vomiting, insomnia, and orthostatic hypotension. Major withdrawal symptoms (convulsions and delirium) may occur within 16 hours and last up to 5 days after abrupt cessation of these drugs. Intensity of withdrawal symptoms gradually declines over a period of approximately 15 days. Individuals susceptible to a barbiturate abuse and dependence include alcoholics and opiate abusers, as well as other sedative-hypnotic and amphetamine abusers.

Drug dependence to barbiturates arises from repeated administration of a barbiturate or agent with barbiturate-like effect on a continuous basis, generally in amounts exceeding therapeutic dose levels. The characteristics of drug dependence to barbiturates include: (a) a strong desire or need to continue taking the drug; (b) a tendency to increase the dose; (c) a psychic dependence on the effects of the drug related to subjective and individual appreciation of those effects; and (d) a physical dependence on the effects of the drug requiring its presence for maintenance of homeostasis and resulting in a definite, characteristic, and self-limited abstinence syndrome when the drug is withdrawn.

Treatment of barbiturate dependence consists of cautious and gradual withdrawal of the drug. Barbiturate-dependent patients can be withdrawn by using a number of different withdrawal regimens. In all cases withdrawal takes an extended period of time. One method involves substituting a 30 mg dose of phenobarbital for each 100 mg to 200 mg dose of barbiturate that the patient has been taking. The total daily amount of phenobarbital is then administered in 3 to 4 divided doses, not to exceed 600 mg daily. Should signs of withdrawal occur on the first day of treatment, a loading dose of 100 mg to 200 mg of phenobarbital may be administered IM in addition to the oral dose. After stabilization on phenobarbital, the total daily dose is decreased by 30 mg a day as long as withdrawal is proceeding smoothly. A modification of this regimen involves initiating treatment at the patient's regular dosage level and decreasing the daily dosage by 10% if tolerated by the patient.

Infants physically dependent on barbiturates may be given phenobarbital 3 mg/kg/day to 10 mg/kg/day. After withdrawal symptoms (hyperactivity, disturbed sleep, tremors, hyperreflexia) are relieved, the dosage of phenobarbital should be gradually decreased and completely withdrawn over a 2-week period.

OVERDOSAGE

The toxic dose of barbiturates varies considerably. In general, an oral dose of 1 g of most barbiturates produces serious poisoning in an adult. Death commonly occurs after 2 g to 10 g of ingested barbiturate. Barbiturate intoxication may be confused with alcoholism, bromide intoxication, and with various neurological disorders.

Acute overdosage with barbiturates is manifested by CNS and respiratory depression which may progress to Cheyne-Stokes respiration, areflexia, constriction of the pupils to a slight degree (though in severe poisoning they may show paralytic dilation), oliguria, tachycardia, hypotension, lowered body temperature, and coma. Typical shock syndrome (apnea, circulatory collapse, respiratory arrest, and death) may occur.

In extreme overdose, all electrical activity in the brain may cease, in which case a "flat" EEG normally equated with clinical death cannot be accepted. This effect is fully reversible unless hypoxic damage occurs. Consideration should be given to the possibility of barbiturate intoxication even in situations that appear to involve trauma.

Complications such as pneumonia, pulmonary edema, cardiac arrhythmias, congestive heart failure, and renal failure may occur. Uremia may increase CNS sensitivity to barbiturates if renal function is impaired. Differential diagnosis should include hypoglycemia, head trauma, cerebrovascular accidents, convulsive states, and diabetic coma.

Treatment of overdosage is mainly supportive and consists of the following:

1. Maintenance of an adequate airway, with assisted respiration and oxygen administration as necessary.
2. Monitoring of vital signs and fluid balance.
3. If the patient is conscious and has not lost the gag reflex, emesis may be induced with ipecac. Care should be taken to prevent pulmonary aspiration of vomitus. After completion of vomiting, 30 g activated charcoal in a glass of water may be administered.
4. If emesis is contraindicated, gastric lavage may be performed with a cuffed endotracheal tube in place with the patient in the face down position. Activated charcoal may be left in the emptied stomach and a saline cathartic administered.
5. Fluid therapy and other standard treatment for shock, if needed.
6. If renal function is normal, forced diuresis may aid in the elimination of the barbiturate. Alkalinization of the urine increases renal excretion of some barbiturates, including mephobarbital (which is metabolized to phenobarbital).
7. Although not recommended as a routine procedure, hemodialysis may be used in severe barbiturate intoxications or if the patient is anuric or in shock.
8. Patient should be rolled from side to side every 30 minutes.
9. Antibiotics should be given if pneumonia is suspected.
10. Appropriate nursing care to prevent hypostatic pneumonia, decubiti aspiration, and other complications of patients with altered states of consciousness.

DOSAGE AND ADMINISTRATION

Epilepsy: Average dose for adults: 400 mg to 600 mg (6 grains to 9 grains) daily; children under 5 years: 16 mg to 32 mg (¼ grain to ½ grain) three or four times daily; children over 5 years: 32 mg to 64 mg (½ grain to 1 grain) three or four times daily. MEBARAL is best taken at bedtime if seizures generally occur at night, and during the day if attacks are diurnal. Treatment should be started with a small dose which is gradually increased over four or five days until the optimum dosage is determined. If the patient has been taking some other antiepileptic drug, it should be tapered off as the doses of MEBARAL are increased, to guard against the temporary marked attacks that may occur when any treatment for epilepsy is changed abruptly. Similarly, when the dose is to be

lowered to a maintenance level or to be discontinued, the amount should be reduced gradually over four or five days.

Special Patient Population. Dosage should be reduced in the elderly or debilitated because these patients may be more sensitive to barbiturates. Dosage should be reduced for patients with impaired renal function or hepatic disease.

Combination with Other Drugs: MEBARAL may be used in combination with phenobarbital, either in the form of alternating courses or concurrently. When the two drugs are used at the same time, the dose should be about one-half the amount of each used alone. The average daily dose for an adult is from 50 mg to 100 mg (¾ grain to 1½ grains) of phenobarbital and from 200 mg to 300 mg (3 grains to 4½ grains) of MEBARAL, brand of mephobarbital tablets. MEBARAL may also be used with phenytoin sodium; in some cases, combined therapy appears to give better results than either agent used alone, since phenytoin sodium is particularly effective for the psychomotor types of seizure but relatively ineffective for petit mal. When the drugs are employed concurrently, a reduced dose of phenytoin sodium is advisable, but the full dose of MEBARAL may be given. Satisfactory results have been obtained with an average daily dose of 230 mg (3½ grains) of phenytoin sodium plus about 600 mg (9 grains) of MEBARAL.

Sedation: Adults: 32 mg to 100 mg (½ grain to 1½ grains)—optimum dose, 50 mg (¾ grain)—three to four times daily. Children: 16 mg to 32 mg (¼ grain to ½ grain) three to four times daily.

HOW SUPPLIED

Tablets

32 mg (½ grain), bottles of 250 (NDC 0024-1231-05)

50 mg (¾ grain), bottles of 250 (NDC 0024-1232-05)

100 mg (1½ grains), bottles of 250 (NDC 0024-1233-05)

NegGram® Caplets®   ℞
brand of nalidixic acid tablets, USP
NegGram® Suspension   ℞
brand of nalidixic acid oral suspension, USP

DESCRIPTION

Nalidixic acid, an oral antibacterial agent, is 1-Ethyl-1, 4-dihydro-7-methyl-4-oxo-1, 8-naphthyridine-3-carboxylic acid. It is a pale yellow, crystalline substance and a very weak organic acid.

Inactive Ingredients.—SUSPENSION: Carbomer 934P, FD&C Red #40, Flavor, Parabens, Purified Water, Saccharin Sodium, Sodium Chloride, Sorbitol Solution. CAPLETS: Hydrogenated Vegetable Oil, Methylcellulose, Microcrystalline Cellulose, Sodium Lauryl Sulfate, Yellow Ferric Oxide.

CLINICAL PHARMACOLOGY

NegGram has marked antibacterial activity against gram-negative bacteria including *Proteus mirabilis, P. morganii, P. vulgaris,* and *P. rettgeri; Escherichia coli;* Enterobacter (Aerobacter), and Klebsiella. Pseudomonas strains are generally resistant to the drug. NegGram is bactericidal and is effective over the entire urinary pH range. Conventional chromosomal resistance to NegGram taken in full dosage has been reported to emerge in approximately 2 to 14 percent of patients during treatment; however, bacterial resistance to NegGram has not been shown to be transferable via R factor.

INDICATIONS AND USAGE

NegGram is indicated for the treatment of urinary tract infections caused by susceptible gram-negative microorganisms, including the majority of Proteus strains, Klebsiella, Enterobacter (Aerobacter), and *E. coli.* Disc susceptibility testing with the 30 µg disc should be performed prior to administration of the drug, and during treatment if clinical response warrants.

CONTRAINDICATIONS

NegGram is contraindicated in patients with known hypersensitivity to nalidixic acid and in patients with a history of convulsive disorders.

WARNINGS

CNS effects including brief convulsions, increased intracranial pressure, and toxic psychosis have been reported rarely. These have occurred in infants and children or in geriatric patients, usually from overdosage or in patients with predisposing factors, and have been completely and rapidly revers-

Continued on next page

This product information was prepared in August 1992. On these and other products of Sanofi Winthrop Pharmaceuticals, detailed information may be obtained on a current basis by direct inquiry to Product Information Services, 90 Park Avenue, New York, NY 10016 (toll free 1-800-446-6267).

Sanofi Winthrop—Cont.

ible upon discontinuation of the drug. If these reactions occur, NegGram should be discontinued and appropriate therapeutic measures instituted; only if rapid disappearance of CNS symptoms does not occur within 48 hours should diagnostic procedures involving risk to the patient be undertaken. (See ADVERSE REACTIONS and OVERDOSAGE.)

PRECAUTIONS

Blood counts and renal and liver function tests should be performed periodically if treatment is continued for more than two weeks. NegGram should be used with caution in patients with liver disease, epilepsy, or severe cerebral arteriosclerosis. While caution should be used in patients with severe renal failure, therapeutic concentrations of NegGram in the urine, without increased toxicity due to drug accumulation in the blood, have been observed in patients on full dosage with creatinine clearances as low as 2 mL/minute to 8 mL/minute.

Patients should be cautioned to avoid undue exposure to direct sunlight while receiving NegGram. Therapy should be discontinued if photosensitivity occurs.

If bacterial resistance to NegGram emerges during treatment, it usually does so within 48 hours, permitting rapid change to another antimicrobial. Therefore, if the clinical response is unsatisfactory or if relapse occurs, cultures and sensitivity tests should be repeated. Underdosage with NegGram during initial treatment (with less than 4 g per day for adults) may predispose to emergence of bacterial resistance. (See DOSAGE AND ADMINISTRATION.)

Drug Interactions. Nitrofurantoin interferes with the therapeutic action of nalidixic acid.

Cross resistance between NegGram and other antimicrobials has been observed only with oxolinic acid.

Nalidixic acid may enhance the effects of oral anticoagulants, warfarin or bishydroxycoumarin, by displacing significant amounts from serum albumin binding sites.

When Benedict's or Fehling's solutions or Clinitest® Reagent Tablets are used to test the urine of patients taking NegGram, a false-positive reaction for glucose may be obtained, due to the liberation of glucuronic acid from the metabolites excreted. However, a colorimetric test for glucose based on an enzyme reaction (eg, with Clinistix® Reagent Strips or Tes-Tape®) does not give a false-positive reaction to the liberated glucuronic acid.

Incorrect values may be obtained for urinary 17-keto and ketogenic steroids in patients receiving NegGram, brand of nalidixic acid, because of an interaction between the drug and the *m*-dinitrobenzene used in the usual assay method. In such cases, the Porter-Silber test for 17-hydroxycorticoids may be used.

Usage in Prepubertal Children. Recent toxicological studies have shown that nalidixic acid and related drugs can produce erosions of the cartilage in weight-bearing joints and other signs of arthropathy in immature animals of most species tested. No such joint lesions have been reported in man to date. Nevertheless, until the significance of this finding is clarified, care should be exercised when prescribing this product for prepubertal children.

Usage in Pregnancy. Safe use of NegGram during the first trimester of pregnancy has not been established. However, the drug has been used during the last two trimesters without producing apparent ill effects in mother or child.

Caution should be used in administering NegGram in the days prior to delivery because of the theoretical risk that exposure to maternal nalidixic acid in utero may lead to significant blood levels of nalidixic acid in the neonate immediately after birth. Patients using NegGram during pregnancy should be advised to discontinue use at the first sign of labor.

ADVERSE REACTIONS

Reactions reported after oral administration of NegGram include *CNS effects:* drowsiness, weakness, headache, and dizziness and vertigo. Reversible subjective visual disturbances without objective findings have occurred infrequently (generally with each dose during the first few days of treatment). These reactions include overbrightness of lights, change in color perception, difficulty in focusing, decrease in visual acuity, and double vision. They usually disappeared promptly when dosage was reduced or therapy was discontinued. Toxic psychosis or brief convulsions have been reported rarely, usually following excessive doses. In general, the convulsions have occurred in patients with predisposing factors such as epilepsy or cerebral arteriosclerosis. In infants and children receiving therapeutic doses of NegGram, increased intracranial pressure with bulging anterior fontanel, papilledema, and headache has occasionally been observed. A few cases of 6th cranial nerve palsy have been reported. Although the mechanisms of these reactions are unknown, the signs and symptoms usually disappeared rapidly with no sequelae when treatment was discontinued. *Gastrointestinal:* abdominal pain, nausea, vomiting, and diarrhea. *Allergic:* rash, pruritus, urticaria, angioedema, eosinophilia, arthralgia with joint stiffness and swelling, and rarely, ana-

phylactoid reaction. Photosensitivity reactions consisting of erythema and bullae on exposed skin surfaces usually resolve completely in 2 weeks to 2 months after NegGram is discontinued; however, bullae may continue to appear with successive exposures to sunlight or with mild skin trauma for up to 3 months after discontinuation of drug. (See PRECAUTIONS.) *Other:* rarely, cholestasis, paresthesia, metabolic acidosis, thrombocytopenia, leukopenia, or hemolytic anemia, sometimes associated with glucose-6-phosphate dehydrogenase deficiency.

DOSAGE AND ADMINISTRATION

Adults. The recommended dosage for initial therapy in adults is 1 g administered four times daily for one or two weeks (total daily dose, 4 g). For prolonged therapy, the total daily dose may be reduced to 2 g after the initial treatment period. Underdosage during initial treatment may predispose to emergence of bacterial resistance.

Children. Until further experience is gained, NegGram should not be administered to infants younger than three months. Dosage in children 12 years of age and under should be calculated on the basis of body weight. The recommended total daily dosage for initial therapy is 25 mg/lb/day (55 mg/kg/day), administered in four equally divided doses. For prolonged therapy, the total daily dose may be reduced to 15 mg/lb/day (33 mg/kg/day). NegGram Suspension or NegGram CAPLETS of 250 mg may be used. One 250 mg tablet is equivalent to one teaspoon (5 mL) of the Suspension.

OVERDOSAGE

Manifestations: Toxic psychosis, convulsions, increased intracranial pressure, or metabolic acidosis may occur in patients taking more than the recommended dosage. Vomiting, nausea, and lethargy may also occur following overdosage.

Treatment: Reactions are short-lived (two to three hours) because the drug is rapidly excreted. If overdosage is noted early, gastric lavage is indicated. If absorption has occurred, increased fluid administration is advisable and supportive measures such as oxygen and means of artificial respiration should be available. Although anticonvulsant therapy has not been used in the few instances of overdosage reported, it may be indicated in a severe case.

HOW SUPPLIED

Suspension (250 mg/5 mL tsp), raspberry flavored, bottles of 1 pint (NDC 0024-1318-06)
CAPLETS of 1 g, scored, bottles of 100 (NDC 0024-1323-04)
CAPLETS of 500 mg, scored, bottles of 56 (NDC 0024-1322-03), 500 (NDC 0024-1322-06)
CAPLETS of 250 mg, scored, bottles of 56 (NDC 0024-1321-03)

PHARMACOLOGY

Following oral administration, NegGram, brand of nalidixic acid, is rapidly absorbed from the gastrointestinal tract, partially metabolized in the liver, and rapidly excreted through the kidneys. Unchanged nalidixic acid appears in the urine along with an active metabolite, hydroxynalidixic acid, which has antibacterial activity similar to that of nalidixic acid. Other metabolites include glucuronic acid conjugates of nalidixic acid and hydroxynalidixic acid, and the dicarboxylic acid derivative. The hydroxy metabolite represents 30 percent of the biologically active drug in the blood and 85 percent in the urine. Peak serum levels of active drug average approximately 20 μg to 40 μg per mL (90 percent protein bound), one to two hours after administration of a 1 g dose to a fasting normal individual, with a half-life of about 90 minutes. Peak urine levels of active drug average approximately 150 μg to 200 μg per mL, three to four hours after administration, with a half-life of about six hours. Approximately four percent of NegGram is excreted in the feces. Traces of nalidixic acid were found in blood and urine of an infant whose mother had received the drug during the last trimester of pregnancy.

ANIMAL PHARMACOLOGY

NegGram (nalidixic acid) and related drugs have been shown to cause arthropathy in juvenile animals of most species tested. (See PRECAUTIONS.)

Hydroxynalidixic acid, the principal metabolite of NegGram, did not produce any oculotoxic effects at any dosage level in seven species of animals including three primate species. However, oral administration of this metabolite in high doses has been shown to have oculotoxic potential, namely in dogs and cats where it produced retinal degeneration upon prolonged administration leading, in some cases, to blindness.

In experiments with NegGram itself, little if any such activity could be elicited in either dogs or cats. Sensitivity to CNS side effects in these species limited the doses of NegGram that could be used; this factor, together with a low conversion rate to the hydroxy metabolite in these species, may explain the absence of these effects.

Shown in Product Identification Section, page 428

NEO-SYNEPHRINE® Hydrochloride   ℞
brand of phenylephrine hydrochloride
injection, USP
1% INJECTION

Well-Tolerated Vasoconstrictor and Pressor

> **WARNING:** PHYSICIANS SHOULD COMPLETELY FAMILIARIZE THEMSELVES WITH THE COMPLETE CONTENTS OF THIS LEAFLET BEFORE PRESCRIBING NEO-SYNEPHRINE.

DESCRIPTION

NEO-SYNEPHRINE hydrochloride, brand of phenylephrine hydrochloride injection, is a vasoconstrictor and pressor drug chemically related to epinephrine and ephedrine. NEO-SYNEPHRINE hydrochloride is a synthetic sympathomimetic agent in sterile form for parenteral injection. Chemically, phenylephrine hydrochloride is (−)-*m*-Hydroxy-α-[(methylamino) methyl] benzyl alcohol hydrochloride.

CLINICAL PHARMACOLOGY

NEO-SYNEPHRINE hydrochloride produces vasoconstriction that lasts longer than that of epinephrine and ephedrine. Responses are more sustained than those to epinephrine, lasting 20 minutes after intravenous and as long as 50 minutes after subcutaneous injection. Its action on the heart contrasts sharply with that of epinephrine and ephedrine, in that it slows the heart rate and increases the stroke output, producing no disturbance in the rhythm of the pulse.

Phenylephrine is a powerful postsynaptic alpha-receptor stimulant with little effect on the beta receptors of the heart. In therapeutic doses, it produces little if any stimulation of either the spinal cord or cerebrum. A singular advantage of this drug is the fact that repeated injections produce comparable effects.

The predominant actions of phenylephrine are on the cardiovascular system. Parenteral administration causes a rise in systolic and diastolic pressures in man and other species. Accompanying the pressor response to phenylephrine is a marked reflex bradycardia that can be blocked by atropine; after atropine, large doses of the drug increase the heart rate only slightly. In man, cardiac output is slightly decreased and peripheral resistance is considerably increased. Circulation time is slightly prolonged, and venous pressure is slightly increased; venous constriction is not marked. Most vascular beds are constricted; renal splanchnic, cutaneous, and limb blood flows are reduced but coronary blood flow is increased. Pulmonary vessels are constricted, and pulmonary arterial pressure is raised.

The drug is a powerful vasoconstrictor, with properties very similar to those of norepinephrine but almost completely lacking the chronotropic and inotropic actions on the heart. Cardiac irregularities are seen only very rarely even with large doses.

INDICATIONS AND USAGE

NEO-SYNEPHRINE is intended for the maintenance of an adequate level of blood pressure during spinal and inhalation anesthesia and for the treatment of vascular failure in shock, shocklike states, and drug-induced hypotension, or hypersensitivity. It is also employed to overcome paroxysmal supraventricular tachycardia, to prolong spinal anesthesia, and as a vasoconstrictor in regional analgesia.

CONTRAINDICATIONS

NEO-SYNEPHRINE hydrochloride should not be used in patients with severe hypertension, ventricular tachycardia, or in patients who are hypersensitive to it.

WARNINGS

If used in conjunction with oxytocic drugs, the pressor effect of sympathomimetic pressor amines is potentiated (see Drug Interaction). The obstetrician should be warned that some oxytocic drugs may cause severe persistent hypertension and that even a rupture of a cerebral blood vessel may occur during the postpartum period.

Contains sodium metabisulfite, a sulfite that may cause allergic-type reactions including anaphylactic symptoms and life-threatening or less severe asthmatic episodes in certain susceptible people. The overall prevalence of sulfite sensitivity in the general population is unknown and probably low. Sulfite sensitivity is seen more frequently in asthmatic than in nonasthmatic people.

PRECAUTIONS

NEO-SYNEPHRINE hydrochloride should be employed only with extreme caution in elderly patients or in patients with hyperthyroidism, bradycardia, partial heart block, myocardial disease, or severe arteriosclerosis.

Drug Interactions—Vasopressors, particularly metaraminol, may cause serious cardiac arrhythmias during halothane anesthesia and therefore should be used only with great caution or not at all.

MAO Inhibitors—The pressor effect of sympathomimetic pressor amines is markedly potentiated in patients receiving

monoamine oxidase inhibitors (MAOI). Therefore, when initiating pressor therapy in these patients, the initial dose should be small and used with due caution. The pressor response of adrenergic agents may also be potentiated by tricyclic antidepressants.

Carcinogenesis, Mutagenesis, Impairment of Fertility—No long-term animal studies have been done to evaluate the potential of NEO-SYNEPHRINE in these areas.

Pregnancy Category C—Animal reproduction studies have not been conducted with NEO-SYNEPHRINE. It is also not known whether NEO-SYNEPHRINE can cause fetal harm when administered to a pregnant woman or can affect reproduction capacity. NEO-SYNEPHRINE should be given to a pregnant woman only if clearly needed.

Labor and Delivery—If vasopressor drugs are either used to correct hypotension or added to the local anesthetic solution, the obstetrician should be cautioned that some oxytocic drugs may cause severe persistent hypertension and that even a rupture of a cerebral blood vessel may occur during the postpartum period (see WARNINGS).

Nursing Mother—It is not known whether this drug is excreted in human milk. Because many are excreted in human milk, caution should be exercised when NEO-SYNEPHRINE hydrochloride, brand of phenylephrine hydrochloride injection, is administered to a nursing woman.

Pediatric Use—To combat hypotension during spinal anesthesia in children, a dose of 0.5 mg to 1 mg per 25 pounds body weight, administered subcutaneously or intramuscularly, is recommended.

ADVERSE REACTIONS

Headache, reflex bradycardia, excitability, restlessness, and rarely arrhythmias.

OVERDOSAGE

Overdosage may induce ventricular extrasystoles and short paroxysms of ventricular tachycardia, a sensation of fullness in the head and tingling of the extremities.

Should an excessive elevation of blood pressure occur, it may be immediately relieved by an α-adrenergic blocking agent, eg, phentolamine.

The oral LD_{50} in the rat is 350 mg/kg, in the mouse 120 mg/kg.

DOSAGE AND ADMINISTRATION

NEO-SYNEPHRINE is generally injected subcutaneously, intramuscularly, slowly intravenously, or in dilute solution as a continuous intravenous infusion. In patients with paroxysmal supraventricular tachycardia and, if indicated, in case of emergency, NEO-SYNEPHRINE is administered directly intravenously. The dose should be adjusted according to the pressor response.

Dosage Calculations

Dose Required	Use NEO-SYNEPHRINE 1%
10 mg	1 mL
5 mg	0.5 mL
1 mg	0.1 mL

For convenience in intermittent intravenous administration, dilute 1 mL NEO-SYNEPHRINE 1% with 9 mL Sterile Water for Injection, USP, to yield 0.1% NEO-SYNEPHRINE.

Dose Required	Use Diluted NEO-SYNEPHRINE (0.1%)
0.1 mg	0.1 mL
0.2 mg	0.2 mL
0.5 mg	0.5 mL

Mild or Moderate Hypotension

Subcutaneously or Intramuscularly: Usual dose, from 2 mg to 5 mg. Range, from 1 mg to 10 mg. Initial dose should not exceed 5 mg.

Intravenously: Usual dose, 0.2 mg. Range, from 0.1 mg to 0.5 mg. Initial dose should not exceed 0.5 mg.

Injections should not be repeated more often than every 10 to 15 minutes. A 5 mg intramuscular dose should raise blood pressure for one to two hours. A 0.5 mg intravenous dose should elevate the pressure for about 15 minutes.

Severe Hypotension and Shock—Including Drug-Related Hypotension

Blood volume depletion should always be corrected as fully as possible before any vasopressor is administered. When, as an emergency measure, intraaortic pressures must be maintained to prevent cerebral or coronary artery ischemia, NEO-SYNEPHRINE hydrochloride, brand of phenylephrine hydrochloride injection, can be administered before and concurrently with blood volume replacement.

Hypotension and occasionally severe shock may result from overdosage or idiosyncrasy following the administration of certain drugs, especially adrenergic and ganglionic blocking agents, rauwolfia and veratrum alkaloids, and phenothiazine tranquilizers. Patients who receive a phenothiazine derivative as preoperative medication are especially susceptible to these reactions. As an adjunct in the management of such episodes, NEO-SYNEPHRINE hydrochloride is a suitable agent for restoring blood pressure.

Higher initial and maintenance doses of NEO-SYNEPHRINE are required in patients with persistent or untreated severe hypotension or shock. Hypotension produced by powerful peripheral adrenergic blocking agents, chlorpromazine, or pheochromocytomectomy may also require more intensive therapy.

Continuous Infusion—Add 10 mg of the drug (1 mL of 1 percent solution) to 500 mL of Dextrose Injection, USP, or Sodium Chloride Injection, USP (providing a 1:50,000 solution). To raise the blood pressure rapidly, start the infusion at about 100 μg to 180 μg per minute (based on 20 drops per mL this would be 100 to 180 drops per minute). When the blood pressure is stabilized (at a low normal level for the individual), a maintenance rate of 40 μg to 60 μg per minute usually suffices (based on 20 drops per mL this would be 40 to 60 drops per minute). If the drop size of the infusion system varies from the 20 drops per mL, the dose must be adjusted accordingly.

If a prompt initial pressor response is not obtained, additional increments of NEO-SYNEPHRINE (10 mg or more) are added to the infusion bottle. The rate of flow is then adjusted until the desired blood pressure level is obtained. (In some cases, a more potent vasopressor, such as norepinephrine bitartrate, may be required.) Hypertension should be avoided. The blood pressure should be checked frequently. Headache and/or bradycardia may indicate hypertension. Arrhythmias are rare.

Spinal Anesthesia—Hypotension

Routine parenteral use of NEO-SYNEPHRINE has been recommended for the prophylaxis and treatment of hypotension during spinal anesthesia. It is best administered subcutaneously or intramuscularly three or four minutes before injection of the spinal anesthetic. The total requirement for high anesthetic levels is usually 3 mg, and for lower levels, 2 mg. For hypotensive emergencies during spinal anesthesia, NEO-SYNEPHRINE may be injected intravenously, using an initial dose of 0.2 mg. Any subsequent dose should not exceed the previous dose by more than 0.1 mg to 0.2 mg and no more than 0.5 mg should be administered in a single dose.

To combat hypotension during spinal anesthesia in children, a dose of 0.5 mg to 1 mg per 25 pounds body weight, administered subcutaneously or intramuscularly, is recommended.

Prolongation of Spinal Anesthesia

The addition of 2 mg to 5 mg of NEO-SYNEPHRINE hydrochloride to the anesthetic solution increases the duration of motor block by as much as approximately 50 percent without any increase in the incidence of complications such as nausea, vomiting, or blood pressure disturbances.

Vasoconstrictor for Regional Analgesia

Concentrations about ten times those employed when epinephrine is used as a vasoconstrictor are recommended. The optimum strength is 1:20,000 (made by adding 1 mg of NEO-SYNEPHRINE hydrochloride to every 20 mL of local anesthetic solution). Some pressor responses can be expected when 2 mg or more are injected.

Paroxysmal Supraventricular Tachycardia

Rapid intravenous injection (within 20 to 30 seconds) is recommended; the initial dose should not exceed 0.5 mg, and subsequent doses, which are determined by the initial blood pressure response, should not exceed the preceding dose by more than 0.1 mg to 0.2 mg, and should never exceed 1 mg.

HOW SUPPLIED

Solution 1 percent

Each 1 mL contains 10 mg of NEO-SYNEPHRINE hydrochloride, 3.5 mg of sodium chloride, 4 mg of sodium citrate, 1 mg of citric acid monohydrate, and not more than 2 mg of sodium metabisulfite.

Uni-Nest™ ampuls of 1 mL, box of 25
(NDC 0024-1342-04).

CARPUJECT® Sterile Cartridge-Needle Unit, 10 mg/mL (1 mL fill in 2 mL cartridge), 22-gauge, 1¼ inch needle, dispensing bins of 50
(NDC 0024-1340-02).

The air in all ampuls and Cartridge-Needle Units has been displaced by nitrogen gas.

Protect from light if removed from carton or dispensing bin.

NW-64-EE

NEO–SYNEPHRINE® Hydrochloride ℞
brand of phenylephrine hydrochloride
ophthalmic solution, USP
Vasoconstrictor and Mydriatic
SOLUTIONS 2.5% AND 10%
VISCOUS SOLUTION 10%

For Use in Ophthalmology

WARNING: PHYSICIANS SHOULD COMPLETELY FAMILIARIZE THEMSELVES WITH THE COMPLETE CONTENTS OF THIS LEAFLET BEFORE PRESCRIBING NEO-SYNEPHRINE.

DESCRIPTION

NEO-SYNEPHRINE hydrochloride, brand of phenylephrine hydrochloride ophthalmic solution, is a sterile solution used as a vasoconstrictor and mydriatic for use in ophthalmology.

NEO-SYNEPHRINE hydrochloride is a synthetic sympathomimetic compound structurally similar to epinephrine and ephedrine.

Phenylephrine hydrochloride is (–)-*m*-Hydroxy-α-[(methylamino)methyl] benzyl alcohol hydrochloride.

CLINICAL PHARMACOLOGY

NEO-SYNEPHRINE possesses predominantly α-adrenergic effects. In the eye, phenylephrine acts locally as a potent vasoconstrictor and mydriatic, by constricting ophthalmic blood vessels and the radial muscle of the iris.

The ophthalmologic usefulness of NEO-SYNEPHRINE hydrochloride is due to its rapid effect and moderately prolonged action, as well as to the fact that it produces no compensatory vasodilatation.

The action of different concentrations of ophthalmic solutions of NEO-SYNEPHRINE hydrochloride is shown in the following table:

Strength of solution (%)	Mydriasis: Maximal (minutes)	Mydriasis: Recovery time (hours)	Paralysis of accommodation
2.5	15-60	3	trace
10	10-60	6	slight

Although rare, systemic absorption of sufficient quantities of phenylephrine may lead to systemic α-adrenergic effects, such as rise in blood pressure which may be accompanied by a reflex atropine-sensitive bradycardia.

INDICATIONS AND USAGE

NEO-SYNEPHRINE hydrochloride is recommended for use as a decongestant and vasoconstrictor and for pupil dilatation in uveitis (posterior synechiae), wide angle glaucoma, prior to surgery, refraction, ophthalmoscopic examination, and diagnostic procedures.

CONTRAINDICATIONS

Ophthalmic solutions of NEO-SYNEPHRINE hydrochloride are contraindicated in persons with narrow angle glaucoma (and in those individuals who are hypersensitive to NEO-SYNEPHRINE). NEO-SYNEPHRINE hydrochloride 10 percent ophthalmic solutions are contraindicated in infants and in patients with aneurysms.

WARNINGS

There have been rare reports associating the use of NEO-SYNEPHRINE 10 percent ophthalmic solutions with the development of serious cardiovascular reactions, including ventricular arrhythmias and myocardial infarctions. These episodes, some ending fatally, have usually occurred in elderly patients with preexisting cardiovascular diseases.

PRECAUTIONS

Exceeding recommended dosages or applying NEO-SYNEPHRINE hydrochloride ophthalmic solutions to the instrumented, traumatized, diseased or postsurgical eye or adnexa, or to patients with suppressed lacrimation, as during anesthesia, may result in the absorption of sufficient quantities of phenylephrine to produce a systemic vasopressor response.

A significant elevation in blood pressure is rare but has been reported following conjunctival instillation of recommended doses of NEO-SYNEPHRINE 10 percent ophthalmic solutions. Caution, therefore, should be exercised in administering the 10 percent solutions to children of low body weight, the elderly, and patients with insulin-dependent diabetes, hypertension, hyperthyroidism, generalized arteriosclerosis, or cardiovascular disease. The posttreatment blood pressure of these patients, and any patients who develop symptoms, should be carefully monitored.

Ordinarily, any mydriatic, including NEO-SYNEPHRINE hydrochloride, brand of phenylephrine hydrochloride ophthalmic solution, is contraindicated in patients with glaucoma, since it may occasionally raise intraocular pressure. However, when temporary dilatation of the pupil may free adhesions or when vasoconstriction of intrinsic vessels may lower intraocular tension, these advantages may temporarily outweigh the danger from coincident dilatation of the pupil.

Continued on next page

This product information was prepared in August 1992. On these and other products of Sanofi Winthrop Pharmaceuticals, detailed information may be obtained on a current basis by direct inquiry to Product Information Services, 90 Park Avenue, New York, NY 10016 (toll free 1-800-446-6267).

Sanofi Winthrop—Cont.

Rebound miosis has been reported in older persons one day after receiving NEO-SYNEPHRINE hydrochloride ophthalmic solutions, and reinstillation of the drug produced a reduction in mydriasis. This may be of clinical importance in dilating the pupils of older subjects prior to retinal detachment or cataract surgery.

Due to a strong action of the drug on the dilator muscle, older individuals may also develop transient pigment floaters in the aqueous humor 30 to 45 minutes following the administration of NEO-SYNEPHRINE hydrochloride ophthalmic solutions. The appearance may be similar to anterior uveitis or to a microscopic hyphema.

To prevent pain, a drop of suitable topical anesthetic may be applied before using the 10 percent ophthalmic solution.

Drug Interaction: As with all other adrenergic drugs, when NEO-SYNEPHRINE 10 percent ophthalmic solutions or 2.5 percent ophthalmic solution is administered simultaneously with, or up to 21 days after, administration of monoamine oxidase (MAO) inhibitors, careful supervision and adjustment of dosages are required since exaggerated adrenergic effects may occur. The pressor response of adrenergic agents may also be potentiated by tricyclic antidepressants, propranolol, reserpine, guanethidine, methyldopa, and atropine-like drugs.

It has been reported that the concomitant use of NEO-SYNEPHRINE 10 percent ophthalmic solutions and systemic beta blockers has caused acute hypertension and, in one case, the rupture of a congenital cerebral aneurysm. NEO-SYNEPHRINE may potentiate the cardiovascular depressant effects of potent inhalation anesthetic agents.

Carcinogenesis, Mutagenesis, Impairment of Fertility: No long-term animal studies have been done to evaluate the potential of NEO-SYNEPHRINE in these areas.

Pregnancy Category C: Animal reproduction studies have not been conducted with NEO-SYNEPHRINE. It is also not known whether NEO-SYNEPHRINE can cause fetal harm when administered to a pregnant woman or can affect reproduction capacity. NEO-SYNEPHRINE should be given to a pregnant woman only if clearly needed.

Nursing Mothers: It is not known whether this drug is excreted in milk; many are. Caution should be exercised when NEO-SYNEPHRINE hydrochloride ophthalmic solution is administered to a nursing woman.

Pediatric Use: NEO-SYNEPHRINE hydrochloride 10 percent ophthalmic solutions are contraindicated in infants. (See CONTRAINDICATIONS.) For use in older children see DOSAGE AND ADMINISTRATION.

Exceeding recommended dosages or applying NEO-SYNEPHRINE hydrochloride ophthalmic solutions to the instrumented, traumatized, diseased or postsurgical eye or adnexa, or to patients with suppressed lacrimation, as during anesthesia, may result in the absorption of sufficient quantities of phenylephrine to produce a systemic vasopressor response.

The hypertensive effects of phenylephrine may be treated with an alpha-adrenergic blocking agent such as phentolamine mesylate, 5 mg to 10 mg intravenously, repeated as necessary.

The oral LD_{50} of phenylephrine in the rat: 350 mg/kg, in the mouse: 120 mg/kg.

DOSAGE AND ADMINISTRATION

Prolonged exposure to air or strong light may cause oxidation and discoloration. Do not use if solution is brown or contains a precipitate.

Vasoconstriction and Pupil Dilatation

NEO-SYNEPHRINE hydrochloride 10 percent ophthalmic solutions are especially useful when rapid and powerful dilatation of the pupil and reduction of congestion in the capillary bed are desired. A drop of a suitable topical anesthetic may be applied, followed in a few minutes by 1 drop of the NEO-SYNEPHRINE hydrochloride 10 percent ophthalmic solution on the upper limbus. The anesthetic prevents stinging and consequent dilution of the solution by lacrimation. It may occasionally be necessary to repeat the instillation after one hour, again preceded by the use of the topical anesthetic.

Uveitis: Posterior Synechiae

NEO-SYNEPHRINE hydrochloride 10 percent ophthalmic solutions may be used in patients with uveitis when synechiae are present or may develop. The formation of synechiae may be prevented by the use of the 10 percent ophthalmic solutions and atropine to produce wide dilatation of the pupil. It should be emphasized, however, that the vasoconstrictor effect of NEO-SYNEPHRINE hydrochloride may be antagonistic to the increase of local blood flow in uveal infection.

To free recently formed posterior synechiae, 1 drop of the 10 percent ophthalmic solutions may be applied to the upper surface of the cornea. On the following day, treatment may be continued if necessary. In the interim, hot compresses should be applied for five or ten minutes three times a day, with 1 drop of a 1 or 2 percent solution of atropine sulfate before and after each series of compresses.

Glaucoma

In certain patients with glaucoma, temporary reduction of intraocular tension may be attained by producing vasoconstriction of the intraocular vessels; this may be accomplished by placing 1 drop of the 10 percent ophthalmic solutions on the upper surface of the cornea. This treatment may be repeated as often as necessary.

NEO-SYNEPHRINE hydrochloride, brand of phenylephrine hydrochloride ophthalmic solution, may be used with miotics in patients with wide angle glaucoma. It reduces the difficulties experienced by the patient because of the small field produced by miosis, and still it permits and often supports the effect of the miotic in lowering the intraocular pressure. Hence, there may be marked improvement in visual acuity after using NEO-SYNEPHRINE hydrochloride in conjunction with miotic drugs.

Surgery

When a short-acting mydriatic is needed for wide dilatation of the pupil before intraocular surgery, the 10 percent ophthalmic solutions or 2.5 percent ophthalmic solution may be applied topically from 30 to 60 minutes before the operation.

Refraction

Prior to determination of refractive errors, NEO-SYNEPHRINE hydrochloride 2.5 percent ophthalmic solution may be used effectively with homatropine hydrobromide, atropine sulfate, or a combination of homatropine and cocaine hydrochloride.

For *adults*, a drop of the preferred cycloplegic is placed in each eye, followed in five minutes by 1 drop of NEO-SYNEPHRINE hydrochloride 2.5 percent ophthalmic solution and in ten minutes by another drop of the cycloplegic. In 50 to 60 minutes, the eyes are ready for refraction.

For *children*, a drop of atropine sulfate 1 percent is placed in each eye, followed in 10 to 15 minutes by 1 drop of NEO-SYNEPHRINE hydrochloride 2.5 percent ophthalmic solution and in five to ten minutes by a second drop of atropine sulfate 1 percent. In one to two hours, the eyes are ready for refraction.

For a "one application method," NEO-SYNEPHRINE hydrochloride 2.5 percent ophthalmic solution may be combined with a cycloplegic to elicit synergistic action. The additive effect varies depending on the patient. Therefore, when using a "one application method," it may be desirable to increase the concentration of the cycloplegic.

Ophthalmoscopic Examination

One drop of NEO-SYNEPHRINE hydrochloride 2.5 percent ophthalmic solution is placed in each eye. Sufficient mydriasis to permit examination is produced in 15 to 30 minutes. Dilatation lasts from one to three hours.

Diagnostic Procedures

Provocative Test for Angle Block in Patients with Glaucoma: The 2.5 percent ophthalmic solution may be used as a provocative test when latent increased intraocular pressure is suspected. Tension is measured before application of NEO-SYNEPHRINE hydrochloride and again after dilatation. A 3 to 5 mm of mercury rise in pressure suggests the presence of angle block in patients with glaucoma; however, failure to obtain such a rise does not preclude the presence of glaucoma from other causes.

Shadow Test (Retinoscopy): When dilatation of the pupil without cycloplegic action is desired for the shadow test, the 2.5 percent ophthalmic solution may be used alone.

Blanching Test: One or 2 drops of the 2.5 percent ophthalmic solution should be applied to the injected eye. After five minutes, examine for perilimbal blanching. If blanching occurs, the congestion is superficial and probably does not indicate iritis.

HOW SUPPLIED

In Mono-Drop ® (plastic dropper) bottle:

Low surface tension solutions

2.5   percent ophthalmic solution — NEO-SYNEPHRINE hydrochloride, brand of phenylephrine hydrochloride ophthalmic solution, 2.5 percent in a sterile, isotonic, buffered, low surface tension vehicle with sodium phosphate, sodium biphosphate, boric acid, and, as antiseptic preservative, benzalkonium chloride, NF, 1:7500. The pH is adjusted with phosphoric acid or sodium hydroxide.

    Bottles of 15 mL (NDC 0024-1358-01)

10   percent ophthalmic solution — NEO-SYNEPHRINE hydrochloride 10 percent in a sterile, buffered, low surface tension vehicle with sodium phosphate, sodium biphosphate, and, as antiseptic preservative, benzalkonium chloride 1:10,000. The pH is adjusted with phosphoric acid or sodium hydroxide.

    Bottles of 5 mL (NDC 0024-1359-01)

Viscous solution

10   percent ophthalmic solution — NEO-SYNEPHRINE hydrochloride 10 percent in a sterile, buffered, viscous vehicle with sodium phosphate, sodium biphosphate, methylcellulose, and, as antiseptic preservative, benzalkonium chloride 1:10,000. The pH is adjusted with phosphoric acid or sodium hydroxide.

    Bottles of 5 mL (NDC 0024-1362-01)

NW-147-CC

NITRONG®   ℞
NITROGLYCERIN
EXTENDED-RELEASE ORAL TABLETS, 2.6 MG AND 6.5 MG

DESCRIPTION

Nitroglycerin is 1,2,3-propanetriol trinitrate, an organic nitrate whose structural formula is:

$$H_2CONO_2$$
$$|$$
$$HCONO_2$$
$$|$$
$$H_2CONO_2$$

and whose molecular weight is 227.09. The organic nitrates are vasodilators, active on both arteries and veins.

Each Nitrong 2.6 mg tablet for oral administration contains 2.6 mg nitroglycerin in extended-release form with light green and white granules containing lactose, calcium stearate, D&C Yellow #10, dicalcium phosphate, synthetic iron oxide, pharmaceutical glaze, sugar spheres, and talc.

Each Nitrong 6.5 mg tablet for oral administration contains 6.5 mg nitroglycerin in extended-release form with light orange and green granules containing lactose, calcium stearate, D&C Yellow #10, dicalcium phosphate, FD&C Yellow #6, synthetic iron oxide, pharmaceutical glaze, povidone, sugar spheres, and talc.

CLINICAL PHARMACOLOGY

The principal pharmacological action of nitroglycerin is relaxation of vascular smooth muscle and consequent dilatation of peripheral arteries and veins, especially the latter. Dilatation of the veins promotes peripheral pooling of blood and decreases venous return to the heart, thereby reducing left ventricular end-diastolic pressure and pulmonary capillary wedge pressure (preload). Arteriolar relaxation reduces systemic vascular resistance, systolic arterial pressure, and mean arterial pressure (afterload). Dilatation of the coronary arteries also occurs. The relative importance of preload reduction, afterload reduction, and coronary dilatation remains undefined.

Dosing regimens for most chronically used drugs are designed to provide plasma concentrations that are continuously greater than a minimally effective concentration. This strategy is inappropriate for organic nitrates. Several well-controlled clinical trials have used exercise testing to assess the antianginal efficacy of continuously-delivered nitrates. In the large majority of these trials, active agents were indistinguishable from placebo after 24 hours (or less) of continuous therapy. Attempts to overcome nitrate tolerance by dose escalation, even to doses far in excess of those used acutely, have consistently failed. Only after nitrates had been absent from the body for several hours was their antianginal efficacy restored.

Pharmacokinetics: The volume of distribution of nitroglycerin is about 3 L/kg, and nitroglycerin is cleared from this volume at extremely rapid rates, with a resulting serum half-life of about 3 minutes. The observed clearance rates (close to 1 L/kg/min) greatly exceed hepatic blood flow; known sites of extrahepatic metabolism include red blood cells and vascular walls.

The first products in the metabolism of nitroglycerin are inorganic nitrate and the 1,2- and 1,3-dinitroglycerols. The dinitrates are less effective vasodilators than nitroglycerin, but they are longer-lived in the serum, and their net contribution to the overall effect of chronic nitroglycerin regimens is not known. The dinitrates are further metabolized to (nonvasoactive) mononitrates and, ultimately, to glycerol and carbon dioxide.

To avoid development of tolerance to nitroglycerin, drug-free intervals of 10–12 hours are known to be sufficient; shorter intervals have not been well studied. In one well-controlled clinical trial, subjects receiving nitroglycerin appeared to exhibit a rebound or withdrawal effect, so that their exercise tolerance at the end of the daily drug-free interval was *less* than that exhibited by the parallel group receiving placebo. Reliable assay techniques for plasma nitroglycerin levels have only recently become available, and studies using these techniques to define the pharmacokinetics of oral nitroglycerin preparations have not been reported. Published studies using older techniques provide results that often differ, in similar experimental settings, by an order of magnitude.

Clinical Trials: Controlled trials of single oral doses of nitroglycerin have demonstrated that nitroglycerin tablets can effectively reduce exercise-related angina for up to 5 hours. Antianginal activity is present about 1 hour after ingestion of a tablet.

Controlled trials of multiple-dose oral nitroglycerin have shown statistically significant antianginal efficacy 2 ½ and 4 hours after a dose when oral nitroglycerin had been administered four times a day for 2 weeks or three times a day for 1 week. As noted above, careful studies with other formulations of nitroglycerin have shown that maintenance of con-

tinuous 24-hour plasma levels of nitroglycerin results in insurmountable tolerance. Presumably, the studied 1-week and 2-week regimens of oral nitroglycerin therapy achieved adequate nitrate-free intervals by non-uniformity of dosing interval, with longer intervals overnight. The investigators did not report how subjects interpreted their dosing instructions, and they similarly did not report which dose of the day was the one after which they obtained the end-of-trial exercise results.

Thus, these studies of oral nitroglycerin should *not* be interpreted as demonstrations that these regimens provide round-the-clock antianginal protection. From large, well-controlled studies of other nitroglycerin formulations, it is reasonable to believe that the maximal achievable daily duration of antianginal effect from Nitrong tablets is about 12 hours.

In some controlled trials of other organic nitrate formulations efficacy has declined with time. Because the controlled, multiple-dose trials of oral nitroglycerin did not include exercise tests before the last day of treatment, it is not known how the efficacy of Nitrong tablets may vary during extended therapy.

INDICATIONS AND USAGE

Nitrong, nitroglycerin, tablets are indicated for the prevention of angina pectoris due to coronary artery disease. The onset of action of oral nitroglycerin is not sufficiently rapid for this product to be useful in aborting an acute anginal episode.

CONTRAINDICATIONS

Allergic reactions to organic nitrates are extremely rare, but they do occur. Nitroglycerin is contraindicated in patients who are allergic to it.

WARNINGS

The benefits of oral nitroglycerin in patients with acute myocardial infarction or congestive heart failure have not been established. If one elects to use nitroglycerin in these conditions, careful clinical or hemodynamic monitoring must be used to avoid the hazards of hypotension and tachycardia. Because the effects of tablets are so difficult to terminate rapidly, tablets are not recommended in these settings.

PRECAUTIIONS

General: Severe hypotension, particularly with upright posture, may occur with even small doses of nitroglycerin. This drug should therefore be used with caution in patients who may be volume depleted or who, for whatever reason, are already hypotensive. Hypotension induced by nitroglycerin may be accompanied by paradoxical bradycardia and increased angina pectoris.

Nitrate therapy may aggravate the angina caused by hypertrophic cardiomyopathy.

As tolerance to other forms of nitroglycerin develops, the effect of sublingual nitroglycerin on exercise tolerance, although still observable, is somewhat blunted.

In industrial workers who have had long-term exposure to unknown (presumably high) doses of organic nitrates, tolerance clearly occurs. Chest pain, acute myocardial infarction, and even sudden death have occurred during temporary withdrawal of nitrates from these workers, demonstrating the existence of true physical dependence.

Some clinical trials in angina patients have provided nitroglycerin for about 12 continuous hours of every 24-hour day. During the nitrate-free intervals in some of these trials, anginal attacks have been more easily provoked than before treatment, and patients have demonstrated hemodynamic rebound and *decreased* exercise tolerance. The importance of these observations to the routine, clinical use of oral nitroglycerin is not known.

Information for Patients: Daily headaches sometimes accompany treatment with nitroglycerin. In patients who get these headaches, the headaches are a marker of the activity of the drug. Patients should resist the temptation to avoid headaches by altering the schedule of their treatment with nitroglycerin, since loss of headache is likely to be associated with simultaneous loss of antianginal efficacy.

Treatment with nitroglycerin may be associated with lightheadedness on standing, especially just after rising from a recumbent or seated position. This effect may be more frequent in patients who have also consumed alcohol.

Drug Interactions: The vasodilating effects of nitroglycerin may be additive with those of other vasodilators. Alcohol, in particular, has been found to exhibit additive effects of this variety.

Marked symptomatic orthostatic hypotension has been reported when calcium channel blockers and organic nitrates were used in combination. Dose adjustments of either class of agents may be necessary.

Carcinogenesis, Mutagenesis, and Impairment of Fertility: Studies to evaluate the carcinogenic or mutagenic potential of nitroglycerin have not been performed. Nitroglycerin's effect upon reproductive capacity is similarly unknown.

Pregnancy Category C: Animal reproduction studies have not been conducted with nitroglycerin. It is also not known whether nitroglycerin can cause fetal harm when administered to a pregnant woman or whether it can affect reproductive capacity. Nitroglycerin should be given to a pregnant woman only if clearly needed.

Nursing Mothers: It is not known whether nitroglycerin is excreted in human milk. Because many drugs are excreted in human milk, caution should be exercised when nitroglycerin is administered to a nursing woman.

Pediatric Use: Safety and effectiveness in children have not been established.

ADVERSE REACTIONS

Adverse reactions to nitroglycerin are generally dose-related, and almost all of these reactions are the result of nitroglycerin's activity as a vasodilator. Headache, which may be severe, is the most commonly reported side effect. Headache may be recurrent with each daily dose, especially at higher doses. Transient episodes of lightheadedness, occasionally related to blood pressure changes, may also occur. Hypotension occurs infrequently, but in some patients it may be severe enough to warrant discontinuation of therapy. Syncope, crescendo angina, and rebound hypertension have been reported but are uncommon.

Allergic reactions to nitroglycerin are also uncommon, and the great majority of those reported have been cases of contact dermatitis or fixed drug eruptions in patients receiving nitroglycerin in ointments or patches. There have been a few reports of genuine anaphylactoid reactions, and these reactions can probably occur in patients receiving nitroglycerin by any route.

Extremely rarely, ordinary doses of organic nitrates have caused methemoglobinemia in normal-seeming patients; for further discussion of its diagnosis and treatment see **OVERDOSAGE.**

Data are not available to allow estimation of the frequency of adverse reactions during treatment with Nitrong, nitroglycerin, tablets.

OVERDOSAGE

Hemodynamic Effects: The ill effects of nitroglycerin overdose are generally the results of nitroglycerin's capacity to induce vasodilatation, venous pooling, reduced cardiac output, and hypotension. These hemodynamic changes may have protean manifestations, including increased intracranial pressure, with any or all of persistent throbbing headache, confusion, and moderate fever; vertigo; palpitations; visual disturbances; nausea and vomiting (possibly with colic and even bloody diarrhea); syncope (especially in the upright posture); air hunger and dyspnea, later followed by reduced ventilatory effort; diaphoresis, with the skin either flushed or cold and clammy; heart block and bradycardia; paralysis; coma; seizures; and death.

Laboratory determinations of serum levels of nitroglycerin and its metabolites are not widely available, and such determinations have, in any event, no established role in the management of nitroglycerin overdose.

No data are available to suggest physiological maneuvers (e.g., maneuvers to change the pH of the urine) that might accelerate elimination of nitroglycerin and its active metabolites. Similarly, it is not known which—if any—of these substances can usefully be removed from the body by hemodialysis.

No specific antagonist to the vasodilator effects of nitroglycerin is known, and no intervention has been subject to controlled study as a therapy of nitroglycerin overdose. Because the hypotension associated with nitroglycerin in overdose is the result of venodilatation and arterial hypovolemia, prudent therapy in this situation should be directed toward increase in central fluid volume. Passive elevation of the patient's legs may be sufficient, but intravenous infusion of normal saline or similar fluid may also be necessary.

The use of epinephrine or other arterial vasoconstrictors in this setting is likely to do more harm than good.

In patients with renal disease or congestive heart failure, therapy resulting in central volume expansion is not without hazard. Treatment of nitroglycerin overdose in these patients may be subtle and difficult, and invasive monitoring may be required.

Methemoglobinemia: Nitrate ions liberated during metabolism of nitroglycerin can oxidize hemoglobin into methemoglobin. Even in patients totally without cytochrome b_5 reductase activity, however, and even assuming that the nitrate moieties of nitroglycerin are quantitatively applied to oxidation of hemoglobin, about 1 mg/kg of nitroglycerin should be required before any of these patients manifests clinically significant ($\geq 10\%$) methemoglobinemia. In patients with normal reductase function, significant production of methemoglobin should require even larger doses of nitroglycerin. In one study in which 36 patients received 2–4 weeks of continuous nitroglycerin therapy at 3.1 to 4.4 mg/hr, the average methemoglobin level measured was 0.2%; this was comparable to that observed in parallel patients who received placebo.

Notwithstanding these observations, there are case reports of significant methemoglobinemia in association with moderate overdoses of organic nitrates. None of the affected patients had been thought to be unusually susceptible.

Methemoglobin levels are available from most clinical laboratories. The diagnosis should be suspected in patients who exhibit signs of impaired oxygen delivery despite adequate cardiac output and adequate arterial pO_2. Classically, methemoglobinemic blood is described as chocolate brown, without color change on exposure to air.

When methemoglobinemia is diagnosed, the treatment of choice is methylene blue, 1 to 2 mg/kg intravenously.

DOSAGE AND ADMINISTRATION

As noted above (CLINICAL PHARMACOLOGY), careful studies with other formulations of nitroglycerin have shown that maintenance of continuous 24-hour plasma levels of nitroglycerin results in tolerance (i.e., loss of clinical response). Every dosing regimen for Nitrong, nitroglycerin, tablets should provide a daily nitrate-free interval to avoid the development of this tolerance. The minimum necessary length of such an interval has not been defined, but studies with other nitroglycerin formulations have shown that 10–12 hours is sufficient. Large controlled studies with other formulations of nitroglycerin show that no dosing regimen with Nitrong tablets should be expected to provide more than about 12 hours of continuous antianginal efficacy per day.

The pharmacokinetics of nitroglycerin tablets, and the clinical effects of multiple-dose regimens, have not been well studied. In clinical trials, the initial regimen of nitroglycerin tablets has been 2.6 to 6.5 mg three times a day, with subsequent upward dose adjustment guided by symptoms and side effects. In one trial, 5 of the 18 subjects were titrated up to a dose of 26 mg four times a day.

HOW SUPPLIED

Nitrong is supplied as scored tablets with a mottled granular appearance.
Tablets of 2.6 mg: green and white in color, imprinted 411 on one side and U_ES on the other, bottles of 100 (NDC 0024-1298-10).
Tablets of 6.5 mg: orange and green in color, imprinted 412 on one side and U_ES on the other, bottles of 100 (NDC 0024-1299-10).
The product has child-resistant closures.
Store at controlled room temperature, between 15°C and 30°C (59°F and 86°F).
CAUTION: Federal (U.S.A.) law prohibits dispensing without prescription.

Distributed by Sanofi Winthrop Pharmaceuticals
New York, NY 10016
Supplied by Rhône-Poulenc Rorer
Collegeville, PA 19426

NSW-1

Shown in Product Identification Section, page 428

NOVOCAIN®   ℞
brand of procaine hydrochloride
injection, USP

DESCRIPTION

Procaine hydrochloride is benzoic acid, 4-amino-, 2-(diethylamino)ethyl ester, monohydrochloride, the ester of diethylaminoethanol and aminobenzoic acid.
It is a white crystalline, odorless powder that is freely soluble in water, but less soluble in alcohol.

HOW SUPPLIED

NOVOCAIN Solution 1 percent
Uni-Nest™, single-dose ampuls of 2 mL, box of 25
NDC 0024-1381-25
Single-dose ampuls of 6 mL, box of 50 NDC 0024-1381-05
Multiple-dose vials of 30 mL, box of 1 NDC 0024-1385-01
NOVOCAIN Solution 2 percent
Multiple-dose vials of 30 mL, box of 1 NDC 0024-1386-01
For complete prescribing information, see package insert or contact Product Information Services.

NW-63-V

Continued on next page

This product information was prepared in August 1992. On these and other products of Sanofi Winthrop Pharmaceuticals, detailed information may be obtained on a current basis by direct inquiry to Product Information Services, 90 Park Avenue, New York, NY 10016 (toll free 1-800-446-6267).

Sanofi Winthrop—Cont.

NOVOCAIN® ℞
brand of procaine hydrochloride
injection, USP
10% Solution for Spinal Anesthesia

DESCRIPTION
NOVOCAIN, brand of procaine hydrochloride, is benzoic acid, 4-amino-, 2-(diethylamino) ethyl ester, monohydrochloride, the ester of diethylaminoethanol and aminobenzoic acid.

It is a white crystalline, odorless powder that is freely soluble in water, but less soluble in alcohol. Each mL contains 100 mg procaine hydrochloride and 4 mg acetone sodium bisulfite as antioxidant. DO NOT USE SOLUTIONS IF CRYSTALS, CLOUDINESS, OR DISCOLORATION IS OBSERVED. EXAMINE SOLUTIONS CAREFULLY BEFORE USE. REAUTOCLAVING INCREASES LIKELIHOOD OF CRYSTAL FORMATION.

CLINICAL PHARMACOLOGY
NOVOCAIN stabilizes the neuronal membrane and prevents the initiation and transmission of nerve impulses, thereby effecting local anesthesia. NOVOCAIN lacks surface anesthetic activity. The onset of action is rapid (2 to 5 minutes) and the duration of action is relatively short (average 1 to 1½ hours), depending upon the anesthetic technique, the type of block, the concentration, and the individual patient.

NOVOCAIN is readily absorbed following parenteral administration and is rapidly hydrolyzed by plasma cholinesterase to aminobenzoic acid and diethylaminoethanol.

A vasoconstrictor may be added to the solution of NOVOCAIN to promote local hemostasis, delay systemic absorption, and increase duration of anesthesia.

INDICATIONS AND USAGE
NOVOCAIN is indicated for spinal anesthesia.

CONTRAINDICATIONS
Spinal anesthesia with NOVOCAIN is contraindicated in patients with generalized septicemia: sepsis at the proposed injection site; certain diseases of the cerebrospinal system, eg, meningitis, syphilis; and a known hypersensitivity to the drug, drugs of a similar chemical configuration, or aminobenzoic acid or its derivatives.

The decision as to whether or not spinal anesthesia should be used in an individual case should be made by the physician after weighing the advantages with the risks and possible complications.

WARNINGS
RESUSCITATIVE EQUIPMENT AND DRUGS SHOULD BE IMMEDIATELY AVAILABLE WHENEVER ANY LOCAL ANESTHETIC DRUG IS USED. Spinal anesthesia should only be administered by those qualified to do so.

Large doses of local anesthetics should not be used in patients with heart block.

Reactions resulting in fatality have occurred on rare occasions with the use of local anesthetics, even in the absence of a history of hypersensitivity.

Usage in Pregnancy. Safe use of NOVOCAIN has not been established with respect to adverse effects on fetal development. Careful consideration should be given to this fact before administering this drug to women of childbearing potential particularly during early pregnancy. This does not exclude the use of the drug at term for obstetrical analgesia.

Vasopressor agents (administered for the treatment of hypotension or added to the anesthetic solution for vasoconstriction) should be used with extreme caution in the presence of oxytocic drugs as they may produce severe, persistent hypertension with possible rupture of a cerebral blood vessel.

Solutions which contain a vasoconstrictor should be used with extreme caution in patients receiving drugs known to produce alterations in blood pressure (ie, monoamine oxidase inhibitors (MAOI), tricyclic antidepressants, phenothiazines, etc), as either severe sustained hypertension or hypotension may occur.

Local anesthetic procedures should be used with caution when there is inflammation and/or sepsis in the region of the proposed injection.

Contains acetone sodium bisulfite, a sulfite that may cause allergic-type reactions including anaphylactic symptoms and life-threatening or less severe asthmatic episodes in certain susceptible people. The overall prevalence of sulfite sensitivity in the general population is unknown and probably low. Sulfite sensitivity is seen more frequently in asthmatic than in nonasthmatic people.

PRECAUTIONS
Standard textbooks should be consulted for specific techniques and precautions for various spinal anesthetic procedures.

The safety and effectiveness of a spinal anesthetic depend upon proper dosage, correct technique, adequate precautions, and readiness for emergencies. The lowest dosage that results in effective anesthesia should be used to avoid high plasma levels and possible adverse effects. Tolerance varies with the status of the patient. Debilitated, elderly patients, or acutely ill patients should be given reduced doses commensurate with their weight and physical status. Reduced dosages are also indicated for obstetric delivery and patients with increased intra-abdominal pressure.

The decision whether or not to use spinal anesthesia in the following disease states depends on the physician's appraisal of the advantages as opposed to the risk: cardiovascular disease (ie, shock, hypertension, anemia, etc), pulmonary disease, renal impairment, metabolic or endocrine disorders, gastrointestinal disorders (ie, intestinal obstruction, peritonitis, etc), or complicated obstetrical deliveries.

NOVOCAIN SHOULD BE USED WITH CAUTION IN PATIENTS WITH KNOWN DRUG ALLERGIES AND SENSITIVITIES. A thorough history of the patient's prior experience with NOVOCAIN or other local anesthetics as well as concomitant or recent drug use should be taken (see CONTRAINDICATIONS). NOVOCAIN should not be used in any condition in which a sulfonamide drug is being employed since aminobenzoic acid inhibits the action of sulfonamides.

Solutions containing a vasopressor should be used with caution in the presence of diseases which may adversely affect the cardiovascular system.

NOVOCAIN, brand of procaine hydrochloride injection, should be used with caution in patients with severe disturbances of cardiac rhythm, shock or heart block.

ADVERSE REACTIONS
Systemic adverse reactions involving the central nervous system and the cardiovascular system usually result from high plasma levels due to excessive dosage, rapid absorption, or inadvertent intravascular injection. In addition, use of inappropriate doses or techniques may result in extensive spinal blockade leading to hypotension and respiratory arrest.

A small number of reactions may result from hypersensitivity, idiosyncrasy, or diminished tolerance to normal dosage. *Excitatory CNS effects* (nervousness, dizziness, blurred vision, tremors) commonly represent the initial signs of local anesthetic systemic toxicity. However, these reactions may be very brief or absent in some patients in which case the first manifestation of toxicity may be drowsiness or convulsions merging into unconsciousness and respiratory arrest. *Cardiovascular system* reactions include depression of the myocardium, hypotension (or sometimes hypertension), bradycardia, and even cardiac arrest.

Allergic reactions are characterized by cutaneous lesions of delayed onset, or urticaria, edema, and other manifestations of allergy. The detection of sensitivity by skin testing is of limited value. As with other local anesthetics, hypersensitivity, idiosyncrasy and anaphylactoid reactions have occurred rarely. The reaction may be abrupt and severe and is not usually dose related.

The following adverse reactions may occur with spinal anesthesia: *Central Nervous System:* postspinal headache, meningismus, arachnoiditis, palsies, or spinal nerve paralysis. *Cardiovascular:* hypotension due to vasomotor paralysis and pooling of the blood in the venous bed. *Respiratory:* respiratory impairment or paralysis due to the level of anesthesia extending to the upper thoracic and cervical segments. *Gastrointestinal:* nausea and vomiting.

Treatment of Reactions. Toxic effects of local anesthetics require symptomatic treatment: there is no specific cure. The physician should be prepared to maintain an airway and to support ventilation with oxygen and assisted or controlled respiration as required. Supportive treatment of the cardiovascular system includes intravenous fluids and, when appropriate, vasopressors (preferably those that stimulate the myocardium, such as ephedrine). Convulsions may be controlled with oxygen and by the intravenous administration of diazepam or ultrashort-acting barbiturates or a short-acting muscle relaxant (succinylcholine). Intravenous anticonvulsant agents and muscle relaxants should only be administered by those familiar with their use and only when ventilation and oxygenation are assured. In spinal and epidural anesthesia, sympathetic blockade also occurs as a pharmacological reaction, resulting in peripheral vasodilation and often *hypotension.* The extent of the hypotension will usually depend on the number of dermatomes blocked. The blood pressure should therefore be monitored in the early phases of anesthesia. If hypotension occurs, it is readily controlled by vasoconstrictors administered either by the intramuscular or the intravenous route, the dosage of which would depend on the severity of the hypotension and the response to treatment.

DOSAGE AND ADMINISTRATION
As with all local anesthetics, the dose of NOVOCAIN, brand of procaine hydrochloride injection, varies and depends upon the area to be anesthetized, the vascularity of the tissues, the number of neuronal segments to be blocked, individual tolerance, and the technique of anesthesia. The lowest dose needed to provide effective anesthesia should be administered. For specific techniques and procedures, refer to standard textbooks.

[See table below.]

The diluent may be sterile normal saline, sterile distilled water, spinal fluid; and for hyperbaric technique, sterile dextrose solution.

The usual rate of injection is 1 mL per 5 seconds. Full anesthesia and fixation usually occur in 5 minutes.

STERILIZATION
The drug in intact ampuls is sterile. The preferred method of destroying bacteria on the exterior of ampuls before opening is heat sterilization (autoclaving). Immersion in antiseptic solution is not recommended.

Autoclave at 15-pound pressure, at 121°C (250°F), for 15 minutes. The diluent dextrose may show some brown discoloration due to caramelization.

HOW SUPPLIED
Uni-Nest™—ampuls of 2 mL (200 mg), box of 25 (NDC 0024-1384-25).

Protect solutions from light.

The air in the ampuls has been displaced by nitrogen gas.

NW 62-Q

PEDIACOF® Ⓥ ℞

DESCRIPTION
Each teaspoon (5 mL) contains:

Codeine phosphate, USP	5.0 mg
(Warning: May be habit forming.)	
Phenylephrine hydrochloride, USP	2.5 mg
Chlorpheniramine maleate, USP	0.75 mg
Potassium iodide, USP	75.0 mg

with sodium benzoate 0.2% as preservative and alcohol 5%.

Inactive Ingredients: Alcohol, Citric Acid, FD&C Red #40, Flavor, Glycerin, Liquid Glucose, Purified Water, Saccharin Sodium, Sodium Benzoate.

HOW SUPPLIED
Bottle of 16 fl oz (NDC 0024-1509-06)
Available on prescription only.
For complete prescribing information see package insert or contact Product Information Services.

PW-295-L

---

pHisoDerm® OTC
(See PDR For Nonprescription Drugs.)

---

pHisoHex® ℞
brand of hexachlorophene detergent cleanser

sudsing antibacterial soapless skin cleanser

DESCRIPTION
pHisoHex, brand of hexachlorophene detergent cleanser, is an antibacterial sudsing emulsion for topical administration. pHisoHex contains a colloidal dispersion of hexachlorophene 3% (w/w) in a stable emulsion consisting of entsufon sodium, petrolatum, lanolin cholesterols, methylcellulose,

RECOMMENDED DOSAGE FOR SPINAL ANESTHESIA

Extent of anesthesia	NOVOCAIN 10% Solution Volume of 10% Solution (mL)	Volume of Diluent (mL)	Total Dose (mg)	Site of Injection (lumbar interspace)
Perineum	0.5	0.5	50	4th
Perineum and lower extremities	1	1	100	3rd or 4th
Up to costal margin	2	1	200	2nd, 3rd or 4th

polyethylene glycol, polyethylene glycol monostearate, lauryl myristyl diethanolamide, sodium benzoate, and water. pH is adjusted with hydrochloric acid. Entsufon sodium is a synthetic detergent.

Chemically, hexachlorophene is Phenol, 2,2′-methylene-bis[3,4,6-trichloro-].

CLINICAL PHARMACOLOGY

pHisoHex is a bacteriostatic cleansing agent. It cleanses the skin thoroughly and has bacteriostatic action against staphylococci and other gram-positive bacteria. Cumulative antibacterial action develops with repeated use. Cleansing with alcohol or soaps containing alcohol removes the antibacterial residue.

Detectable blood levels of hexachlorophene following absorption through intact skin have been found in subjects who regularly scrubbed with hexachlorophene emulsion 3%. (See **WARNINGS** for additional information.)

pHisoHex has the same slight acidity as normal skin (pH value 5.0 to 6.0).

INDICATIONS AND USAGE

pHisoHex is indicated for use as a surgical scrub and a bacteriostatic skin cleanser. It may also be used to control an outbreak of gram-positive infection where other infection control procedures have been unsuccessful. Use only as long as necessary for infection control.

CONTRAINDICATIONS

pHisoHex should not be used on burned or denuded skin. It should not be used as an occlusive dressing, wet pack, or lotion.

It should not be used routinely for prophylactic total body bathing.

It should not be used as a vaginal pack or tampon, or on any mucous membranes.

pHisoHex should not be used on persons with sensitivity to any of its components. It should not be used on persons who have demonstrated primary light sensitivity to halogenated phenol derivatives because of the possibility of cross-sensitivity to hexachlorophene.

WARNINGS

RINSE THOROUGHLY AFTER EACH USE. Patients should be closely monitored and use should be immediately discontinued at the first sign of any of the symptoms described below.

Rapid absorption of hexachlorophene may occur with resultant toxic blood levels when preparations containing hexachlorophene are applied to skin lesions such as ichthyosis congenita, the dermatitis of Letterer-Siwe's syndrome, or other generalized dermatological conditions. Application to burns has also produced neurotoxicity and death.

pHisoHex SHOULD BE DISCONTINUED PROMPTLY IF SIGNS OR SYMPTOMS OF CEREBRAL IRRITABILITY OCCUR.

Infants, especially premature infants or those with dermatoses, are particularly susceptible to hexachlorophene absorption. Systemic toxicity may be manifested by signs of stimulation (irritation) of the central nervous system, sometimes with convulsions.

Infants have developed dermatitis, irritability, generalized clonic muscular contractions and decerebrate rigidity following application of a 6 percent hexachlorophene powder. Examination of brainstems of those infants revealed vacuolization like that which can be produced in newborn experimental animals following repeated topical application of 3 percent hexachlorophene. Moreover, a study of histologic sections of premature infants who died of unrelated causes has shown a positive correlation between hexachlorophene baths and lesions in white matter of brains.

PRECAUTIONS

General

Avoid accidental contact of pHisoHex with the eyes. If contact occurs, promptly rinse thoroughly with water. To assist in the detection of ocular irritation, applications to the head and periorbital skin areas should be performed only in responsive patients with unanesthetized eyes.

RINSE THOROUGHLY AFTER USE, especially from sensitive areas such as the scrotum and perineum.

pHisoHex is intended for external use only. If swallowed, pHisoHex is harmful, especially to infants and children. **pHisoHex should not be poured into measuring cups, medicine bottles, or similar containers since it may be mistaken for baby formula or other medications.**

Carcinogenesis, Mutagenesis, Impairment of Fertility

Carcinogenicity studies in animals: Hexachlorophene was tested in one experiment in rats by oral administration; it had no carcinogenic effect.

Hexachlorophene was not mutagenic in *Salmonella typhimurium* and was negative in a dominant lethal assay in male mice. Cytogenetic tests with cultured human lymphocytes were also negative.

Human data: No case reports or epidemiological studies were available.

Impairment of fertility: Topical exposure of neonatal rats to 3% hexachlorophene solution caused reduced fertility in 7-month-old males, due to inability to ejaculate.

Embryotoxicity and Teratogenicity

Placental transfer of hexachlorophene has been demonstrated in rats.

Hexachlorophene is embryotoxic and produces some teratogenic effects.

Pregnancy Category C

There are no adequate and well-controlled studies in pregnant women. Hexachlorophene should be used during pregnancy only if the potential benefit justifies potential risk to the fetus.

Hexachlorophene has been shown to be teratogenic and embryotoxic in rats when given by mouth or instilled into the vagina in large doses.

Administration of 500 mg/kg diet or 20 to 30 mg/kg bw/day by gavage to rats caused some malformations (angulated ribs, cleft palate, micro- and anophthalmia) and reduction in litter size.

Placental transfer and excretion in milk of hexachlorophene has been demonstrated in rats.

In another study, doses of up to 50 mg/kg diet failed to produce any effects in 3 generations of rats. Hexachlorophene did not interfere with reproduction in hamsters.

Nursing Mothers

It is not known whether this drug is excreted in human milk. Because many drugs are excreted in human milk and because of the potential for serious adverse reactions in nursing infants from hexachlorophene, a decision should be made whether to discontinue nursing or to discontinue the drug taking into account the importance of the drug to the mother.

Pediatric Use

pHisoHex, brand of hexachlorophene detergent cleanser, should not be used routinely for bathing infants. See **WARNINGS.** For premature infants: see **WARNINGS.**

ADVERSE REACTIONS

Adverse reactions to pHisoHex may include dermatitis and photosensitivity. Sensitivity to hexachlorophene is rare; however, persons who have developed photoallergy to similar compounds also may become sensitive to hexachlorophene.

In persons with highly sensitive skin the use of pHisoHex may at times produce a reaction characterized by redness and/or mild scaling or dryness, especially when it is combined with such mechanical factors as excessive rubbing or exposure to heat or cold.

OVERDOSAGE

The accidental ingestion of pHisoHex in amounts from 1 oz to 4 oz has caused anorexia, vomiting, abdominal cramps, diarrhea, dehydration, convulsions, hypotension, and shock, and in several reported instances, fatalities.

If patients are seen early, the stomach should be evacuated by emesis or gastric lavage. Olive oil or vegetable oil (60 mL or 2 fl oz) may then be given to delay absorption of hexachlorophene, followed by a saline cathartic to hasten removal. Treatment is symptomatic and supportive; intravenous fluids (5 percent dextrose in physiologic saline solution) may be given for dehydration. Any other electrolyte derangement should be corrected. If marked hypotension occurs, vasopressor therapy is indicated. Use of opiates may be considered if gastrointestinal symptoms (cramping, diarrhea) are severe. Scheduled medical or surgical procedures should be postponed until the patient's condition has been evaluated and stabilized.

DOSAGE AND ADMINISTRATION

Surgical Hand Scrub

1. Wet hands and forearms with water. Apply approximately 5 mL of pHisoHex over the hands and rub into a copious lather by adding small amounts of water. Spread suds over hands and forearms and scrub well with a wet brush for 3 minutes. Pay particular attention to the nails and interdigital spaces. A separate nail cleaner may be used. *Rinse thoroughly* under running water.

2. Apply 5 mL of pHisoHex to hands again and scrub as above for another 3 minutes. *Rinse thoroughly* with running water and dry.

3. For repeat surgical scrubs during the day, scrub thoroughly with the same amount of pHisoHex for 3 minutes only. *Rinse thoroughly* with water and dry.

Bacteriostatic Cleansing

Wet hands with water. Dispense approximately 5 mL of pHisoHex into the palm, work up a lather with water and apply to area to be cleansed.

Rinse thoroughly after each washing.

INFANT CARE: pHisoHex should not be used routinely for bathing infants. See **WARNINGS.**

PREMATURE INFANTS: See **WARNINGS.**

Use of baby skin products containing alcohol may decrease the antibacterial action of pHisoHex, brand of hexachlorophene detergent cleanser.

HOW SUPPLIED

pHisoHex is available in plastic squeeze bottle of 5 ounces (NDC 0024-1535-02) and 1 pint (NDC 0024-1535-06); in plastic bottle of 1 gallon (NDC 0024-1535-08) and ¼ oz (8 mL) unit packets, box of 50 (NDC 0024-1535-05).

The following, specially constructed, refillable dispensers made with metals and plastics compatible with pHisoHex can also be supplied: 16 oz hand operated wall dispensers; 30 oz pedal operated wall dispensers; 30 oz pedal operated wall dispenser with stand; portable stand with two 30 oz pedal operated dispensers.

Prolonged direct exposure of pHisoHex to strong light may cause brownish surface discoloration but does not affect its antibacterial or detergent properties. Shaking will disperse the color. If pHisoHex is spilled or splashed on porous surfaces, rinse off to avoid discoloration.

> **pHisoHex should not be dispensed from, or stored in, containers with ordinary metal parts. A special type of stainless steel must be used or undesirable discoloration of the product or oxidation of metal may occur. Specially designed dispensers for hospital or office use may be obtained through your local dealer.**

Directions for Cleaning Dispensers: Before initial installation and use, run an antiseptic, such as an aqueous solution of benzalkonium chloride, NF, 1:500 to 1:750, or alcohol, through the working parts; rinse with sterile water. At weekly intervals thereafter, remove dispenser and pour off remainder of pHisoHex emulsion. Rinse empty dispenser with water. Run water through the working parts by operating the dispenser. Sanitize as described above. Rinse thoroughly with sterile water.

ANIMAL TOXICITY

The oral LD_{50} of hexachlorophene in male rats is 66 mg/kg bw, in females 56 mg/kg bw, and in weanling rats 120 mg/kg bw.

In suckling rats (10-days old), it is 9 mg/kg bw.

PW-61-GG

PLAQUENIL® Sulfate   ℞
brand of hydroxychloroquine sulfate tablets, USP

> **WARNING**
> **PHYSICIANS SHOULD COMPLETELY FAMILIARIZE THEMSELVES WITH THE COMPLETE CONTENTS OF THIS LEAFLET BEFORE PRESCRIBING HYDROXY-CHLOROQUINE.**

DESCRIPTION

The compound is a colorless crystalline solid, soluble in water to at least 20 percent; chemically the drug is 2-[[4-[(7-Chloro-4- quinolyl) amino] pentyl] ethylamino] ethanol sulfate (1:1).

Inactive Ingredients: Dibasic Calcium Phosphate, Magnesium Stearate, Starch.

ACTIONS

The drug possesses antimalarial actions and also exerts a beneficial effect in lupus erythematosus (chronic discoid or systemic) and acute or chronic rheumatoid arthritis. The precise mechanism of action is not known.

INDICATIONS

PLAQUENIL is indicated for the suppressive treatment and treatment of acute attacks of malaria due to *Plasmodium vivax, P. malariae, P. ovale,* and susceptible strains of *P. falciparum.* It is also indicated for the treatment of discoid and systemic lupus erythematosus, and rheumatoid arthritis.

CONTRAINDICATIONS

Use of this drug is contraindicated (1) in the presence of retinal or visual field changes attributable to any 4-aminoquinoline compound, (2) in patients with known hypersensitivity to 4-aminoquinoline compounds, and (3) for long-term therapy in children.

WARNINGS, General

PLAQUENIL is not effective against chloroquine-resistant strains of *P. falciparum.*

Children are especially sensitive to the 4-aminoquinoline compounds. A number of fatalities have been reported fol-

Continued on next page

This product information was prepared in August 1992. On these and other products of Sanofi Winthrop Pharmaceuticals, detailed information may be obtained on a current basis by direct inquiry to Product Information Services, 90 Park Avenue, New York, NY 10016 (toll free 1-800-446-6267).

Sanofi Winthrop—Cont.

lowing the accidental ingestion of chloroquine, sometimes in relatively small doses (0.75 g or 1 g in one 3- year-old child). Patients should be strongly warned to keep these drugs out of the reach of children.

Use of PLAQUENIL in patients with psoriasis may precipitate a severe attack of psoriasis. When used in patients with porphyria the condition may be exacerbated. The preparation should not be used in these conditions unless in the judgment of the physician the benefit to the patient outweighs the possible hazard.

Usage in Pregnancy—Usage of this drug during pregnancy should be avoided except in the suppression or treatment of malaria when in the judgment of the physician the benefit outweighs the possible hazard. It should be noted that radioactively-tagged chloroquine administered intravenously to pregnant, pigmented CBA mice passed rapidly across the placenta. It accumulated selectively in the melanin structures of the fetal eyes and was retained in the ocular tissues for five months after the drug had been eliminated from the rest of the body.

PRECAUTIONS, General

Antimalarial compounds should be used with caution in patients with hepatic disease or alcoholism or in conjunction with known hepatotoxic drugs.

Periodic blood cell counts should be made if patients are given prolonged therapy. If any severe blood disorder appears which is not attributable to the disease under treatment, discontinuation of the drug should be considered. The drug should be administered with caution in patients having G-6-PD (glucose-6-phosphate dehydrogenase) deficiency.

OVERDOSAGE

The 4-aminoquinoline compounds are very rapidly and completely absorbed after ingestion, and in accidental overdosage, or rarely with lower doses in hypersensitive patients, toxic symptoms may occur within 30 minutes. These consist of headache, drowsiness, visual disturbances, cardiovascular collapse, and convulsions, followed by sudden and early respiratory and cardiac arrest. The electrocardiogram may reveal atrial standstill, nodal rhythm, prolonged intraventricular conduction time, and progressive bradycardia leading to ventricular fibrillation and/or arrest. Treatment is symptomatic and must be prompt with immediate evacuation of the stomach by emesis (at home, before transportation to the hospital) or gastric lavage until the stomach is completely emptied. If finely powdered, activated charcoal is introduced by the stomach tube, after lavage, and within 30 minutes after ingestion of the tablets, it may inhibit further intestinal absorption of the drug. To be effective, the dose of activated charcoal should be at least five times the estimated dose of hydroxychloroquine ingested. Convulsions, if present, should be controlled before attempting gastric lavage. If due to cerebral stimulation, cautious administration of an ultrashort-acting barbiturate may be tried but, if due to anoxia, it should be corrected by oxygen administration, artificial respiration or, in shock with hypotension, by vasopressor therapy. Because of the importance of supporting respiration, tracheal intubation or tracheostomy, followed by gastric lavage, may also be necessary. Exchange transfusions have been used to reduce the level of 4-aminoquinoline drug in the blood.

A patient who survives the acute phase and is asymptomatic should be closely observed for at least six hours. Fluids may be forced, and sufficient ammonium chloride (8 g daily in divided doses for adults) may be administered for a few days to acidify the urine to help promote urinary excretion in cases of both overdosage and sensitivity.

MALARIA

ACTIONS

Like chloroquine phosphate, USP, PLAQUENIL sulfate is highly active against the erythrocytic forms of *P. vivax* and *malariae* and most strains of *P. falciparum* (but not the gametocytes of *P. falciparum*).

PLAQUENIL sulfate does not prevent relapses in patients with *vivax* or *malariae* malaria because it is not effective against exo-erythrocytic forms of the parasite, nor will it prevent *vivax* or *malariae* infection when administered as a prophylactic. It is highly effective as a suppressive agent in patients with *vivax* or *malariae* malaria, in terminating acute attacks, and significantly lengthening the interval between treatment and relapse. In patients with *falciparum* malaria, it abolishes the acute attack and effects complete cure of the infection, unless due to a resistant strain of *P. falciparum*.

INDICATIONS

PLAQUENIL sulfate, brand of hydroxychloroquine sulfate tablets, is indicated for the treatment of acute attacks and suppression of malaria.

WARNING

In recent years, it has been found that certain strains of *P. falciparum* have become resistant to 4-aminoquinoline compounds (including hydroxychloroquine) as shown by the fact that normally adequate doses have failed to prevent or cure clinical malaria or parasitemia. Treatment with quinine or other specific forms of therapy is therefore advised for patients infected with a resistant strain of parasites.

ADVERSE REACTIONS

Following the administration in doses adequate for the treatment of an acute malarial attack, mild and transient headache, dizziness, and gastrointestinal complaints (diarrhea, anorexia, nausea, abdominal cramps and, on rare occasions, vomiting) may occur.

DOSAGE AND ADMINISTRATION

One tablet of 200 mg of hydroxychloroquine sulfate is equivalent to 155 mg base.

Malaria: Suppression—*In adults,* 400 mg (=310 mg base) on exactly the same day of each week. *In infants and children,* the weekly suppressive dosage is 5 mg, calculated as base, per kg of body weight, but should not exceed the adult dose regardless of weight.

If circumstances permit, suppressive therapy should begin two weeks prior to exposure. However, failing this, in adults an initial double (loading) dose of 800 mg (= 620 mg base), or in children 10 mg base/kg may be taken in two divided doses, six hours apart. The suppressive therapy should be continued for eight weeks after leaving the endemic area.

Treatment of the acute attack—*In adults,* an initial dose of 800 mg (= 620 mg base) followed by 400 mg (= 310 mg base) in six to eight hours and 400 mg (310 mg base) on each of two consecutive days (total 2 g hydroxychloroquine sulfate or 1.55 g base). An alternative method, employing a single dose of 800 mg (= 620 mg base), has also proved effective.

The dosage for adults may also be calculated on the basis of body weight; this method is preferred for infants and children. A total dose representing 25 mg of base per kg of body weight is administered in three days, as follows:

First dose: 10 mg base per kg (but not exceeding a single dose of 620 mg base).

Second dose: 5 mg base per kg (but not exceeding a single dose of 310 mg base) 6 hours after first dose.

Third dose: 5 mg base per kg 18 hours after second dose.

Fourth dose: 5 mg base per kg 24 hours after third dose.

For radical cure of *vivax* and *malariae* malaria concomitant therapy with an 8-aminoquinoline compound is necessary.

LUPUS ERYTHEMATOSUS AND RHEUMATOID ARTHRITIS

INDICATIONS

PLAQUENIL is useful in patients with the following disorders who have not responded satisfactorily to drugs with less potential for serious side effects: lupus erythematosus (chronic discoid and systemic) and acute or chronic rheumatoid arthritis.

WARNINGS

PHYSICIANS SHOULD COMPLETELY FAMILIARIZE THEMSELVES WITH THE COMPLETE CONTENTS OF THIS LEAFLET BEFORE PRESCRIBING PLAQUENIL.

Irreversible retinal damage has been observed in some patients who had received long-term or high-dosage 4-aminoquinoline therapy for discoid and systemic lupus erythematosus, or rheumatoid arthritis. Retinopathy has been reported to be dose related.

When prolonged therapy with any antimalarial compound is contemplated, initial (base line) and periodic (every three months) ophthalmologic examinations (including visual acuity, expert slit-lamp, funduscopic, and visual field tests) should be performed.

If there is any indication of abnormality in the visual acuity, visual field, or retinal macular areas (such as pigmentary changes, loss of foveal reflex), or any visual symptoms (such as light flashes and streaks) which are not fully explainable by difficulties of accommodation or corneal opacities, the drug should be discontinued immediately and the patient closely observed for possible progression. Retinal changes (and visual disturbances) may progress even after cessation of therapy.

All patients on long-term therapy with this preparation should be questioned and examined periodically, including the testing of knee and ankle reflexes, to detect any evidence of muscular weakness. If weakness occurs, discontinue the drug.

In the treatment of rheumatoid arthritis, if objective improvement (such as reduced joint swelling, increased mobility) does not occur within six months, the drug should be discontinued. Safe use of the drug in the treatment of juvenile arthritis has not been established.

PRECAUTIONS

Dermatologic reactions to PLAQUENIL sulfate, brand of hydroxychloroquine sulfate tablets, may occur and, therefore, proper care should be exercised when it is administered to any patient receiving a drug with a significant tendency to produce dermatitis.

The methods recommended for early diagnosis of "chloroquine retinopathy" consist of (1) funduscopic examination of the macula for fine pigmentary disturbances or loss of the foveal reflex and (2) examination of the central visual field with a small red test object for pericentral or paracentral scotoma or determination of retinal thresholds to red. Any unexplained visual symptoms, such as light flashes or streaks should also be regarded with suspicion as possible manifestations of retinopathy.

If serious toxic symptoms occur from overdosage or sensitivity, it has been suggested that ammonium chloride (8 g daily in divided doses for adults) be administered orally three or four days a week for several months after therapy has been stopped, as acidification of the urine increases renal excretion of the 4-aminoquinoline compounds by 20 to 90 percent. However, caution must be exercised in patients with impaired renal function and/or metabolic acidosis.

ADVERSE REACTIONS

Not all of the following reactions have been observed with every 4-aminoquinoline compound during long-term therapy, but they have been reported with one or more and should be borne in mind when drugs of this class are administered. Adverse effects with different compounds vary in type and frequency.

CNS Reactions: Irritability, nervousness, emotional changes, nightmares, psychosis, headache, dizziness, vertigo, tinnitus, nystagmus, nerve deafness, convulsions, ataxia.

Neuromuscular Reactions: Extraocular muscle palsies, skeletal muscle weakness, absent or hypoactive deep tendon reflexes.

Ocular Reactions:

A. *Ciliary body:* Disturbance of accommodation with symptoms of blurred vision. This reaction is dose related and reversible with cessation of therapy.

B. *Cornea:* Transient edema, punctate to lineal opacities, decreased corneal sensitivity. The corneal changes, with or without accompanying symptoms (blurred vision, halos around lights, photophobia), are fairly common, but reversible. Corneal deposits may appear as early as three weeks following initiation of therapy.

The incidence of corneal changes and visual side effects appears to be considerably lower with hydroxychloroquine than with chloroquine.

C. *Retina:*

Macula: Edema, atrophy, abnormal pigmentation (mild pigment stippling to a "bull's-eye" appearance), loss of foveal reflex, increased macular recovery time following exposure to a bright light (photo-stress test), elevated retinal threshold to red light in macular, paramacular and peripheral retinal areas.

Other fundus changes include optic disc pallor and atrophy, attenuation of retinal arterioles, fine granular pigmentary disturbances in the peripheral retina and prominent choroidal patterns in advanced stage.

D. *Visual field defects:* pericentral or paracentral scotoma, central scotoma with decreased visual acuity, rarely field constriction.

The most common visual symptoms attributed to the retinopathy are: reading and seeing difficulties (words, letters, or parts of objects missing), photophobia, blurred distance vision, missing or blacked out areas in the central or peripheral visual field, light flashes and streaks.

Retinopathy appears to be dose related and has occurred within several months (rarely) to several years of daily therapy; a small number of cases have been reported several years after antimalarial drug therapy was discontinued. It has not been noted during prolonged use of weekly doses of the 4-aminoquinoline compounds for suppression of malaria.

Patients with retinal changes may have visual symptoms or may be asymptomatic (with or without visual field changes). Rarely scotomatous vision or field defects may occur without obvious retinal change.

Retinopathy may progress even after the drug is discontinued. In a number of patients, early retinopathy (macular pigmentation sometimes with central field defects) diminished or regressed completely after therapy was discontinued. Paracentral scotoma to red targets (sometimes called "premaculopathy") is indicative of early retinal dysfunction which is usually reversible with cessation of therapy.

A small number of cases of retinal changes have been reported as occurring in patients who received only hydroxychloroquine. These usually consisted of alteration in retinal pigmentation which was detected on periodic ophthalmologic examination; visual field defects were also present in some instances. A case of delayed retinopathy has been reported with loss of vision starting one year after administration of hydroxychloroquine had been discontinued.

Dermatologic Reactions: Bleaching of hair, alopecia, pruritus, skin and mucosal pigmentation, skin eruptions (urticarial, morbilliform, lichenoid, maculopapular, purpuric, erythema annulare centrifugum and exfoliative dermatitis).

Hematologic Reactions: Various blood dyscrasias such as aplastic anemia, agranulocytosis, leukopenia, thrombocytopenia (hemolysis in individuals with glucose-6-phosphate dehydrogenase (G-6-PD) deficiency).

Gastrointestinal Reactions: Anorexia, nausea, vomiting, diarrhea, and abdominal cramps.

Miscellaneous Reactions: Weight loss, lassitude, exacerbation or precipitation of porphyria and nonlight-sensitive psoriasis.

DOSAGE AND ADMINISTRATION

One tablet of hydroxychloroquine sulfate, 200 mg, is equivalent to 155 mg base.

Lupus erythematosus —Initially, the average *adult* dose is 400 mg (=310 mg base) once or twice daily. This may be continued for several weeks or months, depending on the response of the patient. For prolonged maintenance therapy, a smaller dose, from 200 mg to 400 mg (=155 mg to 310 mg base) daily will frequently suffice.

The incidence of retinopathy has been reported to be higher when this maintenance dose is exceeded.

Rheumatoid arthritis —The compound is cumulative in action and will require several weeks to exert its beneficial therapeutic effects, whereas minor side effects may occur relatively early. Several months of therapy may be required before maximum effects can be obtained. If objective improvement (such as reduced joint swelling, increased mobility) does not occur within six months, the drug should be discontinued. Safe use of the drug in the treatment of juvenile rheumatoid arthritis has not been established.

Initial dosage —In *adults,* from 400 mg to 600 mg (=310 mg to 465 mg base) daily, each dose to be taken with a meal or a glass of milk. In a small percentage of patients, troublesome side effects may require temporary reduction of the initial dosage. Later (usually from five to ten days), the dose may gradually be increased to the optimum response level, often without return of side effects.

Maintenance dosage —When a good response is obtained (usually in four to twelve weeks), the dosage is reduced by 50 percent and continued at a usual maintenance level of 200 mg to 400 mg (=155 mg to 310 mg base) daily, each dose to be taken with a meal or a glass of milk. The incidence of retinopathy has been reported to be higher when this maintenance dose is exceeded.

Should a relapse occur after medication is withdrawn, therapy may be resumed or continued on an intermittent schedule if there are no ocular contraindications.

Corticosteroids and salicylates may be used in conjunction with this compound, and they can generally be decreased gradually in dosage or eliminated after the drug has been used for several weeks. When gradual reduction of steroid dosage is indicated, it may be done by reducing every four to five days the dose of cortisone by no more than from 5 mg to 15 mg; of hydrocortisone from 5 mg to 10 mg; of prednisolone and prednisone from 1 mg to 2.5 mg; of methylprednisolone and triamcinolone from 1 mg to 2 mg; and of dexamethasone from 0.25 mg to 0.5 mg.

HOW SUPPLIED

Tablets of 200 mg (equivalent to 155 mg of base), bottle of 100 (NDC 0024-1562-10).

Manufactured by Sterling Pharmaceuticals Inc.
Barceloneta, Puerto Rico 00617
Certain manufacturing operations have been
performed by other firms.

PW-306-T

Shown in Product Identification Section, page 428

PONTOCAINE® Hydrochloride   ℞
brand of tetracaine hydrochloride, USP

Prolonged Spinal Anesthesia

DESCRIPTION

Tetracaine hydrochloride is 2-(Dimethylamino)ethyl *p*-(butylamino) benzoate monohydrochloride. It is a white crystalline, odorless powder that is readily soluble in water, physiologic saline solution, and dextrose solution.

Tetracaine hydrochloride is a local anesthetic of the ester-linkage type, related to procaine.

PONTOCAINE hydrochloride is supplied in two forms for prolonged spinal anesthesia: Niphanoid® and 1% Solution.

NIPHANOID: A sterile, instantly soluble form consisting of a network of extremely fine, highly purified particles, resembling snow.

1% Solution: A sterile, isotonic, isobaric solution, each 1 mL containing 10 mg tetracaine hydrochloride, 6.7 mg sodium chloride, and not more than 2 mg acetone sodium bisulfite. The air in the ampuls has been displaced by nitrogen gas. The pH is 3.2 to 6.

These formulations do not contain preservatives.

CLINICAL PHARMACOLOGY

Parenteral administration of PONTOCAINE stabilizes the neuronal membrane and prevents initiation and transmission of nerve impulses thereby effecting local anesthesia. The onset of action is rapid, and the duration prolonged (up to two or three hours or longer of surgical anesthesia). PONTOCAINE is detoxified by plasma esterases to aminobenzoic acid and diethylaminoethanol.

INDICATIONS AND USAGE

PONTOCAINE is indicated for the production of spinal anesthesia for procedures requiring two to three hours.

CONTRAINDICATIONS

Spinal anesthesia with PONTOCAINE is contraindicated in patients with known hypersensitivity to tetracaine hydrochloride or to drugs of a similar chemical configuration (ester-type local anesthetics), or aminobenzoic acid or its derivatives; and in patients for whom spinal anesthesia as a technique is contraindicated.

The decision as to whether or not spinal anesthesia should be used for an individual patient should be made by the physician after weighing the advantages with the risks and possible complications. Contraindications to spinal anesthesia as a technique can be found in standard reference texts, and usually include generalized septicemia, infection at the site of injection, certain diseases of the cerebrospinal system, uncontrolled hypotension, etc.

WARNINGS

RESUSCITATIVE EQUIPMENT AND DRUGS SHOULD BE IMMEDIATELY AVAILABLE WHENEVER ANY LOCAL ANESTHETIC DRUG IS USED.

Large doses of local anesthetics should not be used in patients with heartblock.

Reactions resulting in fatality have occurred on rare occasions with the use of local anesthetics, even in the absence of a history of hypersensitivity.

Contains acetone sodium bisulfite, a sulfite that may cause allergic-type reactions including anaphylactic symptoms and life-threatening or less severe asthmatic episodes in certain susceptible people. The overall prevalence of sulfite sensitivity in the general population is unknown and probably low. Sulfite sensitivity is seen more frequently in asthmatic than in nonasthmatic people.

PRECAUTIONS

The safety and effectiveness of any spinal anesthetic depend upon proper dosage, correct technique, adequate precautions, and readiness for emergencies. The lowest dosage that results in effective anesthesia should be used to avoid high plasma levels and serious systemic side effects. Tolerance varies with the status of the patient; debilitated, elderly patients or acutely ill patients should be given reduced doses commensurate with their weight, age, and physical status. Reduced doses are also indicated for obstetric patients and those with increased intra-abdominal pressure.

Caution should be used in administering PONTOCAINE to patients with abnormal or reduced levels of plasma esterases.

Blood pressure should be frequently monitored during spinal anesthesia and hypotension immediately corrected.

Spinal anesthetics should be used with caution in patients with severe disturbances of cardiac rhythm, shock, or heartblock.

Drug Interactions: PONTOCAINE should not be used if the patient is being treated with a sulfonamide because aminobenzoic acid inhibits the action of sulfonamides.

Carcinogenesis, Mutagenesis, Impairment of Fertility: Long-term animal studies to evaluate carcinogenic potential and reproduction studies in animals have not been performed. There is no evidence from human data that PONTOCAINE may be carcinogenic or that it impairs fertility.

Pregnancy Category C: Animal reproduction studies have not been conducted with PONTOCAINE. It is not known whether PONTOCAINE can cause fetal harm when administered to a pregnant woman or can affect reproduction capacity. PONTOCAINE should be given to a pregnant woman only if clearly needed and the potential benefits outweigh the risk.

Labor and Delivery: Vasopressor agents administered for the treatment of hypotension resulting from spinal anesthesia may result in severe persistent hypertension and/or rupture of cerebral blood vessels if oxytocic drugs have also been administered; therefore, vasopressors should be used with extreme caution in the presence of oxytocic drugs.

PONTOCAINE has a recognized use during labor and delivery; the effect of the drug on duration of labor, incidence of forceps delivery, status of the newborn, and later growth and development of the child have not been studied.

Nursing Mothers: It is not known whether PONTOCAINE is excreted in human milk; however, it is rapidly metabolized following absorption into the plasma. Because many drugs are excreted in human milk, caution should be exercised when PONTOCAINE, brand of tetracaine hydrochloride, is administered to a nursing woman.

Pediatric Use: Safety and effectiveness of PONTOCAINE in children have not been established.

ADVERSE REACTIONS

Systemic adverse reactions to PONTOCAINE are characteristic of those associated with other local anesthetics and can involve the central nervous system and the cardiovascular system. Systemic reactions usually result from high plasma levels due to excessive dosage, rapid absorption, or inadvertent intravascular injection.

A small number of reactions to PONTOCAINE may result from hypersensitivity, idiosyncrasy, or diminished tolerance to normal dosage.

Central nervous system effects are characterized by excitation or depression. The first manifestation may be nervousness, dizziness, blurred vision, or tremors, followed by drowsiness, convulsions, unconsciousness and possibly respiratory and cardiac arrest. Since excitement may be transient or absent, the first manifestation may be drowsiness, sometimes merging into unconsciousness and respiratory and cardiac arrest. Other central nervous system effects may be nausea, vomiting, chills, constriction of the pupils, or tinnitus.

Cardiovascular system reactions include depression of the myocardium, blood pressure changes (usually hypotension), and cardiac arrest.

Allergic reactions, which may be due to hypersensitivity, idiosyncrasy, or diminished tolerance, are characterized by cutaneous lesions (eg, urticaria), edema, and other manifestations of allergy. Detection of sensitivity by skin testing is of limited value. Severe allergic reactions including anaphylaxis have occurred rarely and are not usually dose-related.

Reactions Associated with Spinal Anesthesia Techniques: *Central Nervous System:* post-spinal headache, meningismus, arachnoiditis, palsies, or spinal nerve paralysis. *Cardiovascular:* hypotension due to vasomotor paralysis and pooling of the blood in the venous bed. *Respiratory:* respiratory impairment or paralysis due to the level of anesthesia extending to the upper thoracic and cervical segments. *Gastrointestinal:* nausea and vomiting.

Treatment of Reactions: Toxic effects of local anesthetics require symptomatic treatment; there is no specific cure. **The most important measure is oxygenation of the patient by maintaining an airway and supporting ventilation.** Supportive treatment of the cardiovascular system includes intravenous fluids and, when appropriate, vasopressors (preferably those that stimulate the myocardium). Convulsions are usually controlled with adequate oxygenation alone but intravenous administration in small increments of a barbiturate (preferably an ultrashort-acting barbiturate such as thiopental and thiamylal) or diazepam can be utilized. Intravenous barbiturates or anticonvulsant agents should only be administered by those familiar with their use and only if ventilation and oxygenation have first been assured. In spinal anesthesia, sympathetic blockade also occurs as a pharmacological action, resulting in peripheral vasodilation and often hypotension. The extent of the hypotension will usually depend on the number of dermatomes blocked. The blood pressure should therefore be monitored in the early phases of anesthesia. If hypotension occurs, it is readily controlled by vasoconstrictors administered either by the intramuscular or the intravenous route, the dosage of which would depend on the severity of the hypotension and the response to treatment.

DOSAGE AND ADMINISTRATION

As with all anesthetics, the dosage varies and depends upon the area to be anesthetized, the number of neuronal segments to be blocked, individual tolerance, and the technique of anesthesia. The lowest dosage needed to provide effective anesthesia should be administered. For specific techniques and procedures, refer to standard textbooks.

[See table on next page.]

The extent and degree of spinal anesthesia depend upon dosage, specific gravity of the anesthetic solution, volume of solution used, force of the injection, level of puncture, position of the patient during and immediately after injection, etc.

When spinal fluid is added to either the NIPHANOID or solution, some turbidity results, the degree depending on the pH of the spinal fluid, the temperature of the solution during mixing, as well as the amount of drug and diluent employed. This cloudiness is due to the release of the *base* from the hydrochloride. Liberation of base (which is completed within the spinal canal) is held to be essential for satisfactory results with any spinal anesthetic.

Continued on next page

This product information was prepared in August 1992. On these and other products of Sanofi Winthrop Pharmaceuticals, detailed information may be obtained on a current basis by direct inquiry to Product Information Services, 90 Park Avenue, New York, NY 10016 (toll free 1-800-446-6267).

Sanofi Winthrop—Cont.

SUGGESTED DOSAGE FOR SPINAL ANESTHESIA

Extent of anesthesia	Using NIPHANOID		Using 1% Solution		Site of injection (lumbar interspace)
	Dose of NIPHANOID (mg)	Volume of spinal fluid (mL)	Dose of solution (mL)	Volume of spinal fluid (mL)	
Perineum	5*	1	0.5 (=5 mg)*	0.5	4th
Perineum and lower extremities	10	2	1 (=10 mg)	1	3d or 4th
Up to costal margin	15 to 20†	3	1.5 to 2 (=15 mg to 20 mg)†	1.5 to 2	2d, 3d, or 4th

*For vaginal delivery (saddle block), from 2 mg to 5 mg in dextrose.
†Doses exceeding 15 mg are rarely required and should be used only in exceptional cases. Inject solution at rate of about 1 mL per 5 seconds.

The specific gravity of spinal fluid at 25°C/25°C varies under normal conditions from 1.0063 to 1.0075. A solution of the instantly soluble form (NIPHANOID) in spinal fluid has only a slightly greater specific gravity. The 1% concentration in saline solution has a specific gravity of 1.0060 to 1.0074 at 25°C/25°C.

A hyperbaric solution may be prepared by mixing equal volumes of the 1% Solution and Dextrose Solution 10% (which is available in ampuls of 3 mL).

If the NIPHANOID form is preferred, it is first dissolved in Dextrose Solution 10% in a ratio of 1 mL dextrose to 10 mg of the anesthetic. Further dilution is made with an equal volume of spinal fluid. The resulting solution now contains 5% dextrose with 5 mg of anesthetic agent per milliliter.

A hypobaric solution may be prepared by dissolving the NIPHANOID in Sterile Water for Injection, USP (1 mg per milliliter). The specific gravity of this solution is essentially the same as that of water, 1.000 at 25°C/25°C.

Examine ampuls carefully before use. Do not use solution if crystals, cloudiness, or discoloration is observed.

These formulations of tetracaine hydrochloride do not contain preservatives; therefore, unused portions should be discarded and the reconstituted NIPHANOID should be used immediately.

STERILIZATION OF AMPULS

The drug in intact ampuls is sterile. The preferred method of destroying bacteria on the exterior of ampuls before opening is heat sterilization (autoclaving). Immersion in antiseptic solution is not recommended.

Autoclave at 15-pound pressure, at 121°C (250°F), for 15 minutes. The NIPHANOID form may also be autoclaved in the same way but may lose its snowlike appearance and tend to adhere to the sides of the ampul. This may slightly decrease the rate at which the drug dissolves but does not interfere with its anesthetic potency.

Autoclaving increases likelihood of crystal formation. Unused autoclaved ampuls should be discarded. Under no circumstance should unused ampuls which have been autoclaved be returned to stock.

HOW SUPPLIED

Protect ampuls from light and store solution under refrigeration.

NIPHANOID (instantly soluble): Ampuls of 20 mg, box of 100.
NDC 0024-1577-06
Uni-Nest ™—1% isotonic isobaric solution: Ampuls of 2 mL, box of 25.
NDC 0024-1574-25

PW-56-Z

TALACEN®   © ℞
Pentazocine hydrochloride, USP,
equivalent to 25 mg base
and acetaminophen, USP, 650 mg

DESCRIPTION

TALACEN is a combination of pentazocine hydrochloride, USP, equivalent to 25 mg base and acetaminophen, USP, 650 mg.

Pentazocine is a member of the benzazocine series (also known as the benzomorphan series). Chemically, pentazocine is 1,2,3,4,5,6-hexahydro-6,11-dimethyl-3-(3-methyl-2-butenyl)-2,6-methano-3-benzazocin-8-ol, a white, crystalline substance soluble in acidic aqueous solutions.

Chemically, acetaminophen is Acetamide, N-(4-hydroxyphenyl)-.

Pentazocine is an analgesic and acetaminophen is an analgesic and antipyretic.

TALACEN is a pale blue, scored caplet for oral administration.

Inactive Ingredients: Colloidal Silicon Dioxide, FD&C Blue

#1, Gelatin, Microcrystalline Cellulose, Potassium Sorbate, Pregelatinized Starch, Sodium Lauryl Sulfate, Sodium Metabisulfite, Sodium Starch Glycolate, Stearic Acid.

CLINICAL PHARMACOLOGY

TALACEN is an analgesic possessing antipyretic actions.

Pentazocine is an analgesic with agonist/antagonist action which when administered orally is approximately equivalent on a mg for mg basis in analgesic effect to codeine.

Acetaminophen is an analgesic and antipyretic.

Onset of significant analgesia with pentazocine usually occurs between 15 and 30 minutes after oral administration, and duration of action is usually three hours or longer. Onset and duration of action and the degree of pain relief are related both to dose and the severity of pretreatment pain. Pentazocine weakly antagonizes the analgesic effects of morphine, meperidine, and phenazocine; in addition, it produces incomplete reversal of cardiovascular, respiratory, and behavioral depression induced by morphine and meperidine. Pentazocine has about 1/50 the antagonistic activity of nalorphine. It also has sedative activity.

Pentazocine is well absorbed from the gastrointestinal tract. Plasma levels closely correspond to the onset, duration, and intensity of analgesia. The mean peak concentration in 24 normal volunteers was 1.7 hours (range 0.5 to 4 hours) after oral administration and the mean plasma elimination half-life was 3.6 hours (range 1.5 to 10 hours).

The action of pentazocine is terminated for the most part by biotransformation in the liver with some free pentazocine excreted in the urine. The products of the oxidation of the terminal methyl groups and glucuronide conjugates are excreted by the kidney. Elimination of approximately 60% of the total dose occurs within 24 hours. Pentazocine passes the placental barrier.

Onset of significant analgesic and antipyretic activity of acetaminophen when administered orally occurs within 30 minutes and is maximal at approximately 2½ hours. The pharmacological mode of action of acetaminophen is unknown at this time.

Acetaminophen is rapidly and almost completely absorbed from the gastrointestinal tract. In 24 normal volunteers the mean peak plasma concentration was 1 hour (range 0.25 to 3 hours) after oral administration and the mean plasma elimination half-life was 2.8 hours (range 2 to 4 hours).

The effect of pentazocine on acetaminophen plasma protein binding or vice versa has not been established. For acetaminophen there is little or no plasma protein binding at normal therapeutic doses. When toxic doses of acetaminophen are ingested and drug plasma levels exceed 90 $\mu g/mL$, plasma binding may vary from 8% to 43%.

Acetaminophen is conjugated in the liver with glucuronic acid and to a lesser extent with sulfuric acid. Approximately 80% of acetaminophen is excreted in the urine after conjugation and about 3% is excreted unchanged. The drug is also conjugated to a lesser extent with cysteine and additionally metabolized by hydroxylation.

If TALACEN is taken every 4 hours over an extended period of time, accumulation of pentazocine and to a lesser extent, acetaminophen, may occur.

INDICATIONS AND USAGE

TALACEN is indicated for the relief of mild to moderate pain.

CONTRAINDICATIONS

TALACEN should not be administered to patients who are hypersensitive to either pentazocine or acetaminophen.

WARNINGS

Contains sodium metabisulfite, a sulfite that may cause allergic-type reactions including anaphylactic symptoms and life-threatening or less severe asthmatic episodes in certain susceptible people. The overall prevalence of sulfite sensitivity in the general population is unknown and probably low. Sulfite sensitivity is seen more frequently in asthmatic than in nonasthmatic people.

Head Injury and Increased Intracranial Pressure. As in the case of other potent analgesics, the potential of pentazocine for elevating cerebrospinal fluid pressure may be attributed to CO_2 retention due to the respiratory depressant effects of the drug. These effects may be markedly exaggerated in the presence of head injury, other intracranial lesions, or a preexisting increase in intracranial pressure. Furthermore, pentazocine can produce effects which may obscure the clinical course of patients with head injuries. In such patients, TALACEN must be used with extreme caution and only if its use is deemed essential.

Acute CNS Manifestations. Patients receiving therapeutic doses of pentazocine have experienced hallucinations (usually visual), disorientation, and confusion which have cleared spontaneously within a period of hours. The mechanism of this reaction is not known. Such patients should be closely observed and vital signs checked. If the drug is reinstituted, it should be done with caution since these acute CNS manifestations may recur.

There have been instances of psychological and physical dependence on parenteral pentazocine in patients with a history of drug abuse, and rarely, in patients without such a history. (See DRUG ABUSE AND DEPENDENCE.)

Due to the potential for increased CNS depressant effects, alcohol should be used with caution in patients who are currently receiving pentazocine.

Pentazocine may precipitate opioid abstinence symptoms in patients receiving courses of opiates for pain relief.

PRECAUTIONS

In prescribing TALACEN for chronic use, the physician should take precautions to avoid increases in dose by the patient.

Myocardial Infarction. As with all drugs, TALACEN should be used with caution in patients with myocardial infarction who have nausea or vomiting.

Certain Respiratory Conditions. Although respiratory depression has rarely been reported after oral administration of pentazocine, the drug should be administered with caution to patients with respiratory depression from any cause, severely limited respiratory reserve, severe bronchial asthma and other obstructive respiratory conditions, or cyanosis.

Impaired Renal or Hepatic Function. Decreased metabolism of the drug by the liver in extensive liver disease may predispose to accentuation of side effects. Although laboratory tests have not indicated that pentazocine causes or increases renal or hepatic impairment, the drug should be administered with caution to patients with such impairment. Since acetaminophen is metabolized by the liver, the question of the safety of its use in the presence of liver disease should be considered.

Biliary Surgery. Narcotic drug products are generally considered to elevate biliary tract pressure for varying periods following their administration. Some evidence suggests that pentazocine may differ from other marketed narcotics in this respect (ie, it causes little or no elevation in biliary tract pressures). The clinical significance of these findings, however, is not yet known.

CNS Effect. Caution should be used when TALACEN is administered to patients prone to seizures; seizures have occurred in a few such patients in association with the use of pentazocine although no cause and effect relationship has been established.

Information for Patients. Since sedation, dizziness, and occasional euphoria have been noted, ambulatory patients should be warned not to operate machinery, drive cars, or unnecessarily expose themselves to hazards. Pentazocine may cause physical and psychological dependence when taken alone and may have additive CNS depressant properties when taken in combination with alcohol or other CNS depressants.

Drug Interactions. Pentazocine is a mild narcotic antagonist. Some patients previously given narcotics, including

methadone for the daily treatment of narcotic dependence, have experienced withdrawal symptoms after receiving pentazocine.

Carcinogenesis, Mutagenesis, Impairment of Fertility. Carcinogenesis, mutagenesis, and impairment of fertility studies have not been done with this combination product.

Pentazocine, when administered orally or parenterally, had no adverse effect on either the reproductive capabilities or the course of pregnancy in rabbits and rats. Embryotoxic effects on the fetuses were not shown.

The daily administration of 4 mg/kg to 20 mg/kg pentazocine subcutaneously to female rats during a 14 day pre-mating period and until the 13th day of pregnancy did not have any adverse effects on the fertility rate.

There is no evidence in long-term animal studies to demonstrate that pentazocine is carcinogenic.

Pregnancy Category C. Animal reproduction studies have not been conducted with TALACEN. It is also not known whether TALACEN can cause fetal harm when administered to pregnant women or can affect reproduction capacity. TALACEN should be given to pregnant women only if clearly needed. However, animal reproduction studies with pentazocine have not demonstrated teratogenic embryotoxic effects.

Nonteratogenic Effects. There has been no experience in this regard with the combination pentazocine and acetaminophen. However, there have been rare reports of possible abstinence syndromes in newborns after prolonged use of pentazocine during pregnancy.

Labor and Delivery. Patients receiving pentazocine during labor have experienced no adverse effects other than those that occur with commonly used analgesics. TALACEN should be used with caution in women delivering premature infants. The effect of TALACEN on the mother and fetus, the duration of labor or delivery, the possibility that forceps delivery or other intervention or resuscitation of the newborn may be necessary, or the effect of TALACEN, on the later growth, development, and functional maturation of the child are unknown at the present time.

Nursing Mothers. It is not known whether this drug is excreted in human milk. Because many drugs are excreted in human milk, caution should be exercised when TALACEN is administered to a nursing woman.

Pediatric Use. Safety and effectiveness in children below the age of 12 have not been established.

ADVERSE REACTIONS

Clinical experience with TALACEN has been insufficient to define all possible adverse reactions with this combination. However, reactions reported after oral administration of pentazocine hydrochloride in 50 mg dosage include *gastrointestinal:* nausea, vomiting, infrequently constipation; and rarely abdominal distress, anorexia, diarrhea. *CNS effects:* dizziness, lightheadedness, hallucinations, sedation, euphoria, headache, confusion, disorientation; infrequently weakness, disturbed dreams, insomnia, syncope, visual blurring and focusing difficulty, depression; and rarely tremor, irritability, excitement, tinnitus. *Autonomic:* sweating; infrequently flushing; and rarely chills. *Allergic:* infrequently rash; and rarely urticaria, edema of the face. *Cardiovascular:* infrequently decrease in blood pressure, tachycardia. *Hematologic:* rarely depression of white blood cells (especially granulocytes), which is usually reversible, moderate transient eosinophilia. *Other:* rarely respiratory depression, urinary retention, paresthesia, toxic epidermal necrolysis, and in one instance, an apparent anaphylactic reaction has been reported.

Numerous clinical studies have shown that acetaminophen, when taken in recommended doses, is relatively free of adverse effects in most age groups, even in the presence of a variety of disease states.

A few cases of hypersensitivity to acetaminophen have been reported, as manifested by skin rashes, thrombocytopenic purpura, rarely hemolytic anemia and agranulocytosis. Occasional individuals respond to ordinary doses with nausea and vomiting and diarrhea.

DRUG ABUSE AND DEPENDENCE

Controlled Substance. TALACEN is a Schedule IV controlled substance.

Abuse and Dependence. There have been some reports of dependence and of withdrawal symptoms with orally administered pentazocine. There have been recorded instances of psychological and physical dependence in patients using parenteral pentazocine. Abrupt discontinuance following the extended use of parenteral pentazocine has resulted in withdrawal symptoms. Patients with a history of drug dependence should be under close supervision while receiving TALACEN. There have been rare reports of possible abstinence syndromes in newborns after prolonged use of pentazocine during pregnancy.

Some tolerance to the analgesic and subjective effects of pentazocine develops with frequent and repeated use.

Drug addicts who are given closely spaced doses of pentazocine (eg, 60 mg to 90 mg every 4 hours) develop physical dependence which is demonstrated by abrupt withdrawal or by administration of naloxone. The withdrawal symptoms exhibited after chronic doses of more than 500 mg of pentazocine per day have similar characteristics, but to a lesser degree, of opioid withdrawal and may be associated with drug seeking behavior.

OVERDOSAGE

Manifestations. Clinical experience with TALACEN has been insufficient to define the signs of overdosage with this product. It may be assumed that signs and symptoms of TALACEN overdose would be a combination of those observed with pentazocine overdose and acetaminophen overdose.

For pentazocine alone in single doses above 60 mg there have been reports of the occurrence of nalorphine-like psychotomimetic effects such as anxiety, nightmares, strange thoughts, and hallucinations. Marked respiratory depression associated with increased blood pressure and tachycardia have also resulted from excessive doses as have dizziness, nausea, vomiting, lethargy, and paresthesias. The respiratory depression is antagonized by naloxone (see *Treatment*).

In acute acetaminophen overdosage, dose-dependent, potentially fatal hepatic necrosis is the most serious adverse effect. Renal tubular necrosis, hypoglycemic coma, and thrombocytopenia may also occur.

In adults, a single dose of 10 g to 15 g (200 mg/kg to 250 mg/kg) of acetaminophen may cause hepatotoxicity. A dose of 25 g or more is potentially fatal. The potential seriousness of the intoxication may not be evident during the first two days of acute acetaminophen poisoning. During the first 24 hours, nausea, vomiting, anorexia, and abdominal pain occur. These may persist for a week or more. Liver injury may become evident the second day, initial signs being elevation of serum transaminase and lactic dehydrogenase activity, increased serum bilirubin concentration, and prolongation of prothrombin time. Serum albumin concentration and alkaline phosphatase activity may remain normal. The hepatotoxicity may lead to encephalopathy, coma, and death. Transient azotemia is evident in a majority of patients and acute renal failure occurs in some.

There have been reports of glycosuria and impaired glucose tolerance, but hypoglycemia may also occur. Metabolic acidosis and metabolic alkalosis have been reported. Cerebral edema and nonspecific myocardial depression have also been noted. Biopsy reveals centrolobular necrosis with sparing of the periportal area. The hepatic lesions are reversible over a period of weeks or months in nonfatal cases.

The severity of the liver injury can be determined by measurement of the plasma half-time of acetaminophen during the first day of acute poisoning. If the half-time exceeds 4 hours, hepatic necrosis is likely and if the half-time is greater than 12 hours, hepatic coma will probably occur. Only minimal liver damage has developed when the serum concentration was below 120 μg/mL at 12 hours after ingestion of the drug. If serum bilirubin concentration is greater than 4 mg/100 mL during the first 5 days, encephalopathy may occur.

The seven day oral LD_{50} value for TALACEN in mice is 3570 mg/kg.

Treatment. Oxygen, intravenous fluids, vasopressors, and other supportive measures should be employed as indicated. Assisted or controlled ventilation should also be considered. For respiratory depression due to overdosage or unusual sensitivity to TALACEN, parenteral naloxone is a specific and effective antagonist.

The toxic effects of acetaminophen may be prevented or minimized by antidotal therapy with N-acetylcysteine. In order to obtain the best possible results, N-acetylcysteine should be administered within approximately 16 hours of ingestion of the overdose.

For complete prescribing information for the approved use of acetylcysteine in the treatment of acetaminophen overdose, see package insert for MUCOMYST® (acetylcysteine) Bristol-Myers Squibb.

Vigorous supportive therapy is required in severe intoxication. Procedures to limit the continuing absorption of the drug must be readily performed since the hepatic injury is dose dependent and occurs early in the course of intoxication. Induction of vomiting or gastric lavage, followed by oral administration of activated charcoal should be done in all cases.

If hemodialysis can be initiated within the first 12 hours, it is advocated for patients with a plasma acetaminophen concentration exceeding 120 μg/mL at 4 hours after ingestion of the drug.

DOSAGE AND ADMINISTRATION

Adult. The usual adult dose is 1 tablet every 4 hours as needed for pain relief, up to a maximum of 6 tablets per day. The usual duration of therapy is dependent upon the condition being treated but in any case should be reviewed regularly by the physician. The effect of meals on the rate and extent of bioavailability of both pentazocine and acetaminophen has not been documented.

HOW SUPPLIED

Caplets®, pale blue, scored, each containing pentazocine hydrochloride equivalent to 25 mg base and acetaminophen 650 mg.

Bottles of 100 (NDC 0024-1937-04).

Unit Dose Dispenser Package of 250 (NDC 0024-1937-14), 10 sleeves of 25 CAPLETS each.

Manufactured by
Sterling Pharmaceuticals Inc.
Barceloneta, Puerto Rico 00617

TW-262-L

Shown in Product Identification Section, page 428

TALWIN® Injection ℭ ℞
brand of pentazocine lactate injection, USP

Analgesic for Parenteral Use

DESCRIPTION

TALWIN injection, brand of pentazocine lactate injection, is a member of the benzazocine series (also known as the benzomorphan series). Chemically, pentazocine lactate is 1, 2, 3, 4, 5, 6-hexahydro-6, 11-dimethyl-3-(3-methyl-2-butenyl)-2,6-methano-3- benzazocin-8-ol lactate, a white, crystalline substance soluble in acidic aqueous solutions.

CLINICAL PHARMACOLOGY

TALWIN is a potent analgesic and 30 mg is usually as effective an analgesic as morphine 10 mg or meperidine 75 mg to 100 mg; however, a few studies suggest the TALWIN to morphine ratio may range from 20 mg to 40 mg TALWIN to 10 mg morphine. The duration of analgesia may sometimes be less than that of morphine. Analgesia usually occurs within 15 to 20 minutes after intramuscular or subcutaneous injection and within 2 to 3 minutes after intravenous injection. TALWIN weakly antagonizes the analgesic effects of morphine, meperidine, and phenazocine; in addition, it produces incomplete reversal of cardiovascular, respiratory, and behavioral depression induced by morphine and meperidine. TALWIN has about 1/50 the antagonistic activity of nalorphine. It also has sedative activity.

INDICATIONS AND USAGE

For the relief of moderate to severe pain. TALWIN may also be used for preoperative or preanesthetic medication and as a supplement to surgical anesthesia.

CONTRAINDICATION

TALWIN should not be administered to patients who are hypersensitive to it.

WARNINGS

Drug Dependence. *Special care should be exercised in prescribing pentazocine for emotionally unstable patients and for those with a history of drug misuse. Such patients should be closely supervised when greater than 4 or 5 days of therapy is contemplated. There have been instances of psychological and physical dependence on TALWIN in patients with such a history and, rarely, in patients without such a history. Extended use of parenteral TALWIN may lead to physical or psychological dependence in some patients. When TALWIN is abruptly discontinued, withdrawal symptoms such as abdominal cramps, elevated temperature, rhinorrhea, restlessness, anxiety, and lacrimation may occur. However, even when these have occurred, discontinuance has been accomplished with minimal difficulty. In the rare patient in whom more than minor difficulty has been encountered, reinstitution of parenteral TALWIN with gradual withdrawal has ameliorated the patient's symptoms. Substituting methadone or other narcotics for TALWIN in the treatment of the pentazocine abstinence syndrome should be avoided. There have been rare reports of possible abstinence syndromes in newborns after prolonged use of TALWIN during pregnancy.*

In prescribing parenteral TALWIN for chronic use, particularly if the drug is to be self-administered, the physician should take precautions to avoid increases in dose and frequency of injection by the patient.

Just as with all medication, the oral form of TALWIN is preferable for chronic administration.

Tissue Damage at Injection Sites. Severe sclerosis of the skin, subcutaneous tissues, and underlying muscle have occurred at the injection sites of patients who have received multiple doses of pentazocine lactate. Constant rotation of injection sites is, therefore, essential. In addition, animal studies have demonstrated that TALWIN is tolerated less

Continued on next page

This product information was prepared in August 1992. On these and other products of Sanofi Winthrop Pharmaceuticals, detailed information may be obtained on a current basis by direct inquiry to Product Information Services, 90 Park Avenue, New York, NY 10016 (toll free 1-800-446-6267).

well subcutaneously than intramuscularly. (See DOSAGE AND ADMINISTRATION.)

Head Injury and Increased Intracranial Pressure. As in the case of other potent analgesics, the potential of TALWIN injection for elevating cerebrospinal fluid pressure may be attributed to CO_2 retention due to the respiratory depressant effects of the drug. These effects may be markedly exaggerated in the presence of head injury, other intracranial lesions, or a preexisting increase in intracranial pressure. Furthermore, TALWIN can produce effects which may obscure the clinical course of patients with head injuries. In such patients, TALWIN must be used with extreme caution and only if its use is deemed essential.

Usage in Pregnancy. Safe use of TALWIN during pregnancy (other than labor) has not been established. Animal reproduction studies have not demonstrated teratogenic or embryotoxic effects. However, TALWIN should be administered to pregnant patients (other than labor) only when, in the judgment of the physician, the potential benefits outweigh the possible hazards. Patients receiving TALWIN during labor have experienced no adverse effects other than those that occur with commonly used analgesics. TALWIN should be used with caution in women delivering premature infants.

Acute CNS Manifestations. Patients receiving therapeutic doses of pentazocine have experienced hallucinations (usually visual), disorientation, and confusion which have cleared spontaneously within a period of hours. The mechanism of this reaction is not known. Such patients should be closely observed and vital signs checked. If the drug is reinstituted, it should be done with caution since these acute CNS manifestations may recur.

Due to the potential for increased CNS depressant effects, alcohol should be used with caution in patients who are currently receiving pentazocine.

Usage in Children. Because clinical experience in children under twelve years of age is limited, the use of TALWIN in this age group is not recommended.

Ambulatory Patients. Since sedation, dizziness, and occasional euphoria have been noted, ambulatory patients should be warned not to operate machinery, drive cars, or unnecessarily expose themselves to hazards.

Myocardial Infarction. Caution should be exercised in the intravenous use of pentazocine for patients with acute myocardial infarction accompanied by hypertension or left ventricular failure. Data suggest that intravenous administration of pentazocine increases systemic and pulmonary arterial pressure and systemic vascular resistance in patients with acute myocardial infarction.

NOTE: Acetone sodium bisulfite, a sulfite that may cause allergic-type reactions including anaphylactic symptoms and life-threatening or less severe asthmatic episodes in certain susceptible people, is contained in both Carpuject® Sterile Cartridge-Needle Unit and multiple-dose vials. The overall prevalence of sulfite sensitivity in the general population is unknown and probably low. Sulfite sensitivity is seen more frequently in asthmatic than in nonasthmatic people.

The ampuls in the Uni-Amp® Pak and the Uni-Nest™ Pak do not contain acetone sodium bisulfite.

PRECAUTIONS

Certain Respiratory Conditions. The possibility that TALWIN may cause respiratory depression should be considered in treatment of patients with bronchial asthma. TALWIN injection, brand of pentazocine lactate injection, should be administered only with caution and in low dosage to patients with respiratory depression (eg, from other medication, uremia, or severe infection), severely limited respiratory reserve, obstructive respiratory conditions, or cyanosis.

Impaired Renal or Hepatic Function. Although laboratory tests have not indicated that TALWIN causes or increases renal or hepatic impairment, the drug should be administered with caution to patients with such impairment. Extensive liver disease appears to predispose to greater side effects (eg, marked apprehension, anxiety, dizziness, sleepiness) from the usual clinical dose, and may be the result of decreased metabolism of the drug by the liver.

Biliary Surgery. Narcotic drug products are generally considered to elevate biliary tract pressure for varying periods following their administration. Some evidence suggests that pentazocine may differ from other marketed narcotics in this respect (ie, it causes little or no elevation in biliary tract pressures). The clinical significance of these findings, however, is not yet known.

Patients Receiving Narcotics. TALWIN is a mild narcotic antagonist. Some patients previously given narcotics, including methadone for the daily treatment of narcotic dependence, have experienced withdrawal symptoms after receiving TALWIN.

CNS Effect. Caution should be used when TALWIN is administered to patients prone to seizures; seizures have occurred in a few such patients in association with the use of TALWIN although no cause and effect relationship has been established.

Use in Anesthesia. Concomitant use of CNS depressants with parenteral TALWIN may produce additive CNS depression. Adequate equipment and facilities should be available to identify and treat systemic emergencies should they occur.

ADVERSE REACTIONS

The most commonly occurring reactions are: nausea, dizziness or lightheadedness, vomiting, euphoria.

Dermatologic Reactions: Soft tissue induration, nodules, and cutaneous depression can occur at injection sites. Ulceration (sloughing) and severe sclerosis of the skin and subcutaneous tissues (and, rarely, underlying muscle) have been reported after multiple doses. Other reported dermatologic reactions include diaphoresis, sting on injection, flushed skin including plethora, dermatitis including pruritus.

Infrequently occurring reactions are—*respiratory:* respiratory depression, dyspnea, transient apnea in a small number of newborn infants whose mothers received TALWIN during labor; *cardiovascular:* circulatory depression, shock, hypertension; *CNS effects:* dizziness, lightheadedness, hallucinations, sedation, euphoria, headache, confusion, disorientation; infrequently weakness, disturbed dreams, insomnia, syncope, visual blurring and focusing difficulty, depression; and rarely tremor, irritability, excitement, tinnitus. *Gastrointestinal:* constipation, dry mouth; *other:* urinary retention, headache, paresthesia, alterations in rate or strength of uterine contractions during labor.

Rarely reported reactions include—*neuromuscular and psychiatric:* muscle tremor, insomnia, disorientation, hallucinations; *gastrointestinal:* taste alteration, diarrhea and cramps; *ophthalmic:* blurred vision, nystagmus, diplopia, miosis; *hematologic:* depression of white blood cells (especially granulocytes), which is usually reversible, moderate transient eosinophilia; *other:* tachycardia, weakness or faintness, chills, allergic reactions including edema of the face, toxic epidermal necrolysis.

See **Acute CNS Manifestations** and **Drug Dependence** under **WARNINGS.**

DOSAGE AND ADMINISTRATION

Adults, Excluding Patients in Labor. The recommended single parenteral dose is 30 mg by intramuscular, subcutaneous, or intravenous route. This may be repeated every 3 to 4 hours. Doses in excess of 30 mg intravenously or 60 mg intramuscularly or subcutaneously are not recommended. Total daily dosage should not exceed 360 mg.

The subcutaneous route of administration should be used only when necessary because of possible severe tissue damage at injection sites (see WARNINGS). When frequent injections are needed, the drug should be administered intramuscularly. In addition, constant rotation of injection sites (eg, the upper outer quadrants of the buttocks, mid-lateral aspects of the thighs, and the deltoid areas) is essential.

Patients in Labor. A single, intramuscular 30 mg dose has been most commonly administered. An intravenous 20 mg dose has given adequate pain relief to some patients in labor when contractions become regular, and this dose may be given two or three times at two-to three-hour intervals, as needed.

Children Under 12 Years of Age. Since clinical experience in children under twelve years of age is limited, the use of TALWIN in this age group is not recommended.

CAUTION. TALWIN should not be mixed in the same syringe with soluble barbiturates because precipitation will occur.

OVERDOSAGE

Manifestations: Clinical experience with TALWIN overdosage has been insufficient to define the signs of this condition.

Treatment: Oxygen, intravenous fluids, vasopressors, and other supportive measures should be employed as indicated. Assisted or controlled ventilation should also be considered. For respiratory depression due to overdosage or unusual sensitivity to TALWIN, brand of pentazocine lactate injection, parenteral naloxone is a specific and effective antagonist.

HOW SUPPLIED

UNI-AMP—Individual unit dose ampuls of 1 mL (30 mg) **NDC 0024-1924-04**, *1.5 mL (45 mg)* **NDC 0024-1925-04**, *and 2 mL (60 mg)* **NDC 0024-1926-04** in box of 25.

UNI-NEST ampuls of 1 mL (30 mg) **NDC 0024-1924-14** *and 2 mL (60 mg)* **NDC 0024-1926-14** in box of 25.

Each 1 mL contains pentazocine lactate equivalent to 30 mg base and 2.8 mg sodium chloride, in Water for Injection.

CARPUJECT **Sterile Cartridge-Needle Unit**, *1 mL (30 mg)* **NDC 0024-1917-02**, *1.5 mL (45 mg)* **NDC 0024-1918-02**, *and 2 mL (60 mg)* **NDC 0024-1919-02, all in 2 mL cartridges**, box of 10. Each 1 mL contains pentazocine lactate equivalent to 30 mg base, 1 mg acetone sodium bisulfite, and 2.2 mg sodium chloride, in Water for Injection.

Multiple-dose vials of 10 mL **NDC 0024-1916-01**, box of 1. Each 1 mL contains pentazocine lactate equivalent to 30 mg base, 2 mg acetone sodium bisulfite, 1.5 mg sodium chloride, and 1 mg methylparaben as preservative, in Water for Injection.

The pH of TALWIN solutions is adjusted between 4 and 5 with lactic acid or sodium hydroxide. The air in the ampuls, vials, and Cartridge-Needle Units has been displaced by nitrogen gas.

TW-109-GG

TALWIN® Compound ©IV ℞

brand of pentazocine hydrochloride and aspirin tablets, USP

DESCRIPTION

TALWIN Compound is a combination of pentazocine hydrochloride, USP, equivalent to 12.5 mg base and aspirin, USP, 325 mg.

Pentazocine is a member of the benzazocine series (also known as the benzomorphan series). Chemically, pentazocine is 1, 2, 3, 4, 5, 6 -hexahydro - 6, 11-dimethyl-3-(3-methyl-2-butenyl)-2, 6-methano-3-benzazocin-8-ol, a white, crystalline substance soluble in acidic aqueous solutions.

Chemically, aspirin is Benzoic acid, 2-(acetyloxy)-,.

Inactive Ingredients: Magnesium Stearate, Microcrystalline Cellulose, Sodium Lauryl Sulfate, Starch.

CLINICAL PHARMACOLOGY

Pentazocine is a potent analgesic which when administered orally is approximately equivalent, on a mg for mg basis, in analgesic effect to codeine. Two Caplets® of TALWIN Compound when administered orally have the additive analgesic effect equivalent to 25 mg of TALWIN plus 650 mg of aspirin. TALWIN Compound provides the analgesic effects of pentazocine and the analgesic, anti-inflammatory, and antipyretic actions of aspirin.

Onset of significant analgesia usually occurs between 15 and 30 minutes after oral administration, and duration of action is usually three hours or longer. Onset and duration of action and the degree of pain relief are related both to dose and the severity of pretreatment pain. Pentazocine weakly antagonizes the analgesic effects of morphine, meperidine, and phenazocine; in addition, it produces incomplete reversal of cardiovascular, respiratory, and behavioral depression induced by morphine and meperidine. Pentazocine has about 1/50 the antagonistic activity of nalorphine. It also has sedative activity.

INDICATION AND USAGE

For the relief of moderate pain

CONTRAINDICATIONS

TALWIN Compound should not be administered to patients who are hypersensitive to either pentazocine or salicylates, or in any situation where aspirin is contraindicated.

WARNINGS

Drug Dependence. There have been instances of psychological and physical dependence on parenteral pentazocine in patients with a history of drug abuse, and rarely, in patients without such a history. Abrupt discontinuance following the extended use of parenteral pentazocine has resulted in withdrawal symptoms. There have been a few reports of dependence and of withdrawal symptoms with orally administered pentazocine. Patients with a history of drug dependence should be under close supervision while receiving TALWIN Compound orally. There have been rare reports of possible abstinence syndromes in newborns after prolonged use of pentazocine during pregnancy.

In prescribing TALWIN Compound for chronic use, the physician should take precautions to avoid increases in dose by the patient and to prevent the use of the drug in anticipation of pain rather than for the relief of pain.

Head Injury and Increased Intracranial Pressure. The respiratory depressant effects of pentazocine and its potential for elevating cerebrospinal fluid pressure may be markedly exaggerated in the presence of head injury, other intracranial lesions, or a preexisting increase in intracranial pressure. Furthermore, pentazocine can produce effects which may obscure the clinical course of patients with head injuries. In such patients, TALWIN Compound must be used with extreme caution and only if its use is deemed essential.

Usage in Pregnancy. Safe use of pentazocine during pregnancy (other than labor) has not been established. Animal reproduction studies have not demonstrated teratogenic or embryotoxic effects. However, TALWIN Compound should be administered to pregnant patients (other than labor) only when, in the judgment of the physician, the potential benefits outweigh the possible hazards. Patients receiving pentazocine during labor have experienced no adverse effects other than those that occur with commonly used analgesics. TALWIN Compound, brand of pentazocine hydrochloride and aspirin tablets, should be used with caution in women delivering premature infants.

Acute CNS Manifestations. Patients receiving therapeutic doses of pentazocine have experienced hallucinations (usually visual), disorientation, and confusion which have

cleared spontaneously within a period of hours. The mechanism of this reaction is not known. Such patients should be closely observed and vital signs checked. If the drug is reinstituted it should be done with caution since these acute CNS manifestations may recur.

Due to the potential for increased CNS depressant effects, alcohol should be used with caution in patients who are currently receiving pentazocine.

Usage in Children. Because clinical experience in children under 12 years of age is limited, administration of TALWIN Compound in this age group is not recommended.

Ambulatory Patients. Since sedation, dizziness, and occasional euphoria have been noted, ambulatory patients should be warned not to operate machinery, drive cars, or unnecessarily expose themselves to hazards.

Other. Because of its aspirin content, TALWIN Compound should be used with caution in the presence of peptic ulcer, in conjunction with anticoagulant therapy, or in any situation where the effects of aspirin may be deleterious.

PRECAUTIONS

Certain Respiratory Conditions. Although respiratory depression has rarely been reported after oral administration of pentazocine, TALWIN Compound, brand of pentazocine hydrochloride and aspirin tablets, should be administered with caution to patients with respiratory depression from any cause, severely limited respiratory reserve, severe bronchial asthma and other obstructive respiratory conditions, or cyanosis.

Impaired Renal or Hepatic Function. Decreased metabolism of the drug by the liver in extensive liver disease may predispose to accentuation of side effects. Although laboratory tests have not indicated that pentazocine causes or increases renal or hepatic impairment, TALWIN Compound should be administered with caution to patients with such impairment.

Myocardial Infarction. As with all drugs, TALWIN Compound should be used with caution in patients with myocardial infarction who have nausea or vomiting.

Biliary Surgery. Narcotic drug products are generally considered to elevate biliary tract pressure for varying periods following administration. Some evidence suggests that pentazocine may differ in this respect (ie, it causes little or no elevation in biliary tract pressures). The clinical significance of these findings, however, is not yet known.

Patients Receiving Narcotics. Pentazocine is a mild narcotic antagonist. Some patients previously given narcotics, including methadone for the daily treatment of narcotic dependence, have experienced withdrawal symptoms after receiving pentazocine.

CNS Effect. Caution should be used when pentazocine is administered to patients prone to seizures. Seizures have occurred in a few such patients in association with the use of pentazocine although no cause and effect relationship has been established.

ADVERSE REACTIONS

Reactions reported after oral administration of pentazocine or TALWIN Compound include *gastrointestinal:* nausea, vomiting; infrequently constipation; and rarely abdominal distress, anorexia, diarrhea. *CNS Effects:* dizziness, lightheadedness, hallucinations, sedation, euphoria, headache, confusion, disorientation; infrequently weakness, disturbed dreams, insomnia, syncope, visual blurring and focusing difficulty, depression; and rarely tremor, irritability, excitement, tinnitus. *Autonomic:* sweating; infrequently flushing; and rarely chills. *Allergic:* infrequently rash; and rarely urticaria, edema of the face, and angioneurotic edema. *Cardiovascular:* infrequently decrease in blood pressure, tachycardia. *Hematologic:* rarely depression of white blood cells (especially granulocytes), which is usually reversible, moderate transient eosinophilia. *Other:* rarely respiratory depression, urinary retention, paresthesia, toxic epidermal necrolysis, and angioneurotic edema.

DOSAGE AND ADMINISTRATION

Adults. The usual adult dose is 2 CAPLETS three or four times a day.

Children Under 12 Years of Age. Since clinical experience in children under 12 years of age is limited, administration of TALWIN Compound in this age group is not recommended.

Duration of Therapy. Patients with chronic pain who receive pentazocine orally for prolonged periods have only rarely been reported to experience withdrawal symptoms when administration was abruptly discontinued (see WARNINGS). Tolerance to the analgesic effect of pentazocine has also been reported only rarely. Significant abnormalities of liver and kidney function tests have not been reported, even after prolonged administration of pentazocine.

OVERDOSAGE

Manifestations: Clinical experience with pentazocine overdosage has been insufficient to define the signs of this condition. Signs of salicylate overdosage include headache, dizziness, confusion, tinnitus, diaphoresis, thirst, nausea, vomiting, diarrhea, tachycardia, tachypnea, Kussmaul breathing, convulsions, and coma. Death is usually from respiratory failure.

Treatment: Treatment for overdosage of TALWIN Compound, brand of pentazocine hydrochloride and aspirin tablets, should include treatment for salicylate poisoning as outlined in standard references.

Oxygen, intravenous fluids, vasopressors, and other supportive measures should be employed as indicated. Assisted or controlled ventilation should also be considered. For respiratory depression due to overdosage or unusual sensitivity to pentazocine, parenteral naloxone is a specific and effective antagonist.

HOW SUPPLIED

CAPLETS, white, each containing pentazocine hydrochloride equivalent to 12.5 mg base and aspirin 325 mg. Bottles of 100 (NDC 0024-1927-04).

Manufactured by Sterling Pharmaceuticals Inc.
Barceloneta, Puerto Rico 00617

TW-225-L(O)

TALWIN® Nx ℂ ℞

brand of pentazocine and naloxone hydrochlorides tablets, USP

Analgesic for Oral Use Only

> TALWIN® Nx is intended for oral use only. Severe, potentially lethal, reactions may result from misuse of TALWIN® Nx by injection either alone or in combination with other substances. (See **DRUG ABUSE AND DEPENDENCE** section.)

DESCRIPTION

TALWIN Nx contains pentazocine hydrochloride, USP, equivalent to 50 mg base and is a member of the benzazocine series (also known as the benzomorphan series), and naloxone hydrochloride, USP, equivalent to 0.5 mg base.

TALWIN Nx is an analgesic for oral administration.

Chemically, pentazocine hydrochloride is 1,2,3,4,5,6-Hexahydro -6,11 -dimethyl -3-(3-methyl-2-butenyl)-2, 6-methano-3-benzazocin-8-ol hydrochloride, a white, crystalline substance soluble in acidic aqueous solutions.

Chemically, naloxone hydrochloride is Morphinan-6-one, 4, 5-epoxy-3, 14-dihydroxy-17-(2-propenyl)-, hydrochloride, (5α)-. It is a slightly off-white powder, and is soluble in water and dilute acids.

Inactive Ingredients: Colloidal Silicon Dioxide, Dibasic Calcium Phosphate, D&C Yellow #10, FD&C Yellow #6, Magnesium Stearate, Microcrystalline Cellulose, Sodium Lauryl Sulfate, Starch.

CLINICAL PHARMACOLOGY

Pentazocine is a potent analgesic which when administered orally in a 50 mg dose appears equivalent in analgesic effect to 60 mg (1 grain) of codeine. Onset of significant analgesia usually occurs between 15 and 30 minutes after oral administration, and duration of action is usually three hours or longer. Onset and duration of action and the degree of pain relief are related both to dose and the severity of pretreatment pain. Pentazocine weakly antagonizes the analgesic effects of morphine and meperidine; in addition, it produces incomplete reversal of cardiovascular, respiratory, and behavioral depression induced by morphine and meperidine. Pentazocine has about 1/50 the antagonistic activity of nalorphine. It also has sedative activity.

Pentazocine is well absorbed from the gastrointestinal tract. Concentrations in plasma coincide closely with the onset, duration, and intensity of analgesia; peak values occur 1 to 3 hours after oral administration. The half-life in plasma is 2 to 3 hours.

Pentazocine is metabolized in the liver and excreted primarily in the urine. Pentazocine passes into the fetal circulation.

Naloxone when administered orally at 0.5 mg has no pharmacologic activity. Naloxone hydrochloride administered parenterally at the same dose is an effective antagonist to pentazocine and a pure antagonist to narcotic analgesics.

TALWIN Nx is a potent analgesic when administered orally. However, the presence of naloxone in TALWIN Nx will prevent the effect of pentazocine if the product is misused by injection.

Studies in animals indicate that the presence of naloxone does not affect pentazocine analgesia when the combination is given orally. If the combination is given by injection the action of pentazocine is neutralized.

INDICATIONS AND USAGE

> TALWIN® Nx is intended for oral use only. Severe, potentially lethal, reactions may result from misuse of TALWIN® Nx by injection either alone or in combination with other substances. (See **DRUG ABUSE AND DEPENDENCE** section.)

TALWIN Nx is indicated for the relief of moderate to severe pain.

TALWIN Nx is indicated for oral use only.

CONTRAINDICATIONS

TALWIN Nx should not be administered to patients who are hypersensitive to either pentazocine or naloxone.

WARNINGS

> TALWIN® Nx is intended for oral use only. Severe, potentially lethal, reactions may result from misuse of TALWIN® Nx by injection either alone or in combination with other substances. (See **DRUG ABUSE AND DEPENDENCE** section.)

Drug Dependence. Pentazocine can cause a physical and psychological dependence. (See **DRUG ABUSE AND DEPENDENCE.**)

Head Injury and Increased Intracranial Pressure. As in the case of other potent analgesics, the potential of pentazocine for elevating cerebrospinal fluid pressure may be attributed to CO_2 retention due to the respiratory depressant effects of the drug. These effects may be markedly exaggerated in the presence of head injury, other intracranial lesions, or a preexisting increase in intracranial pressure. Furthermore, pentazocine can produce effects which may obscure the clinical course of patients with head injuries. In such patients, pentazocine must be used wth extreme caution and only if its use is deemed essential.

Usage with Alcohol. Due to the potential for increased CNS depressant effects, alcohol should be used with caution in patients who are currently receiving pentazocine.

Patients Receiving Narcotics. Pentazocine is a mild narcotic antagonist. Some patients previously given narcotics, including methadone for the daily treatment of narcotic dependence, have experienced withdrawal symptoms after receiving pentazocine.

Certain Respiratory Conditions. Although respiratory depression has rarely been reported after oral administration of pentazocine, the drug should be administered with caution to patients with respiratory depression from any cause, severely limited respiratory reserve, severe bronchial asthma, and other obstructive respiratory conditions, or cyanosis.

Acute CNS Manifestations. Patients receiving therapeutic doses of pentazocine have experienced hallucinations (usually visual), disorientation, and confusion which have cleared spontaneously within a period of hours. The mechanism of this reaction is not known. Such patients should be very closely observed and vital signs checked. If the drug is reinstituted, it should be done with caution since these acute CNS manifestations may recur.

PRECAUTIONS

CNS Effect. Caution should be used when pentazocine is administered to patients prone to seizures; seizures have occurred in a few such patients in association with the use of pentazocine though no cause and effect relationship has been established.

Impaired Renal or Hepatic Function. Decreased metabolism of pentazocine by the liver in extensive liver disease may predispose to accentuation of side effects. Although laboratory tests have not indicated that pentazocine causes or increases renal or hepatic impairment, the drug should be administered with caution to patients with such impairment.

In prescribing pentazocine for long-term use, the physician should take precautions to avoid increases in dose by the patient.

Biliary Surgery. Narcotic drug products are generally considered to elevate biliary tract pressure for varying periods following their administration. Some evidence suggests that pentazocine may differ from other marketed narcotics in this respect (ie, it causes little or no elevation in biliary tract pressures). The clinical significance of these findings, however, is not yet known.

Information for Patients. Since sedation, dizziness, and occasional euphoria have been noted, ambulatory patients should be warned not to operate machinery, drive cars, or unnecessarily expose themselves to hazards. Pentazocine may cause physical and psychological dependence when taken alone and may have additive CNS depressant properties when taken in combination with alcohol or other CNS depressants.

Continued on next page

This product information was prepared in August 1992. On these and other products of Sanofi Winthrop Pharmaceuticals, detailed information may be obtained on a current basis by direct inquiry to Product Information Services, 90 Park Avenue, New York, NY 10016 (toll free 1-800-446-6267).

Sanofi Winthrop—Cont.

Myocardial Infarction. As with all drugs, pentazocine should be used with caution in patients with myocardial infarction who have nausea or vomiting.
Drug Interactions. Usage with Alcohol: See **WARNINGS.**
Carcinogenesis, Mutagenesis, Impairment of Fertility. No long-term studies in animals to test for carcinogenesis have been performed with the components of TALWIN Nx, brand of pentazocine and naloxone hydrochlorides tablets.
Pregnancy Category C. Animal reproduction studies have not been conducted with TALWIN Nx. It is also not known whether TALWIN Nx can cause fetal harm when administered to pregnant women or can affect reproduction capacity. TALWIN Nx should be given to pregnant women only if clearly needed. However, animal reproduction studies with pentazocine have not demonstrated teratogenic embryotoxic effects.
Labor and Delivery. Patients receiving pentazocine during labor have experienced no adverse effects other than those that occur with commonly used analgesics. TALWIN Nx should be used with caution in women delivering premature infants. The effect of TALWIN Nx on the mother and fetus, the duration of labor or delivery, the possibility that forceps delivery or other intervention or resuscitation of the newborn may be necessary, or the effect of TALWIN Nx on the later growth, development, and functional maturation of the child are unknown at the present time.
Nursing Mothers. It is not known whether this drug is excreted in human milk. Because many drugs are excreted in human milk, caution should be exercised when TALWIN Nx is administered to a nursing woman.
Pediatric Use. Safety and effectiveness in children below the age of 12 years have not been established.

ADVERSE REACTIONS

Cardiovascular: Hypotension, tachycardia, syncope.
Respiratory: Rarely, respiratory depression.
Acute CNS Manifestations: Patients receiving therapeutic doses of pentazocine have experienced hallucinations (usually visual), disorientation, and confusion which have cleared spontaneously within a period of hours. The mechanism of this reaction is not known. Such patients should be closely observed and vital signs checked. If the drug is reinstituted it should be done with caution since these acute CNS manifestations may recur.
Other CNS Effects: Dizziness, lightheadedness, hallucinations, sedation, euphoria, headache, confusion, disorientation; infrequently weakness, disturbed dreams, insomnia, syncope, visual blurring and focusing difficulty, depression; and rarely tremor, irritability, excitement, tinnitus.
Autonomic: Sweating; infrequently flushing; and rarely chills.
Gastrointestinal: Nausea, vomiting, constipation, diarrhea, anorexia, rarely abdominal distress.
Allergic: Edema of the face; dermatitis, including pruritus; flushed skin, including plethora; infrequently rash, and rarely urticaria.
Ophthalmic: Visual blurring and focusing difficulty.
Hematologic: Depression of white blood cells (especially granulocytes), which is usually reversible, moderate transient eosinophilia.
Other: Headache, chills, insomnia, weakness, urinary retention, paresthesia.

DRUG ABUSE AND DEPENDENCE

Controlled Substance. TALWIN Nx is a Schedule IV controlled substance.
There have been some reports of dependence and of withdrawal symptoms wth orally administered pentazocine. Patients with a history of drug dependence should be under close supervision while receiving pentazocine orally. There have been rare reports of possible abstinence syndromes in newborns after prolonged use of pentazocine during pregnancy.
There have been instances of psychological and physical dependence on parenteral pentazocine in patients with a history of drug abuse and rarely, in patients without such a history. Abrupt discontinuance following the extended use of parenteral pentazocine has resulted in withdrawal symptoms.
In prescribing pentazocine for chronic use, the physician should take precautions to avoid increases in dose by the patient.
The amount of naloxone present in TALWIN Nx (0.5 mg per tablet) has no action when taken orally and will not interfere with the pharmacologic action of pentazocine. However, this amount of naloxone given by injection has profound antagonistic action to narcotic analgesics.
Severe, even lethal, consequences may result from misuse of tablets by injection either alone or in combination with other substances, such as pulmonary emboli, vascular occlusion, ulceration and abscesses, and withdrawal symptoms in narcotic dependent individuals.
TALWIN Nx, brand of pentazocine and naloxone hydrochlorides tablets, contains an opioid antagonist, naloxone (0.5 mg). Naloxone is inactive when administered orally at this dose, and its inclusion in TALWIN Nx is intended to curb a form of misuse of oral pentazocine. Parenterally, naloxone is an active narcotic antagonist. Thus, TALWIN Nx has a lower potential for parenteral misuse than the previous oral pentazocine formulation TALWIN® 50, brand of pentazocine hydrochloride tablets, USP. However, it is still subject to patient misuse and abuse by the oral route.

OVERDOSAGE

Manifestations. Clinical experience of overdosage with this oral medication has been insufficient to define the signs of this condition.
Treatment. Oxygen, intravenous fluids, vasopressors, and other supportive measures should be employed as indicated. Assisted or controlled ventilation should also be considered. For respiratory depression due to overdosage or unusual sensitivity to pentazocine, parenteral naloxone is a specific and effective antagonist.

DOSAGE AND ADMINISTRATION

> TALWIN® Nx is intended for oral use only. Severe, potentially lethal, reactions may result from misuse of TALWIN® Nx by injection either alone or in combination with other substances. (See **DRUG ABUSE AND DEPENDENCE** section.)

Adults. The usual initial adult dose is 1 tablet every three or four hours. This may be increased to 2 tablets when needed. Total daily dosage should not exceed 12 tablets.
When anti-inflammatory or antipyretic effects are desired in addition to analgesia, aspirin can be administered concomitantly with this product.
Children Under 12 Years of Age. Since clinical experience in children under 12 years of age is limited, administration of this product in this age group is not recommended.
Duration of Therapy. Patients with chronic pain who receive TALWIN Nx orally for prolonged periods have only rarely been reported to experience withdrawal symptoms when administration was abruptly discontinued (see **WARNINGS**). Tolerance to the analgesic effect of pentazocine has also been reported only rarely. However, there is no long-term experience with the oral administration of TALWIN Nx.

HOW SUPPLIED

Tablets (oblong), yellow, scored, each containing pentazocine hydrochloride equivalent to 50 mg base and naloxone hydrochloride equivalent to 0.5 mg base.
Bottles of 100 (NDC 0024-1951-04).
Unit Dose Dispenser Package of 250 (NDC 0024-1951-24), 10 sleeves of 25 tablets each.

Manufactured by
Sterling Pharmaceuticals Inc.
Barceloneta, Puerto Rico 00617

TW-267-I

Shown in Product Identification Section, page 428

TRANCOPAL® ℞

brand of chlormezanone
Nonhypnotic Antianxiety Agent

DESCRIPTION

TRANCOPAL, brand of chlormezanone, is [2-(*p*-Chlorophenyl)tetrahydro-3-methyl-4*H*-1, 3-thiazin-4-one 1, 1-dioxide], a white, virtually tasteless, crystalline powder with a solubility of less than 0.25 percent w/v in water.
Inactive Ingredients—Caplets® **100 mg:** Dibasic Calcium Phosphate, FD&C Yellow #6, Magnesium Stearate, Saccharin Sodium, Starch; CAPLETS **200 mg:** Dibasic Calcium Phosphate, D&C Yellow #10, FD&C Blue #1, Magnesium Stearate, Saccharin Sodium, Starch.

CLINICAL PHARMACOLOGY

TRANCOPAL improves the emotional state by allaying mild anxiety, usually without impairing clarity of consciousness. The relief of symptoms is often apparent in fifteen to thirty minutes after administration and may last up to six hours or longer.

INDICATIONS AND USAGE

TRANCOPAL is indicated for the treatment of mild anxiety and tension states.
The effectiveness of chlormezanone in long-term use, that is, more than 4 months, has not been assessed by systematic clinical studies. The physician should periodically reassess the usefulness of the drug for the individual patient.

CONTRAINDICATION

Contraindicated in patients with a history of a previous hypersensitivity reaction to chlormezanone.

WARNINGS

Should drowsiness occur, the dose should be reduced. As with other CNS-acting drugs, patients receiving chlormezanone should be warned against performing potentially hazardous tasks which require complete mental alertness, such as operating a motor vehicle or dangerous machinery. Patients should also be warned of the possible additive effects which may occur when the drug is taken with alcohol or other CNS-acting drugs.
Usage in Pregnancy. Safe use of this preparation in pregnancy or lactation has not been established, as no animal reproduction studies have been performed; therefore, use of the drug in pregnancy, lactation, or in women of childbearing age requires that the potential benefit of the drug be weighed against its possible hazards to the mother and fetus.

ADVERSE REACTIONS

Adverse effects reported to occur with TRANCOPAL include drowsiness, drug rash, dizziness, flushing, nausea, depression, edema, inability to void, weakness, excitement, tremor, confusion, and headache. Rare instances of erythema multiforme, Stevens-Johnson syndrome, and toxic epidermal necrolysis have been reported. Medication should be discontinued or modified as the case demands.
Jaundice, apparently of the cholestatic type, has been reported as occurring rarely during the use of chlormezanone, but was reversible on discontinuance of therapy.

OVERDOSAGE

Overdose with amounts as low as 7 grams has resulted in coma, hypotension, absence of reflexes, and flaccidity. Ingestion of higher doses may also result in alternation between coma and excitement.

DOSAGE AND ADMINISTRATION

The usual **adult** dosage is 200 mg orally three or four times daily but in some patients 100 mg may suffice. The dosage for **children from 5 to 12 years** is 50 mg to 100 mg three or four times daily. Since the effect of CNS-acting drugs varies, treatment, particularly in children, should begin with the lowest dosage which may be increased as needed.

HOW SUPPLIED

100 mg (peach colored, scored CAPLETS)
bottle of 100 (NDC 0024-1973-04)
200 mg (green colored, scored CAPLETS)
bottle of 100 (NDC 0024-1974-04)

WINSTROL® CIII ℞

brand of stanozolol tablets, USP
For Oral Administration

DESCRIPTION

WINSTROL, brand of stanozolol tablets, is an anabolic steroid, a synthetic derivative of testosterone. Each tablet contains 2 mg of stanozolol. It is designated chemically as 17-methyl-2′*H*-5α-androst-2-eno[3,2-*c*]pyrazol-17β-ol.
Inactive Ingredients: Dibasic Calcium Phosphate, D&C Red #28, FD&C Red #40, Lactose, Magnesium Stearate, Starch.

CLINICAL PHARMACOLOGY

Anabolic steroids are synthetic derivatives of testosterone. Certain clinical effects and adverse reactions demonstrate the androgenic properties of this class of drugs. Complete dissociation of anabolic and androgenic effects has not been achieved. The actions of anabolic steroids are therefore similar to those of male sex hormones with the possibility of causing serious disturbances of growth and sexual development if given to young children. They suppress the gonadotropic functions of the pituitary and may exert a direct effect upon the testes.
WINSTROL has been found to increase low-density lipoproteins and decrease high-density lipoproteins. These changes are not associated with any increase in total cholesterol or triglyceride levels and revert to normal on discontinuation of treatment.
Hereditary angioedema (HAE) is an autosomal dominant disorder caused by a deficient or nonfunctional C1 esterase inhibitor (C1 INH) and clinically characterized by episodes of swelling of the face, extremities, genitalia, bowel wall, and upper respiratory tract.
In small scale clinical studies, stanozolol was effective in controlling the frequency and severity of attacks of angioedema and in increasing serum levels of C1 INH and C4. WINSTROL is not effective in stopping HAE attacks while they are under way. The effect of WINSTROL on increasing serum levels of C1 INH and C4 may be related to an increase in protein anabolism.

INDICATIONS AND USAGE

Hereditary Angioedema. WINSTROL is indicated prophylactically to decrease the frequency and severity of attacks of angioedema.

CONTRAINDICATIONS

The use of WINSTROL is contraindicated in the following:

1. Male patients with carcinoma of the breast, or with known or suspected carcinoma of the prostate.
2. Carcinoma of the breast in females with hypercalcemia; androgenic anabolic steroids may stimulate osteolytic resorption of bone.
3. Nephrosis or the nephrotic phase of nephritis.
4. WINSTROL can cause fetal harm when administered to a pregnant woman.

WINSTROL is contraindicated in women who are or may become pregnant. If this drug is used during pregnancy, or if the patient becomes pregnant while taking this drug, the patient should be apprised of the potential hazard to the fetus.

WARNINGS

PELIOSIS HEPATIS, A CONDITION IN WHICH LIVER AND SOMETIMES SPLENIC TISSUE IS REPLACED WITH BLOOD-FILLED CYSTS, HAS BEEN REPORTED IN PATIENTS RECEIVING ANDROGENIC ANABOLIC STEROID THERAPY. THESE CYSTS ARE SOMETIMES PRESENT WITH MINIMAL HEPATIC DYSFUNCTION, BUT AT OTHER TIMES THEY HAVE BEEN ASSOCIATED WITH LIVER FAILURE. THEY ARE OFTEN NOT RECOGNIZED UNTIL LIFE-THREATENING LIVER FAILURE OR INTRA-ABDOMINAL HEMORRHAGE DEVELOPS. WITHDRAWAL OF DRUG USUALLY RESULTS IN COMPLETE DISAPPEARANCE OF LESIONS.

LIVER CELL TUMORS ARE ALSO REPORTED. MOST OFTEN THESE TUMORS ARE BENIGN AND ANDROGEN-DEPENDENT, BUT FATAL MALIGNANT TUMORS HAVE BEEN REPORTED. WITHDRAWAL OF DRUG OFTEN RESULTS IN REGRESSION OR CESSATION OF PROGRESSION OF THE TUMOR. HOWEVER, HEPATIC TUMORS ASSOCIATED WITH ANDROGENS OR ANABOLIC STEROIDS ARE MUCH MORE VASCULAR THAN OTHER HEPATIC TUMORS AND MAY BE SILENT UNTIL LIFE-THREATENING INTRA-ABDOMINAL HEMORRHAGE DEVELOPS.

BLOOD LIPID CHANGES THAT ARE KNOWN TO BE ASSOCIATED WITH INCREASED RISK OF ATHEROSCLEROSIS ARE SEEN IN PATIENTS TREATED WITH ANDROGENS AND ANABOLIC STEROIDS. THESE CHANGES INCLUDE DECREASED HIGH-DENSITY LIPOPROTEIN AND SOMETIMES INCREASED LOW-DENSITY LIPOPROTEIN. THE CHANGES MAY BE VERY MARKED AND COULD HAVE A SERIOUS IMPACT ON THE RISK OF ATHEROSCLEROSIS AND CORONARY ARTERY DISEASE.

Cholestatic hepatitis and jaundice occur with 17-alpha-alkylated androgens at relatively low doses. If cholestatic hepatitis with jaundice appears, the anabolic steroid should be discontinued. If liver function tests become abnormal, the patient should be monitored closely and the etiology determined. Generally, the anabolic steroid should be discontinued although in cases of mild abnormalities, the physician may elect to follow the patient carefully at a reduced drug dosage.

In patients with breast cancer, anabolic steroid therapy may cause hypercalcemia by stimulating osteolysis. In this case, the drug should be discontinued.

Edema with or without congestive heart failure may be a serious complication in patients with preexisting cardiac, renal, or hepatic disease. Concomitant administration of adrenal cortical steroids or ACTH may add to the edema.

Geriatric male patients treated with androgenic anabolic steroids may be at an increased risk for the development of prostatic hypertrophy and prostatic carcinoma.

In children, anabolic steroid treatment may accelerate bone maturation without producing compensatory gain in linear growth. This adverse effect may result in compromised adult stature. The younger the child, the greater the risk of compromising final mature height. The effect on bone maturation should be monitored by assessing bone age of the wrist and hand every six months.

Anabolic steroids have not been shown to enhance athletic ability.

PRECAUTIONS

General

Anabolic steroids may cause suppression of clotting factors II, V, VII, and X, and an increase in prothrombin time.

Women should be observed for signs of virilization (deepening of the voice, hirsutism, acne, and clitoromegaly). To prevent irreversible change, drug therapy must be discontinued, or the dosage significantly reduced when mild virilism is first detected. Such virilization is usual following androgenic anabolic steroid use at high doses. Some virilizing changes in women are irreversible even after prompt discontinuance of therapy and are not prevented by concomitant use of estrogens. Menstrual irregularities may also occur.

The insulin or oral hypoglycemic dosage may need adjustment in diabetic patients who receive anabolic steroids.

Information for the Patient. The physician should instruct patients to report any of the following side effects of androgens:

Adult or Adolescent Males. Too frequent or persistent erections of the penis, appearance or aggravation of acne.

Women. Hoarseness, acne, changes in menstrual periods, or more hair on the face.

All Patients. Any nausea, vomiting, changes in skin color, or ankle swelling.

Laboratory Tests. Women with disseminated breast carcinoma should have frequent determination of urine and serum calcium levels during the course of androgenic anabolic steroid therapy (see WARNINGS).

Because of the hepatotoxicity associated with the use of 17-alpha-alkylated androgens, liver function tests should be obtained periodically.

Periodic (every 6 months) x-ray examinations of bone age should be made during treatment of prepubertal patients to determine the rate of bone maturation and the effects of androgenic anabolic steroid therapy on the epiphyseal centers.

In common with other anabolic steroids, WINSTROL, brand of stanozolol tablets, has been reported to lower the level of high-density lipoproteins and raise the level of low-density lipoproteins. These changes usually revert to normal on discontinuation of treatment. Increased low-density lipoproteins and decreased high-density lipoproteins are considered cardiovascular risk factors. Serum lipids and high-density lipoprotein cholesterol should be determined periodically.

Hemoglobin and hematocrit should be checked periodically for polycythemia in patients who are receiving high doses of anabolic steroids.

Drug Interaction. Anabolic steroids may increase sensitivity to anticoagulants; therefore, dosage of an anticoagulant may have to be decreased in order to maintain the prothrombin time at the desired therapeutic level.

Drug/Laboratory Test Interferences. Therapy with androgenic anabolic steroids may decrease levels of thyroxine-binding globulin resulting in decreased total T_4 serum levels and increase resin uptake of T_3 and T_4. Free thyroid hormone levels remain unchanged and there is no clinical evidence of thyroid dysfunction.

Carcinogenesis, Mutagenesis, Impairment of Fertility. Animal data: Testosterone has been tested by subcutaneous injection and implantation in mice and rats. The implant induced cervical-uterine tumors in mice, which metastasized in some cases. There is suggestive evidence that injection of testosterone into some strains of female mice increases their susceptibility to hepatoma. Testosterone is also known to increase the number of tumors and decrease the degree of differentiation of chemically-induced carcinomas of the liver in rats.

Human data: There are rare reports of hepatocellular carcinoma in patients receiving long-term therapy with androgens in high doses. Withdrawal of the drugs did not lead to regression of the tumors in all cases.

Geriatric patients treated with androgens may be at an increased risk of developing prostatic hypertrophy and prostatic carcinoma although conclusive evidence to support this concept is lacking.

This compound has not been tested for mutagenic potential. However, as noted above, cacinogenic effects have been attributed to treatment with androgenic hormones. The potential carcinogenic effects likely occur through a hormonal mechanism rather than by a direct chemical interaction mechanism.

Impairment of fertility was not tested directly in animal species. However, as noted under ADVERSE REACTIONS, oligospermia in males and amenorrhea in females are potential adverse effects of treatment with WINSTROL Tablets. Therefore, impairment of fertility is a possible outcome of treatment with WINSTROL.

Pregnancy Category X. See CONTRAINDICATIONS section.

Nursing Mothers. It is not known whether anabolic steroids are excreted in human milk. Many drugs are excreted in human milk and because of the potential for adverse reactions in nursing infants from WINSTROL, a decision should be made whether to discontinue nursing or discontinue the drug, taking into account the importance of the drug to the mother.

Pediatric Use. Anabolic agents may accelerate epiphyseal maturation more rapidly than linear growth in children, and the effect may continue for 6 months after the drug has been stopped. Therefore, therapy should be monitored by x-ray studies at 6 month intervals in order to avoid the risk of compromising the adult height. The safety and efficacy of WINSTROL in children with hereditary angioedema have not been established.

ADVERSE REACTIONS

Hepatic: Cholestatic jaundice with, rarely, hepatic necrosis and death. Hepatocellular neoplasms and peliosis hepatis have been reported in association with long-term androgenic-anabolic steroid therapy (see WARNINGS). Reversible changes in liver function tests also occur including increased bromsulphalein (BSP) retention and increases in serum bilirubin, glutamic oxaloacetic transaminase (SGOT), and alkaline phosphatase.

Genitourinary System: *In men. Prepubertal:* Phallic enlargement and increased frequency of erections.

Postpubertal: Inhibition of testicular function, testicular atrophy and oligospermia, impotence, chronic priapism, epididymitis and bladder irritability.

In women: Clitoral enlargement, menstrual irregularities.

In both sexes: Increased or decreased libido.

CNS: Habituation, excitation, insomnia, depression.

Gastrointestinal: Nausea, vomiting, diarrhea.

Hematologic: Bleeding in patients on concomitant anticoagulant therapy.

Breast: Gynecomastia.

Larynx: Deepening of the voice in women.

Hair: Hirsutism and male pattern baldness in women.

Skin: Acne (especially in women and prepubertal boys).

Skeletal: Premature closure of epiphyses in children (see PRECAUTIONS, **Pediatric Use**).

Fluid and Electrolytes: Edema, retention of serum electrolytes (sodium, chloride, potassium, phosphate, calcium).

Metabolic/Endocrine: Decreased glucose tolerance (see PRECAUTIONS), increased serum levels of low-density lipoproteins and decreased levels of high-density lipoproteins (see PRECAUTIONS, **Laboratory Tests**), increased creatine and creatinine excretion, increased serum levels of creatinine phosphokinase (CPK).

Some virilizing changes in women are irreversible even after prompt discontinuance of therapy and are not prevented by concomitant use of estrogens (see PRECAUTIONS).

DRUG ABUSE AND DEPENDENCE

WINSTROL is classified by the Anabolic Steroids Control Act as a schedule III controlled substance.

DOSAGE AND ADMINISTRATION

The use of anabolic steroids may be associated with serious adverse reactions, many of which are dose related; therefore, patients should be placed on the lowest possible effective dose.

Hereditary Angioedema. The dosage requirements for continuous treatment of hereditary angioedema with WINSTROL should be individualized on the basis of the clinical response of the patient. It is recommended that the patient be started on 2 mg, three times a day. After a favorable initial response is obtained in terms of prevention of episodes of edematous attacks, the proper continuing dosage should be determined by decreasing the dosage at intervals of one to three months to a maintenance dosage of 2 mg a day. Some patients may be successfully managed on a 2 mg alternate day schedule. During the dose adjusting phase, close monitoring of the patient's response is indicated, particularly if the patient has a history of airway involvement.

The prophylactic dose of WINSTROL, brand of stanozolol tablets, to be used prior to dental extraction, or other traumatic or stressful situations has not been established and may be substantially larger.

Attacks of hereditary angioedema are generally infrequent in childhood and the risks from stanozolol administration are substantially increased. Therefore, long-term prophylactic therapy with this drug is generally not recommended in children, and should only be undertaken with due consideration of the benefits and risks involved (see PRECAUTIONS, **Pediatric Use**).

HOW SUPPLIED

Tablets of 2 mg, scored, bottle of 100 (NDC 0024-2253-04)

Manufactured by Sterling Pharmaceuticals Inc.
Barceloneta, Puerto Rico 00617

WW 5-CC

Shown in Product Identification Section, page 428

ZEPHIRAN® CHLORIDE **OTC**

brand of benzalkonium chloride

(See PDR For Nonprescription Drugs.)

This product information was prepared in August 1992. On these and other products of Sanofi Winthrop Pharmaceuticals, detailed information may be obtained on a current basis by direct inquiry to Product Information Services, 90 Park Avenue, New York, NY 10016 (toll free 1-800-446-6267).

Savage Laboratories
a division of Altana Inc.
60 BAYLIS ROAD
MELVILLE, NY 11747

ALPHATREX® ℞
[al"fah-trex']
(betamethasone dipropionate)
Cream, USP 0.05%
Ointment, USP 0.05%
Lotion, USP 0.05%
Potency expressed as betamethasone)
For Dermatologic Use Only–Not for Ophthalmic Use

DESCRIPTION

Alphatrex® Cream, Ointment and Lotion contain Betamethasone Dipropionate USP (Pregna-1, 4-diene-3, 20-dione, 9-fluoro-11-hydroxy-16-methyl-17, 21-bis (1-oxopropoxy)-(11β, 16β)-); it has a molecular formula of $C_{28}H_{37}FO_7$, and a molecular weight of 504.59 (CAS Registry Number 5593-20-4).

Each gram of the 0.05% Cream contains 0.64 mg betamethasone dipropionate (equivalent to 0.5 mg betamethasone) in a soft, white, hydrophilic cream of purified water, mineral oil, white petrolatum, polyethylene glycol 1000 monocetyl ether, cetostearyl alcohol, monobasic sodium phosphate and phosphoric acid or sodium hydroxide; chlorocresol is present as a preservative. Betamethasone Dipropionate Cream contains no parabens.

Each gram of the 0.05% Ointment contains 0.64 mg betamethasone dipropionate (equivalent to 0.5 mg betamethasone) in an ointment base of mineral oil and white petrolatum. Betamethasone Dipropionate Ointment contains no parabens.

Each gram of the 0.05% Lotion contains 0.64 mg of betamethasone dipropionate (equivalent to 0.5 mg betamethasone) in a vehicle of isopropyl alcohol and purified water slightly thickened with carbomer 934P. Phosphoric acid or sodium hydroxide is used to adjust pH.

CLINICAL PHARMACOLOGY

Topical corticosteroids share anti-inflammatory, anti-pruritic and vasoconstrictive actions. The mechanism of anti-inflammatory activity of the topical corticosteroids is unclear. Various laboratory methods, including vasoconstrictor assays, are used to compare and predict potencies and/or clinical efficacies of the topical corticosteroids. There is some evidence to suggest that a recognizable correlation exists between vasoconstrictor potency and therapeutic efficacy in man.

Pharmacokinetics: The extent of percutaneous absorption of topical corticosteroids is determined by many factors including the vehicle, the integrity of the epidermal barrier, and the use of occlusive dressings. Topical corticosteroids can be absorbed from normal intact skin. Inflammation and/or other disease processes in the skin increase percutaneous absorption. Occlusive dressings substantially increase the percutaneous absorption of topical corticosteroids. (See DOSAGE AND ADMINISTRATION) Once absorbed through the skin, topical corticosteroids are handled through pharmacokinetic pathways similar to systemically administered corticosteroids. Corticosteroids are bound to plasma proteins in varying degrees. Corticosteroids are metabolized primarily in the liver and are then excreted by the kidneys. Some of the topical corticosteroids and their metabolites are also excreted into the bile.

INDICATIONS AND USAGE

Topical corticosteroids are indicated for the relief of the inflammatory and pruritic manifestations of corticosteroid-responsive dermatoses.

CONTRAINDICATIONS

Topical corticosteroids are contraindicated in those patients with a history of hypersensitivity to any of the components of the preparation.

PRECAUTIONS

General: Systemic absorption of topical corticosteroids has produced reversible hypothalamic-pituitary-adrenal (HPA) axis suppression, manifestations of Cushing's syndrome, hyperglycemia, and glucosuria in some patients. Conditions which augment systemic absorption include the application of the more potent steroids, use over large surface areas, prolonged use, and the addition of occlusive dressings. (See DOSAGE AND ADMINISTRATION) Therefore, patients receiving a large dose of a potent topical steroid applied to a large surface area should be evaluated periodically for evidence of HPA axis suppression by using the urinary free cortisol and ACTH stimulation tests. If HPA axis suppression is noted, an attempt should be made to withdraw the drug, to reduce the frequency of application, or to substitute a less potent steroid. Recovery of HPA axis function is generally prompt and complete upon discontinuation of the drug. Infrequently, signs and symptoms of steroid withdrawal may occur, requiring supplemental systemic corticosteroids. Children may absorb proportionally larger amounts of topical corticosteroids and thus be more susceptible to systemic toxicity (See PRECAUTIONS-Pediatric Use). If irritation develops topical corticosteroids should be discontinued and appropriate therapy instituted. In the presence of dermatological infections, the use of an appropriate antifungal or antibacterial agent should be instituted. If a favorable response does not occur promptly, the corticosteroid should be discontinued until the infection has been adequately controlled.

Information for the Patient: Patients using topical corticosteroids should receive the following information and instructions:

1. This medication is to be used as directed by the physician. It is for external use only. Avoid contact with the eyes.
2. Patients should be advised not to use this medication for any disorder other than for which it was prescribed.
3. The treated skin area should not be bandaged or otherwise covered or wrapped as to be occlusive. (See DOSAGE AND ADMINISTRATION)
4. Patients should report any signs of local adverse reactions.
5. Parents of pediatric patients should be advised not to use tight fitting diapers or plastic pants on a child being treated in the diaper area, as these garments may constitute occlusive dressings. (See DOSAGE AND ADMINISTRATION)

Laboratory Tests: The following tests may be helpful in evaluating the HPA axis suppression: Urinary free cortisol test; ACTH stimulation test.

Carcinogenesis, Mutagenesis, and Impairment of Fertility: Long-term animal studies have not been performed to evaluate the carcinogenic potential or the effect on fertility of topical corticosteroids. Studies to determine mutagenicity with prednisolone and hydrocortisone have revealed negative results.

Pregnancy Category C: Corticosteroids are generally teratogenic in laboratory animals when administered systemically at relatively low dosage levels. The more potent corticosteroids have been shown to be teratogenic after dermal application in laboratory animals. There are no adequate and well-controlled studies in pregnant women on teratogenic effects from topically applied corticosteroids. Therefore, topical corticosteroids should be used during pregnancy only if the potential benefit justifies the potential risk to the fetus. Drugs of this class should not be used extensively on pregnant patients, in large amounts, or for prolonged periods of time.

Nursing Mothers: It is not known whether topical administration of corticosteroids could result in sufficient systemic absorption to produce detectable quantities in breast milk. Systemically administered corticosteroids are secreted into breast milk in quantities *not* likely to have a deleterious effect on the infant. Nevertheless, caution should be exercised when topical corticosteroids are administered to a nursing woman.

Pediatric Use: *Pediatric patients may demonstrate greater susceptibility to topical corticosteroid-induced HPA axis suppression and Cushing's syndrome than mature patients because of a larger skin surface area to body weight ratio.* Hypothalamic-pituitary-adrenal (HPA) axis suppression, Cushing's syndrome, and intracranial hypertension have been reported in children receiving topical corticosteroids. Manifestations of adrenal suppression in children include linear growth retardation, delayed weight gain, low plasma cortisol levels, and absence of response to ACTH stimulation. Manifestations of intracranial hypertension include bulging fontanelles, headaches, and bilateral papilledema. Administration of topical corticosteroids to children should be limited to the least amount compatible with an effective therapeutic regimen. Chronic corticosteroid therapy may interfere with the growth and development of children.

ADVERSE REACTIONS

The following local adverse reactions are reported infrequently when Alphatrex® products are used as recommended in the DOSAGE AND ADMINISTRATION section. These reactions are listed in an approximate decreasing order of occurrence: burning, itching, irritation, dryness, folliculitis, hypertrichosis, acneiform eruptions, hypopigmentation, perioral dermatitis, allergic contact dermatitis, maceration of the skin, secondary infection, skin atrophy, striae and miliaria.

Systemic absorption of topical corticosteroids has produced reversible hypothalamic-pituitary-adrenal (HPA) axis suppression, manifestations of Cushing's syndrome, hyperglycemia and glucosuria in some patients.

OVERDOSAGE

Topically applied corticosteroids can be absorbed in sufficient amounts to produce systemic effects (See PRECAUTIONS).

DOSAGE AND ADMINISTRATION

Alphatrex® Cream and Ointment are applied to the affected skin areas as a thin film once daily. In some cases, twice daily dosage may be necessary.

Apply a few drops of Alphatrex® Lotion to the affected skin areas and massage lightly until it disappears. Apply twice daily, in the morning and night. If an infection develops, appropriate antimicrobial therapy should be instituted.

Alphatrex® products should not be used with occlusive dressings.

HOW SUPPLIED

Alphatrex® Cream, USP 0.05%
NDC 0281-0055-15, 15 gram tube
NDC 0281-0055-46, 45 gram tube
Alphatrex® Ointment, USP 0.05%
NDC 0281-0056-15, 15 gram tube
NDC 0281-0056-46, 45 gram tube
Alphatrex® Lotion, USP 0.05%
NDC 0281-0057-60, 60 ml bottle

Shake well before using. Store at controlled room temperature 15°–30°C (59°–86°F).

Caution: Federal law prohibits dispensing without prescription.

BETATREX® ℞
[ba"tah-trex']
(betamethasone valerate)
Cream, USP 0.1%
Ointment, USP 0.1%
Lotion, USP 0.1%
Potency expressed as betamethasone
For Dermatologic Use Only—Not for Ophthalmic Use

DESCRIPTION

Betatrex® Cream, Ointment and Lotion contain Betamethasone Valerate USP (Pregna-1,4-diene-3,20-dione, 9-fluoro-11, 21-dihydroxy-16-methyl-17- [(1-oxopentyl)oxy]-, (11β,16β)-); it has a molecular formula of $C_{27}H_{37}FO_6$ and a molecular weight of 476.58 (CAS Registry Number 2152-44-5).

Each gram of the 0.1% cream contains 1.2 mg Betamethasone Valerate (equivalent to 1 mg Betamethasone) in a soft, white hydrophilic cream of Water, Mineral Oil, White Petrolatum, Polyethylene Glycol 1000 Monocetyl Ether, Cetostearyl Alcohol, Monobasic Sodium Phosphate and Phosphoric Acid or Sodium Hydroxide; Chlorocresol is present as a preservative. Betamethasone Valerate Cream contains no parabens.

Each gram of the 0.1% ointment contains 1.2 mg Betamethasone Valerate (equivalent to 1 mg Betamethasone) in an ointment base of White Petrolatum and Mineral Oil. Betamethasone Valerate Ointment contains no parabens.

Each gram of the 0.1% lotion contains 1.2 mg Betamethasone Valerate (equivalent to 1 mg Betamethasone) in a vehicle of Isopropyl Alcohol and Water slightly thickened with Carbomer 934P. Phosphoric Acid or Sodium Hydroxide are used to adjust the pH.

CLINICAL PHARMACOLOGY

Topical corticosteroids share anti-inflammatory, anti-pruritic and vasoconstrictive actions. The mechanism of anti-inflammatory activity of the topical corticosteroids is unclear. Various laboratory methods, including vasoconstrictor assays, are used to compare and predict potencies and/or clinical efficacies of the topical corticosteroids. There is some evidence to suggest that a recognizable correlation exists between vasoconstrictor potency and therapeutic efficacy in man.

Pharmacokinetics: The extent of percutaneous absorption of topical corticosteroids is determined by many factors including the vehicle, the integrity of the epidermal barrier, and the use of occlusive dressings. Topical corticosteroids can be absorbed from normal intact skin. Inflammation and/or other disease processes in the skin increase percutaneous absorption. Occlusive dressings substantially increase the percutaneous absorption of topical corticosteroids. Thus occlusive dressings may be a valuable therapeutic adjunct for treatment of resistant dermatoses (See DOSAGE AND ADMINISTRATION). Once absorbed through the skin, topical corticosteroids are handled through pharmacokinetic pathways similar to systemically administered corticosteroids. Corticosteroids are bound to plasma proteins in varying degrees. Corticosteroids are metabolized primarily in the liver and are then excreted by the kidneys. Some of the topical corticosteroids and their metabolites are also excreted into the bile.

INDICATIONS AND USAGE

Topical corticosteroids are indicated for the relief of the inflammatory and pruritic manifestations of corticosteroid-responsive dermatoses.

CONTRAINDICATIONS

Topical corticosteroids are contraindicated in those patients with a history of hypersensitivity to any of the components of the preparation.

PRECAUTIONS

General: Systemic absorption of topical corticosteroids has produced reversible hypothalamic-pituitary-adrenal (HPA) axis suppression, manifestations of Cushing's syndrome,

hyperglycemia, and glucosuria in some patients. Conditions which augment systemic absorption include the application of the more potent steroids, use over large surface areas, prolonged use, and the addition of occlusive dressings. Therefore, patients receiving a large dose of a potent topical steroid applied to a large surface area or under an occlusive dressing should be evaluated periodically for evidence of HPA axis suppression by using the urinary free cortisol and ACTH stimulation tests. If HPA axis suppression is noted, an attempt should be made to withdraw the drug, to reduce the frequency of application, or to substitute a less potent steroid. Recovery of HPA axis function is generally prompt and complete upon discontinuation of the drug. Infrequently, signs and symptoms of steroid withdrawal may occur, requiring supplemental systemic corticosteroids. Children may absorb proportionally larger amounts of topical corticosteroids and thus be more susceptible to systemic toxicity (See PRECAUTIONS-Pediatric Use). If irritation develops, topical corticosteroids should be discontinued and appropriate therapy instituted. In the presence of dermatological infections, the use of an appropriate antifungal or antibacterial agent should be instituted. If a favorable response does not occur promptly, the corticosteroid should be discontinued until the infection has been adequately controlled.

Information for the Patient: Patients using topical corticosteroids should receive the following information and instructions:

1. This medication is to be used as directed by the physician. It is for external use only. Avoid contact with the eyes.
2. Patients should be advised not to use this medication for any disorder other than for which it was prescribed.
3. The treated skin area should not be bandaged or otherwise covered or wrapped as to be occlusive unless directed by the physician.
4. Patients should report any signs of local adverse reactions especially under occlusive dressing.
5. Parents of pediatric patients should be advised not to use tight fitting diapers or plastic pants on a child being treated in the diaper area, as these garments may constitute occlusive dressings.

Laboratory Tests: The following tests may be helpful in evaluating the HPA axis suppression: Urinary free cortisol test. ACTH stimulation test.

Carcinogenesis, Mutagenesis, and Impairment of Fertility: Long-term animal studies have not been performed to evaluate the carcinogenic potential or the effect on fertility of topical corticosteroids. Studies to determine mutagenicity with prednisolone and hydrocortisone have revealed negative results.

Pregnancy Category C: Corticosteroids are generally teratogenic in laboratory animals when administered systemically at relatively low dosage levels. The more potent corticosteroids have been shown to be teratogenic after dermal application in laboratory animals. There are no adequate and well-controlled studies in pregnant women on teratogenic effects from topically applied corticosteroids. Therefore, topical corticosteroids should be used during pregnancy only if the potential benefit justifies the potential risk to the fetus. Drugs of this class should not be used extensively on pregnant patients, in large amounts, or for prolonged periods of time.

Nursing Mothers: It is not known whether topical administration of corticosteroids could result in sufficient systemic absorption to produce detectable quantities in breast milk. Systemically administered corticosteroids are secreted into breast milk in quantities *not* likely to have a deleterious effect on the infant. Nevertheless, caution should be exercised when topical corticosteroids are administered to a nursing woman.

Pediatric Use: *Pediatric patients may demonstrate greater susceptibility to topical corticosteroid-induced HPA axis suppression and Cushing's syndrome than mature patients because of a larger skin surface area to body weight ratio.* Hypothalamic-pituitary-adrenal (HPA) axis suppression, Cushing's syndrome, and intracranial hypertension have been reported in children receiving topical corticosteroids. Manifestations of adrenal suppression in children include linear growth retardation, delayed weight gain, low plasma cortisol levels, and absence of response to ACTH stimulation. Manifestations of intracranial hypertension include bulging fontanelles, headaches, and bilateral papilledema. Administration of topical corticosteroids to children should be limited to the least amount compatible with an effective therapeutic regimen. Chronic corticosteroid therapy may interfere with the growth and development of children.

ADVERSE REACTIONS

The following local adverse reactions are reported infrequently with topical corticosteroids, but may occur more frequently with the use of occlusive dressings. These reactions are listed in an approximate decreasing order of occurrence: burning, itching, irritation, dryness, folliculitis, hypertrichosis, acneiform eruptions, hypopigmentation, perioral dermatitis, allergic contact dermatitis, maceration of the skin, secondary infection, skin atrophy, striae and miliaria.

OVERDOSAGE

Topically applied corticosteroids can be absorbed in sufficient amounts to produce systemic effects (See PRECAUTIONS).

DOSAGE AND ADMINISTRATION

Betatrex® Cream: Apply a thin film to the affected skin areas one to three times a day. Dosage once or twice a day is often effective.

Betatrex® Ointment: Apply a thin film to the affected skin areas one to three times a day. Dosage once or twice a day is often effective.

Betatrex® Lotion: Apply a few drops of Betatrex® Lotion to the affected area and massage lightly until it disappears. Apply twice daily, in the morning and at night. Dosage may be increased in stubborn cases. Following improvement, apply once daily. For the most effective and economical use, apply nozzle very close to affected area and gently squeeze bottle. Shake well before using. Store at controlled room temperature 15–30°C (59°–86°F).

HOW SUPPLIED

Betatrex® Cream USP, 0.1%
NDC 0281-3510-44, 15 gram tube
NDC 0281-3510-50, 45 gram tube
Betatrex® Ointment USP, 0.1%
NDC 0281-3516-44, 15 gram tube
NDC 0281-3516-50, 45 gram tube
Betatrex® Lotion USP, 0.1%
NDC 0281-3519-46, 60 ml bottle

CAUTION

Federal law prohibits dispensing without prescription.

BREXIN® L.A. Capsules ℞

[*brex 'in*]

(chlorpheniramine maleate, pseudoephedrine hydrochloride)

DESCRIPTION

A red and clear colored capsule containing red and blue colored beads. Each capsule for oral administration contains: chlorpheniramine maleate 8 mg, pseudoephedrine hydrochloride 120 mg in a specially prepared base to provide prolonged action.

This product contains ingredients of the following therapeutic classes: antihistamine and decongestant.

CLINICAL PHARMACOLOGY

Chlorpheniramine maleate is an alkylamine-type antihistamine. This group of antihistamines is among the most active histamine antagonists and is generally effective in relatively low doses. The drugs are not so prone to produce drowsiness and are among the most suitable agents for daytime use: but again, a significant proportion of patients do experience this effect.

Pseudoephedrine hydrochloride is a sympathomimetic which acts predominantly on alpha receptors and has little action on beta receptors. It therefore functions as an oral nasal decongestant with minimal CNS stimulation.

INDICATIONS

For the temporary relief of symptoms of the common cold, allergic rhinitis (hay fever) and sinusitis.

CONTRAINDICATIONS

Hypersensitivity to any of the ingredients. Also contraindicated in patients with severe hypertension, severe coronary artery disease, patients on MAO inhibitor therapy, patients with narrow-angle glaucoma, urinary retention, peptic ulcer and during an asthmatic attack.

Should not be used in children under 12 years, or in nursing mothers.

WARNINGS

Considerable caution should be exercised in patients with hypertension, diabetes mellitus, ischemic heart disease, hyperthyroidism, increased intraocular pressure and prostatic hypertrophy. The elderly (60 years or older) are more likely to exhibit adverse reactions.

Antihistamines may cause excitability, especially in children. At dosages higher than the recommended dose, nervousness, dizziness or sleeplessness may occur.

PRECAUTIONS

General: Caution should be exercised in patients with high blood pressure, heart disease, diabetes or thyroid disease. The antihistamine in this product may exhibit additive effects with other CNS depressants, including alcohol.

Information for Patients: Antihistamines may cause drowsiness and ambulatory patients who operate machinery or motor vehicles should be cautioned accordingly.

Drug Interactions: MAO inhibitors and beta adrenergic blockers increase the effects of sympathomimetics. Sympathomimetics may reduce the antihypertensive effects of methyldopa, mecamylamine, reserpine and veratrum alkaloids. Concomitant use of antihistamines with alcohol and other CNS depressants may have an additive effect.

Pregnancy: The safety of use of this product in pregnancy has not been established.

ADVERSE REACTIONS

Adverse reactions include drowsiness, lassitude, nausea, giddiness, dryness of mouth, blurred vision, cardiac palpitations, flushing, increased irritability or excitement (especially in children).

DOSAGE AND ADMINISTRATION

Adults and children over 12 years of age—1 capsule orally every 12 hours.

HOW SUPPLIED

NDC 0281-1934-53, bottle of 100 capsules.

Store and dispense in tight containers as defined in the USP.

Dispense in child resistant containers.

STORE BETWEEN 15°–30°C (59°–86°F).

CAUTION: Federal law prohibits dispensing without prescription.

Distributed by Savage Laboratories®

Shown in Product Identification Section, page 428

CHROMAGEN® ℞

[*kro "mah-jen*]

Soft Gelatin Capsules

DESCRIPTION

CONTENTS: Each maroon soft gelatin capsule contains: ferrous fumarate USP 200 mg, ascorbic acid USP 250 mg, cyanocobalamin USP 10 mcg, desiccated stomach substance 100 mg.

DISCUSSION: The amount of elemental iron and the absorption of the iron components of commercial iron preparations vary widely. It is further established that certain "accessory components" may be included to enhance absorption and utilization of iron. Chromagen® Capsules are formulated to provide the essential factors for a complete, versatile hematinic.

ACTIONS

HIGH ELEMENTAL IRON CONTENT: Ferrous fumarate, used in Chromagen® Capsules, is an organic iron complex which has a higher elemental iron content than any other hematinic salt—33%. This compares with 20% for ferrous sulfate and 12% for ferrous gluconate.[1,2]

MORE COMPLETE ABSORPTION: It has been repeatedly shown that ascorbic acid, when given in sufficient amounts, can increase the absorption of ferrous iron from the gastrointestinal tract.[3,4,5,6,7,8,9] The absorption-promoting effect is mainly due to the reducing action of ascorbic acid within the gastrointestinal lumen, which helps to prevent or delay the formation of insoluble or less dissociated ferric compounds.[3] Iron absorption has been shown to increase sharply with increasing amounts of ascorbic acid, showing a gain in absorption of approximately 40% at 250 mg. Above 250 mg, the gain becomes insignificant, with an additional gain of only approximately 8% at 500 mg.[3] Each Chromagen® Capsule contains 250 mg of ascorbic acid, believed to be the optimal amount.

PROMOTES MOVEMENT OF PLASMA IRON: Ascorbic acid also plays an important role in the movement of plasma iron to storage depots in the tissues.[10] The action, which leads to the transport of plasma iron to ferritin, presumably involves its reducing effect, converting transferrin iron from the ferric to the ferrous state.[5] There is also evidence that ascorbic acid improves iron utilization, presumably as a further result of its reducing action,[6,9] and some evidence that it may have a direct effect upon erythropoiesis. Ascorbic acid is further alleged to enhance the conversion of folic acid to a more physiologically active form, folinic acid, which would make it even more important in the treatment of anemia since it would aid in the utilization of dietary folic acid.[11]

EXCELLENT ORAL TOLERATION: Ferrous fumarate is used in Chromagen® Capsules because it is less likely to cause the gastric disturbances so often associated with oral iron therapy. Ferrous fumarate has a low ionization constant and high solubility in the entire pH range of the gastrointestinal tract. It does not precipitate proteins or have the astringency of more ionizable forms of iron, and does not interfere with proteolytic or diastatic activities of the digestive system. Because of excellent oral toleration, Chromagen® Capsules can usually be administered between meals when iron absorption is maximal.

FACILITATES ABSORPTION OF VITAMIN B_{12}: It is now known that "Intrinsic Factor" is essential for the adequate alimentary absorption of vitamin B_{12}.[12,13,14,15] The chemical structure of intrinsic factor is still undetermined and it has not yet been isolated in pure form;[16] however, the inclusion of desiccated stomach substance with oral vitamin B_{12} will furnish sufficient intrinsic factor to assure absorption of the vitamin.

Continued on next page

Savage Laboratories—Cont.

TOXICITY: Ferrous fumarate was found to be the least toxic of three popular oral iron salts, with an oral LD_{50} of 630 mg/kg. In the same report, the LD_{50} of ferrous gluconate was reported to be 320 mg/kg and ferrous sulfate 230 mg/kg.[1,17]

INDICATIONS
For the treatment of all anemias responsive to oral iron therapy, such as hypochromic anemia associated with pregnancy, chronic or acute blood loss, dietary restriction, metabolic disease and post-surgical convalescence.

CONTRAINDICATIONS
Hemochromatosis and hemosiderosis are contraindications to iron therapy.

SIDE EFFECTS
Average capsule doses in sensitive individuals or excessive dosage may cause nausea, skin rash, vomiting, diarrhea, precordial pain, or flushing of the face and extremities.

DOSAGE AND ADMINISTRATION
Usual adult dose is 1 soft gelatin capsule daily or as recommended by physician.

HOW SUPPLIED
Chromagen® Capsules:
NDC **0281-4285-53**, bottle of 100
NDC **0281-4285-56**, bottle of 500
Store at controlled room temperature 15°–30°C (59°–86°F).
CAUTION: Federal law prohibits dispensing without prescription.

BIBLIOGRAPHY
[1]Berk, M.S. and Novich, M.A.: "Treatment of Iron Deficiency Anemia With Ferrous Fumarate," Am. J. Obst. & Gynec., 203–206, 1962. [2]Shapleigh, J.B., and Montgomery, A.; Am. Pract & Dig. Treat 10–461, 1959. [3]Brise, H. and Hallberg. L.: "Effect of Ascorbic Acid on Iron Absorption," Acta. Med. Scand. 171:376, 51–58, 1962. [4]New Drugs, p.309, AMA, Chicago, 1966. [5]Mazur, A., Green, S. and Carleton, A.: "Mechanism of Plasma Iron Incorporation into Hepatic Ferritin," J. of Bio. Chem. 3:595–603, 1960. [6]Greenberg, S.M., Tucker, A.E., Mathues, H. and J.D.: "Iron Absorption and Metabolism, I. Interrelationship of Ascorbic Acid and Vitamin E", J. Nutrition 63:19–31, 1957. [7]Moore, C.V., and Dubach, R.: "Observations on the Absorption of Iron From Foods Tagged with Radioiron," Trans. Assoc. Amer. Physic. 64:245, 1951. [8]Steinkamp, R., Dubach, R. and Moore, C.V.: "Studies in Iron Transportation and Metabolism," Arch. Int. Med. 95:181, 1955. [9]Gorten, M.K. and Bradley, J.E.: "The Treatment of Nutritional Anemia in Infancy and Childhood with Oral Iron and Ascorbic Acid," J. Pediatrics, 45:1, 1954. [10]Mazur, A.: "Role of Ascorbic Acid in the Incorportion of Plasma Iron into Ferritin," An. N.Y. Acad. Sci. 92:223–229, 1961. [11]Cox, E.V. et al.: "The Anemia of Scurvy," Amer. J. Med. 42:220–227, 1967. [12]Berk, L. et al.: "Observations on the Etiologic Relationship of Achylia Gastrica to Pernicious Anemia, X," N. Eng. J. Med. 239:911–913, 1948. [13]Hall, B.E.: "Studies on the Nature of the Intrinsic Factor of Castle," Brit. Med. J. 2:585–589, 1950. [14]Wallerstein, R.O. et al.: "Observations on the Etiologic Relationship of Achylia Gastrica to Pernicious Anemia, XV," J. Lab & Clin. Med. 41:363–375, 1953. [15]Castle, W.B.: "Observations on the Etiologic Relationship of Achylia Gastrica to Pernicious Anemia, 1," Am. J. Med. Sc. 178:748–764, 1929. [16]Goodman, L.S. and Gilman, A.: The Pharmacological Basis of Therapeutics, 2 ed., P. 1482, N.Y., 1958. [17]Berenbaum, M.C. et al.: Blood, 15:540, 1960.

Manufactured by R.P. Scherer Corporation, St. Petersburg, Florida 33702
Distributed by
SAVAGE LABORATORIES®
a division of Altana Inc.
MELVILLE, NEW YORK 11747 R9/87

Shown in Product Identification Section, page 428

DILOR® Tablets ℞
[dī'lor]
(dyphylline)

COMPOSITION
Each blue, scored tablet contains dyphylline (dihydroxypropyl theophylline) 200 mg and the following inactive ingredients: colloidal silicon dioxide, corn starch, food starch, povidone, sodium lauryl sulfate, stearic acid and artificial coloring.
Each white scored tablet contains dyphylline (dihydroxypropyl theophylline) 400 mg and the following inactive ingredients: colloidal silicon dioxide, corn starch, food starch, povidone, sodium lauryl sulfate and stearic acid.

DESCRIPTION
Dyphylline [7-(2,3-Dihydroxypropyl) theophylline] [$C_{10}H_{14}N_4O_4$] is a white, extremely bitter, amorphous solid, freely soluble in water and soluble to the extent of 2 gm in 100 ml alcohol.

ACTIONS
As a xanthine derivative, dyphylline possesses the peripheral vasodilator and bronchodilator actions characteristic of theophylline. It has diuretic and myocardial stimulant effects, and is effective orally. Dyphylline may show fewer side effects than aminophylline, but its blood levels and possibly its activity are also lower.

INDICATIONS
For relief of acute bronchial asthma and for reversible bronchospasm associated with chronic bronchitis and emphysema.

CONTRAINDICATIONS
In individuals who have shown hypersensitivity to any of its components. Dyphylline should not be administered concurrently with other xanthine preparations.

WARNINGS
Status asthmaticus is a medical emergency. Excessive doses may be expected to be toxic. In children treated with dyphylline elixir, the alcoholic vehicle of the drug product poses a truly significant factor of drug dependence including all three components of tolerance, physical dependence and compulsive abuse.
Usage in Pregnancy: Safe use in pregnancy has not been established relative to possible adverse effects on fetal development. Therefore, dyphylline should not be used in pregnant women unless, in the judgment of the physician, the potential benefits outweigh the possible hazards.

PRECAUTIONS
Use with caution in patients with severe cardiac disease, hypertension, hyperthyroidism, or acute myocardial injury. Particular caution in dose administration must be exercised in patients with peptic ulcers, since the condition may be exacerbated. Chronic oral administration in high doses (500 to 1,000 mg) is usually associated with gastrointestinal irritation. Great caution should be used in giving dyphylline to patients in congestive heart failure. Such patients have shown markedly prolonged blood level curves which have persisted for long periods following discontinuation of the drug.

ADVERSE REACTIONS
Note: Included in this listing which follows are a few adverse reactions which may not have been reported with this specific drug. However, pharmacological similarities among the xanthine drugs require that each of the reactions be considered when dyphylline is administered. The most consistent adverse reactions are: 1. Gastrointestinal irritation: nausea, vomiting, and epigastric pain, generally preceded by headache, hematemesis, diarrhea. 2. Central nervous system stimulation: irritability, restlessness, insomnia, reflex hyperexcitability, muscle twitching, clonic and tonic generalized convulsions, agitation. 3. Cardiovascular: palpitation, tachycardia, extra systoles, flushing, marked hypotension, and circulatory failure. 4. Respiratory: tachypnea, respiratory arrest. 5. Renal: albuminuria, increased excretion of renal tubule and red blood cells. 6. Others: fever, dehydration.

OVERDOSAGE
Symptoms:
In infants and small children: agitation, headache, hyperreflexia, fasciculations, and clonic and tonic convulsions.
In adults: nervousness, insomnia, nausea, vomiting, tachycardia and extra systoles.
Therapy:
Discontinue drug immediately.
No specific treatment.
Ipecac syrup for oral ingestion.
Avoid sympathomimetics.
Supportive treatment for hypotension, seizure, arrhythmias and dehydration.
Sedatives such as short acting barbiturates will help control central nervous system stimulation.
Restore the acid-base balance with lactate or bicarbonate.
Oxygen and antibiotics provide supportive treatment as indicated.

DRUG INTERACTIONS
Toxic synergism with ephedrine and other sympathomimetic bronchodilator drugs may occur.
Recent controlled studies suggest that the addition of ephedrine to adequate dosage regimens of dyphylline produces no increase in effectiveness over that of dyphylline alone, but does produce an increase in toxic effects.

DOSAGE AND ADMINISTRATION
When administered orally it produces less nausea than aminophylline and other alkaline theophylline compounds. Absorption orally appears to be faster on an empty stomach; preferably the drug is to be given at six hour intervals.
Adults: Usual Adult Dose: 15 mg/kg every 6 hours up to 4 times a day. The dosage should be individualized by titration to the condition and response of the patient.
Pulmonary functional measurements before and after a period of treatment allow an objective assessment of whether or not therapy should be continued in patients with chronic bronchitis and emphysema.

HOW SUPPLIED
Dilor® Tablets

200 mg–	NDC 0281-1115-53, Bottle of 100.
	NDC 0281-1115-57, Bottle of 1000.
	NDC 0281-1115-63, Unit dose, Box of 100
400 mg–	NDC 0281-1116-53, Bottle of 100.
	NDC 0281-1116-57, Bottle of 1000.
	NDC 0281-1116-63, Unit dose, Box of 100

ALSO AVAILABLE
Dilor® Elixir, dyphylline 160 mg/15 ml; and Dilor® Injectable, dyphylline 250 mg/ml.

Shown in Product Identification Section, page 428

DILOR-G® ℞
[dī'lor]
(dyphylline, guaifenesin USP)

COMPOSITION
Each tablet contains dyphylline 200 mg and guaifenesin USP 200 mg. Also contains the following inactive ingredients: colloidal silicon dioxide, corn starch, food starch, povidone, stearic acid and artificial coloring.
Each teaspoonful (5 ml) of the liquid contains dyphylline 100 mg and guaifenesin USP 100 mg in a mint flavored base containing: citric acid, glycerin, saccharin sodium, sorbitol, sucrose, artificial coloring and flavoring, purified water, and sodium hydroxide to adjust pH. Methylparaben and propylparaben are added as preservatives. Contains no alcohol.

DESCRIPTION
Dyphylline is chemically dihydroxypropyl theophylline, an alkylated theophylline molecule. Since it is a molecular modification, rather than a salt or complex of theophylline the usual side effects of theophylline are diminished without affecting activity. The result is less gastric upset than with other theophyllines.
Guaifenesin USP, an ether, is capable of being partially eliminated by way of the expired air, and is therefore able to exert a local expectorant action in the respiratory passages. Guaifenesin USP makes expectoration freer and easier, because the respiratory tract secretions are made more fluid and thereby more easily expelled.
Dyphylline, being a stable, neutral derivative of theophylline, is not precipitated in gastric juice. Investigators, using 5% solutions of dyphylline and aminophylline, observed no precipitation of dyphylline from solution on the addition of simulated gastric juice, but 75% of the theophylline content was precipitated from the aminophylline in six hours.[1]

INDICATIONS
Dilor-G is indicated as a bronchodilator-expectorant for treating bronchial asthma, emphysema, bronchitis, pneumonitis and other related bronchopulmonary insufficiency conditions. Dilor-G acts to dilate bronchioles and liquefy mucus, giving relief from dyspnea, non-productive cough and tracheobronchial irritation.

CONTRAINDICATIONS
As with other theophylline-type drugs, combining dyphylline with ephedrine or other sympathomimetic drugs can cause excessive CNS stimulation. Such combinations are contraindicated in children unless accompanied by sufficient sedation to prevent undue CNS stimulation.

PRECAUTIONS
Due to its myocardial stimulatory effect, this product should be used with caution in cases of acute cardiac disease, severe renal and hepatic disease, severe myocardial damage, hyperthyroidism and glaucoma. Do not use in children under age six. Do not exceed 3 mg of dyphylline per pound of body weight daily in older children. Because the xanthines also act as diuretics, special precaution regarding hydration and avoidance of acidosis should be observed in children. The long term use of xanthine derivatives may result in a cumulative effect with increase in adverse reactions, as well as the development of tolerance.

ADVERSE REACTIONS
This product may cause nausea or headache, but either can usually be controlled by a reduction in dosage. As with other products containing xanthines, large doses of this product may cause excessive CNS stimulation. Large doses of guaifenesin USP may produce emesis, but gastrointestinal upset at ordinary dosage levels is rare.

DOSAGE AND ADMINISTRATION
In tablet form, the usual adult dose is 1 tablet 3 or 4 times a day.
In liquid form, the usual adult dose is 1 or 2 teaspoonfuls of liquid 3 or 4 times a day.

In severe cases, dosage may be doubled or tripled if necessary. Maintenance dosage should be adjusted according to patient response.
USE IN CHILDREN: Although pediatric dosages of dyphylline are established, no firm dosage for a combination of dyphylline and guaifenesin USP can be recommended for children under the age of six. Dosage for children over six may be calculated on the basis of 2 to 3 mg of dyphylline per pound of body weight daily in divided doses.

TOXICITY

Dyphylline was reported to be the least toxic of seven theophylline derivatives, including the piperazine, N,N-diethylamino ethyl and the 2-hydroxy ethyl derivatives.[2] The toxicity of dyphylline is only one-fifth that of aminophylline as determined intraperitoneally in mice, and only one-half as toxic in rats.[3]

HOW SUPPLIED

Dilor-G® Tablets
NDC 0281-1124-53, Tablets, Bottle of 100.
NDC 0281-1124-57, Tablets, Bottle of 1000.
NDC 0281-1124-63, Unit dose, Box of 100.
Dilor-G® Liquid
NDC 0281-1127-74, pint.
NDC 0281-1127-76, gallon.

CAUTION

Federal law prohibits dispensing without prescription.

REFERENCES [1]Maney, P. V. et al.: J Amer. Pharm. Assn. 35:266–272, 1946.[2]Quevauviller and Morin: Presse Med. 61, 1480, 1953. [3]Kjell, Briseid and Jensen: "Respective Toxocity of Dihydroxypropyl Theophylline and Theophylline Ethylene Diamine on the Mouse," Archiv for Pharmacie Og. Chemi. 56, 741–9, 1949.

Shown in Product Identification Section, page 428

DOCTAR™ — OTC

[dock 'tar]
Hair & Scalp
Shampoo and Conditioner

DESCRIPTION

CONTENTS: Amber color gel consisting of Stantar 2%, a purified coal tar extract equivalent to 0.50% coal tar. Also contains demineralized water, sodium laureth sulfate, TEA-lauryl sulfate, cocamidopropyl betaine, PEG-30 glyceryl stearate, polysorbate 80, cocamidopropylamine oxide, cocamide DEA, fragrance.

INDICATIONS

For the relief of scalp itching, irritation, redness, flaking and scaling associated with seborrheic dermatitis, dandruff and psoriasis.

WARNINGS

For external use only. Keep out of reach of children.

PRECAUTIONS

Avoid contact with eyes. If this happens, flush thoroughly with water. If condition worsens or does not improve after regular use as directed, consult a physician. Use caution in exposing skin to sunlight after applying. It may increase your tendency to sunburn up to 24 hours after application.

DOSAGE AND ADMINISTRATION

Wet hair and massage a liberal amount of Doctar™ shampoo into scalp. Rinse well. Re-apply the shampoo and allow lather to remain on scalp five minutes. Rinse thoroughly. Use up to 3 times per week or as physician directs.

HOW SUPPLIED

NDC 0281-0166-10, 100 ml tube

Shown in Product Identification Section, page 428

ETHIODOL® — ℞

[ĕ-thī 'ō 'dŏl]
(brand of ethiodized oil injection)

DESCRIPTION

Ethiodol®, brand of ethiodized oil, is a sterile injectable radio-opaque diagnostic agent for use in hysterosalpingography and lymphography. It contains 37% iodine (475 mg/ml) organically combined with ethyl esters of fatty acids (primarily as ethyl monoiodostearate and ethyl diiodostearate) of poppyseed oil. Stabilized with poppyseed oil, 1%. The precise structure of Ethiodol® is unknown at this time. Ethiodol® is a straw to amber colored, oil fluid, which because of simplified molecular structure, possesses a greatly reduced viscosity (1.280 specific gravity at 15°C yields viscosity of 0.5 to 1.0 poise). This high fluidity provides a new flexibility for radiographic exploration.

HOW SUPPLIED

Ethiodol® (brand of ethiodized oil for injection) is supplied in a box of two 10 ml ampules, NDC 0281-7062-37.

MYTREX® — ℞

[my "trex ']
(nystatin-triamcinolone acetonide)
Cream USP and Ointment USP

For Dermatologic Use Only
Not for Ophthalmic Use

DESCRIPTION

MYTREX® (nystatin-triamcinolone acetonide) Cream and Ointment contain the antifungal agent nystatin and the synthetic corticosteroid triamcinolone acetonide.
Nystatin is a polyene antimycotic obtained from *Streptomyces noursei*. It is a yellow to light tan powder with a cereal-like odor, very slightly soluble in water, and slightly to sparingly soluble in alcohol. It has an empirical formula of $C_{47}H_{75}NO_{17}$ and a molecular weight of 926.13 (CAS Registry Number 1400-61-9).
Triamcinolone Acetonide is designated chemically as Pregna-1, 4-diene-3, 20-dione, 9-fluoro-11, 21-dihydroxy-16,17-[(1-methylethylidene)bis(oxy)]-, (11β, 16α)-; The white to cream crystalline powder has a slight odor, is practically insoluble in water, and very soluble in alcohol. It has an empirical formula of $C_{24}H_{31}FO_6$ and a molecular weight of 434.50 (CAS Registry Number 76-25-5).
Each gram of MYTREX® (nystatin-triamcinolone acetonide) Cream contains 100,000 units of nystatin and 1.0 mg of triamcinolone acetonide in a cream base containing polyoxyethylene fatty alcohol ether, white petrolatum, glyceryl monostearate, polyethylene glycol 400 monostearate, sorbitol solution, simethicone emulsion, propylene glycol, aluminum hydroxide gel, polysorbate 60, titanium dioxide, and purified water with benzyl alcohol as a preservative. Hydrochloric acid or sodium hydroxide to adjust pH.
Each gram of MYTREX® (nystatin-triamcinolone acetonide) Ointment contains 100,000 units of nystatin and 1.0 mg of triamcinolone acetonide in a base of polyethylene and mineral oil.

CLINICAL PHARMACOLOGY

NYSTATIN
Nystatin exerts its antifungal activity against a variety of pathogenic and nonpathogenic yeasts and fungi by binding to sterols in the cell membrane. The binding process renders the cell membrane incapable of functioning as a selective barrier. Nystatin provides specific anticandidal activity to *Candida* (Monilia) *albicans* and other *Candida* species, but it is not active against bacteria, protozoa, trichomonads, or viruses. Nystatin is not absorbed from intact skin or mucous membranes.
TRIAMCINOLONE ACETONIDE
Triamcinolone Acetonide is primarily effective because of its anti-inflammatory, anti-pruritic and vasoconstrictive actions, characteristic of the topical corticosteroid class of drugs. The pharmacological effects of the topical corticosteroids are well known; however, mechanism of their dermatologic actions are unclear. Various laboratory methods, including vasoconstrictor assays, are used to compare and predict potencies and/or clinical efficacies of the topical corticosteroids. There is some evidence to suggest that a recognizable correlation exists between vasoconstrictor potency and therapeutic efficacy in man.
Pharmacokinetics: The extent of percutaneous absorption of topical corticosteroids is determined by many factors including the vehicle, the integrity of the epidermal barrier and the use of occlusive dressings (see DOSAGE AND ADMINISTRATION). Topical corticosteroids can be absorbed from normal intact skin. Inflammation and/or other disease processes in the skin increase percutaneous absorption. Occlusive dressings substantially increase the percutaneous absorption of topical corticosteroids (see DOSAGE AND ADMINISTRATION). Once absorbed through the skin, topical corticosteroids are handled through pharmacokinetic pathways similar to systemically administered corticosteroids. Corticosteroids are bound to plasma proteins in varying degrees. Corticosteroids are metabolized primarily in the liver and then excreted by the kidneys. Some of the topical corticosteroids and their metabolites are also excreted into the bile.
NYSTATIN and TRIAMCINOLONE ACETONIDE
Patients having mild to severe manifestations of cutaneous candidiasis, treated with combined nystatin and triamcinolone acetonide show a faster and more pronounced clearing of erythema and pruritis than patients treated with nystatin or triamcinolone acetonide alone.

INDICATIONS AND USAGE

MYTREX® (nystatin-triamcinolone acetonide) Cream and Ointment is indicated for the treatment of cutaneous candidiasis; it has been demonstrated that the nystatin-steroid combination provides greater benefit than the nystatin component alone during the first few days of treatment.

CONTRAINDICATIONS

This preparation is contraindicated in those patients with a history of hypersensitivity to any of its components.

PRECAUTIONS

General: Systemic absorption of topical corticosteroids has produced reversible hypothalamic-pituitary-adrenal (HPA) axis suppression, manifestations of Cushing's syndrome, hyperglycemia, and glucosuria in some patients. Conditions which augment systemic absorption include the application of the more potent steroids, use over large surface areas, prolonged use, and the addition of occlusive dressings (see DOSAGE AND ADMINISTRATION). Therefore, patients receiving a large dose of any potent topical steroid applied to a large surface area should be evaluated periodically for evidence of HPA axis suppression by using the urinary free cortisol and ACTH stimulation tests, and for impairment of thermal homeostasis. If HPA axis suppression or elevation of the body temperature occurs, an attempt should be made to withdraw the drug, to reduce the frequency of application, or to substitute a less potent steroid. Recovery of HPA axis function and thermal homeostasis are generally prompt and complete upon discontinuation of the drug. Infrequently, signs and symptoms of steroid withdrawal may occur, requiring supplemental systemic corticosteroids. Children may absorb proportionally larger amounts of topical corticosteroids and thus be more susceptible to systemic toxicity (See PRECAUTIONS, Pediatric Use). If irritation or hypersensitivity develops with the combination nystatin and triamcinolone acetonide, treatment should be discontinued and appropriate therapy instituted.
Information for the Patient: Patients using this medication should receive the following information and instructions:
1. This medication is to be used as directed by the physician. It is for external use only. Avoid contact with the eyes.
2. Patients should be advised not to use this medication for any disorder other than for which it was prescribed.
3. The treated skin area should not be bandaged or otherwise covered or wrapped as to be occluded (see DOSAGE AND ADMINISTRATION).
4. Patients should report any signs of local adverse reactions.
5. When using this medication in the inguinal area, patients should be advised to apply cream or ointment sparingly and to wear loose fitting clothing.
6. Parents of pediatric patients should be advised not to use tight-fitting diapers or plastic pants on a child being treated in the diaper area, as these garments may constitute occlusive dressings.
7. Patients should be advised on preventive measures to avoid reinfection.

Laboratory Tests: If there is a lack of therapeutic response, appropriate microbiological studies (e.g., KOH smears and/or cultures) should be repeated to confirm the diagnosis and rule out other pathogens, before instituting another course of therapy. The following tests may be helpful in evaluating hypothalamic-pituitary-adrenal (HPA) axis suppression due to the corticosteroid: Urinary free cortisol test; ACTH stimulation test.
Carcinogenesis, Mutagenesis, and Impairment of Fertility: Long-term animal studies have not been performed to evaluate the carcinogenic or mutagenic potential or possible impairment of fertility in males or females.
Pregnancy Category C: There are no teratogenic studies with combined nystatin and triamcinolone acetonide. Corticosteroids are generally teratogenic in laboratory animals when administered systemically at relatively low dosage levels. The more potent corticosteroids have been shown to be teratogenic after dermal application in laboratory animals. Therefore, any topical corticosteroid preparation should be used during pregnancy only if the potential benefit justifies the potential risk to the fetus. Topical preparations containing corticosteroids should not be used extensively on pregnant patients, in large amounts, or for prolonged periods of time.
Nursing Mothers: It is not known whether any component of this preparation is excreted in human milk. Because many drugs are excreted in human milk, caution should be exercised during use of this preparation by a nursing woman.
Pediatric Use: In clinical studies of a limited number of pediatric patients ranging in age from 2 months through twelve years, Nystatin-Triamcinolone Acetonide Cream cleared or significantly ameliorated the disease state in most patients. *Pediatric patients may demonstrate greater susceptibility to topical corticosteroid-induced hypothalamic-pituitary-adrenal (HPA) axis suppression and Cushing's syndrome than mature patients because of a larger skin surface area to body weight ratio.* HPA axis suppression, Cushing's syndrome, and intracranial hypertension have been reported in children receiving topical corticosteroids. Manifestations of adrenal suppression in children include linear growth retardation, delayed weight gain, low plasma cortisol levels, and absence of response to ACTH stimulation. Manifestations of intracranial hypertension include bulging fontanelles, headaches and bilateral papilledema. Administration of topical corticosteroids to children should be limited to the least amount compatible with an effective therapeutic regimen.

Continued on next page

Savage Laboratories—Cont.

Chronic corticosteroid therapy may interfere with the growth and development of children.

ADVERSE REACTIONS

A single case (approximately one percent of patients studied) of acneiform eruption occurred with the use of combined nystatin and triamcinolone acetonide in clinical studies.
Nystatin is virtually nontoxic and nonsensitizing and is well tolerated by all age groups, even during prolonged use. Rarely, irritation may occur.
The following local adverse reactions are reported infrequently with topical corticosteroids. These reactions are listed in an approximate decreasing order of occurrence: burning, itching, irritation, dryness, folliculitis, hypertrichosis, acneiform eruptions, hypopigmentation, perioral dermatitis, allergic contact dermatitis, maceration of the skin, secondary infection, skin atrophy, striae and miliaria.

OVERDOSAGE

Topically applied corticosteroids can be absorbed in sufficient amounts to produce systemic effects (see PRECAUTIONS, General). However, acute overdosage and serious adverse effects with dermatologic use are unlikely.

DOSAGE AND ADMINISTRATION

Apply MYTREX® (nystatin-triamcinolone acetonide) Cream to the affected area twice daily in the morning and the evening by gently and thoroughly massaging the preparation into the skin. A thin film of MYTREX® Ointment is usually applied to the affected areas twice daily in the morning and evening. The cream or ointment should be discontinued if symptoms persist after 25 days of therapy. (See PRECAUTIONS, Laboratory Tests). MYTREX® (nystatin-triamcinolone acetonide) Cream and Ointment should not be used with occlusive dressings.

HOW SUPPLIED

MYTREX® Cream
12 × 1.5 Gram Foilpac—NDC 0281-0081-08
15 Gram Tube—NDC 0281-0081-15
30 Gram Tube—NDC 0281-0081-30
60 Gram Tube—NDC 0281-0081-60
MYTREX® Ointment
15 gram tube—NDC 0281-0089-15
30 gram tube—NDC 0281-0089-30
60 gram tube—NDC 0281-0089-60
Store at room temperature. Avoid freezing.

CAUTION

Federal law prohibits dispensing without prescription.

Shown in Product Identification Section, page 428

TRYSUL® ℞
[trī'sul]
(triple sulfa vaginal cream, USP)

DESCRIPTION

Trysul® (Triple Sulfa Vaginal Cream, USP) contains sulfathiazole (4-amino-N-2-thiazolylbenzenesulfonamide; N'-2-thiazolylsulfanilamide) 3.42%, sulfacetamide (N-[(4-aminophenyl)sulfonyl]-acetamide; N-sulfanilyl-acetamide) 2.86%, sulfabenzamide (N-[(4-amino-phenyl)sulfonyl]-benzamide; N-sulfanilylbenzamide) 3.7% and urea (carbamide) 0.64%, compounded with glyceryl monostearate, cetyl alcohol, stearic acid, cholesterol, lecithin, peanut oil, propylparaben, propylene glycol, diethylaminoethyl stearamide, phosphoric acid, methylparaben and purified water.

CLINICAL PHARMACOLOGY

The mode of action of Trysul® is not completely known. Trysul® is a topical antibacterial preparation used intravaginally against *Haemophilus (Gardnerella) vaginalis* bacteria. Indirect effects, such as lowering the vaginal pH, may be equally important mechanisms.

INDICATIONS AND USAGE

Trysul® is indicated for the treatment of vaginitis caused by *Haemophilus (Gardnerella) vaginalis* bacteria.
The diagnosis of a *Haemophilus (Gardnerella) vaginalis* vaginitis should be firmly established before initiation of treatment with Trysul®.

CONTRAINDICATIONS

Trysul® is contraindicated in the following circumstances: Kidney disease; hypersensitivity to sulfonamides; in pregnancy at term and during the nursing period because sulfonamides cross the placenta, and are excreted in breast milk and may cause Kernicterus.

WARNINGS

Deaths associated with the administration of sulfonamides have been reported from hypersensitivity reactions, agranulocytosis, aplastic anemia and other blood dyscrasias.
The presence of clinical signs such as sore throat, fever, pallor, purpura or jaundice may be early indications of serious blood disorders.

PRECAUTIONS

Because sulfonamides may be absorbed from the vaginal mucosa, the usual precautions for oral sulfonamides apply. Patients should be observed for skin rash or evidence of systemic toxicity, and if these develop, the medications should be discontinued.

Laboratory Tests: Standard office diagnostic procedures for vaginitis are usually sufficient to establish the diagnosis of *Haemophilus (Gardnerella) vaginalis* and to rule out a trichomonal or monilial infection. These include noting a fish-like odor upon addition of 10% KOH to vaginal discharge and microscopic identification of "clue cells" in a wet mount preparation. If cultures are obtained, care must be taken to use appropriate media and methods for *Haemophilus (Gardnerella) vaginalis.*

Carcinogenesis, Mutagenesis, Impairment of Fertility: The sulfonamides bear certain chemical similarities to some goitrogens. Rats appear to be especially susceptible to the goitrogenic effects of sulfonamides, and long-term administration has produced thyroid malignancies in this species.

Pregnancy:

Teratogenic Effects: Pregnancy Category C: The safe use of sulfonamides in pregnancy has not been established. The teratogenicity potential of most sulfonamides has not been thoroughly investigated in either animals or humans. However, a significant increase in the incidence of cleft palate and other bony abnormalities of offspring has been observed when certain sulfonamides of the short, intermediate and long-acting types were given to pregnant rats and mice at high oral doses (7 to 25 times the human therapeutic dose).

Nursing Mothers: Because of the potential for serious adverse reactions in nursing infants from Trysul®, a decision should be made whether to discontinue nursing or to discontinue the drug, taking into account the importance of the drug to the mother. See CONTRAINDICATIONS.

Pediatric Use: Safety and effectiveness in children have not been established.

ADVERSE REACTIONS

There has been one reported case of agranulocytosis in a patient receiving Triple Sulfa Vaginal Cream, USP. The most frequent adverse reactions to Triple Sulfa Vaginal Cream, USP are localized irritation and/or allergy including rare reports of Stevens Johnson syndrome which may be fatal.

DOSAGE AND ADMINISTRATION

Trysul® (Triple Sulfa Vaginal Cream, USP). One full applicator intravaginally twice daily for four to six days. This course of therapy may be reduced one-half to one-quarter. Store at controlled room temperature 15°–30°C (59°–86°F).

CAUTION

Federal law prohibits dispensing without prescription.

HOW SUPPLIED

Trysul® is available in a 78 g tube (NDC 0281-3790-47) with a measured dose applicator.

Schein Pharmaceutical, Inc.
1800 NORTHERN BLVD.
ROSLYN, NY 11576

InFeD™ ℞
(IRON DEXTRAN INJECTION, USP)

WARNING

THE PARENTERAL USE OF COMPLEXES OF IRON AND CARBOHYDRATES HAS RESULTED IN FATAL ANAPHYLACTIC-TYPE REACTIONS. DEATHS ASSOCIATED WITH SUCH ADMINISTRATION HAVE BEEN REPORTED. THEREFORE, IRON DEXTRAN INJECTION, USP SHOULD BE USED ONLY IN THOSE PATIENTS IN WHOM THE INDICATIONS HAVE BEEN CLEARLY ESTABLISHED AND LABORATORY INVESTIGATIONS CONFIRM AN IRON DEFICIENT STATE NOT AMENABLE TO ORAL IRON THERAPY.

DESCRIPTION

Iron Dextran Injection, a hematinic agent, is a dark brown, slightly viscous liquid complex of ferric hydroxide and dextran for intramuscular or intravenous use.
Each mL contains the equivalent of 50 mg of iron as an iron dextran complex, approximately 0.9% sodium chlroide, in water for injection. Sodium hydroxide and/or hydrochloric acid may have been used to adjust pH. pH range is 5.2 to 6.5. The multiple dose vial also contains 0.5% phenol (for intramuscular use only).

CLINICAL PHARMACOLOGY

The iron dextran complex is dissociated by the reticuloendothelial system, and the ferric iron is transported by transferrin and incorporated into hemoglobin and storage sites.

INDICATIONS AND USAGE

Intravenous or intramuscular injections of Iron Dextran Injection are indicated for treatment of patients with documented iron deficiency in whom oral administration is unsatisfactory or impossible.

CONTRAINDICATIONS

Hypersensitivity to the product. All anemias not associated with iron deficiency.

WARNINGS

Two mL of undiluted iron dextran is the maximum recommended daily dose.
The following pattern of signs/symptoms has been reported as a delayed (1–2 days) reaction at recommended doses: modest-high fever, chills, backache, headache, myalgia, malaise, nausea, vomiting, and dizziness. These reactions have been reported in an unexpectedly high incidence with certain batches. Therefore, in estimating the benefit/risk of treatment for an individual patient, it must be assumed that there is a real possibility that such a delayed reaction may occur.
This preparation should be used with extreme care in the presence of serious impairment of liver function.
A risk of carcinogenesis may attend the intramuscular injection of iron carbohydrate complexes. Such complexes have been found under experimental conditions to produce sarcoma when large doses are injected in rats, mice, and rabbits, and possibly in hamsters.
The long latent period between the injection of a potential carcinogen and the appearance of a tumor makes it impossible to measure the risk in man accurately. There have, however, been several reports in the literature describing tumors at the injection site in humans who had previously received intramuscular injections of iron-carbohydate complexes.

Use in Pregnancy: Animal studies have shown that administration of Iron Dextran Injection during pregnancy caused an increase in the number of stillbirths and fetal anomalies, fetal edema, and a decrease in neonatal survival. In addition, these studies show that the fetus can obtain from 80 to 90% of the iron administered to the pregnant dam during the third trimester of pregnancy. Whether this represents a danger to the fetus and whether the drug is effective in treating maternal iron deficiency under these circumstances is not known.
For these reasons, Iron Dextran Injection should not be used in pregnancy or in women of child-bearing potential unless, in the judgment of the physician, the potential benefits outweigh the possible hazards.

PRECAUTIONS

Unwarranted therapy with parenteral iron will cause excess storage of iron with the consequent possibility of exogenous hemosiderosis. Such iron overload is particularly apt to occur in patients with hemoglobinopathies and other refractory anemias which might be erroneously diagnosed as iron deficiency anemia.
Iron Dextran Injection should be used with caution in individuals with histories of significant allergies and/or asthma. Epinephrine should be immediately available in the event of acute hypersensitivity reactions. (Usual adult dose: 0.5 mL of a 1:1000 solution, by subcutaneous or intramuscular injection.)
Patients with iron deficiency anemia and rheumatoid arthritis may have an acute exacerbation of joint pain and swelling following the intravenous administration of Iron Dextran Injection.

ADVERSE REACTIONS

Anaphylactic reactions including fatal anaphylaxis; other hypersensitivity reactions include dyspnea, urticaria, other rashes and itching, arthralgia and myalgia, and febrile episodes; variable degree of soreness and inflammation at or near injection site, including sterile abscesses (IM injection); brown skin discoloration at injection site (IM injection); lymphadenopathy; local phlebitis at injection site (IV injection); peripheral vascular flushing with overly rapid IV administration; hypotensive reaction; possible arthritic reactivation in patients with quiescent rheumatoid arthritis; leucocytosis, frequently with fever; headache, backache, dizziness, malaise, transitory paresthesias, nausea and shivering.

DOSAGE AND ADMINISTRATION

A. Iron Deficiency Anemia—Dosage: Periodic hematologic determinations should be used as a guide in therapy. It should be recognized that iron storage may lag behind the appearance of normal blood morphology. Although there are significant variations in body build and weight distribution among males and females, the accompanying table and formula represent a simple and convenient means for estimating the total iron required. This total iron requirement reflects the amount of iron needed to restore hemoglobin to normal or near normal levels plus an additional 50% allow-

$$\frac{\text{mg blood iron}}{\text{lb body weight}} = \frac{\text{mL blood}}{\text{lb body weight}} \times \frac{\text{g hemoglobin}}{\text{mL blood}} \times \frac{\text{mg iron}}{\text{g hemoglobin}}$$

a) Blood volume .... 8.5% body weight
b) Normal hemoglobin (males and females)
    over 30 pounds .... 14.8 g/dl
    30 pounds or less .... 12.0 g/dl
c) Iron content of hemoglobin 0.34%
d) Hemoglobin deficit
e) Weight

Based on the above factors, individuals with normal hemoglobin levels will have approximately 20 mg of blood iron per pound of body weight.

$$0.3 \times \text{Body Weight in Pounds} \times \left[100 - \left(\frac{\text{hemoglobin in g/dl} \times 100}{14.8}\right)\right]$$

(To calculate dose in mL of Iron Dextran Injection divide this result by 50.)

ance to provide adequate replenishment of iron stores in most individuals with moderately or severely reduced levels of hemoglobin. Factors contributing to the formula are shown below.

The formula should not be used for patients weighing 30 pounds or less. (Adjustments have been made in the table values to account for the lower normal hemoglobins for those weighing 30 pounds or less.)

Note: The table and accompanying formula are applicable for dosage determinations only in patients with **iron deficiency anemia**; they are not to be used for dosage determinations in patients requiring **iron replacement for blood loss**.

[See table at top of page.]

Total Amount of Iron Dextran Injection Required (to the nearest mL) for Restoration of Hemoglobin and Replacement of Depleted Iron Stores, Based on Observed Hemoglobin and Body Weight

Patient Weight		Milliliter Requirement Based on Observed Hemoglobin of			
lb	kg	4.0 (g/dl)	6.0 (g/dl)	8.0 (g/dl)	10.0 (g/dl)
10	4.5	3 mL	3 mL	2 mL	2 mL
20	9.1	7	6	4	3
30	13.6	10	8	7	5
40	18.1	18	14	11	8
50	22.7	22	18	14	10
60	27.2	26	21	17	12
70	31.8	31	25	19	14
80	36.3	35	28	22	16
90	40.8	39	32	25	18
100	45.4	44	35	28	20
110	49.9	48	39	30	21
120	54.4	53	42	33	23
130	59.0	57	46	36	25
140	63.5	61	50	39	27
150	68.1	66	53	41	29
160	72.6	70	57	44	31
170	77.1	74	60	47	33
180	81.7	79	64	50	35

The total amount of iron (in mg) required to restore hemoglobin to normal levels and to replenish iron stores may be approximated from the formula:

[See second table above.]

Administration: 1. Intravenous Injection—The total amount of Iron Dextran Injection required for the treatment of the iron deficiency anemia is determined from the formula or table (See **Dosage** section above.)

Test dose: Prior to receiving their first Iron Dextran Injection therapeutic dose, all patients should be given an intravenous test dose of 0.5 mL. Although anaphylactic reactions known to occur following Iron Dextran Injection administration are usually evident within a few minutes, or sooner, it is recommended that a period of an hour or longer elapse before the remainder of the initial therapeutic dose is given. Individual doses of 2 mL or less may be given on a daily basis until the calculated total amount required has been reached. Iron Dextran Injection is given undiluted and **slowly** (1 mL or less per minute).

2. Intramuscular Injection—The total amount of Iron Dextran Injection required for the treatment of iron deficiency anemia is determined from the formula or table. (See **Dosage** section above.)

Test dose: Prior to receiving their first Iron Dextran Injection therapeutic dose, all patients should be given an intramuscular test dose of 0.5 mL, administered in the same recommended test site and by the same technique as described in the last paragraph of this section. Although anaphylactic reactions known to occur following Iron Dextran Injection administration are usually evident within a few minutes or sooner, it is recommended that a period of an hour or longer elapse before the remainder of the initial therapeutic dose is given.

If no adverse reactions are observed, the injection can be given according to the following schedule until the calculated total amount required has been reached. Each day's dose should ordinarily not exceed 0.5 mL (25 mg of iron) for infants under 10 lb, 1.0 mL (50 mg of iron) for children under 20 lb, 2.0 mL (100 mg of iron) for other patients.

Iron Dextran Injection should be injected only into the muscle mass of the upper outer quadrant of the buttock—never into the arm or other exposed areas—and should be injected deeply, with a 2-inch or 3-inch 19 or 20 gauge needle. If the patient is standing, he should be bearing his weight on the leg opposite the injection site, or if in bed, he should be in the lateral position with injection site upper-most. To avoid injection or leakage into the subcutaneous tissue, a Z-track technique (displacement of the skin laterally prior to injection) is recommended.

B. Iron Replacement for Blood Loss—Some individuals sustain blood losses on an intermittent or repetitive basis. Such blood losses may occur periodically in patients with hemorrhagic diatheses (familial telangiectasia; hemophilia; gastrointestinal bleeding) and on a repetitive basis from procedures such as renal hemodialysis.

Iron therapy in these patients should be directed toward replacement of the equivalent amount of iron represented in the blood loss. The table and formula described under **A. Iron Deficiency Anemia** are **not** applicable for simple iron replacement values.

Quantitative estimates of the individual's periodic blood loss and hematocrit during the bleeding episode provide a convenient method for the calculation of the required iron dose. The formula shown below is based on the approximation that 1 mL of normocytic, normochromic red cells contains 1 mg of elemental iron:

Replacement iron (in mg) = Blood loss (in mL) × hematocrit
Example: Blood loss of 500 mL with 20% hematocrit
    Replacement Iron = 500 × 0.20 = 100 mg

$$\text{Iron Dextran Injection dose} = \frac{100 \text{ mg}}{50} = 2 \text{ mL}$$

Parenteral drug products should be inspected visually for particulate matter and discoloration prior to administration, whenever the solution and container permit.

HOW SUPPLIED
Iron Dextran Injection, USP, containing 50 mg iron per mL, is available in:
NDC 0364-3012-28 2 mL ampules (for intramuscular or intravenous use) in cartons of 10;
NDC 0364-3011-54 10 mL multiple dose vials (for intramuscular use ONLY) individually boxed or in cartons of 10.
Store at controlled room temperature 15°–30° C (59°–86° F).
CAUTION: Federal law prohibits dispensing without prescription.
Literature revised: March 1991
Product Nos.: 1001-82, 0539-10
910613A6
    Shown in Product Identification Section, page 428

Products are
listed alphabetically
in the
PINK SECTION.

Products are cross-indexed
by product classifications
in the
BLUE SECTION.

Products are cross-indexed by
generic and chemical names
in the
YELLOW SECTION.

Schering Corporation
a wholly-owned subsidiary of Schering-Plough Corporation
GALLOPING HILL ROAD
KENILWORTH, NJ 07033

Product Identification Codes
To provide quick and positive identification of Schering Products, we have imprinted the product identification number of the National Drug Code on most tablets and capsules. In some cases, identification letters also appear. Additionally, the following telephone numbers are provided for inquiries:

Professional Services Department
9:00 AM to 5:00 PM EST
1-800-526-4099
After regular hours and on weekends: (908) 298-4000
For convenience, a complete list of all Schering products and their identification codes, where appropriate, follow:

Product Listing

Product	Code	
CELESTONE®		℞
betamethasone, USP		
Phosphate Injection†		
Soluspan® **Suspension**		
Syrup†		
Tablets 0.6 mg†	011/BDA	
DIPROLENE®		℞
augmented betamethasone dipropionate		
AF Cream 0.05%		
Gel 0.05%		
Lotion 0.05%		
Ointment 0.05%		
DIPROSONE®†		℞
betamethasone dipropionate, USP		
Aerosol 0.1%		
Cream 0.05%		
Lotion 0.05%		
Ointment 0.05%		
ELOCON®		℞
mometasone furoate		
Cream 0.1%		
Lotion 0.1%		
Ointment 0.1%		
ESTINYL® **Tablets**†		℞
estinyl estradiol, USP		
0.02 mg	298	
0.05 mg	070	
0.5 mg	150	
ETRAFON® **Tablets**		℞
perphenazine, USP-amitriptyline hydrochloride, USP		
Tablets (2–10)	ANA/287	
Tablets (2–25)	ANC/598	
A Tablets (4–10)	ANB/119	
Forte Tablets (4–25)	ANE/720	
EULEXIN® **Capsules**		℞
flutamide		
125 mg	525	
FULVICIN® **P/G Tablets**		℞
ultramicrosize griseofulvin, USP		
125 mg	228	
165 mg	654	
250 mg	507	
330 mg	352	
FULVICIN U/F® **Tablets**†		℞
griseofulvin, (microsize), USP		
250 mg	AUF/948	
500 mg	AUG/496	
GARAMYCIN® **Injectables**		℞
gentamicin sulfate, USP		
Disposable Syringes 1.5 ml (60 mg)		
Disposable Syringes 2.0 ml (80 mg)		
Injectable 2 ml vial (80 mg)		
Intrathecal 2 ml (4 mg) ampul		
Pediatric Injectable 2 ml vial (20 mg)		
GARAMYCIN® **Topicals**		℞
gentamicin sulfate, USP		
Cream		
Ointment		
Ophthalmic Ointment		
Ophthalmic Solution		

†For complete prescribing information contact the Schering Professional Services Department.

Information on Schering products appearing on these pages is effective as of August 15, 1992.

Continued on next page

Schering—Cont.

HYPERSTAT® I.V. Injection   ℞
diazoxide injection, USP
INSPIREASE®   ℞
Drug Delivery System for use with
  Metered Dose Inhalers
INTRON® A   ℞
Interferon alfa-2b, recombinant
for Injection
LOTRIMIN®   ℞
clotrimazole, USP
  Cream 1%
  Lotion 1%
  Topical Solution 1%
LOTRISONE® Cream   ℞
clotrimazole, USP, betamethasone
dipropionate, USP
METICORTEN® Tablets†   ℞
prednisone, USP
  1 mg   843
METIMYD®†   ℞
prednisolone acetate, USP/
sulfacetamide sodium, USP
  Ophthalmic Ointment
  Ophthalmic Suspension
MIRADON® Tablets †   ℞
anisindione, USP
NAQUA® Tablets†   ℞
trichlormethiazide, USP
  2 mg   AHG/822
  4 mg   AHH/547
NETROMYCIN®   ℞
netilmicin sulfate
  Injection   100 mg/ml
NORMODYNE®   ℞
labetalol HCl
  Tablets   **100 mg**   244
      200 mg   752
      300 mg   438
  Injection   5 mg/ml
OPTIMINE® Tablets†   ℞
azatadine maleate, USP   282
OPTIMYD® Ophthalmic Solution†   ℞
prednisolone sodium phosphate, USP/
sulfacetamide sodium, USP
ORETON®†   ℞
methyltestosterone, USP
  Methyl Tablets   **10 mg**   311
  Methyl Buccal Tablets   970
OTOBIOTIC® Otic Solution†   ℞
polymyxin B sulfate, USP and
hydrocortisone, USP
PAXIPAM® Tablets ℂ†   ℞
halazepam, USP
  20 mg   251
  40 mg   538
PERMITIL®†   ℞
fluphenazine hydrochloride, USP
  Oral Concentrate
  Tablets   **2.5 mg**   WDR/442
      5 mg   WFF/550
      10 mg   WFG/316
POLARAMINE®†   ℞
dexchlorpheniramine maleate, USP
  Expectorant
  Repetabs® Tablets   **4 mg**   095
      6 mg   148
  Syrup
  Tablets   **2 mg**   AGT/820
PROVENTIL®   ℞
albuterol, USP
  Inhalation Aerosol
PROVENTIL®   ℞
albuterol sulfate, USP
  Solution for Inhalation 0.083%/0.5%
  Syrup
  Repetabs® Tablets   **4 mg**   431
  Tablets   **2 mg**   252
      4 mg   573
SEBIZON® Lotion†   ℞
sulfacetamide sodium, USP 10%
SODIUM SULAMYD®   ℞
sulfacetamide sodium, USP
  Ophthalmic Ointment 10%
  Ophthalmic Solution 10%
  Ophthalmic Solution 30% w/v
SOLGANAL® Suspension   ℞
aurothioglucose, USP
THEOVENT® Long-Acting Capsules†   ℞
theophylline anhydrous, USP
  125 mg   402
  250 mg   753

TRILAFON®   ℞
perphenazine, USP
  Concentrate
  Injection
  Tablets   **2 mg**   ADH/705
      4 mg   ADK/940
      8 mg   ADJ/313
      16 mg   ADM/077
VALISONE®†   ℞
betamethasone valerate, USP
  Cream 0.1%
  Lotion 0.1%
  Ointment 0.1%
  Reduced Strength Cream 0.01%
VANCENASE®   ℞
beclomethasone dipropionate, USP
  Nasal Inhaler
  AQ Nasal Spray 0.042%
VANCERIL® Oral Inhaler   ℞
beclomethasone dipropionate, USP

---

† For complete prescribing information contact the Schering Professional Services Department.

CELESTONE® SOLUSPAN®*   ℞
[se-les 'tōn]
brand of
sterile betamethasone sodium
phosphate and betamethasone
acetate Suspension, USP
6 mg per mL

DESCRIPTION

Each mL of CELESTONE SOLUSPAN* Suspension contains: 3.0 mg betamethasone as betamethasone sodium phosphate; 3.0 mg betamethasone acetate; 7.1 mg dibasic sodium phosphate; 3.4 mg monobasic sodium phosphate; 0.1 mg edetate disodium; and 0.2 mg benzalkonium chloride. It is a sterile, aqueous suspension with a pH between 6.8 and 7.2. The formula for betamethasone sodium phosphate is $C_{22}H_{28}FNa_2O_8P$ with a molecular weight of 516.41. Chemically it is 9-Fluoro-11β,17,21-trihydroxy-16β-methylpregna-1,4-diene-3,20-dione 21-(disodium phosphate).
The formula for betamethasone acetate is $C_{24}H_{31}FO_6$ with a molecular weight of 434.50. Chemically it is 9-Fluoro-11β, 17, 21 -trihydroxy -16β -methylpregna -1, 4-diene-3, 20-dione 21-acetate.
Betamethasone sodium phosphate is a white to practically white, odorless powder, and is hygroscopic. It is freely soluble in water and in methanol, but is practically insoluble in acetone and in chloroform.
Betamethasone acetate is a white to creamy white, odorless powder that sinters and resolidifies at about 165°C, and re-melts at about 200°C–220°C with decomposition. It is practically insoluble in water, but freely soluble in acetone, and is soluble in alcohol and in chloroform.

ACTIONS

Naturally occurring glucocorticoids (hydrocortisone), which also have salt-retaining properties, are used as replacement therapy in adrenocortical deficiency states. Their synthetic analogs are primarily used for their potent anti-inflammatory effects in disorders of many organ systems.
Betamethasone sodium phosphate, a soluble ester, provides prompt activity, while betamethasone acetate is only slightly soluble and affords sustained activity.
Glucocorticoids cause profound and varied metabolic effects. In addition, they modify the body's immune responses to diverse stimuli.

INDICATIONS

When oral therapy is not feasible and the strength, dosage form, and route of administration of the drug reasonably lend the preparation to the treatment of the condition, CELESTONE SOLUSPAN Suspension for intramuscular use is indicated as follows:
Endocrine disorders: Primary or secondary adrenocortical insufficiency (hydrocortisone or cortisone is the drug of choice; synthetic analogs may be used in conjunction with mineralocorticoids where applicable; in infancy, mineralo-corticoid supplementation is of particular importance).
Acute adrenocortical insufficiency (hydrocortisone or cortisone is the drug of choice; mineralocorticoid supplementation may be necessary, particularly when synthetic analogs are used). Preoperatively and in the event of serious trauma or illness, in patients with known adrenal insufficiency or when adrenocortical reserve is doubtful. Shock unresponsive to conventional therapy if adrenocortical insufficiency exists

*Brand of rapid and repository injectable.

---

or is suspected. Congenital adrenal hyperplasia. Nonsuppurative thyroiditis. Hypercalcemia associated with cancer.
Rheumatic disorders: As adjunctive therapy for short-term administration (to tide the patient over an acute episode or exacerbation) in: post-traumatic osteoarthritis; synovitis of osteoarthritis; rheumatoid arthritis, including juvenile rheumatoid arthritis (selected cases may require low-dose maintenance therapy); acute and subacute bursitis; epicondylitis; acute nonspecific tenosynovitis; acute gouty arthritis; psoriatic arthritis; ankylosing spondylitis.
Collagen disease: During an exacerbation or as maintenance therapy in selected cases of: systemic lupus erythematosus; acute rheumatic carditis.
Dermatologic diseases: Pemphigus; severe erythema multiforme (Stevens-Johnson syndrome); exfoliative dermatitis; bullous dermatitis herpetiformis; severe seborrheic dermatitis; severe psoriasis; mycosis fungoides.
Allergic states: Control of severe or incapacitating allergic conditions intractable to adequate trials of conventional treatment in: bronchial asthma; contact dermatitis; atopic dermatitis; serum sickness; seasonal or perennial allergic rhinitis; drug hypersensitivity reactions; urticarial transfusion reactions; acute noninfectious laryngeal edema (epinephrine is the drug of first choice).
Ophthalmic diseases: Severe, acute and chronic allergic and inflammatory processes involving the eye, such as: herpes zoster ophthalmicus; iritis, iridocyclitis; chorioretinitis; diffuse posterior uveitis and choroiditis; optic neuritis; sympathetic ophthalmia; anterior segment inflammation; allergic conjunctivitis; allergic corneal marginal ulcer; keratitis.
Gastrointestinal diseases: To tide the patient over a critical period of disease in: ulcerative colitis—(systemic therapy); regional enteritis—(systemic therapy).
Respiratory diseases: Symptomatic sarcoidosis; berylliosis; fulminating or disseminated pulmonary tuberculosis, when used concurrently with appropriate antituberculous chemotherapy; Loeffler's syndrome not manageable by other means; aspiration pneumonitis.
Hematologic disorders: Acquired (autoimmune) hemolytic anemia. Secondary thrombocytopenia in adults. Erythroblastopenia (RBC anemia). Congenital (erythroid) hypoplastic anemia.
Neoplastic diseases: For palliative management of: leukemias and lymphomas in adults; acute leukemia of childhood.
Edematous state: To induce diuresis or remission of proteinuria in the nephrotic syndrome, without uremia, of the idiopathic type or that due to lupus erythematosus.
Miscellaneous: Tuberculous meningitis with subarachnoid block or impending block when used concurrently with appropriate antituberculous chemotherapy. Trichinosis with neurologic or myocardial involvement.
When the strength and dosage form of the drug lend the preparation to the treatment of the condition, the **intra-articular or soft tissue administration** of CELESTONE SOLUSPAN Suspension is indicated as adjunctive therapy for short-term administration (to tide the patient over an acute episode or exacerbation) in: synovitis of osteoarthritis; rheumatoid arthritis; acute and subacute bursitis; acute gouty arthritis; epicondylitis; acute nonspecific tenosynovitis; post-traumatic osteoarthritis.
When the strength and dosage form of the drug lend the preparation to the treatment of the condition, the **intralesional administration** of CELESTONE SOLUSPAN Suspension is indicated for: keloids; localized hypertrophic, infiltrated, inflammatory lesions of lichen planus, psoriatic plaques, granuloma annulare, and lichen simplex chronicus (neurodermatitis); discoid lupus erythematosus; necrobiosis lipoidica diabeticorum; alopecia areata.
CELESTONE SOLUSPAN Suspension may also be useful in cystic tumors of an aponeurosis or tendon (ganglia).

CONTRAINDICATIONS

CELESTONE SOLUSPAN Suspension is contraindicated in systemic fungal infections.

WARNINGS

CELESTONE SOLUSPAN should not be administered intravenously.
In patients on corticosteroid therapy subjected to any unusual stress, increased dosage of rapidly acting corticosteroids before, during, and after the stressful situation is indicated.
Corticosteroids may mask some signs of infection, and new infections may appear during their use. There may be decreased resistance and inability to localize infection when corticosteroids are used.
Prolonged use of corticosteroids may produce posterior subcapsular cataracts, glaucoma with possible damage to the optic nerves, and may enhance the establishment of secondary ocular infections due to fungi or viruses.
CELESTONE SOLUSPAN contains two betamethasone esters one of which, betamethasone sodium phosphate, disappears rapidly from the injection site. The potential for systemic effect produced by the soluble portion of CELE-

STONE SOLUSPAN should therefore be taken into account by the physician when using the drug.

Average and large doses of cortisone or hydrocortisone can cause elevation of blood pressure, salt and water retention, and increased excretion of potassium. These effects are less likely to occur with the synthetic derivatives except when used in large doses. Dietary salt restriction and potassium supplementation may be necessary. All corticosteroids increase calcium excretion.

While on Corticosteroid Therapy Patients Should Not Be Vaccinated Against Smallpox. Other Immunization Procedures Should Not Be Undertaken in Patients Who Are on Corticosteroids, Especially in High Doses, Because of Possible Hazards of Neurological Complications and Lack of Antibody Response.

Children who are on immunosuppressant drugs are more susceptible to infections than healthy children. Chickenpox and measles, for example, can have a more serious or even fatal course in children on immunosuppressant corticosteroids. In such children, or in adults who have not had these diseases, particular care should be taken to avoid exposure. If exposed, therapy with varicella zoster immune globulin (VZIG) or pooled intravenous immunoglobulin (IVIG), as appropriate, may be indicated. If chickenpox develops, treatment with antiviral agents may be considered.

The use of CELESTONE SOLUSPAN Suspension in active tuberculosis should be restricted to those cases of fulminating or disseminated tuberculosis in which the corticosteroid is used for the management of the disease in conjunction with appropriate antituberculous regimen.

If corticosteroids are indicated in patients with latent tuberculosis or tuberculin reactivity, close observation is necessary as reactivation of the disease may occur. During prolonged corticosteroid therapy, these patients should receive chemoprophylaxis.

Because rare instances of anaphylactoid reactions have occurred in patients receiving parenteral corticosteroid therapy, appropriate precautionary measures should be taken prior to administration, especially when the patient has a history of allergy to any drug.

Usage in pregnancy: Since adequate human reproduction studies have not been done with corticosteroids, the use of these drugs in pregnancy, nursing mothers, or women of childbearing potential requires that the possible benefits of the drug be weighed against the potential hazards to the mother and embryo or fetus. Infants born of mothers who have received substantial doses of corticosteroids during pregnancy should be carefully observed for signs of hypoadrenalism.

PRECAUTIONS

Information for Patients Patients who are on immunosuppressant doses of corticosteroids should be warned to avoid exposure to chickenpox or measles and, if exposed, to obtain medical advice.

General: Drug-induced secondary adrenocortical insufficiency may be minimized by gradual reduction of dosage. This type of relative insufficiency may persist for months after discontinuation of therapy; therefore, in any situation of stress occurring during that period, hormone therapy should be reinstituted. Since mineralocorticoid secretion may be impaired, salt and/or a mineralocorticoid should be administered concurrently.

There is an enhanced effect of corticosteroids in patients with hypothyroidism and in those with cirrhosis.

Corticosteroids should be used cautiously in patients with ocular herpes simplex for fear of corneal perforation.

The lowest possible dose of corticosteroid should be used to control the condition under treatment, and when reduction in dosage is possible, the reduction must be gradual.

Psychic derangements may appear when corticosteroids are used, ranging from euphoria, insomnia, mood swings, personality changes, and severe depression to frank psychotic manifestations. Also, existing emotional instability or psychotic tendencies may be aggravated by corticosteroids.

Aspirin should be used cautiously in conjunction with corticosteroids in hypoprothrombinemia.

Steroids should be used with caution in nonspecific ulcerative colitis, if there is a probability of impending perforation, abscess or other pyogenic infection, also in diverticulitis, fresh intestinal anastomoses, active or latent peptic ulcer, renal insufficiency, hypertension, osteoporosis, and myasthenia gravis.

Growth and development of infants and children on prolonged corticosteroid therapy should be carefully followed.

The following additional precautions also apply for parenteral corticosteroids. **Intra-articular injection of a corticosteroid may produce systemic as well as local effects.**

Appropriate examination of any joint fluid present is necessary to exclude a septic process.

A marked increase in pain accompanied by local swelling, further restriction of joint motion, fever, and malaise are suggestive of septic arthritis. If this complication occurs and the diagnosis of sepsis is confirmed, appropriate antimicrobial therapy should be instituted.

Local injection of a steroid into a previously infected joint is to be avoided.

Corticosteroids should not be injected into unstable joints. The slower rate of absorption by intramuscular administration should be recognized.

ADVERSE REACTIONS

Fluid and electrolyte disturbances: sodium retention; fluid retention; congestive heart failure in susceptible patients; potassium loss; hypokalemic alkalosis; hypertension.

Musculoskeletal: muscle weakness; steroid myopathy; loss of muscle mass; osteoporosis; vertebral compression fractures; aseptic necrosis of femoral and humeral heads; pathologic fracture of long bones.

Gastrointestinal: peptic ulcer with possible subsequent perforation and hemorrhage; pancreatitis; abdominal distention; ulcerative esophagitis.

Dermatologic: impaired wound healing; thin fragile skin; petechiae and ecchymoses; facial erythema; increased sweating; may suppress reactions to skin tests.

Neurological: convulsions; increased intracranial pressure with papilledema (pseudotumor cerebri) usually after treatment; vertigo; headache.

Endocrine: menstrual irregularities; development of cushingoid state; suppression of growth in children; secondary adrenocortical and pituitary unresponsiveness, particularly in times of stress, as in trauma, surgery, or illness; decreased carbohydrate tolerance; manifestations of latent diabetes mellitus; increased requirements for insulin or oral hypoglycemic agents in diabetics.

Ophthalmic: posterior subcapsular cataracts; increased intraocular pressure; glaucoma; exophthalmos.

Metabolic: negative nitrogen balance due to protein catabolism.

The following *additional* adverse reactions are related to parenteral corticosteroid therapy: rare instances of blindness associated with intralesional therapy around the face and head; hyperpigmentation or hypopigmentation; subcutaneous and cutaneous atrophy; sterile abscess; post-injection flare (following intra-articular use); charcot-like arthropathy.

DOSAGE AND ADMINISTRATION

The initial dosage of CELESTONE SOLUSPAN Suspension may vary from 0.5 to 9.0 mg per day depending on the specific disease entity being treated. In situations of less severity, lower doses will generally suffice while in selected patients higher initial doses may be required. Usually the parenteral dosage ranges are one-third to one-half the oral dose given every 12 hours. However, in certain overwhelming, acute, life-threatening situations, administration in dosages exceeding the usual dosages may be justified and may be in multiples of the oral dosages.

The initial dosage should be maintained or adjusted until a satisfactory response is noted. If after a reasonable period of time there is a lack of satisfactory clinical response, CELESTONE SOLUSPAN Suspension should be discontinued and the patient transferred to other appropriate therapy. *It Should Be Emphasized That Dosage Requirements Are Variable and Must Be Individualized on the Basis of the Disease Under Treatment and the Response of the Patient.* After a favorable response is noted, the proper maintenance dosage should be determined by decreasing the initial drug dosage in small decrements at appropriate time intervals until the lowest dosage which will maintain an adequate clinical response is reached. It should be kept in mind that constant monitoring is needed in regard to drug dosage. Included in the situations which may make dosage adjustments necessary are changes in clinical status secondary to remissions or exacerbations in the disease process, the patient's individual drug responsiveness, and the effect of patient exposure to stressful situations not directly related to the disease entity under treatment; in this latter situation it may be necessary to increase the dosage of CELESTONE SOLUSPAN Suspension for a period of time consistent with the patient's condition. If after long-term therapy the drug is to be stopped, it is recommended that it be withdrawn gradually rather than abruptly.

If coadministration of a local anesthetic is desired, CELESTONE SOLUSPAN Suspension may be mixed with 1% or 2% lidocaine hydrochloride, using the formulations which do not contain parabens. Similar local anesthetics may also be used. Diluents containing methylparaben, propylparaben, phenol, etc., should be avoided since these compounds may cause flocculation of the steroid. The required dose of CELESTONE SOLUSPAN Suspension is first withdrawn from the vial into the syringe. The local anesthetic is then drawn in, and the syringe shaken briefly. **Do not inject local anesthetics into the vial of CELESTONE SOLUSPAN Suspension.**

Bursitis, tenosynovitis, peritendinitis. In acute subdeltoid, subacromial, olecranon, and prepatellar bursitis, one intrabursal injection of 1.0 mL CELESTONE SOLUSPAN Suspension can relieve pain and restore full range of movement. Several intrabursal injections of corticosteroids are usually required in recurrent acute bursitis and in acute exacerbations of chronic bursitis. Partial relief of pain and some increase in mobility can be expected in both conditions after one or two injections. Chronic bursitis may be treated with reduced dosage once the acute condition is controlled. In tenosynovitis and tendinitis, three or four local injections at intervals of one to two weeks between injections are given in most cases. Injections should be made into the affected tendon sheaths rather than into the tendons themselves. In ganglions of joint capsules and tendon sheaths, injection of 0.5 mL directly into the ganglion cysts has produced marked reduction in the size of the lesions. *Rheumatoid arthritis and osteoarthritis.* Following intra-articular administration of 0.5 to 2.0 mL of CELESTONE SOLUSPAN Suspension, relief of pain, soreness, and stiffness may be experienced. Duration of relief varies widely in both diseases. Intra-articular Injection—CELESTONE SOLUSPAN Suspension is well tolerated in joints and periarticular tissues. There is virtually no pain on injection, and the "secondary flare" that sometimes occurs a few hours after intra-articular injection of corticosteroids has not been reported with CELESTONE SOLUSPAN Suspension. Using sterile technique, a 20- to 24-gauge needle on an empty syringe is inserted into the synovial cavity, and a few drops of synovial fluid are withdrawn to confirm that the needle is in the joint. The aspirating syringe is replaced by a syringe containing CELESTONE SOLUSPAN Suspension and injection is then made into the joint.

Recommended Doses for Intra-articular Injection

Size of joint	Location	Dose (mL)
Very Large	Hip	1.0-2.0
Large	Knee, Ankle, Shoulder	1.0
Medium	Elbow, Wrist	0.5-1.0
Small (Metacarpophalangeal, interphalangeal) (Sternoclavicular)	Hand Chest	0.25-0.5

A portion of the administered dose of CELESTONE SOLUSPAN Suspension is absorbed systemically following intra-articular injection. In patients being treated concomitantly with oral or parenteral corticosteroids, especially those receiving large doses, the systemic absorption of the drug should be considered in determining intra-articular dosage. *Dermatologic conditions.* In intralesional treatment, 0.2 mL/sq. cm. of CELESTONE SOLUSPAN Suspension is injected intradermally (not subcutaneously) using a tuberculin syringe with a 25-gauge, ½-inch needle. Care should be taken to deposit a uniform depot of medication intradermally. A total of no more than 1.0 mL. at weekly intervals is recommended. *Disorders of the foot.* A tuberculin syringe with a 25-gauge, ¾-inch needle is suitable for most injections into the foot. The following doses are recommended at intervals of three days to a week.

Diagnosis	CELESTONE SOLUSPAN Suspension Dose (mL)
Bursitis	
under heloma durum or heloma molle	0.25-0.5
under calcaneal spur	0.5
over hallux rigidus or digiti quinti varus	0.5
Tenosynovitis, periostitis of cuboid	0.5
Acute gouty arthritis	0.5-1.0

HOW SUPPLIED

CELESTONE SOLUSPAN Suspension, 5 mL multiple-dose vial; box of one (NDC-0085-0566-05). **Shake well before using. Store between 2° and 25°C (36° and 77°F). Protect from light.** Revised 10/91   B-10229758

Continued on next page

Information on Schering products appearing on these pages is effective as of August 15, 1992.

Schering—Cont.

DIPROLENE® ℞
brand of augmented betamethasone dipropionate*
AF CREAM, 0.05 %
OINTMENT, 0.05%
LOTION,0.05%
(Potency expressed as betamethasone)
***Vehicle augments the penetration of the steroid**
For Dermatologic Use Only—Not for Ophthalmic Use

DESCRIPTION

DIPROLENE® products contain betamethasone dipropionate, USP, a synthetic adrenocorticosteroid for dermatologic use. Betamethasone, an analog of prednisolone, has a high degree of corticosteroid activity and a slight degree of mineralocorticoid activity. Betamethasone dipropionate is the 17,21-dipropionate ester of betamethasone.
Chemically, betamethasone dipropionate is 9-fluoro-11β, 17,21-trihydroxy-16β-methylpregna-1,4-diene-3,20-dione 17, 21-dipropionate, with the empirical formula $C_{28}H_{37}FO_7$, and a molecular weight of 504.6.
Betamethasone dipropionate is a white to creamy white, odorless crystalline powder, insoluble in water.
Each gram of DIPROLENE **AF Cream** 0.05% contains: 0.64 mg betamethasone dipropionate, USP (equivalent to 0.5 mg betamethasone), in an emollient cream base of purified water, chlorocresol, propylene glycol, white petrolatum, white wax, cyclomethicone, sorbitol solution, glyceryl monooleate, ceteareth-30, carbomer 940 and sodium hydroxide.
Each gram of DIPROLENE **Lotion** 0.05% contains: 0.64 mg betamethasone dipropionate, USP (equivalent to 0.5 mg betamethasone), in a lotion base of purified water, isopropyl alcohol (30%), hydroxypropylcellulose, propylene glycol, sodium phosphate, phosphoric acid and sodium hydroxide used to adjust the pH to 4.5.
Each gram of DIPROLENE **Ointment** 0.05% contains: 0.64 mg betamethasone dipropionate, USP (equivalent to 0.5 mg betamethasone), in ACTIBASE™, an optimized vehicle of propylene glycol, propylene glycol stearate, white wax and white petrolatum.

CLINICAL PHARMACOLOGY

The corticosteroids are a class of compounds comprising steroid hormones secreted by the adrenal cortex and their synthetic analogs. In pharmacologic doses, corticosteroids are used primarily for their anti-inflammatory and/or immunosuppressive effects.
Topical corticosteroids, such as betamethasone dipropionate, are effective in the treatment of corticosteroid-responsive dermatoses primarily because of their anti-inflammatory, anti-pruritic, and vasoconstrictive actions. However, while the physiologic, pharmacologic, and clinical effects of the corticosteroids are well-known, the exact mechanisms of their actions in each disease are uncertain. Betamethasone dipropionate, a corticosteroid, has been shown to have topical (dermatologic) and systemic pharmacologic and metabolic effects characteristic of this class of drugs.
Pharmacokinetics: The extent of percutaneous absorption of topical corticosteroids is determined by many factors including the vehicle, the integrity of the epidermal barrier, and the use of occlusive dressings. (See **DOSAGE AND ADMINISTRATION** section.)
Topical corticosteroids can be absorbed through normal intact skin. Inflammation and/or other disease processes in the skin may increase percutaneous absorption. Occlusive dressings substantially increase the percutaneous absorption of topical corticosteroids. (See **DOSAGE AND ADMINISTRATION** section.)
Once absorbed through the skin, topical corticosteroids enter pharmacokinetic pathways similar to systemically administered corticosteroids. Corticosteroids are bound to plasma proteins in varying degrees, are metabolized primarily in the liver and excreted by the kidneys. Some of the topical corticosteroids and their metabolites are also excreted into the bile.
DIPROLENE **AF Cream** was applied once daily at 7 grams per day for one week to diseased skin, in patients with psoriasis or atopic dermatitis, to study its effects on the hypothalamic-pituitary-adrenal (HPA) axis. The results suggested that the drug caused a slight lowering of adrenal corticosteroid secretion, although in no case did plasma cortisol levels go below the lower limit of the normal range.
DIPROLENE **Lotion** was applied once daily at 7 mL per day for 21 days to diseased skin (in patients with scalp psoriasis), to study its effects on the hypothalamic-pituitary-adrenal (HPA) axis. In 2 out of 11 patients, the drug lowered plasma cortisol levels below normal limits. Adrenal depression in these patients was transient, and returned to normal within a week. In one of these patients, plasma cortisol levels returned to normal while treatment continued.
At 14 g per day, DIPROLENE **Ointment** was shown to depress the plasma levels of adrenal cortical hormones following repeated application to diseased skin in patients with psoriasis. Adrenal depression in these patients was transient, and rapidly returned to normal upon cessation of treatment. At 7 g per day (3.5 g bid), DIPROLENE **Ointment** was shown to cause minimal inhibition of the hypothalamic-pituitary-adrenal (HPA) axis when applied two times daily for two to three weeks, in normal patients and in patients with psoriasis and eczematous disorders.
With 6 to 7 g of DIPROLENE **Ointment** applied once daily for 3 weeks, no significant inhibition of the HPA axis was observed in patients with psoriasis and atopic dermatitis, as measured by plasma cortisol and 24 hour urinary 17-hydroxycorticosteroid levels.

INDICATIONS AND USAGE

DIPROLENE **AF Cream** and **Ointment** are indicated for relief of the inflammatory and pruritic manifestations of corticosteroid-responsive dermatoses.
DIPROLENE **Lotion** is intended for short-term treatment of the inflammatory and pruritic manifestations of moderate to severe corticosteroid-responsive dermatoses. Treatment beyond two weeks is not recommended for DIPROLENE **Lotion**. The total dosage should not exceed 50 mL per week for DIPROLENE **Lotion** because of potential for the drug to suppress the hypothalamic-pituitary-adrenal axis.

CONTRAINDICATIONS

DIPROLENE products are contraindicated in patients who are hypersensitive to betamethasone dipropionate, to other corticosteroids, or to any ingredient in these preparations.

PRECAUTIONS

General: DIPROLENE **Lotion** is a highly potent topical corticosteroid that has been shown to suppress the HPA axis at 7 mL per day.
Systemic absorption of topical corticosteroids has produced reversible HPA axis suppression, manifestations of Cushing's syndrome, hyperglycemia, and glucosuria in some patients.
Conditions which augment systemic absorption include the application of the more potent corticosteroids, use over large surface areas, prolonged use, and the addition of occlusive dressings. (See **DOSAGE AND ADMINISTRATION** section.)
Therefore, patients receiving a large dose of a potent topical steroid applied to a large surface area should be evaluated periodically for evidence of HPA axis suppression by using the urinary free cortisol and ACTH stimulation tests. If HPA axis suppression is noted, an attempt should be made to withdraw the drug, to reduce the frequency of application, or to substitute a less potent steroid.
Recovery of HPA axis function is generally prompt and complete upon discontinuation of the drug. Infrequently, signs and symptoms of steroid withdrawal may occur, requiring supplemental systemic corticosteroids.
Children may absorb proportionally larger amounts of topical corticosteroids and thus be more susceptible to systemic toxicity. (See **PRECAUTIONS—Pediatric Use.**)
If irritation develops, topical corticosteroids should be discontinued and appropriate therapy instituted.
In the presence of dermatological infections, the use of an appropriate antifungal or antibacterial agent should be instituted. If a favorable response does not occur promptly, the corticosteroid should be discontinued until the infection has been adequately controlled.
Information for Patients: Patients using topical corticosteroids should receive the following information and instructions. This information is intended to aid in the safe and effective use of this medication. It is not a disclosure of all possible adverse or intended effects.

1. This medication is to be used as directed by the physician and should not be used longer than the prescribed time period. It is for external use only. Avoid contact with the eyes.
2. Patients should be advised not to use this medication for any disorder other than that for which it was prescribed.
3. The treated skin areas should not be bandaged or otherwise covered or wrapped so as to be occlusive. (See **DOSAGE AND ADMINISTRATION** section.)
4. Patients should report any sign of local adverse reactions.

Laboratory Tests: The following tests may be helpful in evaluating HPA axis suppression:
Urinary free cortisol test
ACTH stimulation test
Carcinogenesis, Mutagenesis, and Impairment of Fertility: Long-term animal studies have not been performed to evaluate the carcinogenic potential or the effect on fertility of topically applied corticosteroids.
Studies to determine mutagenicity with prednisolone and hydrocortisone have revealed negative results.
Pregnancy Category C: Corticosteroids are generally teratogenic in laboratory animals when administered systemically at relatively low dosage levels. The more potent corticosteroids have been shown to be teratogenic after dermal application in laboratory animals. Betamethasone dipropionate has not been tested for teratogenicity by this route, however, it appears to be fairly well-absorbed percutaneously. There are no adequate and well-controlled studies of the teratogenic effects of topically applied corticosteroids in pregnant women. Therefore, topical corticosteroids should be used during pregnancy only if the potential benefit justifies the potential risk to the fetus. Drugs of this class should not be used extensively on pregnant patients, in large amounts, or for prolonged periods of time.
Nursing Mothers: It is not known whether topical administration of corticosteroids can result in sufficient systemic absorption to produce detectable quantities in breast milk. Systemically administered corticosteroids are secreted into breast milk in quantities not likely to have a deleterious effect on the infant. Nevertheless, a decision should be made whether to discontinue nursing or to discontinue the drug, taking into account the importance of the drug to the mother.
Pediatric Use: Use of DIPROLENE **AF Cream** and DIPROLENE **Ointment** in children under 12 years is not recommended. The safety and efficacy of DIPROLENE **Lotion** when used in children under 12 years of age have not been established.
Pediatric patients may demonstrate greater susceptibility to topical corticosteroid-induced HPA axis suppression and Cushing's syndrome than mature patients because of a larger skin surface area to body weight ratio.
Hypothalamic-pituitary-adrenal (HPA) axis suppression Cushing's syndrome, and intracranial hypertension have been reported in children receiving topical corticosteroids. Manifestations of adrenal suppression in children include linear growth retardation, delayed weight gain, low plasma cortisol levels, and absence of response to ACTH stimulation. Manifestations of intracranial hypertension include bulging fontanelles, headaches, and bilateral papilledema. Chronic corticosteroid therapy may interfere with the growth and development of children.

ADVERSE REACTIONS

The only local adverse reaction reported to be possibly or probably related to treatment with DIPROLENE **AF Cream** during controlled clinical studies was stinging. It occurred in 0.4% of the 242 patients or subjects involved in the studies.
The overall incidence of drug-related adverse reactions in the DIPROLENE **Lotion** clinical studies was 5%. The adverse reactions that were reported to be possibly or probably related to treatment with DIPROLENE **Lotion** during controlled clinical studies involving 327 patients or normal volunteers were as follows: folliculitis occurred in 2%, burning and acneiform papules each occurred in 1%, and hyperesthesia and irritation each occurred in less than 1% of patients.
The local adverse reactions that were reported with DIPROLENE **Ointment** applied either once or twice a day during clinical studies are as follows: erythema, 3 per 767 patients; folliculitis, 2 per 767 patients; pruritus, 2 per 767 patients; vesiculation, 1 per 767 patients.
The following local adverse reactions are reported infrequently when topical corticosteroids are used as recommended. These reactions are listed in approximate decreasing order of occurrence: burning, itching, irritation, dryness, folliculitis, hypertrichosis, acneiform eruptions, hypopigmentation, perioral dermatitis, allergic contact dermatitis, maceration of the skin, secondary infection, skin atrophy, striae, miliaria.

OVERDOSAGE

Topically applied corticosteroids can be absorbed in sufficient amounts to produce systemic effects. (See **PRECAUTIONS.**)

DOSAGE AND ADMINSTRATION

Apply a thin film of DIPROLENE **AF Cream** or DIPROLENE **Ointment** to the affected skin areas once or twice daily. Treatment with either DIPROLENE **AF Cream** or **Ointment** should be limited to 45 g per week.
Apply a few drops of DIPROLENE **Lotion** to the affected area once or twice daily and massage lightly until the lotion disappears. Treatment must be limited to 14 days, and amounts greater than 50 mL per week should not be used.
DIPROLENE products are not to be used with occlusive dressings.

HOW SUPPLIED

DIPROLENE **AF Cream** 0.05% is supplied in 15-(NDC 0085-0517- 01), and 45-gram (NDC 0085-0517-02) tubes; boxes of one.
Store between 2° and 30°C (36° and 86°F).
DIPROLENE **Lotion** 0.05% is supplied in 30 mL (29 g) (NDC 0085- 0962-01), and 60 mL (58 g) (NDC 0085-0962-02), plastic squeeze bottles; boxes of one.
Store between 2° and 30°C (36° and 86°F).
DIPROLENE **Ointment** 0.05% is supplied in 15- (NDC 0085-0575- 02), and 45-gram (NDC 0085-0575-03) tubes; boxes of one.
Store between 2° and 30°C (36° and 86°F).
Revised 6/89

DIPROLENE® ℞
brand of augmented
betamethasone dipropionate*
Gel 0.05%
(potency expressed as
betamethasone)
***Vehicle augments the penetration of the steroid.**
For Dermatologic Use Only—
Not for Ophthalmic Use

DESCRIPTION

DIPROLENE® Gel contains betamethasone dipropionate, USP, a synthetic fluorinated corticosteroid for topical dermatologic use. Betamethasone dipropionate is included in a class of compounds consisting primarily of synthetic corticosteroids for use topically as anti-inflammatory and anti-pruritic agents.
Chemically, betamethasone dipropionate is 9-fluoro-11β, 17,21-trihydroxy-16β-methylpregna-1,4-diene-3,20-dione 17, 21-dipropionate, with the empirical formula $C_{28}H_{37}FO_7$ and a molecular weight of 504.6.
Betamethasone dipropionate is a white to creamy white, odorless crystalline powder, insoluble in water.
Each gram of DIPROLENE Gel contains: 0.64 mg betamethasone dipropionate, USP (equivalent to 0.5 mg betamethasone), in an augmented gel base of purified water, propylene glycol, carbomer 940, and sodium hydroxide.

CLINICAL PHARMACOLOGY

Like other topical corticosteroids, betamethasone dipropionate has anti-inflammatory, anti-pruritic, and vasoconstrictive properties. The mechanism of the anti-inflammatory activity of the topical steroids, in general, is unclear. However, corticosteroids are thought to act by the induction of phospholipase A_2 inhibitory proteins, collectively called lipocortins. It is postulated that these proteins control the biosynthesis of potent mediators of inflammation, such as prostaglandins and leukotrienes, by inhibiting the release of their common precursor, arachidonic acid. Arachidonic acid is released from membrane phospholipids by phospholipase A_2.
Pharmacokinetics: The extent of percutaneous absorption of topical corticosteroids is determined by many factors including the vehicle and the integrity of the epidermal barrier. Occlusive dressings with hydrocortisone for up to 24 hours have not been demonstrated to increase penetration; however, occlusion of hydrocortisone for 96 hours markedly enhances penetration. Topical corticosteroids can be absorbed from normal intact skin. In addition, inflammation and/or other disease processes in the skin may increase percutaneous absorption. Studies performed with DIPROLENE (augmented betamethasone dipropionate) Gel indicate that it is in the super-high range of potency as compared with other topical corticosteroids.

INDICATIONS AND USAGE

DIPROLENE Gel is a super-high potency corticosteroid indicated for the relief of the inflammatory and pruritic manifestations of corticosteroid-responsive dermatoses. Treatment beyond two consecutive weeks is not recommended, and the total dose should not exceed 50 g per week because of potential for the drug to suppress the hypothalamic-pituitary-adrenal (HPA) axis.
This product is not recommended for use in children under 12 years of age.

CONTRAINDICATIONS

DIPROLENE Gel is contraindicated in those patients with a history of hypersensitivity to any of the components of the preparation.

PRECAUTIONS

General: DIPROLENE Gel should not be used in the treatment of rosacea or perioral dermatitis, and it should not be used on the face, groin, or in the axillae.
Systemic absorption of topical corticosteroids can produce reversible hypothalamic-pituitary-adrenal (HPA) axis suppression with the potential for glucocorticosteroid insufficiency after withdrawal of treatment. Manifestations of Cushing's syndrome, hyperglycemia, and glucosuria can also be produced in some patients by systemic absorption of topical corticosteroids while on treatment.
At 7 g per day (applied once daily or as 3.5 g twice daily), DIPROLENE Gel was shown to cause inhibition of the HPA axis following application for one, two or three weeks to diseased skin in some patients with psoriasis or atopic dermatitis. These effects were reversible upon discontinuation of treatment.
Patients receiving DIPROLENE Gel applied to large areas should be evaluated periodically for evidence of HPA axis suppression. This may be done by using the ACTH-stimulation, morning plasma cortisol and urinary free-cortisol tests. Patients should not be treated with DIPROLENE Gel for more than 2 weeks at a time, and amounts greater than 50 g per week should not be used because of the potential for the drug to suppress the HPA axis.
If HPA axis suppression is noted, an attempt should be made to withdraw the drug, to reduce the frequency of application, or to substitute a less potent corticosteroid. Recovery of HPA axis function is generally prompt and complete upon discontinuation of topical corticosteroids. Infrequently, signs and symptoms of glucocorticosteroid insufficiency may occur, requiring supplemental systemic corticosteroids. For information on systemic supplementation, see prescribing information for systemic corticosteroids.
Children may be more susceptible to systemic toxicity from equivalent doses due to their larger skin surface to body mass ratios (see **PRECAUTIONS**—Pediatric Use).
If irritation develops, DIPROLENE Gel should be discontinued and appropriate therapy instituted. Allergic contact dermatitis with corticosteroids is usually diagnosed by observing failure to heal rather than noting clinical exacerbation as with most topical products not containing corticosteroids. Such an observation should be corroborated with appropriate diagnostic patch testing.
If concomitant fungal and/or bacterial skin infections are present or develop, an appropriate antifungal or antibacterial agent should be used. If a favorable response does not occur promptly, use of DIPROLENE Gel should be discontinued until the infection has been adequately controlled.
Information for Patients: Patients using topical corticosteroids should receive the following information and instructions:
1. The medication is to be used as directed by the physician. It is for external use only. Avoid contact with the eyes.
2. The medication should not be used for any disorder other than that for which it was prescribed.
3. The treated skin area should not be bandaged or otherwise covered or wrapped so as to be occlusive.
4. Patients should report to their physician any signs of local adverse reactions.

Laboratory Tests: The following tests may be helpful in evaluating patients for HPA axis suppression:
ACTH-stimulation test
Morning plasma-cortisol test
Urinary free-cortisol test
Carcinogenesis, Mutagenesis, and Impairment of Fertility: Long-term animal studies have not been performed to evaluate the carcinogenic potential of betamethasone dipropionate.
Studies in rabbits, mice and rats using intramuscular doses up to 1.0, 33 and 2.0 mg/kg, respectively, resulted in dose related increases in fetal resorptions in the rabbits and mice.
Pregnancy: Teratogenic Effects: Pregnancy Category C: Corticosteroids have been shown to be teratogenic in laboratory animals when administered systemically at relatively low dosage levels. Some corticosteroids have been shown to be teratogenic after dermal application to laboratory animals.
Betamethasone dipropionate has been shown to be teratogenic in rabbits when given by the intramuscular route at doses of 0.05 mg/kg. This dose is approximately 26 times the human topical dose of DIPROLENE Gel assuming human percutaneous absorption of approximately 3% and the use in a 70 kg person of 7 g per day. The abnormalities observed included umbilical hernias, cephalocele and cleft palate.
There are no adequate and well-controlled studies of the teratogenic potential of betamethasone dipropionate in pregnant women. Therefore, DIPROLENE Gel should be used during pregnancy only if the potential benefit justifies the potential risk to the fetus.
Nursing Mothers: Systemically administered corticosteroids appear in human milk and could suppress growth, interfere with endogenous corticosteroid production, or cause other untoward effects. It is not known whether topical administration of corticosteroids could result in sufficient systemic absorption to produce detectable quantities in human milk. Because many drugs are excreted in human milk, caution should be exercised when DIPROLENE Gel is administered to a nursing woman.
Pediatric Use: Safety and effectiveness of DIPROLENE Gel in children have not been established, therefore its use in children under 12 is not recommended. *Because of a higher ratio of skin surface area to body mass, children are at a greater risk than adults of HPA axis suppression when they are treated with topical corticosteroids. They are, therefore, also at greater risk of glucocorticosteroid insufficiency after withdrawal of treatment and of Cushing's syndrome while on treatment.* Adverse effects, including striae, have been reported with inappropriate use of topical corticosteroids in infants and children.
HPA axis suppression, Cushing's syndrome, and intracranial hypertension have been reported in children receiving topical corticosteroids. Manifestations of adrenal suppression in children include linear growth retardation, delayed weight gain, low plasma cortisol levels, and absence of response to ACTH stimulation. Manifestations of intracranial hypertension include bulging fontanelles, headaches, and bilateral papilledema.

ADVERSE REACTIONS

In controlled clinical trials, the total incidence of adverse events associated with the use of DIPROLENE (augmented betamethasone dipropionate) Gel was 10%. These included stinging or burning in 6% of patients, dry skin in 4% of patients, and pruritus in 2% of patients. Less frequently reported adverse reactions were irritation, skin atrophy, telangiectasia, erythema, cracking/tightening of the skin, follicular rash, and allergic contact dermatitis.
The following additional local adverse reactions are reported infrequently with topical corticosteroids, but may occur more frequently with super-high potency corticosteroids, such as DIPROLENE Gel. These reactions are listed in approximate decreasing order of occurrence: acneiform eruptions, hypopigmentation, perioral dermatitis, secondary infection, striae and miliaria.

OVERDOSAGE

Topically applied DIPROLENE Gel can be absorbed in sufficient amounts to produce systemic effects (see **PRECAUTIONS**).

DOSAGE AND ADMINISTRATION

Apply a thin layer of DIPROLENE Gel to the affected skin once or twice daily and rub in gently and completely.
DIPROLENE Gel is a super-high potency topical corticosteroid; therefore, treatment should be limited to two weeks, and amounts greater than 50 g per week should not be used.
DIPROLENE Gel should not be used with occlusive dressings.

HOW SUPPLIED

DIPROLENE Gel 0.05% is supplied in 15 g (NDC 0085-0634-01), and 45 g (NDC 0085-0634-02) tubes, boxes of one.
Store between 2° and 25°C (36° and 77°F).
Schering Corporation
Kenilworth, NJ 07033 USA
8/91
Copyright© 1991, Schering Corporation.
All rights reserved.

ELOCON® ℞
[el 'ō-con]
brand of mometasone furoate
Cream, 0.1%
Ointment, 0.1%
Lotion, 0.1%
For Dermatologic Use Only
Not for Ophthalmic Use

DESCRIPTION

ELOCON® products contain mometasone furoate for dermatologic use. Mometasone furoate is a synthetic corticosteroid with anti-inflammatory activity.
Chemically, mometasone furoate is 9α,21-Dichloro-11β,17-dihydroxy-16α-methylpregna-1,4-diene-3,20-dione17-(2-furoate), with the empirical formula $C_{27}H_{30}Cl_2O_6$ and a molecular weight of 521.4.
Mometasone furoate is a white to off-white powder practically insoluble in water, slightly soluble in octanol, and moderately soluble in ethyl alcohol. Each gram of ELOCON **Cream** 0.1% contains: 1 mg mometasone furoate in a cream base of hexylene glycol, phosphoric acid, propylene glycol stearate, stearyl alcohol and ceteareth-20, titanium dioxide, aluminum starch octenylsuccinate, white wax, white petrolatum and purified water. Each gram of ELOCON **Ointment** 0.1% contains: 1 mg mometasone furoate in an ointment base of hexylene glycol, propylene glycol stearate, white wax, white petrolatum and purified water. May also contain phosphoric acid. Each gram of ELOCON **Lotion** 0.1% contains: 1 mg of mometasone furoate in a lotion base of isopropyl alcohol (40%), propylene glycol, hydroxypropylcellulose, sodium phosphate and water. May also contain phosphoric acid and sodium hydroxide used to adjust the pH to approximately 4.5.

CLINICAL PHARMACOLOGY

The corticosteroids are a class of compounds comprising steroid hormones secreted by the adrenal cortex and their synthetic analogs. In pharmacologic doses corticosteroids are used primarily for their anti-inflammatory and/or immunosuppressive effects. Topical corticosteroids, such as mometasone furoate, are effective in the treatment of corticosteroid-responsive dermatoses primarily because of their anti-inflammatory, anti-pruritic, and vasoconstrictive actions. However, while the physiologic, pharmacologic, and clinical effects of the corticosteroids are well known, the exact mechanisms of their actions in each disease are uncertain. Mometasone furoate has been shown to have topical (derma-

Continued on next page

Information on Schering products appearing on these pages is effective as of August 15, 1992.

Schering—Cont.

tologic) and systemic pharmacologic and metabolic effects characteristic of this class of drugs.

Pharmacokinetics: The extent of percutaneous absorption of topical corticosteroids is determined by many factors including the vehicle, the integrity of the epidermal barrier, and the use of occlusive dressings. (See **DOSAGE AND ADMINISTRATION.**) Topical corticosteroids can be absorbed from normal intact skin.

The percutaneous absorption of ^{3}H-mometasone furoate was evaluated in rabbits following topical application of both cream (0.1%) and ointment (0.1%) formulations. Approximately 5% of the topically applied dose was systemically absorbed following topical application of the cream and 6% following application of the ointment formulation. Based upon these results, it was concluded that mometasone furoate is absorbed to a similar extent following application of either the cream or ointment formulations. Percutaneous absorption studies of ^{3}H-mometasone furoate ointment in rats and dogs have shown that approximately 2.5% of a topically applied dose was absorbed by rats and 2% by dogs.

The percutaneous absorption of ^{3}H-mometasone furoate was also studied in man following topical application of an ointment (0.1%) formulation. Results showed that only about 0.7% of the steroid was systemically absorbed following 8 hours of contact without occlusion. Minimal absorption would be anticipated with the cream and lotion formulations.

Inflammation and/or other disease processes in the skin increase percutaneous absorption. Occlusive dressings substantially increase the percutaneous absorption of topical corticosteroids. (See **DOSAGE AND ADMINISTRATION.**)

In studies of the effects of mometasone furoate on the hypothalamic-pituitary-adrenal (HPA) axis (one with the cream and one with the ointment), 15 grams were applied twice daily for seven days to six patients with psoriasis or atopic dermatitis. The cream or ointment was applied without occlusion to at least 30% of the body surface. The results suggest that the drug caused a slight lowering of adrenal corticosteroid secretion, although in no case did plasma cortisol levels go below the lower limit of the normal range.

Mometasone furoate lotion was applied at 15 mL twice daily (30 mL per day) to diseased skin (patients with scalp and body psoriasis) of four patients for seven days, to study its effects on the hypothalamic-pituitary-adrenal (HPA) axis. Plasma cortisol levels for each of the four patients remained well within the normal range and changed little from baseline.

Once absorbed through the skin, topical corticosteroids are handled through pharmacokinetic pathways similar to systemically administered corticosteroids. Corticosteroids are bound to plasma proteins in varying degrees. Corticosteroids are metabolized primarily in the liver and are then excreted by the kidneys. Some of the topical corticosteroids and their metabolites are also excreted into the bile.

INDICATIONS AND USAGE

ELOCON products are indicated for the relief of the inflammatory and pruritic manifestations of corticosteroid-responsive dermatoses.

CONTRAINDICATIONS

ELOCON products are contraindicated in patients who are hypersensitive to mometasone furoate, to other corticosteroids, or to any ingredient in these preparations.

PRECAUTIONS

General: Systemic absorption of potent topical corticosteroids has produced reversible hypothalamic-pituitary-adrenal (HPA) axis suppression, manifestations of Cushing's syndrome, hyperglycemia, and glucosuria in some patients. Conditions which augment systemic absorption include application of steroids in optimized vehicles, application of more potent steroids, use over large surface areas, prolonged use, use in areas where the epidermal barrier is disrupted, and the use of occlusive dressings. (See **DOSAGE AND ADMINISTRATION.**)

Patients receiving a large dose of a potent topical steroid applied to a large surface area or under an occlusive dressing should be evaluated periodically for evidence of HPA axis suppression by using the urinary free cortisol and ACTH stimulation tests. If HPA axis suppression is noted, an attempt should be made to withdraw the drug, to reduce the frequency of application, or to substitute a less potent steroid.

Recovery of HPA axis function is generally prompt and complete upon discontinuation of the drug. Infrequently, signs and symptoms of steroid withdrawal may occur, requiring supplemental systemic corticosteroids.

Children may absorb proportionally larger amounts of topical corticosteroids and thus be more susceptible to systemic toxicity. (See **PRECAUTIONS—Pediatric Use.**) If irritation develops, topical corticosteroids should be discontinued and appropriate therapy instituted.

In the presence of dermatological infections, use of an appropriate antifungal or antibacterial agent should be instituted. If a favorable response does not occur promptly, the corticosteroid should be discontinued until the infection has been adequately controlled.

Information for Patients: Patients using topical corticosteroids should receive the following information and instructions. This information is intended to aid in the safe and effective use of this medication. It is not a disclosure of all possible adverse or intended effects.

1. This medication is to be used as directed by the physician. It is for external use only. Avoid contact with the eyes.
2. Patients should be advised not to use this medication for any disorder other than that for which it was prescribed.
3. The treated skin area should not be bandaged or otherwise covered or wrapped so as to be occlusive unless directed by the physician. (See **DOSAGE AND ADMINISTRATION.**)
4. Patients should report any signs of local adverse reactions.
5. Parents of pediatric patients should be advised not to use tight-fitting diapers or plastic pants on a child being treated in the diaper area, as these garments may constitute occlusive dressing. (See **DOSAGE AND ADMINISTRATION.**)

Laboratory Tests: The following tests may be helpful in evaluating HPA axis suppression:
Urinary free cortisol test
ACTH stimulation test

Carcinogenesis, Mutagenesis, and Impairment of Fertility: Long-term animal studies have not been performed to evaluate the carcinogenic potential or the effect on fertility of topical corticosteroids.

Genetic toxicity studies with mometasone furoate, which included the Ames test, mouse lymphoma assay, and a micronucleus test, did not reveal any mutagenic potential.

Pregnancy Category C: Corticosteroids are generally teratogenic in laboratory animals when administered systemically at relatively low dosage levels. Corticosteroids have been shown to be teratogenic after dermal application in laboratory animals. There are no adequate and well-controlled studies of teratogenic effects from topically applied corticosteroids in pregnant women. Therefore, topical corticosteroids should be used during pregnancy only if the potential benefit justifies the potential risk to the fetus. Drugs of this class should not be used extensively on pregnant patients, in large amounts, or for prolonged periods.

Nursing Mothers: It is not known whether topical administration of corticosteroids could result in sufficient systemic absorption to produce detectable quantities in breast milk. Systemically administered corticosteroids are secreted into breast milk in quantities not likely to have a deleterious effect on the infant. Nevertheless, a decision should be made whether to discontinue nursing or to discontinue the drug taking into account the importance of the drug to the mother.

Pediatric Use: *Pediatric patients may demonstrate greater susceptibility to topical corticosteroid-induced HPA axis suppression and Cushing's syndrome than mature patients because of a larger skin surface area to body weight ratio.*

Hypothalamic-pituitary-adrenal (HPA) axis suppression, Cushing's syndrome, and intracranial hypertension have been reported in children receiving topical corticosteroids. Manifestations of adrenal suppression in children include linear growth retardation, delayed weight gain, low plasma cortisol levels, and absence of response to ACTH stimulation. Manifestations of intracranial hypertension include bulging fontanelles, headaches, and bilateral papilledema.

Administration of topical corticosteroids to children should be limited to the least amount compatible with an effective therapeutic regimen. Chronic corticosteroid therapy may interfere with the growth and development of children.

ADVERSE REACTIONS

The following local adverse reactions were reported with ELOCON **Cream** during clinical studies with 319 patients: burning, 1; pruritus, 1; and signs of skin atrophy, 3.

The following local adverse reactions were reported with ELOCON **Ointment** during clinical studies with 812 patients: burning, 13; pruritus, 8; skin atrophy, 8; tingling/stinging, 7; and furunculosis, 3.

The following local adverse reactions were reported with ELOCON **Lotion** during clinical studies with 209 patients; acneiform reaction, 2; burning, 4; and itching, 1. In an irritation/sensitization study with 156 normal subjects, folliculitis was reported in 4.

The following local adverse reactions have been reported infrequently when other topical dermatologic corticosteroids have been used as recommended. These reactions are listed in an approximate decreasing order of occurrence: burning, itching, irritation, dryness, folliculitis, hypertrichosis, acneiform eruptions, hypopigmentation, perioral dermatitis, allergic contact dermatitis, maceration of the skin, secondary infection, skin atrophy, striae, miliaria.

OVERDOSAGE

Topically applied corticosteroids can be absorbed in sufficient amounts to produce systemic effects. (See **PRECAUTIONS.**)

DOSAGE AND ADMINISTRATION

Apply a thin film of ELOCON **Cream** or **Ointment** to the affected skin areas once daily. Do not use occlusive dressings. Apply a few drops of ELOCON **Lotion** to the affected areas once daily and massage lightly until it disappears. For the most effective and economical use, hold the nozzle of the bottle very close to the affected areas and gently squeeze.

HOW SUPPLIED

ELOCON **Cream** 0.1% is supplied in 15 g (NDC 0085-0567-01) and 45 g (NDC 0085-0567-02) tubes; boxes of one.
ELOCON **Ointment** 0.1% is supplied in 15 g (NDC 0085-0370-01) and 45 g (NDC 0085-0370-02) tubes; boxes of one.
ELOCON **Lotion** 0.1% is supplied in 30 mL (27.5 g) (NDC-0085-0854-01) and 60 mL (55 g) (NDC-0085-0854-02) bottles; boxes of one.
Store ELOCON between 2° and 30°C (36° and 86°F).

ETRAFON®   ℞

[ĕ′trah-fon]
brand of perphenazine, USP—amitriptyline hydrochloride, USP

ETRAFON 2–10 TABLETS (2–10)
ETRAFON TABLETS (2–25)
ETRAFON-A TABLETS (4–10)
ETRAFON-FORTE TABLETS (4–25)

DESCRIPTION

ETRAFON Tablets contain perphenazine, USP and amitriptyline hydrochloride, USP. Perphenazine is a piperazinyl phenothiazine having the chemical formula, $C_{21}H_{26}ClN_3OS$. Amitriptyline hydrochloride is a dibenzocycloheptadiene derivative having the chemical formula, $C_{20}H_{23}N\cdot HCl$.

ETRAFON Tablets are available in multiple strengths to afford dosage flexibility for optimum management. They are available as ETRAFON 2-10 Tablets, 2 mg perphenazine and 10 mg amitriptyline hydrochloride; ETRAFON Tablets, 2 mg perphenazine and 25 mg amitriptyline hydrochloride. ETRAFON-A Tablets, 4 mg perphenazine and 10 mg amitriptyline hydrochloride; and ETRAFON-FORTE Tablets, 4 mg perphenazine and 25 mg amitriptyline hydrochloride.

The inactive ingredients for ETRAFON 2-10 Tablets (2-10) include: acacia, butylparaben, calcium phosphate, calcium sulfate, carnauba wax, corn starch, D&C Yellow No. 10 Al Lake, FD&C Yellow No. 6 Al Lake, gelatin, lactose, magnesium stearate, potato starch, sugar, and white wax. May also contain talc.

The inactive ingredients for ETRAFON Tablets (2-25) include: acacia, butylparaben, calcium phosphate, calcium sulfate, carnauba wax, corn starch, D&C Red No. 30 Al Lake, FD&C Yellow No. 6 Al Lake, gelatin, lactose, magnesium stearate, potato starch, sugar, and white wax. May also contain talc.

The inactive ingredients for ETRAFON-A Tablets (4-10) include: acacia, butylparaben, calcium phosphate, calcium sulfate, carnauba wax, corn starch, FD&C Yellow No. 6, gelatin, lactose, magnesium stearate, potato starch, sugar, and white wax. May also contain talc.

The inactive ingredients for ETRAFON-FORTE Tablets (4-25) include: acacia, butylparaben, calcium phosphate, calcium sulfate, carnauba wax, corn starch, FD&C Red No. 40 Al Lake, FD&C Yellow No. 6 Al Lake, gelatin, lactose, magnesium stearate, potato starch, sugar, and white wax. May also contain talc.

ACTIONS

ETRAFON combines the tranquilizing action of perphenazine with the antidepressant properties of amitriptyline hydrochloride. Perphenazine acts on the central nervous system and has a greater behavioral potency than other phenothiazine derivatives whose side chains do not contain a piperazine moiety. Amitriptyline hydrochloride is a tricyclic antidepressant while its mechanism of action in man is not known, it does not act primarily by stimulation of the central nervous system, and is not a monoamine oxidase inhibitor.

INDICATIONS

ETRAFON Tablets are indicated for the treatment of patients with moderate to severe anxiety and/or agitation and depressed mood; patients with depression in whom anxiety and/or agitation are moderate or severe; patients with anxiety and depression associated with chronic physical disease; patients in whom depression and anxiety cannot be clearly differentiated.

Schizophrenic patients who have associated symptoms of depression should be considered for therapy with ETRAFON.

CONTRAINDICATIONS

ETRAFON Tablets are contraindicated in comatose or greatly obtunded patients and in patients receiving large doses of central nervous system depressants (barbiturates, alcohol, narcotics, analgesics, or antihistamines); in the presence of existing blood dyscrasias, bone marrow depression, or liver damage; and in patients who have shown hypersensitivity to ETRAFON Tablets, its components, or related compounds.

ETRAFON Tablets are also contraindicated in patients with suspected or established subcortical brain damage, with or without hypothalamic damage, since a hyperthermic reaction with temperatures in excess of 104°F may occur in such patients, sometimes not until 14 to 16 hours after drug administration. Total body ice-packing is recommended for such a reaction; antipyretics may also be useful.

ETRAFON should not be given concomitantly with a monoamine oxidase inhibiting compound. Hyperpyretic crises, severe convulsions and deaths have occurred in patients receiving tricyclic antidepressant and monoamine oxidase inhibiting drugs simultaneously. In patients who have been receiving a monoamine oxidase inhibitor, it is recommended that two weeks or longer elapse before the start of treatment with ETRAFON Tablets to permit recovery from the effects of the MAO inhibitor and to avoid possible potentiation. Treatment with ETRAFON Tablets should be initiated cautiously in such patients, with gradual increase in dosage until a satisfactory response is obtained.

Amitriptyline hydrochloride is not recommended for use during the acute recovery phase following myocardial infarction.

WARNINGS

Tardive dyskinesia, a syndrome consisting of potentially irreversible, involuntary, dyskinetic movements, may develop in patients treated with neuroleptic (antipsychotic) drugs. Although the prevalence of the syndrome appears to be highest among the elderly, especially elderly women, it is impossible to rely upon prevalence estimates to predict, at the inception of neuroleptic treatment, which patients are likely to develop the syndrome. Whether neuroleptic drug products differ in their potential to cause tardive dyskinesia is unknown.

Both the risk of developing the syndrome and the likelihood that it will become irreversible are believed to increase as the duration of treatment and the total cumulative dose of neuroleptic drugs administered to the patient increase. However, the syndrome can develop, although much less commonly, after relatively brief treatment periods at low doses.

There is no known treatment for established cases of tardive dyskinesia, although the syndrome may remit, partially or completely, if neuroleptic treatment is withdrawn. Neuroleptic treatment itself, however, may suppress (or partially suppress) the signs and symptoms of the syndrome, and thereby may possibly mask the underlying disease process. The effect that symptomatic suppression has upon the long-term course of the syndrome is unknown.

Given these considerations, neuroleptics should be prescribed in a manner that is most likely to minimize the occurrence of tardive dyskinesia. Chronic neuroleptic treatment should generally be reserved for patients who suffer from a chronic illness that, 1) is known to respond to neuroleptic drugs, and, 2) for whom alternative, equally effective, but potentially less harmful treatments are not available or appropriate. In patients who do require chronic treatment, the smallest dose and the shortest duration of treatment producing a satisfactory clinical response should be sought. The need for continued treatment should be reassessed periodically.

If signs and symptoms of tardive dyskinesia appear in a patient on neuroleptics, drug discontinuation should be considered. However, some patients may require treatment despite the presence of the syndrome.

(For further information about the description of tardive dyskinesia and its clinical detection, please refer to **Information for Patients** and **Adverse Reactions.**)

NEUROLEPTIC MALIGNANT SYNDROME (NMS)

A potentially fatal symptom complex sometimes referred to as Neuroleptic Malignant Syndrome (NMS) has been reported in association with antipsychotic drugs. Clinical manifestations of NMS are hyperpyrexia, muscle rigidity, altered mental status and evidence of autonomic instability (irregular pulse or blood pressure, tachycardia, diaphoresis, and cardiac dysrhythmias).

The diagnostic evaluation of patients with this syndrome is complicated. In arriving at a diagnosis, it is important to identify cases where the clinical presentation includes both serious medical illness (e.g., pneumonia, systemic infection, etc.) and untreated or inadequately treated extrapyramidal signs and symptoms (EPS). Other important considerations in the differential diagnosis include central anticholinergic toxicity, heat stroke, drug fever and primary central nervous system (CNS) pathology.

The management of NMS should include 1) immediate discontinuation of antipsychotic drugs and other drugs not essential to concurrent therapy, 2) intensive symptomatic treatment and medical monitoring, and 3) treatment of any concomitant serious medical problems for which specific treatments are available. There is no general agreement about specific pharmacological treatment regimens for uncomplicated NMS.

If a patient requires antipyschotic drug treatment after recovery from NMS, the potential reintroduction of drug therapy should be carefully considered. The patient should be carefully monitored, since recurrences of NMS have been reported.

Patients with cardiovascular disorders should be watched closely. Tricyclic antidepressant drugs, including amitriptyline hydrochloride, particularly when given in high doses, have been reported to produce arrhythmias, sinus tachycardia, and prolongation of the conduction time. Myocardial infarction and stroke have been reported with drugs of this class.

ETRAFON should not be given concomitantly with guanethidine or similarly acting compounds, since amitriptyline, like other tricyclic antidepressants, may block the antihypertensive effect of these compounds.

If hypotension develops, epinephrine should not be administered, since its action is blocked and partially reversed by perphenazine. If a vasopressor is needed, norepinephrine may be used. Severe, acute hypotension has occurred with the use of phenothiazines and is particularly likely to occur in patients with mitral insufficiency or pheochromocytoma. Rebound hypertension may occur in pheochromocytoma patients.

Perphenazine can lower the convulsive threshold in susceptible individuals; it should be used with caution in alcohol withdrawal and in patients with convulsive disorders. If the patient is being treated with an anticonvulsant agent, increased dosage of that agent may be required when ETRAFON Tablets are used concomitantly.

Because of the anticholinergic activity of amitriptyline hydrochloride, ETRAFON should be used with caution in patients with glaucoma, increased intraocular pressure, and those in whom urinary retention is present or anticipated. In patients with angle-closure glaucoma, even average doses may precipitate an attack.

Close supervision is required when amitriptyline hydrochloride is given to hyperthyroid patients or those receiving thyroid medication.

ETRAFON Tablets may impair the mental and/or physical abilities required for the performance of potentially hazardous tasks, such as driving a car or operating machinery, the patient should be warned accordingly.

Usage in Children: Since a dosage for children has not been established, ETRAFON is not recommended for use in children.

Usage in Pregnancy: Safe use of ETRAFON Tablets during pregnancy and lactation has not been established; therefore, in administering the drug to pregnant patients, nursing mothers, or women who may become pregnant, the possible benefits must be weighed against the possible hazards to mother and child.

PRECAUTIONS

The possibility of suicide in depressed patients remains during treatment and until significant remission occurs. This type of patient should not have access to large quantities of this drug.

Perphenazine

As with all phenothiazine compounds, perphenazine should not be used indiscriminately. Caution should be observed in giving it to patients who have previously exhibited severe adverse reactions to other phenothiazines. Some of the untoward actions of perphenazine tend to appear more frequently when high doses are used. However, as with other phenothiazine compounds, patients receiving perphenazine in any dosage should be kept under close supervision.

Neuroleptic drugs elevate prolactin levels; the elevation persists during chronic administration. Tissue culture experiments indicate that approximately one-third of human breast cancers are prolactin dependent *in vitro*, a factor of potential importance if the prescription of these drugs is contemplated in a patient with a previously detected breast cancer. Although disturbances such as galactorrhea, amenorrhea, gynecomastia, and impotence have been reported, the clinical significance of elevated serum prolactin levels is unknown for most patients. An increase in mammary neoplasms has been found in rodents after chronic administration of neuroleptic drugs. Neither clinical studies nor epidemiologic studies conducted to date, however, have shown an association between chronic administration of these drugs and mammary tumorigenesis; the available evidence is considered too limited to be conclusive at this time.

The antiemetic effect of perphenazine may obscure signs of toxicity due to overdosage of other drugs, or render more difficult the diagnosis of disorders such as brain tumors or intestinal obstruction.

A significant, not otherwise explained, rise in body temperature may suggest individual intolerance to perphenazine, in which case ETRAFON should be discontinued.

Patients on large doses of a phenothiazine drug who are undergoing surgery should be watched carefully for possible hypotensive phenomena. Moreover, reduced amounts of anesthetics or central nervous system depressants may be necessary.

Since phenothiazines and central nervous system depressants (opiates, analgesics, antihistamines, barbiturates) can potentiate each other, less than the usual dosage of the added drug is recommended, and caution is advised, when they are administered concomitantly.

Use with caution in patients who are receiving atropine or related drugs because of additive anticholinergic effects and also in patients who will be exposed to extreme heat or organic phosphate insecticides.

The use of alcohol should be avoided, since additive effects and hypotension may occur. Patients should be cautioned that their response to alcohol may be increased while they are being treated with ETRAFON Tablets. The risk of suicide and the danger of overdose may be increased in patients who use alcohol excessively due to its potentiation of the drug's effect.

Blood counts and hepatic and renal functions should be checked periodically. The appearance of signs of blood dyscrasias requires the discontinuance of the drug and institution of appropriate therapy. If abnormalities in hepatic tests occur, phenothiazine treatment should be discontinued. Renal function in patients on long-term therapy should be monitored; if blood urea nitrogen (BUN) becomes abnormal, treatment with the drug should be discontinued.

The use of phenothiazine derivatives in patients with diminished renal function should be undertaken with caution.

Use with caution in patients suffering from respiratory impairment due to acute pulmonary infections, or in chronic respiratory disorders such as severe asthma or emphysema.

In general, phenothiazines do not produce psychic dependence. Gastritis, nausea and vomiting, dizziness, and tremulousness have been reported following abrupt cessation of high-dose therapy. Reports suggest that these symptoms can be reduced by continuing concomitant antiparkinson agents for several weeks after the phenothiazine is withdrawn.

The possibility of liver damage, corneal and lenticular deposits, and irreversible dyskinesias should be kept in mind when patients are on long-term therapy.

Because photosensitivity has been reported, undue exposure to the sun should be avoided during phenothiazine treatment.

Information for Patients: This information is intended to aid in the safe and effective use of this medication. It is not a disclosure of all possible adverse or intended effects.

Given the likelihood that a substantial proportion of patients exposed chronically to neuroleptics will develop tardive dyskinesia, it is advised that all patients in whom chronic use is contemplated be given, if possible, full information about this risk. The decision to inform patients and/or their guardians must obviously take into account the clinical circumstances and the competency of the patients to understand the information provided.

Amitriptyline Hydrochloride

In manic-depressive psychosis, depressed patients may experience a shift toward the manic phase if they are treated with an antidepressant drug. Patients with paranoid symptomatology may have an exaggeration of such symptoms. The tranquilizing effect of ETRAFON has seemed to reduce the likelihood of this effect.

When amitriptyline hydrochloride is given with anticholinergic agents or sympathomimetic drugs, including epinephrine combined with local anesthetics, close supervision and careful adjustment of dosages are required.

Paralytic ileus may occur in patients taking tricyclic antidepressants in combination with anticholinergic-type drugs.

Concurrent use of large doses of ethchlorvynol should be used with caution, since transient delirium has been reported in patients receiving this drug in combination with amitriptyline hydrochloride.

This drug may enhance the response to alcohol and the effects of barbiturates and other CNS depressants.

Concurrent administration of amitriptyline hydrochloride and electroshock therapy may increase the hazards of therapy. Such treatment should be limited to patients for whom it is essential.

Discontinue the drug several days before elective surgery, if possible.

Both elevation and lowering of blood sugar levels have been reported.

The usefulness of amitriptyline in the treatment of depression has been amply demonstrated; however, it should be realized that abuse of amitriptyline among a narcotic-dependent population is not uncommon.

Continued on next page

Information on Schering products appearing on these pages is effective as of August 15, 1992.

Schering—Cont.

Concurrent administration of cimetidine and tricyclic antidepressants can produce clinically significant increases in the plasma concentrations of the tricyclic antidepressant. Serious anticholinergic symptoms (severe dry mouth, urinary retention, blurred vision) have been associated with elevations in the serum levels of the tricyclic antidepressant when cimetidine is added to the drug regimen. Additionally, higher than expected steady-state serum concentrations of the tricyclic antidepressant have been observed when therapy is initiated in patients taking cimetidine.

Alternatively, decreases in the steady-state serum concentration of the tricyclic antidepressant have been reported in well-controlled patients on concurrent therapy upon discontinuance of cimetidine. The therapeutic efficacy of the tricyclic antidepressant may be compromised in these patients as the cimetidine is discontinued.

ADVERSE REACTIONS

Adverse reactions to ETRAFON Tablets are the same as those to its components, perphenazine and amitriptyline hydrochloride. There have been no reports of effects peculiar to the combination of these components in ETRAFON Tablets.

Perphenazine

Not all of the following adverse reactions have been reported with perphenazine; however, pharmacological similarities among various phenothiazine derivatives require that each be considered. With the piperazine group (of which perphenazine is an example), the extrapyramidal symptoms are more common, and others (e.g., sedative effects, jaundice, and blood dyscrasias) are less frequently seen.

CNS Effects: *Extrapyramidal reactions:* opisthotonus, trismus, torticollis, retrocollis, aching and numbness of the limbs, motor restlessness, oculogyric crisis, hyperreflexia, dystonia, including protrusion, discoloration, aching and rounding of the tongue, tonic spasm of the masticatory muscles, tight feeling in the throat, slurred speech, dysphagia, akathisia, dyskinesia, parkinsonism and ataxia. Their incidence and severity usually increase with an increase in dosage, but there is considerable individual variation in the tendency to develop such symptoms. Extrapyramidal symptoms can usually be controlled by the concomitant use of effective antiparkinsonian drugs, such as benztropine mesylate, and/or by reduction in dosage.

In some instances, however, these extrapyramidal reactions may persist after discontinuation of treatment with perphenazine.

Persistent tardive dyskinesia: As with all antipsychotic agents, tardive dyskinesia may appear in some patients on long-term therapy or may appear after drug therapy has been discontinued. Although the risk appears to be greater in elderly patients on high-dose therapy, especially females it may occur in either sex and in children. The symptoms are persistent and in some patients appear to be irreversible. The syndrome is characterized by rhythmical, involuntary movements of the tongue, face, mouth or jaw (eg, protrusion of tongue, puffing of cheeks, puckering of mouth, chewing movements). Sometimes these may be accompanied by involuntary movements of the extremities. There is no known effective treatment for tardive dyskinesia; antiparkinsonism agents usually do not alleviate the symptoms of this syndrome. It is suggested that all antipsychotic agents be discontinued if these symptoms appear. Should it be necessary to reinstitute treatment, or increase the dosage of the agent, or switch to a different antipsychotic agent, the syndrome may be masked. It has been reported that fine, vermicular movements of the tongue may be an early sign of the syndrome, and if the medication is stopped at that time the syndrome may not develop.

Other CNS effects include cerebral edema; abnormality of cerebrospinal fluid proteins; convulsive seizures, particularly in patients with EEG abnormalities or a history of such disorders; and headaches.

Neuroleptic malignant syndrome has been reported in patients treated with neuroleptic drugs (see WARNINGS for further information).

Drowsiness may occur, particularly during the first or second week, after which it generally disappears. If troublesome, lower the dosage. Hypnotic effects appear to be minimal, especially in patients who are permitted to remain active.

Adverse behavioral effects include paradoxical exacerbation of psychotic symptoms, catatonic-like states, paranoid reactions, lethargy, paradoxical excitement, restlessness, hyperactivity, nocturnal confusion, bizarre dreams, and insomnia. Hyperreflexia has been reported in the newborn when a phenothiazine was used during pregnancy.

Autonomic Effects: dry mouth or salivation, nausea, vomiting, diarrhea, anorexia, constipation, obstipation, fecal impaction, urinary retention, frequency or incontinence, polyuria, bladder paralysis, nasal congestion, pallor, myosis, mydriasis, blurred vision, glaucoma, perspiration, hypertension, hypotension, and a change in pulse rate occasionally

may occur. Significant autonomic effects have been infrequent in patients receiving less than 24 mg perphenazine daily.

Adynamic ileus occasionally occurs with phenothiazine therapy and if severe can result in complications and death. It is of particular concern in psychiatric patients, who may fail to seek treatment of the condition.

Allergic Effects: urticaria, erythema, eczema, exfoliative dermatitis, pruritus, photosensitivity, asthma, fever, anaphylactoid reactions, laryngeal edema, and angioneurotic edema; contact dermatitis in nursing personnel administering the drug; and in extremely rare instances, individual idiosyncrasy or hypersensitivity to phenothiazines has resulted in cerebral edema, circulatory collapse, and death.

Endocrine Effects: lactation, galactorrhea, moderate breast enlargement in females and gynecomastia in males on large doses, disturbances in the menstrual cycle, amenorrhea, changes in libido, inhibition of ejaculation, false positive pregnancy tests, hyperglycemia, hypoglycemia, glycosuria, syndrome of inappropriate ADH (antidiuretic hormone) secretion.

Cardiovascular Effects: Postural hypotension, tachycardia (especially with sudden marked increase in dosage), bradycardia, cardiac arrest, faintness, and dizziness. Occasionally the hypotensive effect may produce a shock-like condition. ECG changes, nonspecific, (quinidine-like effect) usually reversible, have been observed in some patients receiving phenothiazine tranquilizers.

Sudden death has occasionally been reported in patients who have received phenothiazines. In some cases the death was apparently due to cardiac arrest; in others the cause appeared to be asphyxia due to failure of the cough reflex. In some patients, the cause could not be determined nor could it be established that the death was due to the phenothiazine.

Hematological Effects: agranulocytosis, eosinophilia, leukopenia, hemolytic anemia, thrombocytopenic purpura, and pancytopenia. Most cases of agranulocytosis have occurred between the fourth and tenth weeks of therapy. Patients should be watched closely especially during that period for the sudden appearance of sore throat or signs of infection. If white blood cell and differential cell counts show significant cellular depression, discontinue the drug and start appropriate therapy. However, a slightly lowered white count is not in itself an indication to discontinue the drug.

Other Effects: Special considerations in long-term therapy include pigmentation of the skin, occurring chiefly in the exposed areas; ocular changes consisting of deposition of fine particulate matter in the cornea and lens, progressing in more severe cases to star-shaped lenticular opacities; epithelial keratopathies; and pigmentary retinopathy. Also noted: peripheral edema, reversed epinephrine effect, increase in PBI not attributable to an increase in thyroxine, parotid swelling (rare), hyperpyrexia, systemic lupus erythematosus-like syndrome, increases in appetite and weight, polyphagia, photophobia, and muscle weakness.

Liver damage (biliary stasis) may occur. Jaundice may occur, usually between the second and fourth weeks of treatment, and is regarded as a hypersensitivity reaction. Incidence is low. The clinical picture resembles infectious hepatitis but with laboratory features of obstructive jaundice. It is usually reversible; however, chronic jaundice has been reported.

Amitriptyline Hydrochloride

Although activation of latent schizophrenia has been reported with antidepressant drugs, including amitriptyline hydrochloride, it may be prevented with ETRAFON Tablets in some cases because of the antipsychotic effect of perphenazine. A few instances of epileptiform seizures have been reported in chronic schizophrenic patients during treatment with amitriptyline hydrochloride.

Note: Included in the listing which follows are a few adverse reactions which have not been reported with this specific drug. However, pharmacological similarities among the tricyclic antidepressant drugs require that each of the reactions be considered when amitriptyline hydrochloride is administered.

Allergic: Rash, pruritus, urticaria, photosensitization, edema of face and tongue.

Anticholinergic: Dry mouth, blurred vision, disturbance of accommodation, constipation, paralytic ileus, urinary retention, dilatation of urinary tract.

Cardiovascular: Hypotension, hypertension, tachycardia, palpitations, myocardial infarction, arrhythmias, heart block, stroke.

CNS and Neuromuscular: Confusional states, disturbed concentration, disorientation, delusions, hallucinations, excitement, jitteriness, anxiety, restlessness, insomnia, nightmares, numbness, tingling, and paresthesias of the extremities, peripheral neuropathy, incoordination, ataxia, tremors, seizures, alteration in EEG patterns, extrapyramidal symptoms, tinnitus.

Endocrine: Testicular swelling and gynecomastia in the male, breast enlargement and galactorrhea in the female, increased or decreased libido, elevation and lowering of blood sugar levels, syndrome of inappropriate ADH (antidiuretic hormone secretion).

Gastrointestinal: Nausea, epigastric distress, heartburn, vomiting, anorexia, stomatitis, peculiar taste, diarrhea, jaundice, parotid swelling, black tongue. Rarely hepatitis has occurred (including altered liver function and jaundice).

Hematologic: Bone marrow depression including agranulocytosis, leukopenia, eosinophilia, purpura, thrombocytopenia.

Other: Dizziness, weakness, fatigue, headache, weight gain or loss, increased perspiration, urinary frequency, mydriasis, drowsiness, alopecia.

Withdrawal Symptoms: Abrupt cessation of treatment after prolonged administration may produce nausea, headache, and malaise. These are not indicative of addiction.

DOSAGE AND ADMINISTRATION

Initial Dosage

In psychoneurotic patients whose anxiety and depression warrant combined therapy, one ETRAFON Tablet (2–25) or one ETRAFON-FORTE Tablet (4–25) three or four times a day is recommended.

In elderly patients, adolescents and other patients as indicated, one ETRAFON-A Tablet (4–10) may be administered three or four times a day as initial dosage. This dosage may be adjusted as required to produce an adequate response.

In more severely ill patients with schizophrenia, two ETRAFON-FORTE Tablets (4–25) three times a day are recommended as the initial dosage. If necessary, a fourth dose may be given at bedtime. The total daily dosage should not exceed eight tablets of any strength.

Maintenance Dosage

Depending on the condition being treated, the onset of therapeutic response may vary from a few days to a few weeks or even longer. After a satisfactory response is noted, dosage should be reduced to the smallest dose which is effective for relief of the symptoms for which ETRAFON Tablets are being administered. A useful maintenance dosage is one ETRAFON Tablet (2–25) or one ETRAFON-FORTE Tablet (4–25) two to four times a day. In some patients, maintenance dosage is required for many months.

ETRAFON 2–10 Tablets (2–10) and ETRAFON-A Tablets (4–10) can be used to increase flexibility in adjusting maintenance dosage to the lowest amount consistent with relief of symptoms.

OVERDOSAGE

In the event of overdosage, emergency treatment should be started immediately. All patients suspected of having taken an overdose should be hospitalized as soon as possible.

Manifestations: Overdosage of perphenazine primarily involves the extrapyramidal mechanism and produces the same side effects described under ADVERSE REACTIONS, but to a more marked degree. It is usually evidenced by stupor or coma; children may have convulsive seizures.

High doses of ETRAFON Tablets may cause temporary confusion, disturbed concentration, or transient visual hallucinations. Overdosage may cause drowsiness; hypothermia; tachycardia and other arrhythmic abnormalities—for example, bundle branch block; ECG evidence of impaired conduction; congestive heart failure; dilated pupils; convulsions; severe hypotension; stupor; and coma. Other symptoms may be agitation, hyperactive reflexes, muscle rigidity, vomiting, hyperpyrexia, or any of the adverse reactions listed for perphenazine or amitriptyline hydrochloride.

Overdosage with tricyclic antidepressants (TCAs), such as imipramine, doxepin, or amitriptyline may result in plasma TCA levels of 1,000 ng/ml or higher. Such levels more accurately define patients who are at risk for major medical complications of overdosage than does the amount of drug ingested based on patient history. In one study, all patients with TCA levels of this magnitude had a QRS duration of 100 msec or more on a routine ECG within the first 24 hours following overdose.

In the absence of TCA blood level determinations, a QRS of 100 msec or more suggests a greater likelihood of serious complications.

Oculomotor paresis (loss of conjugate movement in the so-called doll's eyes maneuver) as a manifestation of amitriptyline overdosage has been reported as being significant in the differential diagnosis of a patient in light coma.

Treatment: Treatment is symptomatic and supportive. There is no specific antidote. The patient should be induced to vomit even if emesis has occurred spontaneously. Pharmacologic vomiting by the administration of ipecac syrup is a preferred method. It should be noted that ipecac has a central mode of action in addition to its local gastric irritant properties, and the central mode of action may be blocked by the antiemetic effect of ETRAFON Tablets. Vomiting should not be induced in patients with impaired consciousness. The action of ipecac is facilitated by physical activity and by the administration of 8 to 12 fluid ounces of water. If emesis does not occur within 15 minutes, the dose of ipecac should be repeated. Precautions against aspiration must be taken, especially in infants and children. Following emesis, any drug remaining in the stomach may be adsorbed by activated charcoal administered as a slurry with water. If vomiting is unsuccessful or contraindicated, gastric lavage should be

performed. Isotonic and one-half isotonic saline are the lavage solutions of choice. Saline cathartics, such as milk of magnesia, draw water into the bowel by osmosis and therefore may be valuable for their action in rapid dilution of bowel content.

Standard measures (oxygen, intravenous fluids, corticosteroids) should be used to manage circulatory shock or metabolic acidosis. An open airway and adequate fluid intake should be maintained. Body temperature should be regulated. Hypothermia is expected, but severe hyperthermia may occur and must be treated vigorously. (See CONTRAINDICATIONS.)

An electrocardiogram should be taken and close monitoring of cardiac function instituted if there is any sign of abnormality. Cardiac arrhythmias may be treated with neostigmine, pyridostigmine, or propranolol. Digitalis should be considered for cardiac failure. Close monitoring of cardiac function is advisable for not less than five days.

Vasopressors such as norepinephrine may be used to treat hypotension, but epinephrine should NOT be used.

The intravenous administration of 1 to 3 mg physostigmine salicylate has been reported to reverse the symptoms of tricyclic antidepressant poisoning and therefore, should be considered in the symptomatic treatment of the central anticholinergic effects due to overdosage with ETRAFON Tablets. Because physostigmine is rapidly metabolized, it should be re-administered as required, especially if life-threatening signs, such as arrhythmias, convulsions, or deep coma recur or persist.

Anticonvulsants (an inhalation anesthetic, diazepam, or paraldehyde) are recommended for control of convulsions, since perphenazine increases the central nervous system depressant action, but not the anticonvulsant action of barbiturates.

If acute parkinson-like symptoms result from perphenazine intoxication, benztropine mesylate or diphenhydramine may be administered.

Central nervous system depression may be treated with nonconvulsant doses of CNS stimulants. Avoid stimulants that may cause convulsions (e.g., picrotoxin and pentylenetetrazol).

Signs of arousal may not occur for 48 hours.

Dialysis is of no value because of low plasma concentrations of the drug.

Since overdosage is often deliberate, patients may attempt suicide by other means during the recovery phase. Deaths by deliberate or accidental overdosage have occurred with this class of drugs.

HOW SUPPLIED

ETRAFON 2–10 Tablets (perphenazine 2 mg and amitriptyline hydrochloride 10 mg): deep yellow, sugar-coated tablets branded in blue-black with the Schering trademark and either product identification letters, ANA, or number, 287; bottles of 100 (NDC 0085-0287-04) and box of 100 for unit-dose dispensing (10 strips of 10 tablets each) (NDC 0085-0287-08).

ETRAFON Tablets (perphenazine 2 mg and amitriptyline hydrochloride 25 mg): pink, sugar-coated tablets branded in red with the Schering trademark and either product identification letters, ANC or number, 598; bottles of 100 (NDC 0085-0598-04) and box of 100 for unit-dose dispensing (10 strips of 10 tablets each) (NDC 0085-0598-08).

ETRAFON-A Tablets (perphenazine 4 mg and amitriptyline hydrochloride 10 mg): orange, sugar-coated tablets branded in blue-black with the Schering trademark and either product identification letters, ANB, or number, 119; bottles of 100 (NDC 0085-0119-04) and box of 100 for unit-dose dispensing (10 strips of 10 tablets each) (NDC 0085-0119-08).

ETRAFON-FORTE Tablets (perphenazine 4 mg and amitriptyline hydrochloride 25 mg): red, sugar-coated tablets branded in blue with the Schering trademark and either product identification letters, ANE, or number, 720; bottles of 100 (NDC 0085-0720-04) and box of 100 for unit-dose dispensing (10 strips of 10 tablets each) (NDC 0085-0720-08).

Store ETRAFON 2-10, 4-10, 2-25 and 4-25 Tablets between 2° and 25°C (36° and 77°F). In addition, protect unit-dose packages from excessive moisture.

Revised 1/91

Shown in Product Identification Section, page 428

EULEXIN® ℞

brand of flutamide
Capsules

DESCRIPTION

EULEXIN Capsules contain flutamide, an acetanilid, nonsteroidal, orally active antiandrogen having the chemical name, 2-methyl-*N*-[4-nitro-3-(trifluoromethyl)phenyl] propanamide.

Each capsule contains 125 mg flutamide. The compound is a buff to yellow powder with a molecular weight of 276.2.

The inactive ingredients for EULEXIN Capsules include: corn starch, lactose, magnesium stearate, povidone, and sodium lauryl sulfate. Gelatin capsule shells may contain methylparaben, propylparaben, butylparaben and the following dye systems: FD&C Blue 1, FD&C Yellow 6 and either FD&C Red 3 or FD&C Red 40 plus D&C Yellow 10, with titanium dioxide and other inactive ingredients.

CLINICAL PHARMACOLOGY

General: In animal studies. flutamide demonstrates potent antiandrogenic effects. It exerts its antiandrogenic action by inhibiting androgen uptake and/or by inhibiting nuclear binding of androgen in target tissues or both. Prostatic carcinoma is known to be androgen-sensitive and responds to treatment that counteracts the effect of androgen and/or removes the source of androgen, e.g., castration.

Pharmacokinetics: Analysis of plasma, urine, and feces following a single oral 200 mg dose of tritium-labeled flutamide to human volunteers showed that the drug is rapidly and completely absorbed. It is excreted mainly in the urine with only 4.2% of the dose excreted in the feces over 72 hours. The composition of plasma radioactivity showed that flutamide is rapidly and extensively metabolized, with flutamide comprising only 2.5% of plasma radioactivity one hour after administration. At least six metabolites have been identified in plasma. The major plasma metabolite is a biologically active alpha-hydroxylated derivative which accounts for 23% of the plasma tritium one hour after drug administration.

The major urinary metabolite is 2-amino-5-nitro-4-(trifluoromethyl)phenol.

Following a single 250 mg oral dose to normal adult volunteers, low plasma levels of varying amounts of flutamide were detected. The biologically active alpha-hydroxylated metabolite reaches maximum plasma levels in about two hours, indicating that it is rapidly formed from flutamide. The plasma half-life for this metabolite is about 6 hours.

Following multiple oral dosing of 250 mg t.i.d. in normal geriatric volunteers, flutamide and its active metabolite approached steady-state plasma levels (based on pharmacokinetic simulations) after the fourth flutamide dose. The half-life of the active metabolite in geriatric volunteers after a single flutamide dose is about 8 hours and at steady-state is 9.6 hours.

Flutamide, *in vivo,* at steady-state plasma concentrations of 24 to 78 ng/mL is 94% to 96% bound to plasma proteins. The active metabolite of flutamide, *in vivo,* at steady-state plasma concentrations of 1556 to 2284 ng/mL, is 92% to 94% bound to plasma proteins.

In male rats neither flutamide nor any of its metabolites is preferentially accumulated in any tissue except the prostate after an oral 5 mg/kg dose of ^{14}C-flutamide. Total drug levels were highest 6 hours after drug administration in all tissues. Levels declined at roughly similar rates to low levels at 18 hours. The major metabolite was present at higher concentrations than flutamide in all tissues studied.

Elevations of plasma testosterone and estradiol levels have been noted following flutamide administration.

Clinical Studies: Flutamide has been demonstrated to interfere with testosterone at the cellular level. This can complement medical castration achieved with leuprolide, which suppresses testicular androgen production by inhibiting luteinizing horome secretion.

To study the effects of combination therapy, 617 patients (311 leuprolide + flutamide, 306 leuprolide + placebo) with previously untreated advanced prostatic carcinoma were enrolled in a large multi-centered, controlled clinical trial. Three and one-half years after the study was initiated, median survival had been reached. The median actuarial survival time was 34.9 months for patients treated with leuprolide and flutamide versus 27.9 months for patients treated with leuprolide alone. This seven month increment represents a 25% improvement in overall survival with the flutamide therapy. Analysis of progression free survival showed a 2.6 month improvement in patients who received leuprolide plus flutamide, a 19% increment over leuprolide and placebo.

INDICATIONS AND USAGE

EULEXIN Capsules are indicated for use in combination with LHRH agonistic analogues (such as leuprolide acetate) for the treatment of metastatic prostatic carcinoma (stage D_2). To achieve the benefit of the adjunctive therapy with EULEXIN, treatment must be started simultaneously using both drugs.

CONTRAINDICATIONS

EULEXIN Capsules are contraindicated in patients who are hypersensitive to flutamide or any component of this preparation.

WARNINGS

Gynecomastia occurred in 9% of patients receiving flutamide together with medical castration.

Flutamide may cause fetal harm when administered to a pregnant woman. There was decreased 24-hour survival in the offspring of rats treated with flutamide at doses of 30, 100, or 200 mg/kg/day (approximately 3, 9, and 19 times the human dose) during pregnancy. A slight increase in minor variations in the development of the sternebrae and vertebrae was seen in fetuses of rats at the two higher doses. Feminization of the males also occurred at the two higher dose levels. There was a decreased survival rate in the offspring of rabbits receiving the highest dose (15 mg/kg/day; equal to 1.4 times the human dose).

Hepatic injury: Since transaminase abnormalities, cholestatic jaundice, hepatic necrosis, and hepatic encephalopathy have been reported with the use of flutamide, periodic liver function tests should be considered. (See **ADVERSE REACTIONS** section.) Appropriate laboratory testing should be done at the first symptom/sign of liver dysfunction (e.g., pruritus, dark urine, persistent anorexia, jaundice, right upper quadrant tenderness or unexplained "flu-like" symptoms). If the patient has jaundice or laboratory evidence of liver injury, in the absence of biopsy-confirmed liver metastases, EULEXIN therapy should be discontinued or the dosage reduced. The hepatic injury is usually reversible after discontinuation of therapy and in some patients, after dosage reduction. However, there have been reports of death following severe hepatic injury associated with use of flutamide.

PRECAUTIONS

Information for Patients: Patients should be informed that EULEXIN Capsules and the drug used for medical castration should be administered concomitantly, and that they should not interrupt their dosing or stop taking these medications without consulting their physician.

Laboratory Tests: See **WARNINGS, Hepatic Injury above.**

Drug Interactions: Interactions between EULEXIN Capsules and leuprolide have not occurred. Increases in prothrombin time have been noted in patients receiving long-term warfarin therapy after flutamide was initiated. Therefore close monitoring of prothrombin time is recommended and adjustment of the anticoagulant dose may be necessary when EULEXIN Capsules are administered concomitantly with warfarin.

Carcinogenesis, Mutagenesis, Impairment of Fertility: No carcinogenicity studies were performed with flutamide. However, daily administration of flutamide to rats for 52 weeks at doses of 30, 90, or 180 mg/kg/day (approximately 3, 8, or 17 times the human dose) produced testicular interstitial cell adenomas at all doses.

Flutamide did not demonstrate DNA modifying activity in the Ames *Salmonella*/microsome Mutagenesis Assay. Dominant lethal tests in rats were negative.

Reduced sperm counts were observed during a six-week study of flutamide monotherapy in normal human volunteers.

Flutamide did not affect estrous cycles or interfere with the mating behavior of male and female rats when the drug was administered at 25 and 75 mg/kg/day prior to mating. Males treated with 150 mg/kg/day (30 times the minimum effective antiandrogenic dose) failed to mate; mating behavior returned to normal after dosing was stopped. Conception rates were decreased in all dosing groups. Suppression of spermatogenesis was observed in rats dosed for 52 weeks at approximately 3, 8, or 17 times the human dose and in dogs dosed for 78 weeks at 1.4, 2.3, and 3.7 times the human dose.

Pregnancy: Pregnancy Category D. See **WARNINGS** section.

ADVERSE REACTIONS

The following adverse experiences were reported during a multicenter clinical trial comparing flutamide + LHRH agonist versus placebo + LHRH agonist.

The most frequently reported (greater than 5%) adverse experiences during treatment with EULEXIN Capsules in combination with a LHRH agonist are listed in the table below. For comparison, adverse experiences seen with a LHRH agonist and placebo are also listed in the following table.

	(n=294) *Flutamide + LHRH agonist % All*	(n=285) *Placebo + LHRH agonist % All*
Hot Flashes	61	57
Loss of Libido	36	31
Impotence	33	29
Diarrhea	12	4
Nausea/Vomiting	11	10
Gynecomastia	9	11
Other	7	9
Other GI	6	4

As shown in the table, for both treatment groups, the most frequently occurring adverse experiences (hot flashes, impotence, loss of libido) were those known to be associated with

Continued on next page

Information on Schering products appearing on these pages is effective as of August 15, 1992.

Schering—Cont.

low serum androgen levels and known to occur with LHRH agonists alone.
The only notable difference was the higher incidence of diarrhea in the flutamide + LHRH agonist group (12%), which was severe in five percent as opposed to the placebo + LHRH agonist (4%), which was severe in less than one percent.
In addition, the following adverse reactions were reported during treatment with flutamide + LHRH agonist. No causal relatedness of these reactions to drug treatment has been made, and some of the adverse experiences reported are those that commonly occur in elderly patients.
Cardiovascular System: hypertension in 1% of patients.
Central Nervous System: CNS (drowsiness/confusion/depression/anxiety/nervousness) reactions occurred in 1% of patients.
Gastrointestinal System: anorexia 4%, and other GI disorders occurred in 6% of patients.
Hematopoietic System: anemia occurred in 6%, leukopenia in 3%, and thrombocytopenia in 1% of patients.
Liver and Biliary System: hepatitis and jaundice in less than 1% of patients.
Skin: irritation at the injection site and rash occurred in 3% of patients.
Other: edema occurred in 4%, genitourinary and neuromuscular symptoms in 2%, and pulmonary symptoms in less than 1% of patients.
In addition, the following spontaneous adverse experiences have been reported during the marketing of flutamide: hemolytic anemia, macrocytic anemia, methemoglobinemia, photosensitivity reactions (including erythema, ulceration, bullous eruptions, and epidermal necrolysis) and urine discoloration. The urine was noted to change to an amber or yellow-green appearance which can be attributed to the flutamide and/or its metabolites. Also reported were cholestatic jaundice, hepatic encephalopathy, and hepatic necrosis. The hepatic conditions were usually reversible after discontinuing therapy; however, there have been reports of death following severe hepatic injury associated with use of flutamide.
Abnormal Laboratory Test Values: Laboratory abnormalities including elevated SGOT, SGPT, bilirubin values. SGGT, BUN and serum creatinine have been reported.

OVERDOSAGE

In animal studies with flutamide alone, signs of overdose included hypoactivity, piloerection, slow respiration, ataxia, and/or lacrimation, anorexia, tranquilization, emesis, and methemoglobinemia.
Clinical trials have been conducted with flutamide in doses up to 1500 mg per day for periods up to 36 weeks with no serious adverse effects reported. Those adverse reactions reported included gynecomastia, breast tenderness and some increases in SGOT. The single dose of flutamide ordinarily associated with symptoms of overdose or considered to be life-threatening has not been established.
Since flutamide is highly protein bound, dialysis may not be of any use as treatment for overdose. As in the management of overdosage with any drug, it should be borne in mind that multiple agents may have been taken. If vomiting does not occur spontaneously, it should be induced if the patient is alert. General supportive care, including frequent monitoring of the vital signs and close observation of the patient, is indicated.

DOSAGE AND ADMINISTRATION

The recommended dosage is two capsules three times a day at eight hour intervals for a total daily dosage of 750 mg.

HOW SUPPLIED

EULEXIN Capsules, 125 mg, are available as opaque, two-toned brown capsules, imprinted with "Schering 525". They are supplied as follows:
NDC 0085-0525-04—Bottles of 100
NDC 0085-0525-05—Bottles of 500
NDC 0085-0525-03—Unit Dose packages of 100 (10 × 10's)
Store between 2° and 30°C (36° and 86°F).
Protect the unit dose packages from excessive moisture.
Rev. 5/91
Copyright © 1989, 1991, Schering Corporation. All rights reserved.
Shown in Product Identification Section, page 428

FULVICIN® P/G ℞

[ful 'vĭ-sin]
brand of ultramicrosize griseofulvin, Tablets, USP

DESCRIPTION

FULVICIN P/G Tablets contain ultramicrosize crystals of griseofulvin, an antibiotic derived from a species of *Penicillium.* Griseofulvin crystals are partly dissolved in polyethylene glycol 6000 and partly dispersed throughout the tablet matrix.
Each FULVICIN P/G Tablet contains 125 mg or 250 mg griseofulvin ultramicrosize.
The inactive ingredients for FULVICIN P/G Tablets, 125 or 250 mg, include: corn starch, lactose, magnesium stearate, PEG, and sodium lauryl sulfate.

ACTIONS

Microbiology Griseofulvin is fungistatic with *in vitro* activity against various species of *Microsporum, Epidermophyton,* and *Trichophyton.* It has no effect on bacteria or on other genera of fungi.
Human Pharmacology: Following oral administration, griseofulvin is deposited in the keratin precursor cells and has a greater affinity for diseased tissue. The drug is tightly bound to the new keratin which becomes highly resistant to fungal invasions.
The efficiency of gastrointestinal absorption of ultramicrocrystalline griseofulvin is approximately one and one-half times that of the conventional microsized griseofulvin. This factor permits the oral intake of two-thirds as much ultramicrocrystalline griseofulvin as the microsize form. However, there is currently no evidence that this lower dose confers any significant clinical differences with regard to safety and/or efficacy.

INDICATIONS

FULVICIN P/G Tablets are indicated for the treatment of ringworm infections of the skin, hair, and nails, namely: tinea corporis, tinea pedis, tinea cruris, tinea barbae, tinea capitis, tinea unguium (onychomycosis) when caused by one or more of the following genera of fungi: *Trichophyton rubrum, Trichophyton tonsurans, Trichophyton mentagrophytes, Trichophyton interdigitale, Trichophyton verrucosum, Trichophyton megninii, Trichophyton gallinae, Trichophyton crateriforme, Trichophyton sulphureum, Trichophyton schoenleinii, Microsporum audouini, Microsporum canis, Microsporum gypseum,* and *Epidermophyton floccosum.*
Note: Prior to therapy, the type of fungi responsible for the infection should be identified.
The use of this drug is not justified in minor or trivial infections which will respond to topical agents alone.
Griseofulvin is not effective in the following: bacterial infections, candidiasis (moniliasis), histoplasmosis, actinomycosis, sporotrichosis, chromoblastomycosis, coccidioidomycosis, North American blastomycosis, cryptococcosis (torulosis), tinea versicolor, and nocardiosis.

CONTRAINDICATIONS

This drug is contraindicated in patients with porphyria, hepatocellular failure, and in individuals with a history of hypersensitivity to griseofulvin.
Rare cases of conjoined twins have been reported in patients taking griseofulvin during the first trimester of pregnancy. Griseofulvin should not be prescribed to pregnant patients or to women contemplating pregnancy.

WARNINGS

Prophylactic Usage: Safety and efficacy of griseofulvin for prophylaxis of fungal infections have not been established.
Animal Toxicology: Chronic feeding of griseofulvin, at levels ranging from 0.5–2.5% of the diet, resulted in the development of liver tumors in several strains of mice, particularly in males. Smaller particle sizes result in an enhanced effect. Lower oral dosage levels have not been tested. Subcutaneous administration of relatively small doses of griseofulvin once a week during the first three weeks of life has also been reported to induce hepatomata in mice. Thyroid tumors, mostly adenomas but some carcinomas, have been reported in male rats receiving griseofulvin at levels of 2.0%, 1.0%, and 0.2% of the diet, and in female rats receiving the two higher dose levels. Although studies in other animal species have not yielded evidence of tumorigenicity, these studies were not of adequate design to form a basis for conclusions in this regard.
In subacute toxicity studies, orally administered griseofulvin produced hepatocellular necrosis in mice, but this has not been seen in other species. Disturbances in porphyrin metabolism have been reported in griseofulvin-treated laboratory animals. Griseofulvin has been reported to have a colchicine-like effect on mitosis and cocarcinogenicity with methylcholanthrene in cutaneous tumor induction in laboratory animals.
Usage in Pregnancy: Griseofulvin should not be prescribed to pregnant patients or to women contemplating pregnancy (see **CONTRAINDICATIONS**).
Animal Reproduction Studies: It has been reported in the literature that griseofulvin was found to be embryotoxic and teratogenic on oral administration to pregnant rats. Pups with abnormalities have been reported in the litters of a few bitches treated with griseofulvin.
Suppression of spermatogenesis has been reported to occur in rats, but investigation in man failed to confirm this.

PRECAUTIONS

Patients on prolonged therapy with any potent medication should be under close observation. Periodic monitoring of organ system function, including renal, hepatic, and hematopoietic, should be done.
Since griseofulvin is derived from species of *Penicillium,* the possibility of cross-sensitivity with penicillin exists; however, known penicillin-sensitive patients have been treated without difficulty.
Since a photosensitivity reaction is occasionally associated with griseofulvin therapy, patients should be warned to avoid exposure to intense natural or artificial sunlight.
Lupus erythematosus or lupus-like syndromes, or exacerbation of existing lupus, have been reported in patients receiving griseofulvin.
Drug Interactions
Griseofulvin decreases the activity of warfarin-type anticoagulants so that patients receiving these drugs concomitantly may require dosage adjustment of the anticoagulant during and after griseofulvin therapy.
Barbiturates usually depress griseofulvin activity, and concomitant administration may require a dosage adjustment of the antifungal agent.
The effects of alcohol may be potentiated by griseofulvin, producing such effects as tachycardia and flush.
Griseofulvin may potentiate an increase in hepatic enzymes that metabolize estrogens at an increased rate, including the estrogen component of oral contraceptives, thereby causing possible decreased contraceptive effects and menstrual irregularities.

ADVERSE REACTIONS

When adverse reactions occur, they are most commonly of the hypersensitivity type, such as skin rashes, urticaria, and rarely, angioneurotic edema, and may necessitate withdrawal of therapy and appropriate countermeasures. Paresthesias of the hands and feet have been reported rarely after extended therapy. Other side effects reported occasionally are oral thrush, nausea, vomiting, epigastric distress, diarrhea, headache, fatigue, dizziness, insomnia, mental confusion, and impairment of performance of routine activities.
Proteinuria, nephrosis, leukopenia, hepatic toxicity, GI bleeding and menstrual irregularities have been reported rarely. Administration of the drug should be discontinued if granulocytopenia occurs.
When rare, serious reactions occur with griseofulvin, they are usually associated with high dosages, long periods of therapy, or both.

DOSAGE AND ADMINISTRATION

Accurate diagnosis of the infecting organism is essential. Identification should be made either by direct microscopic examination of a mounting of infected tissue in a solution of potassium hydroxide or by culture on an appropriate medium.
Medication must be continued until the infecting organism is completely eradicated as indicated by appropriate clinical or laboratory examination. Representative treatment periods are tinea capitis, 4 to 6 weeks; tinea corporis, 2 to 4 weeks; tinea pedis, 4 to 8 weeks; tinea unguium—depending on rate of growth—fingernails, at least 4 months; toenails, at least 6 months.
General measures in regard to hygiene should be observed to control sources of infection or reinfection. Concomitant use of appropriate topical agents is usually required particularly in treatment of tinea pedis. In some forms of athlete's foot, yeasts and bacteria may be involved as well as fungi. Griseofulvin will not eradicate the bacterial or monilial infection.
Adults: Daily administration of 375 mg (as a single dose or in divided amounts) will give a satisfactory response in most patients with tinea corporis, tinea cruris, and tinea capitis.
For those fungus infections more difficult to eradicate, such as tinea pedis and tinea unguium, a divided dose of 750 mg is recommended.
Children: Approximately 3.3 mg per pound of body weight per day of ultramicrosize griseofulvin is an effective dose for most children. On this basis, the following dosage schedule is suggested: Children weighing 35 to 60 pounds—125 mg to 187.5 mg daily. Children weighing over 60 pounds—187.5 mg to 375 mg daily.
Children 2 years of age and younger—dosage has not been established.
Clinical experience with griseofulvin in children with tinea capitis indicates that a single daily dose is effective. Clinical relapse will occur if the medication is not continued until the infecting organism is eradicated.

HOW SUPPLIED

FULVICIN P/G Tablets, 125 mg, white, compressed, scored tablets impressed with the Schering trademark and product identification numbers, 228; bottle of 100 (NDC 0085-0228-03).
FULVICIN P/G Tablets, 250 mg, white, compressed, scored tablets impressed with the Schering trademark and product identification numbers, 507; bottle of 100 (NDC 0085-0507-03).

Store between 15° & 30°C (59° and 86°F).
Revised 5/90
Shown in Product Identification Section, page 428

FULVICIN® P/G 165 and 330   ℞
[*ful'vĭ-sin*]
brand of ultramicrosize griseofulvin
  Tablets, USP

DESCRIPTION
FULVICIN P/G Tablets contain ultramicrosize crystals of griseofulvin, an antibiotic derived from a species of *Penicillium*. Griseofulvin crystals are partly dissolved in polyethylene glycol 8000 and partly dispersed throughout the tablet matrix.
Each FULVICIN P/G Tablet contains 165 mg or 330 mg ultramicrosize griseofulvin, USP.
The inactive ingredients for FULVICIN P/G 165 and 330 Tablets include: corn starch, lactose, magnesium stearate, PEG, and sodium lauryl sulfate.

ACTIONS
Microbiology: Griseofulvin is fungistatic with *in vitro* activity against various species of *Microsporum*, *Epidermophyton*, and *Trichophyton*. It has no effect on bacteria or on other genera of fungi.
Human Pharmacology: Following oral administration, griseofulvin is deposited in the keratin precursor cells and has a greater affinity for diseased tissue. The drug is tightly bound to the new keratin which becomes highly resistant to fungal invasions.
The efficiency of gastrointestinal absorption of ultramicrocrystalline griseofulvin is approximately one and one-half times that of the conventional microsize griseofulvin. This factor permits the oral intake of two-thirds as much ultramicrocrystalline griseofulvin as the microsize form. However, there is currently no evidence that this lower dose confers any significant clinical differences with regard to safety and/or efficacy.

INDICATIONS
FULVICIN P/G Tablets are indicated for the treatment of ringworm infections of the skin, hair, and nails, namely: tinea corporis, tinea pedis, tinea cruris, tinea barbae, tinea capitis, tinea unguium (onychomycosis) when caused by one or more of the following genera of fungi: *Trichophyton rubrum*, *Trichophyton tonsurans*, *Trichophyton mentagrophytes*, *Trichophyton interdigitale*, *Trichophyton verrucosum*, *Trichophyton megninii*, *Trichophyton gallinae*, *Trichophyton crateriforme*, *Trichophyton sulphureum*, *Trichophyton schoenleinii*, *Microsporum audouini*, *Microsporum canis*, *Microsporum gypseum*, and *Epidermophyton floccosum*.
Note: Prior to therapy, the type of fungi responsible for the infection should be identified.
The use of this drug is not justified in minor or trivial infections which will respond to topical agents alone.
Griseofulvin is not effective in the following: bacterial infections, candidiasis (moniliasis), histoplasmosis, actinomycosis, sporotrichosis, chromoblastomycosis, coccidioidomycosis, North American blastomycosis, cryptococcosis (torulosis), tinea versicolor, and nocardiosis.

CONTRAINDICATIONS
This drug is contraindicated in patients with porphyria, hepatocellular failure, and in individuals with a history of hypersensitivity to griseofulvin.
Rare cases of conjoined twins have been reported in patients taking griseofulvin during the first trimester of pregnancy. Griseofulvin should not be prescribed to pregnant patients or to women contemplating pregnancy.

WARNINGS
Prophylactic Usage: Safety and efficacy of griseofulvin for prophylaxis of fungal infections have not been established.
Animal Toxicology: Chronic feeding of griseofulvin, at levels ranging from 0.5–2.5% of the diet, resulted in the development of liver tumors in several strains of mice, particularly in males. Smaller particle sizes result in an enhanced effect. Lower oral dosage levels have not been tested. Subcutaneous administration of relatively small doses of griseofulvin once a week during the first three weeks of life has also been reported to induce hepatomata in mice. Thyroid tumors, mostly adenomas but some carcinomas, have been reported in male rats receiving griseofulvin at levels of 2.0%, 1.0%, and 0.2% of the diet, and in female rats receiving the two higher dose levels. Although studies in other animal species have not yielded evidence of tumorigenicity, these studies were not of adequate design to form a basis for conclusions in this regard.
In subacute toxicity studies, orally administered griseofulvin produced hepatocellular necrosis in mice, but this has not been seen in other species. Disturbances in porphyrin metabolism have been reported in griseofulvin-treated laboratory animals. Griseofulvin has been reported to have a colchicine-like effect on mitosis and cocarcinogenicity with methylcholanthrene in cutaneous tumor induction in laboratory animals.
Usage in Pregnancy: Griseofulvin should not be prescribed to pregnant patients or to women contemplating pregnancy (see *CONTRAINDICATIONS*).
Animal Reproduction Studies: It has been reported in the literature that griseofulvin was found to be embryotoxic and teratogenic on oral administration to pregnant rats. Pups with abnormalities have been reported in the litters of a few bitches treated with griseofulvin.
Suppression of spermatogenesis has been reported to occur in rats, but investigation in man failed to confirm this.

PRECAUTIONS
Patients on prolonged therapy with any potent medication should be under close observation. Periodic monitoring of organ system function, including renal, hepatic, and hematopoietic, should be done.
Since griseofulvin is derived from species of *Penicillium*, the possibility of cross-sensitivity with penicillin exists; however, known penicillin-sensitive patients have been treated without difficulty.
Since a photosensitivity reaction is occasionally associated with griseofulvin therapy, patients should be warned to avoid exposure to intense natural or artificial sunlight.
Lupus erythematosus or lupus-like syndromes, or exacerbation of existing lupus, have been reported in patients receiving griseofulvin.
Drug Interactions: Griseofulvin decreases the activity of warfarin-type anticoagulants so that patients receiving these drugs concomitantly may require dosage adjustment of the anticoagulant during and after griseofulvin therapy.
Barbiturates usually depress griseofulvin activity, and concomitant administration may require a dosage adjustment of the antifungal agent.
The effects of alcohol may be potentiated by griseofulvin, producing such effects as tachycardia and flush.
Griseofulvin may potentiate an increase in hepatic enzymes that metabolize estrogens at an increased rate, including the estrogen component of oral contraceptives, thereby causing possible decreased contraceptive effects and menstrual irregularities.

ADVERSE REACTIONS
When adverse reactions occur, they are most commonly of the hypersensitivity type, such as skin rashes, urticaria, and rarely, angioneurotic edema, and may necessitate withdrawal of therapy and appropriate countermeasures. Paresthesias of the hands and feet have been reported rarely after extended therapy. Other side effects reported occasionally are oral thrush, nausea, vomiting, epigastric distress, diarrhea, headache, fatigue, dizziness, insomnia, mental confusion, and impairment of performance of routine activities. Proteinuria, nephrosis, leukopenia, hepatic toxicity, GI bleeding and menstrual toxicity have been reported rarely. Administration of the drug should be discontinued if granulocytopenia occurs.
When rare, serious reactions occur with griseofulvin, they are usually associated with high dosages, long periods of therapy, or both.

DOSAGE AND ADMINISTRATION
Accurate diagnosis of the infecting organism is essential. Identification should be made either by direct microscopic examination of a mounting of infected tissue in a solution of potassium hydroxide or by culture on an appropriate medium.
Medication must be continued until the infecting organism is completely eradicated as indicated by appropriate clinical or laboratory examination. Representative treatment periods are tinea capitis, 4 to 6 weeks, tinea corporis, 2 to 4 weeks, tinea pedis, 4 to 8 weeks, tinea unguium—depending on rate of growth—fingernails, at least 4 months; toenails, at least 6 months.
General measures in regard to hygiene should be observed to control sources of infection or reinfection. Concomitant use of appropriate topical agents is usually required particularly in treatment of tinea pedis. In some forms of athlete's foot, yeasts and bacteria may be involved as well as fungi. Griseofulvin will not eradicate the bacterial or monilial infection.
Adults: Daily administration of 330 mg (as a single dose or in divided amounts) will give a satisfactory response in most patients with tinea corporis, tinea cruris, and tinea capitis. For those fungus infections more difficult to eradicate, such as tinea pedis and tinea unguium, a divided daily dosage of 660 mg is recommended.
Children: Approximately 3.3 mg per pound of body weight per day is an effective dose for most children. On this basis, the following dosage schedule is suggested: Children weighing 30 to 50 pounds—82.5 mg to 165 mg daily. Children weighing over 50 pounds—165 mg to 330 mg daily.
Children 2 years of age and younger—dosage has not been established.
Clinical experience with griseofulvin in children with tinea capitis indicates that a single daily dose is effective. Clinical relapse will occur if the medication is not continued until the infecting organism is eradicated.

HOW SUPPLIED
FULVICIN P/G 165 Tablets, 165 mg, off-white, oval, compressed, scored tablets impressed with the product name (FULVICIN P/G) and product identification numbers, 654; bottle of 100 (NDC 0085-0654-03).
FULVICIN P/G 330 Tablets, 330 mg, off-white, oval, compressed, scored tablets impressed with the product name (FULVICIN P/G) and product identification numbers, 352; bottle of 100 (NDC 0085-0352-03).
Store between 2° and 30°C (36° and 86°F).
Revised 4/87
Shown in Product Identification Section, page 428

GARAMYCIN®   ℞
[*gar-ah-mī'sin*]
brand of gentamicin sulfate
  Cream, USP 0.1%
  Ointment, USP 0.1%

GARAMYCIN Cream 0.1% (NDC-0085-0008-05) and GARAMYCIN Ointment 0.1% (NDC-0085-0343-05), 15 g tubes.

GARAMYCIN®   ℞
[*gar-ah-mī'sin*]
brand of gentamicin sulfate
  Ophthalmic Solution, USP—Sterile
  Ophthalmic Ointment, USP—Sterile
Each ml or gram contains gentamicin sulfate, USP equivalent to 3.0 mg gentamicin

GARAMYCIN Ophthalmic Solution—Sterile, 5 ml. plastic dropper bottle, box of one (NDC 0085-0899-05).
GARAMYCIN Ophthalmic Ointment—Sterile, 3.5 g, box of one (NDC 0085-0151-05).

GARAMYCIN® Injectable   ℞
[*gar-ah-mī'sin*]
brand of gentamicin sulfate injection, USP
  40 mg per ml
Each ml contains gentamicin sulfate, USP equivalent to 40 mg gentamicin.
For Parenteral Administration

WARNINGS
Patients treated with aminoglycosides should be under close clinical observation because of the potential toxicity associated with their use.
As with other aminoglycosides, GARAMYCIN Injectable is potentially nephrotoxic. The risk of nephrotoxicity is greater in patients with impaired renal function and in those who receive high dosage or prolonged therapy.
Neurotoxicity manifested by ototoxicity, both vestibular and auditory, can occur in patients treated with GARAMYCIN Injectable primarily in those with pre-existing renal damage and in patients with normal renal function treated with higher doses and/or for longer periods than recommended. Aminoglycoside-induced ototoxicity is usually irreversible. Other manifestations of neurotoxicity may include numbness, skin tingling, muscle twitching and convulsions.
Renal and eighth cranial nerve function should be closely monitored, especially in patients with known or suspected reduced renal function at onset of therapy, and also in those whose renal function is initially normal but who develop signs of renal dysfunction during therapy. Urine should be examined for decreased specific gravity, increased excretion of protein, and the presence of cells or casts. Blood urea nitrogen, serum creatinine, or creatinine clearance should be determined periodically. When feasible, it is recommended that serial audiograms be obtained in patients old enough to be tested, particularly high-risk patients. Evidence of ototoxicity (dizziness, vertigo, tinnitus, roaring in the ears or hearing loss) or nephrotoxicity requires dosage adjustment or discontinuance of the drug. As with the other aminoglycosides, on rare occasions changes in renal and eighth cranial nerve function

Continued on next page

Schering—Cont.

may not become manifest until soon after completion of therapy.

Serum concentrations of aminoglycosides should be monitored when feasible to assure adequate levels and to avoid potentially toxic levels. When monitoring gentamicin peak concentrations, dosage should be adjusted so that prolonged levels above 12 mcg/ml are avoided. When monitoring gentamicin trough concentrations, dosage should be adjusted so that levels above 2 mcg/ml are avoided. Excessive peak and/or trough serum concentrations of aminoglycosides may increase the risk of renal and eighth cranial nerve toxicity. In the event of overdose or toxic reactions, hemodialysis may aid in the removal of gentamicin from the blood, especially if renal function is, or becomes, compromised. The rate of removal of gentamicin is considerably less by peritoneal dialysis than by hemodialysis.

Concurrent and/or sequential systemic or topical use of other potentially neurotoxic and/or nephrotoxic drugs, such as cisplatin, cephaloridine, kanamycin, amikacin, neomycin, polymyxin B, colistin, paromomycin, streptomycin, tobramycin, vancomycin, and viomycin, should be avoided. Other factors which may increase patient risk of toxicity are advanced age and dehydration.

The concurrent use of gentamicin with potent diuretics, such as ethacrynic acid or furosemide, should be avoided, since certain diuretics by themselves may cause ototoxicity. In addition, when administered intravenously, diuretics may enhance aminoglycoside toxicity by altering the antibiotic concentration in serum and tissue.

DESCRIPTION

Gentamicin sulfate, USP, a water-soluble antibiotic of the aminoglycoside group, is derived from *Micromonospora purpurea*, an actinomycete. GARAMYCIN Injectable is a sterile, aqueous solution for parenteral administration. Each ml contains gentamicin sulfate, USP equivalent to 40 mg gentamicin base, 1.8 mg methylparaben and 0.2 mg propylparaben as preservatives, 3.2 mg sodium bisulfite, and 0.1 mg edetate disodium.

CLINICAL PHARMACOLOGY

After intramuscular administration of GARAMYCIN Injectable, peak serum concentrations usually occur between 30 and 60 minutes and serum levels are measurable for six to eight hours. When gentamicin is administered by intravenous infusion over a two-hour period, the serum concentrations are similar to those obtained by intramuscular administration.

In patients with normal renal function, peak serum concentrations of gentamicin (mcg/ml) are usually up to four times the single intramuscular dose (mg/kg); for example, a 1.0 mg/kg injection in adults may be expected to result in a peak serum concentration up to 4 mcg/ml; a 1.5 mg/kg dose may produce levels up to 6 mcg/ml. While some variation is to be expected due to a number of variables such as age, body temperature surface area and physiologic differences, the individual patient given the same dose tends to have similar levels in repeated determinations. Gentamicin administered at 1.0 mg/kg every eight hours for the usual 7- to 10-day treatment period to patients with normal renal function does not accumulate in serum.

Gentamicin, like all aminoglycosides, may accumulate in the serum and tissues of patients treated with higher doses and/or for prolonged periods, particularly in the presence of impaired renal function. In adult patients, treatment with gentamicin dosages of 4 mg/kg/day or higher for seven to ten days may result in a slight, progressive rise in both peak and trough concentrations. In patients with impaired renal function, gentamicin is cleared from the body more slowly than in patients with normal renal function. The more severe the impairment, the slower the clearance. (Dosage must be adjusted.)

Since gentamicin is distributed in extracellular fluid, peak serum concentrations may be lower than usual in adult patients who have a large volume of this fluid. Serum concentrations of gentamicin in febrile patients may be lower than those in afebrile patients given the same dose. When body temperature returns to normal, serum concentrations of the drug may rise. Febrile and anemic states may be associated with a shorter than usual serum half-life. (Dosage adjustment is usually not necessary.) In severely burned patients, the half-life may be significantly decreased and resulting serum concentrations may be lower than anticipated from the mg/kg dose.

Protein-binding studies have indicated that the degree of gentamicin binding is low; depending upon the methods used for testing, this may be between 0 and 30%.

After initial administration to patients with normal renal function, generally 70% or more of the gentamicin dose is recoverable in the urine in 24 hours; concentrations in urine above 100 mcg/ml may be achieved. Little, if any, metabolic transformation occurs; the drug is excreted principally by glomerular filtration. After several days of treatment, the amount of gentamicin excreted in the urine approaches the daily dose administered. As with other aminoglycosides, a small amount of the gentamicin dose may be retained in the tissues, especially in the kidneys. Minute quantities of aminoglycosides have been detected in the urine weeks after drug administration was discontinued. Renal clearance of gentamicin is similar to that of endogenous creatinine.

In patients with marked impairment of renal function, there is a decrease in the concentration of aminoglycosides in urine and in their penetration into defective renal parenchyma. This decreased drug excretion, together with the potential nephrotoxicity of aminoglycosides, should be considered when treating such patients who have urinary tract infections.

Probenecid does not affect renal tubular transport of gentamicin.

The endogenous creatinine clearance rate and the serum creatinine level have a high correlation with the half-life of gentamicin in serum. Results of these tests may serve as guides for adjusting dosage in patients with renal impairment (see DOSAGE AND ADMINISTRATION).

Following parenteral administration, gentamicin can be detected in serum, lymph, tissues, sputum, and in pleural, synovial, and peritoneal fluids. Concentrations in renal cortex sometimes may be eight times higher than the usual serum levels. Concentrations in bile, in general, have been low and have suggested minimal biliary excretion. Gentamicin crosses the peritoneal as well as the placental membranes. Since aminoglycosides diffuse poorly into the subarachnoid space after parenteral administration, concentrations of gentamicin in cerebrospinal fluid are often low and dependent upon dose, rate of penetration, and degree of meningeal inflammation. There is minimal penetration of gentamicin into ocular tissues following intramuscular or intravenous administration.

Microbiology: *In vitro* tests have demonstrated that gentamicin is a bactericidal antibiotic which acts by inhibiting normal protein synthesis in susceptible microorganisms. It is active against a wide variety of pathogenic bacteria including *Escherichia coli*, *Proteus* species, (indole-positive and indole-negative), *Pseudomonas aeruginosa*, species of the *Klebsiella-Enterobacter-Serratia* group. *Citrobacter* species and *Staphylococcus* species (including penicillin- and methicillin-resistant strains). Gentamicin is also active *in vitro* against species of *Salmonella* and *Shigella*. The following bacteria are usually resistant to aminoglycoside: *Streptococcus pneumoniae*, most species of streptococci, particularly group D and anaerobic organisms, such as *Bacteroides* species or *Clostridium* species.

In vitro studies have shown that an aminoglycoside combined with an antibiotic that interferes with cell wall synthesis may act synergistically against some group D streptococcal strains. The combination of gentamicin and penicillin G has a synergistic bactericidal effect against virtually all strains of *Streptococcus faecalis* and its varieties (*S. faecalis* var. *liquifaciens*, *S. faecalis* var. *zymogenes*), *S. faecium* and *S. durans*. An enhanced killing effect against many of these strains has also been shown *in vitro* with combinations of gentamicin and ampicillin, carbenicillin, nafcillin, or oxacillin.

The combined effect of gentamicin and carbenicillin is synergistic for many strains of *Pseudomonas aeruginosa*. *In vitro* synergism against other gram-negative organisms has been shown with combinations of gentamicin and cephalosporins. Gentamicin may be active against clinical isolates of bacteria resistant to other aminoglycosides. Bacteria resistant to one aminoglycoside may be resistant to one or more other aminoglycosides. Bacterial resistance to gentamicin is generally developed slowly.

Susceptibility Testing: If the disc method of susceptibility testing used is that described by Bauer *et al* (*Am J Clin Path* 45:493, 1966; *Federal Register* 37:20525-20529, 1972), a disc containing 10 mcg of gentamicin should give a zone of inhibition of 15mm or more to indicate susceptibility of the infecting organism. A zone of 12mm or less indicates that the infecting organism is likely to be resistant. Zones greater than 12mm and less than 15mm indicate intermediate susceptibility. In certain conditions it may be desirable to do additional susceptibility testing by the tube or agar dilution method; gentamicin substance is available for this purpose.

INDICATIONS AND USAGE

GARAMYCIN Injectable is indicated in the treatment of serious infections caused by susceptible strains of the following microorganisms: *Pseudomonas aeruginosa*, *Proteus* species (indole-positive and indole-negative), *Escherichia coli*, *Klebsiella-Enterobacter-Serratia* species, *Citrobacter* species and *Staphylococcus* species (coagulase-positive and coagulase-negative).

Clinical studies have shown GARAMYCIN Injectable to be effective in bacterial neonatal sepsis; bacterial septicemia; and serious bacterial infections of the central nervous system (meningitis), urinary tract, respiratory tract, gastrointestinal tract (including peritonitis), skin, bone and soft tissue (including burns). Aminoglycosides, including gentamicin, are not indicated in uncomplicated initial episodes of urinary tract infections unless the causative organisms are susceptible to these antibiotics and are not susceptible to antibiotics having less potential for toxicity.

Specimens for bacterial culture should be obtained to isolate and identify causative organisms and to determine their susceptibility to gentamicin.

GARAMYCIN may be considered as initial therapy in suspected or confirmed gram-negative infections, and therapy may be instituted before obtaining results of susceptibility testing. The decision to continue therapy with this drug should be based on the results of susceptibility tests, the severity of the infection, and the important additional concepts contained in the "WARNINGS Box" above. If the causative organisms are resistant to gentamicin, other appropriate therapy should be instituted.

In serious infections when the causative organisms are unknown, GARAMYCIN may be administered as initial therapy in conjunction with a penicillin-type or cephalosporin-type drug before obtaining results of susceptibility testing. If anaerobic organisms are suspected as etiologic agents, consideration should be given to using other suitable antimicrobial therapy in conjunction with gentamicin. Following identification of the organism and its susceptibility, appropriate antibiotic therapy should then be continued.

GARAMYCIN has been used effectively in combination with carbenicillin for the treatment of life-threatening infections caused by *Pseudomonas aeruginosa*. It has also been found effective when used in conjunction with a penicillin-type drug for the treatment of endocarditis caused by group D streptococci.

GARAMYCIN Injectable has also been shown to be effective in the treatment of serious staphylococcal infections. While not the antibiotic of first choice, GARAMYCIN Injectable may be considered when penicillins or other less potentially toxic drugs are contraindicated and bacterial susceptibility tests and clinical judgment indicate its use. It may also be considered in mixed infections caused by susceptible strains of staphylococci and gram-negative organisms.

In the neonate with suspected bacterial sepsis or staphylococcal pneumonia, a penicillin-type drug is also usually indicated as concomitant therapy with gentamicin.

CONTRAINDICATIONS

Hypersensitivity to gentamicin is a contraindication to its use. A history of hypersensitivity or serious toxic reactions to other aminoglycosides may contraindicate use of gentamicin because of the known cross-sensitivity of patients to drugs in this class.

WARNINGS

(See boxed **WARNINGS**.) Aminoglycosides can cause fetal harm when administered to a pregnant woman. Aminoglycoside antibiotics cross the placenta, and there have been several reports of total irreversible bilateral congenital deafness in children whose mothers received streptomycin during pregnancy. Serious side effects to mother, fetus, or newborn have not been reported in the treatment of pregnant women with other aminoglycosides. Animal reproduction studies conducted on rats and rabbits did not reveal evidence of impaired fertility or harm to the fetus due to gentamicin sulfate.

It is not known whether gentamicin sulfate can cause fetal harm when administered to a pregnant woman or can affect reproduction capacity. If gentamicin is used during pregnancy or if the patient becomes pregnant while taking gentamicin, she should be apprised of the potential hazard to the fetus.

GARAMYCIN Injectable contains sodium bisulfite, a sulfite that may cause allergic-type reactions including anaphylactic symptoms and life-threatening or less severe asthmatic episodes in certain susceptible people. The overall prevalence of sulfite sensitivity in the general population is unknown and probably low. Sulfite sensitivity is seen more frequently in asthmatic than in nonasthmatic people.

PRECAUTIONS

Neurotoxic and nephrotoxic antibiotics may be absorbed in significant quantities from body surfaces after local irrigation or application. The potential toxic effect of antibiotics administered in this fashion should be considered.

Increased nephrotoxicity has been reported following concomitant administration of aminoglycoside antibiotics and cephalosporins.

Neuromuscular blockade and respiratory paralysis have been reported in the cat receiving high doses (40 mg/kg) of gentamicin. The possibility of these phenomena occurring in man should be considered if aminoglycosides are administered by any route to patients receiving anesthetics, or to patients receiving neuromuscular blocking agents, such as succinylcholine, tubocurarine, or decamethonium, or in patients receiving massive transfusions of citrate-anticoagulated blood. If neuromuscular blockade occurs, calcium salts may reverse it.

Aminoglycosides should be used with caution in patients with neuromuscular disorders, such as myasthenia gravis, since these drugs may aggravate muscle weakness because of their potential curare-like effects on the neuromuscular junction. During or following gentamicin therapy, paresthesias, tetany, positive Chvostek and Trousseau signs, and mental confusion have been described in patients with hypomagnesemia, hypocalcemia, and hypokalemia. When this has occurred in infants, tetany and muscle weakness have been described. Both adults and infants required appropriate corrective electrolyte therapy.

Elderly patients may have reduced renal function which may not be evident in the results of routine screening tests, such as BUN or serum creatinine. A creatinine clearance determination may be more useful. Monitoring of renal function during treatment with gentamicin, as with other aminoglycosides, is particularly important in such patients. A Fanconi-like syndrome, with aminoaciduria and metabolic acidosis, has been reported in some adults and infants being given gentamicin injections.

Cross-allergenicity among aminoglycosides has been demonstrated.

Patients should be well hydrated during treatment.

Although the *in vitro* mixing of gentamicin and carbenicillin results in a rapid and significant inactivation of gentamicin, this interaction has not been demonstrated in patients with normal renal function who received both drugs by different routes of administration. A reduction in gentamicin serum half-life has been reported in patients with severe renal impairment receiving carbenicillin concomitantly with gentamicin.

Treatment with gentamicin may result in overgrowth of nonsusceptible organisms. If this occurs, appropriate therapy is indicated.

See "WARNINGS Box" regarding concurrent use of potent diuretics and regarding concurrent and/or sequential use of other neurotoxic and/or nephrotoxic antibiotics and for other essential information.

Usage in Pregnancy—Safety for use in pregnancy has not been established.

ADVERSE REACTIONS

Nephrotoxicity Adverse renal effects, as demonstrated by the presence of casts, cells, or protein in the urine or by rising BUN, NPN, serum creatinine or oliguria, have been reported. They occur more frequently in patients with a history of renal impairment and in patients treated for longer periods or with larger dosage than recommended.

Neurotoxicity Serious adverse effects on both vestibular and auditory branches of the eighth cranial nerves have been reported, primarily in patients with renal impairment (especially if dialysis is required), and in patients on high doses and/or prolonged therapy. Symptoms include dizziness, vertigo, tinnitus, roaring in the ears and hearing loss, which, as with the other aminoglycosides, may be irreversible. Hearing loss is usually manifested initially by diminution of high-tone acuity. Other factors which may increase the risk of toxicity include excessive dosage, dehydration and previous exposure to other ototoxic drugs.

Peripheral neuropathy or encephalopathy, including numbness, skin tingling, muscle twitching, convulsions, and a myasthenia gravis-like syndrome, have been reported.

Note: The risk of toxic reactions is low in patients with normal renal function who do not receive GARAMYCIN Injectable at higher doses or for longer periods of time than recommended.

Other reported adverse reactions possibly related to gentamicin include: respiratory depression, lethargy, confusion, depression, visual disturbances, decreased appetite, weight loss, and hypotension and hypertension; rash, itching, urticaria, generalized burning, laryngeal edema, anaphylactoid reactions, fever, and headache, nausea, vomiting, increased salivation, and stomatitis; purpura, pseudotumor cerebri, acute organic brain syndrome, pulmonary fibrosis, alopecia, joint pain, transient hepatomegaly, and splenomegaly.

Laboratory abnormalities possibly related to gentamicin include: increased levels of serum transaminase (SGOT, SGPT), serum LDH and bilirubin; decreased serum calcium, magnesium, sodium and potassium; anemia, leukopenia, granulocytopenia, transient agranulocytosis, eosinophilia, increased and decreased reticulocyte counts, and thrombocytopenia. While clinical laboratory test abnormalities may be isolated findings, they may also be associated with clinically related signs and symptoms. For example, tetany and muscle weakness may be associated with hypomagnesemia, hypocalcemia, and hypokalemia.

While local tolerance of GARAMYCIN Injectable is generally excellent, there has been an occasional report of pain at the injection site. Subcutaneous atrophy or fat necrosis suggesting local irritation has been reported rarely.

OVERDOSAGE

In the event of overdose or toxic reactions, hemodialysis may aid in the removal of gentamicin from the blood, and is especially important if renal function is, or becomes, compromised. The rate of removal of gentamicin is considerably less by peritoneal dialysis than it is by hemodialysis.

DOSAGE AND ADMINISTRATION

GARAMYCIN Injectable may be given intramuscularly or intravenously. The patient's pretreatment body weight should be obtained for calculation of correct dosage. The dosage of aminoglycosides in obese patients should be based on an estimate of the lean body mass. It is desirable to limit the duration of treatment with aminoglycosides to short term.

DOSAGE FOR PATIENTS WITH NORMAL RENAL FUNCTION

Adults: The recommended dosage of GARAMYCIN Injectable for patients with serious infections and normal renal function is 3 mg/kg/day, administered in three equal doses every eight hours (Table I).

For patients with life-threatening infections, dosages up to 5 mg/kg/day may be administered in three or four equal doses. This dosage should be reduced to 3 mg/kg/day as soon as clinically indicated (Table I).

It is desirable to measure periodically both peak and trough serum concentrations of gentamicin when feasible during therapy to assure adequate but not excessive drug levels. For example, the peak concentration (at 30 to 60 minutes after intramuscular injection) is expected to be in the range of 4 to 6 mcg/ml. When monitoring peak concentrations after intramuscular or intravenous administration, dosage should be adjusted so that prolonged levels above 12 mcg/ml are avoided. When monitoring trough concentrations (just prior to the next dose), dosage should be adjusted so that levels above 2 mcg/ml are avoided. Determination of the adequacy of a serum level for a particular patient must take into consideration the susceptibility of the causative organism, the severity of the infection, and the status of the patient's host-defense mechanisms.

In patients with extensive burns, altered pharmacokinetics may result in reduced serum concentrations of aminoglycosides. In such patients treated with gentamicin, measurement of serum concentrations is recommended as a basis for dosage adjustment.

TABLE I
DOSAGE SCHEDULE GUIDE FOR ADULTS WITH NORMAL RENAL FUNCTION
(Dosage at Eight-Hour Intervals)
40 mg per ml

Patient's Weight* kg	(lb)	Usual Dose For Serious Infections 1 mg/kg q8h (3 mg/kg/day) mg/dose q8h	ml/dose	Dose for Life-Threatening Infections (Reduce as Soon as Clinically Indicated) 1.7 mg/kg q8h** (5 mg/kg/day) mg/dose q8h	ml/dose
40	(88)	40	1.0	66	1.6
45	(99)	45	1.1	75	1.9
50	(110)	50	1.25	83	2.1
55	(121)	55	1.4	91	2.25
60	(132)	60	1.5	100	2.5
65	(143)	65	1.6	108	2.7
70	(154)	70	1.75	116	2.9
75	(165)	75	1.9	125	3.1
80	(176)	80	2.0	133	3.3
85	(187)	85	2.1	141	3.5
90	(198)	90	2.25	150	3.75
95	(209)	95	2.4	158	4.0
100	(220)	100	2.5	166	4.2

* The dosage of aminoglycosides in obese patients should be based on an estimate of the lean body mass.

** For q6h schedules, dosage should be recalculated.

Children: 6 to 7.5 mg/kg/day. (2.0 to 2.5 mg/kg administered every 8 hours.)

Infants and Neonates: 7.5 mg/kg/day. (2.5 mg/kg administered every 8 hours.)

Premature or Full-Term Neonates One Week of Age or Less: 5 mg/kg/day. (2.5 mg/kg administered every 12 hours).

For further information concerning the use of gentamicin in infants and children, see GARAMYCIN Pediatric Injectable Product Information.

The usual duration of treatment for all patients is seven to ten days. In difficult and complicated infections, a longer course of therapy may be necessary. In such cases, monitoring of renal, auditory, and vestibular functions is recommended, since toxicity is more apt to occur with treatment extended for more than ten days. Dosage should be reduced if clinically indicated.

For Intravenous Administration

The intravenous administration of gentamicin may be particularly useful for treating patients with bacterial septicemia or those in shock. It may also be the preferred route of administration for some patients with congestive heart failure, hematologic disorders, severe burns, or those with reduced muscle mass. For intermittent intravenous administration in adults, a single dose of GARAMYCIN Injectable may be diluted in 50 to 200 ml of sterile isotonic saline solution or in a sterile solution of dextrose 5% in water; in infants and children, the volume of diluent should be less. The solution may be infused over a period of one-half to two hours.

The recommended dosage for intravenous and intramuscular administration is identical.

GARAMYCIN Injectable should not be physically premixed with other drugs, but should be administered separately in accordance with the recommended route of administration and dosage schedule.

DOSAGE FOR PATIENTS WITH IMPAIRED RENAL FUNCTION

Dosage must be adjusted in patients with impaired renal function to assure therapeutically adequate, but not excessive, blood levels. Whenever possible, serum concentrations of gentamicin should be monitored. One method of dosage adjustment is to increase the interval between administration of the usual doses. Since the serum creatinine concentration has a high correlation with the serum half-life of gentamicin, this laboratory test may provide guidance for adjustment of the interval between doses. The interval between doses (in hours) may be approximated by multiplying the serum creatinine level (mg/100 ml) by 8. For example, a patient weighing 60 kg with a serum creatinine level of 2.0 mg/100 ml could be given 60 mg (1 mg/kg) every 16 hours (2×8).

In patients with serious systemic infections and renal impairment, it may be desirable to administer the antibiotic more frequently but in reduced dosage. In such patients, serum concentrations of gentamicin should be measured so that adequate but not excessive levels result. A peak and trough concentration measured intermittently during therapy will provide optimal guidance for adjusting dosage. After the usual initial dose, a rough guide for determining reduced dosage at eight-hour intervals is to divide the normally recommended dose by the serum creatinine level (Table II). For example, after an initial dose of 60 mg (1 mg/kg), a patient weighing 60 kg with a serum creatinine level of 2.0 mg/100 ml could be given 30 mg every eight hours ($60 \div 2$). It should be noted that the status of renal function may be changing over the course of the infectious process. It is important to recognize that deteriorating renal function may require a greater reduction in dosage than that specified in the above guidelines for patients with stable renal impairment.

TABLE II
DOSAGE ADJUSTMENT GUIDE FOR PATIENTS WITH RENAL IMPAIRMENT
(Dosage at Eight-Hour Intervals After the Usual Initial Dose)

Serum Creatinine (mg %)	Approximate Creatinine Clearance Rate (ml/min/1.73M²)	Percent of Usual Doses Shown in Table I
≤ 1.0	> 100	100
1.1–1.3	70–100	80
1.4–1.6	55–70	65
1.7–1.9	45–55	55
2.0–2.2	40–45	50
2.3–2.5	35–40	40
2.6–3.0	30–35	35
3.1–3.5	25–30	30
3.6–4.0	20–25	25
4.1–5.1	15–20	20
5.2–6.6	10–15	15
6.7–8.0	< 10	10

In adults with renal failure undergoing hemodialysis, the amount of gentamicin removed from the blood may vary depending upon several factors including the dialysis method used. An eight-hour hemodialysis may reduce serum concentrations of gentamicin by approximately 50%. The recommended dosage at the end of each dialysis period is 1 to 1.7 mg/kg depending upon the severity of infection. In children, a dose of 2 mg/kg may be administered.

Continued on next page

Information on Schering products appearing on these pages is effective as of August 15, 1992.

Schering—Cont.

The dosage schedules are not intended as rigid recommendations but are provided as guides to dosage when the measurement of gentamicin serum levels is not feasible.
A variety of methods are available to measure gentamicin concentrations in body fluids; these include microbiologic, enzymatic and radioimmunoassay techniques.

HOW SUPPLIED

GARAMYCIN Injectable, 40 mg per ml, for parenteral administration, is supplied in 2 ml (80 mg) vials, boxes of 25 (NDC 0085-0069-04); and in 1.5 ml (60 mg) (NDC 0085-0069-05) and 2 ml (80 mg) (NDC 0085-0069-06) disposable syringes, each in boxes of 1.
Also available, GARAMYCIN Pediatric Injectable, 10 mg per ml, for parenteral administration, supplied in 2 ml (20 mg) vials, boxes of 10 (NDC 0085-0013-06).
GARAMYCIN Injectable is a clear, stable solution that requires no refrigeration.
Store between 2° and 30°C (36° and 86°F).

Schering Corporation
Kenilworth, NJ 07033 USA

Copyright © 1968, 1992, Schering Corporation.
All rights reserved.
Revised 8/91

GARAMYCIN® PEDIATRIC ℞

[*gar-ah-mī′sin*]
Injectable
brand of gentamicin sulfate injection, USP
10 mg per ml
Each ml contains gentamicin sulfate, USP equivalent to 10 mg gentamicin.
For Parenteral Administration

WARNINGS

Patients treated with aminoglycosides should be under close clinical observation because of the potential toxicity associated with their use.
As with other aminoglycosides. GARAMYCIN Pediatric Injectable is potentially nephrotoxic. The risk of nephrotoxicity is greater in patients with impaired renal function and in those who receive high dosage or prolonged therapy.
Neurotoxicity manifested by ototoxicity, both vestibular and auditory, can occur in patients treated with GARAMYCIN Pediatric Injectable, primarily in those with pre-existing renal damage and in patients with normal renal function treated with higher doses and/or for longer periods than recommended. Aminoglycoside-induced ototoxicity is usually irreversible. Other manifestations of neurotoxcity may include numbness, skin tingling, muscle twitching, and convulsions.
Renal and eighth cranial nerve functions should be closely monitored, especially in patients with known or suspected reduced renal function at onset of therapy, and also in those whose renal function is initially normal but who develop signs of renal dysfunction during therapy. Urine should be examined for decreased specific gravity. Increased excretion of protein, and the presence of cells or casts. Blood urea nitrogen, serum creatinine, or creatinine clearance should be determined periodically. When feasible, it is recommended that serial audiograms be obtained in patients old enough to be tested, particularly high-risk patients. Evidence of ototoxicity (dizziness, vertigo, tinnitus, roaring in the ears, or hearing loss) or nephrotoxicity requires dosage adjustment or discontinuance of the drug. As with the other aminoglycosides, on rare occasions changes in renal and eighth cranial nerve function may not become manifest until soon after completion of therapy.
Serum concentrations of aminoglycosides should be monitored when feasible to assure adequate levels and to avoid potentially toxic levels. When monitoring gentamicin peak concentrations, dosage should be adjusted so that prolonged levels above 12 mcg/mL are avoided. When monitoring gentamicin trough concentrations, dosage should be adjusted so that levels above 2 mcg/mL are avoided. Excessive peak and/or trough serum concentrations of aminoglycosides may increase the risk of renal and eighth cranial nerve toxicity. In the event of overdose or toxic reactions, hemodialysis may aid in the removal of gentamicin from the blood, especially if renal function is, or becomes, compromised. The rate of removal of gentamicin is considerably less by peritoneal dialysis than by hemodialysis. In the newborn infant, exchange transfusions may also be considered.
Concurrent and/or sequential systemic or topical use of other potentially neurotoxic and or nephrotoxic drugs, such as cisplatin, cephaloridine, kanamycin, amikacin, neomycin, polymyxin B, colistin, paromomycin, streptomycin, tobramycin, vancomycin, and viomycin, should be avoided. Another factor which may increase patient risk of toxicity is dehydration.
The concurrent use of gentamincin with potent diuretics, such as ethacrynic acid or furosemide, should be avoided, since certain diuretics by themselves may cause ototoxicity. In addition, when administered intravenously, diuretics may enhance aminoglycoside toxicity by altering the antibiotic concentration in serum and tissue.

DESCRIPTION

Gentamicin sulfate, USP, a water-soluble antibiotic of the aminoglycoside group, is derived from *Micromonospora purpurea*, an actinomycete. GARAMYCIN Pediatric Injectable is a sterile, aqueous solution for parenteral administration. Each ml contains gentamicin sulfate, USP equivalent to 10 mg gentamicin base; 1.3 mg methylparaben and 0.2 mg propylparaben as preservatives; 3.2 mg sodium bisulfite and 0.1 mg edetate disodium.

CLINICAL PHARMACOLOGY

After intramuscular administration of GARAMYCIN Pediatric Injectable, peak serum concentrations usually occur between 30 and 60 minutes and serum levels are measurable for 6 to 12 hours. In infants, a single dose of 2.5 mg/kg usually provides a peak serum level in the range of 3 to 5 mcg/mL. When gentamicin is administered by intravenous infusion over a 2-hour period, the serum concentrations are similar to those obtained by intramuscular administration. Age markedly affects the peak concentrations; in one report, a 1 mg/kg dose produced mean peak concentrations of 1.58, 2.03, and 2.81 mcg/mL in patients 6 months to 5 years old, 5 to 10 years old, and over 10 years old, respectively.
In infants 1 week to 6 months of age, the half-life is 3 to 3½ hours. In full-term and large premature infants less than 1 week old, the approximate serum half-life of gentamicin is 5½ hours. In small premature infants, the half-life is inversely related to birth weight. In premature infants weighing less than 1500 grams, the half-life is 11½ hours; in those weighing 1500 to 2000 grams, the half-life is 8 hours; in those weighing over 2000 grams, the half-life is approximately 5 hours. While some variation is to be expected due to a number of variables such as age, body temperature, surface area, and physiologic differences, the individual patient given the same dose tends to have similar levels in repeated determinations.
Gentamicin, like all aminoglycosides, may accumulate in the serum and tissues of patients treated with higher doses and/or for prolonged periods, particularly in the presence of impaired or immature renal function. In patients with immature or impaired renal function, gentamicin is cleared from the body more slowly than in patients with normal renal function. The more severe the impairment, the slower the clearance. (Dosage must be adjusted.)
Since gentamicin is distributed in extracellular fluid, peak serum concentrations may be lower than usual in patients who have a large volume of this fluid. Serum concentrations of gentamicin in febrile patients may be lower than those in afebrile patients given the same dose. When body temperature returns to normal, serum concentrations of the drug may rise. Febrile and anemic states may be associated with a shorter than usual serum half-life. (Dosage adjustment is usually not necessary.) In severely burned patients, the half-life may be significantly decreased and resulting serum concentrations may be lower than anticipated from the mg/kg dose.
Protein-binding studies have indicated that the degree of gentamicin binding is low; depending upon the methods used for testing, this may be between 0 and 30%.
In neonates less than 3 days old, approximately 10% of the administered dose is excreted in 12 hours; in infants 5 to 40 days old, approximately 40% is excreted over the same period. Excretion of gentamicin correlates with postnatal age and creatinine clearance. Thus, with increasing postnatal age and concomitant increase in renal maturity, gentamicin is excreted more rapidly. Little, if any, metabolic transformation occurs; the drug is excreted prinicipally by glomerular filtration. After several days of treatment, the amount of gentamicin excreted in the urine approaches, but does not equal, the daily dose administered. As with other aminoglycosides, a small amount of the gentamicin dose may be retained in the tissues, especially in the kidneys. Minute quantities of aminoglycosides have been detected in the urine of some patients weeks after drug administration was discontinued. Renal clearance of gentamicin is similar to that of endogenous creatinine.
In patients with marked impairment of renal function, there is a decrease in the concentration of aminoglycosides in urine and in their penetration into defective renal parenchyma. This decreased drug execretion, together with the potential nephrotoxicity of aminoglycosides, should be considered when treating such patients who have urinary tract infections.
Probenecid does not affect renal tubular transport of gentamicin.
The endogenous creatinine clearance rate and the serum creatinine level have a high correlation with the half-life of gentamicin in serum. Results of these tests may serve as guides for adjusting dosage in patients with renal impairment (see **DOSAGE AND ADMINISTRATION**).
Following parenteral administration, gentamicin can be detected in serum, lymph, tissues, sputum, and in pleural, synovial, and peritoneal fluids. Concentrations in renal cortex sometimes may be eight times higher than the usual serum levels. Concentrations in bile, in general, have been low and have suggested minimal biliary excretion. Gentamicin crosses the peritoneal as well as the placental membranes. Since aminoglycosides diffuse poorly into the subarachnoid space after parenteral administration, concentrations of gentamicin in cerebrospinal fluid are often low and dependent upon dose, rate of penetration, and degree of meningeal inflammation. There is minimal penetration of gentamicin into ocular tissues following intramuscular or intravenous administration.
Microbiology: *In vitro* tests have demonstrated that gentamicin is a bactericidal antibiotic which acts by inhibiting normal protein synthesis in susceptible microorganisms. It is active against a wide variety of pathogenic bacteria including *Escherichia coli*, *Proteus* species (indole-positive and indole-negative), *Pseudomonas aeruginosa*, species of the *Klebsiella-Enterobacter-Serratia* group, *Citrobacter* species, and *Staphylococcus* species including penicillin- and methicillin-resistant strains). Gentamicin is also active *in vitro* against species of *Salmonella* and *Shigella*. The following bacteria are usually resistant to aminoglycosides: *Streptococcus pneumoniae*, most species of streptolcocci, particularly group D and anaerobic organisms, such as *Bacteroides* species or *Clostridium* species.
In vitro studies have shown that an aminoglycoside combined with an antibiotic that interferes with cell wall synthesis may act synergistically against some group D streptococcal strains. The combination of gentamicin and penicillin G has a synergistic bactericidal effect against virtually all strains of *Streptococcus faecalis* and its varieties (*S. faecalis* var. *liquifaciens*, *S. faecalis* var. *zymogenes*), *S. faecium* and *S. durans*. An enhanced killing effect against many of these strains has also been shown *in vitro* with combinations of gentamicin and ampicillin, carbenicillin, nafcillin, or oxacillin.
The combined effect of gentamicin and carbenicillin is synergistic for many strains of *Pseudomonas aeruginosa*. *In vitro* synergism against other gram-negative organisms has been shown with combinations of gentamicin and cephalosporins.
Gentamicin may be active against clinical isolates of bacteria resistant to other aminoglycosides. Bacteria resistant to one aminoglycoside may be resistant to one or more other aminoglycosides. Bacterial resistance to gentamicin is generally developed slowly.
Susceptibility Testing: If the disc method of susceptibility testing used is that described by Bauer *et al* (*AM J Clin Path* 45:493, 1966; *Federal Register* 37:20525-20529, 1972), a disc containing 10 mcg of gentamicin should give a zone of inhibition of 15 mm or more to indicate susceptibility of the infecting organism. A zone of 12 mm or less indicates that the infecting organism is likely to be resistant. Zones greater than 12 mm and less than 15 mm indicate intermediate susceptibility. In certain conditions it may be desirable to do additional susceptibility testing by the tube or agar dilution method; gentamicin substance is available for this purpose.

INDICATIONS AND USAGE

GARAMYCIN Pediatric Injectable is indicated in the treatment of serious infections caused by susceptible strains of the following microorganisms; *Pseudomonas aeruginosa*, *Proteus* species (indole-positive and indole-negative), *Escherichia coli*, *Klebsiella-Enterobacter-Serratia* species, *Citrobacter* species, and *Staphylococcus* species (coagulase-positive and coagulase-negative).
Clinical studies have shown GARAMYCIN Pediatric Injectable to be effective in bacterial neonatal sepsis; bacterial septicemia; and serious bacterial infections of the central nervous system (meningitis), urinary tract, respiratory tract, gastrointestinal tract (including peritonitis), skin, bone and soft tissue (including burns).
Aminoglycosides, including gentamicin, are not indicated in uncomplicated initial episodes of urinary tract infections unless the causative organisms are susceptible to these antibiotics and are not susceptible to antibiotics having less potential for toxicity.
Specimens for bacterial culture should be obtained to isolate and identify causative organisms and to determine their susceptibility to gentamicin.
GARAMYCIN may be considered as initial therapy in suspected or confirmed gram-negative infections, and therapy may be instituted before obtaining results of susceptibility testing. The decision to continue therapy with this drug should be based on the results of susceptibility tests, the severity of the infection, and the important additional concepts contained in the "**WARNINGS** Box" above. If the causative

organisms are resistant to gentamicin, other appropriate therapy should be instituted.
In serious infections when the causative organisms are unknown, GARAMYCIN may be administered as initial therapy in conjunction with a penicillin-type or cephalosporin-type drug before obtaining results of susceptibility testing. If anaerobic organisms are suspected as etiologic agents, consideration should be given to using other suitable antimicrobial therapy in conjunction with gentamicin. Following identification of the organism and its susceptibility, appropriate antibiotic therapy should then be continued.
GARAMYCIN has been used effectively in combination with carbenicillin for the treatment of life-threatening infections caused by *Pseudomonas aeruginosa*. It has also been found effective when used in conjunction with a penicillin-type drug for the treatment of endocarditis caused by group D streptococci.
GARAMYCIN Pediatric Injectable has also been shown to be effective in the treatment of serious staphyococcal infections. While not the antibiotic of first choice, GARAMYCIN Pediatric Injectable may be considered when penicillins or other less potentially toxic drugs are contraindicated and bacterial susceptibility tests and clinical judgment indicate its use. It may also be considered in mixed infections caused by susceptible strains of staphylococci and gram-negative organisms.
In the neonate with suspected bacterial sepsis or staphylococcal pneumonia, a penicillin-type drug is also usually indicated as concomitant therapy with gentamicin.

CONTRAINDICATIONS

Hypersensitivity to gentamicin is a contraindication to its use. A history of hypersensitivity or serious toxic reactions to other aminoglycosides may contraindicate use of gentamicin because of the known cross-sensitivity of patients to drugs in this class.

WARNINGS

(See boxed **WARNINGS**.) Aminoglycosides can cause fetal harm when administered to a pregnant woman. Aminoglycoside antibiotics cross the placenta, and there have been several reports of total irreversible bilateral congenital deafness in children whose mothers received streptomycin during pregnancy. Serious side effects to mother, fetus, or newborn have not been reported in the treatment of pregnant women with other aminoglycosides. Animal reproduction studies conducted on rats and rabbits did not reveal evidence of impaired fertility or harm to the fetus due to gentamicin sulfate.
It is not known whether gentamicin sulfate can cause fetal harm when administered to a pregnant woman or can affect reproduction capacity. If gentamicin is used during pregnancy or if the patient becomes pregnant while taking gentamicin, she should be apprised of the potential hazard to the fetus.
GARAMYCIN Pediatric Injectable contains sodium bisulfite, a sulfite that may cause allergic-type reactions including anaphylactic symptoms and life-threatening or less severe asthmatic episodes in certain susceptible people. The overall prevalence of sulfite sensitivity in the general population is unknown and probably low. Sulfite sensitivity is seen more frequently in asthmatic than in nonasthmatic people.

PRECAUTIONS

Neurotoxic and nephrotoxic antibiotics may be absorbed in significant quantities from body surfaces after local irrigation or application. The potential toxic effect of antibiotics administered in this fashion should be considered.
Increased nephrotoxicity has been reported following concomitant administration of aminoglycoside antibiotics and cephalosporins.
Neuromuscular blockade and respiratory paralysis have been reported in the cat receiving high doses (40 mg kg) of gentamicin. The possibility of these phenomena occurring in man should be considered if aminoglycosides are administered by any route to patients receiving anesthetics, or to patients receiving neuromuscular blocking agents, such as succinylcholine, tubocurarine, or decamethonium, or in patients receiving massive transfusions of citrate-anticoagulated blood. If neuromuscular blockade occurs, calcium salts may reverse it.
Aminoglycosides should be used with caution in patients with neuromuscular disorders, such as myasthenia gravis, since these drugs may aggravate muscle weakness because of their potential curare-like effects on the neuromuscular junction. During or following gentamicin therapy, paresthesias, tetany, positive Chvostek and Trousseau signs, and mental confusion have been described in patients with hypomagnesemia, hypocalcemia, and hypokalemia. When this has occurred in infants, tetany and muscle weakness has been described. Both adults and infants required appropriate corrective electrolyte therapy.
A Fanconi-like syndrome, with aminoaciduria and metabolic acidosis, has been reported in some adults and infants being given gentamicin injections.
Cross-allergenicity among aminoglycosides has been demonstrated.
Patients should be well hydrated during treatment.
Although the *in vitro* mixing of gentamicin and carbenicillin results in a rapid and significant inactivation of gentamicin, this interaction has not been demonstrated in patients with normal renal function who received both drugs by different routes of administration. A reduction in gentamicin serum half-life has been reported in patients with severe renal impairment receiving carbenicillin concomitantly with gentamicin.
Treatment with gentamicin may result in overgrowth of nonsusceptible organisms. If this occurs, appropriate therapy is indicated.
See "**WARNINGS** Box" regarding concurrent use of potent diuretics and regarding concurrent and/or sequential use of other neurotoxic and or nephrotoxic antibiotics and for other essential information.
Usage in Pregnancy—Safety for use in pregnancy has not been established.

ADVERSE REACTIONS

Nephrotoxicity Adverse renal effects, as demonstrated by the presence of casts, cells, or protein in the urine or by rising BUN, NPN, serum creatinine or oliguria, have been reported. They occur more frequently in patients treated for longer periods or with larger dosages than recommended.
Neurotoxicity Serious adverse effects on both vestibular and auditory branches of the eighth cranial nerves have been reported, primarily in patients with renal impairment (especially if dialysis is required) and in patients on high doses and/or prolonged therapy. Symptoms include dizziness, vertigo, tinnitus, roaring in the ears and hearing loss, which, as with the other aminoglycosides, may be irreversible. Hearing loss is usually manifested initially by diminution of high-tone acuity. Other factors which may increase the risk of toxicity include excessive dosage, dehydration and previous exposure to other ototoxic drugs.
Peripheral neuropathy or encephalopathy, including numbness, skin tingling, muscle twitching, convulsions, and a myasthenia gravis-like syndrome, have been reported.
Note: The risk of toxic reactions is low in neonates, infants, and children with normal renal function who do not receive GARAMYCIN Pediatric Injectable at higher doses or for longer periods of time than recommended.
Other reported adverse reactions possibly related to gentamicin include: respiratory depression, lethargy, confusion, depression, visual disturbances, decreased appetite, weight loss, and hypotension and hypertension; rash, itching, urticaria, generalized burning, laryngeal edema, anaphylactoid reactions, fever, and headache; nausea, vomiting, increased salivation, and stomatitis, purpura, pseudotumor cerebri, acute organic brain syndrome, pulmonary fibrosis, alopecia, joint pain, transient hepatomegaly, and splenomegaly.
Laboratory abnormalities possibly related to gentamicin include: increased levels of serum transaminase (SGOT, SGPT), serum LDH and bilirubin, decreased serum calcium, magnesium, sodium and potassium, anemia, leukopenia, granulocytopenia, transient agranulocytosis, eosinophilia, increased and decreased reticulocyte counts, and thrombocytopenia.
While clinical laboratory test abnormalities may be isolated findings, they may also be associated with clinically related signs and symptoms. For example, tetany and muscle weakness may be associated with hypomagnesemia, hypocalcemia, and hypokalemia.
While local tolerance of GARAMYCIN Pediatric Injectable is generally excellent, there has been an occasional report of pain at the injection site. Subcutaneous atrophy or fat necrosis suggesting local irritation has been reported rarely.

OVERDOSAGE

In the event of overdose or toxic reactions, hemodialysis may aid in the removal of gentamicin from the blood, and is especially important if renal function is, or becomes, compromised. The rate of removal of gentamicin is considerably less by peritoneal dialysis than it is by hemodialysis. In the newborn infant, exchange transfusions may also be considered.

DOSAGE AND ADMINISTRATION

GARAMYCIN Pediatric Injectable may be given intramuscularly or intravenously. The patient's pretreatment body weight should be obtained for calculation of correct dosage. The dosage of aminoglycosides in obese patients should be based on an estimate of the lean body mass. It is desirable to limit the duration of treatment with aminoglycosides to short term.

DOSAGE FOR PATIENTS WITH NORMAL RENAL FUNCTION

Children: 6 to 7.5 mg/kg/day (2.0 to 2.5 mg/kg administered every 8 hours.)

Infants and Neonates: 7.5 mg/kg/day (2.5 mg/kg administered every 8 hours.)

Premature or Full-Term Neonates One Week of Age or Less: 5 mg/kg/day (2.5 mg/kg administered every 12 hours.)

It is desirable to measure periodically both peak and trough serum concentrations of gentamicin when feasible during therapy to assure adequate but not excessive drug levels. For example, the peak concentration (at 30 to 60 minutes after intramuscular injection) is expected to be in the range of 3 to 5 mcg/mL. When monitoring peak concentrations after intramuscular or intravenous administration, dosage should be adjusted so that prolonged levels above 12 mcg/mL are avoided. When monitoring trough concentrations (just prior to the next dose), dosage should be adjusted so that levels above 2 mcg/mL are avoided. Determination of the adequacy of a serum level for a particular patient must take into consideration the susceptibility of the causative organism, the severity of the infection, and the status of the patient's host-defense mechanisms.
In patients with extensive burns, altered pharmacokinetics may result in reduced serum concentrations of aminoglycosides. In such patients treated with gentamicin, measurement of serum concentrations is recommended as a basis for dosage adjustment.
The usual duration of treatment is 7 to 10 days. In difficult and complicated infections, a longer course of therapy may be necessary. In such cases monitoring of renal, auditory, and vestibular functions is recommended, since toxicity is more apt to occur with treatment extended for more than 10 days. Dosage should be reduced if clinically indicated.

For Intravenous Administration

The intravenous administration of gentamicin may be particularly useful for treating patients with bacterial septicemia or those in shock. It may also be the preferred route of administration for some patients with congestive heart failure, hematologic disorders, severe burns, or those with reduced muscle mass.
For intermittent intravenous administration, a single dose of GARAMYCIN Pediatric Injectable may be diluted in sterile isotonic saline solution or in a sterile solution of dextrose 5% in water. The solution may be infused over a period of one-half to two hours.
The recommended dosage for intravenous and intramuscular administration is identical.
GARAMYCIN Pediatric Injectable should not be physically premixed with other drugs, but should be administered separately in accordance with the recommended route of administration and dosage schedule.

DOSAGE FOR PATIENTS WITH IMPAIRED RENAL FUNCTION

Dosage must be adjusted in patients with impaired renal function to assure therapeutically adequate, but not excessive, blood levels. Whenever possible, serum concentrations of gentamicin should be monitored. One method of dosage adjustment is to increase the interval between administration of the usual doses. Since the serum creatinine concentration has a high correlation with the serum half-life of gentamicin, this laboratory test may provide guidance for adjustment of the interval between doses. In adults, the interval between doses (in hours) may be approximated by multiplying the serum creatinine level (mg/100 mL) by 8. For example, a patient weighing 60 kg with a serum creatinine level of 2.0 mg/100 mL could be given 60 mg (1 mg/kg) every 16 hours (2×8). These guidelines may be considered when treating infants and children with serious renal impairment.
In patients with serious systemic infections and renal impairment, it may be desirable to administer the antibiotic more frequently but in reduced dosage. In such patients, serum concentrations of gentamicin should be measured so that adequate but not excessive levels result. A peak and trough concentration measured intermittently during therapy will provide optimal guidance for adjusting dosage. After the usual initial dose, a rough guide for determining reduced dosage at 8-hour intervals is to divide the normally recommended dose by the serum creatinine level (Table 1). For example, after an initial dose of 20 mg (2.0 mg/kg), a child weighing 10 kg with a serum creatinine level of 2.0 mg/100 mL could be given 10 mg every 8 hours ($20 \div 2$). It should be noted that the status of renal function may be changing over the course of the infectious process. It is important to recognize that deteriorating renal function may require a greater reduction in dosage than that specified in the above guidelines for patients with stable renal impairment.
[See table next page.]
In patients with renal failure undergoing hemodialysis, the amount of gentamicin removed from the blood may vary depending upon several factors including the dialysis method used. An 8-hour hemodialysis may reduce serum concentrations of gentamicin by approximately 50%. In chil-

Continued on next page

Information on Schering products appearing on these pages is effective as of August 15, 1992.

Schering—Cont.

TABLE I
DOSAGE ADJUSTMENT GUIDE FOR PATIENTS WITH RENAL IMPAIRMENT
(Dosage at Eight-Hour Intervals After the Usual Initial Dose)

Serum Creatinine (mg %)	Approximate Creatinine Clearance Rate (mL/min/1.73M²)	Percent of Usual Doses Shown Above
≤1.0	>100	100
1.1–1.3	70–100	80
1.4–1.6	55–70	65
1.7–1.9	45–55	55
2.0–2.2	40–45	50
2.3–2.5	35–40	40
2.6–3.0	30–35	35
3.1–3.5	25–30	30
3.6–4.0	20–25	25
4.1–5.1	15–20	20
5.2–6.6	10–15	15
6.7–8.0	<10	10

dren the recommended dose at the end of each dialysis period is 2.0 to 2.5 mg/kg depending upon the severity of infection. The above dosage schedules are not intended as rigid recommendations but are provided as guides to dosage when the measurement of gentamicin serum levels is not feasible.
A variety of methods are available to measure gentamicin concentrations in body fluids; these include microbiologic, enzymatic and radioimmunoassay techniques.

HOW SUPPLIED
GARAMYCIN Pediatric Injectable, 10 mg per mL, for parenteral administration, supplied in 2 mL (20 mg) vials; boxes of 10 (NDC 0085-0013-06).
Also available, GARAMYCIN Injectable, 40 mg per mL, for parenteral administration, supplied in 2 mL (80 mg) vials, boxes of 25 (NDC 0085-0069-04); and in 1.5 mL (60 mg) (NDC 0085-0069-05) and 2 mL (80 mg) (NDC 0085-0069-06) disposable syringes, each in boxes of 1.
GARAMYCIN Pediatric Injectable is a clear, stable solution that requires no refrigeration.
Store between 2° and 30°C (36° and 86°F).
Revised 4/91
Copyright © 1968, 1991, Schering Corporation.
All rights reserved.

GARAMYCIN® Intrathecal   ℞
[gar-ah-mī'sin]
brand of gentamicin sulfate, USP
Injection 2.0 mg/ml
FOR DIRECT ADMINISTRATION INTO THE CEREBROSPINAL FLUID SPACES OF THE CENTRAL NERVOUS SYSTEM

WARNINGS
GARAMYCIN Intrathecal Injection is intended as adjunctive therapy in patients with central nervous system infections.
Since patients considered for treatment with GARAMYCIN Intrathecal Injection will usually be receiving concomitant treatment with intramuscular or intravenous gentamicin sulfate, all warnings and precautions for this or other concomitantly administered agents must be observed. Moreover, when the drug is administered by more than one route, additive effects must be considered. (See GARAMYCIN Injectable or GARAMYCIN Pediatric Injectable Product Information.) Laboratory studies in animals have shown that gentamicin sulfate, when administered directly into the central nervous system, has caused neurologic disturbances, including adverse effects on the eighth cranial nerve. The risk of direct administration of a potentially neurotoxic drug into the cerebrospinal fluid spaces of the central nervous system must be weighed against the potential benefit to be derived from this route of administration.

DESCRIPTION
Gentamicin sulfate, USP, a water-soluble antibiotic of the aminoglycoside group, is derived from *Micromonospora purpurea*, an actinomycete. GARAMYCIN Intrathecal Injection is a sterile, aqueous solution for direct administration into the cerebrospinal fluid spaces of the central nervous system. Each ml contains: gentamicin sulfate, USP equivalent to 2.0 mg gentamicin base; and 8.5 mg sodium chloride.

CLINICAL PHARMACOLOGY
Since gentamicin sulfate and other aminoglycosides diffuse poorly into the subarachnoid space after systemic administration, concentrations of these antibiotics in the lumbar or ventricular cerebrospinal fluid (CSF) are often low. Following intramuscular or intravenous administration of the usual doses, gentamicin concentrations in CSF in the absence of infection are usually less than 1 mcg/ml. In acute meningitis, slightly higher concentrations are obtained but these vary and are usually well below the peak serum concentration. CSF concentrations which are attained following intravenous or intramuscular administration of gentamicin sulfate tend to become lower as meningeal inflammation subsides. GARAMYCIN Intrathecal Injections are intended to increase the concentration of gentamicin in the CSF when used as part of the management of patients with central nervous system infections.
When GARAMYCIN Intrathecal Injection is given concomitantly with systemically administered gentamicin sulfate, the CSF levels are substantially increased depending upon the location of the injection. Peak CSF concentrations which follow intralumbar administration generally occur at 1 to 6 hours after injection.
Factors which affect the concentration of gentamicin in the CSF following injection into cerebrospinal fluid spaces are the dose administered, the site of the injection (intralumbar, intraventricular), the volume in which the dose is diluted, and the presence or absence of obstruction to the CSF flow. There appears to be considerable inter-patient variation.
The half-life of gentamicin in the CSF of adults who received intralumbar injections is approximately 5.5 hours; this is somewhat longer than that in serum.
In one pharmacokinetic study in adults, a 3 to 4 mg intralumbar injection resulted in a mean CSF concentration of 6.2 mcg/ml 24 hours after injection. The mean CSF concentration was noted to decrease with time: during days 1 through 6 of treatment with GARAMYCIN Intrathecal Injection by the intralumbar route, the mean 24-hour concentration was 9.9 mcg/ml, while during days 7 through 13, the mean concentration was 3.7 mcg/ml.
In another study in adults, CSF levels were measured at varying intervals after intralumbar administration of gentamicin sulfate. During days 1 through 6 of treatment, a 4 mg dose produced a mean CSF level of 2.4 mcg/ml 24 hours after injection, while during days 7 through 13, the same dose produced a mean 24-hour level of 0.5 mcg/ml.
Following intralumbar administration there may be limited upward diffusion of the drug, presumably because of the direction of the CSF flow. Intraventricular administration produces high concentrations in the ventricles and throughout the central nervous system. Adequate levels will usually result from dosing every 24 hours, but it is desirable to manage each patient's infection with serial monitoring of gentamicin serum and CSF concentrations.
Microbiology: *In vitro* tests have demonstrated that gentamicin is a bactericidal antibiotic which acts by inhibiting normal protein synthesis in susceptible microorganisms. It is active against a wide variety of pathogenic bacteria including *Escherichia coli*, *Proteus* species (indole-positive and indole-negative), *Pseudomonas aeruginosa*, species of the *Klebsiella-Enterobacter-Serratia* group. *Citrobacter* species, and *Staphylococcus* species (including penicillin- and methicillin-resistant strains). Gentamicin is also active *in vitro* against species of *Salmonella* and *Shigella*. The following bacteria are usually resistant to aminoglycosides: *Streptococcus pneumoniae*, most species of streptococci, particularly group D and anaerobic organisms, such as *Bacteroides* species or *Clostridium* species.
In vitro studies have shown that an aminoglycoside combined with an antibiotic that interferes with cell wall synthesis may act synergistically against some group D streptococcal strains. The combination of gentamicin sulfate and penicillin G has a synergistic bactericidal effect against virtually all strains of *Streptococcus faecalis* and its varieties (*S. faecalis* var. *liquifaciens*, *S. faecalis* var. *zymogenes*), *S. faecium* and *S. durans*. An enhanced killing effect against many of these strains has also been shown *in vitro* with combinations of gentamicin and ampicillin, carbenicillin, nafcillin, or oxacillin.
The combined effect of gentamicin and carbenicillin is synergistic for many strains of *Pseudomonas aeruginosa*.
Gentamicin may be active against clinical isolates of bacteria resistant to other aminoglycosides. However, bacteria resistant to one aminoglycoside may be resistant to one or more other aminoglycosides.
Susceptibility Testing: If the disc method of susceptibility testing used is that described by Bauer *et al* (*Am J Clin Path* **45**:493, 1966; *Federal Register* **37**:20525–20529, 1972), a disc containing 10 mcg of gentamicin, when tested against a bacterial strain susceptible to gentamicin, should give a zone of inhibition of ≥15 mm. A zone of ≤12 mm indicates that the infecting organism is likely to be resistant. Zones greater than 12 mm and less than 15 mm indicate intermediate susceptibility. In certain conditions it may be desirable to do

additional susceptibility testing by the broth or agar dilution method; gentamicin substance is available for this purpose.

INDICATIONS AND USAGE
GARAMYCIN Intrathecal Injection is indicated as adjunctive therapy to systemically administered gentamicin sulfate in the treatment of serious central nervous system infections (meningitis, ventriculitis) caused by susceptible *Pseudomonas* species.
Bacteriologic tests should be performed to determine that the causative organisms are *Pseudomonas* species susceptible to gentamicin.

CONTRAINDICATIONS
Hypersensitivity to gentamicin sulfate is a contraindication to its use. A history of hypersensitivity or serious toxic reactions to aminoglycosides may also contraindicate use of gentamicin sulfate because of the known cross-sensitivity of patients to drugs in this class.

WARNINGS
(See "WARNINGS Box" above and the WARNINGS listed in the Product Information for GARAMYCIN Injectable and GARAMYCIN Pediatric Injectable.)

PRECAUTIONS
See PRECAUTIONS listed in the Product Information for GARAMYCIN Injectable and GARAMYCIN Pediatric Injectable.)
In a patient with a seven-year history of multiple sclerosis who was treated with gentamicin sulfate by intralumbar injection, disseminated microscopic lesions of the brain stem were reported at autopsy. Lesions observed were: tissue rarefaction with loss and marked swelling of axis cylinders with occasional calcification, loss of oligodendroglia and astroglia, and a poor inflammatory response.
Safety and efficacy in children below the age of three months have not been established.

ADVERSE REACTIONS
Local tolerance to GARAMYCIN Intrathecal Injection has been good. Local reactions of arachnoiditis or burning at the injection site have been reported rarely.
Because the recommended dosage of GARAMYCIN Intrathecal Injection is low, the potential for systemic adverse effects is minimal. However, GARAMYCIN Intrathecal Injection is recommended as adjunctive therapy with other antibiotics, such as parenteral gentamicin sulfate, which should be administered in full therapeutic dosages. Evidence of eighth nerve dysfunction, changes in renal function, leg cramps, rash, fever, convulsions, and an increase in cerebrospinal fluid protein have been reported in patients who were treated concomitantly with GARAMYCIN Intrathecal Injection and the parenteral preparation of gentamicin.
Administration of excessive (40 to 160 mg) doses of the parenteral formulation of gentamicin sulfate (which contains a preservative system) by the various intrathecal routes has been reported to produce neuromuscular disturbances, e.g., ataxia, paresis, and incontinence.

DOSAGE AND ADMINISTRATION
GARAMYCIN Intrathecal Injection is intended for administration directly into the cerebrospinal fluid spaces of the central nervous system.
The dosage will vary depending upon factors, such as age and weight of the patient, site of injection, degree of obstruction to cerebrospinal fluid flow and the amount of cerebrospinal fluid estimated to be present. In general, the recommended dose for infants 3 months of age and older (see PRECAUTIONS) and children is 1 to 2 mg once a day. For adults, 4 to 8 mg may be administered once a day.
Administration of GARAMYCIN Intrathecal Injection should be continued as long as sensitive organisms are demonstrated in the cerebrospinal fluid. Since the intralumbar or intraventricular dose is administered immediately after specimens are taken for laboratory study, treatment should usually be continued for at least one day after negative results have been obtained from CSF cultures and/or stained smears.
The suggested method for administering GARAMYCIN Intrathecal Injection into the lumbar area is as follows: the desired quantity of GARAMYCIN Intrathecal Injection is drawn up carefully from the ampule into a 5- or 10-ml sterile syringe. After the lumbar puncture is performed and a specimen of the spinal fluid is removed for laboratory tests, the syringe containing GARAMYCIN Intrathecal Injection is inserted into the hub of the spinal needle. A quantity of cerebrospinal fluid (approximately 10% of the estimated total CSF volume) is allowed to flow into the syringe and mix with the GARAMYCIN Intrathecal Injection. The resultant solution is then injected over a period of 3 to 5 minutes with the bevel of the needle directed upward.
If the cerebrospinal fluid is grossly purulent, or if it is unobtainable, GARAMYCIN Intrathecal Injection may be diluted with sterile normal saline before injection.
GARAMYCIN Intrathecal Injection may also be administered directly into the subdural space or directly into the

ventricles, including administration by use of an implanted reservoir.

HOW SUPPLIED

GARAMYCIN Intrathecal Injection, 2.0 mg per ml, is supplied in 2 ml ampules; box of 25.

Store below 30°C (86°F).

NOTE: This preparation does not contain any preservative. Once opened, contents should be used immediately and unused portions should be discarded.

ANIMAL PHARMACOLOGY AND TOXICOLOGY

In dogs, an 8-hour perfusion of the ventriculosubarchnoid system with a solution containing 40 mcg/ml (~5mg or ~0.3 mg/kg) gentamicin produced no seizure activity or change in vital signs during administration. No morphological changes were observed when the dogs were sacrificed at 10 and 90 days following infusion.

The effects of repeated intrathecal injections of gentamicin at 0.1 and 0.3 mg/kg were evaluated in tranquilized beagle puppies. Transient flaccid paralysis was observed on the first day when the drug was administered rapidly (i.e., in less than 5 seconds), but no adverse effects were observed thereafter when the drug was administered less rapidly (i.e., over a period of approximately 30 seconds). No drug-related changes were found on histological examination of the cerebellum, brain stem or cephalic cord. In cats, gentamicin administered intracisternally at one-hour intervals in doses of up to 50 mg/kg did not produce any abnormalities in the electroencephalogram. In another study in cats, gentamicin sulfate given daily by the intracisternal route for up to 7 days caused neurological disturbances, including adverse effects on the eighth cranial nerve.

In rabbits intracisternal injection of gentamicin at doses 50 and 100 times the therapeutic dose produced peak CSF concentrations of 160 and 180 mcg/ml, respectively. These doses were associated with changes in the myelin sheath predominantly of the lateral columns of the upper cervical cord, and some changes in glial cells and lesions in the medulla oblongata. In addition to a high incidence of mortality, the animals demonstrated weakness, ataxia and paralysis. At doses of one and ten times the therapeutic dose (providing peak levels of 16.5 and 40 mcg/ml CSF), no morphologic changes occurred and there were no drug-related symptoms identified.

Schering Pharmaceutical Corporation (PR)
Manati, Puerto Rico 00701
An Affiliate of Schering Corporation
Kenilworth, NJ 07033

Revised 7/83

HYPERSTAT® I.V. ℞

[hi 'per-stat]

brand of diazoxide, USP
Injection
For Intravenous Use In Hospitalized Patients Only

DESCRIPTION

HYPERSTAT I.V. Injection is a nondiuretic benzothiadiazine antihypertensive agent. Each ampule (20 ml) contains 300 mg diazoxide, USP, in a clear, sterile, colorless aqueous solution; the pH is adjusted to approximately 11.6 with sodium hydroxide.

Diazoxide is 7-chloro-3-methyl-2*H*-1,2,4-benzothiadiazine 1,1-dioxide, with the empirical formula $C_8H_7ClN_2O_2S$, and the molecular weight 230.7. It is a white crystalline powder practically insoluble to sparingly soluble in water.

CLINICAL PHARMACOLOGY

HYPERSTAT I.V. Injection produces a prompt reduction of blood pressure in man by relaxing smooth muscle in the peripheral arterioles. Cardiac output is increased as blood pressure is reduced. Studies in animals demonstrate that coronary blood flow is maintained, while renal blood flow is increased after an initial decrease.

Transient hyperglycemia occurs in the majority of patients treated with HYPERSTAT, but usually requires treatment only in patients with diabetes mellitus. It will respond to the usual management measures, including insulin.

Blood glucose levels should be monitored especially in patients with diabetes and in those requiring multiple injections of diazoxide. Cataracts have been observed in a few animals receiving repeated daily doses of intravenous diazoxide.

Since diazoxide causes sodium retention, repeated injections may precipitate edema and congestive heart failure. Increased volume of extracellular fluid may be a cause of treatment failure in nonresponsive patients. The increase in fluid volume characteristically responds to diuretic agents if adequate renal function exists. Concurrently administered thiazide diuretics may be expected to potentiate the antihypertensive and hyperuricemic actions of diazoxide. (See **Drug Interactions.**)

Diazoxide is extensively bound to serum protein (>90%). The plasma half-life is 28 ± 8.3 hours; however, the duration of its antihypertensive effect is variable, generally lasting less than 12 hours.

INDICATIONS AND USAGE

HYPERSTAT I.V. Injection is indicated for short-term use in the emergency reduction of blood pressure in severe, nonmalignant and malignant hypertension in hospitalized adults; and in acute severe hypertension in hospitalized children, when prompt and urgent decrease of diastolic pressure is required. Treatment with orally effective antihypertensive agents should not be instituted until blood pressure has stabilized. The use of HYPERSTAT I.V. Injection for longer than 10 days is not recommended.

HYPERSTAT I.V. Injection is ineffective against hypertension due to pheochromocytoma.

CONTRAINDICATIONS

HYPERSTAT I.V. Injection should not be used in the treatment of compensatory hypertension, such as that associated with aortic coarctation or arteriovenous shunt, and should not be used in patients hypersensitive to diazoxide, other thiazides, or other sulfonamide-derived drugs.

WARNINGS

Rapid Decrease of Blood Pressure Caution must be observed when reducing severely elevated blood pressure. Diazoxide should only be administered utilizing the new 150 mg minibolus dosage. The use of a 300 mg intravenous dose of diazoxide has been associated with angina and with myocardial and cerebral infarction. One instance of optic nerve infarction was reported when a 100 mmHg reduction in diastolic pressure occurred over ten minutes following a single 300 mg bolus. In one prospective trial conducted in patients with severe hypertension and coexistent coronary artery disease, a 50% incidence of ischemic changes in the electrocardiogram was observed following single 300 mg bolus injections of diazoxide. The desired blood pressure lowering should therefore be achieved over as long a period of time as is compatible with the patient's status. At least several hours and preferably one or two days is tentatively recommended.

Improved safety with equal efficacy can be achieved by administering HYPERSTAT I.V. Injection as a minibolus dose (1 to 3 mg/kg every 5 to 15 minutes up to a maximum of 150 mg in a single injection) until a diastolic blood pressure below 100 mmHg is achieved. HYPERSTAT I.V. Injection should not be administered in a bolus dose of 300 mg since this mode of administration is less predictable and less controllable than the minibolus dosage. If hypotension severe enough to require therapy results from the reduction in blood pressure, it will usually respond to the Trendelenberg maneuver. If necessary, sympathomimetic agents such as dopamine or norepinephrine may be administered.

Special attention is required for patients with diabetes mellitus and those in whom retention of salt and water may present serious problems.

Myocardial Lesions in Animals Intravenous administration of diazoxide in dogs has induced subendocardial necrosis and necrosis of papillary muscles. These lesions, which are also produced by other vasodilator drugs (i.e., hydralazine, minoxidil) and by catecholamines, are presumed to be related to anoxia resulting from a combination of reflex tachycardia and decreased perfusion.

PRECAUTIONS

General: HYPERSTAT (diazoxide) I.V. Injection is an effective antihypertensive agent requiring close monitoring of the patient's blood pressure at frequent intervals. Its administration may occasionally cause hypotension requiring treatment with sympathomimetic drugs. Therefore, HYPERSTAT, I.V. Injection should be used primarily in the hospital or where adequate facilities exist to treat such untoward responses.

HYPERSTAT I.V. Injection should be administered only into a peripheral vein. Because the alkalinity of the solution is irritating to tissue, avoid extravascular injection or leakage. Subcutaneous administration has produced inflammation and pain without subsequent necrosis. If leakage into subcutaneous tissue occurs, the area should be treated with warm compresses and rest.

HYPERSTAT I.V. Injection should be used with care in patients who have impaired cerebral or cardiac circulation, that is, patients in whom abrupt reduction in blood pressure might be detrimental or those in whom mild tachycardia or decreased blood perfusion may be deleterious (see **WARNINGS**). Prolonged hypotension should be avoided so as not to aggravate preexisting renal failure.

Information for Patients: During and immediately following intravenous injection of HYPERSTAT I.V. Injection, the patient should remain supine.

Laboratory Tests: Diagnostic laboratory tests necessary to establish the patient's condition and status should be carried out prior to treatment with HYPERSTAT I.V. Injection. During and following treatment with HYPERSTAT I.V. Injection, laboratory tests to monitor the effects of treatment with this drug and the patient's condition should be done. Among the tests (not necessarily inclusive) are: hematologic (hematocrit, hemoglobin, white blood cell and platelet counts); metabolic (glucose, uric acid, total protein, albumin); electrolyte (sodium, potassium) and osmolality; renal function (creatinine, urine-protein); electrocardiogram.

Drug Interactions: Diazoxide is highly bound to serum protein. It can be expected to displace other substances which are also bound to protein, such as bilirubin or coumarin and its derivatives, resulting in higher blood levels of these substances.

An undesirable hypotension may result when diazoxide is administered to patients who have received other antihypertensive medication within six hours.

One patient in a clinical study exhibited excessive hypotension after concomitant administration of HYPERSTAT with hydralazine and methyldopa. An episode of maternal hypotension and fetal bradycardia occurred in a patient in labor who received both reserpine and hydralazine prior to administration of diazoxide. Neonatal hyperglycemia following intrapartum administration of HYPERSTAT I.V. Injection has also been reported.

HYPERSTAT I.V. Injection should not be administered within six hours of the administration of: hydralazine, reserpine, alphaprodine, methyldopa, beta-blockers, prazosin, minoxidil, the nitrites and other papaverine-like compounds. Concomitant administration with thiazides or other commonly used diuretics may be expected to potentiate the hyperuricemic and antihypertensive effects of diazoxide.

Drug/Laboratory Test Interactions: The hyperglycemic and hyperuricemic effects of diazoxide preclude proper assessment of these metabolic states. Increased renin secretion, IgG concentrations and decreased cortisol secretion have also been noted. Diazoxide inhibits glucagon-stimulated insulin release and will cause a false-negative insulin response to glucagon. In the rat, dog and monkey, diazoxide increased serum free fatty acids and decreased plasma insulin levels.

Carcinogenesis, Mutagenesis, Impairment of Fertility: No long-term animal dosing study has been done to evaluate the carcinogenic potential of diazoxide. No laboratory studies of mutagenic potential or animal studies of effects on fertility have been done.

Pregnancy Category C: Diazoxide has been shown to reduce fetal and/or pup survival; and to reduce fetal growth in rats, rabbits, and dogs at daily doses of 30, 21, or 10 mg/kg, respectively. In rats treated at term, diazoxide, at doses of 10 mg/kg and above, prolonged parturition.

The safety of HYPERSTAT I.V. Injection in pregnancy has not been established.

Non-teratogenic Effects: Diazoxide crosses the placental barrier and appears in cord blood. When given to the mother prior to delivery the drug may produce fetal or neonatal hyperbilirubinemia, thrombocytopenia, altered carbohydrate metabolism, and possibly other side effects that have occurred in adults.

Labor and Delivery: HYPERSTAT I.V. Injection is not indicated for use in pregnancy. Intravenous administration of the drug during labor may cause cessation of uterine contractions, requiring administration of an oxytocic agent.

Nursing Mothers: Information is not available concerning the passage of HYPERSTAT in breast milk. Because many drugs are excreted in human milk and because of the potential for adverse reactions in nursing infants from diazoxide, a decision should be made whether to discontinue nursing or to discontinue the drug, taking into account the importance of the drug to the mother.

Pediatric Use: See **INDICATIONS AND USAGE.**

ADVERSE REACTIONS

It is reasonable to speculate that the currently recommended minibolus dosing regimen, which has replaced the 300 mg bolus dose in clinical practice, will result in adverse effects which are of similar character but of lesser frequency and severity.

In clinical experience with the rapid bolus administration of 300 mg, the most common adverse reactions reported were: hypotension (7%); nausea and vomiting (4%); dizziness and weakness (2%). Additional adverse reactions reported with bolus administration of 300 mg were as follows:

Cardiovascular: sodium and water retention after repeated injections, especially important in patients with impaired cardiac reserve; hypotension to shock levels; myocardial ischemia, usually transient and manifested by angina, atrial and ventricular arrhythmias, and marked electrocardiographic changes, but occasionally leading to myocardial infarction; optic nerve infarction following too rapid decrease in severely elevated blood pressure; supraventricular tachycardia and palpitation; bradycardia; chest discomfort or nonanginal "tightness in the chest."

Continued on next page

Information on Schering products appearing on these pages is effective as of August 15, 1992.

Schering—Cont.

Central Nervous System: cerebral ischemia, usually transient but occasionally leading to infarction and manifested by unconsciousness, convulsions, paralysis, confusion, or focal neurological deficit such as numbness of the hands; vasodilative phenomena, such as orthostatic hypotension, sweating, flushing, and generalized or localized sensations of warmth; various transient neurological findings secondary to alteration in regional blood flow to brain, such as headache (sometimes throbbing), dizziness, lightheadedness, sleepiness (also reported as lethargy, somnolence or drowsiness), euphoria or "funny feeling," ringing in the ears and momentary hearing loss, and weakness of short duration; apprehension or anxiety.

Gastrointestinal: rarely, acute pancreatitis; nausea, vomiting and/or abdominal discomfort; anorexia; alteration in taste; parotid swelling; salivation; dry mouth; lacrimation; ileus; constipation and diarrhea.

Other: hyperglycemia in diabetic patients, especially after repeated injections; hyperosmolar coma in an infant; transient hyperglycemia in nondiabetic patients; transient retention of nitrogenous wastes; various respiratory findings secondary to the relaxation of smooth muscle, such as dyspnea, cough and choking sensation; warmth or pain along the injected vein; cellulitis without sloughing and/or phlebitis at the injection site of extravasation; back pain and increased nocturia; hypersensitivity reactions, such as rash, leukopenia and fever; papilledema induced by plasma volume expansion secondary to the administration of diazoxide reported in a patient who had received eleven injections (300 mg/dose) over a 22-day period; malaise and blurred vision; transient cataract in an infant; hirsutism, and decreased libido.

OVERDOSAGE

Overdosage of HYPERSTAT I.V. Injection may cause an undesirable hypotension. Usually, this can be controlled with the Trendelenberg maneuver. If necessary, sympathomimetic agents, such as dopamine or norepinephrine, may be administered. Failure of blood pressure to rise in response to such agents suggests that the hypotension may have been caused by something other than diazoxide. Excessive hyperglycemia resulting from overdosage will respond to conventional therapy of hyperglycemia.

DOSAGE AND ADMINISTRATION

HYPERSTAT I.V. Injection was originally recommended for use by bolus administration of 300 mg. Recent studies have shown that <u>minibolus administration of HYPERSTAT I.V. Injection</u>, i.e., doses of 1 to 3 mg/kg repeated at intervals of 5 to 15 minutes is as effective in reducing blood pressure. Minibolus administration usually provides a more gradual reduction in blood pressure and thus may be expected to reduce the circulatory and neurological risks associated with acute hypotension.

HYPERSTAT I.V. Injection is administered undiluted and rapidly by intravenous injections of 1 to 3 mg/kg up to a maximum of 150 mg in a single injection. This dose may be repeated at intervals of 5 to 15 minutes until a satisfactory reduction in blood pressure (diastolic pressure below 100 mmHg) has been achieved.

With the patient recumbent, the calculated dose of HYPERSTAT I.V. Injection is administered intravenously in 30 seconds or less.

HYPERSTAT I.V. Injection should only be given into a peripheral vein. Do not administer it intramuscularly, subcutaneously, or into body cavities. Avoid extravasation of the drug into subcutaneous tissues.

Following the use of HYPERSTAT I.V. Injection, the blood pressure should be monitored closely until it has stabilized. Thereafter, measurements taken hourly during the balance of the effect should indicate any unusual response. A further decrease in blood pressure 30 minutes or more after injection should be investigated for causes other than the action of HYPERSTAT I.V. Injection. It is preferable that the patient remain supine for at least one hour after injection. In ambulatory patients, the blood pressure should also be measured with the patient standing before surveillance is ended.

Repeated administration of HYPERSTAT I.V. Injection at intervals of 4 to 24 hours usually will maintain the blood pressure below pretreatment levels until a regimen of oral antihypertensive medication can be instituted. The interval between injections may be adjusted by the duration of the response to each injection. It is usually unnecessary to continue treatment with HYPERSTAT I.V. Injection for more than four to five days.

Since repeated administration of HYPERSTAT I.V. Injection can lead to sodium and water retention, administration of a diuretic may be necessary both for maximal blood pressure reduction and to avoid congestive heart failure. (See **CLINICAL PHARMACOLOGY.**)

Parenteral drug products should be inspected visually for particulate matter and discoloration prior to administration whenever solution and container permit.

HOW SUPPLIED

HYPERSTAT I.V. Injection is supplied in a 20 ml ampule, containing 300 mg diazoxide, in a clear, sterile, colorless, aqueous solution; box of one ampule (NDC 0085-0201-05). **Protect from light and freezing. Store between 2° and 30°C (36° and 86°F).**

Revised 2/85

INSPIREASE®　　　　　　　　　　　　　　　　　　℞
Drug Delivery System for use with metered dose inhalers

DIRECTIONS FOR USE

Your patient should:
1. Connect the mouthpiece to the reservoir bag by lining up the *locking tabs* with the opening in the reservoir bags. Push in and twist to lock.

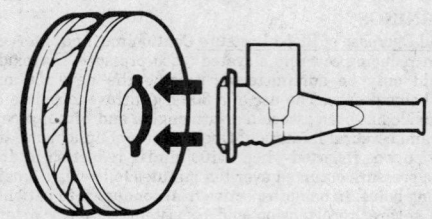

2. Untwist the reservoir bag gently to open it to its full size. Shake "spray inhaler" well before placing its stem into the *mouthpiece*. Make sure the stem sits in the center of the mouthpiece filler. Some inhalers may fit more loosely than others. This will not affect drug delivery.

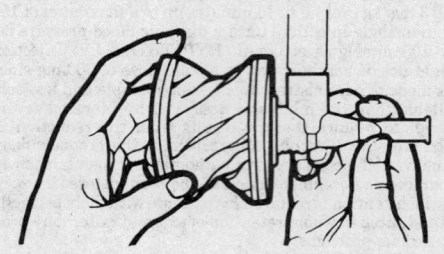

3. Place mouthpiece in mouth and close lips tightly around it.
4. Press down on the "spray inhaler" to release one dose of medication into the bag.
   IMPORTANT NOTE: Follow your doctor's instructions regarding the number of doses you should take and when to take them.

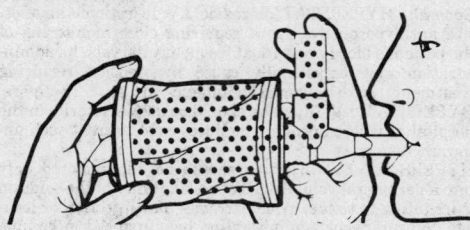

5. Breathe in *slowly* through the mouthpiece. If you hear a whistling sound, breathe slower until no sound can be heard.

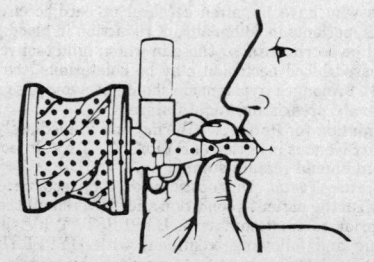

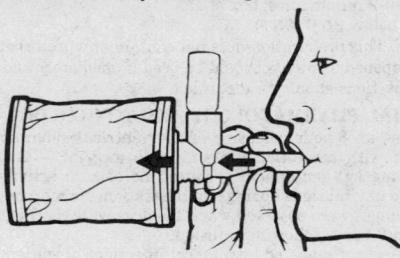

6. Breathe in the entire contents of the bag. You will know to stop when the bag collapses and you cannot breathe in anymore.
7. *Hold his or her breath while slowly counting to five.*
8. Breathe out slowly into the bag.

9. Repeat the inhale/exhale cycle (steps 5 through 8) a second time, keeping lips tightly closed around the mouthpiece.
   IMPORTANT NOTE: Repeat steps 2 through 9 for each dose of medication prescribed by your doctor.
10. Remove the mouthpiece from mouth. Take drug canister off the reservoir bag. Unlock mouthpiece from the bag and store all components in carrying case.

IMPORTANT CLEANING INSTRUCTIONS

Your patients should:
1. Clean only the mouthpiece thoroughly with warm (not hot) running water *at least* once a day. *InspirEase® is not dishwasher safe. Always clean by hand.*
2. The clear plastic reed section of the mouthpiece should not be touched due to potential breakage. We recommend a visual inspection of the reed section for signs of breakage prior to each use. If reed breakage occurs, replace mouthpiece immediately; otherwise replace mouthpiece as needed every six months.
3. After cleaning, wait until mouthpiece is *completely dry* before storing in carrying case. Do not place near artificial heat such as dishwasher or oven.
4. We recommend that the reservoir bag be replaced every two to three weeks or as needed. *However, if there is a hole or tear in it, replace immediately.*

NOTE: You will need a doctor's prescription for replacement bags or a new starter kit.

InspirEase is designed for use with most "spray inhaler" (metered dose inhaler) containers currently available; for single-patient use and single-dose use.

The usual caution should be exercised in dosing medications and evaluating patient response.

The prescribing information for the marketed MDIs varies with respect to dosing, administration, etc. We recommend that these be followed when using InspirEase.

CAUTION: Federal law restricts this device to sale by or on the order of a physician.

Distributed by: Schering Corporation, Kenilworth, NJ 07033 USA

Revised 6/90　　　　　　　　　　　　　　　　　　14379444

INTRON® A　　　　　　　　　　　　　　　　　　℞
Interferon alfa-2b
recombinant
For Injection

DESCRIPTION

INTRON A Interferon alfa-2b, recombinant for intramuscular, subcutaneous or intralesional Injection is a purified sterile, lyophilized recombinant interferon formulation. The 3 million, 5 million, 18 million multidose, 25 million and 50 million IU packages are for use by intramuscular or subcutaneous injection. The 10 million IU package is for intramuscular, subcutaneous, or intralesional injection. (See **WARNINGS** and **PRECAUTIONS.**)

Interferon alfa-2b, recombinant for Injection has been classified as an alfa interferon and is a water soluble protein with a molecular weight of 19,271 daltons produced by recombinant DNA techniques. It is obtained from the bacterial fermentation of a strain of *Escherichia coli* bearing a genetically engineered plasmid containing an interferon alfa-2b gene from human leukocytes. The fermentation is carried out in a defined nutrient medium containing the antibiotic tetracycline hydrochloride at a concentration of 5 to 10 mg/L; the presence of this antibiotic is not detectable in the final product. The specific activity of Interferon alfa-2b, recombinant is approximately 2×10^8 IU/mg protein.

Each INTRON A vial contains either 3 million, 5 million, 10 million, 18 million, 25 million, or 50 million IU of interferon alfa-2b, recombinant, 20 mg glycine, 2.3 mg sodium phosphate dibasic, 0.55 mg sodium phosphate monobasic, and 1.0 mg human albumin are also present. Based on the

specific activity of approximately 2×10^8 IU/mg protein, the corresponding quantities of interferon alfa-2b, recombinant in the vials described above are approximately 0.015 mg, 0.025 mg, 0.05 mg, 0.09 mg, 0.125 mg, and 0.25 mg protein, respectively. Prior to administration, the lyophilized powder is to be reconstituted with the provided Diluent for INTRON A Interferon alfa-2b, recombinant for Injection (bacteriostatic water for injection) containing 0.9% benzyl alcohol as a preservative. (See **DOSAGE AND ADMINISTRATION**.)

Lyophilized INTRON A Interferon alfa-2b, recombinant for Injection is a white to cream colored powder.

CLINICAL PHARMACOLOGY

General The interferons are a family of naturally occurring small proteins and glycoproteins with molecular weights of approximately 15,000 to 27,600 daltons produced and secreted by cells in response to viral infections and to synthetic and biological inducers.

Preclinical Pharmacology Interferons exert their cellular activities by binding to specific membrane receptors on the cell surface. Once bound to the cell membrane, interferons initiate a complex sequence of intracellular events. *In vitro* studies demonstrated that these include the induction of certain enzymes, suppression of cell proliferation, immunomodulating activities such as enhancement of the phagocytic activity of macrophages and augmentation of the specific cytotoxicity of lymphocytes for target cells, and inhibition of virus replication in virus-infected cells.

In a study using human hepatoblastoma cell line, HB 611, the *in vitro* antiviral activity of alpha interferon was demonstrated by its inhibition of hepatitis B virus (HBV) replication.

The correlation between these *in vitro* data and the clinical results is unknown. Any of these activities might contribute to interferon's therapeutic effects.

Pharmacokinetics The pharmacokinetics of INTRON A Interferon alfa-2b, recombinant for Injection were studied in 12 healthy male volunteers following single doses of 5 million IU/m^2 administered intramuscularly, subcutaneously and as a 30-minute intravenous infusion in a crossover design. INTRON A concentrations were determined using a radioimmunoassay (RIA) with a detection limit equal to 10 IU/mL.

The mean serum INTRON A concentrations following intramuscular and subcutaneous injections were comparable. The maximum serum concentrations obtained via these routes were approximately 18 to 116 IU/mL and occurred 3 to 12 hours after administration. The elimination half-life of INTRON A Interferon alfa-2b, recombinant for Injection following both intramuscular and subcutaneous injections was approximately two to three hours. Serum concentrations were below the detection limit by 16 hours after the injections.

After intravenous administration, serum INTRON A concentrations peaked (135 to 273 IU/mL) by the end of the 30-minute infusion, then declined at a slightly more rapid rate than after intramuscular or subcutaneous drug administration, becoming undetectable four hours after the infusion. The elimination half-life was approximately two hours.

Urine INTRON A concentrations following a single dose (5 million IU/m^2) were not detectable after any of the parenteral routes of administration. This result was expected since preliminary studies with isolated and perfused rabbit kidneys have shown that the kidney may be the main site of interferon catabolism.

There are no pharmacokinetic data available for the intralesional route of administration.

Serum Neutralizing Antibodies In INTRON A treated patients tested for antibody activity in clinical trials, serum anti-interferon neutralizing antibodies were detected in 0% (0/90) of patients with hairy cell leukemia, 0.8% (2/260) of patients treated intralesionally for condylomata acuminata, and 4% (1/24) of patients with AIDS-Related Kaposi's Sarcoma. Serum neutralizing antibodies have been detected in <3% of patients treated with higher INTRON A doses in malignancies other than hairy cell leukemia or AIDS-Related Kaposi's Sarcoma. The clinical significance of the appearance of serum anti-interferon neutralizing activity in these indications is not known.

Serum anti-interferon neutralizing antibodies were detected in 15% (7/46) of patients with chronic hepatitis NANB/C and in 13% (6/48) of patients who received INTRON A therapy for chronic hepatitis B at 5 million IU, QD for 4 months, and in 3% (1/33) of patients treated at 10 million IU, TIW. In patients with chronic hepatitis the titers detected were low (≤1:40) and the appearance of serum anti-interferon neutralizing activity did not appear to affect safety or efficacy.

Hairy Cell Leukemia In clinical trials in patients with hairy cell leukemia, there was depression of hematopoiesis during the first 1 to 2 months of INTRON A treatment, resulting in reduced numbers of circulating red and white blood cells, and platelets. Subsequently, both splenectomized and nonsplenectomized patients achieved substantial and sustained improvements in granulocytes, platelets, and hemoglobin levels in 75% of treated patients and at least some improvement (minor responses) occurred in 90%. INTRON A treatment resulted in a decrease in bone marrow hypercellularity and hairy cell infiltrates. The hairy cell index (HCI), which represents the percent of bone marrow cellularity times the percent of hairy cell infiltrate, was greater than or equal to 50% at the beginning of the study in 87% of patients. The percentage of patients with such an HCI decreased to 25% after six months and to 14% after one year. These results indicate that even though hematologic improvement had occurred earlier, prolonged INTRON A treatment may be required to obtain maximal reduction in tumor cell infiltrates in the bone marrow.

The percentage of patients with hairy cell leukemia who required red blood cell or platelet transfusions decreased significantly during treatment and the percentage of patients with confirmed and serious infections declined as granulocyte counts improved. Reversal of splenomegaly and of clinically significant hypersplenism was demonstrated in some patients.

Subsequent follow-up with a median time of approximately 40 months demonstrated an overall survival of 87.8%. In a comparable historical control group followed for 24 months, overall median survival was approximately 40%.

Condylomata Acuminata Condylomata acuminata (venereal or genital warts) are associated with infections of the human papilloma virus (HPV). The safety and efficacy of INTRON A Interferon alfa-2b, recombinant for Injection in the treatment of condylomata acuminata were evaluated in three controlled double-blind clinical trials. In these studies INTRON A doses of 1 milliion IU per lesion were administered intralesionally three times a week (TIW), in ≤5 lesions per patient for 3 weeks. The patients were observed for up to 16 weeks after completion of the full treatment course.

INTRON A treatment of condylomata was significantly more effective than placebo, as measured by disappearance of lesions, decreases in lesion size, and by an overall change in disease status. Of 192 INTRON A treated patients and 206 placebo treated patients who were evaluable for efficacy at the time of best response during the course of the study, 42% of INTRON A patients *versus* 17% of placebo patients experienced clearing of all treated lesions. Likewise 24% of INTRON A patients *versus* 8% of placebo patients experienced marked (≥75% to <100%) reduction in lesion size, 18% *versus* 9% experienced moderate (≥50% to ≤75%) reduction in lesion size, 10% *versus* 42% had a slight (<50%) reduction in lesion size, 5% *versus* 24% had no change in lesion size and 0% *versus* 1% experienced exacerbation ($p<0.001$).

In one of these studies, 43% (54/125) of patients in whom multiple (≤3) lesions were treated, experienced complete clearing of all treated lesions during the course of the study. Of these patients, 81% remained cleared 16 weeks after treatment was initiated.

Patients who did not achieve total clearing of all their treated lesions had these same lesions treated with a second course of therapy. During this second course of treatment, 38% to 67% of patients had clearing of all treated lesions. The overall percentage of patients who had cleared all their treated lesions after 2 courses of treatment ranged from 57% to 85%.

INTRON A treated lesions showed improvement within 2 to 4 weeks after the start of treatment in the above study; maximal response to INTRON A therapy was noted 4 to 8 weeks after initiation of treatment.

The response to INTRON A therapy was better in patients who had condylomata for shorter durations than in patients with lesions for a longer duration.

AIDS-Related Kaposi's Sarcoma The safety and efficacy of INTRON A Interferon alfa-2b, recombinant for Injection in the treatment of Kaposi's Sarcoma (KS), a common manifestation of the Acquired Immune Deficiency Syndrome (AIDS), were evaluated in clinical trials in 144 patients.

In one study, INTRON A doses of 30 million IU/m^2 were administered subcutaneously three times per week (TIW), to patients with AIDS-Related KS. Doses were adjusted for patient tolerance. The average weekly dose delivered in the first 4 weeks was 150 million IU; at the end of 12 weeks this averaged 110 million IU/week; and by 24 weeks averaged 75 million IU/week.

Forty-four percent of asymptomatic patients responded *versus* 7% of symptomatic patients. The median time to response was approximately 2 months and 1 month, respectively, for asymptomatic and symptomatic patients. The median duration of response was approximately 3 months and 1 month, respectively, for the asymptomatic and symptomatic patients. Baseline T4/T8 ratios were 0.46 for responders *versus* 0.33 for nonresponders.

In another study, INTRON A doses of 35 million IU were administered subcutaneously, daily (QD), for 12 weeks. Maintenance treatment, with every other day dosing (QOD), was continued for up to 1 year in patients achieving antitumor and antiviral responses. The median time to response was 2 months and the median duration of response was 5 months in the asymptomatic patients.

In all studies, the likelihood of response was greatest in patients with relatively intact immune systems as assessed by baseline CD4 counts (interchangeable with T4 counts). Results at doses of 30 million IU/m^2 TIW and 35 million IU/QD, subcutaneously were similar and are provided together in TABLE 1. This table demonstrates the relationship of response to baseline CD4 count in both asymptomatic and symptomatic patients in the 30 million IU/m^2 TIW and the 35 million IU/QD treatment groups.

In the 30 million IU study group, 7% (5/72) of patients were complete responders and 22% (16/72) of the patients were partial responders. The 35 million IU study had 13% (3/23) patients) complete responders and 17% (4/23) partial responders.

For patients who received 30 million IU, TIW, the median survival time was longer in patients with CD4 greater than 200 (30.7 months) than in patients with CD4 less than or equal to 200 (8.9 months). Among responders, the median survival time was 22.6 months *versus* 9.7 months in nonresponders.

TABLE 1
*RESPONSE BY BASELINE CD4 COUNT**
IN **AIDS-RELATED KS** *PATIENTS*

	30 million IU/m^2 TIW, SC and 35 million IU QD, SC		
	Asymptomatic		*Symptomatic*
CD4<200	4/14 (29%)		0/19 (0%)
200≤CD4≤400	6/12 (50%)	58%	0/5 (0%)
CD4>400	5/7 (71%)		0/0 (0%)

* Data for CD4, and asymptomatic and symptomatic classification were not available for all patients.

Chronic Hepatitis Non-A, Non-B/C (NANB/C) The safety and efficacy of INTRON A Interferon alfa-2b, recombinant for Injection in the treatment of chronic hepatitis NANB/C were evaluated in 4 randomized controlled clinical studies in which INTRON A doses of 1, 2, or 3 million IU three times a week (TIW), were administered subcutaneously for 6 months (23 or 24 weeks). The patients were 18 years of age or older and had compensated liver disease. Of the 332 patients evaluable for efficacy, 81% had a history of blood or blood product exposure, 8% had a history of intravenous drug abuse, 2% had a history of surgery without blood products, and the remainder had other exposure. Retrospectively, 86% (172/199) of the patients with blood or blood product exposure who were tested were found to be positive for antibody to hepatitis C virus (HCV).

In each of 3 clinical studies, INTRON A therapy at 3 million IU, TIW, resulted in a reduction in serum alanine aminotransferase (ALT) in a statistically significantly greater proportion of patients *versus* control patients (see TABLE 2).

Of the 54% of patients responding to INTRON A therapy at a dose of 3 million IU, 70% achieved reductions in ALT levels to normal, 18% achieved reductions to near normal levels, and 12% achieved partial responses.

Histological improvement was evaluated by comparison of pre- and post-treatment liver biopsies using the semi-quantitative Knodell Histology Activity Index (HAI).[4]

In one of the three studies there was histological improvement in a statistically significantly greater proportion of INTRON A treated patients compared to controls (see TABLE 3). A similar, but not statistically significant trend for improvement was observed in the other two studies.

Subsequent combined analysis of results for the 3 studies showed histological improvement in a statistically significantly greater proportion of patients treated with INTRON A doses of 3 million IU than in control patients ($p=0.04$). The improvement was due primarily to decreases in severity of necrosis and degeneration in the lobular and periportal regions (Knodell HAI Categories I + II), which were observed in 65% (52/80) of patients treated at 3 million IU compared to 46% (32/70) of controls. Diminution of disease activity in these regions of the liver was accompanied by a reduction or normalization of serum ALT in many patients. Disease activity increased in these regions in only 3% of all INTRON A treated patients, whereas an increase was observed in 16% of the controls. No patient achieving an ALT response with 3 million IU INTRON A therapy showed increased periportal or lobular necrosis and degeneration.

Patients were followed for 6 months after the end of INTRON A therapy. During this period the ALT response was maintained in 51% (26/51) of patients who responded at the 3 million IU TIW dose. Of patients who relapsed during the follow-up period and were retreated at this dose, 83% (15/18) responded to retreatment.

Continued on next page

Information on Schering products appearing on these pages is effective as of August 15, 1992.

Schering—Cont.

TABLE 2
ALT RESPONSES†
IN CHRONIC HEPATITIS NANB/C PATIENTS

Study Number	Treatment Group Number of Patients (%) INTRON A 3 million IU		Controls‡		P § Value
1[1]	29/55	(53%)	5/55	(9%)	<0.001
2[2]	10/23	(43%)	3/25	(12%)	0.02
3[3]	12/17	(71%)	3/17	(18%)	0.005
All Studies	**51/95**	**(54%)**	**11/97**	**(11%)**	**<0.001**

† Includes reduction in serum ALT to:
normal,
near normal (≤ 1.5 times the upper limit of normal), or
partial response (> 50% decrease in serum ALT).
‡ Untreated or Placebo
§ INTRON A 3 million IU, TIW, 6 months *versus* control.

TABLE 3
HISTOLOGICAL IMPROVEMENT£
IN CHRONIC HEPATITIS NANB/C PATIENTS

Study Number	Treatment Group Number of Patients (%) INTRON A 3 million IU		Controls**		P †† Value
1	29/45	(64%)	18/36	(50%)	0.26
2	12/19	(63%)	10/18	(56%)	0.75
3	14/16	(88%)	8/15	(53%)	0.054
All Studies	**55/80**	**(69%)**	**36/69**	**(52%)**	**0.04**

£Assessed by the Knodell Histology Activity Index which includes:
Category I—Periportal necrosis
Category II—Intralobular degeneration and necrosis
Category III—Portal inflammation
Category IV—Fibrosis
**Untreated or Placebo
††INTRON A 3 million IU, TIW, 6 months compared to control for improvement *versus* no improvement.

Chronic Hepatitis B The safety and efficacy of INTRON A Interferon alfa-2b, recombinant for Injection in the treatment of chronic hepatitis B were evaluated in three clinical trials in which INTRON A doses of 30 to 35 million IU per week were administered subcutaneously (SC), as either 5 million IU daily (QD), or 10 million IU three times a week (TIW) for 16 weeks *versus* no treatment. All patients were 18 years of age or older with compensated liver disease, and had chronic hepatitis B virus (HBV) infection (serum HBsAg positive for at least 6 months) and HBV replication (serum HBeAg positive). Patients were also serum HBV-DNA positive, an additional indicator of HBV replication, as measured by a research assay.[5,6] All patients had elevated serum alanine aminotransferase (ALT), and liver biopsy findings compatible with the diagnosis of chronic hepatitis. Patients with the presence of antibody to human immunodeficiency virus (anti-HIV) or antibody to hepatitis delta virus (anti-HDV) in the serum were excluded from the studies.
Virologic response to treatment was defined in these studies as a loss of serum markers of HBV replication (HBeAg and HBV-DNA). Secondary parameters of response included loss of serum HBsAg, decreases in serum ALT, and improvement in liver histology.
In each of two randomized controlled studies, a significantly greater proportion of INTRON A treated patients exhibited a virologic response compared with untreated control patients (see TABLE 4). In a third study without a concurrent control group, a similar response rate to INTRON A therapy was observed. Pretreatment with prednisone, evaluated in two of the studies, did not improve the response rate and provided no additional benefit.
The response to INTRON A therapy was durable. No patient responding to INTRON A therapy at a dose of 5 million IU, QD or 10 million IU, TIW, relapsed during the follow-up period which ranged from 2 to 6 months after treatment ended. The loss of serum HBeAg and HBV-DNA was maintained in 100% of 19 responding patients followed for 3.5 to 36 months after the end of therapy.
In a proportion of responding patients, loss of HBeAg was followed by the loss of HBsAg. HBsAg was lost in 27% (4/15) of patients who responded to INTRON A therapy at a dose of 5 million IU, QD, and 35% (8/23) of patients who responded to 10 million IU, TIW. No untreated control patient lost HBsAg in these studies.
In a pilot study, 12 patients responding to INTRON A therapy were followed for 3.8 to 6.6 years after treatment; 100% (12/12) remained serum HBeAg negative and 58% (7/12) lost serum HBsAg.
INTRON A therapy resulted in normalization of serum ALT in a significantly greater proportion of treated patients compared to untreated patients in each of two controlled studies (see TABLE 5). In a third study without a concurrent control group, normalization of serum ALT was observed in 50% (12/24) of patients receiving INTRON A therapy.
Virologic response was associated with a reduction in serum ALT to normal or near normal (≤1.5 times the upper limit of normal) in 87% (13/15) of patients responding to INTRON A therapy at 5 million IU, QD, and 100% (23/23) of patients responding to 10 million IU, TIW.
Improvement in liver histology was evaluated in Studies 1 and 3, by comparison of pre- and 6 month posttreatment liver biopsies using the semi-quantitative Knodell Histology Activity Index.[4] No statistically significant difference in liver histology was observed in treated patients compared to control patients in Study 1. Although statistically significant histological improvement from baseline was observed in treated patients in Study 3 (p ≤ 0.01), there was no control group for comparison. Of those patients exhibiting a virologic response following treatment with 5 million IU, QD or 10 million IU, TIW histological improvement was observed in 85% (17/20) compared to 36% (9/25) of patients who were not virologic responders. The histological improvement was due primarily to decreases in severity of necrosis, degeneration, and inflammation in the periportal, lobular, and portal regions of the liver (Knodell Categories I + II + III). Continued histological improvement was observed in four responding patients who lost serum HBsAg and were followed 2 to 4 years after the end of INTRON A therapy.[7]

TABLE 4
*VIROLOGIC RESPONSE**
IN CHRONIC HEPATITIS B PATIENTS

Study Number	Treatment Group £ Number of Patients (%) INTRON A 5 million IU, QD		INTRON A 10 million IU, TIW		Untreated Controls		P ** Value
1[5]	15/38	(39%)	—	—	3/42	(7%)	0.0009
2	—	—	10/24	(42%)	1/22	(5%)	0.005
3[6]	—	—	13/24‡	(54%)	2/27	(7%)‡	NA‡
All Studies	**15/38**	**(39%)**	**23/48**	**(48%)**	**6/91**	**(7%)**	—

*Loss of HBeAg and HBV-DNA by 6 months posttherapy.
£Patients pretreated with prednisone not shown.
**INTRON A treatment group *versus* untreated control.
‡Untreated control patients evaluated after 24 week observation period. A subgroup subsequently received INTRON A therapy. A direct comparison is not applicable (NA).

TABLE 5
*ALT RESPONSES**
IN CHRONIC HEPATITIS B PATIENTS

Study Number	Treatment Group Number of Patients (%) INTRON A 5 million IU, QD		INTRON A 10 million IU, TIW		Untreated Controls		P** Value
1	16/38	(42%)	—	—	8/42	(19%)	0.03
2	—	—	10/24	(42%)	1/22	(5%)	0.0034
3	—	—	12/24†	(50%)	2/27	(7%)†	NA†
All Studies	**16/38**	**(42%)**	**22/48**	**(46%)**	**11/91**	**(12%)**	—

*Reduction in serum ALT to normal by 6 months posttherapy.
**INTRON A treatment group *versus* untreated control.
†Untreated control patients evaluated after 24 week observation period. A subgroup subsequently received INTRON A therapy. A direct comparison is not applicable (NA).

INDICATIONS AND USAGE

General INTRON A Interferon alfa-2b, recombinant for Injection is indicated in patients 18 years of age or older for the treatment of hairy cell leukemia, selected cases of condylomata acuminata involving external surfaces of the genital and perianal areas, selected patients with AIDS-Related Kaposi's Sarcoma, chronic hepatitis Non-A, Non-B/C (NANB/C) in patients with compensated liver disease who have a history of blood or blood product exposure and/or are HCV antibody positive, and chronic hepatitis B in patients with compensated liver disease and HBV replication (serum HBeAg positive).

Hairy Cell Leukemia INTRON A Interferon alfa-2b, recombinant for Injection is indicated for the treatment of patients 18 years of age or older with hairy cell leukemia. Studies have shown that INTRON A therapy can produce clinically meaningful regression or stabilization of this disease, both in previously splenectomized and non- splenectomized patients. Prior to initiation of therapy, tests should be performed to quantitate peripheral blood hemoglobin, platelets, granulocytes and hairy cells and bone marrow hairy cells. These parameters should be monitored periodically during treatment to determine whether response to treatment has occurred. If a patient does not respond within 6 months, treatment should be discontinued. If a response to treatment does occur, treatment usually should be continued until no further improvement is observed and these laboratory parameters have been stable for about 3 months (see **DOSAGE AND ADMINISTRATION**). It is not known whether continued treatment after that time point is beneficial. Studies are in progress to evaluate this question.

Condylomata Acuminata INTRON A Interferon alfa-2b, recombinant for Injection is indicated for intralesional treatment of selected patients 18 years of age or older with condylomata acuminata involving external surfaces of the genital and perianal areas (see **DOSAGE AND ADMINISTRATION**).
In selecting patients for INTRON A treatment, the physician should consider the nature of the patient's lesion and the patient's past treatment history, in addition to the patient's ability to comply with the treatment regimen. INTRON A therapy offers an additional approach to treatment in condylomata and is particularly useful for those patients who do not respond satisfactorily to other treatment modalities (eg, podophyllin resin, surgery, cryotherapy, chemotherapy, and laser therapy), or whose lesions are more readily treatable by INTRON A Interferon alfa-2b, recombinant for Injection than by other treatments.
The use of this product in adolescents has not been studied. Interferon alpha has been shown to affect the menstrual cycle in non-human primates and to decrease serum estradiol and progesterone levels in women. Consideration should be given as to whether the adolescent patient should be treated.

AIDS-Related Kaposi's Sarcoma INTRON A Interferon alfa-2b, recombinant for Injection is indicated for the treatment of selected patients 18 years of age or older with AIDS-Related Kaposi's Sarcoma. Studies have demonstrated a greater likelihood of response to INTRON A therapy in patients who are without systemic symptoms, who have limited lymphadenopathy and who have a relatively intact immune system.
Lesion measurements and blood counts should be performed prior to initiation of therapy and should be monitored periodically during treatment to determine whether response to treatment or disease stabilization has occurred.
When disease stabilization or a response to treatment occurs, treatment should continue until there is no further evidence of tumor or until discontinuation is required by evidence of a severe opportunistic infection or adverse effect (see **DOSAGE AND ADMINISTRATION**).

Chronic Hepatitis Non-A, Non-B/C (NANB/C) INTRON A Interferon alfa-2b, recombinant for Injection is indicated for the treatment of chronic hepatitis Non-A, Non-B/C (NANB/C) in patients 18 years of age or older with compensated liver disease who have a history of blood or blood product exposure and/or are HCV antibody positive. Studies in these patients demonstrated that INTRON A therapy can produce clinically meaningful effects on this disease, manifested by normalization of serum alanine aminotransferase (ALT) and reduction in liver necrosis and degeneration.
A liver biopsy should be performed to establish the diagnosis of chronic hepatitis. Patients should be tested for the presence of antibody to HCV. Patients with other causes of chronic hepatitis, including autoimmune hepatitis, should be excluded. Prior to initiation of INTRON A therapy, the physician should establish that the patient has compensated liver disease. The following patient entrance criteria for compensated liver disease were used in the clinical studies

and should be considered before INTRON A treatment of patients with chronic hepatitis NANB/C:

- No history of hepatic encephalopathy, variceal bleeding, ascites, or other clinical signs of decompensation
- Bilirubin ≤2 mg/dL
- Albumin Stable and within normal limits
- Prothrombin Time <3 seconds prolonged
- WBC ≥3000/mm^3
- Platelets ≥70,000/mm^3

Serum creatinine should be normal or near normal.

Prior to initiation of INTRON A therapy, CBC and platelet counts should be evaluated in order to establish baselines for monitoring potential toxicity. These tests should be repeated at weeks 1 and 2 following initiation of INTRON A therapy, and monthly thereafter. Serum ALT should be evaluated after 2, 16, and 24 weeks of therapy to assess response to treatment (see **DOSAGE AND ADMINISTRATION**).

Patients with preexisting thyroid abnormalities may be treated if thyroid stimulating hormone (TSH) levels can be maintained in the normal range by medication. TSH levels must be within normal limits upon initiation of INTRON A treatment and TSH testing should be repeated at 3 and 6 months (see **PRECAUTIONS—Laboratory Tests**).

Chronic Hepatitis B INTRON A Interferon alfa-2b, recombinant for Injection is indicated for the treatment of chronic hepatitis B in patients 18 years of age or older with compensated liver disease and HBV replication. Patients must be serum HBsAg positive for at least 6 months and have HBV replication (serum HBeAg positive) with elevated serum ALT. Studies in these patients demonstrated that INTRON A therapy can produce virologic remission of this disease (loss of serum HBeAg), and normalization of serum aminotransferases. INTRON A therapy resulted in the loss of serum HBsAg in some responding patients.

Prior to initiation of INTRON A therapy, it is recommended that a liver biopsy be performed to establish the presence of chronic hepatitis and the extent of liver damage. The physician should establish that the patient has compensated liver disease. The following patient entrance criteria for compensated liver disease were used in the clinical studies and should be considered before INTRON A treatment of patients with chronic hepatitis B:

- No history of hepatic encephalopathy, variceal bleeding, ascites, or other signs of clinical decompensation
- Bilirubin Normal
- Albumin Stable and within normal limits
- Prothrombin Time <3 seconds prolonged
- WBC ≥4000/mm^3
- Platelets ≥100,000/mm^3

Patients with causes of chronic hepatitis other than chronic hepatitis B or chronic hepatitis NANB/C should not be treated with INTRON A Interferon alfa-2b, recombinant for Injection. CBC and platelet counts should be evaluated prior to initiation of INTRON A therapy in order to establish baselines for monitoring potential toxicity. These tests should be repeated at treatment weeks 1, 2, 4, 8, 12, and 16. Liver function tests, including serum ALT, albumin and bilirubin, should be evaluated at treatment weeks 1, 2, 4, 8, 12, and 16. HBeAg, HBsAg, and ALT should be evaluated at the end of therapy, as well as 3 and 6 months posttherapy, since patients may become virologic responders during the 6 month period following the end of treatment. In clinical studies, 39% (15/38) of responding patients lost HBeAg 1 to 6 months following the end of INTRON A therapy. Of responding patients who lost HBsAg, 58% (7/12) did so 1 to 6 months posttreatment.

A transient increase in ALT ≥ 2 times baseline value (flare) can occur during INTRON A therapy for chronic hepatitis B. In clinical trials, this flare generally occurred 8 to 12 weeks after initiation of therapy and was more frequent in responders (63%, 24/38) than in nonresponders (27%, 13/48). However, elevations in bilirubin ≥ 3 mg/dL occurred infrequently (2%, 2/86) during therapy. When ALT flare occurs, in general, INTRON A therapy should be continued unless signs and symptoms of liver failure are observed. During ALT flare, clinical symptomatology and liver function tests including ALT, prothrombin time, alkaline phosphatase, albumin, and bilirubin, should be monitored at approximately 2 week intervals (see **WARNINGS**).

DOSAGE AND ADMINISTRATION

IMPORTANT: INTRON A Interferon alfa-2b, recombinant for Injection dosing regimens are different for each of the following indications described in this section of the product information sheet.

Hairy Cell Leukemia The recommended dosage of INTRON A Interferon alfa-2b, recombinant for Injection for the treatment of hairy cell leukemia is 2 million IU/m^2 administered intramuscularly (see **WARNINGS**) or subcutaneously 3 times a week. The 50 million IU strength is not to be used for the treatment of hairy cell leukemia. Higher doses are not recommended. The normalization of one or more hematologic variables usually begins within 2 months of initiation of therapy. Improvement in all three hematologic variables may require 6 months or more of therapy.

This dosage regimen should be maintained unless the disease progresses rapidly, or severe intolerance is manifested. If severe adverse reactions develop, the dosage should be modified (50% reduction) or therapy should be temporarily discontinued until the adverse reactions abate. If persistent or recurrent intolerance develops following adequate dosage adjustment, or disease progresses, INTRON A treatment should be discontinued. The minimum effective INTRON A dose has not been established.

Condylomata Acuminata The 10 million IU INTRON A vial must be reconstituted with 1 mL of Diluent for INTRON A Interferon alfa-2b, recombinant for Injection (bacteriostatic water for injection), to provide the proper INTRON A concentration for the treatment of condylomata. Do not use the 3, 5, 18 million multidose, or 25 million IU vials for treatment of condylomata acuminata since the dilution required for intralesional treatment would result in a hypertonic solution. The 50 million IU vial is not to be used for the treatment of condylomata. Additionally, do not reconstitute the 10 million IU vial with more than 1 mL of diluent, since the injection would be subpotent.

Inject 1.0 million IU of INTRON A Interferon alfa-2b, recombinant for Injection (0.1 mL of reconstituted INTRON A solution) into each lesion three times per week on alternate days, for three weeks. The injection should be administered intralesionally using a Tuberculin or similar syringe and a 25–30 gauge needle. The needle should be directed at the center of the base of the wart and at an angle almost parallel to the plane of the skin (approximating that in the commonly used PPD test). This will deliver the interferon to the dermal core of the lesion, infiltrating the lesion and causing a small wheal. Care should be taken not to go beneath the lesion too deeply; subcutaneous injection should be avoided, since this area is below the base of the lesion. Do not inject too superficially since this will result in possible leakage, infiltrating only the keratinized layer, and not the dermal core. As many as 5 lesions can be treated at one time. To reduce side effects, INTRON A injections may be administered in the evening, when possible. Additionally, acetaminophen may be administered at the time of injection to alleviate some of the potential side effects.

The maximum response usually occurs four to eight weeks after initiation of the first treatment course. If results at 12 to 16 weeks after the initial treatment course has concluded are not satisfactory, a second course of treatment using the above dosage schedule may be instituted providing that clinical symptoms and signs, or changes in laboratory parameters (liver function tests, WBC and platelets) do not preclude such a course of action.

Patients with six to ten condylomata may receive a second (sequential) course of treatment at the above dosage schedule, to treat up to five additional condylomata per course of treatment. Patients with greater than ten condylomata may receive additional sequences depending on how large a number of condylomata are present.

AIDS-Related Kaposi's Sarcoma The recommended INTRON A dosage is 30 million IU/m^2 three times a week administered subcutaneously or intramuscularly.

The selected dosage regimen should be maintained unless the disease progresses rapidly or severe intolerance is manifested. If severe adverse reactions develop, the dosage should be modified (50% reduction) or therapy should be temporarily discontinued until the adverse reactions abate. When patients initiate therapy at 30 million IU/m^2 TIW, the average dose tolerated at the end of 12 weeks of therapy is 110 million IU/week and 75 million IU/week at the end of 24 weeks of therapy.

When disease stabilization or a response to treatment occurs, treatment should continue until there is no further evidence of tumor or until discontinuation is required by evidence of a severe opportunistic infection or adverse effect.

Chronic Hepatitis Non-A, Non-B/C (NANB/C) The recommended dosage of INTRON A Interferon alfa-2b, recombinant for Injection for the treatment of chronic hepatitis NANB/C is 3 million IU three times a week (TIW) administered subcutaneously or intramuscularly.

Normalization of serum alanine aminotransferase (ALT) may occur in some patients as early as two weeks after initiation of treatment; however, current experience suggests that patients responding to INTRON A therapy with a reduction in serum ALT should complete 6 months (24 weeks) of treatment. The optimal dose and duration of therapy are currently under investigation.

In clinical trials, 54% (51/95) of the patients at a dose of 3 million IU TIW responded with a reduction in serum ALT after 6 months of INTRON A therapy. Since most of these patients (49/51) responded within the first 16 weeks of treatment, consideration could be given to discontinuing INTRON A therapy in patients who fail to respond after 16 weeks. The effect of dose escalation in these patients is under investigation.

If severe adverse reactions develop during INTRON A treatment, the dose should be modified (50% reduction) or therapy should be temporarily discontinued until the adverse reactions abate. If intolerance persists after dose adjustment, INTRON A therapy should be discontinued.

Patients who relapse following INTRON A therapy may be retreated with the same dosage regimen to which they had previously responded.

Chronic Hepatitis B The recommended dosage of INTRON A Interferon alfa-2b, recombinant for Injection for the treatment of chronic hepatitis B is 30 to 35 million IU per week, administered subcutaneously or intramuscularly either as 5 million IU daily (QD), or 10 million IU three times a week (TIW), for 16 weeks.

If severe adverse reactions or laboratory abnormalities develop during INTRON A therapy the dose should be modified (50% reduction), or discontinued if appropriate, until the adverse reactions abate. If intolerance persists after dose adjustment, INTRON A therapy should be discontinued.

For patients with decreases in granulocyte or platelet counts, the following guidelines for dose modification were used in the clinical trials:

INTRON A Dose	*Granulocyte Count*	*Platelet Count*
Reduce 50%	<750/mm^3	<50,000/mm^3
Interrupt	<500/mm^3	<30,000/mm^3

INTRON A therapy was resumed at up to 100% of the initial dose when granulocyte and/or platelet counts returned to normal or baseline values.

At the discretion of the physician, the patient may self-administer the medication. (See illustrated **PATIENT INFORMATION SHEET** for instructions.)

Preparation and Administration of INTRON A Interferon alfa-2b, recombinant for Injection

Reconstitution of lyophilized INTRON A Interferon alfa-2b, recombinant for Injection Inject the amount of Diluent for INTRON A Interferon alfa-2b, recombinant for Injection (bacteriostatic water for injection) stated in the appropriate chart below (diluent is supplied in either a vial or syringe, see **HOW SUPPLIED** below), into the INTRON A vial. Swirl gently to hasten complete dissolution of the powder. The appropriate INTRON A dose should then be withdrawn and injected intramuscularly, subcutaneously, or intralesionally. (See **PATIENT INFORMATION SHEET** for detailed instructions.)

After preparation and administration of the INTRON A injection, it is essential to follow the procedure for proper disposal of syringes and needles. (See **PATIENT INFORMATION SHEET** for detailed instructions.)

Hairy Cell Leukemia

Vial Strength	mL Diluent	Final Concentration
3 million IU	1	3 million IU/mL
5 million IU	1	5 million IU/mL
10 million IU	2	5 million IU/mL
‡18 million IU multidose	3.8	6 million IU/mL
25 million IU	5	5 million IU/mL

‡ This is a multidose vial to deliver 18 million IU of INTRON A Interferon alfa-2b, recombinant for Injection when reconstituted with 3.8 mL of the diluent provided.

Condylomata Acuminata

Vial Strength	mL Diluent	Final Concentration
*10 million IU	1	10 million IU/mL

*IMPORTANT: For patients with condylomata acuminata, reconstitute the 10 million IU vial with only 1 mL of the diluent provided to reach a final concentration of 10 million IU/mL to be administered intralesionally. (See **DOSAGE AND ADMINISTRATION, Condylomata Acuminata.**)

AIDS-Related Kaposi's Sarcoma

Vial Strength	mL Diluent	Final Concentration
50 million IU	1	50 million IU/mL

IMPORTANT: This vial size is to be used only for treatment of patients with AIDS-Related Kaposi's Sarcoma (see **DOSAGE AND ADMINISTRATION, AIDS-Related Kaposi's Sarcoma).**

Chronic Hepatitis Non-A, Non-B/C

Vial Strength	mL Diluent	Final Concentration
3 million IU	1	3 million IU/mL
†18 million IU multidose	3.8	6 million IU/mL

† This is a multidose vial to deliver 18 million IU of INTRON A Interferon alfa-2b, recombinant for Injection when reconstituted with 3.8 mL of the diluent provided.

Chronic Hepatitis B

Vial Strength	mL Diluent	Final Concentration
5 million IU	1	5 million IU/mL
10 million IU	1	10 million IU/mL

Stability INTRON A Interferon alfa-2b, recombinant for Injection provided as lyophilized powder in vials ranging from 3 to 50 million IU per vial, is stable at 45°C (113°F) for up to 7 days. After reconstitution with Diluent for INTRON A Interferon alfa-2b, recominant for Injection (bacteriostatic

Continued on next page

Information on Schering products appearing on these pages is effective as of August 15, 1992.

Schering—Cont.

water for injection) the solution is stable for one month at 2° to 8°C (36° to 46°F). The reconstituted solution is clear and colorless to light yellow.

Parenteral drug products should be inspected visually for particulate matter and discoloration prior to administration, whenever solution and container permit.

INTRON A Interferon alfa-2b, recombinant for Injection may be administered using either sterilized glass or plastic disposable syringes.

CONTRAINDICATIONS

INTRON A Interferon alfa-2b, recombinant for Injection is contraindicated in patients with a history of hypersensitivity to interferon alfa or any component of the injection.

WARNINGS

General Moderate to severe adverse experiences may require modification of the patient's dosage regimen, or in some cases termination of INTRON A therapy. Because of the fever and other "flu-like" symptoms associated with INTRON A administration, it should be used cautiously in patients with debilitating medical conditions, such as those with a history of pulmonary disease (eg, chronic obstructive pulmonary disease), or diabetes mellitus prone to ketoacidosis. Caution should also be observed in patients with coagulation disorders (eg, thrombophlebitis, pulmonary embolism) or severe myelosuppression.

Patients with platelet counts of less than 50,000/mm³ should not be administered INTRON A Interferon alfa-2b, recombinant for Injection intramuscularly, but instead by subcutaneous administration.

INTRON A therapy should be used cautiously in patients with a history of cardiovascular disease such as unstable angina or uncontrolled congestive heart failure. Those patients with a recent history of myocardial infarction and/or previous or current arrhythmic disorder who require INTRON A therapy should be closely monitored (see **Laboratory Tests**). Cardiovascular adverse experiences, which include hypotension, arrhythmia, or tachycardia of 150 beats per minute or greater, and transient reversible cardiomyopathy have been observed in some INTRON A treated patients. Transient reversible cardiomyopathy was reported in approximately 2% of the AIDS-Related Kaposi's Sarcoma patients treated with INTRON A Interferon alfa-2b, recombinant for Injection. The incidence of these complications in patients with preexisting heart disease is unknown. Hypotension may occur during INTRON A administration, or up to two days posttherapy, and may require supportive therapy including fluid replacement to maintain intravascular volume. Supraventricular arrhythmias occurred rarely and appeared to be correlated with preexisting conditions and prior therapy with cardiotoxic agents. These adverse experiences were controlled by modifying the dose or discontinuing treatment, but may require specific additional therapy.

Patients with a preexisting psychiatric condition, especially depression, or a history of severe psychiatric disorder should not be treated with INTRON A Interferon alfa-2b, recombinant for Injection.[8] INTRON A therapy should be discontinued for any patient developing severe depression or other psychiatric disorder during treatment. Central nervous system effects manifested by depression, confusion and other alterations of mental status have been observed in some INTRON A treated patients, and suicidal ideation and attempted suicide have been observed rarely. These adverse effects have occurred in patients treated with recommended doses as well as in patients treated with higher INTRON A doses. More significant obtundation and coma have also been observed in some patients, usually elderly, treated at higher doses. While these effects are usually rapidly reversible upon discontinuation of therapy, full resolution of symptoms has taken up to three weeks in a few severe episodes. Narcotics, hypnotics, or sedatives may be used concurrently with caution and patients should be closely monitored until the adverse effects have resolved.

Patients with preexisting thyroid abnormalities whose thyroid function cannot be maintained in the normal range by medication should not be treated with INTRON A Interferon alfa-2b, recombinant for Injection. Therapy should be discontinued for patients developing thyroid abnormalities during treatment whose thyroid function cannot be normalized by medication.

Hepatotoxicity, including fatality, has been observed rarely in INTRON A treated patients. Any patient developing liver function abnormalities during treatment should be monitored closely and if appropriate, treatment should be discontinued.

The 50 million IU strength is not to be used for the treatment of hairy cell leukemia, condylomata acuminata, chronic hepatitis NANB/C, or chronic hepatitis B. The 3 million, 5 million, 18 million multidose, and 25 million IU strengths are not to be used for the intralesional treatment of condylomata acuminata since the dilution required for the intralesional use would result in a hypertonic solution.

AIDS-Related Kaposi's Sarcoma INTRON A therapy should not be used for patients with rapidly progressive visceral disease (see **CLINICAL PHARMACOLOGY**). Also of note, there may be synergistic adverse effects between INTRON A Interferon alfa-2b, recombinant for Injection and zidovudine. Patients receiving concomitant zidovudine have had a higher incidence of neutropenia than that expected with zidovudine alone. Careful monitoring of the WBC count is indicated in all patients who are myelosuppressed and in all patients receiving other myelosuppressive medications. The effects of INTRON A Interferon alfa-2b, recombinant for Injection when combined with other drugs used in the treatment of AIDS-Related disease are unknown.

Chronic Hepatitis Non-A, Non-B/C (NANB/C) and Chronic Hepatitis B Patients with decompensated liver disease, autoimmune hepatitis or a history of autoimmune disease, and patients who are immunosuppressed transplant recipients should not be treated with INTRON A Interferon alfa-2b, recombinant for Injection. There are reports of worsening liver disease, including jaundice, hepatic encephalopathy, hepatic failure and death following INTRON A therapy in such patients. Therapy should be discontinued for any patient developing signs and symptoms of liver failure. Chronic hepatitis B patients with evidence of decreasing hepatic synthetic functions, such as decreasing albumin levels or prolongation of prothrombin time, may be at increased risk of clinical decompensation in association with a flare of aminotransferases during INTRON A treatment. In considering these patients for INTRON A therapy, the potential risks must be evaluated against the potential benefits of treatment.

PRECAUTIONS

General Acute serious hypersensitivity reactions (eg, urticaria, angioedema, bronchoconstriction, anaphylaxis) have been observed rarely in INTRON A treated patients; if such an acute reaction develops, the drug should be discontinued immediately and appropriate medical therapy instituted. Transient rashes have occurred in some patients following injection, but have not necessitated treatment interruption. While fever may be related to the flu-like syndrome reported commonly in patients treated with interferon, other causes of persistent fever should be ruled out.

There have been reports of interferon exacerbating preexisting psoriasis; therefore, INTRON A therapy should be used in these patients only if the potential benefit justifies the potential risk.

Variations in dosage, routes of administration, and adverse reactions exist among different brands of interferon. Therefore, do not use different brands of interferon in any single treatment regimen.

Drug Interactions Interactions between INTRON A Interferon alfa-2b, recombinant for Injection and other drugs have not been fully evaluated. Caution should be exercised when administering INTRON A therapy in combination with other potentially myelosuppressive agents such as zidovudine.

Information for Patients Patients receiving INTRON A treatment should be directed in its appropriate use, informed of benefits and risks associated with treatment, and referred to the **PATIENT INFORMATION SHEET**. This information is intended to aid in the safe and effective use of this medication. It is not a disclosure of all possible adverse or intended effects.

If home use is prescribed, a puncture-resistant container for the disposal of used syringes and needles should be supplied to the patient. Patients should be thoroughly instructed in the importance of proper disposal and cautioned against any reuse of needles and syringes. The full container should be disposed of according to the directions provided by the physician (see **PATIENT INFORMATION SHEET**).

Patients should be cautioned not to change brands of Interferon without medical consultation as a change in dosage may result.

Patients receiving high INTRON A doses should be cautioned against performing tasks that would require complete mental alertness, such as operating machinery or driving a motor vehicle.

The most common adverse experiences occurring with INTRON A therapy are "flu-like" symptoms, such as fever, headache, fatigue, anorexia, nausea, or vomiting (see **ADVERSE REACTIONS** section) and appear to decrease in severity as treatment continues. Some of these "flu-like" symptoms may be minimized by bedtime administration. Acetaminophen may be used to prevent or partially alleviate the fever and headache. Another common adverse experience is thinning of the hair.

It is advised that patients be well hydrated especially during the initial stages of treatment.

Laboratory Tests In addition to those tests normally required for monitoring patients, the following laboratory tests are recommended for all patients on INTRON A therapy, prior to beginning treatment and then periodically thereafter.

- Standard hematologic tests—including hemoglobin, complete and differential white blood cell counts and platelet count.
- Blood chemistries—electrolytes, liver function tests, and TSH.

Those patients who have preexisting cardiac abnormalities and/or are in advanced stages of cancer, should have electrocardiograms taken prior to and during the course of treatment.

Mild to moderate leukopenia and elevated serum liver enzyme (SGOT) levels have been reported with intralesional administration of INTRON A Interferon alfa-2b, recombinant for Injection (see **ADVERSE REACTIONS** section); therefore, the monitoring of these laboratory parameters should be considered.

Baseline chest X-rays are suggested and should be repeated if clinically indicated.

For specific recommendations in chronic hepatitis NANB/C and chronic hepatitis B, see **INDICATIONS AND USAGE** section.

Carcinogenesis, Mutagenesis, Impairment of Fertility Studies with INTRON A Interferon alfa-2b, recombinant for Injection have not been performed to determine carcinogenicity.

Interferon may impair fertility. In studies of interferon administration in non-human primates, menstrual cycle abnormalities have been observed. Decreases in serum estradiol and progesterone concentrations have been reported in women treated with human leukocyte interferon.[9] Therefore, fertile women should not receive INTRON A therapy unless they are using effective contraception during the therapy period. INTRON A therapy should be used with caution in fertile men.

Mutagenicity studies with INTRON A Interferon alfa-2b, recombinant for Injection revealed no adverse findings.

Studies in mice, rats, and monkeys receiving INTRON A injections for up to one month have revealed no evidence of toxicity. However, due to the known species-specificity of interferon, the effects in animals are unlikely to be predictive of those in man.

Pregnancy Category C INTRON A Interferon alfa-2b, recombinant for Injection has beeen shown to have abortifacient effects in *Macaca mulatta* (rhesus monkeys) in all dose groups studied (7.5 million, 15 million, and 30 million IU/kg), although it was only statistically significant *versus* control at the mid and high dose groups (corresponding to 90 and 180 times the intramuscular or subcutaneous dose of 2 million IU/m²). There are no adequate and well controlled studies in pregnant women. INTRON A therapy should be used during pregnancy only if the potential benefit justifies the potential risk to the fetus.

Nursing Mothers It is not known whether this drug is excreted in human milk. However, studies in mice have shown that mouse interferons are excreted into the milk. Because of the potential for serious adverse reactions from the drug in nursing infants, a decision should be made whether to discontinue nursing or to discontinue INTRON A therapy, taking into account the importance of the drug to the mother.

Pediatric Use Safety and effectiveness have not been established in patients below the age of 18 years.

ADVERSE REACTIONS

General The adverse experiences listed below were reported to be possibly or probably related to INTRON A therapy during clinical trials. Most of these adverse reactions were mild to moderate in severity and were manageable. Some were transient and most diminished with continued therapy.

The most frequently reported adverse reactions were flu-like symptoms, particularly fever, headache, chills, myalgia, and fatigue. More severe toxicities are observed generally at higher doses and may be difficult for patients to tolerate. [See table on next page.]

Hairy Cell Leukemia The adverse reactions most frequently reported during clinical trials in 145 patients with hairy cell leukemia were the flu-like symptoms of fever (68%), fatigue (61%), and chills (46%).

Condylomata Acuminata Eighty-eight percent (311/352) of patients treated with INTRON A Interferon alfa-2b, recombinant for Injection for condylomata acuminata who were evaluable for safety, reported an adverse reaction during treatment. The incidence of the adverse reactions reported increased when the number of treated lesions increased from 1 to 5. All 40 patients who had 5 warts treated, reported some type of adverse reaction during treatment.

Adverse reactions and abnormal laboratory test values reported by patients who were retreated were qualitatively and quantitatively similar to those reported during the initial INTRON A treatment period.

AIDS-Related Kaposi's Sarcoma In patients with AIDS-Related Kaposi's Sarcoma, some type of adverse reaction occurred in 100% of the 74 patients treated with 30 million IU/m² three times a week and in 97% of the 29 patients treated with 35 million IU per day.

TREATMENT-RELATED ADVERSE EXPERIENCES BY INDICATION
Dosing Regimens
Percentage (%) of Patients*

ADVERSE EXPERIENCE	HAIRY CELL LEUKEMIA 2 million IU/m² TIW/SC N=145	CONDYLOMATA ACUMINATA 1 million IU/ lesion N=352	AIDS-RELATED KAPOSI'S SARCOMA 30 million IU/m² TIW/SC N=74	35 million IU/QD/SC N=29	CHRONIC HEPATITIS NANB/C 3 million IU TIW N=159	CHRONIC HEPATITIS B 5 million IU QD N=101	10 million IU TIW N=78
Application-Site Disorders							
injection site inflammation	20	—	—	—	7	3	—
other (<5%)	burning, injection site bleeding, injection site pain, injection site reaction, itching						
Blood Disorders (<5%)	anemia, granulocytopenia, hemolytic anemia, leukopenia, thrombocytopenia						
Body as a Whole							
facial edema	—	<1	—	10	1	3	1
weight decrease	<1	<1	5	3	<1	2	5
other (<5%)	cachexia, dehydration, earache, hypercalcemia, lymphadenopathy, periorbital edema, peripheral edema, thirst, weakness						
Cardiovascular System Disorders (<5%)	arrythmia, atrial fibrillation, bradycardia, cardiac failure, cardiomyopathy, extrasystoles, hypertension, hypotension, palpitations, postural hypotension, tachycardia						
Endocrine System Disorders (<5%)	aggravation of diabetes mellitus, gynecomastia, thyroid disorder, virilism						
Flu-like Symptoms							
fever	68	56	47	55	43	66	86
headache	39	47	36	21	43	61	44
chills	46	45	—	—	—	—	—
myalgia	39	44	34	28	42	59	40
fatigue	61	18	84	48	19	75	69
increased sweating	8	2	4	21	3	1	1
asthenia	7	—	11	—	24	5	15
rigors	—	—	30	14	27	38	42
arthralgia	8	9	—	3	19	19	8
dizziness	12	9	7	24	9	13	10
influenza-like symptoms	37	—	45	79	9	5	—
back pain	19	6	1	3	3	—	—
dry mouth	19	—	22	28	4	6	5
chest pain	<1	<1	1	28	1	4	—
malaise	—	14	5	—	3	9	6
pain (unspecified)	18	3	3	3	—	—	—
other (<5%)	chest pain substernal, rhinitis, rhinorrhea						
Gastrointestinal System Disorders							
diarrhea	18	2	18	45	13	19	8
anorexia	19	1	38	41	13	43	53
nausea	21	17	28	21	23	50	33
taste alteration	13	<1	5	7	1	10	—
abdominal pain	<5	1	5	21	6	5	4
loose stools	—	<1	—	10	3	2	—
vomiting	6	2	11	14	3	7	10
constipation	<1	—	1	10	<1	5	—
gingivitis	—	—	—	14	—	1	—
dyspepsia	—	2	4	—	3	3	8
other (<5%)	abdominal distention, dysphagia, eructation, esophagitis, flatulence, gastric ulcer, gastrointestinal hemorrhage, gastrointestinal mucosal discoloration, gingival bleeding, gum hyperplasia, increased appetite, increased saliva, melena, oral leukoplakia, rectal bleeding after stool, rectal hemorrhage, stomatitis, stomatitis ulcerative, taste loss						
Liver and Biliary System Disorders (<5%)	abnormal hepatic function tests, bilirubinemia, increased transaminases, jaundice, right upper quadrant pain and very rarely, hepatic encephalopathy, hepatic failure, and death						
Musculoskeletal System Disorders							
musculoskeletal pain	—	—	—	—	—	9	1
other (<5%)	arthritis, arthrosis, bone pain, leg cramps, muscle weakness						
Nervous System and Psychiatric Disorders							
depression	6	3	9	28	8	17	6
paresthesia	6	1	3	21	1	6	3
impaired concentration	—	<1	3	14	4	8	5
amnesia	<5	—	—	14	—	—	—
confusion	<5	4	12	10	1	—	—
hypoesthesia	<5	1	—	10	—	—	—
irritability	—	—	—	—	4	16	12
somnolence	<5	3	3	—	1	14	9
anxiety	5	<1	1	3	1	2	—
insomnia	—	<1	3	3	4	11	6
nervousness	—	1	—	3	—	3	1
decreased libido	<5	—	—	—	1	5	1
other (<5%)	abnormal coordination, abnormal dreaming, abnormal gait, abnormal thinking, aggravated depression, aggressive reaction, agitation, apathy, aphasia, ataxia, CNS dysfunction, coma, convulsions, dysphoria, emotional lability, extrapyramidal disorder, feeling of ebriety, flushing, hearing disorder, hot flashes, hyperesthesia, hyperkinesia, hypertonia, hypokinesia, impaired consciousness, migraine, neuropathy, neurosis, paresis, paroniria, parosmia, personality disorder, polyneuropathy, speech disorder, suicide attempt, syncope, tinnitus, tremor, vertigo						
Reproduction System Disorders (<5%)	amenorrhea, impotence, leukorrhea, menorrhagia, uterine bleeding						
Resistance Mechanism Disorders							
moniliasis	—	<1	—	17	—	—	—
herpes simplex	—	1	—	3	—	5	—
other (<5%)	abscess, conjunctivitis, sepsis, stye						

Continued on next page

Information on Schering products appearing on these pages is effective as of August 15, 1992.

TREATMENT-RELATED ADVERSE EXPERIENCES BY INDICATION
Dosing Regimens
Percentage (%) of Patients*

ADVERSE EXPERIENCE	HAIRY CELL LEUKEMIA 2 million IU/m² TIW/SC N=145	CONDYLOMATA ACUMINATA 1 million IU/ lesion N=352	AIDS-RELATED KAPOSI'S SARCOMA 30 million IU/m² TIW/SC N=74	35 million IU/QD/SC N=29	CHRONIC HEPATITIS NANB/C 3 million IU TIW N=159	CHRONIC HEPATITIS B 5 million IU QD N=101	10 million IU TIW N=78
Respiratory System Disorders							
dyspnea	<1	—	1	34	<1	5	—
coughing	<1	—	—	31	<1	4	—
pharyngitis	<5	1	1	31	1	7	1
sinusitis	—	—	—	21	—	—	—
nonproductive coughing	—	—	—	14	—	1	—
nasal congestion	—	1	—	10	—	4	—
other (<5%)	bronchospasm, cyanosis, epistaxis, pleural pain, pneumonia, sneezing, wheezing						
Skin and Appendages Disorders							
dermatitis	8	—	—	—	—	1	—
alopecia	8	—	12	31	17	26	38
pruritus	11	1	7	—	6	6	4
rash	25	—	9	10	6	8	1
dry skin	9	—	9	10	<1	3	—
other (<5%)	abnormal hair texture, acne, cyanosis of the hand, cold and clammy skin, dermatitis lichenoides, epidermal necrolysis, erythema, furunculosis, increased hair growth, lacrimal gland disorder, melanosis, nail disorders, nonherpetic cold sores, peripheral ischemia, photosensitivity, purpura, skin depigmentation, skin discoloration, urticaria, vitiligo						
Urinary System Disorders (<5%)	increased BUN, hematuria, micturition disorder, micturition frequency, nocturia, polyuria						
Vision Disorders (<5%)	abnormal vision, blurred vision, diplopia, dry eyes, eye pain, photophobia						

* Dash (—) indicates not reported

Of these adverse reactions, those classified as severe (World Health Organization grade 3 or 4) were reported in 27% to 55% of patients. Severe adverse reactions in the 30 million IU/m² TIW study included: fatigue (20%), influenza-like symptoms (15%), anorexia (12%), dry mouth (4%), headache (4%), confusion (3%), fever (3%), myalgia (3%), and nausea and vomiting (1% each). Severe adverse reactions for patients who received the 35 million IU QD included: fever (24%), fatigue (17%), influenza-like symptoms (14%), dyspnea (14%), headache (10%), pharyngitis (7%), and ataxia, confusion, dysphagia, GI hemorrhage, abnormal hepatic function, increased SGOT, myalgia, cardiomyopathy, face edema, depression, emotional lability, suicide attempt, chest pain, and coughing (1 patient each). Overall, the incidence of severe toxicity was higher among patients who received the 35 million IU per day dose.

Chronic Hepatitis Non-A, Non-B/C (NANB/C) In patients with chronic hepatitis NANB/C, alopecia, injection site reactions, rash, depression, and irritability apparently increased in incidence with continued treatment; residual mild alopecia persisted posttreatment.

Infrequently, patients receiving INTRON A therapy for chronic hepatitis NANB/C developed thyroid abnormalities, either hypothyroid or hyperthyroid. In clinical trials <1% (4/426) developed thyroid abnormalities. The abnormalities were controlled by conventional therapy for thyroid dysfunction. The mechanism by which INTRON A Interferon alfa-2b, recombinant for Injection may alter thyroid status is unknown. Prior to initiation of INTRON A therapy for the treatment of chronic hepatitis NANB/C, serum TSH should be evaluated. Patients developing symptoms consistent with possible thyroid dysfunction during the course of INTRON A therapy should have their thyroid function evaluated and appropriate treatment instituted. INTRON A treatment may be continued if TSH levels can be maintained in the normal range by medication. Discontinuation of INTRON A therapy has not always reversed thyroid dysfunction occurring during treatment.

Chronic Hepatitis B In patients with chronic hepatitis B, some type of adverse reaction occurred in 98% of the 101 patients treated at 5 million IU, QD and 90% of the 78 patients treated at 10 million IU, TIW. Most of these adverse reactions were mild to moderate in severity, were manageable, and were reversible following the end of therapy.

Adverse reactions classified as severe (causing a significant interference with normal daily activities or clinical state) were reported in 21% to 44% of patients. The severe adverse reactions reported most frequently were the flu-like symptoms of fever (28%), fatigue (15%), headache (5%), myalgia (4%), and rigors (4%), and other severe flu-like symptoms which occurred in 1% to 3% of patients. Other severe adverse reactions occurring in more than one patient were alopecia (8%), anorexia (6%), depression (3%), nausea (3%), and vomiting (2%).

To manage side effects, the dose was reduced, or INTRON A therapy was interrupted in 25% to 38% of patients. Five percent of patients discontinued treatment due to adverse experiences. [See table below.]

HOW SUPPLIED

INTRON A Interferon alfa-2b, recombinant for Injection, 3 million IU per vial and Diluent for INTRON A Interferon alfa-2b, recombinant for Injection (bacteriostatic water for injection) 1 mL per vial or syringe; boxes containing 1 INTRON A vial and 1 vial of Diluent for INTRON A Interferon alfa-2b, recombinant for Injection (bacteriostatic water for injection) (NDC 0085-0647-03), boxes containing 1 INTRON A vial and 1 syringe of Diluent for INTRON A Interferon alfa-2b, recombinant for Injection (bacteriostatic water for injection) (NDC 0085-0647-04).

INTRON A Interferon alfa-2b, recombinant for Injection INTRON® A, Pak-3, containing 6 INTRON A vials, 3 million IU per vial, and 6 syringes of Diluent for INTRON A Interferon alfa-2b, recombinant for Injection (bacteriostatic water for injection) for Chronic Hepatitis Non-A, Non-B/C (NDC 0085-0647-05).

INTRON A Interferon alfa-2b, recombinant for Injection, 5 million IU per vial and Diluent for INTRON A Interferon alfa-2b, recombinant for Injection (bacteriostatic water for injection) 1 mL per vial or syringe; boxes containing 1 INTRON A vial and 1 vial of Diluent for INTRON A Interferon alfa-2b, recombinant for Injection (bacteriostatic water for injection) (NDC 0085-0120-02), boxes containing 1 INTRON A vial and 1 syringe of Diluent for INTRON A Interferon alfa-2b, recombinant for Injection (bacteriostatic water for injection) (NDC 0085-0120-03).

INTRON A Interferon alfa-2b, recombinant for Injection INTRON® A, Pak-5, containing 14 INTRON A vials, 5 million IU per vial, and 14 syringes of Diluent for INTRON A Interferon alfa-2b, recombinant for Injection (bacteriostatic water for injection) for Chronic Hepatitis B (NDC 0085-0120-04).

ABNORMAL LABORATORY TEST VALUES BY INDICATION
Dosing Regimens
Percentage (%) of Patients

Laboratory Tests	HAIRY CELL LEUKEMIA 2 million IU/m² TIW/SC N=145	CONDYLOMATA ACUMINATA 1 million IU lesion N=352	AIDS-RELATED KAPOSI'S SARCOMA 30 million IU/m² TIW/SC N=69-73	35 million IU/QD/SC N=26-28	CHRONIC HEPATITIS NANB/C 3 million IU TIW N=87-158	CHRONIC HEPATITIS B 5 million IU QD N=96-101	10 million IU TIW N=75-103
Hemoglobin	NA	—	1%	15%	15%	32%*	23%*
White Blood Cell Count	NA	17%	10%	22%	18%	68%†	34%†
Platelet Count	NA	—	0%	8%	9%	12%‡	5%‡
Serum Creatinine	0%	—	—	—	2%	3%	0%
Alkaline Phosphatase	4%	—	—	—	3%	8%	4%
Lactate Dehydrogenase	0%	—	—	—	—	—	—
Serum Urea Nitrogen	0%	—	—	—	1%	—	—
SGOT	4%	12%	11%	41%	—	—	—
SGPT	13%	—	10%	15%	—	—	—
Granulocyte Count							
• Total	NA	—	31%	39%	37%§	71%§	61%§
• 1000 – <1500/mm³	—	—	—	—	—	31%	32%
• 750 – <1000/mm³	—	—	—	—	—	23%	18%
• 500 – <750/mm³	—	—	—	—	—	15%	9%
• <500/mm³	—	—	—	—	—	2%	2%

NA—Not Applicable—Patients' initial hematologic laboratory test values were abnormal due to their condition.
* Decrease of ≥ 2 g/dL
† Decrease to < 3000/mm³
‡ Decrease to < 70,000/mm³
§ Neutrophils plus bands

Schering—Cont.

INTRON A Interferon alfa-2b, recombinant for Injection, 10 million IU per vial and Diluent for INTRON A Interferon alfa-2b, recombinant for Injection (bacteriostatic water for injection) 2 mL per vial; boxes containing 1 INTRON A vial and 1 vial of Diluent for INTRON A Interferon alfa-2b, recombinant for Injection (bacteriostatic water for injection) (NDC 0085-0571-02).

INTRON A Interferon alfa-2b, recombinant for Injection INTRON® A, Pak-10, containing 6 INTRON A vials, 10 million IU per vial, and 6 syringes of Diluent for INTRON A Interferon alfa-2b, recombinant for Injection (bacteriostatic water for injection) for Chronic Hepatitis B (NDC 0085-0571-06).

INTRON A Interferon alfa-2b, recombinant for Injection, 18 million IU multidose vial and Diluent for INTRON A Interferon alfa-2b, recombinant for Injection (bacteriostatic water for injection) 3.8 mL per vial; boxes containing 1 multidose vial of INTRON A Interferon alfa-2b, recombinant for Injection and 1 vial of Diluent for INTRON A Interferon alfa-2b, recombinant for Injection (bacteriostatic water for injection) (NDC 0085-0689-01).

INTRON A Interferon alfa-2b, recombinant for Injection, 25 million IU per vial and Diluent for INTRON A Interferon alfa-2b, recombinant for Injection (bacteriostatic water for injection) 5 mL per vial; boxes containing 1 INTRON A vial and 1 vial of Diluent for INTRON A Interferon alfa-2b, recombinant for Injection (bacteriostatic water for injection) (NDC 0085-0285-02).

INTRON A Interferon alfa-2b, recombinant for Injection, 50 million IU per vial and Diluent for INTRON A Interferon alfa-2b, recombinant for Injection (bacteriostatic water for injection) 1 mL per vial; boxes containing 1 INTRON A vial and 1 vial of Diluent for INTRON A Interferon alfa-2b, recombinant for Injection (bacteriostatic water for injection) (NDC 0085-0539-01).

Store INTRON A Interferon alfa-2b, recombinant for Injection both before and after reconstitution between 2° and 8°C (36° and 46°F).

REFERENCES

1. Davis G, et al. *N Engl J Med.* 1989;321:1501–1506.
2. Causse X, et al. *Gastroenterology.* 1991;101:497–502.
3. Marcellin P, et al. *Hepatology.* 1991;13:393–397.
4. Knodell R, et al. *Hepatology.* 1981;1:431–435.
5. Perrillo R, et al. *N Engl J Med.* 1990;323:295–301.
6. Perez V, et al. *J Hepatol.* 1990; 11:S113–S117.
7. Perrillo R, et al. *Ann Intern Med.* 1991;115:113–115.
8. Renault P, et al. *Arch Intern Med.* 1987;147:1577–1580.
9. Kauppila A, et al. *Int J Cancer.* 1982;29:291–294.

Schering Corporation
Kenilworth, NJ 07033 USA

Revised 5/92 B-17374303
U.S. Patents 4,530,901 & 4,496,537
Copyright © 1986, 1988, 1991, 1992, Schering Corporation, Kenilworth, NJ 07033. All rights reserved.

LOTRIMIN® ℞

[lo 'trim-in]
brand of clotrimazole
Cream, USP 1%*
Lotion, USP 1%*
Topical Solution, USP 1%*
For Dermatologic Use Only—
Not For Ophthalmic Use
***These preparations are also available without a prescription as LOTRIMIN AF.**

DESCRIPTION

LOTRIMIN products contain clotrimazole, USP, a synthetic antifungal agent having the chemical name [1-(*o*-Chloro-α,α-diphenylbenzyl)imidazole]; the empirical formula, $C_{22}H_{17}ClN_2$; and a molecular weight of 344.84.

Clotrimazole is an odorless, white crystalline substance. It is practically insoluble in water, sparingly soluble in ether and very soluble in polyethylene glycol 400, ethanol and chloroform.

Each gram of LOTRIMIN **Cream** contains 10 mg clotrimazole, USP in a vanishing cream base of benzyl alcohol, cetearyl alcohol, cetyl esters wax, octyldodecanol, polysorbate, sorbitan monostearate, and water.

Each gram of LOTRIMIN **Lotion** contains 10 mg clotrimazole, USP dispersed in an emulsion vehicle composed of benzyl alcohol, cetearyl alcohol, cetyl esters wax, octyldodecanol, polysorbate, sodium phosphate, sorbitan monostearate, and water.

Each mL of LOTRIMIN **Topical Solution** contains 10 mg clotrimazole, USP in a nonaqueous vehicle of PEG.

CLINICAL PHARMACOLOGY

Clotrimazole is a broad-spectrum antifungal agent that is used for the treatment of dermal infections caused by various species of pathogenic dermatophytes, yeasts, and *Malassezia furfur.* The primary action of clotrimazole is against dividing and growing organisms.

In vitro, clotrimazole exhibits fungistatic and fungicidal activity against isolates of *Trichophyton rubrum, Trichophyton mentagrophytes, Epidermophyton floccosum, Microsporum canis,* and *Candida* species, including *Candida albicans.* In general, the *in vitro* activity of clotrimazole corresponds to that of tolnaftate and griseofulvin against the mycelia of dermatophytes (*Trichophyton, Microsporum,* and *Epidermophyton*), and to that of the polyenes (amphotericin B and nystatin) against budding fungi (*Candida*). Using an *in vivo* (mouse) and an *in vitro* (mouse kidney homogenate) testing system, clotrimazole and miconazole were equally effective in preventing the growth of the pseudomycelia and mycelia of *Candida albicans.*

Strains of fungi having a natural resistance to clotrimazole are rare. Only a single isolate of *Candida guilliermondi* has been reported to have primary resistance to clotrimazole.

No single-step or multiple-step resistance to clotrimazole has developed during successive passages of *Candida albicans* and *Trichophyton mentagrophytes.* No appreciable change in sensitivity was detected after successive passages of isolates of *C. albicans, C. krusei,* or *C. pseudotropicalis* in liquid or solid media containing clotrimazole. Also, resistance could not be developed in chemically induced mutant strains of polyene-resistant isolates of *C. albicans.* Slight, reversible resistance was noted in three isolates of *C. albicans* tested by one investigator. There is a single report that records the clinical emergence of a *C. albicans* strain with considerable resistance to flucytosine and miconazole, and with cross-resistance to clotrimazole; the strain remained sensitive to nystatin and amphotericin B.

In studies of the mechanism of action, the minimum fungicidal concentration of clotrimazole caused leakage of intracellular phosphorus compounds into the ambient medium with concomitant breakdown of cellular nucleic acids and accelerated potassium efflux. Both these events began rapidly and extensively after addition of the drug.

Clotrimazole appears to be well absorbed in humans following oral administration and is eliminated mainly as inactive metabolites. Following topical and vaginal administration, however, clotrimazole appears to be minimally absorbed.

Six hours after the application of radioactive clotrimazole 1% cream and 1% solution onto intact and acutely inflamed skin, the concentration of clotrimazole varied from 100 mcg/cm^3 in the stratum corneum to 0.5 to 1 mcg/cm^3 in the stratum reticulare, and 0.1 mcg/cm^3 in the subcutis. No measurable amount of radioactivity ($\leq$0.001 mcg/ml) was found in the serum within 48 hours after application under occlusive dressing of 0.5 ml of the solution or 0.8 g of the cream. Only 0.5% or less of the applied radioactivity was excreted in the urine.

Following intravaginal administration of 100 mg ^{14}C-clotrimazole vaginal tablets to nine adult females, an average peak serum level, corresponding to only 0.03 μg equivalents/ml of clotrimazole, was reached one to two days after application. After intravaginal administration of 5 g of 1% ^{14}C-clotrimazole vaginal cream containing 50 mg active drug, to five subjects (one with candidal colpitis), serum levels corresponding to approximately 0.01 μg equivalents/ml were reached between 8 and 24 hours after application.

INDICATIONS AND USAGE

Prescription LOTRIMIN (clotrimazole cream, lotion and solution 1%) products are indicated for the topical treatment of candidiasis due to *Candida albicans* and tinea versicolor due to *Malassezia furfur.*

These formulations are also available as the LOTRIMIN AF (clotrimazole cream, lotion and solution 1%) line of nonprescription products which are indicated for the topical treatment of the following dermal infections: tinea pedis, tinea cruris, and tinea corporis due to *Trichophyton rubrum, Trichophyton mentagrophytes, Epidermophyton floccosum,* and *Microsporum canis.*

CONTRAINDICATIONS

LOTRIMIN products are contraindicated in individuals who have shown hypersensitivity to any of their components.

WARNINGS

LOTRIMIN products are not for ophthalmic use.

PRECAUTIONS

General: If irritation or sensitivity develops with the use of clotrimazole, treatment should be discontinued and appropriate therapy instituted.

Information For Patients:
This information is intended to aid in the safe and effective use of this medication. It is not a disclosure of all possible adverse or intended effects.
The patient should be advised to:

1. Use the medication for the full treatment time even though the symptoms may have improved. Notify the physician if there is no improvement after four weeks of treatment.
2. Inform the physician if the area of application shows signs of increased irritation (redness, itching, burning, blistering, swelling, oozing) indicative of possible sensitization.
3. Avoid sources of infection or reinfection.

Laboratory Tests: If there is lack of response to clotrimazole, appropriate microbiological studies should be repeated to confirm the diagnosis and rule out other pathogens before instituting another course of antimycotic therapy.

Drug Interactions: Synergism or antagonism between clotrimazole and nystatin, or amphotericin B, or flucytosine against strains of *C. albicans* has not been reported.

Carcinogenesis, Mutagenesis, Impairment of Fertility: An 18-month oral dosing study with clotrimazole in rats has not revealed any carcinogenic effect.

In tests for mutagenesis, chromosomes of the spermatophores of Chinese hamsters which had been exposed to clotrimazole were examined for structural changes during the metaphase. Prior to testing, the hamsters had received five oral clotrimazole doses of 100 mg/kg body weight. The results of this study showed that clotrimazole had no mutagenic effect.

Usage in Pregnancy: Pregnancy Category B: The disposition of ^{14}C-clotrimazole has been studied in humans and animals. Clotrimazole is very poorly absorbed following dermal application or intravaginal administration to humans. (See **Clinical Pharmacology.**)

In clinical trials, use of vaginally applied clotrimazole in pregnant women in their second and third trimesters has not been associated with ill effects. There are, however, no adequate and well-controlled studies in pregnant women during the first trimester of pregnancy.

Studies in pregnant rats with intravaginal doses up to 100 mg/kg have revealed no evidence of harm to the fetus due to clotrimazole.

High oral doses of clotrimazole in rats and mice ranging from 50 to 120 mg/kg resulted in embryotoxicity (possibly secondary to maternal toxicity), impairment of mating, decreased litter size and number of viable young and decreased pup survival to weaning. However, clotrimazole was not teratogenic in mice, rabbits and rats at oral doses up to 200, 180 and 100 mg/kg, respectively. Oral absorption in the rat amounts to approximately 90% of the administered dose.

Because animal reproduction studies are not always predictive of human response, this drug should be used only if clearly indicated during the first trimester of pregnancy.

Nursing Mothers: It is not known whether this drug is excreted in human milk. Because many drugs are excreted in human milk, caution should be exercised when clotrimazole is used by a nursing woman.

Pediatric Use: Safety and effectiveness in children have been established for clotrimazole when used as indicated and in the recommended dosage.

ADVERSE REACTIONS

The following adverse reactions have been reported in connection with the use of clotrimazole: erythema, stinging, blistering, peeling, edema, pruritus, urticaria, burning, and general irritation of the skin.

OVERDOSAGE

Acute overdosage with topical application of clotrimazole is unlikely and would not be expected to lead to a life-threatening situation.

DOSAGE AND ADMINISTRATION

Gently massage sufficient LOTRIMIN into the affected and surrounding skin areas twice a day, in the morning and evening.

Clinical improvement, with relief of pruritus, usually occurs within the first week of treatment with LOTRIMIN. If the patient shows no clinical improvement after four weeks of treatment with LOTRIMIN, the diagnosis should be reviewed.

HOW SUPPLIED

LOTRIMIN Cream 1% is supplied in 15, 30, 45 and 90-g tubes (NDC 0085-0613-02, 05, 04, 03, respectively); boxes of one.
LOTRIMIN Lotion 1% is supplied in 30 ml bottles (NDC 0085-0707-02); boxes of one.
Shake well before using.
LOTRIMIN Solution 1% is supplied in 10 ml and 30 ml plastic bottles (NDC 0085-0182-02, 04, respectively); boxes of one.
Store LOTRIMIN products between 2° and 30°C (36° and 86°F).
Copyright © 1984, 1991, Schering Corporation, USA.
All rights reserved.
Revised 5/91

Continued on next page

Information on Schering products appearing on these pages is effective as of August 15, 1992.

Schering—Cont.

LOTRISONE®   ℞
[lō'trĭ-sōn]
**brand of clotrimazole
and betamethasone
dipropionate
Cream, USP**

**For Dermatologic Use Only—
Not for Ophthalmic Use**

DESCRIPTION

LOTRISONE Cream contains a combination of clotrimazole, USP, a synthetic antifungal agent, and betamethasone dipropionate, USP, a synthetic corticosteroid, for dermatologic use.

Chemically, clotrimazole is 1-(o-Chloro-α,α-diphenyl benzyl) imidazole, with the empirical formula $C_{22}H_{17}ClN_2$ and a molecular weight of 344.8.

Clotrimazole is an odorless, white crystalline powder, insoluble in water and soluble in ethanol.

Betamethasone dipropionate has the chemical name 9-Fluoro-11β, 17,21-trihydroxy-16β-methylpregna-1,4-diene-3,20-dione 17,21-dipropionate, with the empirical formula $C_{28}H_{37}FO_7$ and a molecular weight of 504.6.

Betamethasone dipropionate is a white to creamy white, odorless crystalline powder, insoluble in water.

Each gram of LOTRISONE Cream contains 10.0 mg clotrimazole, USP, and 0.64 mg betamethasone dipropionate, USP (equivalent to 0.5 mg betamethasone), in a hydrophilic emollient cream consisting of purified water, mineral oil, white petrolatum, cetearyl alcohol, ceteareth-30, propylene glycol, sodium phosphate monobasic, and phosphoric acid; benzyl alcohol as preservative.

LOTRISONE is a smooth, uniform, white to off-white cream.

CLINICAL PHARMACOLOGY

Clotrimazole

Clotrimazole is a broad-spectrum, antifungal agent that is used for the treatment of dermal infections caused by various species of pathogenic dermatophytes, yeasts, and *Malassezia furfur*. The primary action of clotrimazole is against dividing and growing organisms.

In vitro, clotrimazole exhibits fungistatic and fungicidal activity against isolates of *Trichophyton rubrum, Trichophyton mentagrophytes, Epidermophyton floccosum* and *Microsporum canis*. In general, the *in vitro* activity of clotrimazole corresponds to that of tolnaftate and griseofulvin against the mycelia of dermatophytes (*Trichophyton, Microsporum,* and *Epidermophyton*).

In vivo studies in guinea pigs infected with *Trichophyton mentagrophytes* have shown no measurable loss of clotrimazole activity due to combination with betamethasone dipropionate.

Strains of fungi having a natural resistance to clotrimazole have not been reported.

No single-step or multiple-step resistance to clotrimazole has developed during successive passages of *Trichophyton mentagrophytes*.

In studies of the mechanism of action in fungal cultures, the minimum fungicidal concentration of clotrimazole caused leakage of intracellular phosphorous compounds into the ambient medium with concomitant breakdown of cellular nucleic acids, and accelerated potassium efflux. Both of these events began rapidly and extensively after addition of the drug to the cultures.

Clotrimazole appears to be minimally absorbed following topical application to the skin. Six hours after the application of radioactive clotrimazole 1% cream and 1% solution onto intact and acutely inflamed skin, the concentration of clotrimazole varied from 100 mcg/cm³ in the stratum corneum, to 0.5 to 1 mcg/cm³ in the stratum reticulare, and 0.1 mcg/cm³ in the subcutis. No measureable amount of radioactivity (<0.001 mcg/ml) was found in the serum within 48 hours after application under occlusive dressing of 0.5 ml of the solution or 0.8 g of the cream.

Betamethasone dipropionate

Betamethasone dipropionate, a corticosteroid, is effective in the treatment of corticosteroid-responsive dermatoses primarily because of its anti-inflammatory, antipruritic, and vasoconstrictive actions. However, while the physiologic, pharmacologic, and clinical effects of corticosteroids are well-known, the exact mechanisms of their actions in each disease are uncertain. Betamethasone dipropionate, a corticosteroid, has been shown to have topical (dermatologic) and systemic pharmacologic and metabolic effects characteristic of this class of drugs.

Pharmacokinetics: The extent of percutaneous absorption of topical corticosteroids is determined by many factors including the vehicle, the integrity of the epidermal barrier, and the use of occlusive dressings. (See **Dosage and Administration** section.)

Topical corticosteroids can be absorbed from normal intact skin. Inflammation and/or other disease processes in the skin increase percutaneous absorption. Occlusive dressings substantially increase the percutaneous absorption of topical corticosteroids. (See **Dosage and Administration** section.)

Once absorbed through the skin, topical corticosteroids are handled through pharmacokinetic pathways similar to systemically administered corticosteroids. Corticosteroids are bound to plasma proteins in varying degrees. Corticosteroids are metabolized primarily in the liver and are then excreted by the kidneys. Some of the topical corticosteroids and their metabolities are also excreted into the bile.

Clotrimazole and betamethasone dipropionate

In clinical studies of tinea corporis, tinea cruris and tinea pedis, patients treated with LOTRISONE Cream showed a better clinical response at the first return visit than patients treated with clotrimazole cream. In tinea corporis and tinea cruris, the patient returned three days after starting treatment, and in tinea pedis, after one week. Mycological cure rates observed in patients treated with LOTRISONE Cream were as good as or better than in those patients treated with clotrimazole cream.

In these same clinical studies, patients treated with LOTRISONE Cream showed statistically significantly better clinical responses and mycological cure rates when compared with patients treated with betamethasone dipropionate cream.

INDICATIONS AND USAGE

LOTRISONE Cream is indicated for the topical treatment of the following dermal infections: tinea pedis, tinea cruris, and tinea corporis due to *Trichophyton rubrum, Trichophyton mentagrophytes, Epidermophyton floccosum,* and *Microsporum canis*.

CONTRAINDICATIONS

LOTRISONE Cream is contraindicated in patients who are sensitive to clotrimazole, betamethasone dipropionate, other corticosteroids or imidazoles, or to any ingredient in this preparation.

PRECAUTIONS

General: Systemic absorption of topical corticosteroids has produced reversible hypothalamic-pituitary-adrenal (HPA) axis suppression, manifestations of Cushing's syndrome, hyperglycemia, and glucosuria in some patients.

Conditions which augment systemic absorption include the application of the more potent steroids, use over large surface areas, prolonged use, and the addition of occlusive dressings. (See **Dosage and Administration** section.)

Therefore, patients receiving a large dose of a potent topical steroid applied to a large surface area should be evaluated periodically for evidence of HPA axis suppression by using the urinary free cortisol and ACTH stimulation tests. If HPA axis suppression is noted, an attempt should be made to withdraw the drug, to reduce the frequency of application, or to substitute a less potent steroid.

Recovery of HPA axis function is generally prompt and complete upon discontinuation of the drug. Infrequently, signs and symptoms of steroid withdrawal may occur, requiring supplemental systemic corticosteroids.

Children may absorb proportionally larger amounts of topical corticosteroids and thus be more susceptible to systemic toxicity. (See **Precautions-Pediatric Use.**)

If irritation or hypersensitivity develops with the use of LOTRISONE Cream, treatment should be discontinued and appropriate therapy instituted.

Information for Patients Patients using LOTRISONE Cream should receive the following information and instructions:

1. This medication is to be used as directed by the physician. It is for external use only. Avoid contact with the eyes.
2. The medication is to be used for the full prescribed treatment time, even though the symptoms may have improved. Notify the physician if there is no improvement after one week of treatment for tinea cruris or tinea corporis, or after two weeks for tinea pedis.
3. Patients should be advised not to use this medication for any disorder other than for which it was prescribed.
4. The treated skin areas should not be bandaged or otherwise covered or wrapped as to be occluded. (See **Dosage and Administration** section.)
5. When using this medication in the groin area, patients should be advised to use the medication for two weeks only, and to apply the cream sparingly. The physician should be notified if the condition persists after two weeks. Patients should also be advised to wear loose fitting clothing. (See **Dosage and Administration** section.)
6. Patients should report any signs of local adverse reactions.
7. Patients should avoid sources of infection or reinfection.

Laboratory Tests: If there is a lack of response to LOTRISONE Cream, appropriate microbiological studies should be repeated to confirm the diagnosis and rule out other pathogens before instituting another course of antimycotic therapy.

The following tests may be helpful in evaluating HPA axis suppression due to the corticosteroid component:

Urinary free cortisol test
ACTH stimulation test

Carcinogenesis, Mutagenesis, Impairment of Fertility: There are no animal or laboratory studies with the combination clotrimazole and betamethasone dipropionate to evaluate carcinogenesis, mutagenesis or impairment of fertility.

An 18-month oral dosing study with clotrimazole in rats has not revealed any carcinogenic effect.

In tests for mutagenesis, chromosomes of the spermatophores of Chinese hamsters which have been exposed to clotrimazole were examined for structural changes during the metaphase. Prior to testing, the hamsters had received five oral clotrimazole doses of 100 mg/kg body weight. The results of this study showed that clotrimazole had no mutagenic effect.

Pregnancy Category C: There have been no teratogenic studies performed with the combination clotrimazole and betamethasone dipropionate.

Studies in pregnant rats with intravaginal doses up to 100 mg/kg have revealed no evidence of harm to the fetus due to clotrimazole.

High oral doses of clotrimazole in rats and mice ranging from 50 to 120 mg/kg resulted in embryotoxicity (possibly secondary to maternal toxicity), impairment of mating, decreased litter size and number of viable young and decreased pup survival to weaning. However, clotrimazole was not teratogenic in mice, rabbits and rats at oral doses up to 200, 180 and 100 mg/kg, respectively. Oral absorption in the rat amounts to approximately 90% of the administered dose.

Corticosteroids are generally teratogenic in laboratory animals when administered systemically at relatively low dosage levels. The more potent corticosteroids have been shown to be teratogenic after dermal application in laboratory animals.

There are no adequate and well-controlled studies in pregnant women on teratogenic effects from a topically applied combination of clotrimazole and betamethasone dipropionate. Therefore, LOTRISONE Cream should be used during pregnancy only if the potential benefit justifies the potential risk to the fetus.

Drugs containing corticosteroids should not be used extensively on pregnant patients, in large amounts, or for prolonged periods of time.

Nursing Mothers: It is not known whether this drug is excreted in human milk. Because many drugs are excreted in human milk, caution should be exercised when LOTRISONE Cream is used by a nursing woman.

Pediatric Use: Safety and effectiveness in children below the age of 12 have not been established with LOTRISONE Cream.

Pediatric patients may demonstrate greater susceptibility to topical corticosteroid-induced HPA axis suppression and Cushing's syndrome than mature patients because of a larger skin surface area to body weight ratio.

Hypothalamic-pituitary-adrenal (HPA) axis suppression, Cushing's syndrome, and intracranial hypertension have been reported in children receiving topical corticosteroids. Manifestations of adrenal suppression in children include linear growth retardation, delayed weight gain, low plasma cortisol levels, and absence of response to ACTH stimulation. Manifestations of intracranial hypertension include bulging fontanelles, headaches, and bilateral papilledema.

Administration of topical dermatologics containing a corticosteroid to children should be limited to the least amount compatible with an effective therapeutic regimen. Chronic corticosteroid therapy may interfere with the growth and development of children.

The use of LOTRISONE Cream in diaper dermatitis is not recommended.

ADVERSE REACTIONS

The following adverse reactions have been reported in connection with the use of LOTRISONE Cream: paresthesia in 5 of 270 patients, maculopapular rash, edema, and secondary infection, each in 1 of 270 patients.

Adverse reactions reported with the use of clotrimazole are as follows: erythema, stinging, blistering, peeling, edema, pruritus, urticaria, and general irritation of the skin.

The following local adverse reactions are reported infrequently when topical corticosteroids are used as recommended. These reactions are listed in an approximate decreasing order of occurrence: burning, itching, irritation, dryness, folliculitis, hypertrichosis, acneiform eruptions, hypopigmentation, perioral dermatitis, allergic contact dermatitis, maceration of the skin, secondary infection, skin atrophy, striae, and miliaria.

OVERDOSAGE

Acute overdosage with topical application of LOTRISONE Cream is unlikely and would not be expected to lead to a life-threatening situation.

Topically applied corticosteroids can be absorbed in sufficient amounts to produce systemic effects. (See **Precautions.**)

DOSAGE AND ADMINISTRATION

Gently massage sufficient LOTRISONE Cream into the affected and surrounding skin areas twice a day, in the morning and evening for two weeks in tinea cruris and tinea corporis, and for four weeks in tinea pedis. The use of LOTRISONE Cream for longer than four weeks is not recommended.

Clinical improvement, with relief of erythema and pruritus, usually occurs within three to five days of treatment. If a patient with tinea cruris and tinea corporis shows no clinical improvement after one week of treatment with LOTRISONE Cream, the diagnosis should be reviewed. In tinea pedis, the treatment should be applied for two weeks prior to making that decision.

Treatment with LOTRISONE Cream should be discontinued if the condition persists after two weeks in tinea cruris and tinea corporis, and after four weeks in tinea pedis. Alternate therapy may then be instituted with LOTRIMIN Cream, a product containing an antifungal only.

LOTRISONE Cream should not be used with occlusive dressings.

HOW SUPPLIED

LOTRISONE Cream is supplied in 15-gram (NDC 0085-0924-01), and 45-gram tubes (NDC 0085-0924-02); boxes of one.

Store between 2° and 30°C (36° and 86°F).

Revised 1/90

Copyright © 1984, 1986, 1989, 1990 Schering Corporation, USA. All rights reserved.

NETROMYCIN® ℞
brand of netilmicin sulfate
Injection, USP 100 mg/ml

WARNINGS

Patients treated with aminoglycosides should be under close clinical observation because of the potential toxicity associated with the use of these drugs.

Netilmicin has potent neuromuscular blocking potential. Neuromuscular blockade and respiratory paralysis have been reported in animals receiving netilmicin. The possibility of these phenomena occurring in man should be considered if aminoglycosides are administered by any route to patients receiving neuromuscular blocking agents, such as succinylcholine, tubocurarine, or decamethonium, or to patients receiving massive transfusions of citrate-anticoagulated blood. If neuromuscular blockade occurs, calcium salts may lessen it, but mechanical respiratory assistance may also be necessary.

As with other aminoglycosides, netilmicin sulfate injection is potentially nephrotoxic. The risk is greater in patients with impaired renal function, in those who receive high dosage or prolonged therapy, and in the elderly.

Neurotoxicity manifested by ototoxicity, both vestibular and auditory, can occur in patients treated with netilmicin, primarily in those with preexisting renal damage and in patients treated with higher doses and/or for longer periods than recommended. Aminoglycoside-induced ototoxicity is usually irreversible. Other manifestations of aminoglycoside-induced neurotoxicity include numbness, skin tingling, muscle twitching, and convulsions.

Renal and eighth cranial nerve functions should be closely monitored, especially in patients with known or suspected impairment of renal function either at onset of therapy or during therapy. Urine should be examined for increased excretion of protein, the presence of cells or casts, and decreased specific gravity. Serum creatinine concentration or blood urea nitrogen should be determined periodically. A more precise measure of glomerular filtration rate is a carefully conducted determination of creatinine clearance rate or, often more practically, an estimate of creatinine clearance based on published nomograms or equations. (See **DOSAGE AND ADMINISTRATION**.) When feasible it is recommended that serial audiograms be obtained in patients old enough to be tested, particularly in high-risk patients. The dosage of netilmicin should be reduced or administration discontinued if evidence of drug-induced auditory or vestibular toxicity (dizziness, vertigo, tinnitus, nystagmus, or hearing loss) develops during therapy. If evidence of nephrotoxicity occurs, dosage should be adjusted. (See **DOSAGE AND ADMINISTRATION, DOSAGE FOR IMPAIRED RENAL FUNCTION**.) As with the other aminoglycosides, on rare occasions changes in renal and eighth cranial nerve functions may not become manifest until soon after completion of therapy.

Serum concentrations of aminoglycosides should be monitored when feasible to assure adequate levels and to avoid potentially toxic levels. After administration of an appropriate dose of netilmicin, peak serum concentrations occur approximately 30 to 60 minutes after an intramuscular injection or at the end of a one hour intravenous infusion. Dosage should be adjusted so that prolonged peak serum concentrations above 16 mcg/ml are avoided.

When monitoring trough concentrations, dosage should be adjusted so that levels above 4 mcg/ml are avoided. Excessive peak and/or trough serum concentrations of aminoglycosides may increase the risk of renal and eighth cranial nerve toxicity. In the event of overdose or toxic reactions, hemodialysis may aid in removal of netilmicin from the blood, especially if renal function is, or becomes, compromised. Removal of netilmicin by peritoneal dialysis is at a rate considerably less than by hemodialysis.

Concurrent and/or sequential systemic or topical use of other potentially neurotoxic and/or nephrotoxic drugs, such as: cephaloridine, amphotericin B, streptomycin, kanamycin, acyclovir, gentamicin, tobramycin, amikacin, neomycin, vancomycin, bacitracin, polymixin B, colistin, paromomycin, viomycin, or cisplatin should be avoided. The concurrent use of aminoglycosides with potent diuretics, such as ethacrynic acid or furosemide, should be avoided since certain diuretics by themselves may cause ototoxicity. In addition, when administered intravenously, diuretics may enhance aminoglycoside toxicity by altering the antibiotic concentration in the serum and tissues. Other factors which may increase patient risk of toxicity are advanced age and dehydration.

DESCRIPTION

NETROMYCIN Injection contains netilmicin sulfate, USP in clear, sterile aqueous solution with a pH range of 3.5 to 6.0 for intramuscular or intravenous administration.

Netilmicin is a semisynthetic, water-soluble antibiotic of the aminoglycoside group, derived from sisomicin. Its chemical name is: *O*-3-Deoxy-4-*C*-methyl-3-(methylamino)-β-L-arabinopyranosyl-(1→4)-*O*-[2,6-diamino-2,3,4,6-tetradeoxy-α-D-*glycero*-hex-4-enopyranosyl-(1→6)]-2-deoxy-N^3-ethyl-L-streptamine sulfate (2:5) (salt).

Each ml of NETROMYCIN Injection contains netilmicin sulfate, USP equivalent to 100 mg netilmicin; 10 mg benzyl alcohol as a preservative; 0.1 mg edetate disodium; 2.4 mg sodium metabisulfite; 0.8 mg sodium sulfite; and water for injection, q.s.

CLINICAL PHARMACOLOGY

Netilmicin is rapidly and completely absorbed after intramuscular injection. Peak serum levels, after intramuscular injection, usually occur within 30 to 60 minutes and levels are measurable for 12 hours. In adult volunteers with normal renal function, peak serum concentrations of netilmicin in mcg/ml are usually about 3 to 3.5 times the single intramuscular dose in mg/kg. For example, a dose of 2.0 mg/kg may be expected to result in a peak serum concentration of approximately 7 mcg/ml. At eight or more hours after administration of a dose in the recommended range, serum levels are usually less than 3 mcg/ml. When a single dose of netilmicin is administered by 60-minute intravenous infusion, the peak serum concentrations are similar to those obtained by intramuscular administration. Following a rapid intravenous injection of netilmicin, levels in serum may be transiently 2 to 3 times higher than those of the 60-minute infusion. Netilmicin rapidly distributes to tissues.

The half-life of netilmicin after single doses is usually 2 to 2.5 hours, a half-life which is very similar to that of gentamicin, and is independent of the route of administration. The half-life increases as the dose increases (e.g., 2.2 hours after a 1 mg/kg dose to 3 hours after a 3 mg/kg dose). Approximately 80% of the administered dose is excreted in the urine within 24 hours; the urine netilmicin concentration after a dose often exceeds 100 mcg/ml. There is no evidence of metabolic transformation of netilmicin. The drug is excreted principally by glomerular filtration. Probenecid does not affect renal tubular transport of aminoglycosides. The volume of distribution of netilmicin is approximately 20% of body weight; total body clearance is about 80 ml/min and renal clearance is about 60 ml/min. In multiple-dose studies in volunteers when the drug was administered every 12 hours at doses ranging from 1.0 to 4.0 mg/kg, steady-state levels were obtained by the second day.

The serum levels at steady-state were less than 20% higher than those of the first dose. As with other aminoglycosides, the half-life of netilmicin increases, and its renal clearance decreases with decreasing renal function.

The endogenous creatinine clearance rate and the serum creatinine level have a high correlation with the half-life of netilmicin. Results of these tests can serve as a guide for adjusting dosage in patients with renal impairment.

In patients with marked impairment of renal function, there is a decrease in the concentration of aminoglycosides in urine and in their penetration into defective renal parenchyma. This should be considered when treating patients with urinary tract infections. In one study of adults with renal failure undergoing hemodialysis, netilmicin serum levels were reduced by approximately 63% over an 8-hour dialysis session. Shorter dialysis sessions will remove less drug. No hemodialysis information is available for children. Aminoglycosides are also removed by peritoneal dialysis but at a rate considerably less than by hemodialysis.

Since netilmicin is distributed in extracellular fluid, peak serum concentrations may be lower than usual in patients whose extracellular fluid volume is expanded (e.g., patients with edema or ascites). Serum concentrations of aminoglycosides in febrile patients may be lower than those in afebrile patients given the same dose. When body temperature returns to normal, serum concentrations of the drug may rise. Both febrile and anemic states may be associated with a shorter than usual half-life. (Dosage adjustment is usually not necessary.)

In severely burned patients, the half-life of aminoglycosides may be significantly decreased, and serum concentrations resulting from a particular dose may be lower than anticipated.

The elimination half-life of netilmicin in neonates during the first week of life is inversely correlated with body weight, ranging from approximately 8 hours for neonates weighing 1.5 to 2.0 kg to approximately 4.5 hours for 3.0 to 4.0 kg neonates. The elimination half-life of infants and children 6 weeks of age and older is 1.5 to 2.0 hours.

Following parenteral administration, aminoglycosides can be detected in serum, tissues, and sputum and in pericardial, pleural, synovial, and peritoneal fluids. A variety of methods are available to measure netilmicin concentrations in body fluids; these include microbiologic, enzymatic, and radioimmunoassay techniques. Concentrations in renal cortex may be markedly higher than the usual serum levels.

Minute quantities of aminoglycosides have been detected in the urine for up to 30 days after discontinuing administration. Hepatic secretion is minimal. As with all aminoglycosides, netilmicin diffuses poorly into the subarachnoid space after parenteral administration. Concentrations of netilmicin in cerebrospinal fluid are often low and dependent upon dose and the degree of meningeal inflammation. Netilmicin crosses the placenta and has been detected in cord blood and in the fetus. Studies in nursing mothers indicate that small amounts of the drug are excreted in breast milk. Netilmicin is poorly absorbed from the intact gastrointestinal tract after oral administration. As with other aminoglycosides, the binding of netilmicin to serum proteins is low (0–30%).

Microbiology: Netilmicin is a rapidly acting, broad-spectrum bactericidal antibiotic which appears to act by inhibiting normal protein synthesis in susceptible microorganisms.

Netilmicin is active *in vitro* against a wide variety of pathogenic bacteria, primarily gram-negative bacilli and also a few gram-positive organisms including *Citrobacter, Enterobacter, Escherichia coli, Klebsiella* species, *Proteus mirabilis, Pseudomonas aeruginosa, Salmonella* species, *Shigella* species, and *Staphylococcus* species (penicillin- and methicillin-resistant strains).

Netilmicin is also active *in vitro* against some isolates of *Acinetobacter* and *Neisseria* species, indole-positive *Proteus* species, *Pseudomonas* and *Serratia* species. In addition, netilmicin is active *in vitro* against many strains which have acquired resistance to other aminoglycosides. Such resistance is usually caused by aminoglycoside modifying (inactivating) enzymes. In general, netilmicin is active against organisms which inactivate aminoglycosides by either phosphorylation or adenylylation; it has variable activity against acetylating strains, depending on the specific type. For example, the susceptibility of *Serratia* species producing a combination of adenylylating and acetylating enzymes varies according to the level of acetylating enzyme present. Netilmicin is active *in vitro* against certain strains of gram-negative bacteria resistant to gentamicin and tobramycin: *Citrobacter, Enterobacter* species, *Escherichia coli, Klebsiella, Proteus* (indole-positive), *Pseudomonas, Salmonella,* and *Shigella* species. Netilmicin is active *in vitro* against certain staphylococci resistant to amikacin and tobramycin. Like other aminoglycosides, netilmicin is not active against bacteria with reduced permeability to this class of antibiotics.

Most species of streptococci and anaerobic organisms, such as *Bacteroides* and *Clostridium* species, are resistant to aminoglycosides.

The *in vitro* activity of netilmicin and of other aminoglycosides is affected by media pH, protein content, divalent cation concentration, and inoculum size.

Netilmicin acts synergistically *in vitro* with members of the penicillin class of antibiotics against *Streptococcus faecalis.* It also acts synergistically with those penicillins which are active alone against many strains of *Pseudomonas.* In addition, many, but not all isolates of *Serratia* which are resistant to multiple antibiotics, are inhibited by synergistic combina-

Continued on next page

Information on Schering products appearing on these pages is effective as of August 15, 1992.

Schering—Cont.

tions of netilmicin with carbenicillin, azlocillin, mezlocillin, cefamandole, cefotaxime, or moxalactam. Tests for antibiotic synergy are necessary.

Susceptibility Testing: Quantitative methods that require measurements of zone diameters give the most precise estimates of antibiotic susceptibility. One such procedure has been recommended for use with discs to test susceptibility to netilmicin. Interpretation involves correlation of the diameters obtained in the disc test with minimal inhibitory concentration (MIC) values for netilmicin.

Reports from the laboratory giving results of the standardized single disc susceptibility test (Bauer, et al. Am J Clin Path 1966; 45:493 and Federal Register 37:20525–20529, 1972), using a 30 mcg netilmicin disc should be interpreted according to the following criteria:

Organisms producing zones of 15 mm or greater, or MIC's of 8.0 mcg or less are considered susceptible, indicating that the tested organism is likely to respond to therapy.

Resistant organisms produce zones of 12 mm or less or MIC's of 16 mcg or greater. A report of "resistant" from the laboratory indicates that the infecting organism is not likely to respond to therapy.

Zones greater than 12 mm and less than 15 mm, or MIC's of greater than 8.0 mcg and less than 16 mcg, indicate intermediate susceptibility. A report of "intermediate" susceptibility suggests that the organism would be susceptible if the infection is confined to tissues and fluids (e.g., urine), in which high antibiotic levels are attained.

Control organisms are recommended for susceptibility testing. Each time the test is performed one or more of the following organisms should be included: *Escherichia coli* ATCC 25922, *Staphylococcus aureus* ATCC 25923, and *Pseudomonas aeruginosa* ATCC 27853. The control organisms should produce zones of inhibition within the following ranges:

Escherichia coli (ATCC 25922) 22–30 mm
Staphylococcus aureus (ATCC 25923) 22–31 mm
Pseudomonas aeruginosa (ATCC 27853) 17–23 mm

In certain circumstances, particularly with strains of *Pseudomonas aeruginosa*, it may be desirable to do additional susceptibility testing by the tube or agar dilution method. Netilmicin sulfate powder, a diagnostic reagent, is available for this purpose.

The MIC values of netilmicin for the control strains are the following:

Escherichia coli (ATCC 25922) 0.25–0.5 mcg/ml
Staphylococcus aureus (ATCC 25923) 0.125–0.25 mcg/ml
Pseudomonas aeruginosa (ATCC 27853) 4–8 mcg/ml in media supplemented with calcium and magnesium.

INDICATIONS AND USAGE

Netilmicin sulfate injection is indicated for the short-term treatment of patients of all ages, including neonates, infants, and children with serious or life-threatening bacterial infections caused by susceptible strains of the designated microorganisms in the diseases listed below:

COMPLICATED URINARY TRACT infections caused by *Escherichia coli, Klebsiella pneumoniae, Pseudomonas aeruginosa, Enterobacter* species, *Proteus mirabilis, Proteus* species (indole-positive), *Serratia** and *Citrobacter* species, and *Staphylococcus aureus.***

SEPTICEMIA caused by *Escherichia coli, Klebsiella pneumoniae, Pseudomonas aeruginosa, Enterobacter* and *Serratia** species, and *Proteus mirabilis.*

SKIN AND SKIN STRUCTURE infections caused by *Escherichia coli, Klebsiella pneumoniae, Pseudomonas aeruginosa, Enterobacter* and *Serratia** species. *Proteus mirabilis, Proteus* species (indole-positive), and *Staphylococcus aureus*** (pencillinase- and non-penicillinase-producing strains).

INTRA-ABDOMINAL infections including peritonitis and intra-abdominal abscess caused by *Escherichia coli, Klebsiella pneumoniae, Pseudomonas aeruginosa, Enterobacter* species, *Proteus mirabilis, Proteus* species (indole-positive), and *Staphylococcus aureus*** (penicillinase- and non-penicillinase- producing strains).

LOWER RESPIRATORY TRACT infections caused by *Escherichia coli, Klebsiella pneumoniae, Pseudomonas aeruginosa, Enterobacter* and *Serratia** species, *Proteus mirabilis, Proteus* species (indole-positive), and *Staphylococcus aureus*** (penicillinase- and non-penicillinase-producing strains).

Aminoglycosides are indicated for those infections for which less potentially toxic antimicrobial agents are ineffective or contraindicated. They are not indicated in the treatment of uncomplicated initial episodes of urinary tract infection unless the causative organisms are resistant to antimicrobial agents having less potential toxicity.

Netilmicin sulfate injection may be considered as initial therapy in suspected or confirmed gram-negative infections, and therapy may be instituted before obtaining results of susceptibility testing. The decision to continue therapy with netilmicin should be based on the results of susceptibility tests, the severity of the infection, and the important additional concepts contained in the "**WARNINGS** Box" above. If the causative organisms are resistant to netilmicin, other appropriate therapy should be instituted.

In serious infections when the causative organisms are unknown, netilmicin may be administered as initial therapy in conjunction with a penicillin-type or cephalosporin-type drug before obtaining results of susceptibility testing. In neonates with suspected sepsis, a penicillin-type drug is also usually indicated as concomitant therapy with netilmicin. If anaerobic organisms are suspected as etiologic agents, other suitable antimicrobial therapy should also be given. Following identification of the organism and its susceptibility, appropriate antibiotic therapy should then be continued.

Netilmicin sulfate injection has been used effectively in combination with carbenicillin or ticarcillin for the treatment of life-threatening infections caused by *Pseudomonas aeruginosa.*

Clinical studies have shown that netilmicin has been effective in the treatment of serious infections caused by some organisms resistant to other aminoglycosides, *i.e.,* gentamicin, tobramycin, and/or amikacin.

Specimens for bacterial culture should be obtained to isolate and identify causative organisms and to determine their susceptibility to netilmicin.

*(See **Microbiology** Section.)

**While not the antibiotic class of first choice, aminoglycosides, including netilmicin, may be considered for the treatment of serious staphylococcal infections when penicillins or other less potentially toxic drugs are contraindicated and bacterial susceptibility tests and clinical judgment indicate their use. They may also be considered in mixed infections caused by susceptible strains of staphylococci and gram-negative organisms.

CONTRAINDICATION

Hypersensitivity to netilmicin or to any of the ingredients of the preparation is a contraindication to its use. See **WARNINGS** if patient is hypersensitive to another aminoglycoside.

WARNINGS

(See "**WARNINGS** Box" above.) If the patient has a history of hypersensitivity or serious toxic reaction to another aminoglycoside, netilmicin should be used very cautiously, if at all, because cross-sensitivity to drugs in this class has been reported.

Aminoglycosides can cause fetal harm when administered to a pregnant woman. Aminoglycoside antibiotics cross the placenta and there have been several reports of total irreversible bilateral congenital deafness in children whose mothers received streptomycin during pregnancy. Although serious side effects to fetus or newborn have not been reported in the treatment of pregnant women with other aminoglycosides, the potential for harm exists. Reproduction studies in netilmicin have been performed in rats and rabbits using intramuscular and subcutaneous doses approximately 13–15 times the highest adult human dose and have revealed no evidence of impairment of fertility or harm to the fetus. Moreover, there was no evidence of ototoxicity in the offspring of rats treated subcutaneously with netilmicin throughout pregnancy and during the subsequent lactation period. It is not known whether netilmicin sulfate can cause fetal harm when administered to a pregnant women or can affect reproduction capacity. However, if this drug is used during pregnancy, or if the patient becomes pregnant while taking this drug, the patient should be apprised of the potential hazard to the fetus.

NETROMYCIN Injection contains sodium metabisulfite and sodium sulfite, which may cause allergic-type reactions including anaphylactic symptoms and life-threatening or less severe asthmatic episodes in certain susceptible people. The overall prevalence of sulfite sensitivity in the general population is unknown and probably low. Sulfite sensitivity is seen more frequently in asthmatic than in nonasthmatic people.

PRECAUTIONS

General: Neurotoxic and nephrotoxic antibiotics may be almost completely absorbed from body surfaces (except the urinary bladder) after local irrigation and after topical application during surgical procedures. The potential toxic effects of antibiotics administered in this fashion (neuromuscular blockade, respiratory paralysis, oto- and nephrotoxicity) should be considered. (See "**WARNINGS** Box.")

Increased nephrotoxicity has been reported following concomitant administration of aminoglycoside antibiotics with some cephalosporins.

Aminoglycosides should be used with caution in patients with neuromuscular disorders, such as myasthenia gravis, or infant botulism, since these drugs may aggravate muscle weakness because of their potential curare-like effect on the neuromuscular junction.

During or following netilmicin therapy, parasthesias, tetany, positive Chvostek and Trousseau signs, and mental confusion have been described in patients with hypomagnesemia, hypocalcemia, and hypokalemia. When this has occurred in infants, tetany and muscle weakness has been described. Both adults and infants required appropriate corrective electrolyte therapy.

Elderly patients may have reduced renal function which may not be evident in the results of routine screening tests, such as BUN or serum creatinine levels. Determination of creatinine clearance or an estimate based on published nomograms or equations may be more useful. Monitoring of renal function during treatment with netilmicin, as with other aminoglycosides, is particularly important in such patients. A Fanconi-like syndrome, with aminoaciduria and metabolic acidosis, has been reported in some adults and infants being given netilmicin injections.

Patients should be well hydrated during treatment.

Treatment with netilmicin may result in overgrowth of nonsusceptible organisms. If this occurs, appropriate therapy is indicated.

Laboratory Tests: *Tests of renal function:* Urine should be examined periodically for increased excretion of protein and the presence of cells and casts, keeping in mind the effects of the primary illness on these tests. One or more of the following laboratory measurements should be obtained at the onset of therapy, periodically during therapy, and at, or shortly after, the end of therapy:

- creatinine clearance rate (either carefully measured or estimated from published nomograms or equations based on the patient's age, sex, body weight, and serum creatinine concentration) (preferred over BUN);
- serum creatinine concentration (preferred over BUN);
- blood urea nitrogen (BUN).

More frequent testing is desirable if renal function is changing.

See also "**PRECAUTIONS, General**" above regarding elderly patients.

Test of eighth cranial nerve functions: Serial audiometric tests are suggested, particularly when renal function is impaired and/or prolonged aminoglycoside therapy is required; such tests should also be repeated periodically after treatment if there is evidence of a hearing deficit or vestibular abnormality before or during therapy, or when consecutive or concomitant use of other potentially ototoxic drugs is unavoidable.

Drug Interactions: *In vitro* mixing of an aminoglycoside with beta-lactam-type antibiotics (penicillins or cephalosporins) may result in a significant mutual inactivation. Even when an aminoglycoside and a penicillin-type drug are administered separately by different routes, a reduction in aminoglycoside serum half-life or serum levels has been reported in patients with impaired renal function and in some patients with normal renal function. Usually, such inactivation of the aminoglycoside is clinically significant only in patients with severely impaired renal function. (See also "**Drug/Laboratory Test Interactions.**") See "**WARNINGS** Box" regarding concurrent use of potent diuretics, concurrent and/or sequential use of other neurotoxic and/or nephrotoxic antibiotics, and for other essential information.

See also "**PRECAUTIONS, General.**"

Drug/Laboratory Test Interactions: Concomitant cephalosporin therapy may spuriously elevate creatinine determinations.

The inactivation between aminoglycosides and beta-lactam antibiotics described in "**Drug Interactions**" may continue in specimens of body fluids collected for assay, resulting in inaccurate, false low aminoglycoside readings. Such specimens should be properly handled, *i.e.,* assayed promptly, frozen, or treated with beta-lactamase.

Carcinogenesis, Mutagenesis, Impairment of Fertility: Lifetime carcinogenicity tests have been undertaken in the mouse and rat and no drug-related tumors were observed. Similarly, mutagenesis tests with netilmicin have proven negative, and no impairment in fertility has been observed in the rat.

Pregnancy Category D: (See **WARNINGS** Section.)

Nursing Mothers: Clinical studies in nursing mothers indicate that small amounts of netilmicin are excreted in breast milk. Because of the potential for serious adverse reactions from aminoglycosides in nursing infants, a decision should be made whether to discontinue nursing or to discontinue the drug, taking into account the importance of the drug to the mother.

Pediatric Use: Aminoglycosides should be used with caution in prematures and neonates because of the renal immaturity of these patients and the resulting prolongation of serum half-life of these drugs (also see **DOSAGE AND ADMINISTRATION** for use in Neonates and Children).

ADVERSE REACTIONS

Nephrotoxicity—Adverse renal effects due to netilmicin were reported in 7 per 100 patients.

They were demonstrated by a rise in serum creatinine and may have been accompanied by oliguria; the presence of casts, cells or protein in the urine; by rising levels of BUN; or by decreasing creatinine clearance rates. These effects occurred more frequently in the elderly, in patients with a history of renal impairment, and in patients treated for longer periods or with larger doses than recommended. While permanent impairment of renal function may occur following

aminoglycoside therapy, observed renal impairment associated with netilmicin was usually mild and reversible after treatment ended while the drug was being excreted.

Neurotoxicity—Adverse effects on both the auditory and vestibular branches of the eighth cranial nerves have been reported.

Audiometric changes associated with netilmicin occurred in approximately 4 per 100 patients. Subjective netilmicin-related hearing loss occurred in about 1 per 250 patients. Vestibular abnormalities related to netilmicin were seen in 1 per 150 patients. Factors which may increase the risk of aminoglycoside-induced ototoxicity include renal impairment (especially if dialysis is required), excessive dosage, dehydration, concomitant administration of ethacrynic acid or furosemide, or previous exposure to other ototoxic drugs. Peripheral neuropathy or encephalopathy including numbness, skin tingling, muscle twitching, convulsions, and myasthenia gravis-like syndrome have been reported.

Symptoms include dizziness, vertigo, tinnitus, nystagmus, and hearing loss. Aminoglycoside-induced ototoxicity is usually irreversible. Cochlear damage is usually manifested initially by small changes in audiometric test results at the higher frequencies and may not be associated with subjective hearing loss. Vestibular dysfunction is usually manifested by nystagmus, vertigo, nausea, vomiting, or acute Meniere's syndrome.

The risk of toxic reactions is low in patients with normal renal function who do not receive netilmicin injection at higher doses or for longer periods of time than recommended. Some patients who have had previous neurotoxic reactions to other aminoglycosides have been treated with netilmicin without further neurotoxicity.

Neuromuscular blockade manifested as acute muscular paralysis and apnea can occur following treatment with aminoglycosides. (See **"WARNINGS Box."**)

The approximate incidence of other reported adverse reactions to netilmicin injection follows: increased levels of serum transaminase (SGOT or SGPT), alkaline phosphatase, or bilirubin in 15 patients per 1000; rash or itching in 4 or 5 patients per 1000; eosinophilia in 4 patients per 1000; thrombocytosis in 2 patients per 1000; prolonged prothrombin time in 1 patient per 1000; fever in 1 patient per 1000. Fewer than one patient per 1000 was reported to have netilmicin-related anemia, leukopenia, thrombocytopenia, leukemoid reaction, immature circulating white blood cells, hyperkalemia, vomiting, diarrhea, palpitations, hypotension, headache, disorientation, blurred vision, or paresthesias. Local tolerance to intramuscular injection and intravenous infusion of netilmicin is generally excellent, but approximately four patients per 1000 have had severe pain, and similar numbers had induration or hematomas.

OVERDOSAGE

In the event of overdosage or toxic reaction, netilmicin can be removed from the blood by hemodialysis, and is especially important if renal function is, or becomes, compromised. Although there is no specific information concerning removal of netilmicin by peritoneal dialysis, other aminoglycosides are known to be removed by this method but at a rate considerably less than by hemodialysis.

DOSAGE AND ADMINISTRATION

Netilmicin injection may be given intramuscularly or intravenously. (See **CLINICAL PHARMACOLOGY.**) The recommended dosage for both methods of administration is identical.

The patient's pretreatment body weight should be obtained for calculation of correct dosage. The dosage of aminoglycosides in obese patients should be based on an estimate of the lean body mass.

The status of renal function should be estimated by measurement of the serum creatinine concentration or calculation of the endogenous creatinine clearance rate. The blood urea nitrogen (BUN) level is much less reliable for this purpose. Reassessment of renal function should be made periodically during therapy.

In patients with extensive body surface burns, altered pharmacokinetics may result in reduced serum concentrations of aminoglycosides. Measurement of netilmicin serum concentrations is particularly important as a basis for dosage adjustment in such patients.

Duration of Treatment: It is desirable to limit the duration of treatment with aminoglycosides to short-term whenever feasible. The usual duration of treatment for all patients is seven to fourteen days. In complicated infections, a longer course of therapy may be necessary. Although prolonged courses of netilmicin injection have been well tolerated, it is particularly important that patients treated for longer than the usual period be carefully monitored for changes in renal, auditory, and vestibular functions. Dosage should be adjusted if clinically indicated.

Measurement of Serum Concentrations: It is desirable to measure both peak and trough serum concentrations of netilmicin to determine the adequacy and safety of the administered dosage.

Table I
DOSAGE GUIDE FOR ADULTS WITH NORMAL RENAL FUNCTION

Patient's Weight*		For Complicated Urinary Tract Infections, Give 3.0–4.0 mg/kg/day as 1.5–2.0 mg/kg	For Serious Systemic Infections Give 4.0–6.5 mg/kg/day as 1.3–2.2 mg/kg or 2.0–3.25 mg/kg	
		EVERY 12 HOURS	**EVERY 8 HOURS**	**EVERY 12 HOURS**
kg	(lb)	mg/dose	mg/dose	mg/dose
40	(88)	60– 80	52– 88	80–130
45	(99)	68– 90	59– 99	90–146
50	(110)	75–100	65–110	100–163
55	(121)	83–110	72–121	110–179
60	(132)	90–120	78–132	120–195
65	(143)	98–130	85–143	130–211
70	(154)	105–140	91–154	140–228
75	(165)	113–150	98–165	150–244
80	(176)	120–160	104–176	160–260
85	(187)	128–170	111–187	170–276
90	(198)	135–180	117–198	180–293
95	(209)	143–190	124–209	190–309
100	(220)	150–200	130–220	200–325

*The dosage of aminoglycosides in obese patients should be based on an estimate of the lean body mass.

When such measurements are feasible, they should be carried out periodically during therapy. Peak serum concentrations are expected to range from 4 to 12 mcg/ml. Dosage should be adjusted to attain the desired peak and trough concentrations and to avoid prolonged peak serum concentrations above 16 mcg/ml. When monitoring trough concentrations (just prior to the next dose), dosage should be adjusted so that levels above 4 mcg/ml are avoided. Inter-patient variation of aminoglycoside serum concentrations occurs in patients with normal or abnormal renal function. Generally, desirable peak and trough concentrations will be in the range of 6–10 and 0.5–2 mcg/ml, respectively. Determination of the adequacy of a serum level for a particular patient must take into consideration the susceptibility of the causative organism, the severity of the infection, and the status of the patient's host-defense mechanisms.

The dosage recommendations which follow are not intended as rigid schedules, but are provided as guides for initial therapy, or for when the measurement of netilmicin serum levels during therapy is not feasible.

DOSAGE FOR PATIENTS WITH NORMAL RENAL FUNCTION

Table I shows the recommended dosage of netilmicin injection for patients of various ages with normal renal function. Although a causal relationship has not been established, administration of injections preserved with benzyl alcohol has been associated with toxicity in neonates. Caution should be used with NETROMYCIN Injection (100 mg/ml) is administered to neonates and children.

Neonates (less than 6 weeks): 4.0 to 6.5 mg/kg/day given as 2.0 to 3.25 mg/kg every 12 hours.

Infants and Children (6 weeks through 12 years): 5.5 to 8.0 mg/kg/day given either as 1.8 to 2.7 mg/kg every 8 hours, or as 2.7 to 4.0 mg/kg every 12 hours.

DOSAGE FOR PATIENTS WITH IMPAIRED RENAL FUNCTION

Dosage must be individualized in patients with impaired renal function to ensure therapeutic levels are attained. There are several methods of doing this; however, dosage adjustment based upon the measurement of serum drug concentrations during treatment is the most accurate.

If netilmicin serum concentrations are not available and renal function is stable, serum creatinine and creatinine clearance values are the most reliable, readily available indicators of the degree of renal impairment for use as a guide for dosage adjustment.

It is also important to recognize that deteriorating renal function may require a greater reduction in dosage than that specified in the guidelines given below for patients with stable renal impairment.

The initial or loading dose is the same as that for a patient with normal renal function. A number of methods are available to adjust the total daily dosage for the degree of renal impairment. Three suggested methods are:

1) Divide the suggested dosage value for patients with normal renal function from Table I above by the serum creatinine level to obtain the adjusted size of each dose.

2) If the creatinine clearance rate is known or can be estimated from the serum creatinine levels using the formula given below, the adjusted daily dose of netilmicin may be determined by multiplying the dose given in Table I by:

Patient's Creatinine
Clearance Rate
————————
Normal Creatinine
Clearance Rate

3) Alternatively, the following graph may be used to obtain the percentage of the dose selected from Table I, which should be administered at 8-hour intervals:

REDUCED DOSAGE GRAPH

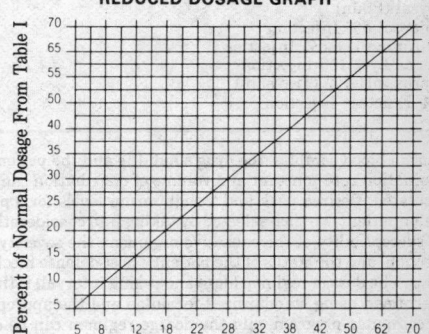

Creatinine Clearance Rate
ml/min/1.73 m^2

Creatinine clearance can be estimated from serum creatinine levels by the following formula for adult males; multiply by 0.85 for adult females (Nephron, 1976; 16:31–41):

$$C_{cr} = \frac{(140 - \text{Age})(\text{Wt. Kg})}{72 \times S_{cr}(\text{mg}/100 \text{ ml})}$$

The adjusted total daily dose may be administered as one dose at 24-hour intervals, or as 2 or 3 equally divided doses at 12-hour or 8-hour intervals, respectively. Generally, each individual dose should not exceed 3.25 mg/kg. In adults with renal failure who are undergoing hemodialysis, the amount of netilmicin removed from the blood may vary depending upon the dialysis equipment and methods used. (See **CLINICAL PHARMACOLOGY.**) In adults, a dose of 2.0 mg/kg at the end of each dialysis period is recommended until the results of tests measuring netilmicin serum levels become available. Dosage should then be appropriately adjusted based on these tests.

ALTERNATE DOSING METHOD FOR PATIENTS WITH NORMAL OR IMPAIRED RENAL FUNCTION

An alternate method of determining a dosage regimen (dose and dosing interval) applicable to all ages and all states of renal function (both normal and abnormal) is to employ pharmacokinetic parameters derived from measurements of serum concentrations.

Following the administration of an initial dose of netilmicin and the determination of drug serum concentrations in post-

Continued on next page

Information on Schering products appearing on these pages is effective as of August 15, 1992.

Schering—Cont.

TABLE II
LARGE VOLUME PARENTERAL SOLUTIONS IN WHICH
NETILMICIN SULFATE IS STABLE

Products/Compositions Tested	Other Trade Names and Manufacturers
	(Solutions of Same Composition)
Sterile Water for Injection	
0.9% Sodium Chloride	
Injection alone or with	
5% Dextrose	
5% or 10% Dextrose Injection	
in Water, or 5% Dextrose in	
Polysal Injection, or 5%	
Dextrose with Electrolyte #48	
or #75	
Ringer's and Lactated	
Ringer's, and Lactated	
Ringer's with 5% Dextrose	
Injection	
10% Travert with Electrolyte	Electrolyte #3 (Cooke &
#2 or #3 Injection	Crowley's Solution) with 10%
(Travenol)	Inverted Sugar Injection (Cutter)
Isolyte E, M, or P with 5%	
Dextrose Injection	
10% Dextran 40 or 6%	
Dextran 75 in 5% Dextrose	
Injection	
Plasma-Lyte 56 or 148	Normosol-M or R in D5-W
Injection with 5% Dextrose	(Abbott), Isolyte H or S with
(Travenol)	5% Dextrose (McGaw), Polyonic
	R-148 or M-56 with 5%
	Dextrose (Cutter)
Plasma-Lyte M Injection 5%	Polysal M with 5% Dextrose
Dextrose (Travenol)	(Cutter)
Ionosol B in D5-W	
5% Amigen Injection alone or	
with 5% Dextrose	
Normosol-R	Polyonic R-148 (Cutter), Isolyte S
	(McGaw) Plasma-Lyte 148
	Injection in Water (Travenol)
Polysal (Plain)	
Aminosol 5% Injection	
Fre-Amine II 8.5% Injection	
Plasma-Lyte 148 Injection	Normosol-R pH 7.4 (Abbott)
(approx. pH 7.4) (Travenol)	
10% Fructose Injection	

infusion blood samples, the drug's half-life and the patient's elimination rate constant and volume of distribution can be calculated. Desired peak and trough serum levels for a particular patient are then selected by taking into consideration the susceptibility of the causative organism, the severity of infection, and the status of the patient's host-defense mechanisms. The dosage regimen (dose and dosing interval) is then determined using standardized formulae and the appropriate computer program, and the dosage regimen can be adjusted to the nearest practical interval and amount.

ADDITION OF NETILMICIN SULFATE TO VARIOUS INTRAVENOUS PREPARATIONS

In adults, a single dose of netilmicin injection may be diluted to 50 to 200 ml of one of the parenteral solutions listed below. In infants and children, the volume of diluent should be less according to the fluid requirements of the patient. The solution may be infused over a period of one-half to two hours. Tested at concentrations of 2.1 to 3.0 mg/ml, netilmicin sulfate has been shown to be stable in the following large volume parenteral solutions for up to 72 hours when stored in glass containers, both when refrigerated and at room temperature. Use after this time period is not recommended.
[See table above.]
Parenteral drug products should be inspected visually for particulate matter and discoloration prior to administration, whenever solution and container permit.

HOW SUPPLIED

NETROMYCIN Injection 100 mg/ml is supplied in 1.5 ml vials, box of 10 (NDC 0085-0264-02). **Store between 2° and 30°C (36°and 86°F).**

ANIMAL PHARMACOLOGY AND/OR ANIMAL TOXICOLOGY

Netilmicin sulfate, administered by the intravenous and intramuscular routes, has been compared to kanamycin, sisomicin, gentamicin, amikacin, and tobramycin in studies ranging in duration from two weeks to three months. Among the aminoglycosides, netilmicin is one of the more potent neuromuscular-blocking agents; however, in six different species, netilmicin sulfate has proven to be the least nephrotoxic and ototoxic of these aminoglycosides, using morphological as well as functional end points. In the clinical trials nephrotoxicity and ototoxicity occurred at about the same

frequency in netilmicin-treated patients as in those treated with other aminoglycosides.

Schering Biochem Corporation,
Manati, Puerto Rico 00701
An Affiliate of Schering Corporation,
Kenilworth, NJ 07033

Revised 1/87

NORMODYNE® ℞
[nŏr-mŏ- dīn]
brand of labetalol hydrochloride
Injection

DESCRIPTION

NORMODYNE (labetalol HCl) is an adrenergic receptor blocking agent that has both selective alpha₁- and nonselective beta-adrenergic receptor blocking actions in a single substance.
Labetalol HCl is 5-[1-hydroxy-2-1[(1-methyl-3- phenylpropyl)amino]ethyl]salicylamide monohydrochloride.
Labetalol HCl has the empirical formula $C_{19}H_{24}N_2O_3HCl$ and a molecular weight of 364.9. It has two asymmetric centers and therefore exists as a molecular complex of two diasteroeisomeric pairs.
Labetalol HCl is a white or off-white crystalline powder, soluble in water.
NORMODYNE (labetalol HCl) Injection is a clear, colorless to light yellow aqueous sterile isotonic solution for intravenous injection. It has a pH range of 3.0 to 4.0. Each mL contains 5 mg labetalol HCl, 45 mg anhydrous dextrose, 0.10 mg edetate disodium; 0.80 mg methylparaben and 0.10 mg propylparaben as preservatives; citric acid monohydrate and sodium hydroxide, as necessary, to bring the solution into the pH range.

CLINICAL PHARMACOLOGY

NORMODYNE (labetalol HCl) combines both selective, competitive alpha₁- adrenergic blocking and nonselective, competitive beta-adrenergic blocking activity in a single substance. In man, the ratios of alpha- to beta-blockade have been estimated to be approximately 1:3 and 1:7 following oral and intravenous administration, respectively. Beta₂-agonist activity has been demonstrated in animals with minimal beta₁- agonist (ISA) activity detected. In animals, at

doses greater than those required for alpha or beta-adrenergic blockade, a membrane stabilizing effect has been demonstrated.
Pharmacodynamics: The capacity of labetalol HCl to block alpha receptors in man has been demonstrated by attenuation of the pressor effect of phen-ylephrine and by a significant reduction of the pressor response caused by immersing the hand in ice-cold water ("cold-pressor test"). Labetalol HCl's beta₁-receptor blockade in man was demonstrated by a small decrease in the resting heart rate, attenuation of tachycardia produced by isoproterenol or exercise, and by attenuation of the reflex tachycardia to the hypotension produced by amyl nitrite. Beta₂-receptor blockade was demonstrated by inhibition of the isoproterenol-induced fall in diastolic blood pressure. Both the alpha- and beta-blocking actions of orally administered labetalol HCl contribute to a decrease in blood pressure in hypertensive patients. Labetalol HCl consistently, in dose-related fashion, blunted increases in exercise-induced blood pressure and heart rate, and in their double product. The pulmonary circulation during exercise was not affected by labetalol HCl dosing.
Single oral doses of labetalol HCl administered in patients with coronary artery disease had no significant effect on sinus rate, intraventricular conduction, or QRS duration. The AV conduction time was modestly prolonged in 2 of 7 patients. In another study, intravenous labetalol HCl slightly prolonged AV nodal conduction time and atrial effective refractory period with only small changes in heart rate. The effects on AV nodal refractoriness were inconsistent.
Labetalol HCl produces dose-related falls in blood pressure without reflex tachycardia and without significant reduction in heart rate, presumably through a mixture of its alpha-blocking and beta-blocking effects. Hemodynamic effects are variable with small nonsignificant changes in cardiac output seen in some studies but not others, and small decreases in total peripheral resistance. Elevated plasma renins are reduced.
Doses of labetalol HCl that controlled hypertension did not affect renal function in mild to severe hypertensive patients with normal renal function.
Due to the alpha₁-receptor blocking activity of labetalol HCl, blood pressure is lowered more in the standing than in the supine position, and symptoms of postural hypotension can occur. During dosing with intravenous labetalol HCl, the contribution of the postural component should be considered when positioning patients for treatment, and patients should not be allowed to move to an erect position unmonitored until their ability to do so is established.
In a clinical pharmacologic study in severe hypertensives, an initial 0.25 mg/kg injection of labetalol HCl, administered to patients in the supine postition, decreased blood pressure by an average of 11/7 mmHg. Additional injections of 0.5 mg/kg at 15-minute intervals up to a total cumulative dose of 1.75 mg/kg. of labetalol HCl caused further dose-related decreases in blood pressure. Some patients required cumulative doses of up to 3.25 mg/kg. The maximal effect of each dose level occurred within 5 minutes. Following discontinuation of intravenous treatment with labetalol HCl, the blood pressure rose gradually and progressively, approaching pretreatment baseline values within an average of 16–18 hours in the majority of patients.
Similar results were obtained in the treatment of patients with severe hypertension requiring urgent blood pressure reduction with an initial dose of 20 mg (which corresponds to 0.25 mg/kg for an 80 kg patient) followed by additional doses of either 40 or 80 mg at 10-minute intervals to achieve the desired effect or up to a cumulative dose of 300 mg.
Labetalol HCl administered as a continuous intravenous infusion, with a mean dose of 136 mg (27 to 300 mg) over a period of 2 to 3 hours (mean of 2 hours and 39 minutes) lowered the blood pressure by an average of 60/35 mmHg.
Exacerbation of angina and, in some cases, myocardial infarction and ventricular dysrhythmias have been reported after abrupt discontinuation of therapy with beta-adrenergic blocking agents in patients with coronary artery disease. Abrupt withdrawal of these agents in patients without coronary artery disease has resulted in transient symptoms, including tremulousness, sweating, palpitation, headache, and malaise. Several mechanisms have been proposed to explain these phenomena, among them increased sensitivity to catecholamines because of increased numbers of beta receptors. Although beta-adrenergic receptor blockade is useful in the treatment of angina and hypertension, there are also situations in which sympathetic stimulation is vital. For example, in patients with severely damaged hearts, adequate ventricular function may depend on sympathetic drive. Beta-adrenergic blockade may worsen AV block by preventing the necessary facilitating effects of sympathetic activity on conduction. Beta₂- adrenergic blockade results in passive bronchial constriction by interfering with endogenous adrenergic bronchodilator activity in patients subject to bronchospasm and may also interfere with exogenous bronchodilators in such patients.
Pharmacokinetics and Metabolism Following intravenous infusion, the elimination half-life is about 5.5 hours and the

total body clearance is approximately 33 mL/min/kg. The plasma half-life of labetalol following oral administration is about six to eight hours. In patients with decreased hepatic or renal function, the elimination half-life of labetalol is not altered, however, the relative bioavailability in hepatically impaired patients is increased due to decreased "first-pass" metabolism.

The metabolism of labetalol is mainly through conjugation to glucuronide metabolites. These metabolites are present in plasma and are excreted in the urine and, via the bile, into the feces. Approximately 55 to 60% of a dose appears in the urine as conjugates or unchanged labetalol within the first 24 hours of dosing.

Labetalol has been shown to cross the placental barrier in humans. Only negligible amounts of the drug crossed the blood-brain barrier in animal studies. Labetalol is approximately 50% protein bound. Neither hemodialysis nor peritoneal dialysis removes a significant amount of labetalol HCl from the general circulation (<1%).

INDICATIONS AND USAGE

NORMODYNE (labetalol HCl) Injection is indicated for control of blood pressure in severe hypertension.

CONTRAINDICATIONS

NORMODYNE (labetalol HCl) Injection is contraindicated in bronchial asthma, overt cardiac failure, greater than first degree heart block, cardiogenic shock, and severe bradycardia. (See **WARNINGS**.)

WARNINGS

Hepatic Injury Severe hepatocellular injury, confirmed by rechallenge in at least one case, occurs rarely with labetalol therapy. The hepatic injury is usually reversible, but hepatic necrosis and death have been reported. Injury has occurred after both short- and long-term treatment and may be slowly progressive despite minimal symptomatology. Appropriate laboratory testing should be done at the first symptom/sign of liver dysfunction (e.g., pruritus, dark urine, persistent anorexia, jaundice, right upper quadrant tenderness, or unexplained "flu-like" symptoms). If the patient has laboratory evidence of liver injury or jaundice, labetalol should be stopped and not restarted.

Cardiac Failure Sympathetic stimulation is a vital component supporting circulatory function in congestive heart failure. Beta blockade carries a potential hazard of further depressing myocardial contractility and precipitating more severe failure. Although beta-blockers should be avoided in overt congestive heart failure, if necessary, labetalol HCl can be used with caution in patients with a history of heart failure who are well-compensated. Congestive heart failure has been observed in patients receiving labetalol HCl. Labetalol HCl does not abolish the inotropic action of digitalis on heart muscle.

In Patients Without a History of Cardiac Failure In patients with latent cardiac insufficiency, continued depression of the myocardium with beta-blocking agents over a period of time can in some cases lead to cardiac failure. At the first sign or symptom of impending cardiac failure, patients should be fully digitalized and/or be given a diuretic, and the response observed closely. If cardiac failure continues, despite adequate digitalization and diuretic, NORMODYNE (labetalol HCl) therapy should be withdrawn (gradually if possible).

Ischemic Heart Disease Angina pectoris has not been reported upon labetalol HCl discontinuation. However, following abrupt cessation of therapy with some beta-blocking agents in patients with coronary artery disease, exacerbations of angina pectoris and, in some cases, myocardial infarction have been reported. Therefore, such patients should be cautioned against interruption of therapy without the physician's advice. Even in the absence of overt angina pectoris, when discontinuation of NORMODYNE (labetalol HCl) is planned, the patient should be carefully observed and should be advised to limit physical activity. If angina markedly worsens or acute coronary insufficiency develops, NORMODYNE (labetalol HCl) administration should be reinstituted promptly, at least temporarily, and other measures appropriate for the management of unstable angina should be taken.

Nonallergic Bronchospasm (e.g., chronic bronchitis and emphysema). Since NORMODYNE (labetalol HCl) Injection at the usual intravenous therapeutic doses has not been studied in patients with nonallergic bronchospastic disease, it should not be used in such patients.

Pheochromocytoma Intravenous labetalol HCl has been shown to be effective in lowering the blood pressure and relieving symptoms in patients with pheochromocytoma; higher than usual doses may be required. However, paradoxical hypertensive responses have been reported in a few patients with this tumor; therefore, use caution when administering labetalol HCl to patients with pheochromocytoma.

Diabetes Mellitus and Hypoglycemia Beta-adrenergic blockade may prevent the appearance of premonitory signs and symptoms (e.g., tachycardia) of acute hypoglycemia. This is especially important with labile diabetics. Beta-blockade also reduces the release of insulin in response to hyperglyce-

mia; it may therefore be necessary to adjust the dose of antidiabetic drugs.

Major Surgery The necessity or desirability of withdrawing beta-blocking therapy prior to major surgery is controversial. Protracted severe hypotension and difficulty in restarting or maintaining a heart beat have been reported with beta-blockers. The effect of labetalol HCl's alpha-adrenergic activity has not been evaluated in this setting.

A synergism between labetalol HCl and halothane anesthesia has been shown (see **Drug Interactions**).

Rapid Decreases of Blood Pressure Caution must be observed when reducing severely elevated blood pressure. Although such findings have not been reported with intravenous labetalol HCl, a number of adverse reactions, including cerebral infarction, optic nerve infarction, angina and ischemic changes in the electrocardiogram, have been reported with other agents when severely elevated blood pressure was reduced over time courses of several hours to as long as one or two days. The desired blood pressure lowering should therefore be achieved over as long a period of time as is compatible with the patient's status.

PRECAUTIONS

General: *Impaired Hepatic Function* may diminish metabolism of NORMODYNE (labetalol HCl) Injection.

Hypotension Symptomatic postural hypotension (incidence 58%) is likely to occur if patients are tilted or allowed to assume the upright position within 3 hours of receiving NORMODYNE (labetalol HCl) Injection. Therefore, the patient's ability to tolerate an upright position should be established before permitting any ambulation.

Risk of Anaphylactic Reaction While taking beta-blockers, patients with a history of severe anaphylactic reaction to a variety of allergens may be more reactive to repeated challenge, either accidental, diagnostic, or therapeutic. Such patients may be unresponsive to the usual doses of epinephrine used to treat allergic reaction.

Jaundice or Hepatic Dysfunction (see **WARNINGS**.)

Information for Patients: The following information is intended to aid in the safe and effective use of this medication. It is not a disclosure of all possible adverse or intended effects. During and immediately following (for up to 3 hours) NORMODYNE Injection, the patient should remain supine. Subsequently, the patient should be advised on how to proceed gradually to become ambulatory, and should be observed at the time of first ambulation.

When the patient is started on NORMODYNE Tablets, following adequate control of blood pressure with NORMODYNE Injection, appropriate directions for titration of dosage should be provided. (See **DOSAGE AND ADMINISTRATION**.)

As with all drugs with beta-blocking activity, certain advice to patients being treated with labetalol HCl is warranted. While no incident of the abrupt withdrawal phenomenon (exacerbation of angina pectoris) has been reported with labetalol HCl, dosing with NORMODYNE Tablets should not be interrupted or discontinued without a physician's advice. Patients being treated with NORMODYNE Tablets should consult a physician at any signs or symptoms of impending cardiac failure or hepatic dysfunction (see **WARNINGS**.) Also transient scalp tingling may occur, usually when treatment with NORMODYNE Tablets is initiated (see **ADVERSE REACTIONS**).

Laboratory Tests: Routine laboratory tests are ordinarily not required before or after intravenous labetalol HCl. In patients with concomitant illnesses, such as impaired renal function, appropriate tests should be done to monitor these conditions.

Drug Interactions: Since NORMODYNE (labetalol HCl) Injection may be administered to patients already being treated with other medications, including other antihypertensive agents, careful monitoring of these patients is necessary to detect and treat promptly any undesired effect from concomitant administration.

In one survey, 2.3% of patients taking labetalol HCl orally in combination with tricyclic antidepressants experienced tremor as compared to 0.7% reported to occur with labetalol HCl alone. The contribution of each of the treatments to this adverse reaction is unknown but the possibility of a drug interaction cannot be excluded.

Drugs possessing beta-blocking properties can blunt the bronchodilator effect of beta-receptor agonist drugs in patients with bronchospasm; therefore, doses greater than the normal anti-asthmatic dose of beta-agonist bronchodilator drugs may be required.

Cimetidine has been shown to increase the bioavailability of labetalol HCl administered orally. Since this could be explained either by enhanced absorption or by an alteration of hepatic metabolism of labetalol HCl, special care should be used in establishing the dose required for blood pressure control in such patients.

Synergism has been shown between halothane anesthesia and intravenously administered labetalol HCl. During controlled hypotensive anesthesia using labetalol HCl in association with halothane, high concentrations (3% or above) of halothane should not be used because the degree of hypoten-

sion will be increased and because of the possibility of a large reduction in cardiac output and an increase in central venous pressure. The anesthesiologist should be informed when a patient is receiving labetalol HCl.

Labetalol HCl blunts the reflex tachycardia produced by nitroglycerin without preventing its hypotensive effect. If labetalol HCl is used with nitroglycerin in patients with angina pectoris, additional antihypertensive effects may occur.

Drug/Laboratory Test Interactions: The presence of labetalol metabolites in the urine may result in falsely elevated levels of urinary catecholamines, metanephrine, normetanephrine, and vanillylmandelic acid (VMA) when measured by fluorimetric or photometric methods. In screening patients suspected of having a pheochromocytoma and being treated with labetalol HCl, a specific method, such as high performance liquid chromatographic assay with solid phase extraction (e.g., *J Chromatogr* 385:241, 1987) should be employed in determining levels of catecholamines.

Labetalol HCl has also been reported to produce a false-positive test for amphetamine when screening urine for the presence of drugs using the commercially available assay methods Toxi-Lab A® (thin-layer chromatographic assay) and Emit-d.a.u.® (radioenzymatic assay). When patients being treated with labetalol have a positive urine test for amphetamine using these techniques, confirmation should be made by using more specific methods, such as a gas chromatographic-mass spectrometer technique.

Carcinogenesis, Mutagenesis, Impairment of Fertility: Long-term oral dosing studies with labetalol HCl for 18 months in mice and for 2 years in rats showed no evidence of carcinogenesis. Studies with labetalol HCl, using dominant lethal assays in rats and mice, and exposing microorganisms according to modified Ames tests, showed no evidence of mutagenesis.

Pregnancy Category C: Teratogenic studies have been performed with labetalol in rats and rabbits at oral doses up to approximately 6 and 4 times the maximum recommended human dose (MRHD), respectively. No reproducible evidence of fetal malformations was observed. Increased fetal resorptions were seen in both species at doses approximating the MRHD. A teratology study performed with labetalol in rabbits at intravenous doses up to 1.7 times the MRHD revealed no evidence of drug related harm to the fetus. There are no adequate and well-controlled studies in pregnant women. Labetalol should be used during pregnancy only if the potential benefit justifies the potential risk to the fetus.

Nonteratogenic Effects: Transient hypotension, bradycardia, and hypoglycemia have been rarely observed in infants of mothers who were treated with labetalol HCl for hypertension during pregnancy. Oral administration of labetalol to rats during late gestation through weaning at doses of 2 to 4 times the MRHD caused a decrease in neonatal survival.

Labor and Delivery: Labetalol HCl given to pregnant women with hypertension did not appear to affect the usual course of labor and delivery.

Nursing Mothers: Small amounts of labetalol (approximately 0.004% of the maternal dose) are excreted in human milk. Caution should be exercised when NORMODYNE (labetalol HCl) Injection is administered to a nursing woman.

Pediatric Use: Safety and effectiveness in children have not been established.

ADVERSE REACTIONS

NORMODYNE (labetalol HCl) Injection is usually well tolerated. Most adverse effects have been mild and transient and in controlled trials involving 92 patients did not require labetalol HCl withdrawal. Symptomatic postural hypotension (incidence 58%) is likely to occur if patients are tilted or allowed to assume the upright position within 3 hours of receiving NORMODYNE (labetalol HCl) Injection. Moderate hypotension occurred in 1 of 100 patients while supine. Increased sweating was noted in 4 of 100 patients, and flushing occurred in 1 of 100 patients.

The following also were reported with NORMODYNE Injection with the incidence per 100 patients as noted:

Cardiovascular System Ventricular arrhythmia in 1.

Central and Peripheral Nervous Systems Dizziness in 9; tingling of the scalp/skin 7; hypoesthesia (numbness), and vertigo 1 each.

Gastrointestinal System Nausea in 13; vomiting 4; dyspepsia and taste distortion, 1 each.

Metabolic Disorders Transient increases in blood urea nitrogen and serum creatinine levels occurred in 8 of 100 patients; these were associated with drops in blood pressure, generally in patients with prior renal insufficiency.

Continued on next page

Information on Schering products appearing on these pages is effective as of August 15, 1992.

Schering—Cont.

Psychiatric Disorders Somnolence/yawning in 3.
Respiratory System Wheezing in 1.
Skin Pruritus in 1.

The incidence of adverse reactions depends upon the dose of labetalol HCl. The largest experience is with oral labetalol HCl (see NORMODYNE Tablet Product Information for details). Certain of the side effects increased with increasing oral dose as shown in the table below which depicts the entire U.S. therapeutic trials data base for adverse reactions that are clearly or possibly dose related. [See table below.]

In addition, a number of other less common adverse events have been reported:

Cardiovascular Hypotension, and rarely, syncope, bradycardia, heart block.

Liver and Biliary System Hepatic necrosis, hepatitis, cholestatic jaundice, elevated liver function tests.

The oculomucocutaneous syndrome associated with the beta-blocker practolol has not been reported with labetalol HCl during investigational use and extensive foreign marketing experience.

Clinical Laboratory Tests: Among patients dosed with NORMODYNE (labetalol HCl) Tablets, there have been reversible increases of serum transaminases in 4% of patients tested, and more rarely, reversible increases in blood urea.

OVERDOSAGE

Overdosage with NORMODYNE (labetalol HCl) Injection causes excessive hypotension that is posture sensitive, and sometimes, excessive bradycardia. Patients should be placed supine and their legs raised if necessary to improve the blood supply to the brain. If overdosage with labetalol HCl follows oral ingestion, gastric lavage or pharmacologically induced emesis (using syrup of ipecac) may be useful for removal of the drug shortly after ingestion. The following additional measures should be employed if necessary: *Excessive bradycardia* —administer atropine or epinephrine. *Cardiac failure* —administer a digitalis glycoside and a diuretic. Dopamine or dobutamine may also be useful. *Hypotension* - —administer vasopressors, eg. norepinephrine. There is pharmacological evidence that norepinephrine may be the drug of choice. *Bronchospasm*- administer epinephrine and/or an aerosolized beta$_2$- agonist. *Seizures* —administer diazepam.

In severe beta-blocker overdose resulting in hypotension and/or bradycardia, glucagon has been shown to be effective when administered in large doses (5 to 10 mg rapidly over 30 seconds, followed by continuous infusion of 5 mg/hr that can be reduced as the patient improves).

Neither hemodialysis nor peritoneal dialysis removes a significant amount of labetalol HCl from the general circulation (<1%).

The oral LD$_{50}$ value of labetalol HCl in the mouse is approximately 600 mg/kg and in the rat is greater than 2 g/kg. The intravenous LD$_{50}$ in these species is 50 to 60 mg/kg.

DOSAGE AND ADMINISTRATION

NORMODYNE (labetalol HCl) Injection is intended for intravenous use in hospitalized patients. DOSAGE MUST BE INDIVIDUALIZED depending upon the severity of hypertension and the repsonse of the patient during dosing.

Patients should always be kept in a supine position during the period of intravenous drug administration. A substantial fall in blood pressure on standing should be expected in these patients. The patient's ability to tolerate an upright position should be established before permitting any ambulation, such as using toilet facilities.

Either of two methods of administration of NORMODYNE Injection may be used: a) repeated intravenous injections, b) slow continuous infusion.

Repeated Intravenous Injection: Initially, NORMODYNE (labetalol HCl) Injection should be given in a dose of 20 mg labetalol HCl (which corresponds to 0.25 mg/kg for an 80 kg patient) by slow intravenous injection over a two-minute period.

Immediately before the injection and at five and ten minutes after injection, supine blood pressure should be measured to evaluate response. Additional injections of 40 mg or 80 mg can be given at ten minute intervals until a desired supine blood pressure is achieved or a total of 300 mg labetalol HCl has been injected. The maximum effect usually occurs within 5 minutes of each injection.

Slow Continuous Infusion: NORMODYNE (labetalol HCl) Injection is prepared for intravenous continuous infusion by diluting the contents with commonly used intravenous fluids (see below). Examples of methods of preparing the infusion solution are:

The contents of either two 20 mL vials (40 mL), or one 40 mL vial, are added to 160 mL of a commonly used intravenous fluid such that the resultant 200 mL of solution contains 200 mg of labetalol HCl, 1 mg/mL. The diluted solution should be administered at a rate of 2 mL/min to deliver 2 mg/min.

Alternatively the contents of either two 20 mL vials (40 mL), or one 40 mL vial, of NORMODYNE (labetalol HCl) Injection are added to 250 mL of a commonly used intravenous fluid. The resultant solution will contain 200 mg of labetalol HCl, approximately 2 mg/3 mL. The diluted solution should be administered at a rate of 3 mL/min to deliver approximately 2 mg/min.

The rate of infusion of the diluted solution may be adjusted according to the blood pressure response, at the discretion of the physician. To facilitate a desired rate of infusion, the diluted solution can be infused using a controlled administration mechanism, e.g., graduated burette or mechanically driven infusion pump.

Since the half life of labetalol is 5 to 8 hours, steady- state blood levels (in the face of a constant rate of infusion) would not be reached during the usual infusion time period. The infusion should be continued until a satisfactory response is obtained and should then be stopped and oral labetalol HCl started (see below). The effective intravenous dose is usually in the range of 50 to 200 mg. A total dose of up to 300 mg may be required in some patients.

Blood Pressure Monitoring: The blood pressure should be monitored during and after completion of the infusion or intravenous injections. Rapid or excessive falls in either systolic or diastolic blood pressure during intravenous treatment should be avoided. In patients with excessive systolic hypertension, the decrease in systolic pressure should be used as indicator of effectiveness in addition to the response of the diastolic pressure.

Initiation of Dosing with NORMODYNE (labetalol HCl) Tablets: Subsequent oral dosing with NORMODYNE (labetalol HCl) Tablets should begin when it has been established that the supine diastolic blood pressure has begun to rise. The recommended initial dose is 200 mg, followed in 6–12 hours by an additional dose of 200 or 400 mg, depending on the blood pressure response. Thereafter, *inpatient titration with NORMODYNE (labetalol HCl) Tablets* may proceed as follows:

Inpatient Titration Instructions

Regimen	Daily Dose*
200 mg bid	400 mg
400 mg bid	800 mg
800 mg bid	1600 mg
1200 mg bid	2400 mg

*If needed, the total daily dose may be given in three divided doses.

While in the hospital, the dosage of NORMODYNE Tablets may be increased at one day intervals to achieve the desired blood pressure reduction.

For subsequent outpatient titration or maintenance dosing see NORMODYNE Tablets Product Information **DOSAGE AND ADMINISTRATION** for additional recommendations.

Compatibility with commonly used intravenous fluids.

Parenteral drug products should be inspected visually for particulate matter and discoloration prior to administration, whenever solution and container permit.

NORMODYNE (labetalol HCl) Injection was tested for compatibility with commonly used intravenous fluids at final concentrations of 1.25 mg to 3.75 mg labetalol HCl per mL of the mixture. NORMODYNE Injection was found to be compatible with and stable (for 24 hours refrigerated or at room temperature) in mixtures with the following solutions:

Ringers Injection, USP
Lactated Ringers Injection, USP
5% Dextrose and Ringers Injection
5% Lactated Ringers and 5% Dextrose Injection
5% Dextrose Injection, USP
0.9% Sodium Chloride Injection, USP
5% Dextrose and 0.2% Sodium Chloride Injection, USP
2.5% Dextrose and 0.45% Sodium Chloride Injection, USP
5% Dextrose and 0.9% Sodium Chloride Injection, USP
5% Dextrose and 0.33% Sodium Chloride Injection, USP

NORMODYNE (labetalol HCl) Injection was NOT compatible with 5% Sodium Bicarbonate Injection, USP.

HOW SUPPLIED

NORMODYNE (labetalol HCl) Injection, 5 mg/mL, is supplied in 20 mL (100 mg) (NDC-0085-0362-07) and 40 mL (200 mg) (NDC-0085- 0362-06) multi-dose vials, boxes of 1; 4 mL (20 mg) (NDC-0085- 0362-08) and 8 mL (40 mg) (NDC-0085-0362-09) single-dose, prefilled, disposable syringes, boxes of 1.

Store between 2° and 30°C (36° and 86°F). Do not freeze. Protect syringe from light.

Note: To insure patient safety, the needle and the prefilled syringes should be handled with care and should be destroyed and discarded if damaged in any manner. If the cannula is bent, no attempt should be made to straighten it. To prevent needle-stick injuries, needles should not be recapped, purposely bent, or broken by hand.

Schering Corporation
Kenilworth, NJ 07033 USA

Revised 4/90 B-14525645

Copyright © 1984, 1990, Schering Corporation. All rights reserved.

Shown in Product Identification Section, page 428

NORMODYNE® ℞

brand of
labetalol hydrochloride
Tablets

DESCRIPTION

NORMODYNE (labetalol HCl) is an adrenergic receptor blocking agent that has both selective alpha$_1$- and nonselective beta-adrenergic receptor blocking actions in a single substance.

Labetalol HCl is 5-[1-hydroxy-2[(1-methyl-3-phenylpropyl) amino] ethyl]salicylamide monohydrochloride.

Labetalol HCl has the empirical formula $C_{19}H_{24}N_2O_3 \cdot HCl$ and a molecular weight of 364.9. It has two asymmetric centers and therefore exists as a molecular complex of two diastereoisomeric pairs.

Labetalol HCl is a white or off-white crystalline powder, soluble in water.

NORMODYNE Tablets contain 100 mg, 200 mg or 300 mg labetalol HCl and are taken orally.

The inactive ingredients for NORMODYNE Tablets, 100 mg, include: corn starch, FD&C Blue No. 2 Al Lake, FD&C Yellow No. 6 Al Lake, hydroxypropyl methylcellulose, lactose, magnesium stearate, methylparaben, PEG and propylparaben. May also contain: potato starch and wheat starch.

The inactive ingredients for NORMODYNE Tablets, 200 mg, include: corn starch, hydroxypropyl methylcellulose, lactose, magnesium stearate, methylparaben, PEG, propylparaben and titanium dioxide. May also contain: potato starch and wheat starch.

The inactive ingredients for NORMODYNE Tablets, 300 mg, include: corn starch, FD&C Blue No. 2 Al Lake, hydroxypropyl methylcellulose, lactose, magnesium stearate, methylparaben, PEG and propylparaben. May also contain: potato starch and wheat starch.

CLINICAL PHARMACOLOGY

NORMODYNE (labetalol HCl) combines both selective, competitive alpha$_1$-adrenergic blocking and nonselective, competitive beta-adrenergic blocking activity in a single substance. In man, the ratios of alpha- to beta-blockade have been estimated to be approximately 1:3 and 1:7 following oral and intravenous administration, respectively. Beta$_2$-agonist activity has been demonstrated in animals with minimal beta$_1$-agonist (ISA) activity detected. In animals, at doses greater than those required for alpha or beta-adrenergic blockade, a membrane-stabilizing effect has been demonstrated.

Pharmacodynamics The capacity of labetalol HCl to block alpha receptors in man has been demonstrated by attenuation of the pressor effect of phenylephrine and by a significant reduction of the pressor response caused by immersing the hand in ice-cold water ("cold-pressor test"). Labetalol HCl's beta$_1$-receptor blockade in man was demonstrated by a small decrease in the resting heart rate, attenuation of tachycardia produced by isoproterenol or exercise, and by attenuation of the reflex tachycardia to the hypotension produced by amyl nitrite. Beta$_2$-receptor blockade was demonstrated by inhibition of the isoproterenol-induced fall in diastolic blood pressure. Both the alpha- and beta-blocking actions of orally administered labetalol HCl contribute to a decrease in blood pressure in hypertensive patients. Labetalol HCl consistently, in dose-related fashion, blunted increases in exer-

Labetalol HCl Daily Dose (mg)	200	300	400	600	800	900	1200	1600	2400
Number of Patients	522	181	606	608	503	117	411	242	175
Dizziness (%)	2	3	3	3	5	1	9	13	16
Fatigue	2	1	4	4	5	3	7	6	10
Nausea	<1	0	1	2	4	0	7	11	19
Vomiting	0	0	<1	<1	<1	0	1	2	3
Dyspepsia	1	0	2	1	1	0	2	2	4
Paresthesias	2	0	2	2	1	1	2	5	5
Nasal Stuffiness	1	1	2	2	2	2	4	5	6
Ejaculation Failure	0	2	1	2	3	0	4	3	5
Impotence	1	1	1	1	2	4	3	4	3
Edema	1	0	1	1	1	0	1	2	2

cise-induced blood pressure and heart rate, and in their double product. The pulmonary circulation during exercise was not affected by labetalol HCl dosing.

Single oral doses of labetalol HCl administered in patients with coronary artery disease had no significant effect on sinus rate, intraventricular conduction, or QRS duration. The AV conduction time was modestly prolonged in 2 of 7 patients. In another study, intravenous labetalol HCl slightly prolonged AV nodal conduction time and atrial effective refractory period with only small changes in heart rate. The effects on AV nodal refractoriness were inconsistent.

Labetalol HCl produces dose-related falls in blood pressure without reflex tachycardia and without significant reduction in heart rate, presumably through a mixture of its alpha-blocking and beta-blocking effects. Hemodynamic effects are variable with small nonsignificant changes in cardiac output seen in some studies but not others, and small decreases in total peripheral resistance. Elevated plasma renins are reduced.

Doses of labetalol HCl that controlled hypertension did not affect renal function in mild to severe hypertensive patients with normal renal function.

Due to the $alpha_1$-receptor blocking activity of labetalol HCl, blood pressure is lowered more in the standing than in the supine position, and symptoms of postural hypotension (2%), including rare instances of syncope, can occur. Following oral administration, when postural hypotension has occurred, it has been transient and is uncommon when the recommended starting dose and titration increments are closely followed (see **DOSAGE AND ADMINISTRATION**). Symptomatic postural hypotension is most likely to occur 2 to 4 hours after a dose, especially following the use of large initial doses or upon large changes in dose.

The peak effects of single oral doses of labetalol HCl occur within 2 to 4 hours. The duration of effect depends upon dose, lasting at least 8 hours following single oral doses of 100 mg and more than 12 hours following single oral doses of 300 mg. The maximum, steady-state blood pressure response upon oral, twice-a-day dosing occurs within 24 to 72 hours.

The antihypertensive effect of labetalol has a linear correlation with the logarithm of labetalol plasma concentration, and there is also a linear correlation between the reduction in exercise-induced tachycardia occurring at two hours after oral administration of labetalol HCl and the logarithm of the plasma concentration.

About 70% of the maximum beta-blocking effect is present for five hours after the administration of a single oral dose of 400 mg, with suggestion that about 40% remains at eight hours.

The anti-anginal efficacy of labetalol HCl has not been studied. In 37 patients with hypertension and coronary artery disease, labetalol HCl did not increase the incidence or severity of angina attacks.

Exacerbation of angina and, in some cases, myocardial infarction and ventricular dysrhythmias have been reported after abrupt discontinuation of therapy with beta-adrenergic blocking agents in patients with coronary artery disease. Abrupt withdrawal of these agents in patients without coronary artery disease has resulted in transient symptoms, including tremulousness, sweating, palpitation, headache, and malaise. Several mechanisms have been proposed to explain these phenomena, among them increased sensitivity to catecholamines because of increased numbers of beta receptors.

Although beta-adrenergic receptor blockade is useful in the treatment of angina and hypertension, there are also situations in which sympathetic stimulation is vital. For example, in patients with severely damaged hearts, adequate ventricular function may depend on sympathetic drive. Beta-adrenergic blockade may worsen AV block by preventing the necessary facilitating effects of sympathetic activity on conduction. $Beta_2$-adrenergic blockade results in passive bronchial constriction by interfering with endogenous adrenergic bronchodilator activity in patients subject to bronchospasm and may also interfere with exogenous bronchodilators in such patients.

Pharmacokinetics and Metabolism Labetalol HCl is completely absorbed from the gastrointestinal tract with peak plasma levels occurring one to two hours after oral administration. The relative bioavailability of labetalol HCl tablets compared to an oral solution is 100%. The absolute bioavailability (fraction of drug reaching systemic circulation) of labetalol when compared to an intravenous infusion is 25%; this is due to extensive "first-pass" metabolism. Despite "first-pass" metabolism there is a linear relationship between oral doses of 100 to 3000 mg and peak plasma levels. The absolute bioavailability of labetalol is increased when administered with food.

The plasma half-life of labetalol following oral administration is about six to eight hours. Steady-state plasma levels of labetalol during repetitive dosing are reached by about the third day of dosing. In patients with decreased hepatic or renal function, the elimination half-life of labetalol is not altered; however, the relative bioavailability in hepatically impaired patients is increased due to decreased "first-pass" metabolism.

The metabolism of labetalol is mainly through conjugation to glucuronide metabolites. These metabolites are present in plasma and are excreted in the urine and, via the bile, into the feces. Approximately 55 to 60% of a dose appears in the urine as conjugates or unchanged labetalol within the first 24 hours of dosing.

Labetalol has been shown to cross the placental barrier in humans. Only negligible amounts of the drug crossed the blood-brain barrier in animal studies. Labetalol is approximately 50% protein bound. Neither hemodialysis nor peritoneal dialysis removes a significant amount of labetalol HCl from the general circulation (<1%).

INDICATIONS AND USAGE

NORMODYNE (labetalol HCl) Tablets are indicated in the management of hypertension. NORMODYNE Tablets may be used alone or in combination with other antihypertensive agents, especially thiazide and loop diuretics.

CONTRAINDICATIONS

NORMODYNE (labetalol HCl) Tablets are contraindicated in bronchial asthma, overt cardiac failure, greater than first degree heart block, cardiogenic shock, and severe bradycardia (see **WARNINGS**).

WARNINGS

Hepatic Injury Severe hepatocellular injury, confirmed by rechallenge in at least one case, occurs rarely with labetalol therapy. The hepatic injury is usually reversible, but hepatic necrosis and death have been reported. Injury has occurred after both short- and long-term treatment and may be slowly progressive despite minimal symptomatology. Appropriate laboratory testing should be done at the first symptom/sign of liver dysfunction (e.g., pruritis, dark urine, persistent anorexia, jaundice, right upper quadrant tenderness, or unexplained "flu-like" symptoms). If the patient has laboratory evidence of liver injury or jaundice, labetalol should be stopped and not restarted.

Cardiac Failure Sympathetic stimulation is a vital component supporting circulatory function in congestive heart failure. Beta blockade carries a potential hazard of further depressing myocardial contractility and precipitating more severe failure. Although beta-blockers should be avoided in overt congestive heart failure, if necessary, labetalol HCl can be used with caution in patients with a history of heart failure who are well-compensated. Congestive heart failure has been observed in patients receiving labetalol HCl. Labetalol HCl does not abolish the inotropic action of digitalis on heart muscle.

In Patients Without a History of Cardiac Failure In patients with latent cardiac insufficiency, continued depression of the myocardium with beta-blocking agents over a period of time can, in some cases, lead to cardiac failure. At the first sign or symptom of impending cardiac failure, patients should be fully digitalized and/or be given a diuretic, and the response observed closely. If cardiac failure continues, despite adequate digitalization and diuretic, NORMODYNE (labetalol HCl) therapy should be withdrawn (gradually if possible).

Exacerbation of Ischemic Heart Disease Following Abrupt Withdrawal Angina pectoris has not been reported upon labetalol HCl discontinuation. However, hypersensitivity to catecholamines has been observed in patients withdrawn from beta-blocker therapy; exacerbation of angina and, in some cases, myocardial infarction have occurred after *abrupt* discontinuation of such therapy. When discontinuing chronically administered NORMODYNE (labetalol HCl), particularly in patients with ischemic heart disease, the dosage should be gradually reduced over a period of one to two weeks and the patient should be carefully monitored. If angina markedly worsens or acute coronary insufficiency develops, NORMODYNE (labetalol HCl) administration should be reinstituted promptly, at least temporarily, and other measures appropriate for the management of unstable angina should be taken. Patients should be warned against interruption or discontinuation of therapy without the physician's advice. Because coronary artery disease is common and may be unrecognized, it may be prudent not to discontinue NORMODYNE (labetalol HCl) therapy abruptly even in patients treated only for hypertension.

Nonallergic Bronchospasm (e.g., chronic bronchitis and emphysema) Patients with bronchospastic disease should, in general, not receive beta-blockers. NORMODYNE may be used with caution, however, in patients who do not respond to, or cannot tolerate, other antihypertensive agents. It is prudent, if NORMODYNE is used, to use the smallest effective dose, so that inhibition of endogenous or exogenous beta-agonists is minimized.

Pheochromocytoma Labetalol HCl has been shown to be effective in lowering the blood pressure and relieving symptoms in patients with pheochromocytoma. However, paradoxical hypertensive responses have been reported in a few patients with this tumor; therefore, use caution when administering labetalol HCl to patients with pheochromocytoma.

Diabetes Mellitus and Hypoglycemia Beta-adrenergic blockade may prevent the appearance of premonitory signs and symptoms (e.g., tachycardia) of acute hypoglycemia. This is especially important with labile diabetics. Beta-blockade also reduces the release of insulin in response to hyperglycemia; it may therefore be necessary to adjust the dose of antidiabetic drugs.

Major Surgery The necessity or desirability of withdrawing beta-blocking therapy prior to major surgery is controversial. Protracted severe hypotension and difficulty in restarting or maintaining a heart beat have been reported with beta-blockers. The effect of labetalol HCl's alpha-adrenergic activity has not been evaluated in this setting.

A synergism between labetalol HCl and halothane anesthesia has been shown (see **Drug Interactions**).

PRECAUTIONS

General: *Impaired Hepatic Function* NORMODYNE (labetalol HCl) Tablets should be used with caution in patients with impaired hepatic function since metabolism of the drug may be diminished.

Jaundice or Hepatic Dysfunction (see **WARNINGS**).

Risk of Anaphylactic Reaction While taking beta-blockers, patients with a history of severe anaphylactic reaction to a variety of allergens may be more reactive to repeated challenge, either accidental, diagnostic, or therapeutic. Such patients may be unresponsive to the usual doses of epinephrine used to treat allergic reaction.

Information for Patients

As with all drugs with beta-blocking activity, certain advice to patients being treated with labetalol HCl is warranted. This information is intended to aid in the safe and effective use of this medication. It is not a disclosure of all possible adverse or intended effects. While no incident of the abrupt withdrawal phenomenon (exacerbation of angina pectoris) has been reported with labetalol HCl, dosing with NORMODYNE Tablets should not be interrupted or discontinued without a physician's advice. Patients being treated with NORMODYNE Tablets should consult a physician at any signs or symptoms of impending cardiac failure or hepatic dysfunction (see **WARNINGS**). Also, transient scalp tingling may occur, usually when treatment with NORMODYNE Tablets is initiated (see **ADVERSE REACTIONS**).

Laboratory Tests

As with any new drug given over prolonged periods, laboratory parameters should be observed over regular intervals. In patients with concomitant illnesses, such as impaired renal function, appropriate tests should be done to monitor these conditions.

Drug Interactions

In one survey, 2.3% of patients taking labetalol HCl in combination with tricyclic antidepressants experienced tremor as compared to 0.7% reported to occur with labetalol HCl alone. The contribution of each of the treatments to this adverse reaction is unknown but the possibility of a drug interaction cannot be excluded.

Drugs possessing beta-blocking properties can blunt the bronchodilator effect of beta-receptor agonist drugs in patients with bronchospasm; therefore, doses greater than the normal anti-asthmatic dose of beta-agonist bronchodilator drugs may be required.

Cimetidine has been shown to increase the bioavailability of labetalol HCl. Since this could be explained either by enhanced absorption or by an alteration of hepatic metabolism of labetalol HCl, special care should be used in establishing the dose required for blood pressure control in such patients.

Synergism has been shown between halothane anesthesia and intravenously administered labetalol HCl. During controlled hypotensive anesthesia using labetalol HCl in association with halothane, high concentrations (3% or above) of halothane should not be used because the degree of hypotension will be increased and because of the possibility of a large reduction in cardiac output and an increase in central venous pressure. The anesthesiologist should be informed when a patient is receiving labetalol HCl.

Labetalol HCl blunts the reflex tachycardia produced by nitroglycerin without preventing its hypotensive effect. If labetalol HCl is used with nitroglycerin in patients with angina pectoris, additional antihypertensive effects may occur.

Drug/Laboratory Test Interactions

The presence of labetalol metabolites in the urine may result in falsely elevated levels of urinary catecholamines, metanephrine, normetanephrine, and vanillylmandelic acid (VMA) when measured by fluorimetric or photometric methods. In screening patients suspected of having a pheochromocytoma and being treated with labetalol HCl, a specific method, such as a high performance liquid chromatographic assay with solid phase extraction (e.g. *J Chromatogr* 385:241,1987) should be employed in determining levels of catecholamines.

Labetalol HCl has also been reported to produce a false-positive test for amphetamine when screening urine for the presence of drugs using the commercially available assay meth-

Continued on next page

Information on Schering products appearing on these pages is effective as of August 15, 1992.

Schering—Cont.

ods Toxi-Lab A® (thin-layer chromatographic assay) and Emit-d.a.u.® (radioenzymatic assay). When patients being treated with labetalol have a positive urine test for amphetamine using these techniques, confirmation should be made by using more specific methods, such as a gas chromatographic-mass spectrometer technique.

Carcinogenesis, Mutagenesis, Impairment of Fertility
Long-term oral dosing studies with labetalol HCl for 18 months in mice and for 2 years in rats showed no evidence of carcinogenesis. Studies with labetalol HCl, using dominant lethal assays in rats and mice, and exposing microorganisms according to modified Ames tests, showed no evidence of mutagenesis.

Pregnancy Category C
Teratogenic studies have been performed with labetalol in rats and rabbits at oral doses up to approximately 6 and 4 times the maximum recommended human dose (MRHD), respectively. No reproducible evidence of fetal malformations was observed. Increased fetal resorptions were seen in both species at doses approximating the MRHD. A teratology study performed with labetalol in rabbits at intravenous doses up to 1.7 times the MRHD revealed no evidence of drug related harm to the fetus. There are no adequate and well-controlled studies in pregnant women. Labetalol should be used during pregnancy only if the potential benefit justifies the potential risk to the fetus.

Nonteratogenic Effects
Transient hypotension, bradycardia, and hypoglycemia have been rarely observed in infants of mothers who were treated with labetalol HCl for hypertension during pregnancy. Oral administration of labetalol to rats during late gestation through weaning at doses of 2 to 4 times the MRHD caused a decrease in neonatal survival.

Labor and Delivery
Labetalol HCl given to pregnant women with hypertension did not appear to affect the usual course of labor and delivery.

Nursing Mothers
Small amounts of labetalol (approximately 0.004% of the maternal dose) are excreted in human milk. Caution should be exercised when NORMODYNE Tablets are administered to a nursing woman.

Pediatric Use
Safety and effectiveness in children have not been established.

ADVERSE REACTIONS

Most adverse effects are mild, transient and occur early in the course of treatment. In controlled clinical trials of 3 to 4 months duration, discontinuation of NORMODYNE (labetalol HCl) Tablets due to one or more adverse effects was required in 7% of all patients. In these same trials, beta-blocker control agents led to discontinuation in 8 to 10% of patients, and a centrally acting alpha-agonist in 30% of patients.

The incidence rates of adverse reactions listed in the following table were derived from multicenter controlled clinical trials, comparing labetalol HCl, placebo, metoprolol and

	Labetalol HCl (N=227) %	Placebo (N=98) %	Propranolol (N=84) %	Metoprolol (N=49) %
Body as a whole				
fatigue	5	0	12	12
asthenia	1	1	1	0
headache	2	1	1	2
Gastrointestinal				
nausea	6	1	1	2
vomiting	<1	0	0	0
dyspepsia	3	1	1	0
abdominal pain	0	0	1	2
diarrhea	<1	0	2	0
taste distortion	1	0	0	0
Central and Peripheral Nervous Systems				
dizziness	11	3	4	4
paresthesias	<1	0	0	0
drowsiness	<1	2	2	2
Autonomic Nervous System				
nasal stuffiness	3	0	0	0
ejaculation failure	2	0	0	0
impotence	1	0	1	3
increased sweating	<1	0	0	0
Cardiovascular				
edema	1	0	0	0
postural hypotension	1	0	0	0
bradycardia	0	0	5	12
Respiratory				
dyspnea	2	0	1	2
Skin				
rash	1	0	0	0
Special Senses				
vision abnormality	1	0	0	0
vertigo	2	1	0	0

Labetalol HCl Daily Dose (mg)	200	300	400	600	800	900	1200	1600	2400
Number of Patients	522	181	606	608	503	117	411	242	175
Dizziness (%)	2	3	3	3	5	1	9	13	16
Fatigue	2	1	4	4	5	3	7	6	10
Nausea	<1	0	1	2	4	0	7	11	19
Vomiting	0	0	<1	<1	<1	0	1	2	3
Dyspepsia	1	0	2	1	1	0	2	2	4
Paresthesias	2	0	2	2	1	1	2	5	5
Nasal Stuffiness	1	1	2	2	2	2	4	5	6
Ejaculation Failure	0	2	1	2	3	0	4	3	5
Impotence	1	1	1	1	2	4	3	4	3
Edema	1	0	1	1	1	0	1	2	2

propranolol, over treatment periods of 3 and 4 months. Where the frequency of adverse effects for labetalol HCl and placebo is similar, causal relationship is uncertain. The rates are based on adverse reactions considered probably drug-related by the investigator. If all reports are considered, the rates are somewhat higher (e.g., dizziness 20%, nausea 14%, fatigue 11%), but the overall conclusions are unchanged. [See table below.]

The adverse effects were reported spontaneously and are representative of the incidence of adverse effects that may be observed in a properly selected hypertensive patient population, (i.e., a group excluding patients with bronchospastic disease, overt congestive heart failure, or other contraindications to beta-blocker therapy.

Clinical trials also included studies utilizing daily doses up to 2400 mg in more severely hypertensive patients. Certain of the side effects increased with increasing dose as shown in the table below which depicts the entire U.S. therapeutic trials data base for adverse reactions that are clearly or possibly drug related. [See table above.]

In addition, a number of other less common adverse events have been reported:

Body as a Whole Fever

Cardiovascular Hypotension, and rarely, syncope, bradycardia, heart block.

Central and Peripheral Nervous Systems Paresthesias, most frequently described as scalp tingling. In most cases, it was mild, transient and usually occurred at the beginning of treatment.

Collagen Disorders Systemic lupus erythematosus; positive antinuclear factor (ANF).

Eyes Dry eyes.

Immunological System Antimitochondrial antibodies.

Liver and Biliary System Hepatic necrosis; hepatitis; cholestatic jaundice, elevated liver function tests.

Musculo-Skeletal System Muscle cramps; toxic myopathy.

Respiratory System Bronchospasm.

Skin and Appendages Rashes of various types, such as generalized maculo-papular; lichenoid; urticarial; bullous lichen planus; psoriaform; facial erythema; Peyronie's disease; reversible alopecia.

Urinary System Difficulty in micturition, including acute urinary bladder retention.

Following approval for marketing in the United Kingdom, a monitored release survey involving approximately 6,800 patients was conducted for further safety and efficacy evaluation of this product. Results of this survey indicate that the type, severity, and incidence of adverse effects were comparable to those cited above.

Potential Adverse Effects
In addition, other adverse effects not listed above have been reported with other beta-adrenergic blocking agents.

Central Nervous System Reversible mental depression progressing to catatonia; an acute reversible syndrome characterized by disorientation for time and place, short-term memory loss, emotional lability, slightly clouded sensorium, and decreased performance on neuropsychometrics.

Cardiovascular Intensification of AV block. See **CONTRA-**

INDICATIONS.

Allergic Fever combined with aching and sore throat; laryngospasm; respiratory distress.

Hematologic Agranulocytosis; thrombocytopenic or nonthrombocytopenic purpura.

Gastrointestinal Mesenteric artery thrombosis; ischemic colitis.

The oculomucocutaneous syndrome associated with the beta-blocker practolol has not been reported with labetalol HCl.

Clinical Laboratory Tests
There have been reversible increases of serum transaminases in 4% of patients treated with labetalol HCl and tested, and more rarely, reversible increases in blood urea.

OVERDOSAGE

Overdosage with NORMODYNE (labetalol HCl) Tablets causes excessive hypotension that is posture sensitive, and sometimes, excessive bradycardia. Patients should be placed supine and their legs raised if necessary to improve the blood supply to the brain. If overdosage with labetalol HCl follows oral ingestion, gastric lavage or pharmacologically induced emesis (using syrup of ipecac) may be useful for removal of the drug shortly after ingestion. The following additional measures should be employed if necessary: *Excessive bradycardia*—administer atropine or epinephrine. *Cardic failure*—administer a digitalis glycoside and a diuretic. Dopamine or dobutamine may also be useful. *Hypotension*—administer vasopressors, e.g., norepinephrine. There is pharmacological evidence that norepinephrine may be the drug of choice. *Bronchospasm*—administer epinephrine and/or an aerosolized beta₂-agonist. *Seizures*—administer diazepam.

In severe beta-blocker overdose resulting in hypotension and/or bradycardia, glucagon has been shown to be effective when administered in large doses (5 to 10 mg rapidly over 30 seconds, followed by continuous infusion of 5 mg/hr that can be reduced as the patient improves).

Neither hemodialysis nor peritoneal dialysis removes a significant amount of labetalol HCl from the general circulation (<1%).

The oral LD_{50} value of labetalol HCl in the mouse is approximately 600 mg/kg and in the rat is greater than 2 g/kg. The intravenous LD_{50} in these species is 50 to 60 mg/kg.

DOSAGE AND ADMINISTRATION

DOSAGE MUST BE INDIVIDUALIZED. The recommended <u>initial</u> dose is 100 mg <u>twice</u> daily whether used alone or added to a diuretic regimen. After 2 or 3 days, using standing blood pressure as an indicator, dosage may be titrated in increments of 100 mg bid every 2 or 3 days. The usual <u>maintenance</u> dosage of labetalol HCl is between 200 and 400 mg <u>twice</u> daily.

Since the full antihypertensive effect of labetalol HCl is usually seen within the first one to three hours of the initial dose or dose increment, the assurance of a lack of an exaggerated hypotensive response can be clinically established in the office setting. The antihypertensive effects of continued dosing can be measured at subsequent visits, approximately 12 hours after a dose, to determine whether further titration is necessary.

Patients with severe hypertension may require from 1200 mg to 2400 mg per day, with or without thiazide diuretics. Should side effects (principally nausea or dizziness) occur with these doses administered bid, the same total daily dose administered bid may improve tolerability and facilitate

further titration. Titration increments should not exceed 200 mg bid.

When a diuretic is added, an additive antihypertensive effect can be expected. In some cases this may necessitate a labetalol HCl dosage adjustment. As with most antihypertensive drugs, optimal dosages of NORMODYNE Tablets are usually lower in patients also receiving a diuretic.

When transferring patients from other antihypertensive drugs, NORMODYNE Tablets should be introduced as recommended and the dosage of the existing therapy progressively decreased.

HOW SUPPLIED

NORMODYNE (labetalol HCl) Tablets, 100 mg, light-brown, round, scored, film-coated tablets engraved on one side with Schering and product identification numbers 244, and on the other side the number 100 for the strength and "NORMODYNE"; bottles of 100 (NDC-0085-0244-04), 500 (NDC-0085-0244-05), bottles of 1000 (NDC-0085-0244-07), and box of 100 for unit-dose dispensing (NDC-0085-0244-08).

NORMODYNE (labetalol HCl) Tablets, 200 mg, white, round, scored, film-coated tablets engraved on one side with Schering and product identification numbers 752, and on the other side the number 200 for the strength and "NORMODYNE"; bottles of 100 (NDC-0085-0752-04), 500 (NDC-0085-0752-05), bottles of 1000 (NDC-0085-0752-07), box of 100 for unit-dose dispensing (NDC-0085-0752-08).

NORMODYNE (labetalol HCl) Tablets, 300 mg, blue, round, film-coated tablets engraved on one side with Schering and product identification numbers 438, and on the other side the number 300 for the strength and "NORMODYNE"; bottles of 100 (NDC-0085-0438-03), 500 (NDC-0085-0438-05), box of 100 for unit-dose dispensing (NDC-0085-0438-06).

NORMODYNE (labetalol HCl) Tablets should be stored between 2° and 30°C (36° and 86°F).

NORMODYNE (labetalol HCl) Tablets in the unit-dose boxes should be protected from excessive moisture.

Schering Corporation
Kenilworth, NJ 07033 USA

Rev. 4/90 B-16098930

Copyright© 1984, 1989, 1990 Schering Corporation. All rights reserved.

Shown in Product Identification Section, page 428

PROVENTIL® Inhalation Aerosol ℞
[pro-ven 'tĭl]
brand of albuterol, USP
Bronchodilator Aerosol
FOR ORAL INHALATION ONLY

DESCRIPTION

The active component of PROVENTIL Inhalation Aerosol is albuterol, USP racemic (α^1-[(*tert*-butylamino) methyl]-4-hydroxy-*m*-xylene-α,α'-diol), a relatively selective beta$_2$-adrenergic bronchodilator.

Albuterol is the official generic name in the United States. The World Health Organization recommended name for the drug is salbutamol. The molecular weight of albuterol is 239.3, and the empirical formula is $C_{13}H_{21}NO_3$. Albuterol is a white to off-white crystalline solid. It is soluble in ethanol, sparingly soluble in water, and very soluble in chloroform.

PROVENTIL Inhalation Aerosol is a metered-dose aerosol unit for oral inhalation. It contains a microcrystalline suspension of albuterol in propellants (trichloromonofluoromethane and dichlorodifluoromethane) with oleic acid. Each actuation delivers from the mouthpiece 90 mcg of albuterol, USP. Each canister provides at least 200 inhalations.

CLINICAL PHARMACOLOGY

In vitro studies and *in vivo* pharmacologic studies have demonstrated that PROVENTIL has a preferential effect on beta$_2$-adrenergic receptors compared with isoproterenol. While it is recognized that beta$_2$-adrenergic receptors are the predominant receptors in bronchial smooth muscle, recent data indicate that there is a population of beta$_2$-receptors in the human heart existing in a concentration between 10–50%. The precise function of these, however, is not yet established. The pharmacologic effects of beta-adrenergic agonist drugs, including PROVENTIL, are at least in part attributable to stimulation through beta-adrenergic receptors of intracellular adenyl cyclase, the enzyme which catalyzes the conversion of adenosine triphosphate (ATP) to cyclic-3', 5'-adenosine monophosphate (c-AMP). Increased c-AMP levels are associated with relaxation of bronchial smooth muscle and inhibition of release of mediators of immediate hypersensitivity from cells, especially from mast cells. Albuterol has been shown in most controlled clinical trials to have more effect on the respiratory tract, in the form of bronchial smooth muscle relaxation, than isoproterenol at comparable doses while producing fewer cardiovascular effects. Controlled clinical studies and other clinical experience have shown that inhaled albuterol, like other beta-adrenergic agonist drugs, can produce a significant cardiovascular effect in some patients, as measured by pulse rate, blood pressure, symptoms, and/or ECG changes.

Albuterol is longer acting than isoproterenol by any route of administration in most patients because it is not a substrate for the cellular uptake processes for catecholamines nor for catechol-*O*-methyl transferase.

Because of its gradual absorption from the bronchi, systemic levels of albuterol are low after inhalation of recommended doses. Studies undertaken with four subjects administered tritiated albuterol, resulted in maximum plasma concentrations occurring within 2 to 4 hours. Due to the sensitivity of the assay method, the metabolic rate and half-life of elimination of albuterol in plasma could not be determined. However, urinary excretion provided data indicating that albuterol has an elimination half-life of 3.8 hours. Approximately 72 percent of the inhaled dose is excreted within 24 hours in the urine, and consists of 28 percent of unchanged drug and 44 percent as metabolite.

Results of animal studies show that albuterol does not pass the blood-brain barrier.

Recent studies in laboratory animals (minipigs, rodents, and dogs) recorded the occurrence of cardiac arrhythmias and sudden death (with histologic evidence of myocardial necrosis) when beta-agonists and methylxanthines were administered concurrently. The significance of these findings when applied to humans is currently unknown.

The effects of rising doses of albuterol and isoproterenol aerosols were studied in volunteers and asthmatic patients. Results in normal volunteers indicated that albuterol is ½ to ¼ as active as isoproterenol in producing increases in heart rate. In asthmatic patients similar cardiovascular differentiation between the two drugs was also seen.

INDICATIONS AND USAGE

PROVENTIL Inhalation Aerosol is indicated for the prevention and relief of bronchospasm in patients with reversible obstructive airway disease, and for the prevention of exercise-induced bronchospasm.

In controlled clinical trials the onset of improvement in pulmonary function was within 15 minutes, as determined by both maximal midexpiratory flow rate (MMEF) and FEV_1. MMEF measurements also showed that near maximum improvement in pulmonary function generally occurs within 60 to 90 minutes following 2 inhalations of albuterol and that clinically significant improvement generally continues for 3 to 4 hours in most patients. In clinical trials, some patients with asthma showed a therapeutic response (defined by maintaining FEV_1 values 15 percent or more above baseline) which was still apparent at 6 hours. Continued effectiveness of albuterol was demonstrated over a 13-week period in these same trials.

In clinical studies, 2 inhalations of albuterol taken approximately 15 minutes prior to exercise prevented exercise-induced bronchospasm, as demonstrated by the maintenance of FEV_1 within 80 percent of baseline values in the majority of patients. One of these studies also evaluated the duration of the prophylactic effect to repeated exercise challenges, which was evident at 4 hours in the majority of patients, and at 6 hours in approximately one third of the patients.

CONTRAINDICATIONS

PROVENTIL Inhalation Aerosol is contraindicated in patients with a history of hypersensitivity to any of its components.

WARNINGS

As with other inhaled beta-adrenergic agonists, PROVENTIL Inhalation Aerosol can produce paradoxical bronchospasm that can be life-threatening. If it occurs, the preparation should be discontinued immediately and alternative therapy instituted.

Fatalities have been reported in association with excessive use of inhaled sympathomimetic drugs. The exact cause of death is unknown, but cardiac arrest following the unexpected development of a severe acute asthmatic crisis and subsequent hypoxia is suspected. Immediate hypersensitivity reactions may occur after administration of albuterol inhalation aerosol, as demonstrated by rare cases of urticaria, angioedema, rash, bronchospasm, anaphylaxis, and oropharyngeal edema.

The contents of PROVENTIL Inhalation Aerosol are under pressure. Do not puncture. Do not use or store near heat or open flame. Exposure to temperatures above 120°F may cause bursting. Never throw container into fire or incinerator. Keep out of reach of children.

PRECAUTIONS

General: Albuterol, as with all sympathomimetic amines, should be used with caution in patients with cardiovascular disorders, especially coronary insufficiency, cardiac arrhythmias, and hypertension, in patients with convulsive disorders, hyperthyroidism, or diabetes mellitus; and in patients who are unusually responsive to sympathomimetic amines.

Large doses of intravenous albuterol have been reported to aggravate preexisting diabetes and ketoacidosis. Additionally, beta-agonists, including albuterol, when given intraveneously may cause a decrease in serum potassium, possibly through intracellular shunting. The relevance of this observation to the use of PROVENTIL Inhalation Aerosol is unknown, since the aerosol dose is much lower than the doses given intravenously.

Although there have been no reports concerning the use of PROVENTIL Inhalation Aerosol during labor and delivery, it has been reported that high doses of albuterol administered intravenously inhibit uterine contractions. Although this effect is extremely unlikely as a consequence of aerosol use, it should be kept in mind.

Information For Patients: The action of PROVENTIL Inhalation Aerosol may last up to six hours and therefore it should not be used more frequently than recommended. Increasing the number or frequency of doses without consulting your physician can be dangerous. If recommended dosage does not provide relief of symptoms or symptoms become worse, seek immediate medical attention. While taking PROVENTIL Inhalation Aerosol, other inhaled medicines should not be used unless prescribed.

See Illustrated Patient Instructions For Use.

Drug Interactions: Other sympathomimetic aerosol bronchodilators should not be used concomitantly with albuterol. If additional adrenergic drugs are to be administered by any route, they should be used with caution to avoid deleterious cardiovascular effects.

Albuterol should be administered with caution to patients being treated with monoamine oxidase inhibitors or tricyclic antidepressants, since the action of albuterol on the vascular system may be potentiated.

Beta-receptor blocking agents and albuterol inhibit the effect of each other.

Carcinogenesis, Mutagenesis, and Impairment of Fertility: In a 2 year study in the rat, albuterol sulfate caused a significant dose-related increase in the incidence of benign leiomyomas of the mesovarium at doses corresponding to 111, 555, and 2,800 times the maximum human inhalational dose. In another study this effect was blocked by the coadministration of propranolol. The relevance of these findings to humans is not known. An 18-month study in mice revealed no evidence of tumorigenicity. Studies with albuterol revealed no evidence of mutagenesis. Reproduction studies in rats revealed no evidence of impaired fertility.

Teratogenic Effects — Pregnancy Category C: Albuterol has been shown to be teratogenic in mice when given in doses corresponding to 14 times the human dose. There are no adequate and well-controlled studies in pregnant women. Albuterol should be used during pregnancy only if the potential benefit justifies the potential risk to the fetus. A reproduction study in CD-1 mice with albuterol (0.025, 0.25, and 2.5 mg/kg, corresponding to 1.4, 14, and 140 times the maximum human inhalational dose) showed cleft palate formation in 5 of 111 (4.5 percent) fetuses at 0.25 mg/kg and in 10 of 108 (9.3 percent) fetuses at 2.5 mg/kg. None were observed at 0.025 mg/kg. Cleft palate also occurred in 22 of 72 (30.5 percent) fetuses treated with 2.5 mg/kg isoproterenol (positive control). A reproduction study in Stride Dutch rabbits revealed cranioschisis in 7 of 19 (37 percent) fetuses at 50 mg/kg, corresponding to 2,800 times the maximum human inhalational dose of albuterol.

Nursing Mothers: It is not known whether this drug is excreted in human milk. Because of the potential for tumorigenicity shown for albuterol in animal studies, a decision should be made whether to discontinue nursing or to discontinue the drug, taking into account the importance of the drug to the mother.

Pediatric Use: Safety and effectiveness in children below the age of 12 years have not been established.

ADVERSE REACTIONS

The adverse reactions of albuterol are similar in nature to those of other sympathomimetic agents, although the incidence of certain cardiovascular effects is less with albuterol. A 13-week double-blind study compared albuterol and isoproterenol aerosols in 147 asthmatic patients. The results of this study showed that the incidence of cardiovascular effects was: palpitations, less than 10 per 100 with albuterol and less than 15 per 100 with isoproterenol; tachycardia, 10 per 100 with both albuterol and isoproterenol; and increased blood pressure, less than 5 per 100 with both albuterol and isoproterenol. In the same study, both drugs caused tremor or nausea in less than 15 patients per 100; dizziness or heartburn in less than 5 per 100 patients. Nervousness occurred in less than 10 per 100 patients receiving albuterol and in less than 15 per 100 patients receiving isoproterenol.

Rare cases of urticaria, angioedema, rash, bronchospasm and oropharyngeal edema have been reported after the use of inhaled albuterol.

In addition, albuterol, like other sympathomimetic agents, can cause adverse reactions such as hypertension, angina,

Continued on next page

Information on Schering products appearing on these pages is effective as of August 15, 1992.

Schering—Cont.

vomiting, vertigo, central nervous system stimulation, insomnia, headache, unusual taste, and drying or irritation of the oropharynx.

OVERDOSAGE

Manifestations of overdosage may include anginal pain, hypertension, hypokalemia, and exaggeration of the pharmacological effects listed in **ADVERSE REACTIONS**.
As with all sympathomimetic aerosol medications, cardiac arrest and even death may be associated with abuse.
The oral LD_{50} in male and female rats and mice was greater than 2,000 mg/kg. The aerosol LD_{50} could not be determined. Dialysis is not appropriate treatment for overdosage of PROVENTIL Inhalation Aerosol. The judicious use of a cardioselective beta-receptor blocker, such as metoprolol tartrate, is suggested, bearing in mind the danger of inducing an asthmatic attack.

DOSAGE AND ADMINISTRATION

For treatment of acute episodes of bronchospasm or prevention of asthmatic symptoms, the usual dosage for adults and children 12 years and older is 2 inhalations repeated every 4 to 6 hours; in some patients, 1 inhalation every 4 hours may be sufficient. More frequent administration or a larger number of inhalations is not recommended. For maintenance therapy or prevention of exacerbation of bronchospasm, 2 inhalations, 4 times a day should be sufficient.
The use of PROVENTIL Inhalation Aerosol can be continued as medically indicated to control recurring bouts of bronchospasm. During this time most patients gain optimal benefit from regular use of the inhaler. Safe usage for periods extending over several years has been documented.
If a previously effective dosage regimen fails to provide the usual relief, medical advice should be sought immediately as this is often a sign of seriously worsening asthma which would require reassessment of therapy.
Exercise-Induced Bronchospasm Prevention: The usual dosage for adults and children 12 years and older is 2 inhalations, 15 minutes prior to exercise.
For treatment, see above.

HOW SUPPLIED

PROVENTIL Inhalation Aerosol, 17.0 g canister; box of one. Each actuation delivers 90 mcg of albuterol from the mouthpiece. It is supplied with an oral adapter and Patient's Instructions (NDC-0085-0614-02). PROVENTIL Inhalation Aerosol REFILL canister, 17.0g, with Patient's Instructions; box of one (NDC-0085-0614-03).
Store between 15° and 30°C (59° and 86°F). Failure to use product within this temperature range may result in improper dosing. Shake well before using.
Copyright© 1981, 1990, 1991, Schering Corporation, USA. All rights reserved.
Revised 3/91
Shown in Product Identification Section, page 428

PROVENTIL®   ℞
brand of albuterol sulfate, USP
Solution for Inhalation 0.5% *
(*Potency expressed as albuterol)

DESCRIPTION

PROVENTIL Solution for Inhalation contains albuterol sulfate, USP, the racemic form of albuterol, and a relatively selective beta$_2$-adrenergic bronchodilator (see **CLINICAL PHARMACOLOGY** section below). Albuterol sulfate has the chemical name α^1-[(*tert*-Butylamino) methyl]-4-hydroxy-m-xylene-α,α'-diol sulfate (2:1) (salt).
Albuterol sulfate has a molecular weight of 576.7 and the empirical formula $(C_{13}H_{21}NO_3)_2 \cdot H_2SO_4$. Albuterol sulfate is a white crystalline powder, soluble in water and slightly soluble in ethanol.
The World Health Organization's recommended name for albuterol base is salbutamol.
PROVENTIL Solution for Inhalation 0.5% solution is in concentrated form. Dilute 0.5 mL of the solution to 3 mL with sterile normal saline solution prior to administration.
Each mL of PROVENTIL Solution for Inhalation 0.5% contains 5 mg of albuterol (as 6.0 mg of albuterol sulfate) in an aqueous solution containing benzalkonium chloride; sulfuric acid is used to adjust the pH between 3 and 5. PROVENTIL Solution for Inhalation 0.5% contains no sulfiting agents. It is supplied in 20 mL bottles.
PROVENTIL Solution for Inhalation is a clear, colorless to light yellow solution.

CLINICAL PHARMACOLOGY

The prime action of beta-adrenergic drugs is to stimulate adenyl cyclase, the enzyme which catalyzes the formation of cyclic-3', 5'-adenosine monophosphate (cyclic AMP) from adenosine triphosphate (ATP). The cyclic AMP thus formed mediates the cellular responses. *In vitro* studies and *in vivo*

pharmacologic studies have demonstrated that albuterol has a preferential effect on beta$_2$-adrenergic receptors compared with isoproterenol. While it is recognized that beta$_2$-adrenergic receptors are the predominant receptors in bronchial smooth muscle, recent data indicate that 10 to 50% of the beta receptors in the human heart may be beta$_2$ receptors. The precise function of these receptors, however, is not yet established. Albuterol has been shown in most controlled clinical trials to have more effect on the respiratory tract, in the form of bronchial smooth muscle relaxation, than isoproterenol at comparable doses while producing fewer cardiovascular effects. Controlled clinical studies and other clinical experience have shown that inhaled albuterol, like other beta-adrenergic agonist drugs, can produce a significant cardiovascular effect in some patients, as measured by pulse rate, blood pressure, symptoms, and/or ECG changes.
Albuterol is longer acting than isoproterenol in most patients by any route of administration because it is not a substrate for the cellular uptake processes for catecholamines nor for catechol-O-methyl transferase.
Studies in asthmatic patients have shown that less than 20% of a single albuterol dose was absorbed following either IPPB or nebulizer administration; the remaining amount was recovered from the nebulizer and apparatus and expired air. Most of the absorbed dose was recovered in the urine 24 hours after drug administration. Following a 3.0 mg dose of nebulized albuterol, the maximum albuterol plasma level at 0.5 hours was 2.1 ng/mL (range 1.4 to 3.2ng/mL). There was a significant dose-related response in FEV_1 and peak flow rate (PFR). It has been demonstrated that following oral administration of 4 mg albuterol, the elimination half-life was 5 to 6 hours.
Animal studies show that albuterol does not pass the blood-brain barrier. Recent studies in laboratory animals (minipigs, rodents, and dogs) recorded the occurrence of cardiac arrhythmias and sudden death (with histologic evidence of myocardial necrosis) when beta-agonists and methylxanthines were administered concurrently. The significance of these findings when applied to humans is currently unknown.
In controlled clinical trials, most patients exhibited an onset of improvement in pulmonary function within 5 minutes as determined by FEV_1. FEV_1 measurements also showed that the maximum average improvement in pulmonary function usually occurred at approximately 1 hour following inhalation of 2.5 mg of albuterol by compressor-nebulizer, and remained close to peak for 2 hours. Clinically significant improvement in pulmonary function (defined as maintenance of a 15% or more increase in FEV_1 over baseline values) continued for 3 to 4 hours in most patients and in some patients continued up to 6 hours.
In repetitive dose studies, continued effectiveness was demonstrated throughout the 3-month period of treatment in some patients.

INDICATIONS AND USAGE

PROVENTIL Solution for Inhalation is indicated for the relief of bronchospasm in patients with reversible obstructive airway disease and acute attacks of bronchospasm.

CONTRAINDICATIONS

PROVENTIL Solution for Inhalation is contraindicated in patients with a history of hypersensitivity to any of its components.

WARNINGS

As with other inhaled beta-adrenergic agonists, PROVENTIL Solution for Inhalation can produce paradoxical bronchospasm, which can be life threatening. If it occurs, the preparation should be discontinued immediately and alternative therapy instituted.
Fatalities have been reported in association with excessive use of inhaled sympathomimetic drugs and with the home use of sympathomimetic nebulizers. It is, therefore, essential that the physician instruct the patient in the need for further evaluation if his/her asthma becomes worse. In individual patients, any beta$_2$-adrenergic agonist, including albuterol solution for inhalation, may have a clinically significant cardiac effect.
Immediate hypersensitivity reactions may occur after administration of albuterol as demonstrated by rare cases of urticaria, angioedema, rash, bronchospasm, and oropharyngeal edema.

PRECAUTIONS

General: Albuterol, as with all sympathomimetic amines, should be used with caution in patients with cardiovascular disorders, especially coronary insufficiency, cardiac arrhythmias and hypertension, in patients with convulsive disorders, hyperthyroidism or diabetes mellitus, and in patients who are unusually responsive to sympathomimetic amines.
Large doses of intravenous albuterol have been reported to aggravate preexisting diabetes mellitus and ketoacidosis. Additionally, beta-agonists, including albuterol, when given intravenously may cause a decrease in serum potassium, possibly through intracellular shunting. The decrease is

usually transient, not requiring supplementation. The relevance of these observations to the use of PROVENTIL Solution for Inhalation is unknown.
Information For Patients: The action of PROVENTIL Solution for Inhalation may last up to 6 hours and therefore it should not be used more frequently than recommended. Do not increase the dose or frequency of medication without medical consultation. If symptoms get worse, medical consultation should be sought promptly. While taking PROVENTIL Solution for Inhalation, other anti-asthma medicines should not be used unless prescribed.
See illustrated "**Patient's Instructions for Use.**"
Drug Interactions: Other sympathomimetic aerosol bronchodilators or epinephrine should not be used concomitantly with albuterol.
Albuterol should be administered with extreme caution to patients being treated with monoamine oxidase inhibitors or tricyclic antidepressants, since the action of albuterol on the vascular system may be potentiated.
Beta-receptor blocking agents and albuterol inhibit the effect of each other.
Carcinogenesis, Mutagenesis, and Impairment of Fertility: Albuterol sulfate, like other agents in its class, caused a significant dose-related increase in the incidence of benign leiomyomas of the mesovarium in a 2-year study in the rat, at oral doses corresponding to 10, 50 and 250 times the maximum human nebulizer dose. In another study, this effect was blocked by the coadministration of propranolol. The relevance of these findings to humans is not known. An 18-month study in mice and a lifetime study in hamsters revealed no evidence of tumorigenicity. Studies with albuterol revealed no evidence of mutagenesis. Reproduction studies in rats revealed no evidence of impaired fertility.
Teratogenic Effects—Pregnancy Category C: Albuterol has been shown to be teratogenic in mice when given subcutaneously in doses corresponding to the human nebulization dose. There are no adequate and well-controlled studies in pregnant women. Albuterol should be used during pregnancy only if the potential benefit justifies the potential risk to the fetus. A reproduction study in CD-1 mice with albuterol (0.025, 0.25 and 2.5 mg/kg subcutaneously, corresponding to 0.1, 1, and 12.5 times the maximum human nebulization dose, respectively) showed cleft palate formation in 5 of 111 (4.5%) of fetuses at 0.25 mg/kg and in 10 of 108 (9.3%) fetuses at 2.5 mg/kg. None were observed at 0.025 mg/kg. Cleft palate also occurred in 22 of 72 (30.5%) fetuses treated with 2.5 mg/kg isoproterenol (positive control). A reproduction study in Stride Dutch rabbits revealed cranioschisis in 7 of 19 (37%) fetuses at 50 mg/kg, corresponding to 250 times the maximum human nebulization dose.
Labor and Delivery: Oral albuterol has been shown to delay preterm labor in some reports. There are presently no well-controlled studies which demonstrate that it will stop preterm labor or prevent labor at term. Therefore, cautious use of PROVENTIL Solution for Inhalation is required in pregnant patients when given for relief of bronchospasm so as to avoid interference with uterine contractibility.
Nursing Mothers: It is not known whether this drug is excreted in human milk. Because of the potential for tumorigenicity shown for albuterol in some animal studies, a decision should be made whether to discontinue nursing or to discontinue the drug, taking into account the importance of the drug to the mother.
Pediatric Use: Safety and effectiveness of albuterol solution for inhalation in children below the age of 12 years have not been established.

ADVERSE REACTIONS

The results of clinical trials with PROVENTIL Solution for Inhalation in 135 patients showed the following side effects which were considered probably or possibly drug related:
Central Nervous System: tremors (20%), dizziness (7%), nervousness (4%), headache (3%), insomnia (1%).
Gastrointestinal: nausea (4%), dyspepsia (1%).
Ear, Nose and Throat: pharyngitis (<1%), nasal congestion (1%).
Cardiovascular: tachycardia (1%), hypertension (1%).
Respiratory: bronchospasm (8%), cough (4%), bronchitis (4%), wheezing (1%).
No clinically relevant laboratory abnormalities related to PROVENTIL Solution for Inhalation administration were determined in these studies.
In comparing the adverse reactions reported for patients treated with PROVENTIL Solution for Inhalation with those of patients treated with isoproterenol during clinical trials of 3 months, the following moderate to severe reactions, as judged by the investigators, were reported. This table does not include mild reactions. [See next page.]
Rare cases of urticaria, angioedema, rash, bronchospasm and oropharyngeal edema have been reported after the use of inhaled albuterol.

OVERDOSAGE

Manifestations of overdosage may include anginal pain, hypertension, hypokalemia, and exaggeration of the pharmacological effects listed in **ADVERSE REACTIONS**.

Percent Incidence of Moderate To Severe Adverse Reactions

Reaction	Albuterol N=65	Isoproterenol N=65
Central Nervous System		
Tremors	10.7%	13.8%
Headache	3.1%	1.5%
Insomnia	3.1%	1.5%
Cardiovascular		
Hypertension	3.1%	3.1%
Arrhythmias	0%	3.0%
*Palpitation	0%	22.0%
Respiratory		
†Bronchospasm	15.4%	18%
Cough	3.1%	5.0%
Bronchitis	1.5%	5.0%
Wheeze	1.5%	1.5%
Sputum Increase	1.5%	1.5%
Dyspnea	1.5%	1.5%
Gastrointestinal		
Nausea	3.1%	0
Dyspepsia	1.5%	0
Systemic		
Malaise	1.5%	0

*The finding of no arrhythmias and no palpitations after albuterol administration in this clinical study should not be interpreted as indicating that these adverse effects cannot occur after the administration of inhaled albuterol.

†In most cases of bronchospasm, this item was generally used to describe exacerbations in the underlying pulmonary disease.

The oral LD_{50} in rats and mice was greater than 2,000 mg/kg. The inhalational LD_{50} could not be determined.
There is insufficient evidence to determine if dialysis is beneficial for overdosage of PROVENTIL Solution for Inhalation.

DOSAGE AND ADMINISTRATION
The usual dosage for adults and children 12 years and older is 2.5 mg of albuterol administered 3 to 4 times daily by nebulization. More frequent administration or higher doses is not recommended. To administer 2.5 mg of albuterol, dilute 0.5 mL of the 0.5% solution for inhalation to a total volume of 3 mL with sterile normal saline solution and administer by nebulization. The flow rate is regulated to suit the particular nebulizer so that the PROVENTIL Solution for Inhalation will be delivered over approximately 5 to 15 minutes.
The use of PROVENTIL Solution for Inhalation can be continued as medically indicated to control recurring bouts of bronchospasm. During treatment, most patients gain optimum benefit from regular use of the nebulizer solution.
If a previously effective dosage regimen fails to provide the usual relief, medical advice should be sought immediately, as this is often a sign of seriously worsening asthma which would require reassessment of therapy.

HOW SUPPLIED
PROVENTIL Solution for Inhalation 0.5%, is a clear, colorless to light yellow solution, and is supplied in bottles of 20 mL (NDC-0085-0208-02) with accompanying calibrated dropper; boxes of one. **Store between 2° and 25°C (36° and 77°F).**
Revised 2/91
Copyright © 1986, 1991, Schering Corporation, Kenilworth, NJ 07033. All rights reserved.

PROVENTIL®   ℞
brand of albuterol sulfate, USP
  Solution for Inhalation 0.083%*
  (*Potency expressed as albuterol)

DESCRIPTION
PROVENTIL Solution for Inhalation contains albuterol sulfate, USP, the racemic form of albuterol, a relatively selective beta₂-adrenergic bronchodilator (see **CLINICAL PHARMACOLOGY** section below). Albuterol sulfate has the chemical name (α^1-[(tert-Bulylamino) methyl]-4-hydroxy-m-xylene-α,α'-diol sulfate (2:1) (salt).
Albuterol sulfate has a molecular weight of 576.7 and the empirical formula $(C_{13}H_{21}NO_3)_2 \cdot H_2SO_4$. Albuterol sulfate is a white crystalline powder, soluble in water and slightly soluble in ethanol.
The World Health Organization recommended name for albuterol base is salbutamol.
Each mL of PROVENTIL Solution for Inhalation 0.083% contains 0.83 mg of albuterol (as 1.0 mg of albuterol sulfate) in an isotonic aqueous solution containing sodium chloride and benzalkonium chloride; sulfuric acid is used to adjust the pH between 3 and 5. The 0.083% solution requires no dilution prior to administration PROVENTIL Solution for Inhalation 0.083% contains no sulfiting agents. It is supplied in 3 mL bottles for unit-dose dispensing.
PROVENTIL Solution for Inhalation is a clear, colorless to light yellow solution.

CLINICAL PHAMACOLOGY
The prime action of beta-adrenergic drugs is to stimulate adenyl cyclase, the enzyme which catalyzes the formation of cyclic-3',5'-adenosine monophosphate (cyclic AMP) from adenosine triphosphate (ATP). The cyclic AMP thus formed mediates the cellular responses. In vitro studies and in vivo pharmacologic studies have demonstrated that albuterol has a preferential effect on beta₂-adrenergic receptors compared with isoproterenol. While it is recognized that beta₂-adrenergic receptors are the predominant receptors in bronchial smooth muscle, recent data indicate that 10 to 50% of the beta receptors in the human heart may be beta₂ receptors. The precise function of these receptors, however, is not yet established. Albuterol has been shown in most controlled clinical trials to have more effect on the respiratory tract, in the form of bronchial smooth muscle relaxation, than isoproterenol at comparable doses while producing fewer cardiovascular effects. Controlled clinical studies and other clinical experience have shown that inhaled albuterol, like other beta-adrenergic agonist drugs, can produce a significant cardiovascular effect in some patients, as measured by pulse rate, blood pressure, symptoms, and/or ECG changes.
Albuterol is longer acting than isoproterenol in most patients by any route of administration because it is not a substrate for the cellular uptake processes for catecholamines nor for catechol-O-methyl transferase.
Studies in asthmatic patients have shown that less than 20% of a single albuterol dose was absorbed following either IPPB or nebulizer administration; the remaining amount was recovered from the nebulizer and apparatus and expired air. Most of the absorbed dose was recovered in the urine 24 hours after drug administration. Following a 3.0 mg dose of nebulized albuterol, the maximum albuterol plasma level at 0.5 hour was 2.1 ng/mL (range 1.4 to 3.2 ng/mL). There was a significant dose-related response in FEV_1 and peak flow rate (PFR). It has been demonstrated that following oral administration of 4 mg albuterol, the elimination half-life was 5 to 6 hours.
Animal studies show that albuterol does not pass the blood-brain barrier. Recent studies in laboratory animals (minipigs, rodents, and dogs) recorded the occurrence of cardiac arrhythmias and sudden death (with histologic evidence of myocardial necrosis) when beta-agonists and methylxanthines were administered concurrently. The significance of these findings when applied to humans is currently unknown.
In controlled clinical trials, most patients exhibited an onset of improvement in pulmonary function within 5 minutes as determined by FEV_1 FEV_1 measurements also showed that the maximum average improvement in pulmonary function usually occurred at approximately 1 hour following inhalation of 2.5 mg of albuterol by compressor-nebulizer, and remained close to peak for 2 hours. Clinically significant improvement in pulmonary function (defined as maintenance of a 15% or more increase in FEV_1 over baseline values) continued for 3 to 4 hours in most patients and in some patients continued up to 6 hours.
In repetitive dose studies, continued effectiveness was demonstrated throughout the 3-month period of treatment in some patients.

INDICATIONS AND USAGE
PROVENTIL Solution for Inhalation is indicated for the relief of bronchospasm in patients with reversible obstructive airway disease and acute attacks of bronchospasm.

CONTRAINDICATIONS
PROVENTIL Solution for Inhalation is contraindicated in patients with a history of hypersensitivity to any of its components.

WARNINGS
As with other inhaled beta-adrenergic agonists, PROVENTIL Solution for Inhalation can produce paradoxical bronchospam, which can be life threatening. If it occurs, the preparation should be discontinued immediately and alternative therapy instituted.
Fatalities have been reported in association with excessive use of inhaled sympathomimetic drugs and with the home use of sympathomimetic nebulizers. It is, therefore, essential that the physician instruct the patient in the need for further evaluation if his/her asthma becomes worse. In individual patients, any beta₂-adrenergic agonist, including albuterol solution for inhalation, may have a clinically significant cardiac effect.
Immediate hypersensitivity reactions may occur after administration of albuterol as demonstrated by rare cases of urticaria, angioedema, rash, bronchospasm, and oropharyngeal edema.

PRECAUTIONS
General: Albuterol, as with all sympathomimetic amines, should be used with caution in patients with cardiovascular disorders, especially coronary insufficiency, cardiac arrhythmias and hypertension, in patients with convulsive disorders, hyperthyroidism or diabetes mellitus, and in patients who are unusually responsive to sympathomimetic amines. Large doses of intravenous albuterol have been reported to aggravate preexisting diabetes mellitus and ketoacidosis. Additionally, beta-agonists, including albuterol, when given intravenously may cause a decrease in serum potassium, possibly through intracellular shunting. The decrease is usually transient, not requiring supplementation. The relevance of these observations to the use of PROVENTIL Solution for Inhalation is unknown.
Information for Patients: The action of PROVENTIL Solution for Inhalation may last up to 6 hours and therefore it should not be used more frequently than recommended. Do not increase the dose or frequency of medication without medical consultation. If symptoms get worse, medical consultation should be sought promptly. While taking PROVENTIL Solution for Inhalation, other anti-asthma medicines should not be used unless prescribed.
See illustrated "Patient's Instructions for Use."
Drug Interactions: Other sympathomimetic aerosol bronchodilators or epinephrine should not be used concomitantly with albuterol.
Albuterol should be administered with extreme caution to patients being treated with monoamine oxidase inhibitors or tricyclic antidepressants, since the action of albuterol in the vascular system may be potentiated.
Beta-receptor blocking agents and albuterol inhibit the effect of each other.
Carcinogenesis, Mutagenesis, and Impairment of Fertility: Albuterol sulfate, like other agents in its class, caused a significant dose-related increase in the incidence of benign leiomyomas of the mesovarium in a 2-year study in the rat, at oral doses corresponding to 10, 50 and 250 times the maximum human nebulizer dose. In another study, this effect was blocked by the coadministration of propranolol. The relevance of these findings to humans is not known. An 18-month study in mice and a lifetime study in hamsters revealed no evidence of tumoriginicity. Studies with albuterol revealed no evidence of mutagenesis. Reproduction studies in rats revealed no evidence of impaired fertility.
Teratogenic Effects—Pregnancy Category C: Albuterol has been shown to be teratogenic in mice when given subcutaneously in doses corresponding to the human nebulization dose. There are no adequate and well-controlled studies in pregnant women. Albuterol should be used during pregnancy only if the potential benefit justifies the potential risk to the fetus. A reproduction study in CD-1 mice with albuterol (0.025, 0.25 and 2.5 mg/kg subcutaneously, corresponding to 0.1, 1, and 12.5 times the maximum human nebulization dose, respectively) showed cleft palate formation in 5 of 111 (4.5%) of fetuses at 0.25 mg/kg and in 10 of 108 (9.3%) fetuses at 2.5 mg/kg. None were observed at 0.025 mg/kg. Cleft palate also occurred in 22 of 72 (30.5%) fetuses treated with 2.5 mg/kg isoproterenol (positive control). A reproduction study in Stride Dutch rabbits revealed cranioschisis in 7 of 19 (37%) fetuses at 50 mg/kg, corresponding to 250 times the maximum human nebulization dose.
Labor and Delivery: Oral albuterol has been shown to delay preterm labor in some reports. There are presently no well-controlled studies which demonstrate that it will stop preterm labor or prevent labor at term. Therefore, cautious use of PROVENTIL Solution for Inhalation is required in pregnant patients when given for relief of bronchospasm so as to avoid interference with uterine contractility.
Nursing Mothers: It is not known whether this drug is excreted in human milk. Because of the potential for tumoriginicity shown for albuterol in some animal studies, a decision should be made whether to discontinue nursing or to discontinue the drug, taking into account the importance of the drug to the mother.
Pediatric Use: Safety and effectiveness of albuterol solution for inhalation in children below the age of 12 years have not been established.

ADVERSE REACTIONS
The results of clinical trials with PROVENTIL Solution for Inhalation in 135 patients showed the following side effects which were considered probably or possibly drug related:
Central Nervous System: tremors (20%), dizziness (7%), nervousness (4%), headache (3%), insomnia (1%).
Gastrointestinal: nausea (4%), dyspepsia (1%).
Ear, Nose and Throat: pharyngitis (<1%), nasal congestion (1%).
Cardiovascular: tachycardia (1%), hypertension (1%).
Respiratory: bronchospasm (8%), cough (4%), bronchitis (4%), wheezing (1%).
No clinically relevant laboratory abnormalities related to PROVENTIL Solution for Inhalation administration were determined in these studies.

Continued on next page

Information on Schering products appearing on these pages is effective as of August 15, 1992.

Schering—Cont.

In comparing the adverse reactions reported for patients treated with PROVENTIL Solution for Inhalation with those of patients treated with isoproterenol during clinical trials of 3 months, the following moderate to severe reactions, as judged by the investigators, were reported. This table does not include mild reactions.

Percent Incidence of Moderate To Severe Reactions

Reaction	Albuterol N=65	Isoproterenol N=65
Central Nervous System		
Tremors	10.7%	13.8%
Headache	3.1%	1.5%
Insomnia	3.1%	1.5%
Cardiovascular		
Hypertension	3.1%	3.1%
Arrhythmias	0%	3.0%
*Palpitation	0%	22.0%
Respiratory		
**Bronchospasm	15.4%	18.0%
Cough	3.1%	5.0%
Bronchitis	1.5%	5.0%
Wheeze	1.5%	1.5%
Sputum Increase	1.5%	1.5%
Dyspnea	1.5%	1.5%
Gastrointestinal		
Nausea	3.1%	0
Dyspepsia	1.5%	0
Systemic		
Malaise	1.5%	0

*The finding of no arrhythmias and no palpitations after albuterol administration in this clinical study should not be interpreted as indicating that these adverse effects can not occur after the administration of inhaled albuterol.

**In most cases of bronchospasm, this item was generally used to describe exacerbations in the underlying pulmonary disease.

Rare cases of urticaria, angioedema, rash, bronchospasm and oropharyngeal edema have been reported after the use of inhaled albuterol.

OVERDOSAGE
Manifestations of overdosage may include anginal pain, hypertension, hypokalemia, and exaggeration of the pharmacological effects listed in **ADVERSE REACTIONS.**
The oral LD_{50} in rats and mice was greater than 2,000 mg/kg. The inhalational LD_{50} could not be determined.
There is insufficient evidence to determine if dialysis is beneficial for overdosage of PROVENTIL Solution for Inhalation.

DOSAGE AND ADMINISTRATION
The usual dosage for adults and children 12 years and older is 2.5 mg of albuterol administered 3 to 4 times daily by nebulization. More frequent administration or higher doses is not recommended. To administer 2.5 mg of albuterol, administer the contents of one unit-dose bottle (3 mL of 0.083% nebulizer solution) by nebulization. The flow rate is regulated to suit the particular nebulizer so that the PROVENTIL Solution for Inhalation will be delivered over approximately 5 to 15 minutes.
The use of PROVENTIL Solution for Inhalation can be continued as medically indicated to control recurring bouts of bronchospasm. During treatment, most patients gain optimum benefit from regular use of the nebulizer solution.
If a previously effective dosage regimen fails to provide the usual relief, medical advice should be sought immediately, as this is often a sign of seriously worsening asthma which would require reassessment of therapy.

HOW SUPPLIED
PROVENTIL Solution for Inhalation, 0.083%, is a clear, colorless to light yellow solution, and is supplied in unit-dose bottles of 3 ml each, boxes of 25 (NDC-0085-0209-01). **Store between 2° and 25°C (36° and 77°F).**
Revised 12/91
Copyright © 1986, 1992, Schering Corporation, Kenilworth, NJ 07033. All rights reserved.

PROVENTIL®   ℞
brand of albuterol sulfate, USP
Syrup

DESCRIPTION
PROVENTIL Syrup contains albuterol sulfate, USP, the racemic form of albuterol and a relatively selective beta$_2$-adrenergic bronchodilator. Albuterol sulfate has the chemical name α^1-[(*tert*-Butylamino)methyl]-4-hydroxy-*m*-xylene-α,α'-diol sulfate (2:1) (salt).
Albuterol sulfate has a molecular weight of 576.7 and the empirical formula $(C_{13}H_{21}NO_3)_2 \cdot H_2SO_4$. Albuterol sulfate is a white crystalline powder, soluble in water and slightly soluble in ethanol.
The World Heatlh Organization recommended name for albuterol base is salbutamol.
PROVENTIL Syrup contains 2 mg of albuterol as 2.4 mg of albuterol sulfate in each teaspoonful (5 ml).
The inactive ingredients for Proventil Syrup include: citric acid, FD&C Yellow No. 6, flavor, hydroxypropyl methylcellulose, saccharin, sodium benzoate, sodium citrate and water.

CLINICAL PHARMACOLOGY
The prime action of beta-adrenergic drugs is to stimulate adenyl cyclase, the enzyme which catalyzes the formation of cyclic-3',5'-adenosine monophosphate (cyclic AMP) from adenosine triphosphate (ATP). The cyclic AMP thus formed mediates the cellular responses. Based on pharmacologic studies in animals, albuterol appears to exert direct and preferential action on beta$_2$-adrenoceptors including those of the bronchial tree and uterus, and may have less cardiac stimulant effect than isoproterenol, when given in the usual recommended dose.
Albuterol is longer acting than isoproterenol in most patients by any route of administration because it is not a substrate for the cellular uptake processes for catecholamines nor for catechol-*O*-methyl transferase.
After oral administration of 10 ml PROVENTIL Syrup (4 mg albuterol) in normal volunteers, albuterol is rapidly absorbed. Maximum plasma albuterol concentrations of about 18 ng/ml are achieved within 2 hours and the drug is eliminated with a half-life of about 5 hours. In other studies, the analysis of urine samples of patients given 8 mg tritiated albuterol orally showed that 76% of the dose was excreted over 3 days, with the majority of the dose being excreted within the first 24 hours. Sixty percent of this radioactivity was shown to be the metabolite. Feces collected over this period contained 4% of the administered dose.
Animal studies show that albuterol does not pass the blood-brain barrier.

INDICATIONS AND USAGE
PROVENTIL Syrup is indicated for the relief of bronchospasm in adults and in children 2 years of age and older with reversible obstructive airway disease.
In controlled clinical trials in patients with asthma, the onset of improvement in pulmonary function, as measured by maximal midexpiratory flow rate (MMEF) and forced expiratory volume in one second (FEV$_1$), was within 30 minutes after a dose of PROVENTIL Syrup. Peak improvement of pulmonary function occurred between 2 to 3 hours. In a controlled clinical trial involving 55 children, clinically significant improvement (defined as maintenance of mean values over baseline of 15% or 20% or more in the FEV$_1$ and MMEF respectively) continued to be recorded up to 6 hours. No decrease in the effectiveness was reported in one uncontrolled study of 32 children who took PROVENTIL Syrup for a 3 month period.

CONTRAINDICATIONS
PROVENTIL Syrup is contraindicated in patients with a history of hypersensitivity to any of its components.

PRECAUTIONS
General: Although albuterol usually has minimal effects on the beta$_1$-adrenoceptors of the cardiovascular system at the recommended dosage, occasionally the usual cardiovascular and CNS stimulatory effects common to all sympathomimetic agents have been seen with patients treated with albuterol necessitating discontinuation. Therefore, albuterol should be used with caution in patients with cardiovascular disorders, including coronary insufficiency and hypertension, in patients with hyperthyroidism or diabetes mellitus, and in patients who are unusually responsive to sympathomimetic amines.
Large doses of intravenous albuterol have been reported to aggravate preexisting diabetes mellitus and ketoacidosis. Additionally, albuterol and other beta-agonists, when given intravenously, may cause a decrease in serum potassium, possibly through intracellular shunting. The decrease is usually transient, not requiring supplementation. The relevance of these observations to the use of PROVENTIL Syrup is unknown.
Information for Patients: The action of PROVENTIL Syrup may last up to 6 hours and therefore it should not be taken more frequently than recommended. Do not increase the dose or frequency of medication without medical consultation. If symptoms get worse, medical consultation should be sought promptly. If pregnant or nursing, consult with your physician.
Drug Interactions: The concomitant use of PROVENTIL Syrup and other oral sympathomimetic agents is not recommended since such combined use may lead to deleterious cardiovascular effects. This recommendation does not preclude the judicious use of an aerosol bronchodilator of the adrenergic stimulant type in patients receiving PROVENTIL Syrup. Such concomitant use, however, should be individualized and not given on a routine basis. If regular coad-

ministration is required, then alternative therapy should be considered.
Albuterol should be administered with extreme caution to patients being treated with monoamine oxidase inhibitors or tricyclic antidepressants since the action of albuterol on the vascular system may be potentiated.
Beta-receptor blocking agents and albuterol inhibit the effect of each other.
Carcinogenesis, Mutagenesis, and Impairment of Fertility: Albuterol sulfate, like other agents in its class, caused a significant dose-related increase in the incidence of benign leiomyomas of the mesovarium in a 2-year study in the rat, at doses corresponding to 2, 9, and 46 times the maximum human (child weighing 21 kg) oral dose. In another study this effect was blocked by the coadministration of propranolol. The relevance of these findings to humans is not known. An 18-month study in mice and a lifetime study in hamsters revealed no evidence of tumorigenicity. Studies with albuterol revealed no evidence of mutagenesis. Reproduction studies in rats revealed no evidence of impaired fertility.
Teratogenic Effects—Pregnancy Category C: Albuterol has been shown to be teratogenic in mice when given subcutaneously in doses corresponding to 0.2 times the maximum human (child weighing 21 kg) oral dose. There are no adequate and well-controlled studies in pregnant women. Albuterol should be used during pregnancy only if the potential benefit justifies the potential risk to the fetus. A reproduction study in CD-1 mice with albuterol showed cleft palate formation in 5 of 111 (4.5%) fetuses at 0.25 mg/kg and in 10 of 108 (9.3%) fetuses at 2.5 mg/kg; none was observed at 0.025 mg/kg. Cleft palate also occurred in 22 of 72 (30.5%) fetuses treated with 2.5 mg/kg isoproterenol (positive control). A reproduction study in Stride Dutch rabbits revealed cranioschisis in 7 of 19 (37%) fetuses at 50 mg/kg, corresponding to 46 times the maximum human (child weighing 21 kg) oral dose of albuterol sulfate.
Labor and Delivery: Oral albuterol has been shown to delay preterm labor in some reports. There are presently no well-controlled studies which demonstrate that it will stop preterm labor or prevent labor at term. Therefore, cautious use of PROVENTIL Syrup is required in pregnant patients when given for relief of bronchospasm so as to avoid interference with uterine contractibility. Use in such patients should be restricted to those patients in whom the benefits clearly outweigh the risks.
Nursing Mothers: It is not know whether this drug is excreted in human milk. Because of the potential for tumorigenicity shown for albuterol in animal studies, a decision should be made whether to discontinue nursing or to discontinue the drug, taking into account the importance of the drug to the mother.
Pediatric Use: Safety and effectiveness in children below the age of 2 years have not yet been adequately demonstrated.

ADVERSE REACTIONS
The adverse reactions to albuterol are similar in nature to those of other sympathomimetic agents. The most frequent adverse reactions to PROVENTIL Syrup in adults and older children were tremor, 10 of 100 patients; nervousness and shakiness, each 9 of 100 patients. Other reported adverse reactions were headache, 4 of 100 patients; dizziness and increased appetite, each 3 of 100 patients; hyperactivity and excitement, each 2 of 100 patients; tachycardia, epistaxis, irritable behavior, and sleeplessness, each 1 of 100 patients. The following adverse effects occurred in less than 1 of 100 patients each: muscle spasm; disturbed sleep, epigastric pain; cough; palpitations; stomach ache; irritable behavior; dilated pupils; sweating; chest pain; weakness.
In young children 2 to 6 years of age, some adverse reactions were noted more frequently than in adults and older children. Excitement was noted in approximately 20% of patients and nervousness in 15%. Hyperkinesia occurred in 4% of patients; insomnia, tachycardia, and gastrointestinal symptoms in 2% each. Anorexia, emotional lability, pallor, fatigue, and conjunctivitis were seen in 1%.
In addition, albuterol, like other sympathomimetic agents, can cause adverse reactions such as hypertension, angina, vomiting, vertigo, central nervous system stimulation, unusual taste, and drying or irritation of the oropharynx.
The reactions are generally transient in nature, and it is usually not necessary to discontinue treatment with PROVENTIL Syrup. In selected cases, however, dosage may be reduced temporarily; after the reaction has subsided, dosage should be increased in small increments to the optimal dosage.

OVERDOSAGE
Manifestations of overdosage include anginal pain, hypertension, hypokalemia, and exaggeration of the effects listed in **Adverse Reactions.**
The oral LD_{50} in rats and mice was greater than 2,000 mg/kg. Dialysis is not appropriate treatment for overdosage of PROVENTIL Syrup. The judicious use of a cardioselective beta-receptor blocker, such as metoprolol tartrate,

is suggested, bearing in mind the danger of inducing an asthmatic attack.

DOSAGE AND ADMINISTRATION

The following dosages of PROVENTIL Syrup are expressed in terms of albuterol base.

Usual Dose: The usual starting dosage for adults and children over age 14 is 2 mg (1 teaspoonful) or 4 mg (2 teaspoonsful) three or four times a day.

The usual starting dosage for children 6 to 14 years of age is 2 mg (1 teaspoonful) three or four times a day.

For children 2 to 6 years of age, dosing should be initiated at 0.1 mg/kg of body weight three times a day. This starting dose should not exceed 2 mg (1 teaspoonful) three times a day.

Dosage Adjustment: For adults and children above age 14, dosage above 4 mg four times a day should be used *only* when the patient fails to respond. If a favorable response does not occur, the dosage may be cautiously increased stepwise, but not to exceed 8 mg four times a day.

For children from 6 to 14 years of age who fail to respond to the initial starting dosage of 2 mg four times a day, the dosage may be cautiously increased stepwise, but not to exceed 24 mg per day (given in divided doses).

For children 2 to 6 years of age who do not respond satisfactorily to the initial dosage, the dose may be increased stepwise to 0.2 mg/kg of body weight three times a day, but not to exceed a maximum of 4 mg (2 teaspoonfuls) given three times a day.

For elderly patients and those sensitive to beta-adrenergic stimulation, the initial dose should be restricted to 2 mg three or four times a day and individually adjusted thereafter.

HOW SUPPLIED

PROVENTIL Syrup, a clear orange-yellow liquid with a strawberry flavor, contains 2 mg albuterol as the sulfate per 5 ml; bottles of 16 fluid ounces (NDC 0085-0315-02).

Store between 2° and 30°C (36° and 86°F).

Revised 3/91

Copyright © 1982, 1991, Schering Corporation, Kenilworth, NJ 07033, USA. All rights reserved.

PROVENTIL®   ℞

[pro-ven 'til]

brand of albuterol sulfate, USP
REPETABS® brand of
    extended-release Tablets
PROVENTIL®
brand of albuterol sulfate, USP
    Tablets

DESCRIPTION

PROVENTIL REPETABS Tablets and PROVENTIL Tablets contain albuterol sulfate, USP, the racemic form of albuterol and a relatively selective beta$_2$-adrenergic bronchodilator. Albuterol sulfate has the chemical name α^1-[(*tert* -Butylamino)methyl]-4-hydroxy-*m* -xylene-α,α'-diol sulfate (2:1) (salt). Albuterol sulfate has a molecular weight of 576.7 and the empirical formula $(C_{13}H_{21}NO_3)_2 \cdot H_2SO_4$. Albuterol sulfate is a white crystalline powder, soluble in water and slightly soluble in ethanol.

The World Health Organization recommended name for albuterol base is salbutamol.

Each PROVENTIL REPETABS Tablet contains a total of 4 mg (2 mg in the coating for immediate release and 2 mg in the core for release after several hours) of albuterol as 4.8 mg of albuterol sulfate.

Each PROVENTIL Tablet contains 2 or 4 mg of albuterol as 2.4 and 4.8 mg of albuterol sulfate, respectively.

The inactive ingredients for PROVENTIL REPETABS Tablets include: acacia, butylparaben, calcium phosphate, calcium sulfate, carnauba wax, corn starch, lactose, magnesium stearate, neutral soap, oleic acid, rosin, sugar, talc, titanium dioxide, white wax, and zein.

The inactive ingredients for PROVENTIL Tablets, 2 and 4 mg include: corn starch, lactose and magnesium stearate.

CLINICAL PHARMACOLOGY

In vitro studies and *in vivo* pharmacologic studies have demonstrated that PROVENTIL has a preferential effect on beta$_2$-adrenergic receptors compared with isoproterenol. While it is recognized that beta$_2$-adrenergic receptors are the predominant receptors in bronchial smooth muscle, recent data indicate that there is a population of beta$_2$-receptors in the human heart, existing in a concentration between 10–50%. The precise function of these receptors, however, is not yet established.

Albuterol is longer acting than isoproterenol in most patients by any route of administration because it is not a substrate for the cellular uptake processes for catecholamines nor for catechol-*O*-methyl transferase.

Albuterol is rapidly and well absorbed following oral administration. In studies involving normal volunteers, the mean steady state peak and trough plasma levels of albuterol were

6.7 and 3.8 ng/ml, respectively, following dosing with a 2 mg PROVENTIL Tablet every 6 hours and 14.8 and 8.6 ng/ml, respectively, following dosing with a 4 mg PROVENTIL Tablet every 6 hours. Maximum albuterol plasma levels are usually obtained between 2 and 3 hours after dosing and the elimination half-life is 5 to 6 hours. These data indicate that albuterol administered orally, is dose proportional and exhibits dose independent pharmacokinetics.

In other studies, the analysis of urine samples of subjects given tritiated albuterol (4–10 mg) orally showed that 65% to 90% of the dose was excreted over 3 days, with the majority of the dose being excreted within the first 24 hours. Sixty percent of this radioactivity was shown to be the metabolite of albuterol. Feces collected over this period contained 4% of the administered dose.

PROVENTIL REPETABS Tablets have been formulated to provide a duration of action of up to 12 hours. In studies conducted in normal volunteers, the mean steady state peak and trough plasma levels of albuterol were 6.5 and 3.0 ng/ml, respectively, following dosing with a 4 mg PROVENTIL REPETABS Tablet every 12 hours. In addition, it has been shown that administration of a 4 mg PROVENTIL REPETABS Tablet every 12 hours is bioequivalent to administration of a 2 mg PROVENTIL Tablet every 6 hours.

Animal studies show that albuterol does not pass the blood-brain barrier. Recent studies in laboratory animals (minipigs, rodents, and dogs) recorded the occurrence of cardiac arrhythmias and sudden death (with histologic evidence of myocardial necrosis) when beta-agonists and methylxanthines were administered concurrently. The significance of these findings when applied to humans is currently unknown.

In controlled clinical trials in patients with asthma, the onset of improvement in pulmonary function, as measured by maximal midexpiratory flow rate, MMEF, was noted within 30 minutes after a dose of PROVENTIL Tablets with peak improvement occurring between 2 to 3 hours. In controlled clinical trials, in which measurements were conducted for 6 hours, significant clinical improvement in pulmonary function (defined as maintaining a 15% or more increase in FEV$_1$ and a 20% or more increase in MMEF over baseline values) was observed in 60% of patients at 4 hours and in 40% at 6 hours. In other single dose, controlled clinical trials, clinically significant improvement was observed in at least 40% of the patients at 8 hours with the 4 mg PROVENTIL Tablet. No decrease in the effectiveness of PROVENTIL Tablets has been reported in patients who received long-term treatment with the drug in uncontrolled studies for periods up to 6 months.

In another controlled clinical study in asthmatic patients, it has been demonstrated that the initiation of therapy with either the 4 mg PROVENTIL REPETABS Tablet dosed every 12 hours, or the 2 mg PROVENTIL Tablet dosed every 6 hours, achieve therapeutically equivalent effects.

INDICATIONS AND USAGE

PROVENTIL REPETABS Tablets and PROVENTIL Tablets are indicated for the relief of bronchospasm in patients with reversible obstructive airway disease.

CONTRAINDICATIONS

PROVENTIL REPETABS Tablets and PROVENTIL Tablets are contraindicated in patients with a history of hypersensitivity to any of their components.

PRECAUTIONS

General: Since albuterol is a sympathomimetic amine, it should be used with caution in patients with cardiovascular disorders, including ischemic heart disease, hypertension or cardiac arrhythmias, in patients with hyperthyroidism or diabetes mellitus, and in patients who are unusually responsive to sympathomimetic amines or who have convulsive disorders. Significant changes in systolic and diastolic blood pressure could be expected to occur in some patients after use of any beta adrenergic bronchodilator.

Large doses of intravenous albuterol have been reported to aggravate preexisting diabetes mellitus and ketoacidosis. Additionally, albuterol and other beta agonists, when given intravenously, may cause a decrease in serum potassium, possibly through intracellular shunting. The decrease is usually transient, not requiring supplementation. The relevance of these observations to the use of PROVENTIL REPETABS Tablets and PROVENTIL Tablets is unknown.

Information for Patients: Patients being treated with PROVENTIL REPETABS Tablets or PROVENTIL Tablets should receive the following information and instructions. This information is intended to aid in the safe and effective use of this medication. It is not a disclosure of all possible adverse or intended effects.

PROVENTIL REPETABS Tablets and PROVENTIL Tablets should not be taken more frequently than recommended. Do not increase the dose or frequency of medication, or add other medications to your therapy without medical consultation. If symptoms get worse, medical consultation should be sought promptly. If pregnant or nursing, consult with your physician.

Drug Interactions: The concomitant use of PROVENTIL REPETABS Tablets or PROVENTIL Tablets and other oral sympathomimetic agents is not recommended since such combined use may lead to deleterious cardiovascular effects. This recommendation does not preclude the judicious use of an aerosol bronchodilator of the adrenergic stimulant type in patients receiving PROVENTIL REPETABS Tablets or PROVENTIL Tablets. Such concomitant use, however, should be individualized and not given on a routine basis. If regular coadministration is required, then alternative therapy should be considered.

Albuterol should be administered with extreme caution to patients being treated with monoamine oxidase inhibitors or tricyclic antidepressants, since the action of albuterol on the vascular system may be potentiated.

Beta-receptor blocking agents and albuterol inhibit the effect of each other.

Carcinogenesis, Mutagenesis, and Impairment of Fertility: Albuterol sulfate, like other agents in its class, caused a significant dose-related increase in the incidence of benign leiomyomas of the mesovarium in a 2-year study in the rat, at doses corresponding to 3, 16, and 78 times the maximum human oral dose. In another study, this effect was blocked by the coadministration of propranolol. The relevance of these findings to humans is not known. An 18-month study in mice and a lifetime study in hamsters revealed no evidence of tumorigenicity.

Studies with albuterol revealed no evidence of mutagenesis. Reproduction studies in rats revealed no evidence of impaired fertility.

Teratogenic Effects—Pregnancy Category C: Albuterol has been shown to be teratogenic in mice when given subcutaneously in doses corresponding to 0.4 times the maximum human oral dose. There are no adequate and well-controlled studies in pregnant women. Albuterol should be used during pregnancy only if the potential benefit justifies the potential risk to the fetus. A reproduction study in CD-1 mice with albuterol showed cleft palate formation in 5 of 111 (4.5%) fetuses at 0.25 mg/kg and in 10 of 108 (9.3%) fetuses at 2.5 mg/kg; none were observed at 0.025 mg/kg. Cleft palate also occurred in 22 of 72 (30.5%) fetuses treated with 2.5 mg/kg isoproterenol (positive control). A reproduction study in Stride Dutch rabbits revealed cranioschisis in 7 of 19 (37%) fetuses at 50 mg/kg, corresponding to 78 times the maximum human oral dose of albuterol.

Labor and Delivery: Oral albuterol has been shown to delay preterm labor in some reports. There are presently no well-controlled studies which demonstrate that it will stop preterm labor or prevent labor at term. Therefore, cautious use of PROVENTIL REPETABS Tablets and PROVENTIL Tablets is required in pregnant patients when given for relief of bronchospasm so as to avoid interference with uterine contractibility.

Nursing Mothers: It is not known whether this drug is excreted in human milk. Because of the potential for tumorigenicity shown for albuterol in some animal studies, a decision should be made whether to discontinue nursing or to discontinue the drug, taking into account the importance of the drug to the mother.

Pediatric Use: Safety and effectiveness in children below the age of 6 years for PROVENTIL Tablets, and below the age of 12 years for PROVENTIL REPETABS Tablets have not been established.

ADVERSE REACTIONS

The adverse reactions to albuterol are similar in nature to those of other sympathomimetic agents. The most frequent adverse reactions to PROVENTIL Tablets were nervousness and tremor, with each occurring in approximately 20 of 100 patients (20%). Other reported reactions were headache, 7 of 100 patients (7%); tachycardia and palpitations, 5 of 100 patients (5%); muscle cramps, 3 of 100 patients (3%); insomnia, nausea, weakness, and dizziness, each occurred in 2 of 100 patients (2%). Drowsiness, flushing, restlessness, irritability, chest discomfort, and difficulty in micturition each occurred in less than 1 of 100 patients (less than 1%).

In a clinical study of one week duration comparing a 4 mg PROVENTIL REPETABS Tablet administered every 12 hours, to a 2 mg PROVENTIL Tablet administered every 6 hours, the following adverse reactions considered to be possibly or probably treatment related were reported: nervousness in 1 of 50 (2%) and 3 of 50 patients (6%) for PROVENTIL REPETABS and PROVENTIL Tablets, respectively; nausea in 2 of 50 (4%) for both; vomiting in 1 of 50 (2%) and 2 of 50 (4%) for PROVENTIL REPETABS and PROVENTIL Tablets, respectively; somnolence in 1 of 50 (2%) for both. The following adverse reactions were reported for PROVENTIL Tablets only, tremor in 3 of 50 patients (6%), tinnitus, dyspepsia, and rash each occurred in 1 of 50 patients (2%).

Continued on next page

Information on Schering products appearing on these pages is effective as of August 15, 1992.

Schering—Cont.

Although not reported for PROVENTIL REPETABS Tablets in the above study, there have been reports of tremor in other trials. When all clinical experience is considered, the incidence of tremor is approximately the same as that seen with PROVENTIL Tablets.

In addition to those adverse reactions reported above, albuterol, like other sympathomimetic agents, can cause adverse reactions such as hypertension, angina, vomiting, vertigo, central nervous system stimulation, unusual taste, and drying or irritation of the oropharynx.

The reactions are generally transient in nature, and it is usually not necessary to discontinue treatment with PROVENTIL REPETABS Tablets or PROVENTIL Tablets. In selected cases, however, dosage may be reduced temporarily; after the reaction has subsided, dosage should be increased in small increments to the optimal dosage.

OVERDOSAGE

Manifestations of overdosage include anginal pain, hypertension, hypokalemia and exaggeration of the pharmacological effects listed in ADVERSE REACTIONS.

The oral LD_{50} in rats and mice was greater than 2,000 mg/kg.

There is insufficient evidence to determine if dialysis is beneficial for overdosage of PROVENTIL REPETABS Tablets or PROVENTIL Tablets.

DOSAGE AND ADMINISTRATION

The following dosages of PROVENTIL REPETABS Tablets and PROVENTIL Tablets are expressed in terms of albuterol base.

PROVENTIL REPETABS Tablets

Usual Dose The usual starting dosage of PROVENTIL REPETABS Tablets for adults and children 12 years and over is 4 or 8 mg (one or two tablets) every 12 hours.

Dosage Adjustment Doses above 8 mg twice a day of PROVENTIL REPETABS Tablets should be used only when the patient fails to respond to lower doses. The dose should be increased cautiously stepwise up to a maximum of 16 mg twice a day if a favorable response does not occur with the 4 mg initial dose.

The total daily dose should not exceed 32 mg in adults and children 12 years and over.

Switching to PROVENTIL REPETABS Tablets Patients currently maintained on PROVENTIL Tablets can be switched to PROVENTIL REPETABS Tablets. For example, the administration of a 4 mg PROVENTIL REPETABS Tablet every 12 hours is equivalent to one 2 mg PROVENTIL Tablet every 6 hours. Multiples of this regimen up to the maximum recommended daily dose also apply.

PROVENTIL Tablets

Usual Dose The usual starting dosage for children 6 to 12 years of age is 2 mg three or four times a day.

The usual starting dosage for adults and children 12 years and over is 2 mg or 4 mg three or four times a day.

Dosage Adjustment For children from 6 to 12 years of age who fail to respond to the initial starting dosage of 2 mg four times a day, the dosage may be cautiously increased stepwise, but not to exceed 24 mg per day (given in divided doses).

For adults and children 12 years and over, a dosage above 4 mg four times a day should be used only when the patient fails to respond to lower doses. The dose should be increased cautiously stepwise up to a maximum of 8 mg four times a day as tolerated if a favorable response does not occur with the 4 mg initial dose.

Elderly Patients and Those Sensitive to Beta-Adrenergic Stimulators An initial dose of 2 mg three or four times a day is recommended for elderly patients and for those with a history of unusual sensitivity to beta-adrenergic stimulators. If adequate bronchodilation is not obtained, dosage may be increased gradually to as much as 8 mg three or four times a day.

The total daily dose should not exceed 32 mg in adults and children 12 years and over.

HOW SUPPLIED

PROVENTIL REPETABS Tablets, 4 mg albuterol as the sulfate (2 mg in the coating for immediate release and 2 mg in the core for release after several hours), white, round, coated tablets, branded in red on one side with the Schering trademark, and product identifications numbers, 431, bottles of 100 (NDC 0085-0431-02) and boxes of 100 for unit dose dispensing (NDC 0085-0431-04).

PROVENTIL Tablets, 2 mg albuterol as the sulfate, white, round, compressed tablets, impressed with the product name (PROVENTIL) and the number 2 on one side, and product identification numbers, 252, and scored on the other, bottles of 100 (NDC 0085-0252-02) and 500 (NDC 0085-0252-03).

PROVENTIL Tablets, 4 mg albuterol as the sulfate, white, round, compressed tablets, impressed with the product name (PROVENTIL) and the number 4 on one side, and product identification numbers, 573, and scored on the other, bottles of 100 (NDC 0085-0573-02) and 500 (NDC 0085-0573-03).

Store PROVENTIL REPETABS Tablets and PROVENTIL Tablets between 2° and 30°C (36° and 86°F). Protect PROVENTIL REPETABS Tablets in the unit dose box from excessive moisture.

Copyright © 1982, 1991, Schering Corporation. All rights reserved.

Shown in Product Identification Section, page 428

Sodium SULAMYD® ℞

[so 'dē-um soo 'lah-mĭd]

brand of sulfacetamide sodium

Ophthalmic Solution, USP 30%—Sterile
Ophthalmic Solution, USP 10%—Sterile
Ophthalmic Ointment, USP 10%—Sterile

DESCRIPTION

Sodium SULAMYD is available in three ophthalmic forms:
Ophthalmic Solution 30% contains in each ml of sterile aqueous solution 300 mg sulfacetamide sodium, USP, 1.5 mg sodium thiosulfate, with 0.5 mg methylparaben and 0.1 mg propylparaben added as preservatives, and monobasic sodium phosphate as buffer.

Ophthalmic Solution 10% contains in each ml of sterile aqueous solution 100 mg sulfacetamide sodium, USP, 3.1 mg sodium thiosulfate, and 5 mg methylcellulose, with 0.5 mg methylparaben and 0.1 mg propylparaben added as preservatives and monobasic sodium phosphate as buffer.

Ophthalmic Ointment 10% is a sterile ointment, each gram containing 100 mg sulfacetamide sodium, USP, with 0.5 mg methylparaben, 0.1 mg propylparaben and 0.25 mg benzalkonium chloride added as preservatives, and sorbitan monolaurate and water in a bland, unctuous, petrolatum base.

ACTIONS

Sodium SULAMYD exerts a bacteriostatic effect against a wide range of gram-positive and gram-negative microorganisms by restricting, through competition with para-aminobenzoic acid, the synthesis of folic acid which bacteria require for growth.

INDICATIONS

Sodium SULAMYD is indicated for the treatment of conjunctivitis, corneal ulcer, and other superficial ocular infections due to susceptible microorganisms, and as adjunctive treatment in systemic sulfonamide therapy of trachoma.

CONTRAINDICATIONS

Sodium SULAMYD is contraindicated in individuals with known or suspected sensitivity to sulfonamides or to any of the ingredients of the preparations.

PRECAUTIONS

Sodium SULAMYD products are incompatible with silver preparations. Ophthalmic ointments may retard corneal healing. Non-susceptible organisms, including fungi, may proliferate with the use of these preparations. Sulfonamides are inactivated by the para-aminobenzoic acid present in purulent exudates.

Sensitization may recur when a sulfonamide is re-administered irrespective of the route of administration, and cross sensitivity between different sulfonamides may occur. If signs of sensitivity or other untoward reactions occur, discontinue use of the preparation.

ADVERSE REACTIONS

Sulfacetamide sodium may cause local irritation, stinging and burning. While the irritation may be transient, occasionally, use of the medication has to be discontinued.

Although sensitivity reactions to sulfacetamide sodium are rare, an isolated incident of Stevens-Johnson syndrome was reported in a patient who had experienced a previous bullous drug reaction to an orally administered sulfonamide and a single instance of local hypersensitivity was reported which progressed to a fatal syndrome resembling systemic lupus erythematosus.

DOSAGE AND ADMINISTRATION

Sodium SULAMYD Ophthalmic Solution 30%. *For conjunctivitis or corneal ulcer:* instill one drop into lower conjunctival sac every two hours or less frequently according to severity of infection. *For trachoma:* Two drops every two hours; concomitant systemic sulfonamide therapy is indicated.

Sodium SULAMYD Ophthalmic Solution 10%. One or two drops into the lower conjunctival sac every two or three hours during the day and less often at night.

Sodium SULAMYD Ophthalmic Ointment 10%. Apply a small amount four times daily and at bedtime. The ointment may be used adjunctively with either of the solution forms.

HOW SUPPLIED

Sodium SULAMYD Ophthalmic Solution 30%, 15 ml dropper bottle (NDC 0085-0717-06), box of one. **Store between 2° and 30°C (36° and 86°F).**

Sodium SULAMYD Ophthalmic Solution 10%, 5 ml dropper bottle (NDC 0085-0946-03), box of 25; 15 ml dropper bottle (NDC 0085-0946-06), box of one. **Store between 2° and 30°C (36° and 86°F).**

Sodium SULAMYD Ophthalmic Ointment 10%, 3.5 g tube (NDC 0085-0066-03), box of one. **Store away from heat.**

On long standing, sulfonamide solutions will darken in color and should be discarded.

Revised 10/84 13227411

Copyright © 1969, 1985, Schering Corporation, USA. All rights reserved.

SOLGANAL® ℞

[sol 'gah-nal]

brand of sterile aurothioglucose
Suspension, USP
FOR INTRAMUSCULAR
INJECTION ONLY—
NOT FOR INTRAVENOUS USE

WARNINGS

Physicians planning to use SOLGANAL Suspension should thoroughly familiarize themselves with its toxicity and its benefits. The possibility of toxic reactions should always be explained to the patient before starting therapy. Patients should be warned to report promptly any symptom suggesting toxicity. Before **each** injection of SOLGANAL Suspension, the physician should review the results of laboratory work and see the patient to determine the presence or absence of adverse reactions, since some of these can be severe or even fatal.

DESCRIPTION

SOLGANAL is a sterile suspension, for **intramuscular injection only.** SOLGANAL Suspension is an antiarthritic agent which is absorbed gradually following intramuscular injection, producing a therapeutically desired prolonged effect.

Each ml contains 50 mg of aurothioglucose, USP in sterile sesame oil with 2% aluminum monostearate; 1 mg propylparaben is added as preservative. Aurothioglucose contains approximately 50% gold by weight.

The empirical formula for aurothioglucose is $C_6H_{11}AuO_5S$; the molecular weight is 392.18. Chemically it is (1-Thio-D-glucopyranosato) gold.

Aurothioglucose is a nearly odorless, yellow powder which is stable in air. An aqueous solution is unstable on long standing. Aurothioglucose is freely soluble in water but practically insoluble in acetone, in alcohol, in chloroform, and in ether.

CLINICAL PHARMACOLOGY

Although the mechanism of action is not well understood, gold compounds have been reported to decrease synovial inflammation and retard cartilage and bone destruction.

Gold is absorbed from injection sites, reaching peak concentration in blood in four to six hours. Following a single intramuscular injection of 50 mg SOLGANAL Suspension in each of two patients, peak serum levels were about 235 mcg/dl in one patient and 450 mcg/dl in the other. In plasma, 95% is bound to the albumin fraction. Approximately 70% of the gold is eliminated in the urine and approximately 30% in the feces. When a standard weekly treatment schedule is followed, approximately 40% of the administered dose is excreted each week, and the remainder is excreted over a longer period. The biological half-life of gold salts following a single 50 mg dose has been reported to range from 3 to 27 days. Following successive weekly doses, the half-life increases and may be 14 to 40 days after the third dose and up to 168 days after the eleventh weekly dose.

After the initial injection, the serum level of gold rises sharply and declines over the next week. Peak levels with aqueous preparations are higher and decline faster than those with oily preparations. Weekly administration produces a continuous rise in the basal value for several months, after which the serum level becomes relatively stable. After a standard weekly dose, considerable individual variation in the levels of gold has been found. A steady decline in gold levels occurs when the interval between injections is lengthened, and small amounts may be found in the serum for months after discontinuance of therapy. The incidence of toxic reactions is apparently unrelated to the plasma level of gold, but it may be related to the cumulative body content of gold.

Storage of gold in human tissues is dependent upon organ mass as well as upon the concentration of gold. Therefore, tissues having the highest gold levels (weight/weight) do not necessarily contain the greatest total amounts of gold. The major depots, in decreasing order of total gold content, are the bone marrow, liver, skin, and bone, accounting for approximately 85% of body gold. The highest concentrations of gold are found in the lymph nodes, adrenal glands, liver, kidneys, bone marrow, and spleen. Relatively small concentrations are found in articular structures.

Gold passes the blood-brain barrier in hamsters.

Transfer of gold across the human placenta at the twentieth week of pregnancy has been documented. The placenta showed numerous gold deposits and smaller amounts were detected in the fetal liver and kidneys; other tissues provided no evidence of gold deposition.

Gold is excreted into human milk in significant amounts and trace amounts can be demonstrated in the blood of nursing infants. (See PRECAUTIONS, "*Nursing Mothers.*")

INDICATIONS AND USAGE

SOLGANAL Suspension is indicated for the adjunctive treatment of early active rheumatoid arthritis (both of the adult and juvenile types) not adequately controlled by other anti-inflammatory agents and conservative measures. In chronic, advanced cases of rheumatoid arthritis, gold therapy is less valuable.

Antirheumatic measures such as salicylates and other anti-inflammatory drugs (both steroidal and non-steroidal) may be continued after initiation of gold therapy. After improvement commences, these measures may be discontinued slowly as symptoms permit.

See Precautions, "*Laboratory Tests*" and **Dosage and Administration**.

CONTRAINDICATIONS

A history of known hypersensitivity to any component of SOLGANAL Suspension contraindicates its use. Gold therapy is contraindicated in patients with uncontrolled diabetes mellitus, severe debilitation, systemic lupus erythematosus, renal disease, hepatic dysfunction, uncontrolled congestive heart failure, marked hypertension, agranulocytosis, other blood dyscrasias, or hemorrhagic diathesis; or if there is a history of infectious hepatitis. Patients who recently have had radiation, and those who have developed severe toxicity from previous exposure to gold or other heavy metals should not receive SOLGANAL Suspension.

Urticaria, eczema, and colitis are also contraindications. Gold therapy is usually contraindicated in pregnancy. (See PRECAUTIONS, "*Usage in Pregnancy*".)

Gold salts should not be used with penicillamine (See MANAGEMENT OF ADVERSE REACTIONS) or antimalarials. The safety of coadministration with immunosuppressive agents other than corticosteroids has not been established.

WARNINGS

The following signs should be considered danger signals of gold toxicity, and no additional injection should be given unless further studies reveal some other cause for their presence: rapid reduction of hemoglobin, leukopenia (WBC below 4000/cu mm), eosinophilia above 5%, platelet count below 100,000/cu mm, albuminuria, hematuria, pruritus, dermatitis, stomatitis, jaundice, and petechiae.

Effects that may occur immediately following an injection, or at any time during gold therapy, include: anaphylactic shock, syncope, bradycardia, thickening of the tongue, difficulty in swallowing and breathing, and angioneurotic edema. If such effects are observed, treatment with SOLGANAL Suspension should be discontinued.

Tolerance to gold usually decreases with advancing age. Diabetes mellitus or congestive heart failure should be under control before gold therapy is instituted.

SOLGANAL Suspension should be used with extreme caution in patients with: skin rash, hypersensitivity to other medications, or a history of renal or liver disease.

PRECAUTIONS

General: Before **each** injection, the physician should personally check the patient for adverse reactions and inquiry should be made regarding pruritus, rash, sore mouth, indigestion, and metallic taste. The patient should be observed for at least 15 minutes following each injection. (See also "*Laboratory Tests*".)

Patients with HLA-D locus histocompatibility antigens DRw2 and DRw3 may have a genetic predisposition to develop certain toxic reactions, such as proteinuria, during treatment with gold or D-penicillamine.

SOLGANAL Suspension should be used with caution in patients with compromised cardiovascular or cerebral circulation.

Information for Patients:
1. Promptly report to the physician any unusual symptoms such as pruritus (itching), rash, sore mouth, indigestion, or metallic taste.
2. Increased joint pain may occur for one or two days after an injection and usually subsides after the first few injections.
3. Exposure to sunlight or artificial ultraviolet light should be minimized.
4. Careful oral hygiene is recommended in conjunction with therapy.
5. Patients should be aware of potential hazards if they become pregnant while receiving gold therapy. (See "*Usage in Pregnancy*".)

Laboratory Tests: Before treatment is started, a complete blood count, platelet count, and urinalysis should be done to serve as reference points. Since gold therapy is usually con-

traindicated in pregnant patients, pregnancy should be ruled out before treatment is started. Throughout the treatment period, urinalysis should be repeated prior to each injection, and complete blood cell and platelet counts should be performed every two weeks. A platelet count is indicated any time that purpura or ecchymosis occurs.

Drug Interactions: Drug interactions have not been reported. (See **Contraindications**.)

Carcinogenesis, Mutagenesis, and Impairment of Fertility: Renal adenomas developed in rats receiving an injectable gold product similar to SOLGANAL Suspension at doses of 2 mg/kg weekly for 46 weeks, followed by 6 mg/kg daily for 47 weeks. These doses were higher and administered more frequently than the recommended human doses. The adenomas were similar histologically to those produced by chronic administration of other gold compounds and heavy metals, such as lead or nickel.

Renal tubular cell neoplasia consisting of renal adenoma and adenocarcinoma were noted in a dose-response relationship in another study in rats using daily intramuscular doses of 3 mg/kg and 6 mg/kg for up to 2 years. These doses were higher and were administered more frequently than the recommended human doses. In this same study, sarcomas at the injection site occurred in some rats but their numbers were not sufficient to demonstrate a dose-response relationship.

No report of renal adenoma or sarcoma at the injection site in man in association with the use of SOLGANAL Suspension has been received.

Gold compounds have not been studied for evaluation of mutagenesis.

Gold sodium thiomalate given subcutaneously did not adversely affect fertility or reproductive performance.

Usage in Pregnancy: Gold therapy is usually contraindicated in pregnant patients. The patient should be warned about the hazards of becoming pregnant while on gold therapy. Rheumatoid arthritis frequently improves when the patient becomes pregnant, thereby eliminating the need for gold therapy. The potential nephrotoxicity of gold should not be superimposed on the increased renal burden which normally occurs in pregnancy and hence, gold therapy should be discontinued upon recognition of pregnancy unless continued use is required in an individual case. The slow excretion of gold and its persistence in body tissues after discontinuation of treatment should be kept in mind when a woman of child-bearing potential being treated with gold plans to become pregnant.

Pregnancy Category C: Gold sodium thiomalate administered subcutaneously, a route not used clinically, has been shown to be teratogenic during the organogenic period in rats and rabbits when given in doses 140 and 175 times, respectively, the usual human dose. Hydrocephalus and microphthalmia were the malformations observed in rats when gold sodium thiomalate was administered at a dose of 25 mg/kg/day from day 6 through day 15 of gestation. In rabbits, limb defects and gastroschisis were the malformations observed when gold sodium thiomalate was administered at doses of 20 to 45 mg/kg/day from day 6 through day 18 of gestation.

Gold compounds administered orally to rabbits from days 6 through 18 of pregnancy resulted in the occurrence of abdominal defects, such as gastroschisis and umbilical hernia; anomalies of the brain, heart, lung, and skeleton; and microphthalmia.

The administration of excessive doses of gold-containing compounds during pregnancy in the above studies was toxic to the mothers and their embryos; the embryotoxic effects probably were secondary to maternal toxicity. Therefore, the significance of these findings in relation to human use is unknown.

There are no adequate and well-controlled studies with SOLGANAL Suspension in pregnant women. Extensive clinical experience with SOLGANAL Suspension has not demonstrated human teratogenicity.

Nursing Mothers: Gold has been demonstated in the milk of lactating mothers. In one patient, a total dose of 135 mg of gold thioglucose was given during the postpartum period. Samples of the maternal milk and urine, and samples of red blood cells and serum of the mother and child were evaluated by atomic absorption spectrophotometry. Trace amounts of gold appeared in the serum and red blood cells of the nursing offspring. It has been postulated that this may be the cause of unexplained rashes, nephritis, hepatitis, and hematologic aberrations in the nursing infants of mothers treated with gold. Because of the potential for serious adverse reactions in nursing infants, a decision should be made whether to discontinue nursing or to discontinue the gold therapy, taking into account the importance of the drug to the mother. The slow excretion of gold and its persistence in the mother after discontinuation of treatment should be kept in mind.

Pediatric Use: Safety and effectiveness in children below the age of six years have not been established.

ADVERSE REACTIONS

Adverse reactions to gold therapy may occur at any time during treatment or many months after therapy has been

discontinued. The incidence of toxic reactions is apparently unrelated to the plasma level of gold, but it may be related to the cumulative body content of gold. Higher than conventional dosage schedules may increase the occurrence and severity of toxicity. Severe effects are most common after 300 to 500 mg have been administered.

Cutaneous Reactions: Dermatitis is the most common reaction. Pruritus should be considered a warning signal of an impending cutaneous reaction. Erythema and occasionally the more severe reactions such as papular, vesicular, and exfoliative dermatitis leading to alopecia and shedding of the nails may occur. Chrysiasis (gray-to-blue pigmentation) has been reported, especially on photoexposed areas. Gold dermatitis may be aggravated by exposure to sunlight, or an actinic rash may develop.

Mucous Membrane Reactions: Stomatitis is the second most common adverse reaction. Shallow ulcers on the buccal membranes, on the borders of the tongue and on the palate, diffuse glossitis, or gingivitis may be preceded by the sensation of metallic taste. Careful oral hygiene is recommended. Inflammation of the upper respiratory tract, pharyngitis, gastritis, colitis, tracheitis, and vaginitis have also been reported. Conjunctivitis is rare.

Renal Reactions: Nephrotic syndrome or glomerulitis with hematuria, which is usually relatively mild, subsides completely if recognized early and treatment is discontinued. These reactions become severe and chronic if gold therapy is continued after their onset. Therefore, it is important to perform a urinalysis before each injection and to discontinue treatment promptly if proteinuria or hematuria develops.

Hematologic Reactions: Although rare, blood dyscrasias, including granulocytopenia, agranulocytosis, thrombocytopenia with or without purpura, leukopenia, eosinophilia, panmyelopathy, hemorrhagic diathesis, and hypoplastic and aplastic anemia, have been reported. These reactions may occur separately or in combination.

Nitritoid and Allergic Reactions: These reactions, which may rarely occur with SOLGANAL Suspension and which resemble anaphylactoid effects, include flushing, fainting, dizziness, sweating, malaise, weakness, nausea, and vomiting.

Miscellaneous Reactions: On rare occasions, gastrointestinal symptoms, i.e., nausea, vomiting, colic, anorexia, abdominal cramps, diarrhea, ulcerative enterocolitis, and headache have been reported.

There have been rare reports of iritis and corneal ulcers. Transient, asymptomatic gold deposits in the cornea or conjunctiva may occur.

Other reported reactions include encephalitis, immunological destruction of the synovia, EEG abnormalities, intrahepatic cholestasis, hepatitis with jaundice, toxic hepatitis, acute yellow atrophy, peripheral neuritis, gold bronchitis, pulmonary injury manifested by interstitial pneumonitis or fibrosis, fever, and partial or complete hair loss.

Less common but more severe effects that may occur shortly after an injection or at any time during gold therapy include: anaphylactic shock, syncope, bradycardia, thickening of the tongue, difficulty in swallowing and breathing, and angioneurotic edema. If they are observed, treatment with SOLGANAL Suspension should be discontinued.

Arthralgia may occur for one or two days after an injection and usually subsides after the first few injections. The mechanism of the transient increase in rheumatic symptoms after injection of gold (the so-called nonvasomotor postinjection reaction) is unknown. These reactions are usually mild but occasionally may be so severe that treatment is stopped prematurely.

MANAGEMENT OF ADVERSE REACTIONS

In the event of toxic reactions, gold therapy should be discontinued immediately.

In the presence of mild reactions, it may be sufficient to discontinue the administration of SOLGANAL Suspension for a short period and then to resume treatment with smaller doses.

Dermatitis and pruritus may respond to soothing lotions, other appropriate antipruritic treatment, or topical glucocorticoids.

If dermatitis or stomatitis becomes severe or spreads, systemic glucocorticoid treatment may be indicated. For renal, hematologic, and most other adverse reactions, glucocorticoids may be required in larger doses and for a longer time than for dermatologic reactions. Often this treatment may be required for many months because of the slow elimination of gold from the body.

If severe adverse reactions do not improve with steroid treatment in patients who receive large doses of gold, a chelating agent, such as dimercaprol (BAL), may be used. In one case, it was reported that penicillamine was beneficial in the treatment of gold-induced thrombocytopenia. Adjunctive

Continued on next page

Information on Schering products appearing on these pages is effective as of August 15, 1992.

Schering—Cont.

use of an anabolic steroid with other drugs (i.e., BAL, penicillamine, and corticosteroids) may contribute to recovery of bone marrow deficiency.
In the presence of severe or idiosyncratic reactions, treatment with SOLGANAL Suspension should not be re-instituted.

OVERDOSAGE

Overdosage resulting from too rapid increases in dosing with SOLGANAL Suspension will be manifested by rapid appearance of toxic reactions, particularly those relating to renal damage, such as hematuria, proteinuria, and to hematologic effects, such as thrombocytopenia and granulocytopenia. Other toxic effects, including fever, nausea, vomiting, diarrhea, and various skin disorders such as papulovesicular lesions, urticaria, and exfoliative dermatitis, all attended with severe pruritus, may develop. Treatment consists of prompt discontinuation of the medication, and early administration of dimercaprol. Specific supportive therapy should be given for the renal and hematologic complications. (See also MANAGEMENT OF ADVERSE REACTIONS above).

DOSAGE AND ADMINISTRATION

Adults—The usual dosage schedule for the intramuscular administration of SOLGANAL is as follows: first dose, 10 mg; second and third doses, 25 mg; fourth and subsequent doses, 50 mg. The interval between doses is one week. The 50 mg dose is continued at weekly intervals until 0.8 to 1.0 g SOLGANAL has been given. If the patient has improved and has exhibited no sign of toxicity, the 50 mg dose may be continued many months longer, at three- to four-week intervals. A weekly dose above 50 mg is usually unnecessary and contraindicated; the tendency in gold therapy is toward lower dosage. With this in mind, it may eventually be established that a 25 mg dose is the one of choice. If no improvement has been demonstrated after a total administration of 1.0 g of SOLGANAL Suspension, the necessity for gold therapy should be reevaluated.
Children 6 to 12 years—one-fourth of the adult dose, governed chiefly by body weight, not to exceed 25 mg per dose.
SOLGANAL Suspension should be injected **intramuscularly,** (preferably intragluteally), **never intravenously.** The patient should be lying down and should remain recumbent for approximately 10 minutes after the injection. The vial should be thoroughly shaken in order to suspend all of the active material. Heating the vial to body temperature (by immersion in warm water) will facilitate drawing the suspension into the syringe. An 18-gauge, 1½-inch needle is recommended for depositing the preparation deep into the muscular tissue. For obese patients, an 18-gauge, 2-inch needle may be used. The site usually selected for injection is the upper outer quadrant of the gluteal region.
NOTE: Shake the vial in horizontal position before the dose is withdrawn. Needle and syringe must be dry. The patient should be observed for at least 15 minutes following each injection.

HOW SUPPLIED

SOLGANAL Suspension is available in 10 ml multiple-dose vials containing 5% (50 mg/ml) aurothioglucose; box of one.
Shake well before using. Store between 0° and 30°C (32° and 86°F). Protect from light. Store in carton until contents are used.
Revised 8/84 B-13288500
Copyright © 1963, 1984, Schering Corporation, USA. All rights reserved.

TRILAFON® ℞

[*tri 'lah-fon*]
brand of perphenazine, USP
Tablets
Concentrate
Injection

DESCRIPTION

TRILAFON products contain perphenazine, USP (4-[3-(2-chlorophenothiazin-10-yl)propyl]-1-piperazineethanol), a piperazinyl phenothiazine having the chemical formula, $C_{21}H_{26}ClN_3OS$. They are available as **Tablets,** 2, 4, 8 and 16 mg; **Concentrate,** 16 mg perphenazine per 5 mL and alcohol less than 0.1%; and **Injection,** perphenazine 5 mg per 1 mL.
The inactive ingredients for TRILAFON **Tablets,** 2, 4, 8 and 16 mg. include: acacia, black iron oxide, butylparaben, calcium phosphate, calcium sulfate, carnauba wax, corn starch, gelatin, lactose, magnesium stearate, potato starch, sugar, titanium dioxide, white wax and other ingredients. May also contain talc.
The inactive ingredients for TRILAFON **Concentrate** include: alcohol, citric acid, flavors, menthol, sodium phosphate, sorbitol, sugar, and water.
The inactive ingredients for TRILAFON **Injection** include: citric acid, sodium bisulfite, sodium hydroxide, and water.

ACTIONS

Perphenazine has actions at all levels of the central nervous system, particularly the hypothalamus. However, the site and mechanism of action of therapeutic effect are not known.

INDICATIONS

Perphenazine is indicated for use in the management of the manifestations of psychotic disorders; and for the control of severe nausea and vomiting in adults.
TRILAFON has not been shown effective for the management of behavioral complications in patients with mental retardation.

CONTRAINDICATIONS

TRILAFON products are contraindicated in comatose or greatly obtunded patients and in patients receiving large doses of central nervous system depressants (barbiturates, alcohol, narcotics, analgesics, or antihistamines); in the presence of existing blood dyscrasias, bone marrow depression, or liver damage; and in patients who have shown hypersensitivity to TRILAFON products, their components, or related compounds.
TRILAFON products are also contraindicated in patients with suspected or established subcortical brain damage, with or without hypothalamic damage, since a hyperthermic reaction with temperatures in excess of 104°F may occur in such patients, sometimes not until 14 to 16 hours after drug administration. Total body ice-packing is recommended for such a reaction; antipyretics may also be useful.

WARNINGS

Tardive dyskinesia, a syndrome consisting of potentially irreversible, involuntary, dyskinetic movements, may develop in patients treated with neuroleptic (antipsychotic) drugs. Although the prevalence of the syndrome appears to be highest among the elderly, especially elderly women, it is impossible to rely upon prevalence estimates to predict, at the inception of neuroleptic treatment, which patients are likely to develop the syndrome. Whether neuroleptic drug products differ in their potential to cause tardive dyskinesia is unknown.
Both the risk of developing the syndrome and the likelihood that it will become irreversible are believed to increase as the duration of treatment and the total cumulative dose of neuroleptic drugs administered to the patient increase. However, the syndrome can develop, although much less commonly, after relatively brief treatment periods at low doses.
There is no known treatment for established cases of tardive dyskinesia, although the syndrome may remit, partially or completely, if neuroleptic treatment is withdrawn. Neuroleptic treatment itself, however, may suppress (or partially suppress) the signs and symptoms of the syndrome, and thereby may possibly mask the underlying disease process. The effect that symptomatic suppression has upon the long-term course of the syndrome is unknown.
Given these considerations, neuroleptics should be prescribed in a manner that is most likely to minimize the occurrence of tardive dyskinesia. Chronic neuroleptic treatment should generally be reserved for patients who suffer from a chronic illness that, 1) is known to respond to neuroleptic drugs, and 2) for whom alternative, equally effective, but potentially less harmful treatments are not available or appropriate. In patients who do require chronic treatment, the smallest dose and the shortest duration of treatment producing a satisfactory clinical response should be sought. The need for continued treatment should be reassessed periodically.
If signs and symptoms of tardive dyskinesia appear in a patient on neuroleptics, drug discontinuation should be considered. However, some patients may require treatment despite the presence of the syndrome.
(For further information about the description of tardive dyskinesia and its clinical detection, please refer to **Information for Patients and Adverse Reactions.**)
TRILAFON **Injection** contains sodium bisulfite, a sulfite that may cause allergic-type reactions including anaphylactic symptoms and life-threatening or less severe asthmatic episodes in certain susceptible people. The overall prevalence of sulfite sensitivity is seen more frequently in asthmatic than in non-asthmatic people.
NEUROLEPTIC MALIGNANT SYNDROME (NMS)
A potentially fatal symptom complex sometimes referred to as Neuroleptic Malignant Syndrome (NMS) has been reported in association with antipsychotic drugs. Clinical manifestations of NMS are hyperpyrexia, muscle rigidity, altered mental status and evidence of autonomic instability (irregular pulse or blood pressure, tachycardia, diaphoresis, and cardiac dysrhythmias).
The diagnostic evaluation of patients with this syndrome is complicated. In arriving at a diagnosis, it is important to identify cases where the clinical presentation includes both serious medical illness (e.g., pneumonia, systemic infection, etc.) and untreated or inadequately treated extrapyramidal signs and symptoms (EPS). Other important considerations in the differential diagnosis include central anticholinergic toxicity, heat stroke, drug fever and primary central nervous system (CNS) pathology.
The management of NMS should include 1) immediate discontinuation of antipsychotic drugs and other drugs not essential to concurrent therapy, 2) intensive symptomatic treatment and medical monitoring, and 3) treatment of any concomitant serious medical problems for which specific treatments are available. There is no general agreement about specific pharmacological treatment regimens for uncomplicated NMS.
If a patient requires antipsychotic drug treatment after recovery from NMS, the potential reintroduction of drug therapy should be carefully considered. The patient should be carefully monitored, since recurrences of NMS have been reported.
If hypotension develops, epinephrine should not be administered since its action is blocked and partially reversed by perphenazine. If a vasopressor is needed, norepinephrine may be used. Severe, acute hypotension has occurred with the use of phenothiazines and is particularly likely to occur in patients with mitral insufficiency or pheochromocytoma. Rebound hypertension may occur in pheochromocytoma patients.
TRILAFON products can lower the convulsive threshold in susceptible individuals; they should be used with caution in alcohol withdrawal and in patients with convulsive disorders. If the patient is being treated with an anticonvulsant agent, increased dosage of that agent may be required when TRILAFON products are used concomitantly.
TRILAFON products should be used with caution in patients with psychic depression.
Perphenazine may impair the mental and/or physical abilities required for the performance of hazardous tasks such as driving a car or operating machinery; therefore, the patient should be warned accordingly.
TRILAFON products are not recommended for children under 12 years of age.
Usage in Pregnancy: Safe use of TRILAFON during pregnancy and lactation has not been established; therefore, in administering the drug to pregnant patients, nursing mothers, or women who may become pregnant, the possible benefits must be weighed against the possible hazards to mother and child.

PRECAUTIONS

The possibility of suicide in depressed patients remains during treatment and until significant remission occurs. This type of patient should not have access to large quantities of this drug.
As with all phenothiazine compounds, perphenazine should not be used indiscriminately. Caution should be observed in giving it to patients who have previously exhibited severe adverse reactions to other phenothiazines. Some of the untoward actions of perphenazine tend to appear more frequently when high doses are used. However, as with other phenothiazine compounds, patients receiving TRILAFON products in any dosage should be kept under close supervision.
Neuroleptic drugs elevate prolactin levels; the elevation persists during chronic administration. Tissue culture experiments indicate that approximately one-third of human breast cancers are prolactin dependent *in vitro*, a factor of potential importance if the prescription of these drugs is contemplated in a patient with a previously detected breast cancer. Although disturbances such as galactorrhea, amenorrhea, gynecomastia, and impotence have been reported, the clinical significance of elevated serum prolactin levels is unknown for most patients. An increase in mammary neoplasms has been found in rodents after chronic administration of neuroleptic drugs. Neither clinical studies nor epidemiologic studies conducted to date, however, have shown an association between chronic administration of these drugs and mammary tumorigenesis, the available evidence is considered too limited to be conclusive at this time.
The antiemetic effect of perphenazine may obscure signs of toxicity due to overdosage of other drugs, or render more difficult the diagnosis of disorders such as brain tumors or intestinal obstruction.
A significant, not otherwise explained, rise in body temperature may suggest individual intolerance to perphenazine, in which case it should be discontinued.
Patients on large doses of a phenothiazine drug who are undergoing surgery should be watched carefully for possible hypotensive phenomena. Moreover, reduced amounts of anesthetics or central nervous system depressants may be necessary.
Since phenothiazines and central nervous system depressants (opiates, analgesics, antihistamines, barbiturates) can potentiate each other, less than the usual dosage of the added drug is recommended, and caution is advised, when they are administered concomitantly.
Use with caution in patients who are receiving atropine or related drugs because of additive anticholinergic effects and also in patients who will be exposed to extreme heat or phosphorus insecticides.

The use of alcohol should be avoided, since additive effects and hypotension may occur. Patients should be cautioned that their response to alcohol may be increased while they are being treated with TRILAFON products. The risk of suicide and the danger of overdose may be increased in patients who use alcohol excessively due to its potentiation of the drug's effect.

Blood counts and hepatic and renal functions should be checked periodically. The appearance of signs of blood dyscrasias requires the discontinuance of the drug and institution of appropriate therapy. If abnormalities in hepatic tests occur, phenothiazine treatment should be discontinued. Renal function in patients on long-term therapy should be monitored; if blood urea nitrogen (BUN) becomes abnormal, treatment with the drug should be discontinued.

The use of phenothiazine derivatives in patients with diminished renal function should be undertaken with caution.

Use with caution in patients suffering from respiratory impairment due to acute pulmonary infections, or in chronic respiratory disorders such as severe asthma or emphysema. In general, phenothiazines, including perphenazine, do not produce psychic dependence. Gastritis, nausea and vomiting, dizziness, and tremulousness have been reported following abrupt cessation of high-dose therapy. Reports suggest that these symptoms can be reduced by continuing concomitant antiparkinson agents for several weeks after the phenothiazine is withdrawn.

The possibility of liver damage, corneal and lenticular deposits, and irreversible dyskinesias should be kept in mind when patients are on long-term therapy.

Because photosensitivity has been reported, undue exposure to the sun should be avoided during phenothiazine treatment.

Information for Patients: This information is intended to aid in the safe and effective use of this medication. It is not a disclosure of all possible adverse or intended effects.

Given the likelihood that a substantial proportion of patients exposed chronically to neuroleptics will develop tardive dyskinesia, it is advised that all patients in whom chronic use is contemplated be given, if possible, full information about this risk. The decision to inform patients and/or their guardians must obviously take into account the clinical circumstances and the competency of the patient to understand the information provided.

ADVERSE REACTIONS

Not all of the following adverse reactions have been reported with this specific drug; however, pharmacological similarities among various phenothiazine derivatives require that each be considered. With the piperazine group (of which perphenazine is an example) the extrapyramidal symptoms are more common, and others (e.g., sedative effects, jaundice, and blood dyscrasias) are less frequently seen.

CNS Effects: *Extrapyramidal reactions:* opisthotonus, trismus, torticollis, retrocollis, aching and numbness of the limbs, motor restlessness, oculogyric crisis, hyperreflexia, dystonia, including protrusion, discoloration, aching and rounding of the tongue, tonic spasm of the masticatory muscles, tight feeling in the throat, slurred speech, dysphagia, akathisia, dyskinesia, parkinsonism, and ataxia. Their incidence and severity usually increase with an increase in dosage, but there is considerable individual variation in the tendency to develop such symptoms. Extrapyramidal symptoms can usually be controlled by the concomitant use of effective antiparkinsonian drugs, such as benztropine mesylate, and/or by reduction in dosage. In some instances, however, these extrapyramidal reactions may persist after discontinuation of treatment with perphenazine.

Persistent tardive dyskinesia: As with all antipsychotic agents, tardive dyskinesia may appear in some patients on long-term therapy or may appear after drug therapy has been discontinued. Although the risk appears to be greater in elderly patients on high-dose therapy, especially females, it may occur in either sex and in children. The symptoms are persistent and in some patients appear to be irreversible. The syndrome is characterized by rhythmical, involuntary movements of the tongue, face, mouth, or jaw (e.g. protrusion of tongue, puffing of cheeks, puckering of mouth, chewing movements). Sometimes these may be accompanied by involuntary movements of the extremities. There is no known effective treatment for tardive dyskinesia; antiparkinsonism agents usually do not alleviate the symptoms of this syndrome. It is suggested that all antipsychotic agents be discontinued if these symptoms appear. Should it be necessary to reinstitute treatment, or increase the dosage of the agent, or switch to a different antipsychotic agent, the syndrome may be masked. It has been reported that fine, vermicular movements of the tongue may be an early sign of the syndrome, and if the medication is stopped at that time the syndrome may not develop.

Other CNS effects include cerebral edema; abnormality of cerebrospinal fluid proteins; convulsive seizures, particularly in patients with EEG abnormalities or a history of such disorders, and headaches.

Neuroleptic malignant syndrome has been reported in patients treated with neuroleptic drugs (see WARNINGS for further information).

Drowsiness may occur, particularly during the first or second week, after which it generally disappears. If troublesome, lower the dosage. Hypnotic effects appear to be minimal, especially in patients who are permitted to remain active.

Adverse behavioral effects include paradoxical exacerbation of psychotic symptoms, catatonic-like states, paranoid reactions, lethargy, paradoxical excitement, restlessness, hyperactivity, nocturnal confusion, bizarre dreams, and insomnia. Hyperreflexia has been reported in the newborn when a phenothiazine was used during pregnancy.

Autonomic Effects: dry mouth or salivation, nausea, vomiting, diarrhea, anorexia, constipation, obstipation, fecal impaction, urinary retention, frequency or incontinence, bladder paralysis, polyuria, nasal congestion, pallor, myosis, mydriasis, blurred vision, glaucoma, perspiration, hypertension, hypotension, and change in pulse rate occasionally may occur. Significant autonomic effects have been infrequent in patients receiving less than 24 mg perphenazine daily.

Adynamic ileus occasionally occurs with phenothiazine therapy and if severe can result in complications and death. It is of particular concern in psychiatric patients, who may fail to seek treatment of this condition.

Allergic Effects: urticaria, erythema, eczema, exfoliative dermatitis, pruritus, photosensitivity, asthma, fever, anaphylactoid reactions, laryngeal edema, and angioneurotic edema; contact dermatitis in nursing personnel administering the drug, and in extremely rare instances, individual idiosyncrasy or hypersensitivity to phenothiazines has resulted in cerebral edema, circulatory collapse, and death.

Endocrine Effects: lactation, galactorrhea, moderate breast enlargement in females and gynecomastia in males on large doses, disturbances in the menstrual cycle, amenorrhea, changes in libido, inhibition of ejaculation, syndrome of inappropriate ADH (antidiuretic hormone) secretion, false positive pregnancy tests, hyperglycemia, hypoglycemia, glycosuria.

Cardiovascular Effects: postural hypotension, tachycardia (especially with sudden marked increase in dosage), bradycardia, cardiac arrest, faintness, and dizziness. Occasionally the hypotensive effect may produce a shock-like condition. ECG changes, nonspecific, (quinidine-like effect) usually reversible, have been observed in some patients receiving phenothiazine tranquilizers.

Sudden death has occasionally been reported in patients who have received phenothiazines. In some cases the death was apparently due to cardiac arrest; in others, the cause appeared to be asphyxia due to failure of the cough reflex. In some patients, the cause could not be determined nor could it be established that the death was due to the phenothiazine.

Hematological Effects: agranulocytosis, eosinophilia, leukopenia, hemolytic anemia, thrombocytopenic purpura, and pancytopenia. Most cases of agranulocytosis have occurred between the fourth and tenth weeks of therapy. Patients should be watched closely especially during that period for the sudden appearance of sore throat or signs of infection. If white blood cell and differential cell counts show significant cellular depression, discontinue the drug and start appropriate therapy. However, a slightly lowered white count is not in itself an indication to discontinue the drug.

Other Effects: Special considerations in long-term therapy include pigmentation of the skin, occurring chiefly in the exposed areas, ocular changes consisting of deposition of fine particulate matter in the cornea and lens, progressing in more severe cases to star-shaped lenticular opacities; epithelial keratopathies; and pigmentary retinopathy. Also noted: peripheral edema, reversed epinephrine effect, increase in PBI not attributable to an increase in thyroxine, parotid swelling (rare), hyperpyrexia, systemic lupus erythematosus-like syndrome, increases in appetite and weight, polyphagia, photophobia, and muscle weakness.

Liver damage (biliary stasis) may occur. Jaundice may occur, usually between the second and fourth weeks of treatment and is regarded as a hypersensitivity reaction. Incidence is low. The clinical picture resembles infectious hepatitis but with laboratory features of obstructive jaundice. It is usually reversible; however, chronic jaundice has been reported.

Side effects with intramuscular TRILAFON Injection have been infrequent and transient. Dizziness or significant hypotension after treatment with TRILAFON Injection is a rare occurrence.

DOSAGE AND ADMINISTRATION

Dosage must be individualized and adjusted according to the severity of the condition and the response obtained. As with all potent drugs, the best dose is the lowest dose that will produce the desired clinical effect. Since extrapyramidal symptoms increase in frequency and severity with increased dosage, it is important to employ the lowest effective dose. These symptoms have disappeared upon reduction of dosage, withdrawal of the drug or administration of an anti-parkinsonian agent.

Prolonged administration of doses exceeding 24 mg daily should be reserved for hospitalized patients or patients under continued observation for early detection and management of adverse reactions. An antiparkinsonian agent, such as trihexyphenidyl hydrochloride or benztropine mesylate, is valuable in controlling drug-induced, extrapyramidal symptoms.

TRILAFON Tablets

Suggested dosages for **Tablets** for various conditions follow:

Moderately disturbed non-hospitalized psychotic patients: **Tablets** 4 to 8 mg t.i.d., initially; reduce as soon as possible to minimum effective dosage.

Hospitalized psychotic patients: **Tablets** 8 to 16 mg b.i.d. to q.i.d.; avoid dosages in excess of 64 mg daily.

Severe nausea and vomiting in adults: **Tablets** 8 to 16 mg daily in divided doses; 24 mg occasionally may be necessary; early dosage reduction is desirable.

TRILAFON INJECTION—Intramuscular Administration

The injection is used when rapid effect and prompt control of acute or intractable conditions is required or when oral administration is not feasible. TRILAFON Injection, administered by deep intramuscular injection, is well tolerated. The injection should be given with the patient seated or recumbent, and the patient should be observed for a short period after administration.

Therapeutic effect is usually evidenced in 10 minutes and is maximal in 1 to 2 hours. The average duration of effective action is 6 hours, occasionally 12 to 24 hours.

Pediatric dosage has not yet been established. Children over 12 years may receive the lowest limit of adult dosage.

The usual initial dose is 5 mg (1 mL). This may be repeated every 6 hours. Ordinarily, the total daily dosage should not exceed 15 mg in ambulatory patients or 30 mg in hospitalized patients. When required for satisfactory control of symptoms in severe conditions, an initial 10 mg intramuscular dose may be given. Patients should be placed on oral therapy as soon as practicable. Generally, this may be achieved within 24 hours. In some instances, however, patients have been maintained on injectable therapy for several months. It has been established that TRILAFON Injection is more potent than TRILAFON Tablets. Therefore, equal or higher dosage should be used when the patient is transferred to oral therapy after receiving the injection.

Psychotic conditions: While 5 mg of the Injection has a definite tranquilizing effect, it may be necessary to use 10 mg doses to initiate therapy in severely agitated states. Most patients will be controlled and amendable to oral therapy within a maximum of 24 to 48 hours. Acute conditions (hysteria, panic reaction) often respond well to a single dose whereas in chronic conditions, several injections may be required. When transferring patients to oral therapy, it is suggested that increased dosage be employed to maintain adequate clinical control. This should be followed by gradual reduction to the minimal maintenance dose which is effective.

Severe nausea and vomiting in adults: To obtain rapid control of vomiting, administer 5 mg (1 mL); in rare instances it may be necessary to increase the dose to 10 mg, in general, higher doses should be given only to hospitalized patients.

TRILAFON Injection—Intravenous Administration

The intravenous administration of TRILAFON Injection is seldom required. This route of administration should be used with particular caution and care and only when absolutely necessary to control severe vomiting, intractable hiccoughs, or acute conditions, such as violent retching during surgery. Its use should be limited to recumbent, hospitalized adults in doses not exceeding 5 mg. When employed in this manner, intravenous injection ordinarily should be given as a diluted solution by either fractional injection or a slow drip infusion. In the surgical patient, slow infusion of no more than 5 mg is preferred. When administered in divided doses, TRILAFON Injection should be diluted to 0.5 mg/mL (1 mL mixed with 9 mL of physiologic saline solution), and not more than 1 mg per injection given at not less than one-to two-minute intervals. Intravenous injection should be discontinued as soon as symptoms are controlled and should not exceed 5 mg. The possibility of hypotensive and extrapyramidal side effects should be considered and appropriate means for management kept available. Blood pressure and pulse should be monitored continuously during intravenous administration. Pharmacologic and clinical studies indicate that intravenous administration of norepinephrine should be useful in alleviating the hypotensive effect.

TRILAFON Concentrate

In hospitalized psychotic patients, the usual dosage range is 8 to 16 mg b.i.d. to q.i.d., depending on the severity of symptoms and individual response. Although a number of investigators have employed higher dosages, a total daily dose of more than 64 mg ordinarily is not required. The **Concentrate**

Continued on next page

Information on Schering products appearing on these pages is effective as of August 15, 1992.

Schering—Cont.

should be diluted only with water, saline, Seven-Up, homogenized milk, carbonated orange drink and pineapple, apricot, prune, orange. V-8, tomato, and grapefruit juices. Trilafon **Concentrate** should not be mixed with beverages containing caffeine (coffee, cola) tannics (tea), or pectinates (apple juice) since physical incompatibility may result. Suggested dilution is approximately two fluid ounces of diluent for each 5 mL (16 mg) teaspoonful of TRILAFON **Concentrate**. For convenience in measuring smaller doses, a graduated dropper marked to measure 8 mg or 4 mg is supplied with each bottle.

OVERDOSAGE

In the event of overdosage, emergency treatment should be started immediately. All patients suspected of having taken an overdose should be hospitalized as soon as possible.

Manifestations: Overdosage of perphenazine primarily involves the extrapyramidal mechanism and produces the same side effects described under ADVERSE REACTIONS, but to a more marked degree. It is usually evidenced by stupor or coma; children may have convulsive seizures.

Treatment: Treatment is symptomatic and supportive. There is no specific antidote. The patient should be induced to vomit even if emesis has occurred spontaneously. Pharmacologic vomiting by the administration of ipecac syrup is a preferred method. It should be noted that ipecac has a central mode of action in addition to its local gastric irritant properties, and the central mode of action may be blocked by the antiemetic effect of TRILAFON products. Vomiting should not be induced in patients with impaired consciousness. The action of ipecac is facilitated by physical activity and by the administration of 8 to 12 fluid ounces of water. If emesis does not occur within 15 minutes, the dose of ipecac should be repeated. Precautions against aspiration must be taken, especially in infants and children. Following emesis, any drug remaining in the stomach may be adsorbed by activated charcoal administered as a slurry with water. If vomiting is unsuccessful or contraindicated, gastric lavage should be performed. Isotonic and one-half isotonic saline are the lavage solutions of choice. Saline cathartics, such as milk of magnesia, draw water into the bowel by osmosis and therefore may be valuable for their action in rapid dilution of bowel content.

Standard measures (oxygen, intravenous fluids, corticosteroids) should be used to manage circulatory shock or metabolic acidosis. An open airway and adequate fluid intake should be maintained. Body temperature should be regulated. Hypothermia is expected, but severe hyperthermia may occur and must be treated vigorously. (See CONTRAINDICATIONS.)

An electrocardiogram should be taken and close monitoring of cardiac function instituted if there is any sign of abnormality. Cardiac arrhythmias may be treated with neostigmine, pyridostigmine, or propranolol. Digitalis should be considered for cadiac failure. Close monitoring of cardiac function is advisable for not less than five days. Vasopressors such as norepinephrine may be used to treat hypotension, but epinephrine should NOT be used.

Anticonvulsants (an inhalation anesthetic, diazepam, or paraldehyde) are recommended for control of convulsions, since perphenazine increases the central nervous system depressant action, but not the anticonvulsant action of barbiturates.

If acute parkinson-like symptoms result from perphenazine intoxication, benztropine mesylate or diphenydramine may be administered.

Central nervous system depression may be treated with nonconvulsant doses of CNS stimulants. Avoid stimulants that may cause convulsions (e.g., picrotoxin and pentylenetetrazol).

Signs of arousal may not occur for 48 hours.

Dialysis is of no value because of low plasma concentrations of the drug.

Since overdosage is often deliberate, patients may attempt suicide by other means during the recovery phase. Deaths by deliberate or accidental overdosage have occurred with this class of drugs.

HOW SUPPLIED

TRILAFON **Tablets** (2 mg): gray, sugar-coated tablets branded in black with the Schering trademark and either product identification letters, ADH, or numbers 705; bottles of 100 (NDC 0085-0705-04) and 500 (NDC 0085-0705-06). Store between 2° and 25°C (36° and 77°F).

TRILAFON **Tablets** (4 mg): gray, sugar-coated tablets branded in green with the Schering trademark and either product identification letters, ADK, or numbers, 940; bottles of 100 (NDC 0085-0940-05) and 500 (NDC 0085-0940-04). Store between 2° and 25°C (36° and 77°F).

TRILAFON **Tablets** (8 mg): gray, sugar-coated tablets branded in blue with the Schering trademark and either product identification letters, ADJ, or numbers 313; bottles of 100 (NDC 0085-0313-05) and 500 (NDC 0085-0313-04). Store between 2° and 25°C (36° and 77°F).

TRILAFON **Tablets** (16 mg): gray, sugar-coated tablets branded in red with the Schering trademark and either product identification letters, ADM, or numbers, 077; bottles of 100 (NDC 0085-0077-05) and 500 (NDC 0085-0077-04). Store between 2° and 25°C (36° and 77°F).

TRILAFON **Concentrate**, 16 mg per 5 mL, 4 fluid ounce (118 mL) bottle with graduated dropper (NDC 0085-0363-02). The **Concentrate** is light-sensitive and should be dispensed in amber bottles. **Protect from light. Store between 2° and 30°C (36° and 86°F). Shake well before using. Store in carton until completely used. Protect from light.**

TRILAFON **Injection**, 5 mg per mL, 1-mL ampul for intramuscular or intravenous use, box of 100 (NDC 0085-0012-04). Keep package closed to protect from light. Exposure may cause discoloration. Slight yellowish discoloration will not alter potency or therapeutic efficacy; if markedly discolored, ampul should be discarded. **Protect from light. Store in carton until contents are used.**

Revised 1/88

Copyright©1969, 1988, Schering Corporation, USA.
All rights reserved.

Shown in Product Identification Section, page 428

VANCENASE® ℞

[van 'sen-ās]

brand of beclomethasone dipropionate, USP
POCKETHALER® Nasal Inhaler
For Nasal Inhalation Only

DESCRIPTION

Beclomethasone dipropionate, USP, the active component of VANCENASE POCKETHALER Nasal Inhaler, is an anti-inflammatory steroid having the chemical name, 9-Chloro-11β,17,21-trihydroxy-16β-methylpregna-1,4-diene-3, 20-dione 17,21-dipropionate, and the following formula:

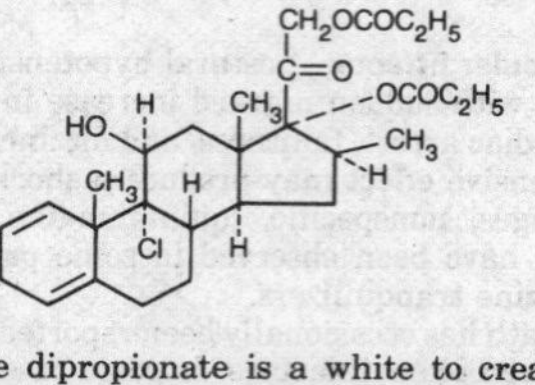

Beclomethasone dipropionate is a white to creamy-white, odorless powder with a molecular weight of 521.25. It is very slightly soluble in water, very soluble in chloroform, and freely soluble in acetone and in alcohol.

VANCENASE POCKETHALER Nasal Inhaler is a metered-dose aerosol unit containing a microcrystalline suspension of beclomethasone dipropionate-trichloromonofluoromethane clathrate in a mixture of propellants (trichloromonofluoromethane and dichlorodifluoromethane) with oleic acid. Each canister contains beclomethasone dipropionate-trichloromonofluoromethane clathrate having a molecular proportion of beclomethasone dipropionate to trichloromonofluoromethane between 3:1 and 3:2. Each actuation delivers from the nasal adapter a quantity of clathrate equivalent to 42 mcg of beclomethasone dipropionate, USP. The contents of one canister provide at least 200 metered doses.

CLINICAL PHARMACOLOGY

Beclomethasone 17,21-dipropionate is a diester of beclomethasone, a synthetic halogenated corticosteroid. Animal studies showed that beclomethasone dipropionate has potent glucocorticoid and weak mineralocorticoid activity. The mechanisms for the anti-inflammatory action of beclomethasone dipropionate are unknown. The precise mechanism of the aerosolized drug's action in the nose is also unknown. Biopsies of nasal mucosa obtained during clinical studies showed no histopathologic changes when beclomethasone dipropionate was administered intranasally.

The effects of beclomethasone dipropionate on hypothalmic-pituitary-adrenal (HPA) function have been evaluated in adult volunteers by other routes of administration. Studies are currently being undertaken with beclomethasone dipropionate by the intranasal route, which may demonstrate that there is more or that there is less absorption by this route of administration. There was no suppression of early morning plasma cortisol concentrations when beclomethasone dipropionate was administered in a dose of 1000 mcg/day for 1 month as an oral aerosol or for 3 days by intramuscular injection. However, partial suppression of plasma cortisol concentration was observed when beclomethasone dipropionate was administered in doses of 2000 mcg/day either by oral aerosol or intramuscularly. Immediate suppression of plasma cortisol concentrations was observed after single doses of 4000 mcg of beclomethasone dipropionate. Suppression of HPA function (reduction of early morning plasma cortisol levels) has been reported in adult patients who received 1600 mcg daily doses of oral beclomethasone dipropionate for one month. In clinical studies using beclomethasone dipropionate intranasally, there was no evidence of adrenal insufficiency.

Beclomethasone dipropionate is sparingly soluble. When given by nasal inhalation in the form of an aqueous or aerosolized suspension, the drug is deposited primarily in the nasal passages. A portion of the drug is swallowed. Absorption occurs rapidly from all respiratory and gastrointestinal tissues. There is no evidence of tissue storage of beclomethasone dipropionate or its metabolites. *In vitro* studies have shown that tissue other than the liver (lung slices) can rapidly metabolize beclomethasone dipropionate to beclomethasone 17-mono-propionate and more slowly to free beclomethasone (which has very weak anti-inflammatory activity). However, irrespective of the route of entry, the principal route of excretion of the drug and its metabolites is the feces. In humans, 12% to 15% of an orally administered dose of beclomethasone dipropionate is excreted in the urine as both conjugated and free metabolites of the drug.

Studies have shown that the degree of binding to plasma proteins is 87%.

INDICATIONS AND USAGE

VANCENASE POCKETHALER Nasal Inhaler is indicated for the relief of the symptoms of seasonal or perennial rhinitis in those cases poorly responsive to conventional treatment.

VANCENASE POCKETHALER Nasal Inhaler is also indicated for the prevention of recurrence of nasal polyps following surgical removal.

Clinical studies in seasonal and perennial rhinitis have shown that improvement is usually apparent within a few days. However, symptomatic relief may not occur in some patients for as long as 2 weeks. Although systemic effects are minimal at recommended doses, VANCENASE treatment should not be continued beyond 3 weeks in the absence of significant symptomatic improvement. VANCENASE treatment should not be used in the presence of untreated, localized infection involving the nasal mucosa.

Clinical studies have shown that treatment of the symptoms associated with nasal polyps may have to be continued for several weeks or more before a therapeutic result can be fully assessed. Recurrence of symptoms due to polyps can occur after stopping treatment, depending on the severity of the disease.

CONTRAINDICATIONS

Hypersensitivity to any of the ingredients of this preparation contraindicates its use.

WARNINGS

The replacement of a systemic corticosteroid with VANCENASE POCKETHALER Nasal Inhaler can be accompanied by signs of adrenal insufficiency.

Careful attention must be given when patients, previously treated for prolonged periods with systemic corticosteroids, are transferred to VANCENASE POCKETHALER Nasal Inhaler. This is particularly important in those patients who have associated asthma or other clinical conditions, where too rapid a decrease in systemic corticosteroids may cause a severe exacerbation of their symptoms.

Studies have shown that the combined administration of alternate day prednisone systemic treatment and orally inhaled beclomethasone increased the likelihood of HPA suppression compared to a therapeutic dose of either one alone. Therefore, VANCENASE treatment should be used with caution in patients already on alternate day prednisone regimens for any disease.

If recommended doses of intranasal beclomethasone are exceeded or if individuals are particularly sensitive or predisposed by virtue of recent systemic steroid therapy, symptoms of hypercorticism may occur, including very rare cases of menstrual irregularities, acneiform lesions, and cushingoid features. If such changes occur, VANCENASE POCKETHALER Nasal Inhaler should be discontinued slowly, consistent with accepted procedures for discontinuing oral steroid therapy.

Children who are on immunosuppressant drugs are more susceptible to infections than healthy children. Chickenpox and measles, for example, can have a more serious or even fatal course in children on immunosuppressant corticosteroids. In such children, or in adults who have not had these diseases, particular care should be taken to avoid exposure. If exposed, therapy with varicella zoster immune globulin (VZIG) or pooled intravenous immunoglobulin (IVIG), as appropriate, may be indicated. If chickenpox develops, treatment with antiviral agents may be considered.

PRECAUTIONS

General: During withdrawal from oral steroids, some patients may experience symptoms of withdrawal, eg, joint and/or muscular pain, lassitude, and depression.

Extremely rare instances of nasal septum perforation and increased intraocular pressure have been reported following the intranasal application of aerosolized corticosteroids.

In clinical studies with beclomethasone dipropionate administered intranasally, the development of localized infections of the nose and pharynx with *Candida albicans* has occurred only rarely. When such an infection develops, it may require treatment with appropriate local therapy or discontinuance of treatment with VANCENASE POCKETHALER Nasal Inhaler.

Beclomethasone dipropionate is absorbed into the circulation. Use of excessive doses of VANCENASE POCKETHALER Nasal Inhaler may suppress HPA function.

VANCENASE treatment should be used with caution, if at all, in patients with active or quiescent tuberculous infections of the respiratory tract, or in untreated fungal, bacterial, systemic viral infections, or ocular herpes simplex.

For VANCENASE POCKETHALER Nasal Inhaler to be effective in the treatment of nasal polyps, the aerosol must be able to enter the nose. Therefore, treatment of nasal polyps with VANCENASE Nasal Inhaler should be considered adjunctive therapy to surgical removal and/or the use of other medications which will permit effective penetration of the VANCENASE product into the nose. Nasal polyps may recur after any form of treatment.

As with any long-term treatment, patients using VANCENASE treatment over several months or longer should be examined periodically for possible changes in the nasal mucosa.

Because of the inhibitory effect of corticosteroids on wound healing, patients who have experienced recent nasal septum ulcers, nasal surgery, or trauma should not use a nasal corticosteroid until healing has occurred.

Although systemic effects have been minimal with recommended doses, this potential increases with excessive doses. Therefore, larger than recommended doses should be avoided.

Information for Patients: Patients should use VANCENASE POCKETHALER Nasal Inhaler at regular intervals since its effectiveness depends on its regular use. The patient should take the medication as directed. It is not acutely effective and the prescribed dosage should not be increased. Instead, nasal vasoconstrictors or oral antihistamines may be needed until the effects of VANCENASE POCKETHALER Nasal Inhaler are fully manifested. One to two weeks may pass before full relief is obtained. The patient should contact the doctor if symptoms do not improve, or if the condition worsens, or if sneezing or nasal irritation occurs. For the proper use of this unit and to attain maximum improvement, the patient should read and follow the accompanying PATIENT'S INSTRUCTIONS carefully.

Patients who are on immunosuppressant doses of corticosteroids should be warned to avoid exposure to chickenpox or measles and, if exposed, to obtain medical advice.

Carcinogenesis, Mutagenesis, Impairment of Fertility: Treatment of rats for a total of 95 weeks, 13 weeks by inhalation and 82 weeks by the oral route, resulted in no evidence of carcinogenic activity. Mutagenic studies have not been performed.

Impairment of fertility, as evidenced by inhibition of the estrus cycle in dogs, was observed following treatment by the oral route. No inhibition of the estrus cycle in dogs was seen following treatment with beclomethasone diproprionate by the inhalation route.

Pregnancy Category C: Like other corticoids, parenteral (subcutaneous) beclomethasone dipropionate has been shown to be tetratogenic and embryocidal in the mouse and rabbit when given in doses approximately ten times the human dose. In these studies, beclomethasone was found to produce fetal resorption, cleft palate, agnathia, microstomia, absence of tongue, delayed ossification, and agenesis of the thymus. No teratogenic or embryocidal effects have been seen in the rat when beclomethasone dipropionate was administered by inhalation at ten times the human dose or orally at 1000 times the human dose. There are no adequate and well-controlled studies in pregnant women. Beclomethasone dipropionate should be used during pregnancy only if the potential benefit justifies the potential risk to the fetus.

Nonteratogenic Effects: Hypoadrenalism may occur in infants born of mothers receiving corticosteroids during pregnancy. Such infants should be carefully observed.

Nursing Mothers: It is not known whether beclomethasone dipropionate is excreted in human milk. Because other corticosteroids are excreted in human milk, caution should be exercised when VANCENASE POCKETHALER Nasal Inhaler is administered to nursing women.

Pediatric Use: Safety and effectiveness in children below the age of 6 years have not been established.

ADVERSE REACTIONS

In general, side effects in clinical studies have been primarily associated with the nasal mucous membranes. Adverse reactions reported in controlled clinical trials and in long-term open studies in patients treated with VANCENASE Nasal Inhaler are described below.

Sensations of irritation and burning in the nose (11 per 100 patients) following the use of VANCENASE Nasal Inhaler have been reported. Also, occasional sneezing attacks (10 per 100 patients) have occurred immediately following the use of the intranasal inhaler. This symptom may be more common in children.

Rhinorrhea may occur occasionally (1 per 100 patients).

Localized infections of the nose and pharynx with *Candida albicans* have occurred rarely. (See **PRECAUTIONS.**)

Transient episodes of epistaxis or bloody discharge from the nose have been reported in 2 per 100 patients. Ulceration of the nasal mucosa has been reported rarely.

Extremely rare instances of nasal septum perforation have been reported following the intranasal application of aerosolized corticosteroids. Rare cases of immediate and delayed hypersensitivity reactions, including urticaria, angioedema, rash, and bronchospasm have been reported following the oral and intranasal inhalation of beclomethasone.

Increased intraocular pressure has been reported rarely. (See **PRECAUTIONS.**)

Systemic corticosteroid side effects were not reported during controlled clinical trials. If recommended doses are exceeded, however, or if individuals are particularly sensitive, symptoms of hypercorticism, ie, Cushing's syndrome could occur.

DOSAGE AND ADMINISTRATION

Adults and Children 12 Years of Age and Over: The usual dosage is one inhalation (42 mcg) in each nostril two to four times a day (total dose 168–336 mcg/day). Patients can often be maintained on a maximum dose of one inhalation in each nostril three times a day (252 mcg/day).

Children 6 to 12 Years of Age: The usual dosage is one inhalation in each nostril three times a day (252 mcg/day).

VANCENASE POCKETHALER Nasal Inhaler is not recommended for children below 6 years of age since safety and efficacy studies have not been conducted in this age group.

In patients who respond to VANCENASE POCKETHALER Nasal Inhaler, an improvement of the symptoms of seasonal or perennial rhinitis usually becomes apparent within a few days after the start of VANCENASE POCKETHALER Nasal Inhaler therapy. However, symptomatic relief may not occur in some patients for as long as 2 weeks. VANCENASE POCKETHALER Nasal Inhaler should not be continued beyond 3 weeks in the absence of significant symptomatic improvement.

The therapeutic effects of corticosteroids, unlike those of decongestants, on seaonsal or perennial rhinitis or on nasal polyps are not immediate. This should be explained to the patient in advance in order to ensure cooperation and continuation of treatment with the prescribed dosage regimen.

VANCENASE POCKETHALER Nasal Inhaler is not recommended for children below 6 years of age.

In the presence of excessive nasal mucus secretion or edema of the nasal mucosa, the drug may fail to reach the site of intended action. In such cases it is advisable to use a nasal vasoconstrictor during the first 2 to 3 days of VANCENASE POCKETHALER Nasal Inhaler therapy.

Directions for Use: Illustrated PATIENT'S INSTRUCTIONS for proper use accompany each package of VANCENASE POCKETHALER Nasal Inhaler.

CONTENTS UNDER PRESSURE. Do not puncture. Do not use or store near heat or open flame. Exposure to temperatures above 120°F may cause bursting. Never throw container into fire or incinerator. Keep out of reach of children.

OVERDOSAGE

When used at excessive doses, systemic corticosteroid effects such as hypercorticism and adrenal suppression may appear. If such changes occur, VANCENASE POCKETHALER Nasal Inhaler should be discontinued slowly consistent with accepted procedures for discontinuing oral steroid therapy.

The oral LD_{50} of beclomethasone dipropionate is greater than 1 g/kg in rodents. One canister of VANCENASE POCKETHALER Nasal Inhaler contains 8.4 mg of beclomethasone dipropionate; therefore acute overdosage is unlikely.

HOW SUPPLIED

VANCENASE POCKETHALER Nasal Inhaler, 7 g canister, box of one. Supplied with nasal adapter and PATIENT'S INSTRUCTIONS (NDC 0085-0649-02).

Store between 15° and 30°C (59° and 86°F).

Failure to use the product within this temperature range may result in improper dosing. Shake well before using.

Revised 3/92

Copyright © 1992, Schering Corporation, Kenilworth, NJ 07033.

All rights reserved.

Shown in Product Identification Section, page 429

VANCENASE® AQ ℞

[van-sen-ase AQ]

brand of beclomethasone dipropionate, monohydrate Nasal Spray 0.042%*

FOR INTRANASAL USE ONLY

***calculated on the dried basis**

DESCRIPTION

Beclomethasone dipropionate, monohydrate, the active component of VANCENASE AQ Nasal Spray, is an anti-inflammatory steroid having the chemical name, 9-Chloro-11β, 17, 21-trihydroxy-16 β -methylpregna-1, 4-diene-3, 20-dione 17,21-dipropionate, monohydrate.

Beclomethasone dipropionate, monohydrate is a white to creamy-white, odorless powder with a molecular weight of 539.06. It is very slightly soluble in water; very soluble in chloroform; and freely soluble in acetone and in alcohol.

VANCENASE AQ Nasal Spray is a metered-dose, manual pump spray unit containing a microcrystalline suspension of beclomethasone dipropionate, monohydrate equivalent to 0.042% w/w beclomethasone dipropionate calculated on the dried basis in an aqueous medium containing microcrystalline cellulose and carboxymethylcellulose sodium, dextrose, benzalkonium chloride, polysorbate 80, and 0.25% v/w phenylethyl alcohol; hydrochloric acid may be added to adjust pH. The pH is between 4.5 and 7.0.

After initial priming (3 to 4 actuations), each actuation of the pump delivers from the nasal adapter 100 mg of suspension containing beclomethasone dipropionate, monohydrate equivalent to 42 mcg beclomethasone dipropionate. Each bottle of VANCENASE AQ Nasal Spray will provide at least 200 metered doses.

CLINICAL PHARMACOLOGY

Beclomethasone 17,21-dipropionate is a diester of beclomethasone, a synthetic halogenated corticosteroid. Animal studies show that beclomethasone dipropionate has potent glucocorticosteroid and weak mineralocorticosteroid activity. The mechanisms for the anti-inflammatory action of beclomethasone dipropionate are unknown. The precise mechanism of the aerosolized drug's action in the nose is also unknown. Biopsies of nasal mucosa obtained during clinical studies showed no histopathologic changes when beclomethasone dipropionate was administered intranasally.

The effects of beclomethasone dipropionate on hypothalamic-pituitary-adrenal (HPA) function have been evaluated in adult volunteers by other routes of administration. Studies with beclomethasone dipropionate by the intranasal route may demonstrate that there is more or that there is less absorption by this route of administration. There was no suppression of early morning plasma cortisol concentrations when beclomethasone dipropionate was administered in a dose of 1000 mcg/day for one month as an oral aerosol or for three days by intramuscular injection. However, partial suppression of plasma cortisol concentration was observed when beclomethasone dipropionate was administered in doses of 2000 mcg/day either by oral aerosol or intramuscular injection. Immediate suppression of plasma cortisol concentrations was observed after single doses of 4000 mcg of beclomethasone dipropionate. Suppression of HPA function (reduction of early morning plasma cortisol levels) has been reported in adult patients who received 1600 mcg daily doses of oral beclomethasone dipropionate for one month. In clinical studies using beclomethasone dipropionate aerosol intranasally, there was no evidence of adrenal insufficiency.

The effect of VANCENASE AQ Nasal Spray on HPA function was not evaluated but would not be expected to differ from intranasal beclomethasone dipropionate aerosol.

In one study in asthmatic children, the administration of inhaled beclomethasone at recommended daily doses for at least one year was associated with a reduction in nocturnal cortisol secretion. The clinical significance of this finding is not clear. It reinforces other evidence, however, that topical beclomethasone may be absorbed in amounts that can have systemic effects and that physicians should be alert for evidence of systemic effects, especially in chronically treated patients (see **PRECAUTIONS**).

Beclomethasone dipropionate is sparingly soluble. When given by nasal inhalation in the form of an aqueous or aerosolized suspension, the drug is deposited primarily in the nasal passages. A portion of the drug is swallowed. Absorption occurs rapidly from all respiratory and gastrointestinal tissues. There is no evidence of tissue storage of beclomethasone dipropionate or its metabolites. *In vitro* studies have shown that tissue other than the liver (lung slices) can rapidly metabolize beclomethasone dipropionate to beclomethasone 17-monopropionate and more slowly to free beclomethasone (which has very weak anti-inflammatory activity). How-

Continued on next page

Information on Schering products appearing on these pages is effective as of August 15, 1992.

Schering—Cont.

ever, irrespective of the route of entry the principal route of excretion of the drug and its metabolites is the feces. In humans, 12% to 15% of an orally administered dose of beclomethasone dipropionate is excreted in the urine as both conjugated and free metabolites of the drug.
Studies have shown that the degree of binding to plasma proteins is 87%.

INDICATIONS AND USAGE

VANCENASE AQ (beclomethasone dipropionate, monohydrate) Nasal Spray is indicated for the relief of the symptoms of seasonal or perennial allergic and non-allergic (vasomotor) rhinitis. Results from two clinical trials have shown that significant symptomatic relief was obtained within three days. However, symptomatic relief may not occur in some patients for as long as two weeks. VANCENASE AQ Nasal Spray should not be continued beyond three weeks in the absence of significant symptomatic improvement. VANCENASE AQ Nasal Spray should not be used in the presence of untreated localized infection involving the nasal mucosa.
VANCENASE AQ Nasal Spray is also indicated for the prevention of recurrence of nasal polyps following surgical removal.
Clinical studies have shown that treatment of the symptoms associated with nasal polyps may have to be continued for several weeks or more before a therapeutic result can be fully assessed. Recurrence of symptoms due to polyps can occur after stopping treatment, depending on the severity of the disease.

CONTRAINDICATIONS

Hypersensitivity to any of the ingredients of this preparation contraindicates its use.

WARNINGS

The replacement of a systemic corticosteroid with VANCENASE AQ Nasal Spray can be accompanied by signs of adrenal insufficiency.
When transferred to VANCENASE AQ Nasal Spray, careful attention must be given to patients previously treated for prolonged periods with systemic corticosteroids. This is particularly important in those patients who have associated asthma or other clinical conditions, where too rapid a decrease in systemic corticosteroids may cause a severe exacerbation of their symptoms.
Studies have shown that the combined administration of alternate day prednisone systemic treatment and orally inhaled beclomethasone increased the likelihood of HPA suppression compared to a therapeutic dose of either one alone. Therefore, VANCENASE AQ Nasal Spray treatment should be used with caution in patients already on alternate day prednisone regimens for any disease.
If recommended doses of intranasal beclomethasone are exceeded or if individuals are particularly sensitive or predisposed by virtue of recent systemic steroid therapy, symptoms of hypercorticism may occur, including very rare cases of menstrual irregularities, acneiform lesions, and cushingoid features. If such changes occur, VANCENASE AQ Nasal Spray should be discontinued slowly, consistent with accepted procedures for discontinuing oral steroid therapy.

PRECAUTIONS

General: During withdrawal from oral steroids, some patients may experience symptoms of withdrawal, e.g., joint and/or muscular pain, lassitude and depression. Rarely, immediate hypersensitivity reactions may occur after the intranasal administration of beclomethasone.
Extremely rare instances of wheezing, nasal septum perforation and increased intraocular pressure have been reported following the intranasal application of aerosolized corticosteroids. Although these have not been observed in clinical trials with VANCENASE AQ Nasal Spray, vigilance should be maintained.
In clinical studies with beclomethasone dipropionate administered intranasally, the development of localized infections of the nose and pharynx with *Candida albicans* has occurred only rarely. When such an infection develops, it may require treatment with appropriate local therapy or discontinuance of treatment with VANCENASE AQ Nasal Spray.
If persistent nasopharyngeal irritation occurs, it may be an indication for stopping VANCENASE AQ Nasal Spray.
Beclomethasone dipropionate is absorbed into the circulation. Use of excessive doses of VANCENASE AQ Nasal Spray may suppress HPA function.
VANCENASE AQ Nasal Spray should be used with caution, if at all, in patients with active or quiescent tuberculous infections of the respiratory tract; in untreated fungal, bacterial, or systemic viral infections; or ocular herpes simplex.
For VANCENASE AQ Nasal Spray to be effective in the treatment of nasal polyps, the spray must be able to enter the nose. Therefore, treatment of nasal polyps with VANCENASE AQ Nasal Spray should be considered adjunctive therapy to surgical removal and/or the use of other medications which will permit effective penetration of VANCENASE AQ Nasal Spray into the nose. Nasal polyps may recur after any form of treatment.
As with any long-term treatment, patients using VANCENASE AQ Nasal Spray over several months or longer should be examined periodically for possible changes in the nasal mucosa.
Because of the inhibitory effect of corticosteroids on wound healing, patients who have experienced recent nasal septal ulcers, nasal surgery, or trauma should not use a nasal corticosteroid until healing has occurred.
Although systemic effects have been minimal with recommended doses, this potential increases with excessive doses. Therefore, larger than recommended doses should be avoided.
Information for Patients: Patients being treated with VANCENASE AQ Nasal Spray should receive the following information and instructions. This information is intended to aid in the safe and effective use of medication. It is not a disclosure of all possible adverse or intended effects. Patients should use VANCENASE AQ Nasal Spray at regular intervals since its effectiveness depends on its regular use. The patient should take the medication as directed. It is not acutely effective and the prescribed dosage should not be increased. Instead, nasal vasoconstrictors or oral antihistamines may be needed until the effects of VANCENASE AQ Nasal Spray are fully manifested. One to two weeks may pass before full relief is obtained. The patient should contact the doctor if symptoms do not improve, or if the condition worsens, or if sneezing or nasal irritation occurs. For the proper use of this unit and to attain maximum improvement, the patient should read and follow the accompanying Patient's Instructions carefully.
Carcinogenesis, Mutagenesis, Impairment or Fertility: Treatment of rats for a total of 95 weeks, 13 weeks by inhalation and 82 weeks by the oral route, resulted in no evidence of carcinogenic activity. Mutagenic studies have not been performed.
Impairment of fertility, as evidenced by inhibition of the estrous cycle in dogs, was observed following treatment by the oral route. No inhibition of the estrous cycle in dogs was seen following treatment with beclomethasone dipropionate by the inhalation route.
Pregnancy Category C: Like other corticosteroids, parenteral (subcutaneous) beclomethasone dipropionate has been shown to be teratogenic and embryocidal in the mouse and rabbit when given in doses approximately ten times the human dose. In these studies beclomethasone was found to produce fetal resorption, cleft palate, agnathia, microstomia, absence of tongue, delayed ossification, and agenesis of the thymus. No teratogenic or embryocidal effects have been seen in the rat when beclomethasone dipropionate was administered by inhalation at ten times the human dose or orally at 1000 times the human dose. There are no adequate and well-controlled studies in pregnant women. Beclomethasone dipropionate should be used during pregnancy only if the potential benefit justifies the potential risk to the fetus.
Nonteratogenic Effects: Hypoadrenalism may occur in infants born of mothers receiving corticosteroids during pregnancy. Such infants should be carefully observed.
Nursing Mothers: It is not known whether beclomethasone dipropionate is excreted in human milk. Because other corticosteroids are excreted in human milk, caution should be exercised when VANCENASE AQ Nasal Spray is administered to nursing women.
Pediatric Use: Safety and effectiveness in children below the age of 6 years have not been established.

ADVERSE REACTIONS

In general, side effects in clinical studies have been primarily associated with irritation of the nasal mucous membranes. Rarely, immediate hypersensitivity reactions may occur after the intranasal administration of beclomethasone dipropionate.
Adverse reactions reported in controlled clinical trials and open studies in patients treated with VANCENASE AQ Nasal Spray are described below.
Mild, transient nasopharyngeal irritation following the use of beclomethasone aqueous nasal spray has been reported in up to 24% of patients treated, including occasional sneezing attacks (about 4%) occurring immediately following use of the inhaler. In patients experiencing these symptoms, none had to discontinue treatment. The incidence of irritation and sneezing was approximately the same in the group of patients who received placebo in these studies, implying that these complaints may be related to vehicle components of the formulation.
Fewer than 5 per 100 patients reported headache, nausea, or lightheadedness following the use of VANCENASE AQ (beclomethasone dipropionate, monohydrate) Nasal Spray. Fewer than 3 per 100 patients reported nasal stuffiness, nosebleeds, rhinorrhea, or tearing eyes.
Extremely rare instances of wheezing, nasal septum perforation and increased intraocular pressure have been reported following the intranasal administration of aerosolized corticosteroids (see **PRECAUTIONS**).

OVERDOSAGE

When used at excessive doses, systemic corticosteroid effects such as hypercorticism and adrenal suppression may appear. If such changes occur, VANCENASE AQ Nasal Spray should be discontinued slowly consistent with accepted procedures for discontinuing oral steroid therapy. The oral LD_{50} of beclomethasone dipropionate is greater than 1 g/kg in rodents. One bottle of VANCENASE AQ Nasal Spray contains beclomethasone dipropionate, monohydrate equivalent to 10.5 mg of beclomethasone dipropionate; therefore, acute overdosage is unlikely.

DOSAGE AND ADMINISTRATION

Adults and Children 6 Years of Age and Older: The usual dosage is 1 or 2 inhalations (42 to 84 mcg) in each nostril 2 times a day (total dose 168 to 336 mcg/day).
In patients who respond to VANCENASE AQ Nasal Spray, an improvement of the symptoms of seasonal or perennial rhinitis usually becomes apparent within a few days after the start of VANCENASE AQ Nasal Spray therapy. However, symptomatic relief may not occur in some patients for as long as two weeks. VANCENASE AQ Nasal Spray should not be continued beyond three weeks in the absence of significant symptomatic improvement.
The therapeutic effects of corticosteroids, unlike those of decongestants on seasonal or perennial rhinitis, or on nasal polyps are not immediate. This should be explained to the patient in advance in order to ensure cooperation and continuation of treatment with the prescribed dosage regimen.
VANCENASE AQ Nasal Spray is not recommended for children below 6 years of age.
In the presence of excessive nasal mucus secretion or edema of the nasal mucosa, the drug may fail to reach the site of intended action. In such cases, it is advisable to use a nasal vasoconstrictor during the first 2 to 3 days of VANCENASE AQ Nasal Spray therapy.
Directions for Use: Illustrated Patient's Instructions for proper use accompany each package of VANCENASE AQ Nasal Spray.

HOW SUPPLIED

VANCENASE AQ (beclomethasone dipropionate, monohydrate) Nasal Spray 0.042%*, 25 g bottle; box of one. Supplied with nasal pump unit and dust cap; and Patient's Instructions (NDC 0085-0259-02).
Store between 2° and 30°C (36° and 86°F).
SHAKE WELL BEFORE EACH USE.
Revised 8/88

*calculated on the dried basis
Shown in Product Identification Section, page 428

VANCERIL® Inhaler ℞

[van 'ser-il]
brand of beclomethasone dipropionate, USP
FOR ORAL INHALATION ONLY

DESCRIPTION

Beclomethasone dipropionate, USP, the active component of VANCERIL Inhaler, is an anti-inflammatory steroid having the chemical name 9-Chloro-11β,17,21-trihydroxy-16 β-methylpregna-1,4-diene-3, 20-dione 17,21-dipropionate.
VANCERIL Inhaler is a metered-dose aerosol unit containing a microcrystalline suspension of beclomethasone dipropionate-trichloromonofluoromethane clathrate in a mixture of propellants (trichloromonofluoromethane and dichlorodifluoromethane) with oleic acid. Each canister contains beclomethasone dipropionate-trichloromonofluoromethane clathrate having a molecular proportion of beclomethasone dipropionate, USP, to trichloromonofluoromethane between 3:1 and 3:2. Each actuation delivers from the mouthpiece a quantity of clathrate equivalent to 42 mcg of beclomethasone dipropionate, USP. The contents of one canister provide at least 200 oral inhalations.

CLINICAL PHARMACOLOGY

Beclomethasone 17,21-dipropionate is a diester of beclomethasone, a synthetic corticosteroid which is chemically related to dexamethasone. Beclomethasone differs from dexamethasone only in having a chlorine at the 9-alpha in place of a fluorine and in having a 16β-methyl group instead of a 16 alpha-methyl group. Animal studies showed that beclomethasone dipropionate has potent anti-inflammatory activity. When administered systemically to mice, the anti-inflammatory activity was accompanied by other typical features of glucocorticoid action including thymic involution, liver glycogen deposition, and pituitary-adrenal suppression. However, after systemic administration to rats, the anti-inflammatory action was associated with little or no effect on other tests of glucocorticoid activity.
Beclomethasone dipropionate is sparingly soluble and is poorly mobilized from subcutaneous or intramuscular injec-

tion sites. However, systemic absorption occurs after all routes of administration. When given to animals in the form of an aerosolized suspension of the trichloromonofluoromethane clathrate, the drug is deposited in the mouth and nasal passages, the trachea and principal bronchi, and in the lung; a considerable portion of the drug is also swallowed. Absorption occurs rapidly from all respiratory and gastrointestinal tissues, as indicated by the rapid clearance of radioactively labeled drug from local tissues and appearance of tracer in the circulation. There is no evidence of tissue storage of beclomethasone dipropionate or its metabolites. Lung slices can metabolize beclomethasone dipropionate rapidly to beclomethasone 17-monopropionate and more slowly to free beclomethasone (which has very weak anti-inflammatory activity). However, irrespective of the route of administration (injection, oral, or aerosol), the principal route of excretion of the drug and its metabolites is the feces. Less than 10% of the drug and its metabolites is excreted in the urine. In humans, 12% to 15% of an orally administered dose of beclomethasone dipropionate was excreted in the urine as both conjugated and free metabolites of the drug.

The mechanisms responsible for the anti-inflammatory action of beclomethasone dipropionate are unknown. The precise mechanism of the aerosolized drug's action in the lung is also unknown.

INDICATIONS

VANCERIL Inhaler is indicated only for patients who require chronic treatment with corticosteroids for control of the symptoms of bronchial asthma. Such patients would include those already receiving systemic corticosteroids, and selected patients who are inadequately controlled on a non-steroid regimen and in whom steroid therapy has been withheld because of concern over potential adverse effects.

VANCERIL Inhaler is NOT indicated:
1. For relief of asthma which can be controlled by bronchodilators and other non-steroid medications.
2. In patients who require systemic corticosteroid treatment infrequently.
3. In the treatment of non-asthmatic bronchitis.

CONTRAINDICATIONS

VANCERIL Inhaler is contraindicated in the primary treatment of status asthmaticus or other acute episodes of asthma where intensive measures are required.

Hypersensitivity to any of the ingredients of this preparation contraindicates its use.

WARNINGS

> Particular care is needed in patients who are transferred from systemically active corticosteroids to VANCERIL Inhaler because deaths due to adrenal insufficiency have occurred in asthmatic patients during and after transfer from systemic corticosteroids to aerosol beclomethasone dipropionate. After withdrawal from systemic corticosteroids, a number of months are required for recovery of hypothalamic-pituitary-adrenal (HPA) function. During this period of HPA suppression, patients may exhibit signs and symptoms of adrenal insufficiency when exposed to trauma, surgery or infections, particularly gastroenteritis. Although VANCERIL Inhaler may provide control of asthmatic symptoms during these episodes, it does NOT provide the systemic steroid which is necessary for coping with these emergencies.
>
> During periods of stress or a severe asthmatic attack, patients who have been withdrawn from systemic corticosteroids should be instructed to resume systemic steroids (in large doses) immediately and to contact their physician for further instruction. These patients should also be instructed to carry a warning card indicating that they may need supplementary systemic steroids during periods of stress or a severe asthma attack. To assess the risk of adrenal insuffficiency in emergency situations, routine tests of adrenal cortical function, including measurement of early morning resting cortisol levels, should be performed periodically in all patients. An early morning resting cortisol level may be accepted as normal only if it falls at or near the normal mean level.

Localized infections with *Candida albicans* or *Aspergillus niger* have occurred frequently in the mouth and pharynx and occasionally in the larynx. Positive cultures for oral *Candida* may be present in up to 75% of patients. Although the frequency of clinically apparent infection is considerably lower, these infections may require treatment with appropriate antifungal therapy or discontinuance of treatment with VANCERIL Inhaler.

VANCERIL Inhaler is not to be regarded as a bronchodilator and is not indicated for rapid relief of bronchospasm.

Patients should be instructed to contact their physician immediately when episodes of asthma which are not responsive to bronchodilators occur during the course of treatment with VANCERIL. During such episodes, patients may require therapy with systemic corticosteroids.

There is no evidence that control of asthma can be achieved by the administration of VANCERIL in amounts greater than the recommended doses.

Transfer of patients from systemic steroid therapy to VANCERIL Inhaler may unmask allergic conditions previously suppressed by the systemic steroid therapy, e.g., rhinitis, conjunctivitis, and eczema.

PRECAUTIONS

During withdrawal from oral steroids, some patients may experience symptoms of systemically active steroid withdrawal, e.g., joint and/or muscular pain, lassitude and depression, despite maintenance or even improvement of respiratory function (See DOSAGE AND ADMINISTRATION for details).

In responsive patients, beclomethasone dipropionate may permit control of asthmatic symptoms without suppression of HPA function, as discussed below (See CLINICAL STUDIES). Since beclomethasone dipropionate is absorbed into the circulation and can be systemically active, the beneficial effects of VANCERIL Inhaler in minimizing or preventing HPA dysfunction may be expected only when recommended dosages are not exceeded.

The long-term effects of beclomethasone dipropionate in human subjects are still unknown. In particular, the local effects of the agent on developmental or immunologic processes in the mouth, pharynx, trachea, and lung are unknown. There is also no information about the possible long-term systemic effects of the agent.

The potential effects of VANCERIL on acute, recurrent, or chronic pulmonary infections, including active or quiescent tuberculosis, are not known. Similarly, the potential effects of long-term administration of the drug on lung or other tissues are unknown.

Pulmonary infiltrates with eosinophilia may occur in patients on VANCERIL Inhaler therapy. Although it is possible that in some patients this state may become manifest because of systemic steroid withdrawal when inhalational steroids are administered, a causative role for beclomethasone dipropionate and/or its vehicle cannot be ruled out.

Use in Pregnancy: Glucocorticoids are known teratogens in rodent species and beclomethasone dipropionate is no exception.

Teratology studies were done in rats, mice, and rabbits treated with subcutaneous beclomethasone dipropionate. Beclomethasone dipropionate was found to produce fetal resorptions, cleft palate, agnathia, microstomia, absence of tongue, delayed ossification and partial agenesis of the thymus. Well-controlled trials relating to fetal risk in humans are not available. Glucocorticoids are secreted in human milk. It is not known whether beclomethasone dipropionate would be secreted in human milk but it is safe to assume that it is likely. The use of beclomethasone dipropionate in pregnancy, nursing mothers, or women of childbearing potential requires that the possible benefits of the drug be weighed against the potential hazards to the mother, embryo, or fetus. Infants born of mothers who have received substantial doses of corticosteroids during pregnancy should be carefully observed for hypoadrenalism.

ADVERSE REACTIONS

Deaths due to adrenal insufficiency have occurred in asthmatic patients during and after transfer from systemic corticosteroids to aerosol beclomethasone dipropionate (See WARNINGS).

Suppression of HPA function (reduction of early morning plasma cortisol levels) has been reported in adult patients who received 1600 mcg daily doses of VANCERIL for one month. A few patients on VANCERIL have complained of hoarseness or dry mouth.

Rare cases of immediate and delayed hypersensitivity reactions, including urticaria, angioedema, rash and bronchospasm have been reported following the oral and intranasal inhalation of beclomethasone.

DOSAGE AND ADMINISTRATION

Adults: The usual recommended dosage is two inhalations (84 mcg) given three or four times a day. Alternatively, four inhalations (168 mcg) given twice daily has been shown to be effective in some patients. In patients with severe asthma, it is advisable to start with 12 to 16 inhalations a day and adjust the dosage downward according to the response of the patient. The maximal daily intake should not exceed 20 inhalations, 840 mcg (0.84 mg), in adults.

Children 6 to 12 years of age: The usual recommended dosage is one or two inhalations (42 to 84 mcg) given three or four times a day according to the response of the patient. Alternatively, four inhalations (168 mcg) given twice daily has been shown to be effective in some patients. The maximal daily intake should not exceed ten inhalations, 420 mcg (0.42 mg), in children 6 to 12 years of age. Insufficient clinical data exist with respect to the administration of VANCERIL Inhaler in children below the age of 6.

Rinsing the mouth after inhalation is advised.

Patients receiving bronchodilators by inhalation should be advised to use the bronchodilator before VANCERIL Inhaler in order to enhance penetration of beclomethasone dipropionate into the bronchial tree. After use of an aerosol bronchodilator, several minutes should elapse before use of the VANCERIL Inhaler to reduce the potential toxicity from the inhaled fluorocarbon propellants in the two aerosols.

Different considerations must be given to the following groups of patients in order to obtain the full therapeutic benefit of VANCERIL Inhaler.

Patients not receiving systemic steroids: The use of VANCERIL Inhaler is straightforward in patients who are inadequately controlled with non-steroid medications but in whom systemic steroid therapy has been withheld because of concern over potential adverse reactions. In patients who respond to VANCERIL, an improvement in pulmonary function is usually apparent within one to four weeks after the start of VANCERIL Inhaler.

Patients receiving systemic steroids: In those patients dependent on systemic steroids, transfer to VANCERIL and subsequent management may be more difficult because recovery from impaired adrenal function is usually slow. Such suppression has been known to last for up to 12 months. Clinical studies, however, have demonstrated that VANCERIL may be effective in the management of these asthmatic patients and may permit replacement or significant reduction in the dosage of systemic corticosteroids.

The patient's asthma should be reasonably stable before treatment with VANCERIL Inhaler is started. Initially, the aerosol should be used concurrently with the patient's usual maintenance dose of systemic steroid. After approximately one week, gradual withdrawal of the systemic steroid is started by reducing the daily or alternate daily dose. The next reduction is made after an interval of one or two weeks, depending on the response of the patient. Generally, these decrements should not exceed 2.5 mg of prednisone or its equivalent. A slow rate of withdrawal cannot be overemphasized. During withdrawal, some patients may experience symptoms of systemically active steroid withdrawal, e.g., joint and/or muscular pain, lassitude and depression, despite maintenance or even improvement of respiratory function. Such patients should be encouraged to continue with the Inhaler but should be watched carefully for objective signs of adrenal insufficiency, such as hypotension and weight loss. If evidence of adrenal insufficiency occurs, the systemic steroid dose should be boosted temporarily and thereafter further withdrawal should continue more slowly. During periods of stress or a severe asthma attack, transfer patients will require supplementary treatment with systemic steroids. Exacerbations of asthma which occur during the course of treatment with VANCERIL Inhaler should be treated with a short course of systemic steroid which is gradually tapered as these symptoms subside. There is no evidence that control of asthma can be achieved by administration of VANCERIL in amounts greater than the recommended doses.

Directions for Use: Illustrated patient instructions for proper use accompany each package of VANCERIL Inhaler. CONTENTS UNDER PRESSURE. Do not puncture. Do not use or store near heat or open flame. Exposure to temperatures above 120°F. may cause bursting. Never throw container into fire or incinerator. Keep out of reach of children.

HOW SUPPLIED

VANCERIL Inhaler 16.8 g canister supplied with an oral adapter and patient's instructions; box of one. (NDC-0085-0736-04).

Store between 15° and 30°C (59° and 86°F). Failure to use the product within this temperature range may result in improper dosing. Shake well before using.

ANIMAL PHARMACOLOGY AND TOXICOLOGY

Studies in a number of animal species including rats, rabbits, and dogs have shown no unusual toxicity during acute experiments. However, the effects of beclomethasone dipropionate in producing signs of glucocorticoid excess during chronic administration by various routes were dose related.

CLINICAL STUDIES

The effects of beclomethasone dipropionate on hypothalamic-pituitary-adrenal (HPA) function have been evaluated in adult volunteers. There was no suppression of early morning plasma cortisol concentrations when beclomethasone dipropionate was administered in a dose of 1000 mcg/day for one month as an aerosol or for three days by intramuscular injection. However, partial suppression of plasma cortisol concentration was observed when beclomethasone dipropionate was administered in doses of 2000 mcg/day either intramuscularly or by aerosol. Immediate suppression of plasma

Continued on next page

Information on Schering products appearing on these pages is effective as of August 15, 1992.

Schering—Cont.

cortisol concentrations was observed after single doses of 4000 mcg of beclomethasone dipropionate.

In one study, the effects of beclomethasone dipropionate on HPA function were examined in patients with asthma. There was no change in basal early morning plasma cortisol concentrations or in the cortisol responses to tetracosactrin (ACTH 1:24) stimulation after daily administration of 400, 800 or 1200 mcg of beclomethasone dipropionate for 28 days. After daily administration of 1600 mcg each day for 28 days, there was a slight reduction in basal cortisol concentrations and a statistically significant (p < .01) reduction in plasma cortisol responses to tetracosactrin stimulation. The effects of a more prolonged period of beclomethasone dipropionate administration on HPA function have not been evaluated. However, a number of investigators have noted that when systemic corticosteroid therapy in asthmatic subjects can be replaced with recommended doses of beclomethasone dipropionate, there is gradual recovery of endogenous cortisol concentrations to the normal range. There is still no documented evidence of recovery from other adverse systemic corticosteroid-induced reactions during prolonged therapy of patients with beclomethasone dipropionate.

Clinical experience has shown that some patients with bronchial asthma who require corticosteroid therapy for control of symptoms can be partially or completely withdrawn from systemic corticosteroid if therapy with beclomethasone dipropionate aerosol is substituted. Beclomethasone dipropionate aerosol is not effective for all patients with bronchial asthma or at all stages of the disease in a given patient.

The early clinical experience has revealed several new problems which may be associated with the use of beclomethasone dipropionate by inhalation for treatment of patients with bronchial asthma:

1. There is a risk of adrenal insufficiency when patients are transferred from systemic corticosteroids to aerosol beclomethasone dipropionate. Although the aerosol may provide adequate control of asthma during the transfer period, it does not provide the systemic steroid which is needed during acute stress situations. Deaths due to adrenal insufficiency have occurred in asthmatic patients during and after transfer from systemic corticosteroids to aerosol beclomethasone dipropionate. (See WARNINGS.)
2. Transfer of patients from systemic steroid therapy to beclomethasone dipropionate aerosol may unmask allergic conditions which were previously controlled by the systemic steroid therapy, e.g., rhinitis, conjunctivitis, and eczema.
3. Localized infections with *Candida albicans* or *Aspergillus niger* have occurred frequently in the mouth and pharynx and occasionally in the larynx. It has been reported that up to 75% of the patients who receive prolonged treatment with beclomethasone dipropionate have positive oral cultures for *Candida albicans*. The incidence of clinically apparent infection is considerably lower but may require therapy with appropriate antifungal agents or discontinuation of treatment with beclomethasone dipropionate aerosol.

The long-term effects of beclomethasone dipropionate in human subjects are still unknown. In particular, the local effects of the agent on developmental or immunologic processes in the mouth, pharynx, trachea and lung are unknown. There is also no information about the possible long-term systemic effects of the agent. The possible relevance of the data in animal studies to results in human subjects cannot be evaluated.

Revised 5/90

Copyright © 1973, 1990, Schering Corporation, USA. All rights reserved.

Shown in Product Identification Section, page 428

Information on Schering products appearing on these pages is effective as of August 15, 1992.

Schering-Plough HealthCare Products

110 ALLEN ROAD
P.O. BOX 276
LIBERTY CORNER, NJ 07938-0276

GYNE–LOTRIMIN®   OTC
Clotrimazole
Vaginal Cream
Antifungal

ACTIVE INGREDIENT
Clotrimazole 1%

INACTIVE INGREDIENTS
Benzyl alcohol, cetearyl alcohol, cetyl esters wax, octyldodecanol, polysorbate 60, purified water, sorbitan monostearate.

INDICATIONS
Gyne-Lotrimin® will cure most recurrent vaginal yeast (Candida) infections. Gyne-Lotrimin® usually starts to relieve the itching and other symptoms of vaginal yeast infection within 3 days. If the patient does not improve in 3 days or if the patient does not get well in 7 days, a condition other than yeast infection may exist. The patient should discontinue use of the product and consult a doctor. Also, if symptoms recur within a 2-month period, patient should consult a doctor.

Important: In order to kill the yeast completely, GYNE-LOTRIMIN must be used the full seven days, even if symptoms are relieved sooner.

WARNINGS
- Do not use if you have abdominal pain, fever, or a foul-smelling vaginal discharge. You may have a condition which is more serious than a yeast infection. Contact your doctor immediately.
- Do not use if this is your first experience with vaginal itch and discomfort. See your doctor.
- If there is no improvement within 3 days, you may have a condition other than a yeast infection. Stop using this product and see your doctor.
- If symptoms recur within a 2-month period, contact your doctor.
- Do not use during pregnancy except under the advice and supervision of a doctor.
- This medication is for vaginal use only. It is not for use in the mouth or the eyes. In case accidentally swallowed, seek professional assistance or contact a Poison Control Center immediately.
- Keep this and all drugs out of reach of children. This product is not to be used on children less than 12 years of age.

DOSAGE
Fill the applicator with the cream and then insert one applicatorful of cream into the vagina every day, preferably at bedtime. Repeat this procedure for seven consecutive days.

Shown in Product Identification Section, page 429

GYNE–LOTRIMIN®   OTC
Clotrimazole
Vaginal Inserts
Antifungal

ACTIVE INGREDIENT
Each insert contains Clotrimazole 100 mg.

INACTIVE INGREDIENTS
Corn starch, lactose, magnesium stearate, povidone.

INDICATIONS
Gyne-Lotrimin® will cure most vaginal yeast (Candida) infections. Gyne-Lotrimin® usually starts to relieve the itching and other symptoms of vaginal yeast infection within 3 days. If the patient does not improve in 3 days or if the patient does not get well in 7 days, a condition other than yeast infection may exist. The patient should discontinue use of the product and consult a doctor. Also, if symptoms recur within a 2-month period, patient should consult a doctor.

Important: In order to kill the yeast completely, GYNE-LOTRIMIN must be used the full seven days, even if symptoms are relieved sooner.

WARNINGS
- Do not use if you have abdominal pain, fever, or a foul-smelling vaginal discharge. You may have a condition which is more serious than a yeast infection. Contact your doctor immediately.
- Do not use if this is your first experience with vaginal itch and discomfort. See your doctor.
- If there is no improvement within 3 days, you may have a condition other than a yeast infection. Stop using this product and see your doctor.
- If symptoms recur within a 2-month period, contact your doctor.
- Do not use during pregnancy except under the advice and supervision of a doctor.
- This medication is for vaginal use only. It is not for use in the mouth or the eyes. In case accidentally swallowed, seek professional assistance or contact a Poison Control Center immediately.
- Keep this and all drugs out of reach of children. This product is not to be used on children less than 12 years of age.

DOSAGE
Using the applicator, place one insert into the vagina, preferably at bedtime. Repeat this procedure for seven consecutive days.

Shown in Product Identification Section, page 429

Schiapparelli Searle
BOX 5110
CHICAGO, IL 60680

Alphabetic Product Listing
Product, ID #, (NDC*), Form, Strength
Banthine, 1501, Tablet, 50 mg
Cyclobenzaprine, (5658), Tablet, 10 mg
Flagyl, I.V., 1804, Vial (partial fill, lyoph. pwd.), 500 mg
Flagyl I.V. RTU, 1847, Plastic Container, 500 mg/100 ml
Haloperidol, 896, Oral Solution, 2 mg/ml, 120 ml
Lactulose, 3036, Syrup USP, 10 g/15 ml
Lactulose, 3056, Syrup USP, 10 g/15 ml
Norethin 1/35E-21, Dispenser, 221, Tablet, 1 mg/35 mcg
Norethin 1/35E-28, Dispenser, 221 (231), Tablet, 1 mg/35 mcg
Norethin 1/50M-21, Dispenser, 431, Tablet, 1 mg/50 mcg
Norethin 1/50M-28, Dispenser, 431 (441), Tablet, 1 mg/50 mcg
Piroxicam USP, 5752, Tablet, 10 mg
Piroxicam USP, 5762, Tablet, 20 mg
Pro-Banthine, 601 (0601), Tablet, 15 mg
Pro-Banthine, Unit Dose, 601 (0601), Tablet, 15 mg
Pro-Banthine, 611 (0611), Tablet, 7½ mg

---

*When the product ID # is not the same as the NDC #, the NDC # appears in parentheses.

Product Information Available on Request
Banthine (methantheline bromide)   ℞
Cyclobenzaprine Tablets USP   ℞
Haloperidol Oral Solution, USP   ℞
Lactulose Syrup USP   ℞

FLAGYL® I.V.   ℞
[flaj'yl]
(metronidazole hydrochloride)
FLAGYL® I.V. RTU   ℞
(metronidazole injection USP) Ready-to-Use
STERILE
For Intravenous Infusion Only

WARNING

Metronidazole has been shown to be carcinogenic in mice and rats (see *Precautions*). Its use, therefore, should be reserved for the conditions described in the *Indications and Usage* section below.

DESCRIPTION
Flagyl I.V., sterile (metronidazole hydrochloride), and Flagyl I.V. RTU, sterile (metronidazole), are parenteral dosage forms of the synthetic antibacterial agents 1-(β-hydroxyethyl)-2-methyl-5-nitroimidazole hydrochloride and 1-(β-hydroxyethyl)-2-methyl-5-nitroimidazole, respectively.

metronidazole hydrochloride   metronidazole

Each single-dose vial of lyophilized Flagyl I.V. contains sterile, nonpyrogenic metronidazole hydrochloride, equivalent to 500 mg metronidazole, and 415 mg mannitol. Each Flagyl I.V. RTU 100-ml single-dose plastic container contains a sterile, nonpyrogenic, isotonic, buffered solution of 500 mg metronidazole, 47.6 mg sodium phosphate, 22.9 mg citric acid, and 790 mg sodium chloride in Water for Injection USP. Flagyl I.V. RTU has a tonicity of 310 mOsm/L

and a pH of 5 to 7. Each container contains 14 mEq of sodium.

The plastic container is fabricated from a specially formulated polyvinyl chloride plastic. Water can permeate from inside the container into the overwrap in amounts insufficient to affect the solution significantly. Solutions in contact with the plastic container can leach out certain of its chemical components in very small amounts within the expiration period, eg, di 2-ethylhexyl phthalate (DEHP), up to 5 parts per million. However, the safety of the plastic has been confirmed in tests in animals according to USP biological tests for plastic containers as well as by tissue culture toxicity studies.

CLINICAL PHARMACOLOGY

Metronidazole is a synthetic antibacterial compound. Disposition of metronidazole in the body is similar for both oral and intravenous dosage forms, with an average elimination half-life in healthy humans of eight hours.

The major route of elimination of metronidazole and its metabolites is via the urine (60–80% of the dose), with fecal excretion accounting for 6–15% of the dose. The metabolites that appear in the urine result primarily from side-chain oxidation [1-(β-hydroxyethyl) -2- hydroxymethyl-5-nitroimidazole and 2-methyl-5-nitroimidazole-1-yl-acetic acid] and glucuronide conjugation, with unchanged metronidazole accounting for approximately 20% of the total. Renal clearance of metronidazole is approximately 10 ml/min/1.73 m^2.

Metronidazole is the major component appearing in the plasma, with lesser quantities of the 2-hydroxymethyl metabolite also being present. Less than 20% of the circulating metronidazole is bound to plasma proteins. Both the parent compound and the metabolite possess *in vitro* bactericidal activity against most strains of anaerobic bacteria.

Metronidazole appears in cerebrospinal fluid, saliva, and breast milk in concentrations similar to those found in plasma. Bactericidal concentrations of metronidazole have also been detected in pus from hepatic abscesses.

Plasma concentrations of metronidazole are proportional to the administered dose. An eight-hour intravenous infusion of 100–4,000 mg of metronidazole in normal subjects showed a linear relationship between dose and peak plasma concentration.

In patients treated with Flagyl I.V., using a dosage regimen of 15 mg/kg loading dose followed six hours later by 7.5 mg/kg every six hours, peak steady-state plasma concentrations of metronidazole averaged 25 mcg/ml with trough (minimum) concentrations averaging 18 mcg/ml.

Decreased renal function does not alter the single-dose pharmacokinetics of metronidazole. However, plasma clearance of metronidazole is decreased in patients with decreased liver function.

In one study newborn infants appeared to demonstrate diminished capacity to eliminate metronidazole. The elimination half-life, measured during the first three days of life, was inversely related to gestational age. In infants whose gestational ages were between 28 and 40 weeks, the corresponding elimination half-lives ranged from 109 to 22.5 hours.

Microbiology: Metronidazole is active *in vitro* against most obligate anaerobes, but does not appear to possess any clinically relevant activity against facultative anaerobes or obligate aerobes. Against susceptible organisms, metronidazole is generally bactericidal at concentrations equal to or slightly higher than the minimal inhibitory concentrations. Metronidazole has been shown to have *in vitro* and clinical activity against the following organisms:

- Anaerobic gram-negative bacilli, including:
  - *Bacteroides* species, including the *Bacteroides fragilis* group (*B. fragilis, B. distasonis, B. ovatus, B. thetaiotaomicron, B. vulgatus*)
  - *Fusobacterium* species.
- Anaerobic gram-positive bacilli, including:
  - *Clostridium* species and susceptible strains of *Eubacterium*
- Anaerobic gram-positive cocci, including:
  - *Peptococcus* species
  - *Peptostreptococcus* species

Susceptibility Tests: Bacteriologic studies should be performed to determine the causative organisms and their susceptibility to metronidazole; however, the rapid, routine susceptibility testing of individual isolates of anaerobic bacteria is not always practical, and therapy may be started while awaiting these results.

Quantitative methods give the most accurate estimates of susceptibility to antibacterial drugs. A standardized agar dilution method and a broth microdilution method are recommended.[1]

Control strains are recommended for standardized susceptibility testing. Each time the test is performed, one or more of the following strains should be included: *Clostridium perfringens* ATCC 13124, *Bacteroides fragilis* ATCC 25285, and *Bacteroides thetaiotaomicron* ATCC 29741. The mode metronidazole MICs for those three strains are reported to be 0.25, 0.25, and 0.5 mcg/ml, respectively.

A clinical laboratory test is considered under acceptable control if the results of the control strains are within one doubling dilution of the mode MICs reported for metronidazole.

A bacterial isolate may be considered susceptible if the MIC value for metronidazole is not more than 16 mcg/ml. An organism is considered resistant if the MIC is greater than 16 mcg/ml. A report of "resistant" from the laboratory indicates that the infecting organism is not likely to respond to therapy.

INDICATIONS AND USAGE

Treatment of Anaerobic Infections

Flagyl I.V. (metronidazole hydrochloride) and Flagyl I.V. RTU (metronidazole) are indicated in the treatment of serious infections caused by susceptible anaerobic bacteria. Indicated surgical procedures should be performed in conjunction with Flagyl I.V. or Flagyl I.V. RTU therapy. In a mixed aerobic and anaerobic infection, antibiotics appropriate for the treatment of the aerobic infection should be used in addition to Flagyl I.V. or Flagyl I.V. RTU.

Flagyl I.V. and Flagyl I.V. RTU are effective in *Bacteroides fragilis* infections resistant to clindamycin, chloramphenicol, and penicillin.

INTRA-ABDOMINAL INFECTIONS, including peritonitis, intra-abdominal abscess, and liver abscess, caused by *Bacteroides* species including the *B. fragilis* group (*B. fragilis, B. distasonis, B. ovatus, B. thetaiotaomicron, B. vulgatus*), *Clostridium* species, *Eubacterium* species, *Peptococcus* species, and *Peptostreptococcus* species.

SKIN AND SKIN STRUCTURE INFECTIONS caused by *Bacteroides* species including the *B. fragilis* group, *Clostridium* species, *Peptococcus* species, *Peptostreptococcus* species, and *Fusobacterium* species.

GYNECOLOGIC INFECTIONS, including endometritis, endomyometritis, tubo-ovarian abscess, and postsurgical vaginal cuff infection, caused by *Bacteroides* species including the *B. fragilis* group, *Clostridium* species, *Peptococcus* species, and *Peptostreptococcus* species.

BACTERIAL SEPTICEMIA caused by *Bacteroides* species including the *B. fragilis* group, and *Clostridium* species.

BONE AND JOINT INFECTIONS, as adjunctive therapy, caused by *Bacteroides* species including the *B. fragilis* group.

CENTRAL NERVOUS SYSTEM (CNS) INFECTIONS, including meningitis and brain abscess, caused by *Bacteroides* species including the *B. fragilis* group.

LOWER RESPIRATORY TRACT INFECTIONS, including pneumonia, empyema, and lung abscess, caused by *Bacteroides* species including the *B. fragilis* group.

ENDOCARDITIS caused by *Bacteroides* species including the *B. fragilis* group.

Prophylaxis

The prophylactic administration of Flagyl I.V. or Flagyl I.V. RTU preoperatively, intraoperatively, and postoperatively may reduce the incidence of postoperative infection in patients undergoing elective colorectal surgery which is classified as contaminated or potentially contaminated.

Prophylactic use of Flagyl I.V. or Flagyl I.V. RTU should be discontinued within 12 hours after surgery. If there are signs of infection, specimens for cultures should be obtained for the identification of the causative organism(s) so that appropriate therapy may be given (see *Dosage and Administration*).

CONTRAINDICATIONS

Flagyl I.V. and Flagyl I.V. RTU are contraindicated in patients with a prior history of hypersensitivity to metronidazole or other nitroimidazole derivatives.

WARNINGS

Convulsive Seizures and Peripheral Neuropathy: Convulsive seizures and peripheral neuropathy, the latter characterized mainly by numbness or paresthesia of an extremity, have been reported in patients treated with metronidazole. The appearance of abnormal neurologic signs demands the prompt evaluation of the benefit/risk ratio of the continuation of therapy.

PRECAUTIONS

General: Patients with severe hepatic disease metabolize metronidazole slowly, with resultant accumulation of metronidazole and its metabolites in the plasma. Accordingly, for such patients, doses below those usually recommended should be administered cautiously.

Administration of solutions containing sodium ions may result in sodium retention. Care should be taken when administering Flagyl I.V. RTU to patients receiving corticosteroids or to patients predisposed to edema.

Known or previously unrecognized candidiasis may present more prominent symptoms during therapy with Flagyl I.V. or Flagyl I.V. RTU and requires treatment with a candicidal agent.

Laboratory Tests: Metronidazole is a nitroimidazole, and Flagyl I.V. or Flagyl I.V. RTU should be used with care in patients with evidence of or history of blood dyscrasia. A mild leukopenia has been observed during its administration; however, no persistent hematologic abnormalities attributable to metronidazole have been observed in clinical studies. Total and differential leukocyte counts are recommended before and after therapy.

Drug Interactions: Metronidazole has been reported to potentiate the anticoagulant effect of warfarin and other oral coumarin anticoagulants, resulting in a prolongation of prothrombin time. This possible drug interaction should be considered when Flagyl I.V. or Flagyl I.V. RTU is prescribed for patients on this type of anticoagulant therapy.

The simultaneous administration of drugs that induce microsomal liver enzymes, such as phenytoin or phenobarbital, may accelerate the elimination of metronidazole, resulting in reduced plasma levels; impaired clearance of phenytoin has also been reported.

The simultaneous administration of drugs that decrease microsomal liver enzyme activity, such as cimetidine, may prolong the half-life and decrease plasma clearance of metronidazole.

Alcoholic beverages should not be consumed during metronidazole therapy because abdominal cramps, nausea, vomiting, headaches, and flushing may occur.

Psychotic reactions have been reported in alcoholic patients who are using metronidazole and disulfiram concurrently. Metronidazole should not be given to patients who have taken disulfiram within the last two weeks.

Drug/Laboratory Test Interactions: Metronidazole may interfere with certain types of determinations of serum chemistry values, such as aspartate aminotransferase (AST, SGOT), alanine aminotransferase (ALT, SGPT), lactate dehydrogenase (LDH), triglycerides, and hexokinase glucose. Values of zero may be observed. All of the assays in which interference has been reported involve enzymatic coupling of the assay to oxidation-reduction of nicotine adenine dinucleotide ($NAD^+ \rightleftarrows NADH$). Interference is due to the similarity in absorbance peaks of NADH (340 nm) and metronidazole (322 nm) at pH 7.

Carcinogenesis, Mutagenesis, Impairment of Fertility: Tumorigenicity in Rodents—Metronidazole has shown evidence of carcinogenic activity in studies involving chronic, oral administration in mice and rats, but similar studies in the hamster gave negative results. Also, metronidazole has shown mutagenic activity in a number of *in vitro* assay systems, but studies in mammals (*in vivo*) failed to demonstrate a potential for genetic damage.

Pregnancy: Teratogenic Effects—Pregnancy Category B. Metronidazole crosses the placental barrier and enters the fetal circulation rapidly. Reproduction studies have been performed in rats at doses up to five times the human dose and have revealed no evidence of impaired fertility or harm to the fetus due to metronidazole. Metronidazole administered intraperitoneally to pregnant mice at approximately the human dose caused fetotoxicity; administered orally to pregnant mice, no fetotoxicity was observed. There are, however, no adequate and well-controlled studies in pregnant women. Because animal reproduction studies are not always predictive of human response, and because metronidazole is a carcinogen in rodents, these drugs should be used during pregnancy only if clearly needed.

Nursing Mothers: Because of the potential for tumorigenicity shown for metronidazole in mouse and rat studies, a decision should be made whether to discontinue nursing or to discontinue the drug, taking into account the importance of the drug to the mother. Metronidazole is secreted in breast milk in concentrations similar to those found in plasma.

Pediatric Use: Safety and effectiveness in children have not been established.

ADVERSE REACTIONS

Two serious adverse reactions reported in patients treated with Flagyl I.V. or Flagyl I.V. RTU have been convulsive seizures and peripheral neuropathy, the latter characterized mainly by numbness or paresthesia of an extremity. Since persistent peripheral neuropathy has been reported in some patients receiving prolonged oral administration of Flagyl® (metronidazole), patients should be observed carefully if neurologic symptoms occur and a prompt evaluation made of the benefit/risk ratio of the continuation of therapy.

The following reactions have also been reported during treatment with Flagyl I.V. (metronidazole hydrochloride) or Flagyl I.V. RTU (metronidazole):

- Gastrointestinal: Nausea, vomiting, abdominal discomfort, diarrhea, and an unpleasant metallic taste.
- Hematopoietic: Reversible neutropenia (leukopenia).
- Dermatologic: Erythematous rash and pruritus.
- Central Nervous System: Headache, dizziness, syncope, ataxia, and confusion.
- Local Reactions: Thrombophlebitis after intravenous infusion. This reaction can be minimized or avoided by avoiding prolonged use of indwelling intravenous catheters.
- Other: Fever. Instances of a darkened urine have also been reported, and this manifestation has been the subject of a special investigation. Although the pigment which is probably responsible for this phenomenon has not been

Continued on next page

Schiapparelli Searle—Cont.

positively identified, it is almost certainly a metabolite of metronidazole and seems to have no clinical significance.

The following adverse reactions have been reported during treatment with oral Flagyl (metronidazole):

Gastrointestinal: Nausea, sometimes accompanied by headache, anorexia, and occasionally vomiting; diarrhea, epigastric distress, abdominal cramping, and constipation.

Mouth: A sharp, unpleasant metallic taste is not unusual. Furry tongue, glossitis, and stomatitis have occurred; these may be associated with a sudden overgrowth of *Candida* which may occur during effective therapy.

Hematopoietic: Reversible neutropenia (leukopenia); rarely, reversible thrombocytopenia.

Cardiovascular: Flattening of the T-wave may be seen in electrocardiographic tracings.

Central Nervous System: Convulsive seizures, peripheral neuropathy, dizziness, vertigo, incoordination, ataxia, confusion, irritability, depression, weakness, and insomnia.

Hypersensitivity: Urticaria, erythematous rash, flushing, nasal congestion, dryness of mouth (or vagina or vulva), and fever.

Renal: Dysuria, cystitis, polyuria, incontinence, a sense of pelvic pressure, and darkened urine.

Other: Proliferation of *Candida* in the vagina, dyspareunia, decrease of libido, proctitis, and fleeting joint pains sometimes resembling "serum sickness." If patients receiving metronidazole drink alcoholic beverages, they may experience abdominal distress, nausea, vomiting, flushing, or headache. A modification of the taste of alcoholic beverages has also been reported. Rare cases of pancreatitis, which abated on withdrawal of the drug, have been reported.

Crohn's disease patients are known to have an increased incidence of gastrointestinal and certain extraintestinal cancers. There have been some reports in the medical literature of breast and colon cancer in Crohn's disease patients who have been treated with metronidazole at high doses for extended periods of time. A cause and effect relationship has not been established. Crohn's disease is not an approved indication for Flagyl I.V. or Flagyl I.V. RTU.

OVERDOSAGE

Use of dosages of Flagyl I.V. (metronidazole hydrochloride) higher than those recommended has been reported. These include the use of 27 mg/kg three times a day for 20 days, and the use of 75 mg/kg as a single loading dose followed by 7.5 mg/kg maintenance doses. No adverse reactions were reported in either of the two cases.

Single oral doses of metronidazole, up to 15 g, have been reported in suicide attempts and accidental overdoses. Symptoms reported include nausea, vomiting, and ataxia.

Oral metronidazole has been studied as a radiation sensitizer in the treatment of malignant tumors. Neurotoxic effects, including seizures and peripheral neuropathy, have been reported after 5 to 7 days of doses of 6 to 10.4 g every other day.

Treatment: There is no specific antidote for overdose; therefore, management of the patient should consist of symptomatic and supportive therapy.

DOSAGE AND ADMINISTRATION

In elderly patients the pharmacokinetics of metronidazole may be altered and therefore monitoring of serum levels may be necessary to adjust the metronidazole dosage accordingly.

Treatment of Anaerobic Infections

The recommended dosage schedule for *adults* is:

Loading dose:

15 mg/kg infused over one hour (approximately 1 g for a 70-kg adult).

Maintenance Dose:

7.5 mg/kg infused over one hour every six hours (approximately 500 mg for a 70-kg adult). The first maintenance dose should be instituted six hours following the initiation of the loading dose.

Parenteral therapy may be changed to oral Flagyl (metronidazole) when conditions warrant, based upon the severity of the disease and the response of the patient to Flagyl I.V. or Flagyl I.V. RTU (metronidazole) treatment. The usual adult oral dosage is 7.5 mg/kg every six hours.

A maximum of 4 g should not be exceeded during a 24-hour period.

Patients with severe hepatic disease metabolize metronidazole slowly, with resultant accumulation of metronidazole and its metabolites in the plasma. Accordingly, for such patients, doses below those usually recommended should be administered cautiously. Close monitoring of plasma metronidazole levels[2] and toxicity is recommended.

In patients receiving Flagyl I.V. or Flagyl I.V. RTU in whom gastric secretions are continuously removed by nasogastric aspiration, sufficient metronidazole may be removed in the aspirate to cause a reduction in serum levels.

The dose of Flagyl I.V. or Flagyl I.V. RTU should not be specifically reduced in anuric patients since accumulated metabolites may be rapidly removed by dialysis.

The usual duration of therapy is 7 to 10 days; however, infections of the bone and joint, lower respiratory tract, and endocardium may require longer treatment.

Prophylaxis

For surgical prophylactic use, to prevent postoperative infection in contaminated or potentially contaminated colorectal surgery, the recommended dosage schedule for adults is:

a. 15 mg/kg infused over 30 to 60 minutes and completed approximately one hour before surgery; followed by
b. 7.5 mg/kg infused over 30 to 60 minutes at 6 and 12 hours after the initial dose.

It is important that (1) administration of the initial preoperative dose be completed approximately one hour before surgery so that adequate drug levels are present in the serum and tissues at the time of initial incision, and (2) Flagyl I.V. or Flagyl I.V. RTU be administered, if necessary, at 6-hour intervals to maintain effective drug levels. Prophylactic use of Flagyl I.V. or Flagyl I.V. RTU should be limited to the day of surgery only, following the above guidelines.

CAUTION: Flagyl I.V. (metronidazole hydrochloride) or Flagyl I.V. RTU (metronidazole) is to be administered by slow intravenous drip infusion only, either as a continuous or intermittent infusion. I.V. admixtures containing metronidazole and other drugs should be avoided. Additives should not be introduced into the Flagyl I.V. RTU solution. If used with a primary intravenous fluid system, the primary solution should be discontinued during metronidazole infusion. DO NOT USE EQUIPMENT CONTAINING ALUMINUM (EG, NEEDLES, CANNULAE) THAT WOULD COME IN CONTACT WITH THE DRUG SOLUTION.

FLAGYL I.V.

Flagyl I.V. <u>cannot</u> be given by direct intravenous injection (I.V. bolus) because of the low pH (0.5 to 2.0) of the reconstituted product. FLAGYL I.V. MUST BE FURTHER DILUTED AND NEUTRALIZED FOR I.V. INFUSION.

Flagyl I.V. is prepared for use in two steps:

NOTE: ORDER OF MIXING IS IMPORTANT

A. Reconstitution
B. Dilution in intravenous solution followed by pH neutralization with sodium bicarbonate injection into the dilution.

Reconstitution: To prepare the solution, add 4.4 ml of one of the following diluents and mix thoroughly: Sterile Water for Injection, USP; Bacteriostatic Water for Injection, USP; 0.9% Sodium Chloride Injection, USP; or Bacteriostatic 0.9% Sodium Chloride Injection, USP. The resultant approximate withdrawal volume is 5.0 ml with an approximate concentration of 100 mg/ml.

The pH of the reconstituted product will be in the range of 0.5 to 2.0. Reconstituted Flagyl I.V. is clear, and pale yellow to yellow-green in color.

Dilution in Intravenous Solutions: Properly reconstituted Flagyl I.V. (metronidazole hydrochloride) may be added to a glass or plastic I.V. container not to exceed a concentration of 8 mg/ml. Any of the following intravenous solutions may be used: 0.9% Sodium Chloride Injection, USP; 5% Dextrose Injection, USP; or Lactated Ringer's Injection, USP.

NEUTRALIZATION IS REQUIRED PRIOR TO ADMINISTRATION.

The final product should be mixed thoroughly and used within 24 hours.

Neutralization For Intravenous Infusion: Neutralize the intravenous solution containing Flagyl I.V. with approximately 5 mEq of sodium bicarbonate injection for each 500 mg of Flagyl I.V. used. Mix thoroughly. The pH of the neutralized intravenous solution will be approximately 6.0 to 7.0. Carbon dioxide gas will be generated with neutralization. It may be necessary to relieve gas pressure within the container.

Note: When the contents of one vial (500 mg) are diluted and neutralized to 100 ml, the resultant concentration is 5 mg/ml. Do not exceed an 8 mg/ml concentration of Flagyl I.V. in the neutralized intravenous solution, since neutralization will decrease the aqueous solubility and precipitation may occur. DO NOT REFRIGERATE NEUTRALIZED SOLUTIONS; otherwise, precipitation may occur.

Storage and Stability: Reconstituted vials of Flagyl I.V. are chemically stable for 96 hours when stored below 86°F (30°C) in room light.

Use diluted and neutralized intravenous solutions containing Flagyl I.V. within 24 hours of mixing.

FLAGYL I.V. RTU

Flagyl I.V. RTU is a ready-to-use isotonic solution. **NO DILUTION OR BUFFERING IS REQUIRED.** Do not refrigerate. Each container of Flagyl I.V. RTU contains 14 mEq of sodium.

Directions for use of plastic container:

CAUTION: Do not use plastic containers in series connections. Such use could result in air embolism due to residual air (approximately 15 ml) being drawn from the primary container before administration of the fluid from the secondary container is complete.

To open. Tear overwrap down side at slit and remove solution container. Some opacity of the plastic due to moisture absorption during the sterilization process may be observed. This is normal and does not affect the solution quality or safety. The opacity will diminish gradually. Check for minute leaks by squeezing inner bag firmly. If leaks are found discard solution as sterility may be impaired.

Preparation for administration:

1. Suspend container from eyelet support.
2. Remove plastic protector from outlet port at bottom of container.
3. Attach administration set. Refer to complete directions accompanying set.

Parenteral drug products should be inspected visually for particulate matter and discoloration prior to administration, whenever solution and container permit. Do not use if cloudy or precipitated or if the seal is not intact.

Use sterile equipment. It is recommended that the intravenous administration apparatus be replaced at least once every 24 hours.

HOW SUPPLIED

FLAGYL I.V.

Flagyl I.V., sterile (metronidazole hydrochloride), is supplied in single-dose lyophilized vials each containing 500 mg metronidazole equivalent, individually packaged in cartons of 10 vials.

Flagyl I.V., prior to reconstitution, should be stored below 86°F (30°C) and protected from light.

FLAGYL I.V. RTU

Flagyl I.V. RTU, sterile (metronidazole), is supplied in 100-ml single-dose plastic containers, each containing an isotonic, buffered solution of 500 mg metronidazole, individually packaged in boxes of 24.

Flagyl I.V. RTU should be stored at controlled room temperature, 59° to 86° F (15° to 30°C), and protected from light during storage.

---

1. Proposed standard: PSM-11—Proposed Reference Dilution Procedure for Antimicrobic Susceptibility Testing of Anaerobic Bacteria, National Committee for Clinical Laboratory Standards; and Sutter, et al.: Collaborative Evaluation of a Proposed Reference Dilution Method of Susceptibility Testing of Anaerobic Bacteria, Antimicrob. Agents Chemother. *16:* 495–502 (Oct.) 1979; and Tally, et al.: *In Vitro* Activity of Thienamycin, Antimicrob. Agents Chemother. *14:* 436–438 (Sept.) 1978.
2. Ralph, E.D., and Kirby, W.M.M.: Bioassay of Metronidazole With Either Anaerobic or Aerobic Incubation, J. Infect. Dis. *132:* 587–591 (Nov.) 1975; or Gulaid, et al.: Determination of Metronidazole and Its Major Metabolites in Biological Fluids by High Pressure Liquid Chromatography, Br. J. Clin. Pharmacol. *6:* 430–432, 1978.

7/9/90●A05034-6

Shown in Product Identification Section, page 428

NORETHIN 1/35E™–21 ℞
NORETHIN 1/35E™–28 ℞

[*nor'ĕ-thin*]

(norethindrone and ethinyl estradiol tablets USP)

NORETHIN 1/50M™–21 ℞
NORETHIN 1/50M™–28 ℞

[*nor'ĕ-thin*]

(norethindrone and mestranol tablets USP)

DESCRIPTION

Norethin 1/35E™-21 and Norethin 1/35E™-28. Each white tablet contains 1 mg of norethindrone and 35 mcg of ethinyl estradiol. Each blue tablet in the Norethin 1/35E™-28 package is a placebo containing inert ingredients.

Norethin 1/50M™-21 and Norethin 1/50M™-28. Each white tablet contains 1 mg of norethindrone and 50 mcg of mestranol. Each blue tablet in the Norethin 1/50M™-28 package is a placebo containing inert ingredients.

In addition to the active ingredients listed with each tablet, all active tablets contain the following inert ingredients: calcium acetate (hydrous), corn starch, dibasic calcium phosphate (anhydrous), hydrogenated castor oil, and povidone. All placebo tablets are composed of calcium sulfate (dihydrate), corn starch, FD&C Blue No. 1 Lake, magnesium stearate, and sucrose.

The chemical name for norethindrone is 17-hydroxy-19-nor-17α-pregn-4-en-20-yn-3-one. The chemical name for ethinyl estradiol is 19-nor-17α-pregna-1,3,5(10)-trien-20-yne-3,17-diol. The chemical name for mestranol is 3-methoxy-19-nor-17α-pregna-1,3,5(10)-trien-20-yn-17-ol. Their structural formulas are as follows:

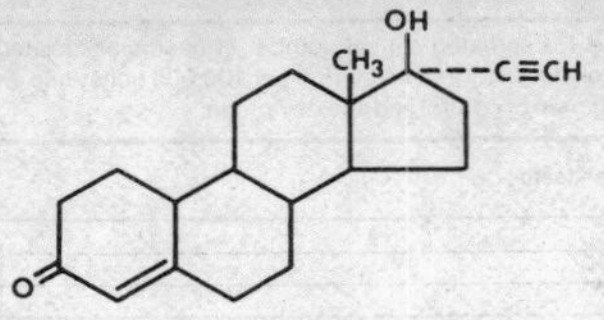

norethindrone

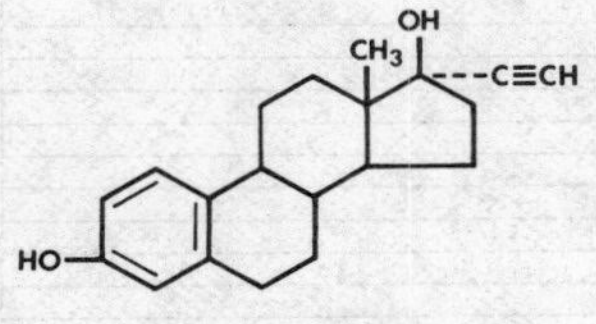

ethinyl estradiol

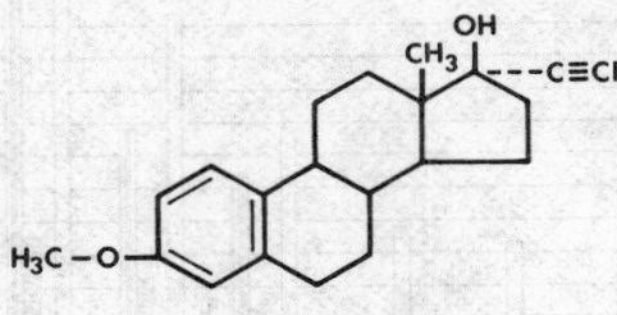

mestranol

Therapeutic Class: Oral contraceptive.

CLINICAL PHARMACOLOGY

Combination oral contraceptives act primarily through the mechanism of gonadotropin suppression due to the estrogenic and progestational activity of their components. Although the primary mechanism of action is inhibition of ovulation, alterations in the genital tract, including changes in the cervical mucus (which reduce sperm penetration) and the endometrium (which reduce the likelihood of implantation) may also contribute to contraceptive effectiveness.

INDICATIONS AND USAGE

Oral contraceptives are indicated for the prevention of pregnancy in women who elect to use oral contraceptives as a method of contraception.

Oral contraceptives are highly effective.[176] The pregnancy rate in women using conventional combination oral contraceptives (containing 35 mcg or more of ethinyl estradiol or 50 mcg or more of mestranol) is generally reported to be less than 1 pregnancy per 100 woman-years of use. Slightly higher rates (somewhat more than 1 pregnancy per 100 woman-years of use) are reported for some combination products containing 35 mcg or less of ethinyl estradiol, and rates on the order of 3 pregnancies per 100 woman-years are reported for the progestogen-only oral contraceptives.

These rates are derived from separate studies conducted by different investigators in several population groups; therefore, a precise comparison cannot be made. Furthermore, pregnancy rates tend to be lower as clinical studies are continued, possibly due to selective retention in the longer studies of those patients who accept the treatment regimen and do not discontinue as a result of adverse reactions, pregnancy, or other reasons. In Table 1 ranges of pregnancy rates as reported in the literature[1] are shown for other means of contraception. The efficacy of these means of contraception, except for the IUD, depends upon the degree of adherence to the method.

Table 1
Pregnancies per 100 Woman-Years

Method	*Range*
IUD	<1 to 6
Diaphragm with spermicidal cream or gel	2 to 20
Condom	3 to 36
Spermicidal aerosol foams	2 to 29
Spermicidal gels and creams	4 to 36
Periodic abstinence (rhythm), all types	<1 to 47
1. Calendar method	14 to 47
2. Temperature method	1 to 20
3. Temperature method (intercourse only in postovulatory phase)	<1 to 7
4. Mucus method	1 to 25
No contraception	60 to 80

Dose-Related Risk of Thromboembolism from Oral Contraceptives: Studies have shown a positive association between the dose of estrogens in oral contraceptives and the risk of thromboembolism[2,96,97] (see *Warning* No. 1). For this reason, it is prudent and in keeping with good principles of therapeutics to minimize exposure to estrogen. The oral contraceptive product prescribed for any given patient should be that product which contains the least amount of estrogen that is compatible with an acceptable pregnancy rate and patient acceptance. It is recommended that new users of oral contraceptives be started on preparations containing 50 mcg or less of estrogen.

CONTRAINDICATIONS

Oral contraceptives should not be used in women with any of the following conditions:

1. Thrombophlebitis or thromboembolic disorders.
2. A past history of deep vein thrombophlebitis or thromboembolic disorders.
3. Cerebral vascular disease, myocardial infarction or coronary artery disease, or a past history of these conditions.
4. Known or suspected carcinoma of the breast.
5. Known or suspected estrogen-dependent neoplasia.
6. Undiagnosed abnormal genital bleeding.
7. Known or suspected pregnancy (see *Warning* No. 5).
8. Past or present, benign or malignant liver tumors among women who developed these tumors during the use of oral contraceptives or other estrogen-containing products (see *Warning* No. 4).

WARNINGS

Cigarette-smoking increases the risk of serious cardiovascular side effects from oral contraceptive use. This risk increases with age and with heavy smoking (15 or more cigarettes per day) and is quite marked in women over 35 years of age. Women who use oral contraceptives should be strongly advised not to smoke.

The use of oral contraceptives is associated with increased risk of several serious conditions including venous and arterial thromboembolism, thrombotic and hemorrhagic stroke, myocardial infarction, visual disorders, liver tumors or other liver lesions, gallbladder disease, hypertension, and fetal abnormalities. Practitioners prescribing oral contraceptives should be familiar with the following information relating to these and other risks.

1. *Thromboembolic Disorders and Other Vascular Problems.* An increased risk of thromboembolic and thrombotic disease associated with the use of oral contraceptives is well established. One study in Great Britain[3] demonstrated an increased relative risk for fatal venous thromboembolism; several British[4,5,14,22,92,156] and U.S.[6–8,23,98–101,126] studies demonstrated an increased relative risk for nonfatal venous thromboembolism. U.S. studies[6,9,10,99,101–103] demonstrated an increased relative risk for stroke, which had not been shown in prior British studies.[3–5] In these studies it was estimated that users of oral contraceptives were 1.9 to 11 times more likely than nonusers to manifest these diseases without evident cause (Table 2). In a British study of idiopathic deep vein thrombosis and pulmonary embolism, the projected annual hospitalization rates for women aged 16–40 were 47 per 100,000 users and 5 for nonusers.[77] In one British mortality study,[3] overall excess mortality due to pulmonary embolism or stroke was on the order of 1.3 to 3.4 deaths annually per 100,000 users and increased with age.

Cerebrovascular Disorders: In a collaborative U.S. study[9,10] of cerebrovascular disorders in women with and without predisposing causes, it was estimated that the risk of hemorrhagic stroke was 2.0 times greater in users than in nonusers, and the risk of thrombotic stroke was 4.0[10] to 9.5[9] times greater in users than in nonusers (Table 2). Analysis of mortality trends in 21 countries indicates that, since oral contraceptives first became available, changes in mortality from nonrheumatic heart disease and hypertension, cerebrovascular disease, and all nonrheumatic cardiovascular disease among women aged 15 to 44 years have been associated with changes in the prevalence of oral contraceptive use in each country.[11]

Table 2. *Summary of Relative Risks of Thromboembolic Disorders and Other Vascular Problems in Oral Contraceptive Users Compared with Nonusers.*

Disorders	*Relative Risk*
Idiopathic thromboembolic disease	2 to 11 times greater
Postsurgery thromboembolic complications	4 to 7 times greater
Thrombotic stroke	4 to 9.5 times greater
Hemorrhagic stroke	2.0 to 2.3 times greater
Myocardial infarction	2 to 12 times greater

In May 1974 the Royal College of General Practitioners[12] issued an interim report of its continuing large-scale prospective study comparing a user group with a nonuser group. It stated: "A statistically significant higher rate of reporting of cerebrovascular accidents in Takers is evident, but the numbers are too small to justify an estimation of the degree of risk." A 1981 analysis of data from this study was reported[13] to show a 4-fold increased mortality from circulatory diseases, mainly from myocardial infarction and hemorrhagic stroke, in users. The excess mortality was associated with age and smoking in users. A 1983 analysis[138] of arterial diseases reported a significantly increased incidence of cerebrovascular disease among current oral contraceptive users. Risk appeared to increase with duration of use up to 8 years. Categories with a significantly increased incidence included cerebral thrombosis or embolism, and transient ischemic attacks, but not hemorrhagic strokes. Incidence of peripheral arterial thromboembolism, Raynaud's disease, and acute myocardial infarction was increased in current users. Women aged 30 years and older had appreciably higher rates of arterial disease than did younger women. Smoking increased the risk for older women in each usage group, the greatest risk being in current users aged 35 years and older who smoked. Expressed as the percentage of women diagnosed as having an arterial disease who died of that disease, the case-fatality rates were 2 to 3 times greater for users who smoked than for women in the other groups.

In October 1976 an interim report was issued on the long-term follow-up study of the British Family Planning Association.[14] There was a highly significant association between oral contraceptive use and stroke, although total numbers were small in this study also. The increase in risk of venous thrombosis and pulmonary embolism among users was about 4-fold and was statistically highly significant. In later reports[15] it was noted that mortality from nonrheumatic heart disease was greater in women who had ever used oral contraceptives. A 1984 report[147] on stroke found pill use to be a significant risk factor for nonhemorrhagic stroke, but not for subarachnoid hemorrhage. Smoking and hypertension were significant risk factors only for the latter.

In the Walnut Creek prospective study,[99,101,102] the risk of subarachnoid hemorrhage was associated with heavy smoking, age, and use of the pill.

Myocardial Infarction: An increased risk of myocardial infarction associated with the use of oral contraceptives has been reported in Great Britain,[16–19,136,138,180] confirming a previously suspected association.[3] The morbidity study[16,17] found that the greater the number of underlying risk factors for coronary artery disease (cigarette-smoking, hypertension, hypercholesterolemia, obesity, diabetes, history of preeclamptic toxemia), the higher the risk of developing myocardial infarction, regardless of whether the patient was an oral contraceptive user or not. Oral contraceptives were considered an additional risk factor.

The annual excess rate of fatal myocardial infarction in British oral contraceptive users was estimated to be approximately 3.5 cases per 100,000 women users in the 30- to 39-year age group and 20 per 100,000 women users in the 40- to 44-year age group.[19] (These estimates are based on British vital statistics, which show acute myocardial infarction death rates 2 to 3 times less than in the U.S. for women in these age groups. In an attempt to extrapolate these figures to U.S. women, it was estimated that the annual excess rates in users are 25.7 cases per 100,000 for women aged 30–39 with predisposing conditions versus 1.5 cases without; corresponding estimates for women aged 40–44 were 86.2 versus 5.1.[78]) The annual excess rate of hospitalization for nonfatal myocardial infarction in married British oral contraceptive users was estimated to be approximately 3.5 per 100,000 women users in the 30- to 39-year age group and 47 per 100,000 women users in the 40- to 44-year age group.[16]

Smoking is considered a major predisposing condition to myocardial infarction. In terms of relative risk, it has been estimated[20] that oral contraceptive users who do not smoke are about twice as likely to have a fatal myocardial infarction as nonusers who do not smoke. Oral contraceptive users who are also smokers have about a 5-fold increased risk of fatal infarction compared to users who do not smoke, but about a 10- to 12-fold increased risk compared to nonusers who do not smoke. Furthermore, the amount of smoking is also an important factor. In determining the importance of these relative risks, however, the baseline rates for various age groups, as shown in Table 3, must be given serious consideration. The importance of other predisposing conditions mentioned above in determining relative and absolute risks has not been quantified; it is likely that the same synergistic action exists, but perhaps to a lesser extent.

Similar findings relating nonfatal and fatal myocardial infarction, oral contraceptives, smoking, and age were subsequently published in the U.S.[91,99,104–108,152] and by the Royal College of General Practitioners in Great Britain.[13,138,190]

[See Table 3 next page.]

Risk of Dose: Reports of thromboembolism following the use of oral contraceptives containing 50 mcg or more of estrogen received by drug safety committees in Great Britain, Sweden, and Denmark were compared with the distribution expected from market research estimates of sales.[2] A positive correlation was found between the dose of estrogen and the reporting of thromboembolism, including coronary thrombosis, in excess of that predicted by sales estimates. Preparations containing 100 mcg or more of estrogen were associated with a higher risk of thromboembolism than those containing 50 to 80 mcg of estrogen. The authors' analysis did suggest, however, that the quantity of estrogen may not be the sole factor involved. Any influence on the part of the

Continued on next page

Schiapparelli Searle—Cont.

Table 3. *Estimated Annual Mortality Rate per 100,000 Women from Myocardial Infarction by Use of Oral Contraceptives, Smoking Habits, and Age in Years*[20]

| Smoking habits | Myocardial infarction | | | |
| | Women aged 30–39 | | Women aged 40–44 | |
	Users	Non-users	Users	Non-users
All smokers	10.2	2.6	62.0	15.9
Heavy*	13.0	5.1	78.7	31.3
Light	4.7	0.9	28.6	5.7
Nonsmokers	1.8	1.2	10.7	7.4
Smokers and nonsmokers	5.4	1.9	32.8	11.7

*15 or more cigarettes per day

progestogens was not considered, which may have been responsible for certain discrepancies in the data. No significant differences were detected between preparations containing the same dose of estrogen nor between the two estrogens ethinyl estradiol and mestranol. A subsequent study of a similar nature in Great Britain found a positive association between the dose of progestogen or estrogen and certain thromboembolic conditions,[96] which is consistent with findings of the Royal College study.[12,92,135] Swedish authorities noted decreased reporting of thromboembolic episodes when higher estrogen preparations were no longer prescribed.[97] Careful epidemiologic studies to determine the degree of thromboembolic risk associated with progestogen-only oral contraceptives have not been performed. Cases of thromboembolic disease have been reported in women using these products, and they should not be presumed to be free of excess risk.

The relative risk of oral contraceptive use one month prior to hospitalization for various types of thromboembolism was calculated in a U.S. retrospective case-control study.[8] If no account is taken of the relative estrogenic potency of different estrogens and if any possible influence of the different progestogenic components is ignored, the products employed may be divided into those containing less than 100 mcg and those containing 100 mcg or more of estrogen. For all cases combined, the larger-dose category was associated with only a slightly higher relative risk; for the idiopathic subgroup, the relative risk was approximately doubled with the larger estrogen content, but the confidence limits overlapped considerably and the differences, therefore, were not statistically significant. Apparently there was less of an increased relative risk for the subgroup with predispositions to thromboembolism.[98]

In the British Family Planning Association study, no non-hemorrhagic strokes occurred during 9,100 woman-years of current use of pills containing less than 50 mcg of estrogen, in contrast to 13 observed during 39,400 woman-years of current use of pills with higher doses.[147] The incidence of venous thromboembolism was greater for those women using pills containing 50 mcg or more of estrogen than for those using pills with less than 50 mcg estrogen.[173]

A decline of serum high density lipoproteins (HDL) has been reported with increasing progestational activity,[165,167,168,182] and decreased HDL has been associated with an increased incidence of ischemic heart disease.[169] The amount of both steroids should be another consideration in the choice of an oral contraceptive.

The risk of thromboembolic and thrombotic disorders, both in users and in nonusers of oral contraceptives, increases with age. Oral contraceptives have been considered an independent risk factor for these events.

Persistence of Risk: A 1977 analysis[13a] of the mortality data from the prospective study of the Royal College of General Practitioners (RCGP) suggested that the risk of circulatory disease increases with the duration of oral contraceptive use and may persist after discontinuation. The ratio of the mortality rate from circulatory disease in former users to that in controls was 4.3 to 1 (P < 0.01), and was still 3.7 to 1 even after excluding the two deaths from malignant hypertension, where use was stopped because of the onset of hypertension. For the category of fatal subarachnoid hemorrhage, the rate ratio comparing former users to controls was also statistically significant.

In 1981, a new analysis of the RCGP mortality data[13] showed significantly increased risk ratios in former users for the categories of all nonrheumatic heart disease plus hypertension (4.6 to 1), cerebrovascular disease (3.6 to 1), as well as the subcategory of subarachnoid hemorrhage (4.5 to 1). Overall, the incidence of fatal circulatory disease for former users was 4.3 times that of the controls.

A 1983 analysis of the incidence of arterial disease in the RCGP study[138] showed that the incidence of all cerebrovascular disease, fatal and nonfatal, was significantly greater in former users than in controls (risk ratio = 2.6) and remained

elevated for at least 6 years after discontinuation of oral contraceptives. Former users had significantly increased rates for cerebral thrombosis (4 vs 0), transient ischemic attacks (8.7 to 1), and "other" cerebrovascular disease (3.8 to 1).

In the Walnut Creek prospective study,[102] former use of oral contraceptives was significantly associated with increased risk of subarachnoid hemorrhage, the relative risk being 5.3.

In a U.S. hospital-based, case-control study,[137] when the duration of oral contraceptive use was considered, the data suggested that the rate of myocardial infarction is increased approximately 2- to 3-fold in older women who had used oral contraceptives for more than 10 years before discontinuation. The excess risk associated with long-term use was evident in subjects who had stopped less than 5 years previously, as well as in those who had stopped 5 to 9 years previously. Whether the excess risk persisted for more than 10 years after discontinuation could not be assessed because of a paucity of data.

In summary, persistence of risk after discontinuation of oral contraceptives has been reported for circulatory disease in general,[13,13a] for nonrheumatic heart disease,[13,137] and for cerebrovascular disease,[13,138] including subarachnoid hemorrhage,[13,13a,102] cerebral thrombosis,[138] and transient ischemic attacks.[138]

Estimate of Excess Mortality from Circulatory Diseases: A large prospective study[13] carried out in the U.K. provided estimates of the mortality rate per 100,000 women per year from diseases of the circulatory system for users and nonusers of oral contraceptives according to age, smoking habits, and duration of use. The overall annual excess death rate from circulatory diseases for oral contraceptive users was estimated at 23 per 100,000 for women of all ages. The rates for nonsmokers and smokers, respectively, were: ages 25–34, 2 and 10 per 100,000; ages 35–44, 15 and 48 per 100,000; and ages 45 and older, 41 and 179 per 100,000. The risk was statistically significant only in cigarette-smokers over age 34. The majority of deaths were due to subarachnoid hemorrhage or ischemic heart disease. Relative risk for women who had ever used oral contraceptives rose with increasing parity, a new observation that needs confirmation.

The available data from a variety of sources have been analyzed[21,163] to estimate the risk of death associated with various methods of contraception. The estimates of risk of death for each method included the combined risk of the contraceptive method (eg, thromboembolic and thrombotic disease in the case of oral contraceptives) plus the risk attributable to pregnancy or abortion in the event of method failure. This latter risk varies with the effectiveness of the contraceptive method. The findings of this analysis are shown in Figure 1.[21] The study concluded that the mortality associated with all methods of birth control is low and below that associated with childbirth, except for that associated with oral contraceptives in women over 40 who smoke. (The rates given for pill only/smokers for each age group are for smokers as a class. For "heavy" smokers [more than 15 cigarettes a day], the rates given would be about double; for "light" smokers [less than 15 cigarettes a day], about 50 percent.[20]) The mortality associated with oral contraceptive use in nonsmokers over 40 is higher than with any other method of contraception in that age group. The lowest mortality is associated with the condom or diaphragm backed up by early legal abortion. [See Figure 1 above.]

The risk of thromboembolic and thrombotic disease associated with oral contraceptives increases with age after approximately age 30 and, for myocardial infarction, is further increased by hypertension, hypercholesterolemia, obesity, diabetes, or history of preeclamptic toxemia, and especially by cigarette-smoking.[20,78,79]

Based on the data currently available, the following table gives a gross estimate of the risk of death from circulatory disorders associated with the use of oral contraceptives:

Table 4. *Smoking Habits and Other Predisposing Conditions—Risk Associated with Use of Oral Contraceptives*

Age	Below 30	30–39	40+
Heavy smokers	C	B	A
Light smokers	D	C	B
Nonsmokers (no predisposing conditions)	D	C,D	C
Nonsmokers (other predisposing conditions)	C	C,B	B,A

A—Use associated with very high risk.
B—Use associated with high risk.
C—Use associated with moderate risk.
D—Use associated with low risk.

The physician and patient should be alert to the earliest manifestations of thromboembolic and thrombotic disorders (eg, thrombophlebitis, pulmonary embolism, cerebrovascu-

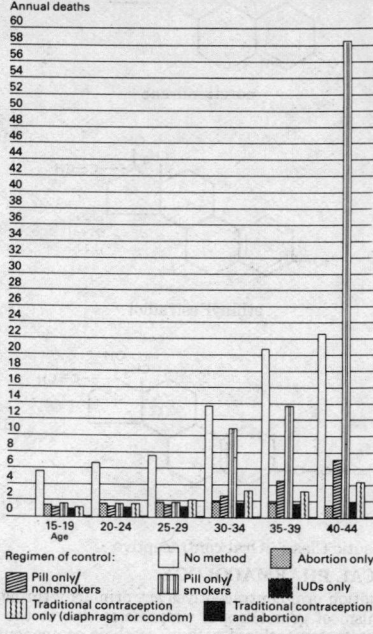

Figure 1. Estimated annual number of deaths associated with control of fertility and no control per 100,000 nonsterile women by regimen of control and age of woman.

Annual deaths

Regimen of control:
- Pill only/nonsmokers
- Pill only/smokers
- No method
- Abortion only
- Traditional contraception only (diaphragm or condom)
- IUDs only
- Traditional contraception and abortion

lar insufficiency, coronary artery disease or myocardial infarction, retinal thrombosis, and mesenteric thrombosis). Should any of these occur or be suspected, the drug should be discontinued immediately.

A 4- to 7-fold increased risk of postsurgery thromboembolic complications has also been reported in oral contraceptive users.[22,23] If feasible, oral contraceptives should be discontinued at least 4 weeks before elective surgery or during periods of prolonged immobilization. The decision as to when to resume oral contraception following major surgery or bed rest should balance the recognized risks of postsurgery thromboembolic complications with the need to reinstate contraceptive practices.

The Royal College of General Practitioners in a large prospective study reported a higher incidence of superficial and deep vein thrombosis in users, the former being correlated with the progestogen dose. The RCGP data suggest that the presence of varicose veins substantially increases the risk of superficial venous thrombosis of the leg, the risk depending upon the severity of the varicosities. The evidence suggests that the presence of varicose veins has little effect on the development of deep vein thrombosis in the leg.[92] Other prospective studies have also reported a higher incidence of venous thrombosis in users.[14,99–101,109]

2. Ocular Lesions. There have been reports of neuro-ocular lesions such as optic neuritis or retinal thrombosis associated with the use of oral contraceptives. Discontinue medication if there is unexplained, gradual or sudden, partial or complete loss of vision; proptosis or diplopia; papilledema; or any evidence of retinal vascular lesions. Appropriate diagnostic and therapeutic measures should be instituted.

3. Carcinoma. Long-term continuous administration of either natural or synthetic estrogens in certain animal species increases the frequency of certain carcinomas, and/or nonmalignant neoplasms, such as those of the breast, uterus, cervix, vagina, ovary, liver, and pituitary. Certain synthetic progestogens, none currently contained in oral contraceptives, have been noted to increase the incidence of mammary nodules, benign and malignant, in dogs.

There is now evidence that estrogens increase the risk of carcinoma of the endometrium in humans. In several independent, retrospective case-control studies,[24–28,80,93] an increased relative risk (2.2 to 13.9 times) was reported, associating endometrial carcinoma with the prolonged use of estrogens in postmenopausal women who took estrogen replacement medication to relieve menopausal symptoms. This risk was independent of the other known risk factors for endometrial cancer and appeared to depend both on duration of treatment[24,27,28] and on estrogen dose.[26–28] These findings are supported by the observation that incidence rates of endometrial cancer have increased sharply since 1969 in 8 different areas of the U.S. with population-based cancer-reporting systems, an increase which may be related to the rapidly expanding use of estrogens during the past decade.[29] There is no evidence at present that "natural"

estrogens are more or less hazardous than "synthetic" estrogens at equiestrogenic doses.

One publication[30] reported on the first 30 cases submitted by physicians to a registry of cases of adenocarcinoma of the endometrium in women under 40 on oral contraceptives. Of the adenocarcinomas found in women without predisposing risk factors for adenocarcinoma of the endometrium (eg, irregular bleeding at the time oral contraceptives were first given, polycystic ovaries), nearly all occurred in women who had used a sequential oral contraceptive. These products are no longer marketed. No statistical association has been reported suggesting an increased risk of endometrial cancer in users of conventional combination or progestogen-only oral contraceptives, although individual cases have been reported.

Several studies[7,31-35,39,99,121,122] have reported no increased risk of breast cancer in women taking oral contraceptives or estrogens; however, several other studies have provided inconsistent data reflecting increased risk in various subgroups. In one study,[36,37] while no overall increased risk of breast cancer was noted in women treated with oral contraceptives, a greater risk was suggested for the subgroups of oral contraceptive users with documented benign breast disease and for long-term (2–4 years) users. Other studies[123,142,175] reported increased risk of breast cancer in women who had used the pill for more than 4 years before their first full-term pregnancy. One other study[38] indicated an increasing risk of breast cancer in women taking menopausal estrogens, which increased with duration of follow-up. Several other studies have also shown oral contraceptives[127-129,133,140,141,144,146,148] or estrogens[130,145] to be associated with breast cancer, particularly in connection with other risk factors[127-129] (eg, family history, previous breast biopsy, late age of first delivery) and long duration of use.[127,128,130,146,161] Several recent studies report increased risk in: nulliparous women aged 20–44 with menarche before age 13 who took the pill for 8 or more years[185]; a two-fold overall increased risk for ever-users, with significant risk for subroups aged 30–39 at interview, for long-term (>5 years) users, and for parous women taking the pill for 1–4 years before the first term pregnancy or for <1 year or >4 years after[186]; age 30–34 at time of diagnosis, and when standardized for age, those who were para 1, and among the latter, those with 2 or more years of use.[187]A reduced occurrence of benign breast tumors in users of oral contraceptives has been well documented.[7,12,14,31,36,39,40,86,99]

Some epidemiologic studies[41,81-84,99,109,120,143,149,150,162,170,189] have suggested an increased risk of cervical dysplasia, intraepithelial neoplasia, erosion, and carcinoma in long-term pill users; however, cause and effect has not been established. There have been other reports of microglandular dysplasia of the cervix in users.

In summary, there is at present no consistent evidence from human studies of an increased risk of cancer associated with oral contraceptives.[42] Close clinical surveillance of all women taking oral contraceptives is, nevertheless, essential. In all cases of undiagnosed persistent or recurrent abnormal vaginal bleeding, nonfunctional causes should be borne in mind and appropriate diagnostic measures should be taken to rule out malignancy. Women who have a strong family history of breast cancer or who have breast nodules, fibrocystic disease, recurrent cystic mastitis, abnormal mammograms, or cervical dysplasia should be monitored with particular care if they elect to use oral contraceptives.

4. *Hepatic Lesions (adenomas, hepatomas, hamartomas, regenerating nodules, focal nodular hyperplasia, hemangiomas, peliosis hepatis, sinusoidal dilatation, hepatocellular carcinoma, etc)*. Benign hepatic adenomas and other hepatic lesions have been associated with the use of oral contraceptives.[43,45,46,85] One study[46] reported that oral contraceptive formulations with high "hormonal potency" were associated with a higher risk than lower-potency formulations, as was age over 30 years. Although benign, these hepatic lesions may rupture and may cause death through intra-abdominal hemorrhage. This has been reported in short-term as well as long-term users of oral contraceptives. Two studies related risk with duration of use of the contraceptive, the risk being much greater after 4 or more years of oral contraceptive use.[45,46] Long-term users of oral contraceptives have an estimated annual incidence of hepatocellular adenoma of 3 to 4 per 100,000.[46] While such hepatic lesions are rare, they should be considered in women presenting with abdominal pain and tenderness, abdominal mass, or shock. Patients with liver tumors have demonstrated variable clinical features, which may make preoperative diagnosis difficult. About one quarter of the cases presented because of abdominal masses; up to one half had signs and symptoms of acute intraperitoneal hemorrhage. Routine radiologic and laboratory studies may not be helpful. Liver scans may clearly show a focal defect. Hepatic arteriography or computed tomography may be useful procedures in diagnosing primary liver neoplasms.

Cases of hepatocellular carcinoma have been reported in women taking oral contraceptives. The relationship of these drugs to this type of malignancy is not known at this time, although epidemiologic studies[157-159] have estimated a relative risk as high as 7 to 20 for users for 8 or more years as compared to nonusers.[158,159] There is also evidence that oral contraceptives are associated with cancer of the bile duct.[172,177-179]

Oral contraceptives are contraindicated if there are past or present, benign or malignant liver tumors among women who developed these tumors during the use of oral contraceptives or other estrogen-containing products.

5. *Use In or Immediately Preceding Pregnancy, Birth Defects in Offspring, and Malignancy in Offspring*. The use of female sex hormones, both estrogens and progestogens, during early pregnancy may seriously damage the offspring. It has been reported that females exposed in utero to diethylstilbestrol and other nonsteroidal estrogens have an increased risk of developing in later life a form of vaginal or cervical cancer that is ordinarily extremely rare.[47,48] This risk has been estimated to be on the order of 1 in 1,000 exposures or less.[49,50,171] The excess incidence for dysplasia and carcinoma in situ has been estimated at 7.8 cases per 1,000 woman-years.[154] Although there is no evidence at the present time that oral contraceptives further enhance the risk of developing this type of malignancy, such patients should be monitored with particular care if they elect to use oral contraceptives instead of other methods of contraception. Furthermore, a high percentage of such exposed women (from 30% to 90%) have been found to have adenosis (epithelial changes) of the vagina and cervix.[51-55] Although these changes are histologically benign, it is not known whether this condition is a precursor of malignancy. DES-exposed daughters appear to have an increased risk of unfavorable outcome of pregnancy.[110-112] DES-exposed male children may develop abnormalities of the urogenital tract[56-58,131] and sperm.[131] Although similar data are not available for the use of other estrogens, it cannot be presumed that they would not induce similar changes.

Several reports suggest an association between fetal exposure to female sex hormones, including oral contraceptives, and congenital anomalies,[59-64,94,113-116,174] including multiple congenital anomalies described by the acronym VACTERL, for vertebral, anal, cardiac, tracheoesophageal, renal, and limb defects.[61,62,113] There appears to be a preferential expression of these defects by exposed male offspring.[63,65,115,124] In one case-control study[63] it was estimated that there was a 4.7-fold increased risk of limb-reduction defects in infants exposed in utero to sex hormones (oral contraceptives, hormonal withdrawal tests for pregnancy, or attempted treatment for threatened abortion). Some of these exposures were very short and involved only a few days of treatment. It is reported that the risk of cardiac anomalies and of limb-reduction defects in exposed fetuses is about 1 in 1,000 live births. In a large prospective study,[64] cardiovascular defects in children born to women who received female hormones, including oral contraceptives, during early pregnancy occurred at a rate of 18.2 per 1,000 births, compared to 7.8 per 1,000 for children not so exposed in utero. These results are statistically significant. Female hormone exposure in utero during the first trimester has been reported to be associated with an increased risk of testicular[183] and ovarian[184] cancer. The incidence of twin births may be increased for women who conceive shortly after discontinuing use of the pill.[14,63,117,118,124]

In the past, female sex hormones have been used during pregnancy in an attempt to treat threatened or habitual abortion. There is considerable evidence that estrogens are ineffective for these indications, and there is no evidence from well-controlled studies that progestogens are effective for these uses. An increased incidence of spontaneous abortion associated with lethal chromosome abnormalities (trisomy, triploidy) was reported with high-dose oral contraceptives.[66] However, a recent study including low-dose oral contraceptives did not confirm this effect.[164] Whether there is an overall increase in spontaneous abortion of pregnancies conceived soon after stopping the oral contraceptives is unknown. A highly significant (P < 0.001) increase of lymphocytic chromosome aberrations in oral contraceptive users has been reported.[160]

The safety of this product in pregnancy has not been demonstrated. Pregnancy should be ruled out before initiating or continuing the contraceptive regimen. Pregnancy should always be considered if withdrawal bleeding does not occur. It is recommended that for any patient who has missed 2 consecutive periods, pregnancy should be ruled out before continuing the contraceptive regimen. If the patient has not adhered to the prescribed schedule, the possibility of pregnancy should be considered at the time of the first missed period, and further use of oral contraceptives should be withheld until pregnancy has been ruled out. If pregnancy is confirmed, oral contraceptive use should not be resumed and the patient should be apprised of the potential risks to the fetus, and the advisability of continuation of the pregnancy should be discussed in the light of these risks.

It is recommended that women who discontinue oral contraceptives with the intent of becoming pregnant use an alternative form of contraception for a period of time before attempting to conceive. Many clinicians recommend 3 months, although no precise information is available on which to base this recommendation.

The administration of progestogen-only or progestogen-estrogen combinations to induce withdrawal bleeding should not be used as a test of pregnancy.

6. *Gallbladder Disease*. Reports of studies[7,8,12,14,33] indicate an increased risk for surgically confirmed gallbladder disease in users of oral contraceptives or estrogens. In one study,[12] an increased risk appeared after 2 years of use and doubled after 4 or 5 years of use. In one of the other studies[7] an increased risk was apparent between 6 and 12 months of use. Bile duct carcinoma has been reported.[172,177-179]

7. *Carbohydrate and Lipid Metabolism*. A decrease in glucose tolerance has been observed in a significant percentage of patients on oral contraceptives. For this reason, prediabetic and diabetic patients should be carefully observed while receiving oral contraceptives. An increase in triglycerides, total phospholipids, and lipoproteins has been observed in patients receiving oral contraceptives.[67,165] The clinical significance of this finding remains to be defined.

8. *Elevated Blood Pressure*. An increase in blood pressure has been reported in patients receiving oral contraceptives.[12,69,109] There is evidence that the degree of hypertension may correlate directly with increasing dosage of progestogen.[86] In some women, hypertension may occur within a few months of beginning oral contraceptive use. The prevalence of hypertension in users is low in the first year of use, and may be no higher than that in a comparable group of nonusers. The prevalence in users increases, however, with longer exposure and, in the fifth year of use, is 2½ to 3 times the reported prevalence in the first year. Age is also strongly correlated with the development of hypertension in oral contraceptive users.

Women with a history of elevated blood pressure (hypertension), preexisting renal disease, a history of toxemia or elevated blood pressure during pregnancy, a familial tendency to hypertension or its consequences, or a history of excessive weight gain or fluid retention during the menstrual cycle may be more likely to develop elevation of blood pressure when given oral contraceptives and, therefore, should be monitored closely.[68] Even though elevated blood pressure may remain within the "normal" range, the clinical implications of elevations should not be ignored and close surveillance is indicated, particularly for women with other risk factors for cardiovascular disease or stroke.[69] High blood pressure may or may not persist after discontinuation of the oral contraceptive.

9. *Headache*. The onset or exacerbation of migraine or development of headache of a new pattern which is recurrent, persistent, or severe, requires discontinuation of oral contraceptives and evaluation of the cause.

10. *Bleeding Irregularities*. Breakthrough bleeding, spotting, and amenorrhea are frequent reasons for discontinuance of oral contraceptives. In breakthrough bleeding, as in all cases of irregular or abnormal vaginal bleeding, nonfunctional causes should be borne in mind. In patients with undiagnosed persistent or recurrent abnormal vaginal bleeding, adequate diagnostic measures are indicated to rule out pregnancy or malignancy. If a pathologic basis has been excluded, passage of time or a change to another formulation may correct the bleeding problem. A change to an oral contraceptive with a higher estrogen content, while potentially useful in minimizing menstrual irregularity, should be made only when considered necessary since this may increase the risk of thromboembolic disease.

Women with a past history of oligomenorrhea or secondary amenorrhea or young women who have not established regular cycles may have a tendency to remain anovulatory or to become amenorrheic after discontinuation of oral contraceptives. Women with these preexisting problems should be informed of these possibilities and encouraged to use other contraceptive methods. Post-use anovulation, possibly prolonged, may also occur in women without previous irregularities. A higher incidence of galactorrhea and of pituitary tumors (eg, adenomas) has been associated with amenorrhea in former users compared with nonusers.[87] One study[70] reported a 16-fold increased prevalence of pituitary prolactin-secreting tumors among patients with postpill amenorrhea when galactorrhea was present. A case-control study[44] reported an increased risk of galactorrhea following discontinuation of oral contraceptives by women who did not have pituitary tumors.

11. *Ectopic Pregnancy*. Contraceptive failure may result in either ectopic or intrauterine pregnancy. In failures with combination-type oral contraceptives, the ratio of ectopic to intrauterine pregnancies is no higher than in women who are not receiving oral contraceptives.

12. *Breast Feeding*. Oral contraceptives given in the postpartum period may interfere with lactation. There may be a decrease in the quantity and quality of the breast milk. Furthermore, a small fraction of the hormonal agents in oral contraceptives has been identified in the milk of mothers

Continued on next page

Schiapparelli Searle—Cont.

receiving these drugs.[71,88,89] The effects, if any, on the breast-fed child have not been determined. If feasible, the use of oral contraceptives should be deferred until the infant has been weaned.

13. *Infertility.* There is evidence of fertility impairment in women discontinuing oral contraceptives in comparison with those discontinuing other methods.[14,90,132,155] While the impairment diminishes with time, there is still an appreciable difference in the results in nulliparous women aged 25 to 29 at 30 months after discontinuation of birth control; the difference is negligible after 48 months. However, among nulliparas aged 30–34, the impairment persists up to 72 months and appears more severe for users for 2 or more years. For parous women aged 25 to 34 the difference is no longer apparent 30 months after cessation of contraception.

PRECAUTIONS

General. 1. A complete medical and family history should be taken and a thorough physical examination should be performed prior to the initiation of oral contraceptives. The pretreatment and periodic physical examinations should include special reference to blood pressure, breasts, abdomen, and pelvic organs, including a Pap smear and relevant laboratory tests. As a general rule, oral contraceptives should not be prescribed for longer than one year without the performance of another physical examination (see *Warnings*).

2. Preexisting uterine leiomyomata may increase in size during oral contraceptive use. While unconfirmed, an increased risk of fibroids with oral contraceptives containing ethynodiol diacetate has been reported.[166]

3. Oral contraceptives appear to be associated with an increased incidence of mental depression. Therefore, patients with a history of depression should be carefully observed and the drug discontinued if depression recurs to a serious degree. Patients becoming significantly depressed while taking oral contraceptives should stop the medication and use an alternative method of contraception in an attempt to determine whether the symptom is drug related.

4. Oral contraceptives may cause some degree of fluid retention. They should be prescribed with caution, and only with careful monitoring, in patients with conditions which might be aggravated by fluid retention, such as convulsive disorders, migraine syndrome, asthma, or cardiac, hepatic, or renal dysfunction.

5. Patients with a past history of jaundice during pregnancy have an increased risk of recurrence of jaundice and should be carefully observed while receiving oral contraceptives. If jaundice develops in any patient receiving such drugs, the medication should be discontinued while the cause is investigated. Cholestatic jaundice has been reported after combined treatment with oral contraceptives and troleandomycin. Hepatotoxicity following a combination of oral contraceptives and cyclosporine has also been reported.

6. Steroid hormones may be poorly metabolized in patients with impaired liver function and should be administered with caution in such patients.

7. Oral contraceptive users may have disturbances in normal tryptophan metabolism, which may result in a relative pyridoxine deficiency. The clinical significance of this is unknown, although megaloblastic anemia has been reported.

8. Serum folate levels may be depressed by oral contraceptive therapy. Since the pregnant woman is predisposed to folate deficiency and the incidence of folate deficiency increases with lengthening gestation, it is possible that if a woman becomes pregnant shortly after stopping oral contraceptives, she may have a greater chance of developing folate deficiency and complications attributable to this deficiency.

9. The pathologist should be advised of oral contraceptive therapy when relevant specimens are submitted.

10. Certain endocrine and liver function tests may be affected by estrogen-containing oral contraceptives. Therefore, it is recommended that any abnormal test be repeated after the drug has been withdrawn for two months. The following alterations in laboratory results have been observed with the use of oral contraceptives:

a. Hepatic function: Increased sulfobromophthalein retention and other abnormalities in tests of liver function.

b. Coagulation tests: Increased prothrombin and coagulation factors VII, VIII, IX, and X; decreased antithrombin III; increased platelet aggregability.

c. Thyroid function: Increased thyroid-binding globulin (TBG) leading to increased circulating total thyroid hormone, as measured by protein-bound iodine (PBI) or T[4] by column or radioimmunoassay. Free T[3] resin uptake is decreased, reflecting the elevated TBG; free T[4] concentration is unaltered.

d. Decreased pregnanediol excretion.

e. Reduced response to metyrapone test.

f. Increased blood transcortin and corticosteroid levels.

g. Increased blood triglyceride and phospholipid concentrations.

h. Reduced serum folate concentration.

i. Impaired glucose tolerance.

j. Altered plasma levels of trace minerals (eg, increased ceruloplasmin).

11. The influence of prolonged oral contraceptive therapy on pituitary, ovarian, adrenal, hepatic, or uterine function, or on the immune response, has not been established.

12. Treatment with oral contraceptives may mask the onset of the climacteric. (See *Warnings* section regarding risks in this age group.)

13. The prevalence of cervical *Chlamydia trachomatis* and *Neisseria gonorrhoeae* in oral contraceptive users is increased several-fold.[151,191] It should not be assumed that oral contraceptives afford protection against pelvic inflammatory disease from *Chlamydia.*[151] HIV seropositivity in female African prostitutes was significantly associated with a history of taking oral medications for the prevention of pregnancy and/or of sexually transmitted diseases.[181,188]

Information for the Patient. See patient labeling printed at end.

Drug Interactions. Oral contraceptives may be rendered less effective and increased incidence of breakthrough bleeding may occur by virtue of drug interaction with rifampin, isoniazid, ampicillin, neomycin, penicillin V, tetracycline, chloramphenicol, sulfonamides, nitrofurantoin, griseofulvin, barbiturates, phenytoin, carbamazepine, primidone, phenylbutazone, analgesics, tranquilizers, and antimigraine preparations.[72,74,95,125,153] Oral contraceptives may alter the effectiveness of other types of drugs, such as oral anticoagulants, anticonvulsants, tranquilizers (eg, diazepam), tricyclic antidepressants, antihypertensive agents (eg, guanethidine), theophylline, caffeine, vitamins, hypoglycemic agents, clofibrate, glucocorticoids, and acetaminophen.[72,119,134,139,153] (See *Precaution* No. 5).

Carcinogenesis. See *Warnings* No. 3 and 4 for information on the carcinogenic potential of oral contraceptives.

Pregnancy. Pregnancy category X. See *Contraindication* No. 7 and *Warning* No. 5.

Nursing Mothers. See *Warning* No. 12.

ADVERSE REACTIONS

An increased risk of the following serious adverse reactions has been associated with the use of oral contraceptives (see *Warnings*):

  Thrombophlebitis and thrombosis
  Pulmonary embolism
  Arterial thromboembolism
  Raynaud's disease
  Myocardial infarction and coronary thrombosis
  Cerebral thrombosis
  Cerebral hemorrhage
  Hypertension
  Gallbladder disease
  Budd-Chiari syndrome
  Benign adenomas and other hepatic lesions, with or without intra-abdominal bleeding
  Hepatocellular carcinoma
  Congenital anomalies

There is evidence of an association between the following conditions and the use of oral contraceptives, although confirmatory studies have not been done:

  Mesenteric thrombosis
  Neuro-ocular lesions (eg, retinal thrombosis and optic neuritis)

The following adverse reactions have been reported in patients receiving oral contraceptives and are believed to be drug related:

  Nausea and vomiting
    (Usually the most common adverse reactions, occurring in approximately 10% or fewer patients during the first cycle. Other reactions, as a general rule, are seen much less frequently or only occasionally.)
  Gastrointestinal symptoms (eg, abdominal cramps and bloating)
  Breakthrough bleeding
  Spotting
  Change in menstrual flow
  Dysmenorrhea
  Amenorrhea during and after use
  Infertility after discontinuation
  Edema
  Chloasma or melasma, which may persist when the drug is discontinued
  Breast changes: tenderness, enlargement, and secretion
  Change in weight (increase or decrease)
  Change in cervical erosion and secretion
  Endocervical hyperplasia
  Possible diminution in lactation when given immediately post partum

  Cholestatic jaundice
  Migraine
  Increase in size of uterine leiomyomata
  Rash (allergic)
  Mental depression
  Reduced tolerance to carbohydrates
  Vaginal candidiasis
  Change in corneal curvature (steepening)
  Intolerance to contact lenses

The following adverse reactions or conditions have been reported in users of oral contraceptives, and the association has been neither confirmed nor refuted:

  Premenstrual-like syndrome
  Cataracts
  Changes in libido
  Chorea
  Changes in appetite
  Cystitis-like syndrome
  Headache
  Paresthesia
  Nervousness
  Dizziness
  Auditory disturbances
  Rhinitis
  Fatigue
  Backache
  Hirsutism
  Loss of scalp hair
  Erythema multiforme
  Erythema nodosum
  Hemorrhagic eruption
  Herpes gestationis
  Hidradenitis suppurativa
  Hemolytic uremic syndrome
  Malignant hypertension
  Impaired renal function
  Acute renal failure, sometimes irreversible
  Itching
  Vaginitis
  Porphyria
  Premature ventricular contractions
  Electrocardiogram abnormalities
  Pulmonary hypertension
  Thrombotic thrombocytopenic purpura
  Anemia
  Pancreatitis
  Hepatitis
  Colitis
  Crohn's disease
  Gingivitis
  Dry socket
  Lupus erythematosus
  Rheumatoid arthritis
  Pituitary tumors (eg, adenoma) with amenorrhea and/or galactorrhea after OC use
  Malignant melanoma
  Endometrial, cervical, breast, and bile duct carcinoma (see *Warning* No. 3)

ACUTE OVERDOSAGE

Serious ill effects have not been reported following the acute ingestion of large doses of oral contraceptives by young children.[75,76] Overdosage may cause nausea, and withdrawal bleeding might occur in females.

DOSAGE AND ADMINISTRATION

Each package contains 21 or 28 tablets in numbered rows of 7 tablets each. The days of the week are printed above the columns.

To achieve maximum contraceptive effectiveness, oral contraceptives must be taken exactly as directed and at intervals of 24 hours.

IMPORTANT: During the first week of *initial* use of oral contraceptives, the patient should be instructed to use an additional method of contraception. The possibility of ovulation and conception prior to initiation of oral contraceptives should be considered.

Dosage Schedules
21-Day Schedules

For use with Norethin 1/35E™-21 and Norethin 1/50M™-21.

Sunday Schedule: The patient starts taking tablets on the first Sunday after the menstrual period begins. If the menstrual period begins on a Sunday, the first tablet is taken that same day. The three rows of tablets are completed, in order, followed by 7 days with no tablets. The next cycle is begun, as before, on a Sunday.

Day-5 Schedule: The patient starts taking tablets on day 5 of the menstrual cycle, counting day 1 as the first day of menstrual flow. The initial tablet is taken in row #1, the day of the week corresponding to day 5 of the cycle. When row #3 has been completed, any tablets remaining in row #1 should be taken. After 7 days of no tablets, the next cycle is begun on the same day of the week as the first cycle.

Postpartum Administration. Norethin 1/35E™-21 and Norethin 1/50M™-21 oral contraceptives may be prescribed

at the first postpartum examination regardless of whether or not the patient has experienced spontaneous menstruation. In non-nursing mothers, administration may be initiated immediately after delivery if desired or on the first Sunday after delivery. If preferred the tablets may be started on the day the patient leaves the hospital. (For nursing mothers, see *Warning* No. 12.) Increased risk of thromboembolism during the postpartum period must be considered. (See *Contraindications, Warnings,* and *Precautions.*)

28-Day Schedules

For use with Norethin 1/35E™-28 and Norethin 1/50M™-28.

Sunday Schedule: The patient starts taking tablets on the first Sunday after the menstrual period begins. If the menstrual period begins on a Sunday, the first tablet is taken that same day. The four rows of tablets are completed in order, and the next cycle is started the next day, Sunday.

If one or more placebo tablets are missed, the next cycle should be started as scheduled on the next Sunday. Risk of pregnancy is not increased by missing placebo tablets, if the schedule of active tablets is followed.

Day-5 Schedule: The patient starts taking white tablets on day 5 of the menstrual cycle, counting day 1 as the first day of menstrual flow. The initial white tablet is in row #1, the day of the week corresponding to day 5 of the cycle. When row #3 has been completed, any white tablets remaining in row #1 should be taken. **The patient must take all of the white tablets before taking any blue placebo tablets in row #4.** After all of the white tablets are used, the patient takes the blue placebo tablets in row #4 for one week (7 days). The patient begins the next cycle on the same day of the week as she began the first cycle.

If one or more placebo tablets are missed, the next cycle should be started as scheduled on the same day of the week as the previous cycle. Risk of pregnancy is not increased by missing placebo tablets, if the schedule of active tablets is followed.

Postpartum Administration. Norethin 1/35E™-28 and Norethin 1/50M™-28 oral contraceptives may be prescribed at the first postpartum examination regardless of whether or not the patient has experienced spontaneous menstruation. In non-nursing mothers, administration may be initiated immediately after delivery if desired or on the first Sunday after delivery. If preferred the tablets may be started on the day the patient leaves the hospital. (For nursing mothers, see *Warning* No. 12.) Increased risk of thromboembolism during the postpartum period must be considered. (See *Contraindications, Warnings,* and *Precautions.*)

Special Notes

Spotting or Breakthrough Bleeding. If spotting (bleeding insufficient to require a pad) or breakthrough bleeding (heavier bleeding similar to a menstrual flow) occurs when these products are used for contraception the patient should continue taking her tablets as directed. The incidence of spotting or breakthrough bleeding is minimal, most frequently occurring in the first cycle. Ordinarily spotting or breakthrough bleeding will stop within a week. Usually the patient will begin to cycle regularly within two or three courses of tablet-taking. In the event of spotting or breakthrough bleeding organic causes should be borne in mind. (See *Warning* No. 10.)

Missed Menstrual Periods. Withdrawal flow will normally occur two or three days after the last active tablet is taken. Failure of withdrawal bleeding ordinarily does not mean that the patient is pregnant, providing the dosage schedule has been correctly followed. (See *Warning* No. 5.)

If the patient has *not* adhered to the prescribed dosage regimen, the possibility of pregnancy should be considered after the first missed period, and oral contraceptives should be withheld until pregnancy has been ruled out.

If the patient has adhered to the prescribed regimen and misses two consecutive periods, pregnancy should be ruled out before continuing the contraceptive regimen.

The first intermenstrual interval after discontinuing the tablets is usually prolonged; consequently, a patient for whom a 28-day cycle is usual might not begin to menstruate for 35 days or longer. Ovulation in such prolonged cycles will occur correspondingly later in the cycle. Posttreatment cycles after the first one, however, are usually typical for the individual woman prior to taking tablets. (See *Warnings* No. 10 and 11.)

Missed Tablets (Contraception). If a woman misses taking one active tablet the missed tablet should be taken as soon as it is remembered. In addition, the next tablet should be taken at the usual time. If two consecutive active tablets are missed the dosage should be doubled for the next two days. The regular schedule should then be resumed, but an additional method of protection is recommended for the remainder of the cycle.

While there is little likelihood of ovulation if only one active tablet is missed, the possibility of spotting or breakthrough bleeding is increased and should be expected if two or more successive active tablets are missed. However, the possibility of ovulation increases with each successive day that scheduled active tablets are missed.

HOW SUPPLIED

Norethin 1/35E:

Each white Norethin 1/35E tablet is round in shape, with a debossed SCS and 221 on one side and 1/35 on the other side, and contains 1 mg of norethindrone and 35 mcg of ethinyl estradiol.

Norethin 1/35E™-21 (NDC 0905-0221-06) is packaged in cartons of six tablet dispensers of 21 tablets each.

Norethin 1/35E™-28 (NDC 0905-0231-06) is packaged in cartons of six tablet dispensers. Each dispenser contains 21 white tablets and 7 blue placebo tablets. (Placebo tablets have a debossed SEARLE on one side and a "P" on the other side.)

Norethin 1/50M:

Each white Norethin 1/50M tablet is round in shape, with a debossed SCS and 431 on one side and 1/50 on the other side, and contains 1 mg of norethindrone and 50 mcg of mestranol.

Norethin 1/50M™-21 (NDC 0905-0431-06) is packaged in cartons of six tablet dispensers of 21 tablets each.

Norethin 1/50M™-28 (NDC 0905-0441-06) is packaged in cartons of six tablet dispensers. Each dispenser contains 21 white tablets and 7 blue placebo tablets. (Placebo tablets have a debossed SEARLE on one side and a "P" on the other side.)

Caution: Federal law prohibits dispensing without prescription.

REFERENCES

1. Population Reports, Series H, No. 2 (May) 1974; Series I, No. 1 (June) 1974; Series B, No. 3 (May) 1979; Series H, No. 3 (Jan.) 1975; Series H, No. 4 (Jan.) 1976; Population Information Program, Geo. Washington U. Medical Center, Washington, D.C. **2.** Inman, W. H. W., et al.: Br. Med. J. *2*:203 (April 25) 1970. **3.** Inman, W. H. W., et al.: Br. Med. J. *2*:193 (April 27) 1968. **4.** Royal College of General Practitioners: J. Coll. Gen. Pract. *13*:267 (May) 1967. **5.** Vessey, M. P., et al.: Br. Med. J. *2*:651 (June 14) 1969. **6.** Sartwell, P. E., et al.: Am. J. Epidemiol. *90*:365 (Nov.) 1969. **7.** Boston Collaborative Drug Surveillance Programme: Lancet *1*:1399 (June 23) 1973. **8.** Stolley, P.D., et al.: Am. J. Epidemiol. *102*:197 (Sept.) 1975. **9.** Collaborative Group for the Study of Stroke in Young Women: N. Engl. J. Med. *288*:871 (April 26) 1973. **10.** Collaborative Group for the Study of Stroke in Young Women: J.A.M.A. *231*:718 (Feb. 17) 1975. **11.** Beral, V.: Lancet *2*:1047 (Nov. 13) 1976. **12.** Royal College of General Practitioners: Oral Contraceptives and Health, New York: Pitman Publ. Corp., May 1974. **13.** Layde, P., et al.: Lancet *1*:541 (March 7) 1981. **13a.** Beral, V., et al.: Lancet *2*:727 (Oct. 8) 1977. **14.** Vessey, M., et al.: J. Biosoc. Sci. *8*:373 (Oct.) 1976. **15.** Vessey, M., et al.: Lancet *2*:731 (Oct. 8) 1977; *1*:549 (March 7) 1981. **16.** Mann, J. I., et al.: Br. Med. J. *2*:241 (May 3) 1975. **17.** Mann, J. I., et al.: Br. Med. J. *3*:631 (Sept. 13) 1975. **18.** Mann, J. I., et al.: Br. Med. J. *2*:245 (May 3) 1975. **19.** Mann, J. I., et al.: Br. Med. J. *2*:445 (Aug. 21) 1976. **20.** Jain, A. K.: Stud. Fam. Plann. *8*:50 (March) 1977. **21.** Tietze, C.: Fam. Plann. Perspect. *9*:74 (March-April) 1977. **22.** Vessey, M. P., et al.: Br. Med. J. *3*:123 (July 18) 1970. **23.** Greene, G. R., et al.: Am. J. Public Health *62*:680 (May) 1972. **24.** Ziel, H. K., et al.: N. Engl. J. Med. *293*:1167 (Dec. 4) 1975. **25.** Smith, D. C., et al.: N. Engl. J. Med. *293*:1164 (Dec. 4) 1975. **26.** Mack, T. M., et al.: N. Engl. J. Med. *294*:1262 (June 3) 1976. **27.** Gray, L. A., et al.: Obstet. Gynecol. *49*:385 (April) 1977. **28.** McDonald, T. W., et al.: Am. J. Obstet. Gynecol. *127*:572 (March 15) 1977. **29.** Weiss, N. S., et al.: N. Engl. J. Med. *294*:1259 (June 3) 1976. **30.** Silverberg, S. G., et al.: Cancer *39*:592 (Feb.) 1977. **31.** Vessey, M. P., et al.: Br. Med. J. *3*:719 (Sept. 23) 1972. **32.** Vessey, M. P., et al.: Lancet *1*:941 (April 26) 1975. **33.** Boston Collaborative Drug Surveillance Program: N. Engl. J. Med. *290*:15 (Jan. 3) 1974. **34.** Arthes, F. G., et al.: Cancer *28*:1391 (Dec.) 1971. **35.** Casagrande, J., et al.: J. Natl. Cancer Inst. *56*:839 (April) 1976. **36.** Fasal, E., et al.: J. Natl. Cancer Inst. *55*:767 (Oct.) 1975. **37.** Paffenbarger, R. S., et al.: Cancer *39*:1887 (April Suppl.) 1977. **38.** Hoover, R., et al.: N. Engl. J. Med. *295*:401 (Aug. 19) 1976. **39.** Kelsey, J. L., et al.: Am. J. Epidemiol. *107*:236 (March) 1978. **40.** Ory, H., et al.: N. Engl. J. Med. *294*:419 (Feb. 19) 1976. **41.** Stern, E., et al.: Science *196*:1460 (June 24) 1977. **42.** Population Reports, Series A, No. 4 (May) 1977: Population Information Program, Geo. Washington U. Medical Center, Washington, D.C. **43.** Baum, J. K., et al.: Lancet *2*:926 (Oct. 27) 1973. **44.** Taler, S.J., et al.: Obstet. Gynecol. *65*:665 (May) 1985. **45.** Edmondson, H. A., et al.: N. Engl. J. Med. *294*:470 (Feb. 26) 1976. **46.** Rooks, J. B., et al.: J.A.M.A. *242*: 644 (Aug. 17) 1979. **47.** Herbst, A. L., et al.: N. Engl. J. Med. *284*:878 (April 22) 1971. **48.** Greenwald, P., et al.: N. Engl. J. Med. *285*:390 (Aug. 12) 1971. **49.** Lanier, A. P., et al.: Mayo Clin. Proc. *48*:793 (Nov.) 1973. **50.** Herbst, A. L., et al.: Am. J. Obstet. Gynecol. *128*:43 (May 1) 1977. **51.** Herbst, A. L., et al.: Obstet. Gynecol. *40*:287 (Sept.) 1972. **52.** Herbst, A. L., et al.: Am. J. Obstet. Gynecol. *118*:607 (March 1) 1974. **53.** Herbst, A. L., et al.: N. Engl. J. Med. *292*:334 (Feb. 13) 1975. **54.** Stafl, A., et al.: Obstet. Gynecol. *43*:118 (Jan.) 1974. **55.** Sherman, A. I., et al.: Obstet. Gynecol. *44*:531 (Oct.) 1974. **56.** Bibbo, M., et al.: J. Reprod. Med. *15*:29 (July) 1975. **57.** Gill, W., et al.: J. Reprod. Med. *16*:147 (April) 1976. **58.** Henderson, B., et al.: Pediatrics *58*:505 (Oct.) 1976. **59.** Gal, I., et al.: Nature *240*:241 (Nov. 24) 1972. **60.** Levy, E. P., et al.: Lancet *1*:611 (March 17) 1973. **61.** Nora, J. J., et al.: Lancet *1*:941 (April 28) 1973. **62.** Nora, A. H., et al.: Arch. Environ. Health *30*:17 (Jan.) 1975; Adv. Plann. Parent. *12*:156, 1978. **63.** Janerich, D. T., et al.: N. Engl. J. Med. *291*:697 (Oct. 3) 1974. **64.** Heinonen, O. P., et al.: N. Engl. J. Med. *296*:67 (Jan. 13) 1977. **65.** Nora, J. J., et al.: N. Engl. J. Med. *291*:731 (Oct. 3) 1974. **66.** Carr, D. H.: Can. Med. Assoc. J. *103*:343 (Aug. 15 & 29) 1970. **67.** Wynn, V., et al.: Lancet *2*:720 (Oct. 1) 1966. **68.** Laragh, J. H.: Am. J. Obstet. Gynecol. *126*:141 (Sept.) 1976. **69.** Fisch, I. R., et al.: J.A.M.A. *237*:2499 (June 6) 1977. **70.** Van Campenhout, J., et al.: Fertil. Steril. *28*:728 (July) 1977. **71.** Laumas, K. R., et al.: Am. J. Obstet. Gynecol. *98*:411 (June 1) 1967. **72.** Stockley, I.: Pharmaceut. J. *216*:140 (Feb. 14) 1976. **73.** Hempel, E., et al.: Drugs *12*:442 (Dec.) 1976. **74.** Bessot, J.-C., et al.: Nouv. Presse Med. *6*:1568 (April 30) 1977. **75.** Francis, W. G., et al.: Can. Med. Assoc. J. *92*:191 (Jan. 23) 1965. **76.** Verhulst, H. L., et al.: J. Clin. Pharmacol. *7*:9 (Jan.-Feb.) 1967. **77.** Vessey, M. P., et al.: Br. Med. J. *2*:199 (April 27) 1968. **78.** Ory, H. W.: J.A.M.A. *237*:2619 (June 13) 1977. **79.** Jain, A. K.: Am. J. Obstet. Gynecol. *126*:301 (Oct. 1) 1976. **80.** Ziel, H. K., et al.: Am. J. Obstet. Gynecol. *124*:735 (April 1) 1976. **81.** Peritz, E., et al.: Am. J. Epidemiol. *106*:462 (Dec.) 1977. **82.** Ory, H. W., et al.: in Garattini, S., and Berendes, H. (eds.): Pharmacology of Steroid Contraceptive Drugs, Raven Press, N.Y., 1977. **83.** Goldacre, M. J., et al.: Br. Med. J. *1*:748 (March 25) 1978. **84.** Meisels, A., et al.: Cancer *40*:3076 (Dec.) 1977. **85.** Klatskin, G.: Gastroenterology *73*:386 (Aug.) 1977. **86.** Kay, C. R.: Lancet *1*:624 (March 19) 1977. **87.** March, C. M., et al.: Fertil. Steril. *28*:346 (March) 1977. **88.** Saxena, B. N., et al.: Contraception *16*:605 (Dec.) 1977. **89.** Nilsson, S., et al.: Contraception *17*:131 (Feb.) 1978. **90.** Vessey, M. P., et al.: Br. Med. J. *1*:265 (Feb. 4) 1978. **91.** Jick, H., et al.: J.A.M.A. *239*:1403, 1407 (April 3) 1978. **92.** Kay, C. R.: J. R. Coll. Gen. Pract. *28*:393 (July) 1978. **93.** Hoogerland, D. L., et al.: Gynecol. Oncol. *6*:451 (Oct.) 1978. **94.** Lorber, C. A., et al.: Fertil. Steril. *31*:21 (Jan.) 1979. **95.** Bacon, J. F., et al.: Br. Med. J. *280*:293 (Feb. 2) 1980. **96.** Meade, T. W., et al.: Br. Med. J. *280*:1157 (May 10) 1980. **97.** Böttiger, L. E., et al.: Lancet *1*:1097 (May 24) 1980. **98.** Maguire, M. G., et al.: Am. J. Epidemiol. *110*:188 (Aug.) 1979. **99.** Ramcharan, S., et al.: The Walnut Creek Contraceptive Drug Study, Vol. 3, U.S. Govt. Ptg. Off., 1981; J. Reprod. Med. *25*:346 (Dec.) 1980. **100.** Petitti, D. B., et al.: Am. J. Epidemiol. *108*:480 (Dec.) 1978. **101.** Petitti, D. B., et al.: J.A.M.A. *242*:1150 (Sept. 14) 1979. **102.** Petitti, D. B., et al.: Lancet *2*:234 (July 29) 1978. **103.** Jick, H., et al.: Ann. Int. Med. *88*:58 (July) 1978. **104.** Jick, H., et al.: J.A.M.A. *240*:2548 (Dec. 1) 1978. **105.** Shapiro, S., et al.: Lancet *1*:743 (April 7) 1979. **106.** Rosenberg, L., et al.: Am. J. Epidemiol. *111*:59 (Jan.) 1980. **107.** Kreuger, D. E., et al.: Am. J. Epidemiol. *111*:655 (June) 1980. **108.** Arthes, F. G., et al.: Chest *70*:574 (Nov.) 1976. **109.** Hoover, R., et al.: Am. J. Public Health *68*:335 (April) 1978. **110.** Herbst, A. L., et al.: J. Reprod. Med. *24*:62 (Feb.) 1980. **111.** Barnes, A. B., et al.: N. Engl. J. Med. *302*:609 (March 13) 1980. **112:** Cousins, L., et al.: Obstet. Gynecol. *56*:70 (July) 1980. **113.** Nora, J. J., et al.: J.A.M.A. *240*:837 (Sept. 1) 1978. **114.** Aarskog, D.: N. Engl. J. Med. *300*:75 (Jan. 11) 1979. **115.** Janerich, D. T., et al.: Am. J. Epidemiol. *112*:73 (July) 1980. **116.** Kasan, P. N., et al.: Br. J. Obstet. Gynaecol. *87*:545 (July) 1980. **117.** Rothman, K. J.: N. Engl. J. Med. *297*:468 (Sept. 1) 1977. **118.** Bracken, M. B.: Am. J. Obstet. Gynecol. *133*:432 (Feb. 15) 1979. **119.** De Teresa, E., et al.: Br. Med. J. *2*:1260 (Nov. 17) 1979. **120.** Swan, S., et al.: Am. J. Obstet. Gynecol. *139*:52 (Jan. 1) 1981. **121.** Kay, C. R.: Br. Med. J. *282*:2089 (June 27) 1981. **122.** Vessey, M. P., et al.: Br. Med. J. *282*:2093 (June 27) 1981. **123.** Pike, M. C., et al.: Br. J. Cancer *43*:72 (Jan.) 1981. **124.** Harlap, S., et al.: Obstet. Gynecol. *55*:447 (April) 1980. **125.** Back, D. J., et al.: Drugs *21*:46 (Jan.) 1981. **126.** Porter, J. B., et al.: Obstet. Gynecol. *66*:1 (July) 1985. **127.** Lees, A.W., et al.: Int. J. Cancer *22*:700, 1978. **128.** Brinton, L. A., et al.: J. Natl. Cancer Inst. (JNCI) *62*:37 (Jan.) 1979. **129.** Black, M. M.: Pathol. Res. Pract. *166*:491, 1980; Cancer *46*:2747 (Dec.) 1980; Cancer *51*: 2147 (June 1) 1983. **130.** Hoover, R., et al.: JNCI *67*:815 (Oct.) 1981. **131.** Gill, W. B., et al.: J. Urol. *122*:36 (July) 1979. **132.** Linn, S., et al.: J.A.M.A. *247*:629 (Feb. 5) 1982. **133.** Clavel, F., et al.: Bull. Cancer (Paris) *68*:449 (Dec.) 1981. **134.** Abernethy, D. R., et al.: N. Engl. J. Med. *306*:791 (April 1) 1982. **135.** Kay, C. R.: Am. J. Obstet. Gynecol. *142*:762 (March 15) 1982. **136.** Adam, S. A., et al.: Br. J. Obstet. Gynaecol. *88*:838 (Aug.) 1981. **137.** Slone, D., et al.: N. Engl. J. Med. *305*:420 (Aug. 20) 1981. **138.** Layde, P.M., et al.: J.R. Coll. Gen. Pract. *33*:75 (Feb.) 1983. **139.** Abernethy, D. R., et al.: Obstet. Gynecol. *60*:338 (Sept.) 1982. **140.** Brinton, L.A., et al.: Int. J. Epidemiol. *11*:316, 1982. **141.** Harris, N.V., et al.: Am. J. Epidemiol. *116*: 643 (Oct.) 1982. **142.** Pike, M.C., et al.: Lancet *2*:926 (Oct. 22) 1983. **143.** Vessey, M.P., et al.: Lancet *2*:930 (Oct. 22) 1983. **144.** Jick, H., et al.: Am. J. Epidemiol. *112*:577 (Nov.) 1980. **145.** Jick, H., et al.: Am. J. Epidemiol. *112*:586 (Nov.) 1980. **146.** McPherson, K., et al.: Lancet *2*:1414 (Dec. 17) 1983. **147.** Vessey, M.P., et al.: Br.

Continued on next page

Schiapparelli Searle—Cont.

Med. J. *289*:530 (Sept. 1) 1984. **148.** Olsson, H., et al.: Lancet *1*:748 (March 30) 1985. **149.** Thomas, D.B., et al.: Br. Med. J. *290*:961 (March 30) 1985. **150.** Dallenbach-Hellweg, G.: Path. Res. Pract. *179*:38, 1984. **151.** Washington, A.E., et al.: J.A.M.A. *253*:2246 (April 19) 1985. **152.** Rosenberg, L., et al.: J.A.M.A. *253*:2965 (May 24/31) 1985. **153.** Baciewicz, A.M.: Therap. Drug Monitor. *7*:26 (March) 1985. **154.** Robboy, S.J., et al.: J.A.M.A. *252*:2979 (Dec. 7) 1984. **155.** Vessey, M.P., et al.: Br. J. Fam. Plann. *11*:120 (Jan.) 1986. **156.** Vessey, M.P., et al.: Br. Med. J. *292*:526 (Feb. 22) 1986. **157.** Henderson, B.E., et al.: Br. J. Cancer *48*:437 (July) 1983. **158.** Neuberger, J., et al.: Br. Med. J. *292*:1355 (May 24) 1986. **159.** Forman, D., et al.: Br. Med. J. *292*:1357 (May 24) 1986. **160.** Pinto, M.R.: Mutat. Res. *169*:149 (March) 1986. **161.** Meirik, O., et al.: Lancet *2*:650 (Sept. 20) 1986. **162.** Brinton, L.A., et al.: Int. J. Cancer *38*:339 (Sept.) 1986. **163.** Ory, H.: Fam. Plann. Perspect. *15*:57 (March-April) 1983. **164.** Harlap, S., et al.: Teratology *31*:381 (June) 1985. **165.** Tikkanen, M.J.: J. Reprod. Med. *31*:898 (Sept.) 1986. **166.** Ross, R.K.: Br. Med. J. *293*:359 (Aug. 9) 1986. **167.** Lipson, A., et al.: Contraception *34*:121 (Aug.) 1986. **168.** Bradley, D. D., et al.: N. Engl. J. Med. *299*:17 (July 6) 1978. **169.** Gordon, T., et al.: Am. J. Med. *62*:707 (May) 1977. **170.** Ebeling, K., et al.: Int. J. Cancer *39*:427 (April) 1987. **171.** Melnick, S., et al.: N. Engl. J. Med. *316*:514 (Feb. 26) 1987. **172.** Ellis, E.F., et al.: Lancet *1*:207 (Jan. 28) 1978. **173.** Vessey, M., et al.: Br. Med. J. *292*:526 (Feb. 22) 1986. **174.** Sainz, M.P., et al.: Med. Clin. (Barcelona) *89*:272, 1987. **175.** McPherson, K., et al.: Br. J. Cancer *56*:653 (Nov.) 1987. **176.** Trussell, J., et al.: Stud. Fam. Plann. *18*:227 (Sept./Oct.) 1987. **177.** Littlewood, E.R., et al.: Lancet *1*:310 (Feb. 4) 1980. **178.** Caggiano, V., et al.: Lancet *2*:365 (Aug. 16) 1980. **179.** Yen, S., et al.: Cancer *59*:2112 (June) 1987. **180.** Mant, D., et al.: J Epidemiol. Commun. Hlth. *41*:215 (Sept.) 1987. **181.** Plummer, F.A., et al.: Second Internat. Symp. AIDS and Assoc. Cancers in Africa, abst. S.9.3, 1987. **182.** Burkman, R.T., et al.: Obstet. Gynecol. *71*:33 (Jan.) 1987. **183.** Depue, R.H., et al.: JNCI *71*:1151 (Dec.) 1983. **184.** Walker, A.H., et al.: Br. J. Cancer *57*:418 (April) 1988. **185.** Stadel, B.V., et al.: Contraception *38*:287 (Sept.) 1988. **186.** Miller, D.R., et al.: Am. J. Epidemiol. *129*:269 (Feb.) 1989. **187.** Kay, C.R., et al.: Br. J. Cancer *58*:675 (Nov.) 1988. **188.** Mann, J.M., et al.: AIDS *2*:249, 1988. **189.** Beral. V., et al.: Lancet *2*:1331 (Dec. 10) 1988. **190.** Croft, P., et al.: Br. Med. J. *298*:165 (Jan. 21) 1989. **191.** Louv, W.C., et al.: Am. J. Obstet. Gynecol. *160*:396 (Feb.) 1989.

BRIEF SUMMARY OF PATIENT LABELING

Cigarette-smoking increases the risk of serious adverse effects on the heart and blood vessels from oral contraceptive use. This risk increases with age and with heavy smoking (15 or more cigarettes per day) and is quite marked in women over 35 years of age. Women who use oral contraceptives should not smoke.

In the detailed leaflet, "What You Should Know About Oral Contraceptives," which you have received, the risks and benefits of oral contraceptives are discussed in much more detail. This leaflet also provides information on other forms of contraception. ***Please take time to read it carefully for it may have been recently revised.***

If you have any questions or problems regarding this information, contact your doctor.

Oral contraceptives taken as directed are about 99% effective in preventing pregnancy. (The mini-pill, however, is somewhat less effective.) Forgetting to take your pills increases the chance of pregnancy.

Women who have or have had clotting disorders, cancer of the breast or sex organs, unexplained vaginal bleeding, stroke, heart attack, chest pains on exertion (angina pectoris), liver tumors associated with the use of the pill or with other estrogen-containing products, or who suspect they may be pregnant should not use oral contraceptives.

Most side effects of the pill are not serious. The most common side effects are nausea, vomiting, bleeding between menstrual periods, weight gain, and breast tenderness. However, proper use of oral contraceptives requires that they be taken under your doctor's continuing supervision, because they can be associated with serious side effects which may be fatal. Fortunately, these are very uncommon, but the risks may persist after use of the pill is discontinued. The serious side effects are:

1. Blood clots in the legs, arms, lungs, brain, heart, eyes, abdomen, or elsewhere in the body.
2. Bleeding in the brain (hemorrhage) as a result of bursting of a blood vessel.
3. Disorders of vision.
4. Liver tumors, which may rupture and cause severe bleeding.
5. Birth defects if the pill is taken during pregnancy.
6. High blood pressure.
7. Gallbladder disease.

The symptoms associated with these serious side effects are discussed in the detailed leaflet given you with your supply of pills. Notify your doctor if you notice any unusual physical disturbance while taking the pill.

Breast cancer and other cancers have developed in certain animals when given the estrogens in oral contraceptives for long periods. These findings suggest that oral contraceptives may also cause cancer in humans. However, studies to date in women taking currently marketed oral contraceptives have not confirmed that oral contraceptives cause cancer in humans.

Caution: Oral contraceptives are of no value in the prevention or treatment of venereal disease.

Various drugs, such as antibiotics, may also decrease the effectiveness of oral contraceptives.

DETAILED PATIENT LABELING: WHAT YOU SHOULD KNOW ABOUT ORAL CONTRACEPTIVES

Please take time to read this booklet carefully for it may have been recently revised.

Oral contraceptives (the pill) are the most effective way (except for sterilization) to prevent pregnancy if you follow the directions for their use and are careful not to skip doses or take them irregularly. They are also convenient and, for most women, free of serious or unpleasant side effects. Oral contraceptives must always be taken under the continuing supervision of a doctor.

It is important that any woman who considers using an oral contraceptive understands the risks involved. Although the oral contraceptives have important advantages over other methods of contraception, they have certain risks that no other method has. Only you can decide whether the advantages are worth these risks. This leaflet will tell you about the most important risks. It will explain how you can help your doctor prescribe the pill as safely as possible by telling him/her about yourself and being alert for the earliest signs of trouble. And it will tell you how to use the pill properly, so that it will be as effective as possible. THERE IS MORE DETAILED INFORMATION AVAILABLE IN THE LEAFLET PREPARED FOR DOCTORS. Your pharmacist can show you a copy; you may need your doctor's help in understanding parts of it.

Caution: Oral contraceptives are of no value in the prevention or treatment of venereal disease.

Cigarette-smoking increases the risk of serious adverse effects on the heart and blood vessels from oral contraceptive use. This risk increases with age and with heavy smoking (15 or more cigarettes per day) and is quite marked in women over 35 years of age. Women who use oral contraceptives should not smoke.

WHO SHOULD NOT USE ORAL CONTRACEPTIVES

You should not use oral contraceptives:

A. If you have any of the following conditions:
   1. Blood clots in the legs, lungs, eyes, or elsewhere in the body.
   2. Chest pains on exertion (angina pectoris).
   3. Known or suspected cancer of the breast or sex organs, such as the womb (uterus), vagina, or cervix.
   4. Unusual vaginal bleeding that has not been diagnosed by your doctor.
   5. Known or suspected pregnancy (one or more menstrual periods missed).

B. If you have had any of the following conditions:
   1. Heart attack or stroke (clots or bleeding in the brain).
   2. Blood clots in the legs, lungs, eyes, or elsewhere in the body.
   3. Liver tumor associated with use of the pill or other estrogen-containing products.

C. If you have scanty or irregular periods or are a young woman without a regular cycle, you should use another method of contraception because, if you use the pill, you may have difficulty becoming pregnant or may fail to have menstrual periods after discontinuing the pill.

DECIDING TO USE ORAL CONTRACEPTIVES

If you do not have any of the conditions listed above and are thinking about using oral contraceptives, to help you decide, you need information about the advantages and risks of oral contraceptives and of other contraceptive methods as well. This leaflet describes the advantages and risks of oral contraceptives. Except for sterilization, the intrauterine device (IUD), and abortion, which have their own specific risks, the only risks of other methods of contraception are those due to pregnancy should the method fail. Your doctor can answer questions you may have with respect to other methods of contraception, and further questions you may have on oral contraceptives after reading this leaflet.

1. *What Oral Contraceptives Are and How They Work.* Oral contraceptives are of two types. The most common, often simply called "the pill," is a *combination* of an estrogen and a progestogen, the two kinds of female hormones. The amount of estrogen and progestogen can vary, but the amount of estrogen is more important because both the effectiveness and some of the dangers of oral contraceptives have been related to the amount of estrogen. This combination oral contraceptive works principally by preventing release of an egg from the ovary during the cycle in which the pills are taken. When the amount of estrogen is 50 micrograms or more, and the pill is taken as directed, oral contraceptives are more than 99% effective (that is, there would be less than 1 pregnancy in 100 women using the pill for one year). Pills that contain 20 to 35 micrograms of estrogen vary slightly in effectiveness, ranging from 98% to more than 99% effective.

The second type of oral contraceptive, often called the mini-pill, contains only a progestogen. It works in part by preventing release of an egg from the ovary, but also by keeping sperm from reaching the egg and by making the womb (uterus) less receptive to any fertilized egg that reaches it. The mini-pill is less effective than the combination oral contraceptive, about 97% effective. In addition, the mini-pill has a tendency to cause irregular bleeding, which may be quite inconvenient, or cessation of bleeding entirely. The mini-pill is used despite its lower effectiveness in the hope that it will prove not to have some of the serious side effects of the estrogen-containing pill, but it is not yet certain that the mini-pill does in fact have fewer serious side effects. The following discussion, while based mainly on information about the combination pills, should be considered to apply as well to the mini-pill.

2. *Other Nonsurgical Ways to Prevent Pregnancy.* As this leaflet will explain, oral contraceptives have several serious risks. Other methods of contraception have lesser risks or none at all. They are also less effective than oral contraceptives, but, used properly, may be effective enough for many women. The following table gives reported pregnancy rates (the number of women out of 100 who would become pregnant in one year) for these methods:

Pregnancies per 100 Women per Year

Method	*Range*
Intrauterine device (IUD)	less than 1 to 6
Diaphragm with spermicidal cream or jelly	2 to 20
Condom (rubber)	3 to 36
Spermicidal aerosol foams	2 to 29
Spermicidal jellies or creams	4 to 36
Periodic abstinence (rhythm), all types	less than 1 to 47
1. Calendar method	14 to 47
2. Temperature method	1 to 20
3. Temperature method (intercourse only in postovulatory phase)	less than 1 to 7
4. Mucus method	1 to 25
No contraception	60 to 80

These figures (except for the IUD) vary widely because people differ in how well they use each method. Very faithful users of the various methods obtain the best results, except for users of the periodic abstinence (rhythm) calendar method. Effective use of these methods, except for the IUD, requires somewhat more effort than simply taking a single pill every day, but it is an effort that many couples undertake successfully. Your doctor can tell you a great deal more about these methods of contraception and their effectiveness.

3. *The Dangers of Oral Contraceptives.*

a. *Circulatory disorders (blood clots, strokes, and heart attacks).* Blood clots occasionally form in the blood vessels of the body and, though rare, are the most common of the serious side effects of oral contraceptives. Clotting can result in a stroke (a clot in the brain), a heart attack (a clot in a blood vessel of the heart), or a pulmonary embolus (a clot that forms in the legs or abdominal region, then breaks off and travels to the lungs), or loss of a limb (a clot in a blood vessel in, or leading to, an arm or leg). Clots can also form in the blood vessels of the intestines or liver. Any of these events can be fatal (lead to death). Clots also occur rarely in the blood vessels of the eye, resulting in blindness or impairment of vision in that eye. There is some evidence that the risk of clotting may increase with higher estrogen doses. It is therefore important for your doctor to keep the dose of estrogen as low as possible, so long as the oral contraceptive used has an acceptable pregnancy rate and doesn't cause unacceptable changes in the menstrual pattern. Higher doses of progestogen have also been suggested as increasing the risk of clotting. Furthermore, cigarette-smoking by oral contraceptive users increases the risk of serious adverse effects on the heart and blood vessels. This risk increases with age and with heavy smoking (15 or more cigarettes per day) and begins to become quite marked in women over 35 years of age. For this reason, women who use oral contraceptives should not smoke.

The risk of abnormal clotting increases with age both in users and in nonusers of oral contraceptives, but the increased risk with the oral contraceptives appears to be present at all ages.

The risks of circulatory disorders may persist or continue after the pill is stopped. This has been reported for circulatory disorders in general, for heart disease or heart attacks, and for strokes caused either by a bursting blood vessel in the brain or by blood clots in the brain.

For oral contraceptive users in general, it has been estimated that in women between the ages of 25 and 34 the risk of death due to circulatory disorders in nonsmokers is about 1 in 23,000 per year. In contrast, for nonusers of the pill the risk is about 1 in 37,000 per year. Estimates of the risk of death due to circulatory disorders can be made, depending upon the woman's age, whether or not she uses oral contraceptives, and whether or not she smokes cigarettes. In the age group 25–34 years, women who use the pill have a risk of 1 in 7,000 (for smokers) to 1 in 23,000 (for nonsmokers) per year. This may be compared to the corresponding risk in women who have not used the pill: 1 in 24,000 (for smokers) to 1 in 37,000 (for nonsmokers) per year. The risks are greater in older women; thus, in the age group 35–44 years, women who use the pill have a risk of 1 in 1,600 (for smokers) to 1 in 4,700 (for nonsmokers) per year. The corresponding risk for women who have not used the pill is 1 in 6,600 (for smokers) to 1 in 16,000 (for nonsmokers) per year.

For women aged 16 to 40 it is estimated that about 1 in 2,000 using oral contraceptives will be hospitalized each year because of abnormal clotting in the veins or lungs. Among nonusers of the same age, about 1 in 20,000 would be hospitalized each year for these disorders.

Disease of the arteries characterized by paleness, numbness, or tingling in the fingers or toes has been reported to be more common in pill users.

Strokes are caused by a bursting blood vessel in the brain (hemorrhage) or a loss of blood circulation to the brain due to blood clots. When they occur, paralysis of all or part of the body may result; death can result. The risk of strokes due to clots or hemorrhages in the brain has been reported to be increased in pill users when compared with nonusers.

It has been estimated that pill users are twice as likely as nonusers to have a stroke due to a bursting blood vessel in the brain. It has further been estimated that pill users are 4 to 10 times as likely as nonusers to have a stroke due to clotting in a blood vessel in or leading to the brain.

It has been reported that women using the pill may have a greater risk of heart attack than nonusers. Even without the pill the risk of having a heart attack increases with age and is also increased by additional risk factors such as high blood pressure, high blood cholesterol, obesity, diabetes, cigarette-smoking, or the occurrence during pregnancy of high blood pressure, swelling of the legs, or protein in the urine. Without any risk factors present, the use of oral contraceptives alone may double the risk of heart attack. However, the combination of cigarette-smoking, especially heavy smoking, and oral contraceptive use greatly increases the risk of heart attack. Oral contraceptive users who smoke are about five times more likely to have a heart attack than users who do not smoke, and about ten times more likely to have a heart attack than nonusers who do not smoke. It has been estimated that users between the ages of 30 and 39 who smoke have about a 1 in 10,000 chance each year of having a fatal heart attack compared to about a 1 in 50,000 chance in users who do not smoke, and about a 1 in 100,000 chance in nonusers who do not smoke. In the age group 40 to 44, the risk is about 1 in 1,700 per year for users who smoke compared to about 1 in 10,000 for users who do not smoke, and to about 1 in 14,000 per year for nonusers who do not smoke. Heavy smoking (about 15 cigarettes or more a day) further increases the risk. If you do not smoke and have none of the other heart attack risk factors described above, you will have a smaller risk than listed. If you have several heart attack risk factors, the risk may be considerably greater than listed.

The above are average figures for Great Britain; comparable estimates for the U.S. have been higher.

Oral contraceptives should never be used at any age by women who have had a stroke, a heart attack, or chest pains on exertion (angina pectoris), or who have had blood clots in the legs, lungs, or elsewhere.

Anyone using the pill who has severe leg or chest pains, coughs up blood, has difficulty in breathing, severe headache or vomiting, dizziness or fainting, disturbances of vision or speech, weakness, numbness, or pain in an arm or leg should call her doctor immediately and stop taking the pill, and use another method of contraception.

b. *Formation of tumors.* When certain animals are given the female sex hormone estrogen (which is an ingredient in oral contraceptives) continuously for long periods, cancers may develop in organs such as the breast, cervix, vagina, liver, womb, ovary, and pituitary.

These findings suggest that oral contraceptives may cause cancer in humans. However, studies to date in women taking currently marketed oral contraceptives have not confirmed that oral contraceptives cause cancer in humans, but it remains possible they will be discovered in the future to do so.

Although several studies have reported no overall increase in breast cancer in oral contraceptive users, other studies have reported increases in certain groups of women who have used oral contraceptives. Such groups reported to be at increased risk have differed from one study to another. Examples of such subgroups are: (a) women aged 20–44 without children who had their first menstrual period before age 13 and who took the pill for 8 or more years; (b) women aged 30–39, users for more than 5 years, and women with children who took the pill for 1–4 years before their first term pregnancy or for less than one year or more than 4 years after delivery; (c) women aged 30–34, and women with one child who took the pill for 2 or more years; (d) women already having benign (noncanceorus) breast disease (for example, cysts); (e) long-term (2–4 years) users; and (f) women having other risk factors (such as family history of breast cancer, a previous breast biopsy, or delay in having a first child). Women with a family history of breast cancer or who have breast nodules (lumps), fibrocystic disease (breast cysts), or abnormal mammograms (x-ray pictures of the breasts), or who were exposed to the estrogen diethylstilbestrol (DES) during their mother's pregnancy, or who have abnormal Pap smears should be followed very closely by their doctors if they choose to use oral contraceptives instead of another method of contraception. Many studies have shown that women taking oral contraceptives have less risk of getting benign (noncancerous) breast disease than those who have not used oral contraceptives. There is strong evidence that estrogens (one component of combination-type oral contraceptives), when given for periods of more than one year to women after the menopause (change-of-life), increase the risk of cancer of the womb (uterus). There is also some evidence that the sequential oral contraceptive, a kind of oral contraceptive that is no longer sold, may increase the risk of cancer of the womb. There is no evidence, however, that the oral contraceptives now available increase the risk of this type of cancer, although some individual cases have been reported. Cancer of the cervix may develop more readily in long-term users of the pill, particularly if they have had preexisting abnormal Pap smears. Cervical erosion and cell abnormalities, as well as chlamydial and gonococcal infections, have been reported to be more frequent in pill users. Unconfirmed observations have reported a greater use of oral contraceptives among African prostitutes testing positive for the AIDS virus.

Very rarely, oral contraceptive users may have a noncancerous tumor of the liver. These tumors do not spread, but they may rupture and cause internal bleeding, which may be fatal. This has been reported in short-term as well as long-term users, although increasing duration of use increases the risk. Long-term users have an estimated annual incidence of 3 to 4 per 100,000. One study reported that oral contraceptive products with a high "hormonal potency" were associated with a higher risk than lower-potency products, as was age over 30 years. Cases of cancer of the liver have been reported in women using oral contraceptives also. Users for 8 or more years were estimated to be 7 to 20 times more likely to develop this cancer than were nonusers. An increased risk of cancer of the bile ducts also has been reported.

A type of skin cancer that has been linked to exposure to sunlight (malignant melanoma) has been reported to be more frequent among pill users. It was not possible to determine what the effect was of greater exposure to sunlight in users.

c. *Dangers to a developing baby if oral contraceptives are used in or immediately preceding pregnancy.* Oral contraceptives should not be taken by pregnant women because they may damage the developing baby. There is an increased risk to the baby of abnormalities of such parts of the body as the backbone, anus, heart, windpipe, esophagus, kidneys, arms, and legs. In addition, the developing female child whose mother has received DES, a synthetic estrogen, during pregnancy has a risk of getting cancer of the vagina or cervix in her teens or young adulthood. This risk is estimated to be about 1 in 1,000 exposures or less. DES-exposed daughters appear to have an increased risk of unfavorable outcome of pregnancy. Abnormalities of the urinary and sex organs and sperm have been reported in DES-exposed male babies as well. It is possible that other estrogens, such as the estrogens in oral contraceptives, could have the same effect in the baby if the mother takes them during pregnancy. It has been reported that there is an increased risk of a type of cancer of the testes and ovaries in people whose mothers received female hormones (including oral contraceptives) during early pregnancy.

Occasionally women who are taking the pill miss periods. It has been reported to occur as frequently as several times each year in some women, depending on various factors such as age and prior history. (Your doctor is the best source of information about this.) The pill should not be used when you are pregnant or suspect you may be pregnant. Very rarely, women who are using the pill as directed become pregnant. The likelihood of becoming pregnant is higher if you occasionally miss one or two pills. Therefore, if you miss a period you should consult your physician before continuing to take the pill. If you miss a period, especially if you have not taken the pill regularly, you should use an alternative method of contraception until pregnancy has been ruled out;

if you have missed more than one pill at any time, you should immediately start using an additional method of contraception and complete your pill cycle.

You should not attempt to become pregnant for at least three months after discontinuing oral contraceptives. Use another method of contraception during this period of time. The reason for this is that during this period there may be an increased risk of miscarriage and deformity to the baby, or an increased chance of having twins. Whether there is an overall increase in miscarriage in women who become pregnant soon after stopping the pill as compared with women who did not use the pill is not known, but it is possible that there may be.

If, however, you do become pregnant soon after stopping oral contraceptives, and do not have a miscarriage, there is no evidence that the baby has an increased risk of being abnormal.

d. *Gallbladder disease.* Women who use oral contraceptives have a greater risk than nonusers of having gallbladder disease requiring surgery. The increased risk may first appear within one year of use and may double after 4 or 5 years of use. Cancer of the ducts that collect bile may be more frequent in pill users.

e. *Other side effects of oral contraceptives.* Some women using oral contraceptives experience unpleasant side effects from the pill which are not dangerous and are not likely to damage their health. Some of these side effects are similar to symptoms women experience in early pregnancy and may be temporary. Your breasts may feel tender, be enlarged, or have a discharge; nausea and vomiting or other stomach or intestinal problems may occur; you may gain or lose weight, and your ankles may swell. A spotty darkening of the skin, particularly of the face, is possible and may persist after the drug is discontinued. An allergic or other type of rash or vaginal yeast infection might occur. You may notice unexpected vaginal bleeding, change in discharge, or changes in your menstrual period. Irregular bleeding is frequently seen when the mini-pill or the combination oral contraceptives containing less than 50 micrograms of estrogen are used. These should all be reported to your doctor.

Other side effects include worsening of migraine, asthma, convulsive disorders (such as epilepsy), and kidney, liver, or heart disease because of a tendency for water to be retained in the body when oral contraceptives are used. Other side effects are painful periods; growth of preexisting fibroid tumors of the womb; mental depression; and liver problems with jaundice (yellowing of the whites of the eyes or of the skin). Your doctor may find that levels of sugar and fatty substances in your blood are elevated; the long-term effects of these changes are not known. Some women develop high blood pressure while taking oral contraceptives, which ordinarily, but not always, returns to the original levels when the oral contraceptive is stopped. The degree of blood pressure rise may be related to the amount of progestogen in the pill. Women with a history of increased blood pressure, kidney disease, or toxemia during pregnancy (increased blood pressure, swelling of the legs, protein in the urine, or convulsions), or a family tendency to high blood pressure or its consequences (stroke, heart disease, kidney disease, blood vessel problems), or a history of excessive weight gain or swelling of the legs during their menstrual cycle, may be more likely to develop increased blood pressure when given oral contraceptives; therefore, they should have their blood pressure taken frequently. High blood pressure predisposes one to stroke, heart attacks, kidney disease, and other diseases of the blood vessels. The effect of prolonged use of oral contraceptives on several of your organs (pituitary, liver, ovaries, womb, and adrenals) or immune system is not known at this time.

Increased damage to the chromosomes of white blood cells has been reported in pill users. The significance for cancer or birth defects is unknown.

Other conditions, although not proved to be caused by oral contraceptives, are occasionally reported. These include more frequent urination and some discomfort when urinating, kidney disease, nervousness, dizziness, hearing problems, inflammation of the nasal passages, loss of scalp hair, an increase in body hair, an increase or decrease in sex drive, appetite changes, gum disease, dry socket, cataracts, a need for a change in contact lens prescription or inability to use contact lenses, tiredness, backache, vaginal infections, itching, anemia, blood cell breakdown with kidney failure, headache, symptoms similar to those you get before a period; breast, womb, cervical, and liver cancer; inflammation of the pancreas, liver, or large or small intestine; chorea (spasmodic movements), burning or prickly sensation, rheumatoid arthritis, pulmonary hypertension, abnormal heart rhythm or electrocardiogram, and a bruising disease caused by decreased blood platelets (TTP).

After you stop using oral contraceptives, there may be a delay before you are able to become pregnant or before you resume having menstrual periods. This is especially true of

Continued on next page

Schiapparelli Searle—Cont.

women who had irregular menstrual cycles prior to the use of oral contraceptives.

One study showed that this delay in becoming pregnant can persist up to 72 months after stopping the pill if you have never had children and are over 30 years old. The delay appears to be more severe if the pill has been used for 2 years or more by such women. For women who have had children, the delay can persist to 30 months, regardless of age. For women who have not had children and who are less than 30, the delay may persist to 48 months. Very rarely there may be secretions from the breast associated with the absence of periods, which might be due to a noncancerous tumor of the pituitary gland requiring surgery. This may occur more frequently in former users of the pill than in nonusers. As discussed previously, you should wait at least three months after stopping the pill before you try to become pregnant. During the first three months after stopping oral contraceptives, use another form of contraception. You should consult your doctor before resuming use of oral contraceptives after childbirth, especially if you plan to nurse your baby. Drugs in oral contraceptives are known to appear in the milk, and the long-range effect on babies is not known at this time. Furthermore, oral contraceptives may cause a decrease in your milk supply as well as in the quality of the milk.

4. *Comparison of the Risks of Oral Contraceptives and Other Contraceptive Methods.*

The many studies on the risks and effectiveness of oral contraceptives and other methods of contraception have been analyzed to estimate the risk of death associated with various methods of contraception. This risk has two parts: (a) the risk of the method itself (for example, the risk that oral contraceptives might cause death due to abnormal blood clotting), and (b) the risk of death due to pregnancy or abortion in the event the method should fail. The results of this analysis are shown in the following bar graph. The height of the bars indicates the number of deaths per 100,000 women each year. There are six sets of bars, each set referring to a specific age group of women. Within each set of bars, there is a single bar for each of the different contraceptive methods.

For oral contraceptives, there are two bars—one for smokers and the other for nonsmokers. The analysis is based on present knowledge and new information could, of course, alter it. The analysis shows that the risk of death from all methods of birth control is low and below that associated with the risks of childbirth, *except for oral contraceptives in women over 40 who smoke.* The risk of death associated with pill use in nonsmokers over 40 is higher than with any other method of contraception in that age group. It shows that the lowest risk of death is associated with the condom or diaphragm (traditional contraception) backed up by early legal abortion in case of failure of the condom or diaphragm to prevent pregnancy. Also, at any age, the risk of death (due to unexpected pregnancy) from use of traditional contraception, even without a backup of abortion, is generally the same as, or less than, that from use of oral contraceptives. [See graph above.]

HOW TO USE ORAL CONTRACEPTIVES AS SAFELY AND EFFECTIVELY AS POSSIBLE, ONCE YOU HAVE DECIDED TO USE THEM

1. *What to Tell Your Doctor.* You can make use of the pill as safe as possible, by telling your doctor if you have any of the following:

a. Conditions that mean you should not use oral contraceptives:

If you *now* have any of the following:

1. Blood clots in the legs, lungs, eyes, or elsewhere in the body.
2. Chest pains on exertion (angina pectoris).
3. Known or suspected cancer of the breast or sex organs, such as the womb (uterus), vagina, or cervix.
4. Unusual vaginal bleeding that has not been diagnosed by your doctor.
5. Known or suspected pregnancy (one or more menstrual periods missed).

If you have *ever* had any of the following:

1. Heart attack or stroke (clots or bleeding in the brain).
2. Blood clots in the legs, lungs, eyes, or elsewhere in the body.
3. Liver tumor associated with use of the pill or other estrogen-containing products.

b. Inform your doctor of the following conditions since s/he will want to watch them closely or they might cause him/her to suggest another method of contraception:

A family history of breast cancer
Breast nodules (lumps), fibrocystic disease (breast cysts), abnormal mammograms (x-ray pictures of the breasts), or abnormal Pap smears
Diabetes
High blood pressure
High blood cholesterol
Cigarette-smoking
Migraine

Figure 1. Estimated annual number of deaths associated with control of fertility and no control per 100,000 nonsterile women by regimen of control and age of woman.

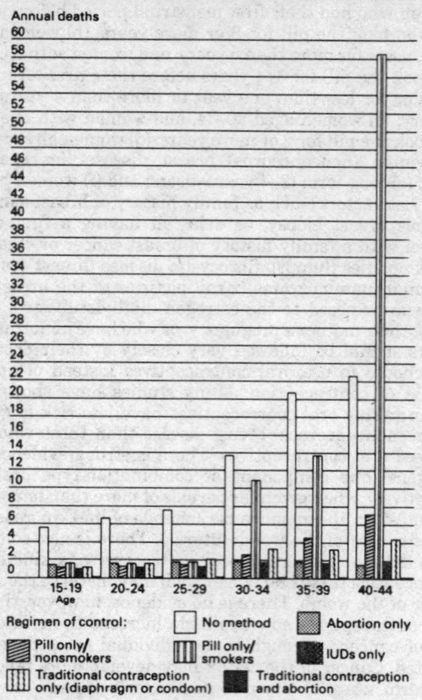

Annual deaths
60
58
56
54
52
50
48
46
44
42
40
38
36
34
32
30
28
26
24
22
20
18
16
14
12
10
8
6
4
2
0
15-19
20-24
25-29
30-34
35-39
40-44
Age
Regimen of control:
No method
Abortion only
Pill only/ nonsmokers
Pill only/ smokers
IUDs only
Traditional contraception only (diaphragm or condom)
Traditional contraception and abortion

Heart or kidney disease
Asthma
Problems during a prior pregnancy
Epilepsy
Mental depression
Fibroid tumors of the womb
History of jaundice (yellowing of the whites of the eyes or of the skin)
Gallbladder disease
Varicose veins
Tuberculosis
Plans for elective surgery
Previous problems with your periods (irregularities)
Use of any of the following kinds of drugs, which might interact with the pill: antibiotics (such as rifampin, ampicillin, and tetracycline), sulfa drugs, drugs for epilepsy or migraine, painkillers, tranquilizers, sedatives or sleeping pills, blood-thinning drugs, cortisone-like drugs, vitamins, drugs being used for the treatment of depression, high blood pressure, high blood sugar (diabetes), elevated blood lipids, or asthma.

c. Once you are using oral contraceptives, you should be alert for signs of a serious adverse effect and call your doctor immediately if any of these occur:

Sharp pain in the chest, coughing up of blood, or sudden shortness of breath (indicating possible clots in the lungs).
Pain in the calf (possible clot in the leg).
Crushing chest pain or heaviness (indicating possible heart attack).
Sudden severe headache or vomiting, dizziness or fainting, disturbance of vision or speech, or weakness or numbness in an arm or leg (indicating a possible stroke).
Sudden partial or complete loss of vision (indicating a possible clot in the blood vessels of the eye).
Abnormal vaginal bleeding.
Breast discharge or lumps (you should ask your doctor to show you how to examine your own breasts).
Severe and/or persistent pain or a mass in the abdomen (indicating a possible tumor of the liver which might have ruptured).
Severe depression.
Yellowing of the whites of the eyes or of the skin (jaundice).
Unusual swelling.
Other unusual conditions.

2. *How to Take the Pill So That It Is Most Effective. Dosage Schedules.* See later sections in this leaflet concerning spotting, breakthrough bleeding, forgotten pills, and missed menstruation.

Each tablet dispenser contains 21 or 28 tablets in numbered rows of 7 tablets each. The days of the week are printed above the columns. To remove a pill, press down on it. The pill will be released through the back of the dispenser.

Read the information below carefully because maximum contraceptive effectiveness of oral contraceptives depends on your taking the pills exactly as directed, every day, and at time intervals of 24 hours. It is recommended that you take your pill at the same time every day.

The first time you take the pill, use another method of contraception in addition, until you have taken the first 7 pills.

21-Day Schedules

For use with Norethin 1/35E™-21 and Norethin 1/50M™-21.

Sunday Schedule: Start taking the pills on the first Sunday after the menstrual period begins. If it begins on a Sunday, start taking the pills that same day. Begin with row #1, Sunday, and take one pill every day, at the same time, in order, for 21 days. Then stop taking the pills for one week (7 days). Begin the next cycle, as before, on Sunday.

Day-5 Schedule: Start taking the pills on day 5 of the menstrual cycle, counting day 1 as the first day of menstrual flow. Begin with row #1 on the day of the week corresponding to day 5. Take a pill every day, at the same time, for 21 days. Complete row #3, then take any pills remaining in row #1. Then stop taking the pill for one week (7 days). Begin the next cycle on the same day of the week as you began the first cycle.

28-Day Schedules

For use with Norethin 1/35E™-28 and Norethin 1/50M™-28.

Sunday Schedule: The first pill in row #1 must be taken on the first Sunday after menstrual flow begins, or on that same day if it begins on Sunday. Take one pill every day, at the same time, and in order. When you finish row #1, begin with Sunday in row #2, and so on. After you have taken 28 pills, begin a new cycle, on Sunday, just as described. Take a pill faithfully every day, even if menstrual flow stops while you are still taking the blue pills in row #4. If you miss one or more of the blue pills (row #4), your chances of becoming pregnant will not increase providing the white pill schedule has been followed.

Day-5 Schedule: Start taking the white pills on day 5 of the menstrual cycle, counting day 1 as the first day of menstrual flow. Begin with row #1 on the day of the week corresponding to day 5. Take a white pill every day, at the same time, for 21 days. Complete row #3, then take any white pills remaining in row #1. **Take all of the white pills before taking any blue placebo pills in row #4.** After all of the white pills are used, take the blue placebo pills in row #4 for one week (7 days). Begin the next cycle on the same day of the week as you began the first cycle. Take a pill faithfully every day, even if menstrual flow stops while you are still taking the blue pills in row #4. If you miss one or more of the blue pills (row #4), your chances of becoming pregnant will not increase providing the white pill schedule has been followed.

Take your pill faithfully every "pill day"!

It is important that you take a pill without fail every pill day, at intervals of 24 hours, for two reasons. First, your ovaries may release an egg and therefore you may become pregnant if you do not take your pills regularly. Second, you may spot or start to flow between your periods. This may be inconvenient.

Take your pill at the same time every day!

You are probably wondering why the same time of day is important. By taking your pill at the same time every day it becomes a good habit, and you are much less likely to forget. You may wish to keep your pills in the medicine cabinet near your toothbrush as a reminder to take them when you brush your teeth at night. The best time to take your daily pill may be either with your evening meal or at bedtime. You may find it helpful to associate your pill-taking with something else you do every day at a particular time.

Another very important reason for you to take your pills as "regular as clockwork" is that you are protected best when you take one every 24 hours; they are made to work that way. Just remember that once every day is not the same as once every 24 hours. Here is why: Suppose you were to take your Monday pill in the morning when you get up, and then not take your Tuesday pill till the evening before you go to bed. True, you will have taken a pill each day, on Monday and on Tuesday—but the time between pill-taking will probably have been more than 36 hours, or more than 1½ days! You might spot. Chances are you would still be protected and would not get pregnant, but why risk it when it is so easy to guarantee yourself maximal protection by taking your pill faithfully every pill day and at the same time every pill day?

In summary, you should take the pills exactly as directed and at intervals of 24 hours in order to achieve maximum contraceptive effectiveness.

Spotting. This is a slight staining between your menstrual periods which may not even require a pad. Some women spot even though they take their pills exactly as directed. Many women spot although they have never taken the pills. Spotting does not mean that your ovaries are releasing an egg. Spotting may be the result of irregular pill-taking. Getting back on schedule will usually stop it.

If you should spot while taking the pills you should not be alarmed because spotting usually stops by itself within a few days. It seldom occurs after the first pill cycle. Consult your

doctor if spotting persists for more than a few days or if it occurs after the second cycle.

Unexpected (Breakthrough) Bleeding. Unexpected (breakthrough) bleeding does not mean your ovaries have released an egg. It seldom occurs, but when it does happen it is most common in the first pill cycle. It is a flow much like a regular period, requiring the use of a pad or tampon.

If you experience breakthrough bleeding use a pad or tampon and continue with your schedule. Usually your periods will become regular within a few cycles. Breakthrough bleeding will seldom bother you again.

Consult your doctor if breakthrough bleeding does not stop within a week or if it occurs after the second cycle.

Forgotten Pills. There is little likelihood of your getting pregnant if only one active pill is missed; however, the possibility increases with each successive day that the scheduled active pills are missed. If you forget to take a pill one day, take two the next day—the one you forgot as soon as you remember and your regular pill at your usual time.

If you forget your pills (except the inactive blue pills in Norethin 1/35E™-28 and Norethin 1/50M™-28) on two consecutive days, do not be surprised if you spot or start to flow. You should take two pills each day for the next two days, and use an additional method of protection for the remainder of the cycle.

If you are using Norethin 1/35E™-28 or Norethin 1/50M™-28 and forget to take one or more blue pills, begin a new cycle on the same day of the week as you began the previous cycle; use a new package and start taking the white pills. Missing the blue pills does not increase your chances of getting pregnant providing the white pill schedule has been followed.

Missed Menstruation. At times there may be no menstrual period after a cycle of pills. Therefore, if you miss one menstrual period but have taken the pills *exactly as you were supposed to,* continue as usual into the next cycle. You may wish to call your doctor. If you have not taken the pills correctly and miss a menstrual period, *you may be pregnant* and should stop taking oral contraceptives until your doctor determines whether or not you are pregnant. Until you can get to your doctor, use another form of contraception. If two consecutive menstrual periods are missed, you should stop taking the pills until it is determined whether you are pregnant. If you do become pregnant while using oral contraceptives, you should discuss the risks to the developing baby with your doctor.

3. *Periodic Examinations.* Your doctor will take a complete medical and family history before prescribing oral contraceptives. At that time and about once a year thereafter, s/he will generally examine your blood pressure, breasts, abdomen, and internal female organs (including a Pap smear test for cancer of the cervix) and perform certain laboratory tests. Certain health problems or conditions in your medical or family history may require that your doctor see you more frequently while you are taking the pill.

SUMMARY

Oral contraceptives are the most effective method, except sterilization, for preventing pregnancy. Other methods, when used conscientiously, are also very effective and have fewer risks. The serious side effects of oral contraceptives are uncommon, but the risk of experiencing them may persist after discontinuing the pill. The pill is a very convenient method for preventing pregnancy.

Women who use oral contraceptives should not smoke.

If you have certain conditions or have had these conditions in the past, you should not use oral contraceptives because of increased risk. These conditions are listed in this leaflet. If you do not have these conditions, and decide to use the pill, please read this leaflet carefully so that you can use the pill safely and effectively.

Based on your doctor's assessment of your medical needs, this drug has been prescribed for you. Do not give it to anyone else.

See your doctor regularly, ask any questions you may have about the use of the pill, and report any special problems that may arise.

Be certain to read new revisions of this leaflet. You may check the date of the most recent revision by phoning the manufacturer toll free at 1-800-323-4204 or by writing to the address below.

Address medical inquiries to:
G.D. Searle & Co.
Medical & Scientific Information Department
4901 Searle Parkway
Skokie, IL 60077 6/25/90•A05604-3

Shown in Product Identification Section, page 429

PIROXICAM CAPSULES USP ℞

[per-ox 'i-cam]

DESCRIPTION

Piroxicam is 4-Hydroxy-2-methyl-*N*-2-pyridinyl-2*H*-1,2-benzothiazine-3-carboxamide 1,1-dioxide, an oxicam.

The molecular and structural formulas are:

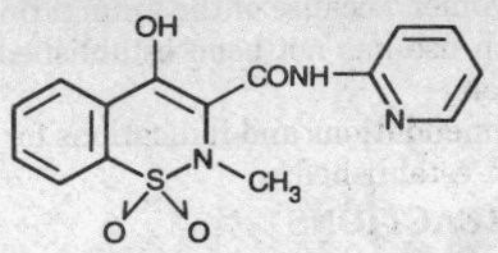

Piroxicam has a molecular weight of 331.35.

Members of the oxicam family are not carboxylic acids, but they are acidic by virtue of the enolic 4-hydroxy substituent. Piroxicam occurs as a white crystalline solid, sparingly soluble in water, dilute acid, and most organic solvents. It is slightly soluble in alcohols and in aqueous alkaline solution. It exhibits a weakly acidic 4-hydroxy proton (pKa 5.1) and a weakly basic pyridyl nitrogen (pKa 1.8).

Each capsule, for oral administration, contains 10 mg or 20 mg piroxicam. In addition, each capsule contains the following inactive ingredients; lactose hydrous; magnesium stearate; sodium lauryl sulfate; corn starch; gelatin and coloring agents titanium dioxide, FD&C Blue 1, and FD&C Red 40.

CLINICAL PHARMACOLOGY

Piroxicam has shown anti-inflammatory, analgesic and antipyretic properties in animals. Edema, erythema, tissue proliferation, fever, and pain can all be inhibited in laboratory animals by the administration of piroxicam. It is effective regardless of the etiology of the inflammation. The mode of action of piroxicam is not fully established at this time. However, a common mechanism for the above effects may exist in the ability of piroxicam to inhibit the biosynthesis of prostaglandins, known mediators of inflammation.

It is established that piroxicam does not act by stimulating the pituitary-adrenal axis.

Piroxicam is well absorbed following oral administration. Drug plasma concentrations are proportional for 10- and 20-mg doses, generally peak within 3 to 5 hours after medication, and subsequently decline with a mean half-life of 50 hours (range of 30 to 86 hours, although values outside of this range have been encountered).

This prolonged half-life results in the maintenance of relatively stable plasma concentrations throughout the day on once-daily doses and to significant drug accumulation upon multiple dosing. A single 20-mg dose generally produces peak piroxicam plasma levels of 1.5 to 2 mcg/mL, while maximum drug plasma concentrations, after repeated daily ingestion of 20 mg piroxicam, usually stabilize at 3 to 8 mcg/mL. Most patients approximate steady-state plasma levels within 7 to 12 days. Higher levels, which approximate steady state at 2 to 3 weeks, have been observed in patients in whom longer plasma half-lives of piroxicam occurred.

Piroxicam and its biotransformation products are excreted in urine and feces, with about twice as much appearing in the urine as in the feces. Metabolism occurs by hydroxylation at the 5 position of the pyridyl side chain and conjugation of this product; by cyclodehydration; and by a sequence of reactions involving hydrolysis of the amide linkage, decarboxylation, ring contraction, and N-demethylation. Less than 5% of the daily dose is excreted unchanged.

Concurrent administration of aspirin (3900 mg/day) and piroxicam (20 mg/day) resulted in a reduction of plasma levels of piroxicam to about 80% of their normal values. The use of piroxicam in conjunction with aspirin is not recommended because data are inadequate to demonstrate that the combination produces greater improvement than that achieved with aspirin alone and the potential for adverse reactions is increased. The effects of impaired renal function or hepatic disease on plasma levels have not been established.

Piroxicam, like salicylates and other nonsteroidal anti-inflammatory agents, is associated with symptoms of gastrointestinal tract irritation (see *Adverse Reactions*). However, in a study utilizing ^{51}Cr-tagged red blood cells, 20 mg of piroxicam administered as a single dose for 4 days did not result in a significant increase in fecal blood loss and did not detectably affect the gastric mucosa. In the same study a total daily dose of 3900 mg of aspirin, ie, 972 mg qid, caused a significant increase in fecal blood loss and mucosal lesions as demonstrated by gastroscopy.

In controlled clinical trials, the effectiveness of piroxicam has been established for both acute exacerbations and long-term management of rheumatoid arthritis and osteoarthritis.

The therapeutic effects of piroxicam are evident early in the treatment of both diseases with a progressive increase in response over several (8 to 12) weeks. Efficacy is seen in terms of pain relief and, when present, subsidence of inflammation.

Doses of 20 mg/day piroxicam display a therapeutic effect comparable to therapeutic doses of aspirin, with a lower incidence of minor gastrointestinal effects and tinnitus.

Piroxicam has been administered concomitantly with fixed doses of gold and corticosteroids. The existence of a "steroid-sparing" effect has not been adequately studied to date.

INDICATIONS AND USAGE

Piroxicam is indicated for acute or long-term use in the relief of signs and symptoms of the following:

1. osteoarthritis
2. rheumatoid arthritis

Dosage recommendations for use in children have not been established.

CONTRAINDICATIONS

Piroxicam should not be used in patients who have previously exhibited hypersensitivity to it, or in individuals with the syndrome comprised of bronchospasm, nasal polyps, and angioedema precipitated by aspirin or other nonsteroidal anti-inflammatory drugs.

WARNINGS

Risk of GI Ulceration, Bleeding and Perforation with NSAID Therapy

Serious gastrointestinal toxicity such as bleeding, ulceration, and perforation can occur at any time, with or without warning symptoms, in patients treated chronically with NSAID therapy. Although minor upper gastrointestinal problems, such as dyspepsia, are common, usually developing early in therapy, the physician should remain alert for ulceration and bleeding in patients treated chronically with NSAIDs even in the absence of previous GI tract symptoms. In patients observed in clinical trials of several months to 2 years duration, symptomatic upper GI ulcers, gross bleeding or perforation appear to occur in approximately 1% of patients treated for 3 to 6 months, and in about 2 to 4% of patients treated for 1 year. Physicians should inform patients about the signs and/or symptoms of serious GI toxicity and what steps to take if they occur.

Studies to date have not identified any subset of patients not at risk of developing peptic ulceration and bleeding. Except for a prior history of serious GI events and other risk factors known to be associated with peptic ulcer disease, such as alcoholism, smoking, etc, no risk factors (eg, age, sex) have been associated with increased risk. Elderly or debilitated patients seem to tolerate ulceration or bleeding less well than other individuals and most spontaneous reports of fatal GI events are in this population. Studies to date are inconclusive concerning the relative risk of various NSAIDs in causing such reactions. High doses of any NSAID probably carry a greater risk of these reactions, although controlled clinical trials showing this do not exist in most cases. In considering the use of relatively large doses (within the recommended dosage range), sufficient benefit should be anticipated to offset the potential increased risk of GI toxicity.

PRECAUTIONS

Renal Effects: As with other nonsteroidal anti-inflammatory drugs, long-term administration of piroxicam to animals has resulted in renal papillary necrosis and other abnormal renal pathology. In humans, there have been reports of acute interstitial nephritis with hematuria, proteinuria, and occasionally, nephrotic syndrome.

A second form of renal toxicity has been seen in patients with prerenal conditions leading to a reduction in renal blood flow or blood volume, where the renal prostaglandins have a supportive role in the maintenance of renal perfusion. In these patients administration of an NSAID may cause a dose-dependent reduction in prostaglandin formation and may precipitate overt renal decompensation. Patients at greatest risk of this reaction are those with impaired renal function, heart failure, liver dysfunction, those taking diuretics, and the elderly. Discontinuation of NSAID therapy is typically followed by recovery to the pretreatment state.

Because of extensive renal excretion of piroxicam and its biotransformation products (less than 5% of the daily dose excreted unchanged, see *Clinical Pharmacology*), lower doses of piroxicam should be anticipated in patients with impaired renal function, and they should be carefully monitored.

Although other nonsteroidal anti-inflammatory drugs do not have the same direct effects on platelets that aspirin does, all drugs inhibiting prostaglandin biosynthesis do interfere with platelet function to some degree; therefore, patients who may be adversely affected by such an action should be carefully observed when piroxicam is administered.

Because of reports of adverse eye findings with nonsteroidal anti-inflammatory agents, it is recommended that patients who develop visual complaints during treatment with piroxicam have ophthalmic evaluation.

As with other nonsteroidal anti-inflammatory drugs, borderline elevations of one or more liver tests may occur in up to 15% of patients. These abnormalities may progress, may remain essentially unchanged, or may be transient with continued therapy. The SGPT (ALT) test is probably the most sensitive indicator of liver dysfunction. Meaningful (three times the upper limit of normal) elevations of SGPT or SGOT (AST) occurred in controlled clinical trials in less than 1% of patients. A patient with symptoms and/or signs suggesting liver dysfunction, or in whom an abnormal liver test has occurred, should be evaluated for evidence of the devel-

Continued on next page

Schiapparelli Searle—Cont.

opment of more severe hepatic reaction while on therapy with piroxicam. Severe hepatic reactions, including jaundice and cases of fatal hepatitis, have been reported with piroxicam. Although such reactions are rare, if abnormal liver tests persist or worsen, if clinical signs and symptoms consistent with liver disease develop, or if systemic manifestations occur (eg, eosinophilia, rash, etc), piroxicam should be discontinued. (See also *Adverse Reactions.*)

Although at the recommended dose of 20 mg/day of piroxicam increased fecal blood loss due to gastrointestinal irritation did not occur (see *Clinical Pharmacology*), in about 4% of the patients treated with piroxicam alone or concomitantly with aspirin, reductions in hemoglobin and hematocrit values were observed. Therefore, these values should be determined if signs or symptoms of anemia occur.

Peripheral edema has been observed in approximately 2% of the patients treated with piroxicam. Therefore, as with other nonsteroidal anti-inflammatory drugs, piroxicam should be used with caution in patients with heart failure, hypertension, or other conditions predisposing to fluid retention, since its usage may be associated with a worsening of these conditions.

A combination of dermatological and/or allergic signs and symptoms suggestive of serum sickness have occasionally occurred in conjunction with the use of piroxicam. These include arthralgias, pruritus, fever, fatigue, and rash including vesiculo bullous reactions and exfoliative dermatitis.

Information for Patients

Piroxicam, like other drugs of its class, is not free of side effects. The side effects of these drugs can cause discomfort and, rarely, there are more serious side effects, such as gastrointestinal bleeding, which may result in hospitalization and even fatal outcomes.

NSAIDs (Nonsteroidal Anti-Inflammatory Drugs) are often essential agents in the management of arthritis, but they also may be commonly employed for conditions which are less serious.

Physicians may wish to discuss with their patients the potential risks (see *Warnings, Precautions,* and *Adverse Reactions* sections) and likely benefits of NSAID treatment, particularly when the drugs are used for less serious conditions where treatment without NSAIDs may represent an acceptable alternative to both the patient and physician.

Laboratory Tests

Because serious GI tract ulceration and bleeding can occur without warning symptoms, physicians should follow chronically treated patients for the signs and symptoms of ulceration and bleeding and should inform them of the importance of this follow-up (see *Risk of GI Ulceration, Bleeding and Perforation with NSAID Therapy*).

Drug Interactions

Piroxicam is highly protein bound, and, therefore, might be expected to displace other protein-bound drugs. Although this has not occurred in in vitro studies with coumarin-type anticoagulants, interactions with coumarin-type anticoagulants have been reported with piroxicam since marketing, therefore, physicians should closely monitor patients for a change in dosage requirements when administering piroxicam to patients on coumarin-type anticoagulants and other highly protein-bound drugs.

Plasma levels of piroxicam are depressed to approximately 80% of their normal values when piroxicam is administered in conjunction with aspirin (3900 mg/day) (see *Clinical Pharmacology*).

Nonsteroidal anti-inflammatory agents, including piroxicam, have been reported to increase steady-state plasma lithium levels. It is recommended that plasma lithium levels be monitored when initiating, adjusting and discontinuing piroxicam.

Carcinogenesis, Chronic Animal Toxicity and Impairment of Fertility

Subacute and chronic toxicity studies have been carried out in rats, mice, dogs, and monkeys.

The pathology most often seen was that characteristically associated with the animal toxicology of anti-inflammatory agents: renal papillary necrosis (see *Precautions*) and gastrointestinal lesions.

In classical studies in laboratory animals piroxicam did not show any teratogenic potential.

Reproductive studies revealed no impairment of fertility in animals.

Pregnancy and Nursing Mothers

Like other drugs which inhibit the synthesis and release of prostaglandins, piroxicam increased the incidence of dystocia and delayed parturition in pregnant animals when piroxicam administration was continued late into pregnancy. Gastrointestinal tract toxicity was increased in pregnant females in the last trimester of pregnancy compared to nonpregnant females or females in earlier trimesters of pregnancy.

Piroxicam is not recommended for use in nursing mothers or in pregnant women because of the animal findings and since safety for such use has not been established in humans.

Use in Children

Dosage recommendations and indications for use in children have not been established.

ADVERSE REACTIONS

The incidence of adverse reactions of piroxicam is based on clinical trials involving approximately 2300 patients, about 400 of whom were treated for more than 1 year and 170 for more than 2 years. About 30% of all patients receiving daily doses of 20 mg of piroxicam experienced side effects. Gastrointestinal symptoms were the most prominent side effects —occurring in approximately 20% of the patients, which in most instances did not interfere with the course of therapy. Of the patients experiencing gastrointestinal side effects, approximately 5% discontinued therapy with an overall incidence of peptic ulceration of about 1%.

Other than the gastrointestinal symptoms, edema, dizziness, headache, changes in hematological parameters, and rash have been reported in a small percentage of patients. Routine ophthalmoscopy and slit-lamp examinations have revealed no evidence of ocular changes in 205 patients followed from 3 to 24 months while on therapy.

Incidence Greater Than 1%

The following adverse reactions occurred more frequently than 1 in 100.

Gastrointestinal: stomatitis, anorexia, epigastric distress,* nausea,* constipation, abdominal discomfort, flatulence, diarrhea, abdominal pain, indigestion.

Hematological: decreases in hemoglobin* and hematocrit* (see *Precautions*), anemia, leucopenia, eosinophilia.

Dermatologic: pruritus, rash.

Central Nervous System: dizziness, somnolence, vertigo.

Urogenital: BUN and creatinine elevations (see *Precautions*).

Body as a Whole: headache, malaise.

Special Senses: tinnitus.

Cardiovascular/Respiratory: edema (see *Precautions*).

Incidence Less Than 1% (Causal Relationship Probable)

The following adverse reactions occurred less frequently than 1 in 100. The probability exists that there is a causal relationship between piroxicam and these reactions.

Gastrointestinal: liver function abnormalities, jaundice, hepatitis (see *Precautions*), vomiting, hematemesis, melena, gastrointestinal bleeding, perforation and ulceration (see *Warnings*), dry mouth.

Hematological: thrombocytopenia, petechial rash, ecchymosis, bone marrow depression including aplastic anemia, epistaxis.

Dermatologic: sweating, erythema, bruising, desquamation, exfoliative dermatitis, erythema multiforme, toxic epidermal necrolysis, Stevens-Johnson syndrome, vesiculo bullous reaction, photoallergic skin reactions.

Central Nervous System: depression, insomnia, nervousness.

Urogenital: hematuria, proteinuria, interstitial nephritis, renal failure, hyperkalemia, glomerulitis, papillary necrosis, nephrotic syndrome (see *Precautions*).

Body as a Whole: pain (colic), fever, flu-like syndrome (see *Precautions*).

Special Senses: swollen eyes, blurred vision, eye irritations.

Cardiovascular/Respiratory: hypertension, worsening of congestive heart failure (see *Precautions*), exacerbation of angina.

Metabolic: hypoglycemia, hyperglycemia, weight increase, weight decrease.

Hypersensitivity: anaphylaxis, bronchospasm, urticaria/angioedema, vasculitis, "serum sickness" (see *Precautions*).

Incidence Less Than 1% (Causal Relationship Unknown)

Other adverse reactions were reported with a frequency of less than 1 in 100, but a causal relationship between piroxicam and the reaction could not be determined.

Gastrointestinal: pancreatitis.

Dermatologic: onycholysis, loss of hair.

Central Nervous System: akathisia, hallucinations, mood alterations, dream abnormalities, mental confusion, paresthesias.

Urogenital System: dysuria.

Body as a Whole: weakness.

Cardiovascular/Respiratory: palpitations, dyspnea.

Hypersensitivity: positive ANA.

Special Senses: transient hearing loss.

Hematological: hemolytic anemia.

OVERDOSAGE

In the event treatment for overdosage is required the long plasma half-life (see *Clinical Pharmacology*) of piroxicam should be considered. The absence of experience with acute overdosage precludes characterization of sequelae and recommendation of specific antidotal efficacy at this time. It is reasonable to assume, however, that the standard measures of gastric evacuation and general supportive therapy would apply. In addition to supportive measures, the use of activated charcoal may effectively reduce the absorption and reabsorption of piroxicam. Experiments in dogs have demonstrated that the use of multiple-dose treatments with activated charcoal could reduce the half-life of piroxicam elimination from 27 hours (without charcoal) to 11 hours and reduce the systemic bioavailability of piroxicam by as much as 37% when activated charcoal is given as late as 6 hours after administration of piroxicam.

*Reactions occurring in 3% to 9% of patients treated with piroxicam. Reactions occurring in 1% to 3% of patients are unmarked.

DOSAGE AND ADMINISTRATION

Rheumatoid Arthritis, Osteoarthritis

It is recommended that piroxicam therapy be initiated and maintained at a single daily dose of 20 mg. If desired the daily dose may be divided. Because of the long half-life of piroxicam, steady-state blood levels are not reached for 7 to 12 days. Therefore, although the therapeutic effects of piroxicam are evident early in treatment, there is a progressive increase in response over several weeks and the effect of therapy should not be assessed for 2 weeks. Dosage recommendations and indications for use in children have not been established.

HOW SUPPLIED

Piroxicam 10-mg capsules have a light blue opaque body imprinted with 5752 and an orange opaque cap imprinted with SCS.

Piroxicam 20-mg capsules have an orange opaque body imprinted with 5762 and an orange opaque cap imprinted with SCS.

Store below 86°F (30°C). Dispense in a tight, light-resistant container with a child-resistant closure.

Caution: Federal law prohibits dispensing without prescription.

4/27/92 ● N252

Manufactured for
Schiapparelli Searle
Box 5110, Chicago IL 60680
by Searle Canada Inc.
Oakville, Ontario L6H 1M5
Canada

Shown in Product Identification Section, page 429

PRO-BANTHĪNE® Tablets ℞

[*prō-ban 'thīne*]
(propantheline bromide)

DESCRIPTION

Pro-Banthīne oral tablets contain 15 mg or 7½ mg of the anticholinergic propantheline bromide, (2-hydroxyethyl)-diisopropylmethylammonium bromide xanthene-9-carboxylate.

The structural formula of Pro-Banthīne is

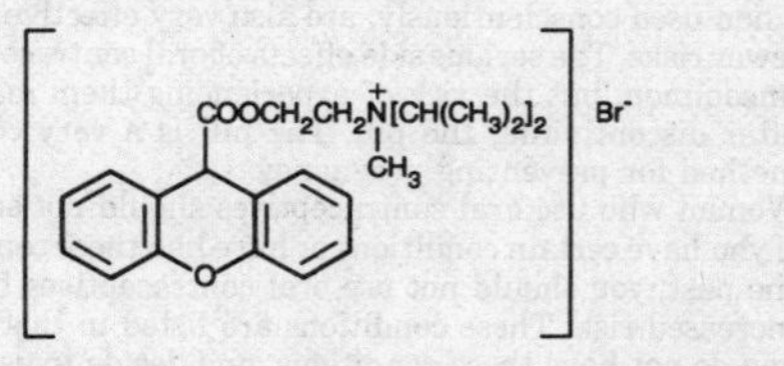
COOCH2CH2N[CH(CH3)2]2
CH3
Br-

Propantheline bromide is very soluble in water, alcohol, and chloroform, but it is practically insoluble in ether and in benzene. Its molecular weight is 448.40.

Inactive ingredients include calcium carbonate, corn starch, edible ink, flavor, lactose, magnesium carbonate, magnesium stearate, sucrose, talc, titanium dioxide, and waxes. The 15-mg tablet also contains red oxide and yellow oxide as coloring agents.

CLINICAL PHARMACOLOGY

Pro-Banthīne inhibits gastrointestinal motility and diminishes gastric acid secretion. The drug also inhibits the action of acetylcholine at the postganglionic nerve endings of the parasympathetic nervous system.

Propantheline bromide is extensively metabolized in man primarily by hydrolysis to the inactive materials xanthene-9-carboxylic acid and (2-hydroxyethyl) diisopropylmethylammonium bromide. After a single 30-mg oral dose given as two 15-mg tablets the mean peak plasma concentration of propantheline was 21 ng/ml at one hour in six healthy subjects.

The plasma elimination half-life of propantheline is about 1.6 hours. Approximately 70% of the dose is excreted in the urine, mostly as metabolites. The urinary excretion of propantheline is about 3% after oral tablet administration.

INDICATIONS AND USAGE

Pro-Banthīne is effective as adjunctive therapy in the treatment of peptic ulcer.

CONTRAINDICATIONS

Pro-Banthīne (propantheline bromide) is contraindicated in patients with:

1. Glaucoma, since mydriasis is to be avoided.
2. Obstructive disease of the gastrointestinal tract (pyloro-duodenal stenosis, achalasia, paralytic ileus, etc.).
3. Obstructive uropathy (eg, bladder-neck obstruction due to prostatic hypertrophy).
4. Intestinal atony of elderly or debilitated patients.
5. Severe ulcerative colitis or toxic megacolon complicating ulcerative colitis.
6. Unstable cardiovascular adjustment in acute hemorrhage.
7. Myasthenia gravis.

WARNINGS

In the presence of a high environmental temperature, heat prostration (fever and heat stroke due to decreased sweating) can occur with the use of Pro-Banthīne.

Diarrhea may be an early symptom of incomplete intestinal obstruction, especially in patients with ileostomy or colostomy. In this instance treatment with Pro-Banthīne would be inappropriate and possibly harmful.

With overdosage, a curare-like action may occur (ie, neuromuscular blockade leading to muscular weakness and possible paralysis).

Pro-Banthīne may cause increased heart rate and, therefore, should be used with caution in patients with heart disease.

PRECAUTIONS

General: Pro-Banthīne (propantheline bromide) should be used with caution in the elderly and in all patients with autonomic neuropathy, hepatic or renal disease, hyperthyroidism, coronary heart disease, congestive heart failure, cardiac tachyarrhythmias, hypertension, or hiatal hernia associated with reflux esophagitis, since anticholinergics may aggravate this condition.

In patients with ulcerative colitis, large doses of Pro-Banthīne may suppress intestinal motility to the point of producing paralytic ileus and, for this reason, may precipitate or aggravate toxic megacolon, a serious complication of the disease.

Information for patients: Pro-Banthīne may produce drowsiness or blurred vision. The patient should be cautioned regarding activities requiring mental alertness, such as operating a motor vehicle or other machinery or performing hazardous work, while taking this drug.

Drug interactions: Anticholinergics may delay absorption of other medication given concomitantly.

Excessive cholinergic blockade may occur if Pro-Banthīne is given concomitantly with belladonna alkaloids, synthetic or semisynthetic anticholinergic agents, narcotic analgesics such as meperidine, Type 1 antiarrhythmic drugs (eg, disopyramide, procainamide, or quinidine), antihistamines, phenothiazines, tricyclic antidepressants, or other psychoactive drugs. Pro-Banthīne may also potentiate the sedative effect of phenothiazines. Increased intraocular pressure may result from concurrent administration of anticholinergics and corticosteroids.

Concurrent use of Pro-Banthīne with slow-dissolving tablets of digoxin may cause increased serum digoxin levels. This interaction can be avoided by using only those digoxin tablets that rapidly dissolve by USP standards.

Carcinogenesis, mutagenesis, impairment of fertility: No long-term fertility, carcinogenicity, or mutagenicity studies have been done with Pro-Banthīne.

Pregnancy: Pregnancy Category C. Animal reproduction studies have not been conducted with Pro-Banthīne. It is also not known whether Pro-Banthīne can cause fetal harm when administered to a pregnant woman or can affect reproduction capacity. Pro-Banthīne should be given to a pregnant woman only if clearly needed.

Nursing mothers: It is not known whether this drug is excreted in human milk. Because many drugs are excreted in human milk, caution should be exercised when Pro-Banthīne is administered to a nursing woman. Suppression of lactation may occur with anticholinergic drugs.

Pediatric use: Safety and effectiveness in children have not been established.

ADVERSE REACTIONS

Varying degrees of drying of salivary secretions may occur as well as decreased sweating. Ophthalmic side effects include blurred vision, mydriasis, cycloplegia, and increased ocular tension. Other reported adverse reactions include urinary hesitancy and retention, tachycardia, palpitations, loss of the sense of taste, headache, nervousness, mental confusion, drowsiness, weakness, dizziness, insomnia, nausea, vomiting, constipation, bloated feeling, impotence, suppression of lactation, and allergic reactions or drug idiosyncrasies, including anaphylaxis, urticaria, and other dermal manifestations.

OVERDOSAGE

The symptoms of overdosage with Pro-Banthīne progress from an intensification of the usual side effects to CNS disturbances (from restlessness and excitement to psychotic behavior), circulatory changes (flushing, fall in blood pressure, circulatory failure), respiratory failure, paralysis, and coma.

Measures to be taken are (1) immediate induction of emesis or lavage of the stomach, (2) injection of physostigmine 0.5 to 2 mg intravenously, repeated as necessary up to a total of 5 mg, and (3) monitoring of vital signs and managing as necessary.

Fever may be treated symptomatically (cooling blanket or alcohol sponging). Excitement of a degree which demands attention may be managed with thiopental sodium 2% solution given slowly intravenously, or diazepam, 5 to 10 mg intravenously or 10 mg intramuscularly. In the event of progression of the curare-like effect to paralysis of the respiratory muscles, mechanical respiration should be instituted and maintained until effective respiratory action returns. The oral LD_{50} of propantheline bromide is 780 mg/kg in the mouse and 370 mg/kg in the rat.

DOSAGE AND ADMINISTRATION

The usual initial adult dosage of Pro-Banthīne tablets is 15 mg taken 30 minutes before each meal and 30 mg at bedtime (a total of 75 mg daily). Subsequent dosage adjustment should be made according to the patient's individual response and tolerance. The administration of one $7\frac{1}{2}$-mg tablet three times a day is convenient for patients with mild manifestations, for geriatric patients, and for those of small stature.

HOW SUPPLIED

Pro-Banthīne 15-mg tablets are round, peach colored, sugar coated, with SCS imprinted on one side and 601 on the other side; bottles of 100 and 500, and cartons containing 100 unit-dose, individually blister-sealed tablets.

Pro-Banthīne $7\frac{1}{2}$-mg tablets are round, white, sugar coated, with SCS imprinted on one side and 611 on the other side; bottles of 100.

Store below 86°F (30°C).

Caution: Federal law prohibits dispensing without prescription.

4/11/91●A05875-2

Schwarz Pharma
Kremers Urban Company
P.O. BOX 2038
5600 W. COUNTY LINE ROAD
MILWAUKEE, WI 53201

CALCIFEROL™ Products
[*kal-si ′fur-ol*]
CALCIFEROL™ Drops　　　　　　　　　　　　　OTC
(ergocalciferol oral solution USP)
8,000 USP Units/mL
CALCIFEROL™ Tablets　　　　　　　　　　　　　℞
(ergocalciferol tablets USP)
50,000 USP Units
CALCIFEROL™ in Oil Injection　　　　　　　　　℞
(ergocalciferol)
500,000 Units/mL

DEPONIT®　　　　　　　　　　　　　　　　　　℞
[*dĕp′ō-nĭt*]
(nitroglycerin transdermal delivery system)

DESCRIPTION

Nitroglycerin is 1,2,3-propanetriol trinitrate, an organic nitrate whose structural formula is:

$$H_2CONO_2$$
$$|$$
$$HCONO_2$$
$$|$$
$$H_2CONO_2$$

and whose molecular weight is 227.09. The organic nitrates are vasodilators, active on both arteries and veins.

The Deponit® transdermal system is a flat unit designed to provide continuous controlled release of nitroglycerin through intact skin. The rate of release of nitroglycerin is linearly dependent upon the area of the applied system; each cm^2 of applied system delivers approximately .013 mg of nitroglycerin per hour. Thus, the 16 cm^2 and 32 cm^2 systems deliver approximately 0.2 and 0.4 mg of nitroglycerin per hour, respectively. The remainder of the nitroglycerin in each system serves as a reservoir and is not delivered in normal use. After 12 hours, for example, each system has delivered 15% of its original content of nitroglycerin. Deponit contains nitroglycerin in a matrix composed of lactose, plasticizer, medical adhesive, polyisobutylene and aluminized plastic for controlled release of the active agent through the skin into the systemic circulation. The 16 cm^2 and 32 cm^2 systems contain 16 mg and 32 mg of nitroglycerin, respectively.

The Deponit system is approximately 0.3 mm thick, insoluble in water, and, as illustrated below, consists of two main elements:

1. A flexible, flesh-colored waterproof covering foil.
2. A multilayered adhesive film that constitutes simultaneously the drug reservoir and the release-control system.

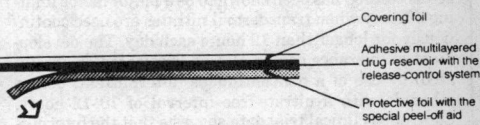

Covering foil
Adhesive multilayered drug reservoir with the release-control system
Protective foil with the special peel-off aid

The system is protected by an aluminum foil which has a patented S-shaped opening to facilitate its removal prior to use of the system. Prior to use the protective foil is removed from the adhesive surface.

CLINICAL PHARMACOLOGY

The principal pharmacological action of nitroglycerin is relaxation of vascular smooth muscle and consequent dilatation of peripheral arteries and veins, especially the latter. Dilatation of the veins promotes peripheral pooling of blood and decreases venous return to the heart, thereby reducing left ventricular end-diastolic pressure and pulmonary capillary wedge pressure (preload). Arteriolar relaxation reduces systemic vascular resistance, systolic arterial pressure, and mean arterial pressure (afterload). Dilatation of the coronary arteries also occurs. The relative importance of preload reduction, afterload reduction and coronary dilatation remains undefined. Dosing regimens for most chronically used drugs are designed to provide plasma concentrations that are continuously greater than a minimally effective concentration. This strategy is inappropriate for organic nitrates. Several well-controlled clinical trials have used exercise testing to assess the anti-anginal efficacy of continuously-delivered nitrates. In the large majority of these trials, active agents were indistinguishable from placebo after 24 hours (or less) of continuous therapy. Attempts to overcome nitrate tolerance by dose escalation, even to doses far in excess of those used acutely, have consistently failed. Only after nitrates have been absent from the body for several hours has their antianginal efficacy been restored.

Pharmacokinetics: The volume of distribution of nitroglycerin is about 3 L/kg, and nitroglycerin is cleared from this volume at extremely rapid rates, with a resulting serum half-life of about 3 minutes. The observed clearance rates (close to 1 L/kg/min) greatly exceed hepatic blood flow; known sites of extrahepatic metabolism include red blood cells and vascular walls. The first products in the metabolism of nitroglycerin are inorganic nitrate and the 1,2- and 1,3-dinitroglycerols. The dinitrates are less effective vasodilators than nitroglycerin, but they are longer-lived in the serum, and their net contribution to the overall effect of chronic nitroglycerin regimens is not known. The dinitrates are further metabolized to (non-vasoactive) mononitrates and, ultimately, to glycerol and carbon dioxide. To avoid development of tolerance to nitroglycerin, drug-free intervals of 10–12 hours are known to be sufficient; shorter intervals have not been well studied. In one well-controlled clinical trial, subjects receiving nitroglycerin appeared to exhibit a rebound or withdrawal effect, so that their exercise tolerance at the end of the daily drug-free interval was *less* than that exhibited by the parallel group receiving placebo. In healthy volunteers, steady-state plasma concentrations of nitroglycerin are reached by about two hours after application of a patch and are maintained for the duration of wearing the system (observations have been limited to 24 hours). Upon removal of the patch, the plasma concentration declines with a half-life of about an hour.

Clinical trials: Regimens in which nitroglycerin patches were worn for 12 hours daily have been studied in well-controlled trials up to 4 weeks in duration. Starting about 2 hours after application and continuing until 10–12 hours after application, patches that deliver at least 0.4 mg of nitroglycerin per hour have consistently demonstrated greater anti-anginal activity than placebo. Lower-dose patches have not been as well studied, but in one large, well-controlled trial in which higher-dose patches were also studied, patches delivering 0.2 mg/hr had significantly *less* anti-anginal activity than placebo. It is reasonable to believe that the rate of nitroglycerin absorption from patches may vary with the site of application, but this relationship has not been adequately studied. The onset of action of transdermal nitroglycerin is not sufficiently rapid for this product to be useful in aborting an acute anginal episode.

Continued on next page

Schwarz Pharma—Cont.

INDICATIONS AND USAGE

This drug product has been conditionally approved by the FDA for the prevention and treatment of angina pectoris due to coronary artery disease. Tolerance to the anti-anginal effects of nitrates (measured by exercise stress testing) has been shown to be a major factor limiting efficacy when transdermal nitrates are used continuously for longer than 12 hours each day. The development of tolerance can be altered (prevented or attenuated) by use of a noncontinuous (intermittent) dosing schedule with a nitrate-free interval of 10–12 hours. Controlled clinical trial data suggests that the intermittent use of nitrates is associated with decreased exercise tolerance, in comparison to placebo, during the last part of the nitrate-free interval; the clinical relevance of this observation is unknown, but the possibility of increased frequency or severity of angina during the nitrate-free interval should be considered. Further investigations of the tolerance phenomenon and best regimen are ongoing. A final evaluation of the effectiveness of the product will be announced by the FDA.

CONTRAINDICATIONS

Allergic reactions to organic nitrates are extremely rare, but they do occur. Nitroglycerin is contraindicated in patients who are allergic to it. Allergy to the adhesives used in nitroglycerin patches has also been reported, and it similarly constitutes a contraindication to the use of this product.

WARNINGS

The benefits of transdermal nitroglycerin in patients with acute myocardial infarction or congestive heart failure have not been established. If one elects to use nitroglycerin in these conditions, careful clinical or hemodynamic monitoring must be used to avoid the hazards of hypotension and tachycardia. A cardioverter/defibrillator should not be discharged through a paddle electrode that overlies a Deponit patch. The arcing that may be seen in this situation is harmless in itself, but it may be associated with local current concentration that can cause damage to the paddles and burns to the patient.

PRECAUTIONS

General:
Severe hypotension, particularly with upright posture, may occur with even small doses of nitroglycerin. This drug should therefore be used with caution in patients who may be volume depleted or who, for whatever reason, are already hypotensive. Hypotension induced by nitroglycerin may be accompanied by paradoxical bradycardia and increased angina pectoris. Nitrate therapy may aggravate the angina caused by hypertrophic cardiomyopathy. As tolerance to other forms of nitroglycerin develops, the effect of sublingual nitroglycerin on exercise tolerance, although still observable, is somewhat blunted. In industrial workers who have had long-term exposure to unknown (presumably high) doses of organic nitrates, tolerance clearly occurs. Chest pain, acute myocardial infarction, and even sudden death have occurred during temporary withdrawal of nitrates from these workers, demonstrating the existence of true physical dependence. Several clinical trials in patients with angina pectoris have evaluated nitroglycerin regimens which incorporated a 10–12 hour nitrate-free interval. In some of these trials, an increase in the frequency of anginal attacks during the nitrate-free interval was observed in a small number of patients. In one trial, patients demonstrated decreased exercise tolerance at the end of the nitrate-free interval. Hemodynamic rebound has been observed only rarely; on the other hand, few studies were so designed that rebound, if it had occurred would have been detected. The importance of these observations to the routine, clinical use of transdermal nitroglycerin is unknown.

Information for Patients:
Daily headaches sometimes accompany treatment with nitroglycerin. In patients who get these headaches, the headaches may be a marker of the activity of the drug. Patients should resist the temptation to avoid headaches by altering the schedule of their treatment with nitroglycerin, since loss of headache may be associated with simultaneous loss of antianginal efficacy. Treatment with nitroglycerin may be associated with lightheadedness on standing, especially just after rising from a recumbent or seated position. This effect may be more frequent in patients who have also consumed alcohol. After normal use, there is enough residual nitroglycerin in discarded patches that they are a potential hazard to children and pets. A patient leaflet is supplied with the systems.

Drug Interactions:
The vasodilating effects of nitroglycerin may be additive with those of other vasodilators. Alcohol, in particular, has been found to exhibit additive effects of this variety.

Carcinogenesis, Mutagenesis, Impairment of Fertility:
No long-term animal studies have examined the carcinogenic or mutagenic potential of nitroglycerin. Nitroglycerin's effect upon reproductive capacity is similarly unknown.

Pregnancy —Pregnancy Category C:
Animal reproduction studies have not been conducted with nitroglycerin. It is also not known whether nitroglycerin can cause fetal harm when administered to a pregnant woman or whether it can affect reproduction capacity. Nitroglycerin should be given to a pregnant woman only if clearly needed.

Nursing Mothers:
It is not known whether nitroglycerin is excreted in human milk. Because many drugs are excreted in human milk, caution should be exercised when nitroglycerin is administered to a nursing woman.

Pediatric use:
Safety and effectiveness in children have not been established.

ADVERSE REACTIONS

Adverse reactions to nitroglycerin are generally dose-related, and almost all of these reactions are the result of nitroglycerin's activity as a vasodilator. Headache, which may be severe, is the most commonly reported side effect. Headache may be recurrent with each daily dose, especially at higher doses. Transient episodes of lightheadedness, occasionally related to blood pressure changes, may also occur. Hypotension occurs infrequently, but in some patients it may be severe enough to warrant discontinuation of therapy. Syncope, crescendo angina, and rebound hypertension have been reported but are uncommon. Extremely rarely, ordinary doses of organic nitrates have caused methemoglobinemia in normal-seeming patients. Methemoglobinemia is so infrequent at these doses that further discussion of its diagnosis and treatment is deferred (see OVERDOSAGE). Application-site irritation may occur but is rarely severe. In two placebo-controlled trials of intermittent therapy with nitroglycerin patches at 0.2 to 0.8 mg/hr, the most frequent adverse reactions among 307 subjects were as follows:

	placebo	patch
headache	18%	63%
lightheadedness	4%	6%
hypotension and/or syncope	0%	4%
increased angina	2%	2%

OVERDOSAGE:

Hemodynamic Effects:
The ill effects of nitroglycerin overdose are generally the results of nitroglycerin's capacity to induce vasodilatation, venous pooling, reduced cardiac output, and hypotension. These hemodynamic changes may have protean manifestations, including increased intracranial pressure, with any or all of persistent throbbing headache, confusion, and moderate fever, vertigo; palpitations; visual disturbances; nausea and vomiting (possibly with colic and even bloody diarrhea); syncope (especially in the upright posture); air hunger and dyspnea, later followed by reduced ventilatory effort; diaphoresis, with the skin either flushed or cold and clammy; heart block and bradycardia; paralysis; coma; seizures; and death. Laboratory determinations of serum levels of nitroglycerin and its metabolites are not widely available, and such determinations have, in any event, no established role in the management of nitroglycerin overdose. No data are available to suggest physiological maneuvers (e.g. maneuvers to change the pH of the urine) that might accelerate elimination of nitroglycerin and its active metabolites. Similarly, it is not known which—if any—of these substances can usefully be removed from the body by hemodialysis. No specific antagonist to the vasodilator effects of nitroglycerin is known, and no intervention has been subject to controlled study as a therapy of nitroglycerin overdose. Because the hypotension associated with nitroglycerin overdose is the result of venodilatation and arterial hypovolemia, prudent therapy in this situation should be directed toward increase in central fluid volume. Passive elevation of the patient's legs may be sufficient, but intravenous infusion of normal saline or similar fluid may also be necessary. The use of epinephrine or other arterial vasoconstrictors in this setting is likely to do more harm than good. In patients with renal disease or congestive heart failure, therapy resulting in central volume expansion is not without hazard. Treatment of nitroglycerin overdose in these patients may be subtle and difficult, and invasive monitoring may be required.

Methemoglobinemia:
Nitrate ions liberated during metabolism of nitroglycerin can oxidize hemoglobin into methemoglobin. Even in patients totally without cytochrome b_5 reductase activity, however, and even assuming that the nitrate moieties of nitroglycerin are quantitatively applied to oxidation of hemoglobin, about 1 mg/kg of nitroglycerin should be required before any of these patients manifests clinically significant ($\geq 10\%$) methemoglobinemia. In patients with normal reductase function, significant production of methemoglobin should require even larger doses of nitroglycerin. In one study in which 36 patients received 2–4 weeks of continuous nitroglycerin therapy at 3.1 to 4.4 mg/hr, the average methemoglobin level measured was 0.2%; this was comparable to that observed in parallel patients who received placebo. Notwithstanding these observations, there are case reports of significant methemoglobinemia in association with moderate overdoses of organic nitrates. None of the affected patients had been thought to be unusually susceptible. Methemoglobin levels are available from most clinical laboratories. The diagnosis should be suspected in patients who exhibit signs of impaired oxygen delivery despite adequate cardiac output and adequate arterial pO_2. Classically, methemoglobinemic blood is described as chocolate brown, without color change on exposure to air. When methemoglobinemia is diagnosed, the treatment of choice is methylene blue, 1–2 mg/kg intravenously.

DOSAGE AND ADMINISTRATION

The suggested starting dose is between 0.2 mg/hr and 0.4 mg/hr. Doses between 0.4 mg/hr and 0.8 mg/hr have shown continued effectiveness for 10–12 hours daily for at least one month (the longest period studied) of intermittent administration. Although the minimum nitrate-free interval has not been defined, data show that a nitrate-free interval of 10–12 hrs is sufficient (see CLINICAL PHARMACOLOGY). Thus, an appropriate dosing schedule for nitroglycerin patches would include a daily patch-on period of 12–14 hours and a daily patch-off period of 10–12 hours. Although some well controlled clinical trials using exercise tolerance testing have shown maintenance of effectiveness when patches are worn continuously, the large majority of such controlled trials have shown the development of tolerance (i.e., complete loss of effect) within the first 24 hours after therapy was initiated. Dose adjustment, even to levels much higher than generally used, did not restore efficacy.

HOW SUPPLIED

Deponit® (nitroglycerin transdermal delivery system) is packaged in cartons containing unit doses of 30 flesh-colored systems on aluminum backings. See table below.
[See table below.]

Nitroglycerin Transdermal Rated Release in vivo	Total Nitroglycerin in System	System Size	Carton Size	NDC
0.2 mg/hr	16 mg	16 cm^2	30	0091-4195-01
0.4 mg/hr	32 mg	32 cm^2	30	0091-4196-01

Store at room temperature not above 25° C (77° F). Do not refrigerate.

CAUTION: Federal law prohibits dispensing without prescription.

US Pat No. 4,524,095 and 4,769,028
Manufactured for
SCHWARZ
PHARMA
Kremers Urban Company
Milwaukee, WI 53201
by Lohmann, Neuwied, West Germany

Shown in Product Identification Section, page 429

FEDAHIST® TIMECAPS™ ℞
FEDAHIST® GYROCAPS® ℞

[fed 'a-hist"]

DESCRIPTION

FEDAHIST® TIMECAPS™ contain 120 mg pseudoephedrine hydrochloride USP and 8 mg chlorpheniramine maleate USP in a timed-release formulation designed for oral b.i.d. dosage.

FEDAHIST® GYROCAPS® contain 65 mg pseudoephedrine hydrochloride USP and 10 mg chlorpheniramine maleate USP in a timed-release formulation designed for oral b.i.d. dosage.

Pseudoephedrine hydrochloride is a nasal decongestant. The empirical formula is $C_{10}H_{15}NO \cdot HCl$ and the molecular weight is 201.70. Chemically, it is benzenemethanol,α-[1-(methylamino)ethyl]-, [S-(R*,R*)]-, hydrochloride. Chlorpheniramine maleate is an antihistamine. The empirical formula is $C_{16}H_{19}ClN_2 \cdot C_4H_4O_4$ and the molecular weight is 390.87. Chemically, it is 2-[p-chloro-α-[2-(dimethylamino)-ethyl]benzyl] pyridine maleate (1:1).

FEDAHIST TIMECAPS also contain as inactive ingredients: FD&C Blue #1, gelatin, pharmaceutical glaze, starch, sucrose, and other ingredients.

FEDAHIST GYROCAPS also contain as inactive ingredients: D&C Yellow #10, FD&C Blue #1, FD&C Blue #2, FD&C Yellow #6, gelatin, pharmaceutical glaze, silicon dioxide, sodium lauryl sulfate, starch, sucrose, titanium dioxide, and other ingredients.

CLINICAL PHARMACOLOGY

Pseudoephedrine is an orally active sympathomimetic amine and exerts a decongestant action on the nasal mucosa. Pseudoephedrine produces peripheral effects similar to those of ephedrine and central effects similar to, but less intense than amphetamines. It has the potential for excitatory side effects. At the recommended oral dosages it has little or no pressor effect in normotensive adults. The serum half-life of pseudoephedrine is approximately 4 to 6 hours. The serum half-life is decreased with increased excretion of drug at urine pH lower than 6 and may be increased with decreased excretion at urine pH higher than 8.

Chlorpheniramine is an antihistamine that possesses anticholinergic and sedative effects. It is considered one of the most effective and least toxic of the histamine antagonists. Chlorpheniramine is a H_1 receptor antagonist. It antagonizes many of the pharmacologic actions of histamine. It prevents released histamine from dilating capillaries and causing edema of the respiratory mucosa. Chlorpheniramine is well absorbed and has a duration of action of 4 to 6 hours (the TIMECAPS and GYROCAPS formulation provide a continuous therapeutic effect for up to 12 hours). Its half-life in serum is 12 to 16 hours. Degradation products of chlorpheniramine's metabolic transformation by the liver are almost completely excreted in 24 hours.

FEDAHIST TIMECAPS release 120 mg pseudoephedrine and 8 mg chlorpheniramine at a controlled and predictable rate for 12 hours. FEDAHIST GYROCAPS release 65 mg pseudoephedrine and 10 mg chlorpheniramine at a controlled and predictable rate for 12 hours. Peak blood levels occur in 4 hours for pseudoephedrine and 6 hours for chlorpheniramine. The apparent plasma half-life is approximately 6 hours for pseudoephedrine and 16 hours for chlorpheniramine. The relative bioavailability of the timed-release dosage form is approximately 85% and 100% for the immediate-release dosage forms for pseudoephedrine and chlorpheniramine, respectively.

INDICATIONS AND USAGE

FEDAHIST is indicated for the relief of nasal congestion and eustachian tube congestion associated with the common cold, sinusitis, and acute upper respiratory infections. FEDAHIST is also indicated for symptomatic relief of perennial and seasonal allergic rhinitis and vasomotor rhinitis. Decongestants in combination with antihistamines have been used to relieve eustachian tube congestion associated with acute eustachian salpingitis, aerotitis, and serous otitis media.

CONTRAINDICATIONS

Sympathomimetic amines are contraindicated in patients with severe hypertension, severe coronary artery disease and in patients on MAO inhibitor therapy. Antihistamines are contraindicated in patients with narrow-angle glaucoma, urinary retention, peptic ulcer, during an asthmatic attack and in patients receiving MAO inhibitors.

Hypersensitivity: Contraindicated in patients with hypersensitivity or idiosyncrasy to sympathomimetic amines. FEDAHIST is also contraindicated in patients hypersensitive to chlorpheniramine and other antihistamines of similar chemical structure.

Nursing Mothers: Contraindicated because of the higher than usual risk for infants from sympathomimetic amines.

Newborn or Premature Infants: FEDAHIST should not be administered to premature or full-term infants.

WARNINGS

Sympathomimetic amines should be used judiciously and sparingly in patients with hypertension, diabetes mellitus, ischemic heart disease, increased intraocular pressure, hyperthyroidism or prostatic hypertrophy (see **CONTRAINDICATIONS**). Sympathomimetics may produce CNS stimulation and convulsions or cardiovascular collapse with accompanying hypotension. Chlorpheniramine maleate has an atropine-like action and should be used with caution in patients with increased intraocular pressure, cardiovascular disease, hypertension or in patients with a history of bronchial asthma (see **CONTRAINDICATIONS**). Antihistamines may cause excitability, especially in children. Do not exceed recommended dosage because at higher doses nervousness, dizziness, or sleeplessness may occur.

Use in the Elderly: The elderly (60 years and older) are more likely to have adverse reactions to sympathomimetics. Overdosage of sympathomimetics in this age group may cause hallucinations, convulsions, CNS depression and death.

PRECAUTIONS

General:

Should be used with caution in patients with diabetes, hypertension, cardiovascular disease and hyperreactivity to ephedrine. The antihistamine may cause drowsiness, therefore ambulatory patients who operate machinery or motor vehicles should be cautioned accordingly.

Information for Patients:

Antihistamines may impair mental and physical abilities required for the performance of potentially hazardous tasks, such as driving a vehicle or operating machinery, and may impair mental alertness in children.

Drug Interactions:

MAO inhibitors and beta adrenergic blockers increase the effect of sympathomimetics. Sympathomimetics may reduce the antihypertensive effects of methyldopa, mecamylamine, reserpine and veratrum alkaloids. Concomitant use of antihistamines with alcohol, tricyclic antidepressants, barbiturates and other CNS depressants may have an additive effect.

Laboratory Test Interactions:

Antihistamines may suppress the wheal and flare reactions to antigen skin testing. Considerable interindividual variation in the extent and duration of suppression have been reported, depending on the antigen and test technique, antihistamine and dosage regimen, time since the last dose and individual response to testing. In one study, usual oral dosages of chlorpheniramine suppressed the wheal response for about 2 days after the last dose. Whenever possible, antihistamines should be discontinued about 4 days prior to skin testing procedures since they may prevent otherwise positive reactions to dermal reactivity indicators.

Carcinogenesis, Mutagenesis, Impairment of Fertility:

No long-term or reproduction studies in animals have been performed with FEDAHIST to evaluate its carcinogenic, mutagenic, and impairment of fertility potential.

Pregnancy—Pregnancy Category C:

Animal reproduction studies have not been conducted with FEDAHIST. It is not known whether FEDAHIST can cause fetal harm when administered to a pregnant woman or can affect reproduction capacity. FEDAHIST may be given to a pregnant woman only if clearly needed.

Nursing Mothers:

Pseudoephedrine is contraindicated in nursing mothers because of the higher than usual risk for infants from sympathomimetic amines.

ADVERSE REACTIONS

Hyperreactive individuals may display ephedrine-like reactions such as tachycardia, palpitations, headache, dizziness or nausea. Patients sensitive to antihistamines may experience mild sedation.

Sympathomimetic drugs have been associated with certain untoward reactions including fear, anxiety, tenseness, restlessness, tremor, weakness, pallor, respiratory difficulty, dysuria, insomnia, hallucinations, convulsions, CNS depression, arrhythmias, and cardiovascular collapse with hypotension.

Possible side effects of antihistamines are drowsiness, restlessness, dizziness, weakness, dry mouth, anorexia, nausea, headache, nervousness, blurring of vision, heartburn, dysuria, and very rarely, dermatitis. Patient idiosyncrasy to adrenergic agents may be manifested by insomnia, dizziness, weakness, tremor or arrhythmias.

OVERDOSAGE

Symptoms: Manifestations of antihistamine overdosage may vary from central nervous system depression (sedation, apnea, cardiovascular collapse) to stimulation (insomnia, hallucinations, tremors or convulsions). Other signs and symptoms may be dizziness, tinnitus, ataxia, blurred vision and hypotension. Stimulation is particularly likely in children, as are atropine-like signs and symptoms (dry mouth, dilated pupils, flushing, hyperthermia, and gastrointestinal symptoms).

Treatment Recommendations: The patient should be induced to vomit even if emesis has occurred spontaneously; however, vomiting should not be induced in patients with impaired consciousness. Precautions against aspiration should be taken, especially in infants and children. Ipecac Syrup is the preferred method for inducing vomiting. The action of ipecac is facilitated by physical activity and the administration of eight to twelve fluid ounces of water. If emesis does not occur in fifteen minutes, the dose of ipecac should be repeated. Following emesis, any drug remaining in the stomach may be absorbed by activated charcoal administered as a slurry with water.

If vomiting is unsuccessful or contraindicated, gastric lavage should be performed. Isotonic and one-half isotonic saline are the lavage solutions of choice. Saline cathartics, such as milk of magnesia, draw water into the bowel by osmosis and, therefore, may be valuable for their action of rapid dilution of bowel content.

Treatment of the signs and symptoms of overdosage is symptomatic and supportive. Vasopressors may be used to treat hypotension. Short-acting barbiturates, diazepam or paraldehyde may be administered to control seizures. Hyperpyrexia, especially in children, may require treatment with tepid water sponge baths or a hypothermic blanket. Apnea is treated with ventilatory support. Stimulants (analeptic agents) should not be used.

The LD_{50} for pseudoephedrine is 202 mg/kg delivered intraperitoneally to rats. When given orally to mice, the LD_{50} for chlorpheniramine is 162 mg/kg.

DOSAGE AND ADMINISTRATION

FEDAHIST TIMECAPS: *Adults and children 12 years of age and older:* One TIMECAP every 12 hours not to exceed 2 TIMECAPS in 24 hours. Not recommended for children under 12 years of age.

FEDAHIST GYROCAPS: *Adults and children 12 years of age and older:* One GYROCAP every 12 hours not to exceed 2 GYROCAPS in 24 hours. Not recommended for children under 12 years of age.

HOW SUPPLIED

FEDAHIST TIMECAPS are clear capsules containing white and blue beadlets and imprinted with "KREMERS URBAN" and "055".

Bottles of 100 capsules   NDC 0091-0055-01

FEDAHIST GYROCAPS are white and yellow capsules containing white and green beadlets and imprinted with "KREMERS URBAN" AND "053".

Bottles of 100 capsules   NDC 0091-1053-01

Store at controlled room temperature 15°–30°C (59°–86°F).

CAUTION

Federal law prohibits dispensing without prescription.

Mfd. by:
Central Pharmaceuticals, Inc.
Seymour, Indiana 47274
For:
SCHWARZ
PHARMA
Kremers Urban Company
Milwaukee, Wisconsin 53201

Shown in Product Identification Section, page 429

KUTAPRESSIN® Injection   ℞
(liver derivative complex)

DESCRIPTION

KUTAPRESSIN® Injection (liver derivative complex) is a sterile solution containing 25.5 mg liver derivative complex per mL in water for injection. KUTAPRESSIN Injection is composed of peptides and amino acids. The product contains no protein, is virtually non-allergenic, and does not exhibit anti-anemia activity.

KUTAPRESSIN Injection also contains as inactive ingredients: phenol 0.5%, water for injection, pH is adjusted with hydrochloric acid or sodium hydroxide when necessary.

CLINICAL PHARMACOLOGY

The specific action of KUTAPRESSIN is to enhance the resolution of inflammation and edema. In the late 1920s it was demonstrated that liver was of benefit to patients suffering from acne vulgaris. As a consequence, various techniques were employed for isolating the active "factor" from liver. Studies published in the late 1930s and early 1940s showed activity in a specially purified liver fraction. During subsequent years refinements in the isolation of the active material led to the marketing of KUTAPRESSIN.

Initially it was thought that the primary action of KUTAPRESSIN was on the capillaries and precapillary sphincters. However, it is now believed that this effect is a secondary one and that the primary action of KUTAPRESSIN is in response to injury at the cellular level. The capillary changes observed following administration of KUTAPRESSIN appear to be part of a more fundamental anti-inflammatory effect. In the normal animal no consistent pharmacodynamic action has been demonstrated for KUTAPRESSIN. In particular there is no effect on the systemic blood pressure, no action on the autonomic nervous system and no alteration in prothrombin, coagulation or bleeding times. It is concluded that the specific action of the product is only apparent when tissues have been subjected to injury and when inflammation and edema are present.

INDICATIONS AND USAGE

A wide variety of dermatological clinical conditions benefit from KUTAPRESSIN therapy. The common denominator in these varied conditions is the presence of inflammation and edema. Favorable response to administration of KUTAPRESSIN in patients with acne vulgaris, herpes zoster, "poison ivy" dermatitis, pityriasis rosea, seborrheic dermatitis, urticaria and eczema, severe sunburn, and rosacea have been reported.

CONTRAINDICATIONS

Contraindicated in patients with hypersensitivity or intolerance to liver or pork products.

WARNING

Use with caution in patients suspected of being hypersensitive to liver or with other allergic diatheses.

Continued on next page

Schwarz Pharma—Cont.

PRECAUTIONS
Drug Interactions:
No clinically significant drug interactions have been reported.
Carcinogenesis, Mutagenesis, Impairment of Fertility:
No long-term animal studies have examined the carcinogenic or mutagenic potential of KUTAPRESSIN. KUTAPRESSIN's effect upon reproductive capacity is similarly unknown.
Pregnancy—Pregnancy Category C:
Animal reproduction studies have not been conducted with KUTAPRESSIN. It is also not known whether KUTAPRESSIN can cause fetal harm when administered to a pregnant woman or can affect reproduction capacity. KUTAPRESSIN should be given to a pregnant woman only if clearly needed.
Nursing Mothers:
It is not known whether this drug is excreted in human milk. Because many drugs are excreted in human milk, caution should be exercised when KUTAPRESSIN is administered to a nursing woman.

ADVERSE REACTIONS
As with all injectable medications, local reactions may occur. Local reactions may include pain, swelling, and erythema.

DRUG ABUSE AND DEPENDENCE
The information on drug abuse and dependence is limited to uncontrolled data derived from marketing experience. Such experience has revealed no evidence of drug abuse and dependence associated with KUTAPRESSIN Injection .

DOSAGE AND ADMINISTRATION
For the management of skin disorders the usual dose of KUTAPRESSIN is 2 mL administered daily or as indicated. The product is given by intramuscular or subcutaneous injection only.
As with all parenteral drug products, KUTAPRESSIN should be inspected visually for particulate matter and discoloration prior to administration, whenever solution and container permit.

HOW SUPPLIED
KUTAPRESSIN Injection (liver derivative complex, 25.5 mg/mL) is a sterile, brown solution.
20 mL multiple-dose vial   NDC 0091-1510-21
Store at controlled room temperature 15°–30°C (59°–86°F).
CAUTION: Federal law prohibits dispensing without prescription.
Mfd. by:
Taylor Pharmacal Company
Decatur, Illinois 62525
For:
SCHWARZ
PHARMA
Kremers Urban Company
Milwaukee, Wisconsin 53201

KUTRASE® Capsules   ℞
[qū'trăs]

DESCRIPTION
KUTRASE® Capsules contain four standardized digestive enzymes: lipase, amylase, protease, cellulase, and hyoscyamine sulfate USP and phenyltoloxamine citrate. Lipase, amylase, protease and cellulase are derived from fungal, plant and animal sources and are oral digestive enzyme supplements. Hyoscyamine sulfate USP is one of the principal anticholinergic/antispasmodic components of belladonna alkaloids. Phenyltoloxamine citrate is a non-barbiturate sedative. Each capsule contains:

lipase	75 mg
amylase	30 mg
protease	6 mg
cellulase	2 mg
hyoscyamine sulfate USP	0.0625 mg
phenyltoloxamine citrate	15 mg

Each capsule also contains as inactive ingredients: D&C Yellow #10, ethylcellulose, FD&C Green #3, FD&C Yellow #6, gelatin, lactose, magnesium stearate, titanium dioxide, vanillin and other ingredients.

CLINICAL PHARMACOLOGY
Diminution of secretions from exocrine glands is often a result of the normal aging process. KUTRASE provides a balanced combination of natural proteolytic, amylolytic, cellulolytic and lipolytic enzymes to enhance digestion of proteins, starch and fat in the gastrointestinal tract. These enzymes do not exert any systemic pharmacologic effects. KUTRASE should be considered an enzyme supplement and not an enzyme replacement therapy. Enzymes in KUTRASE are basically derived from fungal and plant sources and possess a broad spectrum of pH activity. Enzymes are promptly released from the capsule and are bioavailable for digestion of food in the stomach and intestines. Hyoscyamine sulfate provides a potent spasmolytic effect in reducing gastrointestinal hypermotility and intestinal spasm. A mild sedative effect is provided by phenyltoloxamine citrate.

INDICATIONS AND USAGE
KUTRASE is indicated for the relief of the symptoms of functional indigestion devoid of organic pathology commonly referred to as nervous indigestion and colloquially as "butterflies". The symptoms are bloating, gas, and fullness.

CONTRAINDICATIONS
Glaucoma, obstructive uropathy, obstructive disease of the gastrointestinal tract (as in achalasia, pyloroduodenal stenosis); paralytic ileus, intestinal atony of the elderly or debilitated patients; unstable cardiovascular status in acute hemorrhage; severe ulcerative colitis; toxic megacolon complicating ulcerative colitis; myasthenia gravis, or a hypersensitivity to any of the ingredients.

WARNINGS
Do not administer to patients who are allergic to pork products. In the presence of high environmental temperature, heat prostration can occur with drug use (fever and heat stroke due to decreased sweating). Diarrhea may be an early symptom of incomplete intestinal obstruction, especially in patients with ileostomy or colostomy. In this instance, treatment with this drug would be inappropriate. KUTRASE may produce drowsiness or blurred vision. In this event, the patient should be warned not to engage in activities requiring mental alertness such as operating a motor vehicle or other machinery or to perform hazardous work while taking this drug.

PRECAUTIONS
General:
Use with caution in patients with autonomic neuropathy, hyperthyroidism, coronary heart disease, congestive heart failure, cardiac arrhythmias, and hypertension. Investigate any tachycardia before giving any anticholinergic drug since they may increase the heart rate. Use with caution in patients with hiatal hernia associated with reflux esophagitis.
Information for Patients:
If capsules are opened, avoid inhalation of the powder. Sensitive individuals may experience allergic reactions.
Carcinogenesis, Mutagenesis, Impairment of Fertility:
Long-term studies in animals have not been performed to evaluate the carcinogenic, mutagenic or impairment of fertility potential of KUTRASE.
Pregnancy-Pregnancy Category C:
Animal reproduction studies have not been conducted with KUTRASE. It is also not known whether KUTRASE can cause fetal harm when administered to a pregnant woman or can affect reproduction capacity. KUTRASE should be given to a pregnant woman only if clearly needed.
Nursing Mothers:
Hyoscyamine sulfate is excreted in human milk. It is not known whether the enzymes or phenyltoloxamine citrate are excreted in human milk. Caution should be exercised when KUTRASE is administered to a nursing woman.

ADVERSE REACTIONS
Occasionally a slight looseness of the stools may be noticed. If so, dosage should be reduced. Finely powdered pancreatic enzyme may be irritating to the mucous membranes and respiratory tract. Inhalation of the airborne powder may precipitate an asthma attack in sensitive individuals. Other adverse reactions may include dryness of the mouth; urinary hesitancy and retention; blurred vision; tachycardia; palpitations; mydriasis; cycloplegia; increased ocular tension; headache; nervousness; drowsiness; weakness; suppression of lactation; allergic reactions or drug idiosyncrasies; urticaria and other dermal manifestations and decreased sweating.

OVERDOSAGE
The signs and symptoms of overdose are headache, nausea, vomiting, blurred vision, dilated pupils, hot dry skin, dizziness, dryness of the mouth, difficulty in swallowing. Measures to be taken are immediate lavage of the stomach and injection of physostigmine 0.5 to 2 mg intravenously and repeated as necessary up to a total of 5 mg. Fever may be treated symptomatically. Excitement to a degree which demands attention may be managed with sodium thiopental 2% solution given slowly intravenously. In the event of paralysis of the respiratory muscles, artificial respiration should be instituted.

DOSAGE AND ADMINISTRATION
1 or 2 capsules taken with each meal or snack. Dosage may be adjusted according to the conditions and severity of symptoms to assure symptomatic control with a minimum of adverse effects.

HOW SUPPLIED
KUTRASE Capsules are green and white capsules and are imprinted "KREMERS URBAN" and "475."
Bottles of 100 capsules   NDC 0091-3475-01

Store at controlled room temperature 15°–30°C (59°–86°F).

CAUTION
Federal law prohibits dispensing without prescription.
Shown in Product Identification Section, page 429

KU-ZYME® Capsules   ℞
[qū' zīm]

DESCRIPTION
KU-ZYME® Capsules contain four standardized enzymes: lipase, amylase, protease and cellulase. They are derived from fungal, plant and animal sources and are designed for oral digestive enzyme supplement therapy.
Each capsule contains:

lipase	75 mg
amylase	30 mg
protease	6 mg
cellulase	2 mg

Each capsule also contains as inactive ingredients: D&C Yellow #10, FD&C Yellow #6, gelatin, lactose, magnesium stearate, titanium dioxide, vanillin and other ingredients.

CLINICAL PHARMACOLOGY
Diminution of secretions from exocrine glands is often a result of the normal aging process. KU-ZYME provides a balanced combination of natural proteolytic, amylolytic, cellulolytic and lipolytic enzymes to enhance digestion of proteins, starch and fat in the gastrointestinal tract. These enzymes do not exert any systemic pharmacologic effects. KU-ZYME should be considered an enzyme supplement and not an enzyme replacement therapy. Enzymes in KU-ZYME are basically derived from fungal and plant sources and possess a broad spectrum of pH activity. Enzymes are promptly released from the capsule and are bioavailable for digestion of food in the stomach and intestines.

INDICATIONS AND USAGE
For the relief of functional indigestion when due to enzyme deficiency or imbalance. KU-ZYME relieves symptoms due to faulty digestion including the sensation of fullness after meals, dyspepsia, flatulence, abdominal distention and intolerance to certain foods.

CONTRAINDICATIONS
There are no known contraindications to the administration of digestive enzymes. These enzymes do not attack living tissues and do not present any danger to the patient with ulceration or inflammation in the digestive tract.

WARNINGS
Do not administer to patients who are allergic to pork products.

PRECAUTIONS
Information for Patients:
If capsules are opened, avoid inhalation of the powder. Sensitive individuals may experience allergic reactions.
Carcinogenesis, Mutagenesis, Impairment of Fertility:
Long-term studies in animals have not been performed to evaluate carcinogenic, mutagenic or impairment of fertility potential of KU-ZYME.
Pregnancy-Pregnancy Category C:
Animal reproduction studies have not been conducted with KU-ZYME. It is also not known whether KU-ZYME can cause fetal harm when administered to a pregnant woman or can affect reproduction capacity. KU-ZYME should be given to a pregnant woman only if clearly needed.
Nursing Mothers:
It is not known whether KU-ZYME is excreted in human milk. Because many drugs are excreted in human milk, caution should be exercised when KU-ZYME is administered to a nursing woman.

ADVERSE REACTIONS
Virtually unknown. Occasionally, a slight looseness of the stool may be noticed. If so, dosage should be reduced. Finely powdered pancreatic enzyme may be irritating to the mucous membranes and respiratory tract. Inhalation of the airborne powder may precipitate an asthma attack in sensitive individuals.

OVERDOSAGE
No systemic toxicity occurs. Excessive dosage may, however, produce a laxative effect.

DOSAGE AND ADMINISTRATION
1 or 2 capsules taken with each meal or snack. Dosage may be adjusted depending on individual requirements for relief of symptoms due to digestive enzyme deficiency. In patients who experience difficulty in swallowing the capsule, it may be opened and the contents sprinkled on the food. When opening the capsules, avoid inhalation of the powder (see PRECAUTIONS and ADVERSE REACTIONS).

HOW SUPPLIED

KU-ZYME Capsules are yellow and white capsules and are imprinted "KREMERS URBAN" and "522".

   Bottles of 100 capsules   NDC 0091-3522-01

Store at controlled room temperature 15°–30°C (59°–86°F).

CAUTION

Federal law prohibits dispensing without prescription.

Shown in Product Identification Section, page 429

KU-ZYME® HP Capsules   ℞

[qū' zīm]
(pancrelipase capsules USP)

DESCRIPTION

KU-ZYME® HP Capsules (pancrelipase capsules USP) contain standardized lipase, amylase and protease obtained from hog pancreas and are designed for oral digestive enzyme replacement therapy. Each capsule contains:

lipase	8,000 USP units
protease	30,000 USP units
amylase	30,000 USP units

Each capsule also contains as inactive ingredients: gelatin, lactose, magnesium stearate, titanium dioxide and other ingredients.

CLINICAL PHARMACOLOGY

Pancrelipase USP is a pancreatic enzyme concentrate which hydrolyzes fats to glycerol and fatty acids, changes protein into proteoses and derived substances, and converts starch into dextrins and sugars. The administration of pancrelipase reduces the fat and nitrogen content in the stool. Pancreatic enzymes are normally secreted in great excess. Generally, steatorrhea and malabsorption occur only after a 90 percent or greater reduction in secretion of lipase and proteolytic enzymes. It has been estimated that approximately 8,000 units of lipase per hour should be delivered into the duodenum postprandially. Even if all the enzymes taken orally reached the proximal intestine in active form, ingestion of 24,000 units of lipase (8,000 units per hour) for 3 postprandial hours would be required. If one could deliver sufficient pancreatic enzymes to the small intestine, malabsorption could be corrected. It is rarely possible to achieve complete relief of steatorrhea although major improvement in fat absorption can be achieved in most patients.

INDICATIONS

KU-ZYME HP is effective in patients with deficient exocrine pancreatic secretions. Thus, KU-ZYME HP may be used as enzyme replacement therapy in cystic fibrosis, chronic pancreatitis, post pancreatectomy, in ductal obstructions caused by cancer of the pancreas, pancreatic insufficiency and for steatorrhea of malabsorption syndrome and post gastrectomy (Billroth II and Total). May also be used as a presumptive test for pancreatic function, especially in pancreatic insufficiency due to chronic pancreatitis.

CONTRAINDICATIONS

There are no known contraindications for the use of pancrelipase although sensitivity to pork protein may preclude its use.

WARNINGS

Pancreatic exocrine replacement therapy should not delay or supplant treatment of the primary disorder. Use with caution in patients known to be hypersensitive to pork or enzymes.

PRECAUTIONS

Information for Patients:

If capsules are opened, avoid inhalation of the powder. Sensitive individuals may experience allergic reactions.

Drug Interactions:

The serum iron response to oral iron may be decreased by concomitant administration of pancreatic extracts.

Carcinogenesis, Mutagenesis, and Impairment of Fertility:

Long-term studies in animals have not been performed to evaluate the carcinogenic, mutagenic or impairment of fertility potential of KU-ZYME HP.

Pregnancy-Pregnancy Category C:

Animal reproduction studies have not been conducted with KU-ZYME HP. It is also not known whether KU-ZYME HP can cause fetal harm when administered to a pregnant woman or can affect reproduction capacity. KU-ZYME HP should be given to a pregnant woman only if clearly needed.

Nursing Mothers:

It is not known whether KU-ZYME HP is excreted in human milk. Because many drugs are excreted in human milk, caution should be exercised when KU-ZYME HP is administered to a nursing woman.

ADVERSE REACTIONS

High doses may cause nausea, abdominal cramps and/or diarrhea in certain patients. Finely powdered pancreatic enzyme concentrate may be irritating to the mucous membranes and respiratory tract. Inhalation of the airborne powder may precipitate an asthma attack in sensitive individuals. Extremely high doses of exogenous pancreatic enzymes have been associated with hyperuricemia and hyperuricosuria.

DOSAGE AND ADMINISTRATION

1 to 3 capsules taken with each meal or snack. Dosage may be adjusted depending on individual requirements for control of steatorrhea. In severe deficiencies the dose may be increased to 8 capsules with meals or the frequency of administration may increase to hourly intervals if nausea, cramps and/or diarrhea do not occur.

HOW SUPPLIED

KU-ZYME® HP Capsules (pancrelipase capsules USP) are white opaque capsules and are imprinted "KREMERS URBAN" and "525."

   Bottles of 100 capsules   NDC 0091-3525-01

Store at a temperature not exceeding 25°C (77°F).

CAUTION

Federal law prohibits dispensing without prescription.

Shown in Product Identification Section, page 429

LEVSIN® PRODUCTS   ℞

[lev'sin]
(hyoscyamine sulfate USP)
LEVSIN®/SL Tablets
LEVSIN® Tablets
LEVSIN® Elixir
LEVSIN® Drops (Oral Solution)
LEVSIN® Injection
LEVSINEX™ TIMECAPS™

DESCRIPTION

LEVSIN® (hyoscyamine sulfate USP) is one of the principal anticholinergic/antispasmodic components of belladonna alkaloids. The empirical formula is $(C_{17}H_{23}NO_3)_2 \cdot H_2SO_4 \cdot 2H_2O$ and the molecular weight is 712.85. Chemically, it is benzeneacetic acid, α-(hydroxymethyl)-,8-methyl-8-azabicyclo [3.2.1.] oct-3-yl ester, [3(S)-endo]-, sulfate (2:1), dihydrate.

LEVSIN/SL Tablets contain 0.125 mg hyoscyamine sulfate formulated for sublingual administration. However, the tablets may also be chewed or taken orally. Each tablet also contains as inactive ingredients: colloidal silicon dioxide, dextrates, FD&C Green #3, flavor, mannitol, and stearic acid.

LEVSIN Tablets contain 0.125 mg hyoscyamine sulfate formulated for oral administration. Each tablet also contains as inactive ingredients: acacia, confectioner's sugar, corn starch, lactose, powdered cellulose and stearic acid.

LEVSIN Elixir contains 0.125 mg hyoscyamine sulfate per 5 mL (teaspoonful) with 20% alcohol for oral use. LEVSIN Elixir also contains as inactive ingredients: FD&C Red #40, FD&C Yellow #6, flavor, glycerin, purified water, sorbitol solution and sucrose.

LEVSIN Drops, oral solution, contain 0.125 mg hyoscyamine sulfate per mL with 5% alcohol. LEVSIN Drops also contain as inactive ingredients: FD&C Red #40, FD&C Yellow #6, flavor, glycerin, purified water, sodium citrate, sorbitol solution, and sucrose.

LEVSIN Injection is a sterile solution containing 0.5 mg hyoscyamine sulfate per mL. The 1 mL ampuls contain as inactive ingredients: water for injection, pH is adjusted with hydrochloric acid when necessary. The 10 mL multiple-dose vials contain as inactive ingredients: benzyl alcohol 1.5%, sodium metabisulfite 0.1%, isotonic sodium chloride, water for injection, pH is adjusted with hydrochloric acid when necessary.

LEVSINEX TIMECAPS contain 0.375 mg hyoscyamine sulfate in a timed-release formulation designed for oral b.i.d. dosage. Each TIMECAP also contains as inactive ingredients: corn starch, D&C Red #28, FD&C Blue #1, FD&C Blue #2, FD&C Red #40, FD&C Yellow #6, gelatin, sucrose, titanium dioxide and other ingredients.

CLINICAL PHARMACOLOGY

LEVSIN inhibits specifically the actions of acetylcholine on structures innervated by postganglionic cholinergic nerves and on smooth muscles that respond to acetylcholine but lack cholinergic innervation. These peripheral cholinergic receptors are present in the autonomic effector cells of the smooth muscle, cardiac muscle, the sinoatrial node, the atrioventricular node, and the exocrine glands. It is completely devoid of any action in the autonomic ganglia. LEVSIN inhibits gastrointestinal propulsive motility and decreases gastric acid secretion. LEVSIN also controls excessive pharyngeal, tracheal and bronchial secretions.

LEVSIN is absorbed totally and completely by sublingual administration as well as oral administration. Once absorbed, LEVSIN disappears rapidly from the blood and is distributed throughout the entire body. The half-life of LEVSIN is 3 ½ hours. LEVSIN is partly hydrolyzed to tropic acid and tropine but the majority of the drug is excreted in the urine unchanged within the first 12 hours. Only traces of this drug are found in breast milk. LEVSIN passes the blood brain barrier and the placental barrier.

LEVSINEX TIMECAPS release 0.375 mg hyoscyamine sulfate at a controlled and predictable rate for 12 hours. Peak blood levels occur in 2½ hours and the apparent plasma half-life is approximately 7 hours. The relative bioavailability of the timed-release dosage form is approximately 81% that of the immediate-release dosage form. The urinary excretion from both the immediate-release dosage form and the timed-release dosage form is equal and uniform over a 24 hour period.

INDICATIONS AND USAGE

LEVSIN is effective as adjunctive therapy in the treatment of peptic ulcer. It can also be used to control gastric secretion, visceral spasm, and hypermotility in spastic colitis, spastic bladder, cystitis, pylorospasm, and associated abdominal cramps. May be used in functional intestinal disorders to reduce symptoms such as those seen in mild dysenteries, diverticulitis, and acute enterocolitis. For use as adjunctive therapy in the treatment of irritable bowel syndrome (irritable colon, spastic colon, mucous colitis) and functional gastrointestinal disorders. Also as adjunctive therapy in the treatment of neurogenic bladder and neurogenic bowel disturbances including the splenic flexure syndrome and neurogenic colon. Also used in the treatment of infant colic (elixir and drops). LEVSIN is indicated along with morphine or other narcotics in symptomatic relief of biliary and renal colic; as a "drying agent" in the relief of symptoms of acute rhinitis; in the therapy of parkinsonism to reduce rigidity and tremors and to control associated sialorrhea and hyperhidrosis. May be used in the therapy of poisoning by anticholinesterase agents.

Parenterally administered LEVSIN is also effective in reducing duodenal motility to facilitate the diagnostic radiologic procedure, hypotonic duodenography. LEVSIN may be used to reduce pain and hypersecretion in pancreatitis. LEVSIN may also be used in certain cases of partial heart block associated with vagal activity.

IN ANESTHESIA:

LEVSIN Injection is indicated as a pre-operative antimuscarinic to reduce salivary, tracheobronchial, and pharyngeal secretions; to reduce the volume and acidity of gastric secretions, and to block cardiac vagal inhibitory reflexes during induction of anesthesia and intubation. LEVSIN protects against the peripheral muscarinic effects such as bradycardia and excessive secretions produced by halogenated hydrocarbons and cholinergic agents such as physostigmine, neostigmine, and pyridostigmine given to reverse the actions of curariform agents.

IN UROLOGY:

LEVSIN Injection may also be used intravenously to improve radiologic visibility of the kidneys.

CONTRAINDICATIONS

Glaucoma; obstructive uropathy (for example, bladder neck obstruction due to prostatic hypertrophy); obstructive disease of the gastrointestinal tract (as in achalasia, pyloroduodenal stenosis); paralytic ileus, intestinal atony of elderly or debilitated patients; unstable cardiovascular status in acute hemorrhage; severe ulcerative colitis; toxic megacolon complicating ulcerative colitis; myasthenia gravis.

WARNINGS

In the presence of high environmental temperature, heat prostration can occur with drug use (fever and heat stroke due to decreased sweating). Diarrhea may be an early symptom of incomplete intestinal obstruction, especially in patients with ileostomy or colostomy. In this instance, treatment with this drug would be inappropriate and possibly harmful. Like other anticholinergic agents, LEVSIN may produce drowsiness or blurred vision. In this event, the patient should be warned not to engage in activities requiring mental alertness such as operating a motor vehicle or other machinery or to perform hazardous work while taking this drug.

Psychosis has been reported in sensitive individuals given anticholinergic drugs. CNS signs and symptoms inlude confusion, disorientation, short term memory loss, hallucinations, dysarthria, ataxia, coma, euphoria, decreased anxiety, fatigue, insomnia, agitation and mannerisms, and inappropriate affect. These CNS signs and symptoms usually resolve within 12–48 hours after discontinuation of the drug.

The 10 mL multiple-dose vial of LEVSIN Injection contains sodium metabisulfite, a sulfite that may cause allergic-type reactions including anaphylactic symptoms and life-threatening or less severe asthmatic episodes in certain susceptible people. The overall prevalence of sulfite sensitivity in the general population is unknown and probably low. Sulfite sensitivity is seen more frequently in asthmatic than in nonasthmatic people.

Continued on next page

Schwarz Pharma—Cont.

PRECAUTIONS

General:
Use with caution in patients with: autonomic neuropathy, hyperthyroidism, coronary heart disease, congestive heart failure, cardiac arrhythmias, hypertension and renal disease. Investigate any tachycardia before giving any anticholinergic drug since they may increase the heart rate. Use with caution in patients with hiatal hernia associated with reflux esophagitis.
Information for Patients:
LEVSIN may cause drowsiness, dizziness or blurred vision; patients should observe caution before driving, using machinery or performing other tasks requiring mental alertness.
Use of LEVSIN may decrease sweating resulting in heat prostration, fever or heat stroke; febrile patients or those who may be exposed to elevated environmental temperatures should use caution.
Drug Interactions:
Additive adverse effects resulting from cholinergic blockade may occur when LEVSIN is administered concomitantly with other antimuscarinics, amantadine, haloperidol, phenothiazines, monoamine oxidase (MAO) inhibitors, tricyclic antidepressants or some antihistamines.
Antacids may interfere with the absorption of LEVSIN; take LEVSIN before meals and antacids after meals.
Carcinogenesis, Mutagenesis, Impairment of Fertility:
No long term studies in animals have been performed to determine the carcinogenic, mutagenic or impairment of fertility potential of LEVSIN; however, over 30 years of marketing experience shows no demonstrable evidence of a problem.
Pregnancy—Pregnancy Category C:
Animal reproduction studies have not been conducted with LEVSIN. It is also not known whether LEVSIN can cause fetal harm when administered to a pregnant woman or can affect reproduction capacity. LEVSIN should be given to a pregnant woman only if clearly needed.
Nursing Mothers:
LEVSIN is excreted in human milk. Caution should be exercised when LEVSIN is administered to a nursing woman.

ADVERSE REACTIONS

Not all of the following adverse reactions have been reported with hyoscyamine sulfate. The following adverse reactions have been reported for pharmacologically similar drugs with anticholinergic/antispasmodic action. Adverse reactions may include dryness of the mouth; urinary hesitancy and retention; blurred vision; tachycardia; palpitations; mydriasis; cycloplegia; increased ocular tension; loss of taste; headache; nervousness; drowsiness; weakness; dizziness; insomnia; nausea; vomiting; impotence; suppression of lactation; constipation; bloated feeling; allergic reactions or drug idiosyncrasies; urticaria and other dermal manifestations; ataxia; speech disturbance; some degree of mental confusion and/or excitement (especially in elderly persons); and decreased sweating.

OVERDOSAGE

The signs and symptoms of overdose are headache, nausea, vomiting, blurred vision, dilated pupils, hot dry skin, dizziness, dryness of the mouth, difficulty in swallowing and CNS stimulation.
Measures to be taken are immediate lavage of the stomach and injection of physostigmine 0.5 to 2 mg intravenously and repeated as necessary up to a total of 5 mg. Fever may be treated symptomatically (tepid water sponge baths, hypothermic blanket). Excitement to a degree which demands attention may be managed with sodium thiopental 2% solution given slowly intravenously or chloral hydrate (100–200 mL of a 2% solution) by rectal infusion. In the event of progression of the curare-like effect to paralysis of the respiratory muscles, artificial respiration should be instituted and maintained until effective respiratory action returns.
In rats, the LD_{50} for LEVSIN is 375 mg/kg. LEVSIN is dialyzable.

DOSAGE AND ADMINISTRATION

Dosage may be adjusted according to the conditions and severity of symptoms.
LEVSIN/SL Tablets: The tablets may be taken sublingually or orally. *Adults and children 12 years of age and older:* 1 to 2 tablets every four hours or as needed. Do not exceed 12 tablets in 24 hours. *Children 2 to under 12 years of age:* ½ to 1 tablet every four hours or as needed. Do not exceed 6 tablets in 24 hours.
LEVSIN Tablets: The tablets may be taken orally or sublingually. *Adults and children 12 years of age and older:* 1 to 2 tablets every four hours or as needed. Do not exceed 12 tablets in 24 hours.
Children 2 to under 12 years of age: ½ to 1 tablet every four hours or as needed. Do not exceed 6 tablets in 24 hours.
LEVSIN Elixir: *Adults and children 12 years of age and older:* 1 to 2 teaspoonfuls every four hours or as needed. Do not exceed 12 teaspoonfuls in 24 hours.
Children 2 to under 12 years of age: ¼ to 1 teaspoonful every four hours or as needed. Do not exceed 6 teaspoonfuls in 24 hours.
The following dosage guide is based upon body weight. The doses may be repeated every four hours or as needed.

Body Weight	Usual Dose
10 kg (22 lb)	¼ tsp
20 kg (44 lb)	½ tsp
40 kg (88 lb)	¾ tsp
50 kg (110 lb)	1tsp

LEVSIN Drops: *Adults and children 12 years of age and older:* 1 to 2 mL every four hours or as needed. Do not exceed 12 mL in 24 hours.
Children 2 to under 12 years of age: ¼ to 1 mL every four hours or as needed. Do not exceed 6 mL in 24 hours.
Children under 2 years of age: The following dosage guide is based upon body weight. The doses may be repeated every four hours or as needed.

Body Weight	Usual Dose	Do Not Exceed in 24 Hours
2.3 kg (5 lb)	3 drops	18 drops
3.4 kg (7.5 lb)	4 drops	24 drops
5 kg (11 lb)	5 drops	30 drops
7 kg (15 lb)	6 drops	36 drops
10 kg (22 lb)	8 drops	48 drops
15 kg (33 lb)	11 drops	66 drops

LEVSIN Injection: The dose may be administered subcutaneously, intramuscularly, or intravenously without dilution.
Gastrointestinal Disorders: The usual adult recommended dose is 0.5 to 1.0 mL (0.25 to 0.5 mg). Some patients may need only a single dose; others may require administration two, three, or four times a day at four hour intervals.
Hypotonic Duodenography: The usual adult recommended dose is 0.5 to 1.0 mL (0.25 to 0.5 mg) administered 5 to 10 minutes prior to the diagnostic procedure.
Anesthesia: Adults and children over 2 years of age: As a pre-anesthetic medication, the recommended dose is 5 μg (0.005 mg) per kg of body weight. This dose is usually given 30 to 60 minutes prior to the anticipated time of induction of anesthesia or at the time the pre-anesthetic narcotic or sedative is administered.
LEVSIN Injection may be used during surgery to reduce drug-induced bradycardia. It should be administered intravenously in increments of 0.25 mL and repeated as needed.
To achieve reversal of neuromuscular blockade, the recommended dose is 0.2 mg (0.4 mL) LEVSIN Injection for every 1 mg neostigmine or the equivalent dose of physostigmine or pyridostigmine.
Parenteral drug products should be inspected visually for particulate matter and discoloration prior to administration, whenever solution and container permit.
LEVSINEX TIMECAPS: *Adults and children 12 years of age and older:* 1 to 2 TIMECAPS every 12 hours. Dosage may be adjusted to 1 TIMECAP every 8 hours if needed. Do not exceed 4 TIMECAPS in 24 hours.
Children 2 to under 12 years of age: 1 TIMECAP every 12 hours. Do not exceed 2 TIMECAPS in 24 hours.

HOW SUPPLIED

LEVSIN/SL Tablets (hyoscyamine sulfate tablets USP, 0.125 mg) are pale blue-green, peppermint-flavored, octagonal shaped, scored, and embossed with "SCHWARZ" on one side and "532" on the other.
Bottles of 100 tablets NDC 0091-3532-01
Bottles of 500 tablets NDC 0091-3532-05
LEVSIN Tablets (hyoscyamine sulfate tablets USP, 0.125 mg) are white, scored and embossed with "KU" on one side and "531" on the other.
Bottles of 100 tablets NDC 0091-3531-01
Bottles of 500 tablets NDC 0091-3531-05
LEVSIN Elixir (hyoscyamine sulfate elixir USP, 0.125 mg/5mL) is orange colored and orange flavored with 20% alcohol. Pint (473 mL) bottles (NDC 0091-4532-16).
LEVSIN Drops (hyoscyamine sulfate oral solution USP, 0.125 mg/mL) are orange colored, orange flavored and contain 5% alcohol. 15 mL bottle with dropper (NDC 0091-4538-15).
LEVSIN Injection (hyoscyamine sulfate injection USP, 0.5 mg/mL) is a clear, colorless and sterile solution. Box of 5 1-mL ampuls (NDC 0091-1536-05), 10 mL vial (NDC 0091-1536-10).
LEVSINEX TIMECAPS (hyoscyamine sulfate USP, 0.375 mg, timed release) are brown and clear capsules containing brown and white beadlets and imprinted with "KREMERS URBAN" and "537." Bottles of 100 capsules (NDC 0091-3537-01).
LEVSIN with Phenobarbital Products, call Schwarz Pharma (1-800-558-5114) for complete prescribing information.
LEVSIN with Phenobarbital Tablets [0.125 mg hyoscyamine sulfate/15 mg phenobarbital (Warning: May be habit forming)] are pink and scored with "K-U" on one side and "534" on the other.
Bottles of 100 tablets NDC 0091-3534-01
LEVSIN-PB Drops [0.125 mg hyoscyamine sulfate/15 mg phenobarbital (Warning: May be habit forming) per mL] oral solution, is red colored and cherry flavored and contain 5% alcohol. 15 mL bottle with dropper (NDC 0091-4536-15).
Store at controlled room temperature 15°–30°C (59°–86°F).

CAUTION

Federal law prohibits dispensing without prescription.
Shown in Product Identification Section, page 429

PRE-PEN® ℞

[*prē ′pen*]
(benzylpenicilloyl polylysine injection USP)
Skin Test Antigen

DESCRIPTION

PRE-PEN® (benzylpenicilloyl polylysine injection USP) is a skin test antigen used in assessing a patient's allergy status to penicillin.
PRE-PEN is a sterile solution of benzylpenicilloyl polylysine in a concentration of 6.0×10^{-5} M (benzylpenicilloyl) in 0.01 M phosphate buffer and 0.15 M sodium chloride and water for injection. The benzylpenicilloyl polylysine in PRE-PEN is a derivative of poly-l-lysine, where the epsilon amino groups are substituted with benzylpenicilloyl groups (50-70%) forming benzylpenicilloyl alpha amide. Each single dose ampul contains 0.25 mL of PRE-PEN.

CLINICAL PHARMACOLOGY

PRE-PEN reacts specifically with benzylpenicilloyl skin sensitizing antibodies (reagins: IgE class) to initiate release of chemical mediators which produce an immediate wheal and flare reaction at a skin test site. All individuals exhibiting a positive skin test to PRE-PEN possess reagins against the benzylpenicilloyl group which is a haptene. A haptene is a low molecular weight chemical which, when conjugated to a carrier, e.g., poly-l-lysine, has the properties under appropriate conditions of an antigen with the haptene's specificity. It is to be noted that individuals who have previously received therapeutic penicillin may have positive skin test reactions to PRE-PEN as well as to a number of other non-benzylpenicilloyl haptenes. The latter are designated as minor determinants, in that they are present in lesser amounts than the major determinant, benzylpenicilloyl. The minor determinants may nevertheless be associated with examples of significant clinical hypersensitivity.
Virtually everyone who receives penicillin develops specific antibodies to the drug as measured by hemagglutination studies, but (a) positive skin tests to various penicillin and penicillin-derived reagents become positive in less than 10% of patients who have tolerated penicillin in the past and (b) allergic responses are infrequent (less than 1%).
Many individuals reacting positively to PRE-PEN will not develop a systemic allergic reaction on subsequent exposure to therapeutic penicillin. Thus, the PRE-PEN skin test facilitates assessing the local allergic skin reactivity of a patient to benzylpenicilloyl.

INDICATIONS AND USAGE

PRE-PEN is useful as an adjunct in assessing the risk of administering penicillin (benzylpenicillin or penicillin G) when it is the preferred drug of choice in adult patients who have previously received penicillin and have a history of clinical penicillin hypersensitivity. In this situation, a negative skin test to PRE-PEN is associated with an incidence of allergic reactions of less than 5% after the administration of therapeutic penicillin, whereas the incidence may be more than 20% in the presence of a positive skin test to PRE-PEN.
These allergic reactions are predominantly dermatologic. Because of the extremely low incidence of anaphylactic reactions, there are insufficient data at present to document that a decreased incidence of anaphylactic reactions following the administration of penicillin will occur in patients with a negative skin test to PRE-PEN. Similarly, when deciding the risk of proposed penicillin treatment, there are not enough data at present to permit relative weighing in individual cases of a history of clinical penicillin hypersensitivity as compared to positive skin tests to PRE-PEN and/or minor penicillin determinants.
It should be borne in mind that no reagent, test, or combination of tests will completely assure that a reaction to penicillin therapy will not occur.

CONTRAINDICATIONS

PRE-PEN is contraindicated in those patients who have exhibited either a systemic or marked local reaction to its previous administration. Patients known to be extremely hypersensitive to penicillin should not be skin tested.

WARNINGS

There are insufficient data to assess the potential danger of sensitization to repeated skin testing with PRE-PEN.
Rarely, a systemic allergic reaction (see below) may follow a

skin test with PRE-PEN. This can be avoided by making the first application by scratch test and very carefully following the instructions below in administering the intradermal test, using the intradermal route only if the scratch test has been entirely negative.

Skin testing with penicillin and/or other penicillin-derived reagents should not be performed simultaneously.

PRECAUTIONS
General:
There are insufficient data derived from well-controlled studies to determine the value of the PRE-PEN skin test as a means of assessing the risk of administering therapeutic penicillin (when penicillin is the preferred drug of choice) in the following situations:

(1)   Adult patients who give no history of clinical penicillin hypersensitivity.
(2)   Pediatric patients.

In addition, there are no data at present to assess the clinical value of PRE-PEN where exposure to penicillin is suspected as a cause of a drug reaction and in patients who are undergoing routine allergy evaluation.

Furthermore, there are no data relating the clinical value of PRE-PEN skin tests to the risk of administering semi-synthetic penicillins (phenoxymethyl penicillin, ampicillin, carbenicillin, dicloxacillin, methicillin, nafcillin, oxacillin, phenethicillin) and cephalosporin-derived antibiotics.

Recognition that the following clinical outcomes are possible makes it imperative for the physician to weigh risk to benefit in every instance where the decision to administer or not to administer penicillin is based in part on a PRE-PEN skin test.

(1)   An allergic reaction to therapeutic penicillin may occur in a patient with a negative skin test to PRE-PEN.
(2)   It is possible for a patient to have an anaphylactic reaction to therapeutic penicillin in the presence of a negative PRE-PEN skin test and a negative history of clinical penicillin hypersensitivity.
(3)   If penicillin is the absolute drug of choice in a life-threatening situation, successful desensitization with therapeutic penicillin may be possible irrespective of a positive skin test and/or a positive history of clinical penicillin hypersensitivity.

Pregnancy-Pregnancy Category C:
Animal reproduction studies have not been conducted with PRE-PEN. It is not known whether PRE-PEN can cause fetal harm when administered to a pregnant woman or can affect reproduction capacity. The hazards of skin testing in such patients should be weighed against the hazard of penicillin therapy without skin testing.

ADVERSE REACTIONS
Occasionally, patients may develop an intense local inflammatory response at the skin test site. Rarely, patients will develop a systemic allergic reaction, manifested by generalized erythema, pruritus, angioneurotic edema, urticaria, dyspnea, and/or hypotension. The usual methods of treating a skin test antigen-induced reaction—the application of a venous occlusion tourniquet proximal to the skin test site and administration of epinephrine (and, at times, an injection of an antihistamine) — are recommended and will usually control the reaction. As a rule, systemic allergic reactions following skin test procedures are of short duration and controllable, but the patient should be kept under observation for several hours.

DOSAGE AND ADMINISTRATION
SKIN TESTING DOSAGE AND TECHNIQUE
Scratch Testing:
Skin testing is usually performed on the inner volar aspect of the forearm. The skin test material should always be applied first by the scratch technique. After preparing the skin surface, a sterile 20 gauge needle should be used to make a 3–5 mm scratch of the epidermis. Very little pressure is required to break the epidermal continuity. If bleeding occurs, prepare a second site and scratch more lightly with the needle—sufficient to produce a non-bleeding scratched surface. Apply a small drop of PRE-PEN solution to the scratch and rub gently with an applicator, toothpick, or the side of the needle. Observe for the appearance of a wheal, erythema, and the occurrence of itching at the test site during the succeeding 15 minutes at which time the solution over the scratch is wiped off. A positive reaction is unmistakable and consists of the development within 10 minutes of a pale wheal, usually with pseudopods, surrounding the scratch site and varying in diameter from 5 to 15 mm (or more). This wheal may be surrounded by a variable diameter of erythema, and accompanied by a variable degree of itching. The most sensitive individuals develop itching almost instantly, and the wheal and erythema are prompt in their appearance. As soon as a positive response as defined above is clearly evident, the solution over the scratch should be immediately wiped off. If the scratch test is either negative or

equivocally positive (less than 5 mm wheal and little or no erythema, and no itching), an intradermal test may be performed.

The Intradermal Test:
Using a tuberculin syringe with a $\frac{3}{8}''$ to $\frac{5}{8}''$ long, 26 to 30 gauge, short bevel needle, withdraw the contents of the ampul. Prepare a sterile skin test area on the upper, outer arm, sufficiently below the deltoid muscle to permit proximal application of a tourniquet later, if necessary. Be sure to eject all air from the syringe through the needle, then insert the needle, bevel up, immediately below the skin surface. Inject an amount of PRE-PEN sufficient to raise the smallest possible perceptible bleb. This volume will be between 0.01 and 0.02 mL. Using a separate syringe and needle, inject a like amount of saline as a control at least $1\frac{1}{2}$ inches removed from the test site. Most skin reactions will develop within 5–15 minutes and response to the skin test is read as follows:

(—)   Negative response—no increase in size of original bleb and/or no greater reaction than the control site.
(±)   Ambiguous response—wheal being only slightly larger than initial injection bleb, with or without accompanying erythematous flare and larger than the control site.
(+)   Positive response—itching and marked increase in size of original bleb. Wheal may exceed 20 mm in diameter and exhibit pseudopods.

The control site should be completely reactionless. If it exhibits a wheal greater than 2–3 mm, repeat the test, and if the same reaction is observed, a physician experienced with allergy skin testing should be consulted.

Parenteral drug products should be inspected visually for particulate matter and discoloration prior to administration, whenever solution and container permit.

HOW SUPPLIED
PRE-PEN (benzylpenicilloyl polylysine injection USP) is a clear, colorless, sterile solution supplied in ampuls containing 0.25 mL.

   Boxes of five—single dose ampuls........NDC 0091-1640-05
PRE-PEN is stable only when kept under refrigeration. It is, therefore, recommended that test materials subjected to ambient temperatures for over a day be discarded.

CAUTION
Federal law prohibits dispensing without prescription.
Mfd. by:
Taylor Pharmacal Company
Decatur, IL 62525
For:
SCHWARZ PHARMA
Kremers Urban Company
Milwaukee, Wisconsin 53201

Products are cross-indexed by
generic and chemical names
in the
YELLOW SECTION.

G.D. Searle & Co.
BOX 5110
CHICAGO, IL 60680-5110

Alphabetic Product Listing
Product, ID# (NDC*), Form, Strength
Aldactazide, 1011, Tablet, 25 mg/25 mg
Aldactazide, 1021, Tablet, 50 mg/50 mg
Aldactone, 1001, Tablet, 25 mg
Aldactone, 1041, Tablet, 50 mg
Aldactone, 1031, Tablet, 100 mg
Calan, 40 (1771), Tablet, 40 mg
Calan, 80 (1851), Tablet, 80 mg
Calan, 120 (1861), Tablet, 120 mg
Calan SR, 120 (1901), Caplet, 120 mg
Calan SR, 180 (1911), Caplet, 180 mg
Calan SR, 240 (1891), Caplet, 240 mg
Cytotec, 1451, Tablet, 100 mcg
Cytotec, 1461, Tablet, 200 mcg
Demulen 1/35-21, Compack, 151, Tablet, 1 mg/35 mcg
Demulen 1/35-28, Compack, 151 (0161), Tablet, 1 mg/35 mcg
Demulen 1/50-21, Compack, 71, Tablet, 1 mg/50 mcg
Demulen 1/50-28, Compack, 71 (0081), Tablet, 1 mg/50 mcg
Flagyl, 1831, Tablet, 250 mg
Flagyl, 500 (1821), Tablet, 500 mg
Kerlone, 10 (5101), Tablet, 10 mg
Kerlone, 20 (5201), Tablet, 20 mg
Lomotil Ⓒ, 61, Tablet, 2.5 mg/0.025 mg
Lomotil Ⓒ, Liquid, 66, 2.5 mg/0.025 mg per 5 ml
Maxaquin, 400, (1651) Tablet, 400 mg
Nitrodisc, 2058, 0.2 mg/hr (8 cm²)
Nitrodisc, 2078, 0.3 mg/hr (12 cm²)
Nitrodisc, 2068, 0.4 mg/hr (16 cm²)
Norpace, 2752, Capsule, 100 mg
Norpace, 2762, Capsule, 150 mg
Norpace CR, 2732, Capsule, 100 mg
Norpace CR, 2742, Capsule, 150 mg

* When the product ID # is not the same as the NDC #, the NDC # appears in parentheses.

Various educational materials are available for physicians, pharmacists, nurses, physicians' assistants, and patients (through the physician). Please ask your Searle representative for information about these materials.

ALDACTAZIDE®   ℞
[al-dac'tuh "zīde]
(spironolactone with hydrochlorothiazide)

> **WARNING**
> Spironolactone, an ingredient of Aldactazide, has been shown to be a tumorigen in chronic toxicity studies in rats (see *Warnings*). Aldactazide should be used only in those conditions described under *Indications and Usage*. Unnecessary use of this drug should be avoided.
> Fixed-dose combination drugs are not indicated for initial therapy of edema or hypertension. Edema or hypertension requires therapy titrated to the individual patient. If the fixed combination represents the dosage so determined, its use may be more convenient in patient management. The treatment of hypertension and edema is not static but must be reevaluated as conditions in each patient warrant.

DESCRIPTION
Aldactazide oral tablets contain:
spironolactone .... 25 mg
hydrochlorothiazide .... 25 mg
or
spironolactone .... 50 mg
hydrochlorothiazide .... 50 mg

Spironolactone (Aldactone®), an aldosterone antagonist, is 17- hydroxy-7α-mercapto-3-oxo-17α-pregn-4-ene- 21- carboxylic acid γ-lactone acetate and has the following structural formula:

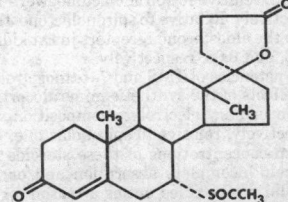

Continued on next page

Searle—Cont.

Spironolactone is practically insoluble in water, soluble in alcohol, and freely soluble in benzene and in chloroform.
Hydrochlorothiazide, a diuretic and antihypertensive, is 6-chloro-3, 4-dihydro-2H-1,2,4-benzothiadiazine-7-sulfonamide 1,1-dioxide and has the following structural formula:
Hydrochlorothiazide is slightly soluble in water and freely soluble in sodium hydroxide solution.

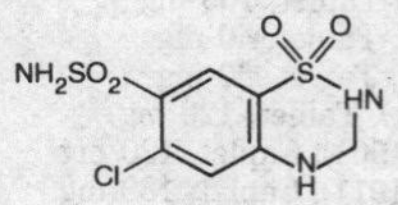

Inactive ingredients include calcium sulfate, corn starch, flavor, hydroxypropyl cellulose, hydroxypropyl methylcellulose, iron oxide, magnesium stearate, polyethylene glycol, povidone, and titanium dioxide.

CLINICAL PHARMACOLOGY

Mechanism of action: Aldactazide is a combination of two diuretic agents with different but complementary mechanisms and sites of action, thereby providing additive diuretic and antihypertensive effects. Additionally, the spironolactone component helps to minimize the potassium loss characteristically induced by the thiazide component.
The diuretic effect of spironolactone is mediated through its action as a specific pharmacologic antagonist of aldosterone, primarily by competitive binding of receptors at the aldosterone-dependent sodium-potassium exchange site in the distal convoluted renal tubule. Hydrochlorothiazide promotes the excretion of sodium and water primarily by inhibiting their reabsorption in the cortical diluting segment of the distal renal tubule.
Aldactazide is effective in significantly lowering the systolic and diastolic blood pressure in many patients with essential hypertension, even when aldosterone secretion is within normal limits.
Both spironolactone and hydrochlorothiazide reduce exchangeable sodium, plasma volume, body weight, and blood pressure. The diuretic and antihypertensive effects of the individual components are potentiated when spironolactone and hydrochlorothiazide are given concurrently.
Pharmacokinetics: Spironolactone is rapidly and extensively metabolized. Sulfur-containing products are the predominant metabolites and are thought to be primarily responsible, together with spironolactone, for the therapeutic effects of the drug. The following pharmacokinetic data were obtained from 12 healthy volunteers following the administration of 100 mg of spironolactone (Aldactone film-coated tablets) daily for 15 days. On the 15th day, spironolactone was given immediately after a low-fat breakfast and blood was drawn thereafter.

	Accumulation Factor: AUC (0–24 hr, day 15)/AUC (0–24 hr, day 1)	Mean Peak Serum Concentration	Mean (SD) Post-Steady State Half-life
7-α-(thiomethyl) spirolactone (TMS)	1.25	391 ng/mL at 3.2 hr	13.8 hr 6.4) (terminal)
6-β-hydroxy-7-α-(thiomethyl) spirolactone (HTMS)	1.50	125 ng/mL at 5.1 hr	15.0 hr (4.0) (terminal)
Canrenone (C)	1.41	181 ng/mL at 4.3 hr	16.5 hr (6.3) (terminal)
Spironolactone	1.30	80 ng/mL at 2.6 hr	Approximately 1.4 hr (0.5) (β half-life)

The pharmacological activity of spironolactone metabolites in man is not known. However, in the adrenalectomized rat the antimineralocorticoid activities of the metabolites C, TMS, and HTMS, relative to spironolactone, were 1.10, 1.28, and 0.32, respectively. Relative to spironolactone, their binding affinities to the aldosterone receptors in rat kidney slices were 0.19, 0.86, and 0.06, respectively.
In humans the potencies of TMS and 7-α-thiospirolactone in reversing the effects of the synthetic mineralocorticoid, fludrocortisone, on urinary electrolyte composition were 0.33 and 0.26, respectively, relative to spironolactone. However, since the serum concentrations of these steroids were not determined, their incomplete absorption and/or first-pass metabolism could not be ruled out as a reason for their reduced *in vivo* activities.
Both spironolactone and canrenone are more than 90% bound to plasma proteins. The metabolites are excreted primarily in the urine and secondarily in bile.
The effect of food on spironolactone absorption (two 100-mg Aldactone tablets) was assessed in a single dose study of 9 healthy, drug-free volunteers. Food increased the bioavailability of unmetabolized spironolactone by almost 100%. The clinical importance of this finding is not known.
Hydrochlorothiazide is rapidly absorbed following oral administration. Onset of action of hydrochlorothiazide is observed within one hour and persists for 6 to 12 hours. Hydrochlorothiazide plasma concentrations attain peak levels at one to two hours and decline with a half-life of four to five hours. Hydrochlorothiazide undergoes only slight metabolic alteration and is excreted in urine. It is distributed throughout the extracellular space, with essentially no tissue accumulation except in the kidney.

INDICATIONS AND USAGE

Spironolactone, an ingredient of Aldactazide, has been shown to be a tumorigen in chronic toxicity studies in rats (see *Warnings* section). Aldactazide should be used only in those conditions described below. Unnecessary use of this drug should be avoided.
Aldactazide is indicated for:
Edematous conditions for patients with:
Congestive heart failure: For the management of edema and sodium retention when the patient is only partially responsive to, or is intolerant of, other therapeutic measures. The treatment of diuretic-induced hypokalemia in patients with congestive heart failure when other measures are considered inappropriate. The treatment of patients with congestive heart failure taking digitalis when other therapies are considered inadequate or inappropriate.
Cirrhosis of the liver accompanied by edema and/or ascites: Aldosterone levels may be exceptionally high in this condition. Aldactazide is indicated for maintenance therapy together with bed rest and the restriction of fluid and sodium.
The nephrotic syndrome: For nephrotic patients when treatment of the underlying disease, restriction of fluid and sodium intake, and the use of other diuretics do not provide an adequate response.
Essential hypertension
For patients with essential hypertension in whom other measures are considered inadequate or inappropriate. In hypertensive patients for the treatment of a diuretic-induced hypokalemia when other measures are considered inappropriate.
Usage in Pregnancy. The routine use of diuretics in an otherwise healthy woman is inappropriate and exposes mother and fetus to unnecessary hazard. Diuretics do not prevent development of toxemia of pregnancy, and there is no satisfactory evidence that they are useful in the treatment of developing toxemia.
Edema during pregnancy may arise from pathologic causes or from the physiologic and mechanical consequences of pregnancy. Aldactazide is indicated in pregnancy when edema is due to pathologic causes just as it is in the absence of pregnancy (however, see *Warnings* section). Dependent edema in pregnancy, resulting from restriction of venous return by the expanded uterus, is properly treated through elevation of the lower extremities and use of support hose; use of diuretics to lower intravascular volume in this case is unsupported and unnecessary. There is hypervolemia during normal pregnancy which is not harmful to either the fetus or the mother (in the absence of cardiovascular disease), but which is associated with edema, including generalized edema, in the majority of pregnant women. If this edema produces discomfort, increased recumbency will often provide relief. In rare instances, this edema may cause extreme discomfort which is not relieved by rest. In these cases, a short course of diuretics may provide relief and may be appropriate.

CONTRAINDICATIONS

Aldactazide is contraindicated in patients with anuria, acute renal insufficiency, significant impairment of renal excretory function, or hyperkalemia, and in patients who are allergic to thiazide diuretics or to other sulfonamide-derived drugs. Aldactazide may also be contraindicated in acute or severe hepatic failure.

WARNINGS

Potassium supplementation, either in the form of medication or as a diet rich in potassium, should not ordinarily be given in association with Aldactazide therapy. Excessive potassium intake may cause hyperkalemia in patients receiving Aldactazide (see *Precautions* section). Aldactazide should not be administered concurrently with other potassium-sparing diuretics. Spironolactone, when used with ACE inhibitors, even in the presence of a diuretic, has been associated with severe hyperkalemia. Extreme caution should be exercised when Aldactazide is given concomitantly with ACE inhibitors (see *Precautions*).
Sulfonamide derivatives, including thiazides, have been reported to exacerbate or activate systemic lupus erythematosus.
Spironolactone has been shown to be a tumorigen in chronic toxicity studies performed in rats, with its proliferative effects manifested on endocrine organs and the liver. In one study using 25, 75, and 250 times the usual daily human dose (2 mg/kg) there was a statistically significant dose-related increase in benign adenomas of the thyroid and testes. In female rats there was a statistically significant increase in malignant mammary tumors at the mid-dose only. In male rats there was a dose-related increase in proliferative changes in the liver. At the highest dosage level (500 mg/kg), the range of effects included hepatocytomegaly, hyperplastic nodules, and hepatocellular carcinoma; the last was not statistically significant at a value of $p = 0.05$. A dose-related (above 20 mg/kg/day) incidence of myelocytic leukemia was observed in rats fed daily doses of potassium canrenoate for a period of one year. In long-term (two-year) oral carcinogenicity studies of potassium canrenoate in the rat, myelocytic leukemia and hepatic, thyroid, testicular, and mammary tumors were observed. Potassium canrenoate did not produce a mutagenic effect in tests using bacteria or yeast. It did produce a positive mutagenic effect in several *in vitro* tests in mammalian cells following metabolic activation. In an *in vivo* mammalian system potassium canrenoate was not mutagenic. Canrenone and canrenoic acid are the major metabolites of potassium canrenoate. Spironolactone is also metabolized to canrenone. An increased incidence of leukemia was not observed in chronic rat toxicity studies conducted with spironolactone at doses up to 500 mg/kg/day.

PRECAUTIONS

Patients receiving Aldactazide therapy should be carefully evaluated for possible disturbances of fluid and electrolyte balance. Hyperkalemia may occur in patients with impaired renal function or excessive potassium intake and can cause cardiac irregularities, which may be fatal. Consequently, no potassium supplement should ordinarily be given with Aldactazide. Hyperkalemia can be treated promptly by the rapid intravenous administration of glucose (20% to 50%) and regular insulin, using 0.25 to 0.5 units of insulin per gram of glucose. This is a temporary measure to be repeated as required. Aldactazide use should be discontinued and potassium intake (including dietary potassium) restricted.
Hypokalemia may develop as a result of profound diuresis, particularly when Aldactazide is used concomitantly with loop diuretics, glucocorticoids, or ACTH. Hypokalemia may exaggerate the effects of digitalis therapy. Potassium depletion may induce signs of digitalis intoxication at previously tolerated dosage levels.
Concomitant administration of potassium-sparing diuretics and ACE inhibitors or indomethacin has been associated with severe hyperkalemia.
Warning signs of possible fluid and electrolyte imbalance include dryness of the mouth, thirst, weakness, lethargy, drowsiness, restlessness, muscle pains or cramps, muscular fatigue, hypotension, oliguria, tachycardia, and gastrointestinal symptoms.
Aldactazide therapy may cause a transient elevation of BUN. This appears to represent a concentration phenomenon rather than renal toxicity, since the BUN level returns to normal after use of Aldactazide is discontinued. Progressive elevation of BUN is suggestive of the presence of preexisting renal impairment.
Reversible hyperchloremic metabolic acidosis, usually in association with hyperkalemia, has been reported to occur in some patients with decompensated hepatic cirrhosis, even in the presence of normal renal function.
Dilutional hyponatremia, manifested by dryness of the mouth, thirst, lethargy, and drowsiness, and confirmed by a low serum sodium level, may be induced, especially when Aldactazide is administered in combination with other diuretics. A true low-salt syndrome may rarely develop with Aldactazide therapy and may be manifested by increasing mental confusion similar to that observed with hepatic coma. This syndrome is differentiated from dilutional hyponatremia in that it does not occur with obvious fluid retention. Its treatment requires that diuretic therapy be discontinued and sodium administered.
Gynecomastia may develop in association with the use of spironolactone; physicians should be alert to its possible onset. The development of gynecomastia appears to be related to both dosage level and duration of therapy and is normally reversible when Aldactazide is discontinued. In rare instances some breast enlargement may persist when Aldactazide is discontinued.
Thiazides have been demonstrated to alter the metabolism of uric acid and carbohydrates, with possible development of hyperuricemia, gout, and decreased glucose tolerance. Thiazides may temporarily exaggerate abnormalities of glucose metabolism in diabetic patients or cause abnormalities to appear in patients with latent diabetes.
The antihypertensive effects of hydrochlorothiazide may be enhanced in patients who have undergone sympathectomy.

Pathologic changes in the parathyroid gland with hypercalcemia and hypophosphatemia have been observed in patients on prolonged thiazide therapy. Thiazides may also decrease serum PBI levels without evidence of alteration of thyroid function.

A determination of serum electrolytes to detect possible electrolyte imbalance should be performed at periodic intervals.

Both spironolactone and hydrochlorothiazide reduce the vascular responsiveness to norepinephrine. Therefore, caution should be exercised in the management of patients subjected to regional or general anesthesia while they are being treated with Aldactazide. Thiazides may also increase the responsiveness to tubocurarine.

Spironolactone has been shown to increase the half-life of digoxin. This may result in increased serum digoxin levels and subsequent digitalis toxicity. It may be necessary to reduce the maintenance and digitalization doses when spironolactone is administered, and the patient should be carefully monitored to avoid over- or underdigitalization.

Hydrochlorothiazide may raise the concentration of blood uric acid. Dosage adjustment of antigout medications may be necessary. Hydrochlorothiazide may also raise blood glucose concentrations. Dosage adjustments of insulin or hypoglycemic medications may be necessary. Concurrent use of diuretics with lithium is not recommended as it may produce lithium toxicity.

Several reports of possible interference with digoxin radioimmunoassays by spironolactone, or its metabolites, have appeared in the literature. Neither the extent nor the potential clinical significance of its interference (which may be assay-specific) has been fully established.

Usage in Pregnancy. Spironolactone or its metabolites may, and hydrochlorothiazide does, cross the placental barrier. Therefore, the use of Aldactazide in pregnant women requires that the anticipated benefit be weighed against possible hazards to the fetus. These hazards include fetal or neonatal jaundice, thrombocytopenia, and possible other adverse reactions which have been reported in the adult.

Nursing Mothers. Canrenone, a metabolite of spironolactone, and hydrochlorothiazide appear in breast milk. If use of these drugs is deemed essential, an alternative method of infant feeding should be instituted.

ADVERSE REACTIONS

Gynecomastia is observed not infrequently. A few cases of agranulocytosis have been reported in patients taking spironolactone. Other adverse reactions that have been reported in association with the use of spironolactone are: gastrointestinal symptoms including cramping and diarrhea, drowsiness, lethargy, headache, maculopapular or erythematous cutaneous eruptions, urticaria, mental confusion, drug fever, ataxia, inability to achieve or maintain erection, irregular menses or amenorrhea, postmenopausal bleeding, hirsutism, deepening of the voice, gastric bleeding, ulceration, gastritis, and vomiting. Carcinoma of the breast has been reported in patients taking spironolactone, but a cause and effect relationship has not been established.

Adverse reactions reported in association with the use of thiazides include: gastrointestinal symptoms (anorexia, nausea, vomiting, diarrhea, abdominal cramps), purpura, thrombocytopenia, leukopenia, agranulocytosis, dermatologic symptoms (cutaneous eruptions, pruritus, erythema multiforme), paresthesia, acute pancreatitis, jaundice, dizziness, vertigo, headache, xanthopsia, photosensitivity, necrotizing angiitis, aplastic anemia, orthostatic hypotension, muscle spasm, weakness, restlessness, and hypokalemia.

Adverse reactions are usually reversible upon discontinuation of Aldactazide.

DOSAGE AND ADMINISTRATION

Optimal dosage should be established by individual titration of the components (see Box Warning).

Edema in adults (*congestive heart failure, hepatic cirrhosis, or nephrotic syndrome*). The usual maintenance dose of Aldactazide is 100 mg each of spironolactone and hydrochlorothiazide daily, administered in a single dose or in divided doses, but may range from 25 mg to 200 mg of each component daily depending on the response to the initial titration. In some instances it may be desirable to administer separate tablets of either Aldactone (spironolactone) or hydrochlorothiazide in addition to Aldactazide in order to provide optimal individual therapy.

The onset of diuresis with Aldactazide occurs promptly and, due to prolonged effect of the spironolactone component, persists for two to three days after Aldactazide is discontinued.

Edema in children. The usual daily maintenance dose of Aldactazide should be that which provides 0.75 to 1.5 mg of spironolactone per pound of body weight (1.65 to 3.3 mg/kg).

Essential hypertension. Although the dosage will vary depending on the results of titration of the individual ingredients, many patients will be found to have an optimal response to 50 mg to 100 mg each of spironolactone and hydrochlorothiazide daily, given in a single dose or in divided doses.

Concurrent potassium supplementation is not recommended when Aldactazide is used in the long-term management of hypertension or in the treatment of most edematous conditions, since the spironolactone content of Aldactazide is usually sufficient to minimize loss induced by the hydrochlorothiazide component.

HOW SUPPLIED

Aldactazide tablets containing 25 mg of spironolactone (Aldactone) and 25 mg of hydrochlorothiazide are round, tan, film coated, with SEARLE and 1011 debossed on one side and ALDACTAZIDE and 25 on the other side, supplied as:

NDC Number	Size
0025-1011-31	bottle of 100
0025-1011-51	bottle of 500
0025-1011-52	bottle of 1000
0025-1011-55	bottle of 2500
0025-1011-34	carton of 100 unit dose

Aldactazide tablets containing 50 mg of spironolactone (Aldactone) and 50 mg of hydrochlorothiazide are oblong, tan, scored, film coated, with SEARLE and 1021 debossed on the scored side and ALDACTAZIDE and 50 on the other side, supplied as:

NDC Number	Size
0025-1021-31	bottle of 100
0025-1021-34	carton of 100 unit dose

Store below 86°F (30°C).

Caution: Federal law prohibits dispensing without prescription.

5/14/92 • A05388-4

Shown in Product Identification Section, page 429

ALDACTONE® ℞

[al-dac'tone]
(spironolactone)

> **WARNING**
> Spironolactone has been shown to be a tumorigen in chronic toxicity studies in rats (see *Warnings*). Aldactone should be used only in those conditions described under *Indications and Usage*. Unnecessary use of this drug should be avoided.

DESCRIPTION

Aldactone oral tablets contain 25 mg, 50 mg, or 100 mg of the aldosterone antagonist spironolactone, 17-hydroxy-7α-mercapto-3-oxo-17α-pregn-4-ene-21-carboxylic acid γ-lactone acetate, which has the following structural formula:

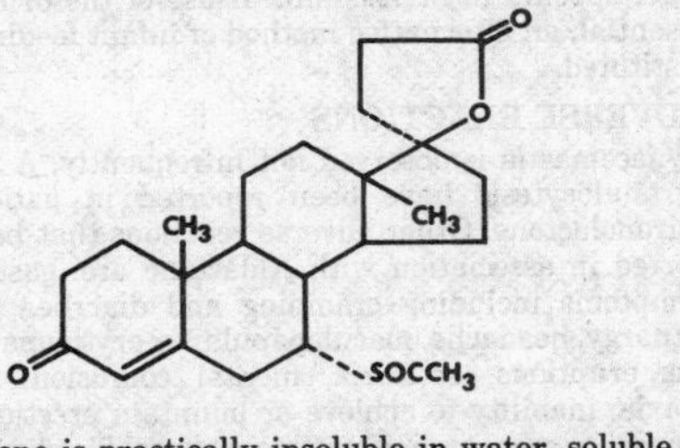

Spironolactone is practically insoluble in water, soluble in alcohol, and freely soluble in benzene and in chloroform.

Inactive ingredients include calcium sulfate, corn starch, flavor, hydroxypropyl methylcellulose, iron oxide, magnesium stearate, polyethylene glycol, povidone, and titanium dioxide.

CLINICAL PHARMACOLOGY

Mechanism of action: Aldactone (spironolactone) is a specific pharmacologic antagonist of aldosterone, acting primarily through competitive binding of receptors at the aldosterone-dependent sodium-potassium exchange site in the distal convoluted renal tubule. Aldactone causes increased amounts of sodium and water to be excreted, while potassium is retained. Aldactone acts both as a diuretic and as an antihypertensive drug by this mechanism. It may be given alone or with other diuretic agents which act more proximally in the renal tubule.

Aldosterone antagonist activity: Increased levels of the mineralocorticoid, aldosterone, are present in primary and secondary hyperaldosteronism. Edematous states in which secondary aldosteronism is usually involved include congestive heart failure, hepatic cirrhosis, and the nephrotic syndrome. By competing with aldosterone for receptor sites, Aldactone provides effective therapy for the edema and ascites in those conditions. Aldactone counteracts secondary aldosteronism induced by the volume depletion and associated sodium loss caused by active diuretic therapy.

Aldactone is effective in lowering the systolic and diastolic blood pressure in patients with primary hyperaldosteronism. It is also effective in most cases of essential hypertension, despite the fact that aldosterone secretion may be within normal limits in benign essential hypertension.

Through its action in antagonizing the effect of aldosterone, Aldactone inhibits the exchange of sodium for potassium in the distal renal tubule and helps to prevent potassium loss.

Aldactone has not been demonstrated to elevate serum uric acid, to precipitate gout, or to alter carbohydrate metabolism.

Pharmacokinetics: Spironolactone is rapidly and extensively metabolized. Sulfur-containing products are the predominant metabolites and are thought to be primarily responsible, together with spironolactone, for the therapeutic effects of the drug. The following pharmacokinetic data were obtained from 12 healthy volunteers following the administration of 100 mg of spironolactone (Aldactone film-coated tablets) daily for 15 days. On the 15th day, spironolactone was given immediately after a low-fat breakfast and blood was drawn thereafter.

	Accumulation Factor: AUC (0–24 hr, day 15)/AUC (0–24 hr, day 1)	Mean Peak Serum Concentration	Mean (SD) Post-Steady State Half-life
7-α-(thiomethyl) spirolactone (TMS)	1.25	391 ng/mL at 3.2 hr	13.8 hr (6.4) (terminal)
6-β-hydroxy-7-α-(thiomethyl) spirolactone (HTMS)	1.50	125 ng/mL at 5.1 hr	15.0 hr (4.0) (terminal)
Canrenone (C)	1.41	181 ng/mL at 4.3 hr	16.5 hr (6.3) (terminal)
Spironolactone	1.30	80 ng/mL at 2.6 hr	Approximately 1.4 hr (0.5) (β half-life)

The pharmacological activity of spironolactone metabolites in man is not known. However, in the adrenalectomized rat the antimineralocorticoid activities of the metabolites C, TMS, and HTMS, relative to spironolactone, were 1.10, 1.28, and 0.32, respectively. Relative to spironolactone, their binding affinities to the aldosterone receptors in rat kidney slices were 0.19, 0.86, and 0.06, respectively.

In humans the potencies of TMS and 7-α-thiospirolactone in reversing the effects of the synthetic mineralocorticoid, fludrocortisone, on urinary electrolyte composition were 0.33 and 0.26, respectively, relative to spironolactone. However, since the serum concentrations of these steroids were not determined, their incomplete absorption and/or first-pass metabolism could not be ruled out as a reason for their reduced *in vivo* activities.

Both spironolactone and canrenone are more than 90% bound to plasma proteins. The metabolites are excreted primarily in the urine and secondarily in bile.

The effect of food on spironolactone absorption (two 100-mg Aldactone tablets) was assessed in a single dose study of 9 healthy, drug-free volunteers. Food increased the bioavailability of unmetabolized spironolactone by almost 100%. The clinical importance of this finding is not known.

INDICATIONS AND USAGE

Aldactone (spironolactone) is indicated in the management of:

Primary hyperaldosteronism for:

- Establishing the diagnosis of primary hyperaldosteronism by therapeutic trial.
- Short-term preoperative treatment of patients with primary hyperaldosteronism.
- Long-term maintenance therapy for patients with discrete aldosterone-producing adrenal adenomas who are judged to be poor operative risks or who decline surgery.
- Long-term maintenance therapy for patients with bilateral micro- or macronodular adrenal hyperplasia (idiopathic hyperaldosteronism).

Edematous conditions for patients with:

- **Congestive heart failure:** For the management of edema and sodium retention when the patient is only partially responsive to, or is intolerant of, other therapeutic measures. Aldactone is also indicated for patients with congestive heart failure taking digitalis when other therapies are considered inappropriate.
- **Cirrhosis of the liver accompanied by edema and/or ascites:** Aldosterone levels may be exceptionally high in this condition. Aldactone is indicated for maintenance therapy together with bed rest and the restriction of fluid and sodium.
- **The nephrotic syndrome:** For nephrotic patients when treatment of the underlying disease, restriction of fluid and sodium intake, and the use of other diuretics do not provide an adequate response.

Continued on next page

Searle—Cont.

Essential hypertension
Usually in combination with other drugs, Aldactone is indicated for patients who cannot be treated adequately with other agents or for whom other agents are considered inappropriate.

Hypokalemia
For the treatment of patients with hypokalemia when other measures are considered inappropriate or inadequate. Aldactone is also indicated for the prophylaxis of hypokalemia in patients taking digitalis when other measures are considered inadequate or inappropriate.

Usage in Pregnancy. The routine use of diuretics in an otherwise healthy woman is inappropriate and exposes mother and fetus to unnecessary hazard. Diuretics do not prevent development of toxemia of pregnancy, and there is no satisfactory evidence that they are useful in the treatment of developing toxemia.

Edema during pregnancy may arise from pathologic causes or from the physiologic and mechanical consequences of pregnancy.

Aldactone is indicated in pregnancy when edema is due to pathologic causes just as it is in the absence of pregnancy (however, see *Warnings* section). Dependent edema in pregnancy, resulting from restriction of venous return by the expanded uterus, is properly treated through elevation of the lower extremities and use of support hose; use of diuretics to lower intravascular volume in this case is unsupported and unnecessary. There is hypervolemia during normal pregnancy which is not harmful to either the fetus or the mother (in the absence of cardiovascular disease), but which is associated with edema, including generalized edema, in the majority of pregnant women. If this edema produces discomfort, increased recumbency will often provide relief. In rare instances, this edema may cause extreme discomfort which is not relieved by rest. In these cases, a short course of diuretics may provide relief and may be appropriate.

CONTRAINDICATIONS
Aldactone is contraindicated for patients with anuria, acute renal insufficiency, significant impairment of renal excretory function, or hyperkalemia.

WARNINGS
Potassium supplementation, either in the form of medication or as a diet rich in potassium, should not ordinarily be given in association with Aldactone therapy. Excessive potassium intake may cause hyperkalemia in patients receiving Aldactone (see *Precautions* section). Aldactone should not be administered concurrently with other potassium-sparing diuretics. Aldactone, when used with ACE inhibitors, even in the presence of a diuretic, has been associated with severe hyperkalemia. Extreme caution should be exercised when Aldactone is given concomitantly with ACE inhibitors (see *Precautions: Drug interactions*).

Spironolactone has been shown to be a tumorigen in chronic toxicity studies performed in rats, with its proliferative effects manifested on endocrine organs and the liver. In one study using 25, 75, and 250 times the usual daily human dose (2 mg/kg) there was a statistically significant dose-related increase in benign adenomas of the thyroid and testes. In female rats there was a statistically significant increase in malignant mammary tumors at the mid-dose only. In male rats there was a dose-related increase in proliferative changes in the liver. At the highest dosage level (500 mg/kg) the range of effects included hepatocytomegaly, hyperplastic nodules, and hepatocellular carcinoma; the last was not statistically significant at a value of $p = 0.05$. A dose-related (above 20 mg/kg/day) incidence of myelocytic leukemia was observed in rats fed daily doses of potassium canrenoate for a period of one year. In long-term (two-year) oral carcinogenicity studies of potassium canrenoate in the rat, myelocytic leukemia and hepatic, thyroid, testicular, and mammary tumors were observed. Potassium canrenoate did not produce a mutagenic effect in tests using bacteria or yeast. It did produce a positive mutagenic effect in several *in vitro* tests in mammalian cells following metabolic activation. In an *in vivo* mammalian system potassium canrenoate was not mutagenic. Canrenone and canrenoic acid are the major metabolites of potassium canrenoate. Spironolactone is also metabolized to canrenone. An increased incidence of leukemia was not observed in chronic rat toxicity studies conducted with spironolactone at doses up to 500 mg/kg/day.

PRECAUTIONS
General: Because of the diuretic action of Aldactone (spironolactone), patients should be carefully evaluated for possible disturbances of fluid and electrolyte balance. Hyperkalemia may occur in patients with impaired renal function or excessive potassium intake and can cause cardiac irregularities, which may be fatal. Consequently, no potassium supplement should ordinarily be given with Aldactone. Hyperkalemia can be treated promptly by the rapid intravenous administration of glucose (20% to 50%) and regular insulin, using 0.25 to 0.5 units of insulin per gram of glucose.

This is a temporary measure to be repeated as required. Aldactone use should be discontinued and potassium intake (including dietary potassium) restricted.

Reversible hyperchloremic metabolic acidosis, usually in association with hyperkalemia, has been reported to occur in some patients with decompensated hepatic cirrhosis, even in the presence of normal renal function.

Hyponatremia, manifested by dryness of the mouth, thirst, lethargy, and drowsiness, and confirmed by a low serum sodium level, may be caused or aggravated, especially when Aldactone is administered in combination with other diuretics.

Gynecomastia may develop in association with the use of spironolactone; physicians should be alert to its possible onset. The development of gynecomastia appears to be related to both dosage level and duration of therapy and is normally reversible when Aldactone is discontinued. In rare instances some breast enlargement may persist when Aldactone is discontinued.

Aldactone therapy may cause a transient elevation of BUN, especially in patients with preexisting renal impairment. Aldactone may cause mild acidosis.

A determination of serum electrolytes to detect possible electrolyte imbalance should be performed at periodic intervals.

Drug interactions: When used in combination with other diuretics or antihypertensive agents, Aldactone potentiates their effects. Therefore, the dosage of such drugs, particularly the ganglionic blocking agents, should be reduced by at least 50% when Aldactone is added to the regimen.

Concomitant administration of potassium-sparing diuretics with ACE inhibitors or indomethacin has been associated with severe hyperkalemia.

Spironolactone reduces the vascular responsiveness to norepinephrine. Therefore, caution should be exercised in the management of patients subjected to regional or general anesthesia while they are being treated with Aldactone.

Spironolactone has been shown to increase the half-life of digoxin. This may result in increased serum digoxin levels and subsequent digitalis toxicity. It may be necessary to reduce the maintenance and digitalization doses when spironolactone is administered, and the patient should be carefully monitored to avoid over- or underdigitalization.

Drug/Laboratory test interactions: Several reports of possible interference with digoxin radioimmunoassays by spironolactone, or its metabolites, have appeared in the literature. Neither the extent nor the potential clinical significance of its interference (which may be assay-specific) has been fully established.

Usage in pregnancy: Spironolactone or its metabolites may cross the placental barrier. Therefore, the use of Aldactone in pregnant women requires that the anticipated benefit be weighed against possible hazard to the fetus.

Nursing mothers: Canrenone, a metabolite of spironolactone, appears in breast milk. If use of the drug is deemed essential, an alternative method of infant feeding should be instituted.

ADVERSE REACTIONS
Gynecomastia is observed not infrequently. A few cases of agranulocytosis have been reported in patients taking spironolactone. Other adverse reactions that have been reported in association with Aldactone are: gastrointestinal symptoms including cramping and diarrhea, drowsiness, lethargy, headache, maculopapular or erythematous cutaneous eruptions, urticaria, mental confusion, drug fever, ataxia, inability to achieve or maintain erection, irregular menses or amenorrhea, postmenopausal bleeding, hirsutism, deepening of the voice, gastric bleeding, ulceration, gastritis, and vomiting. Carcinoma of the breast has been reported in patients taking spironolactone, but a cause and effect relationship has not been established.

Adverse reactions are usually reversible upon discontinuation of the drug.

DOSAGE AND ADMINISTRATION
Primary hyperaldosteronism. Aldactone may be employed as an initial diagnostic measure to provide presumptive evidence of primary hyperaldosteronism while patients are on normal diets.

Long test: Aldactone (spironolactone) is administered at a daily dosage of 400 mg for three to four weeks. Correction of hypokalemia and of hypertension provides presumptive evidence for the diagnosis of primary hyperaldosteronism.

Short test: Aldactone is administered at a daily dosage of 400 mg for four days. If serum potassium increases during Aldactone administration but drops when Aldactone is discontinued, a presumptive diagnosis of primary hyperaldosteronism should be considered.

After the diagnosis of hyperaldosteronism has been established by more definitive testing procedures, Aldactone may be administered in doses of 100 to 400 mg daily in preparation for surgery. For patients who are considered unsuitable for surgery, Aldactone may be employed for long-term maintenance therapy at the lowest effective dosage determined for the individual patient.

Edema in adults (*congestive heart failure, hepatic cirrhosis, or nephrotic syndrome*). An initial daily dosage of 100 mg of Aldactone administered in either single or divided doses is recommended, but may range from 25 to 200 mg daily. When given as the sole agent for diuresis, Aldactone should be continued for at least five days at the initial dosage level, after which it may be adjusted to the optimal therapeutic or maintenance level administered in either single or divided daily doses. If, after five days, an adequate diuretic response to Aldactone has not occurred, a second diuretic which acts more proximally in the renal tubule may be added to the regimen. Because of the additive effect of Aldactone when administered concurrently with such diuretics, an enhanced diuresis usually begins on the first day of combined treatment; combined therapy is indicated when more rapid diuresis is desired. The dosage of Aldactone should remain unchanged when other diuretic therapy is added.

Edema in children. The initial daily dosage should provide approximately 1.5 mg of Aldactone per pound of body weight (3.3 mg/kg) administered in either single or divided doses.

Essential hypertension. For adults, an initial daily dosage of 50 to 100 mg of Aldactone administered in either single or divided doses is recommended. Aldactone may also be given with diuretics which act more proximally in the renal tubule or with other antihypertensive agents. Treatment with Aldactone should be continued for at least two weeks, since the maximum response may not occur before this time. Subsequently, dosage should be adjusted according to the response of the patient.

Hypokalemia. Aldactone in a dosage ranging from 25 mg to 100 mg daily is useful in treating a diuretic-induced hypokalemia, when oral potassium supplements or other potassium-sparing regimens are considered inappropriate.

HOW SUPPLIED
Aldactone 25-mg tablets are round, light yellow, film coated, with SEARLE and 1001 debossed on one side and ALDACTONE and 25 on the other side, supplied as:

NDC Number	Size
0025-1001-31	bottle of 100
0025-1001-51	bottle of 500
0025-1001-52	bottle of 1000
0025-1001-55	bottle of 2500
0025-1001-34	carton of 100 unit dose

Aldactone 50-mg tablets are oval, light orange, scored, film coated, with SEARLE and 1041 debossed on the scored side and ALDACTONE and 50 on the other side, supplied as:

NDC Number	Size
0025-1041-31	bottle of 100
0025-1041-34	carton of 100 unit dose

Aldactone 100-mg tablets are round, peach colored, scored, film coated, with SEARLE and 1031 debossed on the scored side and ALDACTONE and 100 on the other side, supplied as:

NDC Number	Size
0025-1031-31	bottle of 100
0025-1031-34	carton of 100 unit dose

Store below 86°F (30°C).

Caution: Federal law prohibits dispensing without prescription.

5/14/92 ● AO5449-4

Shown in Product Identification Section, page 429

CALAN® Tablets   ℞
[*cal'an*]
(verapamil hydrochloride)

PRODUCT OVERVIEW

KEY FACTS
Calan, a calcium ion antagonist, exerts its pharmacologic effects by modulating the influx of ionic calcium across the cell membrane of the arterial smooth muscle as well as in conductile and contractile myocardial cells. Calan increases myocardial oxygen supply, reduces myocardial oxygen consumption, and is a potent inhibitor of coronary artery spasm, making it an effective antianginal agent. By decreasing the influx of calcium, Calan prolongs the effective refractory period within the AV node and slows AV conduction in a rate-related manner, thereby slowing the ventricular rate in patients with chronic atrial flutter or fibrillation. Calan exerts antihypertensive effects by decreasing systemic vascular resistance, usually without orthostatic decreases in blood pressure or reflex tachycardia.

MAJOR USES
Calan Tablets are indicated for: angina at rest, including vasospastic and unstable angina; chronic stable angina; control (in association with digitalis) of ventricular rate at rest and during stress in patients with chronic atrial flutter and/or atrial fibrillation; prophylaxis of repetitive paroxysmal supraventricular tachycardia; management of essential hypertension.

SAFETY INFORMATION

See complete safety information set forth below.

PRESCRIBING INFORMATION

CALAN® Tablets ℞

[cal'an]

(verapamil hydrochloride)

DESCRIPTION

Calan (verapamil HCl) is a calcium ion influx inhibitor (slow-channel blocker or calcium ion antagonist) available for oral administration in film-coated tablets containing 40 mg, 80 mg, or 120 mg of verapamil hydrochloride.

The structural formula of verapamil HCl is

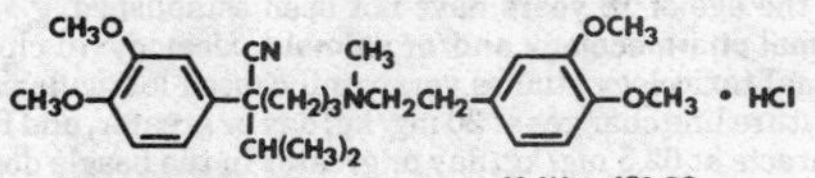

$C_{27}H_{38}N_2O_4 \cdot HCl$ M.W. = 491.08

Benzeneacetonitrile, α-[3-[[2-(3,4-dimethoxyphenyl) ethyl] methylamino]propyl]-3,4-dimethoxy-α-(1-methylethyl) hydrochloride

Verapamil HCl is an almost white, crystalline powder, practically free of odor, with a bitter taste. It is soluble in water, chloroform, and methanol. Verapamil HCl is not chemically related to other cardioactive drugs.

Inactive ingredients include microcrystalline cellulose, corn starch, gelatin, hydroxypropyl cellulose, hydroxypropyl methylcellulose, iron oxide colorant, lactose, magnesium stearate, polyethylene glycol, talc, and titanium dioxide.

CLINICAL PHARMACOLOGY

Calan is a calcium ion influx inhibitor (slow-channel blocker or calcium ion antagonist) that exerts its pharmacologic effects by modulating the influx of ionic calcium across the cell membrane of the arterial smooth muscle as well as in conductile and contractile myocardial cells.

Mechanism of action

Angina: The precise mechanism of action of Calan as an antianginal agent remains to be fully determined, but includes the following two mechanisms:

1. *Relaxation and prevention of coronary artery spasm:* Calan dilates the main coronary arteries and coronary arterioles, both in normal and ischemic regions, and is a potent inhibitor of coronary artery spasm, whether spontaneous or ergonovine-induced. This property increases myocardial oxygen delivery in patients with coronary artery spasm and is responsible for the effectiveness of Calan in vasospastic (Prinzmetal's or variant) as well as unstable angina at rest. Whether this effect plays any role in classical effort angina is not clear, but studies of exercise tolerance have not shown an increase in the maximum exercise rate–pressure product, a widely accepted measure of oxygen utilization. This suggests that, in general, relief of spasm or dilation of coronary arteries is not an important factor in classical angina.
2. *Reduction of oxygen utilization:* Calan regularly reduces the total peripheral resistance (afterload) against which the heart works both at rest and at a given level of exercise by dilating peripheral arterioles. This unloading of the heart reduces myocardial energy consumption and oxygen requirements and probably accounts for the effectiveness of Calan in chronic stable effort angina.

Arrhythmia: Electrical activity through the AV node depends, to a significant degree, upon calcium influx through the slow channel. By decreasing the influx of calcium, Calan prolongs the effective refractory period within the AV node and slows AV conduction in a rate-related manner. This property accounts for the ability of Calan to slow the ventricular rate in patients with chronic atrial flutter or atrial fibrillation.

Normal sinus rhythm is usually not affected, but in patients with sick sinus syndrome, Calan may interfere with sinus-node impulse generation and may induce sinus arrest or sinoatrial block. Atrioventricular block can occur in patients without preexisting conduction defects (see *Warnings*). Calan decreases the frequency of episodes of paroxysmal supraventricular tachycardia.

Calan does not alter the normal atrial action potential or intraventricular conduction time, but in depressed atrial fibers it decreases amplitude, velocity of depolarization, and conduction velocity. Calan may shorten the antegrade effective refractory period of the accessory bypass tract. Acceleration of ventricular rate and/or ventricular fibrillation has been reported in patients with atrial flutter or atrial fibrillation and a coexisting accessory AV pathway following administration of verapamil (see *Warnings*).

Calan has a local anesthetic action that is 1.6 times that of procaine on an equimolar basis. It is not known whether this action is important at the doses used in man.

Essential hypertension: Calan exerts antihypertensive effects by decreasing systemic vascular resistance, usually without orthostatic decreases in blood pressure or reflex tachycardia; bradycardia (rate less than 50 beats/min) is uncommon (1.4%). During isometric or dynamic exercise Calan does not alter systolic cardiac function in patients with normal ventricular function.

Calan does not alter total serum calcium levels. However, one report suggested that calcium levels above the normal range may alter the therapeutic effect of Calan.

Pharmacokinetics and metabolism: More than 90% of the orally administered dose of Calan is absorbed. Because of rapid biotransformation of verapamil during its first pass through the portal circulation, bioavailability ranges from 20% to 35%. Peak plasma concentrations are reached between 1 and 2 hours after oral administration. Chronic oral administration of 120 mg of verapamil HCl every 6 hours resulted in plasma levels of verapamil ranging from 125 to 400 ng/ml, with higher values reported occasionally. A nonlinear correlation between the verapamil dose administered and verapamil plasma levels does exist. No relationship has been established between the plasma concentration of verapamil and a reduction in blood pressure. In early dose titration with verapamil a relationship exists between verapamil plasma concentration and prolongation of the PR interval. However, during chronic administration this relationship may disappear. The mean elimination half-life in single-dose studies ranged from 2.8 to 7.4 hours. In these same studies, after repetitive dosing, the half-life increased to a range from 4.5 to 12.0 hours (after less than 10 consecutive doses given 6 hours apart). Half-life of verapamil may increase during titration. Aging may affect the pharmacokinetics of verapamil. Elimination half-life may be prolonged in the elderly. In healthy men, orally administered Calan undergoes extensive metabolism in the liver. Twelve metabolites have been identified in plasma; all except norverapamil are present in trace amounts only. Norverapamil can reach steady-state plasma concentrations approximately equal to those of verapamil itself. The cardiovascular activity of norverapamil appears to be approximately 20% that of verapamil. Approximately 70% of an administered dose is excreted as metabolites in the urine and 16% or more in the feces within 5 days. About 3% to 4% is excreted in the urine as unchanged drug. Approximately 90% is bound to plasma proteins. In patients with hepatic insufficiency, metabolism is delayed and elimination half-life prolonged up to 14 to 16 hours (see *Precautions*); the volume of distribution is increased and plasma clearance reduced to about 30% of normal. Verapamil clearance values suggest that patients with liver dysfunction may attain therapeutic verapamil plasma concentrations with one third of the oral daily dose required for patients with normal liver function.

After four weeks of oral dosing (120 mg q.i.d.), verapamil and norverapamil levels were noted in the cerebrospinal fluid with estimated partition coefficient of 0.06 for verapamil and 0.04 for norverapamil.

Hemodynamics and myocardial metabolism: Calan reduces afterload and myocardial contractility. Improved left ventricular diastolic function in patients with IHSS and those with coronary heart disease has also been observed with Calan therapy. In most patients, including those with organic cardiac disease, the negative inotropic action of Calan is countered by reduction of afterload, and cardiac index is usually not reduced. However, in patients with severe left ventricular dysfunction (eg, pulmonary wedge pressure above 20 mm Hg or ejection fraction less than 30%), or in patients taking beta-adrenergic blocking agents or other cardiodepressant drugs, deterioration of ventricular function may occur (see *Drug interactions*).

Pulmonary function: Calan does not induce bronchoconstriction and, hence, does not impair ventilatory function.

INDICATIONS AND USAGE

Calan tablets are indicated for the treatment of the following:

Angina

1. Angina at rest, including:
   —Vasospastic (Prinzmetal's variant) angina
   —Unstable (crescendo, pre-infarction) angina
2. Chronic stable angina (classic effort-associated angina)

Arrhythmias

1. In association with digitalis for the control of ventricular rate at rest and during stress in patients with chronic atrial flutter and/or atrial fibrillation (see *Warnings: Accessory bypass tract*)
2. Prophylaxis of repetitive paroxysmal supraventricular tachycardia

Essential hypertension

CONTRAINDICATIONS

Verapamil HCl tablets are contraindicated in:

1. Severe left ventricular dysfunction (see *Warnings*)
2. Hypotension (systolic pressure less than 90 mm Hg) or cardiogenic shock
3. Sick sinus syndrome (except in patients with a functioning artificial ventricular pacemaker)
4. Second- or third-degree AV block (except in patients with a functioning artificial ventricular pacemaker)
5. Patients with atrial flutter or atrial fibrillation and an accessory bypass tract (eg, Wolff-Parkinson-White, Lown-Ganong-Levine syndromes). (See *Warnings*.)
6. Patients with known hypersensitivity to verapamil hydrochloride.

WARNINGS

Heart failure: Verapamil has a negative inotropic effect, which in most patients is compensated by its afterload reduction (decreased systemic vascular resistance) properties without a net impairment of ventricular performance. In clinical experience with 4,954 patients, 87 (1.8%) developed congestive heart failure or pulmonary edema. Verapamil should be avoided in patients with severe left ventricular dysfunction (eg, ejection fraction less than 30%) or moderate to severe symptoms of cardiac failure and in patients with any degree of ventricular dysfunction if they are receiving a beta-adrenergic blocker (see *Drug interactions*). Patients with milder ventricular dysfunction should, if possible, be controlled with optimum doses of digitalis and/or diuretics before verapamil treatment. **(Note interactions with digoxin under *Precautions*.)**

Hypotension: Occasionally, the pharmacologic action of verapamil may produce a decrease in blood pressure below normal levels, which may result in dizziness or symptomatic hypotension. The incidence of hypotension observed in 4,954 patients enrolled in clinical trials was 2.5%. In hypertensive patients, decreases in blood pressure below normal are unusual. Tilt-table testing (60 degrees) was not able to induce orthostatic hypotension.

Elevated liver enzymes: Elevations of transaminases with and without concomitant elevations in alkaline phosphatase and bilirubin have been reported. Such elevations have sometimes been transient and may disappear even with continued verapamil treatment. Several cases of hepatocellular injury related to verapamil have been proven by rechallenge; half of these had clinical symptoms (malaise, fever, and/or right upper quadrant pain), in addition to elevation of SGOT, SGPT, and alkaline phosphatase. Periodic monitoring of liver function in patients receiving verapamil is therefore prudent.

Accessory bypass tract (Wolff-Parkinson-White or Lown-Ganong-Levine): Some patients with paroxysmal and/or chronic atrial fibrillation or atrial flutter and a coexisting accessory AV pathway have developed increased antegrade conduction across the accessory pathway bypassing the AV node, producing a very rapid ventricular response or ventricular fibrillation after receiving intravenous verapamil (or digitalis). Although a risk of this occurring with oral verapamil has not been established, such patients receiving oral verapamil may be at risk and its use in these patients is contraindicated (see *Contraindications*). Treatment is usually DC-cardioversion. Cardioversion has been used safely and effectively after oral Calan.

Atrioventricular block: The effect of verapamil on AV conduction and the SA node may cause asymptomatic first-degree AV block and transient bradycardia, sometimes accompanied by nodal escape rhythms. PR-interval prolongation is correlated with verapamil plasma concentrations especially during the early titration phase of therapy. Higher degrees of AV block, however, were infrequently (0.8%) observed. Marked first-degree block or progressive development to second- or third-degree AV block requires a reduction in dosage or, in rare instances, discontinuation of verapamil HCl and institution of appropriate therapy, depending on the clinical situation.

Patients with hypertrophic cardiomyopathy (IHSS): In 120 patients with hypertrophic cardiomyopathy (most of them refractory or intolerant to propranolol) who received therapy with verapamil at doses up to 720 mg/day, a variety of serious adverse effects were seen. Three patients died in pulmonary edema; all had severe left ventricular outflow obstruction and a past history of left ventricular dysfunction. Eight other patients had pulmonary edema and/or severe hypotension; abnormally high (greater than 20 mm Hg) pulmonary wedge pressure and a marked left ventricular outflow obstruction were present in most of these patients. Concomitant administration of quinidine (see *Drug interactions*) preceded the severe hypotension in 3 of the 8 patients (2 of whom developed pulmonary edema). Sinus bradycardia occurred in 11% of the patients, second-degree AV block in 4%, and sinus arrest in 2%. It must be appreciated that this group of patients had a serious disease with a high mortality rate. Most adverse effects responded well to dose reduction, and only rarely did verapamil use have to be discontinued.

PRECAUTIONS

General

Use in patients with impaired hepatic function: Since verapamil is highly metabolized by the liver, it should be administered cautiously to patients with impaired hepatic function. Severe liver dysfunction prolongs the elimination half-life of verapamil to about 14 to 16 hours; hence, approximately 30% of the dose given to patients with normal liver

Continued on next page

Searle—Cont.

function should be administered to these patients. Careful monitoring for abnormal prolongation of the PR interval or other signs of excessive pharmacologic effects (see *Overdosage*) should be carried out.

Use in patients with attenuated (decreased) neuromuscular transmission: It has been reported that verapamil decreases neuromuscular transmission in patients with Duchenne's muscular dystrophy, and that verapamil prolongs recovery from the neuromuscular blocking agent vecuronium. It may be necessary to decrease the dosage of verapamil when it is administered to patients with attenuated neuromuscular transmission.

Use in patients with impaired renal function: About 70% of an administered dose of verapamil is excreted as metabolites in the urine. Verapamil is not removed by hemodialysis. Until further data are available, verapamil should be administered cautiously to patients with impaired renal function. These patients should be carefully monitored for abnormal prolongation of the PR interval or other signs of overdosage (see *Overdosage*).

Drug interactions

Beta-blockers: Controlled studies in small numbers of patients suggest that the concomitant use of Calan and oral beta-adrenergic blocking agents may be beneficial in certain patients with chronic stable angina or hypertension, but available information is not sufficient to predict with confidence the effects of concurrent treatment in patients with left ventricular dysfunction or cardiac conduction abnormalities. Concomitant therapy with beta-adrenergic blockers and verapamil may result in additive negative effects on heart rate, atrioventricular conduction and/or cardiac contractility.

In one study involving 15 patients treated with high doses of propranolol (median dose, 480 mg/day; range, 160 to 1,280 mg/day) for severe angina, with preserved left ventricular function (ejection fraction greater than 35%), the hemodynamic effects of additional therapy with verapamil HCl were assessed using invasive methods. The addition of verapamil to high-dose beta-blockers induced modest negative inotropic and chronotropic effects that were not severe enough to limit short-term (48 hours) combination therapy in this study. These modest cardiodepressant effects persisted for greater than 6 but less than 30 hours after abrupt withdrawal of beta-blockers and were closely related to plasma levels of propranolol. The primary verapamil/beta-blocker interaction in this study appeared to be hemodynamic rather than electrophysiologic.

In other studies verapamil did not generally induce significant negative inotropic, chronotropic, or dromotropic effects in patients with preserved left ventricular function receiving low or moderate doses of propranolol (less than or equal to 320 mg/day); in some patients, however, combined therapy did produce such effects. Therefore, if combined therapy is used, close surveillance of clinical status should be carried out. Combined therapy should usually be avoided in patients with atrioventricular conduction abnormalities and those with depressed left ventricular function.

Asymptomatic bradycardia (36 beats/min) with a wandering atrial pacemaker has been observed in a patient receiving concomitant timolol (a beta-adrenergic blocker) eyedrops and oral verapamil.

A decrease in metoprolol and propranolol clearance has been observed when either drug is administered concomitantly with verapamil. A variable effect has been seen when verapamil and atenolol were given together.

Digitalis: Clinical use of verapamil in digitalized patients has shown the combination to be well tolerated if digoxin doses are properly adjusted. However, chronic verapamil treatment can increase serum digoxin levels by 50% to 75% during the first week of therapy, and this can result in digitalis toxicity. In patients with hepatic cirrhosis the influence of verapamil on digoxin kinetics is magnified. Verapamil may reduce total body clearance and extrarenal clearance of digitoxin by 27% and 29%, respectively. Maintenance and digitalization doses should be reduced when verapamil is administered, and the patient should be reassessed to avoid over- or underdigitalization. Whenever overdigitalization is suspected, the daily dose of digitalis should be reduced or temporarily discontinued. On discontinuation of Calan use, the patient should be reassessed to avoid underdigitalization.

Antihypertensive agents: Verapamil administered concomitantly with oral antihypertensive agents (eg, vasodilators, angiotensin-converting enzyme inhibitors, diuretics, beta-blockers) will usually have an additive effect on lowering blood pressure. Patients receiving these combinations should be appropriately monitored. Concomitant use of agents that attenuate alpha-adrenergic function with verapamil may result in a reduction in blood pressure that is excessive in some patients. Such an effect was observed in one study following the concomitant administration of verapamil and prazosin.

Antiarrhythmic agents:

Disopyramide: Until data on possible interactions between verapamil and disopyramide are obtained, disopyramide should not be administered within 48 hours before or 24 hours after verapamil administration.

Flecainide: A study in healthy volunteers showed that the concomitant administration of flecainide and verapamil may have additive effects on myocardial contractility, AV conduction, and repolarization. Concomitant therapy with flecainide and verapamil may result in additive negative inotropic effect and prolongation of atrioventricular conduction.

Quinidine: In a small number of patients with hypertrophic cardiomyopathy (IHSS), concomitant use of verapamil and quinidine resulted in significant hypotension. Until further data are obtained, combined therapy of verapamil and quinidine in patients with hypertrophic cardiomyopathy should probably be avoided.

The electrophysiologic effects of quinidine and verapamil on AV conduction were studied in 8 patients. Verapamil significantly counteracted the effects of quinidine on AV conduction. There has been a report of increased quinidine levels during verapamil therapy.

Other:

Nitrates: Verapamil has been given concomitantly with short- and long-acting nitrates without any undesirable drug interactions. The pharmacologic profile of both drugs and the clinical experience suggest beneficial interactions.

Cimetidine: The interaction between cimetidine and chronically administered verapamil has not been studied. Variable results on clearance have been obtained in acute studies of healthy volunteers; clearance of verapamil was either reduced or unchanged.

Lithium: Increased sensitivity to the effects of lithium (neurotoxicity) has been reported during concomitant verapamil-lithium therapy with either no change or an increase in serum lithium levels. However, the addition of verapamil has also resulted in the lowering of serum lithium levels in patients receiving chronic stable oral lithium. Patients receiving both drugs must be monitored carefully.

Carbamazepine: Verapamil therapy may increase carbamazepine concentrations during combined therapy. This may produce carbamazepine side effects such as diplopia, headache, ataxia, or dizziness.

Rifampin: Therapy with rifampin may markedly reduce oral verapamil bioavailability.

Phenobarbital: Phenobarbital therapy may increase verapamil clearance.

Cyclosporin: Verapamil therapy may increase serum levels of cyclosporin.

Theophylline: Verapamil may inhibit the clearance and increase the plasma levels of theophylline.

Inhalation anesthetics: Animal experiments have shown that inhalation anesthetics depress cardiovascular activity by decreasing the inward movement of calcium ions. When used concomitantly, inhalation anesthetics and calcium antagonists, such as verapamil, should each be titrated carefully to avoid excessive cardiovascular depression.

Neuromuscular blocking agents: Clinical data and animal studies suggest that verapamil may potentiate the activity of neuromuscular blocking agents (curare-like and depolarizing). It may be necessary to decrease the dose of verapamil and/or the dose of the neuromuscular blocking agent when the drugs are used concomitantly.

Carcinogenesis, mutagenesis, impairment of fertility: An 18-month toxicity study in rats, at a low multiple (6-fold) of the maximum recommended human dose, and not the maximum tolerated dose, did not suggest a tumorigenic potential. There was no evidence of a carcinogenic potential of verapamil administered in the diet of rats for two years at doses of 10, 35, and 120 mg/kg/day or approximately 1, 3.5, and 12 times, respectively, the maximum recommended human daily dose (480 mg/day or 9.6 mg/kg/day).

Verapamil was not mutagenic in the Ames test in 5 test strains at 3 mg per plate with or without metabolic activation.

Studies in female rats at daily dietary doses up to 5.5 times (55 mg/kg/day) the maximum recommended human dose did not show impaired fertility. Effects on male fertility have not been determined.

Pregnancy: Pregnancy Category C. Reproduction studies have been performed in rabbits and rats at oral doses up to 1.5 (15 mg/kg/day) and 6 (60 mg/kg/day) times the human oral daily dose, respectively, and have revealed no evidence of teratogenicity. In the rat, however, this multiple of the human dose was embryocidal and retarded fetal growth and development, probably because of adverse maternal effects reflected in reduced weight gains of the dams. This oral dose has also been shown to cause hypotension in rats. There are no adequate and well-controlled studies in pregnant women. Because animal reproduction studies are not always predictive of human response, this drug should be used during pregnancy only if clearly needed. Verapamil crosses the placental barrier and can be detected in umbilical vein blood at delivery.

Labor and delivery: It is not known whether the use of verapamil during labor or delivery has immediate or delayed adverse effects on the fetus, or whether it prolongs the duration of labor or increases the need for forceps delivery or other obstetric intervention. Such adverse experiences have not been reported in the literature, despite a long history of use of verapamil in Europe in the treatment of cardiac side effects of beta-adrenergic agonist agents used to treat premature labor.

Nursing mothers: Verapamil is excreted in human milk. Because of the potential for adverse reactions in nursing infants from verapamil, nursing should be discontinued while verapamil is administered.

Pediatric use: Safety and efficacy of Calan in children below the age of 18 years have not been established.

Animal pharmacology and/or animal toxicology: In chronic animal toxicology studies verapamil caused lenticular and/or suture line changes at 30 mg/kg/day or greater, and frank cataracts at 62.5 mg/kg/day or greater in the beagle dog but not in the rat. Development of cataracts due to verapamil has not been reported in man.

ADVERSE REACTIONS

Serious adverse reactions are uncommon when Calan therapy is initiated with upward dose titration within the recommended single and total daily dose. See *Warnings* for discussion of heart failure, hypotension, elevated liver enzymes, AV block, and rapid ventricular response. Reversible (upon discontinuation of verapamil) non-obstructive, paralytic ileus has been infrequently reported in association with the use of verapamil. The following reactions to orally administered verapamil occurred at rates greater than 1.0% or occurred at lower rates but appeared clearly drug-related in clinical trials in 4,954 patients:

Constipation	7.3%	Dyspnea	1.4%
Dizziness	3.3%	Bradycardia	
Nausea	2.7%	(HR < 50/min)	1.4%
Hypotension	2.5%	AV block	
Headache	2.2%	total (1°, 2°, 3°)	1.2%
Edema	1.9%	2° and 3°	0.8%
CHF/Pulmonary		Rash	1.2%
edema	1.8%	Flushing	0.6%
Fatigue	1.7%		

Elevated liver enzymes (see *Warnings*)

In clinical trials related to the control of ventricular response in digitalized patients who had atrial fibrillation or flutter, ventricular rates below 50 at rest occurred in 15% of patients and asymptomatic hypotension occurred in 5% of patients.

The following reactions, reported in 1.0% or less of patients, occurred under conditions (open trials, marketing experience) where a causal relationship is uncertain; they are listed to alert the physician to a possible relationship:

Cardiovascular: angina pectoris, atrioventricular dissociation, chest pain, claudication, myocardial infarction, palpitations, purpura (vasculitis), syncope.

Digestive system: diarrhea, dry mouth, gastrointestinal distress, gingival hyperplasia.

Hemic and lymphatic: ecchymosis or bruising.

Nervous system: cerebrovascular accident, confusion, equilibrium disorders, insomnia, muscle cramps, paresthesia, psychotic symptoms, shakiness, somnolence.

Skin: arthralgia and rash, exanthema, hair loss, hyperkeratosis, macules, sweating, urticaria, Stevens-Johnson syndrome, erythema multiforme.

Special senses: blurred vision.

Urogenital: gynecomastia, galactorrhea/hyperprolactinemia, increased urination, spotty menstruation, impotence.

Treatment of acute cardiovascular adverse reactions: The frequency of cardiovascular adverse reactions that require therapy is rare; hence, experience with their treatment is limited. Whenever severe hypotension or complete AV block occurs following oral administration of verapamil, the appropriate emergency measures should be applied immediately; eg, intravenously administered norepinephrine bitartrate, atropine sulfate, isoproterenol HCl (all in the usual doses), or calcium gluconate (10% solution). In patients with hypertrophic cardiomyopathy (IHSS), alpha-adrenergic agents (phenylephrine HCl, metaraminol bitartrate, or methoxamine HCl) should be used to maintain blood pressure, and isoproterenol and norepinephrine should be avoided. If further support is necessary, dopamine HCl or dobutamine HCl may be administered. Actual treatment and dosage should depend on the severity of the clinical situation and the judgment and experience of the treating physician.

OVERDOSAGE

Overdose with verapamil may lead to pronounced hypotension, bradycardia, and conduction system abnormalities (eg, junctional rhythm with AV dissociation and high degree AV block, including asystole). Other symptoms secondary to hypoperfusion (eg, metabolic acidosis, hyperglycemia, hyperkalemia, renal dysfunction, and convulsions) may be evident.

Treat all verapamil overdoses as serious and maintain observation for at least 48 hours (especially Calan SR), preferably under continuous hospital care. Delayed pharmacodynamic consequences may occur with the sustained-release formulation. Verapamil is known to decrease gastrointestinal transit time. Verapamil cannot be removed by hemodialysis.

Treatment of overdosage should be supportive. Beta-adrenergic stimulation or parenteral administration of calcium solutions may increase calcium ion flux across the slow channel and has been used effectively in treatment of deliberate overdose of verapamil. The following measures may be considered:

Bradycardia and conduction system abnormalities: Atropine, isoproterenol, and cardiac pacing.

Hypotension: Intravenous fluids, vasopressors (eg, dopamine, dobutamine), calcium solutions (eg, 10% calcium chloride solution).

Cardiac failure: Inotropic agents (eg, isoproterenol, dopamine, dobutamine), diuretics.

Asystole should be handled by the usual measures including cardiopulmonary resuscitation.

DOSAGE AND ADMINISTRATION

The dose of verapamil must be individualized by titration. The usefulness and safety of dosages exceeding 480 mg/day have not been established; therefore, this daily dosage should not be exceeded. Since the half-life of verapamil increases during chronic dosing, maximum response may be delayed.

Angina: Clinical trials show that the usual dose is 80 mg to 120 mg three times a day. However, 40 mg three times a day may be warranted in patients who may have an increased response to verapamil (eg, decreased hepatic function, elderly, etc). Upward titration should be based on therapeutic efficacy and safety evaluated approximately eight hours after dosing. Dosage may be increased at daily (eg, patients with unstable angina) or weekly intervals until optimum clinical response is obtained.

Arrhythmias: The dosage in digitalized patients with chronic atrial fibrillation (see *Precautions*) ranges from 240 to 320 mg/day in divided (t.i.d. or q.i.d.) doses. The dosage for prophylaxis of PSVT (non-digitalized patients) ranges from 240 to 480 mg/day in divided (t.i.d or q.i.d.) doses. In general, maximum effects for any given dosage will be apparent during the first 48 hours of therapy.

Essential hypertension: Dose should be individualized by titration. The usual initial monotherapy dose in clinical trials was 80 mg three times a day (240 mg/day). Daily dosages of 360 and 480 mg have been used but there is no evidence that dosages beyond 360 mg provided added effect. Consideration should be given to beginning titration at 40 mg three times per day in patients who might respond to lower doses, such as the elderly or people of small stature. The antihypertensive effects of Calan are evident within the first week of therapy. Upward titration should be based on therapeutic efficacy, assessed at the end of the dosing interval.

HOW SUPPLIED

Calan 40-mg tablets are round, pink, film coated, with CALAN debossed on one side and 40 on the other, supplied as:

NDC Number	Size
0025-1771-31	bottle of 100

Calan 80-mg tablets are oval, peach colored, scored, film coated, with CALAN debossed on one side and 80 on the other, supplied as:

NDC Number	Size
0025-1851-31	bottle of 100
0025-1851-51	bottle of 500
0025-1851-52	bottle of 1,000
0025-1851-34	carton of 100 unit dose

Calan 120-mg tablets are oval, brown, scored, film coated, with CALAN 120 debossed on one side, supplied as:

NDC Number	Size
0025-1861-31	bottle of 100
0025-1861-51	bottle of 500
0025-1861-52	bottle of 1,000
0025-1861-34	carton of 100 unit dose

Store at 59° to 86°F (15° to 30°C) and protect from light. Dispense in tight, light-resistant containers.

Caution: Federal law prohibits dispensing without prescription.

2/13/92 • A05295-6

Shown in Product Identification Section, page 429

CALAN® SR ℞

[cal 'an ess ar]

(verapamil hydrochloride)

Sustained-Release Oral Caplets

PRODUCT OVERVIEW

KEY FACTS

Calan SR, a calcium ion antagonist designed for sustained release in the gastrointestinal tract, exerts an antihypertensive effect by decreasing systemic vascular resistance, usually without orthostatic decreases in blood pressure or reflex tachycardia.

MAJOR USE

Calan SR is indicated for the management of essential hypertension.

SAFETY INFORMATION

See complete safety information set forth below.

PRESCRIBING INFORMATION

CALAN® SR ℞

[cal 'an ess ar]

(verapamil hydrochloride)

Sustained-Release Oral Caplets

DESCRIPTION

Calan SR (verapamil hydrochloride) is a calcium ion influx inhibitor (slow-channel blocker or calcium ion antagonist). Calan SR is available for oral administration as light green, capsule-shaped, scored, film-coated tablets (caplets) containing 240 mg of verapamil hydrochloride; as light pink, oval, scored, film-coated tablets (caplets) containing 180 mg of verapamil hydrochloride; and as light violet, oval, film-coated tablets (caplets) containing 120 mg of verapamil hydrochloride. The caplets are designed for sustained release of the drug in the gastrointestinal tract; sustained-release characteristics are not altered when the caplet is divided in half.

The structural formula of verapamil HCl is

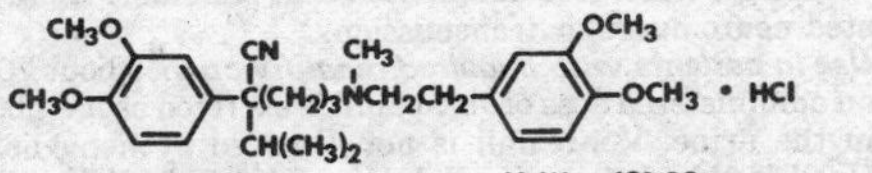

$C_{27}H_{38}N_2O_4 \cdot HCl$ M.W. = 491.08

Benzeneacetonitrile, α-[3-[[2-(3, 4-dimethoxyphenyl) ethyl] methylamino]propyl]-3,4-dimethoxy-α-(1-methylethyl) hydrochloride

Verapamil HCl is an almost white, crystalline powder, practically free of odor, with a bitter taste. It is soluble in water, chloroform, and methanol. Verapamil HCl is not chemically related to other cardioactive drugs.

Inactive ingredients include alginate, carnauba wax, hydroxypropyl methylcellulose, magnesium stearate, microcrystalline cellulose, polyethylene glycol, polyvinyl pyrrolidone, talc, titanium dioxide, and coloring agents: 240-mg—D&C Yellow No. 10 Lake and FD&C Blue No. 2 Lake; 120- and 180-mg—iron oxide.

CLINICAL PHARMACOLOGY

Calan (verapamil HCl) is a calcium ion influx inhibitor (slow-channel blocker or calcium ion antagonist) that exerts its pharmacologic effects by modulating the influx of ionic calcium across the cell membrane of the arterial smooth muscle as well as in conductile and contractile myocardial cells.

Mechanism of action

Essential hypertension: Verapamil exerts antihypertensive effects by decreasing systemic vascular resistance, usually without orthostatic decreases in blood pressure or reflex tachycardia; bradycardia (rate less than 50 beats/min) is uncommon (1.4%). During isometric or dynamic exercise Calan does not alter systolic cardiac function in patients with normal ventricular function.

Calan does not alter total serum calcium levels. However, one report suggested that calcium levels above the normal range may alter the therapeutic effect of Calan.

Other pharmacologic actions of Calan include the following:

Calan dilates the main coronary arteries and coronary arterioles, both in normal and ischemic regions, and is a potent inhibitor of coronary artery spasm, whether spontaneous or ergonovine-induced. This property increases myocardial oxygen delivery in patients with coronary artery spasm and is responsible for the effectiveness of Calan in vasospastic (Prinzmetal's or variant) as well as unstable angina at rest. Whether this effect plays any role in classical effort angina is not clear, but studies of exercise tolerance have not shown an increase in the maximum exercise rate–pressure product, a widely accepted measure of oxygen utilization. This suggests that, in general, relief of spasm or dilation of coronary arteries is not an important factor in classical angina.

Calan regularly reduces the total systemic resistance (afterload) against which the heart works both at rest and at a given level of exercise by dilating peripheral arterioles.

Electrical activity through the AV node depends, to a significant degree, upon calcium influx through the slow channel. By decreasing the influx of calcium, Calan prolongs the effective refractory period within the AV node and slows AV conduction in a rate-related manner.

Normal sinus rhythm is usually not affected, but in patients with sick sinus syndrome, Calan may interfere with sinus-node impulse generation and may induce sinus arrest or sinoatrial block. Atrioventricular block can occur in patients without preexisting conduction defects (see *Warnings*).

Calan does not alter the normal atrial action potential or intraventricular conduction time, but depresses amplitude, velocity of depolarization, and conduction in depressed atrial fibers. Calan may shorten the antegrade effective refractory period of the accessory bypass tract. Acceleration of ventricular rate and/or ventricular fibrillation has been reported in patients with atrial flutter or atrial fibrillation and a coexisting accessory AV pathway following administration of verapamil (see *Warnings*).

Calan has a local anesthetic action that is 1.6 times that of procaine on an equimolar basis. It is not known whether this action is important at the doses used in man.

Pharmacokinetics and metabolism: With the immediate-release formulation, more than 90% of the orally administered dose of Calan is absorbed. Because of rapid biotransformation of verapamil during its first pass through the portal circulation, bioavailability ranges from 20% to 35%. Peak plasma concentrations are reached between 1 and 2 hours after oral administration. Chronic oral administration of 120 mg of verapamil HCl every 6 hours resulted in plasma levels of verapamil ranging from 125 to 400 ng/ml, with higher values reported occasionally. A nonlinear correlation between the verapamil dose administered and verapamil plasma level does exist. In early dose titration with verapamil a relationship exists between verapamil plasma concentration and prolongation of the PR interval. However, during chronic administration this relationship may disappear. The mean elimination half-life in single-dose studies ranged from 2.8 to 7.4 hours. In these same studies, after repetitive dosing, the half-life increased to a range from 4.5 to 12.0 hours (after less than 10 consecutive doses given 6 hours apart). Half-life of verapamil may increase during titration. No relationship has been established between the plasma concentraton of verapamil and a reduction in blood pressure.

Aging may affect the pharmacokinetics of verapamil. Elimination half-life may be prolonged in the elderly. In multiple-dose studies under fasting conditions, the bioavailability, measured by AUC, of Calan SR was similar to Calan (immediate release); rates of absorption were of course different.

In a randomized, single-dose, crossover study using healthy volunteers, administration of 240 mg Calan SR with food produced peak plasma verapamil concentrations of 79 ng/ml; time to peak plasma verapamil concentration of 7.71 hours; and AUC (0–24 hr) of 841 ng·hr/ml). When Calan SR was administered to fasting subjects, peak plasma verapamil concentration was 164 ng/ml; time to peak plasma verapamil concentration was 5.21 hours; and AUC (0–24 hr) was 1,478 ng·hr/ml. Similar results were demonstrated for plasma norverapamil. Food thus produces decreased bioavailability (AUC) but a narrower peak-to-trough ratio. Good correlation of dose and response is not available, but controlled studies of Calan SR have shown effectiveness of doses similar to the effective doses of Calan (immediate release).

In healthy men, orally administered Calan undergoes extensive metabolism in the liver. Twelve metabolites have been identified in plasma; all except norverapamil are present in trace amounts only. Norverapamil can reach steady-state plasma concentrations approximately equal to those of verapamil itself. The cardiovascular activity of norverapamil appears to be approximately 20% that of verapamil. Approximately 70% of an administered dose is excreted as metabolites in the urine and 16% or more in the feces within 5 days. About 3% to 4% is excreted in the urine as unchanged drug. Approximately 90% is bound to plasma proteins. In patients with hepatic insufficiency, metabolism of immediate-release verapamil is delayed and elimination half-life prolonged up to 14 to 16 hours (see *Precautions*); the volume of distribution is increased and plasma clearance reduced to about 30% of normal. Verapamil clearance values suggest that patients with liver dysfunction may attain therapeutic verapamil plasma concentrations with one third of the oral daily dose required for patients with normal liver function.

After four weeks of oral dosing (120 mg q.i.d.), verapamil and norverapamil levels were noted in the cerebrospinal fluid with estimated partition coefficient of 0.06 for verapamil and 0.04 for norverapamil.

Continued on next page

Searle—Cont.

Hemodynamics and myocardial metabolism: Calan reduces afterload and myocardial contractility. Improved left ventricular diastolic function in patients with IHSS and those with coronary heart disease has also been observed with Calan. In most patients, including those with organic cardiac disease, the negative inotropic action of Calan is countered by reduction of afterload, and cardiac index is usually not reduced. However, in patients with severe left ventricular dysfunction (eg, pulmonary wedge pressure above 20 mm Hg or ejection fraction less than 30%), or in patients taking beta-adrenergic blocking agents or other cardiodepressant drugs, deterioration of ventricular function may occur (see *Drug interactions*).

Pulmonary function: Calan does not induce bronchoconstriction and, hence, does not impair ventilatory function.

INDICATIONS AND USAGE

Calan SR is indicated for the management of essential hypertension.

CONTRAINDICATIONS

Verapamil HCl caplets are contraindicated in:
1. Severe left ventricular dysfunction (see *Warnings*)
2. Hypotension (systolic pressure less than 90 mm Hg) or cardiogenic shock
3. Sick sinus syndrome (except in patients with a functioning artificial ventricular pacemaker)
4. Second- or third-degree AV block (except in patients with a functioning artificial ventricular pacemaker)
5. Patients with atrial flutter or atrial fibrillation and an accessory bypass tract (eg, Wolff-Parkinson-White, Lown-Ganong-Levine syndromes). (See *Warnings.*)
6. Patients with known hypersensitivity to verapamil hydrochloride.

WARNINGS

Heart failure: Verapamil has a negative inotropic effect, which in most patients is compensated by its afterload reduction (decreased systemic vascular resistance) properties without a net impairment of ventricular performance. In clinical experience with 4,954 patients, 87 (1.8%) developed congestive heart failure or pulmonary edema. Verapamil should be avoided in patients with severe left ventricular dysfunction (eg, ejection fraction less than 30%) or moderate to severe symptoms of cardiac failure and in patients with any degree of ventricular dysfunction if they are receiving a beta-adrenergic blocker (see *Drug interactions*). Patients with milder ventricular dysfunction should, if possible, be controlled with optimum doses of digitalis and/or diuretics before verapamil treatment. **(Note interactions with digoxin under *Precautions.*)**

Hypotension: Occasionally, the pharmacologic action of verapamil may produce a decrease in blood pressure below normal levels, which may result in dizziness or symptomatic hypotension. The incidence of hypotension observed in 4,954 patients enrolled in clinical trials was 2.5%. In hypertensive patients, decreases in blood pressure below normal are unusual. Tilt-table testing (60 degrees) was not able to induce orthostatic hypotension.

Elevated liver enzymes: Elevations of transaminases with and without concomitant elevations in alkaline phosphatase and bilirubin have been reported. Such elevations have sometimes been transient and may disappear even in the face of continued verapamil treatment. Several cases of hepatocellular injury related to verapamil have been proven by rechallenge; half of these had clinical symptoms (malaise, fever, and/or right upper quadrant pain) in addition to elevation of SGOT, SGPT, and alkaline phosphatase. Periodic monitoring of liver function in patients receiving verapamil is therefore prudent.

Accessory bypass tract (Wolff-Parkinson-White or Lown-Ganong-Levine): Some patients with paroxysmal and/or chronic atrial fibrillation or atrial flutter and a coexisting accessory AV pathway have developed increased antegrade conduction across the accessory pathway bypassing the AV node, producing a very rapid ventricular response or ventricular fibrillation after receiving intravenous verapamil (or digitalis). Although a risk of this occurring with oral verapamil has not been established, such patients receiving oral verapamil may be at risk and its use in these patients is contraindicated (see *Contraindications*). Treatment is usually DC-cardioversion. Cardioversion has been used safely and effectively after oral Calan.

Atrioventricular block: The effect of verapamil on AV conduction and the SA node may cause asymptomatic first-degree AV block and transient bradycardia, sometimes accompanied by nodal escape rhythms. PR-interval prolongation is correlated with verapamil plasma concentrations, especially during the early titration phase of therapy. Higher degrees of AV block, however, were infrequently (0.8%) observed. Marked first-degree block or progressive development to second- or third-degree AV block requires a reduction in dosage or, in rare instances, discontinuation of verapamil HCl

and institution of appropriate therapy, depending upon the clinical situation.

Patients with hypertrophic cardiomyopathy (IHSS): In 120 patients with hypertrophic cardiomyopathy (most of them refractory or intolerant to propranolol) who received therapy with verapamil at doses up to 720 mg/day, a variety of serious adverse effects were seen. Three patients died in pulmonary edema; all had severe left ventricular outflow obstruction and a past history of left ventricular dysfunction. Eight other patients had pulmonary edema and/or severe hypotension; abnormally high (greater than 20 mm Hg) pulmonary wedge pressure and a marked left ventricular outflow obstruction were present in most of these patients. Concomitant administration of quinidine (see *Drug interactions*) preceded the severe hypotension in 3 of the 8 patients (2 of whom developed pulmonary edema). Sinus bradycardia occurred in 11% of the patients, second-degree AV block in 4%, and sinus arrest in 2%. It must be appreciated that this group of patients had a serious disease with a high mortality rate. Most adverse effects responded well to dose reduction, and only rarely did verapamil use have to be discontinued.

PRECAUTIONS

General

Use in patients with impaired hepatic function: Since verapamil is highly metabolized by the liver, it should be administered cautiously to patients with impaired hepatic function. Severe liver dysfunction prolongs the elimination half-life of immediate-release verapamil to about 14 to 16 hours; hence, approximately 30% of the dose given to patients with normal liver function should be administered to these patients. Careful monitoring for abnormal prolongation of the PR interval or other signs of excessive pharmacologic effects (see *Overdosage*) should be carried out.

Use in patients with attenuated (decreased) neuromuscular transmission: It has been reported that verapamil decreases neuromuscular transmission in patients with Duchenne's muscular dystrophy, and that verapamil prolongs recovery from the neuromuscular blocking agent vecuronium. It may be necessary to decrease the dosage of verapamil when it is administered to patients with attenuated neuromuscular transmission.

Use in patients with impaired renal function: About 70% of an administered dose of verapamil is excreted as metabolites in the urine. Verapamil is not removed by hemodialysis. Until further data are available, verapamil should be administered cautiously to patients with impaired renal function. These patients should be carefully monitored for abnormal prolongation of the PR interval or other signs of overdosage (see *Overdosage*).

Drug interactions

Beta-blockers: Concomitant therapy with beta-adrenergic blockers and verapamil may result in additive negative effects on heart rate, atrioventricular conduction and/or cardiac contractility. The combination of sustained-release verapamil and beta-adrenergic blocking agents has not been studied. However, there have been reports of excessive bradycardia and AV block, including complete heart block, when the combination has been used for the treatment of hypertension. For hypertensive patients, the risks of combined therapy may outweigh the potential benefits. The combination should be used only with caution and close monitoring.

Asymptomatic bradycardia (36 beats/min) with a wandering atrial pacemaker has been observed in a patient receiving concomitant timolol (a beta-adrenergic blocker) eyedrops and oral verapamil.

A decrease in metroprolol and propranolol clearance has been observed when either drug is administered concomitantly with verapamil. A variable effect has been seen when verapamil and atenolol were given together.

Digitalis: Clinical use of verapamil in digitalized patients has shown the combination to be well tolerated if digoxin doses are properly adjusted. However, chronic verapamil treatment can increase serum digoxin levels by 50% to 75% during the first week of therapy, and this can result in digitalis toxicity. In patients with hepatic cirrhosis the influence of verapamil on digoxin kinetics is magnified. Verapamil may reduce total body clearance and extrarenal clearance of digitoxin by 27% and 29%, respectively. Maintenance digitalis doses should be reduced when verapamil is administered, and the patient should be carefully monitored to avoid over- or underdigitalization. Whenever overdigitalization is suspected, the daily dose of digitalis should be reduced or temporarily discontinued. On discontinuation of Calan use, the patient should be reassessed to avoid underdigitalization.

Antihypertensive agents: Verapamil administered concomitantly with oral antihypertensive agents (eg, vasodilators, angiotensin-converting enzyme inhibitors, diuretics, beta-blockers) will usually have an additive effect on lowering blood pressure. Patients receiving these combinations should be appropriately monitored. Concomitant use of agents that attenuate alpha-adrenergic function with verapamil may result in a reduction in blood pressure that is excessive in some patients. Such an effect was observed in

one study following the concomitant administration of verapamil and prazosin.

Antiarrhythmic agents:

Disopyramide: Until data on possible interactions between verapamil and disopyramide phosphate are obtained, disopyramide should not be administered within 48 hours before or 24 hours after verapamil administration.

Flecainide: A study in healthy volunteers showed that the concomitant administration of flecainide and verapamil may have additive effects on myocardial contractility, AV conduction, and repolarization. Concomitant therapy with flecainide and verapamil may result in additive negative inotropic effect and prolongation of atrioventricular conduction.

Quinidine: In a small number of patients with hypertrophic cardiomyopathy (IHSS), concomitant use of verapamil and quinidine resulted in significant hypotension. Until further data are obtained, combined therapy of verapamil and quinidine in patients with hypertrophic cardiomyopathy should probably be avoided.

The electrophysiologic effects of quinidine and verapamil on AV conduction were studied in 8 patients. Verapamil significantly counteracted the effects of quinidine on AV conduction. There has been a report of increased quinidine levels during verapamil therapy.

Other:

Nitrates: Verapamil has been given concomitantly with short- and long-acting nitrates without any undesirable drug interactions. The pharmacologic profile of both drugs and the clinical experience suggest beneficial interactions.

Cimetidine: The interaction between cimetidine and chronically administered verapamil has not been studied. Variable results on clearance have been obtained in acute studies of healthy volunteers; clearance of verapamil was either reduced or unchanged.

Lithium: Increased sensitivity to the effects of lithium (neurotoxicity) has been reported during concomitant verapamil-lithium therapy with either no change or an increase in serum lithium levels. However, the addition of verapamil has also resulted in the lowering of serum lithium levels in patients receiving chronic stable oral lithium. Patients receiving both drugs must be monitored carefully.

Carbamazepine: Verapamil therapy may increase carbamazepine concentrations during combined therapy. This may produce carbamazepine side effects such as diplopia, headache, ataxia, or dizziness.

Rifampin: Therapy with rifampin may markedly reduce oral verapamil bioavailability.

Phenobarbital: Phenobarbital therapy may increase verapamil clearance.

Cyclosporin: Verapamil therapy may increase serum levels of cyclosporin.

Theophylline: Verapamil may inhibit the clearance and increase the plasma levels of theophylline.

Inhalation anesthetics: Animal experiments have shown that inhalation anesthetics depress cardiovascular activity by decreasing the inward movement of calcium ions. When used concomitantly, inhalation anesthetics and calcium antagonists, such as verapamil, should each be titrated carefully to avoid excessive cardiovascular depression.

Neuromuscular blocking agents: Clinical data and animal studies suggest that verapamil may potentiate the activity of neuromuscular blocking agents (curare-like and depolarizing). It may be necessary to decrease the dose of verapamil and/or the dose of the neuromuscular blocking agent when the drugs are used concomitantly.

Carcinogenesis, mutagenesis, impairment of fertility: An 18-month toxicity study in rats, at a low multiple (6-fold) of the maximum recommended human dose, and not the maximum tolerated dose, did not suggest a tumorigenic potential. There was no evidence of a carcinogenic potential of verapamil administered in the diet of rats for two years at doses of 10, 35, and 120 mg/kg/day or approximately 1, 3.5, and 12 times, respectively, the maximum recommended human daily dose (480 mg/day or 9.6 mg/kg/day).

Verapamil was not mutagenic in the Ames test in 5 test strains at 3 mg per plate with or without metabolic activation.

Studies in female rats at daily dietary doses up to 5.5 times (55 mg/kg/day) the maximum recommended human dose did not show impaired fertility. Effects on male fertility have not been determined.

Pregnancy: Pregnancy Category C. Reproduction studies have been performed in rabbits and rats at oral doses up to 1.5 (15 mg/kg/day) and 6 (60 mg/kg/day) times the human oral daily dose, respectively, and have revealed no evidence of teratogenicity. In the rat, however, this multiple of the human dose was embryocidal and retarded fetal growth and development, probably because of adverse maternal effects reflected in reduced weight gains of the dams. This oral dose has also been shown to cause hypotension in rats. There are no adequate and well-controlled studies in pregnant women. Because animal reproduction studies are not always predictive of human response, this drug should be used during pregnancy only if clearly needed. Verapamil crosses the pla-

cental barrier and can be detected in umbilical vein blood at delivery.

Labor and delivery: It is not known whether the use of verapamil during labor or delivery has immediate or delayed adverse effects on the fetus, or whether it prolongs the duration of labor or increases the need for forceps delivery or other obstetric intervention. Such adverse experiences have not been reported in the literature, despite a long history of use of verapamil in Europe in the treatment of cardiac side effects of beta-adrenergic agonist agents used to treat premature labor.

Nursing mothers: Verapamil is excreted in human milk. Because of the potential for adverse reactions in nursing infants from verapamil, nursing should be discontinued while verapamil is administered.

Pediatric use: Safety and efficacy of Calan SR in children below the age of 18 years have not been established.

Animal pharmacology and/or animal toxicology: In chronic animal toxicology studies verapamil caused lenticular and/or suture line changes at 30 mg/kg/day or greater, and frank cataracts at 62.5 mg/kg/day or greater in the beagle dog but not in the rat. Development of cataracts due to verapamil has not been reported in man.

ADVERSE REACTIONS

Serious adverse reactions are uncommon when verapamil therapy is initiated with upward dose titration within the recommended single and total daily dose. See *Warnings* for discussion of heart failure, hypotension, elevated liver enzymes, AV block, and rapid ventricular response. Reversible (upon discontinuation of verapamil) non-obstructive, paralytic ileus has been infrequently reported in association with the use of verapamil. The following reactions to orally administered verapamil occurred at rates greater than 1.0% or occurred at lower rates but appeared clearly drug-related in clinical trials in 4,954 patients:

Constipation	7.3%	Dyspnea	1.4%
Dizziness	3.3%	Bradycardia	
Nausea	2.7%	(HR < 50/min)	1.4%
Hypotension	2.5%	AV block	
Headache	2.2%	total (1°, 2°, 3°)	1.2%
Edema	1.9%	2° and 3°	0.8%
CHF, Pulmonary		Rash	1.2%
edema	1.8%	Flushing	0.6%
Fatigue	1.7%		

Elevated liver enzymes (see *Warnings*)

In clinical trials related to the control of ventricular response in digitalized patients who had atrial fibrillation or flutter, ventricular rates below 50/min at rest occurred in 15% of patients and asymptomatic hypotension occurred in 5% of patients.

The following reactions, reported in 1% or less of patients, occurred under conditions (open trials, marketing experience) where a causal relationship is uncertain; they are listed to alert the physician to a possible relationship:

Cardiovascular: angina pectoris, atrioventricular dissociation, chest pain, claudication, myocardial infarction, palpitations, purpura (vasculitis), syncope.

Digestive system: diarrhea, dry mouth, gastrointestinal distress, gingival hyperplasia.

Hemic and lymphatic: ecchymosis or bruising.

Nervous system: cerebrovascular accident, confusion, equilibrium disorders, insomnia, muscle cramps, paresthesia, psychotic symptoms, shakiness, somnolence.

Skin: arthralgia and rash, exanthema, hair loss, hyperkeratosis, macules, sweating, urticaria, Stevens-Johnson syndrome, erythema multiforme.

Special senses: blurred vision.

Urogenital: gynecomastia, galactorrhea/hyperprolactinemia, increased urination, spotty menstruation, impotence.

Treatment of acute cardiovascular adverse reactions: The frequency of cardiovascular adverse reactions that require therapy is rare; hence, experience with their treatment is limited. Whenever severe hypotension or complete AV block occurs following oral administration of verapamil, the appropriate emergency measures should be applied immediately; eg, intravenously administered norepinephrine bitartrate, atropine sulfate, isoproterenol HCl (all in the usual doses), or calcium gluconate (10% solution). In patients with hypertrophic cardiomyopathy (IHSS), alpha-adrenergic agents (phenylephrine HCl, metaraminol bitartrate, or methoxamine HCl) should be used to maintain blood pressure, and isoproterenol and norepinephrine should be avoided. If further support is necessary, dopamine HCl or dobutamine HCl may be administered. Actual treatment and dosage should depend on the severity of the clinical situation and the judgment and experience of the treating physician.

OVERDOSAGE

Overdose with verapamil may lead to pronounced hypotension, bradycardia, and conduction system abnormalities (eg, junctional rhythm with AV dissociation and high degree AV block, including asystole). Other symptoms secondary to hypoperfusion (eg, metabolic acidosis, hyperglycemia, hyperkalemia, renal dysfunction, and convulsions) may be evident.

Treat all verapamil overdoses as serious and maintain observation for at least 48 hours (especially Calan SR), preferably under continuous hospital care. Delayed pharmacodynamic consequences may occur with the sustained-release formulation. Verapamil is known to decrease gastrointestinal transit time. Verapamil cannot be removed by hemodialysis.

Treatment of overdosage should be supportive. Beta-adrenergic stimulation or parenteral administration of calcium solutions may increase calcium ion flux across the slow channel and has been used effectively in treatment of deliberate overdose of verapamil. The following measures may be considered:

Bradycardia and conduction system abnormalities: Atropine, isoproterenol, and cardiac pacing.

Hypotension: Intravenous fluids, vasopressors (eg, dopamine, dobutamine), calcium solutions (eg, 10% calcium chloride solution).

Cardiac failure: Inotropic agents (eg, isoproterenol, dopamine, dobutamine), diuretics.

Asystole should be handled by the usual measures including cardiopulmonary resuscitation.

DOSAGE AND ADMINISTRATION

Essential hypertension: The dose of Calan SR should be individualized by titration and the drug should be administered with food. Initiate therapy with 180 mg of sustained-release verapamil HCl, Calan SR, given in the morning. Lower initial doses of 120 mg a day may be warranted in patients who may have an increased response to verapamil (eg, the elderly or small people). Upward titration should be based on therapeutic efficacy and safety evaluated weekly and approximately 24 hours after the previous dose. The antihypertensive effects of Calan SR are evident within the first week of therapy.

If adequate response is not obtained with 180 mg of Calan SR, the dose may be titrated upward in the following manner:

a) 240 mg each morning,
b) 180 mg each morning plus
180 mg each evening; or
240 mg each morning plus
120 mg each evening,
c) 240 mg every 12 hours.

When switching from immediate-release Calan to Calan SR the total daily dose in milligrams may remain the same.

HOW SUPPLIED

Calan SR 240-mg caplets are light green, capsule shaped, scored, film coated, with CALAN debossed on one side and SR 240 on the other, supplied as:

NDC Number	Size
0025-1891-31	bottle of 100
0025-1891-51	bottle of 500
0025-1891-34	carton of 100 unit dose

Calan SR 180-mg caplets are light pink, oval, scored, film coated, with CALAN debossed on one side and SR 180 on the other, supplied as:

NDC Number	Size
0025-1911-31	bottle of 100
0025-1911-34	carton of 100 unit dose

Calan SR 120-mg caplets are light violet, oval, film-coated, with CALAN debossed on one side and SR 120 on the other, supplied as:

NDC Number	Size
0025-1901-31	bottle of 100
0025-1901-34	carton of 100 unit dose

Store at 59° to 86°F (15° to 30°C) and protect from light and moisture. Dispense in tight, light-resistant containers.

Caution: Federal law prohibits dispensing without prescription.

2/13/92 • A05298-1

Shown in Product Identification Section, page 429

CYTOTEC® ℞

[*sī-tō-tĕc*]

(misoprostol)

CONTRAINDICATIONS AND WARNINGS

Cytotec (misoprostol) is contraindicated, because of its abortifacient property, in women who are pregnant. (See *Precautions.*) Patients must be advised of the abortifacient property and warned not to give the drug to others. Cytotec should not be used in women of childbearing potential unless the patient requires nonsteroidal anti-inflammatory drug (NSAID) therapy and is at high risk of complications from gastric ulcers associated with use of the NSAID, or is at high risk of developing gastric ulceration. In such patients, Cytotec may be prescribed if the patient

- is capable of complying with effective contraceptive measures.
- has received both oral and written warnings of the hazards of misoprostol, the risk of possible contraception failure, and the danger to other women of childbearing potential should the drug be taken by mistake.
- has had a negative *serum* pregnancy test within two weeks prior to beginning therapy.
- will begin Cytotec only on the second or third day of the next normal menstrual period.

DESCRIPTION

Cytotec oral tablets contain either 100 mcg or 200 mcg of misoprostol, a synthetic prostaglandin E_1 analog.

Misoprostol contains approximately equal amounts of the two diastereomers presented below with their enantiomers indicated by (±):

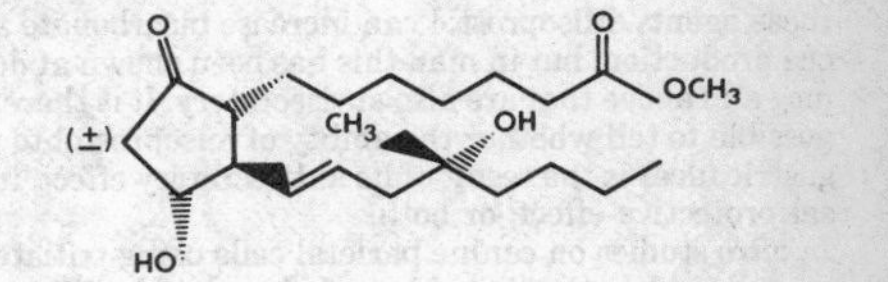

and

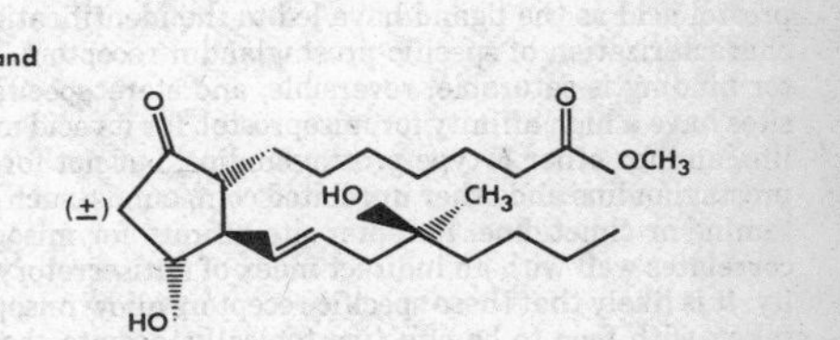

$C_{22}H_{38}O_5$ M.W. = 382.5

(±) methyl 11α, 16-dihydroxy-16-methyl-9-oxoprost-13E-en-1-oate

Misoprostol is a water-soluble, viscous liquid.

Inactive ingredients of tablets are hydrogenated castor oil, hydroxypropyl methylcellulose, microcrystalline cellulose, and sodium starch glycolate.

CLINICAL PHARMACOLOGY

Pharmacokinetics: Misoprostol is extensively absorbed, and undergoes rapid de-esterification to its free acid, which is responsible for its clinical activity and, unlike the parent compound, is detectable in plasma. The alpha side chain undergoes beta oxidation and the beta side chain undergoes omega oxidation followed by reduction of the ketone to give prostaglandin F analogs.

In normal volunteers, Cytotec (misoprostol) is rapidly absorbed after oral administration with a T_{max} of misoprostol acid of 12 ± 3 minutes and a terminal half-life of 20–40 minutes.

There is high variability of plasma levels of misoprostol acid between and within studies but mean values after single doses show a linear relationship with dose over the range of 200–400 mcg. No accumulation of misoprostol acid was noted in multiple dose studies; plasma steady state was achieved within two days.

Maximum plasma concentrations of misoprostol acid are diminished when the dose is taken with food and total availability of misoprostol acid is reduced by use of concomitant antacid. Clinical trials were conducted with concomitant antacid, however, so this effect does not appear to be clinically important.

Mean ± SD	C_{max}(pg/ml)	AUC (0-4) (pg·hr/ml)	T_{max}(min)
Fasting	811 ± 317	417 ± 135	14 ± 8
With Antacid	689 ± 315	349 ± 108*	20 ± 14
With High Fat Breakfast	303 ± 176*	373 ± 111	64 ± 79*

*Comparisons with fasting results statistically significant, $p < 0.05$.

After oral administration of radiolabeled misoprostol, about 80% of detected radioactivity appears in urine. Pharmacokinetic studies in patients with varying degrees of renal impairment showed an approximate doubling of $T_{1/2}$, C_{max}, and AUC compared to normals, but no clear correlation between the degree of impairment and AUC. In subjects over 64 years of age, the AUC for misoprostol acid is increased. No routine dosage adjustment is recommended in older patients or patients with renal impairment, but dosage may need to be reduced if the usual dose is not tolerated.

Cytotec does not affect the hepatic mixed function oxidase (cytochrome P-450) enzyme systems in animals.

Drug interaction studies between misoprostol and several nonsteroidal anti-inflammatory drugs showed no effect on

Continued on next page

Searle—Cont.

the kinetics of ibuprofen or diclofenac, and a 20% decrease in aspirin AUC, not thought to be clinically significant.
Pharmacokinetic studies also showed a lack of drug interaction with antipyrine and propranolol when these drugs were given with misoprostol. Misoprostol given for one week had no effect on the steady state pharmacokinetics of diazepam when the two drugs were administered two hours apart.
The serum protein binding of misoprostol acid is less than 90% and is concentration-independent in the therapeutic range.

Pharmacodynamics: Misoprostol has both antisecretory (inhibiting gastric acid secretion) and (in animals) mucosal protective properties. NSAIDs inhibit prostaglandin synthesis, and a deficiency of prostaglandins within the gastric mucosa may lead to diminishing bicarbonate and mucus secretion and may contribute to the mucosal damage caused by these agents. Misoprostol can increase bicarbonate and mucus production, but in man this has been shown at doses 200 mcg and above that are also antisecretory. It is therefore not possible to tell whether the ability of misoprostol to prevent gastric ulcer is the result of its antisecretory effect, its mucosal protective effect, or both.

In vitro studies on canine parietal cells using tritiated misoprostol acid as the ligand have led to the identification and characterization of specific prostaglandin receptors. Receptor binding is saturable, reversible, and stereospecific. The sites have a high affinity for misoprostol, for its acid metabolite, and for other E type prostaglandins, but not for F or I prostaglandins and other unrelated compounds, such as histamine or cimetidine. Receptor-site affinity for misoprostol correlates well with an indirect index of antisecretory activity. It is likely that these specific receptors allow misoprostol taken with food to be effective topically, despite the lower serum concentrations attained.

Misoprostol produces a moderate decrease in pepsin concentration during basal conditions, but not during histamine stimulation. It has no significant effect on fasting or postprandial gastrin nor on intrinsic factor output.

Effects on gastric acid secretion: Misoprostol, over the range of 50–200 mcg, inhibits basal and nocturnal gastric acid secretion, and acid secretion in response to a variety of stimuli, including meals, histamine, pentagastrin, and coffee. Activity is apparent 30 minutes after oral administration and persists for at least 3 hours. In general, the effects of 50 mcg were modest and shorter lived, and only the 200-mcg dose had substantial effects on nocturnal secretion or on histamine and meal-stimulated secretion.

Uterine effects: Cytotec has been shown to produce uterine contractions that may endanger pregnancy. (See *Contraindications* and *Warnings.*) In studies in women undergoing elective termination of pregnancy during the first trimester, Cytotec caused partial or complete expulsion of the uterine contents in 11% of the subjects and increased uterine bleeding in 41%.

Other pharmacologic effects: Cytotec does not produce clinically significant effects on serum levels of prolactin, gonadotropins, thyroid-stimulating hormone, growth hormone, thyroxine, cortisol, gastrointestinal hormones (somatostatin, gastrin, vasoactive intestinal polypeptide, and motilin), creatinine, or uric acid. Gastric emptying, immunologic competence, platelet aggregation, pulmonary function, or the cardiovascular system are not modified by recommended doses of Cytotec.

Clinical studies: In a series of small short-term (about one week) placebo-controlled studies in healthy human volunteers, doses of misoprostol were evaluated for their ability to prevent NSAID-induced mucosal injury. Studies of 200 mcg q.i.d. of misoprostol with tolmetin and naproxen, and of 100 and 200 mcg q.i.d. with ibuprofen, all showed reduction of the rate of significant endoscopic injury from about 70–75% on placebo to 10–30% on misoprostol. Doses of 25–200 mcg q.i.d. reduced aspirin-induced mucosal injury and bleeding.

Preventing gastric ulcers caused by nonsteroidal anti-inflammatory drugs (NSAIDs): Two 12-week, randomized, double-blind trials in osteoarthritic patients who had gastrointestinal symptoms but no ulcer on endoscopy while taking an NSAID compared the ability of 200 mcg of Cytotec, 100 mcg of Cytotec, and placebo to prevent gastric ulcer (GU) formation. Patients were approximately equally divided between ibuprofen, piroxicam, and naproxen, and continued this treatment throughout the 12 weeks. The 200-mcg dose caused a marked, statistically significant reduction in gastric ulcers in both studies. The lower dose was somewhat less effective, with a significant result in only one of the studies.
[See table below.]

In these trials there were no significant differences between Cytotec and placebo in relief of day or night abdominal pain. No effect of Cytotec in preventing duodenal ulcers was demonstrated, but relatively few duodenal lesions were seen.

In another clinical trial, 239 patients receiving aspirin 650–1300 mg q.i.d. for rheumatoid arthritis who had endoscopic evidence of duodenal and/or gastric inflammation were randomized to misoprostol 200 mcg q.i.d. or placebo for eight weeks while continuing to receive aspirin. The study evaluated the possible interference of Cytotec on the efficacy of aspirin in these patients with rheumatoid arthritis by analyzing joint tenderness, joint swelling, physician's clinical assessment, patient's assessment, change in ARA classification, change in handgrip strength, change in duration of morning stiffness, patient's assessment of pain at rest, movement, interference with daily activity, and ESR. Cytotec did not interfere with the efficacy of aspirin in these patients with rheumatoid arthritis.

INDICATIONS AND USAGE

Cytotec (misoprostol) is indicated for the prevention of NSAID (nonsteroidal anti-inflammatory drugs, including aspirin)-induced gastric ulcers in patients at high risk of complications from gastric ulcer, eg, the elderly and patients with concomitant debilitating disease, as well as patients at high risk of developing gastric ulceration, such as patients with a history of ulcer. Cytotec has not been shown to prevent duodenal ulcers in patients taking NSAIDs. Cytotec should be taken for the duration of NSAID therapy. Cytotec has been shown to prevent gastric ulcers in controlled studies of three months' duration. It had no effect, compared to placebo, on gastrointestinal pain or discomfort associated with NSAID use.

CONTRAINDICATIONS

See boxed *CONTRAINDICATIONS AND WARNINGS.*
Cytotec should not be taken by anyone with a history of allergy to prostaglandins.

Prevention of Gastric Ulcers Induced by Ibuprofen, Piroxicam, or Naproxen
[No. of patients with ulcer(s) (%)]

Therapy	Therapy Duration: 4 weeks	8 weeks	12 weeks	
Study No. 1				
Cytotec 200 mcg q.i.d. (n=74)	1 (1.4)	0	0	1 (1.4)*
Cytotec 100 mcg q.i.d. (n=77)	3 (3.9)	1 (1.3)	1 (1.3)	5 (6.5)*
Placebo (n=76)	11 (14.5)	4 (5.3)	4 (5.3)	19 (25.0)
Study No. 2				
Cytotec 200 mcg q.i.d. (n=65)	1 (1.5)	1 (1.5)	0	2 (3.1)*
Cytotec 100 mcg q.i.d. (n=66)	2 (3.0)	2 (3.0)	1 (1.5)	5 (7.6)
Placebo (n=62)	6 (9.7)	2 (3.2)	3 (4.8)	11 (17.7)
*Studies No. 1 & No. 2***				
Cytotec 200 mcg q.i.d. (n=139)	2 (1.4)	1 (0.7)	0	3 (2.2)*
Cytotec 100 mcg q.i.d. (n=143)	5 (3.5)	3 (2.1)	2 (1.4)	10 (7.0)*
Placebo (n=138)	17 (12.3)	6 (4.3)	7 (5.1)	30 (21.7)

*Statistically significantly different from placebo at the 5% level.
**Combined data from Study No. 1 and Study No. 2.

WARNINGS

See boxed *CONTRAINDICATIONS AND WARNINGS.*

PRECAUTIONS

Information for patients: Cytotec is contraindicated in women who are pregnant, and should not be used in women of childbearing potential unless the patient requires nonsteroidal anti-inflammatory drug (NSAID) therapy and is at high risk of complications from gastric ulcers associated with the use of the NSAID, or is at high risk of developing gastric ulceration. Women of childbearing potential should be told that they must not be pregnant when Cytotec therapy is initiated, and that they must use an effective contraception method while taking Cytotec.
See boxed *CONTRAINDICATIONS AND WARNINGS.*

Patients should be advised of the following:
Cytotec is intended for administration along with nonsteroidal anti-inflammatory drugs (NSAIDs), including aspirin, to decrease the chance of developing an NSAID-induced gastric ulcer.
Cytotec should be taken only according to the directions given by a physician.
If the patient has questions about or problems with Cytotec, the physician should be contacted promptly.
THE PATIENT SHOULD NOT GIVE CYTOTEC TO ANYONE ELSE. Cytotec has been prescribed for the patient's specific condition, may not be the correct treatment for another person, and may be dangerous to the other person if she were to become pregnant.
The Cytotec package the patient receives from the pharmacist will include a leaflet containing patient information. The patient should read the leaflet before taking Cytotec and each time the prescription is renewed because the leaflet may have been revised.
Keep Cytotec out of reach of children.
SPECIAL NOTE FOR WOMEN: Cytotec must not be used by pregnant women. Cytotec may cause miscarriage. Miscarriages caused by Cytotec may be incomplete, which could lead to potentially dangerous bleeding, hospitalization, surgery, infertility, or maternal or fetal death.

Cytotec is available only as a unit-of-use package that includes a leaflet containing patient information. See *Patient Information* at the end of this labeling.

Drug interactions: See *Clinical Pharmacology.* Cytotec has not been shown to interfere with the beneficial effects of aspirin on signs and symptoms of rheumatoid arthritis. Cytotec does not exert clinically significant effects on the absorption, blood levels, and antiplatelet effects of therapeutic doses of aspirin. Cytotec has no clinically significant effect on the kinetics of diclofenac or ibuprofen.

Animal toxicology: A reversible increase in the number of normal surface gastric epithelial cells occurred in the dog, rat, and mouse. No such increase has been observed in humans administered Cytotec for up to one year.
An apparent response of the female mouse to Cytotec in long-term studies at 100 to 1000 times the human dose was hyperostosis, mainly of the medulla of sternebrae. Hyperostosis did not occur in long-term studies in the dog and rat and has not been seen in humans treated with Cytotec.

Carcinogenesis, mutagenesis, impairment of fertility: There was no evidence of an effect of Cytotec on tumor occurrence or incidence in rats receiving daily doses up to 150 times the human dose for 24 months. Similarly, there was no effect of Cytotec on tumor occurrence or incidence in mice receiving daily doses up to 1000 times the human dose for 21 months. The mutagenic potential of Cytotec was tested in several *in vitro* assays, all of which were negative.
Misoprostol, when administered to breeding male and female rats at doses 6.25 times to 625 times the maximum recommended human therapeutic dose, produced dose-related pre- and post-implantation losses and a significant decrease in the number of live pups born at the highest dose. These findings suggest the possibility of a general adverse effect on fertility in males and females.

Pregnancy: Pregnancy Category X. See boxed *CONTRAINDICATIONS AND WARNINGS.*

Nonteratogenic effects: Cytotec may endanger pregnancy (may cause miscarriage) and thereby cause harm to the fetus when administered to a pregnant woman. Cytotec produces uterine contractions, uterine bleeding, and expulsion of the products of conception. Miscarriages caused by Cytotec may be incomplete. In studies in women undergoing elective termination of pregnancy during the first trimester, Cytotec caused partial or complete expulsion of the products of conception in 11% of the subjects and increased uterine bleeding in 41%. If a woman is or becomes pregnant while taking this drug, the drug should be discontinued and the patient apprised of the potential hazard to the fetus.

Teratogenic effects: Cytotec is not fetotoxic or teratogenic in rats and rabbits at doses 625 and 63 times the human dose, respectively.

Nursing mothers: See *Contraindications.* It is unlikely that Cytotec is excreted in human milk since it is rapidly metabolized throughout the body. However, it is not known if the active metabolite (misoprostol acid) is excreted in human

milk. Therefore, Cytotec should not be administered to nursing mothers because the potential excretion of misoprostol acid could cause significant diarrhea in nursing infants.

Pediatric use: Safety and effectiveness in children below the age of 18 years have not been established.

ADVERSE REACTIONS

The following have been reported as adverse events in subjects receiving Cytotec:

Gastrointestinal: In subjects receiving Cytotec 400 or 800 mcg daily in clinical trials, the most frequent gastrointestinal adverse events were diarrhea and abdominal pain. The incidence of diarrhea at 800 mcg in controlled trials in patients on NSAIDs ranged from 14–40% and in all studies (over 5,000 patients) averaged 13%. Abdominal pain occurred in 13–20% of patients in NSAID trials and about 7% in all studies, but there was no consistent difference from placebo.

Diarrhea was dose related and usually developed early in the course of therapy (after 13 days), usually was self-limiting (often resolving after 8 days), but sometimes required discontinuation of Cytotec (2% of the patients). Rare instances of profound diarrhea leading to severe dehydration have been reported. Patients with an underlying condition such as inflammatory bowel disease, or those in whom dehydration, were it to occur, would be dangerous, should be monitored carefully if Cytotec is prescribed. The incidence of diarrhea can be minimized by administering after meals and at bedtime, and by avoiding coadministration of Cytotec with magnesium-containing antacids.

Gynecological: Women who received Cytotec during clinical trials reported the following gynecological disorders: spotting (0.7%), cramps (0.6%), hypermenorrhea (0.5%), menstrual disorder (0.3%) and dysmenorrhea (0.1%). Postmenopausal vaginal bleeding may be related to Cytotec administration. If it occurs, diagnostic workup should be undertaken to rule out gynecological pathology.

Elderly: There were no significant differences in the safety profile of Cytotec in approximately 500 ulcer patients who were 65 years of age or older compared with younger patients.

Additional adverse events which were reported are categorized as follows:

Incidence greater than 1%: In clinical trials, the following adverse reactions were reported by more than 1% of the subjects receiving Cytotec and may be causally related to the drug: nausea (3.2%), flatulence (2.9%), headache (2.4%), dyspepsia (2.0%), vomiting (1.3%), and constipation (1.1%). However, there were no significant diferences between the incidences of these events for Cytotec and placebo.

Causal relationship unknown: The following adverse events were infrequently reported. Causal relationships between Cytotec and these events have not been established but cannot be excluded:

Body as a whole: aches/pains, asthenia, fatigue, fever, rigors, weight changes.

Skin: rash, dermatitis, alopecia, pallor, breast pain.

Special senses: abnormal taste, abnormal vision, conjunctivitis, deafness, tinnitus, earache.

Respiratory: upper respiratory tract infection, bronchitis, bronchospasm, dyspnea, pneumonia, epistaxis.

Cardiovascular: chest pain, edema, diaphoresis, hypotension, hypertension, arrhythmia, phlebitis, increased cardiac enzymes, syncope.

Gastrointestinal: GI bleeding, GI inflammation/infection, rectal disorder, abnormal hepatobiliary function, gingivitis, reflux, dysphagia, amylase increase.

Hypersensitivity: Anaphylaxis.

Metabolic: glycosuria, gout, increased nitrogen, increased alkaline phosphatase.

Genitourinary: polyuria, dysuria, hematuria, urinary tract infection.

Nervous system/Psychiatric: anxiety, change in appetite, depression, drowsiness, dizziness, thirst, impotence, loss of libido, sweating increase, neuropathy, neurosis, confusion.

Musculoskeletal: arthralgia, myalgia, muscle cramps, stiffness, back pain.

Blood/Coagulation: anemia, abnormal differential, thrombocytopenia, purpura, ESR increased.

OVERDOSAGE

The toxic dose of Cytotec in humans has not been determined. Cumulative total daily doses of 1600 mcg have been tolerated, with only symptoms of gastrointestinal discomfort being reported. In animals, the acute toxic effects are diarrhea, gastrointestinal lesions, focal cardiac necrosis, hepatic necrosis, renal tubular necrosis, testicular atrophy, respiratory difficulties, and depression of the central nervous system. Clinical signs that may indicate an overdose are sedation, tremor, convulsions, dyspnea, abdominal pain, diarrhea, fever, palpitations, hypotension, or bradycardia. Symptoms should be treated with supportive therapy.

It is not known if misoprostol acid is dialyzable. However, because misoprostol is metabolized like a fatty acid, it is unlikely that dialysis would be appropriate treatment for overdosage.

DOSAGE AND ADMINISTRATION

The recommended adult oral dose of Cytotec for the prevention of NSAID-induced gastric ulcers is 200 mcg four times daily with food. If this dose cannot be tolerated, a dose of 100 mcg can be used. (See *Clinical Pharmacology: Clinical studies.*) Cytotec should be taken for the duration of NSAID therapy as prescribed by the physician. Cytotec should be taken with a meal, and the last dose of the day should be at bedtime.

Renal impairment: Adjustment of the dosing schedule in renally impaired patients is not routinely needed, but dosage can be reduced if the 200-mcg dose is not tolerated. (See *Clinical Pharmacology.*)

HOW SUPPLIED

Cytotec 100-mcg tablets are white, round, with SEARLE debossed on one side and 1451 on the other side; supplied as:

NDC Number	Size
0025-1451-60	unit-of-use bottle of 60
0025-1451-20	unit-of-use bottle of 120
0025-1451-34	carton of 100 unit dose

Cytotec 200-mcg tablets are white, hexagonal, with SEARLE debossed above and 1461 debossed below the line on one side and a double stomach debossed on the other side; supplied as:

NDC Number	Size
0025-1461-60	unit-of-use bottle of 60
0025-1461-31	unit-of-use bottle of 100
0025-1461-34	carton of 100 unit dose

Store below 86°F (30°C) in a dry area.

Caution: Federal law prohibits dispensing without prescription.

PATIENT INFORMATION

Read this leaflet before taking Cytotec® (misoprostol) and each time your prescription is renewed, because the leaflet may be changed.

Cytotec (misoprostol) is being prescribed by your doctor to decrease the chance of getting stomach ulcers related to the arthritis/pain medication that you take.

Cytotec can cause miscarriage, often associated with potentially dangerous bleeding. This may result in hospitalization, surgery, infertility, or death. **Do not take it if you are pregnant and do not become pregnant while taking this medicine.**

If you become pregnant during Cytotec therapy, stop taking Cytotec and contact your physician immediately. Remember that even if you are on a means of birth control it is still possible to become pregnant. Should this occur, stop taking Cytotec and contact your physician immediately.

Cytotec may cause diarrhea, abdominal cramping, and/or nausea in some people. In most cases these problems develop during the first few weeks of therapy and stop after about a week. You can minimize possible diarrhea by making sure you take Cytotec with food.

Because these side effects are usually mild to moderate and usually go away in a matter of days, most patients can continue to take Cytotec. If you have prolonged difficulty (more than 8 days), or if you have severe diarrhea, cramping and/or nausea, call your doctor.

Take Cytotec only according to the directions given by your physician.

Do not give Cytotec to anyone else. It has been prescribed for your specific condition, may not be the correct treatment for another person, and would be dangerous if the other person were pregnant.

This information sheet does not cover all possible side effects of Cytotec. This patient information leaflet does not address the side effects of your arthritis/pain medication. See your doctor if you have questions.

Keep out of reach of children.

8/12/91 • A05419-2

Shown in Product Identification Section, page 429

DEMULEN® 1/35–21 ℞
DEMULEN® 1/35–28 ℞
DEMULEN® 1/50–21 ℞
DEMULEN® 1/50–28 ℞

[*dem 'ū-len*]

(ethynodiol diacetate with ethinyl estradiol)

PRODUCT OVERVIEW

KEY FACTS

The Searle line of oral contraceptives contains two fixed-dose combination oral contraceptives (DEMULEN 1/35-21 and DEMULEN 1/35-28) containing ethynodiol diacetate (1 mg) with ethinyl estradiol (35 mcg) and two fixed-dose combination oral contraceptives (DEMULEN 1/50-21 and DEMULEN 1/50-28) containing ethynodiol diacetate (1 mg) with ethinyl estradiol (50 mcg). DEMULEN 1/35-21 and DEMULEN 1/50-21 are 21-day dosage regimens. DEMULEN 1/35-28 and DEMULEN 1/50-28 are 28-day dosage regimens (including 7 days of inert tablets). These forms are packaged in Compack® tablet dispensers.

MAJOR USE

DEMULEN 1/35 and DEMULEN 1/50 are highly effective in preventing pregnancy.

SAFETY INFORMATION

See complete safety information set forth below.

PRESCRIBING INFORMATION

DEMULEN® 1/35–21 ℞
DEMULEN® 1/35–28 ℞
DEMULEN® 1/50–21 ℞
DEMULEN® 1/50–28 ℞

[*dem 'ū-len*]

(ethynodiol diacetate with ethinyl estradiol)

DESCRIPTION

Demulen 1/35-21 and Demulen 1/35-28. Each white tablet contains 1 mg of ethynodiol diacetate and 35 mcg of ethinyl estradiol, and the inactive ingredients include calcium acetate, calcium phosphate, corn starch, hydrogenated castor oil, and povidone. Each blue tablet in the Demulen 1/35-28 package is a placebo containing no active ingredients, and the inactive ingredients include calcium sulfate, corn starch, FD&C Blue No. 1 Lake, magnesium stearate, and sucrose.

Demulen 1/50-21 and Demulen 1/50-28. Each white tablet contains 1 mg of ethynodiol diacetate and 50 mcg of ethinyl estradiol, and the inactive ingredients include calcium acetate, calcium phosphate, corn starch, hydrogenated castor oil, and povidone. Each pink tablet in the Demulen 1/50-28 package is a placebo containing no active ingredients, and the inactive ingredients include calcium sulfate, corn starch, FD&C Red No. 3, FD&C Yellow No. 6, magnesium stearate, and sucrose.

The chemical name for ethynodiol diacetate is 19-nor-17α-pregn-4-en-20-yne-3β, 17-diol diacetate, and for ethinyl estradiol it is 19-nor-17α-pregna-1,3,5(10)-trien-20-yne-3, 17-diol. The structural formulas are as follows:

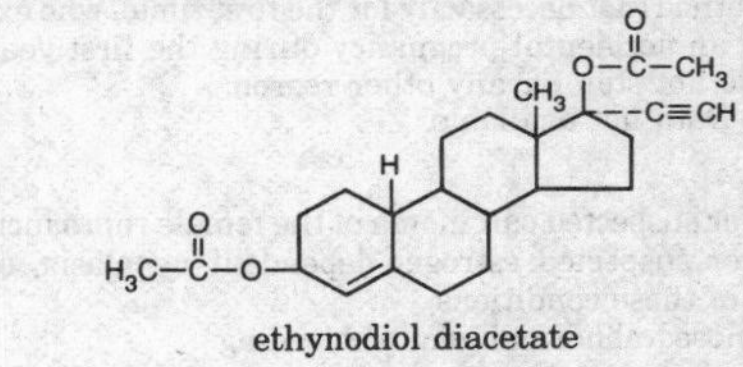

ethynodiol diacetate

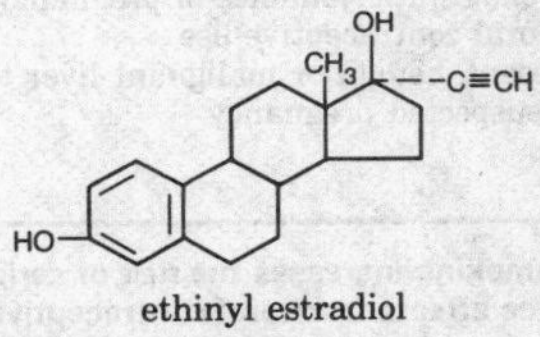

ethinyl estradiol

Therapeutic class: Oral contraceptive.

CLINICAL PHARMACOLOGY

Combination oral contraceptives act primarily by suppression of gonadotropins. Although the primary mechanism of this action is inhibition of ovulation, other alterations in the genital tract, including changes in the cervical mucus (which increase the difficulty of sperm entry into the uterus) and the endometrium (which may reduce the likelihood of implantation) may also contribute to contraceptive effectiveness.

INDICATIONS AND USAGE

Demulen 1/35 and Demulen 1/50 are indicated for the prevention of pregnancy in women who elect to use oral contraceptives as a method of contraception.

Oral contraceptives are highly effective. Table 1 lists the typical accidental pregnancy rates for users of combination oral contraceptives and other methods of contraception. The efficacy of these contraceptive methods, except sterilization, depends upon the reliability with which they are used. Correct and consistent use of methods can result in lower failure rates. [See Table 1 next page.]

CONTRAINDICATIONS

Oral contraceptives should not be used in women who have the following conditions:

- Thrombophlebitis or thromboembolic disorders
- A past history of deep vein thrombophlebitis or thromboembolic disorders
- Cerebral vascular disease, myocardial infarction, or coronary artery disease, or a past history of these conditions
- Known or suspected carcinoma of the breast, or a history of this condition

Continued on next page

Searle—Cont.

Table 1. Lowest expected and typical failure rates during the first year of continuous use of a method. Percent of women experiencing an accidental pregnancy in the first year of continuous use.[1]

Method	Lowest Expected*	Typical**
No contraception	85	85
Oral contraceptives		
Combined	0.1	N/A***
Progestogen only	0.5	N/A***
Diaphragm with spermicidal		
cream or jelly	6	18
Spermicides alone (foam,		
creams, jellies and vaginal		
suppositories)	3	21
Vaginal sponge		
Nulliparous	6	18
Parous	9	28
IUD (medicated)		
Progesterone	2	N/A***
Copper T 380A	0.8	N/A***
Condom without spermicides	2	12
Periodic abstinence (all		
methods)	1–9	20
Female sterilization	0.2	0.4
Male sterilization	0.1	0.15

Adapted from Trussell et al.[1]

* The authors' best guess of the percentage of women expected to experience an accidental pregnancy among couples who initiate a method (not necessarily for the first time) and who use it consistently and correctly during the first year if they do not stop for any other reason.

** This term represents "typical" couples who initiate use of a method (not necessarily for the first time), who experience an accidental pregnancy during the first year if they do not stop for any other reason.

*** N/A—Data not available.

- Known or suspected carcinoma of the female reproductive organs or suspected estrogen-dependent neoplasia, or a history of these conditions
- Undiagnosed abnormal genital bleeding
- History of cholestatic jaundice of pregnancy or jaundice with prior oral contraceptive use
- Past or present, benign or malignant liver tumors
- Known or suspected pregnancy

WARNINGS

> Cigarette smoking increases the risk of serious cardiovascular side effects from oral contraceptive use. This risk increases with age and with heavy smoking (15 or more cigarettes per day) and is quite marked in women over 35 years of age. Women who use oral contraceptives should be strongly advised not to smoke.

The use of oral contraceptives is associated with increased risk of several serious conditions including venous and arterial thromboembolism, thrombotic and hemorrhagic stroke, myocardial infarction, liver tumors or other liver lesions, and gallbladder disease. The risk of morbidity and mortality increases significantly in the presence of other risk factors such as hypertension, hyperlipidemia, obesity, and diabetes mellitus.

Practitioners prescribing oral contraceptives should be familiar with the following information relating to these and other risks.

The information contained herein is principally based on studies carried out in patients who used oral contraceptives with formulations containing higher amounts of estrogens and progestogens than those in common use today. The effect of long-term use of the oral contraceptives with lesser amounts of both estrogens and progestogens remains to be determined.

Throughout this labeling, epidemiological studies reported are of two types: retrospective case-control studies and prospective cohort studies. Case-control studies provide an estimate of the relative risk of a disease, which is defined as the *ratio* of the incidence of a disease among oral contraceptive users to that among nonusers. The relative risk (or odds ratio) does not provide information about the actual clinical occurrence of a disease. Cohort studies provide a measure of both the relative risk and the attributable risk. The latter is the *difference* in the incidence of disease between oral contraceptive users and nonusers. The attributable risk does provide information about the actual occurrence or incidence of a disease in the subject population. For further information, the reader is referred to a text on epidemiological methods.

1. Thromboembolic disorders and other vascular problems.
a. Myocardial infarction. An increased risk of myocardial infarction has been associated with oral contraceptive use.[2-21] This increased risk is primarily in smokers or in women with other underlying risk factors for coronary artery disease such as hypertension, obesity, diabetes, and hypercholesterolemia. The relative risk for myocardial infarction in current oral contraceptive users has been estimated to be 2 to 6. The risk is very low under the age of 30. However, there is the possibility of a risk of cardiovascular disease even in very young women who take oral contraceptives. Smoking in combination with oral contraceptive use has been reported to contribute substantially to the risk of myocardial infarction in women in their mid-thirties or older, with smoking accounting for the majority of excess cases.[22] Mortality rates associated with circulatory disease have been shown to increase substantially in smokers, especially in those 35 years of age and older among women who use oral contraceptives (see Figure 1, Table 2).

Figure 1. Circulatory disease mortality rates per 100,000 woman-years by age, smoking status, and oral contraceptive use.[14]

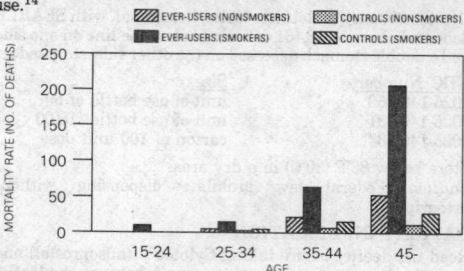

Adapted from Layde and Beral.[14]

Oral contraceptives may compound the effects of well-known cardiovascular risk factors such as hypertension, diabetes, hyperlipidemias, hypercholesterolemia, age, cigarette smoking, and obesity. In particular, some progestogens decrease HDL cholesterol[23-31] and cause glucose intolerance, while estrogens may create a state of hyperinsulinism.[32] Oral contraceptives have been shown to increase blood pressure among some users (see *Warning* No. 9). Similar effects on risk factors have been associated with an increased risk of heart disease.

b. Thromboembolism. An increased risk of thromboembolic and thrombotic disease associated with the use of oral contraceptives is well established.[17,33-51] Case-control studies have estimated the relative risk to be 3 for the first episode of superficial venous thrombosis, 4 to 11 for deep vein thrombosis or pulmonary embolism, and 1.5 to 6 for women with predisposing conditions for venous thromboembolic disease.[34-37,45,46] Cohort studies have shown the relative risk to be somewhat lower, about 3 for new cases (subjects with no past history of venous thrombosis or varicose veins) and about 4.5 for new cases requiring hospitalization.[42,47,48] The risk of venous thromboembolic disease associated with oral contraceptives is not related to duration of use.

A two- to seven-fold increase in relative risk of postoperative thromboembolic complications has been reported with the use of oral contraceptives.[38,39] The relative risk of venous thrombosis in women who have predisposing conditions is about twice that of women without such medical conditions.[43] If feasible, oral contraceptives should be discontinued at least 4 weeks prior to and for 2 weeks after elective surgery of a type associated with an increased risk of thromboembolism, and also during and following prolonged immobilization. Since the immediate postpartum period is also associated with an increased risk of thromboembolism, oral contraceptives should be started no earlier than 4 to 6 weeks after delivery in women who elect not to breast feed.

c. Cerebrovascular diseases. Both the relative and attributable risks of cerebrovascular events (thrombotic and hemorrhagic strokes) have been reported to be increased with oral contraceptive use,[14,17,18,34,42,46,52-59] although, in general, the risk was greatest among older (over 35 years), hypertensive women who also smoked. Hypertension was reported to be a risk factor for both users and nonusers, for both types of strokes, while smoking increased the risk for hemorrhagic strokes.

In one large study,[52] the relative risk for thrombotic stroke was reported as 9.5 times greater in users than in nonusers. It ranged from 3 for normotensive users to 14 for users with severe hypertension.[54] The relative risk for hemorrhagic stroke was reported to be 1.2 for nonsmokers who used oral contraceptives, 1.9 to 2.6 for smokers who did not use oral contraceptives, 6.1 to 7.6 for smokers who used oral contraceptives, 1.8 for normotensive users, and 25.7 for users with severe hypertension. The risk is also greater in older women and among smokers.

d. Dose-related risk of vascular disease with oral contraceptives. A positive association has been reported between the amount of estrogen and progestogen in oral contraceptives

and the risk of vascular disease.[41,43,53,59-64] A decline in serum high density lipoproteins (HDL) has been reported with many progestogens.[23-31] A decline in serum high density lipoproteins has been associated with an increased incidence of ischemic heart disease.[65] Because estrogens increase HDL-cholesterol, the net effect of an oral contraceptive depends on the balance achieved between doses of estrogen and progestogen and the nature and absolute amount of progestogens used in the contraceptives. The amount of both steroids should be considered in the choice of an oral contraceptive.

Minimizing exposure to estrogen and progestogen is in keeping with good principles of therapeutics. For any particular estrogen-progestogen combination, the dosage regimen prescribed should be one that contains the least amount of estrogen and progestogen that is compatible with a low failure rate and the needs of the individual patient. New acceptors of oral contraceptives should be started on preparations containing the lowest estrogen content that produces satisfactory results in the individual.

e. Persistence of risk of vascular disease. There are three studies that have shown persistence of risk of vascular disease for users of oral contraceptives. In a study in the United States, the risk of developing myocardial infarction after discontinuing oral contraceptives persisted for at least 9 years for women 40–49 years old who had used oral contraceptives for 5 or more years, but this increased risk was not demonstrated in other age groups.[16] Another American study reported former use of oral contraceptives was significantly associated with increased risk of subarachnoid hemorrhage.[57] In another study, in Great Britain, the risk of developing nonrheumatic heart disease plus hypertension, subarachnoid hemorrhage, cerebral thrombosis, and transient ischemic attacks persisted for at least 6 years after discontinuation of oral contraceptives, although the excess risk was small.[14,18,66] It should be noted that these studies were performed with oral contraceptive formulations containing 50 mcg or more of estrogens.

2. Estimates of mortality from contraceptive use. One study[67] gathered data from a variety of sources that have estimated the mortality rates associated with different methods of contraception at different ages (Table 2). These estimates include the combined risk of death associated with contraceptive methods plus the risk attributable to pregnancy in the event of method failure. Each method of contraception has its specific benefits and risks. The study concluded that, with the exception of oral contraceptive users 35 and older who smoke and 40 or older who do not smoke, mortality associated with all methods of birth control is low and below that associated with childbirth. The observation of a possible increase in risk of mortality with age for oral contraceptive users is based on data gathered in the 1970's, but not reported until 1983.[67] However, current clinical practice involves the use of lower estrogen dose formulations combined with careful restriction of oral contraceptive use to women who do not have the various risk factors listed in this labeling.

Because of these changes in practice and, also, because of some limited new data that suggest that the risk of cardiovascular disease with the use of oral contraceptives may now be less than previously observed,[48,152] the Fertility and Maternal Health Drugs Advisory Committee was asked to review the topic in 1989. The Committee concluded that, although cardiovascular disease risks may be increased with oral contraceptive use after age 40 in healthy nonsmoking women (even with the newer low-dose formulations), there are greater potential health risks associated with pregnancy in older women and with the alternative surgical and medical procedures that may be necessary if such women do not have access to effective and acceptable means of contraception.

Therefore, the Committee recommended that the benefits of oral contraceptive use by healthy nonsmoking women over 40 may outweigh the possible risks. Of course, older women, as all women who take oral contraceptives, should take the lowest dose formulation that is effective.

3. Carcinoma of the breast and reproductive organs. Numerous epidemiological studies have been performed on the incidence of breast, endometrial, ovarian, and cervical cancer in women using oral contraceptives. While there are conflicting reports, most studies suggest that the use of oral contraceptives is not associated with an overall increase in the risk of developing breast cancer.[17,40,68-78] Some studies have reported an increased relative risk of developing breast cancer, particularly at a young age.[79-102,151] This increased relative risk appears to be related to duration of use.

Some studies suggested that oral contraceptive use was associated with an increase in the risk of cervical intraepithelial neoplasia, dysplasia, erosion, carcinoma, or microglandular dysplasia in some populations of women.[17,50,103-115] However, there continues to be controversy about the extent to which such findings may be due to differences in sexual behavior and other factors.

In spite of many studies of the relationship between oral contraceptive use and breast and cervical cancers, a cause and effect relationship has not been established.

4. Hepatic neoplasia. Benign hepatic adenomas and other hepatic lesions have been associated with oral contraceptive use,[116–121] although the incidence of such benign tumors is rare in the United States. Indirect calculations have estimated the attributable risk to be in the range of 3.3 cases per 100,000 for users, a risk that increases after 4 or more years of use.[120] Rupture of benign, hepatic adenomas or other lesions may cause death through intra-abdominal hemorrhage. Therefore, such lesions should be considered in women presenting with abdominal pain and tenderness, abdominal mass, or shock. About one quarter of the cases presented because of abdominal masses; up to one half had signs and symptoms of acute intraperitoneal hemorrhage.[121] Diagnosis may prove difficult.

Studies from the U.S.,[122,150] Great Britain,[123,124] and Italy[125] have shown an increased risk of hepatocellular carcinoma in long-term (> 8 years; relative risk of 7–20) oral contraceptive users. However, these cancers are rare in the United States, and the attributable risk (the excess incidence) of liver cancers in oral contraceptive users approaches less than 1 per 1,000,000 users.

5. Ocular lesions. There have been reports of retinal thrombosis and other ocular lesions associated with the use of oral contraceptives. Oral contraceptives should be discontinued if there is unexplained, gradual or sudden, partial or complete loss of vision; onset of proptosis or diplopia; papilledema; or any evidence of retinal vascular lesions. Appropriate diagnostic and therapeutic measures should be undertaken immediately.

6. Oral contraceptive use before or during pregnancy. Extensive epidemiological studies have revealed no increased risk of birth defects in women who have used oral contraceptives prior to pregnancy.[126,129] The majority of recent studies also do not suggest a teratogenic effect, particularly insofar as cardiac anomalies and limb reduction defects are concerned,[126–129] when the pill is taken inadvertently during early pregnancy.

The administration of oral contraceptives to induce withdrawal bleeding should not be used as a test for pregnancy. Oral contraceptives should not be used during pregnancy to treat threatened or habitual abortion. It is recommended that for any patient who has missed two consecutive periods, pregnancy should be ruled out before continuing oral contraceptive use. If the patient has not adhered to the prescribed schedule, the possibility of pregnancy should be considered at the time of the first missed period and further use of oral contraceptives should be withheld until pregnancy has been ruled out. Oral contraceptive use should be discontinued if pregnancy is confirmed.

7. Gallbladder disease. Earlier studies reported an increased lifetime relative risk of gallbladder surgery in users of oral contraceptives and estrogens.[40,42,53,70] More recent studies, however, have shown that the relative risk of developing gallbladder disease among oral contraceptive users may be minimal.[130–132] The recent findings of minimal risk may be related to the use of oral contraceptive formulations containing lower doses of estrogens and progestogens.

8. Carbohydrate and lipid metabolic effects. Oral contraceptives have been shown to cause a decrease in glucose tolerance in a significant percentage of users.[32] This effect has been shown to be directly related to estrogen dose.[133] Progestogens increase insulin secretion and create insulin resistance, the effect varying with different progestational agents.[32,134] However, in the nondiabetic woman, oral contraceptives appear to have no effect on fasting blood glucose. Because of these demonstrated effects, prediabetic and diabetic women should be carefully observed while taking oral contraceptives.

Some women may have persistent hypertriglyceridemia while on the pill. As discussed earlier (see *Warnings* 1a and 1d), changes in serum triglycerides and lipoprotein levels have been reported in oral contraceptive users.[23–31,135,136]

9. Elevated blood pressure. An increase in blood pressure has been reported in women taking oral contraceptives[50,53,137–139] and this increase is more likely in older oral contraceptive users[137] and with extended duration of use.[53] Data from the Royal College of General Practitioners[138] and subsequent randomized trials have shown that the incidence of hypertension increases with increasing concentrations of progestogens.

Women with a history of hypertension or hypertension-related diseases, or renal disease[139] should be encouraged to use another method of contraception. If such women elect to use oral contraceptives, they should be monitored closely and if significant elevation of blood pressure occurs, oral contraceptives should be discontinued. For most women, elevated blood pressure will return to normal after stopping oral contraceptives,[137] and there is no difference in the occurrence of hypertension among ever- and never-users.[140]

10. Headache. The onset or exacerbation of migraine or the development of headache of a new pattern that is recurrent, persistent, or severe requires discontinuation of oral contraceptives and evaluation of the cause.

Table 2. Annual number of birth-related or method-related deaths associated with control of fertility per 100,000 nonsterile women, by fertility control method according to age.[67]

	Age					
Method of control	15–19	20–24	25–29	30–34	35–39	40–44
No fertility control methods*	7.0	7.4	9.1	14.8	25.7	28.2
Oral contraceptives						
nonsmoker**	0.3	0.5	0.9	1.9	13.8	31.6
smoker**	2.2	3.4	6.6	13.5	51.1	117.2
IUD**	0.8	0.8	1.0	1.0	1.4	1.4
Condom*	1.1	1.6	0.7	0.2	0.3	0.4
Diaphragm/ spermicide*	1.9	1.2	1.2	1.3	2.2	2.8
Periodic abstinence*	2.5	1.6	1.6	1.7	2.9	3.6

*Deaths are birth-related
**Deaths are method-related
Adapted from Ory.[67]

11. Bleeding irregularities. Breakthrough bleeding and spotting are sometimes encountered in patients on oral contraceptives, especially during the first three months of use. Nonhormonal causes should be considered and adequate diagnostic measures taken to rule out malignancy or pregnancy in the event of breakthrough bleeding, as in the case of any abnormal vaginal bleeding. If a pathologic basis has been excluded, time alone or a change to another formulation may solve the problem. In the event of amenorrhea, pregnancy should be ruled out.

PRECAUTIONS

1. Physical examination and follow-up. A complete medical history and physical examination should be completed prior to the initiation or reinstitution of oral contraceptives and at least annually during the use of oral contraceptives. These physical examinations should include special reference to blood pressure, breasts, abdomen, and pelvic organs, including cervical cytology, and relevant laboratory tests. In case of undiagnosed, persistent, or recurrent abnormal vaginal bleeding, appropriate diagnostic measures should be conducted to rule out malignancy. Women with a strong family history of breast cancer or who have breast nodules should be monitored with particular care.

2. Lipid disorders. Women who are being treated for hyperlipidemias should be followed closely if they elect to use oral contraceptives. Some progestogens may elevate LDL levels and may render the control of hyperlipidemias more difficult.

3. Liver function. If jaundice develops in any woman receiving oral contraceptives, they should be discontinued. Steroids may be poorly metabolized in patients with impaired liver function and should be administered with caution in such patients. Cholestatic jaundice has been reported after combined treatment with oral contraceptives and troleandomycin. Hepatotoxicity following a combination of oral contraceptives and cyclosporine has also been reported.

4. Fluid retention. Oral contraceptives may cause some degree of fluid retention. They should be prescribed with caution, and only with careful monitoring, in patients with conditions that might be aggravated by fluid retention, such as convulsive disorders, migraine syndrome, asthma, or cardiac, hepatic, or renal dysfunction.

5. Emotional disorders. Women with a history of depression should be carefully observed and the drug discontinued if depression recurs to a serious degree.

6. Contact lenses. Contact lens wearers who develop visual changes or changes in lens tolerance should be assessed by an ophthalmologist.

7. Drug interactions. Reduced efficacy and increased incidence of breakthrough bleeding and menstrual irregularities have been associated with concomitant use of rifampin. A similar association, though less marked, has been suggested for barbiturates, phenylbutazone, phenytoin sodium, and possibly with griseofulvin, ampicillin, and tetracyclines.

8. Laboratory test interactions. Certain endocrine and liver function tests and blood components may be affected by oral contraceptives:

a. Increased prothrombin and factors VII, VIII, IX, and X; decreased antithrombin III; increased platelet aggregability.
b. Increased thyroid binding globulin (TBG), leading to increased circulating total thyroid hormone as measured by protein-bound iodine (PBI), T_4 by column or by radioimmunoassay. Free T_3 resin uptake is decreased, reflecting the elevated TBG; free T_4 concentration is unaltered.
c. Other binding proteins may be elevated in the serum.
d. Sex-steroid binding globulins are increased and result in elevated levels of total circulating sex steroids and corticoids; however, free or biologically active levels remain unchanged.
e. Triglycerides and phospholipids may be increased.
f. Glucose tolerance may be decreased.
g. Serum folate levels may be depressed. This may be of clinical significance if a woman becomes pregnant shortly after discontinuing oral contraceptives.
h. Increased sulfobromophthalein and other abnormalities in liver function tests may occur.
i. Plasma levels of trace minerals may be altered.
j. Response to the metyrapone test may be reduced.

9. Carcinogenesis. See *Warnings*.

10. Pregnancy. Pregnancy Category X. See *Contraindications* and *Warnings*.

11. Nursing mothers. Small amounts of oral contraceptive steroids have been identified in the milk of nursing mothers[141–143] and a few adverse effects on the child have been reported, including jaundice and breast enlargement. In addition, oral contraceptives given in the postpartum period may interfere with lactation by decreasing the quantity and quality of breast milk. If possible, the nursing mother should be advised not to use oral contraceptives, but to use other forms of contraception until she has completely weaned her child.

12. Venereal diseases. Oral contraceptives are of no value in the prevention or treatment of venereal disease. The prevalence of cervical *Chlamydia trachomatis* and *Neisseria gonorrhoeae* in oral contraceptive users is increased severalfold.[144,145] It should not be assumed that oral contraceptives afford protection against pelvic inflammatory disease from chlamydia.[144]

13. General.

a. The pathologist should be advised of oral contraceptive therapy when relevant specimens are submitted.
b. Treatment with oral contraceptives may mask the onset of the climacteric. (See *Warnings* regarding risks in this age group.)

INFORMATION FOR THE PATIENT

See patient labeling printed below.

ADVERSE REACTIONS

An increased risk of the following serious adverse reactions has been associated with the use of oral contraceptives (see *Warnings*):

- Thrombophlebitis and thrombosis
- Arterial thromboembolism
- Pulmonary embolism
- Myocardial infarction and coronary thrombosis
- Cerebral hemorrhage
- Cerebral thrombosis
- Hypertension
- Gallbladder disease
- Benign and malignant liver tumors, and other hepatic lesions.

There is evidence of an association between the following conditions and the use of oral contraceptives, although additional confirmatory studies are needed:

- Mesenteric thrombosis
- Neuro-ocular lesions (eg, retinal thrombosis and optic neuritis)

The following adverse reactions have been reported in patients receiving oral contraceptives and are believed to be drug-related:

- Nausea
- Vomiting
- Gastrointestinal symptoms (such as abdominal cramps and bloating)
- Breakthrough bleeding
- Spotting
- Change in menstrual flow
- Amenorrhea during or after use
- Temporary infertility after discontinuation of use

Continued on next page

Searle—Cont.

- Edema
- Chloasma or melasma, which may persist
- Breast changes: tenderness, enlargement, secretion
- Change in weight (increase or decrease)
- Change in cervical erosion or secretion
- Diminution in lactation when given immediately postpartum
- Cholestatic jaundice
- Migraine
- Rash (allergic)
- Mental depression
- Reduced tolerance to carbohydrates
- Vaginal candidiasis
- Change in corneal curvature (steepening)
- Intolerance to contact lenses

The following adverse reactions or conditions have been reported in users of oral contraceptives and the association has been neither confirmed nor refuted:

- Premenstrual syndrome
- Cataracts
- Changes in appetite
- Cystitis-like syndrome
- Headache
- Nervousness
- Dizziness
- Hirsutism
- Loss of scalp hair
- Erythema multiforme
- Erythema nodosum
- Hemorrhagic eruption
- Vaginitis
- Porphyria
- Impaired renal function
- Hemolytic uremic syndrome
- Acne
- Changes in libido
- Colitis
- Budd-Chiari syndrome
- Endocervical hyperplasia or ectropion

OVERDOSAGE

Serious ill effects have not been reported following acute ingestion of large doses of oral contraceptives by young children.[180,181] Overdosage may cause nausea, and withdrawal bleeding may occur in females.

NON-CONTRACEPTIVE HEALTH BENEFITS

The following non-contraceptive health benefits related to the use of oral contraceptives are supported by epidemiological studies that largely utilized oral contraceptive formulations containing estrogen doses exceeding 35 mcg of ethinyl estradiol or 50 mcg of mestranol.[148,149]

Effects on menses:
- Increased menstrual cycle regularity
- Decreased blood loss and decreased risk of iron-deficiency anemia
- Decreased frequency of dysmenorrhea

Effects related to inhibition of ovulation:
- Decreased risk of functional ovarian cysts
- Decreased risk of ectopic pregnancies

Effects from long-term use:
- Decreased risk of fibroadenomas and fibrocystic disease of the breast
- Decreased risk of acute pelvic inflammatory disease
- Decreased risk of endometrial cancer
- Decreased risk of ovarian cancer
- Decreased risk of uterine fibroids

DOSAGE AND ADMINISTRATION

To achieve maximum contraceptive effectiveness, oral contraceptives must be taken exactly as directed and at intervals of 24 hours.
IMPORTANT: The patient should be instructed to use an additional method of protection until after the first week of administration *in the initial cycle.* The possibility of ovulation and conception prior to initiation of use should be considered.

Demulen 1/35-21, Demulen 1/35-28, Demulen 1/50-21, and Demulen 1/50-28 Dosage Schedules
The Demulen 1/35-21 and Demulen 1/50-21 Compack® tablet dispensers contain 21 tablets arranged in three numbered rows of 7 tablets each.
The Demulen 1/35-28 and Demulen 1/50-28 tablet dispensers contain 21 white active tablets arranged in three numbered rows of 7 tablets each, followed by a fourth row of 7 pink (blue for Demulen 1/35-28) placebo tablets.
Days of the week are printed above the tablets, starting with Sunday on the left.
Two dosage schedules are described, one of which may be more convenient or suitable than the other for an individual patient.

Schedule #1: Sunday start. The patient begins taking Demulen 1/35-21, Demulen 1/35-28, Demulen 1/50-21, or Demulen 1/50-28 from the first row of her package, one tablet daily, starting on the first Sunday after the onset of menstruation. If the patient's period begins on a Sunday she takes her first tablet that very same day. The 21st tablet or the 28th tablet, depending on whether the patient is taking the 21- or 28-tablet course, will then be taken on a Saturday.
Subsequent cycles:
21-tablet course—The patient begins a new 21-tablet course on the eighth day, Sunday, after taking her last tablet. All subsequent cycles will also begin on Sunday, one tablet being taken each day for 3 weeks followed by a week of no pill-taking.
28-tablet course—The patient begins a new 28-tablet course on the next day, Sunday, and all subsequent cycles will also begin on Sunday, one tablet being taken each and every day.
With a Sunday-start schedule, a woman whose period begins on the day of or 1 to 4 days before taking the first tablet should expect a diminution of flow and fewer menstrual days. The initial cycle will likely be shortened by from 1 to 5 days. Thereafter, cycles should be about 28 days in length.

Schedule #2: Day 5 start. The patient begins taking Demulen 1/35-21 or Demulen 1/50-21 from the first row of her package, one tablet daily, starting with the pill day which corresponds to day 5 of her menstrual cycle; the first day of menstruation is counted as day 1. After the last (Saturday) tablet in row #3 has been taken, if any remain in the first row, the patient completes her 21-tablet schedule starting with Sunday in row #1.
Subsequent cycles: The patient begins a new 21-tablet course on the eighth day after taking her last tablet, again starting the same day of the week on which she began her first course. All subsequent cycles will also begin on that same day, one tablet being taken each day for 3 weeks followed by a week of no pill-taking.

Special notes
Spotting or breakthrough bleeding: If spotting (bleeding insufficient to require a pad) or breakthrough bleeding (heavier bleeding similar to a menstrual flow) occurs when these products are used for contraception, the patient should continue taking her tablets as directed. The incidence of spotting or breakthrough bleeding is minimal, most frequently occurring in the first cycle. Ordinarily spotting or breakthrough bleeding will stop within a week. Usually the patient will begin to cycle regularly within two or three courses of tablet-taking. In the event of spotting or breakthrough bleeding organic causes should be borne in mind. (See *Warning* No. 11.)
Missed menstrual periods. Withdrawal flow will normally occur 2 or 3 days after the last active tablet is taken. Failure of withdrawal bleeding ordinarily does not mean that the patient is pregnant, providing the dosage schedule has been correctly followed. (See *Warning* No. 6.)
If the patient has *not* adhered to the prescribed dosage regimen, the possibility of pregnancy should be considered after the first missed period, and oral contraceptives should be withheld until pregnancy has been ruled out.
If the patient has adhered to the prescribed regimen and misses two consecutive periods, pregnancy should be ruled out before continuing the contraceptive regimen.
The first intermenstrual interval after discontinuing the tablets is usually prolonged; consequently, a patient for whom a 28-day cycle is usual might not begin to menstruate for 35 days or longer. Ovulation in such prolonged cycles will occur correspondingly later in the cycle. Posttreatment cycles after the first one, however, are usually typical for the individual woman prior to taking tablets. (See *Warning* No. 11.)
Missed tablets: If a woman misses taking one active tablet the missed tablet should be taken as soon as it is remembered. In addition, the next tablet should be taken at the usual time. If two consecutive active tablets are missed the dosage should be doubled for the next 2 days. The regular schedule should then be resumed, but an additional method of protection is recommended for the remainder of the cycle.

While there is little likelihood of ovulation if only one active tablet is missed, the possibility of spotting or breakthrough bleeding is increased and should be expected if two or more successive active tablets are missed. However, the possibility of ovulation increases with each successive day that scheduled active tablets are missed.
If one or more placebo tablets of Demulen 1/35-28 or Demulen 1/50-28 are missed, the Demulen 1/35-28 or Demulen 1/50-28 schedule should be resumed on the following Sunday (the eighth day after the last white tablet was taken). Omission of placebo tablets in the 28-tablet courses does not increase the possibility of conception provided that this schedule is followed.

HOW SUPPLIED

Demulen 1/35:
Each white Demulen 1/35 tablet is round in shape, with a debossed SEARLE on one side and 151 and design on the other side, and contains 1 mg of ethynodiol diacetate and 35 mcg of ethinyl estradiol.
Demulen 1/35-21 is packaged in cartons of 6 and 24 Compack tablet dispensers of 21 tablets each.
Demulen 1/35-28 is packaged in cartons of 6 and 24 Compack tablet dispensers. Each Compack contains 21 white Demulen 1/35 tablets and 7 blue placebo tablets. (Placebo tablets have a debossed SEARLE on one side and a "P" on the other side.)
Demulen 1/50:
Each white Demulen 1/50 tablet is round in shape, with a debossed SEARLE on one side and 71 on the other side, and contains 1 mg of ethynodiol diacetate and 50 mcg of ethinyl estradiol.
Demulen 1/50-21 is packaged in cartons of 6 and 24 Compack tablet dispensers of 21 tablets each.
Demulen 1/50-28 is packaged in cartons of 6 and 24 Compack tablet dispensers. Each Compack contains 21 white Demulen 1/50 tablets and 7 pink placebo tablets. (Placebo tablets have a debossed SEARLE on one side and a "P" on the other side.)

Caution: Federal law prohibits dispensing without prescription.

REFERENCES

1. Trussel J, et al. *Stud Fam Plann.* 1987;18(Sept-Oct):237; and 1990;21(Jan-Feb):51. **2.** Mann JI, et al. *Br Med J.* 1975;2(May 3):241. **3.** Mann JI, et al. *Br Med J.* 1975;3(Sept 13):631. **4.** Mann JI, et al. *Br Med J.* 1975;2(May 3):245. **5.** Mann JI, et al. *Br Med J.* 1976;2(Aug 21):445. **6.** Arthes FG, et al. *Chest.* 1976;70(Nov):574. **7.** Jain AK. *Am J Obstet Gynecol.* 1976;301(Oct 1):126; and *Stud Fam Plann.* 1977;8(March):50. **8.** Ory HW. *JAMA.* 1977;237(June 13):2619. **9.** Jick H, et al. *JAMA.* 1978;239(April 3):1403, 1407. **10.** Jick H, et al. *JAMA.* 1978;240(Dec 1):2548. **11.** Shapiro S, et al. *Lancet.* 1979;1(April 7):743. **12.** Rosenberg L, et al. *Am J Epidemiol.* 1980;111(Jan):59. **13.** Krueger DE, et al. *Am J Epidemiol.* 1980;111(June):655. **14.** Layde P, et al. *Lancet.* 1981;1(March 7):541. **15.** Adam SA, et al. *Br J Obstet Gynaecol.* 1981; 88(Aug):838. **16.** Slone D, et al. *N Engl J Med.* 1981; 305(Aug 20):420. **17.** Ramcharan S, et al. *The Walnut Creek Contraceptive Drug Study.* Vol 3. US Govt Ptg Off; 1981; and *J Reprod Med.* 1980;25(Dec):346. **18.** Layde PM, et al. *J R Coll Gen Pract.* 1983;33(Feb):75. **19.** Rosenberg L, et al. *JAMA.* 1985;253(May 24/31):2965. **20.** Mant D, et al. *J Epidemiol Community Health.* 1987;41(Sept):215. **21.** Croft P, et al. *Br Med J.* 1989;298(Jan 21):165. **22.** Goldbaum GM, et al. *JAMA.* 1987;258(Sept 11):1339. **23.** Bradley DD, et al. *N Engl J Med.* 1978;299(July 6):17. **24** Tikkanen MJ, *J Reprod Med.* 1986;31(Sept suppl):898. **25.** Lipson A, et al. *Contraception.* 1986;34(Aug):121. **26.** Burkman RT, et al. *Obstet Gynecol.* 1988;71(Jan):33. **27.** Knopp RH, *J Reprod Med.* 1986;31(Sept suppl):913. **28.** Krauss RM, et al. *Am J Obstet Gynecol.* 1983; 145(Feb 15):446. **29.** Wahl P, et al. *N Engl J Med.* 1983;308(April 14):862. **30.** Wynn V, et al. *Am J Obstet Gynecol.* 1982;142(March 15):766. **31.** LaRosa JC. *J Reprod Med.* 1986;31(Sept suppl):906. **32.** Wynn V, et al. *J Reprod Med.* 1986;31(Sept suppl):892. **33.** Royal College of General Practitioners. *J R Coll Gen Pract.* 1967;13(May):267. **34.** Inman WHW, et al. *Br Med J.* 1968;2(April 27):193. **35.** Vessey MP, et al. *Br Med J.* 1968;2(April 27):199. **36.** Vessey MP, et al. *Br Med J.* 1969;2(June 14):651. **37.** Sartwell PE, et al. *Am J Epidemiol.* 1969;90(Nov):365. **38.** Vessey MP, et al. *Br Med J.* 1970;3(July 18):123. **39.** Greene GR, et al. *Am J Public Health.* 1972;62(May):680. **40.** Boston Collaborative Drug Surveillance Programme. *Lancet.* 1973;1(June 23):1399. **41.** Stolley PD, et al. *Am J Epidemiol.* 1975;102(Sept):197. **42.** Vessey MP, et al. *J Biosoc Sci.* 1976;8(Oct):373. **43.** Kay CR, *J R Coll Gen Pract.* 1978;28(July):393. **44.** Petitti DB, et al. *Am J Epidemiol.* 1978;108(Dec):480. **45.** Maquire MG, et al. *Am J Epidemiol.* 1979;110(Aug):188. **46.** Petitti DB, et al. *JAMA.* 1979;242(Sept 14):1150. **47.** Porter JB, et al. *Obstet Gynecol.* 1982;59(March):299. **48.** Porter JB, et al. *Obstet Gynecol.* 1985;66(July):1. **49.** Vessey MP, et al. *Br Med J.* 1986;292(Feb 22):526. **50.** Hoover R, et al. *Am J Public Health.* 1978;68(April):335. **51.** Vessey MP. *Br J Fam Plann.* 1980;6(Oct suppl):1. **52.** Collaborative Group for the Study of Stroke in Young Women. *N Engl J Med.* 1973;288(April 26):871. **53.** Royal College of General Practitioners. *Oral Contraceptives and Health.* New York, NY: Pitman Publ Corp; May 1974. **54.** Collaborative Group for the Study of Stroke in Young Women. *JAMA.* 1975;231(Feb 17):718. **55.** Beral V. *Lancet.* 1976;2(Nov 13):1047. **56.** Vessey MP, et al. *Lancet.* 1977;2(Oct 8):731; and 1981;1(March 7):549. **57.** Petitti DB, et al. *Lancet.* 1978;2(July 29):234. **58.** Inman WHW. *Br Med J.* 1979;2(Dec 8):1468. **59.** Vessey MP, et al. *Br Med J.* 1984;289(Sept 1):530. **60.** Inman WHW, et al. *Br Med J.* 1970;2(April 25):203. **61.** Meade TW, et al. *Br Med J.* 1980;280(May 10):1157. **62.** Böttiger LE, et al. *Lancet.* 1980;1(May 24):1097. **63.** Kay CR, *Am J Obstet Gynecol.* 1982;142(March 15):762. **64.** Vessey MP, et al. *Br Med J.* 1986;292(Feb 22):526. **65.** Gordon T, et al. *Am J Med.* 1977;62(May): 707. **66.** Beral V, et al. *Lancet.* 1977;2(Oct 8): 727. **67.** Ory H. *Fam Plann Perspect.* 1983;15(March April):57. **68.** Arthes FG, et al. *Cancer.* 1971;28(Dec):1391. **69.** Vessey MP, et al. *Br Med J.* 1972;3(Sept 23):719. **70.** Boston Collaborative Drug Surveillance Program. *N Engl J Med.* 1974;290(Jan 3):15. **71.** Vessey MP, et al. *Lancet.* 1975;

1(April 26):941. **72.** Casagrande J, et al. *J Natl Cancer Inst.* 1976;56(April):839. **73.** Kelsey JL, et al. *Am J Epidemiol.* 1978;107(March):236. **74.** Kay CR, *Br Med J.* 1981;282(June 27):2089. **75.** Vessey MP, et al. *Br Med J.* 1981;282(June 27):2093. **76.** The Cancer and Steroid Hormone Study of the Centers for Disease Control and the National Institute of Child Health and Human Development. Oral contraceptive use and the risk of breast cancer. *N Engl J Med.* 1986;315(Aug 14):405. **77.** Paul C, et al. *Br Med J.* 1986;293(Sept 20):723. **78.** Miller DR, et al. *Obstet Gynecol.* 1986;68(Dec):863. **79.** Pike MC, et al. *Lancet.* 1983;2(Oct 22):926. **80.** McPherson K, et al. *Br J Cancer.* 1987;56(Nov):653. **81.** Hoover R, et al. *N Engl J Med.* 1976;295(Aug 19):401. **82.** Lees AW, et al. *Int J Cancer.* 1978;22(Dec):700. **83.** Brinton LA, et al. *J Natl Cancer Inst.* 1979;62(Jan):37. **84.** Black MM. *Pathol Res Pract.* 1980;166:491; and *Cancer.* 1980;46(Dec):2747; and *Cancer.* 1983;51(June):2147. **85.** Clavel F, et al. *Bull Cancer (Paris).* 1981;68(Dec):449. **86.** Brinton LA, et al. *Int J Epidemiol.* 1982;11(Dec):316. **87.** Harris NV, et al. *Am J Epidemiol.* 1982;116(Oct):643. **88** Jick H, et al. *Am J Epidemiol.* 1980;112(Nov):577. **89.** McPherson K, et al. *Lancet.* 1983;2(Dec 17):1414. **90.** Hoover R, et al. *J Natl Cancer Inst.* 1981;67(Oct):815. **91.** Jick H, et al. *Am J Epidemiol.* 1980;112(Nov):586. **92.** Meirik O, et al. *Lancet.* 1986;2(Sept 20):650. **93.** Fasal E, et al. *J Natl Cancer Inst.* 1975;55(Oct):767. **94.** Paffenbarger RS, et al. *Cancer.* 1977; 39(April suppl):1887. **95.** Stadel BV, et al. *Contraception.* 1988;38(Sept):287. **96.** Miller DR, et al. *Am J Epidemiol.* 1989;129(Feb):269. **97.** Kay CR, et al. *Br J Cancer.* 1988;58(Nov):675. **98.** Miller DR, et al. *Obstet Gynecol.* 1986;68(Dec):863. **99.** Olsson H, et al. *Lancet.* 1985;1(March 30):748. **100.** Chilvers C, et al. *Lancet.* 1989;1(May 6):973. **101.** Huggins GR, et al. *Fertil Steril.* 1987;47(May):733. **102.** Pike MC, et al. *Br J Cancer.* 1981;43(Jan):72. **103.** Ory H, et al. *Am J Obstet Gynecol.* 1976;124(March 15):573. **104.** Stern E, et al. *Science.* 1977;196(June 24):1460. **105.** Peritz E, et al. *Am J Epidemiol.* 1977;106(Dec):462. **106.** Ory HW, et al. In: Garattini S, Berendes H, eds. *Pharmacology of Steroid Contraceptive Drugs.* New York, NY: Raven Press; 1977:211–224. **107.** Meisels A, et al. *Cancer.* 1977;40(Dec):3076. **108.** Goldacre MJ, et al. *Br Med J.* 1978;1(March 25):748. **109.** Swan SH, et al. *Am J Obstet Gynecol.* 1981;139(Jan 1):52. **110.** Vessey MP, et al. *Lancet.* 1983;2(Oct 22):930. **111.** Dallenbach-Hellweg G. *Pathol Res Pract.* 1984;179:38. **112.** Thomas DB, et al. *Br Med J.* 1985;290(March 30):961. **113.** Brinton LA, et al. *Int J Cancer.* 1986;38(Sept):339. **114.** Ebeling K, et al. *Int J Cancer.* 1987;39(April):427. **115.** Beral V. et al. *Lancet.* 1988;2(Dec 10):1331. **116.** Baum JK, et al. *Lancet.* 1973;2(Oct 27):926. **117.** Edmondson HA, et al. *N Engl J Med.* 1976;294(Feb 26):470. **118.** Bein NN, et al. *Br J Surg.* 1977;64(June):433. **119.** Klatskin G. *Gastroenterology.* 1977;73(Aug):386. **120.** Rooks JB, et al. *JAMA.* 1979;242(Aug 17):644. **121.** Sturtevant FM. In: Moghissi K, ed. *Controversies in Contraception,* Baltimore, MD; Williams & Wilkins; 1979:93–150. **122.** Henderson BE, et al. *Br J Cancer.* 1983;48(July):437. **123.** Neuberger J, et al. *Br Med J.* 1986;292(May 24):1355. **124.** Forman D, et al. *Br Med J.* 1986;292(May 24):1357. **125.** La Vecchia C, et al. *Br J Cancer.* 1989;59(March):460. **126.** Savolainen E, et al. *Am J Obstet Gynecol.* 1981;140(July 1):521. **127.** Ferencz C, et al. *Teratology.* 1980;21(April):225. **128.** Rothman KJ, et al. *Am J Epidemiol.* 1979;109(April):433. **129.** Harlap S, et al. *Obstet Gynecol.* 1980;55(April):447. **130.** Layde PM, et al. *J Epidemiol Community Health.* 1982;36(Dec):274. **131.** Rome Group for the Epidemiology and Prevention of Cholelithiasis (GREPCO). *Am J Epidemiol.* 1984;119(May):796. **132.** Strom BL, et al. *Clin Pharmacol Ther.* 1986;39(March):335. **133.** Wynn V. In: Bardin CE, et al. eds. *Progesterone and Progestins.* New York, NY: Raven Press; 1983:395–410. **134.** Perlman JA, et al. *J Chron Dis.* 1985;38(Oct):857. **135.** Powell MG, et al. *Obstet Gynecol.* 1984;63(June):764. **136.** Wynn V, et al. *Lancet.* 1966;2(Oct 1):720. **137.** Fisch IR, et al. *JAMA.* 1977;237(June 6):2499. **138.** Kay CR, *Lancet.* 1977;1(March 19):624. **139.** Laragh JH. *Am J Obstet Gynecol.* 1976;126(Sept 1):141. **140.** Ramcharan S. In: Garattini S. Berendes HW, eds. *Pharmacology of Steroid Contraceptive Drugs.* New York, NY: Raven Press; 1977:277–288. **141.** Laumas KR, et al. *Am J Obstet Gynecol.* 1967;98(June 1):411. **142.** Saxena BN, et al. *Contraception.* 1977;16(Dec):605. **143.** Nilsson S, et al. *Contraception.* 1978;17(Feb):131. **144.** Washington AE, et al. *JAMA.* 1985;253(April 19):2246. **145.** Louv WC, et al. *Am J Obstet Gynecol.* 1989;160(Feb):396. **146.** Francis WG, et al. *Can Med Assoc J.* 1965;92(Jan 23):191. **147.** Verhulst HL, et al. *J Clin Pharmacol.* 1967;7(Jan-Feb):9. **148.** Ory HW. *Fam Plann Perspect.* 1982;14(July-Aug):182. **149.** Ory HW, et al. *Making Choices: Evaluating the Health Risks and Benefits of Birth Control Methods.* New York, NY: The Alan Guttmacher Institute; 1983. **150.** Palmer JR, et al. *Am J Epidemiol.* 1989;130(Nov):878. **151.** Romieu I, et al. *J Natl Cancer Inst.* 1989;81(Sept):1313. **152.** Porter JB, et al. *Obstet Gynecol.* 1987;70(July):29.

BRIEF SUMMARY OF PATIENT WARNINGS

> Cigarette smoking increases the risk of serious adverse effects on the heart and blood vessels from oral contraceptive use. This risk increases with age and with heavy smoking (15 or more cigarettes per day) and is quite marked in women over 35 years of age. Women who use oral contraceptives are strongly advised not to smoke.

*In the detailed leaflet, "What You Should Know About Oral Contraceptives," which you have received, the risks and benefits of oral contraceptives are discussed in much more detail. That leaflet also provides information on other forms of contraception. **Please take time to read it carefully for it may have been recently revised.***

If you have any questions or problems regarding this information, contact your doctor.

Oral contraceptives, also known as "birth control pills" or "the pill," are taken to prevent pregnancy and, when taken correctly, have a failure rate of about 1% per year when used without missing any pills. The typical failure rate of large numbers of pill users is less than 3% per year when women who miss pills are included. However, forgetting to take pills considerably increases the chances of pregnancy.

For most women, oral contraceptives are free of serious or unpleasant side effects. However, oral contraceptive use is associated with certain serious diseases or conditions that can cause severe disability or death, though rarely. There are some women who are at high risk of developing certain serious diseases that can be life-threatening or may cause temporary or permanent disability. The risks associated with taking oral contraceptives increase significantly if you:

- smoke, or
- have high blood pressure, diabetes, high cholesterol, or are overweight, or
- have or have had clotting disorders, heart attack, stroke, angina pectoris (chest pains on exertion), cancer of the breast or sex organs, jaundice (yellowing of the skin or whites of the eyes), or malignant (cancerous) or benign (noncancerous) liver tumors.

Women should not use oral contraceptives if they suspect they are pregnant or if they have unexplained vaginal bleeding.

Most side effects of the pill are not serious. The most common effects are nausea, vomiting, bleeding between menstrual periods, weight gain, breast tenderness, and difficulty wearing contact lenses. These side effects, especially nausea and vomiting, may subside within the first three months of use.

Proper use of oral contraceptives requires that they be taken under your doctor's continuing supervision, because they can be associated with serious side effects. The serious side effects of the pill occur very infrequently, especially if you are in good health and are young. However, you should know that the following medical conditions have been associated with or made worse by the pill, and that certain of the risks may persist after use of the pill has been discontinued.

1. Blood clots in the legs, arms, lungs, heart (heart attack), eyes, abdomen, or elsewhere in the body. As mentioned above, smoking increases the risk of heart attacks and strokes and subsequent serious medical consequences.
2. Stroke, due to a blood clot, or to bleeding in the brain (hemorrhage) as a result of bursting of a blood vessel. Stroke can lead to paralysis in all or part of the body, or to death.
3. Liver tumors, which may rupture and cause severe bleeding and death. A possible, but not definite, association has also been found with the pill and liver cancer. However, with or without use of the pill, liver cancers are extremely rare in the United States.
4. High blood pressure, although blood pressure ordinarily, but not always, returns to original levels when the pill is stopped.
5. Gallbladder disease, which might require surgery.

The symptoms associated with these serious side effects are discussed in the detailed leaflet given to you with your supply of pills. Notify your doctor or health care provider if you notice any unusual physical disturbances while taking the pill. In addition, you should be aware that drugs such as antiepileptics, antibiotics (especially rifampin), as well as certain other drugs, may decrease oral contraceptive effectiveness.

There is a conflict among studies regarding breast cancer and oral contraceptive use. Some studies have reported an increase in the risk of developing breast cancer, particularly at a younger age. This increased risk appears to be related to duration of use. The majority of studies have found no overall increase in the risk of developing breast cancer. Some studies have found an increase in the incidence of cancer of the cervix in women who use oral contraceptives. However, this finding may be related to factors other than the use of oral contraceptives. There is insufficient evidence to rule out the possibility that pills may cause such cancers.

Taking the pill may provide some important non-contraceptive benefits. These include less painful menstruation, less

menstrual blood loss and anemia, less risk of fibroids, pelvic infections, and noncancerous breast diseases, and less risk of cancer of the ovary and of the lining of the uterus (womb).

Be sure to discuss any medical condition you may have with your health care provider. He or she will take a medical and family history before prescribing oral contraceptives and will also perform a physical examination. You should be reexamined at least once a year while taking oral contraceptives. The detailed patient information leaflet gives you further information that you should read and discuss with your health care provider.

Caution: Oral contraceptives are of no value in the prevention or treatment of venereal disease.

DETAILED PATIENT LABELING: WHAT YOU SHOULD KNOW ABOUT ORAL CONTRACEPTIVES

INTRODUCTION

It is important that any woman who considers using an oral contraceptive understand the risks involved. Although the oral contraceptives have important advantages over other methods of contraception, they have certain risks that no other method has. Only you and your physician can decide whether the advantages are worth these risks. This leaflet will tell you about the most important risks. It will explain how you can help your doctor prescribe the pill as safely as possible by telling him/her about yourself and being alert for the earliest signs of trouble. And it will tell you how to use the pill properly so that it will be as effective as possible. THERE IS MORE DETAILED INFORMATION AVAILABLE IN THE LEAFLET PREPARED FOR DOCTORS. Your pharmacist can show you a copy or you can request one from the manufacturer by phoning toll-free 1-800-323-4204 (within Illinois, call 1-708-982-7000); you may need your doctor's help in understanding parts of it.

This leaflet is not a replacement for a careful discussion between you and your health care provider. You should discuss the information provided in this leaflet with him or her, both when you first start taking the pill and during your revisits. You should also follow your doctor's advice with regard to regular check-ups while you are on the pill.

If you do not have any of the conditions listed below and are thinking about using oral contraceptives, to help you decide, you need information about the advantages and risks of oral contraceptives and of other contraceptive methods as well. This leaflet describes the advantages and risks of oral contraceptives. Except for sterilization, the intrauterine device (IUD), and abortion, which have their own specific risks, the only risks of other methods are those due to pregnancy should the method fail. Your doctor can answer questions you may have with respect to other methods of contraception, and further questions you may have on oral contraceptives after reading this leaflet.

WHAT ARE ORAL CONTRACEPTIVES?

The most common type of oral contraceptive, often simply called "the pill," is a combination of estrogen and progestogen, the two kinds of female hormones. The amount of estrogen and progestogen can vary, but the amount of estrogen is more important because both the effectiveness and some of the dangers of the pill have been related to the amount of estrogen. The pill works principally by preventing release of an egg from the ovary during the cycle in which the pills are taken.

EFFECTIVENESS OF ORAL CONTRACEPTIVES

The pill is more effective in preventing pregnancy than other nonsurgical methods of birth control. When they are taken correctly, without missing any pills, the chance of becoming pregnant is less than 1% (1 pregnancy per 100 women per year of use) when used perfectly, without missing any pills. Typical failure rates are actually 3% per year. The chance of becoming pregnant increases with each missed pill during a menstrual cycle.

In comparison, typical failure rates for other nonsurgical methods of birth control during the first year of use are as follows:

IUD: 3%

Diaphragm with spermicides: 18%

Spermicides alone: 21%

Vaginal sponge: 18% to 28%

Condom alone: 12%

Periodic abstinence (rhythm): 20%

No methods: 85%

WHO SHOULD NOT TAKE ORAL CONTRACEPTIVES

> Cigarette smoking increases the risk of serious adverse effects on the heart and blood vessels from oral contraceptive use. This risk increases with age and with heavy smoking (15 or more cigarettes per day) and is quite

Continued on next page

Searle—Cont.

marked in women over 35 years of age. Women who use oral contraceptives are strongly advised not to smoke.

Some women should not use the pill. For example, you should not take the pill if you are pregnant or think you may be pregnant. You should also not use the pill if you have any of the following conditions:

- Heart attack or stroke (blood clot or hemorrhage in the brain), currently or in the past.
- Blood clots in the legs (thrombophlebitis), lungs (pulmonary embolism), eyes, or elsewhere in the body, currently or in the past.
- Chest pain (angina pectoris), currently or in the past.
- Known or suspected breast cancer or cancer of the lining of the uterus (womb), cervix, or vagina, currently or in the past.
- Unexplained vaginal bleeding (until a diagnosis is reached by your doctor).
- Yellowing of the whites of the eyes or of the skin (jaundice) during pregnancy or during previous use of the pill.
- Liver tumor (whether cancerous or not), currently or in the past.
- Known or suspected pregnancy (one or more menstrual periods missed).

Tell your health care provider if you have ever had any of these conditions. He or she can recommend a safer method of birth control.

OTHER CONSIDERATIONS BEFORE TAKING ORAL CONTRACEPTIVES

Tell your health care provider if you have or have had any of the following conditions, as he or she will want to watch them closely or they might cause him or her to suggest using another method of contraception:

- Breast nodules (lumps), fibrocystic disease (breast cysts), abnormal mammograms (x-ray pictures of the breast), or abnormal Pap smears
- Diabetes
- High blood pressure
- High blood cholesterol or triglycerides
- Migraine or other headaches or epilepsy
- Mental depression
- Gallbladder, heart, or kidney disease
- History of scanty or irregular menstrual periods
- Problems during a prior pregnancy
- Fibroid tumors of the womb
- History of jaundice (yellowing of the whites of the eyes or of the skin)
- Varicose veins
- Tuberculosis
- Plans for elective surgery

Women with any of these conditions should be checked often by their health care provider if they choose to use oral contraceptives.

Also, be sure to inform your doctor if you smoke or are on any medications.

RISKS OF TAKING ORAL CONTRACEPTIVES

1. Risk of developing blood clots. Blood clots and blockage of blood vessels are the most serious side effects of taking oral contraceptives. In particular, a clot in the legs can cause thrombophlebitis and a clot that travels to the lungs can cause a sudden blocking of the vessel carrying blood to the lungs. Rarely, clots occur in the blood vessels of the eye and may cause blindness, double vision, or impaired vision.

If you take oral contraceptives and need elective surgery, need to stay in bed for a prolonged illness, or have recently delivered a baby, you may be at risk of developing blood clots. You should consult your doctor about stopping oral contraceptives 3 to 4 weeks before surgery and not taking oral contraceptives for 2 weeks after surgery or during bed rest. You should also not take oral contraceptives soon after delivery of a baby. It is advisable to wait for at least 4 weeks after delivery if you are not breast feeding. If you are breast feeding, you should wait until you have weaned your child before using the pill. (See also the section on Breast feeding in General Precautions.)

The risk of circulatory disease in oral contraceptive users may be higher in users of high-dose pills and may be greater with longer duration of oral contraceptive use. In addition, some of these increased risks may continue for a number of years after stopping oral contraceptives. The risk of abnormal blood clotting increases with age in both users and nonusers of oral contraceptives, but the increased risk from the oral contraceptive appears to be present at all ages. For women aged 20 to 44 it is estimated that about 1 in 2,000 using oral contraceptives will be hospitalized each year because of abnormal clotting. Among nonusers in the same age group, about 1 in 20,000 would be hospitalized each year. For oral contraceptive users in general, it has been estimated that in women between the ages of 15 and 34, the risk of death due to a circulatory disorder is about 1 in 12,000 per year, whereas for nonusers the rate is about 1 in 50,000 per year. In the age group 35 to 44, the risk is estimated to be about 1 in 2,500 per year for oral contraceptive users and about 1 in 10,000 per year for nonusers.

2. Heart attacks and strokes. Oral contraceptives may increase the tendency to develop strokes (stoppage by blood clots or rupture of blood vessels of the brain) and angina pectoris and heart attacks (blockage of blood vessels of the heart). Any of these conditions can cause death or permanent disability.

Smoking greatly increases the possibility of suffering heart attacks and strokes. Furthermore, smoking and the use of oral contraceptives greatly increase the chances of developing and dying of heart disease.

3. Gallbladder disease. Oral contraceptive users probably have a greater risk than nonusers of having gallbladder disease, although this risk may be related to pills containing high doses of estrogens.

4. Liver tumors. In rare cases, oral contraceptives can cause benign but dangerous liver tumors. These benign tumors can rupture and cause fatal internal bleeding. In addition, a possible but not definite association has been found with the pill and liver cancers in several studies, in which a few women who developed these very rare cancers were found to have used oral contraceptives for long periods. However, liver cancers are rare.

5. Cancer of the reproductive organs and breasts. There is conflict among studies regarding breast cancer and oral contraceptive use. Some studies have reported an increase in the risk of developing breast cancer, particularly at a younger age. This increased risk appears to be related to duration of use. The majority of studies have found no overall increase in the risk of developing breast cancer.

Some studies have found an increase in the incidence of cancer of the cervix in women who use oral contraceptives. However, this finding may be related to factors other than the use of oral contraceptives. There is insufficient evidence to rule out the possibility that pills may cause such cancers.

ESTIMATED RISK OF DEATH FROM A BIRTH CONTROL METHOD OR PREGNANCY

All methods of birth control and pregnancy are associated with a risk of developing certain diseases that may lead to disability or death. An estimate of the number of deaths associated with different methods of birth control and pregnancy has been calculated and is shown in the table below.

In the below table, the risk of death from any birth control method is less than the risk of childbirth, except for oral contraceptive users over the age of 35 who smoke and pill users over the age of 40 even if they do not smoke. It can be seen in the table that for women aged 15 to 39, the risk of death was highest with pregnancy (7–26 deaths per 100,000 women, depending on age). Among pill users who do not smoke, the risk of death was always lower than that associated with pregnancy for any age group, although over the age of 40, the risk increases to 32 deaths per 100,000 women, compared to 28 associated with pregnancy at that age. However, for pill users who smoke and are over the age of 35, the estimated number of deaths exceeds those for other methods of birth control. If a woman is over the age of 40 and smokes, her estimated risk of death is four times higher (117/100,000 women) than the estimated risk associated with pregnancy (28/100,000 women) in that age group.

The suggestion that women over 40 who don't smoke should not take oral contraceptives is based on information from older high-dose pills and on less selective use of pills than is practiced today. An Advisory Committee of the FDA discussed this issue in 1989 and recommended that the benefits of oral contraceptive use by healthy, nonsmoking women over 40 years of age may outweigh the possible risks. However, all women, especially older women, are cautioned to use the lowest dose pill that is effective.

WARNING SIGNALS

If any of these adverse effects occur while you are taking oral contraceptives, call your doctor immediately:

- Sharp chest pain, coughing up of blood, or sudden shortness of breath (indicating a possible clot in the lung)
- Pain in the calf (indicating a possible clot in the leg)
- Crushing chest pain or heaviness in the chest (indicating a possible heart attack)
- Sudden severe headache or vomiting, dizziness or fainting, disturbances of vision or speech, or numbness in an arm or leg (indicating a possible stroke)
- Sudden partial or complete loss of vision (indicating a possible blood clot in the blood vessels of the eye)
- Breast lumps (indicating possible breast cancer or fibrocystic disease of the breast). Ask your doctor or health care provider to show you how to examine your breasts
- Severe pain or tenderness or a mass in the stomach area (indicating a possibly ruptured liver tumor)
- Difficulty in sleeping, weakness, lack of energy, fatigue, or change in mood (possibly indicating severe depression)
- Jaundice or a yellowing of the skin or eyeballs, accompanied frequently by fever, fatigue, loss of appetite, dark-colored urine, or light-colored bowel movements (indicating possible liver problems)
- Unusual swelling
- Other unusual conditions

SIDE EFFECTS OF ORAL CONTRACEPTIVES

1. Vaginal bleeding

Spotting. This is a slight staining between your menstrual periods that may not even require a pad. Some women spot even though they may take their pills exactly as directed. Many women spot although they have never taken the pills. Spotting does not mean that your ovaries are releasing an egg. Spotting may be the result of irregular pill-taking. Getting back on schedule will usually stop it.

If you should spot while taking the pills, you should not be alarmed, because spotting usually stops by itself within a few days. It seldom occurs after the first pill cycle. Consult your doctor if spotting persists for more than a few days or if it occurs after the second cycle.

Unexpected (breakthrough) bleeding. Unexpected (breakthrough) bleeding does not mean that your ovaries have released an egg. It seldom occurs, but when it does happen it is most common in the first pill cycle. It is a flow much like a regular period, requiring the use of a pad or tampon.

If you experience breakthrough bleeding use a pad or tampon and continue with your schedule. Usually your periods will become regular within a few cycles. Breakthrough bleeding will seldom bother you again.

Consult your doctor if breakthrough bleeding is heavy, does not stop within a week, or if it occurs after the second cycle.

2. Contact lenses. If you wear contact lenses and notice a change in vision or an inability to wear your lenses, contact your doctor or health care provider.

3. Fluid retention or raised blood pressure. Oral contraceptives may cause edema (fluid retention), with swelling of the fingers or ankles. If you experience fluid retention, contact your doctor or health care provider. Some women develop high blood pressure while on the pill, which ordinarily, but not always, returns to the original levels when the pill is stopped. High blood pressure predisposes one to strokes, heart attacks, kidney disease, and other diseases of the blood vessels.

4. Melasma. A spotty darkening of the skin is possible, particularly of the face. This may persist after the pill is discontinued.

5. Other side effects. Other side effects may include nausea and vomiting, change in appetite, headache, nervousness, depression, dizziness, loss of scalp hair, rash, and vaginal infections.

If any of these, or other, side effects occur, call your doctor or health care provider.

Annual number of birth-related or method-related deaths associated with control of fertility per 100,000 nonsterile women, by fertility control method according to age.[67]

	Age					
Method of control	15–19	20–24	25–29	30–34	35–39	40–44
No fertility control methods*	7.0	7.4	9.1	14.8	25.7	28.2
Oral contraceptives						
non-smoker**	0.3	0.5	0.9	1.9	13.8	31.6
smoker**	2.2	3.4	6.6	13.5	51.1	117.2
IUD**	0.8	0.8	1.0	1.0	1.4	1.4
Condom*	1.1	1.6	0.7	0.2	0.3	0.4
Diaphragm/ spermicide*	1.9	1.2	1.2	1.3	2.2	2.8
Periodic abstinence*	2.5	1.6	1.6	1.7	2.9	3.6

*Deaths are birth-related

**Deaths are method-related

Adapted from Ory.[67]

GENERAL PRECAUTIONS

1. Missed periods and use of oral contraceptives before or during early pregnancy. Occasionally women who are taking the pill miss periods. It has been reported to occur as frequently as several times each year in some women, depending on various factors such as age and prior history. (Your doctor is the best source of information about this.) The pill should not be used when you are pregnant or suspect you may be pregnant. Very rarely, women who are using the pill as directed become pregnant. The likelihood of becoming pregnant is higher if you occasionally miss one or two pills. Therefore, if you miss a period you should consult your physician before continuing to take the pill. If you miss a period, especially if you have not taken the pill regularly, you should use an alternative method of contraception until pregnancy has been ruled out; if you have missed more than one pill at any time, you should immediately start using an additional method of contraception and complete your pill cycle.
There is no conclusive evidence that oral contraceptive use is associated with an increase in birth defects when taken inadvertently during early pregnancy. Previously, a few studies had reported that oral contraceptives might be associated with birth defects, but these findings have not been seen in more recent studies. Nevertheless, oral contraceptives or any other drugs should not be used during pregnancy unless clearly necessary and prescribed by your doctor. You should check with your doctor about risks to your unborn child of any medication taken during pregnancy.
2. Breast feeding. If you are breast feeding, consult your doctor before starting oral contraceptives. Some of the drug will be passed on to the child in the milk. A few adverse effects on the child have been reported, including yellowing of the skin (jaundice) and breast enlargement. In addition, oral contraceptives may decrease the amount and quality of your milk. If possible, do not use oral contraceptives while breast feeding. You should use another method of contraception since breast feeding provides only partial protection from becoming pregnant and this partial protection decreases significantly as you breast feed for longer periods of time. You should consider starting oral contraceptives only after you have weaned your child completely.
3. Laboratory tests. If you are scheduled for any laboratory tests, tell your doctor you are taking birth control pills. Certain blood tests may be affected by birth control pills.
4. Drug interactions. Certain drugs may interact with birth control pills to make them less effective in preventing pregnancy or cause an increase in breakthrough bleeding. Such drugs include rifampin, drugs used for epilepsy such as barbiturates (for example, phenobarbital) and phenytoin (Dilantin is one brand of this drug), phenylbutazone (Butazolidin is one brand), and possibly certain antibiotics. You may need to use additional contraception when you take drugs that can make oral contraceptives less effective.
Oral contraceptives may have an influence upon the way other drugs act. Check with your doctor if you are taking *any* other drugs while you are on the pill.

HOW TO TAKE ORAL CONTRACEPTIVES

1. General instructions. You must take your pill every day according to the instructions. Oral contraceptives are most effective if taken 24 hours apart. Take your pill at the same time every day so that you are less likely to forget to take it. You will then maintain an effective dose of the oral contraceptive in your body.
When you first begin to use the pill, you should use an additional method of protection until you have taken your first 7 pills.
To remove a pill, press down on it. The pill will drop through a hole in the bottom of the Compack.
The two "three weeks on—one week off" schedules. Your Demulen 1/35-21 or Demulen 1/50-21 Compack contains 21 tablets arranged in three numbered rows with the days of the week printed above them.
Day-5 schedule. If you are to begin on day 5, count the day you start to menstruate as day 1 and determine which day to start. Start in row #1 with the pill under the day that corresponds to day 5 after your flow began. Continue to take one pill each day on consecutive days of the week.
After the last (Saturday) pill in row #3 has been taken, if any remain in the first row, complete your 21-pill schedule by taking one pill daily starting with Sunday in row #1. Then stop for 1 week before starting to take the pills again. Begin your next pill cycle on the same day of the week that you began the first cycle.
Sunday schedule. Start taking the pills on the first Sunday after your period begins unless your period begins on Sunday. If your period begins on Sunday start taking the pill that very same day.
Begin in row #1 and take your pills, one each day on consecutive days, for 3 weeks (21 days), then stop taking them for 1 week (7 days) before starting to take the pills again on Sunday.
Whether you begin on "day 5" or on Sunday, continue taking your pills as directed, month after month, regardless of whether your flow has or has not ceased or whether you may have experienced spotting or unexpected (breakthrough) bleeding during your pill cycle. You will probably have your period about every 28 days.
The "pill-a-day" schedule. Your Demulen 1/35-28 or Demulen 1/50-28 Compack contains 28 pills arranged in four numbered rows of 7 pills each with the days of the week printed above them.
You must take your pills in order, one pill each day. Begin with the Sunday pill in row #1.
1—Start taking the pills on the first Sunday after your period begins unless your period begins on Sunday. *If your period begins on Sunday start taking the pills that very same day.*
2—Continue to take one pill each day on consecutive days of the week.
3—After the Saturday pill in row #1 has been taken begin taking pills in row #2, and so on, until the Saturday pill in row #4 has been taken.
4—Begin a new pill cycle the next day, starting with the Sunday pill in row #1.
You will probably have your period about every 28 days, while you are taking the pink (blue for Demulen 1/35-28) pills.
Continue your pill-a-day schedule, month after month, regardless of whether your flow ceases while you are taking the colored pills, or whether you experience spotting or unexpected (breakthrough) bleeding during a cycle.
Take your pill faithfully every "pill day"!
It is important that you take a pill without fail every pill day, at intervals of 24 hours, for two reasons: First, your ovaries may release an egg and therefore you may become pregnant if you do not take your pills regularly. Second, you may spot or start to flow between your periods. This may be inconvenient.
Take your pill at the same time every day!
You are probably wondering why the same time of day is important. By taking your pill at the same time every day it becomes a good habit, and you are much less likely to forget. You may wish to keep your pills in the medicine cabinet near your toothbrush as a reminder to take them when you brush your teeth at night. The best time to take your daily pill may be at bedtime. You may find it helpful to associate your pill-taking with something else you do every day at a particular time.
Another very important reason for you to take your pills as "regular as clockwork" is that you are protected best when you take one every 24 hours; they are made to work that way. Just remember that once every day is not the same as once every 24 hours. Here is why: Suppose you were to take your Monday pill in the morning when you get up, and then not take your Tuesday pill till the evening before you go to bed. True, you will have taken a pill each day, on Monday and on Tuesday—but the time between pill-taking will probably have been more than 36 hours, or more than $1\frac{1}{2}$ days! You might spot. Chances are you would still be protected and would not get pregnant, but why risk it when it is so easy to guarantee yourself maximal protection by taking your pill faithfully every pill day and at the same time every pill day?

If you are scheduled for surgery, or you need prolonged bed rest, you should tell your doctor that you are on the pill and stop taking the pill 4 weeks before surgery to avoid an increased risk of blood clots. It is also advisable not to start oral contraceptives sooner than 4 weeks after delivery of a baby.
2. If you forget to take your pill. If you miss only one white (active) pill in a cycle, the chance of becoming pregnant is small. Take the missed pill as soon as you realize that you have forgotten it and continue to take your tablets for the rest of that cycle as directed. Since the risk of pregnancy increases with each additional pill you skip, it is very important that you take one pill a day.
If you forget your pills (except the inactive colored pills in Demulen 1/35-28 or Demulen 1/50-28) on 2 consecutive days, do not be surprised if you spot or start to flow. You should take two pills each day for the next 2 days, and use an additional method of protection for the remainder of the cycle.
If you are using Demulen 1/35-28 or Demulen 1/50-28 and forget to take one or more colored pills, begin a new cycle on the next Sunday; use a new package and start taking the white pills. Missing the colored pills does not increase your chances of getting pregnant providing the white pill schedule has been followed.
3. Pregnancy due to pill failure. The incidence of pill failure resulting in pregnancy is approximately 1% (ie, one pregnancy per 100 women per year) if taken every day as directed, but, because some women fail to follow the daily schedule, more typical failure rates are about 3%. If you become pregnant, you should discuss your pregnancy with your doctor.
4. Pregnancy after stopping the pill. There may be some delay in becoming pregnant after you stop using oral contraceptives, especially if you had irregular menstrual cycles before you used oral contraceptives. It may be advisable to postpone conception until you begin menstruating regularly once you have stopped taking the pill and desire pregnancy.

There does not appear to be any increase in birth defects in newborn babies when pregnancy occurs after stopping the pill.
5. Overdosage. Serious ill effects have not been reported following ingestion of large doses of oral contraceptives by young children. Overdosage may cause nausea and withdrawal bleeding in females. In case of overdosage, contact your health care provider, pharmacist, or Poison Control Center.
6. Other information. Your doctor will take a medical and family history before prescribing oral contraceptives. At that time, and about once a year, he or she will generally examine your blood pressure, breasts, abdomen, and internal female organs (including a Pap smear test for cancer of the cervix) and perform certain laboratory tests. Certain health problems or conditions in your medical or family history may require that your doctor see you more frequently while you are taking the pill.
Do not use the drug for any condition other than the one for which it was prescribed. This drug has been prescribed specifically for you; do not give it to others who may want birth control pills.

HEALTH BENEFITS FROM ORAL CONTRACEPTIVES

In addition to preventing pregnancy, use of oral contraceptives may provide certain benefits. They are:
- Menstrual cycles may become more regular
- Blood flow during menstruation may be lighter and less iron may be lost. Therefore, anemia due to iron deficiency is less likely to occur.
- Pain or other symptoms during menstruation may be encountered less frequently
- Ectopic (tubal) pregnancy may occur less frequently
- Noncancerous cysts or lumps in the breast may occur less frequently
- Acute pelvic inflammatory disease may occur less frequently
- Fibroids of the uterus (womb) may occur less frequently
- Oral contraceptive use may provide some protection against developing two forms of cancer: cancer of the ovaries and cancer of the lining of the uterus (womb)

If you want more information about birth control pills, ask your doctor or pharmacist. They have a more technical leaflet called the Professional Labeling, which you may wish to read.
Be certain to read new revisions of this leaflet. You may check the date of the most recent revision by phoning the manufacturer toll-free at 1-800-323-4204 (within Illinois, call 1-708-982-7000), or by writing to the address below.
G.D. Searle & Co.
Medical and Scientific Information Department
4901 Searle Parkway
Skokie, IL 60077

6/27/91 • A05484

These products are shown in the Product Identification Section, page 429

FLAGYL® Tablets ℞
[flaj 'yl]
(metronidazole)

> **WARNING**
> Metronidazole has been shown to be carcinogenic in mice and rats (see *Precautions*). Unnecessary use of the drug should be avoided. Its use should be reserved for the conditions described in the *Indications and Usage* section below.

DESCRIPTION

Flagyl (metronidazole) is an oral synthetic antiprotozoal and antibacterial agent, 1-(β-hydroxyethyl)-2-methyl-5-nitroimidazole, which has the following structural formula:

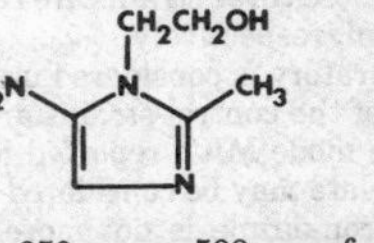

Flagyl tablets contain 250 mg or 500 mg of metronidazole. Inactive ingredients include cellulose, FD&C Blue No. 2 Lake, hydroxypropyl cellulose, hydroxypropyl methylcellulose, polyethylene glycol, stearic acid, and titanium dioxide.

CLINICAL PHARMACOLOGY

Disposition of metronidazole in the body is similar for both oral and intravenous dosage forms, with an average elimination half-life in healthy humans of eight hours.

Continued on next page

Searle—Cont.

The major route of elimination of metronidazole and its metabolites is via the urine (60 to 80% of the dose), with fecal excretion accounting for 6 to 15% of the dose. The metabolites that appear in the urine result primarily from side-chain oxidation [1-(β-hydroxyethyl)-2-hydroxymethyl-5-nitroimidazole and 2-methyl-5-nitroimidazole-1-yl-acetic acid] and glucuronide conjugation, with unchanged metronidazole accounting for approximately 20% of the total. Renal clearance of metronidazole is approximately 10 ml/min/1.73 m^2.

Metronidazole is the major component appearing in the plasma, with lesser quantities of the 2-hydroxymethyl metabolite also being present. Less than 20% of the circulating metronidazole is bound to plasma proteins. Both the parent compound and the metabolite possess *in vitro* bactericidal activity against most strains of anaerobic bacteria and *in vitro* trichomonacidal activity.

Metronidazole appears in cerebrospinal fluid, saliva, and breast milk in concentrations similar to those found in plasma. Bactericidal concentrations of metronidazole have also been detected in pus from hepatic abscesses.

Following oral administration metronidazole is well absorbed, with peak plasma concentrations occurring between one and two hours after administration. Plasma concentrations of metronidazole are proportional to the administered dose. Oral administration of 250 mg, 500 mg, or 2,000 mg produced peak plasma concentrations of 6 mcg/ml, 12 mcg/ml, and 40 mcg/ml, respectively. Studies reveal no significant bioavailability differences between males and females; however, because of weight differences, the resulting plasma levels in males are generally lower.

Decreased renal function does not alter the single-dose pharmacokinetics of metronidazole. However, plasma clearance of metronidazole is decreased in patients with decreased liver function.

Microbiology:

Trichomonas vaginalis, Entamoeba histolytica. Flagyl (metronidazole) possesses direct trichomonacidal and amebacidal activity against *T. vaginalis* and *E. histolytica.* The *in vitro* minimal inhibitory concentration (MIC) for most strains of these organisms is 1 mcg/ml or less.

Anaerobic Bacteria. Metronidazole is active *in vitro* against most obligate anaerobes, but does not appear to possess any clinically relevant activity against facultative anaerobes or obligate aerobes. Against susceptible organisms, metronidazole is generally bactericidal at concentrations equal to or slightly higher than the minimal inhibitory concentrations. Metronidazole has been shown to have *in vitro* and clinical activity against the following organisms:

- Anaerobic gram-negative bacilli, including:
  - *Bacteroides* species including the *Bacteroides fragilis* group (*B. fragilis, B. distasonis, B. ovatus, B. thetaiotaomicron, B. vulgatus)*
  - *Fusobacterium* species
- Anaerobic gram-positive bacilli, including:
  - *Clostridium* species and susceptible strains of *Eubacterium*
- Anaerobic gram-positive cocci, including:
  - *Peptococcus* species
  - *Peptostreptococcus* species

Susceptibility Tests: Bacteriologic studies should be performed to determine the causative organisms and their susceptibility to metronidazole; however, the rapid, routine susceptibility testing of individual isolates of anaerobic bacteria is not always practical, and therapy may be started while awaiting these results.

Quantitative methods give the most precise estimates of susceptibility to antibacterial drugs. A standardized agar dilution method and a broth microdilution method are recommended.[1]

Control strains are recommended for standardized susceptibility testing. Each time the test is performed, one or more of the following strains should be included: *Clostridium perfringens* ATCC 13124, *Bacteroides fragilis* ATCC 25285, and *Bacteroides thetaiotaomicron* ATCC 29741. The mode metronidazole MICs for those three strains are reported to be 0.25, 0.25, and 0.5 mcg/ml, respectively.

A clinical laboratory is considered under acceptable control if the results of the control strains are within one doubling dilution of the mode MICs reported for metronidazole.

A bacterial isolate may be considered susceptible if the MIC value for metronidazole is not more than 16 mcg/ml. An organism is considered resistant if the MIC is greater than 16 mcg/ml. A report of "resistant" from the laboratory indicates that the infecting organism is not likely to respond to therapy.

1. Proposed standard: PSM-11—Proposed Reference Dilution Procedure for Antimicrobic Susceptibility Testing of Anaerobic Bacteria, National Committee for Clinical Laboratory Standards; and Sutter, et al.: Collaborative Evaluation of a Proposed Reference Dilution Method of Susceptibility Testing of Anaerobic Bacteria, Antimicrob. Agents Chemother. *16:* 495–502 (Oct.) 1979; and Tally, et al.: *In Vitro* Activity of Thienamycin, Antimicrob. Agents Chemother. *14:* 436–438 (Sept.) 1978.

INDICATIONS AND USAGE

Symptomatic Trichomoniasis. Flagyl is indicated for the treatment of symptomatic trichomoniasis in females and males when the presence of the trichomonad has been confirmed by appropriate laboratory procedures (wet smears and/or cultures).

Asymptomatic Trichomoniasis. Flagyl is indicated in the treatment of asymptomatic females when the organism is associated with endocervicitis, cervicitis, or cervical erosion. Since there is evidence that presence of the trichomonad can interfere with accurate assessment of abnormal cytological smears, additional smears should be performed after eradication of the parasite.

Treatment of Asymptomatic Consorts. T. vaginalis infection is a venereal disease. Therefore, asymptomatic sexual partners of treated patients should be treated simultaneously if the organism has been found to be present, in order to prevent reinfection of the partner. The decision as to whether to treat an asymptomatic male partner who has a negative culture or one for whom no culture has been attempted is an individual one. In making this decision, it should be noted that there is evidence that a woman may become reinfected if her consort is not treated. Also, since there can be considerable difficulty in isolating the organism from the asymptomatic male carrier, negative smears and cultures cannot be relied upon in this regard. In any event, the consort should be treated with Flagyl in cases of reinfection.

Amebiasis. Flagyl is indicated in the treatment of acute intestinal amebiasis (amebic dysentery) and amebic liver abscess.

In amebic liver abscess, Flagyl therapy does not obviate the need for aspiration or drainage of pus.

Anaerobic Bacterial Infections. Flagyl is indicated in the treatment of serious infections caused by susceptible anaerobic bacteria. Indicated surgical procedures should be performed in conjunction with Flagyl therapy. In a mixed aerobic and anaerobic infection, antibiotics appropriate for the treatment of the aerobic infection should be used in addition to Flagyl.

In the treatment of most serious anaerobic infections, Flagyl I.V. (metronidazole hydrochloride) or Flagyl I.V. RTU® (metronidazole) is usually administered initially. This may be followed by oral therapy with Flagyl (metronidazole) at the discretion of the physician.

INTRA-ABDOMINAL INFECTIONS, including peritonitis, intra-abdominal abscess, and liver abscess, caused by *Bacteroides* species including the *B. fragilis* group (*B. fragilis, B. distasonis, B. ovatus, B. thetaiotaomicron, B. vulgatus), Clostridium* species, *Eubacterium* species, *Peptococcus* species, and *Peptostreptococcus* species.

SKIN AND SKIN STRUCTURE INFECTIONS caused by *Bacteroides* species including the *B. fragilis* group, *Clostridium* species, *Peptococcus* species, *Peptostreptococcus* species, and *Fusobacterium* species.

GYNECOLOGIC INFECTIONS, including endometritis, endomyometritis, tubo-ovarian abscess, and postsurgical vaginal cuff infection, caused by *Bacteroides* species including the *B. fragilis* group, *Clostridium* species, *Peptococcus* species, and *Peptostreptococcus* species.

BACTERIAL SEPTICEMIA caused by *Bacteroides* species including the *B. fragilis* group, and *Clostridium* species.

BONE AND JOINT INFECTIONS, as adjunctive therapy, caused by *Bacteroides* species including the *B. fragilis* group.

CENTRAL NERVOUS SYSTEM (CNS) INFECTIONS, including meningitis and brain abscess, caused by *Bacteroides* species including the *B. fragilis* group.

LOWER RESPIRATORY TRACT INFECTIONS, including pneumonia, empyema, and lung abscess, caused by *Bacteroides* species including the *B. fragilis* group.

ENDOCARDITIS caused by *Bacteroides* species including the *B. fragilis* group.

CONTRAINDICATIONS

Flagyl is contraindicated in patients with a prior history of hypersensitivity to metronidazole or other nitroimidazole derivatives.

In patients with trichomoniasis, Flagyl is contraindicated during the first trimester of pregnancy. (See *Warnings.*)

WARNINGS

Convulsive Seizures and Peripheral Neuropathy: Convulsive seizures and peripheral neuropathy, the latter characterized mainly by numbness or paresthesia of an extremity, have been reported in patients treated with metronidazole. The appearance of abnormal neurologic signs demands the prompt discontinuation of Flagyl therapy. Flagyl should be administered with caution to patients with central nervous system diseases.

PRECAUTIONS

General: Patients with severe hepatic disease metabolize metronidazole slowly, with resultant accumulation of metronidazole and its metabolites in the plasma. Accordingly, for such patients, doses below those usually recommended should be administered cautiously.

Known or previously unrecognized candidiasis may present more prominent symptoms during therapy with Flagyl and requires treatment with a candicidal agent.

Information for patients: Alcoholic beverages should be avoided while taking Flagyl and for at least one day afterward. See *Drug interactions.*

Laboratory tests: Flagyl (metronidazole) is a nitroimidazole and should be used with care in patients with evidence of or history of blood dyscrasia. A mild leukopenia has been observed during its administration; however, no persistent hematologic abnormalities attributable to metronidazole have been observed in clinical studies. Total and differential leukocyte counts are recommended before and after therapy for trichomoniasis and amebiasis, especially if a second course of therapy is necessary, and before and after therapy for anaerobic infection.

Drug interactions: Metronidazole has been reported to potentiate the anticoagulant effect of warfarin and other oral coumarin anticoagulants, resulting in a prolongation of prothrombin time. This possible drug interaction should be considered when Flagyl is prescribed for patients on this type of anticoagulant therapy.

The simultaneous administration of drugs that induce microsomal liver enzymes, such as phenytoin or phenobarbital, may accelerate the elimination of metronidazole, resulting in reduced plasma levels; impaired clearance of phenytoin has also been reported.

The simultaneous administration of drugs that decrease microsomal liver enzyme activity, such as cimetidine, may prolong the half-life and decrease plasma clearance of metronidazole. In patients stabilized on relatively high doses of lithium, short-term Flagyl therapy has been associated with elevation of serum lithium and, in a few cases, signs of lithium toxicity. Serum lithium and serum creatinine levels should be obtained several days after beginning metronidazole to detect any increase that may precede clinical symptoms of lithium intoxication.

Alcoholic beverages should not be consumed during Flagyl therapy and for at least one day afterward because abdominal cramps, nausea, vomiting, headaches, and flushing may occur.

Psychotic reactions have been reported in alcoholic patients who are using metronidazole and disulfiram concurrently. Metronidazole should not be given to patients who have taken disulfiram within the last two weeks.

Drug/Laboratory test interactions: Metronidazole may interfere with certain types of determinations of serum chemistry values, such as aspartate aminotransferase (AST, SGOT), alanine aminotransferase (ALT, SGPT), lactate dehydrogenase (LDH), triglycerides, and hexokinase glucose. Values of zero may be observed. All of the assays in which interference has been reported involve enzymatic coupling of the assay to oxidation-reduction of nicotine adenine dinucleotide ($NAD^+ \rightleftarrows NADH$). Interference is due to the similarity in absorbance peaks of NADH (340 nm) and metronidazole (322 nm) at pH 7.

Carcinogenesis, mutagenesis, impairment of fertility:

Tumorigenicity studies in rodents: Metronidazole has shown evidence of carcinogenic activity in a number of studies involving chronic, oral administration in mice and rats. Prominent among the effects in the mouse was the promotion of pulmonary tumorigenesis. This has been observed in all six reported studies in that species, including one study in which the animals were dosed on an intermittent schedule (administration during every fourth week only). At very high dose levels (approx. 500 mg/kg/day) there was a statistically significant increase in the incidence of malignant liver tumors in males. Also, the published results of one of the mouse studies indicate an increase in the incidence of malignant lymphomas as well as pulmonary neoplasms associated with lifetime feeding of the drug. All these effects are statistically significant.

Several long-term, oral-dosing studies in the rat have been completed. There were statistically significant increases in the incidence of various neoplasms, particularly in mammary and hepatic tumors, among female rats administered metronidazole over those noted in the concurrent female control groups.

Two lifetime tumorigenicity studies in hamsters have been performed and reported to be negative.

Mutagenicity studies: Although metronidazole has shown mutagenic activity in a number of *in vitro* assay systems, studies in mammals (*in vivo*) have failed to demonstrate a potential for genetic damage.

Pregnancy: Teratogenic Effects—Pregnancy Category B. Metronidazole crosses the placental barrier and enters the fetal circulation rapidly. Reproduction studies have been performed in rats at doses up to five times the human dose and have revealed no evidence of impaired fertility or harm to the fetus due to metronidazole. Metronidazole administered intraperitoneally to pregnant mice at approximately

the human dose caused fetotoxicity; administered orally to pregnant mice, no fetotoxicity was observed. There are, however, no adequate and well-controlled studies in pregnant women. Because animal reproduction studies are not always predictive of human response, and because metronidazole is a carcinogen in rodents, this drug should be used during pregnancy only if clearly needed (see *Contraindications*).
Use of Flagyl for trichomoniasis in the second and third trimesters should be restricted to those in whom local palliative treatment has been inadequate to control symptoms.

Nursing mothers: Because of the potential for tumorigenicity shown for metronidazole in mouse and rat studies, a decision should be made whether to discontinue nursing or to discontinue the drug, taking into account the importance of the drug to the mother. Metronidazole is secreted in breast milk in concentrations similar to those found in plasma.

Pediatric use: Safety and effectiveness in children have not been established, except for the treatment of amebiasis.

ADVERSE REACTIONS

Two serious adverse reactions reported in patients treated with Flagyl (metronidazole) have been convulsive seizures and peripheral neuropathy, the latter characterized mainly by numbness or paresthesia of an extremity. Since persistent peripheral neuropathy has been reported in some patients receiving prolonged administration of Flagyl, patients should be specifically warned about these reactions and should be told to stop the drug and report immediately to their physicians if any neurologic symptoms occur.
The most common adverse reactions reported have been referable to the gastrointestinal tract, particularly nausea reported by about 12% of patients, sometimes accompanied by headache, anorexia, and occasionally vomiting; diarrhea; epigastric distress; and abdominal cramping. Constipation has also been reported.
The following reactions have also been reported during treatment with Flagyl (metronidazole):

Mouth: A sharp, unpleasant metallic taste is not unusual. Furry tongue, glossitis, and stomatitis have occurred; these may be associated with a sudden overgrowth of *Candida* which may occur during effective therapy.

Hematopoietic: Reversible neutropenia (leukopenia); rarely, reversible thrombocytopenia.

Cardiovascular: Flattening of the T-wave may be seen in electrocardiographic tracings.

Central Nervous System: Convulsive seizures, peripheral neuropathy, dizziness, vertigo, incoordination, ataxia, confusion, irritability, depression, weakness, and insomnia.

Hypersensitivity: Urticaria, erythematous rash, flushing, nasal congestion, dryness of the mouth (or vagina or vulva), and fever.

Renal: Dysuria, cystitis, polyuria, incontinence, and a sense of pelvic pressure. Instances of darkened urine have been reported by approximately one patient in 100,000. Although the pigment which is probably responsible for this phenomenon has not been positively identified, it is almost certainly a metabolite of metronidazole and seems to have no clinical significance.

Other: Proliferation of *Candida* in the vagina, dyspareunia, decrease of libido, proctitis, and fleeting joint pains sometimes resembling "serum sickness." If patients receiving Flagyl drink alcoholic beverages, they may experience abdominal distress, nausea, vomiting, flushing, or headache. A modification of the taste of alcoholic beverages has also been reported. Rare cases of pancreatitis, which abated on withdrawal of the drug, have been reported.

Crohn's disease patients are known to have an increased incidence of gastrointestinal and certain extraintestinal cancers. There have been some reports in the medical literature of breast and colon cancer in Crohn's disease patients who have been treated with metronidazole at high doses for extended periods of time. A cause and effect relationship has not been established. Crohn's disease is not an approved indication for Flagyl.

OVERDOSAGE

Single oral doses of metronidazole, up to 15 g, have been reported in suicide attempts and accidental overdoses. Symptoms reported include nausea, vomiting, and ataxia.
Oral metronidazole has been studied as a radiation sensitizer in the treatment of malignant tumors. Neurotoxic effects, including seizures and peripheral neuropathy, have been reported after 5 to 7 days of doses of 6 to 10.4 g every other day.
Treatment: There is no specific antidote for Flagyl overdose; therefore, management of the patient should consist of symptomatic and supportive therapy.

DOSAGE AND ADMINISTRATION

In elderly patients the pharmacokinetics of metronidazole may be altered and therefore monitoring of serum levels may be necessary to adjust the metronidazole dosage accordingly.

Trichomoniasis:
In the Female:
One-day treatment—two grams of Flagyl, given either as a single dose or in two divided doses of one gram each given in the same day.
Seven-day course of treatment—250 mg three times daily for seven consecutive days. There is some indication from controlled comparative studies that cure rates as determined by vaginal smears, signs and symptoms, may be higher after a seven-day course of treatment than after a one-day treatment regimen.
The dosage regimen should be individualized. Single-dose treatment can assure compliance, especially if administered under supervision, in those patients who cannot be relied on to continue the seven-day regimen. A seven-day course of treatment may minimize reinfection of the female long enough to treat sexual contacts. Further, some patients may tolerate one course of therapy better than the other.
Pregnant patients should not be treated during the first trimester with either regimen. If treated during the second or third trimester, the one-day course of therapy should not be used, as it results in higher serum levels which reach the fetal circulation. (See *Contraindications* and *Precautions.*)
When repeat courses of the drug are required, it is recommended that an interval of four to six weeks elapse between courses and that the presence of the trichomonad be reconfirmed by appropriate laboratory measures. Total and differential leukocyte counts should be made before and after re-treatment.
In the Male: Treatment should be individualized as for the female.

Amebiasis:
Adults:
For acute intestinal amebiasis (acute amebic dysentery): 750 mg orally three times daily for 5 to 10 days.
For amebic liver abscess: 500 mg or 750 mg orally three times daily for 5 to 10 days.
Children: 35 to 50 mg/kg/24 hours, divided into three doses, orally for 10 days.

Anaerobic Bacterial Infections: In the treatment of most serious anaerobic infections, Flagyl I.V. (metronidazole hydrochloride) or Flagyl I.V. RTU® (metronidazole) is usually administered initially.
The usual adult *oral* dosage is 7.5 mg/kg every six hours (approx. 500 mg for a 70-kg adult). A maximum of 4 g should not be exceeded during a 24-hour period.
The usual duration of therapy is 7 to 10 days; however, infections of the bone and joint, lower respiratory tract, and endocardium may require longer treatment.
Patients with severe hepatic disease metabolize metronidazole slowly, with resultant accumulation of metronidazole and its metabolites in the plasma. Accordingly, for such patients, doses below those usually recommended should be administered cautiously. Close monitoring of plasma metronidazole levels[2] and toxicity is recommended.
The dose of Flagyl should not be specifically reduced in anuric patients since accumulated metabolites may be rapidly removed by dialysis.

HOW SUPPLIED

Flagyl 250-mg tablets are round, blue, film coated, with SEARLE and 1831 debossed on one side and FLAGYL and 250 on the other side; bottles of 50, 100, 250, and 2,500, and cartons of 100 unit-dose individually blister-sealed tablets.
Flagyl 500-mg tablets are oblong, blue, film coated, with FLAGYL debossed on one side and 500 on the other side; bottles of 50, 100, and 500, and cartons of 100 unit-dose individually blister-sealed tablets.
Storage and Stability: Store below 86°F (30°C) and protect from light.

2. Ralph, E.D., and Kirby, W.M.M.: Bioassay of Metronidazole With Either Anaerobic or Aerobic Incubation, J. Infect. Dis. *132:* 587–591 (Nov.) 1975; or Gulaid, et al.: Determination of Metronidazole and Its Major Metabolites in Biological Fluids by High Pressure Liquid Chromatography, Br. J. Clin. Pharmacol. *6:* 430–432, 1978.

7/19/90 • A05709-6
Shown in Product Identification Section, page 429

KERLONE® ℞

[*kur'lōn*]
(betaxolol hydrochloride)

DESCRIPTION

Kerlone (betaxolol hydrochloride) is a β_1-selective (cardioselective) adrenergic receptor blocking agent available as 10-mg and 20-mg tablets for oral administration. Kerlone is chemically described as 2-propanol, 1-[4-[2-(cyclopropylmethoxy)ethyl]phenoxy]-3-[(1-methylethyl)amino]-, hydrochloride, (±). It has the following chemical structure:
[See chemical structure at top of next column.]
Betaxolol hydrochloride is a water-soluble white crystalline powder with a molecular formula of $C_{18}H_{29}NO_3 \cdot HCl$ and a

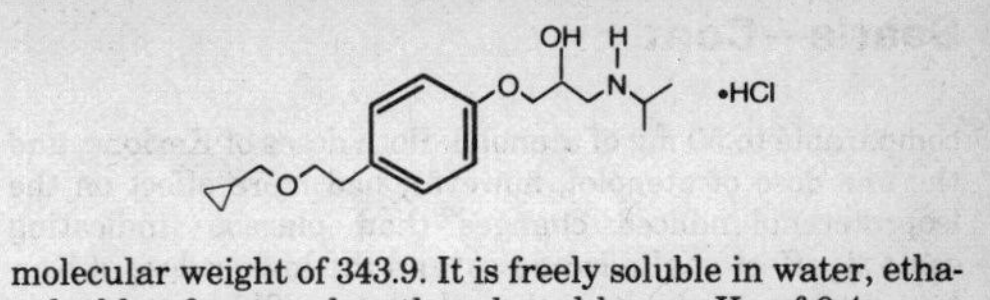

molecular weight of 343.9. It is freely soluble in water, ethanol, chloroform, and methanol, and has a pKa of 9.4.
The inactive ingredients are hydroxypropyl methylcellulose, lactose, magnesium stearate, polyethylene glycol 400, microcrystalline cellulose, colloidal silicon dioxide, sodium starch glycolate, and titanium dioxide.

CLINICAL PHARMACOLOGY

Kerlone is a β_1-selective (cardioselective) adrenergic receptor blocking agent that has weak membrane-stabilizing activity and no intrinsic sympathomimetic (partial agonist) activity. The preferential effect on β_1 receptors is not absolute, however, and some inhibitory effects on β_2 receptors (found chiefly in the bronchial and vascular musculature) can be expected at higher doses.

Pharmacokinetics and metabolism: In man, absorption of an oral dose is complete. There is a small and consistent first-pass effect resulting in an absolute bioavailability of 89 ± 5% that is unaffected by the concomitant ingestion of food or alcohol. Mean peak blood concentrations of 21.6 ng/ml (range 16.3 to 27.9 ng/ml) are reached between 1.5 and 6 (mean about 3) hours after a single oral dose, in healthy volunteers, of 10 mg of Kerlone. Peak concentrations for 20-mg and 40-mg doses are 2 and 4 times that of a 10-mg dose and have been shown to be linear over the dose range of 5 to 40 mg. The peak to trough ratio of plasma concentrations over 24 hours is 2.7. The mean elimination half-life in various studies in normal volunteers ranged from about 14 to 22 hours after single oral doses and is similar in chronic dosing. Steady state plasma concentrations are attained after 5 to 7 days with once-daily dosing in persons with normal renal function.
Kerlone is approximately 50% bound to plasma proteins. It is eliminated primarily by liver metabolism and secondarily by renal excretion. Following oral administration, greater than 80% of a dose is recovered in the urine as betaxolol and its metabolites. Approximately 15% of the dose administered is excreted as unchanged drug, the remainder being metabolites whose contribution to the clinical effect is negligible.
Steady state studies in normal volunteers and hypertensive patients found no important differences in kinetics. In patients with hepatic disease, elimination half-life was prolonged by about 33%, but clearance was unchanged, leading to little change in AUC. Dosage reductions have not routinely been necessary in these patients. In patients with chronic renal failure undergoing dialysis, mean elimination half-life was approximately doubled, as was AUC, indicating the need for a lower initial dosage (5 mg) in these patients. The clearance of betaxolol by hemodialysis was 0.015 L/h/kg and by peritoneal dialysis, 0.010 L/h/kg. In one study patients (n=8) with stable renal failure, not on dialysis, with mean creatinine clearance of 27 ml/min showed slight increases in elimination half-life and AUC, but no change in C_{max}. In a second study of 30 hypertensive patients with mild to severe renal impairment, there was a reduction in clearance of betaxolol with increasing degrees of renal insufficiency. Inulin clearance (mL/min/1.73 m^2) ranged from 70 to 107 in 7 patients with mild impairment, 41 to 69 in 14 patients with moderate impairment, and 8 to 37 in 9 patients with severe impairment. Clearance following oral dosing was reduced significantly in patients with moderate and severe renal impairment (26% and 35%, respectively) when compared with those with mildly impaired renal function. In the severely impaired group, the mean C_{max} and the mean elimination half-life tended to increase (28% and 24%, respectively) when compared with the mildly impaired group. A starting dose of 5 mg is recommended in patients with severe renal impairment. (See *Dosage and Administration.*)
Studies in elderly patients (n=10) gave inconsistent results but suggest some impairment of elimination, with one small study (n=4) finding a mean half-life of 30 hours. A starting dose of 5 mg is suggested in older patients.

Pharmacodynamics: Clinical pharmacology studies have demonstrated the beta-adrenergic receptor blocking activity of Kerlone by (1) reduction in resting and exercise heart rate, cardiac output, and cardiac work load, (2) reduction of systolic and diastolic blood pressure at rest and during exercise, (3) inhibition of isoproterenol-induced tachycardia, and (4) reduction of reflex orthostatic tachycardia.
The β_1 selectivity of Kerlone in man was shown in three ways: (1) In normal subjects, 10- and 40-mg oral doses of Kerlone, which reduced resting heart rate at least as much as 40 mg of propranolol, produced less inhibition of isoproterenol-induced increases in forearm blood flow and finger tremor than propranolol. In this study, 10 mg of Kerlone was at least

Continued on next page

Searle—Cont.

comparable to 50 mg of atenolol. Both doses of Kerlone, and the one dose of atenolol, however, had more effect on the isoproterenol-induced changes than placebo (indicating some β_2 effect at clinical doses) and the higher dose of Kerlone was more inhibitory than the lower. (2) In normal subjects, single intravenous doses of betaxolol and propranolol, which produced equal effects on exercise-induced tachycardia, had differing effects on insulin-induced hypoglycemia, with propranolol, but not betaxolol, prolonging the hypoglycemia compared with placebo. Neither drug affected the maximum extent of the hypoglycemic response. (3) In a single-blind crossover study in asthmatics (n = 10), intravenous infusion over 30 minutes of low doses of betaxolol (1.5 mg) and propranolol (2 mg) had similar effects on resting heart rate but had differing effects on FEV_1 and forced vital capacity, with propranolol causing statistically significant (10% to 20%) reductions from baseline in mean values for both parameters while betaxolol had no effect on mean values. While blood levels were not measured, the dose of betaxolol used in this study would be expected to produce blood concentrations, at the time of the pulmonary function studies, considerably lower than those achieved during antihypertensive therapy with recommended doses of Kerlone. In a randomized double-blind, placebo-controlled crossover (4 × 4 Latin Square) study in 10 asthmatics, betaxolol (about 5 or 10 mg IV) had little effect on isoproterenol-induced increases in FEV_1; in contrast, propranolol (about 7 mg IV) inhibited the response.

Consistent with its negative chronotropic effect, due to beta-blockade of the SA node, and lack of intrinsic sympathomimetic activity, Kerlone increases sinus cycle length and sinus node recovery time. Conduction in the AV node is also prolonged.

Significant reductions in blood pressure and heart rate were observed 24 hours after dosing in double-blind, placebo-controlled trials with doses of 5 to 40 mg administered once daily. The antihypertensive response to betaxolol was similar at peak blood levels (3 to 4 hours) and at trough (24 hours). In a large randomized, parallel dose-response study of 5, 10, and 20 mg, the antihypertensive effects of the 5-mg dose were roughly half of the effects of the 20-mg dose (after adjustment for placebo effects) and the 10-mg dose gave more than 80% of the antihypertensive response to the 20-mg dose. The effect of increasing the dose from 10 mg to 20 mg was thus small. In this study, while the antihypertensive response to betaxolol showed a dose-response relationship, the heart rate response (reduction in HR) was not dose related. In other trials, there was little evidence of a greater antihypertensive response to 40 mg than to 20 mg. The maximum effect of each dose was achieved within 1 or 2 weeks. In comparative trials against propranolol, atenolol, and chlorthalidone, betaxolol appeared to be at least as effective as the comparative agent.

Kerlone has been studied in combination with thiazide-type diuretics and the blood pressure effects of the combination appear additive. Kerlone has also been used concurrently with methyldopa, hydralazine, and prazosin.

The mechanism of the antihypertensive effects of beta-adrenergic receptor blocking agents has not been established. Several possible mechanisms have been proposed, however, including: (1) competitive antagonism of catecholamines at peripheral (especially cardiac) adrenergic-neuronal sites, leading to decreased cardiac output, (2) a central effect leading to reduced sympathetic outflow to the periphery, and (3) suppression of renin activity.

The results from long-term studies have not shown any diminution of the antihypertensive effect of Kerlone with prolonged use.

INDICATIONS AND USAGE

Kerlone is indicated in the management of hypertension. It may be used alone or concomitantly with other antihypertensive agents, particularly thiazide-type diuretics.

CONTRAINDICATIONS

Kerlone is contraindicated in patients with known hypersensitivity to the drug.

Kerlone is contraindicated in patients with sinus bradycardia, heart block greater than first degree, cardiogenic shock, and overt cardiac failure (see *Warnings*).

WARNINGS

Cardiac failure: Sympathetic stimulation may be a vital component supporting circulatory function in congestive heart failure, and beta-adrenergic receptor blockade carries the potential hazard of further depressing myocardial contractility and precipitating more severe heart failure. In hypertensive patients who have congestive heart failure controlled by digitalis and diuretics, beta-blockers should be administered cautiously. Both digitalis and beta-adrenergic receptor blocking agents slow AV conduction.

In patients without a history of cardiac failure: Continued depression of the myocardium with beta-blocking agents over a period of time can, in some cases, lead to cardiac fail-

ure. Therefore, at the first sign or symptom of cardiac failure, discontinuation of Kerlone should be considered. In some cases beta-blocker therapy can be continued while cardiac failure is treated with cardiac glycosides, diuretics, and other agents, as appropriate.

Exacerbation of angina pectoris upon withdrawal: Abrupt cessation of therapy with certain beta-blocking agents in patients with coronary artery disease has been followed by exacerbations of angina pectoris and, in some cases, myocardial infarction has been reported. Therefore, such patients should be warned against interruption of therapy without the physician's advice. Even in the absence of overt angina pectoris, when discontinuation of Kerlone is planned, the patient should be carefully observed and therapy should be reinstituted, at least temporarily, if withdrawal symptoms occur.

Bronchospastic diseases: PATIENTS WITH BRONCHOSPASTIC DISEASE SHOULD NOT IN GENERAL RECEIVE BETA-BLOCKERS. Because of its relative β_1 selectivity (cardioselectivity), low doses of Kerlone may be used with caution in patients with bronchospastic disease who do not respond to or cannot tolerate alternative treatment. Since β_1 selectivity is not absolute and is inversely related to dose, the lowest possible dose of Kerlone should be used (5 to 10 mg once daily) and a bronchodilator should be made available. If dosage must be increased, divided dosage should be considered to avoid the higher peak blood levels associated with once-daily dosing.

Anesthesia and major surgery: The necessity, or desirability, of withdrawal of a beta-blocking therapy prior to major surgery is controversial. Beta-adrenergic receptor blockade impairs the ability of the heart to respond to beta-adrenergically mediated reflex stimuli. While this might be of benefit in preventing arrhythmic response, the risk of excessive myocardial depression during general anesthesia may be increased and difficulty in restarting and maintaining the heart beat has been reported with beta-blockers. If treatment is continued, particular care should be taken when using anesthetic agents which depress the myocardium, such as ether, cyclopropane, and trichloroethylene, and it is prudent to use the lowest possible dose of Kerlone. Kerlone, like other beta-blockers, is a competitive inhibitor of beta-receptor agonists and its effect on the heart can be reversed by cautious administration of such agents (eg, dobutamine or isoproterenol—see *Overdosage*). Manifestations of excessive vagal tone (eg, profound bradycardia, hypotension) may be corrected with atropine 1 to 3 mg IV in divided doses.

Diabetes and hypoglycemia: Beta-blockers should be used with caution in diabetic patients. Beta-blockers may mask tachycardia occurring with hypoglycemia (patients should be warned of this), although other manifestations such as dizziness and sweating may not be significantly affected. Unlike nonselective beta-blockers, Kerlone does not prolong insulin-induced hypoglycemia.

Thyrotoxicosis: Beta-adrenergic blockade may mask certain clinical signs of hyperthyroidism (eg, tachycardia). Abrupt withdrawal of beta-blockade might precipitate a thyroid storm; therefore, patients known or suspected of being thyrotoxic from whom Kerlone is to be withdrawn should be monitored closely (see *Dosage and Administration: Cessation of therapy*).

PRECAUTIONS

General: Beta-adrenoceptor blockade can cause reduction of intraocular pressure. Since betaxolol hydrochloride is marketed as an ophthalmic solution for treatment of glaucoma, patients should be told that Kerlone may interfere with the glaucoma-screening test. Withdrawal may lead to a return of increased intraocular pressure. Patients receiving beta-adrenergic blocking agents orally and beta-blocking ophthalmic solutions should be observed for potential additive effects either on the intraocular pressure or on the known systemic effects of beta-blockade.

Impaired hepatic or renal function: Kerlone is primarily metabolized in the liver to metabolites that are inactive and then excreted by the kidneys; clearance is somewhat reduced in patients with renal failure but little changed in patients with hepatic disease. Dosage reductions have not routinely been necessary when hepatic insufficiency is present (see *Dosage and Administration*) but patients should be observed. Patients with severe renal impairment and those on dialysis require a reduced dose. (See *Dosage and Administration*.)

Information for patients: Patients, especially those with evidence of coronary artery insufficiency, should be warned against interruption or discontinuation of Kerlone therapy without the physician's advice.

Although cardiac failure rarely occurs in appropriately selected patients, patients being treated with beta-adrenergic blocking agents should be advised to consult a physician at the first sign or symptom of failure.

Patients should know how they react to this medicine before they operate automobiles and machinery or engage in other tasks requiring alertness. Patients should contact their physician if any difficulty in breathing occurs, and before surgery of any type. Patients should inform their physicians or dentists that they are taking Kerlone. Patients with diabetes

should be warned that beta-blockers may mask tachycardia occurring with hypoglycemia.

Drug interactions: The following drugs have been coadministered with Kerlone and have not altered its pharmacokinetics: cimetidine, nifedipine, chlorthalidone, and hydrochlorothiazide. Concomitant administration of Kerlone with the oral anticoagulant warfarin has been shown not to potentiate the anticoagulant effect of warfarin.

Catecholamine-depleting drugs (eg, reserpine) may have an additive effect when given with beta-blocking agents. Patients treated with a beta-adrenergic receptor blocking agent plus a catecholamine depletor should therefore be closely observed for evidence of hypotension or marked bradycardia, which may produce vertigo, syncope, or postural hypotension.

Should it be decided to discontinue therapy in patients receiving beta-blockers and clonidine concurrently, the beta-blocker should be discontinued slowly over several days before the gradual withdrawal of clonidine.

Literature reports suggest that oral calcium antagonists may be used in combination with beta-adrenergic blocking agents when heart function is normal, but should be avoided in patients with impaired cardiac function. Hypotension, AV conduction disturbances, and left ventricular failure have been reported in some patients receiving beta-adrenergic blocking agents when an oral calcium antagonist was added to the treatment regimen. Hypotension was more likely to occur if the calcium antagonist were a dihydropyridine derivative, eg, nifedipine, while left ventricular failure and AV conduction disturbances, including complete heart block, were more likely to occur with either verapamil or diltiazem.

Risk of anaphylactic reaction: Although it is known that patients on beta-blockers may be refractory to epinephrine in the treatment of anaphylactic shock, beta-blockers can, in addition, interfere with the modulation of allergic reaction and lead to an increased severity and/or frequency of attacks. Severe allergic reactions including anaphylaxis have been reported in patients exposed to a variety of allergens either by repeated challenge, or accidental contact, and with diagnostic or therapeutic agents while receiving beta-blockers. Such patients may be unresponsive to the usual doses of epinephrine used to treat allergic reaction.

Carcinogenesis, mutagenesis, impairment of fertility: Lifetime studies with betaxolol HCl in mice at oral dosages of 6, 20, and 60 mg/kg/day (up to 90 × the maximum recommended human dose [MRHD] based on 60-kg body weight) and in rats at 3, 12, or 48 mg/kg/day (up to 72 × MRHD) showed no evidence of a carcinogenic effect. In a variety of *in vitro* and *in vivo* bacterial and mammalian cell assays, betaxolol HCl was nonmutagenic. Betaxolol did not adversely affect fertility or mating performance of male or female rats at doses up to 256 mg/kg/day (380 × MRHD).

Pregnancy: Pregnancy Category C. In a study in which pregnant rats received betaxolol at doses of 4, 40, or 400 mg/kg/day, the highest dose (600 × MRHD) was associated with increased postimplantation loss, reduced litter size and weight, and an increased incidence of skeletal and visceral abnormalities, which may have been a consequence of drug-related maternal toxicity. Other than a possible increased incidence of incomplete descent of testes and sternebral reductions, betaxolol at 4 mg/kg/day and 40 mg/kg/day (6 × MRHD and 60 × MRHD) caused no fetal abnormalities. In a second study with a different strain of rat, 200 mg betaxolol/kg/day (300 × MRHD) was associated with maternal toxicity and an increase in resorptions, but no teratogenicity. In a study in which pregnant rabbits received doses of 1, 4, 12, or 36 mg betaxolol/kg/day (54 × MRHD), a marked increase in postimplantation loss occurred at the highest dose, but no drug-related teratogenicity was observed. The rabbit is more sensitive to betaxolol than other species because of higher bioavailability resulting from saturation of the first-pass effect. In a peri- and postnatal study in rats at doses of 4, 32, and 256 mg betaxolol/kg/day (380 × MRHD), the highest dose was associated with a marked increase in total litter loss within 4 days postpartum. In surviving offspring, growth and development were also affected.

There are no adequate and well-controlled studies in pregnant women. Kerlone should be used during pregnancy only if the potential benefit justifies the potential risk to the fetus.

Nursing mothers: Since Kerlone is excreted in human milk in sufficient amounts to have pharmacological effects in the infant, caution should be exercised when Kerlone is administered to a nursing mother.

Pediatric use: Safety and efficacy in children have not been established.

Elderly patients: Kerlone may produce bradycardia more frequently in elderly patients. In general, patients 65 years of age and older had a higher incidence rate of bradycardia (heart rate < 50 BPM) than younger patients in U.S. clinical trials. In a double-blind study in Europe, 19 elderly patients (mean age = 82) received betaxolol 20 mg daily. Dosage reduction to 10 mg or discontinuation was required for 6 patients due to bradycardia (See *Dosage and Administration*).

Table 1

Body System/Adverse Reaction	Betaxolol (N=509) Dose Range 5–40 mg q.d.* (%)	Propranolol (N=73) 40–160 mg b.i.d. (%)	Atenolol (N=75) 25–100 mg q.d. (%)	Placebo (N=109) (%)
Cardiovascular				
Bradycardia				
(heart rate <50 BPM)	8.1	4.1	12.0	0
Symptomatic bradycardia	0.8	1.4	0	0
Edema	1.8	0	0	1.8
Central Nervous System				
Headache	6.5	4.1	5.3	15.6
Dizziness	4.5	11.0	2.7	5.5
Fatigue	2.9	9.6	4.0	0
Lethargy	2.8	4.1	2.7	0.9
Psychiatric				
Insomnia	1.2	8.2	2.7	0
Nervousness	0.8	1.4	2.7	0
Bizarre dreams	1.0	2.7	1.3	0
Depression	0.8	2.7	4.0	0
Autonomic				
Impotence	1.2†	0	0	0
Respiratory				
Dyspnea	2.4	2.7	1.3	0.9
Pharyngitis	2.0	0	4.0	0.9
Rhinitis	1.4	0	4.0	0.9
Upper respiratory infection	2.6	0	0	5.5
Gastrointestinal				
Dyspepsia	4.7	6.8	2.7	0.9
Nausea	1.6	1.4	4.0	0
Diarrhea	2.0	6.8	8.0	0.9
Musculoskeletal				
Chest pain	2.4	1.4	2.7	0.9
Arthralgia	3.1	0	4.0	1.8
Skin				
Rash	1.2	0	0	0

* Five patients received 80 mg q.d.
† N = 336 males; impotence is a known possible adverse effect of this pharmacological class.

ADVERSE REACTIONS

Most adverse reactions have been mild and transient and are typical of beta-adrenergic blocking agents, eg, bradycardia, fatigue, dyspnea, and lethargy. Withdrawal of therapy in U.S. and European controlled clinical trials has been necessary in about 3.5% of patients, principally because of bradycardia, fatigue, dizziness, headache, and impotence. Frequency estimates of adverse events were derived from controlled studies in which adverse reactions were volunteered and elicited in U.S. studies and volunteered and/or elicited in European studies.

In the U.S., the placebo-controlled studies lasted for 4 weeks, while the active-controlled studies had a 22- to 24-week double-blind phase. The following doses were studied: betaxolol—5, 10, 20, and 40 mg once daily; atenolol—25, 50, and 100 mg once daily; and propranolol—40, 80, and 160 mg b.i.d. Kerlone, like other beta-blockers, has been associated with the development of antinuclear antibodies (ANA). In controlled clinical studies, conversion of ANA from negative to positive occurred in 5.3% of the patients treated with betaxolol, 6.3% of the patients treated with atenolol, 4.9% of the patients treated with propranolol, and 3.2% of the patients treated with placebo.

Betaxolol adverse events reported with a 2% or greater frequency, and selected events with lower frequency, in U.S. controlled studies are: [See table above.]

Of the above adverse reactions [listed in Table 1] associated with the use of betaxolol, only bradycardia was clearly dose related, but there was a suggestion of dose relatedness for fatigue, lethargy, and dyspepsia.

In Europe, the placebo-controlled study lasted for 4 weeks, while the comparative studies had a 4- to 52-week double-blind phase. The following doses were studied: betaxolol 20 and 40 mg once daily and atenolol 100 mg once daily.

From European controlled clinical trials, the following adverse events reported by 2% or more patients and selected events with lower frequency are presented:
[See Table 2 below.]

The only adverse event whose frequency clearly rose with increasing dose was bradycardia. Elderly patients were especially susceptible to bradycardia, which in some cases responded to dose-reduction (see *Precautions*).

The following selected (potentially important) adverse events have been reported at an incidence of less than 2% in U.S. controlled hypertension and open, long-term clinical studies, European hypertension controlled clinical trials, or in marketing experience. It is not known whether a causal relationship exists between betaxolol and these events; they are listed to alert the physician to a possible relationship:

Autonomic: flushing, salivation, sweating.
Body as a whole: allergy, fever, malaise, pain, rigors.
Cardiovascular: angina pectoris, arrhythmia, atrioventricular block, heart failure, hypertension, hypotension, myocardial infarction, thrombosis, syncope.
Central and peripheral nervous system: ataxia, neuralgia, neuropathy, numbness, speech disorder, stupor, tremor, twitching.
Gastrointestinal: anorexia, constipation, dry mouth, increased appetite, mouth ulceration, rectal disorders, vomiting, dysphagia.
Hearing and vestibular: earache, labyrinth disorders, tinnitus, deafness.
Hematologic: anemia, leucocytosis, lymphadenopathy, purpura, thrombocytopenia.
Liver and biliary: increased AST, increased ALT.
Metabolic and nutritional: acidosis, diabetes, hypercholesterolemia, hyperglycemia, hyperkalemia, hyperlipemia, hyperuricemia, hypokalemia, weight gain, weight loss, thirst, increased LDH.
Musculoskeletal: arthropathy, neck pain, muscle cramps, tendonitis.
Psychiatric: abnormal thinking, amnesia, impaired concentration, confusion, emotional lability, hallucinations, decreased libido.
Reproductive disorders: Female: breast pain, breast fibroadenosis, menstrual disorder; Male: Peyronie's disease, prostatitis.
Respiratory: bronchitis, bronchospasm, cough, epistaxis, flu, pneumonia, sinusitis.
Skin: alopecia, eczema, erythematous rash, hypertrichosis, pruritus, skin disorders.
Special senses: abnormal taste, taste loss.
Urinary system: cystitis, dysuria, micturition disorder, oliguria, proteinuria, abnormal renal function, renal pain.
Vascular: cerebrovascular disorder, intermittent claudication, leg cramps, peripheral ischemia, thrombophlebitis.
Vision: abnormal lacrimation, abnormal vision, blepharitis, ocular hemorrhage, conjunctivitis, dry eyes, iritis, cataract, scotoma.

Potential adverse effects: Although not reported in clinical studies with betaxolol, a variety of adverse effects have been reported with other beta-adrenergic blocking agents and may be considered potential adverse effects of betaxolol:
Central nervous system: Reversible mental depression progressing to catatonia, an acute reversible syndrome characterized by disorientation for time and place, short-term memory loss, emotional lability with slightly clouded sensorium, and decreased performance on neuropsychometric tests.
Allergic: Fever combined with aching and sore throat, laryngospasm, respiratory distress.
Hematologic: Agranulocytosis, thrombocytopenic purpura, and nonthrombocytopenic purpura.
Gastrointestinal: Mesenteric arterial thrombosis, ischemic colitis.
Miscellaneous: Raynaud's phenomena. There have been reports of skin rashes and/or dry eyes associated with the use of beta-adrenergic blocking drugs. The reported incidence is small, and in most cases, the symptoms have cleared when treatment was withdrawn. Discontinuation of the drug should be considered if any such reaction is not otherwise explicable. Patients should be closely monitored following cessation of therapy.

The oculomucocutaneous syndrome associated with the beta-blocker practolol has not been reported with Kerlone during investigational use and extensive foreign experience. However, dry eyes have been reported.

OVERDOSAGE

No specific information on emergency treatment of overdosage with Kerlone is available. The most common effects expected are bradycardia, congestive heart failure, hypotension, bronchospasm, and hypoglycemia. In one acute overdosage of betaxolol, a 16-year-old female recovered fully after ingesting 460 mg.

Oral LD_{50}s are 350 to 400 mg betaxolol/kg in mice and 860 to 980 mg/kg in rats.

In the case of overdosage, treatment with Kerlone should be stopped and the patient carefully observed. Hemodialysis or peritoneal dialysis does not remove substantial amounts of the drug. In addition to gastric lavage, the following therapeutic measures are suggested if warranted:
Hypotension: Use sympathomimetic pressor drug therapy, such as dopamine, dobutamine, or norepinephrine. In refractory cases of overdosage of other beta-blockers, the use of glucagon hydrochloride has been reported to be useful.
Bradycardia: Atropine should be administered. If there is no response to vagal blockade, isoproterenol should be administered cautiously. In refractory cases the use of a transvenous cardiac pacemaker may be considered.

Table 2

Body System/Adverse Reaction	Betaxolol (N=155) Dose Range 20–40 mg q.d. (%)	Atenolol (N=81) 100 mg q.d. (%)	Placebo (N=60) (%)
Cardiovascular			
Bradycardia			
(heart rate <50 BPM)	5.8	5.0	0
Symptomatic bradycardia	1.9	2.5	0
Palpitation	1.9	3.7	1.7
Edema	1.3	1.2	0
Cold extremities	1.9	0	0
Central Nervous System			
Headache	14.8	9.9	23.3
Dizziness	14.8	17.3	15.0
Fatigue	9.7	18.5	0
Asthenia	7.1	0	16.7
Insomnia	5.0	3.7	3.3
Paresthesia	1.9	2.5	0
Gastrointestinal			
Nausea	5.8	1.2	0
Dyspepsia	3.9	7.4	3.3
Diarrhea	1.9	3.7	0
Musculoskeletal			
Chest pain	7.1	6.2	5.0
Joint pain	5.2	4.9	1.7
Myalgia	3.2	3.7	3.3

Continued on next page

Searle—Cont.

Acute cardiac failure: Conventional therapy including digitalis, diuretics, and oxygen should be instituted immediately.
Bronchospasm: Use a β_2-agonist. Additional therapy with aminophylline may be considered.
Heart block (2nd- or 3rd-degree): Use isoproterenol or a transvenous cardiac pacemaker.

DOSAGE AND ADMINISTRATION

The initial dose of Kerlone in hypertension is ordinarily 10 mg once daily either alone or added to diuretic therapy. The full antihypertensive effect is usually seen within 7 to 14 days. If the desired response is not achieved the dose can be doubled after 7 to 14 days. Increasing the dose beyond 20 mg has not been shown to produce a statistically significant additional antihypertensive effect; but the 40-mg dose has been studied and is well tolerated. An increased effect (reduction) on heart rate should be anticipated with increasing dosage. If monotherapy with Kerlone does not produce the desired response, the addition of a diuretic agent or other antihypertensive should be considered (see *Drug interactions*).

Dosage adjustments for specific patients

Patients with renal failure: In patients with renal impairment, clearance of betaxolol declines with decreasing renal function.
In patients with severe renal impairment and those undergoing dialysis the initial dose of Kerlone is 5 mg once daily. If the desired response is not achieved, dosage may be increased by 5 mg/day increments every 2 weeks to a maximum dose of 20 mg/day.

Patients with hepatic disease: Patients with hepatic disease do not have significantly altered clearance. Dosage adjustments are not routinely needed.

Elderly patients: Consideration should be given to reduction in the starting dose to 5 mg in elderly patients. These patients are especially prone to beta-blocker–induced bradycardia, which appears to be dose related and sometimes responds to reductions in dose.

Cessation of therapy: If withdrawal of Kerlone therapy is planned, it should be achieved gradually over a period of about 2 weeks. Patients should be carefully observed and advised to limit physical activity to a minimum.

HOW SUPPLIED

Kerlone 10-mg tablets are round, white, film coated, with KERLONE 10 debossed on one side and scored on the other, supplied as:

NDC Number	Size
0025-5101-31	bottle of 100
0025-5101-34	carton of 100 unit dose

Kerlone 20-mg tablets are round, white, film coated with KERLONE 20 debossed on one side and β on the other, supplied as:

NDC Number	Size
0025-5201-31	bottle of 100
0025-5201-34	carton of 100 unit dose

Store below 86°F (30°C).

Caution: Federal law prohibits dispensing without prescription.

Manufactured and distributed by
G.D. Searle & Co.
Chicago, IL 60680
by agreement with
Lorex Pharmaceuticals
Skokie, IL

Kerlone is a registered trademark of Synthelabo.

3/6/92 • AO5433-3

Shown in Product Identification Section, page 429

LOMOTIL® Liquid CV
LOMOTIL® Tablets CV
[*lō-mō 'til*]
(diphenoxylate hydrochloride with atropine sulfate)

DESCRIPTION

Each Lomotil tablet and each 5 ml of Lomotil liquid for oral use contains:

diphenoxylate hydrochloride .... 2.5 mg
(Warning—May be habit forming.)
atropine sulfate .... 0.025 mg

Diphenoxylate hydrochloride, an antidiarrheal, is ethyl 1-(3-cyano-3,3-diphenylpropyl)-4-phenylisonipecotate monohydrochloride and has the following structural formula:

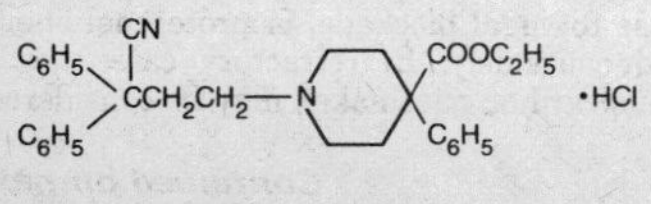

Atropine sulfate, an anticholinergic, is endo-(±)-α-(hydroxymethyl) benzeneacetic acid 8-methyl-8-azabicyclo[3.2.1] oct-3-yl ester sulfate (2:1) (salt) monohydrate and has the following structural formula:

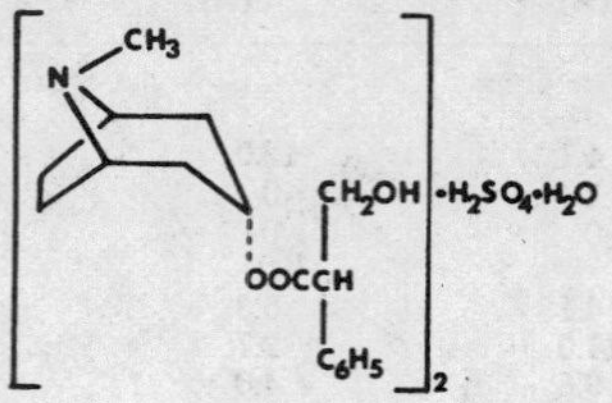

Inactive ingredients of Lomotil tablets include acacia, corn starch, magnesium stearate, sorbitol, sucrose, and talc. Inactive ingredients of Lomotil liquid include cherry flavor, citric acid, ethyl alcohol 15%, FD&C Yellow No. 6, glycerin, sodium phosphate, sorbitol, and water.

IMPORTANT INFORMATION

Lomotil is classified as a Schedule V controlled substance by federal law. Diphenoxylate hydrochloride is chemically related to the narcotic meperidine. Therefore, in case of overdosage, treatment is similar to that for meperidine or morphine intoxication, in which prolonged and careful monitoring is essential. Respiratory depression may be evidenced as late as 30 hours after ingestion and may recur in spite of an initial response to narcotic antagonists. A subtherapeutic amount of atropine sulfate is present to discourage deliberate overdosage. LOMOTIL IS *NOT* AN INNOCUOUS DRUG AND DOSAGE RECOMMENDATIONS SHOULD BE STRICTLY ADHERED TO, ESPECIALLY IN CHILDREN. KEEP THIS AND ALL MEDICATIONS OUT OF REACH OF CHILDREN.

CLINICAL PHARMACOLOGY

Diphenoxylate is rapidly and extensively metabolized in man by ester hydrolysis to diphenoxylic acid (difenoxine), which is biologically active and the major metabolite in the blood. After a 5-mg oral dose of carbon-14 labeled diphenoxylate hydrochloride in ethanolic solution was given to three healthy volunteers, an average of 14% of the drug plus its metabolites was excreted in the urine and 49% in the feces over a four-day period. Urinary excretion of the unmetabolized drug constituted less than 1% of the dose, and diphenoxylic acid plus its glucuronide conjugate constituted about 6% of the dose. In a 16-subject crossover bioavailability study, a linear relationship in the dose range of 2.5 to 10 mg was found between the dose of diphenoxylate hydrochloride (given as Lomotil liquid) and the peak plasma concentration, the area under the plasma concentration-time curve, and the amount of diphenoxylic acid excreted in the urine. In the same study the bioavailability of the tablet compared with an equal dose of the liquid was approximately 90%. The average peak plasma concentration of diphenoxylic acid following ingestion of four 2.5-mg tablets was 163 ng/ml at about 2 hours, and the elimination half-life of diphenoxylic acid was approximately 12 to 14 hours.
In dogs, diphenoxylate hydrochloride has a direct effect on circular smooth muscle of the bowel that conceivably results in segmentation and prolongation of gastrointestinal transit time. The clinical antidiarrheal action of diphenoxylate hydrochloride may thus be a consequence of enhanced segmentation that allows increased contact of the intraluminal contents with the intestinal mucosa.

INDICATIONS AND USAGE

Lomotil is effective as adjunctive therapy in the management of diarrhea.

CONTRAINDICATIONS

Lomotil is contraindicated in patients with
1. Known hypersensitivity to diphenoxylate or atropine.
2. Obstructive jaundice.
3. Diarrhea associated with pseudomembranous enterocolitis or enterotoxin-producing bacteria.

WARNINGS

LOMOTIL IS *NOT* AN INNOCUOUS DRUG AND DOSAGE RECOMMENDATIONS SHOULD BE STRICTLY ADHERED TO, ESPECIALLY IN CHILDREN. LOMOTIL IS NOT RECOMMENDED FOR CHILDREN UNDER 2 YEARS OF AGE. OVERDOSAGE MAY RESULT IN SEVERE RESPIRATORY DEPRESSION AND COMA, POSSIBLY LEADING TO PERMANENT BRAIN DAMAGE OR DEATH (SEE *OVERDOSAGE*). THEREFORE, KEEP THIS MEDICATION OUT OF THE REACH OF CHILDREN.
THE USE OF LOMOTIL SHOULD BE ACCOMPANIED BY APPROPRIATE FLUID AND ELECTROLYTE THERAPY, WHEN INDICATED. IF SEVERE DEHYDRATION OR ELECTROLYTE IMBALANCE IS PRESENT, LOMOTIL SHOULD BE WITHHELD UNTIL APPROPRIATE CORRECTIVE THERAPY HAS BEEN INITIATED. DRUG-INDUCED INHIBITION OF PERISTALSIS MAY RESULT IN FLUID RETENTION IN THE INTESTINE, WHICH MAY FURTHER AGGRAVATE DEHYDRATION AND ELECTROLYTE IMBALANCE.
LOMOTIL SHOULD BE USED WITH SPECIAL CAUTION IN YOUNG CHILDREN BECAUSE THIS AGE GROUP MAY BE PREDISPOSED TO DELAYED DIPHENOXYLATE TOXICITY AND BECAUSE OF THE GREATER VARIABILITY OF RESPONSE IN THIS AGE GROUP.
Antiperistaltic agents may prolong and/or worsen diarrhea associated with organisms that penetrate the intestinal mucosa (toxigenic *E. coli, Salmonella, Shigella*), and pseudomembranous enterocolitis associated with broad-spectrum antibiotics. Antiperistaltic agents should not be used in these conditions.
In some patients with acute ulcerative colitis, agents that inhibit intestinal motility or prolong intestinal transit time have been reported to induce toxic megacolon. Consequently, patients with acute ulcerative colitis should be carefully observed and Lomotil therapy should be discontinued promptly if abdominal distention occurs or if other untoward symptoms develop.
Since the chemical structure of diphenoxylate hydrochloride is similar to that of meperidine hydrochloride, the concurrent use of Lomotil with monoamine oxidase (MAO) inhibitors may, in theory, precipitate hypertensive crisis.
Lomotil should be used with extreme caution in patients with advanced hepatorenal disease and in all patients with abnormal liver function since hepatic coma may be precipitated.
Diphenoxylate hydrochloride may potentiate the action of barbiturates, tranquilizers, and alcohol. Therefore, the patient should be closely observed when any of these are used concomitantly.

PRECAUTIONS

General: Since a subtherapeutic dose of atropine has been added to the diphenoxylate hydrochloride, consideration should be given to the precautions relating to the use of atropine. In children, Lomotil should be used with caution since signs of atropinism may occur even with recommended doses, particularly in patients with Down's syndrome.

Information for patients: INFORM THE PATIENT (PARENT OR GUARDIAN) NOT TO EXCEED THE RECOMMENDED DOSAGE AND TO KEEP LOMOTIL OUT OF THE REACH OF CHILDREN AND IN A CHILD-RESISTANT CONTAINER. INFORM THE PATIENT OF THE CONSEQUENCES OF OVERDOSAGE, INCLUDING SEVERE RESPIRATORY DEPRESSION AND COMA, POSSIBLY LEADING TO PERMANENT BRAIN DAMAGE OR DEATH. Lomotil may produce drowsiness or dizziness. The patient should be cautioned regarding activities requiring mental alertness, such as driving or operating dangerous machinery. Potentiation of the action of alcohol, barbiturates, and tranquilizers with concomitant use of Lomotil should be explained to the patient. The physician should also provide the patient with other information in this labeling, as appropriate.

Drug interactions: Known drug interactions include barbiturates, tranquilizers, and alcohol. Lomotil may interact with MAO inhibitors (see *Warnings*).
In studies with male rats, diphenoxylate hydrochloride was found to inhibit the hepatic microsomal enzyme system at a dose of 2 mg/kg/day. Therefore, diphenoxylate has the potential to prolong the biological half-lives of drugs for which the rate of elimination is dependent on the microsomal drug metabolizing enzyme system.

Carcinogenesis, mutagenesis, impairment of fertility: No long-term study in animals has been performed to evaluate carcinogenic potential. Diphenoxylate hydrochloride was administered to male and female rats in their diets to provide dose levels of 4 and 20 mg/kg/day throughout a three-litter reproduction study. At 50 times the human dose (20 mg/kg/day), female weight gain was reduced and there was a marked effect on fertility as only 4 of 27 females became pregnant in three test breedings. The relevance of this finding to usage of Lomotil in humans is unknown.

Pregnancy: Pregnancy Category C. Diphenoxylate hydrochloride has been shown to have an effect on fertility in rats when given in doses 50 times the human dose (see above discussion). Other findings in this study include a decrease in maternal weight gain of 30% at 20 mg/kg/day and of 10% at 4 mg/kg/day. At 10 times the human dose (4 mg/kg/day), average litter size was slightly reduced.
Teratology studies were conducted in rats, rabbits, and mice with diphenoxylate hydrochloride at oral doses of 0.4 to 20 mg/kg/day. Due to experimental design and small numbers of litters, embryotoxic, fetotoxic, or teratogenic effects cannot be adequately assessed. However, examination of the available fetuses did not reveal any indication of teratogenicity.
There are no adequate and well-controlled studies in pregnant women. Lomotil should be used during pregnancy only if the anticipated benefit justifies the potential risk to the fetus.

Nursing mothers: Caution should be exercised when Lomotil is administered to a nursing woman, since the physico-

chemical characteristics of the major metabolite, diphenoxylic acid, are such that it may be excreted in breast milk and since it is known that atropine is excreted in breast milk.

Pediatric use: Lomotil may be used as an adjunct to the treatment of diarrhea but should be accompanied by appropriate fluid and electrolyte therapy, if needed. LOMOTIL IS NOT RECOMMENDED FOR CHILDREN UNDER 2 YEARS OF AGE. Lomotil should be used with special caution in young children because of the greater variability of response in this age group. See *Warnings* and *Dosage and Administration*. In case of accidental ingestion by children, see *Overdosage* for recommended treatment.

ADVERSE REACTIONS

At *therapeutic* doses, the following have been reported; they are listed in decreasing order of severity, but not of frequency:

Nervous system: numbness of extremities, euphoria, depression, malaise/lethargy, confusion, sedation/drowsiness, dizziness, restlessness, headache.

Allergic: anaphylaxis, angioneurotic edema, urticaria, swelling of the gums, pruritus.

Gastrointestinal system: toxic megacolon, paralytic ileus, pancreatitis, vomiting, nausea, anorexia, abdominal discomfort.

The following atropine sulfate effects are listed in decreasing order of severity, but not of frequency: hyperthermia, tachycardia, urinary retention, flushing, dryness of the skin and mucous membranes. These effects may occur, especially in children.

THIS MEDICATION SHOULD BE KEPT IN A CHILD-RESISTANT CONTAINER AND OUT OF THE REACH OF CHILDREN SINCE AN OVERDOSAGE MAY RESULT IN SEVERE RESPIRATORY DEPRESSION AND COMA, POSSIBLY LEADING TO PERMANENT BRAIN DAMAGE OR DEATH.

DRUG ABUSE AND DEPENDENCE

Controlled substance: Lomotil is classified as a Schedule V controlled substance by federal regulation. Diphenoxylate hydrochloride is chemically related to the narcotic analgesic meperidine.

Drug abuse and dependence: In doses used for the treatment of diarrhea, whether acute or chronic, diphenoxylate has not produced addiction.

Diphenoxylate hydrochloride is devoid of morphine-like subjective effects at therapeutic doses. At high doses it exhibits codeine-like subjective effects. The dose which produces antidiarrheal action is widely separated from the dose which causes central nervous system effects. The insolubility of diphenoxylate hydrochloride in commonly available aqueous media precludes intravenous self-administration. A dose of 100 to 300 mg/day, which is equivalent to 40 to 120 tablets, administered to humans for 40 to 70 days, produced opiate withdrawal symptoms. Since addiction to diphenoxylate hydrochloride is possible at high doses, the recommended dosage should not be exceeded.

OVERDOSAGE

RECOMMENDED DOSAGE SCHEDULES SHOULD BE STRICTLY FOLLOWED. THIS MEDICATION SHOULD BE KEPT IN A CHILD-RESISTANT CONTAINER AND OUT OF THE REACH OF CHILDREN, SINCE AN OVERDOSAGE MAY RESULT IN SEVERE, EVEN FATAL, RESPIRATORY DEPRESSION.

Diagnosis: Initial signs of overdosage may include dryness of the skin and mucous membranes, mydriasis, restlessness, flushing, hyperthermia, and tachycardia followed by lethargy or coma, hypotonic reflexes, nystagmus, pinpoint pupils, and respiratory depression. Respiratory depression may be evidenced as late as 30 hours after ingestion and may recur despite an initial response to narcotic antagonists. TREAT ALL POSSIBLE LOMOTIL OVERDOSAGES AS SERIOUS AND MAINTAIN MEDICAL OBSERVATION FOR AT LEAST 48 HOURS, PREFERABLY UNDER CONTINUOUS HOSPITAL CARE.

Treatment: In the event of overdose, induction of vomiting, gastric lavage, establishment of a patent airway, and possibly mechanically assisted respiration are advised. *In vitro* and animal studies indicate that activated charcoal may significantly decrease the bioavailability of diphenoxylate. In noncomatose patients, a slurry of 100 g of activated charcoal can be administered immediately after the induction of vomiting or gastric lavage.

A pure narcotic antagonist (eg, naloxone) should be used in the treatment of respiratory depression caused by Lomotil. When a narcotic antagonist is administered intravenously, the onset of action is generally apparent within two minutes. It may also be administered subcutaneously or intramuscularly, providing a slightly less rapid onset of action but a more prolonged effect.

To counteract respiratory depression caused by Lomotil overdosage, the following dosage schedule for the narcotic antagonist naloxone hydrochloride should be followed:

Adult dosage: An initial dose of 0.4 mg to 2 mg of naloxone hydrochloride may be administered intravenously. If the desired degree of counteraction and improvement in respiratory function is not obtained, it may be repeated at 2- to 3-minute intervals. If no response is observed after 10 mg of naloxone hydrochloride has been administered, the diagnosis of narcotic-induced or partial narcotic-induced toxicity should be questioned. Intramuscular or subcutaneous administration may be necessary if the intravenous route is not available.

Children: The usual initial dose in children is 0.01 mg/kg body weight given I.V. If this dose does not result in the desired degree of clinical improvement, a subsequent dose of 0.1 mg/kg body weight may be administered. If an I.V. route of administration is not available, naloxone hydrochloride may be administered I.M. or S.C. in divided doses. If necessary, naloxone hydrochloride can be diluted with sterile water for injection.

Following initial improvement of respiratory function, repeated doses of naloxone hydrochloride may be required to counteract recurrent respiratory depression. Supplemental intramuscular doses of naloxone hydrochloride may be utilized to produce a longer-lasting effect.

Since the duration of action of diphenoxylate hydrochloride is longer than that of naloxone hydrochloride, improvement of respiration following administration may be followed by recurrent respiratory depression. Consequently, continuous observation is necessary until the effect of diphenoxylate hydrochloride on respiration has passed. This effect may persist for many hours. The period of observation should extend over at least 48 hours, preferably under continuous hospital care. Although signs of overdosage and respiratory depression may not be evident soon after ingestion of diphenoxylate hydrochloride, respiratory depression may occur from 12 to 30 hours later.

DOSAGE AND ADMINISTRATION

DO NOT EXCEED RECOMMENDED DOSAGE.

Adults: The recommended initial dosage is two Lomotil tablets four times daily or 10 ml (two regular teaspoonfuls) of Lomotil liquid four times daily (20 mg per day). Most patients will require this dosage until initial control has been achieved, after which the dosage may be reduced to meet individual requirements. Control may often be maintained with as little as 5 mg (two tablets or 10 ml of liquid) daily.

Clinical improvement of acute diarrhea is usually observed within 48 hours. If clinical improvement of chronic diarrhea after treatment with a maximum daily dose of 20 mg of diphenoxylate hydrochloride is not observed within 10 days, symptoms are unlikely to be controlled by further administration.

Children: Lomotil is not recommended in children under 2 years of age and should be used with special caution in young children (see *Warnings* and *Precautions*). *The nutritional status and degree of dehydration must be considered. In children under 13 years of age, use Lomotil liquid. Do not use Lomotil tablets for this age group.*

Only the plastic dropper should be used when measuring Lomotil liquid for administration to children.

Dosage schedule for children: The recommended initial total daily dosage of Lomotil liquid for children is 0.3 to 0.4 mg/kg, administered in four divided doses. The following table provides an *approximate* initial daily dosage recommendation for children.

Age (years)	Approximate weight (kg)	(lb)	Dosage in ml (four times daily)
2	11–14	24–31	1.5–3.0
3	12–16	26–35	2.0–3.0
4	14–20	31–44	2.0–4.0
5	16–23	35–51	2.5–4.5
6–8	17–32	38–71	2.5–5.0
9–12	23–55	51–121	3.5–5.0

These pediatric schedules are the best approximation of an average dose recommendation which may be adjusted downward according to the overall nutritional status and degree of dehydration encountered in the sick child. Reduction of dosage may be made as soon as initial control of symptoms has been achieved. Maintenance dosage may be as low as one-fourth of the initial daily dosage. If no response occurs within 48 hours, Lomotil is unlikely to be effective.

KEEP THIS AND ALL MEDICATIONS OUT OF THE REACH OF CHILDREN.

HOW SUPPLIED

Tablets—round, white, with SEARLE debossed on one side and 61 on the other side and containing 2.5 mg of diphenoxylate hydrochloride and 0.025 mg of atropine sulfate, supplied as:

NDC Number	Size
0025-0061-31	bottle of 100
0025-0061-51	bottle of 500
0025-0061-52	bottle of 1,000
0025-0061-55	bottle of 2,500
0025-0061-34	carton of 100 unit dose

Liquid—containing 2.5 mg of diphenoxylate hydrochloride and 0.025 mg of atropine sulfate per 5 ml; bottles of 2 fl oz (NDC Number 0025-0066-02). Dispense only in original container.

A plastic dropper calibrated in increments of ½ ml (¼ mg) with a capacity of 2 ml (1 mg) accompanies each 2-oz bottle of Lomotil liquid. Only this plastic dropper should be used when measuring Lomotil liquid for administration to children.

3/5/90 ● A05758-3

Shown in Product Identification Section, page 429

MAXAQUIN® ℞

[*măx 'ah-kwĭn*]

(lomefloxacin hydrochloride)

Film-coated Tablets

DESCRIPTION

Maxaquin (lomefloxacin HCl) is a synthetic broad-spectrum antimicrobial agent for oral administration. Lomefloxacin HCl, a difluoroquinolone, is the monohydrochloride salt of (±)-1-ethyl-6,8-difluoro-1,4-dihydro-7-(3-methyl-1-piperazinyl)-4-oxo-3-quinolinecarboxylic acid. Its empirical formula is $C_{17}H_{19}F_2N_3O_3 \cdot HCl$, and its structural formula is:

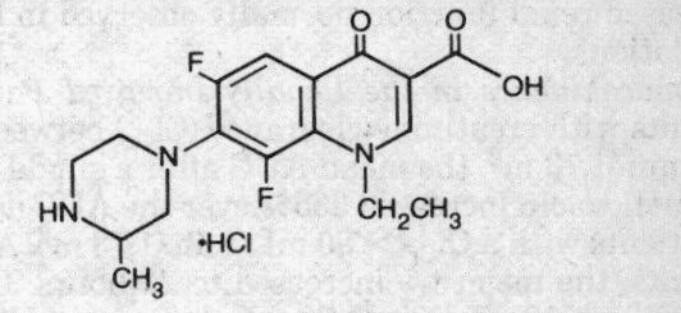

Lomefloxacin HCl is a white to pale yellow powder with a molecular weight of 387.8. It is slightly soluble in water and practically insoluble in alcohol. Lomefloxacin HCl is stable to heat and moisture but is sensitive to light in dilute aqueous solution.

Maxaquin is available as a film-coated tablet formulation containing 400 mg of lomefloxacin base, present as the hydrochloride salt. The base content of the hydrochloride salt is 90.6%. The inactive ingredients are carboxymethylcellulose calcium, hydroxypropyl cellulose, hydroxypropyl methylcellulose, lactose, magnesium stearate, polyethylene glycol, polyoxyl 40 stearate, and titanium dioxide.

CLINICAL PHARMACOLOGY

Pharmacokinetics in Healthy Volunteers: In 6 fasting healthy male volunteers, approximately 95% to 98% of a single oral dose of lomefloxacin was absorbed. Absorption was rapid following single doses of 200 and 400 mg (T_{max} 0.8 to 1.4 hours). Mean plasma concentration increased proportionally between 100 and 400 mg as shown below.

Dose (mg)	Mean Plasma Concentration (μg/mL)	Area Under Curve (AUC) (μg·h/mL)
100	0.8	5.6
200	1.4	10.9
400	3.2	26.1

In 6 healthy male volunteers administered 400 mg of lomefloxacin on an empty stomach q.d. for 7 days, the following mean pharmacokinetic parameter values were obtained:

C_{max}	2.8 μg/mL
C_{min}	0.27 μg/mL
$AUC_{0-24\ h}$	25.9 μg·h/mL
T_{max}	1.5 h
$t_{1/2}$	7.75 h

The elimination half-life in 8 subjects with normal renal function was approximately 8 hours. At 24 hours post dose, subjects with normal renal function receiving single doses of 200 or 400 mg had mean plasma lomefloxacin concentrations of 0.10 and 0.24 μg/mL, respectively. Steady-state concentrations were achieved within 48 hours of initiating therapy with once-a-day dosing. There was no drug accumulation with single daily dosing in patients with normal renal function.

Approximately 65% of an orally administered dose was excreted in the urine as unchanged drug in patients with normal renal function. Following a 400-mg dose of lomefloxacin administered q.d. for 7 days, the mean urine concentration was in excess of 300 μg/mL 4 hours post dose. The mean urine concentration exceeded 35 μg/mL for at least 24 hours after dosing.

Following a single 400-mg dose, lomefloxacin's solubility in urine usually exceeded its peak urinary concentration 2 to 6 fold. In this study, urine pH affected the solubility of lomefloxacin with solubilities ranging from 7.8 mg/mL at pH 5.2, to 2.4 mg/mL at pH 6.5, and 3.03 mg/mL at pH 8.12.

Continued on next page

Searle—Cont.

The urinary excretion of lomefloxacin was virtually complete within 72 hours after cessation of dosing, with approximately 65% of the dose being recovered as parent drug and 9% as its glucuronide metabolite. The mean renal clearance was 145 mL/min in subjects with normal renal function (GFR = 120 mL/min). This may indicate tubular secretion.

Food effect: When lomefloxacin and food were administered concomitantly, the rate of drug absorption was delayed [T_{max} increased to 2 hours (delayed by 41%), C_{max} decreased by 18%], and the extent of absorption (AUC) was decreased by 12%.

Pharmacokinetics in the Geriatric Population: In 16 healthy elderly volunteers (61 to 76 years of age) with normal renal function for their age, lomefloxacin's half-life (mean of 8 hours) and peak plasma concentration (mean of 4.2 µg/mL) following a single 400-mg dose were similar to those in 8 younger subjects dosed with a single 400-mg dose. Thus, drug absorption appears unaffected in the elderly. Plasma clearance was, however, reduced in this elderly population by approximately 25%, and the AUC was increased by approximately 33%. This slower elimination most likely reflects the decreased renal function normally observed in the geriatric population.

Pharmacokinetics in the Renally Impaired Patients: In 8 patients with creatinine clearance (Cl_{Cr}) between 10 and 40 mL/min/1.73 m^2, the mean AUC after a single 400-mg dose of lomefloxacin increased 335% over the AUC demonstrated in patients with a Cl_{Cr} > 80 mL/min/1.73 m^2. Also, in these patients, the mean $t_{1/2}$ increased to 21 hours. In 8 patients with Cl_{Cr} < 10 mL/min/1.73 m^2, the mean AUC after a single 400-mg dose of lomefloxacin increased 700% over the AUC demonstrated in patients with a Cl_{Cr} > 80 mL/min/1.73 m^2. In these patients with Cl_{Cr} < 10 mL/min/1.73 m^2, the mean $t_{1/2}$ increased to 45 hours. The plasma clearance of lomefloxacin was closely correlated with creatinine clearance, ranging from 31 mL/min/1.73 m^2 when creatinine clearance was zero to 271 mL/min/1.73 m^2 at a normal creatinine clearance of 110 mL/min/1.73 m^2. Peak lomefloxacin concentrations were not affected by the degree of renal function when single doses of lomefloxacin were administered. Adjustment of dosage schedules for patients with such decreases in renal function is warranted. (See **Dosage and Administration.**)

Pharmacokinetics in Patients with Cirrhosis: In 12 patients with histologically confirmed cirrhosis, no significant changes in rate or extent of lomefloxacin exposure (C_{max}, T_{max}, $t_{1/2}$ or AUC) were observed when they were administered 400 mg of lomefloxacin as a single dose. No data are available in cirrhotic patients treated with multiple doses of lomefloxacin. Cirrhosis does not appear to reduce the nonrenal clearance of lomefloxacin. There does not appear to be a need for a dosage reduction in cirrhotic patients, provided adequate renal function is present.

Metabolism and Pharmacodynamics of Lomefloxacin: Lomefloxacin is minimally metabolized although 5 metabolites have been identified in human urine. The glucuronide metabolite is found in the highest concentration and accounts for approximately 9% of the administered dose. The other 4 metabolites together account for less than 0.5% of the dose.

Approximately 10% of an oral dose was recovered as unchanged drug in the feces.

Serum protein binding of lomefloxacin is approximately 10%.

The following are mean tissue or fluid to plasma ratios of lomefloxacin following oral administration. Studies have not been conducted to assess the penetration of lomefloxacin into human cerebrospinal fluid.

Tissue or Body Fluid	Mean Tissue or Fluid to Plasma Ratio
Bronchial mucosa	2.1
Bronchial secretions	0.6
Prostatic tissue	2
Sputum	1.3
Urine	140.0

Microbiology: Lomefloxacin is a bactericidal agent with *in vitro* activity against a wide range of gram-negative and gram-positive organisms. The bactericidal action of lomefloxacin results from interference with the activity of the bacterial enzyme DNA gyrase, which is needed for the transcription and replication of bacterial DNA. The minimum bactericidal concentration (MBC) generally does not exceed the minimum inhibitory concentration (MIC) by more than a factor of 2, except for staphylococci, which usually have MBC's 2 to 4 times the MIC.

Lomefloxacin has been shown to be active against most strains of the following organisms both *in vitro* and in clinical infections: (See **Indications and Usage.**)

Gram-positive aerobes
- *Staphylococcus saprophyticus*

Gram-negative aerobes
- *Citrobacter diversus*
- *Enterobacter cloacae*
- *Escherichia coli*
- *Haemophilus influenzae*
- *Klebsiella pneumoniae*
- *Moraxella (Branhamella) catarrhalis*
- *Proteus mirabilis*
- *Pseudomonas aeruginosa* (urinary tract only—See **Indications and Usage** and **Warnings**)

The following *in vitro* data are available; however, their clinical significance is unknown.

Lomefloxacin exhibits *in vitro* MIC's of 2 µg/mL or less against most strains of the following organisms; however, the safety and effectiveness of lomefloxacin in treating clinical infections due to these organisms have not been established in adequate and well-controlled trials:

Gram-positive aerobes
- *Staphylococcus aureus* (including methicillin-resistant strains)
- *Staphylococcus epidermidis* (including methicillin-resistant strains)

Gram-negative aerobes
- *Aeromonas hydrophila*
- *Citrobacter freundii*
- *Enterobacter aerogenes*
- *Enterobacter agglomerans*
- *Haemophilus parainfluenzae*
- *Hafnia alvei*
- *Klebsiella oxytoca*
- *Klebsiella ozaenae*
- *Morganella morganii*
- *Proteus vulgaris*
- *Providencia alcalifaciens*
- *Providencia rettgeri*
- *Serratia liquefaciens*
- *Serratia marcescens*

Other organisms:
- *Legionella pneumophila*

Beta-lactamase production should have no effect on the *in vitro* activity of lomefloxacin.

Most group A, B, D, and G streptococci, *Streptococcus pneumoniae, Pseudomonas cepacia, Ureaplasma urealyticum, Mycoplasma hominis,* and anaerobic bacteria are resistant to lomefloxacin.

Lomefloxacin appears slightly less active *in vitro* when tested at acidic pH. An increase in inoculum size has little effect on the *in vitro* activity of lomefloxacin. *In vitro* resistance to lomefloxacin develops slowly (multiple-step mutation). Rapid one-step development of resistance occurs only rarely ($<10^{-9}$) *in vitro.*

Cross-resistance between lomefloxacin and other quinolone-class antimicrobial agents has been reported; however, cross-resistance between lomefloxacin and members of other classes of antimicrobial agents, such as aminoglycosides, penicillins, tetracyclines, cephalosporins, or sulfonamides has not yet been reported. Lomefloxacin is active *in vitro* against some strains of cephalosporin- and aminoglycoside-resistant gram-negative bacteria.

Susceptibility tests

Diffusion techniques: Quantitative methods that require measurement of zone diameters give the most precise estimate of the susceptibility of bacteria to antimicrobial agents. One such standardized procedure[1] that has been recommended for use with disks to test the susceptibility of organisms to lomefloxacin uses the 10-µg lomefloxacin disk. Interpretation involves correlation of the diameter obtained in the disk test with the MIC for lomefloxacin.

Reports from the laboratory giving results of the standard single-disk susceptibility test with a 10-µg lomefloxacin disk should be interpreted according to the following criteria:

Zone Diameter (mm)	Interpretation
≥22	Susceptible (S)
19–21	Intermediate (I)
≤18	Resistant (R)

A report of "Susceptible" indicates that the pathogen is likely to be inhibited by generally achievable drug concentrations. A report of "Intermediate" indicates that the result should be considered equivocal, and, if the organism is not fully susceptible to alternative clinically feasible drugs, the test should be repeated. This category provides a buffer zone that prevents small uncontrolled technical factors from causing major discrepancies in interpretation. A report of "Resistant" indicates that achievable drug concentrations are unlikely to be inhibitory, and other therapy should be selected.

Standardized susceptibility test procedures require the use of laboratory control organisms. The 10-µg lomefloxacin disk should give the following zone diameters:

Organism	Zone Diameter (mm)
S. aureus (ATCC 25923)	23–29
E. coli (ATCC 25922)	27–33
P. aeruginosa (ATCC 27853)	22–28

Dilution techniques: Use a standardized dilution method[2] (broth, agar, or microdilution) or equivalent with lomefloxacin powder. The MIC values obtained should be interpreted according to the following criteria:

MIC (µg/mL)	Interpretation
≤2	Susceptible (S)
4	Intermediate (I)
≥8	Resistant (R)

As with standard diffusion techniques, dilution methods require the use of laboratory control organisms. Standard lomefloxacin powder should provide the following MIC values:

Organism	MIC (µg/mL)
S. aureus (ATCC 29213)	0.25–2.0
E. coli (ATCC 25922)	0.03–0.12
P. aeruginosa (ATCC 27853)	1.0–4.0

INDICATIONS AND USAGE

TREATMENT:

Maxaquin (lomefloxacin HCl) film-coated tablets are indicated for the treatment of adults with mild to moderate infections caused by susceptible strains of the designated microorganisms in the conditions listed below: (See **Dosage and Administration** for specific dosing recommendations.)

LOWER RESPIRATORY TRACT

Acute Bacterial Exacerbation of Chronic Bronchitis caused by *Haemophilus influenzae* or *Moraxella (Branhamella) catarrhalis**.

NOTE: MAXAQUIN IS NOT INDICATED FOR THE EMPIRIC TREATMENT OF ACUTE BACTERIAL EXACERBATION OF CHRONIC BRONCHITIS WHEN IT IS PROBABLE THAT *S. PNEUMONIAE* IS A CAUSATIVE PATHOGEN. *S. PNEUMONIAE* EXHIBITS *IN VITRO* RESISTANCE TO LOMEFLOXACIN, AND THE SAFETY AND EFFICACY OF LOMEFLOXACIN IN THE TREATMENT OF PATIENTS WITH ACUTE BACTERIAL EXACERBATION OF CHRONIC BRONCHITIS CAUSED BY *S. PNEUMONIAE* HAVE NOT BEEN DEMONSTRATED. IF LOMEFLOXACIN IS TO BE PRESCRIBED FOR GRAM-STAIN GUIDED EMPIRIC THERAPY OF ACUTE BACTERIAL EXACERBATION OF CHRONIC BRONCHITIS, IT SHOULD BE USED ONLY IF SPUTUM GRAM STAIN DEMONSTRATES AN ADEQUATE QUALITY OF SPECIMEN (>25 PMN'S/LPF) AND THERE IS BOTH A PREDOMINANCE OF GRAM NEGATIVE ORGANISMS AND NOT A PREDOMINANCE OF GRAM POSITIVE ORGANISMS.

URINARY TRACT

Uncomplicated Urinary Tract Infections (cystitis) caused by *Escherichia coli, Klebsiella pneumoniae, Proteus mirabilis,* or *Staphylococcus saprophyticus.*

Complicated Urinary Tract Infections caused by *Escherichia coli, Klebsiella pneumoniae, Proteus mirabilis, Pseudomonas aeruginosa, Citrobacter diversus**, or *Enterobacter cloacae**.

NOTE: In clinical trials of complicated urinary tract infections due to *P. aeruginosa*, 12 of 16 patients had the organism eradicated from the urine after therapy with lomefloxacin. No patients had concomitant bacteremia. Serum levels of lomefloxacin do not reliably exceed the MIC of *Pseudomonas* isolates. THE SAFETY AND EFFICACY OF LOMEFLOXACIN IN TREATING PATIENTS WITH *PSEUDOMONAS* BACTEREMIA HAS NOT BEEN ESTABLISHED.

Appropriate culture and susceptibility tests should be performed before antimicrobial treatment in order to isolate and identify organisms causing infection and to determine their susceptibility to lomefloxacin. In patients with urinary tract infections, therapy with Maxaquin film-coated tablets may be initiated before results of these tests are known; once these results become available, appropriate therapy should be continued. In patients with an acute bacterial exacerbation of chronic bronchitis, therapy should not be started empirically with lomefloxacin when there is a probability the causative pathogen is *S. pneumoniae.*

Beta-lactamase production should have no effect on lomefloxacin activity.

* = Although treatment of infections due to this organism in this organ system demonstrated a clinically acceptable overall outcome, efficacy was studied in fewer than 10 infections.

PROPHYLAXIS:

Maxaquin (lomefloxacin HCl) film-coated tablets are indicated pre-operatively to reduce the incidence of urinary tract infections in the early post-operative period (3–5 days post-surgery) in patients undergoing transurethral surgical procedures. Efficacy in decreasing the incidence of infections other than urinary tract infections in the early post-operative period has not been established. Maxaquin, like all drugs for prophylaxis of transurethral surgical procedures, usually should not be used in minor urologic procedures for which prophylaxis is not indicated (e.g., simple cystoscopy or retrograde pyelography).

CONTRAINDICATIONS

Lomefloxacin is contraindicated in patients with a history of hypersensitivity to lomefloxacin or to any of the quinolone group of antimicrobial agents.

WARNINGS

THE SAFETY AND EFFICACY OF LOMEFLOXACIN IN CHILDREN, ADOLESCENTS (UNDER THE AGE OF 18 YEARS), PREGNANT WOMEN, AND LACTATING WOMEN HAVE NOT BEEN ESTABLISHED. (See PRECAUTIONS—*Pregnancy; Nursing Mothers;* and *Pediatric Use.)* The oral administration of multiple doses of lomefloxacin to juvenile dogs at 0.3 and to rats at 5.4 times the recommended adult human dose based on mg/m^2 (0.6 and 34 times the recommended adult human dose based on mg/kg, respectively) caused arthropathy and lameness. Histopathological examination of the weight-bearing joints of these animals revealed permanent lesions of the cartilage. Other quinolones also produce erosions of cartilage of weight-bearing joints and other signs of arthropathy in juvenile animals of various species. (See **Animal Pharmacology**.)

The safety and efficacy of lomefloxacin in the treatment of acute bacterial exacerbation of chronic bronchitis due to *S. pneumoniae* have not been demonstrated. This product should not be used empirically in the treatment of acute bacterial exacerbation of chronic bronchitis when it is probable that *S. pneumoniae* is a causative pathogen.

In clinical trials of complicated urinary tract infections due to *P. aeruginosa*, 12 of 16 patients had the organism eradicated from the urine after therapy with lomefloxacin. No patients had concomitant bacteremia. Serum levels of lomefloxacin do not reliably exceed the MIC of *Pseudomonas* isolates. THE SAFETY AND EFFICACY OF LOMEFLOXACIN IN TREATING PATIENTS WITH *PSEUDOMONAS* BACTEREMIA HAS NOT BEEN ESTABLISHED.

Serious and occasionally fatal hypersensitivity (anaphylactoid or anaphylactic) reactions, some following the first dose, have been reported in patients receiving quinolone therapy. Some reactions were accompanied by cardiovascular collapse, loss of consciousness, tingling, pharyngeal or facial edema, dyspnea, urticaria, or itching. Only a few of these patients had a history of previous hypersensitivity reactions. Serious hypersensitivity reactions have also been reported following treatment with lomefloxacin. If an allergic reaction to lomefloxacin occurs, discontinue the drug. Serious acute hypersensitivity reactions may require immediate emergency treatment with epinephrine. Oxygen, intravenous fluids, antihistamines, corticosteroids, pressor amines, and airway management, including intubation, should be administered as indicated.

Convulsions have been reported in patients receiving lomefloxacin. Whether the convulsions were directly related to lomefloxacin administration has not yet been established. However, convulsions, increased intracranial pressure, and toxic psychoses have been reported in patients receiving other quinolones. Quinolones may also cause central nervous system stimulation, which may lead to tremors, restlessness, lightheadedness, confusion, and hallucinations. If any of these reactions occurs in patients receiving lomefloxacin, the drug should be discontinued and appropriate measures instituted. No evidence of an effect of lomefloxacin on the electrical activity of the brain has been demonstrated. Lomefloxacin does not alter cerebral blood flow or cerebral glucose uptake in the central nervous system based on positron emission tomography. However, until more information becomes available, lomefloxacin, like all other quinolones, should be used with caution in patients with known or suspected central nervous system disorders, such as severe cerebral arteriosclerosis, epilepsy, or other factors that predispose to seizures. (See **Adverse Reactions**.)

Pseudomembranous colitis has been reported with nearly all antibacterial agents, including quinolones, and may range from mild to life-threatening in severity. Therefore, it is important to consider this diagnosis in patients who present with diarrhea subsequent to the administration of antibacterial agents. Treatment with broad-spectrum antibiotics alters the normal flora of the colon and may permit overgrowth of clostridia. Studies indicate that a toxin produced by *Clostridium difficile* is a primary cause of "antibiotic-associated colitis." After the diagnosis of pseudomembranous colitis has been established, therapeutic measures

should be initiated. Mild cases of pseudomembranous colitis usually respond to discontinuation of drug alone. In moderate to severe cases, consideration should be given to management with fluid and electrolytes, protein supplementation, and treatment with an antibacterial drug clinically effective against *C. difficile* colitis.

PRECAUTIONS

General:

Alteration of the dosage regimen is recommended for patients with impairment of renal function (Cl_{Cr} < 40 mL/min/1.73 m^2). (See **Dosage and Administration**.)

Moderate to severe phototoxicity reactions have been observed in patients exposed to excessive sunlight or artificial ultraviolet light while receiving lomefloxacin or some other quinolones. Excessive sunlight and artificial ultraviolet light should be avoided while taking lomefloxacin. Lomefloxacin therapy should be discontinued if phototoxicity occurs.

Information for patients:

Patients should be advised
* to drink fluids liberally,
* that lomefloxacin can be taken without regard to meals,
* that mineral supplements or vitamins with iron or minerals should not be taken within the 2-hour period before or after taking lomefloxacin (see **Drug Interactions**),
* that sucralfate or antacids containing magnesium or aluminum should not be taken within 4 hours before or 2 hours after taking lomefloxacin (see **Drug Interactions**),
* that lomefloxacin can cause dizziness and lightheadedness and, therefore, patients should know how they react to lomefloxacin before they operate an automobile or machinery or engage in activities requiring mental alertness and coordination,
* that lomefloxacin may be associated with hypersensitivity reactions, even following the first dose, and to discontinue the drug at the first sign of a skin rash or other allergic reaction, and
* to avoid excessive sunlight and artificial ultraviolet light while receiving lomefloxacin and to discontinue therapy if phototoxicity occurs.

Drug interactions:

Theophylline: In 3 pharmacokinetic studies including 46 normal, healthy subjects, theophylline clearance and concentration were not significantly altered by the addition of lomefloxacin. In clinical studies where patients were on chronic theophylline therapy, lomefloxacin had no measurable effect on the mean distribution of theophylline concentrations or the mean estimates of theophylline clearance. Though individual theophylline levels fluctuated, there were no clinically significant symptoms of drug interaction.

Antacids and sucralfate: Sucralfate and antacids containing magnesium or aluminum form chelation complexes with lomefloxacin and interfere with its bioavailability. Sucralfate administered 2 hours before lomefloxacin resulted in a slower rate of absorption (mean C_{max} decreased by 30% and mean T_{max} increased by 1 hour) and a lesser extent of absorption (mean AUC decreased by approximately 25%). Magnesium- and aluminum-containing antacids, administered concomitantly with lomefloxacin, significantly decreased the bioavailability (48%) of lomefloxacin. Separating the doses of antacid and lomefloxacin minimizes this decrease in bioavailability; therefore, administration of these agents should precede lomefloxacin dosing by 4 hours or follow lomefloxacin dosing by at least 2 hours.

Caffeine: One hundred mg of caffeine (equivalent to 1 to 3 cups of American coffee) was administered to 16 normal, healthy volunteers who had achieved steady-state blood concentrations of lomefloxacin after being dosed at 400 mg q.d. This did not result in any statistically or clinically relevant changes in the pharmacokinetic parameters of either caffeine or lomefloxacin. No data are available on potential interactions in individuals who consume greater than 100 mg of caffeine per day or in those, such as the geriatric population, who are generally believed to be more susceptible to the development of drug-induced central nervous system-related adverse effects. Other quinolones have demonstrated moderate to marked interference with the metabolism of caffeine, resulting in a reduced clearance, a prolongation of plasma half-life, and an increase in symptoms that accompany high levels of caffeine.

Cimetidine: Cimetidine has been demonstrated to interfere with the elimination of other quinolones. This interference has resulted in significant increases in half-life and AUC. Interaction between lomefloxacin and cimetidine has not been studied.

Cyclosporine: Elevated serum levels of cyclosporine have been reported with concomitant use of cyclosporine with other members of the quinolone class. Interaction between lomefloxacin and cyclosporine has not been studied.

Non-steroidal anti-inflammatory drugs (NSAID's): Concomitant administration of the NSAID, fenbufen, with some quinolones has been reported to increase the risk of CNS stimulation and convulsive seizures.

There was an increase in the incidence of seizures in mice treated with fenbufen, when fenbufen was administered to mice that had been concomitantly treated with a dose of

lomefloxacin equivalent to the recommended human dose on a mg/m^2 basis (10 times the recommended human dose on a mg/kg basis). Fenbufen is not presently an approved drug in the United States. (See **Animal Pharmacology**).

Probenecid: Probenecid slows the renal elimination of lomefloxacin. An increase of 63% in the mean AUC and increases of 50% and 4%, respectively, in the mean T_{max} and mean C_{max} were noted in 1 study of 6 individuals.

Warfarin: Quinolones may enhance the effects of the oral anticoagulant, warfarin, or its derivatives. When these products are administered concomitantly, prothrombin or other suitable coagulation test should be monitored closely.

Carcinogenesis, mutagenesis, impairment of fertility:

Carcinogenesis: Long-term carcinogenicity studies of lomefloxacin in animals have not been performed.

Mutagenesis: One *in vitro* mutagenicity test (CHO/HGPRT assay) was weakly positive at lomefloxacin concentrations of 226 μg/mL and greater and negative at concentrations less than 226 μg/mL. Two other *in vitro* mutagenicity tests (chromosomal aberrations in Chinese hamster ovary cells, chromosomal aberrations in human lymphocytes) and two *in vivo* mouse micronucleus mutagenicity tests were all negative.

Impairment of Fertility: Lomefloxacin did not affect the fertility of male and female rats at oral doses up to 8 times the recommended human dose based on mg/m^2 (34 times the recommended human dose based on mg/kg).

Pregnancy: Teratogenic Effects. Pregnancy Category C.

Reproductive function studies have been performed in rats at doses up to 8 times the recommended human dose based on mg/m^2 (34 times the recommended human dose based on mg/kg), and no impaired fertility or harm to the fetus was reported due to lomefloxacin. Increased incidence of fetal loss in monkeys has been observed at approximately 3 to 6 times the recommended human dose based on mg/m^2 (6 to 12 times the recommended human dose based on mg/kg). No teratogenicity has been observed in rats and monkeys at up to 16 times the recommended human dose exposure. In the rabbit, maternal toxicity and associated fetotoxicity, decreased placental weight, and variations of the coccygeal vertebrae occurred at doses 2 times the recommended human exposure based on mg/m^2. There are, however, no adequate and well-controlled studies in pregnant women. Lomefloxacin should be used during pregnancy only if the potential benefit justifies the potential risk to the fetus.

Nursing mothers:

It is not known whether lomefloxacin is excreted in human milk. However, it is known that other drugs of this class are excreted in human milk and that lomefloxacin is excreted in the milk of lactating rats. Because of the potential for serious adverse reactions from lomefloxacin in nursing infants, a decision should be made whether to discontinue nursing or to discontinue the drug, taking into account the importance of the drug to the mother.

Pediatric use:

The safety and effectiveness of lomefloxacin in children and adolescents below the age of 18 years have not been established. Lomefloxacin causes arthropathy in juvenile animals of several species. (See **Warnings** and **Animal Pharmacology**.)

Geriatric use:

Of the total number of patients in clinical studies of lomefloxacin, 26% were ≥ 65 years of age. No overall differences in effectiveness or safety were observed between these patients and younger patients. (See **Clinical Pharmacology—Pharmacokinetics in the Geriatric Population**.)

ADVERSE REACTIONS

In clinical trials, most of the adverse events reported were mild to moderate in severity and transient in nature. During these clinical investigations, 2869 patients received Maxaquin. In 2.6% of the patients, lomefloxacin was discontinued because of adverse events, primarily involving the gastrointestinal system (0.7%), skin (1.0%), or central nervous system (0.5%).

Adverse Clinical Events: The events with the highest incidence (≥ 1%) in patients, regardless of relationship to drug, were nausea (3.7%), headache (3.2%), photosensitivity (2.4%), dizziness (2.3%), and diarrhea (1.4%).

Additional clinical events reported in less than 1% of patients treated with Maxaquin, regardless of relationship to drug, are listed below:

Autonomic: dry mouth, flushing, increased sweating.

Body as a Whole: fatigue, back pain, malaise, asthenia, chest pain, chills, allergic reaction, face edema, influenza-like symptoms, decreased heat tolerance.

Cardiovascular: hypotension, hypertension, edema, syncope, tachycardia, bradycardia, arrhythmia, extrasystoles, cyanosis, cardiac failure, angina pectoris, myocardial infarction, pulmonary embolism, cerebrovascular disorder, cardiomyopathy, phlebitis.

Central Nervous System: convulsions, coma, hyperkinesia, tremor, vertigo, paresthesias.

Continued on next page

Searle—Cont.

Gastrointestinal: abdominal pain, dyspepsia, vomiting, flatulence, constipation, gastrointestinal inflammation, dysphagia, gastrointestinal bleeding, tongue discoloration.
Hearing: earache, tinnitus.
Hematologic: thrombocytopenia, thrombocythemia, purpura, lymphadenopathy, increased fibrinolysis.
Metabolic: thirst, gout, hypoglycemia.
Musculoskeletal: leg cramps, arthralgia, myalgia.
Ophthalmologic: abnormal vision, conjunctivitis, eye pain.
Psychiatric: somnolence, insomnia, nervousness, anorexia, confusion, anxiety, depression, agitation, increased appetite, depersonalization, paroniria.
Reproductive System: Female: vaginitis, leukorrhea, intermenstrual bleeding, perineal pain, vaginal moniliasis. Male: orchitis, epididymitis.
Respiratory: dyspnea, respiratory infection, epistaxis, respiratory disorder, bronchospasm, cough, increased sputum, stridor.
Skin/Allergic: pruritus, rash, urticaria, eczema, skin exfoliation, skin disorder.
Special Senses: taste perversion.
Urinary: dysuria, hematuria, strangury, micturition disorder, anuria.
Adverse Laboratory Events: Changes in laboratory parameters, listed as adverse events, without regard to drug relationship include:
Hepatic: elevations of ALT (SGPT) (0.4%), AST (SGOT) (0.3%), bilirubin (0.1%), alkaline phosphatase (0.1%).
Hematologic: monocytosis (0.3%), elevated ESR (0.1%).
Renal: elevated BUN (0.1%), decreased potassium (0.1%).
Additional laboratory changes occurring in ≤0.1% in the clinical studies included: elevation of serum gamma glutamyl transferase, decrease in total protein or albumin, prolongation of prothrombin time, anemia, decrease in hemoglobin, leukopenia, eosinophilia, thrombocytopenia, abnormalities of urine specific gravity or serum electrolytes, decrease in blood glucose.
Quinolone-class Adverse Events: Although not reported in completed clinical studies with Maxaquin, a variety of adverse events have been reported with other quinolones.
Clinical adverse events include: anaphylactoid reactions, erythema nodosum, Stevens-Johnson syndrome, exfoliative dermatitis, toxic epidermal necrolysis, hepatic necrosis, possible exacerbation of myasthenia gravis, dysphasia, nystagmus, pseudomembranous colitis, painful oral mucosa, intestinal perforation, hallucinations, manic reaction, ataxia, phobia, hyperpigmentation, diplopia, interstitial nephritis, renal failure, renal calculi, polyuria, urinary retention, acidosis, cardiopulmonary arrest, cerebral thrombosis, laryngeal or pulmonary edema, hiccough, dysgeusia, and photophobia.
Laboratory adverse events include: agranulocytosis, elevation of serum triglycerides, elevation of serum cholesterol, elevation of blood glucose, elevation of serum potassium, albuminuria, candiduria, and crystalluria.

OVERDOSAGE
Information on overdosage in humans is limited. In the event of acute overdosage, the stomach should be emptied by inducing vomiting or by gastric lavage, and the patient should be carefully observed and given supportive treatment. Adequate hydration must be maintained. Hemodialysis or peritoneal dialysis is unlikely to aid in the removal of lomefloxacin as less than 3% is removed by these modalities.
Clinical signs of acute toxicity in rodents progressed from salivation to tremors, decreased activity, dyspnea, and clonic convulsions prior to death. These signs were noted in rats and mice as lomefloxacin doses were increased.

DOSAGE AND ADMINISTRATION
Maxaquin (lomefloxacin HCl) may be taken without regard to meals. (See **Clinical Pharmacology.**)
See **Indications and Usage** for information on appropriate pathogens and patient populations.
TREATMENT:
Patients with Normal Renal Function: The recommended daily dose of Maxaquin is described in the following chart: [See table below.]

Elderly Patients: No dosage adjustment is needed for elderly patients with normal renal function (Cl$_{cr}$ ≥ 40 mL/min/1.73 m^2).
Patients with Impaired Renal Function: Lomefloxacin is primarily eliminated by renal excretion. (See *Clinical Pharmacology.*) Modification of dosage is recommended in patients with renal dysfunction. In patients with a creatinine clearance greater than 10 but less than 40 mL/min/1.73 m^2, the recommended dosage is an initial loading dose of 400 mg followed by daily maintenance doses of 200 mg (½ tablet) once daily for the duration of treatment. It is suggested that serial determinations of lomefloxacin levels be performed to determine any necessary alteration in the appropriate next dosing interval.
If only the serum creatinine is known, the following formula may be used to estimate creatinine clearance.

Men: $\dfrac{\text{(weight in kg)} \times (140 - \text{age})}{(72) \times \text{serum creatinine (mg/dL)}}$

Women: $(0.85) \times$ (calculated value for men)

Dialysis patients: Hemodialysis removes only a negligible amount of lomefloxacin (3% in 4 hours). Hemodialysis patients should receive an initial loading dose of 400 mg followed by daily maintenance doses of 200 mg (½ tablet) once daily for the duration of treatment.
Patients with Cirrhosis: Cirrhosis does not reduce the non-renal clearance of lomefloxacin. The need for a dosage reduction in this population should be based on the degree of renal function of the patient and on the plasma concentrations. (See **Clinical Pharmacology** and **Dosage and Administration**—Impaired Renal Function.)
PROPHYLAXIS:
A single dose of 400 mg of Maxaquin should be administered orally 2 to 6 hours prior to surgery when oral pre-operative prophylaxis for transurethral surgical procedures is considered appropriate.

HOW SUPPLIED
Maxaquin (lomefloxacin HCl) is supplied as a scored, film-coated tablet containing the equivalent of 400 mg of lomefloxacin base present as the hydrochloride. The tablet is oval, white, and film-coated with "MAXAQUIN 400" debossed on one side and scored on the other side and is supplied in:

NDC Number	Size
0025-1651-20	bottle of 20
0025-1651-34	carton of 100 unit dose

Store at 59° to 86°F (15° to 30°C).

Caution: Federal law prohibits dispensing without prescription.

ANIMAL PHARMACOLOGY
Lomefloxacin and other quinolones have been shown to cause arthropathy in juvenile animals. Arthropathy, involving multiple diarthrodial joints, was observed in juvenile dogs administered lomefloxacin at doses as low as 4.5 mg/kg for 7 to 8 days (0.3 times the recommended human dose based on mg/m^2 or 0.6 times the recommended human dose based on mg/kg). In juvenile rats, no changes were observed in the joints with doses up to 91 mg/kg for 7 days (2 times the recommended human dose based on mg/m^2 or 11 times the recommended human dose based on mg/kg). (See **Warnings.**)
In a 13-week oral rat study, gamma globulin decreased when lomefloxacin was administered at less than the recommended human exposure. Beta globulin decreased when lomefloxacin was administered at 0.6 to 2 times the recommended human dose based on mg/m^2. The A/G ratio increased when lomefloxacin was administered at 6 to 20 times the human dose. Following a 4-week recovery period, beta globulins in the females and A/G ratios in the females returned to control values. Gamma globulin values in the females and beta and gamma globulins and A/G ratios in the males were still statistically significantly different from control values. No effects on globulins were seen in oral studies in dogs or monkeys in the limited number of specimens collected.
Twenty-seven NSAID's, administered concomitantly with lomefloxacin, were tested for seizure induction in mice at approximately 2 times the recommended human dose based on mg/m^2. At a dose of lomefloxacin equivalent to the recommended human exposure based on mg/m^2 (10 times the human dose based on mg/kg), only fenbufen, when co-administered, produced an increase in seizures.

Crystalluria and ocular toxicity, seen with some related quinolones, were not observed in any lomefloxacin-treated animals, either in studies designed to look for these effects specifically or in subchronic and chronic toxicity studies in rats, dogs, and monkeys.
Long-term, high-dose systemic use of other quinolones in related animals has caused lenticular opacities; however, this finding was not observed with lomefloxacin.

REFERENCES
1. National Committee for Clinical Laboratory Standards, *Performance Standards for Antimicrobial Disk Susceptibility Tests*—Fourth Edition. Approved Standard NCCLS Document M2-A4, Vol. 10, No. 7, NCCLS, Villanova, PA, 1990. **2.** National Committee for Clinical Laboratory Standards, *Methods for Dilution Antimicrobial Susceptibility Tests for Bacteria that Grow Aerobically*—Second Edition. Approved Standard NCCLS Document M7-A2, Vol. 10, No. 8, NCCLS, Villanova, PA, 1990.

3/2/92 ● A05215

Shown in Product Identification Section, page 429

NITRODISC®   ℞
[nī'trō'disc]
(nitroglycerin transdermal system)
0.2 mg/hr; 0.3 mg/hr; 0.4 mg/hr

DESCRIPTION
Nitroglycerin is 1,2,3-propanetriol trinitrate, an organic nitrate whose structural formula is

$$
\begin{array}{c}
H_2CONO_2 \\
| \\
HCONO_2 \\
| \\
H_2CONO_2
\end{array}
$$

and whose molecular weight is 227.09. The organic nitrates are vasodilators, active on both arteries and veins.
Nitrodisc (nitroglycerin transdermal system) is a unit designed to provide continuous controlled release of nitroglycerin through intact skin. The rate of release of nitroglycerin is linearly dependent upon the active area of the applied system; each cm^2 of applied system delivers approximately 0.026 mg of nitroglycerin per hour. Thus, the 8-, 12-, and 16-cm^2 systems deliver approximately 0.2, 0.3, and 0.4 mg of nitroglycerin per hour, respectively.
The remainder of the nitroglycerin in each system serves as a reservoir and is not delivered in normal use. After 12 hours, for example, each system has delivered 15% of its original content of nitroglycerin.
Inactive ingredients are lactose, isopropyl palmitate, mineral oil, polyethylene glycol, water, silicone rubber, plasticizers, aluminum foil laminate, polyethylene foam, and acrylic adhesive.
Nitrodisc incorporates a patented Microseal Drug Delivery™ system consisting of a solid, nitroglycerin-impregnated polymer bonded to a flexible, nonsensitizing adhesive bandage.

CLINICAL PHARMACOLOGY
The principal pharmacologic action of nitroglycerin is relaxation of vascular smooth muscle and consequent dilatation of peripheral arteries and veins, especially the latter. Dilatation of the veins promotes peripheral pooling of blood and decreases venous return to the heart, thereby reducing left ventricular end-diastolic pressure and pulmonary capillary wedge pressure (preload). Arteriolar relaxation reduces systemic vascular resistance, systolic arterial pressure, and mean arterial pressure (afterload). Dilatation of the coronary arteries also occurs. The relative importance of preload reduction, afterload reduction, and coronary dilatation remains undefined.
Dosing regimens for most chronically used drugs are designed to provide plasma concentrations that are continuously greater than a minimally effective concentration. This strategy is inappropriate for organic nitrates. Several well-controlled clinical trials have used exercise testing to assess the antianginal efficacy of continuously delivered nitrates. In the large majority of these trials, active agents were indistinguishable from placebo after 24 hours (or less) of continuous therapy. Attempts to overcome nitrate tolerance by dose escalation, even to doses far in excess of those used acutely, have consistently failed. Only after nitrates have been absent from the body for several hours has their antianginal efficacy been restored.
Pharmacokinetics: The volume of distribution of nitroglycerin is about 3 L/kg, and nitroglycerin is cleared from this volume at extremely rapid rates, with a resulting serum half-life of about 3 minutes. The observed clearance rates (close to 1 L/kg/min) greatly exceed hepatic blood flow; known sites of extrahepatic metabolism include red blood cells and vascular walls.
The first products in the metabolism of nitroglycerin are inorganic nitrate and the 1,2- and 1,3-dinitroglycerols. The dinitrates are less effective vasodilators than nitroglycerin,

Body System	Infection	Unit Dose	Frequency	Duration	Daily Dose
Lower respiratory tract	Acute bacterial exacerbation of chronic bronchitis	400 mg	q.d.	10 days	400 mg
Urinary tract	Cystitis	400 mg	q.d.	10 days	400 mg
	Complicated Urinary Tract Infections	400 mg	q.d.	14 days	400 mg

but they are longer-lived in the serum, and their net contribution to the overall effect of chronic nitroglycerin regimens is not known. The dinitrates are further metabolized to (nonvasoactive) mononitrates and, ultimately, to glycerol and carbon dioxide.

To avoid development of tolerance to nitroglycerin, drug-free intervals of 10 to 12 hours are known to be sufficient; shorter intervals have not been well studied. In one well-controlled clinical trial, subjects receiving nitroglycerin appeared to exhibit a rebound or withdrawal effect, so that their exercise tolerance at the end of the daily drug-free interval was *less* than that exhibited by the parallel group receiving placebo.

In healthy volunteers, steady-state plasma concentrations of nitroglycerin are reached by about 2 hours after application of a patch and are maintained for the duration of wearing the system (observations have been limited to 24 hours). Upon removal of the patch, the plasma concentration declines with a half-life of about an hour.

Clinical trials: Regimens in which nitroglycerin patches were worn for 12 hours daily have been studied in well-controlled trials up to 4 weeks in duration. Starting about 2 hours after application and continuing until 10 to 12 hours after application, patches that deliver at least 0.4 mg of nitroglycerin per hour have consistently demonstrated greater antianginal activity than placebo. Lower-dose patches have not been as well studied, but in one large, well-controlled trial in which higher-dose patches were also studied, patches delivering 0.2 mg/hr had significantly *less* antianginal activity than placebo.

It is reasonable to believe that the rate of nitroglycerin absorption from patches may vary with the site of application, but this relationship has not been adequately studied.

The onset of action of transdermal nitroglycerin is not sufficiently rapid for this product to be useful in aborting an acute anginal episode.

INDICATIONS AND USAGE

This drug product has been conditionally approved by the FDA for the prevention of angina pectoris due to coronary artery disease. Tolerance to the antianginal effects of nitrates (measured by exercise stress testing) has been shown to be a major factor limiting efficacy when transdermal nitrates are used continuously for longer than 12 hours each day. The development of tolerance can be altered (prevented or attenuated) by use of a noncontinuous (intermittent) dosing schedule with a nitrate-free interval of 10 to 12 hours.

Controlled clinical trial data suggest that the intermittent use of nitrates is associated with decreased exercise tolerance, in comparison to placebo, during the last part of the nitrate-free interval; the clinical relevance of this observation is unknown, but the possibility of increased frequency or severity of angina during the nitrate-free interval should be considered. Further investigations of the tolerance phenomenon and best regimen are ongoing. A final evaluation of the effectiveness of the product will be announced by the FDA.

CONTRAINDICATIONS

Allergic reactions to organic nitrates are extremely rare, but they do occur. Nitroglycerin is contraindicated in patients who are allergic to it. Allergy to the adhesives used in nitroglycerin patches has also been reported, and it similarly constitutes a contraindication to the use of this product.

WARNINGS

The benefits of transdermal nitroglycerin in patients with acute myocardial infarction or congestive heart failure have not been established. If one elects to use nitroglycerin in these conditions, careful clinical or hemodynamic monitoring must be used to avoid the hazards of hypotension and tachycardia.

A cardiovertor/defibrillator should not be discharged through a paddle electrode that overlies a Nitrodisc patch. The arcing that may be seen in this situation is harmless in itself, but it may be associated with local current concentration that can cause damage to the paddles and burns to the patient.

PRECAUTIONS

General: Severe hypotension, particularly with upright posture, may occur with even small doses of nitroglycerin. This drug should, therefore, be used with caution in patients who may be volume depleted or who, for whatever reason, are already hypotensive. Hypotension induced by nitroglycerin may be accompanied by paradoxical bradycardia and increased angina pectoris.

Nitrate therapy may aggravate the angina caused by hypertrophic cardiomyopathy.

As tolerance to other forms of nitroglycerin develops, the effect of sublingual nitroglycerin on exercise tolerance, although still observable, is somewhat blunted.

In industrial workers who have had long-term exposure to unknown (presumably high) doses of organic nitrates, toler-

ance clearly occurs. Chest pain, acute myocardial infarction, and even sudden death have occurred during temporary withdrawal of nitrates from these workers, demonstrating the existence of true physical dependence.

Several clinical trials in patients with angina pectoris have evaluated nitroglycerin regimens which incorporated a 10 to 12 hour nitrate-free interval. In some of these trials, an increase in the frequency of anginal attacks during the nitrate-free interval was observed in a small number of patients. In one trial, patients demonstrated decreased exercise tolerance at the end of the nitrate-free interval. Hemodynamic rebound has been observed only rarely; on the other hand, few studies were so designed that rebound, if it had occurred, would have been detected. The importance of these observations to the routine, clinical use of transdermal nitroglycerin is unknown.

Information for patients: Daily headaches sometimes accompany treatment with nitroglycerin. In patients who get these headaches, the headaches may be a marker of the activity of the drug. Patients should resist the temptation to avoid headaches by altering the schedule of their treatment with nitroglycerin, since loss of headache may be associated with simultaneous loss of antianginal efficacy.

Treatment with nitroglycerin may be associated with lightheadedness on standing, especially just after rising from a recumbent or seated position. This effect may be more frequent in patients who have also consumed alcohol.

After normal use, there is enough residual nitroglycerin in discarded patches that they are a potential hazard to children and pets.

A patient leaflet is supplied with each carton.

Drug interactions: The vasodilating effects of nitroglycerin may be additive with those of other vasodilators. Alcohol, in particular, has been found to exhibit additive effects of this variety.

Carcinogenesis, mutagenesis, and impairment of fertility: No long-term animal studies have examined the carcinogenic or mutagenic potential of nitroglycerin. Nitroglycerin's effect upon reproductive capacity is similarly unknown.

Pregnancy: Pregnancy Category C. Animal reproduction studies have not been conducted with nitroglycerin. It is also not known whether nitroglycerin can cause fetal harm when administered to a pregnant woman or whether it can affect reproductive capacity. Nitroglycerin should be given to a pregnant woman only if clearly needed.

Nursing mothers: It is not known whether nitroglycerin is excreted in human milk. Because many drugs are excreted in human milk, caution should be exercised when nitroglycerin is administered to a nursing woman.

Pediatric use: Safety and effectiveness in children have not been established.

ADVERSE REACTIONS

Adverse reactions to nitroglycerin are generally dose-related, and almost all of these reactions are the result of nitroglycerin's activity as a vasodilator. Headache, which may be severe, is the most commonly reported side effect. Headache may be recurrent with each daily dose, especially at higher doses. Transient episodes of light-headedness, occasionally related to blood pressure changes, may also occur. Hypotension occurs infrequently, but in some patients it may be severe enough to warrant discontinuation of therapy. Syncope, crescendo angina, and rebound hypertension have been reported but are uncommon.

Extremely rarely, ordinary doses of organic nitrates have caused methemoglobinemia in normal-seeming patients. Methemoglobinemia is so infrequent at these doses that further discussion of its diagnosis and treatment is deferred (see *Overdosage*).

Application-site irritation may occur but is rarely severe.

In two placebo-controlled trials of intermittent therapy with nitroglycerin patches at 0.2 to 0.8 mg/hr, the most frequent adverse reactions among 307 subjects were as follows:

	placebo	patch
headache	18%	63%
light-headedness	4%	6%
hypotension and/or syncope	0%	4%
increased angina	2%	2%

OVERDOSAGE

Hemodynamic effects: The ill effects of nitroglycerin overdose are generally the result of nitroglycerin's capacity to induce vasodilatation, venous pooling, reduced cardiac output, and hypotension. These hemodynamic changes may have protean manifestations, including increased intracranial pressure, with any or all of persistent throbbing headache, confusion, and moderate fever; vertigo; palpitations; visual disturbances; nausea and vomiting (possibly with colic and even bloody diarrhea); syncope (especially in the upright posture); air hunger and dyspnea, later followed by reduced ventilatory effort; diaphoresis, with the skin either flushed or cold and clammy; heart block and bradycardia; paralysis; coma; seizures; and death.

Laboratory determinations of serum levels of nitroglycerin and its metabolites are not widely available, and such determinations have, in any event, no established role in the management of nitroglycerin overdose.

No data are available to suggest physiologic maneuvers (eg, maneuvers to change the pH of the urine) that might accelerate elimination of nitroglycerin and its active metabolites. Similarly, it is not known which—if any—of these substances can usefully be removed from the body by hemodialysis.

No specific antagonist to the vasodilator effects of nitroglycerin is known, and no intervention has been subject to controlled study as a therapy of nitroglycerin overdose. Because the hypotension associated with nitroglycerin overdose is the result of venodilatation and arterial hypovolemia, prudent therapy in this situation should be directed toward increase in central fluid volume. Passive elevation of the patient's legs may be sufficient, but intravenous infusion of normal saline or similar fluid may also be necessary.

The use of epinephrine or other arterial vasoconstrictors in this setting is likely to do more harm than good.

In patients with renal disease or congestive heart failure, therapy resulting in central volume expansion is not without hazard. Treatment of nitroglycerin overdose in these patients may be subtle and difficult, and invasive monitoring may be required.

Methemoglobinemia: Nitrate ions liberated during metabolism of nitroglycerin can oxidize hemoglobin into methemoglobin. Even in patients totally without cytochrome b_5 reductase activity, however, and even assuming that the nitrate moieties of nitroglycerin are quantitatively applied to oxidation of hemoglobin, about 1 mg/kg of nitroglycerin should be required before any of these patients manifest clinically significant ($\geq 10\%$) methemoglobinemia. In patients with normal reductase function, significant production of methemoglobin should require even larger doses of nitroglycerin. In one study in which 36 patients received 2 to 4 weeks of continuous nitroglycerin therapy at 3.1 to 4.4 mg/hr, the average methemoglobin level measured was 0.2%; this was comparable to that observed in parallel patients who received placebo.

Notwithstanding these observations, there are case reports of significant methemoglobinemia in association with moderate overdoses of organic nitrates. None of the affected patients had been thought to be unusually susceptible.

Methemoglobin levels are available from most clinical laboratories. The diagnosis should be suspected in patients who exhibit signs of impaired oxygen delivery despite adequate cardiac output and adequate arterial pO_2. Classically, methemoglobinemic blood is described as chocolate brown, without color change on exposure to air.

When methemoglobinemia is diagnosed, the treatment of choice is methylene blue, 1 to 2 mg/kg intravenously.

DOSAGE AND ADMINISTRATION

The suggested starting dose is between 0.2 mg/hr and 0.4 mg/hr. Doses between 0.4 mg/hr and 0.8 mg/hr have shown continued effectiveness for 10 to 12 hours daily for at least 1 month (the longest period studied) of intermittent administration. Although the minimum nitrate-free interval has not been defined, data show that a nitrate-free interval of 10 to 12 hours is sufficient (see *Clinical Pharmacology*). Thus, an appropriate dosing schedule for nitroglycerin patches would include a daily patch-on period of 12 to 14 hours and a daily patch-off period of 10 to 12 hours.

Although some well-controlled clinical trials using exercise tolerance testing have shown maintenance of effectiveness when patches are worn continuously, the large majority of such controlled trials have shown the development of tolerance (ie, complete loss of effect) within the first 24 hours after therapy was initiated. Dose adjustment, even to levels much higher than generally used, did not restore efficacy.

HOW SUPPLIED

Nitroglycerin Transdermal Rated Release *In Vivo*	Total Nitroglycerin In System	System Size	Carton Size
0.2 mg/hr	16 mg	8 cm²	30 Discs NDC 0025-2058-30
			100 Discs* NDC 0025-2058-31
0.3 mg/hr	24 mg	12 cm²	30 Discs NDC 0025-2078-30
			100 Discs* NDC 0025-2078-31
0.4 mg/hr	32 mg	16 cm²	30 Discs NDC 0025-2068-30
			100 Discs* NDC 0025-2068-31

*Institutional Packs

Continued on next page

Searle—Cont.

Store at a controlled room temperature of 59°–86°F (15°–30°C). **Do not refrigerate.** Extremes of temperature and/or humidity should be avoided.
Caution: Federal law prohibits dispensing without prescription.

2/7/91 ● A05582-4

Shown in Product Identification Section, page 429

NORPACE® Capsules ℞
[*nor'pāce*]
(disopyramide phosphate)

NORPACE® CR Capsules ℞
(disopyramide phosphate extended-release)

DESCRIPTION

Norpace (disopyramide phosphate) is an antiarrhythmic drug available for oral administration in immediate-release and controlled-release capsules containing 100 mg or 150 mg of disopyramide base, present as the phosphate. The base content of the phosphate salt is 77.6%. The structural formula of Norpace is:

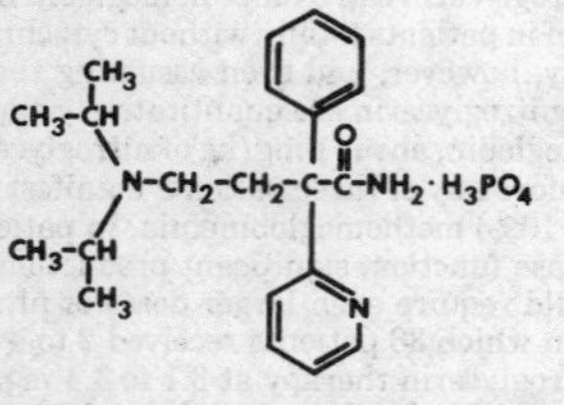

α-[2-(diisopropylamino) ethyl]-α-phenyl-2-pyridine-acetamide phosphate

Norpace is freely soluble in water, and the free base (pKa 10.4) has an aqueous solubility of 1 mg/ml. The chloroform: water partition coefficient of the base is 3.1 at pH 7.2.
Norpace is a racemic mixture of *d*- and *l*-isomers. This drug is not chemically related to other antiarrhythmic drugs.
Norpace CR (controlled-release) capsules are designed to afford a gradual and consistent release of disopyramide. Thus, for maintenance therapy, Norpace CR provides the benefit of less-frequent dosing (every 12 hours) as compared with the every-6-hour dosage schedule of immediate-release Norpace capsules.
Inactive ingredients of Norpace include corn starch, edible ink, FD&C Red No. 3, FD&C Yellow No. 6, gelatin, lactose, talc, and titanium dioxide; the 150-mg capsule also contains FD&C Blue No. 1.
Inactive ingredients of Norpace CR include corn starch, D&C Yellow No. 10, edible ink, ethylcellulose, FD&C Blue No. 1, gelatin, shellac, sucrose, talc, and titanium dioxide; the 150-mg capsule also contains FD&C Red No. 3 and FD&C Yellow No. 6.

CLINICAL PHARMACOLOGY

Mechanisms of Action
Norpace (disopyramide phosphate) is a Type 1 antiarrhythmic drug (ie, similar to procainamide and quinidine). *In animal studies* Norpace decreases the rate of diastolic depolarization (phase 4) in cells with augmented automaticity, decreases the upstroke velocity (phase 0) and increases the action potential duration of normal cardiac cells, decreases the disparity in refractoriness between infarcted and adjacent normally perfused myocardium, and has no effect on alpha- or beta-adrenergic receptors.
Electrophysiology
In man, Norpace at therapeutic plasma levels shortens the sinus node recovery time, lengthens the effective refractory period of the atrium, and has a minimal effect on the effective refractory period of the AV node. Little effect has been shown on AV-nodal and His-Purkinje conduction times or QRS duration. However, prolongation of conduction in accessory pathways occurs.
Hemodynamics
At recommended oral doses, Norpace rarely produces significant alterations of blood pressure in patients without congestive heart failure (see *Warnings*). With intravenous Norpace, either increases in systolic/diastolic or decreases in systolic blood pressure have been reported, depending on the infusion rate and the patient population. Intravenous Norpace may cause cardiac depression with an approximate mean 10% reduction of cardiac output, which is more pronounced in patients with cardiac dysfunction.
Anticholinergic Activity
The *in vitro* anticholinergic activity of Norpace is approximately 0.06% that of atropine; however, the usual dose for Norpace is 150 mg every 6 hours and for Norpace CR 300 mg every 12 hours, compared to 0.4 to 0.6 mg for atropine (see *Warnings* and *Adverse Reactions* for anticholinergic side effects).
Pharmacokinetics
Following oral administration of immediate-release Norpace, disopyramide phosphate is rapidly and almost completely absorbed, and peak plasma levels are usually attained within 2 hours. The usual therapeutic plasma levels of disopyramide base are 2 to 4 mcg/ml, and at these concentrations protein binding varies from 50% to 65%. Because of concentration-dependent protein binding, it is difficult to predict the concentration of the free drug when total drug is measured.
The mean plasma half-life of disopyramide in healthy humans is 6.7 hours (range of 4 to 10 hours). In six patients with impaired renal function (creatinine clearance less than 40 ml/min), disopyramide half-life values were 8 to 18 hours.

After the oral administration of 200 mg of disopyramide to 10 cardiac patients with borderline to moderate heart failure, the time to peak serum concentration of 2.3 ± 1.5 hours (mean ± SD) was increased, and the mean peak serum concentration of 4.8 ± 1.6 mcg/ml was higher than in healthy volunteers. After intravenous administration in these same patients, the mean elimination half-life was 9.7 ± 4.2 hours (range in healthy volunteers of 4.4 to 7.8 hours). In a second study of the oral administration of disopyramide to 7 patients with heart disease, including left ventricular dysfunction, the mean plasma half-life was slightly prolonged to 7.8 ± 1.9 hours (range of 5 to 9.5 hours).
In healthy men, about 50% of a given dose of disopyramide is excreted in the urine as the unchanged drug, about 20% as the mono-N-dealkylated metabolite, and 10% as the other metabolites. The plasma concentration of the major metabolite is approximately one tenth that of disopyramide. Altering the urinary pH in man does not affect the plasma half-life of disopyramide.
In a crossover study in healthy subjects, the bioavailability of disopyramide from Norpace CR capsules was similar to that from the immediate-release capsules. With a single 300-mg oral dose, peak disopyramide plasma concentrations of 3.23 ± 0.75 mcg/ml (mean ± SD) at 2.5 ± 2.3 hours were obtained with two 150-mg immediate-release capsules and 2.22 ± 0.47 mcg/ml at 4.9 ± 1.4 hours with two 150-mg Norpace CR capsules. The elimination half-life of disopyramide was 8.31 ± 1.83 hours with the immediate-release capsules and 11.65 ± 4.72 hours with Norpace CR capsules. The amount of disopyramide and mono-N-dealkylated metabolite excreted in the urine in 48 hours was 128 and 48 mg, respectively, with the immediate-release capsules, and 112 and 33 mg, respectively, with Norpace CR capsules. The differences in the urinary excretion of either constituent were not statistically significant.
Following multiple doses, steady-state plasma levels of between 2 and 4 mcg/ml were attained following either 150 mg every-6-hour dosing with immediate-release capsules or 300 mg every-12-hour dosing with Norpace CR capsules.

INDICATIONS AND USAGE

Norpace and Norpace CR are indicated for the treatment of documented ventricular arrhythmias, such as sustained ventricular tachycardia, that, in the judgment of the physician, are life-threatening. Because of the proarrhythmic effects of Norpace and Norpace CR, their use with lesser arrhythmias is generally not recommended. Treatment of patients with asymptomatic ventricular premature contractions should be avoided.
Initiation of Norpace or Norpace CR treatment, as with other antiarrhythmic agents used to treat life-threatening arrhythmias, should be carried out in the hospital. Norpace CR should not be used initially if rapid establishment of disopyramide plasma levels is desired.
Antiarrhythmic drugs have not been shown to enhance survival in patients with ventricular arrhythmias.

CONTRAINDICATIONS

Norpace and Norpace CR are contraindicated in the presence of cardiogenic shock, preexisting second- or third-degree AV block (if no pacemaker is present), congenital Q-T prolongation, or known hypersensitivity to the drug.

WARNINGS

Mortality:

In the National Heart, Lung and Blood Institute's Cardiac Arrhythmia Suppression Trial (CAST), a long-term, multicentered, randomized, double-blind study in patients with asymptomatic non-life-threatening ventricular arrhythmias who had had myocardial infarctions more than 6 days but less than 2 years previously, an excessive mortality or non-fatal cardiac arrest rate was seen in patients treated with encainide or flecainide (56/730) compared with that seen in patients assigned to matched placebo-treated groups (22/725). The average duration of treatment with encainide or flecainide in this study was 10 months.
The applicability of these results to other populations (eg, those without recent myocardial infarctions) or to other antiarrhythmic drugs is uncertain, but at present it is prudent to consider any antiarrhythmic agent to have a significant risk in patients with structural heart disease.

Negative Inotropic Properties:

Heart Failure/Hypotension
Norpace or Norpace CR may cause or worsen congestive heart failure or produce severe hypotension as a consequence of its negative inotropic properties. Hypotension has been observed primarily in patients with primary cardiomyopathy or inadequately compensated congestive heart failure. Norpace or Norpace CR should not be used in patients with uncompensated or marginally compensated congestive heart failure or hypotension unless the congestive heart failure or hypotension is secondary to cardiac arrhythmia. Patients with a history of heart failure may be treated with Norpace or Norpace CR, but careful attention must be given to the maintenance of cardiac function, including optimal digitalization. If hypotension occurs or congestive heart failure worsens, Norpace or Norpace CR should be discontinued and, if necessary, restarted at a lower dosage only after adequate cardiac compensation has been established.
QRS Widening
Although it is unusual, significant widening (greater than 25%) of the QRS complex may occur during Norpace or Norpace CR administration; in such cases Norpace or Norpace CR should be discontinued.
Q-T Prolongation
As with other Type 1 antiarrhythmic drugs, prolongation of the Q-T interval (corrected) and worsening of the arrhythmia, including ventricular tachycardia and ventricular fibrillation, may occur. Patients who have evidenced prolongation of the Q-T interval in response to quinidine may be at particular risk. As with other Type 1A antiarrhythmics, disopyramide phosphate has been associated with torsade de pointes.
If a Q-T prolongation of greater than 25% is observed and if ectopy continues, the patient should be monitored closely, and consideration be given to discontinuing Norpace or Norpace CR.
Hypoglycemia
In rare instances significant lowering of blood glucose values has been reported during Norpace administration. The physician should be alert to this possibility, especially in patients with congestive heart failure, chronic malnutrition, hepatic, renal, or other diseases, or drugs (eg, beta adrenoceptor blockers, alcohol) which could compromise preservation of the normal glucoregulatory mechanisms in the absence of food. In these patients the blood glucose levels should be carefully followed.
Concomitant Antiarrhythmic Therapy
The concomitant use of Norpace or Norpace CR with other Type 1A antiarrhythmic agents (such as quinidine or procainamide), Type 1C antiarrhythmics (such as encainide, flecainide or propafenone), and/or propranolol should be reserved for patients with life-threatening arrhythmias who are demonstrably unresponsive to single-agent antiarrhythmic therapy. Such use may produce serious negative inotropic effects, or may excessively prolong conduction. This should be considered particularly in patients with any degree of cardiac decompensation or those with a prior history thereof. Patients receiving more than one antiarrhythmic drug must be carefully monitored.
Heart Block
If first-degree heart block develops in a patient receiving Norpace or Norpace CR, the dosage should be reduced. If the block persists despite reduction of dosage, continuation of the drug must depend upon weighing the benefit being obtained against the risk of higher degrees of heart block. Development of second- or third-degree AV block or unifascicular, bifascicular, or trifascicular block requires discontinuation of Norpace or Norpace CR therapy, unless the ventricular rate is adequately controlled by a temporary or implanted ventricular pacemaker.
Anticholinergic Activity
Because of its anticholinergic activity, disopyramide phosphate should not be used in patients with glaucoma, myasthenia gravis, or urinary retention unless adequate overriding measures are taken; these consist of the topical application of potent miotics (eg, pilocarpine) for patients with glaucoma, and catheter drainage or operative relief for patients with urinary retention. Urinary retention may occur in patients of either sex as a consequence of Norpace or Norpace CR administration, but males with benign prostatic hypertrophy are at particular risk. In patients with a family history of glaucoma, intraocular pressure should be measured before initiating Norpace or Norpace CR therapy. Disopyramide phosphate should be used with special care in patients with myasthenia gravis since its anticholinergic properties could precipitate a myasthenic crisis in such patients.

PRECAUTIONS

General

Atrial Tachyarrhythmias
Patients with atrial flutter or fibrillation should be digitalized prior to Norpace or Norpace CR administration to ensure that drug-induced enhancement of AV conduction does not result in an increase of ventricular rate beyond physiologically acceptable limits.

Conduction Abnormalities
Care should be taken when prescribing Norpace or Norpace CR for patients with sick sinus syndrome (bradycardia-tachycardia syndrome), Wolff-Parkinson-White syndrome (WPW), or bundle branch block. The effect of disopyramide phosphate in these conditions is uncertain at present.

Cardiomyopathy
Patients with myocarditis or other cardiomyopathy may develop significant hypotension in response to the usual dosage of disopyramide phosphate, probably due to cardiodepressant mechanisms. Therefore, a loading dose of Norpace should not be given to such patients, and initial dosage and subsequent dosage adjustments should be made under close supervision (see *Dosage and Administration*).

Renal Impairment
More than 50% of disopyramide is excreted in the urine unchanged. Therefore Norpace dosage should be reduced in patients with impaired renal function (see *Dosage and Administration*). The electrocardiogram should be carefully monitored for prolongation of PR interval, evidence of QRS widening, or other signs of overdosage (see *Overdosage*). Norpace CR is not recommended for patients with severe renal insufficiency (creatinine clearance 40 ml/min or less).

Hepatic Impairment
Hepatic impairment also causes an increase in the plasma half-life of disopyramide. Dosage should be reduced for patients with such impairment. The electrocardiogram should be carefully monitored for signs of overdosage (see *Overdosage*).
Patients with cardiac dysfunction have a higher potential for hepatic impairment; this should be considered when administering Norpace or Norpace CR.

Potassium Imbalance
Antiarrhythmic drugs may be ineffective in patients with hypokalemia, and their toxic effects may be enhanced in patients with hyperkalemia. Therefore, potassium abnormalities should be corrected before starting Norpace or Norpace CR therapy.

Drug Interactions
If phenytoin or other hepatic enzyme inducers are taken concurrently with Norpace or Norpace CR, lower plasma levels of disopyramide may occur. Monitoring of disopyramide plasma levels is recommended in such concurrent use to avoid ineffective therapy. Other antiarrhythmic drugs (eg, quinidine, procainamide, lidocaine, propranolol) have occasionally been used concurrently with Norpace. Excessive widening of the QRS complex and/or prolongation of the Q-T interval may occur in these situations (see *Warnings*). In healthy subjects, no significant drug-drug interaction was observed when Norpace was coadministered with either propranolol or diazepam. Concomitant administration of Norpace and quinidine resulted in slight increases in plasma disopyramide levels and slight decreases in plasma quinidine levels. Norpace does not increase serum digoxin levels. Until data on possible interactions between verapamil and disopyramide phosphate are obtained, disopyramide should not be administered within 48 hours before or 24 hours after verapamil administration.

Carcinogenesis, Mutagenesis, Impairment of Fertility
Eighteen months of Norpace administration to rats, at oral doses up to 400 mg/kg/day (about 30 times the usual daily human dose of 600 mg/day, assuming a patient weight of at least 50 kg), revealed no evidence of carcinogenic potential. An evaluation of mutagenic potential by Ames test was negative. Norpace, at doses up to 250 mg/kg/day, did not adversely affect fertility of rats.

Pregnancy
Teratogenic Effects: Pregnancy Category C. Norpace was associated with decreased numbers of implantation sites and decreased growth and survival of pups when administered to pregnant rats at 250 mg/kg/day (20 or more times the usual daily human dose of 12 mg/kg, assuming a patient weight of at least 50 kg), a level at which weight gain and food consumption of dams were also reduced. Increased resorption rates were reported in rabbits at 60 mg/kg/day (5 or more times the usual daily human dose). Effects on implantation, pup growth, and survival were not evaluated in rabbits. There are no adequate and well-controlled studies in pregnant women. Norpace or Norpace CR should be used during pregnancy only if the potential benefit justifies the potential risk to the fetus.
Nonteratogenic Effects: Norpace has been reported to stimulate contractions of the pregnant uterus. Disopyramide has been found in human fetal blood.

Labor and Delivery
It is not known whether the use of Norpace or Norpace CR during labor or delivery has immediate or delayed adverse effects on the fetus, or whether it prolongs the duration of labor or increases the need for forceps delivery or other obstetric intervention.

Nursing Mothers
Studies in rats have shown that the concentration of disopyramide and its metabolites is between one and three times greater in milk than it is in plasma. Following oral administration, disopyramide has been detected in human milk at a concentration not exceeding that in plasma. Because of the potential for serious adverse reactions in nursing infants from Norpace or Norpace CR, a decision should be made whether to discontinue nursing or to discontinue the drug, taking into account the importance of the drug to the mother.

ADVERSE REACTIONS

The adverse reactions which were reported in Norpace clinical trials encompass observations in 1,500 patients, including 90 patients studied for at least 4 years. The most serious adverse reactions are hypotension and congestive heart failure. The most common adverse reactions, which are dose dependent, are associated with the anticholinergic properties of the drug. These may be transitory, but may be persistent or can be severe. Urinary retention is the most serious anticholinergic effect.
The following reactions were reported in 10% to 40% of patients:
> Anticholinergic: dry mouth (32%), urinary hesitancy (14%), constipation (11%)

The following reactions were reported in 3% to 9% of patients:
> Anticholinergic: blurred vision, dry nose/eyes/throat
> Genitourinary: urinary retention, urinary frequency and urgency
> Gastrointestinal: nausea, pain/bloating/gas
> General: dizziness, general fatigue/muscle weakness, headache, malaise, aches/pains

The following reactions were reported in 1% to 3% of patients:
> Genitourinary: impotence
> Cardiovascular: hypotension with or without congestive heart failure, increased congestive heart failure (see *Warnings*), cardiac conduction disturbances (see *Warnings*), edema/weight gain, shortness of breath, syncope, chest pain
> Gastrointestinal: anorexia, diarrhea, vomiting
> Dermatologic: generalized rash/dermatoses, itching
> Central nervous system: nervousness
> Other: hypokalemia, elevated cholesterol/triglycerides

The following reactions were reported in less than 1%:
> Depression, insomnia, dysuria, numbness/tingling, elevated liver enzymes, AV block, elevated BUN, elevated creatinine, decreased hemoglobin/hematocrit

Hypoglycemia has been reported in association with Norpace administration (see *Warnings*).
Infrequent occurrences of reversible cholestatic jaundice, fever, and respiratory difficulty have been reported in association with disopyramide therapy, as have rare instances of thrombocytopenia, reversible agranulocytosis, and gynecomastia. Some cases of LE (lupus erythematosus) symptoms have been reported; most cases occurred in patients who had been switched to disopyramide from procainamide following the development of LE symptoms. Rarely, acute psychosis has been reported following Norpace therapy, with prompt return to normal mental status when therapy was stopped. The physician should be aware of these possible reactions and should discontinue Norpace or Norpace CR therapy promptly if they occur.

OVERDOSAGE

Symptoms
Deliberate or accidental overdosage of oral disopyramide may be followed by apnea, loss of consciousness, cardiac arrhythmias, and loss of spontaneous respiration. Death has occurred following overdosage.
Toxic plasma levels of disopyramide produce excessive widening of the QRS complex and Q-T interval, worsening of congestive heart failure, hypotension, varying kinds and degrees of conduction disturbance, bradycardia, and finally asystole. Obvious anticholinergic effects are also observed.

The approximate oral LD_{50} of disopyramide phosphate is 580 and 700 mg/kg for rats and mice, respectively.

Treatment
Experience indicates that prompt and vigorous treatment of overdosage is necessary, even in the absence of symptoms. Such treatment may be lifesaving. No specific antidote for disopyramide phosphate has been identified. Treatment should be symptomatic and may include induction of emesis or gastric lavage, administration of a cathartic followed by activated charcoal by mouth or stomach tube, intravenous administration of isoproterenol and dopamine, insertion of an intra-aortic balloon for counterpulsation, and mechanically assisted ventilation. Hemodialysis or, preferably, hemoperfusion with charcoal may be employed to lower serum concentration of the drug.

The electrocardiogram should be monitored, and supportive therapy with cardiac glycosides and diuretics should be given as required.
If progressive AV block should develop, endocardial pacing should be implemented. In case of any impaired renal function, measures to increase the glomerular filtration rate may reduce the toxicity (disopyramide is excreted primarily by the kidney).
The anticholinergic effects can be reversed with neostigmine at the discretion of the physician.
Altering the urinary pH in humans does not affect the plasma half-life or the amount of disopyramide excreted in the urine.

DOSAGE AND ADMINISTRATION

The dosage of Norpace or Norpace CR must be individualized for each patient on the basis of response and tolerance. The usual adult dosage of Norpace or Norpace CR is 400 to 800 mg per day given in divided doses. The recommended dosage for most adults is 600 mg/day given in divided doses (either 150 mg every 6 hours for immediate-release Norpace or 300 mg every 12 hours for Norpace CR). For patients whose body weight is less than 110 pounds (50 kg), the recommended dosage is 400 mg/day given in divided doses (either 100 mg every 6 hours for immediate-release Norpace or 200 mg every 12 hours for Norpace CR).
For patients with cardiomyopathy or possible cardiac decompensation, a loading dose, as discussed below, should not be given, and initial dosage should be limited to 100 mg of immediate-release Norpace every 6 to 8 hours. Subsequent dosage adjustments should be made gradually, with close monitoring for the possible development of hypotension and/or congestive heart failure (see *Warnings*).
For patients with moderate renal insufficiency (creatinine clearance greater than 40 ml/min) or hepatic insufficiency, the recommended dosage is 400 mg/day given in divided doses (either 100 mg every 6 hours for immediate-release Norpace or 200 mg every 12 hours for Norpace CR).
For patients with severe renal insufficiency (C_{cr} 40 ml/min or less), the recommended dosage regimen of immediate-release Norpace is 100 mg at intervals shown in the table below, with or without an initial loading dose of 150 mg.

IMMEDIATE-RELEASE NORPACE
DOSAGE INTERVAL FOR PATIENTS
WITH RENAL INSUFFICIENCY

Creatinine clearance (ml/min)	40–30	30–15	less than 15
Approximate maintenance-dosing interval	q 8 hr	q 12 hr	q 24 hr

The above dosing schedules are for Norpace immediate-release capsules; Norpace CR is not recommended for patients with severe renal insufficiency.
For patients in whom rapid control of ventricular arrhythmia is essential, an initial loading dose of 300 mg of immediate-release Norpace (200 mg for patients whose body weight is less than 110 pounds) is recommended, followed by the appropriate maintenance dosage. Therapeutic effects are usually attained 30 minutes to 3 hours after administration of a 300-mg loading dose. If there is no response or evidence of toxicity within 6 hours of the loading dose, 200 mg of immediate-release Norpace every 6 hours may be prescribed instead of the usual 150 mg. If there is no response to this dosage within 48 hours, either Norpace should then be discontinued or the physician should consider hospitalizing the patient for careful monitoring while subsequent immediate-release Norpace doses of 250 mg or 300 mg every 6 hours are given. A limited number of patients with severe refractory ventricular tachycardia have tolerated daily doses of Norpace up to 1600 mg per day (400 mg every 6 hours), resulting in disopyramide plasma levels up to 9 mcg/ml. If such treatment is warranted, it is essential that patients be hospitalized for close evaluation and continuous monitoring.
Norpace CR should not be used initially if rapid establishment of disopyramide plasma levels is desired.

Transferring to Norpace or Norpace CR
The following dosage schedule based on theoretical considerations rather than experimental data is suggested for transferring patients with normal renal function from either quinidine sulfate or procainamide therapy (Type 1 antiarrhythmic agents) to Norpace or Norpace CR therapy:
Norpace or Norpace CR should be started using the regular maintenance schedule **without a loading dose** 6 to 12 hours after the last dose of quinidine sulfate or 3 to 6 hours after the last dose of procainamide.
In patients in whom withdrawal of quinidine sulfate or procainamide is likely to produce life-threatening arrhythmias, the physician should consider hospitalization of the patient.

Continued on next page

Searle—Cont.

When transferring a patient from immediate-release Norpace to Norpace CR, the maintenance schedule of Norpace CR may be started 6 hours after the last dose of immediate-release Norpace.

Pediatric Dosage

Controlled clinical studies have not been conducted in pediatric patients; however, the following suggested dosage table is based on published clinical experience.

Total daily dosage should be divided and equal doses administered orally every 6 hours or at intervals according to individual patient needs. Disopyramide plasma levels and therapeutic response must be monitored closely. Patients should be hospitalized during the initial treatment period, and dose titration should start at the lower end of the ranges provided below.

SUGGESTED TOTAL DAILY DOSAGE*

Age (years)	Disopyramide (mg/kg body weight/day)
Under 1	10 to 30
1 to 4	10 to 20
4 to 12	10 to 15
12 to 18	6 to 15

* Dosage is expressed in milligrams of disopyramide base. Since Norpace (disopyramide phosphate) 100-mg capsules contain 100 mg of disopyramide base, the pharmacist can readily prepare a 1-mg/ml to 10-mg/ml liquid suspension by adding the entire contents of Norpace capsules to cherry syrup, NF. The resulting suspension, when refrigerated, is stable for one month and should be thoroughly shaken before the measurement of each dose. The suspension should be dispensed in an amber glass bottle with a child-resistant closure.

Norpace CR capsules should not be used to prepare the above suspension.

HOW SUPPLIED

Norpace (disopyramide phosphate) is supplied in hard gelatin capsules containing either 100 mg or 150 mg of disopyramide base, present as the phosphate.

Norpace 100-mg capsules are white and orange, with markings SEARLE, 2752, NORPACE, and 100 MG.

NDC Number	Size
0025-2752-31	bottle of 100
0025-2752-51	bottle of 500
0025-2752-52	bottle of 1,000
0025-2752-34	carton of 100 unit dose

Norpace 150-mg capsules are brown and orange, with markings SEARLE, 2762, NORPACE, and 150 MG.

NDC Number	Size
0025-2762-31	bottle of 100
0025-2762-51	bottle of 500
0025-2762-52	bottle of 1,000
0025-2762-34	carton of 100 unit dose

Norpace CR (disopyramide phosphate) Controlled-Release is supplied as specially prepared controlled-release beads in hard gelatin capsules containing either 100 mg or 150 mg of disopyramide base, present as the phosphate.

Norpace CR 100-mg capsules are white and light green, with markings SEARLE, 2732, NORPACE CR, and 100 mg.

NDC Number	Size
0025-2732-31	bottle of 100
0025-2732-51	bottle of 500
0025-2732-34	carton of 100 unit dose

Norpace CR 150-mg capsules are brown and light green, with markings SEARLE, 2742, NORPACE CR, and 150 mg.

NDC Number	Size
0025-2742-31	bottle of 100
0025-2742-51	bottle of 500
0025-2742-34	carton of 100 unit dose

Store below 86°F (30°C).

Caution: Federal law prohibits dispensing without prescription.

7/11/91 ● A05851-6

Shown in Product Identification Section, page 429

Products are cross-indexed by
generic and chemical names in the
YELLOW SECTION.

SERES Laboratories, Inc.
3331 INDUSTRIAL DRIVE
BOX 470
SANTA ROSA, CA 95402

CANTHARONE®   ℞
[kan 'tha-rone]
(cantharidin collodion)
For External Use Only
For Doctor's Use Only

DESCRIPTION

CANTHARONE, cantharidin collodion, is a topical liquid containing 0.7% cantharidin, acetone, pyroxylin, castor oil and camphor.

HOW SUPPLIED

7.5 mL bottles (NDC 50694-096-01). Close tightly immediately after use. Keep away from heat.
Revised July, 1989
Direct inquiries to Kathryn MacLeod, Ph.D.

CANTHARONE® PLUS   ℞
[kan 'tha rone PLUS]
For External Use Only
For Doctor's Use Only

DESCRIPTION

CANTHARONE PLUS is a topical liquid containing 30% salicylic acid, 2% podophyllin B.P., 1% cantharidin, octylphenylpolyethylene glycol, cellosolve, ethocel, pyroxylin, castor oil and acetone.

HOW SUPPLIED

7.5 mL bottles (NDC 50694-097-01). Close tightly immediately after use. Keep away from heat. Do not refrigerate.

SPECIAL WARNING

Do not use for venereal warts.
Do not dispense under any circumstances.
Revised July, 1992
Direct inquiries to Kathryn MacLeod, Ph.D.

NIGHT CAST™ Regular Formula   OTC
(Medicated Acne Mask-lotion)

DESCRIPTION

Contains 4% sulfur, 1.5% salicylic acid and 33% alcohol in a non-comedogenic vehicle.

HOW SUPPLIED

4 fl. oz. in a plastic dispenser bottle.
(NDC 50694-201-04)   Revised July 1991
Currently available only in Canada. For information on inquiries, see below.

NIGHT CAST™ Special Formula   OTC
(Medicated Acne Mask-lotion)

DESCRIPTION

Contains 8% sulfur, 2% resorcinol and 31% alcohol in a non-comedogenic vehicle.

HOW SUPPLIED

4 fl. oz. in a plastic dispenser bottle.
(NDC 50694-202-04)   Revised July 1991
Currently available only in Canada. Direct inquiries to Dormer Laboratories, Point-Claire, Quebec or to Kathryn MacLeod, Ph.D. (SERES)

IDENTIFICATION PROBLEM?
Consult PDR's
Product Identification Section
where you'll find over 1700
products pictured actual size
and in full color.

Serono Laboratories, Inc.
100 LONGWATER CIRCLE
NORWELL, MA 02061

Serono Laboratories, Inc. will be pleased to answer inquiries about the following products:

METRODIN®   ℞
[me 'trō-dēn]
(urofollitropin for injection)
FOR INTRAMUSCULAR USE ONLY

PRODUCT OVERVIEW

KEY FACTS

Metrodin® is a purified, lyophilized preparation of urofollitropin for injection containing 75 IU follicle stimulating hormone activity and less than 1 IU luteinizing hormone activity per ampule. It is administered by intramuscular injection immediately after reconstitution with Sodium Chloride for Injection, USP.

MAJOR USES

Metrodin® is indicated for the induction of ovulation in patients with polycystic ovarian disease, who have an elevated LH/FSH ratio and who have failed to respond adequately to clomiphene citrate therapy. Treatment with Metrodin® alone, in most cases, results only in follicular growth and maturation. Ovulation is induced with human chorionic gonadotropin (hCG: Profasi®).

Metrodin® and hCG may also be used to stimulate the development of multiple oocytes in ovulatory patients participating in an in vitro fertilization program.

SAFETY INFORMATION

Metrodin® should not be administered to patients who have previously demonstrated hypersensitivity to gonadotropins. In rare instances, women may experience the Ovarian Hyperstimulation Syndrome, which may require hospitalization. This risk can be minimized through careful patient monitoring. The patient should be advised of the possibility of multiple gestation occurring with Metrodin® therapy.

PRESCRIBING INFORMATION

METRODIN®   ℞
[me 'trō-dēn]
(urofollitropin for injection)
FOR INTRAMUSCULAR INJECTION

DESCRIPTION

Metrodin® (urofollitropin for injection) is a preparation of gonadotropin extracted from the urine of postmenopausal women. Each ampule of Metrodin® contains 75 IU of follicle-stimulating hormone (FSH) activity in not more than 0.83 mg of extract, plus 10 mg lactose in a sterile, lyophilized form. Metrodin® is administered by intramuscular injection.

Metrodin® contains an acidic, water soluble glycoprotein biologically standardized for FSH gonadotropin activity in terms of the Second International Reference Preparation for Human Menopausal Gonadotropins, established in September, 1964 by the Expert Committee on Biological Standards of the World Health Organization. Negligible amounts (less than 1 IU per 75 IU FSH) of luteinizing hormone (LH) activity are contained in Metrodin®.

Therapeutic Class: Infertility.

CLINICAL PHARMACOLOGY

Metrodin® stimulates ovarian follicular growth in women who do not have primary ovarian failure. Treatment with Metrodin® in most instances results only in follicular growth and maturation. In order to effect ovulation in the absence of an endogenous LH surge, human chorionic gonadotropin (hCG) must be given following the administration of Metrodin® when clinical and laboratory assessment of the patient indicates that sufficient follicular maturation has occurred.

INDICATIONS AND USAGE

Metrodin® and hCG given in a sequential manner are indicated for the induction of ovulation in patients with polycystic ovarian syndrome (PCO) who have an elevated LH/FSH ratio and who have failed to respond to adequate clomiphene citrate therapy.

Metrodin® and hCG may also be used to stimulate the development of multiple oocytes in ovulatory patients participating in an in vitro fertilization program.

Selection of Patients:

1. Before treatment with Metrodin® is instituted, a thorough gynecologic and endocrinologic evaluation must be performed. This should include a hysterosalpingogram (to rule out uterine and tubal pathology) and documentation of anovulation by means of basal body temperature, serial vaginal smears, examination of cervical mucus, determi-

nation of serum (or urinary) progesterone, urinary pregnanediol and endometrial biopsy. Patients with tubal pathology should receive Metrodin® only if enrolled in an in vitro fertilization program.
2. Primary ovarian failure should be excluded by the determination of gonadotropin levels.
3. Careful examination should be made to rule out the presence of early pregnancy.
4. Patients in late reproductive life have a greater predilection to endometrial carcinoma as well as a higher incidence of anovulatory disorders. Cervical dilation and curettage should always be done for diagnosis before starting Metrodin® therapy in such patients who demonstrate abnormal uterine bleeding or other signs of endometrial abnormalities.
5. Evaluation of the husband's fertility potential should be included in the workup.

CONTRAINDICATIONS

Metrodin® is contraindicated in women who exhibit:
1. High levels of FSH indicating primary ovarian failure.
2. Uncontrolled thyroid or adrenal dysfunction.
3. An organic intracranial lesion such as a pituitary tumor.
4. The presence of any cause of infertility other than anovulation, as stated in the "Indications" unless they are candidates for in vitro fertilization.
5. Abnormal bleeding of undetermined origin (see "Selection of Patients").
6. Ovarian cysts or enlargement not due to polycystic ovary syndrome.
7. Prior hypersensitivity to urofollitropin.
8. Metrodin® is contraindicated in women who are pregnant and may cause fetal harm when administered to a pregnant woman. There are limited human data on the effects of Metrodin® when administered during pregnancy.

WARNINGS

Metrodin® is a drug that should only be used by physicians who are thoroughly familiar with infertility problems. It is a potent gonadotropic substance capable of causing mild to severe adverse reactions. Gonadotropin therapy requires a certain time commitment by physicians and supportive health professionals, and its use requires the availability of appropriate monitoring facilities (See "Precautions/Laboratory Tests"). It must be used with a great deal of care.

Overstimulation of the Ovary During Metrodin® Therapy: Ovarian Enlargement: Mild to moderate uncomplicated ovarian enlargement, which may be accompanied by abdominal distension and/or abdominal pain, occurs in approximately 20% of those treated with Metrodin® and hCG, and generally regresses without treatment within two or three weeks.

In order to minimize the hazard associated with the occasional abnormal ovarian enlargement which may occur with Metrodin®-hCG therapy, the lowest dose consistent with expectation of good results should be used. Careful monitoring of ovarian response can further minimize the risk of overstimulation.

If the ovaries are abnormally enlarged on the last day of Metrodin® therapy, hCG should not be administered in this course of therapy. This will reduce the chances of development of the Ovarian Hyperstimulation Syndrome.

The Ovarian Hyperstimulation Syndrome (OHSS): OHSS is a medical event distinct from uncomplicated ovarian enlargement. OHSS may progress rapidly (within 24 hours to several days) to become a serious medical event. It is characterized by an apparent dramatic increase in vascular permeability which can result in a rapid accumulation of fluid in the peritoneal cavity, thorax, and potentially, the pericardium. The early warning signs of development of OHSS are severe pelvic pain, nausea, vomiting, and weight gain. The following symptomatology has been seen with cases of OHSS: abdominal pain, abdominal distension, gastrointestinal symptoms including nausea, vomiting and diarrhea, severe ovarian enlargement, weight gain, dyspnea, and oliguria. Clinical evaluation may reveal hypovolemia, hemoconcentration, electrolyte imbalances, ascites, hemoperitoneum, pleural effusions, hydrothorax, acute pulmonary distress, and thromboembolic events (see "Pulmonary and Vascular Complications").

OHSS occurred in approximately 6.0% of patients treated with Metrodin® therapy in the initial clinical trials, in patients treated for anovulation due to polycystic ovarian syndrome. During studies for in vitro fertilization, four cases of the Ovarian Hyperstimulation Syndrome were reported following 1,586 treatment cycles (0.25%). Cases of OHSS are more common, more severe, and more protracted if pregnancy occurs. OHSS develops rapidly; therefore, patients should be followed for at least two weeks after hCG administration. Most often, OHSS occurs after treatment has been discontinued and reaches its maximum at about seven to ten days following treatment. Usually, OHSS resolves spontaneously with the onset of menses. If there is evidence that OHSS may be developing prior to hCG administration (see "Precautions/Laboratory Tests"), the hCG should be withheld.

If OHSS occurs, treatment should be stopped and the patient should be hospitalized. Treatment is primarily symptomatic and should consist of bed rest, fluid and electrolyte management, and analgesics if needed. The phenomenon of hemoconcentration associated with fluid loss into the peritoneal cavity, pleural cavity, and the pericardial cavity has been seen to occur and should be thoroughly assessed in the following manner: 1) fluid intake and output, 2) weight, 3) hematocrit, 4) serum and urinary electrolytes, 5) urine specific gravity, 6) BUN and creatinine, and 7) abdominal girth. These determinations are to be performed daily or more often if the need arises.

With OHSS there is an increased risk of injury to the ovary. The ascitic, pleural, and pericardial fluid should not be removed unless absolutely necessary to relieve symptoms such as pulmonary distress or cardiac tamponade. Pelvic examination may cause rupture of an ovarian cyst, which may result in hemoperitoneum, and should therefore be avoided. If this does occur, and if bleeding becomes such that surgery is required, the surgical treatment should be designed to control bleeding and to retain as much ovarian tissue as possible. Intercourse should be prohibited in those patients in whom significant ovarian enlargement occurs after ovulation because of the danger of hemoperitoneum resulting from ruptured ovarian cysts.

The management of OHSS may be divided into three phases: the acute, the chronic, and the resolution phases. Because the use of diuretics can accentuate the diminished intravascular volume, diuretics should be avoided except in the late phase of resolution as described below.

Acute Phase: Management during the acute phase should be designed to prevent hemoconcentration due to loss of intravascular volume to the third space and to minimize the risk of thromboembolic phenomena and kidney damage. Treatment is designed to normalize electrolytes while maintaining an acceptable but somewhat reduced intravascular volume. Full correction of the intravascular volume deficit may lead to an unacceptable increase in the amount of third space fluid accumulation. Management includes administration of limited intravenous fluids, electrolytes, and human serum albumin. Monitoring for the development of hyperkalemia is recommended.

Chronic Phase: After stabilizing the patient during the acute phase, excessive fluid accumulation in the third space should be limited by instituting severe potassium, sodium, and fluid restriction.

Resolution Phase: A fall in hematocrit and an increasing urinary output without an increased intake are observed due to the return of third space fluid to the intravascular compartment. Peripheral and/or pulmonary edema may result if the kidneys are unable to excrete third space fluid as rapidly as it is mobilized. Diuretics may be indicated during the resolution phase if necessary to combat pulmonary edema.

Pulmonary and Vascular Complications: The following paragraph describes serious medical events reported following gonadotropin therapy.

Serious pulmonary conditions (e.g., atelectasis, acute respiratory distress syndrome) have been reported. In addition, thromboembolic events both in association with, and separate from the Ovarian Hyperstimulation Syndrome have been reported. Intravascular thrombosis and embolism, which may originate in venous or arterial vessels, can result in reduced blood flow to critical organs or the extremities. Sequelae of such events have included venous thrombophlebitis, pulmonary embolism, pulmonary infarction, cerebral vascular occlusion (stroke), and arterial occlusion resulting in loss of limb. In rare cases, pulmonary complications and/or thromboembolic events have resulted in death.

Multiple Births: Reports of multiple births have been associated with Metrodin®-hCG treatment, including triplet and quintuplet gestations. In clinical studies with Metrodin®, 83% of the pregnancies following therapy resulted in single births and 17% in multiple births. The patient and her husband should be advised of the potential risk of multiple births before starting treatment.

PRECAUTIONS

General: Careful attention should be given to diagnosis in candidates for Metrodin® therapy (see "Indications and Usage/Selection of Patients").

Information for Patients: Prior to the therapy with Metrodin®, patients should be informed of the duration of treatment and monitoring of their condition that will be required. Possible adverse reactions (see "Adverse Reactions") and the risk of multiple births should also be discussed.

Laboratory Tests: In most instances, treatment with Metrodin® results only in follicular growth and maturation. In order to effect ovulation, hCG must be given following the administration of Metrodin® when clinical assessment of the patient indicates that sufficient follicular maturation has occurred. This may be estimated by measuring serum (or urinary) estrogen levels and sonographic visualization of the ovaries. The combination of both estradiol levels and ultrasonography is useful for monitoring the growth and development of follicles, timing hCG administration, as well as minimizing the risk of the Ovarian Hyperstimulation Syndrome and multiple gestation.

Urinary and/or plasma estrogen determinations provide an indirect index of follicular maturity since as the follicles grow and develop, they secrete estrogens in increasing amounts. However, plasma and/or urinary estrogen levels represent the sum of ovarian activity. It is recommended that the number of growing follicles be confirmed using ultrasonography because plasma and/or urinary estrogens do not give an indication of the number of follicles.

Other clinical parameters which may have potential use for monitoring urofollitropin therapy include:
1. Changes in the vaginal cytology,
2. Appearance and volume of the cervical mucus,
3. Spinnbarkeit, and
4. Ferning of the cervical mucus.

The above clinical indices provide an indirect estimate of the estrogenic effect upon the target organs and, therefore, should only be used adjunctively with more direct estimates of follicular development, i.e., serum estradiol and ultrasonography.

The clinical confirmation of ovulation, with the exception of pregnancy, is obtained by direct and indirect indices of progesterone production. The indices most generally used are as follows:
1. A rise in basal body temperature,
2. Increase in serum progesterone, and
3. Menstruation following the shift in basal body temperature.

When used in conjunction with indices of progesterone production, sonographic visualization of the ovaries will assist in determining if ovulation has occurred. Sonographic evidence of ovulation may include the following:
1. Fluid in the cul-de-sac,
2. Ovarian stigmata, and
3. Collapsed follicle.

Because of the subjectivity of the various tests for the determination of follicular maturation and ovulation, it cannot be overemphasized that the physician should choose tests with which he/she is thoroughly familiar.

Drug Interactions: No clinically significant drug/drug or drug/food interactions have been reported during Metrodin® therapy.

Carcinogenesis and Mutagenesis: Carcinogenicity and mutagenicity studies have not been performed.

Pregnancy Category X: See "Contraindications".

Nursing Mothers: It is not known whether this drug is excreted in human milk. Because many drugs are excreted in human milk, caution should be exercised if Metrodin® is administered to a nursing woman.

ADVERSE REACTIONS

The following adverse reactions reported during Metrodin® therapy are listed in decreasing order of potential severity:
1. Pulmonary and vascular complications (see "Warnings"),
2. Ovarian Hyperstimulation Syndrome (see "Warnings"),
3. Mild to moderate ovarian enlargement,
4. Abdominal pain,
5. Sensitivity to Metrodin®,
(Febrile reactions which may be accompanied by chills, musculoskeletal aches, joint pains, malaise, headache, and fatigue have occurred after the administration of Metrodin®. It is not clear whether or not these were pyrogenic responses or possible allergic reactions.)
6. Ovarian cysts,
7. Gastrointestinal symptoms (nausea, vomiting, diarrhea, abdominal cramps, bloating),
8. Pain, rash, swelling and/or irritation at the site of injection,
9. Breast tenderness,
10. Headache,
11. Dermatological symptoms (dry skin, body rash, hair loss, hives).
12. Hemoperitoneum has been reported during menotropins therapy and, therefore, may also occur during Metrodin® therapy.

The following medical events have been reported subsequent to pregnancies resulting from Metrodin® therapy:
1. Ectopic pregnancy
2. Congenital abnormalities
(Three incidents of chromosomal abnormalities and four birth defects have been reported following Metrodin®-hCG or Metrodin®, Pergonal® (menotropins for injection, USP)-hCG therapy in clinical trials for stimulation prior to in vitro fertilization. The aborted pregnancies included one Trisomy 13, one Trisomy 18, and one fetus with multiple congenital anomalies (hydrocephaly, omphalocele, and meningocele). One meningocele, one external ear defect, one dislocated hip and ankle, and one dilated cardiomyopathy in the presence of maternal Systemic Lupus Erythematosus were reported. None of these

Continued on next page

Serono Laboratories—Cont.

events were thought to be drug-related. The incidence does not exceed that found in the general population.)

DRUG ABUSE AND DEPENDENCE
There have been no reports of abuse or dependence with Metrodin®.

OVERDOSAGE
Aside from possible ovarian hyperstimulation and multiple gestations (see "Warnings"), little is known concerning the consequences of acute overdosage with Metrodin®.

DOSAGE AND ADMINISTRATION
Dosage: The dose of Metrodin® to produce maturation of the follicle must be individualized for each patient. It is recommended that the initial dose to any patient should be 75 IU of Metrodin® per day, **ADMINISTERED INTRAMUS-CULARLY**, for seven to twelve days followed by hCG, 5,000 U to 10,000 U, one day after the last dose of Metrodin®. Administration of Metrodin® may exceed 12 days if inadequate follicle development is indicated by estrogen and/or ultrasound measurement. The patient should be treated until indices of estrogenic activity, as indicated under "Precautions," are equivalent to or greater than those of the normal individual. If serum or urinary estradiol determinations or ultrasonographic visualizations are available, they may be useful as a guide to therapy. If the ovaries are abnormally enlarged on the last day of Metrodin® therapy, hCG should not be administered in this course of therapy; this will reduce the chances of development of the Ovarian Hyperstimulation Syndrome. If there is evidence of ovulation but no pregnancy, repeat this dosage regimen for at least two more courses before increasing the dose of Metrodin® to 150 IU of FSH per day for seven to twelve days. As before, this dose should be followed by 5,000 U to 10,000 U of hCG one day after the last dose of Metrodin®. If evidence of ovulation is present, but pregnancy does not ensue, repeat the same dose for two more courses. Doses larger than this are not routinely recommended.

During treatment with both Metrodin® and hCG and during a two week post-treatment period, patients should be examined at least every other day for signs of excessive ovarian stimulation. It is recommended that Metrodin® administration be stopped if the ovaries become abnormally enlarged or abdominal pain occurs. Most instances of OHSS occur after treatment has been discontinued and reach their maximum at about seven to ten days post-ovulation. Patients should be followed for at least two weeks after hCG administration.

The couple should be encouraged to have intercourse daily, beginning on the day prior to the administration of hCG until ovulation becomes apparent from the indices employed for the determination of progestational activity. Care should be taken to insure insemination. In the light of the foregoing indices and parameters mentioned, it should become obvious that, unless a physician is willing to devote considerable time to these patients and be familiar with and conduct the necessary laboratory studies, he/she should not use Metrodin®.

In Vitro Fertilization: For in vitro fertilization, therapy with Metrodin® should be initiated in the early follicular phase (cycle day 2 or 3) at a dose of 150 IU per day, until sufficient follicular development is attained. In most cases, therapy should not exceed ten days.

Administration: Dissolve the contents of one ampule of Metrodin® in one to two mL of sterile saline and **ADMINISTER INTRAMUSCULARLY** immediately. Any unused reconstituted material should be discarded.

Parenteral drug products should be inspected visually, for particulate matter and discoloration prior to administration, whenever solution and container permit.

HOW SUPPLIED
Metrodin® is supplied in a sterile, lyophilized form as a white to off-white powder or pellet in snap-top ampules containing 75 IU FSH activity. The following package combinations are available:
—1 ampule 75 IU Metrodin® and 1 ampule 2 mL Sodium Chloride Injection (USP), NDC 44087-6075-1
—10 ampules 75 IU Metrodin® and 10 ampules 2 mL Sodium Chloride Injection (USP), NDC 44087-6075-3
Lyophilized powder may be stored refrigerated or at room temperature (3°–25°C/37°–77°F). Protect from light. Use immediately after reconstitution. Discard unused material.

CLINICAL STUDIES
The results of the clinical experience and effectiveness of the administration of Metrodin® to 80 PCO patients in 189 courses of therapy are summarized above. All patients had received extensive prior therapy with clomiphene citrate, without success, and many had failed to conceive or hyperstimulated following treatment with Pergonal® (menotropins for injection, USP). [See table above.]

CAUTION: Federal law prohibits dispensing without prescription.

	%
Patients ovulating	88
Patients pregnant	30
Patients aborting	25*
Multiple pregnancies	17*
Hyperstimulation syndrome (% patients)	6

*Based on total pregnancies.

Manufactured for:
SERONO LABORATORIES, INC.
Randolph, MA 02368 USA
by: Laboratoires Serono SA
Aubonne, Switzerland
©SERONO LABORATORIES, INC. 1986, 1990
Revised: April, 1990

PERGONAL®
[per'go-nal]
(menotropins for injection, USP)
FOR INTRAMUSCULAR INJECTION

PRODUCT OVERVIEW
KEY FACTS
Pergonal® is a purified, lyophilized preparation of gonadotropins and contains equal amounts of follicle stimulating hormone and luteinizing hormone. Pergonal® is administered by intramuscular injection immediately after reconstitution with Sodium Chloride for Injection, USP.

MAJOR USES
Women: Pergonal® is used to stimulate follicular development in hypogonadotropic anovulatory women who do not have primary ovarian failure.
Men: Pergonal® is used concomitantly with Profasi® (hCG) to stimulate spermatogenesis in men with infertility due to primary or secondary hypogonadotropic hypogonadism.

SAFETY INFORMATION
Pergonal® is contraindicated in individuals who have previously demonstrated hypersensitivity to the drug. In rare instances, women may experience excessive ovarian enlargement, ascites, and pleural effusion requiring hospitalization. The risk can be minimized through careful patient monitoring. Multiple births, 75% of which are twins, have been reported in 20% of pregnancies resulting from Pergonal® therapy.

PRESCRIBING INFORMATION
PERGONAL®
[per'go-nal]
(menotropins for injection, USP)
FOR INTRAMUSCULAR INJECTION

DESCRIPTION
Pergonal® (menotropins for injection, USP) is a purified preparation of gonadotropins extracted from the urine of postmenopausal women. Each ampule of Pergonal® contains 75 IU or 150 IU of follicle-stimulating hormone (FSH) activity and 75 IU or 150 IU of luteinizing hormone (LH) activity, respectively, plus 10 mg lactose in a sterile, lyophilized form. Pergonal® is administered by intramuscular injection.
Pergonal® is biologically standardized for FSH and LH (ICSH) gonadotropin activities in terms of the Second International Reference Preparation for Human Menopausal Gonadotropins established in September, 1964 by the Expert Committee on Biological Standards of the World Health Organization.
Both FSH and LH are glycoproteins that are acidic and water soluble.
Therapeutic class: Infertility.

CLINICAL PHARMACOLOGY
Women:
Pergonal® administered for seven to twelve days produces ovarian follicular growth in women who do not have primary ovarian failure. Treatment with Pergonal® in most instances results only in follicular growth and maturation. In order to effect ovulation, human chorionic gonadotropin (hCG) must be given following the administration of Pergonal® when clinical assessment of the patient indicates that sufficient follicular maturation has occurred.
Men:
Pergonal® administered concomitantly with human chorionic gonadotropin (hCG) for at least three months induces spermatogenesis in men with primary or secondary pituitary hypofunction who have achieved adequate masculinization with prior hCG therapy.

INDICATIONS AND USAGE
Women:
Pergonal® and hCG given in a sequential manner are indicated for the induction of ovulation and pregnancy in the anovulatory infertile patient, in whom the cause of anovulation is functional and is not due to primary ovarian failure.

Pergonal® and hCG may also be used to stimulate the development of multiple follicles in ovulatory patients participating in an in vitro fertilization program.
Men:
Pergonal® with concomitant hCG is indicated for the stimulation of spermatogenesis in men who have primary or secondary hypogonadotropic hypogonadism.
Pergonal® with concomitant hCG has proven effective in inducing spermatogenesis in men with primary hypogonadotropic hypogonadism due to a congenital factor or prepubertal hypophysectomy and in men with secondary hypogonadotropic hypogonadism due to hypophysectomy, craniopharyngioma, cerebral aneurysm or chromophobe adenoma.

SELECTION OF PATIENTS
Women:
1. Before treatment with Pergonal® is instituted, a thorough gynecologic and endocrinologic evaluation must be performed. Except for those patients enrolled in an in vitro fertilization program, this should include a hysterosalpingogram (to rule out uterine and tubal pathology) and documentation of anovulation by means of basal body temperature, serial vaginal smears, examination of cervical mucus, determination of serum (or urine) progesterone, urinary pregnanediol and endometrial biopsy. Patients with tubal pathology should receive Pergonal® only if enrolled in an in vitro fertilization program.
2. Primary ovarian failure should be excluded by the determination of gonadotropin levels.
3. Careful examination should be made to rule out the presence of an early pregnancy.
4. Patients in late reproductive life have a greater predilection to endometrial carcinoma as well as a higher incidence of anovulatory disorders. Cervical dilation and curettage should always be done for diagnosis before starting Pergonal® therapy in such patients who demonstrate abnormal uterine bleeding or other signs of endometrial abnormalities.
5. Evaluation of the husband's fertility potential should be included in the workup.
Men:
Patient selection should be made based on a documented lack of pituitary function. Prior to hormonal therapy, these patients will have low testosterone levels and low or absent gonadotropin levels. Patients with primary hypogonadotropic hypogonadism will have a subnormal development of masculinization, and those with secondary hypogonadotropic hypogonadism will have decreased masculinization.

CONTRAINDICATIONS
Women:
Pergonal® is contraindicated in women who have:
1. A high FSH level indicating primary ovarian failure.
2. Uncontrolled thyroid and adrenal dysfunction.
3. An organic intracranial lesion such as a pituitary tumor.
4. The presence of any cause of infertility other than anovulation unless they are candidates for in vitro fertilization.
5. Abnormal bleeding of undetermined origin.
6. Ovarian cysts or enlargement not due to polycystic ovary syndrome.
7. Prior hypersensitivity to menotropins.
8. Pergonal® is contraindicated in women who are pregnant and may cause fetal harm when administered to a pregnant woman. There are limited human data on the effects of Pergonal® when administered during pregnancy.
Men:
Pergonal® is contraindicated in men who have:
1. Normal gonadotropin levels indicating normal pituitary function.
2. Elevated gonadotropin levels indicating primary testicular failure.
3. Infertility disorders other than hypogonadotropic hypogonadism.

WARNINGS
Pergonal® is a drug that should only be used by physicians who are thoroughly familiar with infertility problems. It is a potent gonadotropic substance capable of causing mild to severe adverse reactions in women. Gonadotropin therapy requires a certain time commitment by physicians and supportive health professionals, and its use requires the availability of appropriate monitoring facilities (see "Precautions—Laboratory Tests"). In female patients it must be used with a great deal of care.
Overstimulation of the Ovary During Pergonal® Therapy:
Ovarian Enlargement: Mild to moderate uncomplicated ovarian enlargement which may be accompanied by abdominal distension and/or abdominal pain occurs in approximately 20% of those treated with Pergonal® and hCG, and generally regresses without treatment within two or three weeks.
In order to minimize the hazard associated with the occasional abnormal ovarian enlargement which may occur with Pergonal®-hCG therapy, the lowest dose consistent with expectation of good results should be used. Careful monitoring of ovarian response can further minimize the risk of overstimulation.

If the ovaries are abnormally enlarged on the last day of Pergonal® therapy, hCG should not be administered in this course of therapy; this will reduce the chances of development of the Ovarian Hyperstimulation Syndrome.

The Ovarian Hyperstimulation Syndrome (OHSS): OHSS is a medical event distinct from uncomplicated ovarian enlargement. OHSS may progress rapidly to become a serious medical event. It is characterized by an apparent dramatic increase in vascular permeability which can result in a rapid accumulation of fluid in the peritoneal cavity, thorax, and potentially, the pericardium. The early warning signs of development of OHSS are severe pelvic pain, nausea, vomiting, and weight gain. The following symptomatology has been seen with cases of OHSS: abdominal pain, abdominal distension, gastrointestinal symptoms including nausea, vomiting and diarrhea, severe ovarian enlargement, weight gain, dyspnea, and oliguria. Clinical evaluation may reveal hypovolemia, hemoconcentration, electrolyte imbalances, ascites, hemoperitoneum, pleural effusions, hydrothorax, acute pulmonary distress, and thromboembolic events (see "Pulmonary and Vascular Complications" below).

OHSS occurs in approximately 0.4% of patients when the recommended dose is administered and in 1.3% of patients when higher than recommended doses are administered. Cases of OHSS are more common, more severe and more protracted if pregnancy occurs. OHSS develops rapidly; therefore patients should be followed for at least two weeks after hCG administration. Most often, OHSS occurs after treatment has been discontinued and reaches its maximum at about seven to ten days following treatment. Usually, OHSS resolves spontaneously with the onset of menses. If there is evidence that OHSS may be developing prior to hCG administration (see "Precautions—Laboratory Tests"), the hCG should be withheld.

If OHSS occurs, treatment should be stopped and the patient hospitalized. Treatment is primarily symptomatic, consisting of bed rest, fluid and electrolyte management, and analgesics if needed. The phenomenon of hemoconcentration associated with fluid loss into the peritoneal cavity, pleural cavity, and the pericardial cavity has been seen to occur and should be thoroughly assessed in the following manner: 1) fluid intake and output, 2) weight, 3) hematocrit, 4) serum and urinary electrolytes, 5) urine specific gravity, 6) BUN and creatinine, and 7) abdominal girth. These determinations are to be performed daily or more often if the need arises.

With OHSS there is an increased risk of injury to the ovary. The ascitic, pleural, and pericardial fluid should not be removed unless absolutely necessary to relieve symptoms such as pulmonary distress or cardiac tamponade. Pelvic examination may cause rupture of an ovarian cyst, which may result in hemoperitoneum, and should therefore be avoided. If this does occur, and if bleeding becomes such that surgery is required, the surgical treatment should be designed to control bleeding and to retain as much ovarian tissue as possible. Intercourse should be prohibited in those patients in whom significant ovarian enlargement occurs after ovulation because of the danger of hemoperitoneum resulting from ruptured ovarian cysts.

The management of OHSS may be divided into three phases: the acute, the chronic, and the resolution phases. Because the use of diuretics can accentuate the diminished intravascular volume, diuretics should be avoided except in the late phase of resolution as described below.

Acute Phase: Management during the acute phase should be designed to prevent hemoconcentration due to loss of intravascular volume to the third space and to minimize the risk of thromboembolic phenomena and kidney damage. Treatment is designed to normalize electrolytes while maintaining an acceptable but somewhat reduced intravascular volume. Full correction of the intravascular volume deficit may lead to an unacceptable increase in the amount of third space fluid accumulation. Management includes administration of limited intravenous fluids, electrolytes, and human serum albumin. Monitoring for the development of hyperkalemia is recommended.

Chronic Phase: After stabilizing the patient during the acute phase, excessive fluid accumulation in the third space should be limited by instituting severe potassium, sodium, and fluid restriction.

Resolution Phase: A fall in hematocrit and an increasing urinary output without an increased intake are observed due to the return of third space fluid to the intravascular compartment. Peripheral and/or pulmonary edema may result if the kidneys are unable to excrete third space fluid as rapidly as it is mobilized. Diuretics may be indicated during the resolution phase if necessary to combat pulmonary edema.

Pulmonary and Vascular Complications: Serious pulmonary conditions (e.g., atelectasis, acute respiratory distress syndrome) have been reported. In addition, thromboembolic events both in association with, and separate from, the Ovarian Hyperstimulation Syndrome have been reported following Pergonal® therapy. Intravascular thrombosis and embolism, which may originate in venous or arterial vessels, can result in reduced blood flow to critical organs or the extremities. Sequelae of such events have included venous

thrombophlebitis, pulmonary embolism, pulmonary infarction, cerebral vascular occlusion (stroke), and arterial occlusion resulting in loss of limb. In rare cases, pulmonary complications and/or thromboembolic events have resulted in death.

Multiple Births: Data from a clinical trial revealed the following results regarding multiple births: Of the pregnancies following therapy with Pergonal® and hCG, 80% resulted in single births, 15% in twins, and 5% of the total pregnancies resulted in three or more concepti. The patient and her husband should be advised of the frequency and potential hazards of multiple gestation before starting treatment.

PRECAUTIONS

General: Careful attention should be given to diagnosis in the selection of candidates for Pergonal® therapy (see "Indications and Usage—Selection of Patients").

Information for Patients: Prior to therapy with Pergonal®, patients should be informed of the duration of treatment and the monitoring of their condition that will be required. Possible adverse reactions (see "Adverse Reactions" section) and the risk of multiple births should also be discussed.

Laboratory Tests:

Women:

Treatment for Induction of Ovulation

In most instances, treatment with Pergonal® results only in follicular growth and maturation. In order to effect ovulation, hCG must be given following the administration of Pergonal® when clinical assessment of the patient indicates that sufficient follicular maturation has occurred. This may be directly estimated by measuring serum (or urinary) estrogen levels and sonographic visualization of the ovaries. The combination of both estradiol levels and ultrasonography are useful for monitoring the growth and development of follicles, timing hCG administration, as well as minimizing the risk of the Ovarian Hyperstimulation Syndrome and multiple gestation.

Other clinical parameters which may have potential use for monitoring menotropins therapy include:
a) Changes in the vaginal cytology;
b) Appearance and volume of the cervical mucus;
c) Spinnbarkeit; and
d) Ferning of the cervical mucus.

The above clinical indices provide an indirect estimate of the estrogenic effect upon the target organs, and therefore should only be used adjunctively with more direct estimates of follicular development, i.e., serum estradiol and ultrasonography.

The clinical confirmation of ovulation, with the exception of pregnancy, is obtained by direct and indirect indices of progesterone production. The indices most generally used are as follows:
a) A rise in basal body temperature;
b) Increase in serum progesterone; and
c) Menstruation following the shift in basal body temperature.

When used in conjunction with indices of progesterone production, sonographic visualization of the ovaries will assist in determining if ovulation has occurred. Sonographic evidence of ovulation may include the following:
a) Fluid in the cul-de-sac;
b) Ovarian stigmata; and
c) Collapsed follicle.

Because of the subjectivity of the various tests for the determination of follicular maturation and ovulation, it cannot be overemphasized that the physician should choose tests with which he/she is thoroughly familiar.

Drug Interactions: No clinically significant drug/drug or drug/food adverse interactions have been reported during Pergonal® therapy.

Carcinogenesis and Mutagenesis: Long-term toxicity studies in animals have not been performed to evaluate the carcinogenic potential of Pergonal®.

Pregnancy: Pregnancy Category X. See "Contraindications" section.

Nursing Mothers: It is not known whether this drug is excreted in human milk. Because many drugs are excreted in human milk, caution should be exercised if Pergonal® is administered to a nursing woman.

ADVERSE REACTIONS

Women:

The following adverse reactions, reported during Pergonal® therapy, are listed in decreasing order of potential severity:
1. Pulmonary and vascular complications (see "Warnings")
2. Ovarian Hyperstimulation Syndrome (see "Warnings")
3. Hemoperitoneum
4. Mild to moderate ovarian enlargement
5. Ovarian cysts
6. Abdominal pain
7. Sensitivity to Pergonal®
   Febrile reactions after the administration of Pergonal® have occurred. It is not clear whether or not these were pyrogenic responses or possible allergic reactions. In addition, reports of "flu-like symptoms" including fever,

chills, musculoskeletal aches, joint pains, nausea, headache and malaise have been received.
8. Gastrointestinal symptoms (nausea, vomiting, diarrhea, abdominal cramps, bloating)
9. Pain, rash, swelling and/or irritation at the site of injection
10. Body rashes
11. Dizziness, tachycardia, dyspnea, tachypnea

The following medical events have been reported subsequent to pregnancies resulting from Pergonal® therapy:
1. Ectopic pregnancy
2. Congenital abnormalities
   From a study of 287 completed pregnancies following Pergonal®-hCG therapy five incidents of birth defects were reported (1.7%). One infant had multiple congenital anomalies consisting of imperforate anus, aplasia of the sigmoid colon, third degree hypospadias, cecovesicle fistula, bifid scrotum, meningocele, bilateral internal tibial torsion, and right metatarsus adductus. Another infant was born with an imperforate anus and possible congenital heart lesions; another had a supernumerary digit; another was born with hypospadias and exstrophy of the bladder; and the fifth child had Down's syndrome. None of the investigators felt that these defects were drug-related. Subsequently one report of an infant death due to hydrocephalus and cardiac anomalies has been received.

Men:
1. Gynecomastia may occur occasionally during Pergonal®-hCG therapy. This is a known effect of hCG treatment.
2. Erythrocytosis (hct 50%, hgb 17.8 g%) was recorded in one patient.

DRUG ABUSE AND DEPENDENCE

There have been no reports of abuse or dependence with Pergonal®.

OVERDOSAGE

Aside from possible ovarian hyperstimulation (see "Warnings"), little is known concerning the consequences of acute overdosage with Pergonal®.

DOSAGE AND ADMINISTRATION

Women:

1. Dosage:

The dose of Pergonal® to produce maturation of the follicle must be individualized for each patient. It is recommended that the initial dose to any patient should be 75 IU of FSH/LH per day, **ADMINISTERED INTRAMUSCULARLY**, for seven to twelve days followed by hCG, 5,000 U to 10,000 U, one day after the last dose of Pergonal®. Administration of Pergonal® should not exceed 12 days in a single course of therapy. The patient should be treated until indices of estrogenic activity, as indicated under "Precautions" above, are equivalent to or greater than those of the normal individual. If serum or urinary estradiol determinations or ultrasonographic visualizations are available, they may be useful as a guide to therapy. If the ovaries are abnormally enlarged on the last day of Pergonal® therapy, hCG should not be administered in this course of therapy; this will reduce the chances of development of the Ovarian Hyperstimulation Syndrome. If there is evidence of ovulation but no pregnancy, repeat this dosage regime for at least two more courses before increasing the dose of Pergonal® to 150 IU of FSH/LH per day for seven to twelve days. As before, this dose should be followed by 5,000 U to 10,000 U of hCG one day after the last dose of Pergonal®. A Pergonal® dose of 150 IU of FSH/LH per day has proven to be the most effective dose especially for in vitro fertilization. If evidence of ovulation is present, but pregnancy does not ensue, repeat the same dose for two more courses. Doses larger than this are not routinely recommended.

During treatment with both Pergonal® and hCG and during a two-week post-treatment period, patients should be examined at least every other day for signs of excessive ovarian stimulation. It is recommended that Pergonal® administration be stopped if the ovaries become abnormally enlarged or abdominal pain occurs. Most of the Ovarian Hyperstimulation Syndrome occurs after treatment has been discontinued and reaches its maximum at about seven to ten days post-ovulation. Patients should be followed for at least two weeks after hCG administration.

The couple should be encouraged to have intercourse daily, beginning on the day prior to the administration of hCG until ovulation becomes apparent from the indices employed for the determination of progestational activity. Care should be taken to insure insemination. In the light of the foregoing indices and parameters mentioned, it should become obvious that, unless a physician is willing to devote considerable time to these patients and be familiar with and conduct the necessary laboratory studies, he/she should not use Pergonal®.

Continued on next page

Serono Laboratories—Cont.

	% Pts. Ovul.	% Pts. Preg.	% Abort.	% Multi Preg.	% Twins	% 3 or More Concepti	% Hyperstim. Syndr.
Primary Amenorrhea	62	22	14	25	25	0	0
Secondary Amenorrhea	61	28	24	28	18	10	1.9
Secondary Amen. with Galactorrhea	77	42	21	41	31	10	1.2
Polycystic Ovaries	76	26	39	17	17	0	1.1
Anovulatory Cycles	77	24	15	14	9	5	2.0
Miscellaneous	83	20	36	2	2	0	0.1

2. Administration:

Dissolve the contents of one ampule of Pergonal® in one to two ml of sterile saline and **ADMINISTER INTRAMUSCULARLY** immediately. Any unused reconstituted material should be discarded. Parenteral drug products should be inspected visually for particulate matter and discoloration prior to administration, whenever solution and container permit.

Men:

1. Dosage:

Prior to concomitant therapy with Pergonal® and hCG, pretreatment with hCG alone (5,000 U three times a week) is required. Treatment should continue for a period sufficient to achieve serum testosterone levels within the normal range and masculinization as judged by the appearance of secondary sex characteristics. Such pretreatment may require four to six months, then the recommended dose of Pergonal® is 75 IU FSH/LH **ADMINISTERED INTRAMUSCULARLY**, three times a week and the recommended dose of hCG is 2,000 U twice a week. Therapy should be carried on for a minimum of four more months to insure detecting spermatozoa in the ejaculate, as it takes 74± 4 days in the human male for germ cells to reach the spermatozoa stage.

If the patient has not responded with evidence of increased spermatogenesis at the end of four months of therapy, treatment may continue with 75 IU FSH/LH three times a week, or the dose can be increased to 150 IU FSH/LH three times a week, with the hCG dose unchanged.

2. Administration:

Dissolve the contents of one ampule of Pergonal® in one to two ml of sterile saline and **ADMINISTER INTRAMUSCULARLY** immediately. Any unused reconstituted material should be discarded. Parenteral drug products should be inspected visually for particulate matter and discoloration prior to administration, whenever solution and container permit.

HOW SUPPLIED

Pergonal® is supplied in a sterile lyophilized form as a white to off-white powder or pellet in snap-top ampules containing 75 IU or 150 IU FSH/LH activity. The following package combinations are available:
—1 ampule 75 IU Pergonal® and 1 ampule 2 ml Sodium Chloride Injection (USP), NDC 44087-0571-7.
—10 ampules 75 IU Pergonal® and 10 ampules 2 ml Sodium Chloride Injection (USP), NDC 44087-5075-3.
—1 ampule 150 IU Pergonal® and 1 ampule 2 ml Sodium Chloride Injection (USP), NDC 44087-5150-1.
By biological assay, one IU of LH for the Second International Reference Preparation (2nd-IRP) for hMG is biologically equivalent to approximately ½ U of hCG.
Lyophilized powder may be stored refrigerated or at room temperature (3°–25°C/37°–77°F). Protect from light. Use immediately after reconstitution. Discard unused material.

CLINICAL STUDIES

Women:

The results of the clinical experience and effectiveness of the administration of Pergonal® to 1,286 patients in 3,002 courses of therapy are summarized below. The values include patients who were treated with other than the recommended dosage regime. The values for the presently recommended dosage regime are essentially the same.

	%
Patients ovulating	75
Patients pregnant	25
Patients aborting	25*
Multiple pregnancies	20†
Twins	15†
Three or more concepti	5†
Fetal abnormalities	1.7†
Hyperstimulation syndrome	1.3

* Based on total pregnancies
† Based on total deliveries

Results by diagnosis group are summarized below (these values include patients who were treated with other than the present recommended dosage regime):
[See table above.]

Men:

Clinical results of the treatment of men with primary or secondary hypogonadotropic hypogonadism are as follows:
In the Serono Cooperative study, with an adequate treatment period of 3 to 8 months, 60 of 70 men with primary hypogonadotropic hypogonadism and 8 of 11 men with secondary hypogonadotropic hypogonadism responded with mean increases in their sperm counts from less than 5 to 24 million

spermatozoa per milliliter of ejaculate. Forty-one wives of 54 men with primary hypogonadotropic hypogonadism desiring offspring and 7 wives of men with secondary hypogonadotropic hypogonadism conceived. Patients treated with Pergonal® and hCG for less than 3 months or with Pergonal® alone did not respond to therapy.
A world-wide data search revealed that of 160 recorded pregnancies as the result of use of Pergonal®-hCG in men, there were 7 spontaneous abortions, one ectopic pregnancy and 3 congenital anomalies at birth (esophageal atresia in a female infant which was later corrected by surgery, unilateral cryptorchidism, inguinal hernia).
Caution: Federal law prohibits dispensing without prescription.
Manufactured for:
SERONO LABORATORIES, INC.
Randolph, MA 02368 USA
by: Laboratoires Serono, SA
Aubonne, Switzerland
© SERONO LABORATORIES, INC. 1969, 1989
Revised: December, 1989

PROFASI®   ℞
[pro 'fah-se]
(chorionic gonadotropin for injection, USP)
FOR INTRAMUSCULAR INJECTION

PRODUCT OVERVIEW

KEY FACTS

Profasi® is a lyophilized preparation of human chorionic gonadotropin. It is administered by intramuscular injection after reconstitution with Bacteriostatic Water for Injection, USP.

MAJOR USES

Women: Profasi® is used to induce ovulation in women who have been appropriately treated with human menotropins.
Men: Profasi® is used to treat hypogonadotropic males, or to treat prepubertal cryptorchidism not due to anatomical obstruction.

SAFETY INFORMATION

Profasi® should not be administered to patients who have previously demonstrated hypersensitivity to human chorionic gonadotropin. Women who have experienced excessive ovarian enlargement and overstimulation while undergoing human menotropins treatment should not be given HCG. When treating prepubertal cryptorchidism, therapy should be discontinued if signs of precocious puberty occur.

PRESCRIBING INFORMATION

PROFASI®   ℞
[pro 'fah-se]
(chorionic gonadotropin for injection, USP)
FOR INTRAMUSCULAR INJECTION

DESCRIPTION

Human chorionic gonadotropin (HCG), a polypeptide hormone produced by the human placenta, is composed of an alpha and a beta sub-unit. The alpha sub-unit is essentially identical to the alpha sub-units of the human pituitary gonadotropins, luteinizing hormone (LH) and follicle-stimulating hormone (FSH), as well as to the alpha sub-unit of human thyroid-stimulating hormone (TSH). The beta sub-units of these hormones differ in amino acid sequence.
Chorionic Gonadotropin is a water soluble glycoprotein derived from human pregnancy urine. The sterile lyophilized powder is stable. When reconstituted the solution should be refrigerated and should be used within 60 days.
Each vial of chorionic gonadotropin for injection contains: chorionic gonadotropin: 5,000 USP Units or 10,000 USP Units; mannitol 100 mg; with dibasic sodium phosphate and monobasic sodium phosphate to adjust pH.
In addition, when reconstituted with the diluent provided (bacteriostatic water for injection, USP) each vial will contain benzyl alcohol 0.9%.
For intramuscular injection only.

CLINICAL PHARMACOLOGY

The action of HCG is virtually identical to that of pituitary LH, although HCG appears to have a small degree of FSH activity as well. It stimulates production of gonadal steroid hormones by stimulating the interstitial cells (Leydig cells) of the testis to produce androgens and the corpus luteum of the ovary to produce progesterone. Androgen stimulation in the male leads to the development of secondary sex characteristics and may stimulate testicular descent when no anatomical impediment to descent is present. This descent is usually reversible when HCG is discontinued. During the normal menstrual cycle, LH participates with FSH in the development and maturation of the normal ovarian follicle, and the mid-cycle LH surge triggers ovulation. HCG can substitute for LH in this function.
During a normal pregnancy, HCG secreted by the placenta maintains the corpus luteum after LH secretion decreases, supporting continued secretion of estrogen and progesterone and preventing menstruation. HCG HAS NO KNOWN EFFECT ON FAT MOBILIZATION, APPETITE OR SENSE OF HUNGER, OR BODY FAT DISTRIBUTION.

INDICATIONS AND USAGE

HCG HAS NOT BEEN DEMONSTRATED TO BE EFFECTIVE ADJUNCTIVE THERAPY IN THE TREATMENT OF OBESITY. THERE IS NO SUBSTANTIAL EVIDENCE THAT IT INCREASES WEIGHT LOSS BEYOND THAT RESULTING FROM CALORIC RESTRICTION, THAT IT CAUSES A MORE ATTRACTIVE OR "NORMAL" DISTRIBUTION OF FAT, OR THAT IT DECREASES THE HUNGER AND DISCOMFORT ASSOCIATED WITH CALORIE-RESTRICTED DIETS.
1. Prepubertal cryptorchidism not due to anatomical obstruction. In general, HCG is thought to induce testicular descent in situations when descent would have occurred at puberty. HCG thus may help predict whether or not orchiopexy will be needed in the future. Although, in some cases, descent following HCG administration is permanent, in most cases, the response is temporary. Therapy is usually instituted between the ages of 4 and 9.
2. Selected cases of hypogonadotropic hypogonadism (hypogonadism secondary to a pituitary deficiency) in males.
3. Induction of ovulation and pregnancy in the anovulatory, infertile woman in whom the cause of anovulation is secondary and not due to primary ovarian failure, and who has been appropriately pre-treated with human menotropins.

CONTRAINDICATIONS

Precocious puberty, prostatic carcinoma or other androgen-dependent neoplasm, prior allergic reaction to HCG.

WARNINGS

HCG should be used in conjunction with human menopausal gonadotropins only by physicians experienced with infertility problems who are familiar with the criteria for patient selection, contraindications, warnings, precautions, and adverse reactions described in the package insert for menotropins. The principal serious adverse reactions during this use are: (1) Ovarian hyperstimulation, a syndrome of sudden ovarian enlargement, ascites with or without pain, and/or pleural effusion, (2) Rupture of ovarian cysts with resultant hemoperitoneum, (3) Multiple births, and (4) Arterial thromboembolism.

PRECAUTIONS

1. Induction of androgen secretion by HCG may induce precocious puberty in patients treated for cryptorchidism. Therapy should be discontinued if signs of precocious puberty occur.
2. Since androgens may cause fluid retention, HCG should be used with caution in patients with cardiac or renal disease, epilepsy, migraine, or asthma.

ADVERSE REACTIONS

Headache, irritability, restlessness, depression, fatigue, edema, precocious puberty, gynecomastia, pain at the site of injection.

DOSAGE AND ADMINISTRATION

For intramuscular use only. The dosage regimen employed in any particular case will depend upon the indication for use, the age and weight of the patient, and the physician's

preference. The following regimens have been advocated by various authorities.

Prepubertal cryptorchidism not due to anatomical obstruction:
1. 4,000 USP Units three times weekly for three weeks.
2. 5,000 USP Units every second day for four injections.
3. 15 injections of 500 to 1,000 USP Units over a period of six weeks.
4. 500 USP Units three times weekly for four to six weeks. If this course of treatment is not successful, another is begun one month later, giving 1,000 USP Units per injection.

Selected cases of hypogonadotropic hypogonadism in males:
1. 500 to 1,000 USP Units three times a week for three weeks, followed by the same dose twice a week for three weeks.
2. 4,000 USP Units three times weekly for six to nine months, following which the dosage may be reduced to 2,000 USP Units three times weekly for an additional three months.

Induction of ovulation and pregnancy in the anovulatory, infertile woman in whom the cause of anovulation is secondary and not due to primary ovarian failure and who has been appropriately pre-treated with human menotropins (see prescribing information for menotropins for dosage and administration for that drug product):

5,000 to 10,000 USP Units one day following the last dose of menotropins (a dosage of 10,000 USP Units is recommended in the labeling for menotropins).

Parenteral drug products should be inspected visually for particulate matter and discoloration prior to administration, whenever solution and container permit.

DIRECTION FOR RECONSTITUTION

TWO-VIAL PACKAGE: Withdraw sterile air from lyophilized vial and inject into diluent vial. Remove up to 10 mL of diluent and add to lyophilized vial, agitate gently until solution is complete.

HOW SUPPLIED

Chorionic gonadotropin for injection is available as a lyophilized powder in multiple dose vials containing either:
5,000 USP Units per Vial - NDC 44087-8005-3
10,000 USP Units per Vial - NDC 44087-8010-3
with 10 mL vial bacteriostatic water for injection, USP (containing benzyl alcohol 0.9% v/v) and sodium hydroxide and/or hydrochloric acid to adjust pH.

Storage: Store the dry product at controlled room temperature 15°– 30°C (59°– 86°F). AFTER RECONSTITUTION, REFRIGERATE THE PRODUCT AT 2°– 8°C (36°– 46°F) AND USE WITHIN 60 DAYS.

Caution: Federal law prohibits dispensing without prescription.

Manufactured for: SERONO LABORATORIES, INC.
Randolph, MA 02368 USA
Manufactured by: Steris Laboratories, Inc.
Phoenix, AZ 85043 USA
©Serono Laboratories, Inc. 1984, 1991
Revised October 1990

SEROPHENE®   ℞
[se'ro-fēn]
(clomiphene citrate tablets, USP)

PRODUCT OVERVIEW

KEY FACTS

Serophene® is an orally administered, non-steroidal compound with some estrogenic activity. The exact mechanism of action is unknown, although it appears to involve the pituitary by stimulating release of pituitary gonadotropins to mediate ovulation.

MAJOR USES

Serophene® is effective in inducing ovulation in infertile women with physiological indications of normal estrogen

production. Reduced estrogen levels, while less favorable, do not prevent successful therapy.

SAFETY INFORMATION

Serophene® is contraindicated in patients who have previously experienced hypersensitivity to clomiphene citrate. Visual disturbances, vasomotor flushes, and ovarian enlargement occasionally occur. Because the teratogenic potential of clomiphene citrate is unknown, it should not be administered during pregnancy. Multiple births occur in approximately 10% of pregnancies resulting from clomiphene citrate therapy; the vast majority of these are twins.

PRESCRIBING INFORMATION

SEROPHENE®   ℞
[se'ro-fēn]

(clomiphene citrate tablets, USP)

DESCRIPTION

Each scored white tablet contains: clomiphene citrate, USP 50 mg. Clomiphene citrate is designated chemically as 2-[p-(2-chloro-1,2-diphenylvinyl) phenoxy] triethylamine dihydrogen citrate and is represented structurally as:

$$(C_2H_5)_2NCH_2CH_2O—\hspace{-4pt}\bigcirc\hspace{-4pt}—C=C—\hspace{-4pt}\bigcirc\hspace{-4pt}—C_6H_8O_7$$
$$Cl$$

clomiphene citrate, USP (Serophene®)

As shown, one molecule of citric acid is chemically bound with one molecule of the organic base, clomiphene. Clomiphene citrate is a chemical analog of other triarylethylene compounds such as chlorotrianisene and the cholesterol inhibitor, triparanol.

ACTIONS

Clomiphene citrate, an orally-administered, non-steroidal agent, may induce ovulation in selected anovulatory women. It is a drug of considerable pharmacologic potency. Careful evaluation and selection of the patient and close attention to the timing of the dose is mandatory prior to treatment with clomiphene citrate. Conservative selection and management of the patient contribute to successful therapy of anovulation. Clomiphene citrate induces ovulation in most selected anovulatory patients. The various criteria for ovulation include: an ovulation peak of estrogen excretion followed by a biphasic basal body temperature curve, urinary excretion of pregnanediol at post-ovulatory levels, and endometrial histologic findings characteristic of the luteal phase.

A review of eleven publications appearing between 1964 and 1978 showed that pregnancy occurred in 35% of 5154 patients with ovulatory dysfunction who received clomiphene citrate. [See table below.]

Clomiphene citrate therapy appears to mediate ovulation through increased output of pituitary gonadotropins. These stimulate the maturation and endocrine activity of the ovarian follicle which is followed by the development and function of the corpus luteum. Increased urinary excretion of gonadotropins and estrogen suggests involvement of the pituitary.

Studies with ^{14}C labeled clomiphene citrate have shown that it is readily absorbed orally in humans and is excreted principally in the feces. An average of 51% of the administered dose was excreted after 5 days. After intravenous administration, 37% was excreted in 5 days. The appearance of ^{14}C in the feces six weeks after administration suggests that the remaining drug and/or metabolites are slowly excreted from a sequestered enterohepatic recirculation pool.

INDICATIONS

Clomiphene citrate is indicated for the treatment of ovulatory failure in patients desiring pregnancy and whose husbands are fertile and potent. Impediments to this goal must be excluded or adequately treated before beginning therapy. Administration of clomiphene citrate is indicated only in patients with demonstrated ovulatory dysfunction and in whom the following conditions apply:

1. Normal liver function.
2. Physiologic indications of normal endogenous estrogen (as estimated from vaginal smears, endometrial biopsy, assay of serum [or urinary] estrogen, or from bleeding in response to progesterone). Reduced estrogen levels, while less favorable, do not prevent successful therapy.
3. Clomiphene citrate therapy is not effective for those patients with primary pituitary or ovarian failure. It cannot substitute for appropriate therapy of other disturbances leading to ovulatory dysfunction, e.g., diseases of the thyroid or adrenals.
4. Particularly careful evaluation prior to clomiphene citrate therapy should be done in patients with abnormal uterine bleeding. It is most important that neoplastic lesions are detected.

CONTRAINDICATIONS

Pregnancy:
Although no direct effect of clomiphene citrate therapy on the human fetus has been seen established, clomiphene citrate should not be administered in cases of suspected pregnancy as such effects have been reported in animals. To prevent inadvertent clomiphene citrate administration during early pregnancy, the basal body temperature should be recorded throughout all treatment cycles, and therapy should be discontinued if pregnancy is suspected. If the basal body temperature following clomiphene citrate is biphasic and is not followed by menses, the possibility of an ovarian cyst and/or pregnancy should be excluded. Until the correct diagnosis has been determined, the next course of therapy should be delayed.

Clomiphene citrate is also contraindicated in patients who have:
1. Uncontrolled thyroid or adrenal dysfunction.
2. An organic intracranial lesion such as a pituitary tumor.
3. Liver disease or a history of liver dysfunction.
4. Abnormal uterine bleeding of undetermined origin.
5. Ovarian cysts or enlargement not due to polycystic ovarian syndrome.

WARNINGS

Visual Symptoms:
Patients should be warned that blurring and/or other visual symptoms may occur occasionally with clomiphene citrate therapy. These may make activities such as driving or operating machinery more hazardous than usual, particularly under conditions of variable lighting. While their significance is not yet understood (see "Adverse Reactions"), patients having any visual symptoms should discontinue treatment and have a complete ophthalmologic evaluation.

Ovarian Hyperstimulation Syndrome:
The Ovarian Hyperstimulation Syndrome (OHSS) has been reported to occur in patients receiving drug therapy for ovulation induction, including in rare cases patients receiving clomiphene citrate therapy. OHSS is a medical event distinct from uncomplicated ovarian enlargement. OHSS may progress rapidly (within 24 hours to several days) to become a serious medical event. It is characterized by an apparent dramatic increase in vascular permeability which can result in a rapid accumulation of fluid in the peritoneal cavity, thorax, and potentially, the pericardium. The early warning signs of development of OHSS are severe pelvic pain, nausea, vomiting, and weight gain. The following symptomatology has been seen with cases of OHSS: abdominal pain, abdominal distension, gastrointestinal symptoms including nausea, vomiting and diarrhea, severe ovarian enlargement, weight gain, dyspnea, and oliguria. Clinical evaluation may reveal hypovolemia, hemoconcentration, electrolyte imbalances, ascites, hemoperitoneum, pleural effusions, hydrothorax, acute pulmonary distress, and thromboembolic phenomena.

PRECAUTIONS

Diagnosis Prior to Clomiphene Citrate Therapy:
Careful evaluation should be given to candidates for clomiphene citrate therapy. A complete pelvic examination should be performed prior to treatment and repeated before each subsequent course. Clomiphene citrate should not be given to patients with an ovarian cyst, as further ovarian enlargement may result.

Since the incidence of endometrial carcinoma and of ovulatory disorders increases with age, endometrial biopsy should always exclude the former as causative in such patients. If abnormal uterine bleeding is present, full diagnostic measures are necessary.

Ovarian Overstimulation During Treatment with Clomiphene Citrate:
To minimize the hazard associated with the occasional abnormal ovarian enlargement during clomiphene citrate therapy (see "Adverse Reactions"), the lowest dose producing good results should be chosen. Some patients with polycystic ovarian syndrome are unusually sensitive to gonadotropins and may have an exaggerated response to usual doses of clomiphene citrate. Maximal enlargement of the ovary, whether abnormal or physiologic, does not occur until

PREGNANCIES FOLLOWING CLOMIPHENE CITRATE, USP[a]		(Range)
Number of Patients	= 5154	
Percent of Patients Ovulating[b]	= 75	(50-94%)
Percent of Ovulatory Cycles	= 53	(33-69%)
Percent of Patients Pregnant	= 35	(11-52%)
Percent Patients Pregnant	= 46	(22-61%)
Percent Patients Ovulating		
Percent Live Births	= 86	(74-99.8%)
Percent Abortions	= 14	(0.2-26%)
Percent of Single Births	= 90	(67-100%)
Percent Surviving	= 99	(98.2-100%)
Percent of Multiple Births	= 10	(0-33%)
Percent Surviving	= 96	(82-100%)

a) includes patients receiving other than recommended dosage regimen.
b) average from studies.

Continued on next page

Serono Laboratories—Cont.

several days after discontinuation of clomiphene citrate. The patient complaining of pelvic pains after receiving clomiphene citrate should be examined carefully. If enlargement of the ovary occurs, clomiphene citrate therapy should be withheld until the ovaries have returned to pretreatment size, and the dosage or duration of the next course should be reduced. The ovarian enlargement and cyst formation following clomiphene citrate therapy regress spontaneously within a few days or weeks after discontinuing treatment. Therefore, unless a strong indication for laparoscopy (or laparotomy) exists, such cystic enlargement always should be managed conservatively.

Multiple Pregnancy:
In the reviewed publications, the incidence of multiple pregnancies was increased during those cycles in which clomiphene citrate was given. Among the 1,803 pregnancies on which the outcome was reported, 90% were single and 10% twins. Less than 1% of the reported deliveries resulted in triplets or more.
Of these multiple pregnancies, 96-99% resulted in the births of live infants. The patient and her husband should be advised of the frequency and potential hazards of multiple pregnancy before starting treatment.

ADVERSE REACTIONS
At the recommended dosage of clomiphene citrate, side effects occur infrequently and generally do not interfere with treatment. Adverse reactions tend to occur more frequently at higher doses and in the longer treatment courses used in some early studies.
The most frequent adverse reactions to clomiphene citrate include ovarian enlargement (approximately 1 in 7 patients), vasomotor flushes resembling menopausal symptoms which are not usually severe and promptly disappear after treatment is discontinued (approximately 1 in 10 patients), and abdominal discomfort (approximately 1 in 15 patients). Adverse reactions which occur less frequently (approximately 1 in 50 patients or more) include breast tenderness, nausea and vomiting, nervousness, insomnia, and visual disturbances. Other side effects which occur in less than 1 in 100 patients include headache, dizziness and light-headedness, increased urination, depression, fatigue, urticaria and allergic dermatitis, abnormal uterine bleeding, weight gain, ovarian cysts, and reversible hair loss.
Thromboembolic events, such as pulmonary embolism, arterial occlusion, and phlebitis, have been reported rarely in patients treated with clomiphene citrate. It is not clear what, if any, relationship these events have to clomiphene citrate therapy.
When clomiphene citrate is administered at the recommended dose, abnormal ovarian enlargement (see "Precautions") is infrequent, although the usual cyclic variation in ovarian size may be exaggerated. Similarly, mid-cycle ovarian pain (mittelschmerz) may be accentuated.
With prolonged or higher dosage, ovarian enlargement and cyst formation (usually luteal) may occur more often, and the luteal phase of the cycle may be prolonged. Patients with polycystic ovarian syndrome may be unusually sensitive to clomiphene therapy. Rare occurrences of massive ovarian enlargement have been reported, for example, in a patient with polycystic ovarian syndrome whose clomiphene citrate therapy consisted of 100 mg daily for 14 days. Since abnormal ovarian enlargement usually regresses spontaneously, most of these patients should be treated conservatively. The Ovarian Hyperstimulation Syndrome has been reported to occur in rare cases in patients receiving clomiphene citrate therapy (see "Warnings").
The incidence of visual symptoms (see "Warnings" for further recommendations), usually described as "blurring" or spots or flashes (scintillating scotomata), correlates with increasing total dose. Other visual symptoms which may occur include diplopia, phosphenes, photophobia, decreased visual acuity, loss of peripheral vision, and spatial distortion. The symptoms disappear usually within a few days or weeks after clomiphene citrate is discontinued. This may be due to intensification and/or prolongation of after-images. Symptoms often appear first, or are accentuated, upon exposure to a more brightly lit environment.
While measured visual acuity generally has not been affected, in one patient taking 200 mg daily, visual blurring developed on the seventh day of treatment and progressed to severe diminution of visual acuity by the tenth day. No other abnormality was coincident, and the visual acuity was normal by the third day after treatment was stopped. Ophthalmologically definable scotomata and electroretinographic retinal function changes have also been reported.

BSP Laboratory Studies:
Greater than 5% retention of sulfobromophthalein (BSP) has been reported in approximately 10% to 20% of patients in whom it was measured. Retention was usually minimal but was elevated during prolonged clomiphene citrate administration or with apparently unrelated liver disease. In some patients, pre-existing BSP retention decreased even

though clomiphene citrate therapy was continued. Other liver function tests were usually normal.

Other Laboratory Studies:
Clomiphene citrate has not been reported to cause a significant abnormality in hematologic or renal tests, in protein bound iodine, or in serum cholesterol levels.

Birth Defects:
The following medical events have been reported subsequent to pregnancies following ovulation induction therapy with clomiphene citrate: ectopic pregnancy and congenital abnormalities such as syndactyly, polydactyly, congenital heart defects, anencephaly, retinal aplasia, hypospadias, ovarian dysplasia, microcephaly, and cleft lip/palate. One case of congenital abnormality (adactyly) in an infant exposed to clomiphene citrate in utero has been reported.
Of 1,803 births following clomiphene citrate administration, 45 infants with birth defects were reported for a cumulative rate of 2.5%.
Six cases of Down's syndrome, one neonatal death with multiple malformations, and one case of each of the following were reported: club-foot, tibial torsion, blocked tear duct, and hemangioma. The other congenital abnormalities were not described. The investigators did not report that these were presumed to be due to therapy. The cumulative rate of congenital abnormalities does not exceed that reported in the general population.

DOSAGE AND ADMINISTRATION

General Considerations:
Physicians experienced in managing gynecologic or endocrine disorders should supervise the work-up and treatment of candidate patients for clomiphene citrate therapy. Patients should be chosen for clomiphene citrate therapy only after careful diagnostic evaluation (see "Indications"). The plan of therapy should be outlined in advance. Impediments to achieving the goal of therapy must be excluded or adequately treated before beginning clomiphene citrate.
In determining a starting dose schedule, efficacy must be balanced against potential side effects. For example, the available data so far suggest that ovulation and pregnancy are slightly more attainable with 100 mg/day for 5 days than with 50 mg/day for 5 days. As the dosage is increased, however, ovarian overstimulation and other side effects may be expected to increase. Although the data do not yet establish a relationship between dose level and multiple births, it is reasonable that such a correlation exists on pharmacologic grounds.
For these reasons, treatment of the usual patient should initiate with a 50 mg daily dose for 5 days. The dose may be increased only in those patients who do not respond to the first course (see "Recommended Dosage"). Special treatment with lower dosage over shorter duration is particularly recommended if unusual sensitivity to pituitary gonadotropin is suspected, including patients with polycystic ovarian syndrome (see "Precautions").

Recommended Dosage:
The recommended dosage for the first course of clomiphene citrate is 50 mg (1 tablet) daily for 5 days. Therapy may be started at any time if the patient has had no recent uterine bleeding. If progestin-induced bleeding is intended, or if spontaneous uterine bleeding occurs prior to therapy, the regimen of 50 mg daily for 5 days should be started on or about the fifth day of the cycle. When ovulation occurs at this dosage, there is no advantage to increasing the dose in subsequent cycles of treatment. If ovulation does not appear to have occurred after the first course of therapy, a second course of 100 mg daily (two 50 mg tablets given as a single daily dose) for 5 days may be started. This course may begin as early as 30 days after the previous one. It is recommended that the patient be examined for pregnancy, ovarian enlargement, or cyst formation between each treatment cycle. Increasing the dosage or duration of therapy beyond 100 mg/day for 5 days should not be undertaken.
The majority of patients who respond do so during the first course of therapy, and 3 courses constitute an adequate therapeutic trial. If ovulatory menses do not occur, the diagnosis should be re-evaluated. Treatment beyond this is not recommended in the patient who does not exhibit evidence of ovulation.

Pregnancy:
Properly timed coitus is very important for good results. For regularity of cyclic ovulatory response, it is also important that each course of clomiphene citrate be started on or about the fifth day of the cycle, once ovulation has been established. As with other therapeutic modalities, Serophene® therapy follows the rule of diminishing returns, such that the likelihood of conception diminishes with each succeeding course of therapy. If pregnancy has not been achieved after 3 ovulatory responses to Serophene®, further treatment generally is not recommended. Before starting treatment, patients should be advised of the possibility and potential hazards of multiple pregnancy if conception occurs following clomiphene citrate therapy.

Long-Term Cyclic Therapy —Not Recommended:
Since the relative safety of long-term cyclic therapy has not yet been demonstrated conclusively, and since the majority

of patients will ovulate following 3 courses, long-term cyclic therapy is not recommended.

HOW SUPPLIED
Serophene is available as 50 mg scored white tablets in the following package combinations:
- 1 carton 10 tablets, NDC 44087-8090-6
Each carton contains 2 strips of 5 tablets each.
- 1 carton 30 tablets, NDC 44087-8090-1
Each carton contains 3 strips of 10 tablets, each in a 2 × 5 arrangement.
Protect from light, moisture, and excessive heat. Dispense in well-closed, light resistant container as defined in the USP, with child resistant closure. Store at room temperature (15°-30°C/59°-86°F).
Caution: Federal law prohibits dispensing without prescription.

Manufactured for:
SERONO LABORATORIES, INC.
Randolph, MA 02368 USA
©SERONO LABORATORIES, INC. 1982, 1990
Revised: June, 1992

For additional information, please contact:
Serono Laboratories, Inc.
Drug Information and Surveillance Group
100 Longwater Circle
Norwell, MA 02061
800-283-8088 (Toll free)
617-982-9000

EDUCATIONAL MATERIAL

To obtain the Serono Symposia, USA Events and Publications Brochure, a comprehensive overview of the many programs and types of literature that Serono Symposia, USA is sponsoring in 1993, contact Serono Laboratories, Inc.

Sigma-Tau Pharmaceuticals, Inc.
200 ORCHARD RIDGE DRIVE
GAITHERSBURG, MARYLAND 20878

CARNITOR® ℞
[car-nĭt-tor]
(Levocarnitine) Tablets (330 mg)
CARNITOR®
(Levocarnitine) Oral Solution
1 g per 10 mL multidose)
For oral use only.
Not for parenteral use.

DESCRIPTION
CARNITOR® (Levocarnitine) is L-beta-hydroxy-gamma-trimethylamino butyric acid (inner salt). As a bulk drug substance it is a white powder with a melting point of 196–197℃ and is readily soluble in water. The L-isomer of carnitine is the biologically active form. Its chemical structure is:

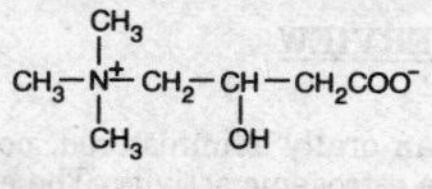

$$CH_3 - \overset{\underset{CH_3}{|}}{\underset{|}{N^+}} - CH_2 - \overset{\underset{OH}{|}}{CH} - CH_2COO^-$$
$$\quad \quad CH_3$$

Each CARNITOR® (Levocarnitine) Tablet contains 330 mg of levocarnitine and the inactive ingredients magnesium stearate, microcrystalline cellulose and povidone.
Each 118 mL container of the CARNITOR® (Levocarnitine) Oral Solution contains 1 g of levocarnitine/10 mL, sucrose syrup, D,L-malic acid, red colors and artificial cherry flavor. Methyl paraben NF and Propylparaben NF are added as preservatives. The pH is approximately 5.

CLINICAL PHARMACOLOGY
CARNITOR® (Levocarnitine) is a naturally occurring substance required in mammalian energy metabolism. It has been shown to facilitate long-chain fatty acid entry into cellular mitochondria, therefore delivering substrate for oxidation and subsequent energy production. Fatty acids are utilized as an energy substrate in all tissues except the brain. In skeletal and cardiac muscle they serve as major fuel. Primary systemic carnitine deficiency is characterized by low plasma, RBC, and/or tissue levels. The resulting impairment in fatty acid metabolism manifests itself as elevated triglycerides and free fatty acids, diminished ketogenesis, and lipid infiltration of liver and muscle. The literature reports that carnitine can promote the excretion of excess organic or

fatty acids in patients with defects in fatty acid metabolism and/or specific organic acidopathies that bioaccumulate acylCoA esters.

Bioavailability

The bioavailability/pharmacokinetics of CARNITOR® (Levocarnitine) Tablets and the Oral Solution preparation have not been determined in well controlled studies.

Metabolism and excretion

The majority of body carnitine is excreted in the urine and feces. In renal failure, carnitine levels may rise.

INDICATIONS AND USAGE

CARNITOR® (Levocarnitine) is indicated in the treatment of primary systemic carnitine deficiency. In the reported cases, the clinical presentation consisted of recurrent episodes of Reye-like encephalopathy, hypoketotic hypoglycemia, and/or cardiomyopathy. Associated symptoms included hypotonia, muscle weakness and failure to thrive. A diagnosis of primary carnitine deficiency requires that serum, red cell and/or tissue carnitine levels be low and that the patient does not have a primary defect in fatty acid or organic acid oxidation (see Clinical Pharmacology). Controlled trials were not conducted, but in some patients, particularly those presenting with cardiomyopathy, carnitine supplementation rapidly alleviated signs and symptoms. Treatment should include, in addition to carnitine, supportive and other therapy as indicated by the condition of the patient.

CONTRAINDICATIONS

None known.

WARNINGS.

None.

PRECAUTIONS

General

CARNITOR® (Levocarnitine) Oral Solution is for oral/internal use only.

Not for parenteral use.

Gastrointestinal reactions may result from too rapid consumption of carnitine. CARNITOR® (Levocarnitine) Oral Solution may be consumed alone, or dissolved in drinks or other liquid foods to reduce taste fatigue. It should be consumed slowly and doses should be spaced evenly throughout the day to maximize tolerance.

Carcinogenesis, mutagenesis, impairment of fertility

Mutagenicity tests have been performed in Salmonella typhimurium, Saccharomyces cerevisiae, and Schizosaccharomyces pombe that do not indicate that CARNITOR® (Levocarnitine) is mutagenic. Long-term animal studies have not been conducted to evaluate the carcinogenicity of the compound.

Usage in pregnancy

Pregnancy Category B Reproductive studies have been performed in rats and rabbits using parenteral administration at doses equivalent on a mg/kg basis to the suggested oral adult dosage and have revealed no harm to the fetus due to CARNITOR® (Levocarnitine). There are, however, no adequate and well controlled studies in pregnant women. Because animal reproduction studies are not always predictive of human response, this drug should be used during pregnancy only if clearly needed.

Nursing mothers

Levocarnitine is a normal component of human milk. Levocarnitine supplementation in nursing mothers has not been studied.

Pediatric use

See Dosage and Administration.

ADVERSE REACTIONS

Various mild gastrointestinal complaints have been reported during the long-term administration of oral L- or D,L-carnitine; these include transient nausea and vomiting, abdominal cramps, and diarrhea. Mild myasthenia has been described only in uremic patients receiving D,L-carnitine. Gastrointestinal adverse reactions with CARNITOR® (Levocarnitine) Oral Solution dissolved in liquids might be avoided by a slow consumption of the solution or by a greater dilution. Decreasing the dosage often diminishes or eliminates drug-related patient body odor or gastrointestinal symptoms when present. Tolerance should be monitored very closely during the first week of administration, and after any dosage increases.

OVERDOSAGE

There have been no reports of toxicity from carnitine overdosage. The oral LD_{50} of levocarnitine in mice is 19.2 g/kg. Carnitine may cause diarrhea. Overdosage should be treated with supportive care.

DOSAGE AND ADMINISTRATION

CARNITOR® (Levocarnitine) Tablets.

Adults: The recommended oral dosage for adults is 990 mg two or three times a day using the 330 mg tablets, depending on clinical response.

Infants and children: The recommended oral dosage for infants and children is between 50 and 100 mg/kg/day in divided doses, with a maximum of 3 g/day. Dosage should begin at 50 mg/kg/day. The exact dosage will depend on clinical reponse.

Monitoring should include periodic blood chemistries, vital signs, plasma carnitine concentrations and overall clinical condition.

CARNITOR® (Levocarnitine) Oral Solution.

For oral use only. **Not for parenteral use.**

Adults: The recommended dosage of levocarnitine is 1 to 3 g/day for a 50 kg subject which is equivalent to 10 to 30 mL/day of Carnitor® (Levocarnitine) Oral Solution. Higher doses should be administered only with caution and only where clinical and biochemical considerations make it seem likely that higher doses will be of benefit. Dosage should start at 1 g/day, (10 mL/day), and be increased slowly while assessing tolerance and therapeutic response. Monitoring should include periodic blood chemistries, vital signs, plasma carnitine concentrations, and overall clinical condition.

Infants and children: The recommended dosage of levocarnitine is 50 to 100 mg/kg/day which is equivalent to 0.5 mL/kg/day CARNITOR® (Levocarnitine) Oral Solution. Higher doses should be administered only with caution and only where clinical and biochemical considerations make it seem likely that higher doses will be of benefit. Dosage should start at 50 mg/kg/day, and be increased slowly to a maximum of 3 g/day (30 mL/day) while assessing tolerance and therapeutic response. Monitoring should include periodic blood chemistries, vital signs, plasma carnitine concentrations, and overall clinical condition.

CARNITOR® (Levocarnitine) Oral Solution may be consumed alone or dissolved in drink or other liquid food. Doses should be spaced evenly throughout the day (every three or four hours) preferably during or following meals and should be consumed slowly in order to maximize tolerance.

HOW SUPPLIED

CARNITOR® (Levocarnitine) Tablets are supplied as 330 mg, individually foil wrapped tablets in boxes of 90 (NDC 54482-144-07). Store at room temperature (25°C/77°F).

CARNITOR® (Levocarnitine) Oral Solution is supplied in 118 mL (4 FL. OZ.) multiple-unit plastic containers. The multiple-unit containers are packaged 24 per case (NDC 54482-145-08). Store at room temperature (25°C/77°F).

CAUTION

Federal (U.S.A.) law prohibits dispensing without prescription.

CARNITOR® (Levocarnitine) Oral Solution manufactured for: Sigma-Tau Pharmaceuticals, Inc. By: Barre-National, Inc. Baltimore, MD 21207-2642.

REFERENCES

1. Bohmer T, Rynding A, Solberg HE: Carnitine levels in human serum in health and disease. **Clin Chim Acta 57**:55–61, 1974.
2. Brooks H, Goldberg L, Holland R et al: Carnitine-induced effects on cardiac and peripheral hemodynamics. **J Clin Pharmacol 17**:561–578, 1977.
3. Christiansen R, Bremer J: Active transport of butyrobetaine and carnitine into isolated liver cells. **Biochem Biophys Acta 448**:562–577, 1977.
4. Lindstedt S, Lindstedt G: Distribution and excretion of carnitine $^{14}CO_2$ in the rat. **Acta Chim Scand 15**:701–702, 1961.
5. Rebouche CJ, Engel AG: Carnitine metabolism and deficiency syndromes. **Mayo Clin Proc 58**:533–540, 1983.
6. Rebouche CJ, Paulson DJ: Carnitine metabolism and function in humans. **Ann Rev Nutr 6**:41–68, 1986.

sigma-tau

PHARMACEUTICALS, INC.

200 Orchard Ridge Drive, Gaithersburg, MD 20878

PREVIOUS EDITION IS OBSOLETE

ST-N18-948-3/92

SmithKline Beecham Consumer Brands

Unit of SmithKline Beecham Inc.
POST OFFICE BOX 1467
PITTSBURGH, PA 15230

A-200® — OTC
Lice Control Spray

PRODUCT OVERVIEW

KEY FACTS

A-200 Lice Control Spray is a pediculicide spray for controlling lice and louse eggs on inanimate objects, to help prevent reinfestation. It contains a highly active synthetic pyrethroid that kills lice and their eggs on inanimate objects. It also controls fleas and ticks.

MAJOR USES

A-200 Lice Control Spray effectively kills lice and louse eggs on garments, bedding, furniture and other inanimate objects that cannot be either laundered or dry cleaned.

SAFETY INFORMATION

A-200 Lice Control Spray is intended for use on inanimate objects only; it is not for use on humans or animals. It is harmful if swallowed. It should not be sprayed in the eyes or on the skin and should not be inhaled. The product should be used only in well ventilated areas; room(s) should be vacated after treatment and ventilated before reoccupying.

PRESCRIBING INFORMATION

A-200
Lice Control Spray

THIS PRODUCT IS NOT FOR USE ON HUMANS OR ANIMALS.

ACTIVE INGREDIENT

(5-Benzyl-3-Furyl)methyl 2,2-dimethyl-3-(2-methyl-propenyl)cyclopropane-carboxylate	0.500%
Related Compounds	0.068%
Aromatic petroleum hydrocarbons	0.664%
Inert Ingredients	98.768%
	100.000%

ACTIONS

A highly active synthetic pyrethroid for the control of lice and louse eggs on garments, bedding, furniture and other inanimate objects.

WARNINGS

HARMFUL IF SWALLOWED or absorbed through the skin. Avoid spraying in eyes. Avoid breathing spray mist. Avoid contact with skin. **THIS PRODUCT IS NOT FOR USE ON HUMANS OR ANIMALS.**

Vacate room after treatment and ventilate before reoccupying. Avoid contamination of feed and foodstuffs. Cover or remove fish bowls.

If lice infestations should occur on humans, consult either your physician or pharmacist for a product for use on humans.

Statement of Practical Treatment:

If inhaled: Remove affected person to fresh air. Apply artificial respiration if indicated.

If in eyes: Flush with plenty of water. Contact physician if irritation persists.

If on skin: Wash affected areas immediately with soap and water.

PHYSICAL AND CHEMICAL HAZARDS

Contents under pressure. Do not use or store near heat or open flame. Do not puncture or incinerate container. Exposure to temperatures above 130°F may cause bursting.

CAUTION: Avoid spraying in eyes. Avoid breathing spray mist. Use only in well ventilated areas. Avoid contact with skin. In case of contact wash immediately with soap and water. Vacate room after treatment and ventilate before reoccupying.

DIRECTIONS FOR USE

It is a violation of Federal law to use this product in a manner inconsistent with its labeling.

Shake well before each use. Remove protective cap. Aim spray opening away from person. Push button to spray.

To kill lice and louse eggs: Spray in an inconspicuous area to test for possible staining or discoloration. Inspect again after drying, then proceed to spray entire area to be treated. Hold container upright with nozzle away from you. Depress valve and spray from a distance of 8 to 10 inches. Spray each square foot for 3 seconds. Spray only those garments, parts of bedding, including mattresses and furniture that cannot be either laundered or dry cleaned. Allow all sprayed articles to dry thoroughly before use. Repeat treatment as necessary.

To kill fleas and ticks: Spray sleeping quarters, bedding, floor, and floor covering where pets are kept. Repeat as necessary. Only use a recommended pet spray on pets.

Buyer assumes all risks of use, storage or handling of this material not in strict accordance with direction given herewith.

DISPOSAL OF CONTAINER

Wrap container and dispose of in trash. Do not incinerate.

HOW SUPPLIED

6 ounce aerosol can. Also available in combination with A-200 Lice Treatment Kit.

Shown in Product Identification Section, page 429

A-200®$_1$ Pediculicide Shampoo Concentrate — OTC

DESCRIPTION

Active Ingredients: Pyrethrins 0..30% and piperonyl butoxide, technical 3.00%, equivalent to 2.4% (butylcarbityl) (6-propylpiperonyl) ether and to 0.6% related compounds. Also contains petroleum distillate 1.20% and benzyl alcohol 2.4% and remaining inert ingredients 93.1%.

Continued on next page

SmithKline Beecham Consumer—Cont.

INDICATIONS

A-200 is indicated for the treatment of head lice, body lice, and pubic (crab) lice.

ACTIONS

A-200 is an effective pediculicide to kill head lice (pediculus humanus capitis), body lice (pediculus humanus corporis), and pubic (crab) lice (phthirus pubis).

WARNING

A-200 should be used with caution by ragweed sensitized-persons.

PRECAUTIONS

This product is for external use on humans only. It is harmful if swallowed. If accidentally swallowed, call a physician or Poison Control Center immediately. It should not be inhaled. It should be kept out of the eyes and contact with mucous membranes should be avoided. If accidental contact with eyes occurs, flush eyes immediately with plenty of water. Call a physician if eye irritation persists. In case of infection or skin irritation, discontinue use immediately and consult a physician. Consult a physician before using this product if infestation of eyebrows or eyelashes occurs. Avoid contamination of feed or foodstuffs. Keep out of reach of children.

STORAGE AND DISPOSAL

Do not contaminate water, food or feed by storage or disposal. Do not transport or store below 32°F. Do not reuse empty container. Wrap in several layers of newspaper and discard in trash.

DIRECTIONS FOR USE

It is a violation of Federal Law to use the product in a manner inconsistent with its labeling. 1. Shake well. Apply undiluted A-200 to dry hair and scalp or any other infested areas and wet entirely. Do not use on eyelashes or eyebrows. 2. Allow A-200 shampoo to remain on area for 10 minutes before washing thoroughly with warm water and soap or regular shampoo. 3. Dead lice and eggs should be removed with special A-200 precision comb provided. 4. Repeat treatment in 7–10 days to kill any newly hatched lice. Do not exceed two consecutive applications within 24 hours.

Since lice infestations are spread by contact, it is important that each family member be examined carefully. If infested, they should be treated promptly to avoid spread or reinfestation of previously treated individuals. To eliminate infestation, all personal head gear, scarfs, coats, and bed linen should be laundered in hot water or dry cleaned. Carpets, upholstery, and mattresses should be vacuumed thoroughly. Combs and brushes should be soaked in hot water (above 130°) for 5 to 10 minutes.

HOW SUPPLIED

In 2 and 4 fl. oz. unbreakable plastic bottles. An A-200 precision comb that removes nits and patient instruction booklet in English and Spanish are included in each carton. Also available in combination with A-200 Lice Treatment Kit.

Shown in Product Identification Section, page 429

ECOTRIN®   OTC
Enteric-Coated Aspirin
Antiarthritic, Antiplatelet

DESCRIPTION

'Ecotrin' is enteric-coated aspirin (acetylsalicylic acid, ASA) available in tablet and caplet forms in 325 mg and 500 mg dosage units.

The enteric coating covers a core of aspirin and is designed to resist disintegration in the stomach, dissolving in the more neutral-to-alkaline environment of the duodenum. Such action helps to protect the stomach from injury that may result from ingestion of plain, buffered or highly buffered aspirin (see SAFETY).

INDICATIONS

'Ecotrin' is indicated for:
- conditions requiring chronic or long-term aspirin therapy for pain and/or inflammation, e.g., rheumatoid arthritis, juvenile rheumatoid arthritis, systemic lupus erythematosus, osteoarthritis (degenerative joint disease), ankylosing spondylitis, psoriatic arthritis, Reiter's syndrome and fibrositis,
- antiplatelet indications of aspirin (see the ANTIPLATELET EFFECT section) and
- situations in which compliance with aspirin therapy may be affected because of the gastrointestinal side effects of plain, i.e., non-enteric-coated, or buffered aspirin.

DOSAGE

For analgesic or anti-inflammatory indications, the OTC maximum dosage for aspirin is 4000 mg per day in divided doses, i.e., 2-325 mg tablets or caplets or 3-325 mg tablets or caplets or 2-500 mg tablets or caplets.

For antiplatelet effect dosage: see the ANTIPLATELET EFFECT section.

Under a physician's direction, the dosage can be increased or otherwise modified as appropriate to the clinical situation. When 'Ecotrin' is used for anti-inflammatory effect, the physician should be attentive to plasma salicylate levels, and may also caution the patient to be alert to the development of tinnitus as an indicator of elevated salicylate levels. It should be noted that patients with a high frequency hearing loss (such as may occur in older individuals) may have difficulty perceiving the tinnitus. Tinnitus would then not be a reliable indicator in such individuals.

INACTIVE INGREDIENTS

Inactive ingredients: Cellulose, Cellulose Acetate Phthalate, D&C Yellow 10, Diethyl Phthalate, FD&C Yellow 6, Pregelatinized Starch, Silicon Dioxide, Sodium Starch Glycolate, Stearic Acid, Titanium Dioxide, and trace amounts of other inactive ingredients.

BIOAVAILABILITY

The bioavailability of aspirin from 'Ecotrin' has been demonstrated in a number of salicylate excretion studies. The studies show levels of salicylate (and metabolites) in urine excreted over 48 hours for 'Ecotrin' do not differ statistically from plain, i.e., non-enteric-coated, aspirin.

Plasma studies, in which 'Ecotrin' has been compared with plain aspirin in steady-state studies over eight days, also demonstrate that 'Ecotrin' provides plasma salicylate levels not statistically different from plain aspirin.

Information regarding salicylate levels over a range of doses was generated in a study in which 24 healthy volunteers (12 male and 12 female) took daily (divided) doses of either 2600 mg, 3900 mg, or 5200 mg of 'Ecotrin'. Plasma salicylate levels generally acknowledged to be anti-inflammatory (15 mg/dL) were attained at daily doses of 5200 mg, on Day 2 by females and Day 3 by males. At 3900 mg, anti-inflammatory levels were attained at Day 3 by females and Day 4 by males. Dissolution of the enteric coating occurs at a neutral-to-basic pH and is therefore dependent on gastric emptying into the duodenum. With continued dosing, appropriate plasma levels are maintained.

SAFETY

The safety of 'Ecotrin' has been demonstrated in a number of endoscopic studies comparing 'Ecotrin', plain aspirin, buffered aspirin, and highly buffered aspirin preparations. In these studies, all forms of aspirin were dosed to the OTC maximum (3900–4000 mg per day) for up to 14 days. The normal healthy volunteers participating in these studies were gastroscoped before and after the courses of treatment and 14-day drug-free periods followed active drug. Compared to all the other preparations, there was less gastric damage at a statistically significant level during the 'Ecotrin' courses. There was also statistically less duodenal damage when compared with the plain i.e., non-enteric-coated aspirin.

Details of studies demonstrating the safety and bioavailability of 'Ecotrin' are available to health care professionals. Write: Professional Services Department, SmithKline Beecham Consumer Brands, P.O. Box 1467, Pittsburgh, Pa. 15230.

WARNING

Consumer Warning: Children and teenagers should not use this medicine for chicken pox or flu symptoms before a doctor is consulted about Reye syndrome, a rare but serious illness. Do not take this product for pain for more than 10 days unless directed by a physician. If pain persists or gets worse, if new symptoms occur, or if redness or swelling is present, consult a physician because these could be signs of a serious condition. Also, consult a physician before using this medicine to treat arthritic or rheumatic conditions affecting children under 12. Discontinue use if dizziness occurs. Do not take this product if you are allergic to aspirin, have asthma, or if you have ulcers or bleeding problems unless directed by a physician. If ringing in the ears or a loss of hearing occurs, consult a physician before taking any more of this product. If you experience persistent or unexplained stomach upset, consult a physician. Keep this and all drugs out of children's reach. In case of accidental overdose, seek professional assistance or contact a poison control center immediately. As with any medicine, if you are pregnant or nursing a baby seek the advice of a health professional before using this product. IT IS ESPECIALLY IMPORTANT NOT TO USE ASPIRIN DURING THE LAST 3 MONTHS OF PREGNANCY UNLESS SPECIFICALLY DIRECTED TO DO SO BY A DOCTOR BECAUSE IT MAY CAUSE PROBLEMS IN THE UNBORN CHILD OR COMPLICATIONS DURING DELIVERY.

Store at controlled room temperature (59°–86°F.).

Drug Interaction Precaution: Do not take this product if you are taking a prescription drug for anticoagulation (thinning of the blood), diabetes, gout, or arthritis unless directed by a physician.

Professional Warning: There have been occasional reports in the literature concerning individuals with impaired gastric emptying in whom there may be retention of one or more 'Ecotrin' tablets over time. This unusual phenomenon may occur as a result of outlet obstruction from ulcer disease alone or combined with hypotonic gastric peristalsis. Because of the integrity of the enteric coating in an acidic environment, these tablets may accumulate and form a bezoar in the stomach. Individuals with this condition may present with complaints of early satiety or of vague upper abdominal distress. Diagnosis may be made by endoscopy or by abdominal films which show opacities suggestive of a mass of small tablets *(Ref.: Bogacz, K. and Caldron, P.: Enteric-coated Aspirin Bezoar: Elevation of Serum Salicylate Level by Barium Study. Amer. J. Med. 1987:83, 783-6.).* Management may vary according to the condition of the patient. Options include: gastrotomy and alternating slightly basic and neutral lavage *(Ref.: Baum, J.: Enteric-Coated Aspirin and the Problem of Gastric Retention. J. Rheum., 1984:11, 250-1.).* While there have been no clinical reports, it has been suggested that such individuals may also be treated with parenteral cimetidine (to reduce acid secretion) and then given sips of slightly basic liquids to effect gradual dissolution of the enteric coating. Progress may be followed with plasma salicylate levels or via recognition of tinnitus by the patient.

It should be kept in mind that individuals with a history of partial or complete gastrectomy may produce reduced amounts of acid and therefore have less acidic gastric pH. Under these circumstances, the benefits offered by the acid-resistant enteric coating may not exist.

ANTIPLATELET EFFECT

FDA approved professional labeling permits the use of aspirin to reduce the risk of death and/or nonfatal myocardial infarction (MI) in patients with a previous infarction or unstable angina pectoris and its use in reducing the risk of transient ischemic attacks in men.

Labeling for both indications follows:

ASPIRIN FOR MYOCARDIAL INFARCTION

Indication: Aspirin is indicated to reduce the risk of death and/or nonfatal myocardial infarction in patients with a previous infarction or unstable angina pectoris.

Clinical Trials: The indication is supported by the results of six, large, randomized multicenter, placebo-controlled studies involving 10,816 predominantly male, post-myocardial infarction (MI) patients and one randomized placebo-controlled study of 1,266 men with unstable angina.[1–7] Therapy with aspirin was begun at intervals after the onset of acute MI varying from less than three days to more than five years and continued for periods of from less than one year to four years. In the unstable angina study, treatment was started within one month after the onset of unstable angina and continued for 12 weeks, and patients with complicating conditions such as congestive heart failure were not included in the study.

Aspirin therapy in MI patients was associated with about a 20 percent reduction in the risk of subsequent death and/or nonfatal reinfarction, a median absolute decrease of 3 percent from the 12 to 22 percent event rates in the placebo groups. In aspirin-treated unstable angina patients, the reduction in risk was about 50 percent, a reduction in event rate of 5% from the 10% in the placebo group over the 12 weeks of the study.

Daily dosage of aspirin in the post-myocardial infarction studies was 300 mg in one study and 900 to 1500 mg in five studies. A dose of 325 mg was used in the study of unstable angina.

Adverse Reactions

Gastrointestinal Reactions: Doses of 1000 mg per day of plain aspirin caused gastrointestinal symptoms and bleeding that in some cases were clinically significant. In the largest postinfarction study (the Aspirin Myocardial Infarction Study [AMIS] with 4,500 people), the percentage incidences of gastrointestinal symptoms of a standard, solid-tablet formulation and placebo-treated subjects, respectively, were: stomach pain (14.5%; 4.4%); heartburn (11.9%; 4.8%); nausea and/or vomiting (7.6%; 2.1%); hospitalization for gastrointestinal disorder (4.9%; 3.5%). In the AMIS and other trials, plain aspirin-treated patients had increased rates of gross gastrointestinal bleeding. Symptoms and signs of gastrointestinal irritation were not significantly increased in subjects treated for unstable angina with buffered aspirin in solution.

Cardiovascular and Biochemical: In the AMIS trial, the dosage of 1000 mg per day of plain aspirin was associated with small increases in systolic blood pressure (BP) (average 1.5 to 2.1 mmHg) and diastolic BP (0.5 to 0.6 mmHg), depending upon whether maximal or last available readings were used. Blood urea nitrogen and uric acid levels were also increased, but by less than 1.0 mg%. Subjects with marked hypertension or renal insufficiency had been excluded from the trial so that the clinical importance of these observations for such subjects or for any subjects treated over more prolonged periods is not known. It is recommended that patients placed on long-term aspirin treatment, even at doses of 300

mg per day, be seen at regular intervals to assess changes in these measurements.

Sodium in Buffered Aspirin for Solution Formulations: One tablet daily of buffered aspirin in solution adds 553 mg of sodium to that in the diet and may not be tolerated by patients with active sodium-retaining states such as congestive heart or renal failure. This amount of sodium adds about 30 percent to the 70 to 90 meq intake suggested as appropriate for dietary hypertension in the 1984 Report of the Joint National Committee on Detection, Evaluation, and Treatment of High Blood Pressure.[8]

Dosage and Administration: Although most of the studies used dosages exceeding 300 mg daily, two trials used only 300 mg and pharmacologic data indicate that this dose inhibits platelet function fully. Therefore, 300 mg or a conventional 325 mg aspirin dose daily is a reasonable, routine dose that would minimize gastrointestinal adverse reactions for both solid oral dosage forms (buffered and plain aspirin) and buffered aspirin in solution.

References:

1. Elwood, P.C., et al.: A Randomized Controlled Trial of Acetylsalicylic Acid in the Secondary Prevention of Mortality from Myocardial Infarction, *Br. Med. J.* 1:436–440, 1974.
2. The Coronary Drug Project Research Group: Aspirin in Coronary Heart Disease, *J. Chronic Dis.* 29:625–642, 1976.
3. Breddin, K., et al.: Secondary Prevention of Myocardial Infarction: A Comparison of Acetylsalicylic Acid, Phenprocoumon or Placebo, *Homeostasis* 470:263–268, 1979.
4. Aspirin Myocardial Infarction Study Research Group: A Randomized Controlled Trial of Aspirin in Persons Recovered from Myocardial Infarction, *J.A.M.A.* 243:661–669, 1980.
5. Elwood, P.C., and Sweetnam, P.M.: Aspirin and Secondary Mortality After Myocardial Infarction, *Lancet* pp. 1313–1315, Dec. 22–29, 1979.
6. The Persantine-Aspirin Reinfarction Study Research Group, Persantine and Aspirin in Coronary Heart Disease, *Circulation* 62:449–469, 1980.
7. Lewis, H.D., et al.: Protective Effects of Aspirin Against Acute Myocardial Infarction and Death in Men with Unstable Angina, Results of a Veterans Administration Cooperative Study, *N. Engl. J. Med.* 309:396–403, 1983.
8. 1984 Report of the Joint National Committee on Detection, Evaluation, and Treatment of High Blood Pressure, "U.S. Department of Health and Human Services and U.S. Public Health Service, National Institutes of Health. NIH Pub. No. 84-1088, 1984."

"ASPIRIN FOR TRANSIENT ISCHEMIC ATTACKS"

Indication

For reducing the risk of recurrent Transient Ischemic Attacks (TIA's) or stroke in men who have had transient ischemia of the brain due to fibrin platelet emboli. There is inadequate evidence that aspirin or buffered aspirin is effective in reducing TIA's in women at the recommended dosage. There is no evidence that aspirin or buffered aspirin is of benefit in the treatment of completed strokes in men or women.

Clinical Trials

The indication is supported by the results of a Canadian study (1) in which 585 patients with threatened stroke were followed in a randomized clinical trial for an average of 26 months to determine whether aspirin or sulfinpyrazone, singly or in combination, was superior to placebo in preventing transient ischemic attacks, stroke or death. The study showed that, although sulfinpyrazone had no statistically significant effect, aspirin reduced the risk of continuing transient ischemic attacks, stroke or death by 19 percent and reduced the risk of stroke or death by 31 percent. Another aspirin study carried out in the United States with 178 patients, showed a statistically significant number of "favorable outcomes," including reduced transient ischemic attacks, stroke and death (2).

Precautions

Patients presenting with signs and/or symptoms of TIA's should have a complete medical and neurologic evaluation. Consideration should be given to other disorders that resemble TIA's. Attention should be given to risk factors: it is important to evaluate and treat, if appropriate, other diseases associated with TIA's and stroke, such as hypertension and diabetes.

Concurrent administration of absorbable antacids at therapeutic doses may increase the clearance of salicylates in some individuals. The concurrent administration of nonabsorbable antacids may alter the rate of absorption of aspirin, thereby resulting in a decreased acetylsalicylic acid/salicylate ratio in plasma. The clinical significance of these decreases in available aspirin is unknown.

Aspirin at dosages of 1,000 milligrams per day has been associated with small increases in blood pressure, blood urea nitrogen, and serum uric acid levels. It is recommended that patients placed on long-term aspirin treatment be seen at regular intervals to assess changes in these measurements.

Adverse Reactions:

At dosages of 1,000 milligrams or higher of aspirin per day, gastrointestinal side effects include stomach pain, heartburn, nausea and/or vomiting, as well as increased rates of gross gastrointestinal bleeding.

Dosage and Administration

Adult dosage for men is 1,300 mg a day, in divided doses of 650 mg twice a day or 325 mg four times a day.

REFERENCES

(1) The Canadian Cooperative Study Group, "Randomized Trial of Aspirin and Sulfinpyrazone in Threatened Stroke," *New England Journal of Medicine*, 299:53–59, 1978.
(2) Fields, W. S., et al., "Controlled Trial of Aspirin in Cerebral Ischemia," *Stroke* 8:301-316, 1977."

SUPPLIED

'Ecotrin' Tablets
  325 mg in bottles of 100*, 250 and 1000.
  500 mg in bottles of 60* and 150.
'Ecotrin' Caplets
  325 mg in bottles of 100.
  500 mg in bottles of 60.
*Without Child-Resistant Caps.

TAMPER-RESISTANT PACKAGE FEATURES FOR YOUR PROTECTION:

- Bottle has imprinted seal under cap.
- The words ECOTRIN REG or ECOTRIN MAX appear on each tablet or caplet (see product illustration printed on carton).
- **DO NOT USE THIS PRODUCT IF ANY OF THESE TAMPER-RESISTANT FEATURES ARE MISSING OR BROKEN.**

Comments or Questions?
Call toll-free 800-245-1040 weekdays.

FEOSOL® CAPSULES   OTC
Hematinic

DESCRIPTION

'Feosol' Capsules provide the body with ferrous sulfate—iron in its most efficient form—for simple iron deficiency and iron-deficiency anemia. The special targeted-release capsule formulation—ferrous sulfate in pellets—reduces stomach upset, a common problem with iron.

FORMULA

Each capsule contains 159 mg. of dried ferrous sulfate USP (50 mg. of elemental iron), equivalent to 250 mg. of ferrous sulfate USP. Inactive Ingredients (listed for individuals with specific allergies): Benzyl Alcohol, Cetylpyridinium Chloride, D&C Red 33, Yellow 10, FD&C Blue 1, D&C Red 7, Red 40, Gelatin, Glyceryl Stearates, Iron Oxide, Polyethylene Glycol, Povidone, Sodium Lauryl Sulfate, Starch, Sucrose, and White Wax.

DOSAGE

Adults: 1 or 2 capsules daily or as directed by a physician. Children: As directed by a physician.

TAMPER-RESISTANT PACKAGE FEATURES:

- Each capsule is encased in a plastic cell with a foil back; do not use if cell or foil is broken.
- Each FEOSOL capsule is protected by a red Perma-Seal™ band which bonds the two capsule halves together; do not use if capsule is broken or band is missing or broken.

WARNING

Do not exceed recommended dosage. The treatment of any anemic condition should be under the advice and supervision of a physician. Iron-containing medication may occasionally cause constipation or diarrhea. Since oral iron products interfere with absorption of oral tetracycline antibiotics, these products should not be taken within two hours of each other. Keep this and all drugs out of the reach of children. In case of accidental overdose, seek professional assistance or contact a poison control center immediately. As with any drug, if you are pregnant or nursing a baby, seek the advice of a health professional before using this product.
Store at controlled room temperature (59°–86°F.).
This carton is protected by a printed overwrap. Do not use if missing or broken.

HOW SUPPLIED

Packages of 30 and 60 capsules, bottle of 500's; in Single Unit Packages of 100 capsules (intended for institutional use only).
Also available in Tablets and Elixir.

FEOSOL® ELIXIR   OTC
Hematinic

DESCRIPTION

'Feosol' Elixir, an unusually palatable iron elixir, provides the body with ferrous sulfate—iron in its most efficient form. The standard elixir for simple iron deficiency and iron-deficiency anemia when the need for such therapy has been determined by a physician. Each 5 ml. (1 teaspoonful) contains ferrous sulfate, USP, 220 mg. (44 mg. of elemental iron); alcohol, 5%.

Inactive Ingredients (listed for individuals with specific allergies): Citric Acid, FD&C Yellow 6 (Sunset Yellow) as a color additive, Flavors, Glucose, Saccharin Sodium, Sucrose, Purified Water.

USUAL DOSAGE

Adults—1 to 2 teaspoonsful three times daily preferably between meals. Children—½ to 1 teaspoonful three times daily preferably between meals. Infants—as directed by physician. Mix with water or fruit juice to avoid temporary staining of teeth; do not mix with milk or wine-based vehicles.

TAMPER-RESISTANT PACKAGE FEATURE:
IMPRINTED SEAL AROUND BOTTLE CAP; DO NOT USE IF BROKEN.

WARNING

The treatment of any anemic condition should be under the advice and supervision of a physician. Since oral iron products interfere with absorption of oral tetracycline antibiotics, these products should not be taken within two hours of each other. Occasional gastrointestinal discomfort (such as nausea) may be minimized by taking with meals and by beginning with one teaspoonful the first day, two the second, etc. until the recommended dosage is reached. Iron-containing medication may occasionally cause constipation or diarrhea, and liquids may cause temporary staining of the teeth (this is less likely when diluted). Keep this and all drugs out of reach of children. In case of accidental overdose, seek professional assistance or contact a poison control center immediately. As with any drug, if you are pregnant or nursing a baby, seek the advice of a health professional before using this product.
Store at controlled room temperature (59°–86°F.).

HOW SUPPLIED

A clear orange liquid in 16 fl. oz. bottles.

ALSO AVAILABLE

'Feosol' Tablets, 'Feosol' Capsules.

FEOSOL® TABLETS   OTC
Hematinic

PRODUCT INFORMATION

'Feosol' Tablets provide the body with ferrous sulfate, iron in its most efficient form, for iron deficiency and iron-deficiency anemia when the need for such therapy has been determined by a physician. The distinctive triangular-shaped tablet has a coating to prevent oxidation and improve palatability.

FORMULA

Active Ingredient: Each tablet contains 200 mg. of dried ferrous sulfate USP (65 mg. of elemental iron), equivalent to 325 mg. (5 grains) of ferrous sulfate USP. Inactive Ingredients (listed for individuals with specific allergies): Calcium Sulfate, D&C Yellow 10, FD&C Blue 2, Glucose, Hydroxypropyl Methylcellulose, Mineral Oil, Polyethylene Glycol, Sodium Lauryl Sulfate, Starch, Stearic Acid, Talc, and Titanium Dioxide.

USUAL DOSAGE

Adults—one tablet 3 to 4 times daily, after meals and upon retiring. Children 6 to 12 years—one tablet three times a day after meals or as directed by a physician. Children under 6 years and infants—use 'Feosol' Elixir.

TAMPER-RESISTANT PACKAGE FEATURES:

- Bottle has printed innerseal beneath cap. Do not use if missing or broken.
- FEOSOL Tablets are triangular shaped (see product illustration printed on carton).

CAUTION: **DO NOT USE THIS PRODUCT IF ANY OF THESE TAMPER-RESISTANT FEATURES ARE MISSING OR BROKEN.**

Comments or Questions?
Call toll-free 800-245-1040 weekdays.

WARNINGS

Do not exceed recommended dosage. The treatment of any anemic condition should be under the advice and supervision of a physician. Since oral iron products interfere with absorption of oral tetracycline antibiotics, these products should not be taken within two hours of each other. Occasional gastrointestinal discomfort (such as nausea) may be minimized by taking with meals and by beginning with one tablet the first day, two the second, etc. until the recommended dosage is reached. Iron-containing medication may occasionally cause constipation or diarrhea. Keep this and all drugs out of reach of children. In case of accidental overdose, seek professional assistance or contact a poison control center immediately. As with any drug, if you are pregnant or

Continued on next page

SmithKline Beecham Consumer—Cont.

nursing a baby, seek the advice of a health professional before using this product.

Store at controlled room temperature (59°–86°F.).

This carton protected by a printed overwrap. Do not use if missing or broken.

HOW SUPPLIED

Bottles of 100 or 1000 tablets; in Single Unit Packages of 100 tablets (intended for institutional use only).

Also available in Capsules and Elixir.

MASSENGILL® Douches   OTC
[*mas 'sen-gil*]

PRODUCT OVERVIEW

KEY FACTS

Massengill is the brand name for a line of douches which are recommended for routine cleansing and for temporary relief of vaginal itching and irritation. Massengill disposable douches are available in two Vinegar & Water formulas (Extra Mild and Extra Cleansing), a Baking Soda formula, four Cosmetic solutions (Country Flowers, Belle-Mai Powder (Fresh Baby Powder Scent), Mountain Breeze, and Spring Rain Freshness), and a Medicated formula (with povidone-iodine). Massengill also is available in a Medicated liquid concentrate (povidone-iodine) and a Non-Medicated liquid concentrate and powder form.

MAJOR USES

Massengill's Vinegar & Water, Baking Soda & Water, and Cosmetic douches are recommended for routine douching, or for cleansing following menstruation, prescribed use of vaginal medication or use of contraceptives. Massengill Medicated is recommended in a seven day regimen for the symptomatic relief of minor itching and irritation associated with vaginitis due to Candida albicans, Trichomonas vaginalis, and Gardnerella vaginalis.

SAFETY INFORMATION

Do not douche during pregnancy unless directed by a physician. Douching does not prevent pregnancy. Do not use this product and consult your physician if you are experiencing any of the following symptoms: unusual vaginal discharge, painful and/or frequent urination, lower abdominal pain, or you or your sex partner has genital sores or ulcers. Massengill Vinegar & Water, Baking Soda & Water, and Cosmetic Douches—If irritation occurs, discontinue use. Massengill Medicated — Women with iodine-sensitivity should not use this product. If symptoms persist after seven days, or if redness, swelling or pain develop, consult a physician. Do not use while nursing unless directed by a physician.

PRODUCT INFORMATION

MASSENGILL®
[*mas 'sen-gil*]
Disposable Douches
MASSENGILL®
Liquid Concentrate
MASSENGILL® Powder

INGREDIENTS

DISPOSABLES: Extra Mild Vinegar and Water—Water and Vinegar.

Extra Cleansing Vinegar and Water—Water, Vinegar, Puraclean™ (Cetylpyridinium Chloride), Diazolidinyl Urea, Disodium EDTA.

Baking Soda and Water—Sanitized Water, Sodium Bicarbonate (Baking Soda).

Belle-Mai Powder (Fresh Baby Powder Scent)—Water, SD Alcohol 40, Lactic Acid, Sodium Lactate, Octoxynol-9, Cetylpyridinium Chloride, Propylene Glycol (and) Diazolidinyl Urea (and) Methyl Paraben (and) Propyl Paraben, Disodium EDTA, Fragrance, FD&C Blue #1.

Country Flowers—Water, SD Alcohol 40, Lactic Acid, Sodium Lactate, Octoxynol-9, Cetylpyridinium Chloride, Propylene Glycol (and) Diazolidinyl Urea (and), Methyl Paraben (and) Propyl Paraben, Disodium EDTA, Fragrance, D&C Red #28, FD&C Blue #1.

Mountain Breeze—Water, SD Alcohol 40, Lactic Acid, Sodium Lactate, Octoxynol-9, Cetylpyridinium Chloride, Propylene Glycol (and) Diazolidinyl Urea (and) Methyl Paraben (and) Propyl Paraben, Disodium EDTA, Fragrance, D&C Yellow #10, FD&C Blue #1.

Spring Rain Freshness—Water, SD Alcohol 40, Lactic Acid, Sodium Lactate, Octoxynol-9, Cetylpyridinium Chloride, Propylene Glycol (and) Diazolidinyl Urea (and Methylparaben (and) Propylparaben, Disodium EDTA, Fragrance.

LIQUID CONCENTRATE: Water, SD Alcohol 40, Lactic Acid, Sodium Bicarbonate, Octoxynol-9, Methyl Salicylate, Liquid Menthol, Eucalyptol, Thymol, D&C Yellow #10, FD&C Yellow #6 (Sunset Yellow).

POWDER: Sodium Chloride, Ammonium alum, PEG-8, Phenol, Methyl Salicylate, Eucalyptus Oil, Menthol, Thymol, D&C Yellow #10, FD&C Yellow #6 (Sunset Yellow).

FLORAL POWDER: Sodium Chloride, Ammonium alum, Octoxynol-9, SD Alcohol 23-A, Fragrance, and FD&C Yellow #6 (Sunset Yellow).

INDICATIONS

Recommended for routine cleansing at the end of menstruation, after use of contraceptive creams or jellies (check the contraceptive package instructions first) or to rinse out the residue of prescribed vaginal medication (as directed by physician).

ACTIONS

The buffered acid solutions of Massengill Douches are valuable adjuncts to specific vaginal therapy following the prescribed use of vaginal medication or contraceptives and in feminine hygiene.

DIRECTIONS

DISPOSABLES: Twist off flat, wing-shaped tab from bottle containing premixed solution, attach nozzle supplied and use. The unit is completely disposable.

LIQUID CONCENTRATE: Fill cap ¾ full, to measuring line, and pour contents into douche bag containing 1 quart of warm water. Mix thoroughly.

POWDER: Dissolve two rounded teaspoonfuls in a douche bag containing 1 quart of warm water. Mix thoroughly.

WARNING

Douching does not prevent pregnancy. If vaginal dryness or irritation occurs discontinue use. Do not use during pregnancy except under the advice and supervision of your physician. If you are experiencing vaginal discharge of an unusual amount, color, or odor, or painful and/or frequent urination, lower abdominal pain or genital sores or ulcers, or have had sex with a partner who has genital symptoms, you may have a serious condition. Do not use this product and contact your doctor immediately.

Use this product only as directed for routine cleansing. You should douche no more than twice a week except on the advice of your doctor.

An association has been reported between frequent douching and pelvic inflammatory disease (PID), a serious infection of the reproductive system. Douches should not be used for self-treatment of sexually transmitted diseases or PID. If you suspect you have one of these infections, stop using this product and see your doctor immediately.

Keep out of reach of children. In case of accidental ingestion, seek professional assistance by contacting your physician, the local poison control center, or the Rocky Mt. Poison Control Center at 303-592-1710 (collect), 24 hours a day.

HOW SUPPLIED

Disposable—6 oz. disposable plastic bottle.

Liquid Concentrate—4 oz., 8 oz., plastic bottles.

Powder—4 oz., 8 oz., 16 oz., Packettes—10's, 12's.

MASSENGILL® Medicated   OTC
[*mas 'sen-gil*]
Disposable Douche
MASSENGILL® Medicated
Liquid Concentrate

ACTIVE INGREDIENT

DISPOSABLE: Cepticin™ (povidone-iodine)

LIQUID CONCENTRATE: Cepticin™ (povidone-iodine)

INDICATIONS

For symptomatic relief of minor vaginal irritation or itching associated with vaginitis due to Candida albicans, Trichomonas vaginalis, and Gardnerella vaginalis.

ACTION

Povidone-iodine is widely recognized as an effective broad spectrum microbicide against both gram negative and gram positive bacteria, fungi, yeasts and protozoa. While remaining active in the presence of blood, serum or bodily secretions, it possesses virtually none of the irritating properties of iodine.

WARNINGS

Douching does not prevent pregnancy. Do not use during pregnancy or while nursing except under the advice and supervision of your physician. If vaginal dryness or irritation occurs discontinue use. If you are experiencing vaginal discharge of an unusual amount, color, or odor or painful and/or frequent urination, lower abdominal pain or genital sores or ulcers, or have had sex with a partner who has genital symptoms, you may have a serious condition. Do not use this product and contact your doctor immediately.

Use this product only as directed. Do not use this product for routine cleansing.

An association has been reported between frequent douching and pelvic inflammatory disease (PID), a serious infection of the reproductive system. Douches should not be used for
self-treatment of sexually transmitted diseases or PID. If you suspect you have one of these infections, stop using this product and see your doctor immediately. Women with iodine sensitivity should not use this product. Keep out of the reach of children. In case of accidental ingestion, seek professional assistance by contacting your physician, the local poison control center, or the Rocky Mt. Poison Control Center at 303-592-1710 (Collect), 24 hours a day.

DOSAGE AND ADMINISTRATION

DISPOSABLE: Dosage is provided as a single unit concentrate to be added to 6 oz. of sanitized water supplied in a disposable bottle. A specially designed nozzle is provided. After use, the unit is discarded. Use one bottle a day. Although symptoms may be relieved earlier, for maximum relief, use for seven days.

LIQUID CONCENTRATE: Pour one capful into douche bag containing one quart of water. Mix thoroughly. Use once daily. Although symptoms may be relieved earlier, for maximum relief, use for seven days.

HOW SUPPLIED

Disposable—6 oz. bottle of sanitized water with 0.17 oz. vial of povidone-iodine and nozzle.

Liquid Concentrate—4 oz., 8 oz. plastic bottles.

MASSENGILL® Medicated   OTC
[*mas 'sen-gil*]
Soft Cloth Towelette

ACTIVE INGREDIENT

Hydrocortisone (0.5%).

INACTIVE INGREDIENTS

Diazolidinyl Urea, DMDM Hydantoin, Isopropyl Myristate, Methylparaben, Polysorbate 60, Propylene Glycol, Propylparaben, Sorbitan Stearate, Steareth-2, Steareth-21, Water.

Also available in non-medicated Baby Powder Scent and Unscented formulas to freshen and cleanse the external vaginal area.

INDICATIONS

For soothing relief of minor external feminine itching or other itching associated with minor skin irritations, inflammation and rashes. Other uses of this product should be only under the advice and supervision of a physician.

ACTION

Massengill Medicated Soft Cloth Towelettes contain hydrocortisone, a proven anti-inflammatory, anti-pruritic ingredient. The towelette delivery system makes the application soothing, soft, and gentle.

WARNINGS

For external use only. Avoid contact with eyes. If condition worsens, symptoms persist for more than seven days, or symptoms recur within a few days, do not use this or any other hydrocortisone product unless you have consulted a physician. If experiencing a vaginal discharge, see a physician. Do not use this product for the treatment of diaper rash.

Keep this and all drugs out of the reach of children. As with any drug, if pregnant or nursing a baby, seek the advice of a health professional before using this product. In case of accidental ingestion, seek professional assistance or contact a Poison Control Center immediately.

DIRECTIONS

Adults and Children two years of age and older—apply to the affected area not more than three to four times daily. Remove towelette from foil packet, gently wipe, and discard. Throw away towelette after it has been used once. Children under 2 years of age: DO NOT USE.

HOW SUPPLIED

Ten individually wrapped, disposable towelettes per carton.

MASSENGILL®   OTC
[*mas 'sen-gil*]
Fragrance-Free Soft Cloth Towelette

INACTIVE INGREDIENTS

Water, Octoxynol-9, Lactic Acid, Sodium Lactate, Potassium Sorbate, Disodium EDTA, and Cetylpyridinium Chloride.

INDICATIONS

For cleansing and refreshing the external vaginal area.

ACTIONS

Massengill Fragrance-Free Soft Cloth Towelettes safely cleanse the external vaginal area and do not contain fragrance. The towelette delivery system makes the application soft and gentle.

WARNINGS

For external use only. Avoid contact with eyes.

DIRECTIONS

Remove towelette from foil packet, unfold, and gently wipe. Throw away towelette after it has been used once.

HOW SUPPLIED

Sixteen individually wrapped, disposable towelettes per carton.

NATURE'S REMEDY® Laxative   OTC
NATURE'S REMEDY® Enema

(See PDR For Nonprescription Drugs.)

OXY–5® Vanishing & Tinted   OTC
OXY–10® Vanishing & Tinted   OTC
Benzoyl Peroxide Lotion 5% and 10%

(See PDR For Nonprescription Drugs.)

OXY-10® DAILY FACE WASH   OTC
Antibacterial Skin Wash

(See PDR For Nonprescription Drugs.)

TELDRIN®   OTC
Chlorpheniramine maleate
Timed-Release Allergy Capsules
Maximum Strength 12 mg.

Antihistamine

FORMULA

Active Ingredient: Each capsule contains Chlorpheniramine Maleate, 12 mg. Inactive Ingredients (listed for individuals with specific allergies): Benzyl Alcohol, Cetylpyridinium Chloride, D&C Red No. 27, D&C Red No. 30, D&C Red No. 33, Ethylcellulose, FD&C Green No. 3, FD&C Red No. 40, FD&C Yellow No. 6, Gelatin, Hydrogenated Castor Oil, Silicon Dioxide, Sodium Lauryl Sulfate, Starch, Sucrose, and trace amounts of other inactive ingredients.

DESCRIPTION

Each 'Teldrin' Timed-Release capsule contains chlorpheniramine maleate, Maximum Strength 12 mg., so formulated that a portion of the antihistamine dose is released initially, and the remaining medication is released gradually over a prolonged period.

INDICATIONS FOR USE

Hay fever and allergies are caused by grass and tree pollen, dust and pollution. 'Teldrin' provides up to 12 hours of relief from hay fever/upper respiratory allergy symptoms; sneezing; runny nose; itchy, watery eyes.

DOSAGE

Adults and children over 12 years of age: Just one capsule in the morning, and one in the evening. Do not give to children under 12 without the advice and consent of a physician. Not to exceed 24 mg. (2 capsules of 12 mg.) in 24 hours.

TAMPER-RESISTANT PACKAGE FEATURES

- Each capsule is encased in a plastic cell with a foil back; do not use if the cell or foil is broken.
- Each 'TELDRIN' capsule is protected by a green PERMA-SEAL™ band which bonds the two capsule halves together; do not use if capsule or band is broken.

WARNINGS

Do not take this product if you have asthma, glaucoma, or difficulty in urination due to enlargement of the prostate gland, except under the advice and supervision of a physician. Do not drive or operate heavy machinery as this preparation may cause drowsiness. Avoid alcoholic beverages while taking this product. May cause excitability, especially in children. Keep this and all drugs out of the reach of children. In case of accidental overdose, seek professional assistance or contact a poison control center immediately. As with any drug, if you are pregnant or nursing a baby, seek the advice of a health professional before using this product. Store at controlled room temperature (59°–86°F.).

HOW SUPPLIED

Packages of 12, 24 and 48 capsules.

TUMS® Antacid Tablets, Regular and   OTC
Extra Strength
TUMS® Plus Antacid + Anti-Gas Tablets   OTC

(See PDR For Nonprescription Drugs.)

┌─────────────────────────────────┐
│   **EDUCATIONAL MATERIAL**   │
└─────────────────────────────────┘

Booklets:

"A Personal Guide to Feminine Freshness"
A 16 page illustrated booklet on vaginal infections, feminine hygiene and douching. Free to physicians, pharmacists and patients in limited quantities by writing SmithKline Beecham Consumer Brands or calling 800-233-2426.
"Myths and Truths About STDS: An Easy Guide For Women"
A 16 page booklet on the common types of STDs and prevention. Free to physicians, pharmacists and patients in limited quantities by sending a SASE to: SmithKline Beecham Consumer Brands or calling 800-233-2426.

Film, Video:

"Feminine Hygiene and You"
This 14 minute color film begins with a simple explanation of how a woman's body works (reproductive system, menstrual cycle, and vaginal secretions) then explains douching. Free loan to physicians, pharmacists and clinics. Available in 16mm, and VHS by writing SmithKline Beecham Consumer Brands or calling 800-233-2426.

SmithKline Beecham Pharmaceuticals
ONE FRANKLIN PLAZA
P.O. BOX 7929
PHILADELPHIA, PA 19101

PRODUCT CODE INDEX

Code	Product, Form and Strength
207	*Anexsia* 5/500 Tablets
188	*Anexsia* 7.5/650 Tablets
189	*Augmentin* 125 mg Chewable Tablets
190	*Augmentin* 250 mg Chewable Tablets
143	*Bactocill* Capsules 250 mg
144	*Bactocill* Capsules 500 mg
185	*Beepen–VK* Tablets 250 mg
186	*Beepen–VK* Tablets 500 mg
169	*Cloxapen* Capsules 250 mg
170	*Cloxapen* Capsules 500 mg
C44	*Compazine* Spansule Capsules 10 mg
C46	*Compazine* Spansule Capsules 15 mg
C47	*Compazine* Spansule Capsules 30 mg
C60	*Compazine* Suppositories 2½ mg
C61	*Compazine* Suppositories 5 mg
C62	*Compazine* Suppositories 25 mg
C66	*Compazine* Tablets 5 mg
C67	*Compazine* Tablets 10 mg
C69	*Compazine* Tablets 25 mg
D14	*Cytomel* Tablets 5 mcg
D16	*Cytomel* Tablets 25 mcg
D17	*Cytomel* Tablets 50 mcg
E12	*Dexedrine* Spansule Capsules 5 mg
E13	*Dexedrine* Spansule Capsules 10 mg
E14	*Dexedrine* Spansule Capsules 15 mg
E19	*Dexedrine* Tablets 5 mg
E33	*Dibenzyline* Capsules 10 mg
165	*Dycill* Capsules 250 mg
166	*Dycill* Capsules 500 mg
J10	*Eskalith* Controlled Release Tablets 450 mg
121	*Livitamin* Capsules
122	*Livitamin* w/Intrinsic Factor Capsules
123	*Livitamin* Chewable Tablets
125	*Menest* Tablets 0.3 mg
126	*Menest* Tablets 0.625 mg
127	*Menest* Tablets 1.25 mg
128	*Menest* Tablets 2.5 mg
182	*Nucofed* Capsules
S03	*Stelazine* Tablets 1 mg
S04	*Stelazine* Tablets 2 mg
S06	*Stelazine* Tablets 5 mg
S07	*Stelazine* Tablets 10 mg
T63	*Thorazine* Spansule Capsules 30 mg
T64	*Thorazine* Spansule Capsules 75 mg
T66	*Thorazine* Spansule Capsules 150 mg
T69	*Thorazine* Spansule Capsules 300 mg
T70	*Thorazine* Suppositories 25 mg
T71	*Thorazine* Suppositories 100 mg
T73	*Thorazine* Tablets 10 mg
T74	*Thorazine* Tablets 25 mg
T76	*Thorazine* Tablets 50 mg
T77	*Thorazine* Tablets 100 mg
T79	*Thorazine* Tablets 200 mg
156	*Tigan* Capsules 100 mg
157	*Tigan* Capsules 250 mg
140	*Totacillin* Capsules 250 mg
141	*Totacillin* Capsules 500 mg

AMOXIL®   ℞
[ā-mŏx 'ĭl]
(amoxicillin trihydrate)
capsules, powder for oral suspension
and chewable tablets

DESCRIPTION

Amoxil (amoxicillin trihydrate) is a semisynthetic antibiotic, an analog of ampicillin, with a broad spectrum of bactericidal activity against many gram-positive and gram-negative microorganisms. Chemically it is D-(-)-α-amino-p-hydroxybenzyl penicillin trihydrate. Inactive Ingredients: Capsules—magnesium stearate and magnesium sulfate. Chewable Tablets—citric acid, corn starch, FD&C Red No. 40, flavorings, glycine, mannitol, magnesium stearate, saccharin sodium, silica gel and sucrose. Oral Suspension—FD&C Red No. 3, flavorings, silica gel, sodium benzoate, sodium citrate, sucrose and xanthan gum.

ACTIONS

PHARMACOLOGY

Amoxicillin is stable in the presence of gastric acid and may be given without regard to meals. It is rapidly absorbed after oral administration. It diffuses readily into most body tissues and fluids, with the exception of brain and spinal fluid, except when meninges are inflamed. The half-life of amoxicillin is 61.3 minutes. Most of the amoxicillin is excreted unchanged in the urine; its excretion can be delayed by concurrent administration of probenecid. Amoxicillin is not highly protein-bound. In blood serum, amoxicillin is approximately 20% protein-bound as compared to 60% for penicillin G. Orally administered doses of 250 mg and 500 mg amoxicillin capsules result in average peak blood levels one to two hours after administration in the range of 3.5 mcg/mL to 5.0 mcg/mL and 5.5 mcg/mL to 7.5 mcg/mL respectively.
Orally administered doses of amoxicillin suspension 125 mg/5 mL and 250 mg/5 mL result in average peak blood levels one to two hours after administration in the range of 1.5 mcg/mL to 3.0 mcg/mL and 3.5 mcg/mL to 5.0 mcg/mL respectively. Amoxicillin chewable tablets, 125 mg and 250 mg, produced blood levels similar to those achieved with the corresponding doses of amoxicillin oral suspensions. Detectable serum levels are observed up to 8 hours after an orally administered dose of amoxicillin. Following a 1 gram dose and utilizing a special skin window technique to determine levels of the antibiotic, it was noted that therapeutic levels were found in the interstitial fluid. Approximately 60 percent of an orally administered dose of amoxicillin is excreted in the urine within six to eight hours.

MICROBIOLOGY

Amoxil (amoxicillin trihydrate) is similar to ampicillin in its bactericidal action against susceptible organisms during the stage of active multiplication. It acts through the inhibition of biosynthesis of cell wall mucopeptide. *In vitro* studies have demonstrated the susceptibility of most strains of the following Gram-positive bacteria: alpha- and beta-hemolytic streptococci, *Diplococcus pneumoniae*, nonpenicillinase-producing staphylococci, and *Streptococcus faecalis*. It is active *in vitro* against many strains of *Haemophilus influenzae*, *Neisseria gonorrhoeae*, *Escherichia coli* and *Proteus mirabilis*. Because it does not resist destruction by penicillinase, it is not effective against penicillinase-producing bacteria, particularly resistant staphylococci. All strains of Pseudomonas and most strains of Klebsiella and Enterobacter are resistant. *DISC SUSCEPTIBILITY TESTS:* Quantitative methods that require measurement of zone diameters give the most precise estimates of antibiotic susceptibility. One such procedure* has been recommended for use with discs for testing susceptibility to ampicillin-class antibiotics. Interpretations correlate diameters of the disc test with MIC values for amoxicillin. With this procedure, a report from the laboratory of "susceptible" indicates that the infecting organism is likely to respond to therapy. A report of "resistant" indicates that the infecting organism is not likely to respond to therapy. A report of "intermediate susceptibility" suggests that the organism would be susceptible if high dosage is used, or if the infection is confined to tissues and fluids (e.g., urine), in which high antibiotic levels are attained.

*Bauer, A. W., Kirby, W. M. M., Sherris, J. C., and Turck, M.: Antibiotic Testing by a Standardized Single Disc Method, Am. J. Clin. Pathol., 45:493, 1966. Standardized Disc Susceptibility Test, FEDERAL REGISTER 37:20527–29, 1972.

Continued on next page

SmithKline Beecham—Cont.

INDICATIONS

Amoxil (amoxicillin trihydrate) is indicated in the treatment of infections due to susceptible strains of the following:

Gram-negative organisms—*H. influenzae, E. coli, P. mirabilis* and *N. gonorrhoeae.*

Gram-positive organisms—Streptococci (including *Streptococcus faecalis), D. pneumoniae* and nonpenicillinase-producing staphylococci.

Therapy may be instituted prior to obtaining results from bacteriological and susceptibility studies to determine the causative organisms and their susceptibility to amoxicillin. Indicated surgical procedures should be performed.

CONTRAINDICATIONS

A history of allergic reaction to any of the penicillins is a contraindication.

WARNINGS

SERIOUS AND OCCASIONALLY FATAL HYPERSENSITIVITY (ANAPHYLACTOID) REACTIONS HAVE BEEN REPORTED IN PATIENTS ON PENICILLIN THERAPY. ALTHOUGH ANAPHYLAXIS IS MORE FREQUENT FOLLOWING PARENTERAL THERAPY, IT HAS OCCURRED IN PATIENTS ON ORAL PENICILLINS. THESE REACTIONS ARE MORE LIKELY TO OCCUR IN INDIVIDUALS WITH A HISTORY OF SENSITIVITY TO MULTIPLE ALLERGENS. THERE HAVE BEEN REPORTS OF INDIVIDUALS WITH A HISTORY OF PENICILLIN HYPERSENSITIVITY WHO HAVE EXPERIENCED SEVERE REACTIONS WHEN TREATED WITH CEPHALOSPORINS. BEFORE THERAPY WITH ANY PENICILLIN, CAREFUL INQUIRY SHOULD BE MADE CONCERNING PREVIOUS HYPERSENSITIVITY REACTIONS TO PENICILLINS, CEPHALOSPORINS, OR OTHER ALLERGENS. IF AN ALLERGIC REACTION OCCURS, APPROPRIATE THERAPY SHOULD BE INSTITUTED AND DISCONTINUANCE OF AMOXICILLIN THERAPY CONSIDERED. **SERIOUS ANAPHYLACTOID REACTIONS REQUIRE IMMEDIATE EMERGENCY TREATMENT WITH EPINEPHRINE. OXYGEN, INTRAVENOUS STEROIDS, AND AIRWAY MANAGEMENT, INCLUDING INTUBATION, SHOULD ALSO BE ADMINISTERED AS INDICATED.**

USAGE IN PREGNANCY

Safety for use in pregnancy has not been established.

PRECAUTIONS

As with any potent drug, periodic assessment of renal, hepatic and hematopoietic function should be made during prolonged therapy.

The possibility of superinfections with mycotic or bacterial pathogens should be kept in mind during therapy. If superinfections occur (usually involving Enterobacter, Pseudomonas or Candida), the drug should be discontinued and/or appropriate therapy instituted.

ADVERSE REACTIONS

As with other penicillins, it may be expected that untoward reactions will be essentially limited to sensitivity phenomena. They are more likely to occur in individuals who have previously demonstrated hypersensitivity to penicillins and in those with a history of allergy, asthma, hay fever or urticaria. The following adverse reactions have been reported as associated with the use of penicillins:

Gastrointestinal: Nausea, vomiting and diarrhea.

Hypersensitivity Reactions: Erythematous maculopapular rashes and urticaria have been reported.

NOTE: Urticaria, other skin rashes and serum sickness-like reactions may be controlled with antihistamines and, if necessary, systemic corticosteroids. Whenever such reactions occur, amoxicillin should be discontinued unless, in the opinion of the physician, the condition being treated is life-threatening and amenable only to amoxicillin therapy.

Liver: A moderate rise in serum glutamic oxaloacetic transaminase (SGOT) has been noted, but the significance of this finding is unknown.

Hemic and Lymphatic Systems: Anemia, thrombocytopenia, thrombocytopenic purpura, eosinophilia, leukopenia and agranulocytosis have been reported during therapy with penicillins. These reactions are usually reversible on discontinuation of therapy and are believed to be hypersensitivity phenomena.

Central Nervous System: Reversible hyperactivity, agitation, anxiety, insomnia, confusion, behavioral changes, and/or dizziness have been reported rarely.

DOSAGE AND ADMINISTRATION

Infections of the ear, nose and throat due to streptococci, pneumococci, nonpenicillinase-producing staphylococci and *H. influenzae;*

Infections of the genitourinary tract due to *E. coli, Proteus mirabilis* and *Streptococcus faecalis;*

Infections of the skin and soft-tissues due to streptococci, susceptible staphylococci and *E. coli:*

USUAL DOSAGE:

Adults: 250 mg every 8 hours.

Children: 20 mg/kg/day in divided doses every 8 hours.

Children weighing 20 kg or more should be dosed according to the adult recommendations.

In severe infections or those caused by less susceptible organisms:

500 mg every 8 hours for adults and 40 mg/kg/day in divided doses every 8 hours for children may be needed.

Infections of the lower respiratory tract due to streptococci, pneumococci, nonpenicillinase-producing staphylococci and *H. influenzae:*

USUAL DOSAGE:

Adults: 500 mg every 8 hours.

Children: 40 mg/kg/day in divided doses every 8 hours.

Children weighing 20 kg or more should be dosed according to the adult recommendations.

Gonorrhea, acute uncomplicated ano-genital and urethral infections due to *N. gonorrhoeae* (males and females):

USUAL DOSAGE:

Adults: 3 grams as a single oral dose.

Prepubertal children: 50 mg/kg amoxicillin combined with 25 mg/kg probenecid as a single dose.

NOTE: SINCE PROBENECID IS CONTRAINDICATED IN CHILDREN UNDER 2 YEARS, THIS REGIMEN SHOULD NOT BE USED IN THESE CASES.

Cases of gonorrhea with a suspected lesion of syphilis should have dark-field examinations before receiving amoxicillin, and monthly serological tests for a minimum of four months. Larger doses may be required for stubborn or severe infections.

The children's dosage is intended for individuals whose weight will not cause a dosage to be calculated greater than that recommended for adults.

It should be recognized that in the treatment of chronic urinary tract infections, frequent bacteriological and clinical appraisals are necessary. Smaller doses than those recommended above should not be used. Even higher doses may be needed at times. In stubborn infections, therapy may be required for several weeks. It may be necessary to continue clinical and/or bacteriological follow-up for several months after cessation of therapy. Except for gonorrhea, treatment should be continued for a minimum of 48 to 72 hours beyond the time that the patient becomes asymptomatic or evidence of bacterial eradication has been obtained. It is recommended that there be at least 10 days' treatment for any infection caused by hemolytic streptococci to prevent the occurrence of acute rheumatic fever or glomerulonephritis.

DOSAGE AND ADMINISTRATION OF PEDIATRIC DROPS

Usual dosage for all indications except infections of the lower respiratory tract:

Under 6 kg (13 lbs): 0.75 mL every 8 hours.

6–7 kg (13–15 lbs): 1.0 mL every 8 hours.

8 kg (16–18 lbs): 1.25 mL every 8 hours.

Infections of the lower respiratory tract:

Under 6 kg (13 lbs): 1.25 mL every 8 hours.

6–7 kg (13–15 lbs): 1.75 mL every 8 hours.

8 kg (16–18 lbs): 2.25 mL every 8 hours.

Children weighing more than 8 kg (18 lbs) should receive the appropriate dose of the Oral Suspension 125 mg or 250 mg/5 mL.

After reconstitution, the required amount of suspension should be placed directly on the child's tongue for swallowing. Alternate means of administration are to add the required amount of suspension to formula, milk, fruit juice, water, ginger ale or cold drinks. These preparations should then be taken immediately. To be certain the child is receiving full dosage, such preparations should be consumed in entirety.

DIRECTIONS FOR MIXING ORAL SUSPENSION

Prepare suspension at time of dispensing as follows: Tap bottle until all powder flows freely. Add approximately ⅓ of the total amount of water for reconstitution (see table below) and shake vigorously to wet powder. Add remainder of the water and again shake vigorously.

125 mg per 5 mL

Bottle Size	Amount of Water Required for Reconstitution
80 mL	62 mL
100 mL	78 mL
150 mL	116 mL

Each teaspoonful (5 mL) will contain 125 mg amoxicillin.

125 mg unit dose	5 mL

250 mg per 5 mL

80 mL	59 mL
100 mL	74 mL
150 mL	111 mL

Each teaspoonful (5 mL) will contain 250 mg amoxicillin.

250 mg unit dose	5 mL

DIRECTIONS FOR MIXING PEDIATRIC DROPS

Prepare pediatric drops at time of dispensing as follows: Add the required amount of water (see table below) to the bottle and shake vigorously. Each mL of suspension will then contain amoxicillin trihydrate equivalent to 50 mg amoxicillin.

Bottle Size	Amount of Water Required for Reconstitution
15 mL	12 mL
30 mL	23 mL

NOTE: SHAKE BOTH ORAL SUSPENSION AND PEDIATRIC DROPS WELL BEFORE USING. Keep bottle tightly closed. Any unused portion of the reconstituted suspension must be discarded after 14 days. Refrigeration preferable, but not required.

HOW SUPPLIED

Amoxil (amoxicillin) **Capsules.** Each capsule contains 250 mg or 500 mg amoxicillin as the trihydrate.

250 mg/Capsule

NDC 0029-6006-30 ....bottles of 100
NDC 0029-6006-32 ....bottles of 500
NDC 0029-6006-31 ....unit dose carton of 100

500 mg/Capsule

NDC 0029-6007-30 ....bottles of 100
NDC 0029-6007-32 ....bottles of 500
NDC 0029-6007-31 ....unit dose carton of 100

Amoxil (amoxicillin) **Chewable Tablets.** Each tablet contains 125 mg or 250 mg amoxicillin as the trihydrate.

125 mg/Tablet

NDC 0029-6004-39 ....bottles of 60

250 mg/Tablet

NDC 0029-6005-30 ....bottles of 100

Amoxil (amoxicillin) **for Oral Suspension.**

125 mg/5 mL

NDC 0029-6008-21 ....80 mL bottle
NDC 0029-6008-23 ....100 mL bottle
NDC 0029-6008-22 ....150 mL bottle

250 mg/5 mL

NDC 0029-6009-21 ....80 mL bottle
NDC 0029-6009-23 ....100 mL bottle
NDC 0029-6009-22 ....150 mL bottle

Each 5 mL of reconstituted suspension contains 125 mg or 250 mg amoxicillin as the trihydrate.

NDC 0029-6008-18 ....125 mg unit dose bottle
NDC 0029-6009-18 ....250 mg unit dose bottle

Amoxil (amoxicillin) **Pediatric Drops for Oral Suspension.** Each mL of reconstituted suspension contains 50 mg amoxicillin as the trihydrate.

NDC 0029-6035-20 ....15 mL bottle
NDC 0029-6038-39 ....30 mL bottle

AM:L2

Shown in Product Identification Section, page 430

ANCEF® ℞

[an-sef']

(brand of sterile cefazolin sodium and cefazolin sodium injection)

DESCRIPTION

Ancef (sterile cefazolin sodium) is a semi-synthetic cephalosporin for parenteral administration. It is the sodium salt of 3-{[(5-methyl-1, 3, 4-thiadiazol-2-yl) thio]-methyl}-8-oxo-7-[2-(1H-tetrazol-1-yl) acetamido]-5-thia-1-azabicyclo [4.2.0] oct-2-ene-2-carboxylic acid.

The sodium content is 46 mg per gram of cefazolin.

Ancef in lyophilized form is supplied in vials equivalent to 500 mg or 1 gram of cefazolin; in "Piggyback" Vials for intravenous admixture equivalent to 1 gram of cefazolin; and in Pharmacy Bulk Vials equivalent to 5 grams or 10 grams of cefazolin.

Ancef is also supplied as a frozen, sterile, nonpyrogenic solution of cefazolin sodium in an iso-osmotic diluent in plastic containers. After thawing, the solution is intended for intravenous use.

The plastic container is fabricated from specially formulated polyvinyl chloride. Solutions in contact with the plastic container can leach out certain of its chemical components in very small amounts within the expiration period, e.g., di 2-ethylhexyl phthalate (DEHP), up to 5 parts per million. However, the suitability of the plastic has been confirmed in tests in animals according to the USP biological tests for plastic containers as well as by tissue culture toxicity studies.

CLINICAL PHARMACOLOGY

Human Pharmacology: After intramuscular administration of *Ancef* to normal volunteers, the mean serum concentrations were 37 mcg/mL at one hour and 3 mcg/mL at eight hours following a 500 mg dose, and 64 mcg/mL at one hour and 7 mcg/mL at eight hours following a 1 gram dose.

Studies have shown that following intravenous administration of *Ancef* to normal volunteers, mean serum concentrations peaked at approximately 185 mcg/mL and were approximately 4 mcg/mL at eight hours for a 1 gram dose.

The serum half-life for *Ancef* is approximately 1.8 hours following I.V. administration and approximately 2.0 hours following I.M. administration.

In a study (using normal volunteers) of constant intravenous infusion with dosages of 3.5 mg/kg for one hour (approximately 250 mg) and 1.5 mg/kg the next two hours (approximately 100 mg), *Ancef* produced a steady serum level at the third hour of approximately 28 mcg/mL.

Studies in patients hospitalized with infections indicate that Ancef (sterile cefazolin sodium) produces mean peak serum levels approximately equivalent to those seen in normal volunteers.

Bile levels in patients without obstructive biliary disease can reach or exceed serum levels by up to five times; however, in patients with obstructive biliary disease, bile levels of *Ancef* are considerably lower than serum levels (< 1.0 mcg/mL).

In synovial fluid, the *Ancef* level becomes comparable to that reached in serum at about four hours after drug administration.

Studies of cord blood show prompt transfer of *Ancef* across the placenta. *Ancef* is present in very low concentrations in the milk of nursing mothers.

Ancef is excreted unchanged in the urine. In the first six hours approximately 60% of the drug is excreted in the urine and this increases to 70%–80% within 24 hours. *Ancef* achieves peak urine concentrations of approximately 2400 mcg/mL and 4000 mcg/mL respectively following 500 mg and 1 gram intramuscular doses.

In patients undergoing peritoneal dialysis (2 l/hr.), *Ancef* produced mean serum levels of approximately 10 and 30 mcg/mL after 24 hours' instillation of a dialyzing solution containing 50 mg/l and 150 mg/l, respectively. Mean peak levels were 29 mcg/mL (range 13–44 mcg/mL) with 50 mg/l (three patients), and 72 mcg/mL (range 26–142 mcg/mL) with 150 mg/l (six patients). Intraperitoneal administration of *Ancef* is usually well tolerated.

Controlled studies on adult normal volunteers, receiving 1 gram 4 times a day for 10 days, monitoring CBC, SGOT, SGPT, bilirubin, alkaline phosphatase, BUN, creatinine and urinalysis, indicated no clinically significant changes attributed to *Ancef*.

Microbiology: *In vitro* tests demonstrate that the bactericidal action of cephalosporins results from inhibition of cell wall synthesis. Ancef (sterile cefazolin sodium) is active against the following organisms *in vitro* and in clinical infections:

Staphylococcus aureus (including penicillinase-producing strains)

Staphylococcus epidermidis

Methicillin-resistant staphylococci are uniformly resistant to cefazolin

Group A beta-hemolytic streptococci and other strains of streptococci (many strains of enterococci are resistant)

Streptococcus pneumoniae

Escherichia coli

Proteus mirabilis

Klebsiella species

Enterobacter aerogenes

Haemophilus influenzae

Most strains of indole positive Proteus (*Proteus vulgaris*), *Enterobacter cloacae*, *Morganella morganii* and *Providencia rettgeri* are resistant. *Serratia, Pseudomonas, Mima, Herellea* species are almost uniformly resistant to cefazolin.

Disk Susceptibility Tests

Disk diffusion technique—Quantitative methods that require measurement of zone diameters give the most precise estimates of antibiotic susceptibility. One such procedure[1] has been recommended for use with disks to test susceptibility to cefazolin.

Reports from a laboratory using the standardized single-disk susceptibility test[1] with a 30 mcg cefazolin disk should be interpreted according to the following criteria:

   Susceptible organisms produce zones of 18 mm or greater, indicating that the tested organism is likely to respond to therapy.

   Organisms of intermediate susceptibility produce zones 15 to 17 mm, indicating that the tested organism would be susceptible if high dosage is used or if the infection is confined to tissues and fluids (e.g., urine), in which high antibiotic levels are attained.

   Resistant organisms produce zones of 14 mm or less, indicating that other therapy should be selected.

For gram-positive isolates, a zone of 18 mm is indicative of a cefazolin-susceptible organism when tested with either the cephalosporin-class disk (30 mcg cephalothin) or the cefazolin disk (30 mcg cefazolin).

Gram-negative organisms should be tested with the cefazolin disk (using the above criteria), since cefazolin has been shown by *in vitro* tests to have activity against certain strains of *Enterobacteriaceae* found resistant when tested with the cephalothin disk. Gram-negative organisms having zones of less than 18 mm around the cephalothin disk may be susceptible to cefazolin.

1 Bauer, A.W.; Kirby, W.M.M.; Sherris, J.C., and Turck, M.: Antibiotic Testing by a Standardized Single Disc Method, Am. J. Clin. Path. 45:493, 1966. Standardized Disc Susceptibility Test, Federal Register 39:19182-19184, 1974.

Standardized procedures require use of control organisms. The 30 mcg cefazolin disk should give zone diameter between 23 and 29 mm for *E. coli* ATCC 25922 and between 29 and 35 mm for *S. aureus* ATCC 25923.

The cefazolin disk should not be used for testing susceptibility to other cephalosporins.

Dilution techniques—A bacterial isolate may be considered susceptible if the minimal inhibitory concentration (MIC) for cefazolin is not more than 16 mcg per mL. Organisms are considered resistant if the MIC is equal to or greater than 64 mcg per mL.

The range of MIC's for the control strains are as follows:
   S. aureus ATCC 25923, 0.25-1.0 mcg/mL
   E. coli ATCC 25922, 1.0-4.0 mcg/mL

INDICATIONS AND USAGE

Ancef (sterile cefazolin sodium) is indicated in the treatment of the following serious infections due to susceptible organisms:

RESPIRATORY TRACT INFECTIONS due to *Streptococcus pneumoniae, Klebsiella* species, *Haemophilus influenzae, Staphylococcus aureus* (penicillin-sensitive and penicillin-resistant) and group A beta-hemolytic streptococci.

Injectable benzathine penicillin is considered to be the drug of choice in treatment and prevention of streptococcal infections, including the prophylaxis of rheumatic fever.

Ancef is effective in the eradication of streptococci from the nasopharynx; however, data establishing the efficacy of *Ancef* in the subsequent prevention of rheumatic fever are not available at present.

URINARY TRACT INFECTIONS due to *Escherichia coli, Proteus mirabilis, Klebsiella* species and some strains of enterobacter and enterococci.

SKIN AND SKIN STRUCTURE INFECTIONS due to *Staphylococcus aureus* (penicillin-sensitive and penicillin-resistant), group A beta-hemolytic streptococci and other strains of streptococci.

BILIARY TRACT INFECTIONS due to *Escherichia coli*, various strains of streptococci, *Proteus mirabilis, Klebsiella* species and *Staphylococcus aureus*.

BONE AND JOINT INFECTIONS due to *Staphylococcus aureus*.

GENITAL INFECTIONS (i.e., prostatitis, epididymitis) due to *Escherichia coli, Proteus mirabilis, Klebsiella* species and some strains of enterococci.

SEPTICEMIA due to *Streptococcus pneumoniae, Staphylococcus aureus* (penicillin-sensitive and penicillin-resistant), *Proteus mirabilis, Escherichia coli* and *Klebsiella* species.

ENDOCARDITIS due to *Staphylococcus aureus* (penicillin-sensitive and penicillin-resistant) and group A beta-hemolytic streptococci.

Appropriate culture and susceptibility studies should be performed to determine susceptibility of the causative organism to *Ancef*.

PERIOPERATIVE PROPHYLAXIS: The prophylactic administration of *Ancef* preoperatively, intraoperatively and postoperatively may reduce the incidence of certain postoperative infections in patients undergoing surgical procedures which are classified as contaminated or potentially contaminated (e.g., vaginal hysterectomy, and cholecystectomy in high-risk patients such as those over 70 years of age, with acute cholecystitis, obstructive jaundice or common duct bile stones).

The perioperative use of *Ancef* may also be effective in surgical patients in whom infection at the operative site would present a serious risk (e.g., during open-heart surgery and prosthetic arthroplasty).

The prophylactic administration of *Ancef* should usually be discontinued within a 24-hour period after the surgical procedure. In surgery where the occurrence of infection may be particularly devastating (e.g., open-heart surgery and prosthetic arthroplasty), the prophylactic administration of *Ancef* may be continued for 3 to 5 days following the completion of surgery.

If there are signs of infection, specimens for cultures should be obtained for the identification of the causative organism so that appropriate therapy may be instituted.
(See DOSAGE AND ADMINISTRATION.)

CONTRAINDICATIONS

ANCEF (STERILE CEFAZOLIN SODIUM) IS CONTRAINDICATED IN PATIENTS WITH KNOWN ALLERGY TO THE CEPHALOSPORIN GROUP OF ANTIBIOTICS.

WARNINGS

BEFORE CEFAZOLIN THERAPY IS INSTITUTED, CAREFUL INQUIRY SHOULD BE MADE CONCERNING PREVIOUS HYPERSENSITIVITY REACTIONS TO CEPHALOSPORINS AND PENICILLIN. CEPHALOSPORIN C DERIVATIVES SHOULD BE GIVEN CAUTIOUSLY IN PENICILLIN-SENSITIVE PATIENTS.
SERIOUS ACUTE HYPERSENSITIVITY REACTIONS MAY REQUIRE EPINEPHRINE AND OTHER EMERGENCY MEASURES.
There is some clinical and laboratory evidence of partial cross-allergenicity of the penicillins and the cephalosporins.

Patients have been reported to have had severe reactions (including anaphylaxis) to both drugs.

Any patient who has demonstrated some form of allergy, particularly to drugs, should receive antibiotics cautiously. No exception should be made with regard to *Ancef*.

Pseudomembranous colitis has been reported with nearly all antibacterial agents, including cefazolin, and has ranged in severity from mild to life-threatening. Therefore, it is important to consider this diagnosis in patients who present with diarrhea subsequent to the administration of antibacterial agents.

Treatment with antibacterial agents alters the normal flora of the colon and may permit overgrowth of clostridia. Studies indicate that a toxin produced by *Clostridium difficile* is one primary cause of "antibiotic-associated colitis."

Mild cases of pseudomembranous colitis usually respond to drug discontinuation alone. In moderate to severe cases, consideration should be given to management with fluids and electrolytes, protein supplementation and treatment with an oral antibiotic drug effective against *C. difficile*.

PRECAUTIONS

General—Prolonged use of Ancef (sterile cefazolin sodium) may result in the overgrowth of nonsusceptible organisms. Careful clinical observation of the patient is essential.

When *Ancef* is administered to patients with low urinary output because of impaired renal function, lower daily dosage is required (see DOSAGE AND ADMINISTRATION).

As with other beta-lactam antibiotics, seizures may occur if inappropriately high doses are administered to patients with impaired renal function (see DOSAGE AND ADMINISTRATION).

Ancef, as with all cephalosporins, should be prescribed with caution in individuals with a history of gastrointestinal disease, particularly colitis.

Drug Interactions—Probenecid may decrease renal tubular secretion of cephalosporins when used concurrently, resulting in increased and more prolonged cephalosporin blood levels.

Drug/Laboratory Test Interactions—A false positive reaction for glucose in the urine may occur with Benedict's solution, Fehling's solution or with Clinitest® tablets, but not with enzyme-based tests such as Clinistix® and Tes-Tape®. Positive direct and indirect antiglobulin (Coombs) tests have occurred; these may also occur in neonates whose mothers received cephalosporins before delivery.

Carcinogenesis/Mutagenesis — Mutagenicity studies and long-term studies in animals to determine the carcinogenic potential of Ancef (sterile cefazolin sodium) have not been performed.

Pregnancy — Teratogenic Effects — Pregnancy Category B. Reproduction studies have been performed in rats, mice and rabbits at doses up to 25 times the human dose and have revealed no evidence of impaired fertility or harm to the fetus due to *Ancef*. There are, however, no adequate and well-controlled studies in pregnant women. Because animal reproduction studies are not always predictive of human response, this drug should be used during pregnancy only if clearly needed.

Labor and Delivery—When cefazolin has been administered prior to caesarean section, drug levels in cord blood have been approximately one quarter to one third of maternal drug levels. The drug appears to have no adverse effect on the fetus.

Nursing Mothers—*Ancef* is present in very low concentrations in the milk of nursing mothers. Caution should be exercised when *Ancef* is administered to a nursing woman.

Pediatric Use—Safety and effectiveness for use in prematures and infants under one month of age have not been established. See DOSAGE AND ADMINISTRATION for recommended dosage in children over one month.

The potential for the toxic effect in children from chemicals that may leach from the single-dose I.V. preparation in plastic has not been determined.

ADVERSE REACTIONS

The following reactions have been reported:

Gastrointestinal: Diarrhea, oral candidiasis (oral thrush), vomiting, nausea, stomach cramps, anorexia and pseudomembranous colitis. Onset of pseudomembranous colitis symptoms may occur during or after antibiotic treatment (see WARNINGS). Nausea and vomiting have been reported rarely.

Allergic: Anaphylaxis, eosinophilia, itching, drug fever, skin rash, Stevens-Johnson syndrome.

Hematologic: Neutropenia, leukopenia, thrombocytopenia, thrombocythemia.

Hepatic and Renal: Transient rise in SGOT, SGPT, BUN and alkaline phosphatase levels has been observed without clinical evidence of renal or hepatic impairment.

Local Reactions: Rare instances of phlebitis have been reported at site of injection. Pain at the site of injection after

Continued on next page

SmithKline Beecham—Cont.

intramuscular administration has occurred infrequently. Some induration has occurred.

Other Reactions: Genital and anal pruritus (including vulvar pruritus, genital moniliasis and vaginitis).

DOSAGE AND ADMINISTRATION
Usual Adult Dosage

Type of Infection	Dose	Frequency
Moderate to severe infections	500 mg to 1 gram	every 6 to 8 hrs.
Mild infections caused by susceptible gram + cocci	250 mg to 500 mg	every 8 hours
Acute, uncomplicated urinary tract infections	1 gram	every 12 hours
Pneumococcal pneumonia	500 mg	every 12 hours
Severe, life-threatening infections (e.g., endocarditis, septicemia)*	1 gram to 1.5 grams	every 6 hours

*In rare instances, doses of up to 12 grams of *Ancef* per day have been used.

Perioperative Prophylactic Use

To prevent postoperative infection in contaminated or potentially contaminated surgery, recommended doses are:

a. 1 gram I.V. or I.M. administered ½ hour to 1 hour prior to the start of surgery.

b. For lengthy operative procedures (e.g., 2 hours or more), 500 mg to 1 gram I.V. or I.M. during surgery (administration modified depending on the duration of the operative procedure).

c. 500 mg to 1 gram I.V. or I.M. every 6 to 8 hours for 24 hours postoperatively.

It is important that (1) the preoperative dose be given just (½ to 1 hour) prior to the start of surgery so that adequate antibiotic levels are present in the serum and tissues at the time of initial surgical incision; and (2) *Ancef* be administered, if necessary, at appropriate intervals during surgery to provide sufficient levels of the antibiotic at the anticipated moments of greatest exposure to infective organisms.

In surgery where the occurrence of infection may be particularly devastating (e.g., open-heart surgery and prosthetic arthroplasty), the prophylactic administration of Ancef (sterile cefazolin sodium) may be continued for 3 to 5 days following the completion of surgery.

Dosage Adjustment for Patients with Reduced Renal Function

Ancef may be used in patients with reduced renal function with the following dosage adjustments: Patients with a creatinine clearance of 55 mL/min. or greater or a serum creatinine of 1.5 mg % or less can be given full doses. Patients with creatinine clearance rates of 35 to 54 mL/min. or serum creatinine of 1.6 to 3.0 mg % can also be given full doses but dosage should be restricted to at least 8 hour intervals. Patients with creatinine clearance rates of 11 to 34 mL/min. or serum creatinine of 3.1 to 4.5 mg % should be given ½ the usual dose every 12 hours. Patients with creatinine clearance rates of 10 mL/min. or less or serum creatinine of 4.6 mg % or greater should be given ½ the usual dose every 18 to 24 hours. All reduced dosage recommendations apply after an initial loading dose appropriate to the severity of the infection. Patients undergoing peritoneal dialysis: See Human Pharmacology.

Pediatric Dosage

In children, a total daily dosage of 25 to 50 mg per kg (approximately 10 to 20 mg per pound) of body weight, divided into three or four equal doses, is effective for most mild to moderately severe infections. Total daily dosage may be increased to 100 mg per kg (45 mg per pound) of body weight for severe infections. Since safety for use in premature infants and in infants under one month has not been established, the use of Ancef (sterile cefazolin sodium) in these patients is not recommended. [See table at top of next column.]

In children with mild to moderate renal impairment (creatinine clearance of 70 to 40 mL/min.), 60 percent of the normal daily dose given in equally divided doses every 12 hours should be sufficient. In patients with moderate impairment (creatinine clearance of 40 to 20 mL/min.), 25 percent of the normal daily dose given in equally divided doses every 12 hours should be adequate. Children with severe renal im-

---

Pediatric Dosage Guide

Weight		25 mg/kg/Day Divided into 3 Doses		25 mg/kg/Day Divided into 4 Doses	
		Approximate Single Dose	Vol. (mL) needed with dilution of 125	Approximate Single Dose	Vol. (mL) needed with dilution of 125
Lbs	Kg	mg/q8h	mg/mL	mg/q6h	mg/mL
10	4.5	40 mg	0.35 mL	30 mg	0.25 mL
20	9.0	75 mg	0.60 mL	55 mg	0.45 mL
30	13.6	115 mg	0.90 mL	85 mg	0.70 mL
40	18.1	150 mg	1.20 mL	115 mg	0.90 mL
50	22.7	190 mg	1.50 mL	140 mg	1.10 mL

Weight		50 mg/kg/Day Divided into 3 Doses		50 mg/kg/Day Divided into 4 Doses	
		Approximate Single Dose	Vol. (mL) needed with dilution of 225	Approximate Single Dose	Vol. (mL) needed with dilution of 225
Lbs	Kg	mg/q8h	mg/mL	mg/q6h	mg/mL
10	4.5	75 mg	0.35 mL	55 mg	0.25 mL
20	9.0	150 mg	0.70 mL	110 mg	0.50 mL
30	13.6	225 mg	1.00 mL	170 mg	0.75 mL
40	18.1	300 mg	1.35 mL	225 mg	1.00 mL
50	22.7	375 mg	1.70 mL	285 mg	1.25 mL

pairment (creatinine clearance of 20 to 5 mL/min.) may be given 10 percent of the normal daily dose every 24 hours. All dosage recommendations apply after an initial loading dose.

RECONSTITUTION
Preparation of Parenteral Solution

Parenteral drug products should be SHAKEN WELL when reconstituted, and inspected visually for particulate matter prior to administration. If particulate matter is evident in reconstituted fluids, the drug solutions should be discarded. When reconstituted or diluted according to the instructions below, Ancef (sterile cefazolin sodium) is stable for 24 hours at room temperature or for 96 hours if stored under refrigeration (5°C or 41°F). Reconstituted solutions may range in color from pale yellow to yellow without a change in potency.

Single-Dose Vials

For I.M. injection, I.V. direct (bolus) injection or I.V. infusion, reconstitute with Sterile Water for Injection according to the following table. SHAKE WELL.

Vial Size	Amount of Diluent	Approximate Concentration	Approximate Available Volume
500 mg	2.0 mL	225 mg/mL	2.2 mL
1 gram	2.5 mL	330 mg/mL	3.0 mL

Pharmacy Bulk Vials

Add Sterile Water for Injection, Bacteriostatic Water for Injection or Sodium Chloride Injection according to the table below. SHAKE WELL.

Vial Size	Amount of Diluent	Approximate Concentration	Approximate Available Volume
5 grams	23 mL	1 gram/5 mL	26 mL
	48 mL	1 gram/10 mL	51 mL
10 grams	45 mL	1 gram/5 mL	51 mL
	96 mL	1 gram/10 mL	102 mL

"Piggyback" Vials

Reconstitute with 50 to 100 mL of Sodium Chloride Injection or other I.V. solution listed under ADMINISTRATION. When adding diluent to vial, allow air to escape by using a small vent needle or by pumping the syringe. SHAKE WELL. Administer with primary I.V. fluids, as a single dose.

ADMINISTRATION

Intramuscular Administration—Reconstitute vials with Sterile Water for Injection according to the dilution table above. Shake well until dissolved. *Ancef* should be injected into a large muscle mass. Pain on injection is infrequent with *Ancef*.

Intravenous Administration—Direct (bolus) injection: Following reconstitution according to the above table, further dilute vials with approximately 5 mL Sterile Water for Injection. Inject the solution slowly over 3 to 5 minutes, directly

or through tubing for patients receiving parenteral fluids (see list below).

Intermittent or continuous infusion: Dilute reconstituted *Ancef* in 50 to 100 mL of one of the following solutions:
Sodium Chloride Injection, USP
5% or 10% Dextrose Injection, USP
5% Dextrose in Lactated Ringer's Injection, USP
5% Dextrose and 0.9% Sodium Chloride Injection, USP
5% Dextrose and 0.45% Sodium Chloride Injection, USP
5% Dextrose and 0.2% Sodium Chloride Injection, USP
Lactated Ringer's Injection, USP
Invert Sugar 5% or 10% in Sterile Water for Injection
Ringer's Injection, USP
5% Sodium Bicarbonate Injection, USP

DIRECTIONS FOR USE OF ANCEF (CEFAZOLIN SODIUM INJECTION) VIAFLEX® PLUS CONTAINER (PL 146® PLASTIC)

Ancef in Viaflex®Plus Container (PL 146®Plastic) is to be administered either as a continuous or intermittent infusion using sterile equipment.

Storage

Store in a freezer capable of maintaining a temperature of −20°C (−4°F)

Thawing of Plastic Container

Thaw frozen container at room temperature (25°C or 77°F) or under refrigeration (5°C or 41°F). (DO NOT FORCE THAW BY IMMERSION IN WATER BATHS OR BY MICROWAVE IRRADIATION.)

Containers may be thawed individually after separation from the frozen shingle. A shingle consists of stacked frozen containers. Remove frozen shingle from carton and allow to rest at room temperature until the containers can be easily separated (approximately 5 minutes). Then grasp the body of the container (not the ports, corner, or tail flap) to separate individual units. *Promptly* return unneeded frozen containers to freezer.

Check for minute leaks by squeezing container firmly. If leaks are detected, discard solution as sterility may be impaired.

Do not add supplementary medication.

The container should be visually inspected. Components of the solution may precipitate in the frozen state and will dissolve upon reaching room temperature with little or no agitation. Potency is not affected. Agitate after solution has reached room temperature. If after visual inspection the solution remains cloudy or if an insoluble precipitate is noted or if any seals or outlet ports are not intact, the container should be discarded.

The thawed solution is stable for 10 days under refrigeration (5°C or 41°F) and 48 hours at room temperature (25°C or 77°F). Do not refreeze thawed antibiotics.

Use sterile equipment. It is recommended that the intravenous administration apparatus be replaced at least once every 48 hours.

CAUTION: Do not use plastic containers in series connections. Such use could result in air embolism due to residual air being drawn from the primary container before administration of the fluid from the secondary container is complete.

Preparation for administration:

1. Suspend container from eyelet support.
2. Remove plastic protector from outlet port at bottom of container.
3. Attach administration set. Refer to complete directions accompanying set.

HOW SUPPLIED

Ancef (sterile cefazolin sodium)—supplied in vials equivalent to 500 mg or 1 gram of cefazolin; in "Piggyback" Vials for intravenous admixture equivalent to 1 gram of cefazolin; and in Pharmacy Bulk Vials equivalent to 5 grams or 10 grams of cefazolin.

Ancef (cefazolin sodium injection) as a frozen, sterile, nonpyrogenic solution in plastic containers—supplied in 50 mL single-dose containers equivalent to 500 mg or 1 gram of cefazolin in 5% Dextrose (D5W). Store at or below −20°C (−4°F). (See DIRECTIONS FOR USE OF ANCEF [CEFAZOLIN SODIUM INJECTION] VIAFLEX® PLUS CONTAINER [PL 146® PLASTIC].)

As with other cephalosporins, *Ancef* tends to darken depending on storage conditions; within the stated recommendations, however, product potency is not adversely affected. Before reconstitution protect from light and store at controlled room temperature 15°–30°C (59°–86°F).

Ancef supplied as a frozen, sterile, nonpyrogenic solution in plastic containers is manufactured for SmithKline Beecham Pharmaceuticals by Baxter Healthcare Corporation, Deerfield, IL 60015.

Viaflex and PL 146 are registered trademarks of Baxter International Inc.

Military—Vial, 5 gram, 100 mL, 10's, 6505-01-058-2046; 10 gram, 100 mL, 6505-01-184-1574.

AF:L47

Shown in Product Identification Section, page 430

ANEXSIA® 5/500 Ⓒ

Hydrocodone Bitartrate and Acetaminophen Tablets

DESCRIPTION

Each tablet contains: hydrocodone bitartrate, 5 mg (**Warning:** May be habit forming); and acetaminophen, 500 mg. **Inactive Ingredients:** Magnesium Stearate, Pregelatinized Starch, Starch (corn), and Stearic Acid.

Hydrocodone bitartrate is an opioid analgesic and antitussive and occurs as fine, white crystals or as a crystalline powder. It is affected by light. The chemical name is: 4,5α-epoxy-3-methoxy-17-methylmorphinan-6-one tartrate (1:1) hydrate (2:5). Its structure is as follows:

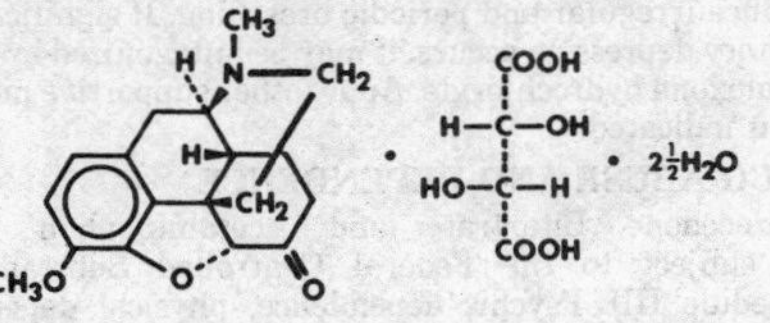

$C_{18}H_{21}NO_3 \cdot C_4H_6O_6 \cdot 2\frac{1}{2}H_2O$ M.W. 494.50

Acetaminophen, 4′-hydroxyacetanilide, is a non-opiate, non-salicylate analgesic and antipyretic which occurs as a white, odorless crystalline powder possessing a slightly bitter taste. Its structure is as follows:

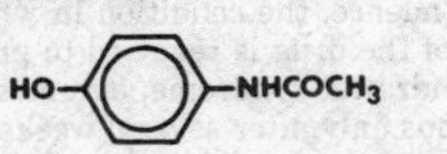

$C_8H_9NO_2$ M.W. 151.16

CLINICAL PHARMACOLOGY

Hydrocodone is a semisynthetic narcotic analgesic and antitussive with multiple actions qualitatively similar to those of codeine. Most of these involve the central nervous system and smooth muscle. The precise mechanism of action of hydrocodone and other opiates is not known, although it is believed to relate to the existence of opiate receptors in the central nervous system. In addition to analgesia, narcotics may produce drowsiness, changes in mood and mental clouding.

Radioimmunoassay techniques have recently been developed for the analysis of hydrocodone in human plasma. After a 10 mg oral dose of hydrocodone bitartrate, a mean peak serum drug level of 23.6 ng/mL and an elimination half-life of 3.8 hours were found.

The analgesic action of acetaminophen involves peripheral and central influences, but the specific mechanism is as yet undetermined. Antipyretic activity is mediated through hypothalamic heat regulating centers. Acetaminophen inhibits prostaglandin synthetase. Therapeutic doses of acetaminophen have negligible effects on the cardiovascular or respiratory systems; however, toxic doses may cause circulatory failure and rapid, shallow breathing. Acetaminophen is rapidly and almost completely absorbed from the gastrointestinal tract, producing maximum serum concentrations within 30 minutes to one hour. The plasma half-life in adults and children ranges from 0.90 hours to 3.25 hours with an average of approximately 2 hours. The drug distributes uniformly in most body fluids and is approximately 25% protein bound. Acetaminophen is conjugated in the liver, with less than 3% of the dose excreted unchanged in 24 hours. The primary metabolic pathway is conjugation to sulfate and glucuronide by-products. A minor oxidative pathway forms cysteine and mercapturic acid. These compounds are subsequently excreted by the kidneys into the urine.

INDICATIONS AND USAGE

For the relief of moderate to moderately severe pain.

CONTRAINDICATIONS

Hypersensitivity to acetaminophen or hydrocodone.

WARNINGS

Respiratory Depression: At high doses or in sensitive patients, hydrocodone may produce dose-related respiratory depression by acting directly on the brain stem respiratory center. Hydrocodone also affects the center that controls respiratory rhythm, and may produce irregular and periodic breathing.

Head Injury and Increased Intracranial Pressure: The respiratory depressant effects of narcotics and their capacity to elevate cerebrospinal fluid pressure may be markedly exaggerated in the presence of head injury, other intracranial lesions or a pre-existing increase in intracranial pressure. Furthermore, narcotics produce adverse reactions which may obscure the clinical course of patients with head injuries.

Acute Abdominal Conditions: The administration of narcotics may obscure the diagnosis or clinical course of patients with acute abdominal conditions.

PRECAUTIONS

Special Risk Patients: As with any narcotic analgesic agent, Hydrocodone Bitartrate and Acetaminophen Tablets should be used with caution in elderly or debilitated patients and those with severe impairment of hepatic or renal function, hypothyroidism, Addison's disease, prostatic hypertrophy or urethral stricture. The usual precautions should be observed and the possibility of respiratory depression should be kept in mind.

Information for Patients: Hydrocodone Bitartrate and Acetaminophen Tablets, like all narcotics, may impair the mental and/or physical abilities required for the performance of potentially hazardous tasks such as driving a car or operating machinery; patients should be cautioned accordingly.

Cough Reflex: Hydrocodone suppresses the cough reflex; as with all narcotics, caution should be exercised when Hydrocodone Bitartrate and Acetaminophen Tablets are used postoperatively and in patients with pulmonary disease.

Drug Interactions: Patients receiving other narcotic analgesics, antipsychotics, antianxiety agents, or other CNS depressants (including alcohol) concomitantly with hydrocodone and acetaminophen tablets may exhibit an additive CNS depression. When combined therapy is contemplated, the dose of one or both agents should be reduced.

The use of MAO inhibitors or tricyclic antidepressants with hydrocodone preparations may increase the effect of either the antidepressant or hydrocodone.

The concurrent use of anticholinergics with hydrocodone may produce paralytic ileus.

Usage in Pregnancy:

Teratogenic Effects: Pregnancy Category C. Hydrocodone has been shown to be teratogenic in hamsters when given in doses 700 times the human dose. There are no adequate and well-controlled studies in pregnant women. Hydrocodone Bitartrate and Acetaminophen Tablets should be used during pregnancy only if the potential benefit justifies the potential risk to the fetus.

Nonteratogenic Effects: Babies born to mothers who have been taking opioids regularly prior to delivery will be physically dependent. The withdrawal signs include irritability and excessive crying, tremors, hyperactive reflexes, increased respiratory rate, increased stools, sneezing, yawning, vomiting, and fever. The intensity of the syndrome does not always correlate with the duration of maternal opioid use or dose. There is no consensus on the best method of managing withdrawal. Chlorpromazine 0.7 to 1 mg/kg q6h, and paregoric 2 to 4 drops/kg q4h, have been used to treat withdrawal symptoms in infants. The duration of therapy is 4 to 28 days, with the dosage decreased as tolerated.

Labor and Delivery: As with all narcotics, administration of Hydrocodone Bitartrate and Acetaminophen Tablets to the mother shortly before delivery may result in some degree of respiratory depression in the newborn, especially if higher doses are used.

Nursing Mothers: It is not known whether this drug is excreted in human milk. Because many drugs are excreted in human milk and because of the potential for serious adverse reactions in nursing infants from Hydrocodone Bitartrate and Acetaminophen Tablets, a decision should be made whether to discontinue nursing or to discontinue the drug, taking into account the importance of the drug to the mother.

Pediatric Use: Safety and effectiveness in children have not been established.

ADVERSE REACTIONS

The most frequently observed adverse reactions include lightheadedness, dizziness, sedation, nausea and vomiting. These effects seem to be more prominent in ambulatory than in nonambulatory patients and some of these adverse reactions may be alleviated if the patient lies down.

Other adverse reactions include:

Central Nervous System: Drowsiness, mental clouding, lethargy, impairment of mental and physical performance, anxiety, fear, dysphoria, psychic dependence, mood changes.

Gastrointestinal System: The antiemetic phenothiazines are useful in suppressing the nausea and vomiting which may occur (see above); however, some phenothiazine derivatives seem to be antianalgesic and to increase the amount of narcotic required to produce pain relief, while other phenothiazines reduce the amount of narcotic required to produce a given level of analgesia. Prolonged administration of Hydrocodone Bitartrate and Acetaminophen Tablets may produce constipation.

Genitourinary System: Ureteral spasm, spasm of vesical sphincters and urinary retention have been reported.

Respiratory Depression: Hydrocodone bitartrate may produce dose-related respiratory depression by acting directly on the brain stem respiratory center. Hydrocodone also affects the center that controls respiratory rhythm, and may produce irregular and periodic breathing. If significant respiratory depression occurs, it may be antagonized by the use of naloxone hydrochloride. Apply other supportive measures when indicated.

DRUG ABUSE AND DEPENDENCE

Hydrocodone Bitartrate and Acetaminophen Tablets are subject to the Federal Controlled Substance Act (Schedule III).

Psychic dependence, physical dependence, and tolerance may develop upon repeated administration of narcotics; therefore, Hydrocodone Bitartrate and Acetaminophen Tablets should be prescribed and administered with caution. However, psychic dependence is unlikely to develop when Hydrocodone Bitartrate and Acetaminophen Tablets are used for a short time for the treatment of pain.

Physical dependence, the condition in which continued administration of the drug is required to prevent the appearance of a withdrawal syndrome, assumes clinically significant proportions only after several weeks of continued narcotic use, although some mild degree of physical dependence may develop after a few days of narcotic therapy. Tolerance, in which increasingly large doses are required in order to produce the same degree of analgesia, is manifested initially by a shortened duration of analgesic effect, and subsequently by decreases in the intensity of analgesia. The rate of development of tolerance varies among patients.

OVERDOSAGE

Acetaminophen

Signs and Symptoms: In acute acetaminophen overdosage, dose-dependent, potentially fatal hepatic necrosis is the most serious adverse effect. Renal tubular necrosis, hypoglycemic coma, and thrombocytopenia may also occur.

In adults, hepatic toxicity has rarely been reported with acute overdoses of less than 10 grams and fatalities with less than 15 grams. Importantly, young children seem to be more resistant than adults to the hepatotoxic effect of an acetaminophen overdose. Despite this, the measures outlined below should be initiated in any adult or child suspected of having ingested an acetaminophen overdose.

Early symptoms following a potentially hepatotoxic overdose may include: nausea, vomiting, diaphoresis and general malaise. Clinical and laboratory evidence of hepatic toxicity may not be apparent until 48 to 72 hours post-ingestion.

Treatment: The stomach should be emptied promptly by lavage or by induction of emesis with syrup of ipecac. Patients' estimates of the quantity of a drug ingested are notoriously unreliable. Therefore, if an acetaminophen overdose is suspected, a serum acetaminophen assay should be obtained as early as possible, but no sooner than four hours following ingestion. Liver function studies should be obtained initially and repeated at 24-hour intervals.

The antidote, N-acetylcysteine, should be administered as early as possible, preferably within 16 hours of the overdose ingestion for optimal results, but in any case, within 24 hours. Following recovery, there are no residual, structural or functional hepatic abnormalities.

Hydrocodone

Signs and Symptoms: Serious overdose with hydrocodone is characterized by respiratory depression (a decrease in respiratory rate and/or tidal volume, Cheyne-Stokes respiration, cyanosis), extreme somnolence progressing to stupor or coma, skeletal muscle flaccidity, cold and clammy skin, and sometimes bradycardia and hypotension. In severe overdose, apnea, circulatory collapse, cardiac arrest and death may occur.

Treatment: Primary attention should be given to the reestablishment of adequate respiratory exchange through provision of a patent airway and the institution of assisted or controlled ventilation. The narcotic antagonist naloxone is a specific antidote against respiratory depression which may result from overdosage or unusual sensitivity to narcotics, including hydrocodone. Therefore, an appropriate dose of naloxone hydrochloride (see package insert) should be administered, preferably by the intravenous route, and simultaneously with efforts at respiratory resuscitation. Since the duration of action of hydrocodone may exceed that of the antagonist, the patient should be kept under continued surveillance and repeated doses of the antagonist should be administered as needed to maintain adequate respiration.

An antagonist should not be administered in the absence of clinically significant respiratory or cardiovascular depression. Oxygen, intravenous fluids, vasopressors and other supportive measures should be employed as indicated.

Gastric emptying may be useful in removing unabsorbed drug.

DOSAGE AND ADMINISTRATION

Dosage should be adjusted according to the severity of pain and the response of the patient. However, it should be kept in mind that tolerance to hydrocodone can develop with continued use and that the incidence of untoward effects is dose related.

The usual adult dosage is one or two tablets every four to six hours as needed for pain. The total 24 hour dose should not exceed 8 tablets.

Continued on next page

SmithKline Beecham—Cont.

HOW SUPPLIED

Hydrocodone Bitartrate and Acetaminophen Tablets
Each tablet contains: hydrocodone bitartrate 5 mg and acetaminophen 500 mg.
They are available as white, round bisected tablets debossed with a logo identified as BMP 207.
Bottles of 100 .... *NDC* 0029-1365-30
Storage: Store at controlled room temperature 15°–30°C. (59°–86°F.).
A Schedule III Narcotic.
0938007 Revised March, 1989
Shown in Product Identification Section, page 430

ANEXSIA® 7.5/650 Ⓒ III

Hydrocodone Bitartrate and Acetaminophen Tablets

DESCRIPTION

Each tablet contains: hydrocodone bitartrate, 7.5 mg (**Warning:** May be habit forming); and acetaminophen, 650 mg.
Inactive Ingredients: Magnesium Stearate, Pregelatinized Starch, Starch (corn), Stearic Acid, and FD&C Yellow No. 6.
Hydrocodone bitartrate is an opioid analgesic and antitussive and occurs as fine, white crystals or as a crystalline powder. It is affected by light. The chemical name is: 4,5α-epoxy-3-methoxy-17-methylmorphinan-6-one tartrate (1:1) hydrate (2:5). Its structure is as follows:

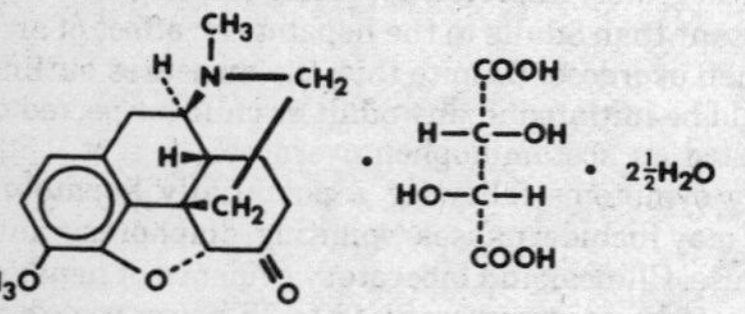

$C_{18}H_{21}NO_3 \cdot C_4H_6O_6 \cdot 2\frac{1}{2}H_2O$ M.W. 494.50

Acetaminophen, 4′-hydroxyacetanilide, is a nonopiate, nonsalicylate analgesic and antipyretic which occurs as a white, odorless crystalline powder possessing a slightly bitter taste. Its structure is as follows:

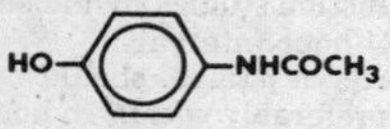

$C_8H_9NO_2$ M.W. 151.16

CLINICAL PHARMACOLOGY

Hydrocodone is a semisynthetic narcotic analgesic and antitussive with multiple actions qualitatively similar to those of codeine. Most of these involve the central nervous system and smooth muscle. The precise mechanism of action of hydrocodone and other opiates is not known, although it is believed to relate to the existence of opiate receptors in the central nervous system. In addition to analgesia, narcotics may produce drowsiness, changes in mood and mental clouding.
Radioimmunoassay techniques have recently been developed for the analysis of hydrocodone in human plasma. After a 10 mg oral dose of hydrocodone bitartrate, a mean peak serum drug level of 23.6 ng/mL and an elimination half-life of 3.8 hours were found.
The analgesic action of acetaminophen involves peripheral and central influences, but the specific mechanism is as yet undetermined. Antipyretic activity is mediated through hypothalamic heat regulating centers. Acetaminophen inhibits prostaglandin synthetase. Therapeutic doses of acetaminophen have negligible effects on the cardiovascular or respiratory systems; however, toxic doses may cause circulatory failure and rapid, shallow breathing. Acetaminophen is rapidly and almost completely absorbed from the gastrointestinal tract, producing maximum serum concentrations within 30 minutes to one hour. The plasma half-life in adults and children ranges from 0.90 hours to 3.25 hours with an average of approximately 2 hours. The drug distributes uniformly in most body fluids and is approximately 25% protein bound. Acetaminophen is conjugated in the liver, with less than 3% of the dose excreted unchanged in 24 hours. The primary metabolic pathway is conjugation to sulfate and glucuronide by-products. A minor oxidative pathway forms cysteine and mercapturic acid. These compounds are subsequently excreted by the kidneys into the urine.

INDICATIONS AND USAGE

For the relief of moderate to moderately severe pain.

CONTRAINDICATIONS

Hypersensitivity to acetaminophen or hydrocodone.

WARNINGS

Respiratory Depression: At high doses or in sensitive patients, hydrocodone may produce dose-related respiratory depression by acting directly on the brain stem respiratory center. Hydrocodone also affects the center that controls respiratory rhythm, and may produce irregular and periodic breathing.
Head Injury and Increased Intracranial Pressure: The respiratory depressant effects of narcotics and their capacity to elevate cerebrospinal fluid pressure may be markedly exaggerated in the presence of head injury, other intracranial lesions or a pre-existing increase in intracranial pressure. Furthermore, narcotics produce adverse reactions which may obscure the clinical course of patients with head injuries.
Acute Abdominal Conditions: The administration of narcotics may obscure the diagnosis or clinical course of patients with acute abdominal conditions.

PRECAUTIONS

Special Risk Patients: As with any narcotic analgesic agent, Hydrocodone Bitartrate and Acetaminophen Tablets should be used with caution in elderly or debilitated patients and those with severe impairment of hepatic or renal function, hypothyroidism, Addison's disease, prostatic hypertrophy or urethral stricture. The usual precautions should be observed and the possibility of respiratory depression should be kept in mind.
Information for Patients: Hydrocodone Bitartrate and Acetaminophen Tablets, like all narcotics, may impair the mental and/or physical abilities required for the performance of potentially hazardous tasks such as driving a car or operating machinery; patients should be cautioned accordingly.
Cough Reflex: Hydrocodone suppresses the cough reflex; as with all narcotics, caution should be exercised when Hydrocodone Bitartrate and Acetaminophen Tablets are used postoperatively and in patients with pulmonary disease.
Drug Interactions: Patients receiving other narcotic analgesics, antipsychotics, antianxiety agents, or other CNS depressants (including alcohol) concomitantly with hydrocodone and acetaminophen tablets may exhibit an additive CNS depression. When combined therapy is contemplated, the dose of one or both agents should be reduced.
The use of MAO inhibitors or tricyclic antidepressants with hydrocodone preparations may increase the effect of either the antidepressant or hydrocodone.
The concurrent use of anticholinergics with hydrocodone may produce paralytic ileus.
Usage in Pregnancy:
Teratogenic Effects: Pregnancy Category C. Hydrocodone has been shown to be teratogenic in hamsters when given in doses 700 times the human dose. There are no adequate and well-controlled studies in pregnant women. Hydrocodone Bitartrate and Acetaminophen Tablets should be used during pregnancy only if the potential benefit justifies the potential risk to the fetus.
Nonteratogenic Effects: Babies born to mothers who have been taking opioids regularly prior to delivery will be physically dependent. The withdrawal signs include irritability and excessive crying, tremors, hyperactive reflexes, increased respiratory rate, increased stools, sneezing, yawning, vomiting, and fever. The intensity of the syndrome does not always correlate with the duration of maternal opioid use or dose. There is no consensus on the best method of managing withdrawal. Chlorpromazine 0.7 to 1 mg/kg q6h, and paregoric 2 to 4 drops/kg q4h, have been used to treat withdrawal symptoms in infants. The duration of therapy is 4 to 28 days, with the dosage decreased as tolerated.
Labor and Delivery: As with all narcotics, administration of Hydrocodone Bitartrate and Acetaminophen Tablets to the mother shortly before delivery may result in some degree of respiratory depression in the newborn, especially if higher doses are used.
Nursing Mothers: It is not known whether this drug is excreted in human milk. Because many drugs are excreted in human milk and because of the potential for serious adverse reactions in nursing infants from Hydrocodone Bitartrate and Acetaminophen Tablets, a decision should be made whether to discontinue nursing or to discontinue the drug, taking into account the importance of the drug to the mother.
Pediatric Use: Safety and effectiveness in children have not been established.

ADVERSE REACTIONS

The most frequently observed adverse reactions include lightheadedness, dizziness, sedation, nausea and vomiting. These effects seem to be more prominent in ambulatory than in nonambulatory patients and some of these adverse reactions may be alleviated if the patient lies down.
Other adverse reactions include:
Central Nervous System: Drowsiness, mental clouding, lethargy, impairment of mental and physical performance, anxiety, fear, dysphoria, psychic dependence, mood changes.
Gastrointestinal System: The antiemetic phenothiazines are useful in suppressing the nausea and vomiting which may occur (see above); however, some phenothiazine derivatives seem to be antianalgesic and to increase the amount of narcotic required to produce pain relief, while other phenothiazines reduce the amount of narcotic required to produce a given level of analgesia. Prolonged administration of Hydrocodone Bitartrate and Acetaminophen Tablets may produce constipation.
Genitourinary System: Ureteral spasm, spasm of vesical sphincters and urinary retention have been reported.
Respiratory Depression: Hydrocodone bitartrate may produce dose-related respiratory depression by acting directly on the brain stem respiratory center. Hydrocodone also affects the center that controls respiratory rhythm, and may produce irregular and periodic breathing. If significant respiratory depression occurs, it may be antagonized by the use of naloxone hydrochloride. Apply other supportive measures when indicated.

DRUG ABUSE AND DEPENDENCE

Hydrocodone Bitartrate and Acetaminophen Tablets are subject to the Federal Controlled Substance Act (Schedule III). Psychic dependence, physical dependence, and tolerance may develop upon repeated administration of narcotics; therefore, Hydrocodone Bitartrate and Acetaminophen Tablets should be prescribed and administered with caution. However, psychic dependence is unlikely to develop when Hydrocodone Bitartrate and Acetaminophen Tablets are used for a short time for the treatment of pain.
Physical dependence, the condition in which continued administration of the drug is required to prevent the appearance of a withdrawal syndrome, assumes clinically significant proportions only after several weeks of continued narcotic use, although some mild degree of physical dependence may develop after a few days of narcotic therapy. Tolerance, in which increasingly large doses are required in order to produce the same degree of analgesia, is manifested initially by a shortened duration of analgesic effect, and subsequently by decreases in the intensity of analgesia. The rate of development of tolerance varies among patients.

OVERDOSAGE

Acetaminophen
Signs and Symptoms: In acute acetaminophen overdosage, dose-dependent, potentially fatal hepatic necrosis is the most serious adverse effect. Renal tubular necrosis, hypoglycemic coma, and thrombocytopenia may also occur.
In adults, hepatic toxicity has rarely been reported with acute overdoses of less than 10 grams and fatalities with less than 15 grams. Importantly, young children seem to be more resistant than adults to the hepatotoxic effect of an acetaminophen overdose. Despite this, the measures outlined below should be initiated in any adult or child suspected of having ingested an acetaminophen overdose.
Early symptoms following a potentially hepatotoxic overdose may include: nausea, vomiting, diaphoresis and general malaise. Clinical and laboratory evidence of hepatic toxicity may not be apparent until 48 to 72 hours post-ingestion.
Treatment: The stomach should be emptied promptly by lavage or by induction of emesis with syrup of ipecac. Patients' estimates of the quantity of a drug ingested are notoriously unreliable. Therefore, if an acetaminophen overdose is suspected, a serum acetaminophen assay should be obtained as early as possible, but no sooner than four hours following ingestion. Liver function studies should be obtained initially and repeated at 24-hour intervals.
The antidote, N-acetylcysteine, should be administered as early as possible, preferably within 16 hours of the overdose ingestion for optimal results, but in any case, within 24 hours. Following recovery, there are no residual, structural or functional hepatic abnormalities.
Hydrocodone
Signs and Symptoms: Serious overdose with hydrocodone is characterized by respiratory depression (a decrease in respiratory rate and/or tidal volume, Cheyne-Stokes respiration, cyanosis), extreme somnolence progressing to stupor or coma, skeletal muscle flaccidity, cold and clammy skin, and sometimes bradycardia and hypotension. In severe overdose, apnea, circulatory collapse, cardiac arrest and death may occur.
Treatment: Primary attention should be given to the re-establishment of adequate respiratory exchange through provision of a patent airway and the institution of assisted or controlled ventilation. The narcotic antagonist naloxone is a specific antidote against respiratory depression which may result from overdosage or unusual sensitivity to narcotics, including hydrocodone. Therefore, an appropriate dose of naloxone hydrochloride (see package insert) should be administered, preferably by the intravenous route, and simultaneously with efforts at respiratory resuscitation. Since the duration of action of hydrocodone may exceed that of the antagonist, the patient should be kept under continued surveillance and repeated doses of the antagonist should be administered as needed to maintain adequate respiration.
An antagonist should not be administered in the absence of clinically significant respiratory or cardiovascular depres-

sion. Oxygen, intravenous fluids, vasopressors and other supportive measures should be employed as indicated.
Gastric emptying may be useful in removing unabsorbed drug.

DOSAGE AND ADMINISTRATION

Dosage should be adjusted according to the severity of pain and the response of the patient. However, it should be kept in mind that tolerance to hydrocodone can develop with continued use and that the incidence of untoward effects is dose related.
The usual adult dosage is one tablet every four to six hours as needed for pain. The total 24 hour dose should not exceed 6 tablets.

HOW SUPPLIED

Hydrocodone Bitartrate and Acetaminophen Tablets
Each tablet contains: hydrocodone bitartrate 7.5 mg and acetaminophen 650 mg.
They are available as peach colored, capsule shaped tablets with a bisecting line and debossed with a BMP 188 identification number.
Bottles of 100 .... *NDC* 0029-1362-30
Storage: Store at controlled room temperature 15°–30°C. (59°–86°F.).
A Schedule III Narcotic.
0937999 Revised March, 1989
Shown in Product Identification Section, page 430

AUGMENTIN® ℞

(amoxicillin/clavulanate potassium)
Tablets, Powder for Oral Suspension and Chewable Tablets

DESCRIPTION

Augmentin is an oral antibacterial combination consisting of the semisynthetic antibiotic amoxicillin and the β-lactamase inhibitor, clavulanate potassium (the potassium salt of clavulanic acid). Amoxicillin is an analog of ampicillin, derived from the basic penicillin nucleus, 6-aminopenicillanic acid. Chemically, amoxicillin is D-(-)-α-amino-p-hydroxybenzyl-penicillin trihydrate and may be represented structurally as:

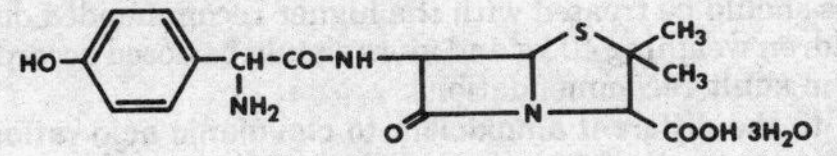

Clavulanic acid is produced by the fermentation of *Streptomyces clavuligerus.* It is a β-lactam structurally related to the penicillins and possesses the ability to inactivate a wide variety of β-lactamases by blocking the active sites of these enzymes. Clavulanic acid is particularly active against the clinically important plasmid mediated β-lactamases frequently responsible for transferred drug resistance to penicillins and cephalosporins. Chemically clavulanate potassium is potassium Z-(3R, 5R)-2-(β-hydroxyethylidene) clavam-3-carboxylate and may be represented structurally as:

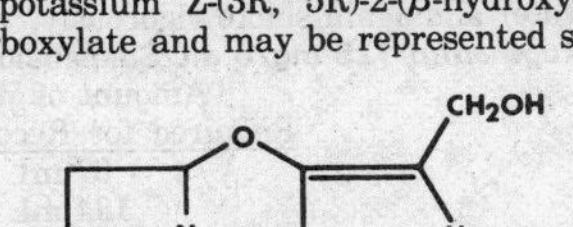

Inactive Ingredients: Tablets—Colloidal silicon dioxide, ethyl cellulose, hydroxypropyl cellulose, hydroxypropyl methylcellulose, magnesium stearate, microcrystalline cellulose, sodium starch glycolate and titanium dioxide. Powder for Oral Suspension—Colloidal silicon dioxide, flavorings, mannitol, silica gel, sodium saccharin, succinic acid and xanthan gum. Chewable Tablets—Colloidal silicon dioxide, D & C Yellow No. 10, glycine, magnesium stearate, mannitol and sodium saccharin.
Augmentin is available in 250 mg and 500 mg white film-coated tablets, 125 mg and 250 mg lemon-lime-flavored chewable tablets, and 125 mg/5 mL banana-flavored and 250 mg/5 mL orange-flavored oral suspensions. Each *Augmentin* 250 mg and 500 mg tablet contains 250 mg and 500 mg amoxicillin as the trihydrate, respectively, together with 125 mg clavulanic acid as the potassium salt. Each 125 mg chewable tablet and each teaspoonful (5 mL) of reconstituted *Augmentin* 125 mg/5 mL oral suspension contain 125 mg amoxicillin and 31.25 mg clavulanic acid as the potassium salt while each 250 mg chewable tablet and each 5 mL of reconstituted *Augmentin* 250 mg/5 mL oral suspension contain 250 mg amoxicillin and 62.5 mg clavulanic acid as the potassium salt.
Each *Augmentin* tablet contains 0.63 mEq potassium. Each 125 mg chewable tablet and each 5 mL of reconstituted *Augmentin* 125 mg/5 mL oral suspension contain 0.16 mEq potassium. Each 250 mg chewable tablet and each 5mL of reconstituted *Augmentin* 250 mg/5 mL oral suspension contain 0.32 mEq potassium.

Recommended *Augmentin* Susceptibility Ranges[1,2]

ORGANISMS	RESISTANT	INTERMEDIATE	SUSCEPTIBLE	MIC[3] CORRELATES mcg/mL R	MIC[3] CORRELATES mcg/mL S
Gram-Negative Enteric Bacteria	≤13 mm	14–17 mm	≥18 mm	≥32/16	≤8/4
Staphylococcus[4] and *Hemophilus* spp.	≤19 mm	—	≥20 mm		≤4/2 ≤4/2

[1] The non-β-lactamase-producing organisms which are normally susceptible to ampicillin, such as streptococci, will have similar zone sizes as for ampicillin disks.
[2] The quality control cultures should have the following assigned daily ranges for *Augmentin*:

		Disks	MIC Range (mcg/mL)
E. coli	(ATCC 25922)	19–25 mm	2/1–8/4
S. aureus	(ATCC 25923)	28–36 mm	0.25/0.12–0.5/0.25
E. coli	(ATCC 35218)	18–22 mm	4/2–16/8

[3] Expressed as concentration of amoxicillin/clavulanic acid.
[4] Organisms which show susceptibility to *Augmentin* but are resistant to methicillin/oxacillin should be considered resistant.

CLINICAL PHARMACOLOGY

Amoxicillin and clavulanate potassium are well absorbed from the gastrointestinal tract after oral administration of *Augmentin. Augmentin* is stable in the presence of gastric acid and may be given without regard to meals.
Oral administration of one *Augmentin* 250 mg or *Augmentin* 500 mg tablet provides average peak serum concentrations one to two hours after dosing of 4.4 mcg/mL and 7.6 mcg/mL, respectively, for amoxicillin and 2.3 mcg/mL for clavulanic acid. The areas under the serum concentration curves obtained during the first 6 hours after dosing were 11.4 mcg/mL.hr. and 20.2 mcg/mL.hr. for amoxicillin, respectively, when one *Augmentin* 250 mg or 500 mg tablet was administered to adult volunteers. The corresponding area under the serum concentration curve for clavulanic acid was 5 mcg/mL.hr. Oral administration of 5 mL of *Augmentin* 250 mg/5 mL suspension or the equivalent dose of 10 mL *Augmentin* 125 mg/5 mL suspension provides average peak serum concentrations approximately one hour after dosing of 6.9 mcg/mL for amoxicillin and 1.6 mcg/mL for clavulanic acid. The areas under the serum concentration curves obtained during the first 6 hours after dosing were 12.6 mcg/mL.hr. for amoxicillin and 2.9 mcg/mL.hr. for clavulanic acid when 5 mL of *Augmentin* 250 mg/5mL suspension or equivalent dose of 10 mL of *Augmentin* 125 mg/5 mL suspension was administered to adult volunteers. One *Augmentin* 250 mg chewable tablet or two *Augmentin* 125 mg chewable tablets are equivalent to 5 mL of *Augmentin* 250 mg/5 mL suspension and provide similar serum levels of amoxicillin and clavulanic acid.
Amoxicillin serum concentrations achieved with *Augmentin* are similar to those produced by the oral administration of equivalent doses of amoxicillin alone. The half-life of amoxicillin after the oral administration of *Augmentin* is 1.3 hours and that of clavulanic acid is 1.0 hour.
Approximately 50–70% of the amoxicillin and approximately 25–40% of the clavulanic acid are excreted unchanged in urine during the first six hours after administration of a single *Augmentin* 250 mg or 500 mg tablet or 10 mL of *Augmentin* 250 mg/5 mL suspension.
Concurrent administration of probenecid delays amoxicillin excretion but does not delay renal excretion of clavulanic acid.
Neither component in *Augmentin* is highly protein-bound; clavulanic acid has been found to be approximately 30% bound to human serum and amoxicillin approximately 20% bound.
Amoxicillin diffuses readily into most body tissues and fluids with the exception of the brain and spinal fluids. The results of experiments involving the administration of clavulanic acid to animals suggest that this compound, like amoxicillin, is well distributed in body tissues.
Two hours after oral administration of a single 35 mg/kg dose of *Augmentin* suspension to fasting children, average concentrations of 3.0 mcg/mL of amoxicillin and 0.5 mcg/mL of clavulanic acid were detected in middle ear effusions.
Microbiology: Amoxicillin is a semisynthetic antibiotic with a broad spectrum of bactericidal activity against many gram-positive and gram-negative microorganisms. Amoxicillin is, however, susceptible to degradation by β-lactamases and therefore the spectrum of activity does not include organisms which produce these enzymes. Clavulanic acid is a β-lactam, structurally related to the penicillins, which possesses the ability to inactivate a wide range of β-lactamase enzymes commonly found in microorganisms resistant to penicillins and cephalosporins. In particular, it has good activity against the clinically important plasmid mediated β-lactamases frequently responsible for transferred drug resistance.
The formulation of amoxicillin with clavulanic acid in *Augmentin* protects amoxicillin from degradation by β-lactamase enzymes and effectively extends the antibiotic spectrum of amoxicillin to include many bacteria normally resistant to amoxicillin and other β-lactam antibiotics. Thus *Augmentin* possesses the distinctive properties of a broad-spectrum antibiotic and a β-lactamase inhibitor.
While *in vitro* studies have demonstrated the susceptibility of most strains of the following organisms, clinical efficacy for infections other than those included in the INDICATIONS AND USAGE section has not been documented:
GRAM-POSITIVE BACTERIA: *Staphylococcus aureus* (β-lactamase and non-β-lactamase producing), *Staphylococcus epidermidis* (β-lactamase and non-β-lactamase producing), *Staphylococcus saprophyticus* (β-lactamase and non-β-lactamase producing), *Streptococcus faecalis* (Enterococcus), Streptococcus pneumoniae* (D. pneumoniae), Streptococcus pyogenes*, Streptococcus viridans**
ANAEROBES: *Clostridium* species*, *Peptococcus* species*, *Peptostreptococcus* species*
*These are non-β-lactamase-producing strains and therefore are susceptible to amoxicillin alone.
GRAM-NEGATIVE BACTERIA: *Hemophilus influenzae* (β-lactamase and non-β-lactamase producing), *Moraxella (Branhamella) catarrhalis* (β-lactamase and non-β-lactamase producing); *Escherichia coli* (β-lactamase and non-β-lactamase producing), *Klebsiella* species (All known strains are β-lactamase producing), *Enterobacter* species (Although most strains of *Enterobacter* species are resistant *in vitro*, clinical efficacy has been demonstrated with *Augmentin* in urinary tract infections caused by these organisms.), *Proteus mirabilis* (β-lactamase and non-β-lactamase producing), *Proteus vulgaris* (β-lactamase and non-β-lactamase producing), *Neisseria gonorrhoeae* (β-lactamase and non-β-lactamase producing), *Legionella* species (β-lactamase and non-β-lactamase producing).
ANAEROBES: *Bacteroides* species, including *B. fragilis* (β-lactamase and non-β-lactamase producing).
SUSCEPTIBILITY TESTING
Diffusion Technique: For Kirby-Bauer method of susceptibility testing, a 30 mcg *Augmentin* (20 mcg amoxicillin + 10 mcg clavulanic acid) diffusion disk should be used. With this procedure, a report from the laboratory of "Susceptible" indicates that the infecting organism is likely to respond to *Augmentin* therapy and a report of "Resistant" indicates that the infecting organism is not likely to respond to therapy. An "intermediate susceptibility" report suggests that the infecting organism would be susceptible to *Augmentin* if the higher dosage is used or if the infection is confined to tissues or fluids (e.g., urine) in which high antibiotic levels are attained.
Dilution Techniques: Broth or agar dilution methods may be used to determine the minimal inhibitory concentration (MIC) value for susceptibility of bacterial isolates to *Augmentin.* Tubes should be inoculated to contain 10^4 to 10^5 organisms/mL or plates "spotted" with 10^3 to 10^4 organisms. The recommended dilution method employs a constant amoxicillin/clavulanic acid ratio of 2 to 1 in all tubes with increasing concentrations of amoxicillin. MICs are reported in terms of amoxicillin concentration in the presence of clavulanic acid at a constant 2 parts amoxicillin to 1 part clavulanic acid.
[See table above.]

INDICATIONS AND USAGE

Augmentin is indicated in the treatment of infections caused by susceptible strains of the designated organisms in the conditions listed below:

Continued on next page

SmithKline Beecham—Cont.

Lower Respiratory Tract Infections—caused by β-lactamase-producing strains of *Hemophilus influenzae* and *Moraxella (Branhamella) catarrhalis.*
Otitis Media—caused by β-lactamase-producing strains of *Hemophilus influenzae* and *Moraxella (Branhamella) catarrhalis.*
Sinusitis—caused by β-lactamase-producing strains of *Hemophilus influenzae* and *Moraxella (Branhamella) catarrhalis.*
Skin and Skin Structure Infections—caused by β-lactamase-producing strains of *Staphylococcus aureus, Escherichia coli* and *Klebsiella* spp.
Urinary Tract Infections—caused by β-lactamase-producing strains of *Escherichia coli, Klebsiella* spp. and *Enterobacter* spp.
While *Augmentin* is indicated only for the conditions listed above, infections caused by ampicillin-susceptible organisms are also amenable to *Augmentin* treatment due to its amoxicillin content. Therefore, mixed infections caused by ampicillin-susceptible organisms and β-lactamase-producing organisms susceptible to *Augmentin* should not require the addition of another antibiotic.
Bacteriological studies, to determine the causative organisms and their susceptibility to *Augmentin,* should be performed together with any indicated surgical procedures.
Therapy may be instituted prior to obtaining the results from bacteriological and susceptibility studies to determine the causative organisms and their susceptibility to *Augmentin* when there is reason to believe the infection may involve any of the β-lactamase-producing organisms listed above. Once the results are known, therapy should be adjusted, if appropriate.

CONTRAINDICATIONS

A history of allergic reactions to any penicillin is a contraindication.

WARNINGS

SERIOUS AND OCCASIONALLY FATAL HYPERSENSITIVITY (ANAPHYLACTOID) REACTIONS HAVE BEEN REPORTED IN PATIENTS ON PENICILLIN THERAPY. ALTHOUGH ANAPHYLAXIS IS MORE FREQUENT FOLLOWING PARENTERAL THERAPY, IT HAS OCCURRED IN PATIENTS ON ORAL PENICILLINS. THESE REACTIONS ARE MORE LIKELY TO OCCUR IN INDIVIDUALS WITH A HISTORY OF PENICILLIN HYPERSENSITIVITY AND/OR A HISTORY OF SENSITIVITY TO MULTIPLE ALLERGENS. THERE HAVE BEEN REPORTS OF INDIVIDUALS WITH A HISTORY OF PENICILLIN HYPERSENSITIVITY WHO HAVE EXPERIENCED SEVERE REACTIONS WHEN TREATED WITH CEPHALOSPORINS. BEFORE INITIATING THERAPY WITH ANY PENICILLIN, CAREFUL INQUIRY SHOULD BE MADE CONCERNING PREVIOUS HYPERSENSITIVITY REACTIONS TO PENICILLINS, CEPHALOSPORINS, OR OTHER ALLERGENS. IF AN ALLERGIC REACTION OCCURS, *AUGMENTIN* SHOULD BE DISCONTINUED AND THE APPROPRIATE THERAPY INSTITUTED. **SERIOUS ANAPHYLACTOID REACTIONS REQUIRE IMMEDIATE EMERGENCY TREATMENT WITH EPINEPHRINE. OXYGEN, INTRAVENOUS STEROIDS, AND AIRWAY MANAGEMENT, INCLUDING INTUBATION, SHOULD ALSO BE ADMINISTERED AS INDICATED.**
Pseudomembranous colitis has been reported with nearly all antibacterial agents, including *Augmentin,* and has ranged in severity from mild to life-threatening. Therefore, it is important to consider this diagnosis in patients who present with diarrhea subsequent to the administration of antibacterial agents.
Treatment with antibacterial agents alters the normal flora of the colon and may permit overgrowth of clostridia. Studies indicate that a toxin produced by *Clostridium difficile* is one primary cause of "antibiotic associated colitis."
Mild cases of pseudomembranous colitis usually respond to drug discontination alone. In moderate to severe cases, consideration should be given to management with fluids and electrolytes, protein supplementation and treatment with an antibacterial drug effective against *C. difficile.*

PRECAUTIONS

General: While *Augmentin* possesses the characteristic low toxicity of the penicillin group of antibiotics, periodic assessment of organ system functions, including renal, hepatic and hematopoietic function, is advisable during prolonged therapy.
A high percentage of patients with mononucleosis who receive ampicillin develop a skin rash. Thus, ampicillin class antibiotics should not be administered to patients with mononucleosis.
The possibility of superinfections with mycotic or bacterial pathogens should be kept in mind during therapy. If superinfections occur (usually involving *Pseudomonas* or *Candida*), the drug should be discontinued and/or appropriate therapy instituted.
Drug Interactions: Probenecid decreases the renal tubular secretion of amoxicillin. Concurrent use with *Augmentin* may result in increased and prolonged blood levels of amoxicillin.
The concurrent administration of allopurinol and ampicillin increases substantially the incidence of rashes in patients receiving both drugs as compared to patients receiving ampicillin alone. It is not known whether this potentiation of ampicillin rashes is due to allopurinol or the hyperuricemia present in these patients. There are no data with *Augmentin* and allopurinol administered concurrently.
Augmentin should not be co-administered with Antabuse® (disulfiram).
Drug/Laboratory Test Interactions: Oral administration of *Augmentin* will result in high urine concentrations of amoxicillin. High urine concentrations of ampicillin may result in false-positive reactions when testing for the presence of glucose in urine using Clinitest®, Benedict's Solution or Fehling's Solution. Since this effect may also occur with amoxicillin and therefore *Augmentin,* it is recommended that glucose tests based on enzymatic glucose oxidase reactions (such as Clinistix® or Tes-Tape®) be used.
Following administration of ampicillin to pregnant women a transient decrease in plasma concentration of total conjugated estriol, estriol-glucuronide, conjugated estrone and estradiol has been noted. This effect may also occur with amoxicillin and therefore *Augmentin.*
Carcinogenesis, Mutagenesis, Impairment of Fertility: Long-term studies in animals have not been performed to evaluate carcinogenic or mutagenic potential.
Pregnancy (Category B): Reproduction studies have been performed in mice and rats at doses up to ten (10) times the human dose and have revealed no evidence of impaired fertility or harm to the fetus due to *Augmentin.* There are, however, no adequate and well-controlled studies in pregnant women. Because animal reproduction studies are not always predictive of human response, this drug should be used during pregnancy only if clearly needed.
Labor and Delivery: Oral ampicillin class antibiotics are generally poorly absorbed during labor. Studies in guinea pigs have shown that intravenous administration of ampicillin decreased the uterine tone, frequency of contractions, height of contractions and duration of contractions. However, it is not known whether the use of *Augmentin* in humans during labor or delivery has immediate or delayed adverse effects on the fetus, prolongs the duration of labor, or increases the likelihood that forceps delivery or other obstetrical intervention or resuscitation of the newborn will be necessary.
Nursing Mothers: Ampicillin class antibiotics are excreted in the milk; therefore, caution should be exercised when *Augmentin* is administered to a nursing woman.

ADVERSE REACTIONS

Augmentin is generally well tolerated. The majority of side effects observed in clinical trials were of a mild and transient nature and less than 3% of patients discontinued therapy because of drug-related side effects. The most frequently reported adverse effects were diarrhea/loose stools (9%), nausea (3%), skin rashes and urticaria (3%), vomiting (1%) and vaginitis (1%). The overall incidence of side effects, and in particular diarrhea, increased with the higher recommended dose. Other less frequently reported reactions include: abdominal discomfort, flatulence and headache.
The following adverse reactions have been reported for ampicillin class antibiotics:
Gastrointestinal: Diarrhea, nausea, vomiting, indigestion, gastritis, stomatitis, glossitis, black "hairy" tongue, enterocolitis and pseudomembranous colitis. Onset of pseudomembranous colitis symptoms may occur during or after antibiotic treatment (see WARNINGS).
Hypersensitivity reactions: Skin rashes, urticaria, angioedema, serum sickness-like reactions (urticaria or skin rash accompanied by arthritis, arthralgia, myalgia and frequently fever), erythema multiforme (rarely Stevens-Johnson Syndrome) and an occasional case of exfoliative dermatitis have been reported. These reactions may be controlled with antihistamines and, if necessary, systemic corticosteroids. Whenever such reactions occur, the drug should be discontinued, unless the opinion of the physician dictates otherwise. Serious and occasional fatal hypersensitivity (anaphylactic) reactions can occur with oral penicillin (See WARNINGS).
Liver: A moderate rise in AST (SGOT) and/or ALT (SGPT) has been noted in patients treated with ampicillin class antibiotics but the significance of these findings is unknown. Hepatic dysfunction, including increases in serum transaminases (AST and/or ALT), serum bilirubin and/or alkaline phosphatase, has been infrequently reported with *Augmentin.* The histologic findings on liver biopsy have consisted of predominantly cholestatic, hepatocellular or mixed cholestatic-hepatocellular changes. The onset of signs/symptoms of hepatic dysfunction may occur during or after therapy. Complete resolution has occurred with time.
Hemic and Lymphatic Systems: Anemia, thrombocytopenia, thrombocytopenic purpura, eosinophilia, leukopenia and agranulocytosis have been reported during therapy with penicillins. These reactions are usually reversible on discontinuation of therapy and are believed to be hypersensitivity phenomena. A slight thrombocytosis was noted in less than 1% of the patients treated with *Augmentin.*
Central Nervous System: Reversible hyperactivity, agitation, anxiety, insomnia, confusion, behavioral changes, and/or dizziness have been reported rarely.

OVERDOSAGE

Amoxicillin may be removed from circulation by hemodialysis.
The molecular weight, degree of protein binding and pharmacokinetic profile of clavulanic acid together with information from a single patient with renal insufficiency all suggest that this compound may also be removed by hemodialysis.

DOSAGE AND ADMINISTRATION

The *Augmentin* 250 mg tablet and the 250 mg chewable tablet do *not* contain the same amount of clavulanic acid (as the potassium salt). The *Augmentin* 250 mg tablet contains 125 mg of clavulanic acid, whereas the 250 mg chewable tablet contains 62.5 mg of clavulanic acid. Therefore, the *Augmentin* 250 mg tablet and the 250 mg chewable tablet should *not be* substituted for each other, as they are not interchangeable.
Since both the *Augmentin* 250 mg and 500 mg tablets contain the same amount of clavulanic acid (125 mg, as the potassium salt), two *Augmentin* 250 mg tablets are not equivalent to one *Augmentin* 500 mg tablet. Therefore, two *Augmentin* 250 mg tablets should not be substituted for one *Augmentin* 500 mg tablet for treatment of more severe infections.
Dosage:
Adults: The usual adult dose is one *Augmentin* 250 mg tablet every eight hours. For more severe infections and infections of the respiratory tract, the dose should be one *Augmentin* 500 mg tablet every eight hours.
Children: The usual dose is 20 mg/kg/day, based on amoxicillin component, in divided doses every eight hours. For otitis media, sinusitis and lower respiratory tract infections, the dose should be 40 mg/kg/day, based on the amoxicillin component, in divided doses every eight hours. Severe infections should be treated with the higher recommended dose. Children weighing 40 kg and more should be dosed according to the adult recommendations.
Due to the different amoxicillin to clavulanic acid ratios in the *Augmentin* 250 mg tablet (250/125) versus the *Augmentin* 250 mg chewable tablet (250/62.5), the *Augmentin* 250 mg tablet should not be used until the child weighs at least 40 kg and more.

DIRECTIONS FOR MIXING ORAL SUSPENSION

Prepare a suspension at time of dispensing as follows: Tap bottle until all the powder flows freely. Add approximately ⅔ of the total amount of water for reconstitution (see table below) and shake vigorously to suspend powder. Add remainder of the water and again shake vigorously.

***Augmentin* 125 mg/5 mL Suspension**

Bottle Size	Amount of Water Required for Reconstitution
75 mL	67 mL
150 mL	134 mL

Each teaspoonful (5 mL) will contain 125 mg amoxicillin and 31.25 mg of clavulanic acid as the potassium salt.

***Augmentin* 250 mg/5 mL Suspension**

Bottle Size	Amount of Water Required for Reconsititution
75 mL	65 mL
150 mL	130 mL

Each teaspoonful (5 mL) will contain 250 mg amoxicillin and 62.5 mg of clavulanic acid as the potassium salt.
Note: SHAKE ORAL SUSPENSION WELL BEFORE USING.
Reconstituted suspension must be stored under refrigeration and discarded after 10 days.
Administration: The absorption of *Augmentin* is unaffected by food. Therefore, *Augmentin* may be administered without regard to meals.

HOW SUPPLIED

***AUGMENTIN* 250 MG TABLETS:** Each white oval film-coated tablet, debossed with AUGMENTIN on one side and 250/125 on the other side, contains 250 mg amoxicillin as the trihydrate and 125 mg clavulanic acid as the potassium salt.
NDC 0029-6075-27 ....bottles of 30
NDC 0029-6075-31 ....Unit Dose (10×10) 100 tablets
***AUGMENTIN* 500 MG TABLETS:** Each white oval film-coated tablet, debossed with AUGMENTIN on one side and 500/125 on the other side, contains 500 mg amoxicillin as the trihydrate and 125 mg clavulanic acid as the potassium salt.
NDC 0029-6080-27 ....bottles of 30
NDC 0029-6080-31 ....Unit Dose (10×10) 100 tablets
***AUGMENTIN* 125 MG/5 ML FOR ORAL SUSPENSION:** Each 5 mL of reconstituted banana-flavored suspension con-

tains 125 mg amoxicillin and 31.25 mg clavulanic acid as the potassium salt.

NDC 0029-6085-39 ....75 mL bottle
NDC 0029-6085-22 ....150 mL bottle

***AUGMENTIN* 250 MG/5 ML FOR ORAL SUSPENSION:** Each 5 mL of reconstituted orange-flavored suspension contains 250 mg amoxicillin and 62.5 mg clavulanic acid as the potassium salt.

NDC 0029-6090-39 ....75 mL bottle
NDC 0029-6090-22 ....150 mL bottle

***AUGMENTIN* 125 MG CHEWABLE TABLETS:** Each yellow mottled round tablet, debossed with BMP 189, contains 125 mg amoxicillin as the trihydrate and 31.25 mg clavulanic acid as the potassium salt.

NDC 0029-6073-47 ....carton of 30 (5×6) tablets

***AUGMENTIN* 250 MG CHEWABLE TABLETS:** Each yellow mottled round tablet, debossed with BMP 190, contains 250 mg amoxicillin as the trihydrate and 62.5 mg clavulanic acid as the potassium salt.

NDC 0029-6074-47 ....carton of 30 (5×6) tablets

Veterans Administration—Tablets, 250 mg/125 mg, 30's, 6505-01-203-6259; 500 mg/125 mg, 30's, 6505-01-206-6228.

Military—Chewable Tablets, 125 mg, 30's 6505-01-282-6332; 250 mg, 30's, 6505-01-264-2366; Tablets 250 mg, 30's, 6505-01-203-6259; 500 mg, 30's, 6505-01-206-6228; Oral Suspension, 125 mg/5 mL, 150 mL, 6505-01-204-5388; 250 mg/5 mL, 150 mL, 6505-01-207-0795; 250 mg/5 mL, 75 mL, 6505-01-207-8205.

AG:L4

Shown in Product Identification Section, page 430

BACTROBAN® ℞

(mupirocin)
Ointment 2%
For Dermatologic Use

DESCRIPTION

Each gram of *Bactroban* Ointment 2% contains 20 mg mupirocin in a bland water miscible ointment base (polyethylene glycol ointment, N.F.) consisting of polyethylene glycol 400 and polyethylene glycol 3350. Mupirocin is a naturally occurring antibiotic. The chemical name is (*E*)-(2*S*,3*R*, 4*R*, 5 *S*)-5-[(2*S*, 3*S*, 4*S*, 5*S*)-2,3-Epoxy-5-hydroxy-4-methylhexyl] tetrahydro -3,4- dihydroxy-*β*-methyl -2*H* -pyran-2-crotonic acid, ester with 9-hydroxynonanoic acid. The chemical structure is:

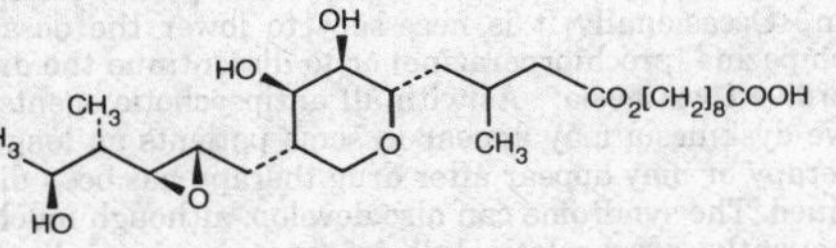

mupirocin

CLINICAL PHARMACOLOGY

Mupirocin is produced by fermentation of the organism *Pseudomonas fluorescens.* Mupirocin inhibits bacterial protein synthesis by reversibly and specifically binding to bacterial isoleucyl transfer-RNA synthetase. Due to this mode of action, mupirocin shows no cross resistance with chloramphenicol, erythromycin, fusidic acid, gentamicin, lincomycin, methicillin, neomycin, novobiocin, penicillin, streptomycin, and tetracycline.

Application of ^{14}C-labeled mupirocin ointment to the lower arm of normal male subjects followed by occlusion for 24 hours showed no measurable systemic absorption (<1.1 nanogram mupirocin per milliliter of whole blood). Measurable radioactivity was present in the stratum corneum of these subjects 72 hours after application.

Microbiology: The following bacteria are susceptible to the action of mupirocin *in vitro:* the aerobic isolates of *Staphylococcus aureus* (including methicillin-resistant and *β*-lactamase producing strains), *Staphylococcus epidermidis, Staphylococcus saprophyticus,* and *Streptococcus pyogenes.*

Only the organisms listed in the INDICATIONS AND USAGE section have been shown to be clinically susceptible to mupirocin.

INDICATIONS AND USAGE

Bactroban (mupirocin) Ointment is indicated for the topical treatment of impetigo due to: *Staphylococcus aureus,* beta hemolytic *Streptococcus**, and *Streptococcus pyogenes.*

CONTRAINDICATIONS

This drug is contraindicated in individuals with a history of sensitivity reactions to any of its components.

WARNINGS

Bactroban Ointment is not for ophthalmic use.

PRECAUTIONS

If a reaction suggesting sensitivity or chemical irritation should occur with the use of *Bactroban* Ointment, treatment should be discontinued and appropriate alternative therapy for the infection instituted.

As with other antibacterial products prolonged use may result in overgrowth of nonsusceptible organisms, including fungi.

Bactroban is not formulated for use on mucosal surfaces. Intranasal use has been associated with isolated reports of stinging and drying.

Polyethylene glycol can be absorbed from open wounds and damaged skin and is excreted by the kidneys. In common with other polyethylene glycol-based ointments, *Bactroban* should not be used in conditions where absorption of large quantities of polyethylene glycol is possible, especially if there is evidence of moderate or severe renal impairment.

Pregnancy Category B: Reproduction studies have been performed in rats and rabbits at systemic doses, i.e., orally, subcutaneously, and intramuscularly, up to 100 times the human topical dose and have revealed no evidence of impaired fertility or harm to the fetus due to mupirocin. There are, however, no adequate and well-controlled studies in pregnant women. Because animal studies are not always predictive of human response, this drug should be used during pregnancy only if clearly needed.

Nursing Mothers: It is not known whether *Bactroban* is present in breast milk. Nursing should be temporarily discontinued while using *Bactroban.*

ADVERSE REACTIONS

The following local adverse reactions have been reported in connection with the use of *Bactroban* Ointment: burning, stinging, or pain in 1.5% of patients; itching in 1% of patients; rash, nausea, erythema, dry skin, tenderness, swelling, contact dermatitis, and increased exudate in less than 1% of patients.

DOSAGE AND ADMINISTRATION

A small amount of *Bactroban* Ointment should be applied to the affected area three times daily. The area treated may be covered with a gauze dressing if desired. Patients not showing a clinical response within 3 to 5 days should be re-evaluated.

HOW SUPPLIED

Bactroban (mupirocin) Ointment 2% is supplied in 1 gram Single Unit Packages of 50 and in 15 gram and 30 gram tubes.

NDC 0029-1525-15 (1 gram SUP)
NDC 0029-1525-22 (15 gram tube)
NDC 0029-1525-25 (30 gram tube)

Store between 15° and 30°C (59° and 86°F).

BC:L3A

* Efficacy for this organism in this organ system was studied in fewer than ten infections.

COMPAZINE® ℞

[*komp'ah-zeen*]
(brand of prochlorperazine)

DESCRIPTION

Tablets—Each round, yellow-green, coated tablet contains prochlorperazine maleate equivalent to prochlorperazine as follows: 5 mg imprinted SKF and C66; 10 mg imprinted SKF and C67; 25 mg imprinted SKF and C69. Inactive ingredients consist of acacia, calcium sulfate, D&C Green No. 5, D&C Yellow No. 10, FD&C Blue No. 1, FD&C Blue No. 2, FD&C Yellow No. 6, FD&C Red No. 40, gelatin, iron oxide, mineral oil, starch, stearic acid, sucrose, talc and trace amounts of other inactive ingredients.

Spansule® sustained release capsules—Each Compazine® *Spansule* capsule is so prepared that an initial dose is released promptly and the remaining medication is released gradually over a prolonged period.

Each capsule, with black cap and natural body, contains prochlorperazine maleate equivalent to prochlorperazine as follows: 10 mg imprinted SKF and C44; 15 mg imprinted SKF and C46; 30 mg imprinted SKF and C47. Inactive ingredients consist of benzyl alcohol, cetylpyridinium chloride, D&C Green No. 5, D&C Yellow No. 10, FD&C Blue No. 1, FD&C Red No. 40, FD&C Yellow No. 6, gelatin, glyceryl monostearate, sodium lauryl sulfate, starch, sucrose, wax and trace amounts of other inactive ingredients.

Ampuls, 2 mL (5 mg/mL)—Each mL contains, in aqueous solution, 5 mg prochlorperazine as the edisylate, 1 mg sodium sulfite, 1 mg sodium bisulfite, 8 mg sodium phosphate and 12 mg sodium biphosphate.

Vials, 2 mL (5 mg/mL) and 10 mL (5 mg/mL)—Each mL contains, in aqueous solution, 5 mg prochlorperazine as the edisylate, 5 mg sodium biphosphate, 12 mg sodium tartrate, 0.9 mg sodium saccharin, and 0.75% benzyl alcohol as preservative.

Disposable Syringes, 2 mL (5 mg/mL)—Each mL contains, in aqueous solution, 5 mg prochlorperazine as the edisylate, 5 mg sodium biphosphate, 12 mg sodium tartrate, 0.9 mg sodium saccharin, and 0.75% benzyl alcohol as preservative.

Suppositories—Each suppository contains 2½ mg, 5 mg, or 25 mg of prochlorperazine; with glycerin, glyceryl monopalmitate, glyceryl monostearate, hydrogenated cocoanut oil fatty acids and hydrogenated palm kernel oil fatty acids.

Syrup—Each 5 mL (one teaspoonful) of clear, yellow-orange, fruit-flavored liquid contains 5 mg of prochlorperazine as the edisylate. Inactive ingredients consist of FD&C Yellow No. 6, flavors, polyoxyethylene polyoxypropylene glycol, sodium benzoate, sodium citrate, sucrose and water.

INDICATIONS

For control of severe nausea and vomiting.

For management of the manifestations of psychotic disorders.

Compazine (prochlorperazine) is effective for the short-term treatment of generalized non-psychotic anxiety. However, *Compazine* is not the first drug to be used in therapy for most patients with non-psychotic anxiety, because certain risks associated with its use are not shared by common alternative treatments (e.g., benzodiazepines).

When used in the treatment of non-psychotic anxiety, *Compazine* should not be administered at doses of more than 20 mg per day or for longer than 12 weeks, because the use of *Compazine* at higher doses or for longer intervals may cause persistent tardive dyskinesia that may prove irreversible (see Warnings).

The effectiveness of *Compazine* as treatment for non-psychotic anxiety was established in four-week clinical studies of outpatients with generalized anxiety disorder. This evidence does not predict that *Compazine* will be useful in patients with other non-psychotic conditions in which anxiety, or signs that mimic anxiety, are found (e.g., physical illness, organic mental conditions, agitated depression, character pathologies, etc.).

Compazine has not been shown effective in the management of behavioral complications in patients with mental retardation.

CONTRAINDICATIONS

Do not use in comatose states or in the presence of large amounts of central nervous system depressants (alcohol, barbiturates, narcotics, etc.).

Do not use in pediatric surgery.

Do not use in children under 2 years of age or under 20 lbs.

Do not use in children for conditions for which dosage has not been established.

WARNINGS

The extrapyramidal symptoms which can occur secondary to Compazine (prochlorperazine) may be confused with the central nervous system signs of an undiagnosed primary disease responsible for the vomiting, e.g., Reye's syndrome or other encephalopathy. The use of *Compazine* and other potential hepatotoxins should be avoided in children and adolescents whose signs and symptoms suggest Reye's syndrome.

Tardive Dyskinesia: Tardive dyskinesia, a syndrome consisting of potentially irreversible, involuntary, dyskinetic movements, may develop in patients treated with neuroleptic (antipsychotic) drugs. Although the prevalence of the syndrome appears to be highest among the elderly, especially elderly women, it is impossible to rely upon prevalence estimates to predict, at the inception of neuroleptic treatment, which patients are likely to develop the syndrome. Whether neuroleptic drug products differ in their potential to cause tardive dyskinesia is unknown.

Both the risk of developing the syndrome and the likelihood that it will become irreversible are believed to increase as the duration of treatment and the total cumulative dose of neuroleptic drugs administered to the patient increase. However, the syndrome can develop, although much less commonly, after relatively brief treatment periods at low doses.

There is no known treatment for established cases of tardive dyskinesia, although the syndrome may remit, partially or completely, if neuroleptic treatment is withdrawn. Neuroleptic treatment itself, however, may suppress (or partially suppress) the signs and symptoms of the syndrome and thereby may possibly mask the underlying disease process. The effect that symptomatic suppression has upon the long-term course of the syndrome is unknown.

Given these considerations, neuroleptics should be prescribed in a manner that is most likely to minimize the occurrence of tardive dyskinesia. Chronic neuroleptic treatment should generally be reserved for patients who suffer from a chronic illness that, 1) is known to respond to neuroleptic drugs, and, 2) for whom alternative, equally effective, but potentially less harmful treatments are *not* available or appropriate. In patients who do require chronic treatment, the smallest dose and the shortest duration of treatment producing a satisfactory clinical response should be sought. The need for continued treatment should be reassessed periodically.

If signs and symptoms of tardive dyskinesia appear in a patient on neuroleptics, drug discontinuation should be considered. However, some patients may require treatment despite the presence of the syndrome.

Continued on next page

SmithKline Beecham—Cont.

For further information about the description of tardive dyskinesia and its clinical detection, please refer to the sections on Precautions and Adverse Reactions.

Neuroleptic Malignant Syndrome (NMS): A potentially fatal symptom complex sometimes referred to as Neuroleptic Malignant Syndrome (NMS) has been reported in association with antipsychotic drugs. Clinical manifestations of NMS are hyperpyrexia, muscle rigidity, altered mental status and evidence of autonomic instability (irregular pulse or blood pressure, tachycardia, diaphoresis, and cardiac dysrhythmias).

The diagnostic evaluation of patients with this syndrome is complicated. In arriving at a diagnosis, it is important to identify cases where the clinical presentation includes both serious medical illness (e.g., pneumonia, systemic infection, etc.) and untreated or inadequately treated extrapyramidal signs and symptoms (EPS). Other important considerations in the differential diagnosis include central anticholinergic toxicity, heat stroke, drug fever and primary central nervous system (CNS) pathology.

The management of NMS should include 1) immediate discontinuation of antipsychotic drugs and other drugs not essential to concurrent therapy, 2) intensive symptomatic treatment and medical monitoring, and 3) treatment of any concomitant serious medical problems for which specific treatments are available. There is no general agreement about specific pharmacological treatment regimens for uncomplicated NMS.

If a patient requires antipsychotic drug treatment after recovery from NMS, the potential reintroduction of drug therapy should be carefully considered. The patient should be carefully monitored, since recurrences of NMS have been reported.

Compazine ampuls contain sodium bisulfite and sodium sulfite, sulfites that may cause allergic-type reactions including anaphylactic symptoms and life-threatening or less severe asthmatic episodes in certain susceptible people. The overall prevalence of sulfite sensitivity in the general population is unknown and probably low. Sulfite sensitivity is seen more frequently in asthmatic than in non-asthmatic people.

Patients with bone marrow depression or who have previously demonstrated a hypersensitivity reaction (e.g., blood dyscrasias, jaundice) with a phenothiazine should not receive any phenothiazine, including *Compazine*, unless in the judgment of the physician the potential benefits of treatment outweigh the possible hazards.

Compazine (prochlorperazine) may impair mental and/or physical abilities, especially during the first few days of therapy. Therefore, caution patients about activities requiring alertness (e.g., operating vehicles or machinery).

Phenothiazines may intensify or prolong the action of central nervous system depressants (e.g., alcohol, anesthetics, narcotics).

Usage in Pregnancy: Safety for the use of *Compazine* during pregnancy has not been established. Therefore, *Compazine* is not recommended for use in pregnant patients except in cases of severe nausea and vomiting that are so serious and intractable that, in the judgment of the physician, drug intervention is required and potential benefits outweigh possible hazards.

There have been reported instances of prolonged jaundice, extrapyramidal signs, hyperreflexia or hyporeflexia in newborn infants whose mothers received phenothiazines.

Nursing Mothers: There is evidence that phenothiazines are excreted in the breast milk of nursing mothers.

PRECAUTIONS

The antiemetic action of Compazine (prochlorperazine) may mask the signs and symptoms of overdosage of other drugs and may obscure the diagnosis and treatment of other conditions such as intestinal obstruction, brain tumor and Reye's syndrome (see Warnings).

When *Compazine* is used with cancer chemotherapeutic drugs, vomiting as a sign of the toxicity of these agents may be obscured by the antiemetic effect of *Compazine*.

Because hypotension may occur, large doses and parenteral administration should be used cautiously in patients with impaired cardiovascular systems. To minimize the occurrence of hypotension after injection, keep patient lying down and observe for at least ½ hour. If hypotension occurs after parenteral or oral dosing, place patient in head-low position with legs raised. If a vasoconstrictor is required, Levophed®* and Neo-Synephrine®† are suitable. Other pressor agents, including epinephrine, should not be used because they may cause a paradoxical further lowering of blood pressure.

Aspiration of vomitus has occurred in a few post-surgical patients who have received *Compazine* as an antiemetic. Although no causal relationship has been established, this

possibility should be borne in mind during surgical aftercare. Deep sleep, from which patients can be aroused, and coma have been reported, usually with overdosage.

Neuroleptic drugs elevate prolactin levels; the elevation persists during chronic administration. Tissue culture experiments indicate that approximately one third of human breast cancers are prolactin-dependent *in vitro*, a factor of potential importance if the prescribing of these drugs is contemplated in a patient with a previously detected breast cancer. Although disturbances such as galactorrhea, amenorrhea, gynecomastia and impotence have been reported, the clinical significance of elevated serum prolactin levels is unknown for most patients. An increase in mammary neoplasms has been found in rodents after chronic administration of neuroleptic drugs. Neither clinical nor epidemiologic studies conducted to date, however, have shown an association between chronic administration of these drugs and mammary tumorigenesis; the available evidence is considered too limited to be conclusive at this time.

Chromosomal aberrations in spermatocytes and abnormal sperm have been demonstrated in rodents treated with certain neuroleptics.

As with all drugs which exert an anticholinergic effect, and/or cause mydriasis, prochlorperazine should be used with caution in patients with glaucoma.

Because phenothiazines may interfere with thermoregulatory mechanisms, use with caution in persons who will be exposed to extreme heat.

Phenothiazines can diminish the effect of oral anticoagulants.

Phenothiazines can produce alpha-adrenergic blockade.

Thiazide diuretics may accentuate the orthostatic hypotension that may occur with phenothiazines.

Antihypertensive effects of guanethidine and related compounds may be counteracted when phenothiazines are used concomitantly.

Concomitant administration of propranolol with phenothiazines results in increased plasma levels of both drugs.

Phenothiazines may lower the convulsive threshold; dosage adjustments of anticonvulsants may be necessary. Potentiation of anticonvulsant effects does not occur. However, it has been reported that phenothiazines may interfere with the metabolism of Dilantin®‡ and thus precipitate *Dilantin* toxicity.

The presence of phenothiazines may produce false positive phenylketonuria (PKU) test results.

Long-Term Therapy: Given the likelihood that some patients exposed chronically to neuroleptics will develop tardive dyskinesia, it is advised that all patients in whom chronic use is contemplated be given, if possible, full information about this risk. The decision to inform patients and/or their guardians must obviously take into account the clinical circumstances and the competency of the patient to understand the information provided.

To lessen the likelihood of adverse reactions related to cumulative drug effect, patients with a history of long-term therapy with *Compazine* and/or other neuroleptics should be evaluated periodically to decide whether the maintenance dosage could be lowered or drug therapy discontinued.

Children with acute illnesses (e.g., chickenpox, C.N.S. infections, measles, gastroenteritis) or dehydration seem to be much more susceptible to neuromuscular reactions, particularly dystonias, than are adults. In such patients, the drug should be used only under close supervision.

Drugs which lower the seizure threshold, including phenothiazine derivatives, should not be used with Amipaque®§. As with other phenothiazine derivatives, Compazine (prochlorperazine) should be discontinued at least 48 hours before myelography, should not be resumed for at least 24 hours postprocedure, and should not be used for the control of nausea and vomiting occurring either prior to myelography with *Amipaque*, or postprocedure.

ADVERSE REACTIONS

Drowsiness, dizziness, amenorrhea, blurred vision, skin reactions and hypotension may occur.

Cholestatic jaundice has occurred. If fever with grippe-like symptoms occurs, appropriate liver studies should be conducted. If tests indicate an abnormality, stop treatment. There have been a few observations of fatty changes in the livers of patients who have died while receiving the drug. No causal relationship has been established.

Leukopenia and agranulocytosis have occurred. Warn patients to report the sudden appearance of sore throat or other signs of infection. If white blood cell and differential counts indicate leukocyte depression, stop treatment and start antibiotic and other suitable therapy.

Neuromuscular (Extrapyramidal) Reactions

These symptoms are seen in a significant number of hospitalized mental patients. They may be characterized by motor restlessness, be of the dystonic type, or they may resemble parkinsonism.

Depending on the severity of symptoms, dosage should be

reduced or discontinued. If therapy is reinstituted, it should be at a lower dosage. Should these symptoms occur in children or pregnant patients, the drug should be stopped and not reinstituted. In most cases barbiturates by suitable route of administration will suffice. (Or, injectable Benadryl®‖ may be useful.) In more severe cases, the administration of an anti-parkinsonism agent, except levodopa, usually produces rapid reversal of symptoms. Suitable supportive measures such as maintaining a clear airway and adequate hydration should be employed.

Motor Restlessness: Symptoms may include agitation or jitteriness and sometimes insomnia. These symptoms often disappear spontaneously. At times these symptoms may be similar to the original neurotic or psychotic symptoms. Dosage should not be increased until these side effects have subsided.

If these symptoms become too troublesome, they can usually be controlled by a reduction of dosage or change of drug. Treatment with anti-parkinsonian agents, benzodiazepines or propranolol may be helpful.

Dystonias: Symptoms may include: spasm of the neck muscles, sometimes progressing to torticollis; extensor rigidity of back muscles, sometimes progressing to opisthotonos; carpopedal spasm, trismus, swallowing difficulty, oculogyric crisis and protrusion of the tongue.

These usually subside within a few hours, and almost always within 24 to 48 hours, after the drug has been discontinued. *In mild cases,* reassurance or a barbiturate is often sufficient. *In moderate cases,* barbiturates will usually bring rapid relief. *In more severe adult cases,* the administration of an anti-parkinsonism agent, except levodopa, usually produces rapid reversal of symptoms. *In children,* reassurance and barbiturates will usually control symptoms. (Or, injectable *Benadryl* may be useful. Note: See *Benadryl* prescribing information for appropriate *children's* dosage.) If appropriate treatment with anti-parkinsonism agents or *Benadryl* fails to reverse the signs and symptoms, the diagnosis should be reevaluated.

Pseudo-parkinsonism: Symptoms may include: mask-like facies; drooling; tremors; pillrolling motion; cogwheel rigidity; and shuffling gait. Reassurance and sedation are important. In most cases these symptoms are readily controlled when an anti-parkinsonism agent is administered concomitantly. Anti-parkinsonism agents should be used only when required. Generally, therapy of a few weeks to two or three months will suffice. After this time patients should be evaluated to determine their need for continued treatment. (Note: Levodopa has not been found effective in pseudo-parkinsonism.) Occasionally it is necessary to lower the dosage of Compazine (prochlorperazine) or to discontinue the drug.

Tardive Dyskinesia: As with all antipsychotic agents, tardive dyskinesia may appear in some patients on long-term therapy or may appear after drug therapy has been discontinued. The syndrome can also develop, although much less frequently, after relatively brief treatment periods at low doses. This syndrome appears in all age groups. Although its prevalence appears to be highest among elderly patients, especially elderly women, it is impossible to rely upon prevalence estimates to predict at the inception of neuroleptic treatment which patients are likely to develop the syndrome. The symptoms are persistent and in some patients appear to be irreversible. The syndrome is characterized by rhythmical involuntary movements of the tongue, face, mouth or jaw (e.g., protrusion of tongue, puffing of cheeks, puckering of mouth, chewing movements). Sometimes these may be accompanied by involuntary movements of extremities. In rare instances, these involuntary movements of the extremities are the only manifestations of tardive dyskinesia. A variant of tardive dyskinesia, tardive dystonia, has also been described.

There is no known effective treatment for tardive dyskinesia; anti-parkinsonism agents do not alleviate the symptoms of this syndrome. It is suggested that all antipsychotic agents be discontinued if these symptoms appear.

Should it be necessary to reinstitute treatment, or increase the dosage of the agent, or switch to a different antipsychotic agent, the syndrome may be masked.

It has been reported that fine vermicular movements of the tongue may be an early sign of the syndrome and if the medication is stopped at that time the syndrome may not develop.

Contact Dermatitis: Avoid getting the Injection solution on hands or clothing because of the possibility of contact dermatitis.

Adverse Reactions Reported with Compazine (prochlorperazine) or Other Phenothiazine Derivatives: Adverse reactions with different phenothiazines vary in type, frequency, and mechanism of occurrence, i.e., some are dose-related, while others involve individual patient sensitivity. Some adverse reactions may be more likely to occur, or occur with greater intensity, in patients with special medical problems, e.g., patients with mitral insufficiency or pheochromocytoma have experienced severe hypotension following recommended doses of certain phenothiazines.

Not all of the following adverse reactions have been observed

---

* norepinephrine bitartrate, Winthrop Pharmaceuticals.

† phenylephrine hydrochloride, Winthrop Pharmaceuticals.

‡ phenytoin, Parke-Davis.

§ metrizamide, Winthrop Pharmaceuticals.

‖ diphenhydramine hydrochloride, Parke-Davis.

with every phenothiazine derivative, but they have been reported with one or more and should be borne in mind when drugs of this class are administered: extrapyramidal symptoms (opisthotonos, oculogyric crisis, hyperreflexia, dystonia, akathisia, dyskinesia, parkinsonism) some of which have lasted months and even years—particularly in elderly patients with previous brain damage; grand mal and petit mal convulsions, particularly in patients with EEG abnormalities or history of such disorders; altered cerebrospinal fluid proteins; cerebral edema; intensification and prolongation of the action of central nervous system depressants (opiates, analgesics, antihistamines, barbiturates, alcohol), atropine, heat, organophosphorus insecticides; autonomic reactions (dryness of mouth, nasal congestion, headache, nausea, constipation, obstipation, adynamic ileus, ejaculatory disorders/impotence, priapism, atonic colon, urinary retention, miosis and mydriasis); reactivation of psychotic processes, catatonic-like states; hypotension (sometimes fatal); cardiac arrest; blood dyscrasias (pancytopenia, thrombocytopenic purpura, leukopenia, agranulocytosis, eosinophilia, hemolytic anemia, aplastic anemia); liver damage (jaundice, biliary stasis); endocrine disturbances (hyperglycemia, hypoglycemia, glycosuria, lactation, galactorrhea, gynecomastia, menstrual irregularities, false positive pregnancy tests); skin disorders (photosensitivity, itching, erythema, urticaria, eczema up to exfoliative dermatitis); other allergic reactions (asthma, laryngeal edema, angioneurotic edema, anaphylactoid reactions); peripheral edema; reversed epinephrine effect; hyperpyrexia; mild fever after large I.M. doses; increased appetite; increased weight; a systemic lupus erythematosus-like syndrome; pigmentary retinopathy; with prolonged administration of substantial doses, skin pigmentation, epithelial keratopathy, and lenticular and corneal deposits.

EKG changes—particularly nonspecific, usually reversible Q and T wave distortions—have been observed in some patients receiving phenothiazine tranquilizers.

Although phenothiazines cause neither psychic nor physical dependence, sudden discontinuance in long-term psychiatric patients may cause temporary symptoms, e.g., nausea and vomiting, dizziness, tremulousness.

Note: There have been occasional reports of sudden death in patients receiving phenothiazines. In some cases, the cause appeared to be cardiac arrest or asphyxia due to failure of the cough reflex.

DOSAGE AND ADMINISTRATION

Notes on Injection: *Stability*—This solution should be protected from light which may cause discoloration. Discard injectable if discolored.

Compatibility—It is recommended that Compazine (prochlorperazine) Injection not be mixed with other agents in the syringe. Do not dilute the contents of *Compazine* ampuls with any diluent that contains parabens as a preservative.

DOSAGE AND ADMINISTRATION—ADULTS

(For children's dosage and administration, see below.) Dosage should be increased more gradually in debilitated or emaciated patients.

Elderly Patients: In general, dosages in the lower range are sufficient for most elderly patients. Since they appear to be more susceptible to hypotension and neuromuscular reactions, such patients should be observed closely. Dosage should be tailored to the individual, response carefully monitored, and dosage adjusted accordingly. Dosage should be increased more gradually in elderly patients.

1. To Control Severe Nausea and Vomiting: Adjust dosage to the response of the individual. Begin with the lowest recommended dosage.

Oral Dosage—Tablets: Usually one 5 mg or 10 mg tablet 3 or 4 times daily. Daily dosages above 40 mg should be used only in resistant cases.

***Spansule* capsules:** Initially, usually one 15 mg capsule on arising or one 10 mg capsule q12h. Some patients may subsequently require one 30 mg capsule in the morning. Daily doses above 40 mg should be used only in resistant cases.

Rectal Dosage: 25 mg twice daily.

I.M. Dosage: Initially 5 to 10 mg (1–2 mL) injected *deeply* into the upper outer quadrant of the buttock. If necessary, repeat every 3 or 4 hours. Total I.M. dosage should not exceed 40 mg per day.

I.V. Dosage: 2½ to 10 mg (½ to 2 mL) by slow I.V. injection or infusion at a rate not to exceed 5 mg per minute. *Compazine* Injection may be administered either undiluted or diluted in isotonic solution. A single dose of the drug should not exceed 10 mg; total I.V. dosage should not exceed 40 mg per day. When administered I.V., do not use bolus injection. Hypotension is a possibility if the drug is given by I.V. injection or infusion.

Subcutaneous administration is not advisable because of local irritation.

2. Adult Surgery (for severe nausea and vomiting): Total parenteral dosage should not exceed 40 mg per day. Hypotension is a possibility if the drug is given by I.V. injection or infusion.

I.M. Dosage: 5 to 10 mg (1–2 mL) 1 to 2 hours before induction of anesthesia (repeat once in 30 minutes, if necessary), or to control acute symptoms during and after surgery (repeat once if necessary).

I.V. Dosage: 5 to 10 mg (1–2 mL) as a slow I.V. injection or infusion 15 to 30 minutes before induction of anesthesia, or to control acute symptoms during or after surgery. Repeat once if necessary. Compazine (prochlorperazine) may be administered either undiluted or diluted in isotonic solution, but a single dose of the drug should not exceed 10 mg. The rate of administration should not exceed 5 mg per minute. When administered I.V., do not use bolus injection.

3. In Adult Psychiatric Disorders: Adjust dosage to the response of the individual and according to the severity of the condition. Begin with the lowest recommended dose. Although response ordinarily is seen within a day or two, longer treatment is usually required before maximal improvement is seen.

Oral Dosage: *Non-Psychotic Anxiety*—Usual dosage is 5 mg 3 or 4 times daily; by *Spansule* capsule, usually one 15 mg capsule on arising or one 10 mg capsule q12h. Do not administer in doses of more than 20 mg per day or for longer than 12 weeks.

Psychotic Disorders—In relatively mild conditions, as seen in private psychiatric practice or in outpatient clinics, dosage is 5 or 10 mg 3 or 4 times daily.

In moderate to severe conditions, for hospitalized or adequately supervised patients, usual starting dosage is 10 mg 3 or 4 times daily. Increase dosage gradually until symptoms are controlled or side effects become bothersome. When dosage is increased by small increments every 2 or 3 days, side effects either do not occur or are easily controlled. Some patients respond satisfactorily on 50 to 75 mg daily.

In more severe disturbances, optimum dosage is usually 100 to 150 mg daily.

I.M. Dosage: For immediate control of severely disturbed adults, inject an initial dose of 10 to 20 mg (2–4 mL) *deeply* into the upper outer quadrant of the buttock. Many patients respond shortly after the first injection. If necessary, however, repeat the initial dose every 2 to 4 hours (or, in resistant cases, every hour) to gain control of the patient. More than 3 or 4 doses are seldom necessary. After control is achieved, switch patient to an oral form of the drug at the same dosage level or higher. If, in rare cases, parenteral therapy is needed for a prolonged period, give 10 to 20 mg (2–4 mL) every 4 to 6 hours. Pain and irritation at the site of injection have seldom occurred.

Subcutaneous administration is not advisable because of local irritation.

DOSAGE AND ADMINISTRATION—CHILDREN

Do not use in pediatric surgery.

Children seem more prone to develop extrapyramidal reactions, even on moderate doses. Therefore, use lowest effective dosage. Tell parents not to exceed prescribed dosage, since the possibility of adverse reactions increases as dosage rises. Occasionally the patient may react to the drug with signs of restlessness and excitement; if this occurs, do not administer additional doses. Take particular precaution in administering the drug to children with acute illnesses or dehydration (see under Dystonias).

When writing a prescription for the 2½ mg size suppository, write "2½," not "2.5"; this will help avoid confusion with the 25 mg adult size.

1. Severe Nausea and Vomiting in Children: Compazine (prochlorperazine) should not be used in children under 20 pounds in weight or two years of age. It should not be used in conditions for which children's dosages have not been established. Dosage and frequency of administration should be adjusted according to the severity of the symptoms and the response of the patient. The duration of activity following intramuscular administration may last up to 12 hours. Subsequent doses may be given by the same route if necessary.

Oral or Rectal Dosage: More than one day's therapy is seldom necessary.

Weight	Usual Dosage	Not to Exceed
under 20 lbs	not recommended	
20-29 lbs	2½ mg 1 or 2 times a day	7.5 mg per day
30-39 lbs	2½ mg 2 or 3 times a day	10 mg per day
40-85 lbs	2½ mg 3 times a day or 5 mg 2 times a day	15 mg per day

I.M. Dosage: Calculate each dose on the basis of 0.06 mg of the drug per lb of body weight; give by deep I.M. injection. Control is usually obtained with one dose.

2. In Psychotic Children:

Oral or Rectal Dosage: For children 2 to 12 years, starting dosage is 2½ mg 2 or 3 times daily. Do not give more than 10 mg the first day. Then increase dosage according to patient's response.

FOR AGES 2–5, total daily dosage usually does not exceed 20 mg.

FOR AGES 6–12, total daily dosage usually does not exceed 25 mg.

I.M. Dosage: For ages under 12, calculate each dose on the basis of 0.06 mg of Compazine (prochlorperazine) per lb of body weight; give by deep I.M. injection. Control is usually obtained with one dose. After control is achieved, switch the patient to an oral form of the drug at the same dosage level or higher.

OVERDOSAGE

(See also Adverse Reactions.)

SYMPTOMS—Primarily involvement of the extrapyramidal mechanism producing some of the dystonic reactions described above.

Symptoms of central nervous system depression to the point of somnolence or coma. Agitation and restlessness may also occur. Other possible manifestations include convulsions, EKG changes and cardiac arrhythmias, fever, and autonomic reactions such as hypotension, dry mouth and ileus.

TREATMENT—It is important to determine other medications taken by the patient since multiple dose therapy is common in overdosage situations. Treatment is essentially symptomatic and supportive. Early gastric lavage is helpful. Keep patient under observation and maintain an open airway, since involvement of the extrapyramidal mechanism may produce dysphagia and respiratory difficulty in severe overdosage. **Do not attempt to induce emesis because a dystonic reaction of the head or neck may develop that could result in aspiration of vomitus.** Extrapyramidal symptoms may be treated with anti-parkinsonism drugs, barbiturates, or *Benadryl*. See prescribing information for these products. Care should be taken to avoid increasing respiratory depression.

If administration of a stimulant is desirable, amphetamine, dextroamphetamine, or caffeine with sodium benzoate is recommended.

Stimulants that may cause convulsions (e.g., picrotoxin or pentylenetetrazol) should be avoided.

If hypotension occurs, the standard measures for managing circulatory shock should be initiated. If it is desirable to administer a vasoconstrictor, *Levophed* and *Neo-Synephrine* are most suitable. Other pressor agents, including epinephrine, are not recommended because phenothiazine derivatives may reverse the usual elevating action of these agents and cause a further lowering of blood pressure.

Limited experience indicates that phenothiazines are *not* dialyzable.

Special note on Spansule *capsules*—Since much of the *Spansule* capsule medication is coated for gradual release, therapy directed at reversing the effects of the ingested drug and at supporting the patient should be continued for as long as overdosage symptoms remain. Saline cathartics are useful for hastening evacuation of pellets that have not already released medication.

HOW SUPPLIED

Tablets—5 and 10 mg, in bottles of 100; in Single Unit Packages of 100 (intended for institutional use only). For use in severe neuropsychiatric conditions, 25 mg, in bottles of 100.

***Spansule* capsules**—10 mg in bottles of 50; 15 mg in bottles of 50 and 500; 30 mg in bottles of 50; 10 and 15 mg in Single Unit Packages of 100 (intended for institutional use only).

Ampuls—2 mL (5 mg/mL), in boxes of 10 and 100.

Vials—2 mL (5 mg/mL), in boxes of 25 and 100 and 10 mL (5 mg/mL), in boxes of 1, 20 and 100.

Disposable Syringes—2 mL (5 mg/mL), in individual cartons.

Suppositories—2½ mg (for young children), 5 mg (for older children) and 25 mg (for adults), in boxes of 12.

Syrup—5 mg/5 mL (1 teaspoonful) in 4 fl oz bottles.

Veterans Administration—Suppositories, 25 mg, 12's, 6505-00-133-5214.

Military—Suppositories, 2.5 mg, 12's, 6505-00-133-5213; 5 mg, 12's, 6505-01-153-2894; 25 mg, 12's, 6505-00-133-5214.

CZ:L78

Shown in Product Identification Section, page 430

CYTOMEL® ℞

[*sigh "toe 'mel*]

(brand of liothyronine sodium)

Tablets

DESCRIPTION

Thyroid hormone drugs are natural or synthetic preparations containing tetraiodothyronine (T_4, levothyroxine) sodium or triiodothyronine (T_3, liothyronine) sodium or both. T_4 and T_3 are produced in the human thyroid gland by the iodination and coupling of the amino acid tyrosine. T_4 contains four iodine atoms and is formed by the coupling of two molecules of diiodotyrosine (DIT). T_3 contains three atoms of iodine and is formed by the coupling of one molecule of DIT

Continued on next page

SmithKline Beecham—Cont.

with one molecule of monoiodotyrosine (MIT). Both hormones are stored in the thyroid colloid as thyroglobulin. Thyroid hormone preparations belong to two categories: (1) natural hormonal preparations derived from animal thyroid, and (2) synthetic preparations. Natural preparations include desiccated thyroid and thyroglobulin. Desiccated thyroid is derived from domesticated animals that are used for food by man (either beef or hog thyroid), and thyroglobulin is derived from thyroid glands of the hog. The United States Pharmacopeia (USP) has standardized the total iodine content of natural preparations. Thyroid USP contains not less than (NLT) 0.17 percent and not more than (NMT) 0.23 percent iodine, and thyroglobulin contains not less than (NLT) 0.7 percent of organically bound iodine. Iodine content is only an indirect indicator of true hormonal biologic activity.

Cytomel (liothyronine sodium) Tablets contain liothyronine (L-triiodothyronine or LT_3), a synthetic form of a natural thyroid hormone, and is available as the sodium salt.

Twenty-five mcg of liothyronine is equivalent to approximately 1 grain of desiccated thyroid or thyroglobulin and 0.1 mg of L-thyroxine.

Each round, white to off-white Cytomel (liothyronine sodium) tablet contains liothyronine sodium equivalent to liothyronine as follows: 5 mcg debossed SKF and D14; 25 mcg scored and debossed SKF and D16; 50 mcg scored and debossed SKF and D17. Inactive ingredients consist of calcium sulfate, gelatin, starch, stearic acid, sucrose and talc.

CLINICAL PHARMACOLOGY

The mechanisms by which thyroid hormones exert their physiologic action are not well understood. These hormones enhance oxygen consumption by most tissues of the body, increase the basal metabolic rate and the metabolism of carbohydrates, lipids and proteins. Thus, they exert a profound influence on every organ system in the body and are of particular importance in the development of the central nervous system.

Pharmacokinetics

Since liothyronine sodium (T_3) is not firmly bound to serum protein, it is readily available to body tissues. The onset of activity of liothyronine sodium is rapid, occurring within a few hours. Maximum pharmacologic response occurs within two or three days, providing early clinical response. The biological half-life is about $2\frac{1}{2}$ days.

T_3 is almost totally absorbed, 95 percent in four hours. The hormones contained in the natural preparations are absorbed in a manner similar to the synthetic hormones.

Liothyronine sodium has a rapid cutoff of activity which permits quick dosage adjustment and facilitates control of the effects of overdosage, should they occur.

The higher affinity of levothyroxine (T_4) for both thyroid-binding globulin and thyroid-binding prealbumin as compared to triiodothyronine (T_3) partially explains the higher serum levels and longer half-life of the former hormone. Both protein-bound hormones exist in reverse equilibrium with minute amounts of free hormone, the latter accounting for the metabolic activity.

INDICATIONS AND USAGE

Thyroid hormone drugs are indicated:

1. As replacement or supplemental therapy in patients with hypothyroidism of any etiology, except transient hypothyroidism during the recovery phase of subacute thyroiditis. This category includes cretinism, myxedema and ordinary hypothyroidism in patients of any age (children, adults, the elderly), or state (including pregnancy); primary hypothyroidism resulting from functional deficiency, primary atrophy, partial or total absence of thyroid gland, or the effects of surgery, radiation, or drugs, with or without the presence of goiter; and secondary (pituitary) or tertiary (hypothalamic) hypothyroidism (See WARNINGS).
2. As pituitary thyroid-stimulating hormone (TSH) suppressants, in the treatment or prevention of various types of euthyroid goiters, including thyroid nodules, subacute or chronic lymphocytic thyroiditis (Hashimoto's) and multinodular goiter.
3. As diagnostic agents in suppression tests to differentiate suspected mild hyperthyroidism or thyroid gland autonomy.

Cytomel (liothyronine sodium) Tablets can be used in patients allergic to desiccated thyroid or thyroid extract derived from pork or beef.

CONTRAINDICATIONS

Thyroid hormone preparations are generally contraindicated in patients with diagnosed but as yet uncorrected adrenal cortical insufficiency, untreated thyrotoxicosis and apparent hypersensitivity to any of their active or extraneous constituents. There is no well-documented evidence from the literature, however, of true allergic or idiosyncratic reactions to thyroid hormone.

WARNINGS

> Drugs with thyroid hormone activity, alone or together with other therapeutic agents, have been used for the treatment of obesity. In euthyroid patients, doses within the range of daily hormonal requirements are ineffective for weight reduction. Larger doses may produce serious or even life-threatening manifestations of toxicity, particularly when given in association with sympathomimetic amines such as those used for their anorectic effects.

The use of thyroid hormones in the therapy of obesity, alone or combined with other drugs, is unjustified and has been shown to be ineffective. Neither is their use justified for the treatment of male or female infertility unless this condition is accompanied by hypothyroidism.

Thyroid hormones should be used with great caution in a number of circumstances where the integrity of the cardiovascular system, particularly the coronary arteries, is suspected. These include patients with angina pectoris or the elderly, in whom there is a greater likelihood of occult cardiac disease. In these patients, liothyronine sodium therapy should be initiated with low doses, with due consideration for its relatively rapid onset of action. Starting dosage of Cytomel (liothyronine sodium) Tablets is 5 mcg daily, and should be increased by no more than 5 mcg increments at two-week intervals. When, in such patients, a euthyroid state can only be reached at the expense of an aggravation of the cardiovascular disease, thyroid hormone dosage should be reduced.

Morphologic hypogonadism and nephrosis should be ruled out before the drug is administered. If hypopituitarism is present, the adrenal deficiency must be corrected prior to starting the drug.

Myxedematous patients are very sensitive to thyroid; dosage should be started at a very low level and increased gradually. Severe and prolonged hypothyroidism can lead to a decreased level of adrenocortical activity commensurate with the lowered metabolic state. When thyroid-replacement therapy is administered, the metabolism increases at a greater rate than adrenocortical activity. This can precipitate adrenocortical insufficiency. Therefore, in severe and prolonged hypothyroidism, supplemental adrenocortical steroids may be necessary.

In rare instances the administration of thyroid hormone may precipitate a hyperthyroid state or may aggravate existing hyperthyroidism.

PRECAUTIONS

General—Thyroid hormone therapy in patients with concomitant diabetes mellitus or insipidus or adrenal cortical insufficiency aggravates the intensity of their symptoms. Appropriate adjustments of the various therapeutic measures directed at these concomitant endocrine diseases are required.

The therapy of myxedema coma requires simultaneous administration of glucocorticoids.

Hypothyroidism decreases and hyperthyroidism increases the sensitivity to oral anticoagulants. Prothrombin time should be closely monitored in thyroid-treated patients on oral anticoagulants and dosage of the latter agents adjusted on the basis of frequent prothrombin time determinations. In infants, excessive doses of thyroid hormone preparations may produce craniosynostosis.

Information for the Patient—Patients on thyroid hormone preparations and parents of children on thyroid therapy should be informed that:

1. Replacement therapy is to be taken essentially for life, with the exception of cases of transient hypothyroidism, usually associated with thyroiditis, and in those patients receiving a therapeutic trial of the drug.
2. They should immediately report during the course of therapy any signs or symptoms of thyroid hormone toxicity, e.g., chest pain, increased pulse rate, palpitations, excessive sweating, heat intolerance, nervousness, or any other unusual event.
3. In case of concomitant diabetes mellitus, the daily dosage of antidiabetic medication may need readjustment as thyroid hormone replacement is achieved. If thyroid medication is stopped, a downward readjustment of the dosage of insulin or oral hypoglycemic agent may be necessary to avoid hypoglycemia. At all times, close monitoring of urinary glucose levels is mandatory in such patients.
4. In case of concomitant oral anticoagulant therapy, the prothrombin time should be measured frequently to determine if the dosage of oral anticoagulants is to be readjusted.
5. Partial loss of hair may be experienced by children in the first few months of thyroid therapy, but this is usually a transient phenomenon and later recovery is usually the rule.

Laboratory Tests—Treatment of patients with thyroid hormones requires the periodic assessment of thyroid status by means of appropriate laboratory tests besides the full clinical evaluation. The TSH suppression test can be used to test

the effectiveness of any thyroid preparation, bearing in mind the relative insensitivity of the infant pituitary to the negative feedback effect of thyroid hormones. Serum T_4 levels can be used to test the effectiveness of all thyroid medications except products containing liothyronine sodium. When the total serum T_4 is low but TSH is normal, a test specific to assess unbound (free) T_4 levels is warranted. Specific measurements of T_4 and T_3 by competitive protein binding or radioimmunoassay are not influenced by blood levels of organic or inorganic iodine and have essentially replaced older tests of thyroid hormone measurements, i.e., PBI, BEI and T_4 by column.

Drug Interactions

Oral Anticoagulants—Thyroid hormones appear to increase catabolism of vitamin K-dependent clotting factors. If oral anticoagulants are also being given, compensatory increases in clotting factor synthesis are impaired. Patients stabilized on oral anticoagulants who are found to require thyroid replacement therapy should be watched very closely when thyroid is started. If a patient is truly hypothyroid, it is likely that a reduction in anticoagulant dosage will be required. No special precautions appear to be necessary when oral anticoagulant therapy is begun in a patient already stabilized on maintenance thyroid replacement therapy.

Insulin or Oral Hypoglycemics—Initiating thyroid replacement therapy may cause increases in insulin or oral hypoglycemic requirements. The effects seen are poorly understood and depend upon a variety of factors such as dose and type of thyroid preparations and endocrine status of the patient. Patients receiving insulin or oral hypoglycemics should be closely watched during initiation of thyroid replacement therapy.

Cholestyramine—Cholestyramine binds both T_4 and T_3 in the intestine, thus impairing absorption of these thyroid hormones. *In vitro* studies indicate that the binding is not easily removed. Therefore, four to five hours should elapse between administration of cholestyramine and thyroid hormones.

Estrogen, Oral Contraceptives—Estrogens tend to increase serum thyroxine-binding globulin (TBg). In a patient with a nonfunctioning thyroid gland who is receiving thyroid replacement therapy, free levothyroxine may be decreased when estrogens are started thus increasing thyroid requirements. However, if the patient's thyroid gland has sufficient function, the decreased free thyroxine will result in a compensatory increase in thyroxine output by the thyroid. Therefore, patients without a functioning thyroid gland who are on thyroid replacement therapy may need to increase their thyroid dose if estrogens or estrogen-containing oral contraceptives are given.

Tricyclic Antidepressants—Use of thyroid products with imipramine and other tricyclic antidepressants may increase receptor sensitivity and enhance antidepressant activity; transient cardiac arrhythmias have been observed. Thyroid hormone activity may also be enhanced.

Digitalis—Thyroid preparations may potentiate the toxic effects of digitalis. Thyroid hormonal replacement increases metabolic rate, which requires an increase in digitalis dosage.

Ketamine—When administered to patients on a thyroid preparation, this parenteral anesthetic may cause hypertension and tachycardia. Use with caution and be prepared to treat hypertension, if necessary.

Levarterenol—Thyroxine increases the adrenergic effect of catecholamines such as epinephrine and norepinephrine. Therefore, injection of these agents into patients receiving thyroid preparations increases the risk of precipitating coronary insufficiency, especially in patients with coronary artery disease. Careful observation is required.

Drug/Laboratory Test Interactions—The following drugs or moieties are known to interfere with laboratory tests performed in patients on thyroid hormone therapy: androgens, corticosteroids, estrogens, oral contraceptives containing estrogens, iodine-containing preparations and the numerous preparations containing salicylates.

1. Changes in TBg concentration should be taken into consideration in the interpretation of T_4 and T_3 values. In such cases, the unbound (free) hormone should be measured. Pregnancy, estrogens and estrogen-containing oral contraceptives increase TBg concentrations. TBg may also be increased during infectious hepatitis. Decreases in TBg concentrations are observed in nephrosis, acromegaly and after androgen or corticosteroid therapy. Familial hyper- or hypo-thyroxine-binding-globulinemias have been described. The incidence of TBg deficiency approximates 1 in 9000. The binding of thyroxine by thyroxine-binding prealbumin (TBPA) is inhibited by salicylates.
2. Medicinal or dietary iodine interferes with all *in vivo* tests of radioiodine uptake, producing low uptakes which may not be reflective of a true decrease in hormone synthesis.
3. The persistence of clinical and laboratory evidence of hypothyroidism in spite of adequate dosage replacement indicates either poor patient compliance, poor absorption, excessive fecal loss, or inactivity of the preparation. Intracellular resistance to thyroid hormone is quite rare.

Carcinogenesis, Mutagenesis and Impairment of Fertility—A reportedly apparent association between prolonged thyroid therapy and breast cancer has not been confirmed and patients on thyroid for established indications should not discontinue therapy. No confirmatory long-term studies in animals have been performed to evaluate carcinogenic potential, mutagenicity, or impairment of fertility in either males or females.

Pregnancy—Category A. Thyroid hormones do not readily cross the placental barrier. The clinical experience to date does not indicate any adverse effect on fetuses when thyroid hormones are administered to pregnant women. On the basis of current knowledge, thyroid replacement therapy to hypothyroid women should not be discontinued during pregnancy.

Nursing Mothers—Minimal amounts of thyroid hormones are excreted in human milk. Thyroid is not associated with serious adverse reactions and does not have a known tumorigenic potential. However, caution should be exercised when thyroid is administered to a nursing woman.

Pediatric Use—Pregnant mothers provide little or no thyroid hormone to the fetus. The incidence of congenital hypothyroidism is relatively high (1:4000) and the hypothyroid fetus would not derive any benefit from the small amounts of hormone crossing the placental barrier. Routine determinations of serum T_4 and/or TSH is strongly advised in neonates in view of the deleterious effects of thyroid deficiency on growth and development.

Treatment should be initiated immediately upon diagnosis and maintained for life, unless transient hypothyroidism is suspected, in which case, therapy may be interrupted for two to eight weeks after the age of three years to reassess the condition. Cessation of therapy is justified in patients who have maintained a normal TSH during those two to eight weeks.

ADVERSE REACTIONS

Adverse reactions, other than those indicative of hyperthyroidism because of therapeutic overdosage, either initially or during the maintenance period are rare (See OVERDOSAGE).

In rare instances, allergic skin reactions have been reported with Cytomel (liothyronine sodium) Tablets.

OVERDOSAGE

Signs and Symptoms—Headache, irritability, nervousness, sweating, tachycardia, increased bowel motility and menstrual irregularities. Angina pectoris or congestive heart failure may be induced or aggravated. Shock may also develop. Massive overdosage may result in symptoms resembling thyroid storm. Chronic excessive dosage will produce the signs and symptoms of hyperthyroidism.

Treatment of Overdosage—Dosage should be reduced or therapy temporarily discontinued if signs and symptoms of overdosage appear. Treatment may be reinstituted at a lower dosage. In normal individuals, normal hypothalamic-pituitary-thyroid axis function is restored in six to eight weeks after thyroid suppression.

Treatment of acute massive thyroid hormone overdosage is aimed at reducing gastrointestinal absorption of the drugs and counteracting central and peripheral effects, mainly those of increased sympathetic activity. Vomiting may be induced initially if further gastrointestinal absorption can reasonably be prevented and barring contraindications such as coma, convulsions, or loss of the gagging reflex. Treatment is symptomatic and supportive. Oxygen may be administered and ventilation maintained. Cardiac glycosides may be indicated if congestive heart failure develops. Measures to control fever, hypoglycemia, or fluid loss should be instituted if needed. Antiadrenergic agents, particularly propranolol, have been used advantageously in the treatment of increased sympathetic activity. Propranolol may be administered intravenously at a dosage of 1 to 3 mg over a 10-minute period or orally, 80 to 160 mg/day, especially when no contraindications exist for its use.

DOSAGE AND ADMINISTRATION

The dosage of thyroid hormones is determined by the indication and must in every case be individualized according to patient response and laboratory findings.

Thyroid hormones are given orally. In acute, emergency conditions, injectable levothyroxine sodium may be given intravenously when oral administration is not feasible or desirable, as in the treatment of myxedema coma or during total parenteral nutrition. Injectable liothyronine sodium is also available from SmithKline Beecham Pharmaceuticals upon request, under investigational status, for the treatment of myxedema coma. Intramuscular administration of these two preparations is not advisable because of reported poor absorption.

With Cytomel (liothyronine sodium) Tablets once-a-day dosage is recommended; although liothyronine sodium has a rapid cutoff, its metabolic effects persist for a few days following discontinuance.

Mild Hypothyroidism: Recommended starting dosage is 25 mcg daily. Daily dosage then may be increased by 12.5 or 25 mcg every one or two weeks. Usual maintenance dose is 25-75 mcg daily. Smaller doses may be fully effective in some patients, while dosage of 100 mcg daily may be required in others.

The rapid onset and dissipation of action of liothyronine sodium (T_3), as compared with levothyroxine sodium (T_4), has led some clinicians to prefer its use in patients who might be more susceptible to the untoward effects of thyroid medication. However, the wide swings in serum T_3 levels that follow its administration and the possibility of more pronounced cardiovascular side effects tend to counterbalance the stated advantages.

Cytomel (liothyronine sodium) Tablets may be used in preference to levothyroxine (T_4) during radioisotope scanning procedures, since induction of hypothyroidism in those cases is more abrupt and can be of shorter duration. It may also be preferred when impairment of peripheral conversion of T_4 and T_3 is suspected.

Myxedema: Recommended starting dosage is 5 mcg daily. This may be increased by 5 to 10 mcg daily every one or two weeks. When 25 mcg daily is reached, dosage may often be increased by 12.5 or 25 mcg every one or two weeks. Usual maintenance dose is 50 to 100 mcg daily.

Myxedema Coma: Myxedema coma is usually precipitated in the hypothyroid patient of long standing by intercurrent illness or drugs such as sedatives and anesthetics and should be considered a medical emergency. A *Cytomel* Injection Kit for the emergency treatment of myxedema coma is available from SmithKline Beecham Pharmaceuticals upon request, under investigational status. Instructions which accompany this kit provide information on administration.

Congenital Hypothyroidism: Recommended starting dosage is 5 mcg daily, with a 5 mcg increment every three to four days until the desired response is achieved. Infants a few months old may require only 20 mcg daily for maintenance. At one year, 50 mcg daily may be required. Above three years, full adult dosage may be necessary (See PRECAUTIONS, Pediatric Use).

Simple (non-toxic) Goiter: Recommended starting dosage is 5 mcg daily. This dosage may be increased by 5 to 10 mcg daily every one or two weeks. When 25 mcg daily is reached, dosage may be increased every week or two by 12.5 or 25 mcg. Usual maintenance dosage is 75 mcg daily.

In the elderly or in children, therapy should be started with 5 mcg daily and increased only by 5 mcg increments at the recommended intervals.

When switching a patient to Cytomel (liothyronine sodium) Tablets from thyroid, L-thyroxine or thyroglobulin, discontinue the other medication, initiate *Cytomel* at a low dosage, and increase gradually according to the patient's response. When selecting a starting dosage, bear in mind that this drug has a rapid onset of action, and that residual effects of the other thyroid preparation may persist for the first several weeks of therapy.

Thyroid Suppression Therapy: Administration of thyroid hormone in doses higher than those produced physiologically by the gland results in suppression of the production of endogenous hormone. This is the basis for the thyroid suppression test and is used as an aid in the diagnosis of patients with signs of mild hyperthyroidism in whom baseline laboratory tests appear normal or to demonstrate thyroid gland autonomy in patients with Graves' ophthalmopathy. ^{131}I uptake is determined before and after the administration of the exogenous hormone. A 50 percent or greater suppression of uptake indicates a normal thyroid-pituitary axis and thus rules out thyroid gland autonomy.

Cytomel (liothyronine sodium) Tablets are given in doses of 75-100 mcg/day for seven days, and radioactive iodine uptake is determined before and after administration of the hormone. If thyroid function is under normal control, the radioiodine uptake will drop significantly after treatment. Cytomel (liothyronine sodium) Tablets should be administered cautiously to patients in whom there is a strong suspicion of thyroid gland autonomy, in view of the fact that the exogenous hormone effects will be additive to the endogenous source.

HOW SUPPLIED

Cytomel (liothyronine sodium) tablets: 5 mcg in bottles of 100; 25 mcg in bottles of 100; and 50 mcg in bottles of 100.

Military—Tablets, 5 mcg, 100's, 6505-00-660-1609.

Manufactured by
Schering Canada, Inc.
3535 Trans-Canada Highway
Pointe Claire, Quebec H9R 1B4 for
SmithKline Beecham Pharmaceuticals
Philadelphia, PA 19101
CY:L33

Shown in Product Identification Section, page 430

DEXEDRINE®

CII

[*dex 'eh-dreen*]
(brand of dextroamphetamine sulfate)
SPANSULE® CAPSULES
brand of sustained release capsules
and TABLETS

WARNING

AMPHETAMINES HAVE A HIGH POTENTIAL FOR ABUSE. THEY SHOULD THUS BE TRIED ONLY IN WEIGHT REDUCTION PROGRAMS FOR PATIENTS IN WHOM ALTERNATIVE THERAPY HAS BEEN INEFFECTIVE. ADMINISTRATION OF AMPHETAMINES FOR PROLONGED PERIODS OF TIME IN OBESITY MAY LEAD TO DRUG DEPENDENCE AND MUST BE AVOIDED. PARTICULAR ATTENTION SHOULD BE PAID TO THE POSSIBILITY OF SUBJECTS OBTAINING AMPHETAMINES FOR NON-THERAPEUTIC USE OR DISTRIBUTION TO OTHERS, AND THE DRUGS SHOULD BE PRESCRIBED OR DISPENSED SPARINGLY.

DESCRIPTION

Dexedrine (dextroamphetamine sulfate) is the dextro isomer of the compound *d,l*-amphetamine sulfate, a sympathomimetic amine of the amphetamine group. Chemically, dextroamphetamine is *d*-alpha-methylphenethylamine, and is present in all forms of *Dexedrine* as the neutral sulfate.

Spansule® capsules

Each *Spansule* sustained release capsule is so prepared that an initial dose is released promptly and the remaining medication is released gradually over a prolonged period.

Each capsule, with brown cap and natural body, contains dextroamphetamine sulfate as follows: 5 mg imprinted SKF and E12, 10 mg imprinted SKF and E13, 15 mg imprinted SKF and E14. Inactive ingredients consist of acacia, benzyl alcohol, calcium sulfate, cetylpyridinium chloride, FD&C Blue No. 1, FD&C Red No. 40, FD&C Yellow No. 5 (tartrazine), FD&C Yellow No. 6, gelatin, glyceryl distearate, glyceryl monostearate, sodium lauryl sulfate, starch, sucrose, wax and trace amounts of other inactive ingredients.

Tablets

Each triangular, orange, scored tablet is debossed SKF and E19 and contains dextroamphetamine sulfate, 5 mg. Inactive ingredients consist of calcium sulfate, FD&C Yellow No. 5 (tartrazine), FD&C Yellow No. 6, gelatin, lactose, mineral oil, starch, stearic acid, sucrose, talc and trace amounts of other inactive ingredients.

CLINICAL PHARMACOLOGY

Amphetamines are non-catecholamine, sympathomimetic amines with CNS stimulant activity. Peripheral actions include elevations of systolic and diastolic blood pressures and weak bronchodilator and respiratory stimulant action.

There is neither specific evidence which clearly establishes the mechanism whereby amphetamines produce mental and behavioral effects in children, nor conclusive evidence regarding how these effects relate to the condition of the central nervous system.

Drugs of this class used in obesity are commonly known as "anorectics" or "anorexigenics." It has not been established, however, that the action of such drugs in treating obesity is primarily one of appetite suppression. Other central nervous system actions, or metabolic effects, may be involved, for example.

Adult obese subjects instructed in dietary management and treated with "anorectic" drugs lose more weight on the average than those treated with placebo and diet, as determined in relatively short-term clinical trials.

The magnitude of increased weight loss of drug-treated patients over placebo-treated patients is only a fraction of a pound a week. The rate of weight loss is greatest in the first weeks of therapy for both drug and placebo subjects and tends to decrease in succeeding weeks. The origins of the increased weight loss due to the various possible drug effects are not established. The amount of weight loss associated with the use of an "anorectic" drug varies from trial to trial, and the increased weight loss appears to be related in part to variables other than the drug prescribed, such as the physician-investigator, the population treated and the diet prescribed. Studies do not permit conclusions as to the relative importance of the drug and nondrug factors on weight loss.

The natural history of obesity is measured in years, whereas the studies cited are restricted to a few weeks' duration; thus, the total impact of drug-induced weight loss over that of diet alone must be considered clinically limited.

Dexedrine (dextroamphetamine sulfate) *Spansule* capsules are formulated to release the active drug substance *in vivo* in a more gradual fashion than the standard formulation, as demonstrated by blood levels. The formulation has not been shown superior in effectiveness over the same dosage of the

Continued on next page

SmithKline Beecham—Cont.

standard, noncontrolled-release formulations given in divided doses.

Pharmacokinetics
Tablet—The single ingestion of two 5 mg tablets by healthy volunteers produced an average peak dextroamphetamine blood level of 29.2 ng/mL at 2 hours post-administration. The average half-life was 10.25 hours. The average urinary recovery was 45% in 48 hours.

Spansule capsule—Ingestion of a *Spansule* capsule containing 15 mg radiolabeled dextroamphetamine sulfate by healthy volunteers produced a peak blood level of radioactivity, on the average, at 8 to 10 hours post-administration with peak urinary recovery seen at 12 to 24 hours.

INDICATIONS AND USAGE
Dexedrine (dextroamphetamine sulfate) is indicated:
1. **In Narcolepsy.**
2. **In Attention Deficit Disorder with Hyperactivity,** as an integral part of a total treatment program which typically includes other remedial measures (psychological, educational, social) for a stabilizing effect in children with a behavioral syndrome characterized by the following group of developmentally inappropriate symptoms: moderate to severe distractibility, short attention span, hyperactivity, emotional lability, and impulsivity. The diagnosis of this syndrome should not be made with finality when these symptoms are only of comparatively recent origin. Nonlocalizing (soft) neurological signs, learning disability, and abnormal EEG may or may not be present, and a diagnosis of central nervous system dysfunction may or may not be warranted.

CONTRAINDICATIONS
Advanced arteriosclerosis, symptomatic cardiovascular disease, moderate to severe hypertension, hyperthyroidism, known hypersensitivity or idiosyncrasy to the sympathomimetic amines, glaucoma.
Agitated states.
Patients with a history of drug abuse.
During or within 14 days following the administration of monoamine oxidase inhibitors (hypertensive crises may result).

WARNING
When tolerance to the "anorectic" effect develops, the recommended dose should not be exceeded in an attempt to increase the effect; rather, the drug should be discontinued.

PRECAUTIONS
General: Caution is to be exercised in prescribing amphetamines for patients with even mild hypertension.
The least amount feasible should be prescribed or dispensed at one time in order to minimize the possibility of overdosage.
These products contain FD&C Yellow No. 5 (tartrazine), which may cause allergic-type reactions (including bronchial asthma) in certain susceptible individuals. Although the overall incidence of FD&C Yellow No. 5 (tartrazine) sensitivity in the general population is low, it is frequently seen in patients who also have aspirin hypersensitivity.
Information for Patients: Amphetamines may impair the ability of the patient to engage in potentially hazardous activities such as operating machinery or vehicles; the patient should therefore be cautioned accordingly.

Drug Interactions
Acidifying agents—Gastrointestinal acidifying agents (guanethidine, reserpine, glutamic acid HCl, ascorbic acid, fruit juices, etc.) lower absorption of amphetamines. Urinary acidifying agents (ammonium chloride, sodium acid phosphate, etc.) increase the concentration of the ionized species of the amphetamine molecule, thereby increasing urinary excretion. Both groups of agents lower blood levels and efficacy of amphetamines.
Adrenergic blockers—Adrenergic blockers are inhibited by amphetamines.
Alkalinizing agents—Gastrointestinal alkalinizing agents (sodium bicarbonate, etc.) increase absorption of amphetamines. Urinary alkalinizing agents (acetazolamide, some thiazides) increase the concentration of the non-ionized species of the amphetamine molecule, thereby decreasing urinary excretion. Both groups of agents increase blood levels and therefore potentiate the actions of amphetamines.
Antidepressants, tricyclic—Amphetamines may enhance the activity of tricyclic or sympathomimetic agents; d-amphetamine with desipramine or protriptyline and possibly other tricyclics cause striking and sustained increases in the concentration of d-amphetamine in the brain; cardiovascular effects can be potentiated.
MAO inhibitors—MAOI antidepressants, as well as a metabolite of furazolidone, slow amphetamine metabolism. This slowing potentiates amphetamines, increasing their effect on the release of norepinephrine and other monoamines from adrenergic nerve endings; this can cause headaches and other signs of hypertensive crisis. A variety of neurologi-

cal toxic effects and malignant hyperpyrexia can occur, sometimes with fatal results.
Antihistamines—Amphetamines may counteract the sedative effect of antihistamines.
Antihypertensives—Amphetamines may antagonize the hypotensive effects of antihypertensives.
Chlorpromazine—Chlorpromazine blocks dopamine and norepinephrine reuptake, thus inhibiting the central stimulant effects of amphetamines, and can be used to treat amphetamine poisoning.
Ethosuximide—Amphetamines may delay intestinal absorption of ethosuximide.
Haloperidol—Haloperidol blocks dopamine and norepinephrine reuptake, thus inhibiting the central stimulant effects of amphetamines.
Lithium carbonate—The antiobesity and stimulatory effects of amphetamines may be inhibited by lithium carbonate.
Meperidine—Amphetamines potentiate the analgesic effect of meperidine.
Methenamine therapy—Urinary excretion of amphetamines is increased, and efficacy is reduced, by acidifying agents used in methenamine therapy.
Norepinephrine—Amphetamines enhance the adrenergic effect of norepinephrine.
Phenobarbital—Amphetamines may delay intestinal absorption of phenobarbital; co-administration of phenobarbital may produce a synergistic anticonvulsant action.
Phenytoin—Amphetamines may delay intestinal absorption of phenytoin; co-administration of phenytoin may produce a synergistic anticonvulsant action.
Propoxyphene—In cases of propoxyphene overdosage, amphetamine CNS stimulation is potentiated and fatal convulsions can occur.
Veratrum alkaloids—Amphetamines inhibit the hypotensive effect of veratrum alkaloids.

Drug/Laboratory Test Interactions
- Amphetamines can cause a significant elevation in plasma corticosteroid levels. This increase is greatest in the evening.
- Amphetamines may interfere with urinary steroid determinations.

Carcinogenesis/Mutagenesis: Mutagenicity studies and long-term studies in animals to determine the carcinogenic potential of Dexedrine (dextroamphetamine sulfate) have not been performed.
Pregnancy—Teratogenic Effects: Pregnancy Category C. *Dexedrine* has been shown to have embryotoxic and teratogenic effects when administered to A/Jax mice and C57BL mice in doses approximately 41 times the maximum human dose. Embryotoxic effects were not seen in New Zealand white rabbits given the drug in doses 7 times the human dose nor in rats given 12.5 times the maximum human dose. There are no adequate and well-controlled studies in pregnant women. *Dexedrine* should be used during pregnancy only if the potential benefit justifies the potential risk to the fetus.
Nonteratogenic Effects: Infants born to mothers dependent on amphetamines have an increased risk of premature delivery and low birth weight. Also, these infants may experience symptoms of withdrawal as demonstrated by dysphoria, including agitation, and significant lassitude.
Nursing Mothers: Amphetamines are excreted in human milk. Mothers taking amphetamines should be advised to refrain from nursing.
Pediatric Use: Long-term effects of amphetamines in children have not been well established.
Amphetamines are not recommended for use as anorectic agents in children under 12 years of age, or in children under 3 years of age with Attention Deficit Disorder with Hyperactivity described under INDICATIONS AND USAGE.
Clinical experience suggests that in psychotic children, administration of amphetamines may exacerbate symptoms of behavior disturbance and thought disorder.
Amphetamines have been reported to exacerbate motor and phonic tics and Tourette's syndrome. Therefore, clinical evaluation for tics and Tourette's syndrome in children and their families should precede use of stimulant medications.
Data are inadequate to determine whether chronic administration of amphetamines may be associated with growth inhibition; therefore, growth should be monitored during treatment.
Drug treatment is not indicated in all cases of Attention Deficit Disorder with Hyperactivity and should be considered only in light of the complete history and evaluation of the child. The decision to prescribe amphetamines should depend on the physician's assessment of the chronicity and severity of the child's symptoms and their appropriateness for his/her age. Prescription should not depend solely on the presence of one or more of the behavioral characteristics.
When these symptoms are associated with acute stress reactions, treatment with amphetamines is usually not indicated.

ADVERSE REACTIONS
Cardiovascular: Palpitations, tachycardia, elevation of blood pressure. There have been isolated reports of cardiomyopathy associated with chronic amphetamine use.
Central Nervous System: Psychotic episodes at recommended doses (rare), overstimulation, restlessness, dizziness, insomnia, euphoria, dyskinesia, dysphoria, tremor, headache, exacerbation of motor and phonic tics and Tourette's syndrome.
Gastrointestinal: Dryness of the mouth, unpleasant taste, diarrhea, constipation, other gastrointestinal disturbances. Anorexia and weight loss may occur as undesirable effects when amphetamines are used for other than the anorectic effect.
Allergic: Urticaria.
Endocrine: Impotence, changes in libido.

DRUG ABUSE AND DEPENDENCE
Dextroamphetamine sulfate is a Schedule II controlled substance.
Amphetamines have been extensively abused. Tolerance, extreme psychological dependence and severe social disability have occurred. There are reports of patients who have increased the dosage to many times that recommended. Abrupt cessation following prolonged high dosage administration results in extreme fatigue and mental depression; changes are also noted on the sleep EEG.
Manifestations of chronic intoxication with amphetamines include severe dermatoses, marked insomnia, irritability, hyperactivity and personality changes. The most severe manifestation of chronic intoxication is psychosis, often clinically indistinguishable from schizophrenia. This is rare with oral amphetamines.

OVERDOSAGE
Individual patient response to amphetamines varies widely. While toxic symptoms occasionally occur as an idiosyncrasy at doses as low as 2 mg, they are rare with doses of less than 15 mg; 30 mg can produce severe reactions, yet doses of 400 to 500 mg are not necessarily fatal.
In rats, the oral LD_{50} of dextroamphetamine sulfate is 96.8 mg/kg.
Manifestations of acute overdosage with amphetamines include restlessness, tremor, hyperreflexia, rhabdomyolysis, rapid respiration, hyperpyrexia, confusion, assaultiveness, hallucinations, panic states.
Fatigue and depression usually follow the central stimulation.
Cardiovascular effects include arrhythmias, hypertension or hypotension and circulatory collapse. Gastrointestinal symptoms include nausea, vomiting, diarrhea and abdominal cramps. Fatal poisoning is usually preceded by convulsions and coma.
TREATMENT—Management of acute amphetamine intoxication is largely symptomatic and includes gastric lavage and sedation with a barbiturate. Experience with hemodialysis or peritoneal dialysis is inadequate to permit recommendation in this regard. Acidification of the urine increases amphetamine excretion. If acute, severe hypertension complicates amphetamine overdosage, administration of intravenous phentolamine (Regitine®, CIBA) has been suggested. However, a gradual drop in blood pressure will usually result when sufficient sedation has been achieved. Chlorpromazine antagonizes the central stimulant effects of amphetamines and can be used to treat amphetamine intoxication.
Since much of the *Spansule* capsule medication is coated for gradual release, therapy directed at reversing the effects of the ingested drug and at supporting the patient should be continued for as long as overdosage symptoms remain. Saline cathartics are useful for hastening the evacuation of pellets that have not already released medication.

DOSAGE AND ADMINISTRATION
Regardless of indication, amphetamines should be administered at the lowest effective dosage and dosage should be individually adjusted. Late evening doses—particularly with the *Spansule* capsule form—should be avoided because of the resulting insomnia.
Narcolepsy: Usual dose 5 to 60 mg per day in divided doses, depending on the individual patient response.
Narcolepsy seldom occurs in children under 12 years of age; however, when it does, Dexedrine (dextroamphetamine sulfate) may be used. The suggested initial dose for patients aged 6–12 is 5 mg daily; daily dose may be raised in increments of 5 mg at weekly intervals until optimal response is obtained. In patients 12 years of age and older, start with 10 mg daily; daily dosage may be raised in increments of 10 mg at weekly intervals until optimal response is obtained. If bothersome adverse reactions appear (e.g., insomnia or anorexia), dosage should be reduced. *Spansule* capsules may be used for once-a-day dosage wherever appropriate. With tablets, give first dose on awakening; additional doses (1 or 2) at intervals of 4 to 6 hours.
Attention Deficit Disorder with Hyperactivity: Not recommended for children under 3 years of age.

In children from 3 to 5 years of age, start with 2.5 mg daily, by tablet; daily dosage may be raised in increments of 2.5 mg at weekly intervals until optimal response is obtained.
In children 6 years of age and older, start with 5 mg once or twice daily; daily dosage may be raised in increments of 5 mg at weekly intervals until optimal response is obtained. Only in rare cases will it be necessary to exceed a total of 40 mg per day.
Spansule capsules may be used for once-a-day dosage wherever appropriate.
With tablets, give first dose on awakening; additional doses (1 or 2) at intervals of 4 to 6 hours.
Where possible, drug administration should be interrupted occasionally to determine if there is a recurrence of behavioral symptoms sufficient to require continued therapy.

HOW SUPPLIED

Dexedrine **Spansule capsules:** Brown cap and natural body as follows: 5 mg imprinted SKF and E12, 10 mg imprinted SKF and E13, 15 mg imprinted SKF and E14. Available: 5 mg, 10 mg and 15 mg in bottles of 50.
Store at controlled room temperature (15° to 30°C; 59° to 86°F). Dispense in a tight, light-resistant container.
5 mg 50's: NDC 0007-3512-15
10 mg 50's: NDC 0007-3513-15
15 mg 50's: NDC 0007-3514-15
Dexedrine (dextroamphetamine sulfate) Tablets: Triangular, orange, scored, debossed SKF and E19. Available: 5 mg in bottles of 100.
Store at controlled room temperature (15° to 30°C; 59° to 86°F). Dispense in a tight, light-resistant container.
5 mg 100's: NDC 0007-3519-20

DX:L42

Shown in Product Identification Section, page 430

DIBENZYLINE® Capsules ℞

[di-benz 'eh-leen]
(brand of phenoxybenzamine hydrochloride)

DESCRIPTION

Each 'DIBENZYLINE' capsule, with red cap and red body, is imprinted SKF and E33 and contains phenoxybenzamine hydrochloride, 10 mg. Inactive ingredients consist of benzyl alcohol, cetylpyridinium chloride, D&C Red No. 33, FD&C Red No. 3, FD&C Yellow No. 6, gelatin, lactose, sodium lauryl sulfate and trace amounts of other inactive ingredients.
'Dibenzyline' is *N*-(2-Chloroethyl)-*N*-(1-methyl-2-phenoxyethyl)benzylamine hydrochloride.
Phenoxybenzamine hydrochloride is a colorless, crystalline powder with a molecular weight of 340.3 which melts between 136° and 141°C. It is soluble in water, alcohol and chloroform; insoluble in ether.

CLINICAL PHARMACOLOGY

Dibenzyline (phenoxybenzamine hydrochloride, SK&F) is a long-acting, adrenergic, *alpha*-receptor blocking agent which can produce and maintain "chemical sympathectomy" by oral administration. It increases blood flow to the skin, mucosa and abdominal viscera, and lowers both supine and erect blood pressures. It has no effect on the parasympathetic system.
Twenty to thirty percent of orally administered phenoxybenzamine appears to be absorbed in the active form.[1]
The half-life of orally administered phenoxybenzamine hydrochloride is not known; however, the half-life of intravenously administered drug is approximately 24 hours. Demonstrable effects with intravenous administration persist for at least three to four days, and the effects of daily administration are cumulative for nearly a week.[1]

INDICATION AND USAGE

Pheochromocytoma, to control episodes of hypertension and sweating. If tachycardia is excessive, it may be necessary to use a beta-blocking agent concomitantly.

CONTRAINDICATIONS

Conditions where a fall in blood pressure may be undesirable.

WARNING

'Dibenzyline'-induced *alpha*-adrenergic blockade leaves *beta*-adrenergic receptors unopposed. Compounds that stimulate both types of receptors may therefore produce an exaggerated hypotensive response and tachycardia.

PRECAUTIONS

General—Administer with caution in patients with marked cerebral or coronary arteriosclerosis or renal damage. Adrenergic blocking effect may aggravate symptoms of respiratory infections.
Drug Interactions[2]—Dibenzyline (phenoxybenzamine hydrochloride, SK&F) may interact with compounds that stimulate both *alpha*- and *beta*-adrenergic receptors (i.e., epinephrine) to produce an exaggerated hypotensive response and tachycardia. (See WARNING.)
'Dibenzyline' blocks hyperthermia production by levarterenol, and blocks hypothermia production by reserpine.
Carcinogenesis, Mutagenesis, Impairment of Fertility—Phenoxybenzamine hydrochloride has shown *in vitro* mutagenic activity in the Ames test and in the mouse lymphoma assay; it has not shown mutagenic activity in the micronucleus test in mice. In rats and mice repeated intraperitoneal administration of phenoxybenzamine hydrochloride resulted in peritoneal sarcomas. Chronic oral dosing in rats has produced malignant tumors in the gastrointestinal tract. The majority of these tumors were found in the nonglandular stomach of the rats.
In chronic oral studies in rats, ulcerative and/or erosive gastritis of the glandular stomach occurred which was probably drug related.
Pregnancy-Teratogenic Effects—Pregnancy Category C. Adequate reproductive studies have not been performed with Dibenzyline (phenoxybenzamine hydrochloride, SK&F). It is also not known whether 'Dibenzyline' can cause fetal harm when administered to a pregnant woman. 'Dibenzyline' should be given to a pregnant woman only if clearly needed.
Nursing Mothers—It is not known whether this drug is excreted in human milk. Because many drugs are excreted in human milk, and because of the potential for serious adverse reactions from phenoxybenzamine hydrochloride, a decision should be made whether to discontinue nursing or to discontinue the drug, taking into account the importance of the drug to the mother.
Pediatric Use—Safety and effectiveness in children have not been established.

ADVERSE REACTIONS

The following adverse reactions have been observed, but there are insufficient data to support an estimate of their frequency:
Autonomic Nervous System*: Postural hypotension, tachycardia, inhibition of ejaculation, nasal congestion, miosis.
Miscellaneous: Gastrointestinal irritation, drowsiness, fatigue.

*These so-called "side effects" are actually evidence of adrenergic blockade and vary according to the degree of blockade.

OVERDOSAGE

SYMPTOMS—These are largely the result of block of the sympathetic nervous system and of the circulating epinephrine. They may include postural hypotension resulting in dizziness or fainting; tachycardia, particularly postural; vomiting; lethargy; shock.
TREATMENT—When symptoms and signs of overdosage exist, discontinue the drug. Treatment of circulatory failure, if present, is a prime consideration. In cases of mild overdosage, recumbent position with legs elevated usually restores cerebral circulation. In the more severe cases, the usual measures to combat shock should be instituted. Usual pressor agents are *not* effective. Epinephrine is contraindicated because it stimulates both *alpha* and *beta* receptors; since *alpha* receptors are blocked, the net effect of epinephrine administration is vasodilation and a further drop in blood pressure (epinephrine reversal).
The patient may have to be kept flat for 24 hours or more in the case of overdose, as the effect of the drug is prolonged. Leg bandages and an abdominal binder may shorten the period of disability.
I.V. infusion of levarterenol bitartrate* may be used to combat severe hypotensive reactions, because it stimulates *alpha* receptors primarily. Although Dibenzyline (phenoxybenzamine hydrochloride, SK&F) is an *alpha* adrenergic blocking agent, a sufficient dose of levarterenol bitartrate will overcome this effect.
The oral LD_{50} for phenoxybenzamine hydrochloride is approximately 2000 mg./kg. in rats and approximately 500 mg./kg. in guinea pigs.

*Available as Levophed® Bitartrate (brand of norepinephrine bitartrate) from Winthrop-Breon.

DOSAGE AND ADMINISTRATION

The dosage should be adjusted to fit the needs of each patient. Small initial doses should be *slowly* increased until the desired effect is obtained or the side effects from blockade become troublesome. *After each increase, the patient should be observed on that level before instituting another increase.* The dosage should be carried to a point where symptomatic relief and/or objective improvement are obtained, but not so high that the side effects from blockade become troublesome. Initially, 10 mg. of Dibenzyline (phenoxybenzamine hydrochloride, SK&F) twice a day. Dosage should be increased every other day, usually to 20 to 40 mg. two or three times a day, until an optimal dosage is obtained, as judged by blood pressure control.

HOW SUPPLIED

Dibenzyline (phenoxybenzamine hydrochloride, SK&F) capsules, 10 mg., in bottles of 100 (*NDC* 0007-3533-20).
Military—Capsules, 10 mg 100's, 6505-00-890-1193.

REFERENCES

1. Weiner, N.: Drugs That Inhibit Adrenergic Nerves and Block Adrenergic Receptors, in Goodman, L., and Gilman, A., *The Pharmacological Basis of Therapeutics*, ed. 6, New York, Macmillan Publishing Co., 1980, p. 179; p. 182.
2. Martin, E.W.: *Drug Interactions Index 1978/1979*, Philadelphia, J.B. Lippincott Co., 1978, pp. 209–210.

DI:L23

Shown in Product Identification Section, page 430

DYAZIDE® Capsules ℞

[dye-uh-zide']
diuretic • antihypertensive

DESCRIPTION

Each *Dyazide* capsule for oral use, with opaque red cap and opaque white body, contains hydrochlorothiazide 25 mg and triamterene 50 mg, and is imprinted with the product name DYAZIDE and SKF. Hydrochlorothiazide is a diuretic/antihypertensive agent and triamterene is an antikaliuretic agent.
Hydrochlorothiazide is slightly soluble in water. It is soluble in dilute ammonia, dilute aqueous sodium hydroxide and dimethylformamide. It is sparingly soluble in methanol.
Hydrochlorothiazide is 6-chloro-3,4-dihydro-2*H*-1,2,4-benzothiadiazine-7-sulfonamide 1,1-dioxide and its structural formula is:

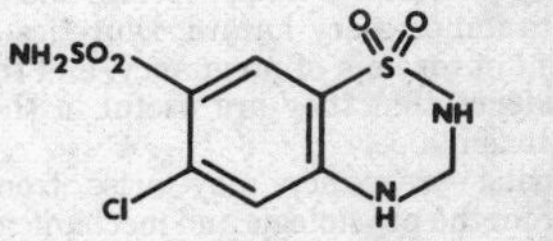

At 50°C, triamterene is practically insoluble in water (less than 0.1%). It is soluble in formic acid, sparingly soluble in methoxyethanol and very slightly soluble in alcohol.
Triamterene is 2,4,7-triamino-6-phenylpteridine and its structural formula is:

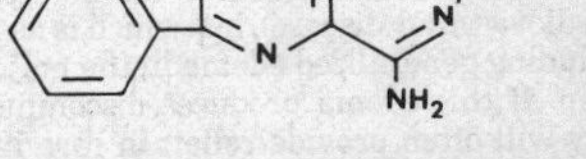

Inactive ingredients consist of benzyl alcohol, cetylpyridinium chloride, D&C Red No. 33, FD&C Yellow No. 6, gelatin, lactose, magnesium stearate, povidone, sodium lauryl sulfate, titanium dioxide and trace amounts of other inactive ingredients.

CLINICAL PHARMACOLOGY

Dyazide is a diuretic/antihypertensive drug product that combines natriuretic and antikaliuretic effects. Each component complements the action of the other. The hydrochlorothiazide component blocks the reabsorption of sodium and chloride ions, and thereby increases the quantity of sodium traversing the distal tubule and the volume of water excreted. A portion of the additional sodium presented to the distal tubule is exchanged there for potassium and hydrogen ions. With continued use of hydrochlorothiazide and depletion of sodium, compensatory mechanisms tend to increase this exchange and may produce excessive loss of potassium, hydrogen and chloride ions. Hydrochlorothiazide also decreases the excretion of calcium and uric acid, may increase the excretion of iodide and may reduce glomerular filtration rate. The exact mechanism of the antihypertensive effect of hydrochlorothiazide is not known.
The triamterene component of *Dyazide* exerts its diuretic effect on the distal renal tubule to inhibit the reabsorption of sodium in exchange for potassium and hydrogen ions. Its natriuretic activity is limited by the amount of sodium reaching its site of action. Although it blocks the increase in this exchange that is stimulated by mineralocorticoids (chiefly aldosterone) it is not a competitive antagonist of aldosterone and its activity can be demonstrated in adrenalectomized rats and patients with Addison's disease. As a result, the dose of triamterene required is not proportionally related to the level of mineralocorticoid activity, but is dictated by the response of the individual patients, and the kaliuretic effect of concomitantly administered drugs. By inhibiting the distal tubular exchange mechanism, triamterene maintains or increases the sodium excretion and reduces the excess loss of potassium, hydrogen, and chloride ions induced by hydrochlorothiazide. As with hydrochlorothiazide, tri-

Continued on next page

SmithKline Beecham—Cont.

amterene may reduce glomerular filtration and renal plasma flow. Via this mechanism it may reduce uric acid excretion although it has no tubular effect on uric acid reabsorption or secretion. Triamterene does not affect calcium excretion. No predictable antihypertensive effect has been demonstrated for triamterene.

Duration of diuretic activity and effective dosage range of the hydrochlorothiazide and triamterene components of *Dyazide* are similar. Onset of diuresis with *Dyazide* takes place within one hour, peaks at two to three hours and tapers off during the subsequent seven to nine hours.

The bioavailability of the hydrochlorothiazide and the triamterene components of *Dyazide* is, in each case, about 50% of that observed with an aqueous suspension of the components. (See PRECAUTIONS, Bioavailability.)

INDICATIONS AND USAGE

This fixed combination drug is not indicated for the initial therapy of edema or hypertension except in individuals in whom the development of hypokalemia cannot be risked.

Dyazide is indicated for the treatment of hypertension or edema in patients who develop hypokalemia on hydrochlorothiazide alone.

Dyazide is also indicated for those patients who require a thiazide diuretic and in whom the development of hypokalemia cannot be risked.

Dyazide may be used alone or as an adjunct to other antihypertensive drugs, such as beta-blockers. Since *Dyazide* may enhance the action of these agents, dosage adjustments may be necessary.

Usage in Pregnancy: The routine use of diuretics in an otherwise healthy woman is inappropriate and exposes mother and fetus to unnecessary hazard. Diuretics do not prevent development of toxemia of pregnancy, and there is no satisfactory evidence that they are useful in the treatment of developed toxemia.

Edema during pregnancy may arise from pathological causes or from the physiologic and mechanical consequences of pregnancy. Diuretics are indicated in pregnancy when edema is due to pathologic causes, just as they are in the absence of pregnancy. Dependent edema in pregnancy resulting from restriction of venous return by the expanded uterus is properly treated through elevation of the lower extremities and use of support hose; use of diuretics to lower intravascular volume in this case is illogical and unnecessary. There is hypervolemia during normal pregnancy which is harmful to neither the fetus nor the mother (in the absence of cardiovascular disease), but which is associated with edema, including generalized edema in the majority of pregnant women. If this edema produces discomfort, increased recumbency will often provide relief. In rare instances this edema may cause extreme discomfort which is not relieved by rest. In these cases a short course of diuretics may provide relief and may be appropriate.

CONTRAINDICATIONS

Antikaliuretic Therapy and Potassium Supplementation

Dyazide should not be given to patients receiving other potassium-conserving agents such as spironolactone, amiloride or other formulations containing triamterene. Concomitant potassium-containing salt substitutes should also not be used.

Potassium supplementation should not be used with *Dyazide* except in severe cases of hypokalemia. Such concomitant therapy can be associated with rapid increases in serum potassium levels. If potassium supplementation is used, careful monitoring of the serum potassium level is necessary.

Impaired Renal Function

Dyazide is contraindicated in patients with anuria, acute and chronic renal insufficiency or significant renal impairment.

Hypersensitivity

Hypersensitivity to either drug in the preparation or to other sulfonamide-derived drugs is a contraindication.

Hyperkalemia

Dyazide should not be used in patients with preexisting elevated serum potassium.

WARNINGS: Hyperkalemia

Abnormal elevation of serum potassium levels (greater than or equal to 5.5 mEq/liter) can occur with all potassium-conserving diuretic combinations, including *Dyazide.* Hyperkalemia is more likely to occur in patients with renal impairment and diabetes (even without evidence of renal impairment), and in the elderly or severely ill. Since uncorrected hyperkalemia may be fatal, serum potassium levels must be monitored at frequent intervals especially in patients first receiving *Dyazide,* when dosages are changed or with any illness that may influence renal function.

If hyperkalemia is suspected (warning signs include paresthesias, muscular weakness, fatigue, flaccid paralysis of the extremities, bradycardia and shock), an electrocardiogram (ECG) should be obtained. However, it is important to monitor serum potassium levels because hyperkalemia may not be associated with ECG changes.

If hyperkalemia is present, *Dyazide* should be discontinued immediately and a thiazide alone should be substituted. If the serum potassium exceeds 6.5 mEq/liter more vigorous therapy is required. The clinical situation dictates the procedures to be employed. These include the intravenous administration of calcium chloride solution, sodium bicarbonate solution and/or the oral or parenteral administration of glucose with a rapid-acting insulin preparation. Cationic exchange resins such as sodium polystyrene sulfonate may be orally or rectally administered. Persistent hyperkalemia may require dialysis.

The development of hyperkalemia associated with potassium-sparing diuretics is accentuated in the presence of renal impairment (see CONTRAINDICATIONS section). Patients with mild renal functional impairment should not receive this drug without frequent and continuing monitoring of serum electrolytes. Cumulative drug effects may be observed in patients with impaired renal function. The renal clearances of hydrochlorothiazide and the pharmacologically active metabolite of triamterene, the sulfate ester of hydroxytriamterene, have been shown to be reduced and the plasma levels increased following *Dyazide* administration to elderly patients and patients with impaired renal function.

Hyperkalemia has been reported in diabetic patients with the use of potassium-conserving agents even in the absence of apparent renal impairment. Accordingly, serum electrolytes must be frequently monitored if *Dyazide* is used in diabetic patients.

Metabolic or Respiratory Acidosis

Potassium-conserving therapy should also be avoided in severely ill patients in whom respiratory or metabolic acidosis may occur. Acidosis may be associated with rapid elevations in serum potassium levels. If *Dyazide* is employed, frequent evaluations of acid/base balance and serum electrolytes are necessary.

PRECAUTIONS

General

Bioavailability: The bioavailability of the hydrochlorothiazide and triamterene components of *Dyazide* is about 50% of the maximum obtainable with oral therapy. Theoretically, a patient transferred from therapy with hydrochlorothiazide with or without triamterene might show an increase in blood pressure, fluid retention, or change in serum potassium. Extensive clinical experience with *Dyazide,* however, suggests that these conditions have not been commonly observed in clinical practice. (See CLINICAL PHARMACOLOGY.)

Impaired Hepatic Function

Thiazides should be used with caution in patients with impaired hepatic function. They can precipitate hepatic coma in patients with severe liver disease. Potassium depletion induced by the thiazide may be important in this connection. Administer *Dyazide* cautiously and be alert for such early signs of impending coma as confusion, drowsiness and tremor; if mental confusion increases discontinue *Dyazide* for a few days. Attention must be given to other factors that may precipitate hepatic coma, such as blood in the gastrointestinal tract or preexisting potassium depletion.

Hypokalemia

Hypokalemia is uncommon with *Dyazide;* but, should it develop, corrective measures should be taken such as potassium supplementation or increased intake of potassium-rich foods. Institute such measures cautiously with frequent determinations of serum potassium levels, especially in patients receiving digitalis or with a history of cardiac arrhythmias. If serious hypokalemia (serum potassium less than 3.0 mEq/L) is demonstrated by repeat serum potassium determinations, *Dyazide* should be discontinued and potassium chloride supplementation initiated. Less serious hypokalemia should be evaluated with regard to other coexisting conditions and treated accordingly.

Electrolyte Imbalance

Electrolyte imbalance, often encountered in such conditions as heart failure, renal disease or cirrhosis of the liver, may also be aggravated by diuretics and should be considered during *Dyazide* therapy when using high doses for prolonged periods or in patients on a salt-restricted diet. Serum determinations of electrolytes should be performed, and are particularly important if the patient is vomiting excessively or receiving fluids parenterally. Possible fluid and electrolyte imbalance may be indicated by such warning signs as: dry mouth, thirst, weakness, lethargy, drowsiness, restlessness, muscle pain or cramps, muscular fatigue, hypotension, oliguria, tachycardia and gastrointestinal symptoms.

Hypochloremia

Although any chloride deficit is generally mild and usually does not require specific treatment except under extraordinary circumstances (as in liver disease or renal disease), chloride replacement may be required in the treatment of metabolic alkalosis. Dilutional hyponatremia may occur in edematous patients in hot weather; appropriate therapy is water restriction, rather than administration of salt, except in rare instances when the hyponatremia is life threatening. In actual salt depletion, appropriate replacement is the therapy of choice.

Renal Stones

Triamterene has been found in renal stones in association with the other usual calculus components. *Dyazide* should be used with caution in patients with a history of renal stones.

Laboratory Tests

Serum Potassium: The normal adult range of serum potassium is 3.5 to 5.0 mEq per liter with 4.5 mEq often being used for a reference point. If hypokalemia should develop, corrective measures should be taken such as potassium supplementation or increased dietary intake of potassium-rich foods. Institute such measures cautiously with frequent determinations of serum potassium levels. Potassium levels persistently above 6 mEq per liter require careful observation and treatment. Serum potassium levels do not necessarily indicate true body potassium concentration. A rise in plasma pH may cause a decrease in plasma potassium concentration and an increase in the intracellular potassium concentration. Discontinue corrective measures for hypokalemia immediately if laboratory determinations reveal an abnormal elevation of serum potassium. Discontinue *Dyazide* and substitute a thiazide diuretic alone until potassium levels return to normal.

Serum Creatinine and BUN: *Dyazide* may produce an elevated blood urea nitrogen level, creatinine level or both. This apparently is secondary to a reversible reduction of glomerular filtration rate or a depletion of intravascular fluid volume (prerenal azotemia) rather than renal toxicity; levels usually return to normal when *Dyazide* is discontinued. If azotemia increases, discontinue *Dyazide.* Periodic BUN or serum creatinine determinations should be made, especially in elderly patients and in patients with suspected or confirmed renal insufficiency.

Serum PBI: Thiazide may decrease serum PBI levels without sign of thyroid disturbance.

Parathyroid Function: Thiazides should be discontinued before carrying out tests for parathyroid function. Calcium excretion is decreased by thiazides. Pathologic changes in the parathyroid glands with hypercalcemia and hypophosphatemia have been observed in a few patients on prolonged thiazide therapy. The common complications of hyperparathyroidism such as bone resorption and peptic ulceration have not been seen.

Drug Interactions

Angiotensin-converting enzyme inhibitors: Potassium-sparing agents should be used with caution in conjunction with angiotensin-converting enzyme (ACE) inhibitors due to an increased risk of hyperkalemia.

Oral hypoglycemic drugs: Concurrent use with chlorpropamide may increase the risk of severe hyponatremia.

Nonsteroidal anti-inflammatory drugs: A possible interaction resulting in acute renal failure has been reported in a few patients on *Dyazide* when treated with indomethacin, a nonsteroidal anti-inflammatory agent. Caution is advised in administering nonsteroidal anti-inflammatory agents with *Dyazide.*

Lithium: Lithium generally should not be given with diuretics because they reduce its renal clearance and increase the risk of lithium toxicity. Read circulars for lithium preparations before use of such concomitant therapy with *Dyazide.*

Surgical considerations: Thiazides have been shown to decrease arterial responsiveness to norepinephrine (an effect attributed to loss of sodium). This diminution is not sufficient to preclude effectiveness of the pressor agent for therapeutic use. Thiazides have also been shown to increase the paralyzing effect of nondepolarizing muscle relaxants such as tubocurarine (an effect attributed to potassium loss); consequently caution should be observed in patients undergoing surgery.

Other Considerations: Concurrent use of hydrochlorothiazide with amphotericin B or corticosteroids or corticotropin (ACTH) may intensify electrolyte imbalance, particularly hypokalemia, although the presence of triamterene minimizes the hypokalemic effect.

Thiazides may add to or potentiate the action of other antihypertensive drugs. See INDICATIONS AND USAGE for concomitant use with other antihypertensive drugs.

The effect of oral anticoagulants may be decreased when used concurrently with hydrochlorothiazide; dosage adjustments may be necessary.

Dyazide may raise the level of blood uric acid; dosage adjustments of antigout medication may be necessary to control hyperuricemia and gout.

The following agents given together with triamterene may promote serum potassium accumulation and possibly result in hyperkalemia because of the potassium-sparing nature of triamterene, especially in patients with renal insufficiency: blood from blood bank (may contain up to 30 mEq of potassium per liter of plasma or up to 65 mEq per liter of whole blood when stored for more than 10 days); low-salt milk (may contain up to 60 mEq of potassium per liter); potassium-containing medications (such as parenteral penicillin G potas-

sium); salt substitutes (most contain substantial amounts of potassium).

Exchange resins, such as sodium polystyrene sulfonate, whether administered orally or rectally, reduce serum potassium levels by sodium replacement of the potassium; fluid retention may occur in some patients because of the increased sodium intake.

Chronic or overuse of laxatives may reduce serum potassium levels by promoting excessive potassium loss from the intestinal tract; laxatives may interfere with the potassium-retaining effects of triamterene.

The effectiveness of methenamine may be decreased when used concurrently with hydrochlorothiazide because of alkalinization of the urine.

Drug/Laboratory Test Interactions

Triamterene and quinidine have similar fluorescence spectra; thus, *Dyazide* will interfere with the fluorescent measurement of quinidine.

Pregnancy: Category C

Teratogenic Effects—The safe use of *Dyazide* in pregnancy has not been established. Animal reproduction studies have not been conducted with *Dyazide*. It is also not known if *Dyazide* can cause fetal harm when administered to a pregnant woman or can affect reproductive capacity. *Dyazide* should be given to a pregnant woman only if clearly needed. *Nonteratogenic Effects*—Thiazides cross the placental barrier and appear in cord blood. The use of thiazides in pregnant women requires that the anticipated benefit be weighed against possible hazards to the fetus. These hazards include fetal or neonatal jaundice, thrombocytopenia, and possible other adverse reactions which have occurred in the adult. Triamterene has been shown to cross the placental barrier and appear in the cord blood of animals. The use of triamterene in pregnant women requires that the anticipated benefit be weighed against possible hazards to the fetus. These possible hazards include adverse reactions which have occurred in the adult.

Nursing Mothers—Thiazides appear and triamterene may appear in breast milk. If use of the drug product is deemed essential, the patient should stop nursing.

Pediatric Use—Safety and effectiveness in children have not been established.

ADVERSE REACTIONS

Adverse effects are listed in decreasing order of frequency; however, the most serious adverse effects are listed first regardless of frequency. The serious adverse effects associated with *Dyazide* have commonly occurred in less than 0.1% of patients treated with this product.

Hypersensitivity: anaphylaxis, rash, urticaria, photosensitivity.

Cardiovascular: arrhythmia, postural hypotension.

Metabolic: diabetes mellitus, hyperkalemia, hyperglycemia, glycosuria, hyperuricemia, hypokalemia, hyponatremia, acidosis, hypochloremia.

Gastrointestinal: jaundice and/or liver enzyme abnormalities, pancreatitis, nausea and vomiting, diarrhea, constipation, abdominal pain.

Renal: acute renal failure, interstitial nephritis, renal stones composed primarily of triamterene, elevated BUN and serum creatinine, abnormal urinary sediment.

Hematologic: leukopenia, thrombocytopenia and purpura, megaloblastic anemia.

Musculoskeletal: muscle cramps.

Central Nervous System: weakness, fatigue, dizziness, headache, dry mouth.

Miscellaneous: impotence, sialadenitis.

Thiazides alone have been shown to cause the following additional adverse reactions:

Central Nervous System: paresthesias, vertigo.

Ophthalmic: xanthopsia, transient blurred vision.

Respiratory: allergic pneumonitis, pulmonary edema, respiratory distress.

Other: necrotizing vasculitis, exacerbation of lupus.

Hematologic: aplastic anemia, agranulocytosis, hemolytic anemia.

Neonate and infancy: thrombocytopenia and pancreatitis—rarely, in newborns whose mothers have received thiazides during pregnancy.

DOSAGE AND ADMINISTRATION

The usual dose of *Dyazide* is one or two capsules given once daily, with appropriate monitoring of serum potassium and of the clinical effect. (See WARNINGS, Hyperkalemia and PRECAUTIONS, Bioavailability.)

OVERDOSAGE

Electrolyte imbalance is the major concern (see WARNINGS section). Symptoms reported include: polyuria, nausea, vomiting, weakness, lassitude, fever, flushed face, and hyperactive deep tendon reflexes. If hypotension occurs, it may be treated with pressor agents such as levarterenol to maintain blood pressure. Carefully evaluate the electrolyte pattern and fluid balance. Induce immediate evacuation of the stomach through emesis or gastric lavage. There is no specific antidote.

Reversible acute renal failure following ingestion of 50 tablets of a product containing a combination of 50 mg triamterene and 25 mg hydrochlorothiazide has been reported. Although triamterene is largely protein-bound (approximately 67%), there may be some benefit to dialysis in cases of overdosage.

HOW SUPPLIED

Capsules containing 25 mg hydrochlorothiazide and 50 mg triamterene, in bottles of 1000 capsules; in Single Unit Packages (unit-dose) of 100 (intended for institutional use only); in Patient-Pak™ unit-of-use bottles of 100.

They are supplied as follows:

NDC 0108-3590-21—Single Unit Packages (unit-dose) of 100 (intended for institutional use only).

NDC 0108-3590-22—in Patient-Pak™ unit-of-use bottles of 100.

NDC 0108-3590-30—bottles of 1000.

Store at controlled room temperature (15°–30°C [59°–86°F]). Protect from light. Dispense in a tight, light-resistant container.

DZ:L61

Shown in Product Identification Section, page 430

DYRENIUM®   ℞

[di-ren'ee-um]
(brand of triamterene)
Capsules
50 mg and 100 mg
potassium-conserving diuretic

DESCRIPTION

Dyrenium (triamterene) is a potassium-conserving diuretic. Triamterene is 2,4,7-triamino-6-phenyl-pteridine. Its molecular weight is 253.27. At 50°C, triamterene is slightly soluble in water. It is soluble in dilute ammonia, dilute aqueous sodium hydroxide and dimethylformamide. It is sparingly soluble in methanol.

Each capsule for oral use, with opaque red cap and body, contains triamterene, 50 or 100 mg, and is imprinted with the product name DYRENIUM, strength (50 or 100) and SKF. Inactive ingredients consist of benzyl alcohol, cetylpyridinium chloride, D&C Red No. 33, FD&C Yellow No. 6, gelatin, lactose, magnesium stearate, povidone, sodium lauryl sulfate, titanium dioxide and trace amounts of other inactive ingredients.

CLINICAL PHARMACOLOGY

Triamterene has a unique mode of action; it inhibits the reabsorption of sodium ions in exchange for potassium and hydrogen ions at that segment of the distal tubule under the control of adrenal mineralocorticoids (especially aldosterone). This activity is not directly related to aldosterone secretion or antagonism; it is a result of a direct effect on the renal tubule.

The fraction of filtered sodium reaching this distal tubular exchange site is relatively small, and the amount which is exchanged depends on the level of mineralocorticoid activity. Thus, the degree of natriuresis and diuresis produced by inhibition of the exchange mechanism is necessarily limited. Increasing the amount of available sodium and the level of mineralocorticoid activity by the use of more proximally acting diuretics will increase the degree of diuresis and potassium conservation.

Triamterene occasionally causes increases in serum potassium which can result in hyperkalemia. It does not produce alkalosis because it does not cause excessive excretion of titratable acid and ammonium.

Triamterene has been shown to cross the placental barrier and appear in the cord blood of animals.

Pharmacokinetics

Onset of action is two to four hours after ingestion. In normal volunteers the mean peak serum levels were 30 ng/mL at three hours. The average percent of drug recovered in the urine (0–48 hours) was 21%. Triamterene is primarily metabolized to the sulfate conjugate of hydroxytriamterene. Both the plasma and urine levels of this metabolite greatly exceed triamterene levels. Triamterene is rapidly absorbed, with somewhat less than 50% of the oral dose reaching the urine. Most patients will respond to Dyrenium (triamterene) during the first day of treatment. Maximum therapeutic effect, however, may not be seen for several days. Duration of diuresis depends on several factors, especially renal function, but it generally tapers off seven to nine hours after administration.

INDICATIONS AND USAGE

Dyrenium (triamterene) is indicated in the treatment of edema associated with congestive heart failure, cirrhosis of the liver, and the nephrotic syndrome; also in steroid-induced edema, idiopathic edema, and edema due to secondary hyperaldosteronism.

Dyrenium may be used alone or with other diuretics either for its added diuretic effect or its potassium-conserving potential. It also promotes increased diuresis when patients

prove resistant or only partially responsive to thiazides or other diuretics because of secondary hyperaldosteronism.

Usage in Pregnancy. The routine use of diuretics in an otherwise healthy woman is inappropriate and exposes mother and fetus to unnecessary hazard. Diuretics do not prevent development of toxemia of pregnancy, and there is no satisfactory evidence that they are useful in the treatment of developed toxemia.

Edema during pregnancy may arise from pathological causes or from the physiologic and mechanical consequences of pregnancy. Diuretics are indicated in pregnancy when edema is due to pathologic causes, just as they are in the absence of pregnancy (however, see Precautions below). Dependent edema in pregnancy, resulting from restriction of venous return by the expanded uterus, is properly treated through elevation of the lower extremities and use of support hose; use of diuretics to lower intravascular volume in this case is illogical and unnecessary. There is hypervolemia during normal pregnancy which is harmful to neither the fetus nor the mother (in the absence of cardiovascular disease), but which is associated with edema, including generalized edema, in the majority of pregnant women. If this edema produces discomfort, increased recumbency will often provide relief. In rare instances, this edema may cause extreme discomfort which is not relieved by rest. In these cases, a short course of diuretics may provide relief and may be appropriate.

CONTRAINDICATIONS

Anuria. Severe or progressive kidney disease or dysfunction with the possible exception of nephrosis. Severe hepatic disease. Hypersensitivity to the drug.

Dyrenium (triamterene) should not be used in patients with pre-existing elevated serum potassium, as is sometimes seen in patients with impaired renal function or azotemia, or in patients who develop hyperkalemia while on the drug. Patients should not be placed on dietary potassium supplements, potassium salts, or potassium-containing salt substitutes in conjunction with *Dyrenium*.

Dyrenium should not be given to patients receiving other potassium-conserving agents such as spironolactone, amiloride hydrochloride, or other formulations containing triamterene. Two deaths have been reported in patients receiving concomitant spironolactone and *Dyrenium* or Dyazide®. Although dosage recommendations were exceeded in one case and in the other serum electrolytes were not properly monitored, these two drugs should not be given concomitantly.

WARNINGS

> Abnormal elevation of serum potassium levels (greater than or equal to 5.5 mEq/liter) can occur with all potassium-conserving agents, including *Dyrenium*. Hyperkalemia is more likely to occur in patients with renal impairment and diabetes (even without evidence of renal impairment), and in the elderly or severely ill. Since uncorrected hyperkalemia may be fatal, serum potassium levels must be monitored at frequent intervals especially in patients receiving *Dyrenium*, when dosages are changed or with any illness that may influence renal function.

There have been isolated reports of hypersensitivity reactions; therefore, patients should be observed regularly for the possible occurrence of blood dyscrasias, liver damage, or other idiosyncratic reactions.

Periodic BUN and serum potassium determinations should be made to check kidney function, especially in patients with suspected or confirmed renal insufficiency. It is particularly important to make serum potassium determinations in elderly or diabetic patients receiving the drug; these patients should be observed carefully for possible serum potassium increases.

If hyperkalemia is present or suspected, an electrocardiogram should be obtained. If the ECG shows no widening of the QRS or arrhythmia in the presence of hyperkalemia, it is usually sufficient to discontinue Dyrenium (triamterene) and any potassium supplementation and substitute a thiazide alone. Sodium polystyrene sulfonate (Kayexalate®, Winthrop) may be administered to enhance the excretion of excess potassium. **The presence of a widened QRS complex or arrhythmia in association with hyperkalemia requires prompt additional therapy.** For tachyarrhythmia, infuse 44 mEq of sodium bicarbonate or 10 mL of 10% calcium gluconate or calcium chloride over several minutes. For asystole, bradycardia, or A-V block transvenous pacing is also recommended.

The effect of calcium and sodium bicarbonate is transient and repeated administration may be required. When indicated by the clinical situation, excess K+ may be removed by dialysis or oral or rectal administration of Kayexalate®. Infusion of glucose and insulin has also been used to treat hyperkalemia.

Continued on next page

SmithKline Beecham—Cont.

PRECAUTIONS

General

Dyrenium (triamterene) tends to conserve potassium rather than to promote the excretion as do many diuretics and, occasionally, can cause increases in serum potassium which, in some instances, can result in hyperkalemia. In rare instances, hyperkalemia has been associated with cardiac irregularities.

Electrolyte imbalance often encountered in such diseases as congestive heart failure, renal disease, or cirrhosis may be aggravated or caused independently by any effective diuretic agent including *Dyrenium*. The use of full doses of a diuretic when salt intake is restricted can result in a low-salt syndrome.

Triamterene can cause mild nitrogen retention which is reversible upon withdrawal of the drug and is seldom observed with intermittent (every-other-day) therapy.

Triamterene may cause a decreasing alkali reserve with the possibility of metabolic acidosis.

By the very nature of their illness, cirrhotics with splenomegaly sometimes have marked variations in their blood pictures. Since triamterene is a weak folic acid antagonist, it may contribute to the appearance of megaloblastosis in cases where folic acid stores have been depleted. Therefore, periodic blood studies in these patients are recommended. They should also be observed for exacerbations of underlying liver disease.

Triamterene has elevated uric acid, especially in persons predisposed to gouty arthritis.

Triamterene has been reported in renal stones in association with other calculus components. *Dyrenium* should be used with caution in patients with histories of renal stones.

Information for Patients

To help avoid stomach upset, it is recommended that the drug be taken after meals.

If a single daily dose is prescribed, it may be preferable to take it in the morning to minimize the effect of increased frequency of urination on nighttime sleep.

If a dose is missed, the patient should not take more than the prescribed dose at the next dosing interval.

Laboratory Tests

Hyperkalemia will rarely occur in patients with adequate urinary output, but it is a possibility if large doses are used for considerable periods of time. If hyperkalemia is observed, Dyrenium (triamterene) should be withdrawn. The normal adult range of serum potassium is 3.5 to 5.0 mEq per liter with 4.5 mEq often being used for a reference point. Potassium levels persistently above 6 mEq per liter require careful observation and treatment. Normal potassium levels tend to be higher in neonates (7.7 mEq per liter) than in adults.

Serum potassium levels do not necessarily indicate true body potassium concentration. A rise in plasma pH may cause a decrease in plasma potassium concentration and an increase in the intracellular potassium concentration. Because *Dyrenium* conserves potassium, it has been theorized that in patients who have received intensive therapy or been given the drug for prolonged periods, a rebound kaliuresis could occur upon abrupt withdrawal. In such patients withdrawal of *Dyrenium* should be gradual.

Drug Interactions

Caution should be used when lithium and diuretics are used concomitantly because diuretic-induced sodium loss may reduce the renal clearance of lithium and increase serum lithium levels with risk of lithium toxicity. Patients receiving such combined therapy should have serum lithium levels monitored closely and the lithium dosage adjusted if necessary.

A possible interaction resulting in acute renal failure has been reported in a few subjects when indomethacin, a nonsteroidal anti-inflammatory agent, was given with triamterene. Caution is advised in administering nonsteroidal anti-inflammatory agents with triamterene.

The effects of the following drugs may be potentiated when given together with triamterene: antihypertensive medication, other diuretics, preanesthetic and anesthetic agents, skeletal muscle relaxants (nondepolarizing).

Potassium-sparing agents should be used with caution in conjunction with angiotensin-converting enzyme (ACE) inhibitors due to an increased risk of hyperkalemia.

The following agents, given together with triamterene, may promote serum potassium accumulation and possibly result in hyperkalemia because of the potassium-sparing nature of triamterene, especially in patients with renal insufficiency: blood from blood bank (may contain up to 30 mEq of potassium per liter of plasma or up to 65 mEq per liter of whole blood when stored for more than 10 days); low-salt milk (may contain up to 60 mEq of potassium per liter); potassium-containing medications (such as parenteral penicillin G potassium); salt substitutes (most contain substantial amounts of potassium).

Dyrenium (triamterene) may raise blood glucose levels; for adult-onset diabetes, dosage adjustments of hypoglycemic agents may be necessary during and after therapy; concurrent use with chlorpropamide may increase the risk of severe hyponatremia.

Drug/Laboratory Test Interactions

Triamterene and quinidine have similar fluorescence spectra; thus, triamterene will interfere with the fluorescent measurement of quinidine.

Carcinogenesis, Mutagenesis, Impairment of Fertility

Long-term studies to determine the carcinogenic potential of triamterene are not available. Studies to determine the mutagenic potential of triamterene are not available. Reproductive studies have been performed in rats at doses up to 30 times the human dose and have revealed no evidence of impaired fertility.

Pregnancy

Teratogenic Effects: Pregnancy Category B: Reproduction studies have been performed in rats at doses up to 30 times the human dose and have revealed no evidence of impaired fertility or harm to the fetus due to triamterene. There are, however, no adequate and well-controlled studies in pregnant women. Because animal reproductive studies are not always predictive of human response, this drug should be used during pregnancy only if clearly needed.

Nonteratogenic Effects: Triamterene has been shown to cross the placental barrier and appear in the cord blood of animals; this may occur in humans. The use of *Dyrenium* in pregnant women requires that the anticipated benefit be weighed against possible hazards to the fetus. These possible hazards include adverse reactions which have occurred in the adult.

Nursing Mothers: Triamterene appears in animal milk; this may occur in humans. If use of the drug is deemed essential, the patient should stop nursing.

Pediatric Use: Safety and effectiveness in children have not been established.

ADVERSE REACTIONS

Adverse effects are listed in decreasing order of frequency; however, the most serious adverse effects are listed first regardless of frequency. All adverse effects occur rarely (that is, one in 1000, or less).

Hypersensitivity: anaphylaxis, rash, photosensitivity.

Metabolic: hyperkalemia, hypokalemia.

Renal: azotemia, elevated BUN and creatinine, renal stones, acute interstitial nephritis (rare).

Gastrointestinal: jaundice and/or liver enzyme abnormalities, nausea and vomiting, diarrhea.

Hematologic: thrombocytopenia, megaloblastic anemia.

Central Nervous System: weakness, fatigue, dizziness, headache, dry mouth.

OVERDOSAGE

In the event of overdosage it can be theorized that electrolyte imbalance would be the major concern, with particular attention to possible hyperkalemia. Other symptoms that might be seen would be nausea and vomiting, other g.i. disturbances, and weakness. It is conceivable that some hypotension could occur. As with an overdose of any drug, immediate evacuation of the stomach should be induced through emesis and gastric lavage. Careful evaluation of the electrolyte pattern and fluid balance should be made. There is no specific antidote.

Reversible acute renal failure following ingestion of 50 tablets of a product containing a combination of 50 mg triamterene and 25 mg hydrochlorothiazide has been reported. The oral LD$_{50}$ in mice is 380 mg/kg. The amount of drug in a single dose ordinarily associated with symptoms of overdose or likely to be life-threatening is not known.

Although triamterene is 67% protein-bound, there may be some benefit to dialysis in cases of overdosage.

DOSAGE AND ADMINISTRATION

Adult Dosage

Dosage should be titrated to the needs of the individual patient. When used alone, the usual starting dose is 100 mg twice daily after meals. When combined with another diuretic or antihypertensive agent, the total daily dosage of each agent should usually be lowered initially and then adjusted to the patient's needs. The total daily dosage should not exceed 300 mg. Please refer to Precautions-General.

When Dyrenium (triamterene) is added to other diuretic therapy or when patients are switched to *Dyrenium* from other diuretics, all potassium supplementation should be discontinued.

HOW SUPPLIED

Capsules: 50 mg in bottles of 100 and in Single Unit Packages of 100 (intended for institutional use only); 100 mg in bottles of 100 and 1000 and in Single Unit Packages of 100 (intended for institutional use only).

Store at controlled room temperature (59°–86°F). Protect from light.

50 mg 100's: NDC 0108-3806-20

50 mg SUP 100's: NDC 0108-3806-21

100 mg 100's: NDC 0108-3807-20

100 mg SUP 100's: NDC 0108-3807-21

100 mg 1000's: NDC 0108-3807-30

Veterans Administration–Capsules, 100 mg, 100's, 6505-00-982-9143.

Military–Capsules, 100 mg, 100's, 6505-00-982-9143.

DY:L39

Shown in Product Identification Section, page 430

EMINASE®   ℞

[em-in-āz]

ANISTREPLASE

DESCRIPTION

Eminase (Anistreplase) is the p-anisoylated derivative of the Lys-Plasminogen-Streptokinase activator complex prepared *in vitro* by acylating human plasma-derived, purified, heat-treated, Lys-Plasminogen and purified Streptokinase from group C β-hemolytic streptococci. *Eminase* has a molecular weight of about 131,000. Each vial of *Eminase* is supplied as a sterile, lyophilized, white to off-white powder containing 30 units of Anistreplase, < 3 mg dimethylsulfoxide, < 0.2 mg sodium hydroxide and the following buffers and stabilizers: 150 μg p-amidinophenyl-p'-anisate (acylating agent), 100 mg mannitol, 46 mg L-lysine, 30 mg Albumin (Human), < 2 mg glycerol, and 1.3 mg ε-aminocaproic acid. *Eminase* is intended only for intravenous (I.V.) injection after reconstitution with **Sterile Water for Injection, USP.** The preparation contains no preservatives and is intended to be used as a single dose. Potency is expressed in units of Anistreplase by using a reference standard which is specific for *Eminase* and is not comparable with units used for other fibrinolytics. The Lys-Plasminogen and the Streptokinase used in the manufacture of *Eminase* are prepared under U.S. license by Oesterreichisches Institut fuer Haemoderivate GmbH and Behringwerke AG, respectively, under shared manufacturing arrangements.

CLINICAL PHARMACOLOGY

Eminase is an inactive derivative of a fibrinolytic enzyme with the catalytic center of the activator complex temporarily blocked by an anisoyl group. The anisoyl group does not decrease the high fibrin-binding ability of the complex. *Eminase* is made *in vitro* from Lys-Plasminogen and Streptokinase. *Eminase* differs from the complex initially formed *in vivo* upon administration of Streptokinase; the latter complex contains predominately glu-plasminogen. Activation of *Eminase* occurs with release of the anisoyl group by deacylation, a non-enzymatic first-order process with a half-life *in vitro* in human blood of about 2 hours. In solution, deacylation of *Eminase* starts immediately and the enzymatically active Lys-Plasminogen-Streptokinase activator complex is progressively formed. The production of plasmin from plasminogen by deacylated *Eminase* can take place in the bloodstream or within the thrombus; the latter process is catalytically more efficient but both may contribute to thrombolysis. The half-life of fibrinolytic activity of the circulating *Eminase* is 70 to 120 minutes (mean 94 minutes).

A number of controlled clinical studies have been performed with *Eminase* to demonstrate benefit. Heparin anticoagulation was administered to all patients routinely following (about 4 to 6 hours) dosing with *Eminase*.

Randomized, controlled studies have demonstrated that *Eminase* reduces mortality when administered within 6 hours of the onset of the symptoms of acute myocardial infarction (AMI). The benefit of mortality reduction occurs acutely and is maintained for at least one year.

In a study of 1258 patients (AIMS trial), mortality at 30 days postinfarction was decreased (47.2%, p = 0.0001) in patients receiving *Eminase* as compared with placebo. At one year, the reduction in mortality was maintained (38%, p = 0.001). The incidence of heart failure was less in patients treated with *Eminase* (17.9%) compared with patients who received placebo (23.3%).[1,2] Similar mortality results were obtained from a smaller, randomized, controlled trial.[1,3]

In a double-blind, randomized trial of *Eminase* compared with heparin bolus, left ventricular function was improved and infarction size reduced. There was significantly (p < 0.01, two sample t-test) higher left ventricular ejection fraction (LVEF) for the *Eminase* treatment group (53%) compared with the heparin treatment group (47.5%) when measured 4 days after treatment (intent-to-treat analysis). This difference was maintained when patients were reexamined by radionuclide ventriculography at day 19, even when patients who experienced successful angioplasty were excluded from the analysis (p = 0.04). About 3 weeks after treatment, mean infarct size was 24% lower in the patients treated with *Eminase* compared with those treated with heparin (n = 188, p = 0.02).[1,4] Similarly, if those patients who experienced successful angioplasty were excluded from the analysis, the mean infarct size in patients treated with *Eminase* was significantly less than that of heparin-treated patients (p < 0.01).

In randomized, comparative studies reperfusion rates of between 50% and 68% have been reported in patients receiv-

ing *Eminase* within 6 hours of symptom onset. However, for maximum rates of reperfusion, treatment should be initiated as soon as possible after onset of symptoms.

In two studies,[1,5,6] *Eminase* and intracoronary (IC) Streptokinase were compared in patients with angiographically proven coronary artery occlusion. Reperfusion occurred about 45 minutes after the start of therapy for both treatment groups. When therapy was initiated within 4 hours of onset of AMI symptoms reperfusion rates of 59% (n = 87) and 68% (n = 41) were observed for *Eminase* compared with 59% (n = 85) and 70% (n = 43) for IC Streptokinase. Of those patients who had coronary artery reperfusion, angiographically demonstrated reocclusion occurred within 24 hours in 3% to 4% of those treated with *Eminase* and in 7% to 12% of those treated with Streptokinase.[1,5,6]

In a well-controlled, randomized study, a patency rate of 72% was obtained with *Eminase* compared with 53% for I.V. Streptokinase. Patency for the 107 patients was determined by posttreatment angiography.[1,7]

Eminase was also found to have a favorable risk/benefit profile in elderly patients (> 65 years, n = 940) who participated in clinical trials. Use of *Eminase* in patients over 75 years old has not been adequately studied.

INDICATIONS AND USAGE

Eminase is indicated for use in the management of acute myocardial infarction (AMI) in adults, for the lysis of thrombi obstructing coronary arteries, the reduction of infarct size, the improvement of ventricular function following AMI, and the reduction of mortality associated with AMI. Treatment should be initiated as soon as possible after the onset of AMI symptoms (**see CLINICAL PHARMACOLOGY**).

CONTRAINDICATIONS

Because thrombolytic therapy increases the risk of bleeding, *Eminase* is contraindicated in the following situations:

- active internal bleeding
- history of cerebrovascular accident
- recent (within 2 months) intracranial or intraspinal surgery or trauma (**see WARNINGS**)
- intracranial neoplasm, arteriovenous malformation, or aneurysm
- known bleeding diathesis
- severe, uncontrolled hypertension

Eminase should not be administered to patients having experienced severe allergic reactions to either this product or Streptokinase.

WARNINGS

Bleeding: (See ADVERSE REACTIONS) The most common complication associated with *Eminase* therapy is bleeding. The types of bleeding associated with thrombolytic therapy can be divided into two broad categories:

1. Internal bleeding involving the gastrointestinal tract, genitourinary tract, retroperitoneal, ocular, or intracranial sites.
2. Superficial or surface bleeding, observed mainly at invaded or disturbed sites (e.g., venous cutdowns, arterial punctures, sites of recent surgical intervention).

The concomitant use of heparin anticoagulation may contribute to the bleeding. Some of the hemorrhagic episodes occurred one or more days after the effects of *Eminase* had dissipated, but while heparin therapy was continuing.

As fibrin is lysed during *Eminase* therapy, bleeding from recent puncture sites may occur. Therefore, thrombolytic therapy requires careful attention to all potential bleeding sites (including catheter insertion sites, arterial and venous puncture sites, cutdown sites, and needle puncture sites).

Intramuscular injections and nonessential handling of the patient should be avoided during treatment with *Eminase*. Venipunctures should be performed carefully and only as required.

Should an arterial puncture be necessary following administration of *Eminase*, it is preferable to use an upper-extremity vessel that is accessible to manual compression. A pressure dressing should be applied, and the puncture site should be checked frequently for evidence of bleeding.

Each patient being considered for therapy with *Eminase* should be carefully evaluated and anticipated benefits should be weighed against potential risks associated with therapy.

In the following conditions, the risks of *Eminase* therapy may be increased and should be weighed against the anticipated benefits:

- recent (within 10 days) major surgery (e.g., coronary artery bypass graft, obstetrical delivery, organ biopsy, previous puncture of noncompressible vessels)
- cerebrovascular disease
- recent gastrointestinal or genitourinary bleeding (within 10 days)
- recent trauma (within 10 days) including cardiopulmonary resuscitation
- hypertension: systolic BP ≥180 mmHg and/or diastolic BP ≥110 mmHg
- high likelihood of left heart thrombus (e.g., mitral stenosis with atrial fibrillation)
- subacute bacterial endocarditis
- acute pericarditis
- hemostatic defects including those secondary to severe hepatic or renal disease
- pregnancy
- age > 75 years (Use of *Eminase* in patients over 75 years old has not been adequately studied.)
- diabetic hemorrhagic retinopathy or other hemorrhagic ophthalmic conditions
- septic thrombophlebitis or occluded AV cannula at seriously infected site
- patients currently receiving oral anticoagulants (e.g., warfarin sodium)
- any other condition in which bleeding constitutes a significant hazard or would be particularly difficult to manage because of its location

Arrhythmias: Coronary thrombolysis may result in arrhythmias associated with reperfusion. These arrhythmias (such as sinus bradycardia, accelerated idioventricular rhythm, ventricular premature depolarizations, ventricular tachycardia) are not different from those often seen in the ordinary course of acute myocardial infarction and may be managed with standard antiarrhythmic measures. It is recommended that antiarrhythmic therapy for bradycardia and/or ventricular irritability be available when injections of *Eminase* are administered.

Hypotension: Hypotension, sometimes severe, not secondary to bleeding or anaphylaxis, has occasionally been observed soon after intravenous *Eminase* administration. Patients should be monitored closely and, should symptomatic or alarming hypotension occur, appropriate symptomatic treatment should be administered.

PRECAUTIONS

General: Standard management of myocardial infarction should be implemented concomitantly with *Eminase* treatment. Invasive procedures should be minimized (**see WARNINGS**). Anaphylactoid reactions have rarely been reported in patients who received *Eminase*. Accordingly, adequate treatment provisions such as epinephrine should be available for immediate use.

Readministration: Because of the increased likelihood of resistance due to antistreptokinase antibody, Eminase (Anistreplase) may not be as effective if administered more than 5 days after prior *Eminase* or Streptokinase therapy or streptococcal infection, particularly between 5 days and 6 months. Increased antistreptokinase antibody levels between 5 days and 6 months after *Eminase* or Streptokinase administration may also increase the risk of allergic reactions.

Repeated administration of *Eminase* within one week of the initial dose has occurred in a small number of patients treated for AMI and non-AMI conditions. The incidence of hematomas/bruising was somewhat greater in those patients who received repeat doses of *Eminase* but otherwise the adverse event profile was similar to those who received one dose.

Laboratory Tests: Intravenous administration of *Eminase* will cause marked decreases in plasminogen and fibrinogen and increases in thrombin time (TT), activated partial thromboplastin time (APTT), and prothrombin time (PT).

Results of coagulation tests and/or measures of fibrinolytic activity performed during *Eminase* therapy may be unreliable unless specific precautions are taken to prevent *in vitro* artifacts. *Eminase*, when present in blood in pharmacologic concentrations, remains active under *in vitro* conditions. This can lead to degradation of fibrinogen in blood samples removed for analysis. Collection of blood samples in the presence of aprotinin (2000 to 3000 KIU/mL) can, to some extent, mitigate this phenomenon.

Drug Interactions: The interaction of *Eminase* with other cardioactive drugs has not been studied. In addition to bleeding associated with heparin and vitamin K antagonists, drugs that alter platelet function (such as aspirin and dipyridamole) may increase the risk of bleeding if administered prior to *Eminase* therapy.

Use of Anticoagulants: *Eminase* alone or in combination with antiplatelet agents and anticoagulants may cause bleeding complications. Therefore, careful monitoring is advised, especially at arterial puncture sites. In clinical studies, a majority of patients treated received anticoagulant therapy postdosing with *Eminase* during their hospital stay and a minority received heparin pretreatment with *Eminase*. The use of antiplatelet agents increased the incidence of bleeding events similarly in patients treated with *Eminase* or non-thrombolytic therapy. There was no evidence of a synergistic effect of combined *Eminase* and antiplatelet agents on bleeding events. In addition, there was no difference in the incidence of hemorrhagic CVAs in *Eminase*-treated patients who did or did not receive aspirin.

Carcinogenesis, Mutagenesis, Impairment of Fertility: Long-term studies in animals have not been performed to evaluate the carcinogenic potential or the effect on fertility. Studies to determine mutagenicity and chromosomal aberration assays in human lymphocytes were negative at all concentrations tested.

Pregnancy (Category C): Animal reproduction studies have not been conducted with *Eminase*. It is also not known whether *Eminase* can cause fetal harm when administered to a pregnant woman or can affect reproduction capacity. *Eminase* should be given to a pregnant woman only if clearly needed.

Nursing Mothers: It is not known whether *Eminase* is excreted in human milk. Because many drugs are excreted in human milk, the physician should decide whether the patient should discontinue nursing or not receive *Eminase*.

Pediatric Use: Safety and effectiveness of *Eminase* in children have not been established.

ADVERSE REACTIONS

Bleeding: The incidence of bleeding (major or minor) varied widely from study to study and may depend on the use of arterial catheterization and other invasive procedures, patient population, and/or concomitant therapy. The overall incidence of bleeding in patients treated with *Eminase* in clinical trials (n = 5275) was 14.6%, with nonpuncture-site bleeding occurring in 10.2%, and puncture-site bleeding occurring in 5.7%, of these patients. Bleeding at the puncture site occurred more frequently in clinical trials in which the patients underwent immediate coronary catheterization (13.3%, n = 637) compared with those who did not (3.0%, n = 2023). The incidence of presumed intracranial bleeding within 7 days postdosing with *Eminase* was 0.57% (n = 5275; 0.34% etiology confirmed hemorrhagic; 0.23% etiology not confirmed) compared to 0.16% (n = 1249) after nonthrombolytic therapy.

In the AIMS trial the overall incidence of bleeding in patients treated with *Eminase* was 14.8% compared with 3.8% for placebo. The incidence of specific bleeding events was:

Type of Bleeding	EMINASE® (n=500)	Placebo (n=501)
Puncture site	4.6%	<1%
Nonpuncture site hematoma	2.8%	<1%
Hematuria/Genitourinary	2.4%	<1%
Hemoptysis	2.2%	<1%
Gastrointestinal hemorrhage	2.0%	1.4%
Intracranial	1.0%	<1%
Gum/Mouth hemorrhage	1.0%	0
Epistaxis	<1%	<1%
Anemia	<1%	<1%
Eye hemorrhage	<1%	<1%
Hemorrhage (unspecified)	<1%	0

In this study there was no difference between *Eminase* and placebo in the incidence of major bleeding events.

Should serious bleeding (not controlled by local pressure) occur in a critical location (intracranial, gastrointestinal, retroperitoneal, pericardial), any concomitant heparin should be terminated immediately and the administration of protamine to reverse heparinization should be considered. If necessary, the bleeding tendency can be reversed with appropriate replacement therapy.

Minor bleeding can be anticipated mainly at invaded or disturbed sites. If such bleeding occurs, local measures should be taken to control the bleeding (**see WARNINGS**).

Cardiovascular: The most frequently reported adverse experiences in *Eminase* clinical trials (n = 5275) were arrhythmia/conduction disorders which were reported in 38% of patients treated with *Eminase* and 46% of nonthrombolytic control patients. Hypotension occurred in 10.4% of patients treated with *Eminase* compared to 7.9% for patients who received nonthrombolytic treatment (**see WARNINGS**).

Allergic-type Reactions: Anaphylactic and anaphylactoid reactions have been observed rarely (0.2%) in patients treated with *Eminase* and are similar in incidence to Streptokinase (0.1% anaphylactic shock in one study). These included symptoms such as bronchospasm or angioedema.

Other milder or delayed effects such as urticaria, itching, flushing, rashes and eosinophilia have been occasionally observed. A delayed purpuric rash appearing one to two weeks after treatment has been reported in 0.3% of patients. The rash may also be associated with arthralgia, ankle edema, gastrointestinal symptoms, mild hematuria and mild proteinuria. This syndrome was self-limiting and without long-term sequelae.

Risk of Viral Transmission: Six batches of *Eminase* (five different batches of Lys-Plasminogen) were used in clinical trials designed specifically to monitor possible hepatitis non-A, non-B transmission. No case of hepatitis was diagnosed in patients receiving *Eminase*. Lys-Plasminogen is derived from human plasma obtained from FDA approved sources and tested for absence of viral contamination, including human immunodeficiency virus type-1 (HIV-1) and hepatitis B surface antigen. The manufacturing process includes a vapor-heat treatment step for inactivation of viruses. The entire manufacturing process has also been validated to yield a cumulative reduction of $\geq 10^{21}$ fold HIV-1 infectious particles, i.e., $\geq 10^{6}$ infectious particles removed by vapor-heat

Continued on next page

SmithKline Beecham—Cont.

treatment and a cumulative total of $\geq 10^{15}$ infectious particles removed by the various steps in the purification process.

Causal Relationship Unknown: Since the following experiences may also be associated with AMI or other therapy, the causal relationship to *Eminase* administration is unknown. The following adverse experiences were infrequently (<10%) reported in clinical trials: **Body as a Whole**—chills, fever, headache, shock; **Cardiovascular**—cardiac rupture, chest pain, emboli; **Dermatology**—purpura, sweating; **Gastrointestinal**—nausea and/or vomiting; **Hemic and Lymphatic**—thrombocytopenia; **Metabolic and Nutritional**—elevated transaminase levels; **Musculoskeletal**—arthralgia; **Nervous**—agitation, dizziness, paresthesia, tremor, vertigo; **Respiratory**—dyspnea, lung edema.

DOSAGE AND ADMINISTRATION

Administer *Eminase* as soon as possible after the onset of symptoms. The recommended dose is 30 units of *Eminase* administered only by intravenous injection over 2 to 5 minutes into an intravenous line or vein.

Reconstitution:

1. Slowly add 5 mL of **Sterile Water for Injection, USP,** by directing the stream of fluid against the side of the vial.
2. Gently roll the vial, mixing the dry powder and fluid. **Do not shake.** Try to minimize foaming.
3. The reconstituted preparation is a colorless to pale yellow transparent solution. Before administration, the product should be visually inspected for particulate matter and discoloration.
4. Withdraw the entire contents of the vial.
5. The reconstituted solution should not be further diluted before administration or added to any infusion fluids. No other medications should be added to the vial or syringe containing *Eminase.*
6. If *Eminase* is not administered within 30 minutes of reconstitution, it should be discarded.

HOW SUPPLIED

Eminase is supplied as a sterile, lyophilized powder in 30-unit vials. NDC 57294-030-20.

Storage: Store lyophilized *Eminase* between 2°–8°C (36°–46°F).

Do not use beyond the expiration date printed on the vial.

REFERENCES

1. Data on File. SmithKline Beecham Pharmaceuticals, Philadelphia.
2. AIMS Trial Study Group. Effect of intravenous APSAC on mortality after acute myocardial infarction: preliminary report of a placebo-controlled clinical trial. Lancet 1988; 1:545–9.
3. Meinertz T, Kasper W, Schumacher M, Just H for the APSAC multicenter trial group. The German multicenter trial of anisoylated plasminogen streptokinase activator complex versus heparin for acute myocardial infarction. Am J Cardiol 1988; 62:347–51.
4. Bassand JP, Machecourt J, Cassagnes J, et al. Multicenter trial of intravenous anisoylated plasminogen streptokinase activator complex (APSAC) in acute myocardial infarction: effects on infarct size and left ventricular function. J Am Coll Cardiol 1989; 13:988–97.
5. Anderson JL, Rothbard RL, Hackworthy RA, et al. Multicenter reperfusion trial of intravenous anisoylated plasminogen streptokinase activator complex (APSAC) in acute myocardial infarction: controlled comparison with intracoronary streptokinase. J Am Coll Cardiol 1988; 11:1153–63.
6. Bonnier HJRM, Visser RF, Klomps HC, Hoffmann HJML and the Dutch Invasive Reperfusion Study Group. Comparison of intravenous anisoylated plasminogen streptokinase activator complex and intracoronary streptokinase in acute myocardial infarction. Am J Cardiol 1988; 62:25–30.
7. Brochier ML, Quilliet L, Kulbertus H, et al. Intravenous anisoylated plasminogen streptokinase activator complex versus intravenous streptokinase in evolving myocardial infarction: preliminary data from a randomized multicentre study. Drugs 1987; 33(Suppl 3):140–5.

0938330

Manufactured by:
Beecham-Wulfing
Neuss, West Germany

Distributed by:
SmithKline Beecham Pharmaceuticals
Philadelphia, PA 19101

U.S. License No. 1097
April, 1991

EM:L1

Shown in Product Identification Section, page 430

ENGERIX-B® ℞

[en 'jur-ix bee]
Hepatitis B Vaccine (Recombinant)

DESCRIPTION

Engerix-B [Hepatitis B Vaccine (Recombinant)] is a noninfectious recombinant DNA hepatitis B vaccine developed and manufactured by SmithKline Beecham Biologicals. It contains purified surface antigen of the virus obtained by culturing genetically engineered *Saccharomyces cerevisiae* cells, which carry the surface antigen gene of the hepatitis B virus. The surface antigen expressed in *Saccharomyces cerevisiae* cells is purified by several physicochemical steps and formulated as a suspension of the antigen adsorbed on aluminum hydroxide. The procedures used to manufacture *Engerix-B* result in a product that contains no more than 5% yeast protein.

No substances of human origin are used in its manufacture.

Engerix-B is supplied as a sterile suspension for intramuscular administration. The vaccine is ready for use without reconstitution; it must be shaken before administration since a fine white deposit with a clear colorless supernatant may form on storage.

Each 1 mL adult dose of vaccine consists of 20 mcg of hepatitis B surface antigen adsorbed on 0.5 mg aluminum as aluminum hydroxide. Each 0.5 mL pediatric dose of vaccine consists of 10 mcg of hepatitis B surface antigen adsorbed on 0.25 mg aluminum as aluminum hydroxide. Both formulations contain 1:20,000 thimerosal (mercury derivative) as a preservative, sodium chloride (9 mg/mL) and phosphate buffers (disodium phosphate dihydrate, 0.98 mg/mL; sodium dihydrogen phosphate dihydrate, 0.71 mg/mL).

CLINICAL PHARMACOLOGY

Several hepatitis viruses are known to cause a systemic infection resulting in major pathologic changes in the liver (e.g., A, B, C, D, E). The estimated lifetime risk of HBV infection in the United States varies from almost 100% for the highest-risk groups to approximately 5% for the population as a whole.[1]

Hepatitis B infection can have serious consequences including acute massive hepatic necrosis, chronic active hepatitis and cirrhosis of the liver. Sixty to 80% of neonates and 6 to 10% of adults who are infected in the United States will become hepatitis B virus carriers.[1] It has been estimated that more than 170 million people in the world today are persistently infected with hepatitis B virus.[2] The Centers for Disease Control (CDC) estimates that there are approximately 0.75 to 1.0 million chronic carriers of hepatitis B virus in the United States.[1] Those patients who become chronic carriers can infect others and are at increased risk of developing primary hepatocellular carcinoma. Among other factors, infection with hepatitis B may be the single most important factor for development of this carcinoma.[1,3] Considering the serious consequences of infection, immunization should be considered for all persons at potential risk of exposure to the hepatitis B virus.

Mothers infected with hepatitis B virus can infect their infants at, or shortly after, birth if they are carriers of the HBsAg antigen or develop an active infection during the third trimester of pregnancy. Infected infants usually become chronic carriers. Therefore, screening of pregnant women for hepatitis B is recommended.[1]

There is no specific treatment for acute hepatitis B infection. However, those who develop anti-HBs antibodies after active infection are usually protected against subsequent infection. Antibody titers ≥10 mIU/mL against HBsAg are recognized as conferring protection against hepatitis B.[4] Seroconversion is defined as antibody titers ≥1 mIU/mL.

Immunogenicity in Healthy Adults and Adolescents: Clinical trials in healthy adult and adolescent subjects have shown that following a course of three doses of 20 mcg *Engerix-B* given according to the Immunization Practices Advisory Committee (ACIP) recommended schedule of injections at months 0, 1 and 6, the seroprotection (antibody titers ≥10 mIU/mL) rate for all individuals was 79% at month 6 and 96% at month 7; the geometric mean antibody titer (GMT) for seroconverters at month 7 was 2,204 mIU/mL. On an alternate schedule (injections at months 0, 1 and 2) designed for certain populations (e.g., neonates born of hepatitis B infected mothers, individuals who have or might have been recently exposed to the virus, and certain travelers to high-risk areas. See INDICATIONS AND USAGE.), 99% of all individuals were seroprotected at month 3 and remained protected through month 12. On the alternate schedule, an additional dose at 12 months produced a GMT for seroconverters at month 13 of 9,163 mIU/mL.

Immunogenicity in Neonates: Immunization with 10 mcg at 0, 1 and 2 months of age produced a seroprotection rate of 96% in infants by month 4, with a GMT among seroconverters of 210 mIU/mL (N=311); an additional dose at month 12 produced a GMT among seroconverters of 2,941 mIU/mL at month 13 (N=126).

Immunization with 10 mcg at 0, 1 and 6 months of age produced seroconversion in 100% of infants by month 7 with a GMT of 713 mIU/mL (N=52), and the seroprotection rate was 97%.

Clinical trials indicate that administration of hepatitis B immune globulin at birth does not alter the response to *Engerix-B.*

Immunogenicity in Children 6 Months to, and Including, 10 Years: In clinical trials with 242 children ages 6 months to, and including, 10 years given 10 mcg at months 0, 1 and 6, the seroprotection rate was 98% one to two months after the third dose; the GMT of seroconverters was 4,023 mIU/mL.

Immunogenicity in Older Subjects: Among older subjects given 20 mcg at months 0, 1 and 6, the seroprotection rate one month after the third dose was 88%. However, as with other hepatitis B vaccines, in adults over 40 years of age, *Engerix-B* vaccine produced anti-HBs titers that were lower than those in younger adults (GMT among seroconverters one month after the third 20 mcg dose with a 0, 1, 6-month schedule: 610 mIU/mL for individuals over 40 years of age, N=50).

Hemodialysis Patients: Hemodialysis patients given hepatitis B vaccines respond with lower titers,[5] which remain at protective levels for shorter durations than in normal subjects. In a study in which patients on chronic hemodialysis (mean time on dialysis was 24 months; N=562) received 40 mcg of the plasma-derived vaccine at months 0, 1 and 6, approximately 50% of patients achieved antibody titers ≥10 mIU/mL.[5]

Since a fourth dose of *Engerix-B* given to healthy adults at month 12 following the 0, 1, 2-month schedule resulted in a substantial increase in the GMT (see above), a four-dose regimen was studied in hemodialysis patients. In a clinical trial of adults who had been on hemodialysis for a mean of 56 months (N=43), 67% of patients were seroprotected two months after the last dose of 40 mcg of *Engerix-B* (two × 20 mcg) given on a 0, 1, 2, 6-month schedule; the GMT among seroconverters was 93 mIU/mL.

Protective Efficacy: Protective efficacy with *Engerix-B* has been demonstrated in a clinical trial in neonates at high risk of hepatitis B infection.[6,7] Fifty-eight neonates born of mothers who were both HBsAg and HBeAg positive were given *Engerix-B* (10 mcg at 0, 1 and 2 months) without concomitant hepatitis B immune globulin. Two infants became chronic carriers in the 12-month follow-up period after initial inoculation. Assuming an expected carrier rate of 70%,[1] the protective efficacy rate against the chronic carrier state during the first 12 months of life was 95%.

Other Clinical Studies: In one study,[8] four of 244 (1.6%) adults (homosexual men) at high risk of contracting hepatitis B virus became infected during the period prior to completion of three doses of *Engerix-B* (20 mcg at 0, 1, 6 months). No additional patients became infected during the 18-month follow-up period after completion of the immunization course.

Interchangeability with Other Hepatitis B Vaccines: Recombinant DNA vaccines are produced in yeast by expression of a hepatitis B virus gene sequence that codes for the hepatitis B surface antigen. Like plasma-derived vaccine, the yeast-derived vaccines are protein particles visible by electron microscopy and have hepatitis B surface antigen epitopes as determined by monoclonal antibody analyses.

Yeast-derived vaccines have been shown by *in vitro* analyses to induce antibodies (anti-HBs) which are immunologically comparable by epitope specificity and binding affinity to antibodies induced by plasma-derived vaccine.[9] In cross absorption studies, no differences were detected in the spectra of antibodies induced in man to plasma-derived or to yeast-derived hepatitis B vaccines.[9]

Additionally, patients immunized approximately three years previously with plasma-derived vaccine and whose antibody titers were <100 mIU/mL (GMT: 35 mIU/mL; range: 9–94) were given a 20 mcg dose of *Engerix-B.* All patients, including two who had not responded to the plasma-derived vaccine, showed a response to *Engerix-B* (GMT: 5,069 mIU/mL; range: 624–15,019).

There have been no clinical studies in which a three-dose vaccine series was initiated with a plasma-derived hepatitis B vaccine and completed with *Engerix-B,* or vice versa. However, because the *in vitro* and *in vivo* studies described above indicate the comparability of the antibody produced in response to plasma-derived vaccine and *Engerix-B,* it should be possible to interchange the use of *Engerix-B* and plasma-derived vaccines (but see CONTRAINDICATIONS).

A controlled study (N=48) demonstrated that completion of a course of immunization with one dose of *Engerix-B* (20 mcg, month 6) following two doses of Recombivax HB®* (10 mcg, months 0 and 1) produced a similar GMT (4,077 mIU/mL) to immunization with three doses of *Recombivax HB* (10 mcg, months 0, 1 and 6; 2,654 mIU/mL). Thus, *Engerix-B* can be used to complete a vaccination course initiated with *Recombivax HB.*

INDICATIONS AND USAGE

Engerix-B is indicated for immunization against infection caused by all known subtypes of hepatitis B virus. As hepati-

* yeast-derived, Hepatitis B Vaccine, MSD.

tis D (caused by the delta virus) does not occur in the absence of hepatitis B infection, it can be expected that hepatitis D will also be prevented by *Engerix-B* vaccination.

Engerix-B will not prevent hepatitis caused by other agents, such as hepatitis A, C and E viruses, or other pathogens known to infect the liver.

Immunization is recommended in persons of all ages, especially those who are, or will be, at increased risk of exposure to hepatitis B virus,[1] for example:

Health Care Personnel
Dentists and oral surgeons.
Dental, medical and nursing students.
Physicians, surgeons and podiatrists.
Nurses.
Paramedical and ambulance personnel and custodial staff who may be exposed to the virus via blood or other patient specimens.
Dental hygienists and dental nurses.
Laboratory and blood-bank personnel handling blood, blood products, and other patient specimens.
Hospital cleaning staff who handle waste.
Selected Patients and Patient Contacts
Patients and staff in hemodialysis units and hematology/ oncology units.
Patients requiring frequent and/or large volume blood transfusions or clotting factor concentrates (e.g., persons with hemophilia, thalassemia, sickle-cell anemia, cirrhosis).
Clients (residents) and staff of institutions for the mentally handicapped.
Classroom contacts of deinstitutionalized mentally handicapped persons who have persistent hepatitis B surface antigenemia and who show aggressive behavior.
Household and other intimate contacts of persons with persistent hepatitis B surface antigenemia.
Infants Born of HBsAg-Positive Mothers Whether HBeAg Positive or Negative (See DOSAGE AND ADMINISTRATION.)
Subpopulations with a Known High Incidence of the Disease, such as:
Alaskan Eskimos.
Pacific Islanders.
Indochinese immigrants.
Haitian immigrants.
Refugees from other HBV endemic areas.
All infants of women born in areas where the infection is highly endemic.
Persons Who May Be Exposed to the Hepatitis B Virus by Travel to High-Risk Areas (See ACIP Guidelines, 1985.)
Military Personnel Identified as Being at Increased Risk
Morticians and Embalmers
Persons at Increased Risk of the Disease Due to Their Sexual Practices, such as:
Persons with more than one sexual partner in a six-month period.
Persons who have contracted a sexually transmitted disease.
Homosexually active males.
Female prostitutes.
Prisoners
Users of Illicit Injectable Drugs
Others:
Police and fire department personnel who render first aid or medical assistance, and any others who, through their work or personal life-style, may be exposed to the hepatitis B virus.
Adoptees from countries of high HBV endemicity.

CONTRAINDICATIONS

Hypersensitivity to yeast or any other component of the vaccine is a contraindication for use of the vaccine.

WARNINGS

Patients experiencing hypersensitivity after an Engerix-B [Hepatitis B Vaccine (Recombinant)] injection should not receive further injections of *Engerix-B*. (See CONTRAINDICATIONS.)

Hepatitis B has a long incubation period. Hepatitis B vaccination may not prevent hepatitis B infection in individuals who had an unrecognized hepatitis B infection at the time of vaccine administration. Additionally, it may not prevent infection in individuals who do not achieve protective antibody titers.

PRECAUTIONS

General

As with any percutaneous vaccine, epinephrine should be available for use in case of anaphylaxis or anaphylactoid reaction.

As with any vaccine, administration of *Engerix-B* should be delayed, if possible, in persons with any febrile illness or active infection.

Pregnancy

Pregnancy Category C: Animal reproduction studies have not been conducted with *Engerix-B*. It is also not known whether *Engerix-B* can cause fetal harm when administered to a pregnant woman or can affect reproduction capacity.

Engerix-B should be given to a pregnant woman only if clearly needed.

Nursing Mothers

It is not known whether *Engerix-B* is excreted in human milk. Because many drugs are excreted in human milk, caution should be exercised when *Engerix-B* is administered to a nursing woman.

Pediatric Use

Engerix-B has been shown to be well tolerated and highly immunogenic in infants and children of all ages. Newborns also respond well; maternally transferred antibodies do not interfere with the active immune response to the vaccine. (See CLINICAL PHARMACOLOGY for seroconversion rates and titers in neonates and children. See DOSAGE AND ADMINISTRATION for recommended pediatric dosage and for recommended dosage for infants born of HBsAg-positive mothers.)

ADVERSE REACTIONS

Engerix-B [Hepatitis B Vaccine (Recombinant)] is generally well tolerated. During clinical studies involving over 10,000 individuals distributed over all age groups, no serious adverse reactions attributable to vaccine administration were reported. As with any vaccine, however, it is possible that expanded commercial use of the vaccine could reveal rare adverse reactions not observed in clinical studies.

Ten double-blind studies involving 2,252 subjects showed no significant difference in the frequency or severity of adverse experiences between *Engerix-B* and plasma-derived vaccines. In 36 clinical studies a total of 13,495 doses of *Engerix-B* were administered to 5,071 healthy adults and children who were initially seronegative for hepatitis B markers, and healthy neonates. All subjects were monitored for 4 days post-administration. Frequency of adverse experiences tended to decrease with successive doses of *Engerix-B*. Using a symptom checklist,[‡] the most frequently reported adverse reactions were injection site soreness (22%) and fatigue[‡] (14%). Other reactions are listed below.

Incidence 1% to 10% of Injections

Local reactions at injection site: Induration; erythema; swelling.
Body as a whole: Fever (> 37.5°C).
Nervous system: Headache[‡]; dizziness.[‡]

Incidence < 1% of Injections

Local reactions at injection site: Pain; pruritus; ecchymosis.
Body as a whole: Sweating; malaise; chills; weakness; flushing; tingling.
Cardiovascular system: Hypotension.
Respiratory system: Influenza-like symptoms; upper respiratory tract illnesses.
Gastrointestinal system: Nausea; anorexia; abdominal pain/cramps; vomiting; constipation; diarrhea.
Lymphatic system: Lymphadenopathy.
Musculoskeletal system: Pain/stiffness in arm, shoulder or neck; arthralgia; myalgia; back pain.
Skin and appendages: Rash; urticaria; petechiae; pruritus; erythema.
Nervous system: Somnolence; insomnia; irritability; agitation.

Additional adverse experiences have been reported with the commercial use of *Engerix-B*. Those listed below are to serve as alerting information to physicians.
Hypersensitivity: Anaphylaxis; erythema multiforme including Stevens-Johnson syndrome; angioedema; arthritis.
Cardiovascular system: Tachycardia/palpitations.
Respiratory system: Bronchospasm including asthma-like symptoms.
Gastrointestinal system: Abnormal liver function tests; dyspepsia.
Nervous system: Migraine; syncope; paresis; neuropathy including hypoesthesia, paresthesia, Guillain-Barré syndrome and Bell's palsy, transverse myelitis; optic neuritis.
Hematologic: Thrombocytopenia.
Skin and appendages: Eczema; purpura; herpes zoster; erythema nodosum.
Special senses: Conjunctivitis; keratitis; visual disturbances; vertigo; tinnitus; earache.
Potential Adverse Experiences: In addition, certain other adverse experiences not observed with *Engerix-B* have been reported with Heptavax-B®[†] and/or *Recombivax HB*. Those listed below are to serve as alerting information to physicians:
Urogenital system: Dysuria.

DOSAGE AND ADMINISTRATION

Injection: *Engerix-B* should be administered by intramuscular injection. *Do not inject intravenously or intradermally.* In adults, the injection should be given in the deltoid region but it may be preferable to inject in the anterolateral thigh in neonates and infants, who have smaller deltoid muscles. *Engerix-B* should not be administered in the gluteal region; such injections may result in suboptimal response.

[‡] Parent or guardian completed forms for children and neonates. Neonatal checklist did not include headache, fatigue or dizziness.
[†] plasma-derived, Hepatitis B Vaccine, MSD.

Engerix-B may be administered subcutaneously to persons at risk of hemorrhage (e.g., hemophiliacs). However, hepatitis B vaccines administered subcutaneously are known to result in lower GMTs. Additionally, when other aluminum-adsorbed vaccines have been administered subcutaneously, an increased incidence of local reactions including subcutaneous nodules has been observed. Therefore, subcutaneous administration should be used only in persons who are at risk of hemorrhage with intramuscular injections.

Preparation for Administration: Shake well before withdrawal and use. Parenteral drug products should be inspected visually for particulate matter or discoloration prior to administration. With thorough agitation, *Engerix-B* is a slightly opaque white suspension. Discard if it appears otherwise.

The vaccine should be used as supplied; no dilution or reconstitution is necessary. The full recommended dose of the vaccine should be used.

Dosing Schedules: The usual immunization regimen consists of 3 doses of vaccine given according to the following schedule:

1st dose: at elected date
2nd dose: 1 month later
3rd dose: 6 months after first dose

There is an alternate schedule with injections at 0, 1 and 2 months designed for certain populations (e.g., neonates born of hepatitis B infected mothers, others who have or might have been recently exposed to the virus, certain travelers to high-risk areas. See INDICATIONS AND USAGE.). On this alternate schedule, an additional dose at 12 months is recommended for infants born of infected mothers and for others for whom prolonged maintenance of protective titers is desired.

dosage for neonates through children up to, and including, 10 years: 10 mcg administered on either schedule.
dosage for other children and adults: 20 mcg administered on either schedule.
schedule and dosage for adult hemodialysis patients: 40 mcg (2 × 20 mcg in one or two injections) at 0, 1, 2 and 6 months. For hemodialysis patients, in whom vaccine-induced protection is less complete and may persist only as long as antibody levels remain above 10 mIU/mL, the need for booster doses should be assessed by annual antibody testing. 40 mcg (two × 20 mcg) booster doses with *Engerix-B* should be given when antibody levels decline below 10 mIU/mL.[1] Data show individuals given a booster with *Engerix-B* achieve high antibody titers. (See CLINICAL PHARMACOLOGY.)
booster vaccinations: Whenever administration of a booster dose is appropriate, the dose of *Engerix-B* is 10 mcg for children 10 years of age and under; 20 mcg for other children and adults. Studies have demonstrated a substantial increase in antibody titers after *Engerix-B* booster vaccination following an initial course with both plasma- and yeast-derived vaccines. (See CLINICAL PHARMACOLOGY.)

See previous section for discussion on booster vaccination for adult hemodialysis patients.

Known or presumed exposure to hepatitis B virus: Unprotected individuals with known or presumed exposure to the hepatitis B virus (e.g., neonates born of infected mothers, others experiencing percutaneous or permucosal exposure) should be given hepatitis B immune globulin (HBIG) in addition to *Engerix-B* in accordance with ACIP recommendations[1] and with the package insert for HBIG. *Engerix-B* can be given on either dosing schedule (see above).

STORAGE

Store between 2° and 8°C (35.6° to 46.6°F). *Do not freeze;* discard if product has been frozen.
Do not dilute to administer.

HOW SUPPLIED

20 mcg/mL in Single-Dose Vials in packages of 1, 10 and 25 vials.
NDC 58160-860-01 (package of 1)
NDC 58160-860-11 (package of 10)
NDC 58160-860-16 (package of 25)
10 mcg/0.5 mL in Single-Dose Vials in packages of 1 vial.
NDC 58160-859-01 (package of 1)

REFERENCES

1. *MMWR:* Recommendations for protection against viral hepatitis. 39(Suppl. 2), Feb. 9, 1990.
2. Robinson, W.S.: Hepatitis B virus and the delta virus. In Mandell, G.L., Douglas, R.G., Bennett, J.E. (eds): *Principles and practice of infectious diseases,* vol. 3, New York, John Wiley & Sons, 1990, pp. 1204–1231.
3. Beasley, R.P., et al.: Efficacy of hepatitis B immune globulin for prevention of perinatal transmission of hepatitis B virus carrier state: final report of a randomized double-blind, placebo-controlled trial. *Hepatology* 3:135–141, 1983.
4. Ambrosch, F.: Persistence of vaccine-induced antibodies to hepatitis B surface antigen—the need for booster vaccina-

Continued on next page

SmithKline Beecham—Cont.

tion in adult subjects. *Postgrad. Med. J.* 63(Suppl. 2):129–135, 1987.

5. Stevens, C.E., et al.: Hepatitis B vaccine in patients receiving hemodialysis. *N. Engl. J. Med.* 311:496–501, 1984.

6. Andre, F.E., and Safary, A.: Clinical experience with a yeast-derived hepatitis B vaccine. In Zuckerman, A.J. (ed): *Viral hepatitis and liver disease,* Alan R. Liss, Inc., 1988, pp. 1025–1030.

7. Poovorawan, Y., et al.: Protective efficacy of a recombinant DNA hepatitis B vaccine in neonates of HBe antigen-positive mothers. *JAMA* 261(22):3278–3281, June 9, 1989.

8. Goilav, C., et al.: Immunization of homosexual men with a recombinant DNA vaccine against hepatitis B: immunogenicity and protection. In Zuckerman, A.J. (ed): *Viral hepatitis and liver disease,* Alan R. Liss, Inc., 1988, pp. 1057–1058.

9. Hauser, P., et al.: Immunological properties of recombinant HBsAg produced in yeast. *Postgrad. Med. J.* 63 (Suppl. 2): 83–91, 1987.

Manufactured by **SmithKline Beecham Biologicals**
Rixensart, Belgium
Distributed by **SmithKline Beecham Pharmaceuticals**
Philadelphia, PA 19101
Engerix-B® is a registered trademark of SmithKline Beecham.

EB:L11A

Shown in Product Identification Section, page 430

ESKALITH®

[*ess-kah 'lith*]
(brand of lithium carbonate)
Capsules, 300 mg
Tablets, 300 mg

ESKALITH CR®

(brand of lithium carbonate)
Controlled Release Tablets, 450 mg

℞

℞

> ### WARNING
> Lithium toxicity is closely related to serum lithium levels, and can occur at doses close to therapeutic levels. Facilities for prompt and accurate serum lithium determinations should be available before initiating therapy (see DOSAGE AND ADMINISTRATION).

DESCRIPTION

Eskalith contains lithium carbonate, a white, light alkaline powder with molecular formula Li_2CO_3 and molecular weight 73.89. Lithium is an element of the alkali-metal group with atomic number 3, atomic weight 6.94 and an emission line at 671 nm on the flame photometer.

Eskalith Capsules: Each capsule, with opaque gray cap and opaque yellow body, is imprinted with the product name ESKALITH and SKF and contains lithium carbonate, 300 mg. Inactive ingredients consist of benzyl alcohol, cetylpyridinium chloride, D&C Yellow No. 10, FD&C Green No. 3, FD&C Red No. 40, FD&C Yellow No. 6, gelatin, lactose, magnesium stearate, povidone, sodium lauryl sulfate, titanium dioxide and trace amounts of other inactive ingredients.

Eskalith Tablets: Each round, gray, scored tablet is debossed SKF and J09 and contains lithium carbonate, 300 mg. Inactive ingredients consist of cellulose, iron oxide, lactose, magnesium stearate and sodium lauryl sulfate.

Eskalith CR Controlled Release Tablets: Each round, buff, scored tablet is debossed SKF and J10 and contains lithium carbonate, 450 mg. Inactive ingredients consist of alginic acid, gelatin, iron oxide, magnesium stearate and sodium starch glycolate.

Eskalith CR tablets 450 mg are designed to release a portion of the dose initially and the remainder gradually; the release pattern of the controlled release tablets reduces the variability in lithium blood levels seen with the immediate release dosage forms.

ACTIONS

Preclinical studies have shown that lithium alters sodium transport in nerve and muscle cells and effects a shift toward intraneuronal metabolism of catecholamines, but the specific biochemical mechanism of lithium action in mania is unknown.

INDICATIONS

Eskalith (lithium carbonate) is indicated in the treatment of manic episodes of manic-depressive illness. Maintenance therapy prevents or diminishes the intensity of subsequent episodes in those manic-depressive patients with a history of mania.

Typical symptoms of mania include pressure of speech, motor hyperactivity, reduced need for sleep, flight of ideas, grandiosity, elation, poor judgment, aggressiveness and possibly hostility. When given to a patient experiencing a manic

episode, *Eskalith* may produce a normalization of symptomatology within 1 to 3 weeks.

WARNINGS

Lithium should generally not be given to patients with significant renal or cardiovascular disease, severe debilitation or dehydration, or sodium depletion, since the risk of lithium toxicity is very high in such patients. If the psychiatric indication is life-threatening, and if such a patient fails to respond to other measures, lithium treatment may be undertaken with extreme caution, including daily serum lithium determinations and adjustment to the usually low doses ordinarily tolerated by these individuals. In such instances, hospitalization is a necessity.

Chronic lithium therapy may be associated with diminution of renal concentrating ability, occasionally presenting as nephrogenic diabetes insipidus, with polyuria and polydipsia. Such patients should be carefully managed to avoid dehydration with resulting lithium retention and toxicity. This condition is usually reversible when lithium is discontinued. Morphologic changes with glomerular and interstitial fibrosis and nephron atrophy have been reported in patients on chronic lithium therapy. Morphologic changes have also been seen in manic-depressive patients never exposed to lithium. The relationship between renal functional and morphologic changes and their association with lithium therapy have not been established.

When kidney function is assessed, for baseline data prior to starting lithium therapy or thereafter, routine urinalysis and other tests may be used to evaluate tubular function (e.g., urine specific gravity or osmolality following a period of water deprivation, or 24-hour urine volume) and glomerular function (e.g., serum creatinine or creatinine clearance). During lithium therapy, progressive or sudden changes in renal function, even within the normal range, indicate the need for reevaluation of treatment.

An encephalopathic syndrome (characterized by weakness, lethargy, fever, tremulousness and confusion, extrapyramidal symptoms, leukocytosis, elevated serum enzymes, BUN and FBS) has occurred in a few patients treated with lithium plus a neuroleptic. In some instances, the syndrome was followed by irreversible brain damage. Because of a possible causal relationship between these events and the concomitant administration of lithium and neuroleptics, patients receiving such combined therapy should be monitored closely for early evidence of neurologic toxicity and treatment discontinued promptly if such signs appear. This encephalopathic syndrome may be similar to or the same as neuroleptic malignant syndrome (NMS).

Lithium toxicity is closely related to serum lithium levels, and can occur at doses close to therapeutic levels (see DOSAGE AND ADMINISTRATION).

Outpatients and their families should be warned that the patient must discontinue lithium carbonate therapy and contact his physician if such clinical signs of lithium toxicity as diarrhea, vomiting, tremor, mild ataxia, drowsiness or muscular weakness occur.

Lithium carbonate may impair mental and/or physical abilities. Caution patients about activities requiring alertness (e.g., operating vehicles or machinery).

Lithium may prolong the effects of neuromuscular blocking agents. Therefore, neuromuscular blocking agents should be given with caution to patients receiving lithium.

Usage in Pregnancy: Adverse effects on implantation in rats, embryo viability in mice and metabolism *in vitro* of rat testes and human spermatozoa have been attributed to lithium, as have teratogenicity in submammalian species and cleft palates in mice.

In humans, lithium carbonate may cause fetal harm when administered to a pregnant woman. Data from lithium birth registries suggest an increase in cardiac and other anomalies, especially Ebstein's anomaly. If this drug is used in women of childbearing potential, or during pregnancy, or if a patient becomes pregnant while taking this drug, the patient should be apprised of the potential hazard to the fetus.

Usage in Nursing Mothers: Lithium is excreted in human milk. Nursing should not be undertaken during lithium therapy except in rare and unusual circumstances where, in the view of the physician, the potential benefits to the mother outweigh possible hazards to the child.

Usage in Children: Since information regarding the safety and effectiveness of lithium carbonate in children under 12 years of age is not available, its use in such patients is not recommended at this time.

There has been a report of a transient syndrome of acute dystonia and hyperreflexia occurring in a 15 kg child who ingested 300 mg of lithium carbonate.

Usage in the Elderly: Elderly patients often require lower lithium dosages to achieve therapeutic serum levels. They may also exhibit adverse reactions at serum levels ordinarily tolerated by younger patients.

PRECAUTIONS

The ability to tolerate lithium is greater during the acute manic phase and decreases when manic symptoms subside (see DOSAGE AND ADMINISTRATION).

Caution should be used when lithium and diuretics are used concomitantly because diuretic-induced sodium loss may reduce the renal clearance of lithium and increase serum lithium levels with risk of lithium toxicity. Patients receiving such combined therapy should have serum lithium levels monitored closely and the lithium dosage adjusted if necessary.

The distribution space of lithium approximates that of total body water. Lithium is primarily excreted in urine with insignificant excretion in feces. Renal excretion of lithium is proportional to its plasma concentration. The half-life of elimination of lithium is approximately 24 hours. Lithium decreases sodium reabsorption by the renal tubules which could lead to sodium depletion. Therefore, it is essential for the patient to maintain a normal diet, including salt, and an adequate fluid intake (2500–3000 mL) at least during the initial stabilization period. Decreased tolerance to lithium has been reported to ensue from protracted sweating or diarrhea and, if such occur, supplemental fluid and salt should be administered under careful medical supervision and lithium intake reduced or suspended until the condition is resolved. In addition to sweating and diarrhea, concomitant infection with elevated temperatures may also necessitate a temporary reduction or cessation of medication.

Previously existing underlying thyroid disorders do not necessarily constitute a contraindication to lithium treatment; where hypothyroidism exists, careful monitoring of thyroid function during lithium stabilization and maintenance allows for correction of changing thyroid parameters, if any; where hypothyroidism occurs during lithium stabilization and maintenance, supplemental thyroid treatment may be used.

Indomethacin and piroxicam have been reported to increase significantly, steady state plasma lithium levels. In some cases, lithium toxicity has resulted from such interactions. There is also some evidence that other nonsteroidal anti-inflammatory agents may have a similar effect. When such combinations are used, increased plasma lithium level monitoring is recommended. Concurrent use of metronidazole with lithium may provoke lithium toxicity due to reduced renal clearance. Patients receiving such combined therapy should be monitored closely.

There is evidence that angiotensin-converting enzyme inhibitors, such as enalapril and captopril, may substantially increase steady-state plasma lithium levels, sometimes resulting in lithium toxicity. When such combinations are used, lithium dosage may need to be decreased, and plasma lithium levels should be measured more often.

Concurrent use of calcium channel blocking agents with lithium may increase the risk of neurotoxicity in the form of ataxia, tremors, nausea, vomiting, diarrhea and/or tinnitus. Caution is recommended.

The following drugs can lower serum lithium concentrations by increasing urinary lithium excretion: acetazolamide, urea, xanthine preparations and alkalinizing agents such as sodium bicarbonate.

ADVERSE REACTIONS

The occurrence and severity of adverse reactions are generally directly related to serum lithium concentrations as well as to individual patient sensitivity to lithium, and generally occur more frequently and with greater severity at higher concentrations.

Adverse reactions may be encountered at serum lithium levels below 1.5 mEq/L. Mild to moderate adverse reactions may occur at levels from 1.5 to 2.5 mEq/L, and moderate to severe reactions may be seen at levels of 2.0 mEq/L and above.

Fine hand tremor, polyuria and mild thirst may occur during initial therapy for the acute manic phase, and may persist throughout treatment. Transient and mild nausea and general discomfort may also appear during the first few days of lithium administration.

These side effects usually subside with continued treatment or a temporary reduction or cessation of dosage. If persistent, cessation of lithium therapy may be required.

Diarrhea, vomiting, drowsiness, muscular weakness and lack of coordination may be early signs of lithium intoxication, and can occur at lithium levels below 2.0 mEq/L. At higher levels, ataxia, giddiness, tinnitus, blurred vision and a large output of dilute urine may be seen. Serum lithium levels above 3.0 mEq/L may produce a complex clinical picture, involving multiple organs and organ systems. Serum lithium levels should not be permitted to exceed 2.0 mEq/L during the acute treatment phase.

The following reactions have been reported and appear to be related to serum lithium levels, including levels within the therapeutic range: **Neuromuscular/Central Nervous System**—tremor, muscle hyperirritability (fasciculations, twitching, clonic movements of whole limbs), hypertonicity, ataxia, choreo-athetotic movements, hyperactive deep tendon reflex, extrapyramidal symptoms including acute dystonia, cogwheel rigidity, blackout spells, epileptiform seizures, slurred speech, dizziness, vertigo, downbeat nystagmus, incontinence of urine or feces, somnolence, psychomotor retardation, restlessness, confusion, stupor, coma, tongue move-

ments, tics, tinnitus, hallucinations, poor memory, slowed intellectual functioning, startled response, worsening of organic brain syndromes; **Cardiovascular**—cardiac arrhythmia, hypotension, peripheral circulatory collapse, bradycardia, sinus node dysfunction with severe bradycardia (which may result in syncope); **Gastrointestinal**—anorexia, nausea, vomiting, diarrhea, gastritis, salivary gland swelling, abdominal pain, excessive salivation, flatulence, indigestion; **Genitourinary**—glycosuria, decreased creatinine clearance, albuminuria, oliguria, and symptoms of nephrogenic diabetes insipidus including polyuria, thirst and polydipsia; **Dermatologic**—drying and thinning of hair, alopecia, anesthesia of skin, acne, chronic folliculitis, xerosis cutis, psoriasis or its exacerbation, generalized pruritus with or without rash, cutaneous ulcers, angioedema; **Autonomic**—blurred vision, dry mouth, impotence/sexual dysfunction; **Thyroid Abnormalities**—euthyroid goiter and/or hypothyroidism (including myxedema) accompanied by lower T_3 and T_4. I^{131} uptake may be elevated. (See PRECAUTIONS.) Paradoxically, rare cases of hyperthyroidism have been reported; **EEG Changes**—diffuse slowing, widening of the frequency spectrum, potentiation and disorganization of background rhythm; **EKG Changes**—reversible flattening, isoelectricity or inversion of T-waves; **Miscellaneous**—fatigue, lethargy, transient scotomata, exophthalmos, dehydration, weight loss, leukocytosis, headache, transient hyperglycemia, hypercalcemia, hyperparathyroidism, excessive weight gain, edematous swelling of ankles or wrists, metallic taste, dysgeusia/taste distortion, salty taste, thirst, swollen lips, tightness in chest, swollen and/or painful joints, fever, polyarthralgia, dental caries.

Some reports of nephrogenic diabetes insipidus, hyperparathyroidism and hypothyroidism which persist after lithium discontinuation have been received.

A few reports have been received of the development of painful discoloration of fingers and toes and coldness of the extremities within one day of the starting of treatment with lithium. The mechanism through which these symptoms (resembling Raynaud's syndrome) developed is not known. Recovery followed discontinuance.

Cases of pseudotumor cerebri (increased intracranial pressure and papilledema) have been reported with lithium use. If undetected, this condition may result in enlargement of the blind spot, constriction of visual fields and eventual blindness due to optic atrophy.

Lithium should be discontinued, if clinically possible, if this syndrome occurs.

DOSAGE AND ADMINISTRATION

Immediate release capsules and tablets are usually given t.i.d. or q.i.d. Doses of controlled release tablets are usually given b.i.d. (approximately 12-hour intervals). When initiating therapy with immediate release or controlled release lithium, dosage must be individualized according to serum levels and clinical response.

When switching a patient from immediate release capsules or tablets to the Eskalith CR (lithium carbonate) Controlled Release Tablets, give the same total daily dose when possible. Most patients on maintenance therapy are stabilized on 900 mg daily, e.g., 450 mg *Eskalith CR* b.i.d. When the previous dosage of immediate release lithium is not a multiple of 450 mg, for example, 1500 mg, initiate *Eskalith CR* dosage at the multiple of 450 mg nearest to, but *below*, the original daily dose, i.e., 1350 mg. When the two doses are unequal, give the larger dose in the evening. In the above example, with a total daily dosage of 1350 mg, generally 450 mg *Eskalith CR* should be given in the morning and 900 mg *Eskalith CR* in the evening. If desired, the total daily dosage of 1350 mg can be given in three equal 450 mg *Eskalith CR* doses. These patients should be monitored at 1–2 week intervals, and dosage adjusted if necessary, until stable and satisfactory serum levels and clinical state are achieved.

When patients require closer titration than that available with *Eskalith CR* doses in increments of 450 mg, immediate release capsules or tablets should be used.

Acute Mania—Optimal patient response to Eskalith (lithium carbonate) can usually be established and maintained with 1800 mg per day in divided doses. Such doses will normally produce the desired serum lithium level ranging between 1.0 and 1.5 mEq/L.

Dosage must be individualized according to serum levels and clinical response. Regular monitoring of the patient's clinical state and serum lithium levels is necessary. Serum levels should be determined twice per week during the acute phase, and until the serum level and clinical condition of the patient have been stabilized.

Long-Term Control—The desirable serum lithium levels are 0.6 to 1.2 mEq/L. Dosage will vary from one individual to another, but usually 900 mg to 1200 mg per day in divided doses will maintain this level. Serum lithium levels in uncomplicated cases receiving maintenance therapy during remission should be monitored at least every two months.

Patients unusually sensitive to lithium may exhibit toxic signs at serum levels below 1.0 mEq/L.

N.B.: Blood samples for serum lithium determinations should be drawn immediately prior to the next dose when lithium concentrations are relatively stable (i.e., 8–12 hours after the previous dose). Total reliance must not be placed on serum levels alone. Accurate patient evaluation requires both clinical and laboratory analysis.

Elderly patients often respond to reduced dosage, and may exhibit signs of toxicity at serum levels ordinarily tolerated by younger patients.

OVERDOSAGE

The toxic levels for lithium are close to the therapeutic levels. It is therefore important that patients and their families be cautioned to watch for early toxic symptoms and to discontinue the drug and inform the physician should they occur. Toxic symptoms are listed in detail under ADVERSE REACTIONS.

Treatment

No specific antidote for lithium poisoning is known. Early symptoms of lithium toxicity can usually be treated by reduction or cessation of dosage of the drug and resumption of the treatment at a lower dose after 24 to 48 hours. In severe cases of lithium poisoning, the first and foremost goal of treatment consists of elimination of this ion from the patient. Treatment is essentially the same as that used in barbiturate poisoning: 1) gastric lavage, 2) correction of fluid and electrolyte imbalance, and 3) regulation of kidney function. Urea, mannitol and aminophylline all produce significant increases in lithium excretion. Hemodialysis is an effective and rapid means of removing the ion from the severely toxic patient. Infection prophylaxis, regular chest X-rays and preservation of adequate respiration are essential.

HOW SUPPLIED

Capsules containing 300 mg lithium carbonate per capsule, in bottles of 100 and 500.

Tablets containing 300 mg lithium carbonate per tablet, in bottles of 100.

Controlled Release Tablets containing 450 mg lithium carbonate per tablet, in bottles of 100.

EL:L36

Shown in Product Identification Section, page 430

FASTIN® Capsules CIV

[*făs'tĭn*]

(phentermine hydrochloride)

DESCRIPTION

Each FASTIN (Phentermine Hydrochloride) capsule contains Phentermine Hydrochloride, 30 mg (equivalent to 24 mg Phentermine).

Phentermine Hydrochloride is a white crystalline powder, very soluble in water and alcohol. Chemically, the product is phenyl-tertiary-butylamine hydrochloride. *Inactive Ingredients:* FD&C Blue 1, Methylcellulose, Polyethylene Glycol, Starch, Titanium Dioxide, Sucrose and Invert Sugar. The branding ink used on the gelatin capsules contains: Ethyl Alcohol, F D & C Blue 1 Aluminum Lake, Isopropyl Alcohol, n-Butyl Alcohol, Propylene Glycol, Pharmaceutical Shellac (modified) or Refined Shellac (Food Grade).

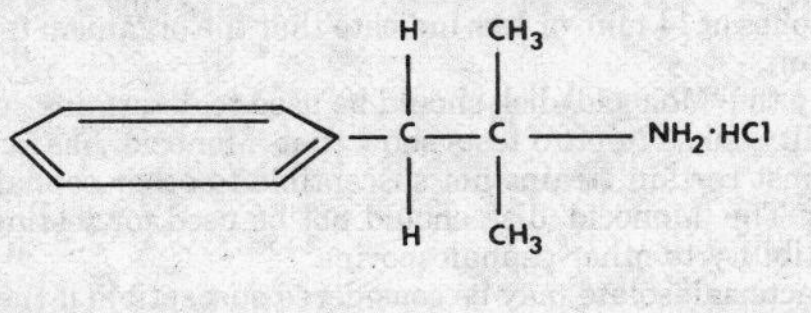

ACTIONS

FASTIN is a sympathomimetic amine with pharmacologic activity similar to the prototype drugs of this class used in obesity, the amphetamines. Actions include central nervous system stimulation and elevation of blood pressure. Tachyphylaxis and tolerance have been demonstrated with all drugs of this class in which these phenomena have been looked for.

Drugs of this class used in obesity are commonly known as "anorectics" or "anorexigenics." It has not been established that the action of such drugs in treating obesity is primarily one of appetite suppression. Other central nervous system actions, or metabolic effects may be involved, for example.

Adult obese subjects instructed in dietary management and treated with "anorectic" drugs, lose more weight on the average than those treated with placebo and diet, as determined in relatively short-term clinical trials.

The magnitude of increased weight loss of drug-treated patients over placebo-treated patients is only a fraction of a pound a week. The rate of weight loss is greatest in the first weeks of therapy for both drug and placebo subjects and tends to decrease in succeeding weeks. The possible origins of the increased weight loss due to the various drug effects are not established. The amount of weight loss associated with the use of an "anorectic" drug varies from trial to trial, and the increased weight loss appears to be related in part to variables other than the drugs prescribed, such as the physician-investigator, the population treated, and the diet prescribed. Studies do not permit conclusions as to the relative importance of the drug and non-drug factors on weight loss. The natural history of obesity is measured in years, whereas the studies cited are restricted to a few weeks duration; thus, the total impact of drug-induced weight loss over that of diet alone must be considered clinically limited.

INDICATION

FASTIN is indicated in the management of exogenous obesity as a short term (a few weeks) adjunct in a regimen of weight reduction based on caloric restriction. The limited usefulness of agents of this class (see ACTIONS) should be measured against possible risk factors inherent in their use such as those described below.

CONTRAINDICATIONS

Advanced arteriosclerosis, symptomatic cardiovascular disease, moderate to severe hypertension, hyperthyroidism, known hypersensitivity, or idiosyncrasy to the sympathomimetic amines, glaucoma.

Agitated states.

Patients with a history of drug abuse.

During or within 14 days following the administration of monoamine oxidase inhibitors (hypertensive crises may result).

WARNINGS

Tolerance to the anorectic effect usually develops within a few weeks. When this occurs, the recommended dose should not be exceeded in an attempt to increase the effect; rather, the drug should be discontinued.

FASTIN may impair the ability of the patient to engage in potentially hazardous activities such as operating machinery or driving a motor vehicle; the patient should therefore be cautioned accordingly.

Drug Dependence: FASTIN is related chemically and pharmacologically to the amphetamines. Amphetamines and related stimulant drugs have been extensively abused, and the possibility of abuse of FASTIN should be kept in mind when evaluating the desirability of including a drug as part of a weight reduction program. Abuse of amphetamines and related drugs may be associated with intense psychological dependence and severe social dysfunction. There are reports of patients who have increased the dosage to many times that recommended. Abrupt cessation following prolonged high dosage administration results in extreme fatigue and mental depression; changes are also noted on the sleep EEG. Manifestations of chronic intoxication with anorectic drugs include severe dermatoses, marked insomnia, irritability, hyperactivity, and personality changes. The most severe manifestation of chronic intoxications is psychosis, often clinically indistinguishable from schizophrenia.

Usage in Pregnancy: Safe use in pregnancy has not been established. Use of FASTIN by women who are or who may become pregnant, and those in the first trimester of pregnancy, requires that the potential benefit be weighed against the possible hazard to mother and infant.

Usage in Children: FASTIN is not recommended for use in children under 12 years of age.

Usage with Alcohol: Concomitant use of alcohol with FASTIN may result in an adverse drug interaction.

PRECAUTIONS

Caution is to be exercised in prescribing FASTIN for patients with even mild hypertension.

Insulin requirements in diabetes mellitus may be altered in association with the use of FASTIN and the concomitant dietary regimen.

FASTIN may decrease the hypotensive effect of guanethidine.

The least amount feasible should be prescribed or dispensed at one time in order to minimize the possibility of overdosage.

ADVERSE REACTIONS

Cardiovascular: Palpitation, tachycardia, elevation of blood pressure.

Central Nervous System: Overstimulation, restlessness, dizziness, insomnia, euphoria, dysphoria, tremor, headache; rarely psychotic episodes at recommended doses.

Gastrointestinal: Dryness of the mouth, unpleasant taste, diarrhea, constipation, other gastrointestinal disturbances.

Allergic: Urticaria.

Endocrine: Impotence, changes in libido.

DOSAGE AND ADMINISTRATION

Exogenous Obesity: One capsule at approximately 2 hours after breakfast for appetite control. Late evening medication should be avoided because of the possibility of resulting insomnia.

Administration of one capsule (30 mg) daily has been found to be adequate in depression of the appetite for twelve to fourteen hours.

FASTIN is not recommended for use in children under 12 years of age.

Continued on next page

SmithKline Beecham—Cont.

OVERDOSAGE

Manifestations of acute overdosage with phentermine include restlessness, tremor, hyperreflexia, rapid respiration, confusion, assaultiveness, hallucinations, panic states. Fatigue and depression usually follow the central stimulation. Cardiovascular effects include arrhythmias, hypertension or hypotension, and circulatory collapse. Gastrointestinal symptoms include nausea, vomiting, diarrhea, and abdominal cramps. Fatal poisoning usually terminates in convulsions and coma.

Management of acute phentermine intoxication is largely symptomatic and includes lavage and sedation with a barbiturate. Experience with hemodialysis or peritoneal dialysis is inadequate to permit recommendations in this regard. Acidification of the urine increases phentermine excretion. Intravenous phentolamine (REGITINE) has been suggested for possible acute, severe hypertension, if this complicates phentermine overdosage.

CAUTION

Federal law prohibits dispensing without prescription.

HOW SUPPLIED

Blue and clear capsules with blue and white beads containing 30 mg phentermine hydrochloride (equivalent to 24 mg phentermine).

NDC 0029-2205-30 ....bottles of 100
NDC 0029-2205-39 ....bottles of 450
NDC 0029-2205-31 ....pack of 30
DGB-0047/6-90 Revised June, 1990

Shown in Product Identification Section, page 430

MONOCID® ℞

[mon 'oh-sid]
brand of sterile cefonicid sodium (lyophilized)

DESCRIPTION

Monocid (sterile cefonicid sodium, SK&F), a sterile, lyophilized, semisynthetic, broad-spectrum cephalosporin antibiotic for intravenous and intramuscular administration, is 5-Thia-1-azabicyclo[4.2.0]oct-2-ene-2-carboxylic acid, 7-[(hydroxyphenyl-acetyl)-amino]-8-oxo-3-[[[1-(sulfomethyl)-1*H*-tetrazol-5-yl]thio] methyl]-disodium salt, [6*R*-[6α, 7β(*R**)]].

Cefonicid sodium contains 85 mg. (3.7 mEq.) sodium per gram of cefonicid activity.

CLINICAL PHARMACOLOGY

Human Pharmacology

The table below demonstrates the levels and duration of Monocid (sterile cefonicid sodium, SK&F) in serum following intravenous and intramuscular administration of 1 gram to normal volunteers.

Serum half-life is approximately 4.5 hours with intravenous and intramuscular administration. 'Monocid' is highly (greater than 90%) and reversibly protein bound.

'Monocid' is not metabolized; 99% is excreted unchanged in the urine in 24 hours. A 500 mg. I.M. dose provides a high (384 mcg./mL.) urinary concentration at 6–8 hours. Probenecid, given concurrently with 'Monocid', slows renal excretion, produces higher peak serum levels and significantly increases the serum half-life of the drug (8.2 hours).

'Monocid' reaches therapeutic levels in the following tissues and fluids:

[See table above.]

Note: Although 'Monocid' reaches therapeutic levels in bile, those levels are lower than those seen with other cephalosporins, and amounts of 'Monocid' released into the gastrointestinal tract are minute. This small amount of 'Monocid' in the gastrointestinal tract is thought to be the reason for the low incidence of gastrointestinal reactions following therapy with 'Monocid'.

No disulfiram-like reactions were reported in a crossover study conducted in healthy volunteers receiving 'Monocid' and alcohol.

Microbiology

The bactericidal action of Monocid (sterile cefonicid sodium, SK&F) results from inhibition of cell-wall synthesis. 'Monocid' is highly resistant to beta-lactamases produced by *Staphylococcus aureus, Hemophilus influenzae, Neisseria gonorrhoeae* and Richmond type I beta-lactamases. 'Monocid' is resistant to degradation by beta-lactamases from certain members of *Enterobacteriaceae*. Active against a wide range of gram-positive and gram-negative organisms, 'Monocid' is usually active against the following organisms *in vitro* and in clinical situations:

Tissue and Body Fluid Levels

Tissue or Body Fluid	Dosage and Route (No. of Patients Sampled)	Time of Sampling After Dose	Average Tissue or Fluid Levels (mcg./g. or/mL.)
Bone	1 g. I.M. (7)	60–90 min.	6.8
	1 g. I.V. (10)	44–99 min.	14.0
Gallbladder	1 g. I.M. (10)	60–70 min.	15.5
Bile	1 g. I.M. (10)	60–70 min.	7.5
Prostate	1 g. I.M. (10)	50–115 min.	13.0
Uterine Tissue	1 g. I.M. (6)	60–90 min.	17.5
Wound Fluid	1 g. I.M. (10)	60–75 min.	37.7
Purulent Wound	1 g. I.M. (9)	60 min.	11.5
Adipose Tissue	1 g. I.M. (5)	60 min.	4.0
Atrial Appendage	1 g. I.M. (7)	77–170 min.	7.5
	2 g. I.M. (7)	105–170 min.	8.7
	15 mg./kg. I.V. (10)	53–160 min.	15.4

Gram-Positive Aerobes: *Staphylococcus aureus* (beta-lactamase producing and non-beta-lactamase producing) and *S. epidermidis* (Note: Methicillin-resistant staphylococci are resistant to cephalosporins, including cefonicid.); *Streptococcus pneumoniae, S. pyogenes* (Group A beta-hemolytic *Streptococcus*), and *S. agalactiae* (Group B *Streptococcus*).

Gram-Negative Aerobes: *Escherichia coli; Klebsiella pneumoniae; Providencia rettgeri* (formerly *Proteus rettgeri*); *Proteus vulgaris; Morganella morganii* (formerly *Proteus morganii*); *Proteus mirabilis;* and *Hemophilus influenzae* (ampicillin-sensitive and -resistant).

In addition to the preceding, 'Monocid' is usually active against the following organisms *in vitro*, but the clinical significance of these data has not been established:

Gram-Negative Aerobes: *Klebsiella oxytoca; Enterobacter aerogenes; Neisseria gonorrhoeae* (penicillin-sensitive and -resistant); *Citrobacter freundii* and *C. diversus.*

Gram-Positive Anaerobes: *Clostridium perfringens; Peptostreptococcus anaerobius; Peptococcus magnus; P. prevotii;* and *Propionibacterium acnes.*

Gram-Negative Anaerobes: *Fusobacterium nucleatum.*

Monocid (sterile cefonicid sodium, SK&F) is usually inactive *in vitro* against most strains of *Pseudomonas, Serratia, Enterococcus* and *Acinetobacter*. Most strains of *B. fragilis* are resistant.

Susceptibility Testing

Results from standardized single-disk susceptibility tests using a 30 mcg. 'Monocid' disk should be interpreted according to the following criteria:

Zones of 18 mm. or greater indicate that the tested organism is susceptible to 'Monocid' and is likely to respond to therapy.

Zones from 15 to 17 mm. indicate that the tested organism is of intermediate (moderate) susceptibility, and is likely to respond to therapy if a higher dosage is used or if the infection is confined to tissues and fluids in which high antibiotic levels are attained.

Zones of 14 mm. or less indicate that the organism is resistant.

Only the 'Monocid' disk should be used to determine susceptibility, since *in vitro* tests show that 'Monocid' has activity against certain strains not susceptible to other cephalosporins. The 'Monocid' disk should not be used for testing susceptibility to other cephalosporins.

A bacterial isolate may be considered susceptible if the MIC value for 'Monocid' is equal to or less than 8 mcg./mL. in accordance with the National Committee for Clinical Laboratory Standards (NCCLS) guidelines. Organisms are considered resistant if the MIC is equal to or greater than 32 mcg./mL. For most organisms the MBC value for 'Monocid' is the same as the MIC value.

The standardized quality control procedure requires use of control organisms. The 30 mcg. 'Monocid' disk should give the zone diameters listed below for the quality control strains.

Organism	ATCC	Zone Size Range
E. coli	25922	25–29 mm.
S. aureus	25923	22–28 mm.

INDICATIONS AND USAGE

Due to the long half-life of 'Monocid', a 1 gram dose results in therapeutic serum levels which provide coverage against susceptible organisms (listed below) for 24 hours.

Studies on specimens obtained prior to therapy should be used to determine the susceptibility of the causative organisms to 'Monocid'. Therapy with 'Monocid' may be initiated pending results of the studies; however, treatment should be adjusted according to study findings.

Treatment

Monocid (sterile cefonicid sodium, SK&F) is indicated in the treatment of infections due to susceptible strains of the microorganisms listed below:

LOWER RESPIRATORY TRACT INFECTIONS, due to *Streptococcus pneumoniae* (formerly *D. pneumoniae*); *Klebsiella pneumoniae**; *Escherichia coli;* and *Hemophilus influenzae* (ampicillin-resistant and ampicillin-sensitive).

URINARY TRACT INFECTIONS, due to *Escherichia coli; Proteus mirabilis* and *Proteus* spp. (which may include the organisms now called *Proteus vulgaris,** *Providencia rettgeri* and *Morganella morganii*); and *Klebsiella pneumoniae.**

SKIN AND SKIN STRUCTURE INFECTIONS, due to *Staphylococcus aureus* and *S. epidermidis; Streptococcus pyogenes* (Group A *Streptococcus*) and *S. agalactiae* (Group B *Streptococcus*).

SEPTICEMIA, due to *Streptococcus pneumoniae* (formerly *D. pneumoniae*) and *Escherichia coli.**

BONE AND JOINT INFECTIONS, due to *Staphylococcus aureus.*

Surgical Prophylaxis

Administration of a single 1 gram dose of 'Monocid' before surgery may reduce the incidence of postoperative infections in patients undergoing surgical procedures classified as contaminated or potentially contaminated (e.g., colorectal surgery, vaginal hysterectomy, or cholecystectomy in high-risk patients), or in patients in whom infection at the operative site would present a serious risk (e.g., prosthetic arthroplasty, open heart surgery). Although cefonicid has been shown to be as effective as cefazolin in prevention of infection following coronary artery bypass surgery, no placebo-controlled trials have been conducted to evaluate any cephalosporin antibiotic in the prevention of infection following coronary artery bypass surgery or prosthetic heart valve replacement.

In cesarean section, the use of 'Monocid' (after the umbilical cord has been clamped) may reduce the incidence of certain postoperative infections.

When administered one hour prior to surgical procedures for which it is indicated, a single 1 gram dose of 'Monocid' provides protection from most infections due to susceptible organisms throughout the course of the procedure. Intraoperative and/or postoperative administrations of 'Monocid' are not necessary. Daily doses of 'Monocid' may be administered for two additional days in patients undergoing prosthetic arthroplasty or open heart surgery.

If there are signs of infection, the causative organisms should be identified and appropriate therapy determined through susceptibility testing.

Before using 'Monocid' concomitantly with other antibiotics, the prescribing information for those agents should be reviewed for contraindications, warnings, precautions and adverse reactions. Renal function should be carefully monitored.

CONTRAINDICATIONS

Monocid (sterile cefonicid sodium, SK&F) is contraindicated in persons who have shown hypersensitivity to cephalosporin antibiotics.

WARNINGS

BEFORE THERAPY WITH MONOCID (STERILE CEFONICID SODIUM, SK&F) IS INSTITUTED, CAREFUL INQUIRY SHOULD BE MADE TO DETERMINE WHETHER THE PATIENT HAS HAD PREVIOUS HYPERSENSITIVITY REACTIONS TO CEPHALOSPORINS, PENICILLINS, OR OTHER DRUGS. THIS PRODUCT SHOULD BE GIVEN CAUTIOUSLY TO PENICILLIN-SENSITIVE PATIENTS. ANTIBIOTICS SHOULD BE ADMINISTERED WITH CAUTION TO ANY PATIENT WHO HAS DEMONSTRATED SOME FORM OF ALLERGY, PARTICULARLY TO DRUGS. SERIOUS ACUTE HYPERSENSITIVITY REAC-

*Efficacy for this organism in this organ system has been demonstrated in fewer than 10 infections.

Serum Concentrations After 1 Gram Administration (mcg./mL.)

Interval	5 min.	15 min.	30 min.	1 hr.	2 hr.	4 hr.	6 hr.	8 hr.	10 hr.	12 hr.	24 hr.
I.V.	221.3	176.4	147.6	124.2	88.9	61.4	40.0	29.3	20.6	15.2	2.6
I.M.	13.5	45.9	73.1	98.6	97.1	77.8	54.9	38.5	28.9	20.6	4.5

TIONS MAY REQUIRE EPINEPHRINE AND OTHER EMERGENCY MEASURES.

Pseudomembranous colitis has been reported with the use of cephalosporins (and other broad-spectrum antibiotics); therefore, it is important to consider that diagnosis in patients who develop diarrhea in association with antibiotic use.

Treatment with broad-spectrum antibiotics alters normal flora of the colon and may permit overgrowth of Clostridia. Studies indicate a toxin produced by *Clostridium difficile* is one primary cause of antibiotic-associated colitis. Cholestyramine and colestipol resins have been shown to bind the toxin *in vitro*.

Mild cases of colitis may respond to drug discontinuance alone.

Moderate to severe cases should be managed with fluid, electrolyte and protein supplementation as indicated.

When the colitis is not relieved by drug discontinuance and when it is severe, oral vancomycin is the treatment of choice for antibiotic-associated pseudomembranous colitis produced by *C. difficile*. Other causes of colitis should also be considered.

PRECAUTIONS

General: With any antibiotic, prolonged use may result in overgrowth of nonsusceptible organisms. Careful observation is essential, and appropriate measures should be taken if superinfection occurs.

Drug Interactions: Nephrotoxicity has been reported following concomitant administration of other cephalosporins and aminoglycosides.

Pregnancy: (Category B.) Reproduction studies have been performed in mice, rabbits and rats at doses up to an equivalent of 40 times the usual adult human dose and have revealed no evidence of impaired fertility or harm to the fetus due to Monocid (sterile cefonicid sodium, SK&F). There are, however, no adequate and well-controlled studies in pregnant women. Because animal reproduction studies are not always predictive of human response, this drug should be used in pregnancy only if clearly needed.

Labor and Delivery: In cesarean section, 'Monocid' should be administered only after the umbilical cord has been clamped.

Nursing Mothers: 'Monocid' is excreted in human milk in low concentrations. Caution should be exercised when 'Monocid' is administered to a nursing woman.

Pediatric Use: Safety and effectiveness in children have not been established.

Beta-lactam antibiotics with methyl-thio-tetrazole side chains have been shown to cause testicular atrophy in prepubertal rats, which persisted into adulthood and resulted in decreased spermatogenesis and decreased fertility. Cefonicid, which contains a methylsulfonic-thio-tetrazole moiety, has no adverse effect on the male reproductive system of prepubertal, juvenile or adult rats when given under identical conditions.

ADVERSE REACTIONS

Monocid (sterile cefonicid sodium, SK&F) is generally well tolerated and adverse reactions have occurred infrequently. The most common adverse reaction has been pain on I.M. injection. On-therapy conditions occurring in greater than 1% of 'Monocid'-treated patients were:

Injection Site Phenomena (5.7%): Pain and/or discomfort on injection; less often, burning, phlebitis at I.V. site.
Increased Platelets (1.7%).
Increased Eosinophils (2.9%).
Liver Function Test Alterations (1.6%): Increased alkaline phosphatase, increased SGOT, increased SGPT, increased GGTP, increased LDH.

Less frequent on-therapy conditions occurring in less than 1% of 'Monocid'-treated patients were:

Hypersensitivity Reactions: Fever, rash, pruritus, erythema, myalgia and anaphylactoid-type reactions have been reported.
Hematology: Decreased WBC, neutropenia, thrombocytopenia, positive Coombs' test.
Renal: Increased BUN and creatinine levels have occasionally been seen. Rare reports of acute renal failure associated with interstitial nephritis, observed with other beta-lactam antibiotics, have also occurred with 'Monocid'.
Diarrhea.

DOSAGE AND ADMINISTRATION

General
The usual adult dosage is 1 gram of Monocid (sterile cefonicid sodium, SK&F) given once every 24 hours, intravenously or by deep intramuscular injection. Doses in excess of 1 gram daily are rarely necessary; however, in exceptional cases dosage of up to 2 grams given once daily have been well tolerated. When administering 2 gram I.M. doses once daily, one-half the dose should be administered in different large muscle masses.

Outpatient Use
'Monocid' has been used (once daily I.M. or I.V.) on an outpatient basis. Individuals responsible for outpatient administration of 'Monocid' should be instructed thoroughly in appropriate procedures for storage, reconstitution and administration.

Surgical Prophylaxis
When administered one hour prior to appropriate surgical procedures (see INDICATIONS AND USAGE) a 1 gram dose of 'Monocid' provides protection from most infections due to susceptible organisms throughout the course of the procedure. Intraoperative and/or postoperative administrations of 'Monocid' are not necessary. Daily doses of 'Monocid' may be administered for two additional days in patients undergoing prosthetic arthroplasty or open heart surgery.
In cesarean section 'Monocid' should be administered only after the umbilical cord has been clamped.

General Guidelines for Dosage of 'Monocid', I.V. or I.M.

Type of Infection	Daily Dose (grams)	Frequency
Uncomplicated Urinary Tract	0.5	once every 24 hours
Mild to Moderate	1	once every 24 hours
Severe or Life-Threatening	2*	once every 24 hours
Surgical Prophylaxis	1	1 hour preoperatively

* When administering 2 gram I.M. doses once daily, one-half the dose should be administered in different large muscle masses.

Impaired Renal Function
Modification of Monocid (sterile cefonicid sodium, SK&F) dosage is necessary in patients with impaired renal function. Following an initial loading dosage of 7.5 mg./kg. I.M. or I.V., the maintenance dosing schedule shown below should be followed. Further dosing should be determined by severity of the infection and susceptibility of the causative organism.
Note: It is not necessary to administer additional dosage following dialysis.

Preparation of Parenteral Solution
Parenteral drug products should be SHAKEN WELL when reconstituted, and inspected visually for particulate matter prior to administration. If particulate matter is evident in reconstituted fluids, the drug solutions should be discarded.

RECONSTITUTION
Single-Dose Vials
For I.M. injection, I.V. direct (bolus) injection, or I.V. infusion, reconstitute with Sterile Water for Injection according to the following table. SHAKE WELL.

Vial Size	Diluent to Be Added	Approx. Avail. Volume	Approx. Avg. Concentration
500 mg.	2.0 mL.	2.2 mL.	225 mg./mL.
1 gram	2.5 mL.	3.1 mL.	325 mg./mL.

These solutions of Monocid (sterile cefonicid sodium, SK&F) are stable 24 hours at room temperature or 72 hours if refrigerated (5°C.). Slight yellowing does not affect potency.
For I.V. infusion, dilute reconstituted solution in 50 to 100 mL. of the parenteral fluids listed under ADMINISTRATION.

Pharmacy Bulk Vials (10 grams)
For I.M. injection, I.V. direct (bolus) injection or I.V. infusion, reconstitute with Sterile Water for Injection, Bacteriostatic Water for Injection, or Sodium Chloride Injection according to the following table:

Amount of Diluent	Approx. Concentration	Approx. Avail. Volume
25 mL.	1 gram/3 mL.	31 mL.
45 mL.	1 gram/5 mL.	51 mL.

These solutions of 'Monocid' are stable 24 hours at room temperature or 72 hours if refrigerated (5°C.). Slight yellowing does not affect potency.
For I.V. infusion add to parenteral fluids listed under ADMINISTRATION.

"Piggyback" Vials
Reconstitute with 50 to 100 mL. of Sodium Chloride Injection or other I.V. solution listed under ADMINISTRATION. Administer with primary I.V. fluids, as a single dose. These solutions of 'Monocid' are stable 24 hours at room temperature or 72 hours if refrigerated (5°C.). Slight yellowing does not affect potency.
A solution of 1 gram of 'Monocid' in 18 mL. of Sterile Water for Injection is isotonic.

ADMINISTRATION
I.M. Injection: Inject well within the body of a relatively large muscle. Aspiration is necessary to avoid inadvertent injection into a blood vessel. When administering 2 gram I.M. doses once daily, one-half the dose should be given in different large muscle masses.

I.V. Administration: For direct (bolus) injection, administer reconstituted 'Monocid' slowly over 3 to 5 minutes, directly or through tubing for patients receiving parenteral fluids (see list below). For infusion, dilute reconstituted 'Monocid' in 50 to 100 mL. of one of the following solutions:
  0.9% Sodium Chloride Injection, USP
  5% Dextrose Injection, USP
  5% Dextrose and 0.9% Sodium Chloride Injection, USP
  5% Dextrose and 0.45% Sodium Chloride Injection, USP
  5% Dextrose and 0.2% Sodium Chloride Injection, USP
  10% Dextrose Injection, USP
  Ringer's Injection, USP
  Lactated Ringer's Injection, USP
  5% Dextrose and Lactated Ringer's Injection
  10% Invert Sugar in Sterile Water for Injection
  5% Dextrose and 0.15% Potassium Chloride Injection
  Sodium Lactate Injection, USP
In these fluids 'Monocid' is stable 24 hours at room temperature or 72 hours if refrigerated (5°C.). Slight yellowing does not affect potency.

HOW SUPPLIED
Monocid (sterile cefonicid sodium, SK&F) is supplied in vials equivalent to 500 mg. and 1 gram of cefonicid; in "Piggyback" Vials for I.V. admixture equivalent to 1 gram of cefonicid; and in Pharmacy Bulk Vials equivalent to 10 grams of cefonicid.

MC:L22

Shown in Product Identification Section, page 430

NUCOFED®   ℞
[nū 'cō-fĕd]
Syrup and Capsules

DESCRIPTION
Nucofed Syrup and Capsules is an antitussive-decongestant containing in each 5 mL (teaspoonful) and each capsule: Codeine Phosphate, 20 mg (Warning: May Be Habit Forming); Pseudoephedrine Hydrochloride, 60 mg. Nucofed Syrup contains no alcohol and contains 2.25 g of sucrose per 5 mL (teaspoonful). Codeine Phosphate and Pseudoephedrine Hydro-

Dosage of 'Monocid' in Adults with Reduced Renal Function

(Monitor renal function and adjust accordingly.)

Creatinine Clearance (ml./min. per 1.73 M²)	Dosage Regimen	
	Mild to Moderate Infections	Severe Infections
79–60	10 mg./kg. (every 24 hours)	25 mg./kg. (every 24 hours)
59–40	8 mg./kg. (every 24 hours)	20 mg./kg. (every 24 hours)
39–20	4 mg./kg. (every 24 hours)	15 mg./kg. (every 24 hours)
19–10	4 mg./kg. (every 48 hours)	15 mg./kg. (every 48 hours)
9–5	4 mg./kg. (every 3 to 5 days)	15 mg./kg. (every 3 to 5 days)
<5	3 mg./kg. (every 3 to 5 days)	4 mg./kg. (every 3 to 5 days)

Continued on next page

SmithKline Beecham—Cont.

chloride may be represented by the following chemical names and structural formulas:

Codeine Phosphate

7,8-didehydro-4,5α-epoxy-3-methoxy-17-methylmorphinan-6α-ol Phosphate (1:1) salt hemihydrate

Pseudoephedrine HCl

[S-(R*,R*)]-α-[1-(methylamino) ethyl]benzene methanol hydrochloride.

Inactive Ingredients, Syrup: Citric Acid, Flavorings, Glycerin, Propylene Glycol, Sodium Benzoate, Sorbitol, Sucrose, D&C Yellow 10, and FD&C Blue 1. **Capsules:** Starch, Lactose, Magnesium Stearate, FD&C Yellow No. 6, FD&C Blue No. 1, and D&C Yellow No. 10.

CLINICAL PHARMACOLOGY

Nucofed Syrup and Capsules
The clinical pharmacology of this formulated product is thought to be due to the action of its ingredients, Codeine Phosphate and Pseudoephedrine Hydrochloride.
Codeine Phosphate. Codeine causes suppression of the cough reflex by a direct effect on the cough center in the medulla and appears to exert a drying effect on respiratory tract mucosa and to increase viscosity of bronchial secretions.
Codeine is well absorbed from the gastrointestinal tract. Following oral administration, peak antitussive effects usually can be expected to occur within 1–2 hours and may persist for a period of four hours. Codeine is metabolized in the liver. The drug undergoes O-demethylation, N-demethylation, and partial conjugation with glucuronic acid, and is excreted mainly in the urine as norcodeine and morphine in the free and conjugated forms.
Codeine appears in breast milk of nursing mothers and has been reported to cross the placental barrier.
Pseudoephedrine Hydrochloride. Pseudoephedrine is a physiologically active stereoisomer of ephedrine which acts directly on *alpha,* and, to a lesser degree, *beta* -adrenergic receptors. The *alpha* -adrenergic effects are believed to result from the reduced production of cyclic adenosine-3',5' monophosphate (cyclic 3',5'-AMP) by inhibition of the enzyme adenyl cyclase, where *beta* -adrenergic effects appear to be caused by the stimulation of adenyl cyclase activity.
Pseudoephedrine acts directly on *alpha* -adrenergic receptors in the respiratory tract mucosa producing vasoconstriction resulting in shrinkage of swollen nasal mucous membranes, reduction of tissue hyperemia, edema, and nasal congestion, and an increase in nasal airway patency. Drainage of sinus secretions is increased and obstructed eustachian ostia may be opened. Relaxation of bronchial smooth muscle by stimulation of *beta* $_2$ adrenergic receptors may also occur. Following oral administration significant bronchodilation has not been demonstrated consistently.
Nasal decongestion usually occurs within 30 minutes and persists for 4–6 hours after oral administration of 60 mg of Pseudoephedrine Hydrochloride.
Although specific information is not available, Pseudoephedrine is presumed to cross the placenta and to enter cerebrospinal fluid. It is incompletely metabolized in the liver by N-demethylation to an inactive metabolite. Both are excreted in the urine with 55%–75% of a dose being unchanged.

INDICATIONS AND USAGE

NUCOFED is indicated for symptomatic relief when both coughing and congestion are associated with upper respiratory infections and related conditions such as common cold, bronchitis, influenza, and sinusitis.

CONTRAINDICATIONS

Hypersensitivity to product's active ingredients.

WARNINGS

Persons with persistent cough such as occurs with smoking, asthma, emphysema, or where cough is accompanied by excessive secretions should not take this product except under the advice and supervision of a physician.

May cause or aggravate constipation.
Do not give this product to children taking other drugs except under the advice and supervision of a physician.
Persons with a chronic pulmonary disease or shortness of breath, high blood pressure, heart disease, diabetes or thyroid disease should not take this product except under the advice and supervision of a physician.
Do not exceed recommended dosage because at higher doses nervousness, dizziness, or sleeplessness may occur.
If symptoms do not improve within 7 days or are accompanied by high fever, consult a physician before continuing use.

PRECAUTIONS

General
Inasmuch as the active ingredients of Nucofed Syrup and Capsules consist of Codeine Phosphate and Pseudoephedrine Hydrochloride, this medication should be used with caution in the presence of the following:
- Cardiovascular disease (of any etiology)
- Diabetes mellitus
- Hypertension (of any severity)
- Abnormal thyroid function
- Prostatic hypertrophy
- Addison's disease
- Chronic ulcerative colitis
- History of drug abuse or dependence
- Chronic respiratory disease or impairment
- Functional impairment of the liver or kidney

Patients taking Nucofed Syrup and Capsules should be cautioned when driving or doing jobs requiring alertness and to get up slowly from a lying or sitting position, or to lie down if nausea occurs.
Possible Drug Interactions
Because of the potential for drug interactions, persons currently taking any of the following medications should take Nucofed Syrup and Capsules on the advice and under the supervision of a physician.
- Beta adrenergic blockers—concurrent use may increase the pressor effect of pseudoephedrine.
- Digitalis glycosides—concurrent use with pseudoephedrine may increase the possibility of cardiac arrhythmias.
- Antihypertensive agents including Veratrum alkaloids—hypotensive effects may be decreased by the concurrent use of pseudoephedrine.
- Monoamine oxidase (MAO) inhibitors—these agents may potentiate the pressor effect of Pseudoephedrine and may result in a hypertensive crisis; pseudoephedrine should not be administered during or within 14 days of MAO inhibitors.
- Sympathomimetics, other—sympathomimetics used concurrently may increase the effects either of these agents or of pseudoephedrine, thereby increasing the potential for side effects.
- Tricyclic antidepressants—the concurrent use of tricyclic antidepressants may antagonize the effects of pseudoephedrine and may increase the effects either of the antidepressants themselves or of the codeine component.
- CNS depressants
- Alcohol
- General anesthetics
- Anticholinergics—concurrent use may result in paralytic ileus.

Drug/Laboratory Test Interactions
- Codeine may cause an elevation in serum amylase levels due to the spasm producing potential of narcotic analgesics on the sphincter of Oddi.

Pregnancy: Category C
Animal reproduction studies of the components of Nucofed Syrup and Capsules (Codeine, Pseudoephedrine) have not been conducted. Thus, it is not known whether these agents can cause fetal harm when administered to pregnant women or whether they affect reproductive capacity. Accordingly, Nucofed Syrup and Capsules should be given to pregnant women only where clearly needed.
Nursing Mothers
Codeine and Pseudoephedrine are excreted in breast milk; therefore, caution should be exercised when this medication is prescribed for a nursing mother.
Pediatric Use
Do not give Nucofed Syrup and Capsules to children under two years of age except on the advice and under the supervision of a physician.

ADVERSE REACTIONS

Based on the composition of Nucofed Syrup and Capsules the following side effects may occur: nervousness, restlessness, trouble in sleeping, drowsiness, difficult or painful urination, dizziness or lightheadedness, headache, nausea and vomiting, constipation, trembling, troubled breathing, increase in sweating, unusual paleness, weakness, changes in heart rate.

DRUG ABUSE AND DEPENDENCE

NUCOFED is placed in Schedule III of the Controlled Substances Act.

OVERDOSAGE

Nucofed Syrup and Capsules contain Codeine Phosphate and Pseudoephedrine Hydrochloride. Overdosage as a result of this product should be treated based upon the symptomatology of the patient as it relates to the individual ingredient. Treatment of acute overdosage would probably be based upon treating the patient for codeine toxicity which may be manifested as:
- Gradual drowsiness, dizziness, heaviness of the head, weariness, diminution of sensibility, loss of pain and other modalities of sensation.
- Nausea and vomiting.
- A transient excitement stage, characterized by extreme restlessness, delirium, and rarely epileptiform convulsions, is sometimes seen in children and rarely in adult women.
- Bilateral miosis, progressing to pinpoint pupils, which do not react to light or accommodation. The pupils may dilate during terminal asphyxia.
- Itching of the skin and nose, sometimes with skin rashes and urticaria.
- Coma, with muscular relaxation and depressed or absent superficial and deep reflexes. A Babinski toe sign may appear.
- Marked slowing of the respiratory rate with inadequate pulmonary ventilation and consequent cyanosis. Breathing becomes stertorous and irregular (Cheyne-Stokes or Biot).
- The pulse is slow and the blood pressure gradually falls to shock levels. Urine formation ceases or is reduced to a very slow rate.

The lethal dose of codeine for an adult is about 0.5–1.0 g. Treatment is as recommended for narcotics.

DOSAGE AND ADMINISTRATION

RECOMMENDED DOSAGE: CAPSULE
Adults: 1 capsule every 6 hours, not to exceed 4 capsules in 24 hours.
RECOMMENDED DOSAGE: SYRUP
Adults: 1 teaspoonful every 6 hours, not to exceed 4 teaspoonfuls in 24 hours.
Children:
  6 to under 12 years: ½ teaspoonful every 6 hours, not to exceed 2 teaspoonfuls in 24 hours.
  2 to under 6 years: ¼ teaspoonful every 6 hours, not to exceed 1 teaspoonful in 24 hours.
Do not give this product to children under 2 years, except under the advice and supervision of a physician.

HOW SUPPLIED

Nucofed Syrup, Green, Mint Flavored
  NDC 0029-3135-34   Pints
Nucofed Capsules, Green Top, Clear Bottom
  NDC 0029-3138-39   Bottles of 60

CAUTION

Federal law prohibits dispensing without prescription.
DGB—0491/1-88
Revised January, 1988
Shown in Product Identification Section, page 431

NUCOFED® EXPECTORANT   Ⓒ ℞
[nū'cō-fĕd]
SYRUP

DESCRIPTION

Nucofed Expectorant is an antitussive-decongestant-expectorant syrup for oral administration containing in each 5 mL (teaspoonful): Codeine Phosphate, 20 mg (Warning: May Be Habit Forming); Pseudoephedrine HCl, 60 mg; Guaifenesin, 200 mg; alcohol, 12.5%
Codeine Phosphate, Pseudoephedrine Hydrochloride and Guaifenesin may be represented by the following chemical names and structural formulas:

Codeine Phosphate

7,8-didehydro-4,5α-epoxy-3-methoxy-17-methylmorphinan-6α-ol Phosphate (1:1) salt hemihydrate

Pseudoephedrine HCl

[S-(R*,R*)]-α-[1-(methylamino) ethyl]benzene methanol hydrochloride

Guaifenesin

3-(O-methoxyphenoxy)-1,2-propanediol

Inactive Ingredients: D & C Yellow 10, F D & C Red 40, Flavoring, Glycerin, Saccharin Sodium, Sodium Chloride and Sucrose.

CLINICAL PHARMACOLOGY

Nucofed Expectorant
The clinical pharmacology of this formulated product is thought to be due to the action of its ingredients, Codeine Phosphate, Pseudoephedrine Hydrochloride and Guaifenesin.
Codeine Phosphate. Codeine causes suppression of the cough reflex by a direct effect on the cough center in the medulla and appears to exert a drying effect on respiratory tract mucosa and to increase viscosity of bronchial secretions.
Codeine is well absorbed from the gastrointestinal tract. Following oral administration, peak antitussive effects usually can be expected to occur within one to two hours and may persist for a period of four hours. Codeine is metabolized in the liver. The drug undergoes O-demethylation, N-demethylation, and partial conjugation with glucuronic acid, and is excreted mainly in the urine as norcodeine and morphine in the free and conjugated forms.
Codeine appears in breast milk of nursing mothers and has been reported to cross the placental barrier.
Pseudoephedrine Hydrochloride. Pseudoephedrine is a physiologically active stereoisomer of ephedrine which acts directly on *alpha*, and to a lesser degree, *beta* -adrenergic receptors. The *alpha* -adrenergic effects are believed to result from the reduced production of cyclic adenosine 3',5' monophosphate (cyclic 3',5'-AMP) by inhibition of the enzyme adenyl cyclase, whereas *beta* -adrenergic effects appear to be caused by the stimulation of adenyl cyclase activity.
Pseudoephedrine acts directly on *alpha* -adrenergic receptors in the respiratory tract mucosa producing vasoconstriction resulting in shrinkage of swollen nasal mucous membranes, reduction of tissue hyperemia, edema, and nasal congestion, and an increase in nasal airway patency. Drainage of sinus secretions is increased and obstructed eustachian ostia may be opened. Relaxation of bronchial smooth muscle by stimulation of *beta* $_2$ adrenergic receptors may also occur. Following oral administration significant bronchodilation has not been demonstrated consistently.
Nasal decongestion usually occurs within 30 minutes and persists for 4-6 hours after oral administration of 60 mg of pseudoephedrine hydrochloride.
Although specific information is not available, pseudoephedrine is presumed to cross the placenta and to enter cerebrospinal fluid. It is incompletely metabolized in the liver by N-demethylation to an inactive metabolite. Both are excreted in the urine with 55%-75% of a dose being unchanged.
Guaifenesin. Guaifenesin, by increasing respiratory tract fluid, reduces the viscosity of tenacious secretions and acts as an expectorant.
Guaifenesin is excreted in the urine mainly as glucuronates and sulfonates.

INDICATIONS AND USAGE

NUCOFED EXPECTORANT is indicated for symptomatic relief when both coughing and congestion are associated with upper respiratory infections and related conditions such as common cold, bronchitis, influenza, and sinusitis.

CONTRAINDICATIONS

Hypersensitivity to product's active ingredients.

WARNINGS

Persons with persistent cough such as occurs with smoking, asthma, emphysema, or where cough is accompanied by excessive secretions should not take this product except under the advice and supervision of a physician.
Do not give this product to children taking other drugs except under the advice and supervision of a physician.
Persons with a chronic pulmonary disease or shortness of breath, high blood pressure, heart disease, diabetes or thyroid disease should not take this product except under the advice and supervision of a physician.
Do not exceed recommended dosage because at higher doses nervousness, dizziness, or sleeplessness may occur.
If symptoms do not improve within 7 days or are accompanied by high fever, consult a physician before continuing use.

PRECAUTIONS

General. Inasmuch as the active ingredients of Nucofed Expectorant consist of Codeine Phosphate, Pseudoephedrine

Hydrochloride and Guaifenesin, this medication should be used with caution in the presence of the following:
- Cardiovascular disease (of any etiology)
- Diabetes mellitus
- Hypertension (of any severity)
- Abnormal thyroid function
- Prostatic hypertrophy
- Addison's disease
- Chronic ulcerative colitis
- History of drug abuse or dependence
- Chronic respiratory disease or impairment
- Functional impairment of the liver or kidney
Patients taking Nucofed Expectorant should be cautioned when driving or doing jobs requiring alertness, and to get up slowly from a lying or sitting position, or to lie down if nausea occurs.
Possible Drug Interactions. Because of the potential for drug interactions, persons currently taking any of the following medications should take Nucofed Expectorant only on the advice and under the supervision of a physician.
- Beta adrenergic blockers—concurrent use may increase the pressor effect of pseudoephedrine.
- Digitalis glycosides—concurrent use with pseudoephedrine may increase the possibility of cardiac arrhythmias.
- Antihypertensive agents including Veratrum alkaloids—hypotensive effects may be decreased by the concurrent use of pseudoephedrine.
- Monoamine oxidase (MAO) inhibitors—these agents may potentiate the pressor effect of pseudoephedrine and may result in a hypertensive crisis; pseudoephedrine should not be administered during or within 14 days of MAO inhibitors.
- Sympathomimetics, other—sympathomimetics used concurrently may increase the effects either of these agents or of pseudoephedrine, thereby increasing the potential for side effects.
- Tricyclic antidepressants—the concurrent use of tricyclic antidepressants may antagonize the effects of pseudoephedrine and may increase the effects either of the antidepressants themselves or of the codeine component.
- CNS depressants
- Alcohol
- General anesthetics
- Anticholinergics—concurrent use may result in paralytic ileus.
Drug/Laboratory Test Interactions
- Codeine may cause an elevation in serum amylase levels due to the spasm producing potential of narcotic analgesics on the sphincter of Oddi.
- Guaifenesin is known to interfere with the colorimetric determination of 5-hydroxyindole-acetic acid (5-HIAA) and vanilmandelic acid (VMA).
Pregnancy: Category C
Animal reproduction studies of the components of Nucofed Expectorant (codeine, pseudoephedrine and guaifenesin) have not been conducted. Thus, it is not known whether these agents can cause fetal harm when administered to pregnant women or whether they affect reproductive capacity. Accordingly, Nucofed Expectorant should be given to pregnant women only where clearly needed.
Nursing Mothers
Codeine and Pseudoephedrine, two of the ingredients in Nucofed Expectorant, are excreted in breast milk; therefore, caution should be exercised when this medication is prescribed for a nursing mother.
Pediatric Use
Do not give Nucofed Expectorant to Children under two years of age except on the advice and under the supervision of a physician.

ADVERSE REACTIONS

Based on the composition of Nucofed Expectorant the following side effects may occur: nervousness, restlessness, trouble in sleeping, drowsiness, difficult or painful urination, dizziness or lightheadedness, headache, nausea or vomiting, constipation, trembling, troubled breathing, increase in sweating, unusual paleness, weakness, changes in heart rate.

DRUG ABUSE AND DEPENDENCE

Nucofed Expectorant has been placed in Schedule III of the Controlled Substances Act.

OVERDOSAGE

Nucofed Expectorant contains Codeine Phosphate, Pseudoephedrine Hydrochloride and Guaifenesin. Overdosage as a result of this product should be treated based upon the symptomatology of the patient as it relates to the individual ingredient. Treatment of acute overdosage would probably be based upon treating the patient for codeine toxicity which may be manifested as:
- Gradual drowsiness, dizziness, heaviness of the head, weariness, diminution of sensibility, loss of pain and other modalities of sensation.
- Nausea and vomiting.
- A transient excitement stage, characterized by extreme restlessness, delirium, and rarely epileptiform convul-

sions, is sometimes seen in children and rarely in adult women.
- Bilateral miosis, progressing to pinpoint pupils, which do not react to light or accommodation. The pupils may dilate during terminal asphyxia.
- Itching of the skin and nose, sometimes with skin rashes and urticaria.
- Coma, with muscular relaxation and depressed or absent superficial and deep reflexes. A Babinski toe sign may appear.
- Marked slowing of the respiratory rate with inadequate pulmonary ventilation and consequent cyanosis. Breathing becomes stertorous and irregular (Cheyne-Stokes or Biot).
- The pulse is slow and the blood pressure gradually falls to shock levels. Urine formation ceases or is reduced to a very low rate.
The lethal dose of codeine for an adult is about 0.5-1.0 g. Treatment is as recommended for narcotics.

DOSAGE AND ADMINISTRATION

RECOMMENDED DOSAGE:
Adults: 1 teaspoonful every 6 hours, not to exceed 4 teaspoonfuls in 24 hours.
Children:
6 to under 12 years: $\frac{1}{2}$ teaspoonful every 6 hours, not to exceed 2 teaspoonfuls in 24 hours.
2 to under 6 years: $\frac{1}{4}$ teaspoonful every 6 hours, not to exceed 1 teaspoonful in 24 hours.
Do not give this product to children under 2 years, except under the advice and supervision of a physician.

HOW SUPPLIED

Red, Wintergreen Flavored Syrup
  NDC 0029-3142-34   Pints

CAUTION

Federal law prohibits dispensing without prescription.
DGB—1266/2-88
Revised February, 1988

NUCOFED®   © ℞
[*nū ' cō-fĕd*]
PEDIATRIC EXPECTORANT
SYRUP

DESCRIPTION

Nucofed Pediatric Expectorant is an antitussive-decongestant-expectorant syrup for oral administration containing in each 5 mL (teaspoonful): Codeine Phosphate, 10 mg (Warning: May Be Habit Forming); Pseudoephedrine HCl, 30 mg; Guaifenesin, 100 mg; alcohol, 6%
Codeine Phosphate, Pseudoephedrine Hydrochloride and Guaifenesin may be represented by the following chemical names and structural formulas:

Codeine Phosphate

$H_2PO_4^-$ · $\frac{1}{2}H_2O$

7,8-didehydro-4,5α-epoxy-3-methoxy-17-methylmorphinan-6α-ol Phosphate (1:1) salt hemihydrate

Pseudoephedrine HCl

[*S-(R*,R*)*]-α-[1-(methylamino) ethyl]benzene methanol hydrochloride

Guaifenesin

3-(O-methoxyphenoxy)-1,2-propanediol

Inactive Ingredients: Edetate Disodium, F D & C Red 40, Flavorings, Glycerin, Potassium Sorbate, Saccharin Sodium, Sodium Chloride and Sucrose.

Continued on next page

SmithKline Beecham—Cont.

CLINICAL PHARMACOLOGY

Nucofed Pediatric Expectorant
The clinical pharmacology of this formulated product is thought to be due to the action of its ingredients, Codeine Phosphate, Pseudoephedrine Hydrochloride and Guaifenesin.

Codeine Phosphate. Codeine causes suppression of the cough reflex by a direct effect on the cough center in the medulla and appears to exert a drying effect on respiratory tract mucosa and to increase viscosity of bronchial secretions.
Codeine is well absorbed from the gastrointestinal tract. Following oral administration, peak antitussive effects usually can be expected to occur within one to two hours and may persist for a period of four hours. Codeine is metabolized in the liver. The drug undergoes O-demethylation, N-demethylation, and partial conjugation with glucuronic acid, and is excreted mainly in the urine as norcodeine and morphine in the free and conjugated forms.
Codeine appears in breast milk of nursing mothers and has been reported to cross the placental barrier.
Pseudoephedrine Hydrochloride. Pseudoephedrine is a physiologically active stereoisomer of ephedrine which acts directly on *alpha*, and to a lesser degree, *beta* -adrenergic receptors. The *alpha* -adrenergic effects are believed to result from the reduced production of cyclic adenosine-3',5' monophosphate (cyclic 3',5'-AMP) by inhibition of the enzyme adenyl cyclase, whereas *beta* -adrenergic effects appear to be caused by the stimulation of adenyl cyclase activity.
Pseudoephedrine acts directly on *alpha* -adrenergic receptors in the respiratory tract mucosa producing vasoconstriction resulting in shrinkage of swollen nasal mucous membranes, reduction of tissue hyperemia, edema, and nasal congestion, and an increase in nasal airway patency. Drainage of sinus secretions is increased and obstructed eustachian ostia may be opened. Relaxation of bronchial smooth muscle by stimulation of *beta$_2$* adrenergic receptors may also occur. Following oral administration significant bronchodilation has not been demonstrated consistently.
Nasal decongestion usually occurs within 30 minutes and persists for 4–6 hours after oral administration of 30 mg of pseudoephedrine hydrochloride.
Although specific information is not available, pseudoephedrine is presumed to cross the placenta and to enter cerebrospinal fluid. It is incompletely metabolized in the liver by N-demethylation to an inactive metabolite. Both are excreted in the urine with 55%–75% of a dose being unchanged.
Guaifenesin. Guaifenesin, by increasing respiratory tract fluid, reduces the viscosity of tenacious secretions and acts as an expectorant.
Guaifenesin is excreted in the urine mainly as glucuronates and sulfonates.

INDICATIONS AND USAGE

NUCOFED PEDIATRIC EXPECTORANT is indicated for symptomatic relief when both coughing and congestion are associated with upper respiratory infections and related conditions such as common cold, bronchitis, influenza, and sinusitis.

CONTRAINDICATIONS

Hypersensitivity to product's active ingredients.

WARNINGS

Persons with persistent cough such as occurs with smoking, asthma, emphysema, or where cough is accompanied by excessive secretions should not take this product except under the advice and supervision of a physician.
Do not give this product to children taking other drugs except under the advice and supervision of a physician.
Persons with a chronic pulmonary disease or shortness of breath, high blood pressure, heart disease, diabetes or thyroid disease should not take this product except under the advice and supervision of a physician.
Do not exceed recommended dosage because at higher doses nervousness, dizziness, or sleeplessness may occur.
If symptoms do not improve within 7 days or are accompanied by high fever, consult a physician before continuing use.

PRECAUTIONS

General. Inasmuch as the active ingredients of Nucofed Pediatric Expectorant consist of Codeine Phosphate, Pseudoephedrine Hydrochloride and Guaifenesin, this medication should be used with caution in the presence of the following:
- Cardiovascular disease (of any etiology)
- Diabetes mellitus
- Hypertension (of any severity)
- Abnormal thyroid function
- Prostatic hypertrophy
- Addison's disease
- Chronic ulcerative colitis
- History of drug abuse or dependence

- Chronic respiratory disease or impairment
- Functional impairment of the liver or kidney
Patients taking Nucofed Pediatric Expectorant should be cautioned when driving or doing jobs requiring alertness and to get up slowly from a lying or sitting position, or to lie down if nausea occurs.
Possible Drug Interactions. Because of the potential for drug interactions, persons currently taking any of the following medications should take Nucofed Pediatric Expectorant only on the advice and under the supervision of a physician.
- Beta adrenergic blockers—concurrent use may increase the pressor effect of pseudoephedrine.
- Digitalis glycosides—concurrent use with pseudoephedrine may increase the possibility of cardiac arrhythmias.
- Antihypertensive agents including Veratrum alkaloids—hypotensive effects may be decreased by the concurrent use of pseudoephedrine.
- Monoamine oxidase (MAO) inhibitors—these agents may potentiate the pressor effect of pseudoephedrine and may result in a hypertensive crisis; pseudoephedrine should not be administered during or within 14 days of MAO inhibitors.
- Sympathomimetics, other—sympathomimetics used concurrently may increase the effects either of these agents or of pseudoephedrine, thereby increasing the potential for side effects.
- Tricyclic antidepressants—the concurrent use of tricyclic antidepressants may antagonize the effects of pseudoephedrine and may increase the effects either of the antidepressants themselves or of the codeine component.
- CNS depressants
- Alcohol
- General anesthetics
- Anticholinergics—concurrent use may result in paralytic ileus.
Drug/Laboratory Test Interactions
- Codeine may cause an elevation in serum amylase levels due to the spasm producing potential of narcotic analgesics on the sphincter of Oddi.
- Guaifenesin is known to interfere with the colorimetric determination of 5-hydroxyindole-acetic acid (5-HIAA) and vanilmandelic acid (VMA).
Pregnancy: Category C
Animal reproduction studies of the components of Nucofed Pediatric Expectorant (codeine, pseudoephedrine and guaifenesin) have not been conducted. Thus, it is not known whether these agents can cause fetal harm when administered to pregnant women or whether they affect reproductive capacity. Accordingly, Nucofed Pediatric Expectorant should be given to pregnant women only where clearly needed.
Nursing Mothers
Codeine and Pseudoephedrine, two of the ingredients in Nucofed Pediatric Expectorant, are excreted in breast milk; therefore, caution should be exercised when this medication is prescribed for a nursing mother.
Pediatric Use
Do not give Nucofed Pediatric Expectorant to Children under two years of age except on the advice and under the supervision of a physician.

ADVERSE REACTIONS

Based on the composition of Nucofed Pediatric Expectorant the following side effects may occur: nervousness, restlessness, trouble in sleeping, drowsiness, difficult or painful urination, dizziness or lightheadedness, headache, nausea or vomiting, constipation, trembling, troubled breathing, increase in sweating, unusual paleness, weakness, changes in heart rate.

DRUG ABUSE AND DEPENDENCE

Nucofed Pediatric Expectorant has been placed in Schedule V of the Controlled Substances Act.

OVERDOSAGE

Nucofed Pediatric Expectorant contains Codeine Phosphate, Pseudoephedrine Hydrochloride and Guaifenesin. Overdosage as a result of this product should be treated based upon the symptomatology of the patient as it relates to the individual ingredient. Treatment of acute overdosage would probably be based upon treating the patient for codeine toxicity which may be manifested as:
- Gradual drowsiness, dizziness, heaviness of the head, weariness, diminution of sensibility, loss of pain and other modalities of sensation.
- Nausea and vomiting.
- A transient excitement stage, characterized by extreme restlessness, delirium, and rarely epileptiform convulsions, is sometimes seen in children and rarely in adult women.
- Bilateral miosis, progressing to pinpoint pupils, which do not react to light or accommodation. The pupils may dilate during terminal asphyxia.
- Itching of the skin and nose, sometimes with skin rashes and urticaria.

- Coma, with muscular relaxation and depressed or absent superficial and deep reflexes. A Babinski toe sign may appear.
- Marked slowing of the respiratory rate with inadequate pulmonary ventilation and consequent cyanosis. Breathing becomes stertorous and irregular (Cheyne-Stokes or Biot).
- The pulse is slow and the blood pressure gradually falls to shock levels. Urine formation ceases or is reduced to a very low rate.
The lethal dose of codeine for an adult is approximately 0.5–1.0 g. Reliable information regarding the lethal dose in children is not available. Treatment is as recommended for narcotics.

DOSAGE AND ADMINISTRATION
RECOMMENDED DOSAGE:
Adults and Children 12 years of age and over: 2 teaspoonfuls every 6 hours, not to exceed 8 teaspoonfuls in 24 hours.
Children:
  6 to under 12 years: 1 teaspoonful every 6 hours, not to exceed 4 teaspoonfuls in 24 hours.
  2 to under 6 years: ½ teaspoonful every 6 hours, not to exceed 2 teaspoonfuls in 24 hours.
Do not give this product to children under 2 years, except under the advice and supervision of a physician.

HOW SUPPLIED
Red, Strawberry Flavored Syrup
NDC 0029-3130-39   Pints

CAUTION
Federal law prohibits dispensing without prescription.
DGB—2010/5-88
Revised May, 1988

ORNADE® SPANSULE® CAPSULES   ℞
[or 'naid]
brand of sustained release capsules

DESCRIPTION
Ornade is a combination of an oral nasal decongestant and an antihistamine.
Each *Ornade* Spansule capsule contains phenylpropanolamine hydrochloride, 75 mg and chlorpheniramine maleate, 12 mg. Inactive ingredients consist of benzyl alcohol, cetylpyridinium chloride, FD&C Blue No. 1, FD&C Red No. 3, FD&C Yellow No. 6, D&C Red No. 27, D&C Red No. 30, gelatin, glyceryl distearate, iron oxide, polyethylene glycol, povidone, silicon dioxide, sodium lauryl sulfate, starch, sucrose, titanium dioxide, wax and trace amounts of other inactive ingredients.
Each *Ornade* Spansule capsule is so prepared that an initial dose is released promptly and the remaining medication is released gradually over a prolonged period.

CLINICAL PHARMACOLOGY
Phenylpropanolamine Hydrochloride
Phenylpropanolamine hydrochloride is a sympathomimetic agent which is closely related to ephedrine in chemical structure and pharmacologic action, but produces less central nervous system stimulation than ephedrine. It is a vasoconstrictor with decongestant action on nasal and upper respiratory tract mucosal membranes.
Chlorpheniramine Maleate
Chlorpheniramine maleate is an antihistamine with anticholinergic (drying) and sedative side effects. Antihistamines appear to compete with histamine for H$_1$ cell receptor sites on effector cells.
Pharmacokinetics
A single *Ornade* Spansule capsule produces blood levels comparable to those produced by administration of three 25 mg doses of phenylpropanolamine hydrochloride and three 4 mg doses of chlorpheniramine maleate in conventional release form given at four-hour intervals. At steady-state conditions, the following peak levels are reached after the oral administration of an *Ornade* Spansule capsule: 21 ng/mL chlorpheniramine maleate in 7.7 hours; 173 ng/mL phenylpropanolamine hydrochloride in 6.1 hours; under these circumstances, the half-lives are approximately 21 and 7 hours, respectively.

INDICATIONS AND USAGE
For the treatment of the symptoms of seasonal and perennial allergic rhinitis and vasomotor rhinitis, including nasal obstruction (congestion); also for the treatment of runny nose, sneezing and nasal congestion associated with the common cold.

CONTRAINDICATIONS
Hypersensitivity to either phenylpropanolamine hydrochloride or chlorpheniramine maleate and other antihistamines of similar chemical structure; severe hypertension; coronary artery disease.
This drug should NOT be used in newborn or premature infants.

Because of the higher risk of antihistamines for infants generally, and for newborns and prematures in particular, antihistamine therapy is contraindicated in nursing mothers. As with any product containing a sympathomimetic, *Ornade* Spansule capsules should NOT be used in patients taking monoamine oxidase (MAO) inhibitors.

WARNINGS

Ornade Spansule capsules may potentiate the effects of alcohol and other CNS depressants. Also, this product should not be taken simultaneously with other products containing phenylpropanolamine hydrochloride or amphetamines.

Ornade Spansule capsules should be used with considerable caution in patients with narrow-angle glaucoma, stenosing peptic ulcer, pyloroduodenal obstruction, symptomatic prostatic hypertrophy, or bladder neck obstruction.

Use in Children: In infants and children, especially, antihistamines in *overdosage* may cause hallucinations, convulsions, or death. As in adults, antihistamines may diminish mental alertness in children. In the young child, particularly, they may produce excitation.

Use in the Elderly (approximately 60 years or older): Antihistamines are more likely to cause dizziness, sedation and hypotension in elderly patients.

PRECAUTIONS

General: Use with caution in patients with lower respiratory disease including asthma, hypertension, cardiovascular disease, hyperthyroidism, increased intraocular pressure, or diabetes.

Information for Patients: Caution patients about activities requiring alertness (e.g., operating vehicles or machinery). Also caution patients about the possible additive effects of alcohol and other CNS depressants (hypnotics, sedatives, tranquilizers, etc.), and not to take simultaneously other products containing phenylpropanolamine hydrochloride or amphetamines. Patients should not take *Ornade* Spansule capsules in conjunction with a monoamine oxidase inhibitor or an oral anticoagulant.

Drug Interactions: *Ornade* Spansule capsules may interact with alcohol and other CNS depressants to potentiate their effects.

This product may have additive effects when taken simultaneously with other products containing phenylpropanolamine hydrochloride or amphetamines.

MAO inhibitors prolong and intensify the anticholinergic (drying) effects of antihistamines and potentiate the pressor effects of sympathomimetics such as phenylpropanolamine hydrochloride (see CONTRAINDICATIONS).

Phenylpropanolamine hydrochloride should not be used with ganglionic blocking drugs—such as mecamylamine—which potentiate reactions of sympathomimetics. It also should not be used with adrenergic blocking drugs, such as guanethidine sulfate or bethanidine, since it antagonizes the hypotensive action of these drugs.

The action of oral anticoagulants may be inhibited by antihistamines.

The CNS depressant and atropine-like effects of anticholinergics may be potentiated by concomitant administration of antihistamines. Concomitant administration of anticholinergics such as trihexyphenidyl, and other drugs with anticholinergic action (such as imipramine), with antihistamines may result in xerostomia.

β-adrenergic blockers may be antagonized by antihistamines.

Concomitant administration of corticosteroids and antihistamines may decrease the effects of the corticosteroids by enzyme induction.

Antihistamines inhibit norepinephrine reuptake by tissues and therefore potentiate the cardiovascular effects of norepinephrine.

Concomitant use of antihistamines with phenothiazines may produce an additive CNS depressant effect; concomitant use also may cause urinary retention or glaucoma.

Carcinogenesis, Mutagenesis, Impairment of Fertility: A long-term oncogenic study in rats with the chlorpheniramine maleate component of *Ornade* Spansule capsules did not produce an increase in the incidence of tumors in the drug-treated groups, as compared with the controls. No evidence of mutagenicity was found when chlorpheniramine maleate was evaluated in a battery of mutagenic studies, including the Ames test.

In an early study in rats with chlorpheniramine maleate a reduction in fertility was observed in female rats at doses approximately 67 times the human dose. More recent studies in rabbits and rats, using more appropriate methodology and doses up to approximately 50 and 85 times the human dose, showed no reduction in fertility.

There are no studies available which indicate whether phenylpropanolamine hydrochloride has carcinogenic or mutagenic effects or impairs fertility.

Pregnancy, Teratogenic Effects, Pregnancy Category B: Reproduction studies have been performed with the components of *Ornade* Spansule capsules. Studies with chlorpheniramine maleate in rabbits and rats at doses up to 50 times and 85 times the human dose, respectively, revealed no

evidence of harm to the fetus. A study with phenylpropanolamine hydrochloride in rats at doses up to 7 times the human dose revealed no evidence of harm to the fetus. There are, however, no adequate and well-controlled studies in pregnant women. Because animal reproduction studies are not always predictive of human response, *Ornade* Spansule capsules should be used during pregnancy only if clearly needed.

Nonteratogenic Effects: Studies of chlorpheniramine maleate in rats showed a decrease in the postnatal survival rate of offspring of animals dosed with 33 and 67 times the human dose.

Nursing Mothers: Small amounts of antihistamines are excreted in breast milk. Because of the higher risk with antihistamines in infants generally, and for newborns and prematures in particular, *Ornade* Spansule capsules should not be administered to a nursing mother (see CONTRAINDICATIONS).

Pediatric Use: The safety and effectiveness of *Ornade* Spansule capsules in children under 12 years of age have not been established.

In infants and children, especially, antihistamines in *overdosage* may cause hallucinations, convulsions, or death. As in adults, antihistamines may diminish mental alertness in children. In the young child, particularly, they may produce excitation. (See WARNINGS.)

ADVERSE REACTIONS

The following adverse reactions have been reported following the use of antihistamines and/or sympathomimetic amines:

General: Anaphylactic shock; chills; drug rash; excessive dryness of mouth, nose and throat; increased intraocular pressure; excessive perspiration; photosensitivity; urticaria; weakness.

Cardiovascular System: Angina pain; extrasystoles; headache; hypertension; hypotension; palpitations; tachycardia.

Hematologic: Agranulocytosis; hemolytic anemia; leukopenia; thrombocytopenia.

Nervous System: Blurred vision; confusion; convulsions; diplopia; disturbed coordination; dizziness; drowsiness; euphoria; excitation; fatigue; hysteria; insomnia; irritability; acute labyrinthitis; nervousness; neuritis; paresthesia; restlessness; sedation; tinnitus; tremor; vertigo.

GI System: Abdominal pain; anorexia; constipation; diarrhea; epigastric distress; nausea; vomiting.

GU System: Dysuria; early menses; urinary frequency; urinary retention.

Respiratory System: Thickening of bronchial secretions; tightness of chest and wheezing; nasal stuffiness.

OVERDOSAGE

In the event of overdosage, emergency treatment should be started immediately.

Symptoms: Effects of antihistamine overdosage may vary from central nervous system depression (sedation, apnea, diminished mental alertness, cardiovascular collapse) to stimulation (insomnia, hallucinations, tremors, or convulsions) to death.

Other signs and symptoms may be dizziness, tinnitus, ataxia, blurred vision and hypotension. Stimulation is particularly likely in children, as are atropine-like signs and symptoms (dry mouth; fixed, dilated pupils; flushing; hyperthermia; and gastrointestinal symptoms). In large doses, sympathomimetics may cause giddiness, headache, nausea, vomiting, sweating, thirst, tachycardia, precordial pain, palpitations, difficulty in micturition, muscular weakness and tenseness, anxiety, restlessness and insomnia. Many patients can present a toxic psychosis with delusions and hallucinations. Some may develop cardiac arrhythmias, circulatory collapse, convulsions, coma and respiratory failure.

Toxicity: In acute oral toxicity tests in rats, the LD_{50} for the ratio of 75 mg phenylpropanolamine hydrochloride and 12 mg chlorpheniramine maleate was 774.2 mg/kg; in mice, the LD_{50} for the formulation was 757.4 mg/kg.

Treatment: The patient should be induced to vomit even if emesis has occurred spontaneously. Pharmacologically induced vomiting by the administration of ipecac syrup is a preferred method. But vomiting should not be induced in patients with impaired consciousness. The action of ipecac is facilitated by physical activity and by the administration of 8 to 12 fluid ounces of water. If emesis does not occur within 15 minutes, the dose of ipecac should be repeated. Precautions against aspiration must be taken, especially in infants and children.

Following emesis, any drug remaining in the stomach may be adsorbed by activated charcoal administered as a slurry with water. If vomiting is unsuccessful or contraindicated, gastric lavage should be performed. Isotonic and one-half isotonic saline are the lavage solutions of choice. Since much of the *Spansule* capsule medication is coated for gradual release, saline cathartics should be administered to hasten evacuation of pellets that have not already released medication. Saline cathartics, such as milk of magnesia, draw water into the bowel by osmosis and therefore may be valuable for their action in rapid dilution of bowel content. Dialysis has not been reported to be effective in the treatment of phenyl-

propanolamine hydrochloride and chlorpheniramine maleate overdosage. After emergency treatment, the patient should continue to be medically monitored.

Treatment of the signs and symptoms of overdosage is symptomatic and supportive. *Stimulants* (analeptic agents) should *not* be used. Vasopressors may be used to treat hypotension. Short-acting barbiturates, diazepam, or paraldehyde may be administered to control seizures. Hyperpyrexia, especially in children, may require treatment with tepid water sponge baths or a hypothermic blanket. Apnea is treated with ventilatory support.

DOSAGE AND ADMINISTRATION

Adults and children 12 years of age and over—one capsule every 12 hours.

Ornade Spansule capsules are not recommended in children under 12.

HOW SUPPLIED

In gelatin capsules with opaque red cap and natural body. Each capsule is imprinted with the product name ORNADE and SKF, and filled with small red, white and gray pellets; in bottles of 50 and 500 capsules, and in Single Unit Packages of 100 capsules (intended for institutional use only). Each capsule contains 75 mg phenylpropanolamine hydrochloride and 12 mg chlorpheniramine maleate. Capsules should be stored at controlled room temperature (59°–86°F).

OR:L38

Shown in Product Identification Section, page 431

PARNATE®   ℞
[*pahr'naight*]
(brand of tranylcypromine sulfate)
Tablets 10 mg

Before prescribing, the physician should be familiar with the entire contents of this prescribing information.

DESCRIPTION

Chemically, tranylcypromine sulfate is (±)-*trans*-2-phenyl-cyclopropylamine sulfate (2:1).

Each round, rose-red, coated tablet is imprinted with the product name PARNATE and SKF and contains tranylcypromine sulfate equivalent to 10 mg of tranylcypromine. Inactive ingredients consist of gelatin, lactose, cellulose, citric acid, croscarmellose sodium, talc, magnesium stearate, iron oxide, D&C Red No. 7, FD&C Blue No. 2, FD&C Yellow No. 6, FD&C Red No. 40, titanium dioxide and trace amounts of other inactive ingredients.

NOTE: Parnate (tranylcypromine sulfate) tablets have been changed from rose-red sugar-coated tablets to rose-red film-coated tablets. The film-coated tablets differ in size from the sugar-coated tablets, but the drug content remains unchanged.

ACTION

Tranylcypromine is a non-hydrazine monoamine oxidase inhibitor with a rapid onset of activity. It increases the concentration of epinephrine, norepinephrine, and serotonin in storage sites throughout the nervous system, and in theory, this increased concentration of monoamines in the brain stem is the basis for its antidepressant activity. When tranylcypromine is withdrawn, monoamine oxidase activity is recovered in 3 to 5 days, although the drug is excreted in 24 hours.

INDICATIONS

For the treatment of Major Depressive Episode Without Melancholia.

Parnate (tranylcypromine sulfate) should be used in adult patients who can be closely supervised. It should rarely be the first antidepressant drug given. Rather, the drug is suited for patients who have failed to respond to the drugs more commonly administered for depression.

The effectiveness of *Parnate* has been established in adult outpatients, most of whom had a depressive illness which would correspond to a diagnosis of Major Depressive Episode Without Melancholia. As described in the American Psychiatric Association's Diagnostic and Statistical Manual, third edition (DSM III), Major Depressive Episode implies a prominent and relatively persistent (nearly every day for at least two weeks) depressed or dysphoric mood that usually interferes with daily functioning and includes at least four of the following eight symptoms: change in appetite, change in sleep, psychomotor agitation or retardation, loss of interest in usual activities or decrease in sexual drive, increased fatigability, feelings of guilt or worthlessness, slowed thinking or impaired concentration, and suicidal ideation or attempts. The effectiveness of *Parnate* in patients who meet the criteria for Major Depressive Episode with Melancholia (endogenous features) has not been established.

SUMMARY OF CONTRAINDICATIONS

Parnate (tranylcypromine sulfate) should not be administered in combination with any of the following: MAO inhibi-

Continued on next page

SmithKline Beecham—Cont.

tors or dibenzazepine derivatives; sympathomimetics (including amphetamines); some central nervous system depressants (including narcotics and alcohol); antihypertensive, diuretic, antihistaminic, sedative or anesthetic drugs; buspirone HCl; dextromethorphan; cheese or other foods with a high tyramine content; or excessive quantities of caffeine.

Parnate (tranylcypromine sulfate) should not be administered to any patient with a confirmed or suspected cerebrovascular defect or to any patient with cardiovascular disease, hypertension or history of headache.

(For complete discussion of contraindications and warnings, see below.)

CONTRAINDICATIONS

Parnate (tranylcypromine sulfate) is contraindicated:

1. In patients with cerebrovascular defects or cardiovascular disorders

Parnate should not be administered to any patient with a confirmed or suspected cerebrovascular defect or to any patient with cardiovascular disease or hypertension. The drug should also be withheld from individuals beyond the age of 60 because of the possibility of existing cerebral sclerosis with damaged vessels.

2. In the presence of pheochromocytoma

Parnate should not be used in the presence of pheochromocytoma since such tumors secrete pressor substances.

3. In combination with MAO inhibitors or with dibenzazepine-related entities

Parnate (tranylcypromine sulfate) should not be administered together or in rapid succession with other MAO inhibitors or with dibenzazepine-related entities. Hypertensive crises or severe convulsive seizures may occur in patients receiving such combinations. [See table above.]

In patients being transferred to *Parnate* from another MAO inhibitor or from a dibenzazepine-related entity, allow a medication-free interval of at least a week, then initiate *Parnate* using half the normal starting dosage for at least the first week of therapy. Similarly, at least a week should elapse between the discontinuance of *Parnate* and the administration of another MAO inhibitor or a dibenzazepine-related entity, or the readministration of *Parnate*.

4. In combination with fluoxetine

There have been reports of serious, sometimes fatal, reactions (including hyperthermia, rigidity, myoclonus, autonomic instability with possible rapid fluctuations of vital signs, and mental status changes that include extreme agitation progressing to delirium and coma) in patients receiving fluoxetine in combination with a monoamine oxidase inhibitor (MAOI), and in patients who have recently discontinued fluoxetine and are then started on an MAOI. Some cases presented with features resembling neuroleptic malignant syndrome. Therefore, fluoxetine (Prozac®, Lilly) should not be used in combination with an MAOI, or within 14 days of discontinuing therapy with an MAOI. Since fluoxetine and its major metabolite have very long elimination half-lives, at least 5 weeks should be allowed after stopping Prozac® before starting an MAOI.

5. In combination with buspirone

Parnate (tranylcypromine sulfate) should not be used in combination with buspirone HCl, since several cases of elevated blood pressure have been reported in patients taking MAO inhibitors who were then given buspirone HCl. At least 10 days should elapse between the discontinuation of *Parnate* and the institution of buspirone HCl.

6. In combination with sympathomimetics

Parnate (tranylcypromine sulfate) should not be administered in combination with sympathomimetics, including amphetamines, and over-the-counter drugs such as cold, hay fever or weight-reducing preparations that contain vasoconstrictors.

During *Parnate* therapy, it appears that certain patients are particularly vulnerable to the effects of sympathomimetics when the activity of certain enzymes is inhibited. Use of sympathomimetics and compounds such as guanethidine, methyldopa, reserpine, dopamine, levodopa and tryptophane with *Parnate* may precipitate hypertension, headache, and related symptoms. In addition, use with tryptophane may precipitate disorientation, memory impairment, and other neurologic and behavioral signs.

7. In combination with meperidine

Do not use meperidine concomitantly with MAO inhibitors or within two or three weeks following MAOI therapy. Serious reactions have been precipitated with concomitant use, including coma, severe hypertension or hypotension, severe respiratory depression, convulsions, malignant hyperpyrexia, excitation, peripheral vascular collapse and death. It is thought that these reactions may be mediated by accumulation of 5-HT (serotonin) consequent to MAO inhibition.

8. In combination with dextromethorphan

The combination of MAO inhibitors and dextromethorphan

Other MAO Inhibitors

Generic Name	Trademark
Furazolidone	Furoxone® (Norwich Eaton)
Isocarboxazid	Marplan® (Roche Laboratories)
Pargyline HCl	Eutonyl® (Abbott Laboratories)
Pargyline HCl and methyclothiazide	Eutron® (Abbott Laboratories)
Phenelzine sulfate	Nardil® (Parke-Davis)
Procarbazine HCl	Matulane® (Roche Laboratories)

Dibenzazepine-Related and Other Tricyclics

Generic Name	Trademark
Amitriptyline HCl	Elavil® (Merck Sharp & Dohme)
	Endep® (Roche Products)
Perphenazine and amitriptyline HCl	Etrafon® (Schering)
	Triavil® (Merck Sharp & Dohme)
Clomipramine hydrochloride	Anafranil® (CIBA-GEIGY)
Desipramine HCl	Norpramin® (Merrell Dow)
	Pertofrane® (Rorer Pharmaceuticals)
Imipramine HCl	Janimine® (Abbott Laboratories)
	Tofranil® (GEIGY Pharmaceuticals)
Nortriptyline HCl	Aventyl® (Eli Lilly & Co.)
	Pamelor® (Sandoz)
Protriptyline HCl	Vivactil® (Merck Sharp & Dohme)
Doxepin HCl	Adapin® (Fisons)
	Sinequan® (Roerig)
Carbamazepine	Tegretol® (GEIGY Pharmaceuticals)
Cyclobenzaprine HCl	Flexeril® (Merck Sharp & Dohme)
Amoxapine	Asendin® (Lederle)
Maprotiline HCl	Ludiomil® (CIBA)
Trimipramine maleate	Surmontil® (Wyeth-Ayerst Laboratories)

has been reported to cause brief episodes of psychosis or bizarre behavior.

9. In combination with cheese or other foods with a high tyramine content

Hypertensive crises have sometimes occurred during *Parnate* therapy after ingestion of foods with a high tyramine content. In general, the patient should avoid protein foods in which aging or protein breakdown is used to increase flavor. In particular, patients should be instructed not to take foods such as cheese (particularly strong or aged varieties), sour cream, Chianti wine, sherry, beer (including nonalcoholic beer), liqueurs, pickled herring, anchovies, caviar, liver, canned figs, raisins, bananas or avocados (particularly if overripe), chocolate, soy sauce, sauerkraut, the pods of broad beans (fava beans), yeast extracts, yogurt, meat extracts or meat prepared with tenderizers.

10. In patients undergoing elective surgery

Patients taking *Parnate* should not undergo elective surgery requiring general anesthesia. Also, they should not be given cocaine or local anesthesia containing sympathomimetic vasoconstrictors. The possible combined hypotensive effects of *Parnate* and spinal anesthesia should be kept in mind. *Parnate* should be discontinued at least 10 days prior to elective surgery. (Withdrawal should be gradual.)

ADDITIONAL CONTRAINDICATIONS

In general, the physician should bear in mind the possibility of a lowered margin of safety when Parnate (tranylcypromine sulfate) is administered in combination with potent drugs.

1. *Parnate* should not be used in combination with some central nervous system depressants such as narcotics and alcohol, or with hypotensive agents. A marked potentiating effect on these classes of drugs has been reported.
2. Anti-parkinsonism drugs should be used with caution in patients receiving *Parnate* since severe reactions have been reported.
3. *Parnate* should not be used in patients with a history of liver disease or in those with abnormal liver function tests.
4. Excessive use of caffeine in any form should be avoided in patients receiving *Parnate*.

WARNING TO PHYSICIANS

Parnate (tranylcypromine sulfate) is a potent agent with the capability of producing serious side effects. *Parnate* is not recommended in those depressive reactions where other antidepressant drugs may be effective. **It should be reserved for patients who can be closely supervised and who have not responded satisfactorily to the drugs more commonly administered for depression.**

Before prescribing, the physician should be completely familiar with the full material on dosage, side effects, and contraindications on these pages, with the principles of MAO inhibitor therapy and the side effects of this class of drugs. Also, the physician should be familiar with the symptomatology of mental depressions and alternate methods of treatment to aid in the careful selection of patients for *Parnate* therapy. In depressed patients, the possibility of suicide should always be considered and adequate precautions taken.

Pregnancy Warning: Use of any drug in pregnancy, during lactation, or in women of childbearing age requires that the potential benefits of the drug be weighed against its possible hazards to mother and child.

Animal reproductive studies show that *Parnate* passes through the placental barrier into the fetus of the rat, and into the milk of the lactating dog. The absence of a harmful action of *Parnate* on fertility or on postnatal development by either prenatal treatment or from the milk of treated animals has not been demonstrated. Tranylcypromine is excreted in human milk.

WARNING TO THE PATIENT

Patients should be instructed to report promptly the occurrence of headache or other unusual symptoms, i.e., palpitation and/or tachycardia, a sense of constriction in the throat or chest, sweating, dizziness, neck stiffness, nausea, or vomiting.

Patients should be warned against eating the foods listed in Section 9 under Contraindications while on Parnate (tranylcypromine sulfate) therapy. Also, they should be told not to drink alcoholic beverages. The patient should also be warned about the possibility of hypotension and faintness, as well as drowsiness sufficient to impair performance of potentially hazardous tasks such as driving a car or operating machinery.

Patients should also be cautioned not to take concomitant medications, whether prescription or over-the-counter drugs such as cold, hay fever or weight-reducing preparations, without the advice of a physician. They should be advised not to consume excessive amounts of caffeine in any form. Likewise, they should inform other physicians, and their dentist, about their use of *Parnate*.

WARNINGS

HYPERTENSIVE CRISES: The most important reaction associated with Parnate (tranylcypromine sulfate) is the occurrence of hypertensive crises which have sometimes been fatal.

These crises are characterized by some or all of the following symptoms: occipital headache which may radiate frontally, palpitation, neck stiffness or soreness, nausea or vomiting, sweating (sometimes with fever and sometimes with cold, clammy skin) and photophobia. Either tachycardia or bradycardia may be present, and associated constricting chest pain and dilated pupils may occur. **Intracranial bleeding, sometimes fatal in outcome, has been reported in association with the paradoxical increase in blood pressure.**

In all patients taking *Parnate* blood pressure should be followed closely to detect evidence of any pressor response. It is emphasized that full reliance should not be placed on blood pressure readings, but that the patient should also be observed frequently.

Therapy should be discontinued immediately upon the occurrence of palpitation or frequent headaches during *Parnate* therapy. These signs may be prodromal of a hypertensive crisis.

**Important:
Recommended treatment in
hypertensive crises**

If a hypertensive crisis occurs, Parnate (tranylcypromine sulfate) should be discontinued and therapy to lower blood pressure should be instituted immediately. Headache tends to abate as blood pressure is lowered. On the basis of present evidence, phentolamine (available as Regitine®*) is recommended. (The dosage reported for phentolamine is 5 mg I.V.) Care should be taken to administer this drug slowly in order to avoid producing an excessive hypotensive effect. Fever should be managed by means of external cooling. Other symptomatic and supportive measures may be desirable in particular cases. Do not use parenteral reserpine.

PRECAUTIONS

Hypotension

Hypotension has been observed during Parnate (tranylcypromine sulfate) therapy. Symptoms of postural hypotension

*phentolamine mesylate USP, CIBA.

are seen most commonly but not exclusively in patients with pre-existent hypertension; blood pressure usually returns rapidly to pretreatment levels upon discontinuation of the drug. At doses above 30 mg daily, postural hypotension is a major side effect and may result in syncope. Dosage increases should be made more gradually in patients showing a tendency toward hypotension at the beginning of therapy. Postural hypotension may be relieved by having the patient lie down until blood pressure returns to normal.
Also, when *Parnate* is combined with those phenothiazine derivatives or other compounds known to cause hypotension, the possibility of additive hypotensive effects should be considered.

OTHER PRECAUTIONS

There have been reports of drug dependency in patients using doses of tranylcypromine significantly in excess of the therapeutic range. Some of these patients had a history of previous substance abuse. The following withdrawal symptoms have been reported: restlessness, anxiety, depression, confusion, hallucinations, headache, weakness and diarrhea.
Drugs which lower the seizure threshold, including MAO inhibitors, should not be used with Amipaque®†. As with other MAO inhibitors, Parnate (tranylcypromine sulfate) should be discontinued at least 48 hours before myelography (Withdrawal should be gradual.) and should not be resumed for at least 24 hours postprocedure.
In depressed patients, the possibility of suicide should always be considered and adequate precautions taken. Exclusive reliance on drug therapy to prevent suicidal attempts is unwarranted, as there may be a delay in the onset of therapeutic effect or an increase in anxiety and agitation. Also, some patients fail to respond to drug therapy or may respond only temporarily.
MAO inhibitors may have the capacity to suppress anginal pain that would otherwise serve as a warning of myocardial ischemia. The usual precautions should be observed in patients with impaired renal function since there is a possibility of cumulative effects in such patients.
Older patients may suffer more morbidity than younger patients during and following an episode of hypertension or malignant hyperthermia. Older patients have less compensatory reserve to cope with any serious adverse reaction. Therefore, *Parnate* should be used with caution in the elderly population.
Although excretion of *Parnate* is rapid, inhibition of MAO may persist up to 10 days following discontinuation.
Because the influence of *Parnate* on the convulsive threshold is variable in animal experiments, suitable precautions should be taken if epileptic patients are treated.
Some MAO inhibitors have contributed to hypoglycemic episodes in diabetic patients receiving insulin or oral hypoglycemic agents. Therefore, *Parnate* should be used with caution in diabetics using these drugs.
Parnate may aggravate coexisting symptoms in depression, such as anxiety and agitation.
Use *Parnate* with caution in hyperthyroid patients because of their increased sensitivity to pressor amines.
Parnate should be administered with caution to patients receiving Antabuse®‡. In a single study, rats given high intraperitoneal doses of *d* or *l* isomers of tranylcypromine sulfate plus disulfiram experienced severe toxicity including convulsions and death. Additional studies in rats given high oral doses of racemic tranylcypromine sulfate (*Parnate*) and disulfiram produced no adverse interaction.

ADVERSE REACTIONS

Overstimulation which may include increased anxiety, agitation and manic symptoms is usually evidence of excessive therapeutic action. Dosage should be reduced, or a phenothiazine tranquilizer should be administered concomitantly.
Patients may experience restlessness or insomnia; may notice some weakness, drowsiness, episodes of dizziness, or dry mouth; or may report nausea, diarrhea, abdominal pain, or constipation. Most of these effects can be relieved by lowering the dosage or by giving suitable concomitant medication.
Tachycardia, significant anorexia, edema, palpitation, blurred vision, chills, and impotence have each been reported.
Headaches without blood pressure elevation have occurred.
Rare instances of hepatitis and skin rash have been reported.
Impaired water excretion compatible with the syndrome of inappropriate secretion of antidiuretic hormone (SIADH) has been reported.
Tinnitus, muscle spasm, tremors, myoclonic jerks, numbness, paresthesia, urinary retention and retarded ejaculation have been reported.
Hematologic disorders including anemia, leukopenia, agranulocytosis, and thrombocytopenia have been reported.

Post-Introduction Reports

The following are spontaneously reported adverse events temporally associated with *Parnate* therapy. No clear relationship between *Parnate* and these events has been established. Localized scleroderma, flare-up of cystic acne, ataxia, confusion, disorientation, memory loss, urinary frequency, urinary incontinence, urticaria, fissuring in corner of mouth, akinesia.

DOSAGE AND ADMINISTRATION

Dosage should be adjusted to the requirements of the individual patient. Improvement should be seen within 48 hours to three weeks after starting therapy.
The usual effective dosage is 30 mg per day, usually given in divided doses. If there are no signs of improvement after a reasonable period (up to two weeks), then the dosage may be increased in 10 mg per day increments at intervals of one to three weeks; the dosage range may be extended to a maximum of 60 mg per day from the usual 30 mg per day.
Withdrawal from Parnate (tranylcypromine sulfate) should be gradual.

OVERDOSAGE

SYMPTOMS: The characteristic symptoms that may be caused by overdosage are usually those described on the preceding pages.
However, an intensification of these symptoms and sometimes severe additional manifestations may be seen, depending on the degree of overdosage and on individual susceptibility. Some patients exhibit insomnia, restlessness and anxiety, progressing in severe cases to agitation, mental confusion and incoherence. Hypotension, dizziness, weakness and drowsiness may occur, progressing in severe cases to extreme dizziness and shock. A few patients have displayed hypertension with severe headache and other symptoms. Rare instances have been reported in which hypertension was accompanied by twitching or myoclonic fibrillation of skeletal muscles with hyperpyrexia, sometimes progressing to generalized rigidity and coma.
TREATMENT: Gastric lavage is helpful if performed early. Treatment should normally consist of general supportive measures, close observation of vital signs and steps to counteract specific symptoms as they occur, since MAO inhibition may persist. The management of hypertensive crises is described under WARNINGS in the HYPERTENSIVE CRISES section.
External cooling is recommended if hyperpyrexia occurs. Barbiturates have been reported to help relieve myoclonic reactions, but frequency of administration should be controlled carefully because Parnate (tranylcypromine sulfate) may prolong barbiturate activity. When hypotension requires treatment, the standard measures for managing circulatory shock should be initiated. If pressor agents are used, the rate of infusion should be regulated by careful observation of the patient because an exaggerated pressor response sometimes occurs in the presence of MAO inhibition. Remember that the toxic effect of *Parnate* may be delayed or prolonged following the last dose of the drug. Therefore, the patient should be closely observed for at least a week. It is not known if tranylcypromine is dialyzable.

HOW SUPPLIED

Tablets, containing tranylcypromine sulfate equivalent to 10 mg of tranylcypromine, in bottles of 100.

PT:L55

Shown in Product Identification Section, page 431

†metrizamide, Winthrop Pharmaceuticals.
‡disulfiram, Wyeth-Ayerst Laboratories.

PENTACEF™ ℞

brand of
ceftazidime for injection
L-arginine formulation

For Intravenous or Intramuscular Use

DESCRIPTION

Ceftazidime is a semisynthetic, broad-spectrum, beta-lactam antibiotic for parenteral administration. It is the pentahydrate of Pyridinium, 1-[[7-[[(2-amino-4-thiazolyl)[(1-carboxy-1-methylethoxy)imino]acetyl]amino]-2-carboxy-8-oxo-5-thia-1-azabicyclo(4.2.0.)oct-2-en-3-yl] methyl]-,hydroxide, inner salt, [6R-(6α, 7β(Z))]. It has the following structural formula:

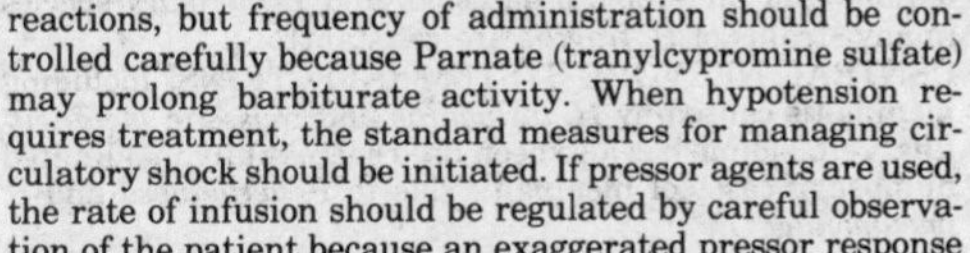

Its molecular formula is $C_{22}H_{22}N_6O_7S_2 \cdot 5H_2O$ and the molecular weight is 636.65.
Pentacef (ceftazidime for injection/L-arginine) is a sterile, dry, powdered mixture of ceftazidime pentahydrate and L-arginine (318 mg/gram of ceftazidime activity). The L-arginine facilitates dissolution. *Pentacef* dissolves without evolution of gas. The product contains no sodium ion. Solutions of *Pentacef* range in color from light yellow to amber, depending upon the diluent and volume used. The pH of freshly reconstituted solutions usually ranges from 5.0 to 7.5.

CLINICAL PHARMACOLOGY

After intravenous administration of 500 mg and 1 gram doses of ceftazidime over five minutes to normal adult male volunteers, mean peak serum concentrations of 45 mcg/mL and 90 mcg/mL, respectively, were achieved. After intravenous infusion of 500 mg, 1 gram and 2 gram doses of ceftazidime over 20 to 30 minutes to normal adult male volunteers, mean peak serum concentrations of 42 mcg/mL, 69 mcg/mL and 170 mcg/mL, respectively, were achieved. The average serum concentrations following intravenous infusion of 500 mg, 1 gram and 2 gram doses to these volunteers over an eight-hour interval are given in Table 1.

Table 1

Ceftazidime I.V. Dosage	Serum Concentrations (mcg/mL) 0.5 hr.	1 hr.	2 hr.	4 hr.	8 hr.
500 mg	42	25	12	6	2
1 gram	60	39	23	11	3
2 grams	129	75	42	13	5

The absorption and elimination of ceftazidime were directly proportional to the size of the dose. The half-life following intravenous administration was approximately 1.9 hours. Less than 10% of ceftazidime was protein bound. The degree of protein binding was independent of concentration. There was no evidence of accumulation of ceftazidime in the serum in individuals with normal renal function following multiple intravenous doses of 1 gram and 2 grams every eight hours for ten days.
Following intramuscular administration of 500 mg and 1 gram doses of ceftazidime to normal adult volunteers, the mean peak serum concentrations were 17 mcg/mL and 39 mcg/mL, respectively, at approximately one hour. Serum concentrations remained above 4 mcg/mL for six and eight hours after the intramuscular administration of 500 mg and 1 gram doses, respectively. The half-life of ceftazidime in these volunteers was approximately two hours.
The presence of hepatic dysfunction had no effect on the pharmacokinetics of ceftazidime in individuals administered 2 grams intravenously every eight hours for five days. Therefore, a dosage adjustment from the normal recommended dosage is not required for patients with hepatic dysfunction, provided renal function is not impaired.
Approximately 80% to 90% of an intramuscular or intravenous dose of ceftazidime is excreted unchanged by the kidneys over a 24-hour period. After the intravenous administration of single 500 mg or 1 gram doses, approximately 50% of the dose appeared in the urine in the first two hours. An additional 20% was excreted between two and four hours after dosing, and approximately another 12% of the dose appeared in the urine between four and eight hours later. The elimination of ceftazidime by the kidneys resulted in high therapeutic concentrations in the urine.
The mean renal clearance of ceftazidime was approximately 100 mL/min. The calculated plasma clearance of approximately 115 mL/min. indicated nearly complete elimination of ceftazidime by the renal route. Administration of probenecid prior to dosing had no effect on the elimination kinetics of ceftazidime. This suggests that ceftazidime is eliminated by glomerular filtration and is not actively secreted by renal tubular mechanisms.
Since ceftazidime is eliminated almost solely by the kidneys, its serum half-life is significantly prolonged in patients with impaired renal function. Consequently, dosage adjustments in such patients as described in the DOSAGE AND ADMINISTRATION section are suggested.
Ceftazidime concentrations achieved in specific body tissues and fluids are depicted in Table 2.
[See table on next page.]

Microbiology

Ceftazidime is bactericidal in action, exerting its effect by inhibition of enzymes responsible for cell-wall synthesis. A wide range of gram-negative organisms is susceptible to ceftazidime *in vitro*, including strains resistant to gentamicin and other aminoglycosides. In addition, ceftazidime has been shown to be active against gram-positive organisms. It is highly stable to most clinically important beta-lactamases, plasmid or chromosomal, which are produced by both gram-negative and gram-positive organisms and, consequently, is active against many strains resistant to ampicillin and other cephalosporins.
Ceftazidime has been shown to be active against the following organisms both *in vitro* and in clinical infections (see INDICATIONS AND USAGE).
Aerobes, Gram-Negative: *Pseudomonas* species (including *Pseudomonas aeruginosa*); *Klebsiella* species (including *Klebsiella pneumoniae*); *Proteus mirabilis*; *Proteus vulgaris*; *Escherichia coli*; *Enterobacter* species, including *Enterobacter clo-*

Continued on next page

SmithKline Beecham—Cont.

acae and *Enterobacter aerogenes; Citrobacter* species, including *Citrobacter freundii* and *Citrobacter diversus; Serratia* species; *Haemophilus influenzae,* including ampicillin-resistant strains; and *Neisseria meningitidis.*

Aerobes, Gram-Positive: *Staphylococcus aureus,* including penicillinase- and non-penicillinase-producing strains; *Streptococcus pyogenes* (group A beta-hemolytic streptococci); *Streptococcus agalactiae* (group B streptococci); and *Streptococcus pneumoniae.*

Anaerobes: *Bacteroides* species (NOTE: Many strains of *Bacteroides fragilis* are resistant).

Ceftazidime has been shown to be active *in vitro* against most strains of the following organisms; however, the clinical significance of this activity is unknown: *Staphylococcus epidermidis; Morganella morganii* (formerly *Proteus morganii*); *Providencia* species (including *Providencia rettgeri,* formerly *Proteus rettgeri*); *Acinetobacter* species; *Salmonella* species; *Clostridium* species (not including *Clostridium difficile*); *Peptococcus* species; *Peptostreptococcus* species; *Neisseria gonorrhoeae; Haemophilus parainfluenzae; Yersinia enterocolitica;* and *Shigella* species.

Ceftazidime and the aminoglycosides have been shown to be synergistic *in vitro* against *P. aeruginosa* and the *Enterobacteriaceae.* Ceftazidime and carbenicillin have also been shown to be synergistic *in vitro* against *P. aeruginosa.*

Ceftazidime is not active *in vitro* against: methicillin-resistant staphylococci; *Streptococcus faecalis* and many other enterococci; *Listeria monocytogenes; Campylobacter* species; or *Clostridium difficile.*

Susceptibility Tests: ***Diffusion Techniques:*** Quantitative methods that require measurement of zone diameters give an estimate of antibiotic susceptibility. One such procedure[1-3] has been recommended for use with disks to test susceptibility to ceftazidime.

Reports from the laboratory giving results of the standard single-disk susceptibility test with a 30 mcg ceftazidime disk should be interpreted according to the following criteria:

Susceptible organisms produce zones of 18 mm or greater, indicating that the test organism is likely to respond to therapy.

Organisms that produce zones of 15 mm to 17 mm are expected to be susceptible if high dosage is used or if the infection is confined to tissues and fluids (e.g., urine) in which high antibiotic levels are attained.

Resistant organisms produce zones of 14 mm or less, indicating that other therapy should be selected.

Organisms should be tested with the ceftazidime disk, since ceftazidime has been shown by *in vitro* tests to be active against certain strains found resistant when other beta-lactam disks are used.

Standardized procedures require the use of laboratory control organisms. The 30 mcg ceftazidime disk should give zone diameters between 25 mm and 32 mm for *E. coli* ATCC 25922. For *P. aeruginosa* ATCC 27853, the zone diameters should be between 22 mm and 29 mm. For *S. aureus* ATCC 25923, the zone diameters should be between 16 mm and 20 mm.

Dilution Techniques: In other susceptibility testing procedures, e.g., ICS agar dilution or the equivalent, a bacterial isolate may be considered susceptible if the MIC value for ceftazidime is not more than 16 mcg/mL. Organisms are considered resistant to ceftazidime if the MIC is equal to or greater than 64 mcg/mL. Organisms having an MIC value of less than 64 mcg/mL but greater than 16 mcg/mL are expected to be susceptible if high dosage is used or if the infection is confined to tissues and fluids (e.g., urine) in which high antibiotic levels are attained.

As with standard diffusion methods, dilution procedures require the use of laboratory control organisms. Standard ceftazidime powder should give MIC values in the range of 4 mcg/mL and 16 mcg/mL for *S. aureus* ATCC 25923. For *E. coli* ATCC 25922, the MIC range should be between 0.125 mcg/mL and 0.5 mcg/mL. For *P. aeruginosa* ATCC 27853, the MIC range should be between 0.5 mcg/mL and 2 mcg/mL.

INDICATIONS AND USAGE

Pentacef (ceftazidime for injection) is indicated for the treatment of patients with infections caused by susceptible strains of the designated organisms in the diseases listed below:

LOWER RESPIRATORY TRACT INFECTIONS, including pneumonia, caused by *P. aeruginosa* and other *Pseudomonas* species; *H. influenzae,* including ampicillin-resistant strains; *Klebsiella* species; *Enterobacter* species, *P. mirabilis; E. coli; Serratia* species; *Citrobacter* species; *S. pneumoniae;* and *S. aureus* (methicillin-susceptible strains).

SKIN AND SKIN STRUCTURE INFECTIONS, caused by *P. aeruginosa, Klebsiella* species; *E. coli; Proteus* species including *P. mirabilis* and indole-positive *Proteus, Enterobacter* species; *Serratia* species; *S. aureus* (methicillin-susceptible strains) and *S. pyogenes* (group A beta-hemolytic streptococci).

URINARY TRACT INFECTIONS, both complicated and uncomplicated, caused by *P. aeruginosa; Enterobacter* species; *Proteus* species, including *P. mirabilis* and indole-positive *Proteus; Klebsiella* species and *E. coli.*

BACTERIAL SEPTICEMIA, caused by *P. aeruginosa, Klebsiella* species; *H. influenzae; E. coli, Serratia* species, *S. pneumoniae* and *S. aureus* (methicillin-susceptible strains).

BONE AND JOINT INFECTIONS, caused by *P. aeruginosa; Klebsiella* species; *Enterobacter* species; and *S. aureus* (methicillin-susceptible strains).

GYNECOLOGIC INFECTIONS, including endometritis, pelvic cellulitis and other infections of the female genital tract caused by *E. coli.*

INTRA-ABDOMINAL INFECTIONS, including peritonitis caused by *E. coli, Klebsiella* species; *S. aureus* (methicillin-susceptible strains), and polymicrobial infections caused by aerobic and anaerobic organisms, and *Bacteroides* species (many strains of *B. fragilis* are resistant).

CENTRAL NERVOUS SYSTEM INFECTIONS, including meningitis caused by *H. influenzae* and *Neisseria meningitidis.* Ceftazidime has also been used successfully in a limited number of cases of meningitis due to *P. aeruginosa* and *S. pneumoniae.*

Specimens for bacterial cultures should be obtained prior to therapy in order to isolate and identify causative organisms and to determine their susceptibility to ceftazidime. Therapy may be instituted before results of susceptibility studies are known; however, once these results become available, the antibiotic treatment should be adjusted accordingly.

Pentacef (ceftazidime for injection) may be used alone in cases of confirmed or suspected sepsis. Ceftazidime has been used successfully in clinical trials as empiric therapy in cases where various concomitant therapies with other antibiotics have been used.

Pentacef may also be used concomitantly with other antibiotics, such as aminoglycosides, vancomycin and clindamycin, in severe and life-threatening infections and in the immunocompromised patient (see COMPATIBILITY AND STABILITY). When such concomitant treatment is appropriate, prescribing information in the labeling for the other antibiotics should be followed. The dose depends on the severity of the infection and the patient's condition.

Table 2. Ceftazidime Concentrations in Body Tissues and Fluids

Tissue or Fluid	Dose/ Route	No. Patients	Time of Sample Post-Dose	Average Tissue or Fluid Level (mcg/mL or mcg/gram)
Urine	500 mg I.M.	6	0–2 hours	2,100
	2 grams I.V.	6	0–2 hours	12,000
Bile	2 grams I.V.	3	90 min.	36.4
Synovial fluid	2 grams I.V.	13	2 hours	25.6
Peritoneal fluid	2 grams I.V.	8	2 hours	48.6
Sputum	1 gram I.V.	8	1 hour	9
Cerebrospinal fluid (inflamed meninges)	2 grams q8h I.V.	5	120 min.	9.8
	2 grams q8h I.V.	6	180 min.	9.4
Aqueous humor	2 grams I.V.	13	1–3 hours	11
Blister fluid	1 gram I.V.	7	2–3 hours	19.7
Lymphatic fluid	1 gram I.V.	7	2–3 hours	23.4
Bone	2 grams I.V.	8	0.67 hour	31.1
Heart muscle	2 grams I.V.	35	30–280 min.	12.7
Skin	2 grams I.V.	22	30–180 min.	6.6
Skeletal muscle	2 grams I.V.	35	30–280 min.	9.4
Myometrium	2 grams I.V.	31	1–2 hours	18.7

CONTRAINDICATIONS

Pentacef is contraindicated in patients who have shown hypersensitivity to ceftazidime or the cephalosporin group of antibiotics.

WARNINGS

BEFORE THERAPY WITH *PENTACEF* IS INSTITUTED, CAREFUL INQUIRY SHOULD BE MADE TO DETERMINE WHETHER THE PATIENT HAS HAD PREVIOUS HYPERSENSITIVITY REACTIONS TO CEFTAZIDIME, CEPHALOSPORINS, PENICILLINS, OR OTHER DRUGS. IF THIS PRODUCT IS GIVEN TO PENICILLIN-SENSITIVE PATIENTS, CAUTION SHOULD BE EXERCISED BECAUSE CROSS-HYPERSENSITIVITY AMONG BETA-LACTAM ANTIBIOTICS HAS BEEN CLEARLY DOCUMENTED AND MAY OCCUR IN UP TO 10% OF PATIENTS WITH A HISTORY OF PENICILLIN ALLERGY. IF AN ALLERGIC REACTION TO *PENTACEF* OCCURS, DISCONTINUE TREATMENT WITH THE DRUG. SERIOUS ACUTE HYPERSENSITIVITY REACTIONS MAY REQUIRE TREATMENT WITH EPINEPHRINE AND OTHER EMERGENCY MEASURES, INCLUDING OXYGEN, I.V. FLUIDS, I.V. ANTIHISTAMINES, CORTICOSTEROIDS, PRESSOR AMINES, AND AIRWAY MANAGEMENT, AS CLINICALLY INDICATED.

Pseudomembranous colitis has been reported with nearly all antibacterial agents, including ceftazidime, and may range in severity from mild to life-threatening. Therefore, it is important to consider this diagnosis in patients who present with diarrhea subsequent to the administration of antibacterial agents.

Treatment with antibacterial agents alters the normal flora of the colon and may permit overgrowth of Clostridia. Studies indicate that a toxin produced by *Clostridium difficile* is the primary cause of "antibiotic-associated colitis."

After the diagnosis of pseudomembranous colitis has been established, therapeutic measures should be initiated. Mild cases of pseudomembranous colitis usually respond to drug discontinuation alone. In moderate to severe cases, consideration should be given to management with fluids and electrolytes, protein supplementation, and treatment with an oral antibacterial drug effective against *C. difficile.*

PRECAUTIONS

General: Ceftazidime has not been shown to be nephrotoxic; however, high and prolonged serum antibiotic concentrations can occur from usual doses in patients with transient or persistent reduction of urinary output because of renal insufficiency. The total daily dosage should be reduced when ceftazidime is administered to patients with renal insufficiency (see DOSAGE AND ADMINISTRATION). In these patients, elevated levels of ceftazidime can lead to seizures, encephalopathy, asterixis, and neuromuscular excitability.

As with other antibiotics, prolonged use of Pentacef (ceftazidime for injection) may result in overgrowth of nonsusceptible organisms. Repeated evaluation of the patient's condition is essential. If superinfection occurs during therapy, appropriate measures should be taken.

Cephalosporins may be associated with a fall in prothrombin activity. Those at risk include patients with renal or hepatic impairment, or poor nutritional state, as well as patients receiving a protracted course of antimicrobial therapy. Prothrombin time should be monitored in patients at risk and exogenous vitamin K administered as indicated.

Pentacef should be prescribed with caution in individuals with a history of gastrointestinal disease, particularly colitis.

Arginine has been shown to alter glucose metabolism and elevate serum potassium transiently when administered at 50 times the recommended dose. The effect of lower dosing is not known.

Drug Interactions: Nephrotoxicity has been reported following concomitant administration of cephalosporins with aminoglycoside antibiotics or potent diuretics, such as furosemide. Renal function should be carefully monitored, especially if higher dosages of the aminoglycosides are to be administered or if therapy is prolonged, because of the potential nephrotoxicity and ototoxicity of aminoglycoside antibiotics. Nephrotoxicity and ototoxicity were not noted when ceftazidime was given alone in clinical trials.

Drug/Laboratory Test Interactions: A false-positive reaction for glucose in the urine may occur with copper reduction tests (Benedict's or Fehling's solution or with Clinitest® tablets), but not with enzyme-based tests for glycosuria (e.g., Clinistix®, Tes-Tape®).

Carcinogenesis, Mutagenesis, Impairment of Fertility: Long-term studies in animals have not been performed to evaluate carcinogenic potential. However, a mouse micronucleus test and an Ames test were both negative for mutagenic effects.

Pregnancy: Teratogenic Effects: **Pregnancy Category B.** Reproduction studies have been performed in mice and rats at doses up to 40 times the human dose and have revealed no evidence of impaired fertility or harm to the fetus due to

Table 3. Recommended Dosage Schedule

	Dose	Frequency
*Adults 12 years and older**		
Usual recommended dosage	**1 gram I.V. or I.M.**	**q8–12h**
Uncomplicated urinary tract infections	250 mg I.V. or I.M.	q12h
Bone and joint infections	2 grams I.V.	q12h
Complicated urinary tract infections	500 mg I.V. or I.M.	q8–12h
Uncomplicated pneumonia; mild skin and skin structure infections	500 mg–1 gram I.V. or I.M.	q8h
Serious gynecological and intra-abdominal infections	2 grams I.V.	q8h
Meningitis	2 grams I.V.	q8h
Very severe life-threatening infections, especially in immunocompromised patients	2 grams I.V.	q8h
Pseudomonal lung infections in patients with cystic fibrosis with normal renal function†	30–50 mg/kg I.V. to a maximum of 6 grams/day	q8h

* This product is for use in patients 12 years and older. If ceftazidime treatment is indicated for pediatric patients, a sodium carbonate formulation should be used.

† Although clinical improvement has been shown, bacteriological cures cannot be expected in patients with chronic respiratory disease and cystic fibrosis.

ceftazidime. Ceftazidime-arginine at 23 times the human dose was not teratogenic or embryotoxic in a rat reproduction study. There are, however, no adequate and well-controlled studies in pregnant women. Because animal reproduction studies are not always predictive of human response, this drug should be used during pregnancy only if clearly needed.

Nursing Mothers: Ceftazidime is excreted in human milk in low concentrations. It is not known whether the arginine component of this product is excreted in human milk. Because many drugs are excreted in human milk and because the safety of the arginine component of Pentacef (ceftazidime for injection) in nursing infants has not been established, a decision should be made whether to discontinue nursing or to discontinue the drug, taking into account the importance of the drug to the mother.

Pediatric Use: Safety in children of the arginine component in *Pentacef* has not been established. This product is for use in patients 12 years and older. If treatment with ceftazidime is indicated for pediatric patients, a sodium carbonate formulation should be used.

ADVERSE REACTIONS

The following adverse effects from clinical trials were considered to be either related to ceftazidime therapy or were of uncertain etiology. The most common were local reactions following I.V. injection and allergic and gastrointestinal reactions. No disulfiram-like reactions were reported.

Local Effects, reported in less than 2% of patients, were phlebitis and inflammation at the site of injection (1 in 69 patients).

Hypersensitivity Reactions, reported in 2% of patients, were pruritus, rash and fever. Immediate hypersensitivity reactions occurred in 1 in 285 patients. Angioedema and anaphylaxis (bronchospasm and/or hypotension) have been reported very rarely.

Gastrointestinal Symptoms, reported in less than 2% of patients, were diarrhea (1 in 78), nausea (1 in 156), vomiting (1 in 500) and abdominal pain (1 in 416).

The onset of pseudomembranous colitis symptoms may occur during or after treatment (see WARNINGS).

Central Nervous System Reactions (less than 1%) include headache, dizziness and paresthesia. Seizures have been reported with several cephalosporins, including ceftazidime (see PRECAUTIONS). In addition, encephalopathy, asterixis and neuromuscular excitability have been reported in renally impaired patients treated with unadjusted dosage regimens of ceftazidime.

Less Frequent Adverse Events (less than 1%) were candidiasis (including oral thrush) and vaginitis.

Laboratory Test Changes noted during ceftazidime clinical trials were transient and included: eosinophilia (1 in 13), positive Coombs' test without hemolysis (1 in 23), thrombocytosis (1 in 45), and slight elevations in one or more of the hepatic enzymes, aspartate aminotransferase (AST, SGOT) (1 in 16), alanine aminotransferase (ALT, SGPT) (1 in 15), LDH (1 in 18), GGT (1 in 19), and alkaline phosphatase (1 in 23). As with some other cephalosporins, transient elevations of blood urea, blood urea nitrogen, and/or serum creatinine were observed occasionally. Transient leukopenia, neutropenia, agranulocytosis, thrombocytopenia, and lymphocytosis were seen very rarely.

In addition to the adverse reactions listed above that have been observed with ceftazidime, the following adverse reactions and altered laboratory tests have been reported for cephalosporin-class antibiotics:

Adverse Reactions: Urticaria, Stevens-Johnson syndrome, erythema multiforme, toxic epidermal necrolysis, colitis, renal dysfunction, toxic nephropathy, hepatic dysfunction including cholestasis, aplastic anemia, hemolytic anemia, hemorrhage.

Altered Laboratory Tests: Prolonged prothrombin time, false-positive test for urinary glucose, elevated bilirubin, pancytopenia.

OVERDOSAGE

Ceftazidime overdosage has occurred in patients with renal failure. Reactions have included seizure activity, encephalopathy, asterixis, and neuromuscular excitability. Patients who receive an acute overdosage should be carefully observed and given supportive treatment. In the presence of renal insufficiency, hemodialysis or peritoneal dialysis may aid in the removal of ceftazidime from the body.

DOSAGE AND ADMINISTRATION

Dosage: The usual adult dosage is 1 gram administered intravenously or intramuscularly every eight or 12 hours. The dosage and route should be determined by the susceptibility of the causative organisms, the severity of infection and the condition and renal function of the patient.

The guidelines for dosage of *Pentacef* are listed in Table 3. The following dosage schedule is recommended.

[See table above.]

Impaired Hepatic Function: No adjustment in dosage is required for patients with hepatic dysfunction.

Impaired Renal Function: Ceftazidime is excreted by the kidneys, almost exclusively by glomerular filtration. Therefore, in patients with impaired renal function (GFR < 50 mL/min.), it is recommended that the dosage of ceftazidime be reduced to compensate for its slower excretion. In patients with suspected renal insufficiency, an initial loading dose of 1 gram of ceftazidime may be given. An estimate of GFR should be made to determine the appropriate maintenance dose. The recommended dosage is presented in Table 4.

Table 4. Recommended Maintenance Doses of Pentacef (ceftazidime for injection) in Renal Insufficiency

NOTE: IF THE DOSE RECOMMENDED IN TABLE 3 ABOVE IS LOWER THAN THAT RECOMMENDED FOR PATIENTS WITH RENAL INSUFFICIENCY AS OUTLINED IN TABLE 4, THE LOWER DOSE SHOULD BE USED.

Creatinine Clearance (mL/min.)	Recommended Unit Dose of *Pentacef*	Frequency of Dosing
50–31	1 gram	q12h
30–16	1 gram	q24h
15–6	500 mg	q24h
<5	500 mg	q48h

When only serum creatinine is available, the following formula (Cockcroft's equation)[4] may be used to estimate creatinine clearance. The serum creatinine should represent a steady state of renal function:

Males:

$$\text{Creatinine clearance (mL/min.)} = \frac{\text{Weight (kg)} \times (140 - \text{age})}{72 \times \text{serum creatinine (mg/dL)}}$$

Females:

0.85 × male value

In patients with severe infections who would normally receive 6 grams of ceftazidime daily were it not for renal insufficiency, the unit dose given in the table above may be increased by 50% or the dosing frequency increased appropri-

ately. Further dosing should be determined by therapeutic monitoring, severity of the infection and susceptibility of the causative organism.

In patients undergoing hemodialysis, a loading dose of 1 gram is recommended, followed by 1 gram after each hemodialysis period.

Pentacef (ceftazidime for injection) can also be used in patients undergoing intraperitoneal dialysis (IPD) and continuous ambulatory peritoneal dialysis (CAPD). In such patients, a loading dose of *Pentacef* 1 gram may be given, followed by 500 mg every 24 hours. It is not known whether or not ceftazidime-arginine can be safely incorporated into dialysis fluid.

NOTE: Generally, *Pentacef* should be continued for two days after the signs and symptoms of infection have disappeared, but in complicated infections longer therapy may be required.

Administration: *Pentacef* may be given intravenously or by deep intramuscular injection into a large muscle mass such as the upper outer quadrant of the gluteus maximus or lateral part of the thigh.

Intramuscular Administration: For intramuscular administration, *Pentacef* should be reconstituted with Sterile Water for Injection. Refer to Table 5.

Intravenous Administration: The I.V. route is preferable for patients with bacterial septicemia, bacterial meningitis, peritonitis, or other severe or life-threatening infections, or for patients who may be poor risks because of lowered resistance resulting from such debilitating conditions as malnutrition, trauma, surgery, diabetes, heart failure or malignancy, particularly if shock is present or pending.

For direct intermittent intravenous administration reconstitute *Pentacef* as directed in Table 5 with Sterile Water for Injection. Slowly inject directly into the vein over a period of three to five minutes or give through the tubing of an administration set while the patient is also receiving one of the compatible intravenous fluids (see COMPATIBILITY AND STABILITY).

For intravenous infusion reconstitute the 1 or 2 gram piggyback vial with 100 mL of Sodium Chloride Injection or one of the compatible intravenous fluids listed under the COMPATIBILITY AND STABILITY section. Alternatively, reconstitute the 1 gram or 2 gram vial and add an appropriate quantity of the resulting solution to an I.V. container with one of the compatible intravenous fluids.

Intermittent intravenous infusion with a Y-type administration set can be accomplished with compatible solutions. However, during infusion of a solution containing *Pentacef* it is advisable to discontinue the other solution.

Solutions of *Pentacef*, like those of most beta-lactam antibiotics, should not be added to solutions of aminoglycoside antibiotics because of potential interaction.

However, if concurrent therapy with *Pentacef* and an aminoglycoside is indicated, each of these antibiotics can be administered separately to the same patient.

RECONSTITUTION

No gas relief needle is required when adding the diluent, except for the "Piggyback" Vials where it is required during the latter stages of addition (in order to preserve product sterility, a gas relief needle should not be inserted until an over-pressure is produced in the vial). No evolution of carbon dioxide gas occurs on constitution.

Single Dose Vials:

For I.M. injection, I.V. direct (bolus) injection, or I.V. infusion, reconstitute with Sterile Water for Injection according to the following table. SHAKE WELL.

Table 5

Vial Size	Diluent to Be Added	Approx. Avail. Volume	Approx. Avg. Concentration
Intramuscular or Intravenous Direct (bolus) Injection			
1 gram	3.0 mL	3.6 mL	280 mg/mL
Intravenous Infusion			
1 gram	10 mL	10.6 mL	95 mg/mL
2 gram	10 mL	11.2 mL	180 mg/mL

Withdraw the total volume of solution into the syringe. For I.V. infusion, constitute the 1 gram or 2 gram vial and add an appropriate quantity of the resulting solution to an I.V. container with one of the compatible I.V. fluids.

"Piggyback" Vials:

Reconstitution should be in two stages. Reconstitute with 10 mL of Sodium Chloride Injection. SHAKE WELL. For ease of reconstitution, vent vial with a gas relief needle and add the remaining 90 mL of Sodium Chloride Injection. Remove the gas relief needle and syringe needle; shake vial and set up for infusion in the normal way. See Table 6 for resulting concentrations.

COMPATIBILITY AND STABILITY

Intramuscular: *Pentacef*, when reconstituted as directed with Sterile Water for Injection, maintains satisfactory po-

Continued on next page

SmithKline Beecham—Cont.

Table 6

Vial Size	Diluent to Be Added	Approx. Avail. Volume	Approx. Avg. Concentration
1 gram	100 mL	100 mL	10 mg/mL
2 gram	100 mL	100 mL	20 mg/mL

tency for 24 hours at room temperature or for seven days under refrigeration (5°C). Solutions in Sterile Water for Injection that are frozen immediately after reconstitution in the original container are stable for three months when stored at −20°C. Components of the solution may precipitate in the frozen state and will dissolve upon reaching room temperature with little or no agitation. Potency is not affected. Frozen solutions should only be thawed at room temperature. Do not force thaw by immersion in water baths or by microwave irradiation. Once thawed, solutions should not be refrozen. Thawed solutions may be stored for up to eight hours at room temperature or for four days in a refrigerator (5°C).

Intravenous: Pentacef (ceftazidime for injection) Vials, when reconstituted as directed with Sterile Water for Injection, maintain satisfactory potency for 24 hours at room temperature or for seven days under refrigeration (5°C). Solutions in Sterile Water for Injection in the original container or in 0.9% Sodium Chloride Injection in Viaflex® small volume containers that are frozen immediately after reconstitution are stable for three months when stored at −20°C. Components of the solution may precipitate in the frozen state and will dissolve upon reaching room temperature with little or no agitation. Potency is not affected. Frozen solutions should only be thawed at room temperature. Do not force thaw by immersion in water baths or by microwave irradiation. For larger volumes where it may be necessary to warm the frozen product (to a maximum of 40°C), care should be taken to avoid heating after thawing is complete. Once thawed, solutions should not be refrozen. Thawed solutions may be stored for up to eight hours at room temperature or for four days in a refrigerator (5°C).

Pentacef is compatible with the more commonly used intravenous infusion fluids. Solutions at concentrations between 1 mg/mL and 40 mg/mL in the following infusion fluids may be stored for up to 24 hours at room temperature or seven days if refrigerated: 0.9% Sodium Chloride Injection; Ringer's Injection USP; Lactated Ringer's Injection USP; 5% Dextrose Injection; 5% Dextrose and 0.225% Sodium Chloride Injection; 5% Dextrose and 0.45% Sodium Chloride Injection; 5% Dextrose and 0.9% Sodium Chloride Injection; 10% Dextrose Injection.

Pentacef is less stable in Sodium Bicarbonate Injection than in other intravenous fluids. It is not recommended as a diluent. Solutions of *Pentacef* in 5% Dextrose and 0.9% Sodium Chloride Injection are stable for at least six hours at room temperature in plastic tubing, drip chambers and volume control devices of common intravenous infusion sets.

Ceftazidime at a concentration of 20 mg/mL has been found compatible for 24 hours at room temperature or seven days under refrigeration in Sterile Water for Injection when admixed with: cefazolin sodium (Ancef®) 330 mg/mL; heparin 1000 units/mL; and cimetidine HCl (Tagamet®) 150 mg/mL.

Ceftazidime at a concentration of 20 mg/mL has been found compatible for 24 hours at room temperature or seven days under refrigeration in 5% Dextrose Injection when admixed with Potassium Chloride 40 mEq/l.

Vancomycin solution exhibits a physical incompatibility when mixed with a number of drugs, including ceftazidime. The likelihood of precipitation with ceftazidime is dependent on the concentrations of vancomycin and ceftazidime present. It is therefore recommended, when both drugs are to be administered by intermittent I.V. infusion, that they be given separately, flushing the I.V. lines (with one of the compatible I.V. fluids) between the administration of these two agents.

Note: Parenteral drug products should be inspected visually for particulate matter prior to administration wherever solution and container permit.

As with other cephalosporins, Pentacef (ceftazidime for injection) powder as well as solutions tends to darken depending on storage conditions; within the stated recommendations, however, product potency is not adversely affected. Before reconstitution, protect from light and store at controlled room temperature 15° to 30°C (59° to 86°F).

HOW SUPPLIED

Vials: equivalent to 1 gram and 2 grams of ceftazidime.
1 gram (tray of 25) NDC 0007-5112-16
2 gram (tray of 10) NDC 0007-5114-11
"Piggyback" Vials for I.V. admixture: equivalent to 1 gram and 2 grams of ceftazidime.
1 gram (tray of 10) NDC 0007-5113-11
2 gram (tray of 10) NDC 0007-5115-11

Also available as:
Pharmacy Bulk Vials: equivalent to 6 grams of ceftazidime. 6 gram (tray of 10) NDC 0007-5116-11

REFERENCES

1. Bauer, A.W.; Kirby, W.M.M., and Sherris, J.C., et al.: Antibiotic susceptibility testing by a standardized single disc method, Am. J. Clin. Pathol. 45:493, 1966. 2. National Committee for Clinical Laboratory Standards, Approved Standard: Performance Standards for Antimicrobial Disc Susceptibility Tests (M2-A3), December, 1984. 3. Standardized disc susceptibility test, Federal Register 39:19182–19184, 1974. 4. Cockcroft, D.W., and Gault, M.H.: Prediction of creatinine clearance from serum creatinine, Nephron 16:31–41, 1976.
Jointly manufactured by
SmithKline Beecham Pharmaceuticals
Philadelphia, PA 19101 and
Bristol-Myers Squibb Co.
New York, NY 10154
PF:L2IV

RELAFEN®   ℞
[rel'ah-fen]
(brand of nabumetone)
Tablets

DESCRIPTION
Relafen (nabumetone) is a naphthylalkanone designated chemically as 4-(6-methoxy-2-naphthalenyl)-2-butanone. It has the following structure:

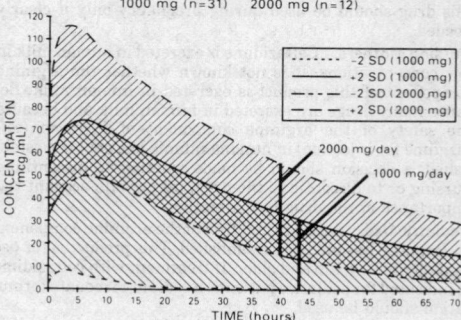

nabumetone

Nabumetone is a white to off-white crystalline substance with a molecular weight of 228.3. It is nonacidic and practically insoluble in water, but soluble in alcohol and most organic solvents. It has an n-octanol:phosphate buffer partition coefficient of 2400 at pH 7.4.

Tablets for Oral Administration: Each oval-shaped, film-coated tablet contains 500 mg or 750 mg of nabumetone. Inactive ingredients consist of hydroxypropyl methylcellulose, microcrystalline cellulose, polyethylene glycol, polysorbate 80, sodium lauryl sulfate, sodium starch glycolate and titanium dioxide. The 750 mg tablets also contain iron oxides.

CLINICAL PHARMACOLOGY
Relafen is a nonsteroidal anti-inflammatory drug (NSAID) that exhibits anti-inflammatory, analgesic and antipyretic properties in pharmacologic studies. As with other nonsteroidal anti-inflammatory agents, its mode of action is not known. However, the ability to inhibit prostaglandin synthesis may be involved in the anti-inflammatory effect.

The parent compound is a prodrug, which undergoes hepatic biotransformation to the active component, 6-methoxy-2-naphthylacetic acid (6MNA), that is a potent inhibitor of prostaglandin synthesis.

6-methoxy-2-naphthylacetic acid (6MNA)

It is acidic and has an n-octanol:phosphate buffer partition coefficient of 0.5 at pH 7.4.

Pharmacokinetics
After oral administration, approximately 80% of a radiolabelled dose of nabumetone is found in the urine, indicating that nabumetone is well absorbed from the gastrointestinal tract. Nabumetone itself is not detected in the plasma because, after absorption, it undergoes rapid biotransformation to the principal active metabolite, 6-methoxy-2-naphthylacetic acid (6MNA). Approximately 35% of a 1000 mg oral dose of nabumetone is converted to 6MNA and 50% is converted into unidentified metabolites which are subsequently excreted in the urine. Following oral administration

of *Relafen*, 6MNA exhibits pharmacokinetic characteristics that generally follow a one-compartment model with first order input and first order elimination.

6MNA is more than 99% bound to plasma proteins. The free fraction is dependent on total concentration of 6MNA and is proportional to dose over the range of 1000 mg to 2000 mg. It is 0.2% to 0.3% at concentrations typically achieved following administration of *Relafen* 1000 mg and is approximately 0.6% to 0.8% of the total concentrations at steady state following daily administration of 2000 mg.

Steady-state plasma concentrations of 6MNA are slightly lower than predicted from single-dose data. This may result from the higher fraction of unbound 6MNA which undergoes greater hepatic clearance.

Coadministration of food increases the rate of absorption and subsequent appearance of 6MNA in the plasma but does not affect the extent of conversion of nabumetone into 6MNA. Peak plasma concentrations of 6MNA are increased by approximately one third.

Coadministration with an aluminum-containing antacid had no significant effect on the bioavailability of 6MNA. [See table below.]

The simulated curves in the graph below illustrate the range of active metabolite plasma concentrations that would be expected from 95% of patients following 1000 mg to 2000 mg doses to steady state. The cross-hatched area represents the expected overlap in plasma concentrations due to intersubject variation following oral administration of 1000 mg to 2000 mg of *Relafen*.

Nabumetone Active Metabolite (6MNA) Plasma Concentrations at Steady State Following Once-Daily Dosing of Nabumetone
1000 mg (n=31)   2000 mg (n=12)

6MNA undergoes biotransformation in the liver, producing inactive metabolites that are eliminated as both free metabolites and conjugates. None of the known metabolites of 6MNA has been detected in plasma. Preliminary *in vivo* and *in vitro* studies suggest that unlike other NSAIDs, there is no evidence of enterohepatic recirculation of the active metabolite. Approximately 75% of a radiolabelled dose was recovered in urine in 48 hours. Approximately 80% was recovered in 168 hours. A further 9% appeared in the feces. In the first 48 hours, metabolites consisted of:

—nabumetone, unchanged	not detectable
—6-methoxy-2-naphthylacetic acid (6MNA), unchanged	<1%
—6MNA, conjugated	11%
—6-hydroxy-2-naphthylacetic acid (6HNA), unchanged	5%
—6HNA, conjugated	7%
—4-(6-hydroxy-2-naphthyl)-butan-2-ol, conjugated	9%
—O-desmethyl-nabumetone, conjugated	7%
—unidentified minor metabolites	34%
Total % Dose:	73%

Following oral administration of dosages of 1000 mg to 2000 mg to steady state, the mean plasma clearance of 6MNA is 20 to 30 mL/min. and the elimination half-life is approximately 24 hours.

Elderly Patients: Steady-state plasma concentrations in elderly patients were generally higher than in young healthy subjects. (See Table 1 for summary of pharmacokinetic parameters.)

Renal Insufficiency: In studies of patients with renal insufficiency, the mean terminal half-life of 6MNA was increased in patients with severe renal dysfunction (creatinine clear-

---

Table 1. Mean pharmacokinetic parameters at steady state following oral administration of 1000 mg or 2000 mg doses of Relafen (nabumetone)

Abbreviation (units)	Young Adults Mean ± SD 1000 mg n=31	Young Adults Mean ± SD 2000 mg n=12	Elderly Mean ± SD 1000 mg n=27
t_{max} (hours)	3.0 (1.0–12.0)	2.5 (1.0–8.0)	4.0 (1.0–10.0)
$t_{1/2}$ (hours)	22.5 ± 3.7	26.2 ± 3.7	29.8 ± 8.1
CL_{SS}/F (mL/min.)	26.1 ± 17.3	21.0 ± 4.0	18.6 ± 13.4
Vd_{SS}/F (L)	55.4 ± 26.4	53.4 ± 11.3	50.2 ± 25.3

ance <30 mL/min./1.73 m^2). In patients undergoing hemodialysis, steady-state plasma concentrations of the active metabolite were similar to those observed in healthy subjects. Due to extensive protein-binding, 6MNA is not dialyzable.

Hepatic Impairment: Data in patients with severe hepatic impairment are limited. Biotransformation of nabumetone to 6MNA and the further metabolism of 6MNA to inactive metabolites is dependent on hepatic function and could be reduced in patients with severe hepatic impairment (history of or biopsy-proven cirrhosis).

Special Studies

Gastrointestinal: Relafen (nabumetone) was compared to aspirin in inducing gastrointestinal blood loss. Food intake was not monitored. Studies utilizing ^{51}Cr-tagged red blood cells in healthy males showed no difference in fecal blood loss after three or four weeks' administration of *Relafen* 1000 mg or 2000 mg daily when compared to either placebo-treated or nontreated subjects. In contrast, aspirin 3600 mg daily produced an increase in fecal blood loss when compared to the *Relafen*-treated, placebo-treated or nontreated subjects. The clinical relevance of the data is unknown.

The following endoscopy trials entered patients who had been previously treated with NSAIDs. These patients had varying baseline scores and different courses of treatment. The trials were not designed to correlate symptoms and endoscopy scores. The clinical relevance of these endoscopy trials, i.e., either G.I. symptoms or serious G.I. events, is not known.

Ten endoscopy studies were conducted in 488 patients who had baseline and post-treatment endoscopy. In five clinical trials that compared a total of 194 patients on *Relafen* 1000 mg daily or naproxen 250 mg or 500 mg twice daily for three to 12 weeks, *Relafen* treatment resulted in fewer patients with endoscopically detected lesions (> 3 mm). In two trials a total of 101 patients on *Relafen* 1000 mg or 2000 mg daily or piroxicam 10 mg to 20 mg for seven to 10 days, there were fewer *Relafen* patients with endoscopically detected lesions. In three trials of a total of 47 patients on *Relafen* 1000 mg daily or indomethacin 100 mg to 150 mg daily for three to four weeks, the endoscopy scores were higher with indomethacin. Another 12-week trial in a total of 171 patients compared the results of treatment with *Relafen* 1000 mg/day to ibuprofen 2400 mg/day and ibuprofen 2400 mg/day plus misoprostol 800 mcg/day. The results showed that patients treated with *Relafen* had a lower number of endoscopically detected lesions (>5 mm) than patients treated with ibuprofen alone but comparable to the combination of ibuprofen plus misoprostol. The results did not correlate with abdominal pain.

Other: In one-week repeat-dose studies in healthy volunteers, *Relafen* 1000 mg daily had little effect on collagen-induced platelet aggregation and no effect on bleeding time. In comparison, naproxen 500 mg daily suppressed collagen-induced platelet aggregation and significantly increased bleeding time.

CLINICAL TRIALS

Osteoarthritis: The use of *Relafen* in relieving the signs and symptoms of osteoarthritis was assessed in double-blind controlled trials in which 1,047 patients were treated for six weeks to six months. In these trials, *Relafen* in a dose of 1000 mg/day administered at night was comparable to naproxen 500 mg/day and to aspirin 3600 mg/day.

Rheumatoid Arthritis: The use of *Relafen* in relieving the signs and symptoms of rheumatoid arthritis was assessed in double-blind, randomized, controlled trials in which 770 patients were treated for three weeks to six months. *Relafen*, in a dose of 1000 mg/day administered at night was comparable to naproxen 500 mg/day and to aspirin 3600 mg/day.

In controlled clinical trials of rheumatoid arthritis patients, *Relafen* has been used in combination with gold, d-penicillamine and corticosteroids.

INDIVIDUALIZATION OF DOSING

There is considerable interpatient variation in response to *Relafen*. Therapy is usually initiated at a *Relafen* dose of 1000 mg daily, then adjusted, if needed, based on clinical response.

In clinical trials with osteoarthritis and rheumatoid arthritis patients, most patients responded to *Relafen* in doses of 1000 mg/day administered nightly; total daily dosages up to 2000 mg were used. In open-labelled studies, 1,490 patients were permitted dosage increases and were followed for approximately one year (mode). Twenty percent of patients (n = 294) were withdrawn for lack of effectiveness during the first year of these open-labelled studies. The following table provides patient-exposure to doses used in the U.S. clinical trials: [See table above.]

As with other NSAIDs, the lowest dose should be sought for each patient. Patients weighing under 50 kg may be less likely to require dosages beyond 1000 mg. Therefore, after observing the response to initial therapy, the dose should be adjusted to meet individual patients' requirements.

Table 2. Clinical double-blind and open-labelled trials of Relafen (nabumetone) in osteoarthritis and rheumatoid arthritis

Relafen Dose	Number of Patients OA	Number of Patients RA	Mean/Mode Duration of Treatment (yrs.) OA	Mean/Mode Duration of Treatment (yrs.) RA
500 mg	17	6	0.4/-	0.2/-
1000 mg	917	701	1.2/1	1.4/1
1500 mg	645	224	2.3/1	1.7/1
2000 mg	15	100	0.6/1	1.3/1

INDICATIONS AND USAGE

Relafen is indicated for acute and chronic treatment of signs and symptoms of osteoarthritis and rheumatoid arthritis.

CONTRAINDICATIONS

Relafen is contraindicated in patients who have previously exhibited hypersensitivity to it.

Relafen is contraindicated in patients in whom *Relafen*, aspirin or other NSAIDs induce asthma, urticaria or other allergic-type reactions. Fatal asthmatic reactions have been reported in such patients receiving NSAIDs.

WARNINGS

Risk of G.I. Ulceration, Bleeding and Perforation with NSAID Therapy: Serious gastrointestinal toxicity such as bleeding, ulceration and perforation can occur at any time, with or without warning symptoms, in patients treated chronically with NSAID therapy. Although minor upper gastrointestinal problems, such as dyspepsia, are common, usually developing early in therapy, physicians should remain alert for ulceration and bleeding in patients treated chronically with NSAIDs even in the absence of previous G.I. tract symptoms. In controlled clinical trials involving 1,677 patients treated with *Relafen* (1,140 followed for one year and 927 for two years), the cumulative incidence of peptic ulcers was 0.3% (95% Cl; 0%, 0.6%) at three to six months, 0.5% (95% Cl; 0.1%, 0.9%) at one year and 0.8% (95% Cl; 0.3%, 1.3%) at two years. Physicians should inform patients about the signs and symptoms of serious G.I. toxicity and what steps to take if they occur. In patients with active peptic ulcer, physicians must weigh the benefits of Relafen (nabumetone) therapy against possible hazards, institute an appropriate ulcer treatment regimen and monitor the patients' progress carefully.

Studies to date have not identified any subset of patients not at risk of developing peptic ulceration and bleeding. Except for a prior history of serious G.I. events and other risk factors known to be associated with peptic ulcer disease, such as alcoholism, smoking, etc., no risk factors (e.g., age, sex) have been associated with increased risk. Elderly or debilitated patients seem to tolerate ulceration or bleeding less well than other individuals and most spontaneous reports of fatal G.I. events are in this population.

High doses of any NSAID probably carry a greater risk of these reactions, although controlled clinical trials showing this do not exist in most cases. In considering the use of relatively large doses (within the recommended dosage range), sufficient benefit should be anticipated to offset the potential increased risk of G.I. toxicity.

PRECAUTIONS

General

Renal Effects: As a class, NSAIDs have been associated with renal papillary necrosis and other abnormal renal pathology during long-term administration to animals.

A second form of renal toxicity often associated with NSAIDs is seen in patients with conditions leading to a reduction in renal blood flow or blood volume, where renal prostaglandins have a supportive role in the maintenance of renal perfusion. In these patients, administration of an NSAID results in a dose-dependent decrease in prostaglandin synthesis and, secondarily, in a reduction of renal blood flow, which may precipitate overt renal decompensation. Patients at greatest risk of this reaction are those with impaired renal function, heart failure, liver dysfunction, those taking diuretics, and the elderly. Discontinuation of NSAID therapy is typically followed by recovery to the pretreatment state.

Because nabumetone undergoes extensive hepatic metabolism, no adjustment of *Relafen* dosage is generally necessary in patients with renal insufficiency. However, as with all NSAIDs, patients with impaired renal function should be monitored more closely than patients with normal renal function (see CLINICAL PHARMACOLOGY, Special Studies). The oxidized and conjugated metabolites of 6MNA are eliminated primarily by the kidneys. The extent to which these largely inactive metabolites may accumulate in patients with renal failure has not been studied. As with other drugs whose metabolites are excreted by the kidneys, the possibility that adverse reactions (not listed in ADVERSE REACTIONS) may be attributable to these metabolites should be considered.

Hepatic Function: As with other NSAIDs, borderline elevations of one or more liver function tests may occur in up to 15% of patients. These abnormalities may progress, may remain essentially unchanged, or may return to normal with continued therapy. The ALT (SGPT) test is probably the most sensitive indicator of liver dysfunction. Meaningful (three times the upper limit of normal) elevations of ALT (SGPT) or AST (SGOT) have occurred in controlled clinical trials of Relafen (nabumetone) in less than 1% of patients. A patient with symptoms and/or signs suggesting liver dysfunction, or in whom an abnormal liver test has occurred, should be evaluated for evidence of the development of a more severe hepatic reaction while on *Relafen* therapy. Severe hepatic reactions, including jaundice and fatal hepatitis, have been reported with other NSAIDs. Although such reactions are rare, if abnormal liver tests persist or worsen, if clinical signs and symptoms consistent with liver disease develop, or if systemic manifestations occur (e.g., eosinophilia, rash, etc.), *Relafen* should be discontinued. Because nabumetone's biotransformation to 6MNA is dependent upon hepatic function, the biotransformation could be decreased in patients with severe hepatic dysfunction. Therefore, *Relafen* should be used with caution in patients with severe hepatic impairment (see Pharmacokinetics, *Hepatic Impairment*).

Fluid Retention and Edema: Fluid retention and edema have been observed in some patients taking *Relafen*. Therefore, as with other NSAIDs, *Relafen* should be used cautiously in patients with a history of congestive heart failure, hypertension or other conditions predisposing to fluid retention.

Photosensitivity: Based on U.V. light photosensitivity testing, *Relafen* may be associated with more reactions to sun exposure than might be expected based on skin tanning types.

Information for Patients: *Relafen*, like other drugs of its class, is not free of side effects. The side effects of these drugs can cause discomfort and, rarely, there are more serious side effects, such as gastrointestinal bleeding, which may result in hospitalization and even fatal outcome.

NSAIDs are often essential agents in the management of arthritis, but they also may be commonly employed for conditions which are less serious. Physicians may wish to discuss with their patients the potential risks (see WARNINGS, PRECAUTIONS and ADVERSE REACTIONS) and likely benefits of NSAID treatment, particularly when the drugs are used for less serious conditions where treatment without NSAIDs may represent an acceptable alternative to both the patient and the physician.

Laboratory Tests: Because severe G.I. tract ulceration and bleeding can occur without warning symptoms, physicians should follow chronically treated patients for signs and symptoms of ulceration and bleeding, and should inform them of the importance of this follow-up (see WARNINGS, Risk of G.I. Ulceration, Bleeding and Perforation with NSAID Therapy).

Drug Interactions: *In vitro* studies have shown that, because of its affinity for protein, 6MNA may displace other protein-bound drugs from their binding site. Caution should be exercised when administering *Relafen* with warfarin since interactions have been seen with other NSAIDs.

Concomitant administration of an aluminum-containing antacid had no significant effect on the bioavailability of 6MNA. When administered with food or milk, there is more rapid absorption; however, the total amount of 6MNA in the plasma is unchanged (see Pharmacokinetics).

Carcinogenesis, Mutagenesis: In two-year studies conducted in mice and rats, nabumetone had no statistically significant tumorigenic effect. Nabumetone did not show mutagenic potential in the Ames test and mouse micronucleus test *in vivo*. However, nabumetone- and 6MNA-treated lymphocytes in culture showed chromosomal aberrations at 80 mcg/mL and higher concentrations (equal to the average human exposure to *Relafen* at the maximum recommended dose).

Impairment of Fertility: Nabumetone did not impair fertility of male or female rats treated orally at doses of 320 mg/kg/day (1888 mg/m^2) before mating.

Pregnancy: Teratogenic Effects. Pregnancy Category C. Nabumetone did not cause any teratogenic effect in rats given up to 400 mg/kg (2360 mg/m^2) and in rabbits up to 300 mg/kg (3540 mg/m^2) orally. However, increased post-implantation loss was observed in rats at 100 mg/kg (590 mg/m^2) orally and at higher doses (equal to the average human exposure to 6MNA at the maximum recommended human dose). There are no adequate, well-controlled studies in pregnant women. This drug should be used during pregnancy only if clearly needed.

Because of the known effect of prostaglandin-synthesis-inhibiting drugs on the human fetal cardiovascular system (closure of ductus arteriosus), use of Relafen (nabumetone) during the third trimester of pregnancy is not recommended.

Continued on next page

SmithKline Beecham—Cont.

Labor and Delivery: The effects of *Relafen* on labor and delivery in women are not known. As with other drugs known to inhibit prostaglandin synthesis, an increased incidence of dystocia and delayed parturition occurred in rats treated throughout pregnancy.

Nursing Mothers: *Relafen* is not recommended for use in nursing mothers because of the possible adverse effects of prostaglandin-synthesis-inhibiting drugs on neonates. It is not known whether nabumetone or its metabolites are excreted in human milk; however, 6MNA is excreted in the milk of lactating rats.

Pediatric Use: *Relafen* is not recommended for use in children because the safety and efficacy in children have not been established.

Geriatric Use: Of the 1,677 patients in U.S. clinical studies who were treated with *Relafen*, 411 patients (24%) were 65 years of age or older; 22 patients (1%) were 75 years of age or older. No overall differences in efficacy or safety were observed between these older patients and younger ones. Similar results were observed in a one-year, non-U.S. postmarketing surveillance study of 10,800 *Relafen* patients, of whom 4,577 patients (42%) were 65 years of age or older.

ADVERSE REACTIONS

Adverse reaction information was derived from blinded-controlled and open-labelled clinical trials and from worldwide marketing experience. In the description below, rates of the more common events (greater than 1%) and many of the less common events (less than 1%) represent results of U.S. clinical studies.

Of the 1,677 patients who received *Relafen* during U.S. clinical trials, 1,524 were treated for at least one month, 1,327 for at least three months, 929 for at least a year and 750 for at least two years. Over 300 patients have been treated for five years or longer.

The most frequently reported adverse reactions were related to the gastrointestinal tract. They were diarrhea, dyspepsia and abdominal pain.

Incidence ≥ 1% — Probably Causally Related

Gastrointestinal: Diarrhea (14%), dyspepsia (13%), abdominal pain (12%), constipation*, flatulence*, nausea*, positive stool guaiac*, dry mouth, gastritis, stomatitis, vomiting.

Central Nervous System: Dizziness*, headache*, fatigue, increased sweating, insomnia, nervousness, somnolence.

Dermatologic: Pruritus*, rash*.

Special Senses: Tinnitus*.

Miscellaneous: Edema*.

*Incidence of reported reaction between 3% and 9%. Reactions occurring in 1% to 3% of the patients are unmarked.

Incidence < 1% — Probably Causally Related†

Gastrointestinal: Anorexia, cholestatic jaundice, duodenal ulcer, dysphagia, gastric ulcer, gastroenteritis, gastrointestinal bleeding, increased appetite, liver function abnormalities, melena.

Central Nervous System: Asthenia, agitation, anxiety, confusion, depression, malaise, paresthesia, tremor, vertigo.

Dermatologic: Bullous eruptions, photosensitivity, urticaria, pseudoporphyria cutanea tarda.

Cardiovascular: Vasculitis.

Metabolic: Weight gain.

Respiratory: Dyspnea, *hypersensitivity pneumonitis.*

Genitourinary: Albuminuria, azotemia, *interstitial nephritis.*

Special Senses: Abnormal vision.

Hypersensitivity: *Anaphylactoid reaction,* angioneurotic edema.

† Adverse reactions reported only in worldwide postmarketing experience or in the literature are italicized.

Incidence < 1% — Causal Relationship Unknown‡

Gastrointestinal: Bilirubinuria, duodenitis, eructation, gallstones, gingivitis, glossitis, pancreatitis, rectal bleeding.

Central Nervous System: Nightmares.

Dermatologic: Acne, alopecia, *erythema multiforme, Stevens-Johnson Syndrome.*

Cardiovascular: Angina, arrhythmia, hypertension, myocardial infarction, palpitations, syncope, thrombophlebitis.

Respiratory: Asthma, cough.

Genitourinary: Dysuria, hematuria, impotence, renal stones.

Special Senses: Taste disorder.

Body as a Whole: Fever, chills.

Hematologic/Lymphatic: Anemia, leukopenia, granulocytopenia, thrombocytopenia.

Metabolic/Nutritional: Hyperglycemia, hypokalemia, weight loss.

‡ Adverse reactions reported only in worldwide postmarketing experience or in the literature are italicized.

OVERDOSAGE

Since only one case of *Relafen* overdose has been reported, the experience is limited. If acute overdose occurs, it is recommended that the stomach be emptied by vomiting or lavage and general supportive measures be instituted, as necessary. In addition, the use of activated charcoal, up to 60 grams, may effectively reduce nabumetone absorption. Coadministration of nabumetone with charcoal to man has resulted in an 80% decrease in maximum plasma concentrations of the active metabolite.

The one overdose occurred in a 17-year-old female patient who had a history of abdominal pain and was hospitalized for increased abdominal pain following ingestion of 30 *Relafen* tablets (15 grams total). Stools were negative for occult blood and there was no fall in serum hemoglobin concentration. The patient had no other symptoms. She was given an H_2-receptor antagonist and discharged from the hospital without sequelae.

DOSAGE AND ADMINISTRATION

Osteoarthritis and Rheumatoid Arthritis

The recommended starting dose is 1000 mg taken as a single dose with or without food. Some patients may obtain more symptomatic relief from 1500 mg to 2000 mg per day. Relafen (nabumetone) can be given in either a single or twice-daily dose. Dosages over 2000 mg per day have not been studied. The lowest effective dose should be used for chronic treatment.

HOW SUPPLIED

Tablets: Oval-shaped, film-coated: 500 mg—white, imprinted with the product name RELAFEN and 500, in bottles of 100 and 500, and in Single Unit Packages of 100 (intended for institutional use only). 750 mg—beige, imprinted with the product name RELAFEN and 750, in bottles of 100 and 500, and in Single Unit Packages of 100 (intended for institutional use only).

Store at controlled room temperature (59° to 86°F) in well-closed container; dispense in light-resistant container.

500 mg 100's: NDC 0029-4851-20
500 mg 500's: NDC 0029-4851-25
500 mg SUP 100's: NDC 0029-4851-21

750 mg 100's: NDC 0029-4852-20
750 mg 500's: NDC 0029-4852-25
750 mg SUP 100's: NDC 0029-4852-21
RL:L3

Shown in Product Identification Section, page 431

RIDAURA® ℞

[ri-door'ah]
(brand of auranofin)
Capsules

> Ridaura (auranofin) contains gold and, like other gold-containing drugs, can cause gold toxicity, signs of which include: fall in hemoglobin, leukopenia below 4,000 WBC/cu mm, granulocytes below 1,500/cu mm, decrease in platelets below 150,000/cu mm, proteinuria, hematuria, pruritus, rash, stomatitis or persistent diarrhea. Therefore, the results of recommended laboratory work (See PRECAUTIONS) should be reviewed before writing each *Ridaura* prescription. Like other gold preparations, *Ridaura* is only indicated for use in selected patients with active rheumatoid arthritis. Physicians planning to use *Ridaura* should be experienced with chrysotherapy and should thoroughly familiarize themselves with the toxicity and benefits of *Ridaura.*
> In addition, the following precautions should be routinely employed:
> 1. The possibility of adverse reactions should be explained to patients before starting therapy.
> 2. Patients should be advised to report promptly any symptoms suggesting toxicity. (See PRECAUTIONS—Information for Patients.)

DESCRIPTION

Ridaura (auranofin) is available in oral form as capsules containing 3 mg auranofin.

Auranofin is (2,3,4,6-tetra-O-acetyl-1-thio-β-D-glucopyranosato-S-) (triethylphosphine) gold.

Auranofin contains 29% gold and has the following chemical structure:

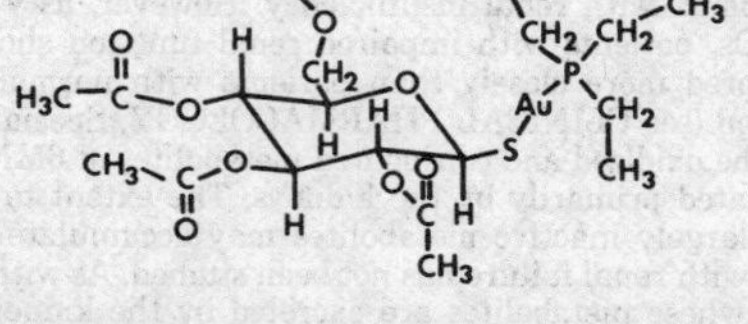

Each *Ridaura* capsule, with opaque brown cap and opaque tan body, contains auranofin, 3 mg, and is imprinted with the product name RIDAURA and SKF. Inactive ingredients consist of benzyl alcohol, cellulose, cetylpyridinium chloride, D&C Red No. 33, FD&C Blue No. 1, FD&C Red No. 40, FD&C Yellow No. 6, gelatin, lactose, magnesium stearate, povidone, sodium lauryl sulfate, sodium starch glycolate, starch, titanium dioxide and trace amounts of other inactive ingredients.

CLINICAL PHARMACOLOGY

The mechanism of action of Ridaura (auranofin) is not understood. In patients with adult rheumatoid arthritis, *Ridaura* may modify disease activity as manifested by synovitis and associated symptoms, and reflected by laboratory parameters such as ESR. There is no substantial evidence, however, that gold-containing compounds induce remission of rheumatoid arthritis.

Pharmacokinetics: Pharmacokinetic studies were performed in rheumatoid arthritis patients, not in normal volunteers. Auranofin is rapidly metabolized and intact auranofin has never been detected in the blood. Thus, studies of the pharmacokinetics of auranofin have involved measurement of gold concentrations. Approximately 25% of the gold in auranofin is absorbed.

The mean terminal plasma half-life of auranofin gold at steady state was 26 days (range 21 to 31 days; n=5). The mean terminal body half-life was 80 days (range 42 to 128; n=5). Approximately 60% of the absorbed gold (15% of the administered dose) from a single dose of auranofin is excreted in urine; the remainder is excreted in the feces.

In clinical studies, steady state blood-gold concentrations are achieved in about three months. In patients on 6 mg auranofin/day, mean steady state blood-gold concentrations were 0.68 ± 0.45 mcg/mL (n=63 patients). In blood, approximately 40% of auranofin gold is associated with red cells, and 60% associated with serum proteins. In contrast, 99% of injectable gold is associated with serum proteins.

Mean blood-gold concentrations are proportional to dose; however, no correlation between blood-gold concentrations and safety or efficacy has been established.

INDICATIONS AND USAGE

Ridaura (auranofin) is indicated in the management of adults with active classical or definite rheumatoid arthritis (ARA criteria) who have had an insufficient therapeutic response to, or are intolerant of, an adequate trial of full doses of one or more nonsteroidal anti-inflammatory drugs. *Ridaura* should be added to a comprehensive baseline program, including non-drug therapies.

Unlike anti-inflammatory drugs, *Ridaura* does not produce an immediate response. Therapeutic effects may be seen after three to four months of treatment, although improvement has not been seen in some patients before six months.

When cartilage and bone damage has already occurred, gold cannot reverse structural damage to joints caused by previous disease. The greatest potential benefit occurs in patients with active synovitis, particularly in its early stage.

In controlled clinical trials comparing *Ridaura* with injectable gold, *Ridaura* was associated with fewer dropouts due to adverse reactions, while injectable gold was associated with fewer dropouts for inadequate or poor therapeutic effect. Physicians should consider these findings when deciding on the use of *Ridaura* in patients who are candidates for chrysotherapy.

CONTRAINDICATIONS

Ridaura (auranofin) is contraindicated in patients with a history of any of the following gold-induced disorders: anaphylactic reactions, necrotizing enterocolitis, pulmonary fibrosis, exfoliative dermatitis, bone marrow aplasia or other severe hematologic disorders.

WARNINGS

Danger signs of possible gold toxicity include fall in hemoglobin, leukopenia below 4,000 WBC/cu mm, granulocytes below 1,500/cu mm, decrease in platelets below 150,000/cu mm, proteinuria, hematuria, pruritus, rash, stomatitis or persistent diarrhea.

Thrombocytopenia has occurred in 1–3% of patients (See ADVERSE REACTIONS) treated with Ridaura (auranofin), some of whom developed bleeding. The thrombocytopenia usually appears to be peripheral in origin and is usually reversible upon withdrawal of *Ridaura.* Its onset bears no relationship to the duration of *Ridaura* therapy and its course may be rapid. While patients' platelet counts should normally be monitored at least monthly (See PRECAUTIONS—Laboratory Tests), the occurrence of a precipitous decline in platelets or a platelet count less than 100,000/cu mm or signs and symptoms (e.g., purpura, ecchymoses or petechiae) suggestive of thrombocytopenia indicates a need to immediately withdraw *Ridaura* and other therapies with the potential to cause thrombocytopenia, and to obtain additional platelet counts. No additional *Ridaura* should be given unless the thrombocytopenia resolves and further studies show it was not due to gold therapy.

Proteinuria has developed in 3–9% of patients (See ADVERSE REACTIONS) treated with *Ridaura.* If clinically significant proteinuria or microscopic hematuria is found (See PRECAUTIONS—Laboratory Tests), *Ridaura* and

other therapies with the potential to cause proteinuria or microscopic hematuria should be stopped immediately.

PRECAUTIONS

General: The safety of concomitant use of Ridaura (auranofin) with injectable gold, hydroxychloroquine, penicillamine, immunosuppressive agents (e.g., cyclophosphamide, azathioprine, or methotrexate) or high doses of corticosteroids has not been established.

Medical problems that might affect the signs or symptoms used to detect *Ridaura* toxicity should be under control before starting Ridaura (auranofin).

The potential benefits of using *Ridaura* in patients with progressive renal disease, significant hepatocellular disease, inflammatory bowel disease, skin rash or history of bone marrow depression should be weighed against 1) the potential risks of gold toxicity on organ systems previously compromised or with decreased reserve, and 2) the difficulty in quickly detecting and correctly attributing the toxic effect.

The following adverse reactions have been reported with the use of gold preparations and require modification of *Ridaura* treatment or additional monitoring. See ADVERSE REACTIONS for the approximate incidence of those reactions specifically reported with *Ridaura*.

Gastrointestinal Reactions: Gastrointestinal reactions reported with gold therapy include diarrhea/loose stools, nausea, vomiting, anorexia and abdominal cramps. The most common reaction to *Ridaura* is diarrhea/loose stools reported in approximately 50% of the patients. This is generally manageable by reducing the dosage (e.g., from 6 mg daily to 3 mg) and in only 6% of the patients is it necessary to discontinue Ridaura (auranofin) permanently.

Ulcerative enterocolitis is a rare serious gold reaction. Therefore, patients with gastrointestinal symptoms should be monitored for the appearance of gastrointestinal bleeding.

Cutaneous Reactions: Dermatitis is the most common reaction to injectable gold therapy and the second most common reaction to *Ridaura*. *Any eruption, especially if pruritic, that develops during treatment should be considered a gold reaction until proven otherwise.* Pruritus often exists before dermatitis becomes apparent, and therefore should be considered to be a warning signal of a cutaneous reaction. Gold dermatitis may be aggravated by exposure to sunlight or an actinic rash may develop. The most serious form of cutaneous reaction reported with injectable gold is generalized exfoliative dermatitis.

Mucous Membrane Reactions: Stomatitis, another common gold reaction, may be manifested by shallow ulcers on the buccal membranes, on the borders of the tongue, and on the palate or in the pharynx. Stomatitis may occur as the only adverse reaction or with a dermatitis. Sometimes diffuse glossitis or gingivitis develops. A metallic taste may precede these oral mucous membrane reactions and should be considered a warning signal.

Renal Reactions: Gold can produce a nephrotic syndrome or glomerulitis with proteinuria and hematuria. These renal reactions are usually relatively mild and subside completely if recognized early and treatment is discontinued. They may become severe and chronic if treatment is continued after the onset of the reaction. *Therefore it is important to perform urinalyses regularly* and to discontinue treatment promptly if proteinuria or hematuria develops.

Hematologic Reactions: Blood dyscrasias including leukopenia, granulocytopenia, thrombocytopenia and aplastic anemia have all been reported as reactions to injectable gold and *Ridaura*. These reactions may occur separately or in combination at anytime during treatment. Because they have potentially serious consequences, *blood dyscrasias should be constantly watched for through regular monitoring (at least monthly) of the formed elements of the blood throughout treatment.*

Miscellaneous Reactions: Rare reactions attributed to gold include cholestatic jaundice; gold bronchitis and interstitial pneumonitis and fibrosis; peripheral neuropathy; partial or complete hair loss; fever.

Information for Patients: Patients should be advised of the possibility of toxicity from *Ridaura* and of the signs and symptoms that they should report promptly. (Patient information sheets are available.)

Women of childbearing potential should be warned of the potential risks of *Ridaura* therapy during pregnancy (See PRECAUTIONS—Pregnancy).

Laboratory Tests: CBC with differential, platelet count, urinalysis, and renal and liver function tests should be performed prior to Ridaura (auranofin) therapy to establish a baseline and to identify any preexisting conditions.

CBC with differential, platelet count and urinalysis should then be monitored at least monthly; other parameters should be monitored as appropriate.

Drug Interactions: In a single patient-report, there is the suggestion that concurrent administration of *Ridaura* and phenytoin may have increased phenytoin blood levels.

Carcinogenesis/Mutagenesis: In a 24-month study in rats, animals treated with auranofin at 0.4, 1.0 or 2.5 mg/kg/day orally (3, 8 or 21 times the human dose) or gold sodium thiomalate at 2 or 6 mg/kg injected twice weekly (4 or 12 times the human dose) were compared to untreated control animals.

There was a significant increase in the frequency of renal tubular cell karyomegaly and cytomegaly and renal adenoma in the animals treated with 1.0 or 2.5 mg/kg/day of auranofin and 2 or 6 mg/kg twice weekly of gold sodium thiomalate. Malignant renal epithelial tumors were seen in the 1.0 mg/kg/day and the 2.5 mg/kg/day auranofin and in the 6 mg/kg twice weekly gold sodium thiomalate-treated animals.

In a 12-month study, rats treated with auranofin at 23 mg/kg/day (192 times the human dose) developed tumors of the renal tubular epithelium, whereas those treated with 3.6 mg/kg/day (30 times the human dose) did not.

In an 18-month study in mice given oral auranofin at doses of 1, 3 and 9 mg/kg/day (8, 24 and 72 times the human dose), there was no statistically significant increase above controls in the instances of tumors.

In the mouse lymphoma forward mutation assay, auranofin at high concentrations (313 to 700 ng/mL) induced increases in the mutation frequencies in the presence of a rat liver microsomal preparation. Auranofin produced no mutation effects in the Ames test (Salmonella), in the *in vitro* assay (Forward and Reverse Mutation Inducement Assay with Saccharomyces), in the *in vitro* transformation of BALB/T3 cell mouse assay or in the Dominant Lethal Assay.

Pregnancy: Teratogenic Effects—Pregnancy Category C. Use of Ridaura (auranofin) by pregnant women is not recommended. Furthermore, women of childbearing potential should be warned of the potential risks of *Ridaura* therapy during pregnancy. (See below.)

Pregnant rabbits given auranofin at doses of 0.5, 3 or 6 mg/kg/day (4.2 to 50 times the human dose) had impaired food intake, decreased maternal weights, decreased fetal weights and an increase above controls in the incidence of resorptions, abortions and congenital abnormalities, mainly abdominal defects such as gastroschisis and umbilical hernia.

Pregnant rats given auranofin at a dose of 5 mg/kg/day (42 times the human dose) had an increase above controls in the incidence of resorptions and a decrease in litter size and weight linked to maternal toxicity. No such effects were found in rats given 2.5 mg/kg/day (21 times the human dose).

Pregnant mice given auranofin at a dose of 5 mg/kg/day (42 times the human dose) had no teratogenic effects.

There are no adequate and well-controlled *Ridaura* studies in pregnant women.

Nursing Mothers: Nursing during *Ridaura* therapy is not recommended. Following auranofin administration to rats and mice, gold is excreted in milk. Following the administration of injectable gold, gold appears in the milk of nursing women; human data on auranofin are not available.

Pediatric Use: Ridaura (auranofin) is not recommended for use in children because its safety and effectiveness have not been established.

ADVERSE REACTIONS

The adverse reactions incidences listed below are based on observations of 1) 4,784 *Ridaura* -treated patients in clinical trials (2,474 U.S., 2,310 foreign), of whom 2,729 were treated more than one year and 573 for more than three years; and 2) postmarketing experience. The highest incidence is during the first six months of treatment; however, reactions can occur after many months of therapy. With rare exceptions, all patients were on concomitant nonsteroidal anti-inflammatory therapy; some of them were also taking low dosages of corticosteroids.

Reactions occurring in more than 1% of *Ridaura*-treated patients

Gastrointestinal: loose stools or diarrhea (47%); abdominal pain (14%); nausea with or without vomiting (10%); constipation; anorexia*; flatulence*; dyspepsia*; dysgeusia.

Dermatological: rash (24%); pruritus (17%); hair loss; urticaria.

Mucous Membrane: stomatitis (13%); conjunctivitis*; glossitis.

Hematological: anemia; leukopenia; thrombocytopenia; eosinophilia.

Renal: proteinuria*; hematuria.

Hepatic: elevated liver enzymes.

*Reactions marked with an asterisk occurred in 3–9% of the patients. The other reactions listed occurred in 1–3%.

Reactions occurring in less than 1% of *Ridaura*-treated patients

Gastrointestinal: dysphagia; gastrointestinal bleeding†; melena†; positive stool for occult blood†; ulcerative enterocolitis.

† Reactions marked with a dagger occurred in 0.1–1% of the patients. The other reactions listed occurred in less than 0.1%.

Dermatological: angioedema.

Mucous Membrane: gingivitis†.

Hematological: aplastic anemia; neutropenia†; agranulocytosis; pure red cell aplasia; pancytopenia.

Hepatic: jaundice.

Respiratory: interstitial pneumonitis.

Neurological: peripheral neuropathy.

Ocular: gold deposits in the lens or cornea unassociated clinically with eye disorders or visual impairment.

Reactions reported with injectable gold preparations, but not with Ridaura (auranofin) (based on clinical trials and on postmarketing experience)

Cutaneous Reactions: generalized exfoliative dermatitis.

Incidence of Adverse Reactions for Specific Categories—18 Comparative Trials

	Ridaura (445 patients)	Injectable Gold (445 patients)
Proteinuria	0.9%	5.4%
Rash	26 %	39 %
Diarrhea	42.5%	13 %
Stomatitis	13 %	18 %
Anemia	3.1%	2.7%
Leukopenia	1.3%	2.2%
Thrombocytopenia	0.9%	2.2%
Elevated liver function tests	1.9%	1.7%
Pulmonary	0.2%	0.2%

OVERDOSAGE

The acute oral LD_{50} for auranofin is 310 mg/kg in adult mice and 265 mg/kg in adult rats. The minimum lethal dose in rats is 30 mg/kg.

In case of acute overdosage, immediate induction of emesis or gastric lavage and appropriate supportive therapy are recommended.

Ridaura overdosage experience is limited. A 50-year-old female, previously on 6 mg *Ridaura* daily, took 27 mg (9 capsules) daily for 10 days and developed an encephalopathy and peripheral neuropathy. *Ridaura* was discontinued and she eventually recovered.

There has been no experience with treating *Ridaura* overdosage with modalities such as chelating agents. However, they have been used with injectable gold and may be considered for *Ridaura* overdosage.

DOSAGE AND ADMINISTRATION

Usual Adult Dosage: The usual adult dosage of Ridaura (auranofin) is 6 mg daily, given either as 3 mg twice daily or 6 mg once daily. Initiation of therapy at dosages exceeding 6 mg daily is not recommended because it is associated with an increased incidence of diarrhea. If response is inadequate after six months, an increase to 9 mg (3 mg three times daily) may be tolerated. If response remains inadequate after a three-month trial of 9 mg daily, *Ridaura* therapy should be discontinued. Safety at dosages exceeding 9 mg daily has not been studied.

Transferring from Injectable Gold: In controlled clinical studies, patients on injectable gold have been transferred to Ridaura (auranofin) by discontinuing the injectable agent and starting oral therapy with *Ridaura*, 6 mg daily. When patients are transferred to *Ridaura*, they should be informed of its adverse reaction profile, in particular the gastrointestinal reactions. (See PRECAUTIONS—Information for Patients.) At six months, control of disease activity of patients transferred to *Ridaura* and those maintained on the injectable agent was not different. Data beyond six months are not available.

HOW SUPPLIED

Capsules, containing 3 mg auranofin, in bottles of 60.

STORAGE AND HANDLING

Store at controlled room temperature (59°–86°F). Dispense in a tight, light-resistant container.

RI:L30

Shown in Product Identification Section, page 431

STELAZINE® ℞

[stel 'ah-zeen]

(brand of trifluoperazine hydrochloride)

DESCRIPTION

Tablets: Each round, blue, film-coated tablet contains trifluoperazine hydrochloride equivalent to trifluoperazine as follows: 1 mg imprinted SKF and S03; 2 mg imprinted SKF and S04; 5 mg imprinted SKF and S06; 10 mg imprinted SKF and S07. Inactive ingredients consist of cellulose, croscarmellose sodium, FD&C Blue No. 2, FD&C Yellow No. 6, FD&C Red No. 40, gelatin, iron oxide, lactose, magnesium

Continued on next page

SmithKline Beecham—Cont.

stearate, talc, titanium dioxide and trace amounts of other inactive ingredients.

Multi-dose Vials, 10 mL (2 mg/mL)—Each mL contains, in aqueous solution, trifluoperazine, 2 mg, as the hydrochloride; sodium tartrate, 4.75 mg; sodium biphosphate, 11.6 mg; sodium saccharin, 0.3 mg; benzyl alcohol, 0.75%, as preservative.

Concentrate —Each mL of clear, yellow, banana-vanilla flavored liquid contains 10 mg of trifluoperazine as the hydrochloride. Inactive ingredients consist of D&C Yellow No. 10, FD&C Yellow No. 6, flavor, sodium benzoate, sodium bisulfite, sucrose and water.

N.B.: The Concentrate is for use in severe neuropsychiatric conditions when oral medication is preferred and other oral forms are considered impractical.

INDICATIONS

For the management of the manifestations of psychotic disorders.

Stelazine (trifluoperazine HCl) is effective for the short-term treatment of generalized non-psychotic anxiety. However, *Stelazine* is not the first drug to be used in therapy for most patients with non-psychotic anxiety because certain risks associated with its use are not shared by common alternative treatments (i.e., benzodiazepines).

When used in the treatment of non-psychotic anxiety, *Stelazine* should not be administered at doses of more than 6 mg per day or for longer than 12 weeks because the use of *Stelazine* at higher doses or for longer intervals may cause persistent tardive dyskinesia that may prove irreversible (see Warnings section).

The effectiveness of *Stelazine* as a treatment for non-psychotic anxiety was established in a four-week clinical multicenter study of outpatients with generalized anxiety disorder (DSM-III). This evidence does not predict that *Stelazine* will be useful in patients with other non-psychotic conditions in which anxiety, or signs that mimic anxiety, are found (i.e., physical illness, organic mental conditions, agitated depression, character pathologies, etc.).

Stelazine (trifluoperazine HCl) has not been shown effective in the management of behavioral complications in patients with mental retardation.

CONTRAINDICATIONS

Comatose or greatly depressed states due to central nervous system depressants, and in cases of existing blood dyscrasias, bone marrow depression and pre-existing liver damage.

WARNINGS

Tardive Dyskinesia: Tardive dyskinesia, a syndrome consisting of potentially irreversible, involuntary, dyskinetic movements, may develop in patients treated with neuroleptic (antipsychotic) drugs. Although the prevalence of the syndrome appears to be highest among the elderly, especially elderly women, it is impossible to rely upon prevalence estimates to predict, at the inception of neuroleptic treatment, which patients are likely to develop the syndrome. Whether neuroleptic drug products differ in their potential to cause tardive dyskinesia is unknown.

Both the risk of developing the syndrome and the likelihood that it will become irreversible are believed to increase as the duration of treatment and the total cumulative dose of neuroleptic drugs administered to the patient increase. However, the syndrome can develop, although much less commonly, after relatively brief treatment periods at low doses.

There is no known treatment for established cases of tardive dyskinesia, although the syndrome may remit, partially or completely, if neuroleptic treatment is withdrawn. Neuroleptic treatment itself, however, may suppress (or partially suppress) the signs and symptoms of the syndrome and thereby may possibly mask the underlying disease process. The effect that symptomatic suppression has upon the long-term course of the syndrome is unknown.

Given these considerations, neuroleptics should be prescribed in a manner that is most likely to minimize the occurrence of tardive dyskinesia. Chronic neuroleptic treatment should generally be reserved for patients who suffer from a chronic illness that 1) is known to respond to neuroleptic drugs, and, 2) for whom alternative, equally effective, but potentially less harmful treatments are *not* available or appropriate. In patients who do require chronic treatment, the smallest dose and the shortest duration of treatment producing a satisfactory clinical response should be sought. The need for continued treatment should be reassessed periodically.

If signs and symptoms of tardive dyskinesia appear in a patient on neuroleptics, drug discontinuation should be considered. However, some patients may require treatment despite the presence of the syndrome.

For further information about the description of tardive dyskinesia and its clinical detection, please refer to the sections on Precautions and Adverse Reactions.

Neuroleptic Malignant Syndrome (NMS)

A potentially fatal symptom complex sometimes referred to as Neuroleptic Malignant Syndrome (NMS) has been reported in association with antipsychotic drugs. Clinical manifestations of NMS are hyperpyrexia, muscle rigidity, altered mental status and evidence of autonomic instability (irregular pulse or blood pressure, tachycardia, diaphoresis, and cardiac dysrhythmias).

The diagnostic evaluation of patients with this syndrome is complicated. In arriving at a diagnosis, it is important to identify cases where the clinical presentation includes both serious medical illness (e.g., pneumonia, systemic infection, etc.) and untreated or inadequately treated extrapyramidal signs and symptoms (EPS). Other important considerations in the differential diagnosis include central anticholinergic toxicity, heat stroke, drug fever and primary central nervous system (CNS) pathology.

The management of NMS should include 1) immediate discontinuation of antipsychotic drugs and other drugs not essential to concurrent therapy, 2) intensive symptomatic treatment and medical monitoring, and 3) treatment of any concomitant serious medical problems for which specific treatments are available. There is no general agreement about specific pharmacological treatment regimens for uncomplicated NMS.

If a patient requires antipsychotic drug treatment after recovery from NMS, the potential reintroduction of drug therapy should be carefully considered. The patient should be carefully monitored, since recurrences of NMS have been reported.

Patients who have demonstrated a hypersensitivity reaction (e.g., blood dyscrasias, jaundice) with a phenothiazine should not be re-exposed to any phenothiazine, including Stelazine (trifluoperazine HCl), unless in the judgment of the physician the potential benefits of treatment outweigh the possible hazard.

Stelazine Concentrate contains sodium bisulfite, a sulfite that may cause allergic-type reactions including anaphylactic symptoms and life-threatening or less severe asthmatic episodes in certain susceptible people. The overall prevalence of sulfite sensitivity in the general population is unknown and probably low. Sulfite sensitivity is seen more frequently in asthmatic than in non-asthmatic people.

Stelazine (trifluoperazine HCl) may impair mental and/or physical abilities, especially during the first few days of therapy. Therefore, caution patients about activities requiring alertness (e.g., operating vehicles or machinery).

If agents such as sedatives, narcotics, anesthetics, tranquilizers, or alcohol are used either simultaneously or successively with the drug, the possibility of an undesirable additive depressant effect should be considered.

Usage in Pregnancy: Safety for the use of *Stelazine* during pregnancy has not been established. Therefore, it is not recommended that the drug be given to pregnant patients except when, in the judgment of the physician, it is essential. The potential benefits should clearly outweigh possible hazards. There are reported instances of prolonged jaundice, extrapyramidal signs, hyperreflexia or hyporeflexia in newborn infants whose mothers received phenothiazines.

Reproductive studies in rats given over 600 times the human dose showed an increased incidence of malformations above controls and reduced litter size and weight linked to maternal toxicity. These effects were not observed at half this dosage. No adverse effect on fetal development was observed in rabbits given 700 times the human dose nor in monkeys given 25 times the human dose.

Nursing Mothers: There is evidence that phenothiazines are excreted in the breast milk of nursing mothers.

PRECAUTIONS

Given the likelihood that some patients exposed chronically to neuroleptics will develop tardive dyskinesia, it is advised that all patients in whom chronic use is contemplated be given, if possible, full information about this risk. The decision to inform patients and/or their guardians must obviously take into account the clinical circumstances and the competency of the patient to understand the information provided.

Thrombocytopenia and anemia have been reported in patients receiving the drug. Agranulocytosis and pancytopenia have also been reported—warn patients to report the sudden appearance of sore throat or other signs of infection. If white blood cell and differential counts indicate cellular depression, stop treatment and start antibiotic and other suitable therapy.

Jaundice of the cholestatic type of hepatitis or liver damage has been reported. If fever with grippe-like symptoms occurs, appropriate liver studies should be conducted. If tests indicate an abnormality, stop treatment.

One result of therapy may be an increase in mental and physical activity. For example, a few patients with angina pectoris have complained of increased pain while taking the drug. Therefore, angina patients should be observed carefully and, if an unfavorable response is noted, the drug should be withdrawn.

Because hypotension has occurred, large doses and parenteral administration should be avoided in patients with impaired cardiovascular systems. To minimize the occurrence of hypotension after injection, keep patient lying down and observe for at least $\frac{1}{2}$ hour. If hypotension occurs from parenteral or oral dosing, place patient in head-low position with legs raised. If a vasoconstrictor is required, Levophed®* and Neo-Synephrine®† are suitable. Other pressor agents, including epinephrine, should not be used as they may cause a paradoxical further lowering of blood pressure. Since certain phenothiazines have been reported to produce retinopathy, the drug should be discontinued if ophthalmoscopic examination or visual field studies should demonstrate retinal changes.

An antiemetic action of Stelazine (trifluoperazine HCl) may mask the signs and symptoms of toxicity or overdosage of other drugs and may obscure the diagnosis and treatment of other conditions such as intestinal obstruction, brain tumor and Reye's syndrome.

With prolonged administration at high dosages, the possibility of cumulative effects, with sudden onset of severe central nervous system or vasomotor symptoms, should be kept in mind.

Neuroleptic drugs elevate prolactin levels; the elevation persists during chronic administration. Tissue culture experiments indicate that approximately one-third of human breast cancers are prolactin-dependent in vitro, a factor of potential importance if the prescribing of these drugs is contemplated in a patient with a previously detected breast cancer. Although disturbances such as galactorrhea, amenorrhea, gynecomastia and impotence have been reported, the clinical significance of elevated serum prolactin levels is unknown for most patients. An increase in mammary neoplasms has been found in rodents after chronic administration of neuroleptic drugs. Neither clinical nor epidemiologic studies conducted to date, however, have shown an association between chronic administration of these drugs and mammary tumorigenesis; the available evidence is considered too limited to be conclusive at this time.

Chromosomal aberrations in spermatocytes and abnormal sperm have been demonstrated in rodents treated with certain neuroleptics.

Because phenothiazines may interfere with thermoregulatory mechanisms, use with caution in persons who will be exposed to extreme heat.

As with all drugs which exert an anticholinergic effect, and/or cause mydriasis, trifluoperazine should be used with caution in patients with glaucoma.

Phenothiazines may diminish the effect of oral anticoagulants.

Phenothiazines can produce alpha-adrenergic blockade.

Concomitant administration of propranolol with phenothiazines results in increased plasma levels of both drugs.

Antihypertensive effects of guanethidine and related compounds may be counteracted when phenothiazines are used concurrently.

Thiazide diuretics may accentuate the orthostatic hypotension that may occur with phenothiazines.

Phenothiazines may lower the convulsive threshold; dosage adjustments of anticonvulsants may be necessary. Potentiation of anticonvulsant effects does not occur. However, it has been reported that phenothiazines may interfere with the metabolism of Dilantin®‡ and thus precipitate *Dilantin* toxicity.

Drugs which lower the seizure threshold, including phenothiazine derivatives, should not be used with Amipaque®§. As with other phenothiazine derivatives, *Stelazine* should be discontinued at least 48 hours before myelography, should not be resumed for at least 24 hours postprocedure, and should not be used for the control of nausea and vomiting occurring either prior to myelography or postprocedure with *Amipaque.*

The presence of phenothiazines may produce false positive phenylketonuria (PKU) test results.

Long-Term Therapy: To lessen the likelihood of adverse reactions related to cumulative drug effect, patients with a history of long-term therapy with Stelazine (trifluoperazine HCl) and/or other neuroleptics should be evaluated periodically to decide whether the maintenance dosage could be lowered or drug therapy discontinued.

ADVERSE REACTIONS

Drowsiness, dizziness, skin reactions, rash, dry mouth, insomnia, amenorrhea, fatigue, muscular weakness, anorexia, lactation, blurred vision and neuromuscular (extrapyramidal) reactions.

Neuromuscular (Extrapyramidal) Reactions

These symptoms are seen in a significant number of hospitalized mental patients. They may be characterized by motor restlessness, be of the dystonic type, or they may resemble parkinsonism.

---

* norepinephrine bitartrate, Winthrop Pharmaceuticals.
† phenylephrine hydrochloride, Winthrop Pharmaceuticals.
‡ phenytoin, Parke-Davis.
§ metrizamide, Winthrop Pharmaceuticals.

Depending on the severity of symptoms, dosage should be reduced or discontinued. If therapy is reinstituted, it should be at a lower dosage. Should these symptoms occur in children or pregnant patients, the drug should be stopped and not reinstituted. In most cases barbiturates by suitable route of administration will suffice. (Or, injectable Benadryl®[ll] may be useful.) In more severe cases, the administration of an anti-parkinsonism agent, except levodopa, usually produces rapid reversal of symptoms. Suitable supportive measures such as maintaining a clear airway and adequate hydration should be employed.

Motor Restlessness: Symptoms may include agitation or jitteriness and sometimes insomnia. These symptoms often disappear spontaneously. At times these symptoms may be similar to the original neurotic or psychotic symptoms. Dosage should not be increased until these side effects have subsided.

If this phase becomes too troublesome, the symptoms can usually be controlled by a reduction of dosage or change of drug. Treatment with anti-parkinsonian agents, benzodiazepines or propranolol may be helpful.

Dystonias: Symptoms may include: spasm of the neck muscles, sometimes progressing to torticollis; extensor rigidity of back muscles, sometimes progressing to opisthotonos; carpopedal spasm, trismus, swallowing difficulty, oculogyric crisis and protrusion of the tongue.

These usually subside within a few hours, and almost always within 24 to 48 hours, after the drug has been discontinued.

In mild cases, reassurance or a barbiturate is often sufficient. *In moderate cases,* barbiturates will usually bring rapid relief. *In more severe adult cases,* the administration of an anti-parkinsonism agent, except levodopa, usually produces rapid reversal of symptoms. Also, intravenous caffeine with sodium benzoate seems to be effective. *In children,* reassurance and barbiturates will usually control symptoms. (Or, injectable *Benadryl* may be useful.) Note: See *Benadryl* prescribing information for appropriate children's dosage. If appropriate treatment with anti-parkinsonism agents or *Benadryl* fails to reverse the signs and symptoms, the diagnosis should be reevaluated.

Pseudo-parkinsonism: Symptoms may include: mask-like facies; drooling; tremors; pill-rolling motion; cogwheel rigidity; and shuffling gait. Reassurance and sedation are important. In most cases these symptoms are readily controlled when an anti-parkinsonism agent is administered concomitantly. Anti-parkinsonism agents should be used only when required. Generally, therapy of a few weeks to two or three months will suffice. After this time patients should be evaluated to determine their need for continued treatment. (Note: Levodopa has not been found effective in pseudo-parkinsonism.) Occasionally it is necessary to lower the dosage of Stelazine (trifluoperazine HCl) or to discontinue the drug.

Tardive Dyskinesia: As with all antipsychotic agents, tardive dyskinesia may appear in some patients on long-term therapy or may appear after drug therapy has been discontinued. The syndrome can also develop, although much less frequently, after relatively brief treatment periods at low doses. This syndrome appears in all age groups. Although its prevalence appears to be highest among elderly patients, especially elderly women, it is impossible to rely upon prevalence estimates to predict at the inception of neuroleptic treatment which patients are likely to develop the syndrome. The symptoms are persistent and in some patients appear to be irreversible. The syndrome is characterized by rhythmical involuntary movements of the tongue, face, mouth or jaw (e.g., protrusion of tongue, puffing of cheeks, puckering of mouth, chewing movements). Sometimes these may be accompanied by involuntary movements of extremities. In rare instances, these involuntary movements of the extremities are the only manifestations of tardive dyskinesia. A variant of tardive dyskinesia, tardive dystonia, has also been described.

There is no known effective treatment for tardive dyskinesia; anti-parkinsonism agents do not alleviate the symptoms of this syndrome. If clinically feasible, it is suggested that all antipsychotic agents be discontinued if these symptoms appear. Should it be necessary to reinstitute treatment, or increase the dosage of the agent, or switch to a different antipsychotic agent, the syndrome may be masked.

It has been reported that fine vermicular movements of the tongue may be an early sign of the syndrome and if the medication is stopped at that time the syndrome may not develop.

Adverse Reactions Reported with Stelazine (trifluoperazine HCl) or Other Phenothiazine Derivatives: Adverse effects with different phenothiazines vary in type, frequency, and mechanism of occurrence, i.e., some are dose-related, while others involve individual patient sensitivity. Some adverse effects may be more likely to occur, or occur with greater intensity, in patients with special medical problems, e.g., patients with mitral insufficiency or pheochromocytoma have experienced severe hypotension following recommended doses of certain phenothiazines.

Not all of the following adverse reactions have been observed with every phenothiazine derivative, but they have been reported with one or more and should be borne in mind when drugs of this class are administered: extrapyramidal symptoms (opisthotonos, oculogyric crisis, hyperreflexia, dystonia, akathisia, dyskinesia, parkinsonism) some of which have lasted months and even years—particularly in elderly patients with previous brain damage; grand mal and petit mal convulsions, particularly in patients with EEG abnormalities or history of such disorders; altered cerebrospinal fluid proteins; cerebral edema; intensification and prolongation of the action of central nervous system depressants (opiates, analgesics, antihistamines, barbiturates, alcohol), atropine, heat, organophosphorus insecticides; autonomic reactions (dryness of mouth, nasal congestion, headache, nausea, constipation, obstipation, adynamic ileus, ejaculatory disorders/impotence, priapism, atonic colon, urinary retention, miosis and mydriasis); reactivation of psychotic processes, catatonic-like states; hypotension (sometimes fatal); cardiac arrest; blood dyscrasias (pancytopenia, thrombocytopenic purpura, leukopenia, agranulocytosis, eosinophilia, hemolytic anemia, aplastic anemia); liver damage (jaundice, biliary stasis); endocrine disturbances (hyperglycemia, hypoglycemia, glycosuria, lactation, galactorrhea, gynecomastia, menstrual irregularities, false positive pregnancy tests); skin disorders (photosensitivity, itching, erythema, urticaria, eczema up to exfoliative dermatitis); other allergic reactions (asthma, laryngeal edema, angioneurotic edema, anaphylactoid reactions); peripheral edema; reversed epinephrine effect; hyperpyrexia; mild fever after large I.M. doses; increased appetite; increased weight; a systemic lupus erythematosus-like syndrome; pigmentary retinopathy; with prolonged administration of substantial doses, skin pigmentation, epithelial keratopathy, and lenticular and corneal deposits.

EKG changes—particularly nonspecific, usually reversible Q and T wave distortions—have been observed in some patients receiving phenothiazine tranquilizers. Although phenothiazines cause neither psychic nor physical dependence, sudden discontinuance in long-term psychiatric patients may cause temporary symptoms, e.g., nausea and vomiting, dizziness, tremulousness.

Note: There have been occasional reports of sudden death in patients receiving phenothiazines. In some cases, the cause appeared to be cardiac arrest or asphyxia due to failure of the cough reflex.

DOSAGE AND ADMINISTRATION—ADULTS

Dosage should be adjusted to the needs of the individual. The lowest effective dosage should always be used. Dosage should be increased more gradually in debilitated or emaciated patients. When maximum response is achieved, dosage may be reduced gradually to a maintenance level. Because of the inherent long action of the drug, patients may be controlled on convenient b.i.d. administration; some patients may be maintained on once-a-day administration.

When Stelazine (trifluoperazine HCl) is administered by intramuscular injection, equivalent oral dosage may be substituted once symptoms have been controlled.

Note: Although there is little likelihood of contact dermatitis due to the drug, persons with known sensitivity to phenothiazine drugs should avoid direct contact.

Elderly Patients: In general, dosages in the lower range are sufficient for most elderly patients. Since they appear to be more susceptible to hypotension and neuromuscular reactions, such patients should be observed closely. Dosage should be tailored to the individual, response carefully monitored, and dosage adjusted accordingly. Dosage should be increased more gradually in elderly patients.

Non-psychotic Anxiety

Usual dosage is 1 or 2 mg twice daily. Do not administer at doses of more than 6 mg per day or for longer than 12 weeks.

Psychotic Disorders

Oral: Usual starting dosage is 2 mg to 5 mg b.i.d. (Small or emaciated patients should always be started on the lower dosage.)

Most patients will show optimum response on 15 mg or 20 mg daily, although a few may require 40 mg a day or more. Optimum therapeutic dosage levels should be reached within two or three weeks.

When the Concentrate dosage form is to be used, it should be added to 60 mL (2 fl oz) or more of diluent *just prior to administration* to insure palatability and stability. Vehicles suggested for dilution are: tomato or fruit juice, milk, simple syrup, orange syrup, carbonated beverages, coffee, tea, or water. Semisolid foods (soup, puddings, etc.) may also be used.

Intramuscular (for prompt control of severe symptoms): Usual dosage is 1 mg to 2 mg (½-1 mL) by deep intramuscular injection q4-6h, p.r.n. More than 6 mg within 24 hours is rarely necessary.

Only in very exceptional cases should intramuscular dosage exceed 10 mg within 24 hours. Injections should not be given at intervals of less than 4 hours because of a possible cumulative effect.

Note: Stelazine (trifluoperazine HCl) Injection has been usually well tolerated and there is little, if any, pain and irritation at the site of injection.

The Injection should be protected from light. Exposure may cause discoloration. Slight yellowish discoloration will not alter potency or efficacy. If markedly discolored, the solution should be discarded.

DOSAGE AND ADMINISTRATION—PSYCHOTIC CHILDREN

Dosage should be adjusted to the weight of the child and severity of the symptoms. These dosages are for children, ages 6 to 12, who are hospitalized or under close supervision.

Oral: The starting dosage is 1 mg administered once a day or b.i.d. Dosage may be increased gradually until symptoms are controlled or until side effects become troublesome.

While it is usually not necessary to exceed dosages of 15 mg daily, some older children with severe symptoms may require higher dosages.

Intramuscular: There has been little experience with the use of Stelazine (trifluoperazine HCl) Injection in children. However, if it is necessary to achieve rapid control of severe symptoms, 1 mg (½ mL) of the drug may be administered intramuscularly once or twice a day.

OVERDOSAGE

(See also under Adverse Reactions.)

SYMPTOMS—Primarily involvement of the extrapyramidal mechanism producing some of the dystonic reactions described above. Symptoms of central nervous system depression to the point of somnolence or coma. Agitation and restlessness may also occur. Other possible manifestations include convulsions, EKG changes and cardiac arrhythmias, fever, and autonomic reactions such as hypotension, dry mouth and ileus.

TREATMENT—It is important to determine other medications taken by the patient since multiple dose therapy is common in overdosage situations. Treatment is essentially symptomatic and supportive. Early gastric lavage is helpful. Keep patient under observation and maintain an open airway, since involvement of the extrapyramidal mechanism may produce dysphagia and respiratory difficulty in severe overdosage. **Do not attempt to induce emesis because a dystonic reaction of the head or neck may develop that could result in aspiration of vomitus.** Extrapyramidal symptoms may be treated with anti-parkinsonism drugs, barbiturates, or *Benadryl.* See prescribing information for these products. Care should be taken to avoid increasing respiratory depression. If administration of a stimulant is desirable, amphetamine, dextroamphetamine, or caffeine with sodium benzoate is recommended. Stimulants that may cause convulsions (e.g., picrotoxin or pentylenetetrazol) should be avoided.

If hypotension occurs, the standard measures for managing circulatory shock should be initiated. If it is desirable to administer a vasoconstrictor, *Levophed* and *Neo-Synephrine* are most suitable. Other pressor agents, including epinephrine, are not recommended because phenothiazine derivatives may reverse the usual elevating action of these agents and cause a further lowering of blood pressure.

Limited experience indicates that phenothiazines are *not* dialyzable.

HOW SUPPLIED

Tablets, 1 mg and 2 mg, in bottles of 100 and 1000; in Single Unit Packages of 100 (intended for institutional use only).

For psychiatric patients who are hospitalized or under close supervision:

Tablets, 5 mg and 10 mg, in bottles of 100 and 1000; in Single Unit Packages of 100 (intended for institutional use only).

Multi-dose Vials, 10 mL (2 mg/mL), in boxes of 1 and 20.

Concentrate (for institutional use), 10 mg/mL, in 2 fl oz bottles and in cartons of 12 bottles.

Each bottle is packaged with a graduated dropper.

The Concentrate form is light-sensitive. For this reason, it should be protected from light and dispensed in amber bottles. *Refrigeration is not required.*

SZ:L65

Shown in Product Identification Section, page 431

TAGAMET® ℞

[tag'ah-met]

(brand of cimetidine tablets cimetidine hydrochloride liquid and cimetidine hydrochloride injection)

DESCRIPTION

Tagamet (cimetidine) is a histamine H_2-receptor antagonist. Chemically it is *N''*-cyano- *N*-methyl-*N'*-[2-[[(5-methyl-1 *H*-imidazol-4-yl) methyl] thio]-ethyl]-guanidine.

The empirical formula for cimetidine is $C_{10}H_{16}N_6S$ and for cimetidine hydrochloride, $C_{10}H_{16}N_6SHCl$; these represent molecular weights of 252.34 and 288.80, respectively.

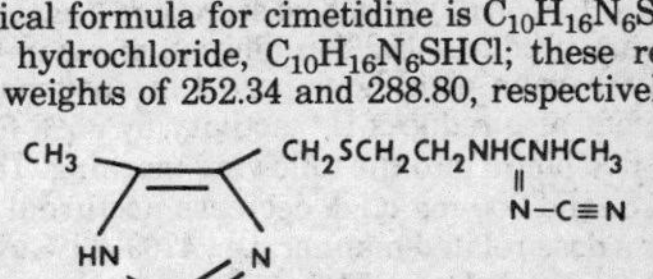

Cimetidine

Continued on next page

[ll] diphenhydramine hydrochloride, Parke-Davis.

SmithKline Beecham—Cont.

Cimetidine contains an imidazole ring, and is chemically related to histamine.
(The liquid and injection dosage forms contain cimetidine as the hydrochloride.)
Cimetidine has a bitter taste and characteristic odor.

Solubility Characteristics: Cimetidine is soluble in alcohol, slightly soluble in water, very slightly soluble in chloroform and insoluble in ether. Cimetidine hydrochloride is freely soluble in water, soluble in alcohol, very slightly soluble in chloroform and practically insoluble in ether.

Tablets for Oral Administration: Each light green, film-coated tablet contains cimetidine as follows: 200 mg—round, imprinted with the product name TAGAMET, SKF and 200; 300 mg—round, imprinted with the product name TAGAMET, SKF and 300; 400 mg—capsule-shaped, imprinted with the product name TAGAMET, SKF and 400; 800 mg—oval Tiltab® tablets, imprinted with the product name TAGAMET, SKF and 800. Inactive ingredients consist of cellulose, D&C Yellow No. 10, FD&C Blue No. 2, FD&C Red No. 40, FD&C Yellow No. 6, hydroxypropyl methylcellulose, iron oxides, magnesium stearate, povidone, propylene glycol, sodium lauryl sulfate, sodium starch glycolate, starch, titanium dioxide and trace amounts of other inactive ingredients.

Liquid for Oral Administration: Each 5 mL (one teaspoonful) of clear, light orange, mint-peach flavored liquid contains cimetidine hydrochloride equivalent to cimetidine, 300 mg; alcohol, 2.8%. Inactive ingredients consist of FD&C Yellow No. 6, flavors, methylparaben, polyoxyethylene polyoxypropylene glycol, propylene glycol, propylparaben, saccharin sodium, sodium chloride, sodium phosphate, sorbitol and water.

Injection:
Single-Dose Vials for Intramuscular or Intravenous Administration: Each 2 mL contains, in sterile aqueous solution (pH range 3.8-6), cimetidine hydrochloride equivalent to cimetidine, 300 mg; phenol, 10 mg.

Multi-Dose Vials for Intramuscular or Intravenous Administration: 8 mL (300 mg/2 mL): Each 2 mL contains, in sterile aqueous solution (pH range 3.8-6), cimetidine hydrochloride equivalent to cimetidine, 300 mg; phenol, 10 mg.

Single-Dose Premixed Plastic Containers for Intravenous Administration: Each 50 mL of sterile aqueous solution (pH range 5–7) contains cimetidine hydrochloride equivalent to 300 mg cimetidine and 0.45 grams sodium chloride. No preservative has been added.
The plastic container is fabricated from specially formulated polyvinyl chloride. The amount of water that can permeate from inside the container into the overwrap is insufficient to affect the solution significantly. Solutions in contact with the plastic container can leach out certain of its chemical components in very small amounts within the expiration period, e.g., di 2-ethylhexyl phthalate (DEHP), up to 5 parts per million. However, the safety of the plastic has been confirmed in tests in animals according to the USP biological tests for plastic containers as well as by tissue culture toxicity studies.

ADD-Vantage®* Vials for Intravenous Administration: Each 2 mL contains, in sterile aqueous solution (pH range 3.8-6), cimetidine hydrochloride equivalent to cimetidine, 300 mg; phenol, 10 mg.
All of the above injection formulations are pyrogen free, and sodium hydroxide N.F. is used as an ingredient to adjust the pH.

CLINICAL PHARMACOLOGY
Tagamet (cimetidine) competitively inhibits the action of histamine at the histamine H_2 receptors of the parietal cells and thus is a histamine H_2-receptor antagonist.
Tagamet is not an anticholinergic agent. Studies have shown that Tagamet inhibits both daytime and nocturnal basal gastric acid secretion. Tagamet also inhibits gastric acid secretion stimulated by food, histamine, pentagastrin, caffeine and insulin.

Antisecretory Activity
1) **Acid Secretion:** Nocturnal: Tagamet 800 mg orally at bedtime reduces mean hourly H^+ activity by greater than 85% over an eight-hour period in duodenal ulcer patients, with no effect on daytime acid secretion. Tagamet 1600 mg orally h.s. produces 100% inhibition of mean hourly H^+ activity over an eight-hour period in duodenal ulcer patients, but also reduces H^+ activity by 35% for an additional five hours into the following morning. Tagamet 400 mg b.i.d. and 300 mg q.i.d. decrease nocturnal acid secretion in a dose-related manner, i.e., 47%–83% over a six- to eight-hour period and 54% over a nine-hour period, respectively.

---
* ADD-Vantage® is a trademark of Abbott Laboratories.

Food Stimulated: During the first hour after a standard experimental meal, oral Tagamet 300 mg inhibited gastric acid secretion in duodenal ulcer patients by at least 50%. During the subsequent two hours Tagamet inhibited gastric acid secretion by at least 75%.
The effect of a 300 mg breakfast dose of Tagamet continued for at least four hours and there was partial suppression of the rise in gastric acid secretion following the luncheon meal in duodenal ulcer patients. This suppression of gastric acid output was enhanced and could be maintained by another 300 mg dose of Tagamet given with lunch.
In another study, Tagamet 300 mg given with the meal increased gastric pH as compared with placebo.

	Mean Gastric pH	
	Tagamet	**Placebo**
1 hour	3.5	2.6
2 hours	3.1	1.6
3 hours	3.8	1.9
4 hours	6.1	2.2

24-Hour Mean H^+ Activity: Tagamet 800 mg h.s., 400 mg b.i.d. and 300 mg q.i.d. all provide a similar, moderate (less than 60%) level of 24-hour acid suppression. However, the 800 mg h.s. regimen exerts its entire effect on nocturnal acid, and does not affect daytime gastric physiology.
Chemically Stimulated: Oral Tagamet (cimetidine) significantly inhibited gastric acid secretion stimulated by betazole (an isomer of histamine), pentagastrin, caffeine and insulin as follows:

Stimulant	Stimulant Dose	Tagamet	% Inhibition
Betazole	1.5mg/kg (sc)	300mg (po)	85% at 2½ hours
Penta-gastrin	6mcg/kg/hr (iv)	100mg/hr (iv)	60% at 1 hour
Caffeine	5mg/kg/hr (iv)	300mg (po)	100% at 1 hour
Insulin	0.03 units/kg/hr (iv)	100mg/hr (iv)	82% at 1 hour

When food and betazole were used to stimulate secretion, inhibition of hydrogen ion concentration usually ranged from 45–75% and the inhibition of volume ranged from 30–65%.
Parenteral administration also significantly inhibits gastric acid secretion. In a crossover study involving patients with active or healed duodenal or gastric ulcers, either continuous I.V. infusion of Tagamet 37.5 mg/hour (900 mg/day) or intermittent injection of Tagamet 300 mg q6h (1200 mg/day) maintained gastric pH above 4.0 for more than 50% of the time under steady-state conditions.
2) **Pepsin:** Oral Tagamet 300 mg reduced total pepsin output as a result of the decrease in volume of gastric juice.
3) **Intrinsic Factor:** Intrinsic factor secretion was studied with betazole as a stimulant. Oral Tagamet 300 mg inhibited the rise in intrinsic factor concentration produced by betazole, but some intrinsic factor was secreted at all times.

Other
Lower Esophageal Sphincter Pressure and Gastric Emptying
Tagamet has no effect on lower esophageal sphincter (LES) pressure or the rate of gastric emptying.

Pharmacokinetics
Tagamet is rapidly absorbed after oral administration and peak levels occur in 45–90 minutes. The half-life of Tagamet is approximately 2 hours. Both oral and parenteral (I.V. or I.M.) administration provide comparable periods of therapeutically effective blood levels; blood concentrations remain above that required to provide 80% inhibition of basal gastric acid secretion for 4–5 hours following a dose of 300 mg.
Steady-state blood concentrations of cimetidine with continuous infusion of Tagamet are determined by the infusion rate and clearance of the drug in the individual patient. In a study of peptic ulcer patients with normal renal function, an infusion rate of 37.5 mg/hour produced average steady-state plasma cimetidine concentrations of about 0.9 mcg/mL. Blood levels with other infusion rates will vary in direct proportion to the infusion rate.
The principal route of excretion of Tagamet is the urine. Following parenteral administration, most of the drug is excreted as the parent compound; following oral administration, the drug is more extensively metabolized, the sulfoxide being the major metabolite. Following a single oral dose, 48% of the drug is recovered from the urine after 24 hours as the parent compound. Following I.V. or I.M. administration, approximately 75% of the drug is recovered from the urine after 24 hours as the parent compound.

CLINICAL TRIALS
Duodenal Ulcer
Tagamet (cimetidine) has been shown to be effective in the treatment of active duodenal ulcer and, at reduced dosage, in maintenance therapy following healing of active ulcers.
Active Duodenal Ulcer: Tagamet accelerates the rate of duodenal ulcer healing. Healing rates reported in U.S. and foreign controlled trials with Tagamet are summarized below, beginning with the regimen providing the lowest nocturnal dose.

Duodenal Ulcer Healing Rates with Various Tagamet Dosage Regimens*

Regimen	300 mg q.i.d.	400 mg b.i.d.	800 mg h.s.	1600 mg h.s.
week 4	68%	73%	80%	86%
week 6	80%	80%	89%	—
week 8	—	92%	94%	—

* Averages from controlled clinical trials.
A U.S., double-blind, placebo-controlled, dose-ranging study demonstrated that all once-daily at bedtime (h.s.) Tagamet regimens were superior to placebo in ulcer healing and that Tagamet 800 mg h.s. healed 75% of patients at four weeks. The healing rate with 800 mg h.s. was significantly superior to 400 mg h.s. (66%) and not significantly different from 1600 mg h.s. (81%).
In the U.S. dose-ranging trial, over 80% of patients receiving Tagamet 800 mg h.s. experienced nocturnal pain relief after one day. Relief from daytime pain was reported in approximately 70% of patients after two days. As with ulcer healing, the 800 mg h.s. dose was superior to 400 mg h.s. and not different from 1600 mg h.s.
In foreign, double-blind studies with Tagamet 800 mg h.s., 79–85% of patients were healed at four weeks.
While short-term treatment with Tagamet (cimetidine) can result in complete healing of the duodenal ulcer, acute therapy will not prevent ulcer recurrence after Tagamet has been discontinued. Some follow-up studies have reported that the rate of recurrence once therapy was discontinued was slightly higher for patients healed on Tagamet than for patients healed on other forms of therapy; however, the Tagamet-treated patients generally had more severe disease.
Maintenance Therapy in Duodenal Ulcer: Treatment with a reduced dose of Tagamet has been proven effective as maintenance therapy following healing of active duodenal ulcers.
In numerous placebo-controlled studies conducted worldwide, the percent of patients with observed ulcers at the end of one year's therapy with Tagamet 400 mg h.s. was significantly lower (10%–45%) than in patients receiving placebo (44%–70%). Thus, from 55% to 90% of patients were maintained free of observed ulcers at the end of one year with Tagamet 400 mg h.s.
Factors such as smoking, duration and severity of disease, gender, and genetic traits may contribute to variations in actual percentages.
Trials of other anti-ulcer therapy, whether placebo-controlled, positive-controlled or open, have demonstrated a range of results similar to that seen with Tagamet.
Active Benign Gastric Ulcer
Tagamet has been shown to be effective in the short-term treatment of active benign gastric ulcer.
In a multicenter, double-blind U.S. study, patients with endoscopically confirmed benign gastric ulcer were treated with Tagamet 300 mg four times a day or with placebo for six weeks. Patients were limited to those with ulcers ranging from 0.5-2.5 cm in size. Endoscopically confirmed healing at six weeks was seen in significantly* more Tagamet-treated patients than in patients receiving placebo, as shown below:

	Tagamet	Placebo
week 2	14/63 (22%)	7/63 (11%)
total at week 6	43/65 (66%)*	30/67 (45%)

*p < 0.05
In a similar multicenter U.S. study of the 800 mg h.s. oral regimen, the endoscopically confirmed healing rates were:

	Tagamet	Placebo
total at week 6	63/83 (76%)*	44/80 (55%)

*p = 0.005
Similarly, in worldwide double-blind clinical studies, endoscopically evaluated benign gastric ulcer healing rates were consistently higher with Tagamet than with placebo.
Gastroesophageal Reflux Disease
In two multicenter, double-blind, placebo-controlled studies in patients with gastroesophageal reflux disease (GERD) and endoscopically proven erosions and/or ulcers, Tagamet was significantly more effective than placebo in healing lesions. The endoscopically confirmed healing rates were:

Trial	Tagamet (800 mg b.i.d.)	Tagamet (400 mg q.i.d.)	Placebo	p-Value (800 mg b.i.d. vs. placebo)
1 Week 6	45%	52%	26%	0.02
Week 12	60%	66%	42%	0.02
2 Week 6	50%		20%	<0.01
Week 12	67%		36%	<0.01

In these trials *Tagamet* was superior to placebo by most measures in improving symptoms of day- and night-time heartburn, with many of the differences statistically significant. The q.i.d. regimen was generally somewhat better than the b.i.d. regimen where these were compared.

Prevention of Upper Gastrointestinal Bleeding in Critically Ill Patients

A double-blind, placebo-controlled randomized study of continuous infusion cimetidine was performed in 131 critically ill patients (mean APACHE II score = 15.99) to compare the incidence of upper gastrointestinal bleeding, manifested as hematemesis or bright red blood which did not clear after adjustment of the nasogastric tube and a 5 to 10 minute lavage, persistent Gastroccult® positive coffee grounds for 8 consecutive hours which did not clear with 100 cc lavage and/or which were accompanied by a drop in hematocrit of 5 percentage points, or melena, with an endoscopically documented upper gastrointestinal source of bleed. 14% (9/65) of patients treated with cimetidine continuous infusion developed bleeding compared to 33% (22/66) of the placebo group. Coffee grounds was the manifestation of bleeding that accounted for the difference between groups. Another randomized, double-blind placebo-controlled study confirmed these results for an end point of upper gastrointestinal bleeding with a confirmed upper gastrointestinal source noted on endoscopy, and by post hoc analyses of bleeding episodes between groups.

Pathological Hypersecretory Conditions
(such as Zollinger-Ellison Syndrome)

Tagamet significantly inhibited gastric acid secretion and reduced occurrence of diarrhea, anorexia and pain in patients with pathological hypersecretion associated with Zollinger-Ellison Syndrome, systemic mastocytosis and multiple endocrine adenomas. Use of *Tagamet* was also followed by healing of intractable ulcers.

INDICATIONS AND USAGE

Tagamet (cimetidine) is indicated in:

(1) **Short-term treatment of active duodenal ulcer.** Most patients heal within 4 weeks and there is rarely reason to use *Tagamet* at full dosage for longer than 6–8 weeks (see Dosage and Administration–Duodenal Ulcer). Concomitant antacids should be given as needed for relief of pain. However, simultaneous administration of *Tagamet* and antacids is not recommended, since antacids have been reported to interfere with the absorption of *Tagamet*.

(2) **Maintenance therapy for duodenal ulcer patients at reduced dosage after healing of active ulcer.** Patients have been maintained on continued treatment with *Tagamet* 400 mg h.s. for periods of up to five years.

(3) **Short-term treatment of active benign gastric ulcer.** There is no information concerning usefulness of treatment periods of longer than 8 weeks.

(4) **Erosive gastroesophageal reflux disease (GERD).** Erosive esophagitis diagnosed by endoscopy. Treatment is indicated for 12 weeks for healing of lesions and control of symptoms. The use of *Tagamet* beyond 12 weeks has not been established (see Dosage and Administration—GERD).

(5) **Prevention of upper gastrointestinal bleeding in critically ill patients.**

(6) **The treatment of pathological hypersecretory conditions** (i.e., Zollinger-Ellison Syndrome, systemic mastocytosis, multiple endocrine adenomas).

CONTRAINDICATIONS

Tagamet is contraindicated for patients known to have hypersensitivity to the product.

PRECAUTIONS

General: Rare instances of cardiac arrhythmias and hypotension have been reported following the rapid administration of Tagamet (cimetidine hydrochloride) Injection by intravenous bolus.

Symptomatic response to *Tagamet* therapy does not preclude the presence of a gastric malignancy. There have been rare reports of transient healing of gastric ulcers despite subsequently documented malignancy.

Reversible confusional states (see Adverse Reactions) have been observed on occasion, predominantly, but not exclusively, in severely ill patients. Advancing age (50 or more years) and preexisting liver and/or renal disease appear to be contributing factors. In some patients these confusional states have been mild and have not required discontinuation of *Tagamet* therapy. In cases where discontinuation was judged necessary, the condition usually cleared within 3-4 days of drug withdrawal.

Drug Interactions: *Tagamet*, apparently through an effect on certain microsomal enzyme systems, has been reported to reduce the hepatic metabolism of warfarin-type anticoagulants, phenytoin, propranolol, nifedipine, chlordiazepoxide, diazepam, certain tricyclic antidepressants, lidocaine, theophylline and metronidazole, thereby delaying elimination and increasing blood levels of these drugs.

Clinically significant effects have been reported with the warfarin anticoagulants; therefore, close monitoring of prothrombin time is recommended, and adjustment of the anticoagulant dose may be necessary when *Tagamet* is administered concomitantly. Interaction with phenytoin, lidocaine and theophylline has also been reported to produce adverse clinical effects.

However, a crossover study in healthy subjects receiving either *Tagamet* 300 mg q.i.d. or 800 mg h.s. concomitantly with a 300 mg b.i.d. dosage of theophylline (Theo-Dur®, Key Pharmaceuticals, Inc.) demonstrated less alteration in steady-state theophylline peak serum levels with the 800 mg h.s. regimen, particularly in subjects aged 54 years and older. Data beyond ten days are not available. (Note: All patients receiving theophylline should be monitored appropriately, regardless of concomitant drug therapy.)

Dosage of the drugs mentioned above and other similarly metabolized drugs, particularly those of low therapeutic ratio or in patients with renal and/or hepatic impairment, may require adjustment when starting or stopping concomitantly administered *Tagamet* to maintain optimum therapeutic blood levels.

Additional clinical experience may reveal other drugs affected by the concomitant administration of *Tagamet*.

Carcinogenesis, Mutagenesis, Impairment of Fertility: In a 24-month toxicity study conducted in rats, at dose levels of 150, 378 and 950 mg/kg/day (approximately 8 to 48 times the recommended human dose), there was a small increase in the incidence of benign Leydig cell tumors in each dose group; when the combined drug-treated groups and control groups were compared, this increase reached statistical significance. In a subsequent 24-month study, there were no differences between the rats receiving 150 mg/kg/day and the untreated controls. However, a statistically significant increase in benign Leydig cell tumor incidence was seen in the rats that received 378 and 950 mg/kg/day. These tumors were common in control groups as well as treated groups and the difference became apparent only in aged rats.

Tagamet (cimetidine) has demonstrated a weak antiandrogenic effect. In animal studies this was manifested as reduced prostate and seminal vesicle weights. However, there was no impairment of mating performance or fertility, nor any harm to the fetus in these animals at doses 8 to 48 times the full therapeutic dose of *Tagamet*, as compared with controls. The cases of gynecomastia seen in patients treated for one month or longer may be related to this effect.

In human studies, *Tagamet* has been shown to have no effect on spermatogenesis, sperm count, motility, morphology or *in vitro* fertilizing capacity.

Pregnancy: Teratogenic Effects. Pregnancy Category B: Reproduction studies have been performed in rats, rabbits and mice at doses up to 40 times the normal human dose and have revealed no evidence of impaired fertility or harm to the fetus due to *Tagamet*. There are, however, no adequate and well-controlled studies in pregnant women. Because animal reproductive studies are not always predictive of human response, this drug should be used during pregnancy only if clearly needed.

Nursing Mothers: Cimetidine is secreted in human milk and, as a general rule, nursing should not be undertaken while a patient is on a drug.

Pediatric Use: Clinical experience in children is limited. Therefore, *Tagamet* therapy cannot be recommended for children under 16, unless, in the judgment of the physician, anticipated benefits outweigh the potential risks. In very limited experience, doses of 20–40 mg/kg per day have been used.

ADVERSE REACTIONS

Adverse effects reported in patients taking *Tagamet* are described below by body system. Incidence figures of 1 in 100 and greater are generally derived from controlled clinical studies.

Gastrointestinal: Diarrhea (usually mild) has been reported in approximately 1 in 100 patients.

CNS: Headaches, ranging from mild to severe, have been reported in 3.5% of 924 patients taking 1600 mg/day, 2.1% of 2,225 patients taking 800 mg/day and 2.3% of 1,897 patients taking placebo. Dizziness and somnolence (usually mild) have been reported in approximately 1 in 100 patients on either 1600 mg/day or 800 mg/day.

Reversible confusional states, e.g., mental confusion, agitation, psychosis, depression, anxiety, hallucinations, disorientation, have been reported predominantly, but not exclusively, in severely ill patients. They have usually developed within 2-3 days of initiation of *Tagamet* therapy and have cleared within 3-4 days of discontinuation of the drug.

Endocrine: Gynecomastia has been reported in patients treated for one month or longer. In patients being treated for pathological hypersecretory states, this occurred in about 4% of cases while in all others the incidence was 0.3% to 1% in various studies. No evidence of induced endocrine dysfunction was found, and the condition remained unchanged or returned toward normal with continuing Tagamet (cimetidine) treatment.

Reversible impotence has been reported in patients with pathological hypersecretory disorders, e.g., Zollinger-Ellison Syndrome, receiving *Tagamet*, particularly in high doses, for at least 12 months (range 12–79 months, mean 38 months). However, in large-scale surveillance studies at regular dosage, the incidence has not exceeded that commonly reported in the general population.

Hematologic: Decreased white blood cell counts in *Tagamet*-treated patients (approximately 1 per 100,000 patients), including agranulocytosis (approximately 3 per million patients), have been reported, including a few reports of recurrence on rechallenge. Most of these reports were in patients who had serious concomitant illnesses and received drugs and/or treatment known to produce neutropenia. Thrombocytopenia (approximately 3 per million patients) and, very rarely, cases of pancytopenia or aplastic anemia have also been reported. As with some other H₂-receptor antagonists, there have been extremely rare reports of immune hemolytic anemia.

Hepatobiliary: Dose-related increases in serum transaminase have been reported. In most cases they did not progress with continued therapy and returned to normal at the end of therapy. There have been rare reports of cholestatic or mixed cholestatic-hepatocellular effects. These were usually reversible. Because of the predominance of cholestatic features, severe parenchymal injury is considered highly unlikely.

There has been reported a single case of biopsy-proven periportal hepatic fibrosis in a patient receiving *Tagamet*.

Rare cases of pancreatitis, which cleared on withdrawal of the drug, have been reported.

Hypersensitivity: Rare cases of fever and allergic reactions including anaphylaxis and hypersensitivity vasculitis, which cleared on withdrawal of the drug, have been reported.

Renal: Small, possibly dose-related increases in plasma creatinine, presumably due to competition for renal tubular secretion, are not uncommon and do not signify deteriorating renal function. Rare cases of interstitial nephritis and urinary retention, which cleared on withdrawal of the drug, have been reported.

Cardiovascular: Rare cases of bradycardia, tachycardia and A-V heart block have been reported with H₂-receptor antagonists.

Musculoskeletal: There have been rare reports of reversible arthralgia and myalgia; exacerbation of joint symptoms in patients with preexisting arthritis has also been reported. Such symptoms have usually been alleviated by a reduction in Tagamet (cimetidine) dosage. Rare cases of polymyositis have been reported, but no causal relationship has been established.

Integumental: Mild rash and, very rarely, cases of severe generalized skin reactions including Stevens-Johnson syndrome, epidermal necrolysis, erythema multiforme, exfoliative dermatitis and generalized exfoliative erythroderma have been reported with H₂-receptor antagonists. Reversible alopecia has been reported very rarely.

OVERDOSAGE

Studies in animals indicate that toxic doses are associated with respiratory failure and tachycardia that may be controlled by assisted respiration and the administration of a beta-blocker.

Reported acute ingestions orally of up to 20 grams have been associated with transient adverse effects similar to those encountered in normal clinical experience. The usual measures to remove unabsorbed material from the gastrointestinal tract, clinical monitoring, and supportive therapy should be employed.

There have been reports of severe CNS symptoms, including unresponsiveness, following ingestion of between 20 and 40 grams of cimetidine, and extremely rare reports following concomitant use of multiple CNS-active medications and ingestion of cimetidine at doses less than 20 grams.

There have been two deaths in adults who were reported to have ingested over 40 grams orally on a single occasion.

DOSAGE AND ADMINISTRATION

Duodenal Ulcer

Active Duodenal Ulcer: Clinical studies have indicated that suppression of nocturnal acid is the most important factor in duodenal ulcer healing (see Clinical Pharmacology—Acid Secretion). This is supported by recent clinical trials (see Clinical Trials—Active Duodenal Ulcer). Therefore, there is no apparent rationale, except for familiarity with use, for treating with anything other than a once-daily at bedtime dosage regimen (h.s.).

Continued on next page

SmithKline Beecham—Cont.

In a U.S. dose-ranging study of 400 mg h.s., 800 mg h.s. and 1600 mg h.s., a continuous dose response relationship for ulcer healing was demonstrated.

However, 800 mg h.s. is the dose of choice for most patients, as it provides a high healing rate (the difference between 800 mg h.s. and 1600 mg h.s. being small), maximal pain relief, a decreased potential for drug interactions (see Precautions—Drug Interactions) and maximal patient convenience. Patients unhealed at four weeks, or those with persistent symptoms, have been shown to benefit from two to four weeks of continued therapy.

It has been shown that patients who both have an endoscopically demonstrated ulcer larger than 1.0 cm and are also heavy smokers (i.e., smoke one pack of cigarettes or more per day) are more difficult to heal. There is some evidence which suggests that more rapid healing can be achieved in this subpopulation with *Tagamet* 1600 mg at bedtime. While early pain relief with either 800 mg h.s. or 1600 mg h.s. is equivalent in all patients, 1600 mg h.s. provides an appropriate alternative when it is important to ensure healing within four weeks for this subpopulation. Alternatively, approximately 94% of all patients will also heal in eight weeks with *Tagamet* 800 mg h.s.

Other *Tagamet* regimens in the U.S. which have been shown to be effective are: 300 mg four times daily, with meals and at bedtime, the original regimen with which U.S. physicians have the most experience, and 400 mg twice daily, in the morning and at bedtime (see Clinical Trials—Active Duodenal Ulcer).

Concomitant antacids should be given as needed for relief of pain. However, simultaneous administration of *Tagamet* and antacids is not recommended, since antacids have been reported to interfere with the absorption of Tagamet (cimetidine).

While healing with *Tagamet* often occurs during the first week or two, treatment should be continued for 4–6 weeks unless healing has been demonstrated by endoscopic examination.

Maintenance Therapy for Duodenal Ulcer: In those patients requiring maintenance therapy, the recommended adult oral dose is 400 mg at bedtime.

Active Benign Gastric Ulcer

The recommended adult oral dosage for short-term treatment of active benign gastric ulcer is 800 mg h.s., or 300 mg four times a day with meals and at bedtime. Controlled clinical studies were limited to six weeks of treatment (see Clinical Trials). 800 mg h.s. is the preferred regimen for most patients based upon convenience and reduced potential for drug interactions. Symptomatic response to *Tagamet* does not preclude the presence of a gastric malignancy. It is important to follow gastric ulcer patients to assure rapid progress to complete healing.

Erosive Gastroesophageal Reflux Disease (GERD)

The recommended adult oral dosage for the treatment of erosive esophagitis that has been diagnosed by endoscopy is 1600 mg daily in divided doses (800 mg b.i.d. or 400 mg q.i.d.) for 12 weeks. The use of *Tagamet* beyond 12 weeks has not been established.

Prevention of Upper Gastrointestinal Bleeding

The recommended adult dosing regimen is continuous I.V. infusion of 50 mg/hour. Patients with creatinine clearance less than 30 cc/min. should receive half the recommended dose. Treatment beyond 7 days has not been studied.

Pathological Hypersecretory Conditions (such as Zollinger-Ellison Syndrome)

Recommended adult oral dosage: 300 mg four times a day with meals and at bedtime. In some patients it may be necessary to administer higher doses more frequently. Doses should be adjusted to individual patient needs, but should not usually exceed 2400 mg per day and should continue as long as clinically indicated.

Parenteral Administration

In hospitalized patients with pathological hypersecretory conditions or intractable ulcers, or in patients who are unable to take oral medication, *Tagamet* may be administered parenterally.

The doses and regimen for parenteral administration in patients with GERD have not been established.

All parenteral drug products should be inspected visually for particulate matter and discoloration prior to administration.

Recommendations for parenteral administration:

Intramuscular injection: 300 mg q 6–8 hours (no dilution necessary). Transient pain at the site of injection has been reported.

Intravenous injection: 300 mg q 6–8 hours. In some patients it may be necessary to increase dosage. When this is necessary, the increases should be made by more frequent administration of a 300 mg dose, but should not exceed 2400 mg per day. Dilute Tagamet (cimetidine hydrochloride) Injection, 300 mg, in Sodium Chloride Injection (0.9%) or another compatible I.V. solution (see Stability of *Tagamet* Injection) to a total volume of 20 mL and inject over a period of not less than 5 minutes (see Precautions).

Intermittent intravenous infusion: 300 mg q 6–8 hours, infused over 15–20 minutes. In some patients it may be necessary to increase dosage. When this is necessary, the increases should be made by more frequent administration of a 300 mg dose, but should not exceed 2400 mg per day. **Vials:** Dilute *Tagamet* Injection, 300 mg, in at least 50 mL of 5% Dextrose Injection, or another compatible I.V. solution (see Stability of *Tagamet* Injection). **Plastic containers:** Use premixed *Tagamet* Injection, 300 mg, in 0.9% Sodium Chloride in 50 mL plastic containers. **ADD-Vantage® Vials:** Dilute contents of one vial in an ADD-Vantage® Diluent Container, available in 50 mL and 100 mL sizes of 0.9% Sodium Chloride Injection, and 5% Dextrose Injection.

Continuous intravenous infusion: 37.5 mg/hour (900 mg/day). For patients requiring a more rapid elevation of gastric pH, continuous infusion may be preceded by a 150 mg loading dose administered by I.V. infusion as described above. Dilute 900 mg *Tagamet* Injection in a compatible I.V. fluid (see Stability of *Tagamet* Injection) for constant rate infusion over a 24-hour period. Note: *Tagamet* may be diluted in 100–1000 mL; however, a volumetric pump is recommended if the volume for 24-hour infusion is less than 250 mL. In one study in patients with pathological hypersecretory states, the mean infused dose of cimetidine was 160 mg/hour with a range of 40–600 mg/hour.

These doses maintained the intragastric acid secretory rate at 10 mEq/hour or less. The infusion rate should be adjusted to individual patient requirements.

DIRECTIONS FOR USE OF TAGAMET (cimetidine hydrochloride) INJECTION IN PLASTIC CONTAINERS

To open: Tear overwrap down side at slit and remove solution containers.

Some opacity of the plastic due to moisture absorption during the sterilization process may be observed. This is normal and does not affect solution quality or safety. The opacity will diminish gradually.

Do not add other drugs to premixed *Tagamet* Injection in plastic containers.

CAUTION: Check for minute leaks by squeezing inner bag firmly. If leaks are found, discard solution as sterility may be impaired. Additives should not be introduced into this solution. Do not use if the solution is cloudy or precipitated or if the seal is not intact.

Do not use plastic containers in series connections. Such use could result in air embolism due to residual air being drawn from the primary container before administration of the fluid from the secondary container is complete.

Use sterile equipment.

Preparation for administration:

1. Suspend container from eyelet support.
2. Remove plastic protector from outlet port at bottom of container.
3. Attach administration set. Refer to complete directions accompanying set.

DIRECTIONS FOR USE OF TAGAMET® INJECTION IN ADD-VANTAGE® VIALS are enclosed in ADD-Vantage® Vial packaging.

Stability of *Tagamet* Injection

When added to or diluted with most commonly used intravenous solutions, e.g., Sodium Chloride Injection (0.9%), Dextrose Injection (5% or 10%), Lactated Ringer's Solution, 5% Sodium Bicarbonate Injection, Tagamet (cimetidine hydrochloride) Injection should not be used after more than 48 hours of storage at room temperature.

Tagamet Injection premixed in plastic containers is stable through the labeled expiration date when stored under the recommended conditions.

Dosage Adjustment for Patients with Impaired Renal Function

Patients with severely impaired renal function have been treated with *Tagamet.* However, such usage has been very limited. On the basis of this experience the recommended dosage is 300 mg q 12 hours orally or by intravenous injection. Should the patient's condition require, the frequency of dosing may be increased to q 8 hours or even further with caution. In severe renal failure, accumulation may occur and the lowest frequency of dosing compatible with an adequate patient response should be used. When liver impairment is also present, further reductions in dosage may be necessary. Hemodialysis reduces the level of circulating *Tagamet.* Ideally, the dosage schedule should be adjusted so that the timing of a scheduled dose coincides with the end of hemodialysis.

Patients with creatinine clearance less than 30 cc/min. who are being treated for prevention of upper gastrointestinal bleeding should receive half the recommended dose.

HOW SUPPLIED

Tablets: Light green, film-coated as follows: 200 mg—round, imprinted with the product name TAGAMET, SKF and 200—tablets in bottles of 100; 300 mg—round, imprinted with the product name TAGAMET, SKF and 300—tablets in bottles of 100 and Single Unit Packages of 100 (intended for institutional use only); 400 mg—capsule-shaped, imprinted with the product name TAGAMET, SKF and 400—tablets in bottles of 60 and Single Unit Packages of 100 (intended for institutional use only); 800 mg—oval-shaped Tiltab®, imprinted with the product name TAGAMET, SKF and 800—tablets in bottles of 30 and Single Unit Packages of 100 (intended for institutional use only).

Store at controlled room temperature (15°–30°C; 59°–86°F); dispense in a tight light-resistant container.

200 mg 100's: NDC 0108-5012-20
300 mg 100's: NDC 0108-5013-20
300 mg SUP 100's: NDC 0108-5013-21
400 mg 60's: NDC 0108-5026-18
400 mg SUP 100's: NDC 0108-5026-21
800 mg 30's: NDC 0108-5027-13
800 mg SUP 100's: NDC 0108-5027-21

Liquid: Clear, light orange, mint-peach flavored, as follows: 300 mg/5 mL, in 8 fl oz (237 mL) amber glass bottles and in single-dose units (300 mg/5 mL), in packages of 10 (intended for institutional use only).

Store at controlled room temperature (15°–30°C; 59°–86°F); dispense in a tight light-resistant container.

300 mg/5 mL 8 fl oz: NDC 0108-5014-48
300 mg/5 mL SUP 10's: NDC 0108-5014-10

Injection:

Vials: 300 mg/2 mL in single-dose vials, in packages of 25, and in 8 mL multi-dose vials, in packages of 10 and 25.

Store at controlled room temperature (15°-30°C; 59°-86°F); do not refrigerate.

300 mg/2 mL Single-Dose Vials: NDC 0108-5017-16 (package of 25 vials)

300 mg/2 mL in 8 mL Multi-Dose Vials:
NDC 0108-5022-11 (package of 10 vials)
NDC 0108-5022-16 (package of 25 vials)

Single-Dose Premixed Plastic Containers: 300 mg in 50 mL of 0.9% Sodium Chloride in single-dose plastic containers, in packages of 4 units. No preservative has been added.

Exposure of the premixed product to excessive heat should be avoided. It is recommended the product be stored at controlled room temperature (15°–30°C; 59°–86°F). Brief exposure up to 40°C does not adversely affect the premixed product.

300 mg/50 mL SUP's: NDC 0108-5029-04

ADD-Vantage® Vials: 300 mg/2 mL in single-dose ADD-Vantage® Vials, in packages of 25.

Store at controlled room temperature (15°–30°C; 59°–86°F); do not refrigerate.

300 mg/2 mL: NDC 0108-5031-16 (package of 25 vials)

Tagamet (cimetidine hydrochloride) Injection premixed in single-dose plastic containers is manufactured for SmithKline Beecham Pharmaceuticals by Baxter Healthcare Corporation, Deerfield, IL 60015.

Military—Tablets, 200 mg, 100's, 6505-01-103-6335; 300 mg, SUP, 100's, 6505-01-050-3546; 300 mg, 100's, 6505-01-050-3547; 300 mg, 500's × 12 Bulk, 6505-01-323-5256; 400 mg, 60's, 6505-01-176-0712; 400 mg, 500's × 12 Bulk, 6505-01-323-5255; Injection, 300 mg/2 mL, 10's, 6505-01-051-4698; 8 mL, 300 mg/2 mL, 10's, 6505-01-069-1661; Liquid, 300 mg/5 mL, 8 fl oz, 6505-01-119-0616.

Veterans Administration—Tablets, 200 mg, 100's, 6505-01-103-6335; 300 mg, 100's, 6505-01-050-3547; 300 mg, SUP, 100's, 6505-01-050-3546; 300 mg, 500's × 12 Bulk, 6505-01-323-5256; 400 mg, 60's, 6505-01-176-0712; 400 mg, 500's × 12 Bulk, 6505-01-323-5255; Liquid, 300 mg/5 mL, 8 fl oz, 6505-01-119-0616; Injection, 300 mg/2 mL, 10's, 6505-01-051-4698; 8 mL, 300 mg/2 mL, 10's, 6505-01-069-1661. TG:L87

Shown in Product Identification Section, page 431

TAZICEF® ℞

[taz'i-sef]

(brand of ceftazidime for injection for intravenous or intramuscular use)

DESCRIPTION

Ceftazidime is a semisynthetic, broad-spectrum, beta-lactam antibiotic for parenteral administration. It is the pentahydrate of Pyridinium, 1-[[7-[[(2-amino-4-thiazolyl)[(1-carboxy-1-methylethoxy) imino]acetyl]amino]-2-carboxy-8-oxo-5-thia-1-azabicyclo (4.2.0.)oct-2-en-3-yl] methyl]-,hydroxide,inner salt, [6R-[6α,7β(Z)]].

Tazicef (ceftazidime for injection) is a sterile, dry, powdered mixture of ceftazidime pentahydrate and sodium carbonate. The sodium carbonate at a concentration of 118 mg/gram of ceftazidime activity has been admixed to facilitate dissolution. The total sodium content of the mixture is approximately 54 mg (2.3 mEq)/gram of ceftazidime activity. Solutions of *Tazicef* range in color from light yellow to amber, depending upon the diluent and volume used. The pH of freshly reconstituted solutions usually ranges from 5.0 to 8.0.

CLINICAL PHARMACOLOGY

After intravenous administration of 500 mg and 1 gram doses of ceftazidime over five minutes to normal adult male volunteers, mean peak serum concentrations of 45 mcg/mL and 90 mcg/mL, respectively, were achieved. After intrave-

nous infusion of 500 mg, 1 gram and 2 gram doses of ceftazidime over 20 to 30 minutes to normal adult male volunteers, mean peak serum concentrations of 42 mcg/mL, 69 mcg/mL and 170 mcg/mL, respectively, were achieved. The average serum concentrations following intravenous infusion of 500 mg, 1 gram and 2 gram doses to these volunteers over an eight-hour interval are given in Table 1.

Table 1

Ceftazidime I.V. Dosage	Serum Concentrations (mcg/mL)				
	0.5 hr.	1 hr.	2 hr.	4 hr.	8 hr.
500 mg	42	25	12	6	2
1 gram	60	39	23	11	3
2 grams	129	75	42	13	5

The absorption and elimination of ceftazidime were directly proportional to the size of the dose. The half-life following intravenous administration was approximately 1.9 hours. Less than 10% of ceftazidime was protein bound. The degree of protein binding was independent of concentration. There was no evidence of accumulation of ceftazidime in the serum in individuals with normal renal function following multiple intravenous doses of 1 gram and 2 grams every eight hours for ten days.

Following intramuscular administration of 500 mg and 1 gram doses of ceftazidime to normal adult volunteers, the mean peak serum concentrations were 17 mcg/mL and 39 mcg/ mL, respectively, at approximately one hour. Serum concentrations remained above 4 mcg/mL for six and eight hours after the intramuscular administration of 500 mg and 1 gram doses, respectively. The half-life of ceftazidime in these volunteers was approximately two hours.

The presence of hepatic dysfunction had no effect on the pharmacokinetics of ceftazidime in individuals administered 2 grams intravenously every eight hours for five days. Therefore, a dosage adjustment from the normal recommended dosage is not required for patients with hepatic dysfunction, provided renal function is not impaired.

Approximately 80%–90% of an intramuscular or intravenous dose of ceftazidime is excreted unchanged by the kidneys over a 24-hour period. After the intravenous administration of single 500 mg or 1 gram doses, approximately 50% of the dose appeared in the urine in the first two hours. An additional 20% was excreted between two and four hours after dosing, and approximately another 12% of the dose appeared in the urine between four and eight hours later. The elimination of ceftazidime by the kidneys resulted in high therapeutic concentrations in the urine.

The mean renal clearance of ceftazidime was approximately 100 mL/min. The calculated plasma clearance of approximately 115 mL/min. indicated nearly complete elimination of ceftazidime by the renal route. Administration of probenecid prior to dosing had no effect on the elimination kinetics of ceftazidime. This suggests that ceftazidime is eliminated by glomerular filtration and is not actively secreted by renal tubular mechanisms.

Since ceftazidime is eliminated almost solely by the kidneys, its serum half-life is significantly prolonged in patients with impaired renal function. Consequently, dosage adjustments in such patients as described in the DOSAGE AND ADMINISTRATION section are suggested.

Therapeutic concentrations of ceftazidime are achieved in the following body tissues and fluid.

[See table above.]

Table 2. Ceftazidime Concentrations in Body Tissues and Fluids

Tissue or Fluid	Dose/ Route	No. Patients	Time of Sample Post-Dose	Average Tissue or Fluid Level (mcg/mL)
Urine	500 mg I.M.	6	0–2 hours	2,100
	2 grams I.V.	6	0–2 hours	12,000
Bile	2 grams I.V.	3	90 min.	36.4
Synovial fluid	2 grams I.V.	13	2 hours	25.6
Peritoneal fluid	2 grams I.V.	8	2 hours	48.6
Sputum	1 gram I.V.	8	1 hour	9
Cerebrospinal fluid	2 grams q8h I.V.	5	120 min.	9.8
(inflamed meninges)	2 grams q8h I.V.	6	180 min.	9.4
Aqueous humor	2 grams I.V.	13	1–3 hours	11
Blister fluid	1 gram I.V.	7	2–3 hours	19.7
Lymphatic fluid	1 gram I.V.	7	2–3 hours	23.4
Bone	2 grams I.V.	8	0.67 hour	31.1
Heart muscle	2 grams I.V.	35	30–280 min.	12.7
Skin	2 grams I.V.	22	30–180 min.	6.6
Skeletal muscle	2 grams I.V.	35	30–280 min.	9.4
Myometrium	2 grams I.V.	31	1–2 hours	18.7

Microbiology

Ceftazidime is bactericidal in action, exerting its effect by inhibition of enzymes responsible for cell-wall synthesis. A wide range of gram-negative organisms is susceptible to ceftazidime *in vitro*, including strains resistant to gentamicin and other aminoglycosides. In addition, ceftazidime has been shown to be active against gram-positive organisms. It is highly stable to most clinically important beta-lactamases, plasmid or chromosomal, which are produced by both gram-negative and gram-positive organisms, and consequently is active against many strains resistant to ampicillin and other cephalosporins.

Ceftazidime has been shown to be active against the following organisms both *in vitro* and in clinical infections (see INDICATIONS AND USAGE).

Aerobes, Gram-Negative: *Pseudomonas* species (including *Pseudomonas aeruginosa*); *Klebsiella* species (including *Klebsiella pneumoniae*); *Proteus mirabilis; Proteus vulgaris; Escherichia coli; Enterobacter* species, including *Enterobacter cloacae* and *Enterobacter aerogenes; Citrobacter* species, including *Citrobacter freundii* and *Citrobacter diversus; Serratia* species; *Haemophilus influenzae,* including ampicillin-resistant strains; and *Neisseria meningitidis.*

Aerobes, Gram-Positive: *Staphylococcus aureus,* including penicillinase- and non-penicillinase-producing strains; *Streptococcus pyogenes* (group A beta-hemolytic streptococci); *Streptococcus agalactiae* (group B streptococci); and *Streptococcus pneumoniae.*

Anaerobes: *Bacteroides* species (NOTE: Many strains of *Bacteroides fragilis* are resistant).

Ceftazidime has also been shown to demonstrate *in vitro* activity against the following microorganisms, although its clinical significance is not known: *Staphylococcus epidermidis; Morganella morganii* (formerly *Proteus morganii*); *Providencia* species (including *Providencia rettgeri,* formerly *Proteus rettgeri*); *Acinetobacter* species; *Salmonella* species; *Clostridium* species (not including *Clostridium difficile*); *Peptococcus* species; *Peptostreptococcus* species; *Neisseria gonorrhoeae; Haemophilus parainfluenzae; Yersinia enterocolitica;* and *Shigella* species.

Ceftazidime and the aminoglycosides have been shown to be synergistic *in vitro* against *P. aeruginosa* and the *Enterobacteriaceae.* Ceftazidime and carbenicillin have also been shown to be synergistic *in vitro* against *P. aeruginosa.*

Ceftazidime is not active *in vitro* against: methicillin-resistant staphylococci; *Streptococcus faecalis* and many other enterococci; *Listeria monocytogenes; Campylobacter* species; or *Clostridium difficile.*

Susceptibility Tests

Quantitative methods that require measurement of zone diameters give the most precise estimate of antibiotic susceptibility. One such procedure[1–3] has been recommended for use with disks to test susceptibility to ceftazidime.

Reports from the laboratory giving results of the standard single-disk susceptibility test with a 30 mcg ceftazidime disk should be interpreted according to the following criteria:

Susceptible organisms produce zones of 18 mm or greater, indicating that the test organism is likely to respond to therapy.

Organisms that produce zones of 15 mm to 17 mm are expected to be susceptible if high dosage is used or if the infection is confined to tissues and fluids (e.g., urine) in which high antibiotic levels are attained.

Resistant organisms produce zones of 14 mm or less, indicating that other therapy should be selected.

Organisms should be tested with the ceftazidime disk, since ceftazidime has been shown by *in vitro* tests to be active against certain strains found resistant when other beta-lactam disks are used.

Standardized procedures require the use of laboratory control organisms. The 30 mcg ceftazidime disk should give zone diameters between 25 mm and 32 mm for *E. coli* ATCC 25922. For *P. aeruginosa* ATCC 27853, the zone diameters should be between 22 mm and 29 mm. For *S. aureus* ATCC 25923, the zone diameters should be between 16 mm and 20 mm.

In other susceptibility testing procedures, e.g, ICS agar dilution or the equivalent, a bacterial isolate may be considered susceptible if the MIC value for ceftazidime is not more than 16 mcg/mL. Organisms are considered resistant to ceftazidime if the MIC is equal to or greater than 64 mcg/mL. Organisms having an MIC value of less than 64 mcg/mL but greater than 16 mcg/mL are expected to be susceptible if high dosage is used or if the infection is confined to tissues and fluids (e.g., urine) in which high antibiotic levels are attained.

As with standard diffusion methods, dilution procedures require the use of laboratory control organisms. Standard ceftazidime powder should give MIC values in the range of 4 mcg/mL and 16 mcg/mL for *S. aureus* ATCC 25923. For *E. coli* ATCC 25922, the MIC range should be between 0.125 mcg/mL and 0.5 mcg/mL. For *P. aeruginosa* ATCC 27853, the MIC range should be between 0.5 mcg/mL and 2 mcg/mL.

INDICATIONS AND USAGE

Tazicef (ceftazidime for injection) is indicated for the treatment of patients with infections caused by susceptible strains of the designated organisms in the diseases listed below:

LOWER RESPIRATORY TRACT INFECTIONS, including pneumonia, caused by *P. aeruginosa* and other *Pseudomonas* species; *H. influenzae,* including ampicillin-resistant strains; *Klebsiella* species; *Enterobacter* species, *P. mirabilis; E. coli; Serratia* species; *Citrobacter* species; *S. pneumoniae;* and *S. aureus* (methicillin-susceptible strains).

SKIN AND SKIN STRUCTURE INFECTIONS, caused by *P. aeruginosa, Klebsiella* species; *E. coli; Proteus* species including *P. mirabilis* and indole-positive *Proteus, Enterobacter* species; *Serratia* species; *S. aureus* (methicillin-susceptible strains) and *S. pyogenes* (group A beta-hemolytic streptococci).

URINARY TRACT INFECTIONS, both complicated and uncomplicated, caused by *P. aeruginosa; Enterobacter* species; *Proteus* species, including *P. mirabilis* and indole-positive *Proteus; Klebsiella* species and *E. coli.*

BACTERIAL SEPTICEMIA, caused by *P. aeruginosa, Klebsiella* species; *H. influenzae; E. coli, Serratia* species, *S. pneumoniae* and *S. aureus* (methicillin-susceptible strains).

BONE AND JOINT INFECTIONS, caused by *P. aeruginosa; Klebsiella* species; *Enterobacter* species; and *S. aureus* (methicillin-susceptible strains).

GYNECOLOGICAL INFECTIONS, including endometritis, pelvic cellulitis and other infections of the female genital tract caused by *E. coli.*

INTRA-ABDOMINAL INFECTIONS, including peritonitis caused by *E. coli, Klebsiella* species; *S. aureus* (methicillin-susceptible strains), and polymicrobial infections caused by aerobic and anaerobic organisms, and *Bacteroides* species (many strains of *B. fragilis* are resistant).

CENTRAL NERVOUS SYSTEM INFECTIONS, including meningitis caused by *H. influenzae* and *Neisseria meningitidis.* Ceftazidime has also been used successfully in a limited number of cases of meningitis due to *P. aeruginosa* and *S. pneumoniae.*

Specimens for bacterial cultures should be obtained prior to therapy in order to isolate and identify causative organisms and to determine their susceptibility to ceftazidime. Therapy may be instituted before results of susceptibility studies are known; however, once these results become available, the antibiotic treatment should be adjusted accordingly.

Tazicef (ceftazidime for injection) may be used alone in cases of confirmed or suspected sepsis. Ceftazidime has been used successfully in clinical trials as empiric therapy in cases where various concomitant therapies with other antibiotics have been used.

Tazicef may also be used concomitantly with other antibiotics, such as aminoglycosides, vancomycin and clindamycin, in severe and life-threatening infections and in the immunocompromised patient. When such concomitant treatment is appropriate, prescribing information in the labeling for the other antibiotics should be followed. The dose depends on the severity of the infection and the patient's condition.

CONTRAINDICATIONS

Tazicef is contraindicated in patients who have shown hypersensitivity to ceftazidime or the cephalosporin group of antibiotics.

WARNINGS

BEFORE THERAPY WITH *TAZICEF* IS INSTITUTED, CAREFUL INQUIRY SHOULD BE MADE TO DETERMINE WHETHER THE PATIENT HAD HAD PREVIOUS HYPERSENSITIVITY REACTIONS TO CEFTAZIDIME, CEPHALOSPORINS, PENICILLINS, OR OTHER DRUGS. ANTIBIOTICS SHOULD BE ADMINISTERED WITH CAU-

Continued on next page

SmithKline Beecham—Cont.

TION TO ANY PATIENT WHO HAS DEMONSTRATED SOME FORM OF ALLERGY, PARTICULARLY TO DRUGS. THIS PRODUCT SHOULD BE GIVEN WITH CAUTION TO PATIENTS WITH TYPE 1 HYPERSENSITIVITY REACTIONS TO PENICILLIN. IF AN ALLERGIC REACTION TO *TAZICEF* OCCURS, DISCONTINUE TREATMENT WITH THE DRUG. SERIOUS ACUTE HYPERSENSITIVITY REACTIONS MAY REQUIRE EPINEPHRINE AND OTHER EMERGENCY MEASURES.

Pseudomembranous colitis has been reported with nearly all antibacterial agents, including ceftazidime, and has ranged in severity from mild to life-threatening. Therefore, it is important to consider this diagnosis in patients who present with diarrhea subsequent to the administration of antibacterial agents.

Treatment with antibacterial agents alters the normal flora of the colon and may permit overgrowth of clostridia. Studies indicate a toxin produced by *C. difficile* is one primary cause of "antibiotic-associated colitis."

Mild cases of pseudomembranous colitis usually respond to drug discontinuation alone. In moderate to severe cases, consideration should be given to management with fluids and electrolytes, protein supplementation and treatment with an oral antibiotic drug effective against *C. difficile.*

PRECAUTIONS

Ceftazidime has not been shown to be nephrotoxic; however, because high and prolonged serum antibiotic concentrations can occur from usual doses in patients with transient or persistent reduction of urinary output because of renal insufficiency, the total daily dosage should be reduced when ceftazidime is administered to such patients (see DOSAGE AND ADMINISTRATION). Continued dosage should be determined by degree of renal impairment, severity of infection and susceptibility of the causative organisms.

As with other antibiotics, prolonged use of Tazicef (ceftazidime for injection) may result in overgrowth of nonsusceptible organisms. Repeated evaluation of the patient's condition is essential. If superinfection occurs during therapy, appropriate measures should be taken.

Tazicef should be prescribed with caution in individuals with a history of gastrointestinal disease, particularly colitis.

Drug Interactions: Nephrotoxicity has been reported following concomitant administration of cephalosporins with aminoglycoside antibiotics or potent diuretics, such as furosemide. Renal function should be carefully monitored, especially if higher dosages of the aminoglycosides are to be administered or if therapy is prolonged, because of the potential nephrotoxicity and ototoxicity of aminoglycoside antibiotics. Nephrotoxicity and ototoxicity were not noted when ceftazidime was given alone in clinical trials.

Carcinogenesis, Mutagenesis, Impairment of Fertility: Long-term studies in animals have not been performed to evaluate carcinogenic potential. However, a mouse micronucleus test and an Ames test were both negative for mutagenic effects.

Usage in Pregnancy: Pregnancy Category B. Reproduction studies have been performed in mice and rats at doses up to 40 times the human dose and have revealed no evidence of impaired fertility or harm to the fetus due to ceftazidime. There are, however, no adequate and well-controlled studies in pregnant women. Because animal reproduction studies are not always predictive of human response, this drug should be used during pregnancy only if clearly needed.

Nursing Mothers: Ceftazidime is excreted in human milk in low concentrations. Caution should be exercised when *Tazicef* is administered to a nursing woman.

ADVERSE REACTIONS

Ceftazidime is generally well tolerated. The incidence of adverse reactions associated with the administration of ceftazidime was low in clinical trials. The most common were local reactions following intravenous injection, and allergic and gastrointestinal reactions. Other adverse reactions were encountered infrequently. No disulfiram-like reactions were reported. The following adverse effects from premarketing clinical trials were considered to be either related to ceftazidime therapy or were of uncertain etiology.

Local Effects, reported in less than 2% of patients, were phlebitis and inflammation at the site of injection (1 in 69 patients).

Hypersensitivity Reactions, reported in 2% of patients, were pruritus, rash and fever. Immediate hypersensitivity reactions occurred in 1 in 285 patients.

Gastrointestinal Symptoms, reported in less than 2% of patients, were diarrhea (1 in 78), nausea (1 in 156), vomiting (1 in 500) and abdominal pain (1 in 416).

Symptoms of pseudomembranous colitis can appear during or after antibiotic treatment (See WARNINGS section).

Less Frequent Adverse Events (less than 1%) were candidiasis and vaginitis; central nervous system events which included headache, dizziness and paresthesia.

Laboratory Test Changes noted during ceftazidime clinical trials were transient and included: eosinophilia (1 in 13), positive Coombs' test without hemolysis (1 in 23), thrombocytosis (1 in 45), and slight elevations in one or more of the hepatic enzymes, SGOT (1 in 16), SGPT (1 in 15), LDH (1 in 18) and alkaline phosphatase (1 in 23). As with some other cephalosporins, transient elevations of blood urea, blood urea nitrogen and/or serum creatinine were observed occasionally. Transient leukopenia, neutropenia, thrombocytopenia and lymphocytosis were seen very rarely.

DOSAGE AND ADMINISTRATION

Dosage: The usual adult dosage is 1 gram administered intravenously or intramuscularly every eight or 12 hours. The dosage and route should be determined by the susceptibility of the causative organisms, the severity of infection and the condition and renal function of the patient.

The guidelines for dosage of *Tazicef* are listed in Table 3. The following dosage schedule is recommended.

Impaired Hepatic Function: No adjustment in dosage is required for patients with hepatic dysfunction.

Impaired Renal Function: Ceftazidime is excreted by the kidneys, almost exclusively by glomerular filtration. Therefore, in patients with impaired renal function (GFR <50 mL/min.), it is recommended that the dosage of ceftazidime be reduced to compensate for its slower excretion. In patients with suspected renal insufficiency, an initial loading dose of 1 gram of ceftazidime may be given. An estimate of GFR should be made to determine the appropriate maintenance dose. The recommended dosage is presented in Table 4.

Table 4. Recommended Maintenance Doses of Tazicef (ceftazidime for injection) in Renal Insufficiency

Creatinine Clearance (mL/min.)	Recommended Unit Dose of Ceftazidime	Frequency of Dosing
50–31	1 gram	q12h
30–16	1 gram	q24h
15–6	500 mg	q24h
<5	500 mg	q48h

When only serum creatinine is available, the following formula (Cockcroft's equation)[4] may be used to estimate creatinine clearance. The serum creatinine should represent a steady state of renal function:

Males:
$$\text{Creatinine clearance (mL/min.)} = \frac{\text{Weight (kg)} \times (140 - \text{age})}{72 \times \text{serum creatinine (mg/dl)}}$$

Females:
$0.85 \times$ above value

In patients with severe infections who would normally receive 6 grams of ceftazidime daily were it not for renal insufficiency, the unit dose given in the table above may be increased by 50% or the dosing frequency increased appropriately. Further dosing should be determined by therapeutic monitoring, severity of the infection and susceptibility of the causative organism.

In children as for adults, the creatinine clearance should be adjusted for body surface area or lean body mass and the dosing frequency reduced in cases of renal insufficiency.

In patients undergoing hemodialysis, a loading dose of 1 gram is recommended, followed by 1 gram after each hemodialysis period.

Tazicef (ceftazidime for injection) can also be used in patients undergoing intra-peritoneal dialysis (IPD) and continuous ambulatory peritoneal dialysis (CAPD). In such patients, a loading dose of *Tazicef* 1 gram may be given, followed by 500 mg every 24 hours. In addition to intravenous use, *Tazicef* can be incorporated in the dialysis fluid at a concentration of 250 mg for 2 liters of dialysis fluid.

NOTE: Generally, *Tazicef* should be continued for two days after the signs and symptoms of infection have disappeared, but in complicated infections longer therapy may be required.

RECONSTITUTION

Single Dose Vials:
For I.M. injection, I.V. direct (bolus) injection, or I.V. infusion, reconstitute with Sterile Water for Injection according to the following table. The vacuum may assist entry of the diluent. SHAKE WELL.

Table 5

Vial Size	Diluent to Be Added	Approx. Avail. Volume	Approx. Avg. Concentration
Intramuscular or Intravenous Direct (bolus) Injection			
1 gram	3.0 mL	3.6 mL	280 mg/mL
Intravenous Infusion			
1 gram	10 mL	10.6 mL	95 mg/mL
2 gram	10 mL	11.2 mL	180 mg/mL

Withdraw the total volume of solution into the syringe (the pressure in the vial may aid withdrawal). The withdrawn solution may contain some bubbles of carbon dioxide.

NOTE: As with the administration of all parenteral products, accumulated gases should be expressed from the syringe immediately before injection of *Tazicef*.

These solutions of *Tazicef* are stable for 18 hours at room temperature or seven days if refrigerated (5°C). Slight yellowing does not affect potency.

For I.V. infusion, dilute reconstituted solution in 50 to 100 mL of one of the parenteral fluids listed under COMPATIBILITY AND STABILITY.

Pharmacy Bulk Vials:
Reconstitute with Sterile Water for Injection according to the following table.

Table 6

Diluent to Be Added	Approx. Avail. Volume	Approx. Avg. Concentration
26 mL	30 mL	1 gram/5 mL
56 mL	60 mL	1 gram/10 mL

The vacuum may assist entry of the diluent. SHAKE WELL. Insert a gas relief needle through the vial closure to relieve the internal pressure. Remove the gas relief needle before extracting any solution.

NOTE: To preserve product sterility, it is important that a gas relief needle is not inserted through the vial closure before the product has dissolved.

These solutions of *Tazicef* are stable for 18 hours at room temperature or seven days if refrigerated (5°C). Slight yellowing does not affect potency. For I.V. infusion add to one of the

Table 3. Recommended Dosage Schedule

	Dose	Frequency
Adults		
Usual recommended dose	1 gram I.V. or I.M.	q8–12h
Uncomplicated urinary tract infections	250 mg I.V. or I.M.	q12h
Bone and joint infections	2 grams I.V.	q12h
Complicated urinary tract infections	500 mg I.V. or I.M.	q8–12h
Uncomplicated pneumonia; mild skin and skin structure infections	500 mg–1 gram I.V. or I.M.	q8h
Serious gynecological and intra-abdominal infections	2 grams I.V.	q8h
Meningitis	2 grams I.V.	q8h
Very severe life-threatening infections, especially in immunocompromised patients	2 grams I.V.	q8h
Pseudomonal lung infections in patients with cystic fibrosis with normal renal function*	30–50 mg/kg I.V. to a maximum of 6 grams/day	q8h
Neonates (0–4 weeks)	30 mg/kg I.V.	q12h
Infants and children (1 month–12 years)	30–50 mg/kg I.V. to a maximum of 6 grams/day†	q8h

* Although clinical improvement has been shown, bacteriological cures cannot be expected in patients with chronic respiratory disease and cystic fibrosis.

† The higher dose should be reserved for immunocompromised children or children with cystic fibrosis or meningitis.

parenteral fluids listed under COMPATIBILITY AND STABILITY.

"Piggyback" Vials:
For I.V. infusion, reconstitute with 10 mL of Sodium Chloride Injection according to the following table. The vacuum may assist entry of the diluent. SHAKE WELL.

Table 7

Vial Size	Diluent to Be Added	Approx. Avail. Volume	Approx. Avg. Concentration
1 gram	100 mL*	100 mL	10 mg/mL
2 gram	100 mL*	100 mL	20 mg/mL

* Addition should be in two stages.

Insert a gas relief needle through the vial closure to relieve the internal pressure. With the gas relief needle in position, add the remaining 90 mL of Sodium Chloride Injection. Remove the gas relief needle and syringe needle; shake the vial and set up for infusion in the normal way.

NOTE: To preserve product sterility, it is important that a gas relief needle is not inserted through the vial closure before the product has dissolved.

These solutions of Tazicef (ceftazidime for injection) are stable for 18 hours at room temperature or seven days if refrigerated (5°C). Slight yellowing does not affect potency.

Administration: Tazicef may be given intravenously or by deep intramuscular injection into a large muscle mass such as the upper outer quadrant of the gluteus maximus or lateral part of the thigh.

Intramuscular Administration: For intramuscular administration, Tazicef should be reconstituted with Sterile Water for Injection. Refer to Table 5.

Intravenous Administration: The I.V. route is preferable for patients with bacterial septicemia, bacterial meningitis, peritonitis, or other severe or life-threatening infections, or for patients who may be poor risks because of lowered resistance resulting from such debilitating conditions as malnutrition, trauma, surgery, diabetes, heart failure or malignancy, particularly if shock is present or pending

For direct intermittent intravenous administration, reconstitute Tazicef as directed in Table 5 with Sterile Water for Injection. Slowly inject directly into the vein over a period of three to five minutes or give through the tubing of an administration set while the patient is also receiving one of the compatible intravenous fluids (See COMPATIBILITY AND STABILITY).

For intravenous infusion, reconstitute the 1 or 2 gram piggyback vial with 100 mL of Sodium Chloride Injection or one of the compatible intravenous fluids listed under the COMPATIBILITY AND STABILITY section. Alternatively, reconstitute the 1 gram or 2 gram vial and add an appropriate quantity of the resulting solution to an I.V. container with one of the compatible intravenous fluids.

Intermittent intravenous infusion with a Y-type administration set can be accomplished with compatible solutions. However, during infusion of a solution containing Tazicef it is advisable to discontinue the other solution.

All vials of Tazicef as supplied are under reduced pressure. When Tazicef is dissolved, carbon dioxide is released and a positive pressure develops. See RECONSTITUTION.

Solutions of Tazicef, like those of most beta-lactam antibiotics, should not be added to solutions of aminoglycoside antibiotics because of potential interaction.

However, if concurrent therapy with Tazicef and an aminoglycoside is indicated, each of these antibiotics can be administered separately to the same patient.

COMPATIBILITY AND STABILITY

Intramuscular: Tazicef, when reconstituted as directed with Sterile Water for Injection, maintains satisfactory potency for 18 hours at room temperature or for seven days under refrigeration (5°C). Solutions in Sterile Water for Injection that are frozen immediately after reconstitution in the original container are stable for three months when stored at −20°C. Once thawed, solutions should not be refrozen. Thawed solutions may be stored for up to eight hours at room temperature or for four days in a refrigerator (5°C).

Intravenous: Tazicef (ceftazidime for injection), when reconstituted as directed with Sterile Water for Injection, maintains satisfactory potency for 18 hours at room temperature or for seven days under refrigeration (5°C). Solutions in Sterile Water for Injection in the original container or in 0.9% Sodium Chloride Injection in Viaflex® small volume containers that are frozen immediately after reconstitution are stable for three months when stored at −20°C. For larger volumes where it may be necessary to warm the frozen product (to a maximum of 40°C), care should be taken to avoid heating after thawing is complete. Once thawed, solutions should not be refrozen. Thawed solutions may be stored for up to eight hours at room temperature or for four days in a refrigerator (5°C).

Tazicef is physically compatible with the more commonly used intravenous infusion fluids. Solutions at concentrations between 1 mg/mL and 40 mg/mL in the following infusion fluids may be stored for up to 18 hours at room temperature or seven days if refrigerated: 0.9% Sodium Chloride Injection; Ringer's Injection USP; Lactated Ringer's Injection USP; 5% Dextrose Injection; 5% Dextrose and 0.225% Sodium Chloride Injection; 5% Dextrose and 0.45% Sodium Chloride Injection; 5% Dextrose and 0.9% Sodium Chloride Injection; 10% Dextrose Injection.

Tazicef is less stable in Sodium Bicarbonate Injection than in other intravenous fluids. It is not recommended as a diluent. Solutions of Tazicef in 5% Dextrose and 0.9% Sodium Chloride Injection are stable for at least six hours at room temperature in plastic tubing, drip chambers and volume control devices of common intravenous infusion sets.

Ceftazidime at a concentration of 20 mg/mL has been found physically compatible for 18 hours at room temperature or seven days under refrigeration in Sterile Water for Injection when admixed with: cefazolin sodium (Ancef®) 330 mg/mL; heparin 1000 units/mL; and cimetidine HCl (Tagamet®) 150 mg/mL.

Ceftazidime at a concentration of 20 mg/mL has been found physically compatible for 18 hours at room temperature or seven days under refrigeration in 5% Dextrose Injection when admixed with potassium chloride 40 mEq/l.

Note: Parenteral drug products should be inspected visually for particulate matter prior to administration wherever solution and container permit.

As with other cephalosporins, Tazicef powder, as well as solutions, tends to darken depending on storage conditions; within the stated recommendations, however, product potency is not adversely affected.

HOW SUPPLIED

Tazicef (ceftazidime for injection) is supplied in vials equivalent to 1 gram and 2 grams of ceftazidime; in "Piggyback" Vials for I.V. admixture equivalent to 1 gram and 2 grams of ceftazidime; and in Pharmacy Bulk Vials equivalent to 6 grams of ceftazidime.

Veterans Administration—Injection, 1 gram/20 mL, 25's, 6505-01-227-3570; 2 gram/60 mL, 10's, 6505-01-228-0009; 6 gram/100 mL, 10's, 6505-01-300-2115.

Military—Injection, 2 gram/100 mL, 10's, 6505-01-231- 4807.

REFERENCES

1. Bauer, A.W.; Kirby, W.M.M., and Sherris, J.C., et al.: Antibiotic susceptibility testing by a standardized single disc method, Am. J. Clin. Pathol. 45:493, 1966. 2. National Committee for Clinical Laboratory Standards, Approved Standard: Performance Standards for Antimicrobial Disc Susceptibility Tests (M2-A3), December, 1984. 3. Standardized disc susceptibility test, Federal Register 39:19182–19184, 1974. 4. Cockcroft, D.W., and Gault, M.H.: Prediction of creatinine clearance from serum creatinine, Nephron 16:31–41, 1976.
TF:L13

Manufactured by
Bristol-Myers Co.
New York, NY
Filled and Distr. by
SmithKline Beecham Pharmaceuticals
Philadelphia, PA 19101
Shown in Product Identification Section, page 431

THORAZINE®　　　　　　　　　　　　　　℞
[thor'ah-zeen]
(brand of chlorpromazine)
tranquilizer · antiemetic

DESCRIPTION

Thorazine (chlorpromazine) is 10-(3-dimethylaminopropyl)-2-chlorphenothiazine, a dimethylamine derivative of phenothiazine. It is present in oral and injectable forms as the hydrochloride salt, and in the suppositories as the base.

Tablets—Each round, orange, coated tablet contains chlorpromazine hydrochloride as follows: 10 mg imprinted SKF and T73; 25 mg imprinted SKF and T74; 50 mg imprinted SKF and T76; 100 mg imprinted SKF and T77; 200 mg imprinted SKF and T79. Inactive ingredients consist of benzoic acid, croscarmellose sodium, D&C Yellow No. 10, FD&C Blue No. 2, FD&C Yellow No. 6, gelatin, hydroxypropyl methylcellulose, lactose, magnesium stearate, methylparaben, polyethylene glycol, propylparaben, talc, titanium dioxide and trace amounts of other inactive ingredients.

Spansule® sustained release capsules—Each Thorazine Spansule® capsule is so prepared that an initial dose is released promptly and the remaining medication is released gradually over a prolonged period.

Each capsule, with opaque orange cap and natural body, contains chlorpromazine hydrochloride as follows: 30 mg imprinted SKF and T63; 75 mg imprinted SKF and T64; 150 mg imprinted SKF and T66. Inactive ingredients consist of benzyl alcohol, calcium sulfate, cetylpyridinium chloride, FD&C Yellow No. 6, gelatin, glyceryl distearate, glyceryl monostearate, iron oxide, povidone, silicon dioxide, sodium lauryl sulfate, starch, sucrose, titanium dioxide, wax and trace amounts of other inactive ingredients.

Ampuls—Each mL contains, in aqueous solution, chlorpromazine hydrochloride, 25 mg; ascorbic acid, 2 mg; sodium bisulfite, 1 mg; sodium chloride, 6 mg; sodium sulfite, 1 mg.

Multi-dose Vials—Each mL contains, in aqueous solution, chlorpromazine hydrochloride, 25 mg; ascorbic acid, 2 mg; sodium bisulfite, 1 mg; sodium chloride, 1 mg; sodium sulfite, 1 mg; benzyl alcohol, 2%, as a preservative.

Syrup—Each 5 mL (one teaspoonful) of clear, orange-custard flavored liquid contains chlorpromazine hydrochloride, 10 mg. Inactive ingredients consist of citric acid, flavors, sodium benzoate, sucrose and water.

Suppositories—Each suppository contains chlorpromazine, 25 or 100 mg, glycerin, glyceryl monopalmitate, glyceryl monostearate, hydrogenated coconut oil fatty acids, and hydrogenated palm kernel oil fatty acids.

Concentrate—Each mL of clear, custard flavored liquid contains chlorpromazine hydrochloride, 30 or 100 mg. Inactive ingredients consist of calcium disodium edetate, citric acid, flavors, hydroxypropyl methylcellulose, propylene glycol, saccharin sodium, sodium benzoate, water and trace amounts of other inactive ingredients.

ACTIONS

The precise mechanism whereby the therapeutic effects of chlorpromazine are produced is not known. The principal pharmacological actions are psychotropic. It also exerts sedative and antiemetic activity. Chlorpromazine has actions at all levels of the central nervous system—primarily at subcortical levels—as well as on multiple organ systems. Chlorpromazine has strong antiadrenergic and weaker peripheral anticholinergic activity; ganglionic blocking action is relatively slight. It also possesses slight antihistaminic and antiserotonin activity.

INDICATIONS

For the management of manifestations of psychotic disorders.
To control nausea and vomiting.
For relief of restlessness and apprehension before surgery.
For acute intermittent porphyria.
As an adjunct in the treatment of tetanus.
To control the manifestations of the manic type of manic-depressive illness.
For relief of intractable hiccups.
For the treatment of severe behavioral problems in children marked by combativeness and/or explosive hyperexcitable behavior (out of proportion to immediate provocations), and in the short-term treatment of hyperactive children who show excessive motor activity with accompanying conduct disorders consisting of some or all of the following symptoms: impulsivity, difficulty sustaining attention, aggressivity, mood lability and poor frustration tolerance.

CONTRAINDICATIONS

Do not use in comatose states or in the presence of large amounts of central nervous system depressants (alcohol, barbiturates, narcotics, etc.).

WARNINGS

The extrapyramidal symptoms which can occur secondary to Thorazine (chlorpromazine) may be confused with the central nervous system signs of an undiagnosed primary disease responsible for the vomiting, e.g., Reye's syndrome or other encephalopathy. The use of Thorazine and other potential hepatotoxins should be avoided in children and adolescents whose signs and symptoms suggest Reye's syndrome.

Tardive Dyskinesia: Tardive dyskinesia, a syndrome consisting of potentially irreversible, involuntary, dyskinetic movements, may develop in patients treated with neuroleptic (antipsychotic) drugs. Although the prevalence of the syndrome appears to be highest among the elderly, especially elderly women, it is impossible to rely upon prevalence estimates to predict, at the inception of neuroleptic treatment, which patients are likely to develop the syndrome. Whether neuroleptic drug products differ in their potential to cause tardive dyskinesia is unknown.

Both the risk of developing the syndrome and the likelihood that it will become irreversible are believed to increase as the duration of treatment and the total cumulative dose of neuroleptic drugs administered to the patient increase. However, the syndrome can develop, although much less commonly, after relatively brief treatment periods at low doses.

There is no known treatment for established cases of tardive dyskinesia, although the syndrome may remit, partially or completely, if neuroleptic treatment is withdrawn. Neuroleptic treatment itself, however, may suppress (or partially suppress) the signs and symptoms of the syndrome and thereby may possibly mask the underlying disease process. The effect that symptomatic suppression has upon the long-term course of the syndrome is unknown.

Given these considerations, neuroleptics should be prescribed in a manner that is most likely to minimize the occurrence of tardive dyskinesia. Chronic neuroleptic treatment should generally be reserved for patients who suffer from a

Continued on next page

SmithKline Beecham—Cont.

chronic illness that, 1) is known to respond to neuroleptic drugs, and, 2) for whom alternative, equally effective, but potentially less harmful treatments are *not* available or appropriate. In patients who do require chronic treatment, the smallest dose and the shortest duration of treatment producing a satisfactory clinical response should be sought. The need for continued treatment should be reassessed periodically.

If signs and symptoms of tardive dyskinesia appear in a patient on neuroleptics, drug discontinuation should be considered. However, some patients may require treatment despite the presence of the syndrome.

For further information about the description of tardive dyskinesia and its clinical detection, please refer to the sections on Precautions and Adverse Reactions.

Neuroleptic Malignant Syndrome (NMS): A potentially fatal symptom complex sometimes referred to as Neuroleptic Malignant Syndrome (NMS) has been reported in association with antipsychotic drugs. Clinical manifestations of NMS are hyperpyrexia, muscle rigidity, altered mental status and evidence of autonomic instability (irregular pulse or blood pressure, tachycardia, diaphoresis, and cardiac dysrhythmias).

The diagnostic evaluation of patients with this syndrome is complicated. In arriving at a diagnosis, it is important to identify cases where the clinical presentation includes both serious medical illness (e.g., pneumonia, systemic infection, etc.) and untreated or inadequately treated extrapyramidal signs and symptoms (EPS). Other important considerations in the differential diagnosis include central anticholinergic toxicity, heat stroke, drug fever and primary central nervous system (CNS) pathology.

The management of NMS should include 1) immediate discontinuation of antipsychotic drugs and other drugs not essential to concurrent therapy, 2) intensive symptomatic treatment and medical monitoring, and 3) treatment of any concomitant serious medical problems for which specific treatments are available. There is no general agreement about specific pharmacological treatment regimens for uncomplicated NMS.

If a patient requires antipsychotic drug treatment after recovery from NMS, the potential reintroduction of drug therapy should be carefully considered. The patient should be carefully monitored, since recurrences of NMS have been reported.

Thorazine (chlorpromazine) ampuls and multi-dose vials contain sodium bisulfite and sodium sulfite, sulfites that may cause allergic-type reactions including anaphylactic symptoms and life-threatening or less severe asthmatic episodes in certain susceptible people. The overall prevalence of sulfite sensitivity in the general population is unknown and probably low. Sulfite sensitivity is seen more frequently in asthmatic than in nonasthmatic people.

Patients with bone marrow depression or who have previously demonstrated a hypersensitivity reaction (e.g., blood dyscrasias, jaundice) with a phenothiazine should not receive any phenothiazine, including *Thorazine*, unless in the judgment of the physician the potential benefits of treatment outweigh the possible hazard.

Thorazine may impair mental and/or physical abilities, especially during the first few days of therapy. Therefore, caution patients about activities requiring alertness (e.g., operating vehicles or machinery).

The use of alcohol with this drug should be avoided due to possible additive effects and hypotension.

Thorazine may counteract the antihypertensive effect of guanethidine and related compounds.

Usage in Pregnancy: Safety for the use of Thorazine (chlorpromazine) during pregnancy has not been established. Therefore, it is not recommended that the drug be given to pregnant patients except when, in the judgment of the physician, it is essential. The potential benefits should clearly outweigh possible hazards. There are reported instances of prolonged jaundice, extrapyramidal signs, hyperreflexia or hyporeflexia in newborn infants whose mothers received phenothiazines.

Reproductive studies in rodents have demonstrated potential for embryotoxicity, increased neonatal mortality and nursing transfer of the drug. Tests in the offspring of the drug-treated rodents demonstrate decreased performance. The possibility of permanent neurological damage cannot be excluded.

Nursing Mothers: There is evidence that chlorpromazine is excreted in the breast milk of nursing mothers.

PRECAUTIONS

Given the likelihood that some patients exposed chronically to neuroleptics will develop tardive dyskinesia, it is advised that all patients in whom chronic use is contemplated be given, if possible, full information about this risk. The decision to inform patients and/or their guardians must obviously take into account the clinical circumstances and the competency of the patient to understand the information provided.

Thorazine (chlorpromazine) should be administered cautiously to persons with cardiovascular, liver or renal disease. There is evidence that patients with a history of hepatic encephalopathy due to cirrhosis have increased sensitivity to the C.N.S. effects of *Thorazine* (i.e., impaired cerebration and abnormal slowing of the EEG).

Because of its C.N.S. depressant effect, *Thorazine* should be used with caution in patients with chronic respiratory disorders such as severe asthma, emphysema and acute respiratory infections, particularly in children.

Because *Thorazine* can suppress the cough reflex, aspiration of vomitus is possible.

Thorazine (chlorpromazine) prolongs and intensifies the action of C.N.S. depressants such as anesthetics, barbiturates and narcotics. When *Thorazine* is administered concomitantly, about ¼ to ½ the usual dosage of such agents is required. When *Thorazine* is not being administered to reduce requirements of C.N.S. depressants, it is best to stop such depressants before starting *Thorazine* treatment. These agents may subsequently be reinstated at low doses and increased as needed.

Note: *Thorazine* does *not* intensify the anticonvulsant action of barbiturates. Therefore, dosage of anticonvulsants, including barbiturates, should *not* be reduced if *Thorazine* is started. Instead, start *Thorazine* at low doses and increase as needed.

Use with caution in persons who will be exposed to extreme heat, organophosphorus insecticides, and in persons receiving atropine or related drugs.

Neuroleptic drugs elevate prolactin levels; the elevation persists during chronic administration. Tissue culture experiments indicate that approximately one third of human breast cancers are prolactin-dependent *in vitro*, a factor of potential importance if the prescribing of these drugs is contemplated in a patient with a previously detected breast cancer. Although disturbances such as galactorrhea, amenorrhea, gynecomastia and impotence have been reported, the clinical significance of elevated serum prolactin levels is unknown for most patients. An increase in mammary neoplasms has been found in rodents after chronic administration of neuroleptic drugs. Neither clinical nor epidemiologic studies conducted to date, however, have shown an association between chronic administration of these drugs and mammary tumorigenesis; the available evidence is considered too limited to be conclusive at this time.

Chromosomal aberrations in spermatocytes and abnormal sperm have been demonstrated in rodents treated with certain neuroleptics.

As with all drugs which exert an anticholinergic effect, and/or cause mydriasis, chlorpromazine should be used with caution in patients with glaucoma.

Chlorpromazine diminishes the effect of oral anticoagulants. Phenothiazines can produce alpha-adrenergic blockade.

Chlorpromazine may lower the convulsive threshold; dosage adjustments of anticonvulsants may be necessary. Potentiation of anticonvulsant effects does not occur. However, it has been reported that chlorpromazine may interfere with the metabolism of Dilantin®* and thus precipitate *Dilantin* toxicity.

Concomitant administration with propranolol results in increased plasma levels of both drugs.

Thiazide diuretics may accentuate the orthostatic hypotension that may occur with phenothiazines.

The presence of phenothiazines may produce false positive phenylketonuria (PKU) test results.

Drugs which lower the seizure threshold, including phenothiazine derivatives, should not be used with Amipaque®†. As with other phenothiazine derivatives, *Thorazine* should be discontinued at least 48 hours before myelography, should not be resumed for at least 24 hours postprocedure, and should not be used for the control of nausea and vomiting occurring either prior to myelography or postprocedure with *Amipaque*.

Long-Term Therapy: To lessen the likelihood of adverse reactions related to cumulative drug effect, patients with a history of long-term therapy with *Thorazine* and/or other neuroleptics should be evaluated periodically to decide whether the maintenance dosage could be lowered or drug therapy discontinued.

Antiemetic Effect: The antiemetic action of *Thorazine* may mask the signs and symptoms of overdosage of other drugs and may obscure the diagnosis and treatment of other conditions such as intestinal obstruction, brain tumor and Reye's syndrome. (See Warnings.)

When *Thorazine* is used with cancer chemotherapeutic drugs, vomiting as a sign of the toxicity of these agents may be obscured by the antiemetic effect of *Thorazine*.

Abrupt Withdrawal: Like other phenothiazines, Thorazine (chlorpromazine) is not known to cause psychic dependence and does not produce tolerance or addiction. There may be, however, following abrupt withdrawal of high-dose therapy, some symptoms resembling those of physical dependence such as gastritis, nausea and vomiting, dizziness and tremulousness. These symptoms can usually be avoided or reduced by gradual reduction of the dosage or by continuing concomitant anti-parkinsonism agents for several weeks after *Thorazine* is withdrawn.

ADVERSE REACTIONS

Note: Some adverse effects of *Thorazine* may be more likely to occur, or occur with greater intensity, in patients with special medical problems, e.g., patients with mitral insufficiency or pheochromocytoma have experienced severe hypotension following recommended doses.

Drowsiness, usually mild to moderate, may occur, particularly during the first or second week, after which it generally disappears. If troublesome, dosage may be lowered.

Jaundice: Overall incidence has been low, regardless of indication or dosage. Most investigators conclude it is a sensitivity reaction. Most cases occur between the second and fourth weeks of therapy. The clinical picture resembles infectious hepatitis, with laboratory features of obstructive jaundice, rather than those of parenchymal damage. It is usually promptly reversible on withdrawal of the medication; however, chronic jaundice has been reported.

There is no conclusive evidence that preexisting liver disease makes patients more susceptible to jaundice. Alcoholics with cirrhosis have been successfully treated with Thorazine (chlorpromazine) without complications. Nevertheless, the medication should be used cautiously in patients with liver disease. Patients who have experienced jaundice with a phenothiazine should not, if possible, be reexposed to *Thorazine* or other phenothiazines.

If fever with grippe-like symptoms occurs, appropriate liver studies should be conducted. If tests indicate an abnormality, stop treatment.

Liver function tests in jaundice induced by the drug may mimic extrahepatic obstruction; withhold exploratory laparotomy until extrahepatic obstruction is confirmed.

Hematological Disorders, including agranulocytosis, eosinophilia, leukopenia, hemolytic anemia, aplastic anemia, thrombocytopenic purpura and pancytopenia have been reported.

Agranulocytosis—Warn patients to report the sudden appearance of sore throat or other signs of infection. If white blood cell and differential counts indicate cellular depression, stop treatment and start antibiotic and other suitable therapy.

Most cases have occurred between the 4th and 10th weeks of therapy; patients should be watched closely during that period.

Moderate suppression of white blood cells is not an indication for stopping treatment unless accompanied by the symptoms described above.

Cardiovascular:

Hypotensive Effects—Postural hypotension, simple tachycardia, momentary fainting and dizziness may occur after the first injection; occasionally after subsequent injections; rarely, after the first oral dose. Usually recovery is spontaneous and symptoms disappear within ½ to 2 hours. Occasionally, these effects may be more severe and prolonged, producing a shock-like condition.

To minimize hypotension after injection, keep patient lying down and observe for at least ½ hour. To control hypotension, place patient in head-low position with legs raised. If a vasoconstrictor is required, Levophed®‡ and Neo-Synephrine®§ are the most suitable. Other pressor agents, including epinephrine, should not be used as they may cause a paradoxical further lowering of blood pressure.

EKG Changes—particularly nonspecific, usually reversible Q and T wave distortions—have been observed in some patients receiving phenothiazine tranquilizers, including Thorazine (chlorpromazine).

Note: Sudden death, apparently due to cardiac arrest, has been reported.

C.N.S. Reactions:

Neuromuscular (Extrapyramidal) Reactions—Neuromuscular reactions include dystonias, motor restlessness, pseudoparkinsonism and tardive dyskinesia, and appear to be dose-related. They are discussed in the following paragraphs:

Dystonias: Symptoms may include spasm of the neck muscles, sometimes progressing to acute, reversible torticollis; extensor rigidity of back muscles, sometimes progressing to opisthotonos; carpopedal spasm, trismus, swallowing difficulty, oculogyric crisis and protrusion of the tongue.

These usually subside within a few hours, and almost always within 24 to 48 hours after the drug has been discontinued. *In mild cases,* reassurance or a barbiturate is often sufficient. *In moderate cases,* barbiturates will usually bring rapid relief. *In more severe adult cases,* the administration of an anti-parkinsonism agent, except levodopa, usually produces rapid reversal of symptoms. *In children,* reassurance and barbiturates will usually control symptoms. (Or, parenteral Bena-

* phenytoin, Parke-Davis.
† metrizamide, Winthrop Pharmaceuticals.

‡ norepinephrine bitartrate, Winthrop Pharmaceuticals.
§ phenylephrine hydrochloride, Winthrop Pharmaceuticals.

dryl®[‖] may be useful. See *Benadryl* prescribing information for appropriate children's dosage.) If appropriate treatment with anti-parkinsonism agents or *Benadryl* fails to reverse the signs and symptoms, the diagnosis should be reevaluated.

Suitable supportive measures such as maintaining a clear airway and adequate hydration should be employed when needed. If therapy is reinstituted, it should be at a lower dosage. Should these symptoms occur in children or pregnant patients, the drug should not be reinstituted.

Motor Restlessness: Symptoms may include agitation or jitteriness and sometimes insomnia. These symptoms often disappear spontaneously. At times these symptoms may be similar to the original neurotic or psychotic symptoms. Dosage should not be increased until these side effects have subsided.

If these symptoms become too troublesome, they can usually be controlled by a reduction of dosage or change of drug. Treatment with anti-parkinsonian agents, benzodiazepines or propranolol may be helpful.

Pseudo-parkinsonism: Symptoms may include: mask-like facies, drooling, tremors, pillrolling motion, cogwheel rigidity and shuffling gait. In most cases these symptoms are readily controlled when an anti-parkinsonism agent is administered concomitantly. Anti-parkinsonism agents should be used only when required. Generally, therapy of a few weeks to two or three months will suffice. After this time patients should be evaluated to determine their need for continued treatment. (Note: Levodopa has not been found effective in neuroleptic-induced pseudo-parkinsonism.) Occasionally it is necessary to lower the dosage of Thorazine (chlorpromazine) or to discontinue the drug.

Tardive Dyskinesia: As with all antipsychotic agents, tardive dyskinesia may appear in some patients on long-term therapy or may appear after drug therapy has been discontinued. The syndrome can also develop, although much less frequently, after relatively brief treatment periods at low doses. This syndrome appears in all age groups. Although its prevalence appears to be highest among elderly patients, especially elderly women, it is impossible to rely upon prevalence estimates to predict at the inception of neuroleptic treatment which patients are likely to develop the syndrome. The symptoms are persistent and in some patients appear to be irreversible. The syndrome is characterized by rhythmical involuntary movements of the tongue, face, mouth or jaw (e.g., protrusion of tongue, puffing of cheeks, puckering of mouth, chewing movements). Sometimes these may be accompanied by involuntary movements of extremities. In rare instances, these involuntary movements of the extremities are the only manifestations of tardive dyskinesia. A variant of tardive dyskinesia, tardive dystonia, has also been described.

There is no known effective treatment for tardive dyskinesia; anti-parkinsonism agents do not alleviate the symptoms of this syndrome. If clinically feasible, it is suggested that all antipsychotic agents be discontinued if these symptoms appear. Should it be necessary to reinstitute treatment, or increase the dosage of the agent, or switch to a different antipsychotic agent, the syndrome may be masked.

It has been reported that fine vermicular movements of the tongue may be an early sign of the syndrome and if the medication is stopped at that time the syndrome may not develop.

Adverse Behavioral Effects—Psychotic symptoms and catatonic-like states have been reported rarely.

Other C.N.S. Effects—Cerebral edema has been reported. Convulsive seizures *(petit mal* and *grand mal)* have been reported, particularly in patients with EEG abnormalities or history of such disorders.

Abnormality of the cerebrospinal fluid proteins has also been reported.

Allergic Reactions of a mild urticarial type or photosensitivity are seen. Avoid undue exposure to sun. More severe reactions, including exfoliative dermatitis, have been reported occasionally.

Contact dermatitis has been reported in nursing personnel; accordingly, the use of rubber gloves when administering *Thorazine* liquid or injectable is recommended.

In addition, asthma, laryngeal edema, angioneurotic edema and anaphylactoid reactions have been reported.

Endocrine Disorders: Lactation and moderate breast engorgement may occur in females on large doses. If persistent, lower dosage or withdraw drug. False-positive pregnancy tests have been reported, but are less likely to occur when a serum test is used. Amenorrhea and gynecomastia have also been reported. Hyperglycemia, hypoglycemia and glycosuria have been reported.

Autonomic Reactions: Occasional dry mouth; nasal congestion; nausea; obstipation; constipation; adynamic ileus; urinary retention; priapism; miosis and mydriasis, atonic colon, ejaculatory disorders/impotence.

Special Considerations in Long-Term Therapy: Skin pigmentation and ocular changes have occurred in some patients taking substantial doses of Thorazine (chlorpromazine) for prolonged periods.

[‖] diphenhydramine hydrochloride, Parke-Davis.

Skin Pigmentation—Rare instances of skin pigmentation have been observed in hospitalized mental patients, primarily females who have received the drug usually for three years or more in dosages ranging from 500 mg to 1500 mg daily. The pigmentary changes, restricted to exposed areas of the body, range from an almost imperceptible darkening of the skin to a slate gray color, sometimes with a violet hue. Histological examination reveals a pigment, chiefly in the dermis, which is probably a melanin-like complex. The pigmentation may fade following discontinuance of the drug.

Ocular Changes—Ocular changes have occurred more frequently than skin pigmentation and have been observed both in pigmented and nonpigmented patients receiving Thorazine (chlorpromazine) usually for two years or more in dosages of 300 mg daily and higher. Eye changes are characterized by deposition of fine particulate matter in the lens and cornea. In more advanced cases, star-shaped opacities have also been observed in the anterior portion of the lens. The nature of the eye deposits has not yet been determined. A small number of patients with more severe ocular changes have had some visual impairment. In addition to these corneal and lenticular changes, epithelial keratopathy and pigmentary retinopathy have been reported. Reports suggest that the eye lesions may regress after withdrawal of the drug.

Since the occurrence of eye changes seems to be related to dosage levels and/or duration of therapy, it is suggested that long-term patients on moderate to high dosage levels have periodic ocular examinations.

Etiology—The etiology of both of these reactions is not clear, but exposure to light, along with dosage/duration of therapy, appears to be the most significant factor. If either of these reactions is observed, the physician should weigh the benefits of continued therapy against the possible risks and, on the merits of the individual case, determine whether or not to continue present therapy, lower the dosage, or withdraw the drug.

Other Adverse Reactions: Mild fever may occur after large I.M. doses. Hyperpyrexia has been reported. Increases in appetite and weight sometimes occur. Peripheral edema and a systemic lupus erythematosus-like syndrome have been reported.

Note: There have been occasional reports of sudden death in patients receiving phenothiazines. In some cases, the cause appeared to be cardiac arrest or asphyxia due to failure of the cough reflex.

DOSAGE AND ADMINISTRATION—ADULTS

Adjust dosage to individual and the severity of his condition, recognizing that the milligram for milligram potency relationship among all dosage forms has not been precisely established clinically. It is important to increase dosage until symptoms are controlled. Dosage should be increased more gradually in debilitated or emaciated patients. In continued therapy, gradually reduce dosage to the lowest effective maintenance level, after symptoms have been controlled for a reasonable period.

In general, dosage recommendations for other oral forms of the drug may be applied to Spansule® brand sustained release capsules on the basis of total daily dosage in milligrams.

The 100 mg and 200 mg tablets are for use in severe neuropsychiatric conditions.

Increase parenteral dosage only if hypotension has not occurred. Before using I.M., see Important Notes on Injection.

Elderly Patients—In general, dosages in the lower range are sufficient for most elderly patients. Since they appear to be more susceptible to hypotension and neuromuscular reactions, such patients should be observed closely. Dosage should be tailored to the individual, response carefully monitored, and dosage adjusted accordingly. Dosage should be increased more gradually in elderly patients.

Psychotic Disorders—Increase dosage gradually until symptoms are controlled. Maximum improvement may not be seen for weeks or even months. Continue optimum dosage for 2 weeks; then gradually reduce dosage to the lowest effective maintenance level. Daily dosage of 200 mg is not unusual. Some patients require higher dosages (e.g., 800 mg daily is not uncommon in discharged mental patients).

HOSPITALIZED PATIENTS: ACUTELY DISTURBED OR MANIC—*I.M.:* 25 mg (1 mL). If necessary, give additional 25 to 50 mg injection in 1 hour. Increase subsequent I.M. doses gradually over several days—up to 400 mg q4-6h in exceptionally severe cases—until patient is controlled. Usually patient becomes quiet and cooperative within 24 to 48 hours and oral doses may be substituted and increased until the patient is calm. 500 mg a day is generally sufficient. While gradual increases to 2,000 mg a day or more may be necessary, there is usually little therapeutic gain to be achieved by exceeding 1,000 mg a day for extended periods. In general, dosage levels should be lower in the elderly, the emaciated and the debilitated. LESS ACUTELY DISTURBED—*Oral:* 25 mg t.i.d. Increase gradually until effective dose is reached —usually 400 mg daily. OUTPATIENTS—*Oral:* 10 mg t.i.d. or q.i.d., or 25 mg b.i.d. or t.i.d. MORE SEVERE CASES —*Oral:* 25 mg t.i.d. After 1 or 2 days, daily dosage may be increased by 20–50 mg at semiweekly intervals until patient becomes calm and cooperative. PROMPT CONTROL OF SEVERE SYMPTOMS—*I.M.:* 25 mg (1 mL). If necessary, repeat in 1 hour. Subsequent doses should be oral, 25–50 mg t.i.d.

Nausea and Vomiting—*Oral:* 10 to 25 mg q4–6h, p.r.n., increased, if necessary. *I.M.:* 25 mg (1 mL). If no hypotension occurs, give 25 to 50 mg q3–4h, p.r.n., until vomiting stops. Then switch to oral dosage. *Rectal:* One 100 mg suppository q6–8h, p.r.n. In some patients, half this dose will do. DURING SURGERY—*I.M.:* 12.5 mg (0.5 mL). Repeat in $\frac{1}{2}$ hour if necessary and if no hypotension occurs. *I.V.:* 2 mg per fractional injection, at 2-minute intervals. Do not exceed 25 mg. Dilute to 1 mg/mL, i.e., 1 mL (25 mg) mixed with 24 mL of saline.

Presurgical Apprehension—*Oral:* 25 to 50 mg, 2 to 3 hours before the operation. *I.M.:* 12.5 to 25 mg (0.5-1 mL), 1 to 2 hours before operation.

Intractable Hiccups—*Oral:* 25 to 50 mg t.i.d. or q.i.d. If symptoms persist for 2-3 days, give 25 to 50 mg (1-2 mL) I.M. Should symptoms persist, use *slow* I.V. infusion with patient flat in bed: 25 to 50 mg (1-2 mL) in 500 to 1,000 mL of saline. Follow blood pressure closely.

Acute Intermittent Porphyria—*Oral:* 25 to 50 mg t.i.d. or q.i.d. Can usually be discontinued after several weeks, but maintenance therapy may be necessary for some patients. *I.M.:* 25 mg (1 mL) t.i.d. or q.i.d. until patient can take oral therapy.

Tetanus—*I.M.:* 25 to 50 mg (1-2 mL) given 3 or 4 times daily, usually in conjunction with barbiturates. Total doses and frequency of administration must be determined by the patient's response, starting with low doses and increasing gradually. *I.V.:* 25 to 50 mg (1-2 mL). Dilute to at least 1 mg per mL and administer at a rate of 1 mg per minute.

DOSAGE AND ADMINISTRATION—CHILDREN

Thorazine (chlorpromazine) should generally not be used in children under 6 months of age except where potentially lifesaving. It should not be used in conditions for which specific children's dosages have not been established.

Severe Behavioral Problems—OUTPATIENTS—Select route of administration according to severity of patient's condition and increase dosage gradually as required. *Oral:* $\frac{1}{4}$ mg/lb body weight q4-6h, p.r.n. (e.g., for 40 lb child —10 mg q4-6h). *Rectal:* $\frac{1}{2}$ mg/lb body weight q6-8h, p.r.n. (e.g., for 20-30 lb child—half a 25 mg suppository q6-8h). *I.M.:* $\frac{1}{4}$ mg/lb body weight q6-8h, p.r.n.

HOSPITALIZED PATIENTS—As with outpatients, start with low doses and increase dosage gradually. In severe behavior disorders or psychotic conditions, higher dosages (50-100 mg daily, and in older children, 200 mg daily or more) may be necessary. There is little evidence that behavior improvement in severely disturbed mentally retarded patients is further enhanced by doses beyond 500 mg per day. *Maximum I.M. Dosage:* Children up to 5 years (or 50 lbs), not over 40 mg/day; 5-12 years (or 50-100 lbs), not over 75 mg/day except in unmanageable cases.

Nausea and Vomiting—Dosage and frequency of administration should be adjusted according to the severity of the symptoms and response of the patient. The duration of activity following intramuscular administration may last up to 12 hours. Subsequent doses may be given by the same route if necessary. *Oral:* $\frac{1}{4}$ mg/lb body weight (e.g., 40 lb child—10 mg q4-6h). *Rectal:* $\frac{1}{2}$ mg/lb body weight q6-8h, p.r.n. (e.g., 20-30 lb child—half of a 25 mg suppository q6-8h). *I.M.:* $\frac{1}{4}$ mg/lb body weight q6-8h, p.r.n. *Maximum I.M. Dosage:* Children up to 5 yrs. (or 50 lbs), not over 40 mg/day; 5-12 yrs. (or 50-100 lbs), not over 75 mg/day except in severe cases. DURING SURGERY—*I.M.:* $\frac{1}{8}$ mg/lb body weight. Repeat in $\frac{1}{2}$ hour if necessary and if no hypotension occurs. *I.V.:* 1 mg per fractional injection at 2-minute intervals and not exceeding recommended I.M. dosage. Always dilute to 1 mg/mL, i.e., 1 mL (25 mg) mixed with 24 mL of saline.

Presurgical Apprehension—$\frac{1}{4}$ mg/lb body weight, either *orally* 2 to 3 hours before operation, or *I.M.* 1 to 2 hours before.

Tetanus—*I.M.* or *I.V.:* $\frac{1}{4}$ mg/lb body weight q6-8h. When given I.V., dilute to at least 1 mg/mL and administer at rate of 1 mg per 2 minutes. In children up to 50 lbs, do not exceed 40 mg daily; 50 to 100 lbs, do not exceed 75 mg, except in severe cases.

IMPORTANT NOTES ON INJECTION

Inject slowly, deep into upper outer quadrant of buttock. Because of possible hypotensive effects, reserve parenteral administration for bedfast patients or for acute ambulatory cases, and keep patient lying down for at least $\frac{1}{2}$ hour after injection. If irritation is a problem, dilute Injection with saline or 2% procaine; mixing with other agents in the syringe is not recommended. Subcutaneous injection is not advised. Avoid injecting undiluted Thorazine (chlorpromazine) into vein. I.V. route is only for severe hiccups, surgery and tetanus.

Because of the possibility of contact dermatitis, avoid getting solution on hands or clothing. Protect from light, or discolor-

Continued on next page

SmithKline Beecham—Cont.

ation may occur. Slight yellowing will not alter potency. Discard if markedly discolored. For information on sulfite sensitivity, see the Warnings section of this labeling.

Note on Concentrate: When the Concentrate is to be used, add the desired dosage of Concentrate to 60 mL (2 fl oz) or more of diluent *just prior to administration.* This will insure palatability and stability. Vehicles suggested for dilution are: tomato or fruit juice, milk, simple syrup, orange syrup, carbonated beverages, coffee, tea, or water. Semisolid foods (soups, puddings, etc.) may also be used. The Concentrate is light sensitive; it should be protected from light and dispensed in amber glass bottles. *Refrigeration is not required.*

OVERDOSAGE

(See also Adverse Reactions.)

SYMPTOMS—Primarily symptoms of central nervous system depression to the point of somnolence or coma. Hypotension and extrapyramidal symptoms.

Other possible manifestations include agitation and restlessness, convulsions, fever, autonomic reactions such as dry mouth and ileus, EKG changes and cardiac arrhythmias.

TREATMENT—It is important to determine other medications taken by the patient since multiple drug therapy is common in overdosage situations. Treatment is essentially symptomatic and supportive. Early gastric lavage is helpful. Keep patient under observation and maintain an open airway, since involvement of the extrapyramidal mechanism may produce dysphagia and respiratory difficulty in severe overdosage. **Do not attempt to induce emesis because a dystonic reaction of the head or neck may develop that could result in aspiration of vomitus.** Extrapyramidal symptoms may be treated with anti-parkinsonism drugs, barbiturates, or *Benadryl.* See prescribing information for these products. Care should be taken to avoid increasing respiratory depression.

If administration of a stimulant is desirable, amphetamine, dextroamphetamine, or caffeine with sodium benzoate is recommended. Stimulants that may cause convulsions (e.g., picrotoxin or pentylenetetrazol) should be avoided.

If hypotension occurs, the standard measures for managing circulatory shock should be initiated. If it is desirable to administer a vasoconstrictor, *Levophed* and *Neo-Synephrine* are most suitable. Other pressor agents, including epinephrine, are not recommended because phenothiazine derivatives may reverse the usual elevating action of these agents and cause a further lowering of blood pressure.

Limited experience indicates that phenothiazines are *not* dializable.

Special note on Spansule® capsules—Since much of the *Spansule* capsule medication is coated for gradual release, therapy directed at reversing the effects of the ingested drug and at supporting the patient should be continued for as long as overdosage symptoms remain. Saline cathartics are useful for hastening evacuation of pellets that have not already released medication.

HOW SUPPLIED

Tablets: 10 mg, in bottles of 100; 25 mg or 50 mg, in bottles of 100 and 1000. For use in severe neuropsychiatric conditions, 100 mg and 200 mg, in bottles of 100 and 1000.

Spansule® brand of sustained release capsules: 30 mg, 75 mg or 150 mg, in bottles of 50.

Ampuls: 1 mL and 2 mL (25 mg/mL), in boxes of 10.

Multi-dose Vials: 10 mL (25 mg/mL), in boxes of 1.

Syrup: 10 mg/5 mL, in 4 fl oz bottles.

Suppositories: 25 mg or 100 mg, in boxes of 12.

Concentrate: Intended for institutional use. 30 mg/mL, in 4 fl oz bottles, and 100 mg/mL, in 8 fl oz bottles, in cartons of 12.

Veterans Administration—Tablets, 25 mg, 1000's, 6505-00-022-1326; Tablets, 50 mg, 1000's, 6505-00-022-1327; Tablets, 100 mg, 1000's, 6505-00-014-1182; Tablets, 200 mg, 1000's 6505-00-014-1186.

TZ:L75

Shown in Product Identification Section, page 431

TICAR®   ℞

[tĭ′kar]

sterile ticarcillin disodium

for Intramuscular or Intravenous Administration

DESCRIPTION

TICAR (Ticarcillin Disodium) is a semisynthetic injectable penicillin derived from the penicillin nucleus, 6-aminopenicillanic acid. Chemically, it is 6-[(Carboxy-3-thienylacetyl)amino] 3,3-dimethyl-7-oxo-4-thia-1-azabicyclo [3.2.0]heptane-2-carboxylic acid disodium salt.

[See Structural Formula at top of next column.]

TICARCILLIN SERUM LEVELS
mcg/ml

Dosage	Route	¼ hr.	½ hr.	1 hr.	2 hr.	3 hr.	4 hr.	6 hr.
Adults:								
500 mg	IM	—	7.7	8.6	6.0	4.0	—	2.9
1 Gm	IM	—	31.0	18.7	15.7	9.7	—	3.4
2 Gm	IM	—	63.6	39.7	32.3	18.9	—	3.4
3 Gm	IV	190.0	140.0	107.0	52.2	31.3	13.8	4.2
5 Gm	IV	327.0	280.0	175.0	106.0	63.0	28.5	9.6
3 Gm + 1 Gm Probenecid	IV Oral	223.0	166.0	123.0	78.0	54.0	35.4	17.1

		½ hr.	1 hr.	1½ hr.	2 hr.	4 hr.	8 hr.
Neonates:							
50 mg/kg	IM	64.0	70.7	63.7	60.1	33.2	11.6

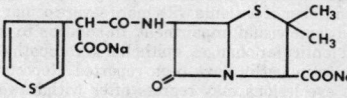

It is supplied as a white to pale yellow powder for reconstitution. The reconstituted solution is clear, colorless or pale yellow, having a pH of 6.0–8.0. Ticarcillin is very soluble in water, its solubility is greater than 600 mg/ml.

ACTIONS

PHARMACOLOGY

Ticarcillin is not absorbed orally, therefore, it must be given intravenously or intramuscularly. Following intramuscular administration, peak serum concentrations occur within ½–1 hour. Somewhat higher and more prolonged serum levels can be achieved with the concurrent administration of probenecid.

The minimum inhibitory concentrations (MIC) for many strains of *Pseudomonas* are relatively high by usual standards; serum levels of 60 mcg/ml or greater are required. However, the low degree of toxicity of Ticarcillin permits the use of doses large enough to achieve inhibitory levels for these strains in serum or tissues. Other susceptible organisms usually require serum levels in the 10–25 mcg/ml range. [See table above.]

As with other penicillins, Ticarcillin is eliminated by glomerular filtration and tubular secretion. It is not highly bound to serum protein (approximately 45%) and is excreted unchanged in high concentrations in the urine. After the administration of a 1–2 Gm I.M. dose, a urine concentration of 2000–4000 mcg/ml may be obtained in patients with normal renal function. The serum half-life of Ticarcillin in normal individuals is approximately 70 minutes.

An inverse relationship exists between serum half-life and creatinine clearance, but the dosage of TICAR need only be adjusted in cases of severe renal impairment (see DOSAGE AND ADMINISTRATION). The administered Ticarcillin may be removed from patients undergoing dialysis; the actual amount removed depends on the duration and type of dialysis.

Ticarcillin can be detected in tissues and interstitial fluid following parenteral administration. Penetration into the cerebrospinal fluid, bile and pleural fluid has been demonstrated.

MICROBIOLOGY

Ticarcillin is bactericidal and demonstrates substantial *in vitro* activity against both Gram-positive and Gram-negative organisms. Many strains of the following organisms were found to be susceptible to Ticarcillin *in vitro:*

Pseudomonas aeruginosa (and other species)
Escherichia coli
Proteus mirabilis
Morganella morganii (formerly Proteus morganii)
Providencia rettgeri (formerly Proteus rettgeri)
Proteus vulgaris
Enterobacter species
Haemophilus influenzae
Neisseria species
Salmonella species
Staphylococcus aureus (non-penicillinase producing)
Staphylococcus epidermidis
Beta-hemolytic streptococci (Group A)
Streptococcus faecalis (Enterococcus)
Streptococcus pneumoniae
Anaerobic bacteria, including:
Bacteroides species including *B. fragilis*
Fusobacterium species
Veillonella species
Clostridium species
Eubacterium species
Peptococcus species
Peptostreptococcus species

In vitro synergism between Ticarcillin and gentamicin sulfate, tobramycin sulfate or amikacin sulfate against certain strains of *Pseudomonas aeruginosa* has been demonstrated. Some strains of such microorganisms as *Mima-Herellea (Acinetobacter), Citrobacter* and *Serratia* have shown susceptibility.

Ticarcillin is not stable in the presence of penicillinase.

Some strains of *Pseudomonas* have developed resistance fairly rapidly.

DISK SUSCEPTIBILITY TESTS

Susceptibility Tests: Ticarcillin disks or powders should be used for testing susceptibility to ticarcillin. However, organisms reportedly susceptible to carbenicillin are susceptible to ticarcillin.

Diffusion Techniques: For the disk diffusion method of susceptibility testing a 75 mcg TICAR DISK should be used. The method for this test is the one outlined in NCCLS publication M2-A3* with the following interpretative criteria:

[See table below.]

Dilution Techniques: Dilution techniques for determining the MIC (minimum inhibitory concentration) are published by NCCLS for the broth and agar dilution procedures. The MIC data should be interpreted in light of the concentrations present in serum, tissue, and body fluids. Organisms with MIC ≤ 64 are considered susceptible when they are in tissue but organisms with MIC ≤ 128 would be susceptible in urine where the TICAR concentrations are much greater. At present, only dilution methods can be recommended for testing antibiotic susceptibility of obligate anaerobes.

Susceptibility testing methods require the use of control organisms. The 75 mcg ticarcillin disk should give zone diameters between 22 and 28 mm for *P. aeruginosa* ATCC 27853 and 24 and 30 mm for *E. Coli* ATCC 25922. Reference strains are available for dilution testing of ticarcillin. 95% of the MIC's should fall within the following MIC ranges and the majority of MIC's should be at values close to the center of the pertinent range. (Reference NCCLS publication M7-A**)

    S. aureus ATCC 29213, 2.0–8.0 mcg/ml; *S. faecalis* ATCC 29212, 16–64 mcg/ml; *E. coli* ATCC 25922, 2.0–8.0 mcg/ml; *P. aeruginosa* ATCC 27853, 8.0–32 mcg/ml.

INDICATIONS

TICAR (Ticarcillin Disodium) is indicated for the treatment of the following infections:

    Bacterial septicemia (†)
    Skin and soft-tissue infections (†)
    Acute and chronic respiratory tract infections (†)(‡)

(†)   caused by susceptible strains of *Pseudomonas aeruginosa, Proteus* species (both indole-positive and indole-negative) and *Escherichia coli.*

(‡)   (Though clinical improvement has been shown, bacteriological cures cannot be expected in patients with chronic respiratory disease or cystic fibrosis.)

    Genitourinary tract infections (complicated and uncomplicated) due to susceptible strains of *Pseudomonas aeruginosa, Proteus* species (both indole-positive and indole-negative), *Escherichia coli, Enterobacter* and *Streptococcus faecalis* (enterococcus).

Ticarcillin is also indicated in the treatment of the following infections due to susceptible anaerobic bacteria:

---

*Performance standards for Antimicrobial Disk Susceptibility Tests, National Committee for Clinical Laboratory Standards, Vol. 4, No. 16, pp. 369–402, 1984.

**Methods for Dilution Antimicrobial Susceptibility Tests for Bacteria That Grow Aerobically, Vol. 5, No. 22, pp. 579–618, 1985.

Culture	Susceptible	Intermediate	Resistant
P. aeruginosa and *Enterobacteriaceae* The MIC correlates are:	≥ 15 mm Resistant > 128 mcg/ml Susceptible ≤ 64 mcg/ml	12–14 mm	≤ 11 mm

1. Bacterial septicemia.
2. Lower respiratory tract infections such as empyema, anaerobic pneumonitis and lung abscess.
3. Intra-abdominal infections such as peritonitis and intra-abdominal abscess (typically resulting from anaerobic organisms resident in the normal gastrointestinal tract).
4. Infections of the female pelvis and genital tract, such as endometritis, pelvic inflammatory disease, pelvic abscess and salpingitis.
5. Skin and soft-tissue infections.

Although Ticarcillin is primarily indicated in Gram-negative infections, its *in vitro* activity against Gram-positive organisms should be considered in treating infections caused by both Gram-negative and Gram-positive organisms (see MICROBIOLOGY).

Based on the *in vitro* synergism between Ticarcillin and gentamicin sulfate, tobramycin sulfate or amikacin sulfate against certain strains of *Pseudomonas aeruginosa*, combined therapy has been successful, using full therapeutic dosages. (For additional prescribing information, see the gentamicin sulfate, tobramycin sulfate and amikacin sulfate package inserts.)

NOTE: Culturing and susceptibilty testing should be performed initially and during treatment to monitor the effectiveness of therapy and the susceptibility of the bacteria.

CONTRAINDICATIONS

A history of allergic reaction to any of the penicillins is a contraindication.

WARNINGS

Serious and occasionally fatal hypersensitivity (anaphylactoid) reactions have been reported in patients receiving penicillin. These reactions are more likely to occur in persons with a history of sensitivity to multiple allergens.

There are reports of patients with a history of penicillin hypersensitivity reactions who experience severe hypersensitivity reactions when treated with a cephalosporin. Before therapy with a penicillin, careful inquiry should be made about previous hypersensitivity reactions to penicillins, cephalosporins, and other allergens. If a reaction occurs, the drug should be discontinued unless, in the opinion of the physician, the condition being treated is life-threatening and amenable only to Ticarcillin therapy. **Serious anaphylactoid reactions require immediate emergency treatment with epinephrine. Oxygen, intravenous steroids, airway management, including intubation, should also be administered as indicated.**

Some patients receiving high doses of Ticarcillin may develop hemorrhagic manifestations associated with abnormalities of coagulation tests, such as bleeding time and platelet aggregation. On withdrawal of the drug, the bleeding should cease and coagulation abnormalities revert to normal. Other causes of abnormal bleeding should also be considered. Patients with renal impairment, in whom excretion of Ticarcillin is delayed, should be observed for bleeding manifestations. Such patients should be dosed strictly according to recommendations (see DOSAGE AND ADMINISTRATION). If bleeding manifestations appear, Ticarcillin treatment should be discontinued and appropriate therapy instituted.

PRECAUTIONS

Although TICAR (Ticarcillin Disodium) exhibits the characteristic low toxicity of the penicillins, as with any other potent agent, it is advisable to check periodically for organ system dysfunction (including renal, hepatic and hematopoietic) during prolonged treatment. If overgrowth of resistant organisms occurs, the appropriate therapy should be initiated.

Since the theoretical sodium content is 5.2 milliequivalents (120 mg) per gram of Ticarcillin, and the actual vial content can be as high as 6.5 mEq/Gm, electrolyte and cardiac status should be monitored carefully.

In a few patients receiving intravenous Ticarcillin, hypokalemia has been reported. Serum potassium should be measured periodically, and, if necessary, corrective therapy should be implemented.

As with any penicillin, the possibility of an allergic response, including anaphylaxis, exists, particularly in hypersensitive patients.

USAGE DURING PREGNANCY

Reproduction studies have been performed in mice and rats and have revealed no evidence of impaired fertility or harm to the fetus due to Ticarcillin. There are no well-controlled studies in pregnant women, but investigational experience does not include any positive evidence of adverse effects on the fetus. Although there is no clearly defined risk, such experience cannot exclude the possibility of infrequent or sub-

DOSAGE AND ADMINISTRATION

Clinical experience indicates that in serious urinary tract and systemic infections, intravenous therapy in the higher doses should be used. Intramuscular injections should not exceed 2 grams per injection.

Adults:

Bacterial Septicemia Respiratory Tract Infections Skin and Soft-Tissue Infections Intra-Abdominal Infections Infections of the Female Pelvis and Genital Tract	200–300 mg/kg/day by I.V. infusion in divided doses every 4 or 6 hours. [The usual dose is 3 gm given every 4 hours (18 gm/day) or 4 gm given every 6 hours (16 gm/day) depending on weight and the severity of the infection.]
Urinary Tract Infections Complicated:	150–200 mg/kg/day by I.V. infusion in divided doses every 4 or 6 hours. [Usual recommended dosage for average (70 kg) adults: 3 grams q.i.d.]
Uncomplicated:	1 gram I.M. or direct I.V. every 6 hours.

Infections complicated by renal insufficiency: (1)
Initial loading dose of 3 grams I.V. followed by I.V. doses, based on creatinine clearance and type of dialysis, as indicated below:

Creatinine clearance ml/min.:	
over 60	3 grams every 4 hours
30–60	2 grams every 4 hours
10–30	2 grams every 8 hours
less than 10	2 grams every 12 hours (or 1 gram I.M. every 6 hours)
less than 10 with hepatic dysfunction	2 grams every 24 hours (or 1 gram I.M. every 12 hours)
patients on peritoneal dialysis	3 grams every 12 hours
patients on hemodialysis	2 grams every 12 hours supplemented with 3 grams after each dialysis

To calculate creatinine clearance* from a serum creatinine value use the following formula:

$$C_{cr} = \frac{(140 - \text{Age}) \ (\text{wt in kg})}{72 \times S_{cr}(\text{mg}/100 \ \text{ml})}$$

This is the calculated creatinine clearance for adult males; for females it is 15% less.

* Cockcroft, D.W., et al, "Prediction of Creatinine Clearance from Serum Creatinine" Nephron 16:31–41 (1976).

(1) The half-life of Ticarcillin in patients with renal failure is approximately 13 hours.

Children: Under 40 kg (88 lbs)

The daily dose for children should not exceed the adult dosage.

Bacterial Septicemia Respiratory Tract Infections Skin and Soft-Tissue Infections Intra-Abdominal Infections Infections of the Female Pelvis and Genital Tract	200–300 mg/kg/day by I.V. infusion in divided doses every 4 or 6 hours.

Urinary Tract Infections
    Complicated:
    Uncomplicated:
	150–200 mg/kg/day by I.V. infusion in divided doses every 4 or 6 hours.
	50–100 mg/kg/day I.M. or direct I.V. in divided doses every 6 or 8 hours.

Infections complicated by renal insufficiency:	Clinical data is insufficient to recommend an optimum dose.

Children weighing more than 40 kg (88 lbs) should receive adult dosages.

Neonates: In the neonate, for severe infections (sepsis) due to susceptible strains of *Pseudomonas*, *Proteus*, and *E. coli*, the following Ticarcillin dosages may be given I.M. or by 10–20 minutes I.V. infusion:

Infants under 2000 grams body weight:		Infants over 2000 grams body weight:	
Aged 0–7 days	75 mg/kg/12 hours (150 mg/kg/day)	Aged 0–7 days	75 mg/kg/8 hours (225 mg/kg/day)
Aged over 7 days	75 mg/kg/8 hours (225 mg/kg/day)	Aged over 7 days	100 mg/kg/8 hours (300 mg/kg/day)

This dosage schedule is intended to produce peak serum concentrations of 125–150 mcg/ml one hour after a dose of Ticarcillin and trough concentrations of 25–50 mcg/ml immediately before the next dose.

NOTE: Gentamicin, tobramycin or amikacin may be used concurrently with Ticarcillin for initial therapy until results of culture and susceptibility studies are known.
Seriously ill patients should receive the higher doses. TICAR has proved to be useful in infections in which protective mechanisms are impaired, such as in acute leukemia and during therapy with immunosuppressive or oncolytic drugs.

SmithKline Beecham—Cont.

tle damage to the fetus. Ticarcillin should be used in pregnant women only when clearly needed.

ADVERSE REACTIONS

The following adverse reactions may occur:

Hypersensitivity Reactions: Skin rashes, pruritus, urticaria, drug fever.

Gastrointestinal Disturbances: Nausea and vomiting.

Hemic and Lymphatic Systems: As with other penicillins, anemia, thrombocytopenia, leukopenia, neutropenia and eosinophilia.

Abnormalities of Blood, Hepatic and Renal Laboratory Studies: As with other semisynthetic penicillins, SGOT and SGPT elevations have been reported. To date, clinical manifestations of hepatic or renal disorders have not been observed which could be ascribed solely to Ticarcillin.

CNS: Patients, especially those with impaired renal function, may experience convulsions or neuromuscular excitability when very high doses of the drug are administered.

Other: Local reactions such as pain (rarely accompanied by induration) at the site of the injection have been reported. Vein irritation and phlebitis can occur, particularly when undiluted solution is directly injected into the vein.

[See table on preceding page.]

DIRECTIONS FOR USE

—1 Gm, 3 Gm and 6 Gm Standard Vials—

INTRAMUSCULAR USE: (Concentration of approximately 385 mg/ml).

For initial reconstitution use Sterile Water for Injection, U.S.P., Sodium Chloride Injection, U.S.P. or 1% Lidocaine Hydrochloride solution* (without epinephrine).

Each gram of Ticarcillin should be reconstituted with 2 ml of Sterile Water for Injection, U.S.P., Sodium Chloride Injection, U.S.P. or 1% Lidocaine Hydrochloride solution* (without epinephrine) and **used promptly**. Each 2.6 ml of the resulting solution will then contain 1 Gm of Ticarcillin.

*[For full product information, refer to manufacturer's package insert for Lidocaine Hydrochloride.]

As with all intramuscular preparations, TICAR (Ticarcillin Disodium) should be injected well within the body of a relatively large muscle using usual techniques and precautions.

INTRAVENOUS ADMINISTRATION: (Concentration of approximately 200 mg/ml).

For initial reconstitution use Sodium Chloride Injection, U.S.P., Dextrose Injection 5% or Lactated Ringer's Injection.

Reconstitute each gram of Ticarcillin with 4 ml of the appropriate diluent. After the addition of 4 ml of diluent per gram of Ticarcillin each 1.0 ml of the resulting solution will have an approximate concentration of 200 mg. Once dissolved, further dilute if desired.

DIRECT INTRAVENOUS INJECTION: In order to avoid vein irritation, administer solution as slowly as possible.

INTRAVENOUS INFUSION: Administer by continuous or intermittent intravenous drip. Intermittent infusion should be administered over a 30 minute to 2 hour period in equally divided doses.

—3 Gm Piggyback Bottles—

DIRECT INTRAVENOUS INJECTION: (Concentrations of approximately 29 mg/ml to 100 mg/ml).

The 3 gram bottle should be reconstituted with a minimum of 30 ml of the desired intravenous solution listed below.

Amount of Diluent	Concentration of Solution
100 ml	1 Gm/34 ml (~29 mg/ml)
60 ml	1 Gm/20 ml (50 mg/ml)
30 ml	1 Gm/10 ml (100 mg/ml)

In order to avoid vein irritation, the solution should be administered as slowly as possible. A dilution of approximately 50 mg/ml or more will further reduce the incidence of vein irritation.

INTRAVENOUS INFUSION: Stability studies in the intravenous solutions listed below indicate that Ticarcillin Disodium will provide sufficient activity at room temperature (70°–75°F) within the stated time periods at concentrations between 10 mg/ml and 50 mg/ml—see Stability Period section below.

After reconstitution and prior to administration TICAR as with other parenteral drugs should be inspected visually for particulate matter and discoloration.

[See table above.]

Refrigerated solutions stored longer than 72 hours should not be used for multidose purposes.

After reconstitution and dilution to a concentration of 10 mg/ml to 100 mg/ml, this solution can be frozen (0°F) and stored for up to 30 days. The thawed solution must be used within 24 hours.

Unused solutions should be discarded after the time periods mentioned above.

It is recommended that TICAR and gentamicin sulfate, tobramycin sulfate or amikacin sulfate not be mixed together in the same I.V. solution due to the gradual inactivation of gentamicin sulfate, tobramycin sulfate or amikacin sulfate under these circumstances. The therapeutic effect of TICAR and these aminoglycoside drugs remains unimpaired when administered separately.

STABILITY PERIOD

Intravenous Solution (concentration of 10 mg/ml to 100 mg/ml)	Room Temperature (70°–75°F)	Refrigeration (40°F)
Sodium Chloride Injection, U.S.P.	72 hours	14 days
Dextrose Injection 5%	72 hours	14 days
Lactated Ringer's Injection	48 hours	14 days

HOW SUPPLIED

TICAR (Sterile Ticarcillin Disodium). Each vial contains Ticarcillin Disodium equivalent to 1 Gm, 3 Gm, 6 Gm Ticarcillin.

NDC 0029-6550-22 ....1 Gm Vial
NDC 0029-6552-26 ....3 Gm Vial
NDC 0029-6555-26 ....6 Gm Vial
NDC 0029-6552-21 ....3 Gm Piggyback Bottle

TICAR is also supplied as:

NDC 0029-6558-21 ....20 Gm Pharmacy Bulk Package
NDC 0029-6559-21 ....30 Gm Pharmacy Bulk Package
NDC 0029-6552-40 ......3 Gm ADD-Vantage® ANTIBIOTIC VIAL

TICAR (Sterile Ticarcillin Disodium). Each vial contains Ticarcillin Disodium equivalent to 20 Gm, 30 Gm, 3 Gm Ticarcillin.

STORE DRY POWDER AT ROOM TEMPERATURE OR BELOW.

Veterans Administration—Vials, 3 g/50 mL, 1's, 6505-01-046-6793; 6 g/50 mL, 1's, 6505-01-069-6303; Pharmacy Bulk Vial, 20 g/100 mL, 1's, 6505-01-123-9172.

June, 1988 7182/C

Shown in Product Identification Section, page 431

TIGAN® ℞

[*tī'găn*]

(trimethobenzamide hydrochloride)
CAPSULES
SUPPOSITORIES
INJECTABLE

DESCRIPTION

Chemically, trimethobenzamide HCl is N-[p-[2-(dimethylamino) -ethoxy] benzyl]-3,4,5-trimethoxybenzamide hydrochloride. It has a molecular weight of 424.93 and the following structural formula:

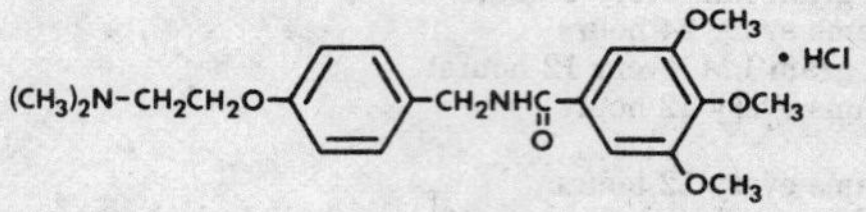

Capsules: Blue, each containing 250 mg trimethobenzamide hydrochloride; blue and white, each containing 100 mg trimethobenzamide hydrochloride.

Inactive Ingredients: Lactose, Magnesium Stearate and Starch.

Suppositories, (200 mg): Each suppository contains 200 mg trimethobenzamide hydrochloride and 2% benzocaine in a base compounded with polysorbate 80, white beeswax and propylene glycol monostearate.

Suppositories, Pediatric (100 mg): Each suppository contains 100 mg trimethobenzamide hydrochloride and 2% benzocaine in a base compounded with polysorbate 80, white beeswax and propylene glycol monostearate.

Ampuls: Each 2-mL ampul contains 200 mg trimethobenzamide hydrochloride compounded with 0.2% parabens (methyl and propyl) as preservatives, 1 mg sodium citrate and 0.4 mg citric acid as buffers and pH adjusted to approximately 5.0 with sodium hydroxide.

Multiple Dose Vials: Each mL contains 100 mg trimethobenzamide hydrochloride compounded with 0.45% phenol as preservative, 0.5 mg sodium citrate and 0.2 mg citric acid as buffers and pH adjusted to approximately 5.0 with sodium hydroxide.

Thera-Ject® (Disposable Syringes): Each 2 mL contains 200 mg trimethobenzamide hydrochloride compounded with 0.45% phenol as preservative, 1 mg sodium citrate and 0.4 mg citric acid as buffers, 0.2 mg disodium edetate as stabilizer and pH adjusted to approximately 5.0 with sodium hydroxide.

ACTIONS

The mechanism of action of Tigan as determined in animals is obscure, but may be the chemoreceptor trigger zone (CTZ), an area in the medulla oblongata through which emetic impulses are conveyed to the vomiting center; direct impulses to the vomiting center apparently are not similarly inhibited. In dogs pretreated with trimethobenzamide HCl, the emetic response to apomorphine is inhibited, while little or no protection is afforded against emesis induced by intragastric copper sulfate.

INDICATIONS

Tigan is indicated for the control of nausea and vomiting.

CONTRAINDICATIONS

The injectable form of Tigan in children, the suppositories in premature or newborn infants, and use in patients with known hypersensitivity to trimethobenzamide are contraindicated. Since the suppositories contain benzocaine they should not be used in patients known to be sensitive to this or similar local anesthetics.

WARNINGS

Caution should be exercised when administering Tigan to children for the treatment of vomiting. Antiemetics are not recommended for treatment of uncomplicated vomiting in children and their use should be limited to prolonged vomiting of known etiology. There are three principal reasons for caution:

1. There has been some suspicion that centrally acting antiemetics may contribute, in combination with viral illnesses (a possible cause of vomiting in children), to development of Reye's syndrome, a potentially fatal acute childhood encephalopathy with visceral fatty degeneration, especially involving the liver. Although there is no confirmation of this suspicion, caution is nevertheless recommended.
2. The extrapyramidal symptoms which can occur secondary to Tigan may be confused with the central nervous system signs of an undiagnosed primary disease responsible for the vomiting, e.g., Reye's syndrome or other encephalopathy.
3. It has been suspected that drugs with hepatotoxic potential, such as Tigan, may unfavorably alter the course of Reye's syndrome. Such drugs should therefore be avoided in children whose signs and symptoms (vomiting) could represent Reye's syndrome. It should also be noted that salicylates and acetaminophen are hepatotoxic at large doses. Although it is not known that at usual doses they would represent a hazard in patients with the underlying hepatic disorder of Reye's syndrome, these drugs, too, should be avoided in children whose signs and symptoms could represent Reye's syndrome, unless alternative methods of controlling fever are not successful.

Tigan may produce drowsiness. Patients should not operate motor vehicles or other dangerous machinery until their individual responses have been determined. Reye's syndrome has been associated with the use of TIGAN and other drugs, including antiemetics, although their contribution, if any, to the cause and course of the disease hasn't been established. This syndrome is characterized by an abrupt onset shortly following a nonspecific febrile illness, with persistent, severe vomiting, lethargy, irrational behavior, progressive encephalopathy leading to coma, convulsions and death.

Usage in Pregnancy: Trimethobenzamide hydrochloride was studied in reproduction experiments in rats and rabbits and no teratogenicity was suggested. The only effects observed were an increased percentage of embryonic resorptions or stillborn pups in rats administered 20 mg and 100 mg/kg and increased resorptions in rabbits receiving 100 mg/kg. In each study these adverse effects were attributed to one or two dams. The relevance to humans is not known. Since there is no adequate experience in pregnant or lactating women who have received this drug, safety in pregnancy or in nursing mothers has not been established.

Usage with Alcohol: Concomitant use of alcohol with Tigan may result in an adverse drug interaction.

PRECAUTIONS

During the course of acute febrile illness, encephalitides, gastroenteritis, dehydration and electrolyte imbalance, especially in children and the elderly or debilitated, CNS reactions such as opisthotonos, convulsions, coma and extrapyramidal symptoms have been reported with and without use of Tigan or other antiemetic agents. In such disorders caution should be exercised in administering Tigan, particularly

to patients who have recently received other CNS-acting agents (phenothiazines, barbiturates, belladonna derivatives). It is recommended that severe emesis should not be treated with an antiemetic drug alone; where possible the cause of vomiting should be established. Primary emphasis should be directed toward the restoration of body fluids and electrolyte balance, the relief of fever and relief of the causative disease process. Overhydration should be avoided since it may result in cerebral edema.

The antiemetic effects of Tigan may render diagnosis more difficult in such conditions as appendicitis and obscure signs of toxicity due to overdosage of other drugs.

ADVERSE REACTIONS

There have been reports of hypersensitivity reactions and Parkinson-like symptoms. There have been instances of hypotension reported following parenteral administration to surgical patients. There have been reports of blood dyscrasias, blurring of vision, coma, convulsions, depression of mood, diarrhea, disorientation, dizziness, drowsiness, headache, jaundice, muscle cramps and opisthotonos. If these occur, the administration of the drug should be discontinued. Allergic-type skin reactions have been observed; therefore, the drug should be discontinued at the first sign of sensitization. While these symptoms will usually disappear spontaneously, symptomatic treatment may be indicated in some cases.

DOSAGE AND ADMINISTRATION

(See WARNINGS and PRECAUTIONS.)

Dosage should be adjusted according to the indication for therapy, severity of symptoms and the response of the patient.

CAPSULES, 250 mg and 100 mg

Usual Adult Dosage

One 250-mg capsule t.i.d. or q.i.d.

Usual Children's Dosage

30 to 90 lbs: One or two 100-mg capsules t.i.d. or q.i.d.

SUPPOSITORIES, 200 mg (Not to be used in premature or newborn infants).

Usual Adult Dosage

One suppository (200 mg) t.i.d. or q.i.d.

Usual Children's Dosage

Under 30 lbs: One-half suppository (100 mg) t.i.d. or q.i.d.

30 to 90 lbs: One-half to one suppository (100 to 200 mg) t.i.d. or q.i.d.

SUPPOSITORIES, PEDIATRIC, 100 mg (Not to be used in premature or newborn infants).

Usual Children's Dosage

Under 30 lbs: One suppository (100 mg) t.i.d. or q.i.d.

30 to 90 lbs: One to two suppositories (100 to 200 mg) t.i.d. or q.i.d.

INJECTABLE, 100 mg/mL (Not recommended for use in children).

Usual Adult Dosage

2 mL (200 mg) t.i.d. or q.i.d. intramuscularly.

Intramuscular administration may cause pain, stinging, burning, redness and swelling at the site of injection. Such effects may be minimized by deep injection into the upper outer quadrant of the gluteal region, and by avoiding the escape of solution along the route.

Note: The injectable form is intended for intramuscular administration only; it is not recommended for intravenous use.

CAUTION

Federal law prohibits dispensing without prescription.

HOW SUPPLIED

Capsules, 250 mg trimethobenzamide hydrochloride each, bottles of 100 and 500; 100 mg trimethobenzamide hydrochloride each, bottles of 100.

Suppositories, 200 mg, boxes of 10 and 50

Suppositories, Pediatric, 100 mg, boxes of 10

Ampuls, 2 mL, boxes of 10

Multiple Dose Vials, 20 mL

Thera-Ject® (Disposable Syringes), 2 mL, boxes of 25

0938212 Revised June, 1990

Shown in Product Identification Section, page 431

TIMENTIN® ℞

[*tī'mĕn-tĭn*]

(brand of sterile ticarcillin disodium and clavulanate potassium) for Intravenous Administration

DESCRIPTION

Timentin is an injectable antibacterial combination consisting of the semisynthetic antibiotic, ticarcillin disodium, and the β-lactamase inhibitor, clavulanate potassium (the potassium salt of clavulanic acid), for intravenous administration. Ticarcillin is derived from the basic penicillin nucleus, 6-amino-penicillanic acid. Chemically, it is 6-[(carboxy-3-thienylacetyl)amino]-3,3-dimethyl-7-oxo-4-thia-1-azabicyclo[3.2.0] heptane-2-carboxylic acid disodium salt and may be represented as:

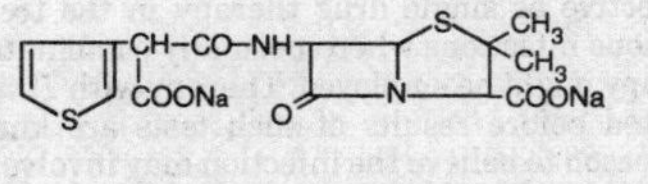

Clavulanic acid is produced by the fermentation of *Streptomyces clavuligerus*. It is a β-lactam structurally related to the penicillins and possesses the ability to inactivate a wide variety of β-lactamases by blocking the active sites of these enzymes. Clavulanic acid is particularly active against the clinically important plasmid-mediated β-lactamases frequently responsible for transferred drug resistance to penicillins and cephalosporins. Chemically, clavulanate potassium is potassium Z-(3R,5R)-2-(β-hydroxyethylidene) clavam-3-carboxylate and may be represented structurally as:

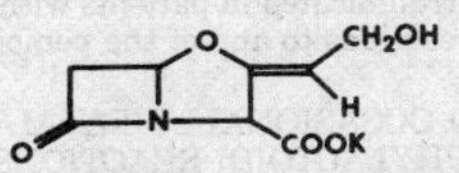

Timentin is supplied as a white to pale yellow powder for reconstitution. *Timentin* is very soluble in water, its solubility being greater than 600 mg/mL. The reconstituted solution is clear, colorless or pale yellow, having a pH of 5.5 to 7.5. For the *Timentin* 3.1 gram and 3.2 gram vials, the theoretical sodium content is 4.75 mEq (109 mg) per gram of *Timentin*. The theoretical potassium content is 0.15 mEq (6 mg) and 0.3 mEq (11.9 mg) per gram of *Timentin* for the 3.1 gram vial and 3.2 gram vial, respectively.

CLINICAL PHARMACOLOGY

After an intravenous infusion (30 min.) of 3.1 grams or 3.2 grams *Timentin*, peak serum concentrations of both ticarcillin and clavulanic acid are attained immediately after completion of infusion. Ticarcillin serum levels are similar to those produced by the administration of equivalent amounts of ticarcillin alone with a mean peak serum level of 330 mcg/mL for the 3.1 gram and 3.2 gram formulations. The corresponding mean peak serum levels for clavulanic acid were 8 mcg/mL and 16 mcg/mL for the 3.1 gram and 3.2 gram formulations, respectively. [See table above.]

SERUM LEVELS IN ADULTS
AFTER A 30-MINUTE I.V. INFUSION OF TIMENTIN®

TICARCILLIN SERUM LEVELS (mcg/mL)

Dose	0	15 min.	30 min.	1 hr.	1.5 hr.	3.5 hr.	5.5 hr.
3.1 gram	324 (293–388)	223 (184–293)	176 (135–235)	131 (102–195)	90 (65–119)	27 (19–37)	6 (5–7)
3.2 gram	336 (301–386)	214 (180–258)	186 (160–218)	122 (108–136)	78 (33–113)	29 (19–44)	10 (5–15)

CLAVULANIC ACID SERUM LEVELS (mcg/mL)

Dose	0	15 min.	30 min.	1 hr.	1.5 hr.	3.5 hr.	5.5 hr.
3.1 gram	8.0 (5.3–10.3)	4.6 (3.0–7.6)	2.6 (1.8–3.4)	1.8 (1.6–2.2)	1.2 (0.8–1.6)	0.3 (0.2–0.3)	0
3.2 gram	15.8 (11.7–21.0)	8.3 (6.4–10.0)	5.2 (3.5–6.3)	3.4 (1.9–4.0)	2.5 (1.3–3.4)	0.5 (0.2–0.8)	0

The mean area under the serum concentration curves for ticarcillin was 485 mcg/mL.hr. for the *Timentin* 3.1 gram and 3.2 gram formulations. The corresponding areas under the serum concentration curves for clavulanic acid were 8.2 mcg/mL.hr. and 15.6 mcg/mL.hr for the *Timentin* 3.1 gram and 3.2 gram formulations, respectively.

The mean serum half-lives of ticarcillin and clavulanic acid in healthy volunteers are 68 minutes and 64 minutes, respectively, following administration of 3.1 grams or 3.2 grams of *Timentin*.

Approximately 60–70% of ticarcillin and approximately 35–45% of clavulanic acid are excreted unchanged in urine during the first six hours after administration of a single dose of *Timentin* to normal volunteers with normal renal function. Two hours after an intravenous injection of 3.1 grams or 3.2 grams *Timentin*, concentrations of ticarcillin in urine generally exceed 1500 mcg/mL. The corresponding concentrations of clavulanic acid in urine generally exceed 40 mcg/mL and 70 mcg/mL following administration of the 3.1 gram and 3.2 gram doses, respectively. By four to six hours after injection, the urine concentrations of ticarcillin and clavulanic acid usually decline to approximately 190 mcg/mL and 2 mcg/mL, respectively, for both doses.

Neither component of *Timentin* is highly protein bound; ticarcillin has been found to be approximately 45% bound to human serum protein and clavulanic acid approximately 9% bound.

Somewhat higher and more prolonged serum levels of ticarcillin can be achieved with the concurrent administration of probenecid; however, probenecid does not enhance the serum levels of clavulanic acid.

Ticarcillin can be detected in tissues and interstitial fluid following parenteral administration.

Penetration of ticarcillin into the bile, pleural fluid and cerebrospinal fluid with inflamed meninges has been demonstrated. The results of experiments involving the administration of clavulanic acid to animals suggest that this compound, like ticarcillin, is well distributed in body tissues.

An inverse relationship exists between the serum half-life of ticarcillin and creatinine clearance. The dosage of *Timentin* need only be adjusted in cases of severe renal impairment (see DOSAGE AND ADMINISTRATION).

Ticarcillin may be removed from patients undergoing dialysis; the actual amount removed depends on the duration and type of dialysis.

MICROBIOLOGY: Ticarcillin is a semisynthetic antibiotic with a broad spectrum of bactericidal activity against many gram-positive and gram-negative aerobic and anaerobic bacteria.

Ticarcillin is, however, susceptible to degradation by β-lactamases and therefore the spectrum of activity does not normally include organisms which produce these enzymes.

Clavulanic acid is a β-lactam, structurally related to the penicillins, which possesses the ability to inactivate a wide range of β-lactamase enzymes commonly found in microorganisms resistant to penicillins and cephalosporins. In particular, it has good activity against the clinically important plasmid-mediated β-lactamases frequently responsible for transferred drug resistance.

The formulation of ticarcillin with clavulanic acid in *Timentin* protects ticarcillin from degradation by β-lactamase enzymes and effectively extends the antibiotic spectrum of ticarcillin to include many bacteria normally resistant to ticarcillin and other β-lactam antibiotics. Thus *Timentin* possesses the distinctive properties of a broad-spectrum antibiotic and a β-lactamase inhibitor.

While *in vitro* studies have demonstrated the susceptibility of most strains of the following organisms, clinical efficacy for infections other than those included in the INDICATIONS AND USAGE section has not been documented:

GRAM-NEGATIVE BACTERIA: *Pseudomonas aeruginosa* (β-lactamase and non-β-lactamase producing), *Pseudomonas* species including *P. maltophilia* (β-lactamase and non-β-lactamase producing), *Escherichia coli* (β-lactamase and non-β-lactamase producing), *Proteus mirabilis* (β-lactamase and non-β-lactamase producing), *Proteus vulgaris* (β-lactamase and non-β-lactamase producing), *Providencia rettgeri* (formerly *Proteus rettgeri*) (β-lactamase and non-β-lactamase producing), *Providencia stuartii* (β-lactamase and non-β-lactamase producing), *Morganella morganii* (formerly *Proteus morganii*) (β-lactamase and non-β-lactamase producing), *Enterobacter* species (Although most strains of *Enterobacter* species are resistant *in vitro*, clinical efficacy has been demonstrated with *Timentin* in urinary tract infections caused by these organisms.), *Acinetobacter* species (β-lactamase and non-β-lactamase producing), *Hemophilus influenzae* (β-lactamase and non-β-lactamase producing), *Branhamella catarrhalis* (β-lactamase and non-β-lactamase producing), *Serratia* species including *S. marcescens* (β-lactamase and non-β-lactamase producing), *Neisseria gonorrhoeae* (β-lactamase and non-β-lactamase producing), *Neisseria meningitidis**, *Salmonella* species (β-lactamase and non-β-lactamase producing), *Klebsiella* species including *K. pneumoniae* (β-lactamase and non-β-lactamase producing), *Citrobacter* species including *C. freundii*, *C. diversus* and *C. amalonaticus* (β-lactamase and non-β-lactamase producing).

GRAM-POSITIVE BACTERIA: *Staphylococcus aureus* (β-lactamase and non-β-lactamase producing), *Staphylococcus saprophyticus*, *Staphylococcus epidermidis* (coagulase-negative staphylococci) (β-lactamase and non-β-lactamase producing), *Streptococcus pneumoniae* * (*D. pneumoniae*), *Streptococcus bovis* *, *Streptococcus agalactiae* * (Group B), *Strepto-*

*These are non-β-lactamase-producing strains and therefore are susceptible to ticarcillin alone. Some of the β-lactamase-producing strains are also susceptible to ticarcillin alone.

Continued on next page

SmithKline Beecham—Cont.

coccus faecalis * (*Enterococcus*), *Streptococcus pyogenes* * (Group A, β-hemolytic), Viridans group streptococci *.

ANAEROBIC BACTERIA: *Bacteroides* species, including *B. fragilis* group (*B. fragilis, B. vulgatus*) (β-lactamase and non-β-lactamase producing), non-*B. fragilis* (*β-melaninogenicus*) (β-lactamase and non-β-lactamase producing), *B. thetaiotaomicron, B. ovatus, B. distasonis,* (β-lactamase and non-β-lactamase producing), *Clostridium* species including *C. perfringens, C. difficile, C. sporogenes, C. ramosum* and *C. bifermentans* *, *Eubacterium* species, *Fusobacterium* species *including F. nucleatum* and *F. necrophorum* *, *Peptococcus* species*, *Peptostreptococcus* species*, *Veillonella* species.

In vitro synergism between *Timentin* and gentamicin, tobramycin or amikacin against multiresistant strains of *Pseudomonas aeruginosa* has been demonstrated.

SUSCEPTIBILITY TESTING:

Diffusion Technique: An 85 mcg *Timentin* (75 mcg ticarcillin plus 10 mcg clavulanic acid) diffusion disk is available for use with the Kirby-Bauer method. Based on the zone sizes given below, a report of "Susceptible" indicates that the infecting organism is likely to respond to *Timentin* therapy, while a report of "Resistant" indicates that the organism is not likely to respond to therapy with this antibiotic. A report of "Intermediate" susceptibility indicates that the organism would be susceptible to *Timentin* at a higher dosage or if the infection is confined to tissues or fluids (e.g., urine) in which high antibiotic levels are attained.

Dilution Technique: Broth or agar dilution methods may be used to determine the minimal inhibitory concentration (MIC) values for bacterial isolates to *Timentin*. Tubes should be inoculated with the test culture containing 10^4 to 10^5 CFU/mL or plates spotted with a test solution containing 10^3 to 10^4 CFU/mL.

The recommended dilution pattern utilizes a constant level of clavulanic acid, 2 mcg/mL, in all tubes together with varying amounts of ticarcillin. MICs are expressed in terms of the ticarcillin concentration in the presence of 2 mcg/mL clavulanic acid.

RECOMMENDED RANGES FOR *Timentin* SUSCEPTIBILITY TESTING[1–3]

Diffusion Method Disk Zone Size, mm		
Res.	Inter.	Susc.
≤11	12–14	≥15

Dilution Method MIC Correlates[4], mcg/mL	
Res.	Susc.
≥128	≤64

[1] The non-β-lactamase-producing organisms which are normally susceptible to ticarcillin will have similar zone sizes as for ticarcillin.

[2] Staphylococci which are susceptible to *Timentin* but resistant to methicillin, oxacillin or nafcillin must be considered as resistant.

[3] The quality control cultures should have the following assigned daily ranges for *Timentin*:

		Disks	MIC Range (mcg/mL)
E. coli	(ATCC 25922)	24–30 mm	2/2–8/2
S. aureus	(ATCC 25923)	32–40 mm	—
Ps. aeruginosa	(ATCC 27853)	20–28 mm	8/2–32/2
E. coli	(ATCC 35218)	21–25 mm	4/2–16/2
S. aureus	(ATCC 29213)	—	0.5/2–2/2

[4] Expressed as concentration of ticarcillin in the presence of a constant 2.0 mcg/mL concentration of clavulanic acid.

INDICATIONS AND USAGE

Timentin is indicated in the treatment of infections caused by susceptible strains of the designated organisms in the conditions listed below:

Septicemia: including bacteremia, caused by β-lactamase-producing strains of *Klebsiella* spp.*, *E. coli**, *Staphylococcus aureus** and *Pseudomonas aeruginosa** (and other *Pseudomonas* species*).

Lower Respiratory Infections: caused by β-lactamase-producing strains of *Staphylococcus aureus, Hemophilus influenzae** and *Klebsiella* spp.*

Bone and Joint Infections: caused by β-lactamase-producing strains of *Staphylococcus aureus.*

Skin and Skin Structure Infections: caused by β-lactamase-producing strains of *Staphylococcus aureus, Klebsiella* spp.* and *E. coli**.

Urinary Tract Infections (complicated and uncomplicated): caused by β-lactamase-producing strains of *E. coli, Klebsiella* spp., *Pseudomonas aeruginosa** (and other *Pseudomonas* spp.*), *Citrobacter* spp.*, *Enterobacter cloacae**, *Serratia marcescens** and *Staphylococcus aureus**.

Gynecologic Infections: endometritis caused by β-lactamase-producing strains of *B. melaninogenicus**, *Enterobacter* spp. (including *E. cloacae**), *Escherichia coli, Klebsiella pneumoniae**, *Staphylococcus aureus* and *Staphylococcus epidermidis.*

Intra-abdominal Infections: peritonitis caused by β-lactamase-producing strains of *Escherichia coli, Klebsiella pneumoniae* and *Bacteroides fragilis** group.

*Efficacy for this organism in this organ system was studied in fewer than 10 infections.

While *Timentin* is indicated only for the conditions listed above, infections caused by ticarcillin-susceptible organisms are also amenable to *Timentin* treatment due to its ticarcillin content. Therefore, mixed infections caused by ticarcillin-susceptible organisms and β-lactamase-producing organisms susceptible to *Timentin* should not require the addition of another antibiotic.

Appropriate culture and susceptibility tests should be performed before treatment in order to isolate and identify organisms causing infection and to determine their susceptibility to *Timentin*. Because of its broad spectrum of bactericidal activity against gram-positive and gram-negative bacteria, *Timentin* is particularly useful for the treatment of mixed infections and for presumptive therapy prior to the identification of the causative organisms. *Timentin* has been shown to be effective as single drug therapy in the treatment of some serious infections where normally combination antibiotic therapy might be employed. Therapy with *Timentin* may be initiated before results of such tests are known when there is reason to believe the infection may involve any of the β-lactamase-producing organisms listed above; however, once these results become available, appropriate therapy should be continued.

Based on the *in vitro* synergism between *Timentin* and aminoglycosides against certain strains of *Pseudomonas aeruginosa,* combined therapy has been successful, especially in patients with impaired host defenses. Both drugs should be used in full therapeutic doses. As soon as results of culture and susceptibility tests become available, antimicrobial therapy should be adjusted as indicated.

CONTRAINDICATIONS

Timentin is contraindicated in patients with a history of hypersensitivity reactions to any of the penicillins.

WARNINGS

SERIOUS AND OCCASIONALLY FATAL HYPERSENSITIVITY (ANAPHYLACTOID) REACTIONS HAVE BEEN REPORTED IN PATIENTS ON PENICILLIN THERAPY. THESE REACTIONS ARE MORE LIKELY TO OCCUR IN INDIVIDUALS WITH A HISTORY OF PENICILLIN HYPERSENSITIVITY AND/OR A HISTORY OF SENSITIVITY TO MULTIPLE ALLERGENS. THERE HAVE BEEN REPORTS OF INDIVIDUALS WITH A HISTORY OF PENICILLIN HYPERSENSITIVITY WHO HAVE EXPERIENCED SEVERE REACTIONS WHEN TREATED WITH CEPHALOSPORINS. BEFORE INITIATING THERAPY WITH *TIMENTIN*, CAREFUL INQUIRY SHOULD BE MADE CONCERNING PREVIOUS HYPERSENSITIVITY REACTIONS TO PENICILLINS, CEPHALOSPORINS OR OTHER DRUGS. IF AN ALLERGIC REACTION OCCURS, *TIMENTIN* SHOULD BE DISCONTINUED AND THE APPROPRIATE THERAPY INSTITUTED. **SERIOUS ANAPHYLACTOID REACTIONS REQUIRE IMMEDIATE EMERGENCY TREATMENT WITH EPINEPHRINE. OXYGEN, INTRAVENOUS STEROIDS AND AIRWAY MANAGEMENT, INCLUDING INTUBATION, SHOULD ALSO BE PROVIDED AS INDICATED.**

Pseudomembranous colitis has been reported with nearly all antibacterial agents, including *Timentin,* and has ranged in severity from mild to life-threatening. Therefore, it is important to consider this diagnosis in patients who present with diarrhea subsequent to the administration of antibacterial agents.

Treatment with antibacterial agents alters the normal flora of the colon and may permit overgrowth of clostridia. Studies indicate that a toxin produced by *Clostridium difficile* is one primary cause of "antibiotic-associated colitis."

Mild cases of pseudomembranous colitis usually respond to drug discontinuation alone. In moderate to severe cases, consideration should be given to management with fluids and electrolytes, protein supplementation and treatment with an oral antibiotic drug effective against *C. difficile.*

PRECAUTIONS

General: While *Timentin* possesses the characteristic low toxicity of the penicillin group of antibiotics, periodic assessment of organ system functions, including renal, hepatic and hematopoietic function is advisable during prolonged therapy.

Bleeding manifestations have occurred in some patients receiving β-lactam antibiotics. These reactions have been associated with abnormalities of coagulation tests such as clotting time, platelet aggregation and prothrombin time and are more likely to occur in patients with renal impairment. If bleeding manifestations appear, *Timentin* treatment should be discontinued and appropriate therapy instituted.

Timentin has only rarely been reported to cause hypokalemia; however, the possibility of this occurring should be kept in mind particularly when treating patients with fluid and electrolyte imbalance. Periodic monitoring of serum potassium may be advisable in patients receiving prolonged therapy.

The theoretical sodium content is 4.75 mEq (109 mg) per gram of *Timentin*. This should be considered when treating patients requiring restricted salt intake.

As with any penicillin, an allergic reaction, including anaphylaxis, may occur during *Timentin* administration, particularly in a hypersensitive individual.

The possibility of superinfections with mycotic or bacterial pathogens should be kept in mind, particularly during prolonged treatment. If superinfections occur, appropriate measures should be taken.

Drug/Laboratory Test Interactions: As with other penicillins, the mixing of *Timentin* with an aminoglycoside in solutions for parenteral administration can result in substantial inactivation of the aminoglycoside.

Probenecid interferes with the renal tubular secretion of ticarcillin, thereby increasing serum concentrations and prolonging serum half-life of the antibiotic.

High urine concentrations of ticarcillin may produce false-positive protein reactions (pseudoproteinuria) with the following methods: sulfosalicylic acid and boiling test, acetic acid test, biuret reaction and nitric acid test. The bromphenol blue (Multi-stix®) reagent strip test has been reported to be reliable.

The presence of clavulanic acid in *Timentin* may cause a nonspecific binding of IgG and albumin by red cell membranes leading to a false-positive Coombs test.

Carcinogenesis, Mutagenesis, Impairment of Fertility: Long-term studies in animals have not been performed to evaluate carcinogenic or mutagenic potential.

Pregnancy (Category B): Reproduction studies have been performed in rats given doses up to 1050 mg/kg/day and have revealed no evidence of impaired fertility or harm to the fetus due to *Timentin*. There are, however, no adequate and well-controlled studies in pregnant women. Because animal reproduction studies are not always predictive of human response, this drug should be used during pregnancy only if clearly needed.

Nursing Mothers: Caution should be exercised when *Timentin* is administered to a nursing woman.

Pediatric Use: The efficacy and safety of *Timentin* have not been established in infants and children under the age of 12.

Drug Abuse and Dependence: Neither *Timentin* abuse nor *Timentin* dependence has been reported.

ADVERSE REACTIONS

As with other penicillins, the following adverse reactions may occur:

Hypersensitivity reactions: skin rash, pruritus, urticaria, arthralgia, myalgia, drug fever, chills, chest discomfort and anaphylactic reactions.

Central nervous system: headache, giddiness, neuromuscular hyperirritability or convulsive seizures.

Gastrointestinal disturbances: disturbances of taste and smell, stomatitis, flatulence, nausea, vomiting and diarrhea, epigastric pain and pseudomembranous colitis. Onset of pseudomembranous colitis symptoms may occur during or after antibiotic treatment (see WARNINGS).

Hemic and Lymphatic systems: thrombocytopenia, leukopenia, neutropenia, eosinophilia and reduction of hemoglobin or hematocrit. Prolongation of prothrombin time and bleeding time.

Abnormalities of hepatic and renal function tests: elevation of serum aspartate aminotransferase (SGOT), serum alanine aminotransferase (SGPT), serum alkaline phosphatase, serum LDH, serum bilirubin. Rarely, transient hepatitis and cholestatic jaundice—as with some other penicillins and some cephalosporins. Elevation of serum creatinine and/or BUN, hypernatremia. Reduction in serum potassium and uric acid.

Local reactions: pain, burning, swelling and induration at the injection site and thrombophlebitis with intravenous administration.

Overdosage: As with other penicillins, *Timentin* in overdosage has the potential to cause neuromuscular hyperirritability or convulsive seizures. Ticarcillin may be removed from circulation by hemodialysis. The molecular weight, degree of protein binding and pharmacokinetic profile of clavulanic acid together with information from a single patient with renal insufficiency all suggest that this compound may also be removed by hemodialysis.

DOSAGE AND ADMINISTRATION

Timentin should be administered by intravenous infusion (30 min.).

Adults: The usual recommended dosage for systemic and urinary tract infections for average (60 kg) adults is 3.1 grams *Timentin* (3.1 gram vial containing 3 grams ticarcillin and 100 mg clavulanic acid) given every four to six hours. For gynecologic infections, *Timentin* should be adminstered as follows: Moderate infections 200 mg/kg/day in divided doses every six hours and for severe infections 300 mg/kg/day in divided doses every four hours. For patients weighing less than 60 kg, the recommended dosage is 200–300 mg/kg/day,

based on ticarcillin content, given in divided doses every four to six hours.
In urinary tract infections, a dosage of 3.2 grams *Timentin* (3.2 gram vial containing 3 grams ticarcillin and 200 mg clavulanic acid) given every eight hours is adequate.
For infections complicated by renal insufficiency[1], an initial loading dose of 3.1 grams should be followed by doses based on creatinine clearance and type of dialysis as indicated below:

Creatinine clearance mL/min.	Dosage
over 60	3.1 grams every 4 hrs.
30–60	2 grams every 4 hrs.
10–30	2 grams every 8 hrs.
less than 10	2 grams every 12 hrs.
Less than 10 with hepatic dysfunction	2 grams every 24 hrs.
patients on peritoneal dialysis	3.1 grams every 12 hrs.
patients on hemodialysis	2 grams every 12 hrs. supplemented with 3.1 grams after each dialysis

To calculate creatinine clearance* from a serum creatinine value use the following formula.

$$C_{cr} = \frac{(140 - \text{Age})\ (\text{wt. in kg})}{72 \times S_{cr}(\text{mg}/100\ \text{mL})}$$

This is the calculated creatinine clearance for adult males; for females it is 15% less.

*Cockcroft, D. W., et al: Prediction of Creatinine Clearance from Serum Creatinine. Nephron 16:31-41, 1976.

Dosage for any individual patient must take into consideration the site and severity of infection the susceptibility of the organisms causing infection and the status of the patient's host defense mechanisms.
The duration of therapy depends upon the severity of infection. Generally, *Timentin* should be continued for at least two days after the signs and symptoms of infection have disappeared. The usual duration is 10 to 14 days; however, in difficult and complicated infections, more prolonged therapy may be required.
Frequent bacteriologic and clinical appraisal is necessary during therapy of chronic urinary tract infection and may be required for several months after therapy has been completed; persistent infections may require treatment for several weeks and doses smaller than those indicated above should not be used.
In certain infections, involving abscess formation, appropriate surgical drainage should be performed in conjunction with antimicrobial therapy.

INTRAVENOUS ADMINISTRATION

DIRECTIONS FOR USE

3.1 gram and 3.2 gram Vials and Piggyback Bottles

The 3.1 gram or 3.2 gram vial should be reconstituted by adding approximately 13 mL of Sterile Water for Injection, USP, or Sodium Chloride Injection, USP, and shaking well. When dissolved, the concentration of ticarcillin will be approximately 200 mg/mL with corresponding concentrations of 6.7 mg/mL and 13.4 mg/mL clavulanic acid for the 3.1 gram and 3.2 gram respective doses. Conversely, each 5.0 mL of the 3.1 gram dose reconstituted with approximately 13 mL of diluent will contain approximately 1 gram of ticarcillin and 33 mg of clavulanic acid. For the 3.2 gram dose reconstituted with 13 mL of diluent, each 5.0 mL will contain 1 gram of ticarcillin and 66 mg of clavulanic acid.
INTRAVENOUS INFUSION: The dissolved drug should be further diluted to desired volume using the recommended solution listed in the COMPATIBILITY AND STABILITY SECTION (STABILITY PERIOD) to a concentration between 10 mg/mL to 100 mg/mL. The solution of reconstituted drug may then be administered over a period of 30 minutes by direct infusion or through a Y-type intravenous infusion set. If this method or the "piggyback" method of administration is used, it is advisable to discontinue temporarily the administration of any other solutions during the infusion of *Timentin*.
Stability—For I.V. solutions, see STABILITY PERIOD below.
When *Timentin* is given in combination with another antimicrobial, such as an aminoglycoside, each drug should be given separately in accordance with the recommended dosage and routes of administration for each drug.
After reconstitution and prior to administration, *Timentin*, as with other parenteral drugs, should be inspected visually for particulate matter. If this condition is evident, the solution should be discarded.
The color of reconstituted solutions of *Timentin* normally ranges from light to dark yellow depending on concentration, duration and temperature of storage while maintaining label claim characteristics.

[1] The half-life of Ticarcillin in patients with renal failure is approximately 13 hours.

COMPATIBILITY AND STABILITY

3.1 gram and 3.2 gram Vials and Piggyback Bottles
(Dilutions derived from a stock solution of 200 mg/mL)
The concentrated stock solution at 200 mg/mL is stable for up to six hours at room temperature (70°–75°F) or up to 72 hours under refrigeration (40°F).
If the concentrated stock solution (200 mg/mL) is held for up to six hours at room temperature (70°–75°F) or up to 72 hours under refrigeration (40°F) and further diluted to a concentration between 10 mg/mL and 100 mg/mL with any of the diluents listed below, then the following stability periods apply.

STABILITY PERIOD
(3.1 gram and 3.2 gram Vials and Piggyback Bottles)

Intravenous Solution (ticarcillin concentrations of 10 mg/mL to 100 mg/mL)	Room Temperature (70°–75°F)	Refrigerated (40°F)
Dextrose Injection 5%, USP	24 hours	3 days
Sodium Chloride Injection, USP	24 hours	7 days
Lactated Ringer's Injection, USP	24 hours	7 days

If the concentrated stock solution (200 mg/mL) is stored for up to six hours at room temperature and then further diluted to a concentration between 10 mg/mL and 100 mg/mL, solutions of Sodium Chloride Injection, USP, and Lactated Ringer's Injection, USP may be stored frozen (0°F) for up to 30 days. Solutions prepared with Dextrose Injection 5%, USP may be stored frozen (0°F) for up to seven days. All thawed solutions should be used within eight hours or discarded. Once thawed, solutions should not be refrozen.
NOTE: *Timentin* is incompatible with Sodium Bicarbonate.
Unused solutions must be discarded after the time periods listed above.

HOW SUPPLIED

Timentin (sterile ticarcillin disodium and clavulanate potassium).
Each 3.1 gram vial contains sterile ticarcillin disodium equivalent to 3 grams ticarcillin and sterile clavulanate potassium equivalent to 0.1 gram clavulanic acid.
NDC 0029-6571-26 ....3.1 gram Vial
NDC 0029-6571-21 ....3.1 gram Piggyback Bottle
Timentin is also supplied as:
NDC 0029-6571-40 ......3.1 gram ADD-Vantage® Antibiotic Vial
NDC 0029-6579-21 ....31 gram Pharmacy Bulk Package
Each 31 gram vial contains sterile ticarcillin disodium equivalent to 30 grams ticarcillin and sterile clavulanate potassium equivalent to 1 gram clavulanic acid.
Timentin vials should be stored at room temperature or below.
TI:L2IV

Shown in Product Identification Section, page 431

TRIOSTAT™ ℞

[try'o-stat]
brand of liothyronine sodium injection (T_3)

DESCRIPTION

Thyroid hormone drugs are natural or synthetic preparations containing tetraiodothyronine (T_4, levothyroxine) sodium or triiodothyronine (T_3, liothyronine) sodium or both. T_4 and T_3 are produced in the human thyroid gland by the iodination and coupling of the amino acid tyrosine. T_4 contains four iodine atoms and is formed by the coupling of two molecules of diiodotyrosine (DIT). T_3 contains three atoms of iodine and is formed by the coupling of one molecule of DIT with one molecule of monoiodotyrosine (MIT). Both hormones are stored in the thyroid colloid as thyroglobulin and released into the circulation. The major source of T_3 has been shown to be peripheral deiodination of T_4. T_3 is bound less firmly than T_4 in the serum, enters peripheral tissues more readily, and binds to specific nuclear receptor(s) to initiate hormonal, metabolic effects. T_4 is the prohormone which is deiodinated to T_3 for hormone activity.
Thyroid hormone preparations belong to two categories: (1) natural hormonal preparations derived from animal thyroid, and (2) synthetic preparations. Natural preparations include desiccated thyroid and thyroglobulin. Desiccated thyroid is derived from domesticated animals that are used for food by man (either beef or hog thyroid), and thyroglobulin is derived from thyroid glands of the hog.
Triostat (liothyronine sodium injection) (T_3) contains liothyronine (L-triiodothyronine or L-T_3), a synthetic form of a natural thyroid hormone, as the sodium salt.
The structural and empirical formulas and molecular weight of liothyronine sodium are given above.

Liothyronine Sodium

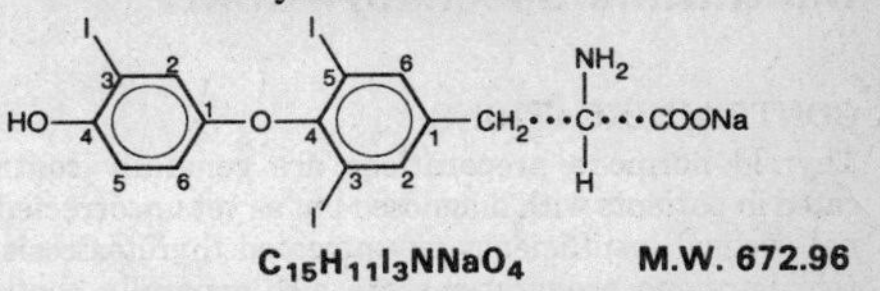

$C_{15}H_{11}I_3NNaO_4$ M.W. 672.96

L-Tyrosine, *O*-(4-hydroxy-3-iodophenyl)-3,5-diiodo-, monosodium salt

In euthyroid patients, 25 mcg of liothyronine is equivalent to approximately 1 grain of desiccated thyroid or thyroglobulin and 0.1 mg of L-thyroxine.
Each mL of *Triostat* in amber-glass vials contains, in sterile non-pyrogenic aqueous solution, sodium liothyronine equivalent to 10 mcg of liothyronine; alcohol, 6.8% by volume; anhydrous citric acid, 0.175 mg; ammonia, 2.19 mg, as ammonium hydroxide.

CLINICAL PHARMACOLOGY

Thyroid hormones enhance oxygen consumption by most tissues of the body and increase the basal metabolic rate and the metabolism of carbohydrates, lipids and proteins. In vitro studies indicate that T_3 increases aerobic mitochondrial function, thereby increasing the rates and synthesis and utilization of myocardial high-energy phosphates. This, in turn, stimulates myosin ATPase and reduces tissue lactic acidosis. Thus, thyroid hormones exert a profound influence on virtually every organ system in the body and are of particular importance in the development of the central nervous system.
While the source of levothyroxine (T_4) and some triiodothyronine (T_3) is via secretion from the thyroid gland, it is now well-established that approximately 80% of circulating T_3 arises predominantly by way of the extrathyroidal conversion of T_4. The membrane-bound enzyme responsible for this reaction is iodothyronine 5′-deiodinase. Activity of the enzyme is greatest in the liver and kidney. A second pathway of T_4 to T_3 conversion occurs via a PTU-insensitive 5′-deiodinase located primarily in the pituitary and central nervous system.
The prohormone T_4 must be converted to T_3 in the body before it can exert biological effects. During periods of illness or stress, this conversion is often inhibited and can be diverted to the inactive reverse T_3 (rT_3) moiety. Therefore, correction of the hypothyroid condition in patients with myxedema coma is facilitated by the parenteral administration of triiodothyronine (T_3). T_3 is bound much less firmly to serum binding proteins and therefore penetrates into the cells much more rapidly than T_4. Also, the binding of T_3 to a nuclear thyroid hormone receptor seems to initiate most of the effects of thyroid hormone in tissues. Although most thyroid hormone analogs, both natural and synthetic, will bind to this protein, the affinity of T_3 for this receptor is roughly 10-fold higher than that of T_4. Thus, T_3 is the biologically active thyroid hormone.

Pharmacodynamics

The clinical features of myxedema coma include depression of the cardiovascular, respiratory, gastrointestinal and central nervous systems, impaired diuresis, and hypothermia. Administration of thyroid hormones reverses or attenuates these conditions. Thyroid hormones increase heart rate, ventricular contractility and cardiac output, as well as decrease total systemic vascular resistance. They also increase the rate and depth of respiration, motility of the gastrointestinal tract, rapidity of cerebration, and vasodilatation. Thyroid hormones correct hypothermia by markedly increasing the basal metabolic rate, as well as the number and activity of mitochondria in almost all cells of the body.

Pharmacokinetics

Since liothyronine sodium (T_3) is not firmly bound to serum protein, it is readily available to body tissues.
Liothyronine sodium has a rapid cutoff of activity which permits quick dosage adjustment and facilitates control of the effects of overdosage, should they occur.
The higher affinity of levothyroxine (T_4) as compared to triiodothyronine (T_3) for both thyroid-binding globulin and thyroid-binding prealbumin partially explains the higher serum levels and longer half-life of the former hormone. Both protein-bound hormones exist in reverse equilibrium with minute amounts of free hormone, the latter accounting for the metabolic activity. T_4 is deiodinated to T_3.
A single dose of liothyronine sodium administered intravenously produces a detectable metabolic response in as little as two to four hours and a maximum therapeutic response within two days. However, no pharmacokinetic studies have been performed with intravenous liothyronine (T_3) in myxedema coma or precoma patients.

INDICATIONS AND USAGE

Triostat (liothyronine sodium injection) (T_3) is indicated in the treatment of myxedema coma/precoma.
Triostat can be used in patients allergic to desiccated thyroid or thyroid extract derived from pork or beef.

Continued on next page

SmithKline Beecham—Cont.

CONTRAINDICATIONS

Thyroid hormone preparations are generally contraindicated in patients with diagnosed but as yet uncorrected adrenal cortical insufficiency or untreated thyrotoxicosis. Thyroid hormone preparations are also generally contraindicated in patients with hypersensitivity to any of the active or extraneous constituents of these preparations; however, there is no well-documented evidence in the literature of true allergic or idiosyncratic reactions to thyroid hormone. Concomitant use of *Triostat* and artificial rewarming of patients is contraindicated. (See PRECAUTIONS.)

WARNINGS

> Drugs with thyroid hormone activity, alone or together with other therapeutic agents, have been used for the treatment of obesity. In euthyroid patients, doses within the range of daily hormonal requirements are ineffective for weight reduction. Larger doses may produce serious or even life-threatening manifestations of toxicity, particularly when given in association with sympathomimetic amines such as those used for their anorectic effects.

The use of thyroid hormones in the therapy of obesity, alone or combined with other drugs, is unjustified and has been shown to be ineffective. Neither is their use justified for the treatment of male or female infertility unless this condition is accompanied by hypothyroidism.

Thyroid hormones should be used with great caution in a number of circumstances where the integrity of the cardiovascular system, particularly the coronary arteries, is suspected. These include patients with angina pectoris or the elderly, in whom there is a greater likelihood of occult cardiac disease. Therefore, in patients with compromised cardiac function, use thyroid hormones in conjunction with careful cardiac monitoring. Although the specific dosage of *Triostat* depends upon individual circumstances, in patients with known or suspected cardiovascular disease the extremely rapid onset of action of *Triostat* may warrant initiating therapy at a dose of 10 mcg to 20 mcg. (See DOSAGE AND ADMINISTRATION.)

Myxedematous patients are very sensitive to thyroid hormones; dosage should be started at a low level and increased gradually as acute changes may precipitate adverse cardiovascular events.

Severe and prolonged hypothyroidism can lead to a decreased level of adrenocortical activity commensurate with the lowered metabolic state. When thyroid-replacement therapy is administered, the metabolism increases at a greater rate than adrenocortical activity. This can precipitate adrenocortical insufficiency. Therefore, in severe and prolonged hypothyroidism, supplemental adrenocortical steroids may be necessary.

In rare instances, the administration of thyroid hormone may precipitate a hyperthyroid state or may aggravate existing hyperthyroidism.

Extreme caution is advised when administering thyroid hormones with digitalis or vasopressors. (See PRECAUTIONS—Drug Interactions.)

Fluid therapy should be administered with great care to prevent cardiac decompensation. (See PRECAUTIONS—Adjunctive Therapy.)

PRECAUTIONS

General

Thyroid hormone therapy in patients with concomitant diabetes mellitus (see PRECAUTIONS—Drug Interactions, Insulin or Oral Hypoglycemics regarding interaction and dose adjustment with insulin) or insipidus or adrenal cortical insufficiency may aggravate the intensity of their symptoms. Appropriate adjustments of the various therapeutic measures directed at these concomitant endocrine diseases are required.

The therapy of myxedema coma requires simultaneous administration of glucocorticoids. (See PRECAUTIONS—Adjunctive Therapy.)

Hypothyroidism decreases and hyperthyroidism increases the sensitivity to anticoagulants. Prothrombin time should be closely monitored in thyroid-treated patients on anticoagulants and dosage of the latter agents adjusted on the basis of frequent prothrombin time determinations.

Oral therapy should be resumed as soon as the clinical situation has been stabilized and the patient is able to take oral medication. If L-thyroxine rather than liothyronine sodium is used in initiating oral therapy, the physician should bear in mind that there is a delay of several days in the onset of L-thyroxine activity and that intravenous therapy should be discontinued gradually.

Adjunctive Therapy

Many investigators recommend that corticosteroids be administered routinely in the initial emergency treatment of

all patients with myxedema coma. Patients with pituitary myxedema should receive adrenocortical hormone replacement therapy at or before the start of *Triostat* therapy. Similarly, patients with primary myxedema may also require adrenocortical hormone replacement therapy since a rapid return to normal body metabolism from a severely hypothyroid state may result in acute adrenocortical insufficiency and shock.

In considering the need to elevate blood pressure, it should be kept in mind that tissue metabolic requirements are markedly reduced in the hypothyroid patient. Because arrhythmias and circulatory collapse have infrequently occurred following the concomitant administration of thyroid hormones and vasopressor therapies, use caution when administering these therapies concomitantly. (See PRECAUTIONS—Drug Interactions, Vasopressors.)

Hyponatremia is frequently present in myxedema coma, but usually resolves without specific therapy as the metabolic status of the patient is improved with thyroid hormone treatment. Fluid therapy should be administered with great care to prevent cardiac decompensation. In addition, some patients with myxedema have inappropriate secretion of ADH and are susceptible to water intoxication.

In some patients, respiratory depression has been a significant factor in the development or persistence of the comatose state. Decreased oxygen saturation and elevated CO_2 levels respond quickly to artificial respiration.

Infection is often present in myxedema coma and should be looked for and treated appropriately.

Concomitant use of *Triostat* and artificial rewarming of patients is contraindicated. Although patients in myxedema coma are often hypothermic, most investigators believe that artificial rewarming is of little value or may be harmful. The peripheral vasodilation produced by external heat serves to further decrease circulation to vital internal organs and to increase shock if present. It has been reported that the administration of liothyronine sodium will restore a normal body temperature in 24 to 48 hours if heat loss is prevented by keeping the patient covered with blankets in a warm room.

Laboratory Tests

Treatment of patients with thyroid hormones requires the periodic assessment of thyroid status by means of appropriate laboratory tests besides the full clinical evaluation. Serum T_3 and TSH levels should be monitored to assess dosage adequacy and biologic effectiveness.

Drug Interactions

Oral Anticoagulants: Thyroid hormones appear to increase catabolism of vitamin K-dependent clotting factors. If oral anticoagulants are also being given, compensatory increases in clotting factor synthesis are impaired. Patients stabilized on oral anticoagulants who are found to require thyroid replacement therapy should be watched very closely when thyroid is started. If a patient is truly hypothyroid, it is likely that a reduction in anticoagulant dosage will be required. No special precautions appear to be necessary when oral anticoagulant therapy is begun in a patient already stabilized on maintenance thyroid replacement therapy.

Insulin or Oral Hypoglycemics: Initiating thyroid replacement therapy may cause increases in insulin or oral hypoglycemic requirements. The effects seen are poorly understood and depend upon a variety of factors such as dose and type of thyroid preparations and endocrine status of the patient. Patients receiving insulin or oral hypoglycemics should be closely watched during initiation of thyroid replacement therapy.

Estrogen, Oral Contraceptives: Estrogens tend to increase serum thyroxine-binding globulin (TBG). In a patient with a nonfunctioning thyroid gland who is receiving thyroid replacement therapy, free levothyroxine may be decreased when estrogens are started thus increasing thyroid requirements. However, if the patient's thyroid gland has sufficient function, the decreased free thyroxine will result in a compensatory increase in thyroxine output by the thyroid. Therefore, patients without a functioning thyroid gland who are on thyroid replacement therapy may need to increase their thyroid dose if estrogens or estrogen-containing oral contraceptives are given.

Tricyclic Antidepressants: Use of thyroid products with imipramine and other tricyclic antidepressants may increase receptor sensitivity and enhance antidepressant activity; transient cardiac arrhythmias have been observed. Thyroid hormone activity may also be enhanced.

Digitalis: Thyroid preparations may potentiate the toxic effects of digitalis. Thyroid hormonal replacement increases metabolic rate, which requires an increase in digitalis dosage.

Ketamine: When administered to patients on a thyroid preparation, this parenteral anesthetic may cause hypertension and tachycardia. Use with caution and be prepared to treat hypertension, if necessary.

Vasopressors: Thyroid hormones increase the adrenergic effect of catecholamines such as epinephrine and norepinephrine. Therefore, use of vasopressors in patients receiving thyroid hormone preparations may increase the risk of precipitating coronary insufficiency, especially in patients

with coronary artery disease. Therefore, use caution when administering vasopressors with liothyronine (T_3).

Drug/Laboratory Test Interactions

The following drugs or moieties are known to interfere with laboratory tests performed in patients on thyroid hormone therapy: androgens, corticosteroids, estrogens, oral contraceptives containing estrogens, iodine-containing preparations and the numerous preparations containing salicylates.

1. Changes in TBG concentration should be taken into consideration in the interpretation of T_4 and T_3 values. In such cases, the unbound (free) hormone should be measured. Pregnancy, estrogens and estrogen-containing oral contraceptives increase TBG concentrations. TBG may also be increased during infectious hepatitis. Decreases in TBG concentrations are observed in nephrosis, acromegaly and after androgen or corticosteroid therapy. Familial hyper- or hypo-thyroxine-binding globulinemias have been described. The incidence of TBG deficiency approximates 1 in 9000. The binding of thyroxine by thyroxine-binding prealbumin (TBPA) is inhibited by salicylates.

2. Medicinal or dietary iodine interferes with all *in vivo* tests of radioiodine uptake, producing low uptakes which may not be reflective of a true decrease in hormone synthesis.

Carcinogenesis, Mutagenesis and Impairment of Fertility

A reportedly apparent association between prolonged thyroid therapy and breast cancer has not been confirmed and patients on thyroid for established indications should not discontinue therapy. No confirmatory long-term studies in animals have been performed to evaluate carcinogenic potential, mutagenicity, or impairment of fertility in either males or females.

Pregnancy

Pregnancy Category A: Thyroid hormones do not readily cross the placental barrier. The clinical experience to date does not indicate any adverse effect on fetuses when thyroid hormones are administered to pregnant women. On the basis of current knowledge, thyroid replacement therapy to hypothyroid women should not be discontinued during pregnancy.

Nursing Mothers

Minimal amounts of thyroid hormones are excreted in human milk. Thyroid hormones are not associated with serious adverse reactions and do not have a known tumorigenic potential. However, caution should be exercised when thyroid hormones are administered to a nursing woman.

Pediatric Use

There is limited experience with *Triostat* in children. Safety and effectiveness have not been established.

ADVERSE REACTIONS

The most frequently reported adverse events were arrhythmia (6% of patients) and tachycardia (3%). Cardiopulmonary arrest, hypotension and myocardial infarction occurred in approximately 2% of patients. The following events occurred in approximately 1% or fewer of patients: angina, congestive heart failure, fever, hypertension, phlebitis and twitching. In rare instances, allergic skin reactions have been reported with liothyronine sodium tablets.

OVERDOSAGE

Signs and Symptoms: Headache, irritability, nervousness, tremor, sweating, increased bowel motility and menstrual irregularities. Angina pectoris, arrhythmia, tachycardia, acute myocardial infarction or congestive heart failure may be induced or aggravated. Shock may also develop if there is untreated pituitary or adrenocortical failure. Massive overdosage may result in symptoms resembling thyroid storm.

Treatment of Overdosage: Dosage should be reduced or therapy temporarily discontinued if signs and symptoms of overdosage appear. Treatment may be reinstituted at a lower dosage. In normal individuals, normal hypothalamic-pituitary-thyroid axis function is restored in six to eight weeks after cessation of therapy following thyroid suppression.

Treatment is symptomatic and supportive. Oxygen may be administered and ventilation maintained. Cardiac glycosides may be indicated if congestive heart failure develops. Beta-adrenergic antagonists have been used advantageously in the treatment of increased sympathetic activity. Measures to control fever, hypoglycemia or fluid loss should be instituted if needed.

DOSAGE AND ADMINISTRATION

Adults

Myxedema coma is usually precipitated in the hypothyroid patient of long standing by intercurrent illness or drugs such as sedatives and anesthetics and should be considered a medical emergency. Therapy should be directed at the correction of electrolyte disturbances, possible infection, or other intercurrent illness in addition to the administration of intravenous liothyronine (T_3). Simultaneous glucocorticosteroids are required.

Triostat (liothyronine sodium injection) (T_3) is for intravenous administration only. It should not be given intramuscularly or subcutaneously.

- Prompt administration of an adequate dose of intravenous liothyronine (T_3) is important in determining clinical outcome.
- Initial and subsequent doses of *Triostat* should be based on continuous monitoring of the patient's clinical status and response to therapy.
- *Triostat* doses should normally be administered at least four hours—and not more than 12 hours—apart.
- Administration of at least 65 mcg/day of intravenous liothyronine (T_3) in the initial days of therapy was associated with lower mortality.
- There is limited clinical experience with intravenous liothyronine (T_3) at total daily doses exceeding 100 mcg/day.

No controlled clinical studies have been done with *Triostat*. The following dosing guidelines have been derived from data analysis of myxedema coma/precoma case reports collected by SmithKline Beecham Pharmaceuticals since 1963 and from scientific literature since 1956.

An initial intravenous *Triostat* dose ranging from 25 mcg to 50 mcg is recommended in the emergency treatment of myxedema coma/precoma in adults. In patients with known or suspected cardiovascular disease, an initial dose of 10 mcg to 20 mcg is suggested (see WARNINGS). However, both the initial dose and subsequent doses should be determined on the basis of continuous monitoring of the patient's clinical condition and response to *Triostat* therapy. Normally at least four hours should be allowed between doses to adequately assess therapeutic response and no more than 12 hours should elapse between doses to avoid fluctuations in hormone levels. Caution should be exercised in adjusting the dose due to the potential of large changes to precipitate adverse cardiovascular events. Review of the myxedema case reports indicates decreased mortality in patients receiving at least 65 mcg/day in the initial days of treatment. However, there is limited clinical experience at total daily doses above 100 mcg. See PRECAUTIONS—Drug Interactions for potential interactions between thyroid hormones and digitalis and vasopressors.

Pediatric Use

There is limited experience with *Triostat* in children. Safety and effectiveness have not been established.

Switching to Oral Therapy

Oral therapy should be resumed as soon as the clinical situation has been stabilized and the patient is able to take oral medication. When switching a patient to liothyronine sodium tablets from *Triostat*, discontinue *Triostat*, initiate oral therapy at a low dosage, and increase gradually according to the patient's response.

If L-thyroxine rather than liothyronine sodium is used in initiating oral therapy, the physician should bear in mind that there is a delay of several days in the onset of L-thyroxine activity and that intravenous therapy should be discontinued gradually.

HOW SUPPLIED

In packages of six 1 mL vials at a concentration of 10 mcg/ mL.
NDC 0007-5210-06
Store between 2° and 8°C.
TS:L1

Shown in Product Identification Section, page 431

TUSS-ORNADE® ℞

[*tuss 'or-naid '*]
LIQUID

DESCRIPTION

Each 5 mL (one teaspoonful) of clear, fruit-flavored *Tuss-Ornade* Liquid contains caramiphen edisylate, 6.7 mg; phenylpropanolamine hydrochloride, 12.5 mg; and alcohol, 5.0%. Inactive ingredients consist of citric acid, flavors, glycerin, menthol, methylparaben, propylparaben, sodium citrate, sorbitol and water.

ACTIONS

The *Tuss-Ornade* formula contains caramiphen edisylate, a synthetic, non-narcotic cough suppressant, and phenylpropanolamine hydrochloride, a vasoconstrictor with decongestant action on nasal and upper respiratory tract mucosal membranes.

INDICATIONS

For the symptomatic relief of coughs and nasal congestion associated with common colds.

N.B.: A final determination has not been made on the effectiveness of this drug combination in accordance with efficacy requirements of the 1962 Amendments to the Food, Drug and Cosmetic Act.

CONTRAINDICATIONS

Hypersensitivity to either of the components; concurrent MAO inhibitor therapy; severe hypertension; bronchial asthma; coronary artery disease.

Do not use *Tuss-Ornade* Liquid in children under 15 pounds or in children less than six months of age.

PRECAUTIONS

Use with caution in patients with cardiovascular disease, glaucoma, prostatic hypertrophy, thyroid disease or diabetes. Use with caution in patients in whom productive cough is desirable to clear excessive secretions from the bronchial tree. Patients taking this medication should be cautioned not to take simultaneously other products containing phenylpropanolamine HCl or amphetamines.

Usage in Pregnancy: Safe use in pregnancy has not been established. This drug should not be used in pregnancy, nursing mothers, or women of childbearing potential unless, in the judgment of the physician, the anticipated benefits outweigh the potential risks.

ADVERSE REACTIONS

Adverse effects associated with products containing a centrally acting antitussive or sympathomimetic amine may occur and include: nausea, gastrointestinal upset, diarrhea, constipation, dizziness, drowsiness, nervousness, insomnia, anorexia, weakness, tightness of chest, angina pain, irritability, palpitations, headache, incoordination, tremor, difficulty in urination, dysuria, hypertension, hypotension, visual disturbances.

DOSAGE AND ADMINISTRATION

Adults and children over 12 years—2 teaspoonfuls every 4 hours; do not exceed 12 teaspoonfuls in 24 hours. Children 6 to 12 years—1 teaspoonful every 4 hours; do not exceed 6 teaspoonfuls in 24 hours. Children 2 to 6 years—½ teaspoonful every 4 hours; do not exceed 3 teaspoonfuls in 24 hours. Data are not available on which to base dosage recommendations for children under 2 years of age. **Do not use in children under 15 pounds or less than 6 months old.**

OVERDOSAGE

Symptoms—May include dryness of mouth, dysphagia, thirst, blurred vision, dilated pupils, photophobia, fever, rapid pulse and respiration, disorientation, dizziness, nausea, fainting, tachycardia, and either excitation or depression of the central nervous system.

Treatment—Immediate evacuation of the stomach should be induced by emesis and gastric lavage, repeated as necessary. Respiratory depression should be treated promptly with oxygen and respiratory stimulants. Do not treat respiratory or CNS depression with analeptics that might precipitate convulsions. If marked excitement occurs, a short-acting barbiturate or chloral hydrate may be used.

SUPPLIED

Liquid containing caramiphen edisylate 6.7 mg; phenylpropanolamine hydrochloride 12.5 mg; and alcohol 5.0% per 5 mL (one teaspoonful), in 8 fl oz bottles.

TOL:L17

TUSS-ORNADE® ℞

[*tuss 'or-naid '*]
SPANSULE® CAPSULES
brand of sustained release capsules

DESCRIPTION

Each *Tuss-Ornade* Spansule capsule, with opaque light blue cap and natural body, is imprinted with the product name TUSS-ORNADE and SKF and contains caramiphen edisylate, 40 mg and phenylpropanolamine hydrochloride,75 mg. Inactive ingredients consist of benzyl alcohol, cetylpyridinium chloride, D&C Red No. 33, FD&C Blue No. 1, FD&C Red No. 3, FD&C Yellow No. 6, D&C Red No. 27, D&C Red No. 30, gelatin, glyceryl distearate, polyethylene glycol, povidone, silicon dioxide, sodium lauryl sulfate, starch, sucrose, titanium dioxide, wax and trace amounts of other inactive ingredients.

Each *Tuss-Ornade* Spansule capsule is so prepared that an initial dose is released promptly and the remaining medication is released gradually over a prolonged period.

ACTIONS

The *Tuss-Ornade* formula contains caramiphen edisylate, a synthetic, non-narcotic cough suppressant, and phenylpropanolamine hydrochloride, a vasoconstrictor with decongestant action on nasal and upper respiratory tract mucosal membranes.

Pharmacokinetics: At steady-state conditions, the following peak levels are reached after the oral administration of a *Spansule* capsule: 24 ng/mL caramiphen in 4.6 hours; 200 ng/mL phenylpropanolamine in 5.5 hours; the half-lives are approximately 11 and 8 hours, respectively.

INDICATIONS

For the symptomatic relief of coughs and nasal congestion associated with common colds.

N.B.: A final determination has not been made on the effectiveness of this drug combination in accordance with efficacy requirements of the 1962 Amendments to the Food, Drug and Cosmetic Act.

CONTRAINDICATIONS

Hypersensitivity to either of the components; concurrent MAO inhibitor therapy; severe hypertension; bronchial asthma; coronary artery disease.

Do not use *Tuss-Ornade* Spansule capsules in children under 12 years of age.

PRECAUTIONS

Use with caution in persons with cardiovascular disease, glaucoma, prostatic hypertrophy, thyroid disease or diabetes. Use with caution in patients in whom productive cough is desirable to clear excessive secretions from the bronchial tree. Patients taking this medication should be cautioned not to take simultaneously other products containing phenylpropanolamine HCl or amphetamines.

Usage in Pregnancy: Safe use in pregnancy has not been established. This drug should not be used in pregnancy, nursing mothers, or women of childbearing potential unless, in the judgment of the physician, the anticipated benefits outweigh the potential risks.

ADVERSE REACTIONS

Adverse effects associated with products containing a centrally acting antitussive or sympathomimetic amine may occur and include: nausea, gastrointestinal upset, diarrhea, constipation, dizziness, drowsiness, nervousness, insomnia, anorexia, weakness, tightness of chest, angina pain, irritability, palpitation, headache, incoordination, tremor, difficulty in urination, dysuria, hypertension, hypotension, visual disturbances.

DOSAGE AND ADMINISTRATION

Tuss-Ornade Spansule capsules: Adults and children 12 years of age and over—one *Tuss-Ornade* Spansule capsule every 12 hours. **Do not use in children under 12 years of age.**

OVERDOSAGE

Symptoms—May include dryness of mouth, dysphagia, thirst, blurred vision, dilated pupils, photophobia, fever, rapid pulse and respiration, disorientation, dizziness, nausea, fainting, tachycardia, and either excitation or depression of the central nervous system.

Treatment—Immediate evacuation of the stomach should be induced by emesis and gastric lavage, repeated as necessary. Respiratory depression should be treated promptly with oxygen and respiratory stimulants. Do not treat respiratory or CNS depression with analeptics that might precipitate convulsions. If marked excitement occurs, a short-acting barbiturate or chloral hydrate may be used.

Since much of the *Spansule* capsule medication is coated for gradual release, saline cathartics should be administered to hasten evacuation of pellets that have not already released medication.

SUPPLIED

Spansule capsules (brand of sustained release capsules) containing caramiphen edisylate 40 mg and phenylpropanolamine hydrochloride 75 mg, in bottles of 50 and 500.

TO:L36

Shown in Product Identification Section, page 431

URISPAS® ℞

[*yore 'eh-spaz*]
(brand of flavoxate HCl)
100 mg. tablets

DESCRIPTION

Urispas (flavoxate HCl, SK&F) tablets contain flavoxate hydrochloride, a synthetic urinary tract spasmolytic.

Chemically, flavoxate hydrochloride is 2-piperidinoethyl 3-methyl -4- oxo-2-phenyl-4H-1-benzopyran -8- carboxylate hydrochloride. The empirical formula of flavoxate hydrochloride is $C_{24}H_{25}NO_4 \cdot HCl$. The molecular weight is 427.94. 'Urispas' is supplied in tablets for oral administration. Each round, white, film-coated 'Urispas' tablet is debossed URISPAS SKF and contains flavoxate hydrochloride, 100 mg. Inactive ingredients consist of calcium phosphate, castor oil, cellulose acetate phthalate, magnesium stearate, polyethylene glycol, starch and talc.

CLINICAL PHARMACOLOGY

Flavoxate hydrochloride counteracts smooth muscle spasm of the urinary tract and exerts its effect directly on the muscle.

In a single study of 11 normal male subjects, the time to onset of action was 55 minutes. The peak effect was observed at 112 minutes. 57% of the flavoxate HCl was excreted in the urine within 24 hours.

INDICATIONS AND USAGE

Urispas (flavoxate HCl, SK&F) is indicated for symptomatic relief of dysuria, urgency, nocturia, suprapubic pain, fre-

Continued on next page

SmithKline Beecham—Cont.

quency and incontinence as may occur in cystitis, prostatitis, urethritis, urethrocystitis/urethrotrigonitis. 'Urispas' is not indicated for definitive treatment, but is compatible with drugs used for the treatment of urinary tract infections.

CONTRAINDICATIONS

Urispas (flavoxate HCl, SK&F) is contraindicated in patients who have any of the following obstructive conditions: pyloric or duodenal obstruction, obstructive intestinal lesions or ileus, achalasia, gastrointestinal hemorrhage, and obstructive uropathies of the lower urinary tract.

WARNINGS

Urispas (flavoxate HCl, SK&F) should be given cautiously in patients with suspected glaucoma.

PRECAUTIONS

Information for Patients: Patients should be informed that if drowsiness and blurred vision occur, they should not operate a motor vehicle or machinery or participate in activities where alertness is required.

Carcinogenesis, Mutagenesis, Impairment of Fertility: Mutagenicity studies and long-term studies in animals to determine the carcinogenic potential of Urispas (flavoxate HCl, SK&F) have not been performed.

Pregnancy: Teratogenic Effects—Pregnancy Category B. Reproduction studies have been performed in rats and rabbits at doses up to 34 times the human dose and revealed no evidence of impaired fertility or harm to the fetus due to flavoxate HCl. There are, however, no well-controlled studies in pregnant women. Because animal reproduction studies are not always predictive of human response, this drug should be used during pregnancy only if clearly needed.

Nursing Mothers: It is not known whether this drug is excreted in human milk. Because many drugs are excreted in human milk, caution should be exercised when 'Urispas' is administered to a nursing woman.

Pediatric Use: Safety and effectiveness in children below the age of 12 years have not been established.

ADVERSE REACTIONS

The following adverse reactions have been observed, but there are not enough data to support an estimate of their frequency.

Gastrointestinal: Nausea, vomiting, dry mouth.

CNS: Vertigo, headache, mental confusion, especially in the elderly, drowsiness, nervousness.

Hematologic: Leukopenia (one case which was reversible upon discontinuation of the drug).

Cardiovascular: Tachycardia and palpitation.

Allergic: Urticaria and other dermatoses, eosinophilia and hyperpyrexia.

Ophthalmic: Increased ocular tension, blurred vision, disturbance in eye accommodation.

Renal: Dysuria.

OVERDOSAGE

The oral LD_{50} for flavoxate HCl in rats is 4273 mg./kg. The oral LD_{50} for flavoxate HCl in mice is 1837 mg./kg.
It is not known whether flavoxate HCl is dialyzable.

DOSAGE AND ADMINISTRATION

Adults and children over 12 years of age: One or two 100 mg. tablets three or four times a day. With improvement of symptoms, the dose may be reduced. This drug cannot be recommended for infants and children under 12 years of age because safety and efficacy have not been demonstrated in this age group.

HOW SUPPLIED

Urispas (flavoxate HCl, SK&F) tablets, 100 mg., in bottles of 100 and in Single Unit Packages of 100 (intended for institutional use only).

Military—Tablets, 100 mg, 100's, 6505-00-172-3420

UR:L16

Shown in Product Identification Section, page 431

VONTROL® ℞

[vohn 'trole]

(brand of diphenidol)

'Vontrol' may cause hallucinations, disorientation, or confusion. For this reason, its use is limited to patients who are hospitalized or under comparable, continuous, close, professional supervision. Even then, the physician should carefully weigh the benefits against the possible risks and give due consideration to alternate therapeutic measures.

DESCRIPTION

Diphenidol, α, α-diphenyl-1-piperidinebutanol, is a compound not related to the antihistamines, phenothiazines, barbiturates, or other agents with antivertigo or antiemetic action.

Each round, orange 'Vontrol' tablet is debossed SKF and 25 and contains diphenidol hydrochloride equivalent to diphenidol, 25 mg. Inactive ingredients consist of acacia, calcium sulfate, cellulose, FD&C Yellow No. 5 (tartrazine), FD&C Yellow No. 6, magnesium stearate and starch.

ACTIONS

'Vontrol' (diphenidol, SK&F) apparently exerts a specific antivertigo effect on the vestibular apparatus to control vertigo and inhibits the chemoreceptor trigger zone to control nausea and vomiting.

INDICATIONS (SEE WARNINGS)

1) VERTIGO—'Vontrol' is indicated in peripheral (labyrinthine) vertigo and associated nausea and vomiting, as seen in such conditions as: Meniere's disease, middle- and inner-ear surgery (labyrinthitis).
2) NAUSEA AND VOMITING—'Vontrol' is indicated in the control of nausea and vomiting, as seen in such conditions as: postoperative states, malignant neoplasms and labyrinthine disturbances.

CONTRAINDICATIONS

Known hypersensitivity to the drug is a contraindication. Anuria is a contraindication. (Since approximately 90% of the drug is excreted in the urine, renal shutdown could cause systemic accumulation.)

WARNINGS

'Vontrol' (diphenidol, SK&F) may cause hallucinations, disorientation or confusion. For this reason, its use is limited to patients who are hospitalized or under comparable, continuous, close, professional supervision. Even then, the physician should carefully weigh the benefits against the possible risks and give due consideration to alternate therapeutic measures.

The incidence of auditory and visual hallucinations, disorientation and confusion appears to be less than ½% or approximately one in 350 patients. The reaction has usually occurred within three days of starting the drug in recommended dosage and has subsided spontaneously usually within three days after discontinuation of the drug. Patients on 'Vontrol' should be observed closely and in the event of such a reaction the drug should be stopped.

Usage in Pregnancy: Use of any drug in pregnancy, lactation or in women of childbearing age requires that the potential benefits of the drug be weighed against its possible hazards to the mother and child.

In animal teratogenesis and reproduction studies of 'Vontrol' (diphenidol, SK&F), there were no significant differences between drug-treated groups and untreated control groups, except as noted under animal Reproduction Studies (see "Pharmacology [animal]").

In 936 patients who received 'Vontrol' during pregnancy, the incidences of normal and abnormal birth were comparable to those reported in the literature for the average population of pregnant patients. And in no instance was there any evidence that 'Vontrol' played a part in birth abnormality (see "In Pregnancy").

'Vontrol' is not indicated for use in nausea and vomiting of pregnancy, since the therapeutic value and safety in this indication have not yet been determined.

PRECAUTIONS

The antiemetic action of 'Vontrol' (diphenidol, SK&F) may mask signs of overdose of drugs (e.g., digitalis) or may obscure diagnosis of conditions such as intestinal obstruction and brain tumor.

Although there have been no reports of blood dyscrasias with 'Vontrol', patients should be observed regularly for any idiosyncratic reactions.

'Vontrol' has a weak peripheral anticholinergic effect and should be used with care in patients with glaucoma, obstructive lesions of the gastrointestinal and genitourinary tracts, such as stenosing peptic ulcer, prostatic hypertrophy, pyloric and duodenal obstruction, and organic cardiospasm.

'Vontrol' Tablets contain FD&C Yellow No. 5 (tartrazine) which may cause allergic-type reactions (including bronchial asthma) in certain susceptible individuals. Although the overall incidence of FD&C Yellow No. 5 (tartrazine) sensitivity in the general population is low, it is frequently seen in patients who also have aspirin hypersensitivity.

Usage in Children

'Vontrol' is not recommended for use in children under 50 pounds. (See Dosage and Administration—Children.)

ADVERSE REACTIONS

Auditory and visual hallucinations, disorientation and confusion have been reported. Drowsiness, overstimulation, depression, sleep disturbance, dry mouth, g.i. irritation (nausea and indigestion), or blurred vision may occur.

Rarely, slight dizziness, skin rash, malaise, headache, or heartburn may occur. Mild jaundice of questionable relationship to the use of 'Vontrol' (diphenidol, SK&F) has been reported. Slight, transient lowering of blood pressure has been reported in a few patients.

(See laboratory studies under "Pharmacology [human]".)

DOSAGE AND ADMINISTRATION (SEE WARNINGS)

ADULTS—FOR VERTIGO OR NAUSEA AND VOMITING: The usual dose is one tablet (25 mg.) every four hours as needed. Some patients may require two tablets (50 mg.).

CHILDREN—FOR NAUSEA AND VOMITING: These recommendations are for nausea and vomiting only. There has been no experience with 'Vontrol' in vertigo in children. Unit doses in children are best calculated by body weight: usually 0.4 mg./lb.

Children's doses usually should not be given more often than every four hours. However, if symptoms persist after the first dose, administration may be repeated after one hour. Thereafter, doses may be given every four hours as needed. The total dose in 24 hours should not exceed 2.5 mg./lb.

NOTE: The drug is not recommended for use in children under 50 pounds. The dosage for children 50 to 100 pounds is one tablet (25 mg.).

OVERDOSAGE

In the event of overdosage, the patient should be managed according to his symptoms. Treatment is essentially supportive, with maintenance of blood pressure and respiration, plus careful observation. Early gastric lavage may be indicated depending on the amount of overdose and nature of symptoms.

HOW SUPPLIED

Tablets containing 25 mg. diphenidol, as the hydrochloride, in bottles of 100.

PHARMACOLOGY (animal): 'Vontrol' (diphenidol, SK&F) exerts its antiemetic effect primarily by inhibiting the chemoreceptor trigger zone, as evidenced by its activity in blocking emesis induced by apomorphine in dogs. In this regard 'Vontrol', as the hydrochloride salt, has a potency equal to the potent phenothiazine antiemetic, chlorpromazine hydrochloride. In animals 'Vontrol' has only weak parasympatholytic activity and no significant sedative, tranquilizing or antihistaminic action or effects on blood pressure, heart rate, respiration or the electrocardiogram.

Subacute and chronic toxicity studies in rats and dogs, in which large doses of 'Vontrol', as the hydrochloride salt, were administered orally and intramuscularly for periods up to one year, revealed no significant effects on hematology, liver function, kidney function or blood glucose determinations. Histological examination of the animals' tissues did not reveal any significant lesions attributable to administration of 'Vontrol'.

Reproduction Studies: Teratogenesis and reproduction studies were carried out in rats and rabbits. In rats, 'Vontrol' (diphenidol, SK&F), as the hydrochloride salt, was fed daily to male and female animals in doses of 20 mg./kg. and 40 mg./kg. (approximately three and six times the maximum recommended daily dose in adult humans) for 60 days before mating, and during mating, gestation and lactation for each of two litters. There were no significant differences between drug-treated and untreated control groups with regard to conception rate, litter size, live birth or viability in either of the two litters. There was no congenital anomaly among the offspring. In rabbits, 'Vontrol', as the hydrochloride salt, was fed in the diets in doses of 5 mg./kg. or 75 mg./kg. (approximately equal to, and 12 times as much as, the maximum recommended daily dose in adult humans) from the first day of gestation through the 26th or 27th day of gestation, when the young were delivered by Cesarean section. There were no significant differences between drug-treated and control groups with regard to number and weight of fetuses, numbers of resorption sites or viable fetuses. There was also no statistically significant difference between drug-treated and control groups with regard to the total percentage of underdeveloped fetuses. However, when data were calculated on the basis of a ratio between underdeveloped fetuses and number of pregnant does, an adverse dose-related effect was observed in the high-dose test group.

PHARMACOLOGY (human): Three double-blind controlled studies comparing 'Vontrol' (diphenidol, SK&F) to placebo were carried out: one in 32 male volunteers over a four-week period; one in 45 volunteers of whom 15 were studied for 12 weeks and 17 for 24 weeks; and one in 48 volunteers of whom 36 were studied for 12 weeks.

In the first study 'Vontrol', as the hydrochloride salt, was given orally in daily doses that were started at 75 mg. during the first week and graduated up to 200 mg. by the fourth week. In the second study, one group received 'Vontrol' orally, as the hydrochloride salt, titrated up to 500 mg. daily, then down to 200 mg. daily; another group received a maximum of 200 mg. daily. In the third study, patients received oral doses of 200 mg. to 300 mg. of 'Vontrol' daily, as the hydrochloride or pamoate salts.

The studies included these laboratory determinations: complete blood counts (including hemoglobin and hematocrit determinations), urinalyses (including microscopic examination), serum alkaline phosphatase, serum bilirubin, and bromsulphalein retention. The studies also included records of weight and blood pressure and, in one, electrocardiograms.

In two of these studies, clinical laboratory changes were seen among volunteers in both treated and control groups. The changes included: extrasystoles, white cells in the urine, increase in prothrombin time, rise in hematocrit, rise in leucocytes, rise in eosinophils, and rise or reduction in neutrophils. At no time in any study did changes in the treated group differ significantly from those in the control group.

'Vontrol', as the hydrochloride salt, was given orally to 17 children (aged five to 15). Total daily doses ranged from 90 to 240 mg. Complete blood counts and, in some patients, urinalyses were done before treatment and after approximately four days of treatment. There was no significant difference between pre- and post-treatment laboratory determinations in any child. No side effects were seen.

EXCRETION: Following oral administration of 'Vontrol' (diphenidol, SK&F) to dogs, as the hydrochloride or pamoate salts, and to humans, as the hydrochloride salt, peak blood concentration of the drug generally occurs in one and a half to three hours. In dogs and rats, virtually all of an oral dose of C^{14}-labeled 'Vontrol' is excreted in the urine and feces within three to four days, as determined by radioactivity counts. Approximately the same percentage of an administered dose appeared in the urine of dogs following either oral administration of the hydrochloride salt or rectal administration of the free base.

IN PREGNANCY: Investigators kept follow-up records on 936 patients who had received 'Vontrol' (diphenidol, SK&F) at some time during pregnancy, primarily during the first trimester.

Of the 936 women, 864 (92%) had normal births of normal infants.

Seventy-two (8%) of the women experienced some birth abnormality. Of the 72, six patients had premature but otherwise normal infants, 40 patients aborted, 10 had stillbirths, and 16 had infants with miscellaneous defects. These included hernias, congenital heart defects, hydrocephalus, internal strabismus, anencephalus, enlarged thyroid, and hypospadia.

These incidences of abnormal birth are lower than those generally reported in the literature for the average population of pregnant patients. And in no instance was there any evidence that the administration of 'Vontrol' played a part in birth abnormality.

VN:L15

Shown in Product Identification Section, page 432

EDUCATIONAL MATERIAL

BOOKLETS

"Essentials of Immune Response, Inflammation and the Pathogenesis of Rheumatoid Arthritis," a 63-page booklet (6½" × 8½"). Reviews current thinking on the pathogenesis of rheumatoid arthritis and, briefly, the basic terminology and principles of immunology and inflammation. Free to physicians and allied health personnel.

"Essentials of a Differential Diagnosis of Rheumatoid Arthritis," a 66-page booklet (6½" × 8½"). Provides a logical stepwise approach to rheumatoid arthritis diagnosis. Free to physicians and allied health personnel.

"Essentials of Managing Rheumatoid Arthritis," a 64-page booklet (6½" × 8½"). Examines the drug and nondrug therapies used to manage rheumatoid arthritis. Free to physicians and allied health personnel.

PATIENT I.D. CARDS

"I am taking Eskalith®/ Eskalith CR® (brand of lithium carbonate)." Packet of 10 wallet-size (2½" × 3½") cards. Provides information to emergency room or other medical personnel about the patient and attending physician and about possible drug-related side effects and their management. Free to physicians.

"I am taking Stelazine® (brand of trifluoperazine hydrochloride)." Packet of 10 wallet-size (2½" × 3½") cards. Provides information to emergency room or other medical personnel about the patient and attending physician and about possible drug-related side effects and their management. Free to physicians.

"I am taking Parnate® (brand of tranylcypromine sulfate)." Packet of 10 wallet-size (2½" × 3½") cards. Provides information to emergency room or other medical personnel about the patient and attending physician and about possible drug-related side effects and their management. Free to physicians.

PATIENT INFORMATION

Patient information on Dyazide® (triamterene and hydrochlorothiazide). Pad (8½" × 11") of 50 sheets. Provides basic information about high blood pressure and *Dyazide*, including special considerations about diet, possible drug interactions, and side effects. These brochures are also available: "Eating Your Way to a Healthier Heart", "High Blood Pressure Is Serious Business", "Fighting Heart Disease" and Patient I.D. Card. Free to physicians.

Instruction sheets for patients on Parnate® (brand of tranylcypromine sulfate). Pad (4¼" × 8") of 24 sheets. Serves as a reminder of principal instructions about *Parnate* therapy, e.g.: the importance of following dosage instructions exactly; the need for consulting before taking any other drugs; what foods and beverages must be avoided; what symptoms should be reported promptly. A carbon copy is provided for the physician's records. Free to physicians.

Patient information on Ridaura® (brand of auranofin). "Understanding Your Treatment of Rheumatoid Arthritis," a 12-page booklet (3"× 6½"). Describes and depicts rheumatoid arthritis and its effects on the body, and discusses how the disease is typically managed. Provides information on what to expect from *Ridaura* therapy with regard to disease control and potential side effects. Emphasizes the importance of cooperating with physician instructions. Free to physicians and other health professionals.

Solvay Pharmaceuticals

901 SAWYER ROAD
MARIETTA, GA 30062

CORTENEMA® ℞

[*kort "en 'a-ma*]
(Hydrocortisone Retention Enema)
Disposable Unit for Rectal Use Only

Each disposable unit (60 mL) contains:
Hydrocortisone, 100 mg in an aqueous solution containing carboxypolymethylene, polysorbate 80, and methylparaben, 0.18% as a preservative.

DESCRIPTION

CORTENEMA® is a convenient disposable single-dose hydrocortisone enema designed for ease of self-administration. Hydrocortisone is a naturally occurring glucocorticoid (adrenal corticosteroid) which, similarly as its acetate and sodium hemisuccinate derivatives, is partially absorbed following rectal administration. Absorption studies in ulcerative colitis patients have shown up to 50% absorption of hydrocortisone administered as CORTENEMA® and up to 30% of hydrocortisone acetate administered in an identical vehicle.

ACTIONS

CORTENEMA® provides the potent anti-inflammatory effect of hydrocortisone. Because this drug is absorbed from the colon, it acts both topically and systemically. Although rectal hydrocortisone, used as recommended for CORTENEMA®, has a low incidence of reported adverse reactions, prolonged use presumably may cause systemic reactions associated with oral dosage forms.

INDICATIONS

CORTENEMA® is indicated as adjunctive therapy in the treatment of ulcerative colitis, especially distal forms, including ulcerative proctitis, ulcerative proctosigmoiditis, and left-sided ulcerative colitis. It has proved useful also in some cases involving the transverse and ascending colons.

CONTRAINDICATIONS

Systemic fungal infections; and ileocolostomy during the immediate or early post-operative period.

WARNINGS

In severe ulcerative colitis, it is hazardous to delay needed surgery while awaiting response to medical treatment.

Damage to the rectal wall can result from careless or improper insertion of an enema tip.

In patients on corticosteroid therapy subjected to unusual stress, increased dosage of rapidly acting corticosteroids before, during, and after the stressful situation is indicated.

Corticosteroids may mask some signs of infection, and new infections may appear during their use. There may be decreased resistance and inability to localize infection when corticosteroids are used.

Prolonged use of corticosteroids may produce posterior subcapsular cataracts, glaucoma with possible damage to the optic nerves, and may enhance the establishment of secondary ocular infections due to fungi or viruses.

Usage in pregnancy: Since adequate human reproduction studies have not been done with corticosteroids, the use of these drugs in pregnancy, nursing mothers or women of childbearing potential requires that the possible benefits of the drug be weighed against the potential hazards to the mother and embryo or fetus. Infants born of mothers who have received substantial doses of corticosteroids during pregnancy should be carefully observed for signs of hypoadrenalism.

Average and large doses of hydrocortisone or cortisone can cause elevation of blood pressure, salt and water retention, and increased excretion of potassium. These effects are less likely to occur with the synthetic derivatives except when used in large doses. Dietary salt restriction and potassium supplementation may be necessary. All corticosteroids increase calcium excretion.

While on corticosteroid therapy patients should not be vaccinated against smallpox. Other immunization procedures should not be undertaken in patients who are on corticosteroids, especially on high dose, because of possible hazards of neurological complications and a lack of antibody response.

If corticosteroids are indicated in patients with latent tuberculosis or tuberculin reactivity, close observation is necessary as reactivation of the disease may occur. During prolonged corticosteroid therapy, these patients should receive chemoprophylaxis.

PRECAUTIONS

CORTENEMA® Hydrocortisone Retention Enema should be used with caution where there is a probability of impending perforation, abscess or other pyogenic infection; fresh intestinal anastomoses; obstruction; or extensive fistulas and sinus tracts. Use with caution in presence of active or latent peptic ulcer; diverticulitis; renal insufficiency; hypertension; osteoporosis; and myasthenia gravis.

Steroid therapy might impair prognosis in surgery by increasing the hazard of infection. If infection is suspected, appropriate antibiotic therapy must be administered, usually in larger than ordinary doses.

Drug-induced secondary adrenocortical insufficiency may occur with prolonged CORTENEMA® therapy. This is minimized by gradual reduction of dosage. This type of relative insufficiency may persist for months after discontinuation of therapy; therefore, in any situation of stress occurring during that period, hormone therapy should be reinstituted. Since mineralocorticoid secretion may be impaired, salt and/ or a mineralocorticoid should be administered concurrently.

There is an enhanced effect of corticosteroids on patients with hypothyroidism and in those with cirrhosis.

Corticosteroid should be used cautiously in patients with ocular herpes simplex because of possible corneal perforation.

The lowest possible dose of corticosteroid should be used to control the conditions under treatment, and when reduction in dosage is possible, the reduction should be gradual.

Psychic derangement may appear when corticosteroids are used, ranging from euphoria, insomnia, mood swings, personality changes, and severe depression, to frank psychotic manifestations. Also, existing emotional instability or psychotic tendencies may be aggravated by corticosteroids.

Aspirin should be used cautiously in conjunction with corticosteroids in hypoprothrombinemia.

Growth and development of infants and children on prolonged corticosteroid therapy should be carefully observed.

ADVERSE REACTIONS

Local pain or burning and rectal bleeding attributed to CORTENEMA® have been reported rarely. Apparent exacerbations or sensitivity reactions also occur rarely. The following adverse reactions should be kept in mind whenever corticosteroids are given by rectal administration.

Fluid and Electrolyte Disturbances: Sodium retention; fluid retention; congestive heart failure in susceptible patients; potassium loss; hypokalemic alkalosis; hypertension. **Musculoskeletal:** Muscle weakness; steroid myopathy; loss of muscle mass; osteoporosis; vertebral compression fractures; aseptic necrosis of femoral and humeral heads; pathologic fracture of long bones. **Gastrointestinal:** Peptic ulcer with possible perforation and hemorrhage; pancreatitis; abdominal distention; ulcerative esophagitis. **Dermatologic:** Impaired wound healing; thin fragile skin; petechiae and ecchymoses; facial erythema; increased sweating; may suppress reactions to skin tests. **Neurological:** Convulsions; increased intracranial pressure with papilledema (pseudo-tumor cerebri) usually after treatment; vertigo; headache. **Endocrine:** Menstrual irregularities; development of Cushingoid state; suppression of growth in children; secondary adrenocortical and pituitary unresponsiveness, particularly in times of stress, as in trauma, surgery or illness; decreased carbohydrate tolerance; manifestations of latent diabetes mellitus; increased requirements for insulin or oral hypoglycemic agents in diabetics. **Ophthalmic:** Posterior subcapsular cataracts; increased intraocular pressure; glaucoma; exophthalmos. **Metabolic:** Negative nitrogen balance due to protein catabolism.

DOSAGE AND ADMINISTRATION

The use of CORTENEMA® Hydrocortisone Retention Enema is predicated upon the concomitant use of modern supportive measures such as rational dietary control, sedatives, anti-diarrheal agents, antibacterial therapy, blood replacement if necessary, etc.

The usual course of therapy is one CORTENEMA® nightly for 21 days, or until the patient comes into remission both clinically and proctologically. Clinical symptoms usually subside promptly within 3 to 5 days. Improvement in the appearance of the mucosa, as seen by sigmoidoscopic examination, may lag somewhat behind clinical improvement. Difficult cases may require as long as 2 or 3 months of COR-

Continued on next page

Solvay—Cont.

TENEMA® treatment. Where the course of therapy extends beyond 21 days, CORTENEMA® should be discontinued gradually by reducing administration to every other night for 2 or 3 weeks.

If clinical or proctologic improvement fail to occur within 2 or 3 weeks after starting CORTENEMA®, discontinue its use.

Symptomatic improvement, evidenced by decreased diarrhea and bleeding; weight gain; improved appetite; lessened fever; and decreased leukocytosis, may be misleading and should not be used as the sole criterion in judging efficacy. Sigmoidoscopic examination and X-ray visualization are essential for adequate monitoring of ulcerative colitis. Biopsy is useful for differential diagnosis.

Patient instructions for administering CORTENEMA® are enclosed in each box of seven units. We recommend that the patient lie on his left side during administration and for 30 minutes thereafter, so that the fluid will distribute throughout the left colon. Every effort should be made to retain the enema for at least an hour and, preferably, all night. This may be facilitated by prior sedation and/or antidiarrheal medication, especially early in therapy, when the urge to evacuate is great.

HOW SUPPLIED

CORTENEMA®, Hydrocortisone 100 mg Retention Enema is supplied as disposable single-dose bottles with lubricated rectal applicator tips, in boxes of seven × 60 mL (NDC 0032-1904-82) and boxes of one × 60 mL (NDC 0032-1904-73). Store at controlled room temperature, 15°–30°C (59°–86°F).

CAUTION

Federal law prohibits dispensing without prescription.

4E Rev. 8/91

SOLVAY PHARAMCEUTICALS
Marietta, GA 30062

CREON®   ℞
[cree 'on]
(PANCREATIN USP)
ENTERIC-COATED MICROSPHERES CAPSULES

DESCRIPTION

CREON capsules are orally administered capsules containing enteric-coated microspheres of pancreatin USP, a standardized concentrate of high lipase which is of porcine pancreatic origin. Each capsule contains Lipase 8,000 USP Units, Amylase 30,000 USP Units, Protease 13,000 USP Units.

Inactive ingredients include hydroxypropylmethylcellulose phthalate, polyethylene glycol, dibutyl phthalate polydimethylsiloxane, liquid paraffin, gelatin, D&C Yellow #10, and FD&C Red #40, black iron oxide, red iron oxide, yellow iron oxide, and titanium dioxide.

CLINICAL PHARMACOLOGY

The pancreatic enzymes in CREON are enteric-coated to resist gastric destruction or inactivation and are designed to be delivered to the duodenum intact. The pancreatic enzymes catalyze the hydrolysis of fats to glycerol and fatty acids, starch into dextrins and short chain sugars, and protein into proteoses and derived substances. The lipase content of CREON is present at a higher level than conventional pancreatin preparations, and therefore effective in controlling steatorrhea and its consequences at low daily dosage levels.

INDICATIONS

CREON capsules are indicated for patients with pancreatic exocrine insufficiency as is often associated with:
- cystic fibrosis
- chronic pancreatitis
- post-pancreatectomy
- post-gastrointestinal bypass surgery (e.g., Billroth II gastroenterostomy)
- ductal obstruction from neoplasm (e.g. of the pancreas or common bile duct)

CONTRAINDICATIONS

CREON is contraindicated in patients known to be hypersensitive to pork protein or in patients with acute pancreatitis.

WARNINGS

Pancreatic exocrine replacement therapy should not delay or supplant treatment of the primary disorder. Should symptoms of sensitivity appear, discontinue medication and initiate symptomatic and supportive therapy if necessary.

PRECAUTIONS

TO PROTECT ENTERIC COATING, MICROSPHERES SHOULD NOT BE CRUSHED OR CHEWED. Where swallowing of capsules is difficult, the capsules may be carefully opened and the microspheres added to a small amount of a soft food, such as applesauce or pudding. The soft food should be swallowed immediately without chewing and followed with a glass of water or juice to ensure complete swallowing. Contact of the microspheres with foods which have a pH greater than 5.5 can dissolve CREON's protective enteric coating.

Carcinogenesis, Mutagenesis, Impairment of Fertility
Long-term studies in animals have not been performed to evaluate carcinogenic potential.

Pregnancy, Category C
Animal reproduction studies have not been conducted with CREON. It is also not known whether CREON can cause fetal harm when administered to a pregnant woman or can affect reproduction capacity. CREON should be given to a pregnant woman only if clearly needed.

Nursing Mothers
It is not known whether this drug is excreted in human milk. Because many drugs are excreted in human milk, caution should be exercised when CREON is administered to a nursing mother.

ADVERSE REACTIONS

The most frequently reported adverse reactions to enzyme-containing products are gastrointestinal such as nausea, cramping, and/or diarrhea which may occur with excessive dosage. Less frequently, allergic-type reactions have also been observed. Very high doses of pancreatin have been associated with hyperuricosuria and hyperuricemia.

DOSAGE AND ADMINISTRATION

Dosage should be adjusted according to the severity of the exocrine pancreatic enzyme deficiency. The number of capsules given with meals and/or snacks should be estimated by assessing which dose minimizes steatorrhea and helps maintain good nutritional status.

Initial starting dosage is one to two capsules with meals or snacks, then adjusting according to the response of the patient and control of steatorrhea.

HOW SUPPLIED

CREON is available in opaque brown/clear yellow hard gelatin capsules imprinted in white with "SOLVAY" and "1200." The capsules contain buff-colored enteric-coated microspheres of pancreatin supplied in bottles of:

100 .... NDC 0032-1200-01
250 .... NDC 0032-1200-07

Store at controlled room temperature, 15°–30°c (59°–86°F). PROTECT FROM MOISTURE. Do not refrigerate. Dispense in tight, light-resistant containers.
Note: For human consumption only, not for use in animal treatment.

Manufactured by Kali-Chemie Pharma GmbH, Hannover, Germany. Marketed by Solvay Pharmaceuticals, Marietta, Georgia, 30062.

4E REV 6/92

Shown in Product Identification Section, page 432

CREON® 25   ℞
(Pancreatin, USP)
Enteric-coated
Microspheres Capsules
Prescribing Information

DESCRIPTION

CREON®25 capsules are orally adminstered capsules containing enteric-coated microspheres of pancreatin USP, a standardized concentrate of high lipase which is of porcine pancreatic origin. Each capsule contains Lipase 25,000 USP Units, Amylase 74,700 USP Units and Protease 62,500 USP Units.

Inactive ingredients include hydroxypropylmethylcellulose phthalate, polythylene glycol, dibutyl, phthalate dimethicone NF, light mineral oil NF, gelatin, D&C Yellow #10, and FD&C Red #40, black iron oxide, red iron oxide, yellow iron oxide, and titanium dioxide.

CLINICAL PHARMACOLOGY

The pancreatic enzymes in CREON 25 are enteric-coated to resist gastric destruction or inactivation and are designed to deliver to the duodenum intact. The pancreatic enzymes catalyze the hydrolysis of fats to glycerol and fatty acids, starch into dextrins and short chain sugars, and protein into proteoses and derived substances. The lipase content of CREON 25 is present at a higher level than conventional pancreatin preparations, and therefore effective in controlling steatorrhea and its consequences at low daily dosage levels.

INDICATIONS

CREON 25 capsules are indicated for patients with pancreatic exocrine insufficiency as is often associated with:
- cystic fibrosis
- chronic pancreatitis
- post-pancreatectomy
- post-gastrointestinal bypass surgery (e.g. Billroth II gastroenterostomy)
- ductal obstruction from neoplasm (e.g. of the pancreas or common bile duct)

CONTRAINDICATIONS

CREON 25 is contraindicated in patients known to be hypersensitive to pork protein or in patients with acute pancreatitis.

WARNINGS

Pancreatic exocrine replacement therapy should not delay or supplant treatment of the primary disorder. Should symptoms of sensitivity appear, discontinue medication and initiate symptomatic and supportive therapy if necessary.

PRECAUTIONS

TO PROTECT ENTERIC COATING, MICROSPHERES SHOULD NOT BE CRUSHED OR CHEWED. Where swallowing of capsules is difficult, the capsules may be carefully opened and the microspheres added to a small amount of soft food, such as applesauce or pudding. The soft food should be swallowed immediately without chewing and followed with a glass of water or juice to insure complete swallowing. Contact of the microspheres with foods having a pH greater than 5.5 can dissolve CREON 25's protective enteric coating.

Carcinogenesis, Mutagenesis, Impairment of Fertility: Long-term studies in the animals have not been performed to evaluate carcinogenic potential.

Pregnancy, Category C: Animal reproduction studies have not been conducted with CREON 25. It is also not known whether CREON 25 can cause fetal harm when administered to a pregnant woman or can affect reproduction capacity. CREON 25 should be given to a pregnant woman only if clearly needed.

Nursing Mothers: It is not known whether this drug is excreted in human milk. Because many drugs are excreted in human milk, caution should be exercised when CREON 25 is administered to a nursing mother.

ADVERSE REACTIONS

The most frequently reported adverse reactions to enzyme-containing products are gastrointestinal such as nausea, cramping, and/or diarrhea may occur with excessive dosage. Less frequently, allergic-type reactions have also been observed. Very high doses of pancreatin have been associated with hyperuricosuria and hyperuricemia.

DOSAGE AND ADMINISTRATION

Dosage should be adjusted according to the severity of the exocrine pancreatic enzyme deficiency. The number of capsules given with meals and/or snacks should be estimated by assessing which dose minimizes steatorrhea and helps maintain good nutritional status.

Initial starting dosage is one capsule with meals or snacks, then adjusting according to the response of the patient and control of steatorrhea.

HOW SUPPLIED

CREON 25 is available in a two-colored gelatin capsule (orange opaque top half, transparent-yellow bottom half) imprinted in white with "SOLVAY" and "1225". Each capsule contain brownish-colored enteric-coated microspheres of pancreatin supplied on bottles of:

100 .... NDC 0032-1225-01

Store at controlled room temperature, 15°–30°C (59°–86°F). PROTECT FROM MOISTURE. Do not refrigerate. Dispense in tight, light-resistant containers.
NOTE:
For human consumption only.
Not for use in animal treatment.
Manufactured By:
Kali-Chemie Pharma GmbH
Hannover, Germany
Marketed by:
SOLVAY PHARMACEUTICALS
MARIETTA, GA 30062

2E REV 7/92

Shown in Product Identification Section, page 432

ESTRATAB®   ℞
[es '-trah-tab]
Esterified Estrogens Tablets, USP
0.3 mg; 0.625 mg; 1.25 mg; 2.5 mg.

WARNING:
1. ESTROGENS HAVE BEEN REPORTED TO INCREASE THE RISK OF ENDOMETRIAL CARCINOMA.
   Three independent case control studies have reported an increased risk of endometrial cancer in postmenopausal women exposed to exogenous estrogens for prolonged periods.[1-3] This risk was independent of the other known risk factors for endometrial cancer. These studies are further supported by the finding that incidence rates of endometrial cancer have increased sharply since 1969 in eight differ-

ent areas of the United States with population-based cancer reporting systems, an increase which may be related to the rapidly expanding use of estrogens during the last decade.[4]

The three case control studies reported that the risk of endometrial cancer in estrogen users was about 4.5 to 13.9 times greater than in nonusers. The risk appears to depend on both duration of treatment[1] and on estrogen dose.[3] In view of these findings, when estrogens are used for the treatment of menopausal symptoms, the lowest dose that will control symptoms should be utilized and medication should be discontinued as soon as possible. When prolonged treatment is medically indicated, the patient should be reassessed on at least a semiannual basis to determine the need for continued therapy. Although the evidence must be considered preliminary, one study suggests that cyclic administration of low doses of estrogen may carry less risk than continuous administration,[3] it therefore appears prudent to utilize such a regimen.

Close clinical surveillance of all women taking estrogens is important. In all cases of undiagnosed persistent or recurring abnormal vaginal bleeding, adequate diagnostic measures should be undertaken to rule out malignancy.

There is no evidence at present that "natural" estrogens are more or less hazardous than "synthetic" estrogens at equiestrogenic doses.

2. ESTROGENS SHOULD NOT BE USED DURING PREGNANCY.

The use of female sex hormones, both estrogens and progestogens, during early pregnancy may seriously damage the offspring. It has been shown that females exposed in utero to diethylstilbestrol, a nonsteroidal estrogen, have an increased risk of developing in later life a form of vaginal or cervical cancer that is ordinarily extremely rare.[5–6] This risk has been estimated as not greater than 4 per 1000 exposures.[7] Furthermore, a high percentage of such exposed women (from 30 to 90 percent) have been found to have vaginal adenosis,[8–12] epithelial changes of the vagina and cervix. Although these changes are histologically benign, it is not known whether they are precursors of malignancy. Although similar data are not available with the use of other estrogens, it cannot be presumed they would not induce similar changes.

Several reports suggest an association between intrauterine exposure to female sex hormones and congenital anomalies, including congenital heart defects and limb reduction defects.[13–16]. One case control study[16] estimated a 4.7 fold increased risk of limb reduction defects in infants exposed in utero to sex hormones (oral contraceptives, hormone withdrawal tests for pregnancy, or attempted treatment for threatened abortion). Some of these exposures were very short and involved only a few days of treatment. The data suggest that the risk of limb reduction defects in exposed fetuses is somewhat less than 1 per 1000.

In the past, female sex hormones have been used during pregnancy in an attempt to treat threatened or habitual abortion. There is considerable evidence that estrogens are ineffective for these indictions, and there is no evidence from well controlled studies that progestogens are effective for these uses.

If ESTRATAB® is used during pregnancy, or if the patient becomes pregnant while taking this drug, she should be apprised of the potential risks to the fetus, and the advisability of pregnancy continuation.

DESCRIPTION

ESTRATAB® (Esterified Estrogens Tablets). Each blue, sugar coated tablet contains 0.3 mg. Each yellow, sugar coated tablet contains 0.625 mg. Each orange-red, sugar coated tablet contains 1.25 mg. Each light purple, sugar coated tablet contains 2.5 mg.

Inactive Ingredients: Acacia, calcium carbonate, carnauba wax, carboxymethylcellulose sodium, citric acid, colloidal silicon dioxide, diacetylated monoglyceride, gelatin, lactose, magnesium stearate, methylparaben, microcrystalline cellulose, pharmaceutical glaze, povidone, propylparaben, shellac, sodium benzoate, sodium bicarbonate, sorbic acid, sucrose, corn starch, talc, titanium dioxide and tribasic calcium phosphate. The 0.3 mg tablet coating contains FD&C Blue #1 Lake; the 0.625 mg tablet coating contains D&C Yellow #10 Lake, FD&C Yellow #6 Lake and FD&C Blue #2 Lake; the 1.25 mg tablet coating contains FD&C Yellow #6 Lake and the 2.5 mg tablet coating contains FD&C Red #40 Lake and FD&C Blue #2 Lake. In addition the tablet imprinting ink for the 0.3 mg, 0.625 mg and the 1.25 mg tablets contain black iron oxide, FD&C Blue #2 Lake, FD&C Red #40 Lake and FD&C Yellow #6 Lake. The 2.5 mg imprinting ink contains Soya lecithin, Dimethyl Polysiloxane, pharmaceutical Shellac and Titanium dioxide.

ESTRATAB® (Esterified Estrogens Tablets) for oral administration is a mixture of the sodium salts of the sulfate esters of the estrogenic substances, principally estrone, that are of the type excreted by pregnant mares. Esterified Estrogens contain not less than 75.0 percent and not more than 85.0 percent of sodium estrone sulfate, and not less than 6.0 percent and not more than 15.0 percent of sodium equilin sulfate, in such proportion that the total of these two components is not less than 90.0 percent.

CLINICAL PHARMACOLOGY

Estrogens are important in the development and maintenance of the female reproductive system and secondary sex characteristics. They promote growth and development of the vagina, uterus, and fallopian tubes, and enlargement of the breasts. Indirectly, they contribute to the shaping of the skeleton, maintenance of tone and elasticity of urogenital structures, changes in the epiphyses of the long bones that allow for the pubertal growth spurt and its termination, growth of axillary and pubic hair, and pigmentation of the nipples and genitals. Decline of estrogenic activity at the end of the menstrual cycle can bring on menstruation, although the cessation of progesterone secretion is the most important factor in the mature ovulatory cycle. However, in the preovulatory or nonovulatory cycle, estrogen is the primary determinant in the onset of menstruation. Estrogens also affect the release of pituitary gonadotropins.

The pharmacologic effects of conjungated estrogens are similar to those of endogenous estrogens. They are soluble in water and are well absorbed from the gastrointestinal tract.

In responsive tissues (female genital organs, breasts, hypothalamus, pituitary) estrogens enter the cell and are transported into the nucleus. As a result of estrogen action, specific RNA and protein synthesis occurs.

Metabolism and inactivation occur primarily in the liver. Some estrogens are excreted into the bile; however they are reabsorbed from the intestine and returned to the liver through the portal venous system. Water soluble estrogen conjugates are strongly acidic and are ionized in body fluids, which favor excretion through the kidneys since tubular reabsorption is minimal.

INDICATIONS AND USAGE

ESTRATAB® is indicated in the treatment of:

1. Moderate to severe *vasomotor* symptoms associated with the menopause. (There is no evidence that estrogens are effective for nervous symptoms or depression which might occur during menopause and they should not be used to treat these conditions).
2. Atrophic vaginitis.
3. Kraurosis vulvae.
4. Female hypogonadism.
5. Female castration.
6. Primary ovarian failure.
7. Breast cancer (for palliation only) in appropriately selected women and men with metastatic disease.
8. Prostatic carcinoma—palliative therapy of advanced disease.

ESTRATAB® HAS NOT BEEN SHOWN TO BE EFFECTIVE FOR ANY PURPOSE DURING PREGNANCY AND ITS USE MAY CAUSE SEVERE HARM TO THE FETUS (SEE BOXED WARNING).

CONTRAINDICATIONS

Estrogens should not be used in women (or men) with any of the following conditions:

1. Known or suspected cancer of the breast except in appropriately selected patients being treated for metastatic disease.
2. Known or suspected estrogen-dependent neoplasia.
3. Known or suspected pregnancy (See Boxed Warning).
4. Undiagnosed abnormal genital bleeding.
5. Active thrombophlebitis or thromboembolic disorders.
6. A past history of thrombophlebitis, thrombosis, or thromboembolic disorders associated with previous estrogen use (except when used in treatment of breast or prostatic malignancy).

WARNINGS

1. **Induction of malignant neoplasms.** Long term continuous administration of natural and synthetic estrogens in certain animal species increases the frequency of carcinomas of the breast, cervix, vagina, and liver. There is now evidence that estrogens increase the risk of carcinoma of the endometrium in humans (See Boxed Warning).

   At the present time there is no satisfactory evidence that estrogens given to postmenopausal women increase the risk of cancer of the breast,[18] although a recent long-term follow up of a single physician's practice has raised this possibility.[18a] Because of the animal data, there is need for caution in prescribing estrogens for women with a strong family history of breast cancer or who have breast nodules, fibrocystic disease, or abnormal mammograms.

2. **Gallbladder disease.** A recent study has reported a 2 to 3-fold increase in the risk of surgically confirmed gallbladder disease in women receiving postmenopausal estrogens,[18] similar to the 2-fold increase previously noted in users of oral contraceptives.[19–24] In the case of oral contraceptives the increased risk appeared after two years of use.[24]

3. **Effects similar to these caused by estrogen-progestogen oral contraceptives.** There are several serious adverse effects of oral contraceptives, most of which have not, up to now, been documented as consequences of postmenopausal estrogen therapy. This may reflect the comparatively low doses of estrogen used in postmenopausal women. It would be expected that the larger doses of estrogen used to treat prostatic or breast cancer or postpartum breast engorgement are more likely to result in these adverse effects, and, in fact, it has been shown that there is an increased risk of thrombosis in men receiving estrogens for prostatic cancer and women for postpartum breast engorgement.[20–23]

   a. **Thromboembolic disease.** It is now well established that users of oral contraceptives have an increased risk of various thomboembolic and thrombotic vascular diseases, such as thrombophlebitis, pulmonary embolism, stroke, and myocardial infarction.[24–31] Cases of retinal thrombosis, mesenteric thrombosis, and optic neuritis have been reported in oral contraceptive users. There is evidence that the risk of several of these adverse reactions is related to the dose of the drug.[32–33] An increased risk of postsurgery thromboembolic complications has also been reported in users of oral contraceptives.[34–35] If feasible, estrogen should be discontinued at least 4 weeks before surgery of the type associated with an increased risk of thromboembolism or during periods of prolonged immobilization.

   While an increased rate of thromboembolic and thrombotic disease in postmenopausal users of estrogens has not been found,[18–36] this does not rule out the possibility that such an increase may be present or that subgroups of women who have underlying risk factors or who are receiving relatively large doses of estrogens may have increased risk. Therefore estrogens should not be used in persons with active thrombophlebitis or thromboembolic disorders, and they should not be used (except in treatment of malignancy) in persons with a history of such disorders in association with estrogen use. They should be used with caution in patients with cerebral vascular or coronary artery disease and only for those in whom estrogens are clearly needed. Large doses of estrogen (5 mg esterified estrogens per day) comparable to those used to treat cancer of the prostate and breast, have been shown in a large prospective clinical trial in men[37] to increase the risk of nonfatal myocardial infarction, pulmonary embolism and thrombophlebitis. When estrogen doses of this size are used, any of the thromboembolic and thrombotic adverse effects associated with oral contraceptive use should be considered a clear risk.

   b. **Hepatic adenoma.** Benign hepatic adenomas appear to be associated with the use of oral contraceptives.[38–40] Although benign and rare, these may rupture and may cause death through intraabdominal hemorrhage. Such lesions have not yet been reported in association with other estrogen or progestogen preparations but should be considered in estrogen users having abdominal pain and tenderness, abdominal mass, or hypovolemic shock. Hepatocellular carcinoma has also been reported in women taking estrogen-containing oral contraceptives.[39] The relationship of this malignancy to these drugs is not known at this time.

   c. **Elevated blood pressure.** Increased blood pressure is not uncommon in women using oral contraceptives. There is now a report that this may occur with use of estrogens in the menopause[41] and blood pressure should be monitored with estrogen use, especially if high doses are used.

   d. **Glucose tolerance.** A worsening of glucose tolerance has been observed in a significant percentage of patients on estrogen-containing contraceptives. For this reason, diabetic patients should be carefully observed while receiving estrogens.

4. **Hypercalcemia.** Administration of estrogens may lead to severe hypercalcemia in patients with breast cancer and bone metastases. If this occurs, the drug should be stopped and appropriate measures taken to reduce the serum calcium level.

PRECAUTIONS

A. General Precautions

1. A complete medical and family history should be taken prior to the initiation of any estrogen therapy. The pretreatment and periodic physical examinations should include special reference to blood pressure, abdomen,

Continued on next page

Solvay—Cont.

and pelvic organs, and should include a Papanicolaou smear. As a general rule, estrogen should not be prescribed for longer than one year without another physical examination being performed.

2. Fluid-retention—Because estrogen may cause some degree of fluid retention, conditions which might be influenced by this factor such as epilepsy, migraine, and cardiac or renal dysfunction, required careful observation.

3. Certain patients may develop undesirable manifestations of excessive estrogenic stimulation, such as abnormal or excessive uterine bleeding, mastodynia, etc.

4. Oral contraceptives appear to be associated with an increased incidence of mental depression.[24] Although it is not clear whether this is due to the estrogenic or progestogenic component of the contraceptive, patients with a history of depression should be carefully observed.

5. Preexisting uterine leiomyomata may increase in size during estrogen use.

6. The pathologist should be advised of estrogen therapy when relevant specimens are submitted.

7. Patients with a past history of jaundice during pregnancy have an increased risk of recurrence of jaundice while receiving estrogen-containing oral contraceptive therapy. If jaundice develops in any patient receiving estrogen, the medication should be discontinued while the cause is investigated.

8. Estrogens may be poorly metabolized in patients with impaired liver functions and they should be administered with caution in such patients.

9. Because estrogens influence the metabolism of calcium and phosphorus, they should be used with caution in patients with metabolic bone diseases that are associated with hypercalcemia or in patients with renal insufficiency.

10. Because of the effects of estrogens on epiphyseal closure, they should be used judiciously in young patients in whom bone growth is not complete.

11. Certain endocrine and liver function tests may be affected by estrogen-containing oral contraceptives. The following similar changes may be expected with larger doses of estrogen:
   a. Increased sulfobromophthalein retention.
   b. Increased prothrombin and factors VII, VIII, IX, and X; decreased antithrombin 3, increased norepinephrine-induced platelet aggregability.
   c. Increased thyroid binding globulin (TBG) leading to increased circulating total thyroid hormone, as measured by PBI, T4 by column, or T4 by radioimmunoassay. Free T3 resin uptake is decreased, reflecting the elevated TBG; free T4 concentration is unaltered.
   d. Impaired glucose tolerance.
   e. Decreased pregnanediol excretion.
   f. Reduced response to metyrapone test.
   g. Reduced serum folate concentration.
   h. Increased serum triglyceride and phospholipid concentration.

12. The lowest effective dose appropriate for the specific indication should be utilized. Studies of the addition of a progestin for seven or more days of a cycle of estrogen administration have reported a lowered incidence of endometrial hyperplasia. Morphological and biochemical studies of endometrium suggest that 10 to 13 days of progestin are needed to provide maximal maturation of the endometrium and to eliminate any hyperplastic changes. Whether this will provide protection from endometrial carcinoma has not been clearly established. There are possible additional risks which may be associated with the inclusion of progestin in estrogen replacement regimes. The potential risks include adverse effects on carbohydrate and lipid metabolism. The choice of progestin and dosage may be important in minimizing these adverse effects.

B. Information for the Patient. See text of Patient Package Insert which appears after the REFERENCES.

C. Pregnancy Category X. See CONTRAINDICATIONS and Boxed WARNING.

D. Nursing Mothers. As a general principle, the administration of any drug to nursing mothers should be done only when clearly necessary since many drugs are excreted in human milk.

ADVERSE REACTIONS
(See Warnings regarding induction of neoplasia, adverse effects on the fetus, increased incidence of gall bladder disease, and adverse effects similar to those of oral contraceptives, including thromboembolism). The following additional adverse reactions have been reported with estrogenic therapy, including oral contraceptives:

1. Genitourinary system.
Breakthrough bleeding, spotting, change in menstrual flow.
Dysmenorrhea.
Premenstrual-like syndrome.
Increase in size of uterine fibromyomata.
Vaginal candidiasis.
Change in cervical erosion and in degree of cervical secretion.
Cystitis-like syndrome.

2. Breasts.
Tenderness, enlargement, secretion.

3. Gastrointestinal.
Nausea, vomiting.
Abdominal cramps, bloating.
Cholestatic jaundice.

4. Skin.
Chloasma or melasma which may persist when drug is discontinued.
Erythema multiforme.
Erythema nodosum.
Hemorrhagic eruption.
Loss of scalp hair.
Hirsutism.

5. Eyes.
Steepening of corneal curvature.
Intolerance to contact lenses.

6. CNS.
Headache, migraine, dizziness.
Mental depression.
Chorea.

7. Miscellaneous.
Increase or decrease in weight.
Reduced carbohydrate tolerance.
Aggravation of porphyria.
Edema.
Changes in libido.

OVERDOSAGE
Numerous reports of ingestion of large doses of estrogen-containing oral contraceptives by young children indicate that serious ill effects do not occur. Overdosage of estrogen may cause nausea, and withdrawal bleeding may occur in females.

DOSAGE AND ADMINISTRATION
1. **Given cyclically for short term use only:**
   For treatment of moderate to severe *vasomotor* symptoms, atrophic vaginitis, or kraurosis vulvae associated with the menopause. The lowest dose that will control symptoms should be chosen and medication should be discontinued as promptly as possible. Administration should be cyclic (e.g., three weeks on and one week off). Attempts to discontinue or taper medication should be made at three to six month intervals.
   Usual dosage ranges.
   Vasomotor symptoms—1.25 mg daily. If the patient has not menstruated within the last two months or more, cyclic administration is started arbitrarily. If the patient is menstruating, cyclic administration is started on day 5 of bleeding.
   Atrophic vaginitis and kraurosis vulvae—0.3 mg to 1.25 mg or more daily, depending upon the tissue response of the individual patient. Administer cyclically.

2. **Given cyclically:** Female hypogonadism; female castration; primary ovarian failure.
   Usual dosage ranges:
   Female hypogonadism—2.5 to 7.5 mg daily, in divided doses for 20 days, followed by a rest period of 10 days' duration. If bleeding does not occur by the end of this period, the same dosage schedule is repeated. The number of courses of estrogen therapy necessary to produce bleeding may vary depending on the responsiveness of the endometrium.
   If bleeding occurs before the end of the 10 day period, begin a 20 day estrogen-progestin cyclic regimen with ESTRATAB® (Esterified Estrogens Tablets, USP), 2.5 to 7.5 mg daily in divided doses, for 20 days. During the last five days of estrogen therapy, give an oral progestin. If bleeding occurs before this regimen is concluded, therapy is discontinued and may be resumed on the fifth day of bleeding.
   Female castration, and primary ovarian failure—1.25 mg daily, cyclically. Adjust dosage upward or downward according to severity of symptoms and response of the patient. For maintenance, adjust dosage to lowest level that will provide effective control.

3. **Given chronically:** Inoperable progressing prostatic cancer—1.25 to 2.5 mg three times daily. The effectiveness of therapy can be judged by phosphatase determinations as well as by symptomatic improvement of the patient. Inoperable progressing breast cancer in appropriately selected men and postmenopausal women. (See INDICATIONS) —Suggested dosage is 10 mg three times daily for a period of at least three months.
   Treated patients with an intact uterus should be monitored closely for signs of endometrial cancer and appropriate diagnosis measures should be taken to rule out malig-

nancy in the event of persistent or recurring abnormal vaginal bleeding.

HOW SUPPLIED
ESTRATAB® (Esterified Estrogens Tablets, USP): Each blue tablet contains 0.3 mg in bottles of 100 (NDC 0032-1014-01) imprinted "SOLVAY 1014" in black.
Each yellow tablet contains 0.625 mg in bottles of 100 (NDC 0032-1022-01) and 1000 (NDC 0032-1022-10) imprinted "SOLVAY 1022" in black.
Each orange-red tablet contains 1.25 mg in bottles of 100 (NDC 0032-1024-01) and 1000 (NDC 0032-1024-10) imprinted "SOLVAY 1024" in black.
Each light purple tablet contains 2.5 mg in bottles of 100 (NDC 0032-1025-01) imprinted "SOLVAY 1025" in white.
STORAGE: Store and dispense in tight, light-resistant containers as defined in the USP. Store below 30°C (86°F). Protect from moisture.

REFERENCES
1. Zeil, H. K. and W. D. Finkle, "Increased Risk of Endometrial Carcinoma Among Users of Conjugated Estrogens." **New England Journal of Medicine,** 293:1167–1170, 1975.
2. Smith, D. C., R. Prentic, D. J. Thompson, and W. L. Hermann, "Association of Exogenous Estrogen and Endometrial Carcinoma," **New England Journal of Medicine,** 293:1164–1167, 1975.
3. Mack, T. M., M. C. Pike, B. E. Henderson, R. I. Pfeffer, V. R. Gerkins, M. Arthur, and S. E. Brown, "Estrogens, and Endometrial Cancer in a Retirement Community." **New England Journal of Medicine,** 284:1262–1267, 1976.
4. Weiss, N. S., D. R. Szekely and D. F. Austin, "Increasing Incidence of Endometrial Cancer in the United States," **New England Journal of Medicine,** 294:1259–1262, 1976.
5. Herbst, A. L., H. Ulfelder and D. C. Poskanzer, "Adenocarcinoma of Vagina," **New England Journal of Medicine,** 284:878–881, 1971.
6. Greenwald, P., J. Barlow, P. Nasca, and W. Burnett, "Vaginal Cancer after Maternal Treatment with Synthetic Estrogens," **New England Journal of Medicine,** 285:390–392, 1971.
7. Lanier, A., K. Noller, D. Decker, L. Elveback, and L. Kurland, "Cancer and Stilbestrol. A Followup of 1719 Persons Exposed to Estrogens in Utero and Born 1943–1959," **Mayo Clinic Proceedings,** 48:793–799, 1973.
8. Herbst, A., R. Kurman, and R. Scully, "Vaginal and Cervical Abnormalities After Exposure to Stilbestrol in Utero," **Obstetrics and Gynecology,** 40:287–298, 1972.
9. Herbst, A., S. Robboy, G. Macdonald, and R. Scully, "The Effects of Local Progesterone on Stilbestrol-Associated Vaginal Adenosis," **American Journal of Obstetrics and Gynecology,** 118:607–615, 1974.
10. Herbst, A., D. Poskanzer, S. Robboy, L. Friedlander, and R. Scully, "Prenatal Exposure to Stilbestrol, A Prospective Comparison of Exposed Female Offspring with Unexposed Controls," **New England Journal of Medicine,** 292:334–339, 1975.
11. Stafl, A. R. Mattingly, D. Foley, and W. Fetherston, "Clinical Diagnosis of Vaginal Adenosis," **Obstetrics and Gynecology,** 43:118–128, 1974.
12. Sherman, A. I., M. Goldrath, A. Berlin, V. Vakhariya, F. Banooni, W. Michaels, P. Goodman, S. Brown, "Cervical-Vaginal Adneosis After In Utero Exposure to Synthetic Estrogens," **Obstetrics and Gynecology,** 44:531–545, 1974.
13. Gal, I., B. Kirman, and J. Stern, "Hormone Pregnancy Tests and Congenital and Malformation," **Nature,** 216:83, 1967.
14. Levy, E. P., A Cohen, and F. C. Fraser, "Hormone Treatment During Pregnancy and Congenital Heart Defects," **Lancet,** 1:611, 1973.
15. Nora, J. and A. Nora, "Birth Defects and Oral Contraceptives," **Lancet,** 1:941–942, 1973.
16. Janerich, D. T., J. M. Piper, and D. M. Glebatis, "Oral Contraceptives and Congenital Limb-Reduction Defects," **New England Journal of Medicine,** 291–697–700, 1974.
17. "Estrogens for Oral or Parental Use," **Federal Register,** 40:8212, 1975.
18. Boston Collaborative Drug Surveillance Program "Surgically Confirmed Gall Bladder Disease, Venous Thromboembolism and Breast Tumors in Relation to Post-Menopausal Estrogen Therapy," **New England Journal of Medicine,** 290:15–19, 1974.
18a. Hoover, R., L. A. Gray, Sr., P. Cole, and B. MacMahon, "Menopausal Estrogens and Breast Cancer," **New England Journal of Medicine,** 295:401–405, 1976.
19. Boston Collaborative Drug Surveillance Program, "Oral Contraceptives and Venous Thromboembolic Disease, Surgically Confirmed Gall Bladder Disease, and Breast Tumors," **Lancet** 1:1399–1404, 1973.
20. Daniel, D., G. H. Campbell, and A. C. Turnbull, "Puerperal Thromboembolism and Suppression of Lactation," **Lancet,** 2:287–289, 1967.

21. The Veterans Administration Cooperative Urological Research Group, "Carcinoma of the Prostate: Treatment Comparisons," **Journal of Urology,** 98:516–522, 1967.

22. Ballar, J.C. "Thromboembolism and Oestrogen Therapy," **Lancet,** 2:560, 1967.

23. Blackard, C., R. Doe, G. Mellinger, and D. Byar, "Incidence of Cardiovascular Disease and Death in Patients Receiving Diethyistilbestrol for Carcinoma of the Prostate," **Cancer,** 26;249–256, 1970.

24. Royal College of General Practioners, "Oral Contraception and Thromboembolic Disease," **Journal of the Royal College of General Practitioners,** 13:267–279, 1967.

25. Inman, W. H. W. and M. P. Veseey, "Investigation of Deaths from Pulmonary, Coronary, and Cerebral Thrombosis and Embolism in Women of Child-Bearing Age,"**British Medical Journal,** 2:193–199, 1968.

26. Vessey, M. P. and R. Doll, "Investigation of Relation Between Use of Oral Contraceptives and Thromboembolic Disease, A Further Report," **British Medical Journal,** 2:651–657, 1969.

27. Sartwell, P. E., A. T. Masi, F. G. Arthes, G. R. Greene, and H. E. Smith, "Thromboembolism and Oral Contraceptives: An Epidemiological Case Control Study," **American Journal of Epidemiology,** 90:365–380, 1969.

28. Collaborative Group for the Study of Stroke in Young Women, "Oral Contraception and Increased Risk of Cerebral Ischemia of Thrombosis," **New England Journal of Medicine,** 288:871–878, 1973.

29. Collaborative Group for the Study of Stroke in Young Women, "Oral Contraceptives and Stroke in Young Women: Associated Risk Factors," **Journal of American Medical Association,** 231:718–722, 1975.

30. Mann, J. I. and W. H. W. Inman, "Oral Contraceptives and Death from Myocardial Infarction," **British Medical Journal,** 2:245–248, 1975.

31. Mann, J. I., M. P. Vessey, M. Thorogood, and R. Doll, "Myocardial Infarction in Young Women with Special Reference to Oral Contraceptive Practice," **British Medical Journal,** 2:241–245, 1975.

32. Inman, W. H., V. P. Vessey, B. Westerholm, and A. Engelund, "Thromboembolic Disease and the Steroidal Content of Oral Contraceptives," **British Medical Journal,** 2:203–209, 1970.

33. Stolley, P. D. J. A. Tonascia, M. S. Tockman, P. E. Sartwell, A. H. Rutledge, and M. P. Jacobs, "Thrombosis with Low-Estrogen Oral Contraceptives," **American Journal of Epidemiology,** 102:197–208, 1975.

34. Vessey, M. P. R. Doll, A. S. Fairbairn, and G. Glober, "Post-Operative Thromboembolism and the Use of the Oral Contraceptives," **British Medical Journal,** 3:123–126, 1970.

35. Greene, G. R. and P. E. Sartwell, "Oral Contraceptives Use in Patients with Thromboembolism Following Surgery, Trauma or Infection," **American Journal of Public Health,** 62:680–685, 1972.

36. Rosenberg, L., M. B. Armstrong and H. Jick, "Myocardial Infarction and Estrogen Therapy in Postmenopausal Women," **New England Journal of Medicine,** 294:1256–1259, 1976.

37. Coronary Drug Project Research Group. The Coronary Drug Project: Initial Findings Leading to Modifications of Its Research Protocol, **Journal of the American Medical Association,** 214:1303–1313, 1970.

38. Baum, J., F. Holtz, J. J. Bookstein, and E. W. Klein, "Possible Association between Benign Hepatomas and Oral Contraceptives," **Lancet,** 2:926–928, 1973.

39. Mays, E. T., W. M. Christopherson, M. M. Mahr, and H. C. Williams, "Hepatic Changes in Young Women Ingesting Contraceptive Steroids, Hepatic Hemorrhage and Primary Hepatic Tumors," **Journal of the American Medical Association,** 235:730–782, 1976.

40. Edmondson, H. A. B. Henderson, and B. Benton, "Liver Cell Adenomas Associated with the Use of Oral Contraceptives," **New England Journal of Medicine,** 294:470–472, 1976.

41. Pfeffer, R. I. and S. Van Den Noore, "Estrogen Use and Stroke Risk in Postmenopausal Women," **American Journal of Epidemiology,** 103:445–456, 1976.

INFORMATION FOR THE PATIENT

WHAT YOU SHOULD KNOW ABOUT ESTROGENS

Estrogens are female hormones produced by the ovaries. The ovaries make several different kinds of estrogens. In addition, scientists have been able to make a variety of synthetic estrogens. As far as we know, all these estrogens have similar properties and therefore much the same usefulness, side effects, and risks. This leaflet is intended to help you understand what estrogens are used for the risks involved in their use, and how to use them as safely as possible.

This leaflet includes the most important information about estrogens, but not all the information. If you want to know more, you can ask your doctor or pharmacist to let you read the package insert prepared for the doctor.

USES OF ESTROGEN

Estrogens are prescribed by doctors for a number of purposes, including:

1. To provide estrogen during a period of adjustment when a woman's ovaries no longer produce it, in order to prevent certain uncomfortable symptoms of estrogen deficiency. (All women normally stop producing estrogens, generally between the ages of 45 and 55; this is called the menopause).
2. To prevent symptoms of estrogen deficiency when a woman's ovaries have been removed surgically before the natural menopause.
3. To prevent pregnancy. (Estrogens are given along with a progestogen, another female hormone; these combinations are called oral contraceptives or birth control pills. Patient labeling is available to women taking oral contraceptives and they will not be discussed in this leaflet).
4. To treat certain cancers in women and men.

THERE IS NO PROPER USE OF ESTROGENS IN A PREGNANT WOMAN.

ESTROGEN IN THE MENOPAUSE

In the natural course of their lives, all women eventually experience a decrease in estrogen production. This usually occurs between ages 45 and 55 but may occur earlier or later. Sometimes the ovaries may need to be removed before natural menopause by an operation, producing a "surgical menopause."

When the amount of estrogen in the blood begins to decrease, many women may develop typical symptoms: Feelings of warmth in the face, neck, and chest or sudden intense episodes of heat and sweating throughout the body (called "hot flashes" or "hot flushes"). These symptoms are sometimes very uncomfortable. A few women eventually develop changes in the vagina (called "atrophic vaginitis") which cause discomfort, especially during and after intercourse. Estrogens can be prescribed to treat these symptoms of the menopause. It is estimated that considerably more than half of all women undergoing the menopause have only mild symptoms or no symptoms at all and therefore do not need estrogens. Other women may need estrogens for a few months, while their bodies adjust to lower estrogen levels. Sometimes the need will be for periods longer than six months. In an attempt to avoid overstimulation of the uterus (womb), estrogens are usually given cyclically during each month of use, that is three weeks of pills followed by one week without pills.

Sometimes women experience nervous symptoms or depression during menopause. There is no evidence that estrogens are effective for such symptoms and they should not be used to treat them, although other treatment may be needed. You may have heard that taking estrogens for long periods (years) after the menopause will keep your skin soft and supple and keep you feeling young. There is no evidence that this is so, however, and such long-term treatment carries important risks.

THE DANGERS OF ESTROGENS

1. **Cancer of the uterus.** If estrogens are used in the postmenopausal period for more than a year, there is an increased risk of **endometrial cancer** (cancer of the uterus). Women taking estrogens have roughly 5 to 10 times as great a change of getting this cancer as women who take no estrogens. To put this another way, while a postmenopausal woman not taking estrogens has 1 chance in 1,000 each year of getting cancer of the uterus, a woman taking estrogens has 5 to 10 chances in 1,000 each year. For this reason **it is important to take estrogens only when you really need them.**

The risk of this cancer is greater the longer estrogens are used and also seems to be greater when larger doses are taken. For this reason **it is important to take the lowest dose of estrogen that will control symptoms and to take it only as long as it is needed.** If estrogens are needed for longer periods of time, your doctor will want to reevaluate your need for estrogens at least every six months. Women using estrogens should report any irregular vaginal bleeding to their doctors; such bleeding may be of no importance, but it can be an early warning of cancer of the uterus. If you have undiagnosed vaginal bleeding, you should not use estrogens until a diagnosis is made and you are certain there is no cancer of the uterus.

2. **Other possible cancers.** Estrogens can cause development of other tumors in animals, such as tumors of the breast, cervix, vagina, or liver, when given for a long time. At present there is no good evidence that women using estrogen in the menopause have an increased risk of such tumors, but there is no way yet to be sure they do not; and one study raises the possibility that use of estrogens in the menopause may increase the risk of breast cancer many years later. This is a further reason to use estrogens only when clearly needed. While you are taking estrogens, it is important that you go to your doctor at least once a year for a physical examination. Also, if members of your family have had breast cancer or if you have breast nodules or abnormal mammograms (breast x-rays), your doctor may

wish to carry out more frequent examinations of your breasts.

3. **Gallbladder disease.** Women who use estrogens after menopause are more likely to develop gallbladder disease needing surgery as women who do not use estrogens. Birth control pills have a similar effect.

4. **Abnormal blood clotting.** Oral contraceptives increase the risk of blood clotting in various parts of the body. This can result in a stroke (if the clot is in the brain), a heart attack (clot in a blood vessel in the heart), or pulmonary embolus (a clot which forms in the legs or pelvis, then breaks off and travels to the lungs). Any of these can be fatal.

At this time use of estrogens in the menopause is not known to cause such blood clotting, but this has not been fully studied and there could still prove to be such a risk. It is recommended that if you have had clotting in the legs or lungs or a heart attack or stroke while you were using estrogens or birth control pills, you should not use estrogens (unless they are being used to treat cancer of the breast or prostate). If you have had a stroke or heart attack or if you have angina pectoris, estrogens should be used with great caution and only if clearly needed (for example, if you have severe symptoms of the menopause). The larger doses of estrogen used to prevent swelling of the breasts after pregnancy have been reported to cause clotting in the legs and lungs.

SPECIAL WARNING ABOUT PREGNANCY. You should not receive estrogen if you are pregnant. If this should occur, there is a greater than usual chance that the developing child will be born with a birth defect, although the possibility remains fairly small. A female child may have an increased risk of developing cancer of the vagina or cervix later in life (in the teens or twenties). Every possible effort should be made to avoid exposure to estrogens during pregnancy. If exposure occurs, see your doctor.

OTHER EFFECTS OF ESTROGENS: In addition to the serious known risks of estrogens described above, estrogens have the following side affects and potential risks.

1. **Nausea and vomiting.** The most common side effect of estrogen therapy in nausea. Vomiting is less common.

2. **Effects on breasts.** Estrogens may cause breast tenderness or enlargement and may cause the breasts to secrete a liquid. These effects are not dangerous.

3. **Effects on the uterus.** Estrogens may cause benign fibroid tumors of the uterus to get larger.

Some women will have menstrual bleeding when estrogens are stopped. But if the bleeding occurs on days you are still taking estrogens you should report this to your doctor.

4. **Effects on liver.** Women taking oral contraceptives develop on rare occasions a benign tumor of the liver which can rupture and bleed into the abdomen. So far, these tumors have not been reported in women using estrogens in the menopause, but you should report any swelling or unusual pain or tenderness in the abdomen to your doctor immediately.

Women with a past history of jaundice (yellowing of the skin and white parts of the eyes) may get jaundice again during estrogen use. If this occurs, stop taking estrogens and see your doctor.

5. **Other effects.** Estrogens may cause excess fluid to be retained in the body. This may make some conditions worse, such as epilepsy, migraine, heart disease, or kidney disease.

SUMMARY

Estrogens have important uses, but they have serious risks as well. You must decide, with your doctor, whether the risks are acceptable to you in view of the benefits of treatment. Except where your doctor has prescribed estrogens for use in special cases of cancer of the breast or prostate, you should not use estrogens if you have cancer of the breast or uterus, are pregnant, have undiagnosed abnormal vaginal bleeding, or have had stroke, heart attack or angina, or clotting in the legs or lungs in the past while your were taking estrogens. You can use estrogens as safely as possible by understanding that your doctor will require regular physical examinations while you are taking them and will try to discontinue the drug as soon as possible and use the smallest dose possible. Be alert for signs of trouble including:

1. Abnormal bleeding from the vagina.
2. Pains in the calves or chest or sudden shortness of breath, or coughing blood (indicating possible clots in the legs, heart, or lungs).
3. Severe headache, dizziness, faintness, or changes in vision (indicating possible developing clots in the brain or eye).
4. Breast lumps (you should ask your doctor how to examine your own breasts).
5. Jaundice (yellowing of the skin).
6. Mental depression.

Based on his or her assessment of your medical needs, your doctor has prescribed this drug for you. Do not give the drug to anyone else.

Continued on next page

Solvay—Cont.

HOW SUPPLIED

ESTRATAB® (Esterified Estrogen Tablets, USP)—Tablets for oral administration.

0.3 mg/Tablet (Blue); 0.625 mg/Tablet (Yellow); 1.25 mg/Tablet (Orange-Red); and 2.5 mg/Tablet (Light Purple).

3E Rev. 6/91

PATIENT INFORMATION
WHAT YOUR SHOULD KNOW ABOUT ESTROGENS

ESTRATAB® (ESTERIFIED ESTROGENS)
WHAT YOU SHOULD KNOW ABOUT ESTROGENS

Estrogens are female hormones produced by the ovaries. The ovaries make several different kinds of estrogens. In addition, scientists have been able to make a variety of synthetic estrogens. As far as we know, all these estrogens have similar properties and therefore much the same usefulness, side effects, and risks. This leaflet is intended to help you understand what estrogens are used for, the risks involved in their use, and how to use them as safely as possible.

This leaflet includes the most important information about estrogens, but not all the information. If you want to know more, you can ask your doctor or pharamcist to let you read the package insert prepared for the doctor.

USES OF ESTROGEN

Estrogens are prescribed by doctors for a number of purposes, including:

1. To provide estrogen during a period of adjustment when a woman's ovaries no longer produce it, in order to prevent certain uncomfortable symptoms of estrogen deficiency. (All women normally stop producing estrogens, generally between the ages of 45 and 55; this is called the menopause).

2. To prevent symptoms of estrogen deficiency when a woman's ovaries have been removed surgically before the natural menopause.

3. To prevent pregnancy. (Estrogens are given along with a progestogen, another female hormone; these combinations are called oral contraceptives or birth control pills. Patient labeling is available to women taking oral contraceptives and they will not be discussed in this leaflet).

4. To treat certain cancers in women and men.

THERE IS NO PROPER USE OF ESTROGENS IN A PREGNANT WOMAN.

ESTROGENS IN THE MENOPAUSE

In the natural course of their lives, all women eventually experience a decrease in estrogen production. This usually occurs between ages 45 and 55 but may occur earlier or later. Sometimes the ovaries may need to be removed before natural menopause by an operation, producing a "surgical menopause."

When the amount of estrogen in the blood begins to decrease, many women may develop typical symptoms: Feelings of warmth in the face, neck, and chest or sudden intense episodes of heat and sweating throughout the body (called "hot flashes" or "hot flushes"). These symptoms are sometimes very uncomfortable. A few women eventually develop changes in the vagina (called "atrophic vaginitis") which cause discomfort, especially during and after intercourse. Estrogens can be prescribed to treat these symptoms of the menopause. It is estimated that considerably more than half of all women undergoing the menopause have only mild symptoms or no symptoms at all and therefore do not need estrogens. Other women may need estrogens for a few months, while their bodies adjust to lower estrogen levels. Sometimes the need will be for periods longer than six months. In an attempt to avoid overstimulation of the uterus (womb), estrogens are usually given cyclically during each month of use, that is three weeks of pills followed by one week without pills.

Sometimes women experience nervous symptoms or depression during menopause. There is no evidence that estrogens are effective for such symptoms and they should not be used to treat them, although other treatment may be needed.

You may have heard that taking estrogens for long periods (years) after the menopause will keep your skin soft and supple and keep you feeling young. There is no evidence that this is so, however, and such long-term treatment carries important risks.

THE DANGERS OF ESTROGENS

1. **Cancer of the uterus.** If estrogens are used in the postmenopausal period for more than a year, there is an increased risk of **endometrial cancer** (cancer of the uterus). Women taking estrogens have roughly 5 to 10 times as great a chance of getting this cancer as women who take no estrogens. To put this another way, while a postmenopausal woman not taking estrogens has 1 chance in 1,000 each year of getting cancer of the uterus, a women taking estrogens has 5 to 10 chances in 1,000 each year. For this reason **it is important to take estrogens only when you really need them.**

The risk of this cancer is greater the longer estrogens are used and also seems to be greater when larger doses are

taken. For this reason **it is important to take the lowest dose of estrogen that will control symptoms and to take it only as long as it is needed.** If estrogens are needed for longer periods of time, your doctor will want to reevaluate your need for estrogens at least every six months.

Women using estrogens should report any irregular vaginal bleeding to their doctors; such bleeding may be of no importance, but it can be an early warning of cancer of the uterus. If you have undiagnosed vaginal bleeding, you should not use estrogens until a diagnosis is made and you are certain there is no cancer of the uterus.

2. **Other possible cancers.** Estrogens can cause development of other tumors in animals, such as tumors of the breast, cervix, vagina, or liver, when given for a long time. At present there is no good evidence that women using estrogen in the menopause have an increased risk of such tumors, but there is no way yet to be sure they do not; and one study raises the possibility that use of estrogens in the menopause may increase the risk of breast cancer many years later. This is a further reason to use estrogens only when clearly needed. While you are taking estrogens, it is important that you go to your doctor at least once a year for a physical examination. Also, if members of your family have had breast cancer or if you have breast nodules or abnormal mammograms (breast x-rays), your doctor may wish to carry out more frequent examinations of your breasts.

3. **Gall bladder disease.** Women who use estrogens after menopause are more likely to develop gall bladder disease needing surgery as women who do not use estrogens. Birth control pills have a similar effect.

4. **Abnormal blood clotting.** Oral contraceptives increase the risk of blood clotting in various parts of the body. This can result in a stroke (if the clot is in the brain), a heart attack (clot in a blood vessel of the heart), or a pulmonary embolus (a clot which forms in the legs or pelvis, then breaks off and travels to the lungs). Any of these can be fatal.

At this time use of estrogens in the menopause is not known to cause such blood clotting, but this has not been fully studied and there could still prove to be such a risk. It is recommended that if you have had clotting in the legs or lungs or a heart attack or stroke while you were using estrogens or birth control pills, you should not use estrogens (unless they are being used to treat cancer of the breast or prostate). If you have had a stroke or heart attack or if you have angina pectoris, estrogens should be used with great caution and only if clearly needed (for example, if you have severe symptoms of the menopause). The larger doses of estrogen used to prevent swelling of the breasts after pregnancy have been reported to cause clotting in the legs and lungs.

SPECIAL WARNING ABOUT PREGNANCY

You should not receive estrogen if you are pregnant. If this should occur, there is a greater than usual chance that the developing child will be born with a birth defect, although the possibility remains fairly small. A female child may have an increased risk of developing cancer of the vagina or cervix later in life (in the teens or twenties). Every possible effort should be made to avoid exposure to estrogens during pregnancy. If exposure occurs, see your doctor.

OTHER EFFECTS OF ESTROGENS

In addition to the serious known risks of estrogens described above, estrogens have the following side effects and potential risks:

1. **Nausea and vomiting.** The most common side effect of estrogen therapy is nausea. Vomiting is less common.

2. **Effects on breasts.** Estrogens may cause breast tenderness or enlargement and may cause the breasts to secrete a liquid. These affects are not dangerous.

3. **Effects on the uterus.** Estrogens may cause benign fibroid tumors of the uterus to get larger. Some women will have menstrual bleeding when estrogens are stopped. But if the bleeding occurs on days you are still taking estrogens you should report this to your doctor.

4. **Effects on liver.** Women taking oral contraceptives develop on rare occasions a benign tumor of the liver which can rupture and bleed into the abdomen. So far, these tumors have not been reported in women using estrogens in the menopause, but you should report any swelling or unusual pain or tenderness in the abdomen to your doctor immediately.

Women with a past history of jaundice (yellowing of the skin and white parts of the eyes) may get jaundice again during estrogen use. If this occurs, stop taking estrogens and see your doctor.

5. **Other effects.** Estrogens may cause excess fluid to be retained in the body. This may make some conditions worse, such as epilepsy, migraine, heart disease, or kidney disease.

SUMMARY

Estrogens have important uses, but they have serious risks as well. You must decide, with your doctor, whether the risks are acceptable to you in view of the benefits of treatment. Except where your doctor has prescribed estrogens for use in special cases of cancer of the breast or prostate, you should

not use estrogens if you have cancer of the breast or uterus, are pregnant, have undiagnosed abnormal bleeding, or have had a stroke, heart attack or angina, or clotting in the legs or lungs in the past while you were taking estrogens.

You can use estrogens as safely as possible by understanding that your doctor will require regular physical examinations while you are taking them and will try to discontinue the drug as soon as possible and use the smallest dose possible. Be alert for signs of trouble including:

1. Abnormal bleeding from the vagina.

2. Pains in the calves or chest or sudden shortness of breath, or coughing blood (indicating possible clots in the legs, heart, or lungs).

3. Severe headache, dizziness, faintness, or changes in vision (indicating possible developing clots in the brain or eye).

4. Breast lumps (you should ask your doctor how to examine your own breasts).

5. Jaundice (yellowing of the skin).

6. Mental depression.

Based on his or her assessment of your medical needs, your doctor has prescribed this drug for you. Do not give the drug to anyone else.

ESTRATAB® (Esterified Estrogen Tablets, USP) —tablets for oral administration.

Each round blue sugar coated tablet contains 0.3 mg.
Each round yellow sugar coated tablet contains 0.625 mg.
Each round orange-red sugar coated tablet contains 1.25 mg.
Each round light purple sugar coated tablet contains 2.5 mg.

4E REV 2/92

SOLVAY PHARMACEUTICALS
MARIETTA, GA 30062

Shown in Product Identification Section, page 432

ESTRATEST®　℞

[es 'trah-test]

ESTRATEST® H.S.　℞

Esterified Estrogens and Methyltestosterone

WARNING

1. ESTROGENS HAVE BEEN REPORTED TO INCREASE THE RISK OF ENDOMETRIAL CARCINOMA.

Three independent case control studies have reported an increased risk of endometrial cancer in postmenopausal women exposed to exogenous estrogens for prolonged periods.[1-3] This risk was independent of the other known risk factors for endometrial cancer. These studies are further supported by the finding that incidence rates of endometrial cancer have increased sharply since 1969 in eight different areas of the United States with population-based cancer reporting systems, an increase which may be related to the rapidly expanding use of estrogens during the last decade.[4]

The three case control studies reported that the risk of endometrial cancer in estrogen users was about 4.5 to 13.9 times greater than in nonusers. The risk appears to depend on both duration of treatment[1] and on estrogen dose.[3] In view of these findings, when estrogens are used for the treatment of menopausal symptoms, the lowest dose that will control symptoms should be utilized and medication should be discontinued as soon as possible. When prolonged treatment is medically indicated, the patient should be reassessed on at least a semiannual basis to determine the need for continued therapy. Although the evidence must be considered preliminary, one study suggests that cyclic administration of low doses of estrogen may carry less risk than continuous administration;[3] it therefore appears prudent to utilize such a regimen.

Close clinical surveillance of all women taking estrogens is important. In all cases of undiagnosed persistent or recurring abnormal vaginal bleeding, adequate diagnostic measures should be undertaken to rule out malignancy.

There is no evidence at present that "natural" estrogens are more or less hazardous than "synthetic" estrogens at equiestrogenic doses.

2. ESTROGENS SHOULD NOT BE USED DURING PREGNANCY.

The use of female sex hormones, both estrogens and progestogens, during early pregnancy may seriously damage the offspring. It has been shown that females exposed in utero to diethylstilbestrol, a non-steroidal estrogen, have an increased risk of developing in later life a form of vaginal or cervical cancer that is ordinarily extremely rare.[5,6] This risk has been estimated as not greater than 4 per 1000 exposures.[7] Furthermore, a high percentage of such exposed women (from 30 to 90 percent) have been found to have vaginal adenosis,[8-12] epithelial changes of the vagina and cervix. Although these changes are histologically benign, it is not known whether they are precursors of malignancy. Although

similar data are not available with the use of other estrogens, it cannot be presumed they would not induce similar changes.
Several reports suggest an association between intrauterine exposure to female sex hormones and congenital anomalies, including congenital heart defects and limb reduction defects.[13–16] One case control study[16] estimated a 4.7 fold increased risk of limb reduction defects in infants exposed in utero to sex hormones (oral contraceptives, hormone withdrawal tests for pregnancy, or attempted treatment for threatened abortion). Some of these exposures were very short and involved only a few days of treatment. The data suggest that the risk of limb reduction defects in exposed fetuses is somewhat less than 1 per 1000.
In the past, female sex hormones have been used during pregnancy in an attempt to treat threatened or habitual abortion. There is considerable evidence that estrogens are ineffective for these indications, and there is no evidence from well controlled studies that progestogens are effective for these uses.
If ESTRATEST® or ESTRATEST® H.S. is used during pregnancy, or if the patient becomes pregnant while taking this drug, she should be apprised of the potential risks to the fetus, and the advisability of pregnancy continuation.

DESCRIPTION

ESTRATEST®: Each dark green, capsule shaped, sugar-coated oral tablet contains: 1.25 mg of Esterified Estrogens, USP and 2.5 mg of Methyltestosterone.
ESTRATEST® H.S. (Half-Strength): Each light green, capsule shaped, sugar-coated oral tablet contains: 0.625 mg of Esterified Estrogens, USP and 1.25 mg of Methyltestosterone.

ESTERIFIED ESTROGENS: Esterified Estrogens, USP is a mixture of the sodium salts of the sulfate esters of the estrogenic substances, principally estrone, that are of the type excreted by pregnant mares. Esterified Estrogens contain not less than 75.0 percent and not more than 85.0 percent of sodium estrone sulfate, and not less than 6.0 percent and not more than 15.0 percent of sodium equilin sulfate, in such proportion that the total of these two components is not less than 90.0 percent.
Category: Estrogens

METHYLTESTOSTERONE: Methyltestosterone is an androgen.
Androgens are derivatives of cyclopentano-perhydrophenanthrene. Endogenous androgens are C-19 steroids with a side chain at C-17, and with two angular methyl groups. Testosterone is the primary endogenous androgen. Fluoxymesterone and methyltestosterone are synthetic derivatives of testosterone.
Methyltestosterone is a white to light yellow crystalline substance that is virtually insoluble in water but soluble in organic solvents. It is stable in air but decomposes in light.
Methyltestosterone structural formula:

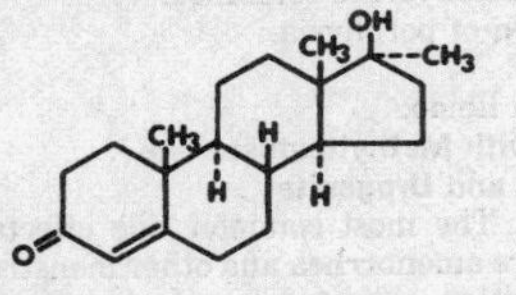

$C_{20}H_{30}O_2$, 302.46
Androst-4-en-3-one, 17-hydroxy-17-methyl-, (17B)-
Category: Androgen.

ESTRATEST® and ESTRATEST® H.S. Tablets also contain the following inactive ingredients: Lactose (hydrous), Microcrystalline Cellulose,, Colloidal Silicon Dioxide, Sodium Bicarbonate and Magnesium Stearate. Ingredients used in the coating for ESTRATEST® and ESTRATEST® H.S. Tablets are: Pharmaceutical Glaze, Povidone, Acetylated Monoglyceride, Talc, Sorbic Acid, Gelatin, Acacia, Sucrose, Calcium Carbonate, Corn Starch, Sodium Benzoate, Citric Acid, Methylparaben, Propylparaben and Carnauba Wax.
The coloring and imprinting material for ESTRATEST® also contains: D&C Yellow No. 10 Aluminum Lake, FD&C Blue No. 1 Aluminum Lake, FD&C Yellow No. 6 Aluminum Lake, Titanium Dioxide, Lecithin, Ethylene Glycol Monoethyl Ether and Dimenthylpolysiloxane.
The coloring and imprinting material for ESTRATEST® H.S. also contains: D&C Yellow No. 10 Aluminum Lake, FD&C Blue No. 1 Aluminum Lake, Black Iron Oxide, FD&C Blue No. 2 Aluminum Lake, FD&C Yellow No. 6 Aluminum Lake, FD&C Red No. 40 Aluminum Lake, Titanium Dioxide and Propylene Glycol.

CLINICAL PHARMACOLOGY

Estrogens: Estrogens are important in the development and maintenance of the female reproductive system and secondary sex characteristics. They promote growth and development of the vagina, uterus, and fallopian tubes, and enlargement of the breasts. Indirectly, they contribute to the shaping of the skeleton, maintenance of tone and elasticity of urogenital structures, changes in the epiphyses of the long bones that allow for the pubertal growth spurt and its termination, growth of axillary and pubic hair, and pigmentation of the nipples and genitals. Decline of estrogenic activity at the end of the menstrual cycle can bring on menstruation, although the cessation of progesterone secretion is the most important factor in the mature ovulatory cycle. However, in the preovulatory or nonovulatory cycle, estrogen is the primary determinant in the onset of menstruation. Estrogens also affect the release of pituitary gonadotropins.
The pharmacologic effects of esterified estrogens are similar to those of endogenous estrogens. They are soluble in water and are well absorbed from the gastrointestinal tract.
In responsive tissues (female genital organs, breasts, hypothalamus, pituitary) estrogens enter the cell and are transported into the nucleus. As a result of estrogen action, specific RNA and protein synthesis occurs.

Estrogen Pharmacokinetics
Metabolism and inactivation occur primarily in the liver. Some estrogens are excreted into the bile; however they are reabsorbed from the intestine and returned to the liver through the portal venous system. Water soluble esterified estrogens are strongly acidic and are ionized in body fluids, which favor excretion through the kidneys since tubular reabsorption is minimal.

Androgens Endogenous androgens are responsible for the normal growth and development of the male sex organs and for maintenance of secondary sex characteristics. These effects include the growth and maturation of prostate, seminal vesicles, penis, and scrotum; the development of male hair distribution, such as beard, pubic, chest, and axillary hair, laryngeal enlargement, vocal cord thickening, alterations in body musculature, and fat distribution. Drugs in this class also cause retention of nitrogen, sodium, potassium, phosphorus, and decreased urinary excretion of calcium. Androgens have been reported to increase protein anabolism and decrease protein catabolism. Nitrogen balance is improved only when there is sufficient intake of calories and protein.
Androgens are responsible for the growth spurt of adolescence and for the eventual termination of linear growth which is brought about by fusion of the epiphyseal growth centers. In children, exogenous androgens accelerate linear growth rates, but may cause a disproportionate advancement in bone maturation. Use over long periods may result in fusion of the epiphyseal growth centers and termination of growth process. Androgens have been reported to stimulate the production of red blood cells by enhancing the production of erythropoietic stimulating factor.

Androgen Pharmacokinetics
Testosterone given orally is metabolized by the gut and 44 percent is cleared by the liver in the first pass. Oral doses as high as 400 mg per day are needed to achieve clinically effective blood levels for full replacement therapy. The synthetic androgens (methyltestosterone and fluoxymesterone) are less extensively metabolized by the liver and have longer half-lives. They are more suitable than testosterone for oral administration.
Testosterone in plasma is 98 percent bound to a specific testosterone-estradiol binding globulin, and about 2 percent is free. Generally, the amount of this sex-hormone binding globulin in the plasma will determine the distribution of testosterone between free and bound forms, and the free testosterone concentration will determine its half-life.
About 90 percent of a dose of testosterone is excreted in the urine as glucuronic and sulfuric acid conjugates of testosterone and its metabolites; about 6 percent of a dose is excreted in the feces, mostly in the unconjugated form. Inactivation of testosterone occurs primarily in the liver. Testosterone is metabolized to various 17-keto steroids through two different pathways. There are considerable variations of the half-life of testosterone as reported in the literature, ranging from 10 to 100 minutes.
In many tissues the activity of testosterone appears to depend on reduction to dihydrotestosterone, which binds to cytosol receptor proteins. The steroid-receptor complex is transported to the nucleus where it initiates transcription events and cellular changes related to androgen action.

INDICATIONS

ESTRATEST® and ESTRATEST® H.S. are indicated in the treatment of:
Moderate to severe *vasomotor* symptoms associated with the menopause in those patients not improved by estrogens alone. (There is no evidence that estrogens are effective for nervous symptoms or depression without associated vasomotor symptoms, and they should not be used to treat such conditions.)
ESTRATEST® AND ESTRATEST® H.S. HAVE NOT BEEN SHOWN TO BE EFFECTIVE FOR ANY PURPOSE DURING PREGNANCY AND ITS USE MAY CAUSE SEVERE HARM TO THE FETUS (SEE BOXED WARNING).

CONTRAINDICATIONS

Estrogens should not be used in women with any of the following conditions:

1. Known or suspected cancer of the breast except in appropriately selected patients being treated for metastatic disease.
2. Known or suspected estrogen-dependent neoplasia.
3. Known or suspected pregnancy (See Boxed Warning).
4. Undiagnosed abnormal genital bleeding.
5. Active thrombophlebitis or thromboembolic disorders.
6. A past history of thrombophlebitis, thrombosis, or thromboembolic disorders associated with previous estrogen use (except when used in treatment of breast malignancy).

Methyltestosterone should not be used in:

1. The presence of severe liver damage.
2. Pregnancy and in breast-feeding mothers because of the possibility of masculinization of the female fetus or breast-fed infant.

WARNINGS

Associated with Estrogens:

1. **Induction of malignant neoplasms.** Long term continuous administration of natural and synthetic estrogens in certain animal species increases the frequency of carcinomas of the breast, cervix, vagina, and liver. There is now evidence that estrogens increase the risk of carcinoma of the endometrium in humans (See Boxed Warning).
   At the present time there is no satisfactory evidence that estrogens given to postmenopausal women increase the risk of cancer of the breast,[18] although a recent long-term follow-up of a single physician's practice has raised this possibility.[18a] Because of the animal data, there is a need for caution in prescribing estrogens for women with a strong family history of breast cancer or who have breast nodules, fibrocystic disease, or abnormal mammograms.
2. **Gallbladder disease.** A recent study has reported a 2 to 3-fold increase in the risk of surgically confirmed gallbladder disease in women receiving postmenopausal estrogens,[18] similar to the 2-fold increase previously noted in users of oral contraceptives.[19–24a] In the case of oral contraceptives the increased risk appeared after two years of use.[24]
3. **Effects similar to those caused by estrogen-progestogen oral contraceptives.** There are several serious adverse effects of oral contraceptives, most of which have not, up to now, been documented as consequences of postmenopausal estrogen therapy. This may reflect the comparatively low doses of estrogen used in postmenopausal women. It would be expected that the larger doses of estrogen used to treat prostatic or breast cancer or postpartum breast engorgement are more likely to result in these adverse effects, and, in fact, it has been shown that there is an increased risk of thrombosis in men receiving estrogens for prostatic cancer and women for postpartum breast engorgement.[20–23]
   a. **Thromboembolic disease.** It is now well established that users of oral contraceptives have an increased risk of various thromboembolic and thrombotic vascular diseases, such as thrombophlebitis, pulmonary embolism, stroke, and myocardial infarction.[24–31] Cases of retinal thrombosis, mesenteric thrombosis, and optic neuritis have been reported in oral contraceptive users. There is evidence that the risk of several of these adverse reactions is related to the dose of the drug.[32,33] An increased risk of postsurgery thromboembolic complications has also been reported in users of oral contraceptives.[34,35] If feasible, estrogen should be discontinued at least 4 weeks before surgery of the type associated with an increased risk of thromboembolism, or during periods of prolonged immobilization.
   While an increased rate of thromboembolic and thrombotic disease in postmenopausal users of estrogens has not been found,[18–36] this does not rule out the possibility that such an increase may be present or that subgroups of women who have underlying risk factors or who are receiving relatively large doses of estrogens may have increased risk. Therefore estrogens should not be used in persons with active thrombophlebitis or thromboembolic disorders, and they should not be used (except in treatment of malignancy) in persons with a history of such disorders in association with estrogen use. They should be used with caution in patients with cerebral vascular or coronary artery disease and only for those in whom estrogens are clearly needed.
   Large doses of estrogen (5 mg esterified estrogens per day), comparable to those used to treat cancer of the prostate and breast, have been shown in a large prospective clinical trial in men[37] to increase the risk of nonfatal myocardial infarction, pulmonary embolism and thrombophlebitis. When estrogen doses of this size are used, any of the thromboembolic and thrombotic adverse effects associated with oral contraceptive use should be considered a clear risk.

Continued on next page

Solvay—Cont.

b. **Hepatic adenoma.** Benign hepatic adenomas appear to be associated with the use of oral contraceptives.[38–40] Although benign and rare, these may rupture and may cause death through intra-abdominal hemorrhage. Such lesions have not yet been reported in association with other estrogen or progestogen preparations but should be considered in estrogen users having abdominal pain and tenderness, abdominal mass, or hypovolemic shock. Hepatocellular carcinoma has also been reported in women taking estrogen-containing oral contraceptives.[39] The relationship of this malignancy to these drugs is not known at this time.

c. **Elevated blood pressure.** Increased blood pressure is not uncommon in women using oral contraceptives. There is now a report that this may occur with use of estrogens in the menopause[41] and blood pressure should be monitored with estrogen use, especially if high doses are used.

d. **Glucose tolerance.** A worsening of glucose tolerance has been observed in a significant percentage of patients on estrogen-containing oral contraceptives. For this reason, diabetic patients should be carefully observed while receiving estrogens.

4. **Hypercalcemia.** Administration of estrogens may lead to severe hypercalcemia in patients with breast cancer and bone metastases. If this occurs, the drug should be stopped and appropriate measures taken to reduce the serum calcium level.

Associated with Methyltestosterone

In patients with breast cancer, androgen therapy may cause hypercalcemia by stimulating osteolysis. In this case, the drug should be discontinued.

Prolonged use of high doses of androgens has been associated with the development of peliosis hepatis and hepatic neoplasms including hepatocellular carcinoma. (See PRECAUTIONS—*Carcinogenesis*). Peliosis hepatis can be a life-threatening or fatal complication.

Cholestatic hepatitis and jaundice occur with 17-alpha-alkylandrogens at a relatively low dose. If cholestatic hepatitis with jaundice appears or if liver function tests become abnormal, the androgen should be discontinued and the etiology should be determined. Drug-induced jaundice is reversible when the medication is discontinued.

Edema with or without heart failure may be a serious complication in patients with preexisting cardiac, renal, or hepatic disease. In addition to discontinuation of the drug, diuretic therapy may be required.

PRECAUTIONS

Associated with Estrogens

A. General Precautions.

1. A complete medical and family history should be taken prior to the initiation of any estrogen therapy. The pretreatment and periodic physical examiniations should include special reference to blood pressure, breasts, abdomen, and pelvic organs, and should include a Papanicolaou smear. As a general rule, estrogen should not be prescribed for longer than one year without another physical examiniation being performed.
2. Fluid retention—Because estrogens may cause some degree of fluid retention, conditions which might be influenced by this factor such as asthma, epilepsy, migraine, and cardiac or renal dysfunction, require careful observation.
3. Certain patients may develop undesirable manifestations of excessive estrogenic stimulation, such as abnormal or excessive uterine bleeding, mastodynia, etc.
4. Oral contraceptives appear to be associated with an increased incidence of mental depression.[24] Although it is not clear whether this is due to the estrogenic or progestogenic component of the contraceptive, patients with a history of depression should be carefully observed.
5. Preexisting uterine leiomyomata may increase in size during estrogen use.
6. The pathologist should be advised of estrogen therapy when relevant specimens are submitted.
7. Patients with a past history of jaundice during pregnancy have an increased risk of recurrence of jaundice while receiving estrogen-containing oral contraceptive therapy. If jaundice develops in any patient receiving estrogen, the medication should be discontinued while the cause is investigated.
8. Estrogens may be poorly metabolized in patients with impaired liver function and they should be administered with caution in such patients.
9. Because estrogens influence the metabolism of calcium and phosphorus, they should be used with caution in patients with metabolic bone diseases that are associated with hypercalcemia or in patients with renal insufficiency.
10. Because of the effects of estrogens on epiphyseal closure, they should be used judiciously in young patients in whom bone growth is not complete.
11. Certain endocrine and liver function tests may be affected by estrogen-containing oral contraceptives. The following similar changes may be expected with larger doses of estrogen:
    a. Increased sulfobromophthalein retention.
    b. Increased prothrombin and factors VII, VIII, IX and X; decreased antithrombin 3; increased norepinephrine-induced platelet aggregability.
    c. Increased thyroid binding globulin (TBG) leading to increased circulating total thyroid hormone, as measured by PBI, T4 by column, or T4 by radioimmunoassay. Free T3 resin uptake is decreased, reflecting the elevated TBG; free T4 concentration is unaltered.
    d. Impaired glucose tolerance.
    e. Decreased pregnanediol excretion.
    f. Reduced response to metyrapone test.
    g. Reduced serum folate concentration.
    h. Increased serum triglyceride and phospholipid concentration.

B. Information for the Patient. See text of Patient Package Insert which appears after the REFERENCES.

C. Pregnancy Category X. See CONTRAINDICATIONS and Boxed WARNING.

D. Nursing Mothers. As a general principle, the administration of any drug to nursing mothers should be done only when clearly necessary since many drugs are excreted in human milk.

Associated with Methyltestosterone:

A. General Precautions

1. Women should be observed for signs of virilization (deepening of the voice, hirsutism, acne, clitoromegaly, and menstrual irregularities). Discontinuation of drug therapy at the time of evidence of mild virilism is necessary to prevent irreversible virilization. Such virilization is usual following androgen use at high doses.
2. Prolonged dosage of androgen may result in sodium and fluid retention. This may present a problem, especially in patients with compromised cardiac reserve or renal disease.
3. Hypersensitivity may occur rarely.
4. PBI may be decreased in patients taking androgens.
5. Hypercalcemia may occur. If this does occur, the drug should be discontinued.

B. Information for the Patient

The physician should instruct patients to report any of the following side effects of androgens:

Women: Hoarseness, acne, changes in menstrual periods, or more hair on the face.

All Patients: Any nausea, vomiting, changes in skin color or ankle swelling.

C. Laboratory tests

1. Women with disseminated breast carcinoma should have frequent determination of urine and serum calcium levels during the course of androgen therapy (See WARNINGS).
2. Because of the hepatotoxicity associated with the use of 17-alpha-alkylated androgens, liver function tests should be obtained periodically.
3. Hemoglobin and hematocrit should be checked periodically for polycythemia in patients who are receiving high doses of androgens.

D. Drug Interactions

1. *Anticoagulants* C-17 substituted derivatives of testosterone, such as methandrostenolone, have been reported to decrease the anticoagulant requirements of patients receiving oral anticoagulants. Patients receiving oral anticoagulant therapy require close monitoring, especially when androgens are started or stopped.
2. *Oxyphenbutazone.* Concurrent administration of oxyphenbutazone and androgens may result in elevated serum levels of oxyphenbutazone.
3. *Insulin.* In diabetic patients the metabolic effects of androgens may decrease blood glucose and insulin requirements.

E. Drug/Laboratory Test Interferences

Androgens may decrease levels of thyroxine-binding globulin, resulting in decreased T_4 serum levels and increased resin uptake of T_3 and T_4. Free thyroid hormone levels remain unchanged, however, and there is no clinical evidence of thyroid dysfunction.

F. Carcinogenesis

Animal Data. Testosterone has been tested by subcutaneous injection and implantation in mice and rats. The implant induced cervical-uterine tumors in mice, which metastasized in some cases. There is suggestive evidence that injection of testosterone into some strains of female mice increases their susceptibility to hepatoma. Testosterone is also known to increase the number of tumors and decrease the degree of differentiation of chemically induced carcinomas of the liver in rats.

Human Data. There are rare reports of hepatocellular carcinoma in patients receiving long-term therapy with androgens in high doses. Withdrawal of the drugs did not lead to regression of the tumors in all cases.

Geriatric patients treated with androgens may be at an increased risk for the development of prostatic hypertrophy and prostatic carcinoma.

G. Pregnancy

Teratogenic Effects. Pregnancy Category X (see CONTRAINDICATIONS).

H. Nursing Mothers

It is not known whether androgens are excreted in human milk. Because many drugs are excreted in human milk and because of the potential for serious adverse reactions in nursing infants from androgens, a decision should be made whether to discontinue nursing or to discontinue the drug, taking into account the importance of the drug to the mother.

ADVERSE REACTIONS

Associated with Estrogens (See Warnings regarding induction of neoplasia, adverse effects on the fetus, increased incidence of gallbladder disease, and adverse effects similar to those of oral contraceptives, including thromboembolism). The following additional adverse reactions have been reported with estrogenic therapy, including oral contraceptives:

1. Genitourinary system.
Breakthrough bleeding, spotting, change in menstrual flow.
Dysmenorrhea.
Premenstrual-like syndrome.
Amenorrhea during and after treatment.
Increase in size of uterine fibromyomata.
Vaginal candidiasis.
Change in cervical erosion and in degree of cervical secretion.
Cystitis-like syndrome.

2. Breasts.
Tenderness, enlargement, secretion.

3. Gastrointestinal.
Nausea, vomiting.
Abdominal cramps, bloating.
Cholestatic jaundice.

4. Skin.
Chloasma or melasma which may persist when drug is discontinued.
Erythema multiforme.
Erythema nodosum.
Hemorrhagic eruption.
Loss of scalp hair.
Hirsutism.

5. Eyes.
Steepening of corneal curvature.
Intolerance to contact lenses.

6. CNS.
Headache, migraine, dizziness.
Mental depression.
Chorea.

7. Miscellaneous.
Increase or decrease in weight.
Reduced carbohydrate tolerance.
Aggravation of porphyria.
Edema.
Changes in libido.

Associated with Methyltestosterone

A. Endocrine and Urogenital

1. *Female:* The most common side effects of androgen therapy are amenorrhea and other menstrual irregularities, inhibition of gonadotropin secretion, and virilization, including deepening of the voice and clitoral enlargement. The latter usually is not reversible after androgens are discontinued. When administered to a pregnant woman androgens cause virilization of external genitalia of the female fetus.
2. *Skin and Appendages:* Hirsutism, male pattern of baldness, and acne.
3. *Fluid and Electrolyte Disturbances:* Retention of sodium, chloride, water, potassium, calcium, and inorganic phosphates.
4. *Gastrointestinal:* Nausea, cholestatic jaundice, alterations in liver function test, rarely hepatocellular neoplasms, and peliosis hepatis (see WARNINGS).
5. *Hematologic:* Suppression of clotting factors II, V, VII, and X, bleeding in patients on concomitant anticoagulant therapy, and polycythemia.
6. *Nervous System:* Increased or decreased libido, headache, anxiety, depression, and generalized paresthesia.
7. *Metabolic:* Increased serum cholesterol.
8. *Miscellaneous:* Inflammation and pain at the site of intramuscular injection or subcutaneous implantation of testosterone containing pellets, stomatitis with buccal preparations, and rarely anaphylactoid reactions.

OVERDOSAGE

Numerous reports of ingestion of large doses of estrogen-containing oral contraceptives by young children indicate that serious ill effects do not occur. Overdosage of estrogen may cause nausea, and withdrawal bleeding may occur in females.

There have been no reports of acute overdosage with the androgens.

DOSAGE AND ADMINISTRATION

1. *Given cyclically for short-term use only:*

For treatment of moderate to severe *vasomotor* symptoms associated with the menopause in patients not improved by estrogen alone.

The lowest dose that will control symptoms should be chosen and medication should be discontinued as promptly as possible.

Administration should be cyclic (e.g., three weeks on and one week off).

Attempts to discontinue or taper medication should be made at three to six month intervals.

Usual Dosage Range: 1 or 2 tablets of ESTRATEST® or ESTRATEST® H.S. daily as recommended by the physician. Treated patients with an intact uterus should be monitored closely for signs of endometrial cancer and appropriate diagnostic measures should be taken to rule out malignancy in the event of persistent or recurring abnormal vaginal bleeding.

HOW SUPPLIED

ESTRATEST® (Imprinted "SOLVAY 1026") in bottles of 100—NDC 0032-1026-01 and 1000—NDC 0032-1026-10.

ESTRATEST® (Dark green, capsule shaped, sugar-coated oral tablets) contains: 1.25 mg of Esterified Estrogens, USP and 2.5 mg of Methyltestosterone, USP.

ESTRATEST® H.S. (Imprinted "SOLVAY 1023") in bottles of 100—NDC 0032-1023-01.

ESTRATEST® H.S. "Half-Strength" (Light green, capsule shaped, sugar-coated oral tablets) contains: 0.625 mg of Esterified Estrogens, USP and 1.25 mg of Methyltestosterone, USP.

Store at controlled room temperature, 15°-30°C (59°-86°F).

REFERENCES

1. Ziel, H.K., *et al.*: N. Engl. J. Med. *293*:1167–1170, 1975.
2. Smith, D.C., *et al.*: N. Engl. J. Med. *293*:1164–1167, 1975.
3. Mack, T.M., *et al.*: N. Engl. J. Med. *294*:1262–1267, 1976.
4. Weiss, N.S., *et al.*: N. Engl. J. Med. *294*:1259–1262, 1976.
5. Herbst, A.L., *et al.*: N. Engl. J. Med. *284*:878–881, 1971.
6. Greenwald, P., *et al.*: N. Engl. J. Med. *285*:390–392, 1971.
7. Lanier, A., *et al.*: Mayo Clin. Proc. *48*:793–799, 1973.
8. Herbst, A., *et al.*: Obstet. Gynecol. *40*:287–298, 1972.
9. Herbst, A., *et al.*: Am. J. Obstet. Gynecol. *118*:607–615, 1974.
10. Herbst, A., *et al.*: N. Engl. J. Med. *292*:334–339, 1975.
11. Stafl, A., *et al.*: Obstet. Gynecol. *43*-128, 1974.
12. Sherman, A.I., *et al.*: Obstet. Gynecol. *44*:531–545, 1974.
13. Gal, I., *et al.*: Nature *216*:83, 1967.
14. Levy, E.P., *et al.*: Lancet *1*:611, 1973.
15. Nora, J., *et al.*: Lancet *1*:941–942, 1973.
16. Janerich, D.T., *et al.*: N. Engl. J. Med. *291*:697–700, 1974.
17. Estrogens for Oral or Parenteral Use: Federal Register *40*:8212, 1975.
18. Boston Collaborative Drug Surveillance Program: N. Engl. J. Med. *290*:15–19, 1974.

18a. Hoover, R., *et al.*: N. Engl. J. Med. *295*:401–405, 1976.

19. Boston Collaborative Drug Surveillance Program: Lancet *1*:1399–1404, 1973.
20. Daniel, D.G., *et al.*: Lancet *2*:287–289, 1967.
21. The Veterans Administration Cooperative Urological Research Group: J. Urol. *98*:516–522, 1967.
22. Bailar, J. C.: Lancet *2*:560, 1967.
23. Blackard, C., *et al.*: Cancer *26*:249–256, 1970.
24. Royal College of General Practitioners: J.R. Coll, Gen. Pract. *13*:267–279, 1967.
25. Inman, W.H.W., *et al.*: Br. Med. J. *2*:193–199, 1968.
26. Vessey, M.P., *et al.*: Br. Med. J. *2*:651–657, 1969.
27. Sartwell, P.E., *et al.*: Am. J. Epidemiol, *90*:365–380, 1969.
28. Collaborative Group for the Study of Stroke in Young Women: N. Engl. J. Med. *288*:871–878, 1973.
29. Collaborative Group for the Study of Stroke in Young Women: J.A.M.A. *231*:718–722, 1975.
30. Mann, J.I., *et al.*: Br. Med. J. *2*:245–248, 1975.
31. Mann, J.I., *et al.*: Br. Med. J. *2*:241–245, 1975.
32. Inman, W.H.W., *et al.*: Br. Med. J. *2*:203–209, 1970.
33. Stolley, P.D., *et al.*: Am. J. Epidemiol, *102*:197–208, 1975.
34. Vessey, M.P., *et al.*: Br. Med. J. *3*:123–126, 1970.
35. Greene, G.R., *et al.*: Am. J. Public Health *62*:680–685, 1972.
36. Rosenberg, L., *et al.*: N. Engl. J. Med. *294*:1256–1259, 1976.
37. Coronary Drug Project Research Group: J.A.M.A. *214*:1303–1313, 1970.
38. Baum, J., *et al.*: Lancet *2*:926–928, 1973.
39. Mays, E.T., *et al.*: J.A.M.A. *235*:730–732, 1976.
40. Edmondson, H.A., *et al.*: N. Engl. J. Med. *294*:470–472, 1976.
41. Pfeffer, R.I., *et al.*: Am. J. Epidemiol, *103*:445–456, 1976.

INFORMATION FOR THE PATIENT:

WHAT YOU SHOULD KNOW ABOUT ESTROGENS: Estrogens are female hormones produced by the ovaries. The ovaries make several different kinds of estrogens. In addition, scientists have been able to make a variety of synthetic estrogens. As far as we know, all these estrogens have similar properties and therefore much the same usefulness, side effects, and risks. This leaflet is intended to help you understand what estrogens are used for, the risks involved in their use, and how to use them as safely as possible.

This leaflet includes the most important information about estrogens, but not all the information. If you want to know more, you can ask your doctor or pharmacist to let you read the package insert prepared for the doctor.

USES OF ESTROGEN:

Estrogens are prescribed by doctors for a number of purposes, including:

1. To provide estrogen during a period of adjustment when a woman's ovaries no longer produce it, in order to prevent certain uncomfortable symptoms of estrogen deficiency. (All women normally stop producing estrogens, generally between the ages of 45 and 55; this is called the menopause).
2. To prevent symptoms of estrogen deficiency when a woman's ovaries have been removed surgically before the natural menopause.
3. To prevent pregnancy. (Estrogens are given along with a progestogen, another female hormone; these combinations are called oral contraceptives or birth controll pills. Patient labeling is available to women taking oral contraceptives and they will not be discussed in this leaflet).
4. To treat certain cancers in women and men.

THERE IS NO PROPER USE OF ESTROGENS IN A PREGNANT WOMAN.

ESTROGENS IN THE MENOPAUSE: In the natural course of their lives, all women eventually experience a decrease in estrogen production. This usually occurs between ages 45 and 55 but may occur earlier or later. Sometimes the ovaries may need to be removed before natural menopause by an operation, producing a "surgical menopause."

When the amount of estrogen in the blood begins to decrease, many women may develop typical symptoms: Feelings of warmth in the face, neck, and chest or sudden intense episodes of heat and sweating throughout the body (called "hot flashes" or "hot flushes"). These symptoms are sometimes very uncomfortable. A few women eventually develop changes in the vagina (called "atrophic vaginitis") which cause discomfort, especially during and after intercourse.

Estrogens can be prescribed to treat these symptoms of the menopause. It is estimated that considerably more than half of all women undergoing the menopause have only mild symptoms or no symptoms at all and therefore do not need estrogens. Other women may need estrogens for a few months, while their bodies adjust to lower estrogen levels. Sometimes the need will be for periods longer than six months. In an attempt to avoid overstimulation of the uterus (womb), estrogens are usually given cyclically during each month of use, that is three weeks of pills followed by one week without pills.

Sometimes women experience nervous symptoms or depression during menopause. There is no evidence that estrogens are effective for such symptoms and they should not be used to treat them, although other treatment may be needed.

You may have heard that taking estrogens for long periods (years) after the menopause will keep your skin soft and supple and keep you feeling young. There is no evidence that this is so, however, and such long-term treatment carries important risks.

THE DANGERS OF ESTROGENS:

1. **Cancer of the uterus.** If estrogens are used in the postmenopausal period for more than a year, there is an increased risk of **endometrial cancer** (cancer of the uterus). Women taking estrogens have roughly 5 to 10 times as great a chance of getting this cancer as women who take no estrogens. To put this another way, while a postmenopausal woman not taking estrogens has 1 chance in 1,000 each year of getting cancer of the uterus, a woman taking estrogens has 5 to 10 chances in 1,000 each year. For this reason **it is important to take estrogens only when you really need them.**

   The risk of this cancer is greater the longer estrogens are used and also seems to be greater when larger doses are taken. For this reason, **It is important to take the lowest dose of estrogen that will control symptoms and to take it only as long as it is needed.** If estrogens are needed for longer periods of time, your doctor will want to reevaluate your need for estrogens at least every six months.

   Women using estrogens should report any irregular vaginal bleeding to their doctors; such bleeding may be of no importance, but it can be an early warning of cancer of the uterus. If you have undiagnosed vaginal bleeding, you should not use estrogens until a diagnosis is made and you are certain there is no cancer of the uterus.
2. **Other possible cancers.** Estrogens can cause development of other tumors in animals, such as tumors of the breast, cervix, vagina, or liver, when given for a long time. At present there is no good evidence that women using estrogen in the menopause have an increased risk of such tumors, but there is no way yet to be sure they do not; and one study raises the possibility that use of estrogens in the menopause may increase the risk of breast cancer many years later. This is a further reason to use estrogens only when clearly needed. While you are taking estrogens, it is important that you go to your doctor at least once a year for a physical examiniation. Also, if members of your family have had breast cancer of if you have had breast nodules or abnormal mammograms (breast x-rays), your doctor may wish to carry out more frequent examinations of your breasts.
3. **Gallbladder disease.** Women who use estrogens after menopause are more likely to develop gall bladder disease needing surgery as women who do not use estrogens. Birth control pills have a similar effect.
4. **Abnormal blood clotting.** Oral contraceptives increase the risk of blood clotting in various parts of the body. This can result in a stroke (if the clot is in the brain), a heart attack (clot in a blood vessel of the heart), or pulmonary embolus (a clot which forms in the legs or pelvis, then breaks off and travels to the lungs). Any of these can be fatal.

   At this time use of estrogens in the menopause is not known to cause such blood clotting, but this has not been fully studied and there could still prove to be such a risk. It is recommended that if you have had clotting in the legs or lungs or a heart attack or stroke while you were using estrogens or birth control pills, you should not use estrogens (unless they are being used to treat cancer of the breast or prostate). If you have had a stroke or heart attack or if you have angina pectoris, estrogens should be used with great caution and only if clearly needed (for example, if you have severe symptoms of the menopause).

   The larger doses of estrogen used to prevent swelling of the breasts after pregnancy have been reported to cause clotting in the legs and lungs.

SPECIAL WARNING ABOUT PREGNANCY: You should not receive estrogen if you are pregnant. If this should occur, there is a greater than usual chance that the developing child will be born with a birth defect, although the possibility remains fairly small. A female child may have an increased risk of developing cancer of the vagina or cervix later in life (in the teens or twenties). Every possible effort should be made to avoid exposure to estrogens during pregnancy. If exposure occurs, see your doctor.

OTHER EFFECTS OF ESTROGENS: In addition to the serious known risks of estrogens described above, estrogens have the following side effects and potential risks:

1. **Nausea and vomiting.** The most common side effect of estrogen therapy is nausea. Vomiting is less common.
2. **Effects on breasts.** Estrogens may cause breast tenderness or enlargement and may cause the breasts to secrete a liquid. These effects are not dangerous.
3. **Effects on the uterus.** Estrogens may cause benign fibroid tumors of the uterus to get larger.

   Some women will have menstrual bleeding when estrogens are stopped. But if the bleeding occurs on days you are still taking estrogens you should report this to your doctor.
4. **Effect on liver.** Women taking oral contraceptives develop on rare occasions a benign tumor of the liver which can rupture and bleed into the abdomen. So far, these tumors have not been reported in women using estrogens in the menopause, but you should report any swelling or unusual pain or tenderness in the abdomen to your doctor immediately.

   Women with a past history of jaundice (yellowing of the skin and white parts of the eyes) may get jaundice again during estrogen use. If this occurs, stop taking estrogens and see your doctor.
5. **Other effects.** Estrogens may cause excess fluid to be retained in the body. This may make some conditions worse, such as epilepsy, migraine, heart disease, or kidney disease.

SUMMARY: Estrogens have important uses, but they have serious risks as well. You must decide, with your doctor, whether the risks are acceptable to you in view of the benefits of treatment. Except where your doctor has prescribed estrogens for use in special cases of cancer of the breast or prostate, you should not use estrogens if you have cancer of the breast or uterus, are pregnant, have undiagnosed abnormal vaginal bleeding, or have had a stroke, heart attack or angina, or clotting in the legs or lungs in the past while you were taking estrogens.

You can use estrogens as safely as possible by understanding that your doctor will require regular physical examinations while you are taking them and will try to discontinue the drug as soon as possible and use the smallest dose possible. Be alert for signs of trouble including:

1. Abnormal bleeding from the vagina.
2. Pains in the calves or chest or sudden shortness of breath, or coughing blood (indicating possible clots in the legs, heart, or lungs).

Continued on next page

Solvay—Cont.

3. Severe headaches, dizziness, faintness, or changes in vision (indicating possible developing clots in the brain or eye).
4. Breast lumps (you should ask your doctor how to examine your own breasts).
5. Jaundice (yellowing of the skin).
6. Mental depression.

Based on his or her assessment of your medical needs, your doctor has prescribed this drug for you. Do not give the drug to anyone else.

HOW SUPPLIED

ESTRATEST® H.S. a combination of Esterified Estrogens and Methyltestosterone. Each capsule-shaped Light Green sugar coated Tablet contains: 0.625 mg of Esterified Estrogens, USP and 1.25 mg of Methyltestosterone, USP.
ESTRATEST® a combination of Esterified Estrogens and Methyltestosterone. Each capsule-shaped Dark Green Sugar Coated Tablet contains: 1.25 mg of Esterified Estrogens, USP and 2.5 mg of Methyltestosterone, USP.

SOLVAY PHARMACEUTICALS
Marietta, GA 30062 3E Rev 11/91
Shown in Product Identification Section, page 432

LITHONATE® Capsules ℞
LITHOTABS™ Tablets ℞
[lĭ'-thō-nāt/lĭ-thō-tăbs]
Brand of Lithium Carbonate

> **WARNING**
> Lithium toxicity is closely related to serum lithium levels, and can occur at doses close to therapeutic levels. Facilities for prompt and accurate serum lithium determinations should be available before initiating therapy.

DESCRIPTION

LITHONATE: Each peach-colored capsule contains 300 mg of lithium carbonate.
LITHOTABS: Each scored, white, film-coated tablet contains 300 mg of lithium carbonate.
Lithium carbonate is a white, light alkaline powder with molecular formula Li_2CO_3 and molecular weight 73.89. Lithium is an element of the alkali-metal group with atomic number 3, atomic weight 6.94 and an emission line at 671 nm on the flame photometer.
Inactive Ingredients: Lithonate 300 mg capsules: FD & C Red No. 40, gelatin, polyethylene glycol, talc and titanium dioxide. Capsule imprinting ink contains red ferric oxide.
Lithotabs 300 mg tablets: Calcium stearate, carnauba wax, cellulose, povidone, propylene glycol, sodium lauryl sulfate and sodium starch glycolate.

INDICATIONS

Lithium is indicated in the treatment of manic episodes of manic depressive illness. Maintenance therapy prevents or diminishes the intensity of subsequent episodes in those manic-depressive patients with a history of mania.
Typical symptoms of mania include pressure of speech, motor hyperactivity, reduced need for sleep, flight of ideas, grandiosity, elation, poor judgment, aggressiveness, and possibly hositility. When given to a patient experiencing a manic episode, lithium may produce a normalization of symptomatology within 1 to 3 weeks.

WARNINGS

Lithium should generally not be given to patients with significant renal or cardiovascular disease, severe debilitation, or dehydration, or sodium depletion, and to patients receiving diuretics, or angiotensin converting enzyme (ACE) inhibitors, since the risk of lithium toxicity is very high in such patients. If the psychiatric indication is life threatening, and if such a patient fails to respond to other measures, lithium treatment may be undertaken with extreme caution, including daily serum lithium determinations and adjustment to the usually low doses ordinarily tolerated by these individuals. In such instances, hospitalization is a necessity.
Lithium Toxicity is closely related to serum lithium levels and can occur at doses close to the therapeutic levels (see DOSAGE AND ADMINISTRATION). Lithium therapy has been reported in some cases to be associated with morphologic changes in the kidneys. The relationship between such changes and renal function has not been established.
Outpatients and their families should be warned that the patient must discontinue lithium therapy and contact his physician if such clinical signs of lithium toxicity as diarrhea, vomiting, tremor, mild ataxia, drowsiness, or muscular weakness occur.
Lithium may prolong the effects of neuromuscular blocking agents. Therefore, neuromuscular blocking agents should be given with caution to patients receiving lithium.
Lithium may impair mental and/or physical abilities. Caution patients about activities requiring alertness (e.g. operating vehicles or machinery).
Usage in Pregnancy: Adverse effects on nidation in rats, embryo viability in mice, and metabolism invitro of rat testis and human spermatozoa have been attributed to lithium, as have teratogenicity in submammalian species and cleft palates in mice. Studies in rats, rabbits and monkeys have shown no evidence of lithium-induced teratology.
There are lithium birth registries in the United States and elsewhere; however, there are at the present time insufficient data to determine the effects of lithium on human fetuses. Therefore at this point lithium should not be used in pregnancy, especially the first trimester, unless in the opinion of the physician, the potential benefits outweigh the possible hazards.
Usage in Nursing Mothers: Lithium is excreted in human milk. Nursing should not be undertaken during lithium therapy except in rare and unusual circumstances where, in the view of the physician, the potential benefits to the mother outweigh possible hazards to the child.
Usage in Children: Since information regarding the safety and effectiveness of lithium in children under 12 years of age is not available, its use in such patients is not recommended at this time.
There has been a report of transient syndrome of acute dystonia and hyperreflexia occurring in a 15 kg child who ingested 300 mg of lithium carbonate.

PRECAUTIONS

The ability to tolerate lithium is greater during the acute manic phase and decreases when manic symptoms subside (see DOSAGE AND ADMINISTRATION).
The distribution of space of lithium approximates that of total body water. Lithium is primarily excreted in urine with insignificant excretion in feces. Renal excretion of lithium is proportional to its plasma concentration. The half-elimination time of lithium is approximately 24 hours. Lithium decreases sodium reabsorption by the renal tubules which could lead to sodium depletion. Therefore, it is essential for the patient to maintain a normal diet, including salt, and an adequate fluid intake (2500–3500 ml) at least during the initial stabilization period. Decreased tolerance to lithium has been reported to ensue from protracted sweating or diarrhea and, if such occur, supplemental fluid and salt should be administered.
In addition to sweating and diarrhea, concomitant infection with elevated temperatures may also necessitate a temporary reduction or cessation of medication. Previously existing underlying disorders do not necessarily constitute a contraindicaton to lithium treatment; where hypothyroidism exists, careful monitoring of thyroid function during lithium stabilization and maintenance allows for correction of changing thyroid parameters, if any, where hypothyroidism occurs during lithium stabilization and maintenance, supplemental thyroid treatment may be used.

DRUG INTERACTIONS

Lithium may prolong or potentiate the effects of neuromuscular blocking agents, such as decamethonium, pancuronium, and succinylcholine. Therefore, neuromuscular blocking agents should be given with caution to patients receiving lithium.
Concomitant use of Diuretics or ACE Inhibitors with lithium carbonate: In general the concomitant use of diuretics or angiotensin converting enzyme (ACE) inhibitors with lithium carbonate should be avoided. In those cases where concomitant use is necessary extreme caution is advised since sodium loss from these drugs may reduce the renal clearance of lithium resulting in increased serum lithium levels with the risk of lithium toxicity. When such combinations are used, the lithium dosage may need to be decreased, and more frequent monitoring of lithium plasma levels is recommended. See WARNINGS for additional caution information.
Concomitant use of haloperidol and lithium: An encephalopathic syndrome (characterized by weakness; lethargy; fever; tremulousness and confusion; extrapyramidal symptoms; leukocytosis; elevated serum enzymes, BUN, and fasting blood sugar), followed by irreversible brain damage, has occurred in a few patients treated with lithium plus haloperidol. A causal relationship between these events and the concomitant administration of lithium and haloperidol has not been established. However, patients receiving such combined therapy should be monitored closely for early evidence of neurological toxicity, and treatment discontinued promptly if such signs appear. The possibility of similar adverse interactions with other antipsychotic medications exists. In addition, concomitant use of lithium with chlorpromazine and possibly other phenothiazines decreases serum chlorpromazine levels as much as 40%.
Concomitant administration of carbamazepine and lithium may increase the risk of neurotoxic side effects.
Aminophylline, caffeine, dyphylline, oxtriphylline, sodium bicarbonate, or theophylline used concomitantly may decrease the therapeutic effect of lithium because of its increased urinary excretion.
Concomitant use of diuretics, especially thiazides with lithium may provoke lithium toxicity due to reduced renal clearance.
Concomitant extended use of iodide preparations, especially potassium iodide, with lithium may produce hypothyroidism, indomeathacin and piroxicam have been reported to increase significantly steady state plasma lithium levels. In some cases lithium toxicity has resulted from such interaction. There is also some evidence that other nonsteroidal, anti-inflammatory agents may have a similar effect. When such combinations are used, increased plasma lithium levels monitoring is recommended.

ADVERSE REACTIONS

Adverse reactions are seldom encountered at serum lithium levels below 1.5mEa/L, except in the occasional patient sensitive to lithium. Mild to moderate toxic reactions may occur at levels from 1.5–2.5 mEq/L, and moderate to severe reactions may be seen at levels from 2.0–2.5 mEq/L, depending upon individual response to the drug.
Fine hand tremor, polyuria and mild thirst may occur during initial therapy for the acute manic phase, and may persist throughout treatment. Transient and mild nausea and general discomfort may also appear during the first few days of lithium administration.
These side effects are an inconvenience rather than a disabling condition, and usually subside with continued treatment or a temporary reduction or cessation of dosage. If persistent, a cessation of dosage is indicated. Diarrhea, vomiting, drowsiness, muscular weakness and lack of coordination may be early signs of lithium intoxication, and can occur at lithium levels below 2.0 mEq/L. At higher levels giddiness, ataxia, blurred vision, tinnitus and a large output of dilute urine may be seen. Serum lithium levels above 3.0 mEq/L may produce a complex clinical picture involving multiple organs and organ systems. Serum lithium levels should not be permitted to exceed 2.0 mEq/L during the acute treatment phase.
The following toxic reactions have been reported and appear to be related to serum lithium levels, including levels within the therapeutic range.
Neuromuscular: tremor, muscle hyperirritability (fasciculations, twitching, clonic movements of whole limbs), ataxia, choreo athetotic movements, hyper-active deep tendon reflexes.
Central Nervous System: blackout spell, epileptiform seizures, slurred speech, dizziness, vertigo, incontinence of urine or feces, somnolence, psychomotor retardation, restlessness, confusion, stupor, coma, acute dystonia, and downbeat nystagmus.
Cases of pseudotumor cerebri (increased intracranial pressure and papilledema) have been reported with lithium use. If undetected, this condition may result in enlargement of the blind spot, constriction of visual fields and eventual blindness due to optic atropy. Lithium should be discontinued, if clinically possible, if this syndrome occurs.
Cardiovascular: cardiac arrhythmia, hypotension, peripheral circulatory collapse.
Gastrointestinal: anorexia, nausea, vomiting, diarrhea.
Genitourinary: albuminuria, oliguria, polyuria, glycosuria.
Dermatologic: drying and thinning of hair, anesthesia of skin, chronic folliculitis, xerosis cutis, alopecia, exacerbation of psoriasis.
Autonomic Nervous System: blurred vision, dry mouth.
Miscellaneous: fatigue, lethargy, tendency to sleep, dehydration, weight loss, transient scotomata.
Thyroid Abnormalities: euthyroid goiter and/or hypothyroidism (including myxedema) accompanied by lower T_3 and T_4. I_{131} Iodine uptake may be elevated (see PRECAUTIONS). Paradoxically, rare cases of hyperthyroidism have been reported.
EEG Changes: diffuse slowing, widening of frequency spectrum, potentiation and disorganization of background rhythm.
EKG Changes: reversible flattening, isoelectricity or inversion of T-waves.
Miscellaneous reactions unrelated to dosage are: transient, electroencephalographic and electrocardiographic changes, leucocytosis, headache, diffuse nontoxic goiter with or without hypothyroidism, transient hyperglycemia, generalized pruritis with or without rash, cutaneous ulcers, albuminuria, worsening of organic brain syndromes, excessive weight gain, edematous swelling of ankles or wrists, and thirst or polyuria, sometimes resembling diabetes insipidus and metallic taste.
A single report has been received of the development of painful discoloration of fingers and toes and coldness of the extremities within one day of the starting of treatment of lithium. The mechanism through which these symptoms (resembling Raynaud's Syndrome) developed is not known. Recovery followed discontinuance.

DOSAGE AND ADMINISTRATION

Acute Mania: Optimal patient response can usually be established and maintained with the following dosages:

LITHONATE .... 600 mg. t.i.d.
LITHOTABS .... 600 mg. t.i.d.

Such doses will normally produce an effective serum lithium level ranging between 1.0 and 1.5 mEq/L. Dosage must be individualized according to serum levels and clinical response. Regular monitoring of the patient's clinical state and of serum lithium levels is necessary. Serum levels should be determined twice per week during the acute phase, and until the serum level and clinical condition of the patient have been stabilized.

Long-Term Control: The desirable serum lithium levels are 0.6 to 1.2 mEq/L. Dosage will vary from one individual to another, but usually the following dosages will maintain this level.

LITHONATE 300 mg. t.i.d. or q.i.d.
LITHOTABS 300 mg. t.i.d. or q.i.d.

Serum lithium levels in uncomplicated cases receiving maintenance therapy during remission should be monitored at least every two months. Patients abnormally sensitive to lithium may exhibit toxic signs at serum levels of 1.0 to 1.5 mEq/L. Elderly patients often respond to reduced dosage, and may exhibit signs of toxicity at serum levels ordinarily tolerated by other patients.

N.B.: Blood samples for serum lithium determinations should be drawn immediately prior to the next dose when lithium concentrations are relatively stable (i.e., 8–12 hours after previous dose). Total reliance must not be placed on serum levels alone. Accurate patient evaluation requires both clinical and laboratory analysis.

OVERDOSAGE

The toxic levels for lithium are close to the therapeutic levels. It is therefore important that patients and their families be cautioned to watch for early toxic symptoms and to discontinue the drug and inform the physician should they occur. Toxic symptoms are listed in detail under ADVERSE REACTIONS.

Treatment: No specific antidote for lithium poisoning is known. Early symptoms of lithium toxicity can usually be treated by reduction or cessation of dosage of the drug and resumption of the treatment at a lower dose after 24 to 48 hours. In severe cases of lithium poisoning, the first and foremost goal of treatment consists of elimination of this ion from the patient.

Treatment is essentially the same as that used in barbiturate poisoning: 1) gastric lavage, 2) correction of fluid and electrolyte imbalance and, 3) regulation of kidney functioning. Urea, mannitol, and aminophyline all produce significant increases in lithium excretion. Hemodialysis is an effective and rapid means of removing the ion from the severely toxic patient. Infection prophylaxis, regular chest X-rays, and preservation of adequate respiration are essential.

HOW SUPPLIED

LITHONATE: (Lithium Carbonate 300 mg) peach colored, No. 3 capsules, imprinted "Solvay 7512" in red.
Bottles of 100 ND 0032-7512-01
Bottles of 1000 NDC 0032-7512-10
Unit Dose Boxes of 100 NDC 0032-7512-11
LITHOTABS (Lithium Carbonate 300 mg) scored, white film-coated tablets imprinted "Solvay 7516."
Bottles of 100 NDC 0032-7516-01
Bottles of 1000 NDC 0032-7516-10
Unit Dose Boxes of 100 NDC 0032-7516-11
Store at controlled room temperature 15°–30°C (59°–86°F)

17E REV 4/92

SOLVAY PHARMACEUTICALS
MARIETTA, GA 30062
Shown in Product Identification Section, page 432

P-V-TUSSIN® Syrup Ⓒ℞
[p-v-tŭs′]

DESCRIPTION

Each 5 mL (one teaspoonful) contains:

Hydrocodone* Bitartrate .... 2.5 mg
(***WARNING:** May be habit forming)
Pseudoephedrine Hydrochloride .... 30 mg
Chlorpheniramine Maleate .... 2 mg
Alcohol 5%

HOW SUPPLIED

P-V-Tussin® Syrup is supplied as an orange, banana-flavored liquid in bottles of 16 fl oz.,
NDC 0032-1083-78 and in 1 gallon bottles,
NDC 0032-1083-79.

P-V-TUSSIN Tablets Ⓒ℞

DESCRIPTION

Each scored tablet contains:

Hydrocodone* Bitartrate .... 5 mg
(***WARNING:** May be habit forming)
Phenindamine Tartrate .... 25 mg
Guaifenesin .... 200 mg

HOW SUPPLIED

P-V-Tussin® Tablets NDC 0032-1088-01, bottles of 100 tablets debossed SOLVAY on one side and 1088 on the other.

ROWASA® ℞
[rō-ă′să]
(mesalamine)
Rectal Suspension-Enema 4.0 grams/unit (60 mL)
Rectal Suppositories 500 mg

DESCRIPTION

The active ingredient in ROWASA® is mesalamine, also known as 5-aminosalicylic acid (5-ASA). Chemically, mesalamine is 5-amino-2-hydroxybenzoic acid, and is classified as an anti-inflammatory drug.

The empirical formula is $C_7H_7NO_3$, representing a molecular weight of 153.14. The structural formula is:

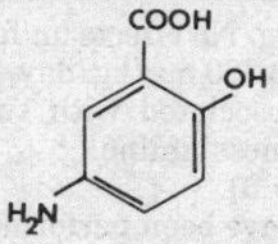

Each rectal suspension enema unit contains 4 grams of mesalamine. In addition to mesalamine the preparation contains the inactive ingredients potassium metabisulfite, carbomer 943P, edetate disodium, potassium acetate, water and xanthan gum. Sodium benzoate is added as a preservative. The disposable unit consists of an applicator tip protected by a polyethylene cover and lubricated with USP white petrolatum. The unit has a one-way valve to prevent back flow of the dispensed product.

Each ROWASA suppository contains 500 mg of mesalamine in a base of saturated vegetable fatty acid esters (Hard Fat, NF). Each suppository is individually wrapped in foil.

CLINICAL PHARMACOLOGY

Sulfasalazine is split by bacterial action in the colon into sulfapyridine (SP) and mesalamine (5-ASA). It is thought that the mesalamine component is therapeutically active in ulcerative colitis [A.K. Azad Khan et al, **Lancet** 2:892–895 (1977)]. The usual oral dose of sulfasalazine for active ulcerative colitis in adults is two to four grams per day in divided doses. Four grams of sulfasalazine provide 1.6 g of free mesalamine to the colon. Each ROWASA enema delivers up to 4 g of mesalamine to the left side of the colon. Each ROWASA suppository delivers 500 mg of mesalamine to the rectum.

The mechanism of action of mesalamine (and sulfasalazine) is unknown, but appears to be topical rather than systemic. Mucosal production of arachidonic acid (AA) metabolites, both through the cyclooxygenase pathways, i.e., prostanoids, and through the lipoxygenase pathways, i.e., leukotrienes (LTs) and hydroxyeicosatetraenoic acids (HETEs) is increased in patients with chronic inflammatory bowel disease, and it is possible that mesalamine diminishes inflammation by blocking cyclooxygenase and inhibiting prostaglandin (PG) production in the colon.

PRECLINICAL TOXICOLOGY

Preclinical studies have shown the kidney to be the major target organ for mesalamine toxicity. Adverse renal function changes were observed in rats after a single 600 mg/kg oral dose, but not after a 200 mg/kg dose. Gross kidney lesions, including papillary necrosis, were observed after a single oral > 900 mg/kg dose, and after i.v. doses of > 214 mg/kg. Mice responded similarly. In a 13-week oral (gavage) dose study in rats, the high dose of 640 mg/kg/day mesalamine caused deaths, probably due to renal failure, and dose-related renal lesions (papillary necrosis and/or multifocal tubular injury) were seen in most rats given the high dose (males and females) as well as in males receiving lower doses 160 mg/kg/day. Renal lesions were not observed in the 160 mg/kg/day female rats. Minimal tubular epithelial damage was seen in the 40 mg/kg/day males and was reversible. In a six-month oral study in dogs, the no-observable dose level of mesalamine was 40 mg/kg/day and doses of 80 mg/kg/day and higher caused renal pathology similar to that described for the rat. The oral preclinical studies were done with a highly bioavailable suspension where absorption throughout the gastrointestinal tract occurred. The human dose of 4 grams represents approximately 80 mg/kg but when mesalamine is given rectally as a suspension, absorption is poor and limited to the distal colon (see **Pharmacokinetics**). Overt renal toxicity has not been observed (see **Adverse Reactions** and **Precautions**), but the potential must be considered.

PHARMACOKINETICS

Mesalamine administered rectally as ROWASA suspension enema is poorly absorbed from the colon and is excreted principally in the feces during subsequent bowel movements. The extent of absorption is dependent upon the retention time of the drug product, and there is considerable individual variation. At steady state, approximatey 10 to 30% of the daily 4-gram dose can be recovered in cumulative 24-hour urine collections. Other than the kidney, the organ distribution and other bioavailability characteristics of absorbed mesalamine in man are not known. It is known that the compound undergoes acetylation but whether this process takes place at colonic or systemic sites has not been elucidated. Whatever the metabolic site, most of the absorbed mesalamine is excreted in the urine as the N-acetyl-5-ASA metabolite. The poor colonic absorption of rectally administered mesalamine is substantiated by the low serum concentration of 5-ASA and N-acetyl-5-ASA seen in ulcerative colitis patients after dosage with mesalamine. Under clinical conditions patients demonstrated plasma levels 10 to 12 hours post mesalamine administration of 2 μg/mL, about two-thirds of which was the N-acetyl metabolite. While the elimination half-life of mesalamine is short (0.5 to 1.5 h), the acetylated metabolite exhibits a half-life of 5 to 10 hours [U. Klotz, **Clin. Pharmacokin.** 10:285–302 (1985)]. In addition, steady state plasma levels demonstrated a lack of accumulation of either free or metabolized drug during repeated daily administrations.

Following single doses of ROWASA 500 mg suppository in normal volunteers, 24-hr urines contained (only) N-acetyl-mesalamine equivalent to 15 to 38% (avg. 24%) of the administered dose. This is commensurate with the finding of 3 to 36% (avg. 10%) in urine in a study of ROWASA 4 g enema in normals. In that study, 40 to 107% (avg. 75%) of the administered dose was recovered in feces. At steady state in ulcerative colitis patients (n=38) being treated with ROWASA enema, 24-hr urines contained 0 to 41% (avg. 8%) of the 4 g daily dose and plasma levels 10 to 12 hr postadministration ranged from 0 to 2.1 mcg/mL (avg. 0.37 mcg/mL) of mesalamine equivalent (84% as N-acetyl metabolite). Multiple dose pharmacokinetic studies have not been conducted with ROWASA suppository nor have plasma levels been reported from single dose studies.

EFFICACY

Rowasa Suspension Enema: In a placebo-controlled, international, multicenter trial of 153 patients with active distal ulcerative colitis, proctosigmoiditis or proctitis, ROWASA suspension enema reduced the overall disease activity index (DAI) and individual components as follows:

[See table at top of next page.]

Differences between ROWASA and placebo were also statistically different in subgroups of patients on concurrent sulfasalazine and in those having an upper disease boundary between 5 and 20 or 20 and 40 cm. Significant differences between ROWASA and placebo were not achieved in those subgroups of patients on concurrent prednisone or with an upper disease boundary between 40 and 50 cm.

Rowasa Suppositories: Two double-blind placebo-controlled, multicenter studies were conducted in North America in patients with active ulcerative proctitis. The primary measures of efficacy were the same in both trials. The main difference between the two studies was the dosage regimen: 500 mg three times daily (1.5 g/d) in Study 1 and 500 mg twice daily (1.0 g/d) in Study 2. A total of 173 patients were studied (Study 1, n=79; Study 2, n=94) Patients were evaluated clinically and sigmoidoscopically after three and six weeks of suppository treatment.

Compared to placebo, ROWASA suppository treatment was statistically ($P<.01$) superior in both trials with respect to stool frequency, rectal bleeding, mucosal appearance, disease severity and overall disease activity after both three and six weeks of treatment. Daily diary records indicated significant improvement in rectal bleeding in the first week of therapy while tenesmus and diarrhea improved significantly within two weeks. Investigators rated patients much improved in 84% and 79% with mesalamine in Studies 1 and 2, respectively compared to 41% and 26% with placebo ($P<.001$, $P<.001$).

Normalization of rectal mucosa was achieved by 62% and 60% of mesalamine-treated patients in Studies 1 and 2 compared to 25% and 10% of placebo-treated patients ($P<.001$, $P<.001$). The effectiveness of ROWASA suppositories was statistically significant irrespective of sex, extent of proctitis, duration, of current episode or duration of disease. Overall the efficacy demonstrated with the twice daily regimen (Study 2) was comparable to that observed with three times daily dosing (Study 1).

Continued on next page

Solvay—Cont.

INDICATIONS AND USAGE

ROWASA suspension enema is indicated for the treatment of active mild to moderate distal ulcerative colitis, proctosigmoiditis or proctitis.

ROWASA suppositories are indicated for the treatment of active ulcerative proctitis.

CONTRAINDICATIONS

ROWASA suspension enema is contraindicated for patients known to have hypersensitivity to the drug or any component of this medication.

ROWASA suppositories are contraindicated for patients known to have hypersensitivity to mesalamine (5-aminosalicylic acid) or to the suppository vehicle [saturated vegetable fatty acid esters (Hard Fat, NF)].

WARNINGS

ROWASA suspension enema contains potassium metabisulfite, a sulfite that may cause allergic-type reactions including anaphylactic symptoms and life-threatening or less severe asthmatic episodes in certain susceptible people. The overall prevalence of sulfite sensitivity in the general population is unknown but probably low. Sulfite sensitivity is seen more frequently in asthmatic or in atopic nonasthmatic persons.

Epinephrine is the preferred treatment for serious allergic or emergency situations even though epinephrine injection contains sodium or potassium metabisulfite with the above-mentioned potential liabilities. The alternatives to using epinephrine in a life-threatening situation may not be satisfactory. The presence of a sulfite(s) in epinephrine injection should not deter the administration of the drug for treatment of serious allergic or other emergency situations.

PRECAUTIONS

Mesalamine has been implicated in the production of an acute intolerance syndrome characterized by cramping, acute abdominal pain and bloody diarrhea, sometimes fever, headache and a rash; in such cases prompt withdrawal is required. The patient's history of sulfasalazine intolerance, if any, should be re-evaluated. If a rechallenge is performed later in order to validate the hypersensitivity it should be carried out under close supervision and only if clearly needed, giving consideration to reduced dosage. In the literature one patient previously sensitive to sulfasalazine was rechallenged with 400 mg oral mesalamine, within eight hours she experienced headache, fever, intensive abdominal colic, profuse diarrhea and was readmitted as an emergency. She responded poorly to steroid therapy and two weeks later a pancolectomy was required.

Although renal abnormalities were not noted in the clinical trials with ROWASA suspension enema, the possibility of increased absorption of mesalamine and concomitant renal tubular damage as noted in the preclinical studies must be kept in mind. Patients on ROWASA suspension enema, especially those on concurrent oral products which liberate mesalamine and those with preexisting renal disease, should be carefully monitored with urinalysis, BUN and creatinine studies.

In a clinical trial most patients who were hypersensitive to sulfasalazine were able to take mesalamine enemas without evidence of any allergic reaction. Nevertheless, caution should be exercised when mesalamine is initially used in patients known to be allergic to sulfasalazine. These patients should be instructed to discontinue therapy if signs of rash or fever become apparent.

While using ROWASA suspension enema some patients have developed pancolitis. However, extension of upper disease boundary and/or flare-ups occurred less often in the ROWASA-treated group than in the placebo-treated group.

Rare instances of pericarditis have been reported with mesalamine containing products including sulfasalazine. Cases of pericarditis have also been reported as manifestations of inflammatory bowel disease. In the cases reported with ROWASA Rectal Suspension Enema there have been positive rechallenges with mesalamine or mesalamine containing products. In one of these cases, however, a second rechallenge with sulfasalazine was negative throughout a 2 month follow-up. Chest pain or dypsnea in patients treated with ROWASA should be investigated with this information in mind. Discontinuation of ROWASA may be warranted in some cases, but rechallenge with mesalamine can be performed under careful clinical observation should the continued therapeutic need for mesalamine be present.

Carcinogenesis, Mutagenesis, Impairment of Fertility

There have been no completed long-term studies of the carcinogenic potential of ROWASA. Mesalamine is not mutagenic to Salmonella typhimurium tester strains TA98, TA100, TA1535, TA1537, TA1538. There were no reverse mutations in an assay using E. coli strain WP2UVRA. There were no effects in an in vivo mouse micronucleus assay at 600 mg/kg and in an in vivo sister chromatid exchange at

doses up to 610 mg/kg. No effects on fertility were observed in rats receiving up to 320 mg/kg/day. The oligospermia and infertility in men associated with sulfasalazine have not been reported with mesalamine.

Pregnancy (Category B)

Teratologic studies have been performed in rats and rabbits at oral doses of up to five and eight times respectively, the maximum recommended human dose, and have revealed no evidence of harm to the embryo or the fetus. There are, however, no adequate and well controlled studies in pregnant women for either sulfasalazine or 5-ASA. Because animal reproduction studies are not always predictive of human response, 5-ASA should be used during pregnancy only if clearly needed.

Nursing Mothers

It is not known whether mesalamine or its metabolite(s) are excreted in human milk. As a general rule, nursing should not be undertaken while a patient is on a drug since many drugs are excreted in human milk.

Pediatric Use

Safety and effectiveness in children have not been established.

ADVERSE REACTIONS

Clinical Adverse Experience

ROWASA suspension enema is usually well tolerated. Most adverse effects have been mild and transient.

EFFECT OF TREATMENT ON SEVERITY OF DISEASE
DATA FROM U.S.-CANADA TRIAL
COMBINED RESULTS OF EIGHT CENTERS
Activity Indices, mean

		n	Baseline	Day 22	End-Point	Change Baseline to End-Point†
Overall DAI	ROWASA	76	7.42	4.05**	3.37***	−55.07%***
	Placebo	77	7.40	6.03	5.83	−21.58%
Stool Frequency	ROWASA		1.58	1.11*	1.01**	−0.57*
	Placebo		1.92	1.47	1.50	−0.41
Rectal Bleeding	ROWASA		1.82	0.59***	0.51***	−1.30***
	Placebo		1.73	1.21	1.11	−0.61
Mucosal inflammation	ROWASA		2.17	1.22**	0.96***	−1.21**
	Placebo		2.18	1.74	1.61	−0.56
Physician's Assessment of Disease Severity	ROWASA		1.86	1.13***	0.88***	−0.97***
	Placebo		1.87	1.62	1.55	−0.30

Each parameter has a 4-point scale with a numerical rating:

0 = normal, 1 = mild, 2 = moderate, 3 = severe. The four parameters are added together to produce a maximum overall DAI of 12.

† Percent change for overall DAI only (calculated by taking the average of the change for each individual patient).
* Significant ROWASA/placebo difference. $p < 0.05$
** Significant ROWASA/placebo difference. $p < 0.01$
*** Significant ROWASA/placebo difference. $p < 0.001$

ADVERSE REACTIONS OCCURRING IN MORE THAN 0.1% OF ROWASA SUSPENSION ENEMA TREATED PATIENTS (COMPARISON TO PLACEBO)

SYMPTOM	ROWASA (n=815) n	%	PLACEBO (n=128) n	%
Abdominal Pain/Cramps/Discomfort	66	8.10	10	7.81
Headache	53	6.50	16	12.50
Gas/Flatulence	50	6.13	5	3.91
Nausea	47	5.77	12	9.38
Flu	43	5.28	1	0.78
Tired/Weak/Malaise/Fatigue	28	3.44	8	6.25
Fever	26	3.19	0	0.00
Rash/Spots	23	2.82	4	3.12
Cold/Sore Throat	19	2.33	9	7.03
Diarrhea	17	2.09	5	3.91
Leg/Joint Pain	17	2.09	1	0.78
Dizziness	15	1.84	3	2.34
Bloating	12	1.47	2	1.56
Back Pain	11	1.35	1	0.78
Pain on Insertion of Enema Tip	11	1.35	1	0.78
Hemorrhoids	11	1.35	0	0.00
Itching	10	1.23	1	0.78
Rectal Pain	10	1.23	0	0.00
Constipation	8	0.98	4	3.12
Hair Loss	7	0.86	0	0.00
Peripheral Edema	5	0.61	11	8.59
UTI/Urinary Burning	5	0.61	4	3.12
Rectal Pain/Soreness/Burning	5	0.61	3	2.34
Asthenia	1	0.12	4	3.12
Insomnia	1	0.12	3	2.34

Hair Loss

Mild hair loss characterized by "more hair in the comb" but no withdrawal from clinical trials has been observed in seven of 815 mesalamine patients but none of the placebo-treated patients. In the literature there are at least six additional patients with mild hair loss who received either mesalamine

or sulfasalazine. Retreatment is not always associated with repeated hair loss.

ADVERSE REACTIONS OCCURRING IN MORE THAN 1% OF ROWASA SUPPOSITORY-TREATED PATIENTS (COMPARISON TO PLACEBO)

SYMPTOM	ROWASA (n=168) n	%	PLACEBO (n=84) n	%
Headache	11	6.5	10	11.9
Flatulence	6	3.6	6	7.1
Abdominal Pain	5	3.0	7	8.3
Diarrhea	5	3.0	5	6.0
Dizziness	5	3.0	2	2.4
Rectal Pain	3	1.8	0	0.0
Upper Resp. Infection	3	1.8	2	2.4
Acne	2	1.2	0	0.0
Asthenia	2	1.2	4	4.8
Colitis	2	1.2	0	0.0
Fever	2	1.2	0	0.0
Generalized Edema	2	1.2	1	1.2
Nausea	2	1.2	6	7.1
Rash	2	1.2	0	0.0

In addition, the following adverse events have been associated with mesalamine containing products: nephrotoxicity, pancreatitis, fibrosing alveolitis and elevated liver enzymes. Cases of pancreatitis and fibrosing alveolitis have been reported as manifestations of inflammatory bowel disease as well.

Overdosage

There have been no documented reports of serious toxicity in man resulting from massive overdosing with mesalamine. Under ordinary circumstances, mesalamine absorption from the colon is limited.

DOSAGE AND ADMINISTRATION

Rowasa Suspension Enema: The usual dosage of ROWASA (mesalamine) suspension enema in 60 mL units is one rectal instillation (4 grams) once a day, preferably at bedtime, and retained for approximately eight hours. While the effect of ROWASA (mesalamine) may be seen within three to twenty-one days, the usual course of therapy would be from three to six weeks depending on symptoms and sigmoidoscopic findings. Studies available to date have not assessed if ROWASA suspension enema will modify relapse rates after the 6-week short-term treatment.

Patients should be instructed to shake the bottle well to make sure the suspension is homogeneous. The patient should remove the protective sheath from the applicator tip. Holding the bottle at the neck will not cause any of the medication to be discharged. The position most often used is obtained by lying on the left side (to facilitate migration into the sigmoid colon); with the lower leg extended and the upper right leg flexed forward for balance. An alternative is the knee-chest position. The applicator tip should be gently inserted in the rectum pointing toward the umbilicus. A steady squeezing of the bottle will discharge most of the preparation. The preparation should be taken at bedtime with the objective of retaining it all night. Patient instructions are included with every seven units.

ROWASA Suppositories: The usual dosage of ROWASA suppositories 500 mg is one rectal suppository 2 times daily. The suppository should be retained for one to three hours or longer, if possible, to achieve the maximum benefit. While the effect of ROWASA suppositories may be seen within

three to twenty-one days, the usual course of therapy would be from three to six weeks depending on symptoms and sigmoidoscopic findings. Studies available to date have not assessed if ROWASA suppositories will modify relapse rates after the six-week short-term treatment.

Patient Instructions:

1. Detach one suppository from strip of suppositories.
2. Hold suppository upright and carefully remove the foil wrapper.
3. Avoid excessive handling of suppository, which is designed to melt at body temperature.
4. Insert suppository completely into rectum with gentle pressure, pointed end first.

HOW SUPPLIED

Rowasa Suspension Enema: ROWASA suspension for rectal administration is an off-white to tan colored suspension. Each disposable enema bottle contains 4.0 grams of mesalamine in 60 mL aqueous suspension. Enema bottles are supplied in boxed, foil-wrapped trays of seven (NDC 0032-1924-82). ROWASA enema are for rectal use only.
Patient instructions are included.
Store at controlled room temperature 15° to 30°C (59° to 86°F). Once the foil-wrapped unit of seven bottles is opened, all enemas should be used promptly as directed by your physician. **Contents of enemas removed from the foil pouch may darken with time. Slight darkening will not affect potency, however enemas with dark brown contents should be discarded.** NOTE: ROWASA suspension enema may cause staining of garments, fabrics, painted surfaces, marble, granite, vinyl or other direct contact surfaces.

ROWASA Suppositories: ROWASA suppositories for rectal administration are available as bullet-shaped, light tan suppositories containing 500 mg mesalamine supplied in boxes of 12 (NDC 0032-1928-46) or boxes of 24 (NDC 0032-1928-24) individually foil-wrapped suppositories. Patient instructions are on back of boxes. Store at 19° to 26°C (66°–79°F).

REFERENCES

1. Williams CN. Efficacy and tolerance of 5-aminosalicylic acid suppositories in the treatment of ulcerative proctitis: A review of two double-blind, placebo controlled trials. *Can J Gastroenterol.* 1990;4(7):472–475.
2. Data on file, Solvay Pharmaceuticals.
3. Hanauer SB. Ulcerative proctitis. *Pract Gastroenterol.* 1990;15(1)(suppl):10–14.
4. Vitti RA, Meyers FA, Knight LC, et al. Colonic distribution of mesalamine enemas. *Treatment Options for Ulcerative Colitis.* NY: McGraw Hill, 1989;pp. 12–18.
5. Robinson MG. Efficacy of 5-aminosalicylic acid enemas in the treatment of distal ulcerative colitis. *Can J Gastroenterol.* 1990;4(7):468–471.
6. McPhee MS, Swan JT, Biddle WL, et al. Proctocolitis unresponsive to conventional therapy: Response to 5-aminosalicylic acid enemas. *Dig Dis Sci.* 1987; 32(12):76S–81S.
7. Greer SD, Foroozan P, Sutherland L, et al. A prospective trial of 5-aminosalicylic acid (5-ASA) enemas in the treatment of distal ulcerative colitis (DUC). *Gastroenterology.* 1986;90:1429. Abstract.
8. Guarino J, Chatzinoff M, Berk T, et al. 5-aminosalicylic acid enemas in refractory distal ulcerative colitis: Long-term results. *Am J Gastroenterol.* 1987;82(8):732–737.
9. Sutherland LR, Martin F, Greer S, et al. 5-aminosalicylic acid enema in the treatment of distal ulcerative colitis, proctosigmoiditis, and proctitis. *Gastroenterology.* 1987;92:1894–1898.
10. Biddle WL, Miner PB. Lifestyle issues: Impact of enema therapy. Presented at a symposium, *Trends in Inflammatory Bowel Disease Therapy,* in Halifax, Nova Scotia, June 1990.

Marketed by:
SOLVAY PHARMACEUTICALS
901 Sawyer Road
Marietta, Georgia 30062 7/91

Shown in Product Identification Section, page 432

ZENATE® ℞

[*ze'nāt*]
Prenatal Multivitamin/Mineral Supplement
Film Coated Tablets

Each tablet contains: [See table above.]

DESCRIPTION

Zenate is a prenatal film coated tablet. Zenate contains the vitamin and mineral components specified above. Zenate may also contain the following inactive ingredients: carnauba wax, cellulose, FD&C Blue No. 1 Aluminum Lake, magnesium stearate, polyethylene glycol, silicon dioxide, sodium starch glycolate, stearic acid, and titanium dioxide.

CLINICAL PHARMACOLOGY

Zenate is a phosphorus free[1] multivitamin/mineral dietary supplement specifically formulated for use during pregnancy and lactation.

VITAMINS:		% U.S. RDA[1] Pregnant or Lactating Women
A (as palmitate)	5,000 I.U.	62.5
D (as calciferol)	400 I.U.	100
E (as dl-alpha tocopheryl acetate)	30 I.U.	100
C (ascorbic acid)	80 mg	133
Folic Acid	1 mg	125
B_1 (as thiamine mononitrate)	3 mg	176
B_2 (riboflavin)	3 mg	150
Niacin (as niacinamide)	20 mg	100
B_6 (as pyridoxine hydrochloride)	10 mg	400
B_{12} (cyanocobalamin)	12 mcg	150
MINERALS:		
Calcium (from calcium carbonate)	300 mg	23
Iodine (from potassium iodide)	175 mcg	117
Iron (from ferrous fumarate)	65 mg	361
Magnesium (from magnesium oxide)	100 mg	22
Zinc (from zinc oxide)	20 mg	133

[1] U.S. Recommended Daily Allowances.

All ingredients covered by a warning or caution for usage in pregnancy have been formulated so as not to exceed maximum recommended strengths. The formulation includes essential vitamins and minerals, including 300 mg of elemental calcium, 65 mg of elemental iron, and 20 mg of elemental zinc. Zenate also offers 1 mg of folic acid to aid in the prevention of megaloblastic anemia.

INDICATIONS

Zenate is a vitamin-mineral dietary adjunct in nutritional stress associated with pregnancy and lactation.

CONTRAINDICATIONS

Zenate is contraindicated in those patients with known hypersensitivity to its use.

PRECAUTIONS

Folic acid in doses above 0.1 mg daily may obscure pernicious anemia in that hematologic remission can occur while neurological manifestations remain progressive. Periodic laboratory studies are considered essential and are recommended. Allergic sensitization has been reported following both oral and parenteral administration of folic acid.

DOSAGE AND ADMINISTRATION

One tablet daily before the first meal, or as directed by the physician.

HOW SUPPLIED

Zenate tablets are baby blue film coated capsule-shaped tablets embossed SOLVAY on one side and 1146 on the other and supplied in bottles of 100 tablets; (NDC 0032-1146-01).
Storage: Store at controlled room temperature, 15°–30°C (59°–86°F).

CAUTION

Federal Law Prohibits Dispensing Without Prescription.

Reference 1. Pitkin, R.M.: Vitamins and Minerals in Pregnancy. Clinics in Perinatology, 2:221–223, 1975.

Rev. 6/91

Shown in Product Identification Section, page 432

Somerset Pharmaceuticals, Inc.

777 SOUTH HARBOUR ISLAND BOULEVARD
SUITE 880
TAMPA, FLORIDA 33602

ELDEPRYL® ℞

[*el'dĕp-rĭl*]
(selegiline hydrochloride)
Tablets

DESCRIPTION

ELDEPRYL (selegiline hydrochloride) is a levorotatory acetylenic derivative of phenethylamine. It is commonly referred to in the clinical and pharmacological literature as L-deprenyl.
The chemical name is: (R)-(-)-N,2-dimethyl-N-2-propynylphenethylamine hydrochloride. It is a white to near white crystalline powder, freely soluble in water, chloroform, and methanol, and has a molecular weight of 223.75. The structural formula is as follows:

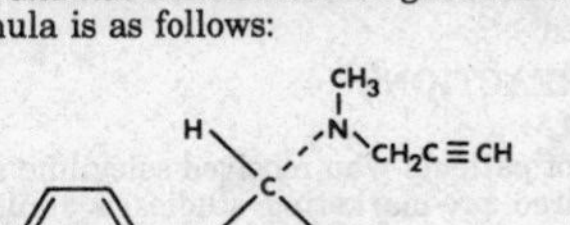

Each round white tablet, debossed on one side with "JU", contains 5 mg selegiline hydrochloride. Inactive ingredients are lactose, starch, povidone, magnesium stearate, and talc.

CLINICAL PHARMACOLOGY

The mechanisms accounting for selegiline's beneficial adjunctive action in the treatment of Parkinson's disease are not fully understood. Inhibition of monoamine oxidase, type B, activity is generally considered to be of primary importance; in addition, there is evidence that selegiline may act through other mechanisms to increase dopaminergic activity.
Selegiline is best known as an irreversible inhibitor of monoamine oxidase (MAO), an intracellular enzyme associated with the outer membrane of mitochondria. Selegiline inhibits MAO by acting as a 'suicide' substrate for the enzyme; that is, it is converted by MAO to an active moiety which combines irreversibly with the active site and/or the enzyme's essential FAD cofactor. Because selegiline has greater affinity for type B than for Type A active sites, it can serve as a selective inhibitor of MAO type B if it is administered at the recommended dose.
MAOs are widely distributed throughout the body; their concentration is especially high in liver, kidney, stomach, intestinal wall, and brain. MAOs are currently subclassified into two types, A and B, which differ in their substrate specificity and tissue distribution. In humans, intestinal MAO is predominantly type A, while most of that in brain is type B.
In CNS neurons, MAO plays an important role in the catabolism of catecholamines (dopamine, norepinephrine and epinephrine) and serotonin. MAOs are also important in the catabolism of various exogenous amines found in a variety of foods and drugs. MAO in the GI tract and liver (primarily type A), for example, is thought to provide vital protection from exogenous amines (e.g., tyramine) that have the capacity, if absorbed intact, to cause a 'hypertensive crisis,' the so-called 'cheese reaction.' (If large amounts of certain exogenous amines gain access to the systemic circulation—e.g., from fermented cheese, red wine, herring, over-the-counter cough/cold medications, etc.—they are taken up by adrenergic neurons and displace norepinephrine from storage sites within membrane bound vesicles. Subsequent release of the displaced norepinephrine causes the rise in systemic blood pressure, etc.)
In theory, therefore, because MAO A of the gut is not inhibited, patients treated with selegiline at a dose of 10 mg a day can take medications containing pharmacologically active amines and consume tyramine-containing foods without risk of uncontrolled hypertension. To date, clinical experience appears to confirm this prediction; cheese reactions have not been reported in selegiline treated patients. The pathophysiology of the 'cheese reaction' is complicated and, in addition to its ability to inhibit MAO B selectively, selegiline's apparent freedom from this reaction has been attributed to an ability to prevent tyramine and other indirect acting sympathomimetics from displacing norepinephrine from adrenergic neurons.
However, until the pathophysiology of the cheese reaction is more completely understood, it seems prudent to assume that selegiline can only be used safely without dietary restrictions at doses where it presumably selectively inhibits MAO B (e.g., 10 mg/day). **In short, attention to the dose dependent nature of selegiline's selectivity is critical if it is to be used without elaborate restrictions being placed on diet and concomitant drug use. (See WARNINGS and PRECAUTIONS).**
It is important to be aware that selegiline may have pharmacological effects unrelated to MAO B inhibition. As noted above, there is some evidence that it may increase dopaminergic activity by other mechanisms, including interfering with dopamine re-uptake at the synapse. Effects resulting from selegiline administration may also be mediated through its metabolites. Two of its three principal metabolites, amphetamine and methamphetamine, have pharmacological actions of their own; they interfere with neuronal uptake and enhance release of several neurotransmitters (e.g., norepinephrine, dopamine, serotonin). However, the extent to which these metabolites contribute to the effects of selegiline are unknown.

Rationale for the Use of a Selective Monoamine Oxidase Type B Inhibitor in Parkinson's Disease

Many of the prominent symptoms of Parkinson's disease are due to a deficiency of striatal dopamine that is the consequence of a progressive degeneration and loss of a population of dopaminergic neurons which originate in the substantia nigra of the midbrain and project to the basal ganglia or striatum. Early in the course of Parkinson's, the deficit in the capacity of these neurons to synthesize dopamine can be overcome by administration of exogenous levodopa, usually given in combination with a peripheral decarboxylase inhibitor (carbidopa).
With the passage of time, due to the progression of the disease and/or the effect of sustained treatment, the efficacy and quality of the therapeutic response of levodopa diminishes. Thus, after several years of levodopa treatment, the response, for a given dose of levodopa, is shorter, has less predictable onset and offset (i.e., there is 'wearing off'), and is

Continued on next page

Somerset—Cont.

often accompanied by side effects (e.g., dyskinesia, akinesias, on-off phenomena, freezing, etc.)

This deteriorating response is currently interpreted as a manifestation of the inability of the ever decreasing population of intact nigrostriatal neurons to synthesize and release adequate amounts of dopamine.

MAO B inhibition may be useful in this setting because, by blocking the catabolism of dopamine, it would increase the net amount of dopamine available (i.e., it would increase the pool of dopamine). Whether or not this mechanism or an alternative one actually accounts for the observed beneficial effects of adjunctive selegiline is unknown.

Selegiline's benefit in Parkinson's disease has only been documented as an adjunct to levodopa/carbidopa. Whether or not it might be effective as a sole treatment is unknown, but past attempts to treat Parkinson's disease with non-selective MAOI monotherapy are reported to have been unsuccessful. It is important to note that attempts to treat Parkinsonian patients with combinations of levodopa and currently marketed non-selective MAO inhibitors were abandoned because of multiple side effects including hypertension, increase in involuntary movement and toxic delirium.

Pharmacokinetic Information (Absorption, Distribution, Metabolism and Elimination—ADME)

Only preliminary information about the details of the pharmacokinetics of selegiline and its metabolites is available.

Data obtained in a study of 12 healthy subjects that was intended to examine the effects of selegiline on the ADME of an oral hypoglycemic agent, however, provides some information. Following the oral administration of a single dose of 10 mg of selegiline hydrochloride to these subjects, serum levels of intact selegiline were below the limit of detection (less than 10 ng/ml). Three metabolites, N-desmethyldeprenyl, the major metabolite (mean half-life 2.0 hours), amphetamine (mean half-life 17.7 hours), and methamphetamine (mean half-life 20.5 hours), were found in serum and urine. Over a period of 48 hours, 45% of the dose administered appeared in the urine as these 3 metabolites.

In an extension of this study intended to examine the effects of steady state conditions, the same subjects were given a 10 mg dose of selegiline hydrochloride for seven consecutive days. Under these conditions, the mean trough serum levels for amphetamine were 3.5 ng/ml and 8.0 ng/ml for methamphetamine; trough levels of N-desmethyldeprenyl were below the levels of detection.

The rate of MAO B regeneration following discontinuation of treatment has not been quantitated. It is this rate, dependent upon de novo protein synthesis, which seems likely to determine how fast normal MAO B activity can be restored.

INDICATIONS AND USAGE

ELDEPRYL is indicated as an adjunct in the management of Parkinsonian patients being treated with levodopa/carbidopa who exhibit deterioration in the quality of their response to this therapy. There is no evidence from controlled studies that selegiline has any beneficial effect in the absence of concurrent levodopa therapy.

Evidence supporting this claim was obtained in randomized controlled clinical investigations that compared the effects of added selegiline or placebo in patients receiving levodopa/carbidopa. Selegiline was significantly superior to placebo on all three principal outcome measures employed; change from baseline in daily levodopa/carbidopa dose, the amount of 'off' time, and patient self-rating of treatment success. Beneficial effects were also observed on other measures of treatment success (e.g., measures of reduced end of dose akinesia, decreased tremor and sialorrhea, improved speech and dressing ability and improved overall disability as assessed by walking and comparison to previous state).

CONTRAINDICATIONS

ELDEPRYL is containdicated in patients with a known hypersensitivity to this drug.

ELDEPRYL is contraindicated for use with meperidine (DEMEROL & other trade names). This contraindication is often extended to other opioids (see Drug Interactions).

WARNINGS

Selegiline should not be used at daily doses exceeding those recommended (10 mg/day) because of the risks associated with non-selective inhibition of MAO. (See CLINICAL PHARMACOLOGY.)

The selectivity of selegiline for MAO B may not be absolute even at the recommended daily dose of 10 mg a day and selectivity is further diminished with increasing daily doses. The precise dose at which selegiline becomes a non-selective inhibitor of all MAO is unknown, but may be in the range of 30 to 40 mg a day.

Definitive clinical data on the concomitant use of ELDEPRYL and fluoxetine hydrochloride (PROZAC) is not available. Death has been reported to occur following the initiation of therapy with nonselective MAOI's (NARDIL, PARNATE) shortly after discontinuation of fluoxetine. To date, this reaction has not been reported with ELDEPRYL; however, since the mechanism of this reaction is not fully understood it seems prudent, in general, to avoid this combination. Because of the long half-lives of fluoxetine and its active metabolite, at least five weeks (approximately 5 half-lives) should elapse between discontinuation of fluoxetine and initiation of MAOI therapy. Based on experience with the combined use of MAOI's and tricyclic antidepressants, at least 14 days should elapse between discontinuation of an MAOI and initiation of treatment with fluoxetine.

PRECAUTIONS

General

Some patients given selegiline may experience an exacerbation of levodopa associated side effects, presumably due to the increased amounts of dopamine reacting with supersensitive post-synaptic receptors. These effects may often be mitigated by reducing the dose of levodopa/carbidopa by approximately 10 to 30%.

The decision to prescribe selegiline should take into consideration that the MAO system of enzymes is complex and incompletely understood and there is only a limited amount of carefully documented clinical experience with selegiline. Consequently, the full spectrum of possible responses to selegiline may not have been observed in pre-marketing evaluation of the drug. It is advisable, therefore, to observe patients closely for atypical responses.

Information for Patients

Patients should be advised of the possible need to reduce levodopa dosage after the initiation of ELDEPRYL therapy.

Patients (or their families if the patient is incompetent) should be advised not to exceed the daily recommended dose of 10 mg. The risk of using higher daily doses of selegiline should be explained, and a brief description of the 'cheese reaction' provided. While hypertensive reactions with selegiline have not been reported, documented experience is limited. Consequently, it may be useful to inform patients (or their families) about the signs and symptoms associated with MAOI induced hypertensive reactions. In particular, patients should be urged to report, immediately, any severe headache or other atypical or unusual symptoms not previously experienced.

Laboratory Tests

No specific laboratory tests are deemed essential for the management of patients on ELDEPRYL. Periodic routine evaluation of all patients, however, is appropriate.

Drug Interactions

The occurrence of stupor, muscular rigidity, severe agitation, and elevated temperature has been reported in a man receiving selegiline and meperidine, as well as other medications. Symptoms resolved over days when the combination was discontinued. This case is typical of the interaction of meperidine and MAOIs. Other serious reactions (including severe agitation, hallucinations, and death) have been reported in patients receiving this combination. While it cannot be said definitively that all of these reactions were caused by this combination, they are all compatible with this well recognized interaction. No other interactions attributed to the combined use of selegiline and other drugs have been reported. However, because the database of documented clinical experience is limited, the level of reassurance provided by this lack of adverse reporting is uncertain. (See WARNINGS and PRECAUTIONS.)

Carcinogenesis, Mutagenesis, and Impairment of Fertility

Studies have not been performed to date to evaluate the carcinogenic potential of selegiline hydrochloride.

Pregnancy

Pregnancy category C. Insufficient animal reproduction studies have been done with selegiline to conclude that selegiline poses no teratogenic risk. However, one rat study carried out at doses as much as 180 fold the recommended human dose revealed no evidence of a teratogenic effect. It is not known whether selegiline can cause fetal harm when administered to a pregnant woman or can affect reproduction capacity. Selegiline should be given to a pregnant woman only if clearly needed.

Nursing Mothers

It is not known whether selegiline hydrochloride is excreted in human milk. Because many drugs are excreted in human milk, consideration should be given to discontinuing the use of all but absolutely essential drug treatments in nursing women.

Pediatric Use

The effects of selegiline hydrochloride in children have not been evaluated.

ADVERSE REACTIONS

Introduction

The number of patients who received selegiline in prospectively monitored pre-marketing studies is limited. While other sources of information about the use of selegiline are available (e.g., literature reports, foreign post-marketing reports, etc.) they do not provide the kind of information necessary to estimate the incidence of adverse events. Thus, overall incidence figures for adverse reactions associated with the use of selegiline cannot be provided. Many of the adverse reactions seen have been also reported as symptoms of dopamine excess.

Moreover, the importance and severity of various reactions reported often cannot be ascertained. One index of relative importance, however, is whether or not a reaction caused treatment discontinuation. In prospective pre-marketing studies, the following events led, in decreasing order of frequency, to discontinuation of treatment with selegiline: nausea, hallucinations, confusion, depression, loss of balance, insomnia, orthostatic hypotension, increased akinetic involuntary movements, agitation, arrhythmia, bradykinesia, chorea, delusions, hypertension, new or increased angina pectoris and syncope. Events reported only once as a cause of discontinuation are ankle edema, anxiety, burning lips/mouth, constipation, drowsiness/lethargy, dystonia, excess perspiration, increased freezing, gastrointestinal bleeding, hair loss, increased tremor, nervousness, weakness and weight loss.

Experience with ELDEPRYL obtained in parallel, placebo controlled, randomized studies provides only a limited basis for estimates of adverse reaction rates. The following reactions that occurred with greater frequency among the 49 patients assigned to selegiline as compared to the 50 patients assigned to placebo in the only parallel, placebo controlled trial performed in patients with Parkinson's disease are shown in the following Table. None of these adverse reactions led to a discontinuation of treatment.

INCIDENCE OF TREATMENT-EMERGENT ADVERSE EXPERIENCES IN THE PLACEBO-CONTROLLED CLINICAL TRIAL

Adverse Event	Number of Patients Reporting Events: selegiline hydrochloride N=49	placebo N=50
Nausea	10	3
Dizziness/Lightheaded/Fainting	7	1
Abdominal Pain	4	2
Confusion	3	0
Hallucinations	3	1
Dry mouth	3	1
Vivid Dreams	2	0
Dyskinesias	2	5
Headache	2	1
The following events were reported once in either or both groups:		
Ache, generalized	1	0
Anxiety/Tension	1	1
Anemia	0	1
Diarrhea	1	0
Hair Loss	0	1
Insomnia	1	1
Lethargy	1	0
Leg pain	1	0
Low back pain	1	0
Malaise	0	1
Palpitations	1	0
Urinary Retention	1	0
Weight Loss	1	0

In all prospectively monitored clinical investigations, enrolling approximately 920 patients, the following adverse events, classified by body system, were reported.

CENTRAL NERVOUS SYSTEM

Motor/Coordination/Extrapyramidal: increased tremor, chorea, loss of balance, restlessness, blephorospasm, increased bradykinesia, facial grimace, falling down, heavy leg, muscle twitch*, myoclonic jerks*, stiff neck, tardive dyskinesia, dystonic symptoms, dyskinesia, involuntary movements, freezing, festination, increased apraxia, muscle cramps.

Mental Status/Behavioral/Psychiatric: hallucinations, dizziness, confusion, anxiety, depression, drowsiness, behavior/mood change, dreams/nightmares, tiredness, delusions, disorientation, lightheadedness, impaired memory*, increased energy*, transient high*, hollow feeling, lethargy/malaise, apathy, overstimulation, vertigo, personality change, sleep disturbance, restlessness, weakness, transient irritability.

Pain/Altered Sensation: headache, back pain, leg pain, tinnitus, migraine, supraorbital pain, throat burning, generalized ache, chills, numbness of toes/fingers, taste disturbance.

AUTONOMIC NERVOUS SYSTEM

dry mouth, blurred vision, sexual dysfunction.

CARDIOVASCULAR

orthostatic hypotension, hypertension, arrhythmia, palpita-

---

*indicates events reported only at doses greater than 10 mg/day.

tions, new or increased angina pectoris, hypotension, tachycardia, peripheral edema, sinus bradycardia, syncope.

GASTROINTESTINAL
nausea/vomiting, constipation, weight loss, anorexia, poor appetite, dysphagia, diarrhea, heartburn, rectal bleeding, bruxism*, gastrointestinal bleeding (exacerbation of preexisting ulcer disease).

GENITOURINARY/GYNECOLOGIC/ENDOCRINE
slow urination, transient anorgasmia*, nocturia, prostatic hypertrophy, urinary hesitancy, urinary retention, decreased penile sensation*, urinary frequency.

SKIN AND APPENDAGES
increased sweating, diaphoresis, facial hair, hair loss, hematoma, rash, photosensitivity.

MISCELLANEOUS
asthma, diplopia, shortness of breath, speech affected.

POSTMARKETING REPORTS
The following experiences were described in spontaneous postmarketing reports. These reports do not provide sufficient information to establish a clear causal relationship with the use of ELDEPRYL.
CNS: Seizure in dialyzed chronic renal failure patient on concomitant medications.

OVERDOSAGE

Selegiline
No specific information is available about clinically significant overdoses with ELDEPRYL. However, experience gained during selegiline's development reveals that some individuals exposed to doses of 600 mg d, l selegiline suffered severe hypotension and psychomotor agitation.
Since the selective inhibition of MAO B by selegiline hydrochloride is achieved only at doses in the range recommended for the treatment of Parkinson's disease (e.g., 10 mg/day), overdoses are likely to cause significant inhibition of both MAO A and MAO B. Consequently, the signs and symptoms of overdose may resemble those observed with marketed non-selective MAO inhibitors [e.g., tranylcypromine (PARNATE), isocarboxazide (MARPLAN), and phenelzine (NARDIL)].

Overdose with Non-Selective MAO Inhibition
NOTE: This section is provided for reference; it does not describe events that have actually been observed with selegiline in overdose.
Characteristically, signs and symptoms of non-selective MAOI overdose may not appear immediately. Delays of up to 12 hours between ingestion of drug and the appearance of signs may occur. Importantly, the peak intensity of the syndrome may not be reached for upwards of a day following the overdose. Death has been reported following overdosage. Therefore, immediate hospitalization, with continuous patient observation and monitoring for a period of at least two days following the ingestion of such drugs in overdose is strongly recommended.
The clinical picture of MAOI overdose varies considerably; its severity may be a function of the amount of drug consumed. The central nervous and cardiovascular systems are prominently involved.
Signs and symptoms of overdosage may include, alone or in combination, any of the following: drowsiness, dizziness, faintness, irritability, hyperactivity, agitation, severe headache, hallucinations, trismus, opisthotonus, convulsions, and coma; rapid and irregular pulse, hypertension, hypotension and vascular collapse; precordial pain, respiratory depression and failure, hyperpyrexia, diaphoresis, and cool, clammy skin.

Treatment Suggestions for Overdose
NOTE: Because there is no recorded experience with selegiline overdose, the following suggestions are offered based upon the assumption that selegiline overdose may be modeled by non-selective MAOI poisoning. In any case, up-to-date information about the treatment of overdose can often be obtained from a certified Regional Poison Control Center. Telephone numbers of certified Poison Control Centers are listed in the *Physicians' Desk Reference (PDR).*
Treatment of overdose with non-selective MAOIs is symptomatic and supportive. Induction of emesis or gastric lavage with instillation of charcoal slurry may be helpful in early poisoning, provided the airway has been protected against aspiration. Signs and symptoms of central nervous system stimulation, including convulsions, should be treated with diazepam, given slowly intravenously. Phenothiazine derivatives and central nervous system stimulants should be avoided. Hypotension and vascular collapse should be treated with intravenous fluids and, if necessary, blood pressure titration with an intravenous infusion of a dilute pressor agent. It should be noted that adrenergic agents may produce a markedly increased pressor response.
Respiration should be supported by appropriate measures, including management of the airway, use of supplemental oxygen, and mechanical ventilatory assistance, as required. Body temperature should be monitored closely. Intensive management of hyperpyrexia may be required. Maintenance of fluid and electrolyte balance is essential.

DOSAGE AND ADMINISTRATION

ELDEPRYL is intended for administration to Parkinsonian patients receiving levodopa/carbidopa therapy who demonstrate a deteriorating response to this treatment. The recommended regimen for the administration of ELDEPRYL is 10 mg per day administered as divided doses of 5 mg each taken at breakfast and lunch. There is no evidence that additional benefit will be obtained from the administration of higher doses. Moreover, higher doses should ordinarily be avoided because of the increased risk of side effects.
After two to three days of selegiline treatment, an attempt may be made to reduce the dose of levodopa/carbidopa. A reduction of 10 to 30% was achieved with the typical participant in the domestic placebo controlled trials who was assigned to selegiline treatment. Further reductions of levodopa/carbidopa may be possible during continued selegiline therapy.

HOW SUPPLIED

Tablets:
5 mg. bottles of 60 tablets, NDC 39506-011-25
Store at controlled room temperature, 59° to 86°F (15° to 30°C).
Caution—Federal (USA) law prohibits dispensing without prescription.
Literature issued December, 1991
011-25-P-105
Shown in Product Identification Section, page 432

E. R. Squibb & Sons, Inc.
A Bristol-Myers Squibb Company
P.O. BOX 4000
PRINCETON, NJ 08543-4000

AZACTAM® FOR INJECTION ℞

[a-zak 'tam]
Aztreonam For Injection USP

DESCRIPTION

AZACTAM (Aztreonam, Squibb) is the first member of a new class of antibiotics developed by the Squibb Institute for Medical Research and classified as monobactams. These agents were originally isolated from *Chromobacterium violaceum.* AZACTAM is a totally synthetic bactericidal antibiotic with activity against a wide spectrum of gram-negative aerobic pathogens.
The monobactams, having a unique monocyclic beta-lactam nucleus, are structurally different from other beta-lactam antibiotics (e.g., penicillins, cephalosporins, cephamycins). The sulfonic acid substituent in the 1-position of the ring activates the beta-lactam moiety; an aminothiazolyl oxime side chain in the 3-position and a methyl group in the 4-position confer the specific antibacterial spectrum and beta-lactamase stability.
Aztreonam is designated chemically as (Z)-2-[[[(2-amino-4-thiazolyl)[[(2S,3S)-2-methyl -4- oxo-1-sulfo-3-azetidinyl]carbamoyl]methylene]amino]oxy]-2-methylpropionic acid.
AZACTAM For Injection (Aztreonam For Injection) is a sterile, nonpyrogenic, sodium-free, white to yellowish-white lyophilized cake containing approximately 780 mg arginine per gram of aztreonam. Following constitution, the product is for intramuscular or intravenous use. Aqueous solutions of the product have a pH in the range of 4.5 to 7.5.

CLINICAL PHARMACOLOGY

Single 30-minute intravenous infusions of 500 mg, 1 g and 2 g doses of AZACTAM in healthy subjects produced peak serum levels of 54, 90 and 204 μg/mL, respectively, immediately after administration; at eight hours, serum levels were 1, 3 and 6 μg/mL, respectively (Figure 1). Single 3-minute intravenous injections of the same doses resulted in serum levels of 58, 125 and 242 μg/mL at five minutes following completion of injection.
Serum concentrations of aztreonam in healthy subjects following completion of single intramuscular injections of 500 mg and 1 g doses are depicted in Figure 1; maximum serum concentrations occur at about one hour. After identical single intravenous or intramuscular doses of AZACTAM, the serum concentrations of aztreonam are comparable at one hour (1.5 hours from start of intravenous infusion) with similar slopes of serum concentrations thereafter.
The serum levels of aztreonam following single 500 mg or 1 g (intramuscular or intravenous) or 2 g (intravenous) doses of AZACTAM (aztreonam) exceed the MIC_{90} for *Neisseria* sp., *H. influenzae* and most genera of the *Enterobacteriaceae* for eight hours (for *Enterobacter* sp., the eight hour serum levels exceed the MIC for 80 percent of strains). For *Ps. aeruginosa*, a single 2 g intravenous dose produces serum levels that exceed the MIC_{90} for approximately four to six hours. All of the above doses of AZACTAM result in average urine levels of aztreonam that exceed the MIC_{90} for the same pathogens for up to 12 hours.

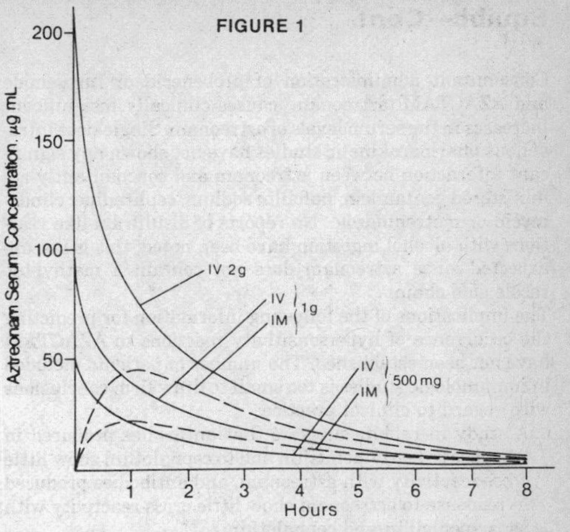

The serum half-life of aztreonam averaged 1.7 hours (1.5 to 2.0) in subjects with normal renal function, independent of the dose and route of administration. In healthy subjects, based on a 70 kg person, the serum clearance was 91 mL/min and renal clearance was 56 mL/min; the apparent mean volume of distribution at steady-state averaged 12.6 liters, approximately equivalent to extracellular fluid volume.
In a study of healthy elderly male subjects (65 to 75 years of age), the average elimination half-life of aztreonam was slightly longer than in young healthy males.
In patients with impaired renal function, the serum half-life of aztreonam is prolonged (see DOSAGE AND ADMINISTRATION, Renal Impairment). The serum half-life of aztreonam is only slightly prolonged in patients with hepatic impairment since the liver is a minor pathway of excretion.
Average urine concentrations of aztreonam were approximately 1100, 3500 and 6600 μg/mL within the first two hours following single 500 mg, 1 g and 2 g intravenous doses of AZACTAM (30-minute infusions), respectively. The range of average concentrations for aztreonam in the 8 to 12 hour urine specimens in these studies was 25 to 120 μg/mL. After intramuscular injection of single 500 mg and 1 g doses of AZACTAM, urinary levels were approximately 500 and 1200 μg/mL, respectively, within the first two hours, declining to 180 and 470 μg/mL in the six to eight hour specimens. In healthy subjects, aztreonam is excreted in the urine about equally by active tubular secretion and glomerular filtration. Approximately 60 to 70 percent of an intravenous or intramuscular dose was recovered in the urine by eight hours. Urinary excretion of a single parenteral dose was essentially complete by 12 hours after injection. About 12 percent of a single intravenous radiolabeled dose was recovered in the feces. Unchanged aztreonam and the inactive beta-lactam ring hydrolysis product of aztreonam were present in feces and urine.
Intravenous or intramuscular administration of a single 500 mg or 1 g dose of AZACTAM (aztreonam) every eight hours for seven days to healthy subjects produced no apparent accumulation of aztreonam or modification of its disposition characteristics; serum protein binding averaged 56 percent and was independent of dose. An average of about 6 percent of a 1 g intramuscular dose was excreted as a microbiologically inactive open beta-lactam ring hydrolysis product (serum half-life approximately 26 hours) of aztreonam in the zero to eight hour urine collection on the last day of multiple dosing.
Renal function was monitored in healthy subjects given aztreonam; standard tests (serum creatinine, creatinine clearance, BUN, urinalysis and total urinary protein excretion) as well as special tests (excretion of N-acetyl-β-glucosaminidase, alanine aminopeptidase and β_2-microglobulin) were used. No abnormal results were obtained.
Aztreonam achieves measurable concentrations in the following body fluids and tissues:
[See table on next page.]
The concentration of aztreonam in saliva at 30 minutes after a single 1 g intravenous dose (9 patients) was 0.2 μg/mL; in breast milk at two hours after a single 1 g intravenous dose (6 patients), 0.2 μg/mL, and at six hours after a single 1 g intramuscular dose (6 patients), 0.3 μg/mL; in amniotic fluid at six to eight hours after a single 1 g intravenous dose (5 patients), 2 μg/mL. The concentration of aztreonam in peritoneal fluid obtained one to six hours after multiple 2 g intravenous doses ranged between 12 and 90 μg/mL in 7 of 8 patients studied.
Aztreonam given intravenously rapidly reaches therapeutic concentrations in peritoneal dialysis fluid; conversely, aztreonam given intraperitoneally in dialysis fluid rapidly produces therapeutic serum levels.

Continued on next page

Squibb—Cont.

Concomitant administration of probenecid or furosemide and AZACTAM (aztreonam) causes clinically insignificant increases in the serum levels of aztreonam. Single-dose intravenous pharmacokinetic studies have not shown any significant interaction between aztreonam and concomitantly administered gentamicin, nafcillin sodium, cephradine, clindamycin or metronidazole. No reports of disulfiram-like reactions with alcohol ingestion have been noted; this is not unexpected since aztreonam does not contain a methyl-tetrazole side chain.

The implications of the following information for predicting the occurrence of hypersensitivity reactions to AZACTAM have not been established. The number of patients included in immunologic studies is too small to draw firm conclusions with regard to clinical practice:

A study in rabbits suggests that antibodies produced in response to benzylpenicillin and to cephalothin show little cross-reactivity with aztreonam, and antibodies produced in response to aztreonam show little cross-reactivity with benzylpenicillin and cephalothin.

In a group of 22 subjects with positive skin tests to penicillin reagents, three also had positive skin tests to aztreonam. One was negative on retesting, one was confirmed as positive, and the third subject refused further evaluation. The 20 subjects with negative aztreonam skin tests were given one injection of AZACTAM 1 g IM. There were no immediate hypersensitivity reactions, but one subject later developed a localized rash that was compatible with a fixed drug eruption.

In 36 subjects receiving multiple doses of AZACTAM over a seven-day period, no IgE antibody response was detectable and only one subject demonstrated an IgG response.

Microbiology

Aztreonam exhibits potent and specific activity *in vitro* against a wide spectrum of gram-negative aerobic pathogens including *Pseudomonas aeruginosa*. The bactericidal action of aztreonam results from the inhibition of bacterial cell wall synthesis due to a high affinity of aztreonam for penicillin binding protein 3 (PBP3). Aztreonam, unlike the majority of beta-lactam antibiotics, does not induce beta-lactamase activity and its molecular structure confers a high degree of resistance to hydrolysis by beta-lactamases (i.e., penicillinases and cephalosporinases) produced by most gram-negative and gram-positive pathogens; it is therefore usually active against gram-negative aerobic organisms that are resistant to antibiotics hydrolyzed by beta-lactamases. Aztreonam maintains its antimicrobial activity over a pH range of 6 to 8 *in vitro*, as well as in the presence of human serum and under anaerobic conditions. Aztreonam is active *in vitro* and is effective in laboratory animal models and clinical infections against most strains of the following organisms, including many that are multiply-resistant to other antibiotics (i.e., certain cephalosporins, penicillins, and aminoglycosides):

Escherichia coli
Enterobacter species
Klebsiella pneumoniae and *K. oxytoca*
Proteus mirabilis
Pseudomonas aeruginosa
Serratia marcescens
Haemophilus influenzae (including ampicillin-resistant and other penicillinase-producing strains)
Citrobacter species

While *in vitro* studies have demonstrated the susceptibility to aztreonam of most strains of the following organisms, clinical efficacy for infections other than those included in the INDICATIONS AND USAGE section has not been documented:

Neisseria gonorrhoeae (including penicillinase-producing strains)
Proteus vulgaris
Morganella morganii (formerly *Proteus morganii*)
Providencia species, including *P. stuartii* and *P. rettgeri* (formerly *Proteus rettgeri*)
Pseudomonas species
Shigella species
Pasteurella multocida
Yersinia enterocolitica
Aeromonas hydrophila
Neisseria meningitidis

Aztreonam and aminoglycosides have been shown to be synergistic in vitro against most strains of Ps. aeruginosa, many strains of Enterobacteriaceae, and other gram-negative aerobic bacilli.

Alterations of the anaerobic intestinal flora by broad spectrum antibiotics may decrease colonization resistance, thus permitting overgrowth of potential pathogens, e.g., *Candida* and Clostridia species. Aztreonam has little effect on the anaerobic intestinal microflora in *in vitro* studies. *Clostridium difficile* and its cytotoxin were not found in animal models following administration of aztreonam (see ADVERSE REACTIONS, Gastrointestinal).

Susceptibility Testing

Diffusion Technique: Quantitative procedures that require measurement of zone diameters give precise estimates of microbial susceptibility to antibiotics. One such method, recommended for use with the aztreonam 30 µg disk, is the National Committee of Clinical Laboratory Standards (NCCLS) approved procedure. Only a 30 µg aztreonam disk should be used; there are no suitable surrogate disks. Results of laboratory tests using 30 µg aztreonam disks should be interpreted using the following criteria:

Zone Diameter (mm)	Interpretation
≥ 22	(S) Susceptible
16–21	(I) Intermediate (Moderate Susceptibility)
≤ 15	(R) Resistant

Dilution Technique: Broth or agar dilution methods may be used to determine the minimal inhibitory concentration (MIC) of aztreonam.

MIC test results should be interpreted according to the concentrations of aztreonam that can be attained in serum, tissues and body fluids.

MIC (µg/mL)	Interpretation
≤ 8	(S) Susceptible
16	(I) Intermediate (Moderate Susceptibility)
≥ 32	(R) Resistant

For any susceptibility test, a report of "susceptible" indicates that the pathogen is likely to respond to AZACTAM therapy; a report of "resistant" indicates that the pathogen is not likely to respond. A report of "intermediate" (moderate susceptibility) indicates that the pathogen is expected to be susceptible to AZACTAM (aztreonam) if high dosages are used, or if the infection is confined to tissues and fluids (e.g., urine, bile) in which high aztreonam levels are attained.

The quality control cultures should have the following assigned daily ranges for aztreonam:

	Disks	Mode MIC (µg/mL)
E. coli (ATCC 25922)	28–36 mm	0.06–0.25
Ps. aeruginosa (ATCC 27853)	23–29 mm	2.0–8.0

INDICATIONS AND USAGE

Before initiating treatment with AZACTAM, appropriate specimens should be obtained for isolation of the causative organism(s) and for determination of susceptibility to aztreonam. Treatment with AZACTAM may be started empirically before results of the susceptibility testing are available; subsequently, appropriate antibiotic therapy should be continued.

AZACTAM For Injection (Aztreonam For Injection) is indicated for the treatment of the following infections caused by susceptible gram-negative microorganisms:

Urinary Tract Infections (complicated and uncomplicated), including pyelonephritis and cystitis (initial and recurrent) caused by *Escherichia coli, Klebsiella pneumoniae, Proteus mirabilis, Pseudomonas aeruginosa, Enterobacter cloacae, Klebsiella oxytoca*, Citrobacter* species* and *Serratia marcescens**.

Lower Respiratory Tract Infections, including pneumonia and bronchitis caused by *Escherichia coli, Klebsiella pneumoniae, Pseudomonas aeruginosa, Haemophilus influenzae, Proteus mirabilis, Enterobacter* species and *Serratia marcescens**.

Septicemia caused by *Escherichia coli, Klebsiella pneumoniae, Pseudomonas aeruginosa, Proteus mirabilis*, Serratia marcescens** and *Enterobacter* species.

Skin and Skin-Structure Infections, including those associated with post-operative wounds, ulcers and burns caused by *Escherichia coli, Proteus mirabilis, Serratia marcescens, Enterobacter* species, *Pseudomonas aeruginosa, Klebsiella pneumoniae* and *Citrobacter* species*.

Intra-abdominal Infections, including peritonitis caused by *Escherichia coli, Klebsiella* species including *K. pneumoniae, Enterobacter* species including *E. cloacae*, Pseudomonas aeruginosa, Citrobacter* species* including *C. freundii** and *Serratia* species* including *S. marcescens**.

Gynecologic Infections, including endometritis and pelvic cellulitis caused by *Escherichia coli, Klebsiella pneumoniae*, Enterobacter* species* including *E. cloacae** and *Proteus mirabilis**.

AZACTAM (aztreonam) is indicated for adjunctive therapy to surgery in the management of infections caused by susceptible organisms, including abscesses, infections complicating hollow viscus perforations, cutaneous infections and infections of serous surfaces. AZACTAM is effective against most of the commonly encountered gram-negative aerobic pathogens seen in general surgery.

Concurrent Therapy

Concurrent initial therapy with other antimicrobial agents and AZACTAM is recommended before the causative organism(s) is known in seriously ill patients who are also at risk of having an infection due to gram-positive aerobic pathogens. If anaerobic organisms are also suspected as etiologic agents, therapy should be initiated using an anti-anaerobic agent concurrently with AZACTAM (see DOSAGE AND ADMINISTRATION). Certain antibiotics (e.g., cefoxitin, imipenem) may induce high levels of beta-lactamase *in vitro* in some gram-negative aerobes such as *Enterobacter* and *Pseudomonas* species, resulting in antagonism to many beta-lactam antibiotics including aztreonam. These *in vitro* findings suggest that such beta-lactamase inducing antibiotics not be used concurrently with aztreonam. Following identification and susceptibility testing of the causative organism(s), appropriate antibiotic therapy should be continued.

CONTRAINDICATIONS

Aztreonam is contraindicated in patients with known allergy to this antibiotic.

WARNINGS

Careful inquiry should be made for a history of hypersensitivity reaction to any antibiotic or other drugs. Antibiotics should be given with caution to any patient who has had

---

EXTRAVASCULAR CONCENTRATIONS OF AZTREONAM AFTER A SINGLE PARENTERAL DOSE[1]

Fluid or Tissue	Dose (g)	Route	Hours Post-injection	Number of Patients	Mean Concentration (µg/mL or µg/g)
Fluids					
bile	1	IV	2	10	39
blister fluid	1	IV	1	6	20
bronchial secretion	2	IV	4	7	5
cerebrospinal fluid (inflamed meninges)	2	IV	0.9–4.3	16	3
pericardial fluid	2	IV	1	6	33
pleural fluid	2	IV	1.1–3.0	3	51
synovial fluid	2	IV	0.8–1.9	11	83
Tissues					
atrial appendage	2	IV	0.9–1.6.	12	22
endometrium	2	IV	0.7–1.9	4	9
fallopian tube	2	IV	0.7–1.9	8	12
fat	2	IV	1.3–2.0	10	5
femur	2	IV	1.0–2.1	15	16
gallbladder	2	IV	0.8–1.3	4	23
kidney	2	IV	2.4–5.6	5	67
large intestine	2	IV	0.8–1.9	9	12
liver	2	IV	0.9–2.0	6	47
lung	2	IV	1.2–2.1	6	22
myometrium	2	IV	0.7–1.9	9	11
ovary	2	IV	0.7–1.9	7	13
prostate	1	IM	0.8–3.0	8	8
skeletal muscle	2	IV	0.3–0.7	6	16
skin	2	IV	0.0–1.0	8	25
sternum	2	IV	1	6	6

[1] Tissue penetration is regarded as essential to therapeutic efficacy, but specific tissue levels have not been correlated with specific therapeutic effects.

---

* Efficacy for this organism in this organ system was studied in fewer than ten infections.

some form of allergy, particularly to drugs. It is recommended that patients who have had immediate hypersensitivity reactions (e.g., anaphylactic or urticarial) to penicillins and/or cephalosporins should be followed with special care. If an allergic reaction to aztreonam occurs, discontinue the drug and institute supportive treatment as appropriate (e.g., maintenance of ventilation, pressor amines, antihistamines, corticosteroids). Serious hypersensitivity reactions may require epinephrine and other emergency measures.

Pseudomembranous colitis has been reported with nearly all antibacterial agents, including aztreonam, and may range in severity from mild to life-threatening. Therefore, it is important to consider this diagnosis in patients who present with diarrhea subsequent to the administration of antibacterial agents.

Treatment with antibacterial agents alters the normal flora of the colon and may permit overgrowth of clostridia. Studies indicate that a toxin produced by *Clostridium difficile* is one primary cause of "antibiotic-associated colitis."

After the diagnosis of pseudomembranous colitis has been established, therapeutic measures should be initiated. Mild cases of pseudomembranous colitis usually respond to drug discontinuation alone. In moderate to severe cases, consideration should be given to management with fluids and electrolytes, protein supplementation, and treatment with an antibacterial drug effective against *C. difficile*.

PRECAUTIONS

General
In patients with impaired hepatic or renal function, appropriate monitoring is recommended during therapy.

If an aminoglycoside is used concurrently with aztreonam, especially if high dosages of the former are used or if therapy is prolonged, renal function should be monitored because of the potential nephrotoxicity and ototoxicity of aminoglycoside antibiotics.

The use of antibiotics may promote the overgrowth of nonsusceptible organisms, including gram-positive organisms (*Staphylococcus aureus* and *Streptococcus faecalis*) and fungi. Should superinfection occur during therapy, appropriate measures should be taken.

Carcinogenesis, Mutagenesis, Impairment of Fertility
Carcinogenicity studies in animals have not been performed. Genetic toxicology studies performed *in vivo* and *in vitro* with aztreonam in several standard laboratory models revealed no evidence of mutagenic potential at the chromosomal or gene level.

Two-generation reproduction studies in rats at daily doses up to 20 times the maximum recommended human dose, prior to and during gestation and lactation, revealed no evidence of impaired fertility. There was a slightly reduced survival rate during the lactation period in the offspring of rats that received the highest dosage, but not in offspring of rats that received five times the maximum recommended human dose.

Pregnancy
Pregnancy Category B
Aztreonam crosses the placenta and enters the fetal circulation.

Studies in pregnant rats and rabbits, with daily doses up to 15 and 5 times, respectively, the maximum recommended human dose, revealed no evidence of embryo- or fetotoxicity or teratogenicity. No drug induced changes were seen in any of the maternal, fetal, or neonatal parameters that were monitored in rats receiving 15 times the maximum recommended human dose of aztreonam during late gestation and lactation.

There are no adequate and well-controlled studies in pregnant women. Because animal reproduction studies are not always predictive of human response, aztreonam should be used during pregnancy only if clearly needed.

Nursing Mothers
Aztreonam is excreted in breast milk in concentrations that are less than 1 percent of concentrations determined in simultaneously obtained maternal serum; consideration should be given to temporary discontinuation of nursing and use of formula feedings.

Pediatric Use
Safety and effectiveness have not been established in infants and children.

ADVERSE REACTIONS

Local reactions such as phlebitis/thrombophlebitis following IV administration, and discomfort/swelling at the injection site following IM administration occurred at rates of approximately 1.9 percent and 2.4 percent, respectively.

Systemic reactions (considered to be related to therapy or of uncertain etiology) occurring at an incidence of 1 to 1.3 percent include diarrhea, nausea and/or vomiting, and rash. Reactions occurring at an incidence of less than 1 percent are listed within each body system in order of decreasing severity:

Hypersensitivity —anaphylaxis, anigioedema, bronchospasm.

Hematologic —pancytopenia, neutropenia, thrombocytopenia, anemia, leukocytosis, thrombocytosis.

Gastrointestinal —abdominal cramps; rare cases of *C. difficile*-associated diarrhea, including pseudomembranous colitis, or gastrointestinal bleeding have been reported. Onset of pseudomembranous colitis symptoms may occur during or after antibiotic treatment (see WARNINGS).

Dermatologic —toxic epidermal necrolysis, purpura, erythema multiforme, exfoliative dermatitis, urticaria, petechiae, pruritus.

Cardiovascular —hypotension, transient ECG changes (ventricular bigeminy and PVC).

Respiratory —one patient experienced flushing, chest pain, and dyspnea.

Hepatobiliary —hepatitis, jaundice.

Nervous System —seizure, confusion, vertigo, paresthesia, insomnia, dizziness.

Musculoskeletal —muscular aches.

Special Senses —tinnitus, diplopia, mouth ulcer, altered taste, numb tongue, sneezing and nasal congestion, halitosis.

Other —vaginal candidiasis, vaginitis, breast tenderness.

Body as a Whole —weakness, headache, fever, malaise, diaphoresis.

Adverse Laboratory Changes
Adverse laboratory changes without regard to drug relationship that were reported during clinical trials were:

Hepatic —elevations of AST (SGOT), ALT (SGPT), and alkaline phosphatase; signs or symptoms of hepatobiliary dysfunction occurred in less than 1 percent of recipients (see above).

Hematologic —increases in prothrombin and partial thromboplastin times, eosinophilia, positive Coombs test.

Renal —increases in serum creatinine.

OVERDOSAGE

If necessary, aztreonam may be cleared from the serum by hemodialysis and/or peritoneal dialysis.

DOSAGE AND ADMINISTRATION

AZACTAM (aztreonam) For Injection may be administered intravenously or by intramuscular injection. Dosage and route of administration should be determined by susceptibility of the causative organisms, severity and site of infection, and the condition of the patient.

AZACTAM DOSAGE GUIDELINES ADULTS

Type of Infection	Dose*	Frequency (hours)
Urinary tract infections	500 mg or 1 g	8 or 12
Moderately severe systemic infections	1 g or 2 g	8 or 12
Severe systemic or life-threatening infections	2 g	6 or 8

*Maximum recommended dose is 8 g per day.

The intravenous route is recommended for patients requiring single doses greater than 1 g or those with bacterial septicemia, localized parenchymal abscess (e.g., intra-abdominal abscess), peritonitis or other severe systemic or life-threatening infections. Because of the serious nature of infections due to *Pseudomonas aeruginosa*, dosage of 2 g every six or eight hours is recommended, at least upon initiation of therapy, in systemic infections caused by this organism.

The duration of therapy depends on the severity of infection. Generally, AZACTAM should be continued for at least 48 hours after the patient becomes asymptomatic or evidence of bacterial eradication has been obtained. Persistent infections may require treatment for several weeks. Doses smaller than those indicated should not be used.

Renal Impairment
Prolonged serum levels of aztreonam may occur in patients with transient or persistent renal insufficiency. Therefore, the dosage of AZACTAM should be halved in patients with estimated creatinine clearances between 10 and 30 mL/min/1.73 m² after an initial loading dose of 1 g or 2 g.

When only the serum creatinine concentration is available, the following formula (based on sex, weight, and age of the patient) may be used to approximate the creatinine clearance (Clcr). The serum creatinine should represent a steady state of renal function.

Males:　Clcr = $\dfrac{\text{weight (kg)} \times (140 - \text{age})}{72 \times \text{serum creatinine (mg/dL)}}$

Females:　0.85 × above value

In patients with severe renal failure (creatinine clearance less than 10 mL/min/1.73 m²), such as those supported by hemodialysis, the usual dose of 500 mg, 1 g or 2 g should be given initially. The maintenance dose should be one-fourth of the usual initial dose given at the usual fixed interval of 6, 8 or 12 hours. For serious or life-threatening infections, in addition to the maintenance doses, one-eighth of the initial dose should be given after each hemodialysis session.

Dosage In The Elderly
Renal status is a major determinant of dosage in the elderly; these patients in particular may have diminished renal func-

tion. Serum creatinine may not be an accurate determinant of renal status. Therefore, as with all antibiotics eliminated by the kidneys, estimates of creatinine clearance should be obtained, and appropriate dosage modifications made if necessary.

Preparation Of Parenteral Solutions
General
Upon the addition of the diluent to the container, contents should be shaken **immediately** and **vigorously**. Constituted solutions are not for multiple-dose use; should the entire volume in the container not be used for a single-dose, the unused solution must be discarded.

Depending upon the concentration of aztreonam and diluent used, constituted AZACTAM (aztreonam) For Injection yields a colorless to light straw yellow solution which may develop a slight pink tint on standing (potency is not affected). Parenteral drug products should be inspected visually for particulate matter and discoloration whenever solution and container permit.

Admixtures With Other Antibiotics
Intravenous infusion solutions of AZACTAM (Aztreonam For Injection) not exceeding 2% w/v prepared with Sodium Chloride Injection USP 0.9% or Dextrose Injection USP 5%, to which clindamycin phosphate, gentamicin sulfate, tobramycin sulfate, or cefazolin sodium have been added at concentrations usually used clinically, are stable for up to 48 hours at room temperature or seven days under refrigeration. Ampicillin sodium admixtures with aztreonam in Sodium Chloride Injection USP 0.9% are stable for 24 hours at room temperature and 48 hours under refrigeration; stability in Dextrose Injection USP 5% is two hours at room temperature and eight hours under refrigeration.

Aztreonam-cloxacillin sodium and aztreonam-vancomycin hydrochloride admixtures are stable in Dianeal® 137 (Peritoneal Dialysis Solution) with 4.25% Dextrose for up to 24 hours at room temperature.

Aztreonam is incompatible with nafcillin sodium, cephradine, and metronidazole.

Other admixtures are not recommended since compatibility data are not available.

Intravenous (IV) Solutions
For Bolus Injection: The contents of an AZACTAM (aztreonam) For Injection 15 mL or 30mL capacity vial should be constituted with 6 to 10 mL Sterile Water for Injection USP.
For Infusion: Contents of the 100 mL capacity bottle should be constituted to a final concentration not exceeding 2 percent w/v (at least 50 mL of any appropriate infusion solution listed below per gram aztreonam). These solutions may be frozen immediately after constitution in the original container (see Stability below).

If the contents of a 15 mL or 30 mL capacity vial are to be transferred to an appropriate infusion solution, each gram of aztreonam should be initially constituted with at least 3 mL Sterile Water for Injection USP. Further dilution may be obtained with one of the following intravenous infusion solutions:

Sodium Chloride Injection USP, 0.9%
Ringer's Injection USP
Lactated Ringer's Injection USP
Dextrose Injection USP, 5% or 10%
Dextrose and Sodium Chloride Injection USP, 5%:0.9%, 5%:0.45% or 5%:0.2%
Sodium Lactate Injection USP (M/6 Sodium Lactate)
Ionosol® B and 5% Dextrose
Isolyte® E
Isolyte® E with 5% Dextrose
Isolyte® M with 5% Dextrose
Normosol®-R
Normosol®-R and 5% Dextrose
Normosol®-M and 5% Dextrose
Mannitol Injection USP, 5% or 10%
Lactated Ringer's and 5% Dextrose Injection
Plasma-Lyte® M and 5% Dextrose
10% Travert® Injection
10% Travert® and Electrolyte No. 1 Injection
10% Travert® and Electrolyte No. 2 Injection
10% Travert® and Electrolyte No. 3 Injection

Intramuscular (IM) Solutions
The contents of an AZACTAM (aztreonam) For Injection 15 mL or 30 mL capacity vial should be consituted with at least 3 mL of an appropriate diluent per gram aztreonam. The following diluents may be used:

Sterile Water for Injection USP
Bacteriostatic Water for Injection USP (with benzyl alcohol or with methyl- and propylparabens)
Sodium Chloride Injection USP, 0.9%
Bacteriostatic Sodium Chloride Injection USP (with benzyl alcohol)

Stability Of IV And IM Solutions
AZACTAM (aztreonam) solutions for IV infusion at concentrations not exceeding 2% w/v must be used within 48 hours following constitution if kept at controlled room tempera-

Continued on next page

Squibb—Cont.

ture (59°–86°F/15°–30°C) or within seven days if refrigerated (36°–46°F/2°–8°C).

Frozen aztreonam infusion solutions may be stored for up to three months at −4°F/−20°C; frozen solutions may be thawed at controlled room temperature or by overnight refrigeration. Solutions that have been thawed and maintained at controlled room temperature or under refrigeration should be used within 24 or 72 hours after removal from the freezer, respectively. Solutions should not be refrozen. AZACTAM solutions at concentrations exceeding 2% w/v, except those prepared with Sterile Water for Injection USP or Sodium Chloride Injection USP, should be used promptly after preparation; the two excepted solutions must be used within 48 hours if stored at controlled room temperature or within seven days if refrigerated.

Intravenous Administration

Bolus Injection: A bolus injection may be used to initiate therapy. The dose should be slowly injected directly into a vein, or the tubing of a suitable administration set, over a period of three to five minutes (see next paragraph regarding flushing of tubing).

Infusion: With any intermittent infusion of aztreonam and another drug with which it is not pharmaceutically compatible, the common delivery tube should be flushed before and after delivery of aztreonam with any appropriate infusion solution compatible with both drug solutions; the drugs should not be delivered simultaneously. Any AZACTAM infusion should be completed within a 20 to 60 minute period. With use of a *Y-type administration set*, careful attention should be given to the calculated volume of aztreonam solution required so that the entire dose will be infused. A *volume control administration set* may be used to deliver an initial dilution of AZACTAM (aztreonam) For Injection (see Preparation Of Parenteral Solutions, For Infusion) into a compatible infusion solution during administration; in this case, the final dilution of aztreonam should provide a concentration not exceeding 2% w/v.

Intramuscular Administration

The dose should be given by deep injection into a large muscle mass (such as the upper outer quadrant of the gluteus maximus or lateral part of the thigh). Aztreonam is well tolerated and should not be admixed with any local anesthetic agent.

HOW SUPPLIED

AZACTAM For Injection (Aztreonam For Injection)—Lyophilized

Single-dose 15 mL capacity vials:

500 mg/vial: Packages of 10 (NDC 0003-2550-10) and 25 (NDC 0003-2550-15)

1 g/vial: Packages of 10 (NDC 0003-2560-10) and 25 (NDC 0003-2560-15)

Single-dose 30 mL capacity vials:

2 g/vial: Packages of 10 (NDC 0003-2570-10) and 25 (NDC 0003-2570-15)

Single-dose 100 mL capacity intravenous infusion bottles with bail bands:

500 mg/bottle: Packages of 10 (NDC 0003-2550-20)

1 g/bottle: Packages of 10 (NDC 0003-2560-20)

2 g/bottle: Packages of 10 (NDC 0003-2570-20)

Storage

Store original packages at room temperature; avoid excessive heat.

(J4-231G/J4-246E)

CAPOTEN® TABLETS ℞

[*kap'o-ten"*]

Captopril Tablets

USE IN PREGNANCY

When used in pregnancy during the second and third trimesters, ACE inhibitors can cause injury and even death to the developing fetus. When pregnancy is detected, CAPOTEN should be discontinued as soon as possible. **See WARNINGS: Fetal/Neonatal Morbidity and Mortality.**

DESCRIPTION

CAPOTEN (captopril) is the first of a new class of antihypertensive agents, a specific competitive inhibitor of angiotensin I-converting enzyme (ACE), the enzyme responsible for the conversion of angiotensin I to angiotensin II. Captopril is also effective in the management of heart failure.

CAPOTEN (captopril) is designated chemically as 1-[(2S)-3-mercapto-2-methylpropionyl]-L-proline [MW 217.29]. Captopril is a white to off-white crystalline powder that may have a slight sulfurous odor; it is soluble in water (approx. 160 mg/mL), methanol, and ethanol and sparingly soluble in chloroform and ethyl acetate.

CAPOTEN (captopril) is available in potencies of 12.5 mg, 25 mg, 50 mg, and 100 mg as scored tablets for oral administration. Inactive ingredients: microcrystalline cellulose, corn starch, lactose, and stearic acid.

CLINICAL PHARMACOLOGY

Mechanism of Action

The mechanism of action of CAPOTEN (captopril) has not yet been fully elucidated. Its beneficial effects in hypertension and heart failure appear to result primarily from suppression of the renin-angiotensin-aldosterone system. However, there is no consistent correlation between renin levels and response to the drug. Renin, an enzyme synthesized by the kidneys, is released into the circulation where it acts on a plasma globulin substrate to produce angiotensin I, a relatively inactive decapeptide. Angiotensin I is then converted by angiotensin converting enzyme (ACE) to angiotensin II, a potent endogenous vasoconstrictor substance. Angiotensin II also stimulates aldosterone secretion from the adrenal cortex, thereby contributing to sodium and fluid retention.

CAPOTEN (captopril) prevents the conversion of angiotensin I to angiotensin II by inhibition of ACE, a peptidyldipeptide carboxy hydrolase. This inhibition has been demonstrated in both healthy human subjects and in animals by showing that the elevation of blood pressure caused by exogenously administered angiotensin I was attenuated or abolished by captopril. In animal studies, captopril did not alter the pressor responses to a number of other agents, including angiotensin II and norepinephrine, indicating specificity of action.

ACE is identical to "bradykininase", and CAPOTEN (captopril) may also interfere with the degradation of the vasodepressor peptide, bradykinin. Increased concentrations of bradykinin or prostaglandin E_2 may also have a role in the therapeutic effect of CAPOTEN.

Inhibition of ACE results in decreased plasma angiotensin II and increased plasma renin activity (PRA), the latter resulting from loss of negative feedback on renin release caused by reduction in angiotensin II. The reduction of angiotensin II leads to decreased aldosterone secretion, and, as a result, small increases in serum potassium may occur along with sodium and fluid loss.

The antihypertensive effects persist for a longer period of time than does demonstrable inhibition of circulating ACE. It is not known whether the ACE present in vascular endothelium is inhibited longer than the ACE in circulating blood.

Pharmacokinetics

After oral administration of therapeutic doses of CAPOTEN (captopril), rapid absorption occurs with peak blood levels at about one hour. The presence of food in the gastrointestinal tract reduces absorption by about 30 to 40 percent; captopril therefore should be given one hour before meals. Based on carbon-14 labeling, average minimal absorption is approximately 75 percent. In a 24-hour period, over 95 percent of the absorbed dose is eliminated in the urine; 40 to 50 percent is unchanged drug; most of the remainder is the disulfide dimer of captopril and captopril-cysteine disulfide.

Approximately 25 to 30 percent of the circulating drug is bound to plasma proteins. The apparent elimination half-life for total radioactivity in blood is probably less than 3 hours. An accurate determination of half-life of unchanged captopril is not, at present, possible, but it is probably less than 2 hours. In patients with renal impairment, however, retention of captopril occurs (see DOSAGE AND ADMINISTRATION).

Pharmacodynamics

Administration of CAPOTEN (captopril) results in a reduction of peripheral arterial resistance in hypertensive patients with either no change, or an increase, in cardiac output. There is an increase in renal blood flow following administration of CAPOTEN (captopril) and glomerular filtration rate is usually unchanged.

Reductions of blood pressure are usually maximal 60 to 90 minutes after oral administration of an individual dose of CAPOTEN (captopril). The duration of effect is dose related. The reduction in blood pressure may be progressive, so to achieve maximal therapeutic effects, several weeks of therapy may be required. The blood pressure lowering effects of captopril and thiazide-type diuretics are additive. In contrast, captopril and beta-blockers have a less than additive effect.

Blood pressure is lowered to about the same extent in both standing and supine positions. Orthostatic effects and tachycardia are infrequent but may occur in volume-depleted patients. Abrupt withdrawal of CAPOTEN has not been associated with a rapid increase in blood pressure.

In patients with heart failure, significantly decreased peripheral (systemic vascular) resistance and blood pressure (afterload), reduced pulmonary capillary wedge pressure (preload) and pulmonary vascular resistance, increased cardiac output, and increased exercise tolerance time (ETT) have been demonstrated. These hemodynamic and clinical effects occur after the first dose and appear to persist for the duration of therapy. Placebo controlled studies of 12 weeks duration in patients who did not respond adequately to di-

uretics and digitalis show no tolerance to beneficial effects on ETT; open studies, with exposure up to 18 months in some cases, also indicate that ETT benefit is maintained. Clinical improvement has been observed in some patients where acute hemodynamic effects were minimal.

Studies in rats and cats indicate that CAPOTEN (captopril) does not cross the blood-brain barrier to any significant extent.

INDICATIONS AND USAGE

Hypertension: CAPOTEN (captopril) is indicated for the treatment of hypertension.

In using CAPOTEN, consideration should be given to the risk of neutropenia/agranulocytosis (see WARNINGS).

CAPOTEN may be used as initial therapy for patients with normal renal function, in whom the risk is relatively low. In patients with impaired renal function, particularly those with collagen vascular disease, captopril should be reserved for hypertensives who have either developed unacceptable side effects on other drugs, or have failed to respond satisfactorily to drug combinations.

CAPOTEN is effective alone and in combination with other antihypertensive agents, especially thiazide-type diuretics. The blood pressure lowering effects of captopril and thiazides are approximately additive.

Heart Failure: CAPOTEN is indicated in the treatment of congestive heart failure in patients who have not responded adequately to treatment with diuretics and digitalis. Although the beneficial effect of captopril in heart failure does not require the presence of digitalis, most controlled clinical trial experience with captopril has been in patients receiving digitalis, as well as diuretic treatment. Consequently, CAPOTEN should generally be added to both of these agents except when digitalis use is poorly tolerated or otherwise not feasible.

CONTRAINDICATIONS

CAPOTEN is contraindicated in patients who are hypersensitive to this product or any other angiotensin-converting enzyme inhibitor (e.g., a patient who has experienced angioedema during therapy with any other ACE inhibitor).

WARNINGS

Angioedema

Angioedema involving the extremities, face, lips, mucous membranes, tongue, glottis or larynx has been seen in patients treated with ACE inhibitors, including captopril. If angioedema involves the tongue, glottis or larynx, airway obstruction may occur and be fatal. Emergency therapy, including but not necessarily limited to, subcutaneous administration of a 1:1000 solution of epinephrine should be promptly instituted.

Swelling confined to the face, mucous membranes of the mouth, lips and extremities has usually resolved with discontinuation of captopril; some cases required medical therapy. (See PRECAUTIONS: Information for Patients and ADVERSE REACTIONS.)

Neutropenia/Agranulocytosis

Neutropenia ($< 1000/mm^3$) with myeloid hypoplasia has resulted from use of captopril. About half of the neutropenic patients developed systemic or oral cavity infections or other features of the syndrome of agranulocytosis.

The risk of neutropenia is dependent on the clinical status of the patient:

In clinical trials in patients with hypertension who have normal renal function (serum creatinine less than 1.6 mg/dL and no collagen vascular disease), neutropenia has been seen in one patient out of over 8,600 exposed.

In patients with some degree of renal failure (serum creatinine at least 1.6 mg/dL) but no collagen vascular disease, the risk of neutropenia in clinical trials was about 1 per 500, a frequency over 15 times that for uncomplicated hypertension. Daily doses of captopril were relatively high in these patients, particularly in view of their diminished renal function. In foreign marketing experience in patients with renal failure, use of allopurinol concomitantly with captopril has been associated with neutropenia but this association has not appeared in U.S. reports.

In patients with collagen vascular diseases (e.g., systemic lupus erythematosus, scleroderma) and impaired renal function, neutropenia occurred in 3.7 percent of patients in clinical trials.

While none of the over 750 patients in formal clinical trials of heart failure developed neutropenia, it has occurred during the subsequent clinical experience. About half of the reported cases had serum creatinine ≥ 1.6 mg/dL and more than 75 percent were in patients also receiving procainamide. In heart failure, it appears that the same risk factors for neutropenia are present.

The neutropenia has usually been detected within three months after captopril was started. Bone marrow examinations in patients with neutropenia consistently showed myeloid hypoplasia, frequently accompanied by erythroid hypoplasia and decreased numbers of megakaryocytes (e.g., hypo-

plastic bone marrow and pancytopenia); anemia and thrombocytopenia were sometimes seen.

In general, neutrophils returned to normal in about two weeks after captopril was discontinued, and serious infections were limited to clinically complex patients. About 13 percent of the cases of neutropenia have ended fatally, but almost all fatalities were in patients with serious illness, having collagen vascular disease, renal failure, heart failure or immunosuppressant therapy, or a combination of these complicating factors.

Evaluation of the hypertensive or heart failure patient should always include assessment of renal function.

If captopril is used in patients with impaired renal function, white blood cell and differential counts should be evaluated prior to starting treatment and at approximately two-week intervals for about three months, then periodically.

In patients with collagen vascular disease or who are exposed to other drugs known to affect the white cells or immune response, particularly when there is impaired renal function, captopril should be used only after an assessment of benefit and risk, and then with caution.

All patients treated with captopril should be told to report any signs of infection (e.g., sore throat, fever). If infection is suspected, white cell counts should be performed without delay.

Since discontinuation of captopril and other drugs has generally led to prompt return of the white count to normal, upon confirmation of neutropenia (neutrophil count < 1000/mm³) the physician should withdraw captopril and closely follow the patient's course.

Proteinuria

Total urinary proteins greater than 1 g per day were seen in about 0.7 percent of patients receiving captopril. About 90 percent of affected patients had evidence of prior renal disease or received relatively high doses of captopril (in excess of 150 mg/day), or both. The nephrotic syndrome occurred in about one-fifth of proteinuric patients. In most cases, proteinuria subsided or cleared within six months whether or not captopril was continued. Parameters of renal function, such as BUN and creatinine, were seldom altered in the patients with proteinuria.

Since most cases of proteinuria occurred by the eighth month of therapy with captopril, patients with prior renal disease or those receiving captopril at doses greater than 150 mg per day, should have urinary protein estimations (dipstick on first morning urine) prior to treatment, and periodically thereafter.

Hypotension

Excessive hypotension was rarely seen in hypertensive patients but is a possible consequence of captopril use in salt/volume depleted persons (such as those treated vigorously with diuretics), patients with heart failure or those patients undergoing renal dialysis. (See PRECAUTIONS: Drug Interactions.)

In heart failure, where the blood pressure was either normal or low, transient decreases in mean blood pressure greater than 20 percent were recorded in about half of the patients. This transient hypotension is more likely to occur after any of the first several doses and is usually well tolerated, producing either no symptoms or brief mild lightheadedness, although in rare instances it has been associated with arrhythmia or conduction defects. Hypotension was the reason for discontinuation of drug in 3.6 percent of patients with heart failure.

BECAUSE OF THE POTENTIAL FALL IN BLOOD PRESSURE IN THESE PATIENTS, THERAPY SHOULD BE STARTED UNDER VERY CLOSE MEDICAL SUPERVISION. A starting dose of 6.25 or 12.5 mg tid may minimize the hypotensive effect. Patients should be followed closely for the first two weeks of treatment and whenever the dose of captopril and/or diuretic is increased.

Hypotension is not *per se* a reason to discontinue captopril. Some decrease of systemic blood pressure is a common and desirable observation upon initiation of CAPOTEN (captopril) treatment in heart failure. The magnitude of the decrease is greatest early in the course of treatment; this effect stabilizes within a week or two, and generally returns to pretreatment levels, without a decrease in therapeutic efficacy, within two months.

Fetal/Neonatal Morbidity and Mortality

ACE inhibitors can cause fetal and neonatal morbidity and death when administered to pregnant women. Several dozen cases have been reported in the world literature. When pregnancy is detected, ACE inhibitors should be discontinued as soon as possible.

The use of ACE inhibitors during the second and third trimesters of pregnancy has been associated with fetal and neonatal injury, including hypotension, neonatal skull hypoplasia, anuria, reversible or irreversible renal failure, and death. Oligohydramnios has also been reported, presumably resulting from decreased fetal renal function; oligohydramnios in this setting has been associated with fetal limb contractures, craniofacial deformation, and hypoplastic lung development. Prematurity, intrauterine growth retardation, and patent ductus arteriosus have also been reported, al-

though it is not clear whether these occurrences were due to the ACE-inhibitor exposure.

These adverse effects do not appear to have resulted from intrauterine ACE-inhibitor exposure that has been limited to the first trimester. Mothers whose embryos and fetuses are exposed to ACE inhibitors only during the first trimester should be so informed. Nonetheless, when patients become pregnant, physicians should make every effort to discontinue the use of captopril as soon as possible.

Rarely (probably less often than once in every thousand pregnancies), no alternative to ACE inhibitors will be found. In these rare cases, the mothers should be apprised of the potential hazards to their fetuses, and serial ultrasound examinations should be performed to assess the intraamniotic environment.

If oligohydramnios is observed, captopril should be discontinued unless it is considered life-saving for the mother. Contraction stress testing (CST), a non-stress test (NST), or biophysical profiling (BPP) may be appropriate, depending upon the week of pregnancy. Patients and physicians should be aware, however, that oligohydramnios may not appear until after the fetus has sustained irreversible injury.

Infants with histories of *in utero* exposure to ACE inhibitors should be closely observed for hypotension, oliguria, and hyperkalemia. If oliguria occurs, attention should be directed toward support of blood pressure and renal perfusion. Exchange transfusion or dialysis may be required as a means of reversing hypotension and/or substituting for disordered renal function. While captopril may be removed from the adult circulation by hemodialysis, there is inadequate data concerning the effectiveness of hemodialysis for removing it from the circulation of neonates or children. Peritoneal dialysis is not effective for removing captopril; there is no information concerning exchange transfusion for removing captopril from the general circulation.

When captopril was given to rabbits at doses about 0.8 to 70 times (on a mg/kg basis) the maximum recommended human dose, low incidences of craniofacial malformations were seen. No teratogenic effects of captopril were seen in studies of pregnant rats and hamsters. On a mg/kg basis, the doses used were up to 150 times (in hamsters) and 625 times (in rats) the maximum recommended human dose.

PRECAUTIONS

General

Impaired Renal Function

Hypertension—Some patients with renal disease, particularly those with severe renal artery stenosis, have developed increases in BUN and serum creatinine after reduction of blood pressure with captopril. Captopril dosage reduction and/or discontinuation of diuretic may be required. For some of these patients, it may not be possible to normalize blood pressure and maintain adequate renal perfusion.

Heart Failure—About 20 percent of patients develop stable elevations of BUN and serum creatinine greater than 20 percent above normal or baseline upon long-term treatment with captopril. Less than 5 percent of patients, generally those with severe preexisting renal disease, required discontinuaton of treatment due to progressively increasing creatinine; subsequent improvement probably depends upon the severity of the underlying renal disease.

See CLINICAL PHARMACOLOGY, DOSAGE AND ADMINISTRATION, ADVERSE REACTIONS: Altered Laboratory Findings.

Hyperkalemia: Elevations in serum potassium have been observed in some patients treated with ACE inhibitors, including captopril. When treated with ACE inhibitors, patients at risk for the development of hyperkalemia include those with: renal insufficiency; diabetes mellitus; and those using concomitant potassium-sparing diuretics, potassium supplements or potassium-containing salt substitutes; or other drugs associated with increases in serum potassium. (See PRECAUTIONS: Information for Patients and Drug Interactions; ADVERSE REACTIONS: Altered Laboratory Findings.)

Cough: Cough has been reported with the use of ACE inhibitors. Characteristically, the cough is nonproductive, persistent and resolves after discontinuation of therapy. ACE inhibitor-induced cough should be considered as part of the differential diagnosis of cough.

Valvular Stenosis: There is concern, on theoretical grounds, that patients with aortic stenosis might be at particular risk of decreased coronary perfusion when treated with vasodilators because they do not develop as much afterload reduction as others.

Surgery/Anesthesia: In patients undergoing major surgery or during anesthesia with agents that produce hypotension, captopril will block angiotensin II formation secondary to compensatory renin release. If hypotension occurs and is considered to be due to this mechanism, it can be corrected by volume expansion.

Information for Patients

Patients should be advised to immediately report to their physician any signs or symptoms suggesting angioedema (e.g., swelling of face, eyes, lips, tongue, larynx and extremi-

ties; difficulty in swallowing or breathing; hoarseness) and to discontinue therapy. (See WARNINGS.)

Patients should be told to report promptly any indication of infection (e.g., sore throat, fever), which may be a sign of neutropenia, or of progressive edema which might be related to proteinuria and nephrotic syndrome.

All patients should be cautioned that excessive perspiration and dehydration may lead to an excessive fall in blood pressure because of reduction in fluid volume. Other causes of volume depletion such as vomiting or diarrhea may also lead to a fall in blood pressure; patients should be advised to consult with the physician.

Patients should be advised not to use potassium-sparing diuretics, potassium supplements or potassium-containing salt substitutes without consulting their physician. (See PRECAUTIONS: General and Drug Interactions; ADVERSE REACTIONS.)

Patients should be warned against interruption or discontinuation of medication unless instructed by the physician.

Heart failure patients on captopril therapy should be cautioned against rapid increases in physical activity.

Patients should be informed that CAPOTEN (captopril) should be taken one hour before meals (see DOSAGE AND ADMINISTRATION).

Pregnancy. Female patients of childbearing age should be told about the consequences of second- and third-trimester exposure to ACE inhibitors, and they should also be told that these consequences do not appear to have resulted from intrauterine ACE-inhibitor exposure that has been limited to the first trimester. These patients should be asked to report pregnancies to their physicians as soon as possible.

Drug Interactions

Hypotension—Patients on Diuretic Therapy: Patients on diuretics and especially those in whom diuretic therapy was recently instituted, as well as those on severe dietary salt restriction or dialysis, may occasionally experience a precipitous reduction of blood pressure usually within the first hour after receiving the initial dose of captopril.

The possibility of hypotensive effects with captopril can be minimized by either discontinuing the diuretic or increasing the salt intake approximately one week prior to initiation of treatment with CAPOTEN (captopril) or initiating therapy with small doses (6.25 or 12.5 mg). Alternatively, provide medical supervision for at least one hour after the initial dose. If hypotension occurs, the patient should be placed in a supine position and, if necessary, receive an intravenous infusion of normal saline. This transient hypotensive response is not a contraindication to further doses which can be given without difficulty once the blood pressure has increased after volume expansion.

Agents Having Vasodilator Activity: Data on the effect of concomitant use of other vasodilators in patients receiving CAPOTEN for heart failure are not available; therefore, nitroglycerin or other nitrates (as used for management of angina) or other drugs having vasodilator activity should, if possible, be discontinued before starting CAPOTEN. If resumed during CAPOTEN therapy, such agents should be administered cautiously, and perhaps at lower dosage.

Agents Causing Renin Release: Captopril's effect will be augmented by antihypertensive agents that cause renin release. For example, diuretics (e.g., thiazides) may activate the renin-angiotensin-aldosterone system.

Agents Affecting Sympathetic Activity: The sympathetic nervous system may be especially important in supporting blood pressure in patients receiving captopril alone or with diuretics. Therefore, agents affecting sympathetic activity (e.g., ganglionic blocking agents or adrenergic neuron blocking agents) should be used with caution. Beta-adrenergic blocking drugs add some further antihypertensive effect to captopril, but the overall response is less than additive.

Agents Increasing Serum Potassium: Since captopril decreases aldosterone production, elevation of serum potassium may occur. Potassium-sparing diuretics such as spironolactone, triamterene, or amiloride, or potassium supplements should be given only for documented hypokalemia, and then with caution, since they may lead to a significant increase of serum potassium. Salt substitutes containing potassium should also be used with caution.

Inhibitors Of Endogenous Prostaglandin Synthesis: It has been reported that indomethacin may reduce the antihypertensive effect of captopril, especially in cases of low renin hypertension. Other nonsteroidal anti-inflammatory agents (e.g., aspirin) may also have this effect.

Lithium: Increased serum lithium levels and symptoms of lithium toxicity have been reported in patients receiving concomitant lithium and ACE inhibitor therapy. These drugs should be coadministered with caution and frequent monitoring of serum lithium levels is recommended. If a diuretic is also used, it may increase the risk of lithium toxicity.

Continued on next page

Squibb—Cont.

Drug/Laboratory Test Interaction
Captopril may cause a false-positive urine test for acetone.
Carcinogenesis, Mutagenesis and Impairment of Fertility
Two-year studies with doses of 50 to 1350 mg/kg/day in mice and rats failed to show any evidence of carcinogenic potential.
Studies in rats have revealed no impairment of fertility.
Animal Toxicology
Chronic oral toxicity studies were conducted in rats (2 years), dogs (47 weeks; 1 year), mice (2 years), and monkeys (1 year). Significant drug related toxicity included effects on hematopoiesis, renal toxicity, erosion/ulceration of the stomach, and variation of retinal blood vessels.
Reductions in hemoglobin and/or hematocrit values were seen in mice, rats, and monkeys at doses 50 to 150 times the maximum recommended human dose (MRHD). Anemia, leukopenia, thrombocytopenia, and bone marrow suppression occurred in dogs at doses 8 to 30 times MRHD. The reductions in hemoglobin and hematocrit values in rats and mice were only significant at 1 year and returned to normal with continued dosing by the end of the study. Marked anemia was seen at all dose levels (8 to 30 times MRHD) in dogs, whereas moderate to marked leukopenia was noted only at 15 and 30 times MRHD and thrombocytopenia at 30 times MRHD. The anemia could be reversed upon discontinuation of dosing. Bone marrow suppression occurred to a varying degree, being associated only with dogs that died or were sacrificed in a moribund condition in the 1 year study. However, in the 47-week study at a dose 30 times MRHD, bone marrow suppression was found to be reversible upon continued drug administration.
Captopril caused hyperplasia of the juxtaglomerular apparatus of the kidneys at doses 7 to 200 times the MRHD in rats and mice, at 20 to 60 times MRHD in monkeys, and at 30 times the MRHD in dogs.
Gastric erosions/ulcerations were increased in incidence at 20 and 200 times MRHD in male rats and at 30 and 65 times MRHD in dogs and monkeys, respectively. Rabbits developed gastric and intestinal ulcers when given oral doses approximately 30 times MRHD for only 5 to 7 days.
In the two-year rat study, irreversible and progressive variations in the caliber of retinal vessels (focal sacculations and constrictions) occurred at all dose levels (7 to 200 times MRHD) in a dose-related fashion. The effect was first observed in the 88th week of dosing, with a progressively increased incidence thereafter, even after cessation of dosing.
Pregnancy Categories C (first trimester) and D (second and third trimesters)
See WARNINGS: Fetal/Neonatal Morbidity and Mortality.
Nursing Mothers
Concentrations of captopril in human milk are approximately one percent of those in maternal blood. Because of the potential for serious adverse reactions in nursing infants from captopril, a decision should be made whether to discontinue nursing or to discontinue the drug, taking into account the importance of CAPOTEN to the mother. (See PRECAUTIONS: Pediatric Use.)
Pediatric Use
Safety and effectiveness in children have not been established. There is limited experience reported in the literature with the use of captopril in the pediatric population; dosage, on a weight basis, was generally reported to be comparable to or less than that used in adults.
Infants, especially newborns, may be more susceptible to the adverse hemodynamic effects of captopril. Excessive, prolonged and unpredictable decreases in blood pressure and associated complications, including oliguria and seizures, have been reported.
CAPOTEN (captopril) should be used in children only if other measures for controlling blood pressure have not been effective.

ADVERSE REACTIONS
Reported incidences are based on clinical trials involving approximately 7000 patients.
Renal: About one of 100 patients developed proteinuria (see WARNINGS).
Each of the following has been reported in approximately 1 to 2 of 1000 patients and are of uncertain relationship to drug use: renal insufficiency, renal failure, nephrotic syndrome, polyuria, oliguria, and urinary frequency.
Hematologic: Neutropenia/agranulocytosis has occurred (see WARNINGS). Cases of anemia, thrombocytopenia, and pancytopenia have been reported.
Dermatologic: Rash, often with pruritus, and sometimes with fever, arthralgia, and eosinophilia, occurred in about 4 to 7 (depending on renal status and dose) of 100 patients, usually during the first four weeks of therapy. It is usually maculopapular, and rarely urticarial. The rash is usually mild and disappears within a few days of dosage reduction, short-term treatment with an antihistaminic agent, and/or discontinuing therapy; remission may occur even if captopril is continued. Pruritus, without rash, occurs in about 2 of 100 patients.

Between 7 and 10 percent of patients with skin rash have shown an eosinophilia and/or positive ANA titers. A reversible associated pemphigoid-like lesion, and photosensitivity, have also been reported.
Flushing or pallor has been reported in 2 to 5 of 1000 patients.
Cardiovascular: Hypotension may occur; see WARNINGS and PRECAUTIONS [Drug Interactions] for discussion of hypotension with captopril therapy.
Tachycardia, chest pain, and palpitations have each been observed in approximately 1 of 100 patients.
Angina pectoris, myocardial infarction, Raynaud's syndrome, and congestive heart failure have each occurred in 2 to 3 of 1000 patients.
Dysgeusia: Approximately 2 to 4 (depending on renal status and dose) of 100 patients developed a diminution or loss of taste perception. Taste impairment is reversible and usually self-limited (2 to 3 months) even with continued drug administration. Weight loss may be associated with the loss of taste.
Angioedema: Angioedema involving the extremities, face, lips, mucous membranes, tongue, glottis or larynx has been reported in approximately one in 1000 patients. Angioedema involving the upper airways has caused fatal airway obstruction. (See WARNINGS and PRECAUTIONS: Information for Patients.)
Cough: Cough has been reported in 0.5–2% of patients treated with captopril in clinical trials (see PRECAUTIONS: General, Cough).
The following have been reported in about 0.5 to 2 percent of patients but did not appear at increased frequency compared to placebo or other treatments used in controlled trials: gastric irritation, abdominal pain, nausea, vomiting, diarrhea, anorexia, constipation, aphthous ulcers, peptic ulcer, dizziness, headache, malaise, fatigue, insomnia, dry mouth, dyspnea, alopecia, paresthesias.
Other clinical adverse effects reported since the drug was marketed are listed below by body system. In this setting, an incidence or causal relationship cannot be accurately determined.
General: Asthenia, gynecomastia.
Cardiovascular: Cardiac arrest, cerebrovascular accident/insufficiency, rhythm disturbances, orthostatic hypotension, syncope.
Dermatologic: Bullous pemphigus, erythema multiforme (including Stevens-Johnson syndrome), exfoliative dermatitis.
Gastrointestinal: Pancreatitis, glossitis, dyspepsia.
Hematologic: Anemia, including aplastic and hemolytic.
Hepatobiliary: Jaundice, hepatitis, including rare cases of necrosis, cholestasis.
Metabolic: Symptomatic hyponatremia.
Musculoskeletal: Myalgia, myasthenia.
Nervous/Psychiatric: Ataxia, confusion, depression, nervousness, somnolence.
Respiratory: Bronchospasm, eosinophilic pneumonitis, rhinitis.
Special Senses: Blurred vision.
Urogenital: Impotence.
As with other ACE inhibitors, a syndrome has been reported which may include: fever, myalgia, arthralgia, interstitial nephritis, vasculitis, rash or other dermatologic manifestations, eosinophilia and an elevated ESR.

Fetal/Neonatal Morbidity and Mortality
See WARNINGS: Fetal/Neonatal Morbidity and Mortality.

Altered Laboratory Findings
Serum Electrolytes: Hyperkalemia: small increases in serum potassium, especially in patients with renal impairment (see PRECAUTIONS).
Hyponatremia: particularly in patients receiving a low sodium diet or concomitant diuretics.
BUN/Serum Creatinine: Transient elevations of BUN or serum creatinine especially in volume or salt depleted patients or those with renovascular hypertension may occur. Rapid reduction of longstanding or markedly elevated blood pressure can result in decreases in the glomerular filtration rate and, in turn, lead to increases in BUN or serum creatinine.
Hematologic: A positive ANA has been reported.
Liver Function Tests: Elevations of liver transaminases, alkaline phosphatase, and serum bilirubin have occurred.

OVERDOSAGE
Correction of hypotension would be of primary concern. Volume expansion with an intravenous infusion of normal saline is the treatment of choice for restoration of blood pressure.
While captopril may be removed from the adult circulation by hemodialysis, there is inadequate data concerning the effectiveness of hemodialysis for removing it from the circulation of neonates or children. Peritoneal dialysis is not effective for removing captopril; there is no information concerning exchange transfusion for removing captopril from the general circulation.

DOSAGE AND ADMINISTRATION
CAPOTEN (captopril) should be taken one hour before meals. Dosage must be individualized.
Hypertension—Initiation of therapy requires consideration of recent antihypertensive drug treatment, the extent of blood pressure elevation, salt restriction, and other clinical circumstances. If possible, discontinue the patient's previous antihypertensive drug regimen for one week before starting CAPOTEN.
The initial dose of CAPOTEN (captopril) is 25 mg bid or tid. If satisfactory reduction of blood pressure has not been achieved after one or two weeks, the dose may be increased to 50 mg bid or tid. Concomitant sodium restriction may be beneficial when CAPOTEN is used alone.
The dose of CAPOTEN in hypertension usually does not exceed 50 mg tid. Therefore, if the blood pressure has not been satisfactorily controlled after one to two weeks at this dose, (and the patient is not already receiving a diuretic), a modest dose of a thiazide-type diuretic (e.g., hydrochlorothiazide, 25 mg daily), should be added. The diuretic dose may be increased at one- to two-week intervals until its highest usual antihypertensive dose is reached.
If CAPOTEN is being started in a patient already receiving a diuretic, CAPOTEN therapy should be initiated under close medical supervision (see WARNINGS and PRECAUTIONS [Drug Interactions] regarding hypotension), with dosage and titration of CAPOTEN as noted above.
If further blood pressure reduction is required, the dose of CAPOTEN may be increased to 100 mg bid or tid and then, if necessary, to 150 mg bid or tid (while continuing the diuretic). The usual dose range is 25 to 150 mg bid or tid. A maximum daily dose of 450 mg CAPOTEN should not be exceeded.
For patients with severe hypertension (e.g., accelerated or malignant hypertension), when temporary discontinuation of current antihypertensive therapy is not practical or desirable, or when prompt titration to more normotensive blood pressure levels is indicated, diuretic should be continued but other current antihypertensive medication stopped and CAPOTEN dosage promptly initiated at 25 mg bid or tid, under close medical supervision.
When necessitated by the patient's clinical condition, the daily dose of CAPOTEN may be increased every 24 hours or less under continuous medical supervision until a satisfactory blood pressure response is obtained or the maximum dose of CAPOTEN is reached. In this regimen, addition of a more potent diuretic, e.g., furosemide, may also be indicated. Beta-blockers may also be used in conjunction with CAPOTEN therapy (see PRECAUTIONS: Drug Interactions), but the effects of the two drugs are less than additive.
Heart Failure—Initiation of therapy requires consideration of recent diuretic therapy and the possibility of severe salt/volume depletion. In patients with either normal or low blood pressure, who have been vigorously treated with diuretics and who may be hyponatremic and/or hypovolemic, a starting dose of 6.25 or 12.5 mg tid may minimize the magnitude or duration of the hypotensive effect (see WARNINGS: Hypotension); for these patients, titration to the usual daily dosage can then occur within the next several days.
For most patients the usual initial daily dosage is 25 mg tid. After a dose of 50 mg tid is reached, further increases in dosage should be delayed, where possible, for at least two weeks to determine if a satisfactory response occurs. Most patients studied have had a satisfactory clinical improvement at 50 or 100 mg tid. A maximum daily dose of 450 mg of CAPOTEN (captopril) should not be exceeded.
CAPOTEN should generally be used in conjunction with a diuretic and digitalis. CAPOTEN therapy must be initiated under very close medical supervision.
Dosage Adjustment in Renal Impairment—Because CAPOTEN (captopril) is excreted primarily by the kidneys, excretion rates are reduced in patients with impaired renal function. These patients will take longer to reach steady-state captopril levels and will reach higher steady-state levels for a given daily dose than patients with normal renal function. Therefore, these patients may respond to smaller or less frequent doses.
Accordingly, for patients with significant renal impairment, initial daily dosage of CAPOTEN (captopril) should be reduced, and smaller increments utilized for titration, which should be quite slow (one- to two-week intervals). After the desired therapeutic effect has been achieved, the dose should be slowly back-titrated to determine the minimal effective dose. When concomitant diuretic therapy is required, a loop diuretic (e.g., furosemide), rather than a thiazide diuretic, is preferred in patients with severe renal impairment.

HOW SUPPLIED
12.5 mg tablets in bottles of 100 (NDC 0003-0450-54) and 1000 (NDC 0003-0450-75), **25 mg tablets** in bottles of 100 (NDC 0003-0452-50) and 1000 (NDC 0003-0452-75), **50 mg tablets** in bottles of 100 (NDC 0003-0482-50) and 1000 (NDC 0003-0482-75), and **100 mg tablets** in bottles of 100 (NDC 0003-0485-50). Bottles contain a desiccant-charcoal canister.

Unimatic® unit-dose packs containing 100 tablets are also available for each potency: **12.5 mg** (NDC 0003-0450-51), **25 mg** (NDC 0003-0452-51), **50 mg** (NDC 0003-0482-51), and **100 mg** (NDC 0003-0485-51).

The **12.5 mg tablet** is a biconvex oval with a partial bisect bar; the **25 mg tablet** is a biconvex rounded square with a quadrisect bar; the **50 and 100 mg tablets** are biconvex ovals with a bisect bar.

All captopril tablets are white and may exhibit a slight sulfurous odor.

Storage

Do not store above 86°F. Keep bottles tightly closed (protect from moisture).

(J3-658Z)

Shown in Product Identification Section, page 432

CAPOZIDE® 25/15
CAPOZIDE® 25/25
CAPOZIDE® 50/15
CAPOZIDE® 50/25
[*kap'o-zīd"*]
Captopril-Hydrochlorothiazide Tablets

USE IN PREGNANCY

When used in pregnancy during the second and third trimesters, ACE Inhibitors can cause injury and even death to the developing fetus. When pregnancy is detected, CAPOZIDE should be discontinued as soon as possible. See **WARNINGS: Captopril, Fetal/Neonatal Morbidity and Mortality.**

DESCRIPTION

CAPOZIDE (Captopril-Hydrochlorothiazide Tablets) for oral administration combines two antihypertensive agents: CAPOTEN (captopril) and hydrochlorothiazide. Captopril, the first of a new class of antihypertensive agents, is a specific competitive inhibitor of angiotensin I-converting enzyme (ACE), the enzyme responsible for the conversion of angiotensin I to angiotensin II. Hydrochlorothiazide is a benzothiadiazide (thiazide) diuretic-antihypertensive.

CAPOZIDE tablets are available in four combinations of captopril with hydrochlorothiazide: 25 mg with 15 mg, 25 mg with 25 mg, 50 mg with 15 mg, and 50 mg with 25 mg. Inactive ingredients: microcrystalline cellulose, colorant (FD&C Yellow No. 6), lactose, magnesium stearate, pregelatinized starch, and stearic acid.

Captopril is designated chemically as 1-[(2S)-3-mercapto-2-methylpropionyl]-L-proline; hydrochlorothiazide is 6-Chloro-3,4-dihydro-2H-1, 2, 4-benzothiadiazine-7-sulfonamide 1,1-dioxide.

Captopril is a white to off-white crystalline powder that may have a slight sulfurous odor; it is soluble in water (approx. 160 mg/mL), methanol, and ethanol and sparingly soluble in chloroform and ethyl acetate.

Hydrochlorothiazide is a white crystalline powder slightly soluble in water but freely soluble in sodium hydroxide solution.

CLINICAL PHARMACOLOGY

Captopril

Mechanism of Action

The mechanism of action of captopril has not yet been fully elucidated. Its beneficial effects in hypertension and heart failure appear to result primarily from suppression of the renin-angiotensin-aldosterone system. However, there is no consistent correlation between renin levels and response to the drug. Renin, an enzyme synthesized by the kidneys, is released into the circulation where it acts on a plasma globulin substrate to produce angiotensin I, a relatively inactive decapeptide. Angiotensin I is then converted by angiotensin converting enzyme (ACE) to angiotensin II, a potent endogenous vasoconstrictor substance. Angiotensin II also stimulates aldosterone secretion from the adrenal cortex, thereby contributing to sodium and fluid retention.

Captopril prevents the conversion of angiotensin I to angiotensin II by inhibition of ACE, a peptidyldipeptide carboxy hydrolase. This inhibition has been demonstrated in both healthy human subjects and in animals by showing that the elevation of blood pressure caused by exogenously administered angiotensin I was attenuated or abolished by captopril. In animal studies, captopril did not alter the pressor responses to a number of other agents, including angiotensin II and norepinephrine, indicating specificity of action.

ACE is identical to "bradykininase", and captopril may also interfere with the degradation of the vasodepressor peptide, bradykinin. Increased concentrations of bradykinin or prostaglandin E$_2$ may also have a role in the therapeutic effect of captopril.

Inhibition of ACE results in decreased plasma angiotensin II and increased plasma renin activity (PRA), the latter resulting from loss of negative feedback on renin release caused by reduction in angiotensin II. The reduction of angiotensin II

leads to decreased aldosterone secretion, and, as a result, small increases in serum potassium may occur along with sodium and fluid loss.

The antihypertensive effects persist for a longer period of time than does demonstrable inhibition of circulating ACE. It is not known whether the ACE present in vascular endothelium is inhibited longer than the ACE in circulating blood.

Pharmacokinetics

After oral administration of therapeutic doses of captopril, rapid absorption occurs with peak blood levels at about one hour. The presence of food in the gastrointestinal tract reduces absorption by about 30 to 40 percent; captopril therefore should be given one hour before meals. Based on carbon-14 labeling, average minimal absorption is approximately 75 percent. In a 24-hour period, over 95 percent of the absorbed dose is eliminated in the urine; 40 to 50 percent is unchanged drug; most of the remainder is the disulfide dimer of captopril and captopril-cysteine disulfide.

Approximately 25 to 30 percent of the circulating drug is bound to plasma proteins. The apparent elimination half-life for total radioactivity in blood is probably less than three hours. An accurate determination of half-life of unchanged captopril is not, at present, possible, but it is probably less than two hours. In patients with renal impairment, however, retention of captopril occurs (see DOSAGE AND ADMINISTRATION).

Pharmacodynamics

Administration of captopril results in a reduction of peripheral arterial resistance in hypertensive patients with either no change, or an increase, in cardiac output. There is an increase in renal blood flow following administration of captopril and glomerular filtration rate is usually unchanged. In patients with heart failure, significantly decreased peripheral (systemic vascular) resistance and blood pressure (afterload), reduced pulmonary capillary wedge pressure (preload) and pulmonary vascular resistance, increased cardiac output, and increased exercise tolerance time (ETT) have been demonstrated.

Reductions of blood pressure are usually maximal 60 to 90 minutes after oral administration of an individual dose of captopril. The duration of effect is dose related and is extended in the presence of a thiazide-type diuretic. The full effect of a given dose may not be attained for 6–8 weeks (see DOSAGE AND ADMINISTRATION). The blood pressure lowering effects of captopril and thiazide-type diuretics are additive. In contrast, captopril and beta-blockers have a less than additive effect.

Blood pressure is lowered to about the same extent in both standing and supine positions. Orthostatic effects and tachycardia are infrequent but may occur in volume-depleted patients. Abrupt withdrawal of captopril has not been associated with a rapid increase in blood pressure.

Studies in rats and cats indicate that captopril does not cross the blood-brain barrier to any significant extent.

Hydrochlorothiazide

Thiazides affect the renal tubular mechanism of electrolyte reabsorption. At maximal therapeutic dosage all thiazides are approximately equal in their diuretic potency.

Thiazides increase excretion of sodium and chloride in approximately equivalent amounts. Natriuresis causes a secondary loss of potassium and bicarbonate.

The mechanism of the antihypertensive effect of thiazides is unknown. Thiazides do not affect normal blood pressure.

The mean plasma half-life of hydrochlorothiazide in fasted individuals has been reported to be approximately 2.5 hours. Onset of diuresis occurs in two hours and the peak effect at about four hours. Its action persists for approximately six to twelve hours. Hydrochlorothiazide is eliminated rapidly by the kidney.

INDICATIONS AND USAGE

CAPOZIDE (Captopril-Hydrochlorothiazide Tablets) is indicated for the treatment of hypertension. The blood pressure lowering effects of captopril and thiazides are approximately additive.

This fixed combination drug may be used as initial therapy or substituted for previously titrated doses of the individual components.

When captopril and hydrochlorothiazide are given together it may not be necessary to administer captopril in divided doses to attain blood pressure control at trough (before the next dose). Also, with such a combination, a daily dose of 15 mg of hydrochlorothiazide may be adequate.

Treatment may, therefore, be initiated with CAPOZIDE 25 mg/15 mg once daily. Subsequent titration should be with additional doses of the components (captopril, hydrochlorothiazide) as single agents or as CAPOZIDE 50 mg/15 mg, 25 mg/25 mg, or 50 mg/25 mg (see DOSAGE AND ADMINISTRATION).

In using CAPOZIDE, consideration should be given to the risk of neutropenia/agranulocytosis (see WARNINGS).

CAPOZIDE may be used for patients with normal renal function, in whom the risk is relatively low. In patients with impaired renal function, particularly those with collagen vascular disease, CAPOZIDE should be reserved for hyperten-

sives who have either developed unacceptable side effects on other drugs, or have failed to respond satisfactorily to other drug combinations.

CONTRAINDICATIONS

Captopril

This product is contraindicated in patients who are hypersensitive to captopril or any other angiotensin-converting enzyme inhibitor (e.g., a patient who has experienced angioedema during therapy with any other ACE inhibitor).

Hydrochlorothiazide

Hydrochlorothiazide is contraindicated in anuria. It is also contraindicated in patients who have previously demonstrated hypersensitivity to hydrochlorothiazide or other sulfonamide-derived drugs.

WARNINGS

Captopril

Angioedema

Angioedema involving the extremities, face, lips, mucous membranes, tongue, glottis or larynx has been seen in patients treated with ACE inhibitors, including captopril. If angioedema involves the tongue, glottis or larynx, airway obstruction may occur and be fatal. Emergency therapy, including but not necessarily limited to, subcutaneous administration of a 1:1000 solution of epinephrine should be promptly instituted.

Swelling confined to the face, mucous membranes of the mouth, lips and extremities has usually resolved with discontinuation of treatment; some cases required medical therapy. (See PRECAUTIONS: Information for Patients and ADVERSE REACTIONS: Captopril.)

Neutropenia/Agranulocytosis

Neutropenia ($<1000/mm^3$) with myeloid hypoplasia has resulted from use of captopril. About half of the neutropenic patients developed systemic or oral cavity infections or other features of the syndrome of agranulocytosis.

The risk of neutropenia is dependent on the clinical status of the patient:

In clinical trials in patients with hypertension who have normal renal function (serum creatinine less than 1.6 mg/dL and no collagen vascular disease), neutropenia has been seen in one patient out of over 8,600 exposed.

In patients with some degree of renal failure (serum creatinine at least 1.6 mg/dL) but no collagen vascular disease, the risk of neutropenia in clinical trials was about 1 per 500, a frequency over 15 times that for uncomplicated hypertension. Daily doses of captopril were relatively high in these patients, particularly in view of their diminished renal function. In foreign marketing experience in patients with renal failure, use of allopurinol concomitantly with captopril has been associated with neutropenia but this association has not appeared in U.S. reports.

In patients with collagen vascular diseases (e.g., systemic lupus erythematosus, scleroderma) and impaired renal function, neutropenia occurred in 3.7 percent of patients in clinical trials.

While none of the over 750 patients in formal clinical trials of heart failure developed neutropenia, it has occurred during the subsequent clinical experience. About half of the reported cases had serum creatinine ≥ 1.6 mg/dL and more than 75 percent were in patients also receiving procainamide. In heart failure, it appears that the same risk factors for neutropenia are present.

The neutropenia has usually been detected within three months after captopril was started. Bone marrow examinations in patients with neutropenia consistently showed myeloid hypoplasia, frequently accompanied by erythroid hypoplasia and decreased numbers of megakaryocytes (e.g., hypoplastic bone marrow and pancytopenia); anemia and thrombocytopenia were sometimes seen.

In general, neutrophils returned to normal in about two weeks after captopril was discontinued, and serious infections were limited to clinically complex patients. About 13 percent of the cases of neutropenia have ended fatally, but almost all fatalities were in patients with serious illness, having collagen vascular disease, renal failure, heart failure or immunosuppressant therapy, or a combination of these complicating factors.

Evaluation of the hypertensive or heart failure patient should always include assessment of renal function.

If captopril is used in patients with impaired renal function, white blood cell and differential counts should be evaluated prior to starting treatment and at approximately two-week intervals for about three months, then periodically.

In patients with collagen vascular disease or who are exposed to other drugs known to affect the white cells or immune response, particularly when there is impaired renal function, captopril should be used only after an assessment of benefit and risk, and then with caution.

All patients treated with captopril should be told to report any signs of infection (e.g., sore throat, fever). If infection is suspected, white cell counts should be performed without delay.

Continued on next page

Squibb—Cont.

Since discontinuation of captopril and other drugs has generally led to prompt return of the white count to normal, upon confirmation of neutropenia (neutrophil count $< 1000/mm^3$) the physician should withdraw captopril and closely follow the patient's course.

Proteinuria

Total urinary proteins greater than 1 g per day were seen in about 0.7 percent of patients receiving captopril. About 90 percent of affected patients had evidence of prior renal disease or received relatively high doses of captopril (in excess of 150 mg/day), or both. The nephrotic syndrome occurred in about one-fifth of proteinuric patients. In most cases, proteinuria subsided or cleared within six months whether or not captopril was continued. Parameters of renal function, such as BUN and creatinine, were seldom altered in the patients with proteinuria.

Since most cases of proteinuria occurred by the eighth month of therapy with captopril, patients with prior renal disease or those receiving captopril at doses greater than 150 mg per day, should have urinary protein estimations (dip-stick on first morning urine) prior to treatment, and periodically thereafter.

Hypotension

Excessive hypotension was rarely seen in hypertensive patients but is a possible consequence of captopril use in salt/volume depleted persons (such as those treated vigorously with diuretics), patients with heart failure or those patients undergoing renal dialysis. (See PRECAUTIONS: Drug Interactions.)

Fetal/Neonatal Morbidity and Mortality

ACE inhibitors can cause fetal and neonatal morbidity and death when administerd to pregnant women. Several dozen cases have been reported in the world literature. When pregnancy is detected, ACE inhibitors should be discontinued as soon as possible.

The use of ACE inhibitors during the second and third trimesters of pregnancy has been associated with fetal and neonatal injury, including hypotension, neonatal skull hypoplasia, anuria, reversible or irreversible renal failure, and death. Oligohydramnios has also been reported, presumably resulting from decreased fetal renal function; oligohydramnios in this setting has been associated with fetal limb contractures, craniofacial deformation, and hypoplastic lung development. Prematurity, intrauterine growth retardation, and patent ductus arteriosus have also been reported, although it is not clear whether these occurrences were due to the ACE-inhibitor exposure.

These adverse effects do not appear to have resulted from intrauterine ACE-inhibitor exposure that has been limited to the first trimester. Mothers whose embryos and fetuses are exposed to ACE-inhibitors only during the first trimester should be so informed. Nonetheless, when patients become pregnant, physicians should make every effort to discontinue the use of captoril as soon as possible.

Rarely (probably less often than once in every thousand pregnancies), no alternative to ACE inhibitors will be found. In these rare cases, the mothers should be apprised of the potential hazards to their fetuses, and serial unltrasound examinations should be performed to assess the intraamniotic environment.

If oligohydramnios is observed, captopril should be discontinued unless it is considered life-saving for the mother. Contraction stress testing (CST), a non-stress test (NST), or biophysical profiling (BPP) may be appropriate, depending upon the week of pregnancy. Patients and physicians should be aware, however, that oligohydramnios may not appear until after the fetus has sustained irreversible injury.

Infants with histories of *in utero* exposure to ACE inhibitors should be closely observed for hypotension, oliguria, and hyperkalemia. If oliguria occurs, attention should be directed toward support of blood pressure and renal perfusion. Exchange transfusion or dialysis may be required as a means of reversing hypotension and/or substituting for disordered renal function. While captopril may be removed from the adult circulation by hemodialysis, there is inadequate data concerning the effectiveness of hemodialysis for removing it from the circulation of neonates or children. Peritoneal dialysis is not effective for removing captopril; there is no information concerning exchange transfusion for removing captopril from the general circulation.

When captopril was given to rabbits at doses about 0.8 to 70 times (on a mg/kg basis) the maximum recommended human dose, low incidences of craniofacial malformations were seen. No teratogenic effects of captopril were seen in studies of pregnant rats and hamsters. On a mg/kg basis, the doses used were up to 150 times (in hamsters) and 625 times (in rats) the maximum recommended human dose.

Hydrochlorothiazide

Thiazides should be used with caution in severe renal disease. In patients with renal disease, thiazides may precipitate azotemia. Cumulative effects of the drug may develop in patients with impaired renal function.

Thiazides should be used with caution in patients with impaired hepatic function or progressive liver disease, since minor alterations of fluid and electrolyte balance may precipitate hepatic coma.

Sensitivity reactions may occur in patients with or without a history of allergy or bronchial asthma.

The possibility of exacerbation or activation of systemic lupus erythematosus has been reported.

In general, lithium should not be given with diuretics (see PRECAUTIONS: Drug Interactions, Hydrochlorothiazide).

PRECAUTIONS

General

Captopril

Impaired Renal Function—Some patients with renal disease, particularly those with severe renal artery stenosis, have developed increases in BUN and serum creatinine after reduction of blood pressure with captopril. Captopril dosage reduction and/or discontinuation of diuretic may be required. For some of these patients, it may not be possible to normalize blood pressure and maintain adequate renal perfusion (see CLINICAL PHARMACOLOGY, DOSAGE AND ADMINISTRATION, ADVERSE REACTIONS: Altered Laboratory Findings).

Hyperkalemia—Elevations in serum potassium have been observed in some patients treated with ACE inhibitors, including captopril. When treated with ACE inhibitors, patients at risk for the development of hyperkalemia include those with: renal insufficiency; diabetes mellitus; and those using concomitant potassium-sparing diuretics, potassium supplements or potassium-containing salt substitutes; or other drugs associated with increases in serum potassium. (See PRECAUTIONS: Information for Patients and Drug Interactions, Captopril; ADVERSE REACTIONS: Altered Laboratory Findings.)

Cough—Cough has been reported with the use of ACE inhibitors. Characteristically, the cough is nonproductive, persistent and resolves after discontinuation of therapy. ACE inhibitor-induced cough should be considered as part of the differential diagnosis of cough.

Surgery/Anesthesia—In patients undergoing major surgery or during anesthesia with agents that produce hypotension, captopril will block angiotensin II formation secondary to compensatory renin release. If hypotension occurs and is considered to be due to this mechanism, it can be corrected by volume expansion.

Hydrochlorothiazide

Periodic determination of serum electrolytes to detect possible electrolyte imbalance should be performed at appropriate intervals.

All patients receiving thiazide therapy should be observed for clinical signs of fluid or electrolyte imbalance, namely: hyponatremia, hypochloremic alkalosis, and hypokalemia. Serum and urine electrolyte determinations are particularly important when the patient is vomiting excessively or receiving parenteral fluids. Warning signs or symptoms of fluid and electrolyte imbalance may include: dryness of mouth, thirst, weakness, lethargy, drowsiness, restlessness, muscle pains or cramps, muscular fatigue, hypotension, oliguria, tachycardia, and gastrointestinal disturbances such as nausea and vomiting.

Hypokalemia may develop, especially with brisk diuresis, or when severe cirrhosis is present. Interference with adequate oral electrolyte intake will also contribute to hypokalemia. Hypokalemia can sensitize or exaggerate the response of the heart to the toxic effects of digitalis (e.g., increased ventricular irritability). Because captopril reduces the production of aldosterone, concomitant therapy with captopril reduces the diuretic-induced hypokalemia. Fewer patients may require potassium supplements and/or foods with a high potassium content (see Drug Interactions, Agents Increasing Serum Potassium).

Any chloride deficit is generally mild and usually does not require specific treatment except under extraordinary circumstances (as in liver disease or renal disease). Dilutional hyponatremia may occur in edematous patients in hot weather; appropriate therapy is water restriction, rather than administration of salt except in rare instances when the hyponatremia is life-threatening. In actual salt depletion, appropriate replacement is the therapy of choice.

Hyperuricemia may occur or frank gout may be precipitated in certain patients receiving thiazide therapy.

Latent diabetes mellitus may become manifest during thiazide administration.

The antihypertensive effect of thiazide diuretics may be enhanced in the postsympathectomy patient.

If progressive renal impairment becomes evident, as indicated by a rising nonprotein nitrogen or blood urea nitrogen (BUN), a careful reappraisal of therapy is necessary with consideration given to withholding or discontinuing diuretic therapy.

Thiazides may decrease serum PBI levels without signs of thyroid disturbance.

Calcium excretion is decreased by thiazides. Pathological changes in the parathyroid gland with hypercalcemia and hypophosphatemia have been observed in a few patients on prolonged thiazide therapy. The common complications of hyperparathyroidism such as renal lithiasis, bone resorption, and peptic ulceration have not been seen. Thiazides should be discontinued before carrying out tests for parathyroid function.

Thiazides have been shown to increase the urinary excretion of magnesium; this may result in hypomagnesemia.

Information for Patients

Patients should be advised to immediately report to their physician any signs or symptoms suggesting angioedema (e.g., swelling of face, eyes, lips, tongue, larynx and extremities; difficulty in swallowing or breathing; hoarseness) and to discontinue therapy. (See WARNINGS: Captopril.)

Patients should be told to report promptly any indication of infection (e.g., sore throat, fever), which may be a sign of neutropenia, or of progressive edema which might be related to proteinuria and nephrotic syndrome.

All patients should be cautioned that excessive perspiration and dehydration may lead to an excessive fall in blood pressure because of reduction in fluid volume. Other causes of volume depletion such as vomiting or diarrhea may also lead to a fall in blood pressure; patients should be advised to consult with the physician.

Patients should be advised not to use potassium-sparing diuretics, potassium supplements or potassium-containing salt substitutes without consulting their physician. (See PRECAUTIONS: General and Drug Interactions, Captopril; ADVERSE REACTIONS: Captopril.)

Patients should be warned against interruption or discontinuation of medication unless instructed by the physician.

Heart failure patients on captopril therapy should be cautioned against rapid increases in physical activity.

Patients should be informed that CAPOZIDE (Captopril-Hydrochlorothiazide Tablets) should be taken one hour before meals (see DOSAGE AND ADMINISTRATION).

Pregnancy. Female patients of childbearing age should be told about the consequences of second- and third-trimester exposure to ACE inhibitors, and they should also be told that these consequences do not appear to have resulted from intrauterine Ace-inhibitor exposure that has been limited to the first trimester. These patients should be asked to report pregnancies to their physicians as soon as possible.

Laboratory Tests

Serum electrolyte levels should be regularly monitored (see WARNINGS: Captopril and Hydrochlorothiazide; PRECAUTIONS: General, Hydrochlorothiazide).

Drug Interactions

Captopril

Hypotension—Patients on Diuretic Therapy: Patients on diuretics and especially those in whom diuretic therapy was recently instituted, as well as those on severe dietary salt restrictions or dialysis, may occasionally experience a precipitous reduction of blood pressure usually within the first hour after receiving the initial dose of captopril.

The possibility of hypotensive effects with captopril can be minimized by either discontinuing the diuretic or increasing the salt intake approximately one week prior to initiation of treatment with captopril or initiating therapy with small doses (6.25 or 12.5 mg). Alternatively, provide medical supervision for at least one hour after the initial dose. If hypotension occurs, the patient should be placed in a supine position and, if necessary, receive an intravenous infusion of normal saline. This transient hypotensive response is not a contraindication to further doses which can be given without difficulty once the blood pressure has increased after volume expansion.

Agents Having Vasodilator Activity: Data on the effect of concomitant use of other vasodilators in patients receiving captopril for heart failure are not available; therefore, nitroglycerin or other nitrates (as used for management of angina) or other drugs having vasodilator activity should, if possible, be discontinued before starting captopril. If resumed during captopril therapy, such agents should be administered cautiously, and perhaps at lower dosage.

Agents Causing Renin Release: Captopril's effect will be augmented by antihypertensive agents that cause renin release. For example, diuretics (e.g., thiazides) may activate the renin-angiotensin-aldosterone system.

Agents Affecting Sympathetic Activity: The sympathetic nervous system may be especially important in supporting blood pressure in patients receiving captopril alone or with diuretics. Therefore, agents affecting sympathetic activity (e.g., ganglionic blocking agents or adrenergic neuron blocking agents) should be used with caution. Beta-adrenergic blocking drugs add some further antihypertensive effect to captopril, but the overall response is less than additive.

Agents Increasing Serum Potassium: Since captopril decreases aldosterone production, elevation of serum potassium may occur. Potassium-sparing diuretics such as spironolactone, triamterene, or amiloride, or potassium supplements, should be given only for documented hypokalemia, and then with caution, since they may lead to a significant increase of serum potassium. Salt substitutes containing potassium should also be used with caution.

Inhibitors Of Endogenous Prostaglandin Synthesis: It has been reported that indomethacin may reduce the antihypertensive effect of captopril, especially in cases of low renin hypertension. Other nonsteroidal anti-inflammatory agents (e.g., aspirin) may also have this effect.

Lithium: Increased serum lithium levels and symptoms of lithium toxicity have been reported in patients receiving concomitant lithium and ACE inhibitor therapy. These drugs should be coadministered with caution and frequent monitoring of serum lithium levels is recommended. If a diuretic is also used, it may increase the risk of lithium toxicity (see PRECAUTIONS: Drug Interactions, Hydrochlorothiazide, Lithium).

Hydrochlorothiazide

When administered concurrently the following drugs may interact with thiazide diuretics:

Alcohol, barbiturates, or narcotics —potentiation of orthostatic hypotension may occur.

Amphotericin B, corticosteroids, or corticotropin (ACTH) —may intensify electrolyte imbalance, particularly hypokalemia. Monitor potassium levels; use potassium replacements if necessary.

Anticoagulants (oral) —dosage adjustments of anticoagulant medication may be necessary since hydrochlorothiazide may decrease their effects.

Antigout medications —dosage adjustments of antigout medication may be necessary since hydrochlorothiazide may raise the level of blood uric acid.

Other antihypertensive medications (e.g., ganglionic or peripheral adrenergic blocking agents) —dosage adjustments may be necessary since hydrochlorothiazide may potentiate their effects.

Antidiabetic drugs (oral agents and insulin) —since thiazides may elevate blood glucose levels, dosage adjustments of antidiabetic agents may be necessary.

Calcium salts —Increased serum calcium levels due to decreased excretion may occur. If calcium must be prescribed monitor serum calcium levels and adjust calcium dosage accordingly.

Cardiac glycosides —enhanced possibility of digitalis toxicity associated with hypokalemia. Monitor potassium levels (see PRECAUTIONS: Drug Interactions, Captopril).

Cholestyramine resin and colestipol HCL —may delay or decrease absorption of hydrochlorothiazide. Sulfonamide diuretics should be taken at least one hour before or four to six hours after these medications.

Diazoxide —enhanced hyperglycemic, hyperuricemic, and antihypertensive effects. Be cognizant of possible interaction; monitor blood glucose and serum uric acid levels.

Lithium —diuretic agents reduce the renal clearance of lithium and increase the risk of lithium toxicity. These drugs should be coadministered with caution and frequent monitoring of serum lithium levels is recommended (see PRECAUTIONS: Drug Interactions, Captopril, Lithium).

MAO inhibitors —dosage adjustments of one or both agents may be necessary since hypotensive effects are enhanced.

Nondepolarizing muscle relaxants, preanesthetics and anesthetics used in surgery (e.g., tubocurarine chloride and gallamine triethiodide) —effects of these agents may be potentiated; dosage adjustments may be required. Monitor and correct any fluid and electrolyte imbalances prior to surgery if feasible.

Nonsteroidal anti-inflammatory agents —in some patients, the administration of a nonsteroidal anti-inflammatory agent can reduce the diuretic, natriuretic, and antihypertensive effect of loop, potassium-sparing or thiazide diuretics. Therefore, when hydrochlorothiazide and nonsteroidal anti-inflammatory agents are used concomitantly, the patient should be observed closely to determine if the desired effect of the diuretic is obtained.

Methenamine —possible decreased effectiveness due to alkalinization of the urine.

Pressor amines (e.g., norepinephrine) —decreased arterial responsiveness, but not sufficient to preclude effectiveness of the pressor agent for therapeutic use. Use caution in patients taking both medications who undergo surgery. Administer preanesthetic and anesthetic agents in reduced dosage, and if possible, discontinue hydrochlorothiazide therapy one week prior to surgery.

Probenecid or sulfinpyrazone —increased dosage of these agents may be necessary since hydrochlorothiazide may have hyperuricemic effects.

Drug/Laboratory Test Interactions

Captopril

Captopril may cause a false-positive urine test for acetone.

Hydrochlorothiazide

Hydrochlorothiazide may cause diagnostic interference of the bentiromide test.

Carcinogenesis, Mutagenesis, Impairment of Fertility

Captopril

Two-year studies with doses of 50 to 1350 mg/kg/day in mice and rats failed to show any evidence of carcinogenic potential.

Studies in rats have revealed no impairment of fertility.

Animal Toxicology

Chronic oral toxicity studies were conducted in rats (2 years), dogs (47 weeks; 1 year), mice (2 years), and monkeys (1 year). Significant drug-related toxicity included effects on hematopoiesis, renal toxicity, erosion/ulceration of the stomach, and variation of retinal blood vessels.

Reductions in hemoglobin and/or hematocrit values were seen in mice, rats, and monkeys at doses 50 to 150 times the maximum recommended human dose (MRHD). Anemia, leukopenia, thrombocytopenia, and bone marrow suppression occurred in dogs at doses 8 to 30 times MRHD. The reductions in hemoglobin and hematocrit values in rats and mice were only significant at 1 year and returned to normal with continued dosing by the end of the study. Marked anemia was seen at all dose levels (8 to 30 times MRHD) in dogs, whereas moderate to marked leukopenia was noted only at 15 and 30 times MRHD and thrombocytopenia at 30 times MRHD. The anemia could be reversed upon discontinuation of dosing. Bone marrow suppression occurred to a varying degree, being associated only with dogs that died or were sacrificed in a moribund condition in the 1 year study. However, in the 47-week study at a dose 30 times MRHD, bone marrow suppression was found to be reversible upon continued drug administration.

Captopril caused hyperplasia of the juxtaglomerular apparatus of the kidneys at doses 7 to 200 times the MRHD in rats and mice, at 20 to 60 times MRHD in monkeys, and at 30 times the MRHD in dogs.

Gastric erosions/ulcerations were increased in incidence at 20 and 200 times MRHD in male rats and at 30 and 65 times MRHD in dogs and monkeys, respectively. Rabbits developed gastric and intestinal ulcers when given oral doses approximately 30 times MRHD for only five to seven days.

In the two-year rat study, irreversible and progressive variations in the caliber of retinal vessels (focal sacculations and constrictions) occurred at all dose levels (7 to 200 times MRHD) in a dose-related fashion. The effect was first observed in the 88th week of dosing, with a progressively increased incidence thereafter, even after cessation of dosing.

Hydrochlorothiazide

Long-term studies in animals have not been performed to evaluate carcinogenic potential, mutagenesis, or whether this drug affects fertility in males or females.

Pregnancy Categories C (first trimester) and D (second and third trimesters)

See WARNINGS: Captopril, Fetal/Neonatal Morbidity and Mortality.

Pregnancy—Nonteratogenic Effects

Hydrochlorothiazide

Thiazides cross the placental barrier and appear in cord blood. The use of thiazides in pregnant women requires that the anticipated benefit be weighed against possible hazards to the fetus. These hazards include fetal or neonatal jaundice, thrombocytopenia, and possibly other adverse reactions which have occurred in the adult.

Nursing Mothers

Both captopril and hydrochlorothiazide are excreted in human milk. Because of the potential for serious adverse reactions in nursing infants from both drugs, a decision should be made whether to discontinue nursing or to discontinue therapy taking into account the importance of CAPOZIDE (Captopril-Hydrochlorothiazide Tablets) to the mother. (See PRECAUTIONS: Pediatric Use.)

Pediatric Use

Safety and effectiveness in children have not been established. There is limited experience reported in the literature with the use of captopril in the pediatric population; dosage, on a weight basis, was generally reported to be comparable to or less than that used in adults.

Infants, especially newborns, may be more susceptible to the adverse hemodynamic effects of captopril. Excessive, prolonged and unpredictable decreases in blood pressure and associated complications, including oliguria and seizures, have been reported.

CAPOZIDE (Captopril-Hydrochlorothiazide Tablets) should be used in children only if other measures for controlling blood pressure have not been effective.

ADVERSE REACTIONS

Captopril

Reported incidences are based on clinical trials involving approximately 7000 patients.

Renal: About one of 100 patients developed proteinuria (see WARNINGS).

Each of the following has been reported in approximately 1 to 2 of 1000 patients and are of uncertain relationship to drug use: renal insufficiency, renal failure, nephrotic syndrome, polyuria, oliguria, and urinary frequency.

Hematologic: Neutropenia/agranulocytosis has occurred (see WARNINGS). Cases of anemia, thrombocytopenia, and pancytopenia have been reported.

Dermatologic: Rash, often with pruritus, and sometimes with fever, arthralgia, and eosinophilia, occurred in about 4 to 7 (depending on renal status and dose) of 100 patients, usually

during the first four weeks of therapy. It is usually maculopapular, and rarely urticarial. The rash is usually mild and disappears within a few days of dosage reduction, short-term treatment with an antihistaminic agent, and/or discontinuing therapy; remission may occur even if captopril is continued. Pruritus, without rash, occurs in about 2 of 100 patients. Between 7 and 10 percent of patients with skin rash have shown eosinophilia and/or positive ANA titers. A reversible associated pemphigoid-like lesion, and photosensitivity, have also been reported.

Flushing or pallor has been reported in 2 to 5 of 1000 patients.

Cardiovascular: Hypotension may occur; see WARNINGS and PRECAUTIONS (Drug Interactions) for discussion of hypotension with captopril therapy.

Tachycardia, chest pain, and palpitations have each been observed in approximately 1 of 100 patients.

Angina pectoris, myocardial infarction, Raynaud's syndrome, and congestive heart failure have each occurred in 2 to 3 of 1000 patients.

Dysgeusia: Approximately 2 to 4 (depending on renal status and dose) of 100 patients developed a diminution or loss of taste perception. Taste impairment is reversible and usually self-limited (2 to 3 months) even with continued drug administration. Weight loss may be associated with the loss of taste.

Angioedema: Angioedema involving the extremities, face, lips, mucous membranes, tongue, glottis or larynx has been reported in approximately one in 1000 patients. Angioedema involving the upper airways has caused fatal airway obstruction. (See WARNINGS: Captopril and PRECAUTIONS: Information for Patients.)

Cough: Cough has been reported in 0.5–2% of patients treated with captopril in clinical trials (see PRECAUTIONS: General, Captopril, Cough).

The following have been reported in about 0.5 to 2 percent of patients but did not appear at increased frequency compared to placebo or other treatments used in controlled trials: gastric irritation, abdominal pain, nausea, vomiting, diarrhea, anorexia, constipation, aphthous ulcers, peptic ulcer, dizziness, headache, malaise, fatigue, insomnia, dry mouth, dyspnea, alopecia, paresthesias.

Other clinical adverse effects reported since the drug was marketed are listed below by body system. In this setting, an incidence or causal relationship cannot be accurately determined.

General: asthenia, gynecomastia.

Cardiovascular: cardiac arrest, cerebrovascular accident/insufficiency, rhythm disturbances, orthostatic hypotension, syncope.

Dermatologic: bullous pemphigus, erythema multiforme (including Stevens-Johnson syndrome), exfoliative dermatitis.

Gastrointestinal: pancreatitis, glossitis, dyspepsia.

Hematologic: anemia, including aplastic and hemolytic.

Hepatobiliary: jaundice, hepatitis, including rare cases of necrosis, cholestasis.

Metabolic: symptomatic hyponatremia.

Musculoskeletal: myalgia, myasthenia.

Nervous/Psychiatric: ataxia, confusion, depression, nervousness, somnolence.

Respiratory: bronchospasm, eosinophilic pneumonitis, rhinitis.

Special Senses: blurred vision.

Urogenital: impotence.

As with other ACE inhibitors, a syndrome has been reported which may include: fever, myalgia, arthralgia, interstitial nephritis, vasculitis, rash or other dermatologic manifestations, eosinophilia and an elevated ESR.

Fetal/Neonatal Morbidity and Mortality

See WARNINGS: Captopril, Fetal/Neonatal Morbidity and Mortality.

Hydrochlorothiazide

Gastrointestinal System: anorexia, gastric irritation, nausea, vomiting, cramping, diarrhea, constipation, jaundice (intrahepatic cholestatic jaundice), pancreatitis, and sialadenitis.

Central Nervous System: dizziness, vertigo, paresthesias, headache, and xanthopsia.

Hematologic: leukopenia, agranulocytosis, thrombocytopenia, aplastic anemia, and hemolytic anemia.

Cardiovascular: orthostatic hypotension.

Hypersensitivity: purpura, photosensitivity, rash, urticaria, necrotizing angiitis (vasculitis; cutaneous vasculitis), fever, respiratory distress including pneumonitis, and anaphylactic reactions.

Other: hyperglycemia, glycosuria, hyperuricemia, muscle spasm, weakness, restlessness, and transient blurred vision. Whenever adverse reactions are moderate or severe, thiazide dosage should be reduced or therapy withdrawn.

Altered Laboratory Findings

Serum Electrolytes: Hyperkalemia: small increases in serum potassium, especially in patients with renal impairment (see PRECAUTIONS: Captopril).

Continued on next page

Squibb—Cont.

Hyponatremia: particularly in patients receiving a low sodium diet or concomitant diuretics.
BUN/Serum Creatinine: Transient elevations of BUN or serum creatinine especially in volume or salt depleted patients or those with renovascular hypertension may occur. Rapid reduction of longstanding or markedly elevated blood pressure can result in decreases in the glomerular filtration rate and, in turn, lead to increases in BUN or serum creatinine.
Hematologic: A positive ANA has been reported.
Liver Function Tests: Elevations of liver transaminases, alkaline phosphatase, and serum bilirubin have occurred.

OVERDOSAGE

Captopril

Correction of hypotension would be of primary concern. Volume expansion with an intravenous infusion of normal saline is the treatment of choice for restoration of blood pressure.
While captopril may be removed from the adult circulation by hemodialysis, there is inadequate data concerning the effectiveness of hemodialysis for removing it from the circulation of neonates or children. Peritoneal dialysis is not effective for removing captopril; there is no information concerning exchange transfusion for removing captopril from the general circulation.

Hydrochlorothiazide

In addition to the expected diuresis, overdosage of thiazides may produce varying degrees of lethargy which may progress to coma within a few hours, with minimal depression of respiration and cardiovascular function and without evidence of serum electrolyte changes or dehydration. The mechanism of thiazide-induced CNS depression is unknown. Gastrointestinal irritation and hypermotility may occur. Transitory increase in BUN has been reported, and serum electrolyte changes may occur, especially in patients with impaired renal function.
In addition to gastric lavage and supportive therapy for stupor or coma, symptomatic treatment of gastrointestinal effects may be needed. The degree to which hydrochlorothiazide is removed by hemodialysis has not been clearly established. Measures as required to maintain hydration, electrolyte balance, respiration, and cardiovascular and renal function should be instituted.

DOSAGE AND ADMINISTRATION

DOSAGE MUST BE INDIVIDUALIZED ACCORDING TO PATIENT'S RESPONSE.
CAPOZIDE may be substituted for the previously titrated individual components.
Alternatively, therapy may be instituted with a single tablet of CAPOZIDE 25 mg/15 mg taken once daily. For patients insufficiently responsive to the initial dose, additional captopril or hydrochlorothiazide may be added as individual components or by using CAPOZIDE 50 mg/15 mg, 25 mg/25 mg or 50 mg/25 mg, or divided doses may be used.
Because the full effect of a given dose may not be attained for 6–8 weeks, dosage adjustments should generally be made at 6 week intervals, unless the clinical situation demands more rapid adjustment.
In general, daily doses of captopril should not exceed 150 mg and of hydrochlorothiazide should not exceed 50 mg.
CAPOZIDE should be taken one hour before meals.
Dosage Adjustment in Renal Impairment—Because captopril and hydrochlorothiazide are excreted primarily by the kidneys, excretion rates are reduced in patients with impaired renal function. These patients will take longer to reach steady-state captopril levels and will reach higher steady-state levels for a given daily dose than patients with normal renal function. Therefore, these patients may respond to smaller or less frequent doses of CAPOZIDE.
After the desired therapeutic effect has been achieved, the dose intervals should be increased or the total daily dose reduced until the minimal effective dose is achieved. When concomitant diuretic therapy is required in patients with severe renal impairment, a loop diuretic (e.g., furosemide), rather than a thiazide diuretic is preferred for use with captopril; therefore, for patients with severe renal dysfunction the captopril-hydrochlorothiazide combination tablet is not usually recommended.

HOW SUPPLIED

CAPOZIDE (Captopril-Hydrochlorothiazide Tablets)
25 mg captopril combined with 15 mg hydrochlorothiazide in bottles of 100 (NDC 0003-0338-50). Tablets are white with distinct orange mottling; they are biconvex rounded squares with quadrisect bars.
25 mg captopril combined with 25 mg hydrochlorothiazide in bottles of 100 (NDC 0003-0349-50). Tablets are peach-colored and may show slight mottling; they are biconvex rounded squares with quadrisect bars.
50 mg captopril combined with 15 mg hydrochlorothiazide in bottles of 100 (NDC 0003-0384-50). Tablets are white with distinct orange mottling; they are biconvex ovals with a bisect bar.
50 mg captopril combined with 25 mg hydrochlorothiazide in bottles of 100 (NDC 0003-0390-50). Tablets are peach-colored and may show slight mottling; they are biconvex ovals with a bisect bar.

STORAGE

Keep bottles tightly closed (protect from moisture); do not store above 86°F.
(J4-005U)

Shown in Product Identification Section, page 432

PRAVACHOL® ℞

[*prăv 'a-cōl*]
Pravastatin Sodium Tablets

DESCRIPTION

PRAVACHOL (pravastatin sodium) is one of a new class of lipid-lowering compounds, the HMG-CoA reductase inhibitors, which reduce cholesterol biosynthesis. These agents are competitive inhibitors of 3-hydroxy-3-methylglutaryl-coenzyme A (HMG-CoA) reductase, the enzyme catalyzing the early rate-limiting step in cholesterol biosynthesis, conversion of HMG-CoA to mevalonate.
Pravastatin sodium is designated chemically as 1-Naphthalene-heptanoic acid, 1,2,6,7,8,8a-hexahydro-β,Δ,6-trihydroxy-2-methyl-8-(2-methyl-1-oxobutoxy)-, monosodium salt, [1S-[1α(βS*,ΔS*),2α,6α,8β(R*),8aα]]-.
Pravastatin sodium is an odorless, white to off-white, fine or crystalline powder. It is a relatively polar hydrophilic compound with a partition coefficient (octanol/water) of 0.59 at a pH of 7.0. It is soluble in methanol and water (> 300 mg/mL), slightly soluble in isopropanol, and practically insoluble in acetone, acetonitrile, chloroform, and ether.
PRAVACHOL is available for oral administration as 10 mg and 20 mg tablets. Inactive ingredients include: croscarmellose sodium, lactose, magnesium stearate, microcrystalline cellulose, and povidone.

CLINICAL PHARMACOLOGY

Mechanism of Action

Cholesterol and triglycerides in the bloodstream circulate as part of lipoprotein complexes. These complexes can be separated by density ultracentrifugation into high (HDL), intermediate (IDL), low (LDL), and very low (VLDL) density lipoprotein fractions. Triglycerides (TG) and cholesterol synthesized in the liver are incorporated into very low density lipoproteins (VLDLs) and released into the plasma for delivery to peripheral tissues. In a series of subsequent steps, VLDLs are transformed into intermediate density lipoproteins (IDLs), and cholesterol-rich low density lipoproteins (LDLs). High density lipoproteins (HDLs), containing apolipoprotein A, are hypothesized to participate in the reverse transport of cholesterol from tissues back to the liver.
PRAVACHOL produces its lipid-lowering effect in two ways. First, as a consequence of its reversible inhibition of HMG-CoA reductase activity, it effects modest reductions in intracellular pools of cholesterol. This results in an increase in the number of LDL-receptors on cell surfaces and enhanced receptor-mediated catabolism and clearance of circulating LDL. Second, pravastatin inhibits LDL production by inhibiting hepatic synthesis of VLDL, the LDL precursor.
Clinical and pathologic studies have shown that elevated levels of total cholesterol (Total-C), low density lipoprotein cholesterol (LDL-C), and apolipoprotein B (a membrane transport complex for LDL) promote human atherosclerosis. Similarly, decreased levels of HDL-cholesterol (HDL-C) and its transport complex, apolipoprotein A, are associated with the development of atherosclerosis. Epidemiologic investigations have established that cardiovascular morbidity and mortality vary directly with the level of Total-C and LDL-C and inversely with the level of HDL-C. In multicenter clinical trials, those pharmacologic and/or non-pharmacologic interventions that simultaneously lowered LDL-C and increased HDL-C reduced the rate of cardiovascular events (both fatal and nonfatal myocardial infarctions). In both normal volunteers and patients with hypercholesterolemia, treatment with PRAVACHOL reduced Total-C, LDL-C, and apolipoprotein B. PRAVACHOL also modestly reduced VLDL-C and TG while producing increases of variable magnitude in HDL-C and apolipoprotein A. The effects of pravastatin on Lp(a), fibrinogen, and certain other independent biochemical risk markers for coronary heart disease are unknown. The effect of pravastatin-induced changes in lipoprotein levels on the evolution of atherosclerosis is also unknown. Although pravastatin is relatively more hydrophilic than other HMG-CoA reductase inhibitors, the effect of relative hydrophilicity, if any, on either efficacy or safety has not been established.

Pharmacokinetics/Metabolism

PRAVACHOL (pravastatin sodium) is administered orally in the active form. In clinical pharmacology studies in man, pravastatin is rapidly absorbed, with peak plasma levels of parent compound attained 1 to 1.5 hours following ingestion. Based on urinary recovery of radiolabeled drug, the average oral absorption of pravastatin is 34% and absolute bioavailability is 17%. While the presence of food in the gastrointestinal tract reduces systemic bioavailability, the lipid-lowering effects of the drug are similar whether taken with, or 1 hour prior, to meals.
Pravastatin undergoes extensive first-pass extraction in the liver (extraction ratio 0.66), which is its primary site of action, and the primary site of cholesterol synthesis and of LDL-C clearance. *In vitro* studies demonstrated that pravastatin is transported into hepatocytes with substantially less uptake into other cells. In view of pravastatin's apparently extensive first-pass hepatic metabolism, plasma levels may not necessarily correlate perfectly with lipid-lowering efficacy. Pravastatin plasma concentrations [including: area under the concentration-time curve (AUC), peak (Cmax), and steady-state minimum (Cmin)] are directly proportional to administered dose. Systemic bioavailability of pravastatin administered following a bedtime dose was decreased 60% compared to that following an AM dose. Despite this decrease in systemic bioavailability, the efficacy of pravastatin administered once daily in the evening, although not statistically significant, was marginally more effective than that after a morning dose. This finding of lower systemic bioavailability suggests greater hepatic extraction of the drug following the evening dose. Steady-state AUCs, Cmax and Cmin plasma concentrations showed no evidence of pravastatin accumulation following once or twice daily administration of PRAVACHOL tablets. Approximately 50% of the circulating drug is bound to plasma proteins. Following single dose administration of ^{14}C-pravastatin, the elimination half-life ($t^{1/2}$) for total radioactivity (pravastatin plus metabolites) in humans is 77 hours.
Pravastatin, like other HMG-CoA reductase inhibitors, has variable bioavailability. The coefficient of variation, based on between-subject variability, was 50% to 60% for AUC.
Approximately 20% of a radiolabeled oral dose is excreted in urine and 70% in the feces. After intravenous administration of radiolabeled pravastatin to normal volunteers, approximately 47% of total body clearance was via renal excretion and 53% by non-renal routes (i.e., biliary excretion and biotransformation). Since there are dual routes of elimination, the potential exists both for compensatory excretion by the alternate route as well as for accumulation of drug and/or metabolites in patients with renal or hepatic insufficiency.
In a study comparing the kinetics of pravastatin in patients with biopsy confirmed cirrhosis (N=7) and normal subjects (N=7), the mean AUC varied 18-fold in cirrhotic patients and 5-fold in healthy subjects. Similarly, the peak pravastatin values varied 47-fold for cirrhotic patients compared to 6-fold for healthy subjects.
Biotransformation pathways elucidated for pravastatin include: (a) isomerization to 6-epi pravastatin and the 3α-hydroxyisomer of pravastatin (SQ 31,906), (b) enzymatic ring hydroxylation to SQ 31,945, (c) δ-1 oxidation of the ester side chain, (d) β-oxidation of the carboxy side chain, (e) ring oxidation followed by aromatization, (f) oxidation of a hydroxyl group to a keto group, and (g) conjugation. The major degradation product is the 3α-hydroxy isomeric metabolite, which has one-tenth to one-fortieth the HMG-CoA reductase inhibitory activity of the parent compound.

Clinical Studies

PRAVACHOL (pravastatin sodium) is highly effective in reducing Total-C and LDL-C in patients with heterozygous familial, presumed familial combined, and non-familial (non-FH) forms of primary hypercholesterolemia. A therapeutic response is seen within 1 week, and the maximum response usually is achieved within 4 weeks. This response is maintained during extended periods of therapy.
A single daily dose administered in the evening (the recommended dosing) is as effective as the same total daily dose given twice a day. Once daily administration in the evening appears to be marginally more effective than once daily administration in the morning, perhaps because hepatic cholesterol is synthesized mainly at night. In multicenter, double-blind, placebo-controlled studies of patients with primary hypercholesterolemia, treatment with pravastatin in daily doses ranging from 10 mg to 40 mg consistently and significantly decreased Total-C, LDL-C, and Total-C/HDL-C and LDL-C/HDL-C ratios; modestly decreased VLDL-C and plasma TG levels; and produced increases in HDL-C of variable magnitude.
[See table at top left of next page.]
In another clinical trial, patients treated with pravastatin in combination with cholestyramine (70% of patients were taking cholestyramine 20 or 24 g per day) had reductions equal to or greater than 50% in LDL-C. Furthermore, pravastatin attenuated cholestyramine-induced increases in TG levels (which are themselves of uncertain clinical significance).

Primary Hypercholesterolemia Study
Dose Response of PRAVACHOL*
Once Daily Administration At Bedtime

Dose	Total-C	LDL-C	HDL-C	TG
10 mg	−16%	−22%	+7%	−15%
20 mg	−24%	−32%	+2%	−11%
40 mg	−25%	−34%	+12%	−24%

*Mean percent change from baseline after 8 weeks

INDICATIONS AND USAGE

Therapy with lipid-altering agents should be considered a component of multiple risk factor intervention in those individuals at increased risk for atherosclerotic vascular disease. PRAVACHOL (pravastatin sodium) is indicated as an adjunct to diet for the reduction of elevated total and LDL-cholesterol levels in patients with primary hypercholesterolemia (Type IIa and IIb)[1] when the response to a diet restricted in saturated fat and cholesterol has not been adequate.

Prior to initiating therapy with pravastatin, secondary causes for hypercholesterolemia (e.g., poorly controlled diabetes mellitus, hypothyroidism, nephrotic syndrome, dysproteinemias, obstructive liver disease, other drug therapy, alcoholism) should be excluded, and a lipid profile performed to measure Total-C, HDL-C, and TG. For patients with triglycerides (TG) <400 mg/dL (<4.5 mmol/L), LDL-C can be estimated using the following equation:

$$LDL\text{-}C = Total\text{-}C - HDL\text{-}C - \tfrac{1}{5}\,TG$$

For TG levels >400 mg/dL (>4.5 mmol/L), this equation is less accurate and LDL-C concentrations should be determined by ultracentrifugation.

Lipid determinations should be performed at intervals of no less than four weeks and dosage adjusted according to the patient's response to therapy.

The National Cholesterol Education Program's Treatment Guidelines† are summarized above: [top right]

	LDL-Cholesterol mg/dL (mmol/L) Initiation Level	LDL-Cholesterol mg/dL (mmol/L) Minimum Goal	Total-Cholesterol mg/dL (mmol/L) Minimum Goal
Without Definite CHD or Two Other Risk Factors*	≥190 (≥4.9)	<160 (<4.1)	<240 (<6.2)
With Definite CHD or Two Other Risk Factors*	≥160 (≥4.1)	<130 (<3.4)	<200 (<5.2)

*Other risk factors for coronary heart disease (CHD) include: male sex, family history of premature CHD, cigarette smoking, hypertension, confirmed HDL-C <35 mg/dL (<0.91 mmol/L), diabetes mellitus, definite cerebrovascular or peripheral vascular disease, or severe obesity.

Since the goal of treatment is to lower LDL-C, the NCEP recommends that LDL-C levels be used to initiate and assess treatment response. Only if LDL-C levels are not available, should the Total-C be used to monitor therapy.

As with other lipid-lowering therapy, PRAVACHOL (pravastatin sodium) is not indicated when hypercholesterolemia is due to hyperalphalipoproteinemia (elevated HDL-C). The efficacy of pravastatin has not been evaluated in patients with combined elevated Total-C and hypertriglyceridemia [>500 mg/dL (>5.7 mmol/L)] or in patients with elevated intermediate density lipoproteins as their primary lipid abnormality.

CONTRAINDICATIONS

Hypersensitivity to any component of this medication.

Active liver disease or unexplained, persistent elevations in liver function tests (see WARNINGS).

Pregnancy and lactation. Atherosclerosis is a chronic process and discontinuation of lipid-lowering drugs during pregnancy should have little impact on the outcome of long-term therapy of primary hypercholesterolemia. Cholesterol and other products of cholesterol biosynthesis are essential components for fetal development (including synthesis of steroids and cell membranes). Since HMG-CoA reductase inhibitors decrease cholesterol synthesis and possibly the synthesis of other biologically active substances derived from cholesterol, they may cause fetal harm when administered to pregnant women. Therefore, HMG-CoA reductase inhibitors are contraindicated during pregnancy and in nursing mothers. **Pravastatin should be administered to women of childbearing age only when such patients are highly unlikely to conceive and have been informed of the potential hazards.** If the patient becomes pregnant while taking this class of drug, therapy should be discontinued and the patient apprised of the potential hazard to the fetus.

[1]**Classification of Hyperlipoproteinemias**

Type		Lipoproteins Elevated	Lipid Elevations major	Lipid Elevations minor
I	(rare)	chylomicrons	TG	↑→C
IIa		LDL	C	—
IIb		LDL, VLDL	C	TG
III	(rare)	IDL	C/TG	—
IV		VLDL	TG	↑→C
V	(rare)	chylomicrons, VLDL	TG	↑→C

C = cholesterol, TG = triglycerides,
LDL = low density lipoprotein,
VLDL = very low density lipoprotein,
IDL = intermediate density lipoprotein.

†For adult diabetic subjects, a modification of these guidelines is recommended—see: American Diabetes Association Consensus Statement: Role of Cardiovascular Risk Factors in Prevention and Treatment of Macrovascular Disease in Diabetes. *Diabetes Care* 12(8):573–579, 1989.

WARNINGS

Liver Enzymes

HMG-CoA reductase inhibitors, like some other lipid-lowering therapies, have been associated with biochemical abnormalities of liver function. Increases of serum transaminase (ALT, AST) values to more than 3 times the upper limit of normal occurring on 2 or more (not necessarily sequential) occasions have been reported in 1.3% of patients treated with pravastatin in the US over an average period of 18 months. These abnormalities were not associated with cholestasis and did not appear to be related to treatment duration. In those patients in whom these abnormalities were believed to be related to pravastatin and who were discontinued from therapy, the transaminase levels usually fell slowly to pretreatment levels. These biochemical findings are usually asymptomatic although worldwide experience indicates that anorexia, weakness, and/or abdominal pain may also be present in rare patients.

As with other lipid-lowering agents, liver function tests should be performed during therapy with pravastatin. Serum aminotransferases, including ALT (SGPT), should be monitored before treatment begins, every six weeks for the first three months, every eight weeks during the remainder of the first year, and periodically thereafter (e.g., at about six-month intervals). Special attention should be given to patients who develop increased transaminase levels. Liver function tests should be repeated to confirm an elevation and subsequently monitored at more frequent intervals. If increases in AST and ALT equal or exceed three times the upper limit of normal and persist, then therapy should be discontinued. Persistence of significant aminotransferase elevations following discontinuation of therapy may warrant consideration of liver biopsy.

Active liver disease or unexplained transaminase elevations are contraindications to the use of pravastatin (see CONTRAINDICATIONS). Caution should be exercised when pravastatin is administered to patients with a history of liver disease or heavy alcohol ingestion (see CLINICAL PHARMACOLOGY: Pharmacokinetics/Metabolism). Such patients should be closely monitored, started at the lower end of the recommended dosing range, and titrated to the desired therapeutic effect.

Skeletal Muscle

Rhabdomyolysis with renal dysfunction secondary to myoglobinuria has been reported with pravastatin and other drugs in this class. Uncomplicated myalgia has been reported in pravastatin-treated patients (see ADVERSE REACTIONS). Myopathy, defined as muscle aching or muscle weakness in conjunction with increases in creatine phosphokinase (CPK) values to greater than 10 times the upper limit of normal was reported to be possibly due to pravastatin in only one patient in clinical trials (<0.1%). Myopathy should be considered in any patient with diffuse myalgias, muscle tenderness or weakness, and/or marked elevation of CPK. Patients should be advised to report promptly unexplained muscle pain, tenderness or weakness, particularly if accompanied by malaise or fever. **Pravastatin therapy should be discontinued if markedly elevated CPK levels occur or myopathy is diagnosed or suspected. Pravastatin therapy should also be temporarily withheld in any patient experiencing an acute or serious condition predisposing to the development of renal failure secondary to rhabdomyolysis, e.g., sepsis; hypotension; major surgery; trauma; severe metabolic, endocrine, or electrolyte disorders; or uncontrolled epilepsy.**

The risk of myopathy during treatment with lovastatin is increased if therapy with either cyclosporine, gemfibrozil, erythromycin, or niacin is administered concurrently. There is no experience with the use of pravastatin together with cyclosporine. Myopathy has not been observed in clinical trials involving small numbers of patients who were treated with pravastatin together with niacin. One trial of limited size involving combined therapy with pravastatin and gemfibrozil showed a trend toward more frequent CPK elevations and patient withdrawals due to musculoskeletal symptoms in the group receiving combined treatment as compared with the groups receiving placebo, gemfibrozil, or pravastatin monotherapy. Myopathy was not reported in this trial (see PRECAUTIONS: Drug Interactions). One patient developed myopathy when clofibrate was added to a previously well tolerated regimen of pravastatin; the myopathy resolved when clofibrate therapy was stopped and pravastatin treatment continued. **The use of fibrates alone may occasionally be associated with myopathy. The combined use of pravastatin and fibrates should generally be avoided.**

PRECAUTIONS

General

Pravastatin may elevate creatine phosphokinase and transaminase levels (see ADVERSE REACTIONS). This should be considered in the differential diagnosis of chest pain in a patient on therapy with pravastatin.

Homozygous Familial Hypercholesterolemia. Pravastatin has not been evaluated in patients with rare homozygous familial hypercholesterolemia. In this group of patients, it has been reported that HMG-CoA reductase inhibitors are less effective because the patients lack functional LDL receptors.

Renal Insufficiency. A single 20 mg oral dose of pravastatin was administered to 24 patients with varying degrees of renal impairment (as determined by creatinine clearance). No effect was observed on the pharmacokinetics of pravastatin or its 3α-hydroxy isomeric metabolite (SQ 31,906). A small increase was seen in mean AUC values and half-life ($t_{1/2}$) for the inactive enzymatic ring hydroxylation metabolite (SQ 31,945). Given this small sample size, the dosage administered, and the degree of individual variability, patients with renal impairment who are receiving pravastatin should be closely monitored.

Information for Patients

Patients should be advised to report promptly unexplained muscle pain, tenderness or weakness, particularly if accompanied by malaise or fever.

Drug Interactions

Immunosuppressive Drugs, Gemfibrozil, Niacin (Nicotinic Acid), Erythromycin: See WARNINGS: Skeletal Muscle.

Antipyrine: Clearance by the cytochrome P450 system was unaltered by concomitant administration of pravastatin. Since pravastatin does not appear to induce hepatic drug-metabolizing enzymes, it is not expected that any significant interaction of pravastatin with other drugs (e.g., phenytoin, quinidine) metabolized by the cytochrome P450 system will occur.

Cholestyramine/Colestipol: Concomitant administration resulted in an approximately 40 to 50% decrease in the mean AUC of pravastatin. However, when pravastatin was administered 1 hour before or 4 hours after cholestyramine or 1 hour before colestipol and a standard meal, there was no clinically significant decrease in bioavailability or therapeutic effect. (See DOSAGE AND ADMINISTRATION: Concomitant Therapy.)

Warfarin: In a study involving 10 healthy male subjects given pravastatin and warfarin concomitantly for 6 days, bioavailability parameters at steady state for pravastatin (parent compound) were not altered. Pravastatin did not alter the plasma protein-binding of warfarin. Concomitant dosing did increase the AUC and Cmax of warfarin but did not produce any changes in its anticoagulant action (i.e., no increase was seen in mean prothrombin time after 6 days of concomitant therapy). However, bleeding and extreme prolongation of prothrombin time has been reported with another drug in this class. Patients receiving warfarin-type anticoagulants should have their prothrombin times closely monitored when pravastatin is initiated or the dosage of pravastatin is changed.

Cimetidine: The AUC_{0-12hr} for pravastatin when given with cimetidine was not significantly different from the AUC for pravastatin when given alone. A significant difference was observed between the AUC's for pravastatin when given with cimetidine compared to when administered with antacid.

Digoxin: In a crossover trial involving 18 healthy male subjects given pravastatin and digoxin concurrently for 9 days, the bioavailability parameters of digoxin were not affected. The AUC of pravastatin tended to increase, but the overall bioavailability of pravastatin plus its metabolites SQ 31,906 and SQ 31,945 was not altered.

Continued on next page

Squibb—Cont.

Gemfibrozil: In a crossover study in 20 healthy male volunteers given concomitant single doses of pravastatin and gemfibrozil, there was a significant decrease in urinary excretion and protein binding of pravastatin. In addition, there was a significant increase in AUC, Cmax, and Tmax for the pravastatin metabolite SQ 31,906. Combination therapy with pravastatin and gemfibrozil is generally not recommended.
In interaction studies with *aspirin, antacids* (1 hour prior to PRAVACHOL), *cimetidine, nicotinic acid,* or *probucol,* no statistically significant differences in bioavailability were seen when PRAVACHOL (pravastatin sodium) was administered.
Other Drugs: During clinical trials, no noticeable drug interactions were reported when PRAVACHOL was added to: diuretics, antihypertensives, digitalis, converting-enzyme inhibitors, calcium channel blockers, beta-blockers, or nitroglycerin.

Endocrine Function
HMG-CoA reductase inhibitors interfere with cholesterol synthesis and lower circulating cholesterol levels and, as such, might theoretically blunt adrenal or gonadal steroid hormone production. Results of clinical trials with pravastatin in males and post-menopausal females were inconsistent with regard to possible effects of the drug on basal steroid hormone levels. In a study of 21 males, the mean testosterone response to human chorionic gonadotropin was significantly reduced ($p < 0.004$) after 16 weeks of treatment with 40 mg of pravastatin. However, the percentage of patients showing a $\geq 50\%$ rise in plasma testosterone after human chorionic gonadotropin stimulation did not change significantly after therapy in these patients. The effects of HMG-CoA reductase inhibitors on spermatogenesis and fertility have not been studied in adequate numbers of patients. The effects, if any, of pravastatin on the pituitary-gonadal axis in pre-menopausal females are unknown. Patients treated with pravastatin who display clinical evidence of endocrine dysfunction should be evaluated appropriately. Caution should be exercised if an HMG-CoA reductase inhibitor or other agent used to lower cholesterol levels is administered to patients also receiving other drugs (e.g., ketoconazole, spironolactone, cimetidine) that may diminish the levels or activity of steroid hormones.

CNS Toxicity
CNS vascular lesions, characterized by perivascular hemorrhage and edema and mononuclear cell infiltration of perivascular spaces, were seen in dogs treated with pravastatin at a dose of 25 mg/kg/day, a dose that produced a plasma drug level about 50 times higher than the mean drug level in humans taking 40 mg/day. Similar CNS vascular lesions have been observed with several other drugs in this class.
A chemically similar drug in this class produced optic nerve degeneration (Wallerian degeneration of retinogeniculate fibers) in clinically normal dogs in a dose-dependent fashion starting at 60 mg/kg/day, a dose that produced mean plasma drug levels about 30 times higher than the mean drug level in humans taking the highest recommended dose (as measured by total enzyme inhibitory activity). This same drug also produced vestibulocochlear Wallerian-like degeneration and retinal ganglion cell chromatolysis in dogs treated for 14 weeks at 180 mg/kg/day, a dose which resulted in a mean plasma drug level similar to that seen with the 60 mg/kg dose.

Carcinogenesis, Mutagenesis, Impairment of Fertility
In a 2-year study in rats fed pravastatin at doses of 10, 30, or 100 mg/kg body weight, there was an increased incidence of hepatocellular carcinomas in males at the highest dose ($p < 0.01$). Although rats were given up to 125 times the human dose (HD) on a mg/kg body weight basis, their serum drug levels were only 6 to 10 times higher than those measured in humans given 40 mg pravastatin as measured by AUC.
The oral administration of 10, 30, or 100 mg/kg (producing plasma drug levels approximately 0.5 to 5.0 times the human drug levels at 40 mg) of pravastatin to mice for 22 months resulted in a statistically significant increase in the incidence of malignant lymphomas in treated females when all treatment groups were pooled and compared to controls ($p < 0.05$). The incidence was not dose-related and male mice were not affected.
A chemically similar drug in this class was administered to mice for 72 weeks at 25, 100, and 400 mg/kg body weight, which resulted in mean serum drug levels approximately 3, 15, and 33 times higher than the mean human serum drug concentration (as total inhibitory activity) after a 40 mg oral dose. Liver carcinomas were significantly increased in high-dose females and mid- and high-dose males, with a maximum incidence of 90 percent in males. The incidence of adenomas of the liver was significantly increased in mid- and high-dose females. Drug treatment also significantly increased the incidence of lung adenomas in mid- and high-dose males and females. Adenomas of the eye Harderian gland (a gland of the eye of rodents) were significantly higher in high-dose mice than in controls.
No evidence of mutagenicity was observed *in vitro,* with or without rat-liver metabolic activation, in the following studies: microbial mutagen tests, using mutant strains of *Salmonella typhimurium* or *Escherichia coli;* a forward mutation assay in L5178YTK +/− mouse lymphoma cells; a chromosomal aberration test in hamster cells; and a gene conversion assay using *Saccharomyces cerevisiae.* In addition, there was no evidence of mutagenicity in either a dominant lethal test in mice or a micronucleus test in mice.
In a study in rats, with daily doses up to 500 mg/kg, pravastatin did not produce any adverse effects on fertility or general reproductive performance. However, in a study with another HMG-CoA reductase inhibitor, there was decreased fertility in male rats treated for 34 weeks at 25 mg/kg body weight, although this effect was not observed in a subsequent fertility study when this same dose was administered for 11 weeks (the entire cycle of spermatogenesis, including epididymal maturation). In rats treated with this same reductase inhibitor at 180 mg/kg/day, seminiferous tubule degeneration (necrosis and loss of spermatogenic epithelium) was observed. Although not seen with pravastatin, two similar drugs in this class caused drug-related testicular atrophy, decreased spermatogenesis, spermatocytic degeneration, and giant cell formation in dogs. The clinical significance of these findings is unclear.

Pregnancy
Pregnancy Category X.
See CONTRAINDICATIONS.
Safety in pregnant women has not been established. Pravastatin was not teratogenic in rats at doses up to 1000 mg/kg daily or in rabbits at doses of up to 50 mg/kg daily. These doses resulted in 20× (rabbit) or 240× (rat) the human exposure based on surface area (mg/meter^2). However, in studies with another HMG-CoA reductase inhibitor, skeletal malformations were observed in rats and mice. PRAVACHOL (pravastatin sodium) should be administered to women of child-bearing potential only when such patients are highly unlikely to conceive and have been informed of the potential hazards. If the woman becomes pregnant while taking PRAVACHOL (pravastatin sodium), it should be discontinued and the patient advised again as to the potential hazards to the fetus.

Nursing Mothers
A small amount of pravastatin is excreted in human breast milk. Because of the potential for serious adverse reactions in nursing infants, women taking PRAVACHOL (pravastatin sodium) should not nurse (see CONTRAINDICATIONS).

Pediatric Use
Safety and effectiveness in individuals less than 18 years old have not been established. Hence, treatment in patients less than 18 years old is not recommended at this time. See also PRECAUTIONS: General.

ADVERSE REACTIONS

Pravastatin is generally well tolerated; adverse reactions have usually been mild and transient. In 4-month long placebo-controlled trials, 1.7% of pravastatin-treated patients and 1.2% of placebo-treated patients were discontinued from treatment because of adverse experiences attributed to study drug therapy; this difference was not statistically significant. In long-term studies, the most common reasons for discontinuation were asymptomatic serum transaminase increases and mild, non-specific gastrointestinal complaints. During clinical trials the overall incidence of adverse events in the elderly was not different than the incidence observed in younger patients.

Adverse Clinical Events
All adverse clinical events (regardless of attribution) reported in more than 2% of pravastatin-treated patients in the placebo-controlled trials are identified in the table below; also shown are the percentages of patients in whom these medical events were believed to be related or possibly related to the drug.

Body System/ Event	All Events: Pravastatin (N = 900) %	All Events: Placebo (N = 411) %	Events Attributed to Study Drug: Pravastatin (N = 900) %	Events Attributed to Study Drug: Placebo (N = 411) %
Cardiovascular				
Cardiac Chest Pain	4.0	3.4	0.1	0.0
Dermatologic				
Rash	4.0*	1.1	1.3	0.9
Gastrointestinal				
Nausea/Vomiting	7.3	7.1	2.9	3.4
Diarrhea	6.2	5.6	2.0	1.9
Abdominal Pain	5.4	6.9	2.0	3.9
Constipation	4.0	7.1	2.4	5.1
Flatulence	3.3	3.6	2.7	3.4
Heartburn	2.9	1.9	2.0	0.7
General				
Fatigue	3.8	3.4	1.9	1.0
Chest Pain	3.7	1.9	0.3	0.2
Influenza	2.4*	0.7	0.0	0.0
Musculoskeletal				
Localized Pain	10.0	9.0	1.4	1.5
Myalgia	2.7	1.0	0.6	0.0
Nervous System				
Headache	6.2	3.9	1.7*	0.2
Dizziness	3.3	3.2	1.0	0.5
Renal/Genitourinary				
Urinary Abnormality	2.4	2.9	0.7	1.2
Respiratory				
Common Cold	7.0	6.3	0.0	0.0
Rhinitis	4.0	4.1	0.1	0.0
Cough	2.6	1.7	0.1	0.0

*Statistically significantly different from placebo.

The following effects have been reported with drugs in this class:
Skeletal: myopathy, rhabdomyolysis.
Neurological: dysfunction of certain cranial nerves (including alteration of taste, impairment of extra-ocular movement, facial paresis), tremor, vertigo, memory loss, paresthesia, peripheral neuropathy, peripheral nerve palsy.
Hypersensitivity Reactions: An apparent hypersensitivity syndrome has been reported rarely which has included one or more of the following features: anaphylaxis, angioedema, lupus erythematous-like syndrome, polymyalgia rheumatica, vasculitis, purpura, thrombocytopenia, leukopenia, hemolytic anemia, positive ANA, ESR increase, arthritis, arthralgia, urticaria, asthenia, photosensitivity, fever, chills, flushing, malaise, dyspnea, toxic epidermal necrolysis, erythema multiforme, including Stevens-Johnson syndrome.
Gastrointestinal: pancreatitis, hepatitis, including chronic active hepatitis, cholestatic jaundice, fatty change in liver, and, rarely, cirrhosis, fulminant hepatic necrosis, and hepatoma; anorexia, vomiting.
Reproductive: gynecomastia, loss of libido, erectile dysfunction.
Eye: progression of cataracts (lens opacities), ophthalmoplegia.

Laboratory Test Abnormalities
Increases in serum transaminase (ALT, AST) values and CPK have been observed (see WARNINGS).
Transient, asymptomatic eosinophilia has been reported. Eosinophil counts usually returned to normal despite continued therapy. Anemia, thrombocytopenia, and leukopenia have been reported with other HMG-CoA reductase inhibitors.

Concomitant Therapy
Pravastatin has been administered concurrently with cholestyramine, colestipol, nicotinic acid, probucol and gemfibrozil. Preliminary data suggest that the addition of either probucol or gemfibrozil to therapy with lovastatin or pravastatin is **not** associated with greater reduction in LDL-cholesterol than that achieved with lovastatin or pravastatin alone. No adverse reactions unique to the combination or in addition to those previously reported for each drug alone

have been reported. Myopathy and rhabdomyolysis (with or without acute renal failure) have been reported when another HMG-CoA reductase inhibitor was used in combination with immunosuppressive drugs, gemfibrozil, erythromycin, or lipid-lowering doses of nicotinic acid. Concomitant therapy with HMG-CoA reductase inhibitors and these agents is generally not recommended. (See WARNINGS: **Skeletal Muscle** and PRECAUTIONS: **Drug Interactions**.)

OVERDOSAGE

There have been no reports of overdoses with pravastatin. Should an accidental overdose occur, treat symptomatically and institute supportive measures as required.

DOSAGE AND ADMINISTRATION

Prior to initiating PRAVACHOL (pravastatin sodium), the patient should be placed on a standard cholesterol-lowering diet (AHA Phase I or NCEP Step 1) for a minimum of 3 to 6 months, depending upon the severity of the lipid elevation. Dietary therapy should be continued during treatment. The recommended starting dose is 10 or 20 mg once daily at bedtime. In primary hypercholesterolemic patients with significant renal or hepatic dysfunction, and in the elderly, a starting dose of 10 mg daily at bedtime is recommended. PRAVACHOL may be taken without regard to meals. Since the maximal effect of a given dose is seen within 4 weeks, periodic lipid determinations should be performed at this time and dosage adjusted according to the patient's response to therapy and established treatment guidelines. The recommended dosage range is generally 10 to 40 mg administered once a day at bedtime. In the elderly, maximum reductions in LDL-cholesterol may be achieved with daily doses of 20 mg or less.

Concomitant Therapy

The lipid-lowering effects of PRAVACHOL (pravastatin sodium) on total and LDL cholesterol are enhanced when combined with a bile-acid-binding resin. When administering a bile-acid-binding resin (e.g., cholestyramine, colestipol) and pravastatin, PRAVACHOL should be given either 1 hour or more before or at least 4 hours following the resin. See also ADVERSE REACTIONS: **Concomitant Therapy**.

HOW SUPPLIED

10 mg tablets: bottles of 100 (NDC 0003-0154-50)
20 mg tablets: bottles of 100 (NDC 0003-0178-50)
Bottles contain a desiccant canister.
Unimatic® unit-dose packs are also available for each potency: **10 mg** (NDC 0003-0154-51), **20 mg** (NDC 0003-0178-51).
Tablets are white to off white, round and biconvex. Tablet identification numbers: **10 mg** 154 and **20 mg** 178.

Storage

Do not store above 86°F (30°C). Keep tightly closed (protect from moisture). Protect from light.

---

[1] Fredrickson classification: Type IIa—elevation of LDL; Type IIb—elevation of LDL and VLDL. Type III (familial dysbetalipoproteinemia)-elevation of IDL. Fredrickson, DS, Fat transport in lipoproteins—an integrated approach to mechanism and disorders, *N Eng J Med* 276:34, 1967. (J4-422A)

Shown in Product Identification Section, page 432

Squibb Diagnostics
A Bristol-Myers Squibb Company
P. O. BOX 4500
PRINCETON, NJ 08543-4500

ISOVUE   ℞

DESCRIPTION

ISOVUE (Iopamidol Injection) formulations are stable, aqueous, sterile, and nonpyrogenic solutions for intravascular administration.
Each mL of ISOVUE-200 (Iopamidol Injection 41%) provides 408 mg iopamidol with 1 mg tromethamine and 0.26 mg edetate calcium disodium. The solution contains approximately 0.029 mg (0.001 mEq) sodium and 200 mg organically bound iodine per mL.
Each mL of ISOVUE-250 (Iopamidol Injection 51%) provides 510 mg iopamidol and 1 mg tromethamine and 0.33 mg edetate calcium disodium. The solution contains approximately 0.036 mg (0.001 mEq) sodium and 250 mg organically bound iodine per mL.
Each mL of ISOVUE-300 (Iopamidol Injection 61%) provides 612 mg iopamidol and 1 mg tromethamine and 0.39 mg ede-

tate calcium disodium. The solution contains approximately 0.043 mg (0.002 mEq) sodium and 300 mg organically bound iodine per mL.
Each mL of ISOVUE-370 (Iopamidol Injection 76%) provides 755 mg iopamidol and 1 mg tromethamine and 0.48 mg edetate calcium disodium. The solution contains approximately 0.053 mg (0.002 mEq) sodium and 370 mg organically bound iodine per mL.
The pH of ISOVUE contrast media has been adjusted to 6.5–7.5 with hydrochloric acid. Pertinent physicochemical data are noted below. ISOVUE (Iopamidol Injection) is hypertonic as compared to plasma and cerebrospinal fluid (approximately 285 and 301 mOsm/kg water, respectively).

Parameter	Iopamidol			
	41%	51%	61%	76%
Concentration (mgI/ml)	200	250	300	370
Osmolality @37°C (mOsm/kg water)	413	524	616	796
Viscosity (cP) @37°C	2.0	3.0	4.7	9.4
@20°C	3.3	5.1	8.8	20.9
Specific Gravity @37°C	1.216	1.281	1.328	1.405

HOW SUPPLIED

ISOVUE-200 (Iopamidol Injection 41%)
  Ten 50mL single dose vials (NDC 0003-1314-30)
  Ten 100mL single dose bottles (NDC 0003-1314-34)
  Ten 200mL single dose bottles (NDC 0003-1314-40)
ISOVUE-250 (Iopamidol Injection 51%)
  Ten 50mL single dose vials (NDC 0003-1317-05)
  Ten 100mL single dose bottles (NDC 0003-1317-02)
  Ten 150mL single dose bottles (NDC 0003-1317-03)
  Ten 200mL single dose bottles (NDC 0003-1317-01)
ISOVUE-300 (Iopamidol Injection 61%)
  Ten 30mL single dose vials (NDC 0003-1315-25)
  Ten 50mL single dose vials (NDC 0003-1315-30)
  Ten 75mL single dose bottles (NDC 0003-1315-47)
  Ten 100mL single dose bottles (NDC 0003-1315-35)
  Ten 150mL single dose bottles (NDC 0003-1315-37)
ISOVUE-370 (Iopamidol Injection 76%)
  Ten 20mL single dose vials (NDC 0003-1316-07)
  Ten 30mL single dose vials (NDC 0003-1316-47)
  Ten 50mL single dose vials (NDC 0003-1316-30)
  Ten 75mL single dose bottles (NDC 0003-1316-52)
  Ten 100mL single dose bottles (NDC 0003-1316-35)
  Ten 150mL single dose bottles (NDC 0003-1316-37)
  Ten 175mL single dose bottles (NDC 0003-1316-44)
  Ten 200mL single dose bottles (NDC 0003-1316-40)

Squibb-Novo, Inc.
(See Novo Nordisk Pharmaceuticals Inc.)

Star Pharmaceuticals, Inc.
1990 N.W. 44TH STREET
POMPANO BEACH, FL 33064-8712

APHRODYNE®   ℞
[af"ro-din']
brand of yohimbine hydrochloride

Each scored aqua caplet contains 5.4 mg yohimbine hydrochloride.

HOW SUPPLIED
Bottles of 100 and 1000.
NDC 0076-0401-03 and 04
Shown in Product Identification Section, page 432

PROSED®/DS   ℞
Tablets/Double Strength

Each dark blue, round sugar-coated tablet contains:
Methenamine ....81.6 mg.
Phenyl Salicylate ....36.2 mg.
Methylene Blue ....10.8 mg.
Benzoic Acid...9.0 mg.
Atropine Sulfate...0.06 mg.
Hyoscyamine Sulfate...................................0.06 mg.

HOW SUPPLIED
Bottles of 100 and 1000
NDC 0076-0108-03 & 04

URO–KP–NEUTRAL®   ℞
[ū'ro-kp-nū'tral]
Phosphorus Supplement

Each peach capsule-shaped, film coated tablet contains:
Phosphorus ....250 mg.
Potassium ....49.4 mg.
Sodium ....250 mg.
Derived from Sodium Phosphate Monobasic Anhydrous, Dipotassium Phosphate Anhydrous, and Disodium Phosphate Anhydrous.

HOW SUPPLIED
Bottles of 100.
NDC 0076-0109-03

UROLENE BLUE®   ℞
[ū'ro-lene blue]
Methylene Blue Tablets

Each blue coated tablet contains Methylene blue USP 65 mg.

HOW SUPPLIED
Bottles of 100 and 1000.
NDC 0076-0501-03 & 04

VIRILON®   ℞ ⓒ
[vir'i-lon]
Methyltestosterone Macro-Beads Capsules
Oral Androgen Macro-Beads

Each capsule contains Methyltestosterone.........USP 10 mg. In a special base. Look for the grey and white seeds in the black and transparent capsule, available only from Star Pharmaceuticals.

HOW SUPPLIED
Bottles of 100 and 1000.
NDC 0076-0301-03 & 04
Shown in Product Identification Section, page 432

VIRILON® IM   ℞ ⓒ
brand of testosterone cypionate
injection sterile solution
200 mg/ml
For Intramuscular Use Only

HOW SUPPLIED
Multiple dose vials of 10 ml containing 200 mg/ml.
NDC 0076-0301-10
Shown in Product Identification Section, page 432

Write for complete prescribing information for all Star products.

EDUCATIONAL MATERIAL

Samples Available to Physicians
APHRODYNE® CAPLETS—4's
  Yohimbine Hydrochloride 5.4 mg
PROSED®/DS—4's
  Methenamine 81.6 mg
  Phenyl Salicylate 36.2 mg
  Methylene Blue 10.8 mg
  Benzoic Acid 9.0 mg
  Atropine Sulfate 0.06 mg
  Hyoscyamine Sulfate 0.06 mg
URO-KP-NEUTRAL CAPLETS—4's
  Orthophosphate Formula
UROLENE® BLUE TABLETS—4's
  Methylene Blue 65 mg
VIRILON® CAPSULES—4's
  Methyltestosterone Macro-Beads 10 mg

IDENTIFICATION PROBLEM?
Consult PDR's
Product Identification Section
where you'll find over 1700
products pictured actual size
and in full color.

Stellar Pharmacal Corp.
1990 N.W. 44TH STREET
POMPANO BEACH, FL 33064-8712

STAR–OTIC® EAR SOLUTION   OTC

(See PDR For Nonprescription Drugs.)

STAR-OPTIC® EYE WASH   OTC

(See PDR For Nonprescription Drugs.)

Stiefel Laboratories, Inc.
2801 PONCE DE LEON BLVD.
CORAL GABLES, FL 33134

BREVOXYL®   ℞
[brĕv-ăhx-il]
(benzoyl peroxide 4%)

DESCRIPTION
Brevoxyl is a topical preparation containing benzoyl peroxide 4% as the active ingredient in a gel vehicle containing purified water, cetyl alcohol, dimethyl isosorbide, fragrance, simethicone, stearyl alcohol and ceteareth-20. The structural formula of benzoyl peroxide is:

CLINICAL PHARMACOLOGY
The exact method of action of benzoyl peroxide in acne vulgaris is not known. Benzoyl peroxide is an antibacterial agent with demonstrated activity against *Propionibacterium acnes*. This action, combined with the mild keratolytic effect of benzoyl peroxide is believed to be responsible for its usefulness in acne.
Benzoyl peroxide is absorbed by the skin where it is metabolized to benzoic acid and excreted as benzoate in the urine.

INDICATIONS AND USAGE
Brevoxyl is indicated for use in the topical treatment of mild to moderate acne vulgaris. Brevoxyl may be used as an adjunct in acne treatment regimens including antibiotics, retinoic acid products, and sulfur/salicylic acid containing preparations.

CONTRAINDICATIONS
Brevoxyl should not be used in patients who have shown hypersensitivity to benzoyl peroxide or to any of the other ingredients in the product.

PRECAUTIONS
General—For external use only. Avoid contact with eyes and mucous membranes. **AVOID CONTACT WITH HAIR, FABRICS OR CARPETING AS BENZOYL PEROXIDE WILL CAUSE BLEACHING.**
Carcinogenesis, Mutagenesis, Impairment of Fertility—Based upon all available evidence, benzoyl peroxide is not considered to be a carcinogen. However, data from a study using mice known to be highly susceptible to cancer suggest that benzoyl peroxide acts as a tumor promoter. The clinical significance of the findings is not known.
Pregnancy: Category C—Animal reproduction studies have not been conducted with benzoyl peroxide. It is also not known whether benzoyl peroxide can cause fetal harm when administered to a pregnant woman or can affect reproduction capacity. Benzoyl peroxide should be used by a pregnant woman only if clearly needed.
Nursing Mothers—It is not known whether this drug is excreted in human milk. Because many drugs are excreted in human milk, caution should be exercised when benzoyl peroxide is administered to a nursing woman.
Pediatric Use—Safety and effectiveness in children below the age of 12 have not been established.

ADVERSE REACTIONS
Contact sensitization reactions are associated with the use of topical benzoyl peroxide products and may be expected to occur in 10 to 25 of 1000 patients. The most frequent adverse reactions associated with benzoyl peroxide use are excessive erythema and peeling which may be expected to occur in 5 of 100 patients. Excessive erythema and peeling most frequently appear during the initial phase of drug use and may normally be controlled by reducing frequency of use.

DOSAGE AND ADMINISTRATION
Brevoxyl should be applied once or twice daily to affected areas. Frequency of use should be adjusted to obtain the desired clinical response. Gentle cleansing of the affected areas

prior to application of Brevoxyl may be beneficial. Clinically visible improvement will normally occur by the third week of therapy. Maximum lesion reduction may be expected after approximately eight to twelve weeks of drug use. Continuing use of the drug is normally required to maintain a satisfactory clinical response.

HOW SUPPLIED
Brevoxyl is supplied in 42.5 g (1.5 oz.) tubes NDC 0145-2374-06.
Store at controlled room temperature 15°–30°C (59°–86°F).

LACTICARE®–HC Lotion 1%, 2½%   ℞
[lăk 'tĭ-kār "]
(hydrocortisone lotion, USP)

CONTAINS
Each ml of LactiCare-HC Lotion 1% and 2½% (hydrocortisone lotion, USP) contains 10 mg and 25 mg respectively of hydrocortisone in a vehicle consisting of carbomer 940, sodium PCA, lactic acid, sodium hydroxide, stearyl alcohol (and) ceteareth-20, glyceryl stearate (and) PEG-100 stearate, cetyl alcohol, isopropyl palmitate, light mineral oil, myristyl lactate, DMDM hydantoin, dehydroacetic acid, fragrance and purified water.

HOW SUPPLIED
2½%—2 fl. oz. bottle NDC 0145-2538-02
1%—4 fl. oz. bottle NDC 0145-2537-04

PANOXYL® 5   ℞
[pan 'ăhx-il]
(benzoyl peroxide 5%)
PANOXYL® 10   ℞
(benzoyl peroxide 10%)

HOW SUPPLIED
PanOxyl 5 and PanOxyl 10 are supplied in 2.0 ounce and 4.0 ounce tubes.
PanOxyl 5
2.0 oz. tube NDC 0145-2372-06
4.0 oz. tube NDC 0145-2372-08
PanOxyl 10
2.0 oz. tube NDC 0145-2373-06
4.0 oz. tube NDC 0145-2373-08
U.S. Patent 4056611

PANOXYL® AQ 2½   ℞
[pan 'ăhx-il]
(benzoyl peroxide 2½%)
PANOXYL® AQ 5   ℞
(benzoyl peroxide 5%)
PANOXYL® AQ 10   ℞
(benzoyl peroxide 10%)

HOW SUPPLIED
PanOxyl AQ 2½, PanOxyl AQ 5, and PanOxyl AQ 10 are supplied in 2.0 ounce and 4.0 ounce tubes.
PanOxyl AQ 2½
2.0 oz. tube NDC 0145-2375-06
4.0 oz. tube NDC 0145-2375-08
PanOxyl AQ 5
2.0 oz. tube NDC 0145-2376-06
4.0 oz. tube NDC 0145-2376-08
PanOxyl AQ 10
2.0 oz. tube NDC 0145-2377-06
4.0 oz. tube NDC 0145-2377-08

SULFOXYL® Lotion Regular   ℞
SULFOXYL® Lotion Strong   ℞
[sul 'fox-ul]

HOW SUPPLIED
Sulfoxyl Lotion Regular and Sulfoxyl Lotion Strong are supplied in 2.0 ounce plastic bottles.

Sulfoxyl Lotion Regular	Sulfoxyl Lotion Strong
NDC 0145-3518-07	NDC 0145-3519-07

Products are cross-indexed by
generic and chemical names in the
YELLOW SECTION.

Stuart Pharmaceuticals
A business unit of ICI Americas Inc.
WILMINGTON, DE 19897 USA

BUCLADIN®-S SOFTAB® Chewable Tablets   ℞
[bu 'cla-din]
(buclizine hydrochloride)

EACH TABLET CONTAINS:
BUCLIZINE HYDROCHLORIDE .... 50 mg

DESCRIPTION
Buclizine hydrochloride is 1-(p-tert-Butylbenzyl) -4- (p-chloro- α -phenylbenzyl) piperazine dihydrochloride. Each tablet contains 50 mg buclizine hydrochloride.
Inactive Ingredients: citric acid, flavor, magnesium stearate, mannitol, microcrystalline cellulose, povidone, starch, Yellow 5 (tartrazine).

ACTIONS
BUCLADIN-S (buclizine hydrochloride) acts centrally to suppress nausea and vomiting.

INDICATIONS
BUCLADIN-S is effective in the management of nausea, vomiting, and dizziness associated with motion sickness.

CONTRAINDICATIONS
Buclizine hydrochloride, when administered to the pregnant rat, induced fetal abnormalities at doses above the human therapeutic range. Clinical data are not adequate to establish nonteratogenicity in early pregnancy. Until such data are available, buclizine hydrochloride is contraindicated for use in early pregnancy.
Buclizine hydrochloride is contraindicated in individuals who have shown a previous hypersensitivity to it.

WARNINGS
Since drowsiness may occur with use of this drug, patients should be warned of this possibility and cautioned against engaging in activities requiring mental alertness, such as driving a car, or operating heavy machinery or appliances. Safe and effective dosage in children has not been established.

PRECAUTION
This product contains Yellow 5 (tartrazine) which may cause allergic-type reactions (including bronchial asthma) in certain susceptible individuals. Although the overall incidence of Yellow 5 (tartrazine) sensitivity in the general population is low, it is frequently seen in patients who also have aspirin hypersensitivity.

ADVERSE REACTIONS
Occasionally drowsiness, dryness of mouth, headache, and jitteriness are encountered.

DOSAGE AND ADMINISTRATION
BUCLADIN-S (buclizine hydrochloride) SOFTAB Tablets can be taken without swallowing water. Place the SOFTAB Tablet in the mouth and allow it to dissolve, or the tablet may be chewed.
ADULTS: One tablet usually serves to alleviate nausea. In severe cases, three tablets a day may be taken. The usual maintenance dosage is one tablet twice daily.
In the prevention of motion sickness, one tablet taken at least ½ hour before beginning travel usually suffices. For extended travel, a second tablet may be taken after 4 to 6 hours.

HOW SUPPLIED
Bottles of 100 scored, yellow, SOFTAB Tablets, embossed front "STUART," reverse "864."
Store at room temperature; avoid excess heat (over 104°F/40°C). Dispense in well-closed light resistant container. NDC 0038-0864.
Manufactured for
Stuart Pharmaceuticals
A business unit of ICI Americas Inc.
Wilmington, DE 19897 USA   Rev G 07/90
Shown in Product Identification Section, page 432

CEFOTAN®   ℞
[cef 'o-tan "]
(cefotetan disodium)
For Intravenous or Intramuscular Use

PRODUCT OVERVIEW

KEY FACTS
CEFOTAN (cefotetan disodium) is a semisynthetic, broad-spectrum, beta-lactamase stable, cephalosporin (cephamycin) antibiotic for parenteral administration. The bactericidal action for cefotetan results from inhibition of cell wall synthesis. Therefore, CEFOTAN is exquisitely active against a wide range of gram-negative aerobes. Like other cephamycins, CEFOTAN exhibits good activity against *Bacteroides*

fragilis and many other anaerobic organisms. The plasma elimination half-life of CEFOTAN is 3 to 4.6 hours after either intravenous or intramuscular administration allowing twice-daily dosing for the treatment of indicated infections and single dose prophylaxis in appropriate surgical procedures.

MAJOR USES

CEFOTAN is indicated for the treatment of the following infections caused by susceptible organisms:
- Gynecologic Infections
- Intra-abdominal Infections
- Skin and Skin Structure Infections

The preoperative administration of CEFOTAN may reduce the incidence of certain postoperative infections in patients undergoing surgical procedures that are classified as clean contaminated or potentially contaminated (eg, cesarean section, abdominal or vaginal hysterectomy, transurethral surgery, biliary tract surgery, and gastrointestinal surgery).

SAFETY INFORMATION

CEFOTAN is contraindicated in patients with known allergy to the cephalosporin group of antibiotics. In patients with renal impairment, dosage adjustment is necessary.

PRESCRIBING INFORMATION

DESCRIPTION

CEFOTAN® (cefotetan disodium) is a sterile, semisynthetic, broad-spectrum, beta-lactamase resistant, cephalosporin (cephamycin) antibiotic for parenteral administration. It is the disodium salt of [6*R*-(6α, 7α)]-7-[[[4-(2-amino-1-carboxy-2-oxoethylidene)-1,3-dithietan-2-yl]carbonyl]amino]-7-methoxy-3-[[(1-methyl-1*H*-tetrazol-5-yl)thio]methyl]-8-oxo-5-thia-1-azabicyclo [4.2.0]oct-2-ene-2-carboxylic acid. Its molecular formula is $C_{17}H_{15}N_7Na_2O_8S_4$ with a molecular weight of 619.56.

Structural Formula

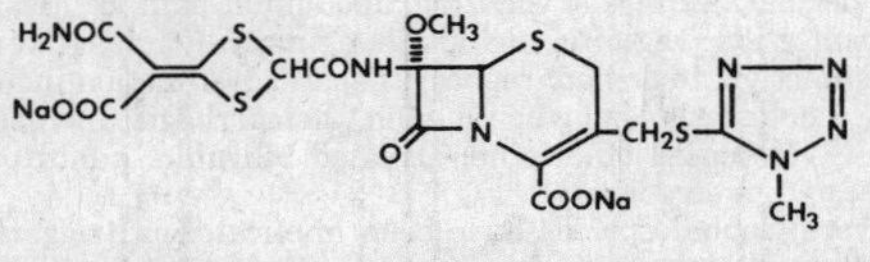

CEFOTAN contains approximately 80 mg (3.5 mEq) of sodium per gram of cefotetan activity. It is a white to pale yellow powder which is very soluble in water. The solution varies from colorless to yellow depending on the concentration. The pH of freshly reconstituted solutions is usually between 4.5 to 6.5.

PHARMACY BULK PACKAGE

This is a container of sterile powder for reconstitution intended for parenteral use and contains many single doses. The contents are intended for use in a pharmacy admixture program and are restricted to the preparation of admixtures for intravenous infusion or the filling of empty sterile syringes for intravenous injection for patients with individualized dosing requirements.

CLINICAL PHARMACOLOGY

High plasma levels of cefotetan are attained after intravenous and intramuscular administration of single doses to normal volunteers.

PLASMA CONCENTRATIONS AFTER 1.0 GRAM IV[a] or IM DOSE
Mean Plasma Concentration (μg/mL)

	Time After Injection						
Route	15 min	30 min	1h	2h	4h	8h	12h
IV	92	158	103	72	42	18	9
IM	34	56	71	68	47	20	9

[a]30-minute infusion

PLASMA CONCENTRATIONS AFTER 2.0 GRAM IV[a] or IM DOSE
Mean Plasma Concentration (μg/mL)

	Time After Injection						
Route	5 min	10 min	1h	3h	5h	9h	12h
IV	237	223	135	74	48	22	12[b]
IM	—	20	75	91	69	33	19

[a] Injected over 3 minutes
[b] Concentrations estimated from regression line

The plasma elimination half-life of cefotetan is 3 to 4.6 hours after either intravenous or intramuscular administration. Repeated administration of CEFOTAN® does not result in accumulation of the drug in normal subjects.

Cefotetan is 88% plasma protein bound.

No active metabolites of cefotetan have been detected; however, small amounts (less than 7%) of cefotetan in plasma and urine may be converted to its tautomer, which has antimicrobial activity similar to the parent drug.

In normal patients, from 51% to 81% of an administered dose of CEFOTAN is excreted unchanged by the kidneys over a 24 hour period, which results in high and prolonged urinary concentrations. Following intravenous doses of 1 gram and 2 grams, urinary concentrations are highest during the first hour and reach concentrations of approximately 1700 and 3500 μg/mL respectively.

In patients with reduced renal function, the plasma half-life of cefotetan is prolonged.

Therapeutic levels of cefotetan are achieved in many body tissues and fluids including:

skin	ureter
muscle	bladder
fat	maxillary sinus mucosa
myometrium	tonsil
endometrium	bile
cervix	peritoneal fluid
ovary	umbilical cord serum
kidney	amniotic fluid

MICROBIOLOGY

The bactericidal action of cefotetan results from inhibition of cell wall synthesis. Cefotetan has *in vitro* activity against a wide range of aerobic and anaerobic gram-positive and gram-negative organisms. The methoxy group in the 7-alpha position provides cefotetan with a high degree of stability in the presence of beta-lactamases including both penicillinases and cephalosporinases of gram-negative bacteria.

Cefotetan has been shown to be active against most strains of the following organisms **both *in vitro* and in clinical infections (see INDICATIONS AND USAGE).**

Gram-Negative Aerobes
Escherichia coli
Haemophilus influenzae (including ampicillin-resistant strains)
Klebsiella species (including *K pneumoniae)*
Morganella morganii
Neisseria gonorrhoeae (nonpenicillinase-producing strains)
Proteus mirabilis
Proteus vulgaris
Providencia rettgeri
Serratia marcescens

NOTE: Approximately one-half of the usually clinically significant strains of *Enterobacter* species, (e.g., *E. aerogenes* and *E. cloacae*) are resistant to cefotetan. Most strains of *Pseudomonas aeruginosa* and *Acinetobacter* species are resistant to cefotetan.

Gram-Positive Aerobes
Staphylococcus aureus (including penicillinase- and nonpenicillinase-producing strains)
Staphylococcus epidermidis
Streptococcus agalactiae (group B beta-hemolytic streptococcus)
Streptococcus pneumoniae
Streptococcus pyogenes (group A beta-hemolytic streptococcus)

NOTE: Methicillin-resistant staphylococci are resistant to cephalosporins, some strains of *Staphylococcus epidermidis* and most strains of enterococci, e.g., *Enterococcus faecalis* (formerly *Streptococcus faecalis*) are resistant to cefotetan.

Anaerobes
Bacteroides bivius
Bacteroides disiens
Bacteroides fragilis
Bacteroides melaninogenicus
Bacteroides vulgatus
Fusobacterium species
Gram-positive bacilli (including *Clostridium* species)

NOTE: Many strains of *C. difficile* are resistant (see WARNINGS).

Peptococcus niger
Peptostreptococcus species

NOTE: Many strains of *B. distasonis, B. ovatus* and *B. thetaiotaomicron* are resistant to cefotetan.

The following *in vitro* data are available but their clinical significance is unknown. Cefotetan has been shown to be active *in vitro* against most strains of the following organisms:

Gram-Negative Aerobes
Citrobacter species (including *C. diversus* and *C. freundii*)
Klebsiella oxytoca
Moraxella (Branhamella) catarrhalis
Neisseria gonorrhoeae (penicillinase-producing strains)
Salmonella species
Serratia species
Shigella species
Yersinia enterocolitica

Anaerobes
Bacteroides asaccharolyticus
Bacteroides oralis
Bacteroides splanchnicus
Clostridium difficile

NOTE: Many strains of *C. difficile* are resistant (see WARNINGS).

Propionbacterium species
Veillonella species

SUSCEPTIBILITY TESTS

Diffusion Technique: Quantitative methods that require measurement of zone diameters give the most precise estimate of antibiotic susceptibility. One such procedure[1] has been recommended for use with disks to test susceptibility to cefotetan. Organisms should be tested with the cefotetan 30 μg disk since cefotetan has been shown to be active *in vitro* against organisms which were found to be resistant to other beta-lactam antibiotics.

Reports from the laboratory with results of standardized single-disk susceptibility tests with a 30 μg cefotetan disk should be interpreted according to the following criteria:

Susceptible organisms produce zone sizes of 16 mm or greater, indicating that the tested organism is likely to respond to therapy.

Moderately susceptible organisms produce zones of 13 to 15 mm indicating the test organism would be susceptible if high dosage is used or if the infection is confined to tissues and fluids (e.g., urine) in which high antibiotic levels are attained.

Resistant organisms produce zones of 12 mm or less, indicating that other therapy should be selected.

Standardized procedures require the use of laboratory control organisms. The 30 μg cefotetan disk should give zone diameters between 17 and 23 mm for *S. aureus* ATCC 25923. For *E. coli* ATCC 25922, the zone diameters should be between 28 to 34 mm.

Dilution Techniques: In other susceptibility testing procedures, e.g., NCCLS broth microdilution or agar dilution methods[2] or equivalent, a bacterial isolate may be considered susceptible if the MIC value for cefotetan is 16 μg/mL or less. Organisms with an MIC of 32 μg/mL are considered moderately susceptible. Organisms are considered resistant to cefotetan if the MIC is equal to or greater than 64 μg/mL. As with standard diffusion methods, dilution procedures require the use of laboratory control organisms. Cefotetan should give MIC values in the range of 4 μg/mL and 16 μg/mL for *S. aureus* ATCC 29213. For *E. coli* ATCC 25922, the MIC range should be between 0.06 μg/mL and 0.25 μg/mL.

INDICATIONS AND USAGE

TREATMENT

CEFOTAN® (cefotetan disodium) is indicated for the therapeutic treatment of the following infections when caused by susceptible strains of the designated organisms:

Urinary Tract Infections caused by *E. coli, Klebsiella* species (including *K. pneumoniae*), *Proteus mirabilis* and *Proteus* sp (which may include the organisms now called *Proteus vulgaris, Providencia rettgeri,* and *Morganella morganii*).

Lower Respiratory Tract Infections caused by *Streptococcus pneumoniae* (formerly *D. pneumoniae*), *Staphylococcus aureus* (penicillinase- and nonpenicillinase-producing strains), *Haemophilus influenzae* (including ampicillin-resistant strains), *Klebsiella* species (including *K. pneumoniae*), *E. coli, Proteus mirabilis,* and *Serratia marcescens**.

Skin and Skin Structure Infections due to *Staphylococcus aureus* (penicillinase- and nonpenicillinase-producing strains), *Staphylococcus epidermidis, Streptococcus pyogenes Streptococcus* species (excluding enterococci), *Escherichia coli, Klebsiella pneumoniae, Peptococcus niger*, and Peptostreptococcus* species.

Gynecologic Infections caused by *Staphylococcus aureus,* (including penicillinase- and nonpenicillinase-producing strains), *Staphylococcus epidermidis, Streptococcus* species (excluding enterococci), *Streptococcus agalactiae, E. coli, Proteus mirabilis, Neisseria gonorrhoeae,* Bacteroides species (excluding *B. distasonis, B. ovatus, B. thetaiotaomicron*), *Fusobacterium* species*, and gram-positive anaerobic cocci (including *Peptococcus niger* and *Peptostreptococcus* species).

Cefotetan, like other cephalosporins, has no activity against *Chlamydia trachomatis.* Therefore, when cephalosporins are used in the treatment of pelvic inflammatory disease, and *C. trachomatis* is one of the suspected pathogens, appropriate antichlamydial coverage should be added.

Intra-abdominal Infections caused by *E. coli, Klebsiella* species (including *K. pneumoniae, Streptococcus* species (excluding enterococci), *Bacteroides* species (excluding *B. distasonis, B. ovatus, B. thetaiotaomicron*) and *Clostridium* species*.

Bone and Joint Infections caused by *Staphylococcus aureus.**

*Efficacy for this organism in this organ system was studied in fewer than ten infections.

Specimens for bacteriological examination should be obtained in order to isolate and identify causative organisms and to determine their susceptibilities to cefotetan. Therapy may be instituted before results of susceptibility studies are known; however, once these results become available, the antibiotic treatment should be adjusted accordingly.

Continued on next page

Stuart—Cont.

In cases of confirmed or suspected gram-positive or gram-negative sepsis or in patients with other serious infections in which the causative organism has not been identified, it is possible to use CEFOTAN® (cefotetan disodium) concomitantly with an aminoglycoside. Cefotetan combinations with aminoglycosides have been shown to be synergistic *in vitro* against many Enterobacteriaceae and also some other gram-negative bacteria. The dosage recommended in the labeling of both antibiotics may be given and depends on the severity of the infection and the patient's condition.

NOTE: If CEFOTAN and an aminoglycoside are used concomitantly, renal function should be carefully monitored, especially if higher dosages of the aminoglycoside are to be administered or if therapy is prolonged, because of the potential nephrotoxicity and ototoxicity of aminoglycosidic antibiotics. Although, to date, nephrotoxicity has not been noted when CEFOTAN was given alone, it is possible that nephrotoxicity may be potentiated if CEFOTAN is used concomitantly with an aminoglycoside.

PROPHYLAXIS

The preoperative administration of CEFOTAN may reduce the incidence of certain postoperative infections in patients undergoing surgical procedures that are classified as clean contaminated or potentially contaminated (eg, cesarean section, abdominal or vaginal hysterectomy, transurethral surgery, biliary tract surgery, and gastrointestinal surgery). The prophylactic dose of CEFOTAN should be administered 30 to 60 minutes prior to surgery. In patients undergoing cesarean section, CEFOTAN should be administered intravenously after the clamping of the umbilical cord.

If there are signs and symptoms of infection, specimens for culture should be obtained for identification of the causative organism so that appropriate therapeutic measures may be initiated.

CONTRAINDICATIONS

CEFOTAN is contraindicated in patients with known allergy to the cephalosporin group of antibiotics.

WARNINGS

BEFORE THERAPY WITH CEFOTAN IS INSTITUTED, CAREFUL INQUIRY SHOULD BE MADE TO DETERMINE WHETHER THE PATIENT HAS HAD PREVIOUS HYPERSENSITIVITY REACTIONS TO CEFOTETAN DISODIUM, CEPHALOSPORINS, PENICILLINS, OR OTHER DRUGS. IF THIS PRODUCT IS TO BE GIVEN TO PENICILLIN-SENSITIVE PATIENTS, CAUTION SHOULD BE EXERCISED BECAUSE CROSS-HYPERSENSITIVITY AMONG BETA-LACTAM ANTIBIOTICS HAS BEEN CLEARLY DOCUMENTED AND MAY OCCUR IN UP TO 10% OF PATIENTS WITH A HISTORY OF PENICILLIN ALLERGY. IF AN ALLERGIC REACTION TO CEFOTAN OCCURS, DISCONTINUE THE DRUG. SERIOUS ACUTE HYPERSENSITIVITY REACTIONS MAY REQUIRE TREATMENT WITH EPINEPHRINE AND OTHER EMERGENCY MEASURES, INCLUDING OXYGEN, INTRAVENOUS FLUIDS, INTRAVENOUS ANTIHISTAMINES, CORTICOSTEROIDS, PRESSOR AMINES AND AIRWAY MANAGEMENT, AS CLINICALLY INDICATED.

Pseudomembranous colitis has been reported with nearly all antibacterial agents, including cefotetan, and may range from mild to life-threatening. Onset of pseudomembranous colitis symptoms may occur during or after antibiotic treatment or surgical prophylaxis. Therefore, it is important to consider this diagnosis in patients who present with diarrhea subsequent to the administration of antibacterial agents.

Treatment with antibacterial agents alters the normal flora of the colon and may permit overgrowth of clostridia. Studies indicate that a toxin produced by *Clostridium difficile* is a primary cause of "antibiotic-associated colitis".

After the diagnosis of pseudomembranous colitis has been established, therapeutic measures should be initiated. Mild cases of pseudomembranous colitis usually respond to discontinuation of the drug alone. In moderate to severe cases, consideration should be given to management with fluids and electrolytes, protein supplementation, and treatment with an oral antibacterial drug effective against *Clostridium difficile*.

In common with many other broad-spectrum antibiotics, CEFOTAN® (cefotetan disodium) may be associated with a fall in prothrombin activity and, possibly, subsequent bleeding. Those at increased risk include patients with renal or hepatobiliary impairment or poor nutritional state, the elderly, and patients with cancer. Prothrombin time should be monitored and exogenous vitamin K administered as indicated.

PRECAUTIONS

General: As with other broad-spectrum antibiotics, prolonged use of CEFOTAN may result in overgrowth of nonsusceptible organisms. Careful observation of the patient is essential. If superinfection does occur during therapy, appropriate measures should be taken.

CEFOTAN should be used with caution in individuals with a history of gastrointestinal disease, particularly colitis.

Information for Patients: As with some other cephalosporins, a disulfiram-like reaction characterized by flushing, sweating, headache, and tachycardia may occur when alcohol (beer, wine, etc) is ingested within 72 hours after CEFOTAN administration. Patients should be cautioned about the ingestion of alcoholic beverages following the administration of CEFOTAN.

Drug Interactions: Although to date nephrotoxicity has not been noted when CEFOTAN was given alone, it is possible that nephrotoxicity may be potentiated if CEFOTAN is used concomitantly with an aminoglycoside.

Drug/Laboratory Test Interactions: The administration of CEFOTAN may result in a false-positive rection for glucose in the urine using Clinitest®†, Benedict's solution, or Fehling's solution. It is recommended that glucose tests based on enzymatic glucose oxidase be used.

As with other cephalosporins, high concentrations of cefotetan may intefere with measurement of serum and urine creatinine levels by Jaffe reaction and produce false increases in the levels of creatinine reported.

Carcinogenesis, Mutagenesis, Impairment of Fertility: Although long-term studies in animals have not been performed to evaluate carcinogenic potential, no mutagenic potential of cefotetan was found in standard laboratory tests. Cefotetan has adverse effects on the testes of prepubertal rats. Subcutaneous administration of 500 mg/kg/day (approximately 8–16 times the usual adult human dose) on days 6–35 of life (thought to be developmentally analogous to late childhood and prepuberty in humans) resulted in reduced testicular weight and seminiferous tubule degeneration in 10 of 10 animals. Affected cells included spermatogonia and spermatocytes; Sertoli and Leydig cells were unaffected. Incidence and severity of lesions were dose-dependent; at 120 mg/kg/day (approximately 2–4 times the usual human dose) only 1 of 10 treated animals was affected, and the degree of degeneration was mild.

Similar lesions have been observed in experiments of comparable design with other methylthiotetrazole-containing antibiotics and impaired fertility has been reported, particularly at high dose levels. No testicular effects were observed in 7-week-old rats treated with up to 1000 mg/kg/day SC for 5 weeks, or in infant dogs (3 weeks old) that received up to 300 mg/kg/day IV for 5 weeks. The relevance of these findings to humans is unknown.

Pregnancy: Teratogenic Effects. Pregnancy Category B: Reproduction studies have been performed in rats and monkeys at doses up to 20 times the human dose and have revealed no evidence of impaired fertility or harm to the fetus due to cefotetan. There are, however, no adequate and well-controlled studies in pregnant women. Because animal re-

productive studies are not always predictive of human response, this drug should be used during pregnancy only if clearly needed.

Nursing Mothers: Cefotetan is excreted in human milk in very low concentrations. Caution should be exercised when cefotetan is administered to a nursing woman.

Pediatric Use: Safety and effectiveness in children have not been established.

ADVERSE REACTIONS

In clinical studies the following adverse effects were considered related to CEFOTAN therapy. Those appearing in italics have been reported during postmarketing experience.

Gastrointestinal symptoms occurred in 1.5% of patients, the most frequent were diarrhea (1 in 80) and nausea (1 in 700); *pseudomembranous colitis.* Onset of pseudomembranous colitis symptoms may occur during or after antibiotic treatment or surgical prophylaxis. (See WARNINGS.)

Hematologic laboratory abnormalities occurred in 1.4% of patients and included eosinophilia (1 in 200), positive direct Coombs' test (1 in 250), and thrombocytosis (1 in 300); *agranulocytosis, hemolytic anemia, leukopenia, thrombocytopenia, and prolonged prothrombin time with or without bleeding.*

Hepatic enzyme elevations occurred in 1.2% of patients and included a rise in SGPT (1 in 150), SGOT (1 in 300), alkaline phosphatase (1 in 700), and LDH (1 in 700).

Hypersensitivity reactions were reported in 1.2% of patients and included rash (1 in 150) and itching (1 in 700); *anaphylactic reactions.*

Local effects were reported in less than 1.0% of patients and included phlebitis at the site of injection (1 in 300), and discomfort (1 in 500).

Miscellaneous: *Fever*

In addition to the adverse reactions listed above which have been observed in patients treated with cefotetan, the following adverse reactions and altered laboratory tests have been reported for cephalosporin-class antibiotics: urticaria, pruritis, Stevens-Johnson syndrome, erythema multiforme, toxic epidermal necrolysis, vomiting, abdominal pain, colitis, superinfection, vaginitis including vaginal candidiasis, renal dysfunction, toxic nephropathy, hepatic dysfunction including cholestasis, aplastic anemia, hemorrhage, increased BUN, increased creatinine, elevated bilirubin, pancytopenia, and neutropenia.

Several cephalosporins have been implicated in triggering seizures, particularly in patients with renal impairment when the dosage was not reduced (see DOSAGE AND ADMINISTRATION and OVERDOSAGE). If seizures associated with drug therapy occur, the drug should be discontinued. Anticonvulsant therapy can be given if clinically indicated.

OVERDOSAGE

Information on overdosage with CEFOTAN® (cefotetan disodium) in humans is not available. If overdosage should occur, it should be treated symptomatically and hemodialysis considered, particularly if renal function is compromised.

DOSAGE AND ADMINISTRATION

TREATMENT

The usual adult dosage is 1 or 2 grams of CEFOTAN administered intravenously or intramuscularly every 12 hours for 5 to 10 days. Proper dosage and route of administration should be determined by the condition of the patient, severity of the infection, and susceptibility of the causative organism. [See table below.]

If *C. trachomatis* is a suspected pathogen in gynecologic infections, appropriate antichlamydial coverage should be added, since cefotetan has no activity against this organism.

PROPHYLAXIS

To prevent postoperative infection in clean contaminated or potentially contaminated surgery in adults, the recommended dosage is 1 or 2 g of CEFOTAN administered once, intravenously 30 to 60 minutes prior to surgery. In patients undergoing cesarean section, the dose should be administered as soon as the umbilical cord is clamped.

IMPAIRED RENAL FUNCTION

When renal function is impaired, a reduced dosage schedule must be employed. The following dosage guidelines may be used.

[See table on top of next page.]

Alternatively, the dosing interval may remain constant at 12 hour intervals, but the dose reduced to one-half the usual recommended dose for patients with a creatinine clearance of 10–30 mL/min, and one-quarter the usual recommended dose for patients with a creatinine clearance of less than 10 mL/min.

When only serum creatinine levels are available, creatinine clearance may be calculated from the following formula. The serum creatinine level should represent a steady state of renal function.

Males: $$\frac{\text{Weight (kg)} \times (140 - \text{age})}{72 \times \text{serum creatinine (mg/100 mL)}}$$

Females: $0.9 \times$ value for males

Cefotetan is dialyzable and it is recommended that for patients undergoing intermittent hemodialysis, one-quarter of

GENERAL GUIDELINES FOR DOSAGE OF CEFOTAN

Type of Infection	Daily Dose	Frequency and Route
Urinary Tract	1–4 grams	500 mg every 12 hours IV or IM 1 or 2 g every 24 hours IV or IM 1 or 2 g every 12 hours IV or IM
Skin & Skin Structure Mild–Moderate[a]	2 grams	2 g every 24 hours IV 1 g every 12 hours IV or IM
Severe	4 grams	2 g every 12 hours IV
Other Sites	2–4 grams	1 or 2 g every 12 hours IV or IM
Severe	4 grams	2 g every 12 hours IV
Life-Threatening	6 grams[b]	3 g every 12 hours IV

[a] *K. pneumoniae* skin and skin skin structure infections should be treated with 1 or 2 grams every 12 hours IV or IM.
[b] Maximum daily dosage should not exceed 6 grams.

DOSAGE GUIDELINES FOR PATIENTS WITH IMPAIRED RENAL FUNCTION

Creatinine Clearance mL/min	Dose	Frequency
> 30	Usual Recommended Dosage*	Every 12 hours
10–30	Usual Recommended Dosage*	Every 24 hours
< 10	Usual Recommended Dosage*	Every 48 hours

*Dose determined by the type and severity of infection, and susceptibility of the causative organism.

the usual recommended dose be given every 24 hours on days between dialysis and one-half the usual recommended dose on the day of dialysis.

PREPARATION OF SOLUTION

For Intravenous Use: Reconstitute with Sterile Water for Injection. Shake to dissolve and let stand until clear.

Vial Size	Amount of Diluent Added (mL)	Approximate Withdrawable Vol (mL)	Approximate Average Concentration (mg/mL)
1 gram	10	10.5	95
2 gram	10–20	11.0–21.0	182–95

Infusion bottles (100 mL) may be reconstituted with 50 to 100 mL of 5% Dextrose Solution or 0.9% Sodium Chloride Solution.

For Intramuscular Use: Reconstitute with Sterile Water for Injection; Bacteriostatic Water for Injection; Normal Saline, USP; 0.5% Lidocaine HCl; or 1.0% Lidocaine HCl. Shake to dissolve and let stand until clear.

Vial Size	Amount of Diluent Added (mL)	Approximate Withdrawable Vol (mL)	Approximate Average Concentration (mg/mL)
1 gram	2	2.5	400
2 gram	3	4.0	500

For Pharmacy Bulk Package: Reconstitute with Sterile Water for Injection; 5% Dextrose Solution; or 0.9% Sodium Chloride Solution. Shake to dissolve and let stand until clear. (See PROPER USE OF PHARMACY BULK PACKAGE) [See table below.]

INTRAVENOUS ADMINISTRATION

The intravenous route is preferable for patients with bacteremia, bacterial septicemia, or other severe or life-threatening infections, or for patients who may be poor risks because of lowered resistance resulting from such debilitating conditions as malnutrition, trauma, surgery, diabetes, heart failure, or malignancy, particularly if shock is present or impending.

For intermittent intravenous administration, a solution containing 1 gram or 2 grams of CEFOTAN® (cefotetan disodium) in Sterile Water for Injection can be injected over a period of three to five minutes. Using an infusion system, the solution may also be given over a longer period of time through the tubing system by which the patient may be receiving other intravenous solutions. Butterfly® or scalp vein-type needles are preferred for this type of infusion. However, during infusion of the solution containing CEFOTAN, it is advisable to discontinue temporarily the administration of other solutions at the same site.

NOTE: Solutions of CEFOTAN must not be admixed with solutions containing aminoglycosides. If CEFOTAN and aminoglycosides are to be administered to the same patient, they must be administered separately and not as a mixed injection.

INTRAMUSCULAR ADMINISTRATION

As with all intramuscular preparations, CEFOTAN® (cefotetan disodium) should be injected well within the body of a relatively large muscle such as the upper outer quadrant of the buttock (ie, gluteus maximus); aspiration is necessary to avoid inadvertent injection into a blood vessel.

COMPATIBILITY AND STABILITY

CEFOTAN reconstituted as described above (PREPARATION OF SOLUTION) maintains satisfactory potency for 24 hours at room temperature (25°C), for 96 hours under refrigeration (5°C), and for at least 1 week in the frozen state. After reconstitution and subsequent storage in disposable glass or plastic syringes, CEFOTAN is stable for 24 hours at room temperature and 96 hours under refrigeration.

Frozen samples should be thawed at room temperature before use. After the periods mentioned above, any unused solutions or frozen materials should be discarded. Do not refreeze.

NOTE: Parenteral drug products should be inspected visually for particulate matter and discoloration prior to administration whenever solution and container permit.

PROPER USE OF PHARMACY BULK PACKAGE

The closure may be penetrated only one time after reconstitution. If necessary, the use of a suitable sterile transfer device or dispensing set which allows measured dispensing of the contents should be considered.

Use of this package is restricted to a suitable work area, such as a laminar flow hood. The aliquotting operation should be completed promptly after reconstitution of the contents (see PREPARATION OF SOLUTION). Product dispensed in this manner should be administered within 24 hours if stored at room temperature, 96 hours if stored under refrigeration (5°C), and 1 week if stored in the frozen state. Any unused portion must be discarded within 24 hours after initial entry.

Vial Size	Amount of Diluent to be Added (mL)	Approximate Withdrawable Vol (mL)	Approximate Average Concentration (mg/mL)
10 g Pharmacy Bulk	50	55	180
10 g Pharmacy Bulk	100	105	95

HOW SUPPLIED

CEFOTAN is a dry, white to pale yellow powder supplied in vials containing cefotetan disodium equivalent to 1 g and 2 g cefotetan activity for intravenous and intramuscular administration. The 1 g dose is available in 10 mL and 100 mL vials, and the 2 g dose is available in 20 mL and 100 mL vials. CEFOTAN is also available in a pharmacy bulk package of 10 g in 100 mL vials. The vials should not be stored at temperatures above 22°C and should be protected from light.

1 g in 10 mL vial (NDC 0038-0376-10)
2 g in 20 mL vial (NDC 0038-0377-20)
1 g in 100 mL vial (NDC 0038-0376-11)
2 g in 100 mL vial (NDC 0038-0377-21)
10 g in 100 mL vial (NDC 0038-0375-10)

[1] National Committee for Clinical Laboratory Standards, Approved Standard: Performance Standards for Antimicrobial Disk Susceptibility Tests, 4th Edition, Vol. 10(7):M2-A4, Villanova, PA, April, 1990.
[2] National Committee for Clinical Laboratory Standards, Tentative Standard: Methods for Dilution Antimicrobial Susceptibility Tests for Bacteria That Grow Aerobically, 2nd Edition, Vol. 10(8):M7-A2, Villanova, PA, April, 1990.

Clinitest®† is a registered trademark of Ames Division, Miles Laboratory, Inc.

Manufactured for
Stuart Pharmaceuticals
A business unit of ICI Americas Inc.
Wilmington, DE 19897 USA
Rev Y 01/92

Shown in Product Identification Section, page 432

DIPRIVAN® (propofol) **Injection** ℞
EMULSION FOR IV ADMINISTRATION

DESCRIPTION

DIPRIVAN® (propofol) Injection is a sterile, nonpyrogenic emulsion containing 10 mg/mL of propofol suitable for intravenous administration. Propofol is chemically described as 2,6-Diisopropylphenol and has a molecular weight of 178.27. The empirical and structural formulas are:

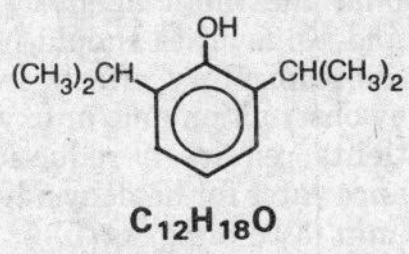
OH
$(CH_3)_2CH$
$CH(CH_3)_2$

$C_{12}H_{18}O$

Propofol is very slightly soluble in water and, thus, is formulated in a white, oil-in-water emulsion. The emulsion is isotonic and has a pH of 7.0–8.5. In addition to the active component, propofol, the formulation also contains soybean oil (100 mg/mL), glycerol (22.5 mg/mL) and egg lecithin (12 mg/mL); with sodium hydroxide to adjust pH.

DIPRIVAN Injection is a single-use parenteral product and contains no antimicrobial preservatives. (See DOSAGE AND ADMINISTRATION, Handling Procedures.)

CLINICAL PHARMACOLOGY

DIPRIVAN Injection is an intravenous sedative hypnotic agent for use in the induction and maintenance of anesthesia or sedation. The pharmacokinetic profile of DIPRIVAN Injection can be characterized as follows: After a single rapid IV bolus dose, two distribution phases are seen, a rapid phase with a half-life of 1.8 to 8.3 min and a slower phase of 34 to 64 min. These distribution phases are associated with the movement of DIPRIVAN from highly perfused tissues (vessel-rich tissues) to less, well-perfused tissues. The terminal elimination half-life of DIPRIVAN ranges from 300 to 700 min. With prolonged administration of DIPRIVAN Injection, the terminal elimination half-life may become extended beyond 700 min. DIPRIVAN has a high metabolic clearance that ranges from 1.6 L/min to 3.4 L/min in healthy 70 kg patients. This metabolic clearance exceeds estimates of hepatic blood flow, suggesting possible extrahepatic metabolism. DIPRIVAN has a large steady state distribution volume that ranges from 150 to 1,000 liters in healthy 70 kg patients. The long terminal elimination half-life of DIPRIVAN is due to the large steady state distribution volume which is presumed to be due to extensive drug partitioning into tissues.

The termination of anesthetic or sedative drug effects of DIPRIVAN after a single IV bolus or a maintenance infusion is due to extensive redistribution from the CNS to other tissues and high metabolic clearance, both of which will decrease blood concentrations. Recovery from anesthesia or sedation is rapid. Following induction (2.0 to 2.5 mg/kg DIPRIVAN Injection) and maintenance (100 to 200 μg/kg/min) of anesthesia for periods up to two hours, the majority of patients are generally awake, responsive to verbal commands, and oriented within 8 minutes. Recovery from the effects of DIPRIVAN Injection occurs due to metabolism and distribution during the first two exponents of the decay curve and is not dependent on the terminal elimination half-life. A study in six subjects showed approximately 70% of the administered radiolabeled DIPRIVAN Injection dose was recovered in the urine in the first 24 hours and approximately 90% of the dose was recovered in the urine within five days. DIPRIVAN is chiefly metabolized by conjugation in the liver to inactive metabolites which are excreted by the kidney. A glucuronide conjugation metabolite accounted for about 50% of the administered dose. The exact metabolic fate of DIPRIVAN and the sites of possible "extrahepatic" metabolism have not been identified.

The pharmacokinetics of DIPRIVAN Injection do not appear to be altered by gender, chronic hepatic cirrhosis or chronic renal failure. The effects of acute hepatic or renal failure on the pharmacokinetics of DIPRIVAN have not been studied.

When given by an infusion for up to two hours, the pharmacokinetics of DIPRIVAN appear to be independent of dose (50 to 150 μg/kg/min) and similar to IV bolus pharmacokinetics. The steady state propofol blood concentrations are proportional to the rate of administration.

With increasing age, the dose of DIPRIVAN Injection needed to achieve a defined anesthetic endpoint (dose-requirement) decreases. This does not appear to be an age-related change of pharmacodynamics or brain sensitivity. With increasing age, distribution pharmacokinetic changes are such that for a given IV bolus dose, higher peak plasma concentrations occur, which explains the decreased dose requirement. These higher peak plasma concentrations in the elderly can predispose patients to cardiorespiratory effects including hypotension, apnea, airway obstruction and/or oxygen desaturation. Total propofol clearance has also been reported to decrease from a mean ±SD of 1.8 ±0.4 L/min in patients aged 18–35 years to 1.4 ±0.4 L/min in patients aged 65–80 years. Age-related distribution pharmacokinetic changes become less prominent at the slow infusion rates. However, lower doses are still recommended for initiation and maintenance of sedation. (See CLINICAL PHARMACOLOGY-Individualization of Dosage.)

Other drugs that cause CNS depression (hypnotics/sedatives, inhalational anesthetics and opiods) can increase the CNS depression induced by DIPRIVAN. Morphine premedication (0.15 mg/kg) with N_2O 67% in oxygen has been shown to decrease the necessary DIPRIVAN Injection maintenance infusion rate and therapeutic blood concentrations when compared to a nonnarcotic (lorazepam) premedication. An alfentanil infusion rate of 50 μg/kg/h has been shown to replace the anesthetic effects of N_2O 67% in oxygen and morphine premedication.

Intravenous injection of a therapeutic dose of DIPRIVAN Injection produces hypnosis rapidly and smoothly with minimal excitation, usually within 40 seconds from the start of an injection (one arm-brain circulation time). As with other rapidly acting intravenous anesthetic agents, the half-time of blood-brain equilibration is approximately 1 to 3 minutes, and this accounts for the rapid induction of anesthesia.

Continued on next page

Stuart—Cont.

Propofol blood concentrations required for maintenance of anesthesia or sedation have not been completely characterized.

When nitrous oxide, oxygen, and propofol are used for maintenance of general anesthesia, supplementation with analgesic agents (eg, narcotics) is generally required; neuromuscular blocking agents may also be required. (See CLINICAL PHARMACOLOGY-Individualization of Dosage.)

The hemodynamic effects of DIPRIVAN Injection during induction of anesthesia vary. If spontaneous ventilation is maintained, the major cardiovascular effects are arterial hypotension (sometimes greater than a 30% decrease) with little or no change in heart rate and no appreciable decrease in cardiac output. If ventilation is assisted or controlled (positive pressure ventilation), the degree and incidence of decrease in cardiac output are accentuated. Addition of a potent opioid (eg, fentanyl) when used as a premedicant further decreases cardiac output.

If anesthesia is continued by infusion of DIPRIVAN Injection, endotracheal intubation and surgical stimulation may return arterial pressure towards normal. However, cardiac output may remain depressed. Comparative clinical studies have shown that the hemodynamic effects of DIPRIVAN during induction are generally more pronounced than with traditional IV induction agents.

Insufficient data are available regarding the cardiovascular effects of DIPRIVAN Injection when used for induction and/or maintenance of anesthesia or sedation in elderly, hypotensive, debilitated patients, patients with severe cardiac disease (ejection fraction <50%) or other ASA III/IV patients. However, limited information suggests that these patients may have more profound adverse cardiovascular responses. It is recommended that if DIPRIVAN Injection is used in these patients, a lower induction dose and a slower maintenance rate of administration of the drug be used. (See DOSAGE AND ADMINISTRATION.)

Clinical and preclinical studies suggest that DIPRIVAN Injection is rarely associated with elevation of plasma histamine levels.

Induction of anesthesia with DIPRIVAN Injection is frequently associated with apnea. In 1573 patients who received DIPRIVAN Injection (2.0 to 2.5 mg/kg), apnea lasted less than 30 seconds in 7% of patients, 30–60 seconds in 24% of patients, and more than 60 seconds in 12% of patients. During maintenance DIPRIVAN Injection (100 to 200 μg/kg/min) causes a decrease in ventilation usually associated with an increase in carbon dioxide tension which may be marked depending upon the rate of administration and other concurrent medications (eg, opioids, sedatives, etc.).

During monitored anesthesia care (MAC) sedation, attention must be given to the cardiorespiratory effects of DIPRIVAN Injection. Hypotension, apnea, airway obstruction, and/or oxygen desaturation can occur, especially with a rapid bolus of DIPRIVAN Injection. During initiation of MAC sedation, slow infusion or slow injection techniques are preferable over rapid bolus administration, and during maintenance of MAC sedation, a variable rate infusion is preferable over intermittent bolus administration in order to minimize undesirable cardiorespiratory effects. In the elderly, debilitated and ASA III or IV patients, rapid (single or repeated) bolus dose administration should not be used for MAC sedation. (See WARNINGS.)

Clinical studies in humans and studies in animals show that DIPRIVAN Injection does not suppress the adrenal response to ACTH.

Preliminary findings in patients with normal intraocular pressure indicate that DIPRIVAN Injection anesthesia produces a decrease in intraocular pressure which may be associated with a concomitant decrease in systemic vascular resistance.

Animal studies and limited experience in susceptible patients have not indicated any propensity of DIPRIVAN Injection to induce malignant hyperthermia.

Individualization of Dosage

General: DIPRIVAN Injection is a potent sedative hypnotic agent which provides clinically useful anesthetic and sedative actions depending upon the dose and technique of administration. Important factors to consider include the types of preinduction and concomitant medications, age, ASA physical classification and level of debilitation of the patient, and ultimately, the dose and rate of administration of DIPRIVAN Injection. Individualization of dose and technique will provide a smooth induction and stable maintenance while reducing potential unwanted side effects. Patients with hypovolemia should have fluid-volume deficits corrected prior to administration of DIPRIVAN Injection.

Induction of Anesthesia: Most adult patients under 55 years of age and classified ASA I or II require 2.0 to 2.5 mg/kg of DIPRIVAN Injection for induction when unpremedicated or when premedicated with oral benzodiazepines or intramuscular opioids. For induction, DIPRIVAN Injection should be titrated (approximately 40 mg every 10

seconds) against the response of the patient until the clinical signs show the onset of anesthesia. As with other sedative hypnotic agents, the amount of intravenous opioid and/or benzodiazepine premedication will influence the response of the patient to an induction dose of DIPRIVAN Injection.

It is important to be familiar with and experienced with the intravenous use of DIPRIVAN Injection before treating elderly, debilitated and ASA III or IV patients. Due to the reduced clearance and higher blood levels, most elderly patients require approximately 1.0 to 1.5 mg/kg (approximately 20 mg every 10 seconds) of DIPRIVAN Injection for induction of anesthesia according to their condition and responses. A rapid bolus should not be used as this will increase the likelihood of undesirable cardiorespiratory depression including hypotension, apnea, airway obstruction and/or oxygen desaturation. (See DOSAGE AND ADMINISTRATION.)

Maintenance of Anesthesia

Anesthesia can be maintained by administering DIPRIVAN Injection by infusion or intermittent IV bolus injection. The patient's clinical response will determine the infusion rate or the amount and frequency of incremental injections.

When administering DIPRIVAN Injection by infusion, syringe pumps or volumetric pumps must be used to provide controlled infusion rates.

Continuous Infusion: DIPRIVAN Injection 100 to 200 μg/kg/min administered in a variable rate infusion with 60%–70% nitrous oxide and oxygen provides anesthesia for patients undergoing general surgery. Maintenance by infusion of DIPRIVAN Injection should immediately follow the induction dose in order to provide satisfactory or continuous anesthesia during the induction phase. During this initial period following the induction dose higher rates of infusion are generally required (150 to 200 μg/kg/min) for the first 10 to 15 minutes. Infusion rates should subsequently be decreased 30%–50% during the first half-hour of maintenance. Changes in vital signs (increases in pulse rate, blood pressure, sweating and/or tearing) that indicate a response to surgical stimulation or lightening of anesthesia may be controlled by the administration of DIPRIVAN Injection 25 mg (2.5 mL) to 50 mg (5.0 mL) incremental boluses and/or by increasing the infusion rate. If vital sign changes are not controlled after a five minute period, other means such as an opioid, barbiturate, vasodilator or inhalation agent therapy should be initiated to control these responses.

For minor surgical procedures (ie, body surface) 60%–70% nitrous oxide can be combined with a variable rate DIPRIVAN infusion to provide satisfactory anesthesia. With more stimulating surgical procedures (ie, intra-abdominal) supplementation with analgesic agents should be considered to provide a satisfactory anesthetic and recovery profile. When supplementation with nitrous oxide is not provided, administration rate(s) of DIPRIVAN Injection and/or opioids should be increased in order to provide adequate anesthesia.

Infusion rates should always be titrated downward in the absence of clinical signs of light anesthesia until a mild response to surgical stimulation is obtained in order to avoid administration of DIPRIVAN Injection at rates higher than are clinically necessary. Generally, rates of 50 to 100 μg/kg/min should be achieved during maintenance in order to optimize recovery times.

Intermittent Bolus: Increments of DIPRIVAN Injection 25 mg (2.5 mL) to 50 mg (5.0 mL) may be administered with nitrous oxide in patients undergoing general surgery. The incremental boluses should be administered when changes in vital signs indicate a response to surgical stimulation or light anesthesia.

DIPRIVAN Injection has been used with a variety of agents commonly used in anesthesia such as atropine, scopolamine, glycopyrrolate, diazepam, depolarizing and nondepolarizing muscle relaxants, and opiod analgesics, as well as with inhalational and regional anesthetic agents.

In the elderly, rapid bolus doses should not be used as this will increase cardiorespiratory effects including hypotension, apnea, airway obstruction and/or oxygen desaturation. Most elderly patients require a reduction of the recommended maintenance rates for healthy adults (<55 years) to 50 to 100 μg/kg/min (3 to 6 mg/kg/h).

MAC Sedation

When DIPRIVAN Injection is administered for sedation, rates of administration should be individualized and titrated to clinical response. In most patients the rates of DIPRIVAN Injection administration will be approximately 25% of those used for maintenance of general anesthesia.

During initiation of MAC sedation, slow infusion or slow injection techniques are preferable over rapid bolus administration. During maintenance of MAC sedation, a variable rate infusion is preferable over intermittent bolus dose administration. In the elderly, debilitated and ASA III or IV patients, rapid (single or repeated) bolus dose administration should not be used for MAC sedation. (See WARNINGS.) **A rapid bolus injection can result in undesirable cardiorespiratory depression including hypotension, apnea, airway obstruction and/or oxygen desaturation.**

Initiation of MAC Sedation:
For initiation of sedation, either an infusion or a slow injection method may be utilized while closely monitoring cardiorespiratory function. With the infusion method, sedation may be initiated by infusing DIPRIVAN Injection at 100 to 150 μg/kg/min (6 to 9 mg/kg/h) for a period of 3 to 5 minutes and titrating to the desired level of sedation while closely monitoring respiratory function. With the slow injection method for initiation, patients will require approximately 0.5 mg/kg administered over 3 to 5 minutes and titrated to clinical responses. When DIPRIVAN Injection is administered slowly over 3 to 5 minutes, most patients will be adequately sedated and the peak drug effect can be achieved while minimizing undesirable cardiorespiratory effects occurring at high plasma levels.

In the elderly, debilitated, and ASA III or IV patients, rapid (single or repeated) bolus dose administration should not be used for MAC sedation. (See WARNINGS.) The rate of administration should be over 3–5 minutes and the dosage of DIPRIVAN Injection should be reduced to approximately 80% of the adult dosage in these patients according to their condition, responses, and changes in vital signs. (See DOSAGE AND ADMINISTRATION.)

Maintenance of MAC Sedation:
For maintenance of sedation, a variable rate infusion method is preferable over an intermittent bolus dose method. With the variable rate infusion method, patients will generally require maintenance rates of 25 to 75 μg/kg/min (1.5 to 4.5 mg/kg/h) during the first 10 to 15 minutes of sedation maintenance. Infusion rates should subsequently be decreased over time to 25 to 50 μg/kg/min and adjusted to clinical responses. In titrating to clinical effect, allow approximately 2 minutes for onset of peak drug effect.

Infusion rates should always be titrated downward in the absence of clinical signs of light sedation until mild responses to stimulation are obtained in order to avoid sedative administration of DIPRIVAN Injection at rates higher than are clinically necessary.

If the intermittent bolus dose method is used, increments of DIPRIVAN Injection 10 mg (1.0 mL) or 20 mg (2.0 mL) can be administered and titrated to desired level of sedation. With the intermittent bolus method of sedation maintenance there is the potential for respiratory depression, transient increases in sedation depth, and/or prolongation of recovery. In the elderly, debilitated, as ASA III or IV patients, rapid (single or repeated) bolus dose administration should not be used for MAC sedation. (See WARNINGS.) The rate of administration and the dosage of DIPRIVAN Injection should be reduced to approximately 80% of the adult dosage in these patients according to their condition, responses, and changes in vital signs. (See DOSAGE AND ADMINISTRATION.)

DIPRIVAN Injection can be administered as the sole agent for maintenance of MAC sedation during surgical/diagnostic procedures. When DIPRIVAN sedation is supplemented with opiod and/or benzodiazepine medications, these agents increase the sedative and respiratory effects of DIPRIVAN and may also result in a slower recovery profile. (See PRECAUTIONS, Drug Interactions.)

INDICATIONS AND USAGE

DIPRIVAN Injection is an IV anesthetic agent that can be used for both induction and/or maintenance of anesthesia as part of a balanced anesthetic technique for inpatient and outpatient surgery.

DIPRIVAN Injection, when administered IV as directed, can be used to initiate and maintain monitored anesthesia care (MAC) sedation during diagnostic procedures. DIPRIVAN Injection may also be used for MAC sedation in conjunction with local/regional anesthesia in patients undergoing surgical procedures. (See PRECAUTIONS.)

DIPRIVAN Injection is not recommended for use at this time in patients with increased intracranial pressure or impaired cerebral circulation because DIPRIVAN Injection may cause substantial decreases in mean arterial pressure, and consequently, substantial decreases in cerebral perfusion pressure. (See PRECAUTIONS.)

DIPRIVAN Injection is not recommended for obstetrics, including cesarean section deliveries. DIPRIVAN Injection crosses the placenta, and as with other general anesthetic agents, the administration of DIPRIVAN Injection may be associated with neonatal depression. (See PRECAUTIONS.)

DIPRIVAN Injection is not recommended for use in nursing mothers because DIPRIVAN Injection has been reported to be excreted in human milk and the effects of oral absorption of small amounts of propofol are not known. (See PRECAUTIONS.)

DIPRIVAN Injection is not recommended for use in pediatric patients because safety and effectiveness have not been established. (See PRECAUTIONS.)

CONTRAINDICATIONS

DIPRIVAN Injection is contraindicated in patients with a known hypersensitivity to DIPRIVAN Injection or its components, or when general anesthesia or sedation are contraindicated.

WARNINGS

For general anesthesia or monitored anesthesia care (MAC) sedation, DIPRIVAN Injection should be administered only by persons trained in the administration of general anesthesia and not involved in the conduct of the surgical/diagnostic procedure. Patients should be continuously monitored and facilities for maintenance of a patent airway, artificial ventilation, and oxygen enrichment and circulatory resuscitation must be immediately available.

In the elderly, debilitated and ASA III or IV patients, rapid (single or repeated) bolus administration should not be used during general anesthesia or MAC sedation in order to minimize undesirable cardiorespiratory depression including hypotension, apnea, airway obstruction and/or oxygen desaturation.

MAC sedation patients should be continuously monitored by persons not involved in the conduct of the surgical or diagnostic procedure; oxygen supplementation should be immediately available and provided where clinically indicated; and oxygen saturation should be monitored in all patients. Patients should be continuously monitored for early signs of hypotension, apnea, airway obstruction and/or oxygen desaturation. These cardiorespiratory effects are more likely to occur following rapid initiation (loading) boluses or during supplemental maintenance boluses, especialy in the elderly, debilitated and ASA III or IV patients.

DIPRIVAN Injection should not be coadministered through the same IV catheter with blood or plasma because compatibility has not been established. In vitro tests have shown that aggregates of the globular component of the emulsion vehicle have occurred with blood/plasma/serum from humans and animals. The clinical significance is not known.

Strict aseptic techniques must always be maintained during handling as DIPRIVAN Injection is a single-use parenteral product and contains no antimicrobial preservatives. The vehicle is capable of supporting rapid growth of microorganisms. (See DOSAGE AND ADMINISTRATION, Handling Procedures.)

Failure to follow aseptic handling procedures may result in microbial contamination causing fever, infection/sepsis and/or other adverse consequences which could lead to life-threatening illness.

PRECAUTIONS

General: A lower induction dose and a slower maintenance rate of administration should be used in elderly, debilitated and ASA III or IV patients. (See CLINICAL PHARMACOLOGY—Individualization of Dosage.) Patients should be continuously monitored for early signs of significant hypotension and/or bradycardia. Treatment may include increasing the rate of intravenous fluid, elevation of lower extremities, use of pressor agents, or administration of atropine. Apnea often occurs during induction and may persist for more than 60 seconds. Ventilatory support may be required. Because DIPRIVAN Injection is an emulsion, caution should be exercised in patients with disorders of lipid metabolism such as primary hyperlipoproteinemia, diabetic hyperlipemia, and pancreatitis.

The clinical criteria for discharge from the recovery/day surgery area established for each institution should be satisfied before discharge of the patient from the care of the anesthesiologist.

When DIPRIVAN Injection is administered to an epileptic patient, there may be a risk of convulsion during the recovery phase.

Transient local pain may occur during intravenous injection, which may be reduced by prior injection of IV lidocaine (1.0 mL of a 1% solution). Venous sequelae (phlebitis or thrombosis) have been reported rarely (< 1%). In two well-controlled clinical studies using dedicated intravenous catheters, no instances of venous sequelae were reported up to 14 days following induction. Pain can be minimized if the larger veins of the forearm or antecubital fossa are used. Accidental clinical extravasation and intentional injection into subcutaneous or perivascular tissues of animals caused minimal tissue reaction. Intra-arterial injection in animals did not induce local tissue effects. Accidental intra-arterial injection has been reported in patients, and other than pain, there were no major sequelae.

Perioperative myoclonia, rarely including convulsions and opisthotonus, has occurred in a temporal relationship in cases in which DIPRIVAN Injection has been administered. Clinical features of anaphylaxis, which may include bronchospasm, erythema and hypotension, occur rarely following DIPRIVAN Injection administration, although use of other drugs in most instances makes the relationship to DIPRIVAN Injection unclear.

There have been rare reports of pulmonary edema in temporal relationship to the administration of DIPRIVAN Injection, although a causal relationship is unknown.

DIPRIVAN Injection has no vagolytic activity and has been associated with reports of bradycardia, occasionally profound, and/or asystole. The intravenous administration of anticholinergic agents (eg, atropine or glycopyrrolate) should be considered to modify potential increases in vagal

tone due to concomitant agents (eg, succinylcholine) or surgical stimuli.

There have been rare reports of cardiac arrest in temporal relationship to the administration of DIPRIVAN Injection.

Neurosurgical Anesthesia: Studies to date indicate that DIPRIVAN Injection decreases cerebral blood flow, cerebral metabolic oxygen consumption, and intracranial pressure, and increases cerebrovascular resistance. DIPRIVAN Injection does not seem to affect cerebrovascular reactivity to changes in arterial carbon dioxide tension. Despite these findings, DIPRIVAN Injection is not recommended for use at this time in patients with increased intracranial pressure or impaired cerbral circulation because DIPRIVAN Injection may cause substantial decreases in mean arterial pressure, and consequently, substantial decreases in cerebral perfusion pressure. Further studies are needed to substantiate what happens to intracranial pressure following DIPRIVAN Injection when decreases in mean arterial and cerebral perfusion are prevented by appropriate measures.

Information for Patients: Patients should be advised that performance of activities requiring mental alertness, such as operating a motor vehicle, or hazardous machinery or signing legal documents may be impaired for some time after general anesthesia or sedation.

Drug Interactions: The induction dose requirements of DIPRIVAN Injection may be reduced in patients with intramuscular or intravenous premedication, particularly with narcotics (eg, morphine, meperidine, and fentanyl) and combinations of opiods and sedatives (eg, benzodiazepines, barbiturates, chloral hydrate, droperidol, etc.). These agents may increase the anesthetic or sedative effects of DIPRIVAN Injection and may also result in more pronounced decreases in systolic, diastolic, and mean arterial pressures and cardiac output.

During maintenance of anesthesia or sedation, the rate of DIPRIVAN Injection administration should be adjusted according to the desired level of anesthesia or sedation and may be reduced in the presence of supplemental analgesic agents (eg, nitrous oxide or opioids). The concurrent administration of potent inhalational agents (eg, isoflurane, enflurane, and halothane) during maintenance with DIPRIVAN Injection has not been extensively evaluated. These inhalational agents can also be expected to increase the anesthetic or sedative and cardiorespiratory effects of DIPRIVAN Injection.

DIPRIVAN Injection does not cause a clinically significant change in onset, intensity or duration of action of the commonly used neuromuscular blocking agents (eg, succinylcholine and nondepolarizing muscle relaxants).

No significant adverse interactions with commonly used premedications or drugs used during anesthesia or sedation (including a range of muscle relaxants, inhalational agents, analgesic agents, and local anesthetic agents) have been observed.

Carcinogenesis, Mutagenesis, Impairment of Fertility: Animal carcinogenicity studies have not been performed with propofol.

In vitro and in vivo animal tests failed to show any potential for mutagenicity by propofol. Tests for mutagenicity included the Ames (using *Salmonella* sp) mutation test, gene mutation/gene conversion using *Saccharomyces cerevisiae*, in vitro cytogenetic studies in Chinese hamsters and a mouse micronucleus test.

Studies in female rats at intravenous doses up to 15 mg/kg/day (6 times the maximum recommended human induction dose) for 2 weeks before pregnancy to day 7 of gestation did not show impaired fertility. Male fertility in rats was not affected in a dominant lethal study at intravenous doses up to 15 mg/kg/day for 5 days.

Pregnancy Category B: Reproduction studies have been performed in rats and rabbits at intravenous doses of 15 mg/kg/day (6 times the recommended human induction dose) and have revealed no evidence of impaired fertility or harm to the fetus due to propofol. Propofol, however, has been shown to cause maternal deaths in rats and rabbits and decreased pup survival during the lactating period in dams treated with 15 mg/kg/day (or 6 times the recommended human induction dose). The pharmacological activity (anesthesia) of the drug on the mother is probably responsible for the adverse effects seen in the offspring. There are, however, no adequate and well-controlled studies in pregnant women. Because animal reproduction studies are not always predictive of human responses, this drug should be used during pregnancy only if clearly needed.

Labor and Delivery: DIPRIVAN Injection is not recommended for obstetrics, including cesarean section deliveries. DIPRIVAN Injection crosses the placenta, and as with other general anesthetic agents, the administration of DIPRIVAN Injection may be associated with neonatal depression.

Nursing Mothers: DIPRIVAN Injection is not recommended for use in nursing mothers because DIPRIVAN has been reported to be excreted in human milk and the effects of oral absorption of small amounts of propofol are not known.

Pediatric Use: DIPRIVAN Injection is not recommended for use in pediatric patients because safety and effectiveness have not been established.

ADVERSE REACTIONS

Adverse event information is derived from controlled clinical trials and worldwide marketing experience. In the description below, rates of the more common events represent US/Canadian clinical study results. Less frequent events are derived principally from publications and marketing experience in over 8 million patients; there are insufficient data to support an accurate estimate of their incidence rates.

The adverse experience profile from reports of 150 patients in the US/Canadian MAC sedation clinical trials is similar to the profile established with DIPRIVAN Injection during anesthesia (see below). During MAC sedation clinical trials, significant respiratory events included cough, upper airway obstruction, apnea, hypoventilation, and dyspnea. The most common adverse events which occurred in more than 3% of the patients receiving DIPRIVAN Injection for MAC sedation included hypotension, nausea, headache, and injection site pain or hotness.

The following estimates of adverse events for DIPRIVAN Injection are derived from reports of 2588 patients included in the US/Canadian studies. These studies were conducted using a variety of premedicants, varying lengths of surgical/diagnostic procedures and various other anesthetic agents. Most adverse events were mild and transient.

The following adverse events were reported in patients treated with DIPRIVAN Injection. They are presented within each body system in order of decreasing frequency.

Incidence Greater than 1%—All events regardless of causality, derived from clinical trials

Body as a Whole: Fever

Cardiovascular: Hypotension* (see also CLINICAL PHARMACOLOGY), Bradycardia, Hypertension, Arrhythmia

Central Nervous System: Movement*, Headache, Dizziness, Twitching

Digestive: Nausea** (15%), Vomiting*, Abdominal Cramping

Injection Site: Pain*, Burning/Stinging*

Respiratory: Hiccough, Cough (see also CLINICAL PHARMACOLOGY)

Skin and Appendages: Rash

Incidence of unmarked events is 1%–3%.

*3% to 9%

**10% or greater

Incidence Less than 1%—Causal Relationship Probable, derived from clinical trials. (Adverse events reported in the literature, not seen in clinical trials, are *italicized*.)

Body as a Whole: Perinatal Disorder, Extremities Pain, Awareness, Chest Pain, Increased Drug Effect, Neck Rigidity/Stiffness, Trunk Pain, *Anaphylaxis/Anaphylactoid Reaction*

Cardiovascular: Tachycardia, Premature Ventricular Contractions, Syncope, Premature Atrial Contractions, Abnormal ECG, ST Segment Depression Bundle Branch Block, Extrasystole, Myocardial Infarction, Heart Block, Atrioventricular Block, Second Degree A-V Block

Central Nervous System: Bucking/Jerking/Thrashing, Clonic/Myoclonic Movement, Hypertonia/Dystonia, Chills/Shivering, Somnolence, Tremor, Agitation, Confusion, Delirium, Paresthesia, Abnormal Dreams, Euphoria, Fatigue, Moaning, Rigidity, Combativeness, Depression

Digestive: Hypersalivation, Dry Mouth, Swallowing, Enlarged Parotid

Injection Site: Tingling/Numbness, Coldness, Discomfort, Phlebitis, Hives/Itching, Redness/Discoloration

Metabolic/Nutritional: Hyperlipemia

Musculoskeletal: Myalgia

Respiratory: Apnea (see also CLINICAL PHARMACOLOGY), Upper Airway Obstruction, Wheezing, Dyspnea, Hypoventilation, Bronchospasm, Burning in Throat, Sneezing, Tachypnea, Hyperventilation, Hypoxia, Pharyngitis

Skin and Appendages: Flushing, Urticaria, Pruritus

Special Senses: Amblyopia, Diplopia, Taste Perversion, Eye Pain, Tinnitus

Urogenital: Abnormal Urine, Urine Retention, *Green Urine*

Incidence Less than 1%—Causal Relationship Unknown, derived from clinical trials.

(Adverse events reported in the literature, not seen in clinical trials, are *italicized*.)

Body as a Whole: *Asthenia*

Cardiovascular: Atrial Fibrillation, Bigeminy, Hemorrhage Edema, Ventricular Fibrillation, Supraventricular Tachycardia, *Myocardial ischemia*

Central Nervous System: Emotional Lability, Anxiety, Hysteria, Insomnia, Generalized and Localized Seizures, *Opisthotonus, Hypotonia, Hallucinations, Neuropathy, Thinking Abnormal*

Digestive: Diarrhea

Hematologic/Lymphatic: Coagulation Disorder

Metabolic/Nutritional: Hyperkalemia

Respiratory: Laryngospasm

Skin and Appendages: Diaphoresis, *Conjunctival Hyperemia*

Continued on next page

Stuart—Cont.

Special Senses: Ear Pain, *Nystagmus*
Urogenital: Oliguria
In addition to those adverse events listed above, the following adverse event has been reported as a result of postmarketing experience: amorous behavior.

DRUG ABUSE AND DEPENDENCE
None known.

OVERDOSAGE
To date, there is no known case of acute overdosage, and no specific information on emergency treatment of overdosage is available. If accidental overdosage occurs, DIPRIVAN Injection administration should be discontinued immediately. Overdosage is likely to cause cardiorespiratory depression. Respiratory depression should be treated by artificial ventilation with oxygen. Cardiovascular depression may require repositioning of the patient by raising the patient's legs, increasing the flow rate of intravenous fluids and administering pressor agents and/or anticholinergic agents.
The intravenous LD_{50} values are 53 mg/kg in mice and 42 mg/kg in rats.

DOSAGE AND ADMINISTRATION
Dosage and rate of administration should be individualized and titrated to the desired effect according to clinically relevant factors including preinduction and concomitant medications, age, ASA physical classification and level of debilitation of the patient.
The following is abbreviated dosage and administration information which is only intended as a general guide in the use of DIPRIVAN Injection. Prior to administering DIPRIVAN Injection, it is imperative that the physician review and be completely familiar with the specific dosage and administration information detailed in the CLINICAL PHARMACOLOGY—Individualization of Dosage section.
In the elderly, debilitated and ASA III or IV patients, rapid bolus doses should not be used in the methods of administration described above. (See WARNINGS.)
[See table above.]

Compatibility and Stability: DIPRIVAN Injection should not be mixed with other therapeutic agents prior to administration.
Dilution Prior to Administration: When DIPRIVAN Injection is diluted prior to administration, it should only be diluted with 5% Dextrose Injection, USP, and it should not be diluted to a concentration less than 2 mg/mL because it is an emulsion. In diluted form it has been shown to be more stable when in contact with glass than with plastic (95% potency after 2 hours of running infusion in plastic.)
Administration Into a Running IV Catheter: Compatibility of DIPRIVAN Injection with the coadministration of blood/serum/plasma has not been established. (See WARNINGS.)
DIPRIVAN Injection has been shown to be compatible with the following intravenous fluids when administered into a running IV catheter.
—5% Dextrose Injection, USP
—Lactated Ringers Injection, USP
—Lactated Ringers and 5% Dextrose Injection
—5% Dextrose and 0.45% Sodium Chloride Injection, USP
—5% Dextrose and 0.2% Sodium Chloride Injection, USP
Handling Procedures: Parenteral drug products should be inspected visually for particulate matter and discoloration prior to administration whenever solution and container permit. DIPRIVAN Injection must not be administered through filters with a pore size less than 5 μm because this could restrict the flow of DIPRIVAN and/or cause the breakdown of the emulsion.
Do not use if there is evidence of separation of the phases of the emulsion.
Strict aseptic techniques must always be maintained during handling as DIPRIVAN Injection is a single-use parenteral product and contains no antimicrobial preservatives. The vehicle is capable of supporting rapid growth of microorganisms.
Failure to follow aseptic handling procedures may result in microbial contamination causing fever, infection/sepsis and/or other adverse consequences which could lead to life-threatening illness.
DIPRIVAN Injection should be prepared for use just prior to initiation of each individual anesthetic/sedative procedure. The ampule neck surface or vial rubber stopper should be disinfected using 70% isopropyl alcohol. DIPRIVAN Injection should be drawn into sterile syringes immediately after ampules or vials are opened. When withdrawing DIPRIVAN Injection from vials, a sterile vent spike should be used. The syringe(s) should be labeled with appropriate information including the date and time the ampule or vial was opened. Administration should commence promptly and be completed within 6 hours after the ampules or vials have been opened.
DIPRIVAN Injection should be prepared for single patient use only. Any unused portions of DIPRIVAN Injection, res-

Induction of Anesthesia	Dosage should be individualized and titrated.
	Adults*: Most patients require 2.0 to 2.5 mg/kg (approximately 40 mg every 10 seconds until induction onset).
	Elderly, Debilitated and ASA III or IV Patients: Most patients require 1.0 to 1.5 mg/kg (approximately 20 mg every 10 seconds until induction onset).
	For complete dosage information, see CLINICAL PHARMACOLOGY—Individualization of Dosage.
Maintenance of Anesthesia: Infusion	Variable rate infusion—titrated to the desired clinical effect.
	Adults*: Most patients require 100 to 200 μg/kg/min (6 to 12 mg/kg/h).
	Elderly, Debilitated and ASA III or IV Patients: Most patients require 50 to 100 μg/kg/min (3 to 6 mg/kg/h).
Maintenance of Anesthesia: Intermittent Bolus	Increments of 25 to 50 mg as needed.
	For complete dosage information, see CLINICAL PHARMACOLOGY—Individualization of Dosage.
Initiation of MAC Sedation	Dosage and rate should be individualized.
	Adults*: Slow infusion or slow injection techniques are preferable over rapid bolus administration. Most patients require an infusion of 100 to 150 μg/kg/min (6 to 9 mg/kg/h) or a slow injection of 0.5 mg/kg over 3 to 5 minutes.
	Elderly, Debilitated and ASA III or IV Patients: Most patients require dosages similar to adults, but must be given as a slow infusion or slow injection and not as a rapid bolus. (See WARNINGS.)
Maintenance of MAC Sedation	Dosage and rate should be titrated to clinical effect.
	Adults*: A variable rate infusion technique is preferable over an intermittent bolus technique. Most patients require an infusion of 25 to 75 μg/kg/min (1.5 to 4.5 mg/kg/h) or incremental bolus doses of 10 mg or 20 mg.
	Elderly, Debilitated and ASA III or IV Patients: Most patients require a 20% reduction of the adult dose. A rapid (single or repeated) bolus dose should not be used. (See WARNINGS.)
	For complete dosage information, see CLINICAL PHARMACOLOGY—Individualization of Dosage.

* Adults—healthy, less than 55 years of age

ervoirs, dedicated administration tubing and/or solutions containing DIPRIVAN Injection must be discarded at the end of the anesthetic procedure or at 6 hours, whichever occurs sooner. The IV line should be flushed every 6 hours and at the end of the anesthetic procedure to remove residual DIPRIVAN Injection.

HOW SUPPLIED
DIPRIVAN Injection is available in ready to use 20 mL ampules and 50 mL infusion vials containing 10 mg/mL of propofol.
20 mL ampules (NDC 0038-0290-20)
50 mL infusion vials (NDC 0038-0290-50)
Store below 22°C (72°F). Do not store below 4°C (40°F). Refrigeration is not recommended. Protect from light. Shake well before use.
Made in Sweden
Manufactured for:
Stuart Pharmaceuticals
A business unit of ICI Americas Inc.
Wilmington, DE 19897 USA
REV B 03/92
Shown in Product Identification Section, page 432

ELAVIL® ℞
(Amitriptyline HCl), Tablets and Injection

DESCRIPTION
Amitriptyline HCl is 3-(10,11-dihydro-5*H*-dibenzo [*a,d*] cycloheptene-5-ylidene)-*N,N*- dimethyl-1-propanamine hydrochloride. Its empirical formula is $C_{20}H_{23}N \cdot HCl$ and its structural formula is:

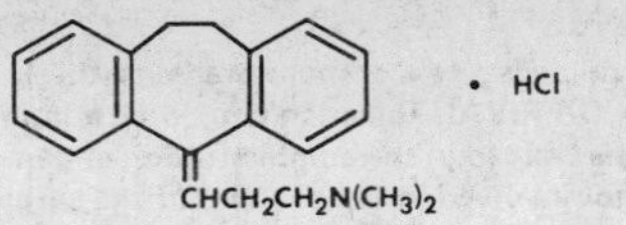

Amitriptyline HCl, a dibenzocycloheptadiene derivative, has a molecular weight of 313.87. It is a white, odorless, crystalline compound which is freely soluble in water.
ELAVIL* (Amitriptyline HCl) is supplied as 10 mg, 25 mg, 50 mg, 75 mg, 100 mg, and 150 mg tablets and as a sterile solution for intramuscular use. Inactive ingredients of the tablets are calcium phosphate, cellulose, colloidal silicon dioxide, hydroxypropyl cellulose, hydroxypropyl methylcellulose, lactose, magnesium stearate, starch, stearic acid, talc, and titanium dioxide. Tablets ELAVIL 10 mg also contain FD&C Blue 1. Tablets ELAVIL 25 mg also contain D&C Yellow 10, FD&C Blue 1, and FD&C Yellow 6. Tablets ELAVIL 50 mg also contain D&C Yellow 10, FD&C Yellow 6 and iron oxide. Tablets ELAVIL 75 mg also contain FD&C Yellow 6. Tablets ELAVIL 100 mg also contain FD&C Blue 2 and FD&C Red 40. Tablets ELAVIL 150 mg also contain FD&C Blue 2 and FD&C Yellow 6. Each milliliter of the sterile solution contains:

Amitriptyline hydrochloride	10 mg
Dextrose	44 mg
Water for Injection, q.s.	1 mL
Added as preservatives:	
Methylparaben	1.5 mg
Propylparaben	0.2 mg

ACTIONS
ELAVIL is an antidepressant with sedative effects. Its mechanism of action in man is not known. It is not a monoamine oxidase inhibitor and it does not act primarily by stimulation of the central nervous system.
Amitriptyline inhibits the membrane pump mechanism responsible for uptake of norepinephrine and serotonin in adrenergic and serotonergic neurons. Pharmacologically this action may potentiate or prolong neuronal activity since reuptake of these biogenic amines is important physiologically in terminating transmitting activity. This interference with the reuptake of norepinephrine and/or serotonin is believed by some to underlie the antidepressant activity of amitriptyline.

INDICATIONS
For the relief of symptoms of depression. Endogenous depression is more likely to be alleviated than are other depressive states.

CONTRAINDICATIONS
ELAVIL is contraindicated in patients who have shown prior hypersensitivity to it.
It should not be given concomitantly with monoamine oxidase inhibitors. Hyperpyretic crises, severe convulsions, and deaths have occurred in patients receiving tricyclic antidepressant and monoamine oxidase inhibiting drugs simultaneously. When it is desired to replace a monoamine oxidase inhibitor with ELAVIL, a minimum of 14 days should be allowed to elapse after the former is discontinued. ELAVIL should then be initiated cautiously with gradual increase in dosage until optimum response is achieved.
This drug is not recommended for use during the acute recovery phase following myocardial infarction.

WARNINGS
ELAVIL may block the antihypertensive action of guanethidine or similarly acting compounds.
It should be used with caution in patients with a history of seizures and, because of its atropine-like action, in patients with a history of urinary retention, angle-closure glaucoma or increased intraocular pressure. In patients with angle-closure glaucoma, even average doses may precipitate an attack.
Patients with cardiovascular disorders should be watched closely. Tricyclic antidepressant drugs, including ELAVIL, particularly when given in high doses, have been reported to produce arrhythmias, sinus tachycardia, and prolongation of the conduction time. Myocardial infarction and stroke have been reported with drugs of this class.
Close supervision is required when ELAVIL is given to hyperthyroid patients or those receiving thyroid medication.
ELAVIL may enhance the response to alcohol and the effects of barbiturates and other CNS depressants. In patients who may use alcohol excessively, it should be borne in mind that the potentiation may increase the danger inherent in any suicide attempt or overdosage. Delirium has been reported with concurrent administration of amitriptyline and disulfiram.
Usage in Pregnancy: Teratogenic effects were not observed in mice, rats, or rabbits when amitriptyline was given orally at doses of 2 to 40 mg/kg/day (up to 13 times the maximum recommended human dose**). Studies in the literature have shown amitriptyline to be teratogenic in mice and hamsters when given by various routes of administration at doses of 28

to 100 mg/kg/day (9 to 33 times the maximum recommended human dose), producing multiple malformations. Another study in the rat reported that an oral dose of 25 mg/kg/day (8 times the maximum recommended human dose) produced delays in ossification of fetal vertebral bodies without other signs of embryotoxicity. In rabbits, an oral dose of 60 mg/kg/day (20 times the maximum recommended human dose) was reported to cause incomplete ossification of the cranial bones.

Amitriptyline has been shown to cross the placenta. Although a causal relationship has not been established, there have been a few reports of adverse events, including CNS effects, limb deformities, or developmental delay, in infants whose mothers had taken amitriptyline during pregnancy.

There are no adequate or well-controlled studies in pregnant women. ELAVIL should be used during pregnancy only if the potential benefit to the mother justifies the potential risk to the fetus.

Nursing Mothers: Amitriptyline is excreted into breast milk. In one report in which a patient received amitriptyline 100 mg/day while nursing her infant, levels of 83–141 ng/mL were detected in the mother's serum. Levels of 135–151 ng/mL were found in the breast milk, but no trace of the drug could be detected in the infant's serum.

Because of the potential for serious adverse reactions in nursing infants from amitriptyline, a decision should be made whether to discontinue nursing or to discontinue the drug, taking into account the importance of the drug to the mother.

Usage in Children: In view of the lack of experience with the use of this drug in children, it is not recommended at the present time for patients under 12 years of age.

PRECAUTIONS

Schizophrenic patients may develop increased symptoms of psychosis; patients with paranoid symptomatology may have an exaggeration of such symptoms. Depressed patients, particularly those with known manic-depressive illness, may experience a shift to mania or hypomania. In these circumstances the dose of amitriptyline may be reduced or a major tranquilizer such as perphenazine may be administered concurrently.

When ELAVIL is given with anticholinergic agents or sympathomimetic drugs, including epinephrine combined with local anesthetics, close supervision and careful adjustment of dosages are required.

Hyperpyrexia has been reported when ELAVIL is administered with anticholingeric agents or with neuroleptic drugs, particularly during hot weather.

Paralytic ileus may occur in patients taking tricyclic antidepressants in combination with anticholinergic-type drugs.

Cimetidine is reported to reduce hepatic metabolism of certain tricyclic antidepressants, thereby delaying elimination and increasing steady-state concentrations of these drugs. Clinically significant effects have been reported with the tricyclic antidepressants when used concomitantly with cimetidine. Increases in plasma levels of tricyclic antidepressants, and in the frequency and severity of side effects, particularly anticholinergic, have been reported when cimetidine was added to the drug regimen. Discontinuation of cimetidine in well-controlled patients receiving tricyclic antidepressants and cimetidine may decrease the plasma levels and efficacy of the antidepressants.

Caution is advised if patients receive large doses of ethchlorvynol concurrently. Transient delirium has been reported in patients who were treated with one gram of ethchlorvynol and 75-150 mg of ELAVIL.

The possibility of suicide in depressed patients remains until significant remission occurs. Potentially suicidal patients should not have access to large quantities of this drug. Prescriptions should be written for the smallest amount feasible.

Concurrent administration of ELAVIL and electroshock therapy may increase the hazards associated with such therapy. Such treatment should be limited to patients for whom it is essential.

When possible, the drug should be discontinued several days before elective surgery.

Both elevation and lowering of blood sugar levels have been reported.

ELAVIL should be used with caution in patients with impaired liver function.

Information for Patients: While on therapy with ELAVIL, patients should be advised as to the possible impairment of mental and/or physical abilities required for performance of hazardous tasks, such as operating machinery or driving a motor vehicle.

ADVERSE REACTIONS

Within each category the following adverse reactions are listed in order of decreasing severity. Included in the listing are a few adverse reactions which have not been reported with this specific drug. However, pharmacological similarities among the tricyclic antidepressant drugs require that each of the reactions be considered when amitriptyline is administered.

Cardiovascular: Myocardial infarction; stroke; nonspecific ECG changes and changes in AV conductor; heart block; arrhythmias; hypotension, particularly orthostatic hypotension; syncope; hypertension; tachycardia; palpitation.

CNS and Neuromuscular: Coma; seizures; hallucinations; delusions; confusional states; disorientation; incoordination; ataxia; tremors; peripheral neuropathy; numbness, tingling, and paresthesias of the extremities; extrapyramidal symptoms including abnormal involuntary movements and tardive dyskinesia; dysarthria; disturbed concentration; excitement; anxiety; insomnia; restlessness; nightmares; drowsiness; dizziness; weakness; fatigue; headache; syndrome of inappropriate ADH (antidiuretic hormone) secretion; tinnitus; alteration in EEG patterns.

Anticholinergic: Paralytic ileus; hyperpyrexia; urinary retention, dilatation of the urinary tract; constipation; blurred vision, disturbance of accommodation, increased intraocular pressure, mydriasis; dry mouth.

Allergic: Skin rash; urticaria; photosensitization; edema of face and tongue.

Hematologic: Bone marrow depression including agranulocytosis, leukopenia, thrombocytopenia; purpura; eosinophilia.

Gastrointestinal: Rarely hepatitis (including altered liver function and jaundice); nausea; epigastric distress; vomiting; anorexia; stomatitis; peculiar taste; diarrhea; parotid swelling; black tongue.

Endocrine: Testicular swelling and gynecomastia in the male; breast enlargement and galactorrhea in the female; increased or decreased libido; impotence; elevation and lowering of blood sugar levels.

Other: Alopecia; edema; weight gain or loss; urinary frequency; increased perspiration.

Withdrawal Symptoms: After prolonged administration, abrupt cessation of treatment may produce nausea, headache, and malaise. Gradual dosage reduction has been reported to produce, within two weeks, transient symptoms including irritability, restlessness, and dream and sleep disturbance. These symptoms are not indicative of addiction. Rare instances have been reported of mania or hypomania occurring within 2–7 days following cessation of chronic therapy with tricyclic antidepressants.

Causal Relationship Unknown: Other reactions, reported under circumstances where a causal relationship could not be established, are listed to serve as alerting information to physicians:

Body as a Whole: Lupus-like syndrome (migratory arthritis, positive ANA and rheumatoid factor).

Digestive: Hepatic failure, ageusia.

DOSAGE AND ADMINISTRATION

Oral Dosage

Dosage should be initiated at a low level and increased gradually, noting carefully the clinical response and any evidence of intolerance.

Initial Dosage for Adults—For outpatients 75 mg of amitriptyline HCl a day in divided doses is usually satisfactory. If necessary, this may be increased to a total of 150 mg per day. Increases are made preferably in the late afternoon and/or bedtime doses. A sedative effect may be apparent before the antidepressant effect is noted, but an adequate therapeutic effect may take as long as 30 days to develop.

An alternate method of initiating therapy in outpatients is to begin with 50 to 100 mg amitriptyline HCl at bedtime. This may be increased by 25 or 50 mg as necessary in the bedtime dose to a total of 150 mg per day.

Hospitalized patients may require 100 mg a day initially. This can be increased gradually to 200 mg a day if necessary. A small number of hospitalized patients may need as much as 300 mg a day.

Adolescent and Elderly Patients—In general, lower dosages are recommended for these patients. Ten mg 3 times a day with 20 mg at bedtime may be satisfactory in adolescent and elderly patients who do not tolerate higher dosages.

Maintenance—The usual maintenance dosage of amitriptyline HCl is 50 to 100 mg per day. In some patients 40 mg per day is sufficient. For maintenance therapy the total daily dosage may be given in a single dose preferably at bedtime. When satisfactory improvement has been reached, dosage should be reduced to the lowest amount that will maintain relief of symptoms. It is appropriate to continue maintenance therapy 3 months or longer to lessen the possibility of relapse.

Intramuscular Dosage

Initially, 20 to 30 mg (2 to 3 mL) four times a day.

When ELAVIL Injection is administered intramuscularly, the effects may appear more rapidly than with oral administration.

When ELAVIL Injection is used for initial therapy in patients unable or unwilling to take ELAVIL tablets, the tablets should replace the injection as soon as possible.

Usage in Children

In view of the lack of experience with the use of this drug in children, it is not recommended at the present time for patients under 12 years of age.

Plasma Levels

Because of the wide variation in the absorption and distribution of tricyclic antidepressants in body fluids, it is difficult to directly correlate plasma levels and therapeutic effect. However, determination of plasma levels may be useful in identifying patients who appear to have toxic effects and may have excessively high levels, or those in whom lack of absorption or noncompliance is suspected. Adjustments in dosage should be made according to the patient's clinical response and not on the basis of plasma levels.***

OVERDOSAGE

Manifestations: High doses may cause temporary confusion, disturbed concentration, or transient visual hallucinations. Overdosage may cause drowsiness; hypothermia; tachycardia and other arrhythmic abnormalities, such as bundle branch block; ECG evidence of impaired conduction; congestive heart failure; dilated pupils; disorders of ocular motility; convulsions; severe hypotension; stupor; coma; and polyradiculoneuropathy. Other symptoms may be agitation, hyperactive reflexes, muscle rigidity, vomiting, hyperpyrexia, or any of those listed under ADVERSE REACTIONS.

There has been a report of fatal dysrhythmia occurring as late as 56 hours after amitriptyline overdose.

All patients suspected of having taken an overdosage should be admitted to a hospital as soon as possible. *Treatment* is symptomatic and supportive. Empty the stomach as quickly as possible by emesis followed by gastric lavage upon arrival at the hospital. Following gastric lavage, activated charcoal may be administered. Twenty to 30 g of activated charcoal may be given every four to six hours during the first 24 to 48 hours after ingestion. An ECG should be taken and close monitoring of cardiac function instituted if there is any sign of abnormality. Maintain an open airway and adequate fluid intake; regulate body temperature.

The intravenous administration of 1–3 mg of physostigmine salicylate is reported to reverse the symptoms of tricyclic antidepressant poisoning. Because physostigmine is rapidly metabolized, the dosage of physostigmine should be repeated as required particularly if life threatening signs such as arrhythmias, convulsions, and deep coma recur or persist after the initial dosage of physostigmine. Because physostigmine itself may be toxic, it is not recommended for routine use.

Standard measures should be used to manage circulatory shock and metabolic acidosis. Cardiac arrhythmias may be treated with neostigmine, pyridostigmine, or propranolol. Should cardiac failure occur, the use of digitalis should be considered. Close monitoring of cardiac function for not less than five days is advisable.

Anticonvulsants may be given to control convulsions. Amitriptyline increases the CNS depressant action but not the anticonvulsant action of barbiturates; therefore, an inhalation anesthetic, diazepam, or paraldehyde is recommended for control of convulsions.

Dialysis is of no value because of low plasma concentrations of the drug.

Since overdosage is often deliberate, patients may attempt suicide by other means during the recovery phase.

Deaths by deliberate or accidental overdosage have occurred with this class of drugs.

HOW SUPPLIED

Tablets ELAVIL, 10 mg, are blue, round, film coated tablets, coded STUART 40. They are supplied as follows:

NDC 0038-0040-10 bottles of 100
NDC 0038-0040-34 bottles of 1000

Tablets ELAVIL, 25 mg, are yellow, round, film coated tablets, coded STUART 45. They are supplied as follows:

NDC 0038-0045-10 bottles of 100
NDC 0038-0045-39 unit dose packages of 100
NDC 0038-0045-34 bottles of 1000
NDC 0038-0045-50 bottles of 5000

Tablets ELAVIL, 50 mg, are beige, round, film coated tablets, coded STUART 41. They are supplied as follows:

NDC 0038-0041-10 bottles of 100
NDC 0038-0041-39 unit dose packages of 100
NDC 0038-0041-34 bottles of 1000

Tablets ELAVIL, 75 mg, are orange, round, film coated tablets, coded STUART 42. They are supplied as follows:

NDC 0038-0042-10 bottles of 100

Tablets ELAVIL, 100 mg, are mauve, round, film coated tablets, coded STUART 43. They are supplied as follows:

NDC 0038-0043-10 bottles of 100

Tablets ELAVIL, 150 mg, are blue, capsule shaped, film coated tablets, coded STUART 47. They are supplied as follows:

NDC 0038-0047-30 bottles of 30
NDC 0038-0047-10 bottles of 100

Injection ELAVIL, 10 mg/mL, is a clear, colorless solution and is supplied as follows:

NDC 0038-0049-10 in 10 mL vials

Storage: Store Tablets ELAVIL in a well-closed container. Avoid storage at temperatures above 30°C (86°F). In addition,

Continued on next page

Stuart—Cont.

tablets ELAVIL 10 mg must be protected from light and stored in a well-closed, light-resistant container.
Protect Injection ELAVIL from freezing and avoid storage above 30°C (86°F).

METABOLISM

Studies in man following oral administration of ^{14}C-labeled drug indicated that amitriptyline is rapidly absorbed and metabolized. Radioactivity of the plasma was practically negligible, although significant amounts of radioactivity appeared in the urine by 4 to 6 hours and one-half to one-third of the drug was excreted within 24 hours.
Amitriptyline is metabolized by N-demethylation and bridge hydroxylation in man, rabbit, and rat. Virtually the entire dose is excreted as glucuronide or sulfate conjugate of metabolites, with little unchanged drug appearing in the urine. Other metabolic pathways may be involved.

REFERENCES

Ayd FJ Jr: Amitriptyline (ELAVIL) therapy for depressive reactions. Psychosomatics 1960;1:320–325.
Diamond S: Human metabolization of amitriptyline tagged with carbon 14. Curr Ther Res, Mar 1965, pp 170–175.
Dorfman W: Clinical experiences with amitriptyline (ELAVIL): A preliminary report. Psychosomatics 1960;1:153–155.
Fallette JM, Stasney CR, Mintz AA: Amitriptyline poisoning treated with physostigmine. South Med J 1970; 63:1492–1493.
Hollister LE, Overall JE, Johnson M, et al: Controlled comparison of amitriptyline, imipramine and placebo in hospitalized depressed patients. J Nerv Ment Dis 1964; 139:370–375.
Hordern A, Burt CG, Holt NF: Depressive states: A pharmacotherapeutic study, Springfield study. Springfield, Ill, Charles C. Thomas, 1965.
Klerman GL, Cole JO: Clinical pharmacology of imipramine and related antidepressant compounds. Int J Psychiatry 1976;3:267–304.
McConaghy N, Joffe AD, Kingston WR, et al: Correlation of clinical features of depressed out-patients with response to amitriptyline and protriptyline. Br J Psychiatry 1968; 114:103–106.
McDonald IM, Perkins M, Marjerrison G, et al: A controlled comparison of amitriptyline and electroconvulsive therapy in the treatment of depression. Am J Psychiatry 1966;122: 1427–1431.
Slovis T, Ott J, Teitelbaum, et al: Physostigmine therapy in acute tricyclic antidepressant poisoning. Clin Toxicol 1971;4: 451–459.
Symposium on depression with special studies of a new antidepressant, amitriptyline. Dis Nerv Syst, (Sect 2) May 1961, pp 5–56.

* Registered trademark of ICI Americas Inc.
** Based on a maximum recommended amitriptyline dose of 150 mg/day or 3 mg/kg/day for a 50 kg patient.
*** Hollister LE: JAMA 1979;241:2350–2533.

Manufactured for
Stuart Pharmaceuticals
A business unit of ICI Americas Inc.
Wilmington, DE 19897 USA
by Merck Sharp & Dohme, Division of Merck & Co., Inc.
Rev C 05/91

Shown in Product Identification Section, page 432

HIBICLENS® Antiseptic/Antimicrobial **OTC**
[hi 'bi-klenz]
Skin Cleanser
(chlorhexidine gluconate)

DESCRIPTION

HIBICLENS is an antiseptic antimicrobial skin cleanser possessing bactericidal activities. HIBICLENS contains 4% w/v HIBITANE® (chlorhexidine gluconate), a chemically unique hexamethylenebis biguanide with inactive ingredients: fragrance, isopropyl alcohol 4%, purified water, Red 40, and other ingredients, in a mild, sudsing base adjusted to pH 5.0–6.5 for optimal activity and stability as well as compatability with the normal pH of the skin.

ACTION

HIBICLENS is bactericidal on contact. It has antiseptic activity and a persistent antimicrobial effect with rapid bactericidal activity against a wide range of microorganisms, including gram-positive bacteria, and gram-negative bacteria such as *Pseudomonas aeruginosa.* The effectiveness of HIBICLENS is not signficantly reduced by the presence of organic matter, such as blood.[1]
In a study[2] simulating surgical use, the immediate bactericidal effect of HIBICLENS after a single six-minute scrub resulted in a 99.9% reduction in resident bacterial flora, with a reduction of 99.98% after the eleventh scrub. Reductions on surgically gloved hands were maintained over the six-hour test period.
HIBICLENS displays persistent antimicrobial action. In one study[2], 93% of a radiolabeled formulation of HIBICLENS remained present on uncovered skin after five hours.
HIBICLENS prevents skin infection thereby reducing the risk of cross-infection.

INDICATIONS

HIBICLENS is indicated for use as a surgical scrub, as a health-care personnel handwash, for patient preoperative showering and bathing, as a patient preoperative skin preparation, and as a skin wound cleanser and general skin cleanser.

SAFETY

The extensive use of chlorhexidine gluconate for over 20 years outside the United States has produced no evidence of absorption of the compound through intact skin. The potential for producing skin reactions is extremely low. HIBICLENS can be used many times a day without causing irritation, dryness, or discomfort. Experimental studies indicate that when used for cleaning superficial wounds, HIBICLENS will neither cause additional tissue injury nor delay healing.

WARNINGS

FOR EXTERNAL USE ONLY. KEEP OUT OF EYES, EARS AND MOUTH. HIBICLENS SHOULD NOT BE USED AS A PREOPERATIVE SKIN PREPARATION OF THE FACE OR HEAD. MISUSE OF HIBICLENS HAS BEEN REPORTED TO CAUSE SERIOUS AND PERMANENT EYE INJURY WHEN IT HAS BEEN PERMITTED TO ENTER AND REMAIN IN THE EYE DURING SURGICAL PROCEDURES. IF HIBICLENS SHOULD CONTACT THESE AREAS, RINSE OUT PROMPTLY AND THOROUGHLY WITH WATER.
Avoid contact with meninges. HIBICLENS should not be used by persons who have a sensitivity to it or its components. Chlorhexidine gluconate has been reported to cause deafness when instilled in the middle ear through perforated ear drums. Irritation, sensitization and generalized allergic reactions have been reported with chlorhexidine-containing products, especially in the genital areas. If adverse reactions occur, discontinue use immediately and if severe, contact a physician. Keep this and all drugs out of the reach of children. In case of accidental ingestion, seek professional assistance or contact a Poison Control Center immediately.
Accidental ingestion: Chlorhexidine gluconate taken orally is poorly absorbed. Treat with gastric lavage using milk, egg white, gelatin or mild soap. Employ supportive measures as appropriate.
Avoid excessive heat (above 104°F).

DIRECTIONS FOR USE

Patient preoperative skin preparation
Apply HIBICLENS liberally to surgical site and swab for at least two minutes. Dry with a sterile towel. Repeat procedure for an additional two minutes and dry with a sterile towel.

Preoperative showering and whole-body bathing
The patient should be instructed to wash the entire body, including the scalp, on two consecutive occasions immediately prior to surgery. Each procedure should consist of two consecutive thorough applications of HIBICLENS followed by thorough rinsing. If the patient's condition allows, showering is recommended for whole-body bathing. The recommended procedure is: Wet the body, including hair. Wash the hair using 25 mL of HIBICLENS and the body with another 25 mL of HIBICLENS. Rinse. Repeat. Rinse thoroughly after second application.

Skin wound and general skin cleansing
Wounds which involve more than the superficial layers of the skin should not be routinely treated with HIBICLENS. HIBICLENS should not be used for repeated general skin cleansing of large body areas except in those patients whose underlying skin condition makes it necessary to reduce the bacterial population of the skin. To use, thoroughly rinse the area to be cleansed with water. Apply the minimum amount of HIBICLENS necessary to cover the skin or wound area and wash gently. Rinse again thoroughly.

HEALTH-CARE PERSONNEL USE

SURGICAL HAND SCRUB

Directions for use of HIBICLENS Liquid: Wet hands and forearms to the elbows with warm water. (Avoid using very cold or very hot water.) Dispense about 5 mL of HIBICLENS into cupped hands. Spread over both hands. Scrub hands and forearms for 3 minutes without adding water, using a brush or sponge. (Avoid using extremely hard-bristled brushes.) While scrubbing, pay particular attention to fingernails, cuticles, and interdigital spaces. (Do not use excessive pressure to produce additional lather.) Rinse thoroughly with warm water. Dispense about 5 mL of HIBICLENS into cupped hands. Wash for an additional 3 minutes. (No need to use brush or sponge.) Then rinse thoroughly. Dry thoroughly.

HAND WASH

Wet hands with warm water. (Avoid using very cold or very hot water.) Dispense about 5 mL of HIBICLENS into cupped hands. Wash for 15 seconds. (Do not use excessive pressure to produce additional lather.) Rinse thoroughly with warm water. Dry thoroughly.

Directions for use of HIBICLENS® Sponge/Brush: Open package and remove nail cleaner. Wet hands. Use nail cleaner under fingernails and to clean cuticles. Wet hands and forearms to the elbow with warm water. (Avoid using very cold or very hot water.) Wet sponge side of sponge/brush. Squeeze and pump immediately to work up adequate lather. Apply lather to hands and forearms using *sponge* side of the product. *Start 3 minute scrub* by using the brush side of the product to scrub *only* nails, cuticles, and interdigital areas. Use sponge side for scrubbing hands and forearms. (Avoid using brush on these more sensitive areas.) Rinse thoroughly with warm water. Scrub for an additional 3 minutes *using sponge side* only. To produce additional lather, add a small amount of water and pump the sponge. (While scrubbing, do not use excessive pressure to produce lather—a small amount of lather is all that is required to adequately cleanse skin with HIBICLENS.) Rinse and dry thoroughly, blotting hands and forearms with a soft sterile towel.

IMPORTANT LAUNDERING ADVICE FOR HOSPITAL STAFF AND OTHER USERS OF ANTISEPTIC PATIENT SKIN PREPARATIONS CONTAINING CHLORHEXIDINE GLUCONATE

Chlorhexidine gluconate is a unique agent that most closely fits the definition of an ideal antimicrobial agent, having (among others) one of the most important characteristics of persistent activity. This persistence is due to chlorhexidine gluconate binding to the protein of the skin and, thus, being available for residual activity over a relatively long period of time.
Chlorhexidine gluconate, however, binds not only to protein of the skin, but also to many fabrics, particularly cotton. Thus, special laundering procedures should be considered when such products contact these fabrics. As a result of such contact, chlorhexidine gluconate may become adsorbed onto the fabric and not be removed by washing. If sufficient available chlorine is present during the washing procedure, a fast brown stain may develop due to a chemical reaction between chlorhexidine gluconate and chlorine.

SUGGESTED LAUNDERING PROCEDURES TO LIMIT STAINING

1. **Not Aging.** Avoid allowing the product to age (set) on unwashed linens.
2. **Flushing and Washing.** A flush operation as the initial step in the wash process is helpful in the laundering of linen exposed to chlorhexidine gluconate. Such flushing is also important in the laundering of linen which contains organic materials such as blood or pus. For best results, warm water flushes (90°–100°F) are recommended. After a number of initial flushings followed by a washing with a low alkaline/nonchlorine detergent, most articles which come in contact with chlorhexidine gluconate should have an acceptable level of whiteness. If a rewash process using bleach is necessary to achieve a greater degree of whiteness, the bleach used should be a nonchlorine bleach.
3. **Not Using Chlorine Bleach.** Modern laundering methods often make the use of chlorine bleach unnecessary. It is worthwhile trying to wash without chlorine to ascertain if the resulting degree of whiteness is acceptable. Omission

Operation	Water Level	Temperature	Time (Min)	Supplies/ 100 lb
Break	Low	180°F	20	1.5 lb oxalic acid
Flush	High	Cold	1	—
Emulsify	Low	160°F	5	18 oz emulsifier
Flush	High	Cold	1	—
Bleach	Low	180°F	20	2 lb alkali builder and 1 lb organic bleach
Rinse	High	Cold	1	—
Antichlor	High	Cold	2	4 oz antichlor
Rinse	High	Cold	1	—
Rinse	High	Cold	1	—
Sour	Low	Cold	4	2 oz rust removing sour

of chlorine from the laundering process can extend the useful life of cotton articles since oxidizing bleaches such as chlorine may cause some damage to cellulose even when used in low concentration.

4. **Changing to a Peroxide-Type Bleach, Such as Sodium Perborate, Sodium Percarbonate or Hydrogen Peroxide.** This should eliminate the reaction which could occur with the use of chlorine bleaches. If a chlorine bleach must be used, a concentration of less than 7 ppm available chlorine ($\frac{1}{10}$ the normal bleach level) is suggested to minimize possible staining.

A NOTE ON LAUNDERING OF PERSONAL CLOTHING
The laundering procedures set forth above using low alkaline, nonchlorinated laundry detergents are also applicable to laundering of uniforms and lab coats. Commercially available laundry detergents which do not contain chlorine include Borax, Borateem, Dreft, Oxydol, and Ivory Snow. These products, however, will not remove stains previously set into the fabric.

RECLAMATION OF STAINED LINENS
For those linens which previously have been stained due to the chemical reaction between chlorhexidine gluconate and chlorine, the following laundering procedure may be helpful in reducing the visible stain:
[See table on next page.]

HOW SUPPLIED
For general handwashing locations: pocket-size, 15 mL foil Packettes; plastic disposable bottles of 4 oz and 8 oz with dispenser caps; and 16 oz filled globes. *For surgical scrub areas:* disposable, unit-of-use 22 mL impregnated Sponge/Brushes with nail cleaner; plastic disposable bottles of 32 oz and 1 gal. The 32-oz bottle is designed for a special foot-operated wall dispenser. A hand-operated wall dispenser is available for the 16-oz globe. Hand pumps are available for 16 oz, 32 oz, and 1 gal sizes. Liquid: NDC 0038-0575. Sponge/Brush: NDC 0038-0577.

REFERENCES
1. Lowbury, EJL and Lilly, HA: The effect of blood on disinfection of surgeons' hands, Brit. J. Surg. 61:19–21 (Jan.) 1974.
2. Peterson AF, Rosenberg A, Alatary SD: Comparative evaluation of surgical scrub preparations, Surg. Gynecol. Obstet. 146:63–65 (Jan.) 1978.
Stuart Pharmaceuticals
A business unit of ICI Americas Inc.
Wilmington, DE 19897 USA
Shown in Product Identification Section, page 432

HIBISTAT® Germicidal Hand Rinse   OTC
HIBISTAT® **TOWELETTE**
Germicidal Handwipe
[*hi'bi-stat*]
(chlorhexidine gluconate)

DESCRIPTION
HIBISTAT is a germicidal hand rinse which provides rapid bactericidal action and has a persistent antimicrobial effect against a wide range of microorganisms. HIBISTAT is a clear, colorless liquid containing 0.5% w/w HIBITANE® (chlorhexidine gluconate) with inactive ingredients: emollients, isopropyl alcohol 70%, purified water.

INDICATIONS
HIBISTAT is indicated for health-care personnel use as a germicidal hand rinse. HIBISTAT is for hand hygiene on physically clean hands. It is used in those situations where hands are physically clean, but in need of degerming, when routine handwashing is not convenient or desirable. HIBISTAT provides rapid germicidal action and has a persistent effect.
HIBISTAT should be used in-between patients and procedures where there are no sinks available or continued return to the sink area is inconvenient. HIBISTAT can be used as an alternative to detergent-based products when hands are physically clean. Also, HIBISTAT is an effective germicidal hand rinse following a soap and water handwash.

WARNINGS
Flammable. This product is alcohol based. Alcohol is extremely flammable. It should be kept away from flame or devices which may generate an electrical spark.
FOR EXTERNAL USE ONLY. KEEP OUT OF EYES, EARS AND MOUTH. HIBISTAT SHOULD NOT BE USED AS A PREOPERATIVE SKIN PREPARATION OF THE FACE OR HEAD. MISUSE OF CHLORHEXIDINE-CONTAINING PRODUCTS HAS BEEN REPORTED TO CAUSE SERIOUS AND PERMANENT EYE INJURY WHEN IT HAS BEEN PERMITTED TO ENTER AND REMAIN IN THE EYE DURING SURGICAL PROCEDURES. IF HIBISTAT SHOULD CONTACT THESE AREAS, RINSE OUT PROMPTLY AND THOROUGHLY WITH WATER. Avoid contact with meninges. HIBISTAT should not be used by persons who have a sensitivity to it or its components. Chlorhexidine gluconate has

been reported to cause deafness when instilled in the middle ear through perforated ear drums. Irritation, sensitization, and generalized allergic reactions have been reported with chlorhexidine-containing products, especially in the genital areas. If adverse reactions occur, discontinue use immediately and if severe, contact a physician. Keep this and all drugs out of the reach of children. In case of accidental ingestion, seek professional assistance or contact a Poison Control Center immediately. Avoid excessive heat (above 104°F).
Accidental ingestion: Chlorhexidine gluconate taken orally is poorly absorbed. Treat with gastric lavage using milk, egg white, gelatin or mild soap avoiding pulmonary aspiration. Do not use apomorphine. Assist respiration if necessary and keep patient warm. Intravenous levulose can accelerate alcohol metabolism. In severe cases, hemodialysis or peritoneal dialysis may be appropriate.

DIRECTIONS FOR USE
HIBISTAT Towelette: Rub hands vigorously with the HIBISTAT Towelette for approximately 15 seconds, paying particular attention to nails and interdigital spaces. HIBISTAT dries rapidly in use. No water or towel drying are necessary. The emollients contained in the HIBISTAT Towelette protect the hands from the potential drying effect of alcohol.
HIBISTAT Liquid: Dispense about 5 mL of HIBISTAT into cupped hands and rub vigorously until dry (about 15 seconds), paying particular attention to nails and interdigital spaces. HIBISTAT dries rapidly in use. No water or toweling are necessary. The emollients contained in HIBISTAT protect the hands from the potential drying effect of alcohol.

LAUNDERING
Chlorhexidine gluconate chemically reacts with chlorine to form a brown stain on fabric. Fabric which has come in contact with chlorhexidine gluconate should be rinsed well and washed without the addition of chlorine products. If bleach is desired, only nonchlorine bleach should be used. Full laundering instructions are packed with each case of HIBISTAT. (Please see HIBICLENS® for full laundering instructions.)

HOW SUPPLIED
In plastic disposable bottles of 4 oz and 8 oz with flip-top cap, and in disposable towelettes containing 5 mL, packaged 50 towelettes to a carton.
NDC 0038-0585 (bottles)
NDC 0038-0587 (towelettes)
Stuart Pharmaceuticals
A business unit of ICI Americas Inc
Wilmington, DE 19897 USA
Shown in Product Identification Section, page 432

KINESED® Tablets   ℞
[*kin'e-sed*]
(belladonna alkaloids and phenobarbital)

DESCRIPTION
Each chewable, fruit-flavored, scored, oval KINESED tablet contains:
Phenobarbital .... 16 mg
      (Warning: May be habit forming)
Hyoscyamine Sulfate
Atropine Sulfate   .... 0.12 mg
Scopolamine Hydrobromide .... 0.007 mg
Inactive ingredients: calcium silicate, citric acid, confectioner's sugar, flavors, glyceryl monostearate, lactose, mannitol, povidone, saccharin calcium, sodium citrate, starch, stearic acid.

ACTIONS
This drug combination provides natural belladonna alkaloids in a specific, fixed ratio combined with phenobarbital to provide peripheral anticholinergic/antispasmodic action and mild sedation.

INDICATIONS
Based on a review of this drug by the National Academy of Sciences—National Research Council and/or other information, FDA has classified the following indications as "possibly" effective:
For use as adjunctive therapy in the treatment of irritable bowel syndrome (irritable colon, spastic colon, mucous colitis) and acute enterocolitis. May also be useful as adjunctive therapy in the treatment of duodenal ulcer. IT HAS NOT BEEN SHOWN CONCLUSIVELY WHETHER ANTICHOLINERGIC/ANTISPASMODIC DRUGS AID IN THE HEALING OF A DUODENAL ULCER, DECREASE THE RATE OF RECURRENCES OR PREVENT COMPLICATIONS.

CONTRAINDICATIONS
Glaucoma, obstructive uropathy (for example, bladder neck obstruction due to prostatic hypertrophy); obstructive dis-

ease of the gastrointestinal tract (as in achalasia, pyloroduodenal stenosis, etc.); paralytic ileus, intestinal atony of the elderly or debilitated patient; unstable cardiovascular status in acute hemorrhage; severe ulcerative colitis, especially if complicated by toxic megacolon; myasthenia gravis; hiatal hernia associated with reflux esophagitis.
KINESED is contraindicated in patients with known hypersensitivity to any of the ingredients. Phenobarbital is contraindicated in acute intermittent porphyria and in those patients in whom phenobarbital produces restlessness and/or excitement.

WARNINGS
In the presence of a high environmental temperature, heat prostration can occur with belladonna alkaloids (fever and heatstroke due to decreased sweating). Diarrhea may be an early symptom of incomplete intestinal obstruction, especially in patients with ileostomy or colostomy. In this instance treatment with this drug would be inappropriate and possibly harmful.
KINESED may produce drowsiness or blurred vision. The patient should be warned, should these occur, not to engage in activities requiring mental alertness, such as operating a motor vehicle or other machinery, and not to perform hazardous work.
Phenobarbital may decrease the effect of anticoagulants, and necessitate larger doses of the anticoagulant for optimal effect. When the phenobarbital is discontinued, the dose of the anticoagulant may have to be decreased. Phenobarbital may be habit forming and should not be administered to individuals known to be addiction prone or those with a history of physical and/or psychological dependence upon drugs. Since barbiturates are metabolized in the liver, they should be used with caution and initial doses should be small in patients with hepatic dysfunction.

PRECAUTIONS
Use with caution in patients with: autonomic neuropathy, hepatic or renal disease, hyperthyroidism, coronary heart disease, congestive heart failure, cardiac arrhythmias, tachycardia, and hypertension.
Belladonna alkaloids may produce a delay in gastric emptying (antral stasis) which would complicate the management of gastric ulcer. Theoretically, with overdosage, a curare-like action may occur.
Carcinogenesis, mutagenesis. Long-term studies in animals have not been performed to evaluate carcinogenic potential.
Pregnancy Category C. Animal reproduction studies have not been conducted with KINESED. It is not known whether KINESED can cause fetal harm when administered to a pregnant woman or can affect reproductive capacity. KINESED should be given to a pregnant woman only if clearly needed.
Nursing mothers. Because belladonna alkaloids are excreted in human milk, caution should be exercised when KINESED is administered to a nursing mother.

ADVERSE REACTIONS
Adverse reactions may include xerostomia; urinary hesitancy and retention; blurred vision; tachycardia; palpitation; mydriasis; cycloplegia; increased ocular tension; loss of taste sense; headache; nervousness; drowsiness; weakness; dizziness; insomnia; nausea; vomiting; impotence; suppression of lactation; constipation; bloated feeling; severe allergic reaction or drug idiosyncrasies, including anaphylaxis, urticaria and other dermal manifestations; and decreased sweating.
Elderly patients may react with symptoms of excitement, agitation, drowsiness, and other untoward manifestations to even small doses of the drug.
Phenobarbital may produce excitement in some patients, rather than a sedative effect. In patients habituated to barbiturates, abrupt withdrawal may produce delirium or convulsions.

DOSAGE AND ADMINISTRATION
The dosage of KINESED chewable tablets should be adjusted to the needs of the individual patient to assure symptomatic control with a minimum of adverse effects.
ADULTS: One or two KINESED tablets, three or four times daily, chewed or swallowed with liquids.
CHILDREN, 2 to 12 years: One-half to one KINESED tablet, three or four times daily, chewed or swallowed with liquids.

OVERDOSAGE
The signs and symptoms of overdose are headache, nausea, vomiting, blurred vision, dilated pupils, hot and dry skin, dizziness, dryness of the mouth, difficulty in swallowing and CNS stimulation. Treatment should consist of gastric lavage, emetics, and activated charcoal. If indicated, parenteral cholinergic agents such as physostigmine or bethanechol chloride should be added.

Continued on next page

Stuart—Cont.

HOW SUPPLIED

Bottles of 100 white scored, oval, fruit-flavored, chewable tablets (embossed front "STUART," reverse "220"). NDC 0038-0220. Store at room temperature; avoid excess heat. Dispense in well-closed, light-resistant container.
Manufactured for
Stuart Pharmaceuticals
A business unit of ICI Americas Inc.
Wilmington, DE 19897 USA

Rev D 10/89

Shown in Product Identification Section, page 432

MULVIDREN®–F SOFTAB® Tablets   ℞
[*mul'vi-dren*]
(fluoride with multivitamins)

DESCRIPTION

MULVIDREN®-F SOFTAB® Tablets are formulated to provide daily, oral supplementation of fluoride and multivitamins. The unique design of the tablet assures delivery of all ingredients whether swallowed whole, chewed, allowed to dissolve in the mouth or crushed and mixed with food.

EACH TABLET CONTAINS

Fluoride (from 2.2 mg sodium fluoride) .... 1 mg
Vitamin A .... 4,000 USP units
Vitamin D (ergocalciferol) .... 400 USP units
Vitamin C (ascorbic acid and
   sodium ascorbate) .... 75 mg
Vitamin B_1 (thiamin mononitrate) .... 1.6 mg
Vitamin B_2 (riboflavin) .... 2 mg
Vitamin B_6 (as pyridoxine hydrochloride) .... 1.0 mg
Vitamin B_{12} (cyanocobalamin) .... 3 mcg
Niacinamide .... 10 mg
Pantothenic Acid .... 2.8 mg
Inactive ingredients: flavors, mannitol, saccharin calcium, starch, Yellow 6.

CLINICAL PHARMACOLOGY

Soluble fluorides such as sodium fluoride are efficiently absorbed from the gastrointestinal tract of man, and some topical absorption occurs on tooth surfaces. The major route of fluoride excretion is by way of the kidneys. Fluoride is also excreted in small amounts in sweat, breast milk and feces. Fluoride provides much of its protective action against dental caries by combining with apatite crystals in the tooth structure, thus, forming the less acid soluble compound fluoroapatite.

Controlled studies show a decrease in the incidence of dental caries in children receiving an optimal nutritional supply of fluoride. To achieve maximal anticariogenic effect, fluoride must be provided throughout the stages of tooth formation and calcification. Thus, fluoride should be provided in adequate amounts from birth through the first 15 years of life. If natural sources are deficient, fluoride should be made available throughout this period by daily dietary supplementation. MULVIDREN-F SOFTAB is a well-accepted and convenient form of administering fluoride for both topical and systemic effects.

INDICATIONS AND USAGE

As an aid in promoting the development of caries-resistant teeth in children from birth through the first 15 years of life, MULVIDREN-F provides a source of daily fluoride supplementation in addition to full nutritional amounts of vitamins.

CONTRAINDICATIONS

Patients living in areas where the drinking water is fluoridated at a concentration of greater than 0.7 ppm and those persons with a known sensitivity to fluoride should not take MULVIDREN-F.

WARNINGS

Dental fluorosis (mottling) may result from exceeding the recommended dose (see Dosage and Administration).

PRECAUTIONS

When prescribing MULVIDREN-F, the physician should make sure the child is not receiving significant amounts of fluoride from other sources (ie, medications, drinking water) (see Dosage and Administration).

ADVERSE REACTIONS

In hypersensitive individuals, fluorides occasionally cause skin eruptions such as atopic dermatitis, eczema or urticaria. Gastric distress, headache and weakness have also been reported. These hypersensitivity reactions usually disappear promptly after discontinuation of the fluoride. In rare cases, a delay in the eruption of teeth has been reported.

DOSAGE AND ADMINISTRATION

The daily fluoride intake from dietary supplements such as MULVIDREN-F must be adjusted according to the fluoride intake from other sources such as drinking water. The following dosage schedules are recommended.

Less than 0.3 ppm fluoride in drinking water:
Infants, birth to 2 years of age—0.25 mg of fluoride daily.
Children 2 to 3 years of age—0.5 mg of fluoride daily or one-half MULVIDREN-F tablet daily.
Children 3 to 16 years of age—1.0 mg of fluoride daily or one MULVIDREN-F tablet daily.
0.3 to 0.7 ppm fluoride in drinking water:
Infants, birth to 2 years of age—no fluoride supplementation recommended.
Children 2 to 3 years of age—0.25 mg of fluoride daily
Children 3 to 16 years of age—0.5 mg of fluoride daily or one-half MULVIDREN-F tablet daily
Greater than 0.7 ppm fluoride in drinking water:
No fluoride supplementation recommended.
MULVIDREN-F tablets may be swallowed, chewed and swallowed, allowed to dissolve in the mouth or crushed and mixed with food.

HOW SUPPLIED

In bottles of 100 orange colored, scored SOFTAB tablets, identified front "Stuart," reverse "710." A childproof safety cap is standard on each 100 tablet bottle as a safeguard against accidental ingestion.
Store at room temperature; avoid excess heat. Dispense in well-closed, light resistant container.
NDC 0038-0710.
Manufactured for
Stuart Pharmaceuticals
A business unit of ICI Americas Inc.
Wilmington, DE 19897 USA

Rev. E 07/90

Shown in Product Identification Section, page 432

STUART PRENATAL® Tablets   OTC
Multivitamin/Multimineral Supplement
As of September 1992, this product was transferred to Wyeth-Ayerst.

ONE TABLET DAILY PROVIDES:

Vitamins	RDA*	
A	90%	4,000 IU
D	100%	400 IU
E	90%	11 mg
C	110%	100 mg
Folic acid	200%	0.8 mg
Thiamin mononitrate	90%	1.5 mg
Riboflavin	90%	1.7 mg
Niacinamide	90%	18 mg
B_6 (pyridoxine)	120%	2.6 mg
B_{12}	150%	4 mcg
Minerals		
Calcium	20%	200 mg
Iron	200%	60 mg
Zinc	130%	25 mg

*Recommended Dietary Allowance (Food and Nutrition Board, NAS/NRC-1989) for pregnant and/or lactating women.

Ingredients:

Active: calcium sulfate, ferrous fumarate, ascorbic acid, dl-alpha tocopheryl acetate, zinc oxide, niacinamide, vitamin A acetate, pyridoxine hydrochloride, riboflavin, thiamin mononitrate, folic acid, cholecalciferol, cyanocobalamin. Inactive: croscarmellose sodium, hydroxpropyl methylcellulose, microcrystalline cellulose, pregelatinized starch, red iron oxide, titanium dioxide.

INDICATIONS

STUART PRENATAL is a nonprescription multivitamin/multimineral supplement for use before, during, and after pregnancy. It provides essential vitamins and minerals, including 60 mg of elemental iron as well-tolerated ferrous fumarate, 200 mg of elemental calcium (non-alkalizing and phosphorus-free), and 25 mg zinc.

DIRECTIONS

Before, during and after pregnancy, one tablet daily, or as directed by a physician.

WARNINGS

As with all medications, keep out of the reach of children. In case of accidental overdose, seek professional assistance or contact a Poison Control Center immediately.

HOW SUPPLIED

Bottles of 100 light pink capsule-shaped tablets imprinted "Stuart 071." A child-resistant safety cap is standard on 100 tablet bottles as a safeguard against accidental ingestion by children.
NDC 0038-0071.
Issued 03/91
Manufactured for
Stuart Pharmaceuticals
A business unit of ICI Americas Inc.
Wilmington, DE 19897 USA

Shown in Product Identification Section, page 432

STUARTNATAL® 1+1 Tablets   ℞
[*stu'art na'tal*]
Multivitamin/Multimineral Supplement
As of September 1992, this product was transferred to Wyeth-Ayerst.

COMPOSITION

One tablet daily provides:

Vitamins	RDA*	
A	90%	4,000 IU
D (cholecalciferol)	100%	400 IU
E	90%	11 mg
C (ascorbic acid)	130%	120 mg
Folic acid	250%	1 mg
Thiamin mononitrate	90%	1.5 mg
Riboflavin	170%	3 mg
Niacinamide	100%	20 mg
B_6 (pyridoxine)	450%	10 mg
B_{12} (cyanocobalamin)	460%	12 mcg
Minerals		
Calcium	20%	200 mg
Copper	NA**	2 mg
Iron	220%	65 mg
Zinc	130%	25 mg

*Recommended Dietary Allowances (Food and Nutrition Board, NAS/NRC-1989) for pregnant and/or lactating women.

**Not Applicable—Because of the uncertainty about the quantitative human requirement for copper, it is not possible to establish an RDA for this trace element. Source: Food and Nutrition Board, NAS/NRC 1989.

INDICATIONS

STUARTNATAL 1+1 is indicated to provide potent vitamin and mineral supplementation throughout pregnancy and during the postnatal period—for both the lactating and non-lactating mother. It is also useful for improving nutritional status prior to conception.
Each tablet provides essential vitamins and minerals, including 1 full grain of elemental iron and 200 mg of elemental calcium (non-alkalizing and phosphorus-free) and 25 mg zinc. STUARTNATAL 1+1 also offers 1 mg folic acid to aid in the prevention of megaloblastic anemia.

PRECAUTION

Federal law prohibits dispensing without prescription.
Folic acid may partially correct the hematological damage due to vitamin B_{12} deficiency of pernicious anemia, while the associated neurological damage progresses.
Store at room temperature; avoid excess heat. Dispense in well-closed, light-resistant container.

DIRECTIONS

Before, during and after pregnancy, one tablet daily, or as directed by a physician.

WARNING

As with all medications, keep out of the reach of children. In case of accidental overdose, seek professional assistance or contact a Poison Control Center immediately.

HOW SUPPLIED

Bottles of 100 and 500 light yellow, capsule-shaped tablets identified "Stuart 021." A child-resistant safety cap is standard on 100 tablet bottles as a safeguard against accidental ingestion by children.
NDC 0038-0021.
Issued 03/91
Manufactured for
Stuart Pharmaceuticals
A business unit of ICI Americas Inc.
Wilmington, DE 19897 USA

Shown in Product Identification Section, page 432

ZESTORETIC®   ℞
(lisinopril, hydrochlorothiazide)

USE IN PREGNANCY
When used in pregnancy during the second and third trimesters, ACE inhibitors can cause injury and death to the developing fetus. When pregnancy is detected, ZESTORETIC should be discontinued as soon as possible. See WARNINGS, Pregnancy, Lisinopril, Fetal/Neonatal Morbidity and Mortality.

DESCRIPTION

ZESTORETIC® (Lisinopril and Hydrochlorothiazide) combines an angiotensin converting enzyme inhibitor, lisinopril, and a diuretic, hydrochlorothiazide.
Lisinopril, a synthetic peptide derivative, is an oral long-acting angiotensin converting enzyme inhibitor. It is chemically described as (S)-1-[N^2-(1-carboxy-3-phenylpropyl)-L-lysyl]-L-proline dihydrate. Its empirical formula is $C_{21}H_{31}N_3O_5 \cdot 2H_2O$ and its structural formula is:
[See chemical structure at top of next page.]

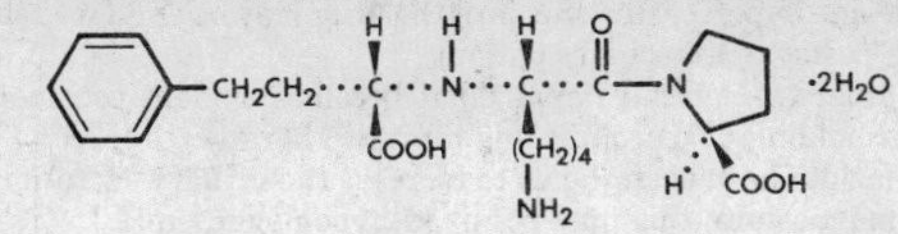

Lisinopril is a white to off-white, crystalline powder, with a molecular weight of 441.53. It is soluble in water, sparingly soluble in methanol, and practically insoluble in ethanol.
Hydrochlorothiazide is 6-chloro-3,4-dihydro-2H-1,2,4-benzothiadiazine-7-sulfonamide 1,1-dioxide. Its empirical formula is $C_7H_8ClN_3O_4S_2$ and its structural formula is:

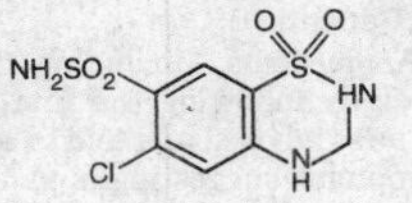

Hydrochlorothiazide is a white, or practically white, crystalline powder with a molecular weight of 297.72, which is slightly soluble in water, but freely soluble in sodium hydroxide solution.
ZESTORETIC is available for oral use in two tablet combinations of lisinopril with hydrochlorothiazide: ZESTORETIC 20-12.5 containing 20 mg lisinopril and 12.5 mg hydrochlorothiazide; and, ZESTORETIC 20-25 containing 20 mg lisinopril and 25 mg hydrochlorothiazide.
Inactive Ingredients:
20-12.5 Tablets—calcium phosphate, magnesium stearate, mannitol, starch.
20-25 Tablets—calcium phosphate, magnesium stearate, mannitol, red ferric oxide, starch, yellow ferric oxide.

CLINICAL PHARMACOLOGY

Lisinopril and Hydrochlorothiazide
As a result of its diuretic effects, hydrochlorothiazide increases plasma renin activity, increases aldosterone secretion, and decreases serum potassium. Administration of lisinopril blocks the renin-angiotensin aldosterone axis and tends to reverse the potassium loss associated with the diuretic.
In clinical studies, the extent of blood pressure reduction seen with the combination of lisinopril and hydrochlorothiazide was approximately additive. The combination appeared somewhat less effective in black patients, but relatively few black patients were studied. In most patients, the antihypertensive effect of ZESTORETIC was sustained for at least 24 hours.
In a randomized, controlled comparison, the mean antihypertensive effects of ZESTORETIC 20-12.5 and ZESTORETIC 20-25 were similar, suggesting that many patients who respond adequately to the latter combination may be controlled with ZESTORETIC 20-12.5. (See DOSAGE AND ADMINISTRATION.)
Concomitant administration of lisinopril and hydrochlorothiazide has little or no effect on the bioavailability of either drug. The combination tablet is bioequivalent to concomitant administration of the separate entities.

Lisinopril
Mechanism of Action: Lisinopril inhibits angiotensin-converting enzyme (ACE) in human subjects and animals. ACE is a peptidyl dipeptidase that catalyzes the conversion of angiotensin I to the vasoconstrictor substance, angiotensin II. Angiotensin II also stimulates aldosterone secretion by the adrenal cortex. Inhibition of ACE results in decreased plasma angiotensin II which leads to decreased vasopressor activity and to decreased aldosterone secretion. The latter decrease may result in a small increase of serum potassium. Removal of angiotensin II negative feedback on renin secretion leads to increased plasma renin activity. In hypertensive patients with normal renal function treated with lisinopril alone for up to 24 weeks, the mean increase in serum potassium was less than 0.1 mEq/L; however, approximately 15 percent of patients had increases greater than 0.5 mEq/L and approximately six percent had a decrease greater than 0.5 mEq/L. In the same study, patients treated with lisinopril plus a thiazide diuretic showed essentially no change in serum potassium. (See PRECAUTIONS.)
ACE is identical to kininase, an enzyme that degrades bradykinin. Whether increased levels of bradykinin, a potent vasodepressor peptide, play a role in the therapeutic effects of lisinopril remains to be elucidated.
While the mechanism through which lisinopril lowers blood pressure is believed to be primarily suppression of the renin-angiotensin-aldosterone system, lisinopril is antihypertensive even in patients with low-renin hypertension. Although lisinopril was antihypertensive in all races studied, black hypertensive patients (usually a low-renin hypertensive population) had a smaller average response to lisinopril monotherapy than nonblack patients.
Pharmacokinetics and Metabolism: Following oral administration of lisinopril, peak serum concentrations occur within about 7 hours. Declining serum concentrations exhibit a prolonged terminal phase which does not contribute to drug accumulation. This terminal phase probably represents saturable binding to ACE and is not proportional to dose. Lisinopril does not appear to be bound to other serum proteins.
Lisinopril does not undergo metabolism and is excreted unchanged entirely in the urine. Based on urinary recovery, the mean extent of absorption of lisinopril is approximately 25 percent, with large intersubject variability (6%–60%) at all doses tested (5–80 mg). Lisinopril absorption is not influenced by the presence of food in the gastrointestinal tract.
Upon multiple dosing, lisinopril exhibits an effective half-life of accumulation of 12 hours.
Impaired renal function decreases elimination of lisinopril, which is excreted principally through the kidneys, but this decrease becomes clinically important only when the glomerular filtration rate is below 30 mL/min. Above this glomerular filtration rate, the elimination half-life is little changed. With greater impairment, however, peak and trough lisinopril levels increase, time to peak concentration increases and time to attain steady state is prolonged. Older patients, on average, have (approximately doubled) higher blood levels and area under the plasma concentration time curve (AUC) than younger patients. (See DOSAGE AND ADMINISTRATION.) Lisinopril can be removed by hemodialysis.
Studies in rats indicate that lisinopril crosses the blood-brain barrier poorly. Multiple doses of lisinopril in rats do not result in accumulation in any tissues. However, milk of lactating rats contains radioactivity following administration of ^{14}C lisinopril. By whole body autoradiography, radioactivity was found in the placenta following administration of labeled drug to pregnant rats, but none was found in the fetuses.
Pharmacodynamics: Administration of lisinopril to patients with hypertension results in a reduction of supine and standing blood pressure to about the same extent with no compensatory tachycardia. Symptomatic postural hypotension is usually not observed although it can occur and should be anticipated in volume and/or salt-depleted patients. (See WARNINGS.)
In most patients studied, onset of antihypertensive activity was seen at one hour after oral administration of an individual dose of lisinopril, with peak reduction of blood pressure achieved by six hours.
In some patients achievement of optimal blood pressure reduction may require two to four weeks of therapy.
At recommended single daily doses, antihypertensive effects have been maintained for at least 24 hours, after dosing, although the effect at 24 hours was substantially smaller than the effect six hours after dosing.
The antihypertensive effects of lisinopril have continued during long term therapy. Abrupt withdrawal of lisinopril has not been associated with a rapid increase in blood pressure; nor with a significant overshoot of pretreatment blood pressure.
In hemodynamic studies in patients with essential hypertension, blood pressure reduction was accompanied by a reduction in peripheral arterial resistance with little or no change in cardiac output and in heart rate. In a study in nine hypertensive patients, following administration of lisinopril, there was an increase in mean renal blood flow that was not significant. Data from several small studies are inconsistent with respect to the effect of lisinopril on glomerular filtration rate in hypertensive patients with normal renal function, but suggest that changes, if any, are not large.
In patients with renovascular hypertension lisinopril has been shown to be well tolerated and effective in controlling blood pressure. (See PRECAUTIONS.)

Hydrochlorothiazide
The mechanism of the antihypertensive effect of thiazides is unknown. Thiazides do not usually affect normal blood pressure.
Hydrochlorothiazide is a diuretic and antihypertensive. It affects the distal renal tubular mechanism of electrolyte reabsorption. Hydrochlorothiazide increases excretion of sodium and chloride in approximately equivalent amounts. Natriuresis may be accompanied by some loss of potassium and bicarbonate.
After oral use diuresis begins within two hours, peaks in about four hours and lasts about 6 to 12 hours.
Hydrochlorothiazide is not metabolized but is eliminated rapidly by the kidney. When plasma levels have been followed for at least 24 hours, the plasma half-life has been observed to vary between 5.6 and 14.8 hours. At least 61 percent of the oral dose is eliminated unchanged within 24 hours. Hydrochlorothiazide crosses the placental but not the blood-brain barrier.

INDICATIONS AND USAGE

ZESTORETIC is indicated for the treatment of hypertension in patients for whom combination therapy is appropriate.
This fixed dose combination is not indicated for initial therapy. Patients already receiving a diuretic when lisinopril is initiated, or given a diuretic and lisinopril simultaneously, can develop symptomatic hypotension. In the initial titration of the individual entities, it is important, if possible, to stop the diuretic for several days before starting lisinopril or, if this is not possible, begin lisinopril at a low initial dose. (See DOSAGE AND ADMINISTRATION.)
In using ZESTORETIC, consideration should be given to the fact that an angiotensin converting enzyme inhibitor, captopril, has caused agranulocytosis, particularly in patients with renal impairment or collagen vascular disease, and that available data are insufficient to show that lisinopril does not have a similar risk. (See WARNINGS.)

CONTRAINDICATIONS

ZESTORETIC is contraindicated in patients who are hypersensitive to any component of this product and in patients with a history of angioedema related to previous treatment with an angiotensin converting enzyme inhibitor. Because of the hydrochlorothiazide component, this product is contraindicated in patients with anuria or hypersensitivity to other sulfonamide-derived drugs.

WARNINGS

Lisinopril
Angioedema: Angioedema of the face, extremities, lips, tongue, glottis and/or larynx has been reported rarely in patients treated with angiotensin converting enzyme inhibitors, including lisinopril. In such cases ZESTORETIC should be promptly discontinued and the appropriate therapy and monitoring should be provided until complete and sustained resolution of signs and symptoms has occurred. In instances where swelling has been confined to the face and lips the condition has generally resolved without treatment, although antihistamines have been useful in relieving symptoms. Angioedema associated with laryngeal edema may be fatal. **Where there is involvement of the tongue, glottis or larynx, likely to cause airway obstruction, subcutaneous epinephrine solution 1:1000 (0.3 mL to 0.5 mL) and/or measures necessary to ensure a patient airway should be promptly provided. (See** ADVERSE REACTIONS.)
Hypotension and Related Effects: Excessive hypotension was rarely seen in uncomplicated hypertensive patients but is a possible consequence of lisinopril use in salt/volume-depleted persons such as those treated vigorously with diuretics or patients on dialysis. (See PRECAUTIONS, Drug Interactions and ADVERSE REACTIONS.)
Syncope has been reported in 0.8 percent of patients receiving ZESTORETIC. In patients with hypertension receiving lisinopril alone, the incidence of syncope was 0.1 percent. The overall incidence of syncope may be reduced by proper titration of the individual components. (See PRECAUTIONS, Drug Interactions, ADVERSE REACTIONS and DOSAGE AND ADMINISTRATION.)
In patients with severe congestive heart failure, with or without associated renal insufficiency, excessive hypotension has been observed and may be associated with oliguria and/or progressive azotemia, and rarely with acute renal failure and/or death. Because of the potential fall in blood pressure in these patients, therapy should be started under very close medical supervision. Such patients should be followed closely for the first two weeks of treatment and whenever the dose of lisinopril and/or diuretic is increased. Similar considerations apply to patients with ischemic heart or cerebrovascular disease in whom an excessive fall in blood pressure could result in a myocardial infarction or cerebrovascular accident.
If hypotension occurs, the patient should be placed in supine position and, if necessary, receive an intravenous infusion of normal saline. A transient hypotensive response is not a contraindication to further doses which usually can be given without difficulty once the blood pressure has increased after volume expansion.
Neutropenia/Agranulocytosis: Another angiotensin converting enzyme inhibitor, captopril, has been shown to cause agranulocytosis and bone marrow depression, rarely in uncomplicated patients but more frequently in patients with renal impairment, especially if they also have a collagen vascular disease. Available data from clinical trials of lisinopril are insufficient to show that lisinopril does not cause agranulocytosis at similar rates. Marketing experience has revealed rare cases of neutropenia and bone marrow deppression in which a causal relationship to lisinopril cannot be excluded. Periodic monitoring of white blood cell counts in patients with collagen vascular disease and renal disease should be considered.

Pregnancy
Lisinopril and Hydrochlorothiazide: Teratogenicity studies were conducted in mice and rats with up to 90 mg/kg/day of lisinopril (56 times the maximum recommended human dose) in combination with 10 mg/kg/day of hydrochlorothiazide (2.5 times the maximum recommended human dose). Maternal of fetotoxic effects were not seen in mice with the combination. In rats decreased maternal weight gain and decreased fetal weight occurred down to 3/10 mg/kg/day (the lowest dose tested). Associated with the decreased fetal weight was a delay in fetal ossification. The

Continued on next page

Stuart—Cont.

decreased fetal weight and delay in fetal ossification were not seen in saline-supplemented animals given $^{90}/_{10}$ mg/kg/day.

If ZESTORETIC is used during pregnancy or if the patient becomes pregnant while taking ZESTORETIC, the patient should be apprised of the potential hazards to the fetus. (See Lisinopril, Fetal/Neonatal Morbidity and Mortality below.)

Lisinopril

Fetal/Neonatal Morbidity and Mortality: ACE inhibitors can cause fetal and neonatal morbidity and death when administered to pregnant women. Several dozen cases have been reported in the world literature. When pregnancy is detected, ACE inhibitor therapy should be discontinued as soon as possible.

The use of ACE inhibitors during the second and third trimesters of pregnancy has been associated with fetal and neonatal injury, including hypotension, neonatal skull hypoplasia, anuria, reversible or irreversible renal failure, and death. Oligohydramnios has also been reported, presumably resulting from decreased fetal renal function; oligohydramnios in this setting has been associated with fetal limb contractures, craniofacial deformation, and hypoplastic lung development. Prematurity, intrauterine growth retardation, and patent ductus arteriosus have also been reported, although it is not clear whether these occurrences were due to the ACE-inhibitor exposure.

These adverse effects do not appear to have resulted from intrauterine ACE-inhibitor exposure that has been limited to the first trimester. Mothers whose embryos and fetuses are exposed to ACE inhibitors only during the first trimester should be so informed. Nonetheless, when patients become pregnant, physicians should make every effort to discontinue the use of ZESTORETIC as soon as possible.

Rarely (probably less often than once in every thousand pregnancies), no alternative to ACE inhibitors will be found. In these rare cases, the mothers should be apprised of the potential hazards to their fetuses, and serial ultrasound examinations should be performed to assess the intraamniotic environment.

If oligohydramnios is observed, ZESTORETIC should be discontinued unless it is considered lifesaving for the mother. Contraction stress testing (CST), a nonstress test (NST), or biophysical profiling (BPP) may be appropriate, depending upon the week of pregnancy. Patients and physicians should be aware, however, that oligohydramnios may not appear until after the fetus has sustained irreversible injury.

Infants with histories of in utero exposure to ACE inhibitors should be closely observed for hypotension, oliguria, and hyperkalemia. If oliguria occurs, attention should be directed toward support of blood pressure and renal perfusion. Exchange transfusion or dialysis may be required as means of reversing hypotension and/or substituting for disordered renal function. Lisinopril, which crosses the placenta, has been removed from neonatal circulation by peritoneal dialysis with some clinical benefit, and theoretically may be removed by exchange transfusion, although there is no experience with the latter procedure.

No teratogenic effects of lisinopril were seen in studies of pregnant rats, mice, and rabbits. On a mg/kg basis, the doses used were up to 625 times (in mice), 188 times (in rats), 0.6 times (in rabbits) the maximum recommended human dose.

Hydrochlorothiazide

Teratogenic Effects: Reproduction studies in the rabbit, the mouse and the rat at doses up to 100 mg/kg/day (50 times the human dose) showed no evidence of external abnormalities of the fetus due to hydrochlorothiazide. Hydrochlorothiazide given in a two-litter study in rats at doses of 4–5.6 mg/kg/day (approximately 1–2 times the usual daily human dose) did not impair fertility or produce birth abnormalities in the offspring. Thiazides cross the placental barrier and appear in cord blood.

Nonteratogenic Effects: These may include fetal or neonatal jaundice, thrombocytopenia, and possibly other adverse reactions have occurred in the adult.

Hydrochlorothiazide

Thiazides should be used with caution in severe renal disease. In patients with renal disease, thiazides may precipitate azotemia. Cumulative effects of the drug may develop in patients with impaired renal function.

Thiazides should be used with caution in patients with impaired hepatic function or progressive liver disease, since minor alterations of fluid and electrolyte balance may precipitate hepatic coma.

Sensitivity reactions may occur in patients with or without a history of allergy or bronchial asthma.

The possibility of exacerbation or activation of systemic lupus erythematosus has been reported.

Lithium generally should not be given with thiazides. (See PRECAUTIONS, Drug Interactions, Lisinopril and Hydrochlorothiazide.)

PRECAUTIONS

General

Lisinopril

Impaired Renal Function: As a consequence of inhibiting the renin-angiotensin-aldosterone system, changes in renal function may be anticipated in susceptible individuals. In patients with severe congestive heart failure whose renal function may depend on the activity of the renin-angiotensin-aldosterone system, treatment with angiotensin converting enzyme inhibitors, including lisinopril, may be associated with oliguria and/or progressive azotemia and rarely with acute renal failure and/or death.

In hypertensive patients with unilateral or bilateral renal artery stenosis, increases in blood urea nitrogen and serum creatinine may occur. Experience with another angiotensin converting enzyme inhibitor suggests that these increases are usually reversible upon discontinuation of lisinopril and/or diuretic therapy. In such patients renal function should be monitored during the first few weeks of therapy. Some hypertensive patients with no apparent pre-existing renal vascular disease have developed increases in blood urea and serum creatinine, usually minor and transient, especially when lisinopril has been given concomitantly with a diuretic. This is more likely to occur in patients with pre-existing renal impairment. Dosage reduction of lisinopril and/or discontinuation of the diuretic may be required.

Evaluation of the hypertensive patient should always include assessment of renal function. (See DOSAGE and ADMINISTRATION.)

Hyperkalemia: In clinical trials hyperkalemia (serum potassium greater than 5.7 mEq/L) occurred in approximately 1.4 percent of hypertensive patients treated with lisinopril plus hydrochlorothiazide. In most cases these were isolated values which resolved despite continued therapy. Hyperkalemia was not a cause of discontinuation of therapy. Risk factors for the development of hyperkalemia include renal insufficiency, diabetes mellitus, and the concomitant use of potassium-sparing diuretics, potassium supplements and/or potassium-containing salt substitutes, which should be used cautiously if at all with ZESTORETIC. (See Drug Interactions.)

Cough: Cough has been reported with the use of ACE inhibitors. Characteristically, the cough is nonproductive, persistent and resolves after discontinuation of therapy. ACE inhibitor-induced cough should be considered as part of the differential diagnosis of cough.

Surgery/Anesthesia: In patients undergoing major surgery or during anesthesia with agents that produce hypotension, lisinopril may block angiotensin II formation secondary to compensatory renin release. If hypotension occurs and is considered to be due to this mechanism, it can be corrected by volume expansion.

Hydrochlorothiazide

Periodic determination of serum electrolytes to detect possible electrolyte imbalance should be performed at appropriate intervals.

All patients receiving thiazide therapy should be observed for clinical signs of fluid or electrolyte imbalance: namely, hyponatremia, hypochloremic alkalosis, and hypokalemia. Serum and urine electrolyte determinations are particularly important when the patient is vomiting excessively or receiving parenteral fluids. Warning signs or symptoms of fluid and electrolyte imbalance, irrespective of cause, include dryness of mouth, thirst, weakness, lethargy, drowsiness, restlessness, muscle pains or cramps, muscular fatigue, hypotension, oliguria, tachycardia, and gastrointestinal disturbances such as nausea and vomiting.

Hypokalemia may develop, especially with brisk diuresis, when severe cirrhosis is present, or after prolonged therapy. Interference with adequate oral electrolyte intake will also contribute to hypokalemia. Hypokalemia may cause cardiac arrhythmia and may also sensitize or exaggerate the response of the heart to the toxic effects of digitalis (eg, increased ventricular irritability). Because lisinopril reduces the production of aldosterone, concomitant therapy with lisinopril attenuates the diuretic-induced potassium loss. (See Drug Interactions, Agents Increasing Serum Potassium.)

Although any chloride deficit is generally mild and usually does not require specific treatment, except under extraordinary circumstances (as in liver disease or renal disease), chloride replacement may be required in the treatment of metabolic alkalosis.

Dilutional hyponatremia may occur in edematous patients in hot weather; appropriate therapy is water restriction, rather than administration of salt except in rare instances when the hyponatremia is life-threatening. In actual salt depletion, appropriate replacement is the therapy of choice.

Hyperuricemia may occur or frank gout may be precipitated in certain patients receiving thiazide therapy.

In diabetic patients dosage adjustments of insulin or oral hypoglycemic agents may be required. Hyperglycemia may occur with thiazide diuretics. Thus latent diabetes mellitus may become manifest during thiazide therapy.

The antihypertensive effects of the drug may be enhanced in the postsympathectomy patient.

If progressive renal impairment becomes evident consider withholding or discontinuing diuretic therapy.

Thiazides have been shown to increase the urinary excretion of magnesium; this may result in hypomagnesemia.

Thiazides may decrease urinary calcium excretion. Thiazides may cause intermittent and slight elevation of serum calcium in the absence of known disorders of calcium metabolism. Marked hypercalcemia may be evidence of hidden hyperparathyroidism. Thiazides should be discontinued before carrying out tests for parathyroid function.

Increases in cholesterol and triglyceride levels may be associated with thiazide diuretic therapy.

Information for Patients

Angioedema: Angioedema, including laryngeal edema, may occur especially following the first dose of lisinopril. Patients should be so advised and told to report immediately any signs or symptoms suggesting angioedema (swelling of face, extremities, eyes, lips, tongue, difficulty in swallowing or breathing) and to take no more drug until they have consulted with the prescribing physician.

Symptomatic Hypotension: Patients should be cautioned to report lightheadedness especially during the first few days of therapy. If actual syncope occurs, the patients should be told to discontinue the drug until they have consulted with the prescribing physician.

All patients should be cautioned that excessive perspiration and dehydration may lead to an excessive fall in blood pressure because of reduction in fluid volume. Other causes of volume depletion such as vomiting or diarrhea may also lead to a fall in blood pressure; patients should be advised to consult with their physician.

Hyperkalemia: Patients should be told not to use salt substitutes containing potassium without consulting their physician.

Neutropenia: Patients should be told to report promptly any indication of infection (eg, sore throat, fever) which may be a sign of neutropenia.

Pregnancy: Female patients of childbearing age should be told about the consequences of second- and third-trimester exposure to ACE inhibitors, and they should also be told that these consequences do not appear to have resulted from intrauterine ACE-inhibitor exposure that has been limited to the first trimester. These patients should be asked to report pregnancies to their physicians as soon as possible.

NOTE: As with many other drugs, certain advice to patients being treated with ZESTORETIC is warranted. This information is intended to aid in the safe and effective use of this medication. It is not a disclosure of all possible adverse or intended effects.

Drug Interactions

Lisinopril

Hypotension—Patients on Diuretic Therapy: Patients on diuretics and especially those in whom diuretic therapy was recently instituted, may occasionally experience an excessive reduction of blood pressure after initiation of therapy with lisinopril. The possibility of hypotensive effects with lisinopril can be minimized by either discontinuing the diuretic or increasing the salt intake prior to initiation of treatment with lisinopril at a dose of 5 mg daily, and provide close medical supervision after the initial dose for at least two hours and until blood pressure has stabilized for at least an additional hour. (See WARNINGS, and DOSAGE AND ADMINISTRATION.) When a diuretic is added to the therapy of a patient receiving lisinopril, an additional antihypertensive effect is usually observed. (See DOSAGE AND ADMINISTRATION.)

Indomethacin: In a study in 36 patients with mild to moderate hypertension where the antihypertensive effects of lisinopril alone were compared to lisinopril given concomitantly with indomethacin, the use of indomethacin was associated with a reduced effect, although the difference between the two regimens was not significant.

Other Agents: Lisinopril has been used concomitantly with nitrates and/or digoxin without evidence of clinically significant adverse interactions. No meaningful clinically important pharmacokinetic interactions occurred when lisinopril was used concomitantly with propranolol, digoxin, or hydrochlorothiazide. The presence of food in the stomach does not alter the bioavailability of lisinopril.

Agents Increasing Serum Potassium: Lisinopril attenuates potassium loss caused by thiazide-type diuretics. Use of lisinopril with potassium-sparing diuretics (eg, spironolactone, triamterene, or amiloride), potassium supplements, or potassium-containing salt substitutes may lead to significant increases in serum potassium. Therefore, if concomitant use of these agents is indicated, because of demonstrated hypokalemia, they should be used with caution and with frequent monitoring of serum potassium.

Lithium: Lithium toxicity has been reported in patients receiving lithium concomitantly with drugs which cause elimination of sodium, including ACE inhibitors. Lithium toxicity was usually reversible upon discontinuation of lithium and the ACE inhibitor. It is recommended that serum

lithium levels be monitored frequently if lisinopril is administered concomitantly with lithium.

Hydrochlorothiazide

When administered concurrently the following drugs may interact with thiazide diuretics.

Alcohol, barbiturates, or narcotics—potentiation of orthostatic hypotension may occur.

Antidiabetic drugs (oral agents and insulin)—dosage adjustment of the antidiabetic drug may be required.

Other antihypertensive drugs—additive effect or potentiation.

Corticosteroids, ACTH—intensified electrolyte depletion, particularly hypokalemia.

Pressor amines (eg, norepinephrine)—possible decreased response to pressor amines but not sufficient to preclude their use.

Skeletal muscle relaxants, nondepolarizing (eg, tubocurarine)—possible increased responsiveness to the muscle relaxant.

Lithium—should not generally be given with diuretics. Diuretic agents reduce the renal clearance of lithium and add a high risk of lithium toxicity. Refer to the package insert for lithium preparations before use of such preparations with ZESTORETIC.

Non-Steroidal Anti-inflammatory Drugs—In some patients, the administration of a non-steroidal anti-inflammatory agent can reduce the diuretic, natriuretic, and antihypertensive effects of loop, potassium-sparing and thiazide diuretics. Therefore, when ZESTORETIC and non-steroidal anti-inflammatory agents are used concomitantly, the patient should be observed closely to determine if the desired effect of ZESTORETIC is obtained.

Carcinogenesis, Mutagenesis, Impairment of Fertility

Lisinopril and Hydrochlorothiazide: Lisinopril in combination with hydrochlorothiazide was not mutagenic in a microbial mutagen test using *Salmonella typhimurium* (Ames test) or *Escherichia coli* with or without metabolic activation or in a forward mutation assay using Chinese hamster lung cells. Lisinopril and hydrochlorothiazide did not produce DNA single strand breaks in an in vitro alkaline elution rat hepatocyte assay. In addition, it did not produce increases in chromosomal aberrations in an in vitro test in Chinese hamster ovary cells or in an in vivo study in mouse bone marrow.

Lisinopril: There was no evidence of a tumorigenic effect when lisinopril was administered for 105 weeks to male and female rats at doses up to 90 mg/kg/day (about 56 times* the maximum recommended daily human dose). Lisinopril has also been administered for 92 weeks to (male and female) mice at doses up to 135 mg/kg/day (about 84 times* the maximum recommended daily human dose) and showed no evidence of carcinogenicity.

Lisinopril was not mutagenic in the Ames microbial mutagen test with or without metabolic activation. It was also negative in a forward mutation assay using Chinese hamster lung cells. Lisinopril did not produce single strand DNA breaks in an in vitro alkaline elution rat hepatocyte assay. In addition, lisinopril did not produce increases in chromosomal aberrations in an in vitro test in Chinese hamster ovary cells or in an in vivo study in mouse bone marrow.

There were no adverse effects on reproductive performance in male and female rats treated with up to 300 mg/kg/day of lisinopril.

Hydrochlorothiazide: Two-year feeding studies in mice and rats conducted under the auspices of the National Toxicology Program (NTP) uncovered no evidence of a carcinogenic potential of hydrochlorothiazide in female mice (at doses of up to approximately 600 mg/kg/day) or in male and female rats (at doses of up to approximately 100 mg/kg/day). The NTP, however, found equivocal evidence for hepatocarcinogenicity in male mice.

Hydrochlorthiazide was not genotoxic in vitro in the Ames mutagenicity assay of *Salmonella typhimurium* strains TA 98, TA 100, TA 1535, TA 1537, and TA 1538 and in the Chinese Hamster Ovary (CHO) test for chromosomal aberrations, or in vivo in assays using mouse germinal cell chromosomes. Chinese hamster bone marrow chromosomes, and the *Drosophila* sex-linked recessive lethal trait gene. Positive test results were obtained only in the in vitro CHO Sister Chromatid Exchange (clastogenicity) and in the Mouse Lymphoma Cell (mutagenicity) assays, using concentrations of hydrochlorothiazide from 43 to 1300 μg/ml, and in the *Aspergillus nidulans* nondisjunction assay at an unspecified concentration.

Hydrochlorothiazide had no adverse effect on the fertility of mice and rats of either sex in studies in wherein these species were exposed via their diet, to doses of up to 100 and 4 mg/kg/day, respectively, prior to conception and throughout gestation.

Pregnancy

Pregnancy Categories C (first trimester) and D (second and third trimesters). See WARNINGS, Pregnancy, Lisinopril, Fetal/Neonatal Morbidity and Mortality.

*Based on patient weight of 50 kg.

Nursing Mothers

It is not known whether lisinopril is excreted in human milk. However, milk of lactating rats contains radioactivity following administration of ^{14}C lisinopril. In another study, lisinopril was present in rat milk at levels similar to plasma levels in the dams. Thiazides do appear in human milk. Because of the potential for serious reactions in nursing infants from hydrochlorothiazide and the unknown effects of lisinopril in infants, a decision should be made whether to discontinue nursing or to discontinue ZESTORETIC, taking into account the importance of the drug to the mother.

Pediatric Use

Safety and effectiveness in children have not been established.

ADVERSE REACTIONS

ZESTORETIC has been evaluated for safety in 930 patients including 100 patients treated for 50 weeks or more.

In clinical trials with ZESTORETIC no adverse experiences peculiar to this combination drug have been observed. Adverse experiences that have occurred have been limited to those that have been previously reported with lisinopril or hydrochlorothiazide.

The most frequent clinical adverse experiences in controlled trials (including open label extensions) with any combination of lisinopril and hydrochlorothiazide were: dizziness (7.5%), headache (5.2%), cough (3.9%), fatigue (3.7%) and orthostatic effects (3.2%) all of which were more common than in placebo-treated patients. Generally, adverse experiences were mild and transient in nature, but see WARNINGS regarding angioedema and excessive hypotension or syncope. Discontinuation of therapy due to adverse effects was required in 4.4% of patients principally because of dizziness, cough, fatigue and muscle cramps.

Adverse experiences occurring in greater than one percent of patients treated with lisinopril plus hydrochlorothiazide in controlled clinical trials are shown below.

Percent of Patients in Controlled Studies

	Lisinopril and Hydrochlorothiazide (n=930) Incidence (discontinuation)		Placebo (n=207) Incidence
Dizziness	7.5	(0.8)	1.9
Headache	5.2	(0.3)	1.9
Cough	3.9	(0.6)	1.0
Fatigue	3.7	(0.4)	1.0
Orthostatic Effects	3.2	(0.1)	1.0
Diarrhea	2.5	(0.2)	2.4
Nausea	2.2	(0.1)	2.4
Upper Respiratory Infection	2.2	(0.0)	0.0
Muscle Cramps	2.0	(0.4)	0.5
Asthenia	1.8	(0.2)	1.0
Paresthesia	1.5	(0.1)	0.0
Hypotension	1.4	(0.3)	0.5
Vomiting	1.4	(0.1)	0.5
Dyspepsia	1.3	(0.0)	0.0
Rash	1.2	(0.1)	0.5
Impotence	1.2	(0.3)	0.0

Clinical adverse experiences occurring in 0.3% to 1.0% of patients in controlled trials included:

Body as a Whole: Chest pain, abdominal pain, syncope, chest discomfort, fever, trauma, virus infection. **Cardiovascular:** Palpitation, orthostatic hypotension. **Digestive:** Gastrointestinal cramps, dry mouth, constipation, heartburn. **Musculoskeletal:** Back pain, shoulder pain, knee pain, back strain, myalgia, foot pain. **Nervous/Psychiatric:** Decreased libido, vertigo, depression, somnolence. **Respiratory:** Common cold, nasal congestion, influenza, bronchitis, pharyngeal pain, dyspnea, pulmonary congestion, chronic sinusitis, allergic rhinitis, pharyngeal discomfort. **Skin:** Flushing, pruritus, skin inflammation, diaphoresis. **Special Senses:** Blurred vision, tinnitus, otalgia. **Urogenital:** Urinary tract infection.

Angioedema: Angioedema of the face, extremities, lips, tongue, glottis and/or larynx has been reported rarely. (See WARNINGS.)

Hypotension: In clinical trials, adverse effects relating to hypotension occurred as follows: hypotension (1.4%), orthostatic hypotension (0.5%), other orthostatic effects (3.2%). In addition syncope occurred in 0.8% of patients. (See WARNINGS.)

Cough: See PRECAUTIONS-Cough.

Clinical Laboratory Test Findings

Serum Electrolytes: (See PRECAUTIONS.)

Creatinine, Blood Urea Nitrogen: Minor reversible increases in blood urea nitrogen and serum creatinine were observed in patients with essential hypertension treated with ZESTORETIC. More marked increases have also been reported and were more likely to occur in patients with renal artery stenosis. (See PRECAUTIONS.)

Serum Uric Acid, Glucose, Magnesium, Cholesterol, Triglycerides and Calcium: (See PRECAUTIONS).

Hemoglobin and Hematocrit: Small decreases in hemoglobin and hematocrit (mean decreases of approximately 0.5 g% and 1.5 vol%, respectively) occurred frequently in hypertensive patients treated with ZESTORETIC but were rarely of clinical importance unless another cause of anemia coexisted. In clinical trials, 0.4% of patients discontinued therapy due to anemia.

Other (Causal Relationship Unknown): Rarely, elevations of liver enzymes and/or serum bilirubin have occurred.

Other adverse reactions that have been reported with the individual components are listed below:

Lisinopril—Lisinopril has been evaluated for safety in 2003 patients. In clinical trials adverse reactions which occurred with lisinopril were also seen with ZESTORETIC. In addition and since lisinopril has been marketed, the following adverse reactions have been reported. **Body as a Whole:** Malaise; **Cardiovascular:** Myocardial infarction or cerebrovascular accident, possibly secondary to excessive hypotension in high risk patients (see WARNINGS, Hypotension); angina pectoris, rhythm disturbances, tachycardia, peripheral edema, vasculitis; **Digestive:** Pancreatitis, hepatitis (hepatocellular or cholestatic jaundice), anorexia, flatulence; **Hematologic:** Rare cases of neutropenia and bone marrow depression have been reported in which a causal relationship to lisinopril cannot be excluded; **Metabolic:** Gout; **Musculoskeletal:** Joint pain; **Nervous System/Psychiatric:** Insomnia, stroke, nervousness, confusion; **Skin:** Urticaria; **Urogenital:** Oliguria, progressive azotemia, acute renal failure.

A symptom complex has been reported which may include a positive ANA, an elevated erythrocyte sedimentation rate, arthralgia/arthritis, myalgia and fever.

Fetal/Neonatal Morbidity and Mortality

See WARNINGS-Pregnancy, Lisinopril, Fetal/Neonatal Morbidity and Mortality.

Hydrochlorothiazide—Body as a Whole: Weakness; **Digestive:** Anorexia, gastric irritation, cramping, jaundice (intrahepatic cholestatic jaundice), pancreatitis, sialodenitis, constipation; **Hematologic:** Leukopenia, agranulocytosis, thrombocytopenia, aplastic anemia, hemolytic anemia; **Musculoskeletal:** Muscle spasm; **Nervous System/Psychiatric:** Restlessness; **Renal:** Renal failure, renal dysfunction, interstitial nephritis (see WARNINGS); **Special Senses:** Xanthopsia; **Hypersensitivity:** Purpura, photosensitivity, urticaria, necrotizing angiitis (vasculitis and cutaneous vasculitis), respiratory distress including pneumonitis and pulmonary edema, anaphylactic reactions.

OVERDOSAGE

No specific information is available on the treatment of overdosage with ZESTORETIC. Treatment is symptomatic and supportive. Therapy with ZESTORETIC should be discontinued and the patient observed closely. Suggested measures include induction of emesis and/or gastric lavage, and correction of dehydration, electrolyte imbalance and hypotension by established procedures.

Lisinopril: The oral LD_{50} of lisinopril is greater than 20 g/kg in mice and rats. The most likely manifestation of overdosage would be hypotension, for which the usual treatment would be intravenous infusion of normal saline solution.

Lisinopril can be removed by hemodialysis.

Hydrochlorothiazide: The oral LD_{50} of hydrochlorothiazide is greater than 10.0 g/kg in both mice and rats. The most common signs and symptoms observed are those caused by electrolyte depletion (hypokalemia, hypochloremia, hyponatremia) and dehydration resulting from excessive diuresis. If digitalis has also been administered, hypokalemia may accentuate cardiac arrhythmias.

DOSAGE AND ADMINISTRATION

DOSAGE MUST BE INDIVIDUALIZED. THE FIXED COMBINATION IS NOT FOR INITIAL THERAPY. IT MAY BE SUBSTITUTED FOR THE TITRATED INDIVIDUAL COMPONENTS. ALTERNATIVELY, PATIENTS WHO HAVE RECEIVED LISINOPRIL MONOTHERAPY 20 OR 40 MG MAY BE GIVEN ZESTORETIC 20-12.5, THEN ZESTORETIC 20-25, THUS TITRATING THE HYDROCHLOROTHIAZIDE COMPONENT USING THE COMBINATION.

The usual dose is one or two tablets of ZESTORETIC 20-12.5 or ZESTORETIC 20-25 once daily. (See INDICATIONS AND USAGE and WARNINGS.) However, because data from a clinical trial suggest that the mean group antihypertensive response is similar when lisinopril 20 mg is combined with hydrochlorothiazide 12.5 mg or 25 mg, patients whose blood pressure is controlled with lisinopril 20 mg plus hydrochlorothiazide 25 mg ordinarily should be given a trial of ZESTORETIC 20-12.5 before ZESTORETIC 20-25 is used. (See CLINICAL PHARMACOLOGY, Lisinopril and Hydrochlorothiazide.)

Patients usually do not require doses in excess of 50 mg of hydrochlorothiazide daily, particularly when it is combined with other antihypertensive agents.

For lisinopril monotherapy the recommended initial dose in patients not on diuretics is 10 mg of lisinopril once a day.

Continued on next page

Stuart—Cont.

Dosage should be adjusted according to blood pressure response. The usual dosage range of lisinopril is 20 to 40 mg administered in a single daily dose; the maximum recommended dose is 80 mg in a single daily dose. Blood pressure should be measured at the interdosing interval to ensure that there is an adequate antihypertensive response at that time. If blood pressure is not controlled with lisinopril alone, a diuretic may be added. Hydrochlorothiazide 12.5 mg has been shown to provide an additive effect. After addition of the diuretic it may be possible to reduce the dose of lisinopril.
In patients who are currently being treated with a diuretic, symptomatic hypotension occasionally may occur following the initial dose of lisinopril. The diuretic should, if possible, be discontinued for two to three days before beginning therapy with lisinopril to reduce the likelihood of hypotension. (See WARNINGS.) If the patient's blood pressure is not controlled with lisinopril alone, diuretic therapy may be resumed.
If the diuretic cannot be discontinued, an initial dose of 5 mg of lisinopril should be used under medical supervision for at least two hours and until blood pressure has stabilized for at least an additional hour. (See WARNINGS AND PRECAUTIONS, Drug Interactions.)
Concomitant administration of ZESTORETIC with potassium supplements, potassium salt substitutes or potassium-sparing diuretics may lead to increases of serum potassium. (See PRECAUTIONS.)
Dosage Adjustment in Renal Impairment: The usual dose of ZESTORETIC is recommended for patients with a creatinine clearance > 30 mL/min (serum creatinine of up to approximately 3 mg/dL).
When concomitant diuretic therapy is required in patients with severe renal impairment, a loop diuretic, rather than a thiazide diuretic is preferred for use with lisinopril; therefore, for patients with severe renal dysfunction the lisinopril and hydrochlorothiazide combination tablet is not recommended.

HOW SUPPLIED

ZESTORETIC 20-12.5 Tablets (NDC 0038-0142) White, round, biconvex, uncoated tablets identified with "STUART" and "142" debossed on one side and "ZESTORETIC" on the other side are supplied in bottles of 100 tablets.
ZESTORETIC 20-25 Tablets (NDC 0038-0145) Peach, round, biconvex, uncoated tablets identified with "STUART" and "145" debossed on one side and "ZESTORETIC" on the other side are supplied in bottles of 100 tablets.
Avoid storage at temperatures above 40°C (104°F). Dispense in a well-closed container.
Rev A 02/92
Stuart Pharmaceuticals
A business unit of ICI Americas Inc.
Wilmington, DE 19897 USA
Shown in Product Identification Section, page 432

ZESTRIL® ℞
(lisinopril-Stuart)

USE IN PREGNANCY
When used in pregnancy during the second and third trimesters, ACE inhibitors can cause injury and death to the developing fetus. When pregnancy is detected, ZESTRIL should be discontinued as soon as possible. See WARNINGS. Fetal/Neonatal Morbidity and Mortality.

DESCRIPTION

ZESTRIL® (lisinopril), a synthetic peptide derivative, is an oral long-acting angiotensin converting enzyme inhibitor. Lisinopril is chemically described as (S)-1-[N^2-(1-Carboxy-3-phenylpropyl)-L-lysyl]-L-proline dihydrate. Its empirical formula is $C_{21}H_{31}N_3O_5 \cdot 2H_2O$ and its structural formula is:

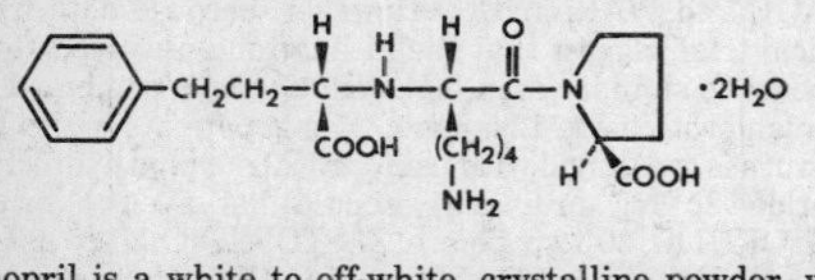

Lisinopril is a white to off-white, crystalline powder, with a molecular weight of 441.53. It is soluble in water and sparingly soluble in methanol and practically insoluble in ethanol.
ZESTRIL is supplied as 5 mg, 10 mg, 20 mg and 40 mg tablets for oral administration.
Inactive Ingredients:
5, 10 and 20 mg tablets—calcium phosphate, magnesium stearate, mannitol, red ferric oxide, starch.
40 mg tablets—calcium phosphate, magnesium stearate, mannitol, starch, yellow ferric oxide.

CLINICAL PHARMACOLOGY

Mechanism of Action: Lisinopril inhibits angiotensin converting enzyme (ACE) in human subjects and animals. ACE is a peptidyl dipeptidase that catalyzes the conversion of angiotensin I to the vasoconstrictor substance, angiotensin II. Angiotensin II also stimulates aldosterone secretion by the adrenal cortex. Inhibition of ACE results in decreased plasma angiotensin II which leads to decreased vasopressor activity and to decreased aldosterone secretion. The latter decrease may result in a small increase of serum potassium. In hypertensive patients with normal renal function treated with ZESTRIL alone for up to 24 weeks, the mean increase in serum potassium was approximately 0.1 mEq/L; however, approximately 15% of patients had increases greater than 0.5 mEq/L and approximately 6% had a decrease greater than 0.5 mEq/L. In the same study, patients treated with ZESTRIL and hydrochlorothiazide for up to 24 weeks had a mean decrease in serum potassium of 0.1 mEq/L; approximately 4% of patients had increases greater than 0.5 mEq/L and approximately 12% had a decrease greater than 0.5 mEq/L. (See PRECAUTIONS.) Removal of angiotensin II negative feedback on renin secretion leads to increased plasma renin activity.
ACE is identical to kininase, an enzyme that degrades bradykinin. Whether increased levels of bradykinin, a potent vasodepressor peptide, play a role in the therapeutic effects of ZESTRIL remains to be elucidated.
While the mechanism through which ZESTRIL lowers blood pressure is believed to be primarily suppression of the renin-angiotensin-aldosterone system, ZESTRIL is antihypertensive even in patients with low-renin hypertension. Although ZESTRIL was antihypertensive in all races studied, black hypertensive patients (usually a low-renin hypertensive population) had a smaller average response to monotherapy than nonblack patients.
Concomitant administration of ZESTRIL and hydrochlorothiazide further reduced blood pressure in black and nonblack patients and any racial differences in blood pressure response were no longer evident.
Pharmacokinetics and Metabolism: Following oral administration of ZESTRIL, peak serum concentrations of lisinopril occur within about 7 hours. Declining serum concentrations exhibit a prolonged terminal phase which does not contribute to drug accumulation. This terminal phase probably represents saturable binding to ACE and is not proportional to dose. Lisinopril does not appear to be bound to other serum proteins.
Lisinopril does not undergo metabolism and is excreted unchanged entirely in the urine. Based on urinary recovery, the mean extent of absorption of lisinopril is approximately 25%, with large intersubject variability (6%–60%) at all doses tested (5–80 mg). Lisinopril absorption is not influenced by the presence of food in the gastrointestinal tract.
Upon multiple dosing, lisinopril exhibits an effective half-life of accumulation of 12 hours.
Impaired renal function decreases elimination of lisinopril, which is excreted principally through the kidneys, but this decrease becomes clinically important only when the glomerular filtration rate is below 30 mL/min. Above this glomerular filtration rate, the elimination half-life is little changed. With greater impairment, however, peak and trough lisinopril levels increase, time to peak concentration increases and time to attain steady state is prolonged. Older patients, on average, have (approximately doubled) higher blood levels and the area under the plasma concentration time curve (AUC) than younger patients. (See DOSAGE AND ADMINISTRATION.) Lisinopril can be removed by hemodialysis.
Studies in rats indicate that lisinopril crosses the blood-brain barrier poorly. Multiple doses of lisinopril in rats do not result in accumulation in any tissues. Milk of lactating rats contains radioactivity following administration of ^{14}C lisinopril. By whole body autoradiography, radioactivity was found in the placenta following administration of labeled drug to pregnant rats, but none was found in the fetuses.
Pharmacodynamics: Administration of ZESTRIL to patients with hypertension results in a reduction of both supine and standing blood pressure to about the same extent with no compensatory tachycardia. Symptomatic postural hypotension is usually not observed although it can occur and should be anticipated in volume and/or salt-depleted patients. (See WARNINGS.) When given together with thiazide-type diuretics, the blood pressure lowering effects of the two drugs are approximately additive.
In most patients studied, onset of antihypertensive activity was seen at one hour after oral administration of an individual dose of ZESTRIL, with peak reduction of blood pressure achieved by 6 hours. Although an antihypertensive effect was observed 24 hours after dosing with recommended single daily doses, the effect was more consistent and the mean effect was considerably larger in some studies with doses of 20 mg or more than with lower doses. However, at all doses studied, the mean antihypertensive effect was substantially smaller 24 hours after dosing than it was 6 hours after dosing.
In some patients achievement of optimal blood pressure reduction may require two to four weeks of therapy.
The antihypertensive effects of ZESTRIL are maintained during long-term therapy. Abrupt withdrawal of ZESTRIL has not been associated with a rapid increase in blood pressure, or a significant increase in blood pressure compared to pretreatment levels.
Two dose-response studies utilizing a once daily regimen were conducted in 438 mild to moderate hypertensive patients not on a diuretic. Blood pressure was measured 24 hours after dosing. An antihypertensive effect of ZESTRIL was seen with 5 mg in some patients. However, in both studies blood pressure reduction occurred sooner and was greater in patients treated with 10, 20 or 80 mg of ZESTRIL. In controlled clinical studies, ZESTRIL 20–80 mg has been compared in patients with mild to moderate hypertension to hydrochlorothiazide 12.5–50 mg and with atenolol 50–200 mg; and in patients with moderate to severe hypertension to metoprolol 100–200 mg. It was superior to hydrochlorothiazide in effects on systolic and diastolic pressure in a population that was 3/4 Caucasian. ZESTRIL was approximately equivalent to atenolol and metoprolol in effects on diastolic blood pressure, and had somewhat greater effects on systolic blood pressure.
ZESTRIL had similar effectiveness and adverse effects in younger and older (> 65 years) patients. It was less effective in blacks than in Caucasians.
In hemodynamic studies in patients with essential hypertension, blood pressure reduction was accompanied by a reduction in peripheral arterial resistance with little or no change in cardiac output and in heart rate. In a study in nine hypertensive patients, following administration of ZESTRIL, there was an increase in mean renal blood flow that was not significant. Data from several small studies are inconsistent with respect to the effect of lisinopril on glomerular filtration rate in hypertensive patients with normal renal function, but suggest that changes, if any, are not large.
In patients with renovascular hypertension ZESTRIL has been shown to be well tolerated and effective in controlling blood pressure. (See PRECAUTIONS.)

INDICATIONS AND USAGE

ZESTRIL is indicated for the treatment of hypertension. It may be used alone as initial therapy or concomitantly with other classes of antihypertensive agents.
In using ZESTRIL, consideration should be given to the fact that another angiotensin converting enzyme inhibitor, captopril, has caused agranulocytosis, particularly in patients with renal impairment or collagen vascular disease, and that available data are insufficient to show that ZESTRIL does not have a similar risk. (See WARNINGS.)

CONTRAINDICATIONS

Zestril is contraindicated in patients who are hypersensitive to this product and in patients with a history of angioedema related to previous treatment with an angiotensin converting enzyme inhibitor.

WARNINGS

Angioedema: Angioedema of the face, extremities, lips, tongue, glottis and/or larynx has been reported in patients treated with angiotensin converting enzyme inhibitors, including ZESTRIL. In such cases, ZESTRIL should be promptly discontinued and appropriate therapy and monitoring should be provided until complete and sustained resolution of signs and symptoms has occurred. In instances where swelling has been confined to the face and lips the condition has generally resolved without treatment, although antihistamines have been useful in relieving symptoms. Angioedema associated with laryngeal edema may be fatal. **Where there is involvement of the tongue, glottis or larynx, likely to cause airway obstruction, appropriate therapy, eg, subcutaneous epinephrine solution 1:1000 (0.3 mL to 0.5 mL) and/or measures necessary to ensure a patent airway should be promptly administered. (See ADVERSE REACTIONS.)**
Hypotension: Excessive hypotension was rarely seen in uncomplicated hypertensive patients but is a possible consequence of use with ZESTRIL in salt/volume-depleted persons, such as those treated vigorously with diuretics or patients on dialysis. (See PRECAUTIONS, Drug Interactions and ADVERSE REACTIONS.) In patients with severe congestive heart failure, with or without associated renal insufficiency, excessive hypotension has been observed and may be associated with oliguria and/or progressive azotemia, and rarely with acute renal failure and/or death. Because of the potential fall in blood pressure in these patients, therapy should be started under very close medical supervision. Such patients should be followed closely for the first two weeks of treatment and whenever the dose of ZESTRIL and/or diuretic is increased. Similar considerations apply to patients with ischemic heart or cerebrovascular disease in whom an excessive fall in blood pressure could result in a myocardial infarction or cerebrovascular accident.

If hypotension occurs, the patient should be placed in supine position and, if necessary, receive an intravenous infusion of normal saline. A transient hypotensive response is not a contraindication to further doses which usually can be given without difficulty once the blood pressure has increased after volume expansion.

Neutropenia/Agranulocytosis: Another angiotensin converting enzyme inhibitor, captopril, has been shown to cause agranulocytosis and bone marrow depression, rarely in uncomplicated patients but more frequently in patients with renal impairment especially if they also have a collagen vascular disease. Available data from clinical trials of ZESTRIL are insufficient to show that ZESTRIL does not cause agranulocytosis at similar rates. Marketing experience has revealed rare cases of neutropenia and bone marrow depression in which a causal relationship to lisinopril cannot be excluded. Periodic monitoring of white blood cell counts in patients with collagen vascular disease and renal disease should be considered.

Fetal/Neonatal Morbidity and Mortality: ACE inhibitors can cause fetal and neonatal morbidity and death when administered to pregnant women. Several dozen cases have been reported in the world literature. When pregnancy is detected, ACE inhibitors should be discontinued as soon as possible.

The use of ACE inhibitors during the second and third trimesters of pregnancy has been associated with fetal and neonatal injury, including hypotension, neonatal skull hypoplasia, anuria, reversible or irreversible renal failure, and death. Oligohydramnios has also been reported, presumably resulting from decreased fetal renal function; oligohydramnios in this setting has been associated with fetal limb contractures, craniofacial deformation, and hypoplastic lung development. Prematurity, intrauterine growth retardation, and patent ductus arteriosus have also been reported, although it is not clear whether these occurrences were due to the ACE-inhibitor exposure.

These adverse effects do not appear to have resulted from intrauterine ACE-inhibitor exposure that has been limited to the first trimester. Mothers whose embryos and fetuses are exposed to ACE inhibitors only during the first trimester should be so informed. Nonetheless, when patients become pregnant, physicians should make every effort to discontinue the use of ZESTRIL as soon as possible.

Rarely (probably less often than once in every thousand pregnancies), no alternative to ACE inhibitors will be found. In these rare cases, the mothers should be apprised of the potential hazards to their fetuses, and serial ultrasound examinations should be performed to assess the intraamniotic environment.

If oligohydramnios is observed, ZESTRIL should be discontinued unless it is considered lifesaving for the mother. Contraction stress testing (CST), a nonstress test (NST), or biophysical profiling (BPP) may be appropriate, depending upon the week of pregnancy. Patients and physicians should be aware, however, that oligohydramnios may not appear until after the fetus has sustained irreversible injury.

Infants with histories of in utero exposure to ACE inhibitors should be closely observed for hypotension, oliguria, and hyperkalemia. If oliguria occurs, attention should be directed toward support of blood pressure and renal perfusion. Exchange transfusion or dialysis may be required as means of reversing hypotension and/or substituting for disordered renal function. Lisinopril, which crosses the placenta, has been removed from neonatal circulation by peritoneal dialysis with some clinical benefit, and theoretically may be removed by exchange transfusion, although there is no experience with the latter procedure.

No teratogenic effects of lisinopril were seen in studies of pregnant rats, mice, and rabbits. On a mg/kg basis, the doses used were up to 625 times (in mice), 188 times (in rats), and 0.6 times (in rabbits) the maximum recommended human dose.

PRECAUTIONS
General
Impaired Renal Function: As a consequence of inhibiting the renin-angiotensin-aldosterone system, changes in renal function may be anticipated in susceptible individuals. In patients with severe congestive heart failure whose renal function may depend on the activity of the renin-angiotensin-aldosterone system, treatment with angiotensin converting enzyme inhibitors, including ZESTRIL, may be associated with oliguria and/or progressive azotemia and rarely with acute renal failure and/or death.

In hypertensive patients with unilateral or bilateral renal artery stenosis, increases in blood urea nitrogen and serum creatinine may occur. Experience with another angiotensin converting enzyme inhibitor suggests that these increases are usually reversible upon discontinuation of ZESTRIL and/or diuretic therapy. In such patients, renal function should be monitored during the first few weeks of therapy. Some hypertensive patients with no apparent pre-existing renal vascular disease have developed increases in blood urea nitrogen and serum creatinine, usually minor and tran-

sient, especially when ZESTRIL has been given concomitantly with a diuretic. This is more likely to occur in patients with pre-existing renal impairment. Dosage reduction of ZESTRIL and/or discontinuation of the diuretic may be required.

Evaluation of the hypertensive patient should always include assessment of renal function. (See DOSAGE AND ADMINISTRATION.)

Hyperkalemia: In clinical trials hyperkalemia (serum potassium greater than 5.7 mEq/L) occurred in approximately 2.2% of hypertensive patients and 4.0% of patients with congestive heart failure. In most cases these were isolated values which resolved despite continued therapy. Hyperkalemia was a cause of discontinuation of therapy in approximately 0.1% of hypertensive patients. Risk factors for the development of hyperkalemia include renal insufficiency, diabetes mellitus, and the concomitant use of potassium-sparing diuretics, potassium supplements and/or potassium-containing salt substitutes, which should be used cautiously, if at all, with ZESTRIL. (See Drug Interactions.)

Cough: Cough has been reported with the use of ACE inhibitors. Characteristically, the cough is nonproductive, persistent and resolves after discontinuation of therapy. ACE inhibitor-induced cough should be considered as part of the differential diagnosis of cough.

Surgery/Anesthesia: In patients undergoing major surgery or during anesthesia with agents that produce hypotension, ZESTRIL may block angiotensin II formation secondary to compensatory renin release. If hypotension occurs and is considered to be due to this mechanism, it can be corrected by volume expansion.

Information for Patients
Angioedema: Angioedema, including laryngeal edema, may occur especially following the first dose of ZESTRIL. Patients should be so advised and told to report immediately any signs or symptoms suggesting angioedema (swelling of face, extremities, eyes, lips, tongue, difficulty in swallowing or breathing) and to take no more drug until they have consulted with the prescribing physician.

Symptomatic Hypotension: Patients should be cautioned to report lightheadedness especially during the first few days of therapy. If actual syncope occurs, the patient should be told to discontinue the drug until they have consulted with the prescribing physician.

All patients should be cautioned that excessive perspiration and dehydration may lead to an excessive fall in blood pressure because of reduction in fluid volume. Other causes of volume depletion such as vomiting or diarrhea may also lead to a fall in blood pressure; patients should be advised to consult with their physician.

Hyperkalemia: Patients should be told not to use salt substitutes containing potassium without consulting their physician.

Neutropenia: Patients should be told to report promptly any indication of infection (eg, sore throat, fever) which may be a sign of neutropenia.

Pregnancy: Female patients of childbearing age should be told about the consequences of second- and third-trimester exposure to ACE inhibitors, and they should also be told that these consequences do not appear to have resulted from intrauterine ACE-inhibitor exposure that has been limited to the first trimester. These patients should be asked to report pregnancies to their physicians as soon as possible.

NOTE: As with many other drugs, certain advice to patients being treated with ZESTRIL is warranted. This information is intended to aid in the safe and effective use of this medication. It is not a disclosure of all possible adverse or intended effects.

DRUG INTERACTIONS

Hypotension—Patients on Diuretic Therapy: Patients on diuretics and especially those in whom diuretic therapy was recently instituted, may occasionally experience an excessive reduction of blood pressure after initiation of therapy with ZESTRIL. The possibility of hypotensive effects with ZESTRIL can be minimized by either discontinuing the diuretic or increasing the salt intake prior to initiation of treatment with ZESTRIL. If it is necessary to continue the diuretic, initiate therapy with ZESTRIL at a dose of 5 mg daily, and provide close medical supervision after the initial dose for at least two hours and until blood pressure has stabilized for at least an additional hour. (See WARNINGS and DOSAGE AND ADMINISTRATION.) When a diuretic is added to the therapy of a patient receiving ZESTRIL, an additional antihypertensive effect is usually observed. Studies with ACE inhibitors in combination with diuretics indicate that the dose of the ACE inhibitor can be reduced when it is given with a diuretic. (See DOSAGE AND ADMINISTRATION.)

Indomethacin: In a study in 36 patients with mild to moderate hypertension where the antihypertensive effects of ZESTRIL alone were compared to ZESTRIL given concomitantly with indomethacin, the use of indomethacin was associated with a reduced effect, although the difference between the two regimens was not significant.

Other Agents: ZESTRIL has been used concomitantly with nitrates and/or digoxin without evidence of clinically significant adverse interactions. No clinically important pharmacokinetic interactions occurred when ZESTRIL was used concomitantly with propranolol or hydrochlorothiazide. The presence of food in the stomach does not alter the bioavailability of ZESTRIL.

Agents Increasing Serum Potassium: ZESTRIL attenuates potassium loss caused by thiazide-type diuretics. Use of ZESTRIL with potassium-sparing diuretics (eg, spironolactone, triamterene or amiloride), potassium supplements, or potassium-containing salt substitutes may lead to significant increases in serum potassium. Therefore, if concomitant use of these agents is indicated because of demonstrated hypokalemia, they should be used with caution and with frequent monitoring of serum potassium.

Lithium: Lithium toxicity has been reported in patients receiving lithium with drugs which cause elimination of sodium, including ACE inhibitors. Lithium toxicity was usually reversible upon discontinuation of both drugs. It is recommended that serum lithium levels be monitored frequently if ZESTRIL is administered concomitantly with lithium.

Carcinogenesis, Mutagenesis, Impairment of Fertility: There was no evidence of a tumorigenic effect when lisinopril was administered for 105 weeks to male and female rats at doses up to 90 mg/kg/day (about 56 times* the maximum recommended daily human dose) or when lisinopril was administered for 92 weeks to (male and female) mice at doses up to 135 mg/kg/day (about 84 times* the maximum recommended daily human dose).

Lisinopril was not mutagenic in the Ames microbial mutagen test with or without metabolic activation. It was also negative in a forward mutation assay using Chinese hamster lung cells. Lisinopril did not produce single strand DNA breaks in an in vitro alkaline elution rat hepatocyte assay. In addition, lisinopril did not produce increases in chromosomal aberrations in an in vitro test in Chinese hamster ovary cells or in an in vivo study in mouse bone marrow. There were no adverse effects on reproductive performance in male and female rats treated with up to 300 mg/kg/day of lisinopril.

Pregnancy
Pregnancy Categories C (first trimester and D (second and third trimesters). (See WARNINGS, Fetal/Neonatal Morbidity and Mortality.

Nursing Mothers: Milk of lactating rats contains radioactivity following administration of ^{14}C lisinopril. It is not known whether this drug is excreted in human milk. Because many drugs are excreted in human milk, caution should be exercised when ZESTRIL is given to a nursing mother.

Pediatric Use: Safety and effectiveness in children have not been established.

ADVERSE REACTIONS
ZESTRIL has been found to be generally well tolerated in controlled clinical trials involving 2003 patients and subjects.

The most frequent clinical adverse experiences in controlled trials with ZESTRIL were dizziness (6.3%), headache (5.3%), fatigue (3.3%), diarrhea (3.2%), upper respiratory symptoms (3.0%), and cough (2.9%), all of which were more frequent than in placebo-treated patients. For the most part, adverse experiences were mild and transient in nature. Discontinuation of therapy was required in 6.0% of patients. In clinical trials, the overall frequency of adverse experiences could not be related to total daily dosage within the recommended therapeutic dosage range.

For adverse experiences which occurred in more than 1% of patients and subjects treated with ZESTRIL or ZESTRIL plus hydrochlorothiazide in controlled clinical trials, comparative incidence data are listed in the table below. [See table on next page.]

Clinical adverse experiences occurring in 0.3% to 1.0% of patients in the controlled trials and rarer, serious, possibly drug related events reported in uncontrolled studies or marketing experience are listed below and, within each category, are in order of decreasing severity.

BODY AS A WHOLE: Chest discomfort, fever, flushing, malaise.

CARDIOVASCULAR: Myocardial infarction or cerebrovascular accident, possibly secondary to excessive hypotension in high risk patients (see WARNINGS, Hypotension); angina pectoris, orthostatic hypotension, rhythm disturbances, tachycardia, peripheral edema, vasculitis, palpitation.

---

*Based on patient weight of 50 kg.

Continued on next page

Stuart—Cont.

DIGESTIVE: Pancreatitis, Hepatitis (hepatocellular or cholestatic jaundice), abdominal pain, anorexia, constipation, flatulence, dry mouth.
METABOLISM: Gout
MUSCULOSKELETAL: Joint pain, shoulder pain.
NERVOUS SYSTEM/PSYCHIATRIC: Depression, somnolence, insomnia, stroke, nervousness, confusion.
RESPIRATORY SYSTEM: Bronchitis, sinusitis, pharyngeal pain.
SKIN: Urticaria, pruritus, diaphoresis.
SPECIAL SENSES: Blurred vision.
UROGENITAL: Oliguria, progressive azotemia, acute renal failure, urinary tract infection.
A symptom complex has been reported which may include a positive ANA, an elevated erythrocyte sedimentation rate, arthalgia/arthritis, myalgia and fever.
ANGIOEDEMA: Angioedema has been reported in patients receiving ZESTRIL (0.1%). Angioedema associated with laryngeal edema may be fatal. If angioedema of the face, extremities, lips, tongue, glottis and/or larynx occurs, treatment with ZESTRIL should be discontinued and appropriate therapy instituted immediately. (See WARNINGS.)
HYPOTENSION: In hypertensive patients, hypotension occurred in 1.2% and syncope occurred in 0.1% of patients. Hypotension or syncope was a cause of discontinuation of therapy in 0.5% of hypertensive patients. (See WARNINGS.) In patients with congestive heart failure, hypotension occurred in 5.0% and syncope occurred in 1.0% of patients. These adverse experiences were causes for discontinuation of therapy in 1.3% of these patients.
Fetal/Neonatal Morbidity and Mortality: See WARNINGS, Fetal/Neonatal Morbidity and Mortality.
Cough: See PRECAUTIONS-Cough.

Clinical Laboratory Test Findings
Serum Electrolytes: Hyperkalemia (See PRECAUTIONS.)
Creatinine, Blood Urea Nitrogen: Minor increases in blood urea nitrogen and serum creatinine, reversible upon discontinuation of therapy, were observed in about 2.0% of patients with essential hypertension treated with ZESTRIL alone. Increases were more common in patients receiving concomitant diuretics and in patients with renal artery stenosis. (See PRECAUTIONS.) Reversible minor increases in blood urea nitrogen and serum creatinine were observed in approximately 9.1% of patients with congestive heart failure on concomitant diuretic therapy. Frequently, these abnormalities resolved when the dosage of the diuretic was decreased.
Hemoglobin and Hematocrit: Small decreases in hemoglobin and hematocrit (mean decreases of approximately 0.4 g% and 1.3 vol%, respectively) occurred frequently in patients treated with ZESTRIL but were rarely of clinical importance in patients without some other cause of anemia. In clinical trials, less than 0.1% of patients discontinued therapy due to anemia.
Other (Causal Relationship Unknown): Rarely, elevations of liver enzymes and/or serum bilirubin have occurred. In marketing experience, rare cases of neutropenia and bone marrow depression have been reported.

Overall, 2.0% of patients discontinued therapy due to laboratory adverse experiences, principally elevations in blood urea nitrogen (0.6%), serum creatinine (0.5%), and serum potassium (0.4%).

OVERDOSAGE

The oral LD_{50} of lisinopril is greater than 20 g/kg in mice and rats. The most likely manifestation of overdosage would be hypotension, for which the usual treatment would be intravenous infusion of normal saline solution.
Lisinopril can be removed by hemodialysis.

DOSAGE AND ADMINISTRATION

Initial Therapy: In patients with uncomplicated essential hypertension not on diuretic therapy, the recommended initial dose is 10 mg once a day. Dosage should be adjusted according to blood pressure response. The usual dosage range is 20–40 mg per day administered in a single daily dose. The antihypertensive effect may diminish toward the end of the dosing interval regardless of the administered dose, but most commonly with a dose of 10 mg daily. This can be evaluated by measuring blood pressure just prior to dosing to determine whether satisfactory control is being maintained for 24 hours. If it is not, an increase in dose should be considered. Doses up to 80 mg have been used but do not appear to give greater effect. If blood pressure is not controlled with ZESTRIL alone, a low dose of a diuretic may be added. Hydrochlorothiazide, 12.5 mg has been shown to provide an additive effect. After the addition of a diuretic, it may be possible to reduce the dose of ZESTRIL.
Diuretic Treated Patients: In hypertensive patients who are currently being treated with a diuretic, symptomatic hypotension may occur occasionally following the initial dose of ZESTRIL. The diuretic should be discontinued, if possible, for two or three days before beginning therapy with ZESTRIL to reduce the likelihood of hypotension. (See WARNINGS.) The dosage of ZESTRIL should be adjusted according to blood pressure response. If the patient's blood pressure is not controlled with ZESTRIL alone, diuretic therapy may be resumed as described above.
If the diuretic cannot be discontinued, an initial dose of 5 mg should be used under medical supervision for at least two hours and until blood pressure has stabilized for at least an additional hour. (See WARNINGS and PRECAUTIONS, Drug Interactions.)
Concomitant administration of ZESTRIL with potassium supplements, potassium salt substitutes, or potassium-sparing diuretics may lead to increases of serum potassium. (See PRECAUTIONS.)
Use in Elderly: In general, blood pressure response and adverse experiences were similar in younger and older patients given similar doses of ZESTRIL. Pharmacokinetic studies, however, indicate that maximum blood levels and area under the plasma concentration time curve (AUC) are doubled in older patients so that dosage adjustments should be made with particular caution.
Dosage Adjustment in Renal Impairment: The usual dose of ZESTRIL (10 mg) is recommended for patients with creatinine clearance > 30 mL/min (serum creatinine of up to ap-

proximately 3 mg/dL). For patients with creatinine clearance ≥ 10 mL/min ≤ 30 mL/min (serum creatinine ≥ 3 mg/dL), the first dose is 5 mg once daily. For patients with creatinine clearance < 10 mL/min (usually on hemodialysis) the recommended initial dose is 2.5 mg. The dosage may be titrated upward until blood pressure is controlled or to a maximum of 40 mg daily.

Renal Status	Creatinine Clearance mL/min	Initial Dose mg/day
Normal Renal Function to Mild Impairment	> 30	10
Moderate to Severe Impairment	≥ 10 ≤ 30	5
Dialysis Patients	< 10	2.5‡

‡ Dosage or dosing interval should be adjusted depending on the blood pressure response.

HOW SUPPLIED

5 mg Tablets (NDC 0038-0130) pink, capsule-shaped, biconvex, bisected, uncoated tablets, identified "ZESTRIL" on one side, and "130" on the other side are supplied in bottles of 100 tablets and 1000 tablets, and unit dose packages of 100 tablets.
10 mg Tablets (NDC 0038-0131) pink, round, biconvex, uncoated tablets identified "ZESTRIL 10" debossed on one side, and "131" debossed on the other side are supplied in bottles of 100 tablets and 1000 tablets, and unit dose packages of 100 tablets.
20 mg Tablets (NDC 0038-0132) red, round, biconvex, uncoated tablets identified "ZESTRIL 20" debossed on one side, and "132" debossed on the other side are supplied in bottles of 100 tablets and 1000 tablets, and unit dose packages of 100 tablets.
40 mg Tablets (NDC 0038-0134) yellow, round, biconvex, uncoated tablets identified "ZESTRIL 40" debossed on one side, and "134" debossed on the other side are supplied in bottles of 100 tablets and unit dose packages of 100 tablets. Store at room temperature. Protect from moisture, freezing and excessive heat. Dispense in a tight container.
Stuart Pharmaceuticals
A business unit of ICI Americas Inc.
Wilmington, DE 19897
Rev B 02/92
Shown in Product Identification Section, page 433

Summit Pharmaceuticals
Division of CIBA-GEIGY Corporation
SUMMIT, NJ 07901

To provide a convenient and accurate means of identifying Summit Pharmaceuticals' solid dosage form products, a code number has been imprinted on all tablets and capsules. To help you quickly identify a Summit Tablet or Capsule by its code number, a numerical listing of codes (with corresponding product names) and an alphabetical listing of products (with corresponding codes and list numbers) have been compiled below.

Summit Product Identification Number	ALPHABETICAL LISTING	National Drug Code Number
	Actigall® ursodiol	
153	CAPSULES, 300 mg (white and pink, hard gelatin)	
	100s	57267-153-30
	Slow-K® potassium chloride USP	
165	TABLETS (round, buff-colored, sugar-coated), each containing 8 mEq (600 mg) potassium chloride	
	100s	57267-165-30
	1000s	57267-165-40
	Accu-Pak® 100s	57267-165-32
	Consumer Pack 100s	57267-165-65
	Ten-K® potassium chloride TABLETS, 750 mg (10 mEq) (white, capsule-shaped, scored)	
146	100s	57267-146-30
	500s	57267-146-35
	100s Unit Dose Pkg.	57267-146-32

Percent of Patients in Controlled Studies

	ZESTRIL (n=2003†) Incidence (discontinuation)	ZESTRIL/ Hydrochlorothiazide (n=644) Incidence (discontinuation)	Placebo (n=207) Incidence
Dizziness	6.3 (0.6)	9.0 (0.9)	1.9
Headache	5.3 (0.2)	4.3 (0.5)	1.9
Fatigue	3.3 (0.2)	3.9 (0.5)	1.0
Diarrhea	3.2 (0.3)	2.6 (0.3)	2.4
Upper Respiratory Symptoms	3.0 (0.0)	4.5 (0.0)	0.0
Cough	2.9 (0.4)	4.5 (0.8)	1.0
Nausea	2.3 (0.3)	2.5 (0.2)	2.4
Hypotension	1.8 (0.8)	1.6 (0.5)	0.5
Rash	1.5 (0.4)	1.6 (0.4)	0.5
Orthostatic Effects	1.4 (0.0)	3.4 (0.2)	1.0
Asthenia	1.3 (0.4)	2.0 (0.2)	1.0
Chest Pain	1.3 (0.1)	1.2 (0.2)	1.4
Vomiting	1.3 (0.2)	1.4 (0.0)	0.5
Dyspnea	1.1 (0.0)	0.5 (0.2)	1.4
Dyspepsia	1.0 (0.0)	1.9 (0.0)	0.0
Paresthesia	0.8 (0.0)	2.0 (0.2)	0.0
Impotence	0.7 (0.2)	1.6 (0.3)	0.0
Muscle Cramps	0.6 (0.0)	2.8 (0.6)	0.5
Back Pain	0.5 (0.0)	1.1 (0.0)	1.4
Nasal Congestion	0.3 (0.0)	1.2 (0.0)	0.0
Decreased Libido	0.2 (0.1)	1.2 (0.0)	0.0
Vertigo	0.1 (0.0)	1.1 (0.2)	0.0

† Includes 420 patients treated for congestive heart failure who were receiving concomitant digitalis and/or diuretic therapy.

Transderm-Nitro®
nitroglycerin

Code	Transderm-Nitro System*	Total Nitroglycerin in System	System Size	National Drug Code Number	Carton Size
902	0.1 mg/hr	12.5 mg	5 cm²	57267-902-26	30 Systems
				57267-902-42	**30 Systems
				57267-902-30	**100 Systems
905	0.2 mg/hr	25 mg	10 cm²	57267-905-26	30 Systems
				57267-905-42	**30 Systems
				57267-905-30	**100 Systems
910	0.4 mg/hr	50 mg	20 cm²	57267-910-26	30 Systems
				57267-910-42	**30 Systems
				57267-910-30	**100 Systems
915	0.6 mg/hr	75 mg	30 cm²	57267-915-26	30 Systems
				57267-915-42	**30 Systems
				57267-915-30	**100 Systems

**Institutional Pack

* Rated release in vivo. Release rates were formerly described in terms of drug delivered per 24 hours. In these terms, the supplied Transderm-Nitro systems would be rated at 2.5 mg/24 hr (0.1 mg/hr), 5 mg/24 hr (0.2 mg/hr), 10 mg/24 hr (0.4 mg/hr), and 15 mg/24 hr (0.6 mg/hr).

Summit Product Identification Number **NUMERICAL LISTING**

Actigall®
ursodiol
153 CAPSULES, 300 mg (white and pink, hard gelatin)
100s

Slow-K®
potassium chloride USP
165 TABLETS (buff colored, sugar-coated), each containing 8 mEq (600 mg) potassium chloride
100s
1000s
Accu-Pak® 100s
Consumer Pack 100s

Ten-K®
potassium chloride
TABLETS, 750 mg (10 mEq) (white, capsule-shaped, scored)
146 100s
500s
100s Unit Dose Pkg.

Transderm-Nitro®
nitroglycerin

902	0.1 mg/hr	30 systems
		*30 systems
		*100 systems
905	0.2 mg/hr	30 systems
		*30 systems
		*100 systems
910	0.4 mg/hr	30 systems
		*30 systems
		*100 systems
915	0.6 mg/hr	30 systems
		*30 systems
		*100 systems

*Institutional Pack

ACTIGALL® ℞
ursodiol
Capsules

SPECIAL NOTE
Gallbladder stone dissolution with Actigall treatment requires months of therapy. Complete dissolution does not occur in all patients and recurrence of stones within 5 years has been observed in up to 50% of patients who do dissolve their stones on bile acid therapy. Patients should be carefully selected for therapy with ursodiol, and alternative therapies should be considered.

DESCRIPTION
Actigall is an agent intended for dissolution of radiolucent gallstones. It is available as 300 mg capsules suitable for oral administration.
Actigall is ursodiol (ursodeoxycholic acid), a naturally occurring bile acid found in small quantities in normal human bile and in larger quantities in the biles of certain species of bears. It is a bitter-tasting, white powder freely soluble in ethanol, and in glacial acetic acid, slightly soluble in chloroform, sparingly soluble in ether, and practically insoluble in water. The chemical name for ursodiol is 3α,7β-dihydroxy-5β-cholan-24-oic acid ($C_{24}H_{40}O_4$). Ursodiol has a molecular weight of 392.56.
Inactive Ingredients: Gelatin; iron oxide; magnesium stearate; colloidal silicon dioxide; starch; and titanium dioxide.

CLINICAL PHARMACOLOGY
About 90% of a therapeutic dose of Actigall is absorbed in the small bowel after oral administration. After absorption, ursodiol enters the portal vein and undergoes efficient extraction from portal blood by the liver (i.e., there is a large "first pass" effect) where it is conjugated with either glycine or taurine and is then secreted into the hepatic bile ducts. Ursodiol in bile is concentrated in the gallbladder and expelled into the duodenum in gallbladder bile via the cystic and common ducts by gallbladder contractions provoked by physiologic responses to eating. Only small quantities of ursodiol appear in the systemic circulation and very small amounts are excreted into urine. The sites of the drug's therapeutic actions are in the liver, bile and gut lumen.
Beyond conjugation, ursodiol is not altered or catabolized appreciably by the liver or intestinal mucosa. A small proportion of orally administered drug undergoes bacterial degradation with each cycle of enterohepatic circulation. Ursodiol can be both oxidized and reduced at the 7-carbon, yielding either 7-keto-lithocholic acid or lithocholic acid, respectively. Further, there is some bacterially catalyzed deconjugation of glyco- and tauro-ursodeoxycholic acid in the small bowel. Free ursodiol, 7-keto-lithocholic acid and lithocholic acid are relatively insoluble in aqueous media and larger proportions of these compounds are lost from the distal gut into the feces. Reabsorbed free ursodiol is reconjugated by the liver. Eighty percent of lithocholic acid formed in the small bowel is excreted in the feces, but the 20% that is absorbed is sulfated at the 3-hydroxyl group in the liver to relatively insoluble lithocholyl conjugates which are excreted into bile and lost in feces. Absorbed 7-keto-lithocholic acid is stereospecifically reduced in the liver to chenodiol.
Lithocholic acid causes cholestatic liver injury and can cause death from liver failure in certain species unable to form sulfate conjugates. Lithocholic acid is formed by 7-dehydroxylation of the dihydroxy bile acids (ursodiol and chenodiol) in the gut lumen. The 7-dehydroxylation reaction appears to be alpha-specific, i.e., chenodiol is more efficiently 7-dehydroxylated than ursodiol and for equimolar doses of ursodiol and chenodiol, levels of lithocholic acid appearing in bile are lower with the former. Man has the capacity to sulfate lithocholic acid. Although liver injury has not been associated with ursodiol therapy, a reduced capacity to sulfate may exist in some individuals, but such a deficiency has not yet been clearly demonstrated.
Pharmacodynamics: Ursodiol suppresses hepatic synthesis and secretion of cholesterol, and also inhibits intestinal absorption of cholesterol. It appears to have little inhibitory effect on synthesis and secretion into bile of endogenous bile acids, and does not appear to affect secretion of phospholipids into bile.
With repeated dosing, bile ursodeoxycholic acid concentrations reach a steady state in about 3 weeks. Although insoluble in aqueous media, cholesterol can be solubilized in at least two different ways in the presence of dihydroxy bile acids. In addition to solubilizing cholesterol in micelles, ursodiol acts by an apparently unique mechanism to cause dispersion of cholesterol as liquid crystals in aqueous media. Thus, even though administration of high doses (e.g., 15–18 mg/kg/day) does not result in a concentration of ursodiol higher than 60% of the total bile acid pool, ursodiol-rich bile effectively solubilizes cholesterol. The overall effect of ursodiol is to increase the concentration level at which saturation of cholesterol occurs.
The various actions of ursodiol combine to change the bile of patients with gallstones from cholesterol-precipitating to cholesterol-solubilizing, thus resulting in bile conducive to cholesterol stone dissolution.
After ursodiol dosing is stopped, the concentration of the bile acid in bile falls exponentially, declining to about 5–10% of its steady state level in about 1 week.
Clinical Results: On the basis of clinical trial results in a total of 868 patients with radiolucent gallstones treated in 8 studies (three in the U.S. involving 282 patients, one in the U.K. involving 130 patients and four in Italy involving 456 patients) for periods ranging from 6–78 months with Actigall doses ranging from about 5 to 20 mg/kg/day, an Actigall dose of about 8–10 mg/kg/day appeared to be the best dose. With an Actigall dose of about 10 mg/kg/day, complete stone dissolution can be anticipated in about 30% of unselected patients with uncalcified gallstones < 20 mm in maximal diameter treated for up to two years. Patients with calcified gallstones prior to treatment, or patients who develop stone calcification or gallbladder nonvisualization on treatment, and patients with stones larger than 20 mm in maximal diameter rarely dissolve their stones. The chance of gallstone dissolution is increased up to 50% in patients with floating or floatable stones (i.e., those with high cholesterol content), and is inversely related to stone size for those less than 20 mm in maximal diameter. Complete dissolution was observed in 81% of patients with stones up to 5 mm in diameter. Age, sex, weight, degree of obesity and serum cholesterol level are not related to the chance of stone dissolution with Actigall.
A nonvisualizing gallbladder by oral cholecystogram prior to the initiation of therapy is not a contraindication to Actigall therapy (the group of patients with nonvisualizing gallbladders in the Actigall studies had complete stone dissolution rates similar to the group of patients with visualizing gallbladders). However, gallbladder nonvisualization developing during ursodiol treatment predicts failure of complete stone dissolution and in such cases therapy should be discontinued.
Partial stone dissolution occurring within 6 months of beginning therapy with Actigall appears to be associated with a > 70% chance of eventual complete stone dissolution with further treatment; partial dissolution observed within one year of starting therapy indicates a 40% probability of complete dissolution.
Stone recurrence after dissolution with Actigall therapy was seen within 2 years in 8/27 (30%) of patients in the U.K. studies. Of 16 patients in the U.K. study whose stones had previously dissolved on chenodiol but later recurred, 11 had complete dissolution on Actigall. Stone recurrence has been observed in up to 50% of patients within 5 years of complete stone dissolution on ursodiol therapy. Serial ultrasonographic examinations should be obtained to monitor for recurrence of stones, bearing in mind that radiolucency of the stones should be established before another course of Actigall is instituted. A prophylactic dose of Actigall has not been established.

ALTERNATIVE THERAPIES
Watchful Waiting: Watchful waiting has the advantage that no therapy may ever be required. For patients with silent or minimally symptomatic stones, the rate of development of moderate to severe symptoms or gallstone complications is estimated to be between 2% and 6% per year, leading to a cumulative rate of 7% to 27% in five years. Presumably the rate is higher for patients already having symptoms.
Cholecystectomy: Surgery offers the advantage of immediate and permanent stone removal, but carries a high risk in some patients. About 5% of cholecystectomized patients have residual symptoms or retained common duct stones. The spectrum of surgical risk varies as a function of age and the presence of disease other than cholelithiasis.

Mortality Rates for Cholecystectomy in the U.S.
(National Halothane Study, JAMA 1966; 197:775–8)
27,600 Cholecystectomies (Smoothed Rates)
Deaths/1000 Operations***

Low Risk Patients*	Age (Yrs)	Cholecystectomy	Cholecystectomy + Common Duct Exploration
Women	0–49	.54	2.13
	50–69	2.80	10.10
Men	0–49	1.04	4.12
	50–69	5.41	19.23
High Risk Patients**			
Women	0–49	12.66	47.62
	50–69	17.24	58.82
Men	0–49	24.39	90.91
	50–69	33.33	111.11

* In good health or with moderate systemic disease.
** With severe or extreme systemic disease.
*** Includes both elective and emergency surgery.

Women in good health or who have only moderate systemic disease, and are under 49 years of age have the lowest surgical mortality rate (0.054); men in all categories have a surgical mortality rate twice that of women. Common duct exploration quadruples the rates in all categories. The rates rise with each decade of life and increase tenfold or more in all categories with severe or extreme systemic disease.

Continued on next page

The full prescribing information for each Summit product is contained herein and is that in effect as of September 1, 1992.

Summit—Cont.

INDICATIONS AND USAGE
Actigall is indicated for patients with radiolucent, noncalcified gallbladder stones <20 mm in greatest diameter in whom elective cholecystectomy would be undertaken except for the presence of increased surgical risk due to systemic disease, advanced age, idiosyncratic reaction to general anesthesia, or for those patients who refuse surgery. Safety of use of Actigall beyond 24 months is not established.

CONTRAINDICATIONS
1. Actigall will not dissolve calcified cholesterol stones, radio-opaque stones or radiolucent bile pigment stones. Hence, patients with such stones are not candidates for Actigall therapy.
2. Patients with compelling reasons for cholecystectomy including unremitting acute cholecystitis, cholangitis, biliary obstruction, gallstone pancreatitis or biliary-gastrointestinal fistula are not candidates for Actigall therapy.
3. Allergy to bile acids.

PRECAUTIONS
Liver Tests: Ursodiol therapy has not been associated with liver damage. Lithocholic acid, a naturally occurring bile acid, is known to be a liver-toxic metabolite. This bile acid is formed in the gut from ursodiol less efficiently and in smaller amounts than that seen from chenodiol. Lithocholic acid is detoxified in the liver by sulfation and although man appears to be an efficient sulfater, it is possible that some patients may have a congenital or acquired deficiency in sulfation, thereby predisposing them to lithocholate-induced liver damage.
Abnormalities in liver enzymes have not been associated with Actigall therapy and in fact Actigall has been shown to decrease liver enzyme levels in liver disease. However, patients given Actigall should have SGOT (AST) and SGPT (ALT) measured at the initiation of therapy and thereafter as indicated by the particular clinical circumstances.
Drug Interactions: Bile acid sequestering agents such as cholestyramine and colestipol may interfere with the action of Actigall by reducing its absorption. Aluminum-based antacids have been shown to adsorb bile acids *in vitro* and may be expected to interfere with Actigall in the same manner as the bile acid sequestering agents. Estrogens, oral contraceptives and clofibrate (and perhaps other lipid-lowering drugs) increase hepatic cholesterol secretion, and encourage cholesterol gallstone formation and hence may counteract the effectiveness of Actigall.
Carcinogenesis, Mutagenesis, and Impairment of Fertility: Ursodeoxycholic acid was tested in two-year oral carcinogenicity studies in CD-1 mice and Sprague-Dawley rats at daily doses of 50, 250, and 1000 mg/kg/day. It was not tumorigenic in mice. In the rat study, it produced statistically significant dose-related increased incidences of pheochromocytomas of adrenal medulla in males ($p = 0.014$, Peto trend test) and females ($p = 0.004$, Peto trend test.)
A 78-week rat study employing intrarectal instillation of lithocholic acid and tauro-deoxycholic acid, metabolites of ursodiol and chenodiol, has been conducted. These bile acids alone did not produce any tumors. A tumor-promoting effect of both metabolites was observed when they were co-administered with a carcinogenic agent. Results of epidemiologic studies suggest that bile acids might be involved in the pathogenesis of human colon cancer in patients who had undergone a cholecystectomy, but direct evidence is lacking. Ursodiol is not mutagenic in the Ames test. Dietary administration of lithocholic acid to chickens is reported to cause hepatic adenomatous hyperplasia.
Pregnancy Category B: Reproduction studies have been performed in rats and rabbits with ursodiol doses up to 200-fold the therapeutic dose and have revealed no evidence of impaired fertility or harm to the fetus at doses of 20 to 100-fold the human dose in rats and at 5-fold the human dose (highest dose tested) in rabbits. Studies employing 100 to 200-fold the human dose in rats have shown some reduction in fertility rate and litter size. There have been no adequate and well-controlled studies of the use of ursodiol in pregnant women, but inadvertent exposure of 4 women to therapeutic doses of the drug in the first trimester of pregnancy during the Actigall trials led to no evidence of effects on the fetus or newborn baby. Although it seems unlikely, the possibility that ursodiol can cause fetal harm cannot be ruled out; hence, the drug is not recommended for use during pregnancy.
Nursing Mothers: It is not known whether ursodiol is excreted in human milk. Because many drugs are excreted in human milk, caution should be exercised when Actigall is administered to a nursing mother.
Pediatric Use: The safety and effectiveness of Actigall in children have not been established.

ADVERSE REACTIONS
Gastrointestinal: Actigall given in doses of 8–10 mg/kg/day rarely causes diarrhea (<1%). One study in which a placebo control was not used was associated with a 6% incidence of mild, transient diarrhea not requiring termination of therapy or lowering of Actigall dose. One patient with ulcerative colitis in the Actigall studies developed diarrhea on therapy. In the National Cooperative Gallstone Study, the incidence of diarrhea was 27.1% in the placebo group.
Dermatological: One patient in the Actigall studies with preexisting psoriasis apparently developed exacerbation of itching on Actigall, which remitted on withdrawal of the drug.
Other: In two ongoing double-blind, placebo-controlled ursodiol studies in the U.S., for which the treatment codes have not yet been broken, the following minor events have been reported:
Pruritus, rash, urticaria, dry skin, sweating, hair thinning, nausea, vomiting, dyspepsia, metallic taste, abdominal pain, biliary pain, cholecystitis, diarrhea, constipation, stomatitis, flatulence, headache, fatigue, anxiety, depression, sleep disorder, arthralgia, myalgia, back pain, cough, rhinitis.
Since these studies are ongoing and blinded, incidence rates in the ursodiol and placebo groups cannot be calculated, nor has it been established whether the reactions listed are associated with ursodiol.

OVERDOSAGE
Neither accidental nor intentional overdosing with Actigall has been reported. Doses of Actigall in the range of 16–20 mg/kg/day have been tolerated for 6–37 months without symptoms by 7 patients. The LD_{50} for ursodiol in rats is over 5,000 mg/kg given over 7–10 days and over 7,500 mg/kg for mice. The most likely manifestation of severe overdose with Actigall would probably be diarrhea, which should be treated symptomatically.

DOSAGE AND ADMINISTRATION
The recommended dose for Actigall treatment of radiolucent gallbladder stones is 8–10 mg/kg/day given in 2 or 3 divided doses.
Ultrasound images of the gallbladder should be obtained at six month intervals for the first year of Actigall therapy to monitor gallstone response. If gallstones appear to have dissolved, Actigall therapy should be continued and dissolution confirmed on a repeat ultrasound examination within one to three months. Most patients who eventually achieve complete stone dissolution will show partial or complete dissolution at the first on-treatment reevaluation. If partial stone dissolution is not seen by 12 months of Actigall therapy, the likelihood of success is greatly reduced.

HOW SUPPLIED
Actigall capsules brand of ursodiol are supplied in a strength of 300 mg. The hard-gelatin capsules are white and pink and printed with the product name and strength. They are supplied as follows:
Capsules 300 mg
Bottles of 100 .... NDC 57267-153-30
Samples, when available, are identified by the word *SAMPLE* appearing on each capsule.
Caution: Federal law prohibits dispensing without prescription.
Do not store above 86°F (30°C).
Dispense in tight container, USP.
C91-54 (Rev. 8/90)

Dist. by:
Summit Pharmaceuticals
Division of CIBA-GEIGY Corporation
Summit, New Jersey 07901
Shown in Product Identification Section, page 433

SLOW-K® ℞
[sloe-kay]
potassium chloride
Extended-Release Tablets USP

DESCRIPTION
Slow-K, potassium chloride extended-release tablets USP, is a sugar-coated (not enteric-coated) tablet for oral administration, containing 600 mg of potassium chloride (equivalent to 8 mEq) in a wax matrix. This formulation is intended to provide an extended release of potassium from the matrix to minimize the likelihood of producing high, localized concentrations of potassium within the gastrointestinal tract.
Slow-K is an electrolyte replenisher. Its chemical name is potassium chloride, and its structural formula is KCl. Potassium chloride USP is a white, granular powder or colorless crystals. It is odorless and has a saline taste. Its solutions are neutral to litmus. It is freely soluble in water and insoluble in alcohol.
Inactive Ingredients. Acacia, cetostearyl alcohol, gelatin, iron oxide, magnesium stearate, polyvinylpyrrolidone, parabens, sodium benzoate, starch, sucrose, talc, and titanium dioxide.

CLINICAL PHARMACOLOGY
The potassium ion is the principal intracellular cation of most body tissues. Potassium ions participate in a number of essential physiological processes, including the maintenance of intracellular tonicity, the transmission of nerve impulses, the contraction of cardiac, skeletal, and smooth muscle, and the maintenance of normal renal function.
In adults normal plasma potassium concentration is 3.5–5.0 mEq/L.
Potassium depletion may occur whenever the rate of potassium loss through renal excretion and/or loss from the gastrointestinal tract exceeds the rate of potassium intake. Such depletion usually develops slowly as a consequence of prolonged therapy with oral diuretics, primary or secondary hyperaldosteronism, diabetic ketoacidosis, severe diarrhea, or inadequate replacement of potassium in patients on prolonged parenteral nutrition. Potassium depletion due to these causes is usually accompanied by a concomitant deficiency of chloride and is manifested by hypokalemia and metabolic alkalosis. Potassium depletion may produce weakness, fatigue, disturbances of cardiac rhythm (primarily ectopic beats), prominent U-waves in the electrocardiogram, and in advanced cases flaccid paralysis and/or impaired ability to concentrate urine.
Potassium depletion associated with metabolic alkalosis is managed by correcting the fundamental causes of the deficiency whenever possible and administering supplemental potassium chloride in the form of high potassium food or potassium chloride solution or tablets.
In rare circumstances (*e.g.,* patients with renal tubular acidosis) potassium depletion may be associated with metabolic acidosis and hyperchloremia. In such patients potassium replacement should be accomplished with potassium salts other than the chloride, such as potassium bicarbonate, potassium citrate, or potassium acetate.
The potassium chloride in Slow-K is completely absorbed before it leaves the small intestine. The wax matrix is not absorbed and is excreted in the feces; in some instances the empty matrices may be noticeable in the stool. When the bioavailability of the potassium ion from Slow-K is compared to that of a true solution the extent of absorption is similar.
The extended-release properties of Slow-K are demonstrated by the finding that a significant increase in time is required for renal excretion of the first 50% of the Slow-K dose as compared to the solution.
Increased urinary potassium excretion is first observed 1 hour after administration of Slow-K, reaches a peak at 4 hours, and extends up to 8 hours. Mean daily steady-state plasma levels of potassium following daily administration of Slow-K cannot be distinguished from those following administration of a potassium chloride solution or from control plasma levels of potassium ion.

INDICATIONS AND USAGE
BECAUSE OF REPORTS OF INTESTINAL AND GASTRIC ULCERATION AND BLEEDING WITH EXTENDED-RELEASE POTASSIUM CHLORIDE PREPARATIONS, THESE DRUGS SHOULD BE RESERVED FOR THOSE PATIENTS WHO CANNOT TOLERATE OR REFUSE TO TAKE LIQUID OR EFFERVESCENT POTASSIUM PREPARATIONS OR FOR PATIENTS IN WHOM THERE IS A PROBLEM OF COMPLIANCE WITH THESE PREPARATIONS.
1. For therapeutic use in patients with hypokalemia with or without metabolic alkalosis; in digitalis intoxication and in patients with hypokalemic familial periodic paralysis.
2. For prevention of potassium depletion when the dietary intake of potassium is inadequate in the following conditions: patients receiving digitalis and diuretics for congestive heart failure; hepatic cirrhosis with ascites; states of aldosterone excess with normal renal function; potassium-losing nephropathy, and certain diarrheal states.
3. The use of potassium salts in patients receiving diuretics for uncomplicated essential hypertension is often unnecessary when such patients have a normal dietary pattern. Serum potassium should be checked periodically, however, and, if hypokalemia occurs, dietary supplementation with potassium-containing foods may be adequate to control milder cases. In more severe cases supplementation with potassium salts may be indicated.

CONTRAINDICATIONS
Potassium supplements are contraindicated in patients with hyperkalemia, since a further increase in serum potassium concentration in such patients can produce cardiac arrest. Hyperkalemia may complicate any of the following conditions: chronic renal failure, systemic acidosis such as diabetic acidosis, acute dehydration, extensive tissue breakdown as in severe burns, adrenal insufficiency, or the administration of a potassium-sparing diuretic (*e.g.,* spironolactone, triamterene) (see OVERDOSAGE).
All solid dosage forms of potassium supplements are contraindicated in any patient in whom there is cause for arrest or delay in tablet passage through the gastrointestinal tract. In

these instances, potassium supplementation should be with a liquid preparation. Wax-matrix potassium chloride preparations have produced esophageal ulceration in certain cardiac patients with esophageal compression due to an enlarged left atrium.

WARNINGS

Hyperkalemia (See OVERDOSAGE.)
In patients with impaired mechanisms for excreting potassium, the administration of potassium salts can produce hyperkalemia and cardiac arrest. This occurs most commonly in patients given potassium by the intravenous route but may also occur in patients given potassium orally. Potentially fatal hyperkalemia can develop rapidly and be asymptomatic.

The use of potassium salts in patients with chronic renal disease, or any other condition which impairs potassium excretion, requires particularly careful monitoring of the serum potassium concentration and appropriate dosage adjustment.

Interaction with Potassium-Sparing Diuretics
Hypokalemia should not be treated by the concomitant administration of potassium salts and a potassium-sparing diuretic (e.g., spironolactone or triamterene), since the simultaneous administration of these agents can produce severe hyperkalemia.

Gastrointestinal lesions
Potassium chloride tablets have produced stenotic and/or ulcerative lesions of the small bowel and deaths. These lesions are caused by a high localized concentration of potassium ion in the region of a rapidly dissolving tablet, which injures the bowel wall and thereby produces obstruction, hemorrhage, or perforation. Slow-K is a wax-matrix tablet formulated to provide an extended- rate of release of potassium chloride and thus to minimize the possibility of a high local concentration of potassium ion near the bowel wall. While the reported frequency of small-bowel lesions is much less with wax-matrix tablets (less than one per 100,000 patient-years) than with enteric-coated potassium chloride tablets (40–50 per 100,000 patient-years) cases associated with wax-matrix tablets have been reported both in foreign countries and in the United States. In addition, perhaps because the wax-matrix preparations are not enteric-coated and release potassium in the stomach, there have been reports of upper gastrointestinal bleeding associated with these products. The total number of gastrointestinal lesions remains approximately one per 100,000 patient-years. Slow-K should be discontinued immediately and the possibility of bowel obstruction or perforation considered if severe vomiting, abdominal pain, distention, or gastrointestinal bleeding occurs.

Metabolic acidosis
Hypokalemia in patients with metabolic *acidosis* should be treated with an alkalinizing potassium salt such as potassium bicarbonate, potassium citrate, or potassium acetate.

PRECAUTIONS

General: The diagnosis of potassium depletion is ordinarily made by demonstrating hypokalemia in a patient with a clinical history suggesting some cause for potassium depletion. In interpreting the serum potassium level, the physician should bear in mind that acute alkalosis *per se* can produce hypokalemia in the absence of a deficit in total body potassium, while acute acidosis *per se* can increase the serum potassium concentration into the normal range even in the presence of a reduced total body potassium.

Information for Patients
Physicians should consider reminding the patient of the following:
To take each dose without crushing, chewing, or sucking the tablets.
To take this medicine only as directed. This is especially important if the patient is also taking both diuretics and digitalis preparations.
To check with the physician if there is trouble swallowing tablets or if the tablets seem to stick in the throat.
To check with the doctor at once if tarry stools or other evidence of gastrointestinal bleeding is noticed.

Laboratory Tests
Regular serum potassium determinations are recommended. In addition, during the treatment of potassium depletion, careful attention should be paid to acid-base balance, other serum electrolyte levels, the electrocardiogram, and the clinical status of the patient, particularly in the presence of cardiac disease, renal disease, or acidosis.

Drug Interactions
Potassium-sparing diuretics: see **WARNINGS**.

Carcinogenesis, Mutagenesis, Impairment of Fertility
Long-term carcinogenicity studies in animals have not been performed.

Pregnancy Category C
Animal reproduction studies have not been conducted with Slow-K. It is also not known whether Slow-K can cause fetal harm when administered to a pregnant woman or can affect reproduction capacity. Slow-K should be given to a pregnant woman only if clearly needed.

Nursing Mothers
The normal potassium ion content of human milk is about 13 mEq/L. It is not known if Slow-K has an effect on this content. Caution should be exercised when Slow-K is administered to a nursing woman.

Pediatric Use
Safety and effectiveness in children have not been established.

ADVERSE REACTIONS
One of the most severe adverse effects is hyperkalemia (see **CONTRAINDICATIONS, WARNINGS** and **OVERDOSAGE**). There also have been reports of upper and lower gastrointestinal conditions including obstruction, bleeding, ulceration, and perforation (see **CONTRAINDICATIONS** and **WARNINGS**); other factors known to be associated with such conditions were present in many of these patients.
The most common adverse reactions to oral potassium salts are nausea, vomiting, abdominal discomfort, and diarrhea. These symptoms are due to irritation of the gastrointestinal tract and are best managed by taking the dose with meals or reducing the dose.
Skin rash has been reported rarely.

OVERDOSAGE
The administration of oral potassium salts to persons with normal excretory mechanisms for potassium rarely causes serious hyperkalemia. However, if excretory mechanisms are impaired or if potassium is administered too rapidly intravenously, potentially fatal hyperkalemia can result (see **CONTRAINDICATIONS** and **WARNINGS**). It is important to recognize that hyperkalemia is usually asymptomatic and may be manifested only by an increased serum potassium concentration (6.5–8.0 mEq/L) and characteristic electrocardiographic changes (peaking of T waves, loss of P wave, depression of S-T segment, and prolongation of the Q-T interval). Late manifestations include muscle paralysis and cardiovascular collapse from cardiac arrest (9–12 mEq/L).
Treatment measures for hyperkalemia include the following: (1) elimination of foods and medications containing potassium and of potassium-sparing diuretics; (2) intravenous administration of 300–500 ml/hr of 10% dextrose solution containing 10–20 units of insulin per 1,000 ml; (3) correction of acidosis, if present, with intravenous sodium bicarbonate; (4) use of exchange resins, hemodialysis, or peritoneal dialysis.
In treating hyperkalemia in patients who have been stabilized on digitalis, too rapid a lowering of the serum potassium concentration can produce digitalis toxicity.

DOSAGE AND ADMINISTRATION
The usual dietary intake of potassium by the average adult is 40–80 mEq per day. Potassium depletion sufficient to cause hypokalemia usually requires the loss of 200 or more mEq of potassium from the total body store. Dosage must be adjusted to the individual needs of each patient but is typically in the range of 20 mEq per day for the prevention of hypokalemia to 40–100 mEq or more per day for the treatment of potassium depletion. Large numbers of tablets should be given in divided doses.

Note: Slow-K extended-release tablets must be swallowed whole and never crushed, chewed, or sucked.

HOW SUPPLIED
Tablets 600 mg potassium chloride (equivalent to 8 mEq)
round, buff colored, sugar-coated (imprinted Slow-K)
   Bottles of 100 .... NDC 57267-165-30
   Bottles of 1000 .... NDC 57267-165-40
   Consumer Pack—One Unit
     12 Bottles—100 tablets each .... NDC 57267-165-65
   Accu-Pak® Unit Dose (Blister pack)
     Box of 100 (strips of 10) .... NDC 57267-165-32
Samples, when available, are identified by the word *SAMPLE* appearing on each tablet.
Do not store above 86°F (30°C). Protect from moisture. Protect from light.
Dispense in tight, light-resistant container (USP).
Dist. by:
Summit Pharmaceuticals
Division of CIBA-GEIGY Corporation
Summit, NJ 07901

C91-27 (Rev. 8/91)
Shown in Product Identification Section, page 433

TEN-K®   ℞
potassium chloride
Extended-Release Tablets USP

DESCRIPTION
Ten-K, potassium chloride extended-release tablets USP, is a multiple-unit tablet for oral administration. Each tablet contains 750 mg of potassium chloride as polymeric-coated crystals (equivalent to 10 mEq of potassium) in a rice starch binder. After ingestion, the tablets disintegrate and disperse rapidly into small particles, each with a polymeric coating, which allows for extended release of potassium and chloride ions over approximately an 8- to 10-hour period. The dispersibility of the coated crystals and the extended release of ions are intended to minimize the likelihood of high localized concentrations of potassium chloride in the gastrointestinal tract.
Potassium chloride has an empirical formula of KCl and a molecular weight of 74.55.
Ten-K as a multiple-unit tablet can be subdivided without significant changes in the release characteristics to improve swallowability. The polymeric coating functions as a water-permeable membrane. Fluids pass through the membrane and gradually dissolve the potassium chloride within the polymeric-coated crystals. The resulting potassium chloride solution slowly diffuses outward through the membrane.
Inactive Ingredients. Acetyl tributyl citrate, cellulose compounds, colloidal silicone dioxide, magnesium stearate, rice starch, talc, and wax.

CLINICAL PHARMACOLOGY
Potassium ion is the principal intracellular cation of most body tissues. Potassium ions participate in a number of essential physiological processes, including the maintenance of intracellular tonicity, the transmission of nerve impulses, the contraction of cardiac, skeletal, and smooth muscle, and the maintenance of normal renal function.
Potassium depletion may occur whenever the rate of potassium loss through renal excretion and/or loss from the gastrointestinal tract exceeds the rate of potassium intake. Such depletion usually develops slowly as a consequence of prolonged therapy with oral diuretics, primary or secondary hyperaldosteronism, diabetic ketoacidosis, severe diarrhea, or inadequate replacement of potassium in patients on prolonged parenteral nutrition. Potassium depletion due to these causes is usually accompanied by a concomitant deficiency of chloride and is manifested by hypokalemia and metabolic alkalosis.
Potassium depletion may produce weakness, fatigue, disturbances of cardiac rhythm (primarily ectopic beats), prominent U waves in the electrocardiogram, and in advanced cases, flaccid paralysis and/or impaired ability to concentrate urine.
Potassium depletion associated with metabolic alkalosis is managed by correcting the fundamental causes of the deficiency whenever possible and administering supplemental potassium chloride in the form of high potassium food or potassium chloride solution, capsules, or tablets. In rare circumstances (e.g., in patients with renal tubular acidosis) potassium depletion may be associated with metabolic acidosis and hyperchloremia. In such patients, potassium replacement should be accomplished with potassium salts other than the chloride, such as potassium bicarbonate, potassium citrate, or potassium acetate.

INDICATIONS AND USAGE
BECAUSE OF REPORTS OF INTESTINAL AND GASTRIC ULCERATION AND BLEEDING WITH EXTENDED-RELEASE POTASSIUM CHLORIDE PREPARATIONS, THESE DRUGS SHOULD BE RESERVED FOR THOSE PATIENTS WHO CANNOT TOLERATE OR REFUSE TO TAKE LIQUID OR EFFERVESCENT POTASSIUM PREPARATIONS OR FOR PATIENTS IN WHOM THERE IS A PROBLEM OF COMPLIANCE WITH THESE PREPARATIONS.
1. For therapeutic use in patients with hypokalemia with or without metabolic alkalosis; in digitalis intoxication and in patients with hypokalemic familial periodic paralysis.
2. For prevention of potassium depletion when the dietary intake of potassium is inadequate in the following conditions: patients receiving digitalis and diuretics for congestive heart failure; hepatic cirrhosis with ascites; states of aldosterone excess with normal renal function; potassium-losing nephropathy; and certain diarrheal states.
3. The use of potassium salts in patients receiving diuretics for uncomplicated essential hypertension is often unnecessary when such patients have a normal dietary pattern. Serum potassium should be checked periodically, however, and if hypokalemia occurs, dietary supplementation with potassium-containing foods may be adequate to control milder cases. In more severe cases, supplementation with potassium salts may be indicated.

CONTRAINDICATIONS
Potassium supplements are contraindicated in patients with hyperkalemia, since a further increase in serum potassium concentration in such patients can produce cardiac arrest. Hyperkalemia may complicate any of the following conditions: chronic renal failure, systemic acidosis such as diabetic acidosis, acute dehydration, extensive tissue breakdown as in severe burns, adrenal insufficiency, or the admin-

Continued on next page

The full prescribing information for each Summit product is contained herein and is that in effect as of September 1, 1992.

Summit—Cont.

istration of a potassium-sparing diuretic (e.g., spironolactone, triamterene, amiloride).

Wax-matrix potassium chloride preparations have produced esophageal ulceration in certain cardiac patients with esophageal compression due to an enlarged left atrium.

All solid dosage forms of potassium supplements are contraindicated in any patients in whom there is cause for arrest or delay in tablet passage through the gastrointestinal tract. In these instances, potassium supplementation should be with a liquid preparation.

WARNINGS

Hyperkalemia
In patients with impaired mechanisms for excreting potassium, the administration of potassium salts can produce hyperkalemia and cardiac arrest. This occurs most commonly in patients given potassium by the intravenous route but may also occur in patients given potassium orally. Potentially fatal hyperkalemia can develop rapidly and be asymptomatic.

The use of potassium salts in patients with chronic renal disease, or any other condition which impairs potassium excretion, requires particularly careful monitoring of the serum potassium concentration and appropriate dosage adjustments.

Interaction With Potassium-Sparing Diuretics
Hypokalemia should not be treated by the concomitant administration of potassium salts and a potassium-sparing diuretic (e.g., spironolactone, triamterene, amiloride), since the simultaneous administration of these agents can produce severe hyperkalemia.

Gastrointestinal Lesions
Potassium chloride tablets have produced stenotic and/or ulcerative lesions of the small bowel and deaths, in addition to upper gastrointestinal bleeding. These lesions are caused by a high localized concentration of potassium ion in the region of a rapidly dissolving tablet, which injures the bowel wall and thereby produces obstruction, hemorrhage, or perforation.

Ten-K tablets consist of polymeric-coated crystals. After ingestion the tablets disintegrate and disperse rapidly in the stomach into subunits, which are formulated to provide extended release of potassium chloride. The dispersibility of the subunits and the extended release of potassium ions from the subunits are intended to minimize the possibility of a high local concentration near the gastrointestinal mucosa and the ability of the potassium chloride to cause stenosis or ulceration. Other means of accomplishing this (e.g., incorporation of potassium chloride into a wax matrix) have reduced the frequency of such lesions to less than one per 100,000 patient-years (compared to 40-50 per 100,000 patient-years with enteric-coated potassium chloride) but have not eliminated them. The frequency of gastrointestinal lesions with Ten-K is at present unknown. Ten-K should be discontinued immediately and the possibility of bowel obstruction or perforation considered if severe vomiting, abdominal pain, distention, or gastrointestinal bleeding occurs.

Metabolic Acidosis
Hypokalemia in patients with metabolic *acidosis* should be treated with an alkalinizing potassium salt such as potassium bicarbonate, potassium citrate, or potassium acetate.

PRECAUTIONS
The diagnosis of potassium depletion is ordinarily made by demonstrating hypokalemia in a patient with a clinical history suggesting some cause for potassium depletion. In interpreting the serum potassium level, the physician should bear in mind that acute alkalosis per se can produce hypokalemia in the absence of a deficit in total body potassium, while acute acidosis per se can increase the serum potassium concentration into the normal range even in the presence of a reduced total body potassium. The treatment of potassium depletion, particularly in the presence of cardiac disease, renal disease, or acidosis, requires careful attention to acid-base balance and appropriate monitoring of serum electrolytes, the electrocardiogram, and the clinical status of the patient.

Carcinogenesis, Mutagenesis, Impairment of Fertility
Long-term carcinogenicity studies in animals have not been performed.

Pregnancy Category C
Animal reproduction studies have not been conducted with Ten-K. It is also not known whether Ten-K can cause fetal harm when administered to a pregnant woman or can affect reproduction capacity. Ten-K should be given to a pregnant woman only if clearly needed.

Nursing Mothers
The normal potassium ion content of human milk is about 13 mEq/L. It is not known if Ten-K has an effect on this content. Caution should be exercised when Ten-K is administered to a nursing woman.

Pediatric Use
Safety and effectiveness in children have not been established.

ADVERSE REACTIONS
The most common adverse reactions to oral potassium salts are nausea, vomiting, abdominal discomfort, and diarrhea. These symptoms are due to irritation of the gastrointestinal tract and may be minimized by taking the dose with meals or by reducing the dose.

Intestinal bleeding, ulceration, perforation, and obstruction have been reported in patients treated with solid dosage forms of potassium salts and may occur with Ten-K (see CONTRAINDICATIONS and WARNINGS). One of the most severe adverse effects of potassium supplementation is hyperkalemia (see CONTRAINDICATIONS, WARNINGS, and OVERDOSAGE).

Skin rash has been reported rarely with potassium preparations.

OVERDOSAGE
The administration of oral potassium salts to persons with normal excretory mechanisms for potassium rarely causes serious hyperkalemia. However, if excretory mechanisms are impaired or if potassium is administered too rapidly intravenously, potentially fatal hyperkalemia can result (see CONTRAINDICATIONS and WARNINGS). It is important to recognize that hyperkalemia is usually asymptomatic and may be manifested only by an increased serum potassium concentration and characteristic electrocardiogram changes (peaking of T-waves, loss of P-wave, depression of S-T segment, and prolongation of the Q-T interval). Late manifestations include muscle paralysis and cardiovascular collapse from cardiac arrest.

Treatment measures for hyperkalemia include the following: (1) elimination of foods and medications containing potassium and of potassium-sparing diuretics; (2) intravenous administration of 300–500 ml/hr of 10% dextrose solution containing 10–20 units of insulin per 1,000 ml; (3) correction of acidosis, if present with intravenous sodium bicarbonate; (4) use of exchange resins, hemodialysis, or peritoneal dialysis.

In treating hyperkalemia, it should be recalled that in patients who have been stabilized on digitalis, too rapid a lowering of the serum potassium concentration can produce digitalis toxicity.

DOSAGE AND ADMINISTRATION
The usual dietary intake of potassium by the average adult is 40–80 mEq per day. Potassium depletion sufficient to cause hyperkalemia usually requires the loss of 200 or more mEq of potassium from the total body store.

Dosage must be adjusted to the individual needs of each patient, but typically is in the range of two to three tablets of Ten-K per day (20–30 mEq of potassium) for the prevention of hypokalemia and four to ten tablets of Ten-K (40–100 mEq of potassium) or more per day for the treatment of potassium depletion. If more than two Ten-K 10 mEq tablets are prescribed per day, the total daily dosage should be divided into two or more separate doses and any single dose should not exceed 20 mEq.

Because Ten-K tablets can be subdivided without a significant change in the dissolution profile and since each crystal of potassium chloride has a polymeric coating, the tablets can be broken in half or crushed, without an unpleasant taste. This mode of administration may be preferred for patients with difficulty in swallowing tablets.

HOW SUPPLIED
Tablets —750 mg of potassium chloride (equivalent to 10 mEq) capsule-shaped, white, scored (imprinted Ten-K)

Bottles of 100	NDC 57267-146-30
Unit Dose (blister pack)	
Box of 100 (strips of 10)	NDC 57267-146-32
Bottles of 500	NDC 57267-146-35

Do not store above 86°F (30°C). Protect from moisture.

ANIMAL TOXICITY
The ulcerogenic potential of polymeric-coated crystals of potassium chloride was studied in monkeys. In monkeys receiving 2400 mEq of potassium chloride as Ten-K for 8½ days, Ten-K showed no tendency to cause intestinal ulceration.

C91-26 (Rev. 8/91)

Dist. by:
Summit Pharmaceuticals
Division of CIBA-GEIGY Corporation
Summit, NJ 07901

Shown in Product Identification Section, page 433

TRANSDERM-NITRO®   ℞
[*trans 'derm nye 'trow*]
nitroglycerin
Transdermal Therapeutic System

Revised Dosage Information

DESCRIPTION
Nitroglycerin is 1,2,3-propanetriol, trinitrate, an organic nitrate whose molecular weight is 227.09. The organic nitrates are vasodilators, active on both arteries and veins. The Transderm-Nitro (nitroglycerin) transdermal system is a flat unit designed to provide continuous controlled release of nitroglycerin through intact skin.

The rate of release of the nitroglycerin is linearly dependent upon the area of the applied system; each cm^2 of applied system delivers approximately 0.02 mg of nitroglycerin per hour. Thus, the 5-, 10-, 20-, and 30-cm^2 systems deliver approximately 0.1, 0.2, 0.4, and 0.6 mg of nitroglycerin per hour, respectively.

The remainder of the nitroglycerin in each system serves as a reservoir and is not delivered in normal use. After 12 hours, for example, each system has delivered 10% of its original content of nitroglycerin.

The Transderm-Nitro system comprises four layers as shown below. Proceeding from the visible surface towards the surface attached to the skin, these layers are: 1) a tan-colored backing layer (aluminized plastic) that is impermeable to nitroglycerin; 2) a drug reservoir containing nitroglycerin adsorbed on lactose, colloidal silicon dioxide, and silicone medical fluid; 3) an ethylene-vinyl acetate copolymer membrane that is permeable to nitroglycerin; and 4) a layer of hypoallergenic silicone adhesive. Prior to use, a protective peel strip is removed from the adhesive surface.

Cross section of the system:

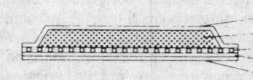

Backing
Drug Reservoir
Semipermeable Membrane
Adhesive
Protective Peel Strip

CLINICAL PHARMACOLOGY
The principal pharmacological action of nitroglycerin is relaxation of vascular smooth muscle, and consequent dilatation of peripheral arteries and veins, especially the latter. Dilatation of the veins promotes peripheral pooling of blood and decreases venous return to the heart, thereby reducing left ventricular end-diastolic pressure and pulmonary capillary wedge pressure (preload). Arteriolar relaxation reduces systemic vascular resistance, systolic arterial pressure, and mean arterial pressure (afterload). Dilatation of the coronary arteries also occurs. The relative importance of preload reduction, afterload reduction, and coronary dilatation remains undefined.

Dosing regimens for most chronically used drugs are designed to provide plasma concentrations that are continuously greater than a minimally effective concentration. This strategy is inappropriate for organic nitrates. Several well-controlled clinical trials have used exercise testing to assess the antianginal efficacy of continuously-delivered nitrates. In the large majority of these trials, active agents were indistinguishable from placebo after 24 hours (or less) of continuous therapy. Attempts to overcome nitrate tolerance by dose escalation, even to doses far in excess of those used acutely, have consistently failed. Only after nitrates had been absent from the body for several hours was their antianginal efficacy restored.

Pharmacokinetics
The volume of distribution of nitroglycerin is about 3L/kg, and nitroglycerin is cleared from this volume at extremely rapid rates, with a resulting serum half-life of about 3 minutes. The observed clearance rates (close to 1L/kg/min) greatly exceed hepatic blood flow, known sites of extrahepatic metabolism include red blood cells and vascular walls. The first products in the metabolism of nitroglycerin are inorganic nitrate and the 1,2- and 1,3-dinitroglycerols. The dinitrates are less effective vasodilators than nitroglycerin, but they are longer-lived in the serum, and their net contribution to the overall effect of chronic nitroglycerin regimens is not known. The dinitrates are further metabolized to (nonvasoactive) mononitrates and, ultimately, to glycerol and carbon dioxide.

To avoid development of tolerance to nitroglycerin, drug-free intervals of 10–12 hours are known to be sufficient; shorter intervals have not been well studied. In one well-controlled clinical trial, subjects receiving nitroglycerin appeared to exhibit a rebound or withdrawal effect, so that their exercise tolerance at the end of the daily drug-free interval was *less* than that exhibited by the parallel group receiving placebo. In healthy volunteers, steady-state plasma concentrations of nitroglycerin are reached by about two hours after application of a patch and are maintained for the duration of wear-

ing the system (observations have been limited to 24 hours). Upon removal of the patch, the plasma concentration declines with a half-life of about an hour.

Clinical Trials

Regimens in which nitroglycerin patches were worn for 12 hours daily have been studied in well-controlled trials up to 4 weeks in duration. Starting about 2 hours after application and continuing until 10–12 hours after application, patches that deliver at least 0.4 mg of nitroglycerin per hour have consistently demonstrated greater antianginal activity than placebo. Lower-dose patches have not been as well studied, but in one large, well-controlled trial in which higher-dose patches were also studied, patches delivering 0.2 mg/hr had significantly less antianginal activity than placebo.

It is reasonable to believe that the rate of nitroglycerin absorption from patches may vary with the site of application, but this relationship has not been adequately studied.

The onset of action of transdermal nitroglycerin is not sufficiently rapid for this product to be useful in aborting an acute anginal episode.

Transderm-Nitro System*	Total Nitroglycerin in System	System Size		Carton Size	
0.1 mg/hr	12.5 mg	5 cm^2	30 Systems	NDC 57267-902-26
			**30 Systems	NDC 57267-902-42
			**100 Systems	NDC 57267-902-30
0.2 mg/hr	25 mg	10 cm^2	30 Systems	NDC 57267-905-26
			**30 Systems	NDC 57267-905-42
			**100 Systems	NDC 57267-905-30
0.4 mg/hr	50 mg	20 cm^2	30 Systems	NDC 57267-910-26
			**30 Systems	NDC 57267-910-42
			**100 Systems	NDC 57267-910-30
0.6 mg/hr	75 mg	30 cm^2	30 Systems	NDC 57267-915-26
			**30 Systems	NDC 57267-915-42
			**100 Systems	NDC 57267-915-30

*Rated release in vivo. Release rates were formerly described in terms of drug delivered per 24 hours. In these terms, the supplied Transderm-Nitro systems would be rated at 2.5 mg/24 hr (0.1 mg/hr), 5 mg/24 hr (0.2 mg/hr), 10 mg/24 hr (0.4 mg/hr), and 15 mg/24 hr (0.6 mg/hr).

**Institutional Pack

Do not store above 86°F (30°C).

C89–46 (Rev. 10/89)

INDICATIONS AND USAGE

This drug product has been conditionally approved by the FDA for the prevention of angina pectoris due to coronary artery disease. Tolerance to the antianginal effects of nitrates (measured by exercise stress testing) has been shown to be a major factor limiting efficacy when transdermal nitrates are used continuously for longer than 12 hours each day. The development of tolerance can be altered (prevented or attenuated) by use of a noncontinuous (intermittent) dosing schedule with a nitrate-free interval of 10–12 hours.

Controlled clinical trial data suggest that the intermittent use of nitrates is associated with decreased exercise tolerance, in comparison to placebo, during the last part of the nitrate-free interval; the clinical relevance of this observation is unknown, but the possibility of increased frequency or severity of angina during the nitrate-free interval should be considered. Further investigations of the tolerance phenomenon and best regimen are ongoing. A final evaluation of the effectiveness of the product will be announced by the FDA.

CONTRAINDICATIONS

Allergic reactions to organic nitrates are extremely rare, but they do occur. Nitroglycerin is contraindicated in patients who are allergic to it. Allergy to the adhesives used in nitroglycerin patches has also been reported, and it similarly constitutes a contraindication to the use of this product.

WARNINGS

The benefits of transdermal nitroglycerin in patients with acute myocardial infarction or congestive heart failure have not been established. If one elects to use nitroglycerin in these conditions, careful clinical or hemodynamic monitoring must be used to avoid the hazards of hypotension and tachycardia.

A cardioverter/defibrillator should not be discharged through a paddle electrode that overlies a Transderm-Nitro patch. The arcing that may be seen in this situation is harmless in itself, but it may be associated with local current concentration that can cause damage to the paddles and burns to the patient.

PRECAUTIONS

General

Severe hypotension, particularly with upright posture, may occur with even small doses of nitroglycerin. This drug should therefore be used with caution in patients who may be volume depleted or who, for whatever reason, are already hypotensive. Hypotension induced by nitroglycerin may be accompanied by paradoxical bradycardia and increased angina pectoris.

Nitrate therapy may aggravate the angina caused by hypertrophic cardiomyopathy.

As tolerance to other forms of nitroglycerin develops, the effect of sublingual nitroglycerin on exercise tolerance, although still observable, is somewhat blunted.

In industrial workers who have had long-term exposure to unknown (presumably high) doses of organic nitrates, tolerance clearly occurs. Chest pain, acute myocardial infarction, and even sudden death have occurred during temporary withdrawal of nitrates from these workers, demonstrating the existence of true physical dependence.

Several clinical trials in patients with angina pectoris have evaluated nitroglycerin regimens which incorporated a 10–12 hour nitrate-free interval. In some of these trials, an increase in the frequency of anginal attacks during the nitrate-free interval was observed in a small number of patients. In one trial, patients demonstrated decreased exercise tolerance at the end of the nitrate-free interval. Hemodynamic rebound has been observed only rarely; on the other hand, few studies were so designed that rebound, if it had occurred, would have been detected. The importance of these

observations to the routine, clinical use of transdermal nitroglycerin is unknown.

Information for Patients

Daily headaches sometimes accompany treatment with nitroglycerin. In patients who get these headaches, the headaches may be a marker of the activity of the drug. Patients should resist the temptation to avoid headaches by altering the schedule of their treatment with nitroglycerin, since loss of headache may be associated with simultaneous loss of antianginal efficacy.

Treatment with nitroglycerin may be associated with lightheadedness on standing, especially just after rising from a recumbent or seated position. This effect may be more frequent in patients who have also consumed alcohol.

After normal use, there is enough residual nitroglycerin in discarded patches that they are a potential hazard to children and pets.

A patient leaflet is supplied with the systems.

Drug Interactions

The vasodilating effects of nitroglycerin may be additive with those of other vasodilators. Alcohol, in particular, has been found to exhibit additive effects of this variety.

Marked symptomatic orthostatic hypotension has been reported when calcium channel blockers and organic nitrates were used in combination. Dose adjustments of either class of agents may be necessary.

Carcinogenesis, Mutagenesis, Impairment of Fertility

No long-term animal studies have examined the carcinogenic or mutagenic potential of nitroglycerin. Nitroglycerin's effect upon reproductive capacity is similarly unknown.

Pregnancy Category C

Animal reproduction studies have not been conducted with nitroglycerin. It is also not known whether nitroglycerin can cause fetal harm when administered to a pregnant woman or whether it can affect reproductive capacity. Nitroglycerin should be given to a pregnant woman only if clearly needed.

Nursing Mothers

It is not known whether nitroglycerin is excreted in human milk. Because many drugs are excreted in human milk, caution should be exercised when nitroglycerin is administered to a nursing woman.

Pediatric Use

Safety and effectiveness in children have not been established.

ADVERSE REACTIONS

Adverse reactions to nitroglycerin are generally dose-related, and almost all of these reactions are the result of nitroglycerin's activity as a vasodilator. Headache, which may be severe, is the most commonly reported side effect. Headache may be recurrent with each daily dose, especially at higher doses. Transient episodes of lightheadedness, occasionally related to blood pressure changes, may also occur. Hypotension occurs infrequently, but in some patients it may be severe enough to warrant discontinuation of therapy. Syncope, crescendo angina, and rebound hypertension have been reported but are uncommon.

Extremely rarely, ordinary doses of organic nitrates have caused methemoglobinemia in normal-seeming patients. Methemoglobinemia is so infrequent at these doses that further discussion of its diagnosis and treatment is deferred (see Overdosage).

Application-site irritation may occur but is rarely severe.

In two placebo-controlled trials of intermittent therapy with nitroglycerin patches at 0.2 to 0.8 mg/hr, the most frequent adverse reactions among 307 subjects were as follows:

	Placebo	Patch
Headache	18%	63%
Lightheadedness	4%	6%
Hypotension, and/or syncope	0%	4%
Increased angina	2%	2%

OVERDOSAGE

Hemodynamic Effects

The ill effects of nitroglycerin overdose are generally the result of nitroglycerin's capacity to induce vasodilatation, venous pooling, reduced cardiac output, and hypotension. These hemodynamic changes may have protean manifestations, including increased intracranial pressure, with any or all of persistent throbbing headache, confusion, and moderate fever; vertigo; palpitations; visual disturbances; nausea and vomiting (possibly with colic and even bloody diarrhea); syncope (especially in the upright posture); air hunger and dyspnea, later followed by reduced ventilatory effort; diaphoresis, with the skin either flushed or cold and clammy; heart block and bradycardia; paralysis; coma; seizures; and death.

Laboratory determinations of serum levels of nitroglycerin and its metabolites are not widely available, and such determinations have, in any event, no established role in the management of nitroglycerin overdose.

No data are available to suggest physiological maneuvers (e.g., maneuvers to change the pH of the urine) that might accelerate elimination of nitroglycerin and its active metabolites. Similarly, it is not known which, if any, of these substances can usefully be removed from the body by hemodialysis.

No specific antagonist to the vasodilator effects of nitroglycerin is known, and no intervention has been subject to controlled study as a therapy of nitroglycerin overdose. Because the hypotension associated with nitroglycerin overdose is the result of venodilatation and arterial hypovolemia, prudent therapy in this situation should be directed toward an increase in central fluid volume. Passive elevation of the patient's legs may be sufficient, but intravenous infusion of normal saline or similar fluid may also be necessary.

The use of epinephrine or other arterial vasoconstrictors in this setting is likely to do more harm than good.

In patients with renal disease or congestive heart failure, therapy resulting in central volume expansion is not without hazard. Treatment of nitroglycerin overdose in these patients may be subtle and difficult, and invasive monitoring may be required.

Methemoglobinemia

Nitrate ions liberated during metabolism of nitroglycerin can oxidize hemoglobin into methemoglobin. Even in patients totally without cytochrome b$_5$ reductase activity, however, and even assuming that the nitrate moieties of nitroglycerin are quantitatively applied to oxidation of hemoglobin, about 1 mg/kg of nitroglycerin should be required before any of these patients manifests clinically significant ($\geq 10\%$) methemoglobinemia. In patients with normal reductase function, significant production of methemoglobin should require even larger doses of nitroglycerin. In one study in which 36 patients received 2–4 weeks of continuous nitroglycerin therapy at 3.1 to 4.4 mg/hr, the average methemoglobin level measured was 0.2%; this was comparable to that observed in parallel patients who received placebo.

Notwithstanding these observations, there are case reports of significant methemoglobinemia in association with moderate overdoses of organic nitrates. None of the affected patients had been thought to be unusually susceptible.

Methemoglobin levels are available from most clinical laboratories. The diagnosis should be suspected in patients who exhibit signs of impaired oxygen delivery despite adequate cardiac output and adequate arterial pO$_2$. Classically, methemoglobinemic blood is described as chocolate brown, without color change on exposure to air.

Continued on next page

The full prescribing information for each Summit product is contained herein and is that in effect as of September 1, 1992.

Summit—Cont.

When methemoglobinemia is diagnosed, the treatment of choice is methylene blue, 1–2 mg/kg intravenously.

DOSAGE AND ADMINISTRATION

The suggested starting dose is between 0.2 mg/hr*, and 0.4 mg/hr*. Doses between 0.4 mg/hr* and 0.8 mg/hr* have shown continued effectiveness for 10–12 hours daily for at least one month (the longest period studied) of intermittent administration. Although the minimum nitrate-free interval has not been defined, data show that a nitrate-free interval of 10–12 hours is sufficient (see CLINICAL PHARMACOLOGY). Thus, an appropriate dosing schedule for nitroglycerin patches would include a daily patch-on period of 12–14 hours and a daily patch-off period of 10–12 hours. Although some well-controlled clinical trials using exercise tolerance testing have shown maintenance of effectiveness when patches are worn continuously, the large majority of such controlled trials have shown the development of tolerance (i.e., complete loss of effect) within the first 24 hours after therapy was initiated. Dose adjustment, even to levels much higher than generally used, did not restore efficacy.

PATIENT INSTRUCTIONS FOR APPLICATION OF SYSTEM

A patient leaflet is supplied with each carton.

HOW SUPPLIED

[See table on next page.]

How to use
TRANSDERM-NITRO®
nitroglycerin
Transdermal Therapeutic System
for the prevention of angina

Transderm-Nitro is easy to use—it has a clear plastic backing, and a special adhesive that keeps the system firmly in place.

Where to place Transderm-Nitro.
Select any area of skin on the body, EXCEPT the extremities below the knee or elbow. The chest is the preferred site. The area should be clean, dry, and hairless. If hair is likely to interfere with system adhesion or removal, it can be clipped, but not shaved. Take care to avoid areas with cuts or irritations. Do NOT apply the system immediately after showering or bathing. It is best to wait until you are certain the skin is completely dry.

How to apply Transderm-Nitro® nitroglycerin
1. Open the package by tearing at the indicated indentations. Carefully pick up the system lengthwise with the tab up, and the clear plastic backing facing you. You should be able to see the white cream containing nitroglycerin. (On very rare occasions, you may find a system without any white medication in it. Do not use it. Simply apply another system.)

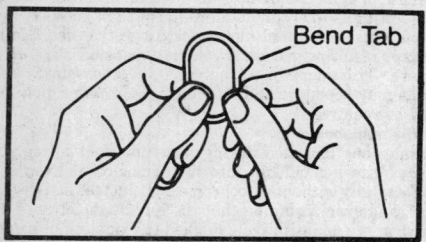

Bend Tab

Figure A.

2. Firmly bend the tab forward with the thumb (Figure A). With both thumbs, begin to remove the clear plastic backing from the system at the tab (Figure B). Do not touch the inside of the exposed system, because the adhesive covers the entire surface.

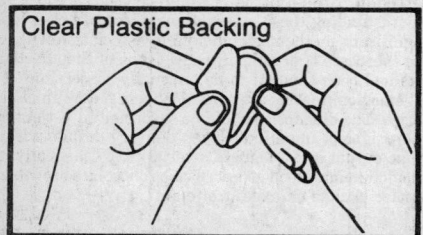

Clear Plastic Backing

Figure B

3. Continue to remove the clear plastic backing slowly along the length of the system, allowing the system to rest on the outside of your fingers (Figure C).

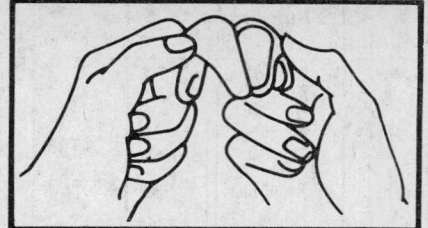

Figure C

4. Place the exposed, adhesive side of the system on the chosen skin site. Press firmly in place with the palm of your hand (Figure D). Once the system is in place, do not test the adhesion by pulling on it.

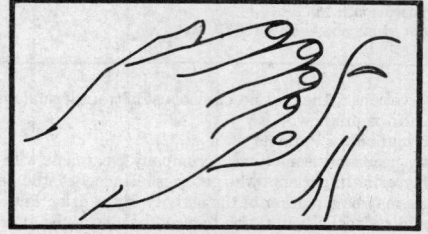

Figure D

When Transderm-Nitro is applied to your body, the nitroglycerin contained in the system begins to flow onto your skin through a unique rate-controlling membrane. This membrane allows the nitroglycerin to be released and available for absorption through your skin at a uniform rate.
5. At the time recommended by your doctor, remove and discard the system.
6. Place a new system on a different skin site, following Steps 1–4, according to your doctor's instructions.
Please note:
Contact with water, as in bathing, swimming, or showering will not affect the system. In the unlikely event that a system falls off, discard it and put a new one on a different skin site.

PRECAUTIONS

The most common side effect is headache, which often decreases as therapy is continued, but may require treatment with a mild analgesic. Although uncommon, faintness, flushing, and dizziness may occur, especially when suddenly rising from the recumbent (lying horizontal) position. If these symptoms occur, remove the system and notify your physician.
Skin irritation may occur. If it persists, consult your physician.
Keep these systems and all drugs out of the reach of children.
Important: Your doctor may decide to increase or decrease the size of the system, or prescribe a combination of systems, to suit your particular needs. The dose may vary depending on your individual response to the system.
This system is to be used for preventing angina, not for treating an acute attack.
DO NOT STORE ABOVE 86°F (30°C).
Dist. by:
Summit Pharmaceuticals
Div. of CIBA-GEIGY Corp.
Summit, NJ 07901

C89-22 (Rev. 6/89)
Shown in Product Identification Section, page 433

Sween Corporation
1940 COMMERCE DRIVE
P.O. BOX 8300
N. MANKATO, MN 56002

ATRAC-TAIN®   OTC
[ütrăc'tān]
Moisturizing
CREAM
with 10% Urea

DESCRIPTION

ATRAC-TAIN CREAM is a moisturizing, vanishing cream consisting of Water, Urea (10%), Lactic Acid, Isopropyl Palmitate, Octyl Palmitate, Stearyl Alcohol, Glyceryl Stearate, Sorbitol, Stearic Acid, Ceteareth-25, Ceteareth-6, and Benzethonium Chloride.

INDICATIONS AND USAGE

ATRAC-TAIN CREAM's dual-action, urea formula moisturizes and softens severely dry, rough skin and thereby, relieves the itching and associated discomforts of many dry skin conditions. Urea increases the water-binding capacity of the stratum corneum by attracting water to the dry skin cells. It also causes a physical softening of the desquamating layer of the epidermis by opening up more areas for H-bonding to water thus partially solubilizing the hard keratins that cause dry skin to feel rough. ATRAC-TAIN CREAM is non-occlusive, contains no petrolatum, mineral oil, parabens, dyes or perfumes.

CONTRAINDICATIONS

Hypersensitivity to any components of the preparation.

PRECAUTIONS AND ADVERSE REACTIONS

For External Use Only. Avoid contact, with eyes. Keep out of reach of children. If irritation occurs, temporarily discontinue use.

DOSAGE AND ADMINISTRATION

1. Cleanse affected area with gentle cleanser and pat dry.
2. Apply ATRAC-TAIN CREAM evenly to affected skin area—massage until absorbed.
3. Reapply CREAM 2–3 times daily.
4. Use once daily to maintain healthy skin.

HOW SUPPLIED

2 ml packets in packages of 100 and 300; 2 oz. and 5 oz. tubes.

ATRAC-TAIN®   OTC
[ütrăc'tān]
Moisturizing
LOTION

DESCRIPTION

ATRAC-TAIN LOTION is a moisturizing lotion containing Water, Urea (5%), Glyceryl Stearate, Sorbitol, Lactic Acid, Isopropyl Palmitate, Octyl Palmitate, Stearyl Alcohol, Stearic Acid, Ceteareth-25, Ceteareth-6, PEG-40 Jojoba Oil, Quaternium-15, EDTA and Benzethonium Chloride.

INDICATIONS AND USAGE

ATRAC-TAIN LOTION's formula enhances the body's normal remoisturizing system offering relief to mild, dry skin conditions. ATRAC-TAIN LOTION also aids in maintaining healthy integrity of the skin once a dry skin condition has improved. Urea increases the water-binding capacity of the stratum corneum by opening up more areas for H-bonding to water thus attracting moisture to the dry skin cells. It also causes a physical softening of the desquamating layer of the epidermis by partially solubilizing the hard keratins that cause dry skin to feel rough.
ATRAC-TAIN LOTION is non-occlusive, contains no petrolatum, mineral oil, parabens, dyes or perfumes.

CONTRAINDICATIONS

Hypersensitivity to any components of the preparation.

PRECAUTIONS AND ADVERSE REACTIONS

For External Use Only. Avoid contact with eyes. Keep out of reach of children. If irritation occurs, temporarily discontinue use.

DOSAGE AND ADMINISTRATION

1. Apply ATRAC-TAIN LOTION evenly to affected area and massage until absorbed.
2. Reapply LOTION as required for soothing relief.

HOW SUPPLIED

2 fl. oz., 4 fl. oz. and 8 fl. oz. bottles with disc-top caps.

BAZA®Cream   OTC
Occlusive Skin Protectant

DESCRIPTION

BAZA Cream contains three active ingredients: Zinc Oxide, Chloroxylenol (PCMX) and Benzethonium Chloride in a rich, soothing, occlusive, water-resistant cream base containing appropriate amounts of natural Vitamins A, D, and E. National Drug Code (NDC) 11701-028.

INDICATIONS AND USAGE

BAZA Cream is a soothing, antimicrobial, antifungal barrier cream designed to function as a skin protectant and to prevent skin from becoming excoriated and denuded due to incontinent conditions. BAZA Cream protects skin from damaging proteolytic enzymes present in urine/feces, caustic fistula, gastric and wound drainage and exudate. The high level of Zinc Oxide in BAZA Cream acts to relieve irritant contact dermatitis associated with perineal inflammation. Its antifungal and antibacterial formulation is effective against numerous fungal and yeast microorganisms, as well as, gram-positive and gram-negative bacteria. BAZA Cream can be used for adjunctive topical treatment of superficial skin infections when oral antibiotic agents are concurrently being administered. BAZA Cream—Barrier, Antimicrobial, Zinc Oxide, Antifungal functions.

CONTRAINDICATIONS
Hypersensitivity to any components of the preparation.

WARNINGS
BAZA is not for ophthalmic, otic, or vaginal use.

PRECAUTIONS
For external use only. If condition does not improve within 7 days, consult a physician. Not to be applied over deep or puncture wounds. Do not use on infants under 2 years of age without consulting physician. Avoid contact with eye.

ADVERSE REACTIONS
BAZA Cream is not considered a primary skin irritant or sensitizer. If irritation or sensitivity develops with the use of BAZA Cream, treatment should be discontinued and appropriate therapy instituted. BAZA Cream is not toxic by oral ingestion.

DOSAGE AND ADMINISTRATION
Cleanse affected area thoroughly. Apply BAZA Cream in thin layer over entire perineal area. Repeat as often as necessary or as directed by physician.

HOW SUPPLIED
2 oz. tube, 5 oz. tube.

CRITIC–AID®   OTC
Antimicrobial Skin Paste

DESCRIPTION
CRITIC-AID contains two active ingredients: Zinc Oxide and Benzethonium Chloride in a soothing, occlusive, moisture-resistant paste. National Drug Code (NDC) 11701-030.

INDICATIONS AND USAGE
CRITIC-AID affords constant protection and conditioning of sensitive, inflamed areas due to contact with caustic diarrhea or enzymatic drainage. It remains intact on inflamed, denuded skin. CRITIC-AID protects traumatized skin from damaging proteolytic enzymes present in urine/feces, caustic fistula, gastric or wound drainage and exudate. Zinc Oxide aids in protecting damaged skin from harmful stimuli and irritations associated with perineal inflammation. Benzethonium Chloride is a proven antimicrobial agent that aids in preventing further skin irritation associated with skin inflammation. It gently soothes and relieves discomfort of denuded skin areas. CRITIC-AID can be used for adjunctive topical treatment of superficial skin infections when oral antibiotic agents are concurrently being administered.

CONTRAINDICATION
Hypersensitivity to any components of the formulation.

WARNINGS
CRITIC-AID is not for ophthalmic, otic or vaginal use.

PRECAUTIONS
For external use only. If condition worsens or does not improve within 7 days, consult a physician. Not to be applied over deep or puncture wounds. Avoid contact with eyes.

ADVERSE REACTIONS
CRITIC-AID is not considered a primary skin irritant or sensitizer. If irritation or sensitivity develops with the use of CRITIC-AID Paste, treatment should be discontinued and appropriate therapy instituted. CRITIC-AID is not toxic by oral ingestion.

DOSAGE AND ADMINISTRATION
Thoroughly cleanse the entire affected area with a very gentle cleanser and pat dry. Apply CRITIC-AID paste and layer as necessary or as directed by a physician.

HOW SUPPLIED
2.5 oz. tube, 6 oz. tube.

MICRO-GUARD®   OTC
[mĭ'crō-gŭard]
Antiseptic, Antifungal Skin Cream

DESCRIPTION
MICRO-GUARD Skin Cream contains the antimicrobial agent, Chloroxylenol (PCMX) in a water washable, vanishing cream base. National Drug Code (NDC) 11701-012.

INDICATIONS AND USAGE
MICRO-GUARD is a soothing antiseptic and antifungal cream. MICRO-GUARD's antifungal action is effective treatment for conditions such as athlete's foot, jock itch and ringworm, while its antiseptic activity helps prevent skin infection. MICRO-GUARD can be used for adjunctive topical treatment of superficial skin infections when oral antibiotic agents are concurrently being administered.

CONTRAINDICATIONS
Hypersensitivity to any components of the preparation.

WARNINGS
MICRO-GUARD is not for ophthalmic, otic or vaginal use.

PRECAUTIONS
For External Use Only. Do not use near eyes. If contact with eye occurs, rinse thoroughly with water and consult physician. Keep out of reach of children. If skin irritation occurs, or if there is no improvement within two weeks, discontinue use and consult physician. Do not use on children under 2 years of age without consulting a physician.

ADVERSE REACTIONS
MICRO-GUARD is not considered a primary skin irritant or sensitizer, but occasional erythema, stinging and eczematous reactions have occurred following its use. If irritation or sensitivity develops with the use of MICRO-GUARD, treatment should be discontinued and appropriate therapy instituted.

DOSAGE AND ADMINISTRATION
Gently and thoroughly cleanse affected area and pat dry. Apply a thin layer of MICRO-GUARD over involved area. Repeat application 2 to 3 times daily or as directed by physician.

HOW SUPPLIED
½ and 2 oz. tubes and 2 oz. jars.

MICRO–GUARD®   OTC
[mĭ'crō gŭard]
Antifungal Powder

DESCRIPTION
MICRO-GUARD Powder contains Chloroxylenol (2.5%) in a Corn Starch base, with Sodium Bicarbonate, Silica and Benzethonium Chloride. NDC 11701-026.

INDICATIONS AND USAGE
MICRO-GUARD Powder is a soothing, antifungal powder. MICRO-GUARD'S antifungal action is an effective treatment for conditions such as jock itch, athletes foot and ringworm. MICRO-GUARD Powder can be used for adjunctive topical treatment of superficial skin infections when oral antibiotic agents are concurrently being administered.

CONTRAINDICATIONS
Hypersensitivity to any components of the preparation.

WARNINGS
MICRO-GUARD Powder is not for ophthalmic, otic or vaginal use.

PRECAUTIONS
For external use only. If irritation occurs or if there is no improvement within two weeks, discontinue use and consult a physician. Keep out of reach of children. Do not use on children under 2 years of age except under the advice and supervision of a physician. Children under 12 years of age should be supervised in the use of this product. This product is not effective on the scalp or nails.

ADVERSE REACTIONS
MICRO-GUARD Powder is not considered a primary skin irritant or sensitizer. If irritation or sensitivity develops with the use of MICRO-GUARD Powder, treatment should be discontinued and appropriate therapy instituted.

DOSAGE AND ADMINISTRATION
Cleanse area and dry. Apply MICRO-GUARD Powder. Smooth over entire area including skin creases and folds. Repeat application 2-3 times daily or as directed by physician.

HOW SUPPLIED
3 oz. container with dispensing top.

PURI-CLENS™   OTC
[pūri-clĕns]
Wound Deodorizer and Cleanser

DESCRIPTION
PURI-CLENS contains a safe and effective, non-irritating, antimicrobial ingredient, Benzethonium Chloride, in a water-washable, soothing base. National Drug Code (NDC) 11701-008.

INDICATIONS AND USAGE
PURI-CLENS deodorizes wounds and aids in the removal of foreign materials and exudates. Will not delay wound healing.

CONTRAINDICATIONS
Hypersensitivity to any components of the preparation.

PRECAUTIONS AND ADVERSE REACTIONS
For External Use Only. Do not use on animal bites or puncture wounds. Do not use for more than ten days without consulting physician. PURI-CLENS is not toxic by oral ingestion and is not considered a primary eye or skin irritant under normal use conditions. Keep out of the reach of children.

DOSAGE AND ADMINISTRATION
Apply PURI-CLENS liberally to a sterile 4″ × 4″ pad. Gently and thoroughly cleanse wound and surrounding area. To aid in removing foreign material and exudates, dab wound carefully with clean 4″ × 4″ pad saturated with PURI-CLENS. May be rinsed with sterile saline, water or hydrogen peroxide solution.

DEODORIZATION
Apply PURI-CLENS directly to wound and cover with a sterile absorbent pad. Do not use solution with occlusive dressing. Repeat one to three times daily to control odors.

HOW SUPPLIED
2 fl. oz. unit dose and 8 fl. oz bottles with disc-top caps.

SWEEN-A-PEEL®   OTC
Wafer Skin Protectant

DESCRIPTION
SWEEN-A-PEEL is a hydrophilic, hydrocolloidal, wafer skin protectant containing the following: WA4 hydrophilic polymer—to provide moisture absorption; high molecular weight synthetic rubber polymers—to provide elasticity and strength; low molecular weight synthetic rubber polymers—to provide adhesion to dry surface; karaya gum powder—to provide adhesion to moist surfaces.

INDICATIONS AND USAGE
SWEEN-A-PEEL wafers applied to the peristomal area in ostomy care or to the area surrounding draining wounds, aid in protecting the skin against contact with exudates. SWEEN-A-PEEL may also be applied to pressure points of immobile patients to help preserve skin integrity and reduce the possible occurrence of decubitus ulcers. SWEEN-A-PEEL has also proven effective when incorporated into a decubitus ulcer treatment procedure.

CONTRAINDICATIONS
Hypersensitivity to any components of the preparation.

PRECAUTIONS
Avoid excess heat and humidity. Store below 77°F (25°C).

ADMINISTRATION
Preparation. 1. Cleanse entire area thoroughly. 2. Remove any residue from weeping, excoriated areas as effectively as possible to assure maximum adherence of SWEEN-A-PEEL. **Ostomy Care.** 1. Use measuring guide to accurately measure stoma base. Transfer pattern to wafer using pencil, then cut. 2. Remove backing paper. Position wafer carefully onto skin. 3. Mold over entire area from stoma base to outer edges. **Wound Care.** 1. Cleanse wound and surrounding area. 2. Measure wound accurately. Use Sween-A-Peel piece large enough to extend 1½″ beyond edge of wound. 3. Remove backing and center over wound. 4. Mold over area from center to outer edges.

HOW SUPPLIED
Individually sealed 4″ × 4″ wafers in cartons of five or twenty, 6″ × 8″ wafers in cartons of three and 12″ × 12″ squares in packages of two and twelve.

SWEEN CREAM®   OTC
[Swēen Crēam]
Protective Cream

DESCRIPTION
A vanishing cream consisting of Water, Lanolin Oil, Cetyl Alcohol, Propylene Glycol, Ichthyo Liver Oil (Natural Vitamins A & D), Stearyl Alcohol, Beeswax, Sodium Lauryl Sulfate, Benzethonium Chloride, Quaternium-15, BHT, and Fragrance. Health Related Item (HRI) 11701-002. Fragrance-Free formulation is also available. Health Related Item (HRI) 11701-019.

INDICATIONS AND USAGE
SWEEN CREAM is an effective preparation for use on skin conditions such as urine scald, diaper rash, rectal itch, psoriasis, minor burns, diarrheal breakdown, chafing and itching. Applied on skin before taping, SWEEN CREAM aids in the prevention of tape burns. SWEEN CREAM is used in long-term care of incontinent, geriatric and para/quadriplegic skin conditions. Also apply to folds of skin subject to perspi-

Continued on next page

Sween—Cont.

ration irritation, to dry or cracked skin and to pressure sensitive areas. For ostomy care, apply a small amount on peristomal skin for protection before attaching appliance. This relieves itching and improves adhesion.

CONTRAINDICATIONS
Hypersensitivity to any components of the preparation.

PRECAUTIONS AND ADVERSE REACTIONS
For External Use Only. Avoid contact with eyes. SWEEN CREAM is not toxic by oral ingestion and is not considered a primary eye or skin irritant under normal use conditions. If infection or other signs develop, discontinue use and consult a physician.

DOSAGE AND ADMINISTRATION
Apply liberally as required.

HOW SUPPLIED
2 ml packets in packages of 300; ½ oz. and 5 oz. tubes; 2-oz. and 9 oz. jars.

SWEEN PREP™   OTC
[Swēen Prĕp]
Protective Skin Barrier Film

DESCRIPTION
SWEEN PREP is a medicated, liquid skin barrier which contains Chloroxylenol (PCMX), a well known antimicrobial agent, in a protective film forming base.

INDICATIONS AND USAGE
SWEEN PREP applies to the skin as a liquid, with the aid of the special "Dab-O-Matic" applicator, the non-aerosol sprayer or the single use wipe. It dries rapidly to form a tough film which provides a visible shield on the skin... a barrier between the skin and irritants. This protective film creates a surface other than the skin itself for the application of tapes, cements and double-faced adhesives.

CONTRAINDICATIONS
Hypersensitivity to any components of the preparation.

PRECAUTIONS AND ADVERSE REACTIONS
For External Use Only. Do not use near eyes. Will cause eye irritation. If contact occurs, flush with water for 15 minutes and consult physician. Keep out of the reach of children. Do not use on children under 6 months of age except under the advice and supervision of a physician.
Flammable. Do not use near open flame or while smoking.

DOSAGE AND ADMINISTRATION
Cleanse the skin area thoroughly, rinse and pat dry. Apply SWEEN PREP liberally to the entire area to be protected (slight stinging may be experienced if the skin is excoriated). Allow to dry (approximately 2 minutes) and apply tapes, adhesives, etc., in the normal manner to the SWEEN PREPPED skin. SWEEN PREP may be removed from the skin with soap and water or, for easier removal, with isopropyl alcohol. Removal is, however, not necessary and the skin may be recoated as frequently as required.

HOW SUPPLIED
Unit dose wipes (NDC 11701-007-20), 2 fl. oz. "Dab-O-Matic" applicator (NDC 11701-007-03) and 4 fl. oz. non-aerosol spray (NDC 11701-006-04).

Important Notice
Before prescribing or administering
any product described in
Physicians' Desk Reference
always consult the PDR Supplement for
possible new or revised information.

Syntex (F.P.) Inc.
HUMACAO, PUERTO RICO 00791

Syntex Laboratories, Inc
3401 HILLVIEW AVE.
P.O. BOX 10850
PALO ALTO, CA 94303

Syntex Puerto Rico, Inc.
HUMACAO, PUERTO RICO 00791

ANADROL®-50   ℞
[an'ă-drawl]
(oxymetholone)
50 mg. Tablets
A product of Syntex Laboratories, Inc.

DESCRIPTION
ANADROL (oxymetholone) tablets for oral administration each contain 50 mg of the steroid oxymetholone, a potent anabolic and androgenic drug.
The chemical name for oxymetholone is 17β-hydroxy-2-(hydroxymethylene)-17-methyl-5α-androstan-3-one.
Inactive Ingredients—lactose, magnesium stearate, povidone, starch

CLINICAL PHARMACOLOGY
Anabolic steroids are synthetic derivatives of testosterone. Nitrogen balance is improved with anabolic agents but only when there is sufficient intake of calories and protein. Whether this positive nitrogen balance is of primary benefit in the utilization of protein-building dietary substances has not been established. Oxymetholone enhances the production and urinary excretion of erythropoietin in patients with anemias due to bone marrow failure and often stimulates erythropoiesis in anemias due to deficient red cell production.
Certain clinical effects and adverse reactions demonstrate the androgenic properties of this class of drugs. Complete dissociation of anabolic and androgenic effects has not been achieved. The actions of anabolic steroids are therefore similar to those of male sex hormones with the possibility of causing serious disturbances of growth and sexual development if given to young children. They suppress the gonadotropic functions of the pituitary and may exert a direct effect upon the testes.

INDICATIONS AND USAGE
ANADROL-50 is indicated in the treatment of anemias caused by deficient red cell production. Acquired aplastic anemia, congenital aplastic anemia, myelofibrosis and the hypoplastic anemias due to the administration of myelotoxic drugs often respond.
ANADROL-50 should not replace other supportive measures such as transfusion, correction of iron, folic acid, vitamin B_{12} or pyridoxine deficiency, antibacterial therapy and the appropriate use of corticosteroids.

CONTRAINDICATIONS
1. Carcinoma of the prostate or breast in male patients.
2. Carcinoma of the breast in females with hypercalcemia; androgenic anabolic steroids may stimulate osteolytic resorption of bones.
3. Oxymetholone can cause fetal harm when administered to pregnant women. It is contraindicated in women who are or may become pregnant. If the patient becomes pregnant while taking the drug, she should be apprised of the potential hazard to the fetus.
4. Nephrosis or the nephrotic phase of nephritis.
5. Hypersensitivity to the drug.
6. Severe hepatic dysfunction.

WARNINGS
The following conditions have been reported in patients receiving androgenic anabolic steroids as a general class of drugs:

Peliosis hepatis, a condition in which liver and sometimes splenic tissue is replaced with blood-filled cysts, has been reported in patients receiving androgenic anabolic steroid therapy. These cysts are sometimes present with minimal hepatic dysfunction, but at other times they have been associated with liver failure. They are often not recognized until life-threatening liver failure or intra-abdominal hemorrhage develops. Withdrawal of drug usually results in complete disappearance of lesions.
Liver cell tumors are also reported. Most often these tumors are benign and androgen-dependent, but fatal malignant tumors have been reported. Withdrawal of drug often results in regression or cessation of progres-

sion of the tumor. However, hepatic tumors associated with androgens or anabolic steroids are much more vascular than other hepatic tumors and may be silent until life-threatening intra-abdominal hemorrhage develops.
Blood lipid changes that are known to be associated with increased risk of atherosclerosis are seen in patients treated with androgens and anabolic steroids. These changes include decreased high density lipoprotein and sometimes increased low density lipoprotein. The changes may be very marked and could have a serious impact on the risk of atherosclerosis and coronary artery disease.

Cholestatic hepatitis and jaundice occur with 17-alpha-alkylated androgens at relatively low doses. Clinical jaundice may be painless, with or without pruritus. It may also be associated with acute hepatic enlargement and right upper-quadrant pain, which has been mistaken for acute (surgical) obstruction of the bile duct. Drug-induced jaundice is usually reversible when the medication is discontinued. Continued therapy has been associated with hepatic coma and death. Because of the hepatotoxicity associated with oxymetholone administration, periodic liver function tests are recommended.
In patients with breast cancer, anabolic steroid therapy may cause hypercalcemia by stimulating osteolysis. In this case, the drug should be discontinued.
Edema with or without congestive heart failure may be a serious complication in patients with pre-existing cardiac, renal or hepatic disease. Concomitant administration with adrenal steroids or ACTH may add to the edema. This is generally controllable with appropriate diuretic and/or digitalis therapy.
Geriatric male patients treated with androgenic anabolic steroids may be at an increased risk for the development of prostate hypertrophy and prostatic carcinoma.
Anabolic steroids have not been shown to enhance athletic ability.

PRECAUTIONS
General:
Women should be observed for signs of virilization (deepening of the voice, hirsutism, acne, and clitoromegaly). To prevent irreversible change, drug therapy must be discontinued when mild virilism is first detected. Such virilization is usual following androgenic anabolic steroid use at high doses. Some virilizing changes in women are irreversible even after prompt discontinuance of therapy and are not prevented by concomitant use of estrogens. Menstrual irregularities, including amenorrhea, may also occur.
The insulin or oral hypoglycemic dosage may need adjustment in diabetic patients who receive anabolic steroids.
Anabolic steroids may cause suppression of clotting factors II, V, VII, and X, and an increase in prothrombin time.
Information for the patient:
The physician should instruct patients to report any of the following side effects of androgens.
Adult or Adolescent Males: Too frequent or persistent erections of the penis, appearance or aggravation of acne.
Women: Hoarseness, acne, changes in menstrual periods, or more hair on the face.
All Patients: Any nausea, vomiting, changes in skin color or ankle swelling.
Laboratory Tests:
Women with disseminated breast carcinoma should have frequent determination of urine and serum calcium levels during the course of androgenic anabolic steroid therapy (see WARNINGS).
Because of the hepatotoxicity associated with the use of 17-alpha-alkylated androgens, liver function tests should be obtained periodically.
Periodic (every 6 months) x-ray examinations of bone age should be made during treatment of prepubertal patients to determine the rate of bone maturation and the effects of androgenic anabolic steroid therapy on the epiphyseal centers.
Anabolic steroids have been reported to lower the level of high-density lipoproteins and raise the level of low-density lipoproteins. These changes usually revert to normal on discontinuation of treatment. Increased low-density lipoproteins and decreased high-density lipoproteins are considered cardiovascular risk factors. Serum lipids and high-density lipoprotein cholesterol should be determined periodically.
Hemoglobin and hematocrit should be checked periodically for polycythemia in patients who are receiving high doses of anabolics.
Because iron deficiency anemia has been observed in some patients treated with oxymetholone, periodic determination of the serum iron and iron binding capacity is recommended. If iron deficiency is detected, it should be appropriately treated with supplementary iron.
Oxymetholone has been shown to decrease 17-ketosteroid excretion.
Drug Interaction:
Anabolic steroids may increase sensitivity to anticoagulants; therefore dosage of an anticoagulant may have to be de-

creased in order to maintain the prothrombin time at the desired therapeutic level.

Drug/Laboratory Test Interferences: Therapy with androgenic anabolic steroids may decrease levels of thyroxine-binding globulin resulting in decreased total T_4 serum levels and increased resin uptake of T_3 and T_4. Free thyroid hormone levels remain unchanged and there is no clinical evidence of thyroid dysfunction. Altered tests usually persist for 2–3 weeks after stopping anabolic therapy.

Anabolic steroids may cause an increase in prothrombin time.

Anabolic steroids have been shown to alter fasting blood sugar and glucose tolerance tests.

Carcinogenesis, Mutagenesis, Impairment of Fertility:
Animal data: Testosterone has been tested by subcutaneous injection and implantation in mice and rats. The implant induced cervical-uterine tumors in mice, which metastasized in some cases. There is suggestive evidence that injection of testosterone into some strains of female mice increases their susceptibility to hepatoma. Testosterone is also known to increase the number of tumors and decrease the degree of differentiation of chemically induced carcinomas of the liver in rats.

Human data: There are rare reports of hepatocellular carcinoma in patients receiving long-term therapy with androgens in high doses. Withdrawal of the drugs did not lead to regression of the tumors in all cases.

Geriatric patients treated with androgens may be at an increased risk of developing prostatic hypertrophy and prostatic carcinoma although conclusive evidence to support this concept is lacking.

This compound has not been tested for mutagenic potential. However, as noted above, carcinogenic effects have been attributed to treatment with androgenic hormones. The potential carcinogenic effects likely occur through a hormonal mechanism rather than by a direct chemical interaction mechanism.

Impairment of fertility was not tested directly in animal species. However, as noted below under ADVERSE REACTIONS, oligospermia in males and amenorrhea in females are potential adverse effects of treatment with ANADROL tablets. Therefore, impairment of fertility is a possible outcome of treatment with ANADROL.

Pregnancy:
Pregnancy category X. See CONTRAINDICATIONS.

Nursing Mothers:
It is not known whether anabolics are excreted in human milk. Because of the potential for serious adverse reactions in nursed infants from anabolics, women who take oxymetholone should not nurse.

Pediatric Use:
Anabolic/androgenic steroids should be used very cautiously in children and only by specialists who are aware of their effects on bone maturation.

Anabolic agents may accelerate epiphyseal maturation more rapidly than linear growth in children, and the effect may continue for 6 months after the drug has been stopped. Therefore, therapy should be monitored by x-ray studies at 6-month intervals in order to avoid the risk of compromising the adult height.

ADVERSE REACTIONS

Hepatic:
Cholestatic jaundice with, rarely, hepatic necrosis and death. Hepatocellular neoplasms and peliosis hepatis have been reported in association with long-term androgenic-anabolic steroid therapy (see WARNINGS).

Genitourinary System:
In Men:
Prepubertal: Phallic enlargement and increased frequency of erections.
Postpubertal: Inhibition of testicular function, testicular atrophy and oligospermia, impotence, chronic priapism, epididymitis, bladder irritability, and decrease in seminal volume.
In Women:
Clitoral enlargement, menstrual irregularities.
In both sexes:
Increased or decreased libido.
CNS: Excitation, insomnia.
Gastrointestinal: Nausea, vomiting, diarrhea.
Hematologic: Bleeding in patients on concomitant anticoagulant therapy, iron-deficiency anemia.

Leukemia has been observed in patients with aplastic anemia treated with oxymetholone. The role, if any, of oxymetholone is unclear because malignant transformation has been seen in blood dyscrasias and leukemia has been reported in patients with aplastic anemia who have not been treated with oxymetholone.

Breast: Gynecomastia.
Larynx: Deepening of the voice in women.
Hair: Hirsutism and male-pattern baldness in women, male-pattern of hair loss in postpubertal males.
Skin: Acne (especially in women and prepubertal boys.)
Skeletal: Premature closure of epiphyses in children (see PRECAUTIONS, Pediatric Use), muscle cramps.

Body as a whole: Chills.
Fluid and Electrolytes: Edema, retention of serum electrolytes (sodium, chloride, potassium, phosphate, calcium).
Metabolic/Endocrine: Decreased glucose tolerance (see PRECAUTIONS), increased serum levels of low-density lipoproteins and decreased levels of high-density lipoproteins (see PRECAUTIONS, Laboratory tests), increased creatine and creatinine excretion, increased serum levels of creatinine phosphokinase (CPK). Reversible changes in liver function tests also occur including increased bromsulphalein (BSP) retention and increases in serum bilirubin, glutamic oxaloacetic transaminase (SGOT), and alkaline phosphatase.

DRUG ABUSE AND DEPENDENCE

Controlled Substance:
ANADROL-50 is considered to be a controlled substance and is listed in Schedule III.

OVERDOSAGE

There have been no reports of acute overdosage with anabolics.

DOSAGE AND ADMINISTRATION

The recommended daily dose in children and adults is 1–5 mg/kg body weight per day. The usual effective dose is 1–2 mg/kg/day but higher doses may be required and the dose should be individualized. Response is not often immediate and a minimum trial of three to six months should be given. Following remission, some patients may be maintained without the drug; others may be maintained on an established lower daily dosage. A continued maintenance dose is usually necessary in patients with congenital aplastic anemia.

HOW SUPPLIED

ANADROL-50 (oxymetholone) is supplied in bottles of 100 white scored tablets imprinted with "2902" and "SYNTEX" (NDC 0033-2902-42).

CAUTION: Federal law prohibits dispensing without prescription.

02-2902-42-06   Revised 4/91
© 1991 Syntex Laboratories, Inc.
Shown in Product Identification Section, page 433

ANAPROX® ℞
[an 'ă-prox]
ANAPROX® DS ℞
(naproxen sodium)
Tablets

Products of Syntex Puerto Rico, Inc.

DESCRIPTION

ANAPROX® (naproxen sodium) filmcoated tablets for oral administration each contain 275 mg of naproxen sodium, which is equivalent to 250 mg naproxen with 25 mg (about 1 mEq) sodium. ANAPROX® DS (naproxen sodium) filmcoated tablets for oral administration each contain 550 mg of naproxen sodium, which is equivalent to 500 mg naproxen with 50 mg (about 2 mEq) sodium. Naproxen sodium is a member of the arylacetic acid group of nonsteroidal anti-inflammatory drugs.

The chemical name of naproxen sodium is 2-naphthaleneacetic acid, 6-methoxy-α-methyl-, sodium salt, (−).

Naproxen sodium is a white to creamy white, crystalline solid, freely soluble in water.

Each ANAPROX 275 mg tablet contains naproxen sodium, the active ingredient, with lactose, magnesium stearate, and microcrystalline cellulose. The coating suspension may contain hydroxypropyl methylcellulose 2910, Opaspray K-1-4210A, polyethylene glycol 8000 or Opadry YS-1-4215. Each ANAPROX DS 550 mg tablet contains naproxen sodium, the active ingredient, with magnesium stearate, microcrystalline cellulose, povidone, and talc. The coating suspension may contain hydroxypropyl methylcellulose 2910, Opaspray K-1-4227, polyethylene glycol 8000 or Opadry YS-1-4216.

CLINICAL PHARMACOLOGY

The sodium salt of naproxen has been developed as an analgesic because it is more rapidly absorbed. Naproxen is a nonsteroidal anti-inflammatory drug with analgesic and antipyretic properties. Naproxen anion inhibits prostaglandin synthesis but beyond this its mode of action is unknown.

Naproxen sodium is rapidly and completely absorbed from the gastrointestinal tract. After administration of naproxen sodium, peak plasma levels of naproxen anion are attained at 1–2 hours with steady-state conditions normally achieved after 4–5 doses. The mean biological half-life of the anion in humans is approximately 13 hours, and at therapeutic levels it is greater than 99% albumin bound. Approximately 95% of the dose is excreted in the urine, primarily as naproxen, 6-0-desmethyl naproxen or their conjugates. The rate of excretion has been found to coincide closely with the rate of drug disappearance from the plasma. The drug does not induce metabolizing enzymes.

In children of 5 to 16 years of age with arthritis, plasma naproxen levels following a 5 mg/kg single dose of naproxen

suspension (see Dosage and Administration) were found to be similar to those found in normal adults following a 500 mg dose. The terminal half-life appears to be similar in children and adults. Pharmacokinetic studies of naproxen were not performed in children of less than 5 years of age.

The drug was studied in patients with mild to moderate pain, and pain relief was obtained within 1 hour. It is not a narcotic and is not a CNS-acting drug. Controlled double-blind studies have demonstrated the analgesic properties of the drug in, for example, post-operative, post-partum, orthopedic and uterine contraction pain and dysmenorrhea. In dysmenorrheic patients, the drug reduces the level of prostaglandins in the uterus, which correlates with a reduction in the frequency and severity of uterine contractions. Analgesic action has been shown by such measures as reduction of pain intensity scores, increase in pain relief scores, decrease in numbers of patients requiring additional analgesic medication, and delay in time for required remedication. The analgesic effect has been found to last for up to 7 hours.

The drug was studied in patients with rheumatoid arthritis, osteoarthritis, juvenile arthritis, ankylosing spondylitis, tendinitis and bursitis, and acute gout. It is not a corticosteroid. Improvement in patients treated for rheumatoid arthritis has been demonstrated by a reduction in joint swelling, a reduction in pain, a reduction in duration of morning stiffness, a reduction in disease activity as assessed by both the investigator and patient, and by increased mobility as demonstrated by a reduction in walking time.

In patients with osteoarthritis, the therapeutic action of the drug has been shown by a reduction in joint pain or tenderness, an increase in range of motion in knee joints, increased mobility as demonstrated by a reduction in walking time, and improvement in capacity to perform activities of daily living impaired by the disease.

In clinical studies in patients with rheumatoid arthritis, osteoarthritis, and juvenile arthritis, the drug has been shown to be comparable to aspirin and indomethacin in controlling the aforementioned measures of disease activity, but the frequency and severity of the milder gastrointestinal adverse effects (nausea, dyspepsia, heartburn) and nervous system adverse effects (tinnitus, dizziness, lightheadedness) were less than in both the aspirin- and indomethacin-treated patients. It is not known whether the drug causes less peptic ulceration than aspirin.

In patients with ankylosing spondylitis, the drug has been shown to decrease night pain, morning stiffness and pain at rest. In double-blind studies the drug was shown to be as effective as aspirin, but with fewer side effects.

In patients with acute gout, a favorable response to the drug was shown by significant clearing of inflammatory changes (e.g., decrease in swelling, heat) within 24–48 hours, as well as by relief of pain and tenderness.

The drug may be used safely in combination with gold salts and/or corticosteroids; however, in controlled clinical trials, when added to the regimen of patients receiving corticosteroids it did not appear to cause greater improvement over that seen with corticosteroids alone. Whether the drug could be used in conjunction with partially effective doses of corticosteroids for a "steroid-sparing" effect has not been adequately studied. When added to the regimen of patients receiving gold salts, the drug did result in greater improvement. Its use in combination with salicylates is not recommended because data are inadequate to demonstrate that the drug produces greater improvement over that achieved with aspirin alone. Further, there is some evidence that aspirin increases the rate of excretion of the drug.

Generally, improvement due to the drug has not been found to be dependent on age, sex, severity or duration of disease. In clinical trials in patients with osteoarthritis and rheumatoid arthritis comparing treatments of 825 mg per day with 1,650 mg per day, there were trends toward increased efficacy with the higher dose and a more clearcut increase in adverse reactions, particularly gastrointestinal reactions severe enough to cause the patient to leave the trial, which approximately doubled.

In ^{51}Cr blood loss and gastroscopy studies with normal volunteers, daily administration of 1,100 mg of naproxen sodium has been demonstrated to cause statistically significantly less gastric bleeding and erosion than 3,250 mg of aspirin.

INDICATIONS AND USAGE

Naproxen sodium is indicated in the relief of mild to moderate pain and for the treatment of primary dysmenorrhea. It is also indicated for the treatment of rheumatoid arthritis, osteoarthritis, juvenile arthritis, ankylosing spondylitis, tendinitis and bursitis, and acute gout.

CONTRAINDICATIONS

The drug is contraindicated in patients who have had allergic reactions to ANAPROX® (naproxen sodium), ANAPROX® DS or to NAPROSYN® (naproxen). It is also contraindicated in patients in whom aspirin or other nonsteroidal anti-inflammatory/analgesic drugs induce the syndrome of asthma, rhinitis, and nasal polyps. Both types of

Continued on next page

Syntex—Cont.

reactions have the potential of being fatal. Anaphylactoid reactions to ANAPROX, ANAPROX DS or NAPROSYN, whether of the true allergic type or the pharmacologic idiosyncratic (e.g., aspirin syndrome) type, usually but not always occur in patients with a known history of such reactions. Therefore, careful questioning of patients for such things as asthma, nasal polyps, urticaria, and hypotension associated with nonsteroidal anti-inflammatory drugs before starting therapy is important. In addition, if such symptoms occur during therapy, treatment should be discontinued.

WARNINGS

Risk of GI Ulceration, Bleeding and Perforation with NSAID Therapy:

Serious gastrointestinal toxicity such as bleeding, ulceration, and perforation, can occur at any time, with or without warning symptoms, in patients treated chronically with NSAID therapy. Although minor upper gastrointestinal problems, such as dyspepsia, are common, usually developing early in therapy, physicians should remain alert for ulceration and bleeding in patients treated chronically with NSAIDs even in the absence of previous GI tract symptoms. In patients observed in clinical trials of several months to two years duration, symptomatic upper GI ulcers, gross bleeding or perforation appear to occur in approximately 1% of patients treated for 3–6 months, and in about 2–4% of patients treated for one year. Physicians should inform patients about the signs and/or symptoms of serious GI toxicity and what steps to take if they occur.

Studies to date have not identified any subset of patients not at risk of developing peptic ulceration and bleeding. Except for a prior history of serious GI events and other risk factors known to be associated with peptic ulcer disease, such as alcoholism, smoking, etc., no risk factors (e.g., age, sex) have been associated with increased risk. Elderly or debilitated patients seem to tolerate ulceration or bleeding less well than other individuals and most spontaneous reports of fatal GI events are in this population. Studies to date are inconclusive concerning the relative risk of various NSAIDs in causing such reactions. High doses of any NSAID probably carry a greater risk of these reactions, although controlled clinical trials showing this do not exist in most cases. In considering the use of relatively large doses (within the recommended dosage range), sufficient benefit should be anticipated to offset the potential increased risk of GI toxicity.

PRECAUTIONS

General:

***ANAPROX* (NAPROXEN SODIUM) or *ANAPROX DS* (NAPROXEN SODIUM) SHOULD NOT BE USED CONCOMITANTLY WITH THE RELATED DRUG *NAPROSYN* (NAPROXEN) SINCE THEY BOTH CIRCULATE IN PLASMA AS THE NAPROXEN ANION.**

Renal Effects: As with other nonsteroidal anti-inflammatory drugs, long-term administration of naproxen to animals has resulted in renal papillary necrosis and other abnormal renal pathology. In humans, there have been reports of acute interstitial nephritis with hematuria, proteinuria, and occasionally nephrotic syndrome.

A second form of renal toxicity has been seen in patients with prerenal conditions leading to a reduction in renal blood flow or blood volume, where the renal prostaglandins have a supportive role in the maintenance of renal perfusion. In these patients, administration of a nonsteroidal anti-inflammatory drug may cause a dose-dependent reduction in prostaglandin formation and may precipitate overt renal decompensation. Patients at greatest risk of this reaction are those with impaired renal function, heart failure, liver dysfunction, those taking diuretics, and the elderly. Discontinuation of nonsteroidal anti-inflammatory therapy is typically followed by recovery to the pretreatment state.

Naproxen sodium and its metabolites are eliminated primarily by the kidneys, therefore the drug should be used with great caution in patients with significantly impaired renal function and the monitoring of serum creatinine and/or creatinine clearance is advised in these patients. Caution should be used if the drug is given to patients with creatinine clearance of less than 20 mL/minute because accumulation of naproxen metabolites has been seen in such patients.

Chronic alcoholic liver disease and probably other forms of cirrhosis reduce the total plasma concentration of naproxen, but the plasma concentration of unbound naproxen is increased. Caution is advised when high doses are required and some adjustment of dosage may be required in these patients. It is prudent to use the lowest effective dose.

Studies indicate that although total plasma concentration of naproxen is unchanged, the unbound plasma fraction of naproxen is increased in the elderly. Caution is advised when high doses are required and some adjustment of dosage may be required in elderly patients. As with other drugs used in the elderly, it is prudent to use the lowest effective dose.

As with other nonsteroidal anti-inflammatory drugs, borderline elevations of one or more liver tests may occur in up to 15% of patients. These abnormalities may progress, may remain essentially unchanged, or may be transient with continued therapy. The SGPT (ALT) test is probably the most sensitive indicator of liver dysfunction. Meaningful (3 times the upper limit of normal) elevations of SGPT or SGOT (AST) occurred in controlled clinical trials in less than 1% of patients. A patient with symptoms and/or signs suggesting liver dysfunction, or in whom an abnormal liver test has occurred, should be evaluated for evidence of the development of more severe hepatic reaction while on therapy with this drug. Severe hepatic reactions, including jaundice and cases of fatal hepatitis, have been reported with this drug as with other nonsteroidal anti-inflammatory drugs. Although such reactions are rare, if abnormal liver tests persist or worsen, if clinical signs and symptoms consistent with liver disease develop, or if systemic manifestations occur (e.g., eosinophilia, rash, etc.), this drug should be discontinued.

If steroid dosage is reduced or eliminated during therapy, the steroid dosage should be reduced slowly and the patients must be observed closely for any evidence of adverse effects, including adrenal insufficiency and exacerbation of symptoms of arthritis.

Patients with initial hemoglobin values of 10 grams or less who are to receive long-term therapy should have hemoglobin values determined periodically.

Peripheral edema has been observed in some patients. Since each naproxen sodium tablet contains approximately 25 mg or 50 mg (about 1 or 2 mEq) of sodium, this should be considered in patients whose overall intake of sodium must be markedly restricted. For these reasons, the drug should be used with caution in patients with fluid retention, hypertension or heart failure.

The antipyretic and anti-inflammatory activities of the drug may reduce fever and inflammation, thus diminishing their utility as diagnostic signs in detecting complications of presumed non-infectious, non-inflammatory painful conditions.

Because of adverse eye findings in animal studies with drugs of this class, it is recommended that ophthalmic studies be carried out if any change or disturbance in vision occurs.

Information for Patients:

Naproxen sodium, like other drugs of its class, is not free of side effects. The side effects of these drugs can cause discomfort and, rarely, there are more serious side effects, such as gastrointestinal bleeding, which may result in hospitalization and even fatal outcomes.

NSAIDs (Nonsteroidal Anti-Inflammatory Drugs) are often essential agents in the management of arthritis and have a major role in the treatment of pain, but they also may be commonly employed for conditions which are less serious. Physicians may wish to discuss with their patients the potential risks (see Warnings, Precautions, and Adverse Reactions sections) and likely benefits of NSAID treatment, particularly when the drugs are used for less serious conditions where treatment without NSAIDs may represent an acceptable alternative to both the patient and physician.

Caution should be exercised by patients whose activities require alertness if they experience drowsiness, dizziness, vertigo or depression during therapy with the drug.

Laboratory Tests:

Because serious GI tract ulceration and bleeding can occur without warning symptoms, physicians should follow chronically treated patients for the signs and symptoms of ulceration and bleeding and should inform them of the importance of this follow-up (see Risk of GI Ulcerations, Bleeding and Perforation with NSAID Therapy).

Drug Interactions:

In vitro studies have shown that naproxen anion, because of its affinity for protein, may displace from their binding sites other drugs which are also albumin-bound. Theoretically, the naproxen anion itself could likewise be displaced. Short-term controlled studies failed to show that taking the drug significantly affects prothrombin times when administered to individuals on coumarin-type anticoagulants. Caution is advised nonetheless, since interactions have been seen with other nonsteroidal agents of this class. Similarly, patients receiving the drug and a hydantoin, sulfonamide or sulfonylurea should be observed for signs of toxicity to these drugs.

The natriuretic effect of furosemide has been reported to be inhibited by some drugs of this class. Inhibition of renal lithium clearance leading to increases in plasma lithium concentrations has also been reported.

This and other nonsteroidal anti-inflammatory drugs can reduce the antihypertensive effect of propranolol and other beta-blockers.

Probenecid given concurrently increases naproxen anion plasma levels and extends its plasma half-life significantly.

Caution should be used if this drug is administered concomitantly with methotrexate. Naproxen and other nonsteroidal anti-inflammatory drugs have been reported to reduce the tubular secretion of methotrexate in an animal model, possibly enhancing the toxicity of that drug.

Drug/Laboratory Test Interactions:

The drug may decrease platelet aggregation and prolong bleeding time. This effect should be kept in mind when bleeding times are determined.

The administration of the drug may result in increased urinary values for 17-ketogenic steroids because of an interaction between the drug and/or its metabolites with m-dinitrobenzene used in this assay. Although 17-hydroxy-corticosteroid measurements (Porter-Silber test) do not appear to be artifactually altered, it is suggested that therapy with the drug be temporarily discontinued 72 hours before adrenal function tests are performed.

The drug may interfere with some urinary assays of 5-hydroxy indoleacetic acid (5HIAA).

Carcinogenesis:

A two-year study was performed in rats to evaluate the carcinogenic potential of the drug. No evidence of carcinogenicity was found.

Pregnancy:

Teratogenic Effects: Pregnancy Category B. Reproduction studies have been performed in rats, rabbits and mice at doses up to six times the human dose and have revealed no evidence of impaired fertility or harm to the fetus due to the drug. There are, however, no adequate and well-controlled studies in pregnant women. Because animal reproduction studies are not always predictive of human response, the drug should not be used during pregnancy unless clearly needed. Because of the known effect of drugs of this class on the human fetal cardiovascular system (closure of ductus arteriosus), use during late pregnancy should be avoided.

Non-teratogenic Effects: As with other drugs known to inhibit prostaglandin synthesis, an increased incidence of dystocia and delayed parturition occurred in rats.

Nursing Mothers:

The naproxen anion has been found in the milk of lactating women at a concentration of approximately 1% of that found in the plasma. Because of the possible adverse effects of prostaglandin-inhibiting drugs on neonates, use in nursing mothers should be avoided.

Pediatric Use:

Safety and effectiveness in children below the age of 2 years have not been established. Pediatric dosing recommendations for juvenile arthritis are based on well-controlled studies. There are no adequate effectiveness or dose-response data for other pediatric conditions, but the experience in juvenile arthritis and other use experience have established that single doses of 2.5–5 mg/kg (as naproxen suspension, see Dosage and Administration), with total daily dose not exceeding 15 mg/kg/day, are safe in children over 2 years of age.

ADVERSE REACTIONS

The following adverse reactions are divided into three parts based on frequency and likelihood of causal relationship to naproxen sodium.

Incidence greater than 1%

Probable Causal Relationship:

Adverse reactions reported in controlled clinical trials in 960 patients treated for rheumatoid arthritis or osteoarthritis are listed below. In general, these reactions were reported 2 to 10 times more frequently than they were in studies in the 962 patients treated for mild to moderate pain or for dysmenorrhea.

A clinical study found gastrointestinal reactions to be more frequent and more severe in rheumatoid arthritis patients taking 1,650 mg naproxen sodium daily compared to those taking 825 mg daily (see Clinical Pharmacology).

In controlled clinical trials with about 80 children and in well monitored open studies with about 400 children with juvenile arthritis, the incidences of rash and prolonged bleeding times were increased, the incidences of gastrointestinal and central nervous system reactions were about the same, and the incidences of other reactions were lower in children than in adults.

Gastrointestinal: The most frequent complaints reported related to the gastrointestinal tract. They were constipation*, heartburn*, abdominal pain*, nausea*, dyspepsia, diarrhea, stomatitis.

Central Nervous System: Headache*, dizziness*, drowsiness*, lightheadedness, vertigo.

Dermatologic: Itching (pruritus)*, skin eruptions*, ecchymoses*, sweating, purpura.

Special Senses: Tinnitus*, hearing disturbances, visual disturbances.

Cardiovascular: Edema*, dyspnea*, palpitations.

General: Thirst.

Incidence less than 1% Probable Causal Relationship:

The following adverse reactions were reported less frequently than 1% during controlled clinical trials and through voluntary reports since marketing. The probability of a causal relationship exists between the drug and these adverse reactions.

Gastrointestinal: Abnormal liver function tests, colitis, gastrointestinal bleeding and/or perforation, hematemesis, jaundice, melena, peptic ulceration with bleeding and/or perforation, vomiting.

---

*Incidence of reported reaction between 3% and 9%. Those reactions occurring in less than 3% of the patients are unmarked.

Renal: Glomerular nephritis, hematuria, hyperkalemia, interstitial nephritis, nephrotic syndrome, renal disease, renal failure, renal papillary necrosis.
Hematologic: Agranulocytosis, eosinophilia, granulocytopenia, leukopenia, thrombocytopenia.
Central Nervous System: Depression, dream abnormalities, inability to concentrate, insomnia, malaise, myalgia and muscle weakness.
Dermatologic: Alopecia, photosensitive dermatitis, skin rashes.
Special Senses: Hearing impairment.
Cardiovascular: Congestive heart failure.
Respiratory: Eosinophilic pneumonitis.
General: Anaphylactoid reactions, menstrual disorders, pyrexia (chills and fever).
Casual Relationship Unknown:
Other reactions have been reported in circumstances in which a causal relationship could not be established. However, in these rarely reported events, the possibility cannot be excluded. Therefore these observations are being listed to serve as alerting information to the physicians.
Hematologic: Aplastic anemia, hemolytic anemia.
Central Nervous System: Aseptic meningitis, cognitive dysfunction.
Dermatologic: Epidermal necrolysis, erythema multiforme, photosensitivity reactions resembling porphyria cutanea tarda and epidermolysis bullosa, Stevens-Johnson syndrome, urticaria.
Gastrointestinal: Non-peptic gastrointestinal ulceration, ulcerative stomatitis.
Cardiovascular: Vasculitis.
General: Angioneurotic edema, hyperglycemia, hypoglycemia.

OVERDOSAGE

Significant overdosage may be characterized by drowsiness, heartburn, indigestion, nausea or vomiting. Because naproxen sodium may be rapidly absorbed, high and early blood levels should be anticipated. A few patients have experienced seizures, but it is not clear whether or not these were drug related. It is not known what dose of the drug would be life threatening. The oral LD_{50} of the drug is 543 mg/kg in rats, 1,234 mg/kg in mice, 4,110 mg/kg in hamsters and greater than 1,000 mg/kg in dogs.
Should a patient ingest a large number of tablets, accidentally or purposefully, the stomach may be emptied and usual supportive measures employed. In animals 0.5 g/kg of activated charcoal was effective in reducing plasma levels of naproxen. Hemodialysis does not decrease the plasma concentration of naproxen because of the high degree of its protein binding.

DOSAGE AND ADMINISTRATION

For Mild to Moderate Pain, Primary Dysmenorrhea and Acute Tendinitis and Bursitis:
The recommended starting dose is 550 mg, followed by 275 mg every 6 to 8 hours, as required. The total daily dose should not exceed 1,375 mg.
For Rheumatoid Arthritis, Osteoarthritis, and Ankylosing Spondylitis:
The recommended dose in adults is 275 mg or 550 mg twice daily (morning and evening). During long-term administration, the dose may be adjusted up or down depending on the clinical response of the patient. A lower daily dose may suffice for long-term administration. The morning and evening doses do not have to be equal in size and the administration of the drug more frequently than twice daily is not necessary.
In patients who tolerate lower doses well, the dose may be increased to 1,650 mg per day for limited periods when a higher level of anti-inflammatory/analgesic activity is required. When treating such patients with the 1,650 mg/day dose, the physician should observe sufficient increased clinical benefits to offset the potential increased risk (see Clinical Pharmacology).
Symptomatic improvement in arthritis usually begins within two weeks. However, if improvement is not seen within this period, a trial for an additional two weeks should be considered.
For Acute Gout:
The recommended starting dose is 825 mg, followed by 275 mg every eight hours until the attack has subsided.
For Juvenile Arthritis:
The recommended total daily dose is approximately 10 mg/kg given in two divided doses. The 275 mg ANAPROX tablet is not well suited to this dosage so use of the related drug NAPROSYN® (naproxen) as the 250 mg scored tablet or the 125 mg/5 mL suspension is recommended for this indication.

HOW SUPPLIED

ANAPROX® (naproxen sodium) is available in filmcoated tablets of 275 mg (light blue), in bottles of 100 tablets (NDC 18393-274-42) (NSN 6505-01-155-5157) and 500 tablets (NDC 18393-274-62) (NSN 6505-01-130-6832) or in cartons of 100 individually blister packed tablets (NDC 18393-274-53). ANAPROX® DS (naproxen sodium) is available in film-coated tablets of 550 mg (dark blue), in bottles of 100 tablets (NDC 18393-276-42) (NSN 6505-01-305-8174)and 500 tablets (NDC 18393-276-62) or in cartons of 100 individually blister packed tablets (NDC 18393-276-53). Store at room temperature in well-closed containers.
CAUTION: Federal law prohibits dispensing without prescription.
U.S. Patent Nos. 4,009,197; 3,998,966 and others.
02-0276-42-04 Revised 9/90
©1990 Syntex Puerto Rico, Inc.
Shown in Product Identification Section, page 433

BREVICON® Tablets ℞
(norethindrone and ethinyl estradiol)

Refer to entry under TRI-NORINYL® tablets (norethindrone and ethinyl estradiol).
Shown in Product Identification Section, page 433

CARDENE® ℞
[*kar'deen*]
(nicardipine hydrochloride)
Capsules

A product of Syntex Laboratories, Inc.

DESCRIPTION

CARDENE® capsules for oral administration each contain 20 mg or 30 mg of nicardipine hydrochloride. CARDENE is a calcium ion influx inhibitor (slow channel blocker or calcium channel blocker).
Nicardipine hydrochloride is a dihydropyridine structure with the IUPAC (International Union of Pure and Applied Chemistry) chemical name 2-(benzyl-methyl amino) ethyl methyl 1,4-dihydro-2,6-dimethyl-4-(*m*-nitrophenyl)-3,5-pyridinedicarboxylate monohydrochloride.
Nicardipine hydrochloride is a greenish-yellow, odorless, crystalline powder that melts at about 169°C. It is freely soluble in chloroform, methanol, and glacial acetic acid, sparingly soluble in anhydrous ethanol, slightly soluble in n-butanol, water, 0.01 M potassium dihydrogen phosphate, acetone, and dioxane, very slightly soluble in ethyl acetate, and practically insoluble in benzene, ether and hexane. It has a molecular weight of 515.99.
CARDENE is available in hard gelatin capsules containing 20 mg or 30 mg nicardipine hydrochloride with magnesium stearate and pregelatinized starch as the inactive ingredients. The 20 mg strength is provided in opaque white-white capsules made tamper evident by a brilliant blue gelatin band while the 30 mg capsules are opaque light blue-powder blue with a brilliant blue gelatin band. The colorants used in the 20 mg capsules are titanium dioxide, D& C Red #7 Calcium Lake and FD&C Blue #1 and the 30 mg capsules use titanium dioxide, FD&C Blue #1, D&C Yellow #10 Aluminum Lake, D&C Red #7 Calcium Lake, and FD&C Blue #2.

CLINICAL PHARMACOLOGY

Mechanism of Action
CARDENE is a calcium entry blocker (slow channel blocker or calcium ion antagonist) which inhibits the transmembrane influx of calcium ions into cardiac muscle and smooth muscle without changing serum calcium concentrations. The contractile processes of cardiac muscle and vascular smooth muscle are dependent upon the movement of extracellular calcium ions into these cells through specific ion channels. The effects of CARDENE are more selective to vascular smooth muscle than cardiac muscle. In animal models, CARDENE produces relaxation of coronary vascular smooth muscle at drug levels which cause little or no negative inotropic effect.
Pharmacokinetics and Metabolism
CARDENE is completely absorbed following oral doses administered as capsules. Plasma levels are detectable as early as 20 minutes following an oral dose and maximal plasma levels are observed within 30 minutes to two hours (mean T_{max} = 1 hour). While CARDENE is completely absorbed, it is subject to saturable first pass metabolism and the systemic bioavailability is about 35% following a 30 mg oral dose at steady state.
When CARDENE was administered one (1) or three (3) hours after a high fat meal, the mean Cmax and mean AUC were lower (20% to 30%) than when CARDENE was given to fasting subjects. These decreases in plasma levels observed following a meal may be significant but the clinical trials establishing the efficacy and safety of CARDENE were done in patients without regard to the timing of meals. Thus the results of these trials reflect the effects of meal-induced variability.
The pharmacokinetics of CARDENE are nonlinear due to saturable hepatic first pass metabolism. Following oral administration, increasing doses result in a disproportionate increase in plasma levels. Steady state Cmax values following 20, 30, and 40 mg doses every 8 hours averaged 36, 88, and 133 ng/mL, respectively. Hence, increasing the dose from 20 to 30 mg every 8 hours more than doubled Cmax and increasing the dose from 20 to 40 mg every 8 hours increased Cmax more than 3-fold. A similar disproportionate increase in AUC with dose was observed. Considerable inter-subject variability in plasma levels was also observed.
Post-absorption kinetics of CARDENE are also non-linear, although there is a reproducible terminal plasma half-life that averaged 8.6 hours following 30 and 40 mg doses at steady state (TID). The terminal half-life represents the elimination of less than 5% of the absorbed drug (measured by plasma concentrations). Elimination over the first 8 hours after dosing is much faster with a half-life of 2–4 hours. Steady state plasma levels are achieved after 2 to 3 days of TID dosing (every 8 hours) and are 2-fold higher than after a single dose.
CARDENE is highly protein bound (>95%) in human plasma over a wide concentration range.
CARDENE is metabolized extensively by the liver; less than 1% of intact drug is detected in the urine. Following a radioactive oral dose in solution, 60% of the radioactivity was recovered in the urine and 35% in feces. Most of the dose (over 90%) was recovered within 48 hours of dosing. CARDENE does not induce its own metabolism and does not induce hepatic microsomal enzymes.
The steady-state pharmacokinetics of CARDENE in elderly hypertensive patients (≥65 years) are similar to those obtained in young normal adults. After one week of CARDENE dosing at 20 mg three times a day, the Cmax, Tmax, AUC, terminal plasma half-life, and the extent of protein binding of CARDENE observed in healthy elderly hypertensive patients did not differ significantly from those observed in young normal volunteers.
CARDENE plasma levels were higher in patients with mild renal impairment (baseline serum creatinine concentration ranged from 1.2 to 5.5 mg/dL) than in normal subjects. After 30 mg CARDENE TID at steady state, Cmax and AUC were approximately 2-fold higher in these patients.
Because CARDENE is extensively metabolized by the liver, the plasma levels of the drug are influenced by changes in hepatic function. CARDENE plasma levels were higher in patients with severe liver disease (hepatic cirrhosis confirmed by liver biopsy or presence of endoscopically-confirmed esophageal varices) than in normal subjects. After 20 mg CARDENE BID at steady state, Cmax and AUC were 1.8 and 4-fold higher, and the terminal half-life was prolonged to 19 hours in these patients.
Hemodynamics
In man, CARDENE produces a significant decrease in systemic vascular resistance. The degree of vasodilation and the resultant hypotensive effects are more prominent in hypertensive patients. In hypertensive patients, nicardipine reduces the blood pressure at rest and during isometric and dynamic exercise. In normotensive patients, a small decrease of about 9 mmHg in systolic and 7 mmHg in diastolic blood pressure may accompany this fall in peripheral resistance. An increase in heart rate may occur in response to the vasodilation and decrease in blood pressure, and in a few patients this heart rate increase may be pronounced. In clinical studies mean heart rate at time of peak plasma levels was usually increased by 5–10 beats per minute compared to placebo, with the greater increases at higher doses, while there was no difference from placebo at the end of the dosing interval. Hemodynamic studies following intravenous dosing in patients with coronary artery disease and normal or moderately abnormal left ventricular function have shown significant increases in ejection fraction and cardiac output with no significant change, or a small decrease, in left ventricular end-diastolic pressure (LVEDP). Although there is evidence that CARDENE increases coronary blood flow, there is no evidence that this property plays any role in its effectiveness in stable angina. In patients with coronary artery disease, intracoronary administration of nicardipine caused no direct myocardial depression. CARDENE does, however, have a negative inotropic effect in some patients with severe left ventricular dysfunction and could, in patients with very impaired function, lead to worsened failure.
"Coronary Steal", the detrimental redistribution of coronary blood flow in patients with coronary artery disease (diversion of blood from underperfused areas toward better perfused areas), has not been observed during nicardipine treatment. On the contrary, nicardipine has been shown to improve systolic shortening in normal and hypokinetic segments of myocardial muscle, and radio-nuclide angiography has confirmed that wall motion remained improved during an increase in oxygen demand. Nonetheless, occasional patients have developed increased angina upon receiving nicardipine. Whether this represents steal in those patients, or is the result of increased heart rate and decreased diastolic pressure, is not clear.
In patients with coronary artery disease nicardipine improves L.V. diastolic distensibility during the early filling phase, probably due to a faster rate of myocardial relaxation in previously underperfused areas. There is little or no effect

Continued on next page

Syntex—Cont.

on normal myocardium, suggesting the improvement is mainly by indirect mechanisms such as afterload reduction, and reduced ischemia. Nicardipine has no negative effect on myocardial relaxation at therapeutic doses. The clinical consequences of these properties are as yet undemonstrated.

Electrophysiologic Effects

In general, no detrimental effects on the cardiac conduction system were seen with the use of CARDENE.

CARDENE increased the heart rate when given intravenously during acute electrophysiologic studies, and prolonged the corrected QT interval to a minor degree. The sinus node recovery times and SA conduction times were not affected by the drug. The PA, AH, and HV intervals* and the functional and effective refractory periods of the atrium were not prolonged by CARDENE and the relative and effective refractory periods of the His-Purkinje system were slightly shortened after intravenous CARDENE.

Renal Function

There is a transient increase in electrolyte excretion, including sodium. CARDENE does not cause generalized fluid retention, as measured by weight changes, although 7–8% of the patients experience pedal edema.

Effects in Angina Pectoris

In controlled clinical trials of up to 12 weeks duration in patients with chronic stable angina, CARDENE increased exercise tolerance and reduced nitroglycerin consumption and the frequency of anginal attacks. The antianginal efficacy of CARDENE (20–40 mg) has been demonstrated in four placebo-controlled studies involving 258 patients with chronic stable angina. In exercise tolerance testing, CARDENE significantly increased time to angina, total exercise duration and time to 1 mm ST segment depression. Included among these four studies was a dose-definition study in which dose-related improvements in exercise tolerance at one and four hours post-dosing and reduced frequency of anginal attacks were seen at doses of 10, 20 and 30 mg TID. Effectiveness at 10 mg TID was, however, marginal. In a fifth placebo-controlled study, the antianginal efficacy of CARDENE was demonstrated at 8 hours post-dose (trough). The sustained efficacy of CARDENE has been demonstrated over long-term dosing. Blood pressure fell in patients with angina by about 10/8 mmHg at peak blood levels and was little different from placebo at trough blood levels.

Effects in Hypertension

CARDENE produced dose-related decreases in both systolic and diastolic blood pressure in clinical trials. The antihypertensive efficacy of CARDENE administered three times daily has been demonstrated in three placebo-controlled studies involving 517 patients with mild to moderate hypertension. The blood pressure responses in the three studies were statistically significant from placebo at peak (1 hour post-dosing) and trough (8 hours post-dosing) although it is apparent that well over half of the antihypertensive effect is lost by the end of the dosing interval. The results from placebo controlled studies of CARDENE given three times daily are shown in the following table: [See table below.]

The responses are shown as differences from the concurrent placebo control group. The large changes between peak and trough effects were not accompanied by observed side effects at peak response times. In a study using 24 hour intra-arterial blood pressure monitoring, the circadian variation in blood pressure remained unaltered, but the systolic and diastolic blood pressures were reduced throughout the whole 24 hours.

When added to beta-blocker therapy, CARDENE further lowers both systolic and diastolic blood pressure.

INDICATIONS AND USAGE

I. Stable Angina

CARDENE is indicated for the management of patients with chronic stable angina (effort-associated angina). CARDENE may be used alone or in combination with beta-blockers.

II. Hypertension

CARDENE is indicated for the treatment of hypertension. CARDENE may be used alone or in combination with other antihypertensive drugs. In administering nicardipine it is important to be aware of the relatively large peak to trough differences in blood pressure effect. (See DOSAGE AND ADMINISTRATION.)

CONTRAINDICATIONS

CARDENE is contraindicated in patients with hypersensitivity to the drug.

Because part of the effect of CARDENE is secondary to reduced afterload, the drug is also contraindicated in patients with advanced aortic stenosis. Reduction of diastolic pressure in these patients may worsen rather than improve myocardial oxygen balance.

WARNINGS

Increased Angina

About 7% of patients in short term placebo-controlled angina trials have developed increased frequency, duration or severity of angina on starting CARDENE or at the time of dosage increases, compared with 4% of patients on placebo. Comparisons with beta-blockers also show a greater frequency of increased angina, 4% vs 1%. The mechanism of this effect has not been established. (See ADVERSE REACTIONS.)

Use in Patients with Congestive Heart Failure

Although preliminary hemodynamic studies in patients with congestive heart failure have shown that CARDENE reduced afterload without impairing myocardial contractility, it has a negative inotropic effect *in vitro* and in some patients. Caution should be exercised when using the drug in congestive heart failure patients, particularly in combination with a beta-blocker.

Beta-Blocker Withdrawal

CARDENE is not a beta-blocker and therefore gives no protection against the dangers of abrupt beta-blocker withdrawal; any such withdrawal should be by gradual reduction of the dose of beta-blocker, preferably over 8–10 days.

PRECAUTIONS

GENERAL

Blood Pressure: Because CARDENE decreases peripheral resistance, careful monitoring of blood pressure during the initial administration and titration of CARDENE is suggested. CARDENE, like other calcium channel blockers, may occasionally produce symptomatic hypotension. Caution is advised to avoid systemic hypotension when administering the drug to patients who have sustained an acute cerebral infarction or hemorrhage. Because of prominent effects at the time of peak blood levels, initial titration should be performed with measurements of blood pressure at peak effect (1–2 hours after dosing) and just before the next dose.

Use in patients with impaired hepatic function: Since the liver is the major site of biotransformation and since CARDENE is subject to first pass metabolism, the drug should be used with caution in patients having impaired liver function or reduced hepatic blood flow. Patients with severe liver disease developed elevated blood levels (4-fold increase in AUC) and prolonged half-life (19 hours) of CARDENE. (See DOSAGE AND ADMINISTRATION.)

Use in patients with impaired renal function: When CARDENE 20 mg or 30 mg TID was given to hypertensive patients with mild renal impairment, mean plasma concentrations, AUC, and Cmax were approximately 2-fold higher in renally impaired patients than in healthy controls. Doses in these patients must be adjusted. (See CLINICAL PHARMACOLOGY and DOSAGE AND ADMINISTRATION.)

DRUG INTERACTIONS

Beta-Blockers

In controlled clinical studies, adrenergic beta-receptor blockers have been frequently administered concomitantly with CARDENE. The combination is well tolerated.

Cimetidine

Cimetidine increases CARDENE plasma levels. Patients receiving the two drugs concomitantly should be carefully monitored.

Digoxin

Some calcium blockers may increase the concentration of digitalis preparations in the blood. CARDENE usually does not alter the plasma levels of digoxin, however, serum digoxin levels should be evaluated after concomitant therapy with CARDENE is initiated.

Maalox

Co-administration of Maalox TC had no effect on CARDENE absorption.

Fentanyl Anesthesia

Severe hypotension has been reported during fentanyl anesthesia with concomitant use of a beta-blocker and a calcium channel blocker. Even though such interactions were not seen during clinical studies with CARDENE, an increased volume of circulating fluids might be required if such an interaction were to occur.

Cyclosporine

Concomitant administration of nicardipine and cyclosporine results in elevated plasma cyclosporine levels. Plasma concentrations of cyclosporine should therefore be closely monitored, and its dosage reduced accordingly, in patients treated with nicardipine.

When therapeutic concentrations of *furosemide, propranolol, dipyridamole, warfarin, quinidine,* or *naproxen* were added to human plasma *(in vitro),* the plasma protein binding of CARDENE was not altered.

Carcinogenesis, Mutagenesis, Impairment of Fertility

Rats treated with nicardipine in the diet (at concentrations calculated to provide daily dosage levels of 5, 15 or 45 mg/kg/day) for two years showed a dose-dependent increase in thyroid hyperplasia and neoplasia (follicular adenoma/carcinoma). One and three month studies in the rat have suggested that these results are linked to a nicardipine-induced reduction in plasma thyroxine (T4) levels with a consequent increase in plasma levels of thyroid stimulating hormone (TSH). Chronic elevation of TSH is known to cause hyperstimulation of the thyroid. In rats on an iodine deficient diet, nicardipine administration for one month was associated with thyroid hyperplasia that was prevented by T4 supplementation. Mice treated with nicardipine in the diet (at concentrations calculated to provide daily dosage levels of up to 100 mg/kg/day) for up to 18 months showed no evidence of neoplasia of any tissue and no evidence of thyroid changes. There was no evidence of thyroid pathology in dogs treated with up to 25 mg nicardipine/kg/day for one year and no evidence of effects of nicardipine on thyroid function (plasma T4 and TSH) in man.

There was no evidence of a mutagenic potential of nicardipine in a battery of genotoxicity tests conducted on microbial indicator organisms, in micronucleus tests in mice and hamsters, or in a sister chromatid exchange study in hamsters.

No impairment of fertility was seen in male or female rats administered nicardipine at oral doses as high as 100 mg/kg/day (50 times the 40 mg TID maximum recommended antianginal or antihypertensive dose in man, assuming a patient weight of 60 kg).

Pregnancy Pregnancy Category C

Nicardipine was embryocidal when administered orally to pregnant Japanese White rabbits, during organogenesis, at 150 mg/kg/day (a dose associated with marked body weight gain suppression in the treated doe) but not at 50 mg/kg/day (25 times the maximum recommended antianginal or antihypertensive dose in man). No adverse effects on the fetus were observed when New Zealand albino rabbits were treated, during organogenesis, with up to 100 mg nicardipine/kg/day (a dose associated with significant mortality in the treated doe). In pregnant rats administered nicardipine orally at up to 100 mg/kg/day (50 times the maximum recommended human dose) there was no evidence of embryolethality or teratogenicity. However, dystocia, reduced birth weights, reduced neonatal survival and reduced neonatal weight gain were noted. There are no adequate and well-controlled studies in pregnant women. CARDENE® should be used during pregnancy only if the potential benefit justifies the potential risk to the fetus.

Nursing Mothers

Studies in rats have shown significant concentrations of CARDENE in maternal milk following oral administration. For this reason it is recommended that women who wish to breast-feed should not take this drug.

Pediatric Use

Safety and efficacy in patients under the age of 18 have not been established.

Use in the Elderly

Pharmacokinetic parameters did not differ between elderly hypertensive patients (≥ 65 years) and healthy controls after one week of CARDENE treatment at 20 mg TID. Plasma CARDENE concentrations in elderly hypertensive patients were similar to plasma concentrations in healthy young adult subjects when CARDENE was administered at doses of 10, 20 and 30 mg TID, suggesting that the pharmacokinetics of CARDENE are similar in young and elderly hypertensive patients. No significant differences in responses to CARDENE have been observed in elderly patients and the general adult population of patients who participated in clinical studies.

ADVERSE REACTIONS

In multiple-dose U.S. and foreign controlled short-term (up to three months) studies 1,910 patients received CARDENE alone or in combination with other drugs. In these studies adverse events were reported spontaneously; adverse experi-

---

*PA = conduction time from high to low right atrium, AH = conduction time from low right atrium to His bundle deflection, or AV nodal conduction time, HV = conduction time through the His bundle and the bundle branch-Purkinje system.

	SYSTOLIC BP (mmHg)					DIASTOLIC BP (mmHg)			
Dose	Number of Patients	Mean Peak Response	Mean Trough Response	Trough/Peak	Dose	Number of Patients	Mean Peak Response	Mean Trough Response	Trough/Peak
20 mg	50	−10.3	−4.9	48%	20 mg	50	−10.6	−4.6	43%
	52	−17.6	−7.9	45%		52	− 9.0	−2.9	32%
30 mg	45	−14.5	−7.2	50%	30 mg	45	−12.8	−4.9	38%
	44	−14.6	−7.5	51%		44	−14.2	−4.3	30%
40 mg	50	−16.3	−9.5	58%	40 mg	50	−15.4	−5.9	38%
	38	−15.9	−6.0	38%		38	−14.8	−3.7	25%

ences were generally not serious but occasionally required dosage adjustment and about 10% of patients left the studies prematurely because of them. Peak responses were not observed to be associated with adverse effects during clinical trials, but physicians should be aware that adverse effects associated with decreases in blood pressure (tachycardia, hypotension, etc.) could occur around the time of the peak effect. Most adverse effects were expected consequences of the vasodilator effects of CARDENE.

Angina

The incidence rates of adverse effects in anginal patients were derived from multicenter, controlled clinical trials. Following are the rates of adverse effects for CARDENE (N = 520) and placebo (N = 310), respectively, that occurred in 0.4% of patients or more. These represent events considered probably drug-related by the investigator (except for certain cardiovascular events which were recorded in a different category). Where the frequency of adverse effects for CARDENE and placebo is similar, causal relationship is uncertain. The only dose-related effects were pedal edema and increased angina.

Percent of Patients with Adverse Effects in Controlled Studies (Incidence of discontinuations shown in parentheses)

Adverse Experience	CARDENE (N=520)	PLACEBO (N=310)
Pedal Edema	7.1 (0)	0.3 (0)
Dizziness	6.9 (1.2)	0.6 (0)
Headache	6.4 (0.6)	2.6 (0)
Asthenia	5.8 (0.4)	2.6 (0)
Flushing	5.6 (0.4)	1.0 (0)
Increased Angina	5.6 (3.5)	4.2 (1.9)
Palpitations	3.3 (0.4)	0.0 (0)
Nausea	1.9 (0)	0.3 (0)
Dyspepsia	1.5 (0.6)	0.6 (0.3)
Dry Mouth	1.4 (0)	0.3 (0)
Somnolence	1.4 (0)	1.0 (0)
Rash	1.2 (0.2)	0.3 (0)
Tachycardia	1.2 (0.2)	0.6 (0)
Myalgia	1.0 (0)	0.0 (0)
Other edema	1.0 (0)	0.0 (0)
Paresthesia	1.0 (0.2)	0.3 (0)
Sustained Tachycardia	0.8 (0.6)	0.0 (0)
Syncope	0.8 (0.2)	0.0 (0)
Constipation	0.6 (0.2)	0.6 (0)
Dyspnea	0.6 (0)	0.0 (0)
Abnormal ECG	0.6 (0.6)	0.0 (0)
Malaise	0.6 (0)	0.0 (0)
Nervousness	0.6 (0)	0.3 (0)
Tremor	0.6 (0)	0.0 (0)

In addition, adverse events were observed which are not readily distinguishable from the natural history of the atherosclerotic vascular disease in these patients. Adverse events in this category each occurred in <0.4% of patients receiving CARDENE and included myocardial infarction, atrial fibrillation, exertional hypotension, pericarditis, heart block, cerebral ischemia and ventricular tachycardia. It is possible that some of these events were drug-related.

Hypertension

The incidence rates of adverse effects in hypertensive patients were derived from multicenter, controlled clinical trials. Following are the rates of adverse effects for CARDENE (N = 1390) and placebo (N = 211), respectively, that occurred in 0.4% of patients or more. These represent events considered probably drug-related by the investigator. Where the frequency of adverse effects for CARDENE and placebo is similar, causal relationship is uncertain. The only dose-related effect was pedal edema.

Percent of Patients with Adverse Effects in Controlled Studies (Incidence of discontinuations shown in parentheses)

Adverse Experience	CARDENE (N=1390)	PLACEBO (N=211)
Flushing	9.7 (2.1)	2.8 (0)
Headache	8.2 (2.6)	4.7 (0)
Pedal Edema	8.0 (1.8)	0.9 (0)
Asthenia	4.2 (1.7)	0.5 (0)
Palpitations	4.1 (1.0)	0.0 (0)
Dizziness	4.0 (1.8)	0.0 (0)
Tachycardia	3.4 (1.2)	0.5 (0)
Nausea	2.2 (0.9)	0.9 (0)
Somnolence	1.1 (0.1)	0.0 (0)
Dyspepsia	0.8 (0.3)	0.5 (0)
Insomnia	0.6 (0.1)	0.0 (0)
Malaise	0.6 (0.1)	0.0 (0)
Other edema	0.6 (0.3)	1.4 (0)
Abnormal dreams	0.4 (0)	0.0 (0)
Dry mouth	0.4 (0.1)	0.0 (0)
Nocturia	0.4 (0)	0.0 (0)
Rash	0.4 (0.4)	0.0 (0)
Vomiting	0.4 (0.4)	0.0 (0)

Rare Events

The following rare adverse events have been reported in clinical trials or the literature:

Body as a Whole: infection, allergic reaction
Cardiovascular: hypotension, postural hypotension, atypical chest pain, peripheral vascular disorder, ventricular extrasystoles, ventricular tachycardia
Digestive: sore throat, abnormal liver chemistries
Musculoskeletal: arthralgia
Nervous: hot flashes, vertigo, hyperkinesia,, impotence, depression, confusion, anxiety
Respiratory: rhinitis, sinusitis
Special Senses: tinnitus, abnormal vision, blurred vision
Urogenital: increased urinary frequency

OVERDOSAGE

Overdosage with a 600 mg single dose (15 to 30 times normal clinical dose) has been reported. Marked hypotension (blood pressure unobtainable) and bradycardia (heart rate 20 bpm in normal sinus rhythm) occurred, along with drowsiness, confusion and slurred speech. Supportive treatment with a vasopressor resulted in gradual improvement with normal vital signs approximately 9 hours post treatment.

Based on results in laboratory animals, overdosage may cause systemic hypotension, bradycardia (following initial tachycardia) and progressive atrioventricular conduction block. Reversible hepatic function abnormalities and sporadic focal hepatic necrosis were noted in some animal species receiving very large doses of nicardipine.

For treatment of overdose standard measures (for example, evacuation of gastric contents, elevation of extremities, attention to circulating fluid volume and urine output) including monitoring of cardiac and respiratory functions should be implemented. The patient should be positioned so as to avoid cerebral anoxia. Frequent blood pressure determinations are essential. Vasopressors are clinically indicated for patients exhibiting profound hypotension. Intravenous calcium gluconate may help reverse the effects of calcium entry blockade.

DOSAGE AND ADMINISTRATION

Angina

The dose should be individually titrated for each patient beginning with 20 mg three times daily. Doses in the range of 20–40 mg three times a day have been shown to be effective. At least three days should be allowed before increasing the CARDENE dose to ensure achievement of steady state plasma drug concentrations.

Concomitant Use With Other Antianginal Agents

1. Sublingual NTG may be taken as required to abort acute anginal attacks during CARDENE therapy.
2. Prophylactic Nitrate Therapy—CARDENE may be safely coadministered with short- and long-acting nitrates.
3. Beta-blockers—CARDENE may be safely coadministered with beta-blockers. (See DRUG INTERACTIONS.)

Hypertension

The dose of CARDENE should be individually adjusted according to the blood pressure response beginning with 20 mg three times daily. The effective doses in clinical trials have ranged from 20 mg to 40 mg three times daily. The maximum blood pressure lowering effect occurs approximately 1–2 hours after dosing. **To assess the adequacy of blood pressure response, the blood pressure should be measured at trough (8 hours after dosing). Because of the prominent peak effects of nicardipine, blood pressure should be measured 1–2 hours after dosing, particularly during initiation of therapy.** (See PRECAUTIONS: Blood Pressures, INDICATIONS and CLINICAL PHARMACOLOGY—Peak/Trough Effects in Hypertension.) At least three days should be allowed before increasing the CARDENE dose to ensure achievement of steady state plasma drug concentrations.

Concomitant use with other Antihypertensive Agents

1. Diuretics—CARDENE may be safely coadministered with thiazide diuretics.
2. Beta-blockers—CARDENE may be safely coadministered with beta-blockers (See DRUG INTERACTIONS.)

Special Patient Populations

Renal Insufficiency—although there is no evidence that CARDENE impairs renal function, careful dose titration beginning with 20 mg TID is advised. (See PRECAUTIONS.)

Hepatic Insufficiency—CARDENE should be administered cautiously in patients with severely impaired hepatic function. A suggested starting dose of 20 mg twice a day is advised with individual titration based on clinical findings maintaining the twice a day schedule. (See PRECAUTIONS.)

Congestive Heart Failure—Caution is advised when titrating CARDENE dosage in patients with congestive heart failure. (See WARNINGS.)

HOW SUPPLIED

CARDENE® 20 mg capsules are available in opaque white-white hard gelatin capsules with a brillant blue band and printed "CARDENE 20 mg" on the cap and "SYNTEX 2437" on the capsule body. These are supplied in bottles of 100 (NDC 0033-2437-42), bottles of 500 (NDC 0033-2437-62) and in foil wrapped cartons of 100 unit dose blister packages (NDC 0033-2437-53).

CARDENE® 30 mg capsules are available in opaque light blue-powder blue hard gelatin capsules with a brillant blue band and printed "CARDENE 30 mg" on the cap and "SYNTEX 2438" on the capsule body. These are supplied in bottles of 100 (NDC 0033-2438-42), bottles of 500 (NDC 0033-2438-62) and in foil wrapped cartons of 100 unit dose blister packages (NDC 0033-2438-53).

Store bottles at room temperature and dispense in light resistant containers.

Store blister packages at room tempertaure and protect from excessive humidity and light. To protect from light, product should remain in manufacturer's package until consumed.

CAUTION: Federal law prohibits dispensing without prescription.

U.S. Patent No. 3,985,758 Revised 2/89
02-2437-42-01 © 1989 Syntex Laboratories, Inc.

Shown in Product Identification Section, page 433

CARDENE® SR ℞

(nicardipine hydrochloride)
Sustained Release Capsules

DESCRIPTION

CARDENE® SR is a sustained release formulation of CARDENE®. CARDENE SR capsules for oral administration each contain 30 mg, 45 mg or 60 mg of nicardipine hydrochloride. Nicardipine hydrochloride is a calcium ion influx inhibitor (slow channel blocker or calcium entry blocker).

Nicardipine hydrochloride is a dihydropyridine derivative with the IUPAC (International Union of Pure and Applied Chemistry) chemical name (±)-2-(benzyl-methyl amino) ethyl methyl 1,4-dihydro-2,6-dimethyl-4-(*m*-nitrophenyl)-3,5-pyridinedicarboxylate monohydrochloride.

Nicardipine hydrochloride is a greenish-yellow, odorless, crystalline powder that melts at about 169°C. It is freely soluble in chloroform, methanol, and glacial acetic acid, sparingly soluble in anhydrous ethanol, slightly soluble in n-butanol, water, 0.01 M potassium dihydrogen phosphate, acetone, and dioxane, very slightly soluble in ethyl acetate, and practically insoluble in benzene, ether and hexane. It has a molecular weight of 515.99.

CARDENE SR is available in hard gelatin capsules containing 30 mg, 45 mg or 60 mg nicardipine hydrochloride. All strengths contain a two component capsule fill. A powder component containing 25% of total nicardipine hydrochloride dose contains pregelatinized starch and magnesium stearate as inactive ingredients. A spherical granule component containing 75% of total nicardipine hydrochloride dose also contains microcrystalline cellulose, starch, lactose and methacrylic acid copolymer Type C as inactive ingredients. The colorants used in the 30 mg capsules are titanium dioxide, FD&C Red No. 40 and Red Iron Oxide and the colorants used in the 45 mg and 60 mg capsules are titanium dioxide and FD&C Blue No. 2.

CLINICAL PHARMACOLOGY

Mechanism of Action

Nicardipine is a calcium entry blocker (slow channel blocker or calcium ion antagonist) which inhibits the transmembrane influx of calcium ions into cardiac muscle and smooth muscle without changing serum calcium concentrations. The contractile processes of cardiac muscle and vascular smooth muscle are dependent upon the movement of extracellular calcium ions into these cells through specific ion channels. The effects of nicardipine are more selective to vascular smooth muscle than cardiac muscle. In animal models, nicardipine produces relaxation of coronary vascular smooth muscle at drug levels which cause little or no negative inotropic effect.

Pharmacokinetics and Metabolism

Nicardipine is completely absorbed following oral doses administered as capsules, and the systemic bioavailability is about 35% following a 30 mg oral dose at steady state. The pharmacokinetics of nicardipine are non-linear due to saturable hepatic first-pass metabolism.

Following oral administration of CARDENE SR, plasma levels are detectable as early as 20 minutes and maximal plasma levels are achieved as a broad peak generally between one and four hours. The average terminal plasma half-life of nicardipine is 8.6 hours. Following oral administration, increasing doses result in disproportionate increases in plasma levels. Steady state Cmax values following 30, 45 and 60 mg doses every 12 hours averaged 13.4, 34.0 and 58.4 ng/ml, respectively. Hence, increasing the dose two-fold increases maximum plasma levels 4-5 fold. A similar disproportionate increase is observed with AUC. In comparison with equivalent daily doses of CARDENE capsules, CARDENE SR shows a significant reduction in Cmax. CARDENE SR also has somewhat lower bioavailability than

Continued on next page

Syntex—Cont.

CARDENE except at the highest dose. Minimum plasma levels produced by equivalent daily doses are similar. CARDENE SR thus exhibits significantly reduced fluctuation in plasma levels in comparison to CARDENE capsules.

When CARDENE SR was administered with a high fat breakfast, mean Cmax was 45% lower, AUC was 25% lower and trough levels were 75% higher than when CARDENE SR was given in the fasting state. Thus, taking CARDENE SR with the meal reduced the fluctuation in plasma levels. Clinical trials establishing the safety and efficacy of CARDENE SR were carried out in patients without regard to the timing of meals.

Nicardipine is highly protein bound (>95%) in human plasma over a wide concentration range.

Nicardipine is metabolized extensively by the liver; less than 1% of intact drug is detected in the urine. Following a radioactive oral dose in solution, 60% of the radioactivity was recovered in the urine and 35% in feces. Most of the dose (over 90%) was recovered within 48 hours of dosing. Nicardipine does not induce its own metabolism and does not induce hepatic microsomal enzymes.

The pharmacokinetics of CARDENE SR in elderly hypertensive patients (mean age 70 years) were compared to those in younger hypertensive patients (mean age 44 years). After a single dose and after one week of dosing with CARDENE SR there were no significant differences in Cmax, Tmax, AUC or clearance between the young and elderly patients. In both groups of patients, steady state plasma levels were significantly higher than following a single dose. In the elderly patients, a disproportional increase in plasma levels with dose was observed similar to that observed in normal subjects.

Nicardipine plasma levels following administration of CARDENE SR in hypertensive patients with moderate renal impairment (creatinine clearance 10–55 ml/min) were significantly higher following a single oral dose and at steady state than in hypertensive patients with mildly impaired renal function (creatinine clearance > 55 ml/min). After 45 mg CARDENE SR b.i.d. at steady state, Cmax and AUC were 2–3 fold higher in the patients with moderate renal impairment. Plasma levels in patients with mildly impaired renal function were similar to those in normal subjects.

In patients with severe renal impairment undergoing routine hemodialysis, plasma levels following a single dose of CARDENE SR were not significantly different from those patients with mildly impaired renal function.

Because nicardipine is extensively metabolized by the liver, the plasma levels of the drug are influenced by changes in hepatic function. Following administration of CARDENE capsules, nicardipine plasma levels were higher in patients with severe liver disease (hepatic cirrhosis confirmed by liver biopsy or presence of endoscopically-confirmed esophageal varices) than in normal subjects. After 20 mg CARDENE b.i.d. at steady state, Cmax and AUC were 1.8 and 4-fold higher, and the terminal half-life was prolonged to 19 hours in these patients. CARDENE SR has not been studied in patients with severe liver disease.

Hemodynamics

In man, nicardipine produces a significant decrease in systemic vascular resistance. The degree of vasodilation and the resultant hypotensive effects are more prominent in hypertensive patients. In hypertensive patients, nicardipine reduces the blood pressure at rest and during isometric and dynamic exercise. In normotensive patients, a small decrease of about 9 mmHg in systolic and 7 mmHg in diastolic blood pressure may accompany this fall in peripheral resistance. An increase in heart rate may occur in response to the vasodilation and decrease in blood pressure, and in a few patients this heart rate increase may be pronounced. In clinical studies mean heart rate at time of peak plasma levels was usually increased by 5–10 beats per minute compared to placebo, with the greater increases at higher doses, while there was no difference from placebo at the end of the dosing interval. Hemodynamic studies following intravenous dosing in patients with coronary artery disease and normal or moderately abnormal left ventricular function have shown significant increases in ejection fraction and cardiac output with no significant change, or a small decrease, in left ventricular end-diastolic pressure (LVEDP). Although there is evidence that nicardipine increases coronary blood flow, there is no evidence that this property plays any role in its effectiveness in stable angina. In patients with coronary artery disease, intracoronary administration of nicardipine caused no direct myocardial depression. CARDENE does, however, have a negative inotropic effect in some patients with severe left ventricular dysfunction and could, in patients with very impaired function, lead to worsened failure.

"Coronary Steal", the detrimental redistribution of coronary blood flow in patients with coronary artery disease (diversion of blood from underperfused areas toward better perfused areas), has not been observed during nicardipine treatment. On the contrary, nicardipine has been shown to improve systolic shortening in normal and hypokinetic segments of myocardial muscle, and radionuclide angiography has confirmed that wall motion remained improved during an increase in oxygen demand. Nonetheless, occasional patients have developed increased angina upon receiving nicardipine. Whether this represents steal in those patients, or is the result of increased heart rate and decreased diastolic pressure, is not clear.

In patients with coronary artery disease nicardipine improves L.V. diastolic distensibility during the early filling phase, probably due to a faster rate of myocardial relaxation in previously underperfused areas. There is little or no effect on normal myocardium, suggesting the improvement is mainly by indirect mechanisms such as afterload reduction, and reduced ischemia. Nicardipine has no negative effect on myocardial relaxation at therapeutic doses. The clinical consequences of these properties are as yet undemonstrated.

Electrophysiologic Effects

In general, no detrimental effects on the cardiac conduction system were seen with the use of CARDENE.

Nicardipine increased the heart rate when given intravenously during acute electrophysiologic studies, and prolonged the corrected QT interval to a minor degree. The sinus node recovery times and SA conduction times were not affected by the drug. The PA, AH, and HV intervals* and the functional and effective refractory periods of the atrium were not prolonged by nicardipine and the relative and effective refractory periods of the His-Purkinje system were slightly shortened after intravenous nicardipine.

Renal Function

There is a transient increase in electrolyte excretion, including sodium. CARDENE does not cause generalized fluid retention, as measured by weight changes.

Effects in Hypertension

CARDENE SR produced decreases in both systolic and diastolic blood pressure throughout the dosing interval in clinical trials. The antihypertensive efficacy of CARDENE SR administered twice daily has been demonstrated using in-clinic blood pressure measures in placebo-controlled trials involving patients with mild to moderate hypertension and in trials using 12 or 24 hour ambulatory blood pressure monitoring.

INDICATIONS AND USAGE

CARDENE SR is indicated for the treatment of hypertension. CARDENE SR may be used alone or in combination with other antihypertensive drugs.

CONTRAINDICATIONS

CARDENE is contraindicated in patients with hypersensitivity to the drug.

Because part of the effect of CARDENE is secondary to reduced afterload, the drug is also contraindicated in patients with advanced aortic stenosis. Reduction of diastolic pressure by any means in these patients may worsen rather than improve myocardial oxygen balance.

WARNINGS

Increased Angina in Patients with Angina: In short-term placebo-controlled angina trials with CARDENE (an immediate release oral dosage form of nicardipine), about 7% of patients on CARDENE (compared with 4% of patients on placebo) have developed increased frequency, duration or severity of angina. Comparisons with beta-blockers also show a greater frequency of increased angina, 4% vs 1%. The mechanism of this effect has not been established.

Use in Patients with Congestive Heart Failure: Although preliminary hemodynamic studies in patients with congestive heart failure have shown that CARDENE reduced afterload without impairing myocardial contractility, it has a negative inotropic effect *in vitro* and in some patients. Caution should be exercised when using the drug in congestive heart failure patients, particularly in combination with a beta-blocker.

Beta-Blocker Withdrawal: CARDENE is not a beta-blocker and therefore gives no protection against the dangers of abrupt beta-blocker withdrawal; any such withdrawal should be by gradual reduction of the dose of beta-blocker, preferably over 8–10 days.

PRECAUTIONS

General

Blood Pressure: Because CARDENE decreases peripheral resistance, careful monitoring of blood pressure during the initial administration and titration of CARDENE is suggested. CARDENE, like other calcium channel blockers, may occasionally produce symptomatic hypotension. Caution is advised to avoid systemic hypotension when administering the drug to patients who have sustained an acute cerebral infarction or hemorrhage.

Use in Patients with Impaired Hepatic Function: Since the liver is the major site of biotransformation and since CARDENE is subject to first-pass metabolism, CARDENE should be used with caution in patients having impaired liver function or reduced hepatic blood flow. Patients with severe liver disease developed elevated blood levels (4-fold increase in AUC) and prolonged half-life (19 hours) of CARDENE.

Use in Patients with Impaired Renal Function: When CARDENE SR 45 mg b.i.d. was given to hypertensive patients with moderate renal impairment, mean AUC and Cmax values were approximately 2–3 fold higher than in patients with mild renal impairment. Doses in these patients must be adjusted. Mean AUC and Cmax values were similar in patients with mildly impaired renal function and normal volunteers. (See CLINICAL PHARMACOLOGY and DOSAGE AND ADMINISTRATION.)

Drug Interactions

Beta-Blockers

In controlled clinical studies, adrenergic beta-receptor blockers have been frequently administered concomitantly with CARDENE. The combination is well tolerated.

Cimetidine

Cimetidine increases CARDENE plasma levels. Patients receiving the two drugs concomitantly should be carefully monitored.

Digoxin

Some calcium blockers may increase the concentration of digitalis preparations in the blood. CARDENE usually does not alter the plasma levels of digoxin, however, serum digoxin levels should be evaluated after concomitant therapy with CARDENE is initiated.

Fentanyl Anesthesia

Severe hypotension has been reported during fentanyl anesthesia with concomitant use of a beta-blocker and a calcium channel blocker. Even though such interactions were not seen during clinical studies with CARDENE, an increased volume of circulating fluids might be required if such an interaction were to occur.

Cyclosporine

Concomitant administration of nicardipine and cyclosporine results in elevated plasma cyclosporine levels. Plasma concentrations of cyclosporine should therefore be closely monitored, and its dosage reduced accordingly, in patients treated with nicardipine.

When therapeutic concentrations of *furosemide, propranolol, dipyridamole, warfarin, quinidine,* or *naproxen* were added to human plasma *(in vitro),* the plasma protein binding of CARDENE was not altered.

Carcinogenesis, Mutagenesis, Impairment of Fertility

Rats treated with nicardipine in the diet (at concentrations calculated to provide daily dosage levels of 5, 15 or 45 mg/kg/day) for two years showed a dose-dependent increase in thyroid hyperplasia and neoplasia (follicular adenoma/carcinoma). One and three month studies in the rat have suggested that these results are linked to a nicardipine-induced reduction in plasma thyroxine (T4) levels with a consequent increase in plasma levels of thyroid stimulating hormone (TSH). Chronic elevation of TSH is known to cause hyperstimulation of the thyroid. In rats on an iodine deficient diet, nicardipine administration for one month was associated with thyroid hyperplasia that was prevented by T4 supplementation. Mice treated with nicardipine in the diet (at concentrations calculated to provide daily dosage levels of up to 100 mg/kg/day) for up to 18 months showed no evidence of neoplasia of any tissue and no evidence of thyroid changes. There was no evidence of thyroid pathology in dogs treated with up to 25 mg nicardipine/kg/day for one year and no evidence of effects of nicardipine on thyroid function (plasma T4 and TSH) in man.

There was no evidence of a mutagenic potential of nicardipine in a battery of genotoxicity tests conducted on microbial indicator organisms, in micronucleus tests in mice and hamsters, or in a sister chromatid exchange study in hamsters.

No impairment of fertility was seen in male or female rats administered nicardipine at oral doses as high as 100 mg/kg/day (50 times the maximum recommended daily dose in man, assuming a patient weight of 60 kg).

Pregnancy

Pregnancy Category C: Nicardipine was embryocidal when administered orally to pregnant Japanese White rabbits, during organogenesis, at 150 mg/kg/day (a dose associated with marked body weight gain suppression in the treated doe) but not at 50 mg/kg/day (25 times the maximum recommended dose in man). No adverse effects on the fetus were observed when New Zealand albino rabbits were treated, during organogenesis, with up to 100 mg nicardipine/kg/day (a dose associated with significant mortality in the treated doe). In pregnant rats administered nicardipine orally at up to 100 mg/kg/day (50 times the maximum recommended human dose) there was no evidence of embryolethality or teratogenicity. However, dystocia, reduced birth weights, reduced neonatal survival and reduced neonatal weight gain were noted. There are no adequate and well-controlled studies in pregnant women. CARDENE® SR should be used during pregnancy only if the potential benefit justifies the potential risk to the fetus.

*PA = conduction time from high to low right atrium,
AH = conduction time from low right atrium to His bundle deflection, or AV nodal conduction time,
HV = conduction time through the His bundle and the bundle branch-Purkinje system.

Nursing Mothers
Studies in rats have shown significant concentrations of nicardipine in maternal milk following oral administration. For this reason it is recommended that women who wish to breast-feed should not take this drug.

Pediatric Use
Safety and efficacy in patients under the age of 18 have not been established.

Use in the Elderly
Pharmacokinetic parameters did not differ significantly between elderly hypertensive patients (mean age 70 years) and younger hypertensive patients (mean age 44 years) after one week of treatment with CARDENE SR. No significant differences in response to CARDENE have been observed in elderly patients and the general adult population of patients who have participated in studies.

ADVERSE EVENTS
In multiple-dose U.S. and foreign controlled studies, 667 patients received CARDENE SR. In these studies adverse events were elicited by nondirected and in some cases directed questioning; adverse events were generally not serious and about 9% of patients withdrew prematurely from the studies because of them.

Hypertension: The incidence rates of adverse events in hypertensive patients were derived from placebo-controlled clinical trials. Following are the rates of adverse events for CARDENE SR (N=322) and placebo (N=140), respectively, that occurred in 0.6% of patients or more on CARDENE SR. These represent events considered probably drug related by the investigator. Where the frequency of adverse events for CARDENE SR and placebo is similar, causal relationship is uncertain. The only dose-related effect was pedal edema.

Percentage of Patients with Probably Drug Related Adverse Events in Placebo-Controlled Studies

Adverse Event	CARDENE SR (N=322)	Placebo (N=140)
Headache	6.2	7.1
Pedal Edema	5.9	1.4
Vasodilatation	4.7	1.4
Palpitation	2.8	1.4
Nausea	1.9	0.7
Dizziness	1.6	0.7
Asthenia	0.9	0.7
Postural Hypotension	0.9	0
Increased Urinary Frequency	0.6	0
Pain	0.6	0
Rash	0.6	0
Sweating Increased	0.6	0
Vomiting	0.6	0

Incidence (%) of Discontinuations Due to Any Adverse Event in Placebo-Controlled Studies

Adverse Event	CARDENE SR (N=322)	Placebo (N=140)
Headache	2.5	1.4
Palpitation	2.2	0.7
Dizziness	1.9	0.7
Asthenia	1.9	0
Pedal Edema	1.2	0
Nausea	1.2	0
Rash	0.9	0.7
Diarrhea	0.9	0
Tachycardia	0.9	0
Blurred Vision	0.6	0
Chest Pain	0.6	0
Face Edema	0.6	0
Myocardial Infarct	0.6	0
Vasodilatation	0.6	0
Vomiting	0.6	0

Uncontrolled experience in over 300 patients with hypertension treated for up to 27.5 months with CARDENE SR has shown no unexpected adverse events or increase in incidence of adverse events compared to the controlled clinical trials.

Rare Events: The following rare adverse events have been reported in clinical trials or the literature:
Body as a Whole: infection, allergic reaction
Cardiovascular: hypotension, atypical chest pain, peripheral vascular disorder, ventricular extrasystoles, ventricular tachycardia, angina pectoris
Digestive: sore throat, abnormal liver chemistries
Musculoskeletal: arthralgia
Nervous: hot flashes, vertigo, hyperkinesia, impotence, depression, confusion, anxiety
Respiratory: rhinitis, sinusitis
Special Senses: tinnitus, abnormal vision, blurred vision

Angina: Data are available from only 91 patients with chronic stable angina pectoris who received CARDENE SR 30–60 mg administered twice daily in open label clinical tri-

als. Fifty-eight of these patients were treated for at least 30 days. The four most frequently reported adverse events thought by the investigators to be probably related to the use of CARDENE SR were vasodilatation (5.5%), pedal edema (4.4%), asthenia (4.4%), and dizziness (3.3%).

OVERDOSAGE
Three overdosages with CARDENE or CARDENE SR have been reported. Two occurred in adults, one of whom ingested 600 mg of CARDENE and the other 2,160 mg of CARDENE SR. Symptoms included marked hypotension, bradycardia, palpitations, flushing, drowsiness, confusion and slurred speech. All symptoms resolved without sequelae. The third overdosage occurred in a one year old child who ingested half of the powder in a 30 mg CARDENE capsule. The child remained asymptomatic.

Based on results obtained in laboratory animals, overdosage may cause systemic hypotension, bradycardia (following initial tachycardia) and progressive atrioventricular conduction block. Reversible hepatic function abnormalities and sporadic focal hepatic necrosis were noted in some animal species receiving very large doses of nicardipine.

For treatment of overdose standard measures (for example, evacuation of gastric contents, elevation of extremities, attention to circulating fluid volume and urine output) including monitoring of cardiac and respiratory functions should be implemented. The patient should be positioned so as to avoid cerebral anoxia. Frequent blood pressure determinations are essential. Vasopressors are clinically indicated for patients exhibiting profound hypotension. Intravenous calcium gluconate may help reverse the effects of calcium entry blockade.

DOSAGE AND ADMINISTRATION
The dose of CARDENE SR should be individually adjusted according to the blood pressure response beginning with 30 mg two times daily. The effective doses in clinical trials have ranged from 30 mg to 60 mg two times daily. The maximum blood pressure lowering effect at steady state is sustained from 2 hours until 6 hours after dosing.

When initiating therapy or upon increasing dose, blood pressure should be measured 2 to 4 hours after the first dose or dose increase, as well as at the end of a dosing interval.

The total daily dose of immediate release nicardipine (CARDENE) may not be a useful guide to judging the effective dose of CARDENE SR. Patients currently receiving immediate release nicardipine may be titrated with CARDENE SR starting at their current total daily dose of immediate release nicardipine and then reexamined to assess the adequacy of blood pressure control.

Concomitant use with other Antihypertensive Agents
1. Diuretics—CARDENE may be safely coadministered with thiazide diuretics.
2. Beta-Blockers—CARDENE may be safely coadministered with beta-blockers. (See DRUG INTERACTIONS.)

Special Patient Populations
Renal Insufficiency—Although there is no evidence that CARDENE SR impairs renal function, careful dose titration beginning with 30 mg CARDENE SR b.i.d. is advised. (See PRECAUTIONS.)
Hepatic Insufficiency—CARDENE SR has not been studied in patients with severe liver impairment. (See PRECAUTIONS.)
Congestive Heart Failure—Caution is advised when titrating CARDENE SR dosage in patients with congestive heart failure. (See WARNINGS.)

HOW SUPPLIED
CARDENE® SR 30 mg capsules are available in opaque pink-pink hard gelatin capsules. The capsule cap is printed with "CARDENE SR 30 mg" and the capsule body is printed with "SYNTEX 2440". These are supplied in bottles of 60 (NDC #0033-2440-40) and bottles of 200 (NDC #0033-2440-60), and in cartons of 100 unit dose blister packages (NDC #0033-2440-53).

CARDENE® SR 45 mg capsules are available in opaque powder blue-powder blue hard gelatin capsules. The capsule cap is printed with "CARDENE SR 45 mg" and the capsule body is printed with "SYNTEX 2441". These are supplied in bottles of 60 (NDC #0033-2441-40) and bottles of 200 (NDC #0033-2441-60), and in cartons of 100 unit dose blister packages (NDC #0033-2441-53).

CARDENE® SR 60 mg capsules are available in opaque light blue-white hard gelatin capsules. The capsule cap is printed with "CARDENE SR 60 mg" and the capsule body is printed with "SYNTEX 2442". These are supplied in bottles of 60 (NDC #0033-2442-40) and bottles of 200 (NDC #0033-2442-60), and in cartons of 100 unit dose blister packages (NDC #0033-2442-53).

Store bottles at room temperature and dispense in light-resistant containers, such as the manufacturer's original container.

Store blister packages at room temperature and protect from excessive humidity and light. To protect from light, product should remain in manufacturer's package until consumed.

CAUTION: Federal law prohibits dispensing without prescription.

U.S. Patent Nos.: 4,940,556; 3,985,758; others pending
SYNTEX LABORATORIES, INC.
PALO ALTO, CA 94304   January 1992
02-2440-40-00   © 1992 SYNTEX LABORATORIES, INC.
Shown in Product Identification Section, page 433

CARMOL® 10   OTC
[kahr 'mawl]
**10% urea lotion
for total body
dry skin care.**

A product of Syntex Laboratories, Inc.
(See PDR For Nonprescription Drugs.)

CARMOL® 20   OTC
[kahr 'mawl]
**20% Urea Cream
Extra strength for
rough, dry skin**

A product of Syntex Laboratories, Inc.
(See PDR For Nonprescription Drugs.)

CARMOL® HC   ℞
[kahr 'mawl]
**(hydrocortisone acetate)
Cream 1%**

Refer to entry under LIDEX® (fluocinonide) Cream 0.05%.

CYTOVENE®   ℞
[si 'tō-veen]
(ganciclovir sodium) Sterile Powder

A product of Syntex Laboratories, Inc.
FOR INTRAVENOUS INFUSION ONLY

> THE CLINICAL TOXICITY OF CYTOVENE INCLUDES GRANULOCYTOPENIA AND THROMBOCYTOPENIA. IN ANIMAL STUDIES CYTOVENE WAS CARCINOGENIC, TERATOGENIC, AND CAUSED ASPERMATOGENESIS. CYTOVENE IS INDICATED FOR USE *ONLY* IN THE TREATMENT OF CYTOMEGALOVIRUS (CMV) RETINITIS IN IMMUNOCOMPROMISED PATIENTS AND FOR THE PREVENTION OF CMV DISEASE IN TRANSPLANT PATIENTS AT RISK FOR CMV DISEASE. (See INDICATIONS AND USAGE section.)

DESCRIPTION
CYTOVENE is the brand name for ganciclovir sodium, an antiviral drug active against cytomegalovirus. Reconstituted CYTOVENE Sterile Powder is for intravenous administration only. Each vial of CYTOVENE Sterile Powder contains the equivalent of 500 mg ganciclovir as the sodium salt (46 mg sodium). CYTOVENE is manufactured as a sterile lyophilized powder. Reconstitution with 10 mL of Sterile Water for Injection, USP, yields a solution with pH 11 and a ganciclovir concentration of approximately 50 mg/mL. Further dilution in an appropriate intravenous solution must be performed before infusion (see DOSAGE AND ADMINISTRATION section). All doses in this insert are specified in terms of ganciclovir. The chemical name of ganciclovir sodium is 9-(1,3-dihydroxy-2-propoxymethyl) guanine, monosodium salt with a molecular formula of $C_9H_{12}N_5NaO_4$ and a molecular weight of 277.21.

Ganciclovir sodium, as a white lyophilized powder, has an aqueous solubility of greater than 50 mg/mL at 25℃. At physiological pH, ganciclovir exists as the unionized form with an aqueous solubility of 3.65 mg/mL at 25℃.

CLINICAL PHARMACOLOGY
Virology
Mechanism of Action: Ganciclovir is a synthetic nucleoside analogue of 2'-deoxyguanosine that inhibits replication of herpesviruses both *in vitro* and *in vivo*. Sensitive human viruses include cytomegalovirus (CMV), herpes simplex virus -1 and -2 (HSV-1, HSV-2), Epstein-Barr virus (EBV) and varicella zoster virus (VZV). Clinical studies have been limited to assessment of efficacy in patients with CMV infection. Available evidence indicates that upon entry into host cells, cytomegaloviruses induce one or more cellular kinases that phosphorylate ganciclovir to its triphosphate. It has been shown that there is approximately a 10-fold greater concentration of ganciclovir-triphosphate in CMV-infected cells

Continued on next page

Syntex—Cont.

than in uninfected cells, indicating a preferential phosphorylation of ganciclovir in virus-infected cells. *In vitro*, ganciclovir-triphosphate is catabolized slowly, with 60 to 70% of the original level remaining in the infected cells 18 hours after removal of ganciclovir from the extracellular medium.[1]
The antiviral activity of ganciclovir-triphosphate is believed to be the result of inhibition of viral DNA synthesis by two known modes: (1) competitive inhibition of viral DNA polymerases (2) direct incorporation into viral DNA, resulting in eventual termination of viral DNA elongation. The cellular DNA polymerase alpha is also inhibited, but at a higher concentration than required for viral DNA polymerase.

Antiviral Activity: Median effective inhibitory doses (ED_{50}) of ganciclovir for human CMV isolates tested *in vitro* in several cell lines ranged from 0.2 to 3.0 µg/mL. The relationship between *in vitro* sensitivity of CMV to ganciclovir and clinical response has not been established. CYTOVENE inhibits mammalian cell proliferation *in vitro* at higher concentrations (10 to 60 µg/mL) with bone marrow colony forming cells being the most sensitive ($ID_{50} \geq 10$ µg/mL) of those cell types tested.
Ganciclovir has shown antiviral activity *in vivo* in several animal CMV infection models. Both normal and immunosuppressed mice had reduced titers of murine CMV when treated with ganciclovir at 5 to 50 mg/kg/day.[2] Normal mice had increased survival as well, when treated with doses of 3 mg/kg/day. Immunosuppressed mice did not show increased survival until they received doses of at least 10 mg/kg/day.[3] In guinea pigs infected with cavian CMV and treated with ganciclovir at 50 mg/kg/day for 7 days, viral titers in the salivary glands were reduced approximately 50% at day 28 post-infection as compared to sham-treated controls.[4]
Of 314 immunocompromised patients enrolled in an open label study of the treatment of life- or sight-threatening CMV disease, 121 patients were identified who had a positive culture for CMV within 7 days prior to treatment and had sequential viral cultures after treatment with CYTOVENE.[5] Post-treatment virologic response was defined as conversion to culture negativity, or a greater than 100-fold decrease in CMV infectious units, as shown in the following table:

Virologic Response

Culture Source	No. Patients Cultured	No. (%) Patients Responding	Median Days to Response
Urine	107	93 (87)	8
Blood	41	34 (83)	8
Throat	21	19 (90)	7
Semen	6	6 (100)	15

The antiviral activity of CYTOVENE has been confirmed in two separate placebo-controlled studies for the prevention of CMV disease in transplant recipients. One hundred forty-nine CMV seropositive heart allograft[6] recipients were randomized to treatment with CYTOVENE (5 mg/kg BID for 14 days followed by 6 mg/kg QD for 5 days/week for an additional 14 days) or placebo. Seventy-two CMV culture positive allogeneic bone marrow[7] transplant recipients were randomized to treatment with CYTOVENE (5 mg/kg BID for 7 days followed by 5 mg/kg QD) or placebo until day 100 post-transplant. CYTOVENE prevented recrudescence of CMV shedding in heart allograft recipients and suppressed CMV shedding in bone marrow allograft recipients. The antiviral effect of CYTOVENE in these patients is summarized in the following table:
[See table below.]

Viral Resistance: Viral resistance has been observed with appreciable frequency (≥8%) in patients receiving prolonged CYTOVENE treatment[8,9,10]. There is also a possibility that some patients may be infected with strains of CMV that are resistant to ganciclovir prior to treatment with CYTOVENE[8]. Viral resistance has been observed in patients receiving prolonged CYTOVENE treatment. In one report, 72 AIDS patients treated with CYTOVENE were prospectively monitored for viral shedding and drug resistance (defined as $ID_{50} \geq 3.0$ µg/mL)[9]. All patients were shedding CYTOVENE-sensitive CMV pre-treatment. During 7 months of therapy with CYTOVENE, approximately 80% of patients were culture negative and 20% continued to shed CMV. No resistant CMV strains were isolated during the first 3 months of treatment. After 3 months, 38% of patients shedding CMV (7.6% of all treated patients) had resistant strains isolated, all of which were associated with clinical progression of CMV retinitis. Therefore, the possibility of viral resistance should be considered in patients who show poor clinical response or experience persistent viral excretion during therapy.

Pharmacokinetics

The pharmacokinetics of CYTOVENE have been evaluated in immunocompromised adults with serious CMV disease. Twenty-two adults with normal renal function, enrolled in open-label treatment at different study centers, received 5 mg/kg doses of CYTOVENE, each dose infused intravenously over one hour. The plasma level of ganciclovir at the end of the first one hour infusion (Cmax) was 8.3 ± 4.0 µg/mL (mean ± SD) and the plasma level 11 hours after the start of infusion (Cmin) was 0.56 ± 0.66 µg/mL. The plasma half-life was 2.9 ± 1.3 hours and the systemic clearance was 3.64 ± 1.86 mL/kg/min (approximately 250 mL/min/1.73M²). Dose-independent kinetics were demonstrated over the range of 1.6 to 5.0 mg/kg. Multiple-dose kinetics were measured in eight patients with normal renal function who received CYTOVENE 5 mg/kg twice daily for 12–14 days. After the first dose and after multiple dosing, plasma levels of ganciclovir at the end of infusion were 7.1 µg/mL (3.1 to 14.0 µg/mL) and 9.5 µg/mL (2.7 to 24.2 µg/mL), respectively. At 7 hours after infusion, plasma levels after the first dose were 0.85 µg/mL (0.2 to 1.8 µg/mL) and were 1.2 µg/mL (0.6 to 1.8 µg/mL) after multiple dosing.
Renal excretion of unchanged drug by glomerular filtration is the major route of elimination of CYTOVENE. In patients with normal renal function, more than 90% of the administered CYTOVENE was recovered unmetabolized in the urine. The pharmacokinetic analysis in 10 patients with renal impairment showed that in 4 patients with mild impairment (creatinine clearance 50 to 79 mL/min/1.73M²) the systemic clearance of CYTOVENE was 128 ± 63 mL/min/1.73M², and the plasma half-life was 4.6 ± 1.4 hours. In 3 patients with moderate impairment (creatinine clearance 25 to 49 mL/min/1.73M²) the systemic clearance of CYTOVENE was 57 ± 8 mL/min/1.73M², and the plasma half-life was 4.4 ± 0.4 hours. In 3 patients with severe impairment (creatinine clearance less than 25 mL/min/1.73M²) the systemic clearance was 30 ± 13 mL/min/1.73M², and the plasma half-life was 10.7 ± 5.7 hours. There was positive correlation between systemic clearance of CYTOVENE and creatinine clearance (r = 0.90).
Data from 4 patients with severe renal impairment showed that hemodialysis reduced plasma drug levels by approximately 50%.

BECAUSE THE MAJOR EXCRETION PATHWAY FOR CYTOVENE IS RENAL, DOSAGE MUST BE REDUCED ACCORDING TO CREATININE CLEARANCE. FOR DOSING INSTRUCTIONS IN RENAL IMPAIRMENT, REFER TO THE SECTION ON DOSAGE AND ADMINISTRATION.

There is limited evidence to suggest that ganciclovir crosses the blood-brain barrier. Cerebrospinal fluid (CSF) concentrations have been measured in three patients who received 2.5 mg/kg ganciclovir intravenously q8 or q12 hours. The results shown in the following table:

CSF Concentrations[11,12]

Patient	CSF Conc. (µg/mL)	Plasma Conc. (µg/mL)	Hr after dose	CSF/ Plasma Ratio
1	0.62	0.92*	5.67	.67
	0.68	2.20*	3.5	.31
	0.51	1.96*	2.75	.26
2	0.50	2.05*	0.25	.24
3	0.31	0.44	5.5	.70

*Estimation (model-predicted values)

Binding of CYTOVENE to plasma proteins is 1–2%. Drug interactions involving binding site displacement are not expected.

INDICATIONS AND USAGE

CYTOVENE is indicated for the treatment of CMV retinitis in immunocompromised individuals, including patients with acquired immunodeficiency syndrome (AIDS). CYTOVENE is also indicated for the prevention of CMV disease in transplant patients at risk for CMV disease (see **Clinical Trials** section below). SAFETY AND EFFICACY OF **CYTOVENE** HAVE NOT BEEN ESTABLISHED FOR CONGENITAL OR NEONATAL CMV DISEASE; NOR FOR TREATMENT OF ESTABLISHED CMV DISEASE OTHER THAN RETINITIS (SUCH AS PNEUMONITIS OR COLITIS); NOR FOR USE IN NON-IMMUNOCOMPROMISED INDIVIDUALS.
The diagnosis of CMV retinitis is ophthalmologic and should be made by indirect ophthalmoscopy. Other conditions in the differential diagnosis of CMV retinitis include candidiasis, toxoplasmosis, histoplasmosis, retinal scars, and cotton wool spots, any of which may produce a retinal appearance similar to CMV. For this reason it is essential that the diagnosis of CMV be established by an ophthalmologist familiar with the retinal presentation of these conditions. The diagnosis of CMV retinitis may be supported by culture of CMV from urine, blood, throat, or other sites, but a negative CMV culture does not rule out CMV retinitis.

CLINICAL TRIALS

1. CMV Retinitis

In a retrospective, non-randomized, single-center analysis[13,14] of 41 patients with AIDS and CMV retinitis, treatment with CYTOVENE resulted in a significant delay in median time to first retinitis progression compared to untreated controls (71 days from diagnosis versus 29 days from diagnosis). Patients in this series received induction treatment of CYTOVENE 5 mg/kg BID for 14–21 days followed by maintenance treatment with either 5 mg/kg once per day, seven days per week or 6 mg/kg once per day, five days each week. (see DOSAGE AND ADMINISTRATION section).

2. Prevention of CMV Disease in Transplant Recipients

CYTOVENE was evaluated in three randomized, controlled trials of prevention of CMV disease in organ transplant recipients.
ICM 1496: In a randomized, double-blind, placebo-controlled study of 149 heart transplant recipients[6] at risk for CMV infection (CMV seropositive, or a seronegative recipient of an organ from a CMV seropositive donor), there was a statistically significant reduction in the overall incidence of CMV disease in CYTOVENE-treated patients. Immediately post-transplant, patients received CYTOVENE 5 mg/kg BID for 14 days followed by 6 mg/kg QD for 5 days/week for an additional 14 days. Twelve of the 76 (16%) CYTOVENE-treated patients versus 31 of the 73 (43%) placebo patients developed CMV disease during the 120 day post-transplant observation period. No significant differences in hematologic toxicities were seen between the two treatment groups. (Refer to table in ADVERSE REACTIONS section).
ICM 1689: In a randomized double-blind, placebo-controlled study of 72 bone marrow transplant recipients[7] with asymptomatic CMV infection (CMV positive culture of urine, throat, or blood) there was a statistically significant reduction in the incidence of CMV disease in CYTOVENE-treated patients. Patients with virologic evidence of CMV infection received CYTOVENE 5 mg/kg BID for 7 days followed by 5 mg/kg QD daily through day 100 post-transplant. One of 37 (3%) of the CYTOVENE-treated patients versus 15 of the 35 (43%) placebo patients developed disease during the study. At six months post-transplant, there continued to be a statistically significant reduction in the incidence of CMV disease in CYTOVENE-treated patients. Six of 37 (16%) of the CYTOVENE-treated patients versus 15 of the 35 (43%) placebo patients developed disease through six months post-transplant. Overall rate of survival was statistically significantly higher in the CYTOVENE-treated group, both at day 100 and day 180 post-transplant. Although the differences in hematologic toxicities were not statistically significant, the incidence of neutropenia was higher in the CYTOVENE-treated group (Refer to table in ADVERSE REACTIONS section).
A second, randomized, unblinded, bone marrow transplant study[15] was performed, evaluating 40 allogenic transplant recipients at risk for CMV disease. Patients underwent bronchoscopy and bronchoalveolar lavage (BAL) on day 35 post-transplant. Patients with histologic, immunologic, or virologic evidence of CMV infection in the lung were then randomized to observation of CYTOVENE treatment (5 mg/kg BID for 14 days followed by 5 mg/kg QD 5 days/week until Day 120). Four of 20 (20%) CYTOVENE patients and 14 of 20 (70%) control patients developed interstitial pneumonia. The incidence of CMV disease was significantly lower in the group treated with CYTOVENE, consistent with the results observed in ICM 1689.

CONTRAINDICATIONS

CYTOVENE is contraindicated in patients with hypersensitivity to ganciclovir or acyclovir.

WARNINGS

Hematologic: CYTOVENE should not be administered if the absolute neutrophil count is less than 500 cells/mm³ or the platelet count is less than 25,000 cells/mm³. Granulocytopenia (neutropenia) and the thrombocytopenia have been observed in CYTOVENE treated patients. The frequency and severity of these events vary widely in different patient populations (see ADVERSE REACTIONS section).
CYTOVENE should, therefore, be used with caution in patients with pre-existing cytopenias, or with a history of cytopenic reactions to other drugs, chemicals or irradiation. Granulocytopenia usually occurs during the first or second

PATIENTS WITH POSITIVE CMV CULTURES

Time	Heart Allograft CYTOVENE	Heart Allograft Placebo	Bone Marrow Allograft CYTOVENE	Bone Marrow Allograft Placebo
Pre-Treatment	2% (1/67)	8% (5/64)	100% (37/37)	100% (35/35)
Week 2	3% (2/75)	16% (11/67)	6% (2/31)	68% (19/28)
Week 4	5% (3/66)	43% (28/66)	0% (0/24)	80% (16/20)

week of treatment, but may occur at any time during treatment. Cell counts usually begin to recover within 3 to 7 days of discontinuing the drug.

Impairment of Fertility: Animal data indicate that administration of CYTOVENE causes inhibition of spermatogenesis and subsequent infertility. These effects were reversible at lower doses and irreversible at higher doses (see Carcinogenesis, Mutagenesis, and Impairment of Fertility sections in PRECAUTIONS). *Although data in humans have not been obtained regarding this effect, it is considered probable that intravenous CYTOVENE at the recommended doses causes temporary or permanent inhibition of spermatogenesis. Animal data also indicate that suppression of fertility in females may occur.*

Teratogenesis: Because of the mutagenic potential of CYTOVENE, women of childbearing potential should be advised to use effective contraception during treatment. Similarly, male patients should be advised to practice barrier contraception during and for at least 90 days following treatment with CYTOVENE (see Pregnancy: Category C).

PRECAUTIONS

General

In clinical studies with CYTOVENE, the maximum single dose administered was 6 mg/kg by intravenous infusion over one hour. It is likely that larger doses, or more rapid infusions, would result in increased toxicity (see OVERDOSAGE section).

Administration of CYTOVENE by intravenous infusion should be accompanied by adequate hydration, since CYTOVENE is excreted by the kidneys and normal clearance depends on adequate renal function. **IF RENAL FUNCTION IS IMPAIRED, DOSAGE ADJUSTMENTS ARE REQUIRED.** Such adjustments should be based on measured or estimated creatinine clearance (see DOSAGE AND ADMINISTRATION section).

Initially reconstituted CYTOVENE solutions have a high pH (pH 11). Despite further dilution in intravenous fluids, phlebitis and/or pain may occur at the site of intravenous infusion. Care must be taken to infuse solutions containing CYTOVENE only into veins with adequate blood flow to permit rapid dilution and distribution (see DOSAGE AND ADMINISTRATION section).

Information for Patients

All patients should be informed that the major toxicities of ganciclovir are granulocytopenia (neutropenia) and thrombocytopenia and that dose modifications may be required, including discontinuation. The importance of close monitoring of blood counts while on therapy should be emphasized.

Patients should be advised that CYTOVENE has caused decreased sperm production in animals and may cause infertility in humans. Women of childbearing potential should be advised that CYTOVENE causes birth defects in animals and should not be used during pregnancy. Women of child bearing potential should be advised to use effective contraception during CYTOVENE treatment. Similarly, men should be advised to practice barrier contraception during and for at least 90 days following CYTOVENE treatment.

Patients should be advised that CYTOVENE causes tumors in animals. Although there is no information from human studies, CYTOVENE should be considered a potential carcinogen.

Patients with AIDS and CMV Retinitis: CYTOVENE is not a cure for CMV retinitis, and immunocompromised patients may continue to experience progression of retinitis during or following treatment. Patients should be advised to have ophthalmologic follow-up examinations at a minimum of every six weeks while being treated with CYTOVENE. (Many patients will require more frequent follow-up.)

Patients with AIDS may be receiving zidovudine (Retrovir). Patients should be counseled that treatment with both CYTOVENE and zidovudine simultaneously will not be tolerated by many patients, and may result in severe granulocytopenia (neutropenia).

Transplant Recipients: Transplant recipients should be counseled regarding the high frequency of impaired renal function in transplant recipients who received CYTOVENE in controlled clinical trials, particularly in patients receiving concomitant administration of nephrotoxic agents such as cyclosporine and amphotericin B. Although the specific mechanism of this transient toxicity has not been determined, the higher rate of renal impairment in patients receiving CYTOVENE compared to those who received placebo in the same trials may indicate that CYTOVENE played a significant role.

Laboratory Testing

Due to the frequency of granulocytopenia and thrombocytopenia in patients receiving CYTOVENE (see ADVERSE REACTIONS section), it is recommended that neutrophil counts and platelet counts be performed every two days during BID dosing of CYTOVENE and at least weekly thereafter. Neutrophil counts should be monitored daily in patients in whom CYTOVENE or other nucleoside analogues have previously resulted in leukopenia, or in whom neutrophil counts are less than 1,000 cells/mm^3 at the beginning of treatment. Because dosing must be modified in patients with renal impairment, patients should have serum creatinine or creatinine clearance monitored at least once every two weeks.

Drug Interactions

It is possible that probenecid, as well as other drugs that inhibit renal tubular secretion or resorption, may reduce renal clearance of CYTOVENE. It is also possible that drugs that inhibit replication of rapidly dividing cell populations such as bone marrow, spermatogonia, and germinal layers of skin and gastrointestinal mucosa may have additive toxicity when administered concomitantly with CYTOVENE. Therefore, drugs such as dapsone, pentamidine, flucytosine, vincristine, vinblastine, adriamycin, amphotericin B, trimethoprim/sulfa combinations or other nucleoside analogues, should be considered for concomitant use with CYTOVENE only if the potential benefits are judged to outweigh the risks.

Patients with AIDS may be receiving, or have received, treatment with zidovudine (Retrovir). *Since both zidovudine and CYTOVENE have the potential to cause granulocytopenia (neutropenia), many patients will not tolerate combination therapy with those two drugs at full dosage strength.* Data from 41 patients indicate that treatment with ganciclovir plus zidovudine at the recommended doses is not tolerated.[16]

Generalized seizures have been reported in seven patients who received CYTOVENE and imipenem-cilastatin. These drugs should not be used concomitantly with CYTOVENE unless the potential benefits outweigh the risks.

No formal drug interaction studies of CYTOVENE and drugs commonly used in transplant recipients have been conducted. Allograft recipients treated with CYTOVENE in three controlled clinical studies also received a variety of concomitant medications, including amphotericin B, azathioprine, cyclosporine, muromonab-CD3 (OKT3), and/or prednisone. Increases in serum creatinine were observed in patients treated with CYTOVENE plus either cyclosporine or amphotericin B, drugs with known potential for nephrotoxicity (see ADVERSE REACTIONS section).

Carcinogensis, Mutagenesis*

Ganciclovir was carcinogenic in the mouse at oral doses of 20 and 1000 mg/kg/day (approximately 0.1x and 1.4x, respectively, the mean drug exposure in humans following the recommended intravenous dose of 5 mg/kg, based on area under the plasma concentration curve (AUC) comparisons). At the dose of 1000 mg/kg/day there was a significant increase in the incidence of tumors of the preputial gland in males, forestomach (nonglandular mucosa) in males and females, and reproductive tissues, (ovaries, uterus, mammary gland, clitoral gland and vagina) and liver in females. At the dose of 20 mg/kg/day, a slightly increased incidence of tumors was noted in the preputial and harderian glands in males, forestomach in males and females, and liver in females. No carcinogenic effect was observed in mice administered ganciclovir at 1 mg/kg/day (estimated as 0.01x the human dose based on AUC comparison). Except for histiocytic sarcoma of the liver, ganciclovir induced tumors were generally of epithelial or vascular origin. Although the preputial and clitoral glands, forestomach, and harderian glands of mice do not have human counterparts, CYTOVENE should be considered a potential carcinogen in humans.

Ganciclovir increased mutations in mouse lymphoma cells and DNA damage in human lymphocytes in vitro at concentrations between 50–500 and 250–2000 μg/mL, respectively. In the mouse micronucleus assay, ganciclovir was clastogenic at doses of 150 and 500 mg/kg (IV) (2.8–10x human exposure based on AUC) but not 50 mg/kg (exposure approximately comparable to the human based on AUC). Ganciclovir was not mutagenic in the Ames Salmonella assay at concentrations of 500–5000 μg/mL.

Impairment of Fertility*

Ganciclovir caused decreased mating behavior, decreased fertility, and an increased incidence of embryolethality in female mice following intravenous doses of 90 mg/kg/day (approximately 1.7x the mean drug exposure in humans following the dose of 5 mg/kg, based on AUC comparisons). Ganciclovir caused decreased fertility in male mice and hypospermatogenesis in mice and dogs following daily oral or intravenous administration of doses ranging from 0.2–10 mg/kg. Systemic drug exposure (AUC) at the lowest dose showing toxicity in each species ranged from 0.03–0.1x the AUC of the recommended human intravenous dose.

Pregnancy: Category C*

CYTOVENE has been shown to be embryotoxic in rabbits and mice following intravenous administration. Fetal resorptions were present in at least 85% of rabbits and mice administered 60 mg/kg/day and 108 mg/kg/day (2x the human exposure based on AUC comparisons), respectively. Effects observed in rabbits included: fetal growth retardation, embryolethality, teratogenicity, and/or maternal toxicity. Teratogenic changes included cleft palate, anophthalmia/microphthalmia, aplastic organs (kidney and pancreas), hydrocephaly, and brachygnathia. In mice, effects observed were maternal/fetal toxicity and embryolethality.

Daily intravenous dose of 90 mg/kg administered to female mice prior to mating, during gestation, and during lactation caused hypoplasia of the testes and seminal vesicles in the month-old male offspring, as well as pathologic changes in the nonglandular region of the stomach (see Carcinogensis, Mutagenesis section). The drug exposure in mice as estimated by the AUC was approximately 1.7x the human AUC.

CYTOVENE may be teratogenic or embryotoxic at dose levels recommended for human use. There are no adequate and well-controlled studies in pregnant women. CYTOVENE should be used during pregnancy only if the potential benefits justify the potential risk to the fetus.

Nursing Mothers

It is not known if CYTOVENE is excreted in human milk. However, many drugs are excreted in human milk and, because carcinogenic and teratogenic effects occurred in animals treated with ganciclovir, the possibility of serious adverse reactions from ganciclovir in nursing infants is considered likely (see Pregnancy: Category C section). Mothers should be instructed to discontinue nursing if they are receiving CYTOVENE. The minimum interval before nursing can safely be resumed after the last dose of CYTOVENE is unknown.

Pediatric Use

SAFETY AND EFFICACY OF CYTOVENE IN CHILDREN HAVE NOT BEEN ESTABLISHED. THE USE OF *CYTOVENE* IN CHILDREN WARRANTS EXTREME CAUTION DUE TO THE PROBABILITY OF LONG-TERM CARCINOGENICITY AND REPRODUCTIVE TOXICITY. ADMINISTRATION TO CHILDREN SHOULD BE UNDERTAKEN ONLY AFTER CAREFUL EVALUATION AND ONLY IF THE POTENTIAL BENEFITS OF TREATMENT OUTWEIGH THE RISKS.

Adverse events reported in 120 immunocompromised children with serious CMV infections receiving ganciclovir were similar to those reported in adults. Granulocytopenia (17%) and thrombocytopenia (10%) were the most common adverse events reported.

There has been very limited clinical experience in treating cytomegalovirus retinitis in patients under the age of 12 years. Two children (ages 9 and 5 years) showed improvement or stabilization of retinitis for 23 and 9 months, respectively. These children received induction treatment with 2.5 mg/kg TID followed by maintenance therapy with 6–6.5 mg/kg once per day, five to seven days per week. When retinitis progressed during once daily maintenance therapy, both children were treated with 5 mg/kg BID regimen. Two other children (ages 2.5 and 4 years) who received similar induction regimens showed only partial or no response to treatment. Another child, a six year old with T-cell dysfunction, showed stabilization of retinitis for 3 months while receiving continuous infusions of CYTOVENE at doses of 2–5 mg/kg/24 hours. Continuous infusion treatment was discontinued due to granulocytopenia. Pharmacokinetic data have not been obtained in pediatric patients.

Eleven of the 72 patients in the placebo-controlled trial in bone marrow transplant recipients were children, ranging in age from 3 to 10 years of age (5 CYTOVENE-treated and 6 placebo-treated). All of the CYTOVENE treated pediatric patients received CYTOVENE 5 mg/kg BID for 7 days and then 5 mg/kg QD until day 100 post-transplant. Results were similar to those observed in the CYTOVENE treated adult transplant recipients. Two of the 6 placebo-treated pediatric patients developed CMV pneumonia, versus none of the 5 CYTOVENE-treated patients. Toxicity in the pediatric group was similar to that observed in the adult patients.

Use in Patients with Renal Impairment

CYTOVENE should be used with caution in patients with impaired renal function because the plasma half-life and peak plasma levels of CYTOVENE will be increased due to reduced renal clearance (see DOSAGE AND ADMINISTRATION and ADVERSE REACTIONS: Renal Toxicity sections).

Data from 4 patients indicate that CYTOVENE plasma levels are reduced approximately 50% following hemodialysis.

Use in the Elderly

No studies of the efficacy or safety of CYTOVENE in elderly patients have been conducted. Since elderly individuals frequently have reduced glomerular filtration, particular attention should be paid to assessing renal function before and during CYTOVENE administration (see DOSAGE AND ADMINISTRATION section).

ADVERSE REACTIONS

During clinical trials, CYTOVENE was withdrawn or interrupted in approximately 32% of patients because of adverse events. In some instances treatment was restarted and the

Continued on next page

FOOTNOTE

* All dose comparisons presented in the Carcinogenesis and Mutagenesis, Impairment of Fertility, and Pregnancy: Category C sections are based on the human AUC following administration of a single 5 mg/kg intravenous infusion as used during the maintenance phase of treatment. Because human exposure is approximately doubled during the induction phase of treatment (5 mg/kg, BID) the cross-species dose comparisons should be divided by 2.

Syntex—Cont.

reappearance of adverse events again necessitated withdrawal or interruption.

Hematologic Toxicity: The most frequent adverse events seen in patients treated with CYTOVENE are granulocytopenia/neutropenia and thrombocytopenia.

In most cases, withdrawal of CYTOVENE resulted in increased neutrophil or platelet counts. While granulocytopenia was generally reversible with discontinuation of treatment, some patients experienced irreversible neutropenia or died with severe bacterial or fungal infections during neutropenia episodes.

The following table shows the frequency of granulocytopenia and thrombocytopenia observed in CYTOVENE clinical trials.

[See table below.]

Adverse events other than granulocytopenia and thrombocytopenia were reported as "probably related", "probably not related", and "unknown" in relationship to CYTOVENE therapy. Evaluation of these reports was difficult because of the protean manifestations of the underlying disease, and because most patients received numerous concomitant medications.

Renal Toxicity: In a placebo-controlled clinical trial (ICM 1496) conducted in heart allograft recipients treated with CYTOVENE, patients receiving CYTOVENE had more elevation of serum creatinine to values exceeding 2.5 mg/dL than patients receiving placebo (18% vs. 4%, respectively). These increases in serum creatinine, up to 5.5 mg/dL in one patient, were transient and occurred primarily during the first week of CYTOVENE treatment. In another randomized, but unblinded study of CYTOVENE in bone marrow allograft recipients, more CYTOVENE-treated patients than untreated patients experienced serum creatinine values exceeding 1.5 mg/dL (70% vs. 35%, respectively). These elevations in serum creatinine, up to 3.2 mg/dL in one patient, were transient and occurred intermittently throughout the 3 month study. Most patients in these studies received cyclosporine. The mechanism of impairment of renal function (whether it is the result of an interaction between CYTOVENE and cyclosporine or other nephrotoxic agents) is not known. However, careful monitoring of renal function during CYTOVENE therapy is essential, especially for those patients receiving concomitant agents that may cause nephrotoxicity.

CNS Toxicity: In two placebo-controlled trials in transplant recipients, headache (17% vs. 11%, respectively), and confusion (6% vs. 1%, respectively) were noted to occur more frequently in CYTOVENE-treated patients than in placebo-treated patients.

Other Toxicities: In the same two studies, sepsis was observed more frequently in the CYTOVENE-treated patients than in the placebo-treated patients (6% vs 2%, respectively).

Retinal Detachment
Retinal detachment has been observed in patients with CMV retinitis both before and after initiation of CYTOVENE therapy. The relationship of retinal detachment to CYTOVENE therapy is unknown. Patients with CMV retinitis should have frequent ophthalmologic evaluations to monitor the status of their retinitis and detect any other retinal lesions.

General: Other than leukopenia and thrombocytopenia, the most frequent adverse events observed in over 5,000 patients who received CYTOVENE were anemia, fever, rash, and abnormal liver function values, each of which was reported in approximately 2% of treated patients. Adverse events that were thought to be possibly related to drug and oc-

curred in 1% or fewer patients who received CYTOVENE were:
Body as a Whole: chills, edema, infections, malaise
Cardiovascular System: arrhythmia, hypertension, hypotension
Central Nervous System: abnormal thoughts or dreams, ataxia, coma, confusion, dizziness, headache, nervousness, paresthesia, psychosis, somnolence, tremor (Overall, neurologic system events occurred in 5% of patients.)
Digestive System: nausea, vomiting, anorexia, diarrhea, hemorrhage, abdominal pain
Hematologic System: eosinophilia
Laboratory Abnormalities: decrease in blood glucose
Respiratory System: dyspnea
Skin and Appendages: alopecia, pruritus, urticaria
Urogenital System: hematuria, increased blood urea nitrogen (BUN)
Injection Site: Inflammation, pain, phlebitis

OVERDOSAGE

Overdosage with CYTOVENE has been reported in eleven patients. In three of these patients, no adverse events were observed after the overdosage. (The doses received were: 7 doses of 11 mg/kg over a 3-day period, 9 mg/kg BID for 3 days, and 2 doses of 500 mg given to a 21 month old child.) An eighteen month old child received a single dose of approximately 60 mg/kg and was given an exchange transfusion. No adverse events were noted. A four month old child received a 500 mg dose (72.5 mg/kg) and no adverse events were noted. The child underwent 48 hours of peritoneal dialysis and was doing well at the completion.

Irreversible pancytopenia was reported following overdose in one 28 year old AIDS patient with CMV colitis and abdominal pain who inadvertently received 3000 mg of CYTOVENE on each of two consecutive days. After the second dosage the patient became anorexic and had more severe abdominal pain, substernal pain, vomiting and lethargy. The patient was dialyzed twice for acute renal failure. Two weeks following the overdose he was noted to be pancytopenic. The patient continued to have persistent bone marrow suppression and pancytopenia, until his death from a malignancy several months later.

Reversible neutropenia was reported following overdoses in three patients: one patient had a history of bone marrow depression prior to treatment and received CYTOVENE 5 mg/kg BID for 14 days followed by 8 mg/kg given as single daily doses for 4 days; one patient received a single dose of 1,675 mg (approximately 24 mg/kg); and a 60 year old man with preexisting neutropenia received a single dose of 20 mg/kg CYTOVENE. In all cases the neutropenia was reversible (after 17 days, 1 day, and 9 days, respectively) following discontinuation of CYTOVENE.

A nineteen year old patient with a history of renal insufficiency and hematuria received a single dose of 500 mg CYTOVENE and developed a worsening of the hematuria, which resolved in 2 days. During evaluation for renal insufficiency (creatinine 5.2 mg/dL), a 33 year old patient reported that 4 days prior to the evaluation, he had intentionally self administered a single dose of 5 to 7 g of CYTOVENE; no hematologic abnormalities were noted and the relationship of the overdosage to his renal insufficiency is unknown.

Hemodialysis and hydration may be of benefit in reducing drug plasma levels in patients who receive an overdosage of CYTOVENE.

Creatinine clearance for males = $\dfrac{(140 - \text{age [yrs]}) (\text{body wt [kg]})}{(72) (\text{serum creatinine [mg/dL]})}$

Creatinine clearance for females = $0.85 \times \text{male value}$

DOSAGE AND ADMINISTRATION

CAUTION—DO NOT ADMINISTER *CYTOVENE* BY RAPID OR BOLUS INTRAVENOUS INJECTION. THE TOXICITY OF *CYTOVENE* MAY BE INCREASED AS A RESULT OF EXCESSIVE PLASMA LEVELS.
CAUTION—INTRAMUSCULAR OR SUBCUTANEOUS INJECTION OF RECONSTITUTED *CYTOVENE* MAY RESULT IN SEVERE TISSUE IRRITATION DUE TO HIGH pH (11).
Dosage
THE RECOMMENDED DOSAGE, FREQUENCY, OR INFUSION RATES SHOULD NOT BE EXCEEDED.

For Treatment of CMV Rentinitis:
1. **Induction Treatment.** The recommended initial dose for patients with normal renal function is 5 mg/kg (given intravenously at a constant rate over 1 hour) every 12 hours for 14–21 days.
2. **Maintenance Treatment.** Following induction treatment the recommended dose of CYTOVENE is 5 mg/kg given as an intravenous infusion over one hour once per day on seven days each week, or 6 mg/kg once per day on five days each week. Patients who experience progression of retinitis while receiving maintenance therapy may be retreated with the BID regimen.

For the Prevention of CMV Disease in Transplant Recipients
The recommended initial dose for patients with normal renal function is 5 mg/kg (given intravenously at the constant rate over 1 hour) every 12 hours for 7 to 14 days, followed by 5 mg/kg once per day on seven days each week, or 6 mg/kg once per day on five days each week.

The duration of treatment with CYTOVENE in transplant recipients is dependent upon the duration and degree of immunosuppression. In controlled clinical trials in bone marrow allograft recipients, treatment was continued until day 100 to 120 post-transplantation. CMV disease occurred in several patients who discontinued treatment with CYTOVENE prematurely. In heart allograft recipients, the onset of newly diagnosed CMV disease occurred after CYTOVENE treatment was stopped at day 28 post-transplant, suggesting that continued dosing may be necessary to prevent late occurrence of CMV disease in this patient population. (See Indications and Usage section for a more detailed discussion.)

Renal Impairment
For patients with impairment of renal function, refer to the table below for recommended doses during the induction phase of treatment, and adjust the dosing interval as indicated.

Creatinine Clearance* (mL/min)	CYTOVENE Dose (mg/kg)	Dosing Interval (hours)
≥80	5.0	12
50–79	2.5	12
25–49	2.5	24
<25	1.25	24

*Creatinine clearance can be related to serum creatinine by the following formulae: [See table above.]

The optimal maintenance dose for patients with renal impairment is not known. Physicians may elect to reduce the dose to 50% of the induction dose and monitor the patient for disease progression.

	Uncontrolled Trials		Controlled Trials—Transplant Recipients			
	Persons w/AIDS	Transplant Recipients	Heart Allograft*		Bone Marrow Allograft**	
	CYTOVENE (n=532)	CYTOVENE (n=207)	CYTOVENE (n=76)	Placebo (n=73)	CYTOVENE (n=57)	Control (n=55)
Granulocytopenia/Neutropenia						
ANC <500/µL	18%	11%	4%	3%	12%	6%
ANC 500–1000/µL	24%	10%	3%	8%	29%	17%
TOTAL ANC ≤1,000 µL	42%	21%	7%	11%	41%	23%
Thrombocytopenia						
Platelet counts <25,000/µL	4%	22%	3%	1%	32%	28%
Platelet counts 25,000–50,000/µL	9%	23%	5%	3%	25%	37%
TOTAL Platelets ≤50,000 µL	13%	45%	8%	4%	57%	65%

*Mean duration of treatment = 28 days
**Mean duration of treatment = 45 days
(See discussion of clinical trials under **INDICATIONS AND USAGE** section.)

Only limited data are available on CYTOVENE elimination in patients undergoing hemodialysis. Dosing for these patients should not exceed 1.25 mg/kg/24 hours. On days when hemodialysis is performed, the dose should be given shortly after the completion of the hemodialysis session, since hemodialysis has been shown to reduce plasma levels by approximately 50%. Neutrophil and platelet counts should be monitored daily.

Patient Monitoring
Due to the frequency of granulocytopenia and thrombocytopenia in patients receiving CYTOVENE (see ADVERSE REACTIONS section), it is recommended that neutrophil counts and platelet counts be performed every two days during BID dosing of CYTOVENE and at least weekly thereafter. In patients in whom CYTOVENE or other nucleoside analogues have previously resulted in leukopenia, or in whom neutrophil counts are less than 1,000 cells/mm³ at the beginning of treatment, neutrophil counts should be monitored daily. Because dosing must be modified in patients with renal impairment, all patients should have serum creatinine or creatinine clearance monitored at least once every two weeks.

Reduction of Dose
The most frequently observed adverse event following treatment with CYTOVENE is leukopenia/neutropenia (see ADVERSE REACTION section).
Therefore, frequent white blood cell counts should be performed. Severe neutropenia (ANC less than 500/mm³) or severe thrombocytopenia (platelets less than 25,000/mm³) requires a dose interruption until evidence of marrow recovery is observed (ANC ≥ 750/mm³).

Method of Preparation
Each 10 mL clear glass vial contains ganciclovir sodium equivalent to 500 mg of the free base form of CYTOVENE and 46 mg of sodium. The contents of the vial should be prepared for administration in the following manner:

1. Reconstituted Solution:
  a. Lyophilized CYTOVENE should be reconstituted by injecting 10 mL of Sterile Water for Injection, USP, into the vial.
DO NOT USE BACTERIOSTATIC WATER FOR INJECTION CONTAINING PARABENS. IT IS INCOMPATIBLE WITH *CYTOVENE* STERILE POWDER AND MAY CAUSE PRECIPITATION.
  b. The vial should be shaken to dissolve the drug.
  c. Reconstituted solution should be inspected visually for particulate matter and discoloration prior to proceeding with infusion solution. If particulate matter or discoloration is observed, the vial should be discarded.
  d. Reconstituted solution in the vial is stable at room temperature for 12 hours. It should not be refrigerated.

2. Infusion Solution
Based on patient weight, the appropriate calculated dose volume should be removed from the vial (ganciclovir concentration 50 mg/mL) and added to an acceptable (see below) infusion fluid (typically 100 mL) for delivery over the course of one hour. Infusion concentrations greater than 10 mg/mL are not recommended. The following infusion fluids have been determined to be chemically and physically compatible with CYTOVENE: 0.9% Sodium Chloride, 5% Dextrose, Ringer's Injection, and Lactated Ringer's Injection, USP.
Note: Because non-bacteriostatic infusion fluid must be used with CYTOVENE, the infusion solution must be used within 24 hours of dilution to reduce the risk of bacterial contamination. The infusion solution should be refrigerated. Freezing is not recommended.

Handling and Disposal
Caution should be exercised in the handling and preparation of CYTOVENE solutions. CYTOVENE solutions are alkaline (pH 11). Avoid direct contact with the skin or mucous membranes. If such contact occurs, wash thoroughly with soap and water; rinse eyes thoroughly with plain water. Because CYTOVENE shares some of the properties of antitumor agents (i.e., carcinogenicity and mutagenicity), consideration should be given to handling and disposal according to guidelines issued for antineoplastic drugs. Several guidelines on this subject have been published.[17-22]
There is no general agreement that all of the procedures recommended in the guidelines are necessary or appropriate.

HOW SUPPLIED
CYTOVENE® (ganciclovir sodium) Sterile Powder is supplied in 10 mL sterile vials, each containing ganciclovir sodium equivalent to 500 mg of ganciclovir, in cartons of 25 (NDC 0033-2903-48).
Store below 40°C (104°F).
CAUTION: Federal law prohibits dispensing without prescription.

REFERENCES
1. Smee D.F., Boehme R., Chernow M., et al: Intracellular metabolism and enzymatic phosphorylation of 9-(1,3-dihydroxy-2-propoxymethyl) guanine and acyclovir in herpes simplex virus-infected and uninfected cells. *Biochemical Pharmacol* 1985; 34:1049–1056.
2. Shanley J.D., Morningstar J., Jordan M.C.: Inhibition of murine cytomegalovirus lung infection and interstitial pneumonitis by acyclovir and 9-(1,3-dihydroxy-2-propoxymethyl) guanine. *Antimicrob Agents Chemother* 1985; 28: 172–175.
3. Wilson E. J., Medearis D.N. Jr., Hansen L.A., et al: 9-(1,3-dihydroxy-2-propoxymethyl) guanine prevents death but not immunity in murine cytomegalovirus-infected normal and immunosuppressed BALB/c mice, *Antimicrob Agents Chemother* 1987; 31:1017–1020.
4. Fong C.K.Y., Cohen S.D., McCormick S., Hsiung G.D.: Antiviral Effect of 9-(1,3-dihydroxy-2-propoxymethyl) guanine against cytomegalovirus infection in a guinea pig model. *Antiviral Res* 1987; 7: 11–23.
5. Buhles W.C., Mastre B.J., Tinker A.J., et al: Ganciclovir Treatment of Life- or Sight-Threatening Cytomegalovirus Infection: Experience in 314 immunocompromised Patients. *Rev Inf Dis* 1988; 10:495–506.
6. Merigan, T.C., Renlund, D.G., et al: A Controlled Trial of Ganciclovir to Prevent Cytomegalovirus Disease After Heart Transplantation. *NEJM* 1992; 326: 1182–1186.
7. Goodrich, J.M., Mori, M., et al: Early Treatment With Ganciclovir To Prevent Cytomegalovirus Disease After Allogenic Bone Marow Transplantation. *NEJM* 1991; 325: 1601–1607.
8. Erice A., Chou S., Byron K.K., et al: Progressive disease due to ganciclovir-resistant cytomegalovirus in immunocompromised patients. *NEJM* 1989; 320:289–293.
9. Drew, W.L., Miner, R.C., et al: Prevalence of Resistance In Patients Receiving Ganciclovir For Serious Cytomegalovirus Infection. *J. Infect. Dis.* 1991; 163: 716–719.
10. Jacobson, M.A., Drew, W.L., Feinberg, J., et al.: Foscarnet Therapy for Ganciclovir-Resistant Cytomegalovirus Retinitis in AIDS. *J. Infect. Dis.* 1991; 163: 1348–1351.
11. Fletcher C., Balfour H.: Evaluation of ganciclovir for cytomegalovirus disease. *DICP, Ann Pharmacother* 1989; 23:5–12.
12. Fletcher C., Sawchuk R., Chinnock B., et al: Human pharmacokinetics of the antiviral drug DHPG. *Clin Pharmacol Ther* 1986; 40:281–286.
13. Jabs D., Enger E., Bartlett J.: Cytomegalovirus retinitis and acquired immunodeficiency syndrome. *Arch Ophthalmol* 1989; 107:75–80.
14. Updated unpublished data on file with Syntex Corp.
15. Schmidt, G., Horak, D., et al: A Randomized, Controlled Trial of Prophylactic Ganciclovir For Cytomegalovirus Pulmonary Infection In Recipients of Allogenic Bone Marrow Transplants. *NEJM* 1991; 15: 1005–1011.
16. Hochster, H., et al: Toxicity of Combined Ganciclovir and Zidovudine for Cytomegalovirus Disease Associated with AIDS. *Annals of Internal Medicine,* 1990; 113: 111–117.
17. Recommendations for the Safe Handling of Parenteral Antineoplastic Drugs. NIH Publication No. 83-2621. For sale by the Superintendent of Documents, U.S. Government Printing Office, Washington, D.C. 20402.
18. AMA Council Report. Guidelines for Handling Parenteral Antineoplastics. *JAMA*, March 15, 1985.
19. National Study Commission on Cytotoxic Exposure-Recommendations for Handling Cytotoxic Agents. Available from Louis P. Jeffrey, Sc. D., Director of Pharmacy Services, Rhode Island Hospital, 593 Eddy Street, Providence, Rhode Island 02902.
20. Clinical Oncological Society of Australia: Guidelines and recommendations for safe handling of antineoplastic agents. *Med J Australia* 1983; 1:426–428.
21. Jones R.B., et al. Safe handling of chemotherapeutic agents: A report from the Mount Sinai Medical Center, CA—*A Cancer Journal for Clinicians* 1983; 33: 258–263.
22. American Society of Hospital Pharmacists technical assistance bulletin on handling cytotoxic drugs in hospitals. *Am J Hosp Pharm* 1985; 42:131–137.

Mfd. for Syntex Labortories, Inc. Palo Alto, CA 94304
Mfd. by Ben Venue Laboratories, Inc. Bedford, OH 44146
U.S. Patent No. 4,355,032; 4,507,305 and others.
02-2903-48-04
© 1992 Syntex Laboratories, Inc.   Revised June 1992
Shown in Product Identification Section, page 433

FEMSTAT®   ℞
[fem 'stat]
(butoconazole nitrate)
Vaginal Cream 2%

A product of Syntex Laboratories, Inc.

DESCRIPTION
FEMSTAT Vaginal Cream contains butoconazole nitrate 2%, an imidazole derivative with antifungal activity. Its chemical name is (±)-1-[4-(*p* -Chlorophenyl)-2-[(2,6-dichlorophenyl) thio]butyl] imidazole mononitrate.
Butoconazole nitrate is a white to off-white crystalline powder with a molecular weight of 474.79. It is sparingly soluble in methanol; slightly soluble in chloroform, methylene chloride, acetone and ethanol; very slightly soluble in ethyl acetate; and practically insoluble in water. It melts at about 159°C with decomposition.
FEMSTAT Vaginal Cream contains butoconazole nitrate 2% in a water-washable emollient cream of cetyl alcohol, glyceryl stearate (and) PEG-100 stearate, methylparaben and propylparaben (preservatives), mineral oil, polysorbate 60, propylene glycol, sorbitan monostearate, stearyl alcohol and water (purified).

CLINICAL PHARMACOLOGY
Butoconazole nitrate is an imidazole derivative that has fungicidal activity *in vitro* against *Candida, Trichophyton, Microsporum,* and *Epidermophyton.* It is also active *in vitro* against some gram positive bacteria. Clinically, it is highly effective against vaginal infections induced by strains of *Candida albicans, Candida tropicalis,* and other species of this genus.
The primary site of action of imidazoles appears to be the cell membrane. The permeability of the cell membrane is altered, resulting in a reduced osmotic resistance and viability of the fungus. The exact mechanism of the antifungal activity of butoconazole nitrate is not known.
Following vaginal administration of butoconazole nitrate, 5.5% of the dose is absorbed on average. After vaginal administration peak plasma levels of the drug and its metabolites are attained at 24 hours and the plasma half-life is approximately 21–24 hours.

INDICATIONS AND USAGE
FEMSTAT Vaginal Cream is indicated for the local treatment of vulvovaginal mycotic infections caused by *Candida* species. The diagnosis should be confirmed by KOH smears and/or cultures.
FEMSTAT Vaginal Cream can be used in association with oral contraceptive and antibiotic therapy. FEMSTAT is effective in both non-pregnant and pregnant women, but in pregnant women it should be used only during the second and third trimesters.

CONTRAINDICATIONS
FEMSTAT Vaginal Cream 2% is contraindicated in patients with a history of hypersensitivity to any of the components of the cream.

PRECAUTIONS
General
If clinical symptoms persist, microbiological tests should be repeated to rule out other pathogens and to confirm the diagnosis.
If sensitization or irritation is reported during use, the treatment should be discontinued.
Information for the Patient
The patient should be cautioned against premature discontinuation of the medication during menstruation or in response to relief of symptoms.
Carcinogenesis
Long-term studies in animals have not been performed to evaluate the carcinogenic potential of this drug.
Mutagenesis
Butoconazole nitrate was not mutagenic when tested on microbial indicator organisms.
Impairment of Fertility
No impairment of fertility was seen in rabbits or rats administered butoconazole nitrate in oral doses up to 30 mg/kg/day or 100 mg/kg/day respectively.
Pregnancy
Pregnancy Category C.
In pregnant rats administered 6 mg/kg/day (3–7 times the human dose) butoconazole nitrate intravaginally during the period of organogenesis, there was an increase in resorption rate and decrease in litter size, but no teratogenicity. Butoconazole nitrate had no apparent adverse effect when administered orally to pregnant rats throughout organogenesis, at dose levels up to 50 mg/kg/day. Daily oral doses of 100, 300, or 750 mg/kg resulted in fetal malformations (abdominal wall defects, cleft palate), but maternal stress was evident at these higher dose levels. There were no adverse effects on litters of rabbits receiving butoconazole nitrate orally, even at maternally stressful dose levels (e.g., 150 mg/kg). There are no adequate and well-controlled studies in pregnant women during the first trimester.
Butoconazole nitrate, like other azole antimycotic agents, causes dystocia in rats when treatment is extended through parturition. However, this effect was not apparent in rabbits treated with as much as 100 mg/kg/day orally.
In clinical studies, over 200 pregnant patients have used butoconazole nitrate cream 2% for 3 or 6 days during the second or third trimester and the drug had no adverse effect on the course of pregnancy. Follow-up reports available on infants born to these women reveal no adverse effects or complications that were attributable to the drug.

Continued on next page

Syntex—Cont.

Nursing Mothers
It is not known whether this drug is excreted in human milk. Because many drugs are excreted in human milk, caution should be exercised when butoconazole nitrate is administered to a nursing woman.
Pediatric Use
Safety and effectiveness in children have not been established.

ADVERSE REACTIONS
Of the 561 patients treated with butoconazole nitrate cream 2% for 3 or 6 days in controlled clinical trials, 13 (2.3%) reported complaints probably related to therapy. Vulvar/vaginal burning occurred in 2.3%, vulvar itching in 0.9%, and discharge, soreness, swelling, and itching of the fingers each occurred in 0.2%. Nine patients (1.6%) discontinued because of these complaints.

DOSAGE AND ADMINISTRATION
Non-pregnant Patients: The recommended dose is one applicatorful of cream (approximately 5 grams) intravaginally at bedtime for three days. Treatment can be extended for an additional three days if necessary.
Pregnant Patients (2nd and 3rd trimesters only): The recommended dose is one applicatorful of cream (approximately 5 grams) intravaginally at bedtime for six days.

HOW SUPPLIED
FEMSTAT® (butoconazole nitrate) Vaginal Cream 2% is available in a 28-gram tube with 3 disposable measured-dose applicators (NDC 0033-2280-14).
Store at room temperature. Avoid excessive heat, above 40°C (104°F), and avoid freezing.
Caution: Federal law prohibits dispensing without prescription.
U.S. Patent No. 4,078,071   Revised 3/90
02-2280-72-00

© 1988 Syntex Laboratories, Inc.
Shown in Product Identification Section, page 433

FEMSTAT® PREFILL   ℞
(butoconazole nitrate)
Vaginal Cream 2%
Prefilled Applicator

A product of Syntex Laboratories, Inc.
DESCRIPTION
FEMSTAT Vaginal Cream contains butoconazole nitrate 2%, an imidazole derivative with antifungal activity. Its chemical name is (±)-1-[4-(*p*-Chlorophenyl)-2-[(2,6-dichlorophenyl) thio]butyl] imidazole mononitrate.
Butoconazole nitrate is a white to off-white crystalline powder with a molecular weight of 474.79. It is sparingly soluble in methanol; slightly soluble in chloroform, methylene chloride, acetone and ethanol; very slightly soluble in ethyl acetate; and practically insoluble in water. It melts at about 159°C with decomposition.
FEMSTAT Vaginal Cream contains butoconazole nitrate 2% in a water-washable emollient cream of stearyl alcohol, propylene glycol, cetyl alcohol, sorbitan monostearate, glyceryl stearate (and) PEG-100 stearate, mineral oil, polysorbate 60, purified water, with methylparaben and propylparaben as preservatives.

CLINICAL PHARMACOLOGY
Butoconazole nitrate is an imidazole derivative that has fungicidal activity *in vitro* against *Candida, Trichophyton, Microsporum,* and *Epidermophyton.* It is also active against some gram positive bacteria. Clinically, it is highly effective against vaginal infections induced by strains of *Candida albicans, Candida tropicalis,* and other species of this genus. The primary site of action of imidazoles appears to be the cell membrane. The permeability of the cell membrane is altered, resulting in a reduced osmotic resistance and viability of the fungus. The exact mechanism of antifungal activity of butoconazole nitrate is not known.
Following vaginal administration of butoconazole nitrate, 5.5% of the dose is absorbed on average. After vaginal administration peak plasma levels of the drug and its metabolites are attained at 24 hours and the plasma half-life is approximately 21–24 hours.

INDICATIONS AND USAGE
FEMSTAT Vaginal Cream is indicated for the local treatment of vulvovaginal mycotic infections caused by *Candida* species. The diagnosis should be confirmed by KOH smears and/or cultures.
FEMSTAT Vaginal Cream can be used in association with oral contraceptive and antibiotic therapy. FEMSTAT is effective in both non-pregnant and pregnant women, but in pregnant women it should be used only during the second and third trimesters.

CONTRAINDICATIONS
FEMSTAT Vaginal Cream 2% is contraindicated in patients with a history of hypersensitivity to any of the components of the cream.

PRECAUTIONS
General:
If clinical symptoms persist, microbiological tests should be repeated to rule out other pathogens and to confirm the diagnosis.
If sensitization or irritation is reported during use, the treatment should be discontinued.
Information for the Patient:
The patient should be cautioned against premature discontinuation of the medication during menstruation or in response to relief of symptoms.
Carcinogenesis:
Long-term studies in animals have not been performed to evaluate the carcinogenic potential of this drug.
Mutagenesis:
Butoconazole nitrate was not mutagenic when tested on microbial indicator organisms.
Impairment of Fertility:
No impairment of fertility was seen in rabbits or rats administered butoconazole nitrate in oral doses up to 30 mg/kg/day or 100 mg/kg/day respectively.
Pregnancy:
Pregnancy Category C. In pregnant rats administered 6 mg/kg/day (3–7 times the human dose) butoconazole nitrate intravaginally during the period of organogenesis, there was an increase in resorption rate and decrease in litter size, but no teratogenicity. Butoconazole nitrate had no apparent adverse effect when administered orally to pregnant rats throughout organogenesis, at dose levels up to 50 mg/kg/day. Daily oral doses of 100, 300, or 750 mg/kg resulted in fetal malformations (abdominal wall defects, cleft palate), but maternal stress was evident at these higher dose levels. There were no adverse effects on litters of rabbits receiving butoconazole nitrate orally, even at maternally stressful dose levels (e.g., 150 mg/kg). There are no adequate and well-controlled studies in pregnant women during the first trimester.
Butoconazole nitrate, like other azole antimycotic agents, causes dystocia in rats when treatment is extended through parturition. However, this effect was not apparent in rabbits treated with as much as 100 mg/kg/day orally.
In clinical studies, over 200 pregnant patients have used butoconazole nitrate cream 2% for 3 or 6 days during the second or third trimester and the drug had no adverse effect on the course of pregnancy. Follow-up reports available on infants born to these women reveal no adverse effects or complications that were attributable to the drug.
Nursing Mothers:
It is not known whether this drug is excreted in human milk. Because many drugs are excreted in human milk, caution should be exercised when butoconazole nitrate is administered to a nursing woman.
Pediatric Use:
Safety and effectiveness in children have not been established.

ADVERSE REACTIONS
Of the 561 patients treated with butoconazole nitrate cream 2% for 3 or 6 days in controlled clinical trials, 13 (2.3%) reported complaints probably related to therapy. Vulvar/vaginal burning occurred in 2.3%, vulvar itching in 0.9%, and discharge, soreness, swelling, and itching of the fingers each occurred in 0.2%. Nine patients (1.6%) discontinued because of these complaints.

DOSAGE AND ADMINISTRATION
Non-pregnant Patients: The recommended dose is one applicatorful of cream (approximately 5 grams) intravaginally at bedtime for three days. Treatment can be extended for an additional three days if necessary.
Pregnant Patients (2nd and 3rd trimesters only): The recommended dose is one applicatorful of cream (approximately 5 grams) intravaginally at bedtime for six days.

HOW SUPPLIED
FEMSTAT® PREFILL (butoconazole nitrate) Vaginal Cream 2% is available in cartons containing 3 single dose prefilled disposable applicators (NDC 0033-2280-16).
Store at room temperature. Avoid excessive heat, above 40°C (104°F), and avoid freezing.
CAUTION: Federal law prohibits dispensing without prescription.
U.S. Patent Nos. 4,078,071 and 4,636,202   March 1988
02-2280-16-03

© 1988 Syntex Laboratories, Inc.
Shown in Product Identification Section, page 433

LIDEX®   ℞
[*li'dex*]
(fluocinonide)
Cream 0.05%
Gel 0.05%
Ointment 0.05%
Topical Solution 0.05%

LIDEX–E®   ℞
(fluocinonide)
Cream 0.05%

CARMOL® HC   ℞
[*kahr'mawl*]
(hydrocortisone acetate)
Cream 1%

NEO-SYNALAR® Cream   ℞
[*ne"o sin'ă-lahr*]
[neomycin sulfate 0.5% (0.35% neomycin base), fluocinolone acetonide 0.025%]

SYNACORT®   ℞
[*sin'ă-cort*]
(hydrocortisone)
Cream 1%
Cream 2.5%

SYNALAR®   ℞
[*sin'ă-lahr*]
(fluocinolone acetonide)
Cream 0.025%
Cream 0.01%
Ointment 0.025%
Topical Solution 0.01%

SYNALAR–HP®   ℞
(fluocinolone acetonide)
Cream 0.2%

SYNEMOL®   ℞
[*sin'ĕ-mol*]
(fluocinolone acetonide)
Cream 0.025%

Products of Syntex Laboratories, Inc.

DESCRIPTION
These preparations are all intended for topical administration.
LIDEX preparations have as their active component the corticosteroid fluocinonide, which is the 21-acetate ester of fluocinolone acetonide and has the chemical name pregna-1,4-diene-3,20-dione, 21-(acetyloxy)-6,9-difluoro-11-hydroxy-16,17-[(1-methylethylidene)bis(oxy)]-, (6α,11β, 16α)-.
LIDEX cream contains fluocinonide 0.5 mg/g in FAPG® cream, a specially formulated cream base consisting of citric acid, 1,2,6-hexanetriol, polyethylene glycol 8000, propylene glycol and stearyl alcohol. This white cream vehicle is greaseless, non-staining, anhydrous and completely water miscible. The base provides emollient and hydrophilic properties. In this formulation the active ingredient is totally in solution.
LIDEX gel contains fluocinonide 0.5 mg/g in a specially formulated gel base consisting of carbomer 940, edetate disodium, propyl gallate, propylene glycol, sodium hydroxide and/or hydrochloric acid (to adjust the pH), and water (purified). This clear, colorless thixotropic vehicle is greaseless, non-staining and completely water miscible. In this formulation the active ingredient is totally in solution.
LIDEX ointment contains fluocinonide 0.5 mg/g in a specially formulated ointment base consisting of glyceryl monostearate, white petrolatum, propylene carbonate, propylene glycol, and white wax. It provides the occlusive and emollient effects desirable in an ointment. In this formulation the active ingredient is totally in solution.
LIDEX topical solution contains fluocinonide 0.5 mg/mL in a solution of alcohol (35%), citric acid, diisopropyl adipate, and propylene glycol. In this formulation the active ingredient is totally in solution.
LIDEX-E cream contains fluocinonide 0.5 mg/g in a water-washable aqueous emollient base of cetyl alcohol, citric acid, mineral oil, polysorbate 60, propylene glycol, sorbitan monostearate, stearyl alcohol, and water (purified).
CARMOL HC Cream has the corticosteroid hydrocortisone acetate, which has the chemical name pregn-4-ene-3,20-dione,21-(acetyloxy)-11,17-dihydroxy-,(11β)-, as its active component. CARMOL HC contains micronized hydrocortisone acetate, USP, 10 mg/g, in a water-washable vanishing cream containing carbomer 940, cetyl alcohol, edetate disodium, isopropyl myristate, isopropyl palmitate, PPG-26 oleate, propylene glycol, sodium metabisulfite, sodium laureth sulfate, stearic acid, trolamine, urea (10%), water (purified), and xanthan gum; scented with hypoallergenic perfume.
CARMOL HC is non-lipid, non-occlusive and hypoallergenic; it contains no mineral oil, petrolatum, lanolin or parabens.

NEO-SYNALAR cream contains neomycin sulfate 5 mg/g (3.5 mg/g neomycin base) and fluocinolone acetonide 0.25 mg/g in a water-washable aqueous base of butylated hydroxytoluene, cetyl alcohol, citric acid, edetate disodium, methylparaben and propylparaben (preservatives), mineral oil, polyoxyl 20 cetostearyl ether, propylene glycol, simethicone, stearyl alcohol, water (purified), and white wax.

SYNACORT creams have as their active component the corticosteroid hydrocortisone, which has the chemical name pregn-4-ene-3,20-dione, 11,17,21-trihydroxy-,(11β)-.

SYNACORT creams contain hydrocortisone, USP, 10 mg/g or 25 mg/g in a cream containing cetyl alcohol, citric acid, mineral oil, polysorbate 60, propylene glycol, sorbitan monostearate, stearyl alcohol, and water (purified).

SYNALAR preparations, SYNALAR-HP cream, and SYNEMOL cream have as their active component the corticosteroid fluocinolone acetonide, which has the chemical name pregna-1,4-diene-3,20-dione,6,9-difluoro-11,21-dihydroxy-16,17-[(1-methylethylidene)bis(oxy)]-,(6α,11β, 16α)-.

SYNALAR creams contains fluocinolone acetonide 0.25 mg/g or 0.1 mg/g in a water-washable aqueous base of stearyl alcohol, propylene glycol, cetyl alcohol, polyoxyl 20 cetostearyl ether, mineral oil, white wax, simethicone, butylated hydroxytoluene, edetate disodium, citric acid, and purified water, with methylparaben and propylparaben as preservatives.

SYNALAR ointment contains fluocinolone acetonide 0.25 mg/g in a white petrolatum USP vehicle.

SYNALAR solution contains fluocinolone acetonide 0.1 mg/mL in a water-washable base of citric acid and propylene glycol.

SYNALAR-HP cream contains fluocinolone acetonide 2 mg/g in a water-washable aqueous base of cetyl alcohol, citric acid, methylparaben and propylparaben (preservatives), mineral oil, polysorbate 60, propylene glycol, sorbitan monostearate, stearyl alcohol, and water (purified).

SYNEMOL cream contains fluocinolone acetonide 0.25 mg/g in a water-washable aqueous emollient base of cetyl alcohol, citric acid, mineral oil, polysorbate 60, propylene glycol, sorbitan monostearate, stearyl alcohol, and water (purified).

CLINICAL PHARMACOLOGY

Topical corticosteroids share anti-inflammatory, antipruritic and vasoconstrictive actions.

The mechanism of anti-inflammatory activity of the topical corticosteroids is unclear. Various laboratory methods, including vasoconstrictor assays, are used to compare and predict potencies and/or clinical efficacies of the topical corticosteroids. There is some evidence to suggest that a recognizable correlation exists between vasoconstrictor potency and therapeutic efficacy in man.

PHARMACOKINETICS

The extent of percutaneous absorption of topical corticosteroids is determined by many factors including the vehicle, the integrity of the epidermal barrier, and the use of occlusive dressings. A significantly greater amount of fluocinonide is absorbed from the solution than from the cream or gel formulations.

Topical corticosteroids can be absorbed from normal intact skin. Inflammation and/or other disease processes in the skin increase percutaneous absorption. Occlusive dressings substantially increase the percutaneous absorption of topical corticosteroids. Thus, occlusive dressings may be a valuable therapeutic adjunct for treatment of resistant dermatoses. (See DOSAGE AND ADMINISTRATION).

Once absorbed through the skin, topical corticosteroids are handled through pharmacokinetic pathways similar to systemically administered corticosteroids. Corticosteroids are bound to plasma proteins in varying degrees. Corticosteroids are metabolized primarily in the liver and are then excreted by the kidneys. Some of the topical corticosteroids and their metabolites are also excreted into the bile.

INDICATIONS AND USAGE

These products are indicated for the relief of the inflammatory and pruritic manifestations of corticosteroid-responsive dermatoses.

NEO-SYNALAR is indicated for the treatment of corticosteroid-responsive dermatoses with secondary infection. It has not been demonstrated that this steroid-antibiotic combination provides greater benefit then the steroid component alone after 7 days of treatment (see WARNINGS).

CONTRAINDICATIONS

Topical corticosteroids are contraindicated in those patients with a history of hypersensitivity to any of the components of the preparation. NEO-SYNALAR should not be used in the external auditory canal if the eardrum is perforated.

Warnings for NEO-SYNALAR: If local infection should continue or become severe, or in the presence of systemic infection, appropriate systemic antibacterial therapy, based on susceptibility testing, should be considered.

Because of the concern of nephrotoxicity and ototoxicity associated with neomycin, this combination product should not be used over a wide area or for extended periods of time.

There are articles in the current medical literature that indicate an increase in the prevalence of persons sensitive to neomycin.

Warnings for CARMOL HC: Contains sodium metabisulfite, a sulfite that may cause allergic-type reactions including anaphylactic symptoms and life-threatening or less severe asthmatic episodes in certain susceptible people. The overall prevalence of sulfite sensitivity in the general population is unknown and probably low. Sulfite sensitivity is seen more frequently in asthmatic than in nonasthmatic people.

PRECAUTIONS

General: It is recommended that NEO-SYNALAR cream not be used under occlusive dressing.

Systemic absorption of topical corticosteroids has produced reversible hypothalamic-pituitary-adrenal (HPA) axis suppression, manifestations of Cushing's syndrome, hyperglycemia, and glucosuria in some patients.

Conditions which augment systemic absorption include the application of the more potent steroids, use over large surface areas, prolonged use, the addition of occlusive dressings, and dosage form.

Therefore, patients receiving a large dose of a potent topical steroid applied to a large surface area or under an occlusive dressing should be evaluated periodically for evidence of HPA axis suppression by using the urinary free cortisol and ACTH stimulation tests. If HPA axis suppression is noted, an attempt should be made to withdraw the drug, to reduce the frequency of application, or to substitute a less potent steroid.

Recovery of HPA axis function is generally prompt and complete upon discontinuation of the drug. Infrequently, signs and symptoms of steroid withdrawal may occur, requiring supplemental systemic corticosteroids.

Children may absorb proportionally larger amounts of topical corticosteroids and thus be more susceptible to systemic toxicity. (See PRECAUTIONS—Pediatric Use).

Not for ophthalmic use. Severe irritation is possible if fluocinonide solution contacts the eye. If that should occur, immediate flushing of the eye with a large volume of water is recommended.

If irritation develops, topical corticosteroids should be discontinued and appropriate therapy instituted.

As with any topical corticosteroid product, prolonged use may produce atrophy of the skin and subcutaneous tissues. When used on intertriginous or flexor areas, or on the face, this may occur even with short-term use.

In the presence of dermatological infections, the use of an appropriate antifungal or antibacterial agent should be instituted. If a favorable response does not occur promptly, the corticosteroid should be discontinued until the infection has been adequately controlled.

As with all antibiotics, prolonged use of NEO-SYNALAR may result in over-growth of nonsusceptible organisms. If superinfection occurs, appropriate measures should be taken.

SYNALAR-HP cream should not be used for prolonged periods and the quantity per day should not exceed 2 g. of formulated material.

Information for the Patient: Patients using topical corticosteroids should receive the following information and instructions:

1. This medication is to be used as directed by the physician. It is for external use only. Avoid contact with the eyes. If there is contact with the eyes and severe irritation occurs, immediately flush with a large volume of water.
2. Patients should be advised not to use this medication for any disorder other than for which it was prescribed.
3. The treated skin area should not be bandaged or otherwise covered or wrapped as to be occlusive unless directed by the physician.
4. Patients should report any signs of local adverse reactions especially under occlusive dressing.
5. Parents of pediatric patients should be advised not to use tight-fitting diapers or plastic pants on a child being treated in the diaper area, as these garments may constitute occlusive dressings.

Laboratory Tests: The following tests may be helpful in evaluating HPA axis suppression: Urinary free cortisol test and ACTH stimulation test.

Carcinogenesis, Mutagenesis, and Impairment of Fertility: Long-term animal studies have not been performed to evaluate the carcinogenic potential or the effect on fertility of topical corticosteroids.

Studies to determine mutagenicity with prednisolone and hydrocortisone have revealed negative results.

Pregnancy Category C: Corticosteroids are generally teratogenic in laboratory animals when administered systemically at relatively low dosage levels. The more potent corticosteroids have been shown to be teratogenic after dermal application in laboratory animals. There are no adequate and well-controlled studies in pregnant women on teratogenic effects from topically applied corticosteroids. Therefore, topical corticosteroids should be used during pregnancy only if the potential benefit justifies the potential risk to the fe-

tus. Drugs of this class should not be used extensively on pregnant patients, in large amounts, or for prolonged periods of time.

Nursing Mothers: It is not known whether topical administration of corticosteroids could result in sufficient systemic absorption to produce detectable quantities in breast milk. Systemically administered corticosteroids are secreted into breast milk in quantities *not* likely to have a deleterious effect on the infant. Nevertheless, caution should be exercised when topical corticosteroids are administered to a nursing woman.

Pediatric Use: SYNALAR-HP cream 0.2% should not be used on infants up to 2 years of age.

Pediatric patients may demonstrate greater susceptibility to topical corticosteroid-induced HPA axis suppression and Cushing's syndrome than mature patients because of a larger skin surface area to body weight ratio.

Hypothalamic-pituitary-adrenal (HPA) axis suppression, Cushing's syndrome, and intracranial hypertension have been reported in children receiving topical corticosteroids. Manifestations of adrenal suppression in children include linear growth retardation, delayed weight gain, low plasma cortisol levels, and absence of response to ACTH stimulation. Manifestations of intracranial hypertension include bulging fontanelles, headaches, and bilateral papilledema.

Administration of topical corticosteroids to children should be limited to the least amount compatible with an effective therapeutic regimen. Chronic corticosteroid therapy may interfere with the growth and development of children.

ADVERSE REACTIONS

The following local adverse reactions are reported infrequently with topical corticosteroids, but may occur more frequently with the use of occlusive dressings. These reactions are listed in an approximate decreasing order of occurrence: burning, itching, irritation, dryness, folliculitis, hypertrichosis, acneiform eruptions, hypopigmentation, perioral dermatitis, allergic contact dermatitis, maceration of the skin, secondary infection, skin atrophy, striae, miliaria. The following reactions have been reported with the topical use of neomycin: ototoxicity and nephrotoxicity.

OVERDOSAGE

Topically applied corticosteroids can be absorbed in sufficient amounts to produce systemic effects (See PRECAUTIONS).

DOSAGE AND ADMINISTRATION

Topical corticosteroids are generally applied to the affected area as a thin film from two to four times daily depending on the severity of the condition. In hairy sites, the hair should be parted to allow direct contact with the lesion.

Occlusive dressings may be used for the management of psoriasis or recalcitrant conditions. Some plastic films may be flammable and due care should be exercised in their use. Similarly, caution should be employed when such films are used on children or left in their proximity, to avoid the possibility of accidental suffocation.

If an infection develops, the use of occlusive dressings should be discontinued and appropriate antimicrobial therapy instituted.

HOW SUPPLIED

LIDEX® (fluocinonide) cream 0.05%—15 g Tube (NDC 0033-2511-13), 30 g Tube (NDC 0033-2511-14), 60 g Tube (NDC 0033-2511-17), and 120 g Tube (NDC 0033-2511-22). Store at room temperature. Avoid excessive heat, above 40°C (104°F).

LIDEX® (fluocinonide) gel 0.05%—15 g Tube (NDC 0033-2507-13), 30 g Tube (NDC 0033-2507-14), 60 g Tube (NDC 0033-2507-17), and 120 g Tube (NDC 0033-2507-22). Store at controlled room temperature, 15–30°C (59–86°F).

LIDEX® (fluocinonide) ointment 0.05%—15 g Tube (NDC 0033-2514-13), 30 g Tube (NDC 0033-2514-14), 60 g Tube (NDC 0033-2514-17), and 120 g Tube (NDC 0033-2514-22). Store at room temperature. Avoid temperature above 30°C (86°F).

LIDEX® (fluocinonide) topical solution 0.05%—Plastic squeeze bottles: 20 cc (NDC 0033-2517-44) and 60 cc (NDC 0033-2517-46). Store at room temperature. Avoid excessive heat, above 40°C (104°F).

LIDEX-E® (fluocinonide) cream 0.05%—15 g Tube (NDC 0033-2513-13), 30 g Tube (NDC 0033-2513-14), 60 g Tube (NDC 0033-2513-17), and 120 g Tube (NDC 0033-2513-22). Store at room temperature. Avoid excessive heat, above 40°C (104°F).

CARMOL® HC (hydrocortisone acetate) cream 1%—1 oz. Tube (NDC 0033-2550-15) and 4 oz. Jar (NDC 0033-2550-11). Store at room temperature. Avoid excessive heat, above 40°C (104°F). Dispense in well-closed containers.

NEO-SYNALAR® cream—15 g Tube (NDC 0033-2505-13), 30 g Tube (NDC 0033-2505-14), 60 g Tube (NDC 0033-2505-17). Store at room temperature. Avoid freezing and excessive heat, above 40°C (104°F).

SYNACORT® (hydrocortisone) cream 1%—15 g Tube (NDC 0033-2519-13), 30 g Tube (NDC 0033-2519-14), and 60 g Tube

Continued on next page

Syntex—Cont.

(NDC 0033-2519-17). SYNACORT® (hydrocortisone) cream 2.5%—30 g Tube (NDC 0033-2520-14). Store at room temperature. Avoid excessive heat, above 40°C (104°F).

SYNALAR® (fluocinolone acetonide) cream 0.025%—15 g Tube (NDC 0033-2501-13), 30 g Tube (NDC 0033-2501-14), 60 g Tube (NDC 0033-2501-17), and 425 g Jar (NDC 0033-2501-23). Store tubes at room temperature. Avoid freezing and excessive heat, above 40°C (104°F). Store jars at controlled room temperature, 15°–30°C (59°–86°F).

SYNALAR® (fluocinolone acetonide) cream 0.01%—15 g Tube (NDC 0033-2502-13), 30 g Tube (NDC 0033-2502-14), 60 g Tube (NDC 0033-2502-17), and 425 g Jar (NDC 0033-2502-23). Store tubes at room temperature. Avoid freezing and excessive heat, above 40°C (104°F). Store jars at controlled room temperature, 15°–30°C (59°–86°F).

SYNALAR® (fluocinolone acetonide) ointment 0.025%—15 g Tube (NDC 0033-2504-13), 30 g Tube (NDC 0033-2504-14), 60 g Tube (NDC 0033-2504-17), and 425 g Jar (NDC 0033-2504-23). Store at room temperature. Avoid excessive heat, above 40°C (104°F).

SYNALAR® (fluocinolone acetonide) topical solution 0.01%—20 cc (NDC 0033-2506-44) and 60 cc (NDC 0033-2506-46). Store at room temperature. Avoid freezing.

SYNALAR-HP® (fluocinolone acetonide) cream 0.2%—12 g Tube (NDC 0033-2503-12). Store at room temperature. Avoid excessive heat, above 40°C (104°F).

SYNEMOL® (fluocinolone acetonide) cream 0.025%—15 g Tube (NDC 0033-2509-13), 30 g Tube (NDC 0033-2509-14), 60 g Tube (NDC 0033-2509-17). Store at room temperature. Avoid excessive heat, above 40°C (104°F).

CAUTION: Federal law prohibits dispensing without a prescription.

LIDEX ointment: U.S. Patent No. 4,017,615
LIDEX cream: U.S. Patent Nos. 3,592,930 and 3,888,995

Revised 4/91

© 1990 Syntex Laboratories, Inc.

NAPROSYN® ℞

[nă'pro-sin]
(naproxen)
Tablets and Suspension

Products of Syntex Puerto Rico, Inc.

DESCRIPTION

NAPROSYN® (naproxen) tablets for oral administration each contain 250 mg, 375 mg or 500 mg of naproxen. NAPROSYN suspension for oral administration contains 125 mg/5 mL of naproxen. NAPROSYN is a member of the arylacetic acid group of nonsteroidal anti-inflammatory drugs.

The chemical name for naproxen is 2-naphthaleneacetic acid, 6-methoxy-α-methyl-,(+).

Naproxen is an odorless, white to off-white crystalline substance. It is lipid soluble, practically insoluble in water at low pH and freely soluble in water at high pH.

Each tablet contains naproxen, the active ingredient, with the following inactive ingredients: Croscarmellose sodium, iron oxides, magnesium stearate and povidone.

NAPROSYN suspension for oral administration contains 125 mg/5 mL of naproxen, the active ingredient, in a vehicle of FD&C Yellow #6, fumaric acid, imitation orange flavor, imitation pineapple flavor, magnesium aluminum silicate, methylparaben, purified water, sodium chloride, sorbitol solution and sucrose.

CLINICAL PHARMACOLOGY

NAPROSYN (naproxen) is a nonsteroidal anti-inflammatory drug with analgesic and antipyretic properties. Naproxen sodium, the sodium salt of naproxen, has been developed as an analgesic because it is more rapidly absorbed. The naproxen anion inhibits prostaglandin synthesis but beyond this its mode of action is unknown.

Naproxen is rapidly and completely absorbed from the gastrointestinal tract. After administration of naproxen, peak plasma levels of naproxen anion are attained in 2 to 4 hours, with steady-state conditions normally achieved after 4–5 doses. The mean biological half-life of the anion in humans is approximately 13 hours, and at therapeutic levels it is greater than 99% albumin bound. At doses of naproxen greater than 500 mg/day there is a lack of dose proportionality due to an increase in clearance caused by saturation of plasma proteins at higher doses. Approximately 95% of the dose is excreted in the urine, primarily as naproxen, 6-0-desmethyl naproxen or their conjugates. The rate of excretion has been found to coincide closely with the rate of drug disappearance from the plasma. The drug does not induce metabolizing enzymes.

In children of 5 to 16 years of age with arthritis, plasma naproxen levels following a 5 mg/kg single dose of suspension were found to be similar to those found in normal adults fol-

lowing a 500 mg dose. The terminal half-life appears to be similar in children and adults. Pharmacokinetic studies of naproxen were not performed in children of less than 5 years of age.

The drug was studied in patients with rheumatoid arthritis, osteoarthritis, juvenile arthritis, ankylosing spondylitis, tendinitis and bursitis, and acute gout. It is not a corticosteroid. Improvement in patients treated for rheumatoid arthritis has been demonstrated by a reduction in joint swelling, a reduction in pain, a reduction in duration of morning stiffness, a reduction in disease activity as assessed by both the investigator and patient, and by increased mobility as demonstrated by a reduction in walking time.

In patients with osteoarthritis, the therapeutic action of the drug has been shown by a reduction in joint pain or tenderness, an increase in range of motion in knee joints, increased mobility as demonstrated by a reduction in walking time, and improvement in capacity to perform activities of daily living impaired by the disease.

In clinical studies in patients with rheumatoid arthritis, osteoarthritis, and juvenile arthritis, the drug has been shown to be comparable to aspirin and indomethacin in controlling the aforementioned measures of disease activity, but the frequency and severity of the milder gastrointestinal adverse effects (nausea, dyspepsia, heartburn) and nervous system adverse effects (tinnitus, dizziness, lightheadedness) were less than in both the aspirin- and indomethacin-treated patients. It is not known whether the drug causes less peptic ulceration than aspirin.

In patients with ankylosing spondylitis, the drug has been shown to decrease night pain, morning stiffness and pain at rest. In double-blind studies the drug was shown to be as effective as aspirin, but with fewer side effects.

In patients with acute gout, a favorable response to the drug was shown by significant clearing of inflammatory changes (e.g., decrease in swelling, heat) within 24–48 hours, as well as by relief of pain and tenderness.

The drug may be used safely in combination with gold salts and/or corticosteroids; however, in controlled clinical trials, when added to the regimen of patients receiving corticosteroids it did not appear to cause greater improvement over that seen with corticosteroids alone. Whether the drug could be used in conjunction with partially effective doses of corticosteroid for a "steroid-sparing" effect has not been adequately studied. When added to the regimen of patients receiving gold salts the drug did result in greater improvement. Its use in combination with salicylates is not recommended because data are inadequate to demonstrate that the drug produces greater improvement over that achieved with aspirin alone. Further, there is some evidence that aspirin increases the rate of excretion of the drug.

Generally, improvement due to the drug has not been found to be dependent on age, sex, severity or duration of disease.

In clinical trials in patients with osteoarthritis and rheumatoid arthritis comparing treatments of 750 mg per day with 1,500 mg per day, there were trends toward increased efficacy with the higher dose and a more clearcut increase in adverse reactions, particularly gastrointestinal reactions severe enough to cause the patient to leave the trial, which approximately doubled.

The drug was studied in patients with mild to moderate pain, and pain relief was obtained within 1 hour. It is not a narcotic and is not a CNS-acting drug. Controlled double-blind studies have demonstrated the analgesic properties of the drug in, for example, post-operative, post-partum, orthopedic and uterine contraction pain and dysmenorrhea. In dysmenorrheic patients, the drug reduces the level of prostaglandins in the uterus, which correlates with a reduction in the frequency and severity of uterine contractions. Analgesic action has been shown by such measures as a reduction of pain intensity scores, increase in pain relief scores, decrease in numbers of patients requiring additional analgesic medication, and delay in time for required remedication. The analgesic effect has been found to last for up to 7 hours.

In ^{51}Cr blood loss and gastroscopy studies with normal volunteers, daily administration of 1000 mg of the drug has been demonstrated to cause statistically significantly less gastric bleeding and erosion than 3250 mg of aspirin.

INDICATIONS AND USAGE

NAPROSYN (naproxen) is indicated for the treatment of rheumatoid arthritis, osteoarthritis, juvenile arthritis, ankylosing spondylitis, tendinitis and bursitis, and acute gout. It is also indicated in the relief of mild to moderate pain and for the treatment of primary dysmenorrhea.

CONTRAINDICATIONS

The drug is contraindicated in patients who have had allergic reactions to NAPROSYN® (naproxen), ANAPROX® (naproxen sodium) or ANAPROX® DS (naproxen sodium). It is also contraindicated in patients in whom aspirin or other nonsteroidal anti-inflammatory/analgesic drugs induce the syndrome of asthma, rhinitis, and nasal polyps. Both types of reactions have the potential of being fatal. Anaphylactoid reactions to NAPROSYN, ANAPROX, or ANAPROX DS, whether of the true allergic type or the phar-

macologic idiosyncratic (e.g., aspirin syndrome) type, usually but not always occur in patients with a known history of such reactions. Therefore, careful questioning of patients for such things as asthma, nasal polyps, urticaria, and hypotension associated with nonsteroidal anti-inflammatory drugs before starting therapy is important. In addition, if such symptoms occur during therapy, treatment should be discontinued.

WARNINGS

Risk of GI Ulceration, Bleeding and Perforation with NSAID Therapy:

Serious gastrointestinal toxicity such as bleeding, ulceration, and perforation, can occur at any time, with or without warning symptoms, in patients treated chronically with NSAID therapy. Although minor upper gastrointestinal problems, such as dyspepsia, are common, usually developing early in therapy, physicians should remain alert for ulceration and bleeding in patients treated chronically with NSAIDs even in the absence of previous GI tract symptoms. In patients observed in clinical trials of several months to two years duration, symptomatic upper GI ulcers, gross bleeding or perforation appear to occur in approximately 1% of patients treated for 3–6 months, and in about 2–4% of patients treated for one year. Physicians should inform patients about the signs and/or symptoms of serious GI toxicity and what steps to take if they occur.

Studies to date have not identified any subset of patients not at risk of developing peptic ulceration and bleeding. Except for a prior history of serious GI events and other risk factors known to be associated with peptic ulcer disease, such as alcoholism, smoking, etc., no risk factors (e.g., age, sex) have been associated with increased risk. Elderly or debilitated patients seem to tolerate ulceration or bleeding less well than other individuals and most spontaneous reports of fatal GI events are in this population. Studies to date are inconclusive concerning the relative risk of various NSAIDs in causing such reactions. High doses of any NSAID probably carry a greater risk of these reactions, although controlled clinical trials showing this do not exist in most cases. In considering the use of relatively large doses (within the recommended dosage range), sufficient benefit should be anticipated to offset the potential increased risk of GI toxicity.

PRECAUTIONS

General:

NAPROSYN (NAPROXEN) SHOULD NOT BE USED CONCOMITANTLY WITH THE RELATED DRUG ANAPROX OR ANAPROX DS (NAPROXEN SODIUM) SINCE THEY BOTH CIRCULATE IN PLASMA AS THE NAPROXEN ANION.

Renal Effects: As with other nonsteroidal anti-inflammatory drugs, long-term administration of naproxen to animals has resulted in renal papillary necrosis and other abnormal renal pathology. In humans, there have been reports of acute interstitial nephritis with hematuria, proteinuria, and occasionally nephrotic syndrome.

A second form of renal toxicity has been seen in patients with prerenal conditions leading to the reduction in renal blood flow or blood volume, where the renal prostaglandins have a supportive role in the maintenance of renal perfusion. In these patients, administration of a nonsteroidal anti-inflammatory drug may cause a dose-dependent reduction in prostaglandin formation and may precipitate overt renal decompensation. Patients at greatest risk of this reaction are those with impaired renal function, heart failure, liver dysfunction, those taking diuretics, and the elderly. Discontinuation of nonsteroidal anti-inflammatory therapy is typically followed by recovery to the pretreatment state.

NAPROSYN and its metabolites are eliminated primarily by the kidneys, therefore the drug should be used with great caution in patients with significantly impaired renal function and the monitoring of serum creatinine and/or creatinine clearance is advised in these patients. Caution should be used if the drug is given to patients with creatinine clearance of less than 20 mL/minute because accumulation of naproxen metabolites has been seen in such patients.

Chronic alcoholic liver disease and probably other forms of cirrhosis reduce the total plasma concentration of naproxen, but the plasma concentration of unbound naproxen is increased. Caution is advised when high doses are required and some adjustment of dosage may be required in these patients. It is prudent to use the lowest effective dose.

Studies indicate that although total plasma concentration of naproxen is unchanged, the unbound plasma fraction of naproxen is increased in the elderly. Caution is advised when high doses are required and some adjustment of dosage may be required in elderly patients. As with other drugs used in the elderly, it is prudent to use the lowest effective dose.

As with other nonsteroidal anti-inflammatory drugs, borderline elevations of one or more liver tests may occur in up to 15% of patients. These abnormalities may progress, may remain essentially unchanged, or may be transient with continued therapy. The SGPT (ALT) test is probably the most sensitive indicator of liver dysfunction. Meaningful (3 times the upper limit of normal) elevations of SGPT or SGOT (AST) occurred in controlled clinical trials in less than 1% of patients. A patient with symptoms and/or signs suggesting

liver dysfunction, or in whom an abnormal liver test has occurred, should be evaluated for evidence of the development of more severe hepatic reaction while on therapy with this drug. Severe hepatic reactions, including jaundice and cases of fatal hepatitis, have been reported with this drug as with other nonsteroidal anti-inflammatory drugs. Although such reactions are rare, if abnormal liver tests persist or worsen, if clinical signs and symptoms consistent with liver disease develop, or if systemic manifestations occur (e.g. eosinophilia, rash, etc.), this drug should be discontinued.

If steroid dosage is reduced or eliminated during therapy, the steroid dosage should be reduced slowly and the patients must be observed closely for any evidence of adverse effects, including adrenal insufficiency and exacerbation of symptoms of arthritis.

Patients with initial hemoglobin values of 10 grams or less who are to receive long-term therapy should have hemoglobin values determined periodically.

Peripheral edema has been observed in some patients. For this reason, the drug should be used with caution in patients with fluid retention, hypertension or heart failure.

Naprosyn suspension contains 8 mg/mL of sodium. This should be considered in patients whose overall intake of sodium must be restricted.

The antipyretic and anti-inflammatory activities of the drug may reduce fever and inflammation, thus diminishing their utility as diagnostic signs in detecting complications of presumed non-infectious, non-inflammatory painful conditions.

Because of adverse eye findings in animal studies with drugs of this class, it is recommended that ophthalmic studies be carried out if any change or disturbance in vision occurs.

Information for Patients:

Naproxen, like other drugs of its class, is not free of side effects. The side effects of these drugs can cause discomfort and, rarely, there are more serious side effects, such as gastrointestinal bleeding, which may result in hospitalization and even fatal outcomes.

NSAIDs (Nonsteroidal Anti-Inflammatory Drugs) are often essential agents in the management of arthritis and have a major role in the treatment of pain, but they also may be commonly employed for conditions which are less serious.

Physicians may wish to discuss with their patients the potential risks (see Warnings, Precautions, and Adverse Reactions sections) and likely benefits of NSAID treatment, particularly when the drugs are used for less serious conditions where treatment without NSAIDs may represent an acceptable alternative to both the patient and physician.

Caution should be exercised by patients whose activities require alertness if they experience drowsiness, dizziness, vertigo or depression during therapy with the drug.

Laboratory Tests:

Because serious GI tract ulceration and bleeding can occur without warning symptoms, physicians should follow chronically treated patients for the signs and symptoms of ulceration and bleeding and should inform them of the importance of this follow-up (see Risk of GI Ulcerations, Bleeding and Perforation with NSAID Therapy).

Drug Interactions:

In vitro studies have shown that naproxen anion, because of its affinity for protein, may displace from their binding sites other drugs which are also albumin-bound. Theoretically, the naproxen anion itself could likewise be displaced. Short-term controlled studies failed to show that taking the drug significantly affects prothrombin times when administered to individuals on coumarin-type anticoagulants. Caution is advised nonetheless, since interactions have been seen with other nonsteroidal agents of this class. Similarly, patients receiving the drug and a hydantoin, sulfonamide or sulfonylurea should be observed for signs of toxicity to these drugs.

The natriuretic effect of furosemide has been reported to be inhibited by some drugs of this class. Inhibition of renal lithium clearance leading to increases in plasma lithium concentrations has also been reported.

This and other nonsteroidal anti-inflammatory drugs can reduce the antihypertensive effect of propranolol and other beta-blockers.

Probenecid given concurrently increases naproxen anion plasma levels and extends its plasma half-life significantly.

Caution should be used if this drug is administered concomitantly with methotrexate. Naproxen and other nonsteroidal anti-inflammatory drugs have been reported to reduce the tubular secretion of methotrexate in an animal model, possibly enhancing the toxicity of that drug.

Drug/Laboratory Test Interactions:

The drug may decrease platelet aggregation and prolong bleeding time. This effect should be kept in mind when bleeding times are determined.

The administration of the drug may result in increased urinary values for 17-ketogenic steroids because of an interaction between the drug and/or its metabolites with m-dinitrobenzene used in this assay. Although 17-hydroxy-corticosteroid measurements (Porter-Silber test) do not appear to be artifactually altered, it is suggested that therapy with the drug be temporarily discontinued 72 hours before adrenal function tests are performed.

The drug may interfere with some urinary assays of 5-hydroxy indoleacetic acid (5HIAA).

Carcinogenesis:

A two-year study was performed in rats to evaluate the carcinogenic potential of the drug. No evidence of carcinogenicity was found.

Pregnancy:

Teratogenic Effects: Pregnancy Category B. Reproduction studies have been performed in rats, rabbits and mice at doses up to six times the human dose and have revealed no evidence of impaired fertility or harm to the fetus due to the drug. There are, however, no adequate and well-controlled studies in pregnant women. Because animal reproduction studies are not always predictive of human response, the drug should not be used during pregnancy unless clearly needed. Because of the known effect of drugs of this class on the human fetal cardiovascular system (closure of ductus arteriosus), use during late pregnancy should be avoided.

Non-teratogenic Effects: As with other drugs known to inhibit prostaglandin synthesis, an increased incidence of dystocia and delayed parturition occurred in rats.

Nursing Mothers:

The naproxen anion has been found in the milk of lactating women at a concentration of approximately 1% of that found in the plasma. Because of the possible adverse effects of prostaglandin-inhibiting drugs on neonates, use in nursing mothers should be avoided.

Pediatric Use:

Safety and effectiveness in children below the age of 2 years have not been established. Pediatric dosing recommendations for juvenile arthritis are based on well-controlled studies (see Dosage and Administration). There are no adequate effectiveness or dose-response data for other pediatric conditions, but the experience in juvenile arthritis and other use experience have established that single doses of 2.5–5 mg/kg, with total daily dose not exceeding 15 mg/kg/day, are safe in children over 2 years of age.

ADVERSE REACTIONS

The following adverse reactions are divided into 3 parts based on frequency and likelihood of causal relationship to naproxen.

Incidence greater than 1%

Probable Causal Relationship:

Adverse reactions reported in controlled clinical trials in 960 patients treated for rheumatoid arthritis or osteoarthritis are listed below. In general, these reactions were reported 2 to 10 times more frequently than they were in studies in the 962 patients treated for mild to moderate pain or for dysmenorrhea.

A clinical study found gastrointestinal reactions to be more frequent and more severe in rheumatoid arthritis patients taking 1,500 mg naproxen daily compared to those taking 750 mg daily (see Clinical Pharmacology).

In controlled clinical trials with about 80 children and in well-monitored open studies with about 400 children with juvenile arthritis, the incidences of rash and prolonged bleeding times were increased, the incidences of gastrointestinal and central nervous system reactions were about the same, and the incidences of other reactions were lower in children than in adults.

Gastrointestinal: The most frequent complaints reported related to the gastrointestinal tract. They were: constipation*, heartburn*, abdominal pain*, nausea*, dyspepsia, diarrhea, stomatitis.

Central Nervous System: Headache*, dizziness*, drowsiness*, lightheadedness, vertigo.

Dermatologic: Itching (pruritus)*, skin eruptions*, ecchymoses*, sweating, purpura.

Special Senses: Tinnitus*, hearing disturbances, visual disturbances.

Cardiovascular: Edema*, dyspnea*, palpitations.

General: Thirst.

Incidence less than 1%

Probable Causal Relationship:

The following adverse reactions were reported less frequently than 1% during controlled clinical trials and through voluntary reports since marketing. The probability of a causal relationship exists between the drug and these adverse reactions:

Gastrointestinal: Abnormal liver function tests, colitis, gastrointestinal bleeding and/or perforation, hematemesis, jaundice, melena, peptic ulceration with bleeding and/or perforation, vomiting.

Renal: Glomerular nephritis, hematuria, hyperkalemia, interstitial nephritis, nephrotic syndrome, renal disease, renal failure, renal papillary necrosis.

Hematologic: Agranulocytosis, eosinophilia, granulocytopenia, leukopenia, thrombocytopenia.

Central Nervous System: Depression, dream abnormalities, inability to concentrate, insomnia, malaise, myalgia and muscle weakness.

* Incidence of reported reactions between 3% and 9%. Those reactions occurring in less than 3% of the patients are unmarked.

Dermatologic: Alopecia, photosensitive dermatitis, skin rashes.

Special Senses: Hearing impairment.

Cardiovascular: Congestive heart failure.

Respiratory: Eosinophilic pneumonitis.

General: Anaphylactoid reactions, menstrual disorders, pyrexia (chills and fever).

Causal Relationship Unknown:

Other reactions have been reported in circumstances in which a causal relationship could not be established. However, in these rarely reported events, the possibility cannot be excluded. Therefore, these observations are being listed to serve as alerting information to the physicians:

Hematologic: Aplastic anemia, hemolytic anemia.

Central Nervous System: Aseptic meningitis, cognitive dysfunction.

Dermatologic: Epidermal necrolysis, erythema multiforme, photosensitivity reactions resembling porphyria cutanea tarda and epidermolysis bullosa, Stevens-Johnson syndrome, urticaria.

Gastrointestinal: Non-peptic gastrointestinal ulceration, ulcerative stomatitis.

Cardiovascular: Vasculitis.

General: Angioneurotic edema, hyperglycemia, hypoglycemia.

OVERDOSAGE

Significant overdosage may be characterized by drowsiness, heartburn, indigestion, nausea or vomiting. A few patients have experienced seizures, but it is not clear whether or not these were drug related. It is not known what dose of the drug would be life threatening. The oral LD_{50} of the drug is 543 mg/kg in rats, 1234 mg/kg in mice, 4110 mg/kg in hamsters and greater than 1000 mg/kg in dogs.

Should a patient ingest a large number of tablets or a large volume of suspension, accidentally or purposefully, the stomach may be emptied and usual supportive measures employed. In animals 0.5 g/kg of activated charcoal was effective in reducing plasma levels of naproxen. Hemodialysis does not decrease the plasma concentration of naproxen because of the high degree of its protein binding.

DOSAGE AND ADMINISTRATION

A measuring cup marked in ½ teaspoon and 2.5 milliliter increments is provided with the suspension. This cup or a teaspoon may be used to measure the appropriate dose.

For Rheumatoid Arthritis, Osteoarthritis, and Ankylosing Spondylitis:

The recommended dose of NAPROSYN® (naproxen) in adults is 250 mg (10 mL or 2 tsp of suspension), 375 mg (15 mL or 3 tsp), or 500 mg (20 mL or 4 tsp) twice daily (morning and evening). During long-term administration, the dose may be adjusted up or down depending on the clinical response of the patient. A lower daily dose may suffice for long-term administration. The morning and evening doses do not have to be equal in size and the administration of the drug more frequently than twice daily is not necessary. In patients who tolerate lower doses well, the dose may be increased to 1,500 mg per day for limited periods when a higher level of anti-inflammatory/analgesic activity is required. When treating such patients with the 1,500 mg/day dose, the physician should observe sufficient increased clinical benefits to offset the potential increased risk (see Clinical Pharmacology).

Symptomatic improvement in arthritis usually begins within 2 weeks. However, if improvement is not seen within this period, a trial for an additional 2 weeks should be considered.

For Juvenile Arthritis:

The recommended total daily dose of NAPROSYN is approximately 10 mg/kg given in 2 divided doses. One half of the 250 mg tablet may be used to approximate this dose. The following table may be used as a guide for the suspension:

Child's Weight	Dose
13 kg (29 lb)	2.5 mL (½ tsp) b.i.d.
25 kg (55 lb)	5 mL (1 tsp) b.i.d.
38 kg (84 lb)	7.5 mL (1½ tsp) b.i.d.

For Acute Gout:

The recommended starting dose of NAPROSYN is 750 mg (30 mL or 6 tsp), followed by 250 mg (10 mL or 2 tsp) every 8 hours until the attack has subsided.

For Mild to Moderate Pain, Primary Dysmenorrhea and Acute Tendinitis and Bursitis:

The recommended starting dose of NAPROSYN is 500 mg (20 mL or 4 tsp), followed by 250 mg (10 mL or 2 tsp) every 6 to 8 hours as required. The total daily dose should not exceed 1,250 mg (50 mL or 10 tsp).

HOW SUPPLIED

NAPROSYN® (naproxen) is available as yellow 250 mg tablets in light-resistant bottles of 100 tablets (NDC 18393-272-42) (NSN 6505-01-026-9730) and 500 tablets (NDC 18393-272-62) (NSN 6505-01-046-0126) or in cartons of 100 individually blister-packed tablets (NDC 18393-272-53) (NSN 6505-01-097-9611). Peach 375 mg tablets are available in light-

Continued on next page

Syntex—Cont.

resistant bottles of 100 tablets (NDC 18393-273-42) (NSN 6505-01-135-8462) and 500 tablets (NDC 18393-273-62) (NSN 6505-01-204-5297) or in cartons of 100 individually blister-packed tablets (NDC 18393-273-53) (NSN 6505-01-204-5298). Yellow 500 mg tablets are available in light-resistant bottles of 100 tablets (NDC 18393-277-42) (NSN 6505-01-200-2474) and 500 tablets (NDC 18393-277-62) (NSN 6505-01-186-8758) or in cartons of 100 individually blister-packed tablets (NDC 18393-277-53). Store at room temperature in well-closed containers; dispense in light-resistant containers.
NAPROSYN® suspension is available in 1 pint (474 mL) light-resistant bottles (NDC 18393-278-20). Measuring cups are provided so that one can be dispensed with each prescription. Store at room temperature; avoid excessive heat, above 40°C (104° F). Dispense in light-resistant container.
CAUTION: Federal law prohibits dispensing without prescription.
U.S. Patent Nos. 3,904,682; 3,998,966 and others.
02-0273-53-02 Revised 9/90
©1990 Syntex Puerto Rico, Inc.
Shown in Product Identification Section, page 433

NASALIDE® ℞
[na 'ză-lide]
(flunisolide)
Nasal Solution
0.025%
For Nasal Use Only

A product of Syntex Laboratories, Inc.

DESCRIPTION

NASALIDE® (flunisolide) nasal solution is intended for administration as a spray to the nasal mucosa. Flunisolide, the active component of NASALIDE nasal solution, is an anti-inflammatory steroid with the chemical name: 6α-fluoro-11β, 16α, 17,21-tetrahydroxypregna-1,4-diene-3,20-dione cyclic 16,17-acetal with acetone (USAN).
Flunisolide is a white to creamy white crystalline powder with a molecular weight of 434.49. It is soluble in acetone, sparingly soluble in chloroform, slightly soluble in methanol, and practically insoluble in water. It has a melting point of about 245°C.
Each 25 mL spray bottle contains flunisolide 6.25 mg (0.25 mg/mL) in a solution of propylene glycol, polyethylene glycol 3350, citric acid, sodium citrate, butylated hydroxyanisole, edetate disodium, benzalkonium chloride, and purified water, with NaOH and/or HCl added to adjust the pH to approximately 5.3. It contains no fluorocarbons.
After priming the delivery system for NASALIDE, each actuation of the unit delivers a metered droplet spray containing approximately 25 mcg of flunisolide. The size of the droplets produced by the unit is in excess of 8 microns to facilitate deposition on the nasal mucosa. The contents of one nasal spray bottle deliver at least 200 sprays.

CLINICAL PHARMACOLOGY

NASALIDE® (flunisolide) has demonstrated potent glucocorticoid and weak mineralocorticoid activity in classical animal test systems. As a glucocorticoid it is several hundred times more potent than the cortisol standard. Clinical studies with flunisolide have shown therapeutic activity on nasal mucous membranes with minimal evidence of systemic activity at the recommended doses.
A study in approximately 100 patients which compared the recommended dose of flunisolide nasal solution with an oral dose providing equivalent systemic amounts of flunisolide has shown that the clinical effectiveness of NASALIDE, when used topically as recommended, is due to its direct local effect and not to an indirect effect through systemic absorption.
Following administration of flunisolide to man, approximately half of the administered dose is recovered in the urine and half in the stool; 65–70% of the dose recovered in urine is the primary metabolite, which has undergone loss of the 6α fluorine and addition of a 6β hydroxy group. Flunisolide is well absorbed but is rapidly converted by the liver to the much less active primary metabolite and to glucuronate and/or sulfate conjugates. Because of first-pass liver metabolism, only 20% of the flunisolide reaches the systemic circulation when it is given orally whereas 50% of the flunisolide administered intranasally reaches the systemic circulation unmetabolized. The plasma half-life of flunisolide is 1–2 hours.
The effects of flunisolide on hypothalamic-pituitary-adrenal (HPA) axis function have been studied in adult volunteers. NASALIDE was administered intranasally as a spray in total doses over 7 times the recommended dose (2200 mcg, equivalent to 88 sprays/day) in 2 subjects for 4 days, about 3 times the recommended dose (800 mcg, equivalent to 32 sprays/day) in 4 subjects for 4 days, and over twice the recommended dose (700 mcg, equivalent to 28 sprays/day) in 6 subjects for 10 days. Early morning plasma cortisol concentrations and 24-hour urinary 17-ketogenic steroids were measured daily. There was evidence of decreased endogenous cortisol production at all three doses.
In controlled studies, NASALIDE was found to be effective in reducing symptoms of stuffy nose, runny nose and sneezing in most patients. These controlled clinical studies have been conducted in 488 adult patients at doses ranging from 8 to 16 sprays (200–400 mcg) per day and 127 children at doses ranging from 6 to 8 sprays (150–200 mcg) per day for periods as long as 3 months. In 170 patients who had cortisol levels evaluated at baseline and after 3 months or more of flunisolide treatment, there was no unequivocal flunisolide-related depression of plasma cortisol levels.
The mechanisms responsible for the anti-inflammatory action of corticosteroids and for the activity of the aerosolized drug on the nasal mucosa are unknown.

INDICATIONS

NASALIDE® (flunisolide) is indicated for the topical treatment of the symptoms of seasonal or perennial rhinitis when effectiveness of or tolerance to conventional treatment is unsatisfactory.
Clinical studies have shown that improvement is based on a local effect rather than systemic absorption, and is usually apparent within a few days after starting NASALIDE. However, symptomatic relief may not occur in some patients for as long as two weeks. Although systemic effects are minimal at recommended doses, NASALIDE should not be continued beyond 3 weeks in the absence of significant symptomatic improvement.
NASALIDE should not be used in the presence of untreated localized infection involving nasal mucosa.

CONTRAINDICATIONS

Hypersensitivity to any of the ingredients.

WARNINGS

The replacement of a systemic corticosteroid with a topical corticoid can be accompanied by signs of adrenal insufficiency, and in addition some patients may experience symptoms of withdrawal, e.g., joint and/or muscular pain, lassitude and depression. Patients previously treated for prolonged periods with systemic corticosteroids and transferred to NASALIDE® (flunisolide) should be carefully monitored to avoid acute adrenal insufficiency in response to stress.
When transferred to NASALIDE, careful attention must be given to patients previously treated for prolonged periods with systemic corticosteroids. This is particularly important in those patients who have associated asthma or other clinical conditions, where too rapid a decrease in systemic corticosteroids may cause a severe exacerbation of their symptoms.
The use of NASALIDE with alternate-day prednisone systemic treatment could increase the likelihood of HPA suppression compared to a therapeutic dose of either one alone. Therefore, NASALIDE treatment should be used with caution in patients already on alternate-day prednisone regimens for any disease.

PRECAUTIONS

General: In clinical studies with flunisolide administered intranasally, the development of localized infections of the nose and pharynx with *Candida albicans* has occurred only rarely. When such an infection develops it may require treatment with appropriate local therapy or discontinuance of treatment with NASALIDE® (flunisolide).
Flunisolide is absorbed into the circulation. Use of excessive doses of NASALIDE may suppress hypothalamic-pituitary-adrenal function.
Flunisolide should be used with caution, if at all, in patients with active or quiescent tuberculosis infections of the respiratory tract or in untreated fungal, bacterial or systemic viral infections or ocular herpes simplex.
Because of the inhibitory effect of corticosteroids on wound healing, in patients who have experienced recent nasal septal ulcers, recurrent epistaxis, nasal surgery or trauma, a nasal corticosteroid should be used with caution until healing has occurred.
Although systemic effects have been minimal with recommended doses, this potential increases with excessive dosages. Therefore, larger than recommended doses should be avoided.
Information for Patients: Patients should use NASALIDE at regular intervals since its effectiveness depends on its regular use. The patient should take the medication as directed. It is not acutely effective and the prescribed dosage should not be increased. Instead, nasal vasoconstrictors or oral antihistamines may be needed until the effects of NASALIDE are fully manifested. One to two weeks may pass before full relief is obtained. The patient should contact the physician if symptoms do not improve, or if the condition worsens, or if sneezing or nasal irritation occurs.
For the proper use of this unit and to attain maximum improvement, the patient should read and follow the accompanying Patient Instructions carefully.
Carcinogenesis: Long-term studies were conducted in mice and rats using oral administration to evaluate the carcinogenic potential of the drug. There was an increase in the incidence of pulmonary adenomas in mice, but not in rats.
Female rats receiving the highest oral dose had an increased incidence of mammary adenocarcinoma compared to control rats. An increased incidence of this tumor type has been reported for other corticosteroids.
Impairment of fertility: Female rats receiving high doses of flunisolide (200 mcg/kg/day) showed some evidence of impaired fertility. Reproductive performance in the low (8 mcg/kg/day) and mid-dose (40 mcg/kg/day) groups was comparable to controls.
Pregnancy: Teratogenic effects: Pregnancy Category C. As with other corticosteroids, flunisolide has been shown to be teratogenic in rabbits and rats at doses of 40 and 200 mcg/kg/day respectively. It was also fetotoxic in these animal reproductive studies. There are no adequate and well-controlled studies in pregnant women. Flunisolide should be used during pregnancy only if the potential benefit justifies the potential risk to the fetus.
Nursing Mothers: It is not known whether this drug is excreted in human milk. Because other corticosteroids are excreted in human milk, caution should be exercised when flunisolide is administered to nursing women.

ADVERSE REACTIONS

Adverse reactions reported in controlled clinical trials and long-term open studies in 595 patients treated with NASALIDE are described below. Of these patients, 409 were treated for 3 months or longer, 323 for 6 months or longer, 259 for 1 year or longer, and 91 for 2 years or longer.
In general, side effects elicited in the clinical studies have been primarily associated with the nasal mucous membranes. The most frequent complaints were those of mild transient nasal burning and stinging, which were reported in approximately 45% of the patients treated with NASALIDE in placebo-controlled and long-term studies. These complaints do not usually interfere with treatment; in only 3% of patients was it necessary to decrease dosage or stop treatment because of these symptoms. Approximately the same incidence of mild transient nasal burning and stinging was reported in patients on placebo as was reported in patients treated with NASALIDE in controlled studies, implying that these complaints may be related to the vehicle or the delivery system. The incidence of complaints of nasal burning and stinging decreased with increasing duration of treatment.
Other side effects reported at a frequency of 5% or less were: nasal congestion, sneezing, epistaxis and/or bloody mucus, nasal irritation, watery eyes, sore throat, nausea and/or vomiting, headaches and loss of sense of smell and taste. As is the case with other nasally inhaled corticosteroids, nasal septal perforations have been observed in rare instances.
Systemic corticosteroid side effects were not reported during the controlled clinical trials. If recommended doses are exceeded, or if individuals are particularly sensitive, symptoms of hypercorticism, i.e., Cushing's syndrome, could occur.

OVERDOSAGE

I.V. flunisolide in animals at doses up to 4 mg/kg showed no effect. One spray bottle contains 6.25 mg of NASALIDE; therefore acute overdosage is unlikely.

DOSAGE AND ADMINISTRATION

The therapeutic effects of corticosteroids, unlike those of decongestants, are not immediate. This should be explained to the patient in advance in order to ensure cooperation and continuation of treatment with the prescribed dosage regimen. Full therapeutic benefit requires regular use, and is usually evident within a few days. However, a longer period of therapy may be required for some patients to achieve maximum benefit (up to 3 weeks). If no improvement is evident by that time, NASALIDE® (flunisolide) should not be continued.
Patients with blocked nasal passages should be encouraged to use a decongestant just before NASALIDE administration to ensure adequate penetration of the spray. Patients should also be advised to clear their nasal passages of secretions prior to use.
Adults: The recommended starting dose of NASALIDE is 2 sprays (50 mcg) in each nostril 2 times a day (total dose 200 mcg/day). If needed, this dose may be increased to 2 sprays in each nostril 3 times a day (total dose 300 mcg/day).
Children 6 to 14 years: The recommended starting dose of NASALIDE is one spray (25 mcg) in each nostril 3 times a day or two sprays (50 mcg) in each nostril 2 times a day (total dose 150-200 mcg/day). NASALIDE is not recommended for use in children less than 6 years of age as safety and efficacy studies, including possible adverse effects on growth, have not been conducted.
Maximum total daily doses should not exceed 8 sprays in each nostril for adults (total dose 400 mcg/day) and 4 sprays in each nostril for children under 14 years of age (total dose 200 mcg/day). Since there is no evidence that exceeding the maximum recommended dosage is more effective and increased systemic absorption would occur, higher doses should be avoided.

After the desired clinical effect is obtained, the maintenance dose should be reduced to the smallest amount necessary to control the symptoms. Approximately 15% of patients with perennial rhinitis may be maintained on as little as 1 spray in each nostril per day.

HOW SUPPLIED

Each 25 mL NASALIDE® (flunisolide) nasal solution spray bottle (NDC 0033-2906-40) (NSN 6505-01-132-9979) contains 6.25 mg (0.25 mg/mL) of flunisolide and is supplied in a nasal pump dispenser with dust cover and a patient leaflet of instructions.

Store at controlled room temperature, 15°–30°C (59°–86°F)
CAUTION: Federal law prohibits dispensing without prescription.

02-2906-42-00   Revised 7/88
© 1988 Syntex Laboratories, Inc.
Shown in Product Identification Section, page 433

NORINYL® 1+35 Tablets   ℞
(norethindrone and ethinyl estradiol)
NORINYL® 1+50 Tablets   ℞
(norethindrone and mestranol)

Refer to entry under TRI-NORINYL® Tablets (norethindrone and ethinyl estradiol).
Shown in Product Identification Section, page 433

NOR-QD®   ℞
(norethindrone)
Tablets

Refer to entry under TRI-NORINYL® Tablets (norethindrone and ethinyl estradiol).
Shown in Product Identification Section, page 433

SYNACORT®   ℞
(hydrocortisone)
Cream 1%
Cream 2.5%
SYNALAR®   ℞
(fluocinolone acetonide)
Cream 0.025%
Cream 0.01%
Ointment 0.025%
Topical Solution 0.01%
SYNALAR-HP®   ℞
(fluocinolone acetonide)
Cream 0.2%
SYNEMOL®   ℞
(fluocinolone acetonide)
Cream 0.025%

Refer to entry under LIDEX® (fluocinonide) Cream 0.05%.

SYNAREL®   ℞
[*sin'er-el*]
(nafarelin acetate)
Nasal Solution 2 mg/mL
(as nafarelin base)

A product of Syntex Laboratories, Inc.

DESCRIPTION

SYNAREL (nafarelin acetate) Nasal Solution is intended for administration as a spray to the nasal mucosa. Nafarelin acetate, the active component of SYNAREL Nasal Solution, is a decapeptide with the chemical name: 5-oxo-*L*-prolyl-*L*-histidyl-*L*-tryptophyl-*L*-seryl-*L*-tyrosyl -3- (2- naphthyl)-*D*-alanyl- *L*- leucyl- *L*-arginyl- *L* -prolyl-glycinamide acetate. Nafarelin acetate is a synthetic analog of the naturally occuring gonadotropin releasing hormone (GnRH).

SYNAREL Nasal Solution contains nafarelin acetate (2 mg/mL, content expressed as nafarelin base) in a solution of benzalkonium chloride, glacial acetic acid, sodium hydroxide or hydrochloric acid (to adjust pH), sorbitol, and purified water.

After priming the pump unit for SYNAREL, each actuation of the unit delivers approximately 100 μL of the spray containing approximately 200 μg nafarelin base. The contents of one spray bottle are intended to deliver at least 60 sprays.

CLINICAL PHARMACOLOGY

Nafarelin acetate is a potent agonistic analog of gonadotropin releasing hormone (GnRH). At the onset of administration, nafarelin stimulates the release of the pituitary gonadotropins, LH and FSH, resulting in a temporary increase of ovarian steroidogenesis. Repeated dosing abolishes the stimulatory effect on the pituitary gland. Twice daily administration leads to decreased secretion of gonadal steroids by about

4 weeks; consequently, tissues and functions that depend on gonadal steroids for their maintenance become quiescent. Nafarelin acetate is rapidly absorbed into systemic circulation after intranasal administration. Maximum serum concentrations (measured by RIA) are achieved between 10 and 40 minutes. Following a single dose of 200 μg base, the observed average peak concentration is 0.6 ng/mL, whereas following a single dose of 400 μg base, the observed average peak concentration is 1.8 ng/mL. Bioavailability from a 400 μg dose averaged 2.8%. The average serum half-life of nafarelin following intranasal administration is approximately 3 hours. About 80% of nafarelin acetate is bound to plasma proteins at 4°C.

After subcutaneous administration of ^{14}C-nafarelin acetate, 44–55% of the dose was recovered in urine and 18.5–44.2% was recovered in feces. Approximately 3% of the administered dose appears as unchanged nafarelin in urine. The ^{14}C serum half-life of the metabolites is about 85.5 hours. Six metabolites of nafarelin have been identified of which the major metabolite is Tyr-D(2)-Nal-Leu-Arg-Pro-Gly-NH$_2$(5-10). The activity of the metabolites, the metabolism of nafarelin by nasal mucosa, and the pharmacokinetics of the drug in hepatic- and renal-impaired patients have not been determined.

The effect of rhinitis or a topical decongestant on SYNAREL has not been determined.

In controlled clinical studies, SYNAREL at doses of 400 and 800 μg/day for 6 months was shown to be comparable to danazol, 800 mg/day, in relieving the clinical symptoms of endometriosis (pelvic pain, dysmenorrhea, and dyspareunia) and in reducing the size of endometrial implants as determined by laparoscopy. The clinical significance of a decrease in endometriotic lesions is not known at this time and in addition, laparoscopic staging of endometriosis does not necessarily correlate with severity of symptoms.

SYNAREL 400 μg daily induced amenorrhea in approximately 65%, 80%, and 90% of the patients after 60, 90, and 120 days, respectively. In the first, second, and third post-treatment months, normal menstrual cycles resumed in 4%, 82%, and 100%, respectively, of those patients who did not become pregnant.

At the end of treatment, 60% of patients who received SYNAREL, 400 μg/day, were symptom free, 32% had mild symptoms, 7% had moderate symptoms and 1% had severe symptoms. Of the 60% of patients who had complete relief of symptoms at the end of treatment, 17% had moderate symptoms 6 months after treatment was discontinued, 33% had mild symptoms, 50% remained symptom free, and no patient had severe symptoms.

During the first two months of SYNAREL use, some women experience vaginal bleeding of variable duration and intensity. In all likelihood, this bleeding represents estrogen withdrawal bleeding, and is expected to stop spontaneously. If vaginal bleeding continues, the possibility of lack of compliance with the dosing regimen should be considered. If the patient is complying carefully with the regimen, an increase in dose to 400 μg twice a day should be considered.

There is no evidence that pregnancy rates are enhanced or adversely affected by the use of SYNAREL.

INDICATIONS AND USAGE

SYNAREL is indicated for management of endometriosis, including pain relief and reduction of endometriotic lesions. Experience with SYNAREL for the management of endometriosis has been limited to women 18 years of age and older treated for 6 months.

CONTRAINDICATIONS

1. Hypersensitivity to GnRH, GnRH agonist analogs or any of the excipients in SYNAREL;
2. Undiagnosed abnormal vaginal bleeding;
3. Use in pregnancy or in women who may become pregnant while receiving the drug. SYNAREL may cause fetal harm when administered to a pregnant woman. Major fetal abnormalities were observed in rats, but not in mice or rabbits after administration of SYNAREL throughout gestation. There was a dose-related increase in fetal mortality and a decrease in fetal weight in rats (see Pregnancy Section). The effects on rat fetal mortality are expected consequences of the alterations in hormonal levels brought about by the drug. If this drug is used during pregnancy or if the patient becomes pregnant while taking this drug, she should be apprised of the potential hazard to the fetus;
4. Use in women who are breast feeding (see Nursing Mothers Section).

WARNINGS

Safe use of nafarelin acetate in pregnancy has not been established clinically. Before starting treatment with SYNAREL, pregnancy must be excluded.

When used regularly at the recommended dose, SYNAREL usually inhibits ovulation and stops menstruation. Contraception is not insured, however, by taking SYNAREL, particularly if patients miss successive doses. Therefore, patients should use nonhormonal methods of contraception. Patients should be advised to see their physician if they believe they

may be pregnant. If a patient becomes pregnant during treatment, the drug must be discontinued and the patient must be apprised of the potential risk to the fetus.

PRECAUTIONS

General
As with other drugs in this class, ovarian cysts have been reported to occur in the first two months of therapy with SYNAREL. Many, but not all, of these events occurred in patients with polycystic ovarian disease. These cystic enlargements may resolve spontaneously, generally by about four to six weeks of therapy, but in some cases may require discontinuation of drug and/or surgical intervention.

Information for Patients
An information pamphlet for patients is included with the product. Patients should be aware of the following information:

1. Since menstruation should stop with effective doses of SYNAREL, the patient should notify her physician if regular menstruation persists. The cause of vaginal spotting, bleeding or menstruation could be non-compliance with the treatment regimen, or it could be that a higher dose of the drug is required to achieve amenorrhea. The patient should be questioned regarding her compliance. If she is careful and compliant, and menstruation persists to the second month, consideration should be given to doubling the dose of SYNAREL. If the patient has missed several doses, she should be counseled on the importance of taking SYNAREL regularly as prescribed.
2. Patients should not use SYNAREL if they are pregnant, breast feeding, have undiagnosed abnormal vaginal bleeding, or are allergic to any of the ingredients in SYNAREL.
3. Safe use of the drug in pregnancy has not been established clinically. Therefore, a nonhormonal method of contraception should be used during treatment. Patients should be advised that if they miss successive doses of SYNAREL, breakthrough bleeding or ovulation may occur with the potential for conception. If a patient becomes pregnant during treatment, she should discontinue treatment and consult her physician.
4. Those adverse events occurring most frequently in clinical studies with SYNAREL are associated with hypoestrogenism; the most frequently reported are hot flashes, headaches, emotional lability, decreased libido, vaginal dryness, acne, myalgia, and reduction in breast size. Estrogen levels returned to normal after treatment was discontinued. Nasal irritation occurred in about 10% of all patients who used intranasal nafarelin.
5. The induced hypoestrogenic state results in a small loss in bone density over the course of treatment, some of which may not be reversible. During one six-month treatment period, this bone loss should not be important. In patients with major risk factors for decreased bone mineral content such as chronic alcohol and/or tobacco use, strong family history of osteoporosis, or chronic use of drugs that can reduce bone mass such as anticonvulsants or corticosteroids, SYNAREL therapy may pose an additional risk. In these patients the risks and benefits must be weighed carefully before therapy with SYNAREL is instituted. Repeated courses of treatment with gonadotropin-releasing hormone analogs are not advisable in patients with major risk factors for loss of bone mineral content.
6. Patients with intercurrent rhinitis should consult their physician for the use of a topical nasal decongestant. If the use of a topical nasal decongestant is required during treatment with SYNAREL, the decongestant must be used at least 30 minutes after SYNAREL dosing to decrease the possibility of reducing drug absorption.
7. Retreatment cannot be recommended since safety data beyond 6 months are not available.

Drug Interactions
No pharmacokinetic-based drug-drug interaction studies have been conducted with SYNAREL. However, because nafarelin acetate is a peptide that is primarily degraded by peptidase and not by cytochrome P-450 enzymes, and the drug is only about 80% bound to plasma proteins at 4°C, drug interations would not be expected to occur.

Drug/Laboratory Test Interactions
Administration of SYNAREL in therapeutic doses results in suppression of the pituitary-gonadal system. Normal function is usually restored within 4 to 8 weeks after treatment is discontinued. Therefore, diagnostic tests of pituitary gonadotropic and gonadal functions conducted during treatment and up to 4 to 8 weeks after discontinuation of SYNAREL therapy may be misleading.

Carcinogenesis, Mutagenesis, Impairment of Fertility
Carcinogenicity studies of nafarelin were conducted in rats (24 months) at doses up to 100 μg/kg/day and mice (18 months) at doses up to 500 μg/kg/day using intramuscular doses (up to 110 times and 560 times the maximum recommended human intranasal dose, respectively). These multiples of the human dose are based on the relative bioavailability of the drug by the two routes of administration. As seen with other GnRH agonists, nafarelin acetate given to labora-

Continued on next page

Syntex—Cont.

tory rodents at high doses for prolonged periods induced proliferative responses (hyperplasia and/or neoplasia) of endocrine organs. At 24 months, there was an increase in the incidence of pituitary tumors (adenoma/carcinoma) in high-dose female rats and a dose-related increase in male rats. There was an increase in pancreatic islet cell adenomas in both sexes, and in benign testicular and ovarian tumors in the treated groups. There was a dose-related increase in benign adrenal medullary tumors in treated female rats. In mice, there was a dose-related increase in Harderian gland tumors in males and an increase in pituitary adenomas in high-dose females. No metastases of these tumors were observed. It is known that tumorigenicity in rodents is particularly sensitive to hormonal stimulation.

Mutagenicity studies have been performed with nafarelin acetate using bacterial, yeast, and mammalian systems. These studies provided no evidence of mutagenic potential. Reproduction studies in male and female rats have shown full reversibility of fertility suppression when drug treatment was discontinued after continuous administration for up to 6 months.

Pregnancy, Teratogenic Effects
Pregnancy Category X. See 'Contraindications'. Intramuscular SYNAREL was administered to rats throughout gestation at 0.4, 1.6, and 6.4 µg/kg/day (about 0.5, 2, and 7 times the maximum recommended human intranasal dose based on the relative bioavailability by the two routes of administration). An increase in major fetal abnormalities was observed in 4/80 fetuses at the highest dose. A similar, repeat study at the same doses in rats and studies in mice and rabbits at doses up to 600 µg/kg/day and 0.18 µg/kg/day, respectively, failed to demonstrate an increase in fetal abnormalities after administration throughout gestation. In rats and rabbits, there was a dose-related increase in fetal mortality and a decrease in fetal weight with the highest dose.

Nursing Mothers
It is not known whether SYNAREL is excreted in human milk. Because many drugs are excreted in human milk, and because the effects of SYNAREL on lactation and/or the breastfed child have not been determined, SYNAREL should not be used by nursing mothers.

Pediatric Use
Safety and effectiveness in children have not been established.

ADVERSE REACTIONS
As would be expected with a drug which lowers serum estradiol levels, the most frequently reported adverse reactions were those related to hypoestrogenism.

In controlled studies comparing SYNAREL (400 µg/day) and danazol (600 or 800 mg/day), adverse reactions most frequently reported and thought to be drug-related are shown in the figure below.

In addition, less than 1% of patients experienced paresthesia, palpitations, chloasma, maculopapular rash, eye pain, urticaria, asthenia, lactation, breast engorgement, and arthralgia. In formal clinical trials, immediate hypersensitiv-

ity thought to be possibly or probably related to nafarelin occurred in 3 (0.2%) of 1509 healthy subjects or patients.

Changes in Bone Density
After six months of treatment with SYNAREL, vertebral trabecular bone density and total vertebral bone mass, measured by quantitative computed tomography (QCT), decreased by an average of 8.7% and 4.3%, respectively, compared to pretreatment levels. There was partial recovery of bone density in the post-treatment period; the average trabecular bone density and total bone mass were 4.9% and 3.3% less than the pretreatment levels, respectively. Total vertebral bone mass, measured by dual photon absorptiometry (DPA), decreased by a mean of 5.9% at the end of treatment. Mean total vertebral mass, re-examined by DPA six months after completion of treatment, was 1.4% below pretreatment levels. There was little, if any, decrease in the mineral content in compact bone of the distal radius and second metacarpal. Use of SYNAREL for longer than the recommended six months or in the presence of other known risk factors for decreased bone mineral content may cause additional bone loss.

Changes in Laboratory Values During Treatment
Plasma enzymes. During clinical trials with SYNAREL, regular laboratory monitoring revealed that SGOT and SGPT levels were more than twice the upper limit of normal in only one patient each. There was no other clinical or laboratory evidence of abnormal liver function and levels returned to normal in both patients after treatment was stopped.

Lipids. At enrollment, 9% of the patients in the SYNAREL 400 µg/day group and 2% of the patients in the danazol group had total cholesterol values above 250 mg/dL. These patients also had cholesterol values above 250 mg/dL at the end of treatment.

Of those patients whose pretreatment cholesterol values were below 250 mg/dL, 6% in the SYNAREL group and 18% in the danazol group, had post-treatment values above 250 mg/dL.

The mean (±SEM) pretreatment values for total cholesterol from all patients were 191.8 (4.3) mg/dL in the SYNAREL group and 193.1 (4.6) mg/dL in the danazol group. At the end of treatment, the mean values for total cholesterol from all patients were 204.5 (4.8) mg/dL in the SYNAREL group and 207.7 (5.1) mg/dL in the danazol group. These increases from the pretreatment values were statistically significant (p < 0.05) in both groups.

Triglycerides were increased above the upper limit of 150 mg/dL in 12% of the patients who received SYNAREL and in 7% of the patients who received danazol.

At the end of treatment, no patients receiving SYNAREL had abnormally low HDL cholesterol fractions (less than 30 mg/dL) compared with 43% of patients receiving danazol. None of the patients receiving SYNAREL had abnormally high LDL cholesterol fractions (greater than 190 mg/dL) compared with 15% of those receiving danazol. There was no increase in the LDL/HDL ratio in patients receiving SYNAREL, but there was approximately a 2-fold increase in the LDL/HDL ratio in patients receiving danazol.

Other changes. In comparative studies, the following changes were seen in approximately 10% to 15% of patients. Treatment with SYNAREL was associated with elevations of

plasma phosphorus and eosinophil counts, and decreases in serum calcium and WBC counts. Danazol therapy was associated with an increase of hematocrit and WBC.

OVERDOSAGE
In experimental animals, a single subcutaneous administration of up to 60 times the recommended human dose (on a µg/kg basis, not adjusted for bioavailability) had no adverse effects. At present, there is no clinical evidence of adverse effects following overdosage of GnRH analogs.

Based on studies in monkeys, SYNAREL is not absorbed after oral administration.

DOSAGE AND ADMINISTRATION
For the management of endometriosis, the recommended daily dose of SYNAREL is 400 µg. This is achieved by one spray (200 µg) into one nostril in the morning and one spray into the other nostril in the evening. Treatment should be started between days 2 and 4 of the menstrual cycle.

In an occasional patient, the 400 µg daily dose may not produce amenorrhea. For these patients with persistent regular menstruation after 2 months of treatment, the dose of SYNAREL may be increased to 800 µg daily. The 800 µg dose is administered as one spray into each nostril in the morning (a total of two sprays) and again in the evening. The recommended duration of administration is six months.

Retreatment cannot be recommended since safety data for retreatment are not available. If the symptoms of endometriosis recur after a course of therapy, and further treatment with SYNAREL is contemplated, it is recommended that bone density be assessed before retreatment begins to ensure that values are within normal limits.

If the use of a topical nasal decongestant is necessary during treatment with SYNAREL, the decongestant should not be used until at least 30 minutes after SYNAREL dosing.

At 400 µg/day, a bottle of SYNAREL provides a 30-day (about 60 sprays) supply. If the daily dose is increased, increase the supply to the patient to ensure uninterrupted treatment for the recommended duration of therapy.

HOW SUPPLIED
Each 0.5 ounce bottle (NDC 0033-2260-40) contains 10 mL SYNAREL (nafarelin acetate) Nasal Solution 2 mg/mL (as nafarelin base), and is supplied with a metered spray pump that delivers 200 µg of nafarelin per spray. A dust cover and a leaflet of patient instructions are also included.

Store upright at room temperature. Avoid heat above 30°C (86°F). Protect from light. Protect from freezing.

CAUTION: Federal law prohibits dispensing without prescription.

U.S. Patent No. 4,234,571
02-2260-40-03   Revised 4/91
© 1991 Syntex Laboratories, Inc.
Shown in Product Identification Section, page 433

TICLID® Tablets   ℞
[tye'klid]
(ticlopidine hydrochloride)

A product of Syntex Laboratories, Inc.

DESCRIPTION
TICLID® (ticlopidine hydrochloride) is a platelet aggregation inhibitor. Chemically it is 5-[(2-chlorophenyl)methyl]-4,5,6,7-tetrahydrothieno[3,2-c] pyridine hydrochloride.

Ticlopidine hydrochloride is a white crystalline solid. It is freely soluble in water and self buffers to a pH of 3.6. It also dissolves freely in methanol, is sparingly soluble in methylene chloride and ethanol, slightly soluble in acetone, and insoluble in a buffer solution of pH 6.3. It has a molecular weight of 300.25.

TICLID tablets for oral administration are provided as white, oval, film coated, blue imprinted tablets containing 250 mg of ticlopidine hydrochloride. Each tablet also contains citric acid, magnesium stearate, microcrystalline cellulose, povidone, starch and stearic acid as inactive ingredients. The white film coating contains hydroxypropylmethyl cellulose, polyethylene glycol and titanium dioxide. Each tablet is printed with blue ink which includes FD&C Blue #1 aluminum lake as the colorant. The tablets are identified with "Ticlid" on one side and "250" on the reverse side.

CLINICAL PHARMACOLOGY
Mechanism of Action
When taken orally, ticlopidine hydrochloride causes a time and dose-dependent inhibition of both platelet aggregation and release of platelet granule constituents, as well as a prolongation of bleeding time. The intact drug has no significant *in vitro* activity at the concentrations attained *in vivo*, and, although analysis of urine and plasma indicates at least twenty metabolites, no metabolite which accounts for the activity of ticlopidine has been isolated.

Ticlopidine hydrochloride, after oral ingestion, interferes with platelet membrane function by inhibiting ADP-induced platelet-fibrinogen binding and subsequent platelet-platelet interactions. The effect on platelet function is irreversible

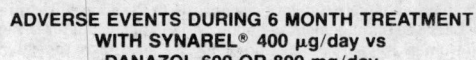

ADVERSE EVENTS DURING 6 MONTH TREATMENT
WITH SYNAREL® 400 µg/day vs
DANAZOL 600 OR 800 mg/day

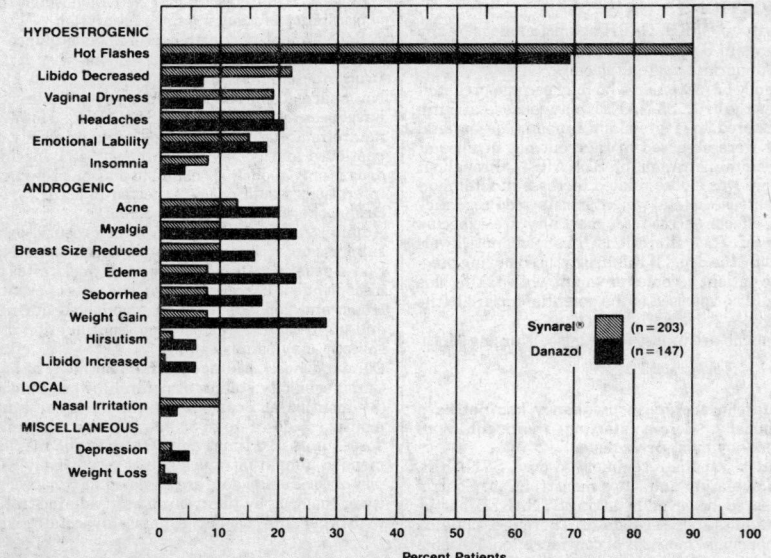

for the life of the platelet, as shown both by persistent inhibition of fibrinogen binding after washing platelets ex vivo and by inhibition of platelet aggregation after resuspension of platelets in buffered medium.

Pharmacokinetics and Metabolism

After oral administration of a single 250 mg dose, ticlopidine hydrochloride is rapidly absorbed, with peak plasma levels occurring at approximately 2 hours after dosing, and is extensively metabolized. Absorption is greater than 80%. Administration after meals results in a 20% increase in the AUC of ticlopidine.

Ticlopidine hydrochloride displays non-linear pharmacokinetics and clearance decreases markedly on repeated dosing. In older volunteers the apparent half-life of ticlopidine after a single 250 mg dose is about 12.6 hours, with repeat dosing at 250 mg BID, the terminal elimination half-life rises to 4-5 days and steady state levels of ticlopidine hydrochloride in plasma are obtained after approximately 14–21 days.

Ticlopidine hydrochloride binds reversibly (98%) to plasma proteins, mainly to serum albumin and lipoproteins. The binding to albumin and lipoproteins is nonsaturable over a wide concentration range. Ticlopidine also binds to alpha-1 acid glycoprotein. At concentrations attained with the recommended dose, only 15% or less ticlopidine in plasma is bound to this protein.

Ticlopidine hydrochloride is metabolized extensively by the liver; only trace amounts of intact drug are detected in the urine. Following an oral dose of radioactive ticlopidine hydrochloride administered in solution, 60% of the radioactivity is recovered in the urine and 23% in the feces. Approximately, ⅓ of the dose excreted in the feces is intact ticlopidine hydrochloride, possibly excreted in the bile. Ticlopidine hydrochloride is a minor component in plasma (5%) after a single dose, but at steady state is the major component (15%). Approximately 40–50% of the radioactive metabolites circulating in plasma are covalently bound to plasma proteins, probably by acylation.

Clearance of ticlopidine decreases with age. Steady state trough values in elderly patients (mean age 70 years) are about twice those in young volunteer populations.

Hepatically Impaired Patients: The effect of decreased hepatic function on the pharmacokinetics of TICLID was studied in 17 patients with advanced cirrhosis. The average plasma concentration of ticlopidine in these subjects was slightly higher than that seen in older subjects in a separate trial. (See Contraindications)

Renally Impaired Patients: Patients with mildly (Ccr 50–80 ml/min) or moderately (Ccr 20–50 ml/min) impaired renal function were compared to normal subjects (Ccr 80–150 ml/min) in a study of the pharmacokinetic and platelet pharmacodynamic effects of TICLID (250 mg BID) for 11 days. Concentrations of unchanged TICLID were measured after a single 250 mg dose and after the final 250 mg dose on Day 11. AUC values of ticlopidine increased by 28 and 60% in mild and moderately impaired patients respectively and plasma clearance decreased by 37 and 52% respectively, but there were no statistically significant differences in ADP-induced platelet aggregation. In this small study (26 patients) bleeding times showed significant prolongation only in the moderately impaired patients.

Pharmacodynamics

In healthy volunteers over the age of 50 substantial inhibition (over 50%) of ADP-induced platelet aggregation is detected within 4 days after administration of ticlopidine hydrochloride 250 mg BID and maximum platelet aggregation inhibition (60–70%) is achieved after 8 to 11 days. Lower doses cause less, and more delayed, platelet aggregation inhibition, while doses above 250 mg BID give little additional effect on platelet aggregation, but an increased rate of adverse effects. The dose of 250 mg BID is the only dose that has been evaluated in controlled clinical trials.

After discontinuation of ticlopidine hydrochloride, bleeding time and other platelet function tests return to normal within two weeks in the majority of patients.

At the recommended therapeutic dose (250 mg BID), ticlopidine hydrochloride has no known significant pharmacological actions in man other than inhibition of platelet function and prolongation of the bleeding time.

CLINICAL TRIALS

The effect of ticlopidine on the risk of stroke and cardiovascular events was studied in two multi-center randomized double-blind trials.

1. Study in patients experiencing stroke precursors: In a trial comparing ticlopidine and aspirin (The Ticlopidine Aspirin Stroke Study or TASS), 3069 patients (1987 men, 1082 women) who had experienced such stroke precursors as transient ischemic attack (TIA), transient monocular blindness (amaurosis fugax), reversible ischemic neurological deficit, or minor stroke were randomized to ticlopidine 250 mg BID or aspirin 650 mg BID. The study was designed to follow patients for at least 2 and up to 5 years.

Over the duration of the study, TICLID significantly reduced the risk of fatal and nonfatal stroke by 24% (p=.011) from 18.1 to 13.8 per 100 patients followed for five years, compared to aspirin. During the first year, when the risk of stroke is greatest, the reduction in risk of stroke (fatal and nonfatal) compared to aspirin was 48%, the reduction was similar in men and women.

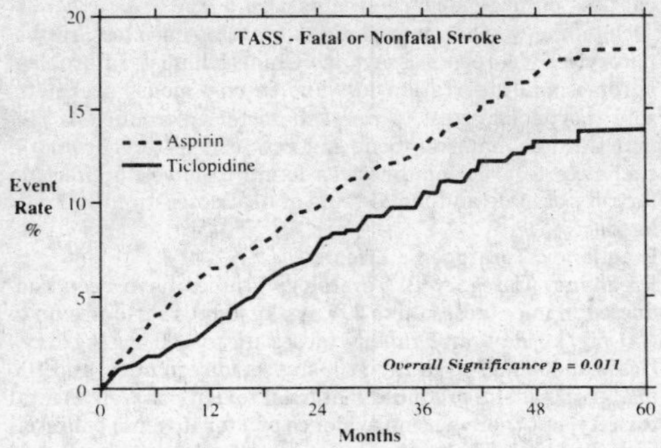

2. Study in patients who had a completed atherothrombotic stroke: In a trial comparing ticlopidine with placebo (The Canadian American Ticlopidine Study, or CATS) 1073 patients who had experienced a previous atherothrombotic stroke were treated with TICLID 250 mg BID or placebo for up to 3 years.

TICLID significantly reduced the overall risk of stroke by 24% (p=.017) from 24.6 to 18.6 per 100 patients followed for three years, compared to placebo. During the first year the reduction in risk of fatal and nonfatal stroke over placebo was 33%.

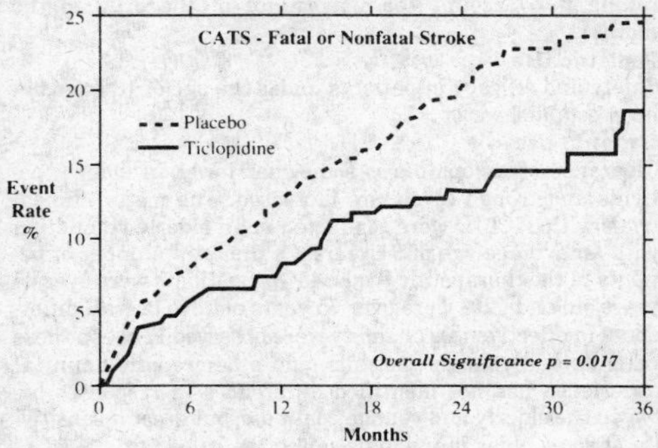

INDICATIONS AND USAGE

TICLID is indicated to reduce the risk of thrombotic stroke (fatal or nonfatal) in patients who have experienced stroke precursors, and in patients who have had a completed thrombotic stroke.

Because TICLID is associated with a risk of neutropenia/agranulocytosis, which may be life-threatening (See Warnings), TICLID should be reserved for patients who are intolerant to aspirin therapy where indicated to prevent stroke.

CONTRAINDICATIONS

The use of TICLID® is contraindicated in the following conditions:

- Hypersensitivity to the drug.
- Presence of hematopoietic disorders such as neutropenia and thrombocytopenia.
- Presence of a hemostatic disorder or active pathological bleeding (such as bleeding peptic ulcer or intracranial bleeding).
- Patients with severe liver impairment.

WARNINGS

Neutropenia

Neutropenia defined in these studies as an ANC < 1200 neutrophilis/mm³ occurred in 50 of 2,048 (2.4%) stroke patients who received TICLID in clinical trials.

Severe Neutropenia (< 450 neutrophils/mm³):

Severe neutropenia and/or agranulocytosis occurred in 17 of the 2,048 (0.8%) patients who received TICLID. When the drug was discontinued in these patients, the neutrophil counts returned to normal (> 1200 neutrophils/mm³) within 1–3 weeks.

Mild to Moderate Neutropenia (451–1200 neutrophils/mm³):

Mild to moderate neutropenia occurred in 33 of the 2,048 (1.6%) patients who received TICLID. Eleven of the patients discontinued treatment and recovered within a few days. In the remaining 22 patients, the neutropenia was transient and did not require discontinuation of therapy.

The onset of severe neutropenia occurred 3 weeks to 3 months after the start of therapy with TICLID, with no documented cases of severe neutropenia beyond that time in the large controlled trials. The bone marrow typically showed a reduction in myeloid precursors.

It is therefore essential that CBCs and white cell differentials be performed every two weeks starting from the second week to the end of the third month of therapy with TICLID, but more frequent monitoring is necessary for patients whose absolute neutrophil counts have been consistently declining or are 30% less than the baseline count.

Neutropenia (an absolute neutrophil count (ANC) of less than 1200 neutrophils/mm³) is calculated as follows: ANC = WBC × % neutrophils. If clinical evaluation and repeat laboratory testing confirm the presence of neutropenia (< 1200/mm³), the drug should be discontinued.

In clinical trials, when therapy was discontinued immediately upon detection of neutropenia, the neutrophil counts returned to normal within 1–3 weeks.

After the first three months of therapy, CBCs need be obtained only for patients with signs or symptoms suggestive of infection.

Thrombocytopenia

Rarely, thrombocytopenia may occur in isolation or together with neutropenia.

If clinical evaluation and repeat laboratory testing confirm the presence of thrombocytopenia (<80,000 cells/mm³), the drug should be discontinued.

Cholesterol Elevation

TICLID® therapy causes increased serum cholesterol and triglycerides. Serum total cholesterol levels are increased 8–10% within one month of therapy and persist at that level. The ratios of the lipoprotein subfractions are unchanged.

Other Hematological Effects

Rare cases of pancytopenia and thrombotic thrombocytopenic purpura, some of which have been fatal, have been reported in Post-Marketing Surveillance.

Anticoagulant Drugs

The tolerance and safety of coadministration of TICLID with heparin, oral anticoagulants, or fibrinolytic agents has not been established. If a patient is switched from an anticoagulant or fibrinolytic drug to TICLID, the former drug should be discontinued prior to TICLID administration.

PRECAUTIONS

General

TICLID should be used with caution in patients who may be at risk of increased bleeding from trauma, surgery, or pathological conditions. If it is desired to eliminate the antiplatelet effects of TICLID prior to elective surgery, the drug should be discontinued 10–14 days prior to surgery. Several controlled clinical studies have found increased surgical blood loss in patients undergoing surgery during treatment with ticlopidine. In TASS and CATS it was recommended that patients have ticlopidine discontinued prior to elective surgery. Several hundred patients underwent surgery during the trials, and no excessive surgical bleeding was reported.

Prolonged bleeding time is normalized within two hours after administration of 20 mg methylprednisolone i.v. Platelet transfusions may also be used to reverse the effect of TICLID on bleeding.

GI Bleeding

TICLID prolongs template bleeding time. The drug should be used with caution in patients who have lesions with a propensity to bleed (such as ulcers). Drugs that might induce such lesions should be used with caution in patients on TICLID. (See Contraindications.)

Use in Hepatically Impaired Patients

Because of limited experience in patients with severe hepatic disease, who may have bleeding diatheses, the use of TICLID is not recommended in this population. (See Clinical Pharmacology and Contraindications.)

Use in Renally Impaired Patients

There is limited experience in patients with renal impairment. In controlled clinical trials, no unexpected problems have been encountered in patients having mild renal impairment and there is no experience with dosage adjustment in patients with greater degrees of renal impairment. Nevertheless, for renally impaired patients it may be necessary to reduce the dosage of ticlopidine or discontinue it altogether, if hemorrhagic or hematopoietic problems are encountered. (See Clinical Pharmacology)

Information for the Patient (See PPI)

Patients should be told that a decrease in the number of white blood cells (neutropenia) can occur with TICLID®, especially during the first three months of treatment, and that if neutropenia is severe, it could result in an increased risk of infection. They should be told it is critically important to obtain the scheduled blood tests to detect neutropenia. Patients should also be reminded to contact their physicians if they experience any indication of infection such as fever, chills, and sore throat, all of which may be consequences of neutropenia.

Continued on next page

Syntex—Cont.

All patients should be told that it may take them longer than usual to stop bleeding when they take TICLID and that they should report any unusual bleeding to their physician. Patients should tell physicians and dentists that they are taking TICLID before any surgery is scheduled and before any new drug is prescribed.

Patients should be told to report promptly side effects of TICLID such as severe or persistent diarrhea, skin rashes, or subcutaneous bleeding, or any signs of cholestasis, such as yellow skin or sclera, dark urine, or light colored stools. Patients should be told to take TICLID with food or just after eating in order to minimize gastrointestinal discomfort.

Laboratory Tests

Liver Function: TICLID therapy has been associated with elevations of alkaline phosphatase and transaminases which generally occurred within 1–4 months of therapy initiation. In controlled clinical trials, the incidence of elevated alkaline phosphatase (greater than 2 times upper limit of normal) was 7.6% in ticlopidine patients, 6.0% in placebo patients and 2.5% in aspirin patients. The incidence of elevated AST (SGOT) (greater than 2 times upper limit of normal) was 3.1% in ticlopidine patients, 4.0% in placebo patients and 2.1% in aspirin patients. No progressive increases were observed in closely monitored clinical trials (e.g. no transaminase greater than 10 times the upper limit of normal was seen), but most patients with these abnormalities had therapy discontinued. Occasionally patients had developed minor elevations in bilirubin.

Based on post-marketing and clinical trials experiences, liver function testing should be considered whenever liver dysfunction is suspected, particularly during the first four months of treatment.

Drug Interactions

Therapeutic doses of TICLID caused a 30% increase in the plasma half-life of antipyrine and may cause analogous effect on similarly metabolized drugs. Therefore the dose of drugs metabolized by hepatic microsomal enzymes with low therapeutic ratios, or being given to patients with hepatic impairment, may require adjustment to maintain optimal therapeutic blood levels when starting or stopping concomitant therapy with ticlopidine. Studies of specific drug interactions yielded the following results:

Aspirin: Aspirin did not modify the ticlopidine-mediated inhibition of ADP-induced platelet aggregation, but ticlopidine potentiated the effect of aspirin on collagen-induced platelet aggregation. The safety of this combination has not been established and concomitant use of aspirin and ticlopidine is not recommended. (See Precautions—GI Bleeding).

Antacids: Administration of TICLID after antacids resulted in an 18% decrease in plasma levels of ticlopidine.

Cimetidine: Chronic administration of cimetidine reduced the clearance of a single dose of TICLID by 50%.

Digoxin: Co-administration of TICLID with digoxin resulted in a slight decrease (approximately 15%) in digoxin plasma levels. Little or no change in therapeutic efficacy of digoxin would be expected.

Theophylline: In normal volunteers, concomitant administration of TICLID resulted in a significant increase in the theophylline elimination half-life from 8.6 to 12.2 hr and a comparable reduction in total plasma clearance of theophylline.

Phenobarbital: In six normal volunteers, the inhibitory effects of TICLID on platelet aggregation were not altered by chronic administration of phenobarbital.

Phenytoin: In vitro studies demonstrated that ticlopidine does not alter the plasma protein binding of phenytoin. However, the protein binding interactions of ticlopidine and its metabolites have not been studies in vivo. Caution should be exercised in coadministering this drug with TICLID and it may be useful to remeasure phenytoin blood concentrations.

Propranolol: In vitro studies demonstrated that ticlopidine does not alter the plasma protein binding of propranolol. However, the protein binding interactions of ticlopidine and its metabolites have not been studies in vivo. Caution should be exercised in coadministering this drug with TICLID.

Other Concomitant Therapy: Although specific interaction studies were not performed, in clinical studies, TICLID was used concomitantly with beta blockers, calcium channel blockers, diuretics, and nonsteroidal anti-inflammatory drugs without evidence of clinically significant adverse interactions. (See Precautions.)

Food Interaction: The oral bioavailability of ticlopidine is increased by 20% when taken after a meal. Administration of TICLID with food is recommended to maximize gastrointestinal tolerance. In controlled trials, TICLID was taken with meals.

Carcinogenesis, Mutagenesis, Impairment of Fertility

In a two-year oral carcinogenicity study in rats, ticlopidine at daily doses of up to 100 mg/kg (610 mg/m^2) was not tumorigenic. For a 70 kg person (1.73m^2 body surface area), the dose represents 14 times the recommended clinical dose on a mg/kg basis and 2 times the clinical dose on body surface area basis. In a 78 week oral carcinogenicity study in mice ticlopidine at daily doses up to 275 mg/kg (1180 mg/m^2) was not tumorigenic. The dose represents 40 times the recommended clinical dose on a mg/kg basis and 4 times the clinical dose on body surface area basis.

Ticlopidine was not mutagenic in *in vitro* Ames test, rat hepatocyte DNA-repair assay, and Chinese hamster fibroblast chromosomal aberration test and *in vivo* mouse spermatozoid morphology test, Chinese hamster micronucleus test and Chinese hamster bone marrow cell sister chromatid exchange test. Ticlopidine was found to have no effect on fertility of male and female rats at oral doses up to 400 mg/kg/day.

Pregnancy: Teratogenic Effects

Pregnancy Category B. Teratology studies have been conducted in mice (doses up to 200 mg/kg/day), rats (doses up to 400 mg/kg/day) and rabbits (doses up to 200 mg/kg/day). Doses of 400 mg/kg in rats, 200 mg/kg/day in mice, and 100 mg/kg in rabbits produced maternal toxicity as well as fetal toxicity, but there was no evidence of a teratogenic potential of ticlopidine. There are, however, no adequate and well-controlled studies in pregnant women. Because animal reproduction studies are not always predictive of a human response, this drug should be used during pregnancy only if clearly needed.

Nursing Mothers

Studies in rats have shown ticlopidine is excreted in the milk. It is not known whether this drug is excreted in human milk. Because many drugs are excreted in human milk and because of the potential for serious adverse reactions in nursing infants from ticlopidine, a decision should be made whether to discontinue nursing or to discontinue the drug, taking into account the importance of the drug to the mother.

Pediatric Use

Safety and efficacy in patients under the age of 18 have not been established.

Geriatric Use

Clearance of ticlopidine is somewhat lower in elderly patients and trough levels are increased. The major clinical trials with TICLID were conducted in an elderly population with an average age of 64 years. Of the total number of patients in the therapeutic trials, 45% of patients were over 65 years old and 12% were over 75 years old. No overall differences in effectiveness or safety were observed between these patients and younger patients, and other reported clinical experience has not identified differences in responses between the elderly and younger patients, but greater sensitivity of some older individuals cannot be ruled out.

ADVERSE REACTIONS

Adverse reactions were relatively frequent, with over 50% of patients reporting at least one. Most (30 to 40%) involved the gastrointestinal tract. Most adverse effects are mild, but 21% of patients discontinued therapy because of an adverse event, principally diarrhea, rash, nausea, vomiting, G.I. pain, and neutropenia. Most adverse effects occur early in the course of treatment, but a new onset of adverse effects can occur after several months.

The incidence rates of adverse events listed in the following table were derived from multicenter, controlled clinical trials described above comparing TICLID, placebo, and aspirin over study periods of up to 5.8 years. Adverse events considered by the investigator to probably drug-related that occurred in at least one percent of patients treated with TICLID are shown in the following table:

Percent of Patients with Adverse Events in Controlled Studies

Event	TICLID (n=2048) Incidence	Aspirin (n=1527) Incidence	Placebo (n=536) Incidence
Any Events	*60.0 (20.9)*	*53.2 (14.5)*	*34.3 (6.1)*
Diarrhea	12.5 (6.3)	5.2 (1.8)	4.5 (1.7)
Nausea	7.0 (2.6)	6.2 (1.9)	1.7 (0.9)
Dyspepsia	7.0 (1.1)	9.0 (2.0)	0.9 (0.2)
Rash	5.1 (3.4)	1.5 (0.8)	0.6 (0.9)
GI Pain	3.7 (1.9)	5.6 (2.7)	1.3 (0.4)
Neutropenia	2.4 (1.3)	0.8 (0.1)	1.1 (0.4)
Purpura	2.2 (0.2)	1.6 (0.1)	0.0 (0.0)
Vomiting	1.9 (1.4)	1.4 (0.9)	0.9 (0.4)
Flatulence	1.5 (0.1)	1.4 (0.3)	0.0 (0.0)
Pruritus	1.3 (0.8)	0.3 (0.1)	0.0 (0.0)
Dizziness	1.1 (0.4)	0.5 (0.4)	0.0 (0.0)
Anorexia	1.0 (0.4)	0.5 (0.3)	0.0 (0.0)
Abnormal Liver Function test	1.0 (0.7)	0.3 (0.3)	0.0 (0.0)

Incidence of discontinuation, regardless of relationship therapy, is shown in parentheses

Neutropenia/Thrombocytopenia

See Warnings.

Gastrointestinal

TICLID therapy has been associated with a variety of gastrointestinal complaints including diarrhea and nausea. The majority of cases are mild, but about 13% of patients discontinued therapy because of these. They usually occur within 3 months of initiation of therapy and typically are resolved within 1–2 weeks without discontinuation of therapy. If the effect is severe or persistent, therapy should be discontinued.

Hemorrhagic

TICLID has been associated with a number of bleeding complications such as ecchymosis, epistaxis, hematuria, conjunctival hemorrhage, gastrointestinal bleeding and perioperative bleeding.

Intracerebral bleeding was rare in clinical trials with TICLID, with an incidence no greater than that seen with comparator agents. (Ticlopidine 0.5%, aspirin 0.6%, placebo 0.75%.)

Rash

Ticlopidine has been associated with a maculopapular or urticarial rash (often with pruritus). Rash usually occurs within 3 months of initiation of therapy, with a mean onset time of 11 days. If drug is discontinued, recovery occurs within several days. Many rashes do not recur on drug rechallenge. There have been rare reports of severe rashes.

Less Frequent Adverse Reactions (Probably Related)

Clinical adverse experiences occurring in 0.5 to 1.0 percent of patients in the controlled trials include:

Digestive System: GI fullness.
Skin and Appendages: urticaria.
Nervous System: headache.
Body as a Whole: asthenia, pain.
Hemostatic System: epistaxis.
Special Senses: tinnitus.

In addition, rarer, relatively serious events have also been reported, mainly from foreign post marketing experience: Pancytopenia, hemolytic anemia with reticulocytosis, allergic pneumonitis, systemic lupus (positive ANA), peripheral neuropathy, vasculitis, serum sickness, arthropathy, hepatitis, cholestatic jaundice, nephrotic syndrome, myositis, hyponatremia, immune thrombocytopenia and thrombocytopenic thrombotic purpura (TTP).

OVERDOSAGE

One case of deliberate overdosage with TICLID has been reported by foreign postmarketing surveillance program. A 38 year old male took a single 6000 mg dose of TICLID (equivalent to 24 standard 250 mg tablets). The only abnormalities reported were increased bleeding time and increased SGPT. No special therapy was instituted and the patient recovered without sequelae.

Single oral doses of ticlopidine at 1600 mg/kg and 500 mg/kg were lethal to rats and mice, respectively. Symptoms of acute toxicity were GI hemorrhage, convulsions, hypothermia, dyspnea, loss of equilibrium and abnormal gait.

DOSAGE AND ADMINISTRATION

The recommended dose of TICLID is 250 mg BID taken with food. Other doses have not been studied in controlled trials for these indications.

HOW SUPPLIED

TICLID is available in white oval film coated 250 mg tablets, printed in blue with "TICLID" on one side and "250" on the other. They are provided in unit of use bottles of 30 (NDC #0033-0431-38) and in cartons of 100 blister packed tablets (NDC #0033-0431-53). Store at 15–30°C (59–86°F).

CAUTION: Federal law prohibits dispensing without prescription.

IMPORTANT INFORMATION ABOUT TICLID (ticlopidine HCl) Tablets

The information in this leaflet is intended to help you use TICLID safely. Please read the leaflet carefully. Although it does not contain all the detailed medical information that is provided to your doctor, it provides facts about TICLID that are important for you to know. If you still have questions after reading this sheet or if you have questions at any time during your treatment with TICLID, check with your doctor.

Special Warning for Users of TICLID/Necessary Blood Tests

Your doctor has prescribed TICLID tablets (250 mg) to help reduce your risk of having a stroke, either because you have had a stroke already (to decrease the chance of another one) or because a stroke is threatening.

TICLID is recommended only for patients who cannot take aspirin, which also can decrease the risk of stroke. This is because TICLID can on occasion, cause a serious white blood cell abnormality. A small percentage of people who take TICLID (about 1.0%) develop a large fall in the number of their white cells (a condition called neutropenia) that can be life-threatening because it leaves them unable to fight infection. If neutropenia occurs, it almost always does so during the first three months of treatment.

To make sure you don't develop this problem, your doctor will arrange for you to have your blood tested every two weeks for the first three months you are on TICLID. If de-

tected, neutropenia can almost always be reversed, but if left untreated, neutropenia can lead to fatal infection. It is therefore essential that you keep your appointments for the blood tests and that you call your doctor immediately if you have any sign of an infection, such as fever, chills, or sore throat, because these can mean that you have neutropenia.

Other Warnings and Precautions
A few people may develop jaundice while being treated with TICLID. The signs of jaundice are yellowing of the skin or the whites of the eyes, or consistent darkening in the color of urine or lightening in the color of stools. **If these symptoms occur, contact your doctor immediately.**

TICLID should be used only as directed by your doctor. Do not give TICLID to anyone else. **Keep TICLID out of reach of children!**

Some people may have such side effects as diarrhea, skin rash, stomach or intestinal discomfort. If any of these problems are persistent, or if you are concerned about them, bring them to your doctor's attention.

It may take longer than usual to stop bleeding when taking TICLID. Tell your doctor if you have any more bleeding or bruising than usual, and be sure to let your doctor know that you are taking TICLID if you have emergency surgery. Also, tell your doctor well in advance of any planned surgery (including tooth extraction), because he or she may recommend that you stop taking TICLID temporarily.

How TICLID Works
A stroke occurs when a clot (or thrombus) forms in a blood vessel in the brain or forms in another part of the body and breaks off, then travels to the brain (an embolus). In both cases the blood supply to part of the brain is blocked and that part of the brain is damaged. TICLID works by making the blood less likely to clot, although not so much less that it causes you to become likely to bleed, unless you have a bleeding disorder or some injury (such as a bleeding ulcer of the stomach or intestine) that is especially likely to bleed.

Who Should Not Take TICLID?
Contact your doctor immediately and do not take TICLID if
• you have an allergic reaction to TICLID
• you have a blood disorder or a serious bleeding problem, such as a bleeding stomach ulcer
• you have severe liver disease or other liver problems
• you are pregnant or you are planning to become pregnant
• you are breast-feeding
U.S. Patent Nos. 4,051,141; 4,591,592
02-0431-00-00
NOVEMBER 1991
©1991 SYNTEX LABORATORIES, INC.
Shown in Product Identification Section, page 433

TORADOL® IM AND TORADOL® ORAL
[tō rah-dol]
(ketorolac tromethamine)
    ℞

A product of Syntex Laboratories, Inc.

DESCRIPTION
TORADOL (ketorolac tromethamine) is a member of the pyrrolo-pyrrole group of nonsteroidal anti-inflammatory drugs (NSAIDs). The chemical name for ketorolac tromethamine is (±)-5-benzoyl-2,3-dihydro-1$\underline{H}$-pyrrolizine-1-carboxylic acid, 2-amino-2-(hydroxymethyl)-1,3-propanediol.
TORADOL is a racemic mixture of R-(+)- and S-(−)- ketorolac tromethamine. Ketorolac tromethamine may exist in three crystal forms. All forms are equally soluble in water. Ketorolac tromethamine has a pKa of 3.5 and an n-octanol/water partition coefficient of 0.26. The molecular weight of ketorolac tromethamine is 376.41.
TORADOL^{IM} is available for intramuscular (IM) administration as: 15 mg in 1 mL (1.5%), 30 mg in 1 mL (3%), or 60 mg in 2 mL (3%) of ketorolac tromethamine in sterile solution. The 15 mg/mL solution contains 10% (w/v) alcohol, USP, and 6.68 mg of sodium chloride in sterile water. The 30 mg/mL solution contains 10% (w/v) alcohol, USP, and 4.35 mg sodium chloride in sterile water. The pH is adjusted with sodium hydroxide or hydrochloric acid and solutions are packaged with nitrogen. The sterile solutions are clear and slightly yellow in color.
TORADOL^{ORAL} is available as round, white, film-coated red-print tablets. Each tablet contains 10 mg ketorolac tromethamine, the active ingredient, with lactose, magnesium stearate, and microcrystalline cellulose. The white film-coating contains hydroxypropyl methylcellulose, polyethylene glycol, and titanium dioxide.
The tablets are printed with red ink which includes FD&C Red #40 Aluminum lake as the colorant. The tablets are identified as follows:
[See table at top of next column.]

CLINICAL PHARMACOLOGY
Pharmacodynamics
Ketorolac is a nonsteroidal anti-inflammatory drug (NSAID) that exhibits analgesic, anti-inflammatory, and antipyretic

	Side 1	Side 2
Trade:	TORADOL*	SYNTEX*
Sample:	TORADOL*	SAMPLE*

*Printed with a bold horizontal line above lettering and a bold vertical line centered below, forming a large T.

activity. Ketorolac inhibits synthesis of prostaglandins and may be considered a peripherally acting analgesic. As with other NSAIDs, the biological activity of ketorolac is associated with the S form. Ketorolac does not have any known effects on opiate receptors.
Pain relief, following extraction of impacted third molars, is clinically evident when steady state plasma levels average approximately 0.3 µg/mL, while side effects are frequent above concentrations of 5 µg/mL. Pain relief is comparable following IM or oral administration. Pain relief is statistically different from that following placebo at ½ hour (the first time point at which it was measured) following the largest recommended doses of ketorolac and by 1 hour following the smallest recommended dose. The peak analgesic effect occurs at 2 to 3 hours and is not statistically significantly different over the recommended dosage range of ketorolac. The greatest difference between large and small doses of TORADOL by either route is in the duration of analgesia. In controlled clinical trials 75% of patients receiving 90 mg of TORADOL^{IM} or 100 mg TORADOL^{ORAL} did not request remedication at 6 hours as compared to 56% of those patients receiving 10 mg of TORADOL^{IM} or 10 to 12.5 mg TORADOL^{ORAL}. [See table next column.]

Table of Estimated Pharmacodynamic Parameters Following Oral or Intramuscular Doses of TORADOL

$C_{50}est^1$	0.3 µg/mL
$C_{toxic}est^2$	5 µg/mL

[1] Estimated concentration required to obtain 50% decreases in pain intensity scores in dental surgery pain
[2] Estimated concentration above which side effects are frequent

Pharmacokinetics (see Tables and Graph)
The pharmacokinetics of ketorolac in humans, following single or multiple intramuscular or oral doses, are apparently linear, i.e., plasma levels are approximately proportional to dosage. Steady state plasma levels are achieved after dosing every 6 hours for one day. No changes in clearance occur with chronic dosing. More than 99% of the ketorolac in plasma is protein bound over a wide concentration range.
The pharmacokinetic profiles of IM and oral doses are very similar. Following IM administration, some individuals have slower absorption which is reflected below in the two tables showing results of studies of 15, 30, and 60 mg of TORADOL^{IM} and 10 mg of TORADOL^{ORAL}. Note that the studies used different but comparable subject populations. The tables show slightly longer times to peak plasma levels and slightly longer apparent half-lives following IM administration.
TORADOL^{IM} is completely absorbed following intramuscular administration with mean peak plasma concentrations of 2.2–3.0 µg/mL occurring an average of 50 minutes after a

Table of Approximate Average Pharmacokinetic Parameters Following Intramuscular and Oral Doses of TORADOL

Pharmacokinetic Parameter (units)	Oral†		Intramuscular*	
	10 mg	15 mg	30 mg	60 mg
Bioavailability (extent)	100%	100%	100%	100%
T_{max}^1 (min)	20–60	30–60	30–60	30–60
C_{max}^2 (µg/mL) [single dose]	0.7–1.1	1.0–1.4	2.2–3.0	4.0–4.5
C_{max} (µg/mL) [steady state qid]	0.7–1.2	1.1–1.7	2.3–3.5	N/A††
C_{min}^3 (µg/mL) [steady state qid]	0.2–0.3	0.2–0.3	0.3–0.7	N/A
C_{ave}^4 (µg/mL) [steady state qid]	0.3–0.6	0.6–0.8	1.3–1.5	N/A
$Vd(\beta)^5$ (L/kg)	0.15–0.33			

% Dose metabolized = <50   % Dose excreted in feces = 6
% Dose excreted in urine = 91   % Plasma protein binding = 99

* Derived from IM pharmacokinetic studies in 32 normal volunteers.
† Derived from PO pharmacokinetic studies in 23 normal fasted volunteers.
†† Not applicable because 60 mg is only recommended as a loading dose
[1] Time to peak plasma concentration
[2] Peak plasma concentration
[3] Trough plasma concentration
[4] Average plasma concentration
[5] Volume of distribution (calculated from mean clearance and terminal half-life)

The Influence of Age, Liver and Kidney Function on the Clearance and Terminal Half-life of TORADOL^{IM1} and ^{ORAL2}

Type of Subjects	Total Clearance [in L/h/kg]^3		Terminal Half-life [in hours]	
	IM mean (range)	Oral mean (range)	IM mean (range)	Oral mean (range)
Normal subjects IM (n=54), Oral (n=77)	0.023 (0.010–0.046)	0.025 (0.013–0.050)	5.3 (3.5–9.2)	5.3 (2.4–9.0)
Healthy elderly subjects IM (n=13), Oral (n=12) (mean age=72, range=65–78)	0.019 (0.013–0.034)	0.024 (0.018–0.034)	7.0 (4.7–8.6)	6.1 (4.3–7.6)
Patients with Hepatic Dysfunction IM and Oral (n=7)	0.029 (0.013–0.066)	0.033 (0.019–0.051)	5.4 (2.2–6.9)	4.5 (1.6–7.6)
Patients with Renal Impairment IM and Oral (n=9) (serum creatinine 1.9–5.0 mg/dL)	0.014 (0.007–0.043)	0.016 (0.007–0.052)	10.3 (8.1–15.7)	10.8 (3.4–18.9)
Renal Dialysis Patients IM (n=9)	0.016 (0.003–0.036)	—	13.6 (8.0–39.1)	—

1. Estimated from 30 mg single IM doses of ketorolac tromethamine
2. Estimated from 10 mg single oral doses of ketorolac tromethamine
3. Liters/hour/kilogram

Continued on next page

Syntex—Cont.

single 30 mg dose. The terminal plasma half-life is 3.5–9.2 hours in young adults and 4.7–8.6 hours in elderly subjects (mean age 72).

TORADOL^{ORAL} is completely absorbed following oral administration with a mean peak plasma concentration of 0.7–1.1 μg/mL occurring an average of 44 minutes after a single 10 mg dose in fasted subjects. The terminal plasma half-life is 2.4–9.0 hours in young adults and 4.3–7.6 hours in elderly subjects (mean age 72).

A high fat meal decreased the peak and delayed the time to peak concentration, but did not affect the extent of absorption, while antacid had no effect upon absorption of TORADOL^{ORAL}.

Ketorolac, following intravenous, intramuscular and oral administration, displays characteristics of a two-compartment model. In order to minimize the time delay in achieving adequate analgesic effect, an IM or oral loading dose equal to twice the maintenance dose is recommended. This is based upon the pharmacokinetic principle that when the dosing interval is near the drug's half-life, the target steady-state plasma level is achieved faster if the first dose is twice the maintenance dose. Due to the two-compartment characteristics of ketorolac, the loading dose results in plasma levels during the first dosing interval that are higher than in subsequent intervals (see graph of IM dosing which illustrates this).

Metabolism and Excretion

The primary route of excretion of ketorolac and its metabolites (conjugates and a para-hydroxy metabolite) is in the urine (mean 91.4%) and the remainder (mean 6.1%) is excreted in the feces. In patients with serum creatinine values ranging from 1.9 to 5.0 mg/dL, the rate of ketorolac clearance was reduced to approximately two-thirds of normal. Decreases in serum albumin, such as encountered in liver cirrhosis, would be expected to change ketorolac clearance. However, in a study of 7 patients with liver cirrhosis, no correlation was found between serum albumin concentration and ketorolac clearance.

Hemodynamics of anesthetized patients were not altered by parenteral administration of ketorolac. Unlike opiate analgesics such as morphine, ketorolac does not cause respiratory depression.

Ketorolac poorly penetrates the blood-brain barrier (levels in the cerebrospinal fluid were found to be 0.002 times or less than those in plasma).

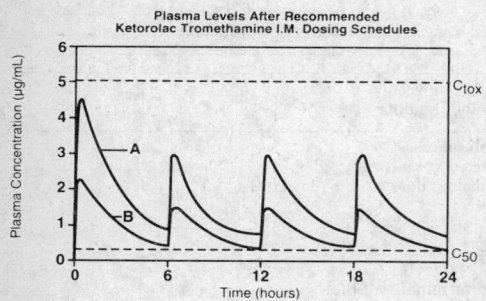

Plasma Levels After Recommended Ketorolac Tromethamine I.M. Dosing Schedules

A = Ketorolac tromethamine 60 mg followed by 30 mg doses (q6h)
B = Ketorolac tromethamine 30 mg followed by 15 mg doses (q6h)
C_{tox} = Estimated concentration above which side effects are frequent
C₅₀ = Estimated concentration required to obtain 50% decreases in pain intensity scores in dental surgery pain

Clinical Studies

The analgesic efficacy of intramuscularly and orally administered ketorolac was investigated in two postoperative pain models: general surgery (orthopedic, gynecologic and abdominal) and oral surgery (removal of impacted third molars). The studies were primarily double-blind, single dose, parallel trial designs in patients with moderate to severe pain at baseline. TORADOL^{IM} was compared to meperidine or morphine administered intramuscularly. TORADOL^{ORAL} was compared to naproxen, ibuprofen, aspirin, acetaminophen and aspirin with codeine.

Short Term Use (up to 5 days)

In the comparisons of intramuscular administration during the first hour, the onset of analgesic action was similar to TORADOL and the narcotics. TORADOL 30 or 90 mg intramuscularly gave pain relief comparable to meperidine 100 mg or morphine 12 mg. TORADOL 10 mg was comparable to 50 mg of meperidine or 6 mg morphine. The duration of analgesia was longer with all three doses of TORADOL. The percentage of patients who did not remedicate by 6 hours, i.e., by the end of the studies, was roughly 70%, 60% and 50% for

TORADOL 90, 30 and 10 mg respectively, as compared to 30% and 20% for the high and low doses of the two narcotics. In a multi-dose, postoperative (general surgery) double-blind trial of TORADOL 30 mg versus morphine 6 and 12 mg, each drug given on an "as needed" basis for up to 5 days, the overall analgesic effect of TORADOL 30 mg was in between that of morphine 6 and 12 mg. TORADOL 30 mg caused less drowsiness, nausea and vomiting than morphine 12 mg. The majority of patients treated with either TORADOL or morphine were dosed for up to 3 days; a small percentage of patients received 5 days of dosing.

In the first hour, the comparisons of TORADOL^{ORAL} in dental surgery studies, 10 or 20 mg of TORADOL^{ORAL} gave comparable pain relief to ibuprofen 400 mg, aspirin 650 mg, acetaminophen 600 mg and acetaminophen 600 mg combined with codeine 60 mg. The peak effects of the 2 TORADOL^{ORAL} doses and ibuprofen were comparable and beyond 2 to 3 hours, the patients who received those 3 treatments had statistically significantly better pain relief than patients who received the other 3 treatments. The percentage of patients who required remedication after 3 hours were as follows:

Treatment	4 hr	5 hr	6 hr
Ketorolac 10 mg	20%	35%	46%
Ketorolac 20 mg	23%	41%	54%
Ibuprofen 400 mg	35%	41%	65%
Aspirin 650 mg	38%	62%	76%
Acetaminophen 600 mg	50%	69%	78%
Acetaminophen 600 mg with codeine 60 mg	46%	69%	74%

In the comparisons of TORADOL^{ORAL} in post-operative patients following other surgical procedures, 10 mg of TORADOL^{ORAL} resulted in comparable pain relief to aspirin 650 mg combined with codeine 60 mg and naproxen sodium 550 mg in onset, duration and peak effect. The percentage of patients who required remedication after 3 hours were as follows:

Treatment	4 hr	5 hr	6 hr
Ketorolac 10 mg	24%	37%	43%
Aspirin 650 mg	27%	39%	51%
Aspirin 650 mg with codeine 60 mg	20%	27%	38%
Naproxen 500 mg or naproxen sodium 550 mg	13%	16%	19%

Limited Duration Use of TORADOL^{IM} Followed by TORADOL^{ORAL} prn for Acute Post-Surgical Pain

The use of TORADOL^{ORAL} (10 mg) following TORADOL^{IM} (30 mg) therapy after surgery was evaluated in 210 patients in a double-blind trial compared to IM meperidine 100 mg followed by oral acetaminophen 600 mg with codeine 60 mg. The use of both IM and oral treatment in this study was prn. Patients received TORADOL^{IM} for a median duration of 2 days (median dose 60 mg/day) followed by TORADOL^{ORAL} for a median duration of 8 days (median dose 25 mg/day). The efficacy of the ketorolac was comparable to the meperidine/acetaminophen plus codeine regimen. The adverse events are shown in the following table:

[See table at top of next column.]

There were no serious adverse reactions reported during this study or in other studies of 490 additional patients who received TORADOL^{IM} 10 or 30 mg single dose or qid prn followed by TORADOL^{ORAL} 10 mg qid prn for 3–10 days.

Long-Term Use of TORADOL

TORADOL^{IM} is not recommended for use beyond 5 days at recommended doses because of the increase in side effects which may occur.

In a clinical trial in 823 patients with chronic pain states comparing TORADOL^{ORAL} 10 mg qid (553 patients) with aspirin 650 mg qid (270 patients), during the first week there was a 2.4% dropout rate because of upper GI complaints in the TORADOL^{ORAL} treated patients as compared with a 0.4% rate in the aspirin treated group. After the first 2 weeks, the dropout rates due to GI pain or discomfort were comparable in both treatment groups. The time-adjusted percentages of patients who developed ulcers or upper GI bleeding are as follows:

[See table at right.]

Table of Differences in Adverse Events

Body System and Term	Meperidine IM followed by Acetaminophen + Codeine (n=104)	Ketorolac IM followed by Ketorolac oral (n=106)
Gastrointestinal		
Nausea	66%	39%
Constipation	24%	8%
Diarrhea	3%	9%
Nervous System		
Dizziness	28%	8%
Somnolence	28%	8%
Dry Mouth	20%	9%
Insomnia	9%	14%
Nervousness	2%	6%
Tremor	5%	0%
Skin		
Pruritus	10%	4%
Rash	6%	3%
Urogenital		
Urinary Retention	8%	0%

PHYSICIANS SHOULD CAREFULLY WEIGH THE POTENTIAL RISKS AND BENEFITS OF TORADOL^{ORAL} USE ON A LONG-TERM BASIS. PATIENTS SHOULD BE INSTRUCTED TO WATCH FOR SIGNS OF SERIOUS GI ADVERSE EVENTS AND THEY SHOULD BE MONITORED MORE CLOSELY THAN IF THEY WERE ON ANOTHER NSAID.

Individualization of Dosage: *Suggestions for using TORADOL^{IM} on a PRN schedule.*

Since the half-life of TORADOL is approximately 6 hours, an assessment of the size of a repeat dose can be based on the duration of pain relief from the previous dose. For example, if pain returns within 3 to 5 hours of a maintenance dose (15 or 30 mg), the next dose could be increased by up to 50% [Note: The recommended maximum total daily dose is 120 mg (150 mg on the first day); an alternative would be to use morphine or meperidine concomitantly (see INDICATIONS and DRUG INTERACTIONS)]. Alternatively, if pain does not return for 8 to 12 hours, the next dose could be decreased by as much as 50%, or the dosage interval could be increased to 8 to 12 hours.

Note: The initial intramuscular loading dose (30 or 60 mg) should be given only once, unless therapy has been interrupted for 3 half-lives (15–40 hours, see half-life of TORADOL^{IM} in Table in CLINICAL PHARMACOLOGY).

TORADOL^{IM} is only recommended for short-term therapy (not over 5 days), because adverse reactions may increase with longer use at recommended doses (see WARNINGS and PRECAUTIONS).

The lower end of the dosage range is recommended for patients under 50 kg (110 pounds) of body weight, for patients over 65 years of age, and for patients with reduced renal function (see CLINICAL PHARMACOLOGY and PRECAUTIONS).

If management by regular scheduled doses is elected, see DOSAGE AND ADMINISTRATION for dosing recommendations.

The most logical use of TORADOL^{ORAL} is in patients who have benefited from TORADOL^{IM} without limiting side effects. They can be continued on analgesic treatment with TORADOL^{ORAL} (see DOSAGE AND ADMINISTRATION—Transition from TORADOL^{IM} to TORADOL^{ORAL}). It is recommended to use the lowest effective dose of TORADOL^{IM} at the transition to TORADOL^{ORAL} and to continue treatment with TORADOL^{ORAL} for as short a time as possible (see WARNINGS and ADVERSE REACTIONS).

INDICATIONS AND USAGE

TORADOL^{IM} is indicated for the short-term management (up to 5 days) of pain (see "Clinical Studies" in CLINICAL PHARMACOLOGY). TORADOL^{IM} is not recommended for longer use (more than 5 days) because of the possibility of increased frequency and severity of adverse reactions associated with the recommended doses (see WARNINGS, DOSAGE AND ADMINISTRATION and ADVERSE REACTIONS).

TORADOL^{IM} is not recommended as a pre-operative medication for support of anesthesia, because it inhibits platelet aggregation and may prolong bleeding time (see PRECAUTIONS—Hematologic Effects) and because it possesses no sedative or anxiolytic properties.

Cumulative Occurrence

Interval	Ketorolac	Aspirin
≤3 month	0.69	0
≤6 months	1.59	0.73

TORADOL^{IM} is not recommended in obstetric analgesia because it has not been adequately studied for such use and because of the known effects of drugs that inhibit prostaglandin synthesis on uterine contraction and fetal circulation.

TORADOL^{IM} has been used concomitantly with morphine and meperidine without apparent adverse effects.

TORADOL^{ORAL} is indicated for limited duration prn use in the management of pain (see WARNINGS, ADVERSE REACTIONS and CLINICAL PHARMACOLOGY—Clinical Studies Sections for details about relative risks associated with TORADOL^{ORAL}).

TORADOL^{ORAL} is not recommended for long-term use in patients with chronic painful conditions.

TORADOL$^{IM \text{ and } ORAL}$ are not recommended for concurrent use with other nonsteroidal anti-inflammatory drugs (NSAIDs) because of the potential for additive side effects. The protein-binding of ketorolac is affected by aspirin (see PRECAUTIONS) but not by acetaminophen, ibuprofen, naproxen or piroxicam; studies with other nonsteroidals have not been performed.

CONTRAINDICATIONS

TORADOL should not be used in patients with previously demonstrated hypersensitivity to ketorolac tromethamine, or in individuals with the complete or partial syndrome of nasal polyps, angioedema, bronchospastic reactivity (e.g., asthma) or other allergic manifestations to aspirin or other nonsteroidal anti-inflammatory drugs (NSAIDs). Severe anaphylactic-like reactions to TORADOL have been reported in such patients. Therefore, before starting therapy, careful questioning of patients for such things as asthma, nasal polyps, urticaria, and hypotension associated with nonsteroidal anti-inflammatory drugs is important. In addition, if such symptoms occur during therapy, treatment should be discontinued.

WARNINGS

The most serious risks associated with TORADOL are: *gastrointestinal* ulcerations, bleeding and perforation (see PRECAUTIONS); *renal* events ranging from interstitial nephritis to acute renal failure (see PRECAUTIONS), especially in patients with pre-existing kidney problems; *hemorrhage,* especially in patients where strict hemostasis is critical (see PRECAUTIONS); *hypersensitivity reactions* such as anaphylaxis, bronchospasm, vascular collapse, urticaria, angioedema, Stevens-Johnson syndrome and vesicular bullous rash. Anaphylactoid reactions may occur in patients with a history of hypersensitivity to aspirin, other nonsteroidal anti-inflammatory drugs, or TORADOL. They may, however, also occur in patients without a known previous exposure or hypersensitivity to these agents. Both types of reactions may be fatal.

The use of TORADOL^{IM} at recommended doses for more than 5 days is associated with an increased frequency and severity of adverse events.

The use of TORADOL^{ORAL} 10 mg on a long-term basis is associated with more GI tract adverse effects than aspirin 650 mg qid (see CLINICAL PHARMACOLOGY—Clinical Studies). Long-term treatment is not recommended (see INDICATIONS AND USAGE).

High oral doses (e.g., 80 or 120 mg/day) are not recommended because risks of serious adverse events are greater with daily doses exceeding the recommended 40 mg oral per day (see ADVERSE REACTIONS).

PRECAUTIONS

Physicians should be alert to the pharmacologic similarity of TORADOL to other nonsteroidal anti-inflammatory drugs (NSAIDs) that inhibit cyclo-oxygenase.

General Precautions

Risk of Gastrointestinal Ulcerations, Bleeding and Perforation: Serious gastrointestinal toxicity, such as bleeding, ulceration, and perforation, can occur at any time, with or without warning symptoms, in patients treated with NSAIDs.

Studies to date with NSAIDs have not identified any subset of patients not at risk of developing peptic ulceration and bleeding. Except for a prior history of serious GI events and other risk factors known to be associated with peptic ulcer disease, such as alcoholism, smoking, etc., no other factors have been associated with increased risk. Elderly or debilitated patients seem to tolerate ulcertion or bleeding less well than other individuals, and most spontaneous reports of fatal GI events are in this population. Postmarketing experience with TORADOL^{IM} suggests that there may be a greater risk of gastrointestinal ulcerations, bleeding and perforation in the elderly.

Studies so far are inconclusive concerning the relative risk of various nonsteroidal anti-inflammatory drugs (NSAIDs) in causing such reactions. High doses of any such agent probably carry a greater risk of these reactions, although this is rarely established in controlled clinical trials. In considering the intramuscular use of relatively large doses (within the recommended dosage range), or treatment with TORADOL^{IM} for a duration longer than 5 days, sufficient benefit should be anticipated to offset the potential increased risk of GI toxicity.

The risks of gastrointestinal side effects associated with long-term use of TORADOL^{ORAL} are described under CLINICAL PHARMACOLOGY—Clinical Studies (Long-Term Use of TORADOL).

Impaired Renal or Hepatic Function: As with other nonsteroidal anti-inflammatory drugs (NSAIDs), TORADOL should be used with caution in patients with impaired renal or hepatic function, or a history of kidney or liver disease.

Renal Effects: As with other nonsteroidal anti-inflammatory drugs (NSAIDs), administration of ketorolac tromethamine to animals resulted in renal papillary necrosis and other abnormal renal pathology. In humans, there have been reports of hematuria, proteinuria, glomerular nephritis, interstitial nephritis, renal papillary necrosis, nephrotic syndrome, and acute renal failure.

Another, equally important, renal toxicity has been seen in patients with conditions leading to a reduction in blood volume and/or renal blood flow, where renal prostaglandins have a supportive role in the maintenance of renal perfusion. In these patients, administration of a nonsteroidal anti-inflammatory drug (NSAID) may cause a dose-dependent reduction in renal prostaglandin formation and may precipitate acute renal failure. Patients at greatest risk of this reaction are those with impaired renal function, heart failure, liver dysfunction, those taking diuretics and the elderly. Discontinuation of NSAID therapy is usually followed by recovery to the pretreatment state.

TORADOL and its metabolities are eliminated primarily by the kidneys which, in patients with reduced creatinine clearance, will result in diminished clearance of the drug (see CLINICAL PHARMACOLOGY). Therefore, TORADOL should be used with caution in patients with impaired renal function (see WARNINGS and DOSAGE AND ADMINISTRATION) and such patients should be followed closely.

Fluid Retention and Edema: As with other nonsteroidal anti-inflammatory drugs (NSAIDs) that inhibit prostaglandin biosynthesis, fluid retention, edema, retention of NaCl, oliguria, elevations of serum urea nitrogen and creatinine have been reported in clinical trials with TORADOL. Therefore, TORADOL should be used with caution in patients with acute renal failure, cardic decompensation, hypertension, or similar conditions.

Hepatic Effects: As with other nonsteroidal anti-inflammatory drugs (NSAIDs) treatment with TORADOL may cause elevations of liver enzymes, and in patients with pre-existing liver dysfunction, it may lead to the development of a more severe hepatic reaction. The ALT (SGPT) test is probably the most sensitive indicator of liver injury. In patients with symptoms and signs suggesting liver dysfunction, or in whom an abnormal liver test has occurred as a result of TORADOL therapy, the administration of the drug should be discontinued.

Hematologic Effects: TORADOL inhibits platelet aggregation and may prolong bleeding time. Unlike aspirin, the inhibition of platelet function by TORADOL disappears within 24 to 48 hours after the drug is discontinued. TORADOL does not appear to affect platelet count, prothrombin time (PT) or partial thromboplastin time (PTT). In controlled clinical studies where TORADOL was administered intramuscularly or intravenously postoperatively, the incidence of clinically significant postoperative bleeding was 0.4% for TORADOL compared to 0.2% in the control groups receiving narcotic analgesics.

Because prostaglandins play an important role on hemostasis, NSAIDs affect platelet aggregation as well, use of TORADOL in patients who have coagulation disorders should be undertaken with caution, and those patients should be carefully monitored. Patients on therapeutic doses of anticoagulants (e.g., heparin or dicumarol derivatives) have an increased risk of bleeding complications if given TORADOL concurrently; physicians should administer such concomitant therapy with extreme caution. The concurrent use of TORADOL and prophylatic, low-dose heparin (2500–5000 units q12h) has not been studied extensively, but may also be associated with an increased risk of bleeding. Physicians should weigh the benefits against the risk, and exercise caution in using such concomitant therapy in these patients. In patients who receive anticoagulants for any reason, there is an increased risk of intramuscular hematoma formation from TORADOL^{IM} injections (see PRECAUTIONS—Drug Interactions).

In postmarketing experience, postoperative hematomas and other signs of wound bleeding have been reported in association with the perioperative use of TORADOL^{IM}. Caution should be used, therefore, when TORADOL is administered pre- or intra-operatively. Perioperative use of TORADOL should be undertaken with caution when strict hemostasis is critical.

Information for Patients

TORADOL, like other drugs of its class, is not free of side effects. The side effects of these drugs can cause discomfort and, rarely, there are more serious side effects, such as gastrointestinal bleeding, which may result in hospitalization and even fatal outcomes.

Physicians may wish to discuss with their patients the potential risks (see WARNINGS, PRECAUTIONS, and ADVERSE

REACTIONS Sections) and likely benefits of TORADOL treatment, particularly when it is used for less serious conditions when lengthy treatment is anticipated and when acceptable alternatives to both the patient and physician may be available.

Laboratory Tests

Because serious GI tract ulceration and bleeding can occur without warning symptoms, physicians should follow patients for the signs and symptoms of ulceration and bleeding and should inform them of the importance of this follow-up (see PRECAUTIONS—Risk of GI Ulceration, Bleeding and Perforation).

Drug Interactions

TORADOL is highly bound to human plasma protein (mean 99.2%) and binding is independent of concentration.

The *in vitro* binding of **warfarin** to plasma proteins is only slightly reduced by TORADOL (99.5% control vs 99.3%) with TORADOL plasma concentrations of 5 to 10 μg/mL. TORADOL does not alter **digoxin** protein binding.

In vitro studies indicate that, at therapeutic plasma concentrations of **salicylate** (300 μg/mL), the binding of TORADOL was reduced from approximately 99.2% to 97.5%, representing a potential two-fold increase in unbound TORADOL plasma levels; hence, TORADOL should be used with caution (or at a reduced dosage) in patients being treated with high-dose salicylate regimens. Therapeutic concentrations of **digoxin, warfarin, ibuprofen, naproxen, piroxicam, acetaminophen, phenytoin,** and **tolbutamide** did not alter TORADOL protein binding.

In a study involving 12 volunteers, oral TORADOL was co-administered with a single dose of 25 mg **warafin,** causing no significant changes in pharmacokinetics or pharmacodynamics of warfarin. In another study, intramuscular TORADOL (following oral dosing) was given with two doses of 5000 U of **heparin** to 11 healthy volunteers, resulting in a mean template bleeding time of 6.4 minutes (3.2–11.4 min) compared to a mean of 6.0 minutes (3.4–7.5 min) for heparin alone and 5.1 minutes (3.8–8.5 min) for placebo. Although these results do not indicate significant interaction between TORADOL and warfarin or heparin, the administration of TORADOL, or other NSAIDs, to patients taking anticoagulants should be done with caution and patients should be closely monitored (see PRECAUTIONS—Hematologic Effects).

Intramuscular TORADOL reduced the diuretic response to **furosemide** in normovolemic healthy subjects by approximately 20% (mean sodium and urinary output decreased 17%).

Concomitant administration of oral TORADOL and **probenecid** resulted in decreased clearance of ketorolac and significant increases in ketorolac plasma levels (total AUC increased approximately 3-fold from 5.4 to 17.8 μg·h/mL) and terminal half-life (increased approximately 2-fold from 6.6 to 15.1 hours).

Inhibition of renal **lithium** clearance, leading to increase in plasma lithium concentration, has been reported with some prostaglandin sysnthesis inhibiting drugs. The effect of TORADOL on plasma lithium has not been studied.

Concomitant administration of **methotrexate** and some NSAIDs has been reported to reduce the clearance of methotrexate, enhancing the toxicity of methotrexate. The effect of TORADOL on methotrexate clearance has not been studied.

In post-marketing experience, there have been three reports of a possible interaction between TORADOL^{IM} and **nondepolarizing muscle relaxants,** appearing to enhance the effect of the muscle relaxant. The concurrent use of TORADOL with muscle relaxants has not been formally studied.

Intramuscular TORADOL has been administered concurrently with **morphine** in several clinical trials of postoperative pain without evidence of adverse interactions.

There is no evidence, in animal or human studies, that TORADOL induces or inhibits hepatic enzymes capable of metabolizing itself or other drugs.

Carcinogenesis, Mutagenesis, and Impairment of Fertility

An 18-month study in mice at oral doses of ketorolac tromethamine equal to the parenteral MRHD (Maximum Recommended Human Dose) and a 24-month study in rats at oral doses 2.5 times the parenteral MRHD, showed no evidence of tumorigenicity.

Ketorolac tromethamine was not mutagenic in Ames test, unscheduled DNA synthesis and repair, and in forward mutation assays. Ketorolac did not cause chromosome breakage in the *in vivo* mouse micronucleus assay. At 1590 μg/mL (approximately 1000 times the average human plasma levels) and at higher concentrations, ketorolac tromethamine increased the incidence of chromosomal aberrations in Chinese hamster ovarian cells.

Impairment of fertility did not occur in male or female rats at oral doses of 9 mg/kg (53.1 mg/m^2) and 16 mg/kg (94.4 mg/m^2), respectively.

Continued on next page

Syntex—Cont.

Pregnancy:

Pregnancy Category C.

Reproduction studies have been performed in rabbits, using daily oral doses at 3.6 mg/kg (42.35 mg/m^2) and in rats at 10 mg/kg (59 mg/m^2) during organogenesis. Results of these studies did not reveal evidence of teratogenicity to the fetus. Oral doses of ketorolac tromethamine at 1.5 mg/kg (8.8 mg/m^2), which was half of the human oral exposure, administered after gestation day 17 caused dystocia and higher pup mortality in rats. There are no adequate and well-controlled studies in pregnant women. Ketorolac tromethamine should be used during pregnancy only if the potential benefit justifies the potential risk to the fetus.

Labor and Delivery

TORADOL is not recommended for use during labor and delivery (see INDICATIONS).

Lactation and Nursing

After a single oral administration of 10 mg of TORADOL^{ORAL} to humans, the maximum milk concentration observed was 7.3 ng/mL and the maximum milk-to-plasma ratio was 0.037. After one day of dosing (qid), the maximum milk concentration was 7.9 ng/mL and the maximum milk-to-plasma ratio was 0.025. Caution should be exercised when TORADOL$^{IM\ or\ ORAL}$ is administered to a nursing woman.

Pediatric Use

Safety and efficacy in children have not been established. Therefore, TORADOL is not recommended for use in children.

Use in the Elderly

Because ketorolac tromethamine is cleared somewhat more slowly by the elderly (see CLINICAL PHARMACOLOGY) who are also more sensitive to the renal effects of NSAIDs (see PRECAUTIONS—Renal Effects), extra caution and reduced dosages (see DOSAGE AND ADMINISTRATION) should be used when treating the elderly with TORADOL.

ADVERSE REACTIONS

Adverse reaction rates from short-term use of NSAIDs are generally from $^1/_{10}$ to $^1/_2$ the rates associated with long-term use. This is also true for TORADOL. Adverse reaction rates also may increase with higher doses of TORADOL (see WARNINGS and DOSAGE AND ADMINISTRATION).

TORADOL^{IM} is indicated for short-term use. Physicians using TORADOL^{IM} should be alert for the usual complications of NSAID treatment, and should be aware that with longer use (exceeding 5 days) of TORADOL^{IM}, the frequency and severity of adverse reactions may increase.

Physicians using TORADOL^{ORAL} should be alert to the relative risks associated with dose and dose duration as described in CLINICAL PHARMACOLOGY—Clinical Studies.

Physicians using TORADOL should be alert for the usual complications of NSAID treatment.

The adverse reactions listed below were reported in clinical trials with TORADOL in which patients received up to 20 doses, in 5 days, of TORADOL^{IM} 30 mg or up to 4 doses a day from long-term studies of TORADOL^{ORAL} 10 mg qid. In addition, adverse reactions that were reported from TORADOL^{IM} post-marketing surveillance are included in "Incidence 1% or Less."

Incidence Greater than 1% (probably causally related)

Body as a Whole: EDEMA*

Cardiovascular: HYPERTENSION

Dermatologic: RASH, pruritus*

Gastrointestinal: NAUSEA (12%), DYSPEPSIA (12%), GASTROINTESTINAL PAIN (13%), constipation, diarrhea*, flatulence, gastrointestinal fullness, vomiting, STOMATITIS

Hemic and Lymphatic: purpura

Nervous System: drowsiness*, dizziness*, HEADACHE (17%), sweating

Injection site pain was reported by 2% of patients in multidose studies (vs. 5% for morphine control group).

Incidence 1% or Less (probably causally related)

Body as a Whole: hypersensitivity reactions such as *anaphylaxis*[1], *bronchospasm, laryngeal edema, tongue edema, hypotension*, and *flushing*, weight gain, fever

Cardiovascular: flushing, palpitation, pallor, *hypotension*, syncope

Dermatologic: *Lyell's syndrome, Stevens-Johnson syndrome, exfoliative dermatitis, muculo-papular rash*, urticaria

Gastrointestinal: *peptic ulceration, GI hemorrhage, GI perforation* (see WARNINGS and PRECAUTIONS), *melena*, rectal bleeding, gastritis, eructation, anorexia, increased appetite

Hemic and Lymphatic: *postoperative wound hemorrhage*, rarely requiring blood transfusion (see WARNINGS and PRECAUTIONS), *thrombocytopenia*, epistaxis, anemia

*Incidence of reported reaction between 3% and 9%. Those reactions occurring in less than 3% of the patients are unmarked. Reactions reported predominantly from long-term TORADOL^{ORAL} studies are CAPITALIZED.

[1] *Italics* denote reactions reported from *postmarketing experience.*

Nervous System: *convulsions*, vertigo, tremors, abnormal dreams, hallucinations, euphoria

Respiratory: dyspnea, *asthma*, pulmonary edema

Urogenital: *acute renal failure* (see WARNINGS and PRECAUTIONS), *flank pain with or without hematuria and/or azotemia*, oliguria, nephritis

Other Adverse Events (causal relationship unknown)[2]

Body as a Whole: asthenia

Gastrointestinal: *pancreatitis*

Hemic and Lymphatic: *leukopenia*, EOSINOPHILIA

Nervous System: paresthesia, depression, insomnia, nervousness, excessive thrist, dry mouth, abnormal thinking, inability to concentrate, hyperkinesia, stupor

Respiratory: RHINITIS, COUGH, dyspnea

Special Senses: abnormal taste, abnormal vision, blurred vision, tinnitus, HEARING LOSS

Urogenital: polyuria, increased urinary frequency

DRUG ABUSE AND PHYSICAL DEPENDENCE

TORADOL is not a narcotic agonist or antagonist. Subjects did not show any subjective symptoms or objective signs of drug withdrawal upon abrupt discontinuation of intravenous or intramuscular dosing. Patients receiving TORADOL^{ORAL} for long-term therapy have not developed tolerance to the drug and there is no pharmacologic basis to expect addiction. Ketorolac did not exhibit activity in classical animal studies which are reasonable predictors of opiate analgesic action. *In vitro*, ketorolac does not bind to opiate receptors. These studies demonstrate that kerorolac does not have central opiate-like activity.

OVERDOSAGE

The absence of experience with acute overdosage precludes characterization of sequelae and assessment of antidotal efficacy at this time. At single oral doses greater than 100 mg/kg in rats, mice and monkeys, symptoms such as decreased activity, diarrhea, pallor, labored breathing, rales, and vomiting were observed.

DOSAGE AND ADMINISTRATION

TORADOL^{IM} may be used on a regular schedule or prn ("as needed"), based on the return of pain. For the short-term management of pain on a regular schedule (see CLINICAL PHARMACOLOGY for details of clinical trials), the recommended initial dose is 30 or 60 mg IM, as a loading dose, followed by half of the loading dose, i.e., 15 or 30 mg, every 6 hours. The maximum recommended daily dose is 150 mg for the first day and 120 mg/day thereafter. It is recommended that intramuscular TORADOL be limited to short-term therapy (not over 5 days) because the frequency and severity of adverse events may increase with longer use at recommended doses (see WARNINGS and PRECAUTIONS).

Note: The initial intramuscular loading dose should be given only once, unless therapy has been interrupted for 3 half-lives (15–40 hours, see half-life of TORADOL^{IM} in Table in CLINICAL PHARMACOLOGY).

The lower end of the dosage range is recommended for patients under 50 kg (110 pounds) of body weight, for patients over 65 years of age, and for patients with reduced renal function (see CLINICAL PHARMACOLOGY and PRECAUTIONS).

If prn management is elected, see Individualization of Dosage in CLINICAL PHARMACOLOGY for suggestions.

Parenteral drug products should be inspected visually for particulate matter and discoloration prior to administration, whenever solution and container permit.

Pharmaceutical Compatibility of TORADOL^{IM}

TORADOL^{IM} should not be mixed in smal volume (e.g., in a syringe) with morphine sulfate, meperidine hydrochloride, promethazine hydrochloride or hydrolyzine hydrochloride; this will result in precipitation of kerorolac from solution.

TORADOL^{ORAL} is indicated for the management of pain. The recommended oral dose is 10 mg prn every 4 to 6 hours for limited duration. Doses of 10 mg qid chronically are not recommended (see WARNINGS, ADVERSE REACTIONS and CLINICAL PHARMACOLOGY—Clinical Studies Sections for details about relative risks associated with TORADOL^{ORAL}).

Transition From TORADOL^{IM} to TORADOL^{ORAL}

When TORADOL^{ORAL} is used as follow-on therapy to TORADOL^{IM}, the total combined dose should not exceed 120 mg on the day of transition, including a maximum of 40 mg orally. Subsequent oral dosing should not exceed recommended daily maximum of 40 mg.

HOW SUPPLIED

TORADOL®^{IM}

TORADOL^{IM} (ketorolac tromethamine) for single-dose intramuscular use is available in a Cartrix® syringe or a TUBEX® Cartridge-Needle Unit:

[2] Reactions occurred under circumstances where causal relationship to TORADOL treatment has not been clearly established; they are presented as alerting information for physicians. Reactions reported predominantly from long-term TORADOL^{ORAL} studies are CAPITALIZED.

15 mg: 15 mg/mL, 1 mL Cartrix® syringe (box of 10) NDC #0033-2443-40

30 mg: 30 mg/mL, 1 mL Cartrix® syringe (box of 10) NDC #0033-2434-40

60 mg: 30 mg/mL, 2 mL Cartrix® syringe (box of 10) NDC #0033-2444-40

Mfd. for Syntex Laboratories, Inc.
Palo Alto, CA 94304
by Survival Technology, Inc.
Rockville, MD 20850

15 mg: 15 mg/mL, 1 mL TUBEX® Sterile Cartridge-Needle Unit (22 gauge × 1-$^1/_4$ inch needle) (box of 10) NDC #0033-2443-50

30 mg: 30 mg/mL, 1 mL TUBEX® Sterile Cartridge-Needle Unit (22 gauge × 1-$^1/_4$ inch needle) (box of 10) NDC #0033-2434-50

60 mg: 30 mg/mL, 2 mL TUBEX® Sterile Cartridge-Needle Unit (22 gauge × 1-$^1/_4$ inch needle) (box of 10) NDC #0033-2444-50

Mfd. for Syntex Laboratories, Inc.
Palo Alto, CA 94304
by Wyeth Laboratories, Inc.
Philadelphia, PA 19101

Store at controlled room temperature 15°–30°C (59°–86°F) with protection from light.

See the TORADOL^{IM} carton and package insert for DIRECTIONS FOR USE of the Cartrix® syringe and TUBEX® Cartridge-Needle Unit.

TORADOL®^{ORAL}

TORADOL^{ORAL} 10 mg tablets are available in bottles of 100 tablets (NDC #0033-2435-42) and in cartons of 100 blister-packed tablets (NDC #0033-2435-53).

Store bottles at controlled room temperature, 15°–30°C (59°–86°F). Store blister packages at controlled room temperature, 15°–30°C (59°–86°F). Protect from excessive humidity and light.

DIRECTIONS FOR USE

TUBEX® Injector

NOTE: The TUBEX® Injector is reusable: do not discard.

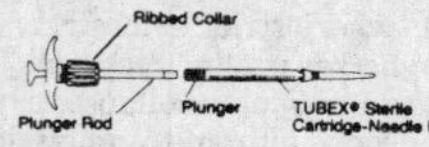

To load a TUBEX® Sterile Cartridge-Needle Unit into the TUBEX® Injector

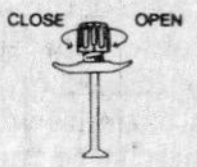

1. Turn the ribbed collar to the "OPEN" position until it stops.

2. Hold the Injector with the open end up and fully insert the TUBEX® Sterile Cartridge-Needle Unit. Firmly tighten the ribbed collar in the direction of the "CLOSE" arrow.

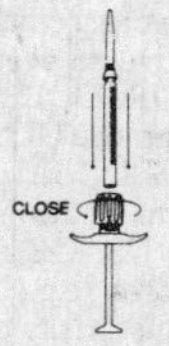

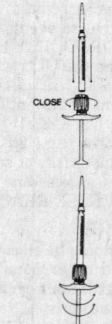

3. Thread the plunger rod into the plunger of the TUBEX® Sterile Cartridge-Needle Unit until slight resistance is felt. The Injector is now ready for use in the usual manner.

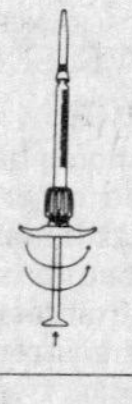

To administer

Method of administration is the same as with conventional syringe. Remove needle cover by grasping it securely; twist and pull. Introduce needle into patient, aspirate by pulling back slightly on the plunger, and inject.

To remove the empty TUBEX® Cartridge-Needle Unit and dispose into a vertical needle disposal container

1. Do not recap the needle. Disengage the plunger rod.
2. Hold the Injector, needle down, over a vertical needle disposal container and loosen the ribbed collar. TUBEX® Cartridge-Needle Unit will drop into the container.

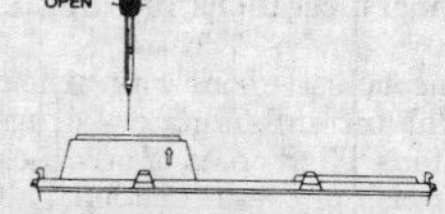

3. Discard the needle cover.

To remove the empty TUBEX® Cartridge-Needle Unit and dispose into a horizontal (mailbox) needle disposal container.

1. Do not recap the needle. Disengage the plunger rod.
2. Open the horizontal (mailbox) needle disposal container. Insert TUBEX® Cartridge-Needle Unit, needle pointing

down, halfway into container. Close the container lid on cartridge. Loosen ribbed collar; TUBEX® Cartridge Unit will drop into the container.

3. Discard the needle cover.
The TUBEX® Injector is reusable and should not be disdcarded.
Used TUBEX® Cartridge-Needle Units should not be employed for successive injections or as multiple-dose containers. They are intended to be used only once and discarded.

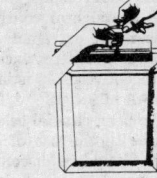

NOTE: Any graduated markings on TUBEX® Sterile Cartridge-Needle Units are to be used only as a guide in mixing, withdrawing, or administering measured doses.
Wyeth does not recommend and will not accept responsibility for the use of any cartridge-needle units other than TUBEX® Cartridge-Needle Units in the TUBEX® Injector. Directions for Use of the TUBEX® Injector have been reproduced with permission of Wyeth Laboratories.

CAUTION: Federal law prohibits dispensing without prescription.
U.S. Patent No. 4,089,969 and others.
02-2435-00-01
4/92
©1991 Syntex Laboratories, Inc.
Shown in Product Identification Section, page 433

TRI-NORINYL® Tablets   ℞
(norethindrone and
ethinyl estradiol)

BREVICON® Tablets   ℞
[*brev 'ĭ-kahn*]
(norethindrone and
ethinyl estradiol)

NORINYL® 1 + 35 Tablets   ℞
[*nor 'ĭ-nil*]
(norethindrone and
ethinyl estradiol)

NORINYL® 1 + 50 Tablets   ℞
(norethindrone and mestranol)

NOR-QD® Tablets   ℞
(norethindrone)
Tablets 0.35 mg.

Products of Syntex (F.P.) Inc.

DESCRIPTION

TRI-NORINYL 21-DAY Tablets provide an oral contraceptive regimen of 7 blue tablets followed by 9 yellow-green tablets and 5 more blue tablets. Each blue tablet contains norethindrone 0.5 mg and ethinyl estradiol 0.035 mg and each yellow-green tablet contains norethindrone 1 mg and ethinyl estradiol 0.035 mg.
TRI-NORINYL 28-DAY Tablets provide a continuous oral contraceptive regimen of 7 blue tablets, 9 yellow-green tablets, 5 more blue tablets, and then 7 orange tablets. Each blue tablet contains norethindrone 0.5 mg and ethinyl estradiol 0.035 mg, each yellow-green tablet contains norethindrone 1.0 mg and ethinyl estradiol 0.035 mg, and each orange tablet contains inert ingredients.
BREVICON 21-DAY Tablets provide an oral contraceptive regimen consisting of 21 blue tablets containing norethindrone 0.5 mg and ethinyl estradiol 0.035 mg.
BREVICON 28-DAY Tablets provide a continuous oral contraceptive regimen consisting of 21 blue tablets containing norethindrone 0.5 mg and ethinyl estradiol 0.035 mg and 7 orange tablets containing inert ingredients.
NORINYL 1 + 35 21-DAY Tablets provide an oral contraceptive regimen consisting of 21 yellow-green tablets containing norethindrone 1 mg and ethinyl estradiol 0.035 mg.
NORINYL 1 + 35 28-DAY Tablets provide a continuous oral contraceptive regimen consisting of 21 yellow-green tablets containing norethindrone 1 mg and ethinyl estradiol 0.035 mg and 7 orange tablets containing inert ingredients.
NORINYL 1 + 50 21-DAY Tablets provide an oral contraceptive regimen consisting of 21 white tablets containing norethindrone 1 mg and mestranol 0.05 mg.
NORINYL 1 + 50 28-DAY Tablets provide a continuous oral contraceptive regimen consisting of 21 white tablets containing norethindrone 1 mg and mestranol 0.05 mg and 7 orange tablets containing inert ingredients.
NOR-QD Tablets provide a continuous oral contraceptive regimen of one yellow norethindrone 0.35 mg tablet daily. Norethindrone is a potent progestational agent with the chemical name 17-hydroxy-19-nor-17α-pregn-4-en-20-yn-

3-one. Ethinyl estradiol is an estrogen with the chemical name 19-nor-17α-pregna-1, 3, 5(10) -trien-20-yne-3, 17-diol. Mestranol is an estrogen with the chemical name 3-methoxy-19-nor-17α-pregna-1, 3, 5(10) -trien-20-yn-17-ol.
Inactive Ingredients: Each tablet contains the following inactive ingredients: lactose, magnesium stearate, povidone, starch, and one or more of the following dyes; D&C Green No. 5, D&C Yellow No. 10, FD&C Blue No. 1, FD&C Yellow No. 6.

CLINICAL PHARMACOLOGY

Combination oral contraceptives act by suppression of gonadotrophins. Although the primary mechanism of this action is inhibition of ovulation, other alterations include changes in the cervical mucus (which increase the difficulty of sperm entry into the uterus) and the endometrium (which may reduce the likelihood of implantation).

INDICATIONS AND USAGE

Oral contraceptives are indicated for the prevention of pregnancy in women who elect to use these products as a method of contraception.
Oral contraceptives are highly effective. Table I lists the typical accidental pregnancy rates for users of combination oral contraceptives and other methods of contraception.[1] The efficacy of these contraceptive methods, except sterilization, depends upon the reliability with which they are used. Correct and consistent use of methods can result in lower failure rates.

TABLE I: LOWEST EXPECTED AND TYPICAL
FAILURE RATES DURING THE FIRST YEAR OF
CONTINUOUS USE OF A METHOD
% of Women Experiencing an Accidental Pregnancy
in the First Year of Continuous Use

Method	Lowest Expected[a]	Typical[b]
(No contraception)	(89)	(89)
Oral contraceptives		3
combined	0.1	N/A[c]
progestogen only	0.5	N/A[c]
Diaphragm with spermicidal cream or jelly	3	18
Spermicides alone (foam, creams, jellies and vaginal suppositories)	3	21
Vaginal sponge		
Nulliparous	5	18
Multiparous	>8	>28
IUD (medicated)	1	6[d]
Condom without spermicides	2	12
Periodic abstinence (all methods)	2–10	20
Female sterilization	0.2	0.4
Male sterilization	0.1	0.15

Adapted from J. Trussell and K. Kost, Table II [1]
[a] The authors' best guess of the percentage of women expected to experience an accidental pregnancy among couples who initiate a method (not necessarily for the first time) and who use it consistently and correctly during the first year if they do not stop for any other reason.
[b] This term represents "typical" couples who initiate use of a method (not necessarily for the first time), who experience an accidental pregnancy during the first year if they do not stop use for any other reason. The authors derive these data largely from the National Surveys of Family Growth (NSFG), 1976 and 1982.
[c] N/A—Data not available from the NSFG, 1976 and 1982.
[d] Combined typical rate for both medicated and non-medicated IUD. The rate for medicated IUD alone is not available.

CONTRAINDICATIONS

Oral contraceptives should not be used in women who have the following conditions:
● Thrombophlebitis or thromboembolic disorders
● A past history of deep vein thrombophlebitis or thromboembolic disorders
● Cerebral vascular or coronary artery disease
● Known or suspected carcinoma of the breast
● Carcinoma of the endometrium, and known or suspected estrogen-dependent neoplasia
● Undiagnosed abnormal genital bleeding
● Cholestatic jaundice of pregnancy or jaundice with prior pill use
● Hepatic adenomas, carcinomas or benign liver tumors
● Known or suspected pregnancy

WARNINGS

Cigarette smoking increases the risk of serious cardio-vascular side effects from oral contraceptive use. This risk increases with age and with heavy smoking (15 or

more cigarettes per day) and is quite marked in women over 35 years of age. Women who use oral contraceptives should be strongly advised not to smoke.

The use of oral contraceptives is associated with increased risks of several serious conditions including myocardial infarction, thromboembolism, stroke, hepatic neoplasia and gallbladder disease, although the risk of serious morbidity and mortality increases significantly in the presence of other underlying risk factors such as hypertension, hyperlipidemias, hypercholesterolemia, obesity and diabetes.[2-5] Practitioners prescribing oral contraceptives should be familiar with the following information relating to these risks. The information contained in this package insert is principally based on studies carried out in patients who used oral contraceptives with formulations containing 0.05 mg or higher of estrogen.[6-11] The effects of long-term use with lower dose formulations of both estrogens and progestogens remain to be determined.
Throughout this labeling, epidemiological studies reported are of two types: retrospective or case control studies and prospective or cohort studies. Case control studies provide a measure of the relative risk of a disease. Relative risk, the *ratio* of the incidence of a disease among oral contraceptive users to that among nonusers, cannot be assessed directly from case control studies, but the odds ratio obtained is a measure of relative risk. The relative risk does not provide information on the actual clinical occurrence of a disease. Cohort studies provide not only a measure of the relative risk but a measure of attributable risk, which is the *difference* in the incidence of disease between oral contraceptive users and nonusers. The attributable risk does provide information about the actual occurrence of a disease in the population.[12-13]

1. THROMBOEMBOLIC DISORDERS AND OTHER VASCULAR PROBLEMS
a. Myocardial Infarction
An increased risk of myocardial infarction has been attributed to oral contraceptive use. This risk is primarily in smokers or women with other underlying risk factors for coronary artery disease such as hypertension, hypercholesterolemia, morbid obesity, and diabetes.[2-5,13] The relative risk of heart attack for current oral contraceptive users has been estimated to be 2 to 6.[2,14-19] The risk is very low under the age of 30. However, there is the possibility of a risk of cardiovascular disease even in very young women who take oral contraceptives.
Smoking in combination with oral contraceptive use has been shown to contribute substantially to the incidence of myocardial infarctions in women 35 or older, with smoking accounting for the majority of excess cases.[20]
Mortality rates associated with circulatory disease have been shown to increase substantially in smokers over the age of 35 and non-smokers over the age of 40 among women who use oral contraceptives (See Table II).[16]

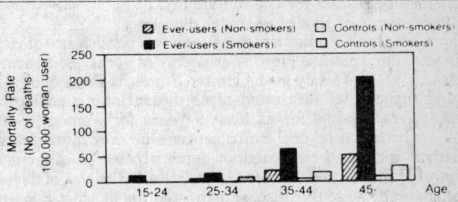

TABLE II: CIRCULATORY DISEASE MORTALITY RATES PER 100 000 WOMAN YEARS BY AGE, SMOKING STATUS AND ORAL CONTRACEPTIVE USE

Adapted from P.M. Layde and V. Beral, Table V[16]

Oral contraceptives may compound the effects of well-known risk factors for coronary artery disease, such as hypertension, diabetes, hyperlipidemias, hypercholesterolemia, age and obesity.[3,13,21] In particular, some progestogens are known to decrease HDL cholesterol and impair oral glucose tolerance, while estrogens may create a state of hyperinsulinism.[21-25] Oral contraceptives have been shown to increase blood pressure among users (see **WARNINGS**, section 9). Similar effects on risk factors have been associated with an increased risk of heart disease. Oral contraceptives must be used with caution in women with cardiovascular disease risk factors.
b. Thromboembolism
An increased risk of thromboembolic and thrombotic disease associated with the use of oral contraceptives is well established. Case control studies have found the relative risk of users compared to non-users to be 3 for the first episode of superficial venous thrombosis, 4 to 11 for deep vein thrombosis or pulmonary embolism, and 1.5 to 6 for women with predisposing conditions for venous thromboembolic disease.[12,13,26-31] One cohort study has shown the relative risk

Continued on next page

Syntex—Cont.

to be somewhat lower, about 3 for new cases (subjects with no past history of venous thrombosis or varicose veins) and about 4.5 for new cases requiring hospitalization.[32] The risk of thromboembolic disease due to oral contraceptives is not related to length of use and disappears after pill use is stopped.[12]

A 2-to 6-fold increase in relative risk of post-operative thromboembolic complications has been reported with the use of oral contraceptives.[18] If feasible, oral contraceptives should be discontinued at least 4 weeks prior to and for 2 weeks after elective surgery and during and following prolonged immobilization. Since the immediate postpartum period is also associated with an increased risk of thromboembolism, oral contraceptives should be started no earlier than 4 to 6 weeks after delivery in women who elect not to breast feed.[33]

c. Cerebrovascular diseases

An increase in both the relative and attributable risks of cerebrovascular events (thrombotic and hemorrhagic strokes) has been shown in users of oral contraceptives. In general, the risk is greatest among older (> 35 years), hypertensive women who also smoke. Hypertension was found to be a risk factor for both users and non-users for both types of strokes while smoking interacted to increase the risk for hemorrhagic strokes.[34]

In a large study, the relative risk of thrombotic strokes has been shown to range from 3 for normotensive users to 14 for users with severe hypertension.[35] The relative risk of hemorrhagic stroke is reported to be 1.2 for non-smokers who used oral contraceptives, 2.6 for smokers who did not use oral contraceptives, 7.6 for smokers who used oral contraceptives, 1.8 for normotensive users and 25.7 for users with severe hypertension.[35] The attributable risk also is greater in women 35 or older and among smokers.[13]

d. Dose-related risk of vascular disease from oral contraceptives

A positive association has been observed between the amount of estrogen and progestogen in oral contraceptives and the risk of vascular disease.[36–38] A decline in serum high density lipoproteins (HDL) has been reported with some progestational agents.[22–24] A decline in serum high density lipoproteins has been associated with an increased incidence of ischemic heart disease.[39] Because estrogens increase HDL cholesterol, the net effect of an oral contraceptive depends on a balance achieved between doses of estrogen and progestogen and the nature and absolute amount of progestogens used in the contraceptives. The amount of both hormones should be considered in the choice of an oral contraceptive.[37] Minimizing exposure to estrogen and progestogen is in keeping with good principles of therapeutics. For any particular estrogen/progestogen combination, the dosage regimen prescribed should be one which contains the least amount of estrogen and progestogen that is compatible with a low failure rate and the needs of the individual patient. New acceptors of oral contraceptive agents should be started on preparations containing the lowest estrogen content that produces satisfactory results for the individual.

e. Persistence of risk of vascular disease

There are three studies which have shown persistence of risk of vascular disease for ever-users of oral contraceptives.[17,34,40] In a study in the United States, the risk of developing myocardial infarction after discontinuing oral contraceptives persists for at least 9 years for women 40–49 years who had used oral contraceptives for 5 or more years, but this increased risk was not demonstrated in other age groups.[17] In another study in Great Britain, the risk of developing cerebrovascular disease persisted for at least 6 years after discontinuation of oral contraceptives, although excess risk was very small.[40] Subarachnoid hemorrhage also has a significantly increased relative risk after termination of use of oral contraceptives.[34] However, these studies were performed with oral contraceptive formulations containing 0.05 mg or higher of estrogen.

2. ESTIMATES OF MORTALITY FROM CONTRACEPTIVE USE

One study gathered data from a variety of sources which have estimated the mortality rates associated with different methods of contraception at different ages (see Table III).[41] These estimates include the combined risk of death associated with contraceptive methods plus the risk attributable to pregnancy in the event of method failure. Each method of contraception has its specific benefits and risks. The study concluded that with the exception of oral contraceptive users 35 and older who smoke and 40 and older who do not smoke, mortality associated with all methods of birth control is low and below that associated with childbirth. The observation of a possible increase in risk of mortality with age for oral contraceptive users is based on data gathered in the 1970's—but not reported in the U.S. until 1983.[16,41] However, current clinical practice involves the use of lower estrogen dose formulations combined with careful restriction of oral contraceptive use to women who do not have the various risk factors listed in this labeling.

Because of these changes in practice and, also, because of some limited new data which suggest that the risk of cardiovascular disease with the use of oral contraceptives may now be less than previously observed[78,79], the Fertility and Maternal Health Drugs Advisory Committee was asked to review the topic in 1989. The Committee concluded that although cardiovascular disease risks may be increased with oral contraceptive use after age 40 in healthy non-smoking women (even with the newer low-dose formulations), there are greater potential health risks associated with pregnancy in older women and with the alternative surgical and medical procedures which may be necessary if such women do not have access to effective and acceptable means of contraception.

Therefore, the Committee recommended that the benefits of oral contraceptive use by healthy non-smoking women over 40 may outweigh the possible risks. Of course, older women, as all women who take oral contraceptives, should take the lowest possible dose formulation that is effective.[80]

[See table below.]

3. CARCINOMA OF THE BREAST AND REPRODUCTIVE ORGANS

Numerous epidemiological studies have been performed on the incidence of breast, endometrial, ovarian and cervical cancer in women using oral contraceptives. The evidence in the literature suggests that use of oral contraceptives is not associated with an increase in the risk of developing breast cancer, regardless of the age and parity of first use or with most of the marketed brands and doses.[42,43] The Cancer and Steroid Hormone study also showed no latent effect on the risk of breast cancer for at least a decade following long-term use.[43] A few studies have shown a slightly increased relative risk of developing breast cancer,[44–47] although the methodology of these studies, which included differences in examination of users and non-users and differences in age at start of use, has been questioned.[47–49] Some studies have reported an increased relative risk of developing breast cancer, particularly at a younger age. This increased relative risk appears to be related to duration of use.[81,82]

Some studies suggest that oral contraceptive use has been associated with an increase in the risk of cervical intraepithelial neoplasia in some populations of women.[50–53] However, there continues to be controversy about the extent to which such findings may be due to differences in sexual behavior and other factors.

In spite of many studies of the relationship between oral contraceptive use and breast or cervical cancers, a cause and effect relationship has not been established.

4. HEPATIC NEOPLASIA

Benign hepatic adenomas are associated with oral contraceptive use although the incidence of benign tumors is rare in the United States. Indirect calculations have estimated the attributable risk to be in the range of 3.3 cases per 100,000 for users, a risk that increases after 4 or more years of use.[54]

Rupture of rare, benign, hepatic adenomas may cause death through intra-abdominal hemorrhage.[55–56]

Studies in the United States and Britain have shown an increased risk of developing hepatocellular carcinoma in long-term (> 8 years) oral contraceptive users.[57–59] However, these cancers are extremely rare in the United States and the attributable risk (the excess incidence) of liver cancers in oral contraceptive users is less than 1 per 1,000,000 users.

5. OCULAR LESIONS

There have been clincial case reports of retinal thrombosis associated with the use of oral contraceptives. Oral contraceptives should be discontinued if there is unexplained partial or complete loss of vision; onset of proptosis or diplopia; papilledema; or retinal vascular lesions. Appropriate diagnostic and therapeutic measures should be undertaken immediately.

6. ORAL CONTRACEPTIVE USE BEFORE OR DURING EARLY PREGNANCY

Extensive epidemiological studies have revealed no increased risk of birth defects in women who have used oral contraceptives prior to pregnancy.[60–62] More recent studies do not suggest a teratogenic effect, particularly insofar as cardiac anomalies and limb reduction defects are concerned, when taken inadvertently during early pregnancy.[60,61,63,64]

The administration of oral contraceptives to induce withdrawal bleeding should not be used as a test for pregnancy. Oral contraceptives should not be used during pregnancy to treat threatened or habitual abortion.

It is recommended that for any patient who has missed 2 consecutive periods, pregnancy should be ruled out before continuing oral contraceptive use. If the patient has not adhered to the prescribed schedule, the possibility of pregnancy should be considered at the time of the first missed period. Oral contraceptive use should be discontinued if pregnancy is confirmed.

7. GALLBLADDER DISEASE

Earlier studies have reported an increased lifetime relative risk of gallbladder surgery in users of oral contraceptives and estrogens.[65–66] More recent studies, however, have shown that the relative risk of developing gallbladder disease among oral contraceptive users may be minimal.[67] The recent findings of minimal risk may be related to the use of oral contraceptive formulations containing lower hormonal doses of estrogens and progestogens.[68]

8. CARBOHYDRATE AND LIPID METABOLIC EFFECTS

Oral contraceptives have been shown to impair oral glucose tolerance.[69] Oral contraceptives containing greater than 0.075 mg of estrogen cause glucose intolerance with impaired insulin secretion, while lower doses of estrogen may produce less glucose intolerance.[70] Progestogens increase insulin secretion and create insulin resistance, this effect varying with different progestational agents.[25,71] However, in the non-diabetic woman, oral contraceptives appear to have no effect on fasting blood glucose.[69] Because of these demonstrated effects, prediabetic and diabetic women should be carefully observed while taking oral contraceptives.

Some women may develop persistent hypertriglyceridemia while on the pill.[72] As discussed earlier (see **WARNINGS** sections 1a. and 1d.), changes in serum triglycerides and lipoprotein levels have been reported in oral contraceptive users.[23]

9. ELEVATED BLOOD PRESSURE

An increase in blood pressure has been reported in women taking oral contraceptives. The incidence of risk also was reported to increase with continued use and among older women.[66] Data from the Royal College of General Practitioners and subsequent randomized trials have shown that the incidence of hypertension increases with increasing concentrations of progestogens.

Women with a history of hypertension or hypertension-related diseases, or renal disease should be encouraged to use another method of contraception. If women elect to use oral contraceptives, they should be monitored closely and if significant elevation of blood pressure occurs, oral contraceptives should be discontinued. For most women, elevated blood pressure will return to normal after stopping oral contraceptives, and there is no difference in the occurrence of hypertension among ever-and never-users.[73–75]

10. HEADACHE

The onset or exacerbation of migraine or development of headache with a new pattern which is recurrent, persistent or severe requires discontinuation of oral contraceptives and evaluation of the cause.

11. BLEEDING IRREGULARITIES

Breakthrough bleeding and spotting are sometimes encountered in patients on oral contraceptives, especially during the first 3 months of use. Non-hormonal causes should be considered and adequate diagnostic measures taken to rule out malignancy or pregnancy in the event of breakthrough bleeding, as in the case of any abnormal vaginal bleeding. If pathology has been excluded, time or a change to another formulation may solve the problem. In the event of amenorrhea, pregnancy should be ruled out.

TABLE III: ESTIMATED ANNUAL NUMBER OF BIRTH-RELATED OR METHOD-RELATED DEATHS ASSOCIATED WITH CONTROL OF FERTILITY PER 100,000 NONSTERILE WOMEN, BY FERTILITY CONTROL METHOD ACCORDING TO AGE

Method of control and outcome	15–19	20–24	25–29	30–34	35–39	40–44
No fertility control methods*	7.0	7.4	9.1	14.8	25.7	28.2
Oral contraceptives non-smoker**	0.3	0.5	0.9	1.9	13.8	31.6
Oral contraceptives smoker**	2.2	3.4	6.6	13.5	51.1	117.2
IUD**	0.8	0.8	1.0	1.0	1.4	1.4
Condom*	1.1	1.6	0.7	0.2	0.3	0.4
Diaphragm/Spermicide*	1.9	1.2	1.2	1.3	2.2	2.8
Periodic abstinence*	2.5	1.6	1.6	1.7	2.9	3.6

* Deaths are birth related
** Deaths are method related

Estimates adapted from H.W. Ory, Table 3[41]

Some women may encounter post-pill amenorrhea or oligomenorrhea, especially when such a condition was pre-existent.

PRECAUTIONS

1. PHYSICAL EXAMINATION AND FOLLOW UP

A complete medical history and physical examination should be taken prior to the initiation or reinstitution of oral contraceptives and at least annually during use of oral contraceptives. These physical examinations should include special reference to blood pressure, breasts, abdomen and pelvic organs, including cervical cytology, and relevant laboratory tests. In case of undiagnosed, persistent or recurrent abnormal vaginal bleeding, appropriate diagnostic measures should be conducted to rule out malignancy. Women with a strong family history of breast cancer or who have breast nodules should be monitored with particular care.

2. LIPID DISORDERS

Women who are being treated for hyperlipidemias should be followed closely if they elect to use oral contraceptives. Some progestogens may elevate LDL levels and may render the control of hyperlipidemias more difficult.

3. LIVER FUNCTION

If jaundice develops in any woman receiving oral contraceptives, the medication should be discontinued. Steroid hormones may be poorly metabolized in patients with impaired liver function.

4. FLUID RETENTION

Oral contraceptives may cause some degree of fluid retention. They should be prescribed with caution, and only with careful monitoring, in patients with conditions which might be aggravated by fluid retention.

5. EMOTIONAL DISORDERS

Women with a history of depression should be carefully observed and the drug discontinued if depression recurs to a serious degree.

6. CONTACT LENSES

Contact lens wearers who develop visual changes or changes in lens tolerance should be assessed by an ophthalmologist.

7. DRUG INTERACTIONS

Reduced efficacy and increased incidence of breakthrough bleeding and menstrual irregularities have been associated with concomitant use of rifampin. A similar association, though less marked, has been suggested with barbiturates, phenylbutazone, phenytoin sodium, and possibly with griseofulvin, ampicillin and tetracyclines.[76]

8. INTERACTIONS WITH LABORATORY TESTS

Certain endocrine and liver function tests and blood components may be affected by oral contraceptives:

a. Increased prothrombin and factors VII, VIII, IX, and X; decreased antithrombin 3; increased norepinephrine-induced platelet aggregability.

b. Increased thyroid binding globulin (TBG) leading to increased circulating total thyroid hormone, as measured by protein-bound iodine (PBI), T4 by column or by radioimmunoassay. Free T3 resin uptake is decreased, reflecting the elevated TBG. Free T4 concentration is unaltered.

c. Other binding proteins may be elevated in serum.

d. Sex steroid binding globulins are increased and result in elevated levels of total circulating sex steroids and corticoids; however, free or biologically active levels remain unchanged.

e. Triglycerides may be increased.

f. Glucose tolerance may be decreased.

g. Serum folate levels may be depressed by oral contraceptive therapy. This may be of clinical significance if a woman becomes pregnant shortly after discontinuing oral contraceptives.

9. CARCINOGENESIS

See **WARNINGS** section.

10. PREGNANCY

Pregnancy Category X. See **CONTRAINDICATIONS** and **WARNINGS** sections.

11. NURSING MOTHERS

Small amounts of oral contraceptive steroids have been identified in the milk of nursing mothers and a few adverse effects on the child have been reported, including jaundice and breast enlargement. In addition, oral contraceptives given in the postpartum period may interfere with lactation by decreasing the quantity and quality of breast milk. If possible, the nursing mother should be advised not to use oral contraceptives but to use other forms of contraception until she has completely weaned her child.

INFORMATION FOR THE PATIENT

See **Patient Labeling** printed below

ADVERSE REACTIONS

An increased risk of the following serious adverse reactions has been associated with the use of oral contraceptives (see **WARNINGS** section):

- Thrombophlebitis
- Arterial thromboembolism
- Pulmonary embolism
- Myocardial infarction
- Cerebral hemorrhage
- Cerebral thrombosis

- Hypertension
- Gallbladder disease
- Hepatic adenomas, carcinomas or benign liver tumors

There is evidence of an association between the following conditions and the use of oral contraceptives, although additional confirmatory studies are needed:

- Mesenteric thrombosis
- Retinal thrombosis

The following adverse reactions have been reported in patients receiving oral contraceptives and are believed to be drug-related:

- Nausea
- Vomiting
- Gastrointestinal symptoms (such as abdominal cramps and bloating)
- Breakthrough bleeding
- Spotting
- Change in menstrual flow
- Amenorrhea
- Temporary infertility after discontinuation of treatment
- Edema
- Melasma which may persist
- Breast changes: tenderness, enlargement, secretion
- Change in weight (increase or decrease)
- Change in cervical erosion and secretion
- Diminution in lactation when given immediately postpartum
- Cholestatic jaundice
- Migraine
- Rash (allergic)
- Mental depression
- Reduced tolerance to carbohydrates
- Vaginal candidiasis
- Change in corneal curvature (steepening)
- Intolerance to contact lenses

The following adverse reactions have been reported in users of oral contraceptives and the association has been neither confirmed nor refuted:

- Pre-menstrual syndrome
- Cataracts
- Changes in appetite
- Cystitis-like syndrome
- Headache
- Nervousness
- Dizziness
- Hirsutism
- Loss of scalp hair
- Erythema multiforme
- Erythema nodosum
- Hemorrhagic eruption
- Vaginitis
- Porphyria
- Impaired renal function
- Hemolytic uremic syndrome
- Budd-Chiari syndrome
- Acne
- Changes in libido
- Colitis

OVERDOSAGE

Serious ill effects have not been reported following acute ingestion of large doses of oral contraceptives by young children. Overdosage may cause nausea, and withdrawal bleeding may occur in females.

NON-CONTRACEPTIVE HEALTH BENEFITS

The following non-contraceptive health benefits related to the use of oral contraceptives are supported by epidemiological studies which largely utilized oral contraceptive formulations containing estrogen doses exceeding 0.035 mg of ethinyl estradiol or 0.05 mg of mestranol.[6-11]

Effects on menses:

- Increased menstrual cycle regularity
- Decreased blood loss and decreased incidence of iron deficiency anemia
- Decreased incidence of dysmenorrhea

Effects related to inhibition of ovulation:

- Decreased incidence of functional ovarian cysts
- Decreased incidence of ectopic pregnancies

Effects from long-term use:

- Decreased incidence of fibroadenomas and fibrocystic disease of the breast
- Decreased incidence of acute pelvic inflammatory disease
- Decreased incidence of endometrial cancer
- Decreased incidence of ovarian cancer

DOSAGE AND ADMINISTRATION

To achieve maximum contraceptive effectiveness, oral contraceptives must be taken exactly as described and at intervals not exceeding 24 hours.

21-Day Schedule for TRI-NORINYL: The first blue tablet is taken on the first Sunday after menstrual flow begins. If menstrual flow begins on Sunday, the first blue tablet is taken on that day. One blue tablet is taken each evening at bedtime for 7 days, then one yellow-green tablet each evening for 9 days, then one blue tablet each evening for 5 days. No tablets are taken for 7 days; then, whether bleeding has

stopped or not, a new sequence of tablets is started for 21 days. This institutes a three weeks on, one week off dosage regimen.

28-Day Schedule for TRI-NORINYL: The first blue tablet is taken on the first Sunday after menstrual flow begins. If menstrual flow begins on Sunday, the first blue tablet is taken on that day. One blue tablet is taken each evening at bedtime for 7 days, then one yellow-green tablet each evening for 9 days, then one blue tablet each evening for 5 days, then one orange (inert) tablet each evening for 7 days. After all 28 tablets have been taken, whether bleeding has stopped or not, the same dosage schedule is repeated beginning on the following day.

21-Day Schedule for BREVICON, NORINYL 1 + 35, NORINYL 1 + 50, For the initial cycle of therapy the first tablet may be taken on Day 5 of the menstrual cycle, counting the first day of menstrual flow as Day 1 (DAY 5 START), or the first tablet may be taken on the first Sunday after menstrual flow begins (SUNDAY START). For SUNDAY START when menstrual flow begins on Sunday, the first tablet is taken on that day. With either DAY 5 START or SUNDAY START, one tablet is taken each day at the same time for 21 days. No tablets are taken for 7 days, then, whether bleeding has stopped or not, a new course is started of one tablet a day for 21 days. This institutes a three weeks on, one week off dosage regimen.

28-Day Schedule for BREVICON, NORINYL 1 + 35, NORINYL 1 + 50, For the initial cycle of therapy the first tablet may be taken on Day 5 of the menstrual cycle, counting the first day of menstrual flow as Day 1 (DAY 5 START), or the first tablet may be taken on the first Sunday after menstrual flow begins (SUNDAY START). For SUNDAY START when menstrual flow begins on Sunday, the first tablet is taken on that day. With either DAY 5 START or SUNDAY START, one white, blue, or yellow-green tablet is taken each day at the same time for 21 days. Then the orange tablets are taken, one each day at the same time for 7 days. After all 28 tablets have been taken, whether bleeding has stopped or not, repeat the same dosage schedule beginning on the following day.

NOR-QD® (norethindrone) is administered as a continuous daily dosage regimen starting on the first day of menstruation, i.e., one tablet each day, every day. Tablets should be taken at the same time each day and continued daily, without interruption, whether bleeding occurs or not. This is especially important for patients new to progestogen-only oral contraception. The patient should be advised that if prolonged bleeding occurs, she should consult her physician.

INSTRUCTIONS TO PATIENTS

- To achieve maximum contraceptive effectiveness, the oral contraceptive pill must be taken exactly as directed and at intervals not exceeding 24 hours.
- Important: Women should be instructed to use an additional method of protection until after the first 7 days of administration *in the initial cycle.*
- Due to the normally increased risk of thromboembolism occurring postpartum, women should be instructed not to initiate treatment with oral contraceptives earlier than 4 weeks after a full-term delivery. If pregnancy is terminated in the first 12 weeks, the patient should be instructed to start oral contraceptives immediately or within 7 days. If pregnancy is terminated after 12 weeks, the patient should be instructed to start oral contraceptives after 2 weeks.[33,77]
- If spotting or breakthrough bleeding should occur, the patient should continue the medication according to the schedule. Should spotting or breakthrough bleeding persist, the patient should notify her physician.
- If the patient misses 1 pill, she should be instructed to take it as soon as she remembers and then take the next pill at the regular time. If the patient has missed 2 pills, she should take 1 of the missed pills as soon as she remembers and discard the other missed pill. She should then take her next pill at the regular time. Furthermore, she should use an additional method of contraception in addition to taking her pills for the remainder of the cycle.
- If the patient has missed more than 2 pills, she should be instructed to discontinue taking the remaining pills and to use an alternative method of contraception until pregnancy has been ruled out.
- Use of oral contraceptives in the event of a missed menstrual period:
  1. If the patient has not adhered to the prescribed dosage regimen, the possibility of pregnancy should be considered after the first missed period and oral contraceptives should be withheld until pregnancy has been ruled out.
  2. If the patient has adhered to the prescribed regimen and misses 2 consecutive periods, pregnancy should be ruled out before continuing the contraceptive regimen.

HOW SUPPLIED

TRI-NORINYL® 21-DAY Tablets and TRI-NORINYL® 28-DAY Tablets (norethindrone and ethinyl estradiol) are avail-

Continued on next page

Syntex—Cont.

able in 21-pill or 28-pill blister cards with a WALLETTE® pill dispenser, BREVICON® 21-DAY Tablets and BREVICON® 28-DAY Tablets (norethindrone and ethinyl estradiol), NORINYL® 1 + 35 21-DAY Tablets and NORINYL® 1 + 35 28-DAY Tablets (norethindrone and ethinyl estradiol), NORINYL® 1 + 50 21-DAY Tablets and NORINYL® 1 + 50 28-DAY Tablets (norethindrone and mestranol). Each 28-pill card contains 7 orange inert pills. NOR-QD® (norethindrone) tablets are available in 42-tablet dispensers.

CAUTION: Federal law prohibits dispensing without prescription.

REFERENCES

1. Trussell, J., et al: *Stud Fam Plann* 18(5):237–283, 1987. **2.** Mann, J., et al.: *Br Med J* 2(5956):241–245, 1975. **3.** Knopp, R.H.: *J Reprod Med* 31(9):913–921, 1986. **4.** Mann, J.I., et al.: *Br Med J* 2:445–447, 1976. **5.** Ory, H.: *JAMA* 237:2619–2622, 1977. **6.** The Cancer and Steroid Hormone Study of the Centers for Disease Control: *JAMA* 249(2):1596–1599, 1983. **7.** The Cancer and Steroid Hormone Study of the Centers for Disease Control: *JAMA* 257(6):796–800, 1987. **8.** Ory, H.W.: *JAMA* 228(1):68–69, 1974. **9.** Ory, H.W., et al.: *N Engl J Med* 294:419–422, 1976. **10.** Ory, H.W.: *Fam Plann Perspect* 14:182–184, 1982. **11.** Ory, H.W., et al.: *Making Choices*, New York, The Alan Guttmacher Institute, 1983. **12.** Stadel, B.: *N Engl J Med* 305(11):612–618, 1981. **13.** Stadel, B: *N Engl J Med* 305(12):672–677, 1981. **14.** Adam, S., et al.: *Br J Obstet Gynaecol* 88:838–845, 1981. **15.** Mann, J., et al.: *Br Med J* 2(5965):245–248, 1975. **16.** Royal College of General Practitioners' Oral Contraceptive Study: *Lancet* 1:541–546, 1981. **17.** Slone, D., et al.: *N Engl J Med* 305(8):420–424, 1981. **18.** Vessey, M.P.: *Br J Fam Plann* 6 (supplement:1–12, 1980. **19.** Russell-Briefel, R., et al.: *Prev Med* 15:352–362, 1986. **20.** Goldbaum, G., et al.: *JAMA* 258(10):1339–1342, 1987. **21.** LaRosa, J.C.: *J Reprod Med* 31(9):906–912, 1986. **22.** Krauss, R.M., et al.: *Am J Obstet Gynecol* 145:446–452, 1983. **23.** Wahl, P., et al.: *N Engl J Med* 308(15):862–867, 1983. **24.** Wynn, V., et al.: *Am J Obstet Gynecol* 142(6):766–771, 1982. **25.** Wynn V., et al.: *J Reprod Med* 31(9):892–897, 1986. **26.** Inman, W.H., et al.: *Br Med J* 2(5599):193–199, 1968. **27.** Maguire, M.G., et al.: *Am J Epidemiol* 110(2):188–195, 1979. **28.** Petitti, D., et al.: *JAMA* 242(11):1150–1154, 1979. **29.** Vessey, M.P., et al.: *Br Med J* 2(5599):199–205, 1968. **30.** Vessey, M.P., et al.: *Br Med J* 2(5658):651–657, 1969. **31.** Porter, J.B., et al.: *Obstet Gynecol* 59(3):299–302, 1982. **32.** Vessey, M.P., et al.: *J Biosoc Sci* 8:373–427, 1976. **33.** Mishell, D.R., et al.: *Reproductive Endocrinology*, Philadelphia, F.A. Davis Co., 1979. **34.** Petitti, D.B., et al.: *Lancet* 2:234–236, 1978. **35.** Collaborative Group for the Study of Stroke in Young Women: *JAMA* 231(7):718–722, 1975. **36.** Inman, W.H., et al.: *Br Med J* 2:203–209, 1970. **37.** Meade, T.W., et al.: *Br Med J* 280 (6224):1157–1161, 1980. **38.** Kay, C.R.: *Am J Obstet Gynecol* 142(6):762–765, 1982. **39.** Gordon, T., et al.: *Am J Med* 62:707–714, 1977. **40.** Royal College of General Practitioners' Oral Contraception Study: *J Coll Gen Pract* 33:75–82, 1983. **41.** Ory, H.W.: *Fam Plann Perspect* 15(2):57–63, 1983. **42.** Paul, C., et al.: *Br Med J* 293:723–725, 1986. **43.** The Cancer and Steroid Hormone Study of the Centers for Disease Control: *N Engl J Med* 315(7):405–411, 1986. **44.** Pike, M.C., et al.: *Lancet* 2:926–929, 1983. **45.** Miller, D.R., et al.: *Obstet Gynecol* 68:863–868, 1986. **46.** Olsson, H., et al.: *Lancet* 2:748–749, 1985. **47.** McPherson, K., et al.: *Br J Cancer* 56:653–660, 1987. **48.** Huggins, G.R., et al.: *Fertil Steril* 47(5):733–761, 1987. **49.** McPherson, K., et al.: *Br Med J* 293:709–710, 1986. **50.** Ory, H., et al.: *Am J Obstet Gynecol* 124(6):573–577, 1976. **51.** Vessey, M.P., et al.: *Lancet* 2:930, 1983. **52.** Brinton, L.A., et al.: *Int J Cancer* 38:339–344, 1986. **53.** WHO Collaborative Study of Neoplasia and Steroid Contraceptives: *Br Med J* 290:961–965, 1985. **54.** Rooks, J.B., et al.: *JAMA* 242(7):644–648, 1979. **55.** Bein, N.N., et al.: *Br J Surg* 64:433–435, 1977. **56.** Klatskin, G.: *Gastroenterology* 73:386–394, 1977. **57.** Henderson, B.E., et al.: *Br J Cancer* 48:437–440, 1983. **58.** Neuberger, J., et al.: *Br Med J* 292:1355–1357, 1986. **59.** Forman, D., et al.: *Br Med J* 292:1357–1361, 1986. **60.** Harlap, S., et al.: *Obstet Gynecol* 55(4):447–452, 1980. **61.** Savolainen, E., et al.: *Am J Obstet Gynecol* 140(5):521–524, 1981. **62.** Janerich, D.T., et al.: *Am J Epidemiol* 112(1):73–79, 1980. **63.** Ferencz, C., et al.: *Teratology* 21:225–239, 1980. **64.** Rothman, K.J., et al.: *Am J Epidemiol* 109(4):433–439, 1979. **65.** Boston Collaborative Drug Surveillance Program: *Lancet* 1:1399–1404, 1973. **66.** Royal College of General Practitioners: *Oral contraceptives and health*. New York, Pittman, 1974. **67.** Rome Group for the Epidemiology and Prevention of Cholelithiasis: *Am J Epidemiol* 119(5):796–805, 1984. **68.** Strom, B.L., et al.: *Clin Pharmacol Ther* 39(3):335–341, 1986. **69.** Perlman, J.A., et al.: *J Chornic Dis* 38(10):857–864, 1985. **70.** Wynn, V., et al.: *Lancet* 1:1045–1049, 1979. **71.** Wynn, V.: *Progesterone and Progestin*, New York, Raven Press, 1983. **72.** Wynn, V., et al.: *Lancet* 2:720–723, 1966. **73.** Fisch, I.R., et al.: *JAMA* 237(23):2499–2503, 1977. **74.** Laragh, J.J.: *Am J Obstet Gynecol* 126(1):141–147, 1976. **75.** Ramcharan, S., et al.: *Pharmacology of Steroid Contraceptive Drugs*, New York, Raven Press, 1977. **76.** Stockley, I.: *Pharm J* 216:140–143, 1976. **77.** Dickey, R.P.: *Managing Contraceptive Pill Patients*, Oklahoma, Creative Informatics Inc., 1984. **78.** Porter JB, Hunter J, Jick H, et al: *Obstet Gynecol* 1985;66:1–4. **79.** Porter JB, Hershel J, Walker AM.: *Obstet Gynecol* 1987;70:29–32. **80.** Fertility and Maternal Health Drugs Advisory Committee, F.D.A., October, 1989. **81.** Schlesselman J, Stadel BV, Murray P, Lai S.: *Breast cancer in relation to early use of oral contraceptives.* *JAMA* 1988;259:1828–1833. **82.** Hennekens CH, Speizer FE, Lipnick RJ, Rosner B, Bain C, Belanger C, Stampfer NJ, Willett W, Peto R.: *A case-control study of oral contraceptive use and breast cancer.* *JNCl* 1984:72:39–42.

DETAILED PATIENT LABELING

INTRODUCTION

Any woman who considers using oral contraceptives ("birth control pills" or "the pill") should understand the benefits and risks of using this form of birth control. This leaflet will give you much of the information you will need to make this decision and will also help you determine if you are at risk of developing any of the serious side effects of the pill. It will tell you how to use the pill properly so that it will be as effective as possible. However, this leaflet is not a replacement for a careful discussion between you and your health care provider. You should discuss the information provided in this leaflet with him or her, both when you first start taking the pill and during your regular visits. You also should follow the advice of your health care provider with regard to regular check-ups while you are on the pill.

EFFECTIVENESS OF ORAL CONTRACEPTIVES

Oral contraceptives are used to prevent pregnancy and are more effective than other non-surgical methods of birth control. When they are taken correctly, without missing any pills, the chance of becoming pregnant is less than 1% (1 pregnancy per 100 women per year of use). Typical failure rates are actually 3% per year. The chance of becoming pregnant increases with each missed pill during a menstrual cycle.

In comparison, typical failure rates for other non-surgical methods of birth control during the first year of use are as follows:

IUD: 6%
Diaphragm with spermicides: 18%
Spermicides alone: 21%
Vaginal sponge: 18% to 30%
Condom alone: 12%
Periodic abstinence: 20%
No methods: 89%

WHO SHOULD NOT TAKE ORAL CONTRACEPTIVES

> **Cigarette smoking increases the risk of serious cardiovascular side effects from oral contraceptive use. This risk increases with age and with heavy smoking (15 or more cigarettes per day) and is quite marked in women over 35 years of age. Women who use oral contraceptives are strongly advised not to smoke.**

Some women should not use the pill. For example, you should not take the pill if you are pregnant or think you may be pregnant. You should also not use the pill if you have any of the following conditions:

- A history of heart attack or stroke
- Blood clots in the legs (thrombophlebitis), brain (stroke), lungs (pulmonary embolism), or eyes
- A history of blood clots in the deep veins of your legs
- Chest pain (angina pectoris)
- Known or suspected breast cancer or cancer of the lining of the uterus, cervix or vagina
- Unexplained vaginal bleeding (until a diagnosis is reached by your doctor)
- Yellowing of the whites of the eyes or of the skin (jaundice) during pregnancy or during previous use of the pill
- Liver tumor (benign or cancerous)
- Known or suspected pregnancy

Tell your health care provider if you have ever had any of these conditions. Your health care provider can recommend a safer method of birth control.

OTHER CONSIDERATIONS BEFORE TAKING ORAL CONTRACEPTIVES

Tell your health care provider if you have or have had:

- Breast nodules, fibrocystic disease of the breast, an abnormal breast x-ray or mammogram
- Diabetes
- Elevated cholesterol or triglycerides
- High blood pressure
- Migraine or other headaches or epilepsy
- Mental depression
- Gallbladder, heart or kidney disease
- History of scanty or irregular menstrual periods

Women with any of these conditions should be checked often by their health care provider if they choose to use oral contraceptives.

Also, be sure to inform your doctor or health care provider if you smoke or are on any medications.

RISKS OF TAKING ORAL CONTRACEPTIVES

1. Risk of developing blood clots

Blood clots and blockage of blood vessels are the most serious side effects of taking oral contraceptives. In particular, a clot in the legs can cause thrombophlebitis and a clot that travels to the lungs can cause a sudden blocking of the vessel carrying blood to the lungs. Rarely, clots occur in the blood vessels of the eye and may cause blindness, double vision, or impaired vision.

If you take oral contraceptives and need elective surgery, need to stay in bed for a prolonged illness or have recently delivered a baby, you may be at risk of developing blood clots. You should consult your doctor about stopping oral contraceptives three to four weeks before surgery and not taking oral contraceptives for two weeks after surgery or during bed rest. You should also not take oral contraceptives soon after delivery of a baby. It is advisable to wait for at least four weeks after delivery if you are not breast feeding. If you are breast feeding, you should wait until you have weaned your child before using the pill (see **GENERAL PRECAUTIONS, While Breast Feeding**).

2. Heart attacks and strokes

Oral contraceptives may increase the tendency to develop strokes (stoppage or rupture of blood vessels in the brain) and angina pectoris and heart attacks (blockage of blood vessels in the heart). Any of these conditions can cause death or temporary or permanent disability.

Smoking greatly increases the possibility of suffering heart attacks and strokes. Furthermore, smoking and the use of oral contraceptives greatly increase the chances of developing and dying of heart disease.

3. Gallbladder disease

Oral contraceptive users may have a greater risk than non-users of having gallbladder disease, although this risk may be related to pills containing high doses of estrogen.

4. Liver tumors

In rare cases, oral contraceptives can cause benign but dangerous liver tumors. These benign liver tumors can rupture and cause fatal internal bleeding. In addition, a possible but not definite association has been found with the pill and liver cancers in 2 studies, in which a few women who developed these very rare cancers were found to have used oral contraceptives for long periods. However, liver cancers are extremely rare.

5. Cancer of the breast and reproductive organs

There is, at present, no confirmed evidence that oral contraceptives increase the risk of cancer of the reproductive organs in human studies. Several studies have found no overall increase in the risk of developing breast cancer. However, women who use oral contraceptives and have a strong family history of breast cancer or who have breast nodules or abnormal mammograms should be followed closely by their doctors. Some studies have reported an increase in the risk of developing breast cancer, particularly at a younger age. This increased risk appears to be related to duration of use. Some studies have found an increase in the incidence of cancer of the cervix in women who use oral contraceptives. However, this finding may be related to factors other than the use of oral contraceptives.

ESTIMATED RISK OF DEATH FROM A BIRTH CONTROL METHOD OR PREGNANCY

All methods of birth control and pregnancy are associated with a risk of developing certain diseases which may lead to disability or death. An estimate of the number of deaths associated with different methods of birth control and pregnancy has been calculated and is shown in the following table. [See table on next page.]

In the above table, the risk of death from any birth control method is less than the risk of childbirth except for oral contraceptive users over the age of 35 who smoke and pill users over the age of 40 even if they do not smoke. It can be seen from the table that for women aged 15 to 39 the risk of death is highest with pregnancy (7–26 deaths per 100,000 women, depending on age). Among pill users who do not smoke the risk of death is always lower than that associated with pregnancy for any age group, although over the age of 40 the risk increases to 32 deaths per 100,000 women compared to 28 associated with pregnancy at that age. However, for pill users who smoke and are over the age of 35 the estimated number of deaths exceeds those for other methods of birth control. If a woman is over the age of 40 and smokes, her estimated risk of death is 4 times higher (117/100,000 women) than the estimated risk associated with pregnancy (28/100,000 women) in that age group.

The suggestion that women over 40 who don't smoke should not take oral contraceptives is based on information from older high-dose pills and on less selective use of pills than is practiced today. An Advisory Committee of the FDA discussed this issue in 1989 and recommended that the benefits of oral contraceptive use by healthy, non-smoking women over 40 years of age may outweigh the possible risks. However, all women, especially older women, are cautioned to use the lowest dose pill that is effective.

WARNING SIGNALS

If any of these adverse effects occur while you are taking oral contraceptives, call your doctor immediately:

- Sharp chest pain, coughing of blood or sudden shortness of breath (indicating a possible clot in the lung)
- Pain in the calf (indicating a possible clot in the leg)
- Crushing chest pain or heaviness in the chest (indicating a possible heart attack)
- Sudden severe headache or vomiting, dizziness or fainting, disturbances of vision or speech, weakness, or numbness in an arm or leg (indicating a possible stroke)
- Sudden partial or complete loss of vision (indicating a possible clot in the eye)
- Breast lumps (indicating possible breast cancer or fibrocystic disease of the breast: ask your doctor or health care provider to show you how to examine your breasts)
- Severe pain or tenderness in the stomach area (indicating a possible ruptured liver tumor)
- Difficulty in sleeping, weakness, lack of energy, fatigue or change in mood (possibly indicating severe depression)
- Jaundice or a yellowing of the skin or eyeballs, accompanied frequently by fever, fatigue, loss of appetite, dark colored urine or light colored bowel movements (indicating possible liver problems)

SIDE EFFECTS OF ORAL CONTRACEPTIVES

1. Vaginal bleeding

Irregular vaginal bleeding or spotting may occur while you are taking the pill. Irregular bleeding may vary from slight staining between menstrual periods to breakthrough bleeding which is a flow much like a regular period. Irregular bleeding occurs most often during the first few months of oral contraceptive use but may also occur after you have been taking the pill for some time. Such bleeding may be temporary and usually does not indicate any serious problem. It is important to continue taking your pills on schedule. If the bleeding occurs in more than 1 cycle or lasts for more than a few days, talk to your doctor or health care provider.

2. Contact lenses

If you wear contact lenses and notice a change in vision or an inability to wear your lenses, contact your doctor or health care provider.

3. Fluid retention

Oral contraceptives may cause edema (fluid retention) with swelling of the fingers or ankles and may raise your blood pressure. If you experience fluid retention, contact your doctor or health care provider.

4. Melasma (Mask of Pregnancy)

A spotty darkening of the skin is possible, particularly of the face.

5. Other side effects

Other side effects may include change in appetite, headache, nervousness, depression, dizziness, loss of scalp hair, rash, and vaginal infections.

If any of these side effects occur, contact your doctor or health care provider.

GENERAL PRECAUTIONS

1. Missed periods and use of oral contraceptives before or during early pregnancy

At times you may not menstruate regularly after you have completed taking a cycle of pills. If you have taken your pills regularly and miss 1 menstrual period, continue taking your pills for the next cycle but be sure to inform your health care provider before doing so. If you have not taken the pills daily as instructed and miss 1 menstrual period, or if you miss 2 consecutive menstrual periods, you may be pregnant. You should stop taking oral contraceptives until you are sure you are not pregnant and continue to use another method of contraception.

There is no conclusive evidence that oral contraceptive use is associated with an increase in birth defects when taken inadvertently during early pregnancy. Previously, a few studies had reported that oral contraceptives might be associated with birth defects but these studies have not been confirmed. Nevertheless, oral contraceptives or any other drugs should not be used during pregnancy unless clearly necessary and prescribed by your doctor. You should check with your doctor about risks to your unborn child from any medication taken during pregnancy.

2. While breast feeding

If you are breast feeding, consult your doctor before starting oral contraceptives. Some of the drug will be passed on to the child in the milk. A few adverse effects on the child have been reported, including yellowing of the skin (jaundice) and breast enlargement. In addition, oral contraceptives may decrease the amount and quality of your milk. If possible, use another method of contraception while breast feeding. You should consider starting oral contraceptives only after you have weaned your child completely.

3. Laboratory tests

If you are scheduled for any laboratory tests, tell your doctor you are taking birth control pills. Certain blood tests may be affected by birth control pills.

ESTIMATED ANNUAL NUMBER OF BIRTH-RELATED OR METHOD-RELATED DEATHS ASSOCIATED WITH CONTROL OF FERTILITY PER 100,000 NONSTERILE WOMEN, BY FERTILITY CONTROL METHOD ACCORDING TO AGE

Method of control and outcome	15–19	20–24	25–29	30–34	35–39	40–44
No fertility control methods*	7.0	7.4	9.1	14.8	25.7	28.2
Oral contraceptives non-smoker**	0.3	0.5	0.9	1.9	13.8	31.6
Oral contraceptives smoker**	2.2	3.4	6.6	13.5	51.1	117.2
IUD**	0.8	0.8	1.0	1.0	1.4	1.4
Condom*	1.1	1.6	0.7	0.2	0.3	0.4
Diaphragm/Spermicide*	1.9	1.2	1.2	1.3	2.2	2.8
Periodic abstinence*	2.5	1.6	1.6	1.7	2.9	3.6

*Deaths are birth-related
**Deaths are method-related

4. Drug interactions

Certain drugs may interact with birth control pills to make them less effective in preventing pregnancy or cause an increase in breakthrough bleeding. Such drugs include rifampin, drugs used for epilepsy such as barbiturates (for example, phenobarbital) and phenytoin (Dilantin is one brand of this drug), phenylbutazone (Butazolidin is one brand of this drug) and possibly certain antibiotics. You may need to use additional contraception when you take drugs which can make oral contraceptives less effective.

HOW TO TAKE ORAL CONTRACEPTIVES

1. General instructions

- You must take your pill every day according to the instructions. Oral contraceptives are most effective if taken no more than 24 hours apart. Take your pill at the same time every day so that you are less likely to forget to take it. You will then maintain the proper amount of drug in your body.
- If you are scheduled for surgery or you need prolonged bed rest you should advise your doctor that you are on the pill and stop taking the pill 4 weeks before surgery to avoid an increased risk of blood clots. It is also advisable not to start oral contraceptives sooner than 4 weeks after delivery of a baby.
- When you first begin to use the pill, you should use an additional method of protection until you have taken your first 7 pills.

Your physician has prescribed one of the following dosage schedules. Please follow the instructions appropriate for your schedule.

- 21-Day Schedule for TRI-NORINYL: Take the first blue pill on the first Sunday after menstrual flow begins. If menstrual flow begins on Sunday, take the first blue pill on that day. Take 1 blue pill the same time each day, preferably at bedtime, for the first 7 days, 1 yellow-green pill daily for the next 9 days, and then 1 blue pill each day for 5 days. Wait for 7 days, during which time a menstrual period usually occurs, then begin a new cycle of pills on the eighth day after you took your last pill, whether or not the menstrual flow has stopped. This cycle of 21 days on pills and 7 days off pills is repeated until the time for your visit with your physician or health care provider.
- 28-Day Schedule for TRI-NORINYL: Take the first blue pill on the first Sunday after the menstrual flow begins. If menstrual flow begins on Sunday, take the blue pill on that day. Take 1 blue pill the same time each day, preferably at bedtime, for the first 7 days, 1 yellow-green pill daily for the next 9 days, and then 1 blue pill each day for 5 days. Take 1 orange pill daily for the next 7 days and expect a menstrual period during this week. The orange pills contain no active drug and are included simply for your convenience—to eliminate the need for counting days. After all 28 pills have been taken, whether bleeding has stopped or not, take the first blue pill of the next cycle without any interruption. With the 28-day package, a pill is taken every day with no gap between cycles until the time for your visit with your physician or health care provider.
- 21-Day Schedule for BREVICON, NORINYL 1 + 35, NORINYL 1 + 50 Tablets: You may start taking the pill on Day 5 of your menstrual cycle or on Sunday. To start on Day 5, count the first day of menstrual flow as Day 1 and take the first pill on Day 5 of the menstrual cycle whether or not the flow has stopped. To start on Sunday, take the first pill on the first Sunday after your menstrual period begins. If it begins on Sunday, take the first pill that day. Whether you start on Day 5 or on Sunday, take another pill the same time each day, preferably at bedtime, for 21 days. Then wait for 7 days, during which time a menstrual period usually occurs, and begin taking 1 pill every day on the eighth day after you took your last pill, whether or not the menstrual flow has stopped. This cycle of 21 days on pills and 7 days off pills is repeated until the time for your visit with your physician or health care provider.
- 28-Day Schedule for BREVICON, NORINYL 1 + 35, NORINYL 1 + 50 Tablets: You may start taking the pill on Day 5 of your menstrual cycle or on Sunday. To start on Day 5, count the first day of menstrual flow as Day 1 and take the first white, yellow-green, or blue pill on Day 5 of the menstrual cycle whether or not the flow has stopped. To start on Sunday, take the first white, yellow-green, or blue pill on the first Sunday after your menstrual period begins. If it begins on Sunday, take the first pill that day. Whether you start on Day 5 or on Sunday, follow the sequence around the card and continue taking another pill at the same time each day, preferably at bedtime, for 21 days. Then take an orange pill from the bottom of the card each day for 7 days and expect a menstrual period during this week. The orange pills contain no active drug and are included simply for your convenience—to eliminate the need for counting days. After all 28 pills have been taken, whether bleeding has stopped or not, take the first white, yellow-green, or blue pill of the next cycle without any interruption. With the 28-day package, pills are taken every day with no gap between cycles until the time for your visit with your physician or health care provider.
- NOR-QD Tablets 0.35 mg Schedule: Take the first pill on the first day of the menstrual flow, and take another pill each day, every day until the time for your visit with your physician or health care provider. The pill should be taken at the same time of day, preferably at bedtime, and continued daily without interruption whether bleeding occurs or not. If prolonged bleeding occurs, you should consult your physician.

2. Missed periods/breakthrough bleeding

At times, there may be no menstrual period after you complete a cycle of pills. If you miss 1 menstrual period but have taken the pills *exactly as you were supposed to,* continue as usual into the next cycle. If you have not taken the pills correctly, and have missed a menstrual period, *you may be pregnant* and you should stop taking oral contraceptives until your doctor determines whether or not you are pregnant. Until you can get to your doctor, use another form of contraception. If you miss 2 consecutive menstrual periods, you should stop taking the pills until it is determined that you are not pregnant.

Even if spotting or breakthrough bleeding should occur, continue the medication according to the schedule. Should spotting or breakthrough bleeding persist, you should notify your physician.

3. If you forget to take your pill

If you miss only 1 pill in a cycle, the chance of becoming pregnant is small. Take the missed pill as soon as you realize that you have forgotten it. Since the risk of pregnancy increases with each additional pill you skip, it is very important that you take each pill according to schedule.

If you miss 2 pills in a row, you should take 1 of the missed pills as soon as you remember, discard the other missed pill and take your regular pill for that day at the proper time. Furthermore, you should use an additional method of contraception in addition to taking your pills for the remainer of the cycle. If more than 2 pills in a row have been missed, discontinue taking your pills immediately and use an additional method of contraception until you have a period or your doctor determines that you are not pregnant. Missing orange pills in the 28-day schedule does not increase your chances of becoming pregnant.

4. Pregnancy due to pill failure

When taken correctly, the incidence of pill failure resulting in pregnancy is approximately 1% (i.e., 1 pregnancy per 100 women per year). If failure occurs, the risk to the fetus is minimal. The typical failure rate of large numbers of pill users is less than 3% when women who miss pills are included. If you become pregnant, you should discuss your pregnancy with your doctor.

5. Pregnancy after stopping the pill

There may be some delay in becoming pregnant after you stop using oral contraceptives, especially if you had irregular menstrual cycles before you used oral contraceptives. It may be advisable to postpone conception until you begin menstruating regularly once you have stopped taking the pill and desire pregnancy.

Continued on next page

Syntex—Cont.

There does not appear to be any increase in birth defects in newborn babies when pregnancy occurs soon after stopping the pill.

6. Overdosage
Serious ill effects have not been reported following ingestion of large doses of oral contraceptives by young children. Overdosage may cause nausea and withdrawal bleeding in females. In case of overdosage, contact your health care provider or pharmacist.

7. Other information
Your health care provider will take a medical and family history and will examine you before prescribing oral contraceptives. You should be reexamined at least once a year. Be sure to inform your health care provider if there is a family history of any of the conditions listed previously in this leaflet. Be sure to keep all appointments with your health care provider because this is a time to determine if there are early signs of side effects of oral contraceptive use.

Do not use the drug for any condition other than the one for which it was prescribed. This drug has been prescribed specifically for you: do not give it to others who may want birth control pills.

If you want more information about birth control pills, ask your doctor or health care provider. They have a more technical leaflet called **PHYSICIAN LABELING** which you may wish to read.

NON-CONTRACEPTIVE HEALTH BENEFITS

In addition to preventing pregnancy, use of oral contraceptives may provide certain non-contraceptive benefits:
- Menstrual cycles may become more regular
- Blood flow during menstruation may be lighter and less iron may be lost. Therefore, anemia due to iron deficiency is less likely to occur.
- Pain or other symptoms during menstruation may be encountered less frequently
- Ectopic (tubal) pregnancy may occur less frequently
- Non-cancerous cysts or lumps in the breast may occur less frequently
- Acute pelvic inflammatory disease may occur less frequently
- Oral contraceptive use may provide some protection against developing two forms of cancer: cancer of the ovaries and cancer of the lining of the uterus.

BRIEF SUMMARY

PATIENT PACKAGE INSERT
Oral contraceptives, also known as "birth control pills" or "the pill," are taken to prevent pregnancy and, when taken correctly, have a failure rate of about 1% per year when used without missing any pills. The typical failure rate of large numbers of pill users is less than 3% per year when women who miss pills are included. For most women, oral contraceptives are also free of serious or unpleasant side effects. However, forgetting to take oral contraceptives considerably increases the chances of pregnancy.

For the majority of women, oral contraceptives can be taken safely, but there are some women who are at high risk of developing certain serious diseases that can be life-threatening or may cause temporary or permanent disability. The risks associated with taking oral contraceptives increase significantly if you:
- Smoke
- Have high blood pressure, diabetes, or high cholesterol
- Have or have had clotting disorders, heart attack, stroke, angina pectoris, cancer of the breast or sex organs, jaundice or malignant or benign liver tumors

You should not take the pill if you suspect you are pregnant or have unexplained vaginal bleeding.

Cigarette smoking increases the risk of serious cardiovascular side effects from oral contraceptive use. This risk increases with age and with heavy smoking (15 or more cigarettes per day) and is quite marked in women over 35 years of age. Women who use oral contraceptives are strongly advised not to smoke.

Most side effects of the pill are not serious. The most common such effects are nausea, vomiting, bleeding between menstrual periods, weight gain, breast tenderness, and difficulty wearing contact lenses. These side effects, especially nausea and vomiting, may subside within the first 3 months of use. The serious side effects of the pill occur very infrequently, especially if you are in good health and are young. However, you should know that the following medical conditions have been associated with or made worse by the pill:

1. Blood clots in the legs (thrombophlebitis) or lungs (pulmonary embolism), stoppage or rupture of a blood vessel in the brain (stroke), blockage of blood vessels in the heart (heart attack or angina pectoris), eye or other organs of the

body. As mentioned above, smoking increases the risk of heart attacks and strokes and subsequent serious medical consequences.

2. Liver tumors, which may rupture and cause severe bleeding. A possible but not definite association has been found with the pill and liver cancer. However, liver cancers are extremely rare.

3. High blood pressure, although blood pressure usually returns to normal when the pill is stopped.

The symptoms associated with these serious side effects are discussed in the detailed leaflet given to you with your supply of pills. Notify your doctor or health care provider if you notice any unusual physical disturbances while taking the pill. In addition, drugs such as rifampin, as well as some anticonvulsants and some antibiotics, may decrease oral contraceptive effectiveness.

Studies to date of women taking the pill have not shown an increase in the incidence of cancer of the breast or cervix. There is, however, insufficient evidence to rule out the possibility that the pill may cause such cancers. Some studies have reported an increase in the risk of developing breast cancer, particularly at a younger age. This increased risk appears to be related to duration of use.

Taking the pill may provide some important non-contraceptive benefits. These include less painful menstruation, less menstrual blood loss and anemia, fewer acute pelvic infections, and fewer cancers of the ovary and the lining of the uterus.

Be sure to discuss any medical condition you may have with your health care provider. Your health care provider will take a medical and family history before prescribing oral contraceptives and will examine you. You should be reexamined at least once a year while taking oral contraceptives. The detailed patient information leaflet gives you further information which you should read and discuss with your health care provider.

U.S. Patent No. 4,390,531 (for TRI-NORINYL® tablets only)
02-0100-97-01,02-0114-97-00
©1990 Syntex (F.P.) Inc.   Revised 3/90
Shown in Product Identification Section, page 433

TAP Pharmaceuticals Inc.
DEERFIELD, IL 60015

LUPRON®   ℞
[lu 'pron]
(leuprolide acetate) Injection

DESCRIPTION

LUPRON (leuprolide acetate) Injection is a synthetic nonapeptide analog of naturally occurring gonadotropin releasing hormone (GnRH or LH-RH). The analog possesses greater potency than the natural hormone. The chemical name is 5-Oxo-L-prolyl-L-histidyl-L-tryptophyl-L-seryl-L-tyrosyl-D-leucyl-L-leucyl-L-arginyl-N-ethyl-L-prolinamide acetate (salt) with the following structural formula:
[See below.]
LUPRON is a sterile, aqueous solution intended for subcutaneous injection. It is available in a 2.8 ml multiple-dose vial containing 5 mg/ml of leuprolide acetate, sodium chloride for tonicity adjustment, 9 mg/ml of benzyl alcohol as a preservative and water for injection. The pH may have been adjusted with sodium hydroxide and/or acetic acid.

CLINICAL PHARMACOLOGY

Leuprolide acetate, an LH-RH agonist, acts as a potent inhibitor of gonadotropin secretion when given continuously and

in therapeutic doses. Animal and human studies indicate that following an initial stimulation, chronic administration of leuprolide acetate results in suppression of ovarian and testicular steroidogenesis. This effect is reversible upon discontinuation of drug therapy. Administration of leuprolide acetate has resulted in inhibition of the growth of certain hormone dependent tumors (prostatic tumors in Noble and Dunning male rats and DMBA-induced mammary tumors in female rats) as well as atrophy of the reproductive organs. In humans, subcutaneous administration of single daily doses of leuprolide acetate results in an initial increase in circulating levels of luteinizing hormone (LH) and follicle stimulating hormone (FSH), leading to a transient increase in levels of the gonadal steroids (testosterone and dihydrotestosterone in males, and estrone and estradiol in pre-menopausal females). However, continuous daily administration of leuprolide acetate results in decreased levels of LH and FSH in all patients. In males, testosterone is reduced to castrate levels. In pre-menopausal females, estrogens are reduced to post-menopausal levels. These decreases occur within two to four weeks after initiation of treatment, and castrate levels of testosterone in prostatic cancer patients have been demonstrated for periods of up to five years. Leuprolide acetate is not active when given orally. Bioavailability by subcutaneous administration is comparable to that by intravenous administration. Leuprolide acetate has a plasma half-life of approximately three hours. The metabolism, distribution and excretion of leuprolide acetate in man have not been determined.

INDICATIONS AND USAGE

LUPRON (leuprolide acetate) Injection is indicated in the palliative treatment of advanced prostatic cancer. It offers an alternative treatment of prostatic cancer when orchiectomy or estrogen administration are either not indicated or unacceptable to the patient. In a controlled study comparing LUPRON 1 mg/day given subcutaneously to DES (diethylstilbestrol), 3 mg/day, the survival rate for the two groups was comparable after two years treatment. The objective response to treatment was also similar for the two groups.

CONTRAINDICATIONS

A report of an anaphylactic reaction to synthetic GnRH (Factrel) has been reported in the medical literature.[1]
LUPRON is contraindicated in women who are or may become pregnant while receiving the drug. When administered on day 6 of pregnancy at test dosages of 0.00024, 0.0024, and 0.024 mg/kg (1/600 to 1/6 the human dose) to rabbits, LUPRON produced a dose related increase in major fetal abnormalities. Similar studies in rats failed to demonstrate an increase in fetal malformations. There was increased fetal mortality and decreased fetal weights with the two higher doses of LUPRON in rabbits and with the highest dose in rats. The effects on fetal mortality are logical consequences of the alterations in hormonal levels brought about by this drug. Therefore, the possibility exists that spontaneous abortion may occur if the drug is administered during pregnancy.

WARNINGS

Isolated cases of worsening of signs and symptoms during the first weeks of treatment have been reported. Worsening of symptoms may contribute to paralysis with or without fatal complications.

PRECAUTIONS

Patients with metastatic vertebral lesions and/or with urinary tract obstruction should be closely observed during the first few weeks of therapy (see "ADVERSE REACTIONS" section).
Patients with known allergies to benzyl alcohol, an ingredient of the drug's vehicle, may present symptoms of hypersen-

sitivity, usually local, in the form of erythema and induration at the injection site.

Information for Patients: See Information for Patients which appears after the "HOW SUPPLIED" section.

Laboratory Tests: Response to leuprolide acetate should be monitored by measuring serum levels of testosterone and acid phosphatase. In the majority of patients, testosterone levels increased above baseline during the first week, declining thereafter to baseline levels or below by the end of the second week of treatment. Castrate levels were reached within two to four weeks and once attained were maintained for as long as drug administration continued. Transient increases in acid phosphatase levels occurred sometimes early in treatment. However, by the fourth week, the elevated levels usually decreased to values at or near baseline.

Drug Interactions: None have been reported.

Carcinogenesis, Mutagenesis, Impairment of Fertility: Two-year carcinogenicity studies were conducted in rats and mice. In rats, a dose-related increase of benign pituitary hyperplasia and benign pituitary adenomas was noted at 24 months when the drug was administered subcutaneously at high daily doses (0.6 to 4 mg/kg). In mice no pituitary abnormalities were observed at a dose as high as 60 mg/kg for two years. Patients have been treated with leuprolide acetate for up to three years with doses as high as 10 mg/day and for two years with doses as high as 20 mg/day without demonstrable pituitary abnormalities.

Mutagenicity studies have been performed with leuprolide acetate using bacterial and mammalian systems. These studies provided no evidence of a mutagenic potential.

Clinical and pharmacologic studies with leuprolide acetate and similar analogs have shown full reversibility of fertility suppression when the drug is discontinued after continuous administration for periods of up to 24 weeks. However, no clinical studies have been conducted with leuprolide acetate to assess the reversibility of fertility suppression.

Pregnancy Category X. See "CONTRAINDICATIONS" section.

ADVERSE REACTIONS

In the majority of patients testosterone levels increased above baseline during the first week, declining thereafter to baseline levels or below by the end of the second week of treatment. This transient increase was occasionally associated with a temporary worsening of signs and symptoms, usually manifested by an increase in bone pain (See "WARNINGS" section). In a few cases a temporary worsening of existing hematuria and urinary tract obstruction occurred during the first week. Temporary weakness and paresthesia of the lower limbs have been reported in a few cases.

Potential exacerbations of signs and symptoms during the first few weeks of treatment is a concern in patients with vertebral metastases and/or urinary obstruction which, if aggravated, may lead to neurological problems or increase the obstruction.

In a comparative trial of LUPRON (leuprolide acetate) Injection versus DES, in 5% or more of the patients receiving either drug, the following adverse reactions were reported to have a possible or probable relationship to drug as ascribed by the treating physician. Often, causality is difficult to assess in patients with metastatic prostate cancer. Reactions considered not drug related are excluded.

[See table above.]

In this same study, the following adverse reactions were reported in less than 5% of the patients on Lupron.

Cardiovascular System—Angina, Cardiac arrhythmias, Myocardial infarction, Pulmonary emboli; *Gastrointestinal System*—Diarrhea, Dysphagia, Gastrointestinal bleeding, Gastrointestinal disturbance, Peptic ucler, Rectal polyps; *Endocrine System*—Libido decrease, Thyroid enlargement; *Musculoskeletal System*—Joint pain; *Central/Peripheral Nervous System*—Anxiety, Blurred vision, Lethargy, Memory disorder, Mood swings, Nervousness, Numbness, Paresthesia, Peripheral neuropathy, Syncope/blackouts, Taste disorders; *Respiratory System*—Cough, Pleural rub, Pneumonia, Pulmonary fibrosis; *Integumentary System*—Carcinoma of skin/ear, Dry skin, Ecchymosis, Hair loss, Itching, Local skin reactions, Pigmentation, Skin lesions; *Urogenital System*—Bladder spasms, Dysuria, Incontinence, Testicular pain, Urinary obstruction; *Miscellaneous*—Depression, Diabetes, Fatigue, Fever/chills, Hypoglycemia, Increased BUN, Increased calcium, Increased creatinine, Infection/inflammation, Ophthalmologic disorders, Swelling (temporal bone).

The following additional adverse reactions have been reported with LUPRON or LUPRON DEPOT (leuprolide acetate for depot suspension) during other clinical trials and/or during postmarketing surveillance. Reactions considered as nondrug related by the treating physician are excluded.

Cardiovascular System—Hypotension, Transient ischemic attack/stroke; *Gastrointestinal System*—Hepatic dysfunction; *Endocrine System*—Libido increase; *Hemic and Lymphatic System*—Decreased WBC, Hemoptysis; *Musculoskeletal System*—Ankylosing spondylosis, Pelvic fibrosis; *Central/Peripheral Nervous System*—Hearing disorder, Peripheral neuropathy, Spinal fracture/paralysis; *Respiratory System*—Pulmonary infiltrate, Respiratory disorders; Integumentary System—Hair growth; *Urogenital System*—Penile swelling, Prostate pain; *Miscellaneous*—Hypoproteinemia, Hard nodule in throat, Weight gain, Increased uric acid.

	LUPRON (N = 98)	DES (N = 101)
	Number of Reports	
Cardiovascular System		
Congestive heart failure	1	5
ECG changes/ischemia	19	22
High blood pressure	8	5
Murmur	3	8
Peripheral edema	12	30
Phlebitis/thrombosis	2	10
Gastrointestinal System		
Anorexia	6	5
Constipation	7	9
Nausea/vomiting	5	17
Endocrine System		
Decreased testicular size	7	11
Gynecomastia/breast tenderness or pain	7	63
Hot flashes	55	12
Impotence	4	12
Hemic and Lymphatic System		
Anemia	5	5
Musculoskeletal System		
Bone pain	5	2
Myalgia	3	9
Central/Peripheral Nervous System		
Dizziness/lightheadedness	5	7
General pain	13	13
Headache	7	4
Insomnia/sleep disorders	7	5
Respiratory System		
Dyspnea	2	8
Sinus congestion	5	6
Integumentary System		
Dermatitis	5	8
Urogenital System		
Frequency/urgency	6	8
Hematuria	6	4
Urinary tract infection	3	7
Miscellaneous		
Asthenia	10	10

*Physiologic effect of decreased testosterone.

OVERDOSAGE

In rats subcutaneous administration of 250 to 500 times the recommended human dose, expressed on a per body weight basis, resulted in dyspnea, decreased activity, and local irritation at the injection site. There is no evidence at present that there is a clinical counterpart of this phenomenon. In early clinical trials with leuprolide acetate doses as high as 20 mg/day for up to two years caused no adverse effects differing from those observed with the 1 mg/day dose.

DOSAGE AND ADMINISTRATION

The recommended dose is 1 mg (0.2 ml) administered as a single daily subcutaneous injection. As with other drugs administered chronically by subcutaneous injection, the injection site should be be varied periodically.

NOTE: As with all parenteral products, inspect container's solution for discoloration and particulate matter before each use.

HOW SUPPLIED

LUPRON (leuprolide acetate) Injection is a sterile solution supplied in a 2.8 ml multiple-dose vial, **NDC** 0300-3626-28. Refrigerate until dispensed. Patient may store unrefrigerated below 86°F. Avoid freezing. Protect from light—store vial in carton until use.

Each 0.2 ml contains 1 mg of leuprolide acetate, sodium chloride for tonicity adjustment, 1.8 mg of benzyl alcohol as preservative and water for injection. The pH may have been adjusted with sodium hydroxide and/or acetic acid.

Caution: Federal (U.S.A.) law prohibits dispensing without a prescription.

Revised: February, 1990.

U.S. Patent Nos. 4,005,063 and 4,005,194.

Reference: 1. MacLeod TL, Eisen A, Sussman GL, et al: Anaphylactic reaction to synthetic luteinizing hormone-releasing hormone. *Fertil Steril* 1987 Sept;48 (3):500–502.

INFORMATION FOR PATIENTS

NOTE: Be sure to consult your physician with any questions you may have or for information about LUPRON (leuprolide acetate) Injection and its use.

WHAT IS LUPRON?

LUPRON (leuprolide acetate) Injection is chemically similar to gonadotropin releasing hormone (GnRH or LH-RH), a hormone which occurs naturally in your body.

Normally, your body releases small amounts of LH-RH, and this leads to events which stimulate the production of sex hormones.

However, when you inject LUPRON Injection, the normal events that lead to sex hormone production are interrupted and testosterone is no longer produced by the testes.

LUPRON must be injected because, like insulin which is injected by diabetics, LUPRON is inactive when taken by mouth.

If you were to discontinue the drug for any reason, your body would begin making testosterone again.

DIRECTIONS FOR USING LUPRON

1. Wash hands thoroughly with soap and water.
2. If using a new bottle for the first time, flip off the plastic cover to expose the gray rubber stopper. Wipe metal ring and rubber stopper with an alcohol wipe each time you use LUPRON. Check the liquid in the container. If it is not clear or has particles in it, DO NOT USE IT. Exchange it at your pharmacy for another container.
3. Remove outer wrapping from one syringe. Pull plunger back until the tip of the plunger is at the .2 mark.
4. Take cover off needle and push the cover into the appropriate hole in the Daily Dose Reminder area. Push the needle through the center of the rubber stopper on the LUPRON bottle.
5. Push the plunger all the way in to inject air into the bottle.
6. Keep the needle in the bottle and turn the bottle upside down. Check to make sure the tip of the needle is in the liquid. Slowly pull back on the plunger, until the syringe fills to the .2 mark.
7. Toward the end of a two-week period, the amount of LUPRON left in the bottle will be small. Take special care to hold the bottle straight and to keep the needle tip in liquid while pulling back on the plunger.
8. Keeping the needle in the bottle and the bottle upside down, check for air bubbles in the syringe. If you see any, push the plunger *slowly* in to push the air bubble back into the bottle. Keep the tip of the needle in the liquid and pull the plunger back again to fill to the .2 mark.
9. Do this again if necessary to eliminate air bubbles. Remove needle from bottle and lay syringe down on the syringe rest. DO NOT TOUCH THE NEEDLE OR ALLOW THE NEEDLE TO TOUCH ANY SURFACE.
10. To protect your skin, inject each daily dose at a different body spot.
11. Choose an injection spot. Cleanse the injection spot with another alcohol wipe.
12. Hold the syringe in one hand. Hold the skin taut, or pull up a little flesh with the other hand, as you were instructed.
13. Holding the syringe as you would a pencil, thrust the needle all the way into the skin at a 90° angle.
14. Hold an alcohol wipe down on your skin where the needle is inserted and withdraw the needle at the same angle it was inserted.
15. Use the disposable syringe only once and dispose of it properly as you were instructed. A waste area is provided in the LUPRON Patient Administration Kit. Needles thrown into a garbage bag could accidentally stick someone. NEVER LEAVE SYRINGES, NEEDLES OR DRUGS WHERE CHILDREN CAN REACH THEM.

SOME SPECIAL ADVICE

- You may experience hot flashes when using LUPRON (leuprolide acetate) Injection. During the first few weeks of treatment you may experience increased bone pain, increased difficulty in urinating, and less commonly but most importantly, you may experience the onset or aggravation of nerve symptoms. In any of these events, discuss the symptoms with your doctor.
- You may experience some irritation at the injection site, such as burning, itching or swelling. These reactions are usually mild and go away. If they do not, tell your doctor.
- Do not stop taking your injections because you feel better. You need an injection every day to make sure LUPRON keeps working for you.
- If you need to use an alternate syringe, low-dose insulin syringes should be utilized.
- When the drug level gets low, take special care to hold the bottle straight up and down and to keep the needle tip in liquid while pulling back on the plunger.
- Do not try to get every last drop out of the bottle. This will increase the possibility of drawing air into the syringe and getting an incomplete dose. Some extra drug has been provided so that you can withdraw the recommended number of doses.
- Tell your pharmacist when you will need your next LUPRON kit so it will be at the pharmacy when you need it.
- This drug may be stored at room temperature (not above 86°F). Do not store near a radiator or other very warm place.
- Do not leave your drug or hypodermic syringes where anyone can pick them up.

Continued on next page

TAP—Cont.

- Keep this and all other medications out of reach of children.

Manufactured for TAP Pharmaceuticals Inc.
Deerfield, IL 60015, U.S.A.
by Abbott Laboratories
North Chicago, IL 60064
(New)—Rev. January 1990

LUPRON DEPOT® 3.75 mg   ℞
[lu 'pron dē 'pō]
(leuprolide acetate for depot suspension)

DESCRIPTION
Leuprolide acetate is a synthetic nonapeptide analog of naturally occurring gonadotropin releasing hormone (GnRH or LH-RH). The analog possesses greater potency than the natural hormone. The chemical name is 5-Oxo-L-prolyl-L-histidyl-L- tryptophyl-L-seryl-L- tyrosol-D- leucyl-L-leucyl-L-arginyl-N-ethyl-L-prolinamide acetate (salt) with the following structural formula:
[See below.]
LUPRON DEPOT is supplied in a vial containing sterile lyophilized microspheres, which when mixed with diluent, become a suspension, which is intended as a monthly intramuscular injection.
The single-dose vial of LUPRON DEPOT 3.75 mg contains leuprolide acetate (3.75 mg), purified gelatin (0.65 mg), DL-lactic and glycolic acids copolymer (33.1 mg), and D-mannitol (6.6 mg). The accompanying ampule of diluent contains carboxymethylcellulose sodium (7.5 mg), D-mannitol (75 mg), polysorbate 80 (1.5 mg), water for injection, USP, and acetic acid, NF to control pH.

CLINICAL PHARMACOLOGY
Leuprolide acetate is a long acting GnRH analog. A single monthly injection of leuprolide acetate results in an initial stimulation followed by a prolonged suppression of pituitary gonadotropins. Repeated dosing at monthly intervals results in decreased secretion of gonadal steroids; consequently, tissues and functions that depend on gonadal steroids for their maintenance become quiescent. This effect is reversible on discontinuation of drug therapy.
Leuprolide acetate is not active when given orally. Intramuscular injection of the depot formulation provides plasma concentrations of leuprolide acetate over a period of one month.
In males receiving a single dose of LUPRON DEPOT 7.5 mg IM, there was an initial burst of leuprolide acetate in plasma. Mean plasma leuprolide levels of about 0.80 ng/mL were maintained which slowly declined over a period of several weeks. In most of the patient volunteers, plasma leuprolide concentrations were undetected eight weeks after injection. However, three of these men had low, but detectable levels up to 12 weeks.
Absolute bioavailability from a 7.5 mg dose was estimated to be about 90%.
The metabolism, distribution and excretion of leuprolide acetate in humans have not been fully determined.
The pharmacokinetics of the drug in hepatic- and renal-impaired patients have not been determined.
In controlled clinical studies, LUPRON DEPOT 3.75 mg monthly for 6 months was shown to be comparable to danazol, 800 mg/day in relieving the clinical symptoms of endometriosis (pelvic pain, dysmenorrhea, dyspareunia, pelvic tenderness, and induration) and in reducing the size of endometrial implants as evidenced by laparoscopy. The clinical significance of a decrease in endometriotic lesions is not known at this time and in addition, laparoscopic staging of endometriosis does not necessarily correlate with the severity of symptoms.

FIGURE 1
PERCENT OF PATIENTS WITH SYMPTOMS AT BASELINE, FINAL TREATMENT VISIT, AND AFTER 6 AND 12 MONTHS OF FOLLOW–UP

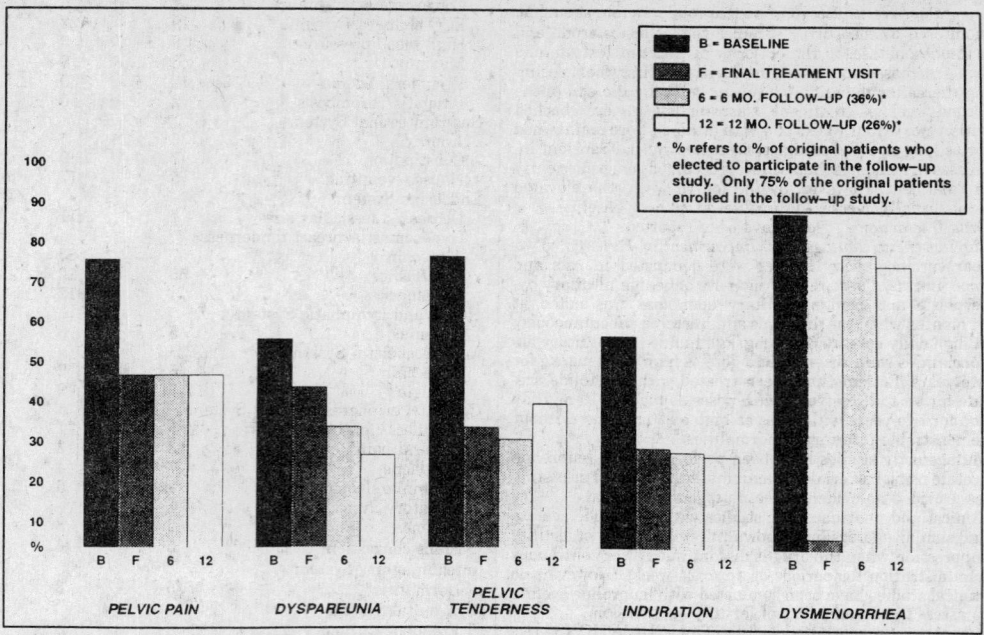

LUPRON DEPOT 3.75 mg monthly induced amenorrhea in 74% and 98% of the patients after the first and second treatment months respectively. Most of the remaining patients reported episodes of only light bleeding or spotting. In the first, second and third post-treatment months, normal menstrual cycles resumed in 7%, 71% and 95% respectively, of those patients who did not become pregnant.
Figure 1 illustrates the percent of patients with symptoms at baseline, final treatment visit and sustained relief at 6 and 12 months following discontinuation of treatment for the various symptoms evaluated during the study. This included all patients at end of treatment and those who elected to participate at the follow-up periods. This might provide a slight bias in the results at follow-up as 75% of the original patients entered the follow-up study, and 36% were evaluated at 6 months and 26% at 12 months respectively.
There is no evidence that pregnancy rates are enhanced or adversely affected by the use of LUPRON DEPOT.

INDICATIONS AND USAGE
LUPRON DEPOT (leuprolide acetate for depot suspension) is indicated for management of endometriosis, including pain relief and reduction of endometriotic lesions. Experience with LUPRON DEPOT for the management of endometriosis has been limited to women 18 years of age and older treated for 6 months.

CONTRAINDICATIONS
1. Hypersensitivity to GnRH, GnRH agonist analogs or any of the excipients in LUPRON DEPOT.
2. Undiagnosed abnormal vaginal bleeding.
3. LUPRON DEPOT is contraindicated in women who are or may become pregnant while receiving the drug. LUPRON DEPOT may cause fetal harm when administered to a pregnant woman. Major fetal abnormalities were observed in rabbits but not in rats after administration of LUPRON DEPOT throughout gestation. There was in-

creased fetal mortality and decreased fetal weights in rats and rabbits (see Pregnancy Section). The effects on fetal mortality are expected consequences of the alterations in hormonal levels brought about by the drug. If this drug is used during pregnancy or if the patient becomes pregnant while taking this drug, she should be apprised of the potential hazard to the fetus.
4. Use in women who are breast feeding (see Nursing Mothers Section).
5. A report of an anaphylactic reaction to synthetic GnRH (Factrel) has been reported in the medical literature.[1]

WARNINGS
Safe use of leuprolide acetate in pregnancy has not been established clinically. Before starting treatment with LUPRON DEPOT, pregnancy must be excluded.
When used monthly at the recommended dose, LUPRON DEPOT usually inhibits ovulation and stops menstruation. Contraception is not insured, however, by taking LUPRON DEPOT. Therefore, patients should use nonhormonal methods of contraception. Patients should be advised to see their physician if they believe they may be pregnant. If a patient becomes pregnant during treatment, the drug must be discontinued and the patient must be apprised of the potential risk to the fetus.
During the early phase of therapy, sex steroids temporarily rise above baseline because of the physiologic effect of the drug. Therefore, an increase in clinical signs and symptoms may be observed during the initial days of therapy, but these will dissipate with continued therapy.

PRECAUTIONS
Information for Patients: An information pamphlet for patients is included with the product. Patients should be aware of the following information:
1. Since menstruation should stop with effective doses of LUPRON DEPOT, the patient should notify her physician if regular menstruation persists. Patients missing successive doses of LUPRON DEPOT may experience breakthrough bleeding.
2. Patients should not use LUPRON DEPOT if they are pregnant, breast feeding, have undiagnosed abnormal vaginal bleeding, or are allergic to any of the ingredients in LUPRON DEPOT.
3. Safe use of the drug in pregnancy has not been established clinically. Therefore, a nonhormonal method of contraception should be used during treatment. Patients should be advised that if they miss successive doses of LUPRON DEPOT, breakthrough bleeding or ovulation may occur with the potential for conception. If a patient becomes pregnant during treatment, she should discontinue treatment and consult her physician.
4. Those adverse events occurring in clinical studies with LUPRON DEPOT are associated with hypoestrogenism; like hot flashes, headaches, emotional lability, decreased libido, acne, myalgia, reduction in breast size, and vaginal dryness. Estrogen levels returned to normal after treatment was discontinued.

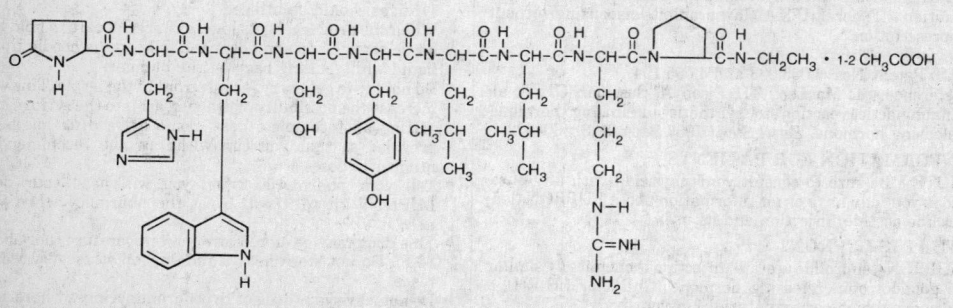

5. The induced hypoestrogenic state results in a small loss in bone density over the course of treatment, some of which may not be reversible. During one six-month treatment period, this bone loss should not be important. In patients with major risk factors for decreased bone mineral content such as chronic alcohol and/or tobacco use, strong family history of osteoporosis, or chronic use of drugs that can reduce bone mass such as anticonvulsants or corticosteroids, LUPRON DEPOT therapy may pose an additional risk. In these patients the risks and benefits must be weighed carefully before therapy with LUPRON DEPOT is instituted. Repeated courses of treatment with gonadotropin-releasing hormone analogs are not advisable in patients with major risk factors for loss of bone mineral content.

6. Retreatment cannot be recommended since safety data beyond 6 months are not available.

Drug Interactions: No pharmacokinetic-based drug-drug interaction studies have been conducted with LUPRON DEPOT. However, because leuprolide acetate is a peptide that is primarily degraded by peptidase and not by cytochrome P-450 enzymes as noted in specific studies, and the drug is only about 46% bound to plasma proteins, drug interactions would not be expected to occur.

Drug/Laboratory Test Interactions: Administration of LUPRON DEPOT (leuprolide acetate for depot suspension) in therapeutic doses results in suppression of the pituitary-gonadal system. Normal function is usually restored within 4 to 12 weeks after treatment is discontinued. Therefore, diagnostic tests of pituitary gonadotropic and gonadal functions conducted during treatment and up to 4 to 8 weeks after discontinuation of LUPRON DEPOT therapy may be misleading.

Carcinogenesis, Mutagenesis, Impairment of Fertility: A two-year carcinogenicity study was conducted in rats and mice. In rats, a dose-related increase of benign pituitary hyperplasia and benign pituitary adenomas was noted at 24 months when the drug was administered subcutaneously at high daily doses (0.6 to 4 mg/kg). There was a significant but not dose-related increase of pancreatic islet-cell adenomas in females and of testes interstitial cell adenomas in males (highest incidence in the low dose group). In mice, no leuprolide acetate-induced tumors or pituitary abnormalities were observed at a dose as high as 60 mg/kg for two years. Patients have been treated with leuprolide acetate for up to three years with doses as high as 10 mg/day and for two years with doses as high as 20 mg/day without demonstrable pituitary abnormalities.

Mutagenicity studies have been performed with leuprolide acetate using bacterial and mammalian systems. These studies provided no evidence of a mutagenic potential.

Clinical and pharmacologic studies in adults with leuprolide acetate and similar analogs have shown full reversibility of fertility suppression when the drug is discontinued after continuous administration for periods of up to 24 weeks. No clinical studies have been completed with leuprolide acetate in children to assess the reversibility of fertility suppression.

Pregnancy, Teratogenic Effects: Pregnancy Category X. See "Contraindications" section. When administered on day 6 of pregnancy at test dosages of 0.00024, 0.0024, and 0.024 mg/kg (¹/₃₀₀ to ¹/₃ the human dose) to rabbits, LUPRON DEPOT produced a dose-related increase in major fetal abnormalities. Similar studies in rats failed to demonstrate an increase in fetal malformations. There was increased fetal mortality and decreased fetal weights with the two higher doses of LUPRON DEPOT in rabbits and with the highest dose (0.024 mg/kg) in rats.

Nursing Mothers: It is not known whether LUPRON DEPOT (leuprolide acetate for depot suspension) is excreted in human milk. Because many drugs are excreted in human milk, and because the effects of LUPRON DEPOT on lactation and/or the breastfed child have not been determined, LUPRON DEPOT should not be used by nursing mothers.

Pediatric Use: Safety and effectiveness in children have not been established.

ADVERSE REACTIONS

Estradiol levels may increase during the first weeks following the initial injection, but then decline to postmenopausal levels. This transient increase in estradiol can be associated with a temporary worsening of signs and symptoms (See "Warnings" Section).

As would be expected with a drug that lowers serum estradiol levels, the most frequently reported adverse reactions were those related to hypoestrogenism.

In controlled studies comparing LUPRON DEPOT, 3.75 mg monthly and danazol (800 mg/day), or placebo, adverse reactions most frequently reported and thought to be possibly or probably drug-related are shown in Figure 2.

Cardiovascular System —Palpitations, Syncope, Tachycardia; *Gastrointestinal System* —Dry mouth, Thirst, Appetite changes; *Central/Peripheral Nervous System* —Anxiety,* Personality disorder, Memory disorder, Delusions; *Integumentary System* —Ecchymosis, Alopecia, Hair disorder; *Uro-*

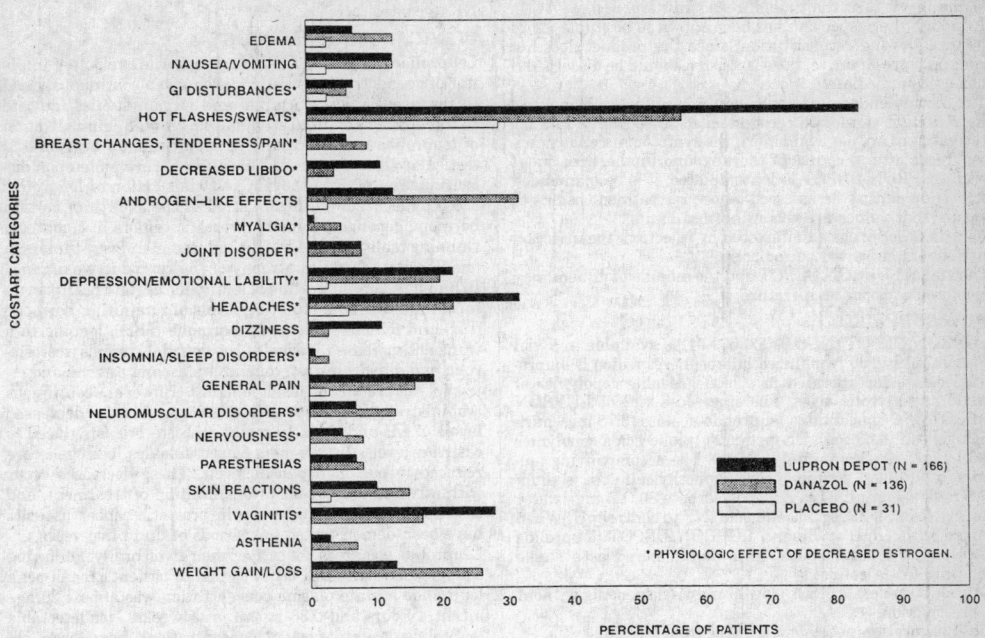

FIGURE 2
ADVERSE EVENTS REPORTED DURING 6 MONTHS OF TREATMENT
WITH LUPRON DEPOT 3.75 MG

genital System —Dysuria,* Lactation; *Miscellaneous* —Ophthalmologic disorders,* Lymphadenopathy.

In other clinical trials involving patients with prostate cancer and during postmarketing surveillance, the following adverse reactions were reported to have a possible, probable, or unknown relationship to LUPRON as ascribed by the treating physician. Often, it is difficult to assess causality in patients with prostate cancer. Reactions considered not drug related have been excluded.

Cardiovascular System —Congestive heart failure, ECG changes/ischemia, High blood pressure, Murmur, Phlebitis/thrombosis, Angina, Cardiac arrhythmias, Myocardial infarction, Pulmonary emboli, Hypotension, Transient ischemic attack/stroke; *Gastrointestinal System* —Dysphagia, Gastrointestinal bleeding, Peptic ulcer, Rectal polyps, Hepatic dysfunction; *Endocrine System* —Decreased testicular size, Gynecomastia, Impotence, Libido increase, *Hemic and Lymphatic System* —Anemia, Decreased WBC, Hemoptysis; *Musculoskeletal System* —Bone pain; *Central/Peripheral Nervous System* —Peripheral neuropathy, Syncope/blackouts, Hearing disorder, Spinal fracture/paralysis; *Respiratory System* —Dyspnea, Sinus congestion, Cough, Pleural rub, Pneumonia, Pulmonary fibrosis, Respiratory disorders; *Urogenital System* —Frequency/urgency, Hematuria, Urinary tract infection, Bladder spasms, Incontinence, Testicular pain, Urinary obstruction, Penile swelling, Prostate Pain; *Miscellaneous* —Diabetes, Fever, Hypoglycemia, Increased BUN, Increased calcium, Increased creatinine, Inflammation.

Changes in Bone Density:
After six months of LUPRON DEPOT (leuprolide acetate for depot suspension) treatment, vertebral trabecular bone density measured by quantitative computed tomography (QCT) decreased by an average of 13.5% compared to pretreatment levels. A small number of original patients were retested at 6 and 12 months after completion of treatment. At 6 months, 9 patients had an average bone density change from baseline by QCT of −3.2%. At 12 months after completion of treatment, 6 patients had an average bone density change from baseline of −2.4%. These results show that there was partial to complete recovery of bone density in the post-treatment period in a small number of original patients who were retested. Use of LUPRON DEPOT for longer than the recommended six months or in the presence of other known risk factors for decreased bone mineral content may cause additional bone loss.

Changes in Laboratory Values During Treatment:
Plasma enzymes: During clinical trials with LUPRON DEPOT, regular laboratory monitoring revealed that SGOT levels were more than twice the upper limit of normal in only one patient. There was no other clinical or laboratory evidence of abnormal liver function.

Lipids: At enrollment, 4% of the LUPRON DEPOT patients and 1% of the danazol patients had total cholesterol values above the normal range. These patients also had cholesterol values above the normal range at the end of treatment.

Of those patients whose pretreatment cholesterol values were in the normal range, 7% of the LUPRON DEPOT patients and 9% of the danazol patients had post-treatment values above the normal range.

The mean (±SEM) pretreatment values for total cholesterol from all patients were 178.8 (2.9) mg/dL in the LUPRON DEPOT group and 175.3 (3.0) mg/dL in the danazol group. At the end of treatment, the mean values for total cholesterol from all patients were 193.3 mg/dL in the LUPRON DEPOT group and 194.4 mg/dL in the danazol group. These increases from the pretreatment values were statistically significant (p < 0.03) in both groups.

Triglycerides were increased above the upper limit of normal in 12% of the patients who received LUPRON DEPOT and in 6% of the patients who received danazol.

At the end of treatment, HDL cholesterol fractions decreased below the lower limit of the normal range in 2% of the LUPRON DEPOT patients compared with 54% of those receiving danazol. LDL cholesterol fractions increased above the upper limit of the normal range in 6% of the patients receiving LUPRON DEPOT compared with 23% of those receiving danazol. There was no increase in the LDL/HDL ratio in patients receiving LUPRON DEPOT, but there was approximately a two-fold increase in the LDL/HDL ratio in patients receiving danazol.

Other changes: In comparative studies, the following changes were seen in approximately 5% to 8% of patients. LUPRON DEPOT was associated with elevations of LDH and phosphorus, and decreases in WBC counts. Danazol therapy was associated with increases in hematocrit, platelet count, and LDH.

OVERDOSAGE

In rats subcutaneous administration of 250 to 500 times the recommended human dose, expressed on a per body weight basis, resulted in dyspnea, decreased activity, and local irritation at the injection site. There is no evidence at present that there is a clinical counterpart of this phenomenon. In early clinical trials using daily subcutaneous leuprolide acetate in patients with prostate cancer, doses as high as 20 mg/day for up to two years caused no adverse effects differing from those observed with the 1 mg/day dose.

DOSAGE AND ADMINISTRATION

LUPRON DEPOT Must Be Administered Under The Supervision Of A Physician.

The recommended dose of LUPRON DEPOT (leuprolide acetate for depot suspension) is 3.75 mg, incorporated in a depot formulation. The lyophilized microspheres are to be reconstituted and administered monthly as a single intramuscular injection, in accord with the following directions:

1. Using a syringe with a 22 gauge needle, withdraw 1 mL of diluent from the ampule, and inject it into the vial. (Extra diluent is provided; any remaining should be discarded.)
2. Shake well to thoroughly disperse particles to obtain a uniform suspension. The suspension will appear milky.

Continued on next page

TAP—Cont.

3. Withdraw the entire contents of the vial into the syringe and inject it at the time of reconstitution.

Although the suspension has been shown to be stable for 24 hours following reconstitution, since the product does not contain a preservative, the suspension should be discarded if not used immediately.

The recommended duration of administration is six months. Retreatment cannot be recommended since safety data for retreatment are not available. If the symptoms of endometriosis recur after a course of therapy, and further treatment with LUPRON DEPOT is contemplated, it is recommended that bone density be assessed before retreatment begins to ensure that values are within normal limits.

As with other drugs administered by injection, the injection site should be varied periodically.

The vial of LUPRON DEPOT and the ampule of diluent may be stored at room temperature.

HOW SUPPLIED

LUPRON DEPOT (NDC 0300-3639-01) is available in a vial containing sterile lyophilized microspheres which is leuprolide acetate incorporated in a biodegradable copolymer of lactic and glycolic acids. The singe-dose vial of LUPRON DEPOT 3.75 mg contains leuprolide acetate (3.75 mg), purified gelatin (0.65 mg), DL-lactic & glycolic acids copolymer (33.1 mg), and D-mannitol (6.6 mg). The accompanying ampule of diluent contains carboxymethylcellulose sodium (7.5 mg), D-mannitol (75 mg), polysorbate 80 (1.5 mg), water for injection, USP, and acetic acid, NF to control pH. When mixed with 1 mL of diluent, LUPRON DEPOT (leuprolide acetate for depot suspension) is administered as a single monthly IM injection.

Caution: Federal (U.S.A.) law prohibits dispensing without a prescription.

No refrigeration necessary. Protect from freezing.

Revised: October 1990

REFERENCE

1. MacLeod TL, et al. Anaphylactic reaction to synthetic luteinizing hormone-releasing hormone. *Fertil Steril* 1987 Sept;48(3):500–502.

U.S. Patent Nos. 4,005,063; 4,005,194; 4,652,441; 4,677,191; 4,728,721 and 4,849,228.

TAP Pharmaceuticals Inc.
Deerfield, Illinois 60015-1595, U.S.A.
LUPRON DEPOT manufactured by Takeda Chemical Industries, Ltd. Osaka, JAPAN 541
®—Registered Trademark
Shown in Product Identification Section, page 433

LUPRON DEPOT® 7.5 mg
[lu ′pron dē ′pō]
(leuprolide acetate for depot suspension)

DESCRIPTION

Leuprolide acetate is a synthetic nonapeptide analog of naturally occurring gonadotropin releasing hormone (GnRH or LH-RH). The analog possesses greater potency than the natural hormone. The chemical name is 5-Oxo-L-prolyl-L-histidyl-L-tryptophyl-L-seryl-L-tyrosyl-D-leucyl-L-leucyl-L-arginyl-N-ethyl-L-prolinamide acetate (salt) with the following structural formula:
[See below.]

LUPRON DEPOT is available in a vial containing sterile lyophilized microspheres, which when mixed with diluent, become a suspension, which is intended as a monthly intramuscular injection.

The single-dose vial of LUPRON DEPOT contains leuprolide acetate (7.5 mg), purified gelatin (1.3 mg), DL-lactic and gly-

colic acids copolymer (66.2 mg), and D-mannitol (13.2 mg). The accompanying ampule of diluent contains carboxymethylcellulose sodium (7.5 mg), D-mannitol (75 mg), polysorbate 80 (1.5 mg), water for injection, USP and acetic acid, NF to control pH.

CLINICAL PHARMACOLOGY

Leuprolide acetate, an LH-RH agonist, acts as a potent inhibitor of gonadotropin secretion when given continuously and in therapeutic doses. Animal and human studies indicate that following an initial stimulation, chronic administration of leuprolide acetate results in suppression of ovarian and testicular steroidogenesis. This effect is reversible upon discontinuation of drug therapy. Administration of leuprolide acetate has resulted in inhibition of the growth of certain hormone dependent tumors (prostatic tumors in Noble and Dunning male rats and DMBA-induced mammary tumors in female rats) as well as atrophy of the reproductive organs. In humans, administration of leuprolide acetate results in an initial increase in circulating levels of luteinizing hormone (LH) and follicle stimulating hormone (FSH), leading to a transient increase in levels of the gonadal steroids (testosterone and dihydrotestosterone in males, and estrone and estradiol in pre-menopausal females). However, continuous administration of leuprolide acetate results in decreased levels of LH and FSH. In males, testosterone is reduced to castrate levels. In pre-menopausal females, estrogens are reduced to post-menopausal levels. These decreases occur within two to four weeks after initiation of treatment, and castrate levels of testosterone in prostatic cancer patients have been demonstrated for periods of up to five years.

Leuprolide acetate is not active when given orally. Following a single LUPRON DEPOT injection to patients, mean peak leuprolide acetate plasma concentration was almost 20 ng/mL at 4 hours and 0.36 ng/mL at 4 weeks. Nondetectable leuprolide acetate plasma concentrations have been observed during chronic LUPRON DEPOT administration, but testosterone levels appear to be maintained at castrate levels. The metabolism, distribution, and excretion of leuprolide acetate in humans have not been determined.

INDICATIONS AND USAGE

LUPRON DEPOT is indicated in the palliative treatment of advanced prostatic cancer. It offers an alternative treatment of prostatic cancer when orchiectomy or estrogen administration are either not indicated or unacceptable to the patient. In clinical trials, the safety and efficacy of LUPRON DEPOT does not differ from that of the original daily subcutaneous injection.

CONTRAINDICATIONS

A report of an anaphylactic reaction to synthetic GnRH (Factrel) has been reported in the medical literature.[1]

LUPRON DEPOT is contraindicated in women who are or may become pregnant while receiving the drug. When administered on day 6 of pregnancy at test dosages of 0.00024, 0.0024, and 0.024 mg/kg ($\frac{1}{600}$ to $\frac{1}{6}$ the human dose) to rabbits, LUPRON DEPOT produced a dose related increase in major fetal abnormalities. Similar studies in rats failed to demonstrate an increase in fetal malformations. There was increased fetal mortality and decreased fetal weights with the two higher doses of LUPRON DEPOT (leuprolide acetate for depot suspension) in rabbits and with the highest dose in rats. The effects on fetal mortality are logical consequences of the alterations in hormonal levels brought about by this drug. Therefore, the possibility exists that spontaneous abortion may occur if the drug is administered during pregnancy.

WARNINGS

Isolated cases of worsening of signs and symptoms during the first weeks of treatment have been reported with LH-RH analogs. Worsening of symptoms may contribute to paralysis with or without fatal complications. For patients at risk, the physician may consider initiating therapy with daily

LUPRON® (leuprolide acetate) Injection for the first two weeks to facilitate withdrawal of treatment if that is considered necessary.

PRECAUTIONS

Patients with metastatic vertebral lesions and/or with urinary tract obstruction should be closely observed during the first few weeks of therapy (see "WARNINGS" section).

Laboratory Tests: Response to leuprolide acetate should be monitored by measuring serum levels of testosterone and acid phosphatase. In the majority of patients, testosterone levels increased above baseline during the first week, declining thereafter to baseline levels or below by the end of the second week. Castrate levels were reached within two to four weeks and once achieved were maintained for as long as the patients received their monthly injection on time. Transient increases in acid phosphatase levels may occur sometime early in treatment. However, by the fourth week, the elevated levels can be expected to decrease to values at or near baseline.

Drug Interactions: None have been reported.

Carcinogenesis, Mutagenesis, Impairment of Fertility: Two-year carcinogenicity studies were conducted in rats and mice. In rats, a dose-related increase of benign pituitary hyperplasia and benign pituitary adenomas was noted at 24 months when the drug was administered subcutaneously at high daily doses (0.6 to 4 mg/kg). In mice no pituitary abnormalities were observed at a dose as high as 60 mg/kg for two years. Patients have been treated with leuprolide acetate for up to three years with doses as high as 10 mg/day and for two years with doses as high as 20 mg/day without demonstrable pituitary abnormalities.

Mutagenicity studies have been performed with leuprolide acetate using bacterial and mammalian systems. These studies provided no evidence of a mutagenic potential.

Clinical and pharmacologic studies with leuprolide acetate and similar analogs have shown reversibility of fertility suppression when the drug is discontinued after continuous administration for periods of up to 24 weeks.

Pregnancy Category X. See "CONTRAINDICATIONS" section.

ADVERSE REACTIONS

In the majority of patients testosterone levels increased above baseline during the first week, declining thereafter to baseline levels or below by the end of the second week of treatment.

Potential exacerbations of signs and symptoms during the first few weeks of treatment is a concern in patients with vertebral metastases and/or urinary obstruction or hematuria which, if aggravated, may lead to neurological problems such as temporary weakness and/or paresthesia of the lower limbs or worsening of urinary symptoms (see "WARNINGS" section).

In a clinical trial of LUPRON DEPOT, the following adverse reactions were reported to have a possible or probable relationship to drug as ascribed by the treating physician in 5% or more of the patients receiving the drug. Often, causality is difficult to assess in patients with metastatic prostate cancer. Reactions considered not drug related are excluded.

	LUPRON DEPOT N = 56	(Percent)
Cardiovascular System		
Edema	7	(12.5%)
Gastrointestinal System		
Nausea/vomiting	3	(5.4%)
Endocrine System		
*Decreased testicular size	3	(5.4%)
*Hot flashes/sweats	33	(58.9%)
*Impotence	3	(5.4%)
Central/Peripheral Nervous System		
General pain	4	(7.1%)
Respiratory System		
Dyspnea	3	(5.4%)
Miscellaneous		
Asthenia	3	(5.4%)

*Physiologic effect of decreased testosterone.

Laboratory: Elevations of certain parameters were observed, but it is difficult to assess these abnormalities in this population.

SGOT (>2N)	4	(5.4%)
LDH (>2N)	11	(19.6%)
Alkaline phos (>1.5N)	4	(5.4%)

In this same study, the following adverse reactions were reported in less than 5% of the patients on LUPRON DEPOT.

Cardiovascular System —Angina, Cardiac arrhythmia; *Gastrointestinal System* —Anorexia, Diarrhea; *Endocrine System* —Gynecomastia, Libido decrease; *Musculoskeletal System* —Bone pain, Myalgia; *Central/Peripheral Nervous System* —Paresthesia, Insomnia; *Respiratory System* —Hemoptysis; *Integumentary System* —Dermatitis, Local skin reactions, hair growth; *Urogenital System* —Dysuria, Fre-

quency/urgency, Hematuria, Testicular pain; *Miscellaneous* —Diabetes, Fever/chills, hard nodule in throat, Increased calcium, Weight gain, Increased uric acid.
The following additional adverse reactions have been reported with LUPRON (leuprolide acetate) Injection. Reactions considered by the treating physician as nondrug related are not included.
Cardiovascular System —Congestive heart failure, ECG changes/ischemia, High blood pressure, Hypotension, Myocardial infarction, Murmur, Phlebitis/thrombosis, Pulmonary emboli, Transient ischemic attack/stroke; *Gastrointestinal System* —Constipation, Dysphagia, Gastrointestinal bleeding, Gastrointestinal disturbance, Hepatic dysfunction, Peptic ulcer, Rectal polyps; *Endocrine System* —Breast tenderness or pain, Libido increase, Thyroid enlargement; *Hemic and Lymphatic System* —Anemia, Decreased WBC; *Musculoskeletal System* —Ankylosing spondylosis, Joint pain, Pelvic fibrosis; *Central/Peripheral Nervous System* —Anxiety, Blurred vision, Dizziness/lightheadedness, Headache, Hearing disorder, Sleep disorders, Lethargy, Memory disorder, Mood swings, Nervousness, Numbness, Peripheral neuropathy, Spinal fracture/paralysis, Syncope/blackouts, Taste disorders; *Respiratory System* —Cough, Pleural rub, Pneumonia, Pulmonary fibrosis, Pulmonary infiltrate, Respiratory disorders, Sinus congestion; *Integumentary System* —Carcinoma of skin/ear, Dry skin, Ecchymosis, Hair loss, Itching, Pigmentation, Skin lesions; *Urogenital System* —Bladder spasms, Incontinence, Penile swelling, Prostate pain, Urinary obstruction, Urinary tract infection; *Miscellaneous* —Depression, Hypoglycemia, Hypoproteinemia, Increased BUN, Increased creatinine, Infection/inflammation, Ophthalmologic disorders, Swelling (temporal bone).

OVERDOSAGE

In rats, subcutaneous administration of 250 to 500 times the recommended human dose, expressed on a per body weight basis, resulted in dyspnea, decreased activity, and local irritation at the injection site. There is no evidence at present that there is a clinical counterpart of this phenomenon. In early clinical trials with daily subcutaneous leuprolide acetate, doses as high as 20 mg/day for up to two years caused no adverse effects differing from those observed with the 1 mg/day dose.

DOSAGE AND ADMINISTRATION

LUPRON DEPOT Must Be Administered Under The Supervision Of A Physician.
The recommended dose of LUPRON DEPOT is 7.5 mg, incorporated in a depot formulation. The lyophilized microspheres are to be reconstituted and administered monthly as a single intramuscular injection, in accord with the following directions:
1. Using a syringe with a 22 gauge needle, withdraw 1 mL of diluent from the ampule, and inject it into the vial. (Extra diluent is provided; any remaining should be discarded.)
2. Shake well to thoroughly disperse particles to obtain a uniform suspension. The suspension will appear milky.
3. Withdraw the entire contents of the vial into the syringe and inject it at the time of reconstitution.
Although the solution has been shown to be stable for 24 hours following reconstitution, since the product does not contain a preservative, the suspension should be discarded if not used immediately.
As with other drugs administered by injection, the injection site should be varied periodically.
The vial of LUPRON DEPOT and the ampule of diluent may be stored at room temperature.

HOW SUPPLIED

LUPRON DEPOT (NDC 0300-3629-01) is available in a vial containing sterile lyophilized microspheres which is leuprolide acetate incorporated in a biodegradable copolymer of lactic and glycolic acids. The single-dose vial of LUPRON DEPOT contains leuprolide acetate (7.5 mg), purified gelatin (1.3 mg), DL-lactic & glycolic acids copolymer (66.2 mg), and D-mannitol (13.2 mg). The accompanying ampule of diluent contains carboxymethylcellulose sodium (7.5 mg), D-mannitol (75 mg), polysorbate 80 (1.5 mg), water for injection, USP and acetic acid, NF to control pH. When mixed with 1 mL of diluent, LUPRON DEPOT is administered as a single monthly IM injection.
No refrigeration necessary. Protect from freezing.
Caution: Federal (U.S.A.) law prohibits dispensing without a prescription.
U.S. Patent Nos. 4,005,063; 4,005,194; 4,728,721; and 4,849,228.
Reference:
1. MacLeod TL, Eisen A, Sussman GL, et al: Anaphylactic reaction to synthetic luteinizing hormone-releasing hormone. *Fertil Steril* 1987 Sept;48(3):500-502.

TAP Pharmaceuticals Inc.
Deerfield, IL 60015 U.S.A.
LUPRON DEPOT manufactured by
Takeda Chemical Industries Ltd.
Osaka, Japan
(New)—Rev. January 1990
Shown in Product Identification Section, page 433

EDUCATIONAL MATERIAL

All Free to the medical profession
Lupron® Injection
"Introduction to Lupron® (leuprolide acetate) Injection"—product monograph.
"Information for Patient Instruction"—a brochure to help professionals answer patients' questions about Lupron and to aid in subcutaneous self-injection.
Lupron Depot® 3.75 mg
"Lupron Depot 3.75 mg: the First Once-A-Month GnRH Agonist for the Treatment of Endometriosis –product monograph.
"Lupron Depot 3.75 mg: Patient Information on the Treatment of Endometriosis –a patient brochure that discusses the use of Lupron Depot 3.75 mg in the management of endometriosis.
"Endometriosis: The Disease and Its Treatment"—a brochure for the patient that discusses the etiology of the disease, its symptoms and diagnosis, and treatment options.
Lupron Depot® 7.5 mg
"An Introduction: Lupron Depot the Next Generation of GnRH Agonist Analogs"—product monograph.
"Questions and Answers on Lupron Depot the First Once-a-Month GnRH Agonist"—a brochure that answers many common questions posed by the health professional.
"Your Choice for Treating Prostate Cancer"—a brochure for the patient that briefly describes prostate cancer and how Lupron Depot is used to treat it.
"Prostate Cancer: What Everyone Should Know"—a patient brochure that discusses the symptoms, detection, and treatment of prostate cancer.

Taro Pharmaceuticals U.S.A., Inc.
SIX SKYLINE DRIVE
HAWTHORNE, NY 10532

[See table below.]

Rx Product/Brand Name	Sizes	NDC #
Betamethasone Valerate Cream, USP 0.1%	15 gram tube	51672-1269-01
	45 gram tube	51672-1269-06
Betamethasone Dipropionate Cream, USP 0.05%	15 gram tube	51672-1274-01
	45 gram tube	51672-1274-06
Carbamazepine Tablets, USP 200 mg.	100's	51672-1268-01
Desonide Cream, 0.05%	15 gram tube	51672-1280-01
	60 gram tube	51672-1280-03
Desoximetasone Cream, USP 0.25%	15 gram tube	51672-1270-01
	60 gram tube	51672-1270-03
Desoximetasone Cream, USP 0.05%	15 gram tube	51672-1271-01
	60 gram tube	51672-1271-03
Fluocinonide Cream, USP 0.05%	15 gram tube	51672-1254-01
	30 gram tube	51672-1254-02
	60 gram tube	51672-1254-03
	15 gram tube	51672-1253-01
	30 gram tube	51672-1253-02
	60 gram tube	51672-1253-03
	120 gram tube	51672-1253-04
Nystatin & Triamcinolone Acetonide Cream	15 gram tube	51672-1263-01
	30 gram tube	51672-1263-02
	60 gram tube	51672-1263-03
Triamcinolone Acetonide Dental Paste, 0.1%	5 gram tube	51672-1267-05
Hydrocortisone ½% cream	½ oz. tube	51672-20101
	1 oz. tube	51672-20102
Hydrocortisone ½% ointment	½ oz. tube	51672-20151
	1 oz. tube	51672-20152
Hydrocortisone 1% cream	½ oz. tube	51672-20131
	1 oz. tube	51672-20132
Hydrocortisone 1% ointment	½ oz. tube	51672-20181
	1 oz. tube	51672-20182
Taro lubricating jelly	4¼ oz. tube	63691-11751
Miconazole Nitrate 2% cream	½ oz. tube	51672-20011
	1 oz. tube	51672-20012
Tolnaftate 1% cream	½ oz. tube	51672-20201

Tsumura Medical
Division of Tsumura International Inc.
1000 VALLEY PARK DR
SHAKOPEE, MN 55379

GLANDOSANE®   OTC
Synthetic Saliva

DESCRIPTION
Glandosane® spray is an aqueous solution. Each 50 mL contains:

Sodium Carboxymethylcellulose	0.500 g
Sorbitol	1.500 g
Sodium chloride	0.042 g
Potassium chloride	0.060 g
Calcium chloride, dihydrate	0.007 g
Magnesium chloride	0.003 g
Dipotassium hydrogen phosphate	0.017 g

Propellant: Carbon dioxide (CO_2)

ACTIONS
Glandosane spray moistens the mucosa of the mouth, tongue and throat and maintains moistness up to 2 hours after each application. It relieves diffuse dryness and fissuring of the oral mucosa, as well as painful tongue conditions due to hyposalivation.
As a replacement saliva, Glandosane spray facilitates chewing and speaking; loosens tough mucus immediately; prevents mucus membranes from sticking together; improves adherence of dentures in patients suffering from dryness of the mouth and also relieves bad taste.

INDICATIONS
Glandosane spray is indicated for dryness of the mouth or throat (hyposalivation, xerostomia), regardless of the cause and regardless of whether the condition is temporary or permanent.
Glandosane spray is indicated for relief of dryness when hyposalivation results from surgery or radiotherapy near the salivary glands; infection or dysfunction of the salivary glands as a side effect of drug therapy*; inflammation of the mouth or throat; fever; emotional factors such as fear or anxiety; and obstruction of the salivary ducts. It is useful in Sjögren's syndrome and Bell's Palsy when these conditions cause xerostomia.
Glandosane spray may prove especially useful when dryness of the oral mucosa is due to drugs such as antihistamines, atropine or other anticholinergic agents that suppress salivary secretion.

PRECAUTIONS
Avoid spraying near the eyes. Keep out of the reach of children.

*Pharmacy chart listing common drugs which can cause dry mouth/throat is available.

Continued on next page

Tsumura Medical—Cont.

CAUTION: Contents under pressure. Do not puncture or incinerate. Protect from direct sunlight. Protect from heat. Do not store above 120°F (50°C).
Do not spray into flames or upon hot objects.

DOSAGE AND ADMINISTRATION
Glandosane spray should be held approximately one inch or less from the mouth and directed carefully into the mouth or throat. Spray for 1 to 2 seconds, using it as often as needed to maintain moistness, or as instructed by physician.
The Glandosane spray can should always be held upright, with nozzle pointed into the mouth (or nostril, if instructed by the physician). The nozzle should be pushed down for 1 to 2 seconds. The valve opening should be cleaned if it clogs.

WARNING
Glandosane spray contains sodium. If restricted to a low sodium diet, consult a physician before use.

HOW SUPPLIED
Glandosane spray is available as the following:
Natural flavor 50 mL   (HRIC #8192-1660-05)
Lemon flavor 50 mL   (HRIC #8192-1661-05)
Peppermint flavor 50 mL   (HRIC #8192-1662-05)
Natural flavor 100 mL   (HRIC #8192-1660-10)
Distributed by:
TSUMURA MEDICAL
Quality Dermatology Products for the Health Care Industry
1000 Valley Park Drive
Shakopee, MN 55379
(612) 496-4700
(800) 345-8084

TRANS–VER–SAL®   OTC
Salicylic Acid USP, 15%
WART REMOVER
DERMAL PATCH DELIVERY SYSTEM
TRANS–PLANTAR®   OTC
Salicylic Acid USP, 21%
PLANTAR WART REMOVER
DERMAL PATCH DELIVERY SYSTEM

DESCRIPTION
The TRANS-VER-SAL® Dermal Patch Delivery System contains Salicylic Acid USP, 15%. TRANS-PLANTAR® Dermal Patch Delivery System contains Salicylic Acid USP, 21%. Both products' active ingredient is evenly dispersed in an adhesive patch composed of natural, non-sensitizing Karaya, Polyethylene Glycol-300 USP, Propylene Glycol USP and Quaternium-15. The system is designed to be applied topically to wart tissue and provide sustained release of the active drug over an eight-hour treatment period. Each patch is covered with a polyethylene moisture barrier which creates a beneficial occlusive effect.
TRANS-VER-SAL® and TRANS-PLANTAR® patches are sealed in moisture resistant, polyester-foil-polyethylene laminate. Upon application, the patches are held in place with skin-compatible adhesive tapes provided in the kit. A cleaning file is also supplied to aid in the removal of the wart tissue.

CLINICAL PHARMACOLOGY
The pharmacologic activity of the TRANS-VER-SAL® and TRANS-PLANTAR® delivery systems is attributed to Salicylic Acid USP. The structural formula of Salicylic Acid is:

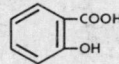

While the exact mode of action of Salicylic Acid in wart treatment is unknown, its activity appears to be due to a keratolytic action which results in mechanical removal of stratum corneum cells infected with the papilloma virus. The application of Salicylic Acid by a dermal patch delivery system provides for a more steady release of the drug into the stratum corneum than traditional collodion formulas which tend to unload their concentration of Salicylic Acid after the solvents evaporate.
A moisture barrier which covers each patch maintains an occluded, hydrated environment to allow for better penetration of the active drug and increased sloughing of keratolized wart tissue.

INDICATIONS AND USAGE
The TRANS-VER-SAL® delivery system is clinically proven effective for the treatment of common warts. The TRANS-PLANTAR® delivery system is clinically proven effective for the removal of plantar warts. See DOSAGE AND ADMINISTRATION for information on frequency and duration of use.

WARNINGS
For external use only. Do not use these products on irritated skin, or any area that is infected or reddened, if you are a diabetic or if your have poor blood circulation. If discomfort persists, see your doctor. Do not use on moles, birthmarks, warts with hair growing from them, genital warts or warts on the face or mucous membranes.
Patient Instructions: *These are provided on the back panel of dispensing package.*

ADVERSE REACTIONS
Localized irritation will occur if TRANS-VER-SAL® or TRANS-PLANTAR® patches are applied in contact with normal skin surrounding wart tissue. In the event of such a reaction, the irritation should be allowed to subside by temporarily discontinuing treatment. Upon resuming treatment, TRANS-VER-SAL® and TRANS-PLANTAR® patches should be carefully trimmed so as to contact only wart tissue.

DOSAGE AND ADMINISTRATION
TRANS-VER-SAL® and TRANS-PLANTAR® patches are applied once each day before retiring. The wart tissue should first be cleaned of debris with the emery file provided and then moistened with warm water using a cotton tipped applicator. The patch is then removed from the clear strip, trimmed to size (if necessary), and applied to the wart with the occlusive top film facing up. The patch is then secured with the adhesive tape provided.
The TRANS-VER-SAL® or TRANS-PLANTAR® patch should be left in place overnight and discarded in the morning. This procedure is to be repeated each day until wart resolution is complete, for up to 12 weeks. Generally, visible clinical improvement will occur during the first several days of treatment. Complete resolution may be expected after six to twelve weeks of therapy.
TRANS-VER-SAL®:   Store below 100°F (37.8°C).
TRANS-PLANTAR®:   Store between 40–100°F (4–37.8°C), DO NOT FREEZE.
KEEP THIS AND ALL DRUGS OUT OF THE REACH OF CHILDREN.
IN CASE OF ACCIDENTAL INGESTION, SEEK PROFESSIONAL ASSISTANCE OR CONTACT A POISON CONTROL CENTER IMMEDIATELY.
For a more detailed user instruction sheet, call 1-800-345-8084.

HOW SUPPLIED
TRANS-VER-SAL® 6mm: 6mm patches, 40 ea., complete with 42 tapes and one file NDC #53309-202-04
TRANS-VER-SAL® 12mm: 12mm patches, 40 ea., complete with 42 tapes and one file NDC #55309-202-06
TRANS-PLANTAR®:   20mm patches, 25 ea; complete with 25 tapes, one file NDC #53309-203-04
Patches may be trimmed to accommodate various sizes of warts.
For further information, please contact:
TSUMURA MEDICAL
Division of Tsumura International Inc
1000 Valley Park Drive, Shakopee, MN 55379
(612) 496-4700 ● (800) 345-8084
*U.S. Patent 4,778,786 Tsumura International Inc. Licensed Under U.S. Patent 4,675,009 ● LecTec Corporation
Rev 3/91

Shown in Product Identification Section, page 433

Products are cross-indexed
by product classifications
in the
BLUE SECTION.

Tyson & Associates, Inc.
12832 CHADRON AVENUE
HAWTHORNE, CA 90250

AMINOMINE™	OTC
(Excitatory neurotransmitters)	700mg/cap
AMINOLETE™	OTC
(Athletic Endurance/P.E.R.)	700mg/cap
AMINOPLEX®	OTC
(Anti-stress/Nitrogen balance)	740mg/cap
AMINOSTASIS®	OTC
(Branched Chain formula)	700mg/cap
AMINOTATE®	OTC
(Glycogenic formula)	700mg/cap
AMINOVIROX™	OTC
(Arginine-free formula)	700mg/cap
AMINOXIN®	OTC
(Enteric Pyridoxal-5'-Phosphate)	20mg/tab
ATP	OTC
(Enteric Adenosine Triphosphate)	20mg/tab
L–CARNITINE	OTC
(Fatty Acid Combustion)	250mg/cap
ENDORPHENYL®	OTC
(Enkephalinase inhibitor D-Phenylalanine)	500mg/cap
RIBO-2™	OTC
(Enteric Riboflavin 5'Phosphate)	5mg/tab
RXOSINE	OTC
(L-tyrosine depression, narcolepsy)	800mg/cap
THIAMILATE®	OTC
(Enteric Thiamine Pyrophosphate)	20mg/tab

AMINOPLEX®   OTC

DESCRIPTION
U.S.P. crystalline amino acid formulation. Formula contains 740 mg Anhydrous of 18 crystalline L-amino acids including neurotransmitter precursors and sulfur amino acids, and supplies 130 mg Nitrogen per capsule. Balanced formulation replacement based on quantitative Amino Acid Fractionation.

COMPOSITION
L-Lysine, L-Arginine, L-Isoleucine, L-Leucine, L-Alamine, L-Threonine, L-Histidine, L-Cystine, L-Methionine, L-Glutamine, L-Tyrosine, L-Aspartic Acid, L-Valine, L-Glutamic Acid, L-Phenylalamine, Glycine, L-Serine, L-Cysteine HCl.

DOSAGE AND ADMINISTRATION
1–3 capsules half an hour before meals.

HOW SUPPLIED
Bottles of 100 capsules—NDC 53335-701-14

CATEMINE®   OTC
(Catecholamine Precursor)

DESCRIPTION
Enterically coated preparation of 800 mg L-Tyrosine and 10 mg pyridoxal-5'-phosphate.

ACTIONS AND USES
Biochemical precursor of dopamine and norepinephrine.

DOSAGE AND ADMINISTRATION
2 tablets b.i.d. in between meals.

HOW SUPPLIED
Bottles of 60—NDC 53335-056-12
Samples upon request.

THREOSTAT™   OTC
(L-Threonine USP)

DESCRIPTION
Encapsulated U.S.P. Crystalline powder of 500 mg L-Threonine.

ACTIONS AND USES
May be helpful in reducing some symptoms of ALS.

DOSAGE AND ADMINISTRATION
4 to 8 capsules per day divided t.i.d. taken 60 minutes before meals or as directed.

UAD Laboratories
8339 HIGHWAY 18
JACKSON, MS 39209

AEROBID®   ℞
[air'ōbid]
(flunisolide)

DESCRIPTION
Each canister contains one hundred metered inhalations of Flunisolide.
NDC #0456-0672-99
See Product Information Under Forest Pharmaceuticals, Inc.

AEROCHAMBER®
Aerosol holding chamber for use with metered-dose inhalers.

See Product Information Under Forest Pharmaceuticals, Inc.

AEROCHAMBER® W/Mask
Aerosol holding chamber for use with metered-dose inhalers

See Product Information Under Forest Pharmaceuticals, Inc.

DALALONE D.P.® INJECTION   ℞
[dal 'ä-lone]

DESCRIPTION
Dexamethasone Acetate Suspension
Equivalent to Dexamethasone 16 mg/mL
NDC #0785-9080-05
See Product Information Under Forest Pharmaceuticals, Inc.

ENDAL™-HD   ⅢR ℞
[ĕn dăl-HD]

DESCRIPTION
Each 5mL contains:
Hydrocodone Bitartrate .... 1.67 mg
  (WARNING: May Be Habit Forming)
Phenylephrine Hydrochloride .... 5 mg
Chlorpheniramine Maleate .... 2 mg

HOW SUPPLIED
Endal-HD is supplied in bottles of one pint (473 mL) NDC# 0785-6200-16.

LORCET®-HD   ⅢR ℞
[lōr-sét h d]

DESCRIPTION
Each Lorcet-HD capsule contains 5 mg Hydrocodone Bitartrate (WARNING: May be habit forming) and 500 mg Acetaminophen.

HOW SUPPLIED
Lorcet-HD capsules are opaque maroon capsules imprinted with the UAD logo on cap and "1120" on body of capsule. Each capsule contains 5 mg Hydrocodone Bitartrate (WARNING: May Be Habit Forming) and 500 mg Acetaminophen (APAP). Supplied in bottles of 100 capsules, NDC# 0785-1120-01.

LORCET® PLUS   ⅢR ℞
[lōr-sét plus]

DESCRIPTION
Each Lorcet Plus tablet contains:
Hydrocodone Bitartrate .... 7.5 mg
    (WARNING: May be habit forming)
Acetaminophen .... 650 mg

HOW SUPPLIED
Each tablet contains 7.5 hydrocodone bitartrate (WARNING: May Be Habit Forming) and 650 mg acetaminophen, and is a white, capsule-shaped, scored tablet debossed "U " on one side and "201" on the other side. Supplied in containers of 20 tablets, NDC #0785-1122-30, containers of 100 tablets, NDC #0785-1122-01, containers of 500 tablets, NDC

#0785-1122-50, and in hospital unit-dose cartons of 100 tablets (4 cards of 25 tablets per card), NDC #0785-1122-63.
Shown in Product Identification Section, page 433

LORCET® 10/650   ⅢR ℞
[lōr sét]
**Hydrocodone Bitartrate
and Acetaminophen Tablets
10 mg/650 mg**

DESCRIPTION
Each Lorcet® 10/650 tablet contains:
Hydrocodone* Bitartrate .... 10 mg
    *(WARNING: May be habit forming)
Acetaminophen .... 650 mg
Also contains colloidal silicon dioxide, croscarmellose sodium, crospovidone, microcrystalline cellulose, povidone, pregelatinized starch, stearic acid and FD&C Blue #1 Lake. Hydrocodone bitartrate is an opioid analgesic and antitussive which occurs as fine, white crystals or as a crystalline powder. It is affected by light. The chemical name is: 4, 5α-epoxy-3-methoxy-17-methylmorphinan-6-one tartrate (1:1) hydrate (2:5).
Its structure is as follows:

$$C_{18}H_{21}NO_3 \cdot C_4H_6O_6 \cdot 2\frac{1}{2}\ H_2O \qquad \text{M.W. } 494.50$$

Acetaminophen, 4'-hydroxyacetanilide, is a non-opiate, non-salicylate analgesic and antipyretic which occurs as a white, odorless, crystalline powder possessing a slightly bitter taste. Its structure is as follows:

$$C_8H_9NO_2 \qquad \text{M.W. } 151.16$$

CLINICAL PHARMACOLOGY
Hydrocodone is a semisynthetic narcotic analgesic and antitussive with multiple actions qualitatively similar to those of codeine. Most of these involve the central nervous system and smooth muscle. The precise mechanism of action of hydrocodone and other opiates is not known, although it is believed to relate to the existence of opiate receptors in the central nervous system. In addition to analgesia, narcotics may produce drowsiness, changes in mood and mental clouding.
Radioimmunoassay techniques have recently been developed for the analysis of hydrocodone in human plasma. After a 10 mg oral dose of hydrocodone bitartrate, a mean peak serum drug level of 23.6 ng/mL and an elimination half-life of 3.8 hours were found.
The analgesic action of acetaminophen involves peripheral and central influences, but the specific mechanism is as yet undetermined. Antipyretic activity is mediated through hypothalamic heat regulating centers. Acetaminophen inhibits prostaglandin synthetase. Therapeutic doses of acetaminophen have negligible effects on the cardiovascular or respiratory systems; however, toxic doses may cause circulatory failure and rapid, shallow breathing. Acetaminophen is rapidly and almost completely absorbed from the gastrointestinal tract, producing maximum serum concentrations within 30 minutes to one hour. The plasma half-life in adults and children ranges from 0.90 hours to 3.25 hours with an average of approximately 2 hours. The drug distributes uniformly in most body fluids and is approximately 25% protein bound. Acetaminophen is conjugated in the liver, with less than 3% of the dose excreted unchanged in 24 hours. The primary metabolic pathway is conjugation to sulfate and glucuronide by-products. A minor oxidative pathway forms cysteine and mercapturic acid. These compounds are subsequently excreted by the kidneys into the urine.

INDICATIONS AND USAGE
For the relief of moderate to moderately severe pain.

CONTRAINDICATIONS
Hypersensitivity to acetaminophen or hydrocodone.

WARNINGS
Respiratory Depression:
At high doses or in sensitive patients, hydrocodone may produce dose-related respiratory depression by acting directly on the brain stem respiratory center. Hydrocodone also affects the center that controls respiratory rhythm, and may produce irregular and periodic breathing.

Head Injury and Increased Intracranial Pressure:
The respiratory depressant effects of narcotics and their capacity to elevate cerebrospinal fluid pressure may be markedly exaggerated in the presence of head injury, other intracranial lesions or a preexisting increase in intracranial pressure. Furthermore, narcotics produce adverse reactions which may obscure the clinical course of patients with head injuries.

Acute Abdominal Conditions:
The administration of narcotics may obscure the diagnosis or clinical course of patients with acute abdominal conditions.

PRECAUTIONS
Special Risk Patients:
As with any narcotic analgesic agent, Lorcet® 10/650 should be used with caution in elderly or debilitated patients and those with severe impairment of hepatic or renal function, hypothyroidism, Addison's disease, prostatic hypertrophy or urethral stricture. The usual precautions should be observed and the possibility of respiratory depression should be kept in mind.

Information for Patients:
Lorcet® 10/650, like all narcotics, may impair the mental and/or physical abilities required for the performance of potentially hazardous tasks such as driving a car or operating machinery; patients should be cautioned accordingly.

Cough Reflex:
Hydrocodone suppresses the cough reflex; as with all narcotics, caution should be exercised when Lorcet® 10/650 is used postoperatively and in patients with pulmonary disease.

Drug Interactions:
Patients receiving other narcotic analgesics, antipsychotics, antianxiety agents, or other CNS depressants (including alcohol) concomitantly with Lorcet® 10/650 may exhibit an additive CNS depression. When combined therapy is contemplated, the dose of one or both agents should be reduced.
The use of MAO inhibitors or tricyclic antidepressants with hydrocodone preparations may increase the effect of either the antidepressant or hydrocodone.
The concurrent use of anticholinergics with hydrocodone may produce paralytic ileus.

Usage in Pregnancy:
Teratogenic Effects: Pregnancy Category C. Hydrocodone has been shown to be teratogenic in hamsters when given in doses 700 times the human dose. There are no adequate and well-controlled studies in pregnant women. Lorcet® 10/650 should be used during pregnancy only if the potential benefit justifies the potential risk to the fetus.
Nonteratogenic Effects: Babies born to mothers who have been taking opioids regularly prior to delivery will be physically dependent. The withdrawal signs include irritability and excessive crying, tremors, hyperactive reflexes, increased respiratory rate, increased stools, sneezing, yawning, vomiting, and fever. The intensity of the syndrome does not always correlate with the duration of maternal opioid use or dose. There is no consensus on the best method of managing withdrawal. Chlorpromazine 0.7 to 1 mg/kg q6h, and paregoric 2 to 4 drops/kg q4h, have been used to treat withdrawal symptoms in infants. The duration of therapy is 4 to 28 days, with the dosage decreased as tolerated.

Labor and Delivery:
As with all narcotics, administration of Lorcet® 10/650 to the mother shortly before delivery may result in some degree of respiratory depression in the newborn, especially if higher doses are used.

Nursing Mothers:
It is not known whether this drug is excreted in human milk. Because many drugs are excreted in human milk and because of the potential for serious adverse reactions in nursing infants from Lorcet® 10/650, a decision should be made whether to discontinue nursing or to discontinue the drug, taking into account the importance of the drug to the mother.

Pediatric Use:
Safety and effectiveness in children have not been established.

ADVERSE REACTIONS
The most frequently observed adverse reactions include lightheadedness, dizziness, sedation, nausea and vomiting. These effects seem to be more prominent in ambulatory than in nonambulatory patients and some of these adverse reactions may be alleviated if the patient lies down.
Other adverse reactions include:
Central Nervous System:
Drowsiness, mental clouding, lethargy, impairment of mental and physical performance, anxiety, fear, dysphoria, psychic dependence, mood changes.
Gastrointestinal System:
The antiemetic phenothiazines are useful in suppressing the nausea and vomiting which may occur (see above); however, some phenothiazine derivatives seem to be antianalgesic and to increase the amount of narcotic required to produce pain

Continued on next page

UAD Laboratories—Cont.

relief, while other phenothiazines reduce the amount of narcotic required to produce a given level of analgesia. Prolonged administration of Lorcet® 10/650 may produce constipation.

Genitourinary System:

Ureteral spasm, spasm of vesical sphincters and urinary retention have been reported.

Respiratory Depression:

Hydrocodone bitartrate may produce dose-related respiratory depression by acting directly on the brain stem respiratory center. Hydrocodone also affects the center that controls respiratory rhythm, and may produce irregular and periodic breathing. If significant respiratory depression occurs, it may be antagonized by the use of naloxone hydrochloride. Apply other supportive measures when indicated.

DRUG ABUSE AND DEPENDENCE

Lorcet® 10/650 is subject to the Federal Controlled Substances Act (Schedule III).

Psychic dependence, physical dependence, and tolerance may develop upon repeated administration of narcotics; therefore, Lorcet® 10/650 should be prescribed and administered with caution. However, psychic dependence is unlikely to develop when Lorcet® 10/650 is used for a short time for the treatment of pain.

Physical dependence, the condition in which continued administration of the drug is required to prevent the appearance of a withdrawal syndrome, assumes clinically significant proportions only after several weeks of continued narcotic use, although some mild degree of physical dependence may develop after a few days of narcotic therapy. Tolerance, in which increasingly large doses are required in order to produce the same degree of analgesia, is manifested initially by a shortened duration of analgesic effect, and subsequently by decreases in the intensity of analgesia. The rate of development of tolerance varies among patients.

OVERDOSAGE

Acetaminophen:

Signs and Symptoms: In acute acetaminophen overdosage, dose-dependent, potentially fatal hepatic necrosis is the most serious adverse effect. Renal tubular necrosis, hypoglycemic coma, and thrombocytopenia may also occur.

In adults, hepatic toxicity has rarely been reported with acute overdoses of less than 10 grams and fatalities with less than 15 grams. Importantly, young children seem to be more resistant than adults to the hepatotoxic effect of an acetaminophen overdose. Despite this, the measures outlined below should be initiated in any adult or child suspected of having ingested an acetaminophen overdose.

Early symptoms following a potentially hepatotoxic overdose may include: nausea, vomiting, diaphoresis and general malaise. Clinical and laboratory evidence of hepatic toxicity may not be apparent until 48 to 72 hours post-ingestion.

Treatment: The stomach should be emptied promptly by lavage or by induction of emesis with syrup of ipecac. Patients' estimates of the quantity of a drug ingested are notoriously unreliable. Therefore, if an acetaminophen overdose is suspected, a serum acetaminophen assay should be obtained as early as possible, but no sooner than four hours following ingestion. Liver function studies should be obtained initially and repeated at 24-hour intervals.

The antidote, N-acetylcysteine, should be administered as early as possible, preferably within 16 hours of the overdose ingestion for optimal results, but in any case, within 24 hours. Following recovery, there are no residual, structural or functional hepatic abnormalities.

Hydrocodone:

Signs and Symptoms: Serious overdose with hydrocodone is characterized by respiratory depression (a decrease in respiratory rate or tidal volume, Cheyne-Stokes respiration, cyanosis), extreme somnolence progressing to stupor or coma, skeletal muscle flaccidity, cold and clammy skin, and sometimes bradycardia and hypotension. In severe overdosage, apnea, circulatory collapse, cardiac arrest and death may occur.

Treatment: Primary attention should be given to the reestablishment of adequate respiratory exchange through provision of a patent airway and the institution of assisted or controlled ventilation. The narcotic antagonist naloxone is a specific antidote against respiratory depression which may result from overdosage or unusual sensitivity to narcotics, including hydrocodone. Therefore, an appropriate dose of naloxone hydrochloride (see package insert) should be administered, preferably by the intravenous route, and simultaneously with efforts at respiratory resuscitation. Since the duration of action of hydrocodone may exceed that of the antagonist, the patient should be kept under continued surveillance and repeated doses of the antagonist should be administered as needed to maintain adequate respiration.

An antagonist should not be administered in the absence of clinically significant respiratory or cardiovascular depres-

sion. Oxygen, intravenous fluids, vasopressors and other supportive measures should be employed as indicated. Gastric emptying may be useful in removing unabsorbed drug.

DOSAGE AND ADMINISTRATION

Dosage should be adjusted according to the severity of the pain and the response of the patient. However, it should be kept in mind that tolerance to hydrocodone can develop with continued use and that the incidence of untoward effects is dose related.

The usual adult dosage is one tablet every four to six hours as needed for pain. The total 24 hour dose should not exceed 6 tablets.

HOW SUPPLIED

Lorcet® 10/650, Hydrocodone* Bitartrate and Acetaminophen Tablets 10 mg/650 mg, each tablet of which contains hydrocodone* bitartrate 10 mg *(**WARNING:** May be habit forming) and acetaminophen 650 mg, are light-blue, capsule-shaped, scored tablets, debossed "UAD" on one side and "63 50" on the other side, and are supplied in containers of 20 tablets, NDC 0785-6350-30, in containers of 100 tablets, NDC 0785-6350-01 and containers of unit dose (4 × 25's), NDC 0785-6350-63.

Storage: Store at controlled room temperature 15°–30°C (59°–86°F).

Dispense in a tight, light-resistant container, with a child-resistant closure.

CAUTION: Federal law prohibits dispensing without prescription.

A Schedule CIII Controlled Substance.

Manufactured by: MIKART, INC. ATLANTA, GA 30318

Manufactured for
UAD Laboratories
Division of Forest Pharmaceuticals, Inc.
Jackson, MS 39209

Revised 6/92

Shown in Product Identification Section, page 433

TESSALON® PERLES　　　　　　　　　　　　　　R

[tess'-ä-lon]

DESCRIPTION

Each Tessalon Perle contains:

Benzonatate U.S.P., 100 mg

See Product Information Under Forest Pharmaceuticals, Inc.

ZONE–A CREAM 1%　　　　　　　　　　　　　　R

[zōn'a]

DESCRIPTION

A topical preparation containing Hydrocortisone acetate 1% and Pramoxine HCl 1% in a hydrophilic cream base containing stearic acid, cetyl alcohol, aquaphor, isopropyl palmitate, polyoxyl 40 stearate, propylene glycol, potassium sorbate 0.1%, sorbic acid 0.1%, triethanolamine lauryl sulfate and water.

HOW SUPPLIED

1 oz. tube.

ZONE-A LOTION 1%　　　　　　　　　　　　　　R

[zōn'ā]

DESCRIPTION

Zone-A Lotion is a topical preparation containing Hydrocortisone acetate 1% and Pramoxine HCl 1% in a hydrophilic lotion base containing stearic acid, cetyl alcohol, forlan-L, glycerine, triethanolamine, polyoxyl 40 stearate, di-isopropyl adipate, povidone, silicone fluid-200, potassium sorbate 0.1%, sorbic acid 0.1% and water. Topical corticosteroids are anti-inflammatory and antipruritic agents.

HOW SUPPLIED

2 fl. oz.

Products are cross-indexed by
generic and chemical names
in the
YELLOW SECTION.

U.S. Bioscience, Inc.

ONE TOWER BRIDGE
100 FRONT STREET
WEST CONSHOHOCKEN, PA 19428

HEXALEN　　　　　　　　　　　　　　　　　　　R

[hex'a-len]
(ALTRETAMINE)
CAPSULES
50 mg

WARNINGS

1. HEXALEN® should only be given under the supervision of a physician experienced in the use of antineoplastic agents.

2. Peripheral blood counts should be monitored at least monthly, prior to the initiation of each course of HEXALEN, and as clinically indicated (see Adverse Reactions).

3. Because of the possibility of HEXALEN-related neurotoxicity, neurologic examination should be performed regularly during HEXALEN administration (see Adverse Reactions).

DESCRIPTION

HEXALEN (altretamine) is a synthetic cytotoxic antineoplastic s-triazine derivative. HEXALEN capsules contain 50 mg of altretamine for oral administration. Inert ingredients include lactose, anhydrous and calcium stearate. Altretamine, known chemically as $N,N,N'N'N''N''$-hexamethyl-1,3,5-triazine-2,4,6-triamine, with the following structural formula:

$$(CH_3)_2N - \text{triazine} - N(CH_3)_2$$
$$N(CH_3)_2$$

Its empirical formula is $C_9H_{18}N_6$ with a molecular weight of 210.28. Altretamine is a white crystalline powder, melting at $172° \pm 1°C$. Altretamine is practically insoluble in water but increasingly soluble at pH 3 and below.

CLINICAL PHARMACOLOGY

The precise mechanism by which HEXALEN exerts its cytotoxic effect is unknown, although a number of theoretical possibilities have been studied. Structurally, HEXALEN resembles the alkylating agent triethylenemelamine, yet *in vitro* tests for alkylating activity of HEXALEN and its metabolites have been negative. HEXALEN has been demonstrated to be efficacious for certain ovarian tumors resistant to classical alkylating agents. Metabolism of altretamine is a requirement for cytotoxicity. Synthetic monohydroxymethylmelamines, and products of altretamine metabolism, *in vitro* and *in vivo*, can form covalent adducts with tissue macromolecules including DNA, but the relevance of these reactions to antitumor activity is unknown.

HEXALEN is well-absorbed following oral administration in humans, but undergoes rapid and extensive demethylation in the liver, producing variation in altretamine plasma levels. The principal metabolites are pentamethylmelamine and tetramethylmelamine.

Pharmacokinetic studies were performed in a limited number of patients and should be considered preliminary. After oral administration of HEXALEN to 11 patients with advanced ovarian cancer in doses of 120–300 mg/m², peak plasma levels (as measured by gas-chromatographic assay) were reached between 0.5 and 3 hours, varying from 0.2 to 20.8 mg/l. Half-life of the β-phase of elimination ranged from 4.7 to 10.2 hours. Altretamine and metabolites show binding to plasma proteins. The free fractions of altretamine, pentamethylmelamine and tetramethylmelamine are 6%, 25% and 50%, respectively.

Following oral administration of ${}^{14}C$-ring-labeled altretamine (4 mg/kg), urinary recovery of radioactivity was 61% at 24 hours and 90% at 72 hours. Human urinary metabolites were N-demethylated homologues of altretamine with <1% unmetabolized altretamine excreted at 24 hours.

After intraperitoneal administration of ${}^{14}C$-ring-labeled altretamine to mice, tissue distribution was rapid in all organs, reaching a maximum at 30 minutes. The excretory organs (liver and kidney) and the small intestine showed high concentrations of radioactivity, whereas relatively low concentrations were found in other organs, including the brain.

There have been no formal pharmacokinetic studies in patients with compromised hepatic and/or renal function, though HEXALEN has been administered both concurrently and following nephrotoxic drugs such as cisplatin.

HEXALEN has been administered in 4 divided doses, with meals and at bedtime, though there is no pharmacokinetic

data on this schedule nor information from formal interaction studies about the effect of food on its bioavailability or pharmacokinetics.

In two studies in patients with persistent or recurrent ovarian cancer following first-line treatment with cisplatin and/or alkylating agent-based combinations, HEXALEN was administered as a single agent for 14 or 21 days of a 28 day cycle. In the 51 patients with measurable or evaluable disease, there were 6 clinical complete responses, 1 pathologic complete response, and 2 partial responses for an overall response rate of 18%. The duration of these responses ranged from 2 months in a patient with a palpable pelvic mass to 36 months in a patient who achieved a pathologic complete response. In some patients, tumor regression was associated with improvement in symptoms and performance status.

INDICATIONS AND USAGE

HEXALEN (altretamine) is indicated for use as a single agent in the palliative treatment of patients with persistent or recurrent ovarian cancer following first-line therapy with a cisplatin and/or alkylating agent-based combination.

CONTRAINDICATIONS

HEXALEN is contraindicated in patients who have shown hypersensitivity to it. HEXALEN should not be employed in patients with preexisting severe bone marrow depression or severe neurologic toxicity. HEXALEN has been administered safely, however, to patients heavily pretreated with cisplatin and/or alkylating agents, including patients with preexisting cisplatin neuropathies. Careful monitoring of neurologic function in these patients is essential.

WARNINGS

See boxed Warnings.

Concurrent administration of HEXALEN and antidepressants of the monoamine oxidase (MAO) inhibitor class may cause severe orthostatic hypotension. Four patients, all over 60 years of age, were reported to have experienced symptomatic hypotension after 4 to 7 days of concomitant therapy with HEXALEN and MAO inhibitors.

HEXALEN causes mild to moderate myelosuppression and neurotoxicity. Blood counts and a neurologic examination should be performed prior to the initiation of each course of therapy and the dose of HEXALEN adjusted as clinically indicated (see Dosage and Administration).

Pregnancy: Category D

HEXALEN has been shown to be embryotoxic and teratogenic in rats and rabbits when given at doses 2 and 10 times the human dose. HEXALEN may cause fetal damage when administered to a pregnant woman. If HEXALEN is used during pregnancy, or if the patient becomes pregnant while taking the drug, the patient should be appraised of the potential hazard to the fetus. Women of childbearing potential should be advised to avoid becoming pregnant.

PRECAUTIONS

General

Neurologic examination should be performed regularly (see Adverse Reactions).

Laboratory Tests

Peripheral blood counts should be monitored at least monthly, prior to the initiation of each course of HEXALEN, and as clinically indicated (see Adverse Reactions).

Drug Interactions

Concurrent administration of HEXALEN and antidepressants of the MAO inhibitor class may cause severe orthostatic hypotension (see Warnings section). Cimetidine, an inhibitor of microsomal drug metabolism, increased altretamine's half-life and toxicity in a rat model.

Data from a randomized trial of HEXALEN and cisplatin plus or minus pyridoxine in ovarian cancer indicated that pyridoxine significantly reduced neurotoxicity; however, it adversely affected response duration suggesting that pyridoxine should not be administered with HEXALEN and/or cisplatin (1).

Carcinogenesis, Mutagenesis and Impairment of Fertility

The carcinogenic potential of HEXALEN has not been studied in animals, but drugs with similar mechanisms of action have been shown to be carcinogenic. HEXALEN was weakly mutagenic when tested in strain TA100 of *Salmonella typhimurium*. HEXALEN administered to female rats 14 days prior to breeding through the gestation period had no adverse effect on fertility, but decreased post-natal survival at 120 mg/m^2/day and was embryocidal at 240 mg/m^2/day. Administration of 120 mg/m^2/day HEXALEN to male rats for 60 days prior to mating resulted in testicular atrophy, reduced fertility and a possible dominant lethal mutagenic effect. Male rats treated with HEXALEN at 450 mg/m^2/day for 10 days had decreased spermatogenesis, atrophy of testes, seminal vesicles and ventral prostate.

Pregnancy

Pregnancy Category D: see Warnings section.

Nursing Mothers

It is not known whether altretamine is excreted in human milk. Because there is a possibility of toxicity in nursing infants secondary to HEXALEN treatment of the mother, it is recommended that breast feeding be discontinued if the mother is treated with HEXALEN.

Pediatric Use

The safety and effectiveness of HEXALEN in children have not been established.

ADVERSE REACTIONS

Gastrointestinal

With continuous high-dose daily HEXALEN, nausea and vomiting of gradual onset occur frequently. Although in most instances these symptoms are controllable with antiemetics, at times the severity requires HEXALEN dose reduction or, rarely, discontinuation of HEXALEN therapy. In some instances, a tolerance of these symptoms develops after several weeks of therapy. The incidence and severity of nausea and vomiting are reduced with moderate-dose administration of HEXALEN. In 2 clinical studies of single-agent HEXALEN utilizing a moderate, intermittent dose and schedule, only 1 patient (1%) discontinued HEXALEN due to severe nausea and vomiting.

Neurotoxicity

Peripheral neuropathy and central nervous system symptoms (mood disorders, disorders of consciousness, ataxia, dizziness, vertigo) have been reported. They are more likely to occur in patients receiving continuous high-dose daily HEXALEN than moderate-dose HEXALEN administered on an intermittent schedule. Neurologic toxicity has been reported to be reversible when therapy is discontinued. Data from a randomized trial of HEXALEN and cisplatin plus or minus pyridoxine in ovarian cancer indicated that pyridoxine significantly reduced neurotoxicity; however, it adversely affected response duration suggesting that pyridoxine should not be administered with HEXALEN and/or cisplatin (1).

Hematologic

HEXALEN (altretamine) causes mild to moderate dose-related myelosuppression. Leukopenia below 3000 WBC/mm^3 occurred in < 15% of patients on a variety of intermittent or continuous dose regimens. Less than 1% had leukopenia below 1000 WBC/mm^3. Thrombocytopenia below 50,000 platelets/mm^3 was seen in < 10% of patients. When given in doses of 8–12 mg/kg/day over a 21 day course, nadirs of leukocyte and platelet counts were reached by 3–4 weeks, and normal counts were regained by 6 weeks. With continuous administration at doses of 6–8 mg/kg/day, nadirs are reached in 6–8 weeks (median).

Data in the following table are based on the experience of 76 patients with ovarian cancer previously treated with a cisplatin-based combination regimen who received single-agent HEXALEN. In one study, HEXALEN, 260 mg/m^2/day, was administered for 14 days of a 28 day cycle. In another study, HEXALEN, 6–8 mg/kg/day, was administered for 21 days of a 28 day cycle.

ADVERSE EXPERIENCES IN 76 PREVIOUSLY TREATED OVARIAN CANCER PATIENTS RECEIVING SINGLE-AGENT HEXALEN

	%
Gastrointestinal	
Nausea and Vomiting	33
Mild to Moderate	32
Severe	1
Increased Alkaline Phosphatase	9
Neurologic	
Peripheral Sensory Neuropathy	31
Mild	22
Moderate to Severe	9
Anorexia and Fatigue	1
Seizures	1
Hematologic	
Leukopenia	5
WBC 2000–2999/mm^3	4
WBC < 2000/mm^3	1
Thrombocytopenia	9
Platelets 75,000–99,000/mm^3	6
Platelets < 75,000/mm^3	3
Anemia	33
Mild	20
Moderate to Severe	13
Renal	
Serum Creatinine 1.6–3.75 mg/dl	7
BUN	9
25–40 mg%	5
41–60 mg%	3
> 60 mg%	1

Additional adverse reaction information is available from 13 single-agent altretamine studies (total of 1014 patients) conducted under the auspices of the National Cancer Institute. The treated patients had a variety of tumors and many were heavily pretreated with other chemotherapies; most of these trials utilized high, continuous daily doses of altretamine

(6–12 mg/kg/day). In general, adverse reaction experiences were similar in the two trials described above. Additional toxicities, not reported in the above table, included hepatic toxicity, skin rash, pruritus and alopecia, each occurring in < 1% of patients.

OVERDOSAGE

No case of acute overdosage in humans has been described. The oral LD50 dose in rats was 1050 mg/kg and 437 mg/kg in mice.

DOSAGE AND ADMINISTRATION

HEXALEN is administered orally. Doses are calculated on the basis of body surface area.

HEXALEN may be administered either for 14 or 21 consecutive days in a 28 day cycle at a dose of 260 mg/m^2/day. The total daily dose should be given as 4 divided oral doses after meals and at bedtime. There is no pharmacokinetic information supporting this dosing regimen and the effect of food on HEXALEN bioavailability or pharmacokinetics has not been evaluated.

HEXALEN should be temporarily discontinued (for 14 days or longer) and subsequently restarted at 200 mg/m^2/day for any of the following situations:

1) Gastrointestinal intolerance unresponsive to symptomatic measures;
2) White blood count < 2000/mm^3 or granulocyte count < 1000/mm^3;
3) Platelet count < 75,000/mm^3;
4) Progressive neurotoxicity.

If neurologic symptoms fail to stabilize on the reduced dose schedule, HEXALEN should be discontinued indefinitely. Procedures for proper handling and disposal of anticancer drugs should be considered. Several guidelines on this subject have been published (2–8). There is no general agreement that all of the procedures recommended in the guidelines are necessary or appropriate.

HOW SUPPLIED

HEXALEN (altretamine) is available in 50 mg clear, hard gelatin capsules in bottles of 100 (**NDC** 58178-001-70). The capsules are imprinted with the following inscription: USB001 HEXALEN 50 mg. Store at controlled room temperature 15°–30°C (59°–86°F).

REFERENCES

1. Wiernik PH, et al. Hexamethylmelamine and Low or Moderate Dose Cisplatin With or Without Pyridoxine for Treatment of Advanced Ovarian Carcinoma: A Study of the Eastern Cooperative Oncology Group. *Cancer Investigation* 10(1): 1–9, 1992.
2. Recommendations for the Safe Handling of Parenteral Antineoplastic Drugs. NIH Publication No. 83-2621. For sale by the Superintendent of Documents, U.S. Government Printing Office, Washington, D.C. 20402.
3. AMA Council Report. Guidelines for Handling Parenteral Antineoplastics. *Journal of the American Medical Association* March 15, 1985.
4. National Study Commission on Cytotoxic Exposure—Recommendation for Handling Cytotoxic Agents. Available from Louis P. Jeffrey, Sc.D., Director of Pharmacy Services, Rhode Island Hospital, 593 Eddy Street, Providence, Rhode Island 02902.
5. Clinical Oncological Society of Australia: Guidelines and Recommendations for Safe Handling of Antineoplastic Agents. *Medical Journal of Australia* 1:426–428, 1983.
6. Jones, RB, et al. Safe Handling of Chemotherapeutic Agents: A Report from the Mount Sinai Medical Center. *CA—A Cancer Journal for Clinicians* Sept/Oct, 258–263, 1983.
7. American Society of Hospital Pharmacists Technical Assistance Bulletin on Handling Cytotoxic Drugs in Hospitals. *American Journal of Hospital Pharmacy* 42:131–137, 1985.
8. OSHA Work Practice Guidelines for Personnel Dealing with Cytotoxic (Antineoplastic) Drugs. *American Journal of Hospital Pharmacy* 43:1193–1204, 1986.

Manufactured by:
Applied Analytical Industries, Inc.
Wilmington, NC 28405
For: **U.S. Bioscience**
One Tower Bridge
100 Front Street
West Conshohocken, PA 19428
Revision Date 5/92   **PE**
Shown in Product Identification Section, page 433

Products are
listed alphabetically
in the
PINK SECTION.

U.S. Pharmaceutical Corporation
2401-C MELLON COURT
DECATUR, GA 30035

HEMOCYTE™ Tablets   OTC
(ferrous fumarate 324 mg.)

HOW SUPPLIED
Bottles of 100 NDC 52747-307-60

HEMOCYTE PLUS ELIXIR   ℞
Iron-Vitamin-Mineral Complex

DESCRIPTION:
Dexpanthenol	10 mg
Niacinamide	40 mg
Pyridoxine HCl (B₆)	4 mg
Cyanocobalamin (B₁₂)	12 mcg
Folic Acid	1 mg
Iron (Polysaccharide Iron Complex)	36 mg
Zinc (as Zinc Sulfate)	15 mg
Manganese (as Manganese Sulfate)	4 mg
Alcohol	13%

HOW SUPPLIED
Bottles of one pint (473 mL) NDC 52747-309-90

HEMOCYTE PLUS™ Tabules   ℞
Iron-Vitamin-Mineral Complex

DESCRIPTION
Each tabule contains:
Ferrous Fumarate (anhydrous)	324	mg.
[Equivalent to about 106 mg. of Elemental Iron]		
Sodium Ascorbate (Vit. C)	200	mg.
Vit. B-1—Thiamine Mononitrate	10	mg.
Vit. B-2—Riboflavin	6	mg.
Vit. B-6—Pyridoxine HCl	5	mg.
Vit. B-12—Cyanocobalamin Concentrate	15	mcg.
Folic Acid	1	mg.
Niacinamide	30	mg.
Calcium Pantothenate	10	mg.
Zinc (as Zinc Sulfate)	18.2	mg.
Magnesium (as Magnesium Sulfate)	6.9	mg.
Manganese (as Manganese Sulfate)	1.3	mg.
Copper (as Copper Sulfate)	0.8	mg.

HOW SUPPLIED
Bottles of 100 NDC 52747-308-60

HEMOCYTE–C Tablets   OTC
(Chewable Iron/Vitamin C)

DESCRIPTION
Each tablet contains:
Iron (elemental) (as Ferrous Fumarate)	50 mg
Ascorbic Acid (as Ascorbic Acid and Sodium Ascorbate)	250 mg

HOW SUPPLIED
Tablets: Bottles of 50 NDC 52747-303-50

HEMOCYTE–F TABLETS   ℞

DESCRIPTION
Each tablet contains:
Ferrous Fumarate (anhydrous)	324 mg.
Folic Acid	1 mg.

HOW SUPPLIED
Bottles of 100 NDC 52747-306-60

ISOVEX® Capsules   ℞
(ethaverine hydrochloride 100 mg.)

HOW SUPPLIED
Bottles of 100 NDC 52747-204-60
Bottles of 1000 NDC 52747-204-80

MAGSAL™ TABLETS   ℞

DESCRIPTION
Each tablet contains:
Magnesium Salicylate	600 mg.
Phenyltoloxamine Dihydrogen Citrate	25 mg.

HOW SUPPLIED
Bottles of 100 NDC 52747-321-60

MEDIGESIC® Capsules/Tablets   ℞

DESCRIPTION
Each capsule or tablet contains:
Butalbital*	50 mg
*WARNING: May be habit forming.	
Acetaminophen	325 mg
Caffeine	40 mg

HOW SUPPLIED
Capsules: Bottles of 100 NDC 52747-212-60
Tablets: Bottles of 100 NDC 52747-311-60

The Upjohn Company
KALAMAZOO, MI 49001

PRODUCT IDENTIFICATION
Prescription capsules and tablets manufactured by The Upjohn Company are imprinted with one or a combination of the following: (1) Product trademark (2) Dosage strength (3) "Upjohn" or "U" (4) That portion of the National Drug Code (NDC) number which indicates product and strength. A list of oral solid dosage forms with NDC product identification numbers is provided below.

Code #	Product	Strength
10	**HALCION®** Tablets (triazolam tablets, USP) *See Product Identification Section*	0.125 mg
11	**FEMINONE®** Tablets (ethinyl estradiol tablets, USP)	0.05 mg
12	**CORTEF®** Tablets (hydrocortisone tablets, USP)	5 mg
14	**HALOTESTIN®** Tablets (fluoxymesterone tablets, USP) *See Product Identification Section*	2 mg
15	**CORTISONE ACETATE** Tablets, USP	5 mg
17	**HALCION®** Tablets (triazolam tablets, USP) *See Product Identification Section*	0.25 mg
18	**DIDREX®** Tablets (benzphetamine hydrochloride) *See Product Identification Section*	25 mg
19	**HALOTESTIN®** Tablets (fluoxymesterone tablets, USP) *See Product Identification Section*	5 mg
22	**MEDROL®** Tablets (methylprednisolone tablets, USP) *See Product Identification Section*	8 mg
23	**CORTISONE ACETATE** Tablets, USP	10 mg
24	**DIDREX®** Tablets (benzphetamine hydrochloride) *See Product Identification Section*	50 mg
29	**XANAX®** Tablets (alprazolam tablets, USP) *See Product Identification Section*	0.25 mg
31	**CORTEF®** Tablets (hydrocortisone tablets, USP)	10 mg
32	**DELTASONE®** Tablets (prednisone tablets, USP) *See Product Identification Section*	2.5 mg.
34	**CORTISONE ACETATE** Tablets, USP	25 mg
36	**HALOTESTIN®** Tablets (fluoxymesterone tablets, USP) *See Product Identification Section*	10 mg
38	**HALODRIN®** Tablets (fluoxymesterone and ethinyl estradiol)	
44	**CORTEF®** Tablets (hydrocortisone tablets, USP)	20 mg
45	**DELTASONE®** Tablets (prednisone tablets, USP) *See Product Identification Section*	5 mg
49	**MEDROL®** Tablets (methylprednisolone tablets, USP) *See Product Identification Section*	2 mg
50	**PROVERA®** Tablets (medroxyprogesterone acetate tablets, USP) *See Product Identification Section*	10 mg
55	**XANAX®** Tablets (alprazolam tablets, USP) *See Product Identification Section*	0.5 mg
56	**MEDROL®** Tablets (methylprednisolone tablets, USP) *See Product Identification Section*	4 mg
61	**PAMINE®** Tablets (methscopamine bromide tablets, USP)	2.5 mg
64	**PROVERA®** Tablets (medroxyprogesterone acetate tablets, USP) *See Product Identification Section*	2.5 mg
70	**TOLINASE®** Tablets (tolazamide tablets, USP) *See Product Identification Section*	100 mg
73	**MEDROL®** Tablets (methylprednisolone tablets, USP) *See Product Identification Section*	16 mg
90	**XANAX®** Tablets (alprazolam tablets, USP) *See Product Identification Section*	1 mg
94	**XANAX®** Tablets (alprazolam tablets, USP) *See Product Identification Section*	2 mg
100	**ORINASE®** Tablets (tolbutamide tablets, USP) *See Product Identification Section*	500 mg
101	**ALBAMYCIN®** Capsules (novobiocin sodium)	250 mg
114	**TOLINASE®** Tablets (tolazamide tablets, USP) *See Product Identification Section*	250 mg
115	**ADEFLOR M®** Tablets Vitamins and minerals with fluoride *See Product Identification Section*	
121	**LONITEN®** Tablets (minoxidil tablets, USP) *See Product Identification Section*	2.5 mg
131	**MICRONASE®** Tablets (glyburide) *See Product Identification Section*	1.25 mg
137	**LONITEN®** Tablets (minoxidil tablets, USP) *See Product Identification Section*	10 mg
141	**MICRONASE®** Tablets (glyburide) *See Product Identification Section*	2.5 mg
155	**MEDROL®** Tablets (methylprednisolone tablets, USP) *See Product Identification Section*	24 mg
165	**DELTASONE®** Tablets (prednisone tablets, USP) *See Product Identification Section*	20 mg
170	**ANSAID®** Tablets (flurbiprofen) *See Product Identification Section*	50 mg
171	**MICRONASE®** Tablets (glyburide) *See Product Identification Section*	5 mg
176	**MEDROL®** Tablets (methylprednisolone tablets, USP) *See Product Identification Section*	32 mg
193	**DELTASONE®** Tablets (prednisone tablets, USP) *See Product Identification Section*	10 mg
225	**CLEOCIN HCl®** Capsules (clindamycin hydrochloride capsules, USP) *See Product Identification Section*	150 mg
286	**PROVERA®** Tablets (medroxyprogesterone acetate tablets, USP) *See Product Identification Section*	5 mg
305	**ANSAID®** Tablets (flurbiprofen) *See Product Identification Section*	100 mg
331	**CLEOCIN HCl®** Capsules (clindamycin hydrochloride capsules, USP) *See Product Identification Section*	75 mg
336	**LINCOCIN®** Pediatric Capsules (lincomycin hydrochloride capsules, USP)	250 mg
	GLYNASE™ PresTab™ Tablets (glyburide) *See Product Identification Section*	1.5 mg
	GLYNASE™ PresTab™ Tablets (glyburide) *See Product Identification Section*	3 mg
388	**DELTASONE®** Tablets (prednisone tablets, USP) *See Product Identification Section*	50 mg
395	**CLEOCIN HCl®** Capsules (clindamycin hydrochloride capsules, USP) *See Product Identification Section*	300 mg

412	**MAOLATE**® Tablets (chlorphenesin carbamate)	400 mg
477	**TOLINASE**® Tablets (tolazamide tablets, USP) *See Product Identification Section*	500 mg
500	**LINCOCIN**® Capsules (lincomycin hydrochloride capsules, USP)	500 mg
701	**ORINASE**® Tablets (tolbutamide tablets, USP) *See Product Identification Section*	250 mg
725	**MOTRIN**® Tablets (ibuprofen tablets, USP) *See Product Identification Section*	800 mg
733	**MOTRIN**® Tablets (ibuprofen tablets, USP) *See Product Identification Section*	300 mg
742	**MOTRIN**® Tablets (ibuprofen tablets, USP) *See Product Identification Section*	600 mg
750	**MOTRIN**® Tablets (ibuprofen tablets, USP) *See Product Identification Section*	400 mg
782	**PANMYCIN**® Capsules (tetracycline hydrochloride capsules, USP)	250 mg
949	**URACIL MUSTARD** Capsules, USP	1 mg

ADEFLOR M® ℞

brand of vitamin and mineral tablets with fluoride

COMPOSITION

Each ADEFLOR M tablet for oral use contains:

Fluoride (as sodium fluoride)	**1 mg**
Vitamin A	6000 Int. Units
Vitamin D (ergocalciferol)	400 Int. Units
Thiamine Mononitrate	1.5 mg
Riboflavin	2.5 mg
Ascorbic Acid (as sodium ascorbate)	100 mg
Niacinamide	20 mg
Pyridoxine Hydrochloride	10 mg
Calcium Pantothenate	10 mg
Cyanocobalamin	2 mcg
Calcium (as calcium carbonate)	250 mg
Iron (from 91.27 mg ferrous fumarate)	30 mg

INACTIVE INGREDIENTS

Acetylated monoglycerides, calcium carbonate, calcium sulfate, carnauba wax, colloidal silicon dioxide, corn starch, dibasic calcium phosphate, erythrosine sodium, FD & C blue No. 1, gelatin, magnesium stearate, polyethylene glycol, sesame oil, shellac, simethicone, sodium benzoate, sorbic acid, sorbitol, stearate emulsifiers, sucrose, terra alba, titanium dioxide.

HOW SUPPLIED

Bottles of 100 (elliptical, pink) NDC 0009-0115-01

Shown in Product Identification Section, page 433

ANSAID® ℞

brand of flurbiprofen tablets

50 mg, 100's	**NSN 6505-01-302-0807**
50 mg, 500's	**NSN 6505-01-301-0806**
100 mg, 100's	**NSN 6505-01-301-0804**
100 mg, 500's	**NSN 6505-01-301-0805**

DESCRIPTION

ANSAID Tablets contain flurbiprofen, a nonsteroidal anti-flammatory agent. Flurbiprofen is a phenylalkanoic acid derivative designated chemically as [1,1′-biphenyl]-4-acetic acid, 2-fluoro-alphamethyl-, (±)-. The empirical formula is $C_{15}H_{13}FO_2$, with a molecular weight of 244.26. Flurbiprofen is a white or slightly yellow crystalline powder. It is slightly soluble in water at pH 7.0 and readily soluble in most polar solvents. Its structural formula is:

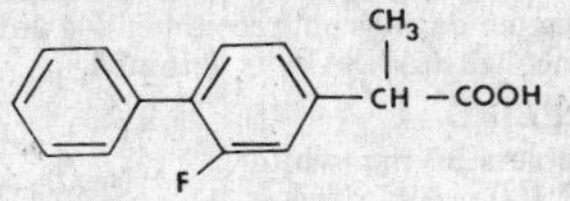

ANSAID is available as 50 mg and 100 mg tablets for oral administration. Inactive ingredients for both strengths are carnauba wax, colloidal silicon dioxide, croscarmellose sodium, hydroxypropyl methylcellulose, lactose, magnesium stearate, microcrystalline cellulose, propylene glycol, and titanium dioxide. In addition, the 100 mg tablet contains FD&C blue No. 2.

CLINICAL PHARMACOLOGY

Flurbiprofen is a nonsteroidal anti-inflammatory agent which has shown anti-inflammatory, analgesic, and antipyretic properties in pharmacologic studies. As with other such drugs, its mode of action is not known. However, it is a potent prostaglandin synthesis inhibitor, and this property may be involved in its anti-inflammatory effect.

Flurbiprofen is well absorbed after oral administration, reaching peak blood levels in approximately 1.5 hours (range 0.5 to 4 hours). Administration with food alters the rate of absorption but does not affect the extent of drug availability. The elimination half-life is 5.7 hours with 90% of the half-life values from 3 to 9 hours. Individual half-life values ranged from 2.8 to 12 hours. There is no evidence of drug accumulation and flurbiprofen does not induce enzymes that alter its metabolism. Excretion of flurbiprofen is 88% to 98% complete 24 hours after the last dose.

Flurbiprofen is extensively metabolized and excreted primarily in the urine, about 20% as free and conjugated drug and about 50% as hydroxylated metabolites. About 90% of the flurbiprofen in urine is present as conjugates. The major metabolite, 4′-hydroxyl-flurbiprofen, has been detected in human plasma, but in animal models of inflammation this metabolite showed little anti-inflammatory activity. Flurbiprofen is more than 99% bound to human serum proteins.

The average maximum serum concentration of flurbiprofen, following a 100 mg oral dose of ANSAID Tablets in normal volunteers (n=184), was 15.2 μg/ml, with 90% of the values between 10 and 22 μg/ml. In geriatric subjects (n=7) between the ages of 58 and 77 years, 100 mg ANSAID Tablets resulted in an average peak drug level of 18.0 μg/ml and an average elimination half-life of 6.5 hours (range 3–10 hours). In geriatric rheumatoid arthritis patients (n=13) between the ages of 65 and 83 years receiving 100 mg ANSAID Tablets, the average maximum blood level was 12.7 μg/ml and the average elimination half-life was 5.6 hours (range 4–10 hours).

In a study assessing flurbiprofen pharmacokinetics in end stage renal disease (ESRD), mean urinary recovery of a 100 mg dose was 73% in 48 hours for 9 normal subjects and 17% in 96 hours for 8 ESRD patients undergoing continuous ambulatory peritoneal dialysis. Plasma concentrations of flurbiprofen were about 40% lower in the ESRD patients; the elimination half-life of flurbiprofen was unchanged. Elimination of the 4′-hydroxy-flurbiprofen metabolite was markedly reduced in the ESRD patients. The pharmacokinetics of flurbiprofen in patients with decreased renal function but not ESRD have not been determined.

The pharmacokinetics of flurbiprofen in patients with hepatic disease have not been determined.

The efficacy of ANSAID has been demonstrated in patients with rheumatoid arthritis and osteoarthritis. Using standard assessments of therapeutic response, ANSAID (200–300 mg/day) demonstrated effectiveness comparable to aspirin (2000–4000 mg/day), ibuprofen (2400–3200 mg/day), and indomethacin (75–150 mg/day).

In patients with rheumatoid arthritis, ANSAID may be used in combination with gold salts or corticosteroids.

INDICATIONS AND USAGE

ANSAID Tablets are indicated for the acute or long-term treatment of the signs and symptoms of rheumatoid arthritis and osteoarthritis.

CONTRAINDICATIONS

ANSAID Tablets are contraindicated in patients who have previously demonstrated hypersensitivity to it. ANSAID should not be given to patients in whom ANSAID, aspirin, or other nonsteroidal anti-inflammatory drugs induce asthma, urticaria, or other allergic-type reactions. Fatal asthmatic reactions have been reported in such patients receiving this type of drug.

WARNINGS

Risk of Gastrointestinal (GI) Ulcerations, Bleeding and Perforation with Nonsteroidal Anti-inflammatory Therapy

Serious gastrointestinal toxicity, such as bleeding, ulceration, and perforation, can occur at any time, with or without warning symptoms, in patients treated chronically with nonsteroidal anti-inflammatory drugs. Although minor upper GI problems, such as dyspepsia, are common, usually developing early in therapy, physicians should remain alert for ulceration and bleeding in patients treated chronically with nonsteroidal anti-inflammatory drugs, even in the absence of previous GI tract symptoms. In patients observed in clinical trials of such agents for several months to two years, symptomatic upper GI ulcers, gross bleeding, or perforation appear to occur in approximately 1% of patients treated for 3–6 months, and in about 2–4% of patients treated for one year. Physicians should inform patients about the signs and/fd,50 or symptoms of serious GI toxicity and what steps to take if they occur.

Studies to date have not identified any subset of patients not at risk of developing peptic ulceration and bleeding. Except for a prior history of serious GI events and other risk factors known to be associated with peptic ulcer disease, such as alcoholism, smoking, etc., no risk factors (e.g., age, sex) have been associated with increased risk. Elderly or debilitated patients seem to tolerate ulceration or bleeding less well than other individuals and most spontaneous reports of fatal GI events are in this population. Studies to date are inconclusive concerning the relative risk of various nonsteroidal anti-inflammatory agents in causing such reactions. High doses of any such agent probably carry a greater risk of these reactions, although controlled clinical trials showing this do not exist in most cases. In considering the use of relatively large doses (within the recommended dosage range), sufficient benefit should be anticipated to off-set the potential increased risk of GI toxicity.

Because serious GI tract ulceration and bleeding can occur without warning symptoms, physicians should follow chronically treated patients for the signs and symptoms of ulceration and bleeding and should inform the patients of the importance of this follow-up.

PRECAUTIONS

General Precautions

Impaired Renal or Hepatic Function: As with other nonsteroidal anti-inflammatory drugs, ANSAID Tablets should be used with caution in patients with impaired renal or hepatic function, or a history of kidney or liver disease. Studies to assess the pharmacokinetics of ANSAID in patients with decreased liver function have not been done.

Renal Effects: Toxicology studies in rats have shown renal papillary necrosis at dosage levels equivalent on a mg/kg basis to those used clinically in humans. Similar findings were seen in monkeys given high doses (50–100 mg/kg, or approximately 20–40 times the human therapeutic dose) for 90 days.

In Upjohn clinical studies, kidney function tests were done at least monthly in patients taking ANSAID. In these studies, renal effects of ANSAID were similar to those seen with other nonsteroidal anti-inflammatory drugs.

A second form of renal toxicity has been seen in patients with prerenal conditions leading to a reduction in renal blood flow or blood volume, where the renal prostaglandins have a supportive role in the maintenance of renal perfusion. In these patients administration of a nonsteroidal anti-inflammatory drug may cause a dose-dependent reduction in prostaglandin formation, which may precipitate overt renal decompensation. Patients at greatest risk of this reaction are those with impaired renal function, heart failure, liver dysfunction, those taking diuretics, and the elderly. Discontinuation of nonsteroidal anti-inflammatory drug therapy is typically followed by recovery of the pretreatment state. Those patients at high risk who chronically take ANSAID should have renal function monitored if they have signs or symptoms that may be consistent with mild azotemia, such as malaise, fatigue, loss of appetite, etc. Occasional patients may develop some elevation of serum creatinine and BUN levels without signs or symptoms.

The elimination half-life of flurbiprofen was unchanged in patients with end stage renal disease (ESRD). Flurbiprofen metabolites are primarily eliminated by the kidneys and elimination of 4-hydroxy-flurbiprofen was markedly reduced in ESRD patients. Therefore, patients with significantly impaired renal function may require a reduction of dosage to avoid accumulation of flurbiprofen metabolites and should be monitored. (See also the CLINICAL PHARMACOLOGY section.)

Liver Tests: As with other nonsteroidal anti-inflammatory drugs, borderline elevations of one or more liver tests may occur in up to 15% of patients. These abnormalities may progress, may remain essentially unchanged, or may disappear with continued therapy. The ALT (SGPT) test is probably the most sensitive indicator of liver injury. Meaningful (3 times the upper limit of normal) elevations of ALT or AST (SGOT) have been reported in controlled clinical trials in less than 1% of patients. A patient with symptoms and/or signs suggesting liver dysfunction, or in whom an abnormal liver test has occurred, should be evaluated for evidence of the development of a more severe hepatic reaction while on therapy with flurbiprofen.

Anemia: Anemia is commonly observed in rheumatoid arthritis and is sometimes aggravated by nonsteroidal anti-inflammatory drugs, which may produce fluid retention or minor gastrointestinal blood loss in some patients. Therefore, patients who have initial hemoglobin values of 10 g/dL or less, and who are to receive long-term therapy, should have hemoglobin values determined periodically.

Fluid Retention and Edema: Fluid retention and edema have been reported; therefore, ANSAID should be used with caution in patients with cardiac decompensation, hypertension, or similar conditions.

Vision Changes: Blurred and/or diminished vision has been reported with the use of ANSAID and other nonsteroi-

Continued on next page

Information on these Upjohn products is based on labeling in effect June 1, 1992. Further information concerning these and other Upjohn products may be obtained by direct inquiry to Medical Information, The Upjohn Company, Kalamazoo, Michigan 49001.

Upjohn—Cont.

dal anti-inflammatory drugs. Patients experiencing eye complaints should have ophthalmologic examinations.

Effect on Platelets and Coagulation: Flurbiprofen inhibits collagen-induced platelet aggregation. Prolongation of bleeding time by flurbiprofen has been demonstrated in humans after single and multiple oral doses. Patients who may be adversely affected by prolonged bleeding time should be carefully observed when ANSAID is administered.

Information for Patients: ANSAID, like other drugs of its class, is not free of side effects. The side effects of these drugs can cause discomfort and, rarely, there are more serious side effects, such as gastrointestinal bleeding, which may result in hospitalization and even fatal outcomes. Nonsteroidal anti-inflammatory drugs are often essential agents in the management of arthritis, but they also may be commonly employed for conditions which are less serious. Physicians may wish to discuss with their patients the potential risks (see WARNINGS, PRECAUTIONS, and ADVERSE REACTIONS sections) and likely benefits of nonsteroidal anti-inflammatory drug treatment, particularly when the drugs are used for less serious conditions where treatment without such agents may represent an acceptable alternative to both the patient and the physician.

Drug Interactions

Antacids: Administration of ANSAID to volunteers under fasting conditions, or with antacid suspension, yielded similar serum flurbiprofen-time profiles in young subjects (n=12). In geriatric subjects (n=7) there was a reduction in the rate but not the extent of flurbiprofen absorption.

Anticoagulants: Flurbiprofen, like other nonsteroidal anti-inflammatory drugs, has been shown to affect bleeding parameters in patients receiving anticoagulants, and serious clinical bleeding has been reported. The physician should be cautious when administering ANSAID to patients taking anticoagulants.

Aspirin: Concurrent administration of aspirin and flurbiprofen resulted in 50% lower serum flurbiprofen concentrations. This effect of aspirin (which also lowers serum concentrations of other nonsteroidal anti-inflammatory drugs given with it) has been demonstrated in patients with rheumatoid arthritis (n=15) as well as normal volunteers (n=16). Concurrent use of ANSAID and aspirin is therefore not recommended.

Beta-adrenergic Blocking Agents: The effect of flurbiprofen on blood pressure response to propranolol and atenolol was evaluated in men with mild uncomplicated hypertension (n=10). Flurbiprofen pretreatment attenuated the hypotensive effect of a single dose of propranolol but not atenolol. Flurbiprofen did not appear to affect the beta-blocker-mediated reduction in heart rate. Flurbiprofen did not affect the pharmacokinetic profile of either drug, and the mechanism underlying the interference with propranolol's hypotensive effect is unknown. Patients taking both flurbiprofen and a beta-blocker should be monitored to ensure that a satisfactory hypotensive effect is achieved.

Cimetidine, Ranitidine: In normal volunteers (n=9), pretreatment with cimetidine or ranitidine did not affect flurbiprofen pharmacokinetics, except that a small (13%) but statistically significant increase in the area under the serum concentration curve of flurbiprofen resulted with cimetidine.

Digoxin: Studies of concomitant administration of flurbiprofen and digoxin to healthy men (n=14) did not show a change in the steady state serum levels of either drug.

Diuretics: Studies in normal volunteers have shown that flurbiprofen, like other nonsteroidal anti-inflammatory drugs, can interfere with the effects of furosemide. Although results have varied from study to study, effects have been shown on furosemide-stimulated diuresis, natriuresis, and kaliuresis. Other nonsteroidal anti-inflammatory drugs that inhibit prostaglandin synthesis have been shown to interfere with thiazide diuretics in some studies, and with potassium-sparing diuretics. Patients receiving ANSAID and furosemide or other diuretics should be observed closely to determine if the desired effect is obtained.

Oral Hypoglycemia Agents: In one study, flurbiprofen was given to adult diabetics who were already receiving glyburide (n=4), metformin (n=2), chlorpropamide with phenformin (n=3), or glyburide with phenformin (n=6). Although there was a slight reduction in blood sugar concentrations during concomitant administration of flurbiprofen and hypoglycemic agents, there were no signs or symptoms of hypoglycemia.

Carcinogenesis, Mutagenesis, impairment of Fertility

An 80-week study in mice at doses of 2, 5, and 12/mg/kg/day and a 2-year study in rats at doses of 0.5, 2, and 4 mg/kg/day did not show evidence of carcinogenicity at maximum tolerated doses of flurbiprofen.

Flurbiprofen did not impair the fertility of male or female rats treated orally at 2.25 mg/kg/day for 65 days and 16 days, respectively, before mating.

Teratogenic Effects: Pregnancy Category B

In teratology studies flurbiprofen, given to mice in doses up to 12 mg/kg/day, to rats in doses up to 25 mg/kg/day, and to rabbits in doses up to 7.5 mg/kg/day, showed no teratogenic effects.

Because there re no adequate and well-controlled studies in pregnant women, and animal teratology studies do not always predict human response, ANSAID is not recommended for use in pregnancy.

Labor and Delivery: The effects of ANSAID on labor and delivery in women are not known. As with other drugs known to inhibit prostaglandin synthesis, an increased incidence of dystocia and delayed parturition occurred in rats treated throughout pregnancy. Because of the known effects of prostaglandin-inhibiting drugs on the fetal cardiovascular system (closure of the ductus arteriosus), use of ANSAID during late pregnancy is not recommended.

Nursing Mothers: Concentrations of flurbiprofen in breast milk and plasma of nursing mothers suggested that a nursing infant could receive approximately 0.10 mg flurbiprofen per day in the established milk of a woman taking 200 mg/day. Because of possible adverse effects of prostaglandin-inhibiting drugs on neonates, ANSAID is not recommended for use in nursing mothers.

Pediatric Use: Safety and effectiveness in children have not been established.

ADVERSE REACTIONS

Adverse reaction information was derived from patients who received flurbiprofen in blinded-controlled and open-label clinical trials, and from worldwide marketing experience and from publications. In the description below, rates of the more common events (greater than 1%) and many of the less common events (less than 1%) represent clinical study results. For rarer events that were derived principally from worldwide marketing experience and the literature (printed in *italics*), accurate rate estimates are generally impossible. Of the 4123 patients in premarketing studies, 2954 were treated for at least 1 month, 1448 for at least 3 months, 948 for at least 6 months, 356 for at least 1 year, and 100 for at least 2 years. Of the 4123 patients, 9.4% dropped out of the studies because of an adverse drug reaction, principally involving the gastrointestinal tract (5.8%) central nervous system and special senses (1.4%), skin (0.6%) and genitourinary tract (0.5%).

Incidence Greater Than 1%

An asterisk after a reaction identifies reactions which occurred in 3–9% of patients treated with flurbiprofen. Reactions occurring in 1–3% of the patients are unmarked.

Gastrointestinal: Dyspepsia*, diarrhea*, abdominal pain*, nausea*, constipation, GI bleeding, flatulence, elevated liver enzymes, and vomiting.

Central Nervous System: Headache*, nervousness, and other manifestations of CNS "stimulation" (e.g., anxiety, insomnia, reflexes increased, and tremor), and symptoms associated with CNS "inhibition" (e.g., amnesia, asthenia, somnolence, malaise, and depression).

Respiratory: Rhinitis.

Dermatological: Rash.

Special Senses: Dizziness, tinnitus, and changes in vision.

Genitourinary: Signs and symptoms suggesting urinary tract infection*.

Body as a Whole: Edema*.

Metabolic/Nutritional: Body weight changes.

Incidence Less than 1%
(Causal Relationship Probable)

The reactions listed in this category occurred in <1% of patients in the clinical trials or were reported during postmarketing experience from other countries. Adverse reactions reported only in worldwide postmarketing experience or the literture (which presumably indicates that they are rarer) are italicized.

Gastrointestinal: Peptic ulcer disease (see also **WARNINGS, Risk of Gastrointestinal (GI) Ulcerations, Bleeding and Perforation with Nonsteroidal Anti-inflammatory Therapy)**, gastritis, bloody diarrhea, stomatitis, esophageal disease, hematemesis, and hepatitis; *cholestatic and non-cholestatic jaundice.*

Central Nervous System: Ataxia, cerebrovascular ischemia, confusion, parethesia, and twitching.

Hematologic: Decrease in hemoglobin and hematocrit, iron deficiency anemia, *hemolytic anemia* and *aplastic anemia*; leukopenia; eosinophilia; ecchymosis and *thrombocytopenia.* (See also **PRECAUTIONS, Effect On Platelets and Coagulation.)**

Respiratory: Asthma and epistaxis.

Dermatological: Angioedema, urticaria, eczema, and pruritus; *photosensitivity, toxic epidermal necrolysis,* and *exfoliative dermatitis.*

Special Senses: Conjunctivitis and parosmia.

Genitourinary: Hematuria and renal failure; *interstititial nephritis.*

Body as a Whole: Chills and fever; *anaphylactic reaction.*

Metabolic/Nutritional: Hyperuricemia.

Cardiovascular: Heart failure, hypertension, vascular diseases and vasodilation.

Incidence Less than 1% (Causal Relationship Unknown)

The following reactions have been reported in patients taking flurbiprofen under circumstances that do not permit a clear attribution of the reaction to flurbiprofen. These reactions are being included as alerting information for physicians. Adverse reactions reported only in worldwide postmarketing experience or the literature (which presumably indicates that they are rarer) are italicized.

Gastrointestinal: Periodontal abscess, appetite changes, cholecystitis, and dry mouth.

Central Nervous System: Convulsion, meningitis, hypertonia, cerebrovascular accident, emotional lability, and subarachnoid hemorrhage.

Hematologic: Lymphadenopathy.

Respiratory: Bronchitis, laryngitis, dyspnea, pulmonary embolism, pulmonary infarct, and hyperventilation.

Dermatological: Alopecia, nail disorder, herpes simplex, zoster, dry skin, and sweating.

Special Senses: Ear disease, corneal opacity, glaucoma, retrobulbar neuritis, changes in taste, and transient hearing loss; *retinal hemorrhage.*

Genitourinary: Menstrual disturbances, vaginal and uterine hemorrhage, vulvovaginitis, and prostate disease.

Metabolic/Nutritional: Hyperkalemia.

Cardiovascular: Arrhythmias, angina pectoris, and myocardial infarction.

Musculoskeletal: Myasthenia.

DRUG ABUSE AND DEPENDENCE

No drug abuse or drug dependence has been observed with ANSAID.

OVERDOSAGE

Information on overdosage is available for 13 children and 12 adults. Nine of the 13 children were less than 6 years old. Drowsiness occurred after doses of 150 to 800 mg in 3 of these young children (with dilated pupils in 1), and in a 2-year-old who also had semi-consciousness, pinpoint pupils, diminished tone, and elevated liver enzymes. Other children who ingested doses of 200 mg to 2.5 g showed no symptoms.

Among the adults, a 70-year-old man with a history of chronic obstructive airway disease died. Toxicological analysis showed acute flurbiprofen overdose and a blood ethanol concentration of 100 mg/dL. In the other cases, symptoms were as follows: coma and respiratory depression after 3–6 g; drowsiness, nausea and epigastric pain after 2.5–5 g; epigastric pain and dizziness after 3 g; headache and nausea after ≤ 2 g; agitation after 1.5 g; and drowsiness after 1.0 g. One patient, who took 200–400 mg flurbiprofen and 2.4 g fenoprofen, had disorientation and diplopia. Three adults had no symptoms after 3–5 g flurbiprofen.

Treatment of an overdose: the stomach should be emptied by vomiting or lavage, though little drug will likely be recovered if more than an hour has elapsed since ingestion. Supportive treatment should be instituted as necessary. Some patients have been given supplemental oral or intravenous fluids and required no other treatment.

In mice, the flurbiprofen LD_{50} was 750 mg/kg when administered orally and 200 mg/kg when administered intraperitoneally. The primary signs of toxicity were prostration, ataxia, loss of righting reflex, labored respiration, twitches, convulsions, CNS depression, and splayed hind limbs. In rats, the flurbiprofen LD_{50} was 160 mg/kg when administered orally and 400 mg/kg when administered intraperitoneally. The primary signs of toxicity were tremors, convulsions, labored respiration, and prostration. These were observed mostly in the intraperitoneal studies.

DOSAGE AND ADMINISTRATION

ANSAID Tablets are administered orally.

Rheumatoid arthritis and osteoarthritis: Recommended starting dose is 200 to 300 mg total daily dose administered BID, TID, or QID. (Most experience in rheumatoid arthritis has been with TID or QID dosage.) The largest recommended single dose in a multiple-dose daily regimen is 100 mg. The dose should be tailored to each patient according to the severity of the symptoms and the response to therapy.

Although a few patients have received higher doses, doses above 300 mg per day are not recommended until more clinical experience with ANSAID is obtained.

HOW SUPPLIED

ANSAID Tablets 50 mg (white)

Bottles of 100	NDC 0009-0170-07
Bottles of 500	NDC 0009-0170-09
Unit Dose (blister pack) packages of 100	NDC 0009-0170-08

ANSAID Tablets 100 mg (blue)

Bottles of 100	NDC 0009-0305-03
Bottles of 500	NDC 0009-0305-05
Unit Dose (blister pack) packages of 100	NDC 0009-0305-06

Store at controlled room temperature 15°-30°C (59°-86°F).

Code 813 094 002

Shown in Product Identification Section, page 433

ATGAM®   ℞

brand of lymphocyte immune globulin, anti-thymocyte globulin [equine] sterile solution

For Intravenous Use Only

WARNING

Only physicians experienced in immunosuppressive therapy in the management of renal transplant or aplastic anemia patients should use ATGAM.

Patients receiving ATGAM should be managed in facilities equipped and staffed with adequate laboratory and supportive medical resources.

DESCRIPTION

ATGAM Sterile Solution contains lymphocyte immune globulin, anti-thymocyte globulin [equine]. It is the purified, concentrated, and sterile gamma globulin, primarily monomeric IgG, from hyperimmune serum of horses immunized with human thymus lymphocytes. ATGAM is a transparent to slightly opalescent aqueous protein solution. It may appear colorless to faintly pink or brown and is nearly odorless. It may develop a slight granular or flaky deposit during storage. (For information about in-line filters, see Infusion Instructions in the DOSAGE AND ADMINISTRATION SECTION).

Before release for clinical use, each lot of ATGAM is tested to assure its ability to inhibit rosette formation between human peripheral lymphocytes and sheep red blood cells *in vitro*. In each lot, antibody activity against human red blood cells and platelets is also measured and determined to be within acceptable limits. Only lots that test negative for antihuman serum protein antibody, antiglomerular basement membrane antibody and pyrogens are released.

Each milliliter of ATGAM contains 50 mg of horse gamma globulin stabilized in 0.3 molar glycine to a pH of approximately 6.8; preserved with thimerosal (mercury derivative) 1:10,000 (0.01%).

CLINICAL AND ANIMAL PHARMACOLOGY

ATGAM Sterile Solution is a lymphocyte-selective immunosuppressant as is demonstrated by its ability to reduce the number of circulating, thymus-dependent lymphocytes that form rosettes with sheep erythrocytes. This antilymphocytic effect is believed to reflect an alteration of the function of the T-lymphocytes, which are responsible in part for cell-mediated immunity and are involved in humoral immunity. In addition to its antilymphocytic activity, ATGAM contains low concentrations of antibodies against other formed elements of the blood. In rhesus and cynomolgus monkeys, ATGAM reduces lymphocytes in the thymus-dependent areas of the spleen and lymph nodes. It also decreases the circulating sheep-erythrocyte-rosetting lymphocytes that can be detected, but ordinarily ATGAM does not cause severe lymphopenia.

In general, when ATGAM is given with other immunosuppressive therapy, such as antimetabolites and corticosteroids, the patient's own antibody response to horse gamma globulin is minimal. In a small clinical study, ATGAM administered with other immunosuppressive therapy and measured as horse IgG had a serum half-life of 5.7 ± 3 days.

INDICATIONS AND USAGE

Renal Transplantation

ATGAM Sterile Solution is indicated for the management of allograft rejection in renal transplant patients. When administered with conventional therapy at the time of rejection, it increases the frequency of resolution of the acute rejection episode. The drug has also been administered as an adjunct to other immunosuppressive therapy to delay the onset of the first rejection episode. Data accumulated to date have not consistently demonstrated improvement in functional graft survival associated with therapy to delay the onset of the first rejection episode.

Aplastic Anemia

ATGAM is indicated for the treatment of moderate to severe aplastic anemia in patients who are unsuitable for bone marrow transplantation.

When administered with a regimen of supportive care, ATGAM may induce partial or complete hematologic remission. In a controlled trial, patients receiving ATGAM showed a statistically significant higher improvement rate compared to standard supportive care at 3 months. Improvement was defined in terms of sustained increase in peripheral blood counts and reduced transfusion needs.

Clinical trials conducted at two centers evaluated the one year survival rate for patients with severe and moderate to severe aplastic anemia. Seventy-four of the 83 patients enrolled were evaluable based on response to treatment. The treatment groups studied consisted of: 1) ATGAM and supportive care, 2) ATGAM administered following 3 months of supportive care alone, 3) ATGAM, mismatched marrow infusion, androgens and supportive care, or 4) ATGAM, androgens and supportive care. There were no statistically signifi-

cant differences between the treatment groups. The one year survival rate for the pooled treatment groups was 69%. These survival results can be compared to a historical survival rate of about 25% for patients receiving standard supportive care alone.

The usefulness of ATGAM has not been demonstrated in patients with aplastic anemia who are suitable candidates for bone marrow transplantation or in patients with aplastic anemia secondary to neoplastic disease, storage disease, myelofibrosis, Fanconi's syndrome or in patients known to have been exposed to myelotoxic agents or radiation.

To date, safety and efficacy have not been established in circumstances other than renal transplantation and aplastic anemia.

Skin Testing

Before the first infusion of ATGAM, The Upjohn Company strongly recommends that patients be tested with an intradermal injection of 0.1 mL of a 1:1000 dilution (5μg horse IgG) of ATGAM in Sodium Chloride Injection, USP and a contralateral Sodium Chloride Injection control. Use only freshly diluted ATGAM for skin testing. The patient and specifically the skin test should be observed every 15 to 20 minutes over the first hour after intradermal injection. A local reaction of 10 mm or greater with a wheal or erythema or both with or without pseudopod formation and itching or a marked local swelling should be considered a positive test. Note: The predictive value of this test has not been proven clinically. Allergic reactions such as anaphylaxis have occurred in patients whose skin test is negative. In the presence of a locally positive skin test to ATGAM, serious consideration to alternative forms of therapy should be given. The risk to benefit ratio must be carefully weighed. If therapy with ATGAM is deemed appropriate following a locally positive skin test, treatment should be administered in a setting where intensive life support facilities are immediately available and with a physician familiar with the treatment of potentially life threatening allergic reactions in attendance. **A systemic reaction such as a generalized rash, tachycardia, dyspnea, hypotension, or anaphylaxis precludes any additional administration of ATGAM.**

SEE WARNINGS, PRECAUTIONS, AND ADVERSE REACTIONS.

CONTRAINDICATIONS

Do not administer ATGAM Sterile Solution to a patient who has had a severe systemic reaction during prior administration of ATGAM or any other equine gamma globulin preparation.

WARNINGS

Only physicians experienced in immunosuppressive therapy in the management of renal transplant or aplastic anemia patients should use ATGAM.

Patients receiving ATGAM should be managed in facilities equipped and staffed with adequate laboratory and supportive medical resources.

Precise methods of determining the potency of ATGAM have not been established, thus activity may potentially vary from lot to lot.

Discontinue treatment with ATGAM if any of the following occurs:

1. Symptoms of anaphylaxis (See ADVERSE REACTIONS)
2. Severe and unremitting thrombocytopenia in renal transplant patients
3. Severe and unremitting leukopenia in renal transplant patients

In common with products derived from, or purified with human blood components, the possibility of transmission of infectious agents exists.

PRECAUTIONS

Because ATGAM Sterile Solution is an immunosuppressive agent ordinarily given with corticosteroids and antimetabolites, watch patients carefully for signs of leukopenia, thrombocytopenia or concurrent infection. Several studies have suggested an increase in the incidence of cytomegalovirus infection in patients receiving ATGAM. In one study it has been found that it may be possible to reduce this risk by decreasing the dosage of other immunosuppressive agents administered concomitantly with ATGAM. If infection occurs, institute appropriate adjunctive therapy promptly. On the basis of the clinical circumstances, a physician should decide whether or not therapy with ATGAM will continue.

Pregnancy category C: ATGAM has not been evaluated in either pregnant or lactating women. Animal reproduction studies have not been conducted with ATGAM. It is also not known whether ATGAM can cause fetal harm when administered to a pregnant woman or can affect reproduction capacity. Administration of ATGAM to pregnant women is not recommended and should be considered only under exceptional circumstances.

The safety and effectiveness of ATGAM have been demonstrated only in renal transplant patients who receive concomitant immunosuppressive therapy.

Experience with children has been limited. ATGAM has been administered safely to a small number of pediatric renal allograft recipients and pediatric aplastic anemia patients at dosage levels comparable to those in adults.

Dilution of ATGAM in Dextrose Injection, USP, is not recommended, as low salt concentrations may result in precipitation. The use of highly acidic infusion solutions is also not recommended because of possible physical instability over time.

DRUG INTERACTIONS

We do not recommend the dilution of ATGAM Sterile Solution in Dextrose Injection, USP, as low salt concentrations may cause precipitation. The use of highly acidic infusion solutions is also not recommended because of possible physical instability over time. When the dose of corticosteroids and other immunosuppressants is being reduced, some previously masked reactions to ATGAM may appear. Under these circumstances, observe patients especially carefully during therapy with ATGAM.

ADVERSE REACTIONS

Renal Transplantation

The primary clinical experience with ATGAM Sterile Solution has been in renal allograft patients who were also receiving concurrent standard immunosuppressive therapy (azathioprine, corticosteroids). In controlled trials, investigators frequently reported the following adverse reactions: fever in 1 patient in 3; chills in 1 patient in 7; leukopenia in 1 patient in 7; thrombocytopenia in 1 patient in 9; and dermatological reactions, such as rash, pruritus, urticaria, wheal, and flare, in 1 patient in 8. The following reactions were reported in more than 1% but less than 5% of the patients: arthralgia, chest or back pain or both, clotted A/V fistula, diarrhea, dyspnea, headache, hypotension, nausea or vomiting or both, night sweats, pain at the infusion site, peripheral thrombophlebitis, and stomatitis.

Reactions reported in less than 1% of the patients in the controlled trials were anaphylaxis, dizziness, weakness or faintness, edema, herpes simplex reactivation, hiccoughs or epigastric pain, hyperglycemia, hypertension, iliac vein obstruction, laryngospasm, localized infection, lymphadenopathy, malaise, myalgia, paresthesia, possible serum sickness, pulmonary edema, renal artery thrombosis, seizures, systemic infection, tachycardia, toxic epidermal necrosis, and wound dehiscence.

Aplastic Anemia

In premarketing clinical trials with ATGAM in the treatment of aplastic anemia, patients were also being concurrently managed with support therapy (transfusions, steroids, antibiotics, antihistamines).

In these trials most patients experienced fever and skin reactions. Other frequently reported adverse reactions were chills, 1 patient in 2; arthralgia, 1 patient in 2; headache, 1 patient in 6; myalgia, 1 patient in 10; nausea, 1 patient in 15; chest pain, 1 patient in 15 and phlebitis, 1 patient in 20.

The following reactions were reported by at least 1 patient, and less than 5% of the total patients: diaphoresis, joint stiffness, periorbital edema, aches, edema, muscle ache, vomiting, agitation/lethargy, listlessness, lightheadedness, seizures, diarrhea, bradycardia, myocarditis, cardiac irregularity, hepatosplenomegaly, possible encephalitis or post viral encephalopathy, hypotension, congestive heart failure, hypertension, burning soles/palms, foot sole pain, lymphadenopathy, post-cervical lymphadenopathy, tender lymph nodes, bilateral pleural effusion, respiratory distress, anaphylactic reaction, and proteinuria.

In other support studies in patients with aplastic anemia and other hematologic abnormalities who have received ATGAM, abnormal tests of liver function (SGOT, SGPT, alkaline phosphatase) and renal function (serum creatinine) have been observed. In some trials, clinical and laboratory findings of serum sickness were seen in a majority of patients.

Post-Marketing Experience

During approximately five years of post-approval marketing experience, the frequency of adverse reactions in voluntarily reported cases is as follows: fever 51%; chills 16%; thrombocytopenia 30%; leukopenia 14%; rashes 27%; systemic infection 13%. Events reported in 5 to 10% of reported cases include: abnormal renal function tests, serum sickness-like symptoms, dyspnea/apnea, arthralgia, chest, back or flank pain, diarrhea and nausea and/or vomiting. Events reported with a frequency of less than 5% include: hypertension, Herpes Simplex infection, pain, swelling or redness at infusion site, eosinophilia, headache, myalgias or leg pains, hypotension, anaphylaxis, tachycardia, edema, localized infection, malaise, seizures, GI bleeding or perforation, deep vein

Continued on next page

Information on these Upjohn products is based on labeling in effect June 1, 1992. Further information concerning these and other Upjohn products may be obtained by direct inquiry to Medical Information, The Upjohn Company, Kalamazoo, Michigan 49001.

Upjohn—Cont.

thrombosis, sore mouth/throat, hyperglycemia, acute renal failure, abnormal liver function tests, confusion or disorientation, cough, neutropenia or granulocytopenia, anemia, thrombophlebitis, dizziness, epigastric or stomach pain, lymphadenopathy, pulmonary edema or congestive heart failure, abdominal pain, nosebleed, vasculitis, aplasia or pancytopenia, abnormal involuntary movement or tremor, rigidity, sweating, laryngospasm/edema, hemolysis or hemolytic anemia, viral hepatitis, faintness, enlarged or ruptured kidney, paresthesias and renal artery thrombosis.

The recommended management for some of the adverse reactions that could occur with treatment with ATGAM follows:

1. **Anaphylaxis** is uncommon but serious and may occur at any time during therapy with ATGAM. Stop infusion of ATGAM immediately; administer 0.3 mL aqueous epinephrine (1:1000 solution) intramuscularly. Administer steroids, assist respiration, and provide other resuscitative measures. DO NOT resume therapy with ATGAM.
2. **Hemolysis** can usually be detected only in the laboratory. Clinically significant hemolysis has been reported rarely. Appropriate treatment of hemolysis may include transfusion of erythrocytes; if necessary, administer intravenous mannitol, furosemide, sodium bicarbonate, and fluids. Severe and unremitting hemolysis may require discontinuation of therapy with ATGAM.
3. **Thrombocytopenia** is usually transient in renal transplant patients; platelet counts generally return to adequate levels without discontinuing therapy with ATGAM. Platelet transfusions may be necessary in patients with aplastic anemia. (See PRECAUTIONS, WARNINGS and DOSAGE AND ADMINISTRATION.)
4. **Respiratory distress** may indicate an anaphylactoid reaction. Discontinue infusion of ATGAM. If distress persists, administer an antihistamine or epinephrine or corticosteroids or some combination of the three.
5. **Pain in chest, flank or back** may indicate anaphylaxis or hemolysis. Treatment is that indicated above for those conditions.
6. **Hypotension** may indicate anaphylaxis. Stop infusion of ATGAM and stabilize blood pressure with pressors if necessary.
7. **Chills and fever** occur frequently in patients receiving ATGAM. ATGAM may release endogenous leukocyte pyrogens. Prophylactic and/or therapeutic administration of antihistamines, antipyretics or corticosteroids generally controls this reaction.
8. **Chemical phlebitis** can be caused by infusion of ATGAM through peripheral veins. This can often be avoided by administering the infusion solution into a high-flow vein. A subcutaneous arterialized vein produced by a Brescia fistula is also a useful administration site.
9. **Itching and erythema** probably result from the effect of ATGAM on blood elements. Antihistamines generally control the symptoms.
10. **Serum sickness-like symptoms** in aplastic anemia patients have been treated with oral or IV corticosteroids. Resolution of symptoms has generally been prompt and long-term sequelae have not been observed. Prophylactic administration of corticosteroids may decrease the frequency of this reaction.

OVERDOSAGE

Because of its mode of action and because it is a biologic substance, the maximal tolerated dose of ATGAM Sterile Solution would be expected to vary from patient to patient. To date, the largest single daily dose administered to a patient, a renal transplant recipient, was 7000 mg administered at a concentration of approximately 10 mg/mL Sodium Chloride Injection, USP, approximately 7 times the recommended total dose and infusion concentration. In this patient, administration of ATGAM was not associated with any signs of acute intoxication.

The greatest number of doses (10 to 20 mg/kg/dose) that can be administered to a single patient has not yet been determined. Some renal transplant patients have received up to 50 doses in 4 months, and others have received 28-day courses of 21 doses followed by as many as 3 more courses for the treatment of acute rejection. The incidence of toxicologic manifestations did not increase with any of these regimens.

DOSAGE AND ADMINISTRATION

Renal Allograft Recipients
Adult renal allograft patients have received ATGAM Sterile Solution at the dosage of 10 to 30 mg/kg of body weight daily. The few children studied received 5 to 25 mg/kg daily. ATGAM has been used to delay the onset of the first rejection episodes[1-4] and at the time of the first rejection episode.[5-9] Most patients who received ATGAM for the treatment of acute rejection had not received it starting at the time of transplantation.

Usually, ATGAM is used concomitantly with azathioprine and corticosteroids, which are commonly used to suppress

the immune response. Exercise caution during repeat courses of ATGAM; carefully observe patients for signs of allergic reactions.

Delaying the Onset of Allograft Rejection: Give a fixed dose of 15 mg/kg daily for 14 days, then every other day for 14 days for a total of 21 doses in 28 days. Administer the first dose within 24 hours before or after the transplant.

Treatment of Rejection: The first dose of ATGAM can be delayed until the diagnosis of the first rejection episode. The recommended dose is 10 to 15 mg/kg daily for 14 days. Additional alternate-day therapy up to a total of 21 doses can be given.

Aplastic Anemia
The recommended dosage regimen is 10 to 20 mg/kg daily for 8 to 14 days. Additional alternate-day therapy up to a total of 21 doses can be administered[10-12]. Because thrombocytopenia can be associated with the administration of ATGAM, patients receiving it for the treatment of aplastic anemia may need prophylactic platelet transfusions to maintain platelets at clinically acceptable levels.

Preparation of Solution
Parenteral drug products should be inspected visually for particulate matter and discoloration prior to administration whenever solution and container permit. However, because ATGAM is a gamma globulin product, it can be transparent to slightly opalescent, colorless to faintly pink or brown and may develop a slight granular or flaky deposit during storage. ATGAM (diluted or undiluted) should not be shaken because excessive foaming and/or denaturation of the protein may occur.

Dilute ATGAM for intravenous infusion in an inverted bottle of sterile vehicle so the undiluted ATGAM does not contact the air inside. Add the total daily dose of ATGAM to the sterile vehicle (see Compatibility and Stability). The concentration should not exceed 4 mg of ATGAM per mL. The diluted solution should be gently rotated or swirled to effect thorough mixing.

Administration
The diluted ATGAM should be allowed to reach room temperature before infusion. ATGAM is appropriately administered into a vascular shunt, arterial venous fistula, or a high-flow central vein through an in-line filter with a pore size of 0.2 to 1.0 micron. The in-line filter should be used with all infusions of ATGAM to prevent the administration of any insoluble material that may develop in the product during storage. The use of high-flow veins will minimize the occurrence of phlebitis and thrombosis. Do not infuse a dose of ATGAM in less than 4 hours. Always keep appropriate resuscitation equipment at the patient's bedside while ATGAM is being administered. Observe the patient continuously for possible allergic reactions throughout the infusions (See ADVERSE REACTIONS).

Compatibility and Stability
ATGAM, once diluted, has been shown to be physically and chemically stable for up to 24 hours at concentrations of up to 4 mg per mL in the following diluents: 0.9% Sodium Chloride Injection, 5% Dextrose and 0.225% Sodium Chloride Injection, and 5% Dextrose and 0.45% Sodium Chloride Injection.

Adding ATGAM to Dextrose Injection is not recommended, as low salt concentrations can cause precipitation. Highly acidic infusion solutions can also contribute to physical instability over time. It is recommended that diluted ATGAM be stored in a refrigerator if it is prepared prior to the time of infusion. Even if it is stored in a refrigerator, the total time in dilution should not exceed 24 hours (including infusion time).

HOW SUPPLIED
ATGAM Sterile Solution is supplied in 5 mL ampoules containing 50 mg of horse gamma globulin/mL, NDC 0009-0926-04.

STORAGE
Store in a refrigerator at 2° to 8° C. **DO NOT FREEZE.**

CAUTION
Federal law prohibits dispensing without prescription.

ANIMAL TOXICOLOGY
During the development of ATGAM Sterile Solution, aliquots of the various clinical lots were infused intravenously in either *Macaca mulatta* or *Macaca irus* monkeys. The dosage used was 100 mg/kg on day 0, 200 mg/kg on day 2 and 400 mg/kg on day 4. A 3-week observation period followed. Currently, all marketed lots are similarly tested using a dosage of 50 mg/kg on days 0, 2, 4 and 7 followed by a 3-week observation period.

Many of the changes observed could have been anticipated on the basis of the antilymphocytic activity of ATGAM. They are decreased peripheral blood lymphocytes and increased total leukocyte and neutrophil counts occurring within 24 hours after infusion, decreased thymus size with involution or atrophy or both, and decreased lymphocyte populations in the thymus-dependent areas of the spleen and lymph nodes. The atrophy was particularly common in the animals receiving the higher doses. In animals receiving either dosage regi-

men, packed cell volume, total erythrocyte counts, and hemoglobin concentrations have decreased and reticulocytes and nucleated erythrocytes have increased enough to be classified as anemia. An occasional animal death believed to have resulted from anemia has occurred. Transient decreases in blood platelet counts have also occurred. Thrombus formation occurred frequently along the routes of infusion, ie, the saphenous and femoral veins. However, the incidence of thrombi has dropped since in-line filters have been used during infusion. In these animals, definitive evidence of DIC (disseminated intravascular coagulation) has not been observed.

REFERENCES
1. Cosimi AB, Wortis HH, Delmonico FL, Russell PS: Randomized clinical trial of antithymocyte globulin in cadaver renal allograft recipients: importance of T cell monitoring. Surg 80: 155–163 (1976)
2. Wechter WJ, Brodie JA, Morrell RM, Rafi M, Schultz JR: Antithymocyte globulin (ATGAM) in renal allograft recipients. Trans 28(4):294–302 (1979)
3. Kountz SL, Butt KHM, Rao TKS, Zielinski CM, Rafi M, Schultz JR: Antithymocyte globulin (ATG) dosage and graft survival in renal transplantation. Trans Proc 9:1023–1025 (1977)
4. Butt KMH, Zielinski CM, Parsa I, Elberg AJ, Wechter WJ, Kountz SL: Trends in immunosuppression for kidney transplantation. Kidney Int 13(Suppl 8): S95–S98 (1978)
5. Filo RS, Smith EJ, Leapman SB: Reversal of acute renal allograft rejection with adjunctive ATG therapy. Trans Proc 13(1): 482–490 (1981)
6. Nowygrod R, Appel G, Hardy M: Use of ATG for reversal of acute allograft rejection. Trans Proc 13(1): 469–472 (1981).
7. Hardy MA, Nowygrod R, Elberg A, Appel G: Use of ATG in treatment of steroid-resistant rejection. Trans 29:162–164 (1980)
8. Shield CH, Cosimi AB, Tolkoff-Rubin N, Rubin R, Herrin J, Russell PS: Use of antithymocyte globulin for reversal of acute allograft rejection. Trans 28(6): 461–464 (1979)
9. Cosimi AB: The clinical value of antilymphocyte antibodies. Trans Proc 13(1): 462–468 (1981)
10. Cosimi AB, Peters C, Harmon D, Ellman L: Treatment of severe aplastic anemia with a prolonged course of antithymocyte globulin. Trans Proc 14:761–764 (1982)
11. Champlin R, Ho W, Gale R: Antithymocyte globulin treatment in patients with aplastic anemia. NEJM 308(3):113–118 (1983)
12. Doney K, Dahlberg S, Monroe D et al: Therapy of severe aplastic anemia with anti-human thymocyte globulin and androgens: The effect of HLA-haploidentical marrow infusion. Blood 63(2):342–348 (1984)
13. Rubin RH, Cosimi AB, Hirsch MS, Herrin JT: Effects of antithymocyte globulin on cytomegalovirus infection in renal transplant recipients. Trans 31(2):143–145 (1981)

Code 811 700 007

CLEOCIN HCl®   ℞
brand of clindamycin hydrochloride capsules, USP

150 mg (100's):
NSN 6505-00-159-4892 (M)

> ### WARNING
> Clindamycin therapy has been associated with severe colitis which may end fatally. Therefore, it should be reserved for serious infections where less toxic antimicrobial agents are inappropriate, as described in the Indications section. It should not be used in patients with nonbacterial infections, such as most upper respiratory tract infections. Studies indicate a toxin(s) produced by *Clostridia* is one primary cause of antibiotic associated colitis. Cholestyramine and colestipol resins have been shown to bind the toxin *in vitro*. See WARNINGS section. The colitis is usually characterized by severe, persistent diarrhea and severe abdominal cramps and may be associated with the passage of blood and mucus. Endoscopic examination may reveal pseudomembranous colitis. Stool culture for *Clostridium difficile* and stool assay for *C. difficile* toxin may be helpful diagnostically.
> When significant diarrhea occurs, the drug should be discontinued or, if necessary, continued only with close observation of the patient. Large bowel endoscopy has been recommended.
> Antiperistaltic agents such as opiates and diphenoxylate with atropine (Lomotil) may prolong and/or worsen the condition. Vancomycin has been found to be effective in the treatment of antibiotic associated pseudomembranous colitis produced by *Clostridium difficile*. The usual adult dosage is 500 milligrams to 2 grams of vancomycin orally per day in three to four divided doses administered for 7 to 10 days. Cholestyramine or coles-

tipol resins bind vancomycin *in vitro*. If both a resin and vancomycin are to be administered concurrently, it may be advisable to separate the time of administration of each drug.
Diarrhea, colitis, and pseudomembranous colitis have been observed to begin up to several weeks following cessation of therapy with clindamycin.

DESCRIPTION

Clindamycin hydrochloride is the hydrated hydrochloride salt of clindamycin. Clindamycin is a semisynthetic antibiotic produced by a 7(S)-chloro-substitution of the 7(R)-hydroxyl group of the parent compound lincomycin.
CLEOCIN HCl Capsules contain clindamycin hydrochloride equivalent to 75 mg, 150 mg or 300 mg of clindamycin.
Inactive ingredients: **75 mg**—corn starch, erythrosine sodium, FD&C blue no. 1, FD&C yellow no. 5, gelatin, lactose, magnesium stearate and talc; **150 mg**—corn starch, erythrosine sodium, FD&C blue no. 1, FD&C yellow no. 5, gelatin, lactose, magnesium stearate, talc and titanium dioxide; **300 mg**—corn starch, erythrosine sodium, FD&C blue no. 1, gelatin, lactose, magnesium, stearate, talc and titanium dioxide.
The chemical name for clindamycin hydrochloride is Methyl 7-chloro-6,7,8-trideoxy-6-(1-methyl-*trans* -4-propyl-L-2-pyrrolidinecarboxamido)-1-thio-L-*threo* -*a* -D-*galacto* -octopyranoside monohydrochloride.

CLINICAL PHARMACOLOGY

Microbiology: Clindamycin has been shown to have *in vitro* activity against isolates of the following organisms:
Aerobic gram-positive cocci, including:
Staphylococcus aureus
Staphylococcus epidermidis
(penicillinase and nonpenicillinase producing strains). When tested by *in vitro* methods some staphylococcal strains originally resistant to erythromycin rapidly develop resistance to clindamycin.
Streptococci (except *Streptococcus faecalis*)
Pneumococci
Anaerobic gram-negative bacilli, including:
Bacteroides species (including *Bacteroides fragilis* group and *Bacteroides melaninogenicus* group)
Fusobacterium species
Anaerobic gram-positive nonsporeforming bacilli, including;
Propionibacterium
Eubacterium
Actinomyces species
Anaerobic and microaerophilic gram-positive cocci, including:
Peptococcus species
Peptostreptococcus species
Microaerophilic streptococci
Clostridia: Clostridia are more resistant than most anaerobes to clindamycin. Most *Clostridium perfringens* are susceptible, but other species, eg, *Clostridium sporogenes* and *Clostridium tertium,* are frequently resistant to clindamycin. Susceptibility testing should be done.
Cross resistance has been demonstrated between clindamycin and lincomycin.
Antagonism has been demonstrated between clindamycin and erythromycin.
Human Pharmacology. Serum level studies with a 150 mg oral dose of clindamycin hydrochloride in 24 normal adult volunteers showed that clindamycin was rapidly absorbed after oral administration. An average peak serum level of 2.50 mcg/mL was reached in 45 minutes; serum levels averaged 1.51 mcg/mL at 3 hours and 0.70 mcg/mL at 6 hours. Absorption of an oral dose is virtually complete (90%), and the concomitant administration of food does not appreciably modify the serum concentrations; serum levels have been uniform and predictable from person to person and dose to dose. Serum level studies following multiple doses of CLEOCIN HCl Capsules (clindamycin hydrochloride) for up to 14 days show no evidence of accumulation or altered metabolism of drug.
Serum half-life of clindamycin is increased slightly in patients with markedly reduced renal function. Hemodialysis and peritoneal dialysis are not effective in removing clindamycin from the serum.
Concentrations of clindamycin in the serum increased linearly with increased dose. Serum levels exceed the MIC (minimum inhibitory concentration) for most indicated organisms for at least six hours following administration of the usually recommended doses. Clindamycin is widely distributed in body fluids and tissues (including bones). The average biological half-life is 2.4 hours. Approximately 10% of the bio-activity is excreted in the urine and 3.6% in the feces; the remainder is excreted as bio-inactive metabolites.
Doses of up to 2 grams of clindamycin per day for 14 days have been well tolerated by healthy volunteers, except that the incidence of gastrointestinal side effects is greater with the higher doses.
No significant levels of clindamycin are attained in the cerebrospinal fluid, even in the presence of inflamed meninges.

INDICATIONS AND USAGE

Clindamycin is indicated in the treatment of serious infections caused by susceptible anaerobic bacteria.
Clindamycin is also indicated in the treatment of serious infections due to susceptible strains of streptococci, pneumococci, and staphylococci. Its use should be reserved for penicillin-allergic patients or other patients for whom, in the judgment of the physician, a penicillin is inappropriate. Because of the risk of colitis, as described in the WARNING box, before selecting clindamycin the physician should consider the nature of the infection and the suitability of less toxic alternatives (eg, erythromycin).
Anaerobes: Serious respiratory tract infections such as empyema, anaerobic pneumonitis and lung abscess; serious skin and soft tissue infections; septicemia; intra-abdominal infections such as peritonitis and intra-abdominal abscess (typically resulting from anaerobic organisms resident in the normal gastrointestinal tract); infections of the female pelvis and genital tract such as endometritis, nongonococcal tubo-ovarian abscess, pelvic cellulitis and postsurgical vaginal cuff infection.
Streptococci: Serious respiratory tract infections; serious skin and soft tissue infections.
Staphylococci: Serious respiratory tract infections; serious skin and soft tissue infections.
Pneumococci: Serious respiratory tract infections.
Bacteriologic studies should be performed to determine the causative organisms and their susceptibility to clindamycin.
In Vitro Susceptibility Testing: A standardized disk testing procedure* is recommended for determining susceptibility of aerobic bacteria to clindamycin. A description is contained in the CLEOCIN® Susceptibility Disk (clindamycin) insert. Using this method, the laboratory can designate isolates as resistant, intermediate, or susceptible. Tube or agar dilution methods may be used for both anaerobic and aerobic bacteria. When the directions in the CLEOCIN® Susceptibility Powder insert are followed, an MIC of 1.6 mcg/mL may be considered susceptible; MICs of 1.6 to 4.8 mcg/mL may be considered intermediate and MICs greater than 4.8 mcg/mL may be considered resistant.
CLEOCIN Susceptibility Disks 2 mcg. See package insert for use.
CLEOCIN Susceptibility Powder 20 mg. See package insert for use.
For anaerobic bacteria the minimal inhibitory concentration (MIC) of clindamycin can be determined by agar dilution and broth dilution (including microdilution) techniques. If MICs are not determined routinely, the disk broth method is recommended for routine use. THE KIRBY-BAUER DISK DIFFUSION METHOD AND ITS INTERPRETIVE STANDARDS ARE NOT RECOMMENDED FOR ANAEROBES.

CONTRAINDICATIONS

CLEOCIN HCl Capsules (clindamycin hydrochloride) are contraindicated in individuals with a history of hypersensitivity to preparations containing clindamycin or lincomycin.

WARNINGS

See WARNING box. Studies indicate a toxin(s) produced by *Clostridia* is one primary cause of antibiotic associated colitis.[1-5] Cholestyramine and colestipol resins have been shown to bind the toxin *in vitro*. Mild cases of colitis may respond to drug discontinuance alone. Moderate to severe cases should be managed with fluid, electrolyte and protein supplementation as indicated. Vancomycin has been found to be effective in the treatment of antibiotic associated pseudomembranous colitis produced by *Clostridium difficile*. The usual adult dosage is 500 milligrams to 2 grams of vancomycin orally per day in three to four divided doses administered for 7 to 10 days. Cholestyramine or colestipol resins bind vancomycin *in vitro*. If both a resin and vancomycin are to be administered concurrently, it may be advisable to separate the time of administration of each drug. Systemic corticoids and corticoid retention enemas may help relieve the colitis. Other causes of colitis should also be considered.
A careful inquiry should be made concerning previous sensitivities to drugs and other allergens.

*Bauer, AW, Kirby, WMM, Sherris, JC, et al; Antibiotic susceptibility testing by a standardized single disc method, *Am J Clin Path* 45:493-496, 1966. Standardized disc susceptibility test, *Federal Register* 37:20527-29, 1972.

1. Bartlett JG, et al: Antibiotic associated Pseudomembranous Colitis Due to Toxin-producing *Clostridia. N Engl J Med* 298(10):531-534, 1978.
2. George RH, et al: Identification of *Clostridium difficile* as a cause of Pseudomembranous Colitis. *Br Med J* 6114:669-671, 1978.
3. Larson HE, Price AB: Pseudomembranous Colitis Presence of Clostridial Toxin, *Lancet* 8052/3:1312-1314, 1977.
4. Rifkin GD, Fekety FR, Silva J: Antibiotic-induced Colitis Implication of a Toxin Neutralized by *Clostridium sordellii* Antitoxin. *Lancet* 8048:1103-1106, 1977.
5. Bailey WR, Scott EG: Diagnostic Microbiology. The CV Mosby Company, St. Louis, 1978.

Usage in Pregnancy - Safety for use in pregnancy has not been established.
Usage in Newborns and Infants: When CLEOCIN HCl Capsules (clindamycin hydrochloride) are administered to newborns and infants, appropriate monitoring of organ system functions is desirable.
Nursing Mothers—Clindamycin has been reported to appear in breast milk in ranges of 0.7 to 3.8 mcg/mL.
Usage in Meningitis: Since clindamycin does not diffuse adequately into the cerebrospinal fluid, the drug should not be used in the treatment of meningitis.
Antagonism has been demonstrated between clindamycin and erythromycin *in vitro*. Because of possible clinical significance, these two drugs should not be administered concurrently.

PRECAUTIONS

Review of experience to date suggests that a subgroup of older patients with associated severe illness may tolerate diarrhea less well. When clindamycin is indicated in these patients, they should be carefully monitored for change in bowel frequency.
CLEOCIN HCl Capsules (clindamycin hydrochloride) should be prescribed with caution in individuals with a history of gastrointestinal disease, particularly colitis.
CLEOCIN HCl should be prescribed with caution in atopic individuals.
During prolonged therapy, periodic liver and kidney function tests and blood counts should be performed.
Indicated surgical procedures should be performed in conjunction with antibiotic therapy.
The use of CLEOCIN HCl occasionally results in overgrowth of nonsusceptible organisms—particularly yeasts. Should superinfections occur, appropriate measures should be taken as indicated by the clinical situation.
Patients with very severe renal disease and/or very severe hepatic disease accompanied by severe metabolic aberrations should be dosed with caution, and serum clindamycin levels monitored during high-dose therapy.
Clindamycin has been shown to have neuromuscular blocking properties that may enhance the action of other neuromuscular blocking agents. Therefore, it should be used with caution in patients receiving such agents.
The 75 mg and 150 mg capsules contain FD&C Yellow No. 5 (tartrazine) which may cause allergic-type reactions (including bronchial asthma) in certain susceptible individuals. Although the overall incidence of FD&C Yellow No. 5 (tartrazine) sensitivity in the general population is low, it is frequently seen in patients who also have aspirin hypersensitivity.

ADVERSE REACTIONS

The following reactions have been reported with the use of clindamycin.
Gastrointestinal: Abdominal pain, esophagitis, nausea, vomiting and diarrhea. (See **Warning** Box)
Hypersensitivity Reactions: Maculopapular rash and urticaria have been observed during drug therapy. Generalized mild to moderate morbilliform-like skin rashes are the most frequently reported of all adverse reactions. Rare instances of erythema multiforme, some resembling Stevens-Johnson syndrome, have been associated with clindamycin. A few cases of anaphylactoid reactions have been reported. If a hypersensitivity reaction occurs, the drug should be discontinued. The usual agents (epinephrine, corticosteroids, antihistamines) should be available for emergency treatment of serious reactions.
Liver: Jaundice and abnormalities in liver function tests have been observed during clindamycin therapy.
Renal: Although no direct relationship of clindamycin to renal damage has been established, renal dysfunction as evidenced by azotemia, oliguria, and/or proteinuria has been observed in rare instances.
Hematopoietic: Transient neutropenia (leukopenia) and eosinophilia have been reported. Reports of agranulocytosis and thrombocytopenia have been made. No direct etiologic relationship to concurrent clindamycin therapy could be made in any of the foregoing.
Musculoskeletal: Rare instances of polyarthritis have been reported.

DOSAGE AND ADMINISTRATION

If significant diarrhea occurs during therapy, this antibiotic should be discontinued. (See **Warning** box).
Adults: *Serious infections* —150 to 300 mg every 6 hours. *More severe infections* —300 to 450 mg every 6 hours.
Children: *Serious infections* —8 to 16 mg/kg/day (4 to 8 mg/lb/day) divided into three or four equal doses. *More severe*

Continued on next page

Information on these Upjohn products is based on labeling in effect June 1, 1992. Further information concerning these and other Upjohn products may be obtained by direct inquiry to Medical Information, The Upjohn Company, Kalamazoo, Michigan 49001.

Upjohn—Cont.

infections —16 to 20 mg/kg/day (8 to 10 mg/lb/day) divided into three or four equal doses.

To avoid the possibility of esophageal irritation, CLEOCIN HCl Capsules (clindamycin hydrochloride) should be taken with a full glass of water.

Serious infections due to anaerobic bacteria are usually treated with CLEOCIN PHOSPHATE® Sterile Solution (clindamycin phosphate). However, in clinically appropriate circumstances, the physician may elect to initiate treatment or continue treatment with CLEOCIN HCl Capsules.

In cases of β-hemolytic streptococcal infections, treatment should continue for at least 10 days.

HOW SUPPLIED

CLEOCIN HCl Capsules (clindamycin hydrochloride) are available in the following strengths, colors and sizes:

75 mg Lavender:	
Bottles of 100	*NDC 0009-0331-02*
150 mg Lavender and Maroon:	
Bottles of 16	*NDC 0009-0225-01*
Bottles of 100	*NDC 0009-0225-02*
Unit Dose Package (100)	*NDC 0009-0225-03*
300 mg Maroon:	
Bottles of 16	*NDC 0009-0395-13*
Bottles of 100	*NDC 0009-0395-14*
Unit dose package of 100	*NDC 0009-0395-02*

Store at controlled room temperature 15°–30°C (59°–86°F).

TOXICOLOGY

Animal toxicity studies showed the following:

LD_{50} I.P. Administration— Mouse	361 mg/kg
LD_{50} I.V. Administration— Mouse	245 mg/kg
LD_{50} Oral Administration— Rat	2,618 mg/kg

One year oral toxicity studies in Spartan Sprague-Dawley rats and Beagle dogs at levels of 30, 100 and 300 mg/kg/day (3 grams/day per dog) have shown CLEOCIN HCl to be well tolerated. No appreciable difference in pathological findings has been obtained in groups of animals treated with CLEOCIN HCl from comparable control groups. Rats receiving clindamycin hydrochloride at 600 mg/kg/day for six months tolerated the drug well; however, dogs dosed at this level vomited, would not eat, and lost weight.

Code 810 570 614

Shown in Product Identification Section, page 434

CLEOCIN PEDIATRIC® ℞

brand of clindamycin palmitate hydrochloride flavored granules
(clindamycin palmitate hydrochloride for oral solution, USP)
Not for Injection

WARNING

Clindamycin therapy has been associated with severe colitis which may end fatally. Therefore, it should be reserved for serious infections where less toxic antimicrobial agents are inappropriate, as described in the Indications Section. It should not be used in patients with nonbacterial infections, such as most upper respiratory tract infections. Studies indicate a toxin(s) produced by *Clostridia* is one primary cause of antibiotic associated colitis. Cholestyramine and colestipol resins have been shown to bind the toxin *in vitro*. See WARNINGS section. The colitis is usually characterized by severe, persistent diarrhea and severe abdominal cramps and may be associated with the passage of blood and mucus. Endoscopic examination may reveal pseudomembranous colitis. Stool culture for *Clostridium difficile* and stool assay for *C. difficile* toxin may be helpful diagnostically.

When significant diarrhea occurs, the drug should be discontinued or, if necessary, continued only with close observation of the patient. Large bowel endoscopy has been recommended.

Antiperistaltic agents such as opiates and diphenoxylate with atropine (Lomotil) may prolong and/or worsen the condition. Vancomycin has been found to be effective in the treatment of antibiotic associated pseudomembranous colitis produced by *Clostridium difficile*. The usual adult dosage is 500 milligrams to 2 grams of vancomycin orally per day in three to four divided doses administered for 7 to 10 days. Cholestyramine or colestipol resins bind vancomycin *in vitro*. If both a resin and vancomycin are to be administered concurrently, it may be advisable to separate the time of administration of each drug.

Diarrhea, colitis, and pseudomembranous colitis have been observed to begin up to several weeks following cessation of therapy with clindamycin.

DESCRIPTION

Clindamycin palmitate hydrochloride is a water soluble hydrochloride salt of the ester of clindamycin and palmitic acid. Clindamycin is a semisynthetic antibiotic produced by a 7(S)-chloro-substitution of the 7(R)-hydroxyl group of the parent compound lincomycin.

The chemical name for clindamycin palmitate hydrochloride is Methyl 7-chloro-6,7,8-trideoxy-6-(1-methyl-*trans*-4-propyl-L-2-pyrrolidinecarboxamido)-1-thio-L-*threo*-*a*-D-*galacto*-octopyranoside 2-palmitate monohydrochloride.

CLEOCIN PEDIATRIC Flavored Granules contain clindamycin palmitate hydrochloride for reconstitution. Each 5 mL contains the equivalent of 75 mg clindamycin. Inactive ingredients: artificial cherry flavor, dextrin, ethylparaben, pluronic F68, polymethylsiloxane, sucrose.

CLINICAL PHARMACOLOGY

Microbiology: Although clindamycin palmitate HCl is inactive *in vitro*, rapid *in vivo* hydrolysis converts this compound to the antibacterially active clindamycin.

Clindamycin has been shown to have *in vitro* activity against isolates of the following organisms:

Aerobic gram positive cocci, including:
- *Staphylococcus aureus*
- *Staphylococcus epidermidis* (penicillinase and non-penicillinase producing strains). When tested by *in vitro* methods some staphylococcal strains originally resistant to erythromycin rapidly develop resistance to clindamycin.
- Streptococci (except *Streptococcus faecalis*)
- Pneumococci

Anaerobic gram negative bacilli, including:
- Bacteroides species (including *Bacteroides fragilis* group and *Bacteroides melaninogenicus* group)
- Fusobacterium species

Anaerobic gram positive nonsporeforming bacilli, including:
- Propionibacterium
- Eubacterium
- Actinomyces species

Anaerobic and microaerophilic gram positive cocci, including:
- Peptococcus species
- Peptostreptococcus species
- Microaerophilic streptococci

Clostridia: Clostridia are more resistant than most anaerobes to clindamycin. Most *Clostridium perfringens* are susceptible, but other species, eg, *Clostridium sporogenes* and *Clostridium tertium* are frequently resistant to clindamycin. Susceptibility testing should be done.

Cross resistance has been demonstrated between clindamycin and lincomycin.

Antagonism has been demonstrated between clindamycin and erythromycin.

Human Pharmacology: Blood level studies comparing clindamycin palmitate HCl with clindamycin hydrochloride show that both products reach their peak active serum levels at the same time, indicating a rapid hydrolysis of the palmitate to the clindamycin.

Clindamycin is widely distributed in body fluids and tissues (including bones). Approximately 10% of the biological activity is excreted in the urine. The average biological half-life after doses of clindamycin is approximately two hours in children.

Serum half-life of clindamycin is increased slightly in patients with markedly reduced renal function. Hemodialysis and peritoneal dialysis do not appreciably affect the half-life of clindamycin in the serum.

Serum level studies with clindamycin palmitate HCl in normal children weighing 50-100 lbs given 2, 3 or 4 mg/kg every 6 hours (8, 12 or 16 mg/kg/day) demonstrated mean peak clindamycin serum levels of 1.24, 2.25 and 2.44 mcg/mL respectively, one hour after the first dose. By the fifth dose, the 6-hour serum concentration had reached equilibrium. Peak serum concentrations after this time would be about 2.46, 2.98 and 3.79 mcg/mL with doses of 8, 12, 16 mg/kg/day, respectively. Serum levels have been uniform and predictable from person to person and dose to dose. Multiple-dose studies in newborns and infants up to 6 months of age show that the drug does not accumulate in the serum and is excreted rapidly. Serum levels exceed the MICs for most indicated organisms for at least six hours following administration of the usually recommended doses of CLEOCIN PEDIATRIC in adults and children.

No significant levels of clindamycin are attained in the cerebrospinal fluid, even in the presence of inflamed meninges.

INDICATIONS AND USAGE

CLEOCIN PEDIATRIC Flavored Granules (clindamycin palmitate HCl) are indicated in the treatment of serious infections caused by susceptible anaerobic bacteria.

Clindamycin is also indicated in the treatment of serious infections due to susceptible strains of streptococci, pneumococci, and staphylococci. Its use should be reserved for penicillin-allergic patients or other patients for whom, in the judgment of the physician, a penicillin is inappropriate. Because of the risk of colitis, as described in the WARNING box, before selecting clindamycin the physician should consider the nature of the infection and the suitability of less toxic alternatives (eg, erythromycin).

Anaerobes: Serious respiratory tract infections such as empyema, anaerobic pneumonitis and lung abscess; serious skin and soft tissue infections; septicemia; intra-abdominal infections such as peritonitis and intra-abdominal abscess (typically resulting from anaerobic organisms resident in the normal gastrointestinal tract); infections of the female pelvis and genital tract such as endometritis, nongonococcal tubo-ovarian abscess, pelvic cellulitis and postsurgical vaginal cuff infection.

Streptococci: Serious respiratory tract infections; serious skin and soft tissue infections.

Staphylococci: Serious respiratory tract infections; serious skin and soft tissue infections.

Pneumococci: Serious respiratory tract infections.

Bacteriologic studies should be performed to determine the causative organisms and their susceptibility to clindamycin.

In Vitro Susceptibility Testing: A standardized disk testing procedure* is recommended for determining susceptibility of aerobic bacteria to clindamycin. A description is contained in the CLEOCIN® Susceptibility Disk (clindamycin) insert. Using this method, the laboratory can designate isolates as resistant, intermediate, or susceptible. Tube or agar dilution methods may be used for both anaerobic and aerobic bacteria. When the directions in the CLEOCIN Susceptibility Powder insert are followed, an MIC (minimal inhibitory concentration) of 1.6 mcg/mL may be considered susceptible; MICs of 1.6 to 4.8 mcg/mL may be considered intermediate and MICs greater than 4.8 mcg/mL may be considered resistant.

CLEOCIN Susceptibility Disks 2 mcg. See package insert for use.

CLEOCIN Susceptibility Powder 20 mg. See package insert for use.

For anaerobic bacteria the minimal inhibitory concentration (MIC) of clindamycin can be determined by agar dilution and broth dilution (including microdilution) techniques. If MICs are not determined routinely, the disk broth method is recommended for routine use. THE KIRBY-BAUER DISK DIFFUSION METHOD AND ITS INTERPRETIVE STANDARDS ARE NOT RECOMMENDED FOR ANAEROBES.

CONTRAINDICATIONS

This drug is contraindicated in individuals with a history of hypersensitivity to preparations containing clindamycin or lincomycin.

WARNINGS

See WARNING box. Studies indicate a toxin(s) produced by *Clostridia* is one primary cause of antibiotic associated colitis.[1–5] Cholestyramine and colestipol resins have been shown to bind the toxin *in vitro*. Mild cases of colitis may respond to drug discontinuance alone. Moderate to severe cases should be managed promptly with fluid, electrolyte and protein supplementation as indicated. Vancomycin has been found to be effective in the treatment of antibiotic associated pseudomembranous colitis produced by *Clostridium difficile*. The usual adult dosage is 500 milligrams to 2 grams of vancomycin orally per day in three to four divided doses administered for 7 to 10 days. Cholestyramine or colestipol resins bind vancomycin *in vitro*. If both a resin and vancomycin are to be administered concurrently, it may be advisable to separate the time of administration of each drug. Systemic corticoids and corticoid retention enemas may help relieve the colitis. Other causes of colitis should also be considered.

A careful inquiry should be made concerning previous sensitivities to drugs and other allergens.

Usage in Pregnancy—Safety for use in pregnancy has not been established.

Usage in Newborns and Infants: When CLEOCIN PEDIATRIC Flavored Granules (clindamycin palmitate

---

*Bauer, AW, Kirby, WMM, Sherris, JC, Turck, M.: Antibiotic susceptibility testing by a standardized single disc method, *Am J Clin Path*, **45**:493-496, 1966. Standardized Disc Susceptibility Test, *Federal Register* **37**:20527-29, 1972.

1. Bartlett JG, et al: Antibiotic associated Pseudomembranous Colitis Due to Toxin-producing *Clostridia. N Engl J Med* 298(10):531-534, 1978.
2. George RH, et al: Identification of *Clostridium difficile* as a cause of Pseudomembranous Colitis. *Br Med J* 6114:669-671, 1978.
3. Larson HE, Price AB: Pseudomembranous Colitis Presence of Clostridial Toxin. *Lancet* 8052/3:1312-1314, 1977.
4. Rifkin GD, Fekety FR, Silva J: Antibiotic-induced Colitis Implication of a Toxin Neutralized by *Clostridium sordellii* Antitoxin. *Lancet* 8048:1103-1106, 1977.
5. Bailey WR, Scott EG: Diagnostic Microbiology. The CV Mosby Company, St. Louis, 1978.

HCl) are administered to newborns and infants, appropriate monitoring of organ system functions is desirable.

Nursing Mothers—Clindamycin has been reported to appear in breast milk in ranges of 0.7 to 3.8 mcg/mL.

Usage in Meningitis: Since clindamycin does not diffuse adequately into the cerebrospinal fluid, the drug should not be used in the treatment of meningitis.

Antagonism has been demonstrated between clindamycin and erythromycin *in vitro*. Because of possible clinical significance, these two drugs should not be administered concurrently.

PRECAUTIONS

Review of experience to date suggests that a subgroup of older patients with associated severe illness may tolerate diarrhea less well. When clindamycin is indicated in these patients, they should be carefully monitored for change in bowel frequency.

CLEOCIN PEDIATRIC Flavored Granules (clindamycin palmitate HCl) should be prescribed with caution in individuals with a history of gastrointestinal disease, particularly colitis.

CLEOCIN PEDIATRIC should be prescribed with caution in atopic individuals.

During prolonged therapy periodic liver and kidney function tests and blood counts should be performed.

Indicated surgical procedures should be performed in conjunction with antibiotic therapy.

The use of CLEOCIN PEDIATRIC may result in overgrowth of nonsusceptible organisms—particularly yeasts. Should superinfections occur, appropriate measures should be taken as indicated by the clinical situation.

Patients with very severe renal disease and/or very severe hepatic disease accompanied by severe metabolic aberrations should be dosed with caution, and serum clindamycin levels monitored during high-dose therapy.

Clindamycin has been shown to have neuromuscular blocking properties that may enhance the action of other neuromuscular blocking agents. Therefore, it should be used with caution in patients receiving such agents.

ADVERSE REACTIONS

The following reactions have been reported with the use of clindamycin.

Gastrointestinal: Abdominal pain, nausea, vomiting and diarrhea. (See **Warning** box)

Hypersensitivity Reactions: Maculopapular rash and urticaria have been observed during drug therapy. Generalized mild to moderate morbilliform-like skin rashes are the most frequently reported of all adverse reactions. Rare instances of erythema multiforme, some resembling Stevens-Johnson syndrome, have been associated with clindamycin. A few cases of anaphylactoid reactions have been reported. If a hypersensitivity reaction occurs, the drug should be discontinued. The usual agents (epinephrine, corticosteroids, antihistamines) should be available for emergency treatment of serious reactions.

Liver: Jaundice and abnormalities in liver function tests have been observed during clindamycin therapy.

Renal: Although no direct relationship of clindamycin to renal damage has been established, renal dysfunction as evidenced by azotemia, oliguria, and/or proteinuria has been observed in rare instances.

Hematopoietic: Transient neutropenia (leukopenia) and eosinophilia have been reported. Reports of agranulocytosis and thrombocytopenia have been made. No direct etiologic relationship to concurrent clindamycin therapy could be made in any of the foregoing.

Musculoskeletal: Rare instances of polyarthritis have been reported.

DOSAGE AND ADMINISTRATION

If significant diarrhea occurs during therapy, this antibiotic should be discontinued. (See **Warning** box.) Concomitant administration of food does not adversely affect the absorption of clindamycin palmitate HCl contained in CLEOCIN PEDIATRIC Flavored Granules.

Serious infections: 8-12 mg/kg/day (4-6 mg/lb/day) divided into 3 or 4 equal doses.

Severe infections: 13-16 mg/kg/day (6.5-8 mg/lb/day) divided into 3 or 4 equal doses.

More severe infections: 17-25 mg/kg/day (8.5-12.5 mg/lb/day) divided into 3 or 4 equal doses.

In children weighing 10 kg or less, ½ teaspoon (37.5 mg) three times a day should be considered the minimum recommended dose.

Serious infections due to anaerobic bacteria are usually treated with CLEOCIN PHOSPHATE® Sterile Solution (clindamycin phosphate). However, in clinically appropriate circumstances, the physician may elect to initiate treatment or continue treatment with CLEOCIN PEDIATRIC.

NOTE: In cases of β-hemolytic streptococcal infections, treatment should be continued for at least 10 days.

Reconstitution instructions:

When reconstituted with water as follows, each 5 mL (teaspoon) of solution contains clindamycin palmitate HCl equivalent to 75 mg clindamycin.

Reconstitute bottles of 100 mL with **75 mL** of water. Add a large portion of the water and shake vigorously; add the remainder of the water and shake until the solution is uniform.

Storage conditions:

Store unreconstituted product at controlled room temperature 15°-30°C (59°-86°F).

Do **NOT** refrigerate the reconstituted solution; when chilled, the solution may thicken and be difficult to pour. The solution is stable for 2 weeks at room temperature.

HOW SUPPLIED

CLEOCIN PEDIATRIC Flavored Granules (clindamycin palmitate HCl) for oral solution is available in bottles of 100 mL *NDC 0009-0760-04*

When reconstituted as directed, each bottle yields a solution containing 75 mg of clindamycin per 5 mL.

Code 810 568 009

CLEOCIN PHOSPHATE® ℞

brand of clindamycin phosphate sterile solution and clindamycin phosphate IV Solution)
(clindamycin phosphate injection, USP and clindamycin phosphate injection in 5% dextrose)
Sterile Solution is for Intramuscular and Intravenous Use
CLEOCIN PHOSPHATE in the ADD-Vantage‡ Vial is For Intravenous Use Only

WARNING

Clindamycin therapy has been associated with severe colitis which may end fatally. Therefore, it should be reserved for serious infections where less toxic antimicrobial agents are inappropriate, as described in the Indications and Usage Section. It should not be used in patients with nonbacterial infections, such as most upper respiratory tract infections. Studies indicate a toxin(s) produced by *Clostridia* is one primary cause of antibiotic-associated colitis. Cholestyramine and colestipol resins have been shown to bind the toxin *in vitro*. See WARNINGS section. The colitis is usually characterized by severe, persistent diarrhea and severe abdominal cramps and may be associated with the passage of blood and mucus. Endoscopic examination may reveal pseudomembranous colitis. Stool culture for *Clostridium difficile* and stool assay for *C. difficile* toxin may be helpful diagnostically.

When significant diarrhea occurs, the drug should be discontinued or, if necessary, continued only with close observation of the patient. Large bowel endoscopy has been recommended.

Antiperistaltic agents such as opiates and diphenoxylate with atropine (Lomotil) may prolong and/or worsen the condition. Vancomycin has been found to be effective in the treatment of antibiotic associated pseudomembranous colitis produced by *Clostridium difficile*. The usual adult dosage is 500 milligrams to 2 grams of vancomycin orally per day in three to four divided doses administered for 7 to 10 days. Cholestyramine or colestipol resins bind vancomycin *in vitro*. If both a resin and vancomycin are to be administered concurrently, it may be advisable to separate the time of administration of each drug.

Diarrhea, colitis, and pseudomembranous colitis have been observed to begin up to several weeks following cessation of therapy with clindamycin.

DESCRIPTION

CLEOCIN PHOSPHATE Sterile Solution in vials contains clindamycin phosphate, a water soluble ester of clindamycin and phosphoric acid. Each mL contains the equivalent of 150 mg clindamycin, 0.5 mg disodium edetate and 9.45 mg benzyl alcohol added as preservative in each mL. Clindamycin is a semisynthetic antibiotic produced by a 7(S)-chloro-substitution of the 7(R)-hydroxyl group of the parent compound lincomycin.

The chemical name of clindamycin phosphate is L-*threo*-α-D-*galacto*-Octopyranoside, methyl 7-chloro-6,7,8-trideoxy-6-[[(1-methyl-4-propyl-2-pyrrolidinyl) carbonyl] amino]-1-thio-, 2-(dihydrogen phosphate), (2S-*trans*)-.

The molecular formula is $C_{18}H_{34}ClN_2O_8PS$ and the molecular weight is 504.96.

CLEOCIN PHOSPHATE in the ADD-Vantage Vial is intended for intravenous use only after further dilution with appropriate volume of ADD-Vantage diluent base solution.

CLEOCIN PHOSPHATE IV Solution in the Galaxy® plastic container for intravenous use is composed of clindamycin phosphate equivalent to 300, 600 and 900 mg of clindamycin premixed with 5% dextrose as a sterile solution. Disodium edetate has been added at a concentration of 0.04 mg/mL. The pH has been adjusted with sodium hydroxide and/or hydrochloric acid.

The plastic container is fabricated from a specially designed multilayer plastic, PL 2501. Solutions in contact with the plastic container can leach out certain of its chemical components in very small amounts within the expiration period. The suitability of the plastic has been confirmed in tests in animals according to the USP biological tests for plastic containers, as well as by tissue culture toxicity studies.

‡ ADD-Vantage is a registered trademark of Abbott Laboratories.

CLINICAL PHARMACOLOGY

Biologically inactive clindamycin phosphate is rapidly converted to active clindamycin.

By the end of short-term intravenous infusion, peak serum levels of active clindamycin are reached. Biologically inactive clindamycin phosphate disappears rapidly from the serum; the average disappearance half-life is 6 minutes; however, the serum disappearance half-life of active clindamycin is about 3 hours in adults and 2 ½ hours in children.

After intramuscular injection of clindamycin phosphate, peak levels of active clindamycin are reached within 3 hours in adults and 1 hour in children. Serum level curves may be constructed from IV peak serum levels as given in Table 1 by application of disappearance half-lives listed above.

Serum levels of clindamycin can be maintained above the *in vitro* minimum inhibitory concentrations for most indicated organisms by administration of clindamycin phosphate every 8-12 hours in adults and every 6-8 hours in children, or by continuous intravenous infusion. An equilibrium state is reached by the third dose.

The disappearance half-life of clindamycin is increased slightly in patients with markedly reduced renal or hepatic function. Hemodialysis and peritoneal dialysis are not effective in removing clindamycin from the serum. Dosage schedules need not be modified in the presence of mild or moderate renal or hepatic disease.

No significant levels of clindamycin are attained in the cerebrospinal fluid, even in the presence of inflamed meninges.

Serum assays for active clindamycin require an inhibitor to prevent *in vitro* hydrolysis of clindamycin phosphate.

[See table on next page.]

Microbiology: Although clindamycin phosphate is inactive *in vitro*, rapid *in vivo* hydrolysis converts this compound to the antibacterially active clindamycin.

Clindamycin has been shown to have *in vitro* activity against isolates of the following organisms:

Aerobic gram positive cocci, including:
- *Staphylococcus aureus*
- *Staphylococcus epidermidis* (penicillinase and nonpenicillinase producing strains). When tested by *in vitro* methods some staphylococcal strains originally resistant to erythromycin rapidly develop resistance to clindamycin.
- Streptococci (except *Enterococcus faecalis*)
- Pneumococci

Anaerobic gram negative bacilli, including:
- Bacteroides species (including *Bacteroides fragilis* group and *Bacteroides melaninogenicus* group)
- Fusobacterium species

Anaerobic gram positive nonsporeforming bacilli, including:
- Propionibacterium
- Eubacterium
- Actinomyces species

Anaerobic and microaerophilic gram positive cocci, including:
- Peptococcus species
- Peptostreptococcus species
- Microaerophilic streptococci

Clostridia: Clostridia are more resistant than most anaerobes to clindamycin. Most *Clostridium perfringens* are susceptible, but other species, eg, *Clostridium sporogenes* and *Clostridium tertium* are frequently resistant to clindamycin. Susceptibility testing should be done.

Cross resistance has been demonstrated between clindamycin and lincomycin.

Antagonism has been demonstrated between clindamycin and erythromycin.

In vitro Susceptibility Testing:

Disk diffusion technique—Quantitative methods that require measurement of zone diameters give the most precise estimates of antibiotic susceptibility. One such procedure[1] has been recommended for use with disks to test susceptibility to clindamycin.

Continued on next page

Information on these Upjohn products is based on labeling in effect June 1, 1992. Further information concerning these and other Upjohn products may be obtained by direct inquiry to Medical Information, The Upjohn Company, Kalamazoo, Michigan 49001.

Upjohn—Cont.

Reports from a laboratory using the standardized single-disk susceptibility test[1] with a 2 mcg clindamycin disk should be interpreted according to the following criteria:

Susceptible organisms produce zones of 17 mm or greater, indicating that the tested organism is likely to respond to therapy.

Organisms of intermediate susceptibility produce zones of 15–16 mm, indicating that the tested organism would be susceptible if a high dosage is used or if the infection is confined to tissues and fluids (e.g., urine), in which high antibiotic levels are attained.

Resistant organisms produce zones of 14 mm or less, indicating that other therapy should be selected.

Standardized procedures require the use of control organisms. The 2 mcg clindamycin disk should give a zone diameter between 24 and 30 mm for *S. aureus* ATCC 25923.

Dilution techniques—A bacterial isolate may be considered susceptible if the minimum inhibitory concentration (MIC) for clindamycin is not more than 1.6 mcg/mL. Organisms are considered moderately susceptible if the MIC is greater than 1.6 mcg/mL and less than or equal to 4.8 mcg/mL. Organisms are considered resistant if the MIC is greater than 4.8 mcg per mL.

The range of MIC's for the control strains are as follows:
S. aureus ATCC 29213, 0.06–0.25 mcg/mL.
E. faecalis ATCC 29212, 4.0–16 mcg/mL.

For anaerobic bacteria the minimum inhibitory concentration (MIC) of clindamycin can be determined by agar dilution and broth dilution (including microdilution) techniques.[2] If MICs are not determined routinely, the disk broth method is recommended for routine use. THE KIRBY-BAUER DISK DIFFUSION METHOD AND ITS INTERPRETIVE STANDARDS ARE NOT RECOMMENDED FOR ANAEROBES.

INDICATIONS AND USAGE

CLEOCIN PHOSPHATE products are indicated in the treatment of serious infections caused by susceptible anaerobic bacteria.

CLEOCIN PHOSPHATE products are also indicated in the treatment of serious infections due to susceptible strains of streptococci, pneumococci, and staphylococci. Its use should be reserved for penicillin-allergic patients or other patients for whom, in the judgment of the physician, a penicillin is inappropriate. Because of the risk of antibiotic-associated pseudomembranous colitis, as described in the WARNING box, before selecting clindamycin the physician should consider the nature of the infection and the suitability of less toxic alternatives (e.g., erythromycin).

Bacteriologic studies should be performed to determine the causative organisms and their susceptibility to clindamycin.

Indicated surgical procedures should be performed in conjunction with antibiotic therapy.

CLEOCIN PHOSPHATE is indicated in the treatment of serious infections caused by susceptible strains of the designated organisms in the conditions listed below:

Lower respiratory tract infections including pneumonia, empyema, and lung abscess caused by anaerobes, *Streptococcus pneumoniae*, other streptococci (except *E. faecalis*), and *Staphylococcus aureus*.

Skin and skin structure infections caused by *Streptococcus pyogenes, Staphylococcus aureus*, and anaerobes.

Gynecological infections including endometritis, nongonococcal tubo-ovarian abscess, pelvic cellulitis, and postsurgical vaginal cuff infection caused by susceptible anaerobes.

Intra-abdominal infections including peritonitis and intra-abdominal abscess caused by susceptible anaerobic organisms.

Septicemia caused by *Staphylococcus aureus*, streptococci (except *Enterococcus faecalis*), and susceptible anaerobes.

Bone and joint infections including acute hematogenous osteomyelitis caused by *Staphylococcus aureus* and as adjunctive therapy in the surgical treatment of chronic bone and joint infections due to susceptible organisms.

CONTRAINDICATIONS

This drug is contraindicated in individuals with a history of hypersensitivity to preparations containing clindamycin or lincomycin.

WARNINGS

See WARNING box. Studies indicate a toxin(s) produced by Clostridia is one primary cause of antibiotic associated colitis.[3–7] Cholestyramine and colestipol resins have been shown to bind the toxin *in vitro*. Mild cases of colitis may respond to drug discontinuance alone. Moderate to severe cases should be managed promptly with fluid, electrolyte and protein supplementation as indicated. Vancomycin has been found to be effective in the treatment of antibiotic-associated pseudomembranous colitis produced by *Clostridium difficile*. The usual adult dosage is 500 milligrams to 2 grams of vancomycin orally per day in three to four divided doses administered for 7 to 10 days. Cholestyramine or colestipol resins bind vancomycin *in vitro*. If both a resin and vancomycin are to be administered concurrently, it may be advisable to separate the time of administration of each drug. Systemic corticoids and corticoid retention enemas may help relieve the colitis. Other causes of colitis should also be considered.

A careful inquiry should be made concerning previous sensitivities to drugs and other allergens.

This product contains benzyl alcohol as a preservative. Benzyl alcohol has been associated with a fatal "Gasping Syndrome" in premature infants. (See PRECAUTIONS—Pediatric Use).

Usage in Meningitis: Since clindamycin does not diffuse adequately into the cerebrospinal fluid, the drug should not be used in the treatment of meningitis.

SERIOUS ANAPHYLACTOID REACTIONS REQUIRE IMMEDIATE EMERGENCY TREATMENT WITH EPINEPHRINE. OXYGEN AND INTRAVENOUS CORTICOSTEROIDS SHOULD ALSO BE ADMINISTERED AS INDICATED.

PRECAUTIONS

General

Review of experience to date suggests that a subgroup of older patients with associated severe illness may tolerate diarrhea less well. When clindamycin is indicated in these patients, they should be carefully monitored for change in bowel frequency.

CLEOCIN PHOSPHATE products should be prescribed with caution in individuals with a history of gastrointestinal disease, particularly colitis.

CLEOCIN PHOSPHATE should be prescribed with caution in atopic individuals.

Certain infections may require incision and drainage or other indicated surgical procedures in addition to antibiotic therapy.

The use of CLEOCIN PHOSPHATE may result in overgrowth of nonsusceptible organisms—particularly yeasts. Should superinfections occur, appropriate measures should be taken as indicated by the clinical situation.

CLEOCIN PHOSPHATE should not be injected intravenously undiluted as a bolus, but should be infused over at least 10–60 minutes as directed in the DOSAGE AND ADMINISTRATION section.

Patients with very severe renal disease and/or very severe hepatic disease accompanied by severe metabolic aberrations should be dosed with caution, and serum clindamycin levels monitored during high-dose therapy (see OVERDOSAGE).

Laboratory Tests

During prolonged therapy periodic liver and kidney function tests and blood counts should be performed.

Drug Interactions

Clindamycin has been shown to have neuromuscular blocking properties that may enhance the action of other neuromuscular blocking agents. Therefore, it should be used with caution in patients receiving such agents.

Antagonism has been demonstrated between clindamycin and erythromycin *in vitro*. Because of possible clinical significance, the two drugs should not be administered concurrently.

Usage in Pregnancy: Safety for use in pregnancy has not been established.

Nursing Mothers

Clindamycin has been reported to appear in breast milk in the range of 0.7 to 3.8 mcg/mL at dosages of 150 mg orally to 600 mg intravenously. Because of the potential for adverse reactions due to clindamycin in neonates (see Pediatric Use), the decision to discontinue the drug should be made, taking into account the importance of the drug to the mother.

Pediatric Use

When CLEOCIN PHOSPHATE Sterile Solution is administered to newborns, infants, and children, appropriate monitoring of organ system functions is desirable.

Usage in Newborns and Infants

The product contains benzyl alcohol as a preservative. Benzyl alcohol has been associated with a fatal "Gasping Syndrome" in premature infants.

The potential for the toxic effect in children from chemicals that may leach from the single dose premixed IV preparation in plastic has not been evaluated.

ADVERSE REACTIONS

The following reactions have been reported with the use of clindamycin.

Gastrointestinal: Abdominal pain, nausea, vomiting and diarrhea (See **Warnings**). An unpleasant or metallic taste occasionally has been reported after intravenous administration of the higher doses of clindamycin phosphate.

Hypersensitivity Reactions: Maculopapular rash and urticaria have been observed during drug therapy. Generalized mild to moderate morbilliform-like skin rashes are the most frequently reported of all adverse reactions. Rare instances of erythema multiforme, some resembling Stevens-Johnson syndrome, have been associated with clindamycin. A few cases of anaphylactoid reactions have been reported.

If a hypersensitivity reaction occurs, the drug should be discontinued. The usual agents (epinephrine, corticosteroids, antihistamines) should be available for emergency treatment of serious reactions.

Liver: Jaundice and abnormalities in liver function tests have been observed during clindamycin therapy.

Renal: Although no direct relationship of clindamycin to renal damage has been established, renal dysfunction as evidenced by azotemia, oliguria, and/or proteinuria has been observed in rare instances.

Hematopoietic: Transient neutropenia (leukopenia) and eosinophilia have been reported. Reports of agranulocytosis and thrombocytopenia have been made. No direct etiologic relationship to concurrent clindamycin therapy could be made in any of the foregoing.

Local Reactions: Pain, induration and sterile abscess have been reported after intramuscular injection and thrombophlebitis after intravenous infusion. Reactions can be minimized or avoided by giving deep intramuscular injections and avoiding prolonged use of indwelling intravenous catheters.

Musculoskeletal: Rare instances of polyarthritis have been reported.

Cardiovascular: Rare instances of cardiopulmonary arrest and hypotension have been reported following too rapid intravenous administration. (See DOSAGE AND ADMINISTRATION Section)

OVERDOSAGE

Hemodialysis and peritoneal dialysis are not effective in removing clindamycin from the serum.

Table 1. Average Peak Serum Concentrations After Dosing with Clindamycin Phosphate

CLEOCIN PHOSPHATE Dosage Regimen	Clindamycin mcg/mL	Clindamycin Phosphate mcg/mL
Healthy Adult Males (Post equilibrium)		
300 mg IV in 10 min, q8h	7	15
600 mg IV in 20 min, q8h**	10	23
900 mg IV in 30 min, q12h**	11	29
1200 mg IV in 45 min, q12h	14	49
300 mg IM q8h	6	3
600 mg IM q12h*	9	3
Children (first dose)*		
5-7 mg/kg IV in 1 hr	10	
3-5 mg/kg IM	4	
5-7 mg/kg IM	8	

*Data in this group from patients being treated for infection
**CLEOCIN PHOSPHATE in the ADD-Vantage Vial is For Intravenous Use Only.

[1] Bauer, AW, Kirby, WMM, Sherris, JC, Turck, M: Antibiotic susceptibility testing by a standardized single disc method, *Am J Clin Path*, **45**:493–496, 1966. Standardized Disc Susceptibility Test, *Federal Register* **37**:20527–29, 1972.

[2] National Committee for Clinical Lab. Standards. Methods for Antimicrobial Susceptibility Testing of Anaerobic Bacteria—Second Edition; Tentative Standard. NCCLS publication M11-T2. Villanova, PA; NCCLS; 1988.

[3] Bartlett JG, et al: Antibiotic associated pseudomembranous colitis due to toxin-producing *Clostridia*. *N Engl J Med* **298**(10):531–534, 1978.

[4] George RH, et al: Identification of *Clostridium difficile* as a cause of pseudomembranous colitis. *Br Med J* **6114**:669–671, 1978.

[5] Larson HE, Price AB: Pseudomembranous colitis presence of clostridial toxin. *Lancet* **8052/3**:1312–1314, 1977.

[6] Rifkin GD, Fekety FR, Silva J: Antibiotic-induced colitis implication of a toxin neutralized by *Clostridium sordellii* antitoxin. *Lancet* **8048**:1103–1106, 1977.

[7] Bailey WR, Scott EG: Diagnostic Microbiology. The CV Mosby Company, St. Louis, 1978.

CLEOCIN PHOSPHATE

To maintain serum clindamycin levels	Rapid infusion rate	Maintenance infusion rate
Above 4 mcg/mL	10 mg/min for 30 min	0.75 mg/min
Above 5 mcg/mL	15 mg/min for 30 min	1.00 mg/min
Above 6 mcg/mL	20 mg/min for 30 min	1.25 mg/min

DOSAGE AND ADMINISTRATION

If diarrhea occurs during therapy, this antibiotic should be discontinued. (See **Warning** box).

Adults

Parenteral (IM or IV Administration):

Serious infections due to aerobic gram-positive cocci and the more susceptible anaerobes (NOT generally including *Bacteroides fragilis, Peptococcus* species and *Clostridium* species other than *Clostridium perfringens*):

600–1200 mg/day in 2, 3 or 4 equal doses.

More severe infections, particularly those due to proven or suspected *Bacteroides fragilis Peptococcus* species, or *Clostridium* species other than *Clostridium perfringens*:

1200–2700 mg/day in 2, 3 or 4 equal doses

For more serious infections, these doses may have to be increased. In life threatening situations due to aerobes or anaerobes, these doses may be increased. Doses of as much as 4800 mg daily have been given intravenously to adults. See **Dilution and Infusion Rates** section below.

Single intramuscular injections of greater than 600 mg are not recommended.

Alternatively, drug may be administered in the form of a single rapid infusion of the first dose followed by continuous IV infusion as follows: [See table above.]

Neonates (less than 1 month):

15 to 20 mg/kg/day in 3 to 4 equal doses. The lower dosage may be adequate for small prematures.

Children (over 1 month of age): Parenteral (IM or IV) administration: 20 to 40 mg/kg/day in 3 or 4 equal doses. The higher doses would be used for more severe infections. As an alternative to dosing on a body weight basis, children may be dosed on the basis of square meters body surface: 350 mg/m²/day for serious infections and 450 mg/m²/day for more severe infections.

Parenteral therapy may be changed to oral CLEOCIN PEDIATRIC® Flavored Granules (clindamycin palmitate hydrochloride) or CLEOCIN HCl® Capsules (clindamycin hydrochloride) when the condition warrants and at the discretion of the physician.

In cases of β-hemolytic streptococcal infections, treatment should be continued for at least 10 days.

Dilution and Infusion Rates

Clindamycin phosphate must be diluted prior to IV administration. The concentration of clindamycin in diluent for infusion should not exceed 18 mg per mL. Infusion rates should not exceed 30 mg per minute. The usual infusion dilutions and rates are as follows:

Dose	Diluent	Time
300 mg	50 mL	10 min
600 mg	50 mL	20 min
900 mg	100 mL	30 min
1200 mg	100 mL	40 min

Administration of more than 1200 mg in a single 1-hour infusion is not recommended.

Parenteral drug products should be inspected visually for particulate matter and discoloration prior to administration, whenever solution and container permit.

Dilution and Compatibility: Physical and biological compatibility studies monitored for 24 hours at room temperature have demonstrated no inactivation or incompatibility with the use of CLEOCIN PHOSPHATE Sterile Solution (clindamycin phosphate) in IV solutions containing sodium chloride, glucose, calcium or potassium, and solutions containing vitamin B complex in concentrations usually used clinically. No incompatibility has been demonstrated with the antibiotics cephalothin, kanamycin, gentamicin, penicillin or carbenicillin.

The following drugs are physically incompatible with clindamycin phosphate: ampicillin sodium, phenytoin sodium, barbiturates, aminophylline, calcium gluconate, and magnesium sulfate.

The compatibility and duration of stability of drug admixtures will vary depending on concentration and other conditions. For current information regarding compatibilities of clindamycin phosphate under specific conditions, please contact the Medical Correspondence Unit, The Upjohn Company.

Physico-Chemical Stability of diluted solutions of CLEOCIN PHOSPHATE

Room temperature: 6, 9 and 12 mg/mL (equivalent to clindamycin base) in dextrose 5% in water, sodium chloride 0.9%, or Lactated Ringers in glass bottles or minibags, demonstrated physical and chemical stability for at least 16 days at 25°C. Also, 18 mg/mL (equivalent to clindamycin base) in dextrose 5% in water, in minibags, demonstrated physical and chemical stability for at least 16 days at 25°C.

Refrigeration: 6, 9 and 12 mg/mL (equivalent to clindamycin base) in dextrose 5% in water, sodium chloride 0.9%, or Lactated Ringers in glass bottles or minibags, demonstrated physical and chemical stability for at least 32 days at 4°C.

Frozen: 6,9 and 12 mg/mL (equivalent to clindamycin base) in dextrose 5% in water, sodium chloride 0.9%, or Lactated Ringers in minibags demonstrated physical and chemical stability for at least eight weeks at −10°C.

Frozen solutions should be thawed at room temperature and not refrozen.

DIRECTIONS FOR DISPENSING:

Pharmacy Bulk Package—Not for Direct Infusion

The Pharmacy Bulk Package is for use in a Pharmacy Admixture Service only under a laminar flow hood. Entry into the vial should be made with a small diameter sterile transfer set or other small diameter sterile dispensing device, and contents dispensed in aliquots using aseptic technique. Multiple entries with a needle and syringe are not recommended. AFTER ENTRY USE ENTIRE CONTENTS OF VIAL PROMPTLY. ANY UNUSED PORTION MUST BE DISCARDED WITHIN 24 HOURS AFTER INITIAL ENTRY.

DIRECTIONS FOR USE

CLEOCIN PHOSPHATE IV Solution in Galaxy Plastic Container

Premixed CLEOCIN PHOSPHATE IV Solution is for intravenous administration using sterile equipment. Check for minute leaks prior to use by squeezing bag firmly. If leaks are found, discard solution as sterility may be impaired. Do not add supplementary medication. Parenteral drug products should be inspected visually for particulate matter and discoloration prior to administration whenever solution and container permit. Do not use unless solution is clear and seal is intact.

Caution: Do not use plastic containers in series connections. Such use could result in air embolism due to residual air being drawn from the primary container before administration of the fluid from the secondary container is complete.

Preparation for Administration:

1. Suspend container from eyelet support.
2. Remove protector from outlet port at bottom of container.
3. Attach administration set. Refer to complete directions accompanying set.

Preparation of CLEOCIN PHOSPHATE in ADD-Vantage‡-System-For IV Use Only. CLEOCIN PHOSPHATE 600 mg and 900 mg may be reconstituted in 50 ml or 100 ml, respectively, of 5% Dextrose or 0.9% Sodium Chloride in the ADD-diluent container. Refer to separate instructions for ADD-Vantage System.

HOW SUPPLIED

Each ml of CLEOCIN PHOSPHATE Sterile Solution contains clindamycin phosphate equivalent to 150 mg clindamycin; 0.5 mg disodium edetate; 9.45 mg benzyl alcohol added as preservative. When necessary, pH is adjusted with sodium hydroxide and/or hydrochloric acid.

CLEOCIN PHOSPHATE is available in the following packages:

25-2 mL vials	NDC 0009-0870-21
25-4 mL vials	NDC 0009-0775-20
25-6 mL vials	NDC 0009-0902-11
1–60 mL Pharmacy Bulk Package	NDC 0009-0728-05

CLEOCIN PHOSPHATE is supplied in ADD-Vantage vials as follows:

NDC#	Vial Size	Total Clindamycin Phosphate/vial	Amount of Diluent
0009-3124-01	4 mL	600 mg	50 mL
0009-3447-01	6 mL	900 mg	100 mL

Store at controlled room temperature 15°–30°C (59°–86°F).

CLEOCIN PHOSPHATE IV Solution in Galaxy plastic containers is a sterile solution of clindamycin phosphate with 5% dextrose. The single dose Galaxy plastic containers are available as follows:

24—300 mg/50 mL containers	NDC 0009-3381-01
24—600 mg/50 mL containers	NDC 0009-3375-01
24—900 mg/50 mL containers	NDC 0009-3382-01

Exposure of pharmaceutical products to heat should be minimized. It is recommended that Galaxy plastic containers be stored at room temperature (25° C). Avoid temperatures above 30° C.

Code 810 020 127

CLEOCIN PHOSPHATE IV Solution in the Galaxy plastic containers is manufactured for The Upjohn Company by Baxter-Healthcare Corporation, Deerfield, IL 60015. Galaxy® is a registered trademark of Baxter International, Inc.

Shown in Product Identification Section, page 434

CLEOCIN T®   ℞

brand of clindamycin phosphate topical solution, topical gel and topical lotion

For External Use

30 mL bottle
NSN 6505-01-140-6450 (M)
60 mL bottle
NSN 6505-01-116-5655 (M & VA)

DESCRIPTION

CLEOCIN T Topical Solution , CLEOCIN T Topical Gel and CLEOCIN T Topical Lotion contain clindamycin phosphate, USP, at a concentration equivalent to 10 mg clindamycin per milliliter.

Clindamycin phosphate is a water soluble ester of the semi-synthetic antibiotic produced by a 7(S)-chloro-substitution of the 7(R)-hydroxyl group of the parent antibiotic lincomycin.

The solution contains isopropyl alcohol 50% v/v, propylene glycol, and water.

The gel contains allantoin, carbomer 934P, methylparaben, polyethylene glycol 400, propylene glycol, sodium hydroxide, and purified water.

The lotion contains cetostearyl alcohol (2.5%); glycerin; glyceryl stearate SE (with potassium monostearate); isostearyl alcohol (2.5%); methylparaben (0.3%); sodium lauroyl sarcosinate; stearic acid; and purified water.

The chemical name for clindamycin phosphate is 7(S)-chloro-7-deoxylincomycin-2-phosphate. (MW = 504.96.)

CLINICAL PHARMACOLOGY

Although clindamycin phosphate is inactive *in vitro*, rapid *in vivo* hydrolysis converts this compound to the antibacterially active clindamycin.

Clindamycin has been shown to have *in vivo* activity against isolates of *Propionibacterium acnes*. This may account for its usefulness in acne.

Cross resistance has been demonstrated between clindamycin and lincomycin.

Antagonism has been demonstrated between clindamycin and erythromycin.

Following multiple topical applications of clindamycin phosphate at a concentration equivalent to 10 mg clindamycin per mL in an isopropyl alcohol and water solution, very low levels of clindamycin are present in the serum (0–3 ng/mL) and less than 0.2% of the dose is recovered in urine as clindamycin.

Clindamycin activity has been demonstrated in comedones from acne patients. The mean concentration of antibiotic activity in extracted comedones after application of CLEOCIN T Topical Solution for 4 weeks was 597 mcg/g of comedonal material (range 0–1490). Clindamycin *in vitro* inhibits all *Propionibacterium acnes* cultures tested (MICs 0.4 mcg/mL). Free fatty acids on the skin surface have been decreased from approximately 14% to 2% following application of clindamycin.

INDICATIONS AND USAGE

CLEOCIN T Topical Solution, CLEOCIN T Topical Gel and CLEOCIN T Topical Lotion are indicated in the treatment of acne vulgaris. In view of the potential for diarrhea, bloody diarrhea and pseudomembranous colitis, the physician should consider whether other agents are more appropriate. (See CONTRAINDICATIONS, WARNINGS and ADVERSE REACTIONS.)

CONTRAINDICATIONS

CLEOCIN T Topical Solution, CLEOCIN T Topical Gel and CLEOCIN T Topical Lotion are contraindicated in individuals with a history of hypersensitivity to preparations containing clindamycin or lincomycin, a history of regional enteritis or ulcerative colitis, or a history of antibiotic-associated colitis.

WARNINGS

Orally and parenterally administered clindamycin has been associated with severe colitis which may end fatally. Use of the topical formulation results in absorption of the antibiotic from the skin surface. Diarrhea, bloody diarrhea, and colitis (including pseudomembranous colitis) have been reported

Continued on next page

Information on these Upjohn products is based on labeling in effect June 1, 1992. Further information concerning these and other Upjohn products may be obtained by direct inquiry to Medical Information, The Upjohn Company, Kalamazoo, Michigan 49001.

Upjohn—Cont.

with the use of topical and systemic clindamycin. Symptoms can occur after a few days, weeks or months following initiation of clindamycin therapy. They have also been observed to begin up to several weeks after cessation of therapy with clindamycin. Studies indicate a toxin(s) produced by *Clostridium difficile* is one primary cause of antibiotic-associated colitis. The colitis is usually characterized by severe persistent diarrhea and severe abdominal cramps and may be associated with the passage of blood and mucus. Endoscopic examination may reveal pseudomembranous colitis.

When significant diarrhea occurs, the drug should be discontinued. Large bowel endoscopy should be considered in cases of severe diarrhea.

Antiperistaltic agents such as opiates and diphenoxylate with atropine (Lomotil) may prolong and /or worsen the condition. Vancomycin has been found to be effective in the treatment of antibiotic-associated pseudomembranous colitis produced by *Clostridium difficile*. The usual adult dosage is 500 mg to 2 grams of vancomycin orally per day in three to four divided doses administered for 7 to 10 days.

Mild cases of colitis may respond to discontinuance of clindamycin. Moderate to severe cases should be managed promptly with fluid, electrolyte, and protein supplementation as indicated. Cholestyramine and colestipol resins have been shown to bind the toxin *in vitro*. If both a resin and vancomycin are to be administered concurrently, it may be advisable to separate the time of administration of each drug. Systemic corticoids and corticoid retention enemas may help relieve the colitis. Other causes of colitis should also be considered. A careful inquiry should be made concerning previous sensitivities to drugs and other allergens.

PRECAUTIONS

CLEOCIN T Topical Solution contains an alcohol base which will cause burning and irritation of the eye. In the event of accidental contact with sensitive surfaces (eye, abraded skin, mucous membranes), bathe with copious amounts of cool tap water. The solution has an unpleasant taste and caution should be exercised when applying medication around the mouth.

CLEOCIN T should be prescribed with caution in atopic individuals.

Pregnancy Category B

Reproduction studies have been performed in rats and mice using subcutaneous and oral doses of clindamycin ranging from 100 to 600 mg/kg/day and have revealed no evidence of impaired fertility or harm to the fetus due to clindamycin. There are, however, no adequate and well-controlled studies in pregnant women. Because animal reproduction studies are not always predictive of human response, this drug should be used during pregnancy only if clearly needed.

Nursing Mothers

It is not known whether clindamycin is excreted in human milk following use of CLEOCIN T. However, orally and parenterally administered clindamycin has been reported to appear in breast milk. As a general rule, nursing should not be undertaken while a patient is on a drug since many drugs are excreted in human milk.

Pediatric Use

Safety and effectiveness in children under the age of 12 has not been established.

ADVERSE REACTIONS

Skin dryness is the most common adverse reaction seen with the solution.

Clindamycin has been associated with severe colitis which may end fatally (See WARNINGS).

Cases of diarrhea, bloody diarrhea and colitis (including pseudomembranous colitis) have been reported as adverse reactions in patients treated with topical formulations of clindamycin.

Other effects which have been reported in association with the use of topical formulations of clindamycin include:

Local Effects	Systemic Effects
Contact dermatitis	Abdominal pain
Irritation (e.g., erythema,	Gastrointestinal
peeling, and burning)	disturbances
Oily skin	
Gram-negative folliculitis	

DOSAGE AND ADMINISTRATION

Apply a thin film of CLEOCIN T Topical Solution, CLEOCIN T Topical Lotion or CLEOCIN T Topical Gel twice daily to affected area.

Lotion: Shake well immediately before using. Keep all dosage form containers tightly closed.

HOW SUPPLIED

CLEOCIN T Topical Solution containing clindamycin phosphate equivalent to 10 mg clindamycin per milliliter is available in the following sizes:

30 mL applicator bottle—NDC 0009-3116-01
60 mL applicator bottle—NDC 0009-3116-02
16 oz (473 mL) bottle—NDC 0009-3116-04

CLEOCIN T Topical Gel containing clindamycin phosphate equivalent to 10 mg clindamycin per milliliter is available in the following sizes:

7.5 gram tube—NDC 0009-3331-03
30 gram tube—NDC 0009-3331-02

CLEOCIN T Topical Lotion containing clindamycin phosphate equivalent to 10 mg clindamycin per milliliter is available in the following size:

60 mL plastic squeeze bottle—NDC 0009-3329-01

Store at controlled room temperature 15°–30°C (59°–86°F). Protect from freezing.
Code 811 373 221

Shown in Product Identification Section, page 434

COLESTID®   ℞

brand of colestipol hydrochloride granules
(colestipol hydrochloride for oral suspension, USP)

Box of 30-5 gram packets
                NSN 6505-01-051-4697 (M & VA)
Box of 90-5 gram packets
                NSN 6505-01-292-8929 (M & VA)
300 gram   NSN 6505-01-336-6194 (M & VA)
500 gram   NSN 6505-01-244-5511 (M & VA)

DESCRIPTION

COLESTID Granules consist of colestipol hydrochloride, which is a lipid lowering agent for oral use. COLESTID is an insoluble, high molecular weight basic anion-exchange copolymer of diethylenetriamine and 1-chloro-2,3-epoxypropane, with approximately 1 out of 5 amine nitrogens protonated (chloride form). It is a light yellow resin which is hygroscopic and swells when placed in water or aqueous fluids. COLESTID is tasteless and odorless. Inactive ingredient: Silicon dioxide.

CLINICAL PHARMACOLOGY

Cholesterol is the major, and probably the sole precursor of bile acids. During normal digestion, bile acids are secreted via the bile from the liver and gall bladder into the intestines. Bile acids emulsify the fat and lipid materials present in food, thus facilitating absorption. A major portion of the bile acids secreted is reabsorbed from the intestines and returned via the portal circulation to the liver, thus completing the enterohepatic cycle. Only very small amounts of bile acids are found in normal serum.

COLESTID Granules (colestipol hydrochloride) bind bile acids in the intestine forming a complex that is excreted in the feces. This nonsystemic action results in a partial removal of the bile acids from the enterohepatic circulation, preventing their reabsorption. Since colestipol hydrochloride is an anion exchange resin, the chloride anions of the resin can be replaced by other anions, usually those with a greater affinity for the resin than chloride ion.

Colestipol hydrochloride is hydrophilic, but it is virtually water insoluble (99.75%) and it is not hydrolyzed by digestive enzymes. The high molecular weight polymer in COLESTID apparently is not absorbed. Less than 0.05% of ^{14}C-labeled colestipol hydrochloride is excreted in the urine.

The increased fecal loss of bile acids due to administration of COLESTID leads to an increased oxidation of cholesterol to bile acids. This results in an increase in the number of LDL receptors, increased hepatic uptake of LDL and a decrease in beta lipoprotein or low density lipoprotein serum levels, and a decrease in serum cholesterol levels. Although COLESTID produces an increase in the hepatic synthesis of cholesterol in man, serum cholesterol levels fall.

There is evidence to show that this fall in cholesterol is secondary to an increased rate of cholesterol rich lipoproteins (beta or low density lipoproteins) from the plasma. Serum triglyceride levels may increase or remain unchanged in colestipol treated patients.

The decline in serum cholesterol levels with treatment with COLESTID is usually evident by one month. When COLESTID is discontinued, serum cholesterol levels usually return to baseline levels within one month. Periodic determinations of serum cholesterol levels as outlined in the National Cholesterol Education Program (NCEP) guidelines should be done to confirm a favorable initial and long-term response.[1]

In patients with heterozygous familial hypercholesterolemia who have not obtained an optimal response to colestipol hydrochloride alone in maximal doses, the combination of colestipol hydrochloride and nicotinic acid has been shown to provide effective further lowering of serum cholesterol, triglyceride, and LDL cholesterol values. Simultaneously, HDL cholesterol values increased significantly. In many such patients it is possible to normalize serum lipid values.[1–3]

Preliminary evidence suggests that the cholesterol-lowering effects of lovastatin and the bile acid sequestrant, colestipol, are additive.

The effect of intensive lipid-lowering therapy on coronary atherosclerosis has been assessed by arteriography in hyperlipidemic patients. In these randomized, controlled clinical trials, patients were treated for two to four years by either conventional measures (diet, placebo, or in some cases low-dose resin), or with intensive combination therapy using diet plus COLESTID Granules plus either nicotinic acid or lovastatin. When compared to conventional measures, intensive lipid-lowering combination therapy significantly reduced the frequency of progression and increased the frequency of regression of coronary atherosclerotic lesions in patients with or at risk for coronary artery disease.[5–8]

INDICATIONS AND USAGE

Since no drug is innocuous, strict attention should be paid to the indications and contraindications, particularly when selecting drugs for chronic long-term use.

COLESTID Granules (colestipol hydrochloride) are indicated as adjunctive therapy to diet for the reduction of elevated serum total and low-density lipoprotein (LDL) cholesterol in patients with primary hypercholesterolemia (elevated low density lipoproteins [LDL] cholesterol) who do not respond adequately to diet. Generally, COLESTID has no clinically significant effect on serum triglycerides, but with its use triglyceride levels may be raised in some patients.

In a large, placebo-controlled, multiclinic study, the LRC-CPPT[4], hypercholesterolemic subjects treated with cholestyramine, a bile acid sequestrant with a mechanism of action and an effect on serum cholesterol similar to that of COLESTID, had reductions in total and low-density lipoprotein cholesterol (LDL-C). Over the seven-year study period the cholestyramine group experienced a 19% reduction in the combined rate of coronary heart disease death plus nonfatal myocardial infarction (cumulative incidences of 7% cholestyramine and 8.6% placebo). The subjects included in the study were middle-aged men (age 35-59) with serum cholesterol levels above 265 mg/dl, LDL-C above 175 mg/dL on a moderate cholesterol lowering diet, and no history of heart disease. It is not clear to what extent these findings can be extrapolated to other segments of the hypercholesterolemic population not studied.

Treatment for elevated serum cholesterol (> 200 mg/dL) should begin with dietary therapy and be carried out in two steps (i.e., Step-One and Step-Two Diets). A minimum of six months of intensive dietary therapy and counseling should be carried out prior to initiation of drug therapy. Shorter periods can be considered in patients with severe elevations of LDL-cholesterol (> 225 mg/dL) or with definite CHD.

CONTRAINDICATIONS

COLESTID Granules (colestipol hydrochloride) are contraindicated in those individuals who have shown hypersensitivity to any of its components.

WARNINGS

TO AVOID ACCIDENTAL INHALATION OR ESOPHAGEAL DISTRESS, COLESTID GRANULES (colestipol hydrochloride) SHOULD NOT BE TAKEN IN ITS DRY FORM. ALWAYS MIX COLESTID WITH WATER OR OTHER FLUIDS BEFORE INGESTING.

PRECAUTIONS

Before instituting therapy with COLESTID Granules (colestipol hydrochloride), diseases contributing to increased blood cholesterol such as hypothyroidism, diabetes mellitus, nephrotic syndrome, dysproteinemias and obstructive liver disease should be looked for and specifically treated. The patient's current medications should be reviewed for their potential to increase serum LDL-cholesterol or total cholesterol. It should be verified that an elevated LDL-C level is responsible for high total cholesterol, especially in those patients with marked elevations of high density lipoprotein (HDL) cholesterol and those with triglycerides over 400 mg/dL whose total cholesterol elevation may be due to very low density lipoprotein (VLDL) cholesterol rather than LDL-C. In most patients, LDL-C may be estimated according to the following equation:

LDL-C = total cholesterol − [0.16 × (triglycerides) + HDL-C]

When the total triglycerides are greater than 400, this equation is less accurate.

Because it sequesters bile acids, COLESTID may interfere with normal fat absorption and thus may prevent absorption of fat soluble vitamins such as A, D, and K.

Chronic use of COLESTID may be associated with an increased bleeding tendency due to hypoprothrombinemia from vitamin K deficiency. This will usually respond promptly to parenteral vitamin K_1 and recurrences can be prevented by oral administration of vitamin K_1.

Serum cholesterol and triglyceride levels should be determined periodically based on NCEP guidelines to confirm a favorable initial and adequate long-term response.

COLESTID may produce or severely worsen pre-existing constipation. The dosage should be increased gradually in patients to minimize the risk of developing fecal impaction. In patients with preexisting constipation, the starting dose should be 5 grams (1 packet or 1 scoop) once daily for 5–7

days, increasing to 5 grams twice daily with monitoring of constipation and of serum lipoproteins, at least twice, 4–6 weeks apart. Increased fluid and fiber intake should be encouraged to alleviate constipation and a stool sofener may occasionally be indicated. If the initial dose is well tolerated, the dose may be increased as needed by a further 5 grams/day (at monthly intervals) with periodic monitoring of serum lipoproteins. If constipation worsens or the desired therapeutic response is not achieved at 5–30 grams/day, combination therapy or alternate therapy should be considered. Particular effort should be made to avoid constipation in patients with symptomatic coronary artery disease. Constipation associated with COLESTID may aggravate hemorrhoids.

While there have been no reports of hypothyroidism induced in individuals with normal thyroid function, the theoretical possibility exists, particularly in patients with limited thyroid reserve.

Since COLESTID is a chloride form of an anion exchange resin, there is a possibility that prolonged use may lead to development of hyperchloremic acidosis.

Carcinogenesis, mutagenesis and impairment of fertility

Since COLESTID is a chloride form of an anion exchange resin, there is a possibility that prolonged use may lead to the development of hyperchloremic acidosis.

In studies conducted in rats in which cholestyramine resin (a bile acid sequestering agent similar to colestipol hydrochloride) was used as a tool to investigate the role of various intestinal factors, such as fat, bile salts and microbial flora, in the development of intestinal tumors induced by potent carcinogens, the incidence of such tumors was observed to be greater in cholestyramine resin treated rats than in control rats.

The relevance of this laboratory observation from studies in rats with cholestyramine resin to the clinical use of COLESTID is not known. In the LRC-CPPT study referred to above, the total incidence of fatal and non-fatal neoplasms was similar in both treatment groups. When the many different categories of tumors are examined, various alimentary system cancers were somewhat more prevalent in the cholestyramine group. The small numbers and the multiple categories prevent conclusions from being drawn. Further follow-up of the LRC-CPPT participants by the sponsors of that study is planned for cause-specific mortality and cancer morbidity.

When COLESTID was administered in the diet to rats for 18 months, there was no evidence of any drug related intestinal tumor formation. In the Ames assay, COLESTID was not mutagenic.

Use in Pregnancy

The use of COLESTID in pregnancy or lactation or by women of childbearing age requires that the potential benefits of drug therapy be weighed against the possible hazards to the mother and child. The safe use of the resin in COLESTID by pregnant women has not been established.

Use in Children

Safety and effectiveness in children have not been established.

DRUG INTERACTIONS

Since colestipol hydrochloride is an anion exchange resin, it may have a strong affinity for anions other than the bile acids. Therefore, colestipol hydrochloride resin may delay or reduce the absorption of concomitant oral medication. The interval between the administration of COLESTID and any other medication should be as long as possible. Patients should take other drugs at least one hour before or four hours after COLESTID to avoid impeding their absorption.

Human studies have demonstrated that COLESTID may decrease propranolol absorption. Effects on the absorption of other beta-blockers have not been determined. Therefore, patients on propranolol should be observed when COLESTID is either added or deleted from a therapeutic regimen.

In vitro studies have indicated that COLESTID binds a number of drugs. Studies in humans show that the absorption of chlorothiazide as reflected in urinary excretion is markedly decreased even when administered one hour before COLESTID. The absorption of tetracycline, furosemide, penicillin G and gemfibrozil was significantly decreased when given simultaneously with COLESTID; these drugs were not tested to determine the effect of administration one hour before COLESTID.

No depressant effect on blood levels in humans was noted when COLESTID was administered with any of the following drugs: aspirin, clindamycin, clofibrate, methyldopa, tolbutamide, phenytoin or warfarin. Particular caution should be observed with digitalis preparations since there are conflicting results for the effect of COLESTID on the availability of digoxin and digitoxin. The potential for binding of these drugs if given concomitantly is present. Discontinuing COLESTID could pose a hazard to health if a potentially toxic drug that is significantly bound to the resin has been titrated to a maintenance level while the patient was taking COLESTID.

ADVERSE REACTIONS

1. *Gastrointestinal*

   The most common adverse reactions are confined to the gastrointestinal tract. To achieve minimal GI disturbance with an optimal LDL-cholesterol lowering effect, a gradual increase of dosage starting with 5 grams once daily is recommended. Constipation, reported by about one patient in 10, is the major single complaint and at times is severe and occasionally accompanied by impaction. Most instances of constipation are mild, transient, and controlled with standard treatment. Increased fluid intake and inclusion of additional dietary fiber should be the first step; a stool softener may be added if needed. Some patients require decreased dosage or discontinuation of therapy. Hemorrhoids may be aggravated.

   Less frequent gastrointestinal complaints occurring in about one in 30 to one in 100 patients, are abdominal discomfort (abdominal pain and distention), belching, flatulence, nausea, vomiting, and diarrhea. Peptic ulceration, gastrointestinal irritation and bleeding, cholecystitis, and cholelithiasis have been reported by fewer than one in 500 patients and are not necessarily drug related.
2. *Hypersensitivity*

   Urticaria and dermatitis were noted in fewer than one in 1,000 patients. Asthma and wheezing were not reported in the studies with COLESTID but have been noted during treatment with other cholesterol-lowering agents.
3. *Musculoskeletal*

   Muscle and joint pains, and arthritis have had a reported incidence of less than one in 1,000 patients.
4. *Neurologic*

   Headache and dizziness were noted in about one in 300 patients; anxiety, vertigo, and drowsiness were reported in fewer than one in 1,000.
5. *Miscellaneous*

   Anorexia, fatigue, weakness, and shortness of breath have been seen in 1–3 patients in 1,000. Transient and modest elevations of serum glutamic oxaloacetic transaminase and of alkaline phosphatase were observed in one or more occasions in various patients treated with COLESTID Granules (colestipol hydrochloride). Some patients have shown an increase in serum phosphorus and chloride with a decrease in sodium and potassium.

OVERDOSE

Overdosage of COLESTID Granules (colestipol hydrochloride) has not been reported. Should overdosage occur, however, the chief potential harm would be obstruction of the gastrointestinal tract. The location of such potential obstruction, the degree of obstruction and the presence or absence of normal gut motility would determine treatment.

DOSAGE AND ADMINISTRATION

For adults, COLESTID Granules (colestipol hydrochloride) are recommended in doses of 5–30 grams/day given once or in divided doses. The starting dose should be 5 grams once or twice daily with a daily increment of 5 grams at one- or two-month intervals. Appropriate use of lipid profiles as per NCEP guidelines including LDL-cholesterol and trigycerides is advised so that optimal, but not excessive doses are used to obtain the desired therapeutic effect on LDL-cholesterol level. If the desired therapeutic effect is not obtained at a dose of 5–30 grams/day with good compliance and acceptable side effects, combined therapy or alternate treatment should be considered.

To avoid accidental inhalation or esophageal distress, COLESTID should not be taken in its dry form. COLESTID should always be mixed with water or other fluids before ingesting. Patients should take other drugs at least one hour before or four hours after COLESTID to minimize possible interference with their absorption. (See DRUG INTERACTIONS).

Before Administration of COLESTID

1. Define the type of hyperlipoproteinemia, as described in NCEP guidelines.
2. Institute a trial of diet and weight reduction.
3. Establish baseline serum total and LDL-cholesterol and triglyceride levels.

During Administration of COLESTID

1. The patient should be carefully monitored clinically, including serum cholesterol and triglyceride levels. Periodic determinations of serum cholesterol levels is outlined in the NCEP guidelines should be done to confirm a favorable initial and long-term response.
2. Failure of total or LDL-cholesterol to fall within the desired range should lead one to first examine dietary and drug compliance. If these are deemed acceptable, combined therapy or alternate treatment should be considered.
3. Significant rise in triglyceride level should be considered as indication for dose reduction, drug discontinuation, or combined or alternate therapy.

Mixing and Administration Guide

COLESTID Granules (colestipol hydrochloride) should always be taken mixed in a liquid such as orange or tomato juice, milk, carbonated beverage, or water. It may also be taken in soups or with cereals or pulpy fruits. COLESTID *should never be taken in its dry form.*

With beverages

1. Add the prescribed amount of COLESTID to a glassful (three ounces or more) of water, milk, flavored drink, or a favorite juice (orange, tomato, pineapple, or other fruit juice). A heavy or pulpy juice may minimize complaints relative to consistency. An unsweetened juice may improve palatability.
2. Stir the mixture until the medication is completely mixed. (COLESTID will not dissolve in the liquid.) COLESTID may also be mixed with carbonated beverages, slowly stirred in a large glass; however, this mixture may be associated with GI complaints.

   Rinse the glass with a small amount of additional beverage to make sure all the medication is taken.

With cereals, soups, and fruits

COLESTID may be taken mixed with milk in hot or regular breakfast cereals, or even mixed in soups that have a high fluid content (tomato or chicken noodle soup). It may also be added to fruits that are pulpy such as crushed pineapple, pears, peaches, or fruit cocktail.

HOW SUPPLIED

COLESTID Granules (colestipol hydrochloride) are available as follows:

Cartons of 30 foil packets—	*NDC 0009-0260-01*
Cartons of 90 foil packets—	*NDC 0009-0260-04*
Bottles of 300 grams with scoop—	*NDC 0009-0260-17*
Bottles of 500 grams with scoop—	*NDC 0009-0260-02*

Each packet or each level scoop supplies 5 grams of COLESTID.

Store at controlled room temperature 15°-30°C (59°-86°F).

REFERENCES

1. National Cholesterol Education Program (NCEP), The Expert Panel. Report of the National Cholesterol Education Program Expert Panel on Detection, Evaluation, and Treatment of High Blood Cholesterol in Adults. *Arch Intern Med* 148:36–69, 1988.
2. Kane JP, Malloy MJ, Tun P et al: Normalization of low-density-lipoprotein levels in heterozygous familial hypercholesterolemia with a combined drug regimen. *N. Engl J. Med* 304:251–258, 1981.
3. Illingworth DR, Phillipson BE, JH Rapp et al: Colestipol plus nicotinic acid in treatment of heterozygous familial hypercholesterolemia. *Lancet* 1:296–298, 1981.
4. Kuo PT, Kostis JB, Moreyra AE et al: Familial type II hyperlipoproteinemia with coronary heart disease: Effect of diet-colestipol-nicotinic acid treatment. *Chest* 79:286–291, 1981.
5. Blankenhorn DH, et al. Beneficial Effects of Combined Colestipol-Niacin Therapy on Coronary Atherosclerosis and Coronary Venous Bypass Grafts. *JAMA* 257(23):3233–3240, 1987.
6. Cashin-Hemphill L, et al. Beneficial Effects of Colestipol-Niacin on Coronary Atherosclerosis: A 4-Year Follow-up. *JAMA* 264:3013–3017, 1990.
7. Brown G, et al. Regression of Coronary Artery Disease as a Result of Intensive Lipid-Lowering Therapy in Men with High Levels of Apolipoprotein B. *N Engl. J. Med* 323:1289–1298, 1990.
8. Kane JP, Malloy MJ, et al. Regression of Coronary Atherosclerosis During Treatment of Familial Hypercholesterolemia with Combined Drug Regimens. *JAMA* 264:3007–3012, 1990.
9. Lipid Metabolism-Atherogenesis Branch, National Heart, Lung, and Blood Institute, Bethesda, MD: The Lipid Research Clinics Coronary Primary Prevention Trial Results. I. Reduction in Incidence of Coronary Heart Disease, *JAMA* 251:351–364, 1984.

Caution: Federal law prohibits dispensing without prescription.

Code 810 307 008

Shown in Product Identification Section, page 434

Continued on next page

Information on these Upjohn products is based on labeling in effect June 1, 1992. Further information concerning these and other Upjohn products may be obtained by direct inquiry to Medical Information, The Upjohn Company, Kalamazoo, Michigan 49001.

Upjohn—Cont.

CYTOSAR-U® ℞
brand of cytarabine sterile powder
(sterile cytarabine, USP)
For intravenous, Intrathecal and Subcutaneous Use Only

100 mg vial	NSN 6505-01-314-4278
500 mg vial	NSN 6505-01-315-3730

WARNING
Only physicians experienced in cancer chemotherapy should use CYTOSAR-U Sterile Powder.
For induction therapy patients should be treated in a facility with laboratory and supportive resources sufficient to monitor drug tolerance and protect and maintain a patient compromised by drug toxicity. The main toxic effect of CYTOSAR-U is bone marrow suppression with leukopenia, thrombocytopenia and anemia. Less serious toxicity includes nausea, vomiting, diarrhea and abdominal pain, oral ulceration, and hepatic dysfunction.
The physician must judge possible benefit to the patient against known toxic effects of this drug in considering the advisability of therapy with CYTOSAR-U. Before making this judgment or beginning treatment, the physician should be familiar with the following text.

DESCRIPTION
CYTOSAR-U Sterile Powder (cytarabine), commonly known as ara-C, an antineoplastic, is a sterile lyophilized material for reconstitution and intravenous, intrathecal or subcutaneous administration. It is available in multi-dose vials containing 100 mg, 500 mg, 1 g or 2 g sterile cytarabine. The pH of CYTOSAR-U was adjusted, when necessary, with hydrochloric acid and/or sodium hydroxide.
Cytarabine is chemically 4-amino-1-β-D-arabinofuranosyl-2(1H)-pyrimidinone.
Cytarabine is an odorless, white to off-white, crystalline powder which is freely soluble in water and slightly soluble in alcohol and in chloroform.

PHARMACOLOGY
Cell Culture Studies
Cytarabine is cytotoxic to a wide variety of proliferating mammalian cells in culture. It exhibits cell phase specificity, primarily killing cells undergoing DNA synthesis (S-phase) and under certain conditions blocking the progression of cells from the G_1 phase to the S-phase. Although the mechanism of action is not completely understood, it appears that cytarabine acts through the inhibition of DNA polymerase. A limited, but significant, incorporation of cytarabine into both DNA and RNA has also been reported. Extensive chromosomal damage, including chromatoid breaks, have been produced by cytarabine and malignant transformation of rodent cells in culture has been reported. Deoxycytidine prevents or delays (but does not reverse) the cytotoxic activity. Cell culture studies have shown an antiviral effect.[1] However, efficacy against herpes zoster or smallpox could not be demonstrated in controlled clinical trials.[2–4]
Cellular Resistance and Sensitivity
Cytarabine is metabolized by deoxycytidine kinase and other nucleotide kinases to the nucleotide triphosphate, an effective inhibitor of DNA polymerase; it is inactivated by a pyrimidine nucleoside deaminase which converts it to the nontoxic uracil derivative. It appears that the balance of kinase and deaminase levels may be an important factor in determining sensitivity or resistance of the cell to cytarabine.
Animal Studies
In experimental studies with mouse tumors, cytarabine was most effective in those tumors with a high growth fraction. The effect was dependent on the treatment schedule; optimal effects were achieved when the schedule (multiple closely spaced doses or constant infusion) ensured contact of the drug with the tumor cells when the maximum number of cells were in the susceptible S-phase. The best results were obtained when courses of therapy were separated by intervals sufficient to permit adequate host recovery.
Human Pharmacology
Cytarabine is rapidly metabolized and is not effective orally; less than 20 percent of the orally administered dose is absorbed from the gastrointestinal tract.
Following rapid intravenous injection of cytarabine with tritium, the disappearance from plasma is biphasic. There is an initial distributive phase with a half-life of about 10 minutes, followed by a second elimination phase with a half-life of about 1 to 3 hours. After the distributive phase, more than 80 percent of plasma radioactivity can be accounted for by the inactive metabolite 1-β-D-arabinofuranosyluracil (ara-U). Within 24 hours about 80 percent of the administered radioactivity can be recovered in the urine, approximately 90 percent of which is excreted as ara-U.
Relatively constant plasma levels can be achieved by continuous intravenous infusion.
After subcutaneous or intramuscular administration of cytarabine labeled with tritium, peak-plasma levels of radioactivity are achieved about 20 to 60 minutes after injection and are considerably lower than those after intravenous administration.
Cerebrospinal fluid levels of cytarabine are low in comparison to plasma levels after single intravenous injection. However, in one patient in whom cerebrospinal levels were examined after 2 hours of constant intravenous infusion, levels approached 40 percent of the steady state plasma level. With intrathecal administration, levels of cytarabine in the cerebrospinal fluid declined with a first order half-life of about 2 hours. Because cerebrospinal fluid levels of deaminase are low, little conversion to ara-U was observed.
Immunosuppressive Action
CYTOSAR-U Sterile Powder is capable of obliterating immune responses in man during administration with little or no accompanying toxicity.[5,6] Suppression of antibody responses to E-coli-VI antigen and tetanus toxoid have been demonstrated. This suppression was obtained during both primary and secondary antibody responses.
CYTOSAR-U also suppressed the development of cell-mediated immune responses such as delayed hypersensitivity skin reaction to dinitrochlorobenzene. However, it had no effect on already established delayed hypersensitivity reactions.
Following 5-day courses of intensive therapy with CYTOSAR-U the immune response was suppressed, as indicated by the following parameters: macrophage ingress into skin windows; circulating antibody response following primary antigenic stimulation; lymphocyte blastogenesis with phytohemagglutinin. A few days after termination of therapy there was a rapid return to normal.[7]

INDICATIONS AND USAGE
CYTOSAR-U Sterile Powder in combination with other approved anticancer drugs is indicated for remission induction in acute non-lymphocytic leukemia of adults and children. It has also been found useful in the treatment of acute lymphocytic leukemia and the blast phase of chronic myelocytic leukemia. Intrathecal administration of CYTOSAR-U is indicated in the prophylaxis and treatment of meningeal leukemia.

CONTRAINDICATIONS
CYTOSAR-U Sterile Powder is contraindicated in those patients who are hypersensitive to the drug.

WARNINGS (See boxed WARNING)
Cytarabine is a potent bone marrow suppressant. Therapy should be started cautiously in patients with pre-existing drug-induced bone marrow suppression. Patients receiving this drug must be under close medical supervision and, during induction therapy, should have leukocyte and platelet counts performed daily. Bone marrow examinations should be performed frequently after blasts have disappeared from the peripheral blood. Facilities should be available for management of complications, possibly fatal, of bone marrow suppression (infection resulting from granulocytopenia and other impaired body defenses, and hemorrhage secondary to thrombocytopenia). One case of anaphylaxis that resulted in acute cardiopulmonary arrest and required resuscitation has been reported. This occurred immediately after the intravenous administration of CYTOSAR-U Sterile Powder.
Severe and at times fatal CNS, GI and pulmonary toxicity (different from that seen with conventional therapy regimens of CYTOSAR-U) has been reported following some experimental dose schedules of CYTOSAR-U.[8–11] These reactions include reversible corneal toxicity, and hemorrhagic conjunctivitis, which may be prevented or diminished by prophylaxis with a local corticosteroid eye drop; cerebral and cerebellar dysfunction, including personality changes, somnolence and coma, usually reversible; severe gastrointestinal ulceration, including pneumatosis cystoides intestinalis leading to peritonitis; sepsis and liver abscess; pulmonary edema, liver damage with increased hyperbilirubinemia; bowel necrosis; and necrotizing colitis. Rarely, severe skin rash, leading to desquamation has been reported. Complete alopecia is more commonly seen with experimental high dose therapy than with standard treatment programs for CYTOSAR-U. If experimental high dose therapy is used, do not use a diluent containing benzyl alcohol.
An increase in cardiomyopathy with subsequent death has been reported following experimental high dose therapy with cytarabine in combination with cyclophosphamide when used for bone marrow transplant preparation.[12]
A syndrome of sudden respiratory distress, rapidly progressing to pulmonary edema and radiographically pronounced cardiomegaly has been reported following experimental high dose therapy with cytarabine used for the treatment of relapsed leukemia from one institution in 16/72 patients. The outcome of this syndrome can be fatal.[13]
Benzyl alcohol is contained in the diluent for this product. Benzyl alcohol has been reported to be associated with a fatal "Gasping Syndrome" in premature infants.
Two patients with childhood acute myelogenous leukemia who received intrathecal and intravenous CYTOSAR-U at conventional doses (in addition to a number of other concomitantly administered drugs) developed delayed progressive ascending paralysis resulting in death in one of the two patients.[14]
Use in Pregnancy
CYTOSAR-U can cause fetal harm when administered to a pregnant woman. (See ANIMAL TOXICOLOGY). There are no adequate and well-controlled studies in pregnant women. If CYTOSAR-U is used during pregnancy, or if the patient becomes pregnant while taking CYTOSAR-U, the patient should be apprised of the potential hazard to the fetus. Women of childbearing potential should be advised to avoid becoming pregnant.

PRECAUTIONS
1. General Precautions
Patients receiving CYTOSAR-U Sterile Powder must be monitored closely. Frequent platelet and leukocyte counts and bone marrow examinations are mandatory. Consider suspending or modifying therapy when drug-induced marrow depression has resulted in a platelet count under 50,000 or a polymorphonuclear granulocyte count under 1000/mm^3. Counts of formed elements in the peripheral blood may continue to fall after the drug is stopped and reach lowest values after drug-free intervals of 12 to 24 days. When indicated, restart therapy when definite signs of marrow recovery appear (on successive bone marrow studies). Patients whose drug is withheld until "normal" peripheral blood values are attained may escape from control.
When large intravenous doses are given quickly, patients are frequently nauseated and may vomit for several hours postinjection. This problem tends to be less severe when the drug is infused.
The human liver apparently detoxifies a substantial fraction of an administered dose. Use the drug with caution and at reduced dose in patients whose liver function is poor.
Periodic checks of bone marrow, liver and kidney functions should be performed in patients receiving CYTOSAR-U.
Like other cytotoxic drugs, CYTOSAR-U may induce hyperuricemia secondary to rapid lysis of neoplastic cells. The clinician should monitor the patient's blood uric acid level and be prepared to use such supportive and pharmacologic measures as might be necessary to control this problem.
Acute pancreatitis has been reported to occur in patients being treated with CYTOSAR-U who have had prior treatment with L-asparaginase.[15]
2. Information for patient
Not applicable.
3. Laboratory tests
See General Precautions
4. Drug Interactions
Reversible decreases in steady-state plasma digoxin concentrations and renal glycoside excretion were observed in patients receiving beta-acetyldigoxin and chemotherapy regimens containing cyclophosphamide, vincristine and prednisone with or without CYTOSAR-U or procarbazine.[39] Steady-state plasma digitoxin concentrations did not appear to change. Therefore, monitoring of plasma digoxin levels may be indicated in patients receiving similar combination chemotherapy regimens. The utilization of digitoxin for such patients may be considered as an alternative.
An *in vitro* interaction study between gentamicin and cytarabine showed a cytarabine related antagonism for the susceptibility of *K. pneumoniae* strains. This study suggests that in patients on cytarabine being treated with gentamicin for a *K. pneumoniae* infection, the lack of a prompt therapeutic response may indicate the need for reevaluation of antibacterial therapy.[40]
Clinical evidence in one patient showed possible inhibition of fluorocytosine efficacy during therapy with CYTOSAR-U.[41] This may be due to potential competitive inhibition of its uptake.[42]
5. Carcinogenesis, mutagenesis, impairment of fertility
Extensive chromosomal damage, including chromatoid breaks have been produced by cytarabine and malignant transformation of rodent cells in culture has been reported.
6. Pregnancy
Pregnancy Category D. See WARNINGS.
A review of the literature has shown 32 reported cases where CYTOSAR-U was given during pregnancy, either alone or in combination with other cytotoxic agents:
Eighteen normal infants were delivered. Four of these had first trimester exposure. Five infants were premature or low birth weight. Twelve of the 18 normal infants were followed up at ages ranging from six weeks to seven years, and showed no abnormalities. One apparently normal infant died at 90 days of gastroenteritis.

Two cases of congenital abnormalities have been reported, one with upper and lower distal limb defects,[16] and the other with extremity and ear deformities.[17] Both of these cases had first trimester exposure.

There were seven infants with various problems in the neonatal period, including pancytopenia; transient depression of WBC, hematocrit or platelets; electrolyte abnormalities; transient eosinophilia; and one case of increased IgM levels and hyperpyrexia possibly due to sepsis. Six of the seven infants were also premature. The child with pancytopenia died at 21 days of sepsis.

Therapeutic abortions were done in five cases. Four fetuses were grossly normal, but one had an enlarged spleen and another showed Trisomy C chromosome abnormality in the chorionic tissue.

Because of the potential for abnormalities with cytotoxic therapy, particularly during the first trimester, a patient who is or who may become pregnant while on CYTOSAR-U should be apprised of the potential risk to the fetus and the advisability of pregnancy continuation. There is a definite, but considerably reduced risk if therapy is initiated during the second or third trimester. Although normal infants have been delivered to patients treated in all three trimesters of pregnancy, follow-up of such infants would be advisable.

7. Labor and delivery
Not applicable

8. Nursing mothers
It is now known whether this drug is excreted in human milk. Because many drugs are excreted in human milk and because of the potential for serious adverse reactions in nursing infants from cytarabine, a decision should be made whether to discontinue nursing or to discontinue the drug, taking into account the importance of the drug to the mother.

9. Pediatric use
See INDICATIONS AND USAGE

ADVERSE REACTIONS

Expected Reactions
Because cytarabine is a bone marrow suppressant, anemia, leukopenia, thrombocytopenia, megaloblastosis and reduced reticulocytes can be expected as a result of administration with CYTOSAR-U Sterile Powder. The severity of these reactions are dose and schedule dependent.[18] Cellular changes in the morphology of bone marrow and peripheral smears can be expected.[19]

Following 5-day constant infusions or acute injections of 50 mg/m[2] to 600 mg/m[2], white cell depression follows a biphasic course. Regardless of initial count, dosage level, or schedule, there is an initial fall starting the first 24 hours with a nadir at days 7–9. This is followed by a brief rise which peaks around the twelfth day. A second and deeper fall reaches nadir at days 15–24. Then there is rapid rise to above baseline in the next 10 days. Platelet depression is noticeable at 5 days with a peak depression occurring between days 12–15. Thereupon, a rapid rise to above baseline occurs in the next 10 days.[20]

Infectious Complications
Infection: Viral, bacterial, fungal, parasitic, or saprophytic infections, in any location in the body may be associated with the use of CYTOSAR-U alone or in combination with other immunosuppressive agents following immunosuppressant doses that affect cellular or humoral immunity. The infections may be mild, but can be severe and at time fatal.

The Cytarabine (Ara-C) Syndrome
A cytarabine syndrome has been described by Castleberry.[21] It is characterized by fever, myalgia, bone pain, occasionally chest pain, maculopapular rash, conjunctivitis and malaise. It usually occurs 6–12 hours following drug administration. Corticosteroids have been shown to be beneficial in treating or preventing this syndrome. If the symptoms of the syndrome are deemed treatable, corticosteroids should be contemplated as well as continuation of therapy with CYTOSAR-U.

Most Frequent Adverse Reactions
anorexia
nausea
vomiting
diarrhea
oral and anal inflammation or ulceration
hepatic dysfunction
fever
rash
thrombophlebitis
bleeding (all sites)
Nausea and vomiting are most frequent following rapid intravenous injection.

Less Frequent Adverse Reactions
sepsis
pneumonia
cellulitis at injection site
skin ulceration
urinary retention
renal dysfunction
neuritis
neural toxicity
sore throat
esophageal ulceration
esophagitis
chest pain
bowel necrosis
abdominal pain
freckling
jaundice
conjunctivitis (may occur with rash)
dizziness
alopecia
anaphylaxis (See WARNINGS)
allergic edema
pruritus
shortness of breath
urticaria
headache

Experimental Doses
Severe and at times fatal CNS, GI and pulmonary toxicity (different from that seen with conventional therapy regimens of CYTOSAR-U) has been reported following some experimental dose schedules of CYTOSAR-U.[8–11] These reactions include reversible corneal toxicity and hemorrhagic conjunctivitis, which may be prevented or diminished by prophylaxis with a local corticosteroid eye drop; cerebral and cerebellar dysfunction, including personality changes, somnolence and coma, usually reversible; severe gastrointestinal ulceration, including pneumatosis cystoides intestinalis leading to peritonitis; sepsis and liver abscess; pulmonary edema, liver damage with increased hyperbilirubinemia; bowel necrosis; and necrotizing colitis. Rarely, severe skin rash, leading to desquamation has been reported. Complete alopecia is more commonly seen with experimental high dose therapy than with standard treatment programs of CYTOSAR-U. If experimental high dose therapy is used, do not use a diluent containing benzyl alcohol.

An increase in cardiomyopathy with subsequent death has been reported following experimental high dose therapy with cytarabine in combination with cyclophosphamide when used for bone marrow transplant preparation.[12] **This cardiac toxicity may be schedule dependent[45]**.

A syndrome of sudden respiratory distress, rapidly progressing to pulmonary edema and radiographically pronounced cardiomegaly has been reported following experimental high dose therapy with cytarabine used for the treatment of relapsed leukemia from one institution in 16/72 patients. The outcome of this syndrome can be fatal.[13]

Two patients with adult acute non-lymphocytic leukemia developed peripheral motor and sensory neuropathies after consolidation with high-dose CYTOSAR-U, daunorubicin, and asparaginase. Patients treated with high-dose CYTOSAR-U should be observed for neuropathy since dose schedule alterations may be needed to avoid irreversible neurologic disorders.[22]

Ten patients treated with experimental intermediate doses of CYTOSAR-U (1 g/m[2]) with and without other chemotherapeutic agents (meta-AMSA, daunorubicin, etoposide) at various dose regimes developed a diffuse interstitial pneumonitis without clear cause that may have been related to the CYTOSAR-U.[45]

Two cases of pancreatitis have been reported following experimental doses of CYTOSAR-U and numerous other drugs. CYTOSAR-U could have been the causative agent.[46]

OVERDOSAGE

There is no antidote for overdosage of CYTOSAR-U. Doses of 4.5 g/m[2] by intravenous infusion over 1 hour every 12 hours for 12 doses has caused an unacceptable increase in irreversible CNS toxicity and death.[9]

Single doses as high as 3 g/m[2] have been administered by rapid intravenous infusion without apparent toxicity.[23]

DOSAGE AND ADMINISTRATION

CYTOSAR-U Sterile Powder is not active orally. The schedule and method of administration varies with the program of therapy to be used. CYTOSAR-U may be given by intravenous infusion or injection, subcutaneously or intrathecally. Thrombophlebitis has occurred at the site of drug injection or infusion in some patients, and rarely patients have noted pain and inflammation at subcutaneous injection sites. In most instances, however, the drug has been well tolerated.

Patients can tolerate higher total doses when they receive the drug by rapid intravenous injection as compared with slow infusion. This phenomenon is related to the drug's rapid inactivation and brief exposure of susceptible normal and neoplastic cells to significant levels after rapid injection. Normal and neoplastic cells seem to respond in somewhat parallel fashion to these different modes of administration and no clear-cut clinical advantage has been demonstrated for either.

In the induction therapy of acute non-lymphocytic leukemia, the usual cytarabine dose in combination with other anticancer drugs is 100 mg/m[2] day by continuous IV infusion (Days 1–7) or 100 mg/m[2] IV every 12 hours (Days 1–7).

The literature should be consulted for the current recommendations for use in acute lymphocytic leukemia.

Intrathecal Use in Meningeal Leukemia
CYTOSAR-U has been used intrathecally in acute leukemia in doses ranging from 5 mg/m[2] to 75 mg/m[2] of body surface area. The frequency of administration varied from once a day for 4 days to once every 4 days. The most frequently used dose was 30 mg/m[2] every 4 days until cerebrospinal fluid findings were normal, followed by one additional treatment.[24–28] The dosage schedule is usually governed by the type and severity of central nervous system manifestations and the response to previous therapy.

If used intrathecally, do not use a diluent containing benzyl alcohol. Many clinicians reconstitute with autologous spinal fluid or preservative-free 0.9% Sodium Chloride, USP, for Injection and use immediately.

CYTOSAR-U given intrathecally may cause systemic toxicity and careful monitoring of the hemopoietic system is indicated. Modification of other anti-leukemia therapy may be necessary. Major toxicity is rare. The most frequently reported reactions after intrathecal administration were nausea, vomiting and fever; these reactions are mild and self-limiting. Paraplegia has been reported.[29] Necrotizing leukoencephalopathy occurred in 5 children; these patients had also been treated with intrathecal methotrexate and hydrocortisone, as well as by central nervous system radiation.[30] Isolated neurotoxicity has been reported.[31] Blindness occurred in two patients in remission whose treatment had consisted of combination systemic chemotherapy, prophylactic central nervous system radiation and intrathecal CYTOSAR-U.[32]

Focal leukemic involvement of the central nervous system may not respond to intrathecal CYTOSAR-U and may better be treated with radiotherapy.

The 100 mg vial may be reconstituted with 5 ml of Bacteriostatic Water for Injection with Benzyl Alcohol 0.945% w/v added as preservative. The resulting solution contains 20 mg of cytarabine per ml. (Do not use Bacteriostatic Water for Injection with Benzyl Alcohol 0.945% w/v as a diluent for intrathecal use. See WARNINGS).

The 500 mg vial may be reconstituted with 10 ml Bacteriostatic Water for Injection with Benzyl Alcohol 0.945% w/v added as preservative. The resulting solution contains 50 mg of cytarabine per ml. (Do not use Bacteriostatic Water for Injection with Benzyl Alcohol 0.945% w/v as a diluent for intrathecal use. See WARNINGS).

The 1 gram vial may be reconstituted with 10 ml of Bacteriostatic Water for Injection with Benzyl Alcohol 0.945% w/v added as preservative. The resulting solution contains 100 mg of cytarabine per ml. (Do not use Bacteriostatic Water for Injection with Benzyl Alcohol 0.945% w/v as a dilient for intrathecal use. See WARNINGS).

The 2 gram vial may be reconstituted with 20 ml of Bacteriostatic Water for Injection with Benzyl Alcohol 0.945% w/v added as preservative. The resulting solution contains 100 mg of cytarabine per ml. (Do not use Bacteriostatic Water for Injection with Benzyl Alcohol 0.945% w/v as a diluent for intrathecal use. See WARNINGS).

If used intrathecally many clinicians reconstitute with preservative-free 0.9% Sodium Chloride for Injection and use immediately.

The pH of the reconstituted solutions is about 5. Solutions reconstituted with Bacteriostatic Water for Injection with Benzyl Alcohol 0.945% w/v may be stored at controlled room temperature, 15°–30°C (59°–86°F) for 48 hours. Discard any solutions in which a slight haze develops.

Solutions reconstituted without a preservative should be used immediately.

Chemical Stability of Infusion Solutions:
Chemical stability studies were performed by ultraviolet assay on infusion solutions of CYTOSAR-U. These studies showed that when reconstituted CYTOSAR-U was added to Water for Injection, 5% Dextrose in Water or Sodium Chloride Injection, 94 to 96 percent of the cytarabine was present after 192 hours storage at room temperature.

Parenteral drugs should be inspected visually for particulate matter and discoloration, prior to administration, whenever solution and container permit.

Procedures for proper handling and disposal of anticancer drugs should be considered. Several guidelines on this subject have been published.[33–38] There is no general agreement that all of the procedures recommended in the guidelines are necessary or appropriate.

HOW SUPPLIED

CYTOSAR-U Sterile Powder (sterile cytarabine) is available in multi-dose vials of four sizes:

Continued on next page

Information on these Upjohn products is based on labeling in effect June 1, 1992. Further information concerning these and other Upjohn products may be obtained by direct inquiry to Medical Information, The Upjohn Company, Kalamazoo, Michigan 49001.

Upjohn—Cont.

100 mg vial, NDC 0009-3063-01
100 mg vial, NDC 0009-0373-01
500 mg vial, NDC 0009-3070-01
500 mg vial, NDC 0009-0473-01
1 g vial, NDC 0009-3295-01
2 g vial, NDC 0009-3296-01
Store the product at controlled room temperature 15°–30°C
(59°–86°F.)

REFERENCES

1. Zaky DA, Betts RF, Douglas RG, et al: Varicella-Zoster Virus and Subcutaneous Cytarabine: Correlation of In Vitro Sensitivities to Blood Levels, *Antimicrob Agents Chemother* 1975; 7:229–232
2. Davis CM, VanDersarl JV, Coltman CA Jr: Failure of Cytarabine in Varicella-Zoster Infections, *JAMA* 1973; 224:122–123
3. Betts RF, Zaky DA, Douglas RG, et al: Ineffectiveness of Subcutaneous Cytosine Arabinoside in Localized Herpes Zoster, *Ann Intern Med* 1975; 82:778–783
4. Dennis DT, Doberstyn EB, Awoke S, et al: Failure of Cytosine Arabinoside in Treatment Smallpox; A Double-blind Study, *Lancet* 1974; 2:377–379
5. Gray GD: ARA-C and Derivatives as Examples of Immunosuppressive Nucleoside Analogs, *Ann NY Acad Sci* 1975; 255:372–379
6. Mitchell MS, Wade ME, DeConti RC, et al: Immunosuppressive Effects of Cytosine Arabinoside and Methotrexate in Man, *Ann Intern Med* 1969; 70:535–547
7. Frei E, Ho DHW, Bodey GP, et al: Pharmacologic and Cytokinetic Studies of Arabinosyl Cytosine. In *Unifying Concepts of Leukemia, Bibl. Hematol.* No. 39. Karger, Basel 1973, pp 1085–1097
8. Hopen G, Mondino BJ, Johnson BL, et al: Corneal Toxicity with Systemic Cytarabine, *Am J Ophthalmol* 1981; 91:500–504
9. Lazarus HM, Herzig RH, Herzig GP, et al; Central Nervous System Toxicity of High-Dose Systemic Cytosine Arabinoside, *Cancer* 1981; 48:2577–2582
10. Slavin RE, Dias MA, Soral R: Cytosine Arabinoside Induced Gastrointestinal Toxic Alterations in Sequential Chemotherapeutic Protocols—A Clinical Pathologic Study of 33 Patients, *Cancer* 1978; 42:1747–1759
11. Haupt HM, Hutchins GM, Moore GW; Ara-C Lung: Non-cardiogenic Pulmonary Edema Complicating Cytosine Arabinoside Therapy of Leukemia, *Am J Med* 1981; 70:256–261
12. Takvorian T, Anderson K, Ritz J: A Fatal Cardiomyopathy Associated with High Dosage Ara-C (HiDAC) and Cyclophosphamide (CTX) in Bone Marrow Transplantation (BMTx). (Abstract submitted for 1985 AACR Meetings in Houston, Texas.)
13. Andersson BS, Cogan B, Keating MJ, Estey EH, et al: Subacute Pulmonary Failure Complicating Therapy with High-Dose Ara-C in Acute Leukemia, *Cancer* 1985; 56:2181–2184
14. Dunton SF, Ruprecht N, Spruce W, et al: Progressive Ascending Paralysis Following Administration of Intrathecal and Intravenous Cytosine Arabinoside, *Cancer* 1986; 57:1083–1088
15. Altman AJ, Dinndorf P, Quinn JJ: Acute Pancreatitis in Association with Cytosine Arabinoside Therapy, *Cancer* 1982; 49:1384–1386
16. Shafer AI: Teratogenic Effects of Antileukemic Chemotherapy, *Arch Intern Med* 1981; 141:514–515
17. Wagner VM, et al: Congenital Abnormalities in Baby Born to Cytarabine Treated Mother, *Lancet* 1980; 2:98–99
18. Frei E III, Bickers JN, Hewlett JS, et al: Dose Schedule and Antitumor Studies of Arabinosyl Cytosine (NSC 63878), *Cancer Res* 1969; 29:1325–1332
19. Bell WR, Wang JJ, Carbone PP, et al: Cytogenetic and Morphologic Abnormalities in Human Bone Marrow Cells during Cytosine Arabinoside Therapy, *J Hematol* 1966; 27:771–781
20. Burke PJ, Serpick AA, Carbone PP, et al: A Clinical Evaluation of Dose and Schedule of Administration of Cytosine Arabinoside (NSC 63878), *Cancer Res* 1968; 28:274–279
21. Castleberry RP, Crist WM, Holbrook T, et al: The Cytosine Arabinoside (Ara-C) Syndrome, *Med Pediatr Oncol* 1981; 9:257–264
22. Powell BL, Capizzi RL, Lyerly EW, et al: Peripheral Neuropathy After High-Dose Cytosine Arabinoside, Daunorubicin, and Asparaginase Consolidation for Acute Nonlymphocytic Leukemia, *J Clin Oncol* 1986; 4(1):95–97
23. Rudnick SA, et al: High Dose Cytosine Arabinoside (HDARAC) in Refractory Acute Leukemia, *Cancer* 1979; 44:1189–1193
24. Proceedings of the Chemotherapy Conference on ARA-C: Development and Application (Cytosine Arabinoside Hydrochloride—NSC 63878), Oct. 10, 1969
25. Lay HN, Colebatch JH, Ekert H: Experiences with Cytosine Arabinoside in Childhood Leukaemia and Lymphoma, *Med J Aust* 1971; 2:187–192
26. Halikowski B, Cyklis R, Armata J, et al: Cytosine Arabinoside Administered Intrathecally in Cerebromeningeal Leukemia, *Acta Paediat Scand* 1970; 59:164–168
27. Wang JJ, Pratt CB: Intrathecal Arabinosyl Cytosine in Meningeal Leukemia, *Cancer* 1970; 25:531–534
28. Band PR, Holland JF, Bernard J, et al: Treatment of Central Nervous System Leukemia with Intrathecal Cytosine Arabinoside, *Cancer* 1973; 32:744–748
29. Saiki JH, Thompson S, Smith F, et al: Paraplegia Following Intrathecal Chemotherapy, *Cancer* 1972; 29:370–374
30. Rubinstein LJ, Herman MM, Long TF, et al: Disseminated Necrotizing Leukoencephalopathy: A Complication of Treated Central System Leukemia and Lymphoma, *Cancer* 1975; 35:291–305
31. Marmont AM, Damasio EE: Neurotoxicity of Intrathecal Chemotherapy for Leukaemia, *Brit Med J* 1973; 4:47
32. Margileth DA, Poplack DG, Pizzo PA, et al: Blindness During Remission in Two Patients with Acute Lymphoblastic Leukemia, *Cancer* 1977; 39:58–61
33. Recommendations for the Safe Handling of Parenteral Antineoplastic Drugs. NIH Publication No. 83-2621. For sale by the Superintendent of Documents, US Government Printing Office, Washington, DC 20402.
34. AMA Council Report. Guidelines for Handling Parenteral Antineoplastics. *JAMA*, March 15, 1985.
35. National Study Commission on Cytotoxic Exposure-Recommendations for Handling Cytotoxic Agents. Available from Louis P. Jeffrey, ScD, Director of Pharmacy Services, Rhode Island Hospital, 593 Eddy Street, Providence, Rhode Island 02902.
36. Clinical Oncological Society of Australia: Guidelines and recommendations for safe handling of antineoplastic agents. *Med J Australia* 1983; 1:426–428.
37. Jones, RB, et al. Safe handling of chemotherapeutic agents: A report from the Mount Sinai Medical Center CA-A *Cancer Journal for Clinicians* Sept/Oct., 1983, pp. 258–263.
38. American Society of Hospital Pharmacists Technical assistance bulletin on handling cytotoxic drugs in hospitals. *Am J Hosp Pharm* 1985; 42:131–137.
39. Kuhlman J: Inhibition of Digoxin Absorption but not of Digitoxin During Cytostatic Drug Therapy. *Arzneim Forsch* 1982; 32:698–704.
40. Moody MR, Morris JJ, Yang VM, et al: Effect of Two Cancer Chemotherapeutic Agents on the Antibacterial Activity of Three Antimicrobial Agents. *Antimicrob Agents Chemother* 1978; 14:737–742.
41. Holt RJ: Clinical Problems with 5-Fluorocytosine. *Mykosen* 1978; 21(11):363–369.
42. Polak A, Grenson M: Interference Between the Uptake of Pyrimidines and Purines in Yeasts. *Path Microbiol* 1973; 39:37–38.
43. Peters WG, Willemze R, Colly LP: Results of Induction and Consolidation Treatment with Intermediate and High-Dose Ara-C and m-AMSA Containing Regimens in Patients with Primarily Failed or Relapsed Acute Leukemia and Non-Hodgkin's Lymphoma. *Scan J Hemat* 1986; 36 (Suppl 44):7–16.
44. Siemers RF, Friedenberg WR, Norfleet RG: High-Dose Cytosine Arabinoside-Associated Pancreatitis. *Cancer* 1985; 56:1940–1942.
45. Paul S, et al: "High Dose Ara-C Does Not Increase the Cardiotoxicity of cyclophosphamide—Total Body Irradiation Conditioning Regimes for Bone Marrow Transplantation". *Proceeding of ASCO* 1989; 8:16, abstract 60.

ANIMAL TOXICOLOGY

Toxicity of cytarabine in experimental animals, as well as activity, is markedly influenced by the schedule of administration. For example, in mice the LD_{10} for single intraperitoneal administration is greater than 6000 mg/m^2. However, when administered in 8 doses, each separated by 3 hours, the LD_{10} is less than 750 mg/m^2 total dose. Similarly, although a total dose of 1920 mg/m^2 administered as 12 injections at 6-hour intervals was lethal to beagle dogs (severe bone marrow hypoplasia with evidence of liver and kidney damage), dogs receiving the same total dose administered in 8 injections (again at 6-hour intervals) over a 48-hour period survived with minimal signs of toxicity. The most consistent observation in surviving dogs was elevated transaminase levels. In all experimental species the primary limiting toxic effect is marrow suppression with leukopenia. In addition, cytarabine causes abnormal cerebellar development in the neonatal hamster and is teratogenic to the rat fetus.
Code 810 126 016

DELTASONE®   ℞
brand of prednisone tablets, USP

DESCRIPTION

DELTASONE Tablets contain prednisone which is a glucocorticoid. Glucocorticoids are adrenocortical steroids, both naturally occurring and synthetic, which are readily absorbed from the gastrointestinal tract. Prednisone is a white to practically white, odorless, crystalline powder. It is very slightly soluble in water; slightly soluble in alcohol, in chloroform, in dioxane, and in methanol.
The chemical name for prednisone is pregna-1,4-diene-3,11,20-trione, 17,21-dihydroxy- and its molecluar weight is 358.43.
The structural formula is represented below:

DELTASONE Tablets are available in 5 strengths: 2.5 mg, 5 mg, 10 mg, 20 mg and 50 mg. Inactive Ingredients: **2.5 mg**—Calcium Stearate, Corn Starch, Erythrosine Sodium, Lactose, Mineral Oil, Sorbic Acid and Sucrose. **5 mg**—Calcium Stearate, Corn Starch, Lactose, Mineral Oil, Sorbic Acid and Sucrose. **10 mg**—Calcium Stearate, Corn Starch, Lactose, Sorbic Acid and Sucrose. **20 mg**—Calcium Stearate, Corn Starch, FD&C Yellow No. 6, Lactose, Sorbic Acid and Sucrose. **50 mg**—Corn Starch, Lactose, Magnesium Stearate, Sorbic Acid, Sucrose, and Talc.

ACTIONS

Naturally occurring glucocorticoids (hydrocortisone and cortisone), which also have salt-retaining properties, are used as replacement therapy in adrenocortical deficiency states. Their synthetic analogs are primarily used for their potent anti-inflammatory effects in disorders of many organ systems.
Glucocorticoids cause profound and varied metabolic effects. In addition, they modify the body's immune responses to diverse stimuli.

INDICATIONS

DELTASONE Tablets are indicated in the following conditions:

1. Endocrine Disorders
Primary or secondary adrenocortical insufficiency (hydrocortisone or cortisone is the first choice; synthetic analogs may be used in conjunction with mineralocorticoids where applicable; in infancy mineralocorticoid supplementation is of particular importance)
Congenital adrenal hyperplasia
Hypercalcemia associated with cancer
Nonsuppurative thyroiditis

2. Rheumatic Disorders
As adjunctive therapy for short-term administration (to tide the patient over an acute episode or exacerbation) in:
Psoriatic arthritis
Rheumatoid arthritis, including juvenile rheumatoid arthritis (selected cases may require low-dose maintenance therapy)
Ankylosing spondylitis
Acute and subacute bursitis
Acute nonspecific tenosynovitis
Acute gouty arthritis
Post-traumatic osteoarthritis
Synovitis of osteoarthritis
Epicondylitis

3. Collagen Diseases
During an exacerbation or as maintenance therapy in selected cases of:
Systemic lupus erythematosus
Systemic dermatomyositis (polymyositis)
Acute rheumatic carditis

4. Dermatologic Diseases
Pemphigus
Bullous dermatitis herpetiformis
Severe erythema multiforme
(Stevens-Johnson syndrome)
Exfoliative dermatitis
Mycosis fungoides
Severe psoriasis
Severe seborrheic dermatitis

5. Allergic States
Control of severe or incapacitating allergic conditions intractable to adequate trials of conventional treatment:
Seasonal or perennial allergic rhinitis
Bronchial asthma
Contact dermatitis
Atopic dermatitis
Serum sickness
Drug hypersensitivity reactions

6. Ophthalmic Diseases
Severe acute and chronic allergic and inflammatory processes involving the eye and its adnexa such as:
Allergic corneal marginal ulcers
Herpes zoster ophthalmicus
Anterior segment inflammation
Diffuse posterior uveitis and choroiditis
Sympathetic ophthalmia
Allergic conjunctivitis
Keratitis
Chorioretinitis
Optic neuritis
Iritis and iridocyclitis

7. Respiratory Diseases
Symptomatic sarcoidosis
Loeffler's syndrome not manageable by other means
Berylliosis
Fulminating or disseminated pulmonary tuberculosis when used concurrently with appropriate antituberculous chemotherapy
Aspiration pneumonitis

8. Hematologic Disorders
Idiopathic thrombocytopenic purpura in adults
Secondary thrombocytopenia in adults
Acquired (autoimmune) hemolytic anemia
Erythroblastopenia (RBC anemia)
Congenital (erythroid) hypoplastic anemia

9. Neoplastic Diseases
For palliative management of:
Leukemias and lymphomas in adults
Acute leukemia of childhood

10. Edematous States
To induce a diuresis or remission of proteinuria in the nephrotic syndrome, without uremia, of the idiopathic type or that due to lupus erythematosus

11. Gastrointestinal Diseases
To tide the patient over a critical period of the disease in:
Ulcerative colitis
Regional enteritis

12. Nervous System
Acute exacerbations of multiple sclerosis

13. Miscellaneous
Tuberculous meningitis with subarachnoid block or impending block when used concurrently with appropriate antituberculous chemotherapy
Trichinosis with neurologic or myocardial involvement

CONTRAINDICATIONS
Systemic fungal infections and known hypersensitivity to components.

WARNINGS
In patients on corticosteroid therapy subjected to unusual stress, increased dosage of rapidly acting corticosteroids before, during, and after the stressful situation is indicated.
Corticosteroids may mask some signs of infection, and new infections may appear during their use. There may be decreased resistance and inability to localize infection when corticosteroids are used.
Prolonged use of corticosteroids may produce posterior subcapsular cataracts, glaucoma with possible damage to the optic nerves, and may enhance the establishment of secondary ocular infections due to fungi or viruses.
Usage in pregnancy: Since adequate human reproduction studies have not been done with corticosteroids, the use of these drugs in pregnancy, nursing mothers or women of childbearing potential requires thhat the possible benefits of the drug be weighed against the potential hazards to the mother and embryo or fetus. Infants born of mothers who have received substantial doses of corticosteroids during pregnancy, should be carefully observed for signs of hypoadrenalism.
Average and large doses of hydrocortisone or cortisone can cause elevation of blood pressure, salt and water retention, and increased excretion of potassium. These effects are less likely to occur with the synthetic derivatives except when used in large doses. Dietary salt restriction and potassium supplementation may be necessary. All corticosteroids increase calcium excretion.
While on corticosteroid therapy patients should not be vaccinated against smallpox. Other immunization procedures should not be undertaken in patients who are on corticosteroids, especially on high dose, because of possible hazards of neurological complications and a lack of antibody response.
The use of DELTASONE Tablets in active tuberculosis should be restricted to those cases of fulminating or disseminated tuberculosis in which the corticosteroid is used for the management of the disease in conjunction with an appropriate anti-tuberculous regimen.
If corticosteroids are indicated in patients with latent tuberculosis or tuberculin reactivity, close observation is necessary as reactivation of the disease may occur. During prolonged corticosteroid therapy, these patients should receive chemoprophylaxis.

Children who are on immunosuppressant drugs are more susceptible to infections than healthy children. Chickenpox and measles, for example, can have a more serious or even fatal course in children on immunosuppressant corticosteroids. In such children, or in adults who have not had these diseases, particular care should be taken to avoid exposure. If exposed, therapy with varicella zoster immune globulin (VZIG) or pooled intravenous immunoglobin (IVIG), as appropriate, may be indicated. If chickenpox develops, treatment with antiviral agents may be considered.

PRECAUTIONS
Drug-induced secondary adrenocortical insufficiency may be minimized by gradual reduction of dosage. This type of relative insufficiency may persist for months after discontinuation of therapy; therefore, in any situation of stress occurring during that period, hormone therapy should be reinstituted. Since mineralocorticoid secretion may be impaired, salt and/or a mineralocorticoid should be administered concurrently.
There is an enhanced effect of corticosteroids on patients with hypothyroidism and in those with cirrhosis.
Corticosteroids should be used cautiously in patients with ocular herpes simplex because of possible corneal perforation.
The lowest possible dose of corticosteroid should be used to control the condition under treatment, and when reduction in dosage is possible, the reduction should be gradual.
Psychic derangements may appear when corticosteroids are used, ranging from euphoria, insomnia, mood swings, personality changes, and severe depression, to frank psychotic manifestations. Also, existing emotional instability or psychotic tendencies may be aggravated by corticosteroids.
Aspirin should be used cautiously in conjunction with corticosteroids in hypoprothrombinemia.
Steroids should be used with caution in nonspecific ulcerative colitis, if there is a probability of impending perforation, abscess or other pyogenic infection; diverticulitis; fresh intestinal anastomoses; active or latent peptic ulcer; renal insufficiency; hypertension; osteoporosis; and myasthenia gravis.
Growth and development of infants and children on prolonged corticosteroid therapy should be carefully observed.
Although controlled clinical trials have shown corticosteroids to be effective in speeding the resolution of acute exacerbations of multiple sclerosis, they do not show that corticosteroids affect the ultimate outcome or natural history of the disease. The studies do show that relatively high doses of corticosteroids are necessary to demonstrate a significant effect. (See DOSAGE AND ADMINISTRATION).
Since complications of treatment with glucocorticoids are dependent on the size of the dose and the duration of treatment, a risk/benefit decision must be made in each individual case as to dose and duration of treatment and as to whether daily or intermittent therapy should be used.
Convulsions have been reported with concurrent use of methylprednisolone and cyclosporin. Since concurrent use of these agents results in a mutual inhibition of metabolism, it is possible that adverse events associated with the individual use of either drug may be more apt to occur.

Information for the Patient
Patients who are on immunosuppressant doses of corticosteroids should be warned to avoid exposure to chickenpox or measles and, if exposed, to obtain medical advice.

ADVERSE REACTIONS
Fluid and Electrolyte Disturbances
Sodium retention
Fluid retention
Congestive heart failure in susceptible patients
Potassium loss
Hypokalemic alkalosis
Hypertension
Musculoskeletal
Muscle weakness
Steroid myopathy
Loss of muscle mass
Osteoporosis
Vertebral compression fractures
Aseptic necrosis of femoral and humeral heads
Pathologic fracture of long bones
Gastrointestinal
Peptic ulcer with possible perforation and hemorrhage
Pancreatitis
Abdominal distention
Ulcerative esophagitis
Dermatologic
Impaired wound healing
Thin fragile skin
Petechiae and ecchymoses
Facial erythema
Increased sweating
May suppress reactions to skin tests

Metabolic
Negative nitrogen balance due to protein catabolism
Neurological
Increased intracranial pressure with papilledema (pseudotumor cerebri) usually after treatment
Convulsions
Vertigo
Headache
Endocrine
Menstrual irregularities
Development of Cushingoid state
Secondary adrenocortical and pituitary unresponsiveness, particularly in times of stress, as in trauma, surgery or illness.
Suppression of growth in children
Decreased carbohydrate tolerance
Manifestations of latent diabetes mellitus
Increased requirements for insulin or oral hypoglycemic agents in diabetics
Ophthalmic
Posterior subcapsular cataracts
Increased intraocular pressure
Glaucoma
Exophthalmos
Additional Reactions
Urticaria and other allergic, anaphylactic or hypersensitivity reactions

DOSAGE AND ADMINISTRATION
The initial dosage of DELTASONE Tablets may vary from 5 mg to 60 mg of prednisone per day depending on the specific disease entity being treated. In situations of less severity lower doses will generally suffice while in selected patients higher initial doses may be required. The initial dosage should be maintained or adjusted until a satisfactory response is noted. If after a reasonable period of time there is a lack of satisfactory clinical response, DELTASONE should be discontinued and the patient transferred to other appropriate therapy. **IT SHOULD BE EMPHASIZED THAT DOSAGE REQUIREMENTS ARE VARIABLE AND MUST BE INDIVIDUALIZED ON THE BASIS OF THE DISEASE UNDER TREATMENT AND THE RESPONSE OF THE PATIENT.** After a favorable response is noted, the proper maintenance dosage should be determined by decreasing the initial drug dosage in small decrements at appropriate time intervals until the lowest dosage which will maintain an adequate clinical response is reached. It should be kept in mind that constant monitoring is needed in regard to drug dosage. Included in the situations which may make dosage adjustments necessary are changes in clinical status secondary to remissions or exacerbations in the disease process, the patient's individual drug responsiveness, and the effect of patient exposure to stressful situations not directly related to the disease entity under treatment; in this latter situation, it may be necessary to increase the dosage of DELTASONE for a period of time consistent with the patient's condition. If after long-term therapy the drug is to be stopped, it is recommended that it be withdrawn gradually rather than abruptly.

Multiple Sclerosis
In the treatment of acute exacerbations of multiple sclerosis daily doses of 200 mg of prednisolone for a week followed by 80 mg every other day for 1 month have been shown to be effective. (Dosage range is the same for prednisone and prenisolone).

ADT® (Alternate Day Therapy)
ADT is a corticosteroid dosing regimen in which twice the usual daily dose of corticoid is administered every other morning. The purpose of this mode of therapy is to provide the patient requiring long-term pharmacologic dose treatment with the beneficial effects of corticoids while minimizing certain undesirable effects, including pituitary-adrenal suppression, the Cushingoid state, corticoid withdrawal symptoms, and growth suppression in children.
The rationale for this treatment schedule is based on two major premises: (a) the anti-inflammatory or therapeutic effect of corticoids persists longer than their physical presence and metabolic effects and (b) administration of the corticosteroid every other morning allows for re-establishment of more nearly normal hypothalamic-pituitary-adrenal (HPA) activity on the off-steroid day.
A brief review of the HPA physiology may be helpful in understanding this rationale. Acting primarily through the hypothalamus a fall in free cortisol stimulates the pituitary gland to produce increasing amounts of corticotropin (ACTH) while a rise in free cortisol inhibits ACTH secretion. Normally the HPA system is characterized by diurnal (circa-

Continued on next page

Information on these Upjohn products is based on labeling in effect June 1, 1992. Further information concerning these and other Upjohn products may be obtained by direct inquiry to Medical Information, The Upjohn Company, Kalamazoo, Michigan 49001.

Upjohn—Cont.

dian) rhythm. Serum levels of ACTH rise from a low point about 10 pm to a peak level about 6 am. Increasing levels of ACTH stimulate adrenocortical activity resulting in a rise in plasma cortisol with maximal levels occurring between 2 am and 8 am. This rise in cortisol dampens ACTH production and in turn adrenocortical activity. There is a gradual fall in plasma corticoids during the day with lowest levels occurring about midnight.

The diurnal rhythm of the HPA axis is lost in Cushing's disease, a syndrome of adrenocortical hyperfunction characterized by obesity with centripetal fat distribution, thinning of the skin with easy bruisability, muscle wasting with weakness, hypertension, latent diabetes, osteoporosis, electrolyte imbalance, etc. The same clinical findings of hyperadrenocorticism may be noted during long-term pharmacologic dose corticoid therapy administered in conventional daily divided doses. It would appear, then, that a disturbance in the diurnal cycle with maintenance of elevated corticoid values during the night may play a significant role in the development of undesirable corticoid effects. Escape from these constantly elevated plasma levels for even short periods of time may be instrumental in protecting against undesirable pharmacologic effects.

During conventional pharmacologic dose corticosteroid therapy. ACTH production is inhibited with subsequent suppression of cortisol production by the adrenal cortex. Recovery time for normal HPA activity is variable depending upon the dose and duration of treatment. During this time the patient is vulnerable to any stressful situation. Although it has been shown that there is considerably less adrenal suppression following a single morning dose of prednisolone (10 mg) as opposed to a quarter of that dose administered every 6 hours, there is evidence that some suppressive effect on adrenal activity may be carrried over into the following day when pharmacologic doses are used. Further, it has been shown that a single dose of certain corticosteroids will produce adrenocortical suppression for two or more days. Other corticoids, including methylprednisolone, hydrocortisone, prednisone, and prednisolone, are considered to be short acting (producing adrenocortical suppression for 1¼ to 1½ days following a single dose) and thus are recommended for alternate day therapy.

The following should be kept in mind when considering alternate day therapy:

1) Basic principles and indications for corticosteroid therapy should apply. The benefits of ADT should not encourage the indiscriminate use of steroids.

2) ADT is a therapeutic technique primarily designed for patients in whom long-term pharmacologic corticoid therapy is anticipated.

3) In less severe disease processes in which corticoid therapy is indicated, it may be possible to initiate treatment with ADT. More severe disease states usually will require daily divided high dose therapy for initial control of the disease process. The initial suppressive dose level should be continued until satisfactory clinical response is obtained, usually four to ten days in the case of many allergic and collagen diseases. It is important to keep the period of initial suppressive dose as brief as possible particularly when subsequent use of alternate day therapy is intended.

Once control has been established, two courses are available: (a) change to ADT and then gradually reduce the amount of corticoid given every other day **or** (b) following control of the disease process reduce the daily dose of corticoid to the lowest effective level as rapidly as possible and then change over to an alternate day schedule. Theoretically, course (a) may be preferable.

4) Because of the advantages of ADT, it may be desirable to try patients on this form of therapy who have been on daily corticoids for long periods of time (eg, patients with rheumatoid arthritis). Since these patients may already have a suppressed HPA axis, establishing them on ADT may be difficult and not always successful. However, it is recommended that regular attempts be made to change them over. It may be helpful to triple or even quadruple the daily maintenance dose and administer this every other day rather than just doubling the daily dose if difficulty is encountered. Once the patient is again controlled, an attempt should be made to reduce this dose to a minimum.

5) As indicated above, certain corticosteroids, because of their prolonged suppressive effect on adrenal activity, are not recommended for alternate day therapy (eg, dexamethasone and betamethasone).

6) The maximal activity of the adrenal cortex is between 2 am and 8 am, and it is minimal between 4 pm and midnight. Exogenous corticosteroids suppress adrenocortical activity the least, when given at the time of maximal activity (am).

7) In using ADT it is important, as in all therapeutic situations to individualize and tailor the therapy to each patient. Complete control of symptoms will not be possible in all patients. An explanation of the benefits of ADT will help the patient to understand and tolerate the possible flare-up in symptoms which may occur in the latter part of the off-steroid day. Other symptomatic therapy may be added or increased at this time if needed.

8) In the event of an acute flare-up of the disease process, it may be necessary to return to a full suppressive daily corticoid dose for control. Once control is again established alternate day therapy may be re-instituted.

9) Although many of the undesirable features of corticosteroid therapy can be minimized by ADT, as in any therapeutic situation, the physician must carefully weigh the benefit-risk ratio for each patient in whom corticoid therapy is being considered.

HOW SUPPLIED

DELTASONE Tablets are available as scored, compressed tablets in the following strengths and sizes:

2.5 mg	Bottles of 100	**NDC** 0009-0032-01
5 mg	Bottles of 100	**NDC** 0009-0045-01
	Bottles of 500	**NDC** 0009-0045-02
	Bottles of 1000	**NDC** 0009-0045-16
	DOSEPAK™ Unit-of-Use (21 tablets)	**NDC** 0009-0045-04
	Unit Dose Packages (100)	**NDC** 0009-0045-05
10 mg	Bottles of 100	**NDC** 0009-0193-01
	Bottles of 500	**NDC** 0009-0193-02
	Unit Dose Packages (100)	**NDC** 0009-0193-03
20 mg	Bottles of 100	**NDC** 0009-0165-01
	Bottles of 500	**NDC** 0009-0165-02
	Unit Dose Packages (100)	**NDC** 0009-0165-03
50 mg	Bottles of 100	**NDC** 0009-0388-01

Code 810 324 812

Shown in Product Identification Section, page 434

DEPO-MEDROL® ℞

brand of methylprednisolone acetate sterile aqueous suspension (sterile methylprednisolone acetate suspension, USP)
Not for Intravenous Use

40 mg/ml (1 ml vial):
NSN 6505-00-952-0267 (M)

DESCRIPTION

DEPO-MEDROL Sterile Aqueous Suspension contains methylprednisolone acetate which is the 6-methyl derivative of prednisolone. Methylprednisolone acetate is a white or practically white, odorless, crystalline powder which melts at about 215° with some decomposition. It is soluble in dioxane, sparingly soluble in acetone, in alcohol, in chloroform, and in methanol, and slightly soluble in ether. It is practically insoluble in water.

The chemical name for methylprednisolone acetate is pregna-1,4-diene-3,20-dione,21-(acetyloxy)-11,17-dihydroxy-6-methyl-,(6α, 11β)- and the molecular weight is 416.51.

DEPO-MEDROL is an anti-inflammatory glucocorticoid for intramuscular, intrasynovial, soft tissue or intralesional injection. It is available in three strengths: 20 mg/mL; 40 mg/mL; 80 mg/mL.

Each mL of these preparations contains: [See table below.] When necessary, pH was adjusted with sodium hydroxide and/or hydrochloric acid.

The pH of the finished product remains within the USP specified range; ie, 3.5 to 7.0.

ACTIONS

Naturally occurring glucocorticoids (hydrocortisone), which also have salt retaining properties, are used in replacement therapy in adrenocortical deficiency states. Their synthetic analogs are used primarily for their potent anti-inflammatory effects in disorders of many organ systems.

Glucocorticoids cause profound and varied metabolic effects. In addition, they modify the body's immune response to diverse stimuli.

As of November, 1990, the formulation for DEPO-MEDROL Sterile Aqueous Suspension was revised. In a bioavailability study with thirty subjects, the new formulation was found to be more bioavailable than the previous formulation. An increase in the extent of methylprednisolone absorption was observed for the new formulation as indicated by significantly increased values for area under the serum methylprednisolone concentration curve and maximum serum methylprednisolone concentration (see table below). No difference in elimination half-life ($t_{1/2}$, calculated from the mean terminal elimination rate) was observed between the two formulations. No medically meaningful differences between the two formulations were seen in relation to vital signs, safety laboratory analyses, formulation effects, local tolerance, or side effects. This increase in absorption is not considered clinically significant.

	Previous Formulation	*Current Formulation*
AUC 0–240 hrs (ng × hr/mL)	1053 (47.3)* [133–2297]**	1286 (39.2) [208–2225]
C_{max} (ng/mL)	8.98 (65.9) [0–28.5]	11.8 (44.1) [3.37–23.4]
$t_{1/2}$ (hr)	139 [46–990]	139 [58–866]

*Coefficient of variation (%)
**Range of values

INDICATIONS

A. FOR INTRAMUSCULAR ADMINISTRATION

When oral therapy is not feasible and the strength, dosage form, and route of administration of the drug reasonably lend the preparation to the treatment of the condition, the intramuscular use of DEPO-MEDROL Sterile Aqueous Suspension (methylprednisolone acetate) is indicated as follows:

1. **Endocrine Disorders**
   - Primary or secondary adrenocortical insufficiency (hydrocortisone or cortisone is the drug of choice; synthetic analogs may be used in conjunction with mineralocorticoids where applicable; in infancy, mineralocorticoid supplementation is of particular importance)
   - Acute adrenocortical insufficiency (hydrocortisone or cortisone is the drug of choice; mineralocorticoid supplementation may be necessary, particularly when synthetic analogs are used)
   - Preoperatively and in the event of serious trauma or illness, in patients with known adrenal insufficiency or when adrenocortical reserve is doubtful
   - Congenital adrenal hyperplasia
   - Hypercalcemia associated with cancer
   - Nonsuppurative thyroiditis
2. **Rheumatic Disorders**
   As adjunctive therapy for short-term administration (to tide the patient over an acute episode or exacerbation) in:
   - Post-traumatic osteoarthritis
   - Synovitis of osteoarthritis
   - Rheumatoid arthritis, including juvenile rheumatoid arthritis (selected cases may require low-dose maintenance therapy)
   - Acute and subacute bursitis
   - Epicondylitis
   - Acute nonspecific tenosynovitis
   - Acute gouty arthritis
   - Psoriatic arthritis
   - Ankylosing spondylitis
3. **Collagen Diseases**
   During an exacerbation or as maintenance therapy in selected cases of:
   - Systemic lupus erythematosus
   - Systemic dermatomyositis (polymyositis)
   - Acute rheumatic carditis
4. **Dermatologic Diseases**
   - Pemphigus
   - Severe erythema multiforme (Stevens-Johnson syndrome)
   - Exfoliative dermatitis
   - Bullous dermatitis herpetiformis
   - Severe seborrheic dermatitis
   - Severe psoriasis
   - Mycosis fungoides
5. **Allergic States**
   Control of severe or incapacitating allergic conditions intractable to adequate trials of conventional treatment in:
   - Bronchial asthma
   - Contact dermatitis
   - Atopic dermatitis
   - Serum sickness
   - Seasonal or perennial allergic rhinitis
   - Drug hypersensitivity reactions
   - Urticarial transfusion reactions
   - Acute noninfectious laryngeal edema (epinephrine is the drug of first choice)
6. **Ophthalmic Diseases**
   Severe acute and chronic allergic and inflammatory processes involving the eye, such as:

Methylprednisolone acetate	20 mg	40 mg	80 mg
Polyethylene glycol 3350	29.5 mg	29.1 mg	28.2 mg
Polysorbate 80	1.97 mg	1.94 mg	1.88 mg
Monobasic sodium phosphate	6.9 mg	6.8 mg	6.59 mg
Dibasic sodium phosphate USP	1.44 mg	1.42 mg	1.37 mg
Benzyl alcohol added as a preservative	9.3 mg	9.16 mg	8.88 mg

Sodium Chloride was added to adjust tonicity.

Herpes zoster ophthalmicus
Iritis, iridocyclitis
Chorioretinitis
Diffuse posterior uveitis and choroiditis
Optic neuritis
Sympathetic ophthalmia
Anterior segment inflammation
Allergic conjunctivitis
Allergic corneal marginal ulcers
Keratitis

7. **Gastrointestinal Diseases**
To tide the patient over a critical period of the disease in:
Ulcerative colitis (systemic therapy)
Regional enteritis (systemic therapy)

8. **Respiratory Diseases**
Symptomatic sarcoidosis
Berylliosis
Fulminating or disseminated pulmonary tuberculosis when used concurrently with appropriate antituberculous chemotherapy
Loeffler's syndrome not manageable by other means
Aspiration pneumonitis

9. **Hematologic Disorders**
Acquired (autoimmune) hemolytic anemia
Secondary thrombocytopenia in adults
Erythroblastopenia (RBC anemia)
Congenital (erythroid) hypoplastic anemia

10. **Neoplastic Diseases**
For palliative management of:
Leukemias and lymphomas in adults
Acute leukemia of childhood

11. **Edematous States**
To induce diuresis or remission of proteinuria in the nephrotic syndrome, without uremia, of the idiopathic type or that due to lupus erythematosus

12. **Nervous System**
Acute exacerbations of multiple sclerosis

13. **Miscellaneous**
Tuberculous meningitis with subarachnoid block or impending block when used concurrently with appropriate antituberculous chemotherapy
Trichinosis with neurologic or myocardial involvement

B. FOR INTRASYNOVIAL OR SOFT TISSUE ADMINISTRATION (see WARNINGS)
DEPO-MEDROL is indicated as adjunctive therapy for short-term administration (to tide the patient over an acute episode or exacerbation) in:
Synovitis of osteoarthritis
Rheumatoid arthritis
Acute and subacute bursitis
Acute gouty arthritis
Epicondylitis
Acute nonspecific tenosynovitis
Post-traumatic osteoarthritis

C. FOR INTRALESIONAL ADMINISTRATION
DEPO-MEDROL is indicated for intralesional use in the following conditions:
Keloids
Localized hypertrophic, infiltrated,
inflammatory lesions of:
lichen planus, psoriatic plaques, granuloma annulare, and lichen simplex chronicus (neurodermatitis)
Discoid lupus erythematosus
Necrobiosis lipodica diabeticorum
Alopecia areata
DEPO-MEDROL also may be useful in cystic tumors of an aponeurosis or tendon (ganglia).

CONTRAINDICATIONS

DEPO-MEDROL Sterile Aqueous Suspension is contraindicated for intrathecal administration. Reports of severe medical events have been associated with this route of administration. DEPO-MEDROL is contraindicated for use in premature infants because the formulation contains benzyl alcohol. Benzyl alcohol has been reported to be associated with a fatal "gasping syndrome" in premature infants. DEPO-MEDROL is also contraindicated in systemic fungal infections and known hypersensitivity to the product and its constituents.

WARNINGS

This product contains benzyl alcohol which is potentially toxic when administered locally to neural tissue.
Multidose use of DEPO-MEDROL Sterile Aqueous Suspension from a single vial requires special care to avoid contamination
Although initially sterile, any multidose use of vials may lead to contamination unless strict aseptic technique is observed. Particular care, such as use of disposable sterile syringes and needles is necessary.
While crystals of adrenal steroids in the dermis suppress inflammatory reactions, their presence may cause disintegration of the cellular elements and physiochemical changes in the ground substance of the connective tissue. The resul-

tant infrequently occurring dermal and/or subdermal changes may form depressions in the skin at the injection site. The degree to which this reaction occurs will vary with the amount of adrenal steroid injected. Regeneration is usually complete within a few months or after all crystals of the adrenal steroid have been absorbed.
In order to minimize the incidence of dermal and subdermal atrophy, care must be exercised not to exceed recommended doses in injections. Multiple small injections into the area of the lesion should be made whenever possible. The technique of intrasynovial and intramuscular injection should include precautions against injection or leakage into the dermis. Injection into the deltoid muscle should be avoided because of a high incidence of subcutaneous atrophy.
It is critical that, during administration of DEPO-MEDROL, appropriate technique be used and care taken to assure proper placement of drug.
In patients on corticosteroid therapy subjected to any unusual stress, increased dosage of rapidly acting corticosteroids before, during, and after the stressful situation is indicated.
Corticosteroids may mask some signs of infection, and new infections may appear during their use. There may be decreased resistance and inability to localize infection when corticosteroids are used. Do not use intra-articularly, intrabursally or for intratendinous administration for *local* effect in the presence of acute infection.
Prolonged use of corticosteroids may produce posterior subcapsular cataracts, glaucoma with possible damage to the optic nerves, and may enhance the establishment of secondary ocular infections due to fungi or viruses.
Usage in pregnancy. Since adequate human reproduction studies have not been done with corticosteroids, the use of these drugs in pregnancy, nursing mothers, or women of childbearing potential requires that the possible benefits of the drug be weighed against the potential hazards to the mother and embryo or fetus. Infants born of mothers who have received substantial doses of corticosteroids during pregnancy should be carefully observed for signs of hypoadrenalism.
Average and large doses of cortisone or hydrocortisone can cause elevation of blood pressure, salt and water retention, and increased excretion of potassium. These effects are less likely to occur with the synthetic derivatives except when used in large doses. Dietary salt restriction and potassium supplementation may be necessary. All corticosteroids increase calcium excretion.
While on corticosteroid therapy patients should not be vaccinated against smallpox. Other immunization procedures should not be undertaken in patients who are on corticosteroids, especially in high doses, because of possible hazards of neurological complications and lack of antibody response.
The use of DEPO-MEDROL in active tuberculosis should be restricted to those cases of fulminating or disseminated tuberculosis in which the corticosteroid is used for the management of the disease in conjunction with appropriate antituberculous regimen.
If corticosteroids are indicated in patients with latent tuberculosis or tuberculin reactivity, close observation is necessary as reactivation of the disease may occur. During prolonged corticosteroid therapy, these patients should receive chemoprophylaxis.
Because rare instances of anaphylactoid reactions have occurred in patients receiving parenteral corticosteroid therapy, appropriate precautionary measures should be taken prior to administration especially when the patient has a history of allergy to any drug.
Children who are on immunosuppressant drugs are more susceptible to infections than healthy children. Chickenpox and measles, for example, can have a more serious or even fatal course in children on immunosuppressant corticosteroids. In such children, or in adults who have not had these diseases, particular care should be taken to avoid exposure. If exposed, therapy with varicella zoster immune globulin (VZIG) or pooled intravenous immunoglobin (IVIG), as appropriate, may be indicated. If chickenpox develps, treatment with antiviral agents may be considered.

PRECAUTIONS

Drug-induced secondary adrenocortical insufficiency may be minimized by gradual reduction of dosage. This type of relative insufficiency may persist for months after discontinuation of therapy; therefore, in any situation of stress occurring during that period, hormone therapy should be reinstituted. Since mineralocorticoid secretion may be impaired, salt and/or a mineralocorticoid should be administered concurrently.
When multidose vials are used, special care to prevent contamination of the contents is essential. There is some evidence that benzalkonium chloride is not an adequate antiseptic for sterilizing DEPO-MEDROL Sterile Aqueous Suspension multidose vials. A povidone-iodine solution or similar product is recommended to cleanse the vial top prior to aspiration of contents. (See WARNINGS).
There is an enhanced effect of corticosteroids in patients with hypothyroidism and in those with cirrhosis.

Corticosteroids should be used cautiously in patients with ocular herpes simplex for fear of corneal perforation.
The lowest possible dose of corticosteroid should be used to control the condition under treatment, and when reduction in dosage is possible, the reduction must be gradual.
Psychic derangements may appear when corticosteroids are used, ranging from euphoria, insomnia, mood swings, personality changes, and severe depression to frank psychotic manifestations. Also, existing emotional instability or psychotic tendencies may be aggravated by corticosteroids.
Aspirin should be used cautiously in conjunction with corticosteroids in hypoprothrombinemia.
Steroids should be used with caution in nonspecific ulcerative colitis, if there is a probability of impending perforation, abscess or other pyogenic infection. Caution must also be used in diverticulitis, fresh intestinal anastomoses, active or latent peptic ulcer, renal insufficiency, hypertension, osteoporosis, and myasthenia gravis, when steroids are used as direct or adjunctive therapy.
Growth and development of infants and children on prolonged corticosteroid therapy should be carefully followed.
The following additional precautions apply for parenteral corticosteroids. Intrasynovial injection of a corticosteroid may produce systemic as well as local effects.
Appropriate examination of any joint fluid present is necessary to exclude a septic process.
A marked increase in pain accompanied by local swelling, further restriction of joint motion, fever, and malaise are suggestive of septic arthritis. If this complication occurs and the diagnosis of sepsis is confirmed, appropriate antimicrobial therapy should be instituted.
Local injection of a steroid into a previously infected joint is to be avoided.
Corticosteroids should not be injected into unstable joints.
The slower rate of absorption by intramuscular administration should be recognized.
Although controlled clinical trials have shown corticosteroids to be effective in speeding the resolution of acute exacerbations of multiple sclerosis, they do not show that corticosteroids affect the ultimate outcome or natural history of the disease. The studies do show that relatively high doses of corticosteroids are necessary to demonstrate a significant effect. (See **Dosage And Administration**).
Since complications of treatment with glucocorticoids are dependent on the size of the dose and the duration of treatment, a risk/benefit decision must be made in each individual case as to dose and duration of treatment and as to whether daily or intermittent therapy should be used.
Convulsions have been reported with concurrent use of methylprednisolone and cyclosporin. Since concurrent use of these agents results in a mutual inhibition of metabolism, it is possible that adverse events associated with the individual use of either drug may be more apt to occur.
Information for the Patient
Patients who are on immunosuppressant doses of corticosteroids should be warned to avoid exposure to chickenpox or measles and, if exposed, to obtain medical advice.

ADVERSE REACTIONS

Fluid and electrolyte disturbances:
Sodium retention
Fluid retention
Congestive heart failure in susceptible patients
Potassium loss
Hypokalemic alkalosis
Hypertension
Musculoskeletal:
Muscle weakness
Steroid myopathy
Loss of muscle mass
Osteoporosis
Vertebral compression fractures
Aseptic necrosis of femoral and humeral heads
Pathologic fracture of long bones
Gastrointestinal:
Peptic ulcer with possible subsequent perforation and hemorrhage
Pancreatitis
Abdominal distention
Ulcerative esophagitis
Dermatologic:
Impaired wound healing
Thin fragile skin
Petechiae and ecchymoses
Facial erythema
Increased sweating
May suppress reactions to skin tests

Continued on next page

Information on these Upjohn products is based on labeling in effect June 1, 1992. Further information concerning these and other Upjohn products may be obtained by direct inquiry to Medical Information, The Upjohn Company, Kalamazoo, Michigan 49001.

Upjohn—Cont.

Neurological:
- Convulsions
- Increased intracranial pressure with papilledema (pseudotumor cerebri) usually after treatment
- Vertigo
- Headache

Endocrine:
- Menstrual irregularities
- Development of Cushingoid state
- Suppression of growth in children
- Secondary adrenocortical and pituitary unresponsiveness, particularly in times of stress, as in trauma, surgery or illness
- Decreased carbohydrate tolerance
- Manifestations of latent diabetes mellitus
- Increased requirements for insulin or oral hypoglycemic agents in diabetes

Ophthalmic:
- Posterior subcapsular cataracts
- Increased intraocular pressure
- Glaucoma
- Exophthalmos

Metabolic:
- Negative nitrogen balance due to protein catabolism

The following *additional* adverse reactions are related to parenteral corticosteroid therapy:
- Anaphylactic reaction
- Allergic or hypersensitivity reactions
- Urticaria
- Hyperpigmentation or hypopigmentation
- Subcutaneous and cutaneous atrophy
- Sterile abscess
- Injection site infections following non-sterile administration (see WARNINGS)
- Postinjection flare, following intra-articular use
- Charcot-like arthropathy

Adverse Reactions Reported with the Following Routes of Administration

Intrathecal/Epidural
- Arachnoiditis
- Meningitis
- Paraparesis/paraplegia
- Sensory disturbances
- Bowel/bladder dysfunction
- Headache
- Seizures

Intranasal
- Temporary/permanent visual impairment including blindness
- Allergic reactions
- Rhinitis

Ophthalmic
- Temporary/permanent visual impairment including blindness
- Increased intraocular pressure
- Ocular and periocular inflammation including allergic reactions
- Infection
- Residue or slough at injection site

Miscellaneous injection sites (scalp, tonsillar fauces, sphenopalatine ganglion)-blindness

DOSAGE AND ADMINISTRATION

Because of possible physical incompatibilities, DEPO-MEDROL Sterile Aqueous Suspension (methylprednisolone acetate) should not be diluted or mixed with other solutions.

A. Administration for Local Effect

Therapy with DEPO-MEDROL does not obviate the need for the conventional measures usually employed. Although this method of treatment will ameliorate symptoms, it is in no sense a cure and the hormone has no effect on the cause of the inflammation.

1. Rheumatoid and Osteoarthritis. The dose for intra-articular administration depends upon the size of the joint and varies with the severity of the condition in the individual patient. In chronic cases, injections may be repeated at intervals ranging from one to five or more weeks depending upon the degree of relief obtained from the initial injection. The doses in the following table are given as a general guide: [See table above.]

Size of Joint	*Examples*	*Range of Dosage*
Large	Knees Ankles Shoulders	20 to 80 mg
Medium	Elbows Wrists	10 to 40 mg
Small	Metacarpophalangeal Interphalangeal Sternoclavicular Acromioclavicular	4 to 10 mg

Procedure: It is recommended that the anatomy of the joint involved be reviewed before attempting intra-articular injection. In order to obtain the full anti-inflammatory effect it is important that the injection be made into the synovial space. Employing the same sterile technique as for a lumbar puncture, a sterile 20 to 24 gauge needle (on a dry syringe) is quickly inserted into the synovial cavity. Procaine infiltration is elective. The aspiration of only a few drops of joint fluid proves the joint space has been entered by the needle. *The injection site for each joint is determined by that location where the synovial cavity is most superficial and most free of large vessels and nerves.* With the needle in place, the aspirating syringe is removed and replaced by a second syringe containing the desired amount of DEPO-MEDROL Sterile Aqueous Suspension. The plunger is then pulled outward slightly to aspirate synovial fluid and to make sure the needle is still in the synovial space. After injection, the joint is moved gently a few times to aid mixing of the synovial fluid and the suspension. The site is covered with a small sterile dressing.

Suitable sites for intra-articular injection are the knee, ankle, wrist, elbow, shoulder, phalangeal, and hip joints. Since difficulty is not infrequently encountered in entering the hip joint, precautions should be taken to avoid any large blood vessels in the area. Joints not suitable for injection are those that are anatomically inaccessible such as the spinal joints and those like the sacroiliac joints that are devoid of synovial space. Treatment failures are most frequently the result of failure to enter the joint space. Little or no benefit follows injection into surrounding tissue. If failures occur when injections into the synovial spaces are certain, as determined by aspiration of fluid, repeated injections are usually futile.

Local therapy does not alter the underlying disease process, and whenever possible comprehensive therapy including physiotherapy and orthopedic correction should be employed.

Following intra-articular steroid therapy, care should be taken to avoid overuse of joints in which symptomatic benefit has been obtained. Negligence in this matter may permit an increase in joint deterioration that will more than offset the beneficial effects of the steroid.

Unstable joints should not be injected. Repeated intra-articular injection may in some cases result in instability of the joint. X-ray follow-up is suggested in selected cases to detect deterioration.

If a local anesthetic is used prior to injection of DEPO-MEDROL the anesthetic package insert should be read carefully and all the precautions observed.

2. Bursitis. The area around the injection site is prepared in a sterile way and a wheal at the site made with 1 percent procaine hydrochloride solution. A 20 to 24 gauge needle attached to a dry syringe is inserted into the bursa and the fluid aspirated. The needle is left in place and the aspirating syringe changed for a small syringe containing the desired dose. After injection, the needle is withdrawn and a small dressing applied.

3. Miscellaneous: Ganglion, Tendinitis, Epicondylitis. In the treatment of conditions such as tendinitis or tenosynovitis, care should be taken, following application of a suitable antiseptic to the overlying skin, to inject the suspension into the tendon sheath rather than into the substance of the tendon. The tendon may be readily palpated when placed on a stretch. When treating conditions such as epicondylitis, the area of greatest tenderness should be outlined carefully and the suspension infiltrated into the area. For ganglia of the tendon sheaths, the suspension is injected directly into the cyst. In many cases, a single injection causes a marked decrease in the size of the cystic tumor and may effect disappearance. The usual sterile precautions should be observed, of course, with each injection.

The dose in the treatment of the various conditions of the tendinous or bursal structures listed above varies with the condition being treated and ranges from 4 to 30 mg. In recurrent or chronic conditions, repeated injections may be necessary.

4. Injections for Local Effect in Dermatologic Conditions. Following cleansing with an appropriate antiseptic such as 70% alcohol, 20 to 60 mg of the suspension is injected into the lesion. It may be necessary to distribute doses ranging from 20 to 40 mg by repeated local injections in the case of large lesions. Care should be taken to avoid injection of sufficient material to cause blanching since this may be followed by a small slough. One to four injections are usually employed, the intervals between injections varying with the type of lesion being treated and the duration of improvement produced by the initial injection.

When multidose vials are used, special care to prevent contamination of the contents is essential (See WARNINGS).

B. Administration for Systemic Effect

The intramuscular dosage will vary with the condition being treated. When employed as a temporary substitute for oral therapy, a single injection during each 24-hour period of a dose of the suspension equal to the total daily oral dose of MEDROL® Tablets (methylprednisolone) is usually sufficient. When a prolonged effect is desired, the weekly dose may be calculated by multiplying the daily oral dose by 7 and given as a single intramuscular injection.

Dosage must be individualized according to the severity of the disease and response of the patient. For infants and children, the recommended dosage will have to be reduced, but dosage should be governed by the severity of the condition rather than by strict adherence to the ratio indicated by age or body weight.

Hormone therapy is an adjunct to, and not a replacement for, conventional therapy. Dosage must be decreased or discontinued gradually when the drug has been administered for more than a few days. The severity, prognosis and expected duration of the disease and the reaction of the patient to medication are primary factors in determining dosage. If a period of spontaneous remission occurs in a chronic condition, treatment should be discontinued. Routine laboratory studies, such as urinalysis, two-hour postprandial blood sugar, determination of blood pressure and body weight, and a chest X-ray should be made at regular intervals during prolonged therapy. Upper GI X-rays are desirable in patients with an ulcer history or significant dyspepsia.

In patients with the **adrenogenital syndrome,** a single intramuscular injection of 40 mg every two weeks may be adequate. For maintenance of patients with **rheumatoid arthritis,** the weekly intramuscular dose will vary from 40 to 120 mg. The usual dosage for patients with **dermatologic lesions** benefited by systemic corticoid therapy is 40 to 120 mg of methylprednisolone acetate administered intramuscularly at weekly intervals for one to four weeks. In acute severe dermatitis due to poison ivy, relief may result within 8 to 12 hours following intramuscular administration of a single dose of 80 to 120 mg. In chronic contact dermatitis repeated injections at 5 to 10 day intervals may be necessary. In seborrheic dermatitis, a weekly dose of 80 mg may be adequate to control the condition.

Following intramuscular administration of 80 to 120 mg to asthmatic patients, relief may result within 6 to 48 hours and persist for several days to two weeks. Similarly in patients with allergic rhinitis (hay fever) an intramuscular dose of 80 to 120 mg may be followed by relief of coryzal symptoms within six hours persisting for several days to three weeks.

If signs of stress are associated with the condition being treated, the dosage of the suspension should be increased. If a rapid hormonal effect of maximum intensity is required, the intravenous administration of highly soluble methylprednisolone sodium succinate is indicated.

Multiple Sclerosis

In treatment of acute exacerbations of multiple sclerosis daily doses of 200 mg of prednisolone for a week followed by 80 mg every other day for 1 month have been shown to be effective (4 mg of methylprednisolone is equivalent to 5 mg of prednisolone).

HOW SUPPLIED

DEPO-MEDROL Sterile Aqueous Suspension (methylprednisolone acetate) is available in the following strengths and package sizes:

20 mg/mL	5 mL vial	*NDC 0009-0274-01*
40 mg/mL	5 mL vial	*NDC 0009-0280-02*
	25-5 mL vials	*NDC 0009-0280-32*
	10 mL vial	*NDC 0009-0280-03*
	25-10 mL vials	*NDC 0009-0280-33*
80 mg/mL	5 mL vial	*NDC 0009-0306-02*
	25–5 mL vials	*NDC 0009-0306-10*

Store at controlled room temperature 15°–30° C (59°–86° F)
Code 810 341 118

Shown in Product Identification Section, page 434

DEPO–PROVERA® ℞

brand of medroxyprogesterone acetate
sterile aqueous suspension
(sterile medroxyprogesterone acetate suspension, USP)

100 mg/mL, 5 mL	**NSN 6505-00-207-7965 (M)**
400 mg/mL, 2.5 mL	**NSN 6505-01-059-9006 (M)**

WARNING

THE USE OF *DEPO-PROVERA* Sterile Aqueous Suspension (medroxyprogesterone acetate) DURING THE FIRST FOUR MONTHS OF PREGNANCY IS NOT RECOMMENDED.

Progestational agents have been used beginning with the first trimester of pregnancy in an attempt to prevent habitual abortion. There is no adequate evidence that such use is effective when such drugs are given during the first four months of pregnancy. Furthermore, in the vast majority of women, the cause of abortion is a defective ovum, which progestational agents could not be expected to influence. In addition, the use of progestational agents, with their uterine-relaxant properties, in patients with fertilized defective ova may

cause a delay in spontaneous abortion. Therefore, the use of such drugs during the first four months of pregnancy is not recommended.

Several reports suggest an association between intrauterine exposure to progestational drugs in the first trimester of pregnancy and genital abnormalities in male and female fetuses. The risk of hypospadias, 5 to 8 per 1,000 male births in the general population, may be approximately doubled with exposure to these drugs. There are insufficient data to quantify the risk to exposed female fetuses, but insofar as some of these drugs induce mild virilization of the external genitalia of the female fetus, and because of the increased association of hypospadias in the male fetus, it is prudent to avoid the use of these drugs during the first trimester of pregnancy.

If the patient is exposed to DEPO-PROVERA Sterile Aqueous Suspension (medroxyprogesterone acetate) during the first four months of pregnancy or if she becomes pregnant while taking this drug, she should be apprised of the potential risks to the fetus.

DESCRIPTION

DEPO-PROVERA Sterile Aqueous Suspension contains medroxyprogesterone acetate which is a derivative of progesterone and is active by the parenteral and oral routes of administration. It is a white to off-white, odorless crystalline powder, stable in air, melting between 200 and 210° C. It is freely soluble in chloroform, soluble in acetone and dioxane, sparingly soluble in alcohol and methanol, slightly soluble in ether and insoluble in water.

The chemical name for medroxyprogesterone acetate is Pregn-4-ene-3,20-dione, 17-(acetyloxy)-6-methyl-, (6α)-.

DEPO-PROVERA for intramuscular injection is available in 2 strengths, 100 mg/mL and 400 mg/mL medroxyprogesterone acetate.

Each mL of the **100 mg/mL** suspension contains:

Medroxyprogesterone Acetate	100 mg

Also

Polyethylene glycol 3350	27.6 mg
Polysorbate 80	1.84 mg
Sodium chloride	8.3 mg

with

Methylparaben	1.75 mg
Propylparaben	0.194 mg

added as preservatives

Each mL of the **400 mg/mL** suspension contains:

Medroxyprogesterone acetate	400 mg
Polyethylene glycol 3350	20.3 mg
Sodium sulfate anhydrous	11 mg

with

Myristyl-gamma-picolinium chloride	1.69 mg

added as preservative

When necessary, pH was adjusted with sodium hydroxide and/or hydrochloric acid.

ACTIONS

Medroxyprogesterone acetate administered parenterally in the recommended doses to women with adequate endogenous estrogen transforms proliferative endometrium into secretory endometrium.

Medroxyprogesterone acetate inhibits (in the usual dose range) the secretion of pituitary gonadotropin which, in turn, prevents follicular maturation and ovulation.

Because of its prolonged action and the resulting difficulty in predicting the time of withdrawal bleeding following injection, medroxyprogesterone acetate is not recommended in secondary amenorrhea or dysfunctional uterine bleeding. In these conditions oral therapy is recommended.

INDICATIONS AND USAGE

Adjunctive therapy and palliative treatment of inoperable, recurrent, and metastatic endometrial or renal carcinoma.

CONTRAINDICATIONS

1. Thrombophlebitis, thromboembolic disorders, cerebral apoplexy or patients with a past history of these conditions.
2. Carcinoma of the breast.
3. Undiagnosed vaginal bleeding.
4. Missed abortion.
5. As a diagnostic test for pregnancy.
6. Known sensitivity to DEPO-PROVERA Sterile Aqueous Suspension.

WARNINGS

1. The physician should be alert to the earliest manifestations of thrombotic disorders (thrombophlebitis, cerebrovascular disorders, pulmonary embolism, and retinal thrombosis). Should any of these occur or be suspected, the drug should be discontinued immediately.
2. Long term toxicology studies in the monkey, dog and rat disclose:
    1) Beagle dogs receiving 75 mg/kg and 3 mg/kg every 90 days developed mammary nodules, as did some of the control animals. The nodules appearing in the

control animals were intermittent in nature, whereas the nodules in the drug treated animals were larger, more numerous, persistent, and there were two high dose animals that developed breast malignancies.
    2) Two of the monkeys receiving 150 mg/kg every 90 days developed undifferentiated carcinoma of the uterus. No uterine malignancies were found in monkeys receiving 30 mg/kg, 3 mg/kg, or placebo every 90 days. Transient mammary nodules were found during the study in the control, 3 mg/kg and 30 mg/kg groups, but not in the 150 mg/kg group. At sacrifice, the only nodules extant were in three of the monkeys in the 30 mg/kg group. Upon histopathologic examination these nodules have been determined to be hyperplastic.
    3) No uterine or breast abnormalities were revealed in the rat.

The relevance of any of these findings with respect to humans has not been established.
3. The use of DEPO-PROVERA Sterile Aqueous Suspension (medroxyprogesterone acetate) for contraception is investigational since there are unresolved questions relating to its safety for this indication. Therefore, this is not an approved indication.
4. Discontinue medication pending examination if there is sudden partial or complete loss of vision, or if there is a sudden onset of proptosis, diplopia or migraine. If examination reveals papilledema or retinal vascular lesions, medication should be withdrawn.
5. Usage in pregnancy (See WARNING Box).
6. Retrospective studies of morbidity and mortality in Great Britain and studies of morbidity in the United States have shown a statistically significant association between thrombophlebitis, pulmonary embolism, and cerebral thrombosis and embolism and the use of oral contraceptives.[1-4] The estimate of the relative risk of thromboembolism in the study by Vessey and Doll[3] was about sevenfold, while Sartwell and associates[4] in the United States found a relative risk of 4.4, meaning that the users are several times as likely to undergo thromboembolic disease without evident cause as non-users. The American study also indicated that the risk did not persist after discontinuation of administration, and that it was not enhanced by long continued administration. The American study was not designed to evaluate a difference between products.
7. Following repeated injections, amenorrhea and infertility may persist for periods up to 18 months and occasionally longer.
8. The physician should be alert to the earliest manifestations of impaired liver function. Should these occur or be suspected, the drug should be discontinued and the patient's status re-evaluated.

PRECAUTIONS

1. The pretreatment physical examination should include special reference to breast and pelvic organs, as well as Papanicolaou smear.
2. Because progestogens may cause some degree of fluid retention, conditions which might be influenced by this factor, such as epilepsy, migraine, asthma, cardiac or renal dysfunction, require careful observation.
3. In cases of breakthrough bleeding, as in all cases of irregular bleeding per vaginum, nonfunctional causes should be borne in mind. In cases of undiagnosed vaginal bleeding, adequate diagnostic measures are indicated.
4. Patients who have a history of psychic depression should be carefully observed and the drug discontinued if the depression recurs to a serious degree.
5. Any possible influence of prolonged progestin therapy on pituitary, ovarian, adrenal, hepatic or uterine functions awaits further study.
6. A decrease in glucose tolerance has been observed in a small percentage of patients on estrogen-progestin combination drugs. The mechanism of this decrease is obscure. For this reason, diabetic patients should be carefully observed while receiving progestin therapy.
7. The age of the patient constitutes no absolute limiting factor although treatment with progestins may mask the onset of the climacteric.
8. The pathologist should be advised of progestin therapy when relevant specimens are submitted.
9. Because of the occasional occurrence of thrombotic disorders, (thrombophlebitis, pulmonary embolism, retinal thrombosis, and cerebrovascular disorders) in patients taking estrogen-progestin combinations and since the mechanism is obscure, the physician should be alert to the earliest manifestation of these disorders.
10. Aminoglutethimide administered concomitantly with DEPO-PROVERA may significantly depress the bioavailability of DEPO-PROVERA.

Information for the Patient
See Patient Information at end of insert.
The patient insert should be given to all premenopausal women, except those in whom childbearing is impossible.

ADVERSE REACTIONS

(See WARNING Box for possible adverse effects on the fetus).

In a few instances there have been undesirable sequelae at the site of injection, such as residual lump, change in color of skin or sterile abscess.

The following adverse reactions have been associated with the use of DEPO-PROVERA Sterile Aqueous Suspension.

Breast—In a few instances, breast tenderness or galactorrhea have occurred.

Psychic—An occasional patient has experienced nervousness, insomnia, somnolence, fatigue or dizziness.

Thromboembolic Phenomena—Thromboembolic phenomena including thrombophlebitis and pulmonary embolism have been reported.

Skin and Mucous Membranes—Sensitivity reactions ranging from pruritus, urticaria, angioneurotic edema to generalized rash and anaphylaxis and/or anaphylactoid reactions have occasionally been reported. Acne, alopecia, or hirsutism have been reported in a few cases.

Gastrointestinal—Rarely, nausea has been reported. Jaundice, including neonatal jaundice, has been noted in a few instances.

Miscellaneous—Rare cases of headache and hyperpyrexia have been reported.

The following adverse reactions have been observed in women taking progestins including DEPO-PROVERA:
breakthrough bleeding
spotting
change in menstrual flow
amenorrhea
edema
change in weight
    (increase or decrease)
changes in cervical erosion and
    cervical secretions
cholestatic jaundice
rash (allergic) with and
    without pruritus
melasma or chloasma
mental depression

A statistically significant association has been demonstrated between use of estrogen-progestin combination drugs and the following serious adverse reactions: thrombophlebitis; pulmonary embolism and cerebral thrombosis and embolism. For this reason patients on progestin therapy should be carefully observed.

Although available evidence is suggestive of an association, such a relationship has been neither confirmed nor refuted for the following serious adverse reactions: neuro-ocular lesions, eg, retinal thrombosis and optic neuritis.

The following adverse reactions have been observed in patients receiving estrogen-progestin combination drugs:
rise in blood pressure in susceptible individuals
premenstrual-like syndrome
changes in libido
changes in appetite
cystitis-like syndrome
headache
nervousness
dizziness
fatigue
backache
hirsutism
loss of scalp hair
erythema multiforme
erythema nodosum
hemorrhagic eruption
itching

In view of these observations, patients on progestin therapy should be carefully observed.

The following laboratory results may be altered by the use of estrogen-progestin combination drugs:
Increased sulfobromophthalein retention and other hepatic function tests.
Coagulation tests: increase in prothrombin factors VII, VIII, IX and X.
Metyrapone test.
Pregnanediol determination.
Thyroid function: increase in PBI, and butanol extractable protein bound iodine and decrease in T[3] uptake values.

DOSAGE AND ADMINISTRATION

The suspension is intended for intramuscular administration only.

Continued on next page

Information on these Upjohn products is based on labeling in effect June 1, 1992. Further information concerning these and other Upjohn products may be obtained by direct inquiry to Medical Information, The Upjohn Company, Kalamazoo, Michigan 49001.

Upjohn—Cont.

Endometrial or renal carcinoma—doses of 400 mg to 1000 mg of DEPO-PROVERA Sterile Aqueous Suspension per week are recommended initially. If improvement is noted within a few weeks or months and the disease appears stabilized, it may be possible to maintain improvement with as little as 400 mg per month. Medroxyprogesterone acetate is not recommended as primary therapy, but as adjunctive and palliative treatment in advanced inoperable cases including those with recurrent or metastatic disease.

HOW SUPPLIED

DEPO-PROVERA Sterile Aqueous Suspension is available in 2 strengths:

100 mg/mL: 5 mL vials	NDC 0009-0248-02
400 mg/mL:	
2.5 mL vial	NDC 0009-0626-01
10 mL vial	NDC 0009-0626-02

REFERENCES

1. Royal College of General Practitioners: Oral contraception and thromboembolic disease. J Coll Gen Pract *13*:267–279, 1967.
2. Inman WHW, Vessey MP: Investigation of deaths from pulmonary, coronary, and cerebral thrombosis and embolism in women of child-bearing age. Br Med J *2*:193–199, 1968.
3. Vessey MP, Doll R: Investigation of relation between use of oral contraceptives and thromboembolic disease. A further report. Br Med J *2*:651–657, 1969.
4. Sartwell PE, Masi AT, Arthes FG, et al: Thromboembolism and oral contraceptives: An epidemiological case-control study. Am J Epidemiol *90*:365–380, 1969.

The text of the patient insert for progesterone and progesterone-like drugs is set forth below.

PATIENT INFORMATION

DEPO-PROVERA Sterile Aqueous Suspension contains medroxyprogesterone acetate. The information below is that which the U.S. Food and Drug Administration requires be provided for all patients taking progesterones. The information below relates only to the risk to the unborn child associated with use of progesterone during pregnancy. For further information on the use, side effects and other risks associated with this product, ask your doctor.

WARNING FOR WOMEN

Progesterone or progesterone-like drugs have been used to prevent miscarriage in the first few months of pregnancy. No adequate evidence is available to show that they are effective for this purpose. Furthermore, most cases of early miscarriage are due to causes which could not be helped by these drugs.

There is an increased risk of minor birth defects in children whose mothers take this drug during the first 4 months of pregnancy. Several reports suggest an association between mothers who take these drugs in the first trimester of pregnancy and genital abnormalities in male and female babies. The risk to the male baby is the possibility of being born with a condition in which the opening of the penis is on the underside rather than the tip of the penis (hypospadias). Hypospadias occurs in about 5 to 8 per 1,000 male births and is about doubled with exposure to these drugs. There is not enough information to quantify the risk to exposed female fetuses, but enlargement of the clitoris and fusion of the labia may occur, although rarely.

Therefore, since drugs of this type may induce mild masculinization of the external genitalia of the female fetus, as well as hypospadias in the male fetus, it is wise to avoid using the drug during the first trimester of pregnancy.

These drugs have been used as a test for pregnancy but such use is no longer considered safe because of possible damage to a developing baby. Also, more rapid methods for testing for pregnancy are now available.

If you take DEPO-PROVERA Sterile Aqueous Suspension and later find you were pregnant when you took it, be sure to discuss this with your doctor as soon as possible.

Code 810 597 006

DEPO®-TESTOSTERONE Ⓒ℞

brand of testosterone cypionate sterile solution (testosterone cypionate injection, USP)
For Intramuscular Use Only

HOW SUPPLIED

DEPO-Testosterone Sterile Solution is available in the following packages:

100 mg per mL. Each mL contains 100 mg testosterone cypionate, 0.1 mL benzyl benzoate, 736 mg cottonseed oil, and 9.45 mg benzyl alcohol (as preservative).

10 mL vial *NDC 0009-0347-02*

200 mg per mL. Each mL contains 200 mg testosterone cypionate, 0.2 mL benzyl benzoate, 560 mg cottonseed oil, and 9.45 mg benzyl alcohol (as preservative).

1 mL vial *NDC 0009-0417-01*
10 mL vial *NDC 0009-0417-02*

DIDREX® Ⓒ℞

brand of benzphetamine hydrochloride tablets

DESCRIPTION

DIDREX Tablets contain the anorectic agent benzphetamine hydrochloride. Benzphetamine hydrochloride is a white crystalline powder readily soluble in water and 95% ethanol. The chemical name for benzphetamine hydrochloride is *d*-N,α-Dimethyl-N-(phenylmethyl)-benzeneethanamine hydrochloride and its molecular weight is 275.82.

Each DIDREX tablet, for oral administration, contains 25 or 50 mg of benzphetamine hydrochloride.

Inactive Ingredients

25 mg—Calcium Stearate, Corn Starch, FD & C Yellow No. 5, Lactose, Povidone, Sorbital.

50 mg—Calcium Stearate, Corn Starch, Erythrosine Sodium, FD & C Yellow No. 6, Lactose, Povidone, Sorbital.

CLINICAL PHARMACOLOGY

Benzphetamine hydrochloride is a sympathomimetic amine with pharmacologic activity similar to the prototype drugs of this class used in obesity, the amphetamines. Actions include central nervous system stimulation and elevation of blood pressure. Tachyphylaxis and tolerance have been demonstrated with all drugs of this class in which these phenomena have been looked for.

Drugs of this class used in obesity are commonly known as "anorectics" or "anorexigenics." It has not been established, however, that the action of such drugs in treating obesity is primarily one of appetite suppression. Other central nervous system actions, or metabolic effects, may be involved.

Adult obese subjects instructed in dietary management and treated with "anorectic" drugs, lose more weight on the average than those treated with placebo and diet, as determined in relatively short term clinical trials.

The magnitude of increased weight loss of drug treated patients over placebo treated patients is only a fraction of a pound a week. The rate of weight loss is greatest in the first weeks of therapy for both drug and placebo subjects and tends to decrease in succeeding weeks. The possible origins of the increased weight loss due to the various drug effects are not established. The amount of weight loss associated with the use of an "anorectic" drug varies from trial to trial, and the increased weight loss appears to be related in part to variables other than the drug prescribed, such as the physician-investigator, the population treated, and the diet prescribed. Studies do not permit conclusions as to the relative importance of the drug and nondrug factors on weight loss.

The natural history of obesity is measured in years, whereas the studies cited are restricted to a few weeks duration; thus, the total impact of drug induced weight loss over that of diet alone must be considered to be clinically limited.

Pharmacokinetic data in humans are not available.

INDICATIONS AND USAGE

DIDREX Tablets (benzphetamine hydrochloride) are indicated in the management of exogenous obesity as a short term adjunct (a few weeks) in a regimen of weight reduction based on caloric restriction. The limited usefulness of agents of this class (see **Clinical Pharmacology**) should be weighed against possible risks inherent in their use such as those described below.

CONTRAINDICATIONS

DIDREX Tablets (benzphetamine hydrochloride) are contraindicated in patients with advanced arteriosclerosis, symptomatic cardiovascular disease, moderate to severe hypertension, hyperthyroidism, known hypersensitivity or idiosyncrasy to sympathomimetic amines, and glaucoma. Benzphetamine should not be given to patients who are in an agitated state or who have a history of drug abuse.

Hypertensive crises have resulted when sympathomimetic amines have been used concomitantly or within 14 days following use of monamine oxidase inhibitors. DIDREX should not be used concomitantly with other CNS stimulants.

DIDREX may cause fetal harm when administered to a pregnant woman. Amphetamines have been shown to be teratogenic and embryotoxic in mammals at high multiples of the human dose. DIDREX is contraindicated in women who are or may become pregnant. If this drug is used during pregnancy, or if the patient becomes pregnant while taking this drug, the patient should be apprised of the potential hazard to the fetus.

WARNINGS

When tolerance to the anorectic effect develops, the recommended dose should not be exceeded in an attempt to increase the effect; rather, the drug should be discontinued.

PRECAUTIONS

General: Insulin requirements in diabetes mellitus may be altered in association with use of anorexigenic drugs and the concomitant dietary restrictions.

Psychological disturbances have been reported in patients who receive an anorectic agent together with a restrictive dietary regime.

Caution is to be exercised in prescribing amphetamines for patients with even mild hypertension. The least amount feasible should be prescribed or dispensed at one time in order to minimize the possibility of overdosage.

DIDREX Tablets, 25 mg, contain FD&C Yellow No. 5 (tartrazine) which may cause allergic-type reactions (including bronchial asthma) in certain susceptible individuals. Although the overall incidence of FD&C Yellow No. 5 (tartrazine) sensitivity in the general population is low, it is frequently seen in patients who also have aspirin hypersensitivity.

INFORMATION FOR PATIENTS

Amphetamines may impair the ability of the patient to engage in potentially hazardous activities such as operating machinery or driving a motor vehicle; the patient should therefore be cautioned accordingly.

DRUG INTERACTIONS

Hypertensive crises have resulted when sympathomimetic amines have been used concomitantly or within 14 days following use of monoamine oxidase inhibitors. DIDREX should not be used concomitantly with other CNS stimulants.

Amphetamines may decrease the hypotensive effect of antihypertensives. Amphetamines may enhance the effects of tricyclic antidepressants.

Urinary alkalinizing agents increase blood levels and decrease excretion of amphetamines. Urinary acidifying agents decrease blood levels and increase excretion of amphetamines.

Carcinogenesis, Mutagenesis, Impairment of Fertility: Animal studies to evaluate the potential for carcinogenesis, mutagenesis or impairment of fertility have not been performed by The Upjohn Company.

Pregnancy: Pregnancy Category X. (See CONTRAINDICATIONS section).

Nursing Mothers: Amphetamines are excreted in human milk. Mothers taking amphetamines should be advised to refrain from nursing.

Pediatric Use: Use of benzphetamine hydrochloride is not recommended in children under 12 years of age.

ADVERSE REACTIONS

The following have been associated with the use of benzphetamine hydrochloride:

Cardiovascular

Palpitation, tachycardia, elevation of blood pressure. There have been isolated reports of cardiomyopathy associated with chronic amphetamine use.

CNS

Overstimulation, restlessness, dizziness, insomnia, tremor, sweating, headache; rarely, psychotic episodes at recommended doses; depression following withdrawal of the drug.

Gastrointestinal

Dryness of the mouth, unpleasant taste, nausea, diarrhea, other gastrointestinal disturbances.

Allergic

Urticaria and other allergic reactions involving the skin.

Endocrine

Changes in libido.

DRUG ABUSE AND DEPENDENCE

Benzphetamine is a controlled substance under the Controlled Substance Act by the Drug Enforcement Administration and has been assigned to Schedule III.

Benzphetamine hydrochloride is related chemically and pharmacologically to the amphetamines. Amphetamines and related stimulant drugs have been extensively abused and the possibility of abuse of DIDREX Tablets should be kept in mind when evaluating the desirability of including a drug as part of a weight reduction program. Abuse of amphetamines and related drugs may be associated with intense psychological dependence and severe social dysfunction. There are reports of patients who have increased the dosage to many times that recommended. Abrupt cessation following prolonged high dosage administration results in extreme fatigue and mental depression; changes are also noted on the sleep EEG. Manifestations of chronic intoxication with anorectic drugs include severe dermatoses, marked insomnia, irritability, hyperactivity, and personality changes. The most severe manifestation of chronic intoxication is psychosis, often clinically indistinguishable from schizophrenia.

OVERDOSAGE

Manifestations of Overdosage:

Acute overdosage with amphetamines may result in restlessness, tremor, tachypnea, confusion, assaultiveness and panic states. Fatigue and depression usually follow the central stimulation. Cardiovascular effects include arrhythmias, hypertension or hypotension, and circulatory collapse. Gastrointestinal symptoms include nausea, vomiting, diarrhea, and abdominal cramps. Hyperpyrexia and rhabdomyolysis have been reported and can lead to a number of associated

complications. Fatal poisoning is usually preceded by convulsions and coma.

TREATMENT OF OVERDOSAGE

(See **Warnings**) Information concerning the effects of overdosage with DIDREX Tablets (benzphetamine hydrochloride) is extremely limited. The following is based on experience with other anorexiants.

Management of acute amphetamine intoxication is largely symptomatic and includes sedation with a barbiturate. If hypertension is marked, the use of a nitrite or rapidly acting alpha receptor blocking agent should be considered. Experience with hemodialysis or peritoneal dialysis is inadequate to permit recommendations in this regard.

Acidification of the urine increases amphetamine excretion. The oral LD_{50} is 174 mg/kg in mice and 104 mg/kg in rats. The intraperitoneal LD_{50} in mice is 153 mg/kg.

DOSAGE AND ADMINISTRATION

Dosage should be individualized according to the response of the patient. The suggested dosage ranges from 25 to 50 mg one to three times daily. Treatment should begin with 25 to 50 mg once daily with subsequent increase in individual dose or frequency according to response. A single daily dose is preferably given in mid-morning or mid-afternoon, according to the patient's eating habits. In an occasional patient it may be desirable to avoid late afternoon administration. Use of benzphetamine hydrochloride is not recommended in children under 12 years of age.

HOW SUPPLIED

DIDREX Tablets (benzphetamine hydrochloride) are available in the following strengths and colors:

25 mg (yellow)
Bottles of 100 *NDC 0009-0018-01*

50 mg (peach, scored)
Bottles of 100 *NDC 0009-0024-01*
Bottles of 500 *NDC 0009-0024-02*

Store at controlled room temperature 15°–30°C (59°–86°F).
Code 810 735 409

Shown in Product Identification Section, page 434

GELFOAM® ℞

brand of absorbable gelatin sterile sponge
(absorbable gelatin sponge, USP)

Size 12-7 mm:	**NSN 6510-00-080-2053 (M & VA)**
Size 100:	**NSN 6510-00-080-2054 (M & VA)**
Size 200:	**NSN 6510-00-655-8522 (VA)**
Size 100 Compressed:	**NSN 6510-01-066-8966 (VA)**
Dental Packs, Size 4:	**NSN 6510-00-064-4858 (M)**

DESCRIPTION

GELFOAM Sterile Sponge is a medical device intended for application to bleeding surfaces as a hemostatic. It is a water-insoluble, off-white, nonelastic, porous, pliable product prepared from purified pork Skin Gelatin USP Granules and Water for Injection, USP. It may be cut without fraying and is able to absorb and hold within its interstices, many times its weight of blood and other fluids.

ACTION

GELFOAM Sterile Sponge has hemostatic properties. While its mode of action is not fully understood, its effect appears to be more physical than the result of altering the blood clotting mechanism.

When not used in excessive amounts, GELFOAM is absorbed completely, with little tissue reaction. This absorption is dependent on several factors, including the amount used, degree of saturation with blood or other fluids, and the site of use. When placed in soft tissues, GELFOAM is usually absorbed completely in from four to six weeks, without inducing excessive scar tissue. When applied to bleeding nasal, rectal or vaginal mucosa, it liquefies within two to five days.

HEMOSTASIS: GELFOAM Sterile Sponge, used dry or saturated with sterile sodium chloride solution, is indicated in surgical procedures as a hemostatic device, when control of capillary, venous, and arteriolar bleeding by pressure, ligature, and other conventional procedures is either ineffective or impractical.

DIRECTIONS FOR USE

Sterile technique should always be used to remove GELFOAM Sterile Sponge from its packaging. Cut to the desired size, a piece of GELFOAM, either dry or saturated with sterile, isotonic sodium chloride solution (sterile saline), can be applied with pressure directly to the bleeding site. When applied dry, a single piece of GELFOAM should be manually compressed before application to the bleeding site, and then held in place with moderate pressure until hemostasis results. When used with sterile saline, GELFOAM should be first immersed in the solution and then withdrawn, squeezed between gloved fingers to expel air bubbles, and then replaced in saline until needed. The GELFOAM sponge should promptly return to its original size and shape in the solution. If it does not, it should be removed again and kneaded vigorously until all air is expelled and it does expand to its original size and shape when returned to the sterile saline.

GELFOAM is used wet or blotted to dampness on gauze before application to the bleeding site. It should be held in place with moderate pressure, using a pledget of cotton or small gauze sponge until hemostasis results. Removal of the pledget or gauze is made easier by wetting it with a few drops of sterile saline, to prevent pulling up the GELFOAM which by then should enclose a firm clot. Use of suction applied over the pledget of cotton or gauze to draw blood into the GELFOAM is unnecessary, as the GELFOAM will draw up sufficient blood by capillary action. The first application of GELFOAM will usually control bleeding, but if not, additional applications may be made using fresh pieces, prepared as described above.

Use only the minimum amount of GELFOAM, cut to appropriate size, necessary to produce hemostasis. The GELFOAM may be left in place at the bleeding site, when necessary. Since GELFOAM causes little more cellular reaction than does the blood clot, the wound may be closed over it. GELFOAM may be left in place when applied to mucosal surfaces until it liquifies.

CONTRAINDICATIONS

GELFOAM Sterile Sponge should not be used in closure of skin incisions because it may interfere with healing of the skin edges. This is due to mechanical interposition of gelatin and is not secondary to intrinsic interference with wound healing.

GELFOAM should not be placed in intravascular compartments, because of the risk of embolization.

WARNINGS

GELFOAM Sterile Sponge is not intended as a substitute for meticulous surgical technique and the proper application of ligatures, or other conventional procedures for hemostasis.

GELFOAM is supplied as a sterile product and cannot be resterilized. Unused, opened envelopes of GELFOAM should be discarded.

Only the minimum amount of GELFOAM necessary to achieve hemostatis should be used. Once hemostatis is attained, excess GELFOAM should be carefully removed.

The use of GELFOAM is not recommended in the presence of infection. GELFOAM should be used with caution in contaminated areas of the body. If signs of infection or abscess develop where GELFOAM has been positioned, reoperation may be necessary in order to remove the infected material and allow drainage.

The hemostatic property of GELFOAM has not been shown to be enhanced by the addition of exogenous thrombin. Because thrombin is antigenic, it should not be combined with GELFOAM.

While packing a cavity for hemostasis is sometimes surgically indicated, GELFOAM should not be used in this manner unless excess product not needed to maintain hemostasis is removed.

Whenever possible, it should be removed after use in laminectomy procedures and from foramina in bone, once hemostasis is achieved. This is because GELFOAM may swell to its original size on absorbing fluids, and produce nerve damage by pressure within confined bony spaces.

The packing or wadding of GELFOAM, particularly within bony cavities, should be avoided, since swelling to original size may interfere with normal function and/or possibly result in compression necrosis of surrounding tissues.

PRECAUTIONS

Use only the minimum amount of GELFOAM Sterile Sponge needed for hemostasis, holding it at the site until bleeding stops, then removing the excess.

GELFOAM should **not** be used for controlling postpartum hemorrhage or menorrhagia.

It has been demonstrated that fragments of microfibrillar collagen pass through the 40μ transfusion filters of blood scavenging systems. Although not the same product, GELFOAM should also not be used in conjunction with autologous blood salvage circuits.

Microfibrillar collagen has been reported to reduce the strength of methylmethacrylate adhesives used to attach prosthetic devices to bone surfaces. As a precaution, GELFOAM should not be used in conjunction with such adhesives.

GELFOAM is not recommended for the primary treatment of coagulation disorders.

It is not recommended that GELFOAM be saturated with an antibiotic solution or dusted with antibiotic powder.

ADVERSE REACTIONS

There have been reports of fever associated with the use of GELFOAM, without demonstrable infection. GELFOAM Sterile Sponge may serve as a nidus for infection and abscess formation[1], and has been reported to potentiate bacterial growth. Giant-cell granuloma has been reported at the implantation site of absorbable gelatin product in the brain[2], as has compression of the brain and spinal cord resulting from the accumulation of sterile fluid.[3]

Foreign body reactions, "encapsulation" of fluid and hematoma have also been reported.

When GELFOAM was used in laminectomy operations, multiple neurologic events were reported, including but not limited to cauda equina syndrome, spinal stenosis, meningitis, arachnoiditis, headaches, paresthesias, pain, bladder and bowel dysfunction, and impotence.

Excessive fibrosis and prolonged fixation of a tendon have been reported when absorbable gelatin products were used in severed tendon repair.

Toxic shock syndrome has been reported in association with the use of GELFOAM in nasal surgery.

Fever, failure of absorption, and hearing loss have been reported in association with the use of GELFOAM during tympanoplasty.

ADVERSE REACTIONS REPORTED FROM UNAPPROVED USES

GELFOAM is not recommended for use other than as an adjunct for hemostasis.

While some adverse medical events following the unapproved use of GELFOAM have been reported to The Upjohn Company (see Adverse Reactions), other hazards associated with such use may not have been reported.

When GELFOAM has been used during intravascular catheterization for the purpose of producing vessel occlusion, the following adverse events have been reported; fever, duodenal and pancreatic infarct, embolization of lower extremity vessels, pulmonary embolization, splenic abscess, necrosis of specific anatomic areas, asterixis, and death.

These adverse medical events have been associated with the use of GELFOAM for repair of dural defects encountered during laminectomy and craniotomy operations: fever, infection, leg paresthesias, neck and back pain, bladder and bowel incontinence, cauda equina syndrome, neurogenic bladder, impotence, and paresis.

DOSAGE AND ADMINISTRATION

Sterile technique should always be used in removing the inner envelope containing the GELFOAM Sterile Sponge from the outer printed sealed envelope. The minimum amount of GELFOAM of appropriate size and shape should be applied (dry or wet, see DIRECTIONS FOR USE) to the bleeding site and held firmly in place until hemostasis is observed. Opened envelopes of unused GELFOAM should always be discarded.

HOW SUPPLIED

GELFOAM Sterile Sponge (absorbable gelatin sponge) is available in the following sizes:

Size 12—3 mm 20 mm × 60 mm (12 sq cm × 3 mm [3/4 in × 2 3/8 in (1 2/4 sq in) × 1/8 in] *in boxes of 4 sponges in individual envelopes.*
NDC 0009-0301-01

Size 12—7 mm 20 mm × 60 mm (12 sq cm) × 7 mm [3/4 in × 2 3/8 in (1 3/4 sq in) × 1/4 in] *in boxes of 12 sponges in individual envelopes, and in jars of 4 sponges.*
Box NDC 0009-0315-03
Jar NDC 0009-0315-02

Size 50, 80 mm × 62.5 mm (50 sq cm) × 10 mm [3 1/8 in × 2 1/2 in (7 7/8 sq in) × 3/8 in] *in boxes of 4 sponges in individual envelopes.*
NDC 0009-0323-01

Size 100, 80 mm × 125 mm (100 sq cm) × 100 mm [3 1/8 in × 5 in (15 5/8 sq in) × 3/8 in] *in boxes of 6 sponges in individual envelopes.*
NDC 0009-0342-01

Size 200, 80 mm × 250 mm (200 sq cm) × 10 mm (3 1/8 in × 10 in (31 1/4 sq in) × 3/8 in] *in boxes of 6 sponges in individual envelopes.*
NDC 0009-0349-01

Size 2 cm (approximately 40 cm × 2 cm) [15 3/4 in × 3/4 in] *packaged in individual jars.*
NDC 0009-0364-01

Size 6 cm (approximately 40 cm × 6 cm) [15 3/4 in × 2 3/8 in] *packaged in cartons of six sponges in individual envelopes.*
NDC 0009-0371-01

STORAGE AND HANDLING

GELFOAM Sterile Sponge (absorbable gelatin sponge) should be stored at controlled room temperature 15°–30°C (59°–86°F). Once the package is opened, contents are subject to contamination. It is recommended that GELFOAM be used as soon as the package is opened and unused contents discarded.

CAUTION

Federal law restricts this device to sale by or on the order of a physician.

Continued on next page

Information on these Upjohn products is based on labeling in effect June 1, 1992. Further information concerning these and other Upjohn products may be obtained by direct inquiry to Medical Information, The Upjohn Company, Kalamazoo, Michigan 49001.

Upjohn—Cont.

CLINICAL STUDIES

GELFOAM Sterile Sponge is a water-soluble, hemostatic device prepared from purified skin gelatin, and capable of absorbing up to 45 times its weight of whole blood.[4] The absorptive capacity of GELFOAM is a function of its physical size, increasing as the size of the gelatin sponge increases.[5] The mechanism of action of surface-mediated hemostatic devices is supportive and mechanical.[5] Surface-acting devices, when applied directly to bleeding surfaces, arrest bleeding by the formation of an artifical clot and by producing a mechanical matrix that facilitates clotting.[6] Jenkins et al[7] have theorized that the clotting effect of GELFOAM may be due to release of thromboplastin from platelets, occurring when platelets entering the sponge become damaged by contact with the walls of its myriad of interstices. Thromboplastin interacts with prothrombin and calcium to produce thrombin, and this sequence of events initiates the clotting reaction. The authors suggest that the physiologic formation of thrombin in the sponge is sufficient to produce formation of a clot, by its action on the fibrinogen in blood.[7] The spongy physical properties of the gelatin sponge hasten clot formation and provide structural support for the forming clot.[6,8]
Several investigators have claimed that GELFOAM becomes liquefied within a week or less and is completely absorbed in four to six weeks, without inducing excessive scar formation.[4,7,9,10,11] Barnes[10] reviewed experiences with GELFOAM in gynecologic surgery. No excessive scar tissue, attributable to the absorption of GELFOAM, could be palpated at postoperative examination.

ANIMAL PHARMACOLOGY

Surface-acting hemostatic devices, when applied directly to bleeding surfaces, arrest bleeding by providing a mechanical matrix that facilitates clotting,[6,8,15,16] Due to their bulk, surface-acting hemostatic agents slow the flow of blood, protect the forming clot, and offer a framework for deposition of the cellular elements of blood.[6,7,8,15]
MacDonald and Mathews[14] studied GELFOAM implants in canine kidneys and reported that it assisted in healing, with no marked inflammatory or foreign-body reactions.
Jenkins and Janda[15] studied the use of GELFOAM in canine liver resections and noted that the gelatin sponge appeared to offer a protective cover and provide structural support for the reparative process.
Correll et al[16] studied the histology of GELFOAM Sterile Sponge when implanted in rat muscle and reported no significant tissue reaction.

REFERENCES

1. Lindstrom, PA: Complications from the use of absorbable hemostatic sponges. *AMA Arch Surg* 1956;73:133–141.
2. Knowlson GTG: Gel-foam granuloma in the brain. *J Neuro Neurosurg Psychiatry* 1974;37:971–973.
3. Herndon JH, Grillo HC, Riseborough EJ, et al: Compression of the brain and spinal cord following use of GELFOAM. *Arch Surg* 1972;104:107.
4. Council on Pharmacy and Chemistry: Absorbable Gelatin sponge—new and nonofficial remedies. *JAMA* 1947;135:921.
5. Goodman LS, Gilman A: Surface-acting drugs, in The Pharmacologic Basis of Therapeutics, ed 6. *New York, MacMillan Publishing Co.* 1980, p955.
6. Guralnick W, Berg L: GELFOAM in oral surgery. *Oral Surg* 1948;1:629–632.
7. Jenkins HP, Senz EH, Owen H, et al: Present status of gelatin sponge for control of hemorrhage. *JAMA* 1946;132:614–619.
8. Jenkins HP, Janda R, Clarke J: Clinical and experimental observations on the use of gelatin sponge or foam. *Surg* 1946;20:124–132.
9. Treves N: Prophylaxis of post mammectomy lymphedema by the use of GELFOAM laminated rolls. *Cancer* 1952;5:73–83.
10. Barnes AC: The use of gelatin foam sponges in obstetrics and gynecology. *Am J Obstet Gynecol* 1963;86:105–107.
11. Rarig HR: Successful use of gelatin foam sponge in surgical restoration of fertility. *Am J Obstet Gynecol* 1963;86:136.
12. Jacobs BJ, Rafel SS: Pharmacology and Therapeutics: Absorbable hemostatic agents. *Oral Surg* 1950;2:356–377.
13. Nishimura S: The fate of a gelatin sponge introduced into the fourth ventricle: Experiments in dogs. *Arch Jap Chir* 1954; 23:310–319.
14. MacDonald SA, Mathews WH: Fibrin foam and GELFOAM in experimental kidney wounds. *Annual American Urological Association,* July 1946.
15. Jenkins HP, Janda R: Studies on the use of gelatin sponge or foam as a hemostatic agent in experimental liver resections and injuries to large veins. *Ann Surg* 1946;124:952–961.
16. Correll JT, Prentice HR, Wise EC: Biologic investigations of a new absorbable sponge. *Surg Gynecol Obstet* 1945;181:585–589.

Code 812 250 005
Also available:
GELFOAM Sterile Compressed Sponge (absorbable gelatin sponge, USP) Size 100. For application in dry state. Sponges measure 80 mm × 125 mm and are available in boxes of 6 sponges in individual envelopes.
NDC 0009-0353-01

GELFOAM Sterile Dental Pack (absorbable gelatin sponge, USP), Size 4. Each measures approximately 20 × 20 × 7 mm; packaged in jars of 15 packs.
Size 4 NDC 0009-0396-01

GELFOAM Sterile Prostatectomy Cones, (absorbable gelatin sponge, USP) Size 13 cm or 18 cm (for use with Foley bag catheter). Each cone diameter measures 13 cm or 18 cm, respectively; packaged in boxes of 6 cones in individual envelopes.
Size 13 cm NDC 0009-0449-01
Size 18 cm NDC 0009-0457-01

GELFOAM® ℞
brand of absorbable gelatin sterile powder
(absorbable gelatin powder)

HOW SUPPLIED

GELFOAM Sterile Powder (absorbable gelatin powder) is supplied in jars containing 1 gram.
NDC 0009-0433-01

GLYNASE™ PresTab™ Tablets ℞
brand of
glyburide tablets
1.5 and 3 mg

DESCRIPTION

GLYNASE PresTab Tablets contain micronized (smaller particle size) glyburide, which is an oral blood-glucose-lowering drug of the sulfonylurea class. Glyburide is a white, crystalline compound, formulated as GLYNASE PresTab Tablets of 1.5 and 3 mg strengths for oral administration. Inactive ingredients: colloidal silicon dioxide, corn starch, lactose, magnesium stearate. In addition, the **3 mg** strength contains aluminum oxide and FD&C Blue No. 1. The chemical name for glyburide is 1-[[p-[2-(5-chloro-o-anisamido) ethyl]phenyl]-sulfonyl]-3-cyclohexylurea and the molecular weight is 493.99. The structural formula is represented below.

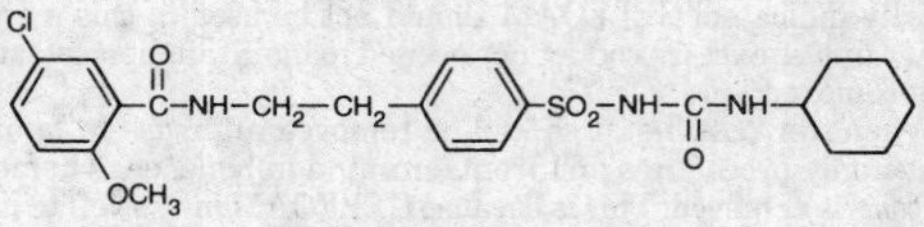

CLINICAL PHARMACOLOGY

Actions

Glyburide appears to lower the blood glucose acutely by stimulating the release of insulin from the pancreas, an effect dependent upon functioning beta cells in the pancreatic islets. The mechanism by which glyburide lowers blood glucose during long-term administration has not been clearly established. With chronic administration in Type II diabetic patients, the blood glucose lowering effect persists despite a gradual decline in the insulin secretory response to the drug. Extrapancreatic effects may be involved in the mechanism of action of oral sulfonylurea hypoglycemic drugs.
Some patients who are initially responsive to oral hypoglycemic drugs, including glyburide, may become unresponsive or poorly responsive over time. Alternatively, glyburide may be effective in some patients who have become unresponsive to one or more other sulfonylurea drugs.
In addition to its blood glucose lowering actions, glyburide produces a mild diuresis by enhancement of renal free water clearance. Disulfiram-like reactions have very rarely been reported in patients treated with glyburide.

Pharmacokinetics

Single dose studies with GLYNASE PresTab Tablets in normal subjects demonstrate significant absorption of glyburide within one hour, peak drug levels at about two to three hours, and low but detectable levels at twenty-four hours.
Bioavailability studies have demonstrated that GLYNASE PresTab Tablets 3 mg provide serum glyburide concentrations that are not bioequivalent to those from MICRONASE® Tablets 5 mg. Therefore, the patient should be retitrated.
In a single-dose bioavailability study (see Figure A) in which subjects received GLYNASE PresTab Tablets 3 mg and MICRONASE Tablets 5 mg with breakfast, the peak of the mean serum glyburide concentration-time curve was 97.2 ng/mL for GLYNASE PresTab Tablets 3 mg and 87.5 ng/mL for MICRONASE Tablets 5 mg. The mean of the individual maximum serum concentration values of glyburide (Cmax) from GLYNASE PresTab Tablets 3 mg was 106 ng/mL and that from MICRONASE Tablets 5 mg was 104 ng/mL. The mean glyburide area under the serum concentration-time curve (AUC) for this study was 568 ng × hr/mL for GLYNASE PresTab Tablets 3 mg and 746 ng × hr/mL for MICRONASE Tablets 5 mg.

Figure A

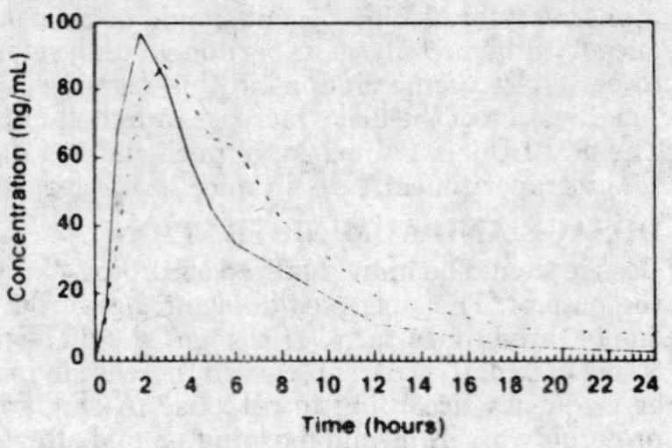

——— GLYNASE PresTab Tablets 3 mg
.... MICRONASE Tablets 5 mg

In a single-dose study, in fasting healthy subjects, two GLYNASE PresTab Tablets 1.5 mg were shown to be bioequivalent to one GLYNASE PresTab Tablet 3 mg.
Mean serum levels of glyburide, as reflected by areas under the serum concentration-time curve, increase in proportion to corresponding increases in dose. Multiple dose studies with glyburide in diabetic patients demonstrate drug level concentration-time curves similar to single dose studies, indicating no buildup of drug in tissue depots.
The serum concentration of glyburide in normal subjects decreased with a half-life of about four hours.
In single dose studies in fasting normal subjects, the degree and duration of blood glucose lowering is proportional to the dose administered and to the area under the drug level concentration-time curve. The blood glucose lowering effect persists for 24 hours following single morning doses in nonfasting diabetic patients. Under conditions of repeated administration in diabetic patients, however, there is no reliable correlation between blood drug levels and fasting blood glucose levels. A one year study of diabetic patients treated with glyburide showed no reliable correlation between administered dose and serum drug level.
The major metabolite of glyburide is the 4-trans-hydroxy derivative. A second metabolite, the 3-cis-hydroxy derivative, also occurs. These metabolites probably contribute no significant hypoglycemic action in humans since they are only weakly active (1/400th and 1/40th as active, respectively, as glyburide) in rabbits.
Glyburide is excreted as metabolites in the bile and urine, approximately 50% by each route. This dual excretory pathway is qualitatively different from that of other sulfonylureas, which are excreted primarily in the urine.
Sulfonylurea drugs are extensively bound to serum proteins. Displacement from protein binding sites by other drugs may lead to enhanced hypoglycemic action. *In vitro,* the protein binding exhibited by glyburide is predominantly non-ionic, whereas that of other sulfonylureas (chlorpropamide, tolbutamide, tolazamide) is predominantly ionic. Acidic drugs such as phenylbutazone, warfarin, and salicylates displace the ionic-binding sulfonylureas from serum proteins to a far greater extent than the non-ionic binding glyburide. It has not been shown that this difference in protein binding will result in fewer drug-drug interactions with glyburide in clinical use.

INDICATIONS AND USAGE

GLYNASE PresTab Tablets are indicated as an adjunct to diet to lower the blood glucose in patients with non-insulin-dependent diabetes mellitus (Type II) whose hyperglycemia cannot be satisfactorily controlled by diet alone.
In initiating treatment for non-insulin-dependent diabetes, diet should be emphasized as the primary form of treatment. Caloric restriction and weight loss are essential in the obese diabetic patient. Proper dietary management alone may be effective in controlling the blood glucose and symptoms of hyperglycemia. The importance of regular physical activity should also be stressed, and cardiovascular risk factors should be identified and corrective measures taken where possible. If this treatment program fails to reduce symptoms and/or blood glucose, the use of an oral sulfonylurea or insulin should be considered. Use of GLYNASE PresTab must be viewed by both the physician and patient as a treatment in addition to diet and not as a substitution or as a convenient mechanism for avoiding dietary restraint. Furthermore, loss of blood glucose control on diet alone may be transient, thus requiring only short-term administration of GLYNASE PresTab.
During maintenance programs, GLYNASE PresTab should be discontinued if satisfactory lowering of blood glucose is no

longer achieved. Judgment should be based on regular clinical and laboratory evaluations.

In considering the use of GLYNASE PresTab in asymptomatic patients, it should be recognized that controlling blood glucose in non-insulin-dependent diabetes has not been definitely established to be effective in preventing the long-term cardiovascular or neural complications of diabetes.

CONTRAINDICATIONS

GLYNASE PresTab Tablets are contraindicated in patients with:

1. Known hypersensitivity or allergy to the drug.
2. Diabetic ketoacidosis, with or without coma. This condition should be treated with insulin.
3. Type I diabetes mellitus, as sole therapy.

SPECIAL WARNING ON INCREASED RISK OF CARDIOVASCULAR MORTALITY

The administration of oral hypoglycemic drugs has been reported to be associated with increased cardiovascular mortality as compared to treatment with diet alone or diet plus insulin. This warning is based on the study conducted by the University Group Diabetes Program (UGDP), a long-term prospective clinical trial designed to evaluate the effectiveness of glucose-lowering drugs in preventing or delaying vascular complications in patients with non-insulin-dependent diabetes. The study involved 823 patients who were randomly assigned to one of four treatment groups (*Diabetes*, 19 (Suppl. 2):747–830, 1970).

UGDP reported that patients treated for 5 to 8 years with diet plus a fixed dose of tolbutamide (1.5 grams per day) had a rate of cardiovascular mortality approximately 2½ times that of patients treated with diet alone. A significant increase in total mortality was not observed, but the use of tolbutamide was discontinued based on the increase in cardiovascular mortality, thus limiting the opportunity for the study to show an increase in overall mortality. Despite controversy regarding the interpretation of these results, the findings of the UGDP study provide an adequate basis for this warning. The patient should be informed of the potential risks and advantages of GLYNASE PresTab and of alternative modes of therapy.

Although only one drug in the sulfonylurea class (tolbutamide) was included in this study, it is prudent from a safety standpoint to consider that this warning may also apply to other oral hypoglycemic drugs in this class, in view of their close similarities in mode of action and chemical structure.

PRECAUTIONS

Bioavailability studies have demonstrated that GLYNASE PresTab Tablets 3 mg provide serum glyburide concentrations that are not bioequivalent to those from MICRONASE Tablets 5 mg. Therefore, patients should be retitrated when transferred from MICRONASE or Diabeta or other oral hypoglycemic agents.

General

Hypoglycemia: All sulfonylureas are capable of producing severe hypoglycemia. Proper patient selection and dosage and instructions are important to avoid hypoglycemic episodes. Renal or hepatic insufficiency may cause elevated drug levels of glyburide and the latter may also diminish gluconeogenic capacity, both of which increase the risk of serious hypoglycemic reactions. Elderly, debilitated or malnourished patients, and those with adrenal or pituitary insufficiency, are particularly susceptible to the hypoglycemic action of glucose-lowering drugs. Hypoglycemia may be difficult to recognize in the elderly and in people who are taking beta-adrenergic blocking drugs. Hypoglycemia is more likely to occur when caloric intake is deficient, after severe or prolonged exercise, when alcohol is ingested, or when more than one glucose lowering drug is used.

Loss of Control of Blood Glucose: When a patient stabilized on any diabetic regimen is exposed to stress such as fever, trauma, infection or surgery, a loss of control may occur. At such times it may be necessary to discontinue GLYNASE PresTab and administer insulin.

The effectiveness of any hypoglycemic drug, including GLYNASE PresTab, in lowering blood glucose to a desired level decreases in many patients over a period of time which may be due to progression of the severity of diabetes or to diminished responsiveness to the drug. This phenomenon is known as secondary failure, to distinguish it from primary failure in which the drug is ineffective in an individual patient when GLYNASE PresTab is first given. Adequate adjustment of dose and adherence to diet should be assessed before classifying a patient as a secondary failure.

Information for Patients: Patients should be informed of the potential risks and advantages of GLYNASE PresTab and of alternative modes of therapy. They also should be informed about the importance of adherence to dietary instructions, of a regular exercise program, and of regular testing of urine and/or blood glucose.

The risks of hypoglycemia, its symptoms and treatment, and conditions that predispose to its development should be explained to patients and responsible family members. Primary and secondary failure also should be explained.

Laboratory Tests

Therapeutic response to GLYNASE PresTab Tablets should be monitored by frequent urine glucose tests and periodic blood glucose tests. Measurement of glycosylated hemoglobin levels may be helpful in some patients.

Drug Interactions

The hypoglycemic action of sulfonylureas may be potentiated by certain drugs including nonsteroidal anti-inflammatory agents and other drugs that are highly protein bound, salicylates, sulfonamides, chloramphenicol, probenecid, coumarins, monoamine oxidase inhibitors, and beta adrenergic blocking agents. When such drugs are administered to a patient receiving glyburide, the patient should be observed closely for hypoglycemia. When such drugs are withdrawn from a patient receiving glyburide, the patient should be observed closely for loss of control.

Certain drugs tend to produce hyperglycemia and may lead to loss of control. These drugs include the thiazides and other diuretics, corticosteroids, phenothiazines, thyroid products, estrogens, oral contraceptives, phenytoin, nicotinic acid, sympathomimetics, calcium channel blocking drugs, and isoniazid. When such drugs are administered to a patient receiving glyburide, the patient should be closely observed for loss of control. When such drugs are withdrawn from a patient receiving glyburide, the patient should be observed closely for hypoglycemia.

A potential interaction between oral miconazole and oral hypoglycemic agents leading to severe hypoglycemia has been reported. Whether this interaction also occurs with the intravenous, topical or vaginal preparations of miconazole is not known.

Carcinogenesis, Mutagenesis, and Impairment of Fertility

Studies in rats at doses up to 300 mg/kg/day for 18 months showed no carcinogenic effects. Glyburide is nonmutagenic when studied in the Salmonella microsome test (Ames test) and in the DNA damage/alkaline elution assay.

No drug-related effects were noted in any of the criteria evaluated in the two-year oncogenicity study of glyburide in mice.

Pregnancy

Teratogenic Effects: Pregnancy Category B

Reproduction studies have been performed in rats and rabbits at doses up to 500 times the human dose and have revealed no evidence of impaired fertility or harm to the fetus due to glyburide. There are, however, no adequate and well controlled studies in pregnant women. Because animal reproduction studies are not always predictive of human response, this drug should be used during pregnancy only if clearly needed.

Because recent information suggests that abnormal blood glucose levels during pregnancy are associated with a higher incidence of congenital abnormalities, many experts recommend that insulin be used during pregnancy to maintain blood glucose as close to normal as possible.

Nonteratogenic Effects: Prolonged severe hypoglycemia (4 to 10 days) has been reported in neonates born to mothers who were receiving a sulfonylurea drug at the time of delivery. This has been reported more frequently with the use of agents with prolonged half-lives. If GLYNASE PresTab is used during pregnancy, it should be discontinued at least two weeks before the expected delivery date.

Nursing Mothers

Although it is not known whether glyburide is excreted in human milk, some sulfonylurea drugs are known to be excreted in human milk. Because the potential for hypoglycemia in nursing infants may exist, a decision should be made whether to discontinue nursing or to discontinue the drug, taking into account the importance of the drug to the mother. If the drug is discontinued, and if diet alone is inadequate for controlling blood glucose, insulin therapy should be considered.

Pediatric Use

Safety and effectiveness in children have not been established.

ADVERSE REACTIONS

Hypoglycemia: See PRECAUTIONS and OVERDOSAGE Sections.

Gastrointestinal Reactions: Cholestatic jaundice and hepatitis may occur rarely; GLYNASE PresTab Tablets should be discontinued if this occurs.

Liver function abnormalities, including isolated transaminase elevations, have been reported.

Gastrointestinal disturbances, *eg*, nausea, epigastric fullness, and heartburn are the most common reactions, having occurred in 1.8% of treated patients during clinical trials. They tend to be dose related and may disappear when dosage is reduced.

Dermatologic Reactions: Allergic skin reactions, *eg*, pruritus, erythema, urticaria, and morbilliform or maculopapular eruptions occurred in 1.5% of treated patients during clinical trials. These may be transient and may disappear despite continued use of glyburide. If skin reactions persist, the drug should be discontinued.

Porphyria cutanea tarda and photosensitivity reactions have been reported with sulfonylureas.

Hematologic Reactions: Leukopenia, agranulocytosis, thrombocytopenia, hemolytic anemia, aplastic anemia, and pancytopenia have been reported with sulfonylureas.

Metabolic Reactions: Hepatic porphyria and disulfiram-like reactions have been reported with sulfonylureas; however, hepatic porphyria has not been reported with glyburide and disulfiram-like reactions have been reported very rarely.

Cases of hyponatremia have been reported with glyburide and all other sulfonylureas, most often in patients who are on other medications or have medical conditions known to cause hyponatremia or increase release of antidiuretic hormone. The syndrome of inappropriate antidiuretic hormone (SIADH) secretion has been reported with certain other sulfonylureas, and it has been suggested that these sulfonylureas may augment the peripheral (antidiuretic) action of ADH and/or increase release of ADH.

Other Reactions: Changes in accommodation and/or blurred vision have been reported with glyburide and other sulfonylureas. These are thought to be related to fluctuation in glucose levels.

In addition to dermatologic reactions, allergic reactions such as angioedema, arthralgia, myalgia and vasculitis have been reported.

OVERDOSAGE

Overdosage of sulfonylureas, including glyburide, can produce hypoglycemia. Mild hypoglycemic symptoms, without loss of consciousness or neurological findings, should be treated aggressively with oral glucose and adjustments in drug dosage and/or meal patterns. Close monitoring should continue until the physician is assured that the patient is out of danger. Severe hypoglycemic reactions with coma, seizure, or other neurological impairment occur infrequently but constitute medical emergencies requiring immediate hospitalization. If hypoglycemic coma is diagnosed or suspected, the patient should be given a rapid intravenous injection of concentrated (50%) glucose solution. This should be followed by a continuous infusion of a more dilute (10%) glucose solution at a rate which will maintain the blood glucose at a level above 100 mg/dL. Patients should be closely monitored for a minimum of 24 to 48 hours, since hypoglycemia may recur after apparent clinical recovery.

DOSAGE AND ADMINISTRATION

Patients should be retitrated when transferred from MICRONASE or Diabeta or other oral hypoglycemic agents.

There is no fixed dosage regimen for the management of diabetes mellitus with GLYNASE PresTab Tablets or any other hypoglycemic agent. In addition to the usual monitoring of urinary glucose, the patient's blood glucose must also be monitored periodically to determine the minimum effective dose for the patient; to detect primary failure, *ie*, inadequate lowering of blood glucose at the maximum recommended dose of medication; and to detect secondary failure, *ie*, loss of adequate blood glucose lowering response after an initial period of effectiveness. Glycosylated hemoglobin levels may also be of value in monitoring the patient's response to therapy.

Short-term administration of GLYNASE PresTab may be sufficient during periods of transient loss of control in patients usually controlled well on diet.

Usual Starting Dose

The suggested starting dose of GLYNASE PresTab is 1.5 to 3 mg daily, administered with breakfast or the first main meal. Those patients who may be more sensitive to hypoglycemic drugs should be started at 0.75 mg daily. (See PRECAUTIONS Section for patients at increased risk.) Failure to follow an appropriate dosage regimen may precipitate hypoglycemia. Patients who do not adhere to their prescribed dietary and drug regimen are more prone to exhibit unsatisfactory response to therapy.

Transfer From Other Hypoglycemic Therapy; Patients Receiving Other Oral Antidiabetic Therapy: Patients should be retitrated when transferred from MICRONASE or other oral hypoglycemic agents. The initial daily dose should be 1.5 to 3 mg. When transferring patients from oral hypoglycemic agents other than chlorpropamide to GLYNASE PresTab, no transition period and no initial or priming dose are necessary. When transferring patients from chlorpropamide, particular care should be exercised during the first two weeks because the prolonged retention of chlorpropamide in the body and subsequent overlapping drug effects may provoke hypoglycemia.

Patients Receiving Insulin: Some Type II diabetic patients being treated with insulin may respond satisfactorily to GLYNASE PresTab. If the insulin dose is less than 20 units

Continued on next page

Information on these Upjohn products is based on labeling in effect June 1, 1992. Further information concerning these and other Upjohn products may be obtained by direct inquiry to Medical Information, The Upjohn Company, Kalamazoo, Michigan 49001.

Upjohn—Cont.

daily, substitution of GLYNASE PresTab 1.5 to 3 mg as a single daily dose may be tried. If the insulin dose is between 20 and 40 units daily, the patient may be placed directly on GLYNASE PresTab Tablets 3 mg daily as a single dose. If the insulin dose is more than 40 units daily, a transition period is required for conversion to GLYNASE PresTab. In these patients, insulin dosage is decreased by 50% and GLYNASE PresTab Tablets 3 mg daily is started. Please refer to Titration to Maintenance Dose for further explanation.

Titration to Maintenance Dose

The usual maintenance dose is in the range of 0.75 to 12 mg daily, which may be given as a single dose or in divided doses (See Dosage Interval Section). Dosage increases should be made in increments of no more than 1.5 mg at weekly intervals based upon the patient's blood glucose response.

No exact dosage relationship exists between GLYNASE PresTab and the other oral hypoglycemic agents, including MICRONASE or Diabeta. Although patients may be transferred from the maximum dose of other sulfonylureas, the maximum starting dose of 3 mg of GLYNASE PresTab Tablets should be observed. A maintenance dose of 3 mg of GLYNASE PresTab Tablets provides approximately the same degree of blood glucose control as 250 to 375 mg chlorpropamide, 250 to 375 mg tolazamide, 5 mg of glyburide (nonmicronized tablets), 500 to 750 mg acetohexamide, or 1000 to 1500 mg tolbutamide.

When transferring patients receiving more than 40 units of insulin daily, they may be started on a daily dose of GLYNASE PresTab Tablets 3 mg concomitantly with a 50% reduction in insulin dose. Progressive withdrawal of insulin and increase of GLYNASE PresTab in increments of 0.75 to 1.5 mg every 2 to 10 days is then carried out. During this conversion period when both insulin and GLYNASE PresTab are being used, hypoglycemia may rarely occur. During insulin withdrawal, patients should test their urine for glucose and acetone at least three times daily and report results to their physician. The appearance of persistent acetonuria with glycosuria indicates that the patient is a Type I diabetic who requires insulin therapy.

Maximum Dose

Daily doses of more than 12 mg are not recommended.

Dosage Interval

Once-a-day therapy is usually satisfactory. Some patients, particularly those receiving more than 6 mg daily, may have a more satisfactory response with twice-a-day dosage.

Specific Patient Populations

GLYNASE PresTab Tablets are not recommended for use in pregnancy or for use in children.

In elderly patients, debilitated or malnourished patients, and patients with impaired renal or hepatic function, the initial and maintenance dosing should be conservative to avoid hypoglycemic reactions. (See PRECAUTIONS Section.)

HOW SUPPLIED

GLYNASE PresTab Tablets are supplied as follows:

GLYNASE PresTab Tablets 1.5 mg	(white, ovoid, PresTab™, contour, scored)
Plastic Bottles of 30	NDC 0009-0341-06
Plastic Bottles of 60	NDC 0009-0341-07
Plastic Bottles of 100	NDC 0009-0341-01
Plastic Bottles of 500	NDC 0009-0341-03
Plastic Bottles of 1000	NDC 0009-0341-04
Unit Dose Package of 100	NDC 0009-0341-02
GLYNASE PresTab Tablets 3 mg	(blue, ovoid, PresTab™, contour, scored)
Plastic Bottles of 30	NDC 0009-0352-06
Plastic Bottles of 60	NDC 0009-0352-07
Plastic Bottles of 90	NDC 0009-0352-08
Plastic Bottles of 100	NDC 0009-0352-01
Plastic Bottles of 500	NDC 0009-0352-03
Plastic Bottles of 1000	NDC 0009-0352-04
Unit Dose Package of 100	NDC 0009-0352-02

The PresTab Tablet can be easily divided in half for a more flexible dosing regimen. Press gently on the score and the PresTab Tablet will split in even halves.

Caution: Federal law prohibits dispensing without prescription. Store at controlled room temperature 15°-30°C (59°-86°F). Dispensed in well closed containers with safety closures. Keep container tightly closed.

GLYNASE is a trademark of The Upjohn Company
PresTab is a trademark of The Upjohn Company
Diabeta is a trademark of Hoechst-Roussel Pharmaceuticals, Inc.

The Upjohn Company
Kalamazoo, MI 49001, USA
March 1992

814 930 001
691015

Shown in Product Identification Section, page 434

HALCION® Ⓒ ℞

brand of triazolam tablets, USP

DESCRIPTION

HALCION Tablets contain triazolam, a triazolobenzodiazepine hypnotic agent.

Triazolam is a white crystalline powder, soluble in alcohol and poorly soluble in water. It has a molecular weight of 343.21.

The chemical name for triazolam is 8-chloro- 6- (o-chlorophenyl) -1- methyl-4H-s-triazolo- [4,3-α] [1,4] benzodiazepine.

The structural formula is represented below:

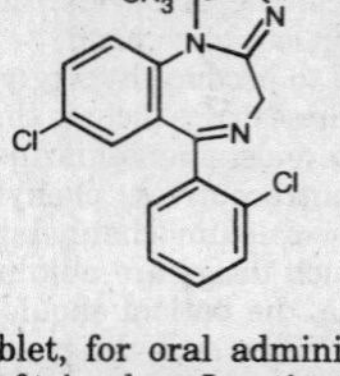

Each HALCION tablet, for oral administration, contains 0.125 mg or 0.25 mg of triazolam. Inactive ingredients: **0.125 mg**—cellulose, corn starch, docusate sodium, lactose, magnesium stearate, silicon dioxide, sodium benzoate; **0.25 mg**—cellulose, corn starch, docusate sodium, FD&C Blue No. 2, lactose, magnesium stearate, silicon dioxide, sodium benzoate.

CLINICAL PHARMACOLOGY

Triazolam is a hypnotic with a short mean plasma half-life reported to be in the range of 1.5 to 5.5 hours. In normal subjects treated for 7 days with four times the recommended dosage, there was no evidence of altered systemic bioavailability, rate of elimination, or accumulation. Peak plasma levels are reached within 2 hours following oral administration. Following recommended doses of HALCION, triazolam peak plasma levels in the range of 1 to 6 ng/mL are seen. The plasma levels achieved are proportional to the dose given.

Triazolam and its metabolites, principally as conjugated glucuronides, which are presumably inactive, are excreted primarily in the urine. Only small amounts of unmetabolized triazolam appear in the urine. The two primary metabolites accounted for 79.9% of urinary excretion. Urinary excretion appeared to be biphasic in its time course.

HALCION Tablets 0.5 mg, in two separate studies, did not affect the prothrombin times or plasma warfarin levels in male volunteers administered sodium warfarin orally.

Extremely high concentrations of triazolam do not displace bilirubin bound to human serum albumin *in vitro*.

Triazolam ^{14}C was administered orally to pregnant mice. Drug-related material appeared uniformly distributed in the fetus with ^{14}C concentrations approximately the same as in the brain of the mother.

In sleep laboratory studies, HALCION Tablets significantly decreased sleep latency, increased the duration of sleep, and decreased the number of nocturnal awakenings. After 2 weeks of consecutive nightly administration, the drug's effect on total wake time is decreased, and the values recorded in the last third of the night approach baseline levels. On the first and/or second night after drug discontinuance (first or second post-drug night), total time asleep, percentage of time spent sleeping, and rapidity of falling asleep frequently were significantly less than on baseline (predrug) nights. This effect is often called "rebound" insomnia.

The type and duration of hypnotic effects and the profile of unwanted effects during administration of benzodiazepine drugs may be influenced by the biologic half-life of administered drug and any active metabolites formed. When half-lives are long, the drug or metabolites may accumulate during periods of nightly administration and be associated with impairments of cognitive and motor performance during waking hours; the possibility of interaction with other psychoactive drugs or alcohol will be enhanced. In contrast, if half-lives are short, the drug and metabolites will be cleared before the next dose is ingested, and carry-over effects related to excessive sedation or CNS depression should be minimal or absent. However, during nightly use for an extended period pharmacodynamic tolerance or adaptation to some effects of benzodiazepine hypnotics may develop. If the drug has a short half-life of elimination, it is possible that a relative deficiency of the drug or its active metabolites (ie, in relationship to the receptor site) may occur at some point in the interval between each night's use. This sequence of events may account for two clinical findings reported to occur after several weeks of nightly use of rapidly eliminated benzodiazepine hypnotics: 1) increased wakefulness during the last third of the night and 2) the appearance of increased daytime anxiety after 10 days of continuous treatment.

INDICATIONS AND USAGE

HALCION is indicated for the short-term treatment of insomnia (generally 7–10 days). Use for more than 2–3 weeks requires complete reevaluation of the patient (see WARNINGS).

Prescriptions for HALCION should be written for short-term use (7–10 days) and it should not be prescribed in quantities exceeding a 1-month supply.

CONTRAINDICATIONS

HALCION Tablets are contraindicated in patients with known hypersensitivity to this drug or other benzodiazepines.

Benzodiazepines may cause fetal damage when administered during pregnancy. An increased risk of congenital malformations associated with the use of diazepam and chlordiazepoxide during the first trimester of pregnancy has been suggested in several studies. Transplacental distribution has resulted in neonatal CNS depression following the ingestion of therapeutic doses of a benzodiazepine hypnotic during the last weeks of pregnancy.

HALCION is contraindicated in pregnant women. If there is a likelihood of the patient becoming pregnant while receiving HALCION, she should be warned of the potential risk to the fetus. Patients should be instructed to discontinue the drug prior to becoming pregnant. The possibility that a woman of childbearing potential may be pregnant at the time of institution of therapy should be considered.

WARNINGS

Sleep disturbance may be the presenting manifestation of a physical and/or psychiatric disorder. Consequently, a decision to initiate symptomatic treatment of insomnia should only be made after the patient has been carefully evaluated.

The failure of insomnia to remit after 7–10 days of treatment may indicate the presence of a primary psychiatric and/or medical illness.

Worsening of insomnia or the emergence of new abnormalities of thinking or behavior may be the consequence of an unrecognized psychiatric or physical disorder. These have also been reported to occur in association with the use of HALCION.

Because some of the adverse effects of HALCION appear to be dose related (see PRECAUTIONS and DOSAGE AND ADMINISTRATION), it is important to use the smallest possible effective dose. Elderly patients are especially susceptible to dose related adverse effects.

An increase in daytime anxiety has been reported for HALCION after as few as 10 days of continuous use. In some patients this may be a manifestation of interdose withdrawal (see CLINICAL PHARMACOLOGY). If increased daytime anxiety is observed during treatment, discontinuation of treatment may be advisable.

A variety of abnormal thinking and behavior changes have been reported to occur in association with the use of benzodiazepine hypnotics including HALCION. Some of these changes may be characterized by decreased inhibition, eg, aggressiveness and extroversion that seem excessive, similar to that seen with alcohol and other CNS depressants (eg, sedative/hypnotics). Other kinds of behavioral changes have also been reported, for example, bizarre behavior, agitation, hallucinations, depersonalization. In primarily depressed patients, the worsening of depression, including suicidal thinking, has been reported in association with the use of benzodiazepines.

It can rarely be determined with certainty whether a particular instance of the abnormal behaviors listed above is drug induced, spontaneous in origin, or a result of an underlying psychiatric or physical disorder. Nonetheless, the emergence of any new behavioral sign or symptom of concern requires careful and immediate evaluation.

Because of its depressant CNS effects, patients receiving triazolam should be cautioned against engaging in hazardous occupations requiring complete mental alertness such as operating machinery or driving a motor vehicle. For the same reason, patients should be cautioned about the concomitant ingestion of alcohol and other CNS depressant drugs during treatment with HALCION Tablets.

As with some, but not all benzodiazepines, anterograde amnesia of varying severity and paradoxical reactions have been reported following therapeutic doses of HALCION. Data from several sources suggest that anterograde amnesia may occur at a higher rate with HALCION than with other benzodiazepine hypnotics.

PRECAUTIONS

General: In elderly and/or debilitated patients it is recommended that treatment with HALCION Tablets be initiated at 0.125 mg to decrease the possibility of development of oversedation, dizziness, or impaired coordination.

Some side effects reported in association with the use of HALCION appear to be dose related. These include drowsiness, dizziness, light-headedness, and amnesia.

The relationship between dose and what may be more serious behavioral phenomena is less certain. Specifically, some evidence, based on spontaneous marketing reports, suggests that confusion, bizarre or abnormal behavior, agitation, and hallucinations may also be dose related; but this evidence is inconclusive. In accordance with good medical practice it is

recommended that therapy be initiated at the lowest effective dose. (see DOSAGE AND ADMINISTRATION).

Cases of "traveler's amnesia" have been reported by individuals who have taken HALCION to induce sleep while traveling, such as during an airplane flight. In some of these cases, insufficient time was allowed for the sleep period prior to awakening and before beginning activity. Also, the concomitant use of alcohol may have been a factor in some cases.

Caution should be exercised if HALCION is prescribed to patients with signs or symptoms of depression that could be intensified by hypnotic drugs. Suicidal tendencies may be present in such patients and protective measures may be required. Intentional overdosage is more common in these patients, and the least amount of drug that is feasible should be available to the patient at any one time.

The usual precautions should be observed in patients with impaired renal or hepatic function, chronic pulmonary insufficiency, and sleep apnea. In patients with compromised respiratory function, respiratory depression and apnea have been reported infrequently.

Information for patients: The text of a patient package insert is printed at the end of this insert. To assure safe and effective use of HALCION, the information and instructions provided in this package insert should be discussed with patients.

Laboratory tests: Laboratory tests are not ordinarily required in otherwise healthy patients.

Drug interactions: Both pharmacodynamic and pharmacokinetic interactions have been reported with benzodiazepines. *In particular, triazolam produces additive* CNS depressant effects when co-administered with other psychotropic medications, anticonvulsants, antihistamines, ethanol, and other drugs which themselves produce CNS depression.

Pharmacokinetic interactions can occur when triazolam is administered along with drugs that interfere with its metabolism. Specific examples, documented with evidence from controlled trials, show that the co-administration of either cimetidine or erythromycin with triazolam causes an approximate doubling of the elimination half-life and plasma levels of triazolam. Consequently, consideration of dose reduction may be appropriate in patients treated concomitantly with either cimetidine or erythromycin and triazolam.

Carcinogenesis, mutagenesis, impairment of fertility: No evidence of carcinogenic potential was observed in mice during a 24-month study with HALCION Tablets in doses up to 4,000 times the human dose.

Pregnancy:

1. Teratogenic effects: Pregnancy category X (see CONTRAINDICATIONS).
2. Non-teratogenic effects: It is to be considered that the child born of a mother who is on benzodiazepines may be at some risk for withdrawal symptoms from the drug, during the postnatal period. Also, neonatal flaccidity has been reported in an infant born of a mother who had been receiving benzodiazepines.

Nursing mothers: Human studies have not been performed; however, studies in rats have indicated that HALCION and its metabolites are secreted in milk. Therefore, administration of HALCION to nursing mothers is not recommended.

Pediatric use: Safety and efficacy of HALCION in children below the age of 18 have not been established.

ADVERSE REACTIONS

During placebo-controlled clinical studies in which 1,003 patients received HALCION Tablets, the most troublesome side effects were extensions of the pharmacologic activity of triazolam, eg, drowsiness, dizziness, or lightheadedness.

The figures cited below are estimates of untoward clinical event incidence among subjects who participated in the relatively short duration (ie, 1 to 42 days) placebo-controlled clinical trials of HALCION. The figures cannot be used to predict precisely the incidence of untoward events in the course of usual medical practice where patient characteristics and other factors often differ from those in the clinical trials. These figures cannot be compared with those obtained from other clinical studies involving related drug products and placebo, as each group of drug trials is conducted under a different set of conditions.

Comparison of the cited figures, however, can provide the prescriber with some basis for estimating the relative contributions of drug and nondrug factors to the untoward event incidence rate in the population studied. Even this use must be approached cautiously, as a drug may relieve a symptom in one patient while inducing it in others. (For example, an anticholinergic, anxiolytic drug may relieve dry mouth [a sign of anxiety] in some subjects but induce it [an untoward event] in others.)

	HALCION	Placebo
Number of Patients	1003	997
% of Patients Reporting:		
Central Nervous System		
Drowsiness	14.0	6.4
Headache	9.7	8.4
Dizziness	7.8	3.1
Nervousness	5.2	4.5
Light-headedness	4.9	0.9
Coordination disorders/ataxia	4.6	0.8
Gastrointestinal		
Nausea/vomiting	4.6	3.7

In addition to the relatively common (ie, 1% or greater) untoward events enumerated above, the following adverse events have been reported less frequently (ie, 0.9% to 0.5%): euphoria, tachycardia, tiredness, confusional states/memory impairment, cramps/pain, depression, visual disturbances.

Rare (ie, less than 0.5%) adverse reactions included constipation, taste alterations, diarrhea, dry mouth, dermatitis/allergy, dreaming/nightmares, insomnia, paresthesia, tinnitus, dysesthesia, weakness, congestion, death from hepatic failure in a patient also receiving diuretic drugs.

In addition to these untoward events for which estimates of incidence are available, the following adverse events have been reported in association with the use of HALCION and other benzodiazepines: amnestic symptoms (anterograde amnesia with appropriate or inappropriate behavior), confusional states (disorientation, derealization, depersonalization, and/or clouding of consciousness), dystonia, anorexia, fatigue, sedation, slurred speech, jaundice, pruritus, dysarthria, changes in libido, menstrual irregularities, incontinence, and urinary retention. Other factors may contribute to some of these reactions, eg, concomitant intake of alcohol or other drugs, sleep deprivation, an abnormal premorbid state, etc.

Other events reported include: paradoxical reactions such as stimulation, mania, an agitational state (restlessness, irritability, and excitation), increased muscle spasticity, sleep disturbances, hallucinations, delusions, aggressiveness, falling, somnambulism, syncope, inappropriate behavior, and other adverse behavioral effects. Should these occur, use of the drug should be discontinued.

The following events have also been reported: chest pain, burning tongue/glossitis/stomatitis.

Laboratory analyses were performed on all patients participating in the clinical program for HALCION. The following incidences of abnormalities were observed in patients receiving HALCION and the corresponding placebo group. None of these changes were considered to be of physiological significance. [See table below.]

	HALCION		Placebo	
Number of patients	380		361	
% of Patients Reporting:	Low	High	Low	High
Hematology				
Hematocrit	*	*	*	*
Hemoglobin	*	*	*	*
Total WBC count	1.7	2.1	*	1.3
Neutrophil count	1.5	1.5	3.3	1.0
Lymphocyte count	2.3	4.0	3.1	3.8
Monocyte count	3.6	*	4.4	1.5
Eosinophil count	10.2	3.2	9.8	3.4
Basophil count	1.7	2.1	*	1.8
Urinalysis				
Albumin	—	1.1	—	*
Sugar	—	*	—	*
RBC/HPF	—	2.9	—	2.9
WBC/HPF	—	11.7	—	7.9
Blood chemistry				
Creatinine	2.4	1.9	3.6	1.5
Bilirubin	*	1.5	1.0	*
SGOT	*	5.3	*	4.5
Alkaline phosphatase	*	2.2	*	2.6

*Less than 1%

When treatment with HALCION is protracted, periodic blood counts, urinalysis, and blood chemistry analyses are advisable.

Minor changes in EEG patterns, usually low-voltage fast activity, have been observed in patients during therapy with HALCION and are of no known significance.

DRUG ABUSE AND DEPENDENCE

Controlled Substance: Triazolam is a controlled substance under the Controlled Substance Act, and HALCION Tablets have been assigned to Schedule IV.

Abuse, Dependence and Withdrawal: Withdrawal symptoms, similar in character to those noted with barbiturates and alcohol (convulsions, tremor, abdominal and muscle cramps, vomiting, sweating, dysphoria, perceptual disturbances and insomnia), have occurred following abrupt discontinuance of benzodiazepines, including HALCION. The more severe symptoms are usually associated with higher dosages and longer usage, although patients at therapeutic dosages given for as few as 1–2 weeks can also have withdrawal symptoms and in some patients there may be withdrawal symptoms (daytime anxiety, agitation) between nightly doses (see CLINICAL PHARMACOLOGY). Consequently, abrupt discontinuation should be avoided and a gradual dosage tapering schedule is recommended in any patient taking more than the lowest dose for more than a few weeks. The recommendation for tapering is particularly important in any patient with a history of seizure.

The risk of dependence is increased in patients with a history of alcoholism, drug abuse, or in patients with marked personality disorders. Such dependence-prone individuals should be under careful surveillance when receiving HALCION. As with all hypnotics, repeat prescriptions should be limited to those who are under medical supervision.

OVERDOSAGE

Because of the potency of triazolam, some manifestations of overdosage may occur at 2 mg, four times the maximum recommended therapeutic dose (0.5 mg).

Manifestations of overdosage with HALCION Tablets include somnolence, confusion, impaired coordination, slurred speech, and ultimately, coma. Respiratory depression and apnea have been reported with overdosages of HALCION. Seizures have occasionally been reported after overdosages.

Death has been reported in association with overdoses of triazolam by itself, as it has with other benzodiazepines. In addition, fatalities have been reported in patients who have overdosed with a combination of a single benzodiazepine, including triazolam, and alcohol; benzodiazepine and alcohol levels seen in some of these cases have been lower than those usually associated with reports of fatality with either substance alone.

As in all cases of drug overdosage, respiration, pulse, and blood pressure should be monitored and supported by general measures when necessary. Immediate gastric lavage should be performed. An adequate airway should be maintained. Intravenous fluids may be administered.

Experiments in animals have indicated that cardiopulmonary collapse can occur with massive intravenous doses of triazolam. This could be reversed with positive mechanical respiration and the intravenous infusion of norepinephrine bitartrate or metaraminol bitartrate. Hemodialysis and forced diuresis are probably of little value. As with the management of intentional overdosage with any drug, the physician should bear in mind that multiple agents may have been ingested by the patient.

The oral LD_{50} in mice is greater than 1,000 mg/kg and in rats is greater than 5,000 mg/kg.

DOSAGE AND ADMINISTRATION

It is important to individualize the dosage of HALCION Tablets for maximum beneficial effect and to help avoid significant adverse effects.

The recommended dose for most adults is 0.25 mg before retiring. A dose of 0.125 mg may be found to be sufficient for some patients (eg, low body weight). A dose of 0.5 mg should be used only for exceptional patients who do not respond adequately to a trial of a lower dose since the risk of several adverse reactions increases with the size of the dose administered. A dose of 0.5 mg should not be exceeded.

In geriatric and/or debilitated patients the recommended dosage range is 0.125 mg to 0.25 mg. Therapy should be initiated at 0.125 mg in this group and the 0.25 mg dose should be used only for exceptional patients who do not respond to a trial of the lower dose. A lower dose of 0.25 mg should not be exceeded in these patients.

As with all medications, the lowest effective dose should be used.

Continued on next page

Information on these Upjohn products is based on labeling in effect June 1, 1992. Further information concerning these and other Upjohn products may be obtained by direct inquiry to Medical Information, The Upjohn Company, Kalamazoo, Michigan 49001.

Upjohn—Cont.

HOW SUPPLIED

HALCION Tablets are available in the following strengths and package sizes:
0.125 mg (white):
Unit of Use (10's)
NDC 0009-0010-06
Unit Dose Pkg (100)
NDC 0009-0010-22
VISIPAK® Reverse Numbered Pack (100)
NDC 0009-0010-04
Bottles of 500
NDC 0009-0010-11
0.25 mg (powder blue, scored):
Unit of Use (10's)
NDC 0009-0017-11
Unit Dose Pkg (100)
NDC 0009-0017-08
VISIPAK Reverse Numbered Pack (100)
NDC 0009-0017-17
Bottles of 500
NDC 0009-0017-02
Store at controlled room temperature 15°–30°C (59°–86°F).
Caution: Federal law prohibits dispensing without prescription.
US Patent No. 3,987,052
The text of the patient insert for HALCION is set forth below.

PATIENT INFORMATION

INTRODUCTION

HALCION is intended to help you sleep. It is one of several benzodiazepine sleeping pills that have generally similar properties. Anyone who is considering using one of these medications should be aware of both their benefits and several important risks and limitations, including diminishing effectiveness with continued use and the possible development of dependence (addiction) and possibly mental changes particularly when the drugs are used for more than a few days to a week. This patient information statement is intended to provide you with knowledge about this class of medications in general and about HALCION in particular that will be useful to guide you in the safe use of this product, BUT IT SHOULD NOT REPLACE A DISCUSSION BETWEEN YOU AND YOUR PHYSICIAN ABOUT THE RISKS AND BENEFITS OF HALCION.
This leaflet will focus on the beneficial and adverse effects of all members of this class of medications, as well as some specific information about HALCION. There are some differences among these products, and your physician may wish to discuss any specific advantages and disadvantages of particular members of this drug class with you.

EFFECTIVENESS OF BENZODIAZEPINE SLEEPING PILLS

Benzodiazepine sleeping pills are effective medications and are relatively free of serious problems when they are used for short-term management of sleep problems (insomnia). Insomnia is not always the same. It may be reflected in difficulty in falling asleep, frequent awakening during the night, and/or early morning awakening. Insomnia is often transient in nature, responding to brief treatment with sleeping pills. Use for more than a short while requires discussion with your physician about the risks and benefits of prolonged use.

SIDE EFFECTS

Common Side Effects
The most common side effects of benzodiazepine sleeping pills are related to the ability of the medications to make you sleepy; drowsiness, dizziness, lightheadedness, and difficulty with coordination. Users must be cautious about engaging in hazardous activities requiring complete mental alertness, eg, operating machinery or driving a motor vehicle. Do not take alcohol while using HALCION. Benzodiazepine sleeping pills should not be used with other medications or substances that may cause drowsiness, without discussing said use with your physician.
How sleepy you are the day after you use one of these sleep medications depends on your individual response and on how quickly the product is eliminated from your body. The larger the dose, the more likely an individual will experience next day residual effects such as drowsiness. For this reason, it is important to use the lowest effective dose for each individual patient. Benzodiazepines that are eliminated rapidly, eg, HALCION, tend to cause less next day drowsiness but may cause more withdrawal problems the day after use (see below).

Special Concerns
Memory Problems
All benzodiazepine sleeping pills can cause a special type of amnesia (memory loss) in which a person may not recall events occurring during some period of time, usually several

hours, after taking a drug. This is ordinarily not a problem, because the person taking a sleeping pill intends to be asleep during this vulnerable period of time. It can be a problem when the drugs are taken to induce sleep while traveling, such as during an airplane flight, because the person may awake before the effect of the drug is gone. This has been called "traveler's amnesia". HALCION is more likely than other members of the class to cause this problem.
Tolerance/Withdrawal Phenomena
Some loss of effectiveness or adaptation to the sleep inducing effects of these medications may develop after nightly use for more than a few weeks and there may be a degree of dependence that develops. For the benzodiazepine sleeping pills that are eliminated quickly from the body, a relative deficiency of the drug may occur at some point in the interval between each night's use. This can lead to (1) increased wakefulness during the last third of the night, and (2) the appearance of increased signs of daytime anxiety or nervousness. These two events have been reported in particular for HALCION.
There can be more severe withdrawal effects when a benzodiazepine sleeping pill is stopped. Such effects can occur after discontinuing these drugs following use for only a week or two, but may be more common and more severe after longer periods of continuous use. One type of withdrawal phenomenon is the occurrence of what is known as 'rebound insomnia'. That is, on the first few nights after the drug is stopped, insomnia is actually worse than before the sleeping pill was given. Other withdrawal phenomena following abrupt stopping of benzodiazepine sleeping pills range from mild unpleasant feelings to a major withdrawal syndrome which may include abdominal and muscle cramps, vomiting, sweating, tremor, and rarely, convulsions. These more severe withdrawal phenomena are uncommon.
Dependence/Abuse Phenomena
All benzodiazepine sleeping pills can cause dependence (addiction), especially when used regularly for more than a few weeks or at higher doses. Some people develop a need to continue taking these drugs, either at the prescribed dose or at increasing doses, not so much for continued therapeutic effect, but rather, to avoid withdrawal phenomena and/or to achieve nontherapeutic effects. Individuals who have been dependent on alcohol or other drugs may be at particular risk of becoming dependent on drugs in this class, but all people appear to be at some risk. This possibility must be considered before extending the use of these drugs for more than a few weeks.
Mental and Behavioral Changes
A variety of abnormal thinking and behavior changes have been reported to occur in association with the use of benzodiazepine sleeping pills. Some of these changes are like the release of inhibition seen in association with alcohol, eg, aggressiveness and extroversion that seem out of character. Others, however, can be more unusual and more extreme, such as confusion, bizarre behavior, agitation, hallucinations, depersonalization, and worsening of depression, including suicidal thinking. It is rarely clear whether such events are induced by the drug being taken, are caused by some underlying illness or are simply spontaneous happenings. In fact, worsened insomnia may in some cases be associated with illnesses that were present before the medication was used. In any event, the most important fact is to understand that regardless of the cause, users of these medications should promptly report any mental or behavioral changes to their doctor.
Effects on Pregnancy
Certain benzodiazepines have been linked to birth deffects when administered during the early months of pregnancy. In addition, the administration of benzodiazepines during the last weeks of pregnancy has been associated with sedation of the fetus. Consequently, the use of this drug should be avoided at any time during pregnancy.

SAFE USE OF BENZODIAZEPINE SLEEPING PILLS

To assure the safe and effective use of HALCION, you should adhere to the following cautions:
1. HALCION is a prescription medication, and, therefore, should be used only as directed by your doctor. Follow your doctor's advice about how to take it, when to take it, and how long to take it. As with other prescription medication, HALCION should be taken only by the individual for whom it is prescribed.
2. Do not extend your use of HALCION beyond 7–10 days without first consulting your physician.
3. If you develop any unusual and disturbing thoughts or behavior during treatment with HALCION, you should discuss such problems with your physician.
4. Inform your physician about any alcohol consumption and medicine you are taking now, including drugs you may buy without a prescription. Do not use alcohol while taking HALCION.
5. Do not take HALCION in circumstances where a full night's sleep and elimination of the drug from the body are not possible before you would again need to be active and functional, eg, an overnight flight of less than 7–8 hours,

because amnestic episodes have been reported in such situations.
6. Do not increase the prescribed dose except on the advice of your physician.
7. Until you experience how this medication affects you, do not drive a car or operate potentially dangerous machinery, etc.
8. Be aware that you may experience an increase in sleep difficulties (rebound insomnia) on the first night or two after discontinuing HALCION.
9. Inform you physician if you are planning to become pregnant, if you are pregnant, or if you become pregnant while you are taking this medicine. The use of HALCION should be avoided at any time during pregnancy.
The Upjohn Company
Kalamazoo, Michigan 49001, USA
Revised December 1991   812 110 523
                 691157

Shown in Product Identification Section, page 434

HALOTESTIN®   Ⓒ℔ ℞
brand of fluoxymesterone tablets, USP

10 mg-100s
NSN 6505-01-041-8165 (M & VA)

DESCRIPTION

HALOTESTIN Tablets contain fluoxymesterone, an androgenic hormone.
Fluoxymesterone is a white or practically white odorless, crystalline powder, melting at about 240° C. with some decomposition. It is practically insoluble in water, sparingly soluble in alcohol and slightly soluble in chloroform.
The chemical name for fluoxymesterone is androst-4-en-3-one, 9-fluoro -11, 17- dihydroxy-17- methyl-,(11β,17β). The molecular formula is $C_{20}H_{29}FO_3$ and the molecular weight 336.45.
Each HALOTESTIN tablet, for oral administration, contains 2 mg, 5 mg or 10 mg fluoxymesterone. Inactive ingredients: calcium stearate, corn starch, FD&C yellow no. 5, lactose, sorbic acid, sucrose, tragacanth. In addition, the **2 mg** tablet contains FD&C yellow no. 6 and the **5 mg** and **10 mg** contain FD&C blue no. 2.

CLINICAL PHARMACOLOGY

Endogenous androgens are responsible for normal growth and development of the male sex organs and for maintenance of secondary sex characteristics. These effects include growth and maturation of the prostate, seminal vesicles, penis, and scrotum; development of male hair distribution, such as beard, pubic, chest, and axillary hair; laryngeal enlargement, vocal cord thickening, and alterations in body musculature and fat distribution. Drugs in this class also cause retention of nitrogen, sodium, potassium, and phosphorus, and decreased urinary excretion of calcium. Androgens have been reported to increase protein anabolism and decrease protein catabolism. Nitrogen balance is improved only when there is sufficient intake of calories and protein. Androgens are responsible for the growth spurt of adolescence and for eventual termination of linear growth, brought about by fusion of the epiphyseal growth centers. In children, exogenous androgens accelerate linear growth rates, but may cause disproportionate advancement in bone maturation. Use over long periods may result in fusion of the epiphyseal growth centers and termination of the growth process. Androgens have been reported to stimulate production of red blood cells by enhancing production of erythropoietic stimulation factor.
During exogenous administration of androgens, endogenous testosterone release is inhibited through feedback inhibition of pituitary luteinizing hormone (LH). At large doses of exogenous androgen, spermatogenesis may also be suppressed through feedback inhibition of pituitary follicle stimulating hormone (FSH).
Inactivation of testosterone occurs primarily in the liver.
The half-life of fluoxymesterone after oral administration is approximately 9.2 hours.

INDICATIONS AND USAGE

In the male—HALOTESTIN Tablets (fluoxymesterone) are indicated for:
1. Replacement therapy in conditions associated with symptoms of deficiency or absence of endogenous testosterone:
a. Primary hypogonadism (congenital or acquired)—testicular failure due to cryptorchidism, bilateral torsion, orchitis, vanishing testis syndrome; or orchidectomy.
b. Hypogonadotropic hypogonadism (congenital or acquired)—idiopathic gonadotropin or LHRH deficiency, or pituitary-hypothalamic injury from tumors, trauma, or radiation.
2. Delayed puberty, provided it has been definitely established as such, and is not just a familial trait.
In the female—HALOTESTIN Tablets are indicated for palliation of androgen-responsive recurrent mammary cancer

in women who are more than one year but less than five years postmenopausal, or who have been proven to have a hormone-dependent tumor as shown by previous beneficial response to castration.

CONTRAINDICATIONS

1. Known hypersensitivity to the drug
2. Males with carcinoma of the breast
3. Males with known or suspected carcinoma of the prostate gland
4. Women known or suspected to be pregnant
5. Patients with serious cardiac, hepatic or renal disease

WARNINGS

Hypercalcemia may occur in immobilized patients and in patients with breast cancer. If this occurs, the drug should be discontinued.

Prolonged use of high doses of androgens (principally the 17-α alkyl-androgens) has been associated with development of hepatic adenomas, hepatocellular carcinoma, and peliosis hepatis—all potentially life-threatening complications.

Cholestatic hepatitis and jaundice may occur with 17-α-alkyl-androgens. Should this occur, the drug should be discontinued. This is reversible with discontinuation of the drug. Geriatric patients treated with androgens may be at an increased risk of developing prostatic hypertrophy and prostatic carcinoma although conclusive evidence to support this concept is lacking.

Edema, with or without congestive heart failure, may be a serious complication in patients with pre-existing cardiac, renal or hepatic disease.

Gynecomastia may develop and occasionally persists in patients being treated for hypogonadism.

Androgen therapy should be used cautiously in males with delayed puberty. Androgens can accelerate bone maturation without producing compensatory gain in linear growth. The effect on bone maturation should be monitored by assessing bone age of the wrist and hand every six months.

This drug has not been shown to be safe and effective for the enhancement of athletic performance. Because of the potential risk of serious adverse health effects, this drug should not be used for such purpose.

PRECAUTIONS

General

Women should be observed for signs of virilization which is usual following androgen use at high doses. Discontinuation of drug therapy at the time of evidence of mild virilism is necessary to prevent irreversible virilization. A decision may be made by the patient and the physician that some virilization will be tolerated during treatment for breast carcinoma. Patients with benign prostatic hypertrophy may develop acute urethral obstruction. Priapism or excessive sexual stimulation may develop. Oligospermia may occur after prolonged administration or excessive dosage. If any of these effects appear, the androgen should be stopped and if restarted, a lower dosage should be utilized.

This product contains FD&C Yellow No. 5 (tartrazine) which may cause allergic-type reactions (including bronchial asthma) in certain susceptible individuals. Although the overall incidence of FD&C Yellow No. 5 (tartrazine) sensitivity in the general population is low, it is frequently seen in patients who also have aspirin hypersensitivity.

Information for patients

Patients should be instructed to report any of the following: nausea, vomiting, changes in skin color, and ankle swelling. Males should be instructed to report too frequent or persistent erections of the penis and females any hoarseness, acne, changes in menstrual periods or increase in facial hair.

Laboratory tests

Women with disseminated breast carcinoma should have frequent determination of urine and serum calcium levels during the course of androgen therapy (See WARNINGS). Because of the hepatotoxicity associated with the use of 17-alpha-alkylated androgens, liver function tests should be obtained periodically.

Periodic (every six months) x-ray examinations of bone age should be made during treatment of prepubertal males to determine the rate of bone maturation and the effects of androgen therapy on the epiphyseal centers.

Hemoglobin and hematocrit levels (to detect polycythemia) should be checked periodically in patients receiving long-term androgen administration.

Serum cholesterol may increase during androgen therapy.

DRUG INTERACTIONS

Androgens may increase sensitivity to oral anticoagulants. Dosage of the anticoagulant may require reduction in order to maintain satisfactory therapeutic hypoprothrombinemia. Concurrent administration of oxyphenbutazone and androgens may result in elevated serum levels of oxyphenbutazone.

In diabetic patients, the metabolic effects of androgens may decrease blood glucose and, therefore, insulin requirements.

Drug/Laboratory test interferences

Androgens may decrease levels of thyroxine-binding globulin, resulting in decreased total T_4 serum levels and in-

creased resin uptake of T_3 and T_4. Free thyroid hormone levels remain unchanged, however, and there is no clinical evidence of thyroid dysfunction.

Carcinogenesis, mutagenesis, impairment of fertility

Animal data: Testosterone has been tested by subcutaneous injection and implantation in mice and rats. The implant induced cervical-uterine tumors in mice, which metastasized in some cases. There is suggestive evidence that injection of testosterone into some strains of female mice increases their susceptibility to hepatoma. Testosterone is also known to increase the number of tumors and decrease the degree of differentiation of chemically-induced carcinomas of the liver in rats.

Human data: There are rare reports of hepatocellular carcinoma in patients receiving long-term therapy with androgens in high doses. Withdrawal of the drugs did not lead to regression of the tumors in all cases.

Geriatric patients treated with androgens may be at an increased risk of developing prostatic hypertrophy and prostatic carcinoma although conclusive evidence to support this concept is lacking.

This compound has not be tested for mutagenic potential. However, as noted above, carcinogenic effects have been attributed to treatment with androgenic hormones. The potential carcinogenic effects likely occur through a hormonal mechanism rather than by a direct chemical interaction mechanism.

Impairment of fertility was not tested directly in animal species. However, as noted below under Adverse Reactions, oligospermia in males and amenorrhea in females are potential adverse effects of treatment with HALOTESTIN Tablets. Therefore, impairment of fertility is a possible outcome of treatment with HALOTESTIN.

Pregnancy

Teratogenic effects: Pregnancy Category X. (See CONTRAINDICATIONS.)

Nursing mothers

HALOTESTIN Tablets (fluoxymesterone) are not recommended for use in nursing mothers.

Pediatric use

Androgen therapy should be used very cautiously in children and only by specialists aware of the adverse effects on bone maturation. Skeletal maturation must be monitored every six months by an x-ray of the hand and wrist (See WARNINGS).

ADVERSE REACTIONS

Endocrine and urogenital

Female: The most common side effects of androgen therapy are amenorrhea and other menstrual irregularities; inhibition of gonadotropin secretion; and virilization, including deepening of the voice and clitoral enlargement. The latter usually is not reversible after androgens are discontinued. When administered to a pregnant woman, androgens can cause virilization of external genitalia of the female fetus.

Male: Gynecomastia, and excessive frequency and duration of penile erections. Oligospermia may occur at high dosage.

Skin and appendages

Hirsutism, male pattern of baldness, seborrhea, and acne.

Fluid and electrolyte disturbances

Retention of sodium, chloride, water, potassium, calcium, and inorganic phosphates.

Gastrointestinal

Nausea, cholestatic jaundice, alterations in liver function tests, rarely hepatocellular neoplasms and peliosis hepatis (see WARNINGS).

Hematologic

Suppression of clotting factors II, V, VII, and X, bleeding in patients on concomitant anticoagulant therapy, and polycythemia.

Nervous system

Increased or decreased libido, headache, anxiety, depression, and generalized paresthesia.

Allergic

Hypersensitivity, including skin manifestations and anaphylactoid reactions.

DRUG ABUSE AND DEPENDENCE

Controlled Substance Class: Fluoxymesterone is a controlled substance under the Anabolic Steroids Control Act, and HALOTESTIN Tablets has been assigned to Schedule III.

OVERDOSAGE

There have been no reports of acute overdosage with the androgens.

DOSAGE AND ADMINISTRATION

The dosage will vary depending upon the individual, the condition being treated, and its severity. The total daily oral dose may be administered singly or in divided (three or four) doses.

Male hypogonadism: For complete replacement in the hypogonadal male, a daily dose of 5 to 20 mg will suffice in the majority of patients. It is usually preferable to begin treatment with full therapeutic doses which are later ad-

justed to individual requirements. Priapism is indicative of excessive dosage and is indication for temporary withdrawal of the drug.

Delayed puberty: Dosage should be carefully titrated utilizing a low dose, appropriate skeletal monitoring, and by limiting the duration of therapy to four to six months.

Inoperable carcinoma of the breast in the female: The recommended total daily dose for palliative therapy in advanced inoperable carcinoma of the breast is 10 to 40 mg. Because of its short action, fluoxymesterone should be administered to patients in divided, rather than single, daily doses to ensure more stable blood levels. In general, it appears necessary to continue therapy for at least one month for a satisfactory subjective response, and for two to three months for an objective response.

HOW SUPPLIED

HALOTESTIN Tablets (fluoxymesterone), scored, are available in the following strengths and colors:

2 mg (peach)
    Bottles of 100   NDC 0009-0014-01

5 mg (light green)
    Bottles of 100   NDC 0009-0019-06

10 mg (green)
    Bottles of 30   NDC 0009-0036-03
    Bottles of 100   NDC 0009-0036-04

Code 810 804 304

Shown in Product Identification Section, page 434

HEPARIN SODIUM INJECTION, USP   ℞
Sterile Solution

DESCRIPTION

Heparin is a heterogenous group of straight-chain anionic mucopolysaccharides, called glycosaminoglycans having anticoagulant properties. Although others may be present, the main sugars occurring in heparin are: (1) α-L-iduronic acid 2-sulfate, (2) 2-deoxy-2-sulfamino-α-D-glucose 6-sulfate, (3) β-D-glucoronic acid, (4) 2-acetamido-2-deoxy-α-D-glucose, and (5) α-L-iduronic acid. These sugars are present in decreasing amounts, usually in the order (2) > (1) > (4) > (3) > (5), and are joined by glycosidic linkages, forming polymers of varying sizes. Heparin is strongly acidic because of its content of covalently linked sulfate and carboxylic acid groups. In heparin sodium, the acidic protons of the sulfate units are partially replaced by sodium ions.

Heparin Sodium Injection, USP is a sterile solution of heparin sodium derived from bovine lung tissue, standardized for anticoagulant activity. It is to be administered by intravenous or deep subcutaneous routes. The potency is determined by a biological assay using a USP reference standard based on units of heparin activity per milligram. Heparin is pyrogen-free.

Each ml of the 1,000 and 5,000 USP Units per ml preparations contains: Heparin sodium 1,000 or 5,000 USP Units; 9 mg sodium chloride; 9.45 mg benzyl alcohol added as preservative. Each ml of the 10,000 USP Units per ml preparations contains: heparin sodium 10,000 USP Units; 9.45 mg benzyl alcohol added as preservative.

When necessary, the pH of Heparin Sodium Injection, USP was adjusted with hydrochloric acid and/or sodium hydroxide. The pH range is 5.0-7.5.

CLINICAL PHARMACOLOGY

Heparin inhibits reactions that lead to the clotting of blood and the formation of fibrin clots both *in vitro* and *in vivo*. Heparin acts at multiple sites in the normal coagulation system. Small amounts of heparin in combination with antithrombin III (heparin cofactor) can inhibit thrombosis by inactivating activated Factor X and inhibiting the conversion of prothrombin to thrombin. Once active thrombosis has developed, larger amounts of heparin can inhibit further coagulation by inactivating thrombin and preventing the conversion of fibrinogen to fibrin. Heparin also prevents the formation of a stable fibrin clot by inhibiting the activation of the fibrin stabilizing factor.

Bleeding time is usually unaffected by heparin. Clotting time is prolonged by full therapeutic doses of heparin; in most cases, it is not measurably affected by low doses of heparin. Peak plasma levels of heparin are achieved 2–4 hours following subcutaneous administration, although there are considerable individual variations. Loglinear plots of heparin plasma concentrations with time for a wide range of dose levels are linear which suggests the absence of zero order processes. Liver and the reticulo-endothelial system are the

Continued on next page

Information on these Upjohn products is based on labeling in effect June 1, 1992. Further information concerning these and other Upjohn products may be obtained by direct inquiry to Medical Information, The Upjohn Company, Kalamazoo, Michigan 49001.

Upjohn—Cont.

site of biotransformation. The biphasic elimination curve, a rapidly declining alpha phase ($t\frac{1}{2} = 10$ minutes) and after the age of 40 a slower beta phase, indicates uptake in organs. The absence of a relationship between anticoagulant half-life and concentration half-life may reflect factors such as protein binding of heparin.

Heparin does not have fibrinolytic activity; therefore, it will not lyse existing clots.

INDICATIONS AND USAGE

Heparin Sodium Injection is indicated for:

Anticoagulant therapy in prophylaxis and treatment of venous thrombosis and its extension;

(In a low-dose regimen) for prevention of postoperative deep venous thrombosis and pulmonary embolism in patients undergoing major abdomino-thoracic surgery or who for other reasons are at risk of developing thromboembolic disease (see DOSAGE AND ADMINISTRATION);

Prophylaxis and treatment of pulmonary embolism;

Atrial fibrillation with embolization;

Diagnosis and treatment of acute and chronic consumption coagulopathies (disseminated intravascular coagulation);

Prevention of clotting in arterial and heart surgery;

Prophylaxis and treatment of peripheral arterial embolism;

As an anticoagulant in blood transfusions, extracorporeal circulation, and dialysis procedures and in blood samples for laboratory purposes.

CONTRAINDICATIONS

Heparin sodium should not be used in patients:

With severe thrombocytopenia;

In whom suitable blood coagulation tests—e.g., the whole-blood clotting time, partial thromboplastin time, etc.—cannot be performed at appropriate intervals (this contraindication refers to full-dose heparin; there is usually no need to monitor coagulation parameters in patients receiving low-dose heparin);

With an uncontrollable active bleeding state (see WARNINGS), except when this is due to disseminated intravascular coagulation.

WARNINGS

Heparin is not intended for intramuscular use.

Hypersensitivity: Patients with documented hypersensitivity to heparin should be given the drug only in clearly life-threatening situations.

Hemorrhage: Hemorrhage can occur at virtually any site in patients receiving heparin. An unexplained fall in hematocrit, fall in blood pressure, or any other unexplained symptom should lead to serious consideration of a hemorrhagic event.

Heparin sodium should be used with extreme caution in disease states in which there is increased danger of hemorrhage. Some of the conditions in which increased danger of hemorrhage exists are:

Cardiovascular—Subacute bacterial endocarditis. Severe hypotension.

Surgical—During and immediately following (a) spinal tap or spinal anesthesia or (b) major surgery, especially involving the brain, spinal cord, or eye.

Hematologic—Conditions associated with increased bleeding tendencies, such as hemophilia, thrombocytopenia, and some vascular purpuras.

Gastrointestinal—Ulcerative lesions and continuous tube drainage of the stomach or small intestine.

Other—Menstruation, liver disease with impaired hemostasis.

Coagulation Testing: When heparin sodium is administered in therapeutic amounts, its dosage should be regulated by frequent blood coagulation tests. If the coagulation test is unduly prolonged or if hemorrhage occurs, heparin sodium should be discontinued promptly (see OVERDOSAGE).

Thrombocytopenia: Thrombocytopenia has been reported to occur in patients receiving heparin with a reported incidence of 0 to 30%. Mild thrombocytopenia (count greater than 100,000/mm³) may remain stable or reverse even if heparin is continued. However, thrombocytopenia of any degree should be monitored closely. If the count falls below 100,000/mm³ or if recurrent thrombosis develops (see White Clot Syndrome, PRECAUTIONS), the heparin product should be discontinued. If continued heparin therapy is essential, administration of heparin from a different organ source can be reinstituted with caution.

Miscellaneous: This product contains benzyl alcohol as preservative: Benzyl alcohol has been reported to be associated with a fatal "Gasping Syndrome" in premature infants.

PRECAUTIONS

1. General

a. White Clot Syndrome

It has been reported that patients on heparin may develop new thrombus formation in association with thrombocytopenia resulting from irreversible aggregation of platelets induced by heparin, the so-called "white clot syndrome."

The process may lead to severe thromboembolic complications like skin necrosis, gangrene of the extremities that may lead to amputation, myocardial infarction, pulmonary embolism, stroke, and possibly death. Therefore, heparin administration should be promptly discontinued if a patient develops new thrombosis in association with thrombocytopenia.

b. Heparin Resistance

Increased resistance to heparin is frequently encountered in fever, thrombosis, thrombophlebitis, infections with thrombosing tendencies, myocardial infarction, cancer and in postsurgical patients.

c. Increased Risk in Older Women:

A higher incidence of bleeding has been reported in women over 60 years of age.

2. Laboratory Tests: Periodic platelet counts, hematocrits, and tests for occult blood in stool are recommended during the entire course of heparin therapy, regardless of the route of administration (see DOSAGE AND ADMINISTRATION).

3. Drug Interactions:

Oral anticoagulants: Heparin sodium may prolong the one-stage prothrombin time. Therefore, when heparin sodium is given with dicumarol or warfarin sodium, a period of at least 5 hours after the last intravenous dose or 24 hours after the last subcutaneous dose should elapse before blood is drawn if a valid prothrombin time is to be obtained.

Platelet inhibitors: Drugs such as acetylsalicylic acid, dextran, phenylbutazone, ibuprofen, indomethacin, dipyridamole, hydroxychloroquine and others that interfere with platelet-aggregation reactions (the main hemostatic defense of heparinized patients) may induce bleeding and should be used with caution in patients receiving heparin sodium.

Other interactions: Digitalis, tetracyclines, nicotine, or antihistamines may partially counteract the anticoagulant action of heparin sodium.

4. Drug/Laboratory Tests Interactions:

Hyperaminotransferasemia: Significant elevations of aminotransferase (SGOT [S-AST] and SPT [S-ALT])levels have occurred in a high percentage of patients (and healthy subjects) who have received heparin. Since aminotransferase determinations are important in the differential diagnosis of myocardial infarction, liver disease, and pulmonary emboli, rises that might be caused by drugs (like heparin) should be interpreted with caution.

5. Carcinogenesis, Mutagenesis, Impairment of Fertility: No long-term studies in animals have been performed to evaluate carcinogenic potential of heparin. Also, no reproduction studies in animals have been performed concerning mutagenesis or impairment of fertility.

6. Pregnancy:

Teratogenic Effects: Pregnancy Category C. Animal reproduction studies have not been conducted with heparin sodium. It is also not known whether heparin sodium can cause fetal harm when administered to a pregnant woman or can affect reproduction capacity. Heparin sodium should be given to a pregnant woman only if clearly needed.

Nonteratogenic Effects: Heparin does not cross the placental barrier.

7. Nursing Mothers: Heparin is not excreted in human milk.

8. Pediatric Use: See DOSAGE AND ADMINISTRATION.

ADVERSE REACTIONS

1. Hemorrhage. Hemorrhage is the chief complication that may result from heparin therapy (see WARNINGS). An overly prolonged clotting time or minor bleeding during therapy can usually be controlled by withdrawing the drug (see OVERDOSAGE). **It should be appreciated that gastrointestinal or urinary tract bleeding during anticoagulant therapy may indicate the presence of an underlying occult lesion.** Bleeding can occur at any site but certain specific hemorrhagic complications may be difficult to detect.

a. Adrenal hemorrhage, with resultant acute adrenal insufficiency, has occurred during anticoagulant therapy. Therefore, such treatment should be discontinued in patients who develop signs and symptoms of acute adrenal hemorrhage and insufficiency. Initiation of corrective therapy should not depend on laboratory confirmation of the diagnosis, since any delay in an acute situation may result in the patient's death.

b. Ovarian (corpus luteum) hemorrhage developed in a number of women of reproductive age receiving short- or long-term anticoagulant therapy. This complication if unrecognized may be fatal.

c. Retroperitoneal hemorrhage.

2. Local irritation. Local irritation, erythema, mild pain, hematoma or ulceration may follow deep subcutaneous (intrafat) injection of heparin sodium. These complications are much more common after intramuscular use, and such use is not recommended.

3. Hypersensitivity. Generalized hypersensitivity reactions have been reported, with chills, fever, and urticaria as the most usual manifestations, and asthma, rhinitis, lacrimation, headache, nausea and vomiting, and anaphylactoid reactions, including shock, occurring more rarely. Itching

---

and burning, especially on the plantar site of the feet, may occur.

Thrombocytopenia has been reported to occur in patients receiving heparin with a reported incidence of 0–30%. While often mild and of no obvious clinical significance, such thrombocytopenia can be accompanied by severe thromboembolic complications such as skin necrosis, gangrene of the extremities, that may lead to amputation, myocardial infarction, pulmonary embolism, stroke, and possibly death. (See WARNINGS, PRECAUTIONS.)

Certain episodes of painful, ischemic, and cyanosed limbs have in the past been attributed to allergic vasospastic reactions. Whether these are in fact identical to the thrombocytopenia associated complications remains to be determined.

4. Miscellaneous. Osteoporosis following long-term administration of high doses of heparin, cutaneous necrosis after systemic administration, supression of aldosterone synthesis, delayed transient alopecia, priapism, and rebound hyperlipemia on discontinuation of heparin sodium have also been reported.

Significant elevations of aminotransferase (SGOT [S-AST] and SGPT [S-ALT]) levels have occurred in a high percentage of patients (and healthy subjects) who have received heparin.

OVERDOSAGE

Symptoms: Bleeding is the chief sign of heparin overdosage. Nosebleeds, blood in urine or tarry stools may be noted as the first sign of bleeding. Easy bruising or petechial formations may precede frank bleeding.

Treatment: Neutralization of heparin effect. When clinical circumstances (bleeding) require reversal of heparinization, protamine sulfate (1% solution) by slow infusion will neutralize heparin sodium. **No more than 50 mg should be administered, very slowly,** in any 10 minute period. Each mg of protamine sulfate neutralizes approximately 100 USP heparin units. The amount of protamine required decreases over time as heparin is metabolized. Although the metabolism of heparin is complex, it may, for the purpose of choosing a protamine dose, be assumed to have a half-life of about $\frac{1}{2}$ hour after intravenous injection.

Administration of protamine sulfate can cause severe hypotensive and anaphylactoid reactions. Because fatal reactions often resembling anaphylaxis have been reported, the drug should be given only when resuscitation techniques and treatment of anaphylactoid shock are readily available.

For additional information the labeling of Protamine Sulfate Injection, USP products should be consulted.

DOSAGE AND ADMINISTRATION

Parenteral drug products should be inspected visually for particulate matter and discoloration prior to administration, whenever solution and container permit. Slight discoloration does not alter potency.

When heparin is added to an infusion solution for continuous intravenous administration, the container should be inverted at least six times to insure adequate mixing and prevent pooling of the heparin in the solution.

Heparin sodium is not effective by oral administration and should be given by intermittent intravenous injection, intravenous infusion, or deep subcutaneous (intrafat, i.e., above the iliac crest or abdominal fat layer) injection. **The intramuscular route of administration should be avoided because of the frequent occurrence of hematoma at the injection site.** The dosage of heparin soldium should be adjusted according to the patient's coagulation test results. When heparin is given by continuous intravenous infusion, the coagulation time should be determined approximately every 4 hours in the early stages of treatment. When the drug is administered intermittently by intravenous injection, coagulation tests should be performed before each injection during the early stages of treatment and at appropriate intervals thereafter. Dosage is considered adequate when the activated partial thromboplastin time (APTT) is 1.5 to 2 times normal or when the whole blood clotting time is elevated approximately 2.5 to 3 times the control value. After deep subcutaneous (intrafat) injections, tests for adequacy of dosage are best performed on samples drawn 4–6 hours after the injections.

Periodic platelet counts, hematocrits, and tests for occult blood in stool are recommended during the entire course of heparin therapy, regardless of the route of administration. Heparin Sodium Injection should not be mixed with Adriamycin (doxorubicin) or Inapsine (droperidol) since it has been reported that these drugs are incompatible with heparin and a precipitate may form.

Converting to Oral Anticoagulant: When an oral anticoagulant of the coumarin or similar type is to be begun in patients already receiving heparin sodium, baseline and subsequent tests of prothrombin activity must be determined at a time when heparin activity is too low to affect the prothrombin time. This is about 5 hours after the last I.V. bolus and 24 hours after the last subcutaneous dose. If continuous I.V. heparin infusion is used, prothrombin time can usually be measured at any time.

In converting from heparin to an oral anticoagulant, the dose of the oral anticoagulant should be the usual initial

METHOD OF ADMINISTRATION	FREQUENCY	RECOMMENDED DOSE*
Deep Subcutaneous (Intrafat) Injection	Initial Dose	5,000 units by I.V. injection, followed by 10,000–20,000 units of a concentrated solution, subcutaneously
A different site should be used for each injection to prevent the development of massive hematoma.	Every 8 hours	8,000 –10,000 units of a concentrated solution
	or Every 12 hours	15,000–20,000 units of a concentrated solution
Intermittent Intravenous Injection	Initial Dose	10,000 units, either undiluted or in 50–100 ml of 0.9% Sodium Chloride Injection, USP
	Every 4 to 6 hours	5,000–10,000 units, either diluted or in 50–100 ml of 0.9% Sodium Chloride Injection, USP
Continuous intravenous Infusion	Initial Dose	5,000 units by I.V. injection
	Continuous	20,000–40,000 units/24 hours in 1,000 ml of 0.9% Sodium Chloride Injection, USP (or in any compatible solution) for infusion

* Based on 150-lb. (68-kg) patient.

amount and thereafter prothrombin time should be determined at the usual intervals. To ensure continuous anticoagulation, it is advisable to continue full heparin therapy for several days after the prothrombin time has reached the therapeutic range. Heparin therapy may then be discontinued without tapering.

Therapeutic Anticoagulant Effect with Full-Dose Heparin. Although dosage must be adjusted for the individual patient according to the results of suitable laboratory tests, the following dosage schedules may be used as guidelines: [See table above.]

Pediatric Use: Follow recommendations of appropriate pediatric reference texts. In general, the following dosage schedule may be used as a guideline:

Initial Dose: 50 units/kg (I.V., drip)
Maintenance Dose: 100 units/kg (I.V., drip) every four hours, or 20,000 units/M²/24 hours continuously

Surgery of the Heart and Blood Vessels: Patients undergoing total body perfusion for open-heart surgery should receive an initial dose of not less than 150 units of heparin sodium per kilogram of body weight. Frequently, a dose of 300 units per kilogram is used for procedures estimated to last less than 60 minutes or 400 units per kilogram for those estimated to last longer than 60 minutes.

Low-Dose Prophylaxis of Postoperative Thromboembolism: A number of well-controlled clinical trials have demonstrated that low-dose heparin prophylaxis, given just prior to and after surgery, will reduce the incidence of postoperative deep vein thrombosis in the legs (as measured by the I-125 fibrinogen technique and venography) and of clinical pulmonary embolism. The most widely used dosage has been 5,000 units 2 hours before surgery and 5,000 units every 8 to 12 hours thereafter for 7 days or until the patient is fully ambulatory, whichever is longer. The heparin is given by deep subcutaneous (intrafat, i.e., above the iliac crest or abdominal fat layer, arm or thigh) injection with a fine (25 to 26 - gauge) needle to minimize tissue trauma. A concentrated solution of heparin sodium is recommended. Such prophylaxis should be reserved for patients over the age of 40 who are undergoing major surgery. Patients with bleeding disorders and those having brain or spinal cord surgery, spinal anesthesia, eye surgery, or potentially sanguineous operations should be excluded, as should patients receiving oral anticoagulants or platelet-active drugs (see WARNINGS). The value of such prophylaxis in hip surgery has not been established. The possibility of increased bleeding during surgery or postoperatively should be borne in mind. If such bleeding occurs, discontinuation of heparin and neutralization with protamine sulfate are advisable. If clinical evidence of thromboembolism develops despite low-dose prophylaxis, full therapeutic doses of anticoagulants should be given unless contraindicated. Prior to initiating heparinization the physician should rule out bleeding disorders by ap-

propriate history and laboratory tests, and appropriate coagulations tests should be repeated just prior to surgery. Coagulation tests values should be normal or only slightly elevated at these times.

Extracorporeal Dialysis: Follow equipment manufacturers' operating directions carefully.

Blood Transfusion: Addition of 400 to 600 USP units per 100 ml of whole blood is usually employed to prevent coagulation. Usually, 7,500 USP units of heparin sodium are added to 100 ml of 0.9% Sodium Chloride Injection, USP (or 75,000 USP units per 1,000 ml of 0.9% Sodium Chloride Injection, USP) and mixed; from this sterile solution, 6 to 8 ml are added per 100 ml of whole blood.

Laboratory Samples: Addition of 70 to 150 units of heparin sodium per 10 to 20 ml sample of whole blood is usually employed to prevent coagulation of the sample. Leukoycte counts should be performed on heparinized blood within 2 hours after addition of the heparin. Heparinized blood should not be used for isoagglutinin, complement, or erythrocyte fragility tests or platelet counts.

HOW SUPPLIED

Heparin Sodium Injection, USP derived **from beef lung** is available in the following strengths and package sizes:

1,000 units per ml
     10 ml vials   NDC 0009-0268-01
    25–10 ml vials   NDC 0009-0268-07
    30 ml vials   NDC 0009-0268-02
5,000 units per ml
     1 ml vials   NDC 0009-0291-02
    10 ml vials   NDC 0009-0291-01
10,000 units per ml
     1 ml vials   NDC 0009-0317-01
    25–1 ml vials   NDC 0009-0317-08
     4 ml vials   NDC 0009-0317-02
    25–4 ml vials   NDC 0009-0317-09

Store the product at controlled room temperature 15°–30°C (59°–86°F).

Code 810 670 016

LINCOCIN®   ℞

brand of lincomycin hydrochloride capsules and lincomycin hydrochloride sterile solution (lincomycin hydrochloride capsules, USP, and lincomycin hydrochloride injection, USP)

WARNING

Lincomycin therapy has been associated with severe colitis which may end fatally. Therefore, it should be reserved for serious infections where less toxic antimicrobial agents are inappropriate, as described in the Indications Section. It should not be used in patients with nonbacterial infections, such as most upper respiratory tract infections. Studies indicate a toxin(s) produced by *Clostridia* is one primary cause of antibiotic

associated colitis. The colitis is usually characterized by severe, persistent diarrhea and severe abdominal cramps and may be associated with the passage of blood and mucus. Endoscopic examination may reveal pseudomembranous colitis.

When significant diarrhea occurs, the drug should be discontinued or, if necessary, continued only with close observation of the patient. Large bowel endoscopy has been recommended.

Antiperistaltic agents such as opiates and diphenoxylate with atropine (Lomotil) may prolong and/or worsen the condition. Vancomycin has been found to be effective in the treatment of antibiotic associated pseudomembranous colitis produced by *Clostridium difficile*. The usual adult dose is 500 milligrams to 2 grams of vancomycin orally per day in three to four divided doses administered for 7 to 10 days. Cholestyramine or colestipol resins bind vancomycin *in vitro*. If both a resin and vancomycin are to be administered concurrently, it may be advisable to separate the time of administration of each drug.

Diarrhea, colitis, and pseudomembranous colitis have been observed to begin up to several weeks following cessation of therapy with lincomycin.

DESCRIPTION

LINCOCIN Capsules and LINCOCIN Sterile Solution contain lincomycin hydrochloride which is the monohydrated salt of lincomycin, a substance produced by the growth of a member of the *lincolnensis* group of *Streptomyces lincolnensis* (Fam. *Streptomycetaceae*). It is a white, or practically white, crystalline powder and is odorless or has a faint odor. Its solutions are acid and are dextrorotatory. Lincomycin hydrochloride is freely soluble in water; soluble in dimethylformamide and very slightly soluble in acetone.

LINCOCIN Capsules contain the following inactive ingredients: erythrosine sodium, FD&C blue No. 1, gelatin, lactose, magnesium stearate, talc and titanium dioxide.

CLINICAL PHARMACOLOGY

Microbiology—Lincomycin has been shown to be effective against most of the common gram-positive pathogens. Depending on the sensitivity of the organism and concentration of the antibiotic, it may be either bactericidal or bacteriostatic. Cross resistance has not been demonstrated with penicillin, chloramphenicol, ampicillin, cephalosporins or the tetracyclines. Despite chemical differences, lincomycin exhibits antibacterial activity similar but not identical to the macrolide antibiotics (eg erythromycin). Some cross resistance (with erythromycin) including a phenomenon known as dissociated cross resistance or macrolide effect has been reported. Microorganisms have not developed resistance to lincomycin rapidly when tested by *in vitro* or *in vivo* methods. Staphylococci develop resistance to lincomycin in a slow, step-wise manner based on *in vitro*, serial subculture experiments. This pattern of resistance development is unlike that shown for streptomycin.

Studies indicate that lincomycin does not share antigenicity with penicillin compounds.

Biological Studies—*In vitro* studies indicate that the spectrum of activity includes *Staphylococcus aureus, Staphylococcus albus, β-hemolytic Streptococcus, Streptococcus viridans, Diplococcus pneumoniae, Clostridium tetani, Clostridium perfringens, Corynebacterium diphtheriae* and *Corynebacterium acnes*.

NOTE: The drug is not active against most strains of *Streptococcus faecalis*, nor against *Neisseria gonorrhoeae, Neisseria meningitidis, Hemophilus influenzae*, or other gram-negative organisms or yeasts.

Human Pharmacology—Lincomycin is absorbed rapidly after a 500 mg oral dose, reaching peak levels in 2 to 4 hours. Levels are maintained above the MIC (minimum inhibitory concentration) for most gram-positive organisms for 6 to 8 hours. Urinary recovery of drug in a 24-hour period ranges from 1.0 to 31 percent (mean: 4.0) after a single oral dose of 500 mg of lincomycin. Tissue level studies indicate that bile is an important route of excretion. Significant levels have been demonstrated in the majority of body tissues. Although the drug is not present in significant amounts in the spinal fluid of normal volunteers, it has been demonstrated in the spinal fluid of one patient with pneumococcal meningitis. Intramuscular administration of a single dose of 600 mg produces a peak serum level at 30 minutes with detectable levels persisting for 24 hours. Urinary excretion after this dose ranges from 1.8 to 24.8 percent (mean: 17.3).

Continued on next page

Information on these Upjohn products is based on labeling in effect June 1, 1992. Further information concerning these and other Upjohn products may be obtained by direct inquiry to Medical Information, The Upjohn Company, Kalamazoo, Michigan 49001.

Upjohn—Cont.

The intravenous infusion over a 2-hour interval of 600 mg of lincomycin hydrochloride in 500 mL of 5 percent glucose in distilled water yields therapeutic levels for 14 hours. Urinary excretion ranges from 4.9 to 30.3 percent (mean: 13.8).
The biological half-life, after oral, intramuscular or intravenous administration is 5.4 ± 1.0 hours.
Hemodialysis and peritoneal dialysis do not effectively remove lincomycin from the blood.

INDICATIONS AND USAGE

LINCOCIN preparations (lincomycin) are indicated in the treatment of serious infections due to susceptible strains of streptococci, pneumococci, and staphylococci. Its use should be reserved for penicillin-allergic patients or other patients for whom, in the judgment of the physician, a penicillin is inappropriate. Because of the risk of colitis, as described in the WARNING box, before selecting lincomycin the physician should consider the nature of the infection and the suitability of less toxic alternatives (eg, erythromycin).
Lincomycin has been demonstrated to be effective in the treatment of staphylococcal infections resistant to other antibiotics and susceptible to lincomycin. Staphylococcal strains resistant to LINCOCIN have been recovered; culture and susceptibility studies should be done in conjunction with therapy with LINCOCIN. In the case of macrolides, partial but not complete cross resistance may occur (see **Microbiology**). The drug may be administered concomitantly with other antimicrobial agents when indicated.

CONTRAINDICATIONS

This drug is contraindicated in patients previously found to be hypersensitive to lincomycin or clindamycin. It is not indicated in the treatment of minor bacterial infections or viral infections.

WARNINGS

(See WARNING box). Studies indicate a toxin(s) produced by *Clostridia* is one primary cause of antibiotic associated colitis.[1–5] Mild cases of colitis may respond to drug discontinuance alone. Moderate to severe cases should be managed promptly with fluid, electrolyte and protein supplementation as indicated. Vancomycin has been found to be effective in the treatment of antibiotic associated pseudomembranous colitis produced by *Clostridium difficile*. The usual adult dosage is 500 milligrams to 2 grams of vancomycin orally per day in three to four divided doses administered for 7 to 10 days. Cholestyramine or colestipol resins bind vancomycin *in vitro*. If both a resin and vancomycin are to be administered concurrently, it may be advisable to separate the time of administration of each drug. Systemic corticoids and corticoid retention enemas may help relieve the colitis. Other causes of colitis should also be considered.
A careful inquiry should be made concerning previous sensitivities to drugs and other allergens.
Usage in Pregnancy—Safety for use in pregnancy has not been established.
Usage in Newborn—Until further clinical experience is obtained, LINCOCIN preparations (lincomycin) are not indicated in the newborn.
Nursing Mothers—LINCOCIN has been reported to appear in breast milk in ranges of 0.5 to 2.4 mcg/mL.
LINCOCIN Sterile Solution contains benzyl alcohol which has been associated with a fatal gasping syndrome in infants.

1. Bailey, WR, Scott, EG, *Diagnostic Microbiology* CV Mosby Company, St. Louis, 1978.
2. Bartlett, JG, et al, "Clindamycin-associated Colitis due to a Toxin-producing Species of *Clostridium* in Hamsters" *J. Inf. Dis.* **136**(5): 701–705, (November) 1977.
3. Larson, HE, Price, AB, "Pseudomembranous Colitis: Presence of Clostridial Toxin," *Lancet*, 1312–1314 (December) 24 and 31, 1977.
4. Lusk, RH, et al, "Clindamycin-Induced Enterocolitis in Hamsters", *J. Inf. Dis.* **137**(4): 464–474 (April) 1978.
5. "Antibiotic-associated Colitis: A Progress Report", *British Med. J.* **1**:669–671 (March 18) 1978.

PRECAUTIONS

Review of experience to date suggests that a subgroup of older patients with associated severe illness may tolerate diarrhea less well. When LINCOCIN preparations (lincomycin) are indicated in these patients, they should be carefully monitored for change in bowel frequency.
LINCOCIN should be prescribed with caution in individuals with a history of gastrointestinal disease, particularly colitis.
LINCOCIN, like any drug, should be used with caution in patients with a history of asthma or significant allergies.
The use of antibiotics occasionally results in overgrowth of nonsusceptible organisms—particularly yeasts. Should superinfections occur, appropriate measures should be taken. When patients with pre-existing monilial infections require therapy with LINCOCIN, concomitant antimonilial treatment should be given.
During prolonged therapy with LINCOCIN, periodic liver and renal function studies and blood counts should be performed.
Since adequate data are not yet available in patients with pre-existing liver disease, its use in such patients is not recommended at this time unless special clinical circumstances so indicate.
Lincomycin has been shown to have neuromuscular blocking properties that may enhance the action of other neuromuscular blocking agents. Therefore, it should be used with caution in patients receiving such agents.
Indicated surgical procedures should be performed in conjunction with antibiotic therapy.

ADVERSE REACTIONS

Gastrointestinal—Glossitis, stomatitis, nausea, vomiting. Persistent diarrhea, enterocolitis and pruritus ani. (See **Warning** box)
Hematopoietic: Neutropenia, leukopenia, agranulocytosis and thrombocytopenic purpura have been reported. There have been rare reports of aplastic anemia and pancytopenia in which LINCOCIN preparations (lincomycin hydrochloride) could not be ruled out as the causative agent.
Hypersensitivity Reactions—Hypersensitivity reactions such as angioneurotic edema, serum sickness and anaphylaxis have been reported, some of these in patients known to be sensitive to penicillin. Rare instances of erythema multiforme, some resembling Stevens-Johnson syndrome, have been associated with LINCOCIN. If an allergic reaction should occur, the drug should be discontinued and the usual agents (epinephrine, corticosteroids, antihistamines) should be available for emergency treatment.
Skin and Mucous Membranes—Skin rashes, urticaria and vaginitis and rare instances of exfoliative and vesiculobullous dermatitis have been reported.
Liver—Although no direct relationship of LINCOCIN to liver dysfunction has been established, jaundice and abnormal liver function tests (particularly elevations of serum transaminase) have been observed in a few instances.
Renal—Although no direct relationship of lincomycin to renal damage has been established, renal dysfunction as evidenced by azotemia, oliguria, and/or proteinuria has been observed in rare instances.
Cardiovascular—After too rapid intravenous administration, rare instances of cardiopulmonary arrest and hypotension have been reported. (See **Dosage and Administration**).
Special Senses—Tinnitus and vertigo have been reported occasionally.
Local Reactions—Patients have demonstrated excellent local tolerance to intramuscularly administered LINCOCIN. Reports of pain following injection have been infrequent. Intravenous administration of LINCOCIN in 250 to 500 mL of 5 percent glucose in distilled water or normal saline produced no local irritation or phlebitis.

DOSAGE AND ADMINISTRATION

If significant diarrhea occurs during therapy, this antibiotic should be discontinued. (See **Warning** box).
***Oral*—Adults:** *Serious infections*—500 mg 3 times per day (500 mg approximately every 8 hours). *More severe infections*—500 mg or more 4 times per day (500 mg or more approximately every 6 hours). **Children over 1 month of age:** *Serious infections*—30 mg/kg/day (15 mg/lb/day) divided into 3 or 4 equal doses. *More severe infections*—60 mg/kg/day (30 mg/lb/day) divided into 3 or 4 equal doses.
With β-hemolytic streptococcal infections, treatment should continue for at least 10 days to diminish the likelihood of subsequent rheumatic fever or glomerulonephritis.
NOTE: For optimal absorption it is recommended that nothing be given by mouth except water for a period of one to two hours before and after oral administration of LINCOCIN preparations (lincomycin).
***Intramuscular*—Adults:** *Serious infections*—600 mg (2 mL) intramuscularly every 24 hours. *More severe infections*—600 mg (2 mL) intramuscularly every 12 hours or more often.
Children over 1 month of age: *Serious infections*—one intramuscular injection of 10 mg/kg (5 mg/lb) every 24 hours. *More severe infections*—one intramuscular injection of 10 mg/kg (5 mg/lb) every 12 hours or more often.
***Intravenous*—Adults:** The intravenous dose will be determined by the severity of the infection. For serious infections doses of 600 mg of lincomycin (2 mL of LINCOCIN Sterile Solution) to 1 gram are given every 8-12 hours. For more severe infections these doses may have to be increased. In life-threatening situations daily intravenous doses of as much as 8 grams have been given. **Intranvenous doses are given on the basis of 1 gram of lincomycin diluted in not less than 100 mL of appropriate solution (see PHYSICAL COMPATIBILITIES) and infused over a period of not less than one hour.**

Dose	Vol. Diluent	Time
600 mg	100 mL	1 hr
1 gram	100 mL	1 hr
2 grams	200 mL	2 hr
3 grams	300 mL	3 hr
4 grams	400 mL	4 hr

These doses may be repeated as often as required to the limit of the maximum recommended daily dose of 8 grams of lincomycin.
Children over 1 month of age: 10-20 mg/kg/day (5-10 mg/lb/day) depending on the severity of the infection may be infused in divided doses as described above for adults.
NOTE: Severe cardiopulmonary reactions have occurred when this drug has been given at greater than the recommended concentration and rate.
Subconjunctival Injection—0.25 mL (75 mg) injected subconjunctivally will result in ocular fluid levels of antibiotic (lasting for at least 5 hours) with MIC's sufficient for most susceptible pathogens.
Patients with diminished renal function: *When therapy with LINCOCIN is required in individuals with severe impairment of renal function, an appropriate dose is 25 to 30% of that recommended for patients with normally functioning kidneys.*

HOW SUPPLIED

LINCOCIN Capsules (lincomycin) are available in the following strengths and package sizes:
250 mg Pediatric (blue):
Bottles of 24 *NDC 0009-0336-01*
500 mg (powder blue and dark blue):
Bottles of 24 *NDC 0009-0500-01*
Bottles of 100 *NDC 0009-0500-02*
LINCOCIN Capsules contain lincomycin hydrochloride equivalent to 250 mg or 500 mg of lincomycin.
LINCOCIN Sterile Solution is available in the following strength and package sizes:
300 mg
2 mL Syringe—NDC 0009-0600-01
2 mL Vials—NDC 0009-0555-01
10 mL Vials—NDC 0009-0555-02
Each mL of LINCOCIN Sterile Solution contains lincomycin hydrochloride equivalent to lincomycin 300 mg; also benzyl alcohol, 9.45 mg added as preservative.
Store at controlled room temperature 15°-30°C (59°-86°F).

ANIMAL PHARMACOLOGY

In vivo experimental animal studies demonstrated the effectiveness of LINCOCIN preparations (lincomycin) in protecting animals infected with *Streptococcus viridans*, *β-hemolytic Streptococcus*, *Staphylococcus aureus*, *Diplococcus pneumoniae* and *Leptospira pomona*. It was ineffective in *Klebsiella*, *Pasteurella*, *Pseudomonas*, *Salmonella* and *Shigella* infections.

CLINICAL STUDIES

Experience with 345 obstetrical patients receiving this drug revealed no ill effects related to pregnancy.
Physical Compatibilities:
Physically compatible for 24 hours at room temperature unless otherwise indicated.
Infusion Solutions
Dextrose in Water, 5% and 10%
Dextrose in Saline, 5% and 10%
Ringer's Solution
Sodium Lactate 1/6 Molar
Travert 10%—Electrolyte No. 1
Dextran in Saline 6% w/v
Vitamins in Infusion Solutions
B-Complex
B-Complex with Ascorbic Acid
Antibiotics in Infusion Solutions
Penicillin G Sodium (Satisfactory for 4 hours)
Cephalothin
Tetracycline HCl
Cephaloridine
Colistimethate (Satisfactory for 4 hours)
Ampicillin
Methicillin
Chloramphenicol
Polymyxin B Sulfate
Physically Incompatible with:
Novobiocin
Kanamycin
IT SHOULD BE EMPHASIZED THAT THE COMPATIBLE AND INCOMPATIBLE DETERMINATIONS ARE PHYSICAL OBSERVATIONS ONLY, NOT CHEMICAL DETERMINATIONS. ADEQUATE CLINICAL EVALUATION OF THE SAFETY AND EFFICACY OF THESE COMBINATIONS HAS NOT BEEN PERFORMED.
Code 810 174 006

LONITEN® ℞
brand of minoxidil tablets, USP

WARNINGS
LONITEN Tablets contain the powerful antihypertensive agent, minoxidil, which may produce serious adverse effects. It can cause pericardial effusion, occasion-

ally progressing to tamponade, and angina pectoris may be exacerbated. LONITEN should be reserved for hypertensive patients who do not respond adequately to maximum therapeutic doses of a diuretic and two other antihypertensive agents.
In experimental animals, minoxidil caused several kinds of myocardial lesions as well as other adverse cardiac effects (see Cardiac Lesions in Animals).
LONITEN must be administered under close supervision, usually concomitantly with therapeutic doses of a beta-adrenergic blocking agent to prevent tachycardia and increased myocardial workload. It must also usually be given with a diuretic, frequently one acting in the ascending limb of the loop of Henle, to prevent serious fluid accumulation. Patients with malignant hypertension and those already receiving guanethidine (see Warnings) should be hospitalized when LONITEN is first administered so that they can be monitored to avoid too rapid, or large orthostatic, decreases in blood pressure.

DESCRIPTION
LONITEN Tablets contain minoxidil, an antihypertensive peripheral vasodilator. Minoxidil occurs as a white or off-white, odorless, crystalline solid that is soluble in water to the extent of approximately 2 mg/ml; is readily soluble in propylene glycol or ethanol; and is almost insoluble in acetone, chloroform or ethyl acetate. The chemical name for minoxidil is 2,4-pyrimidinediamine, 6-(1-piperidinyl)-, 3-oxide (mw = 209.25).
LONITEN Tablets for oral administration contain either 2.5 mg or 10 mg of minoxidil. Inactive ingredients: cellulose, corn starch, lactose, magnesium stearate, silicon dioxide.

CLINICAL PHARMACOLOGY
1. General Pharmacologic Properties
Minoxidil is an orally effective direct acting peripheral vasodilator that reduces elevated systolic and diastolic blood pressure by decreasing peripheral vascular resistance. Microcirculatory blood flow in animals is enhanced or maintained in all systemic vascular beds. In man, forearm and renal vascular resistance decline; forearm blood flow increases while renal blood flow and glomerular filtration rate are preserved.
Because it causes peripheral vasodilation, minoxidil elicits a number of predictable reactions. Reduction of peripheral arteriolar resistance and the associated fall in blood pressure trigger sympathetic, vagal inhibitory, and renal homeostatic mechanisms, including an increase in renin secretion, that lead to increased cardiac rate and output and salt and water retention. These adverse effects can usually be minimized by concomitant administration of a diuretic and a beta-adrenergic blocking agent or other sympathetic nervous system suppressant.
Minoxidil does not interfere with vasomotor reflexes and therefore does not produce orthostatic hypotension. The drug does not enter the central nervous system in experimental animals in significant amounts, and it does not affect CNS function in man.
2. Effects on Blood Pressure and Target Organs
The extent and time-course of blood pressure reduction by minoxidil do not correspond closely to its concentration in plasma. After an effective single oral dose, blood pressure usually starts to decline within one-half hour, reaches a minimum between 2 and 3 hours and recovers at an arithmetically linear rate of about 30%/day. The total duration of effect is approximately 75 hours. When minoxidil is administered chronically, once or twice a day, the time required to achieve maximum effect on blood pressure with a given daily dose is inversely related to the size of the dose. Thus, maximum effect is achieved on 10 mg/day within 7 days, on 20 mg/day within 5 days, and on 40 mg/day within 3 days.
The blood pressure response to minoxidil is linearly related to the logarithm of the dose administered. The slope of this log-linear dose-response relationship is proportional to the extent of hypertension and approaches zero at a supine diastolic blood pressure of approximately 85 mmHg.
When used in severely hypertensive patients resistant to other therapy, frequently with an accompanying diuretic and beta-blocker, LONITEN Tablets (minoxidil) usually decreased the blood pressure and reversed encephalopathy and retinopathy."
3. Absorption and Metabolism
Minoxidil is at least 90% absorbed from the GI tract in experimental animals and man. Plasma levels of the parent drug reach maximum within the first hour and decline rapidly thereafter. The average plasma half-life in man is 4.2 hours. Approximately 90% of the administered drug is metabolized, predominantly by conjugation with glucuronic acid at the N-oxide position in the pyrimidine ring, but also by conversion to more polar products. Known metabolites exert much less pharmacologic effect than minoxidil itself; all are excreted principally in the urine. Minoxidil does not bind to plasma proteins, and its renal clearance corresponds to the glomerular filtration rate. In the absence of functional renal tissue, minoxidil and its metabolites can be removed by hemodialysis.
4. Cardiac Lesions in Animals
Minoxidil produced two types of cardiac lesions in non-primate species:
(a) Dog atrial lesion—
Daily oral doses of 0.5 mg/kg for several days to 1 month or longer produced a grossly visible hemorrhagic lesion of the right atrium of the dog. This lesion has not been seen in other species. Microscopic examination showed replacement of myocardial cells by proliferating fibroblasts and angioblasts; phagocytosis; and hemosiderin accumulation in macrophages.
(b) Papillary muscle lesion—
Short term treatment (about 3 days) in several species (dog, rat, minipig) produced necrosis of the papillary muscles, and, in some cases subendocardial areas of the left ventricle, lesions similar to those produced by other peripheral dilators and by beta-adrenergic receptor agonists such as isoproterenol and epinephrine. These are thought to result from myocardial ischemia resulting from reflex sympathetic or vagal withdrawal-induced tachycardia in combination with hypotension. These lesions were reduced in incidence and severity by beta-adrenergic receptor blockade.
(c) *Hemorrhagic lesions* were seen in many parts of the heart, mainly in the epicardium, endocardium, and walls of small coronary arteries and arterioles, after acute minoxidil treatment in dogs, and left atrial hemorrhagic lesions were seen in minipigs.
In addition to these lesions, longer term studies in rats, dogs, and monkeys showed cardiac hypertrophy and (in rats) cardiac dilation. In monkeys, hydrochlorothiazide partly reversed the increased heart weight, suggesting it may be related to fluid overload. In a one-year dog study, serosanguinous pericardial fluid was seen.
Autopsies of 79 patients who died from various causes and who had received minoxidil did not reveal right atrial or other hemorrhagic pathology of the kind seen in dogs. Instances of necrotic areas in the papillary muscles were seen, but these occurred in the presence of known pre-existing ischemic heart disease and did not appear different from, or more common than, lesions seen in patients never exposed to minoxidil. Studies to date cannot rule out the possibility that minoxidil can be associated with cardiac damage in humans.

INDICATIONS AND USAGE
Because of the potential for serious adverse effects, LONITEN Tablets (minoxidil) are indicated only in the treatment of hypertension that is symptomatic or associated with target organ damage and is not manageable with maximum therapeutic doses of a diuretic plus two other antihypertensive drugs. At the present time use in milder degrees of hypertension is not recommended because the benefit-risk relationship in such patients has not been defined.
LONITEN reduced supine diastolic blood pressure by 20 mm Hg or to 90 mm Hg or less in approximately 75% of patients, most of whom had hypertension that could not be controlled by other drugs.

CONTRAINDICATIONS
LONITEN Tablets (minoxidil) are contraindicated in pheochromocytoma, because minoxidil may stimulate secretion of catecholamines from the tumor through its antihypertensive action.

WARNINGS
1. Salt and Water Retention; Congestive Heart Failure—concomitant use of an adequate diuretic is required—LONITEN Tablets (minoxidil) must usually be administered concomitantly with a diuretic adequate to prevent fluid retention and possible congestive heart failure; a high ceiling (loop) diuretic is *almost always* required. Body weight should be monitored closely. If LONITEN is used without a diuretic, retention of several hundred milli-equivalents of salt and corresponding volumes of water can occur within a few days, leading to increased plasma and interstitial fluid volume and local or generalized edema. Diuretic treatment alone, or in combination with restricted salt intake, will usually minimize fluid retention, although reversible edema did develop in approximately 10% of nondialysis patients so treated. Ascites has also been reported. Diuretic effectiveness was limited mostly by disease-related impaired renal function. The condition of patients with preexisting congestive heart failure occasionally deteriorated in association with fluid retention although because of the fall in blood pressure (reduction of afterload), more than twice as many improved than worsened. Rarely, refractory fluid retention may require discontinuation of LONITEN. Provided that the patient is under close medical supervision, it may be possible to resolve refractory salt retention by discontinuing LONITEN for 1 or 2 days and then resuming treatment in conjunction with vigorous diuretic therapy.
2. Concomitant Treatment to Prevent Tachycardia is Usually Required—LONITEN increases the heart rate. Angina may worsen or appear for the first time during treatment with LONITEN, probably because of the increased oxygen demands associated with increased heart rate and cardiac output. The increase in rate and the occurrence of angina generally can be prevented by the concomitant administration of a beta-adrenergic blocking drug or other sympathetic nervous system suppressant. The ability of beta-adrenergic blocking agents to minimize papillary muscle lesions in animals is further reason to utilize such an agent concomitantly. Round-the-clock effectiveness of the sympathetic suppressant should be ensured.
3. Pericarditis, Pericardial Effusion and Tamponade—There have been reports of pericarditis occurring in association with the use of LONITEN. The relationship of this association to renal status is uncertain. Pericardial effusion, occasionally with tamponade, has been observed in about 3% of treated patients not on dialysis, especially those with inadequate or compromised renal function. Although in many cases, the pericardial effusion was associated with a connective tissue disease, the uremic syndrome, congestive heart failure, or marked fluid retention, there have been instances in which these potential causes of effusion were not present. Patients should be observed closely for any suggestion of a pericardial disorder, and echocardiographic studies should be carried out if suspicion arises. More vigorous diuretic therapy, dialysis, pericardiocentesis, or surgery may be required. If the effusion persists, withdrawal of LONITEN should be considered in light of other means of controlling the hypertension and the patient's clinical status.
4. *Interaction with Guanethidine:*
Although minoxidil does not itself cause orthostatic hypotension, its administration to patients already receiving guanethidine can result in profound orthostatic effects. If at all possible, guanethidine should be discontinued well before minoxidil is begun. Where this is not possible, minoxidil therapy should be started in the hospital and the patient should remain institutionalized until severe orthostatic effects are no longer present or the patient has learned to avoid activities that provoke them.
5. *Hazard of Rapid Control of Blood Pressure:*
In patients with very severe blood pressure elevation, too rapid control of blood pressure, especially with intravenous agents, can precipitate syncope, cerebrovascular accidents, myocardial infarction and ischemia of special sense organs with resulting decrease or loss of vision or hearing. Patients with compromised circulation or cryoglobulinemia may also suffer ischemic episodes of the affected organs. Although such events have not been unequivocally associated with minoxidil use, total experience is limited at present.
Any patient with malignant hypertension should have initial treatment with minoxidil carried out in a hospital setting, both to assure that blood pressure is falling and to assure that it is not falling more rapidly than intended.

PRECAUTIONS
1. General Precautions—(a) **Monitor fluid and electrolyte balance and body weight** (see **Warnings:** Salt and Water Retention).
(b) **Observe patients for signs and symptoms of pericardial effusion** (see **Warnings:** Pericardial Effusion and Tamponade).
(c) **Use after myocardial infarction—**LONITEN Tablets (minoxidil) have not been used in patients who have had a myocardial infarction within the preceding month. It is possible that a reduction of arterial pressure with LONITEN might further limit blood flow to the myocardium, although this might be compensated by decreased oxygen demand because of lower blood pressure.
(d) **Hypersensitivity—**Possible hypersensitivity to LONITEN, manifested as a skin rash, has been seen in less than 1% of patients; whether the drug should be discontinued when this occurs depends on treatment alternatives.
(e) **Renal failure or dialysis patients** may require smaller doses of LONITEN and should have close medical supervision to prevent exacerbation of renal failure or precipitation of cardiac failure.
2. Information for patient—The patient should be made fully aware of the importance of continuing all of his antihypertensive medications and of the nature of symptoms that would suggest fluid overload. A patient brochure has been prepared and is included with each package of LONITEN. The text of this brochure is reprinted at the end of the insert.
3. Laboratory tests
Those laboratory tests which are abnormal at the time of initiation of minoxidil therapy, such as urinalysis, renal function tests, EKG, chest x-ray, echocardiogram, etc., should be repeated at intervals to ascertain whether im-

Continued on next page

Information on these Upjohn products is based on labeling in effect June 1, 1992. Further information concerning these and other Upjohn products may be obtained by direct inquiry to Medical Information, The Upjohn Company, Kalamazoo, Michigan 49001.

Upjohn—Cont.

provement or deterioration is occuring under minoxidil therapy. Initially, such tests should be performed frequently, eg, 1–3 month intervals; later as stabilization occurs, at intervals of 6–12 months.

4. Drug Interactions
See "Interaction with guanethidine" under **WARNINGS**.

5. Carcinogenesis, Mutagenesis and Impairment of Fertility—Twenty-two month carcinogenicity studies in rats at doses 15 times the human dose did not provide evidence of tumorigenicity. The drug was not mutagenic in the Salmonella (Ames) test.
Rats receiving up to five times the human dose of minoxidil had a reduction in conception rate, possibly related to drug treatment. There was no evidence of increased fetal resorptions in rats but they did occur in rabbits.

6. Pregnancy-Teratogenic Effects—Pregnancy Category C. Minoxidil has been shown to reduce the conception rate in rats and to show evidence of increased fetal absorption in rabbits when administered at five times the human dose. There was no evidence of teratogenic effects in rats and rabbits. There are no adequate and well controlled studies in pregnant women. LONITEN should be used during pregnancy only if the potential benefit justifies the potential risk to the fetus.

7. Labor and delivery
The effects on labor and delivery are unknown.

8. Nursing Mothers—Minoxidil has been reported to be secreted in human milk. As a general rule, nursing should not be undertaken while a patient is on LONITEN.

9. Pediatric Use—Use in children has been limited to date, particularly in infants. The recommendations under **Dosage and Administration** can be considered only a rough guide at present and careful titration is essential.

10. Unapproved Use—Use of LONITEN Tablets, in any formulation, to promote hair growth is not an approved indication. Clinical trials are in progress and are designed to determine efficacy, dosage, duration of treatment, and actual side effects. Pending completion and analysis of these trials, efficacy, dose and duration of the therapy are not known. Because systemic absorption of topically applied drug may occur and is dependent on vehicle and/or method of use, extemporaneous topical formulations made from LONITEN should be considered to share in the full range of CONTRAINDICATIONS, WARNINGS, PRECAUTIONS, and ADVERSE REACTIONS listed in this insert. In addition, skin intolerance to drug and/or vehicle may occur.

ADVERSE REACTIONS

1. Salt and Water Retention (see **Warnings:** Concomitant Use of Adequate Diuretic is Required) —Temporary edema developed in 7% of patients who were not edematous at the start of therapy.

2. Pericarditis, Pericardial Effusion and **Tamponade** (see **Warnings**).

3. Dermatologic—Hypertrichosis—Elongation, thickening, and enhanced pigmentation of fine body hair are seen in about 80% of patients taking LONITEN Tablets (minoxidil). This develops within 3 to 6 weeks after starting therapy. It is usually first noticed on the temples, between the eyebrows, between the hairline and the eyebrows, or in the side-burn area of the upper lateral cheek, later extending to the back, arms, legs, and scalp. Upon discontinuation of LONITEN, new hair growth stops, but 1 to 6 months may be required for restoration to pretreatment appearance. No endocrine abnormalities have been found to explain the abnormal hair growth; thus, it is hypertrichosis without virilism. Hair growth is especially disturbing to children and women and such patients should be thoroughly informed about this effect before therapy with LONITEN is begun.
Allergic—Rashes have been reported, including rare reports of bullous eruptions, and Stevens-Johnson Syndrome.

4. Hematologic—Thrombocytopenia and leukopenia (WBC < 3000/mm^3) have rarely been reported.

5. Gastrointestinal—Nausea and/or vomiting has been reported. In clinical trials the incidence of nausea and vomiting associated with the underlying disease has shown a decrease from pretrial levels.

6. Miscellaneous—Breast tenderness—This developed in less than 1% of patients.

7. Altered Laboratory Findings—(a) ECG changes—changes in direction and magnitude of the ECG T-waves occur in approximately 60% of patients treated with LONITEN. In rare instances a large negative amplitude of the T-wave may encroach upon the S-T segment, but the S-T segment is not independently altered. These changes usually disappear with continuance of treatment and revert to the pretreatment state if LONITEN is discontinued. No symptoms have been associated with these changes, nor have there been alterations in blood cell counts or in plasma enzyme concentrations that would suggest myocardial damage. Long-term treatment of patients manifesting such changes has provided no evidence of deteriorating cardiac function. At present the changes appear to be nonspecific and without identifiable clinical significance. (b) Effects of hemodilution—hematocrit, hemoglobin and erythrocyte count usually fall about 7% initially and then recover to pretreatment levels. (c) Other—Alkaline phosphatase increased varyingly without other evidence of liver or bone abnormality. Serum creatinine increased an average of 6% and BUN slightly more, but later declined to pretreatment levels.

OVERDOSAGE

There have been only a few instances of deliberate or accidental overdosage with LONITEN Tablets (minoxidil). One patient recovered after taking 50 mg of minoxidil together with 500 mg of a barbiturate. When exaggerated hypotension is encountered, it is most likely to occur in association with residual sympathetic nervous system blockade from previous therapy (guanethidine-like effects or alpha-adrenergic blockage), which prevents the usual compensatory maintenance of blood pressure. Intravenous administration of normal saline will help to maintain blood pressure and facilitate urine formation in these patients. Sympathomimetic drugs such as norepinephrine or epinephrine should be avoided because of their excessive cardiac stimulating action. Phenylephrine, angiotensin II, vasopressin, and dopamine all reverse hypotension due to LONITEN, but should only be used if underperfusion of a vital organ is evident.
Radioimmunoassay can be performed to determine the concentration of minoxidil in the blood. At the maximum adult dosage of 100 mg/day, peak blood levels of 1641 ng/ml and 2441 ng/ml were observed in two patients, respectively. Due to patient-to-patient variation in blood levels, it is difficult to establish an overdosage warning level. In general, a substantial increase above 2000 ng/ml should be regarded as overdosage, unless the physician is aware that the patient has taken no more than the maximum dose.
Oral LD_{50} in rats has ranged from 1321–3492 mg/kg; in mice, 2456-2648 mg/kg.

DOSAGE AND ADMINISTRATION

Patients over 12 years of age: The recommended initial dosage of LONITEN Tablets (minoxidil) is 5 mg given as a single daily dose. Daily dosage can be increased to 10, 20 and then to 40 mg in single or divided doses if required for optimum blood pressure control. The effective dosage range is usually 10 to 40 mg per day. The maximum recommended dosage is 100 mg per day.

Patients under 12 years of age: The initial dosage is 0.2 mg/kg minoxidil as a single daily dose. The dosage may be increased in 50 to 100% increments until optimum blood pressure control is achieved. The effective dosage range is usually 0.25 to 1.0 mg/kg/day. The maximum recommended dosage is 50 mg daily. (see **9. Pediatric Use** under **Precautions**).

Dose frequency: The magnitude of within-day fluctuation of arterial pressure during therapy with LONITEN is directly proportional to the extent of pressure reduction. If supine diastolic pressure has been reduced less than 30 mmHg, the drug need be administered only once a day; if supine diastolic pressure has been reduced more than 30 mmHg, the daily dosage should be divided into two equal parts.

Frequency of dosage adjustment: Dosage must be titrated carefully according to individual response. Intervals between dosage adjustments normally should be at least 3 days since the full response to a given dose is not obtained for at least that amount of time. **Where a more rapid management of hypertension is required, dose adjustments can be made every 6 hours if the patient is carefully monitored.**

Concomitant therapy: Diuretic and beta-blocker or other sympathetic nervous system supressant.

Diuretics: LONITEN must be used in conjunction with a diuretic in patients relying on renal function for maintaining salt and water balance. Diuretics have been used at the following dosages when starting therapy with LONITEN: hydrochlorothiazide (50 mg, b.i.d.) or other thiazides at equieffective dosage; chlorthalidone (50 to 100 mg, once daily); furosemide (40 mg, b.i.d.). If excessive salt and water retention results in a weight gain of more than 5 pounds, diuretic therapy should be changed to furosemide; if the patient is already taking furosemide, dosage should be increased in accordance with the patient's requirements.

Beta-blocker or other sympathetic nervous system suppressants: When therapy with LONITEN is begun, the dosage of a beta-adrenergic receptor blocking drug should be the equivalent of 80 to 160 mg of propranolol per day in divided doses.
If beta-blockers are contraindicated, methyldopa (250 to 750 mg, b.i.d.) may be used instead. Methyldopa must be given for at least 24 hours before starting therapy with LONITEN because of the delay in the onset of methyldopa's action. Limited clinical experience indicates that clonidine may also be used to prevent tachycardia induced by LONITEN; the usual dosage is 0.1 to 0.2 mg twice daily.
Sympathetic nervous system suppressants may not completely prevent an increase in heart rate due to LONITEN but usually do prevent tachycardia. Typically, patients receiving a beta-blocker prior to initiation of therapy with LONITEN have a bradycardia and can be expected to have an increase in heart rate toward normal when LONITEN is added. When treatment with LONITEN and beta-blocker or other sympathetic nervous system suppressant are begun simultaneously, their opposing cardiac effects usually nullify each other, leading to little change in heart rate.

HOW SUPPLIED

LONITEN Tablets (minoxidil) are available as round, scored, white tablets. Dosage strengths are imprinted on one convex surface. The following strengths and container sizes are available:

Strength	Container and Size	NDC Number
2.5 mg	Unit of Use bottles of 100,	0009-0121-01
10 mg	Unit of Use bottles of 100,	0009-0137-01
	bottles of 500	0009-0137-02

Store at controlled room temperature 15°–30°C (59°–86°F).

Patient Information: LONITEN Tablets contain minoxidil, a medicine for the treatment of high blood pressure in the patient who has not been controlled or is experiencing unacceptable side effects with other medications. It must usually be taken with other medicines.
Be absolutely sure to take all of your medicines for high blood pressure according to your doctor's instructions. Do not stop taking LONITEN unless your doctor tells you to. Do not give any of your medicine to other people.
It is important that you look for the warning signals of certain undesired effects of LONITEN. Call your doctor if they occur. Your doctor will need to see you regularly while you are taking LONITEN. Be sure to keep all your appointments or to arrange for new ones if you must miss one.
Do not hesitate to call your doctor if any discomforts or problems occur.
The information here is intended to help you take LONITEN properly. It does not tell you all there is to know about LONITEN. There is a more technical leaflet that you may request from the pharmacist; you may need your doctor's help in understanding parts of that leaflet.

What is LONITEN?
LONITEN Tablets contain minoxidil which is a drug for lowering the blood pressure. It works by relaxing and enlarging certain small blood vessels so that blood flows through them more easily.

Why lower blood pressure?
Your doctor has prescribed LONITEN to lower your blood pressure and protect vital parts of your body. Uncontrolled blood pressure can cause stroke, heart failure, blindness, kidney failure, and heart attacks.
Most people with high blood pressure need to take medicines to treat it for their whole lives.

Who should take LONITEN?
There are many people with high blood pressure, but most of them do not need LONITEN. LONITEN is used ONLY when your doctor decides that:

1. your high blood pressure is severe;
2. your high blood pressure is causing symptoms or damage to vital organs; and
3. other medicines did not work well enough or had very disturbing side effects.

LONITEN should be taken only when a doctor prescribes it. Never give any of your LONITEN Tablets, or any other high blood pressure medicine, to a friend or relative.

Pregnancy: In some cases doctors may prescribe LONITEN for women who are pregnant or who are planning to have children. However, its safe use in pregnancy has not been established. Laboratory animals had a reduced ability to become pregnant and a reduced survival of offspring while taking LONITEN. If you are pregnant or are planning to become pregnant, be sure to tell your doctor.

How to take LONITEN.
Usually, your doctor will prescribe two other medicines along with LONITEN. These will help lower blood pressure and will help prevent undesired effects of LONITEN.
Often, when a medicine like LONITEN lowers blood pressure, your body tries to return the blood pressure to the original, higher level. It does this by holding on to water and salt (so there will be more fluid to pump) and by making your heart beat faster. To prevent this, your doctor will usually prescribe a water tablet to remove the extra salt and water from your body (a diuretic dye-u-RET-tic) and another medicine to slow your heart beat.
You must follow your doctor's instructions exactly, taking all the prescribed medicines, in the right amounts, each day. These medicines will help keep your blood pressure down. The water tablet and heart beat medicine will help prevent the undesired effects of LONITEN.
LONITEN Tablets come in two strengths (2 ½ milligrams and 10 milligrams) that are marked on each tablet. Pay close attention to the tablet markings to be sure you are taking the correct strength. Your doctor may prescribe half a tablet; the tablets are scored (partly cut on one side) so that you can easily break them.
When you first start taking LONITEN, your doctor may need to see you often in order to adjust your dosage. Take all your medicine according to the schedule prescribed by your

doctor. Do not skip any doses. **If you should forget a dose of LONITEN, wait until it is time for your next dose, then continue with your regular schedule. Remember: do not stop taking LONITEN,** or any of your other high blood pressure medicines, without checking with your doctor. Make sure that any doctor treating or examining you knows that you are taking high blood pressure medicines, including LONITEN.

WARNING SIGNALS

Even if you take all your medicines correctly, LONITEN Tablets may cause undesired effects. Some of these are serious and you should be on the lookout for them. **If any of the following warning signals occur, you must call your doctor immediately:**

1. Increase in heart rate—You should measure your heart rate by counting your pulse rate **while you are resting.** If you have an increase of 20 beats or more a minute over your normal pulse, contact your doctor immediately. If you do not know how to take your pulse rate, ask your doctor. Also ask your doctor how often to check your pulse.

2. Rapid weight gain of more than 5 pounds—You should weigh yourself daily. If you quickly gain five or more pounds, or if there is any swelling or puffiness in the face, hands, ankles, or stomach area, this could be a sign that you are retaining body fluids. Your doctor may have to change your drugs or change the dose of your drugs. You may also need to reduce the amount of salt you eat. A smaller weight gain (2 to 3 pounds) often occurs when treatment is started. You may lose this extra weight with continued treatment.

3. Increased difficulty in breathing, especially when lying down. This too may be due to an increase of body fluids. It can also happen because your high blood pressure is getting worse. In either case, you might require treatment with other medicines.

4. New or worsening of pain in the chest, arm, or shoulder or signs of severe indigestion — These could be signs of serious heart problems.

5. Dizziness, lightheadedness or fainting — These can be signs of high blood pressure or they may be side effects from one of the medicines. Your doctor may need to change or adjust the dosage of the medicines you are taking.

OTHER UNDESIRED EFFECTS

LONITEN Tablets can cause other undesired effects such as nausea and/or vomiting that are annoying but not dangerous. Do not stop taking the drug because of these other undesired effects without talking to your doctor.

Hair growth: About 8 out of every 10 patients who have taken LONITEN noticed that fine **body hair grew darker or longer** on certain parts of the body. This happened about three to six weeks after beginning treatment. The hair may first be noticed on the forehead and temples, between the eyebrows, or on the upper part of the cheeks. Later, hair may grow on the back, arms, legs, or scalp. Although hair growth may not be noticeable to some patients, it often is bothersome in women and children. **Unwanted hair can be controlled with a hair remover or by shaving.** The extra hair is not permanent, it disappears within 1 to 6 months of stopping LONITEN. Nevertheless, **you should not stop taking LONITEN without first talking to your doctor.**

A few patients have developed a rash or breast tenderness while taking LONITEN Tablets (minoxidil), but this is unusual.

Code 810 384 212

Shown in Product Identification Section, page 434

MEDROL® ℞
brand of methylprednisolone tablets, USP

4 mg, 21's Dosepak	NSN 6505-01-131-5619 (M)
4 mg, 100's	NSN 6505-01-134-6647 (M)
4 mg, 500's	NSN 6505-00-050-3068

DESCRIPTION

MEDROL Tablets contain methylprednisolone which is a glucocorticoid. Glucocorticoids are adrenocortical steroids, both naturally occurring and synthetic, which are readily absorbed from the gastrointestinal tract. Methylprednisolone occurs as a white to practically white, odorless, crystalline powder. It is sparingly soluble in alcohol, in dioxane, and in methanol, slightly soluble in acetone, and in chloroform, and very slightly soluble in ether. It is practically insoluble in water.

The chemical name for methylprednisolone is pregna-1, 4-diene-3, 20-dione,11, 17, 21-trihydroxy-6-methyl-,(6α, 11β)- and the molecular weight is 374.48.

Each MEDROL tablet for oral administration contains 2 mg, 4 mg, 8 mg, 16 mg, 24 mg, or 32 mg of methylprednisolone.

Inactive ingredients:

2 mg	4 and 16 mg
Calcium Stearate	Calcium Stearate
Corn Starch	Corn Starch
Erythrosine Sodium	Lactose
Lactose	Mineral Oil
Mineral Oil	Sorbic Acid
Sorbic Acid	Sucrose
Sucrose	

8 and 32 mg	24 mg
Calcium Stearate	Calcium Stearate
Corn Starch	Corn Starch
F D & C Yellow No. 6	F D & C Yellow No. 5
Lactose	Lactose
Mineral Oil	Mineral Oil
Sorbic Acid	Sorbic Acid
Sucrose	Sucrose

ACTIONS

Naturally occurring glucocorticoids (hydrocortisone and cortisone), which also have salt-retaining properties, are used as replacement therapy in adrenocortical deficiency states. Their synthetic analogs are primarily used for their potent anti-inflammatory effects in disorders of many organ systems.

Glucocorticoids cause profound and varied metabolic effects. In addition, they modify the body's immune responses to diverse stimuli.

INDICATIONS

MEDROL Tablets (methylprednisolone) are indicated in the following conditions:

1. Endocrine Disorders
Primary or secondary adrenocortical insufficiency (hydrocortisone or cortisone is the first choice; synthetic analogs may be used in conjunction with mineralocorticoids where applicable; in infancy mineralocorticoid supplementation is of particular importance).
Congenital adrenal hyperplasia
Nonsuppurative thyroiditis
Hypercalcemia associated with cancer

2. Rheumatic Disorders
As adjunctive therapy for short-term administration (to tide the patient over an acute episode or exacerbation) in:
Psoriatic arthritis
Rheumatoid arthritis, including juvenile rheumatoid arthritis (selected cases may require low-dose maintenance therapy)
Ankylosing spondylitis
Acute and subacute bursitis
Acute nonspecific tenosynovitis
Acute gouty arthritis
Post-traumatic osteoarthritis
Synovitis of osteoarthritis
Epicondylitis

3. Collagen Diseases
During an exacerbation or as maintenance therapy in selected cases of:
Systemic lupus erythematosus
Acute rheumatic carditis
Systemic dermatomyositis (polymyositis)

4. Dermatologic Diseases
Pemphigus
Bullous dermatitis herpetiformis
Severe erythema multiforme (Stevens-Johnson syndrome)
Exfoliative dermatitis
Mycosis fungoides
Severe psoriasis
Severe seborrheic dermatitis

5. Allergic States
Control of severe or incapacitating allergic conditions intractable to adequate trials of conventional treatment:
Seasonal or perennial allergic rhinitis
Serum sickness
Bronchial asthma
Drug hypersensitivity reactions
Contact dermatitis
Atopic dermatitis

6. Ophthalmic Diseases
Severe acute and chronic allergic and inflammatory processes involving the eye and its adnexa such as:
Allergic corneal marginal ulcers
Herpes zoster ophthalmicus
Anterior segment inflammation
Diffuse posterior uveitis and choroiditis
Sympathetic ophthalmia
Allergic conjunctivitis
Keratitis
Chorioretinitis
Optic neuritis
Iritis and iridocyclitis

7. Respiratory Diseases
Symptomatic sarcoidosis
Loeffler's syndrome not manageable by other means
Berylliosis
Fulminating or disseminated pulmonary tuberculosis when used concurrently with appropriate antituberculous chemotherapy
Aspiration pneumonitis

8. Hematologic Disorders
Idiopathic thrombocytopenic purpura in adults
Secondary thrombocytopenia in adults
Acquired (autoimmune) hemolytic anemia
Erythroblastopenia (RBC anemia)
Congenital (erythroid) hypoplastic anemia

9. Neoplastic Diseases
For palliative management of:
Leukemias and lymphomas in adults
Acute leukemia of childhood

10. Edematous States
To induce a diuresis or remission of proteinuria in the nephrotic syndrome, without uremia, of the idiopathic type or that due to lupus erythematosus.

11. Gastrointestinal diseases
To tide the patient over a critical period of the disease in:
Ulcerative colitis
Regional enteritis

12. Nervous System
Acute exacerbations of multiple sclerosis

13. Miscellaneous
Tuberculous meningitis with subarachnoid block or impending block when used concurrently with appropriate antituberculous chemotherapy.
Trichinosis with neurologic or myocardial involvement

CONTRAINDICATIONS

Systemic fungal infections and known hypersensitivity to components.

WARNINGS

In patients on corticosteroid therapy subjected to unusual stress, increased dosage of rapidly acting corticosteroids before, during, and after the stressful situation is indicated.

Corticosteroids may mask some signs of infection and new infections may appear during their use. There may be decreased resistance and inability to localize infection when corticosteroids are used.

Prolonged use of corticosteroids may produce posterior subcapsular cataracts, glaucoma with possible damage to the optic nerves, and may enhance the establishment of secondary ocular infections due to fungi or viruses.

Usage in pregnancy: Since adequate human reproduction studies have not been done with corticosteroids, the use of these drugs in pregnancy, nursing mothers or women of childbearing potential requires that the possible benefits of the drug be weighed against the potential hazards to the mother and embryo or fetus. Infants born of mothers who have received substantial doses of corticosteroids during pregnancy should be carefully observed for signs of hypoadrenalism.

Average and large doses of hydrocortisone or cortisone can cause elevation of blood pressure, salt and water retention, and increased excretion of potassium. These effects are less likely to occur with the synthetic derivatives except when used in large doses. Dietary salt restriction and potassium supplementation may be necessary. All corticosteroids increase calcium excretion.

While on corticosteroid therapy patients should not be vaccinated against smallpox. Other immunization procedures should not be undertaken in patients who are on corticosteroids, especially on high dose, because of possible hazards of neurological complications and a lack of antibody response. The use of MEDROL Tablets (methylprednisolone) in active tuberculosis should be restricted to those cases of fulminating or disseminated tuberculosis in which the corticosteroid is used for the management of the disease in conjunction with an appropriate antituberculous regimen.

If corticosteroids are indicated in patients with latent tuberculosis or tuberculin reactivity, close observation is necessary as reactivation of the disease may occur. During prolonged corticosteroid therapy, these patients should receive chemoprophylaxis.

Children who are on immunosuppressant drugs are more susceptible to infections than healthy children. Chickenpox and measles, for example, can have a more serious or even fatal course in children on immunosuppressant corticoste-

Continued on next page

Information on these Upjohn products is based on labeling in effect June 1, 1992. Further information concerning these and other Upjohn products may be obtained by direct inquiry to Medical Information, The Upjohn Company, Kalamazoo, Michigan 49001.

Upjohn—Cont.

roids. In such children, or in adults who have not had these diseases, particular care should be taken to avoid exposure. If exposed, therapy with varicella zoster immune globulin (VZIG) or pooled intravenous immunoglobin (IVIG), as appropriate, may be indicated. If chickenpox develops, treatment with antiviral agents may be considered.

PRECAUTIONS

Drug-induced secondary adrenocortical insufficiency may be minimized by gradual reduction of dosage. This type of relative insufficiency may persist for months after discontinuation of therapy; therefore, in any situation of stress occurring during that period, hormone therapy should be reinstituted. Since mineralocorticoid secretion may be impaired, salt and/ or a mineralocorticoid should be administered concurrently. There is an enhanced effect of corticosteroids on patients with hypothyroidism and in those with cirrhosis.

Corticosteroids should be used cautiously in patients with ocular herpes simplex because of possible corneal perforation.

The lowest possible dose of corticosteroid should be used to control the condition under treatment, and when reduction in dosage is possible, the reduction should be gradual.

Psychic derangements may appear when corticosteroids are used, ranging from euphoria, insomnia, mood swings, personality changes and severe depression, to frank psychotic manifestations. Also, existing emotional instability or psychotic tendencies may be aggravated by corticosteroids.

Aspirin should be used cautiously in conjunction with corticosteroids in hypoprothrombinemia.

Steroids should be used with caution in nonspecific ulcerative colitis, if there is a probability of impending perforation, abscess or other pyogenic infection; diverticulitis; fresh intestinal anastomoses; active or latent peptic ulcer; renal insufficiency; hypertension; osteoporosis; and myasthenia gravis.

Growth and development of infants and children on prolonged corticosteroid therapy should be carefully observed. Although controlled clinical trials have shown corticosteroids to be effective in speeding the resolution of acute exacerbations of multiple sclerosis, they do not show that corticosteroids affect the ultimate outcome or natural history of the disease. The studies do show that relatively high doses of corticosteroids are necessary to demonstrate a significant effect. (See **Dosage and Administration**)

Since complications of treatment with glucocorticoids are dependent on the size of the dose and the duration of treatment, a risk/benefit decision must be made in each individual case as to dose and duration of treatment and as to whether daily or intermittent therapy should be used.

The 24 mg tablet contains FD&C Yellow No. 5 (tartrazine) which may cause allergic-type reactions (including bronchial asthma) in certain susceptible individuals. Although the overall incidence of FD&C Yellow No. 5 (tartrazine) sensitivity in the general population is low, it is frequently seen in patients who also have aspirin hypersensitivity.

Convulsions have been reported with concurrent use of methylprednisolone and cyclosporin. Since concurrent use of these agents results in a mutual inhibition of metabolism, it is possible that adverse events associated with the individual use of either drug may be more apt to occur.

Information for the Patient

Patients who are on immunosuppressant doses of corticosteroids should be warned to avoid exposure to chickenpox or measles and, if exposed, to obtain medical care.

ADVERSE REACTIONS

Fluid and Electrolyte Disturbances
- Sodium retention
- Fluid retention
- Congestive heart failure in susceptible patients
- Potassium loss
- Hypokalemic alkalosis
- Hypertension

Musculoskeletal
- Muscle weakness
- Steroid myopathy
- Loss of muscle mass
- Osteoporosis
- Vertebral compression fractures
- Aseptic necrosis of femoral and humeral heads
- Pathologic fracture of long bones

Gastrointestinal
- Peptic ulcer with possible perforation and hemorrhage
- Pancreatitis
- Abdominal distention
- Ulcerative esophagitis

Dermatologic
- Impaired wound healing
- Thin fragile skin
- Petechiae and ecchymoses
- Facial erythema
- Increased sweating
- May suppress reactions to skin tests

Neurological
- Increased intracranial pressure with papilledema (pseudotumor cerebri) usually after treatment
- Convulsions
- Vertigo
- Headache

Endocrine
- Development of Cushingoid state
- Suppression of growth in children
- Secondary adrenocortical and pituitary unresponsiveness, particularly in times of stress, as in trauma, surgery or illness.
- Menstrual irregularities
- Decreased carbohydrate tolerance
- Manifestations of latent diabetes mellitus
- Increased requirements for insulin or oral hypoglycemic agents in diabetics

Ophthalmic
- Posterior subcapsular cataracts
- Increased intraocular pressure
- Glaucoma
- Exophthalmos

Metabolic
- Negative nitrogen balance due to protein catabolism

The following additional reactions have been reported following oral as well as parenteral therapy: Urticaria and other allergic, anaphylactic or hypersensitivity reactions.

DOSAGE AND ADMINISTRATION

The initial dosage of MEDROL Tablets (methylprednisolone) may vary from 4 mg to 48 mg per day depending on the specific disease entity being treated. In situations of less severity lower doses will generally suffice while in selected patients higher initial doses may be required. The initial dosage should be maintained or adjusted until a satisfactory response is noted. If after a reasonable period of time there is a lack of satisfactory clinical response, MEDROL should be discontinued and the patient transferred to other appropriate therapy. **IT SHOULD BE EMPHASIZED THAT DOSAGE REQUIREMENTS ARE VARIABLE AND MUST BE INDIVIDUALIZED ON THE BASIS OF THE DISEASE UNDER TREATMENT AND THE RESPONSE OF THE PATIENT.** After a favorable response is noted, the proper maintenance dosage should be determined by decreasing the initial drug dosage in small decrements at appropriate time intervals until the lowest dosage which will maintain an adequate clinical response is reached. It should be kept in mind that constant monitoring is needed in regard to drug dosage. Included in the situations which may make dosage adjustments necessary are changes in clinical status secondary to remissions or exacerbations in the disease process, the patient's individual drug responsiveness, and the effect of patient exposure to stressful situations not directly related to the disease entity under treatment; in this latter situation it may be necessary to increase the dosage of MEDROL for a period of time consistent with the patient's condition. If after long-term therapy the drug is to be stopped, it is recommended that it be withdrawn gradually rather than abruptly.

Multiple Sclerosis

In treatment of acute exacerbations of multiple sclerosis daily doses of 200 mg of prednisolone for a week followed by 80 mg every other day for 1 month have been shown to be effective (4 mg of methylprednisolone is equivalent to 5 mg of prednisolone).

ADT® (Alternate Day Therapy)

Alternate day therapy is a corticosteroid dosing regimen in which twice the usual daily dose of corticoid is administered every other morning. The purpose of this mode of therapy is to provide the patient requiring long-term pharmacologic dose treatment with the beneficial effects of corticoids while minimizing certain undesirable effects, including pituitary-adrenal suppression, the Cushingoid state, corticoid withdrawal symptoms, and growth suppression in children.

The rationale for this treatment schedule is based on two major premises: (a) the anti-inflammatory or therapeutic effect of corticoids persists longer than their physical presence and metabolic effects and (b) administration of the corticosteroid every other morning allows for re-establishment of more nearly normal hypothalamic-pituitary-adrenal (HPA) activity on the off-steroid day.

A brief review of the HPA physiology may be helpful in understanding this rationale. Acting primarily through the hypothalamus a fall in free cortisol stimulates the pituitary gland to produce increasing amounts of corticotropin (ACTH) while a rise in free cortisol inhibits ACTH secretion. Normally the HPA system is characterized by diurnal (circadian) rhythm. Serum levels of ACTH rise from a low point about 10 pm to a peak level about 6 am. Increasing levels of ACTH stimulate adrenal cortical activity resulting in a rise in plasma cortisol with maximal levels occurring between 2 am and 8 am. This rise in cortisol dampens ACTH production and in turn adrenal cortical activity. There is a gradual fall in plasma corticoids during the day with lowest levels occurring about midnight.

The diurnal rhythm of the HPA axis is lost in Cushing's disease, a syndrome of adrenal cortical hyperfunction characterized by obesity with centripetal fat distribution, thinning of the skin with easy bruisability, muscle wasting with weakness, hypertension, latent diabetes, osteoporosis, electrolyte imbalance, etc. The same clinical findings of hyperadrenocorticism may be noted during long-term pharmacologic dose corticoid therapy administered in conventional daily divided doses. It would appear, then, that a disturbance in the diurnal cycle with maintenance of elevated corticoid values during the night may play a significant role in the development of undesirable corticoid effects. Escape from these constantly elevated plasma levels for even short periods of time may be instrumental in protecting against undesirable pharmacologic effects.

During conventional pharmacologic dose corticosteroid therapy, ACTH production is inhibited with subsequent suppression of cortisol production by the adrenal cortex. Recovery time for normal HPA activity is variable depending upon the dose and duration of treatment. During this time the patient is vulnerable to any stressful situation. Although it has been shown that there is considerably less adrenal suppression following a single morning dose of prednisolone (10 mg) as opposed to a quarter of that dose administered every 6 hours, there is evidence that some suppressive effect on adrenal activity may be carried over into the following day when pharmacologic doses are used. Further, it has been shown that a single dose of certain corticosteroids will produce adrenal cortical suppression for two or more days. Other corticoids, including methylprednisolone, hydrocortisone, prednisone, and prednisolone, are considered to be short acting (producing adrenal cortical suppression for $1\frac{1}{4}$ to $1\frac{1}{2}$ days following a single dose) and thus are recommended for alternate day therapy.

The following should be kept in mind when considering alternate day therapy:

1) Basic principles and indications for corticosteroid therapy should apply. The benefits of ADT should not encourage the indiscriminate use of steroids.

2) ADT is a therapeutic technique primarily designed for patients in whom long-term pharmacologic corticoid therapy is anticipated.

3) In less severe disease processes in which corticoid therapy is indicated, it may be possible to initiate treatment with ADT. More severe disease states usually will require daily divided high dose therapy for initial control of the disease process. The initial suppressive dose level should be continued until satisfactory clinical response is obtained, usually four to ten days in the case of many allergic and collagen diseases. It is important to keep the period of initial suppressive dose as brief as possible particularly when subsequent use of alternate day therapy is intended.

Once control has been established, two courses are available: (a) change to ADT and then gradually reduce the amount of corticoid given every other day *or* (b) following control of the disease process reduce the daily dose of corticoid to the lowest effective level as rapidly as possible and then change over to an alternate day schedule. Theoretically, course (a) may be preferable.

4) Because of the advantages of ADT, it may be desirable to try patients on this form of therapy who have been on daily corticoids for long periods of time (eg, patients with rheumatoid arthritis). Since these patients may already have a suppressed HPA axis, establishing them on ADT may be difficult and not always successful. However, it is recommended that regular attempts be made to change them over. It may be helpful to triple or even quadruple the daily maintenance dose and administer this every other day rather than just doubling the daily dose if difficulty is encountered. Once the patient is again controlled, an attempt should be made to reduce this dose to a minimum.

5) As indicated above, certain corticosteroids, because of their prolonged suppressive effect on adrenal activity, are not recommended for alternate day therapy (eg, dexamethasone and betamethasone).

6) The maximal activity of the adrenal cortex is between 2 am and 8 am, and it is minimal between 4 pm and midnight. Exogenous corticosteroids suppress adrenocortical activity the least, when given at the time of maximal activity (am).

7) In using ADT it is important, as in all therapeutic situations, to individualize and tailor the therapy to each patient. Complete control of symptoms will not be possible in all patients. An explanation of the benefits of ADT will help the patient to understand and tolerate the possible flare-up in symptoms which may occur in the latter part of the off-steroid day. Other symptomatic therapy may be added or increased at this time if needed.

8) In the event of an acute flare-up of the disease process, it may be necessary to return to a full suppressive daily divided corticoid dose for control. Once control is again established alternate day therapy may be reinstituted.

9) Although many of the undesirable features of corticosteroid therapy can be minimized by ADT, as in any therapeutic situation, the physician must carefully weigh the benefit-risk ratio for each patient in whom corticoid therapy is being considered.

HOW SUPPLIED

MEDROL Tablets (methylprednisolone), elliptical and scored, are available in the following strengths and sizes:

2 mg (pink)
Bottles of 100   NDC 0009-0049-02
4 mg (white)
Bottles of 30   NDC 0009-0056-01
Bottles of 100   NDC 0009-0056-02
Bottles of 500   NDC 0009-0056-03
Unit Dose
Package (100)   NDC 0009-0056-05
Dosepak ™ Unit of Use
(21 tablets)   NDC 0009-0056-04
8 mg (peach)
Bottles of 25   NDC 0009-0022-01
16 mg (white)
Bottles of 50   NDC 0009-0073-01
ADT Pak ®
(14 tablets) Unit of Use
     NDC 0009-0073-02
24 mg (yellow)
Bottles of 25   NDC 0009-0155-01
32 mg (peach)
Bottles of 25   NDC 0009-0176-01

Store at controlled room temperature 15°–30°C (59°–86°F).
Code 810 487 613

Shown in Product Identification Section, page 434

MICRONASE®   ℞
brand of glyburide tablets
(1.25, 2.5, and 5 mg)

2.5 mg, 100's	NSN 6505-01-216-6289 (M & VA)
5 mg, 30's	NSN 6505-01-259-7117 (VA)
5 mg, 60's	NSN 6505-01-263-4532 (VA)
5 mg, 90's	NSN 6505-01-263-4533 (VA)
5 mg, 100's	NSN 6505-01-204-5417 (M & VA)
5 mg, 100's, Unit Dose	NSN 6505-01-243-4103 (VA)
5 mg, 500's	NSN 6505-01-216-6288 (M & VA)
5 mg, 1000's	NSN 6505-01-219-7968 (M & VA)

DESCRIPTION

MICRONASE Tablets contain glyburide, which is an oral blood-glucose-lowering drug of the sulfonylurea class. Glyburide is a white, crystalline compound, formulated as MICRONASE Tablets of 1.25, 2.5, and 5 mg strengths for oral administration. Inactive ingredients: colloidal silicon dioxide, dibasic calcium phosphate, magnesium stearate, microcrystalline cellulose, sodium alginate, talc. In addition, the **2.5 mg** contains aluminum oxide and FD&C red no. 40 and the **5 mg** contains aluminum oxide and FD&C blue no. 1. The chemical name for glyburide is 1-[[p-[2-(5-chloro-o-anisamido)ethyl]phenyl]-sulfonyl]-3-cyclohexylurea and the molecular weight is 493.99.

CLINICAL PHARMACOLOGY
Actions

Glyburide appears to lower the blood glucose acutely by stimulating the release of insulin from the pancreas, an effect dependent upon functioning beta cells in the pancreatic islets. The mechanism by which glyburide lowers blood glucose during long-term administration has not been clearly established. With chronic administration in Type II diabetic patients, the blood glucose lowering effect persists despite a gradual decline in the insulin secretory response to the drug. Extrapancreatic effects may be involved in the mechanism of action of oral sulfonylurea hypoglycemic drugs.

Some patients who are initially responsive to oral hypoglycemic drugs, including MICRONASE Tablets (glyburide), may become unresponsive or poorly responsive over time. Alternatively, MICRONASE may be effective in some patients who have become unresponsive to one or more other sulfonylurea drugs.

In addition to its blood glucose lowering actions, glyburide produces a mild diuresis by enhancement of renal free water clearance. Disulfiram-like reactions have very rarely been reported in patients treated with MICRONASE Tablets.

Pharmacokinetics

Single dose studies with MICRONASE Tablets in normal subjects demonstrate significant absorption of glyburide within one hour, peak drug levels at about four hours, and low but detectable levels at twenty-four hours. Mean serum levels of glyburide, as reflected by areas under the serum concentration-time curve, increase in proportion to corresponding increases in dose. Multiple dose studies with MICRONASE in diabetic patients demonstrate drug level concentration-time curves similar to single dose studies, indicating no buildup of drug in tissue depots. The decrease of glyburide in the serum of normal healthy individuals is biphasic; the terminal half-life is about 10 hours. In single dose studies in fasting normal subjects, the degree and duration of blood glucose lowering is proportional to the dose administered and to the area under the drug level concentration-time curve. The blood glucose lowering effect persists

for 24 hours following single morning doses in nonfasting diabetic patients. Under conditions of repeated administration in diabetic patients, however, there is no reliable correlation between blood drug levels and fasting blood glucose levels. A one year study of diabetic patients treated with MICRONASE showed no reliable correlation between administered dose and serum drug level.

The major metabolite of glyburide is the 4-trans-hydroxy derivative. A second metabolite, the 3-cis-hydroxy derivative, also occurs. These metabolites probably contribute no significant hypoglycemic action in humans since they are only weakly active (1/400th and 1/40th as active, respectively, as glyburide) in rabbits.

Glyburide is excreted as metabolites in the bile and urine, approximately 50% by each route. This dual excretory pathway is qualitatively different from that of other sulfonylureas, which are excreted primarily in the urine.

Sulfonylurea drugs are extensively bound to serum proteins. Displacement from protein binding sites by other drugs may lead to enhanced hypoglycemic action. *In vitro*, the protein binding exhibited by glyburide is predominantly non-ionic, whereas that of other sulfonylureas (chlorpropamide, tolbutamide, tolazamide) is predominantly ionic. Acidic drugs such as phenylbutazone, warfarin, and salicylates displace the ionic-binding sulfonylureas from serum proteins to a far greater extent than the non-ionic binding glyburide. It has not been shown that this difference in protein binding will result in fewer drug-drug interactions with MICRONASE Tablets in clinical use.

INDICATIONS AND USAGE

MICRONASE Tablets (glyburide) are indicated as an adjunct to diet to lower the blood glucose in patients with non-insulin-dependent diabetes mellitus (type II) whose hyperglycemia cannot be satisfactorily controlled by diet alone.

In initiating treatment for non-insulin-dependent diabetes, diet should be emphasized as the primary form of treatment. Caloric restriction and weight loss are essential in the obese diabetic patient. Proper dietary management alone may be effective in controlling the blood glucose and symptoms of hyperglycemia. The importance of regular physical activity should also be stressed, and cardiovascular risk factors should be identified and corrective measures taken where possible. If this treatment program fails to reduce symptoms and/or blood glucose, the use of an oral sulfonylurea or insulin should be considered. Use of MICRONASE must be viewed by both the physician and patient as a treatment in addition to diet and not as a substitution or as a convenient mechanism for avoiding dietary restraint. Furthermore, loss of blood glucose control on diet alone may be transient, thus requiring only short-term administration of MICRONASE. During maintenance programs, MICRONASE should be discontinued if satisfactory lowering of blood glucose is no longer achieved. Judgment should be based on regular clinical and laboratory evaluations.

In considering the use of MICRONASE in asymptomatic patients, it should be recognized that controlling blood glucose in non-insulin-dependent diabetes has not been definitely established to be effective in preventing the long-term cardiovascular or neural complications of diabetes.

CONTRAINDICATIONS

MICRONASE Tablets (glyburide) are contraindicated in patients with:

1. Known hypersensitivity or allergy to the drug.
2. Diabetic ketoacidosis, with or without coma. This condition should be treated with insulin.
3. Type I diabetes mellitus, as sole therapy.

Special Warning on Increased Risk of Cardiovascular Mortality: The administration of oral hypoglycemic drugs has been reported to be associated with increased cardiovascular mortality as compared to treatment with diet alone or diet plus insulin. This warning is based on the study conducted by the University Group Diabetes Program (UGDP), a long-term prospective clinical trial designed to evaluate the effectiveness of glucose-lowering drugs in preventing or delaying vascular complications in patients with non-insulin-dependent diabetes. The study involved 823 patients who were randomly assigned to one of four treatment groups (*Diabetes,* 19 (Suppl. 2):747–830, 1970).

UGDP reported that patients treated for 5 to 8 years with diet plus a fixed dose of tolbutamide (1.5 grams per day) had a rate of cardiovascular mortality approximately 2½ times that of patients treated with diet alone. A significant increase in total mortality was not observed, but the use of tolbutamide was discontinued based on the increase in cardiovascular mortality, thus limiting the opportunity for the study to show an increase in overall mortality. Despite controversy regarding the interpretation of these results, the findings of the UGDP study provide an adequate basis for this warning. The patient should be informed of the potential risks and advantages of MICRONASE and of alternative modes of therapy.

Although only one drug in the sulfonylurea class (tolbutamide) was included in this study, it is prudent from a safety standpoint to consider that this warning may also apply to

other oral hypoglycemic drugs in this class, in view of their close similarities in mode of action and chemical structure.

PRECAUTIONS
General

Hypoglycemia: All sulfonylureas are capable of producing severe hypoglycemia. Proper patient selection and dosage and instructions are important to avoid hypoglycemic episodes. Renal or hepatic insufficiency may cause elevated drug levels of glyburide and the latter may also diminish gluconeogenic capacity, both of which increase the risk of serious hypoglycemic reactions. Elderly, debilitated or malnourished patients, and those with adrenal or pituitary insufficiency, are particularly susceptible to the hypoglycemic action of glucose-lowering drugs. Hypoglycemia may be difficult to recognize in the elderly and in people who are taking beta-adrenergic blocking drugs. Hypoglycemia is more likely to occur when caloric intake is deficient, after severe or prolonged exercise, when alcohol is ingested, or when more than one glucose lowering drug is used.

Loss of Control of Blood Glucose: When a patient stabilized on any diabetic regimen is exposed to stress such as fever, trauma, infection or surgery, a loss of control may occur. At such times it may be necessary to discontinue MICRONASE Tablets (glyburide) and administer insulin.

The effectiveness of any hypoglycemic drug, including MICRONASE, in lowering blood glucose to a desired level decreases in many patients over a period of time which may be due to progression of the severity of diabetes or to diminished responsiveness to the drug. This phenomenon is known as secondary failure, to distinguish it from primary failure in which the drug is ineffective in an individual patient when MICRONASE is first given. Adequate adjustment of dose and adherence to diet should be assessed before classifying a patient as a secondary failure.

Information for Patients: Patients should be informed of the potential risks and advantages of MICRONASE and of alternative modes of therapy. They also should be informed about the importance of adherence to dietary instructions, of a regular exercise program, and of regular testing of urine and/or blood glucose.

The risks of hypoglycemia, its symptoms and treatment, and conditions that predispose to its development should be explained to patients and responsible family members. Primary and secondary failure also should be explained.

Laboratory Tests

Therapeutic response to MICRONASE Tablets should be monitored by frequent urine glucose tests and periodic blood glucose tests. Measurement of glycosylated hemoglobin levels may be helpful in some patients.

Drug Interactions

The hypoglycemic action of sulfonylureas may be potentiated by certain drugs including nonsteroidal anti-inflammatory agents and other drugs that are highly protein bound, salicylates, sulfonamides, chloramphenicol, probenecid, coumarins, monoamine oxidase inhibitors, and beta adrenergic blocking agents. When such drugs are administered to a patient receiving MICRONASE, the patient should be observed closely for hypoglycemia. When such drugs are withdrawn from a patient receiving MICRONASE, the patient should be observed closely for loss of control.

Certain drugs tend to produce hyperglycemia and may lead to loss of control. These drugs include the thiazides and other diuretics, corticosteroids, phenothiazines, thyroid products, estrogens, oral contraceptives, phenytoin, nicotinic acid, sympathomimetics, calcium channel blocking drugs, and isoniazid. When such drugs are administered to a patient receiving MICRONASE, the patient should be closely observed for loss of control. When such drugs are withdrawn from a patient receiving MICRONASE, the patient should be observed closely for hypoglycemia.

A potential interaction between oral miconazole and oral hypoglycemic agents leading to severe hypoglycemia has been reported. Whether this interaction also occurs with the intravenous, topical or vaginal preparations of miconazole is not known.

Carcinogenesis, Mutagenesis, and Impairment of Fertility

Studies in rats at doses to 300 mg/kg/day for 18 months showed no carcinogenic effects. Glyburide is non-mutagenic when studied in the Salmonella microsome test (Ames test) and in the DNA damage/alkaline elution assay.

Pregnancy

Teratogenic Effects: Pregnancy Category B

Reproduction studies have been performed in rats and rabbits at doses up to 500 times the human dose and have revealed no evidence of impaired fertility or harm to the fetus due to glyburide. There are, however, no adequate and well

Continued on next page

Information on these Upjohn products is based on labeling in effect June 1, 1992. Further information concerning these and other Upjohn products may be obtained by direct inquiry to Medical Information, The Upjohn Company, Kalamazoo, Michigan 49001.

Upjohn—Cont.

controlled studies in pregnant women. Because animal reproduction studies are not always predictive of human response, this drug should be used during pregnancy only if clearly needed.

Because recent information suggests that abnormal blood glucose levels during pregnancy are associated with a higher incidence of congenital abnormalities, many experts recommend that insulin be used during pregnancy to maintain blood glucose as close to normal as possible.

Nonteratogenic Effects: Prolonged severe hypoglycemia (4 to 10 days) has been reported in neonates born to mothers who were receiving a sulfonylurea drug at the time of delivery. This has been reported more frequently with the use of agents with prolonged half-lives. If MICRONASE is used during pregnancy, it should be discontinued at least two weeks before the expected delivery date.

Nursing Mothers

Although it is not known whether glyburide is excreted in human milk, some sulfonylurea drugs are known to be excreted in human milk. Because the potential for hypoglycemia in nursing infants may exist, a decision should be made whether to discontinue nursing or to discontinue the drug, taking into account the importance of the drug to the mother. If the drug is discontinued, and if diet alone is inadequate for controlling blood glucose, insulin therapy should be considered.

Pediatric Use

Safety and effectiveness in children have not been established.

ADVERSE REACTIONS

Hypoglycemia: See Precautions and Overdosage Sections.

Gastrointestinal Reactions: Cholestatic jaundice and hepatitis may occur rarely; MICRONASE Tablets (glyburide) should be discontinued if this occurs.

Liver function abnormalities, including isolated transaminase elevations, have been reported.

Gastrointestinal disturbances, *e.g.*, nausea, epigastic fullness, and heartburn are the most common reactions, having occurred in 1.8% of treated patients during clinical trials. They tend to be dose related and may disappear when dosage is reduced.

Dermatologic Reactions: Allergic skin reactions, *e.g.*, pruritus, erythema, urticaria, and morbilliform or maculopapular eruptions occurred in 1.5% of treated patients during clinical trials. These may be transient and may disappear despite continued use of MICRONASE; if skin reactions persist, the drug should be discontinued.

Porphyria cutanea tarda and photosensitivity reactions have been reported with sulfonylureas.

Hematologic Reactions: Leukopenia, agranulocytosis, thrombocytopenia, hemolytic anemia, aplastic anemia, and pancytopenia have been reported with sulfonylureas.

Metabolic Reactions: Hepatic porphyria and disulfiram-like reactions have been reported with sulfonylureas; however, hepatic porphyria has not been reported with MICRONASE and disulfiram-like reactions have been reported very rarely.

Cases of hyponatremia have been reported with glyburide and all other sulfonylureas, most often in patients who are on other medications or have medical conditions known to cause hyponatremia or increase release of antidiuretic hormone. The syndrome of inappropriate antidiuretic hormone (SIADH) secretion has been reported with certain other sulfonylureas, and it has been suggested that these sulfonylureas may augment the peripheral (antidiuretic) action of ADH and/or increase release of ADH.

Other Reactions: Changes in accommodation and/or blurred vision have been reported with glyburide and other sulfonylureas. These are thought to be related to fluctuation in glucose levels.

In addition to dermatologic reactions, allergic reactions such as angioedema, arthralgia, myalgia and vasculitis have been reported.

OVERDOSAGE

Overdosage of sulfonylureas, including MICRONASE Tablets (glyburide), can produce hypoglycemia. Mild hypoglycemic symptoms, without loss of consciousness or neurological findings, should be treated aggressively with oral glucose and adjustments in drug dosage and/or meal patterns. Close monitoring should continue until the physician is assured that the patient is out of danger. Severe hypoglycemic reactions with coma, seizure, or other neurological impairment occur infrequently, but constitute medical emergencies requiring immediate hospitalization. If hypoglycemic coma is diagnosed or suspected, the patient should be given a rapid intravenous injection of concentrated (50%) glucose solution. This should be followed by a continuous infusion of a more dilute (10%) glucose solution at a rate which will maintain the blood glucose at a level above 100 mg/dL. Patients should be closely monitored for a minimum of 24 to 48 hours, since hypoglycemia may recur after apparent clinical recovery.

DOSAGE AND ADMINISTRATION

There is no fixed dosage regimen for the management of diabetes mellitus with MICRONASE Tablets (glyburide) or any other hypoglycemic agent. In addition to the usual monitoring of urinary glucose, the patient's blood glucose must also be monitored periodically to determine the minimum effective dose for the patient; to detect primary failure, *i.e.*, inadequate lowering of blood glucose at the maximum recommended dose of medication; and to detect secondary failure, *i.e.*, loss of adequate blood glucose lowering response after an initial period of effectiveness. Glycosylated hemoglobin levels may also be of value in monitoring the patient's response to therapy.

Short-term administration of MICRONASE may be sufficient during periods of transient loss of control in patients usually controlled well on diet.

Usual Starting Dose

The usual starting dose of MICRONASE Tablets is 2.5 to 5.0 mg daily, administered with breakfast or the first main meal. Those patients who may be more sensitive to hypoglycemic drugs should be started at 1.25 mg daily. (See Precautions Sections for patients at increased risk.) Failure to follow an appropriate dosage regimen may precipitate hypoglycemia. Patients who do not adhere to their prescribed dietary and drug regimen are more prone to exhibit unsatisfactory response to therapy.

Transfer From Other Hypoglycemic Therapy

Patients Receiving Other Oral Antidiabetic Therapy: Transfer of patients from other oral antidiabetic regimens to MICRONASE should be done conservatively and the initial daily dose should be 2.5 to 5 mg. When transferring patients from oral hypoglycemic agents other than chlorpropamide to MICRONASE, no transition period and no initial or priming dose are necessary. When transferring patients from chlorpropamide, particular care should be exercised during the first two weeks because the prolonged retention of chlorpropamide in the body and subsequent overlapping drug effects may provoke hypoglycemia.

Patients Receiving Insulin: Some type II diabetic patients being treated with insulin may respond satisfactorily to MICRONASE. If the insulin dose is less than 20 units daily, substitution of MICRONASE Tablets 2.5 to 5.0 mg as a single daily dose may be tried. If the insulin dose is between 20 and 40 units daily, the patient may be placed directly on MICRONASE Tablets 5.0 mg daily as a single dose. If the insulin dose is more than 40 units daily, a transition period is required for conversion to MICRONASE. In these patients, insulin dosage is decreased by 50% and MICRONASE Tablets 5 mg daily is started. Please refer to Titration to Maintenance Dose for further explanation.

Titration to Maintenance Dose

The usual maintenance dose is in the range of 1.25 to 20 mg daily, which may be given as a single dose or in divided doses (See Dosage Interval Section). Dosage increases should be made in increments of no more than 2.5 mg at weekly intervals based upon the patient's blood glucose response.

No exact dosage relationship exists between MICRONASE and the other oral hypoglycemic agents. Although patients may be transferred from the maximum dose of other sulfonylureas, the maximum starting dose of 5.0 mg of MICRONASE Tablets should be observed. A maintenance dose of 5 mg of MICRONASE Tablets provides approximately the same degree of blood glucose control as 250 to 375 mg chlorpropamide, 250 to 375 mg tolazamide, 500 to 750 mg acetohexamide, or 1000 to 1500 mg tolbutamide.

When transferring patients receiving more than 40 units of insulin daily, they may be started on a daily dose of MICRONASE Tablets 5 mg concomitantly with a 50% reduction in insulin dose. Progressive withdrawal of insulin and increase of MICRONASE in increments of 1.25 to 2.5 mg every 2 to 10 days is then carried out. During this conversion period when both insulin and MICRONASE are being used, hypoglycemia may rarely occur. During insulin withdrawal, patients should test their urine for glucose and acetone at least three times daily and report results to their physician. The appearance of persistent acetonuria with glycosuria indicates that the patient is a type I diabetic who requires insulin therapy.

Maximum Dose

Daily doses of more than 20 mg are not recommended.

Dosage Interval

Once-a-day therapy is usually satisfactory. Some patients, particularly those receiving more than 10 mg daily, may have a more satisfactory response with twice-a-day dosage.

Specific Patient Populations

MICRONASE is not recommended for use in pregnancy or for use in children.

In elderly patients, debilitated or malnourished patients, and patients with impaired renal or hepatic function, the initial and maintenance dosing should be conservative to avoid hypoglycemic reactions. (See Precautions Section.)

HOW SUPPLIED

MICRONASE Tablets (glyburide) are supplied as follows:

MICRONASE Tablets 1.25 mg (White, Round, Scored)

Bottles of 100	NDC 0009-0131-01

MICRONASE Tablets 2.5 mg (Dark Pink, Round, Scored)

Bottles of 30	NDC 0009-0141-06
Bottles of 60	NDC 0009-0141-07
Bottles of 100	NDC 0009-0141-01
Unit Dose Pkg of 100	NDC 0009-0141-02

MICRONASE Tablets 5 mg (Blue, Round, Scored)

Plastic bottles of 30	NDC 0009-0171-11
Plastic bottles of 60	NDC 0009-0171-12
Plastic bottles of 90	NDC 0009-0171-13
Plastic bottles of 100	NDC 0009-0171-05
Plastic bottles of 500	NDC 0009-0171-06
Plastic bottles of 1000	NDC 0009-0171-07
Unit Dose Pkg of 100	NDC 0009-0171-03

Caution: Federal law prohibits dispensing without prescription. Store at controlled room temperature 15°–30° C (59°–86° F). Dispensed in well closed containers with safety closures. Keep container tightly closed.

Code 811 985 315

Shown in Product Identification Section, page 434

MOTRIN® ℞

brand of ibuprofen tablets, USP

DESCRIPTION

MOTRIN Tablets contain the active ingredient ibuprofen, which is (±)-2-(*p*-isobutylphenyl) propionic acid. Ibuprofen is a white powder with a melting point of 74–77°C and is very slightly soluble in water (< 1 mg/ml) and readily soluble in organic solvents such as ethanol and acetone.

The structural formula is represented below:

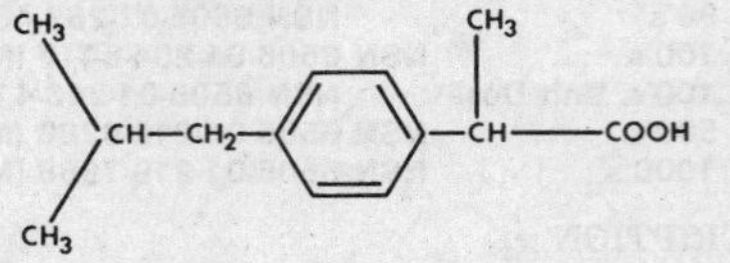

MOTRIN, a nonsteroidal anti-inflammatory agent, is available in 300 mg, 400 mg, 600 mg, and 800 mg tablets for oral administration.

Inactive ingredients: **300 mg**—acacia, acetylated monoglyceride, calcium sulfate, carboxymethylcellulose sodium, carnauba wax, colloidal silicon dioxide, corn starch, povidone, pregelatinized starch, sesame oil, shellac, stearic acid, sucrose, white wax; may contain hydroxypropyl methylcellulose and propylene glycol. **400 mg**—acacia, acetylated monoglyceride, calcium sulfate, carboxymethylcellulose sodium, carnauba wax, colloidal silicon dioxide, corn starch, FD&C yellow no. 6, pregelatinized starch, povidone, sesame oil, shellac, sodium benzoate, stearic acid, sucrose, titanium dioxide, white wax; may contain hydroxypropyl cellulose, hydroxypropyl methylcellulose and propylene glycol. **600 mg**—carnauba wax, colloidal silicon dioxide, corn starch, FD&C yellow no. 6, hydroxypropyl cellulose, hydroxypropyl methylcellulose, pregelatinized starch, propylene glycol, stearic acid, titanium dioxide; may contain hydroxypropyl cellulose. **800 mg**—carnauba wax, colloidal silicon dioxide, croscarmellose sodium, FD&C yellow no. 6, hydroxypropyl methylcellulose, magnesium stearate, microcrystalline cellulose, propylene glycol, talc, titanium dioxide.

CLINICAL PHARMACOLOGY

MOTRIN Tablets contain ibuprofen which possesses analgesic and antipyretic activities. Its mode of action, like that of other nonsteroidal anti-inflammatory agents, is not completely understood, but may be related to prostaglandin synthetase inhibition.

In clinical studies in patients with rheumatoid arthritis and osteoarthritis, MOTRIN has been shown to be comparable to aspirin in controlling pain and inflammation and to be associated with a statistically significant reduction in the milder gastrointestinal side effects (see ADVERSE REACTIONS). MOTRIN may be well tolerated in some patients who have had gastrointestinal side effects with aspirin, but these patients when treated with MOTRIN should be carefully followed for signs and symptoms of gastrointestinal ulceration and bleeding. Although it is not definitely known whether MOTRIN causes less peptic ulceration than aspirin, in one study involving 885 patients with rheumatoid arthritis treated for up to one year, there were no reports of gastric ulceration with MOTRIN whereas frank ulceration was reported in 13 patients in the aspirin group (statistically significant $p < .001$).

Gastroscopic studies at varying doses show an increased tendency toward gastric irritation at higher doses. However, at comparable doses, gastric irritation is approximately half that seen with aspirin. Studies using ^{51}Cr-tagged red cells indicate that fecal blood loss associated with MOTRIN Tab-

lets in doses up to 2400 mg daily did not exceed the normal range, and was significantly less than that seen in aspirin-treated patients.

In clinical studies in patients with rheumatoid arthritis, MOTRIN has been shown to be comparable to indomethacin in controlling the signs and symptoms of disease activity and to be associated with a statistically significant reduction of the milder gastrointestinal (see ADVERSE REACTIONS) and CNS side effects.

MOTRIN may be used in combination with gold salts and/or corticosteroids.

Controlled studies have demonstrated that MOTRIN is a more effective analgesic than propoxyphene for the relief of episiotomy pain, pain following dental extraction procedures, and for the relief of the symptoms of primary dysmenorrhea.

In patients with primary dysmenorrhea, MOTRIN has been shown to reduce elevated levels of prostaglandin activity in the menstrual fluid and to reduce resting and active intrauterine pressure, as well as the frequency of uterine contractions. The probable mechanism of action is to inhibit prostaglandin synthesis rather than simply to provide analgesia. The ibuprofen in MOTRIN is rapidly absorbed when administered orally. Peak serum ibuprofen levels are generally attained one to two hours after administration. With single doses up to 800 mg, a linear relationship exists between amount of drug administered and the integrated area under the serum drug concentration vs time curve. Above 800 mg, however, the area under the curve increases less than proportional to increases in dose. There is no evidence of drug accumulation or enzyme induction.

The administration of MOTRIN Tablets either under fasting conditions or immediately before meals yields quite similar serum ibuprofen concentration-time profiles. When MOTRIN is administered immediately after a meal, there is a reduction in the rate of absorption but no appreciable decrease in the extent of absorption. The bioavailability of the drug is minimally altered by the presence of food.

A bioavailability study has shown that there was no interference with the absorption of ibuprofen when MOTRIN was given in conjunction with an antacid containing both aluminum hydroxide and magnesium hydroxide.

Ibuprofen is rapidly metabolized and eliminated in the urine. The excretion of ibuprofen is virtually complete 24 hours after the last dose. The serum half-life is 1.8 to 2.0 hours.

Studies have shown that following ingestion of the drug, 45% to 79% of the dose was recovered in the urine within 24 hours as metabolite A (25%), (+) - 2 - [p - (2hydroxymethyl-propyl)- phenyl] propionic acid and metabolite B (37%), (+)-2-[p-(2carboxypropyl)-phenyl] propionic acid; the percentages of free and conjugated ibuprofen were approximately 1% and 14%, respectively.

INDICATIONS AND USAGE

MOTRIN Tablets (ibuprofen) are indicated for relief of the signs and symptoms of rheumatoid arthritis and osteoarthritis.

MOTRIN is indicated for relief of mild to moderate pain.

MOTRIN is also indicated for the treatment of primary dysmenorrhea.

Since there have been no controlled clinical trials to demonstrate whether or not there is any beneficial effect or harmful interaction with the use of MOTRIN in conjunction with aspirin, the combination cannot be recommended (see **Drug Interactions**).

Controlled clinical trials to establish the safety and effectiveness of MOTRIN in children have not been conducted.

CONTRAINDICATIONS

MOTRIN Tablets (ibuprofen) should not be used in patients who have previously exhibited hypersensitivity to the drug, or in individuals with the syndrome of nasal polyps, angioedema and bronchospastic reactivity to aspirin or other nonsteroidal anti-inflammatory agents. Anaphylactoid reactions have occurred in such patients.

WARNINGS

Risk of GI Ulceration, Bleeding and Perforation with Nonsteroidal Anti-inflammatory Therapy:

Serious gastrointestinal toxicity such as bleeding, ulceration, and perforation, can occur at any time, with or without warning symptoms, in patients treated chronically with nonsteroidal anti-inflammatory drugs. Although minor upper gastrointestinal problems, such as dyspepsia, are common, usually developing early in therapy, physicians should remain alert for ulceration and bleeding in patients treated chronically with nonsteroidal anti-inflammatory drugs even in the absence of previous GI tract symptoms. In patients observed in clinical trials of several months to two years duration, symptomatic upper GI ulcers, gross bleeding or perforation appear to occur in approximately 1% of patients treated for 3-6 months, and in about 2-4% of patients treated for one year. Physicians should inform patients about the signs and/or symptoms of serious GI toxicity and what steps to take if they occur.

Studies to date have not identified any subset of patients not at risk of developing peptic ulceration and bleeding. Except for a prior history of serious GI events and other risk factors known to be associated with peptic ulcer disease, such as alcoholism, smoking, etc., no risk factors (eg, age, sex) have been associated with increased risk. Elderly or debilitated patients seem to tolerate ulceration or bleeding less well than other individuals and most spontaneous reports of fatal GI events are in this population. Studies to date are inconclusive concerning the relative risk of various nonsteroidal anti-inflammatory agents in causing such reactions. High doses of any such agents probably carry a greater risk of these reactions, although controlled clinical trials showing this do not exist in most cases. In considering the use of relatively large doses (within the recommended dosage range), sufficient benefit should be anticipated to offset the potential increased risk of GI toxicity.

PRECAUTIONS

Blurred and/or diminished vision, scotomata, and/or changes in color vision have been reported. If a patient develops such complaints while receiving MOTRIN Tablets (ibuprofen), the drug should be discontinued and the patient should have an ophthalmologic examination which includes central visual fields and color vision testing.

Fluid retention and edema have been reported in association with MOTRIN; therefore, the drug should be used with caution in patients with a history of cardiac decompensation or hypertension.

MOTRIN, like other nonsteroidal anti-inflammatory agents, can inhibit platelet aggregation but the effect is quantitatively less and of shorter duration than that seen with aspirin. MOTRIN has been shown to prolong bleeding time (but within the normal range) in normal subjects. Because this prolonged bleeding effect may be exaggerated in patients with underlying hemostatic defects, MOTRIN should be used with caution in persons with intrinsic coagulation defects and those on anticoagulant therapy.

Patients on MOTRIN should report to their physicians signs or symptoms of gastrointestinal ulceration or bleeding, blurred vision or other eye symptoms, skin rash, weight gain, or edema.

In order to avoid exacerbation of disease or adrenal insufficiency, patients who have been on prolonged corticosteroid therapy should have their therapy tapered slowly rather than discontinued abruptly when MOTRIN is added to the treatment program.

The antipyretic and anti-inflammatory activity of ibuprofen may reduce fever and inflammation, thus diminishing their utility as diagnostic signs in detecting complications of presumed noninfectious noninflammatory painful conditions.

As with other nonsteroidal anti-inflammatory drugs, borderline elevations of one or more liver tests may occur in up to 15% of patients. These abnormalities may progress, may remain essentially unchanged, or may be transient with continued therapy. The SGPT (ALT) test is probably the most sensitive indicator of liver dysfunction. Meaningful (3 times the upper limit of normal) elevations of SGPT or SGOT (AST) occurred in controlled clinical trials in less than 1% of patients. A patient with symptoms and/or signs suggesting liver dysfunction, or in whom an abnormal liver test has occurred, should be evaluated for evidence of the development of more severe hepatic reaction while on therapy with MOTRIN. Severe hepatic reactions, including jaundice and cases of fatal hepatitis, have been reported with ibuprofen as with other nonsteroidal anti-inflammatory drugs. Although such reactions are rare, if abnormal liver tests persist or worsen, if clinical signs and symptoms consistent with liver disease develop, or if systemic manifestations occur (eg, eosinophilia, rash, etc.), MOTRIN should be discontinued.

In cross-study comparisons with doses ranging from 1200 mg to 3200 mg daily for several weeks, a slight dose-response decrease in hemoglobin/hematocrit was noted. This has been observed with other nonsteroidal anti-inflammatory drugs; the mechanism is unknown. With daily doses of 3200 mg, the total decrease in hemoglobin may exceed 1 gram; if there are no signs of bleeding, it is probably not clinically important. In two postmarketing clinical studies the incidence of a decreased hemoglobin level was greater than previously reported. Decrease in hemoglobin of 1 gram or more was observed in 17.1% of 193 patients on 1600 mg ibuprofen daily (osteoarthritis), and in 22.8% of 189 patients taking 2400 mg of ibuprofen daily (rheumatoid arthritis). Positive stool occult blood tests and elevated serum creatinine levels were also observed in these studies.

Aseptic Meningitis: Aseptic meningitis with fever and coma has been observed on rare occasions in patients on ibuprofen therapy. Although it is probably more likely to occur in patients with systemic lupus erythematosus and related connective tissue diseases, it has been reported in patients who do not have an underlying chronic disease. If signs or symptoms of meningitis develop in a patient on MOTRIN, the possibility of its being related to MOTRIN should be considered.

Renal Effects: As with other nonsteroidal anti-inflammatory drugs, long term administration of ibuprofen to animals

has resulted in renal papillary necrosis and other abnormal renal pathology. In humans, there have been reports of acute interstitial nephritis with hematuria, proteinuria, and occasionally nephrotic syndrome.

A second form of renal toxicity has been seen in patients with prerenal conditions leading to a reduction in renal blood flow or blood volume, where the renal prostaglandins have a supportive role in the maintenance of renal perfusion. In these patients administration of a nonsteroidal anti-inflammatory drug may cause a dose dependent reduction in prostaglandin formation and may precipitate overt renal decompensation. Patients at greatest risk of this reaction are those with impaired renal function, heart failure, liver dysfunction, those taking diuretics and the elderly. Discontinuation of nonsteroidal anti-inflammatory drug therapy is typically followed by recovery to the pretreatment state. Those patients at high risk who chronically take MOTRIN should have renal function monitored if they have signs or symptoms which may be consistent with mild azotemia, such as malaise, fatigue, loss of appetite, etc. Occasional patients may develop some elevation of serum creatinine and BUN levels without signs or symptoms.

Since ibuprofen is eliminated primarily by the kidneys, patients with significantly impaired renal function should be closely monitored; and a reduction in dosage should be anticipated to avoid drug accumulation. Prospective studies on the safety of ibuprofen in patients with chronic renal failure have not been conducted.

Information for Patients

MOTRIN, like other drugs of its class, is not free of side effects. The side effects of these drugs can cause discomfort and, rarely, there are more serious side effects, such as gastrointestinal bleeding, which may result in hospitalization and even fatal outcomes.

Nonsteroidal anti-inflammatory drugs are often essential agents in the management of arthritis and have a major role in the treatment of pain, but they also may be commonly employed for conditions which are less serious.

Physicians may wish to discuss with their patients the potential risks (see WARNINGS, PRECAUTIONS, and ADVERSE REACTIONS) and likely benefits of nonsteroidal anti-inflammatory drug treatment, particularly when the drugs are used for less serious conditions where treatment without such agents may represent an acceptable alternative to both the patient and physician.

Laboratory Tests

Because serious GI tract ulcerations and bleeding can occur without warning symptoms, physicians should follow chronically treated patients for the signs and symptoms of ulcerations and bleeding and should inform them of importance of this follow-up (see Risk of GI Ulceration, Bleeding and Perforation with Nonsteroidal Anti-inflammatory therapy).

Drug Interactions: *Coumarin-type anticoagulants.* Several short-term controlled studies failed to show that MOTRIN significantly affected prothrombin times or a variety of other clotting factors when administered to individuals on coumarin-type anticoagulants. However, because bleeding has been reported when MOTRIN and other nonsteroidal anti-inflammatory agents have been administered to patients on coumarin-type anticoagulants, the physician should be cautious when administering MOTRIN to patients on anticoagulants.

Aspirin: Animal studies show that aspirin given with nonsteroidal anti-inflammatory agents, including MOTRIN, yields a net decrease in anti-inflammatory activity with lowered blood levels of the non-aspirin drug. Single dose bioavailability studies in normal volunteers have failed to show an effect of aspirin on ibuprofen blood levels. Correlative clinical studies have not been done.

Methotrexate: Ibuprofen, as well as other nonsteroidal anti-inflammatory drugs, probably reduces the tubular secretion of methotrexate based on *in-vitro* studies in rabbit kidney slices. This may indicate that ibuprofen could enhance the toxicity of methotrexate. Caution should be used if MOTRIN is administered concomitantly with methotrexate.

H-2 Antagonists: In studies with human volunteers, co-administration of cimetidine or ranitidine with ibuprofen had no substantive effect on ibuprofen serum concentrations.

Furosemide: Clinical studies, as well as random observations, have shown that ibuprofen can reduce the natriuretic effect of furosemide and thiazides in some patients. This response has been attributed to inhibition of renal prostaglandin synthesis. During concomitant therapy with ibuprofen, the patient should be observed closely for signs of renal fail-

Continued on next page

Information on these Upjohn products is based on labeling in effect June 1, 1992. Further information concerning these and other Upjohn products may be obtained by direct inquiry to Medical Information, The Upjohn Company, Kalamazoo, Michigan 49001.

Upjohn—Cont.

ure (See PRECAUTIONS, Renal Effects) as well as to assure diuretic efficacy.

Lithium: Ibuprofen produced an elevation of plasma lithium levels and a reduction in renal lithium clearance in a study of eleven normal volunteers. The mean minimum lithium concentration increased 15% and the renal clearance of lithium was decreased by 19% during this period of concomitant drug administration. This effect has been attributed to inhibition of renal prostaglandin synthesis by ibuprofen. Thus, when ibuprofen and lithium are administered concurrently, subjects should be observed carefully for signs of lithium toxicity. (Read circulars for lithium preparation before use of such concurrent therapy.)

Pregnancy: Reproductive studies conducted in rats and rabbits at doses somewhat less than the maximal clinical dose did not demonstrate evidence of developmental abnormalities. However, animal reproduction studies are not always predictive of human response. As there are no adequate and well-controlled studies in pregnant women, this drug should be used during pregnancy only if clearly needed. Because of the known effects of nonsteroidal anti-inflammatory drugs on the fetal cardiovascular system (closure of ductus arteriosus), use during late pregnancy should be avoided. As with other drugs known to inhibit prostaglandin synthesis, an increased incidence of dystocia and delayed parturition occurred in rats. Administration of MOTRIN is not recommended during pregnancy.

Nursing Mothers: In limited studies, an assay capable of detecting 1 mcg/ml did not demonstrate ibuprofen in the milk of lactating mothers. However, because of the limited nature of the studies, and the possible adverse effects of prostaglandin-inhibiting drugs on neonates, MOTRIN is not recommended for use in nursing mothers.

ADVERSE REACTIONS

The most frequent type of adverse reaction occurring with MOTRIN Tablets (ibuprofen) is gastrointestinal. In controlled clinical trials the percentage of patients reporting one or more gastrointestinal complaints ranged from 4% to 16%.

In controlled studies when MOTRIN was compared to aspirin and indomethacin in equally effective doses, the overall incidence of gastrointestinal complaints was about half that seen in either the aspirin- or indomethacin-treated patients. Adverse reactions observed during controlled clinical trials at an incidence greater than 1% are listed in the table. Those reactions listed in Column one encompass observations in approximately 3,000 patients. More than 500 of these patients were treated for periods of at least 54 weeks.

Still other reactions occurring less frequently than 1 in 100 were reported in controlled clinical trials and from marketing experience. These reactions have been divided into two categories: Column two of the following table lists reactions with therapy with MOTRIN where the probability of a causal relationship exists: for the reactions in Column three, a causal relationship with MOTRIN has not been established. Reported side effects were higher at doses of 3200 mg/day than at doses of 2400 mg or less per day in clinical trials of patients with rheumatoid arthritis. The increases in incidence were slight and still within the ranges reported in the table below.

OVERDOSAGE

Approximately $1\frac{1}{2}$ hours after the reported ingestion of from 7 to 10 MOTRIN Tablets (ibuprofen) (400 mg), a 19-month old child weighing 12 kg was seen in the hospital emergency room, apneic and cyanotic, responding only to painful stimuli. This type of stimulus, however, was sufficient to induce respiration. Oxygen and parenteral fluids were given; a greenish-yellow fluid was aspirated from the stomach with no evidence to indicate the presence of ibuprofen. Two hours after ingestion the child's condition seemed stable; she still responded only to painful stimuli and continued to have periods of apnea lasting from 5 to 10 seconds. She was admitted to intensive care and sodium bicarbonate was administered as well as infusions of dextrose and normal saline. By four hours post-ingestion she could be aroused easily, sit by herself and respond to spoken commands. Blood level of ibuprofen was 102.9 µg/ml approximately $8\frac{1}{2}$ hours after accidental ingestion. At 12 hours she appeared to be completely recovered.

In two other reported cases where children (each weighing approximately 10 kg) accidentally, acutely ingested approximately 120 mg/kg, there were no signs of acute intoxication or late sequelae. Blood level in one child 90 minutes after ingestion was 700 µg/ml—about 10 times the peak levels seen in absorption-excretion studies.

A 19-year old male who had taken 8,000 mg of ibuprofen over a period of a few hours complained of dizziness, and nystagmus was noted. After hospitalization, parenteral hydration and three days' bed rest, he recovered with no reported sequelae.

In cases of acute overdosage, the stomach should be emptied by vomiting or lavage, though little drug will likely be recovered if more than an hour has elapsed since ingestion. Because the drug is acidic and is excreted in the urine, it is theoretically beneficial to administer alkali and induce diuresis. In addition to supportive measures the use of oral activated charcoal may help to reduce the absorption and reabsorption of ibuprofen in MOTRIN.

DOSAGE AND ADMINISTRATION

Do not exceed 3200 mg total daily dose. If gastrointestinal complaints occur, administer MOTRIN Tablets (ibuprofen) with meals or milk.

Rheumatoid arthritis and osteoarthritis, including flare-ups of chronic disease:

Suggested Dosage: 1200 mg-3200 mg daily (300 mg qid; 400 mg, 600 mg or 800 mg tid or qid). Individual patients may show a better response to 3200 mg daily, as compared with 2400 mg, although in well-controlled clinical trials patients on 3200 mg did not show a better mean response in terms of efficacy. Therefore, when treating patients with 3200 mg/day, the physician should observe sufficient increased clinical benefits to offset potential increased risk.

The dose should be tailored to each patient, and may be lowered or raised depending on the severity of symptoms either at time of initiating drug therapy or as the patient responds or fails to respond.

MOTRIN

Incidence Greater than 1% (but less than 3%) Probable Causal Relationship	Precise Incidence Unknown (but less than 1%) Probable Causal Relationship**	Precise Incidence Unknown (but less than 1%) Causal Relationship Unknown**
GASTROINTESTINAL Nausea*, epigastric pain*, heartburn*, diarrhea, abdominal distress, nausea and vomiting, indigestion, constipation, abdominal cramps or pain, fullness of GI tract (bloating and flatulence)	Gastric or duodenal ulcer with bleeding and/or perforation, gastrointestinal hemorrhage, melena, gastritis, hepatitis, jaundice, abnormal liver function tests; pancreatis	
CENTRAL NERVOUS SYSTEM Dizziness*, headache, nervousness	Depression, insomnia, confusion, emotional lability, somnolence, aseptic meningitis with fever and coma	Paresthesias, hallucinations, dream abnormalities, pseudotumor cerebri
DERMATOLOGIC Rash* (including maculopapular type), pruritis	Vesiculobullous eruptions, urticaria, erythema multiforme, Stevens-Johnson syndrome, alopecia	Toxic epidermal necrolysis, photoallergic skin reactions
SPECIAL SENSES Tinnitus	Hearing loss, amblyopia (blurred and/or diminished vision, scotomata and/or changes in color vision) (see PRECAUTIONS)	Conjunctivitis, diplopia, optic neuritis, cataracts
HEMATOLOGIC	Neutropenia, agranulocytosis, aplastic anemia, hemolytic anemia (sometimes Coombs positive), thrombocytopenia with or without purpura, eosinophilia, decreases in hemoglobin and hematocrit (see PRECAUTIONS)	Bleeding episodes (eg epistaxis, menorrhagia)
METABOLIC/ENDOCRINE Decreased appetite		Gynecomastia, hypoglycemic reaction, acidosis
CARDIOVASCULAR Edema, fluid retention (generally responds promptly to drug discontinuation; see PRECAUTIONS)	Congestive heart failure in patients with marginal cardiac function, elevated blood pressure, palpitations	Arrhythmias (sinus tachycardia, sinus bradycardia)
ALLERGIC	Syndrome of abdominal pain, fever, chills, nausea and vomiting; anaphylaxis; bronchospasm (see CONTRAINDICATIONS)	Serum sickness, lupus erythematosus syndrome, Henoch-Schönlein vasculitis, angioedema
RENAL	Acute renal failure (see PRECAUTIONS), decreased creatinine clearance, polyuria, azotemia, cystitis, hematuria	Renal papillary necrosis
MISCELLANEOUS	Dry eyes and mouth, gingival ulcer, rhinitis	

* Reactions occurring in 3% to 9% of patients treated with MOTRIN. (Those reactions occurring in less than 3% of the patients are unmarked).

** Reactions are classified under "*Probable Causal Relationship (PCR)*" if there has been one positive rechallenge or if three or more cases occur which might be causally related. Reactions are classified under "*Causal Relationship Unknown*" if seven or more events have been reported but the criteria for PCR have not been met.

In general, patients with rheumatoid arthritis seem to require higher doses of MOTRIN than do patients with osteoarthritis.

The smallest dose of MOTRIN that yields acceptable control should be employed. A linear blood level dose-response relationship exists with single doses up to 800 mg (See CLINICAL PHARMACOLOGY for effects of food on rate of absorption).

The availability of four tablet strengths facilitates dosage adjustment.

In chronic conditions, a therapeutic response to therapy with MOTRIN is sometimes seen in a few days to a week but most often is observed by two weeks. After a satisfactory response has been achieved, the patient's dose should be reviewed and adjusted as required.

Mild to moderate pain:

400 mg every 4 to 6 hours as necessary for relief of pain. In controlled analgesic clinical trials, doses of MOTRIN greater than 400 mg were no more effective than the 400 mg dose.

Dysmenorrhea:

For the treatment of dysmenorrhea, beginning with the earliest onset of such pain, MOTRIN should be given in a dose of 400 mg every 4 hours as necessary for the relief of pain.

HOW SUPPLIED

MOTRIN Tablets (ibuprofen) are supplied as follows:

MOTRIN Tablets, 300 mg (white)

Unit of Use bottles of 60	NDC 0009-0733-01
Bottles of 500	NDC 0009-0733-02

MOTRIN Tablets, 400 mg (orange)

Unit of Use bottles of 100	NDC 0009-0750-25
Unit-dose package of 100	NDC 0009-0750-06
Unit of Use bottles of 120	NDC 0009-0750-26
Bottles of 500	NDC 0009-0750-02

MOTRIN Tablets, 600 mg (peach)

Unit of Use bottles of 90	NDC 0009-0742-08
Unit of Use bottles of 100	NDC 0009-0742-03
Unit-dose package of 100	NDC 0009-0742-05
Bottles of 500	NDC 0009-0742-02

MOTRIN Tablets, 800 mg (apricot)

Unit of Use bottles of 90	NDC 0009-0725-08
Unit of Use bottles of 100	NDC 0009-0725-01
Unit-dose package of 100	NDC 0009-0725-02
Bottles of 500	NDC 0009-0725-03
Code 810 015 530	

Shown in Product Identification Section, page 434

ORINASE® ℞

brand of tolbutamide tablets, USP
0.5 gram, 100's, Unit Dose   NSN 6505-00-131-9268 (M)

DESCRIPTION

ORINASE Tablets contain tolbutamide, an oral blood glucose lowering drug of the sulfonylurea category. Tolbutamide is a pure white crystalline compound practically insoluble in water but forming water-soluble salts with alkalies. The chemical names for tolbutamide are (1) Benzenesulfonamide, N-[(butylamino) carbonyl]-4-methyl; (2) 1-Butyl-3-(p-tolylsulfonyl)urea and its molecular weight is 270.35.

Each ORINASE Tablet for oral administration contains 250 mg or 500 mg tolbutamide. Inactive ingredients: colloidal silicon dioxide, crosscarmellose sodium, magnesium stearate, pregelatinized starch.

CLINICAL PHARMACOLOGY

Actions

Tolbutamide appears to lower blood glucose acutely by stimulating the release of insulin from the pancreas, an effect dependent upon functioning beta cells in the pancreatic islets. The mechanism by which tolbutamide lowers blood glucose during long-term administration has not been clearly established. With chronic administration in Type II diabetic patients, the blood glucose lowering effect persists despite a gradual decline in the insulin secretory response to the drug. Extrapancreatic effects may be involved in the mechanism of action of oral sulfonylurea hypoglycemic drugs.

Some patients who are initially responsive to oral hypoglycemic drugs, including ORINASE, may become unresponsive or poorly responsive over time. Alternatively, ORINASE may be effective in some patients who have become unresponsive to one or more other sulfonylurea drugs.

Pharmacokinetics

When administered orally, the tolbutamide in ORINASE Tablets is readily absorbed from the gastrointestinal tract. Absorption is not impaired and glucose lowering and insulin releasing effects are not altered if the drug is taken with food. Detectable levels are present in the plasma within twenty minutes after oral ingestion of a 500 mg ORINASE tablet, with peak levels occurring at three to four hours and only small amounts detectable at 24 hours. The half-life of tolbutamide is 4.5 to 6.5 hours. As tolbutamide has no p-amino group, it cannot be acetylated, which is one of the common modes of metabolic degradation for the antibacterial

sulfonamides. However, the presence of the p-methyl group renders tolbutamide susceptible to oxidation, and this appears to be the principal manner of its metabolic degradation in man. The p-methyl group is oxidized to form a carboxyl group, converting tolbutamide into the totally inactive metabolite 1-butyl-3-p-carboxy-phenylsulfonylurea, which can be recovered in the urine within 24 hours in amounts accounting for up to 75% of the administered dose.

The major tolbutamide metabolite has been found to have no hypoglycemic or other action when administered orally and IV to both normal and diabetic subjects. This tolbutamide metabolite is highly soluble over the critical acid range of urinary pH values, and its solubility increases with increase in pH. Because of the marked solubility of the tolbutamide metabolite, crystalluria does not occur. A second metabolite, 1-butyl-3-(p-hydroxymethyl) phenyl sulfonylurea also occurs to a limited extent. It is an inactive metabolite.

The administration of 3 grams of tolbutamide to either nondiabetic or tolbutamide-responsive diabetic subjects will, in both instances, occasion a gradual lowering of blood glucose. Increasing the dose to 6 grams does not usually cause a response which is significantly different from that produced by the 3 gram dose. Following the administration of a 3 gram dose of ORINASE solution, nondiabetic fasting adults exhibit a 30% or greater reduction in blood glucose within one hour, following which the blood glucose gradually returns to the fasting level over six to twelve hours. Following the administration of a 3 gram dose of ORINASE solution, tolbutamide responsive diabetic patients show a gradually progressive blood glucose lowering effect, the maximal response being reached between five to eight hours after ingestion of a single 3 gram dose. The blood glucose then rises gradually and by the 24th hour has usually returned to pretest levels. The magnitude of the reduction, when expressed in terms of percent of the protest blood glucose, tends to be similar to the response seen in the nondiabetic subject.

INDICATIONS AND USAGE

ORINASE Tablets (tolbutamide) are indicated as an adjunct to diet to lower the blood glucose in patients with noninsulin-dependent diabetes whose hyperglycemia cannot be satisfactorily controlled by diet alone. In initiating treatment for noninsulin-dependent diabetes, diet should be emphasized as the primary form of treatment. Caloric restriction and weight loss are essential in the obese diabetic patient. Proper dietary management alone may be effective in controlling the blood glucose and symptoms of hyperglycemia. The importance of regular physical activity should also be stressed and cardiovascular risk factors should be identified and corrective measures taken where possible.

If this treatment program fails to reduce symptoms and/or blood glucose, the use of an oral sulfonylurea or insulin should be considered. Use of ORINASE must be viewed by both the physician and patient as a treatment in addition to diet, and not as a substitute for diet or as a convenient mechanism for avoiding dietary restraint. Furthermore, loss of blood glucose control on diet alone may be transient, thus requiring only short-term administration of ORINASE.

During maintenance programs, ORINASE should be discontinued if satisfactory lowering of blood glucose is no longer achieved. Judgments should be based on regular clinical and laboratory evaluations.

In considering the use of ORINASE in asymptomatic patients, it should be recognized that controlling the blood glucose in noninsulin-dependent diabetes has not been definitely established to be effective in preventing the long-term cardiovascular or neural complications of diabetes.

CONTRAINDICATIONS

ORINASE Tablets (tolbutamide) are contraindicated in patients with: 1) known hypersensitivity or allergy to ORINASE; 2) diabetic ketoacidosis, with or without coma. This condition should be treated with insulin. 3) Type I diabetes, as sole therapy.

Special Warning on Increased Risk of Cardiovascular Mortality: The administration of oral hypoglycemic drugs has been reported to be associated with increased cardiovascular mortality as compared to treatment with diet alone or diet plus insulin. This warning is based on the study conducted by the University Group Diabetes Program (UGDP), a long-term prospective clinical trial designed to evaluate the effectiveness of glucose-lowering drugs in preventing or delaying vascular complications in patients with noninsulin-dependent diabetes. The study involved 823 patients who were randomly assigned to one of four treatment groups (Diabetes, 19 (supp. 2):747-830, 1970.)

UGDP reported that patients treated for five to eight years with diet plus a fixed dose of tolbutamide (1.5 grams per day) had a rate of cardiovascular mortality approximately 2½ times that of patients with diet alone. A significant increase in total mortality was not observed, but the use of tolbutamide was discontinued based on the increase in cardiovascular mortality, thus limiting the opportunity for the study to show an increase in overall mortality. Despite controversy regarding the interpretation of these results, the findings of the UGDP study provide an adequate basis for this warning.

The patient should be informed of the potential risks and advantages of ORINASE and of alternative modes of therapy.

Although only one drug in the sulfonylurea class (tolbutamide) was included in this study, it is prudent from a safety standpoint to consider that this warning may also apply to other oral hypoglycemic drugs in this class, in view of their close similarities in mode of action and chemical structure.

PRECAUTIONS

General

Hypoglycemia—All sulfonylurea drugs are capable of producing severe hypoglycemia. Proper patient selection and dosage and instructions are important to avoid hypoglycemic episodes. Renal or hepatic insufficiency may cause elevated blood levels of tolbutamide and the latter may also diminish gluconeogenic capacity, both of which increase the risk of serious hypoglycemic reactions. Elderly, debilitated or malnourished patients and those with adrenal or pituitary insufficiency are particularly susceptible to the hypoglycemic action of glucose lowering drugs. Hypoglycemia may be difficult to recognize in the elderly and people who are taking beta-adrenergic blocking drugs. Hypoglycemia is more likely to occur when caloric intake is deficient, after severe or prolonged exercise, when alcohol is ingested, or when more than one glucose lowering drug is used.

Loss of Control of Blood Glucose—When a patient stabilized on any diabetic regimen is exposed to stress such as fever, trauma, infection, or surgery, loss of blood glucose control may occur. At such times it may be necessary to discontinue ORINASE and administer insulin.

The effectiveness of any hypoglycemic drug, including ORINASE, in lowering blood glucose to a desired level decreases in patients over a period of time, which may be due to progression of the severity of the diabetes or to diminished responsiveness to the drug. This phenomenon is known as secondary drug failure to distinguish it from primary failure in which the drug is ineffective in an individual patient when first given. Adequate adjustment of dose and adherence to diet should be assessed before classifying a patient as a secondary failure.

Information for Patients

Patients should be informed of the potential risks and advantages of ORINASE Tablets (tolbutamide) and of alternative modes of therapy. They should also be informed about the importance of adherence to dietary instructions, of a regular exercise program, and of regular testing of urine and/or blood glucose.

The risks of hypoglycemia, its symptoms and treatment, and conditions that predispose to its development should be explained to patients and responsible family members. Primary and secondary failure should also be explained.

Laboratory Tests

Blood and urine glucose should be monitored periodically. Measurement of glycosylated hemoglobin may be useful in some patients.

A metabolite of tolbutamide in urine may give a false positive reaction for albumin if measured by the acidification-after-boiling test, which causes the metabolite to precipitate. There is no interference with the sulfosalicylic acid test.

Drug Interactions

The hypoglycemic action of sulfonylureas may be potentiated by certain drugs including nonsteroidal anti-inflammatory agents and other drugs that are highly protein bound, salicylates, sulfonamides, chloramphenicol, probenecid, coumarins, monoamine oxidase inhibitors, and beta adrenergic blocking agents. When such drugs are administered to a patient receiving ORINASE, the patient should be closely observed for hypoglycemia. When such drugs are withdrawn from a patient receiving ORINASE, the patient should be observed closely for loss of control.

Certain drugs tend to produce hyperglycemia and may lead to loss of control. These drugs include the thiazides and other diuretics, corticosteroids, phenothiazines, thyroid products, estrogens, oral contraceptives, phenytoin, nicotinic acid, sympathomimetics, calcium channel blocking drugs and isoniazid. When such drugs are administered to a patient receiving ORINASE, the patient should be closely observed for loss of control of blood glucose. When such drugs are withdrawn from a patient receiving ORINASE, the patient should be observed closely for hypoglycemia.

A potential interaction between oral miconazole and oral hypoglycemic agents leading to severe hypoglycemia has been reported. Whether this interaction also occurs with the intravenous, topical or vaginal preparations of miconazole is not known.

Continued on next page

Information on these Upjohn products is based on labeling in effect June 1, 1992. Further information concerning these and other Upjohn products may be obtained by direct inquiry to Medical Information, The Upjohn Company, Kalamazoo, Michigan 49001.

Upjohn—Cont.

Carcinogenesis and Mutagenicity
Bioassay for carcinogenicity was performed in both sexes of rats and mice following ingestion of tolbutamide for 78 weeks. No evidence of carcinogenicity was found.
Tolbutamide has also been demonstrated to be nonmutagenic in the Ames salmonella/mammalian microsome mutagenicity test.
Pregnancy
Teratogenic Effects
Pregnancy Category C. ORINASE has been shown to be teratogenic in rats given in doses 25 to 100 times the human dose. In some studies, pregnant rats given high doses of tolbutamide have shown increased mortality in offspring and ocular and bony abnormalities. Repeat studies in other species (rabbits) have not demonstrated a teratogenic effect. There are no adequate and well controlled studies in pregnant women. ORINASE is not recommended for the treatment of pregnant diabetic patients. Serious consideration should also be given to the possible hazards of the use of ORINASE in women of child-bearing age and in those who might become pregnant while using the drug.
Because recent information suggests that abnormal blood glucose levels during pregnancy are associated with a higher incidence of congenital abnormalities, many experts recommend that insulin be used during pregnancy to maintain blood glucose levels as close to normal as possible.
Nonteratogenic Effects
Prolonged severe hypoglycemia (four to ten days) has been reported in neonates born to mothers who were receiving a sulfonylurea drug at the time of delivery. This has been reported more frequently with the use of agents with prolonged half lives. If ORINASE is used during pregnancy, it should be discontinued at least two weeks before the expected delivery date.
Nursing Mothers
Although it is not known whether tolbutamide is excreted in human milk, some sulfonylurea drugs are known to be excreted in human milk. Because the potential for hypoglycemia in nursing infants may exist, a decision should be made whether to discontinue nursing or to discontinue the drug, taking into account the importance of the drug to the mother. If the drug is discontinued and if diet alone is inadequate for controlling blood glucose, insulin therapy should be considered.
Pediatric Use
Safety and effectiveness in children have not been established.

ADVERSE REACTIONS
Hypoglycemia — See **Precautions** and **Overdosage** sections.
Gastrointestinal Reactions: Cholestatic jaundice may occur rarely; ORINASE Tablets (tolbutamide) should be discontinued if this occurs. Gastrointestinal disturbances, eg, nausea, epigastric fullness, and heartburn, are the most common reactions and occurred in 1.4% of patients treated during clinical trials. They tend to be dose-related and may disappear when dosage is reduced.
Dermatologic Reactions: Allergic skin reactions, eg, pruritus, erythema, urticaria, and morbilliform or maculopapular eruptions, occurred in 1.1% of patients treated during clinical trials. These may be transient and may disappear despite continued use of ORINASE; if skin reactions persist, the drug should be discontinued.
Porphyria cutanea tarda and photosensitivity reactions have been reported with sulfonylureas.
Hematologic Reactions: Leukopenia, agranulocytosis, thrombocytopenia, hemolytic anemia, aplastic anemia, and pancytopenia have been reported with sulfonylureas.
Metabolic Reactions: Hepatic porphria and disulfiram-like reactions have been reported with sulfonylureas.
Endocrine Reactions: Cases of hyponatremia and the syndrome of inappropriate antidiuretic hormone (SIADH) secretion have been reported with this and other sulfonylureas.
Miscellaneous Reactions: Headache and taste alterations have occasionally been reported with tolbutamide administration.

OVERDOSAGE
Overdosage of sulfonylureas, including ORINASE Tablets, can produce symptoms of hypoglycemia.
Mild hypoglycemic symptoms without loss of consciousness or neurologic findings should be treated aggressively with oral glucose and adjustments in drug dosage and/or meal patterns. Close monitoring should continue until the physician is assured the patient is out of danger. Severe hypoglycemic reactions with coma, seizure, or other neurological impairment occur infrequently but constitute medical emergencies requiring immediate hospitalization. If hypoglycemic coma is suspected or diagnosed, the patient should be given a rapid intravenous injection of concentrated (50%) glucose solution. This should be followed by a continuous infusion of a more dilute (10%) glucose solution at a rate which will maintain the blood glucose level above 100 mg/dl. Patients should be closely monitored for a minimum of 24 to 48 hours, since hypoglycemia may recur after apparent clinical recovery.

DOSAGE AND ADMINISTRATION
There is no fixed dosage regimen for the management of diabetes mellitus with ORINASE Tablets (tolbutamide) or any other hypoglycemic agent. In addition to the usual monitoring of urinary glucose, the patient's blood glucose must also be monitored periodically to determine the minimum effective dose for the patient; to detect primary failure, ie, inadequate lowering of blood glucose at the maximum recommended dose of medication; and to detect secondary failure, ie, loss of adequate blood glucose response after an initial period of effectiveness. Glycosylated hemoglobin levels may also be of value in monitoring the patient's response to therapy.
Short-term administration of ORINASE may be sufficient during periods of transient loss of control in patients usually controlled well on diet.
Usual Starting Dose
The usual starting dose is 1 to 2 grams daily. This may be increased or decreased depending on individual patient response. Failure to follow an appropriate dosage regimen may precipitate hyoglycemia. Patients who do not adhere to their prescribed dietary regimens are more prone to exhibit unsatisfactory response to drug therapy.
Transfer From Other Hypoglycemic Therapy
Patients Receiving Other Oral Antidiabetic Therapy—Transfer of patients from other oral antidiabetes regimens to ORINASE should be done conservatively. When transferring patients from oral hypoglycemic agents other than chlorpropamide to ORINASE, no transition period and no initial or priming doses are necessary. When transferring patients from chlorpropamide, however, particular care should be exercised during the first two weeks because of the prolonged retention of chlorpropamide in the body and the possibility that subsequent overlapping drug effects might provoke hypoglycemia.
Patients Receiving Insulin—Patients requiring 20 units or less of insulin daily may be placed directly on ORINASE and insulin abruptly discontinued. Patients whose insulin requirement is between 20 and 40 units daily may be started on therapy with ORINASE with a concurrent 30 to 50% reduction in insulin dose, with further daily reduction of the insulin when response to tolbutamide is observed. In patients requiring more than 40 units of insulin daily, therapy with ORINASE may be initiated in conjunction with a 20% reduction in insulin dose the first day, with further careful reduction of insulin as response is observed. Occasionally, conversion to ORINASE in the hospital may be advisable in candidates who require more than 40 units of insulin daily. During this conversion period when both insulin and ORINASE are being used, hypoglycemia may rarely occur. During insulin withdrawal, patients should test their urine for glucose and acetone at least three times daily and report results to their physician. The appearance of persistent acetonuria with glycosuria indicates that the patient is a Type 1 diabetic patient who requires insulin therapy.
Maximum Dose
Daily doses of greater than 3 grams are not recommended.
Usual Maintenance Dose
The maintenance dose is in the range of 0.25 - 3 grams daily. Maintenance doses above 2 grams are seldom required.
Dosage Interval
The total daily dose may be taken either in the morning or in divided doses through the day. While either schedule is usually effective, the divided dose system is preferred by some clinicians from the standpoint of digestive tolerance.
In elderly, debilitated or malnourished patients and patients with impaired renal or hepatic function, the initial and maintenance dosing should be conservative to avoid hypoglycemic reactions (see **Precautions** section).

HOW SUPPLIED
ORINASE Tablets (tolbutamide) are available in the following strengths and package sizes:

250 mg (scored, round, white)

Unit-of-Use bottles of 100	NDC 0009-0701-01

500 mg (scored, round, white)

Bottles of 200	NDC 0009-0100-02
Bottles of 500	NDC 0009-0100-03
Bottles of 1000	NDC 0009-0100-05
Unit-of-Use bottles of 100	NDC 0009-0100-11
Unit-Dose package of 100	NDC 0009-0100-06

Store at controlled room temperature 15–30°C (59–86°F).
Code 811 646 210
Shown in Product Identification Section, page 434

PAMINE® ℞
brand of methscopolamine bromide tablets, USP

HOW SUPPLIED
Each tablet contains 2.5 mg methscopolamine bromide.
Bottles of 100 *NDC 0009-0061-01*

PROSTIN VR PEDIATRIC® ℞
brand of alprostadil sterile solution
(alprostadil injection, USP)
500 micrograms per ml

WARNING
Apnea is experienced by about 10 to 12% of neonates with congenital heart defects treated with PROSTIN VR PEDIATRIC Sterile Solution (alprostadil). Apnea is most often seen in neonates weighing less than 2 kg at birth and usually appears during the first hour of drug infusion. Therefore, respiratory status should be monitored throughout treatment, and PROSTIN VR PEDIATRIC should be used where ventilatory assistance is immediately available.

DESCRIPTION
PROSTIN VR PEDIATRIC Sterile Solution for intravascular infusion contains 500 micrograms alprostadil, more commonly known as prostaglandin E_1, in 1.0 ml dehydrated alcohol.
The chemical name for alprostadil is (11α, 13E, 15S)-11,15 dihydroxy-9-oxoprost-13-en-1-oic acid, and the molecular weight is 354.49.
Alprostadil is a white to off-white crystalline powder with a melting point between 110° and 116°C. Its solubility at 35°C is 8000 micrograms per 100 ml double distilled water.

CLINICAL PHARMACOLOGY
Alprostadil (prostaglandin E_1) is one of a family of naturally occurring acidic lipids with various pharmacologic effects. Vasodilation, inhibition of platelet aggregation, and stimulation of intestinal and uterine smooth muscle are among the most notable of these effects. Intravenous doses of 1 to 10 micrograms of alprostadil per kilogram of body weight lower the blood pressure in mammals by decreasing peripheral resistance. Reflex increases in cardiac output and rate accompany the reduction in blood pressure.
Smooth muscle of the ductus arteriosus is especially sensitive to alprostadil, and strips of lamb ductus markedly relax in the presence of the drug. In addition, administration of alprostadil reopened the closing ductus of newborn rats, rabbits, and lambs. These observations led to the investigation of alprostadil in infants who had congenital defects which restricted the pulmonary or systemic blood flow and who depended on a patent ductus arteriosus for adequate blood oxygenation and lower body perfusion.
In infants with restricted pulmonary blood flow, about 50% responded to alprostadil infusion with at least a 10 torr increase in blood pO_2 (mean increase about 14 torr and mean increase in oxygen saturation about 23%). In general, patients who responded best had low pretreatment blood pO_2 and were 4 days old or less.
In infants with restricted systemic blood flow, alprostadil often increased pH in those having acidosis, increased systemic blood pressure, and decreased the ratio of pulmonary artery pressure to aortic pressure.
Alprostadil must be infused continuously because it is very rapidly metabolized. As much as 80% of the circulating alprostadil may be metabolized in one pass through the lungs, primarily by β- and ω-oxidation. The metabolites are excreted primarily by the kidney, and excretion is essentially complete within 24 hours after administration. No unchanged alprostadil has been found in the urine, and there is no evidence of tissue retention of alprostadil or its metabolites.

INDICATIONS AND USAGE
PROSTIN VR PEDIATRIC Sterile Solution (alprostadil) is indicated for palliative, not definitive, therapy to temporarily maintain the patency of the ductus arteriosus until corrective or palliative surgery can be performed in neonates who have congenital heart defects and who depend upon the patent ductus for survival. Such congenital heart defects include pulmonary atresia, pulmonary stenosis, tricuspid atresia, tetralogy of Fallot, interruption of the aortic arch, coarctation of the aorta, or transposition of the great vessels with or without other defects.
In infants with restricted pulmonary blood flow, the increase in blood oxygenation is inversely proportional to pretreatment pO_2 values; that is, patients with low pO_2 values respond best, and patients with pO_2 values of 40 torr or more usually have little response.

PROSTIN VR PEDIATRIC should be administered only by trained personnel in facilities that provide pediatric intensive care.

CONTRAINDICATIONS
None.

WARNINGS
See WARNING box.

Note: PROSTIN VR PEDIATRIC Sterile Solution (alprostadil) must be diluted before it is administered. See dilution instructions in DOSAGE AND ADMINISTRATION section.

PRECAUTIONS

General Precautions
Cortical proliferation of the long bones, first observed in dogs, has also been observed in infants during long-term infusions of alprostadil. The cortical proliferation in infants regressed after withdrawal of the drug.

In infants treated with PROSTIN VR PEDIATRIC at the usual doses for 10 hours to 12 days and who died of causes unrelated to ductus structural weakness, tissue sections of the ductus and pulmonary arteries have shown intimal lacerations, a decrease in medial muscularity and disruption of the medial and internal elastic lamina. Localized and aneurysmal dilatations and vessel wall edema also were seen compared to a series of pathological specimens from infants not treated with PROSTIN VR PEDIATRIC. The incidence of such structural alterations has not been defined.

PROSTIN VR PEDIATRIC Sterile Solution (alprostadil) should be infused for the shortest time and at the lowest dose that will produce the desired effects. The risks of long-term infusion of PROSTIN VR PEDIATRIC should be weighed against the possible benefits that critically ill infants may derive from its administration.

Because alprostadil inhibits platelet aggregation, use PROSTIN VR PEDIATRIC cautiously in neonates with bleeding tendencies.

PROSTIN VR PEDIATRIC should not be used in neonates with respiratory distress syndrome. A differential diagnosis should be made between respiratory distress syndrome (hyaline membrane disease) and cyanotic heart disease (restricted pulmonary blood flow). If full diagnostic facilities are not immediately available, cyanosis (pO_2 less than 40 torr) and restricted pulmonary blood flow apparent on an X-ray are appropriate indicators of congenital heart defects.

Necessary Monitoring: In all neonates, arterial pressure should be monitored intermittently by umbilical artery catheter, auscultation, or with a Doppler transducer. *Should arterial pressure fall significantly, decrease the rate of infusion immediately.*

In infants with restricted pulmonary blood flow, measure efficacy of PROSTIN VR PEDIATRIC by monitoring improvement in blood oxygenation. In infants with restricted systemic blood flow, measure efficacy by monitoring improvement of systemic blood pressure and blood pH.

Drug Interactions: No drug interactions have been reported between PROSTIN VR PEDIATRIC and the therapy standard in neonates with restricted pulmonary or systemic blood flow. Standard therapy includes antibiotics, such as penicillin and gentamicin; vasopressors, such as dopamine and isoproterenol; cardiac glycosides; and diuretics, such as furosemide.

Carcinogenesis, Mutagenesis, and Impairment of Fertility: Long-term carcinogenicity studies and fertility studies have not been done. The Ames and Alkaline Elution assays reveal no potential for mutagenesis.

ADVERSE REACTIONS
Central Nervous System: Apnea has been reported in about 12% of the neonates treated. (See WARNING box.) Other common adverse reactions reported have been fever in about 14% of the patients treated and seizures in about 4%. The following reactions have been reported in less than 1% of the patients: cerebral bleeding, hyperextension of the neck, hyperirritability, hypothermia, jitteriness, lethargy, and stiffness.

Cardiovascular System: The most common adverse reactions reported have been flushing in about 10% of patients (more common after intraarterial dosing), bradycardia in about 7%, hypotension in about 4%, tachycardia in about 3%, cardiac arrest in about 1%, and edema in about 1%. The following reactions have been reported in less than 1% of the patients: congestive heart failure, hyperemia, second degree heart block, shock, spasm of the right ventricle infundibulum, supraventricular tachycardia, and ventricular fibrillation.

Respiratory System: The following reactions have been reported in less than 1% of the patients: bradypnea, bronchial wheezing, hypercapnia, respiratory depression, respiratory distress, and tachypnea.

Gastrointestinal System: The most common adverse reaction reported has been diarrhea in about 2% of the patients. The following reactions have been reported in less than 1% of the patients; gastric regurgitation, and hyperbilirubinemia.

Hematologic System: The most common hematologic event reported has been disseminated intravascular coagulation in about 1% of the patients. The following events have been reported in less than 1% of the patients: anemia, bleeding, and thrombocytopenia.

Excretory System: Anuria and hematuria have been reported in less than 1% of the patients.

Skeletal System: Cortical proliferation of the long bones has been reported. See PRECAUTIONS.

Miscellaneous: Sepsis has been reported in about 2% of the patients. Peritonitis has been reported in less than 1% of the patients. Hypokalemia has been reported in about 1%, and hypoglycemia and hyperkalemia have been reported in less than 1% of the patients.

OVERDOSAGE
Apnea, bradycardia, pyrexia, hypotension, and flushing may be signs of drug overdosage. If apnea or bradycardia occurs, discontinue the infusion, and provide appropriate medical treatment. Caution should be used in restarting the infusion. If pyrexia or hypotension occurs, reduce the infusion rate until these symptoms subside. Flushing is usually a result of incorrect intraarterial catheter placement, and the catheter should be repositioned.

DOSAGE AND ADMINISTRATION
The preferred route of administration for PROSTIN VR PEDIATRIC Sterile Solution (alprostadil) is continuous intravenous infusion into a large vein. Alternatively, PROSTIN VR PEDIATRIC may be administered through an umbilical artery catheter placed at the ductal opening. Increases in blood pO_2 (torr) have been the same in neonates who received the drug by either route of administration.

Begin infusion with 0.05 to 0.1 micrograms alprostadil per kilogram of body weight per minute. A starting dose of 0.1 micrograms per kilogram of body weight per minute is the recommended starting dose based on clinical studies; however, adequate clinical response has been reported using a starting dose of 0.05 micrograms per kilogram of body weight per minute. After a therapeutic response is achieved (increased pO_2 in infants with restricted pulmonary blood flow or increased systemic blood pressure and blood pH in infants with restricted systemic blood flow), reduce the infusion rate to provide the lowest possible dosage that maintains the response. This may be accomplished by reducing the dosage from 0.1 to 0.05 to 0.025 to 0.01 micrograms per kilogram of body weight per minute. If response to 0.05 micrograms per kilogram of body weight per minute is inadequate, dosage can be increased up to 0.4 micrograms per kilogram of body weight per minute although, in general, higher infusion rates do not produce greater effects.

Dilution instructions: To prepare infusion solutions, dilute 1 ml of PROSTIN VR PEDIATRIC Sterile Solution with Sodium Chloride Injection USP or Dextrose Injection USP. Dilute to volumes appropriate for the pump delivery system available. Prepare fresh infusion solutions every 24 hours. *Discard any solution more than 24 hours old.*

Sample Dilutions and Infusion Rates to
Provide a Dosage of 0.1 Micrograms per
Kilogram of Body Weight per Minute

Add 1 ampoule (500 micrograms) alprostadil to:	Approximate concentration of resulting solution (micrograms/ml)	Infusion rate (ml/min per kg of body weight)
250 ml	2	0.05
100 ml	5	0.02
50 ml	10	0.01
25 ml	20	0.005

Example: To provide 0.1 micrograms/kilogram of body weight per minute to an infant weighing 2.8 kilograms using a solution of 1 ampoule PROSTIN VR PEDIATRIC in 100 ml of saline or dextrose: INFUSION RATE = 0.02 ml/min per kg × 2.8 kg = 0.056 ml/min or 3.36 ml/hr.

HOW SUPPLIED
PROSTIN VR PEDIATRIC Sterile Solution (alprostadil) is available in packages of 5—1 ml ampoules (NDC 0009-3169-01). Each ml contains 500 micrograms alprostadil in dehydrated alcohol.

Store PROSTIN VR PEDIATRIC Sterile Solution in a refrigerator at 2°–8°C (36°–46°F).

Code 811 987 004

PROVERA®
brand of medroxyprogesterone acetate tablets, USP   ℞

WARNING

THE USE OF PROVERA (MEDROXYPROGESTERONE ACETATE) DURING THE FIRST FOUR MONTHS OF PREGNANCY IS NOT RECOMMENDED.

Progestational agents have been used beginning with the first trimester of pregnancy in an attempt to prevent habitual abortion. There is no adequate evidence that such use is effective when such drugs are given during the first four months of pregnancy. Furthermore, in the vast majority of women, the cause of abortion is a defective ovum, which progestational agents could not be expected to influence. In addition, the use of progestational agents with their uterine-relaxant properties, in patients with fertilized defective ova may cause a delay in spontaneous abortion. Therefore, the use of such drugs during the first four months of pregnancy is not recommended.

Several reports suggest an association between intrauterine exposure to progestational drugs in the first trimester of pregnancy and genital abnormalities in male and female fetuses. The risk of hypospadias, 5 to 8 per 1,000 male births in the general population, may be approximately doubled with exposure to these drugs. There are insufficient data to quantify the risk to exposed female fetuses, but insofar as some of these drugs induce mild virilization of the external genitalia of the female fetus, and because of the increased association of hypospadias in the male fetus, it is prudent to avoid the use of these drugs during the first trimester of pregnancy.

If the patient is exposed to PROVERA Tablets (medroxyprogesterone acetate) during the first four months of pregnancy or if she becomes pregnant while taking this drug, she should be apprised of the potential risks to the fetus.

DESCRIPTION
PROVERA Tablets contain medroxyprogesterone acetate, which is a derivative of progesterone. It is a white to off-white, odorless crystalline powder, stable in air, melting between 200 and 210° C. It is freely soluble in chloroform, soluble in acetone and in dioxane, sparingly soluble in alcohol and in methanol, slightly soluble in ether, and insoluble in water.

The chemical name for medroxyprogesterone acetate is Pregn-4-ene-3,20-dione, 17-(acetyloxy)-6-methyl-, (6α)-. The structural formula is:

Each PROVERA tablet for oral administration contains 2.5 mg, 5 mg or 10 mg of medroxyprogesterone acetate. Inactive ingredients: calcium stearate, corn starch, lactose, mineral oil, sorbic acid, sucrose, talc. The 2.5 mg tablet contains FD&C Yellow no. 6.

ACTIONS
Medroxyprogesterone acetate, administered orally or parenterally in the recommended doses to women with adequate endogenous estrogen, transforms proliferative into secretory endometrium. Androgenic and anabolic effects have been noted, but the drug is apparently devoid of significant estrogenic activity. While parenterally administered medroxyprogesterone acetate inhibits gonadotropin production, which in turn prevents follicular maturation and ovulation, available data indicate that this does not occur when the usually recommended oral dosage is given as single daily doses.

Continued on next page

Information on these Upjohn products is based on labeling in effect June 1, 1992. Further information concerning these and other Upjohn products may be obtained by direct inquiry to Medical Information, The Upjohn Company, Kalamazoo, Michigan 49001.

Upjohn—Cont.

INDICATIONS AND USAGE

Secondary amenorrhea; abnormal uterine bleeding due to hormonal imbalance in the absence of organic pathology, such as fibroids or uterine cancer.

CONTRAINDICATIONS

1. Thrombophlebitis, thromboembolic disorders, cerebral apoplexy or patients with a past history of these conditions.
2. Liver dysfunction or disease.
3. Known or suspected malignancy of breast or genital organs.
4. Undiagnosed vaginal bleeding.
5. Missed abortion.
6. As a diagnostic test for pregnancy.
7. Known sensitivity to PROVERA Tablets.

WARNINGS

1. The physician should be alert to the earliest manifestations of thrombotic disorders (thrombophlebitis, cerebrovascular disorders, pulmonary embolism, and retinal thrombosis). Should any of these occur or be suspected, the drug should be discontinued immediately.
2. Beagle dogs treated with medroxyprogesterone acetate developed mammary nodules some of which were malignant. Although nodules occasionally appeared in control animals, they were intermittent in nature, whereas the nodules in the drug-treated animals were larger, more numerous, persistent, and there were some breast malignancies with metastases. Their significance with respect to humans has not been established.
3. Discontinue medication pending examination if there is sudden partial or complete loss of vision, or if there is a sudden onset of proptosis, diplopia or migraine. If examination reveals papilledema or retinal vascular lesions, medication should be withdrawn.
4. Detectable amounts of progestin have been identified in the milk of mothers receiving the drug. The effect of this on the nursing infant has not been determined.
5. Usage in pregnancy is not recommended (See WARNING Box).
6. Retrospective studies of morbidity and mortality in Great Britain and studies of morbidity in the United States have shown a statistically significant association between thrombophlebitis, pulmonary embolism, and cerebral thrombosis and embolism and the use of oral contraceptives.[1-4] The estimate of the relative risk of thromboembolism in the study by Vessey and Doll[3] was about sevenfold, while Sartwell and associates[4] in the United States found a relative risk of 4.4, meaning that the users are several times as likely to undergo thromboembolic disease without evident cause as nonusers. The American study also indicated that the risk did not persist after discontinuation of administration, and that it was not enhanced by long continued administration. The American study was not designed to evaluate a difference between products.

PRECAUTIONS

1. The pretreatment physical examination should include special reference to breast and pelvic organs, as well as Papanicolaou smear.
2. Because progestogens may cause some degree of fluid retention, conditions which might be influenced by this factor, such as epilepsy, migraine, asthma, cardiac or renal dysfunction, require careful observation.
3. In cases of breakthrough bleeding, as in all cases of irregular bleeding per vaginum, nonfunctional causes should be borne in mind. In cases of undiagnosed vaginal bleeding, adequate diagnostic measures are indicated.
4. Patients who have a history of psychic depression should be carefully observed and the drug discontinued if the depression recurs to a serious degree.
5. Any possible influence of prolonged progestin therapy on pituitary, ovarian, adrenal, hepatic or uterine functions awaits further study.
6. A decrease in glucose tolerance has been observed in a small percentage of patients on estrogen-progestin combination drugs. The mechanism of this decrease is obscure. For this reason, diabetic patients should be carefully observed while receiving progestin therapy.
7. The age of the patient constitutes no absolute limiting factor although treatment with progestins may mask the onset of the climacteric.
8. The pathologist should be advised of progestin therapy when relevant specimens are submitted.
9. Because of the occasional occurrence of thrombotic disorders, (thrombophlebitis, pulmonary embolism, retinal thrombosis, and cerebrovascular disorders) in patients taking estrogen-progestin combinations and since the mechanism is obscure, the physician should be alert to the earliest manifestation of these disorders.
10. Studies of the addition of a progestin product to an estrogen replacement regimen for seven or more days of a

cycle of estrogen administration have reported a lowered incidence of endometrial hyperplasia. Morphological and biochemical studies of endometrium suggest that 10–13 days of a progestin are needed to provide maximal maturation of the endometrium and to eliminate any hyperplastic changes. Whether this will provide protection from endometrial carcinoma has not been clearly established. There are possible additional risks which may be associated with the inclusion of progestin in estrogen replacement regimen. The potential risks include adverse effects on carbohydrate and lipid metabolism. The dosage used may be important in minimizing these adverse effects.
11. Aminoglutethimide administered concomitantly with PROVERA may significantly depress the bioavailability of PROVERA.

Carcinogenesis, Mutagenesis, Impairment of Fertility.
Long-term intramuscular administration of PROVERA has been shown to produce mammary tumors in beagle dogs (see WARNINGS). There was no evidence of a carcinogenic effect associated with the oral administration of PROVERA to rats and mice. Medroxyprogesterone acetate was not mutagenic in a battery of in vitro or in vivo genetic toxicity assays. Medroxyprogesterone acetate at high doses is an antifertility drug and high doses would be expected to impair fertility until the cessation of treatment.

Information for the Patient
See Patient Information at the end of insert.

ADVERSE REACTIONS

Pregnancy—(See WARNING Box for possible adverse effects on the fetus).
Breast—Breast tenderness or galactorrhea has been reported rarely.
Skin—Sensitivity reactions consisting of urticaria, pruritus, edema and generalized rash have occurred in an occasional patient. Acne, alopecia and hirsutism have been reported in a few cases.
Thromboembolic Phenomena—Thromboembolic phenomena including thrombophlebitis and pulmonary embolism have been reported.
The following adverse reactions have been observed in women taking progestins including PROVERA Tablets:
breakthrough bleeding
spotting
change in menstrual flow
amenorrhea
edema
change in weight (increase or decrease)
changes in cervical erosion and cervical secretions
cholestatic jaundice
anaphylactoid reactions and anaphylaxis
rash (allergic) with and without pruritus
mental depression
pyrexia
insomnia
nausea
somnolence
A statistically significant association has been demonstrated between use of estrogen-progestin combination drugs and the following serious adverse reactions: thrombophlebitis; pulmonary embolism and cerebral thrombosis and embolism. For this reason patients on progestin therapy should be carefully observed.
Although available evidence is suggestive of an association, such a relationship has been neither confirmed nor refuted for the following serious adverse reactions:
neuro-ocular lesions, eg, retinal thrombosis and optic neuritis.
The following adverse reactions have been observed in patients receiving estrogen-progestin combination drugs:
rise in blood pressure in susceptible individuals
premenstrual-like syndrome
changes in libido
changes in appetite
cystitis-like syndrome
headache
nervousness
fatigue
backache
hirsutism
loss of scalp hair
erythema multiforme
erythema nodosum
hemorrhagic eruption
itching
dizziness
In view of these observations, patients on progestin therapy should be carefully observed.
The following laboratory results may be altered by the use of estrogen-progestin combination drugs:
Increased sulfobromophthalein retention and other hepatic function tests.
Coagulation tests: increase in prothrombin factors VII, VIII, IX and X.

Metyrapone test.
Pregnanediol determination.
Thyroid function: increase in PBI, and butanol extractable protein bound iodine and decrease in T[3] uptake values.

DOSAGE AND ADMINISTRATION

Secondary Amenorrhea—PROVERA Tablets may be given in dosages of 5 to 10 mg daily for from 5 to 10 days. A dose for inducing an optimum secretory transformation of an endometrium that has been adequately primed with either endogenous or exogenous estrogen is 10 mg of PROVERA daily for 10 days. In cases of secondary amenorrhea, therapy may be started at any time. Progestin withdrawal bleeding usually occurs within three to seven days after discontinuing PROVERA therapy.
Abnormal Uterine Bleeding Due to Hormonal Imbalance in the Absence of Organic Pathology—Beginning on the calculated 16th or 21st day of the menstrual cycle, 5 to 10 mg of medroxyprogesterone acetate may be given daily for from 5 to 10 days. To produce an optimum secretory transformation of an endometrium that has been adequately primed with either endogenous or exogenous estrogen, 10 mg of medroxyprogesterone acetate daily for 10 days beginning on the 16th day of the cycle is suggested. Progestin withdrawal bleeding usually occurs within three to seven days after discontinuing therapy with PROVERA. Patients with a past history of recurrent episodes of abnormal uterine bleeding may benefit from planned menstrual cycling with PROVERA.

HOW SUPPLIED

PROVERA Tablets are available in the following strengths and package sizes:
2.5 mg (scored, round, orange)

Bottles of 30	NDC 0009-0064-06
Bottles of 100	NDC 0009-0064-04

5 mg (scored, hexagonal, white)

Bottles of 30	NDC 0009-0286-32
Bottles of 100	NDC 0009-0286-03

10 mg (scored, round, white)

Bottles of 30	NDC 0009-0050-09
Bottles of 100	NDC 0009-0050-02
Bottles of 500	NDC 0009-0050-11
DOSEPAK™ Unit of Use (10)	NDC 0009-0050-12

Store at controlled room temperature 15°–30°C (59°–86°F).

REFERENCES

1. Royal College of General Practitioners: Oral contraception and thromboembolic disease. J Coll Gen Pract **13**:267–279, 1967.
2. Inman WHW, Vessey MP: Investigation of deaths from pulmonary, coronary, and cerebral thrombosis and embolism in women of child-bearing age. Br Med J **2**:193–199, 1968.
3. Vessey MP, Doll R: Investigation of relation between use of oral contraceptives and thromboembolic disease. A further report. Br Med J **2**:651–657, 1969.
4. Sartwell PE, Masi AT, Arthes FG, et al: Thromboembolism and oral contraceptives: An epidemiological case-control study. Am J Epidemiol **90**:365–380, 1969.

The text of the patient insert for progesterone and progesterone-like drugs is set forth below.

PATIENT INFORMATION

PROVERA Tablets contain medroxyprogesterone acetate, a progesterone. The information below is that which the U.S. Food and Drug Administration requires be provided for all patients taking progesterones. The information below relates only to the risk to the unborn child associated with use of progesterone during pregnancy. For further information on the use, side effects and other risks associated with this product, ask your doctor.

WARNING FOR WOMEN

Progesterone or progesterone-like drugs have been used to prevent miscarriage in the first few months of pregnancy. No adequate evidence is available to show that they are effective for this purpose. Furthermore, most cases of early miscarriage are due to causes which could not be helped by these drugs.
There is an increased risk of minor birth defects in children whose mothers take this drug during the first 4 months of pregnancy. Several reports suggest an association between mothers who take these drugs in the first trimester of pregnancy and genital abnormalities in male and female babies. The risk to the male baby is the possibility of being born with a condition in which the opening of the penis is on the underside rather than the tip of the penis (hypospadias). Hypospadias occurs in about 5 to 8 per 1,000 male births and is about doubled with exposure to these drugs. There is not enough information to quantify the risk to exposed female fetuses, but enlargement of the clitoris and fusion of the labia may occur, although rarely.
Therefore, since drugs of this type may induce mild masculinization of the external genitalia of the female fetus, as well as hypospadias in the male fetus, it is wise to avoid using the drug during the first trimester of pregnancy.
These drugs have also been used as a test for pregnancy but such use is no longer considered safe because of possible dam-

age to a developing baby. Also, more rapid methods for testing for pregnancy are now available.

If you take PROVERA and later find you were pregnant when you took it, be sure to discuss this with your doctor as soon as possible.

Caution: Federal law prohibits dispensing without prescription.

The Upjohn Company
Kalamazoo, MI 49001, USA
Revised January 1992 812 584 409
691015

Shown in Product Identification Section, page 434

ROGAINE® ℞
brand of minoxidil topical solution
2%
For Topical Use
2%, 60 ml bottle **NSN 6505-01-290-4660**

DESCRIPTION

ROGAINE Topical Solution is a hair growth stimulant. ROGAINE contains the active ingredient minoxidil. Minoxidil appears as a white or off-white, odorless crystalline solid that is soluble in water to the extent of approximately 2 mg/mL, is readily soluble in propylene glycol or ethanol, and is almost insoluble in acetone, chloroform or ethyl acetate.

The chemical name for minoxidil is 2,4-pyrimidinediamine, 6-(l-piperidinyl)-, 3-oxide (MW = 209.25). The structural formula is represented below:

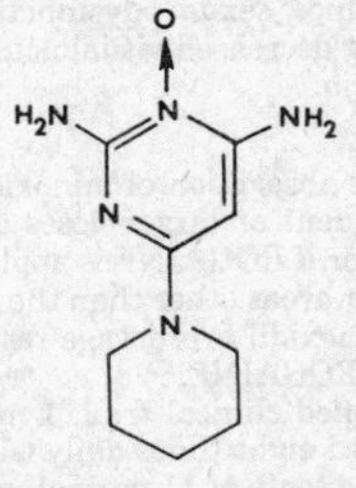

ROGAINE Topical Solution is available at a concentration of 2% (20 mg minoxidil per milliliter) in a solution of alcohol 60% v/v, propylene glycol, and water.

CLINICAL PHARMACOLOGY

Pharmacologic Properties and Pharmacokinetics

ROGAINE Topical Solution stimulates hair growth in individuals with androgenetic alopecia, expressed in males as baldness of the vertex of the scalp and in females as diffuse hair loss or thinning of the frontoparietal areas. The mechanism by which minoxidil stimulates hair growth is not known but like minoxidil some other arterial dilating drugs also stimulate hair growth when given systemically.

Because of its serious side effects oral minoxidil is indicated only for the treatment of hypertension that is symptomatic or associated with target organ damage and is not manageable with maximum therapeutic doses of a diuretic plus two other antihypertensive drugs. It is a direct acting peripheral arterial dilator that reduces blood pressure by decreasing peripheral vascular resistance. Reduction of peripheral arteriolar resistance and the resulting fall in blood pressure trigger sympathetic, vagal inhibitory, and renal homeostatic mechanisms, including increased renin secretion, that lead to increased heart rate and cardiac output and salt and water retention.

The major side effects of oral minoxidil, aside from unwelcome generalized hair growth, result from fluid retention, often profound, and tachycardia, and require that minoxidil be administered in most cases with a beta-blocker or other agent to reduce heart rate and a diuretic, almost always a high ceiling (loop) diuretic. Fluid retention can lead to marked weight gain, local or generalized edema, heart failure, and pleural or pericardial effusion, including cardiac tamponade. Pericarditis has been reported, usually in patients with renal failure or collagen vascular disease, but in some cases these causes of pericarditis do not seem to have been present. The tachycardia and increased cardiac output caused by minoxidil can lead to exacerbation of existing angina or the onset of angina in persons with compromised coronary circulation. It is these serious side effects that have restricted use of oral minoxidil to patients with severe hypertension not controllable with other agents.

In placebo controlled trials involving over 3500 male patients given topical minoxidil for 4 months (longer treatment was given after the placebo group was discontinued), and in over 300 female patients given topical minoxidil for eight months, the typical systemic effects of oral minoxidil (weight gain, edema, tachycardia, fall in blood pressure, and their more serious consequences) were not seen more frequently in patients given topical minoxidil than in those given topical placebo (See ADVERSE REACTIONS). The mean changes from baseline in weight, heart rate, and blood pressure in the treated and placebo groups were similar, and the number of patients experiencing significant changes, such as a blood pressure decrease of 15 mmHg or more diastolic or 30 mmHg or more systolic, a heart rate increase of 15 beats/minute or more, or weight gain of at least 5 pounds, was also similar.

In an effort to explore the potential for systemic effects of topical minoxidil, three concentrations of topical minoxidil (1, 2 and 5%) applied twice daily were compared to low oral doses (2.5 and 5 mg given once daily), and placebo in hypertensive patients (normotensive patients have little or no blood pressure response to minoxidil at dose of 10 mg per day) in a double-blind controlled trial. The 5 mg oral dose had readily detectable effects, a fall in diastolic pressure of about 5 mmHg and an increase in heart rate of 7 beats/minute. No other group had a clear effect, although there was some evidence of a weak and inconsistent effect in the 2.5 mg oral, and possibly the 5% topical, treatments.

The failure to detect evidence of systemic effects during treatment with topical minoxidil reflects the poor absorption of topical minoxidil, which averages about 1.4% (range 0.3 to 4.5%) from normal intact scalp, and was about 2% in the hypertensive patients, whose scalps were shaved.

In a comparison of topical and oral absorption, peak serum levels of unchanged minoxidil after 1 mL b.i.d. of 2% minoxidil solution (the maximum recommended dose) averaged 5.8% (range 1.4% to 12.7%) of the level observed after 2.5 mg b.i.d. oral doses (5 mg is the recommended starting dose of oral minoxidil). Similarly, in the hypertension study, where patients had shaved scalps, mean minoxidil concentrations after 1 mL b.i.d. of 2% topical minoxidil (1.7 ng/mL) were 1/20 the concentrations seen after daily oral doses of 2.5 mg (32.8 ng/mL) or 5 mg (59.2 ng/mL). Blood levels obtained in the large controlled hair growth trials averaged less than 2 ng/mL for the 2% solution. There were, however, occasional values that were higher; about 1% of the patients on 2% minoxidil had serum levels of 5 ng/mL or greater and a few approached 30 ng/mL. It is possible, therefore, that if more than the recommended dose were applied to inflamed skin in an individual with relatively high absorption, blood levels with systemic effects might rarely be obtained. Physicians and patients need to be aware of the possibility.

Serum minoxidil levels resulting from administration of ROGAINE are governed by the drug's percutaneous absorption rate. Following cessation of topical dosing of ROGAINE approximately 95% of systemically absorbed minoxidil is eliminated within four days. The metabolic biotransformation of minoxidil absorbed following administration of ROGAINE has not been fully determined.

Minoxidil absorbed following oral administration is metabolized predominantly by conjugation with glucuronic acid at the N-oxide position in the pyrimidine ring but also by conversion to more polar products. Known metabolites exert much less pharmacologic effect than the parent compound. Minoxidil and its metabolites are excreted principally in the urine. Minoxidil does not bind to plasma proteins and its renal clearance corresponds to the glomerular filtration rate. Minoxidil does not enter the central nervous system (CNS) of experimental animals in significant amounts and it does not affect CNS function in man.

Cardiac Lesions in Animals

Minoxidil produces several cardiac lesions in animals. Some are characteristic of agents that cause tachycardia and diastolic hypotension (beta-agonists like isoproterenol, arterial dilators like hydralazine) while others are produced by a narrower range of agents with arterial dilating properties. The significance of these lesions for humans is not clear, as they have not been recognized in patients treated with oral minoxidil at systemically active doses, despite formal review of over 150 autopsies of treated patients.

(a) Papillary muscle/subendocardial necrosis
The most characteristic lesion of minoxidil, seen in rat, dog, and minipig (but not monkeys) is focal necrosis of the papillary muscle and subendocardial areas of the left ventricle. These lesions appear rapidly, within a few days of treatment with doses of 0.5 to 10 mg/kg/day in the dog and minipig, and are not progressive, although they leave residual scars. They are similar to lesions produced by other peripheral arterial dilators, by theobromine, and by beta-adrenergic receptor agonists such as isoproterenol, epinephrine, and albuterol. The lesions are thought to reflect ischemia provoked by increased oxygen demand (tachycardia, increased cardiac output) and relative decrease in coronary flow (decreased diastolic pressure and decreased time in diastole) caused by the vasodilatory effects of these agents coupled with reflex or directly induced tachycardia.

(b) Hemorrhagic lesions
After acute oral minoxidil treatment (0.5 to 10 mg/kg/day) in dogs and minipigs, hemorrhagic lesions are seen in many parts of the heart, mainly in the epicardium, endocardium, and walls of small coronary arteries and arterioles. In minipigs the lesions occur primarily in the left atrium while in dogs they are most prominent in the right atrium, frequently appearing as grossly visible hemorrhagic lesions. With exposure of 1–20 mg/kg/day in the dog for 30 days or longer, there is replacement of myocardial cells by proliferating fibroblasts and angioblasts, hemorrhage and hemosiderin accumulation. These lesions can be produced by topical minoxidil administration that gives systemic absorption of 0.5 to 1 mg/kg/day. Other peripheral dilators, including an experimental agent, nicorandil, and theobromine, have produced similar lesions.

(c) Epicarditis
A less fully studied lesion is focal epicarditis, seen in dogs after 2 days of oral minoxidil. More recently, chronic proliferative epicarditis was observed in dogs treated topically twice a day for 90 days. In a one year oral dog study, serosanguinous percardial fluid was seen.

(d) Hypertrophy and Dilation
Oral and topical studies in rats, dogs, monkeys (oral only), and rabbits (dermal only) show cardiac hypertrophy and dilation. This is presumed to represent the consequences of prolonged fluid overload; there is preliminary evidence in monkeys that diuretics partly reverse these effects.

Autopsies of over 150 patients who died of various causes after receiving oral minoxidil for hypertension have not revealed the characteristics hemorrhagic (especially atrial) lesions seen in dogs and minipigs. While areas of papillary muscle and subendocardial necrosis were occasionally seen, they occurred in the presence of known pre-existing coronary artery disease and were also seen in patients never exposed to minoxidil in another series using similar, but not identical, autopsy methods.

CLINICAL TRIAL EXPERIENCE—MALES

In clinical trials in **males**, three main parameters of efficacy were used: hair counts in a one inch diameter circle on the vertex of the scalp; investigator evaluation of terminal hair regrowth; and patient evaluation of hair regrowth. At the end of four-month placebo-controlled portions of 12-month clinical studies (ie, baseline to Month 4), ROGAINE Topical Solution (20 mg minoxidil per mL) demonstrated the following efficacy:

A. Hair Counts
ROGAINE was significantly more effective than placebo in producing hair regrowth as assessed by hair counts. Patients using ROGAINE had a mean increase from baseline of 72 non-vellus hairs in the one inch diameter circle compared with a mean increase of 39 non-vellus hairs in patients using the placebo ($P < 0.0005$).

B. Investigator Evaluation
Based on the investigators' evaluation, there was no statistically significant difference in terminal hair regrowth between treatment groups. Eight percent (8%) of the patients using ROGAINE demonstrated moderate to dense terminal hair regrowth compared with 4% using the placebo. During the initial four months of treatment, however, very little regrowth of terminal hair can be expected. Although most patients did not demonstrate cosmetically significant regrowth of hair, 26% of the patients showed minimal terminal hair regrowth using ROGAINE compared with 16% of those using placebo as assessed by the investigator.

C. Patient Evaluation
Based on the patients' self-evaluation, 26% using ROGAINE demonstrated moderate to dense hair regrowth compared with 11% using the placebo ($P < 0.0005$).

Patients who continued on ROGAINE during the remaining eight months of the 12-month clinical studies (ie, the non-placebo-controlled portion of the studies) continued to sustain a regrowth response as evaluated by hair counts, investigator evaluation, and patient evaluation.

At the end of the eight month non-placebo-controlled portion of the 12-month clinical studies (ie, Months 4 to 12), the following results were obtained.

A. Hair Count
Patients using ROGAINE had a mean increase of 112 non-vellus hairs in the same one inch diameter circle as compared to Month 4 ($P < 0.0005$).

B. Investigator Evaluation
Based on the investigators' evaluation, 39% of the patients achieved moderate to dense terminal hair by Month 12.

C. Patient Evaluation
Based on the patients' assessment, 48% felt they had achieved moderate to dense hair regrowth at Month 12.

Trends in the data suggest that those patients who are older, who have been balding for a longer period of time, or who have a larger area of baldness, may do less well.

Continued on next page

Information on these Upjohn products is based on labeling in effect June 1, 1992. Further information concerning these and other Upjohn products may be obtained by direct inquiry to Medical Information, The Upjohn Company, Kalamazoo, Michigan 49001.

Upjohn—Cont.

CLINICAL TRIAL EXPERIENCE—FEMALES

In clinical trials in **females** (age range 18–45 years, 90% who were Caucasian) with Ludwig grade I and II diffuse frontoparietal hair thinning, the main parameters of efficacy were: non-vellus hair counts in a designated 1.0 cm^2 site on the frontoparietal areas of the scalp; investigator evaluation of hair regrowth; and patient evaluation of hair regrowth. Data demonstrate that 44% to 63% (investigators' evaluation from the international and US multicenter trials, respectively) of women with androgenetic alopecia will have discernible growth of non-vellus hair when treated with ROGAINE for 32 weeks versus 29% to 39% for vehicle control treated women.

Two 8-month placebo-controlled studies in females (US multicenter trial and an international multicenter trial) produced the following results:

A. Hair Counts. ROGAINE was significantly more effective than placebo in producing hair regrowth as assessed by hair counts in both studies. Patients using ROGAINE had a mean increase from baseline of 22.7 and 33.2 non-vellus hairs, respectively, in the same 1.0 cm^2 site compared with a mean increase of 11.0 and 19.1 non-vellus hairs, respectively, in patients using placebo (p=0.0004 and p=0.0001, respectively).

B. Investigator Evaluation. Based on the investigators' evaluation 63% (13% moderate and 50% minimal) and 44% (12% moderate and 32% minimal), respectively, of the patients using ROGAINE in the two studies achieved hair regrowth at Week-32, compared with 39% (6% moderate and 33% minimal) and 29% (5% moderate and 24% minimal), respectively, of those using placebo (p < 0.0005 and p=0.008, respectively).

C. Patient Evaluation. Based on the patients' self evaluation, 59% (19% moderate and 40% minimal) and 55% (1% dense, 24% moderate, and 30% minimal), respectively, of the patients using ROGAINE reported hair regrowth at Week-32, compared with 40% (7% moderate and 33% minimal) and 41% (12% moderate and 29% minimal), respectively, of those using placebo (p=0.002 and p=0.013, respectively).

Hair growth was defined as follows:

Investigator Evaluation of Growth:
No visible new hair growth
Minimal growth: Definite growth but no substantial covering of thinning areas.
Moderate growth: New growth partially covering thinning areas, less dense than non-thinning areas (readily discernible)
Dense Growth: Full covering of thinning areas; density of hair similar to non-thinning areas

Patient Evaluation of Growth:
No visible hair growth
Minimal hair growth: Barely discernible
Moderate new hair growth: Readily discernible
Dense new hair growth

INDICATIONS AND USAGE

ROGAINE Topical Solution is indicated for the treatment of androgenetic alopecia, expressed in males as baldness of the vertex of the scalp and in females as diffuse hair loss or thinning of the frontoparietal areas. At least four months of twice daily applications of ROGAINE are generally required before evidence of hair growth can be expected.

CONTRAINDICATIONS

ROGAINE Topical Solution is contraindicated in those patients with a history of hypersensitivity to any of the components of the preparation.

WARNINGS

1. Need for normal scalp
The majority of clinical studies included only healthy patients with normal scalps and no cardiovascular disease. Before starting a patient on ROGAINE, the physician should ascertain that the patient has a healthy, normal scalp. Local abrasion or dermatitis may increase absorption and hence increase the risk of side effects.
2. Potential adverse effects
Although extensive use of topical minoxidil has not revealed evidence that enough minoxidil is absorbed to have systemic effects, greater absorption because of misuse or individual variability or unusual sensitivity could lead, at least theoretically, to a systemic effect, and physicians and patients need to be aware of this.
Experience with oral minoxidil has shown the following major cardiovascular effects (the package insert for LONITEN®, minoxidil tablets, should be reviewed for details):

—salt and water retention, generalized and local edema
—pericardial effusion, pericarditis, tamponade
—tachycardia
—increased frequency of angina or new onset of angina
If systemic effects were to occur, patients with underlying heart disease, including coronary artery disease and congestive heart failure, would be at particular risk. Minoxidil could also have additive effects with other therapy in patients being treated for hypertension.
Patients being considered for ROGAINE Topical Solution should have a history and physical examination. Patients should be advised of the potential risk and a decision should be made by the patient and physician that the benefits outweigh the risks. Patients with a history of underlying heart disease should be aware that adverse effects in them might be especially serious. Patients should be alerted to the possibility of tachycardia and fluid retention and should watch for, and be monitored for, increased heart rate and weight gain or other systemic effects.

PRECAUTIONS

General Precautions
Patients treated with ROGAINE Topical Solution should be monitored one month after starting ROGAINE and at least every six months thereafter. If systemic effects should occur, discontinue use of ROGAINE.
ROGAINE contains an alcohol base which will cause burning and irritation of the eye. In the event of accidental contact with sensitive surfaces (eye, abraded skin, and mucous membranes), the area should be bathed with large amounts of cool tap water.
Inhalation of the spray mist should be avoided.
ROGAINE should not be used in conjunction with other topical agents including topical corticosteroids, retinoids, and petrolatum or agents that are known to enhance cutaneous drug absorption.
ROGAINE is for Topical Use Only. Each milliliter of ROGAINE contains 20 mg minoxidil. Accidental ingestion of the solution could lead to possible adverse systemic effects (see OVERDOSAGE.)
As is the case with other topically applied drugs, decreased integrity of the epidermal barrier caused by inflammation or disease processes in the skin (eg, excoriations of the scalp, scalp psoriasis, or severe sunburn) may increase percutaneous absorption of minoxidil.

Information for the Patient
A patient information leaflet has been prepared and is included with each package of ROGAINE. The text of the leaflet is printed at the end of this insert.

Drug Interactions
There are currently no known drug interactions associated with the use of ROGAINE Topical Solution. Although it has not been clinically demonstrated, there exists the theoretical possibility of absorbed minoxidil potentiating orthostatic hypotension in patients concurrently taking guanethidine.

Carcinogenesis, Mutagenesis, and Impairment of Fertility
No evidence of carcinogenicity was detected in rats and rabbits when ROGAINE Topical Solution was applied to the skin for up to one year. Dietary administration of minoxidil to mice for up to 24 months was associated with an increased incidence of malignant lymphomas in females and an increased incidence of hepatic nodules in males. The lymphoma incidence was unrelated to dose levels and at all doses was within the range seen in control groups from other studies employing mice from the same colony. The incidence of hepatic nodules was dose dependent, with a significant increase observed at 63 but not at 25 or 10 mg/kg/day. There was no effect of drug on the incidence of malignant tumors of the liver. As with the lymphomas, the incidence of hepatic nodules was within the historical control range for the subject mouse colony. No evidence of carcinogenic potential was obtained from a dietary administration study of minoxidil in rats. However, the rat study involved only ⅓ the number of animals and half the maximum dosage level evaluated in the mouse experiment, and shorter durations of administration (up to 15 months in males and up to 22 months in females). Minoxidil was not mutagenic in the salmonella (Ames) test, the DNA damage/alkaline elution assay or the rat micronucleus test.
In a study in which male and female rats received one or five times the maximum recommended human oral antihypertensive dose of minoxidil (multiples based on a 50 kg patient) there was a dose-dependent reduction in conception rate.

Pregnancy
Pregnancy Category C. Adequate and well-controlled studies have not been conducted in pregnant women treated with ROGAINE Topical Solution nor in pregnant women treated with oral minoxidil for hypertension. Oral administration of minoxidil has been associated with evidence of increased fetal resorption in rabbits, but not rats, when administered at five times the oral antihypertensive human dose. There was no evidence of teratogenic effects of ORALLY administered minoxidil in rats or rabbits. Subcutaneous administration of minoxidil to pregnant rats at 80 mg/kg/day (approximately 2000 times the maximal systemic human exposure from daily topical administration) was maternally toxic but

not teratogenic. Higher subcutaneous doses produced evidence of developmental toxicity. ROGAINE should not be administered to pregnant women.

Labor and Delivery
The effects on labor and delivery are unknown.

Nursing Mothers
There has been one report of minoxidil excretion in the breast milk of a woman treated with 5 mg oral minoxidil twice daily for hypertension. Because of the potential for adverse effects in nursing infants from minoxidil absorption, ROGAINE should not be administered to a nursing woman.

Pediatric Use
Safety and effectiveness in patients under 18 years of age have not been established.

Post-Menopausal Use
Efficacy in post-menopausal women has not been studied.

ADVERSE REACTIONS

ROGAINE Topical Solution has been used by 3,857 patients (347 females) enrolled in placebo-controlled trials. The rate of adverse events, grouped by body system, is shown in the following table. Except dermatologic events, which were more common in the minoxidil group, no individual reaction or body system grouping seemed to be increased in the minoxidil-treated group.
[See table on next page.]
Patients have been followed for up to 5 years and there has been no change in incidence or severity of reported reactions. Additional events reported in postmarketing clinical experience include:

eczema, hypertrichosis, local erythema, pruritus, dry skin/scalp flaking, sexual dysfunction, visual disturbances including decreased visual acuity, exacerbation of hair loss, alopecia.

OVERDOSAGE

Increased systemic absorption of minoxidil may potentially occur if more frequent or larger doses of ROGAINE (than directed) are used or if ROGAINE is applied to large surface areas of the body or areas other than the scalp. There are no known cases of minoxidil overdosage resulting from topical administration of ROGAINE.
In a 14-day controlled clinical trial, 1 mL of 3% minoxidil solution was applied eight times daily (six times the recommended dose) to the scalp of 11 normal male volunteers and to the chest of 11 other volunteers. No significant systemic effects were observed in these subjects when compared with a similar number of placebo-treated subjects. All subjects in the study were monitored for vital sign, electrocardiographic, and echocardiographic changes.
In a reported case of accidental ingestion, a 3-year-old male swallowed 1 to 2 mL of a 3% concentration of topical minoxidil solution. After vomiting he was treated in an emergency room. The child was found to be alert and active with no obvious signs of distress. His temperature was 37° C, pulse 152 bpm, respiration 32, and systolic blood pressure 110 by palpation. Cardiovascular, chest, lungs, abdomen, head, skin, and neurological examinations were normal. Blood levels taken indicated a total minoxidil level (glucuronide and unchanged) of 320.6 ng/mL. The child was discharged without sequelae.
Because of the high concentration of minoxidil in ROGAINE Topical Solution, accidental ingestion has the potential of producing systemic effects related to the pharmacologic action of the drug (5 mL of ROGAINE Topical Solution contains 100 mg minoxidil, the maximum adult dose for oral minoxidil administration when used to treat hypertension). Signs and symptoms of minoxidil overdosage would most likely be cardiovascular effects associated with fluid retention and tachycardia. Fluid retention can be managed with appropriate diuretic therapy. Clinically significant tachycardia can be controlled by administration of a beta-adrenergic blocking agent. If encountered, hypotension should be treated by intravenous administration of normal saline. Sympathomimetic drugs, such as norepinephrine and epinephrine, should be avoided because of their excessive cardiac stimulating activity.
Oral LD$_{50}$ in rats has ranged from 1321 to 3492 mg/kg; in mice 2457 to 2648 mg/kg. Minoxidil and its metabolites are hemodialyzable.

DOSAGE AND ADMINISTRATION

Hair and scalp should be dry prior to topical application of ROGAINE Topical Solution. A dose of 1 mL ROGAINE Topical Solution should be applied to the total affected areas of the scalp twice daily. The total daily dosage should not exceed 2 mL. If finger tips are used to facilitate drug application, hands should be washed afterwards. Twice daily application for four months or longer may be required before evidence of hair regrowth is observed. Onset and degree of hair regrowth may be variable among patients. If hair regrowth is realized, twice daily applications of ROGAINE appear necessary for additional or continued hair regrowth. Some anecdotal patient reports indicate that regrown hair and the balding process return to their untreated state three to four months following cessation of the drug.

HOW SUPPLIED

ROGAINE Topical Solution is a clear, colorless to light yellow solution containing 20 mg minoxidil per mL in a 60 mL bottle and is available as:

one—60 mL bottle with applicators ....NDC 0009-3367-05
three—60 mL bottles with applicators ...NDC 0009-3367-19
Store at controlled room temperature: 15° to 30° C (59°–86° F).

CAUTION

Federal law prohibits dispensing without a prescription.

IMPORTANT INFORMATION ABOUT—
ROGAINE® Topical Solution (minoxidil 2%)

Your doctor has prescribed ROGAINE Topical Solution for you to use as a hair regrowth stimulant to treat alopecia androgenetica (hair loss). ROGAINE is a prescription medication and therefore should be used only as directed by your doctor.

Please read this booklet thoroughly. It will help you to understand ROGAINE Topical Solution and what to expect from its use. If you have any questions after reading this booklet, or anytime during treatment with ROGAINE, you should consult your doctor or ask your pharmacist.

What is ROGAINE?

ROGAINE Topical Solution, discovered and made by The Upjohn Company, is a standardized topical (for use only on the skin) prescription medication proved effective for the treatment of alopecia androgenetica (hair loss).

ROGAINE is a topical solution of minoxidil. Minoxidil in tablet form has been used since 1980 to lower blood pressure. The use of *minoxidil tablets* is limited to treatment of patients with severe high blood pressure. When a high enough dosage in tablet form is used to lower blood pressure, certain effects that merit your attention may occur. These effects appear to be dose related. (See [What are the potential side effects on the heart and circulation when using ROGAINE?])

Persons who use ROGAINE Topical Solution have a low level of absorption of minoxidil, much lower than that of persons being treated with *minoxidil tablets* for high blood pressure. Therefore, the likelihood that a person using ROGAINE Topical Solution will develop the effects associated with *minoxidil tablets* is very small. In fact, none of these effects has been directly attributed to ROGAINE in clinical studies.

Exactly how ROGAINE works to stimulate hair regrowth in some people is not known. Upjohn scientists are doing research in this area.

How effective is ROGAINE?
Males

Clinical studies with ROGAINE were conducted by physicians in 27 U.S. medical centers involving over 2,300 patients with male pattern baldness involving the top (vertex) of the head. At the end of four months, hair counts showed that on average, the patients using ROGAINE Topical Solution had significantly more hair regrowth than those who used placebo (a similar solution without the active medication).

Based on the patients' self evaluation at the end of four months, 59% of the patients using ROGAINE had minimal to dense hair growth compared with 42% of those using placebo. Below is a bar chart illustrating patients' self evaluation of hair regrowth.

Male Results
Patient Self Evaluation of
Hair Regrowth at 4 Months
Combined Results of
27 U.S. Medical Centers

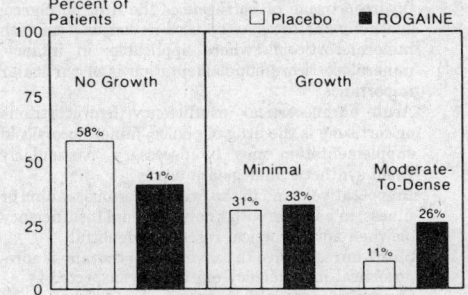

By the end of one year, 48% of the people who continued in the study using ROGAINE rated their hair growth as moderate or better.

Females

Clinical studies with ROGAINE were conducted by physicians in eleven U.S. and ten European medical centers involving over 600 female patients with hair loss. Based on actual hair counts, the women using ROGAINE had significantly more hair regrowth at the end of eight months than those who used placebo (a similar solution without the active medication).

MEDICAL EVENT PERCENT OCCURRENCE BY BODY SYSTEM IN THE PLACEBO-CONTROL CLINICAL TRIALS INVOLVING MINOXIDIL TOPICAL SOLUTION—ALL PATIENTS ENROLLED

BODY SYSTEM	MINOXIDIL SOLN N=3857 (4–8 months) # PATS.	% OCC.	PLACEBO N=2717 (4–8 months) # PATS.	% OCC.
DERMATOLOGICAL (irritant dermatitis, allergic contact dermatitis)	284	7.36	1.47	5.41
RESPIRATORY (bronchitis, upper respiratory infection, sinusitis)	276	7.16	233	8.58
GASTROINTESTINAL (diarrhea, nausea, vomiting)	167	4.33	178	6.55
NEUROLOGY (headache, dizziness, faintness, lightheadedness)	132	3.42	94	3.46
MUSCULOSKELETAL (fractures, back pain, tendinitis, aches and pains)	100	2.59	60	2.21
CARDIOVASCULAR (edema, chest pain, blood pressure increases/decreases, palpitations, pulse rate increases/decreases)	59	1.53	42	1.55
ALLERGY (non-specific allergic reactions, hives, allergic rhinitis, facial swelling, and sensitivity)	49	1.27	26	0.96
METABOLIC-NUTRITIONAL (edema, weight gain)	48	1.24	35	1.29
SPECIAL SENSES (conjunctivitis, ear infections, vertigo)	45	1.17	33	1.21
GENITAL TRACT (prostatitis, epididymitis, pregnancy, vaginitis, vulvitis, vaginal discharge and itching)	35	0.91	22	0.81
URINARY TRACT (urinary tract infections, renal calculi, urethritis)	36	0.93	31	1.14
ENDOCRINE (menstrual changes, breast symptoms)	18	0.47	14	0.52
PSYCHIATRIC (anxiety, depression, fatigue)	14	0.36	26	0.96
HEMATOLOGY (lymphadenopathy, thrombocytopenia, anemia)	12	0.31	15	0.55

Based on the patients' self evaluation, 59% of the U.S. patients using ROGAINE reported hair regrowth at Week 32 compared with 40% of those using placebo. Of the 59% reporting hair regrowth, 19% reported moderate and 40% reported minimal hair growth. In the European study, the percentage of patients reporting hair regrowth at Week 32 was 55% among the ROGAINE users compared with 41% among the placebo patients. Of the 55% reporting hair regrowth, 1% reported dense, 24% reported moderate and 30% reported minimal hair growth.

In the combined results of the U.S. and European studies, 57% of the women using ROGAINE evaluated their hair regrowth as minimal or moderate after 32 weeks compared to 40% of those using placebo. Below is a bar chart illustrating patients' self evaluation of hair regrowth.

Female Results
Patient Self Evaluation of
Hair Regrowth at 32 Weeks
Combined Results of U.S. &
European Studies

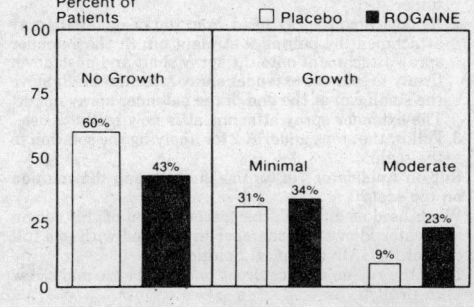

How soon can I expect results from using ROGAINE?
Studies have shown that the response to treatment with ROGAINE may vary widely. If you respond to treatment, it usually will take four months or longer before there is evidence of hair growth.

Some patients receiving ROGAINE may see faster results than others; others may respond with a slower rate of hair growth. You should not expect visible growth in less than four months.

If I respond to ROGAINE, what will the hair look like?
If you have very little hair and respond to treatment, your first hair growth may be soft, downy, colorless hair that is barely visible. After further treatment the new hair should be the same color and thickness as the other hair on your scalp. If you start with substantial hair, the new hair should be of the same color and thickness as the rest of your hair.

How long do I need to use ROGAINE?
ROGAINE is a treatment, not a cure. If you respond to treatment, you will need to continue using ROGAINE to maintain or increase hair growth. If you do not begin to show a response to treatment with ROGAINE after a reasonable period of time (at least four months or more), your doctor may advise you to discontinue using ROGAINE.

What happens if I stop using ROGAINE? Will I keep the new hair?
If you stop using ROGAINE, you will probably shed the new hair within a few months after stopping treatment.

Continued on next page

Information on these Upjohn products is based on labeling in effect June 1, 1992. Further information concerning these and other Upjohn products may be obtained by direct inquiry to Medical Information, The Upjohn Company, Kalamazoo, Michigan 49001.

Upjohn—Cont.

What is the dosage of ROGAINE?

You should apply a 1 mL dose of ROGAINE two times a day, once in the morning and once at night. Each bottle should last about 26–30 days. A bottle of ROGAINE is ¾ full. This fill level is intentional so that if the rub-on applicator is used, the tube is not submerged in the solution when the bottle is inverted for dosage administration. The applicators in each package of ROGAINE are designed to apply the correct amount of ROGAINE with each application. *Please refer to the Instructions for Use.*

What if I miss a dose or forget to use ROGAINE?

If you miss one or two daily applications of ROGAINE, you should restart your twice-daily application and return to your usual schedule. You should not attempt to make up for missed applications.

Can I use ROGAINE more than twice a day? Will it work faster?

No. Studies by The Upjohn Company have been carefully conducted to determine the correct amount of ROGAINE to use to obtain the most satisfactory results. More frequent applications or use of larger doses (more than one mL twice a day) have not been shown to speed up the process of hair growth and may increase the possibility of side effects.

What are the most common side effects reported in clinical studies with ROGAINE?

Studies of patients using ROGAINE have shown that the most common adverse effects directly attributable to ROGAINE Topical Solution were itching and other skin irritations of the treated area of the scalp.

Other side effects, including light-headedness, dizziness, and headaches were reported by patients using ROGAINE or placebo (a similar solution without the active medication). The frequency of these side effects was similar in the ROGAINE and placebo groups. For further information about side effects please ask your doctor.

ROGAINE Topical Solution contains alcohol, which could cause burning or irritation of the eyes, mucous membranes, or sensitive skin areas. If ROGAINE accidentally gets into these areas, bathe the area with large amounts of cool tap water. Contact your doctor if irritation persists.

What are the potential side effects on the heart and circulation when using ROGAINE?

Although serious side effects have not been attributed to ROGAINE in clinical studies, there is a possibility that they could occur because the active ingredient in ROGAINE Topical Solution is the same as in *minoxidil tablets.*

Minoxidil tablets are used to treat high blood pressure. *Minoxidil tablets* lower blood pressure by relaxing the arteries, an effect called vasodilation. Vasodilation leads to retention of fluid and increased heart rate. The following effects have occurred in some patients taking *minoxidil tablets* for high blood pressure:

1) Increased heart rate. Some patients have reported that their resting heart rate increased by more than 20 beats per minute.

2) Rapid weight gain of more than 5 pounds or swelling (edema) of the face, hands, ankles, or stomach area.

3) Difficulty in breathing, especially when lying down, a result of an increase in body fluids or fluid around the heart.

4) Worsening of, or new onset of, angina pectoris.

When ROGAINE Topical Solution is used on normal skin very little minoxidil is absorbed and these effects are not expected. If, however, you experience any of the above, discontinue use of ROGAINE and consult your doctor.

Presumably, such effects would be most likely if greater absorption occurred, eg, because ROGAINE was used on damaged or inflamed skin or in greater than recommended amounts.

In animal studies, minoxidil, in doses higher than would be obtained from topical use in people, has caused important heart structure damage. This kind of damage has not been seen in humans given *minoxidil tablets* for high blood pressure at effective doses.

What factors may increase the risk of serious side effects with ROGAINE?

Individuals with known or suspected underlying coronary artery disease, or the presence of or predisposition to heart failure would be at particular risk if systemic effects (that is, increased heart rate or fluid retention) of minoxidil were to occur. Physicians, and patients with these kinds of underlying diseases, should be conscious of the potential risk of treatment if they choose to use ROGAINE.

Because absorption of minoxidil may be increased and the risk of side effects may become greater, ROGAINE should be applied only to the scalp and should not be used on other parts of the body. You should not use ROGAINE if your scalp becomes irritated or is sunburned, and you should not use it along with another topical treatment medication on your scalp.

Can people with high blood pressure use ROGAINE?

Individuals with hypertension, including those under treatment with antihypertensive agents, can use ROGAINE but

should be monitored closely by their doctor. Patients taking guanethidine for high blood pressure should not use ROGAINE.

Will ROGAINE change my menstrual cycle?

No. Carefully conducted studies have shown that the use of ROGAINE will not increase the length of the menstrual cycle (interval between periods) or change the amount of flow or duration of the menstrual period. However, if your menstrual period does not occur at the expected time, you should discontinue the use of ROGAINE and consult your doctor as soon as possible.

Should I continue to use ROGAINE if I desire to become pregnant?

If you plan to become pregnant, you should discontinue using ROGAINE at least one month before you discontinue your birth control. Adequate and well-controlled studies have not been conducted in pregnant women treated with ROGAINE or in pregnant women taking oral minoxidil for the treatment of high blood pressure.

Can nursing mothers use ROGAINE?

No. We do not have any data from clinical trials or voluntary reports on minoxidil being reported in the breast milk following use of ROGAINE. It should be noted, however, that there has been one report of minoxidil excretion in the breast milk of a woman treated with 5 mg oral minoxidil twice daily for hypertension. Consequently, ROGAINE should not be administered to a nursing woman.

Instructions for Use

Please read this information before using ROGAINE Topical Solution. One mL (or 1 dose) of ROGAINE should be applied to the total affected areas of the scalp twice daily. The hair and scalp should be dry before application of ROGAINE. Each prescription of ROGAINE comes with three complimentary, disposable applicators to accommodate your individual preference and needs. You may wish to change the applicator if the condition of your hair changes.

Each applicator is designed to deliver a measured amount (1 mL, or 1 dose) of solution when used as directed. This amount of ROGAINE has been used in extensive clinical studies and determined to be the proper amount for the treatment of alopecia androgenetica (hair loss).

You must understand that twice-daily application for four months or longer may be required before hair regrowth may be observed.

Like all medications, keep ROGAINE out of the reach of children. In the event of accidental ingestion, contact your doctor. If, after reading this information, you have any questions, consult your doctor or ask your pharmacist.

DIRECTIONS FOR USE

Remove the large outer cap; remove the small inside child-resistant tamper-evident cap with a firm downward counter-clockwise motion. Both caps should be retained for reuse. If small children are present in the household, the child-resistant cap should be reapplied with a firm, clockwise motion until tight. If the product is not accessible to children, the spray and rub-on applicators do not need to be removed after each use. Once properly applied, they are designed not to leak even during travel. The extender spray attachment should be removed during travel and replaced with the spray tip or the child-resistant cap. If the applicators are removed and the child-resistant cap is reapplied after each use, some loss of product will occur as a result of product hang-up in the applicator. This may result in the bottle lasting fewer than the expected 26–30 days.

A. Metered Spray Attachment for applying the solution to large areas of the scalp

1. Insert spray assembly into bottle and screw on firmly. The spray attachment is now ready to use.

2. With the bottle held in an upright position, pump the spray attachment six times (for one full dose of 1 mL), pausing after each pump to massage the solution into the scalp area to be treated. Be careful not to inhale the spray mist. Place the clear plastic cap and the large outer cap on bottle when not in use.

B. Extender Spray Attachment for applying the solution on scalp areas under the hair

1. The metered spray attachment (A) must be on the bottle to use the extender spray attachment. Follow steps under A. 1.

2. Remove small spray head from top of metered spray attachment by pulling it straight off; fit the extender spray attachment onto the spray shaft and push down firmly to seat the extender spray attachment. Remove the small cap at the end of the extender spray nozzle. The extender spray attachment is now ready to use.

3. Follow the steps under A.2 for applying the solution to the scalp.

C. Rub-on Applicator Tip for use in spreading the solution on the scalp

When used as directed, the special design of this rub-on applicator allows the chamber to be filled with one full dose of ROGAINE Topical Solution.

1. Fit the rub-on applicator tip onto the bottle and screw on firmly.

2. Holding the bottle upright, squeeze the bottle to fill the upper chamber to the black line. Release pressure on the bottle. Any excess solution will drain into the bottle. The metered applicator tip now contains one full dose (1 mL) and is ready to use.

3. Holding the bottle upside down without squeezing the bottle, rub the applicator on the scalp area to be treated until the chamber is empty. Place large outer cap on bottle when not in use.

Code 813 264 010

Shown in Product Identification Section, page 434

SOLU-CORTEF® ℞

brand of hydrocortisone sodium succinate sterile powder
(hydrocortisone sodium succinate
for injection, USP)
For Intravenous or Intramuscular
Administration

DESCRIPTION

SOLU-CORTEF Sterile Powder contains hydrocortisone sodium succinate as the active ingredient. Hydrocortisone sodium succinate is a white or nearly white, odorless, hygroscopic amorphous solid. It is very soluble in water and in alcohol, very slightly soluble in acetone and insoluble in chloroform. The chemical name is pregn-4-ene-3,20-dione,21-(3-carboxy-1-oxopropoxy)-11,17-dihydroxy-, monosodium salt, (11β)-and its molecular weight is 484.52.

Hydrocortisone sodium succinate is an anti-inflammatory adrenocortical steroid. This highly water-soluble sodium succinate ester of hydrocortisone permits the immediate intravenous administration of high doses of hydrocortisone in a small volume of diluent and is particularly useful where high blood levels of hydrocortisone are required rapidly.

SOLU-CORTEF Sterile Powder (hydrocortisone sodium succinate) is available in several packages for intravenous or intramuscular administration.

100 mg Plain—Vials containing hydrocortisone sodium succinate equivalent to 100 mg hydrocortisone, also 0.8 mg monobasic sodium phosphate anhydrous, 8.73 mg dibasic sodium phosphate dried.

ACT-O-VIAL® System (Single-Dose Vial) in four strengths:
[See table on next page.]

ACTIONS

Hydrocortisone sodium succinate has the same metabolic and anti-inflammatory actions as hydrocortisone. When given parenterally and in equimolar quantities, the two compounds are equivalent in biologic activity. Following the intravenous injection of hydrocortisone sodium succinate, demonstrable effects are evident within one hour and persist for a variable period. Excretion of the administered dose is nearly complete within 12 hours. Thus, if constantly high blood levels are required, injections should be made every 4 to 6 hours. This preparation is also rapidly absorbed when administered intramuscularly and is excreted in a pattern similar to that observed after intravenous injection.

INDICATIONS

When oral therapy is not feasible, and the strength, dosage form and route of administration of the drug reasonably lend the preparation to the treatment of the condition, SOLU-CORTEF Sterile Powder (hydrocortisone sodium succinate) is indicated for intravenous or intramuscular use in the following conditions:

1. **Endocrine Disorders**

   Primary or secondary adrenocortical insufficiency (hydrocortisone or cortisone is the drug of choice; synthetic analogs may be used in conjunction with mineralocorticoids where applicable; in infancy, mineralocorticord supplementation is of particular importance)

   Acute adrenocortical insufficiency (hydrocortisone or cortisone is the drug of choice; mineralocorticoid supplementation may be necessary, particularly when synthetic analogs are used)

   Preoperatively and in the event of serious trauma or illness, in patients with known adrenal insufficiency or when adrenocortical reserve is doubtful

   Shock unresponsive to conventional therapy if adrenocortical insufficiency exists or is suspected

   Congenital adrenal hyperplasia

   Hypercalcemia associated with cancer

   Nonsuppurative thyroiditis

2. **Rheumatic Disorders**

   As adjunctive therapy for short-term administration (to tide the patient over an acute episode or exacerbation) in:

   Post-traumatic osteoarthritis

   Synovitis of osteoarthritis

   Rheumatoid arthritis, including juvenile rheumatoid arthritis (selected cases may require low-dose maintenance therapy)

SOLU-CORTEF	100 mg (ACT-O-VIAL)® Each 2 mL contains: (when mixed)	250 mg (ACT-O-VIAL) Each 2 mL contains: (when mixed)	500 mg (ACT-O-VIAL) Each 4 mL contains: (when mixed)	1000 mg (ACT-O-VIAL) Each 8 mL contains: (when mixed)
Hydrocortisone sodium succinate	equiv. to 100 mg hydrocortisone	equiv. to 250 mg hydrocortisone	equiv. to 500 mg hydrocortisone	equiv. to 1000 mg hydrocortisone
Monobasic sodium phosphate anhydrous	0.8 mg	2 mg	4 mg	8 mg
Diabasic sodium phosphate dried	8.76 mg	21.8 mg	44 mg	87.32 mg
Benzyl alcohol added as preservative	18.1 mg	16.4 mg	33.4 mg	66.9 mg

When necessary, the pH of each formula was adjusted with sodium hydroxide so that the pH of the reconstituted solution is within the USP specified range of 7 to 8.

Acute and subacute bursitis
Epicondylitis
Acute nonspecific tenosynovitis
Acute gouty arthritis
Psoriatic arthritis
Ankylosing spondylitis
3. **Collagen Diseases**
During an exacerbation or as maintenance therapy in selected cases of:
Systemic lupus erythematosus
Systemic dermatomyositis (polymyositis)
Acute rheumatic carditis
4. **Dermatologic Diseases**
Pemphigus
Severe erythema multiforme (Stevens-Johnson syndrome)
Exfoliative dermatitis
Bullous dermatitis herpetiformis
Severe seborrheic dermatitis
Severe psoriasis
Mycosis fungoides
5. **Allergic States**
Control of severe or incapacitating allergic conditions intractable to adequate trials of conventional treatment in:
Bronchial asthma
Contact dermatitis
Atopic dermatitis
Serum sickness
Seasonal or perennial allergic rhinitis
Drug hypersensitivity reactions
Urticarial transfusion reactions
Acute noninfectious laryngeal edema (epinephrine is the drug of first choice)
6. **Ophthalmic Diseases**
Severe acute and chronic allergic and inflammatory processes involving the eye, such as:
Herpes zoster ophthalmicus
Iritis, iridocyclitis
Chorioretinitis
Diffuse posterior uveitis and choroiditis
Optic neuritis
Sympathetic ophthalmia
Anterior segment inflammation
Allergic conjunctivitis
Allergic corneal marginal ulcers
Keratitis
7. **Gastrointestinal Diseases**
To tide the patient over a critical period of the disease in:
Ulcerative colitis (systemic therapy)
Regional enteritis (systemic therapy)
8. **Respiratory Diseases**
Symptomatic sarcoidosis
Berylliosis
Fulminating or disseminated pulmonary tuberculosis when used concurrently with appropriate antituberculous chemotherapy
Loeffler's syndrome not manageable by other means
Aspiration pneumonitis
9. **Hematologic Disorders**
Acquired (autoimmune) hemolytic anemia
Idiopathic thrombocytopenic purpura in adults (IV only; IM administration is contraindicated)
Secondary thrombocytopenia in adults
Erythroblastopenia (RBC anemia)
Congenital (erythroid) hypoplastic anemia
10. **Neoplastic Diseases**
For palliative mangement of:
Leukemias and lymphomas in adults
Acute leukemia of childhood
11. **Edematous States**
To induce diuresis or remission of proteinuria in the nephrotic syndrome, without uremia, of the idiopathic type or that due to lupus erythematosus

12. **Nervous System**
Acute exacerbations of multiple sclerosis
13. **Miscellaneous**
Tuberculous meningitis with subarachnoid block or impending block when used concurrently with appropriate antituberculous chemotherapy
Trichinosis with neurologic or myocardial involvement

CONTRAINDICATIONS
The use of SOLU-CORTEF Sterile Powder is contraindicated in premature infants because the 100 mg, 250 mg, 500 mg and 1000 mg ACT-O-VIAL System and MIX-O-VIAL Two-Compartment Vial contain benzyl alcohol. Benzyl alcohol has been reported to be associated with a fatal "Gasping Syndrome" in premature infants. SOLU-CORTEF Sterile Powder is also contraindicated in systemic fungal infections and patients with known hypersensitivity to the product and its constituents.

WARNINGS
In patients on corticosteroid therapy subjected to unusual stress, increased dosage of rapidly acting corticosteroids before, during, and after the stressful situation is indicated.
Corticosteroids may mask some signs of infection, and new infections may appear during their use. There may be decreased resistance and inability to localize infection when corticosteroids are used.
Prolonged use of corticosteroids may produce posterior subcapsular cataracts, glaucoma with possible damage to the optic nerves, and may enhance the establishment of secondary ocular infections due to fungi or viruses.
Usage in pregnancy. Since adequate human reproduction studies have not been done with corticosteroids, the use of these drugs in pregnancy, nursing mothers, or women of childbearing potential requires that the possible benefits of the drug be weighed against the potential hazards to the mother and embryo or fetus. Infants born of mothers who have received substantial doses of corticosteroids during pregnancy should be carefully observed for signs of hypoadrenalism.
Average and large doses of hydrocortisone can cause elevation of blood pressure, salt and water retention, and increased excretion of potassium. These effects are less likely to occur with the synthetic derivatives except when used in large doses. Dietary salt restriction and potassium supplementation may be necessary. All corticosteroids increase calcium excretion.
While on corticosteroid therapy patients should not be vaccinated against smallpox. Other immunization procedures should not be undertaken in patients who are on corticosteroids, especially on high dose, because of possible hazards of neurological complications and a lack of antibody response.
The use of SOLU-CORTEF Sterile Powder (hydrocortisone sodium succinate) in active tuberculosis should be restricted to those cases of fulminating or disseminated tuberculosis in which the corticosteroid is used for the management of the disease in conjunction with appropriate antituberculous regimen.
If corticosteroids are indicated in patients with latent tuberculosis or tuberculin reactivity, close observation is necessary as reactivation of the disease may occur. During prolonged corticosteroid therapy, these patients should receive chemoprophylaxis.
Because rare instances of anaphylactoid reactions (eg, bronchospasm) have occurred in patients receiving parenteral corticosteroid therapy, appropriate precautionary measures should be taken prior to administration, especially when the patient has a history of allergy to any drug.
Children who are on immunosuppressant drugs are more susceptible to infections than healthy children. Chickenpox and measles, for example, can have a more serious or even fatal course in children on immunosuppressant corticosteroids. In such children, or in adults who have not had these diseases, particular care should be taken to avoid exposure. If exposed, therapy with varicella zoster immune globulin (VZIG) or pooled intravenous immunoglobin (IVIG), as ap-

propriate, may be indicated. If chickenpox develops, treatment with antiviral agents may be considered.

PRECAUTIONS
Drug-induced secondary adrenocortical insufficiency may be minimized by gradual reduction of dosage. This type of relative insufficiency may persist for months after discontinuation of therapy; therefore, in any situation of stress occurring during that period, hormone therapy should be reinstituted. Since mineralocorticoid secretion may be impaired, salt and/or a mineralocorticoid should be administered concurrently.
There is an enhanced effect of corticosteroids in patients with hypothyroidism and in those with cirrhosis.
Corticosteroids should be used cautiously in patients with ocular herpes simplex for fear of corneal perforation.
The lowest possible dose of corticosteroid should be used to control the condition under treatment, and when reduction in dosage is possible, the reduction must be gradual.
Psychic derangements may appear when corticosteroids are used, ranging from euphoria, insomnia, mood swings, personality changes, and severe depression to frank psychotic manifestations. Also, existing emotional instability or psychotic tendencies may be aggravated by corticosteroids.
Aspirin should be used cautiously in conjunction with corticosteroids in hypoprothrombinemia.
Steroids should be used with caution in nonspecific ulcerative colitis, if there is a probability of impending perforation, abscess or other pyogenic infection, also in diverticulitis, fresh intestinal anastomoses, active or latent peptic ulcer, renal insufficiency, hypertension, osteoporosis, and myasthenia gravis.
Growth and development of infants and children on prolonged corticosteroid therapy should be carefully followed. Although controlled clinical trials have shown corticosteroids to be effective in speeding the resolution of acute exacerbations of multiple sclerosis, they do not show that corticosteroids affect the ultimate outcome or natural history of the disease. The studies do show that relatively high doses of corticosteroids are necessary to demonstrate a significant effect. (See **Administration and Dosage**).
Since complications of treatment with glucocorticoids are dependent on the size of the dose and the duration of treatment, a risk/benefit decision must be made in each individual case as to dose and duration of treatment and as to whether daily or intermittent therapy should be used.

Information for the Patient
Patients who are on immunosuppressant doses of corticosteroids should be warned to avoid exposure to chickenpox or measles and, if exposed, to obtain medical advice.

ADVERSE REACTIONS
Fluid and Electrolyte Disturbances
Sodium retention
Fluid retention
Congestive heart failure in susceptible patients
Potassium loss
Hypokalemic alkalosis
Hypertension
Musculoskeletal
Muscle weakness
Steroid myopathy
Loss of muscle mass
Osteoporosis
Vertebral compression fractures
Aseptic necrosis of femoral and humeral heads
Pathologic fracture of long bones
Gastrointestinal
Peptic ulcer with possible perforation and hemorrhage
Pancreatitis
Abdominal distention
Ulcerative esophagitis
Dermatologic
Impaired wound healing
Thin fragile skin
Petechiae and ecchymoses
Facial erythema
Increased sweating
May suppress reactions to skin tests
Neurological
Convulsions
Increased intracranial pressure with papilledema (pseudotumor cerebri) usually after treatment
Vertigo
Headache

Continued on next page

Upjohn—Cont.

Endocrine
Menstrual irregularities
Development of Cushingoid state
Suppression of growth in children
Secondary adrenocortical and pituitary unresponsiveness, particularly in times of stress, as in trauma, surgery, or illness
Decreased carbohydrate tolerance
Manifestations of latent diabetes mellitus
Increased requirements for insulin or oral hypoglycemic agents in diabetics

Ophthalmic
Posterior subcapsular cataracts
Increased intraocular pressure
Glaucoma
Exophthalmos

Metabolic
Negative nitrogen balance due to protein catabolism

The following additional reactions are related to parenteral corticosteroid therapy:
Allergic, anaphylactic or other hypersensitivity reactions
Hyperpigmentation or hypopigmentation
Subcutaneous and cutaneous atrophy
Sterile abscess

ADMINISTRATION AND DOSAGE

This preparation may be administered by intravenous injection, by intravenous infusion, or by intramuscular injection, the preferred method for initial emergency use being intravenous injection. Following the initial emergency period, consideration should be given to employing a longer acting injectable preparation or an oral preparation.

Therapy is initiated by administering SOLU-CORTEF Sterile Powder (hydrocortisone sodium succinate) intravenously over a period of 30 seconds (eg, 100 mg) to 10 minutes (eg, 500 mg or more). In general, high dose corticosteroid therapy should be continued only until the patient's condition has stabilized—usually not beyond 48 to 72 hours. Although adverse effects associated with high dose, short-term corticoid therapy are uncommon, peptic ulceration may occur. Prophylactic antacid therapy may be indicated.

When high dose hydrocortisone therapy must be continued beyond 48–72 hours, hypernatremia may occur. Under such circumstances it may be desirable to replace SOLU-CORTEF with a corticoid such as methylprednisolone sodium succinate which causes little or no sodium retention.

The initial dose of SOLU-CORTEF Sterile Powder is 100 mg to 500 mg, depending on the severity of the condition. This dose may be repeated at intervals of 2, 4 or 6 hours as indicated by the patient's response and clinical condition. While the dose may be reduced for infants and children, it is governed more by the severity of the condition and response of the patient than by age or body weight but should not be less than 25 mg daily.

Patients subjected to severe stress following corticosteroid therapy should be observed closely for signs and symptoms of adrenocortical insufficiency.

Corticoid therapy is an adjunct to, and not a replacement for, conventional therapy.

Preparation of Solutions

100 mg Plain—For intravenous or intramuscular injection, prepare solution by aseptically adding **not more than 2 ml** of Bacteriostatic Water for Injection or Bacteriostatic Sodium Chloride Injection to the contents of one vial. **For intravenous infusion,** first prepare solution by adding **not more than 2 ml** of Bacteriostatic Water for Injection to the vial; this solution may then be added to 100 to 1000 ml (but not less than 100 ml) of the following: 5% dextrose in water (or isotonic saline solution or 5% dextrose in isotonic saline solution if patient is not on sodium restriction).

Directions for using MIX-O-VIAL Two-Compartment Vial
1. Remove protective cap, give the plunger-stopper a quarter-turn and press to force diluent into the lower compartment.
2. Gently agitate to effect solution.
3. Sterilize top of plunger-stopper with a suitable germicide.
4. Insert needle **squarely through center** of plunger-stopper until tip is just visible. Invert vial and withdraw dose.

Directions for using the ACT-O-VIAL System
1. Press down on plastic activator to force diluent into the lower compartment.
2. Gently agitate to effect solution.
3. Remove plastic tab covering center of stopper.
4. Sterilize top of stopper with a suitable germicide.
5. Insert needle **squarely through center** of stopper until tip is just visible. Invert vial and withdraw dose.

Further dilution is not necessary for intravenous or intramuscular injection. For intravenous infusion, first prepare solution as just described. The **100 mg** solution may then be added to 100 to 1000 ml of 5% dextrose in water (or isotonic saline solution or 5% dextrose in isotonic saline solution if patient is not on sodium restriction). The **250 mg** solution may be added to 250 to 1000 ml, the **500 mg** solution may be added to 500 to 1000 ml and the **1000 mg** solution to 1000 ml of the same diluents. In cases where administration of a small volume of fluid is desirable, 100 mg to 3000 mg of SOLU-CORTEF Sterile Powder may be added to 50 ml of the above diluents. The resulting solutions are stable for at least 4 hours and may be administered either directly or by IV piggyback.

When reconstituted as directed, pH's of the solutions range from 7 to 8 and the tonicities are: 100 mg MIX-O-VIAL (ACT-O-VIAL), .36 osmolar; 250 mg MIX-O-VIAL (ACT-O-VIAL), 500 mg MIX-O-VIAL (ACT-O-VIAL), and the 1000 mg MIX-O-VIAL (ACT-O-VIAL), .57 osmolar. (Isotonic saline = .28 osmolar.)

HOW SUPPLIED

SOLU-CORTEF Sterile Powder (hydrocortisone sodium succinate) is available in the following packages:

100 mg Plain—NDC 0009-0825-01
100 mg ACT-O-VIAL (Single-Dose Vial)
2 mL—NDC 0009-0900-13
25-2 mL—NDC 0009-0900-15
250 mg ACT-O-VIAL (Single-Dose Vial)
2 mL—NDC 0009-0909-08
25-2 mL—NDC 0009-0909-09
500 mg ACT-O-VIAL (Single-Dose Vial)—NDC 0009-0912-05
1000 mg ACT-O-VIAL (Single-Dose Vial)—NDC 0009-0920-03

STORAGE CONDITIONS

Store unreconstituted product at controlled room temperature 15°–30°C (59°–86°F).

Store solution at controlled room temperature 15°–30°C (59°–86°F) and protect from light. Use solution only if it is clear. Unused solution should be discarded after 3 days.

Code 810 379 016

SOLU–MEDROL® ℞

brand of methylprednisolone sodium succinate sterile powder
(methylprednisolone sodium succinate for injection, USP)
For Intravenous or Intramuscular Administration

DESCRIPTION

SOLU-MEDROL Sterile Powder contains methylprednisolone sodium succinate as the active ingredient. Methylprednisolone sodium succinate, USP, occurs as a white, or nearly white, odorless hygroscopic, amorphous solid. It is very soluble in water and in alcohol; it is insoluble in chloroform and is very slightly soluble in acetone.

The chemical name for methylprednisolone sodium succinate is pregna-1,4-diene-3,20-dione,21-(3-carboxy-1-oxopropoxy)-11,17-dihydroxy-6-methyl-,monosodium salt, (6α, 11β), and the molecular weight is 496.53.

Methylprednisolone sodium succinate is so extremely soluble in water that it may be administered in a small volume of diluent and is especially well suited for intravenous use in situations in which high blood levels of methylprednisolone are required rapidly.

SOLU-MEDROL is available in several strengths and packages for intravenous or intramuscular administration.

40 mg ACT-O-VIAL® System (Single-Dose Vial)—Each mL (when mixed) contains methylprednisolone sodium succinate equivalent to 40 mg methylprednisolone; also 1.6 mg monobasic sodium phosphate anhydrous; 17.46 mg dibasic sodium phosphate dried; 25 mg lactose hydrous; 8.8 mg benzyl alcohol added as preservative.

125 mg ACT-O-VIAL System (Single-Dose Vial)—Each 2 mL (when mixed) contains methylprednisolone sodium succinate equivalent to 125 mg methylprednisolone; also 1.6 mg monobasic sodium biphosphate anhydrous; 17.4 mg dibasic sodium phosphate dried; 17.6 mg benzyl alcohol added as preservative.

500 mg Vial—Each 8 mL (when mixed as directed) contains methylprednisolone sodium succinate equivalent to 500 mg methylprednisolone; also 6.4 mg monobasic sodium biphosphate anhydrous; 69.6 mg dibasic sodium phosphate dried.

500 mg Vial with Diluent—Each 8 mL (when mixed as directed) contains methylprednisolone sodium succinate equivalent to 500 mg methylprednisolone; also 6.4 mg monobasic sodium phosphate anhydrous; 69.6 mg dibasic sodium phosphate dried; 70.2 mg benzyl alcohol added as preservative.

1 gram Vial—Each 16 mL (when mixed as directed) contains methylprednisolone sodium succinate equivalent to 1 gram methylprednisolone; also 12.8 mg monobasic sodium phosphate anhydrous; 139.2 mg dibasic sodium phosphate dried.

1 gram Vial with Diluent—Each 16 mL (when mixed as directed) contains methylprednisolone sodium succinate equivalent to 1 gram methylprednisolone; also 12.8 mg monobasic sodium phosphate anhydrous; 139.2 mg dibasic sodium phosphate dried; 141 mg benzyl alcohol added as preservative.

1 gram ACT-O-VIAL System (Single-Dose Vial)—Each 8 mL (when mixed) contains methylprednisolone sodium succinate equivalent to 1 gram methylprednisolone: also 12.8 mg monobasic sodium phosphate anhydrous: 139.2 mg dibasic sodium phosphate dried: 66.8 mg benzyl alcohol added as preservative.

2 gram Vial with Diluent—Each 30.6 mL (when mixed as directed) contains methylprednisolone sodium succinate equivalent to 2 grams methylprednisolone; also 25.6 mg monobasic sodium phosphate anhydrous; 278 mg dibasic sodium phosphate dried; 273 mg benzyl alcohol added as preservative.

When necessary, the pH of each formula was adjusted with sodium hydroxide so that the pH of the reconstituted solution is within the USP specified range of 7 to 8 and the tonicities are, for the 40 mg per mL solution, 0.50 osmolar; for the 125 mg per 2 mL, 500 mg per 8 mL and 1 gram per 16 mL solutions, 0.40 osmolar; for the 2 gram per 30.6 mL solutions, 0.42 osmolar. (Isotonic saline = 0.28 osmolar).

IMPORTANT—Use only the accompanying diluent or Bacteriostac Water For Injection with Benzyl Alcohol when reconstituting SOLU-MEDROL.

Use within 48 hours after mixing

ACTIONS

Methylprednisolone is a potent anti-inflammatory steroid synthesized in the Research Laboratories of The Upjohn Company. It has a greater anti-inflammatory potency than prednisolone and even less tendency than prednisolone to induce sodium and water retention.

Methylprednisolone sodium succinate has the same metabolic and anti-inflammatory actions as methylprednisolone. When given parenterally and in equimolar quantities, the two compounds are equivalent in biologic activity. The relative potency of SOLU-MEDROL Sterile Powder (methylprednisolone sodium succinate) and hydrocortisone sodium succinate, as indicated by depression of eosinophil count, following intravenous administration, is at least four to one. This is in good agreement with the relative oral potency of methylprednisolone and hydrocortisone.

INDICATIONS

When oral therapy is not feasible, and the strength, dosage form and route of administration of the drug reasonably lend the preparation to the treatment of the condition, SOLU-MEDROL Sterile Powder (methylprednisolone sodium succinate) is indicated for intravenous or intramuscular use in the following conditions:

1. Endocrine Disorders
Primary or secondary adrenocortical insufficiency (hydrocortisone or cortisone is the drug of choice; synthetic analogs may be used in conjunction with mineralocorticoids where applicable; in infancy, mineralocorticoid supplementation is of particular importance)
Acute adrenocortical insufficiency (hydrocortisone or cortisone is the drug of choice; mineralocorticoid supplementation may be necessary, particularly when synthetic analogs are used)
Preoperatively and in the event of serious trauma or illness, in patients with known adrenal insufficiency or when adrenocortical reserve is doubtful
Shock unresponsive to conventional therapy if adrenocortical insufficiency exists or is suspected
Congenital adrenal hyperplasia
Hypercalcemia associated with cancer
Nonsuppurative thyroiditis

2. Rheumatic Disorders
As adjunctive therapy for short-term administration (to tide the patient over an acute episode or exacerbation) in:
Post-traumatic osteoarthritis
Synovitis of osteoarthritis
Rheumatoid arthritis, including juvenile rheumatoid arthritis (selected cases may require low-dose maintenance therapy)
Acute and subacute bursitis
Epicondylitis
Acute nonspecific tenosynovitis
Acute gouty arthritis
Psoriatic arthritis
Ankylosing spondylitis

3. Collagen Diseases
During an exacerbation or as maintenance therapy in selected cases of:
Systemic lupus erythematosus
Systemic dermatomyositis (polymyositis)
Acute rheumatic carditis

4. Dermatologic Diseases
Pemphigus
Severe erythema multiforme (Stevens-Johnson syndrome)
Exfoliative dermatitis
Bullous dermatitis herpetiformis
Severe seborrheic dermatitis
Severe psoriasis
Mycosis fungoides

5. **Allergic States**
Control of severe or incapacitating allergic conditions intractable to adequate trials of conventional treatment in:
Bronchial asthma
Contact dermatitis
Atopic dermatitis
Serum sickness
Seasonal or perennial allergic rhinitis
Drug hypersensitivity reactions
Urticarial transfusion reactions
Acute noninfectious laryngeal edema (epinephrine is the drug of first choice)

6. **Ophthalmic Diseases**
Severe acute and chronic allergic and inflammatory processes involving the eye, such as:
Herpes zoster ophthalmicus
Iritis, iridocyclitis
Chorioretinitis
Diffuse posterior uveitis and choroiditis
Optic neuritis
Sympathetic ophthalmia
Anterior segment inflammation
Allergic conjunctivitis
Allergic corneal marginal ulcers
Keratitis

7. **Gastrointestinal Diseases**
To tide the patient over a critical period of the disease in:
Ulcerative colitis (systemic therapy)
Regional enteritis (systemic therapy)

8. **Respiratory Diseases**
Symptomatic sarcoidosis
Berylliosis
Fulminating or disseminated pulmonary tuberculosis when used concurrently with appropriate antituberculous chemotherapy
Loeffler's syndrome not manageable by other means
Aspiration pneumonitis

9. **Hematologic Disorders**
Acquired (autoimmune) hemolytic anemia
Idiopathic thrombocytopenic purpura in adults (IV only; IM administration is contraindicated)
Secondary thrombocytopenia in adults
Erythroblastopenia (RBC anemia)
Congenital (erythroid) hypoplastic anemia

10. **Neoplastic Diseases**
For palliative management of:
Leukemias and lymphomas in adults
Acute leukemia of childhood

11. **Edematous Diseases**
To induce diuresis or remission of proteinuria in the nephrotic syndrome, without uremia, of the idiopathic type or that due to lupus erythematosus

12. **Nervous System**
Acute exacerbations of multiple sclerosis

13. **Miscellaneous**
Tuberculous meningitis with subarachnoid block or impending block when used concurrently with appropriate antituberculous chemotherapy
Trichinosis with neurologic or myocardial involvement

CONTRAINDICATIONS

The use of SOLU-MEDROL Sterile Powder is contraindicated in premature infants because the **40 mg ACT-O-VIAL,** the **125 mg ACT-O-VIAL,** the **1 gram ACT-O-VIAL System,** and the accompanying diluent for the 500 mg, 1 gram, and 2 gram vials contain benzyl alcohol. Benzyl alcohol has been reported to be associated with a fatal "Gasping Syndrome" in premature infants. SOLU-MEDROL Sterile Powder is also contraindicated in systemic fungal infections and patients with known hypersensitivity to the product and its constituents.

WARNINGS

In patients on corticosteroid therapy subjected to any unusual stress, increased dosage of rapidly acting corticosteroids before, during, and after the stressful situation is indicated.
Corticosteroids may mask some signs of infection, and new infections may appear during their use. There may be decreased resistance and inability to localize infection when corticosteroids are used.
A study has failed to establish the efficacy of SOLU-MEDROL in the treatment of sepsis syndrome and septic shock. The study also suggests that treatment of these conditions with SOLU-MEDROL may increase the risk of mortality in certain patients (ie, patients with elevated serum creatinine levels or patients who develop secondary infections after SOLU-MEDROL).
Prolonged use of corticosteroids may produce posterior subcapsular cataracts, glaucoma with possible damage to the optic nerves, and may enhance the establishment of secondary ocular infections due to fungi or viruses.

Usage in pregnancy. Since adequate human reproduction studies have not been done with corticosteroids, the use of these drugs in pregnancy, nursing mothers, or women of childbearing potential requires that the possible benefits of the drug be weighed against the potential hazards to the mother and embryo or fetus. Infants born of mothers who have received substantial doses of corticosteroids during pregnancy should be carefully observed for signs of hypoadrenalism.
Average and large doses of cortisone or hydrocortisone can cause elevation of blood pressure, salt and water retention, and increased excretion of potassium. These effects are less likely to occur with the synthetic derivatives except when used in large doses. Dietary salt restriction and potassium supplementation may be necessary. All corticosteroids increase calcium excretion.
While on corticosteroid therapy patients should not be vaccinated against smallpox. Other immunization procedures should not be undertaken in patients who are on corticosteroids, especially on high dose, because of possible hazards of neurological complications and a lack of antibody response.
The use of SOLU-MEDROL Sterile Powder (methylprednisolone sodium succinate) in active tuberculosis should be restricted to those cases of fulminating or disseminated tuberculosis in which the corticosteroid is used for the management of the disease in conjunction with appropriate antituberculous regimen.
If corticosteroids are indicated in patients with latent tuberculosis or tuberculin reactivity, close observation is necessary as reactivation of the disease may occur. During prolonged corticosteroid therapy, these patients should receive chemoprophylaxis.
Because rare instances of anaphylactic (eg, bronchospasm) reactions have occurred in patients receiving parenteral corticosteroid therapy, appropriate precautionary measures should be taken prior to administration, especially when the patient has a history of allergy to any drug.
There are reports of cardiac arrhythmias and/or circulatory collapse and/or cardiac arrest following the rapid administration of large IV doses of SOLU-MEDROL (greater than 0.5 gram administered over a period of less than 10 minutes). Bradycardia has been reported during or after the administration of large doses of methylprednisolone sodium succinate, and may be unrelated to the speed or duration of infusion.
Children who are on immunosuppressant drugs are more susceptible to infections than healthy children. Chickenpox and measles, for example, can have a more serious or even fatal course in children on immunosuppressant corticosteroids. In such children, or in adults who have not had these diseases, particular care should be taken to avoid exposure. If exposed, therapy with varicella zoster immune globulin (VZIG) or pooled intravenous immunoglobin (IVIG), as appropriate, may be indicated. If chickenpox develops, treatment with antiviral agents may be considered.

PRECAUTIONS

Drug-induced secondary adrenocortical insufficiency may be minimized by gradual reduction of dosage. This type of relative insufficiency may persist for months after discontinuation of therapy; therefore, in any situation of stress occurring during that period, hormone therapy should be reinstituted. Since mineralocorticoid secretion may be impaired, salt and/or a mineralocorticoid should be administered concurrently. There is an enhanced effect of corticosteroids on patients with hypothyroidism and in those with cirrhosis.
Corticosteroids should be used cautiously in patients with ocular herpes simplex because of possible corneal perforation.
The lowest possible dose of corticosteroid should be used to control the condition under treatment, and when reduction in dosage is possible, the reduction should be gradual.
Psychic derangements may appear when corticosteroids are used, ranging from euphoria, insomnia, mood swings, personality changes and severe depression, to frank psychotic manifestations. Also, existing emotional instability or psychotic tendencies may be aggravated by corticosteroids.
Aspirin should be used cautiously in conjunction with corticosteroids in hypoprothrombinemia.
Steroids should be used with caution in nonspecific ulcerative colitis, if there is a probability of impending perforation, abscess or other pyogenic infection; diverticulitis; fresh intestinal anastomoses; active or latent peptic ulcer; renal insufficiency; hypertension; osteoporosis; and myasthenia gravis.
Growth and development of infants and children on prolonged corticosteroid therapy should be carefully observed. Although controlled clinical trials have shown corticosteroids to be effective in speeding the resolution of acute exacerbations of multiple sclerosis, they do not show that corticosteroids affect the ultimate outcome or natural history of the disease. The studies do show that relatively high doses of corticosteroids are necessary to demonstrate a significant effect. (See DOSAGE AND ADMINISTRATION).
Since complications of treatment with glucocorticoids are dependent on the size of the dose and the duration of treat-

ment, a risk/benefit decision must be made in each individual case as to dose and duration of treatment and as to whether daily or intermittent therapy should be used.
Convulsions have been reported with concurrent use of methylprednisolone and cyclosporin. Since concurrent use of these agents results in a mutual inhibition of metabolism, it is possible that adverse events associated with the individual use of either drug may be more apt to occur.

Information for the Patient
Patients who are on immunosuppressant doses of corticosteroids should be warned to avoid exposure to chickenpox or measles and, if exposed, to obtain medical advice.

ADVERSE REACTIONS

Fluid and Electrolyte Disturbances
Sodium retention
Fluid retention
Congestive heart failure in susceptible patients
Potassium loss
Hypokalemic alkalosis
Hypertension
Musculoskeletal
Muscle weakness
Steroid myopathy
Loss of muscle mass
Severe arthralgia
Vertebral compression fractures
Aseptic necrosis of femoral and humeral heads
Pathologic fracture of long bones
Osteoporosis
Gastrointestinal
Peptic ulcer with possible perforation and hemorrhage
Pancreatitis
Abdominal distention
Ulcerative esophagitis
Dermatologic
Impaired wound healing
Thin fragile skin
Petechiae and ecchymoses
Facial erythema
Increased sweating
May suppress reactions to skin tests
Neurological
Increased intracranial pressure with papilledema (pseudotumor cerebri) usually after treatment
Convulsions
Vertigo
Headache
Endocrine
Development of Cushingoid state
Suppression of growth in children
Secondary adrenocortical and pituitary unresponsiveness, particularly in times of stress, as in trauma, surgery or illness
Menstrual irregularities
Decreased carbohydrate tolerance
Manifestations of latent diabetes mellitus
Increased requirements for insulin or oral hypoglycemic agents in diabetics
Ophthalmic
Posterior subcapsular cataracts
Increased intraocular pressure
Glaucoma
Exophthalmos
Metabolic
Negative nitrogen balance due to protein catabolism
The following *additional* adverse reactions are related to parenteral corticosteroid therapy:
Hyperpigmentation or hypopigmentation
Subcutaneous and cutaneous atrophy
Sterile abscess
Anaphylactic reaction with or without circulatory collapse, cardiac arrest, bronchospasm
Urticaria
Nausea and vomiting
Cardiac arrhythmias; hypotension or hypertension

DOSAGE AND ADMINISTRATION

When high dose therapy is desired, the recommended dose of SOLU-MEDROL Sterile Powder (methylprednisolone sodium succinate) is 30 mg/kg administered intravenously over at least 30 minutes. This dose may be repeated every 4 to 6 hours for 48 hours.
In general, high dose corticosteroid therapy should be continued only until the patient's condition has stabilized; usually not beyond 48 to 72 hours.

Continued on next page

Information on these Upjohn products is based on labeling in effect June 1, 1992. Further information concerning these and other Upjohn products may be obtained by direct inquiry to Medical Information, The Upjohn Company, Kalamazoo, Michigan 49001.

Upjohn—Cont.

Although adverse effects associated with high dose short-term corticoid therapy are uncommon, peptic ulceration may occur. Prophylactic antacid therapy may be indicated. In other indications initial dosage will vary from 10 to 40 mg of methylprednisolone depending on the clinical problem being treated. The larger doses may be required for short-term management of severe, acute conditions. The initial dose usually should be given intravenously over a period of one to several minutes. Subsequent doses may be given intravenously or intramuscularly at intervals dictated by the patient's response and clinical condition. Corticoid therapy is an adjunct to, and not replacement for conventional therapy.

Dosage may be reduced for infants and children but should be governed more by the severity of the condition and response of the patient than by age or size. It should not be less than 0.5 mg per kg every 24 hours.

Dosage must be decreased or discontinued gradually when the drug has been administered for more than a few days. If a period of spontaneous remission occurs in a chronic condition, treatment should be discontinued. Routine laboratory studies, such as urinalysis, two-hour postprandial blood sugar, determination of blood pressure and body weight, and a chest X-ray should be made at regular intervals during prolonged therapy. Upper GI X-rays are desirable in patients with an ulcer history or significant dyspepsia.

SOLU-MEDROL may be administered by intravenous or intramuscular injection or by intravenous infusion, the preferred method for initial emergency use being intravenous injection. To administer by intravenous (or intramuscular) injection, prepare solution as directed. The desired dose may be administered intravenously over a period of several minutes. Subsequent doses may be withdrawn and administered similarly. If desired, the medication may be administered in diluted solutions by adding Water for Injection or other suitable diluent (see below) to the ACT-O-VIAL and withdrawing the indicated dose.

To prepare solutions for intravenous infusion, first prepare the solution for injection as directed. This solution may then be added to indicated amounts of 5% dextrose in water, isotonic saline solution or 5% dextrose in isotonic saline solution.

Multiple Sclerosis

In treatment of acute exacerbations of multiple sclerosis, daily doses of 200 mg of prednisolone for a week followed by 80 mg every other day for 1 month have been shown to be effective (4 mg of methylprednisolone is equivalent to 5 mg of prednisolone).

Directions for Using the ACT-O-VIAL System

1. Press down on plastic activator to force diluent into the lower compartment.
2. Gently agitate to effect solution.
3. Remove plastic tab covering center of stopper.
4. Sterilize top of stopper with a suitable germicide.
5. Insert needle squarely through center of stopper until tip is just visible. Invert vial and withdraw dose.

STORAGE CONDITIONS

Store unreconstituted product at controlled room temperature 15°–30°C (59°–86°F).

Store solution at controlled room temperature 15°–30°C (59°–86°F).

Use solution within 48 hours after mixing.

HOW SUPPLIED

SOLU-MEDROL Sterile Powder (methylprednisolone sodium succinate) is available in the following packages:

  40 mg ACT-O-VIAL System
    1 mL NDC 0009-0113-12
    25—1 mL NDC 0009-0113-13
  125 mg ACT-O-VIAL System
    2 mL NDC 0009-0190-09
    25—2 mL NDC 0009-0190-10
  500 mg Vial NDC 0009-0758-01
  500 mg Vial with Diluent NDC 0009-0887-01
  1 gram Vial NDC 0009-0698-01
  1 gram ACT-O-VIAL System
    8 mL NDC 0009-3389-01
  2 gram Vial NDC 0009-0988-01
  2 gram Vial with Diluent NDC 0009-0796-01
                Code 810 431 023
Shown in Product Identification Section, page 434

TOLINASE®
brand of tolazamide tablets, USP   ℞

DESCRIPTION

TOLINASE Tablets contain tolazamide, an oral blood glucose lowering drug of the sulfonylurea class. Tolazamide is a white or creamy-white powder with a melting point of 165° to 173° C. The solubility of tolazamide at pH 6.0 (mean urinary pH) is 27.8 mg per 100 ml.

The chemical names for tolazamide are (1) Benzenesulfonamide, N-[[(hexahydro-1H-azepin-1-yl)amino]-carbonyl]-4-methyl-; (2) 1-(Hexahydro-1H-azepin-1-yl)-3-(p-tolylsulfonyl)-urea and its molecular weight is 311.40.

TOLINASE Tablets for oral administration are available as scored, white tablets containing 100 mg, 250 mg or 500 mg tolazamide. Inactive ingredients: calcium sulfate, docusate sodium, magnesium stearate, methylcellulose, sodium alginate.

CLINICAL PHARMACOLOGY

Actions

Tolazamide appears to lower the blood glucose acutely by stimulating the release of insulin from the pancreas, an effect dependent upon functioning beta cells in the pancreatic islets. The mechanism by which tolazamide lowers blood glucose during long-term administration has not been clearly established. With chronic administration in type II diabetic patients, the blood glucose lowering effect persists despite a gradual decline in the insulin secretory response to the drug. Extrapancreatic effects may be involved in the mechanism of action of oral sulfonylurea hypoglycemic drugs.

Some patients who are initially responsive to oral hypoglycemic drugs, including TOLINASE Tablets (tolazamide), may become unresponsive or poorly responsive over time. Alternatively, TOLINASE may be effective in some patients who have become unresponsive to one or more sulfonylurea drugs.

In addition to its blood glucose lowering actions, tolazamide produces a mild diuresis by enhancement of renal free water clearance.

Pharmacokinetics

Tolazamide is rapidly and well absorbed from the gastrointestinal tract. Peak serum concentrations occur at three to four hours following a single oral dose of the drug. The average biological half-life of the drug is seven hours. The drug does not continue to accumulate in the blood after the first four to six doses are administered. A steady or equilibrium state is reached during which the peak and nadir values do not change from day to day after the fourth to sixth doses. Tolazamide is metabolized to five major metabolites ranging in hypoglycemic activity from 0–70%. They are excreted principally in the urine. Following a single oral dose of tritiated tolazamide, 85% of the dose was excreted in the urine and 7% in the feces over a five-day period. Most of the urinary excretion of the drug occurred within the first 24 hours postadministration.

When nomal fasting nondiabetic subjects are given a single 500 mg dose of tolazamide orally, a hypoglycemic effect can be noted within 20 minutes after ingestion with a peak hypoglycemic effect occurring in two to four hours. Following a single oral dose of 500 mg tolazamide, a statistically significant hypoglycemic effect was demonstrated in fasted nondiabetic subjects 20 hours after administration. With fasting diabetic patients, the peak hypoglycemic effect occurs at four to six hours. The duration of maximal hypoglycemic effect in fed diabetic patients is about ten hours, with the onset occurring at four to six hours and with the blood glucose levels beginning to rise at 14 to 16 hours. Single dose potency of tolazamide in normal subjects has been shown to be 6.7 times that of tolbutamide on a milligram basis. Clinical experience in diabetic patients has demonstrated tolazamide to be approximately five times more potent than tolbutamide on a milligram basis, and approximately equivalent in milligram potency to chlorpropamide.

INDICATIONS AND USAGE

TOLINASE Tablets (tolazamide) are indicated as an adjunct to diet to lower the blood glucose in patients with noninsulin dependent diabetes mellitus (Type II) whose hyperglycemia cannot be satisfactorily controlled by diet alone.

In initiating treatment for noninsulin-dependent diabetes, diet should be emphasized as the primary form of treatment. Caloric restriction and weight loss are essential in the obese diabetic patient. Proper dietary management alone may be effective in controlling the blood glucose and symptoms of hyperglycemia. The importance of regular physical activity should also be stressed and cardiovascular risk factors should be identified and corrective measures taken where possible.

If this treatment program fails to reduce symptoms and/or blood glucose, the use of an oral sulfonylurea or insulin should be considered. Use of TOLINASE must be viewed by both the physician and patient as a treatment in addition to diet and not as a substitute for diet or as a convenient mechanism for avoiding dietary restraint. Furthermore, loss of blood glucose control on diet alone may be transient thus requiring only short-term administration of TOLINASE.

During maintenance programs, TOLINASE should be discontinued if satisfactory lowering of blood glucose is no longer achieved. Judgments should be based on regular clinical and laboratory evaluations.

In considering the use of TOLINASE in asymptomatic patients, it should be recognized that controlling the blood glucose in noninsulin-dependent diabetes has not been definitely established to be effective in preventing the long-term cardiovascular or neural complications of diabetes.

CONTRAINDICATIONS

TOLINASE Tablets (tolazamide) are contraindicated in patients with: 1) known hypersensitivity or allergy to TOLINASE; 2) diabetic ketoacidosis, with or without coma. This condition should be treated with insulin; 3) Type I diabetes, as sole therapy.

Special Warning on Increased Risk of Cardiovascular Mortality: The administration of oral hypoglycemic drugs has been reported to be associated with increased cardiovascular mortality as compared to treatment with diet alone or diet plus insulin. This warning is based on the study conducted by the University Group Diabetes Program (UGDP), a long-term prospective clinical trial designed to evaluate the effectiveness of glucose-lowering drugs in preventing or delaying vascular complications in patients with noninsulin-dependent diabetes. The study involved 823 patients who were randomly assigned to one of four treatment groups (DIABETES, 19 (supp. 2):747–830, 1970.)

UGDP reported that patients treated for five to eight years with diet plus a fixed dose of tolbutamide (1.5 grams per day) had a rate of cardiovascular mortality approximately 2½ times that of patients with diet alone. A significant increase in total mortality was not observed, but the use of tolbutamide was discontinued based on the increase on cardiovascular mortality, thus limiting the opportunity for the study to show an increase in overall mortality. Despite controversy regarding the interpretation of these results, the findings of the UGDP study provide an adequate basis for this warning. The patient should be informed of the potential risks and advantages of TOLINASE and of alternative modes of therapy.

Although only one drug in the sulfonylurea class (tolbutamide) was included in this study, it is prudent from a safety standpoint to consider that this warning may also apply to other oral hypoglycemic drugs in this class, in view of their close similarities in mode of action and chemical structure.

PRECAUTIONS

General

Hypoglycemia—All sulfonylurea drugs are capable of producing severe hypoglycemia. Proper patient selection and dosage and instructions are important to avoid hypoglycemic episodes. Renal or hepatic insufficiency may cause elevated blood levels of TOLINASE Tablets (tolazamide) and the latter may also diminish gluconeogenic capacity, both of which increase the risk of serious hypoglycemic reactions. Elderly, debilitated, or malnourished patients and those with adrenal or pituitary insufficiency are particularly susceptible to the hypoglycemic action of glucose lowering drugs. Hypoglycemia may be difficult to recognize in the elderly and in people who are taking beta-adrenergic blocking drugs. Hypoglycemia is more likely to occur when caloric intake is deficient, after severe or prolonged exercise, when alcohol is ingested, or when more than one glucose-lowering drug is used.

Loss of Control of Blood Glucose—When a patient stabilized on any diabetic regimen is exposed to stress such as fever, trauma, infection, or surgery, loss of control of blood glucose may occur. At such times it may be necessary to discontinue TOLINASE and administer insulin.

The effectiveness of any hypoglycemic drug, including TOLINASE, in lowering blood glucose to a desired level decreases in many patients over a period of time, which may be due to progression of the severity of the diabetes or to diminished responsiveness to the drug. This phenomenon is known as secondary failure to distinguish it from primary failure in which the drug is ineffective in an individual patient when first given. Adequate adjustment of dose and adherence to diet should be assessed before classifying a patient as a secondary failure.

Information for Patients

Patients should be informed of the potential risks and advantages of TOLINASE Tablets (tolazamide) and of alternative modes of therapy. They should also be informed about the importance of adherence to dietary instructions, of a regular exercise program, and of regular testing of urine and/or blood glucose.

The risks of hypoglycemia, its symptoms and treatment, and conditions that predispose to its development should be explained to patients and responsible family members. Primary and secondary failure should also be explained.

Laboratory Tests

Blood and urine glucose should be monitored periodically. Measurement of glycosylated hemoglobin may be useful in some patients.

Drug Interactions

The hypoglycemia action of sulfonylureas may be potentiated by certain drugs including nonsteroidal anti-inflammatory agents and other drugs that are highly protein bound, salicylates, sulfonamides, chloramphenicol, probenecid, coumarins, monoamine oxidase inhibitors, and beta-adren-

ergic blocking agents. When such drugs are administered to a patient receiving TOLINASE, the patient should be closely observed for hypoglycemia. When such drugs are withdrawn from a patient receiving TOLINASE, the patient should be observed closely for loss of control.

Certain drugs tend to produce hyperglycemia and may lead to loss of control. These drugs include the thiazides and other diuretics, corticosteroids, phenothiazines, thyroid products, estrogens, oral contraceptives, phenytoin, nicotinic acid, sympathomimetics, calcium channel blocking drugs, and isoniazid. When such drugs are administered to a patient receiving TOLINASE, the patient should be closely observed for loss of control. When such drugs are withdrawn from a patient receiving TOLINASE, the patient should be observed closely for hypoglycemia.

A potential interaction between oral miconazole and oral hypoglycemic agents leading to severe hypoglycemia has been reported. Whether this interaction also occurs with the intravenous, topical or vaginal preparations of miconazole is not known.

Carcinogenicity

In a bioassay for carcinogenicity, rats and mice of both sexes were treated with tolazamide for 103 weeks at low and high doses. No evidence of carcinogenicity was found.

Pregnancy

Teratogenic Effects:

Pregnancy Category C. TOLINASE, administered to pregnant rats at ten times the human dose, decreased litter size but did not produce teratogenic effects in the offspring. In rats treated at a daily dose of 14 mg/kg no reproductive aberrations or drug related fetal anomalies were noted. At an elevated dose of 100 mg/kg per day there was a reduction in the number of pups born and an increased perinatal mortality. There are, however, no adequate and well-controlled studies in pregnant women. Because animal reproduction studies are not always predictive of human response, TOLINASE is not recommended for the treatment of the pregnant diabetic patient. Serious consideration should also be given to the possible hazards of the use of TOLINASE in women of child bearing age and in those who might become pregnant while using the drug.

Because recent information suggests that abnormal blood glucose levels during pregnancy are associated with a higher incidence of congenital abnormalities, many experts recommend that insulin be used during pregnancy to maintain blood glucose levels as close to normal as possible.

Nonteratogenic Effects:

Prolonged severe hypoglycemia (four to ten days) has been reported in neonates born to mothers who were receiving a sulfonylurea drug at the time of delivery. This has been reported more frequently with the use of agents with prolonged half-lives. If TOLINASE is used during pregnancy, it should be discontinued at least two weeks before the expected delivery date.

Nursing Mothers

Altough it is not known whether tolazamide is excreted in human milk, some sulfonylurea drugs are known to be excreted in human milk. Because the potential for hypoglycemia in nursing infants may exist, a decision should be made whether to discontinue nursing or to discontinue the drug, taking into account the importance of the drug to the mother. If the drug is discontinued and if diet alone is inadequate for controlling blood glucose, insulin therapy should be considered.

Pediatric Use

Safety and effectiveness in children have not been established.

ADVERSE REACTIONS

TOLINASE Tablets (tolazamide) have generally been well tolerated. In clinical studies in which more than 1,784 diabetic patients were specifically evaluated for incidence of side effects, only 2.1% were discontinued from therapy because of side effects.

Hypoglycemia: See **Precautions** and **Overdosage** sections.

Gastrointestinal Reactions: Cholestatic jaundice may occur rarely; TOLINASE Tablets should be discontinued if this occurs. Gastrointestinal disturbances, eg, nausea, epigastric fullness, and heartburn, are the most common reactions and occurred in 1% of patients treated during clinical trials. They tend to be dose-related and may disappear when dosage is reduced.

Dermatologic Reactions: Allergic skin reactions, eg, pruritus, erythema, urticaria, and morbilliform or maculopapular eruptions, occurred in 0.4% of patients treated during clinical trials. These may be transient and may disappear despite continued use of TOLINASE; if skin reactions persist, the drug should be discontinued.

Porphyria cutanea tarda and photosensitivity reactions have been reported with sulfonylureas.

Hematologic Reactions: Leukopenia, agranulocytosis, thrombocytopenia, hemolytic anemia, aplastic anemia, and pancytopenia have been reported with sulfonylureas.

Metabolic Reactions: Hepatic porphyria and disulfiram-like reactions have been reported with sulfonylureas; however, disulfiram-like reactions with TOLINASE have been reported very rarely.

Cases of hyponatremia have been reported with tolazamide and all other sulfonylureas, most often in patients who are on other medications or have medical conditions known to cause hyponatremia or increase release of antidiuretic hormone. The syndrome of inappropriate antidiuretic hormone (SIADH) secretion has been reported with certain other sulfonylureas, and it has been suggested that these sulfonylureas may augment the peripheral (antidiuretic) action of ADH and/or increase release of ADH.

Miscellaneous: Weakness, fatigue, dizziness, vertigo, malaise and headache were reported infrequently in patients treated during clinical trials. The relationship to therapy with TOLINASE is difficult to assess.

OVERDOSAGE

Overdosage of sulfonylureas, including TOLINASE Tablets (tolazamide), can produce hypoglycemia.

Mild hypoglycemic symptoms without loss of consciousness or neurologic findings should be treated aggressively with oral glucose and adjustment in drug dosage and/or meal patterns. Close monitoring should continue until the physician is assured the patient is out of danger. Severe hypoglycemic reactions with coma, seizure, or other neurological impairment occur infrequently, but constitute medical emergencies requiring immediate hospitalization. If hypoglycemic coma is suspected or diagnosed, the patient should be given a rapid intravenous injection of concentrated (50%) glucose solution. This should be followed by a continuous infusion of a more dilute (10%) glucose solution at a rate which will maintain the blood glucose at a level above 100 mg/dl. Patients should be closely monitored for a minimum of 24 to 48 hours since hypoglycemia may recur after apparent clinical recovery.

DOSAGE AND ADMINISTRATION

There is no fixed dosage regimen for the management of diabetes mellitus with TOLINASE Tablets (tolazamide) or any other hypoglycemic agent. In addition to the usual monitoring of urinary glucose, the patient's blood glucose must also be monitored periodically to determine the minimum effective dose for the patient; to detect primary failure, ie, inadequate lowering of blood glucose at the maximum recommended dose of medication; and to detect secondary failure, ie, loss of adequate blood glucose response after an initial period of effectiveness. Glycosylated hemoglobin levels may also be of value in monitoring the patient's response to therapy.

Short-term administration of TOLINASE may be sufficient during periods of transient loss of control in patients usually controlled well on diet.

Usual Starting Dose

The usual starting dose of TOLINASE Tablets for the mild to moderately severe Type II diabetic patient is 100–250 mg daily administered with breakfast or the first main meal. Generally, if the fasting blood glucose is less than 200 mg/dl, the starting dose is 100 mg/day as a single daily dose. If the fasting blood glucose value is greater than 200 mg/dl, the starting dose is 250 mg/day as a single dose. If the patient is malnourished, underweight, elderly, or not eating properly, the initial therapy should be 100 mg once a day. Failure to follow an appropriate dosage regimen may precipitate hypoglycemia. Patients who do not adhere to their prescribed dietary regimen are more prone to exhibit unsatisfactory response to drug therapy.

Transfer From Other Hypoglycemic Therapy

Patients Receiving Other Oral Antidiabetic Therapy—Transfer of patients from other oral antidiabetes regimens to TOLINASE should be done conservatively. When transferring patients from oral hypoglycemic agents other than chlorpropamide to TOLINASE, no transition period or initial or priming dose is necessary. When transferring from chlorpropamide, particular care should be exercised to avoid hypoglycemia.

Tolbutamide: If receiving less than 1 gm/day, begin at 100 mg of tolazamide per day. If receiving 1 gm or more per day, initiate at 250 mg of tolazamide per day as a single dose.

Chlorpropamide: 250 mg of chlorpropamide may be considered to provide approximately the same degree of blood glucose control as 250 mg of tolazamide. The patient should be observed carefully for hypoglycemia during the transition period from chlorpropamide to TOLINASE (one to two weeks) due to the prolonged retention of chlorpropamide in the body and the possibility of a subsequent overlapping drug effect.

Acetohexamide: 100 mg of tolazamide may be considered to provide approximately the same degree of blood glucose control as 250 mg of acetohexamide.

Patients Receiving Insulin—Some Type II diabetic patients who have been treated only with insulin may respond satisfactorily to therapy with TOLINASE. If the patient's previous insulin dosage has been less than 20 units, substitution of 100 mg of tolazamide per day as a single daily dose may be tried. If the previous insulin dosage was less than 40 units, but more than 20 units, the patient should be placed directly on 250 mg of tolazamide per day as a single dose. If the previous insulin dosage was greater than 40 units, the insulin dosage should be decreased by 50% and 250 mg of tolazamide per day started. The dosage of TOLINASE should be adjusted weekly (or more often in the group previously requiring more than 40 units of insulin). During this conversion period when both insulin and TOLINASE are being used, hypoglycemia may rarely occur. During insulin withdrawal, patients should test their urine for glucose and acetone at least three times daily and report results to their physician. The appearance of persistent acetonuria with glycosuria indicates that the patient is a Type I diabetic who requires insulin therapy.

Maximum Dose

Daily doses of greater than 1000 mg are not recommended. Patients will generally have no further response to doses larger than this.

Usual Maintenance Dose

The usual maintenance dose is in the range of 100–1000 mg/day with the average maintenance dose being 250–500 mg/day. Following initiation of therapy, dosage adjustment is made in increments of 100 mg to 250 mg at weekly intervals based on the patient's blood glucose response.

Dosage Interval

Once a day therapy is usually satisfactory. Doses up to 500 mg/day should be given as a single dose in the morning. 500 mg once daily is as effective as 250 mg twice daily. When a dose of more than 500 mg/day is required, the dose may be divided and given twice daily.

In elderly patients, debilitated or malnourished patients, and patients with impaired renal or hepatic function, the initial and maintenance dosing should be conservative to avoid hypoglycemic reactions (see **PRECAUTIONS** section).

HOW SUPPLIED

TOLINASE Tablets (tolazamide) are available in the following strengths and package sizes:

100 mg (scored, round, white)
Unit-of-Use bottles of 100 NDC 0009-0070-02
250 mg (scored, round, white)
Bottles of 200 NDC 0009-0114-04
Bottles of 1000 NDC 0009-0114-02
Unit-of-Use bottles of 100 NDC 0009-0114-05
Unit-Dose package of 100 NDC 0009-0114-06
500 mg (scored, round, white)
Unit-of-Use bottles of 100 NDC 0009-0477-06

Store at controlled room temperature 15–30° C (59–86° F).
Code 811 417 407

Shown in Product Identification Section, page 434

TROBICIN® ℞

brand of spectinomycin hydrochloride sterile powder (sterile spectinomycin hydrochloride for suspension, USP)
For Intramuscular Injection

2 Gm vial NSN 6505-00-079-7611 (M)
4 Gm vial NSN 6505-00-079-7643 (M)

DESCRIPTION

TROBICIN Sterile Powder contains spectinomycin hydrochloride which is an aminocyclitol antibiotic produced by a species of soil microorganism designated as *Streptomyces spectabilis*. Sterile spectinomycin hydrochloride is the pentahydrated dihydrochloride salt of spectinomycin.

Spectinomycin hydrochloride is isolated as a white to pale buff crystalline dihydrochloride pentahydrate powder, molecular weight 495, and is stable in the dry state for 36 months.

CLINICAL PHARMACOLOGY

Spectinomycin hydrochloride is an inhibitor of protein synthesis in the bacterial cell; the site of action is the 30S ribosomal subunit.

In vitro studies have shown spectinomycin hydrochloride to be active against most strains of *Neisseria gonorrhoeae* (minimum inhibitory concentration < 7.5 to 20 mcg/ml).

Definitive *in vitro* studies have shown no cross-resistance of *N. gonorrhoeae* between spectinomycin hydrochloride and penicillin. The antibiotic is not significantly bound to plasma protein.

INDICATIONS AND USAGE

TROBICIN Sterile Powder (spectinomycin hydrochloride) is indicated in the treatment of acute gonorrheal urethritis and proctitis in the male and acute gonorrheal cervicitis and

Continued on next page

Information on these Upjohn products is based on labeling in effect June 1, 1992. Further information concerning these and other Upjohn products may be obtained by direct inquiry to Medical Information, The Upjohn Company, Kalamazoo, Michigan 49001.

Upjohn—Cont.

proctitis in the female when due to susceptible strains of *Neisseria gonorrhoeae*. Men and women with known recent exposure to gonorrhea should be treated as those known to have gonorrhea.
The *in vitro* susceptibility of *Neisseria gonorrhoeae* to spectinomycin hydrochloride can be tested by agar dilution methods. TROBICIN Susceptibility Powder is available for this purpose, and its package insert should be consulted for details.

CONTRAINDICATIONS

The use of TROBICIN Sterile Powder (spectinomycin hydrochloride) is contraindicated in patients previously found hypersensitive to it.

WARNINGS

Spectinomycin hydrochloride is not effective in the treatment of syphilis. Antibiotics used in high doses for short periods of time to treat gonorrhea may mask or delay the symptoms of incubating syphilis. Since the treatment of syphilis demands prolonged therapy with any effective antibiotic, patients being treated for gonorrhea should be closely observed clinically. All patients with gonorrhea should have a serologic test for syphilis at the time of diagnosis. Patients treated with spectinomycin hydrochloride should have a follow-up serologic test for syphilis after three months.
Usage in pregnancy: Safety for use in pregnancy has not been established.
Usage in infants and children: Safety for use in infants and children has not been established.
The diluent provided with this product contains benzyl alcohol which has been associated with a fatal gasping syndrome in infants.

PRECAUTIONS

The usual precautions should be observed with atopic individuals.
The clinical effectiveness of TROBICIN Sterile Powder (spectinomycin hydrochloride) should be monitored to detect evidence of development of resistance by *Neisseria gonorrhoeae*.

ADVERSE REACTIONS

The following reactions were observed during the single dose clinical trials: soreness at the injection site, urticaria, dizziness, nausea, chills, fever and insomnia.
During multiple dose subchronic tolerance studies in normal human volunteers, the following were noted: a decrease in hemoglobin, hematocrit and creatinine clearance; elevation of alkaline phosphatase, BUN and SGPT. In single and multiple dose studies in normal volunteers, a reduction in urine output was noted. Extensive renal function studies demonstrated no consistent changes indicative of renal toxicity.
Although no clearly defined case of anaphylaxis has been reported with TROBICIN Sterile Powder, the possibility of such reactions should be considered particularly when using antibiotics.
A few cases of anaphylaxis or anaphylactoid reactions have been reported. If serious allergic reactions occur, the usual agents (epinephrine, corticosteroids, and/or antihistamines) should be available for emergency use. In cases of severe anaphylaxis, airway support and oxygen may also be required.

DOSAGE AND ADMINISTRATION

Preparation of Drug for Intramuscular Injection
TROBICIN Sterile Powder, 2 grams (spectinomycin hydrochloride): reconstitute with 3.2 ml of the accompanying diluent.*
TROBICIN Sterile Powder, 4 grams: reconstitute with 6.2 ml of the accompanying diluent.*
Shake vials vigorously immediately after adding diluent and before withdrawing dose. It is recommended that disposable syringes and needles be used to avoid contamination with penicillin residue, especially when treating patients known to be highly sensitive to penicillin. **Use of 20 gauge needle is recommended.**
Dosage
Intramuscular injections should be made deep into the upper outer quadrant of the gluteal muscle.
Adults (Men and Women)—Inject 5 ml intramuscularly for a 2 gram dose. This is also the recommended dose for patients being treated after failure of previous antibiotic therapy.
In geographic areas where antibiotic resistance is known to be prevalent, initial treatment with 4 grams (10 ml) intramuscularly is preferred. The 10 ml injection may be divided between two gluteal injection sites.

STORAGE CONDITIONS

Store unreconstituted product at controlled room temperature 15°– 30°C (59°–86°F). Store prepared suspension at controlled room temperature 15°–30°C (59°–86°F) and use within 24 hours.

*Bacteriostatic Water for Injection with Benzyl Alcohol 0.945% w/v added as preservative.

HOW SUPPLIED

TROBICIN Sterile Powder (spectinomycin hydrochloride) is available as:
TROBICIN Sterile Powder, 2 gram vial—with one ampoule of Bacteriostatic Water for Injection with Benzyl Alcohol 0.945% w/v added as preservative. When reconstituted with 3.2 ml of the accompanying diluent, each vial yields a sufficient quantity for withdrawal of 5 ml of a suspension containing 400 mg spectinomycin per ml (as the hydrochloride). 5 ml provides 2 grams spectinomycin. For intramuscular use only.
NDC 0009-0566-01
TROBICIN Sterile Powder 4 gram vial—with one ampoule of Bacteriostatic Water for Injection with Benzyl Alcohol 0.945% w/v added as preservative. When reconstituted with 6.2 ml of the accompanying diluent, each vial yields a sufficient quantity for withdrawal of 10 ml of a suspension containing spectinomycin hydrochloride equivalent to 400 mg spectinomycin per ml. 10 ml provides 4 grams spectinomycin. For intramuscular use only.
NDC 0009-0592-01
TROBICIN Susceptibility Powder—100 mg. See package insert for *in vitro* testing procedure.

HUMAN PHARMACOLOGY

TROBICIN Sterile Powder (spectinomycin hydrochloride) is rapidly absorbed after intramuscular injection. A single, two gram injection produces peak serum concentrations averaging about 100 mcg/ml at one hour; a single, four gram injection produces peak serum concentrations averaging 160 mcg/ml at two hours. Average serum concentrations of 15 mcg/ml for the two gram dose and 31 mcg/ml for the four gram dose were present eight hours after dosing.
Code 810 130 007

XANAX® Ⓒ ℞

brand of alprazolam tablets, USP

0.25 mg, 100's Unit Dose	**NSN 6505-01-188-7936 (VA)**
0.25 mg, 100's	**NSN 6505-01-143-9269 (M & VA)**
0.25 mg, 500's	**NSN 6505-01-197-3966**
0.5 mg, 100's Unit Dose	**NSN 6505-01-140-3201 (M & VA)**
0.5 mg, 100's	**NSN 6505-01-140-3199 (M & VA)**
0.5 mg, 500's	**NSN 6505-01-196-9501**
1.0 mg, 100's Unit Dose	**NSN 6505-01-140-3202 (VA)**
1.0 mg, 100's	**NSN 6505-01-140-3200 (M & VA)**
1.0 mg, 500's	**NSN 6505-01-197-9003**
2.0 mg, 100's	**NSN 6505-01-336-6197**
2.0 mg, 500's	**NSN 6505-01-336-6198**

DESCRIPTION

XANAX Tablets contain alprazolam which is a triazolo analog of the 1,4 benzodiazepine class of central nervous system-active compounds.
The chemical name of alprazolam is 8-Chloro-1-methyl-6-phenyl-4H-s-triazolo[4,3-α] [1,4] benzodiazepine.
The structural formula is represented below.

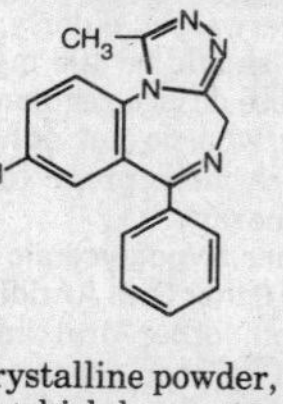

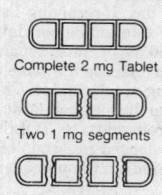

Alprazolam is a white crystalline powder, which is soluble in methanol or ethanol but which has no appreciable solubility in water at physiological pH.
Each XANAX tablet, for oral administration, contains 0.25, 0.5, 1 or 2 mg of alprazolam.
XANAX Tablets, 2 mg, are multi-scored and may be divided as shown below:

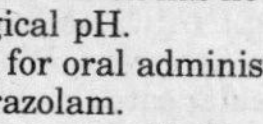

Complete 2 mg Tablet

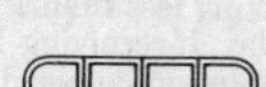

Two 1 mg segments

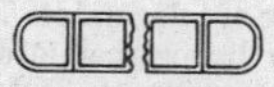

Four 0.5 mg segments

Inactive ingredients: cellulose, corn starch, docusate sodium, lactose, magnesium stearate, silicon dioxide and sodium benzoate. In addition, the 0.5 mg tablet contains FD&C Yellow No. 6 and the 1 mg tablet contains FD&C Blue No. 2.

CLINICAL PHARMACOLOGY

CNS agents of the 1,4 benzodiazepine class presumably exert their effects by binding at stereo specific receptors at several sites within the central nervous system. Their exact mechanism of action is unknown. Clinically, all benzodiazepines cause a dose-related central nervous system depressant activity varying from mild impairment of task performance to hypnosis.
Following oral administration, alprazolam is readily absorbed. Peak concentrations in the plasma occur in one to two hours following administration. Plasma levels are proportionate to the dose given; over the dose range of 0.5 to 3.0 mg, peak levels of 8.0 to 37 ng/ml were observed. Using a specific assay methodology, the mean plasma elimination half-life of alprazolam has been found to be about 11.2 hours (range: 6.3–26.9 hours) in healthy adults.
The predominant metabolites are α-hydroxy-alprazolam and a benzophenone derived from alprazolam. The biological activity of α-hydroxy-alprazolam is approximately one-half that of alprazolam. The benzophenone metabolite is essentially inactive. Plasma levels of these metabolites are extremely low, thus precluding precise pharmacokinetic description. However, their half-lives appear to be of the same order of magnitude as that of alprazolam. Alprazolam and its metabolites are excreted primarily in the urine.
The ability of alprazolam to induce human hepatic enzyme systems has not yet been determined. However, this is not a property of benzodiazepines in general. Further, alprazolam did not affect the prothrombin or plasma warfarin levels in male volunteers administered sodium warfarin orally.
In vitro, alprazolam is bound (80 percent) to human serum protein.
Changes in the absorption, distribution, metabolism and excretion of benzodiazepines have been reported in a variety of disease states including alcoholism, impaired hepatic function and impaired renal function. Changes have also been demonstrated in geriatric patients. A mean half-life of alprazolam of 16.3 hours has been observed in healthy elderly subjects (range: 9.0–26.9 hours, n=16) compared to 11.0 hours (range: 6.3–15.8 hours, n=16) in healthy adult subjects. The co-administration of oral contraceptives to healthy women increased the half-life of alprazolam as compared to that in healthy control women (mean: 12.4 hours, n=11 versus 9.6 hours, n=9). There was a prolongation in the mean half-life of alprazolam from 12.4 hours (range: 7.2–18.4 hours, n=9) to 16.6 hours (range: 10.0–24.3 hours, n=9) by the co-administration of cimetidine to the same healthy adults. In patients with alcoholic liver disease the half-life of alprazolam ranged between 5.8 and 65.3 hours (mean: 19.7 hours, n=17) as compared to between 6.3 and 26.9 hours (mean=11.4 hours, n=17) in healthy subjects. In an obese group of subjects the half-life of alprazolam ranged between 9.9 and 40.4 hours (mean=21.8 hours, n=12) as compared to between 6.3 and 15.8 hours (mean=10.6 hours, n=12) in healthy subjects.
Because of its similarity to other benzodiazepines, it is assumed that alprazolam undergoes transplacental passage and that it is excreted in human milk.

INDICATIONS AND USAGE

XANAX Tablets (alprazolam) are indicated for the management of anxiety disorder (a condition corresponding most closely to the APA Diagnostic and Statistical Manual [DSM-III-R] diagnosis of generalized anxiety disorder) or the short-term relief of symptoms of anxiety. Anxiety or tension associated with the stress of everyday life usually does not require a treatment with an anxiolytic.
Generalized anxiety disorder is characterized by unrealistic or excessive anxiety and worry (apprehensive expectation) about two or more life circumstances, for a period of six months or longer, during which the person has been bothered more days than not by these concerns. At least 6 of the following 18 symptoms are often present in these patients: *Motor Tension* (trembling, twitching, or feeling shaky; muscle tension, aches, or soreness; restlessness; easy fatigability); *Autonomic Hyperactivity* (shortness of breath or smothering sensations; palpitations or accelerated heart rate; sweating, or cold clammy hands; dry mouth; dizziness or lightheadedness; nausea, diarrhea, or other abdominal distress; flushes or chills; frequent urination; trouble swallowing or 'lump in throat'); *Vigilance and Scanning* (feeling keyed up or on edge; exaggerated startle response; difficulty concentrating or 'mind going blank' because of anxiety; trouble falling or staying asleep; irritability). These symptoms must not be secondary to another psychiatric disorder or caused by some organic factor.
Anxiety associated with depression is responsive to XANAX.
XANAX is also indicated for the treatment of panic disorder, with or without agoraphobia.
Studies supporting this claim were conducted in patients whose diagnoses corresponded closely to the DSM-III-R criteria for panic disorder (See CLINICAL STUDIES).
Panic disorder is an illness characterized by recurrent panic attacks. The panic attacks, at least initially, are unexpected. Later in the course of this disturbance certain situations, eg, driving a car or being in a crowded place, may become associated with having a panic attack. These panic attacks are not triggered by situations in which the person is the focus of others' attention (as in social phobia). The diagnosis requires four such attacks within a four week period, or one or more

attacks followed by at least a month of persistent fear of having another attack. The panic attacks must be characterized by at least four of the following symptoms: dyspnea or smothering sensations; dizziness, unsteady feelings, or faintness; palpitations or tachycardia; trembling or shaking; sweating; choking; nausea or abdominal distress; depersonalization or derealization; paresthesias; hot flashes or chills; chest pain or discomfort; fear of dying; fear of going crazy or of doing something uncontrolled. At least some of the panic attack symptoms must develop suddenly, and the panic attack symptoms must not be attributable to some known organic factors. Panic disorder is frequently associated with some symptoms of agoraphobia.

Demonstrations of the effectiveness of XANAX by systematic clinical study are limited to four months duration for anxiety disorder and four to ten weeks duration for panic disorder; however, patients with panic disorder have been treated on an open basis for up to eight months without apparent loss of benefit. The physician should periodically reassess the usefulness of the drug for the individual patient.

CONTRAINDICATIONS

XANAX Tablets are contraindicated in patients with known sensitivity to this drug or other benzodiazepines. XANAX may be used in patients with open angle glaucoma who are receiving appropriate therapy, but is contraindicated in patients with acute narrow angle glaucoma.

WARNINGS

Dependence and withdrawal reactions, including seizures:
Certain adverse clinical events, some life-threatening, are a direct consequence of physical dependence to XANAX. These include a spectrum of withdrawal symptoms; the most important is seizure (see DRUG ABUSE AND DEPENDENCE). Even after relatively short-term use at the doses recommended for the treatment of transient anxiety and anxiety disorder (ie, 0.75 to 4.0 mg per day), there is some risk of dependence. Post-marketing surveillance data suggest that the risk of dependence and its severity appear to be greater in patients treated with relatively high doses (above 4 mg per day) and for long periods (more than 8–12 weeks).

The importance of dose and the risks of XANAX as a treatment for panic disorder,
Because the management of panic disorder often requires the use of average daily doses of XANAX above 4 mg, the risk of dependence among panic disorder patients may be higher than that among those treated for less severe anxiety. Experience in randomized placebo-controlled discontinuation studies of patients with panic disorder showed a high rate of rebound and withdrawal symptoms in patients treated with XANAX compared to placebo treated patients.

Relapse or return of illness was defined as a return of symptoms characteristic of panic disorder (primarily panic attacks) to levels approximately equal to those seen at baseline before active treatment was initiated. Rebound refers to a return of symptoms of panic disorder to a level substantially greater in frequency, or more severe in intensity than seen at baseline. Withdrawal symptoms were identified as those which were generally not characteristic of panic disorder and which occurred for the first time more frequently during discontinuation than at baseline.

In a controlled clinical trial in which 63 patients were randomized to XANAX and where withdrawal symptoms were specifically sought, the following were identified as symptoms of withdrawal: heightened sensory perception, impaired concentration, dysosmia, clouded sensorium, paresthesias, muscle cramps, muscle twitch, diarrhea, blurred vision, appetite decrease and weight loss. Other symptoms, such as anxiety and insomnia, were frequently seen during discontinuation, but it could not be determined if they were due to return of illness, rebound or withdrawal.

In a larger database comprised of both controlled and uncontrolled studies in which 641 patients received XANAX, discontinuation-emergent symptoms which occurred at a rate of over 5% in patients treated with XANAX and at a greater rate than the placebo treated group were as follows:
[See table above.]

DISCONTINUATION-EMERGENT SYMPTOM INCIDENCE
Percentage of 641 XANAX-Treated Panic Disorder Patients Reporting Events

Body System/Event	
Neurologic	
Insomnia	29.5
Lightheadedness	19.3
Abnormal involuntary movement	17.3
Headache	17.0
Muscular twitching	6.9
Impaired Coordination	6.6
Muscle tone disorders	5.9
Weakness	5.8
Psychiatric	
Anxiety	19.2
Fatigue and Tiredness	18.4
Irritability	10.5
Cognitive disorder	10.3
Memory impairment	5.5
Depression	5.1
Confusional state	5.0
Gastrointestinal	
Nausea/Vomiting	16.5
Diarrhea	13.6
Decreased salivation	10.6
Metabolic-Nutritional	
Weight loss	13.3
Decreased appetite	12.8
Dermatological	
Sweating	14.4
Cardiovascular	
Tachycardia	12.2
Special Senses	
Blurred vision	10.0

From the studies cited, it has not been determined whether these symptoms are clearly related to the dose and duration of therapy with XANAX in patients with panic disorder.

In two controlled trials of six to eight weeks duration where the ability of patients to discontinue medication was measured, 71%–93% of patients treated with XANAX tapered completely off therapy compared to 89%–96% of placebo treated patients. The ability of patients to completely discontinue therapy with XANAX after long-term therapy has not been reliably determined.

Seizures attributable to XANAX were seen after drug discontinuance or dose reduction in 8 of 1980 patients with panic disorder or in patients participating in clinical trials where doses of XANAX greater than 4 mg daily for over 3 months were permitted. Five of these cases clearly occurred during abrupt dose reduction, or discontinuation from daily doses of 2 to 10 mg. Three cases occurred in situations where there was not a clear relationship to abrupt dose reduction or discontinuation. In one instance, seizure occurred after discontinuation from a single dose of 1 mg after tapering at a rate of 1 mg every three days from 6 mg daily. In two other instances, the relationship to taper is indeterminate; in both of these cases the patients had been receiving doses of 3 mg daily prior to seizure. The duration of use in the above 8 cases ranged from 4 to 22 weeks. There have been occasional voluntary reports of patients developing seizures while apparently tapering gradually from XANAX. The risk of seizure seems to be greatest 24–72 hours after discontinuation (see DOSAGE and ADMINISTRATION for recommended tapering and discontinuation schedule).

Status epilepticus and its treatment:
The medical event voluntary reporting system shows that withdrawal seizures have been reported in association with the discontinuation of XANAX. In most cases, only a single seizure was reported; however, multiple seizures and status epilepticus were reported as well. Ordinarily, the treatment of status epilepticus of any etiology involves use of intravenous benzodiazepines plus phenytoin or barbiturates, maintenance of a patent airway and adequate hydration. For additional details regarding therapy, consultation with an appropriate specialist may be considered.

Interdose Symptoms:
Early morning anxiety and emergence of anxiety symptoms between doses of XANAX have been reported in patients with panic disorder taking prescribed maintenance doses of XANAX. These symptoms may reflect the development of tolerance or a time interval between doses which is longer than the duration of clinical action of the administered dose. In either case, it is presumed that the prescribed dose is not sufficient to maintain plasma levels above those needed to prevent relapse, rebound or withdrawal symptoms over the entire course of the interdosing interval. In these situations, it is recommended that the same total daily dose be given divided as more frequent administrations (See DOSAGE AND ADMINISTRATION).

Risk of dose reduction:
Withdrawal reactions may occur when dosage reduction occurs for any reason. This includes purposeful tapering, but also inadvertent reduction of dose (eg. the patient forgets, the patient is admitted to a hospital, etc.). Therefore, the dosage of XANAX should be reduced or discontinued gradually (See DOSAGE AND ADMINISTRATION).

XANAX Tablets are not of value in the treatment of psychotic patients and should not be employed in lieu of appropriate treatment for psychosis. Because of its CNS depressant effects, patients receiving XANAX should be cautioned against engaging in hazardous occupations or activities requiring complete mental alertness such as operating machinery or driving a motor vehicle. For the same reason, patients should be cautioned about the simultaneous ingestion of alcohol and other CNS depressant drugs during treatment with XANAX.

Benzodiazepines can potentially cause fetal harm when administered to pregnant women. If XANAX is used during pregnancy, or if the patient becomes pregnant while taking this drug, the patient should be apprised of the potential hazard to the fetus. Because of experience with other members of the benzodiazepine class, XANAX is assumed to be capable of causing an increased risk of congenital abnormalities when administered to a pregnant woman during the first trimester. Because use of these drugs is rarely a matter of urgency, their use during the first trimester should almost always be avoided. The possibility that a woman of childbearing potential may be pregnant at the time of institution of therapy should be considered. Patients should be advised that if they become pregnant during therapy or intend to become pregnant they should communicate with their physicians about the desirability of discontinuing the drug.

PRECAUTIONS

General: If XANAX Tablets are to be combined with other psychotropic agents or anticonvulsant drugs, careful consideration should be given to the pharmacology of the agents to be employed, particularly with compounds which might potentiate the action of benzodiazepines (See DRUG INTERACTIONS).

As with other psychotropic medications, the usual precautions with respect to administration of the drug and size of the prescription are indicated for severely depressed patients or those in whom there is reason to expect concealed suicidal ideation or plans.

It is recommended that the dosage be limited to the smallest effective dose to preclude the development of ataxia or oversedation which may be a particular problem in elderly or debiliated patients. (See DOSAGE AND ADMINISTRATION). The usual precautions in treating patients with impaired renal, hepatic or pulmonary function should be observed. There have been rare reports of death in patients with severe puolmonary disease shortly after the initiation of treatment with XANAX. A decreased systemic alprazolam elimination rate (eg, increased plasma half-life) has been observed in both alcoholic liver disease patients and obese patients receiving XANAX (See CLINICAL PHARMACOLOGY)

Episodes of hypomania and mania have been reported in association with the use of XANAX in patients with depression.

Alprazolam has a weak uricosuric effect. Although other medications with weak uricosuric effect have been reported to cause acute renal failure, there have been no reported instances of acute renal failure attributable to therapy with XANAX.

Information for Patients:
For all users of XANAX.
To assure safe and effective use of benzodiazepines, all patients prescribed XANAX should be provided with the following guidance. In addition, panic disorder patients, for whom higher doses are typically prescribed, should be advised about the risks associated with the use of higher doses.

1. Inform your physician about any alcohol consumption and medicine you are taking now, including medication you may buy without a prescription. Alcohol should generally not be used during treatment with benzodiazepines.
2. Not recommended for use in pregnancy. Therefore, inform your physician if you are pregnant, if you are planning to have a child, or if you become pregnant while you are taking this medication.
3. Inform your physician if you are nursing.
4. Until you experience how this medication affects you, do not drive a car or operate potentially dangerous machinery, etc.
5. Do not increase the dose even if you think the mediciation "does not work anymore" without consulting your physician. Benzodiazepines, even when used as recommended, may produce emotional and/or physical dependence.
6 Do not stop taking the drug abruptly or decrease the dose without consulting your physician, since withdrawal symptoms can occur.

Additional advice for panic disorder patients:
The use of XANAX at the high doses (above 4 mg per day), often necessary to treat panic disorder, is accompanied by risks that you may need to carefully consider. When used at

Continued on next page

Information on these Upjohn products is based on labeling in effect June 1, 1992. Further information concerning these and other Upjohn products may be obtained by direct inquiry to Medical Information, The Upjohn Company, Kalamazoo, Michigan 49001.

Upjohn—Cont.

high doses for long intervals, which may or may not be required for your treatment, XANAX has the potential to cause severe emotional and physical dependence in some patients and these patients may find it exceedingly difficult to terminate treatment. In two controlled trials of six to eight weeks duration where the ability of patients to discontinue medication was measured, 7 to 29% of patients treated with XANAX did not completely taper off therapy. The ability of patients to completely discontinue therapy with XANAX after long-term therapy has not been reliably determined. In all cases, it is important that your physician help you discontinue this medication in a careful and safe manner to avoid overly extended use of XANAX.

In addition, the extended use at high doses appears to increase the incidence and severity of withdrawal reactions when XANAX is discontinued. These are generally minor but seizure can occur, especially if you reduce the dose too rapidly or discontinue the medication abruptly. Seizure can be life-threatening.

Laboratory Tests: Laboratory tests are not ordinarily required in otherwise healthy patients.

Drug Interactions: The benzodiazepines, including alprazolam, produce additive CNS depressant effects when co-administered with other psychotropic medications, anticonvulsants, antihistaminics, ethanol and other drugs which themselves produce CNS depression.

The steady state plasma concentrations of imipramine and desipramine have been reported to be increased an average of 31% and 20%, respectively, by the concomitant administration of XANAX Tablets in doses up to 4 mg/day. The clinical significance of these changes is unknown.

Pharmacokinetic interactions of benzodiazepines with other drugs have been reported. For example, the clearance of alprazolam and certain other benzodiazepines can be delayed by the co-administration of cimetidine. The clearance of alprazolam can also be delayed by the co-administration of oral contraceptives (See CLINICAL PHARMACOLOGY). The clinical significance of these interactions is unclear.

Drug/Laboratory Test Interactions: Although interactions between benzodiazepines and commonly employed clinical laboratory tests have occasionally been reported, there is no consistent pattern for a specific drug or specific test.

Carcinogenesis, Mutagenesis, Impairment of Fertility: No evidence of carcinogenic potential was observed during 2-year bioassay studies of alprazolam in rats at doses up to 30 mg/kg/day (150 times the maximum recommended daily human dose of 10 mg/day) and in mice at doses up to 10 mg/

kg/day (50 times the maximum recommended daily human dose).

Alprazolam was not mutagenic in the rat micronucleus test at doses up to 100 mg/kg, which is 500 times the maximum recommended daily human dose of 10 mg/day. Alprazolam also was not mutagenic in vitro in the DNA Damage/Alkaline Elution Assay or the Ames Assay.

Alprazolam produced no impairment of fertility in rats at doses up to 5 mg/kg/day, which is 25 times the maximum recommended daily human dose of 10 mg/day.

Pregnancy: Teratogenic Effects: Pregnancy Category D: (See WARNINGS Section)

Nonteratogenic Effects: It should be considered that the child born of a mother who is receiving benzodiazepines may be at some risk for withdrawal symptoms from the drug during the postnatal period. Also, neonatal flaccidity and respiratory problems have been reported in children born of mothers who have been receiving benzodiazepines.

Labor and Delivery: XANAX has no established use in labor or delivery.

Nursing Mothers: Benzodiazepines are known to be excreted in human milk. It should be assumed that alprazolam is as well. Chronic administration of diazepam to nursing mothers has been reported to cause their infants to become lethargic and to lose weight. As a general rule, nursing should not be undertaken by mothers who must use XANAX.

Pediatric Use: Safety and effectiveness in children below the age of 18 years have not been established.

ADVERSE REACTIONS

Side effects to XANAX Tablets, if they occur, are generally observed at the beginning of therapy and usually disappear upon continued medication. In the usual patient, the most frequent side effects are likely to be an extension of the pharmacological activity of alprazolam, eg, drowsiness or lightheadedness.

The data cited in the two tables below are estimates of untoward clinical event incidence among patients who participated under the following clinical conditions: relatively short duration (ie, four weeks) placebo-controlled clinical studies with dosages up to 4 mg/day of XANAX (for the management of anxiety disorders or for the short-term relief of the symptoms of anxiety) and short-term (up to ten weeks) placebo-controlled clinical studies with dosages up to 10 mg/day of XANAX in patients with panic disorder, with or without agoraphobia.

These data cannot be used to predict precisely the incidence of untoward events in the course of usual medical practice where patient characteristics, and other factors often differ from those in clinical trials. These figures cannot be com-

PANIC DISORDER

	Treatment-Emergent Symptom Incidence*	
	XANAX	Placebo
Number of Patients	1388	1231
% of Patients Reporting:		
Central Nervous System		
Drowsiness	76.8	42.7
Fatigue and Tiredness	48.6	42.3
Impaired Coordination	40.1	17.9
Irritability	33.1	30.1
Memory Impairment	33.1	22.1
Lightheadness/Dizziness	29.8	36.9
Insomnia	29.4	41.8
Headache	29.2	35.6
Cognitive Disorder	28.8	20.5
Dysarthria	23.3	6.3
Anxiety	16.6	24.9
Abnormal Involuntary Movement	14.8	21.0
Decreased Libido	14.4	8.0
Depression	13.8	14.0
Confusional State	10.4	8.2
Muscular Twitching	7.9	11.8
Increased Libido	7.7	4.1
Change in Libido (Not Specified)	7.1	5.6
Weakness	7.1	8.4
Muscle Tone Disorders	6.3	7.5
Syncope	3.8	4.8
Akathisia	3.0	4.3
Agitation	2.9	2.6
Disinhibition	2.7	1.5
Paresthesia	2.4	3.2
Talkativeness	2.2	1.0
Vasomotor Disturbances	2.0	2.6
Derealization	1.9	1.2
Dream Abnormalities	1.8	1.5
Fear	1.4	1.0
Feeling Warm	1.3	0.5
Gastrointestinal		
Decreased Salivation	32.8	34.2
Constipation	26.2	15.4
Nausea/Vomiting	22.0	31.8
Diarrhea	20.6	22.8
Abdominal Distress	18.3	21.5
Increased Salivation	5.6	4.4
Cardio-Respiratory		
Nasal Congestion	17.4	16.5
Tachycardia	15.4	26.8
Chest Pain	10.6	18.1
Hyperventilation	9.7	14.5
Upper Respiratory Infection	4.3	3.7
Sensory		
Blurred Vision	21.0	21.4
Tinnitus	6.6	10.4
Musculoskeletal		
Muscular Cramps	2.4	2.4
Muscle Stiffness	2.2	3.3
Cutaneous		
Sweating	15.1	23.5
Rash	10.8	8.1
Other		
Increased Appetite	32.7	22.8
Decreased Appetite	27.8	24.1
Weight Gain	27.2	17.9
Weight Loss	22.6	16.5
Micturition Difficulties	12.2	8.6
Menstrual Disorders	10.4	8.7
Sexual Dysfunction	7.4	3.7
Edema	4.9	5.6
Incontinence	1.5	0.6
Infection	1.3	1.7

Events reported by 1% or more of patients on XANAX are included.

ANXIETY DISORDERS

	Treatment-Emergent Symptom Incidence†		Incidence of Intervention Because of Symptom
	XANAX	Placebo	XANAX
Number of Patients	565	505	565
% of Patients Reporting:			
Central Nervous System			
Drowsiness	41.0	21.6	15.1
Light-headedness	20.8	19.3	1.2
Depression	13.9	18.1	2.4
Headache	12.9	19.6	1.1
Confusion	9.9	10.0	0.9
Insomnia	8.9	18.4	1.3
Nervousness	4.1	10.3	1.1
Syncope	3.1	4.0	*
Dizziness	1.8	0.8	2.5
Akathisia	1.6	1.2	*
Tiredness/Sleepiness	*	*	1.8
Gastrointestinal			
Dry Mouth	14.7	13.3	0.7
Constipation	10.4	11.4	0.9
Diarrhea	10.1	10.3	1.2
Nausea/Vomiting	9.6	12.8	1.7
Increased Salivation	4.2	2.4	*
Cardiovascular			
Tachycardia/Palpitations	7.7	15.6	0.4
Hypotension	4.7	2.2	*
Sensory			
Blurred Vision	6.2	6.2	0.4
Musculoskeletal			
Rigidity	4.2	5.3	*
Tremor	4.0	8.8	0.4
Cutaneous			
Dermatitis/Allergy	3.8	3.1	0.6
Other			
Nasal			
Congestion	7.3	9.3	*
Weight Gain	2.7	2.7	*
Weight Loss	2.3	3.0	*

* *None reported*
† *Events reported by 1% or more of patients on XANAX are included.*

pared with those obtained from other clinical studies involving related drug products and placebo as each group of drug trials are conducted under a different set of conditions.

Comparison of the cited figures, however, can provide the prescriber with some basis for estimating the relative contributions of drug and non-drug factors to the untoward event incidence in the population studied. Even this use must be approached cautiously, as a drug may relieve a symptom in one patient but induce it in others. (For example, an anxiolytic drug may relieve dry mouth [a symptom of anxiety] in some subjects but induce it [an untoward event] in others.) Additionally, for anxiety disorders the cited figures can provide the prescriber with an indication as to the frequency with which physician intervention (eg, increased surveillance, decreased dosage or discontinuation of drug therapy) may be necessary because of the untoward clinical event. [See table at left.]

In addition to the relatively common (i.e., greater than 1%) untoward events enumerated above, the following adverse events have been reported in association with the use of ben-

zodiazepines: dystonia, irritability, concentration difficulties, anorexia, transient amnesia or memory impairment, loss of coordination, fatigue, seizures, sedation, slurred speech, jaundice, musculoskeletal weakness, pruritus, diplopia, dysarthria, changes in libido, menstrual irregularities, incontinence and urinary retention.

[See table at top of preceding page.]

In addition to the relatively common (ie, greater than 1%) untoward events enumerated in the table above, the following adverse events have been reported in association with the use of XANAX: seizures, hallucinations, depersonalization, taste alterations, diplopia, elevated bilirubin, elevated hepatic enzymes, and jaundice.

There have also been reports of withdrawal seizures upon rapid decrease or abrupt discontinuation of XANAX Tablets (See WARNINGS).

To discontinue treatment in patients taking XANAX, the dosage should be reduced slowly in keeping with good medical practice. It is suggested that the daily dosage of XANAX be decreased by no more than 0.5 mg every three days (See DOSAGE AND ADMINISTRATION). Some patients may require an even slower dosage reduction.

Panic disorder has been associated with primary and secondary major depressive disorders and increased reports of suicide among untreated patients. Therefore, the same precaution must be exercised when using the higher doses of XANAX in treating patients with panic disorder as is exercised with the use of any psychotropic drug in treating depressed patients or those in whom there is reason to expect concealed suicidal ideation or plans.

As with all benzodiazepines, paradoxical reactions such as stimulation, agitation, rage, increased muscle spasticity, sleep disturbances, hallucinations and other adverse behavioral effects may occur in rare instances and in a random fashion. Should these occur, use of the drug should be discontinued.

Laboratory analyses were performed on all patients participating in the clinical program for XANAX. The following incidences of abnormalities shown below were observed in patients receiving XANAX and in patients in the corresponding placebo group. Few of these abnormalities were considered to be of physiological significance.

	XANAX		Placebo	
	Low	High	Low	High
Hematology				
Hematocrit	*	*	*	*
Hemoglobin	*	*	*	*
Total WBC Count	1.4	2.3	1.0	2.0
Neutrophil Count	2.3	3.0	4.2	1.7
Lymphocyte Count	5.5	7.4	5.4	9.5
Monocyte Count	5.3	2.8	6.4	*
Eosinophil Count	3.2	9.5	3.3	7.2
Basophil Count	*	*	*	*
Urinalysis				
Albumin	—	*	—	*
Sugar	—	*	—	*
RBC/HPF	—	3.4	—	5.0
WBC/HPF	—	25.7	—	25.9
Blood Chemistry				
Creatinine	2.2	1.9	3.5	1.0
Bilirubin	*	1.6	*	*
SGOT	*	3.2	1.0	1.8
Alkaline Phosphatase	*	1.7	*	1.8

**Less than 1%*

When treatment with XANAX is protracted, periodic blood counts, urinalysis and blood chemistry analyses are advisable.

Minor changes in EEG patterns, usually low-voltage fast activity have been observed in patients during therapy with XANAX and are of no known significance.

Post Introduction Reports: Various adverse drug reactions have been reported in association with the use of XANAX since market introduction. The majority of these reactions were reported through the medical event voluntary reporting system. Because of the spontaneous nature of the reporting of medical events and the lack of controls, a causal relationship to the use of XANAX cannot be readily determined. Reported events include: liver enzyme elevations, gynecomastia and galactorrhea.

DRUG ABUSE AND DEPENDENCE

Physical and Psychological Dependence: Withdrawal symptoms similar in character to those noted with sedative/hypnotics and alcohol have occurred following abrupt discontinuance of benzodiazepines, including XANAX. The symptoms can range from mild dysphoria and insomnia to a major syndrome that may include abdominal and muscle cramps, vomiting, sweating, tremors and convulsions. Distinguishing between withdrawal emergent signs and symptoms and the recurrence of illness is often difficult in patients undergoing dose reduction. The long term strategy for treatment of these phenomena will vary with their cause and the therapeutic goal. When necessary, immediate management of withdrawal symptoms requires re-institution of treatment at doses of XANAX sufficient to suppress symptoms. There have been reports of failure of other benzodiazephines to fully suppress these withdrawal symptoms. These failures have been attributed to incompete cross-tolerance but may also reflect the use of an inadequate dosage regimen of the substituted benzodiazepine or the effects of concomitant medications.

While it is difficult to distinguish withdrawal and recurrence for certain patients, the time course and the nature of the symptoms may be helpful. A withdrawal symdrome typically includes the occurence of new symptoms, tends to appear toward the end of the taper or shortly after discontinuation, and will decrease with time. In recurring panic disorder, symptoms similar to those observed before treatment may recur either early or late, and they will persist.

While the severity and incidence of withdrawal phenomena appear to be related to dose and duration of treatment, withdrawal symptoms, including seizures, have been reported after only brief therapy with XANAX at doses within the recommended range for the treatment of anxiety (eg, 0.75 to 4 mg/day). Signs and symptoms of withdrawal are often more prominent after rapid decrease of dosage or abrupt discontinuance. The risk of withdrawal seizures may be increased at doses above 4 mg/day (See WARNINGS).

Patients, especially individuals with a history of seizures or epilepsy, should not be abruptly discontinued from any CNS depressant agent, including XANAX. It is recommended that all patients on XANAX who require a dosage reduction be gradually tapered under close supervision (See WARNINGS and DOSAGE AND ADMINISTRATION).

Psychological dependence is a risk with all benzodiazepines, including XANAX. The risk of psychological dependence may also be increased at higher doses and with longer term use, and this risk is further increased in patient with a history of alcohol or drug abuse. Some patients have experienced considerable difficulty in tapering and discontinuing from XANAX, especially those receiving higher doses for extended periods. Addiction-prone individuals should be under careful surveillance when receiving XANAX. As with all anxiolytics, repeat prescriptions should be limited to those who are under medical supervision.

Controlled Substance Class: Alprazolam is a controlled substance under the Controlled Substance Act by the Drug Enforcement Administration and XANAX Tablets have been assigned to Schedule IV.

OVERDOSAGE

Manifestations of alprazolam overdosage include somnolence, confusion, impaired coordination, diminished reflexes and coma. Death has been reported in association with overdoses of alprazolam by itself, as it has with other benzodiazepines. In addition, fatalities have been reported in patients who have overdosed with a combination of a single benzodiazepine, including alprazolam, and alcohol; alcohol levels seen in some of these patients have been lower than those usually associated with alcohol-induced fatality.

The acute oral LD_{50} in rats is 331–2171 mg/kg. Other experiments in animals have indicated that cardiopulmonary collapse can occur following massive intravenous doses of alprazolam (over 195 mg/kg; 975 times the maximum recommended daily human dose of 10 mg/day). Animals could be resuscitated with positive mechanical ventilation and the intravenous infusion of norepinephrine bitartrate.

Animal experiments have suggested that forced diuresis or hemodialysis are probably of little value in treating overdosage.

General Treatment of Overdose: Overdosage reports with XANAX Tablets are limited. As in all cases of drug overdosage, respiration, pulse rate, and blood pressure should be monitored. General supportive measures should be employed, along with immediate gastric lavage. Intravenous fluids should be administered and an adequate airway maintained. If hypotension occurs, it may be combated by the use of vasopressors. Dialysis is of limited value. As with the management of intentional overdosing with any drug, it should be borne in mind that multiple agents may have been ingested.

DOSAGE AND ADMINISTRATION

Dosage should be individualized for maximum beneficial effect. While the usual daily dosages given below will meet the needs of most patients, there will be some who require higher doses. In such cases, dosage should be increased cautiously to avoid adverse effects.

Anxiety disorders and transient symptoms of anxiety:

Treatment for patients with anxiety should be initiated with a dose of 0.25 to 0.5 mg given three times daily. The dose may be increased to achieve a maximum therapeutic effect, at intervals of 3 to 4 days, to a maximum daily dose of 4 mg, given in divided doses. The lowest possible effective dose should be employed and the need for continued treatment reassessed frequently. The risk of dependence may increase with dose and duration of treatment.

In elderly patients, in patients with advanced liver disease or in patients with debilitating disease, the usual starting dose is 0.25 mg, given two or three times daily. This may be gradually increased if needed and tolerated. The elderly may be especially sensitive to the effects of benzodiazepines.

If side effects occur at the recommended starting dose, the dose may be lowered.

In all patients, dosage should be reduced gradually when discontinuing therapy or when decreasing the daily dosage. Although there are no systematically collected data to support a specific discontinuation schedule, it is suggested that the daily dosage be decreased by no more than 0.5 mg every three days. Some patients may require an even slower dosage reduction.

Panic disorder:

The successful treatment of many panic disorder patients has required the use of XANAX at doses greater than 4 mg daily. In controlled trials conducted to establish the efficacy of XANAX in panic disorder, doses in the range of 1 to 10 mg daily were used. The mean dosage employed was approximately 5 to 6 mg daily. Among the approximately 1700 patients participating in the panic disorder development program, about 300 received maximum XANAX dosages of greater than 7 mg/day, including approximately 100 patients who received maximum dosages of greater than 9 mg/day. Occasional patients required as much as 10 mg a day to achieve a successful response.

However, in the absence of systematic studies evaluating the dose response relationship, the dosing regimen for the administration of XANAX to patients with panic disorder must be based on generic principles. Generally, therapy should be initiated at a low dose to minimize the risk of adverse responses in patients especially sensitive to the drug. Thereafter, the dose can be increased at intervals equal to at least 5 times the elimination half-life (about 11 hours in young patients, about 16 hours in elderly patients). Longer titration intervals should probably be used because the maximum therapeutic response may not occur until after the plasma levels achieve steady state. Dose should be advanced until an acceptable therapeutic response (ie, a substantial reduction in or total elimination of panic attacks) is achieved, intolerance occurs, or the maximum recommended dose is attained.

Because of the danger of withdrawal, abrupt discontinuation of treatment should be avoided (See WARNINGS, PRECAUTIONS, DRUG ABUSE AND DEPENDENCE).

The following regimen is one that follows the principles outlined above:

Treatment may be initiated with a dose of 0.5 mg three times daily. Depending on the response, the dose may be increased at intervals of 3 to 4 days in increments of no more than 1 mg per day. Slower titration to the higher dose levels may be advisable to allow full expression of the pharmacodynamic effect of XANAX. To lessen the possibility of interdose symptoms, the times of administration should be distributed as evenly as possible throughout the waking hours, that is, on a three or four times per day schedule.

The necessary duration of treatment for panic disorder patients responding to XANAX is unknown. After a period of extended freedom from attacks, a carefully supervised tapered discontinuation may be attempted, but there is evidence that this may often be difficult to accomplish without recurrence of symptoms and/or the manifestation of withdrawal phenomena.

In any case, reduction of dose must be undertaken under close supervision and must be gradual. If significant withdrawal symptoms develop, the previous dosing schedule should be reinstituted and, only after stabilization, should a less rapid schedule of discontinuation be attempted. Although no experimental studies have been conducted to assess the comparative benefits of various discontinuation regimens, a possible approach is to reduce the dose by no more than 0.5 mg every three days, with the understanding that some patients may require an even more gradual discontinuation. Some patients may prove resistant to all discontinuation regimens.

HOW SUPPLIED

XANAX Tablets are available as follows:

0.25 mg (white, oval, scored)

Bottles of 100	**NDC** 0009-0029-01
Unit-Dose Pkg (100)	**NDC** 0009-0029-09
VISIPAK® Reverse Numbered Pack (100)	**NDC** 0009-0029-20
Bottles of 500	**NDC** 0009-0029-02

0.5 mg (peach, oval, scored)

Bottles of 100	**NDC** 0009-0055-01
Unit-Dose Pkg (100)	**NDC** 0009-0055-02
VISIPAK® Reverse Numbered Pack (100)	**NDC** 0009-0055-22
Bottles of 500	**NDC** 0009-0055-03

Continued on next page

Information on these Upjohn products is based on labeling in effect June 1, 1992. Further information concerning these and other Upjohn products may be obtained by direct inquiry to Medical Information, The Upjohn Company, Kalamazoo, Michigan 49001.

Upjohn—Cont.

1 mg (blue, oval, scored)
Bottles of 100 **NDC** 0009-0090-01
Unit-Dose Pkg (100) **NDC** 0009-0090-02
VISIPAK® Reverse Numbered
Pack (100) **NDC** 0009-0090-17
Bottles of 500 **NDC** 0009-0090-04
2 mg (white, oblong, multi-scored)
Bottles of 100 **NDC** 0009-0094-01
Unit Dose Pkg (100) **NDC** 0009-0094-02
VISIPAK® Reverse Numbered
Pack (100) **NDC** 0009-0094-07
Bottles of 500 **NDC** 0009-0094-03
Store at controlled room temperature 15°–30°C (59°–86°F).
Caution: Federal law prohibits dispensing without prescription.

ANIMAL STUDIES

When rats were treated with alprazolam at 3, 10, and 30 mg/kg/day (15 to 150 times the maximum recommended human dose) orally for 2 years, a tendency for a dose related increase in the number of cataracts was observed in females and a tendency for a dose related increase in corneal vascularization was observed in males. These lesions did not appear until after 11 months of treatment.

CLINICAL STUDIES

Anxiety Disorders:
XANAX Tablets were compared to placebo in double blind clinical studies (doses up to 4 mg/day) in patients with a diagnosis of anxiety or anxiety with associated depressive symptomatology. XANAX was significantly better than placebo at each of the evaluation periods of these four week studies as judged by the following psychometric instruments: Physician's Global Impressions, Hamilton Anxiety Rating Scale Target Symptoms, Patient's Global Impressions and Self-Rating Symptom Scale.
Panic Disorder:
Support for the effectiveness of XANAX in the treatment of panic disorder came from three short-term, placebo controlled studies (up to 10 weeks) in patients with diagnoses closely corresponding to DSM-III-R criteria for panic disorder.
The average dose of XANAX was 5–6 mg/day in two of the studies, and the doses of XANAX were fixed at 2 and 6 mg/day in the third study. In all three studies, XANAX was superior to placebo on a variable defined as "the number of patients with zero panic attacks" (range, 37–83% met this criterion), as well as on a global improvement score. In two of the three studies, XANAX was superior to placebo on a variable defined as "change from baseline on the number of panic attacks per week" (range, 3.3–5.2), and also on a phobia rating scale. A subgroup of patients who were improved on XANAX during short-term treatment in one of these trials was continued on an open basis up to eight months, without apparent loss of benefit.
Code 811 557 620

Shown in Product Identification Section, page 434

ZANOSAR® ℞
brand of streptozocin sterile powder

WARNING

ZANOSAR Sterile Powder should be administered under the supervision of a physician experienced in the use of cancer chemotherapeutic agents.
A patient need not be hospitalized but should have access to a facility with laboratory and supportive resources sufficient to monitor drug tolerance and to protect and maintain a patient compromised by drug toxicity. Renal toxicity is dose-related and cumulative and may be severe or fatal. Other major toxicities are nausea and vomiting which may be severe and at times treatment-limiting. In addition, liver dysfunction, diarrhea, and hematological changes have been observed in some patients. Streptozocin is mutagenic. When administered parenterally, it has been found to be tumorigenic or carcinogenic in some rodents.
The physician must judge the possible benefit to his patient against the known toxic effects of this drug in considering the advisability of therapy with ZANOSAR. He should be familiar with the following text before making his judgment and beginning treatment.

DESCRIPTION

Each vial of ZANOSAR Sterile Powder contains 1 g of the active ingredient streptozocin 2 - deoxy - 2 - [[(methylnitrosoamino)carbonyl]amino]- α(and β) - D - glucopyranose and 220 mg citric acid anhydrous. ZANOSAR is available as a sterile, pale yellow, freeze-dried preparation for intravenous administration. The pH was adjusted with sodium hydroxide. When reconstituted as directed, the pH of the solution will be between 3.5 and 4.5. Streptozocin is a synthetic antineoplastic agent that is chemically related to other nitrosoureas used in cancer chemotheraphy. Streptozocin is an ivory-colored crystalline powder with a molecular weight of 265.2. It is very soluble in water or physiological saline and is soluble in alcohol.

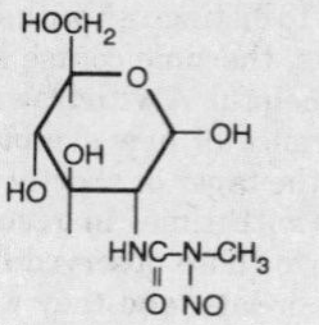

CLINICAL PHARMACOLOGY

Streptozocin inhibits DNA snythesis in bacterial and mammalian cells. In bacterial cells, a specific interaction with cytosine moieties leads to degradation of DNA. The biochemical mechanism leading to mammalian cell death has not been definitely established; streptozocin inhibits cell proliferation at a considerably lower level than that needed to inhibit precursor incorporation into DNA or to inhibit several of the enzymes involved in DNA synthesis. Although streptozocin inhibits the progression of cells into mitosis, no specific phase of the cell cycle is particularly sensitive to its lethal effects.
Streptozocin is active in the L1210 leukemic mouse over a fairly wide range of parenteral dosage schedules. In experiments in many animal species, streptozocin induced a diabetes that resembles human hyperglycemic nonketotic diabetes mellitus. This phenomenon, which has been extensively studied, appears to be mediated through a lowering of beta cell nicotinamide adenine dinucleotide (NAD) and consequent histopathologic alteration of pancreatic islet beta cells.
The metabolism and the chemical dissociation of streptozocin that occurs under physiologic conditions has not been extensively studied. When administered intravenously to a variety of experimental animals, streptozocin disappears from the blood very rapidly. In all species tested, it was found to concentrate in the liver and kidney. As much as 20% of the drug (or metabolites containing an N-nitrosourea group) is metabolized and/or excreted by the kidney. Metabolic products have not yet been identified.

INDICATIONS AND USAGE

ZANOSAR Sterile Powder is indicated in the treatment of metastatic islet cell carcinoma of the pancreas. Responses have been obtained with both functional and nonfunctional carcinomas. Because of its inherent renal toxicity, therapy with this drug should be limited to patients with symptomatic or progressive metastatic disease.

WARNINGS

Renal Toxicity
Many patients treated with ZANOSAR Sterile Powder have experienced renal toxicity, as evidenced by azotemia, anuria hypophosphatemia, glycosuria and renal tubular acidosis. **Such toxicity is dose-related and cumulative and may be severe or fatal.** Renal function must be monitored before and after each course of therapy. Serial urinalysis, blood urea nitrogen, plasma creatinine, serum electrolytes and creatinine clearance should be obtained prior to, at least weekly during, and for four weeks after drug administration. Serial urinalysis is particularly important for the early detection of proteinuria and should be quantitated with a 24 hour collection when proteinuria is detected. Mild proteinuria is one of the first signs of renal toxicity and may herald further deterioration of renal function. Reduction of the dose of ZANOSAR or discontinuation of treatment is suggested in the presence of significant renal toxicity.
Use of ZANOSAR in patients with preexisting renal disease requires a judgment by the physician of potential benefit as opposed to the known risk of serious renal damage.
This drug should not be used in combination with or concomitantly with other potential nephrotoxins.
When exposed dermally, some rats developed benign tumors at the site of application of streptozocin. Consequently, streptozocin may pose a carcinogenic hazard following topical exposure if not properly handled (see DOSAGE AND ADMINISTRATION).
See additional warnings at the beginning of this insert.

PRECAUTIONS

Laboratory Tests: Patients who are treated with ZANOSAR Sterile Powder must be monitored closely, particularly for evidence of renal, hepatic, and hematopoietic toxicity. Renal function tests are described in the WARNINGS section. Patients should also be monitored closely for evidence of hematopoietic and hepatic toxicities. Complete blood counts and liver function tests should be done at least weekly. Dosage adjustments or discontinuance of the drug may be indicated, depending upon the degree of toxicity noted.
Mutagenesis, Carcinogenesis, Impairment of Fertility: Streptozocin is mutagenic in bacteria, plants, and mammalian cells. When administered parenterally, it has been shown to induce renal tumors in rats and to induce liver tumors and other tumors in hamsters. Stomach and pancreatic tumors were observed in rats treated orally with streptozocin. Streptozocin has also been shown to be carcinogenic in mice.
Streptozocin adversely affected fertility when administered to male and female rats.
Pregnancy Category C: Reproduction studies revealed that streptozocin is teratogenic in the rat and has abortifacient effects in rabbits. When administered intravenously to pregnant monkeys, it appears rapidly in the fetal circulation. There are no studies in pregnant women. ZANOSAR should be used during pregnancy only if the potential benefit justifies the potential risk to the fetus.
Nursing Mothers: It is not known whether streptozocin is excreted in human milk. Because many drugs are excreted in human milk and because of the potential for serious adverse reactions in nursing infants, nursing should be discontinued in patients receiving ZANOSAR.

ADVERSE REACTIONS

Renal: See WARNINGS.
Gastrointestinal: Most patients treated with ZANOSAR Sterile Powder have experienced severe nausea and vomiting, occasionally requiring discontinuation of drug therapy. Some patients experienced diarrhea. A number of patients have experienced hepatic toxicity, as characterized by elevated liver enzyme (SGOT and LDH) levels and hypoalbuminemia.
Hematological: Hematological toxicity has been rare, most often involving mild decreases in hematocrit values. However, **fatal hematological toxicity with substantial reductions in leukocyte and platelet count** has been observed.
Metabolic: Mild to moderate abnormalities of glucose tolerance have been noted in some patients treated with ZANOSAR. These have generally been reversible, but insulin shock with hypoglycemia has been observed.
Genitourinary: Two cases of nephrogenic diabetes insipidus following therapy with ZANOSAR have been reported. One had spontaneous recovery and the second responded to indomethacin.

OVERDOSAGE

No specific antidote for ZANOSAR is known.

DOSAGE AND ADMINISTRATION

ZANOSAR Sterile Powder should be administered intravenously. It is not active orally. Although it has been administered intra-arterially, this is not recommended pending further evaluation of the possibility that adverse renal effects may be evoked more rapidly by this route of administration.
Two different dosage schedules have been employed successfully with ZANOSAR.
Daily Schedule—The recommended dose for daily intravenous administration is 500 mg/m^2 of body surface area for five consecutive days every six weeks until maximum benefit or until treatment-limiting toxicity is observed. Dose escalation on this schedule is not recommended.
Weekly Schedule—The recommended initial dose for weekly intravenous administration is 1000 mg/m^2 of body surface area at weekly intervals for the first two courses (weeks). In subsequent courses, drug doses may be escalated in patients who have not achieved a therapeutic response and who have not experienced significant toxicity with the previous course of treatment. However A SINGLE DOSE OF 1500 mg/m^2 BODY SURFACE AREA SHOULD NOT BE EXCEEDED as a greater dose may cause azotemia. When administered on this schedule, the median time to onset of response is about 17 days and the median time to maximum response is about 35 days. The median **total** dose to onset of response is about 2000 mg/m^2 body surface area and the median **total** dose to maximum response is about 4000 mg/m^2 body surface area.
The ideal duration of maintenance therapy with ZANOSAR has not yet been clearly established for either of the above schedules.
For patients with functional tumors, serial monitoring of fasting insulin levels allows a determination of biochemical response to therapy. For patients with either functional or nonfunctional tumors, response to therapy can be determined by measurable reductions of tumor size (reduction of organomegaly, masses, or lymph nodes).
Reconstitute ZANOSAR with 9.5 ml of Dextrose Injection USP, or 0.9% Sodium Chloride Injection USP. The resulting pale-gold solution will contain 100 mg of streptozocin and 22 mg of citric acid per ml. Where more dilute infusion solutions are desirable, further dilution in the above vehicles is recommended. The total storage time for streptozocin after it has been placed in solution should not exceed 12 hours. This product contains no preservatives and is not intended as a multiple-dose vial.
Caution in the handling and preparation of the powder and solution should be exercised, and the use of gloves is recommended. If ZANOSAR Sterile Powder or a solution prepared

from ZANOSAR contacts the skin or mucosae, immediately wash the affected area with soap and water.

Procedures for proper handling and disposal of anticancer drugs should be considered. Several guidelines on this subject have been published.[4-9] There is no general agreement that all of the procedures recommended in the guidelines are necessary or appropriate.

HOW SUPPLIED

ZANOSAR Sterile Powder is supplied in 1 gram vials (NDC 0009-0844-01). Unopened vials of ZANOSAR should be stored at refrigeration temperatures (2°–8° C) and protected from light (preferably stored in carton).

REFERENCES

1. Broder LE and Carter SK: *Ann Int Med, 79*:101–118, 1972.
2. Schein PS, O'Connell MJ, Blom J, Hubbard S, Magrath IT, Bergevin P, Wiernik PH, Ziegler TL, and DeVita VT: *Cancer, 34*:993–1000, 1974.
3. Moertel CG, *et al: Cancer Chemother Rep, 55*:303–307, 1972.
4. Recommendations for the Safe Handling of Parenteral Antineoplastic Drugs, NIH Publication No. 83-2621. For sale by the Superintendent of Documents, US Government Printing Office, Washington, DC 20402.
5. AMA Council Report. Guidelines for Handling Parenteral Antineoplastics. JAMA, March 15, 1985.
6. National Study Commission on Cytotoxic Exposure-Recommendations for Handling Cytotoxic Agents. Available from Louis P. Jeffrey, ScD, Director of Pharmacy Services, Rhode Island Hospital, 593 Eddy Street, Providence, Rhode Island 02902.
7. Clinical Oncological Society of Australia: Guidelines and recommendations for safe handling of antineoplastic agents. *Med J Australia 1*:426–428, 1983.
8. Jones RB, et al, Safe handling of chemotherapeutic agents: A report from the Mount Sinai Medical Center CA-A Cancer Journal for Clinicians Sept/Oct., 1983, pp. 258–263.
9. American Society of Hospital Pharmacists Technical assistance bulletin on handling cytotoxic drugs in hospitals. *AmJ Hosp Pharm 42*:131–137, 1985.

Code 812 350 004

ZEFAZONE® ℞

brand of cefmetazole sodium sterile powder (cefmetazole sodium)

For Intravenous Use

DESCRIPTION

ZEFAZONE Sterile Powder contains cefmetazole sodium, a semisynthetic, cephem antibiotic for intravenous administration. It was originally derived from cephyamycin C, produced by *Streptomyces jumonjinensis*. It is now synthetically produced from 7-amino-cephalosporanic acid. It is the sodium salt of (6R-cis)-7-[[[(cyanomethyl)thio]acetyl]amino]-7-methoxy-3-[[(1-methyl-1H-tetrazol-5-yl)thio]methyl]-8-oxo-5-thia-1-azabicyclo;[4.2.0]oct-2-ene-2-carboxylic acid. The empirical formula is $C_{15}H_{16}N_7O_5S_3Na$ and the structural formula is represented below:

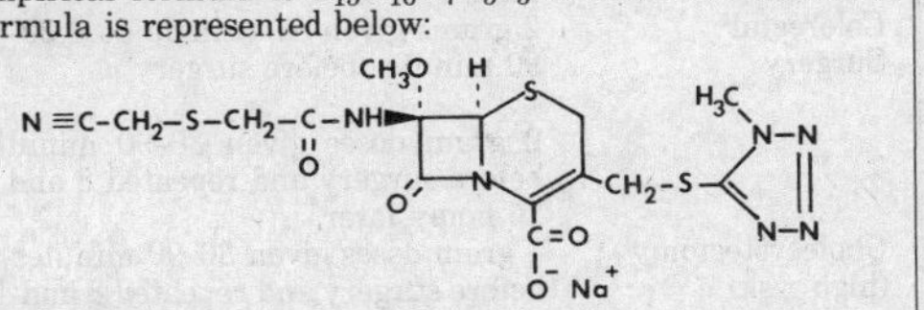

The molecular weight of cefmetazole sodium is 493.51.

ZEFAZONE contains 49 mg (2 milliequivalents) of sodium per gram of cefmetazole activity. Solutions of cefmetazole sodium range from colorless to light amber. The pH of freshly reconstituted solutions ranges from 4.2 to 6.2.

CLINICAL PHARMACOLOGY

Following an intravenous dose of 2 grams administered over 60 minutes to normal volunteers, the mean maximum serum concentration of cefmetazole was 143 mcg/mL.

SERUM LEVELS (mcg/mL) AFTER INITIAL 60 MINUTE I.V. INFUSIONS

	Time after beginning of infusion					
Dose	**30 min**	**1 hr**	**2 hr**	**4 hr**	**6 hr**	**8 hr**
1 gram	44	73	31	9	3	—
2 gram	92	143	70	20	6	2

Following repeated administration of 2 grams every 6 hours, the mean maximum and trough serum levels of cefmetazole were 138 and 6 mcg/mL, respectively.

After a 5 minute intravenous infusion of 2 grams to normal volunteers, the mean maximum serum concentration of cefmetazole was 290 mcg/mL.

SERUM LEVELS (mcg/mL) AFTER 5 MINUTE I.V. INFUSIONS

	Time after beginning of infusion				
Dose	**10 min**	**20 min**	**1 hr**	**2 hr**	**4 hr**
1 gram	129	90	43	25	8
2 gram	214	156	91	52	17

The mean plasma or serum elimination half-life after intravenous infusion is approximately 1.2 hours, and the mean plasma clearance is 121 mL/min. Cefmetazole is 65% bound to serum proteins at a concentration of 100 mcg/mL.

Approximately 85% of a dose of cefmetazole is excreted unchanged in the urine over a 12-hour period resulting in high urinary concentrations. Mean urinary concentrations over collection intervals ranged from 9828 to 52 mcg/mL (mean urine volumes = 104 mL and 645 mL, respectively) in a 12 hour period following a 1 hour I.V. infusion of 2 grams. After a 5 minute I.V. infusion of 2 grams, analogous mean urinary concentrations ranged from 5138 to 46 mcg/mL (mean urine volumes = 183 mL and 575 mL, respectively).

Cefmetazole is excreted by tubular secretion. Probenecid doubles the half-life and increases the duration of measurable plasma concentrations of cefmetazole; however, the maximum plasma concentrations remain unchanged. In patients with reduced renal function, the plasma clearance is decreased and the half-life of cefmetazole is prolonged (see DOSAGE AND ADMINISTRATION).

After a 1 gram I.V. dose, mean concentrations in the gallbladder wall and the bile at 2.8 hours were 130 mcg/g and 310 mcg/mL, respectively.

After a 1 gram I.V. dose, vaginal, uterine and adnexal tissue concentrations were variable and lower than serum concentrations, ranging from 2.7 to 62.5 mcg/g at 0.1 to 2 hours after the dose.

After a 2 gram dose, the mean maximum concentration in interstitial fluid was 4.5 mcg/mL at one hour after administration and was less than 2 mcg/mL by 4 hours after administration.

Data on CSF levels of cefmetazole are not available.

Microbiology

The bactericidal action of cefmetazole results from inhibition of cell wall synthesis. Cefmetazole is active *in vitro* against a wide range of aerobic and anaerobic gram-positive and gram-negative organisms. The methoxy group in the 7α position provides cefmetazole sodium with a high degree of stability in the presence of beta-lactamases, both penicillinases and cephalosporinases. Cefmetazole is usually active against the following organisms *in vitro* and in clinical infections (see INDICATIONS AND USAGE).

Gram-positive [a]

- *Staphylococcus aureus* [b] (including penicillinase- and non-penicillinase-producing strains)
- *Staphylococcus epidermidis* [b]
- *Streptococcus pneumoniae*
- *Streptococcus agalactiae*
- *Streptococcus pyogenes*

Gram-negative [c]

- *Escherichia coli*
- *Klebsiella pneumoniae*
- *Klebsiella oxytoca*
- *Haemophilus influenzae* (non-penicillinase-producing strains)
- *Proteus mirabilis*
- *Proteus vulgaris*
- *Morganella morganii*
- *Providencia stuartii*

Anaerobic organisms

- *Bacteroides fragilis*
- *Bacteroides melaninogenicus*
- *Clostridium perfringens*

ZEFAZONE has been shown to be active *in vitro* against most strains of the following organisms; however clinical efficacy has not been established.

Gram-negative

- *Citrobacter diversus*
- *Haemophilus influenzae* (penicillinase-producing strains)
- *Moraxella (Branhamella) catarrhalis*
- *Neisseria gonorrhoeae* (penicillinase- and non-penicillinase-producing strains)
- *Providencia rettgeri*
- *Salmonella species*
- *Shigella species*

Anaerobic organisms

- *Bacteroides bivius*
- *Bacteroides disiens*
- *Bacteroides intermedius*
- *Bacteroides ureolyticus*
- *Peptococcus* species
- *Peptostreptococcus* species

NOTE:

[a] Most strains of enterococci, e.g., *Enterococcus faecalis* (formerly *Streptococcus faecalis*) are resistant to cefmetazole.

[b] ZEFAZONE Sterile Powder should not be used for treatment of infections caused by methicillin-resistant staphylococci.

[c] Cefmetazole is inactive *in vitro* against most strains of *Pseudomonas aeruginosa* and many strains of *Enterobacter* species.

Susceptibility Testing

Susceptibility Tests: Diffusion Techniques

Quantitative method that require measurement of zone diameters give an estimate of antibiotic susceptibility. One such procedure[1] has been recommended for use with disks to test susceptiblity to cefmetazole. Interpretation involves correlation of the diameters obtained in the disk test with the minimum inhibitory concentration (MIC) values for cefmetazole.

Reports from the laboratory giving results of the standardized single disk susceptibility test using a 30 mcg cefmetazole disk should be interpreted according to the following criteria:

Zone diameter (mm)	Interpretation
≥ 16	(S) Susceptible
13–15	(MS) Moderately Susceptible
≤ 12	(R) Resistant

A report of "Susceptible" indicates that the pathogen is likely to be inhibited by generally achievable blood levels. A report of "Moderately Susceptible" indicates that inhibitory concentrations of the antibiotic may well be achieved if high dosage is used or if the infection is confined to tissues and fluids (e.g., urine) in which high antibiotic levels are attained. A report of "Resistant" indicates that achievable concentrations of the antibiotic are unlikely to be inhibitory and other therapy should be selected.

Standardized procedures require the use of laboratory control organisms. The 30 mcg disk should give the following zone diameters:

Organism	Zone diameter (mm)
E. coli ATCC 25922	26–32
S. aureus ATCC 25923	25–34

Cephalosporin class disks should not be used to test for cefmetazole susceptibility.

Dilution Techniques

In other susceptibility testing procedures, e.g., NCCLS broth microdilution or agar dilution methods[2] or equivalent, a bacterial isolate may be considered susceptible if the MIC value for cefmetazole is 16 mcg/mL or less. Organisms with an MIC of 32 mcg/mL are considered moderately susceptible. Organisms are considered resistant to cefmetazole if the MIC is equal to or greater than 64 mcg/mL.

As with standard diffusion methods, dilution procedures require the use of laboratory control organisms. Standard cefmetazole powder should give MIC values in the range of 0.25–2.0 mcg/mL for *E. coli* ATCC 25922 and in the range of 0.5–2.0 mcg/mL for *S. aureus* ATCC 29213.

INDICATIONS AND USAGE

Treatment

ZEFAZONE Sterile Powder is indicated for the treatment of serious infections caused by susceptible strains of the designated mincroorganisms in the following diseases:

Urinary Tract Infections. Complicated or uncomplicated urinary tract infections caused by *Escherichia coli.*

Lower Respiratory Tract Infections. Pneumonia and bronchitis caused by *Streptococcus pneumoniae, Staphylococcus aureus* (penicillinase- and non-penicillinase-producing strains), *Escherichia coli*, and *Haemophilus influenzae* (non-penicillinase producing strains).

Skin and Skin Structure Infections caused by *Staphylococcus aureus* (penicillinase- and non-penicillinase-producing strains), *Staphylococcus epidermidis, Streptococcus pyogenes, Streptococcus agalactiae, Escherichia coli, Proteus mirabilis, Proteus vulgaris*, Morganella morganii*, Providencia stuartii*, Klebsiella pneumoniae, Klebsiella oxytoca*, Bacteroides fragilis,* and *Bacteroides melaninogenicus**.

Intraabdominal Infections caused by *Escherichia coli, Klebsiella pneumoniae*, Klebsiella oxytoca*, Bacteroides fragilis,* and *Clostridium perfringens**.

Appropriate specimens for bacteriological examination should be obtained in order to isolate and identify causative organisms and to determine their susceptibility to cefmetazole sodium. Therapy with ZEFAZONE may be instituted before results of susceptibility studies are known; however, once these results become available, antibiotic treatment should be adjusted accordingly.

Prophylaxis

Preoperative administrative of ZEFAZONE may reduce the incidence of certain postoperative infections in patients who undergo cesarean section, abdominal or vaginal hysterec-

*Efficacy for this organism in this organ system was studied in fewer than 20 infections.

Continued on next page

Information on these Upjohn products is based on labeling in effect June 1, 1992. Further information concerning these and other Upjohn products may be obtained by direct inquiry to Medical Information, The Upjohn Company, Kalamazoo, Michigan 49001.

Upjohn—Cont.

tomy, cholecystectomy (high risk patients), and colorectal surgery. These procedures are classified as clean contaiminated or potentially contaminated surgery.

If signs and symptoms of an infection develop after surgery, the causative organism should be identified by culture and appropriate therapeutic measures initiated.

CONTRAINDICATIONS

ZEFAZONE Sterile Powder is contraindicated in patients with known allergy to cefmetazole or to the cephalosporin group of antibiotics.

WARNINGS

BEFORE THERAPY WITH *ZEFAZONE* STERILE POWDER IS INSTITUTED, CAREFUL INQUIRY SHOULD BE MADE TO DETERMINE WHETHER THE PATIENT HAS HAD PREVIOUS HYPERSENSITIVTY REACTIONS TO CEFMETAZOLE, CEPHALOSPORINS, PENICILLINS, OR OTHER DRUGS. IF THIS PRODUCT IS TO BE GIVEN TO PENICILLIN-SENSITIVE PATIENTS, CAUTION SHOULD BE EXERCISED BECAUSE CROSS HYPERSENSITIVITY AMONG BETA-LACTAM ANTIBIOTICS HAS BEEN CLEARLY DOCUMENTED AND MAY OCCUR IN UP TO 10% OF PATIENTS WITH A HISTORY OF PENICILLIN ALLERGY. IF AN ALLERGIC REACTION TO *ZEFAZONE* OCCURS, DISCONTINUE THE DRUG. SERIOUS ACUTE HYPERSENSITIVITY REACTIONS MAY REQUIRE TREATMENT WITH EPINEPHRINE AND OTHER EMERGENCY MEASURES, INCLUDING OXYGEN, INTRAVENOUS FLUIDS, INTRAVENOUS ANTIHISTAMINES, CORTICOSTEROIDS, PRESSOR AMINES, AND AIRWAY MANAGEMENT, AS CLINICALLY INDICATED.

Pseudomembranous colitis has been reported with nearly all antibacterial agents, including ZEFAZONE, and may range in severity from mild to life-threatening. Therefore, it is important to consider this diagnosis in patients who present with diarrhea subsequent to the administration of antibacterial agents.

Treatment with antibacterial agents alters the normal flora of the colon and may permit overgrowth of clostridia. Studies indicate that a toxin produced by *Clostridium difficile* is the primary cause of "antibiotic-associated colitis".

After the diagnosis of pseudomembranous colitis has been established, therapeutic measures should be initiated. Mild cases of pseudomembranous colitis usually respond to drug discontinuation alone. In moderate to severe cases, consideration should be given to management with fluids and electrolytes, protein supplementation and treatment with an oral antibacterial drug effective against *C. difficile.*

PRECAUTIONS

General

In patients with transient or persistent reduction in urinary output due to renal insufficiency, the total daily dose of ZEFAZONE Sterile Powder should be reduced (see DOSAGE AND ADMINISTRATION), because high and prolonged serum antibiotic concentrations can occur in such individuals following usual doses.

As with other antibiotics, prolonged use of ZEFAZONE may result in overgrowth of nonsusceptible organisms. Repeated evaluation of the patient's condition is essential. If superinfection occurs during therapy, appropriate measures should be taken.

As with some other cephalosporins, ZEFAZONE may be associated with a fall in prothrombin activity. Those at risk include patients with renal or hepatic impairment, or poor nutritional state, as well as patients receiving a protracted course of antimicrobial therapy. Prothrombin time should be monitored for patients at risk and exogenous Vitamin K administered as indicated.

A disulfiram-like reaction has been reported after ingestion of alcohol (see Drug Interactions). Therefore, patients should be advised against the ingestion of alcohol-containing beverages during and for 24 hours after the administration of ZEFAZONE.

Antibiotics, including cephalosporins, should be prescribed with caution to individuals with a history of gastrointestinal disease, particularly colitis.

Drug Interactions

A disulfiram-like reaction, characterized by flushing, sweating, headache, and tachycardia, has been reported when alcohol was ingested after cefmetazole sodium administration. A similar reaction has been reported with other structurally-related cephalosporins.

Although nephrotoxicity has not been noted when ZEFAZONE was given alone, it is possible that nephrotoxicity may be potentiated if ZEFAZONE is used concomitantly with an aminoglycoside.

Drug/Laboratory Test Interactions

Patients receiving cefmetazole may show a false positive result for glucose in the urine with tests that use Benedict's or Fehling's solution.

Carcinogenesis, Mutagenesis, Impairment of Fertility

Long-term carcinogenesis studies of cefmetazole sodium have not been performed in animals. Mutagenesis studies of cefmetazole sodium, including the Ames test, the unscheduled DNA synthesesis test, the mammalian cell foward gene mutation assay, and the dominant lethal test, were all negative. When administered subcutaneously for 35 days to young (6-41 days of age) rats at dosages of 300 mg/kg/day or 1,000 mg/kg/day, cefmetazole was associated with a reduced number of mature spermatids in the testis and a slight, dose-related reduction of testicular weight. These effects were completely reversible; rats examined 5 and 10 weeks after cessation of the 35 day cefmetazole treatment regimen at the above doses had normal testicular weights and normal spermatogenesis. In an extension of this study, all aspects of reproductive function were normal in male rats allowed to mate at either 4 to 5 weeks or 7 to 8 weeks after cessation of the 300 or 1,000 mg/kg/day cefmetazole sodium treatment regimen. In separate studies, there were no adverse effects on the testicles when cefmetazole sodium was given for 30 days to sexually mature male rats at doses up to 2,500 mg/kg/day. The effects of cefmetazole sodium on the testes of sexually immature rats are probably due to the methylthiotetrazole side chain which is released from the parent compound by nonenzymatic hydrolysis in the intestine. Rats metabolize the parent compound to release the methylthiotetrazole side chain at a greater rate than humans. There are also species differences in age at onset of spermatogenesis and rate of reproductive maturation. The significance for humans of these testicular changes in sexually immature rats treated with high doses of cefmetazole sodium is unknown.

Pregnancy: Pregnancy Category B

Cefmetazole sodium was not teratogenic or embryocidal when administered to rats or mice at doses up to 2,000 mg/kg/day (approximately 12.5 times the maximum human dose) during the period of organogenesis. There are, however, no adequate and well-controlled studies of cefmetazole use in pregnant women. Because animal reproduction studies are not always predictive of human response, this drug should be used during pregnancy only if clearly needed.

Nursing Mothers

Trace concentractions of cefmetazole are excreted in human milk: therefore, consideration should be given to temporarily discontinuing nursing during therapy with ZEFAZONE.

Pediatric Use

Safety and effectiveness in children have not been established. For information concerning testicular changes in prepubertal rats, see the Carcinogenesis, Mutagenesis, Impairment of Fertility subsection.

ADVERSE REACTIONS

ZEFAZONE was generally well-tolerated. Adverse reactions that were reported as possibly or probably related to theraphy with ZEFAZONE were:

Gastrointestinal: Diarrhea (3.6%), nausea (1.0%), vomiting, epigastric pain, candidiasis, bleeding. There have been rare reports of pseudomembranous colitis in patients receiving ZEFAZONE. The onset of pseudomembranous colitis symptoms may occur during or after antibiotic treatment (see WARNINGS).

Hypersensitivity: Allergic reactions including anaphylaxis and urticaria.

Dermatologic: Rash (1.1%), pruritus, generalized erythema.

Local: Pain and/or swelling at the injection site, phlebitis, thrombophlebitis.

Cardiovascular: Shock, hypotension.

Central Nervous System: Headache, hot flashes.

Respiratory Tract: Pleural effusion, dyspnea, epistaxis, respiratory distress.

Special Senses: Alteration in color perception.

Musculoskeletal: Joint pain and inflammation.

Other: Fever, superinfection, vaginitis.

Adverse Laboratory Changes

Adverse laboratory changes that have been reported, without regard to drug relationship, were:

Hepatic: Transient increases in AST (SGOT), ALT (SGPT), alkaline phosphatase, bilirubin, and LDH.

Hematologic: Eosinophillia, leucocytosis, lymphocytosis, granulocytosis, basophilia, monocytosis, thrombocytosis, decreased hemoglobin, decreased hematocrit, decreased RBC, leucopenia, neutropenia, lymphocytopenia, thrombocytopenia, positive Coombs test, prolonged PT and PTT.

Serum Chemistry: Increase glucose, decreased serum albumin, decreased total serum protein.

Renal: Increased BUN, increased creatinine.

In addition to the adverse reactions listed above which have been observed in patients treated with ZEFAZONE, the following adverse reactions and altered laboratory tests have been reported for cephalosporin class antibiotics:

Adverse reactions: Allergic reactions including Stevens-Johnson syndrome, erythema multiforme, toxic epidermal necrolysis, renal dysfunction, toxic nephropathy, hepatic dysfunction including cholestasis, aplastic anemia, hemolytic anemia, hemorrhage.

Several cephalosporins have been implicated in triggering seizures, paraticularly in patients with renal impairment when the dosage was not reduced (see DOSAGE AND ADMINISTRATION and OVERDOSAGE). If seizures associated with drug therapy occur, the drug should be discontinued. Anticonvulsant theraphy can be given if clinically indicated.

Abnormal Laboratory Tests: Agranulocytosis, pancytopenia.

OVERDOSAGE

Information on overdosage in humans is not available. In the event of serious toxic reactions for overdosage, hemodialysis or peritoneal dialysis may aid in the removal of cefmetazole from the body, particular if renal function is compromised. In 7 anuric patients, mean hemodialysis clearance for cefmetazole was 104 mL/min.

DOSAGE AND ADMINISTRATION

Treatment

The usual adult dosage is 2 grams of ZEFAZONE Sterile Powder (cefmetazole sodium) administrative intravenously every 6 to 12 hours for 5 to 14 days. Proper dosage should be determined by the condition of the patient, location and severity of the infection, and susceptibility of the causative organisms.

General Guidelines for Dosage of ZEFAZONE Sterile Powder

Type of Infection	Daily Dose	Frequency
URINARY TRACT	4 grams	2 grams every 12 hours I.V.
OTHER SITES		
Mild to Moderate	6 grams	2 grams every 8 hours I.V.
Severe to Life-Threatening	8 grams	2 grams every 6 hours I.V.

Prophylaxis

To reduce the incidence of postoperative infection following vaginal hysterectomy, abdominal hysterectomy, cesarean section, colorectal surgery, or cholecystectomy (high risk) in adults, the recommended doses are:

Surgery	Dosing Regimen
Vaginal Hysterectomy	2 grams given as a single dose 30–90 minutes before surgery or 1 gram doses given 30– 90 minutes before surgery and repeated 8 and 16 hours later
Abdominal Hysterectomy	1 gram doses given 30–90 minutes before surgery and repeated 8 and 16 hours later
Cesarean Section	2 grams given as a single dose after clamping the cord or 1 gram doses given after clamping the cord and repeated 8 and 16 hours later
Colorectal[a] Surgery	2 grams given as a single dose 30–90 minutes before surgery or 2 gram doses given 30–90 minutes before surgery and repeated 8 and 16 hours later
Cholecystectomy (high risk)	1 gram doses given 30–90 minutes before surgery and repeated 8 and 16 hours later

[a] All patients studied received preoperative bowel preparation with mechanical cleansing, oral neomycin or kanamycin and oral erythromycin.

If surgery lasts more than 4 hours, the preoperative dose should be repeated.

Impaired Renal Function

For patients with impaired renal function, a reduced dosage schedule should be employed. The following dosage guidelines are derived from clinical pharmacology studies:

Dosage Guidelines for ZEFAZONE Sterile Powder in Adults With Impaired Renal Function

Renal Function	Creatinine Clearance ($mL/min/1.73M^2$)	Dose (grams)	Frequency
Mild Impairment	90–50	1–2	Q 12 h
Moderate Impairment	49–30	1–2	Q 16 h
Severe Impairment	29–10	1–2	Q 24 h
Essentially No Function	<10	1–2	Q 48 h*

*administered after hemodialysis

When only the serum creatinine level is available, the following formula (based on sex, weight, and age of the patient) may be used to convert this value into creatinine clearance. The serum creatinine level should represent a steady state of renal function.

Males: $\dfrac{\text{Weight (kg)} \times (140 - \text{age})}{72 \times \text{serum creatinine (mg/100 mL)}}$

Females: $0.85 \times$ above value

Preparation of Solution

General Reconstitution Procedures

Reconstitute with Sterile Water for Injection, Bacteriostatic Water for Injection, or 0.9 Percent Sodium Chloride Injection. Shake to dissolve and let stand until clear.

Vial Size	Amount of Dulent to be Added (mL)	Approximate Withdrawable Volume (mL)	Approximate Average Concentration (mg/mL)
1 gram	10	10.4	100
1 gram	3.7	4.1	250
2 gram	15	16	125
2 gram	7	8	250

Intravenous Administration

A solution containing 1 gram or 2 grams of ZEFAZONE Sterile Powder in Sterile Water for Injection, Bacteriostatic Water for Injection, or 0.9 Percent Sodium Chloride Injection can be administered by IV infusion over 10 to 60 minutes. For otherwise healthy patients undergoing elective surgical procedures, a solution containing 1 gram or 2 grams of ZEFAZONE Sterile Powder in Sterile Water for Injection, Bacteriostatic Water for Injection, or 0.9 Percent Sodium Chloride Injection can also be injected over three to five minutes. During infusion of the solution containing cefmetazole sodium, it is necessary to temporarily discontinue administration of other solutions at the same site.

Solutions of cefmetazole sodium, like those of most beta-lactam antibiotics, should not be added to aminoglycoside solutions. If cefmetazole sodium and aminoglycosides are to be administered to the same patient, they must be administered separately and not admixed.

Compatibility And Stability

When reconstituted as described above (Preparation of Solution), ZEFAZONE Sterile Powder maintains satisfactory potency for 24 hours at room temperature (25°C, 77°F), for 7 days under refrigeration (8°C, 46°F), and for 6 weeks in the frozen state (at or below −20°C, −4°F).

Primary cefmetazole solutions (as described in Preparation of Solution) may be further diluted to concentrations of 1.0 to 20 mg/mL in the following diluents and maintain potency for 24 hours at room temperature (25°C, 77°F), for 7 days under refrigeration (8°C, 46°F), and for 6 weeks in the frozen state (at or below −20°C, −4°F).

  0.9 percent Sodium Chloride Injection
  5 percent Dextrose Injection
  Lactated Ringer's Injection

Reconstituted cefmetazole sodium solutions may be stored in glass, Viaflex* PL146 or McGaw‡ PAB flexible plastic parenteral solution containers.

Do not refreeze thawed solutions.

At the end of the time periods specified above, any unused solutions or frozen material should be discarded.

DIRECTIONS FOR USE OF PLASTIC CONTAINERS

Storage

Use an appropriate storage module in order to avoid unnecessary handling and to prevent surface contact between bags. Store in a freezer capable of maintaining a temperature of −20°C (−4°F).

Thawing Of Plastic Containers

Thaw frozen bag at temperature (25°C, 77°F). [DO NOT FORCE THAW BY IMMERSION IN WATER BATHS OR BY MICROWAVE IRRADIATION.] Check for minute leaks by squeezing bag firmly. If leaks are detected, discard solution as sterility may be impaired.

The bag should be visually inspected. Components of the solution may precipitate in the frozen state and will dissolve upon reaching room temperature with little or no agitation. If after visual inspection the solution remains cloudy or if an insoluble precipitate is noted or if any seals or outlet parts are not intact, the bag should be discarded.

The thawed solution is stable for 24 hours under either refrigeration (8°C, 46°F) or at room temperature (25°C, 77°F). Do not refreeze thawed antibiotics.

Caution: Do not use plastic containers in series connections. Such use could result in an embolism due to residual air being drawn from the primary container before administration of the fluid from the secondary container is complete.

Preparation for Administration:

a. Suspend container(s) from eyelet support.

b. Remove protector from outlet part at bottom of container.

c. Attach adminsitration set. Refer to complete directions accompanying set.

HOW SUPPLIED

ZEFAZONE Sterile Powder (cefmetazole sodium) is a dry, white to pale yellow powder supplied in vials containing cef-

* Viaflex is a registered trademark of Baxter Travenol Laboratories, Inc.

‡ McGaw is a registered trademark of Kendall McGaw Laboratories

metazole sodium equivalent to 1 gram and 2 grams cefmetazole activity for intravenous administration. The vials should be stored at controlled room temperature 15°–30°C (59°–86°F).

1 gram vial   NDC 0009-3471-01
2 gram vial   NDC 0009-3477-01

REFERENCES

1. National Committee for Clinical Laboratory Standards Approved Standard: *Performance Standards for Antimicrobial Disk Susceptibility Tests*, 3rd Edition, Vol. 4(**16**):M2–A3, Villanova, PA, December, 1985.
2. National Committee for Clinical Laboratory Standards, Tentative Standard: *Methods for Dilution Antimicrobial Susceptibility Tests for Bacteria That Grow Aerobically*, 2nd Edition, Vol. 8(**8**):M7–T2, Villanova, PA, December 1988.

Manufactured by and licensed from Sankyo Company, Ltd., Japan for

The Upjohn Company
Kalamazoo, Michigan 49001, USA

Code 814 341 000

Upsher-Smith Laboratories, Inc.
14905 23RD AVE. NORTH
MINNEAPOLIS, MN 55447

FEVERALL® SPRINKLE CAPS®   OTC
[fē′ver-all spring′kel kaps]
acetaminophen taste-free powder
80 mg Children's Strength
160 mg Junior Strength

DESCRIPTION

Each Feverall® Sprinkle Cap® contains 80 mg or 160 mg of acetaminophen. The fine powder is taste-free and does not contain artificial colors or dyes so it will not stain clothing or cause adverse reactions sometimes associated with dyes.

DOSING

All dosages may be repeated every 4 hours, but not to exceed more than 5 times daily, or as directed by a physician. Administer to children under 2 years only on the advice of a physician.

80 mg Children's Strength Dosing

Four–23 months or 12–23 pounds: 1 Sprinkle Cap. 2–3 years or 24–35 pounds: 2 Sprinkle Caps. 4–5 years or 36–47 pounds: 3 Sprinkle Caps. 6–8 years or 48–59 pounds: 4 Sprinkle Caps. 9–10 years or 60–71 pounds: 5 Sprinkle Caps. 11 years or 72–95 pounds: 6 Sprinkle Caps.

160 mg Junior Strength Dosing

Two–5 years or 24–47 pounds: 1 Sprinkle Cap. 6–10 years or 48–71 pounds: 2 Sprinkle Caps. 11 years or 72–95 pounds: 3 Sprinkle Caps. 12–14 years or over 96 pounds: 4 Sprinkle Caps.

WARNINGS

Keep this and all drugs out of the reach of children. In the case of accidental overdose seek professional assistance or contact a poison control center immediately. Prompt medical attention is critical even if you do not notice any signs or symptoms. Do not give this product for pain for more than 5 days or for fever for more than 3 days unless directed by a physician. If pain or fever persists or gets worse, if new symptoms occur, or if redness or swelling is present, consult a physician because these could be signs of a serious condition. As with any drug, if you are pregnant or nursing a baby, seek the advice of a health professional before using this product.

HOW SUPPLIED

Feverall® Sprinkle Caps® are available in both strengths, in packages of 20 Sprinkle Caps.
NDC 0245–0175–20 (80 mg); white with clear cap
NDC 0245–0176–20 (160 mg); red with clear cap

FEVERALL® Suppositories   OTC
[fē′ver-all]
acetaminophen rectal suppositories
120 mg Children's Strength
325 mg Junior Strength

DESCRIPTION

Feverall® Suppositories are supplied in 120 mg and 325 mg strengths. Feverall® Suppositories are unit dose labeled.

INDICATIONS

For the temporary relief of fever, minor aches, pains and headaches. For rectal administration.

DOSING

120 mg:
Children (3 to 6 years)—One suppository every 4 to 6 hours. No more than a total of 6 suppositories in any 24 hour period.
Children (under 3 years)—Consult a physician.

325 mg:
Adults—Two suppositories every 4 to 6 hours. No more than a total of 12 suppositories in any 24 hour period. Children (6 to 12 years)—One suppository every 4 to 6 hours. No more than a total of 8 suppositories in any 24 hour period.

WARNINGS

Severe or recurrent pain or high or continued fever may be indicative of serious illness. If fever persists for more than 3 days (72 hours), or recurs, consult your physician. Do not use consistently for more than 10 days except on the advice of a physician. Keep this and all drugs out of the reach of children. In case of accidental ingestion, seek professional assistance or contact a Poison Control Center immediately.
Caution: As with any drug, if you are pregnant or nursing a baby, seek the advice of a health professional before using this product.

HOW SUPPLIED

Feverall® Suppositories are available in packages of 6 suppositories.
NDC 0245-0116-06 (120 mg)
NDC 0245-0117-06 (325 mg)

KLOR–CON® POWDER   ℞
[klōr′kon]
Potassium Chloride for Oral Solution, USP
20 mEq. (1.5 g) per packet

DESCRIPTION

Each packet contains 1.5 g potassium chloride providing potassium 20 mEq and chloride 20 mEq. Fruit-flavored with artificial color and sweetener (saccharin) added.

HOW SUPPLIED

KLOR-CON® Powder 20 mEq (1.5 g Potassium Chloride). In cartons of 30 and 100 packets.
30's   NDC 0245-0035-30,   100's   NDC 0245-0035-01

KLOR–CON®/25 POWDER   ℞
[klōr′kon]
Potassium Chloride for Oral Solution, USP
25 mEq. (1.875 g) per packet

DESCRIPTION

Each packet contains 1.875 g potassium chloride providing potassium 25 mEq and chloride 25 mEq. Fruit-flavored with artificial color and sweetener (saccharin) added.

HOW SUPPLIED

Cartons of 30, 100 and 250 packets.
30's   NDC 0245-0037-30,   100's   NDC 0245-0037-01
250's   NDC 0245-0037-25

KLOR–CON® 8/KLOR–CON® 10   ℞
[klōr′kon]
Potassium Chloride
Extended–release Tablets, USP
8 mEq and 10 mEq

DESCRIPTION

KLOR-CON® Extended-release Tablets, USP are a solid oral dosage form of potassium chloride. Each contains 600 mg or 750 mg of potassium chloride equivalent to 8 mEq or 10 mEq of potassium in a wax matrix tablet. This formulation is intended to slow the release of potassium so that the likelihood of a high localized concentration of potassium chloride within the gastrointestinal tract is reduced.

Klor-Con® Extended-release Tablets are an electrolyte replenisher. The chemical name is potassium chloride, and the structural formula is KCl. Potassium chloride USP occurs as a white, granular powder or as colorless crystals. It is odorless and has a saline taste. Its solutions are neutral to litmus. It is freely soluble in water and insoluble in alcohol.

Inactive Ingredients: Castor oil, hydroxypropyl methylcellulose 2910, magnesium stearate, polyethylene glycol 3350, propylene glycol, synthetic iron oxide, titanium dioxide, and other ingredients. Yellow tablets also contain FD& C Yellow No. 10 aluminum lake and FD & C Yellow No. 6 aluminum lake. Blue tablets also contain FD & C Blue No. 1 aluminum lake.

Continued on next page

Upsher-Smith Laboratories—Cont.

CLINICAL PHARMACOLOGY

The potassium ion is the principal intracellular cation of most body tissues. Potassium ions participate in a number of essential physiological processes, including the maintenance of intracellular tonicity, the transmission of nerve impulses, the contraction of cardiac, skeletal, and smooth muscle, and the maintenance of normal renal function.

The intracellular concentration of potassium is approximately 150 to 160 mEq per liter. The normal adult plasma concentration is 3.5 to 5 mEq per liter. An active ion transport system maintains this gradient across the plasma membrane.

Potassium is a normal dietary constituent and under steady state conditions the amount of potassium absorbed from the gastrointestinal tract is equal to the amount excreted in the urine. The usual dietary intake of potassium is 50 to 100 mEq per day.

Potassium depletion will occur whenever the rate of potassium loss through renal excretion and/or loss from the gastrointestinal tract exceeds the rate of potassium intake. Such depletion usually develops as a consequence of therapy with diuretics, primary or secondary hyperaldosteronism, diabetic ketoacidosis, or inadequate replacement of potassium in patients on prolonged parenteral nutrition. Depletion can develop rapidly with severe diarrhea, especially if associated with vomiting. Potassium depletion due to these causes is usually accompanied by a concomitant loss of chloride and is manifested by hypokalemia and metabolic alkalosis. Potassium depletion may produce weakness, fatigue, disturbances of cardiac rhythm (primarily ectopic beats), prominent U-waves in the electrocardiogram, and, in advanced cases, flaccid paralysis and/or impaired ability to concentrate urine.

If potassium depletion associated with metabolic alkalosis cannot be managed by correcting the fundamental cause of the deficiency (e.g., where the patient requires long term diuretic therapy) supplemental potassium in the form of high potassium food or potassium chloride may be able to restore normal potassium levels.

In rare circumstances (e.g., patients with renal tubular acidosis) potassium depletion may be associated with metabolic acidosis and hyperchloremia. In such patients potassium replacement should be accomplished with potassium salts other than the chloride, such as potassium bicarbonate, potassium citrate, potassium acetate, or potassium gluconate.

INDICATIONS AND USAGE

BECAUSE OF REPORTS OF INTESTINAL AND GASTRIC ULCERATION AND BLEEDING WITH CONTROLLED RELEASE POTASSIUM CHLORIDE PREPARATIONS, THESE DRUGS SHOULD BE RESERVED FOR THOSE PATIENTS WHO CANNOT TOLERATE OR REFUSE TO TAKE LIQUIDS OR EFFERVESCENT POTASSIUM PREPARATIONS OR FOR PATIENTS IN WHOM THERE IS A PROBLEM OF COMPLIANCE WITH THESE PREPARATIONS.

1. For the treatment of patients with hypokalemia, with or without metabolic alkalosis; in digitalis intoxication; and patients with hypokalemic familial periodic paralysis. If hypokalemia is the result of diuretic therapy, consideration should be given to the use of a lower dose of diuretic, which may be sufficient without leading to hypokalemia.

2. For the prevention of hypokalemia in patients who would be at particular risk if hypokalemia were to develop, e.g., digitalized patients or patients with significant cardiac arrhythmias.

The use of potassium salts in patients receiving diuretics for uncomplicated essential hypertension is often unnecessary when such patients have a normal dietary pattern and when low doses of the diuretic are used. Serum potassium should be checked periodically, however, and if hypokalemia occurs, dietary supplementation with potassium-containing foods may be adequate to control milder cases. In more severe cases, and if dose adjustment of the diuretic is ineffective or unwarranted, supplementation with potassium salts may be indicated.

CONTRAINDICATIONS

Potassium supplements are contraindicated in patients with hyperkalemia since a further increase in serum potassium concentration in such patients can produce cardiac arrest. Hyperkalemia may complicate any of the following conditions: chronic renal failure, systemic acidosis such as diabetic acidosis, acute dehydration, extensive tissue breakdown as in severe burns, adrenal insufficiency, or the administration of a potassium-sparing diuretic (e.g., spironolactone, triamterene or amiloride) (see OVERDOSAGE).

Controlled release formulations of potassium chloride have produced esophageal ulceration in certain cardiac patients with esophageal compression due to an enlarged left atrium. Potassium supplementation, when indicated in such patients, should be given as a liquid preparation.

All solid oral dosage forms of potassium chloride are contraindicated in any patients in whom there is structural, pathological (e.g., diabetic gastroparesis) or pharmacologic (use of anticholinergic agents or other agents with anticholinergic properties at sufficient doses to exert anticholinergic effects) cause for arrest or delay in tablet passage through the gastrointestinal tract.

WARNINGS

Hyperkalemia (see Overdosage):

In patients with impaired mechanisms for excreting potassium, the administration of potassium salts can produce hyperkalemia and cardiac arrest. This occurs most commonly in patients given potassium by the intravenous route but may also occur in patients given potassium orally. Potentially fatal hyperkalemia can develop rapidly and be asymptomatic. The use of potassium salts in patients with chronic renal disease, or any other condition which impairs potassium excretion, requires particularly careful monitoring of the serum potassium concentration and appropriate dosage adjustment.

Interaction with Potassium-Sparing Diuretics:

Hypokalemia should not be treated by the concomitant administration of potassium salts and a potassium-sparing diuretic (e.g., spironolactone, triamterene, or amiloride), since the simultaneous administration of these agents can produce severe hyperkalemia.

Interaction with Angiotensin Converting Enzyme Inhibitors:

Angiotensin coverting enzyme (ACE) inhibitors (e.g., captopril, enalapril) will produce some potassium retention by inhibiting aldosterone production. Potassium supplements should be given to patients receiving ACE inhibitors only with close monitoring.

Gastrointestinal Lesions: Solid oral dosage forms of potassium chloride can produce ulcerative and/or stenotic lesions of the gastrointestinal tract. Based on spontaneous adverse reaction reports, enteric coated preparations of potassium chloride are associated with an increased frequency of small bowel lesions (40–50 per 100,000 patient years) compared to sustained release wax matrix formulations (less than one per 100,000 patient years). Because of the lack of extensive marketing experience with microencapsulated products, a comparison between such products and wax matrix or enteric coated products is not available. KlorCon® Extended-release Tablets are wax matrix tablets formulated to provide a controlled rate of release of potassium chloride and thus to minimize the possibility of high local concentration of potassium near the gastrointestinal wall.

Prospective trials have been conducted in normal human volunteers in which the upper gastrointestinal tract was evaluated by endoscopic inspection before and after one week of solid oral potassium chloride therapy. The ability of this model to predict events occurring in usual clinical practice is unknown. Trials which approximated usual clinical practice did not reveal any clear differences between the wax matrix and microencapsulated dosage forms. In contrast, there was a higher incidence of gastric and duodenal lesions in subjects receiving a high dose of a wax matrix controlled release formulation under conditions which did not resemble usual or recommended clinical practice (i.e., 96 mEq per day in divided doses of potassium chloride administered to fasted patients, in the presence of an anticholinergic drug to delay gastric emptying). The upper gastrointestinal lesions observed by endoscopy were asymptomatic and were not accompanied by evidence of bleeding (hemoccult testing). The relevance of these findings to the usual conditions (i.e., nonfasting, no anticholinergic agent, smaller doses) under which controlled release potassium chloride products are used is uncertain; epidemiologic studies have not identified an elevated risk, compared to microencapsulated products, for upper gastrointestinal lesions in patients receiving wax matrix formulations. Klor-Con® Extended-release Tablets should be discontinued immediately and the possibility of ulceration, obstruction, or perforation considered if severe vomiting, abdominal pain, distention, or gastrointestinal bleeding occurs.

Metabolic Acidosis:

Hypokalemia in patients with metabolic acidosis should be treated with an alkalinizing potassium salt such as potassium bicarbonate, potassium citrate, potassium acetate, or potassium gluconate.

PRECAUTIONS

General: The diagnosis of potassium depletion is ordinarily made by demonstrating hypokalemia in a patient with a clinical history suggesting some cause for potassium depletion. In interpreting the serum potassium level, the physician should bear in mind that acute alkalosis per se can produce hypokalemia in the absence of a deficit in total body potassium, while acute acidosis per se can increase the serum potassium concentration into the normal range even in the presence of a reduced total body potassium. The treatment of potassium depletion, particularly in the presence of cardiac disease, renal disease, or acidosis, requires careful attention to acid-base balance and appropriate monitoring of serum electrolytes, the electrocardiogram, and the clinical status of the patient.

Information for Patients: Physicians should consider reminding the patient of the following:

To take each dose without crushing, chewing or sucking the tablets.

To take each dose with meals and with a full glass of water or other liquid.

To take this medicine following the frequency and amount prescribed by the physician. This is especially important if the patient is also taking diuretics and/or digitalis preparations.

To check with the physician if there is trouble swallowing the tablets or if the tablets seem to stick in the throat.

To check with the physician at once if tarry stools or other evidence of gastrointestinal bleeding is noticed.

To be aware that the expended matrix is not absorbed and may be excreted intact in the stool.

Laboratory Tests: When blood is drawn for analysis of plasma potassium it is important to recognize that artifactual elevations can occur after improper venipuncture technique or as a result of in vitro hemolysis of the sample.

Drug Interactions: Potassium-sparing diuretic, angiotensin converting enzyme inhibitors: see WARNINGS.

Carcinogenesis, Mutagenesis, Impairment of Fertility: Carcinogenicity, mutagenicity, and fertility studies in animals have not been performed. Potassium is a normal dietary constituent.

Pregnancy Catetory C: Animal reproduction studies have not been conducted with Klor-Con® Extended-release Tablets. It is unlikely that potassium supplementation that does not lead to hyperkalemia would have an adverse effect on the fetus or would affect reproductive capacity.

Nursing Mothers: The normal potassium ion content of human milk is about 13 mEq per liter. Since oral potassium becomes part of the body potassium pool, so long as body potassium is not excessive, the contribution of potassium chloride supplementation should have little or no effect on the level in human milk.

Pediatric Use: Safety and effectiveness in children have not been established.

ADVERSE REACTIONS

One of the most severe adverse effects is hyperkalemia (see CONTRAINDICATIONS, WARNINGS, and OVERDOSAGE). There also have been reports of upper and lower gastrointestinal conditions including obstruction, bleeding, ulceration, and perforation (see CONTRAINDICATIONS and WARNINGS).

The most common adverse reactions to the oral potassium salts are nausea, vomiting, flatulence, abdominal pain/discomfort, and diarrhea. These symptoms are due to irritation of the gastrointestinal tract and are best managed by diluting the preparation further, taking the dose with meals, or reducing the amount taken at one time.

OVERDOSAGE

The administration of oral potassium salts to persons with normal excretory mechanisms for potassium rarely causes serious hyperkalemia. However, if excretory mechanisms are impaired, or if potassium is administered too rapidly intravenously, potentially fatal hyperkalemia can result (see CONTRAINDICATIONS and WARNINGS). It is important to recognize that hyperkalemia is usually asymptomatic and may be manifested only by an increased serum potassium concentration (6.5–8.0 mEq/L) and characteristic electrocardiographic changes (peaking of T-waves, loss of P-wave, depression of S-T segment, and prolongation of the QT interval). Late manifestations include muscle paralysis and cardiovascular collapse from cardiac arrest (9–12 mEq./L).

Treatment measures for hyperkalemia include the following:

1. Elimination of foods and medications containing potassium and of any agents with potassium-sparing properties;
2. Intravenous administration of 300 to 500 ml/hr of 10% dextrose solution containing 10–20 units of crystalline insulin per 1,000 ml;
3. Correction of acidosis, if present, with intravenous sodium bicarbonate;
4. Use of exchange resins, hemodialysis, or peritoneal dialysis.

In treating hyperkalemia, it should be recalled that in patients who have been stabilized on digitalis, too rapid a lowering of the serum potassium concentration can produce digitalis toxicity.

DOSAGE AND ADMINISTRATION

The usual dietary potassium intake by the average adult is 50 to 100 mEq per day. Potassium depletion sufficient to cause hypokalemia usually requires the loss of 200 or more mEq of potassium from the total body store.

Dosage must be adjusted to the individual needs of each patient. The dose for the prevention of hypokalemia is typically in the range of 20 mEq per day. Doses of 40–100 mEq per day or more are used for the treatment of potassium depletion. Dosage should be divided if more than 20 mEq per day is

given such that no more than 20 mEq is given in a single dose.

Each Klor-Con® Extended-release Tablet provides 8 mEq or 10 mEq of potassium chloride.

Klor-Con® Extended-release Tablets should be taken with meals and with a glass of water or other liquid. This product should not be taken on an empty stomach because of its potential for gastric irritation (see WARNINGS).

NOTE: Klor-Con® Extended-release Tablets must be swallowed whole. Take each dose without crushing, chewing or sucking the tablets.

HOW SUPPLIED

Film coated, Klor-Con® 8 (blue), Klor-Con® 10 (yellow), imprinted round tablets containing:

600 mg potassium chloride (equivalent to 8 mEq) in bottles of 100 (NDC 0245-0040-11), bottles of 500 (NDC 0245-0040-15), and unit-dose packages of 100 (NDC 0245-0040-01); 750 mg potassium chloride (equivalent to 10 mEq) in bottles of 100 (NDC 0245-0041-11), bottles of 500 (NDC 0245-0041-15), and unit-dose packages of 100 (NDC 0245-0041-01).

Protect from light and moisture. Store at controlled room temperature 59°–86°F (15°–30°C). Dispense in container with child resistant closure.

CAUTION: Federal law prohibits dispensing without prescription.

Shown in Product Identification Section, page 434

KLOR-CON®/EF 25mEq   ℞
[klōr'kon]
Potassium Bicarbonate Effervescent Tablets for Oral Solution, USP

DESCRIPTION

Each effervescent tablet in solution provides 25 mEq (978 mg) potassium as bicarbonate and citrate. KLOR-CON®/EF tablets are sugar-free and orange flavored.

HOW SUPPLIED

KLOR-CON®/EF 25 mEq effervescent tablets in cartons of 30 and 100 individually wrapped tablets.
30's NDC 0245-0039-30, 100's NDC 0245-0039-01

LUBRIN® Vaginal Lubricating Inserts   OTC
[lu'brin]

DESCRIPTION

Vaginal dryness can occur due to a variety of reasons including: menopause, stress, medication use, side effects from cancer treatment, or even after the use of a tampon. Lubrin® Inserts are the first premeasured, easy-to-use inserts specifically designed for vaginal dryness. Lubrin® Inserts are unscented, colorless, water-soluble inserts that provide long lasting lubrication. Lubrin® Inserts quickly liquefy within the vagina to simulate natural lubrication for several hours.

HOW SUPPLIED

Lubrin® Inserts are available in packages of five and twelve inserts.
5's List No.: 0245-0118-19, 12's List No.: 0245-0118-12.

NIACOR®   ℞
[nī'akor]
Niacin Tablets, 500 mg

DESCRIPTION

Niacor® Tablets (immediate-release niacin) are white scored tablets with "NIACOR" imprinted on one side, containing 500 mg of niacin (nicotinic acid). The structure is shown below. The tablets also contain acacia, corn starch, lactose anhydrous, magnesium stearate, methanol, P.V.P., stearic acid and water.

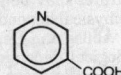

CLINICAL PHARMACOLOGY

Niacin functions in the body as a component of two hydrogen transporting coenzymes: Coenzyme I (Nicotinamide Adenine Dinucleotide [NAD], sometimes called Diphosphopyridine Nucleotide [DPN]) and Coenzyme II (Nicotinamide Adenine Dinucleotide Phosphate [NADP], sometimes called Triphosphopyridine Nucleotide [TPN]). Niacin, in addition to its functions as a vitamin, exerts several distinctive pharmacological effects which vary according to the dosage level employed. Niacin, in large doses, causes a reduction in serum lipids. The exact mechanism of this action is unknown.

INDICATIONS

Since no drug is innocuous, strict attention should be paid to the indications and contraindications, particularly when selecting drugs for long term use. Niacor® Tablets are indicated as adjunctive therapy in patients with significant hyperlipidemia (elevated cholesterol and/or triglycerides) who do not respond adequately to diet and weight loss.

Notice: It has not been established whether the drug-induced lowering of serum cholesterol or triglyceride levels has a beneficial effect, no effect, or a detrimental effect on the morbidity or mortality due to atherosclerosis including coronary heart disease. Investigations now in progress may yield an answer to this question.

CONTRAINDICATIONS

Niacor® Tablets are contraindicated in patients with a known idiosyncrasy to niacin, with hepatic dysfunction, with active peptic ulcer or with arterial bleeding.

WARNINGS

Use of this drug in pregnancy, lactation or in women of child-bearing age requires that the potential benefits of the drug be weighed against its possible hazards to the mother and child. Although fetal abnormalities have not been reported with this drug, its use as an antilipidemic agent requires high dosages, and animal reproduction or teratology studies have not been done. There are insufficient studies done for usage in children.

KEEP OUT OF REACH OF CHILDREN.

PRECAUTIONS

Great caution must be exercised when niacin is used in patients with coronary disease or gallbladder disease. Patients with a past history of jaundice, liver disease or peptic ulcer should be observed closely while taking the medication. Frequent monitoring of liver function tests and blood glucose should be performed during therapy to ascertain that the drug has no adverse effects on these organ systems. Antihypertensive drugs of the adrenergic-blocking type may have an additive vasodilating effect and produce postural hypotension. Elevated uric acid levels have occurred, therefore use with caution in patients predisposed to gout.

Drug Interactions: Antihypertensive drugs may have an additive vasodilating effect and produce postural hypotension. Diabetic or potential diabetic patients should be observed closely in the event of decreased glucose tolerance. Adjustment of diet and/or hypoglycemic therapy may be necessary.

ADVERSE REACTIONS

Atrial fibrillation and other cardiac arrhythmias
Severe generalized flushing
Decreased glucose tolerance
Activaton of peptic ulcers
Abnormalities of hepatic functional tests
Jaundice
Gastrointestinal disorders
Dryness of the skin
Acanthosis Nigricans
Pruritus
Hyperuricemia
Toxic amblyopia
Hypotension
Transient headache

OVERDOSAGE

High doses of nicotinic acid may produce temporary flushing, pruritus, and gastrointestinal distress.

DOSAGE AND ADMINISTRATION

Usually Recommended Adult Dosage—1 to 2 grams three times a day. The dosage must be adjusted to the response of the patient. Start with two tablets (1 g) three times a day with food or after meals, taken with cold liquids, if necessary, to facilitate swallowing. Since low dosages may control hyperlipidemia in some patients, the dosage should be individualized according to the effect on serum lipid levels. If the plasma cholesterol and/or triglyceride level does not show a decrease after a reasonable time at this dosage, an increase in dosage may be considered but requires careful titration and observation of the patient for unwanted effects. The dosage may be increased every 2 to 4 weeks, but in no case should the dosage exceed 6 grams/day.

Since flushing, pruritis and gastrointestinal distress appear frequently and tend to be dose-related, increase the dosage gradually in increments of 500 mg (1 tablet) while carefully observing the patient and monitoring the plasma cholesterol and/or triglyceride level for therapeutic response and for adverse effects. Where the observed adverse reactions or potential hazards exceed the benefits of use, dosage should be reduced to the minimum recommended dosage and, where necessary, discontinued entirely.

HOW SUPPLIED

White scored tablets with "NIACOR" imprinted on one side, containing 500 mg niacin each, in bottles of 100, (NDC 0245-0066-11). Dispense in tight container as defined in the USP. Store at controlled room temperature, 15°–30°C (59°–86°F).

CAUTION: Federal law prohibits dispensing without a prescription.

Manufactured for
UPSHER-SMITH LABORATORIES, INC.
Minneapolis, MN
55447
by
Halsey Drug Co., Inc.
Brooklyn, NY USA
11233-3599

OMS® Concentrate   ℃ ℞
Morphine Sulfate (Immediate Release) Concentrated Oral Solution

DESCRIPTION

Each ml of OMS® Concentrate contains:
Morphine Sulfate .... 20 mg
(WARNING: May be habit forming)

HOW SUPPLIED

OMS® Concentrate
(Morphine Sulfate Immediate Release, Concentrated Oral Solution)
20 mg per ml
NDC 0245–0167–31: Bottle of 30 ml with calibrated dropper.
NDC 0245–0167–04: Bottle of 120 ml with calibrated dropper.

RMS® Suppositories   ℃ ℞
Rectal Morphine Sulfate

WARNING—MAY BE HABIT FORMING

DESCRIPTION

Suppositories contain 5, 10, 20, or 30 mg of morphine sulfate.

HOW SUPPLIED

RMS® Suppositories are individually sealed and unit dose labeled. 12 suppositories per carton.
 5 mg NDC 0245-0160-12, 10 mg NDC 0245-0161-12
20 mg NDC 0245-0162-12, 30 mg NDC 0245-0163-12

SSKI®   ℞
Potassium Iodide Oral Solution, USP

DESCRIPTION

SSKI® (potassium iodide oral solution, USP) is a saturated solution of potassium iodide containing 1 g of potassium iodide per ml.

HOW SUPPLIED

SSKI® (potassium iodide oral solution, USP) is supplied in 1 fluid ounce (30 ml) bottles (NDC 0245-0003-31) with a calibrated dropper marked to deliver 0.3 ml and 0.6 ml; and 8 fluid ounces (237 ml) bottles (NDC 0245-0003-08).

SALSITAB®   ℞
[sal'si"tab]
(salsalate)
Tablets

DESCRIPTION

Salsitab® (salsalate) Tablets are a nonsteroidal anti-inflammatory agent for oral administration.

Each round, blue, film coated Salsitab® Tablet contains 500 mg salsalate. Each capsule-shaped, blue, scored, film coated Salsitab® Tablet contains 750 mg salsalate.

HOW SUPPLIED

500 mg tablets in bottles of 100 (NDC 0245-0153-11)
500 mg tablets in bottles of 500 (NDC 0245-0153-15)
500 mg tablets in cartons of 100 unit dose (NDC 0245-0153-01)
750 mg tablets in bottles of 100 (NDC 0245-0154-11)
750 mg tablets in bottles of 500 (NDC 0245-0154-15)
750 mg tablets in cartons of 100 unit dose (NDC 0245-0154-01)

Continued on next page

Upsher-Smith Laboratories—Cont.

SLO–NIACIN®   OTC

[slō "nī'-a-sin]
polygel™ controlled-release niacin tablets
(Nicotinic Acid)
250, 500, and 750 mg

DESCRIPTION

Slo-Niacin® Tablets are manufactured utilizing a unique, patent pending, polygel™ controlled-release delivery system. This exclusive technology assures the gradual and measured release of niacin and is designed to significantly reduce the incidence of flushing and itching commonly associated with niacin use. Slo-Niacin® Tablets are available in 250, 500, and 750 mg strengths.

USES

Slo-Niacin® Tablets are used in all those conditions in which niacin supplementation is indicated. It has the advantage of a slower release of niacin than conventional tablet dosage forms. This may permit its use by those who do not tolerate immediate-release tablets.

CAUTIONS

Niacin may cause flushing, itching and skin reddening. The effects are temporary and usually disappear. Persons taking niacin supplements for prolonged periods of time should do so under the care of a physician. Slo-Niacin® Tablets should not be used by persons with a known sensitivity to niacin (nicotinic acid, vitamin B_3) and by persons with heart or gallbladder disease, gout, arterial bleeding, glaucoma, diabetes, impaired liver function, peptic ulcer, or by pregnant or lactating women. Patients taking anti-hypertensive drugs should consult a physician before taking niacin tablets.

SIDE EFFECTS

Temporary flushing and feeling of warmth may be expected. These seldom reach levels so as to necessitate discontinuance. Temporary headache, itching and tingling, gastric disturbances, skin rash, and allergies may occur. If these symptoms persist, discontinue use and consult a physician.

DOSAGE

Usual Adult Dose:
250 mg—One Slo-Niacin® Tablet morning and evening or as directed by physician.
500 mg—One Slo-Niacin® Tablet morning or evening, or one-half Slo-Niacin® Tablet morning and evening or as directed by physician.
750 mg—One-half Slo-Niacin® Tablet morning or evening or as directed by physician.
Before using 500 mg or more daily, consult physician.
NOTE: Slo-Niacin® Tablets may be broken on the score line but should not be crushed or chewed. The expended matrix is not absorbed and may be excreted intact in the stool. Keep out of reach of children.

HOW SUPPLIED

250 mg tablets in bottles of 100: List No. 0245–0062–11
500 mg tablets in bottles of 100: List No. 0245–0063–11
750 mg tablets in bottles of 100: List No. 0245–0064–11
Polygel is a trademark of Upsher-Smith Laboratories, Inc.
Shown in Product Identifications Section, page 434

Vitaline Formulas
722 JEFFERSON AVE
ASHLAND, OR 97520

3mg BIOTIN FORTE®   OTC

3mg (3000mcg) Biotin, Folic Acid with other B-Complex Vitamins, Vitamin C and Zinc.

and

Extra Stength 5mg BIOTIN FORTE®   OTC

5mg (5000mcg) Biotin, Folic Acid, with other B-Complex Vitamins and Vitamin C. No Zinc.

CAL-LACTATE   OTC

Calcium Lactate Scored Caplets 1100mg
(170mg elemental calcium)

L-CARNITINE   OTC
250mg tablets
L-CARNITINE   OTC
660mg tablets

COENZYME Q₁₀ (Ubiquinone)   OTC
25mg & 60mg tablets

High Lipase
8X PANCREATIN 900mg USP   OTC
Equivalent to pancreatin 7200mg USP
Pancreatic Enzyme Replacement

Each Tablet Provides:
Lipase 22,500 USP units, Protease 180,000 USP units, Amylase 180,000 USP units.

PRECAUTIONS
Use with caution in patients known to be allergic to pork protein.
Suggested Use
Usual dosage: 1 or 2 tablets with each meal or as directed by physician.

TOTAL FORMULA–2   OTC
High Potency Multivitamin/Multimineral
Supplement with micro-trace elements.
An iron free formula is also available.

Each Tablet Contains:

VITAMINS: Beta Carotene, Vitamins A, C, D, E, K, B_1,B_2,B_3,B_5,B_6,B_{12},Biotin, Folic Acid, Choline, Hesperidin Complex, Citrus Bioflavonoids, Rutin, Inositol and PABA.
MINERALS: Calcium, Magnesium, Phosphorus, Potassium, Iron, Zinc, Copper, Manganese, Iodine, Chromium, Selenium, Molybdenum, Silicon and Vanadium.

Wallace Laboratories
P.O. BOX 1001
CRANBURY, NJ 08512

AQUATENSEN®   ℞
(methyclothiazide tablets, USP 5 mg)
Tablets

BUTISOL SODIUM®   ℅ ℞
(butabarbital sodium)
Tablets and Elixir

DESCRIPTION

BUTISOL SODIUM (butabarbital sodium) is a nonselective central nervous system depressant which is used as a sedative or hypnotic (WARNING: May be habit-forming). It is available for oral administration as *Tablets* containing 15 mg, 30 mg, 50 mg or 100 mg butabarbital sodium; and as *Elixir* containing 30 mg/5 mL, with alcohol (by volume) 7%. Other ingredients in the Tablets are: calcium stearate, corn starch, dibasic calcium phosphate, FD&C Blue No. 1 (15 mg and 30 mg only), FD&C Blue No. 2 (100 mg only); FD&C Red No. 3 (15 mg and 100 mg only), FD&C Yellow No. 5 (30 mg and 50 mg only)—see Precautions), FD&C Yellow No. 6 (100 mg only). Other ingredients in the Elixir are: D&C Green No. 5, edetate disodium, FD&C Yellow No. 5 (see Precautions), flavors (natural and artificial), propylene glycol, purified water, saccharin sodium, sodium benzoate. Butabarbital sodium occurs as a white, bitter powder which is freely soluble in water and alcohol, but practically insoluble in benzene and ether.
The structural formula for butabarbital sodium is:

$$\text{NaO} \quad \begin{array}{c} \text{H} \\ \text{N} \\ \end{array} \quad \begin{array}{c} \text{O} \\ \text{CH}_2\text{CH}_3 \\ \text{CHCH}_2\text{CH}_3 \\ \text{O} \\ \end{array}$$

Sodium 5-*sec*-butyl-5-ethylbarbiturate

CLINICAL PHARMACOLOGY

BUTISOL SODIUM (butabarbital sodium), like other barbiturates, is capable of producing all levels of CNS mood alteration from excitation to mild sedation, to hypnosis, and deep coma. Overdosage can produce death. Barbiturates depress the sensory cortex, decrease motor activity, alter cerebellar function, and produce drowsiness, sedation, and hypnosis.
Barbiturate-induced sleep differs from physiological sleep. Sleep laboratory studies have demonstrated that barbiturates reduce the amount of time spent in the rapid eye movement (REM) phase of sleep or dreaming stage. Also, Stages III and IV sleep are decreased. Following abrupt cessation of barbiturates used regularly, patients may experience markedly increased dreaming, nightmares, and/or insomnia. Therefore, withdrawal of a single therapeutic dose over 5 or 6 days has been recommended to lessen the REM rebound and disturbed sleep which contribute to drug withdrawal syndrome (for example, decrease the dose from 3 to 2 doses a day for 1 week).
In studies, secobarbital sodium and pentobarbital sodium have been found to lose most of their effectiveness for both inducing and maintaining sleep by the end of 2 weeks of continued drug administration even with the use of multiple doses. As with secobarbital sodium and pentobarbital sodium, other barbiturates might be expected to lose their effectiveness for inducing and maintaining sleep after about 2 weeks. The short-, intermediate-, and, to a lesser degree, long-acting barbiturates have been widely prescribed for treating insomnia. Although the clinical literature abounds with claims that the short-acting barbiturates are superior for producing sleep while the intermediate-acting compounds are more effective in maintaining sleep, controlled studies have failed to demonstrate these differential effects. Therefore, as sleep medications, the barbiturates are of limited value beyond the short-term use.
Barbiturates are respiratory depressants. The degree of respiratory depression is dependent upon dose. With hypnotic doses, respiratory depression produced by barbiturates is similar to that which occurs during physiologic sleep with slight decrease in blood pressure and heart rate.
Barbiturates do not impair normal hepatic function, but have been shown to induce liver microsomal enzymes, thus increasing and/or altering the metabolism of barbiturates and other drugs (see Precautions—*Drug interactions*).
Pharmacokinetics: BUTISOL SODIUM (butabarbital sodium) is the sodium salt of a weak acid. Barbiturates are weak acids that are absorbed and rapidly distributed to all tissues and fluids with high concentrations in the brain, liver, and kidneys. Barbiturates are bound to plasma and tissue proteins. The rate of absorption is increased if it is ingested as a dilute solution or taken on an empty stomach. Barbiturates are metabolized primarily by the hepatic microsomal enzyme system, and most metabolic products are excreted in the urine. The excretion of unchanged butabarbital in the urine is negligible. BUTISOL SODIUM (butabarbital sodium) is classified as an intermediate-acting barbiturate. The average plasma half-life for butabarbital is 100 hours in the adult.
Although variable from patient to patient, butabarbital has an onset of action of about ¾ to 1 hour, and a duration of action of about 6 to 8 hours.

INDICATIONS AND USAGE

BUTISOL SODIUM (butabarbital sodium) is indicated for use as a sedative or hypnotic.
Since barbiturates appear to lose their effectiveness for sleep induction and sleep maintenance after 2 weeks, use of BUTISOL SODIUM in treating insomnia should be limited to this time (see Clinical Pharmacology above).

CONTRAINDICATIONS

Barbiturates are contraindicated in patients with known barbiturate sensitivity. Barbiturates are also contraindicated in patients with a history of manifest or latent porphyria.

WARNINGS

Habit forming: Barbiturates may be habit forming. Tolerance, psychological and physical dependence may occur with continued use (see Drug Abuse and Dependence below). Patients who have psychological dependence on barbiturates may increase the dosage or decrease the dosage interval without consulting a physician and may subsequently develop a physical dependence on barbiturates. To minimize the possibility of overdosage or the development of dependence, the prescribing and dispensing of sedative-hypnotic barbiturates should be limited to the amount required for the interval until the next appointment. Abrupt cessation after prolonged use in the dependent person may result in withdrawal symptoms, including delirium, convulsions, and possibly death. Barbiturates should be withdrawn gradually from any patient known to be taking excessive dosage over long periods of time. (See Drug Abuse and Dependence below.)

Acute or chronic pain: Caution should be exercised when barbiturates are administered to patients with acute or chronic pain, because paradoxical excitement could be induced, or important symptoms could be masked. However, the use of barbiturates as sedatives in the postoperative surgical period, and as adjuncts to cancer chemotherapy, is well established.

Use in pregnancy: Barbiturates can cause fetal damage when administered to a pregnant woman. Retrospective, case-controlled studies have suggested a connection between the maternal consumption of barbiturates and a higher than expected incidence of fetal abnormalities. Following oral administration, barbiturates readily cross the placental barrier and are distributed throughout fetal tissues with highest concentrations found in the placenta, fetal liver, and brain. Withdrawal symptoms occur in infants born to mothers who receive barbiturates throughout the last trimester of pregnancy (see Drug Abuse and Dependence). If this drug is used during pregnancy, or if the patient becomes pregnant while taking this drug, the patient should be apprised of the potential hazard to the fetus.

PRECAUTIONS

General: Barbiturates should be administered with caution, if at all, to patients who are mentally depressed, have suicidal tendencies, or a history of drug abuse.

Elderly or debilitated patients may react to barbiturates with marked excitement, depression, and confusion. In some persons, barbiturates repeatedly produce excitement rather than depression.

In patients with hepatic damage, barbiturates should be administered with caution and initially in reduced doses. Barbiturates should not be administered to patients showing the premonitory signs of hepatic coma.

BUTISOL SODIUM (butabarbital sodium) Tablets, 30 mg and 50 mg, and Elixir contain FD&C Yellow No. 5 (tartrazine) which may cause allergic-type reactions (including bronchial asthma) in certain susceptible individuals. Although the overall incidence of FD&C Yellow No. 5 (tartrazine) sensitivity in the general population is low, it is frequently seen in patients who also have aspirin hypersensitivity.

Information for Patients: Practitioners should give the following information and instructions to patients receiving barbiturates.

The use of barbiturates carries with it an associated risk of psychological and/or physical dependence. The patient should be warned against increasing the dose of the drug without consulting a physician.

Barbiturates may impair mental and/or physical abilities required for the performance of potentially hazardous tasks, such as driving or operating machinery.

Alcohol should not be consumed while taking barbiturates. Concurrent use of the barbiturates with other CNS depressants, including other sedatives or hypnotics, alcohol, narcotics, tranquilizers, and antihistamines, may result in additional CNS depressant effects.

Laboratory tests: Prolonged therapy with barbiturates should be accompanied by periodic laboratory evaluation of organ systems, including hematopoietic, renal, and hepatic systems (see Precautions—*General* and Adverse Reactions).

Drug interactions: Most reports of clinically significant drug interactions occurring with the barbiturates have involved phenobarbital. However, the application of these data to other barbiturates appears valid and warrants serial blood level determinations of the relevant drugs when there are multiple therapies.

1. *Anticoagulants.* Phenobarbital lowers the plasma levels of dicumarol and causes a decrease in anticoagulant activity as measured by the prothrombin time. Barbiturates can induce hepatic microsomal enzymes resulting in increased metabolism and decreased anticoagulant response of oral anticoagulants (e.g., warfarin, acenocoumarol, dicumarol, and phenprocoumon). Patients stabilized on anticoagulant therapy may require dosage adjustments if barbiturates are added to or withdrawn from their dosage regimen.
2. *Corticosteroids.* Barbiturates appear to enhance the metabolism of exogenous corticosteroids probably through the induction of hepatic microsomal enzymes. Patients stabilized on corticosteroid therapy may require dosage adjustments if barbiturates are added to or withdrawn from their dosage regimen.
3. *Griseofulvin.* Phenobarbital appears to interfere with the absorption of orally administered griseofulvin, thus decreasing its blood level. The effect of the resultant decreased blood levels of griseofulvin on therapeutic response has not been established. However, it would be preferable to avoid concomitant administration of these drugs.
4. *Doxycycline.* Phenobarbital has been shown to shorten the half-life of doxycycline for as long as 2 weeks after barbiturate therapy is discontinued. The mechanism is probably through the induction of hepatic microsomal enzymes that metabolize the antibiotic. If phenobarbital and doxycycline are administered concurrently, the clinical response to doxycycline should be monitored closely.
5. *Phenytoin, sodium valproate, valproic acid.* The effect of barbiturates on the metabolism of phenytoin appears to be variable. Some investigators report an accelerating effect, while others report no effect. Because the effect of barbiturates on the metabolism of phenytoin is not predictable, phenytoin and barbiturate blood levels should be monitored more frequently if these drugs are given concurrently. Sodium valproate and valproic acid appear to decrease barbiturate metabolism; therefore, barbiturate blood levels should be monitored and appropriate adjustments made as indicated.
6. *Central nervous system.* The concomitant use of other central nervous system depressants, including other sedatives or hypnotics, antihistamines, tranquilizers, or alcohol, may produce additive depressant effects.
7. *Monoamine oxidase inhibitors (MAOI).* MAOI prolong the effects of barbiturates probably because metabolism of the barbiturate is inhibited.
8. *Estradiol, estrone, progesterone and other steroid hormones.* Pretreatment with or concurrent administration of phenobarbital may decrease the effect of estradiol by increasing its metabolism. There have been reports of patients treated with antiepileptic drugs (e.g. phenobarbital) who become pregnant while taking oral contraceptives. An alternate contraceptive method might be suggested to women taking phenobarbital.

Carcinogenesis, mutagenesis, impairment of fertility: No long-term studies in animals have been performed with butabarbital sodium to determine carcinogenic and mutagenic potential, or effects on fertility.

Pregnancy: Teratogenic effects—Pregnancy Category D (See Warnings—*Use in pregnancy* above).

Nonteratogenic effects—Infants suffering from long-term barbiturate exposure *in utero* may have an acute withdrawal syndrome of seizures and hyperirritability from birth to a delayed onset of up to 14 days (see Drug Abuse and Dependence).

Labor and delivery: Hypnotic doses of barbiturates do not appear to significantly impair uterine activity during labor. Administration of sedative-hypnotic barbiturates to the mother during labor may result in respiratory depression in the newborn. Premature infants are particularly susceptible to the depressant effects of barbiturates. If barbiturates are used during labor and delivery, resuscitation equipment should be available.

Nursing mothers: Caution should be exercised when a barbiturate is administered to a nursing woman since small amounts of some barbiturates are excreted in the milk.

ADVERSE REACTIONS

The following adverse reactions have been observed with the use of barbiturates in hospitalized patients. Because such patients may be less aware of certain of the milder adverse effects of barbiturates, the incidence of these reactions may be somewhat higher in fully ambulatory patients.

More than 1 in 100 patients. The most common adverse reaction, somnolence, is estimated to occur at a rate of 1 to 3 patients per 100.

Less than 1 in 100 patients. The most common adverse reactions estimated to occur at a rate of less than 1 in 100 patients listed below, grouped by organ system, and by decreasing order of occurrence are:

Central nervous system/psychiatric: Agitation, confusion, hyperkinesia, ataxia, CNS depression, nightmares, nervousness, psychiatric disturbance, hallucinations, insomnia, anxiety, dizziness, thinking abnormality.

Respiratory: Hypoventilation, apnea.

Cardiovascular: Bradycardia, hypotension, syncope.

Gastrointestinal: Nausea, vomiting, constipation.

Other reported reactions: Headache, hypersensitivity (angioedema, skin rashes, exfoliative dermatitis), fever, liver damage.

DRUG ABUSE AND DEPENDENCE

Controlled substance: Schedule III.

Abuse and dependence: Barbiturates may be habit-forming. Tolerance, psychological dependence, and physical dependence may occur especially following prolonged use of high doses of barbiturates. Daily administration in excess of 400 milligrams (mg) of pentobarbital or secobarbital for approximately 90 days is likely to produce some degree of physical dependence. A dosage of from 600 to 800 mg taken for at least 35 days is sufficient to produce withdrawal seizures. The average daily dose for the barbiturate addict is usually about 1.5 grams. As tolerance to barbiturates develops, the amount needed to maintain the same level of intoxication increases; tolerance to a fatal dosage, however, does not increase more than two-fold. As this occurs, the margin between an intoxicating dosage and fatal dosage becomes smaller.

Symptoms of acute intoxication with barbiturates include unsteady gait, slurred speech, and sustained nystagmus. Mental signs of chronic intoxication include confusion, poor judgment, irritability, insomnia, and somatic complaints. Symptoms of barbiturate dependence are similar to those of chronic alcoholism.

If an individual appears to be intoxicated with alcohol to a degree that is radically disproportionate to the amount of alcohol in his or her blood, the use of barbiturates should be suspected. The lethal dose of a barbiturate is far less if alcohol is also ingested.

The symptoms of barbiturate withdrawal can be severe and may cause death. Minor withdrawal symptoms may appear 8 to 12 hours after the last dose of a barbiturate. These symptoms usually appear in the following order: anxiety, muscle twitching, tremor of hands and fingers, progressive weakness, dizziness, distortion in visual perception, nausea, vomiting, insomnia, and orthostatic hypotension. Major withdrawal symptoms (convulsions and delirium) may occur within 16 hours and last up to 5 days after abrupt cessation of these drugs. Intensity of withdrawal symptoms gradually declines over a period of approximately 15 days.

Drug dependence to barbiturates arises from repeated administration of a barbiturate or agent with barbiturate-like effect on a continuous basis, generally in amounts exceeding the therapeutic dose levels. The characteristics of drug dependence to barbiturates include: (a) a strong desire or need to continue taking the drug; (b) a tendency to increase the dose; (c) a psychic dependence on the effects of the drug related to subjective and individual appreciation for those effects; and (d) a physical dependence on the effects of the drug requiring its presence for maintenance of homeostasis and resulting in a definite, characteristic, and self-limited abstinence syndrome when the drug is withdrawn.

Treatment of barbiturate dependence consists of cautious and gradual withdrawal of the drug. Barbiturate-dependent patients can be withdrawn by using a number of different withdrawal regimens. In all cases, withdrawal takes an extended period of time. One method involves initiating treatment at the patient's regular dosage level, in 3 to 4 divided doses, and decreasing the daily dose by 10 percent if tolerated by the patient.

Infants physically dependent on barbiturates may be given phenobarbital 3 to 10 mg/kg/day. After withdrawal symptoms (hyperactivity, disturbed sleep, tremors, hyperreflexia) are relieved, the dosage of phenobarbital should be gradually decreased and completely withdrawn over a 2-week period.

OVERDOSAGE

Signs and symptoms: The toxic dose of barbiturates varies considerably. In general, an oral dose of 1 gram of most barbiturates produces serious poisoning in an adult. Death commonly occurs after 2 to 10 grams of ingested barbiturates. Symptoms of acute intoxication with barbiturates include unsteady gait, slurred speech, and sustained nystagmus. Mental signs of chronic intoxication include confusion, poor judgment, irritability, insomnia, and somatic complaints. Barbiturate intoxication may be confused with alcoholism, bromide intoxication, and with various neurological disorders.

Acute overdosage with barbiturates is manifested by CNS and respiratory depression which may progress to Cheyne-Stokes respiration, areflexia, constriction of the pupils to a slight degree (though in severe poisoning they may show paralytic dilation), oliguria, tachycardia, hypotension, lowered body temperature, and coma. Typical shock syndrome (apnea, circulatory collapse, respiratory arrest, and death) may occur.

In extreme overdose, all electrical activity in the brain may cease, in which case a "flat" EEG normally equated with clinical death cannot be accepted. This effect is fully reversible unless hypoxic damage occurs. Consideration should be given to the possibility of barbiturate intoxication even in situations that appear to involve trauma.

Complications: Pneumonia, pulmonary edema, cardiac arrhythmias, congestive heart failure, and renal failure may occur. Uremia may increase CNS sensitivity to barbiturates if renal function is impaired. Differential diagnosis should include hypoglycemia, head trauma, cerebrovascular accidents, convulsive states, and diabetic coma.

Treatment: Treatment of overdosage is mainly supportive and consists of the following:

1. Maintenance of an adequate airway, with assisted respiration and oxygen administration as necessary.
2. Monitoring of vital signs and fluid balance.
3. If the patient is conscious and has not lost the gag reflex, emesis may be induced with ipecac. Care should be taken to prevent pulmonary aspiration of vomitus. After completion of vomiting, 30 grams activated charcoal in a glass of water may be administered.
4. If emesis is contraindicated, gastric lavage may be performed with a cuffed endotracheal tube in place with the patient in the face down position. Activated charcoal may be left in the emptied stomach and a saline cathartic administered.
5. Fluid therapy and other standard treatment for shock, if needed.
6. If renal function is normal, forced diuresis may aid in the elimination of the barbiturate.

Continued on next page

Wallace Laboratories—Cont.

7. Although not recommended as a routine procedure, hemodialysis may be used in severe barbiturate intoxications or if the patient is anuric or in shock.
8. Appropriate nursing care, including rolling patients from side-to-side every 30 minutes, to prevent hypostatic pneumonia, decubiti, aspiration, and other complications of patients with altered states of consciousness.
9. Antibiotics should be given if pneumonia is suspected.

DOSAGE AND ADMINISTRATION

Usual adult dosage:
Daytime sedative—15 to 30 mg, 3 or 4 times daily.
Bedtime hypnotic—50 to 100 mg.
Preoperative sedative—50 to 100 mg, 60 to 90 minutes before surgery.
Usual pediatric dosage:
Preoperative sedative—2 to 6 mg/kg maximum 100 mg.
Special patient population:
Dosage should be reduced in the elderly or debilitated because these patients may be more sensitive to barbiturates. Dosage should be reduced for patients with impaired renal function or hepatic disease (see Precautions).

HOW SUPPLIED

BUTISOL SODIUM® (butabarbital sodium) Tablets:
15 mg—colored lavender, scored, imprinted "BUTISOL SODIUM" and $^{37}{}_{112}$ in bottles of 100 (NDC 0037-0112-60) and 1000 (NDC 0037-0112-80).
30 mg*—colored green, scored, imprinted "BUTISOL SODIUM" and $^{37}{}_{113}$ in bottles of 100 (NDC 0037-0113-60) and 1000 (NDC 0037-0113-80).
50 mg*—colored orange, scored, imprinted "BUTISOL SODIUM" and $^{37}{}_{114}$ in bottles of 100 (NDC 0037-0114-60).
100 mg—colored pink, scored, imprinted "BUTISOL SODIUM" and $^{37}{}_{115}$ in bottles of 100 (NDC 0037-0115-60).
BUTISOL SODIUM® (butabarbital sodium) Elixir*: 30 mg/5 mL, alcohol (by volume) 7%—colored green in bottles of one pint (NDC 0037-0110-16) and one gallon (NDC 0037-0110-28).
Storage: Tablets and *Elixir*—Store at room temperature. Keep bottle tightly closed.

*Contains FD&C Yellow No. 5 (see Precautions).

Rev. 2/85

Shown in Product Identification Section, page 434

DEPEN® ℞
(penicillamine tablets, USP)
Titratable Tablets

> Physicians planning to use penicillamine should thoroughly familiarize themselves with its toxicity, special dosage considerations, and therapeutic benefits. Penicillamine should never be used casually. Each patient should remain constantly under the close supervision of the physician. Patients should be warned to report promptly any symptoms suggesting toxicity.

DESCRIPTION

Penicillamine is 3-mercapto-D-valine, a disease modifying antirheumatic drug. It is a white or practically white, crystalline powder, freely soluble in water, slightly soluble in alcohol, and insoluble in ether, acetone, benzene, and carbon tetrachloride. Although its configuration is D, it is levorotatory as usually measured:

$$[\alpha]\ 25^\circ_D = -62.5^\circ \pm 2.0^\circ\ (C = 1, 1N\ NaOH)$$

The empirical formula is $C_5H_{11}NO_2S$, giving it a molecular weight of 149.21. The structural formula is:

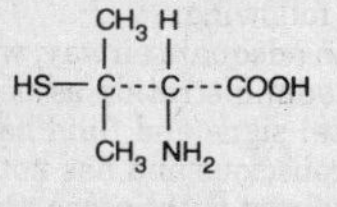

It reacts readily with formaldehyde or acetone to form a thiazolidine-carboxylic acid.
Depen® Titratable Tablets (penicillamine tablets, USP) for oral administration contain 250 mg of penicillamine.
Other ingredients (inactive): edetate disodium, hydroxypropyl methylcellulose, lactose, magnesium stearate, magnesium trisilicate, polyethylene glycol, povidone, simethicone emulsion, starch, and stearic acid.

CLINICAL PHARMACOLOGY

Penicillamine is a chelating agent recommended for the removal of excess copper in patients with Wilson's disease. From *in vitro* studies which indicate that one atom of copper combines with two molecules of penicillamine, it would appear that one gram of penicillamine should be followed by the excretion of about 200 milligrams of copper; however, the actual amount excreted is about one percent of this.
Penicillamine also reduces excess cystine excretion in cystinuria. This is done, at least in part, by disulfide interchange between penicillamine and cystine, resulting in formation of penicillamine-cysteine disulfide, a substance that is much more soluble than cystine and is excreted readily.
Penicillamine interferes with the formation of cross-links between tropocollagen molecules and cleaves them when newly formed.
The mechanism of action of penicillamine in rheumatoid arthritis is unknown, although it appears to suppress disease activity. Unlike cytotoxic immunosuppressants, penicillamine markedly lowers IgM rheumatoid factor but produces no significant depression in absolute levels of serum immunoglobulins. Also unlike cytotoxic immunosuppressants, which act on both, penicillamine *in vitro* depresses T-cell activity but not B-cell activity.
In vitro, penicillamine dissociates macroglobulins (rheumatoid factor) although the relationship of the activity to its effect in rheumatoid arthritis is not known.
In rheumatoid arthritis, the onset of therapeutic response to DEPEN may not be seen for two or three months. In those patients who respond, however, the first evidence of suppression of symptoms such as pain, tenderness, and swelling usually is generally apparent within three months. The optimum duration of therapy has not been determined. If remissions occur, they may last from months to years but usually require continued treatment (see DOSAGE AND ADMINISTRATION).
In all patients receiving penicillamine, it is important that DEPEN be given on an empty stomach, at least one hour before meals or two hours after meals, and at least one hour apart from any other drug, food or milk. This permits maximum absorption and reduces the likelihood of inactivation by metal binding in the gastrointestinal tract.
Methodology for determining the bioavailability of penicillamine is not available; however, penicillamine is known to be a very soluble substance.

INDICATIONS

DEPEN is indicated in the treatment of Wilson's disease, cystinuria, and in patients with severe, active rheumatoid arthritis who have failed to respond to an adequate trial of conventional therapy. Available evidence suggests that DEPEN is not of value in ankylosing spondylitis.
Wilson's Disease—Wilson's disease (hepatolenticular degeneration) results from the interaction of an inherited defect and an abnormality in copper metabolism. The metabolic defect, which is the consequence of the autosomal inheritance of one abnormal gene from each parent, manifests itself in a greater positive copper balance than normal. As a result, copper is deposited in several organs and appears eventually to produce pathologic effects most prominently seen in the brain, where degeneration is widespread; in the liver, where fatty infiltration, inflammation, and hepatocellular damage progress to postnecrotic cirrhosis; in the kidney, where tubular and glomerular dysfunction results; and in the eye, where characteristic corneal copper deposits are known as Kayser-Fleischer rings.
Two types of patients require treatment for Wilson's disease: (1) the symptomatic, and (2) the asymptomatic in whom it can be assumed the disease will develop in the future if the patient is not treated.
Diagnosis, suspected on the basis of family or individual history, physical examination, or a low serum concentration of ceruloplasmin,* is confirmed by the demonstration of Kayser-Fleischer rings or, particularly in the asymptomatic patient, by the quantitative demonstration in a liver biopsy specimen of a concentration of copper in excess of 250 mcg/g dry weight.
Treatment has two objectives:
(1) to minimize dietary intake and absorption of copper.
(2) to promote excretion of copper deposited in tissues.
The first objective is attained by a daily diet that contains no more than one or two milligrams of copper. Such a diet should exclude, most importantly, chocolate, nuts, shellfish, mushrooms, liver, molasses, broccoli, and cereals enriched with copper, and be composed to as great an extent as possible of foods with a low copper content. Distilled or demineralized water should be used if the patient's drinking water contains more than 0.1 mg of copper per liter.
For the second objective, a copper chelating agent is used.
In symptomatic patients, this treatment usually produces marked neurologic improvement, fading of Kayser-Fleischer rings, and gradual amelioration of hepatic dysfunction and psychic disturbances.

* For quantitative test for serum ceruloplasmin see: Morell, A. G.; Windsor, J.; Sternlieb, I.; Scheinberg, I. H.: Measurement of the concentration of ceruloplasmin in serum by determination of its oxidase activity, in "Laboratory Diagnosis of Liver Disease," F. W. Sunderman; F. W Sunderman, Jr. (eds.), St. Louis, Warren H. Green, Inc., 1968, pp. 193–195.

Clinical experience to date suggests that life is prolonged with the above regimen.
Noticeable improvement may not occur for one to three months. Occasionally, neurologic symptoms become worse during initiation of therapy with DEPEN. Despite this, the drug should not be discontinued permanently. Although temporary interruption may result in clinical improvement of the neurological symptoms, it carries an increased risk of developing a sensitivity reaction upon resumption of therapy (See WARNINGS).
Treatment of asymptomatic patients has been carried out for over ten years. Symptoms and signs of the disease appear to be prevented indefinitely if daily treatment with DEPEN can be continued.
Cystinuria—Cystinuria is characterized by excessive urinary excretion of the dibasic amino acids, arginine, lysine, ornithine, and cystine, and the mixed disulfide of cysteine and homocysteine. The metabolic defect that leads to cystinuria is inherited as an autosomal, recessive trait. Metabolism of the affected amino acids is influenced by at least two abnormal factors: (1) defective gastrointestinal absorption and (2) renal tubular dysfunction.
Arginine, lysine, ornithine, and cysteine are soluble substances, readily excreted. There is no apparent pathology connected with their excretion in excessive quantities.
Cystine, however, is so slightly soluble at the usual range of urinary pH that it is not excreted readily, and so crystallizes and forms stones in the urinary tract. Stone formation is the only known pathology in cystinuria. Normal daily output of cystine is 40 to 80 mg. In cystinuria, output is greatly increased and may exceed 1 g/day. At 500 to 600 mg/day, stone formation is almost certain. When it is more than 300 mg/day, treatment is indicated.
Conventional treatment is directed at keeping urinary cystine diluted enough to prevent stone formation, keeping the urine alkaline enough to dissolve as much cystine as possible, and minimizing cystine production by a diet low in methionine (the major dietary precursor of cystine). Patients must drink enough fluid to keep urine specific gravity below 1.010, take enough alkali to keep urinary pH at 7.5 to 8, and maintain a diet low in methionine. This diet is not recommended in growing children and probably is contraindicated in pregnancy because of its low protein content (see PRECAUTIONS).
When these measures are inadequate to control recurrent stone formation, DEPEN may be used as additional therapy.
When patients refuse to adhere to conventional treatment, DEPEN may be a useful substitute. It is capable of keeping cystine excretion to near normal values, thereby hindering stone formation and the serious consequences of pyelonephritis and impaired renal function that develop in some patients.
Bartter and colleagues depict the process by which penicillamine interacts with cystine to form penicillamine-cysteine mixed disulfide as:

CSSC	+	PS′	⇄	CS′ + CSSP
PSSP	+	CS′	⇄	PS′ + CSSP
CSSC	+	PSSP	⇄	2 CSSP

CSSC	=	cystine
CS′	=	deprotonated cysteine
PSSP	=	penicillamine
PS′	=	deprotonated penicillamine sulfhydryl
CSSP	=	penicillamine-cysteine mixed disulfide

In this process, it is assumed that the deprotonated form of penicillamine, PS′, is the active factor in bringing about the disulfide interchange.
Rheumatoid Arthritis—Because DEPEN can cause severe adverse reactions, its use in rheumatoid arthritis should be restricted to patients who have severe, active disease and who have failed to respond to an adequate trial of conventional therapy. Even then, benefit-to-risk ratio should be carefully considered. Other measures, such as rest, physiotherapy, salicylates and corticosteroids should be used, when indicated, in conjunction with DEPEN (see PRECAUTIONS).

CONTRAINDICATIONS

Except for treatment of Wilson's disease or certain cases of cystinuria, use of penicillamine during pregnancy is contraindicated (see WARNINGS).
Although breast milk studies have not been reported in animals or humans, mothers on therapy with penicillamine should not nurse their infants.
Patients with a history of penicillamine-related aplastic anemia or agranulocytosis should not be restarted on penicillamine (see WARNINGS and ADVERSE REACTIONS).
Because of its potential for causing renal damage, penicillamine should not be administered to rheumatoid arthritis patients with a history or other evidence of renal insufficiency.

WARNINGS

The use of penicillamine has been associated with fatalities due to certain diseases, such as aplastic anemia, agranulocytosis, thrombocytopenia, Goodpasture's syndrome, and myasthenia gravis.

Because of the potential for serious hematological and renal adverse reactions to occur at any time, routine urinalysis, white and differential blood cell count, hemoglobin determination, and direct platelet count must be done every two weeks for at least the first six months of penicillamine therapy and monthly thereafter. Patients should be instructed to report promptly the development of signs and symptoms of granulocytopenia and/or thrombocytopenia such as fever, sore throat, chills, bruising or bleeding. The above laboratory studies should then be promptly repeated.

Leukopenia and thrombocytopenia have been reported to occur in up to five percent of patients during penicillamine therapy. Leukopenia is of the granulocytic series and may or may not be associated with an increase in eosinophils. A confirmed reduction in WBC below 3500 per cubic mL mandates discontinuance of penicillamine therapy. Thrombocytopenia may be on an idiosyncratic basis with decreased or absent megakaryocytes in the marrow, when it is part of an aplastic anemia. In other cases the thrombocytopenia is presumably on an immune basis since the number of megakaryocytes in the marrow has been reported to be normal or sometimes increased. The development of a platelet count below 100,000 per cubic mL, even in the absence of clinical bleeding, requires at least temporary cessation of penicillamine therapy. A progressive fall in either platelet count or WBC in three successive determinations, even though values are still within the normal range, likewise requires at least temporary cessation.

Proteinuria and/or hematuria may develop during therapy and may be warning signs of membranous glomerulopathy which can progress to a nephrotic syndrome. Close observation of these patients is essential. In some patients the proteinuria disappears with continued therapy; in others penicillamine must be discontinued. When a patient develops proteinuria or hematuria the physician must ascertain whether it is a sign of drug-induced glomerulopathy or is unrelated to penicillamine.

Rheumatoid arthritis patients who develop moderate degrees of proteinuria may be continued cautiously on penicillamine therapy, provided that quantitative 24-hour urinary protein determinations are obtained at intervals of one to two weeks. Penicillamine dosage should not be increased under these circumstances. Proteinuria which exceeds 1 g/24 hours, or proteinuria which is progressively increasing requires either discontinuance of the drug or a reduction in the dosage. In some patients, proteinuria has been reported to clear following reduction in dosage.

In rheumatoid arthritis patients, penicillamine should be discontinued if unexplained gross hematuria or persistent microscopic hematuria develops.

In patients with Wilson's disease or cystinuria the risks of continued penicillamine therapy in patients manifesting potentially serious urinary abnormalities must be weighed against the expected therapeutic benefits.

When penicillamine is used in cystinuria, an annual x-ray for renal stones is advised. Cystine stones form rapidly, sometimes in six months.

Up to one year or more may be required for any urinary abnormalities to disappear after penicillamine has been discontinued.

Because of rare reports of intrahepatic cholestasis and toxic hepatitis, liver function tests are recommended every six months for the duration of therapy.

Goodpasture's syndrome has occurred rarely. The development of abnormal urinary findings associated with hemoptysis and pulmonary infiltrates on x-ray requires immediate cessation of penicillamine.

Obliterative bronchiolitis has been reported rarely. The patient should be cautioned to report immediately pulmonary symptoms such as exertional dyspnea, unexplained cough or wheezing. Pulmonary function studies should be considered at that time.

Myasthenic syndrome sometimes progressing to myasthenia gravis has been reported. Ptosis and diplopia, with weakness of the extraocular muscles, are often early signs of myasthenia. In the majority of cases, symptoms of myasthenia have receded after withdrawal of penicillamine.

Most of the various forms of pemphigus have occurred during treatment with penicillamine. Pemphigus vulgaris and pemphigus foliaceus are reported most frequently, usually as a late complication of therapy. The seborrhea-like characteristics of pemphigus foliaceus may obscure an early diagnosis. When pemphigus is suspected, DEPEN should be discontinued. Treatment has consisted of high doses of corticosteroids alone or, in some cases, concomitantly with an immunosuppressant. Treatment may be required for only a few weeks or months, but may need to be continued for more than a year.

Once instituted for Wilson's disease or cystinuria, treatment with penicillamine should, as a rule, be continued on a daily basis. Interruptions for even a few days have been followed by sensitivity reactions after reinstitution of therapy.

Use in Pregnancy—Penicillamine has been shown to be teratogenic in rats when given in doses 6 times higher than the highest dose recommended for human use (based on a standard weight of 50 kg). Skeletal defects, cleft palates and fetal toxicity (resorptions) have been reported.

There are no controlled studies on the use of penicillamine in pregnant women. Although normal outcomes have been reported, characteristic congenital cutis laxa and associated birth defects have been reported in infants born of mothers who received therapy with penicillamine during pregnancy. Penicillamine should be used in women of childbearing potential only when the expected benefits outweigh the possible hazards. Women on therapy with penicillamine who are of childbearing potential should be apprised of this risk, advised to report promptly any missed menstrual periods or other indications of possible pregnancy, and followed closely for early recognition of pregnancy.

Wilson's Disease—Reported experience* shows that continued treatment with penicillamine throughout pregnancy protects the mother against relapse of the Wilson's disease, and that discontinuation of penicillamine has deleterious effects on the mother.

If penicillamine is administered during pregnancy to patients with Wilson's disease, it is recommended that the daily dosage be limited to 1 g. If cesarean section is planned, the daily dosage should be limited to 250 mg during the last six weeks of pregnancy and postoperatively until wound healing is complete.

Cystinuria—If possible, penicillamine should not be given during pregnancy to women with cystinuria (see CONTRAINDICATIONS). There are reports of women with cystinuria on therapy with penicillamine who gave birth to infants with generalized connective tissue defects who died following abdominal surgery. If stones continue to form in these patients, the benefits of therapy to the mother must be evaluated against the risk to the fetus.

Rheumatoid Arthritis—Penicillamine should not be administered to rheumatoid arthritis patients who are pregnant (see CONTRAINDICATIONS) and should be discontinued promptly in patients in whom pregnancy is suspected or diagnosed.

There is a report that a woman with rheumatoid arthritis treated with less than one gram a day of penicillamine during pregnancy gave birth (cesarean delivery) to an infant with growth retardation, flattened face with broad nasal bridge, low set ears, short neck with loose skin folds, and unusually lax body skin.

PRECAUTIONS

Some patients may experience drug fever, a marked febrile response to penicillamine, usually in the second or third week following initiation of therapy. Drug fever may sometimes be accompanied by a macular cutaneous eruption.

In the case of drug fever in patients with Wilson's disease or cystinuria, penicillamine should be temporarily discontinued until the reaction subsides. Then penicillamine should be reinstituted with a small dose that is gradually increased until the desired dosage is attained. Systemic steroid therapy may be necessary, and is usually helpful, in such patients in whom toxic reactions develop a second or third time.

In the case of drug fever in rheumatoid arthritis patients, because other treatments are available, penicillamine should be discontinued and another therapeutic alternative tried, since experience indicates that the febrile reaction will recur in a very high percentage of patients upon readministration of penicillamine.

The skin and mucous membranes should be observed for allergic reactions. Early and late rashes have occurred. Early rash occurs during the first few months of treatment and is more common. It is usually a generalized pruritic, erythematous, maculopapular or morbilliform rash and resembles the allergic rash seen with other drugs. Early rash usually disappears within days after stopping penicillamine and seldom recurs when the drug is restarted at a lower dosage. Pruritus and early rash may often be controlled by the concomitant administration of antihistamines. Less commonly, a late rash may be seen, usually after six months or more of treatment, and requires discontinuation of penicillamine. It is usually on the trunk, is accompanied by intense pruritus, and is usually unresponsive to topical corticosteroid therapy. Late rash may take weeks to disappear after penicillamine is stopped and usually recurs if the drug is restarted.

The appearance of drug eruption accompanied by fever, arthralgia, lymphadenopathy or other allergic manifestations usually requires discontinuation of penicillamine.

Certain patients will develop a positive antinuclear antibody (ANA) test and some of these may show a lupus erythematosus-like syndrome similar to drug-induced lupus associated with other drugs. The lupus erythematosus-like syndrome is not associated with hypocomplementemia and may be present without nephropathy. The development of a positive ANA test does not mandate discontinuance of the drug; however, the physician should be alerted to the possibility that a lupus erythematosus-like syndrome may develop in the future.

* Scheinberg, I. H., Sternlieb, I.: *N Engl J Med 293:* 1300–1302, December 18, 1975.

Some patients may develop oral ulcerations which in some cases have the appearance of aphthous stomatitis. The stomatitis usually recurs on rechallenge but often clears on a lower dosage. Although rare, cheilosis, glossitis and gingivostomatitis have also been reported. These oral lesions are frequently dose-related and may preclude further increase in penicillamine dosage or require discontinuation of the drug.

Hypogeusia (a blunting or diminution in taste perception) has occurred in some patients. This may last two to three months or more and may develop into a total loss of taste; however, it is usually self-limited, despite continued penicillamine treatment. Such taste impairment is rare in patients with Wilson's disease.

Penicillamine should not be used in patients who are receiving concurrently gold therapy, antimalarial or cytotoxic drugs, oxyphenbutazone or phenylbutazone because these drugs are also associated with similar serious hematologic and renal adverse reactions. Patients who have had gold salt therapy discontinued due to a major toxic reaction may be at greater risk of serious adverse reactions with penicillamine, but not necessarily of the same type.

Patients who are allergic to penicillin may theoretically have cross-sensitivity to penicillamine. The possibility of reactions from contamination of penicillamine by trace amounts of penicillin has been eliminated now that penicillamine is being produced synthetically rather than as a degradation product of penicillin.

Because of their dietary restrictions, patients with Wilson's disease and cystinuria should be given 25 mg/day of pyridoxine during therapy, since penicillamine increases the requirement for this vitamin. Patients also may receive benefit from a multivitamin preparation, although there is no evidence that deficiency of any vitamin other than pyridoxine is associated with penicillamine. In Wilson's disease, multivitamin preparations must be copper-free.

Rheumatoid arthritis patients whose nutrition is impaired should also be given a daily supplement of pyridoxine. Mineral supplements should not be given, since they may block the response to penicillamine.

Iron deficiency may develop, especially in children and in menstruating women. In Wilson's disease, this may be a result of adding the effects of the low copper diet, which is probably also low in iron, and the penicillamine to the effects of blood loss or growth. In cystinuria, a low methionine diet may contribute to iron deficiency, since it is necessarily low in protein. If necessary, iron may be given in short courses, but a period of two hours should elapse between administration of penicillamine and iron, since orally administered iron has been shown to reduce the effects of penicillamine.

Penicillamine causes an increase in the amount of soluble collagen. In the rat this results in inhibition of normal healing and also a decrease in tensile strength of intact skin. In man this may be the cause of increased skin friability at sites especially subject to pressure or trauma, such as shoulders, elbows, knees, toes, and buttocks. Extravasations of blood may occur and may appear as purpuric areas, with external bleeding if the skin is broken, or as vesicles containing dark blood. Neither type is progressive. There is no apparent association with bleeding elsewhere in the body and no associated coagulation defect has been found. Therapy with penicillamine may be continued in the presence of these lesions. They may not recur if dosage is reduced. Other reported effects probably due to the action of penicillamine on collagen are excessive wrinkling of the skin and development of small, white papules at venipuncture and surgical sites.

The effects of penicillamine on collagen and elastin make it advisable to consider a reduction in dosage to 250 mg/day when surgery is contemplated. Reinstitution of full therapy should be delayed until wound healing is complete.

Carcinogenesis—Long-term animal carcinogenicity studies have not been done with penicillamine. There is a report that five of ten autoimmune disease-prone NZB hybrid mice developed lymphocytic leukemia after 6 months' intraperitoneal treatment with a dose of 400 mg/kg penicillamine 5 days per week.

Nursing Mothers—See CONTRAINDICATIONS.

Usage in Children—The efficacy of DEPEN in juvenile rheumatoid arthritis has not been established.

ADVERSE REACTIONS

Penicillamine is a drug with a high incidence of untoward reactions, some of which are potentially fatal. Therefore, it is mandatory that patients receiving penicillamine therapy remain under close medical supervision throughout the period of drug administration (see WARNINGS and PRECAUTIONS).

Reported incidences (%) for the most commonly occurring adverse reactions in rheumatoid arthritis patients are noted, based on 17 representative clinical trials reported in the literature (1270 patients).

Allergic—Generalized pruritus, early and late rashes (5%), pemphigus (see WARNINGS), and drug eruptions which may be accompanied by fever, arthralgia or lymphadenopa-

Continued on next page

Wallace Laboratories—Cont.

thy have occurred (see WARNINGS and PRECAUTIONS). Some patients may show a lupus erythematosus-like syndrome similar to drug-induced lupus produced by other pharmacological agents (see PRECAUTIONS).
Urticaria and exfoliative dermatitis have occurred.
Thyroiditis has been reported; hypoglycemia in association with anti-insulin antibodies has been reported. These reactions are extremely rare.
Some patients may develop a migratory polyarthralgia, often with objective synovitis (see DOSAGE and ADMINISTRATION).
Gastrointestinal—Anorexia, epigastric pain, nausea, vomiting or occasional diarrhea may occur (17%).
Isolated cases of reactivated peptic ulcer have occurred, as have hepatic dysfunction and pancreatitis. Intrahepatic cholestasis and toxic hepatitis have been reported rarely. There have been a few reports of increased serum alkaline phosphatase, lactic dehydrogenase, and positive cephalin flocculation and thymol turbidity tests.
Some patients may report a blunting, diminution or total loss of taste perception (12%); or may develop oral ulcerations. Although rare, cheilosis, glossitis and gingivostomatitis have been reported (see PRECAUTIONS).
Gastrointestinal side effects are usually reversible following cessation of therapy.
Hematological—Penicillamine can cause bone marrow depression (see WARNINGS). Leukopenia (2%) and thrombocytopenia (4%) have occurred. Fatalities have been reported as a result of thrombocytopenia, agranulocytosis, aplastic anemia, and sideroblastic anemia.
Thrombotic thrombocytopenic purpura, hemolytic anemia, red cell aplasia, monocytosis, leukocytosis, eosinophilia, and thrombocytosis have also been reported.
Renal—Patients on penicillamine therapy may develop proteinuria (6%) and/or hematuria which, in some, may progress to the development of the nephrotic syndrome as a result of an immune complex membranous glomerulopathy (see WARNINGS).
Central Nervous System—Tinnitus, optic neuritis and peripheral sensory and motor neuropathies (including polyradiculoneuropathy), i.e., Guillain-Barré Syndrome) have been reported. Muscular weakness may or may not occur with the peripheral neuropathies.
Neuromuscular—Myasthenia gravis (see WARNINGS).
Other—Adverse reactions that have been reported rarely include thrombophlebitis; hyperpyrexia (see PRECAUTIONS); falling hair or alopecia; lichen planus; polymyositis; dermatomyositis; mammary hyperplasia; elastosis perforans serpiginosa; toxic epidermal necrolysis; anetoderma (cutaneous macular atrophy); and Goodpasture's syndrome, a severe and ultimately fatal glomerulonephritis associated with intra-alveolar hemorrhage (see WARNINGS). Fatal renal vasculitis has also been reported. Allergic alveolitis, obliterative bronchiolitis, interstitial pneumonitis and pulmonary fibrosis have been reported in patients with severe rheumatoid arthritis, some of whom were receiving penicillamine. Bronchial asthma has also been reported.
Increased skin friability, excessive wrinkling of skin, and development of small, white papules at venipuncture and surgical sites have been reported (see PRECAUTIONS).
The chelating action of the drug may cause increased excretion of other heavy metals such as zinc, mercury and lead.
There have been reports associating penicillamine with leukemia. However, circumstances involved in these reports are such that a cause and effect relationship to the drug has not been established.

DOSAGE AND ADMINISTRATION

In all patients receiving penicillamine, it is important that DEPEN be given on an empty stomach, at least one hour before meals or two hours after meals, and at least one hour apart from any other drug, food, or milk. Because penicillamine increases the requirement for pyridoxine, patients may require a daily supplement of pyridoxine (see PRECAUTIONS).
Wilson's Disease—Optimal dosage can be determined by measurement of urinary copper excretion and the determination of free copper in the serum. The urine must be collected in copper-free glassware, and should be quantitatively analyzed for copper before and soon after initiation of therapy with DEPEN.
Determination of 24-hour urinary copper excretions is of greatest value in the first week of therapy with penicillamine. In the absence of any drug reaction, a dose between 0.75 and 1.5 g that results in an initial 24-hour cupriuresis of over 2 mg should be continued for about three months, by which time the most reliable method of monitoring maintenance treatment is the determination of free copper in the serum. This equals the difference between quantitatively determined total copper and ceruloplasmin-copper. Adequately treated patients will usually have less than 10 mcg free copper/dL of serum. It is seldom necessary to exceed a dosage of 2 g/day. If the patient is intolerant to therapy with DEPEN, alternative treatment is trientine hydrochloride.
In patients who cannot tolerate as much as 1 g/day initially, initiating dosage with 250 mg/day, and increasing gradually to the requisite amount, gives closer control of the effects of the drug and may help to reduce the incidence of adverse reactions.
Cystinuria—It is recommended that DEPEN be used along with conventional therapy. By reducing urinary cystine, it decreases crystalluria and stone formation. In some instances, it has been reported to decrease the size of, and even to dissolve, stones already formed.
The usual dosage of DEPEN in the treatment of cystinuria is 2 g/day for adults, with a range of 1 to 4 g/day. For children, dosage can be based on 30 mg/kg/day. The total daily amount should be divided into four doses. If four equal doses are not feasible, give the larger portion at bedtime. If adverse reactions necessitate a reduction in dosage, it is important to retain the bedtime dose.
Initiating dosage with 250 mg/day, and increasing gradually to the requisite amount, gives closer control of the effects of the drug and may help to reduce the incidence of adverse reactions.
In addition to taking DEPEN, patients should drink copiously. It is especially important to drink about a pint of fluid at bedtime and another pint once during the night when urine is more concentrated and more acid than during the day. The greater the fluid intake, the lower the required dosage of DEPEN.
Dosage must be individualized to an amount that limits cystine excretion to 100–200 mg/day in those with no history of stones, and below 100 mg/day in those who have had stone formation and/or pain. Thus, in determining dosage, the inherent tubular defect, the patient's size, age, and rate of growth, and his diet and water intake all must be taken into consideration.
The standard nitroprusside cyanide test has been reported useful as a qualitative measure of the effective dose*: Add 2 mL of freshly prepared 5 percent sodium cyanide to 5 ml of a 24-hour aliquot of protein-free urine and let stand ten minutes. Add 5 drops of freshly prepared 5 percent sodium nitroprusside and mix. Cystine will turn the mixture magenta. If the result is negative, it can be assumed that cystine excretion is less than 100 mg/g creatinine.
Although penicillamine is rarely excreted unchanged, it also will turn the mixture magenta. If there is any question as to which substance is causing the reaction, a ferric chloride test can be done to eliminate doubt: Add 3 percent ferric chloride dropwise to the urine. Penicillamine will turn the urine an immediate and quickly fading blue. Cystine will not produce any change in appearance.
Rheumatoid Arthritis—The principal rule of treatment with DEPEN in rheumatoid arthritis is patience. The onset of therapeutic response is typically delayed. Two or three months may be required before the first evidence of a clinical response is noted (see CLINICAL PHARMACOLOGY).
When treatment with DEPEN has been interrupted because of adverse reactions or other reasons, the drug should be reintroduced cautiously by starting with a lower dosage and increasing slowly.
Initial Therapy—The currently recommended dosage regimen in rheumatoid arthritis begins with a single daily dose of 125 mg or 250 mg which is thereafter increased at one to three month intervals, by 125 mg or 250 mg/day, as patient response and tolerance indicate. If a satisfactory remission of symptoms is achieved, the dose associated with the remission should be continued (see Maintenance Therapy). If there is no improvement and there are no signs of potentially serious toxicity after two to three months of treatment with doses of 500–750 mg/day, increases of 250 mg/day at two to three month intervals may be continued until a satisfactory remission occurs (see Maintenance Therapy) or signs of toxicity develop (see WARNINGS and PRECAUTIONS). If there is no discernible improvement after three to four months of treatment with 1000 to 1500 mg of penicillamine/day, it may be assumed the patient will not respond and DEPEN should be discontinued.
Maintenance Therapy—The maintenance dosage of DEPEN must be individualized, and may require adjustment during the course of treatment. Many patients respond satisfactorily to a dosage within the 500–750 mg/day range. Some need less.
Changes in maintenance dosage levels may not be reflected clinically or in the erythrocyte sedimentation rate for two to three months after each dosage adjustment.
Some patients will subsequently require an increase in the maintenance dosage to achieve maximal disease suppression. In those patients who do respond, but who evidence incomplete suppression of their disease after the first six to nine months of treatment, the daily dosage of DEPEN may be increased by 125 mg or 250 mg/day at three-month intervals. It is unusual in current practice to employ a dosage in excess of 1 g/day, but up to 1.5 g/day has sometimes been required.
Management of Exacerbations—During the course of treatment some patients may experience an exacerbation of disease activity following an initial good response. These may be self-limited and can subside within twelve weeks. They are usually controlled by the addition of nonsteroidal anti-inflammatory drugs, and only if the patient has demonstrated a true "escape" phenomenon (as evidenced by failure of the flare to subside within this time period) should an increase in the maintenance dose ordinarily be considered.
In the rheumatoid patient, migratory polyarthralgia due to penicillamine is extremely difficult to differentiate from an exacerbation of the rheumatoid arthritis. Discontinuance or a substantial reduction in the dosage of DEPEN for up to several weeks will usually determine which of these processes is responsible for the arthralgia.
Duration of Therapy—The optimum duration of DEPEN therapy in rheumatoid arthritis has not been determined. If the patient has been in remission for six months or more, a gradual, stepwise dosage reduction in decrements of 125 mg or 250 mg/day at approximately three month intervals may be attempted.
Concomitant Drug Therapy—DEPEN should not be used in patients who are receiving gold therapy, antimalarial or cytotoxic drugs, oxyphenbutazone or phenylbutazone (see PRECAUTIONS). Other measures, such as salicylates, other nonsteroidal anti-inflammatory drugs or systemic corticosteroids may be continued when DEPEN is initiated. After improvement commences, analgesic and anti-inflammatory drugs may be slowly discontinued as symptoms permit. Steroid withdrawal must be done gradually, and many months of DEPEN treatment may be required before steroids can be completely eliminated.
Dosage Frequency—Based on clinical experience, dosages up to 500 mg/day can be given as a single daily dose. Dosages in excess of 500 mg/day should be administered in divided doses.

* Lotz, M., Potts, J. T. and Bartter, F. C.: *Brit Med J* 2:521, August 28, 1965 (in Medical Memoranda).

HOW SUPPLIED

DEPEN® Titratable Tablets: 250 mg scored, oval, white tablets debossed with 37-4401 and Wallace; available in bottles of 100 (NDC 0037-4401-01).
Storage: Store at controlled room temperature 15°–30°C (59°–86°F). Protect from moisture.

WALLACE LABORATORIES
Division of
CARTER-WALLACE, INC.
Cranbury, New Jersey 08512
Manufactured under license from ASTA Pharma AG, Frankfurt, Federal Republic of Germany

Rev. 6/90

Shown in Product Identification Section, page 434

DEPROL® Ⓒ ℞

(meprobamate 400 mg + benactyzine hydrochloride 1 mg)

DESCRIPTION

'Deprol' is available as light pink, scored tablets, each containing meprobamate, U.S.P., 400 mg and benactyzine hydrochloride 1 mg.
Other ingredients: alginic acid, D&C Red #30 Aluminum Lake, FD&C Yellow #5 Aluminum Lake, purified stearic acid, starch, talc.

ACTIONS

'Deprol'* (meprobamate + benactyzine hydrochloride) combines the tranquilizing action of meprobamate with the antidepressant action of benactyzine hydrochloride.

Benactyzine hydrochloride
Benactyzine hydrochloride is a mild antidepressant and anticholinergic agent which in animals has been shown to reduce the autonomic response to emotion-provoking stress.
Meprobamate
Meprobamate is a carbamate derivative which has been shown in animal studies to have effects at multiple sites in the central nervous system, including the thalamus and limbic system.

*U.S. Patent No. 3,090,726 covers the ingredients combination.

INDICATIONS

Based on a review of this drug by the National Academy of Sciences—National Research Council and/or other information, FDA has classified the indication as follows:
"Possibly" effective: in the management of depression, both acute (reactive) and chronic. It is particularly useful in the less severe depressions and where the depression is accompanied by anxiety, insomnia, agitation, or rumination. It is also useful for management of depres-

sion and associated anxiety accompanying or related to organic illnesses. Final classification of this indication requires further investigation.

CONTRAINDICATIONS

Benactyzine hydrochloride
Glaucoma and allergic or idiosyncratic reactions to benactyzine hydrochloride or related compounds.

Meprobamate
Acute intermittent porphyria as well as allergic or idiosyncratic reactions to meprobamate or related compounds such as carisoprodol, mebutamate, tybamate, or carbromal.

WARNINGS

The following information on meprobamate pertains to 'Deprol' (meprobamate + benactyzine hydrochloride):

Meprobamate

Drug Dependence—Physical dependence, psychological dependence, and abuse have occurred. When chronic intoxication from prolonged use occurs, it usually involves ingestion of greater than recommended doses and is manifested by ataxia, slurred speech, and vertigo. Therefore, careful supervision of dose and amounts prescribed is advised, as well as avoidance of prolonged administration, especially for alcoholics and other patients with a known propensity for taking excessive quantities of drugs.

Sudden withdrawal of the drug after prolonged and excessive use may precipitate recurrence of pre-existing symptoms, such as anxiety, anorexia, or insomnia, or withdrawal reactions, such as vomiting, ataxia, tremors, muscle twitching, confusional states, hallucinosis, and, rarely, convulsive seizures. Such seizures are more likely to occur in persons with central nervous system damage or pre-existent or latent convulsive disorders. Onset of withdrawal symptoms occurs usually within 12 to 48 hours after discontinuation of meprobamate; symptoms usually cease within the next 12 to 48 hours.

When excessive dosage has continued for weeks or months, dosage should be reduced gradually over a period of one or two weeks rather than abruptly stopped. Alternatively, a short-acting barbiturate may be substituted, then gradually withdrawn.

Potentially Hazardous Tasks—Patients should be warned that this drug may impair the mental and/or physical abilities required for the performance of potentially hazardous tasks such as driving a motor vehicle or operating machinery.

Additive Effects—Since the effects of meprobamate and alcohol or meprobamate and other CNS depressants or psychotropic drugs may be additive, appropriate caution should be exercised with patients who take more than one of these agents simultaneously.

Usage in Pregnancy and Lactation

An increased risk of congenital malformations associated with the use of minor tranquilizers (meprobamate, chlordiazepoxide, and diazepam) during the first trimester of pregnancy has been suggested in several studies. Because use of these drugs is rarely a matter of urgency, their use during this period should almost always be avoided. The possibility that a woman of childbearing potential may be pregnant at the time of institution of therapy should be considered. Patients should be advised that if they become pregnant during therapy or intend to become pregnant they should communicate with their physicians about the desirability of discontinuing the drug.

Meprobamate passes the placental barrier. It is present both in umbilical cord blood at or near maternal plasma levels and in breast milk of lactating mothers at concentrations two to four times that of maternal plasma. When use of meprobamate is contemplated in breast-feeding patients, the drug's higher concentrations in breast milk as compared to maternal plasma levels should be considered.

Usage in Children—This combination is not intended for use in children.

PRECAUTIONS

Meprobamate—The lowest effective dose should be administered, particularly to elderly and/or debilitated patients, in order to preclude oversedation.

The possibility of suicide attempts should be considered and the least amount of drug feasible should be dispensed at any one time.

Meprobamate is metabolized in the liver and excreted by the kidney; to avoid its excess accumulation, caution should be exercised in administration to patients with compromised liver or kidney function.

Meprobamate occasionally may precipitate seizures in epileptic patients.

This product contains FD&C Yellow No. 5 (tartrazine) which may cause allergic-type reactions (including bronchial asthma) in certain susceptible individuals. Although the overall incidence of FD&C Yellow No. 5 (tartrazine) sensitivity in the general population is low, it is frequently seen in patients who also have aspirin hypersensitivity.

ADVERSE REACTIONS

Side effects have included nausea, dryness of mouth, and other gastrointestinal symptoms; syncope; and one case each of severe nervousness and loss of power of concentration.

The following side effects, which have occurred after administration of its components alone, have either occurred or might occur when the combination is taken.

Benactyzine Hydrochloride
Benactyzine hydrochloride alone, particularly in high dosage, may produce dizziness, thought-blocking, a sense of depersonalization, aggravation of anxiety, or disturbance of sleep patterns, and a subjective feeling of muscle relaxation. There may also be anticholinergic effects such as blurred vision, dryness of mouth, or failure of visual accommodation. Other reported side effects have included gastric distress, allergic response, ataxia, and euphoria.

Meprobamate

Central Nervous System—Drowsiness, ataxia, dizziness, slurred speech, headache, vertigo, weakness, paresthesias, impairment of visual accommodation, euphoria, overstimulation, paradoxical excitement, fast EEG activity.

Gastrointestinal—Nausea, vomiting, diarrhea.

Cardiovascular—Palpitations, tachycardia, various forms of arrhythmia, transient ECG changes, syncope; also, hypotensive crises (including one fatal case).

Allergic or Idiosyncratic—Allergic or idiosyncratic reactions are usually seen within the period of the first to fourth dose in patients having had no previous contact with the drug. Milder reactions are characterized by an itchy, urticarial, or erythematous maculopapular rash which may be generalized or confined to the groin. Other reactions have included leukopenia, acute nonthrombocytopenic purpura, petechiae, ecchymoses, eosinophilia, peripheral edema, adenopathy, fever, fixed drug eruption with cross reaction to carisoprodol, and cross sensitivity between meprobamate/mebutamate and meprobamate/carbromal.

More severe hypersensitivity reactions, rarely reported, include hyperpyrexia, chills, angioneurotic edema, bronchospasm, oliguria, and anuria. Also, anaphylaxis, erythema multiforme, exfoliative dermatitis, stomatitis, proctitis, Stevens-Johnson syndrome, and bullous dermatitis, including one fatal case of the latter following administration of meprobamate in combination with prednisolone.

In case of allergic or idiosyncratic reactions to meprobamate, discontinue the drug and initiate appropriate symptomatic therapy, which may include epinephrine, antihistamines, and in severe cases corticosteroids. In evaluating possible allergic reactions, also consider allergy to excipients (information on excipients is available to physicians on request).

Hematologic (See also **Allergic or Idiosyncratic.**)—Agranulocytosis and aplastic anemia have been reported, although no causal relationship has been established. These cases rarely were fatal. Rare cases of thrombocytopenic purpura have been reported.

Other—Exacerbation of porphyric symptoms.

DOSAGE AND ADMINISTRATION

The usual adult starting dosage of 'Deprol' (meprobamate + benactyzine hydrochloride) is one tablet three or four times daily, which may be increased gradually to six tablets daily and gradually reduced to maintenance levels upon establishment of relief. Doses above six tablets daily are not recommended, even though higher doses have been used by some clinicians to control depression, and in chronic psychotic patients.

OVERDOSAGE

Overdosage of 'Deprol' (meprobamate + benactyzine hydrochloride) has not differed substantially from meprobamate overdosage:

Meprobamate
Suicidal attempts with meprobamate have resulted in drowsiness, lethargy, stupor, ataxia, coma, shock, vasomotor and respiratory collapse. Some suicidal attempts have been fatal. The following data on meprobamate tablets have been reported in the literature and from other sources. These data are not expected to correlate with each case (considering factors such as individual susceptibility and length of time from ingestion to treatment), but represent the *usual ranges* reported.

Acute simple overdose (meprobamate alone): Death has been reported with ingestion of as little as 12 gm meprobamate and survival with as much as 40 gm.

Blood Levels:
0.5–2.0 mg% represents the usual blood level range of meprobamate after therapeutic doses. The level may occasionally be as high as 3.0 mg%.
3–10 mg% usually corresponds to findings of mild to moderate symptoms of overdosage, such as stupor or light coma.
10–20 mg% usually corresponds to deeper coma, requiring more intensive treatment. Some fatalities occur.
At levels greater than 20 mg%, more fatalities than survivals can be expected.

Acute combined overdose (meprobamate with alcohol or other CNS depressants or psychotropic drugs): Since effects can be additive, a history of ingestion of a low dose of meprobamate plus any of these compounds (or of a relatively low blood or tissue level) cannot be used as a prognostic indicator.

In cases where excessive doses have been taken, sleep ensues rapidly and blood pressure, pulse, and respiratory rates are reduced to basal levels. Any drug remaining in the stomach should be removed and symptomatic therapy given. Should respiration or blood pressure become compromised, respiratory assistance, central nervous system stimulants, and pressor agents should be administered cautiously as indicated. Meprobamate is metabolized in the liver and excreted by the kidney. Diuresis, osmotic (mannitol) diuresis, peritoneal dialysis, and hemodialysis have been used successfully. Careful monitoring of urinary output is necessary and caution should be taken to avoid overhydration. Relapse and death, after initial recovery, have been attributed to incomplete gastric emptying and delayed absorption. Meprobamate can be measured in biological fluids by two methods: colorimetric (Hoffman, A.J. and Ludwig, B.J.: *J Amer Pharm Assn 48:* 740, 1959) and gas chromatographic (Douglas, J.F. et al: *Anal Chem 39:* 956, 1967).

HOW SUPPLIED

Bottles of 100 (NDC 0037-3001-01). Bottles of 500 (NDC 0037-3001-03).

WALLACE LABORATORIES
Division of
CARTER-WALLACE, INC.
Cranbury, New Jersey 08512

Rev. 4/86

DIUTENSEN®-R ℞
(methyclothiazide and reserpine)
Tablets

DORAL® Ⓒ
(quazepam)
Tablets

DESCRIPTION

DORAL (brand of quazepam) Tablets contain quazepam, a trifluoroethyl benzodiazepine hypnotic agent, having the chemical name 7-chloro-5-(o-fluorophenyl)-1,3-dihydro-1-(2,2,2-trifluoroethyl)-2*H*-1,4-benzodiazepine-2-thione and the following structural formula:

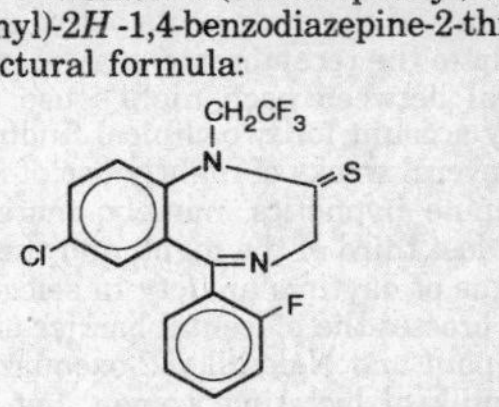

Quazepam has the empirical formula $C_{17}H_{11}ClF_4N_2S$, and a molecular weight of 386.8. It is a white crystalline compound, soluble in ethanol and insoluble in water. Each DORAL Tablet contains either 7.5 or 15 mg of quazepam. The inactive ingredients for DORAL Tablets 7.5 or 15 mg include cellulose, corn starch, FD&C Yellow No. 6 Al Lake, lactose, magnesium stearate, silicon dioxide, and sodium lauryl sulfate.

CLINICAL PHARMACOLOGY

Central nervous system agents of the 1,4-benzodiazepine class presumably exert their effects by binding to stereospecific receptors at several sites within the central nervous system (CNS). Their exact mechanism of action is unknown.

In a sleep laboratory study, DORAL Tablets significantly decreased sleep latency and total wake time, and significantly increased total sleep time and percent sleep time, for one or more nights. Quazepam 15 mg was effective on the first night of administration. Sleep latency, total wake time and wake time after sleep onset were still decreased and percent sleep time was still increased for several nights after the drug was discontinued. Percent slow wave sleep was decreased, and REM sleep was essentially unchanged. No transient sleep disturbance, such as "rebound insomnia," was observed after withdrawal of the drug in sleep laboratory studies in 12 patients using 15 mg doses.

In outpatient studies. DORAL Tablets improved all subjective measures of sleep including sleep induction time, duration of sleep, number of nocturnal awakenings, occurrence of early morning awakening, and sleep quality. Some effects were evident on the first night of administration of DORAL Tablets (sleep induction time, number of nocturnal awakenings, and duration of sleep). Residual medication effects ("hangover") were minimal.

Quazepam is rapidly (absorption half-life of about 30 minutes) and well absorbed from the gastrointestinal tract. The

Continued on next page

Wallace Laboratories—Cont.

peak plasma concentration of quazepam is approximately 20 ng/ml after a 15 mg dose and is obtained at about 2 hours. Quazepam, the active parent compound, is extensively metabolized in the liver; two of the plasma metabolites are 2-oxoquazepam and N-desalkyl-2-oxoquazepam. All three compounds show pharmacological central nervous system activity in animals.

Following administration of ^{14}C-quazepam, approximately 31% of the dose appears in the urine and 23% in the feces over a five-day period; only trace amounts of unchanged drug are present in the urine.

The mean elimination half-life of quazepam and 2-oxoquazepam is 39 hours and that of N-desalkyl-2-oxoquazepam is 73 hours. Steady-state levels of quazepam and 2-oxoquazepam are attained by the seventh daily dose and that of N-desalkyl-2-oxoquazepam by the thirteenth daily dose.

The pharmacokinetics of quazepam and 2-oxoquazepam in geriatric subjects are comparable to those seen in young adults; as with desalkyl metabolites of other benzodiazepines, the elimination half-life of N-desalkyl-2-oxoquazepam in geriatric patients is about twice that of young adults.

The degree of plasma protein binding for quazepam and its two major metabolites is greater than 95%. The absorption, distribution, metabolism, and excretion of benzodiazepines may be altered in various disease states including alcoholism, impaired hepatic function, and impaired renal function. The type and duration of hypnotic effects and the profile of unwanted effects during administration of benzodiazepine drugs may be influenced by the biologic half-life of administered drug and any active metabolites formed. When half-lives are long, drug or metabolites may accumulate during periods of nightly administration and be associated with impairments of cognitive and/or motor performance during waking hours; the possibility of interaction with other psychoactive drugs or alcohol will be enhanced. In contrast, if half-lives are short, drug and metabolites will be cleared before the next dose is ingested, and carry-over effects related to excessive sedation or CNS depression should be minimal or absent. However, during nightly use for an extended period, pharmacodynamic tolerance or adaptation to some effects of benzodiazepine hypnotics may develop. If the drug has a short half-life of elimination, it is possible that a relative deficiency of the drug or its active metabolites (i.e., in relationship to the receptor site) may occur at some point in the interval between each night's use. This sequence of events may account for two clinical findings reported to occur after several weeks of nightly use of rapidly eliminated benzodiazepine hypnotics, namely, increased wakefulness during the last third of the night, and the appearance of increased signs of daytime anxiety in selected patients.

Quazepam crosses the placental barrier of mice. Quazepam, 2-oxoquazepam and N-desalkyl-2-oxoquazepam are present in breast milk of lactating women, but the total amount found in the milk represents only about 0.1% of the administered dose.

INDICATIONS AND USAGE

DORAL Tablets are indicated for the treatment of insomnia characterized by difficulty in falling asleep, frequent nocturnal awakenings, and/or early morning awakenings. The effectiveness of DORAL has been established in placebo-controlled clinical studies of 5 nights duration in acute and chronic insomnia. The sustained effectiveness of DORAL has been established in chronic insomnia in a sleep lab (polysomnographic) study of 28 nights duration.

Because insomnia is often transient and intermittent, the prolonged administration of DORAL Tablets is generally not necessary or recommended. Since insomnia may be a symptom of several other disorders, the possibility that the complaint may be related to a condition for which there is a more specific treatment should be considered.

CONTRAINDICATIONS

DORAL Tablets are contraindicated in patients with known hypersensitivity to this drug or other benzodiazepines, and in patients with established or suspected sleep apnea.

Usage in Pregnancy: Benzodiazepines may cause fetal damage when administered during pregnancy. An increased risk of congenital malformations associated with the use of diazepam and chlordiazepoxide during the first trimester of pregnancy has been suggested in several studies. Transplacental distribution has resulted in neonatal CNS depression following the ingestion of therapeutic doses of a benzodiazepine hypnotic during the last weeks of pregnancy.

DORAL Tablets are contraindicated in pregnancy because the potential risks outweigh the possible advantages of their use during this period. If there is a likelihood of the patient becoming pregnant while receiving DORAL, she should be warned of the potential risk to the fetus. Patients should be instructed to discontinue the drug prior to becoming pregnant. The possibility that a woman of childbearing potential may be pregnant at the time of institution of therapy should be considered. (See **Pregnancy, Teratogenic Effects: Pregnancy Category X.**)

WARNINGS

Patients receiving benzodiazepines should be cautioned about possible combined effects with alcohol and other CNS depressants. Also, caution patients that an additive effect may occur if alcoholic beverages are consumed during the day following the use of benzodiazepines for nighttime sedation. The potential for this interaction continues for several days following their discontinuance until serum levels of psychoactive metabolites have declined.

Patients should also be cautioned about engaging in hazardous occupations requiring complete mental alertness, such as operating machinery or driving a motor vehicle, after ingesting benzodiazepines, including potential impairment of the performance of such activities which may occur the day following ingestion.

Withdrawal symptoms of the type associated with sedatives/hypnotics (e.g., barbiturates, bromides, etc.) and alcohol have been reported after the discontinuation of benzodiazepines. While these symptoms have been more frequently reported after the discontinuation of excessive benzodiazepine doses, there have also been controlled studies demonstrating the occurrence of such symptoms after discontinuation of therapeutic doses of benzodiazepines, generally following prolonged use (but in some instances after periods as brief as six weeks). It is generally believed that the gradual reduction of dosage will diminish the occurrence of such symptoms (see **Drug Abuse and Dependence**).

PRECAUTIONS

General: Impaired motor and/or cognitive performance attributable to the accumulation of benzodiazepines and their active metabolites following several days of repeated use at their recommended doses is a concern in certain vulnerable patients (e.g., those especially sensitive to the effects of benzodiazepines or those with a reduced capacity to metabolize and eliminate them). Consequently, elderly or debilitated patients and those with impaired renal or hepatic function should be cautioned about the risk and advised to monitor themselves for signs of excessive sedation or impaired coordination.

The possibility of respiratory depression in patients with chronic pulmonary insufficiency should be considered.

When benzodiazepines are administered to depressed patients, there is a risk that the signs and symptoms of depression may be intensified. Consequently, appropriate precautions (e.g., limiting the total prescription size and increased monitoring for suicidal ideation) should be considered.

Information for Patients: It is suggested that physicians discuss the following information with patients. This information is intended to aid in the safe and effective use of this medication. It is not a disclosure of all possible adverse or intended effects.

1. Inform your physician about any alcohol consumption and medicine you are taking now, including drugs you may buy without a prescription. Alcohol should generally not be used during treatment with hypnotics.
2. Inform your physician if you are planning to become pregnant, if you are pregnant, or if you become pregnant while you are taking this medicine.
3. Inform your physician if you are nursing.
4. Until you experience how this medicine affects you, do not drive a car or operate potentially dangerous machinery, etc.
5. Benzodiazepines may cause daytime sedation, which may persist for several days following drug discontinuation.
6. Patients should be told not to increase the dose on their own and should inform their physician if they believe the drug "does not work anymore."
7. If benzodiazepines are taken on a prolonged and regular basis (even for periods as brief as six weeks), patients should be advised not to stop taking them abruptly or to decrease the dose without consulting their physician, because withdrawal symptoms may occur.

Laboratory Tests: Laboratory tests are not ordinarily required in otherwise healthy patients when quazepam is used as recommended.

Drug Interactions: The benzodiazepines, including DORAL Tablets, produce additive CNS depressant effects when co-administered with psychotropic medications, anticonvulsants, antihistaminics, ethanol, and other drugs which produce CNS depression.

Carcinogenesis, Mutagenesis, Impairment of Fertility: Quazepam showed no evidence of carcinogenicity or other significant pathology in oral oncogenicity studies in mice and hamsters.

Quazepam was tested for mutagenicity using the L5178Y TK +/− Mouse Lymphoma Mutagenesis Assay and Ames Test. The L5178Y TK +/−Assay was equivocal and the Ames Test did not show mutagenic activity.

Reproduction studies in mice conducted with quazepam at doses equal to 60 and 180 times the human dose of 15 mg, and with diazepam at 67 times the human dose, produced slight reductions in the pregnancy rate. Similar reduction in preg-

nancy rates have been reported in mice dosed with other benzodiazepines, and is believed to be related to the sedative effects of these drugs at high doses.

Pregnancy: Teratogenic Effects: Pregnancy Category X (See **CONTRAINDICATIONS, Usage in Pregnancy** section.) Reproduction studies of quazepam in mice at doses up to 400 times the human dose revealed no major drug-related malformations. Minor developmental variations that occurred were delayed ossification of the sternum, vertebrae, distal phalanges and supraoccipital bones, at doses of 66 and 400 times the human dose. Studies with diazepam at 200 times the human dose showed a similar or greater incidence than quazepam. A reproduction study of quazepam in New Zealand rabbits at doses up to 134 times the human dose demonstrated no effect on fetal morphology or development of offspring.

Nonteratogenic Effects: The child born of a mother who is taking benzodiazepines may be at some risk of withdrawal symptoms from the drug during the postnatal period. Neonatal flaccidity has been reported in children born of mothers who had been receiving benzodiazepines.

Labor and Delivery: DORAL Tablets have no established use in labor or delivery.

Nursing Mothers: Quazepam and its metabolites are excreted in the milk of lactating women. Therefore, administration of DORAL Tablets to nursing women is not recommended.

Pediatric Use: Safety and effectiveness in children below the age of 18 years have not been established.

ADVERSE REACTIONS

Adverse events most frequently encountered in patients treated with quazepam are drowsiness and headache.

Accurate estimates of the incidence of adverse events associated with the use of any drug are difficult to obtain. Estimates are influenced by drug dose, detection technique, setting, physician judgments, etc. Consequently, the table below is presented solely to indicate the relative frequency of adverse events reported in representative controlled clinical studies conducted to evaluate the safety and efficacy of quazepam. The figures cited cannot be used to predict precisely the incidence of such events in the course of usual medical practice. These figures, also, cannot be compared with those obtained from other clinical studies involving related drug products and placebo.

The figures cited below are estimates of untoward clinical event incidences of 1% or greater among subjects who participated in the relatively short duration placebo-controlled clinical trials of quazepam.

	DORAL*	PLACEBO
NUMBER OF PATIENTS	267	268
% OF PATIENTS REPORTING		
Central Nervous System		
Daytime Drowsiness	12.0	3.3
Headache	4.5	2.2
Fatigue	1.9	0
Dizziness	1.5	<1
Autonomic Nervous System		
Dry Mouth	1.5	<1
Gastrointestinal System		
Dyspepsia	1.1	<1
*Doral 15 mg		

The following incidences of laboratory abnormalities occurred at a rate of 1% or greater in patients receiving quazepam and the corresponding placebo group. None of these changes were considered to be of physiological significance. [See table next page.]

The following additional events occurred among individuals receiving quazepam at doses equivalent to or greater than those recommended during its clinical testing and development. There is no way to establish whether or not the administration of DORAL caused these events.

Hypokinesia, ataxia, confusion, incoordination, hyperkinesia, speech disorder and tremor were reported.

Also, depression, nervousness, agitation, amnesia, anorexia, anxiety, apathy, euphoria, impotence, decreased libido, paranoid reaction, nightmares, abnormal thinking, abnormal taste perception, abnormal vision, and cataract were reported.

Also reported were urinary incontinence, palpitations, nausea, constipation, diarrhea, abdominal pain, pruritus, rash, asthenia, and malaise.

The following list provides an overview of adverse experiences that have been reported and are considered to be reasonably related to the administration of benzodiazepines: incontinence, slurred speech, urinary retention, jaundice, dysarthria, dystonia, changes in libido, irritability, and menstrual irregularities.

As with all benzodiazepines, paradoxical reactions such as stimulation, agitation, increased muscle spasticity, sleep disturbances, hallucinations, and other adverse behavioral

	DORAL		PLACEBO	
NUMBER OF PATIENTS	234		244	
% of Patients Reporting	Low	High	Low	High
Hematology				
Hemoglobin	1.4	0	1.2	0
Hematocrit	1.5	0	1.7	0
Lymphocyte	1.3	1.6	1.2	1.9
Eosinophil	*	1.5	*	1.3
SEG	1.1	*	1.6	*
Monocyte	*	1.1	*	*
Blood Chemistry				
Glucose	*	*	*	1.2
SGOT	*	1.3	*	1.1
Urinalysis				
Specific Gravity	*	*	*	1.1
WBC	0	2.6	0	3.0
RBC	0	*	0	1.1
Epithelial Cells	0	2.5	0	3.2
Crystals	0	*	0	1.0

*These laboratory abnormalities occurred in less than 1% of patients. In addition, abnormalities in the following laboratory tests were observed in less than 1% of the patients evaluated: WBC count, platelet count, total protein, albumin, BUN, creatinine, total bilirubin, alkaline phosphatase and SGPT.

effects may occur in rare instances and in a random fashion. Should these occur, use of the drug should be discontinued. There have been reports of withdrawal signs and symptoms of the type associated with withdrawal from CNS depressant drugs following the rapid decrease or the abrupt discontinuation of benzodiazepines (see **Drug Abuse and Dependence** section).

DRUG ABUSE AND DEPENDENCE

Controlled Substance: DORAL is a controlled substance under the Controlled Substance Act and has been assigned by the Drug Enforcement Administration to Schedule IV.
Abuse and Dependence: Withdrawal symptoms similar in character to those noted with barbiturates and alcohol (e.g., convulsions, tremor, abdominal and muscle cramps, vomiting and sweating) have occurred following abrupt discontinuance of benzodiazepines. The more severe withdrawal symptoms have usually been limited to those patients who received excessive doses over an extended period of time. Generally milder withdrawal symptoms (e.g., dysphoria and insomnia) have been reported following abrupt discontinuance of benzodiazepines taken continuously at therapeutic levels for several months. Consequently, after extended therapy, abrupt discontinuation should generally be avoided and a gradual dosage tapering schedule followed. Addiction-prone individuals (such as drug addicts or alcoholics) should be under careful surveillance when receiving quazepam or other psychotropic agents because of the predisposition of such patients to habituation and dependence.

OVERDOSAGE

Manifestations of overdosage seen with other benzodiazepines include somnolence, confusion, and coma. In the event that an overdose occurs, the following is the recommended treatment. Respiration, pulse, and blood pressure should be monitored, as in all cases of drug overdosage. General supportive measures should be employed, along with immediate gastric lavage. Intravenous fluids should be administered and an adequate airway maintained. Hypotension may be treated with the use of norepinephrine bitartrate or metaraminol bitartrate. Dialysis is of limited value. Animal experiments suggest that forced diuresis or hemodialysis are probably of little value in treating overdosage. As with the management of intentional overdosing with any drug, it should be borne in mind that multiple agents may have been ingested.
The oral LD_{50} in mice was greater than 5,000 mg/kg.

DOSAGE AND ADMINISTRATION

Adults: Initiate therapy at 15 mg until individual responses are determined. In some patients, the dose may then be reduced to 7.5 mg.
Elderly and debilitated patients: Because the elderly and debilitated may be more sensitive to benzodiazepines, attempts to reduce the nightly dosage after the first one or two nights of therapy are suggested.

HOW SUPPLIED

DORAL Tablets, 7.5 mg, unscored, capsule-shaped, light orange, slightly white speckled tablets, impressed with the product identification number 7.5 on one side of the tablet, and the product name (DORAL) on the other.
7.5 mg   Bottles of 100   NDC 0037-9000-01
      Unit-dose pkg.   NDC 0037-9000-02
      (10 strips of 10)
DORAL Tablets, 15 mg, unscored, capsule-shaped, light orange, slightly white speckled tablets, impressed with the product identification number 15 on one side of the tablet, and the product name (DORAL) on the other.

15 mg   Bottles of 100   NDC 0037-9002-01
      Unit-dose pkg.   NDC 0037-9002-02
      (10 strips of 10)
Store DORAL Tablets between 2°–30°C (36°–86°F). Protect unit doses from excessive moisture.
Distributed by
WALLACE LABORATORIES
Division of Carter-Wallace, Inc.
Cranbury, NJ 08512
Under license from Baker Cummins Pharmaceuticals, Inc.
Manufactured by Schering Corporation
Kenilworth, NJ 07033
©1989, 1990 Carter-Wallace, Inc.
Printed in U.S.A.   Rev. 8/91
Shown in Product Identification Section, page 435

LUFYLLIN®   ℞
(dyphylline)
Elixir

LUFYLLIN® Injection   ℞
(dyphylline injection USP)
FOR INTRAMUSCULAR USE ONLY

LUFYLLIN® Tablets   ℞
(dyphylline tablets, USP, 200 mg)
LUFYLLIN®–400 Tablets   ℞
(dyphylline tablets, USP, 400 mg)

DESCRIPTION

LUFYLLIN (dyphylline), a xanthine derivative, is a bronchodilator available for oral administration as tablets containing 200 mg and 400 mg of dyphylline. Other ingredients: magnesium stearate, microcrystalline cellulose.
Chemically, dyphylline is 7-(2,3-dihydroxypropyl)-theophylline, a white, extremely bitter, amorphous powder that is freely soluble in water and soluble in alcohol to the extent of 2 g/100 ml. Dyphylline forms a neutral solution that is stable in gastrointestinal fluids over a wide range of pH.
The molecular formula for dyphylline is $C_{10}H_{14}N_4O_4$ with a molecular weight of 254.25. Its structural formula is:

CLINICAL PHARMACOLOGY

Dyphylline is a xanthine derivative with pharmacologic actions similar to theophylline and other members of this class of drugs. Its primary action is that of bronchodilation, but it also exhibits peripheral vasodilatory and other smooth muscle relaxant activity to a lesser degree. The bronchodilatory action of dyphylline, as with other xanthines, is thought to be mediated through competitive inhibition of phosphodiesterase with a resulting increase in cyclic AMP producing relaxation of bronchial smooth muscle.
LUFYLLIN is well tolerated and produces less nausea than aminophylline and other alkaline theophylline compounds when administered orally. Unlike the hydrolyzable salts of theophylline, dyphylline is not converted to free theophylline *in vivo*. It is absorbed rapidly in therapeutically active form and in healthy volunteers reaches a mean peak plasma concentration of 17.1 mcg/ml in approximately 45 minutes following a single oral dose of 1000 mg of LUFYLLIN.
Dyphylline exerts its bronchodilatory effects directly and, unlike theophylline, is excreted unchanged by the kidneys without being metabolized by the liver. Because of this, dyphylline pharmacokinetics and plasma levels are not influenced by various factors that affect liver function and hepatic enzyme activity, such as smoking, age, congestive heart failure or concomitant use of drugs which affect liver function.
The elimination half-life of dyphylline is approximately two hours (1.8–2.1 hr) and approximately 88% of a single oral dose can be recovered from the urine unchanged. The renal clearance would be correspondingly reduced in patients with impaired renal function. In anuric patients, the half-life may be increased 3 to 4 times normal.
Dyphylline plasma levels are dose-related and generally predictable. The range of plasma levels within which dyphyl-

line can be expected to produce effective bronchodilation has not been determined.
Dyphylline plasma concentrations can be accurately determined using high pressure liquid chromatography (HPLC)* or gas-liquid chromatography (GLC).

INDICATIONS AND USAGE

For relief of acute bronchial asthma and for reversible bronchospasm associated with chronic bronchitis and emphysema.

CONTRAINDICATIONS

Hypersensitivity to dyphylline or related xanthine compounds.

WARNINGS

LUFYLLIN is not indicated in the management of status asthmaticus, which is a serious medical emergency.
Although the relationship between plasma levels of dyphylline and appearance of toxicity is unknown, excessive doses may be expected to be associated with an increased risk of adverse effects.

PRECAUTIONS

General: Use LUFYLLIN with caution in patients with severe cardiac disease, hypertension, hyperthyroidism, acute myocardial injury or peptic ulcer.
Drug interactions: Synergism between xanthine bronchodilators (e.g., theophylline), ephedrine and other sympathomimetic bronchodilators has been reported. This should be considered whenever these agents are prescribed concomitantly. Concurrent administration of dyphylline and probenecid, which competes for tubular secretion, has been shown to increase the plasma half-life of dyphylline (see Clinical Pharmacology).
Carcinogenesis, mutagenesis, impairment of fertility: No long-term animal studies have been performed with LUFYLLIN.
Pregnancy: Teratogenic effects—Pregnancy Category C. Animal reproduction studies have not been conducted with LUFYLLIN. It is also not known if LUFYLLIN can cause fetal harm when administered to a pregnant woman or can affect reproduction capacity. LUFYLLIN should be given to a pregnant woman only if clearly needed.
Nursing mothers: Dyphylline is present in human milk at approximately twice the maternal plasma concentration. Caution should be exercised when LUFYLLIN is administered to a nursing woman.
Pediatric use: Safety and effectiveness in children have not been established.

ADVERSE REACTIONS

Adverse reactions with the use of LUFYLLIN have been infrequent, relatively mild, and rarely required reduction in dosage or withdrawal of therapy.
The following adverse reactions which have been reported with other xanthine bronchodilators, and which have most often been related to excessive drug plasma levels, should be considered as potential adverse effects when dyphylline is administered:
Gastrointestinal: nausea, vomiting, epigastric pain, hematemesis, diarrhea.
Central nervous system: headache, irritability, restlessness, insomnia, hyperexcitability, agitation, muscle twitching, generalized clonic and tonic convulsions.
Cardiovascular: palpitation, tachycardia, extrasystoles, flushing, hypotension, circulatory failure, ventricular arrhythmias.
Respiratory: tachypnea.
Renal: albuminuria, gross and microscopic hematuria, diuresis.
Other: hyperglycemia, inappropriate ADH syndrome.

OVERDOSAGE

There have been no reports, in the literature, of overdosage with LUFYLLIN. However, the following information based on reports of theophylline overdosage are considered typical of the xanthine class of drugs and should be kept in mind.
Signs and symptoms: Restlessness, anorexia, nausea, vomiting, diarrhea, insomnia, irritability, and headache. Marked overdosage with resulting severe toxicity has produced agitation, severe vomiting, dehydration, excessive thirst, tinnitus, cardiac arrhythmias, hyperthermia, diaphoresis, and generalized clonic and tonic convulsions. Cardiovascular collapse has also occcurred, with some fatalities. Seizures have occurred in some cases associated with very high theophylline plasma concentrations, without any premonitory symptoms of toxicity.
Treatment: There is no specific antidote for overdosage with drugs of the xanthine class. Symptomatic treatment and general supportive measures should be instituted with

*See Valia, et al. J. Chromatogr. **221:** 170 (1980). Small quantities of pure dyphylline powder may be obtained from Wallace Laboratories, Cranbury, N.J. The internal standard, β-hydroxyethyltheophylline, may be obtained from companies supplying analytical chemicals.

Continued on next page

Wallace Laboratories—Cont.

careful monitoring and maintenance of vital signs, fluids and electrolytes. The stomach should be emptied by inducing emesis if the patient is conscious and responsive, or by gastric lavage, taking care to protect against aspiration, especially in stuporous or comatose patients. Maintenance of an adequate airway is essential in case oxygen or assisted respiration is needed. Sympathomimetic agents should be avoided but sedatives such as short-acting barbiturates may be useful.

Dyphylline is dialyzable and, although not recommended as a routine procedure in overdosage cases, hemodialysis may be of some benefit when severe intoxication is present or when the patient has not responded to general supportive and symptomatic treatment.

DOSAGE AND ADMINISTRATION

Dosage should be individually titrated according to the severity of the condition and the response of the patient.

Usual adult dosage: Up to 15 mg/kg every six hours.

Appropriate dosage adjustments should be made in patients with impaired renal function (see Clinical Pharmacology).

HOW SUPPLIED

LUFYLLIN Tablets: Available as white, rectangular, monogrammed tablets containing 200 mg dyphylline in bottles of 100 (NDC 0037-0521-92) and 1000 (NDC 0037-0521-97), and individually film-sealed tablets in unit-dose boxes of 100 (NDC 0037-0521-85).

LUFYLLIN-400 Tablets: Available as white, capsule-shaped, monogrammed tablets containing 400 mg dyphylline in bottles of 100 (NDC 0037-0731-92) and 1000 (NDC 0037-0731-97), and individually film-sealed tablets in unit-dose boxes of 100 (NDC 0037-0731-85).

Storage: Store at controlled room temperature.

CAUTION: Federal law prohibits dispensing without prescription.

WALLACE LABORATORIES
Division of
CARTER-WALLACE, INC.
Cranbury, New Jersey 08512

8/87

Shown in Product Identification Section, page 435

LUFYLLIN®-GG ℞

(dyphylline and guaifenesin tablets and elixir, USP) Tablets and Elixir

DESCRIPTION

LUFYLLIN®-GG is a bronchodilator/expectorant combination available for oral administration as *Tablets* and *Elixir.*

Each Tablet contains:

Dyphylline	200 mg
Guaifenesin	200 mg

Other ingredients: corn starch, D&C Yellow No. 10, magnesium aluminium silicate, magnesium stearate, microcrystalline cellulose.

Each 15 mL (one tablespoonful) of Elixir contains:

Dyphylline	100 mg
Guaifenesin	100 mg
Alcohol (by volume)	17%

Other ingredients: citric acid, FD&C Yellow No. 6, flavor (artificial), purified water, saccharin sodium, sodium citrate, sucrose.

Dyphylline is 7-(2,3-dihydroxypropyl)-theophylline, a white, extremely bitter, amorphous powder that is fully soluble in water and soluble in alcohol to the extent of 2 g/100 mL. Dyphylline forms a neutral solution that is stable in gastrointestinal fluids over a wide range of pH.

CLINICAL PHARMACOLOGY

Dyphylline is a xanthine derivative with pharmacologic actions similar to theophylline and other members of this class of drugs. Its primary action is that of bronchodilation, but it also exhibits peripheral vasodilatory and other smooth muscle relaxant activity to a lesser degree. The bronchodilatory action of dyphylline, as with as other xanthines, is thought to be mediated through competitive inhibition of phosphodiesterase with a resulting increase in cyclic AMP producing relaxation of bronchial smooth muscle.

Dyphylline in LUFYLLIN-GG is well tolerated and produces less nausea than aminophylline and other alkaline theophylline compounds when administered orally. Unlike the hydrolyzable salts of theophylline, dyphylline is not converted to free theophylline *in vivo.* It is absorbed rapidly in therapeutically active form and in healthy volunteers reaches a mean peak plasma concentration of 17.1 mcg/mL in approximately 45 minutes following a single oral dose of 1000 mg of dyphylline.

Dyphylline exerts its bronchodilatory effects directly and, unlike theophylline, is excreted unchanged by the kidneys without being metabolized by the liver. Because of this, dyphylline pharmacokinetics and plasma levels are not influenced by various factors that affect liver function and hepatic enzyme activity, such as smoking, age, or concomitant use of drugs which affect liver function.

The elimination half-life of dyphylline is approximately two hours (1.8–2.1 hr) and approximately 88% of a single oral dose can be recovered from the urine unchanged. The renal clearance would be correspondingly reduced in patients with impaired renal function. In anuric patients, the half-life may be increased 3 to 4 times normal.

Dyphylline plasma levels are dose-related and generally predictable. The therapeutic range of plasma levels within which dyphylline can be expected to produce effective bronchodilation has not been determined.

Dyphylline plasma concentrations can be accurately determined using high pressure liquid chromatography (HPLC)* or gas-liquid chromatography (GLC).

Guaifenesin is an expectorant whose action helps increase the output of thin respiratory tract fluid to facilitate mucociliary clearance and removal of inspissated mucus.

INDICATIONS AND USAGE

For relief of acute bronchial asthma and for reversible bronchospasm associated with chronic bronchitis and emphysema.

CONTRAINDICATIONS

Hypersensitivity to any of the ingredients or related compounds.

WARNINGS

LUFYLLIN-GG is not indicated in the management of status asthmaticus, which is a serious medical emergency.

Although the relationship between plasma levels of dyphylline and appearance of toxicity is unknown, excessive doses may be expected to be associated with an increased risk of adverse effects.

PRECAUTIONS

General: Use LUFYLLIN-GG with caution in patients with severe cardiac disease, hypertension, hyperthyroidism, acute myocardial injury or peptic ulcer.

Drug interactions: Synergism between xanthine bronchodilators (e.g., theophylline), ephedrine and other sympathomimetic bronchodilators has been reported. This should be considered whenever these agents are prescribed concomitantly. Concurrent administration of dyphylline and probenecid, which competes for tubular secretion, has been shown to increase plasma half-life of dyphylline (see Clinical Pharmacology).

Carcinogenesis, mutagenesis, impairment of fertility: No long-term animal studies have been performed with LUFYLLIN-GG.

Pregnancy: Teratogenic effects—Pregnancy Category C. Animal reproduction studies have not been conducted with LUFYLLIN-GG. It is also not known whether this product can cause fetal harm when administered to a pregnant woman or can affect reproduction capacity. LUFYLLIN-GG should be given to a pregnant woman only if clearly needed.

Nursing mothers: Dyphylline is present in human milk at approximately twice the maternal plasma concentration. Caution should be exercised when LUFYLLIN-GG is administered to a nursing woman.

Pediatric use: Safety and effectiveness in children below the age of six have not been established. Use caution when administering to children six years of age or older.

ADVERSE REACTIONS

LUFYLLIN-GG may cause nausea, headache, cardiac palpitation and CNS stimulation. Postprandial administration may help avoid gastric discomfort.

The following adverse reactions which have been reported with other xanthine bronchodilators, and which have most often been related to excessive drug plasma levels, should be considered as potential adverse effects when dyphylline is administered:

Gastrointestinal: nausea, vomiting, epigastric pain, hematemesis, diarrhea.

Central nervous system: headache, irritability, restlessness, insomnia, hyperexcitability, agitation, muscle twitching, generalized clonic and tonic convulsions.

Cardiovascular: palpitation, tachycardia, extrasystoles, flushing, hypotension, circulatory failure, ventricular arrhythmias.

Respiratory: tachypnea.

Renal: albuminuria, gross and microscopic hematuria, diuresis.

Other: hyperglycemia, inappropriate ADH syndrome.

OVERDOSAGE

There have been no reports, in the literature, of overdosage with LUFYLLIN-GG. However, the following information based on reports of theophylline overdosage are considered typical of the xanthine class of drugs and should be kept in mind.

Signs and symptoms: Restlessness, anorexia, nausea, vomiting, diarrhea, insomnia, irritability, and headache. Marked overdosage with resulting severe toxicity has produced agitation, severe vomiting, dehydration, excessive thirst, tinnitus, cardiac arrhythmias, hyperthermia, diaphoresis, and generalized clonic and tonic convulsions. Cardiovascular collapse has also occurred, with some fatalities. Seizures have occurred in some cases associated with very high theophylline plasma concentrations, without any premonitory symptoms of toxicity.

Treatment: There is no specific antidote for overdosage with drugs of the xanthine class. Symptomatic treatment and general supportive measures should be instituted with careful monitoring and maintenance of vital signs, fluids and electrolytes. The stomach should be emptied by inducing emesis if the patient is conscious and responsive, or by gastric lavage, taking care to protect against aspiration, especially in stuporous or comatose patients. Maintenance of an adequate airway is essential in case oxygen or assisted respiration is needed. Sympathomimetic agents should be avoided but sedatives such as short-acting barbiturates may be useful.

Dyphylline is dialyzable and, although not recommended as a routine procedure in overdosage cases, hemodialysis may be of some benefit when severe intoxication is present or when the patient has not responded to general supportive and symptomatic treatment.

DOSAGE AND ADMINISTRATION

Dosage should be individually titrated according to the severity of the condition and the response of the patient.

Usual adult dosage:

1 tablet or 30 mL (2 tablespoonfuls) Elixir, four times daily.

Children above age six:

½ to 1 tablet or 15 to 30 mL (1 to 2 tablespoonfuls) Elixir, 3 or 4 times daily.

Not recommended for use in children below age six: (see Precautions).

HOW SUPPLIED

LUFYLLIN-GG Tablets: round, light yellow, monogrammed tablets, scored on one side, in bottles of 100 (NDC 0037-0541-92) and 1000 (NDC 0037-0541-97) and boxes of 100 unit-dose, individually film-sealed tablets (NDC 0037-0541-85).

LUFYLLIN-GG Elixir: clear, light yellow-orange liquid with a mild wine-like odor and taste, in bottles of one pint (NDC 0037-0545-68) and one gallon (NDC 0037-0545-69).

Storage:

Tablets—Avoid excessive heat—above 40°C (104°F).

Elixir—Store below 30°C (86°F).

CAUTION: Federal law prohibits dispensing without prescription.

WALLACE LABORATORIES
Division of
CARTER-WALLACE, INC.
Cranbury, New Jersey 08512

Rev. 10/89

Shown in Product Identification Section, page 435

MALTSUPEX® OTC

(malt soup extract)
Powder, Liquid, Tablets

(See PDR For Nonprescription Drugs.)

MEPROSPAN® Ⓒ ℞

(meprobamate, sustained-release capsules)

MILTOWN® Ⓒ ℞

(meprobamate tablets, U.S.P.)

DESCRIPTION

Meprobamate is a white powder with a *characteristic odor* and a bitter taste. It is slightly soluble in water, freely soluble in acetone and alcohol, and sparingly soluble in ether. The structural formula of meprobamate is:

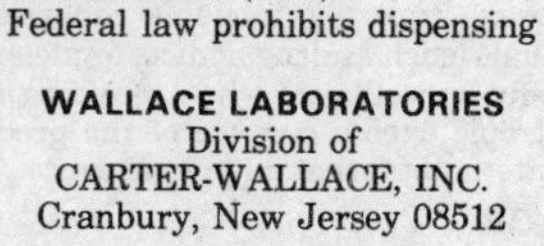
CH3
NH2COOCH2—C—CH2OOCNH2
CH2CH2CH3

'Miltown'-200 contains 200 mg meprobamate per tablet. Other ingredients: acacia, carnauba wax, corn starch, gelatin, magnesium carbonate, magnesium stearate, methylcel-

---

*See Valia, *et al, J Chromatogr.* **221**: 170 (1980). Small quantities of pure dyphylline powder may be obtained from Wallace Laboratories, Cranbury, N.J. The internal standard, β-hydroxyethyltheophylline, may be obtained from companies supplying analytical chemicals.

lulose, shellac, sugar, talc, titanium dioxide, white wax and other ingredients.

'Miltown'-400 contains 400 mg meprobamate per tablet. Other ingredients: corn starch, magnesium stearate, methylcellulose.

'Miltown'-600 contains 600 mg meprobamate per tablet. Other ingredients: alginic acid, corn starch, ethylcellulose, magnesium stearate, purified stearic acid.

ACTIONS

Meprobamate is a carbamate derivative which has been shown in animal studies to have effects at multiple sites in the central nervous system, including the thalamus and limbic system.

INDICATIONS

'Miltown' (meprobamate) is indicated for the management of anxiety disorders or for the short-term relief of the symptoms of anxiety. Anxiety or tension associated with the stress of everyday life usually do not require treatment with an anxiolytic.

The effectiveness of 'Miltown' in long-term use, that is, more than 4 months, has not been assessed by systematic clinical studies. The physician should periodically reassess the usefulness of the drug for the individual patient.

CONTRAINDICATIONS

Acute intermittent porphyria as well as allergic or idiosyncratic reactions to meprobamate or related compounds such as carisoprodol, mebutamate, tybamate or carbromal.

WARNINGS

Drug Dependence

Physical dependence, psychological dependence, and abuse have occurred. When chronic intoxication from prolonged use occurs, it usually involves ingestion of greater than recommended doses and is manifested by ataxia, slurred speech, and vertigo. Therefore, careful supervision of dose and amounts prescribed is advised, as well as avoidance of prolonged administration, especially for alcoholics and other patients with a known propensity for taking excessive quantities of drugs.

Sudden withdrawal of the drug after prolonged and excessive use may precipitate recurrence of pre-existing symptoms, such as anxiety, anorexia, or insomnia, or withdrawal reactions, such as vomiting, ataxia, tremors, muscle twitching, confusional states, hallucinosis, and, rarely, convulsive seizures. Such seizures are more likely to occur in persons with central nervous system damage or pre-existent or latent convulsive disorders. Onset of withdrawal symptoms occurs usually within 12 to 48 hours after discontinuation of meprobamate; symptoms usually cease within the next 12 to 48 hours.

When excessive dosage has continued for weeks or months, dosage should be reduced gradually over a period of one or two weeks rather than abruptly stopped. Alternatively, a short-acting barbiturate may be substituted, then gradually withdrawn.

Potentially Hazardous Tasks

Patients should be warned that this drug may impair the mental and/or physical abilities required for the performance of potentially hazardous tasks such as driving a motor vehicle or operating machinery.

Additive Effects

Since the effects of meprobamate and alcohol or meprobamate and other CNS depressants or psychotropic drugs may be additive, appropriate caution should be exercised with patients who take more than one of these agents simultaneously.

Usage in Pregnancy and Lactation

An increased risk of congenital malformations associated with the use of minor tranquilizers (meprobamate, chlordiazepoxide, and diazepam) during the first trimester of pregnancy has been suggested in several studies. Because use of these drugs is rarely a matter of urgency, their use during this period should almost always be avoided. The possibility that a woman of childbearing potential may be pregnant at the time of institution of therapy should be considered. Patients should be advised that if they become pregnant during therapy or intend to become pregnant they should communicate with their physician about the desirability of discontinuing the drug.

Meprobamate passes the placental barrier. It is present both in umbilical cord blood at or near maternal plasma levels and in breast milk of lactating mothers at concentrations two to four times that of maternal plasma. When use of meprobamate is contemplated in breast-feeding patients, the drug's higher concentration in breast milk as compared to maternal plasma levels should be considered.

Usage in Children

'Miltown'-200 and 'Miltown'-400 should not be administered to children under age six, since there is a lack of documented evidence for safety and effectiveness in this age group.

'Miltown'-600 is not intended for use in children.

PRECAUTIONS

The lowest effective dose should be administered, particularly to elderly and/or debilitated patients, in order to preclude oversedation.

The possibility of suicide attempts should be considered and the least amount of drug feasible should be dispensed at any one time.

Meprobamate is metabolized in the liver and excreted by the kidney; to avoid its excess accumulation, caution should be exercised in administration to patients with compromised liver or kidney function.

Meprobamate occasionally may precipitate seizures in epileptic patients.

ADVERSE REACTIONS

Central Nervous System

Drowsiness, ataxia, dizziness, slurred speech, headache, vertigo, weakness, paresthesias, impairment of visual accomodation, euphoria, overstimulation, paradoxical excitement, fast EEG activity.

Gastrointestinal

Nausea, vomiting, diarrhea.

Cardiovascular

Palpitations, tachycardia, various forms of arrhythmia, transient ECG changes, syncope; also, hypotensive crises (including one fatal case).

Allergic or Idiosyncratic

Allergic or idiosyncratic reactions are usually seen within the period of the first to fourth dose in patients having had no previous contact with the drug. Milder reactions are characterized by an itchy, urticarial, or erythematous maculopapular rash which may be generalized or confined to the groin. Other reactions have included leukopenia, acute non-thrombocytopenic purpura, petechiae, ecchymoses, eosinophilia, peripheral edema, adenopathy, fever, fixed drug eruption with cross reaction to carisoprodol, and cross sensitivity between meprobamate/mebutamate and meprobamate/carbromal.

More severe hypersensitivity reactions, rarely reported, include hyperpyrexia, chills, angioneurotic edema, bronchospasm, oliguria, and anuria. Also, anaphylaxis, erythema multiforme, exfoliative dermatitis, stomatitis, proctitis, Stevens-Johnson syndrome, and bullous dermatitis, including one fatal case of the latter following administration of meprobamate in combination with prednisolone.

In case of allergic or idiosyncratic reactions to meprobamate, discontinue the drug and initiate appropriate symptomatic therapy, which may include epinephrine, antihistamines, and in severe cases corticosteroids. In evaluating possible allergic reactions, also consider allergy to excipients.

Hematologic

(See also **Allergic or Idiosyncratic**.) Agranulocytosis and aplastic anemia have been reported. These cases rarely were fatal. Rare cases of thrombocytopenic purpura have been reported.

Other

Exacerbation of porphyric symptoms.

DOSAGE AND ADMINISTRATION

'Miltown'-200 and 400:

The usual adult daily dosage is 1200 mg to 1600 mg, in three or four divided doses; a daily dosage above 2400 mg is not recommended. The usual daily dosage for children ages six to twelve is 200 mg to 600 mg, in two or three divided doses.

Not recommended for children under age 6 (see **Usage in Children**).

'Miltown'-600:

Adults—One tablet twice a day. Doses of meprobamate above 2400 mg daily are not recommended.

Not recommended for use in children (see **Usage in Children**).

OVERDOSAGE

Suicidal attempts with meprobamate have resulted in drowsiness, lethargy, stupor, ataxia, coma, shock, vasomotor and respiratory collapse. Some suicidal attempts have been fatal. The following data on meprobamate tablets have been reported in the literature and from other sources. These data are not expected to correlate with each case (considering factors such as individual susceptibility and length of time from ingestion to treatment), but represent the **usual ranges** reported.

Acute simple overdose (meprobamate alone): Death has been reported with ingestion of as little as 12 gm meprobamate and survival with as much as 40 gm.

Blood Levels:

0.5–2.0 mg% represents the usual blood level range of meprobamate after therapeutic doses. The level may occasionally be as high as 3.0 mg%.

3–10 mg% usually corresponds to findings of mild to moderate symptoms of overdosage, such as stupor or light coma.

10–20 mg% usually corresponds to deeper coma, requiring more intensive treatment. Some fatalities occur.

At levels greater than 20%, more fatalities than survivals can be expected.

Acute combined overdose (meprobamate with alcohol or other CNS depressants or psychotropic drugs): Since effects can be additive, a history of ingestion of a low dose of meprobamate plus any of these compounds (or of a relative low blood or tissue level) cannot be used as a prognostic indicator. In cases where excessive doses have been taken, sleep ensues rapidly and blood pressure, pulse, and respiratory rates are reduced to basal levels. Any drug remaining in the stomach should be removed and symptomatic therapy given. Should respiration or blood pressure become compromised, respiratory assistance, central nervous system stimulants, and pressor agents should be administered cautiously as indicated. Meprobamate is metabolized in the liver and excreted by the kidney. Diuresis, osmotic (mannitol) diuresis, peritoneal dialysis, and hemodialysis have been used successfully. Careful monitoring of urinary output is necessary and caution should be taken to avoid overhydration. Relapse and death, after initial recovery, have been attributed to incomplete gastric emptying and delayed absorption. Meprobamate can be measured in biological fluids by two methods: colorimetric (Hoffman, A.J. and Ludwig, B.J.: *J Amer Pharm Assn 48:* 740, 1959) and gas chromatographic (Douglas, J.F. et al.: *Anal Chem 39:* 956, 1967).

HOW SUPPLIED

'Miltown'-200: 200 mg white, sugar-coated tablets in bottles of 100 (NDC 0037-1101-01).

'Miltown'-400: 400 mg white, scored tablets in bottles of 100 (NDC 0037-1001-01), 500 (NDC 0037-1001-03), and 1000 (NDC 0037-1001-02).

'Miltown'-600: 600 mg white, capsule-shaped tablets in bottles of 100 (NDC 0037-1601-01).

Storage: Store at controlled room temperature 15°–30°C (59°–86°F). Dispense in a tight container.

WALLACE LABORATORIES
Division of
CARTER-WALLACE, INC.
Cranbury, New Jersey 08512

Rev. 12/90.

Shown in Product Identification Section, page 435

ORGANIDIN®   ℞
(iodinated glycerol)
Tablets, Elixir, Solution

DESCRIPTION

ORGANIDIN® (iodinated glycerol), a mucolytic-expectorant, contains a mixture of several iodinated compounds formed by the reaction of iodine and glycerin. The major iodinated compounds are 3-iodo-1,2-propanediol and a mixture of diastereomers of 1,5,6-trihydroxy-2-iodomethyl-3-oxahexane. Iodinated glycerol is an amber liquid and is stable in an acid medium.

ORGANIDIN is available for oral administration as:

Tablets —each containing 30 mg ORGANIDIN (15 mg organically bound iodine). Other ingredients: corn starch, dibasic calcium phosphate, FD&C Red No. 40, magnesium stearate, microcrystalline cellulose, tribasic calcium phosphate.

Elixir —containing 60 mg ORGANIDIN (30 mg organically bound iodine) per 5 mL (teaspoonful), and alcohol, 21.75% by volume. Other ingredients: flavors (natural and artificial), liquid glucose, purified water, saccharin sodium.

Solution —containing 50 mg ORGANIDIN (25 mg organically bound iodine) per mL. Other ingredients: caramel, glycerin, purified water.

CLINICAL PHARMACOLOGY

ORGANIDIN increases the output of thin respiratory tract fluid and helps liquefy tenacious mucus in the bronchial tree. Iodides are readily absorbed from the gastrointestinal tract and concentrated primarily in the secretions of the respiratory tract, but their mechanism of action as mucolytic-expectorants is not clear.

INDICATIONS AND USAGE

ORGANIDIN is indicated for adjunctive treatment as a mucolytic-expectorant in respiratory tract conditions such as bronchitis and asthma.

DURATION OF TREATMENT

The effects of mucolytic therapy may be seen early after the initiation of therapy; however, at least four weeks may be needed to demonstrate an effect for those patients responding. Patients not responding within four weeks should not be continued on this therapy. Continuation of therapy beyond eight weeks cannot currently be recommended unless in the experience and/or opinion of the physician, the ongoing condition or clinical status of the patient warrants such continuation. It should be recognized that chronic pulmonary diseases are intermittently marked by exacerbations and that the adjunctive use of ORGANIDIN during these exacerba-

Continued on next page

Wallace Laboratories—Cont.

tions is the most appropriate form of therapy as opposed to long-term, continuous use.

CONTRAINDICATIONS

History of marked sensitivity to inorganic iodides; hypersensitivity to any of the ingredients or related compounds; pregnancy; newborns; and nursing mothers.

The human fetal thyroid begins to concentrate iodine in the 12th to 14th week of gestation and the use of inorganic iodides in pregnant women during this period and thereafter has rarely been reported to induce fetal goiter (with or without hypothyroidism) with the potential for airway obstruction. If the patient becomes pregnant while taking ORGANIDIN, the drug should be discontinued and the patient should be apprised of the potential risk to the fetus.

WARNINGS

Discontinue use if rash or other evidence of hypersensitivity appears. Use with caution or avoid use in patients with history or evidence of thyroid disease.

PRECAUTIONS

General: Iodides have been reported to cause a flare-up of adolescent acne. Children with cystic fibrosis appear to have an exaggerated susceptibility to the goitrogenic effect of iodides.

Dermatitis and other reversible manifestations of iodism have been reported with chronic use of inorganic iodides. Although these have not been reported to be a problem clinically with ORGANIDIN, they should be kept in mind in patients receiving these preparations for prolonged periods.

Laboratory Tests: Chronic administration of pharmacologic doses of iodide does not affect the normal thyroid; the excess iodide is excreted by the kidneys. Reversible, mild to moderately elevated TSH (thyrotropin) levels with or without depressed serum T_4 and T_3 levels have been noted sporadically in patients (usually elderly) receiving iodide therapy for prolonged periods; in most such cases, no pretreatment thyroid function tests were available. Iodide-induced 'biochemical hypothyroidism' (i.e., subclinical hypothyroidism manifested only by depressed serum T_4 or T_3 levels and/or elevated TSH) may be noted in patients with underlying thyroid dysfunction (where the thyroid homeostatic mechanism does not function normally). Iodide-induced 'biochemical hypothyroidism' typically reverses to pretreatment levels (in weeks or months) usually spontaneously. Patients with 'functional' hypothyroidism may receive iodotherapy, provided thyroid hormone (e.g., Synthroid-levothyroxine) is administered concomitantly in replacement doses. Radioactive iodine (I^{131}) and iodide transport tests are depressed during iodide therapy; these tests could be expected to return to basal levels two or three days after stopping treatment with ORGANIDIN.

Pediatric Use: Due to the developmental nature of many organ systems in this age group, the physician must weigh the perceived benefit against any potential risk in using iodide in children.

Drug Interactions: Iodides may potentiate the hypothyroid effect of lithium and other antithyroid drugs.

CARCINOGENESIS, MUTAGENESIS, IMPAIRMENT OF FERTILITY:

Twenty-four (24) month carcinogenicity studies were conducted by the National Toxicology Program (NTP) in rats and mice using doses of iodinated glycerol that ranged between 13 and 52 times the recommended human dose. The conclusions of the NTP under the conditions of these gavage studies were species and sex specific and included the following: (1) no evidence of carcinogenicity in female F344/N rats; some evidence in male F344/N rats, based on increased incidences of a) mononuclear cell leukemia and b) follicular cell carcinomas of the thyroid gland. (There were no other chemical related nonneoplastic lesions of the thyroid gland in male or female rats.) (2) No evidence of carcinogenicity in male B6C3F1 mice; some evidence in female B6C3F1 mice, based on increased incidences of a) adenomas of the pituitary gland and b) neoplasms of the Harderian gland. The latter tumors were not found in the male mouse or in male or female rats. (There are no known human equivalents to mononuclear cell leukemia in the rat and Harderian gland neoplasms in the mouse.) The relevance of these findings to humans is not known. Both positive and negative results were found with iodinated glycerol in a standard battery of *in vitro* mutagenicity assays that were conducted with or without microsomal activation. In the only *in vivo* mutagenicity study that was conducted, the results were negative for genotoxic effects, in that no increase in micronucleated polychromatic erythrocytes was observed in the bone marrow of B6C3F1 mice after administration of either iodinated glycerol or 3-iodo-1,2-propanediol. The relevance of these findings to humans is not known. No long-term animal studies on impairment of fertility have been performed with ORGANIDIN.

Pregnancy: Teratogenic effects: Pregnancy Category X (see Contraindications).

Nursing Mothers: ORGANIDIN should not be administered to a nursing woman.

ADVERSE REACTIONS

Reports of gastrointestinal irritation, rash, hypersensitivity, thyroid gland enlargement, and acute parotitis have been rare.

OVERDOSAGE

Acute overdosage experience with ORGANIDIN has been rare and there have been no reports of any serious problems.

DOSAGE AND ADMINISTRATION

Note: Add *Solution* to fruit juice or other liquid. One drop *Solution* equals approximately 3 mg ORGANIDIN.

Adults: *Tablets*—2 tablets 4 times a day, with liquid.
        Elixir—1 teaspoonful (5 mL) 4 times a day.
        Solution—20 drops 4 times a day.

Children: Up to one-half the adult dosage, based on the child's weight.

HOW SUPPLIED

ORGANIDIN is available as:

Tablets—round, flat faced, bevel-edged, one side scored, other side imprinted 37-WALLACE 4224, mottled, rose-colored tablets, each containing 30 mg ORGANIDIN (15 mg organically bound iodine), in bottles of 100 (NDC 0037-4224-40) and 500 (NDC 0037-4224-03).

Elixir—clear amber liquid, each teaspoonful (5 mL) containing 60 mg ORGANIDIN (30 mg organically bound iodine), in bottles of one pint (NDC 0037-4213-30) and one gallon (NDC 0037-4213-40).

Solution—clear amber liquid, containing 50 mg ORGANIDIN (25 mg organically bound iodine) per mL, in 30 mL dropper bottles (NDC 0037-4211-10).

Storage: ORGANIDIN Tablets—Store at controlled room temperature 15°–30°C (59°–86°F). Protect from moisture. ORGANIDIN Elixir and Solution—Store at controlled room temperature 15°–30°C (59°–86°F).

ORGANIDIN *Tablets* are manufactured by:
WALLACE LABORATORIES
Division of CARTER-WALLACE, INC.
Cranbury, New Jersey 08512
ORGANIDIN *Elixir* and *Solution* are
distributed by:
WALLACE LABORATORIES
Division of CARTER-WALLACE, INC.
Cranbury, New Jersey 08512
Manufactured by:
DENVER CHEMICAL (Puerto Rico), Inc.
Subsidiary of CARTER-WALLACE, INC.
Humacao, Puerto Rico 00661
Based on IN-046T2-06
(Rev. 4/92)

                                   Rev. 4/92

Shown in Product Identification Section, page 435

RYNA® (Liquid)
RYNA–C®   ℂ
(Liquid)
RYNA–CX®   ℂ
(Liquid)

(See PDR For Nonprescription Drugs.)

RYNATAN®   ℞
Tablets
Pediatric Suspension
RYNATAN®-S*
Pediatric Suspension

DESCRIPTION

RYNATAN® is an antihistamine/nasal decongestant combination available for oral administration as **Tablets** and as **Pediatric Suspension**. Each tablet contains:

Phenylephrine Tannate	25 mg
Chlorpheniramine Tannate	8 mg
Pyrilamine Tannate	25 mg

Other ingredients: corn starch, dibasic calcium phosphate, magnesium stearate, methylcellulose, polygalacturonic acid, talc.

Each 5 mL (teaspoonful) of the Pediatric Suspension contains:

Phenylephrine Tannate	5 mg
Chlorpheniramine Tannate	2 mg
Pyrilamine Tannate	12.5 mg

Other ingredients: benzoic acid, FD&C Red No. 3, flavors (natural and artificial), glycerin, kaolin, magnesium aluminum silicate, methylparaben, pectin, purified water, saccharin sodium, sucrose.

* Patent Pending

CLINICAL PHARMACOLOGY

RYNATAN combines the sympathomimetic decongestant effect of phenylephrine with the antihistaminic actions of chlorpheniramine and pyrilamine.

INDICATIONS AND USAGE

RYNATAN is indicated for symptomatic relief of the coryza and nasal congestion associated with the common cold, sinusitis, allergic rhinitis and other upper respiratory tract conditions. Appropriate therapy should be provided for the primary disease.

CONTRAINDICATIONS

RYNATAN is contraindicated for newborns, nursing mothers and patients sensitive to any of the ingredients or related compounds.

WARNINGS

Use with caution in patients with hypertension, cardiovascular disease, hyperthyroidism, diabetes, narrow angle glaucoma or prostatic hypertrophy. Use with caution or avoid use in patients taking monoamine (MAO) inhibitors. This product contains antihistamines which may cause drowsiness and may have additive central nervous system (CNS) effects with alcohol or other CNS depressants (e.g., hypnotics, sedatives, tranquilizers).

PRECAUTIONS

General: Antihistamines are more likely to cause dizziness, sedation and hypotension in elderly patients. Antihistamines may cause excitation, particularly in children, but their combination with sympathomimetics may cause either mild stimulation or mild sedation.

Information for Patients: Caution patients against drinking alcoholic beverages or engaging in potentially hazardous activities requiring alertness, such as driving a car or operating machinery while using this product.

Drug Interactions: MAO inhibitors may prolong and intensify the anticholinergic effects of antihistamines and the overall effects of sympathomimetic agents.

Carcinogenesis, Mutagenesis, Impairment of Fertility: No long-term animal studies have been performed with RYNATAN®.

Pregnancy: Teratogenic Effects: Pregnancy Category C. Animal reproduction studies have not been conducted with RYNATAN. It is also not known whether RYNATAN can cause fetal harm when administered to a pregnant woman or can affect reproduction capacity. RYNATAN should be given to a pregnant woman only if clearly needed.

Nursing mothers: RYNATAN should not be administered to a nursing woman.

ADVERSE REACTIONS

Adverse effects associated with RYNATAN at recommended doses have been minimal. The most common have been drowsiness, sedation, dryness of mucous membranes, and gastrointestinal effects. Serious side effects with oral antihistamines or sympathomimetics have been rare.

OVERDOSAGE

Signs and Symptoms: May vary from CNS depression to stimulation (restlessness to convulsions). Antihistamine overdosage in young children may lead to convulsions and death. Atropine-like signs and symptoms may be prominent.

Treatment: Induce vomiting if it has not occurred spontaneously. Precautions must be taken against aspiration especially in infants, children and comatose patients. If gastric lavage is indicated, isotonic or half-isotonic saline solution is preferred. Stimulants should not be used. If hypotension is a problem, vasopressor agents may be considered.

DOSAGE AND ADMINISTRATION

Administer the recommended dose every 12 hours.

RYNATAN Tablets: Adults—1 or 2 tablets.

RYNATAN Pediatric Suspension: **Children over six years of age**—5 to 10 mL (1 to 2 teaspoonfuls); **Children two to six years of age**—2.5 to 5 mL (½ to 1 teaspoonful); **Children under two years of age**—Titrate dose individually.

HOW SUPPLIED

RYNATAN® Tablets: buff, capsule-shaped, compressed tablets in bottles of 100 (NDC 0037-0713-92), 500 (NDC 0037-0713-96), and 2000 (NDC 0037-0713-95).

RYNATAN® Pediatric Suspension: pink with strawberry-currant flavor, in 4 fl. oz. bottles (NDC 0037-0715-67, labeled RYNATAN®-S*) and in pint bottles (NDC 0037-0715-68).

Storage

RYNATAN® Tablets—Store at controlled room temperature 15°–30°C (59°–86°F).

RYNATAN® Pediatric Suspension—Store at controlled room temperature 15°–30°C (59°–86°F).

Dispense in a tight container.

RYNATAN®-S is RYNATAN Pediatric Suspension either in a 4 fl. oz. unit of use container with a 10 mL calibrated oral syringe (patent pending) or in a 15 mL sample container.

WALLACE LABORATORIES
Division of
CARTER-WALLACE, INC.
Cranbury, New Jersey 08512

Rev. 11/91

Shown in Product Identification Section, page 435

RYNATUSS®
Tablets
Pediatric Suspension

℞

DESCRIPTION

RYNATUSS® is an antitussive/ antihistaminic/ decongestant/ bronchodilator combination available for oral administration as *Tablets* and as *Pediatric Suspension*.
Each tablet contains:

Carbetapentane Tannate .... 60 mg
Chlorpheniramine Tannate .... 5 mg
Ephedrine Tannate .... 10 mg
Phenylephrine Tannate .... 10 mg
Other ingredients: corn starch, dibasic calcium phosphate, FD&C Blue No. 1, FD&C Red No. 40, magnesium stearate, methylcellulose, polygalacturonic acid, povidone, talc.
Each 5 ml (one teaspoonful) of the Pediatric Suspension contains:

Carbetapentane Tannate .... 30 mg
Chlorpheniramine Tannate .... 4 mg
Ephedrine Tannate .... 5 mg
Phenylephrine Tannate .... 5 mg
Other ingredients: benzoic acid, FD&C Blue No. 1, FD&C Red No. 3, FD&C Red No. 40, FD&C Yellow #5, flavors (natural and artificial), glycerin, kaolin, magnesium aluminum silicate, methylparaben, pectin, purified water, saccharin sodium, sucrose.

CLINICAL PHARMACOLOGY

RYNATUSS combines the antitussive action of carbetapentane, the sympathomimetic decongestant effect of phenylephrine, the antihistaminic action of chlorpheniramine, and the bronchodilator action of ephedrine.

INDICATIONS AND USAGE

RYNATUSS is indicated for the symptomatic relief of cough associated with respiratory tract conditions such as the common cold, bronchial asthma, acute and chronic bronchitis. Appropriate therapy should be provided for the primary disease.

CONTRAINDICATIONS

RYNATUSS is contraindicated for newborns, nursing mothers and patients who are sensitive to any of the ingredients or related compounds.

WARNINGS

Use with caution in patients with hypertension, cardiovascular disease, hyperthyroidism, diabetes, narrow angle glaucoma or prostatic hypertrophy. Use with caution or avoid use in patients taking monoamine oxidase (MAO) Inhibitors. This product contains antihistamines which may cause drowsiness and may have additive central nervous system (CNS) effects with alcohol or other CNS depressants (e.g., hypnotics, sedatives, tranquilizers).

PRECAUTIONS

For RYNATUSS Pediatric Suspension only: This product contains FD&C Yellow No. 5 (tartrazine) which may cause allergic-type reactions (including bronchial asthma) in certain susceptible individuals. Although the overall incidence of FD&C Yellow No. 5 (tartrazine) sensitivity in the general population is low, it is frequently seen in patients who also have aspirin hypersensitivity.
General: Antihistamines are more likely to cause dizziness, sedation and hypotension in elderly patients. Antihistamines may cause excitation, particularly in children, but their combination with sympathomimetics may cause either mild stimulation or mild sedation.
Information for patients: Caution patients against drinking alcoholic beverages or engaging in potentially hazardous activities requiring alertness, such as driving a car or operating machinery, while using this product.
Drug interactions: MAO inhibitors may prolong and intensify the anticholinergic effects of antihistamines and the overall effects of sympathomimetic agents.
Carcinogenesis, mutagenesis, impairment of fertility: No long term animal studies have been performed with RYNATUSS.
Pregnancy: Teratogenic Effects: Pregnancy Category C. Animal reproduction studies have not been conducted with RYNATUSS. It is also not known whether RYNATUSS can cause fetal harm when administered to a pregnant woman or can affect reproduction capacity. RYNATUSS should be given to a pregnant woman only if clearly needed.
Nursing mothers: RYNATUSS should not be administered to a nursing woman.

ADVERSE REACTIONS

Adverse effects associated with RYNATUSS at recommended doses have been minimal. The most common have been drowsiness, sedation, dryness of mucous membranes, and gastrointestinal effects. Serious side effects with oral antihistamines or sympathomimetics have been rare.

OVERDOSAGE

Signs and Symptoms: May vary from CNS depression to stimulation (restlessness to convulsions). Antihistamine overdosage in young children may lead to convulsions and death. Atropine-like signs and symptoms may be prominent.
Treatment: Induce vomiting if it has not occurred spontaneously. Precautions must be taken against aspiration especially in infants, children and comatose patients. If gastric lavage is indicated, isotonic or half-isotonic saline solution is preferred. Stimulants should not be used. If hypotension is a problem, vasopressor agents may be considered.

DOSAGE AND ADMINISTRATION

Administer the recommended dose every 12 hours.
RYNATUSS Tablets: Adults—1 to 2 tablets.
RYNATUSS Pediatric Suspension: Children over six years of age—5 to 10 mL (1 to 2 teaspoonfuls); *Children two to six years of age*—2.5 to 5 mL (½ to 1 teaspoonful); *Children under two years of age*—Titrate dose individually.

HOW SUPPLIED

RYNATUSS® Tablets: mauve, capsule-shaped, compressed tablets in bottles of 100 (NDC 0037-0717-92) and bottles of 500 (NDC 0037-0717-96).
RYNATUSS® Pediatric Suspension: pink with strawberry-currant flavor, in bottles of 8 fl oz (NDC 0037-0718-67) and one pint (NDC 0037-0718-68).

STORAGE

RYNATUSS Tablets: Store at room temperature; avoid excessive heat—above 40°C (104°F).
RYNATUSS Pediatric Suspension: Store at controlled room temperature—between 15°C-30°C (59°F-86°F); protect from freezing.

WALLACE LABORATORIES
Division of
CARTER WALLACE, INC.
Cranbury, N.J. 08512   2/85
Shown in Product Identification Section, page 435

SOMA®
(carisoprodol tablets, USP)
350 mg

℞

DESCRIPTION

'Soma' (carisoprodol) is available as 350 mg round, white tablets. Carisoprodol is N-isopropyl-2-methyl-2-propyl-1,3-propanediol dicarbamate.
Other ingredients: alginic acid, magnesium stearate, potassium sorbate, starch, tribasic calcium phosphate.

ACTIONS

Carisoprodol produces muscle relaxation in animals by blocking interneuronal activity in the descending reticular formation and spinal cord. The onset of action is rapid and effects last four to six hours.

INDICATIONS

Carisoprodol is indicated as an adjunct to rest, physical therapy, and other measures for the relief of discomfort associated with acute, painful musculoskeletal conditions. The mode of action of this drug has not been clearly identified, but may be related to its sedative properties. Carisoprodol does not directly relax tense skeletal muscles in man.

CONTRAINDICATIONS

Acute intermittent porphyria as well as allergic or idiosyncratic reactions to carisoprodol or related compounds such as meprobamate, mebutamate, or tybamate.

WARNINGS

Idiosyncratic Reactions—On very rare occasions, the first dose of carisoprodol has been followed by idiosyncratic symptoms appearing within minutes or hours. Symptoms reported include: extreme weakness, transient quadriplegia, dizziness, ataxia, temporary loss of vision, diplopia, mydriasis, dysarthria, agitation, euphoria, confusion, and disorientation. Symptoms usually subside over the course of the next several hours. Supportive and symptomatic therapy, including hospitalization, may be necessary.
Usage in Pregnancy and Lactation—Safe usage of this drug in pregnancy or lactation has not been established. Therefore, use of this drug in pregnancy, in nursing mothers, or in women of childbearing potential requires that the potential benefits of the drug be weighed against the potential hazards to mother and child. Carisoprodol is present in breast milk of lactating mothers at concentrations two to four times that of maternal plasma. This factor should be taken into account when use of the drug is contemplated in breast-feeding patients.

Usage in Children—Because of limited clinical experience, 'Soma' is not recommended for use in patients under 12 years of age.
Potentially Hazardous Tasks—Patients should be warned that this drug may impair the mental and/or physical abilities required for the performance of potentially hazardous tasks such as driving a motor vehicle or operating machinery.
Additive Effects—Since the effects of carisoprodol and alcohol or carisoprodol and other CNS depressants or psychotropic drugs may be additive, appropriate caution should be exercised with patients who take more than one of these agents simultaneously.
Drug Dependence—In dogs, no withdrawal symptoms occurred after abrupt cessation of carisoprodol from dosages as high as 1 gm/kg/day. In a study in man, abrupt cessation of 100 mg/kg/day (about five times the recommended daily adult dosage) was followed in some subjects by mild withdrawal symptoms such as abdominal cramps, insomnia, chilliness, headache, and nausea. Delirium and convulsions did not occur. In clinical use, psychological dependence and abuse have been rare, and there have been no reports of significant abstinence signs. Nevertheless, the drug should be used with caution in addiction-prone individuals.

PRECAUTIONS

Carisoprodol is metabolized in the liver and excreted by the kidney; to avoid its excess accumulation, caution should be exercised in administration to patients with compromised liver or kidney function.

ADVERSE REACTIONS

Central Nervous System—Drowsiness and other CNS effects may require dosage reduction. Also observed: dizziness, vertigo, ataxia, tremor, agitation, irritability, headache, depressive reactions, syncope, and insomnia. (See also Idiosyncratic Reactions under "Warnings.")
Allergic or Idiosyncratic—Allergic or idiosyncratic reactions occasionally develop. They are usually seen within the period of the first to fourth dose in patients having had no previous contact with the drug. Skin rash, erythema multiforme, pruritus, eosinophilia, and fixed drug eruption with cross reaction to meprobamate have been reported with carisoprodol. Severe reactions have been manifested by asthmatic episodes, fever, weakness, dizziness, angioneurotic edema, smarting eyes, hypotension, and anaphylactoid shock. (See also Idiosyncratic Reactions under "Warnings.") In case of allergic or idiosyncratic reactions to carisoprodol, discontinue the drug and initiate appropriate symptomatic therapy, which may include epinephrine, antihistamines, and in severe cases corticosteroids. In evaluating possible allergic reactions, also consider allergy to excipients (information on excipients is available to physicians on request).
Cardiovascular—Tachycardia, postural hypotension, and facial flushing.
Gastrointestinal—Nausea, vomiting, hiccup, and epigastric distress.
Hematologic—Leukopenia, in which other drugs or viral infection may have been responsible, and pancytopenia, attributed to phenylbutazone, have been reported. No serious blood dyscrasias have been attributed to carisoprodol.

DOSAGE AND ADMINISTRATION

The usual adult dosage of 'Soma' (carisoprodol) is one 350 mg tablet, three times daily and at bedtime. Usage in patients under age 12 is not recommended.

OVERDOSAGE

Overdosage of carisoprodol has produced stupor, coma, shock, respiratory depression, and, very rarely, death. The effects of an overdosage of carisoprodol and alcohol or other CNS depressants or psychotropic agents can be additive even when one of the drugs has been taken in the usual recommended dosage. Any drug remaining in the stomach should be removed and symptomatic therapy given. Should respiration or blood pressure become compromised, respiratory assistance, central nervous system stimulants, and pressor agents should be administered cautiously as indicated. Carisoprodol is metabolized in the liver and excreted by the kidney. Although carisoprodol overdosage experience is limited, the following types of treatment have been used successfully with the related drug meprobamate: diuresis, osmotic (mannitol) diuresis, peritoneal dialysis, and hemodialysis (carisoprodol is dialyzable). Careful monitoring of urinary output is necessary and caution should be taken to avoid overhydration. Observe for possible relapse due to incomplete gastric emptying and delayed absorption. Carisoprodol can be measured in biological fluids by gas chromatography (Douglas, J. F. et al: *J Pharm Sci 58:* 145, 1969).

HOW SUPPLIED

'Soma': Bottles of 100 (NDC 0037-2001-01) and 500 (NDC 0037-2001-03), and Unit Dose packages of 100 (NDC 0037-2001-85).
Storage: Store at controlled room temperature 15–30°C (59–86°F).

Continued on next page

Wallace Laboratories—Cont.

Rev. 4/91

WALLACE LABORATORIES
Division of CARTER-WALLACE, INC.
Cranbury, New Jersey 08512
Shown in Product Identification Section, page 435

SOMA ® COMPOUND†   ℞
(carisoprodol and aspirin tablets, USP)
carisoprodol 200 mg + aspirin 325 mg
TABLETS

DESCRIPTION

'Soma' Compound is a combination product containing carisoprodol, a centrally-acting muscle relaxant, plus aspirin, an analgesic with antipyretic and anti-inflammatory properties. It is available as a two-layered, white and orange, round tablet for oral administration. Each tablet contains carisoprodol 200 mg and aspirin 325 mg. Chemically, carisoprodol is N-isopropyl-2-methyl-2-propyl-1,3-propanediol dicarbamate. Its empirical formula is $C_{12}H_{24}N_2O_4$, with a molecular weight of 260.33. The structural formula is:

$$
\begin{array}{c}
CH_2CH_2CH_3 \\
| \\
H_2NCOOCH_2CCH_2OOCNHCH(CH_3)_2 \\
| \\
CH_3
\end{array}
$$

Other ingredients: croscarmellose sodium, FD&C Red #40, FD&C Yellow #6, hydroxypropyl methylcellulose, magnesium stearate, microcrystalline cellulose, povidone, starch, stearic acid.

CLINICAL PHARMACOLOGY

Carisoprodol: Carisoprodol is a centrally-acting muscle relaxant that does not directly relax tense skeletal muscles in man. The mode of action of carisoprodol in relieving acute muscle spasm of local origin has not been clearly identified, but may be related to its sedative properties. In animals, carisoprodol has been shown to produce muscle relaxation by blocking interneuronal activity and depressing transmission of polysynaptic neurons in the spinal cord and in the descending reticular formation of the brain. The onset of action is rapid and lasts four to six hours.
Carisoprodol is metabolized in the liver and is excreted by the kidneys. It is dialyzable by peritoneal and hemodialysis.
Aspirin: Aspirin is a non-narcotic analgesic with anti-inflammatory and antipyretic activity. Inhibition of prostaglandin biosynthesis appears to account for most of its anti-inflammatory and for at least part of its analgesic and antipyretic properties.
Aspirin is rapidly absorbed and almost totally hydrolyzed to salicylic acid following oral administration. Although aspirin has a half-life of only about 15 minutes, the apparent biologic half-life of salicylic acid in the therapeutic plasma concentration range is between 6 and 12 hours. Salicylic acid is eliminated by renal excretion and by biotransformation to inactive metabolites. Clearance of salicylic acid in the high-dose range is sensitive to urinary pH (see *Drug Interactions*) and is reduced by renal dysfunction.

INDICATIONS AND USAGE

'Soma' Compound is indicated as an adjunct to rest, physical therapy, and other measures for the relief of pain, muscle spasm, and limited mobility associated with acute, painful musculoskeletal conditions.

CONTRAINDICATIONS

Acute intermittent porphyria; bleeding disorders; allergic or idiosyncratic reactions to carisoprodol, aspirin or related compounds.

WARNINGS

On very rare occasions, the first dose of carisoprodol has been followed by an idiosyncratic reaction with symptoms appearing within minutes or hours. These may include extreme weakness, transient quadriplegia, dizziness, ataxia, temporary loss of vision, diplopia, mydriasis, dysarthia, agitation, euphoria, confusion, and disorientation. Although symptoms usually subside over the course of the next several hours, discontinue 'Soma' Compound and initiate appropriate supportive and symptomatic therapy, which may include epinephrine and/or antihistamines. In severe cases, corticosteroids may be necessary. Severe reactions have been manifested by asthmatic episodes, fever, weakness, dizziness, angioneurotic edema, smarting eyes, hypotension, and anaphylactoid shock.
The effects of carisoprodol with agents such as alcohol, other CNS depressants, or psychotropic drugs may be additive. Appropriate caution should be exercised with patients who

†Patent No. 4534973

---

may take one or more of these agents simultaneously with 'Soma' Compound.

PRECAUTIONS

General: To avoid excessive accumulation of carisoprodol, aspirin, or their metabolites, use 'Soma' Compound with caution in patients with compromised liver or kidney function, or in elderly or debilitated patients (see CLINICAL PHARMACOLOGY).
Use with caution in patients with history of gastritis or peptic ulcer, in patients on anticoagulant therapy, and in addiction-prone individuals.
Information for Patients: Caution patients that this drug may impair the mental and/or physical abilities required for the performance of potentially hazardous tasks such as driving a motor vehicle or operating machinery.
Caution patients with a predisposition for gastrointestinal bleeding that concomitant use of aspirin and alcohol may have an additive effect in this regard.
Caution patients that dosage of medications used for gout, arthritis, or diabetes may have to be adjusted when aspirin is administered or discontinued (see *Drug Interactions*).
Drug Interactions: Clinically important interactions may occur when certain drugs are administered concomitantly with aspirin or aspirin-containing drugs.
1. *Oral anticoagulants*—By interfering with platelet function or decreasing plasma prothrombin concentration, aspirin enhances the potential for bleeding in patients on anticoagulants.
2. *Methotrexate*—aspirin enhances the toxic effects of this drug.
3. *Probenecid and Sulfinpyrazone*—large doses of aspirin reduce the uricosuric effect of both drugs. Renal excretion of salicylate may also be reduced.
4. *Oral Antidiabetic Drugs*—enhancement of hypoglycemia may occur.
5. *Antacids*—to the extent that they raise urinary pH, antacids may substantially decrease plasma salicylate concentrations; conversely, their withdrawal can result in a substantial increase.
6. *Ammonium Chloride*—this and other drugs that acidify a relatively alkaline urine can elevate plasma salicylate concentrations.
7. *Ethyl Alcohol*—enhanced aspirin-induced fecal blood loss has been reported.
8. *Corticosteroids*—salicylate plasma levels may be decreased when adrenal corticosteroids are given, and may be increased substantially when they are discontinued.
Carcinogenesis, Mutagenesis, Impairment of Fertility: No long-term studies have been done with 'Soma' Compound.
Pregnancy—Teratogenic Effects: Pregnancy Category C. Adequate animal reproduction studies have not been conducted with 'Soma' Compound. It is also not known whether 'Soma' Compound can cause fetal harm when administered to a pregnant woman or can affect reproduction capacity. 'Soma' Compound should be given to a pregnant woman only if clearly needed.
Studies in rodents have shown salicylates to be teratogenic when given in early gestation, and embryocidal when given in later gestation in doses considerably greater than usual therapeutic doses in humans. Studies in women who took aspirin during pregnancy have not demonstrated an increased incidence of congenital abnormalities in the offspring.
Labor and Delivery: Ingestion of aspirin near term or prior to delivery may prolong delivery or lead to bleeding in mother, fetus, or neonate.
Nursing Mothers: Carisoprodol is excreted in human milk in concentrations two-to-four times that in maternal plasma. Aspirin is excreted in human milk in moderate amounts and can produce a bleeding tendency in nursing infants. Because of the potential for serious adverse reactions in nursing infants, a decision should be made whether to discontinue nursing or the drug, taking into account the importance of the drug to the mother.
Pediatric Use: Safety and effectiveness in children below the age of twelve have not been established.

ADVERSE REACTIONS

If severe reactions occur, discontinue 'Soma' Compound and initiate appropriate symptomatic and supportive therapy. The following side effects which have occurred with the administration of the individual ingredients alone may also occur with the combination.
Carisoprodol: *Central Nervous System*—Drowsiness is the most frequent complaint and along with other CNS effects may require dosage reduction. Observed less frequently are dizziness, vertigo and ataxia. Tremor, agitation, irritability, headache, depressive reactions, syncope, and insomnia have been infrequent or rare.
Idiosyncratic—Idiosyncratic reactions are very rare. They are usually seen within the period of the first to fourth dose in patients having had no previous contact with the drug (see WARNINGS).
Allergic—Skin rash, erythema multiforme, pruritus, eosinophilia, and fixed drug eruptions with cross-reaction to mep-

---

robamate have been reported. If allergic reactions occur, discontinue 'Soma' Compound and treat symptomatically. In evaluating possible allergic reactions, also consider allergy to excipients (information on excipients is available to physicians on request).
Cardiovascular—Tachycardia, postural hypotension, and facial flushing.
Gastrointestinal—Nausea, vomiting, epigastric distress and hiccup.
Hematologic—No serious blood dyscrasias have been attributed to carisoprodol alone. Leukopenia and pancytopenia have been reported, very rarely, in situations in which other drugs or viral infections may have been responsible.
Aspirin: The most common adverse reactions associated with the use of aspirin have been gastrointestinal, including nausea, vomiting, gastritis, occult bleeding, constipation and diarrhea. Gastric erosion, angioedema, asthma, rash, pruritus and urticaria have been reported less commonly. Tinnitus is a sign of high serum salicylate levels (see OVERDOSAGE).
Aspirin Intolerance—Allergic type reactions in aspirin-sensitive individuals may involve the respiratory tract or the skin. Symptoms of the former range from rhinorrhea and shortness of breath to severe asthma, and the latter may consist of urticaria, edema, rash, or angioedema (giant hives). These may occur independently or in combination.

DRUG ABUSE AND DEPENDENCE

Abuse: In clinical use, abuse has been rare.
Dependence: In clinical use, dependence with 'Soma' Compound has been rare and there have been no reports of significant abstinence signs. Nevertheless, the following information on the individual ingredients should be kept in mind.
Carisoprodol—In dogs, no withdrawal symptoms occurred after abrupt cessation of carisoprodol from dosages as high as 1 gm/kg/day. In a study in man, abrupt cessation of 100 mg/kg/day (about five times the recommended daily adult dosage) was followed in some subjects by mild withdrawal symptoms such as abdominal cramps, insomnia, chills, headache, and nausea. Delirium and convulsions did not occur (see PRECAUTIONS).

OVERDOSAGE

Signs and Symptoms: Any of the following which have been reported with the individual ingredients may occur and may be modified to a varying degree by the effects of the other ingredients present in 'Soma' Compound.
Carisoprodol—Stupor, coma, shock, respiratory depression and, very rarely, death. Overdosage with carisoprodol in combination with alcohol, other CNS depressants, or psychotropic agents can have additive effects, even when one of the agents has been taken in the usually recommended dosage.
Aspirin—Headache, tinnitus, hearing difficulty, dim vision, dizziness, lassitude, hyperpnea, rapid breathing, thirst, nausea, vomiting, sweating and occasionally diarrhea are characteristic of mild to moderate salicylate poisoning. Salicylate poisoning should be considered in children with symptoms of vomiting, hyperpnea, and hyperthermia.
Hyperpnea is an early sign of salicylate poisoning, but dyspnea supervenes at plasma levels above 50 mg/dl. These respiratory changes eventually lead to serious acid-base disturbances. Metabolic acidosis is a constant finding in infants but occurs in older children only with severe poisoning; adults usually exhibit respiratory alkalosis initially and acidosis terminally.
Other symptoms of severe salicylate poisoning include hyperthermia, dehydration, delirium, and mental disturbances. Skin eruptions, GI hemorrhage, or pulmonary edema are less common. Early CNS stimulation is replaced by increasing depression, stupor, and coma. Death is usually due to respiratory failure or cardiovascular collapse.
Treatment: *General* Provide symptomatic and supportive treatment, as indicated. Any drug remaining in the stomach should be removed using appropriate procedures and caution to protect the airway and prevent aspiration, especially in the stuporous or comatose patient. Incomplete gastric emptying with delayed absorption of carisoprodol has been reported as a cause for relapse. Should respiration or blood pressure become compromised, respiratory assistance, central nervous system stimulants, and pressor agents should be administered cautiously, as indicated.
Carisoprodol—The following have been used successfully in overdosage with the related drug meprobamate: diuretics, osmotic (mannitol) diuresis, peritoneal dialysis, and hemodialysis (see CLINICAL PHARMACOLOGY). Careful monitoring of urinary output is necessary and caution should be taken to avoid overhydration. Carisoprodol can be measured in biological fluid by gas chromatography (Douglas, J. F., et al: *J Pharm Sci 58:* 145, 1969).
Aspirin—Since there are no specific antidotes for salicylate poisoning, the aim of treatment is to enhance elimination of salicylate and prevent or reduce further absorption; to correct any fluid, electrolyte or metabolic imbalance; and to provide general and cardiorespiratory support. If acidosis is present, intravenous sodium bicarbonate must be given, along with adequate hydration, until salicylate levels de-

crease to within the therapeutic range. To enhance elimination, forced diuresis and alkalinization of the urine may be beneficial. The need for hemoperfusion or hemodialysis is rare and should be used only when other measures have failed.

DOSAGE AND ADMINISTRATION

Usual Adult Dosage: 1 or 2 tablets, four times daily. Not recommended for use in children under age twelve (see PRECAUTIONS).

HOW SUPPLIED

'Soma' Compound Tablets: In bottles of 100 (NDC 0037-2103-01) and 500 (NDC 0037-2103-03) and Unit dose packages of 100 (NDC 0037-2103-85).

Storage: Store at controlled room temperature 15–30°C (59–86°F). Protect from moisture.

WALLACE LABORATORIES
Division of CARTER-WALLACE, INC.
Cranbury, New Jersey 08512

Rev. 4/91

Shown in Product Identification Section, page 435

SOMA® COMPOUND with CODEINE†   ℞
(carisoprodol, aspirin and codeine phosphate tablets, USP)
carisoprodol 200 mg †
aspirin 325 mg †
codeine phosphate 16 mg·
Warning: May be habit-forming.
TABLETS

DESCRIPTION

'Soma' Compound with Codeine is a combination product containing carisoprodol, a centrally-acting muscle relaxant, plus aspirin, an analgesic with antipyretic and anti-inflammatory properties and codeine phosphate, a centrally-acting narcotic analgesic. It is available as a two-layered, white and yellow, oval-shaped tablet for oral administration. Each tablet contains carisoprodol 200 mg, aspirin 325 mg, and codeine phosphate 16 mg. Chemically, carisoprodol is N-isopropyl-2-methyl-2-propyl-1,3-propanediol dicarbamate. Its empirical formula is $C_{12}H_{24}N_2O_4$, with a molecular weight of 260.33. The structural formula is:

$$CH_2CH_2CH_3$$
$$|$$
$$H_2NCOOCH_2CCH_2OOCNHCH(CH_3)_2$$
$$|$$
$$CH_3$$

Other ingredients: croscarmellose sodium, D&C Yellow #10, hydroxypropyl methylcellulose, magnesium stearate, microcrystalline cellulose, povidone, sodium metabisulfite, starch, stearic acid.

CLINICAL PHARMACOLOGY

Carisoprodol: Carisoprodol is a centrally-acting muscle relaxant that does not directly relax tense skeletal muscles in man. The mode of action of carisoprodol in relieving acute muscle spasm of local origin has not been clearly identified, but may be related to its sedative properties. In animals, carisoprodol has been shown to produce muscle relaxation by blocking interneuronal activity and depressing transmission of polysynaptic neurons in the spinal cord and in the descending reticular formation of the brain. The onset of action is rapid and lasts four to six hours.

Carisoprodol is metabolized in the liver and is excreted by the kidneys. It is dialyzable by peritoneal and hemodialysis.

Aspirin: Aspirin is a non-narcotic analgesic with anti-inflammatory and antipyretic activity. Inhibition of prostaglandin biosynthesis appears to account for most of its anti-inflammatory and for at least part of its analgesic and antipyretic activity.

Aspirin is rapidly absorbed and almost totally hydrolyzed to salicylic acid following oral administration. Although aspirin has a half-life of only about 15 minutes, the apparent biologic half-life of salicylic acid in the therapeutic plasma concentration range is between 6 and 12 hours. Salicylic acid is eliminated by renal excretion and by biotransformation to inactive metabolites. Clearance of salicylic acid in the high-dose range is sensitive to urinary pH (see *Drug Interactions*) and is reduced by renal dysfunction.

Codeine Phosphate: Codeine phosphate is a centrally-acting narcotic-analgesic. Its actions are qualitatively similar to morphine, but its potency is substantially less.

Clinical studies have shown that combining aspirin and codeine produces a significant additive effect in analgesic efficacy.

INDICATIONS AND USAGE

'Soma' Compound with Codeine is indicated as an adjunct to rest, physical therapy, and other measures for the relief of pain, muscle spasm, and limited mobility associated with acute, painful musculoskeletal conditions when the additional action of codeine is desired.

† Patent No. 4534974

CONTRAINDICATIONS

Acute intermittent porphyria; bleeding disorders; allergic or idiosyncratic reactions to carisoprodol, aspirin, codeine, or related compounds.

WARNINGS

On very rare occasions, the first dose of carisoprodol has been followed by idiosyncratic reactions, with symptoms appearing within minutes or hours. These may include extreme weakness, transient quadriplegia, dizziness, ataxia, temporary loss of vision, diplopia, mydriasis, dysarthria, agitation, euphoria, confusion, and disorientation. Although symptoms usually subside over the course of the next several hours, discontinue 'Soma' Compound with Codeine and initiate appropriate supportive and symptomatic therapy, which may include epinephrine and/or antihistamines. In severe cases, corticosteroids may be necessary. Severe reactions have been manifested by asthmatic episodes, fever, weakness, dizziness, angioneurotic edema, smarting eyes, hypotension, and anaphylactoid shock.

The effects of carisoprodol with agents such as alcohol, other CNS depressants, or psychotropic drugs may be additive. Appropriate caution should be exercised with patients who take one or more of these agents simultaneously with Soma Compound with Codeine.

Contains sodium metabisulfite, a sulfite that may cause allergic-type reactions including anaphylactic symptoms and life-threatening or less severe asthmatic episodes in certain susceptible people. The overall prevalence of sulfite sensitivity in the general population is unknown and probably low. Sulfite sensitivity is seen more frequently in asthmatic than in nonasthmatic people.

PRECAUTIONS

General: To avoid excessive accumulation of carisoprodol, aspirin, or their metabolites, use 'Soma' Compound with Codeine with caution in patients with compromised liver or kidney function, or in elderly or debilitated patients (see CLINICAL PHARMACOLOGY).

Use with caution in patients with history of gastritis or peptic ulcer, in patients on anticoagulant therapy, and in addiction-prone individuals.

Information for Patients: Caution patients that this drug may impair the mental and/or physical abilities required for the performance of potentially hazardous tasks such as driving a motor vehicle or operating machinery.

Caution patients with a predisposition for gastrointestinal bleeding that concomitant use of aspirin and alcohol may have an additive effect in this regard.

Caution patients that dosage of medications used for gout, arthritis, or diabetes may have to be adjusted when aspirin is administered or discontinued (see *Drug Interactions*).

Drug Interactions: Clinically important interactions may occur when certain drugs are administered concomitantly with aspirin or aspirin-containing drugs.

1. *Oral Anticoagulants* —By interfering with platelet function or decreasing plasma prothrombin concentration, aspirin enhances the potential for bleeding in patients on anticoagulants.

2. *Methotrexate* —aspirin enhances the toxic effects of this drug.

3. *Probenecid and Sulfinpyrazone* —large doses of aspirin reduce the uricosuric effect of both drugs. Renal excretion of salicylate may also be reduced.

4. *Oral Antidiabetic Drugs* —enhancement of hypoglycemia may occur.

5. *Antacids* —to the extent that they raise urinary pH, antacids may substantially decrease plasma salicylate concentrations; conversely, their withdrawal can result in a substantial increase.

6. *Ammonium Chloride* —this and other drugs that acidify a relatively alkaline urine can elevate plasma salicylate concentrations.

7. *Ethyl Alcohol* —enhanced aspirin-induced fecal blood loss has been reported.

8. *Corticosteroids* —salicylate plasma levels may be decreased when adrenal corticosteroids are given, and may be increased substantially when they are discontinued.

Carcinogenesis, Mutagenesis, Impairment of Fertility: No long-term studies have been done with 'Soma' Compound with Codeine.

Pregnancy—Teratogenic Effects: **Pregnancy Category C.** Adequate animal reproduction studies have not been conducted with 'Soma' Compound with Codeine. It is also not known whether 'Soma' Compound with Codeine can cause fetal harm when administered to a pregnant woman or can affect reproduction capacity. 'Soma' Compound with Codeine should be given to a pregnant woman only if clearly needed. Studies in rodents have shown salicylates to be teratogenic when given in early gestation, and embryocidal when given in later gestation in doses considerably greater than usual therapeutic doses in humans. Studies in women who took aspirin during pregnancy have not demonstrated an increased incidence of congenital abnormalities in the offspring.

Labor and Delivery: Ingestion of aspirin near term or prior to delivery may prolong delivery or lead to bleeding in mother, fetus, or neonate.

Nursing Mothers: Carisoprodol is excreted in human milk in concentrations two-to-four times that in maternal plasma. Aspirin is excreted in human milk in moderate amounts and can produce a bleeding tendency in nursing infants. Because of the potential for serious adverse reactions in nursing infants, a decision should be made whether to discontinue nursing or the drug, taking into account the importance of the drug to the mother.

Pediatric Use: Safety and effectiveness in children below the age of twelve have not been established.

ADVERSE REACTIONS

If severe reactions occur, discontinue 'Soma' Compound with Codeine and initiate appropriate symptomatic and supportive therapy.

The following side effects which have occurred with the administration of the individual ingredients alone may also occur with the combination.

Carisoprodol: Central Nervous System—Drowsiness is the most frequent complaint and along with other CNS effects may require dosage reduction. Observed less frequently are dizziness, vertigo and ataxia. Tremor, agitation, irritability, headache, depressive reactions, syncope, and insomnia have been infrequent or rare.

Idiosyncratic—Idiosyncratic reactions are very rare. They are usually seen within the period of the first to fourth dose in patients having had no previous contact with the drug (see WARNINGS).

Allergic—Skin rash, erythema multiforme, pruritus, eosinophilia, and fixed drug eruptions with cross-reaction to meprobamate have been reported. If allergic reactions occur, discontinue 'Soma' Compound with Codeine and treat symptomatically. In evaluating possible allergic reactions, also consider allergy to excipients (information on excipients is available to physicians on request).

Cardiovascular—Tachycardia, postural hypotension, and facial flushing.

Gastrointestinal—Nausea, vomiting, epigastric distress and hiccup.

Hematologic—No serious blood dyscrasias have been attributed to carisoprodol alone. Leukopenia and pancytopenia have been reported, very rarely, in situations in which other drugs or viral infections may have been responsible.

Aspirin: The most common adverse reactions associated with the use of aspirin have been gastrointestinal, including nausea, vomiting, gastritis, occult bleeding, constipation and diarrhea. Gastric erosion, angioedema, asthma, rash, pruritus and urticaria have been reported less commonly. Tinnitus is a sign of high serum salicylate levels (see OVERDOSAGE).

Aspirin Intolerance—Allergic type reactions in aspirin-sensitive individuals may involve the respiratory tract or the skin. Symptoms of the former range from rhinorrhea and shortness of breath to severe asthma, and the latter may consist of urticaria, edema, rash, or angioedema (giant hives). These may occur independently or in combination.

Codeine Phosphate: Nausea, vomiting, constipation, miosis, sedation, and dizziness have been reported.

DRUG ABUSE AND DEPENDENCE

Controlled Substance: Schedule C-III (see PRECAUTIONS).

Abuse: In clinical use, abuse has been rare.

Dependence: In clinical use, dependence with 'Soma' Compound with Codeine has been rare and there have been no reports of significant abstinence signs. Nevertheless, the following information on the individual ingredients should be kept in mind.

Carisoprodol—In dogs, no withdrawal symptoms occurred after abrupt cessation of carisoprodol from dosages as high as 1 gm/kg/day. In a study in man, abrupt cessation of 100 mg/kg/day (about five times the recommended daily adult dosage) was followed in some subjects by mild withdrawal symptoms such as abdominal cramps, insomnia, chills, headache, and nausea. Delirium and convulsions did not occur (see PRECAUTIONS).

Codeine Phosphate—Drug dependence of the morphine type may result.

OVERDOSAGE

Signs and Symptoms: Any of the following which have been reported with the individual ingredients may occur and may be modified to a varying degree by the effects of the other ingredients present in 'Soma' Compound with Codeine.

Carisoprodol—Stupor, coma, shock, respiratory depression and, very rarely, death. Overdosage with carisoprodol in combination with alcohol, other CNS depressants, or psychotropic agents can have additive effects, even when one of the agents has been taken in the usually recommended dose.

Aspirin—Headache, tinnitus, hearing difficulty, dim vision, dizziness, lassitude, hyperpnea, rapid breathing, thirst, nausea, vomiting, sweating and occasionally diarrhea are characteristic of mild to moderate salicylate poisoning. Salicylate

Continued on next page

Wallace Laboratories—Cont.

poisoning should be considered in children with symptoms of vomiting, hyperpnea, and hyperthermia.

Hyperpnea is an early sign of salicylate poisoning, but dyspnea supervenes at plasma levels above 50 mg/dl. These respiratory changes eventually lead to serious acid-base disturbances. Metabolic acidosis is a constant finding in infants but occurs in older children only with severe poisoning; adults usually exhibit respiratory alkalosis initially and acidosis terminally.

Other symptoms of severe salicylate poisoning include hyperthermia, dehydration, delirium, and mental disturbances. Skin eruptions, GI hemorrhage, or pulmonary edema are less common. Early CNS stimulation is replaced by increasing depression, stupor, and coma. Death is usually due to respiratory failure or cardiovascular collapse.

Codeine Phosphate—pinpoint pupils, CNS depression, coma, respiratory depression, and shock.

Treatment: *General*—Provide symptomatic and supportive treatment, as indicated. Any drug remaining in the stomach should be removed using appropriate procedures and caution to protect the airway and prevent aspiration, especially in the stuporous or comatose patient. Incomplete gastric emptying with delayed absorption of carisoprodol has been reported as a cause for relapse. Should respiration or blood pressure become compromised, respiratory assistance, central nervous system stimulants, and pressor agents should be administered cautiously, as indicated.

Carisoprodol—The following have been used successfully in overdosage with the related drug meprobamate: diuretics, osmotic (mannitol) diuresis, peritoneal dialysis, and hemodialysis (see CLINICAL PHARMACOLOGY). Careful monitoring of urinary output is necessary and caution should be taken to avoid overhydration. Carisoprodol can be measured in biological fluid by gas chromatography (Douglas, J. F., et al: *J Pharm Sci 58:* 145, 1969).

Aspirin—Since there are no specific antidotes for salicylate poisoning, the aim of treatment is to enhance elimination of salicylate and prevent or reduce further absorption; to correct any fluid, electrolyte or metabolic imbalance; and to provide general and cardiorespiratory support. If acidosis is present, intravenous sodium bicarbonate must be given, along with adequate hydration, until salicylate levels decrease to within the therapeutic range. To enhance elimination, forced diuresis and alkalinization of the urine may be beneficial. The need for hemoperfusion or hemodialysis is rare and should be used only when other measures have failed.

Codeine Phosphate—Narcotic antagonists, such as nalorphine and levallorphan, may be indicated.

DOSAGE AND ADMINISTRATION

Usual Adult Dosage: 1 or 2 tablets, four times daily.
Not recommended for use in children under age twelve.

HOW SUPPLIED

'Soma' Compound with Codeine Tablets: In bottles of 100 (NDC 0037-2403-01).

Storage: Store at controlled room temperature 15–30°C (59–86°F). Protect from moisture.

WALLACE LABORATORIES
Division of CARTER-WALLACE, INC.
Cranbury, New Jersey 08512

Rev. 4/91

Shown in Product Identification Section, page 435

TUSSI–ORGANIDIN® Liquid ℂ ℞
TUSSI–ORGANIDIN®-S† Liquid ℂ ℞
TUSSI–ORGANIDIN® DM Liquid ℞
TUSSI–ORGANIDIN® DM-S† Liquid ℞

DESCRIPTION

TUSSI-ORGANIDIN® and TUSSI-ORGANIDIN® DM are antitussive/mucolytic-expectorant combinations available for oral administration as liquids.

TUSSI-ORGANIDIN—each 5 mL (teaspoonful) contains ORGANIDIN® (iodinated glycerol) 30 mg (15 mg organically bound iodine) and codeine phosphate (**Warning:** May be habit-forming) 10 mg. ORGANIDIN® (iodinated glycerol), a mucolytic-expectorant, contains a mixture of several iodinated compounds formed by the reaction of iodine and glycerin. The major iodinated compounds are 3-iodo-1,2-propanediol and a mixture of diastereomers of 1,5,6-trihydroxy-2-iodomethyl-3-oxahexane. Iodinated glycerol is an amber liquid which contains virtually no free iodine and is stable in an acid medium.

Other ingredients: citric acid, FD&C Red #40, flavor (artificial), glycerin, propylene glycol, purified water, saccharin sodium, sodium benzoate, sorbitol solution.

TUSSI-ORGANIDIN DM—as for TUSSI-ORGANIDIN; codeine phosphate is replaced by dextromethorphan hydrobromide, 10 mg per 5 mL.

†Patent Pending

Other ingredients: citric acid, D&C Yellow #10, FD&C Red #40, flavor (artificial), glycerin, propylene glycol, purified water, saccharin sodium, sodium benzoate, sorbitol solution.

CLINICAL PHARMACOLOGY

TUSSI-ORGANIDIN combines the antitussive action of codeine with the mucolytic-expectorant action of ORGANIDIN.

TUSSI-ORGANIDIN DM combines the non-narcotic antitussive action of dextromethorphan with the mucolytic-expectorant action of ORGANIDIN.

INDICATIONS AND USAGE

TUSSI-ORGANIDIN and TUSSI-ORGANIDIN DM are indicated for the symptomatic relief of irritating, nonproductive cough associated with respiratory tract conditions such as bronchitis and asthma. Appropriate therapy should be provided for the primary disease.

DURATION OF TREATMENT

The antitussive therapy is directed at the symptomatic relief of the irritating cough. The effects of mucolytic therapy may be seen early after the initiation of therapy; however, at least three to four weeks may be needed to demonstrate maximum effects for those patients responding. Patients not responding within four weeks should not be continued on this therapy. Continuation of therapy beyond eight weeks cannot currently be recommended unless in the experience and/or opinion of the physician, the ongoing condition or clinical status of the patient warrants such continuation. It should be recognized that chronic pulmonary diseases are intermittently marked by exacerbations and that the adjunctive use of TUSSI-ORGANIDIN or TUSSI-ORGANIDIN DM during these exacerbations is the most appropriate form of therapy as opposed to long-term, continuous use.

CONTRAINDICATIONS

History of marked sensitivity to inorganic iodides; hypersensitivity to any of the ingredients or related compounds; pregnancy; newborns; and nursing mothers.

The human fetal thyroid begins to concentrate iodine in the 12th to 14th week of gestation and the use of inorganic iodides in pregnant women during this period and thereafter has rarely been reported to induce fetal goiter (with or without hypothyroidism) with the potential for airway obstruction. If the patient becomes pregnant while taking any of these products, the drug should be discontinued and the patient should be apprised of the potential risk to the fetus.

WARNINGS

Discontinue use if rash or other evidence of hypersensitivity appears. Use with caution or avoid use in patients with history or evidence of thyroid disease.

PRECAUTIONS

General—Iodides have been reported to cause a flare-up of adolescent acne. Children with cystic fibrosis appear to have an exaggerated susceptibility to the goitrogenic effect of iodides.

Dermatitis and other reversible manifestations of iodism have been reported with chronic use of inorganic iodides. Although these have not been a problem clinically with ORGANIDIN formulations, they should be kept in mind in patients receiving these preparations for prolonged periods.

Laboratory Tests—Chronic administration of pharmacologic doses of iodide does not affect the normal thyroid; the excess iodide is excreted by the kidneys. Reversible, mild to moderately elevated TSH (thyrotropin) levels with or without depressed serum T_4 and T_3 levels have been noted sporadically in patients (usually elderly) receiving iodide therapy for prolonged periods; in most such cases, no pretreatment thyroid function tests were available. Iodide-induced 'biochemical hypothyroidism' (i.e., subclinical hypothyroidism manifested only by depressed serum T_4 or T_3 levels and/or elevated TSH) may be noted in patients with underlying thyroid dysfunction (where the thyroid homeostatic mechanism does not function normally). Iodide-induced 'biochemical hypothyroidism' typically reverses to pretreatment levels (in weeks or months) usually spontaneously. Patients with 'functional' hypothyroidism may receive iodotherapy, provided thyroid hormone (e.g., Synthroid-levothyroxine) is administered concomitantly in replacement doses. Radioactive iodine (I^{131}) and iodide transport tests are depressed during iodide therapy; these tests could be expected to return to basal levels two or three days after stopping treatment with TUSSI-ORGANIDIN or TUSSI-ORGANIDIN DM.

Pediatric Use—Due to the developmental nature of many organ systems in this age group, the physician must weigh the perceived benefit against any potential risk in using iodide in children.

Drug Interactions: Iodides may potentiate the hypothyroid effect of lithium and other antithyroid drugs. TUSSI-ORGANIDIN DM—potential for a drug interaction exists between dextromethorphan and monoamine oxidase inhibitors (MAOIs).

CARCINOGENESIS, MUTAGENESIS, IMPAIRMENT OF FERTILITY: Twenty-four (24) month carcinogenicity studies were conducted by the National Toxicology Program (NTP) in rats and mice using doses of iodinated glycerol that ranged between 13 and 52 times the recommended human dose. The conclusions of the NTP under the conditions of these gavage studies were species and sex specific and included the following: (1) no evidence of carcinogenicity in female F344/N rats; some evidence in male F344/N rats, based on increased incidences of a) mononuclear cell leukemia and b) follicular cell carcinomas of the thyroid gland. (There were no other chemical related nonneoplastic lesions of the thyroid gland in male or female rats.) (2) No evidence of carcinogenicity in male B6C3F1 mice; some evidence in female B6C3F1 mice, based on increased incidences of a) adenomas of the pituitary gland and b) neoplasms of the Harderian gland. The latter tumors were not found in the male mouse or in male or female rats. (There are no known human equivalents to mononuclear cell leukemia in the rat and Harderian gland neoplasms in the mouse.) The relevance of these findings to humans is not known. Both positive and negative results were found with iodinated glycerol in a standard battery of in vitro mutagenicity assays that were conducted with or without microsomal activation. In the only in vivo mutagenicity study that was conducted, the results were negative for genotoxic effects, in that no increase in micronucleated polychromatic erythrocytes was observed in the bone marrow of B6C3F1 mice after administration of either iodinated glycerol or 3-iodo-1, 2-propanediol. The relevance of these findings to humans is not known. No long-term animal studies on impairment of fertility have been performed with these products.

Pregnancy—Teratogenic effects: Pregnancy Category X (see **CONTRAINDICATIONS**).

Nursing Mothers—These products should not be administered to a nursing woman.

ADVERSE REACTIONS

Side effects have been rare, including those which may occur with the individual active ingredients and which may be modified as a result of their combination.

ORGANIDIN—Rare side effects include gastrointestinal irritation, rash, hypersensitivity, thyroid gland enlargement, and acute parotitis.

Codeine—(TUSSI-ORGANIDIN only): Nausea, vomiting, constipation, drowsiness, dizziness, and miosis have been reported.

Dextromethorphan—(TUSSI-ORGANIDIN DM only): Rarely produces drowsiness or gastrointestinal disturbances.

DRUG ABUSE AND DEPENDENCE

(TUSSI-ORGANIDIN only)

Controlled Substance—Schedule V

Dependence—Codeine may be habit-forming.

OVERDOSAGE

Acute overdosage experience with ORGANIDIN formulations has been rare and there have been no reports of any serious problems.

DOSAGE AND ADMINISTRATION

TUSSI-ORGANIDIN and TUSSI-ORGANIDIN DM:

Adults—1 to 2 teaspoonfuls (5–10 mL) every 4 hours.

Children—½ to 1 teaspoonful (2½–5 mL) every 4 hours.

HOW SUPPLIED

TUSSI-ORGANIDIN Liquid—clear red liquid, each 5 mL (teaspoonful) contains ORGANIDIN® (iodinated glycerol) 30 mg (15 mg organically bound iodine) and codeine phosphate 10 mg (Warning: May be habit-forming), in 4 fl. oz. bottles (NDC 0037-4812-01, labeled TUSSI-ORGANIDIN® and NDC 0037-4812-50, labeled TUSSI-ORGANIDIN®–S†) and in bottles of one pint (NDC 0037-4812-10) and one gallon (NDC 0037-4812-20).

TUSSI-ORGANIDIN DM Liquid—clear yellow liquid, each 5 mL (teaspoonful) contains ORGANIDIN® (iodinated glycerol) 30 mg (15 mg organically bound iodine) and dextromethorphan 10 mg, in 4 fl. oz. bottles (NDC 0037-4712-01, labeled TUSSI-ORGANIDIN® DM and NDC 0037-4712-50, labeled TUSSI-ORGANIDIN® DM-S†) and in bottles of one pint (NDC 0037-4712-10) and one gallon (NDC 0037-4712-20).

Storage: Store at controlled room temperature 15°–30°C (59°–86°F).

TUSSI-ORGANIDIN®-S and TUSSI-ORGANIDIN® DM-S are TUSSI-ORGANIDIN® and TUSSI-ORGANIDIN® DM Liquids, respectively, either in 4 fl. oz. unit of use containers with a 10 mL graduated, oral syringe (patent pending) or in 30 mL sample containers.

TUSSI-ORGANIDIN Liquid and TUSSI-ORGANIDIN DM Liquid are distributed by:
Wallace Laboratories
Division of Carter-Wallace, Inc.,
Cranbury, New Jersey 08512
Manufactured by: Denver Chemical (Puerto Rico), Inc.
Subsidiary of Carter-Wallace, Inc.
Humacao, Puerto Rico 00661
Based on IN-ORG30-08 (Rev. 4/92) Rev. 6/92

Shown in Product Identification Section, page 435

VASCOR®
brand of bepridil hydrochloride
Tablets

Marketed jointly by McNeil Pharmaceutical and Wallace Laboratories. See McNeil Pharmaceutical for product information.

Shown in Product Identification Section, page 435

VoSoL®   ℞
(acetic acid otic solution, USP)
OTIC SOLUTION

VoSoL® HC   ℞
(hydrocortisone and acetic acid otic solution, USP)
OTIC SOLUTION

DESCRIPTION
VoSoL (acetic acid otic solution, USP) is a solution of acetic acid (2%), in a propylene glycol vehicle containing propylene glycol diacetate (3%), benzethonium chloride (0.02%), and sodium acetate (0.015%).

VoSoL HC (hydrocortisone and acetic acid otic solution, USP) also contains hydrocortisone (1%) and citric acid (0.2%). The empirical formulas for acetic acid and hydrocortisone are CH_3COOH and $C_{21}H_{30}O_5$, with a molecular weight of 60.05 and 362.46, respectively. The structural formulas are:

Acetic Acid

Chemically, hydrocortisone is:
Pregn-4-ene-3,20-dione,
11,17,21-trihydroxy-(11β)-.

VoSoL and VoSoL HC are available as nonaqueous otic solutions buffered at pH 3 for use in the external ear canal.

CLINICAL PHARMACOLOGY
Acetic acid is anti-bacterial and anti-fungal; propylene glycol is hydrophilic and provides a low surface tension; benzethonium chloride is a surface active agent that promotes contact of the solution with tissues; hydrocortisone (in VoSoL HC) is anti-inflammatory, anti-allergic and anti-pruritic.

INDICATIONS AND USAGE
VoSoL—For the treatment of superficial infections of the external auditory canal caused by organisms susceptible to the action of the antimicrobial.

VoSoL HC—For the treatment of superficial infections of the external auditory canal caused by organisms susceptible to the action of the antimicrobial, complicated by inflammation.

CONTRAINDICATIONS
Hypersensitivity to any of the ingredients. VoSoL HC is contraindicated in vaccinia and varicella. Perforated tympanic membrane is considered a contraindication to the use of any medication in the external ear canal.

WARNINGS
Discontinue promptly if sensitization or irritation occurs.

PRECAUTIONS
Transient stinging or burning may be noted occasionally when the solution is first instilled into the acutely inflamed ear.

ADVERSE REACTIONS
Stinging or burning may be noted occasionally; local irritation has occurred very rarely.

DOSAGE AND ADMINISTRATION
Carefully remove all cerumen and debris to allow VoSoL to contact infected surfaces directly. To promote continuous contact, insert a wick saturated with VoSoL or VoSoL HC into the ear canal; the wick may also be saturated after insertion. Instruct the patient to keep the wick in for at least 24 hours and to keep it moist by adding 3 to 5 drops of VoSoL or VoSoL HC every 4 to 6 hours. The wick may be removed after 24 hours but the patient should continue to instill 5 drops of VoSoL 3 or 4 times daily thereafter, for as long as indicated.

HOW SUPPLIED
VoSoL Otic Solution, 15 mL volume (NDC 0037-3611-10) and 30 mL volume (NDC 0037-3611-30) in measured drop, safety-tip plastic bottles.

VoSoL HC Otic Solution, 10 mL volume in measured-drop, safety-tip plastic bottle (NDC 0037-3811-12).

Storage: Store at controlled room temperature 15°C–30°C (59°F–86°F).

Distributed by
WALLACE LABORATORIES
Division of
CARTER-WALLACE, INC.
Cranbury, New Jersey 08512
Manufactured by Denver Chemical (Puerto Rico), Inc.
Subsidiary of Carter-Wallace, Inc.
Humaco, Puerto Rico 00661
Rev. 12/89
Shown in Product Identification Section, page 435

Warner Chilcott Laboratories
Division of Warner-Lambert Company
201 TABOR ROAD
MORRIS PLAINS, NJ 07950

NDC #	PRODUCT	
0640	Acetaminophen Tablets, USP 325 mg	OTC
0759	Acetaminophen Caplets 500 mg	OTC
0634	Acetaminophen with Codeine Phosphate Tablets No. 2	ℭ/℞
0635	Acetaminophen with Codeine Phosphate Tablets No. 3	ℭ/℞
0637	Acetaminophen with Codeine Phosphate Tablets No. 4	ℭ/℞
0956	Albuterol Sulfate Tablets, 2 mg	℞
0957	Albuterol Sulfate Tablets, 4 mg	℞
0515	Allopurinol Tablets, 100 mg	℞
0517	Allopurinol Tablets, 300 mg	℞
0853	Amantadine HCl Capsules, USP 100 mg	℞
0832	Amiloride HCl and Hydrochlorothiazide Tablets 5 mg/150 mg	℞
	Amoxapine Tablets, 25 mg	℞
	Amoxapine Tablets, 50 mg	℞
	Amoxapine Tablets, 100 mg	℞
	Amoxapine Tablets, 150 mg	℞
0730	Amoxicillin Capsules, USP 250 mg	℞
0731	Amoxicillin Capsules, USP 500 mg	℞
2500	Amoxicillin for Oral Suspension, USP 125 mg/5 mL	℞
2501	Amoxicillin for Oral Suspension, USP 250 mg/5 mL	℞
0402	Ampicillin Capsules, USP 250 mg	℞
0404	Ampicillin Capsules, USP 500 mg	℞
2301	Ampicillin for Oral Suspension, USP 125 mg/5 mL	℞
2302	Ampicillin for Oral Suspension, USP 250 mg/5 mL	℞
0606	Aspirin Tablets, USP 5 gr	OTC
0611	Baclofen Tablets 10 mg	℞
0612	Baclofen Tablets 20 mg	℞
2909	Bromarest DX Cough Syrup (brompheniramine maleate 2 mg/5 mL pseudoephedrine HCl 30 mg/5 mL dextromethorphan HBr 10 mg/5 mL)	OTC
0242	Carbamazepine Chewable Tablets, 100 mg	℞
0938	Cephalexin Capsules, USP 250 mg	℞
0939	Cephalexin Capsules, USP 500 mg	℞
2375	Cephalexin for Oral Suspension, USP 125 mg/5 mL	℞
2376	Cephalexin for Oral Suspension, USP 250 mg/5 mL	℞
0808	Cephradine Capsules, USP 250 mg	℞
0809	Cephradine Capsules, USP 500 mg	℞
0443	Clonidine HCl Tablets, USP 0.1 mg	℞
0444	Clonidine HCl Tablets, USP 0.2 mg	℞
0445	Clonidine HCl Tablets, USP 0.3 mg	℞
0451	Clorazepate Dipotassium Tablets 3.75 mg	℞
0452	Clorazepate Dipotassium Tablets 7.5 mg	℞
0453	Clorazepate Dipotassium Tablets 15 mg	℞
0949	Cloxacillin Sodium Capsules, USP 250 mg	℞
0950	Cloxacillin Sodium Capsules, USP 500 mg	℞
2995	Cloxacillin for Oral Solution 125 mg/5 mL	℞
4119	Cyanocobalamin Injection, USP	℞
	Cyclobenzaprine Tablets 10 mg	℞
3998	DermUspray™	℞
0594	Desipramine Tablets 25 mg	℞
0595	Desipramine Tablets 50 mg	℞
0596	Desipramine Tablets 75 mg	℞
0141	Diazepam Tablets, USP 2 mg	ℭ/℞
0142	Diazepam Tablets, USP 5 mg	ℭ/℞
0143	Diazepam Tablets, USP 10 mg	ℭ/℞
0945	Dicloxacillin Sodium Capsules, USP 250 mg	℞
0946	Dicloxacillin Sodium Capsules, USP 500 mg	℞
0247	Docusate Sodium Capsules, USP (D-S-S)	OTC
0248	Docusate Sodium with Casanthranol Capsules (D-S-S Plus)	OTC
2623	Doxepin HCl Oral Solution 10 mg/mL	℞
0829	Doxycycline Hyclate Capsules, USP 50 mg	℞
0830	Doxycycline Hyclate Capsules, USP 100 mg	℞
0813	Doxycycline Hyclate Tablets, USP 100 mg	℞
0850	Duraquin® Tablets (quinidine gluconate)	℞
0081	Fenoprofen Calcium Capsules 300 mg	℞
0077	Fenoprofen Calcium Tablets 600 mg	℞
0988	Flurazepam HCl Capsules, USP 15 mg	ℭ/℞
0989	Flurazepam HCl Capsules, USP 30 mg	ℭ/℞
0440	Furosemide Tablets, USP 20 mg	℞
0441	Furosemide Tablets, USP 40 mg	℞
0442	Furosemide Tablets, USP 80 mg	℞
2913	Haloperidol Concentrate (haloperidol oral solution, USP) 2 mg/mL	℞
	Hydrocodone w/APAP 5.0/500 mg	ℭ/℞
2902	Hydroxyzine Syrup	℞
0516	Ibuprofen Tablets, 400 mg	℞
0922	Ibuprofen Tablets, 600 mg	℞
0914	Ibuprofen Tablets, 800 mg	℞
0887	Indomethacin Capsules, USP 25 mg	℞
0888	Indomethacin Capsules, USP 50 mg	℞
0875	Indomethacin Extended-Release Capsules, USP 75 mg	℞
0431	Lorazepam Tablets 0.5 mg	ℭ/℞
0432	Lorazepam Tablets 1 mg	ℭ/℞
0433	Lorazepam Tablets 2 mg	ℭ/℞
0621	Loxapine Capsules 5 mg	℞
0632	Loxapine Capsules 10 mg	℞
0650	Loxapine Capsules 25 mg	℞
0651	Loxapine Capsules 50 mg	℞
0790	Maprotiline Tablets 25 mg	℞
0791	Maprotiline Tablets 50 mg	℞
0795	Maprotiline Tablets 75 mg	℞
0874	Medroxyprogesterone Tablets 10 mg	℞
0865	Methyldopa Tablets, USP 250 mg	℞
0866	Methyldopa Tablets, USP 500 mg	℞
0030	Methyldopa and Hydrochlorothiazide Tablets, USP 250 mg/15 mg	℞
0031	Methyldopa and Hydrochlorothiazide Tablets, USP 250 mg/25 mg	℞
0032	Methyldopa and Hydrochlorothiazide Tablets, USP 500 mg/30 mg	℞
0033	Methyldopa and Hydrochlorothiazide Tablets, USP 500 mg/50 mg	℞
2996	Metoclopramide HCl Syrup 5 mg/5 mL	℞
0878	Metoclopramide HCl Tablets 10 mg	℞
0615	Minocycline HCl Capsules 50 mg	℞
0616	Minocycline HCl Capsules 100 mg	℞
0930/ 0927	Nelova™ 1/35E (norethindrone 1 mg and ethinyl estradiol 35 mcg)	℞
0929/ 0926	Nelova™ 0.5/35E (norethindrone 0.5 mg and ethinyl estradiol 35 mcg)	℞
0941/ 0944	Nelova™ 10/11	℞
0942/ 0947	Nelova™ 1/50M (norethindrone 1 mg and mestranol 50 mcg)	℞
0078	Nifedipine Capsules 10 mg	℞
0079	Nifedipine Capsules 20 mg	℞
2922	Nystatin Oral Suspension, USP	℞
0690	Oxazepam Capsules 10 mg	ℭ/℞
0665	Oxazepam Capsules 15 mg	ℭ/℞
0667	Oxazepam Capsules 30 mg	ℭ/℞
0551	Oxazepam Tablets, USP 15 mg	ℭ/℞
0648	Penicillin V Potassium Tablets, USP 250 mg	℞
0673	Penicillin V Potassium Tablets, USP 500 mg	℞
2449	Penicillin VK for Oral Solution, USP 125 mg/ 5 mL	℞
2506	Penicillin VK for Oral Solution, USP 250 mg/5 mL	℞
0699	Phenobarbital Tablets, USP 15 mg	ℭ/℞
0700	Phenobarbital Tablets, USP 30 mg	ℭ/℞
0607	Phenobarbital Tablets, USP 60 mg	ℭ/℞
0698	Phenobarbital Tablets, USP 100 mg	ℭ/℞
0951	Potassium Chloride Extended-Release Tablets, USP 8 mEq (600 mg)	℞
0843	Prazosin Capsules 1 mg	℞
0844	Prazosin Capsules 2 mg	℞
0845	Prazosin Capsules 5 mg	℞

Continued on next page

Warner Chilcott—Cont.

2890 Promethazine VC with Codeine Ⓒ/℞
0980 Propoxyphene Napsylate and Acetaminophen Ⓒ/℞
Tablets, USP 100 mg/650 mg
0070 Propranolol HCl Tablets, USP 10 mg ℞
0071 Propranolol HCl Tablets, USP 20 mg ℞
0072 Propranolol HCl Tablets, USP 40 mg ℞
0073 Propranolol HCl Tablets, USP 60 mg ℞
0074 Propranolol HCl Tablets, USP 80 mg ℞
0014 Propranolol HCl and Hydrochlorothiazide ℞
Tablets 40 mg/25 mg
0015 Propranolol HCl and Hydrochlorothiazide ℞
Tablets 80 mg/25 mg
0617 Quinidine Gluconate Tablets 324 mg ℞
0849 Quinidine Sulfate Tablets, USP ℞
0420 Quinine Sulfate Capsules, USP OTC
2885 R-Tannate Pediatric Suspension ℞
0940 R-Tannate Tablets ℞
phenylephrine tannate 25 mg
chlorpheniramine tannate 8 mg
pyrilamine tannate 25 mg
0773 Sulindac Tablets, USP 150 mg ℞
0774 Sulindac Tablets, USP 200 mg ℞
2903 Sulfamethoxazole and Trimethoprim ℞
Oral Suspension, USP
0977 Temazepam Capsules, 15 mg Ⓒ/℞
0978 Temazepam Capsules, 30 mg Ⓒ/℞
0407 Tetracycline HCl Capsules, USP 250 mg ℞
0697 Tetracycline HCl Capsules, USP 500 mg ℞
0657 Theophylline Controlled-Release ℞
Tablets 100 mg
0659 Theophylline Controlled-Release ℞
Tablets 200 mg
0592 Theophylline Controlled-Release ℞
Tablets 300 mg
2912 Theophylline Elixir, 80 mg/15 mL ℞
0835 Transdermal-NTG ℞
(nitroglycerin transdermal system) 0.2 mg/hour
0837 Transdermal-NTG ℞
(nitroglycerin transdermal system) 0.4 mg/hour
0577 Trazodone HCl Tablets 50 mg ℞
0578 Trazodone HCl Tablets 100 mg ℞
0716 Trazodone HCl Tablets 150 mg ℞
0833 Triamterene and Hydrochlorothiazide ℞
Tablets, 75 mg/50 mg
2935 Trifluoperazine HCl Syrup, ℞
USP (Concentrate) 10 mg/mL
3122 Unibase OTC
0557 Verapamil HCl Tablets 80 mg ℞
0573 Verapamil HCl Tablets 120 mg ℞

Webcon Pharmaceuticals

Division of
ALCON (Puerto Rico) INC.
P.O. BOX 3000
HUMACAO, PUERTO RICO 00661

SUPPRETTES®, Webcon's identifying trademark for suppository medication in the NEOCERA® base, a unique blend of water-soluble Carbowaxes* that release drugs by hydrophilic action.
*TM Union Carbide.

ANESTACON® ℞
(2% lidocaine hydrochloride viscous solution for topical use)

DESCRIPTION

A sterile anesthetic for endourethral use. Each mL contains: Active: Lidocaine Hydrochloride 20 mg (2%). Vehicle: Hydroxypropyl Methylcellulose 10 mg (1%). Preservative: Benzalkonium Chloride 0.1 mg (0.01%). Inactive: Sodium Chloride, Hydrochloric Acid and/or Sodium Hydroxide (to adjust pH), Purified Water. DM-00

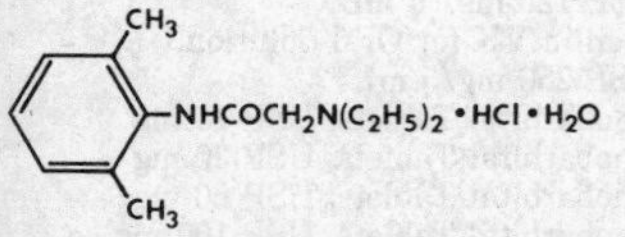

Established Name: Lidocaine Hydrocloride
Chemical Name: 2-(diethylamino)-N-(2,6-dimethylphenyl) acetamide monohydrochloride monohydrate

CLINICAL PHARMACOLOGY

Mechanism of Action: Lidocaine HCl acts on surface mucous membranes of the urethra to produce local anesthesia by altering the permeability of the nerve cell membrane to sodium and potassium ions, resulting in an increased threshold for electrical excitability and a decreased conduction of impulses whereby depolarization and ion exchanges are inhibited. The anesthetic effect usually begins within two to five minutes and lasts for at least 15 minutes.

HEMODYNAMICS

Excessive blood levels may cause changes in cardiac output, total peripheral resistance, and mean arterial pressure. These changes may be attributable to a direct depressant effect of the local anesthetic agent on various components of the cardiovascular system. The net effect is normally a modest hypotension when the recommended dosages are not exceeded.

PHARMACOKINETICS AND METABOLISM

Lidocaine is absorbed following topical administration to mucous membranes, its rate and extent of absorption being dependent upon concentration and total dose administered, the specific site of application, and duration of exposure. In general, the rate of absorption of local anesthetic agents following topical application occurs most rapidly after intratracheal administration. Lidocaine is also well-absorbed from the urethra, but little intact drug appears in the circulation because of biotransformation in the liver.

The plasma binding of lidocaine is dependent on drug concentration, and the fraction bound decreases with increasing concentration. At concentrations of 1 to 4 μg of free base per mL, 60 to 80 percent of lidocaine is protein bound. Binding is also dependent on the plasma concentration of the alpha-1-acid glycoprotein.

Lidocaine crosses the blood-brain and placental barriers, presumably by passive diffusion.

Lidocaine is metabolized rapidly by the liver, and metabolites and unchanged drug are excreted by the kidneys. Biotransformation includes oxidative N-dealkylation, ring hydroxylation, cleavage of the amide linkage, and conjugation. N-dealkylation, a major pathway of biotransformation, yields the metabolites monoethylglycinexylidide and glycinexylidide. The pharmacological/toxicological actions of these metabolites are similar to, but less potent than, those of lidocaine. Approximately 90% of lidocaine administered is excreted in the form of various metabolites, and less than 10% is excreted unchanged. The primary metabolite in urine is a conjugate of 4-hydroxy-2, 6-dimethylaniline.

The elimination half-life of lidocaine following an intravenous bolus injection is typically 1.5 to 2.0 hours. Because of the rapid rate at which lidocaine is metabolized, any condition that affects liver function may alter lidocaine kinetics. The half-life may be prolonged two-fold or more in patients with liver dysfunction. Renal dysfunction does not affect lidocaine kinetics but may increase the accumulation of metabolites.

Factors such as acidosis and the use of CNS stimulants and depressants affect the CNS levels of lidocaine required to produce overt systemic effects. Objective adverse manifestations become increasingly apparent with increasing venous plasma levels above 6.0 μg free base per mL. In the rhesus monkey arterial blood levels of 18–21 μg/mL have been shown to be threshold for convulsive activity.

INDICATIONS AND USAGE

For prevention and control of pain in procedures involving the male and female urethra and for topical treatment of painful urethritis.

CONTRAINDICATIONS

Contraindicated in patients with a known sensitivity (allergy) to lidocaine or other drugs of a similar chemical nature, or to other components of the formulation.

WARNINGS

EXCESSIVE DOSAGE, OR SHORT INTERVALS BETWEEN DOSES, CAN RESULT IN HIGH PLASMA LEVELS AND SERIOUS ADVERSE EFFECTS. PATIENTS SHOULD BE INSTRUCTED TO STRICTLY ADHERE TO THE RECOMMENDED DOSAGE AND ADMINISTRATION GUIDELINES AS SET FORTH IN THIS PACKAGE INSERT.

THE MANAGEMENT OF SERIOUS ADVERSE REACTIONS MAY REQUIRE THE USE OF RESUSCITATIVE EQUIPMENT, OXYGEN, AND OTHER RESUSCITATIVE DRUGS.

LIDOCAINE SHOULD BE USED WITH EXTREME CAUTION ON TRAUMATIZED MUCOSA OR IN A REGION OF SEPSIS. **NOT FOR OPHTHALMIC USE OR INJECTION.**

NOTE: After initial use of the 15 mL single-dose container, the remaining contents of the container should be discarded. The 240 mL container should be used for only an individual patient. See CAUTION under DOSAGE AND ADMINISTRATION.

PRECAUTIONS

General: The safety and effectiveness of lidocaine depend on proper dosage, correct technique, adequate precautions, and readiness for emergencies (See WARNINGS and ADVERSE REACTIONS). The lowest dosage that results in effective anesthesia should be used to avoid high plasma levels and serious adverse effects. Repeated doses of lidocaine may cause significant increases in blood levels with each repeated dose because of slow accumulation of the drug and/or its metabolites. Tolerance varies with the status of the patient. Debilitated, elderly patients, acutely ill patients, and children should be given reduced doses commensurate with their age, weight and physical condition. Lidocaine should also be used with caution in patients with severe shock or heart block. ANESTACON should be used with caution in persons with known drug sensitivities. Patients allergic to para-aminobenzoic acid derivatives (procaine, tetracaine, benzocaine, etc.) are not likely to show cross sensitivity to lidocaine.

PATIENTS SHOULD BE INSTRUCTED TO STRICTLY ADHERE TO DOSING INSTRUCTIONS, AND TO KEEP THE SUPPLY OF MEDICATION OUT OF THE REACH OF CHILDREN.

CARCINOGENESIS, MUTAGENESIS, IMPAIRMENT OF FERTILITY: Studies of lidocaine in animals to evaluate the carcinogenic and mutagenic potential or the effect on fertility have not been conducted.

PREGNANCY CATEGORY C: Animal reproduction studies have not been conducted with ANESTACON®. It is also not known whether ANESTACON can cause fetal harm when administered to a pregnant woman or can affect reproduction capacity. ANESTACON should be administered to a pregnant woman only if clearly needed.

NURSING MOTHERS: It is not known whether this drug is excreted in human milk. Because many drugs are excreted in human milk, caution should be exercised when ANESTACON is administered to a nursing mother.

ADVERSE REACTIONS

Adverse experiences following the administration of lidocaine are similar in nature to those observed with other amide local anesthetic agents. These adverse experiences are, in general, dose-related and may result from high plasma levels caused by excessive dosage or rapid absorption, or may result from a hypersensitivity, idiosyncrasy or diminished tolerance on the part of the patient. Serious adverse experiences are generally systemic in nature. The following types are those most commonly reported:

CENTRAL NERVOUS SYSTEM: CNS manifestations are excitatory and/or depressant and may be characterized by light-headedness, nervousness, apprehension, euphoria, confusion, dizziness, drowsiness, tinnitus, blurred or double vision, vomiting, sensations of heat, cold or numbness, twitching, tremors, convulsions, unconsciousness, respiratory depression and arrest. The excitatory manifestations may be very brief or may not occur at all, in which case manifestation of toxicity may be drowsiness merging into unconsciousness and respiratory arrest.

Drowsiness following the administration of lidocaine is usually an early sign of a high blood level of the drug and may occur as a consequence of rapid absorption.

CARDIOVASCULAR SYSTEM: Cardiovascular manifestations are usually depressant and are characterized by bradycardia, hypotension, and cardiovascular collapse, which may lead to cardiac arrest.

ALLERGIC: Allergic reactions are characterized by cutaneous lesions of delayed onset, urticaria, edema or other manifestations of allergy. Allergic reactions as a result of sensitivity to lidocaine are rare and, if they occur, should be managed by conventional means. The detection of sensitivity by skin testing is of doubtful value.

OVERDOSAGE

Acute emergencies from local anesthetics are generally related to high plasma levels encountered during therapeutic use of local anesthetics. (See ADVERSE REACTIONS, WARNINGS, and PRECAUTIONS.)

DOSAGE AND ADMINISTRATION

Dosage varies and depends upon the area to be anesthetized, vascularity of the tissues, individual tolerance, and the technique of anesthesia. The least volume of the drug needed to provide effective anesthesia should be administered. For specific techniques and procedures refer to standard texts. Avoid forceful injection in the presence of known stricture, as this may cause intravascular injection. THE USUAL ADULT DOSE SHOULD NOT EXCEED 600 mg OR 30 mL OF ANESTACON IN ANY TWELVE HOUR PERIOD. THE **CHILD** DOSE SHOULD BE REDUCED COMMENSURATE WITH AGE, WEIGHT AND PHYSICAL CONDITION.

15 ML SINGLE-DOSE CONTAINER: ADULT MALES: Immediately before use, remove the label and cap and firmly insert the sterile tip into the urethral orifice. Slowly instill 5 mL to 15 mL by exerting pressure on opposite sides of the container—the full dose should be administered in a single action without removing the tip. While waiting two to five minutes for induction of anesthesia, the urethra should be occluded with a penile clamp or by manual compression. ADULT FEMALES: The sterile tip may be used to insert about 1 mL.

240 ML CONTAINER: This is for use for an individual patient only. CAUTION: Care should be taken to prevent con-

tamination of bottle contents (e.g., aspiration of urethral contents into the container when using insertion tip). **ADULT MALES:** Instill slowly into the urethra 5 mL to 15 mL and allow two to five minutes for induction of anesthesia. Optimal anesthesia is attained after 5 minutes. The medication is retained in the urethra by means of a penile clamp or by manual compression of the distal urethra. **ADULT FEMALES:** Apply liberal amount of medication on a cotton swab and insert into urethra for two to five minutes, or a dropper may be employed to insert about 1 mL.

STORAGE
Store at room temperature.

HOW SUPPLIED
In 15 mL single-dose and 240 mL multiple-dose disposable containers for single patient use.
STRENGTH: 2% (20 mg/mL) Lidocaine Hydrochloride
15 mL: **NDC** 0998-0300-10
240 mL: **NDC** 0998-0300-20

A URICEUTICAL® Specialty of
WEBCON™
Mfd. for: ALCON (Puerto Rico) INC.
Humacao, P.R. 00661
Mfd. by: Alcon Laboratories, Inc.
Fort Worth, Texas 76134 USA

B & O SUPPRETTES®   C II R
No. 15A and No. 16A
(Belladonna and Opium) Rectal Suppositories

DESCRIPTION
Each B&O SUPPRETTE® contains (in the water-soluble NEOCERA® Suppository Base for rectal administration):
B&O No. 15A: Powdered opium* 30 mg (½ gr) and Powdered Belladonna Extract 16.2 mg (equivalent to 0.21 mg or 0.0035 gr alkaloid of belladonna).
B&O No. 16A: Powdered opium* 60 mg (1 gr) and Powdered Belladonna Extract 16.2 mg (equivalent to 0.21 mg or 0.0035 gr alkaloid of belladonna).
NEOCERA® Base is a blend of Polyethylene Glycol 400, 1450, 8000 and Polysorbate 60.
This drug falls into the pharmacologic/therapeutic class of narcotic analgesic/antispasmotic agents.
The pharmacologically active principles present in the belladonna extract component of B&O SUPPRETTES are:

Established Name: Atropine
Chemical Name: dl Tropyl Tropate

Established Name: Scopolamine
Chemical Name: dl Scopolamine

Opium contains more than a score of alkaloids, the principal ones being morphine (10%), narcotine (6%), papaverine (1%) and codeine (0.5%). The major pharmacologically active principle of the powdered opium component of B&O SUPPRETTES, however is:

Established Name: Morphine
Chemical Name: 7,8-Didehydro-4,5-epoxy-17-methyl-morphinan-3,6-diol

CLINICAL PHARMACOLOGY
Through its parasympatholytic action, atropine relaxes smooth muscle resulting from parasympathetic stimulation. It is the dl isomer of l-hyoscyamine and therefore exhibits the same clinical effects. It is, however, approximately one-half as active peripherally as l-hyoscyamine, the latter being the major active plant alkaloid. The dl isomer atropine is

*See "Warnings".

---

formed during the process of isolation of the belladonna extract.[1]
Morphine, the major active principle of powdered opium, is responsible for the action of powdered opium although the other alkaloids present also contribute to it. The sedative and analgesic action of morphine, the effect desired by inclusion in B&O SUPPRETTES of powdered opium, are thought to be due to its depressant effect on the cerebral cortex, hypothalamus and medullary centers. In large doses, the opiates and their analogs also inhibit synaptic conduction in the spinothalamic tracts, depress the function of the reticular formation, the lemniscus and the thalamic relays, and inhibit spinal synaptic reflexes; but these inhibitor actions are not elicited with therapeutic doses of the drug. Moderate doses of powdered opium should not alter the electroencephalogram.
The action of morphine consists mainly of a descending depression of the central nervous system. It exerts its analgesic action by increasing the pain threshold or the magnitude of stimulus required to evoke pain and by dulling the sensibility or reaction to pain. In addition to its action in abolishing pain, morphine induces a sense of well-being (euphoria) facilitating certain mental processes while retarding others. Upon absorption of morphine, oxidative dealkylation to produce nor-compounds appears to be the first step in the reaction sequence which imparts analgesia. Morphine is conjugated in the liver to form the 3-glucuronide which passes into the bile and is reabsorbed and excreted in the urine. The atropine effect of the belladonna extract serves to eliminate morphine induced smooth muscle spasm without affecting the sedative analgesic action of powdered opium.[2]

INDICATIONS AND USAGE
B&O SUPPRETTES are used for relief of moderate to severe pain associated with ureteral spasm not responsive to non-narcotic analgesics and to space intervals between injections of opiates.

CONTRAINDICATIONS
Do not use B&O SUPPRETTES in patients suffering from glaucoma, severe hepatic or renal disease, bronchial asthma, narcotic idiosyncrasies, respiratory depression, convulsive disorders, acute alcoholism, delirium tremens and premature labor.

WARNINGS
True addiction may result from opium usage. These preparations are not recommended for use in children.

PRECAUTIONS
Administer with caution to persons with a known idiosyncrasy to atropine or atropine-like compounds; to persons known to be sensitive to or addicted to morphine or morphine-like drugs; to persons with cardiac disease, incipient glaucoma or prostatic hypertrophy. Caution should be used in the administration of this drug to old and debilitated patients and patients with increased intracranial pressure, toxic psychosis and myxedema.
Pregnancy Category C. Animal studies have not been conducted with B&O SUPPRETTES. It is also not known whether B&O SUPPRETTES 15A and 16A can affect reproduction capacity. The active principles of B&O SUPPRETTES, atropine and morphine, are known to enter the fetal circulation. Regular use of opium alkaloids during pregnancy has resulted in addiction of the fetus leading to withdrawal symptoms in the neonate. B&O SUPPRETTES therefore should be used by a pregnant woman with caution and only when clearly indicated.
Nursing Mothers: It is not known whether this drug is excreted in human milk. Because many drugs are excreted in human milk, caution should be exercised when B&O SUPPRETTES are administered to a nursing woman.

ADVERSE REACTIONS
Belladonna may cause drowsiness, dry mouth, urinary retention, photophobia, rapid pulse, dizziness and blurred vision. Opium usage may result in constipation, nausea or vomiting. Pruritis and urticaria may occasionally occur.

DRUG ABUSE AND DEPENDENCE
Because of their content of opium, B&O SUPPRETTES are considered as Schedule II drugs by the Drug Enforcement Administration. No data exists on chronic abuse effects or dependence characteristics of B&O SUPPRETTES.

OVERDOSAGE
As with morphine and related narcotics, overdosage is characterized by respiratory depression, pinpoint pupils and coma. Respiratory depression may be reversed by intravenous administration of naloxone hydrochloride. In addition, supportive measures such as oxygenation, intravenous fluids and vasopressors should be used as indicated. As with atropine derivatives, hot, dry, flushed skin; dry mouth and hyperpyrexia may occur.

1. Gilman, A. G., Goodman, L. S. & Gilman, A. 6th Edition, *The Pharmacological Basis of Therapeutics*, MacMillan Pub. Co., N.Y. 1980, pp. 121-127.
2. Ibid, pp. 494-513.

DOSAGE AND ADMINISTRATION
Adults: One B&O SUPPRETTE No. 15A or No. 16A rectally once or twice daily, not to exceed four doses daily or as recommended by the physician. Moisten finger and SUPPRETTE with water before inserting. Not recommended for use in children 12 and under. Absorption is dependent on body hydration and not on body temperature. Store at room temperature. DO NOT refrigerate.

HOW SUPPLIED
In strip packaged units of 12 (scored for ½ dosage), DEA order required (Schedule II).
B&O SUPPRETTES No. 15A NDC 0998-5015-75.
B&O SUPPRETTES No. 16A NDC 0998-5016-75.
WEBCON™
ALCON (Puerto Rico) INC.
Humacao, Puerto Rico 00661

CYSTOSPAZ®   R
(hyoscyamine) Tablets
CYSTOSPAZ-M®   R
(hyoscyamine sulfate) Timed-Release Capsules

DESCRIPTION
CYSTOSPAZ® is a pale blue uncoated compressed tablet for oral administration. It contains the parasympatholytic agent hyoscyamine as the free base. Each tablet contains: Active: hyoscyamine 0.15 mg. Inactive: FD&C Blue No. 2, Lactose, Magnesium Stearate, Povidone, Starch and Talc. CYSTOSPAZ-M® is a light blue timed-release capsule containing hyoscyamine sulfate 0.375 mg.

Established name:
Hyoscyamine
Chemical name:
λ tropyl tropate

CLINICAL PHARMACOLOGY
Through its parasympatholytic action, hyoscyamine relaxes smooth muscle spasm resulting from parasympathetic stimulation. It is the λ-isomer of atropine and therefore exhibits the same clinical effects as atropine. It is, however, approximately twice as active peripherally as atropine, since the latter is the racemic (dλ) form of hyoscyamine and d-hyoscyamine possesses only a very weak anti-cholinergic action. Since only one-half the atropine dose is required for λ-hyoscyamine, it has only one-half the unwanted central effects of atropine.[1]

INDICATIONS AND USAGE
In the management of disorders of the lower urinary tract associated with hypermotility. Although specific therapy is often required to remove the underlying cause of spasm, CYSTOSPAZ Tablets and CYSTOSPAZ-M Capsules are offered as antispasmodic agent dosage forms which may be combined with other forms of therapy where indicated.

CONTRAINDICATIONS
Glaucoma, urinary bladder neck or pyloric obstruction, duodenal obstruction and cardiospasm. Hypersensitivity to any of the ingredients.

PRECAUTIONS
Administer with caution to persons with known idiosyncrasy to atropine-like compounds and to patients suffering cardiac disease.
Pregnancy Category C—Animal reproduction studies have not been conducted with CYSTOSPAZ Tablets or CYSTOSPAZ-M Capsules. It is also not known whether CYSTOSPAZ Tablets or CYSTOSPAZ-M Capsules can cause fetal harm when administered to a pregnant woman or can affect reproduction capacity. CYSTOSPAZ Tablets and CYSTOSPAZ-M Capsules should be taken by a pregnant woman only if clearly needed.
Nursing Mothers—It is not known whether this drug is excreted in human milk. Because many drugs are excreted in human milk, caution should be exercised when CYSTOSPAZ® Tablets or CYSTOSPAZ-M® Capsules are administered to a nursing woman.

ADVERSE REACTIONS
The side effects encountered with this class of antispasmodic-antisecretory agents (drowsiness, dryness of the mouth, photophobia, constipation, urinary retention and allergic reactions) may also be seen with this drug. If rapid pulse, dizziness or blurring of vision occurs, discontinue use immediately. Acute urinary retention may be precipitated in

Continued on next page

Webcon—Cont.

prostatic hypertrophy. **Note:** Slight dryness of the mouth is an indication that parasympathetic blockage is effective.

DRUG ABUSE AND DEPENDENCE

A dependence on the use of CYSTOSPAZ Tablets or CYSTOSPAZ-M Capsules has not been reported and due to the nature of their ingredients, abuse of CYSTOSPAZ Tablets or CYSTOSPAZ-M Capsules is not expected.

OVERDOSAGE

Symptoms of overdosage include severe dryness of the mouth, nose, throat, and hot dry flushed skin, hyperpyrexia (especially in children), difficulty or inability to swallow, difficult speech, dilated pupils until iris almost disappears, restlessness and garrulity indicating an irritability of the brain, marked tremors, convulsions, respiratory failure, death.[1] In adults, symptoms of overdosage may begin in the range of ingestion of 0.6 to 1 mg with doses exceeding 1–2 mg eliciting more profound toxicity.

DOSAGE AND ADMINISTRATION

Adults: CYSTOSPAZ Tablets—One or two tablets four times daily or fewer if needed. CYSTOSPAZ-M Capsules—One capsule every twelve hours.
Children (12 and under): Reduce dosage in proportion to age and weight.

HOW SUPPLIED

CYSTOSPAZ Tablets— Bottles of 100 light blue tablets **NDC 0998-2225-10.** Tablets are imprinted with a "**W 2225**". CYSTOSPAZ-M Capsules—Bottles of 100 light blue timed-release capsules **NDC 0998-2260-10.** Capsules are identified with "**W 2260**" printed in black.

STORAGE

Store in a dry place at room temperature.

REFERENCES

1. Gilman, A. L., Goodman, L.S. & Gilman, A., *The Pharmacological Basis of Therapeutics*, 6th Edition, p. 127.
CYSTOSPAZ-M Capsules are manufactured by:
K. V. Pharmaceutical Company
St. Louis, Mo. 63144
A URICEUTICAL® Specialty of
WEBCON™
ALCON (Puerto Rico) INC.
Humacao, Puerto Rico 00661

URISED®   ℞

DESCRIPTION

URISED® is a purple, round, sugar coated tablet for oral administration. It is a combination of antiseptics (Methenamine, Methylene Blue, Phenyl Salicylate, Benzoic Acid) and parasympatholytics (Atropine Sulfate, Hyoscyamine). The active ingredients are represented by the chemical structures:

Established name:
Methenamine
Chemical name:
Hexamethylenetetramine

Established name:
Phenyl Salicylate
Chemical name:
2-Hydroxybenzoic acid phenyl ester

Established name:
Methylene Blue
Chemical name:
Methylthionine chloride

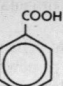

Established name:
Benzoic Acid
Chemical name:
Benzenecarboxylic acid

Established name:
AtropineSulfate
Chemical name:
***dl* tropyl tropate**

Established name:
Hyoscyamine
Chemical name:
***l*-tropyl tropate**

Each tablet contains: Methenamine 40.8 mg, Phenyl Salicylate 18.1 mg, Methylene Blue 5.4 mg, Benzoic Acid 4.5 mg, Atropine Sulfate 0.03 mg and Hyoscyamine 0.03 mg.

CLINICAL PHARMACOLOGY

Methenamine itself does not have antiseptic, irritant, or toxic properties in the urine. Methenamine, in an acid urine (pH 6 or below), hydrolyzes into formaldehyde within the urinary tract providing mild antiseptic activity[1]. When given as directed and the daily urine volume is 1000 to 1500 mL, a daily dose of 2 grams will yield a urinary concentration of 18–60 mcg/mL of free formaldehyde in the urine. This is more than the minimal inhibitory dose of formaldehyde which must be available for most urinary tract pathogens. Methenamine is readily absorbed from the gastrointestinal tract and is rapidly excreted almost entirely in the urine. Methylene Blue and Benzoic Acid are mild but effective antiseptics which contribute to the antiseptic properties of Methenamine. Phenyl Salicylate is a mild analgesic and antipyretic with weak antiseptic activity. All of these compounds are readily absorbed from the gastrointestinal tract and excreted in the urine. Through parasympatholytic action, atropine and hyoscyamine relax smooth muscle spasms resulting from parasympathetic stimulation.[2]

INDICATIONS AND USAGE

URISED is indicated for the relief of discomfort of the lower urinary tract caused by hypermotility resulting from inflammation or diagnostic procedures and in the treatment of cystitis, urethritis, and trigonitis when caused by organisms which maintain or produce an acid urine and are susceptible to formaldehyde.

CONTRAINDICATIONS

Glaucoma, urinary bladder neck obstruction, pyloric or duodenal obstruction, or cardiospasm. Hypersensitivity to any of the ingredients.

WARNINGS

Do not exceed recommended dose. Methenamine may combine with sulfonamides in the urine to give mutual antagonism and should not be used with sulfonamides.

PRECAUTIONS

Administer with caution to persons with known idiosyncrasy to atropine-like compounds and to patients suffering from cardiac disease. Bacteriological studies of the urine may be helpful in following the patient response. Methylene Blue interferes with the analysis for some urinary components such as free formaldehyde. Drugs and/or foods which produce an alkaline urine should be restricted.[3]
Patient should be advised that the urine may become blue to blue-green and the feces may be discolored as a result of excretion of Methylene Blue. Methenamine preparations should not be given to patients taking sulfonamides since insoluble precipitates may form with formaldehyde in the urine. No known long-term animal studies have been performed to evaluate carcinogenic potential.
Pregnancy Category C. Animal reproduction studies have not been conducted with URISED® tablets. It is also not known whether URISED tablets can cause fetal harm when

---

administered to a pregnant woman or can affect reproduction capacity. URISED tablets should be given to a pregnant woman only if clearly needed.
Nursing Mothers: It is not known whether this drug is excreted in human milk. Because many drugs are excreted in human milk, caution should be exercised when URISED tablets are administered to a nursing woman.
Prolonged Use: There have been no studies to establish the safety of prolonged use in humans.

ADVERSE REACTIONS

Prolonged use may result in a generalized skin rash, pronounced dryness of the mouth, flushing, difficulty in initiating micturition, rapid pulse, dizziness or blurring of vision. If any of these reactions occurs, discontinue use immediately. Acute urinary retention may be precipitated in prostatic hypertrophy. See "OVERDOSAGE."

DRUG ABUSE AND DEPENDENCE

A dependence on the use of URISED has not been reported and due to the nature of its ingredients, abuse of URISED is not expected.

OVERDOSAGE

By exceeding the recommended dosage of URISED, symptomology related to the overdose of its individual active ingredients may be expected as follows:
Atropine Sulfate, Hyoscyamine: Symptoms associated with an overdosage of URISED will most probably be manifested in the symptoms related to overdosage of the alkaloids Atropine Sulfate and Hyoscyamine. Such symptoms as dryness of mucous membranes; dilatation of pupils; hot, dry, flushed skin; hyperpyrexia; tachycardia; palpitations; elevated blood pressure; coma; circulatory collapse and death from respiratory failure can occur due to overdosage of these alkaloids.
Methenamine: If large amounts of the drug (2–8 gm daily) are used over extended periods (3–4 weeks), bladder and gastrointestinal irritation, painful and frequent micturition, albuminuria and gross hematuria may be expected.
Methylene Blue: Symptoms of Methylene Blue overdosage associated with the overdosage of URISED are not expected to be discernible from those associated with the other active ingredients in URISED.
Benzoic Acid: Symptoms of Benzoic Acid overdosage associated with the overdosage of URISED are not expected to be discernible from those associated with the other active ingredients in URISED.
Phenyl Salicylate: Symptoms of Phenyl Salicylate overdosage include burning pain in throat and mouth, white necrotic lesions in the mouth, abdominal pain, vomiting, bloody diarrhea, pallor, sweating, weakness, headache, dizziness and tinnitus. The symptoms, however, are not expected to be discernible from those associated with the other active ingredients in URISED.

DOSAGE AND ADMINISTRATION

Adults: Two tablets four times daily. See "PRECAUTIONS."
Usual pediatric dosage: Children up to 6 years of age—Use is not recommended. Children 6 years of age and older—Dosage must be individualized by physician.

HOW SUPPLIED

Bottles of 100 (NDC 0998-2183-10) and 500 (NDC 0998-2183-20) tablets. Tablets are imprinted with a "**W 2183**".

STORAGE

Store in a dry place at room temperature.

REFERENCES

1. Gollamudi, R., Straughn, A.B., and Meyer, M.C., "Urinary Excretion of Methenamine and Formaldehyde: Evaluation of 10 Methenamine Products in Humans," J. Pharm. Sci., 70, 596, 1981.
2. Goodman, L. S. and Gilman, G., *The Pharmacological Basis of Therapeutics*, Sixth Edition, Macmillan Pub. Co. 121, 971, 980, 1119 (1980).
3. *AMA Drug Evaluation*, Fifth Edition, 1745 (1983).
A URICEUTICAL® Specialty of
WEBCON™
Alcon (Puerto Rico) Inc.
Humacao, Puerto Rico 00661

Westwood-Squibb Pharmaceuticals Inc.
100 FOREST AVENUE
BUFFALO, NY 14213

CAPITROL®   ℞
(chloroxine 2%)
Shampoo

CAUTION
Federal law prohibits dispensing without a prescription.

DESCRIPTION
CAPITROL is an antibacterial shampoo containing 2% (w/w) chloroxine (each gram contains 20 mg chloroxine) suspended in a base of sodium octoxynol-2 ethane sulfonate, water, PEG-6 lauramide, dextrin, sodium lauryl sulfoacetate, sodium dioctyl sulfosuccinate, 1% benzyl alcohol, PEG-14M, magnesium aluminum silicate, fragrance, EDTA, and color. May contain citric acid to adjust pH.
Chloroxine is a synthetic antibacterial compound that is effective in the treatment of dandruff and seborrheic dermatitis when incorporated in a shampoo.
The chemical name of chloroxine is 5,7-dichloro-8-hydroxyquinoline. The chemical structure of chloroxine is:

CLINICAL PHARMACOLOGY
Well controlled studies demonstrate Capitrol effectively reduces the excess scaling in patients with dandruff or seborrheic dermatitis. Though the cause of dandruff is not known, it is thought to be the result of accelerated mitotic activity in the epidermis. The presumed mechanism of action to reduce scaling would be to slow down the mitotic activity.
The role of microbes in seborrheic dermatitis is not known; however, *Staphylococcus aureus* and *Pityrosporon* species are often present in increased numbers during the course of the disease. Chloroxine is antibacterial, inhibiting the growth of Gram-positive as well as some Gram-negative organisms. Antifungal activity against some dermatophytes and yeasts also has been shown.
The absorption, metabolism and pharmacokinetics of Capitrol in humans have not been studied.

INDICATIONS AND USAGE
Capitrol is indicated in the treatment of dandruff and mild-to-moderately severe seborrheic dermatitis of the scalp. Clinical studies indicate that improvement may be observed after 14 days of therapy.

CONTRAINDICATIONS
Capitrol is contraindicated in those patients with a history of hypersensitivity to any of the listed ingredients.

WARNINGS
Capitrol should not be used on acutely inflamed (exudative) lesions of the scalp.

PRECAUTIONS
Information for patients: Exercise care to prevent Capitrol from entering the eyes. If contact occurs, the patient should flush eyes with cool water. Discoloration of light-colored hair (e.g. blond, gray or bleached) may follow use of this preparation.
Irritation and a burning sensation on the scalp and adjacent areas have been reported.
Drug/Laboratory Test Interactions: There is no known interference of Capitrol with laboratory tests.
Carcinogenesis, Mutagenesis: No long term studies in animals have been performed to evaluate the carcinogenic potential of Capitrol.
Results of the *in vitro* Ames Salmonella/Microsome Plate test show that Capitrol does not demonstrate genetic activity and is considered non-mutagenic.
Pregnancy Category C: Animal reproduction studies have not be conducted with Capitrol. It is also not known whether Capitrol can cause fetal harm when administered to a pregnant woman or can affect reproduction capacity. Capitrol should be given to a pregnant woman only if clearly needed.
Nursing Mothers: It is not known whether this drug is excreted in human milk. Because many drugs are excreted in human milk, caution should be exercised when Capitrol is administered to a nursing woman.
Pediatric Use: Specific studies to demonstrate the safety and effectiveness for use of Capitrol in children have not been conducted.

ADVERSE REACTION
One patient out of 225 in clinical studies was reported to have contact dermatitis.

OVERDOSAGE
The acute oral LD_{50} in mice was found to be 200 mg/kg and in rats 450 mg/kg. On the basis of these animal studies, Capitrol may be considered practically non-toxic.

DOSAGE AND ADMINISTRATION
Capitrol should be massaged thoroughly onto the wet scalp, avoiding contact with the eyes. Lather should remain on the scalp for approximately three minutes, then rinsed. The application should be repeated and the scalp rinsed thoroughly. Two treatments per week are usually sufficient.

HOW SUPPLIED
Capitrol shampoo contains 2% (w/w) chloroxine (20 mg chloroxine per gram) and is supplied in 4 oz. plastic bottles (NDC 0072-6850-04).
Store at room temperature.

WATER BASE   ℞
DESQUAM-E™ 2.5 Emollient Gel
(2.5% benzoyl peroxide)

WATER BASE   ℞
DESQUAM-E™ 5 Emollient Gel
(5% benzoyl peroxide)

WATER BASE   ℞
DESQUAM-E™ 10 Emollient Gel
(10% benzoyl peroxide)

WATER BASE   ℞
DESQUAM-X® 2.5 Gel
(2.5% Benzoyl Peroxide)

WATER BASE   ℞
DESQUAM-X® 5 Gel
(5% Benzoyl Peroxide)

WATER BASE   ℞
DESQUAM-X® 10 Gel
(10% Benzoyl Peroxide)

WATER BASE   ℞
DESQUAM-X® 5 Wash
(5% benzoyl peroxide)

WATER BASE
DESQUAM-X 10 ® Wash
(10% benzoyl peroxide)

DESQUAM-X® 10 Bar   ℞
(10% benzoyl peroxide)

CAUTION
Federal law prohibits dispensing without prescription.

DESCRIPTION
DESQUAM-E 2.5, DESQUAM-E 5 and DESQUAM-E 10 brand topical anti-acne gels contain benzoyl peroxide (2.5, 5 and 10%) in a water-base vehicle of carbomer 940, diisopropanolamine, disodium edetate, docusate sodium, methyl gluceth-20 and polyquaternium-7.
DESQUAM-X 2.5, DESQUAM-X 5 and DESQUAM-X 10 brand topical anti-acne gels contain benzoyl peroxide (2.5, 5 and 10%), in a water-base vehicle of carbomer 940, disodium edetate and laureth-4. May contain diisopropanolamine or triethanolamine to adjust pH.
DESQUAM-X[5] and DESQUAM-X[10] brand topical therapeutic anti-acne cleansers contain benzoyl peroxide (5% and 10%) in a lathering water base of sodium octoxynol-3 sulfonate, dioctyl sodium sulfosuccinate, magnesium aluminum silicate, methylcellulose and EDTA.
DESQUAM-X10 brand therapeutic anti-acne BAR contains 10% benzoyl peroxide, boric acid, cellulose gum, dextrin (may contain wheat starch), disodium EDTA, docusate sodium, lactic acid, PEG-14M, sodium lauryl sulfoacetate (or sodium dodecyl benzene sulfonate and trisodium sulfosuccinate), sorbitol, urea and water.

Benzoyl Peroxide

CLINICAL PHARMACOLOGY
The effectiveness of benzoyl peroxide in the treatment of acne vulgaris is primarily attributable to its antibacterial activity, especially with respect to *Propionibacterium acnes*, the predominant organism in sebaceous follicles and comedones. The antibacterial activity of this compound is presumably due to the release of active or free-radical oxygen capable of oxidizing bacterial proteins. In acne patients treated topically with benzoyl peroxide, resolution of the acne usually coincides with reduction in the level of *P. acnes* and free fatty acids (FFA). Mild desquamation is another observed action of topically applied benzoyl peroxide and may also play a role in the drug's effectiveness in acne. Studies also indicate that topical benzoyl peroxide may exert a sebostatic effect with a resultant reduction of skin surface lipids. Benzoyl peroxide has been shown to be absorbed by the skin, where it is metabolized to benzoic acid and then excreted as benzoate in the urine.

INDICATIONS AND USAGE
DESQUAM-E (2..5, 5 or 10) EMOLLIENT GEL is indicated for the topical treatment of mild to moderate acne vulgaris and as an adjunct in therapeutic regimens including antibiotics, retinoic acid products and sulfur/salicylic acid-containing preparations. DESQUAM-E EMOLLIENT GEL has been shown effective in the treatment of the following acne lesion types: papules, pustules, open and closed comedones. Clinical studies have demonstrated therapeutic response after two to three weeks.
DESQUAM-X (2.5, 5 or 10) GEL is indicated for the topical treatment of mild to moderate acne vulgaris and as an adjunct in therapeutic regimens including antibiotics, retinoic acid products and sulfur/salicylic acid-containing preparations. DESQUAM-X GEL has been shown effective in the treatment of the following acne lesion types: papules, pustules, open and closed comedones. Clinical studies have demonstrated therapeutic response after two to three weeks. DESQUAM-X GEL may also be used as adjunctive treatment for nodulo-cystic acne (acne conglobata), although its effectiveness for this condition has not been proven.
DESQUAM-X (5 or 10) WASH is indicated for the topical treatment of mild to moderate acne. In more severe cases, it may be used as an adjunct in therapeutic regimens including benzoyl peroxide gels, antibiotics, retinoic acid products and sulfur/salicylic acid-containing preparations. The improvement of the treated condition is dependent on the degree and type of acne, the frequency of use of DESQUAM-X WASH and the nature of other therapies employed.
DESQUAM-X10 BAR is indicated for the topical treatment of acne. It may be used as an adjunct in therapeutic regimens including benzoyl peroxide gels, antibiotics, retinoic acid products and sulfur/salicylic acid-containing preparations. The improvement of the treated condition is dependent on the degree and type of acne, the frequency of use of DESQUAM-X10 BAR and the nature of other therapies employed.

CONTRAINDICATIONS
This product should not be used in patients known to be sensitive to benzoyl peroxide or any of the other listed ingredients.

PRECAUTIONS
General: Avoid contact with eyes and other mucous membranes. For external use only. In patients known to be sensitive to the following substances, there is a possibility of cross-sensitization: benzoic acid derivatives (including certain topical anesthetics) and cinnamon.
Information for Patients: This product may bleach colored fabric or hair. Concurrent use with PABA-containing sunscreens may result in transient discoloration of the skin.
Carcinogenesis, Mutagenesis, Impairment of Fertility: Based upon considerable evidence, benzoyl peroxide is not considered to be a carcinogen. However, in one study, using mice known to be highly susceptible to cancer, there was evidence for benzoyl peroxide as a tumor promoter. Benzoyl peroxide has been found to be inactive as a mutagen in the *Ames Salmonella* and other assays, including the mouse dominant lethal assay. This assay is frequently used to assess the effect of substances on spermatogenesis.
Pregnancy (Category C): Animal reproduction studies have not been conducted with benzoyl peroxide. It is also not known whether benzoyl peroxide can cause fetal harm when administered to a pregnant woman or can affect reproductive capacity. Benzoyl peroxide should be given to a pregnant woman only if clearly needed.
Nursing Mothers: It is not known whether this drug is excreted in human milk. Caution should be exercised when benzoyl peroxide is administered to a nursing woman.
Pediatric Use: Safety and effectiveness in children below the age of 12 have not been established.

ADVERSE REACTIONS
Adverse reactions which may be encountered with topical benzoyl peroxide include excessive drying (manifested by marked peeling, erythema and possible edema), and allergic contact sensitization.
Excessive dryness would appear to occur in approximately 2 patients in 50.
Pertinent literature indicates that allergic sensitization to benzoyl peroxide may occur in 10 to 25 patients in 1,000. There is one reference that reports an occurrence of sensitization in 5 of 100 patients.

Continued on next page

Westwood-Squibb—Cont.

OVERDOSAGE

In the event that excessive scaling, erythema or edema occur, the use of this preparation should be discontinued. If the reaction is judged to be due to excessive use and not allergenicity, after symptoms and signs subside, a reduced dosage schedule may be cautiously tried.

To hasten resolution of the adverse effects, emollients, cool compresses and/or topical corticosteroid preparations may be used.

DOSAGE AND ADMINISTRATION

DESQUAM-E EMOLLIENT GEL should be gently rubbed into all affected areas once or twice daily. Suitable cleansing of the affected area should precede application. In fair-skinned individuals or under excessively drying conditions, it is suggested that therapy be initiated with one application daily. The degree of drying or peeling may be controlled by modification of dose frequency or drug concentration. The use of DESQUAM-E EMOLLIENT GEL may be continued as long as deemed necessary.

DESQUAM-X GEL should be gently rubbed into all affected areas once or twice daily. Suitable cleansing of the affected area should precede application. In fair-skinned individuals or under excessively drying conditions, it is suggested that therapy be initiated with one application daily. The degree of drying or peeling may be controlled by modification of dose frequency or drug concentration. The use of DESQUAM-X GEL may be continued as long as deemed necessary.

DESQUAM-X (5 or 10) WASH—
Shake well before use. Wash affected areas once or twice daily, avoiding contact with eyes or mucous membranes. Wet skin areas to be treated prior to administration; apply DESQUAM-X WASH, work to a full lather, rinse thoroughly and pat dry. The amount of drying or peeling may be controlled by modification of dose frequency or drug concentration.

DESQUAM-X 10 BAR—
Wash entire area gently with fingertips for 1 to 2 minutes 2 or 3 times daily or as physician directs. Rinse well. The desired degree of dryness and peeling may be obtained by regulating frequency of use.

HOW SUPPLIED

DESQUAM-E 2.5 EMOLLIENT GEL
1.5 oz. (42.5g)   Plastic Tubes   NDC 0072-6003-45
DESQUAM-E 5 EMOLLIENT GEL
1.5 oz. (42.5g)   Plastic Tubes   NDC 0072-6103-45
DESQUAM-E 10 EMOLLIENT GEL
1.5 oz. (42.5g)   Plastic Tubes   NDC 0072-6203-45
     Store at controlled room temperature (59°–86°F).

DESQUAM-X 2.5 GEL
1.5 oz. (42.5 g)   Plastic Tubes   NDC 0072-6300-01
DESQUAM-X 5 GEL
1.5 oz. (42.5 g)   Plastic Tubes   NDC 0072-6621-01
3 oz. (85 g)   Plastic Tubes   NDC 0072-6621-03
DESQUAM-X 10 GEL
1.5 oz. (42.5 g)   Plastic Tubes   NDC 0072-6721-01
3 oz. (85 g)   Plastic Tubes   NDC 0072-6721-03
     Store at controlled room temperature (59°–86° F).

DESQUAM-X WASH (5%)
5 oz.   Plastic Bottle   NDC 0072-6905-05
DESQUAM-X WASH (10%)
5 oz.   Plastic Bottle   NDC 0072-7000-05
     Store at controlled room temperature (59°–86°F; 15°–30°C).

DESQUAM-X BAR (10%):
3.75 oz.   carton   NDC 0072-2000-04
     Store at controlled room temperature (59°–86°F).

EURAX®

(crotamiton USP)
Lotion/Cream
Scabicide/Antipruritic

CAUTION

Federal law prohibits dispensing without prescription.

DESCRIPTION

EURAX, crotamiton USP, is a scabicidal and antipruritic agent available as a cream or lotion for topical use only. EURAX provides 10% (w/w) of the synthetic, crotamiton USP, in a vanishing-cream or emollient-lotion base containing: water, petrolatum, propylene glycol, steareth-2, cetyl alcohol, dimethicone, laureth-23, fragrance, magnesium aluminum silicate, carbomer-934, sodium hydroxide, diazolidinyl urea, methylchloroisothiazolinone, methylisothiazolinone and magnesium nitrate. In addition, the cream contains glyceryl stearate. Crotamiton is N-ethyl-N-(o-methylphenyl)-2-butenamide and its structural formula is:

$$CH_3 \; CH = CHCONCH_2 \; CH_3$$

Crotamiton USP is a colorless to slightly yellowish oil, having a faint amine-like odor. It is miscible with alcohol and with methanol. Crotamiton is a mixture of the *cis* and *trans* isomers. Its molecular weight is 203.28.

CLINICAL PHARMACOLOGY

EURAX has scabicidal and antipruritic actions. The mechanisms of these actions are not known.

INDICATIONS AND USAGE

For eradication of scabies (*Sarcoptes scabiei*) and for symptomatic treatment of pruritic skin.

CONTRAINDICATIONS

EURAX should not be applied topically to patients who develop a sensitivity or are allergic to it or who manifest a primary irritation response to topical medications.

WARNINGS

If severe irritation or sensitization develops, treatment with this product should be discontinued and appropriate therapy instituted.

PRECAUTIONS

General: EURAX should not be applied in the eyes or mouth because it may cause irritation. It should not be applied to acutely inflamed skin or raw or weeping surfaces until the acute inflammation has subsided.

Information for Patients: See "Directions for patients with scabies".

Drug Interactions: None known.

Carcinogenesis, Mutagenesis, Impairment of Fertility: Long-term carcinogenicity studies in animals have not been conducted.

Pregnancy (Category C): Animal reproduction studies have not been conducted with EURAX. It is also not known whether EURAX can cause fetal harm when applied topically to a pregnant woman or can affect reproduction capacity. EURAX should be given to a pregnant woman only if clearly needed.

Pediatric Use: Safety and effectiveness in children have not been established.

ADVERSE REACTIONS

Allergic sensitivity or primary irritation reactions may occur in some patients.

OVERDOSAGE

There is no specific information on the effect of overtreatment with repeated topical applications in humans. Acute toxicity (after accidental oral administration in children): Highest known doses ingested: Cream: children—2g (age 1½ years); Lotion: 1 ounce (age 2 years). A death was reported but cause was not confirmed.

Oral LD$_{50}$ in animals (mg/kg): rats, 2212; mice, 2011.

Signs and symptoms (of oral ingestion): Burning sensation in the mouth, irritation of the buccal, esophageal and gastric mucosa, nausea, vomiting, abdominal pain.

Treatment: There is no specific antidote if taken orally. General measures to eliminate the drug and reduce its absorption, combined with symptomatic treatment, are recommended.

DOSAGE AND ADMINISTRATION

LOTION: Shake well before using—*In Scabies:* Thoroughly massage into the skin of the whole body from the chin down, paying particular attention to all folds and creases. A second application is advisable 24 hours later. Clothing and bed linen should be changed the next morning. A cleansing bath should be taken 48 hours after the last application. *In Pruritus:* Massage gently into affected areas until medication is completely absorbed. Repeat as needed.

DIRECTIONS FOR PATIENTS WITH SCABIES

1. Take a routine bath or shower. Thoroughly massage EURAX cream or lotion into the skin from the chin to the toes including folds and creases.
2. A second application is advisable 24 hours later.
3. This 60 gram tube or bottle is sufficient for two applications.
4. Clothing and bed linen should be changed the next day. Contaminated clothing and bed linen may be dry-cleaned, or washed in the hot cycle of the washing machine.
5. A cleansing bath should be taken 48 hours after the last application.

HOW SUPPLIED

Cream: 60g tubes (NDC 0072-2103-60; NSN 6505-00-116-0200).

Lotion: 60g (2 oz.) bottles (NDC 0072-2203-60, NSN 6505-01-153-4423).

    454 g (16 oz.) bottles (NDC 0072-2203-16).

Store at room temperature.

EXELDERM®

(sulconazole nitrate)
Cream, 1.0%
For topical use only. Not for ophthalmic use.

CAUTION

Federal law prohibits dispensing without prescription.

DESCRIPTION

EXELDERM (sulconazole nitrate) CREAM, 1.0% is a broad-spectrum antifungal agent intended for topical application. Sulconazole nitrate, the active ingredient in EXELDERM CREAM, is an imidazole derivative with in vitro antifungal and antiyeast activity. Its chemical name is (±)-1-[2.4-dichloro-β-[(p-chlorobenzyl)-thio]-phenethyl] imidazole mononitrate and it has the following chemical structure:

Sulconazole nitrate is a white to off-white crystalline powder with a molecular weight of 460.77. It is freely soluble in pyridine; slightly soluble in ethanol, acetone, and chloroform; and very slightly soluble in water. It has a melting point of about 130°C.

EXELDERM CREAM contains sulconazole nitrate 10 mg/g in an emollient cream base consisting of propylene glycol, stearyl alcohol, isopropyl myristate, cetyl alcohol, polysorbate 60, sorbitan monostearate, glyceryl stearate (and) PEG-100 stearate, ascorbyl palmitate, and purified water, with sodium hydroxide and/or nitric acid added to adjust the pH.

CLINICAL PHARMACOLOGY

Sulconazole nitrate is an imidazole derivative with broad-spectrum antifungal activity that inhibits the growth in vitro of the common pathogenic dermatophytes including *Trichophyton rubrum*, *Trichophyton mentagrophytes*, *Epidermophyton floccosum* and *Microsporum canis*. It also inhibits (*in vitro*) the organism responsible for tinea versicolor, *Malassezia furfur*. Sulconazole nitrate has been shown to be active *in vitro* against the following microorganisms, although clinical efficacy has not been established: *Candida albicans* and certain gram positive bacteria.

A modified Draize test showed no allergic contact dermatitis and a phototoxicity study showed no phototoxic or photoallergic reaction to sulconazole nitrate cream. Maximization tests with sulconazole nitrate cream showed no evidence of contact sensitization or irritation.

INDICATIONS AND USAGE

EXELDERM (sulconazole nitrate) CREAM, 1.0% is an antifungal agent indicated for the treatment of tinea pedis (athlete's foot), tinea cruris, and tinea corporis caused by *Trichophyton rubrum*, *Trichophyton mentagrophytes*, *Epidermophyton floccosum*, and *Microsporum canis*,* and for the treatment of tinea versicolor.

CONTRAINDICATIONS

EXELDERM (sulconazole nitrate) CREAM, 1.0% is contraindicated in patients who have a history of hypersensitivity to any of its ingredients.

PRECAUTIONS

General: EXELDERM (sulconazole nirate) CREAM, 1.0% is for external use only. Avoid contact with the eyes. If irritation develops, the cream should be discontinued and appropriate therapy instituted.

Information for Patients: Patients should be told to use EXELDERM CREAM as directed by the physician, to use it externally only, and to avoid contact with the eyes.

Carcinogenesis, Mutagenesis, Impairment of Fertility: Long-term animal studies to determine carcinogenic potential have not been performed. In vitro studies have shown no mutagenic activity.

Pregnancy (Category C): There are no adequate and well controlled studies in pregnant women. Sulconazole nitrate should be used during pregnancy only if clearly needed. Sulconazole nitrate has been shown to be embryotoxic in rats when given in doses of 125 times the adult human dose (in mg/kg). The drug was not teratogenic in rats or rabbits at oral doses of 50 mg/kg/day.

Sulconazole nitrate given orally to rats at a dose 125 times the human dose resulted in prolonged gestation and dystocia. Several females died during the prenatal period, most likely due to labor complications.

Nursing Mothers: It is not known whether sulconazole nitrate is excreted in human milk. Caution should be exercised when sulconazole nitrate is administered to a nursing woman.

* Efficacy for this organism in the organ system was studied in fewer than ten infections.

Pediatric Use: Safety and effectiveness in children have not been established.

ADVERSE REACTIONS

There were no systemic effects and only infrequent cutaneous adverse reactions in 1185 patients treated with sulconazole nitrate cream in controlled clinical trials. Approximately 3% of these patients reported itching, 3% burning or stinging, and 1% redness. These complaints did not usually interfere with treatment.

CLINICAL STUDIES

In a vehicle-controlled study for the treatment of tinea pedis (moccasin type) due to *T. rubrum,* after 4–6 weeks of treatment 69% of patients on the active drug and 19% of patients on the drug vehicle had become KOH and culture negative. In addition, 68% of patients on the active drug and 20% of patients on the drug vehicle showed a good or excellent clinical response.

DOSAGE AND ADMINISTRATION

A small amount of cream should be gently massaged into the affected and surrounding skin areas once or twice daily, except in tinea pedis, where administration should be twice daily.

Early relief of symptoms is experienced by the majority of patients and clinical improvement may be seen fairly soon after treatment is begun; however, tinea corporis/cruris and tinea versicolor should be treated for 3 weeks and tinea pedis for 4 weeks to reduce the possibility of recurrence.

If significant clinical improvement is not seen after 4 to 6 weeks of treatment, an alternate diagnosis should be considered.

HOW SUPPLIED

EXELDERM (sulconazole nitrate) CREAM, 1.0%:
15 g tube—NDC 0072-8200-15
30 g tube—NDC 0072-8200-30
60 g tube—NDC 0072-8200-60
Avoid excessive heat, above 40°C (104°F).

EXELDERM® ℞
(sulconazole nitrate)
Solution, 1.0%
For topical use only. Not for ophthalmic use.

CAUTION

Federal law prohibits dispensing without prescription.

DESCRIPTION

EXELDERM (sulconazole nitrate) SOLUTION, 1.0% is a broad-spectrum antifungal agent intended for topical application. Sulconazole nitrate, the active ingredient in EXELDERM SOLUTION, is an imidazole derivative with antifungal and antiyeast activity. Its chemical name is (±)-1-[2.4-dichloro-β-[(p-chlorobenzyl)-thio]-phenethyl] imidazole mononitrate and it has the following chemical structure:

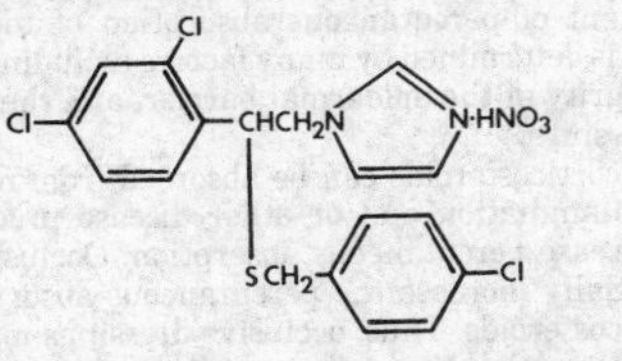

Sulconazole nitrate is a white to off-white crystalline powder with a molecular weight of 460.77. It is freely soluble in pyridine; slightly soluble in ethanol, acetone, and chloroform; and very slightly soluble in water. It has a melting point of about 130°C.

EXELDERM SOLUTION contains sulconazole nitrate 10 mg/mL in a solution of propylene glycol, poloxamer 407, polysorbate 20, butylated hydroxyanisole, and purified water, with sodium hydroxide and, if necessary, nitric acid added to adjust the pH.

CLINICAL PHARMACOLOGY

Sulconazole nitrate is an imidazole derivative that inhibits the growth of the common pathogenic dermatophytes including *Trichophyton rubrum, Trichophyton mentagrophytes, Epidermophyton floccosum,* and *Microsporum canis.* It also inhibits the organism responsible for tinea versicolor, *Malassezia furfur,* and certain gram positive bacteria.

A maximization test with sulconazole nitrate solution showed no evidence of irritation or contact sensitization.

INDICATIONS AND USAGE

EXELDERM (sulconazole nitrate) SOLUTION, 1.0% is a broad-spectrum antifungal agent indicated for the treatment of tinea cruris and tinea corporis caused by *Trichophyton rubrum, Trichophyton mentagrophytes, Epidermophyton floccosum,* and *Microsporum canis;* and for the treatment of tinea versicolor. Effectiveness has not been proven in tinea pedis (athlete's foot).

Symptomatic relief usually occurs within a few days after starting EXELDERM SOLUTION and clinical improvement usually occurs within one week.

CONTRAINDICATIONS

EXELDERM (sulconazole nitrate) SOLUTION, 1.0% is contraindicated in patients who have a history of hypersensitivity to any of the ingredients.

PRECAUTIONS

General: EXELDERM (sulconazole nitrate) SOLUTION, 1.0% is for external use only. Avoid contact with the eyes. If irritation develops, the solution should be discontinued and appropriate therapy instituted.

Information for Patients: Patients should be told to use EXELDERM SOLUTION as directed by the physician, to use it externally only, and to avoid contact with the eyes.

Carcinogenesis, Mutagenesis, Impairment of Fertility: Long-term animal studies to determine carcinogenic potential have not been performed. In vitro studies have shown no mutagenic activity.

Pregnancy: Pregnancy Category C: Sulconazole nitrate has been shown to be embryotoxic in rats when given in doses 125 times the human dose (in mg/kg). The drug at this dose given orally to rats also resulted in prolonged gestation and dystocia. Several females died during the perinatal period, most likely due to labor complications. Sulconazole nitrate was not teratogenic in rats or rabbits at oral doses of 50 mg/kg/day.

There are no adequate and well-controlled studies in pregnant women. Sulconazole nitrate should be used during pregnancy only if the potential benefit justifies the potential risk to the fetus.

Nursing Mothers: It is not known whether this drug is excreted in human milk. Because many drugs are excreted in human milk, caution should be exercised when sulconazole nitrate is administered to a nursing woman.

Pediatric Use: Safety and effectiveness in children have not been established.

ADVERSE REACTIONS

There were no systemic effects and only infrequent cutaneous adverse reactions in 370 patients treated with sulconazole nitrate solution in controlled clinical trials. Approximately 1% of these patients reported itching and 1% burning or stinging. These complaints did not usually interfere with treatment.

DOSAGE AND ADMINISTRATION

A small amount of the solution should be gently massaged into the affected and surrounding skin areas once or twice daily.

Symptomatic relief usually occurs within a few days after starting EXELDERM (sulconazole nitrate) SOLUTION, 1.0%, and clinical improvement usually occurs within one week. To reduce the possibility of recurrence, tinea cruris, tinea corporis, and tinea versicolor should be treated for 3 weeks.

If significant clinical improvement is not seen after 4 weeks of treatment, an alternate diagnosis should be considered.

HOW SUPPLIED

EXELDERM SOLUTION, 1.0%

30 mL	Plastic Bottle	NDC 0072-8400-30

Avoid excessive heat, above 40°C (104°F), and protect from light.

HALOG CREAM ℞
Halcinonide Cream USP 0.1%
HALOG Ointment ℞
Halcinonide Ointment USP 0.1%
HALOG Solution ℞
Halcinonide Topical Solution USP 0.1%
HALOG-E Cream ℞
Halcinonide Cream USP 0.1%
For dermatologic use only.
Not for ophthalmic use.

DESCRIPTION

The topical corticosteroids constitute a class of primarily synthetic steroids used as anti-inflammatory and antipruritic agents. The steroids in this class include halcinonide. Halcinonide is designated chemically as 21-Chloro-9-fluoro-11β, 16α, 17-trihydroxypregn-4-ene-3,20-dione cyclic 16,17-acetal with acetone.

Each gram of 0.1% HALOG Cream (Halcinonide Cream) contains 1 mg halcinonide in a specially formulated cream base consisting of glyceryl monostearate NF XII, cetyl alcohol, isopropyl palmitate, dimethicone 350, polysorbate 60, titanium dioxide, propylene glycol, and purified water.

Each gram of 0.1% **HALOG Ointment (Halcinonide Ointment)** contains 1 mg halcinonide in Plastibase® (Plasticized Hydrocarbon Gel), a polyethylene and mineral oil gel base with polyethylene glycol 400, polyethylene glycol 6000 distearate, polyethylene glycol 300, polyethylene glycol 1450, and butylated hydroxytoluene as an antioxidant.

Each mL of 0.1% **HALOG Solution (Halcinonide Topical Solution)** contains 1 mg halcinonide with edetate disodium, polyethylene glycol 300, purified water, and butylated hydroxytoluene as an antioxidant.

Each gram of 0.1% **HALOG-E Cream (Halcinonide Cream)** contains 1 mg halcinonide in a hydrophilic vanishing cream base consisting of propylene glycol, dimethicone 350, castor oil, cetearyl alcohol (and) ceteareth-20, propylene glycol stearate, white petrolatum, and purified water. This formulation is water-washable, greaseless, and nonstaining, with moisturizing and emollient properties.

CLINICAL PHARMACOLOGY

Topical corticosteroids share anti-inflammatory, antipruritic and vasoconstrictive actions.

The mechanism of anti-inflammatory activity of the topical corticosteroids is unclear. Various laboratory methods, including vasoconstrictor assays, are used to compare and predict potencies and/or clinical efficacies of the topical corticosteroids. There is some evidence to suggest that a recognizable correlation exists between vasoconstrictor potency and therapeutic efficacy in man.

PHARMACOKINETICS

The extent of percutaneous absorption of topical corticosteroids is determined by many factors including the vehicle, the integrity of the epidermal barrier, and the use of occlusive dressings.

Topical corticosteroids can be absorbed from normal intact skin. Inflammation and/or other disease processes in the skin increase percutaneous absorption. Occlusive dressings substantially increase the percutaneous absorption of topical corticosteroids. Thus, occlusive dressings may be a valuable therapeutic adjunct for treatment of resistant dermatoses (see DOSAGE AND ADMINISTRATION).

Once absorbed through the skin, topical corticosteroids are handled through pharmacokinetic pathways similar to systemically administered corticosteroids. Corticosteroids are bound to plasma proteins in varying degrees. Corticosteroids are metabolized primarily in the liver and are then excreted by the kidneys. Some of the topical corticosteroids and their metabolites are also excreted into the bile.

INDICATIONS AND USAGE

HALOG (Halcinonide) preparations are indicated for the relief of the inflammatory and pruritic manifestations of corticosteroid-responsive dermatoses.

CONTRAINDICATIONS

Topical corticosteroids are contraindicated in those patients with a history of hypersensitivity to any of the components of the preparations.

PRECAUTIONS

General

Systemic absorption of topical corticosteroids has produced reversible hypothalamic-pituitary-adrenal (HPA) axis suppression, manifestations of Cushing's syndrome, hyperglycemia, and glucosuria in some patients.

Conditions which augment systemic absorption include the application of the more potent steroids, use over large surface areas, prolonged use, and the addition of occlusive dressings.

Therefore, patients receiving a large dose of any potent topical steroid applied to a large surface area or under an occlusive dressing should be evaluated periodically for evidence of HPA axis suppression by using the urinary free cortisol and ACTH stimulation tests, and for impairment of thermal homeostasis. If HPA axis suppression or elevation of the body temperature occurs, an attempt should be made to withdraw the drug, to reduce the frequency of application, substitute a less potent steroid, or use a sequential approach when utilizing the occlusive technique.

Recovery of HPA axis function and thermal homeostasis are generally prompt and complete upon discontinuation of the drug. Infrequently, signs and symptoms of steroid withdrawal may occur, requiring supplemental systemic corticosteroids. Occasionally, a patient may develop a sensitivity reaction to a particular occlusive dressing material or adhesive and a substitute material may be necessary.

Children may absorb proportionally larger amounts of topical corticosteroids and thus be more susceptible to systemic toxicity (see PRECAUTIONS, Pediatric Use).

If irritation develops, topical corticosteroids should be discontinued and appropriate therapy instituted.

In the presence of dermatological infections, the use of an appropriate antifungal or antibacterial agent should be instituted. If a favorable response does not occur promptly, the

Continued on next page

Westwood-Squibb—Cont.

corticosteroid should be discontinued until the infection has been adequately controlled.

These preparations are not for ophthalmic use.

Information for the Patient

Patients using topical corticosteroids should receive the following information and instructions:

1. These medications are to be used as directed by the physician. They are for dermatologic use only. Avoid contact with the eyes.
2. Patients should be advised not to use these medications for any disorder other than for which it was prescribed.
3. The treated skin area should not be bandaged or otherwise covered or wrapped as to be occlusive unless directed by the physician.
4. Patients should report any signs of local adverse reactions especially under occlusive dressing.
5. Parents of pediatric patients should be advised not to use tight-fitting diapers or plastic pants on a child being treated in the diaper area, as these garments may constitute occlusive dressings.

Laboratory Tests

A urinary free cortisol test and ACTH stimulation test may be helpful in evaluating HPA axis suppression.

Carcinogenesis, Mutagenesis, and Impairment of Fertility

Long-term animal studies have not been performed to evaluate the carcinogenic potential or the effect on fertility of topical corticosteroids. Studies to determine mutagenicity with prednisolone and hydrocortisone showed negative results.

Pregnancy: Teratogenic Effects

Category C. Corticosteroids are generally teratogenic in laboratory animals when administered systemically at relatively low dosage levels. The more potent corticosteroids have been shown to be teratogenic after dermal application in laboratory animals. There are no adequate and well-controlled studies in pregnant women on teratogenic effects from topically applied corticosteroids. Therefore, topical corticosteroids should be used during pregnancy only if the potential benefit justifies the potential risk to the fetus. Drugs of this class should not be used extensively on pregnant patients, in large amounts, or for prolonged periods of time.

Nursing Mothers

It is not known whether topical administration of corticosteroids could result in sufficient systemic absorption to produce detectable quantities in breast milk. Systemically administered corticosteroids are secreted into breast milk in quantities **not** likely to have a deleterious effect on the infant. Nevertheless, caution should be exercised when topical corticosteroids are administered to a nursing woman.

Pediatric Use

Pediatric patients may demonstrate greater susceptibility to topical corticosteroid-induced HPA axis suppression and Cushing's syndrome than mature patients because of a larger skin surface area to body weight ratio.

HPA axis suppression, Cushing's syndrome, and intracranial hypertension have been reported in children receiving topical corticosteroids. Manifestations of adrenal suppression in children include linear growth retardation, delayed weight gain, low plasma cortisol levels, and absence of response to ACTH stimulation. Manifestations of intracranial hypertension include bulging fontanelles, headaches, and bilateral papilledema.

Administration of topical corticosteroids to children should be limited to the least amount compatible with an effective therapeutic regimen. Chronic corticosteroid therapy may interfere with the growth and development of children.

ADVERSE REACTIONS

The following local adverse reactions are reported infrequently with topical corticosteroids, but may occur more frequently with the use of occlusive dressings (reactions are listed in an approximate decreasing order of occurrence): burning, itching, irritation, dryness, folliculitis, hypertrichosis, acneiform eruptions, hypopigmentation, perioral dermatitis, allergic contact dermatitis, maceration of the skin, secondary infection, skin atrophy, striae, and miliaria.

OVERDOSAGE

Topically applied corticosteroids can be absorbed in sufficient amounts to produce systemic effects (see PRECAUTIONS, General).

DOSAGE AND ADMINISTRATION

HALOG Creams (Halcinonide Cream): Apply the 0.1% HALOG Cream (Halcinonide Cream) to the affected area two to three times daily. Rub in gently.

HALOG Ointment (Halcinonide Ointment): Apply a thin film of 0.1% HALOG Ointment (Halcinonide Ointment) to the affected area two to three times daily.

HALOG Solution (Halcinonide Topical Solution): Apply HALOG Solution (Halcinonide Topical Solution) 0.1% to the affected area two to three times daily.

HALOG-E Cream (Halcinonide Cream): Apply HALOG-E Cream (Halcinonide Cream) 0.1% to the affected area one to three times daily. Rub in gently.

Occlusive Dressing Technique

Occlusive dressings may be used for the management of psoriasis or other recalcitrant conditions.

HALOG Cream (Halcinonide Cream) 0.1% and HALOG-E Cream (Halcinonide Cream) 0.1%: Gently rub a small amount of the cream into the lesion until it disappears. Reapply the preparation leaving a thin coating on the lesion, cover with a pliable nonporous film, and seal the edges. If needed, additional moisture may be provided by covering the lesion with a dampened clean cotton cloth before the nonporous film is applied or by briefly wetting the affected area with water immediately prior to applying the medication. The frequency of changing dressings is best determined on an individual basis. It may be convenient to apply HALOG/HALOG-E Cream under an occlusive dressing in the evening and to remove the dressing in the morning (i.e., 12-hour occlusion). When utilizing the 12-hour occlusion regimen, additional cream should be applied, without occlusion, during the day. Reapplication is essential at each dressing change.

If an infection develops, the use of occlusive dressings should be discontinued and appropriate antimicrobial therapy instituted.

HALOG Ointment (Halcinonide Ointment) 0.1%: Apply a thin film of the ointment to the lesion, cover with a pliable nonporous film, and seal the edges. If needed, additional moisture may be provided by covering the lesion with a dampened clean cotton cloth before the nonporous film is applied or by briefly wetting the affected area with water immediately prior to applying the medication. The frequency of changing dressings is best determined on an individual basis. It may be convenient to apply HALOG Ointment under an occlusive dressing in the evening and to remove the dressing in the morning (i.e., 12-hour occlusion). When utilizing the 12-hour occlusion regimen, additional ointment should be applied, without occlusion, during the day. Reapplication is essential at each dressing change.

If an infection develops, the use of occlusive dressings should be discontinued and appropriate antimicrobial therapy instituted.

HALOG Solution (Halcinonide Topical Solution) 0.1%: Apply the solution to the lesion, cover with a pliable nonporous film, and seal the edges. If needed, additional moisture may be provided by covering the lesion with a dampened clean cotton cloth before the nonporous film is applied or by briefly wetting the affected area with water immediately prior to applying the medication. The frequency of changing dressings is best determined on an individual basis. It may be convenient to apply HALOG solution under an occlusive dressing in the evening and to remove the dressing in the morning (i.e., 12-hour occlusion). When utilizing the 12-hour occlusion regimen, additional solution should be applied, without occlusion, during the day. Reapplication is essential at each dressing change.

If an infection develops, the use of occlusive dressings should be discontinued and appropriate antimicrobial therapy instituted.

HOW SUPPLIED

HALOG Cream (Halcinonide Cream USP)

0.1%: tubes containing 15 g (NDC 0003-1482-15), 30 g (NDC 0003-1482-20), 60 g (NDC 0003-1482-30); and jars containing 240 g (NDC 0003-1482-40) of cream.

HALOG Ointment (Halcinonide Ointment USP)

0.1%: tubes containing 15 g (NDC 0003-0248-15), 30 g (NDC 0003-0248-20), and 60 g (NDC 0003-0248-30); and jars containing 240 g (NDC 0003-0248-40) of ointment.

HALOG Solution (Halcinonide Topical Solution USP)

0.1%: plastic squeeze bottles containing 20 mL (NDC 0003-0249-15) and 60 mL (NDC 0003-0249-20) of solution.

HALOG-E Cream (Halcinonide Cream USP)

0.1%: tubes containing 15 g (NDC 0003-1494-14), 30 g (NDC 0003-1494-21), and 60 g (NDC 0003-1494-31) of cream.

Storage

HALOG Cream (Halcinonide Cream USP)

Store at room temperature; avoid excessive heat (104°F).

HALOG Ointment (Halcinonide Ointment USP)

Store at room temperature; avoid excessive heat (104°F).

HALOG Solution (Halcinonide Topical Solution USP)

Store at room temperature; avoid freezing and temperatures above 104°F.

HALOG-E Cream (Halcinonide Cream USP)

Store at room temperature; avoid freezing and refrigeration.

KENALOG® Creams ℞

Triamcinolone Acetonide Cream USP
0.025%, 0.1% and 0.5%

KENALOG® Lotions ℞

Triamcinolone Acetonide Lotion USP
0.025% and 0.1%

KENALOG® Ointments ℞

Triamcinolone Acetonide Ointment USP
0.025%, 0.1% and 0.5%

KENALOG® Spray ℞

Triamcinolone Acetonide Topical Aerosol USP
For dermatologic use only.
Not for ophthalmic use.

DESCRIPTION

The topical corticosteroids constitute a class of primarily synthetic steroids used as anti-inflammatory and antipruritic agents. The steroids in this class include triamcinolone acetonide. Triamcinolone acetonide is designated chemically as 9-Fluoro-11β, 16α, 17, 21-tetrahydroxypregna-1,4-diene-3, 20-dione cyclic 16, 17-acetal with acetone.

Each gram of 0.025%, 0.1%, and 0.5% **KENALOG Cream** (Triamcinolone Acetonide Cream) provides 0.25 mg, 1 mg, or 5 mg triamcinolone acetonide, respectively, in a vanishing cream base containing propylene glycol, cetearyl alcohol (and) ceteareth-20, white petrolatum, sorbitol solution, glyceryl monostearate, polyethylene glycol monostearate, simethicone, sorbic acid, and purified water.

Each mL of 0.025% and 0.1% **KENALOG Lotion** (Triamcinolone Acetonide Lotion) provides 0.25 mg and 1 mg triamcinolone acetonide, respectively, in a lotion base containing propylene glycol, cetyl alcohol, stearyl alcohol, sorbitan monopalmitate, polysorbate 20, simethicone, and purified water.

Each gram of 0.1% **KENALOG Ointment** (Triamcinolone Acetonide Ointment) provides 1 mg triamcinolone acetonide in Plastibase® (Plasticized Hydrocarbon Gel), a polyethylene and mineral oil gel base.

KENALOG Spray (Triamcinolone Acetonide Topical Aerosol) is **for dermatologic use only.** A two-second application, which covers an area approximately the size of the hand, delivers an amount of triamcinolone acetonide not exceeding 0.2 mg. After spraying, the nonvolatile vehicle remaining on the skin contains approximately 0.2% triamcinolone acetonide. Each gram of spray provides 0.147 mg triamcinolone acetonide in a vehicle of isopropyl palmitate, dehydrated alcohol (10.3%), and isobutane propellant.

CLINICAL PHARMACOLOGY

Topical corticosteroids share anti-inflammatory, antipruritic and vasoconstrictive actions.

The mechanism of anti-inflammatory activity of the topical corticosteroids is unclear. Various laboratory methods, including vasoconstrictor assays, are used to compare and predict potencies and/or clinical efficacies of the topical corticosteroids. There is some evidence to suggest that a recognizable correlation exists between vasoconstrictor potency and therapeutic efficacy in man.

Pharmacokinetics

The extent of percutaneous absorption of topical corticosteroids is determined by many factors including the vehicle, the integrity of the epidermal barrier, and the use of occlusive dressings.

Topical corticosteroids can be absorbed from normal intact skin. Inflammation and/or other disease processes in the skin increase percutaneous absorption. Occlusive dressings substantially increase the percutaneous absorption of topical corticosteroids. Thus, occlusive dressings may be a valuable therapeutic adjunct for treatment of resistant dermatoses (see DOSAGE AND ADMINISTRATION).

Once absorbed through the skin, topical corticosteroids are handled through pharmacokinetic pathways similar to systemically administered corticosteroids. Corticosteroids are bound to plasma proteins in varying degrees. Corticosteroids are metabolized primarily in the liver and are then excreted by the kidneys. Some of the topical corticosteroids and their metabolites are also excreted into the bile.

INDICATIONS AND USAGE

KENALOG (Triamcinolone Acetonide) topical preparations are indicated for relief of the inflammatory and pruritic manifestations of corticosteroid-responsive dermatoses.

CONTRAINDICATIONS

Topical corticosteroids are contraindicated in those patients with a history of hypersensitivity to any of the components of the preparations.

PRECAUTIONS

General

Systemic absorption of topical corticosteroids has produced reversible hypothalamic-pituitary-adrenal (HPA) axis suppression, manifestations of Cushing's syndrome, hyperglycemia, and glucosuria in some patients.

Conditions which augment systemic absorption include the application of the more potent steroids, use over large surface areas, prolonged use, and the addition of occlusive dressings.

Therefore, patients receiving a large dose of any potent topical steroid applied to a large surface area or under an occlusive dressing should be evaluated periodically for evidence of HPA axis suppression by using the urinary free cortisol and ACTH stimulation tests, and for impairment of thermal homeostasis. If HPA axis suppression or elevation of the body temperature occurs, an attempt should be made to withdraw the drug, to reduce the frequency of application, substitute a less potent steroid, or use a sequential approach when utilizing the occlusive technique.

Recovery of HPA axis function and thermal homeostasis are generally prompt and complete upon discontinuation of the drug. Infrequently, signs and symptoms of steroid withdrawal may occur, requiring supplemental systemic corticosteroids. Occasionally, a patient may develop a sensitivity reaction to a particular occlusive dressing material or adhesive and a substitute material may be necessary.

Children may absorb proportionally larger amounts of topical corticosteroids and thus be more susceptible to systemic toxicity (see PRECAUTIONS, Pediatric Use).

If irritation develops, topical corticosteroids should be discontinued and appropriate therapy instituted.

In the presence of dermatological infections, the use of an appropriate antifungal or antibacterial agent should be instituted. If a favorable response does not occur promptly, the corticosteroid should be discontinued until the infection has been adequately controlled.

These preparations are not for ophthalmic use.

Information for the Patient
Patients using topical corticosteroids should receive the following information and instructions:

1. These medications are to be used as directed by the physician. They are for dermatologic (external) use only. Avoid contact with the eyes. Avoid inhalation of the spray.
2. Patients should be advised not to use these medications for any disorder other than for which they are prescribed.
3. The treated skin area should not be bandaged or otherwise covered or wrapped as to be occlusive unless directed by the physician.
4. Patients should report any signs of local adverse reactions especially under occlusive dressing.
5. Parents of pediatric patients should be advised not to use tight-fitting diapers or plastic pants on a child being treated in the diaper area, as these garments may constitute occlusive dressings.

Laboratory Tests
A urinary free cortisol test and ACTH stimulation test may be helpful in evaluating HPA axis suppression.

Carcinogenesis, Mutagenesis, and Impairment of Fertility
Long-term animal studies have not been performed to evaluate the carcinogenic potential or the effect on fertility of topical corticosteroids.

Studies to determine mutagenicity with prednisolone and hydrocortisone showed negative results.

Pregnancy: Teratogenic Effects
Category C. Corticosteroids are generally teratogenic in laboratory animals when administered systemically at relatively low dosage levels. The more potent corticosteroids have been shown to be teratogenic after dermal application in laboratory animals. There are no adequate and well-controlled studies in pregnant women on teratogenic effects from topically applied corticosteroids. Therefore, topical corticosteroids should be used during pregnancy only if the potential benefit justifies the potential risk to the fetus. Drugs of this class should not be used extensively on pregnant patients, in large amounts, or for prolonged periods of time.

Nursing Mothers
It is not known whether topical administration of corticosteroids could result in sufficient systemic absorption to produce detectable quantities in breast milk. Systemically administered corticosteroids are secreted into breast milk in quantities not likely to have a deleterious effect on the infant. Nevertheless, caution should be exercised when topical corticosteroids are administered to a nursing woman.

Pediatric Use
Pediatric patients may demonstrate greater susceptibility to topical corticosteroid-induced HPA axis suppression and Cushing's syndrome than mature patients because of a larger skin surface area to body weight ratio.

HPA axis suppression, Cushing's syndrome, and intracranial hypertension have been reported in children receiving topical corticosteroids. Manifestations of adrenal suppression in children include linear growth retardation, delayed weight gain, low plasma cortisol levels, and absence of response to ACTH stimulation. Manifestations of intracranial hypertension include bulging fontanelles, headaches, and bilateral papilledema.

Administration of topical corticosteroids to children should be limited to the least amount compatible with an effective therapeutic regimen. Chronic corticosteroid therapy may interfere with the growth and development of children.

ADVERSE REACTIONS
The following local adverse reactions are reported infrequently with topical corticosteroids, but may occur more frequently with the use of occlusive dressings (reactions are listed in an approximate decreasing order of occurrence): burning, itching, irritation, dryness, folliculitis, hypertrichosis, acneiform eruptions, hypopigmentation, perioral dermatitis, allergic contact dermatitis, maceration of the skin, secondary infection, skin atrophy, striae, and miliaria.

OVERDOSAGE
Topically applied corticosteroids can be absorbed in sufficient amounts to produce systemic effects (see PRECAUTIONS, General).

DOSAGE AND ADMINISTRATION
KENALOG Cream (Triamcinolone Acetonide Cream) 0.025%: Apply to the affected area two to four times daily. Rub in gently.

KENALOG Cream (Triamcinolone Acetonide Cream) 0.1% or 0.5%: Apply, as appropriate, to the affected area two to three times daily. Rub in gently.

KENALOG Lotion (Triamcinolone Acetonide Lotion) 0.025%: Apply to the affected area two to four times daily. Rub in gently.

KENALOG Lotion (Triamcinolone Acetonide Lotion) 0.1%: Apply to the affected area two to three times daily. Rub in gently.

KENALOG Ointment (Triamcinolone Acetonide Ointment) 0.1%: Apply a thin film, as appropriate, to the affected area two to three times daily.

KENALOG Spray (Triamcinolone Acetonide Topical Aerosol): Directions for use of the spray can are provided on the label. The preparation may be applied to any area of the body, but when it is sprayed about the face, care should be taken to see that the eyes are covered, and that inhalation of the spray is avoided.

Three or four applications daily of KENALOG Spray (Triamcinolone Acetonide Topical Aerosol) are generally adequate.

Occlusive Dressing Technique
KENALOG Cream (Triamcinolone Acetonide Cream) 0.025%, 0.1%, and 0.5% and KENALOG Lotion (Triamcinolone Acetonide Lotion) 0.025% and 0.1%: Occlusive dressings may be used for the management of psoriasis or other recalcitrant conditions. Gently rub a small amount of the preparation into the lesion until it disappears. Reapply the preparation leaving a thin coating on the lesion, cover with a pliable nonporous film, and seal the edges. If needed, additional moisture may be provided by covering the lesion with a dampened clean cotton cloth before the nonporous film is applied or by briefly wetting the affected area with water immediately prior to applying the medication. The frequency of changing dressings is best determined on an individual basis. It may be convenient to apply the preparation under an occlusive dressing in the evening and to remove the dressing in the morning (i.e., 12-hour occlusion). When utilizing the 12-hour occlusion regimen, additional preparation should be applied, without occlusion, during the day. Reapplication is essential at each dressing change.

If an infection develops, the use of occlusive dressings should be discontinued and appropriate antimicrobial therapy instituted.

KENALOG Ointment (Triamcinolone Acetonide Ointment) 0.1% and KENALOG Spray (Triamcinolone Acetonide Topical Aerosol): Occlusive dressings may be used for the management of psoriasis or other recalcitrant conditions. Apply a thin coating of the preparation or spray a small amount of the preparation onto the lesion, cover with a pliable nonporous film, and seal the edges. If needed, additional moisture may be provided by covering the lesion with a dampened clean cotton cloth before the nonporous film is applied or by briefly wetting the affected area with water immediately prior to applying the medication. The frequency of changing dressings is best determined on an individual basis. It may be convenient to apply the preparation under an occlusive dressing in the evening and to remove the dressing in the morning (i.e., 12-hour occlusion). When utilizing the 12-hour occlusion regimen, additional preparation should be applied, without occlusion, during the day. Reapplication is essential at each dressing change.

If an infection develops, the use of occlusive dressings should be discontinued and appropriate antimicrobial therapy instituted.

HOW SUPPLIED
KENALOG Cream (Triamcinolone Acetonide Cream USP)
0.025%: tubes containing 15 g (NDC 0003-0172-22) and 80 g (NDC 0003-0172-68) of cream.
0.1%: tubes containing 15 g (NDC 0003-0506-20), 60 g (NDC 0003-0506-46), and 80 g (NDC 0003-0506-49) and jars containing 2.38 kg (NDC 0003-0506-89) of cream.
0.5%: tubes containing 20 g (NDC 0003-1483-20) of cream.
KENALOG Lotion (Triamcinolone Acetonide Lotion USP)
0.025%: plastic squeeze bottles containing 60 mL (NDC 0003-0173-60) of lotion.

0.1%: plastic squeeze bottles containing 15 mL (NDC 0003-0502-20) and 60 mL (NDC 0003-0502-70) of lotion.
KENALOG Ointment (Triamcinolone Acetonide Ointment USP)
0.1%: tubes containing 15 g (NDC 0003-0508-20) and 60 g (NDC 0003-0508-56) and jars containing 240 g (NDC 0003-0508-60) of ointment.
KENALOG Spray (Triamcinolone Acetonide Topical Aerosol USP)
63 g (NDC 0003-0501-62) aerosol cans.
Storage
KENALOG Cream (Triamcinolone Acetonide Cream USP)
Store at room temperature; avoid freezing.
KENALOG Lotion (Triamcinolone Acetonide Lotion USP)
Store at room temperature; avoid freezing.
KENALOG Ointment (Triamcinolone Acetonide Ointment USP)
Store at room temperature
KENALOG Spray (Triamcinolone Acetonide Topical Aerosol USP)
Store at room temperature; avoid excessive heat.

KENALOG®-10 INJECTION　　　　　　　　℞
[ken 'ah-log "]
Sterile Triamcinolone Acetonide Suspension USP
For Intra-articular, Intrabursal or Intradermal Use
NOT FOR INTRAVENOUS OR INTRAMUSCULAR USE

DESCRIPTION
KENALOG-10 Injection (Sterile Triamcinolone Acetonide Suspension USP) provides triamcinolone acetonide, a synthetic corticosteroid with marked anti-inflammatory action, in a sterile aqueous suspension suitable for intradermal, intra-articular, and intrabursal injection and for injection into tendon sheaths. This preparation is NOT suitable for intravenous or intramuscular use. Each mL of the sterile aqueous suspension provides 10 mg triamcinolone acetonide, with sodium chloride for isotonicity, 0.9% (w/v) benzyl alcohol as a preservative, 0.75% carboxymethylcellulose sodium, and 0.04% polysorbate 80; sodium hydroxide or hydrochloric acid may have been added to adjust pH between 5.0 and 7.5. At the time of manufacture, the air in the container is replaced by nitrogen.

The chemical name for triamcinolone acetonide is 9-fluoro-11β, 16α, 17, 21-tetrahydroxypregna-1,4-diene-3,20-dione cyclic 16, 17-acetal with acetone.

CLINICAL PHARMACOLOGY
Naturally occurring glucocorticoids (hydrocortisone), which also have salt-retaining properties, are used as replacement therapy in adrenocortical deficiency states. Their synthetic analogs are primarily used for their potent anti-inflammatory effects in disorders of many organ systems. Glucocorticoids cause profound and varied metabolic effects. In addition, they modify the body's immune responses to diverse stimuli.

INDICATIONS AND USAGE
Intra-Articular
KENALOG-10 Injection (Sterile Triamcinolone Acetonide Suspension USP) is indicated for intra-articular or intrabursal administration, and for injection into tendon sheaths, as adjunctive therapy for short-term administration (to tide the patient over an acute episode or exacerbation) in: synovitis of osteoarthritis, rheumatoid arthritis, acute and subacute bursitis, acute gouty arthritis, epicondylitis, acute nonspecific tenosynovitis, and post-traumatic osteoarthritis.
Intradermal
Intralesional administration of KENALOG-10 Injection is indicated for the treatment of keloids, discoid lupus erythematosus, necrobiosis lipoidica diabeticorum, alopecia areata, and localized hypertrophic, infiltrated, inflammatory lesions of: lichen planus, psoriatic plaques, granuloma annulare, and lichen simplex chronicus (neurodermatitis). KENALOG-10 Injection also may be useful in cystic tumors of an aponeurosis or tendon (ganglia).

CONTRAINDICATIONS
Corticosteroids are contraindicated in patients with systemic fungal infections.

WARNINGS
Because it is a suspension, the preparation should *not* be administered intravenously. Strict aseptic technique is mandatory.

When patients who are receiving corticosteroid therapy are subjected to unusual stress, increased dosage of rapidly acting corticosteroids is indicated before, during, and after the stressful situation. KENALOG-10 Injection (Sterile Triam-

Continued on next page

Westwood-Squibb—Cont.

cinolone Acetonide Suspension USP), as a long-acting preparation, is *not* suitable for use in acute stress situations.

Corticosteroids may mask some signs of infection, and new infections may appear during their use. There may be decreased resistance and inability to localize infection when corticosteroids are used. If an infection occurs during corticosteroid therapy, it should be promptly controlled by suitable antimicrobial therapy (see PRECAUTIONS).

Prolonged use of corticosteroids may produce posterior subcapsular cataracts, glaucoma with possible damage to the optic nerves, and may enhance the establishment of secondary ocular infections due to fungi or viruses.

Average and large doses of hydrocortisone or cortisone can cause elevation of blood pressure, salt and water retention, and increased excretion of potassium. These effects are less likely to occur with the synthetic derivatives except when they are used in large doses; dietary salt restriction and potassium supplementation may be necessary (see PRECAUTIONS). All corticosteroids increase calcium excretion.

Children who are on immunosuppressant drugs are more susceptible to infections than healthy children. Chickenpox and measles, for example, can have a more serious or even fatal course in children on immunosuppressant corticosteriods. In such children, or in adults who have not had these diseases, particular care should be taken to avoid exposure. If exposed, therapy with varicella zoster immune globulin (VZIG) or pooled intravenous immunoglobulin (IVIG), as appropriate, may be indicated. If chickenpox develops, treatment with antiviral agents may be considered.

Patients should not be vaccinated against smallpox while on corticosteroid therapy. Other immunization procedures should not be undertaken in patients who are on corticosteroids, especially on high dose, because of possible hazards of neurological complications and a lack of antibody response.

The use of triamcinolone acetonide in patients with active tuberculosis should be restricted to those cases of fulminating or disseminated tuberculosis in which the corticosteroid is used for the management of the disease in conjunction with an appropriate antituberculous regimen. If corticosteroids are indicated in patients with latent tuberculosis or tuberculin reactivity, close observation is necessary since reactivation of the disease may occur. During prolonged corticosteroid therapy these patients should receive chemoprophylaxis.

Because rare instances of anaphylactoid reactions have occurred in patients receiving parenteral corticosteroid therapy, appropriate precautionary measures should be taken prior to administration, especially when the patient has a history of allergy to any drug.

Safety of use of KENALOG-10 Injection (Sterile Triamcinolone Acetonide Suspension USP) by intraturbinal, subconjunctival, subtenons, and retrobulbar injection has not been established.

Usage in Pregnancy

Since adequate human reproduction studies have not been done with corticosteroids, the use of these drugs in pregnancy, nursing mothers, or women of child-bearing potential requires that the possible benefits of the drug be weighed against the potential hazards to the mother and the embryo, fetus, or nursing infant. Infants born of mothers who have received substantial doses of corticosteroids during pregnancy should be carefully observed for signs of hypoadrenalism.

PRECAUTIONS

Drug-induced secondary adrenocortical insufficiency may be minimized by a gradual reduction of dosage. This type of relative insufficiency may persist for months after discontinuation of therapy; therefore, in any situation of stress (such as trauma, surgery, or severe illness) occurring during that period, hormone therapy should be reinstituted. Since mineralocorticoid secretion may be impaired, salt and/or a mineralocorticoid should be administered concurrently.

There is an enhanced corticosteroid effect in patients with hypothyroidism and in those with cirrhosis.

Corticosteroids should be used cautiously in patients with ocular herpes simplex because of possible corneal perforation.

The lowest possible dose of corticosteroid should be used to control the condition being treated. A gradual reduction in dosage should be made when possible.

Psychic derangements may appear when corticosteroids are used. These may range from euphoria, insomnia, mood swings, personality changes, and severe depression, to frank psychotic manifestations. Existing emotional instability or psychotic tendencies may also be aggravated by corticosteroids.

Aspirin should be used cautiously in conjunction with corticosteroids in patients with hypoprothrombinemia.

Corticosteroids should be used with caution in patients with nonspecific ulcerative colitis if there is a probability of impending perforation, abscess, or other pyogenic infection. Corticosteroids should also be used cautiously in patients with diverticulitis, fresh intestinal anastomoses, active or latent peptic ulcer, renal insufficiency, hypertension, osteoporosis, and myasthenia gravis.

Patients who are on immunosuppressant doses of corticosteroids should be warned to avoid exposure to chickenpox or measles and, if exposed, to obtain medical advice.

Growth and development of infants and children on prolonged corticosteroid therapy should be carefully observed.

Although therapy with KENALOG-10 Injection (Sterile Triamcinolone Acetonide Suspension USP) may ameliorate symptoms, it is in no sense a cure and the hormone has no effect on the cause of the inflammation. Therefore, this method of treatment does not obviate the need for the conventional measures usually employed.

Intra-articular injection of a corticosteroid may produce systemic as well as local effects. The inadvertent injection of the suspension into the soft tissues surrounding a joint is not harmful, but is the most common cause of failure to achieve the desired local results.

Following intra-articular steroid therapy, patients should be specifically warned to avoid overuse of joints in which symptomatic benefit has been obtained. Negligence in this matter may permit an increase in joint deterioration that will more than offset the beneficial effects of the steroid. To detect deterioration follow-up x-ray examination is suggested in selected cases.

Overdistention of the joint capsule and deposition of steroid along the needle track should be avoided in intra-articular injection since this may lead to subcutaneous atrophy.

Corticosteroids should not be injected into unstable joints.

Repeated intra-articular injection may in some cases result in instability of the joint. In selected cases, particularly when repeated injections are given, x-ray follow-up is suggested.

An increase in joint discomfort has seldom occurred. A marked increase in pain accompanied by local swelling, further restriction of joint motion, fever, and malaise are suggestive of a septic arthritis. If these complications should appear, and the diagnosis of septic arthritis is confirmed, administration of triamcinolone acetonide should be stopped, and antimicrobial therapy should be instituted immediately and continued for 7 to 10 days after all evidence of infection has disappeared. Appropriate examination of any joint fluid present is necessary to exclude a septic process.

Local injection of a steroid into a previously infected joint is to be avoided.

KENALOG-10 Injection (Sterile Triamcinolone Acetonide Suspension USP) should be administered only with full knowledge of characteristic activity of, and varied responses to, adrenocortical hormones. Like other potent corticosteroids, triamcinolone acetonide should be used under close clinical supervision. Triamcinolone acetonide can cause elevation of blood pressure, salt and water retention, and increased potassium and calcium excretion necessitating dietary salt restriction and potassium supplementation. Edema may occur in the presence of renal disease with a fixed or decreased glomerular filtration rate.

During prolonged therapy, *a liberal protein intake is essential* for counteracting the tendency to gradual weight loss sometimes associated with negative nitrogen balance, wasting and weakness of skeletal muscles.

When local or systemic microbial infections are present, therapy with triamcinolone acetonide is not recommended, but may be employed with caution and only in conjunction with appropriate antibiotic or chemotherapeutic medication. Triamcinolone acetonide may mask signs of infection and enhance dissemination of the infecting organism. Hence, all patients receiving triamcinolone acetonide should be watched for evidence of intercurrent infection. Should infection occur, vigorous, appropriate anti-infective therapy should be initiated. If possible, abrupt cessation of steroids should be avoided because of the danger of superimposing adrenocortical insufficiency on the infectious process.

Menstrual irregularities may occur, and this possibility should be mentioned to female patients past menarche.

In peptic ulcer, recurrence may be asymptomatic until perforation or hemorrhage occurs. X-rays should be taken in peptic ulcer patients complaining of gastric distress, or when therapy is prolonged. Whether or not changes are observed, an ulcer regimen is recommended.

As with other corticosteroids, the possibility of other severe reactions should be considered. If such reactions should occur, appropriate corrective measures should be instituted and use of the drug discontinued.

Continued supervision of the patient after termination of triamcinolone acetonide therapy is essential, since there may be a sudden reappearance of severe manifestations of the disease for which the patient was treated.

ADVERSE REACTIONS

Undesirable reactions following intra-articular administration of the preparation have included postinjection flare, transient pain, occasional local irritation at the injection site, sterile abscesses, hyper- and hypopigmentation, charcot-like arthropathy, and occasional brief increase in joint discomfort; following intradermal administration, rare instances of blindness associated with intralesional therapy around the face and head, transient local discomfort, sterile abscesses, hyper- and hypopigmentation, and subcutaneous and cutaneous atrophy (which usually disappears, unless the basic disease process is itself atrophic) have occurred.

Since systemic absorption may occasionally occur with intra-articular or other local administration, patients should be watched closely for the following adverse reactions which may be associated with any corticosteroid therapy:

Fluid and electrolyte disturbances—sodium retention, fluid retention, congestive heart failure in susceptible patients, potassium loss, cardiac arrythmias or ECG changes due to potassium deficiency, hypokalemic alkalosis, and hypertension.

Musculoskeletal—muscle weakness, fatigue, steroid myopathy, loss of muscle mass, osteoporosis, vertebral compression fractures, delayed healing of fractures, aseptic necrosis of femoral and humeral heads, pathologic fractures of long bones, and spontaneous fractures.

Gastrointenstinal—peptic ulcer with possible subsequent perforation and hemorrhage, pancreatitis, abdominal distention, and ulcerative esophagitis.

Dermatologic—impaired wound healing, thin fragile skin, petechiae and ecchymoses, facial erythema, increased sweating, purpura, striae, hirsutism, acneiform eruptions, lupus erythematosus-like lesions and suppressed reactions to skin tests.

Neurological—convulsions, increased intracranial pressure with papilledema (pseudo-tumor cerebri) usually after treatment, vertigo, headache, neuritis or paresthesias, and aggravation of pre-existing psychiatric conditions.

Endocrine—menstrual irregularities; development of the cushingoid state; suppression of growth in children; secondary adrenocortical and pituitary unresponsiveness, particularly in times of stress (e.g., trauma, surgery, or illness); decreased carbohydrate tolerance; manifestations of latent diabetes mellitus; and increased requirements for insulin or oral hypoglycemic agents in diabetics.

Ophthalmic—posterior subcapsular cataracts, increased intraocular pressure, glaucoma, and exophthalmos.

Metabolic—hyperglycemia, glycosuria, and negative nitrogen balance due to protein catabolism.

Others—necrotizing angiitis, thrombophlebitis, thromboembolism, aggravation or masking of infections, insomnia, syncopal episodes, and anaphylactoid reactions.

DOSAGE AND ADMINISTRATION

Dosage

The initial dose of KENALOG-10 Injection (Sterile Triamcinolone Acetonide Suspension USP) for intra-articular or intrabursal administration and for injection into tendon sheaths may vary from 2.5 mg to 5 mg for smaller joints and from 5 to 15 mg for larger joints depending on the specific disease entity being treated. Single injections into several joints for multiple locus involvement, up to a total of 20 mg or more, have been given without incident. For intradermal administration, the initial dose of triamcinolone acetonide will vary depending upon the specific disease entity being treated but should be limited to 1.0 mg (0.1 mL) per injection site, since larger volumes are more likely to produce cutaneous atrophy. Multiple sites (separated by one centimeter or more) may be so injected, keeping in mind that the greater the *total* volume employed the more corticosteroid becomes available for possible systemic absorption and subsequent corticosteroid effects. Such injections may be repeated, if necessary, at weekly or less frequent intervals.

The lower dosages in the initial dosage range of triamcinolone acetonide may produce the desired effect when the corticosteroid is administered to provide a localized concentration. The site of the injection and the volume of the injection should be carefully considered when triamcinolone acetonide is administered for this purpose. The initial dosage should be maintained or adjusted until a satisfactory response is noted. If after a reasonable period of time there is a lack of satisfactory clinical response, KENALOG-10 Injection should be discontinued and the patient transferred to other appropriate therapy. IT SHOULD BE EMPHASIZED THAT DOSAGE REQUIREMENTS ARE VARIABLE AND MUST BE INDIVIDUALIZED ON THE BASIS OF THE DISEASE UNDER TREATMENT AND THE RESPONSE OF THE PATIENT. After a favorable response is noted, the proper maintenance dosage should be determined by decreasing the initial drug dosage in small increments at appropriate time intervals until the lowest dosage which will maintain an adequate clinical response is reached. It should be kept in mind that constant monitoring is needed in regard to drug dosage. Included in the situations which may make dosage adjustments necessary are changes in clinical status secondary to remissions or exacerbations in the disease process, the patient's individual drug responsiveness, and the effect of patient exposure to stressful situations not directly related to the disease entity under treatment; in this latter situation it may be necessary to increase the dosage of KENALOG-10 Injection (Sterile Triamcinolone Acetonide Suspension USP) for a period of time consistent with the patient's condition. If the drug is to be stopped after long-term

therapy, it is recommended that it be withdrawn gradually rather than abruptly.

Administration

Shake the vial before use to insure a uniform suspension. Prior to withdrawal, inspect suspension for clumping or granular appearance (agglomeration). An agglomerated product results from exposure to freezing temperatures and should not be used. After withdrawal, inject without delay to prevent settling in the syringe. Careful technique should be employed to avoid the possibility of entering a blood vessel or introducing infection.

Routine laboratory studies, such as urinalysis, two-hour postprandial blood sugar, determination of blood pressure and body weight, and a chest x-ray should be made at regular intervals during prolonged therapy. Upper GI x-rays are desirable in patients with an ulcer history or significant dyspepsia.

For treatment of joints, the usual intra-articular injection technique, as described in standard textbooks, should be followed. If an excessive amount of synovial fluid is present in the joint, some, but not all, should be aspirated to aid in the relief of pain and to prevent undue dilution of the steroid. With intra-articular or intrabursal administration, and with injection of KENALOG-10 Injection into tendon sheaths, the use of a local anesthetic may often be desirable. When a local anesthetic is used, its package insert should be read with care and all the precautions connected with its use should be observed. It should be injected into the surrounding soft tissues prior to the injection of the corticosteroid. A small amount of the anesthetic solution may be instilled into the joint.

In treating acute nonspecific tenosynovitis, care should be taken to insure that the injection of KENALOG-10 Injection is made into the tendon sheath rather than the tendon substance. Epicondylitis (tennis elbow) may be treated by infiltrating the preparation into the area of greatest tenderness. For treatment of dermal lesions, KENALOG-10 Injection is injected directly into the lesion, i.e., intradermally or sometimes subcutaneously. For accuracy of dosage measurement and ease of administration, it is preferable to employ a tuberculin syringe and a small bore needle (23 to 25 gauge). Ethyl chloride spray may be used to alleviate the discomfort of the injection.

HOW SUPPLIED

KENALOG-10 Injection (Sterile Triamcinolone Acetonide Suspension USP) is supplied in 5 mL multiple dose vials (NDC 0003-0494-20) providing 10 mg triamcinolone acetonide per mL.

Storage

Store at room temperature; avoid freezing; protect from light.

KENALOG®-40 INJECTION   ℞

[ken 'ah-log"]

Sterile Triamcinolone Acetonide Suspension
USP
NOT FOR INTRAVENOUS OR
INTRADERMAL USE

DESCRIPTION

KENALOG-40 Injection (Sterile Triamcinolone Acetonide Suspension USP) provides a synthetic corticosteroid with marked anti-inflammatory action. Each mL of the sterile aqueous suspension provides 40 mg of triamcinolone acetonide, with sodium chloride for isotonicity, 0.9% (w/v) benzyl alcohol as a preservative, 0.75% carboxymethylcellulose sodium and 0.04% polysorbate 80. Sodium hydroxide or hydrochloric acid may be present to adjust pH to 5.0–7.5. At the time of manufacture, the air in the container is replaced by nitrogen.

ACTIONS

Naturally occurring glucocorticoids (hydrocortisone), which also have salt-retaining properties, are used as replacement therapy in adrenocortical deficiency states. Their synthetic analogs are primarily used for their potent anti-inflammatory effects in disorders of many organ systems.

Glucocorticoids cause profound and varied metabolic effects. In addition, they modify the body's immune responses to diverse stimuli.

KENALOG-40 Injection has an extended duration of effect which may be permanent, or sustained over a period of several weeks. Studies indicate that following a single intramuscular dose of 60 to 100 mg of triamcinolone acetonide, adrenal suppression occurs within 24 to 48 hours and then gradually returns to normal, usually in 30 to 40 days. This finding correlates closely with the extended duration of therapeutic action achieved with the drug.

INDICATIONS

Intramuscular

Where oral therapy is not feasible or is temporarily undesirable in the judgment of the physician, KENALOG-40 Injection is indicated for intramuscular use as follows:

1. *Endocrine disorders*—Nonsuppurative thyroiditis.
2. *Rheumatic disorders*—As adjunctive therapy for short-term administration (to tide the patient over an acute episode or exacerbation) in: post-traumatic osteoarthritis; synovitis of osteoarthritis; rheumatoid arthritis; acute and subacute bursitis; epicondylitis; acute nonspecific tenosynovitis; acute gouty arthritis; psoriatic arthritis; ankylosing spondylitis; juvenile rheumatoid arthritis.
3. *Collagen diseases*—During an exacerbation or as maintenance therapy in selected cases of: systemic lupus erythematosus; acute rheumatic carditis.
4. *Dermatologic diseases*—Pemphigus; severe erythema multiforme (Stevens-Johnson syndrome); exfoliative dermatitis; bullous dermatitis herpetiformis; severe seborrheic dermatitis; severe psoriasis.
5. *Allergic states*—Control of severe or incapacitating allergic conditions intractable to adequate trials of conventional treatment in: bronchial asthma; contact dermatitis; atopic dermatitis; seasonal or perennial allergic rhinitis.
6. *Ophthalmic diseases*—Severe chronic allergic and inflammatory processes involving the eye, such as: herpes zoster ophthalmicus; iritis; iridocyclitis; chorioretinitis; diffuse posterior uveitis and choroiditis; optic neuritis; sympathetic ophthalmia; anterior segment inflammation.
7. *Gastrointestinal diseases*—To tide the patient over a critical period of disease in: ulcerative colitis (systemic therapy); regional enteritis (systemic therapy).
8. *Respiratory diseases*—Symptomatic sarcoidosis; berylliosis; aspiration pneumonitis.
9. *Hematologic disorders*—Acquired (autoimmune) hemolytic anemia.
10. *Neoplastic diseases*—For palliative management of: leukemias and lymphomas in adults; acute leukemia of childhood.
11. *Edematous state*—To induce diuresis or remission of proteinuria in the nephrotic syndrome, without uremia, of the idiopathic type or that due to lupus erythematosus.

Intra-Articular

KENALOG-40 Injection (Sterile Triamcinolone Acetonide Suspension USP) is indicated for intra-articular or intrabursal administration, and for injections into tendon sheaths, as adjunctive therapy for short-term administration (to tide the patient over an acute episode or exacerbation) in: synovitis of osteoarthritis; rheumatoid arthritis; acute and subacute bursitis; acute gouty arthritis; epicondylitis; acute nonspecific tenosynovitis; post-traumatic osteoarthritis.

CONTRAINDICATIONS

Corticosteroids are contraindicated in patients with systemic fungal infections. Intramuscular corticosteroid preparations are contraindicated for idiopathic thrombocytopenic purpura.

WARNINGS

Because it is a suspension, the preparation should **not** be administered intravenously. Strict aseptic technique is mandatory. This preparation is not recommended for children under six years of age.

Adequate studies to demonstrate the safety of administration of KENALOG-40 Injection (Sterile Triamcinolone Acetonide Suspension USP) by intraturbinal, subconjunctival, subtenon and retrobulbar injections have not been performed. Several instances of blindness have been reported following injection of corticosteroid suspensions into the nasal turbinates and intralesional injection about the head. When patients who are receiving corticosteroid therapy are subjected to unusual stress, increased dosage of rapidly acting corticosteroids is indicated before, during and after the stressful situation.

Corticosteroids may mask some signs of infection, and new infections may appear during their use. There may be decreased resistance and inability to localize infection when corticosteroids are used. If an infection occurs during corticosteroid therapy, it should be promptly controlled by suitable antimicrobial therapy (see PRECAUTIONS).

Children who are on immunosuppressant drugs are more susceptible to infections than healthy children. Chickenpox and measles, for example, can have a more serious or even fatal course in children on immunosuppressant corticosteroids. In such children, or in adults who have not had these diseases, particular care should be taken to avoid exposure. If exposed, therapy with varicella zoster immune globulin (VZIG) or pooled intravenous immunoglobulin (IVIG), as appropriate, may be indicated. If chickenpox develops, treatment with antiviral agents may be considered.

Prolonged use of corticosteroids may produce posterior subcapsular cataracts, glaucoma with possible damage to the optic nerves, and may enhance the establishment of secondary ocular infections due to fungi or viruses.

Average and large doses of hydrocortisone or cortisone can cause elevation of blood pressure, salt and water retention and increased excretion of potassium. These effects are less likely to occur with the synthetic derivatives except when they are used in large doses; dietary salt restriction and potassium supplementation may be necessary (see PRECAUTIONS). All corticosteroids increase calcium excretion.

Patients should not be vaccinated against smallpox while on corticosteroid therapy. Other immunization procedures should not be undertaken in patients who are on corticosteroids, especially on high dose, because of possible hazards of neurological complications and a lack of antibody response. The use of corticosteroids in patients with active tuberculosis should be restricted to those cases of fulminating or disseminated tuberculosis in which the corticosteroid is used for the management of the disease in conjunction with an appropriate antituberculous regimen. If corticosteroids are indicated in patients with latent tuberculosis or tuberculin reactivity, close observation is necessary since reactivation of the disease may occur. During prolonged corticosteroid therapy these patients should receive chemoprophylaxis.

Because rare instances of anaphylactoid reactions have occurred in patients receiving parenteral corticosteroid therapy, appropriate precautionary measures should be taken prior to administration, especially when the patient has a history of allergy to any drug.

Unless a **deep** intramuscular injection is given, local atrophy is likely to occur. (For recommendations on injection techniques, see DOSAGE AND ADMINISTRATION.) Due to the significantly higher incidence of local atrophy when the material is injected into the deltoid area, this injection site should be avoided in favor of the gluteal area. Only very unusual circumstances would warrant injection into the deltoid area.

USAGE IN PREGNANCY

Since adequate human reproduction studies have not been done with corticosteroids, the use of these drugs in pregnancy, nursing mothers, or women of childbearing potential requires that the possible benefits of the drug be weighed against the potential hazards to the mother and the embryo, fetus, or nursing infant. Infants born of mothers who have received substantial doses of corticosteroids during pregnancy should be carefully observed for signs of hypoadrenalism.

PRECAUTIONS

Drug-induced secondary adrenocortical insufficiency may be minimized by a gradual reduction of dosage. This type of relative insufficiency may persist for months after discontinuation of therapy; therefore, in any situation of stress (such as trauma, surgery or severe illness) occurring during that period, hormone therapy should be reinstituted. Since mineralocorticoid secretion may be impaired, salt and/or a mineralocorticoid should be administered concurrently.

There is an enhanced corticosteroid effect in patients with hypothyroidism and in those with cirrhosis.

Corticosteroids should be used cautiously in patients with ocular herpes simplex because of possible corneal perforation.

The lowest possible dose of corticosteroid should be used to control the condition being treated. A gradual reduction in dosage should be made when possible.

Psychic derangements may appear when corticosteroids are used. These may range from euphoria, insomnia, mood swings, personality changes and severe depression to frank psychotic manifestations. Existing emotional instability or psychotic tendencies may also be aggravated by corticosteroids.

Aspirin should be used cautiously in conjunction with corticosteroids in patients with hypoprothrombinemia.

Corticosteroids should be used with caution in patients with nonspecific ulcerative colitis if there is a probability of impending perforation, abscess, or other pyogenic infection. Corticosteroids should also be used cautiously in patients with diverticulitis, fresh intestinal anastomoses, active or latent peptic ulcer, renal insufficiency, hypertension, osteoporosis, acute glomerulonephritis, vaccinia, varicella, exanthema, Cushing's syndrome, antibiotic resistant infections, diabetes mellitus, congestive heart failure, chronic nephritis, thromboembolitic tendencies, thrombophlebitis, convulsive disorders, metastatic carcinoma, and myasthenia gravis.

Patients who are on immunosuppressant doses of corticosteroids should be warned to avoid exposure to chickenpox or measles and, if exposed, to obtain medical advice.

Growth and development of infants and children on prolonged corticosteroid therapy should be carefully observed. Although therapy with KENALOG-40 Injection (Sterile Triamcinolone Acetonide Suspension USP) will ameliorate symptoms, it is in no sense a cure and the hormone has no effect on the cause of the inflammation. Therefore, this method of treatment does not obviate the need for the conventional measures usually employed.

Intra-articular injection of a corticosteroid may produce systemic as well as local effects. The inadvertent injection of the suspension into the soft tissues surrounding a joint is not harmful, but may lead to the occurrence of systemic effects, and is the most common cause of failure to achieve the desired local results.

Continued on next page

Westwood-Squibb—Cont.

Following intra-articular steroid therapy, patients should be specifically warned to avoid overuse of joints in which symptomatic benefit has been obtained. Negligence in this matter may permit an increase in joint deterioration that will more than offset the beneficial effects of the steroid. To detect deterioration, follow-up x-ray examination is suggested in selected cases.

Overdistention of the joint capsule and deposition of steroid along the needle track should be avoided in intra-articular injection since this may lead to subcutaneous atrophy.

Corticosteroids should not be injected into unstable joints. Repeated intra-articular injection may in some cases result in instability of the joint. In selected cases, particularly when repeated injections are given, x-ray follow-up is suggested.

An increase in joint discomfort has seldom occurred. A marked increase in pain accompanied by local swelling, further restriction of joint motion, fever and malaise are suggestive of a septic arthritis. If these complications should appear, and the diagnosis of septic arthritis is confirmed, administration of triamcinolone acetonide should be stopped, and antimicrobial therapy should be instituted immediately and continued for 7 to 10 days after all evidence of infection has disappeared. Appropriate examination of any joint fluid present is necessary to exclude a septic process. Local injection of a steroid into a previously infected joint is to be avoided.

KENALOG-40 Injection (Sterile Triamcinolone Acetonide Suspension USP) should be administered only with full knowledge of characteristic activity of, and varied responses to, adrenocortical hormones. Like other potent corticosteroids, triamcinolone acetonide should be used under close clinical supervision. Triamcinolone acetonide can cause elevation of blood pressure, salt and water retention, and increased potassium and calcium excretion necessitating dietary salt restriction and potassium supplementation. Edema may occur in the presence of renal disease with a fixed or decreased glomerular filtration rate.

During prolonged therapy, **a liberal protein intake is essential** for counteracting the tendency to gradual weight loss sometimes associated with negative nitrogen balance, wasting and weakness of skeletal muscles.

When local or systemic microbial infections are present, therapy with triamcinolone acetonide is not recommended, but may be employed with caution and only in conjunction with appropriate antibiotic or chemotherapeutic medication. Triamcinolone acetonide may mask signs of infection and enhance dissemination of the infecting organism. Hence, all patients receiving triamcinolone acetonide should be watched for evidence of intercurrent infection. Should infection occur, vigorous, appropriate anti-infective therapy should be initiated. If possible, abrupt cessation of steroids should be avoided because of the danger of superimposing adrenocortical insufficiency on the infectious process.

Menstrual irregularities may occur, and this possibility should be mentioned to female patients past menarche.

In peptic ulcer, recurrence may be asymptomatic until perforation or hemorrhage occurs. Long-term adrenocorticoid therapy may evoke hyperacidity or peptic ulcer; therefore, as a prophylactic measure, an ulcer regimen and the administration of an antacid are highly recommended. X-rays should be taken in peptic ulcer patients complaining of gastric distress, or when therapy is prolonged. Whether or not changes are observed, an ulcer regimen is recommended.

As with other corticosteroids, the possibility of other severe reactions should be considered. If such reactions should occur, appropriate corrective measures should be instituted and use of the drug discontinued.

Continued supervision of the patient after termination of triamcinolone acetonide therapy is essential, since there may be a sudden reappearance of severe manifestations of the disease for which the patient was treated.

ADVERSE REACTIONS

Following Administration by Any Route — Patients should be watched closely for the following adverse reactions which may be associated with any corticosteroid therapy:

Fluid and electrolyte disturbances — sodium retention, fluid retention, congestive heart failure in susceptible patients, potassium loss, cardiac arrhythmias or ECG changes due to potassium deficiency, hypokalemic alkalosis and hypertension.

Musculoskeletal — muscle weakness, fatigue, steroid myopathy, loss of muscle mass, osteoporosis, vertebral compression fractures, delayed healing of fractures, aseptic necrosis of femoral and humeral heads, pathologic fractures of long bones, and spontaneous fractures.

Gastrointestinal — peptic ulcer with possible subsequent perforation and hemorrhage, pancreatitis, abdominal distention, and ulcerative esophagitis.

Dermatologic — impaired wound healing, thin fragile skin, petechiae and ecchymoses, facial erythema, increased sweating, purpura, striae, hirsutism, acneiform eruptions, lupus

erythematosus-like lesions and suppressed reactions to skin tests.

Neurological — convulsions, increased intracranial pressure with papilledema (pseudo-tumor cerebri) usually after treatment, vertigo, headache, neuritis or paresthesias and aggravation of preexisting psychiatric conditions.

Endocrine — menstrual irregularities; development of the cushingoid state; suppression of growth in children; secondary adrenocortical and pituitary unresponsiveness, particularly in times of stress (e.g., trauma, surgery or illness); decreased carbohydrate tolerance; manifestations of latent diabetes mellitus and increased requirements for insulin or oral hypoglycemic agents in diabetics.

Ophthalmic — posterior subcapsular cataracts, increased intraocular pressure, glaucoma and exophthalmos.

Metabolic — hyperglycemia, glycosuria and negative nitrogen balance due to protein catabolism.

Others — necrotizing angiitis, thrombophlebitis, thromboembolism, aggravation or masking of infections, insomnia, syncopal episodes and anaphylactoid reactions.

Following Intramuscular Administration

Severe pain has been reported in a few cases. Sterile abscess formation, subcutaneous and cutaneous atrophy, hyperpigmentation and hypopigmentation and charcot-like arthropathy have also occurred.

Following Intra-Articular Administration

Undesirable reactions have included postinjection flare, transient pain, occasional irritation at the injection site, sterile abscess formation, hyperpigmentation and hypopigmentation, charcot-like arthropathy and occasional brief increase in joint discomfort.

DOSAGE AND ADMINISTRATION

General

The initial dose of KENALOG-40 Injection (Sterile Triamcinolone Acetonide Suspension USP) may vary from 2.5 to 60 mg per day depending on the specific disease entity being treated (see **Dosage** section below). In situations of less severity, lower doses will generally suffice while in selected patients higher initial doses may be required. Usually the parenteral dosage ranges are one-third to one-half the oral dose given every 12 hours. However, in certain overwhelming, acute, life-threatening situations, administration of dosages exceeding the usual dosages may be justified and may be in multiples of the oral dosages.

The initial dosage should be maintained or adjusted until a satisfactory response is noted. If after a reasonable period of time there is a lack of satisfactory clinical response, KENALOG-40 Injection should be discontinued and the patient transferred to other appropriate therapy. IT SHOULD BE EMPHASIZED THAT DOSAGE REQUIREMENTS ARE VARIABLE AND MUST BE INDIVIDUALIZED ON THE BASIS OF THE DISEASE UNDER TREATMENT AND THE RESPONSE OF THE PATIENT. After a favorable response is noted, the proper maintenance dosage should be determined by decreasing the initial drug dosage in small increments at appropriate time intervals until the lowest dosage which will maintain an adequate clinical response is reached. It should be kept in mind that constant monitoring is needed in regard to drug dosage. Included in the situations which may make dosage adjustments necessary are changes in clinical status secondary to remissions or exacerbations in the disease process, the patient's individual drug responsiveness, and the effect of patient exposure to stressful situations not directly related to the disease entity under treatment; in this latter situation it may be necessary to increase the dosage of KENALOG-40 Injection for a period of time consistent with the patient's condition. If after long-term therapy the drug is to be stopped, it is recommended that it be withdrawn gradually rather than abruptly.

Dosage

Systemic

Although KENALOG-40 Injection may be administered intramuscularly for initial therapy, most physicians prefer to adjust the dose orally until adequate control is attained. Intramuscular administration provides a sustained or depot action which can be used to supplement or replace initial oral therapy. With intramuscular therapy, greater supervision of the amount of steroid used is made possible in the patient who is inconsistent in following an oral dosage schedule. In maintenance therapy, the patient-to-patient response is not uniform and, therefore, the dose must be individualized for optimal control.

For **adults and children over 12 years of age,** the suggested initial dose is 60 mg, **injected deeply into the gluteal muscle.** Subcutaneous fat atrophy may occur if care is not taken to inject the preparation intramuscularly. Dosage is usually adjusted within the range of 40 to 80 mg, depending upon patient response and duration of relief. However, some patients may be well controlled on dosages as low as 20 mg or less. Patients with hay fever or pollen asthma who are not responding to pollen administration and other conventional therapy may obtain a remission of symptoms lasting throughout the pollen season after one injection of 40 to 100 mg.

For **children from 6 to 12 years of age,** the suggested initial dose is 40 mg, although dosage depends more on the severity of symptoms than on age or weight. There is insufficient clinical experience with KENALOG-40 Injection (Sterile Triamcinolone Acetonide Suspension USP) to recommend its use in children under six years of age.

Local

For intra-articular or intrabursal administration and for injection into tendon sheaths, the initial dose of KENALOG-40 Injection may vary from 2.5 to 5 mg for smaller joints and from 5 to 15 mg for larger joints depending on the specific disease entity being treated. (A more dilute form of Sterile Triamcinolone Acetonide Suspension USP is available—see ALSO AVAILABLE.) For adults, doses up to 10 mg for smaller areas and up to 40 mg for larger areas have usually been sufficient to alleviate symptoms. Single injections into several joints for multiple locus involvement, up to a total of 80 mg, have been given without undue reactions. A single local injection of triamcinolone acetonide is frequently sufficient, but several injections may be needed for adequate relief of symptoms. The lower dosages in the initial dosage range of triamcinolone acetonide may produce the desired effect when the corticosteroid is administered to provide a localized concentration. The site of the injection and the volume of the injection should be carefully considered when triamcinolone acetonide is administered for this purpose.

Administration

General

Shake the vial before use to insure a uniform suspension. Prior to withdrawal, inspect suspension for clumping or granular appearance (agglomeration). An agglomerated product results from exposure to freezing temperatures and should not be used. After withdrawal, inject without delay to prevent settling in the syringe. Careful technique should be employed to avoid the possibility of entering a blood vessel or introducing infection.

Routine laboratory studies, such as urinalysis, two-hour postprandial blood sugar, determination of blood pressure and body weight and a chest x-ray should be made at regular intervals during prolonged therapy. Upper GI x-rays are desirable in patients with an ulcer history or significant dyspepsia.

Systemic

For systemic therapy, injection should be made **deeply into the gluteal muscle** to insure intramuscular delivery (see WARNINGS). For adults, a minimum needle length of 1 ½ inches is recommended. In obese patients, a longer needle may be required. Use alternate sites for subsequent injections.

Local

For treatment of joints, the usual intra-articular injection technique, as described in standard textbooks, should be followed. If an excessive amount of synovial fluid is present in the joint, some, but not all, should be aspirated to aid in the relief of pain and to prevent undue dilution of the corticosteroid.

With intra-articular or intrabursal administration, and with injection of the drug into tendon sheaths, the use of a local anesthetic may often be desirable. When a local anesthetic is used, its package insert should be read with care and all the precautions connected with its use should be observed. It should be injected into the surrounding soft tissues prior to the injection of the corticosteroid. A small amount of the anesthetic solution may be instilled into the joint. Care should be taken with intra-articular and intrabursal injections (particularly in the deltoid region) and with injection into tendon sheaths to avoid injecting the suspension into the tissues surrounding the site since this may lead to tissue atrophy.

In treating acute nonspecific tenosynovitis, care should be taken to insure that the injection of the corticosteroid is made into the tendon sheath rather than the tendon substance. Epicondylitis (tennis elbow) may be treated by infiltrating the preparation into the area of greatest tenderness.

HOW SUPPLIED

KENALOG-40 Injection (Sterile Triamcinolone Acetonide Suspension USP) is supplied in vials providing 40 mg triamcinolone acetonide per mL.

ALSO AVAILABLE

KENALOG-10 Injection (Sterile Triamcinolone Acetonide Suspension USP) providing 10 mg triamcinolone acetonide per mL, with sodium chloride for isotonicity, 0.9% (w/v) benzyl alcohol as a preservative, 0.75% carboxymethylcellulose sodium, and 0.04% polysorbate 80. See package insert for full information.

Storage

Store at room temperature; avoid freezing. Protect from light.

LAC–HYDRIN® 12%*   ℞
(ammonium lactate)
Lotion

PRODUCT OVERVIEW

KEY FACTS
Lac-Hydrin® is a therapeutic lotion which is active in the treatment of moderate to severe xerosis and ichthyosis vulgaris. The active ingredient, ammonium lactate, helps improve the stratum corneum to provide a sustained effect in the treatment of dry skin.

MAJOR USES
Lac-Hydrin has been shown to be clinically effective for cases of moderate to severe xerosis and ichthyosis vulgaris.

SAFETY INFORMATION
Contact with eyes, lips or mucous membranes should be avoided. A mild transient stinging may occur on application to abraded or inflamed areas or in individuals with sensitive skin.

PRESCRIBING INFORMATION

LAC–HYDRIN® 12%*   ℞
(ammonium lactate)
Lotion
For topical use only. Not for ophthalmic use.

CAUTION
Federal law prohibits dispensing without a prescription.

DESCRIPTION*
LAC-HYDRIN, specially formulates 12% lactic acid neutralized with ammonium hydroxide, as ammonium lactate to provide a lotion pH of 4.5–5.5. LAC-HYDRIN also contains light mineral oil, glyceryl stearate, PEG-100 stearate, propylene glycol, polyoxyl 40 stearate, glycerin, magnesium aluminum silicate, laureth-4, cetyl alcohol, methyl and propylparabens, methylcellulose, fragrance, quaternium-15 and water. Lactic acid is a racemic mixture of 2-hydroxypropanoic acid and has the following structural formula:

$$\begin{array}{c} COOH \\ | \\ CHOH \\ | \\ CH_3 \end{array}$$

CLINICAL PHARMACOLOGY
It is generally accepted that the water content of the stratum corneum is a controlling factor in maintaining skin flexibility. When the stratum corneum contains more than 10% water it remains soft and pliable; however, when the water content drops below 10% the stratum corneum becomes less flexible and rough, and may exhibit scaling and cracking and the underlying skin may become irritated.
Symptomatic relief of dry skin is provided by skin protectants containing hygroscopic substances (humectants) which increase skin moisture. Lactic acid, an α-hydroxy acid, is reported to be one of the most effective naturally occurring humectants in the skin. The α-hydroxy acids (and their salts), in addition to having beneficial effects on dry skin, have also been shown to reduce excessive epidermal keratinization in patients with hyperkeratotic conditions (e.g., ichthyosis).
Pharmacokinetics: The mechanism of action of topically applied neutralized lactic acid is not yet known.

INDICATIONS AND USAGE
LAC-HYDRIN is indicated for the treatment of dry, scaly skin (xerosis) and ichthyosis vulgaris and for temporary relief of itching associated with these conditions.

CONTRAINDICATIONS
Known hypersensitivity to any of the label ingredients.

PRECAUTIONS
General: For external use only. Avoid contact with eyes, lips or mucous membranes. Caution is advised when used on the face of fair-skinned individuals since irritation may occur. A mild, transient stinging may occur on application to abraded or inflamed areas or in individuals with sensitive skin.
Carcinogenesis, Mutagenesis, Impairment of Fertility: LAC-HYDRIN was nonmutagenic in the Ames/Salmonella/ Microsome Plate Assay. Reproductive studies in rats given lactic acid orally showed no effect on the sex ratio of the offspring.
Pregnancy (Category C): Animal reproduction studies have not been conducted with LAC-HYDRIN. It is also not known whether LAC-HYDRIN can cause fetal harm when administered to a pregnant woman or can affect reproduction capacity. LAC-HYDRIN should be given to a pregnant woman only if clearly needed.
Nursing Mothers: Although lactic acid is a normal constituent of blood and tissues, it is not known to what extent this drug affects normal lactic acid levels in human milk. Because many drugs are excreted in human milk, caution

should be exercised when LAC-HYDRIN is administered to a nursing woman.
Pediatric Use: Safety and effectiveness of LAC-HYDRIN have been demonstrated in infants and children. No unusual toxic effects were reported.

ADVERSE REACTIONS
The most frequent adverse experiences in patients with xerosis are transient stinging (1 in 30 patients), burning (1 in 30 patients), erythema (1 in 50 patients) and peeling (1 in 60 patients). Other adverse reactions which occur less frequently are irritation, eczema, petechiae, dryness and hyperpigmentation.
Due to the more severe initial skin conditions associated with ichthyosis, there was a higher incidence of transient stinging, burning and erythema (each occurring in 1 in 10 patients).

OVERDOSAGE
The oral administration of LAC-HYDRIN to rats and mice showed this drug to be practically non-toxic ($LD_{50} >$ 15 ml/kg).

DOSAGE AND ADMINISTRATION
Shake well. Apply to the affected areas and rub in thoroughly. Use twice daily or as directed by a physician.

HOW SUPPLIED
8 oz. (NDC 0072-5712-08; NSN 6505-01-216-6274) plastic bottle and 14 oz. (NDC 0072-5712-14) plastic bottle.
Store at controlled room temperature (15°–30°C; 59°–86°F).

MOISTUREL® CREAM   OTC
Fragrance Free Skin Protectant—Moisturizer

COMPOSITION
Active Ingredients: Dimethicone 1%, petrolatum 30%. Also contains: Water, glycerin, PG dioctanoate, cetyl alcohol, steareth-2, PVP/hexadecene copolymer, laureth-23, magnesium aluminum silicate, diazolidinyl urea, carbomer-934, sodium hydroxide, methylchloroisothiazolinone and methylisothiazolinone.

ACTIONS AND USES
A highly effective, concentrated formula clinically proven to relieve dry skin and designed not to cause acne or blemishes. Ideal for sensitive skin. Free of lanolins, fragrances, and parabens that can sensitize or irritate skin.
Helps prevent and temporarily protects chafed, chapped, cracked or windburned skin. For temporary protection of minor cuts, scrapes, burns and sunburn. Helps treat and prevent minor skin irritation due to diaper rash and helps seal out wetness.

WARNINGS
For external use only. Avoid contact with the eyes. Not to be applied over puncture wounds or infections.

ADMINISTRATION AND DOSAGE
Apply liberally as often as needed. If used for diaper rash, change wet diapers promptly, cleanse the diaper area and allow to dry. Apply cream liberally with each changing.

HOW SUPPLIED
4 oz. (NDC 0072-9500-04) and 16 oz. (NDC 0072-9500-16) plastic jars.

MOISTUREL® LOTION   OTC
Skin Protectant—Moisturizer

COMPOSITION
Active Ingredient: Dimethicone 3%. Also contains: Water, petrolatum, glycerin, steareth-2, cetyl alcohol, benzyl alcohol, laureth-23, magnesium aluminum silicate, carbomer-934, sodium hydroxide, quaternium-15.

ACTION AND USES
Quick absorbing, long lasting formula that leaves the skin feeling smooth and soft. Clinically proven to relieve dry skin and designed not to cause acne. Free of lanolins and parabens that can irritate sensitive skin.
Generalized dry skin. Helps prevent and temporarily protects chafed, chapped, cracked or windburned skin. Helps treat and prevent minor skin irritation due to diaper rash and helps seal out wetness.

WARNINGS
For external use only. Avoid contact with the eyes. Not to be applied over puncture wounds or infections.

ADMINISTRATION AND DOSAGE
Apply liberally as often as needed to soothe and soften sensitive skin. If used for diaper rash, change wet diapers promptly, cleanse the diaper area and allow to dry. Apply lotion liberally with each changing.

HOW SUPPLIED
8 oz. (NDC 0072-9100-08) and 12 oz. (NDC 0072-9100-12) plastic bottles.

MYCOLOG®-II   ℞
[mĭk 'ō-log "]
Nystatin and Triamcinolone Acetonide Cream USP
Nystatin and Triamcinolone Acetonide Ointment USP
For Dermatologic Use Only
Not for Ophthalmic Use

DESCRIPTION
MYCOLOG-II Cream and Ointment (Nystatin and Triamcinolone Acetonide Cream and Ointment) for dermatologic use contains the antifungal agent nystatin and the synthetic corticosteroid triamcinolone acetonide.
Nystatin is a polyene antimycotic obtained from *Streptomyces noursei*. It is a yellow to light tan powder with a cereal-like odor, very slightly soluble in water, and slightly to sparingly soluble in alcohol.
Triamcinolone acetonide is designated chemically as 9-fluoro-11β, 16α, 17,21-tetrahydroxypregna-1,4-diene-3,20-dione cyclic 16,17-acetal with acetone. The white to cream crystalline powder has a slight odor, is practically insoluble in water, and very soluble in alcohol.
MYCOLOG-II Cream (Nystatin and Triamcinolone Acetonide Cream) is a soft, smooth, cream having a light yellow to buff color. Each gram provides 100,000 USP nystatin units and 1 mg triamcinolone acetonide in an aqueous perfumed vanishing cream base with aluminum hydroxide concentrated wet gel, titanium dioxide, glyceryl monostearate, polyethylene glycol monostearate, simethicone, sorbic acid, propylene glycol, white petrolatum, cetearyl alcohol (and) ceteareth-20, and sorbitol solution.
MYCOLOG-II Ointment (Nystatin and Triamcinolone Acetonide Ointment) provides, in each gram, 100,000 USP nystatin units and 1 mg triamcinolone acetonide in a protective ointment base, Plastibase® (Plasticized Hydrocarbon Gel), a polyethylene and mineral oil gel base.

CLINICAL PHARMACOLOGY
Nystatin
Nystatin exerts its antifungal activity against a variety of pathogenic and nonpathogenic yeasts and fungi by binding to sterols in the cell membrane. The binding process renders the cell membrane incapable of functioning as a selective barrier. Nystatin provides specific anticandidal activity to *Candida* (Monilia) *albicans* and other *Candida* species, but is not active against bacteria, protozoa, trichomonads, or viruses.
Nystatin is not absorbed from intact skin or mucous membranes.
Triamcinolone Acetonide
Triamcinolone acetonide is primarily effective because of its anti-inflammatory, antipruritic and vasoconstrictive actions, characteristic of the topical corticosteroid class of drugs. The pharmacologic effects of the topical corticosteroids are well-known; however, the mechanisms of their dermatologic actions are unclear. Various laboratory methods, including vasoconstrictor assays, are used to compare and predict potencies and/or clinical efficacies of the topical corticosteroids. There is some evidence to suggest that a recognizable correlation exists between vasoconstrictor potency and therapeutic efficacy in man.
Pharmacokinetics
The extent of percutaneous absorption of topical corticosteroids is determined by many factors including the vehicle, the integrity of the epidermal barrier, and the use of occlusive dressings (see DOSAGE AND ADMINISTRATION).
Topical corticosteroids can be absorbed from normal intact skin. Inflammation and/or disease processes in the skin increase percutaneous absorption. Occlusive dressings substantially increase the percutaneous absorption of topical corticosteroids (see DOSAGE AND ADMINISTRATION). Once absorbed through the skin, topical corticosteroids are handled through pharmacokinetic pathways similar to systemically administered corticosteroids. Corticosteroids are bound to plasma proteins in varying degrees. Corticosteroids are metabolized primarily in the liver and are then excreted by the kidneys. Some of the topical corticosteroids and their metabolites are also excreted into the bile.
Nystatin and Triamcinolone Acetonide
During clinical studies of mild to severe manifestations of cutaneous candidiasis, patients treated with combined nystatin and triamcinolone acetonide showed a faster and more pronounced clearing of erythema and pruritus than patients treated with nystatin or triamcinolone acetonide alone.

INDICATIONS AND USAGE
MYCOLOG-II Cream and Ointment (Nystatin and Triamcinolone Acetonide Cream and Ointment) are indicated for the treatment of cutaneous candidiasis; it has been demon-

Continued on next page

Westwood-Squibb—Cont.

strated that the nystatin-steroid combination provides greater benefit than the nystatin component alone during the first few days of treatment.

CONTRAINDICATIONS

These preparations are contraindicated in those patients with a history of hypersensitivity to any of their components.

PRECAUTIONS

General

Systemic absorption of topical corticosteroids has produced reversible hypothalamic-pituitary-adrenal (HPA) axis suppression, manifestations of Cushing's syndrome, hyperglycemia, and glucosuria in some patients.

Conditions that augment systemic absorption include application of the more potent steroids, use over large surface areas, prolonged use, and the addition of occlusive dressings (see DOSAGE AND ADMINISTRATION).

Therefore, patients receiving a large dose of any potent topical steroid applied to a large surface area should be evaluated periodically for evidence of HPA axis suppression by using the urinary free cortisol and ACTH stimulation tests, and for impairment of thermal homeostasis. If HPA axis suppression or elevation of the body temperature occurs, an attempt should be made to withdraw the drug, to reduce the frequency of application, or to substitute a less potent steroid.

Recovery of HPA axis function and thermal homeostasis are generally prompt and complete upon discontinuation of the drug. Infrequently, signs and symptoms of steroid withdrawal may occur, requiring supplemental systemic corticosteroids.

Children may absorb proportionally larger amounts of topical corticosteroids and thus be more susceptible to systemic toxicity (see PRECAUTIONS, Pediatric Use).

If irritation or hypersensitivity develops with the combination nystatin and triamcinolone acetonide, treatment should be discontinued and appropriate therapy instituted.

Information for the Patient

Patients using these medications should receive the following information and instructions:

1. These medications are to be used as directed by the physician. They are for dermatologic use only. Avoid contact with the eyes.
2. Patients should be advised not to use these medication for any disorder other than for which it was prescribed.
3. The treated skin area should not be bandaged or otherwise covered or wrapped as to be occluded (see DOSAGE AND ADMINISTRATION).
4. Patients should report any signs of local adverse reactions.
5. When using these medications in the inguinal area, patients should be advised to apply the cream or ointment sparingly and to wear loose-fitting clothing.
6. Parents of pediatric patients should be advised not to use tight-fitting diapers or plastic pants on a child being treated in the diaper area, as these garments may constitute occlusive dressings.
7. Patients should be advised on preventive measures to avoid reinfection.

Laboratory Tests

If there is a lack of therapeutic response, appropriate microbiological studies (e.g., KOH smears and/or cultures) should be repeated to confirm the diagnosis and rule out other pathogens, before instituting another course of therapy.

A urinary free cortisol test and ACTH stimulation test may be helpful in evaluating hypothalamic-pituitary-adrenal (HPA) axis suppression due to corticosteroid.

Carcinogenesis, Mutagenesis, and Impairment of Fertility

Long-term animal studies have not been performed to evaluate carcinogenic or mutagenic potential, or possible impairment of fertility in males or females.

Pregnancy Category C

There are no teratogenic studies with combined nystatin and triamcinolone acetonide. Corticosteroids are generally teratogenic in laboratory animals when administered systemically at relatively low dosage levels. The more potent corticosteroids have been shown to be teratogenic after dermal application in laboratory animals. Therefore, any topical corticosteroid preparation should be used during pregnancy only if the potential benefit justifies the potential risk to the fetus.

Topical preparations containing corticosteroids should not be used extensively on pregnant patients, in large amounts, or for prolonged periods of time.

Nursing Mothers

It is not known whether any component of these preparations are excreted in human milk. Because many drugs are excreted in human milk, caution should be exercised during use of these preparations by a nursing woman.

Pediatric Use

In clinical studies of a limited number of pediatric patients ranging in age from two months through 12 years, nystatin-triamcinolone cream formulation cleared or significantly ameliorated the disease state in most patients.

Pediatric patients may demonstrate greater susceptibility to topical corticosteroid-induced hypothalamic-pituitary-adrenal (HPA) axis suppression and Cushing's syndrome than mature patients because of a larger skin surface area to body weight ratio.

HPA axis suppression, Cushing's syndrome, and intracranial hypertension have been reported in children receiving topical corticosteroids. Manifestations of adrenal suppression in children include linear growth retardation, delayed weight gain, low plasma cortisol levels, and absence of response to ACTH stimulation. Manifestations of intracranial hypertension include bulging fontanelles, headaches, and bilateral papilledema.

Administration of topical corticosteroids to children should be limited to the least amount compatible with an effective therapeutic regimen. Chronic corticosteroid therapy may interfere with the growth and development of children.

ADVERSE REACTIONS

A single case (approximately one percent of patients studied) of acneform eruption occurred with use of combined nystatin and triamcinolone acetonide in clinical studies.

Nystatin is virtually nontoxic and nonsensitizing and is well tolerated by all age groups, even during prolonged use. Rarely, irritation may occur.

The following local adverse reactions are reported infrequently with topical corticosteroids (reactions are listed in an approximate decreasing order of occurrence): burning, itching, irritation, dryness, folliculitis, hypertrichosis, acneform eruptions, hypopigmentation, perioral dermatitis, allergic contact dermatitis, maceration of the skin, secondary infection, skin atrophy, striae, and miliaria.

OVERDOSAGE

Topically applied corticosteroids can be absorbed in sufficient amounts to produce systemic effects (see PRECAUTIONS, General); however, acute overdosage and serious adverse effects with dermatologic use are unlikely.

DOSAGE AND ADMINISTRATION

MYCOLOG-II Cream (Nystatin and Triamcinolone Acetonide Cream) is usually applied to the affected areas twice daily in the morning and evening by gently and thoroughly massaging the preparation into the skin. The cream should be discontinued if symptoms persist after 25 days of therapy (see PRECAUTIONS, Laboratory Tests).

MYCOLOG-II Cream should *not* be used with occlusive dressings.

A thin film of **MYCOLOG-II Ointment (Nystatin and Triamcinolone Acetonide Ointment)** is usually applied to the affected areas twice daily in the morning and evening.

The preparation should be discontinued if symptoms persist after 25 days of therapy (see PRECAUTIONS, Laboratory Tests).

MYCOLOG-II Ointment should *not* be used with occlusive dressings.

HOW SUPPLIED

MYCOLOG-II Cream (Nystatin and Triamcinolone Acetonide Cream USP) is supplied in 15 g (NDC 0003-0566-30, NSN 6505-01-210-9506), 30 g (NDC 0003-0566-60), and 60 g (NDC 0003-0566-65) tubes and 120 g (NDC 0003-0566-50) jars.

MYCOLOG-II Ointment (Nystatin and Triamcinolone Acetonide Ointment) is supplied in 15 g (NDC 0003-0466-30, NSN 6505-01-210-9507), 30 g (NDC 0003-0466-60), and 60 g (NDC 0003-0466-65) tubes and 120 g (NDC 0003-0466-50) jars.

Storage

Store at room temperature; avoid freezing cream.

MYCOSTATIN® CREAM ℞

[*mīk 'ō-stat "in*]

Nystatin Cream USP

MYCOSTATIN® TOPICAL POWDER ℞

Nystatin Topical Powder USP

MYCOSTATIN® OINTMENT ℞

Nystatin Ointment USP

For topical use only.

Not for ophthalmic use.

DESCRIPTION

MYCOSTATIN Cream (Nystatin Cream), MYCOSTATIN Topical Powder (Nystatin Topical Powder), and MYCOSTATIN Ointment (Nystatin Ointment) are for dermatologic use.

MYCOSTATIN Cream contains the antifungal antibiotic nystatin at a concentration of 100,000 USP nystatin units per gram in an aqueous, perfumed vanishing cream base containing aluminum hydroxide concentrated wet gel, titanium dioxide, propylene glycol, cetearyl alcohol (and) ceteareth-20, white petrolatum, sorbitol solution, glyceryl monostearate, polyethylene glycol monostearate, sorbic acid and simethicone.

MYCOSTATIN Topical Powder provides, in each gram, 100,000 USP nystatin units dispersed in talc.

MYCOSTATIN Ointment provides 100,000 USP nystatin units per gram in Plastibase® (Plasticized Hydrocarbon Gel), a polyethylene and mineral oil gel base.

CLINICAL PHARMACOLOGY

Nystatin is an antifungal antibiotic which is both fungistatic and fungicidal *in vitro* against a wide variety of yeasts and yeast-like fungi. It probably acts by binding to sterols in the cell membrane of the fungus with a resultant change in membrane permeability allowing leakage of intracellular components. Nystatin is a polyene antibiotic of undetermined structural formula that is obtained from *Streptomyces noursei*, and is the first well tolerated antifungal antibiotic of dependable efficacy for the treatment of cutaneous, oral and intestinal infections caused by *Candida* (Monilia) *albicans* and other Candida species. It exhibits no appreciable activity against bacteria.

Nystatin provides specific therapy for all localized forms of candidiasis. Symptomatic relief is rapid, often occurring within 24 to 72 hours after the initiation of treatment. Cure is effected both clinically and mycologically in most cases of localized candidiasis.

INDICATIONS AND USAGE

MYCOSTATIN (nystatin) topical preparations are indicated in the treatment of cutaneous or mucocutaneous mycotic infections caused by *Candida* (Monilia) *albicans* and other Candida species.

CONTRAINDICATIONS

MYCOSTATIN topical preparations are contraindicated in patients with a history of hypersensitivity to any of their components.

PRECAUTIONS

Should a reaction of hypersensitivity occur the drug should be immediately withdrawn and appropriate measures taken. These preparations are not for ophthalmic use.

ADVERSE REACTIONS

Nystatin is virtually nontoxic and nonsensitizing and is well tolerated by all age groups including debilitated infants, even on prolonged administration. If irritation on topical application should occur, discontinue medication.

DOSAGE AND ADMINISTRATION

The cream and the ointment should be applied liberally to affected areas twice daily or as indicated until healing is complete. The powder should be applied to candidal lesions two or three times daily until lesions have healed. For fungal infection of the feet caused by Candida species, the powder should be dusted freely on the feet as well as in shoes and socks. The cream is usually preferred to the ointment in candidiasis involving intertriginous areas; very moist lesions, however, are best treated with the topical dusting powder.

The preparations do not stain skin or mucous membranes and they provide a simple, convenient means of treatment.

HOW SUPPLIED

MYCOSTATIN Cream (Nystatin Cream USP) is supplied in 15g (NDC 0003-0579-20) and 30g (NDC 0003-0579-31) tubes providing 100,000 USP nystatin units per gram in an aqueous, perfumed vanishing cream base.

MYCOSTATIN Topical Powder (Nystatin Topical Powder USP) is supplied in 15g (NDC 0003-0593-20) plastic squeeze bottles providing, in each gram, 100,000 USP nystatin units.

MYCOSTATIN Ointment (Nystatin Ointment USP) is supplied in 15g (NDC 0003-0584-40) and 30g (NDC 0003-0584-30) tubes providing 100,000 USP nystatin units per gram.

Storage

MYCOSTATIN Cream (Nystatin Cream USP)

Store at room temperature; avoid freezing.

MYCOSTATIN Topical Powder (Nystatin Topical Powder USP)

Store at room temperature; avoid excessive heat (40°C; 104°F).

Keep tightly closed.

MYCOSTATIN Ointment (Nystatin Ointment USP)

Store at room temperature.

T-STAT® ℞

(erythromycin) 2.0% Topical Solution and Pads

For topical use only. Not for ophthalmic use.

CAUTION

Federal law prohibits dispensing without prescription.

DESCRIPTION

Erythromycin is an antibiotic produced from a strain of Streptomyces erythraeus. It is basic and readily forms salts with acids. Each ml of T-STAT (erythromycin). 2.0% Topical Solution contains 20 mg of erythromycin base in a vehicle consisting of alcohol (71.2%), propylene glycol and fragrance. It may contain citric acid to adjust pH.

ACTIONS
Although the mechanism by which T-STAT Solution acts in reducing inflammatory lesions of acne vulgaris is unknown, it is presumably due to its antibiotic action.

INDICATIONS
T-STAT Solution is indicated for the topical control of acne vulgaris.

CONTRAINDICATIONS
T-STAT Solution is contraindicated in persons who have shown hypersensitivity to any of its ingredients.

WARNING
The safe use of T-STAT (erythromycin) 2.0% Solution during pregnancy or lactation has not been established.

PRECAUTIONS
General —The use of antibiotic agents may be associated with the overgrowth of antibiotic-resistant organisms. If this occurs, administration of this drug should be discontinued and appropriate measures taken.
Information for Patients —T-STAT Solution is for external use only and should be kept away from the eyes, nose, mouth, and other mucous membranes. Concomitant topical acne therapy should be used with caution because a cumulative irritant effect may occur, especially with the use of peeling, desquamating, or abrasive agents.
Carcinogensis, Mutagenesis, Impairment of Fertility —Long-term animal studies to evaluate carcinogenic potential, mutagenicity, or the effect on fertility of erythromycin have not been performed.
Pregnancy: Pregnancy Category C. —Animal reproduction studies have not been conducted with erythromycin. It is also not known whether erythromycin can cause fetal harm when administered to a pregnant woman or can affect reproduction capacity. Erythromycin should be given to a pregnant woman only if clearly needed.
Nursing Mothers —Erythromycin is excreted in breast milk. Caution should be exercised when erythromycin is administered to a nursing woman.

ADVERSE REACTIONS
Adverse conditions reported include dryness, tenderness, pruritus, desquamation, erythema, oiliness, and burning sensation. Irritation of the eyes has also been reported. A case of generalized urticarial reaction, possibly related to the drug, which required the use of systemic steroid therapy has been reported.

DOSAGE AND ADMINISTRATION
T-STAT Solution or Pads should be applied over the affected area twice a day after the skin is thoroughly washed with warm water and soap and patted dry. Acne lesions on the face, neck, shoulder, chest, and back may be treated in this manner. Additional pads may be used, if needed.
This medication should be applied with applicator top or the disposable applicator pads. If fingertips or pads are used, wash hands after application. Drying and peeling may be controlled by reducing the frequency of applications.

HOW SUPPLIED
T-STAT Solution, 60 ml plastic bottle with optional applicator, NDC 0072-8300-60. T-STAT Pads, 60 disposable premoistened applicator pads in a plastic jar. NDC 0072-8303-60. Store in a dry place at temperatures between 15°C and 25°C (59°F and 77°F).

ULTRAVATE® ℞
(halobetasol propionate)
Cream, 0.05%
For Dermatological Use Only. Not for Ophthalmic Use.

CAUTION: Federal law prohibits dispensing without a prescription.

DESCRIPTION
ULTRAVATE (halobetasol propionate) Cream contains the active compound halobetasol propionate, a synthetic corticosteroid for topical dermatological use.
Chemically, halobetasol propionate is 21-chloro-6α,9α-difluoro-11β,17-dihydroxy-16β-methylpregna-1,4-diene-3-20-dione, 17-propionate, with the empirical formula $C_{25}H_{31}ClF_2O_5$, a molecular weight of 485, and the following structural formula:

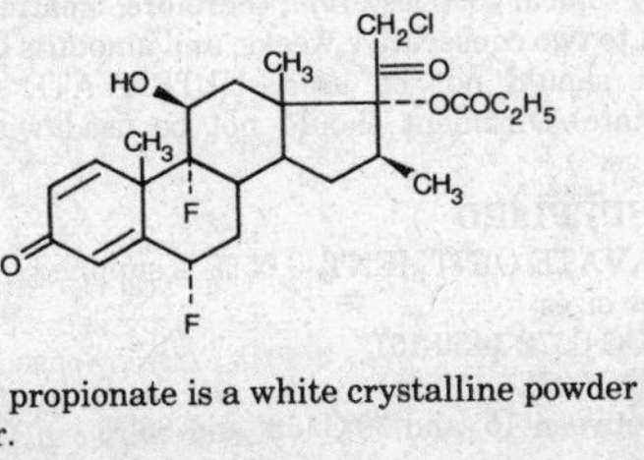

Halobetasol propionate is a white crystalline powder insoluble in water.
ULTRAVATE Cream contains halobetasol propionate 0.5 mg/g in a cream base of cetyl alcohol, glycerin, isopropyl isostearate, isopropyl palmitate, steareth-21, diazolidinyl urea, methylchloroisothiazolinone (and) methylisothiazolinone and water.

CLINICAL PHARMACOLOGY
Like other topical corticosteroids, halobetasol propionate has anti-inflammatory, anti-pruritic and vasoconstrictive actions. The mechanism of the anti-inflammatory activity of the topical corticosteroids, in general, is unclear. However, corticosteroids are thought to act by the induction of phospholipase A_2 inhibitory proteins, collectively called lipocortins. It is postulated that these proteins control the biosynthesis of potent mediators of inflammation such as prostaglandins and leukotrienes by inhibiting the release of their common precursor arachidonic acid. Arachidonic acid is released from membrane phospholipids by phospholipase A_2.
Pharmacokinetics —The extent of percutaneous absorption of topical corticosteroids is determined by many factors, including the vehicle and the integrity of the epidermal barrier. Occlusive dressings with hydrocortisone for up to 24 hours have not been demonstrated to increase penetration; however, occlusion of hydrocortisone for 96 hours markedly enhances penetration. Topical corticosteroids can be absorbed from normal intact skin while inflammation and/or other disease processes in the skin may increase percutaneous absorption.
Human and animal studies indicate that approximately 2% of the applied dose of halobetasol propionate enters the circulation within 96 hours following topical administration of the cream.
Studies performed with ULTRAVATE (halobetasol propionate) Ointment indicate that is is in the super-high range of potency as compared with other topical corticosteroids. In one of three studies conducted with ULTRAVATE (halobetasol propionate) Cream, its potency was comparable to ULTRAVATE Ointment. However, in two other studies, ULTRAVATE Cream did not appear to be as potent as ULTRAVATE Ointment.

INDICATIONS AND USAGE
ULTRAVATE (halobetasol propionate) Cream 0.05% is a high to super-high potency corticosteroid (See CLINICAL PHARMACOLOGY) indicated for the relief of the inflammatory and pruritic manifestations of corticosteroid-responsive dermatoses. Treatment beyond two consecutive weeks is not recommended, and the total dosage should not exceed 50g/week because of the potential for the drug to suppress the hypothalamic-pituitary-adrenal (HPA) axis.

CONTRAINDICATIONS
ULTRAVATE (halobetasol propionate) Cream is contraindicated in those patients with a history of hypersensitivity to any of the components of the preparation.

PRECAUTIONS
General —Systemic absorption of topical corticosteroids can produce reversible hypothalamic-pituitary-adrenal (HPA) axis suppression with the potential for glucocorticosteroid insufficiency after withdrawal of treatment. Manifestations of Cushing's syndrome, hyperglycemia, and glucosuria can also be produced in some patients by systemic absorption of topical corticosteroids while on treatment.
Patients receiving a large dose of a higher potency topical steroid applied to a large surface area or under an occlusive dressing should be evaluated periodically for evidence of HPA axis suppression. This may be done by using the ACTH stimulation, A.M. plasma cortisol, and urinary free-cortisol tests. Patients receiving super-potent corticosteroids should not be treated for more than 2 weeks at a time and only small areas should be treated at any one time due to the increased risk of HPA suppression.
ULTRAVATE (halobetasol propionate) Ointment produced HPA axis suppression when used in divided doses at 7 grams per day for one week in patients with psoriasis. These effects were reversible upon discontinuation of treatment.
If HPA axis suppression is noted, an attempt should be made to withdraw the drug, to reduce the frequency of application, or to substitute a less potent corticosteroid. Recovery of HPA axis function is generally prompt and complete upon discontinuation of topical corticosteroids. Infrequently, signs and symptoms of glucocorticosteroid insufficiency may occur, requiring supplemental systemic corticosteroids. For information on systemic supplementation, see prescribing information for those products.
Children may be more susceptible to systemic toxicity from equivalent doses due to their larger skin surface to body mass ratios (see PRECAUTIONS: Pediatric Use).
If irritation develops ULTRAVATE (halobetasol propionate) Cream should be discontinued and appropriate therapy instituted. Allergic contact dermatitis with corticosteroids is usually diagnosed by observing failure to heal rather than noting a clinical exacerbation as with most topical products not containing corticosteroids. Such an observation should be corroborated with appropriate diagnostic patch testing.
If concomitant skin infections are present or develop, an appropriate antifungal or antibacterial agent should be used. If a favorable response does not occur promptly, use of ULTRAVATE (halobetasol propionate) Cream should be discontinued until the infection has been adequately controlled.
ULTRAVATE (halobetasol propionate) Cream should not be used in the treatment of rosacea or perioral dermatitis, and it should not be used on the face, groin, or axillae.
Information for Patients: Patients using topical corticosteroids should receive the following information and instructions:

1. The medication is to be used as directed by the physician. It is for external use only. Avoid contact with the eyes.
2. The medication should not be used for any disorder other than that for which it was prescribed.
3. The treated skin area should not be bandaged or otherwise covered or wrapped so as to be occlusive unless directed by the physician.
4. Patients should report to their physician any signs of local adverse reactions.

Laboratory Tests: The following tests may be helpful in evaluating patients for HPA axis suppression: ACTH-stimulation test; A.M. plasma-cortisol test; Urinary free-cortisol test.
Carcinogenesis, Mutagenesis and Impairment of Fertility: Long-term animal studies have not been performed to evaluate the carcinogenic potential of halobetasol propionate.
Studies in the rat following oral administration at dose levels up to 50 μg/kg/day indicated no impairment of fertility or general reproductive performance.
Positive mutagenicity effects were observed in two genotoxicity assays. Halobetasol propionate was positive in a Chinese hamster micronucleus test, and a mouse lymphoma gene mutation assay *in vitro*.
In other genotoxicity testing halobetasol propionate was not found to be genotoxic in the Ames/Salmonella assay, in the sister chromatid exchange test in somatic cells of the Chinese hamster, in chromosome aberration studies of germinal and somatic cells of rodents, and in a mammalian spot test to determine point mutations.
Pregnancy: Teratogenic effects: Pregnancy Category C: Corticosteroids have been shown to be teratogenic in laboratory animals when administered systemically at relatively low dosage levels. Some corticosteroids have been shown to be teratogenic after dermal application to laboratory animals.
Halobetasol propionate has been shown to be teratogenic in SPF rats and chinchilla-type rabbits when given systemically during gestation at doses of 0.04 to 0.1 mg/kg in rats and 0.01 mg/kg in rabbits. These doses are approximately 13, 33 and 3 times, respectively, the human topical dose of ULTRAVATE (halobetasol propionate) Cream. Halobetasol propionate was embryotoxic in rabbits but not in rats.
Cleft palate was observed in both rats and rabbits. Omphalocele was seen in rats, but not in rabbits.
There are no adequate and well-controlled studies of the teratogenic potential of halobetasol propionate in pregnant women. Therefore, ULTRAVATE (halobetasol propionate) Cream should be used during pregnancy only if the potential benefit justifies the potential risk to the fetus.
Nursing Mothers: Systemically administered corticosteroids appear in human milk and could suppress growth, interfere with endogenous corticosteroid production, or cause other untoward effects. It is not known whether topical administration of corticosteroids could result in sufficient systemic absorption to produce detectable quantities in human milk. Because many drugs are excreted in human milk, caution should be exercised when ULTRAVATE (halobetasol propionate) Cream is administered to a nursing woman.
Pediatric Use —Safety and effectiveness of ULTRAVATE (halobetasol propionate) Cream in children have not been established. Because of a higher ratio of skin surface area to body mass, children are at a greater risk than adults of HPA-axis suppression when they are treated with topical corticosteroids. They are therefore also at greater risk of glucocorticosteroid insufficiency after withdrawal of treatment and of Cushing's syndrome while on treatment. Adverse effects including striae have been reported with inappropriate use of topical corticosteroids in infants and children. (See PRECAUTIONS.)
HPA axis suppression, Cushing's syndrome, and intracranial hypertension have been reported in children receiving topical corticosteroids. Manifestations of adrenal suppression in children include linear growth retardation, delayed weight gain, low plasma cortisol levels, and absence of response to ACTH stimulation. Manifestations of intracranial hypertension include bulging fontanelles, headaches, and bilateral papilledema.

ADVERSE REACTIONS
In controlled clinical trials, the most frequent adverse events reported for ULTRAVATE (halobetasol propionate) Cream included stinging, burning or itching in 4.4% of the patients.

Continued on next page

Westwood-Squibb—Cont.

Less frequently reported adverse reactions were dry skin, erythema, skin atrophy, leukoderma, vesicles and rash.
The following additional local adverse reactions are reported infrequently with topical corticosteroids, but may occur more frequently with high potency corticosteroids, such as ULTRAVATE (halobetasol propionate) Cream. These reactions are listed in an approximate decreasing order of occurrence: folliculitis, hypertrichosis, acneiform eruptions, hypopigmentation, perioral dermatitis, allergic contact dermatitis, secondary infection, striae, and miliaria.

OVERDOSAGE

Topically applied ULTRAVATE (halobetasol propionate) Cream can be absorbed in sufficient amounts to produce systemic effects (see PRECAUTIONS).

DOSAGE AND ADMINISTRATION

Apply a thin layer of ULTRAVATE (halobetasol propionate) Cream to the affected skin once or twice daily, as directed by your physician, and rub in gently and completely.
ULTRAVATE (halobetasol propionate) Cream is a high potency topical corticosteroid; therefore, treatment should be limited to two weeks, and amounts greater than 50g/wk should not be used. ULTRAVATE (halobetasol propionate) Cream should not be used with occlusive dressings.

HOW SUPPLIED

ULTRAVATE CREAM, 0.05% is supplied in the following tube sizes:
15 g (NDC 0072-1400-15)
45 g (NDC 0072-1400-45)
Store between 15° and 30°C (59° and 86°F).

ULTRAVATE® ℞
(halobetasol propionate)
Ointment, 0.05%
For Dermatological Use Only. Not for Ophthalmic Use.

CAUTION: Federal law prohibits dispensing without a prescription.

DESCRIPTION

ULTRAVATE (halobetasol propionate) Ointment contains the active halobetasol propionate, a synthetic corticosteroid for topical dermatological use.
Chemically, halobetasol proportionate is 21-chloro-6α, 9-difluoro-11β, 17 dihydroxy-16β-methyl-pregna-1, 4-diene-3-20-dione, 17-propionate, with the empirical formula $C_{25}H_{31}ClF_2O_5$, a molecular weight of 485, and the following stuctural formula:

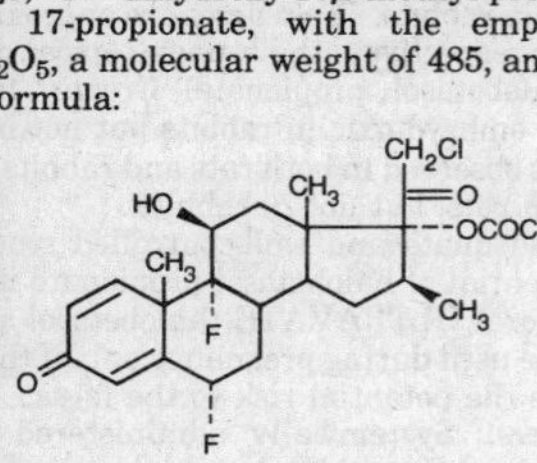

Halobetasol propionate is a white crystalline powder insoluble in water.
ULTRAVATE Ointment contains halobetasol propionate 0.5 mg/g in a base of aluminum stearate, beeswax, pentaerythritol cocoate, petrolatum, propylene glycol, sorbitan sesquioleate, and stearyl citrate.

CLINICAL PHARMACOLOGY

Like other topical corticosteroids, halobetasol propionate has anti-inflammatory, anti-pruritic and vasoconstrictive actions. The mechanism of the anti-inflammatory activity of the topical corticosteroids, in general, is unclear. However, corticosteroids are thought to act by the induction of phospholipase A_2 inhibitory proteins, collectively called lipocortins. It is postulated that these proteins control the biosynthesis of potent mediators of inflammation such as prostaglandins and leukotrienes by inhibiting the release of their common precursor arachidonic acid. Arachidonic acid is released from membrane phospholipids by phospholipase A_2.
Pharmacokinetics—The extent of percutaneous absorption of topical corticosteroids is determined by many factors, including the vehicle and the integrity of the epidermal barrier. Occlusive dressings with hydrocortisone for up to 24 hours have not been demonstrated to increase penetration; however, occlusion of hydrocortisone for 96 hours markedly enhances penetration. Topical corticosteroids can be absorbed from normal intact skin while inflammation and/or other disease processes in the skin may increase percutaneous absorption.
Human and animal studies indicate that approximately 3% of the applied dose of halobetasol propionate enters the circulation within 96 hours following topical administration of the ointment.
Studies performed with ULTRAVATE (halobetasol propionate) Ointment indicate that it is in the super-high range of potency as compared with other topical corticosteroids.

INDICATIONS AND USAGE

ULTRAVATE (halobetasol propionate) Ointment 0.05% is a super-high potency corticosteroid indicated for the relief of the inflammatory and pruritic manifestations of corticosteroid-responsive dermatoses. Treatment beyond two consecutive weeks is not recommended, and the total dosage should not exceed 50g/week because of the potential for the drug to suppress the hypothalamic-pituitary-adrenal (HPA) axis.

CONTRAINDICATIONS

ULTRAVATE (halobetasol propionate) Ointment is contraindicated in those patients with a history of hypersensitivity to any of the components of the preparation.

PRECAUTIONS

General—Systemic absorption of topical corticosteroids can produce reversible hypothalamic-pituitary-adrenal (HPA) axis suppression with the potential for glucocorticosteroid insufficiency after withdrawal of treatment. Manifestations of Cushing's syndrome, hyperglycemia, and glucosuria can also be produced in some patients by systemic absorption of topical corticosteroids while on treatment.
Patients receiving a large dose of a higher potency topical steroid applied to a large surface area or under an occlusive dressing should be evaluated periodically for evidence of HPA axis suppression. This may be done by using the ACTH stimulation, A.M. plasma cortisol, and urinary free-cortisol tests. Patients receiving super-potent corticosteroids should not be treated for more than 2 weeks at a time and only small areas should be treated at any one time due to the increased risk of HPA suppression.
ULTRAVATE (halobetasol propionate) Ointment produced HPA axis suppression when used in divided doses at 7 grams per day for one week in patients with psoriasis. These effects were reversible upon discontinuation of treatment.
If HPA axis suppression is noted, an attempt should be made to withdraw the drug, to reduce the frequency of application, or to substitute a less potent corticosteroid. Recovery of HPA axis function is generally prompt and complete upon discontinuation of topical corticosteroids. Infrequently, signs and symptoms of glucocorticosteroid insufficiency may occur, requiring supplemental systemic corticosteroids. For information on systemic supplementation, see prescribing information for those products.
Children may be more susceptible to systemic toxicity from equivalent doses due to their larger skin surface to body mass ratios (see PRECAUTIONS: Pediatric Use).
If irritation develops, ULTRAVATE (halobetasol propionate) Ointment should be discontinued and appropriate therapy instituted. Allergic contact dermatitis with corticosteroids is usually diagnosed by observing failure to heal rather than noting a clinical exacerbation as with most topical products not containing corticosteroids. Such an observation should be corroborated with appropriate diagnostic patch testing.
If concomitant skin infections are present or develop, an appropriate antifungal or antibacterial agent should be used. If a favorable response does not occur promptly, use of ULTRAVATE (halobetasol propionate) Ointment should be discontinued until the infection has been adequately controlled.
ULTRAVATE (halobetasol propionate) Ointment should not be used in the treatment of rosacea or perioral dermatitis, and it should not be used on the face, groin, or axillae.
Information for Patients: Patients using topical corticosteroids should receive the following information and instructions:

1. The medication is to be used as directed by the physician. It is for external use only. Avoid contact with the eyes.
2. The medication should not be used for any disorder other than that for which it was prescribed.
3. The treated skin area should not be bandaged or otherwise covered or wrapped so as to be occlusive unless directed by the physician.
4. Patients should report to their physician any signs of local adverse reactions.

Laboratory Tests: The following tests may be helpful in evaluating patients for HPA axis suppression: ACTH-stimulation test; A.M. plasma-cortisol test; urinary free-cortisol test.
Carcinogenesis, Mutagenesis and Impairment of Fertility: Long-term animal studies have not been performed to evaluate the carcinogenic potential of halobetasol propionate.
Studies in the rat following oral administration at dose levels up to 50 μg/kg/day indicated no impairment of fertility or general reproductive performance.
Positive mutagenicity effects were observed in two genotoxicity assays. Halobetasol propionate was positive in a Chinese hamster micronucleus test, and a mouse lymphoma gene mutation assay *in vitro*.
In other genotoxicity testing halobetasol propionate was not found to be genotoxic in the Ames/Salmonella assay, in the sister chromatid exchange test in somatic cells of the Chinese hamster, in chromosome aberration studies of germinal and somatic cells of rodents, and in a mammalian spot test to determine point mutations.
Pregnancy: Teratogenic effects: Pregnancy Category C: Corticosteroids have been shown to be teratogenic in laboratory animals when administered systemically at relatively low dosage levels. Some corticosteroids have been shown to be teratogenic after dermal application to laboratory animals.
Halobetasol propionate has been shown to be teratogenic in SPF rats and chinchilla-type rabbits when given systemically during gestation at doses of 0.04 to 0.1 mg/kg in rats and 0.01 mg/kg in rabbits. These doses are approximately 13, 33 and 3 times, respectively, the human topical dose of ULTRAVATE (halobetasol propionate) Ointment. Halobetasol propionate was embryotoxic in rabbits but not in rats.
Cleft palate was observed in both rats and rabbits. Omphalocele was seen in rats, but not in rabbits.
There are no adequate and well-controlled studies of the teratogenic potential of halobetasol propionate in pregnant women. Therefore, ULTRAVATE (halobetasol propionate) Ointment should be used during pregnancy only if the potential benefit justifies the potential risk to the fetus.
Nursing Mothers: Systemically administered corticosteroids appear in human milk and could suppress growth, interfere with endogenous corticosteroid production, or cause other untoward effects. It is not known whether topical administration of corticosteroids could result in sufficient systemic absorption to produce detectable quantities in human milk. Because many drugs are excreted in human milk, caution should be exercised when ULTRAVATE (halobetasol propionate) Ointment is administered to a nursing woman.
Pediatric Use—Safety and effectiveness of ULTRAVATE (halobetasol propionate) Ointment in children have not been established. Because of higher ratio of skin surface area to body mass, children are at a greater risk than adults of HPA-axis suppression when they are treated with topical corticosteroids. They are therefore also at greater risk of glucocorticosteroid insufficiency after withdrawal of treatment and of Cushing's syndrome while on treatment. Adverse effects including striae have been reported with inappropriate use of topical corticosteroids in infants and children. (See PRECAUTIONS.)
HPA axis suppression, Cushing's syndrome, and intracranial hypertension have been reported in children receiving topical corticosteroids. Manifestations of adrenal suppression in children include linear growth retardation, delayed weight gain, low plasma cortisol levels, and absence of response to ACTH stimulation. Manifestations of intracranial hypertension include bulging fontanelles, headaches, and bilateral papilledema.

ADVERSE REACTIONS

In controlled clinical trials, the most frequent adverse events reported for ULTRAVATE (halobetasol propionate) Ointment included stinging or burning in 2.4% of the patients. Less frequently reported adverse reactions were pustulation, erythema, skin atrophy, leukoderma, acne, itching, secondary infection, telangiectasia, urticaria, dry skin, miliaria, paresthesia, tingling, and rash.
The following additional local adverse reactions are reported infrequently with topical corticosteroids, but may occur more frequently with high potency corticosteroids, such as ULTRAVATE (halobetasol propionate) Ointment. These reactions are listed in an approximate decreasing order of occurrence: folliculitis, hypertrichosis, hypopigmentation, perioral dermatitis, allergic contact dermatitis, irritation, and striae.

OVERDOSAGE

Topically applied ULTRAVATE (halobetasol propionate) Ointment can be absorbed in sufficient amounts to produce systemic effects (see PRECAUTIONS).

DOSAGE AND ADMINISTRATION

Apply a thin layer of ULTRAVATE (halobetasol propionate) Ointment to the affected skin once or twice daily, as directed by your physician, and rub in gently and completely.
ULTRAVATE (halobetasol propionate) Ointment is a high potency topical corticosteroid; therefore, treatment must be limited to two consecutive weeks, and amounts greater than 50g/wk should not be used. ULTRAVATE (halobetasol propionate) Ointment should not be used with occlusive dressings.

HOW SUPPLIED

ULTRAVATE OINTMENT, 0.05% is supplied in the following tube sizes:
15g (NDC 0072-1450-15)
45g (NDC 0072-1450-45)
Store between 15° and 30°C (59° and 86°F).

WESTCORT® ℞

(hydrocortisone valerate)
Cream/Ointment, 0.2%
For topical use only. Not for use in eyes.

Caution: Federal law prohibits dispensing without a prescription.

DESCRIPTION

WESTCORT is a topical formulation containing hydrocortisone valerate, a non-fluorinated steroid. It has the chemical name Pregn-4-ene-3, 20-dione, 11, 21-dihydroxy-17-[(1-oxopentyl) oxy]-, (11β)-; the empirical formula is: $C_{26}H_{38}O_6$; the molecular weight is 446.58, and the CAS registry number is: 57524-89-7. The structural formula is:

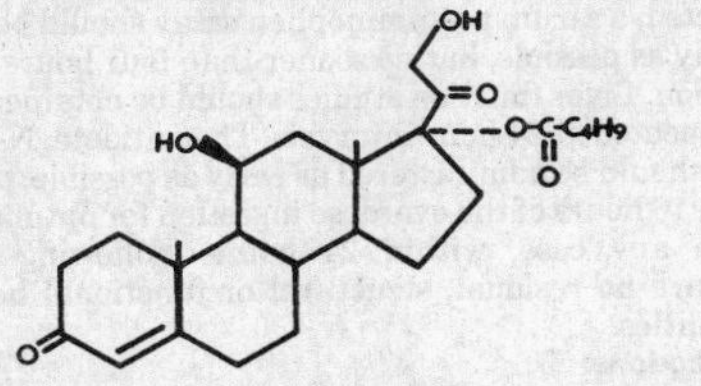

Each gram of WESTCORT CREAM contains 2.0 mg hydrocortisone valerate in a hydrophilic base composed of white petrolatum, stearyl alcohol, propylene glycol, amphoteric-9, carbomer-940, dried sodium phosphate, sodium lauryl sulfate, sorbic acid and water.
Each gram of Westcort Ointment contains 2.0 mg hydrocortisone valerate in a hydrophilic base composed of white petrolatum, stearyl alcohol, propylene glycol, sorbic acid, sodium lauryl sulfate, carbomer-934, dried sodium phosphate, mineral oil, steareth-2, steareth-100, and water.

CLINICAL PHARMACOLOGY

Topical corticosteroids share anti-inflammatory, anti-pruritic and vasoconstrictive actions.
The mechanism of anti-inflammatory activity of the topical corticosteroids is unclear. Various laboratory methods, including vasoconstrictor assays, are used to compare and predict potencies and/or clinical efficacies of the topical corticosteroids. There is some evidence to suggest that a recognizable correlation exists between vasoconstrictor potency and therapeutic efficacy in man.
Pharmacokinetics: The extent of percutaneous absorption of topical corticosteroids is determined by many factors including the vehicle, the integrity of the epidermal barrier, and the use of occlusive dressings.
Topical corticosteroids can be absorbed from normal intact skin. Inflammation and/or other disease processes in the skin increase percutaneous absorption. Occlusive dressings substantially increase the percutaneous absorption of topical corticosteroids. Thus, occlusive dressings may be a valuable therapeutic adjunct for treatment of resistant dermatoses (see DOSAGE AND ADMINISTRATION).
Once absorbed through the skin, topical corticosteroids are handled through pharmacokinetic pathways similar to systemically administered corticosteroids. Corticosteroids are bound to plasma proteins in varying degrees. Corticosteroids are metabolized primarily in the liver and are then excreted by the kidneys. Some of the topical corticosteroids and their metabolites are also excreted into the bile.

INDICATIONS AND USAGE

WESTCORT is indicated for the relief of the inflammatory and pruritic manifestations of the corticosteroid-responsive dermatoses.

CONTRAINDICATIONS

Topical corticosteroids are contraindicated in those patients with a history of hypersensitivity to any of the components of the preparation.

PRECAUTIONS

General: Systemic absorption of topical corticosteroids has produced reversible hypothalamic-pituitary-adrenal (HPA) axis suppression, manifestations of Cushing's syndrome, hyperglycemia, and glucosuria in some patients. Conditions which augment systemic absorption include the application of the more potent steroids, use over large surface areas, prolonged use, and the addition of occlusive dressings.
Therefore, patients receiving a large dose of a potent topical steroid applied to a large surface area or under an occlusive dressing should be evaluated periodically for evidence of HPA axis suppression by using the urinary free cortisol and ACTH stimulation tests. If HPA axis suppression is noted, an attempt should be made to withdraw the drug, to reduce the frequency of application, or to substitute a less potent steroid.
Recovery of HPA axis function is generally prompt and complete upon discontinuation of the drug. Infrequently, signs and symptoms of steroid withdrawal may occur, requiring supplemental systemic corticosteroids.
Children may absorb proportionally larger amounts of topical corticosteroids and thus be more susceptible to systemic toxicity (see PRECAUTIONS—Pediatric Use).
If irritation develops, topical corticosteroids should be discontinued and appropriate therapy instituted.
In the presence of dermatological infections, the use of an appropriate antifungal or antibacterial agent should be instituted. If a favorable response does not occur promptly, the corticosteroids should be discontinued until the infection has been adequately controlled.
Information for the Patient: Patients using topical corticosteroids should receive the following information and instructions:

1. This medication is to be used as directed by the physician. It is for external use only. Avoid contact with the eyes.
2. Patients should be advised not to use this medication for any disorder other than for which it was prescribed.
3. The treated skin area should not be bandaged or otherwise covered or wrapped as to be occlusive unless directed by the physician.
4. Patients should report any signs of local adverse reactions especially under occlusive dressing.
5. Parents of pediatric patients should be advised not to use tight-fitting diapers or plastic pants on a child being treated in the diaper area, as these garments may constitute occlusive dressing.

Laboratory Tests: The following tests may be helpful in evaluating the HPA axis suppression:
Urinary free cortisol test
ACTH stimulation test
Carcinogenesis, Mutagenesis, and Impairment of Fertility: Long-term animal studies have not been performed to evaluate the carcinogenic potential or the effect on fertility of topical corticosteroids.
Studies to determine mutagenicity with prednisolone and hydrocortisone have revealed negative results.
Pregnancy Category C: Corticosteroids are generally teratogenic in laboratory animals when administered systemically at relatively low dosage levels. The more potent corticosteroids have been shown to be teratogenic after dermal application in laboratory animals. There are no adequate and well-controlled studies in pregnant women on teratogenic effects from topically applied corticosteroids. Therefore, topical corticosteroids should be used during pregnancy only if the potential benefit justifies the potential risk to the fetus. Drugs of this class should not be used extensively on pregnant patients, in large amounts, or for prolonged periods of time.
Nursing Mothers: It is not known whether topical administration of corticosteroids could result in sufficient systemic absorption to produce detectable quantities in breast milk. Systemically administered corticosteroids are secreted into breast milk in quantities *not* likely to have a deleterious effect on the infant. Nevertheless, caution should be exercised when topical corticosteroids are administered to a nursing woman.
Pediatric Use: Pediatric patients may demonstrate greater susceptibility to topical corticosteroid-induced HPA axis suppression and Cushing's syndrome than mature patients because of a larger skin surface area to body weight ratio.
Hypothalamic-pituitary-adrenal (HPA) axis suppression, Cushing's syndrome, and intracranial hypertension have been reported in children receiving topical corticosteroids. Manifestations of adrenal suppression in children include linear growth retardation, delayed weight gain, low plasma cortisol levels, and absence of response to ACTH stimulation. Manifestations of intracranial hypertension include bulging fontanelles, headaches, and bilateral papilledema.
Administration of topical corticosteroids to children should be limited to the least amount compatible with an effective therapeutic regimen. Chronic corticosteroid therapy may interfere with the growth and development of children.

ADVERSE REACTIONS

The following local adverse reactions are reported infrequently with topical corticosteroids, but may occur more frequently with the use of occlusive dressings. These reactions are listed in an approximate decreasing order of occurrence: burning; itching; irritation; dryness; folliculitis; hypertrichosis; acneiform eruptions; hypopigmentation; perioral dermatitis; allergic contact dermatitis; maceration of the skin; secondary infection; skin atrophy; striae; miliaria.

OVERDOSAGE

Topically applied corticosteroids can be absorbed in sufficient amounts to produce systemic effects (see PRECAUTIONS).

DOSAGE AND ADMINISTRATION

WESTCORT should be applied to the affected area as a thin film two or three times daily depending on the severity of the condition.
Occlusive dressings may be used for the management of psoriasis or recalcitrant conditions.
If an infection develops, the use of occlusive dressings should be discontinued and appropriate antimicrobial therapy instituted.

HOW SUPPLIED

WESTCORT CREAM, 0.2% is supplied in the following tube sizes:
15 g NDC 0072-8100-15; 6505-01-093-9901.
45 g NDC 0072-8100-45; 6505-01-083-9395.
60 g NDC 0072-8100-60; 6505-01-121-0118.
WESTCORT OINTMENT, 0.2% is supplied in the following tube sizes:
15 g NDC 0072-7800-15; 6505-01-224-0178
45 g NDC 0072-7800-45; 6505-01-204-1835
60 g NDC 0072-7800-60; 6505-01-224-0177
Store below 78°F (26°C).

Whitby Pharmaceuticals, Inc.

1211 SHERWOOD AVENUE
P.O. BOX 85054
RICHMOND, VA 23261-5054

LORTAB® Tablets Ⓒ ℞
LORTAB® Liquid Ⓒ ℞
[*lŏr'tab*]

DESCRIPTION

Each LORTAB® 2.5/500 tablet contains:
Hydrocodone Bitartrate* .... 2.5 mg
***WARNING:** May be habit forming.
Acetaminophen .... 500 mg
Also contains colloidal silicon dioxide, croscarmellose sodium, crospovidone, microcrystalline cellulose, povidone, starch, stearic acid and sugar spheres which are composed of starch (derived from corn), sucrose and FD&C Red #3.
Each LORTAB® 5/500 tablet contains:
Hydrocodone Bitartrate* .... 5 mg
***WARNING:** May be habit forming.
Acetaminophen .... 500 mg
Also contains cornstarch, FD&C Blue #1, gelatin, magnesium stearate, microcrystalline cellulose, sugar spheres, povidone, pregelatinized starch, sodium starch glycolate.
Each LORTAB® 7.5/500 tablet contains:
Hydrocodone Bitartrate* .... 7.5 mg
***WARNING:** May be habit forming.
Acetaminophen .... 500 mg
Also contains colloidal silicon dioxide, croscarmellose sodium, crospovidone, microcrystalline cellulose, povidone, pregelatinized starch, stearic acid and sugar spheres which are composed of starch (derived from corn), sucrose, FD&C Blue #1 and D&C Yellow #10.
Each 5cc (1 teaspoonful) LORTAB® LIQUID contains:
Hydrocodone Bitartrate* .... 2.5 mg
***WARNING:** May be habit forming.
Acetaminophen .... 120 mg
Alcohol 7%
Also contains citric acid, glycerin, methylparaben, propylene glycol, propylparaben, purified water, saccharin sodium, sorbitol solution, and sucrose with natural and artificial flavor, and the following coloring agents: D&C Yellow #10 and FD&C Blue #1.
Hydrocodone bitartrate is an opioid analgesic and antitussive which occurs as fine, white crystals or as a crystalline powder. It is affected by light. The chemical name is: 4,5α-epoxy-3-methoxy-17-methylmorphinan-6-one tartrate (1:1) hydrate (2:5). Its structure is as follows:

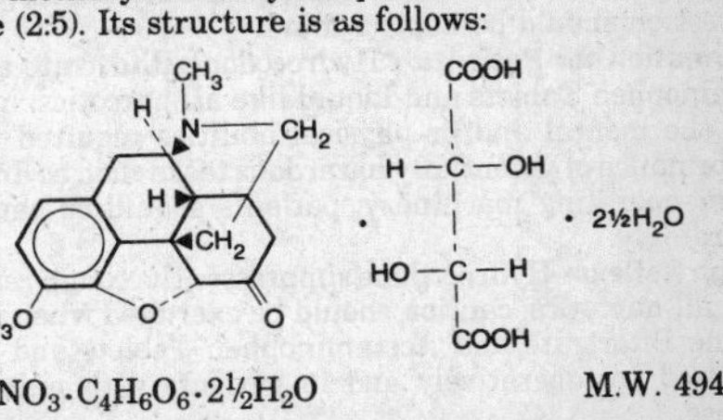

$C_{18}H_{21}NO_3 \cdot C_4H_6O_6 \cdot 2\frac{1}{2}H_2O$ M.W. 494.50

Acetaminophen, 4'-hydroxyacetanilide is a non-opiate, non-salicylate analgesic, and antipyretic which occurs as a white, odorless crystalline powder, possessing a slightly bitter taste. Its structure is as follows:

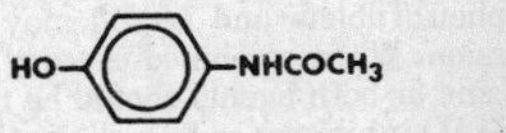

$C_8H_9NO_2$ M.W. 151.16

CLINICAL PHARMACOLOGY

Hydrocodone is a semisynthetic narcotic analgesic and antitussive with multiple actions qualitatively similar to those of codeine. Most of these involve the central nervous system

Continued on next page

Whitby—Cont.

and smooth muscle. The precise mechanism of action of hydrocodone and other opiates is not known, although it is believed to relate to the existence of opiate receptors in the central nervous system. In addition to analgesia, narcotics may produce drowsiness, changes in mood and mental clouding.

Radioimmunoassay techniques have recently been developed for the analysis of hydrocodone in human plasma. After a 10 mg oral dose of hydrocodone bitartrate, a mean peak serum drug level of 23.6 ng/mL and an elimination half-life of 3.8 hours were found.

The analgesic action of acetaminophen involves peripheral and central influences, but the specific mechanism is as yet undetermined. Antipyretic activity is mediated through hypothalamic heat regulating centers. Acetaminophen inhibits prostaglandin synthetase. Therapeutic doses of acetaminophen have negligible effects on the cardiovascular or respiratory systems; however, toxic doses may cause circulatory failure and rapid, shallow breathing. Acetaminophen is rapidly and almost completely absorbed from the gastrointestinal tract, producing maximum serum concentrations within 30 minutes to one hour. The plasma half-life in adults and children ranges from 0.90 hours to 3.25 hours with an average of approximately 2 hours. The drug distributes uniformly in most body fluids and is approximately 25% protein bound. Acetaminophen is conjugated in the liver, with less than 3% of the dose excreted unchanged in 24 hours. The primary metabolic pathway is conjugation to sulfate and glucuronide by-products. A minor oxidative pathway forms cysteine and mercapturic acid. These compounds are subsequently excreted by the kidneys into the urine.

INDICATIONS AND USAGE
For the relief of moderate to moderately severe pain.

CONTRAINDICATIONS
Hypersensitivity or intolerance to hydrocodone or acetaminophen.

WARNINGS
Respiratory Depression: At high doses or in sensitive patients, hydrocodone may produce dose-related respiratory depression by acting directly on the brain stem respiratory center. Hydrocodone also affects the center that controls respiratory rhythm, and may produce irregular and periodic breathing.

Head Injury and Increased Intracranial Pressure: The respiratory depressant effects of narcotics and their capacity to elevate cerebrospinal fluid pressure may be markedly exaggerated in the presence of head injury, other intracranial lesions or a pre-existing increase in intracranial pressure. Furthermore, narcotics produce adverse reactions which may obscure the clinical course of patients with head injuries.

Acute Abdominal Conditions: The administration of narcotics may obscure the diagnosis or clinical course of patients with acute abdominal conditions.

PRECAUTIONS
Special Risk Patients: As with any narcotic analgesic agent, Hydrocodone Bitartrate and Acetaminophen Tablets and Liquid should be used with caution in elderly or debilitated patients and those with severe impairment of hepatic or renal function, hypothyroidism, Addison's disease, prostatic hypertrophy or urethral stricture. The usual precautions should be observed and the possibility of respiratory depression should be kept in mind.

Information for Patients: Hydrocodone Bitartrate and Acetaminophen Tablets and Liquid like all narcotics, may impair the mental and/or physical abilities required for the performance of potentially hazardous tasks such as driving a car or operating machinery; patients should be cautioned accordingly.

Cough Reflex: Hydrocodone suppresses the cough reflex; as with all narcotics, caution should be exercised when Hydrocodone Bitartrate and Acetaminophen Tablets and Liquid are used postoperatively and in patients with pulmonary disease.

Drug Interactions:
Patients receiving other narcotic analgesics, antipsychotics, antianxiety agents, or other CNS depressants (including alcohol) concomitantly with Hydrocodone Bitartrate and Acetaminophen Tablets and Liquid may exhibit additive CNS depression. When combined therapy is contemplated, the dose of one or both agents should be reduced.

The use of MAO inhibitors or tricyclic antidepressants with hydrocodone preparations may increase the effect of either the antidepressant or hydrocodone.

The concurrent use of anticholinergics with hydrocodone, as with all narcotics, may produce paralytic ileus.

Pregnancy:
Teratogenic Effects: Pregnancy Category C.
Hydrocodone has been shown to be teratogenic in hamsters when given in doses 700 times the human dose. There are no

adequate and well-controlled studies in pregnant women. Hydrocodone Bitartrate and Acetaminophen Tablets and Liquid should be used during pregnancy only if the potential benefit justifies the potential risk to the fetus.

Nonteratogenic Effects:
Babies born to mothers who have been taking opioids regularly prior to delivery will be physically dependent. The withdrawal signs include irritability and excessive crying, tremors, hyperactive reflexes, increased respiratory rate, increased stools, sneezing, yawning, vomiting, and fever. The intensity of the syndrome does not always correlate with the duration of maternal opioid use or dose. There is no consensus on the best method of managing withdrawal. Chlorpromazine 0.7 to 1 mg/kg q6h, and paregoric 2 to 4 drops/kg q4h, have been used to treat withdrawal symptoms in infants. The duration of therapy is 4 to 28 days, with the dosage decreased as tolerated.

Labor and Delivery: As with all narcotics, administration of Hydrocodone Bitartrate and Acetaminophen Tablets and Liquid to the mother shortly before delivery may result in some degree of respiratory depression in the newborn, especially if higher doses are used.

Nursing Mothers: It is not known whether hydrocodone is excreted in human milk. Because many drugs are excreted in human milk and because of the potential for serious adverse reactions in nursing infants from Hydrocodone Bitartrate and Acetaminophen Tablets and Liquid, a decision should be made whether to discontinue nursing or to discontinue the drug, taking into account the importance of the drug to the mother.

Pediatric Use: Safety and effectiveness in children have not been established.

ADVERSE REACTIONS
The most frequently observed adverse reactions include lightheadedness, dizziness, sedation, nausea and vomiting. These effects seem to be more prominent in ambulatory than in nonambulatory patients and some of these adverse reactions may be alleviated if the patient lies down.
Other adverse reactions include:

Central Nervous System:
Drowsiness, mental clouding, lethargy, impairment of mental and physical performance, anxiety, fear, dysphoria, dizziness, psychic dependence, mood changes.

Gastrointestinal System:
The antiemetic phenothiazines are useful in suppressing the nausea and vomiting which may occur (see above); however, some phenothiazine derivatives seem to be antianalgesic and to increase the amount of narcotic required to produce pain relief, while other phenothiazines reduce the amount of narcotic required to produce a given level of analgesia. Prolonged administration of Hydrocodone Bitartrate and Acetaminophen Tablets and Liquid may produce constipation.

Genitourinary System:
Ureteral spasm, spasm of vesical sphincters and urinary retention have been reported.

Respiratory Depression:
Hydrocodone bitartrate may produce dose-related respiratory depression by acting directly on the brain stem respiratory center. Hydrocodone also affects the center that controls respiratory rhythm, and may produce irregular and periodic breathing.
If significant respiratory depression occurs, it may be antagonized by the use of naloxone hydrochloride. Apply other supportive measures when indicated.

DRUG ABUSE AND DEPENDENCE
Hydrocodone Bitartrate and Acetaminophen Tablets and Liquid are subject to the Federal Controlled Substance Act [Schedule CIII].
Psychic dependence, physical dependence, and tolerance may develop upon repeated administration of narcotics; therefore, Hydrocodone Bitartrate and Acetaminophen Tablets and Liquid should be prescribed and administered with caution. However, psychic dependence is unlikely to develop when Hydrocodone Bitartrate and Acetaminophen Tablets and Liquid are used for a short time for the treatment of pain.
Physical dependence, the condition in which continued administration of the drug is required to prevent the appearance of a withdrawal syndrome, assumes clinically significant proportions only after several weeks of continued narcotic use, although some mild degree of physical dependence may develop after a few days of narcotic therapy. Tolerance, in which increasingly large doses are required in order to produce the same degree of analgesia, is manifested initially by shortened duration of analgesic effect, and subsequently by decreases in the intensity of analgesia. The rate of development of tolerance varies among patients.

OVERDOSAGE
Acetaminophen:
Signs and Symptoms: In acute acetaminophen overdosage, dose-dependent, potentially fatal hepatic necrosis is the most serious adverse effect. Renal tubular necrosis, hypoglycemic coma, and thrombocytopenia may also occur.

In adults, hepatic toxicity has rarely been reported with acute overdoses of less than 10 grams and fatalities with less than 15 grams. Importantly, young children seem to be more resistant than adults to the hepatotoxic effect of an acetaminophen overdose. Despite this, the measures outlined below should be initiated in any adult or child suspected of having ingested an acetaminophen overdosage.

Early symptoms following a potentially hepatotoxic overdose may include: nausea, vomiting, diaphoresis and general malaise. Clinical and laboratory evidence of hepatic toxicity may not be apparent until 48 to 72 hours post-ingestion.

Treatment: The stomach should be emptied promptly by lavage or by induction of emesis with syrup of ipecac. Patients' estimates of the quantity of a drug ingested are notoriously unreliable. Therefore, if an acetaminophen overdose is suspected, a serum acetaminophen assay should be obtained as early as possible, but no sooner than four hours following ingestion. Liver function studies should be obtained initially and repeated at 24-hour intervals. The antidote, N-acetylcysteine, should be administered as early as possible, preferably within 16 hours of the overdose ingestion for optimal results, but in any case, within 24 hours. Following recovery, there are no residual, structural or functional hepatic abnormalities.

Hydrocodone:
Signs and Symptoms: Serious overdose with hydrocodone is characterized by respiratory depression (a decrease in respiratory rate and/or tidal volume, Cheyne-Stokes respiration, cyanosis), extreme somnolence progressing to stupor or coma, skeletal muscle flaccidity, cold and clammy skin, and sometimes bradycardia and hypotension. In severe overdosage, apnea, circulatory collapse, cardiac arrest and death may occur.

Treatment: Primary attention should be given to the reestablishment of adequate respiratory exchange through provision of a patent airway and the institution of assisted or controlled ventilation. The narcotic antagonist naloxone is a specific antidote against respiratory depression which may result from overdosage or unusual sensitivity to narcotics, including hydrocodone. Therefore, an appropriate dose of naloxone hydrochloride (see package insert) should be administered, preferably by the intravenous route, and simultaneously with efforts at respiratory resuscitation. Since the duration of action of hydrocodone may exceed that of the antagonist, the patient should be kept under continued surveillance and repeated doses of the antagonist should be administered as needed to maintain adequate respiration.
A narcotic antagonist should not be administered in the absence of clinically significant respiratory or cardiovascular depression. Oxygen, intravenous fluids, vasopressors and other supportive measures should be employed as indicated. Gastric emptying may be useful in removing unabsorbed drug.

DOSAGE AND ADMINISTRATION
Dosage should be adjusted according to the severity of the pain and the response of the patient. However, tolerance to hydrocodone can develop with continued use and the incidence of untoward effects is dose related.
The usual adult dosage for LORTAB® 2.5/500 tablets is one or two tablets every four to six hours as needed for pain. The total 24 hour dose should not exceed 8 tablets.
The usual adult dosage for LORTAB® 5/500 tablets is one or two tablets every four to six hours as needed for pain. The total 24 hour dose should not exceed 8 tablets.
The usual adult dosage for LORTAB® 7.5/500 tablets is one tablet every four to six hours as needed for pain. The total 24 hour dose should not exceed 6 tablets.
The usual adult dosage for LORTAB® Liquid is for adults: 1 tablespoonful (15 cc) every 4 hours as needed (up to 6 tablespoonfuls in 24 hours).

HOW SUPPLIED
LORTAB® 2.5/500 tablets (hydrocodone bitartrate and acetaminophen tablets) contain hydrocodone bitartrate (Warning: May Be Habit Forming) 2.5 mg and acetaminophen 500 mg. They are supplied as white with pink specks, capsule-shaped, bisected tablets, debossed "WHITBY 901" in containers of 24 tablets (NDC 50474-925-24) and in containers of 100 tablets (NDC 50474-925-01).
LORTAB® 5/500 tablets (hydrocodone bitartrate and acetaminophen tablets) contain hydrocodone bitartrate (Warning: May Be Habit Forming) 5 mg and acetaminophen 500 mg. They are supplied as white with blue specks, capsule-shaped, bisected tablets, debossed "WHITBY 902" in bottles of 100 (NDC 50474-902-01), 500 (NDC 50474-902-50) and in hospital unit-dose packages of 100 (NDC 50474-902-60).
LORTAB® 7.5/500 tablets (hydrocodone bitartrate and acetaminophen tablets) contain hydrocodone bitartrate (Warning: May Be Habit Forming) 7.5 mg and acetaminophen 500 mg. They are supplied as white with green specks, capsule-shaped, bisected tablets, debossed "WHITBY 903" in containers of 24 tablets (NDC 50474-907-24), in containers of 100 tablets (NDC 50474-907-01), in containers of 500 tablets (NDC 50474-907-50) and in hospital unit-dose packages of 100 (NDC 50474-907-60).

LORTAB® Liquid, (colored green, tropical punch flavored), contains hydrocodone bitartrate (Warning: May Be Habit Forming) 2.5 mg and acetaminophen 120 mg with 7% alcohol per 5 ml. It is supplied in bottles of 1 pint (NDC 50474-905-16) and 4 oz. (NDC 50474-905-04).

STORAGE

Store at controlled room temperature, 15°–30°C (59°–86°F). DISPENSE IN A TIGHT, LIGHT-RESISTANT CONTAINER AS DEFINED IN THE USP/NF WITH A CHILD-RESISTANT CLOSURE.

CAUTION

Federal law prohibits dispensing without prescription.

Schedule CIII Controlled Substances (Narcotic).

Manufactured For:
WHITBY PHARMACEUTICALS, INC.
Richmond, VA 23220

Lortab 2.5/500, Lortab 7.5/500 and Lortab Liquid Manufactured By:

MIKART, INC.
Atlanta, GA 30318

Lortab 5/500 Manufactured By:
D. M. GRAHAM LABORATORIES, INC.
Hobart, NY 13788

Revised 5/92

Shown in Product Identification Section, page 435

LORTAB® ASA ℞

[*lŏr'tab*]

Hydrocodone Bitartrate and Aspirin Tablets

5 mg/500 mg

DESCRIPTION

Each tablet contains:
Hydrocodone Bitartrate* .... 5 mg
***WARNING:** May be habit forming.
Aspirin .... 500 mg

Hydrocodone bitartrate is an opioid analgesic and antitussive and occurs as fine, white crystals or as a crystalline powder. It is affected by light. The chemical name is: 4,5α-epoxy-3-methoxy-17-methylmorphinan-6-one tartrate (1:1) hydrate (2:5). Its structure is as follows:

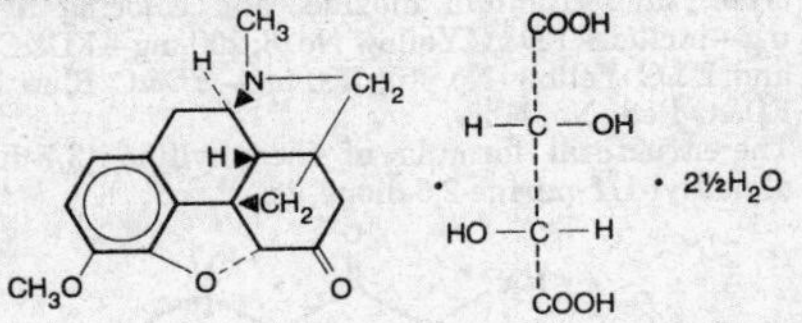

$C_{18}H_{21}NO_3 \cdot C_4H_6O_6 \cdot 2\frac{1}{2}H_2O$ M.W. 494.50

Aspirin, salicylic acid acetate, is a nonopiate, salicylate analgesic, anti-inflammatory, and antipyretic which occurs as a white, crystalline tabular or needle like powder and is odorless or has a faint odor. Its structure is as follows:

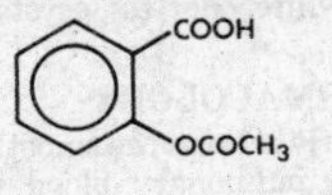

$C_9H_8O_4$ M.W. 180.16

Inactive Ingredients: D&C Red #7 Lake, Pregelatinized Starch and Stearic Acid.

CLINICAL PHARMACOLOGY

Hydrocodone: Hydrocodone is a semisynthetic narcotic analgesic and antitussive with multiple actions qualitatively similar to those of codeine. Most of these involve the central nervous system and smooth muscle. The precise mechanism of action of hydrocodone and other opiates is not known, although it is believed to relate to the existence of opiate receptors in the central nervous system. In addition to analgesia, narcotics may produce drowsiness, changes in mood and mental clouding.

Radioimmunoassay techniques have recently been developed for the analysis of hydrocodone in human plasma. After a 10 mg oral dose of hydrocodone bitartrate, a mean peak serum drug level of 23.6 ng/ml and an elimination half-life of 3.8 hours were found.

Aspirin: The analgesic, anti-inflammatory and antipyretic effects of aspirin are believed to result from inhibition of the synthesis of certain prostaglandins. Aspirin interferes with clotting mechanisms primarily by diminishing platelet aggregation; at high doses prothrombin synthesis can be inhibited.

Aspirin in solution is rapidly absorbed from the stomach and from the upper small intestine. About 50 percent of an oral dose is absorbed in 30 minutes and peak plasma concentrations are reached in about 40 minutes. Higher than normal stomach pH or the presence of food slightly delays absorption.

Once absorbed, aspirin is mainly hydrolyzed to salicylic acid and distributed to all body tissues and fluids, including fetal tissue, breast milk and the central nervous system (CNS). Highest concentrations are found in plasma, liver, renal cortex, heart and lung.

From 50 to 80 percent of salicylic acid and it metabolites in plasma are loosely bound to protein. The plasma half-life of total salicylate is about 3.0 hours, with a 650 mg dose. Higher doses of aspirin cause increases in plasma salicylate half-life. Almost all of a therapeutic dose of aspirin is excreted through the kidneys, either as salicylic acid or it metabolites. Renal clearance of salicylate is greatly augmented by an alkaline urine, as is produced by concurrent administration of sodium bicarbonate or potassium citrate.

Toxic salicylate blood levels are usually above 30 mg/100 ml. The single lethal dose of aspirin in normal adults is approximatey 25–30 g, but patients have recovered from much larger doses with appropriate treatment.

INDICATIONS AND USAGE

For the relief of moderate to moderately severe pain.

CONTRAINDICATIONS

Hydrocodone Bitartrate and Aspirin Tablets are contraindicated under the following conditions:

(1) hypersensitivity or intolerance to hydrocodone or aspirin.
(2) severe bleeding, disorders of coagulation or primary hemostasis, including hemophilia, hypoprothrombinemia, von Willebrand's disease, thrombocytopenias, thrombasthenia and other ill-defined hereditary platelet dysfunctions, severe vitamin K deficiency and severe liver damage.
(3) anticoagulant therapy.
(4) peptic ulcer, or other serious gasrointestinal lesions.

WARNINGS

Hydrocodone: Respiratory Depression: At high doses or in sensitive patients, hydrocodone may produce dose-related respiratory depression by acting directly on the brain stem respiratory center. Hydrocodone also affects the center that controls respiratory rhythm, and may produce irregular and periodic breathing.

Head Injury and Increased Intracranial Pressure: The respiratory depressant effects of narcotics and their capacity to elevate cerebrospinal fluid pressure may be markedly exaggerated in the presence of head injury, other intracranial lesions or a pre-existing increase in intracranial pressure. Furthermore, narcotics produce adverse reactions which may obscure the clinical course of patients with head injuries.

Acute Abdominal Conditions: The administration of narcotics may obscure the diagnosis or clinical course of patients with acute abdominal conditions.

Aspirin: Allergic Reactions: Therapeutic doses of aspirin can cause anaphylactic shock and other severe allergic reactions. A history of allergy is often lacking.

Bleeding: Significant bleeding can result from aspirin therapy in patients with peptic ulcer or other gastrointestinal lesions, and in patients with bleeding disorders. Aspirin administered preoperatively may prolong bleeding time.

PRECAUTIONS

Special Risk Patients: As with any narcotic analgesic agent, Hydrocodone Bitartrate and Aspirin Tablets should be used with caution in elderly or debilitated patients and those with severe impairment of hepatic or renal function, gallbladder disease or gallstones, respiratory impairment, cardiac arrhythmias, inflammatory disorders of the gastrointestinal tract, hypothyroidism, Addison's disease, prostatic hypertrophy or urethral stricture, coagulation disorders, head injuries or acute abdominal conditions. The usual precautions should be observed and the possibility of respiratory depression should not be overlooked.

Precautions should be taken when administering salicylates to persons with known allergies. Hypersensitivity to aspirin is particularly likely in patients with nasal polyps, and relatively common with asthma.

Information for Patients: Hydrocodone Bitartrate and Aspirin Tablets, like all narcotics, may impair the mental and/or physical abilities required for the performance of potentially hazardous tasks such as driving a car or operating machinery; patients should be cautioned accordingly.

Cough Reflex: Hydrocodone suppresses the cough reflex; as with all narcotics, caution should be exercised when Hydrocodone Bitartrate and Aspirin Tablets are used postoperatively and in patients with pulmonary disease.

Laboratory Tests: Hypersensitivity to aspirin cannot be detected by skin testing or radioimmunoassay procedures.

Drug Interactions

Hydrocodone: Patients receiving other narcotic analgesics, antipsychotics, antianxiety agents, or other CNS depressants (including alcohol) concomitantly with Hydrocodone Bitartrate and Aspirin Tablets may exhibit additive CNS depression. When combined therapy is contemplated, the dose of one or both agents should be reduced.

The use of MAO inhibitors or tricyclic antidepressants with hydrocodone preparations may increase the effect of either the antidepressant or hydrocodone.

The concurrent use of anticholinergics with hydrocodone, as with all narcotics, may produce paralytic ileus.

Aspirin: Aspirin may *enhance* the effects of:

(1) oral anticoagulants, causing bleeding by inhibiting prothrombin formation in the liver and displacing anticoagulants from plasma protein binding sites.
(2) oral antidiabetic agents and insulin, causing hypoglycemia by contributing an additive effect, and by displacing the oral antidiabetic agents from secondary binding sites.
(3) 6-mercaptopurine and methotrexate, causing bone marrow toxicity and blood dyscrasias by displacing these drugs from secondary binding sites.
(4) non-steroidal anti-inflammatory agents increasing the risk of peptic ulceration and bleeding by contributing additive effects.
(5) corticosteroids, potentiating anti-inflammatory effects by displacing steroids from protein binding sites. Aspirin intoxication may occur with corticosteroid withdrawal because steroids promote renal clearance of salicylates.

Aspirin may *diminish* the effects of uricosuric agents, such as probenecid and sulfinpyrazone, in the treatment of gout by competing for protein binding sites.

Drug/Laboratory Test Interactions:

Aspirin: Aspirin may interfere with the following laboratory determinations.

In blood: serum amylase, fasting blood glucose, carbon dioxide, cholesterol, protein, protein bound iodine, uric acid, prothrombin time, bleeding time and spectrophotometric detection of barbiturates.

In urine: glucose, 5-hydroxyindoleacetic acid, Gerhardt ketone, vanillylmandelic acid (VMA), protein, uric acid, and diacetic acid.

Pregnancy:

Teratogenic Effects: Pregnancy Category C.

Hydrocodone: Hydrocodone has been shown to be teratogenic in hamsters when given in doses 700 times the human dose. There are no adequate and well-controlled studies in pregnant women. Hydrocodone Bitartrate and Aspirin Tablets should be used during pregnancy only if the potential benefit justifies the potential risk to the fetus.

Aspirin: Reproductive studies in rats and mice have shown aspirin to be teratogenic and embryocidal at four to six times the human therapeutic dose. Studies in pregnant women, however, have not shown that aspirin increases the risk of abnormalities when administered during the first trimester of pregnancy. In controlled studies involving 41,337 pregnant women and their offspring, there was no evidence that aspirin taken during pregnancy caused stillbirth, neonatal death or reduced birthweight. In controlled studies of 50,282 pregnant women and their offspring, aspirin administration in moderate and heavy doses during the first four months of pregnancy showed no teratogenic effect.

Nonteratogenic Effects:

Hydrocodone: Babies born to mothers who have been taking opioids regularly prior to delivery will be physically dependent. The withdrawal signs include irritability and excessive crying, tremors, hyperactive reflexes, increased respiratory rate, increased stools, sneezing, yawning, vomiting, and fever. The intensity of the syndrome does not always correlate with the duration of maternal opioid use or dose. There is no consensus on the best method of managing withdrawal. Chlorpromazine 0.7 to 1 mg/kg q6h, and paregoric 2 to 4 drops/kg q4h, have been used to treat withdrawal symptoms in infants. The duration of therapy is 4 to 28 days, with the dosage decreased as tolerated.

Aspirin: Therapeutic doses of aspirin in pregnant women close to term may cause bleeding in the mother, fetus, or neonate. During the last six months of pregnancy, regular use of aspirin in high doses may prolong pregnancy and delivery.

Labor and Delivery: As with all narcotics, administration of Hydrocodone Bitartrate and Aspirin Tablets to the mother shortly before delivery may result in some degree of respiratory depression in the newborn, especially if higher doses are used. Ingestion of aspirin prior to delivery may prolong delivery or lead to bleeding in the mother or neonate.

Nursing Mothers: Aspirin is excreted in human milk in a small amount; the significance of its effect on nursing infants is not known. It is not known whether hydrocodone is excreted in human milk. Because many drugs are excreted in human milk and because of the potential for serious adverse reactions in nursing infants, a decision should be made whether to discontinue nursing or to discontinue the drug, taking into account the importance of the drug to the mother.

Continued on next page

Whitby—Cont.

Pediatric Use: Safety and effectiveness in children have not been established.

ADVERSE REACTIONS

The most frequently observed adverse reactions include lightheadedness, dizziness, sedation, nausea and vomiting. These effects seem to be more prominent in ambulatory than in nonambulatory patients and some of these adverse reactions may be alleviated if the patient lies down.

Other adverse reactions include:

Central Nervous System:

Hydrocodone: Drowsiness, mental clouding, lethargy, impairment of mental and physical performance, anxiety, fear, dysphoria, psychic dependence, mood changes.

Aspirin: Headache, drowsiness and mental confusion can occur in response to chronic use of large doses.

Gastrointestinal System:

Hydrocodone: The antiemetic phenothiazines are useful in suppressing the nausea and vomiting which may occur (see above); however, some phenothiazine derivatives seem to be antianalgesic and to increase the amount of narcotic required to produce pain relief, while other phenothiazines reduce the amount of narcotic required to produce a given level of analgesia. Prolonged administration of Hydrocodone Bitartrate and Aspirin Tablets may produce constipation.

Aspirin: Some patients are unable to take aspirin or other salicylates without developing nausea or vomiting. Occasional patients respond to aspirin (usually large doses) with dyspepsia or heartburn, which may be accompanied by occult bleeding. Excessive bruising or bleeding is sometimes seen in patients with mild disorders or primary hemostasis who regularly use low doses of aspirin.

Prolonged use of aspirin can cause painless erosion of gastric mucosa, occult bleeding and infrequently, iron-deficiency anemia. High doses of aspirin can exacerbate symptoms of peptic ulcer and, occasionally, cause extensive bleeding. Excessive bleeding can follow injury or surgery in patients with or without known bleeding disorders who have taken therapeutic doses of aspirin within the preceding 10 days. Hepatotoxicity has been reported in association with prolonged use of large doses of aspirin in patients with lupus erythematosus, rheumatoid arthritis and rheumatic disease.

Hematologic:

Aspirin: Bone marrow depression, manifested by weakness, fatigue or abnormal bruising or bleeding, has occasionally been reported with aspirin.

In patients with glucose-6-phosphate dehydrogenase deficiency, aspirin can cause a mild degree of hemolytic anemia.

Respiratory:

Hydrocodone: Hydrocodone bitartrate may produce dose-related respiratory depression by acting directly on the brain stem respiratory center. Hydrocodone also affects centers that control repiratory rhythm, and may produce irregular and periodic breathing.

If significant respiratory depression occurs, it may be antagonized by the use of naloxone hydrochloride. Apply other supportive measures when indicated.

Aspirin: Hyperpnea and hyperventilation can occur in response to chronic use of large doses.

Cardiovascular:

Aspirin: Tachycardia can occur in response to chronic use of large doses of aspirin.

Genitourinary:

Hydrocodone: Ureteral spasm, spasm of vesical sphincters and urinary retention have been reported.

Metabolic:

Aspirin: In hyperuricemic persons, low doses of aspirin may reduce the effectiveness of uricosuric therapy or precipitate an attack of gout.

Allergic:

Aspirin: Therapeutic doses of aspirin can induce mild or severe allergic reactions manifested by skin rashes, urticaria, angioedema, rhinorrhea, asthma, abdominal pain, nausea, vomiting, or anaphylactic shock. A history of allergy is often lacking, and allergic reactions may occur even in patients who have previously taken aspirin without any ill effects. Allergic reactions to aspirin are most likely to occur in patients with a history of allergic disease, especially in patients with nasal polyps or asthma.

Other:

Aspirin: Sweating and thirst can occur in response to chronic use of large doses of aspirin.

DRUG ABUSE AND DEPENDENCE

Hydrocodone Bitartrate and Aspirin Tablets are subject to the Federal Controlled Substance Act [Schedule CIII].

Psychic dependence, physical dependence, and tolerance may develop upon repeated administration of narcotics; therefore, Hydrocodone Bitartrate and Aspirin Tablets should be prescribed and administered with caution. However, psychic dependence is unlikely to develop when Hydrocodone Bitartrate and Aspirin Tablets are used for a short time for the treatment of pain.

Physical dependence, the condition in which continued administration of the drug is required to prevent the appearance of a withdrawal syndrome, assumes clinically significant proportions only after several weeks of continued narcotic use, although some mild degree of physical dependence may develop after a few days of narcotic therapy. Tolerance, in which increasingly large doses are required in order to produce the same degree of analgesia, is manifested initially by shortened duration of analgesic effect, and subsequently by decreases in the intensity of analgesia. The rate of development of tolerance varies among patients.

OVERDOSAGE

Hydrocodone:

Signs and Symptoms: Serious overdose with hydrocodone is characterized by respiratory depression (a decrease in respiratory rate and/or tidal volume, Cheyne-Stokes respiration, cyanosis), extreme somnolence progressing to stupor or coma, skeletal muscle flaccidity, cold and clammy skin, and sometimes bradycardia and hypotension. In severe overdosage, apnea, circulatory collapse, cardiac arrest and death may occur.

Treatment: Primary attention should be given to the reestablishment of adequate respiratory exchange through provision of a patent airway and institution of assisted or controlled ventilation. If significant respiratory depression occurs, it may be antagonized by the use of naloxone hydrochloride intravenously (see package insert for dosage and full information). Naloxone promptly reverses the effects of morphine-like opioid antagonists such as hydrocodone. In patients who are physically dependent, small doses of naloxone may be sufficient not only to antagonize respiratory depression, but also to precipitate withdrawal phenomena. The dose of naloxone should therefore be adjusted accordingly in such patients. Since the duration of action of hydrocodone may exceed that of the antagonist, the patient should be kept under continued surveillance and repeated doses of the antagonist should be administered as needed to maintain adequate respiration.

A narcotic antagonist should not be administered in the absence of clinically significant respiratory or cardiovascular depression. Oxygen, intravenous fluids, vasopressors and other supportive measures should be employed as indicated. Gastric emptying may be useful in removing unabsorbed drug.

Aspirin:

Signs and Symptoms: The most severe manifestations from aspirin results from cardiovascular and respiratory insufficiency secondary to acid-base and electrolyte disturbances, complicated by hyperthermia and dehydration.

Respiratory alkalosis is characteristic of the early phase of intoxication with aspirin while hyperventilation is occurring, but is quickly followed by metabolic acidosis in most people with severe intoxication.

Concentrations of aspirin in plasma above 30 mg/100 ml are associated with toxicity (See Clinical Pharmacology Section for information on factors influencing aspirin blood levels.) The single lethal dose of aspirin in adults is probably about 25–30 g. but is not known with certainty.

Hemodialysis and peritoneal dialysis can be performed to reduce the body aspirin content.

Treatment: Treatment consists primarily of supporting vital functions, increasing salicylate elimination, and correcting the acid-base imbalance due primarily to salicylism. Gastric emptying (Syrup of Ipecac) and/or lavage is recommended as soon as possible after ingestion, even if the patient has vomited spontaneously. Administration of activated charcoal as a slurry is beneficial after lavage and/or emesis, if less than three hours have passed since ingestion. Charcoal adsorption should *not* be employed prior to emesis or lavage.

Severity of aspirin intoxication is determined by measuring the blood salicylate level. Acid-base status should be closely followed with serial blood gas and serum pH measurements. Fluid and electrolyte balance should also be regularly monitored.

In severe cases, hyperthermia and hypovolemia are the major immediate threats to life. Children should be sponged with tepid water. Replacement fluid should be administered intravenously and augmented with sufficient bicarbonate to correct acidosis, with monitoring of plasma electrolytes and pH, to promote alkaline diuresis of salicylate if renal function is normal. Complete control may also require infusion of glucose to control hypoglycemia.

In patients with renal insufficiency or in cases of life-threatening intoxication, dialysis is usually required. Peritoneal dialysis or exchange transfusion is indicated in infants and young children and hemodialysis in older patients.

DOSAGE AND ADMINISTRATION

Dosage should be adjusted according to the severity of the pain and the response of the patient. However, tolerance to hydrocodone can develop with continued use and the incidence of untoward effects is dose related.

The usual adult dosage is one or two tablets every four to six hours as needed for pain. The total 24 hour dose should not exceed 8 tablets.

Hydrocodone Bitartrate 5mg and Aspirin 500mg Tablets should be taken with food or a full glass of milk or water to lessen gastric irritation.

HOW SUPPLIED

Dark pink capsule shaped tablet containing 5mg of Hydrocodone Bitartrate (WARNING: may be habit forming) and 500mg Aspirin. Each tablet is debossed with the Whitby logo on one side and the number 500 on the other side.

Supplied in bottles of 100 tablets (NDC 50474-500-01).

STORAGE

Store at controlled room temperature, 15°–30°C (59°–86°F). Protect from moisture.

DISPENSE IN A TIGHT, LIGHT-RESISTANT CONTAINER AS DEFINED IN THE USP/NF WITH A CHILD-RESISTANT CLOSURE.

CAUTION

Federal law prohibits dispensing without prescription.

A Schedule CIII Controlled Substance (Narcotic).

Manufactured For:

WHITBY PHARMACEUTICALS, INC.

Richmond, VA 23220

Manufactured By:

CENTRAL PHARMACEUTICALS, INC.

Seymour, IN 47274

Revised August 1991

Shown in Product Identification Section, page 435

THEO–24®   ℞

[*thē'ō-24*]

(theophylline anhydrous)

DESCRIPTION

Theo-24 oral capsules contain 100 mg, 200 mg, or 300 mg of anhydrous theophylline, a xanthine bronchodilator, in a extended-release formulation which allows a 24-hour dosing interval for appropriate patients.

Inactive ingredients are edible ink, ethylcellulose, gelatin, pharmaceutical glaze, colloidal silicon dioxide, starch, sucrose, talc, titanium dioxide, and coloring agents: 100-mg—includes FD&C Yellow No. 6; 200-mg—FD&C Red No. 3 and D&C Yellow No. 10; 300-mg—FD&C Blue No. 1 and FD&C Red. No. 40.

The structural formula of theophylline (3,7-dihydro-1,3-dimethyl-1H-purine-2,6-dione, is:

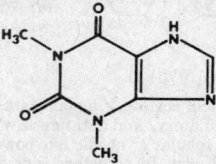

Theophylline is a white, odorless, crystalline powder having a bitter taste.

CLINICAL PHARMACOLOGY

Theophylline directly relaxes the smooth muscle of the bronchial airways and pulmonary blood vessels, thus acting mainly as a bronchodilator and smooth muscle relaxant. It has also been demonstrated that aminophylline has a potent effect on diaphragmatic contractility in normal persons and may then be capable of reducing fatigability and thereby improve contractility in patients with chronic obstructive airways disease. The exact mode of action remains unsettled. Although theophylline causes inhibition of phosphodiesterase with a resultant increase in intracellular cyclic adenosine monophosphate (AMP), other agents similarly inhibit the enzyme, producing a rise of cyclic AMP, but are unassociated with any demonstrable bronchodilation. Other mechanisms proposed include an effect on translocation of intracellular calcium, prostaglandin antagonism, stimulation of endogenous catecholamines, inhibition of cyclic guanosine monophosphate metabolism, and adenosine receptor antagonism. None of these mechanisms has been proved, however.

In vitro, theophylline has been shown to act synergistically with beta agonists, and there are data that demonstrate an additive effect *in vivo* with combined use.

Pharmacokinetics: The half-life of theophylline is influenced by a number of known variables. It may be prolonged in chronic alcoholics, particularly those with liver disease (cirrhosis or alcoholic liver disease), in patients with congestive heart failure, and in patients taking certain other drugs (see *Precautions: Drug interactions*). Newborns have extremely slow clearance rates compared to older infants and children, ie, those over 1 year. Older children have rapid clearance rates while most nonsmoking adults have clearance rates

between these two extremes. In premature neonates the decreased clearance is related to undeveloped oxidative pathways.

Theophylline Elimination Characteristics

	Half-Life (in hours)	
	Range	Mean
Children	1 to 9	3.7
Adults	3 to 15	7.7

In cigarette smokers (1 to 2 packs/day) the mean half-life is 4 to 5 hours, much shorter than in nonsmokers. The increase in clearance associated with smoking is presumably due to stimulation of the hepatic metabolic pathway by components of cigarette smoke. The duration of this effect after cessation of smoking is unknown but may require 6 months to 2 years before the rate approaches that of the nonsmoker.

Theo-24 capsules contain hundreds of coated beads of theophylline. Each bead is an individual extended-release delivery system. After dissolution of the capsules these beads are released and distributed in the gastrointestinal tract, thus minimizing the probability of high local concentrations of theophylline at any particular site.

In a 6-day multiple-dose study involving 18 subjects (with theophylline clearance rates between 0.57 and 1.02 ml/kg/min) who had fasted overnight and 2 hours after morning dosing, Theo-24 given once daily in a dose of 1500 mg produced serum theophylline levels that ranged between 5.7 mcg/ml and 22 mcg/ml. The mean minimum and maximum values were 11.6 mcg/ml and 18.1 mcg/ml, respectively, with an average peak-trough difference of 6.5 mcg/ml. The mean percent fluctuation $[(Cmax - Cmin/Cmin) \times 100]$ equals 80%. A 24-hour single-dose study demonstrated an approximately proportional increase in serum levels as the dose was increased from 600 to 1500 mg.

Taking Theo-24 with a high-fat-content meal may result in a significant increase in the peak serum level and in the extent of absorption of theophylline as compared to administration in the fasted state (see *Precautions: Drug/Food interactions*).

Following the single-dose administration (8 mg/kg) of Theo-24 to 20 normal subjects who had fasted overnight and 2 hours after morning dosing, peak serum theophylline concentrations of 4.8 ± 1.5 (SD) mcg/ml were obtained at 13.3 ± 4.7 (SD) hours. The amount of the dose absorbed was approximately 13% at 3 hours, 31% at 6 hours, 55% at 12 hours, 70% at 16 hours, and 88% at 24 hours. The extent of theophylline bioavailability from Theo-24 was comparable to the most widely used 12-hour extended-release product when both products were administered every 12 hours.

INDICATIONS AND USAGE

Theo-24 is indicated for relief and/or prevention of symptoms from asthma and for reversible bronchospasm associated with chronic bronchitis and emphysema.

CONTRAINDICATIONS

Theo-24 is contraindicated in patients with a history of hypersensitivity to theophylline. It is also contraindicated in patients with active peptic ulcer disease and in patients with underlying seizure disorders (unless receiving appropriate anticonvulsant medication).

WARNINGS

Serum levels above 20 mcg/ml are rarely found after appropriate administration of the recommended doses. However, in individuals in whom theophylline plasma clearance is reduced *for any reason*, even conventional doses may result in increased serum levels and potential toxicity. Reduced theophylline clearance has been documented in the following readily identifiable groups: (1) patients with impaired liver function; (2) patients over 55 years of age, particularly males and those with chronic lung disease; (3) patients with cardiac failure from any cause; (4) patients with sustained high fever; (5) infants under 1 year of age; and (6) patients taking certain drugs (see *Precautions: Drug/Drug interactions*). Frequently, such patients have markedly prolonged theophylline serum levels following discontinuation of the drug.

Reduction of dosage and laboratory monitoring is especially appropriate in the above individuals.

Serious side effects such as ventricular arrhythmias, convulsions, or even death may appear as the first sign of toxicity without any previous warning. Less serious signs of theophylline toxicity (ie, nausea and restlessness) may occur frequently when initiating therapy, but are usually transient; when such signs are persistent during maintenance therapy, they are often associated with serum concentrations above 20 mcg/ml. *Serious toxicity is not reliably preceded by less severe side effects.* A serum concentration measurement is the most reliable method of predicting potentially life-threatening toxicity.

Many patients who require theophylline may exhibit tachycardia due to their underlying disease process so that the cause/effect relationship to elevated serum theophylline concentrations may not be recognized.

Theophylline products may cause arrhythmia and/or worsen preexisting arrhythmias. Any significant change in rate and/or rhythm warrants monitoring and further investigation. Halothane anesthesia in the presence of theophylline may produce sinus tachycardia or ventricular arrhythmias.

Studies in laboratory animals (minipigs, rodents, and dogs) recorded the occurrence of cardiac arrhythmias and sudden death (with histologic evidence of necrosis of the myocardium) when theophylline and beta agonists were administered concomitantly. The significance of these findings when applied to humans is unknown.

PRECAUTIONS

General: On the average, theophylline's half-life is shorter in cigarette and marijuana smokers than in nonsmokers, but smokers can have half-lives as long as nonsmokers. Theophylline should not be administered concomitantly with other xanthines. Use with caution in patients with hypoxemia, hypertension, or those with a history of peptic ulcer. Theophylline may occasionally act as a local irritant to the gastrointestinal tract when administered orally, although gastrointestinal symptoms are more commonly centrally mediated and associated with serum drug concentrations over 20 mcg/ml.

Information for patients: Patients should be instructed to take this medication in the morning, at approximately the same time each day, and not to exceed the prescribed dose.

Patients who require a relatively high dose of theophylline (ie, a dose equal to or greater than 900 mg or 13 mg/kg, whichever is less) should be informed of important considerations relating to time of drug administration and meal content (see *Precautions: Drug/Food interactions;* and *Dosage and Administration*).

As with any extended-release theophylline product the patient should alert the physician if symptoms occur repeatedly, especially near the end of a dosing interval.

Laboratory tests: Serum levels should be monitored periodically to determine the theophylline level associated with observed clinical response and as the method of predicting toxicity. For such measurements, the serum sample should be obtained at the time of peak concentrations, approximately 12 hours after administration of a morning dose. It is important that the patient has not missed or taken additional doses during the previous 72 hours and that dosing intervals have been reasonably consistent. Dose adjustment based on measurements when these instructions have not been followed may result in toxicity (see *Dosage and Administration*).

Drug interactions

Drug/Drug interactions: Toxic synergism has been documented with ephedrine and may occur with other sympathomimetic bronchodilators. Halothane anesthesia in the presence of theophylline may produce sinus tachycardia or ventricular arrhythmias.

In addition, the following drug interactions have been demonstrated with theophylline:

Lithium carbonate	Increased renal excretion of lithium
Allopurinol (high-dose)	Increased serum theophylline levels
Cimetidine	Increased serum theophylline levels
Erythromycin, troleandomycin	Increased serum theophylline levels
Oral contraceptive steroids	Increased serum theophylline levels
Ciprofloxacin	Increased serum theophylline levels
Propranolol	Increased serum theophylline levels
Phenytoin	Decreased theophylline and phenytoin serum levels
Carbamazepine	Decreased serum theophylline levels
Phenobarbital	Decreased serum theophylline levels
Rifampin	Decreased serum theophylline levels

Drug/Food interactions: Taking Theo-24 less than one hour before a high-fat-content meal, such as 8 oz whole milk, 2 fried eggs, 2 bacon strips, 2 oz hashed brown potatoes, and 2 slices of buttered toast (about 985 calories, including approximately 71 g of fat) may result in a significant increase in peak serum level and in the extent of absorption of theophylline as compared to administration in the fasted state. In some cases (especially with doses of 900 mg or more taken less than one hour before a high-fat-content meal) serum theophylline levels may exceed the 20 mcg/ml level, above which theophylline toxicity is more likely to occur.

Drug/Laboratory test interactions: Currently available analytical methods, including high pressure liquid chromatography and immunoassay techniques, for measuring serum theophylline levels are specific. Metabolites and other drugs generally do not affect the results. Other new analytical methods are in use. The physician should be aware of the laboratory method used and whether other drugs will interfere with the assay for theophylline.

Carcinogenesis, mutagenesis, and impairment of fertility: Long-term carcinogenicity studies have not been performed with theophylline. Theophylline has been shown to be mutagenic in *Escherichia coli* and other lower organisms (*Euglena gracilis* and *Ophiostoma multiannulatum*). Chromosome-breaking activity was detected in human cell cultures at concentrations of theophylline up to 50 times the therapeutic serum concentration in humans. Theophylline was not mutagenic in the dominant lethal assay in male mice given theophylline intraperitoneally in doses up to 30 times the maximum daily human oral dose. Studies to determine the effect on fertility have not been performed with theophylline.

Pregnancy: Pregnancy Category C. Limited animal studies have shown teratogenic activity of theophylline in mice and rats. There are no adequate and well-controlled studies in pregnant women. Theophylline should be used during pregnancy only if the potential benefit justifies the potential risk to the fetus.

Nursing mothers: Theophylline is distributed into breast milk and may cause irritability or other signs of toxicity in nursing infants. Because of the potential for serious adverse reactions in nursing infants from theophylline, a decision should be made whether to discontinue nursing or to discontinue the drug, taking into account the importance of the drug to the mother.

Pediatric use: Safety and effectiveness in children under 12 years of age have not been established with this product.

ADVERSE REACTIONS

The following adverse reactions have been observed, but there has not been enough systematic collection of data to support an estimate of their frequency. The most consistent adverse reactions are usually due to overdosage.

Gastrointestinal: nausea, vomiting, epigastric pain, hematemesis, diarrhea.

Central nervous system: headaches, irritability, restlessness, insomnia, reflex hyperexcitability, muscle twitching, clonic and tonic generalized convulsions.

Cardiovascular: palpitation, tachycardia, extrasystoles, flushing, hypotension, circulatory failure, ventricular arrhythmias.

Respiratory: tachypnea.

Renal: potentiation of diuresis.

Other: alopecia, hyperglycemia, inappropriate ADH (antidiuretic hormone) syndrome, rash.

OVERDOSAGE

Management

It is suggested that the management principles (consistent with the clinical status of the patient when first seen) outlined below be instituted and that simultaneous contact with a Regional Poison Control Center be established. In this way both updated information and individualization regarding required therapy may be provided.

When potential oral overdose is established and seizure has not occurred:

A. If patient is alert and seen within the early hours after ingestion, induction of emesis may be of value. Gastric lavage has been demonstrated to be of no value in influencing outcome in patients who present more than 1 hour after ingestion.

B. Administer a cathartic. Sorbitol solution is reported to be of value.

C. Administer repeated doses of activated charcoal and monitor theophylline serum levels.

D. Prophylactic administration of phenobarbital has been shown to increase the seizure threshold in laboratory animals and administration of this drug can be considered.

If patient presents with a seizure:

A. Establish an airway.

B. Administer oxygen.

C. Treat the seizure with intravenous diazepam, 0.1 to 0.3 mg/kg up to 10 mg. If seizures cannot be controlled, the use of general anesthesia should be considered.

D. Monitor vital signs, maintain blood pressure, and provide adequate hydration.

If postseizure coma is present:

A. Maintain airway and oxygenation.

B. If a result of oral medication, follow above recommendations to prevent absorption of the drug, but intubation and lavage will have to be performed instead of inducing emesis, and the cathartic and charcoal will need to be introduced via a large bore gastric lavage tube.

Continued on next page

Whitby—Cont.

C. Continue to provide full supportive care and adequate hydration until the drug is metabolized. In general, drug metabolism is sufficiently rapid so as not to warrant dialysis. If repeated oral activated charcoal is ineffective (as noted by stable or rising serum levels) charcoal hemoperfusion may be indicated.

DOSAGE AND ADMINISTRATION

Patients who require a relatively high dose of theophylline (ie, a dose equal to or greater than 900 mg or 13 mg/kg, whichever is less) should not take Theo-24 less than 1 hour before a high-fat-content meal since this may result in a significant increase in peak serum level and in the extent of absorption of theophylline as compared to administration in the fasted state (see *Precautions: Drug/Food interactions*).

Effective use of theophylline (ie, the concentration of drug in the serum associated with optimal benefit and minimal risk of toxicity) is considered to occur when the theophylline concentration is maintained from 10 to 20 mcg/ml. The early studies from which these levels were derived were carried out in patients immediately or shortly after recovery from acute exacerbations of their disease (some hospitalized with status asthmaticus).

Although the 20 mcg/ml level remains appropriate as a critical value (above which toxicity is more likely to occur) for safety purposes, additional data are now available that indicate that the serum theophylline concentrations required to produce maximum physiologic benefit may, in fact, fluctuate with the degree of bronchospasm present and are variable. Therefore, the physician should individualize the range appropriate to the patient's requirements, based on both symptomatic response and improvement in pulmonary function. It should be stressed that serum theophylline concentrations maintained at the upper level of the 10 to 20 mcg/ml range may be associated with potential toxicity when factors known to reduce theophylline clearance are operative. (See *Warnings* and *Precautions*.)

Theo-24, like other extended-release theophylline products, is intended for patients with relatively continuous or recurring symptoms who have a need to maintain therapeutic serum levels of theophylline. It is not intended for patients experiencing an acute episode of bronchospasm (associated with asthma, chronic bronchitis, or emphysema). Such patients require rapid relief of symptoms and should be treated with an immediate-release or intravenous theophylline preparation (or other bronchodilators) and not with extended-release products.

Patients who metabolize theophylline at a normal or slow rate are reasonable candidates for once-daily dosing with Theo-24. Patients who metabolize theophylline rapidly (eg, the young, smokers, and some nonsmoking adults) and who have symptoms repeatedly at the end of a dosing interval, will require either increased doses given once a day or preferably, are likely to be better controlled by a schedule of twice-daily dosing. Those patients who require increased daily doses are more likely to experience relatively wide peak-trough differences and may be candidates for twice-a-day dosing with Theo-24.

Patients should be instructed to take this medication each morning at approximately the same time and not to exceed the prescribed dose.

Recent studies suggest that dosing of extended-release theophylline products at night (after the evening meal) results in serum concentrations of theophylline which are not identical to those recorded during waking hours and may be characterized by early trough and delayed peak levels. This appears to occur whether the drug is given as an immediate-release, extended-release, or intravenous product. To avoid this phenomenon when two doses per day are prescribed, it is recommended that the second dose be given 10 to 12 hours after the morning dose and before the evening meal.

Food and posture, along with changes associated with circadian rhythm, may influence the rate of absorption and/or clearance rates of theophylline from extended-release dosage forms administered at night. The exact relationship of these and other factors to nighttime serum concentrations and the clinical significance of such findings require additional study. Therefore, it is not recommended that Theo-24 (when used as a once-a-day product) be administered at night.

Since there is a wide variation from patient to patient in the total dose of theophylline required to attain the desired level in the serum, it is essential that the dose be titrated and that serum levels be monitored before and after transfer to any sustained-release product.

When serum levels are not measured, the initial dosage should be restricted to the amount recommended below (see *Initiation of therapy*).

As a practical consideration, it is not always possible to obtain serum level determinations. Under such conditions, restriction of the daily dose (in otherwise healthy adults) to not greater than 13 mg/kg/day (or 900 mg, whichever is lower) will result in relatively few patients exceeding serum

levels of 20 mcg/ml, thereby reducing the risk of developing toxicity.

Dosage Guidelines

WARNING: DO NOT ATTEMPT TO MAINTAIN ANY DOSE THAT IS NOT TOLERATED. Dosage guidelines are approximations only, and the wide range of clearance of theophylline among individuals (particularly those with concomitant disease) makes indiscriminate usage hazardous.

Because a high-fat-content meal may significantly increase the peak level and extent of absorption of theophylline from Theo-24, patients receiving large single doses (ie, equal to or greater than 900 mg or 13 mg/kg, whichever is less) should be instructed to avoid eating a high-fat-content morning meal or to take their medication at least 1 hour before eating. If the physician cannot be assured that the patient will follow the regimen, then the patient should be placed on a twice-daily dosing regimen.

For patients receiving lower once-daily single doses (less than 900 mg), very high peak levels are less likely to occur when Theo-24 is taken with food. With close monitoring, patients less certain to observe the fasting requirements could be treated with once-daily dosing.

It is recommended that dosing be considered in three stages: (I) initiation of therapy with Theo-24, (II) titration and adjustment, and (III) chronic maintenance.

I. Initiation of therapy with Theo-24

A. *Transfer of patients* already on established daily doses of theophylline (whether stabilized on immediate- or extended-release products) can be accomplished by administering the total daily dosage as a single dose given in the morning (eg, 300 mg of an immediate-release product given t.i.d. should be given as 900 mg of Theo-24). The initial transfer should not be made at doses exceeding 900 mg/day or 13 mg/kg/day, whichever is less. Subsequent dose titration should be done on the basis of serum levels and with appropriate attention to the time of drug administration and meal content as noted above.

It must be recognized that the peak and trough serum theophylline levels produced by once-daily dosing may vary (usually wider peak-trough differences) from those produced by the previous product and/or dosage regimen.

B. *For initiation of therapy with Theo-24* in patients who are not currently taking a theophylline product, the total daily dose, administered in the morning, must be established in accordance with the following guidelines:

Body Weight	Daily Dose
Children	
35 kg and above	400 mg
Adults	400 mg

Theophylline does not distribute into fatty tissue. Therefore, dosage should be calculated on the basis of lean (ideal) body weight where mg/kg doses are used.

If appropriate serum theophylline concentrations or adequate improvement in pulmonary function is not obtained after 3 days, the instructions in Part II (below) should be followed.

II. Titration and adjustment of dose

This phase of adjustment should be implemented either by the use of serum concentration measurements or by empiric principles when serum level determinations are not available.

A. If serum levels can be measured:

After 3 days' therapy with Theo-24, serum levels should be determined for peak concentration (sample obtained 12 hours after the morning dose) and trough concentration (24 hours after the morning dose). It is important that the patient has not missed or added any dose during the 72-hour period and that dosing intervals have been reasonably consistent. Dose adjustment based on measurements when these instructions have not been followed may result in toxicity.

Based on the results of the peak-trough values obtained, three possibilities exist:

1. The values of serum theophylline concentration fall within the desired range. If this result is obtained, the dosage should be maintained if it is tolerated.
2. If the serum theophylline concentration is too high, the dosage should be reduced as follows:
   a. If the values are between 20 and 25 mcg/ml, the daily dose may be reduced by about 10% and serum theophylline levels should be rechecked after 3 days.
   b. If the values are between 25 and 30 mcg/ml, the next dose should be skipped and the daily dose reduced by about 25%. The serum concentration should be rechecked after 3 days.
   c. If the values are over 30 mcg/ml, the next dose should be skipped and the daily dose reduced by

50%. The serum concentration should be rechecked after 3 days.
3. If the serum theophylline concentration is too low, the dosage should be increased at 3-day intervals by 100 mg or 200 mg (but not greater than 25% of the current dose), depending upon the desired goal. The serum concentration may be rechecked at appropriate intervals, but at least at the end of this adjustment period.

B. If serum levels cannot be measured:
1. If the clinical response is satisfactory then the total daily dose should be maintained.
2. If the response is unsatisfactory (due to persistence of symptoms or minimal improvement in measured function) after 3 days, then the dose may be increased by 100-mg increments. Reevaluation should be undertaken every 3 days.
3. If the response is still unsatisfactory and there are no adverse reactions, the dose may be cautiously adjusted upward in increments of 100 mg/day at 3- to 5-day intervals up to 900 mg (or 13 mg/kg/day, whichever is less).
4. If a response is accompanied by adverse reactions, then the next dose should be withheld or reduced by 25% depending on the severity of the reactions.

III. Chronic maintenance

After the dose is established, theophylline serum concentrations usually remain stable. However, as noted elsewhere (see *Warnings* and *Precautions*), certain exogenous and endogenous factors alter theophylline elimination (including concomitant disease and drug interactions) which require drug monitoring and adjustments in total daily dose requirements while such factors are operative.

Older adults, those with cor pulmonale, congestive heart failure, and/or liver disease may have unusually low dosage requirements and thus may experience toxicity at the minimal dosage recommended above.

If the patient's condition is otherwise clinically stable and none of the recognized factors that alter elimination is present, measurement of serum levels need be repeated only every 6 to 12 months.

HOW SUPPLIED

Theo-24 (theophylline anhydrous) is supplied in extended-release capsules containing 100, 200, or 300 mg of anhydrous theophylline.

Theo-24 100-mg capsules are yellow-orange and clear, with markings Theo-24, 100 mg, WHITBY, and 2832, supplied as:

NDC Number	Size
50474-2832-6	bottle of 100
50474-2832-4	carton of 100 unit dose

Theo-24 200-mg capsules are red-orange and clear, with markings Theo-24, 200 mg, WHITBY, and 2842, supplied as:

NDC Number	Size
50474-2842-6	bottle of 100
50474-2842-8	bottle of 500
50474-2842-4	carton of 100 unit dose

Theo-24 300-mg capsules are red and clear, with markings Theo-24, 300 mg, WHITBY, and 2852, supplied as:

NDC Number	Size
50474-2852-6	bottle of 100
50474-2852-8	bottle of 500
50474-2852-4	carton of 100 unit dose

Caution: Federal law prohibits dispensing without prescription.

5/92

Manufactured for Whitby Pharmaceuticals, Inc. by G.D. Searle & Co., Chicago, IL 60680

Shown in Product Identification Section, page 435

TRINSICON®   ℞

[tren 'sa-kon]
Hematinic Concentrate
With Intrinsic Factor
A Highly Potent Oral Antianemia Preparation

DESCRIPTION

Each TRINSICON® capsule contains:

Special liver-stomach concentrate (containing intrinsic factor)	240 mg
Vitamin B$_{12}$ (activity equivalent)	15 mcg
Iron, elemental (as ferrous fumarate)	110 mg
Ascorbic acid (vitamin C)	75 mg
Folic acid	0.5 mg

with other factors of vitamin B complex present in the liver-stomach concentrate.

Each capsule also contains the inactive ingredients FD&C Blue No. 1, D&C Red No. 28, FD&C Red No. 40, D&C

Yellow No. 10, gelatin, silicon dioxide, sodium lauryl sulfate and titanium dioxide.

CLINICAL PHARMACOLOGY

Vitamin B$_{12}$ with Intrinsic Factor: When secretion of intrinsic factor in gastric juice is inadequate or absent (eg, in Addisonian pernicious anemia or after gastrectomy), vitamin B$_{12}$ in physiologic doses is absorbed poorly, if at all. The resulting deficiency of vitamin B$_{12}$ leads to the clinical manifestations of pernicious anemia. Similar megaloblastic anemias may develop in fish tapeworm (*Diphyllobothrium latum*) infection or after a surgically created small-bowel blind loop; in these situations, treatment requires freeing the host of the parasites or bacteria that appear to compete for the available vitamin B$_{12}$. Strict vegetarianism and malabsorption syndromes may also lead to vitamin B$_{12}$ deficiency. In the latter case, parenteral therapy, or oral therapy with so-called massive doses of vitamin B$_{12}$, may be necessary for adequate treatment of the patient.

Potency of intrinsic factor concentrates is determined physiologically, ie, by their use in patients with pernicious anemia. The liver-stomach concentrate with intrinsic factor and the vitamin B$_{12}$ contained in two TRINSICON® (hematinic concentrate with intrinsic factor) capsules provide 1½ times the minimum amount of therapeutic agent, which, when given daily in an uncomplicated case of pernicious anemia, will produce a satisfactory reticulocyte response and relief of anemia and symptoms.

Concentrates of intrinsic factor derived from hog gastric, pyloric, and duodenal mucosa have been used successfully in patients who lack intrinsic factor. For example, Fouts et al maintained patients with pernicious anemia in clinical remission with oral therapy (liver extracts or intrinsic factor concentrate with vitamin B$_{12}$) for as long as 29 years. After total gastrectomy, Ficarra found multifactor preparations taken orally to be "just as effective in maintaining blood levels as any medication that has to be administered parenterally." His study was based on 24 patients who had survived for five years after total gastrectomy for cancer and who had been taking two TRINSICON capsules daily.

Folic Acid: Folic acid deficiency is the immediate cause of most, if not all, cases of nutritional megaloblastic anemia and of the megaloblastic anemias of pregnancy and infancy; usually, it is also at least partially responsible for the megaloblastic anemias of malabsorption syndromes, eg, tropical and nontropical sprue.

It is apparent that in vitamin B$_{12}$ deficiency (eg, pernicious anemia), lack of this vitamin results in impaired utilization of folic acid. There are other evidences of the close folic acid-vitamin B$_{12}$ interrelationship: (1) B$_{12}$ influences the storage, absorption, and utilization of folic acid, and (2) as a deficiency of B$_{12}$ progresses, the requirement for folic acid increases. However, folic acid does not change the requirement for vitamin B$_{12}$.

Iron: A very common anemia is that due to iron deficiency. In most cases, the response to iron salts is prompt, safe, and predictable. Within limits, the response is quicker and more certain to large doses of iron than to small doses.

Each TRINSICON capsule furnishes 110 mg of elemental iron (as ferrous fumarate) to provide a maximum response.

Ascorbic Acid: Vitamin C plays a role in anemia therapy. It augments the conversion of folic acid to its active form, folinic acid. In addition, ascorbic acid promotes the reduction of ferric iron in food to the more readily absorbed ferrous form. Severe and prolonged vitamin C deficiency is associated with an anemia that is usually hypochromic but occasionally megaloblastic in type.

INDICATIONS AND USAGE

TRINSICON® (hematinic concentrate with intrinsic factor) is a multifactor preparation effective in the treatment of anemias that respond to oral hematinics, including pernicious anemia and other megaloblastic anemias and also iron-deficiency anemia. Therapeutic quantities of hematopoietic factors that are known to be important are present in the recommended daily dose.

CONTRAINDICATIONS

Hemochromatosis and hemosiderosis are contraindications to iron therapy.

PRECAUTIONS

General: Anemia is a manifestation that requires appropriate investigation to determine its cause or causes. Folic acid *alone* is unwarranted in the treatment of pure vitamin B$_{12}$ deficiency states, such as pernicious anemia.

Folic acid may obscure pernicious anemia in that the blood picture may revert to normal while neurolological manifestations remain progressive.

As with all preparations containing intrinsic factor, resistance may develop in some cases of pernicious anemia to the potentiation of absorption of physiologic doses of vitamin B$_{12}$. If resistance occurs, parenteral therapy or oral therapy with so-called massive doses of vitamin B$_{12}$ may be necessary for adequate treatment of the patient. No single regimen fits all cases, and the status of the patient observed in follow-up is the final criterion for adequacy of therapy. Periodic clini-

cal and laboratory studies are considered essential and are recommended.

Pregnancy: *Pregnancy Category C:* Animal reproduction studies have not been conducted with TRINSICON® (hematinic concentrate with intrinsic factor). It is also not known whether these products can cause fetal harm when administered to a pregnant woman or can affect reproduction capacity. These products should be given to a pregnant woman only if clearly needed.

Nursing Mothers: It is not known whether these drugs are excreted in human milk. Because many drugs are excreted in human milk, caution should be exercised when TRINSICON is administered to a nursing woman.

Pediatric Use: Safety and effectiveness in children below the age of 10 have not been established.

ADVERSE REACTIONS

Rarely, iron in therapeutic doses produces gastrointestinal reactions, such as diarrhea or constipation. Reducing the dose and administering it with meals will minimize these effects in the iron-sensitive patient.

In extremely rare instances, skin rash suggesting allergy has been noted following the oral administration of liver-stomach material. Allergic sensitization has been reported following both oral and parenteral administration of folic acid.

OVERDOSAGE

Symptoms: Those of iron intoxication, which may include pallor and cyanosis, vomiting, hematemesis, diarrhea, melena, shock, drowsiness, and coma.

Treatment: For specific therapy, exchange transfusion and chelating agents. For general management, gastric and rectal lavage with sodium bicarbonate solution or milk, administration of intravenous fluids and electrolytes, and use of oxygen.

DOSAGE AND ADMINISTRATION

One capsule twice a day. (Two capsules daily produce a standard response in the average uncomplicated case of pernicious anemia.)

HOW SUPPLIED

Dark pink and dark red capsules imprinted "WHITBY/TRINSICON" in bottles of 60 (NDC 50474-364-22) and 500 (NDC 50474-364-24) and unit dose packages of 100 (NDC 50474-364-27).

Manufactured for
WHITBY PHARMACEUTICALS, INC.
Richmond, VA 23220
By D.M. Graham Laboratories, Inc.
Hobart, NY 13788

Revised 3/92
Shown in Product Identification Section, page 435

VICON FORTE® Capsules   ℞
[vī'kon for'tā]
(Therapeutic Vitamins-Minerals)

DESCRIPTION

Each black and orange VICON FORTE® capsule for oral administration contains:

Vitamin A .... 8,000 IU
Vitamin E .... 50 IU
Ascorbic acid .... 150 mg
Zinc sulfate, USP* .... 80 mg
Magnesium sulfate, USP† .... 70 mg
Niacinamide .... 25 mg
Thiamine mononitrate .... 10 mg
d-Calcium pantothenate .... 10 mg
Riboflavin .... 5 mg
Manganese chloride .... 4 mg
Pyridoxine hydrochloride .... 2 mg
Folic acid .... 1 mg
Vitamin B$_{12}$ (Cyanocobalamin) .... 10 mcg

* As 50 mg dried zinc sulfate.
† As 50 mg dried magnesium sulfate.

Each capsule also contains FD&C Blue No. 1, FD&C Red No. 40, FD&C Yellow No. 6, gelatin, lactose, magnesium stearate, sodium propionate, and titanium dioxide.

INDICATIONS AND USAGE

VICON FORTE® is indicated for the treatment and/or prevention of vitamin and mineral deficiencies associated with restricted diets, improper food intake, alcoholism, and decreased absorption. VICON FORTE is also indicated in patients with increased requirements for vitamins and minerals due to chronic disease, infection, and burns and in persons using alcohol to excess. Preoperative and postoperative use of VICON FORTE can provide the increased amounts of vitamins and minerals necessary for optimal recovery from the stress of surgery.

CONTRAINDICATIONS
None known.

PRECAUTIONS

General: Folic acid in doses above 0.1 mg daily may obscure pernicious anemia in that hematologic remission can occur while neurological manifestations remain progressive.

DOSAGE AND ADMINISTRATION

One capsule daily or as directed by physician.

HOW SUPPLIED

Orange and black capsules imprinted with "WHITBY" and "316" in bottles of 60 (NDC 50474-316-22) and 500 (NDC 50474-316-24) and unit dose packs of 100 (NDC 50474-316-27). Dispense in tight, light-resistant containers as defined in the USP/NF.

Manufactured for Whitby Pharmaceuticals, Inc., Richmond, VA 23220 by D.M. Graham Laboratories, Inc., Hobart, NY 13788

Revised 10/91
Shown in Product Identification Section, page 435

Whitehall Laboratories Inc.
Division of American Home
    Products Corporation
685 THIRD AVENUE
NEW YORK, NY 10017

ADVIL®   **OTC**
Ibuprofen Tablets, USP
Ibuprofen Caplets
Pain Reliever/Fever Reducer

WARNING

ASPIRIN SENSITIVE PATIENTS. Do not take this product if you have had a severe allergic reaction to aspirin, e.g. —asthma, swelling, shock or hives, because even though this product contains no aspirin or salicylates, cross-reactions may occur in patients allergic to aspirin.

INDICATIONS

For the temporary relief of minor aches and pains associated with the common cold, headache, toothache, muscular aches, backache, for the minor pain of arthritis, for the pain of menstrual cramps and for reduction of fever.

DOSAGE AND ADMINISTRATION

Adults: Take one tablet every 4 to 6 hours while symptoms persist. If pain or fever does not respond to one tablet, two tablets may be used but do not exceed six tablets in 24 hours unless directed by a doctor. The smallest effective dose should be used. Take with food or milk if occasional and mild heartburn, upset stomach, or stomach pain occurs with use. Consult a doctor if these symptoms are more than mild or if they persist. **Children:** Do not give this product to children under 12 except under the advice and supervision of a doctor.

WARNINGS

Do not take for pain for more than 10 days or for fever for more than 3 days unless directed by a doctor. If pain or fever persists or gets worse, if new symptoms occur, or if the painful area is red or swollen, consult a doctor. These could be signs of serious illness. If you are under a doctor's care for any serious condition, consult a doctor before taking this product. As with aspirin and acetaminophen, if you have any condition which requires you to take prescription drugs or if you have had any problems or serious side effects from taking any non-prescription pain reliever, do not take this product without first discussing it with your doctor. **IF YOU EXPERIENCE ANY SYMPTOMS WHICH ARE UNUSUAL OR SEEM UNRELATED TO THE CONDITION FOR WHICH YOU TOOK IBUPROFEN, CONSULT A DOCTOR BEFORE TAKING ANY MORE OF IT.** Although ibuprofen is indicated for the same conditions as aspirin and acetaminophen, it should not be taken with them except under a doctor's direction. Do not combine this product with any other ibuprofen-containing product. As with any drug, if you are pregnant or nursing a baby, seek the advice of a health professional before using this product. IT IS ESPECIALLY IMPORTANT NOT TO USE IBUPROFEN DURING THE LAST 3 MONTHS OF PREGNANCY UNLESS SPECIFICALLY DIRECTED TO DO SO BY A DOCTOR BECAUSE IT MAY CAUSE PROBLEMS IN THE UNBORN CHILD OR COMPLICATIONS DURING DELIVERY.

Keep this and all drugs out of the reach of children. In case of accidental overdose, seek professional assistance or contact a poison control center immediately.

Continued on next page

Whitehall Laboratories—Cont.

ACTIVE INGREDIENT
Each tablet contains Ibuprofen 200 mg.

INACTIVE INGREDIENTS
Acacia, Acetylated Monoglycerides, Beeswax or Carnauba Wax, Calcium Sulfate, Colloidal Silicon Dioxide, Dimethicone, Iron Oxide, Lecithin, Pharmaceutical Glaze, Povidone, Sodium Benzoate, Sodium Carboxymethylcellulose, Starch, Stearic Acid, Sucrose, Titanium Dioxide.

PROFESSIONAL LABELING
Same as stated under Indications.

HOW SUPPLIED
Coated tablets in bottles of 8, 24, 50 (non-child resistant size), 100, 165 and 250.
Coated caplets in bottles of 8, 24, 50 (non-child resistant size), 100, 165, and 250.
Coated tablets in thermoform packaging of 8.

STORAGE
Store at room temperature; avoid excessive heat 40°C (104°F).
Shown in Product Identification Section, page 435

ADVIL® COLD & SINUS (formerly CoADVIL®) OTC
[ad'vil kŏld si-nus]
Ibuprofen/Pseudoephedrine Caplets*
Pain Reliever/Fever Reducer/Nasal Decongestant
*Oval-Shaped tablets

WARNING
ASPIRIN SENSITIVE PATIENTS. Do not take this product if you have had a severe allergic reaction to aspirin, e.g. —asthma, swelling, shock or hives, because even though this product contains no aspirin or salicylates, cross-reactions may occur in patients allergic to aspirin.

INDICATIONS
For temporary relief of symptoms associated with the common cold, sinusitis or flu including nasal congestion, headache, fever, body aches, and pains.

DIRECTIONS
Adults: Take 1 caplet every 4 to 6 hours while symptoms persist. If symptoms do not respond to 1 caplet, 2 caplets may be used but do not exceed 6 caplets in 24 hours unless directed by a doctor. The smallest effective dose should be used. Take with food or milk if occasional and mild heartburn, upset stomach, or stomach pain occurs with use. Consult a doctor if these symptoms are more than mild or if they persist. Children: Do not give this product to children under 12 years of age except under the advice and supervision of a doctor.

WARNINGS
Do not take for colds for more than 7 days or for fever for more than 3 days unless directed by a doctor. If the cold or fever persists or gets worse, or if new symptoms occur, consult a doctor. These could be signs of serious illness. As with aspirin and acetaminophen, if you have any condition which requires you to take prescription drugs or if you have had any problems or serious side effects from taking any nonprescription pain reliever, do not take this product without first discussing it with your doctor. IF YOU EXPERIENCE ANY SYMPTOMS WHICH ARE UNUSUAL OR SEEM UNRELATED TO THE CONDITION FOR WHICH YOU TOOK THIS PRODUCT, CONSULT A DOCTOR BEFORE TAKING ANY MORE OF IT. If you are under a doctor's care for any serious condition, consult a doctor before taking this product.
Do not exceed recommended dosage because at higher doses nervousness, dizziness or sleeplessness may occur. Do not take this product if you have high blood pressure, heart disease, diabetes, thyroid disease or difficulty in urination due to enlargement of the prostate gland, except under the advice and supervision of a doctor.
Drug Interaction Precaution: Do not take this product if you are presently taking a prescription drug for high blood pressure or depression without first consulting your doctor. Do not combine this product with other non-prescription pain relievers. Do not combine this product with any other ibuprofen-containing product. As with any drug, if you are pregnant or nursing a baby, seek the advice of a health professional before using this product.
IT IS ESPECIALLY IMPORTANT NOT TO USE THIS PRODUCT DURING THE LAST 3 MONTHS OF PREGNANCY UNLESS SPECIFICALLY DIRECTED TO DO SO BY A DOCTOR BECAUSE IT MAY CAUSE PROBLEMS IN THE UNBORN CHILD OR COMPLICATIONS DURING DELIVERY. Keep this and all drugs out of the reach of children. In case of accidental overdose, seek professional assistance or contact a poison control center immediately.

ACTIVE INGREDIENTS: Each caplet contains Ibuprofen 200 mg and Pseudoephedrine HCl 30 mg.
INACTIVE INGREDIENTS: Carnauba or Equivalent Wax, Croscarmellose Sodium, Iron Oxides, Methylparaben, Microcrystalline Cellulose, Propylparaben, Silicon Dioxide, Sodium Benzoate, Sodium Lauryl Sulfate, Starch, Stearic Acid, Sucrose, Titanium Dioxide.

HOW SUPPLIED
Advil®Cold & Sinus is an oval-shaped tan-colored caplet supplied in consumer bottles of 40, and Blister Packs of 20. Medical samples are available in a 2's Pouch Dispenser.
STORAGE: Store at room temperature; avoid excessive heat (40°C, 104°F).
Shown in Product Identification Section, page 435

Children's Advil® Suspension ℞

See Wyeth-Ayerst Laboratories for full prescribing information.

Maximum Strength OTC
ANBESOL® Gel and Liquid
Antiseptic Anesthetic
Regular Strength
ANBESOL® Gel and Liquid OTC
[ăn'bă-sŏl "]
Antiseptic Anesthetic

DESCRIPTION
Anbesol is an antiseptic anesthetic which is available in a Maximum Strength and Regular Strength gel and liquid product.
The Maximum Strength formulations contain Benzocaine 20% and Alcohol 60%.
The Regular Strength formulations contain Benzocaine 6.3%, Phenol 0.5%, and Alcohol 70%.

INDICATIONS
Maximum Strength and Regular Strength Anbesol are indicated for the fast temporary relief of pain due to toothache, braces, denture and orthodontic irritation, sore gums, cold and canker sores and fever blisters. Regular Strength Anbesol is also indicated for the fast temporary relief of teething pain.

ACTIONS
Temporarily deadens sensations of nerve endings to provide relief of pain and discomfort; reduces oral bacterial flora temporarily as an aid in oral hygiene.

WARNINGS
Flammable. Keep away from fire or flame. Avoid smoking during application and until product has dried. Do not use near eyes. Localized allergic reactions may occur after prolonged or repeated use. Keep this and all medicines out of the reach of children.

PRECAUTIONS
Not for prolonged use. If the condition persists or irritation develops, discontinue use and consult a physician or dentist. FOR GEL ONLY: NOT FOR USE UNDER DENTURES OR OTHER DENTAL WORK.

DOSAGE AND ADMINISTRATION
Apply topically to the affected area on or around the lips, or within the mouth. FOR DENTURE IRRITATION: Apply thin layer of gel to affected area and do not reinsert dental work until irritation/pain is relieved. Rinse mouth before reinserting dentures. If irritation/pain persists, contact your dentist.

INACTIVE INGREDIENTS
Maximum Strength Gel: Carbomer 934P, D&C Yellow #10, FD&C Red #40, FD&C Blue #1, Flavor, Polyethylene Glycol, Saccharin. Maximum Strength Liquid: D&C Yellow #10, FD&C Blue #1, FD&C Red #40, Flavor, Polyethylene Glycol, Saccharin.
Regular Gel: Camphor, Carbomer 934P, D&C Red #33, D&C Yellow #10, FD&C Blue #1, FD&C Yellow #6, Flavor, Glycerin. Regular Liquid: Camphor, Glycerin, Menthol, Potassium Iodide, Povidone Iodine.

HOW SUPPLIED
Maximum Strength Gel in .25 oz (7.2 g) tube, Maximum Strength Liquid in .31 fl oz (9 mL) bottle.
Regular Gel in .25 oz. (7.2 g) tube. Regular Liquid in two sizes—.31 fl. oz. (9 mL) and .74 fl. oz. (22 mL) bottles.
Shown in Product Identification Section, page 435

BABY ANBESOL® OTC
[ăn'bă-sŏl "]
Oral Anesthetic Gel

DESCRIPTION
Baby Anbesol Gel contains Benzocaine 7.5%, a safe and effective anesthetic which soothes the sore gums of an infant by providing temporary relief from teething pain.

INDICATIONS
Baby Anbesol Gel is indicated for fast, temporary relief from the pain and irritation associated with teething.

ACTIONS
Temporarily numbs nerve endings to provide relief from pain and discomfort.

WARNINGS
Avoid getting into eyes. For persistent or excessive teething pain, consult a physician or dentist. Localized allergic reactions may occur after prolonged or repeated use. Keep this and all medicines out of the reach of children. In case of accidental overdose, seek professional assistance or contact a poison control center immediately.

DOSAGE AND ADMINISTRATION
Apply a small amount of Baby Anbesol on the infant's irritated gums with cotton swab or finger tip no more than 4 times a day.

INACTIVE INGREDIENTS
Carbomer 934P, D&C Red No. 33, Disodium Edetate, Flavor, Glycerin, Polyethylene Glycol, Saccharin, Water.

HOW SUPPLIED
Clear gel in .25 oz. (7.2 g) tube.
Shown in Product Identification Section, page 435

Maximum Strength
ARTHRITIS PAIN FORMULA™ OTC
[är'thrīt-is 'pān 'for-mye-la]
By the Makers of Anacin® Analgesic
Tablets

DESCRIPTION
Each caplet contains 500 mg microfined aspirin and two buffers, 27 mg Aluminum Hydroxide and 100 mg Magnesium Hydroxide.
Arthritis Pain Formula is a buffered analgesic and antipyretic with microfined aspirin.

INDICATIONS AND ACTIONS
Arthritis Pain Formula provides hours of relief from minor aches and pains of arthritis and rheumatism and low back pain. Also relieves the pain of headache, neuralgia, neuritis, sprains, muscular aches, discomforts and fever of colds, pain caused by tooth extraction and toothache, and menstrual discomfort.

WARNINGS
Children and teenagers should not use this medicine for chicken pox or flu symptoms before a doctor is consulted about Reye syndrome, a rare but serious illness reported to be associated with aspirin. As with any drug, if you are pregnant or nursing a baby, seek the advice of a health professional before using this product. IT IS ESPECIALLY IMPORTANT NOT TO USE ASPIRIN DURING THE LAST 3 MONTHS OF PREGNANCY UNLESS SPECIFICALLY DIRECTED TO DO SO BY A DOCTOR BECAUSE IT MAY CAUSE PROBLEMS IN THE UNBORN CHILD OR COMPLICATIONS DURING DELIVERY. Keep this and all medications out of children's reach. In case of accidental overdose, contact a physician immediately.

PRECAUTIONS
If pain persists for more than 10 days, or redness is present or in arthritic or rheumatic conditions affecting children under 12, consult a physician immediately.

DOSAGE AND ADMINISTRATION
Adult Dosage: 2 caplets, 3 or 4 times a day. Do not exceed 8 caplets in any 24-hour period. For children under 12, consult a physician.

INACTIVE INGREDIENTS
Hydrogenated Vegetable Oil, Microcrystalline Cellulose, Starch, Surfactant.

HOW SUPPLIED
In plastic bottles of 40 (non-child-resistant size), 100 and 175 caplets.
Shown in Product Identification Section, page 435

COMPOUND W®   OTC
[kam-paund w]
Liquid and Gel

DESCRIPTION
Compound W is a salicylic acid (17% W/W) preparation available as a liquid or gel.

INDICATION
Compound W is indicated for the removal of common warts. The common wart is easily recognized by the rough "cauliflower-like" appearance of the surface.

ACTIONS
Warts are common benign skin lesions which appear mainly on the back of hands and on fingers, but can also appear on other parts of the body. They are caused by an infectious virus which stimulates mitosis in the basal cell layer of the skin resulting in the production of elevated epithelial growths. The keratolytic action of salicylic acid in a flexible collodion vehicle causes the cornified epithelium to swell, soften, macerate and then desquamate.

WARNINGS
For external use only. Do not use this product on irritated skin, on any area that is infected or reddened, if you are diabetic, or if you have poor blood circulation. If discomfort persists, see your doctor. Do not use on moles, birthmarks, warts with hair growing from them, or warts on the face, near the eyes or on mucous membranes (inside mouth, nose, anus, genitals, or on lips). Extremely flammable. Keep away from fire or flame. Cap bottle or tube tightly and store at room temperature away from heat. Avoid smoking during application and until product has dried. If product gets into the eye, flush with water for 15 minutes. Avoid inhaling vapors. Keep this and all drugs out of the reach of children. In case of accidental ingestion, seek professional assistance or contact a poison control center immediately.

PRECAUTIONS
If redness or irritation occurs, discontinue product for 2 days and then reapply. Should stinging or irritation recur, discontinue use.

DOSAGE AND ADMINISTRATION
Wash affected area. May soak wart in warm water for 5 minutes. Dry area thoroughly. Apply 1 drop at a time to sufficiently cover each wart by using the plastic rod provided with the liquid or by squeezing the tube. Let dry. Repeat this procedure once or twice daily as needed (until wart is removed) for up to 12 weeks.

INACTIVE INGREDIENTS
Liquid: Alcohol 21.2%, Camphor, Castor Oil, Collodion, Ether 63.6%, Ethylcellulose, Hypophosphorous Acid, Menthol, Polysorbate 80. *Gel:* Alcohol 67.5% by vol., Camphor, Castor Oil, Collodion, Colloidal Silicon Dioxide, Hydroxypropyl Cellulose, Hypophosphorous Acid, Polysorbate 80.

HOW SUPPLIED
Compound W Liquid is available in .31 fluid oz. clear bottles with plastic applicators. Compound W Gel is available in .25 oz. tubes. Store at room temperature.

DENOREX®   OTC
[den'ō-reks]
Medicated Shampoo
DENOREX®   OTC
Mountain Fresh Herbal Scent
Medicated Shampoo
DENOREX®   OTC
Medicated Shampoo and Conditioner
DENOREX®   OTC
Extra Strength Medicated Shampoo
DENOREX®   OTC
Extra Strength Medicated Shampoo with Conditioners

DESCRIPTION
The Shampoo (Regular and Mt. Fresh Herbal) and the Shampoo and Conditioner contain Coal Tar Solution 9.0%. The Extra Strength Shampoo and the Extra Strength Shampoo with Conditioners contain Coal Tar Solution 12.5%.

ACTIONS
Denorex Shampoo is an antiseborrheic and antipruritic which loosens and softens scales and crusts. Coal tar helps correct abnormalities of keratinization by decreasing epidermal proliferation and dermal infiltration.

INDICATIONS
Relieves and helps eliminate the itching, flaking, scaling and irritation associated with dandruff, seborrheic dermatitis and psoriasis.

WARNINGS
For external use only. Avoid contact with eyes. If contact occurs, rinse eyes thoroughly with water. If condition wors-

ens or does not improve after regular use of this product as directed, consult a doctor. Use caution in exposing skin to sunlight after applying this product. It may increase your tendency to sunburn for up to 24 hours after application. Do not use for prolonged periods without consulting a doctor. Do not use this product with other forms of psoriasis therapy such as ultraviolet radiation or prescription drugs unless directed to do so by a doctor. If condition covers a large area of the body, consult your doctor before using this product. Keep this and all drugs out of the reach of children. In case of accidental ingestion, seek professional assistance or contact a poison control center immediately.

DIRECTIONS
Lather, rinse thoroughly; repeat. The scalp may tingle slightly during treatment. For best results use at least twice a week or as directed by a doctor.

INACTIVE INGREDIENTS
Shampoo: Chloroxylenol, Lauramide DEA, Menthol, Stearic Acid, TEA-Lauryl Sulfate, Water, and Alcohol 7.5% by volume (plus Fragrance and Hydroxypropyl Methylcellulose in Mountain Fresh Herbal Scent Formula).
Shampoo with Conditioner: Chloroxylenol, Citric Acid, Fragrance, Hydroxypropyl Methylcellulose, Lauramide DEA, Menthol, PEG-27 Lanolin, Polyquaternium-11, TEA-Lauryl Sulfate, Water, and Alcohol 7.5% by volume.
Extra Strength: Chloroxylenol, FD&C Red #40, Fragrance, Glycol Distearate, Hydroxypropyl Methylcellulose, Lauramide DEA, Menthol, TEA-Lauryl Sulfate, Water, and Alcohol 10.4% by volume.
Extra Strength Shampoo and Conditioner: Chloroxylenol, Citric Acid, Cocodimonium Hydrolyzed Protein, FD&C Red #40, Fragrance, Glycol Distearate, Hydroxypropyl Methylcellulose, Lauramide DEA, Menthol, PEG-27 Lanolin, Polyquaternium-6, TEA-Lauryl Sulfate, Water, and Alcohol 10.4% by volume.

HOW SUPPLIED
Available in: 4 oz., 8 oz. and 12 oz. bottles.
Shown in Product Identification Section, page 435

DERMOPLAST® LOTION   OTC
[der'mō-plăst]
Anesthetic Pain Relief Lotion

DESCRIPTION
DERMOPLAST Lotion contains benzocaine 8% and menthol 0.5%.

ACTIONS
DERMOPLAST is a topical anesthetic and antipruritic.

INDICATIONS
DERMOPLAST is indicated for the fast, temporary relief of pain and itching from sunburn, insect bites, minor cuts, abrasions, minor burns, and minor skin irritations.

WARNINGS
FOR EXTERNAL USE ONLY.
In case of accidental ingestion, seek professional assistance or contact a Poison Control Center. Avoid contact with eyes. If symptoms persist, or if rash or irritation develops, discontinue use and consult physician. Keep this and all drugs out of the reach of children.

DIRECTIONS
Apply freely over sunburned or irritated skin. Repeat three or four times daily, as needed.

INACTIVE INGREDIENTS
Aloe Vera Gel, Carbomer 934P, Ceteth-16, Glycerin, Glyceryl Stearate, Laneth-16, Methylparaben, Oleth-16, Propylparaben, Simethicone, Steareth-16, Triethanolamine, Water.

HOW SUPPLIED
DERMOPLAST Anesthetic Pain Relief Lotion, in Net Wt 3 fl oz. plastic squeeze bottle.

DERMOPLAST® SPRAY   OTC
[der'mō-plăst]
Anesthetic Pain Relief Spray

DESCRIPTION
DERMOPLAST is an aerosol containing benzocaine 20% and menthol 0.5%.

INDICATIONS
DERMOPLAST is indicated for the fast, soothing temporary relief of skin pain and itching due to sunburn, insect bites, minor cuts, abrasions, minor burns, and skin irritations.

CAUTIONS
For external use only. In case of accidental ingestion, seek professional assitance or contact a poison control center immediately. Avoid spraying in eyes or inhaling. Intentional misuse can be harmful or fatal. If condition persists, or if rash or irritation develops, discontinue use and consult a physician.

WARNINGS
Contents under pressure. Do not puncture or incinerate. Do not expose to heat or temperatures above 120°F. Do not use near open flame. Keep this and all drugs out of the reach of children.

DIRECTIONS FOR USE
Hold can 6-12 inches away from affected area. Point spray nozzle and press button. To apply to face, spray in palm of hand. May be administered three or four times daily, or as directed by physician.

INACTIVE INGREDIENTS
Acetylated Lanolin Alcohol, Aloe Vera Oil, Butane, Cetyl Acetate, Hydrofluorocarbon, Methylparaben, PEG-8 Laurate, Polysorbate 85.

HOW SUPPLIED
DERMOPLAST Anesthetic Pain Relief Spray, in Net Wt 2 oz (57 g) and Net Wt 2¾ oz (78 g). Store at room temperature.

DRISTAN PRODUCTS

[See table on next page.]

DRISTAN®   OTC
[drĭs'tăn]
Nasal Spray
Nasal Spray with metered dose pump
Menthol Nasal Spray

DESCRIPTION
Dristan Nasal Spray contains Phenylephrine HCl 0.5%, Pheniramine Maleate 0.2%.

ACTIONS
Phenylephrine HCl is a sympathomimetic agent that constricts the smaller arterioles of the nasal passages producing a gentle and predictable decongesting effect.

INDICATIONS
Dristan Nasal Spray provides prompt temporary relief of nasal congestion due to colds, sinusitis, hay fever or other upper respiratory allergies.

WARNINGS
Do not exceed recommended dosage because symptoms may occur such as burning, stinging, sneezing, or increase of nasal discharge. Do not use this product for more than 3 days. If symptoms persist, consult a physician. The use of this dispenser by more than one person may spread infection. For adult use only. Do not give this product to children under 12 years except under the advice and supervision of a physician. Keep these and all drugs out of the reach of children. In case of accidental ingestion, seek professional assistance or contact a Poison Control Center immediately.

DOSAGE AND ADMINISTRATION
(Squeeze bottle) with head upright, insert nozzle in nostril. Spray quickly, firmly and sniff deeply. (Metered Dose Pump) prime the metered dose pump by depressing pump firmly several times. With head upright, insert nozzle in nostril. Depress pump 2 or 3 times, all the way down, with a firm even stroke and sniff deeply. Adults: Spray 2 or 3 times into each nostril. Repeat every 4 hours as needed. Children under 12 years of age: As directed by a physician.

INACTIVE INGREDIENTS
Dristan Nasal Spray: Alcohol 0.4%, Benzalkonium Chloride 1:5000 in buffered isotonic aqueous solution, Eucalyptol, Hydroxypropyl Methylcellulose, Menthol, Sodium Chloride, Sodium Phosphate, Thimerosal Preservative 0.002%, and Water.
Dristan Menthol Nasal Spray: Benzalkonium Chloride 1:5000 in buffered isotonic aqueous solution, Camphor, Eucalyptol, Hydroxypropyl Methylcellulose, Menthol, Methyl Salicylate; Polysorbate 80, Sodium Chloride, Sodium Phosphate, Thimerosal Preservative 0.002%, and Water.

HOW SUPPLIED
Dristan Nasal Spray: 15 mL and 30 mL plastic squeeze bottles, and 15 mL metered dose pumps.
Dristan Menthol Nasal Spray: 15 mL and 30 mL plastic squeeze bottles.
Shown in Product Identification Section, page 435

Continued on next page

Whitehall Laboratories—Cont.

DRISTAN® ALLERGY   OTC
Nasal Decongestant/Antihistamine Caplets

[See table.]

DESCRIPTION
Each Dristan Allergy Coated Caplet contains: Pseudoephedrine Hydrochloride 60 mg and Brompheniramine Maleate 4 mg.

ACTIONS
Pseudoephedrine HCl is an oral nasal decongestant and is effective in relieving nasal/sinus congestion. Brompheniramine maleate is an antihistamine effective in the control of the runny nose, sneezing, and watery eyes associated with elevated histamine levels in disorders of the respiratory tract.

INDICATIONS
DRISTAN ALLERGY CAPLETS provide hours of effective relief of symptoms associated with allergies, hay fever or other upper respiratory problems. DRISTAN ALLERGY CAPLETS are indicated for relief of nasal congestion, sinus pressure, swollen nasal passages, sneezing, runny nose, and itchy/watery eyes. Each caplet is coated for easy swallowing.

DIRECTIONS
ADULTS and CHILDREN over 12 years of age: 1 caplet every 4 to 6 hours, not to exceed 4 caplets in 24 hours.

WARNINGS
Avoid alcoholic beverages and driving a motor vehicle or operating heavy machinery while taking this product. May cause drowsiness or excitability especially in children. Persons with asthma, glaucoma, high blood pressure, diabetes, heart or thyroid disease, difficulty in urination due to an enlarged prostate gland, or taking an antidepressant drug, should use only as directed by a physician. Do not exceed recommended dosage because at higher doses nervousness, dizziness, or sleeplessness may occur.
If symptoms do not improve within 7 days or are accompanied by high fever, discontinue use and see a physician.
As with an drug, if you are pregnant or nursing a baby, seek the advice of a health professional before using this product. Do not give to children under 12 years of age. Keep this and all drugs out of the reach of children. In case of accidental overdose, seek professional assistance or contact a poison control center immediately.

INACTIVE INGREDIENTS
Ammonium Hydroxide, Calcium Stearate, D&C Yellow #10 Lake, FD&C Blue #1 Lake, Hydrogenated Vegetable Oil, Hydroxypropyl Methylcellulose, Iron Oxide, Microcrystalline Cellulose, Pharmaceutical Glaze, Polyethylene Glycol, Polysorbate 80, Potassium Hydroxide, Propylene Glycol, Silica and Titanium Dioxide.

HOW SUPPLIED
Green coated caplets in blister packs of 20 and bottles of 40. Store at room temperature.
Shown in Product Identification Section, page 435

DRISTAN®   OTC
[drĭs'tăn]
12-hr Nasal Spray
12-hr Nasal Spray with metered dose pump
12-hr Menthol Nasal Spray

DESCRIPTION
Dristan 12-hr nasal spray contains Oxymetazoline HCl 0.05%.

ACTIONS
The sympathomimetic action of Dristan 12-hr nasal spray and Dristan 12-hr menthol nasal spray constricts the smaller arterioles of the nasal passages, and produces a prolonged (up to 12 hours), gentle and predictable decongesting effect.

INDICATIONS
Dristan 12-hr nasal spray and Dristan 12-hr menthol nasal spray provide prompt temporary relief of nasal congestion due to colds, sinusitis, hay fever, or other upper respiratory allergies for up to 12 hours.

WARNINGS
Do not exceed recommended dosage because symptoms may occur, such as burning, stinging, sneezing, or increase of nasal discharge. Do not use this product for more than 3 days. If symptoms persist, consult a physician. The use of the dispenser by more than one person may spread infection. Keep

	Dristan Cold & Flu Hot Drink Mix—Packet	Dristan Juice Mix-In Packet	Max. Str. Dristan Cold* Gel Caplet	Max. Str. Dristan Cold** Coated Caplet	Dristan Cold Coated Tablet	Dristan Allergy Coated Caplet	Dristan Sinus Coated Caplet
Analgesic							
Acetaminophen	500 mg	500 mg	500 mg	500 mg	325 mg	—	—
Ibuprofen	—	—	—	—	—	—	200 mg
Nasal Decongestant							
Pseudoephedrine HCl	60 mg	60 mg	30 mg	30 mg	—	60 mg	30 mg
Phenylephrine HCl	—	—	—	—	5 mg	—	—
Antihistamine							
Brompheniramine Maleate	—	—	2 mg	—	—	4 mg	—
Chlorpheniramine Maleate	4 mg	—	—	—	2 mg	—	—
Cough Suppressant							
Dextromethorphan HBr	20 mg	20 mg	—	—	—	—	—

* Multi-Symptom Formula
** No Drowsiness Formula

these and all drugs out of the reach of children. In case of accidental ingestion, seek professional assistance or contact a Poison Control Center immediately.

DOSAGE AND ADMINISTRATION
Squeeze bottle-with head upright, insert nozzle in nostril. Spray quickly, firmly and sniff deeply.
Metered Dose Pump-prime the metered dose pump by depressing pump firmly several times. With head upright, insert nozzle in nostril. Depress pump 2 or 3 times, all the way down, with a firm even stroke and sniff deeply.
Adults and children 6 years of age and over: spray 2 or 3 times into each nostril. Repeat twice daily—morning and evening. Not recommended for children under six years of age.

INACTIVE INGREDIENTS
Dristan 12-hr nasal spray—Benzalkonium Chloride 1:5000 in buffered isotonic aqueous solution, Hydroxypropyl Methylcellulose, Potassium Phosphate, Sodium Chloride, Sodium Phosphate, Thimerosal Preservative 0.002%, and Water.
Dristan 12-hr menthol nasal spray—Benzalkonium Chloride 1:5000 in buffered isotonic aqueous solution, Camphor, Eucalyptol, Hydroxypropyl Methylcellulose Menthol, Potassium Phosphate, Sodium Chloride, Sodium Phosphate, Thimerosal Preservative 0.002%, Water, and Alcohol 0.4%.

HOW SUPPLIED
Dristan 12-hr nasal spray: 15 mL and 30 mL plastic squeeze bottles, and 15 mL metered dose pump.
Dristan 12-hr menthol nasal spray: 15 mL plastic squeeze bottle.
Shown in Product Identification Section, page 435

DRISTAN® Cold   OTC
[drĭs'tăn kŏld]
Nasal Decongestant/Antihistamine/Analgesic Coated Tablets

DESCRIPTION
Each Dristan Cold Coated Tablet contains: Phenylephrine HCl 5 mg, Chlorpheniramine Maleate 2 mg, Acetaminophen 325 mg.

ACTIONS
Acetaminophen, an antipyretic and an analgesic, reduces elevated body temperature and relieves headache, minor sore throat pain, and body aches associated with a cold.
Phenylephrine HCl, an oral nasal decongestant (sympathomimetic amine), reduces nasal/sinus congestion, sinus pressure, and swollen nasal passages. Phenylephrine produces little or no central nervous system stimulation.
Chlorpheniramine maleate, an antihistamine, controls rhinorrhea, sneezing and lacrimation associated with elevated histamine levels in disorders of the respiratory tract.

INDICATIONS
Dristan Cold is indicated for effective multi-symptom relief of colds, sinusitis, flu, hay fever, or other upper respiratory allergies: nasal congestion, sneezing, runny nose, fever, headache and minor aches and pains.

WARNINGS
Avoid alcoholic beverages and driving a motor vehicle or operating heavy machinery while taking this product. May cause drowsiness or excitability, especially in children. Persons with asthma, glaucoma, high blood pressure, diabetes, heart or thyroid disease, difficulty in urination due to enlarged prostate gland, or taking an antidepressant drug, should use only as directed by a physician. Do not exceed

recommended dosage because at higher doses nervousness, dizziness, or sleeplessness may occur. If symptoms do not improve within 7 days or are accompanied by high fever, discontinue use and see a physician. As with any drug, if you are pregnant or nursing a baby, seek the advice of a health professional before using this product.
Do not give to children under 6 years of age. Keep this and all drugs out of the reach of children. In case of accidental overdose, seek professional assistance or contact a poison control center immediately.

DOSAGE AND ADMINISTRATION
Adults: Two tablets every four hours, not to exceed 12 tablets in 24 hours. Children (6–12): One tablet every four hours, not to exceed six tablets in 24 hours.

INACTIVE INGREDIENTS
Calcium Stearate, Croscarmellose Sodium, D&C Yellow #10 Lake, FD&C Yellow #6 Lake, Hydroxypropyl Methylcellulose, Microcrystalline Cellulose, Polyethylene Glycol, Povidone, Starch, Stearic Acid.

HOW SUPPLIED
Yellow/White coated tablets in tins of 12, blister packages of 20, and bottles of 40 and 75.
Shown in Product Identification Section, page 435

DRISTAN® COLD & FLU   OTC

[See table.]

DESCRIPTION
A lemon flavored hot drink mix containing Acetaminophen 500 mg, Pseudoephedrine HCl 60 mg, Chlorpheniramine Maleate 4 mg, and Dextromethorphan HBr 20 mg.

ACTIONS
Acetaminophen is both an analgesic and an antipyretic. Pseudoephedrine HCl is an oral nasal decongestant. Chlorpheniramine Maleate is an antihistamine effective in the control of symptoms caused by elevated histamine levels in disorders of the respiratory tract. Dextromethorphan HBr is a cough suppressant that provides temporary relief of cough due to colds.

INDICATIONS
DRISTAN COLD & FLU provides soothing hot liquid medication for hours of effective relief of cold and flu symptoms. DRISTAN COLD & FLU contains a **cough suppressant** to relieve irritating coughs; a **decongestant** to relieve nasal congestion, sinus pressure and reduce swollen nasal passages; an **antihistamine** to relieve sneezing, runny nose, and watery eyes; and an **analgesic** to relieve headache, body aches, minor sore throat pain and reduce fever.

DIRECTIONS
Adults and children 12 years of age: Dissolve one packet in 6 oz. cup of hot water. Sip while hot. Sweeten to taste if desired. May repeat every 4 hours, not to exceed 4 doses in 24 hours. Children under 12 years should use only as directed by a physician.

WARNINGS
Avoid alcoholic beverages and driving a motor vehicle or operating heavy machinery while taking this product. May cause drowsiness or excitability especially in children. Do not take this product for persistent cough such as occurs with smoking, asthma or emphysema, or if cough is accompanied by excessive secretions (mucus), unless directed by a physician. A persistent cough may be a sign of a serious condition. If cough persists for more than 1 week, recurs, or if accompanied by fever, rash or persistent headache, consult

a physician. Persons with asthma, glaucoma, high blood pressure, diabetes, heart or thyroid disease, difficulty in urination due to an enlarged prostate gland, or taking an antidepressant drug, should use only as directed by a physician. Do not exceed recommended dosage because at higher doses nervousness, dizziness, or sleeplessness may occur. If symptoms do not improve within 7 days or are accompanied by high fever, discontinue use and see a physician. As with any drug, if you are pregnant or nursing a baby, seek the advice of a health professional before using this product. Do not give to children under 12 years of age. Keep this and all drugs out of the reach of children. In case of accidental overdose, seek professional assistance or contact a poison control center immediately.

INACTIVE INGREDIENTS
Ascorbic Acid, Citric Acid, Corn Syrup, D&C Yellow #10 Lake, FD&C Yellow #6 Lake, Flavor, Sodium Citrate, Starch, Sucrose, Titanium Dioxide, Tricalcium Phosphate.

HOW SUPPLIED
Dristan Cold and Flu is supplied as boxes of 6 or 12 individual use packets.
Store at room temperature.
Shown in Product Identification Section, page 435

DRISTAN® JUICE MIX-IN™   OTC
Nasal Decongestant/Analgesic/Cough Suppressant

[See table on preceding page.]
DESCRIPTION
Each packet contains: Acetaminophen 500mg, Pseudoephedrine HCl 60 mg, and Dextromethorphan HBr 20 mg.

INDICATIONS
DRISTAN® JUICE MIX-IN™ contains a **cough suppressant** to temporarily relieve irritating coughs; a **decongestant** to temporarily relieve nasal congestion and sinus pressure and reduce swollen nasal passages; and an **analgesic** to temporarily relieve headache, body aches, minor sore throat pain and reduce fever.

ACTIONS
Acetaminophen is an analgesic and antipyretic. Pseudoephedrine HCl is an oral nasal decongestant. Dextromethorphan HBr is a cough suppressant.

WARNINGS
Do not take this product for persistent cough such as occurs with smoking, asthma or emphysema, or if cough is accompanied by excessive secretions (mucus), unless directed by a physician. A persistent cough may be a sign of a serious condition. If cough persists for more than 1 week, recurs, or is accompanied by fever, rash or persistent headache, consult a physician. Persons with asthma, glaucoma, diabetes, heart or thyroid disease or difficulty in urination due to enlarged prostate gland, should use only as directed by a physician. *Drug Interaction Precaution:* Do not take this product if you are presently taking a prescription drug for high blood pressure or depression, or a monoamine oxidase inhibitor, unless directed by a doctor. Do not exceed recommended dosage because at higher doses nervousness, dizziness, or sleeplessness may occur. If symptoms do not improve within 7 days or are accompanied by high fever, discontinue use and see a physician. If sore throat is severe, persists for more than 2 days, is accompanied or followed by fever, headache, rash, nausea or vomiting, consult a doctor promptly. As with any drug, if you are pregnant or nursing a baby, seek the advice of a health professional before using this product. Do not give to children under 12. Keep this and all drugs out of the reach of children. In case of accidental overdose, seek professional assistance or contact a poison control center immediately. Prompt medical attention is critical for adults as well as for children even if you do not notice any signs or symptoms.
Do not mix with any juice to which you have had an allergic reaction in the past.

DIRECTIONS
Adults and Children 12 years of age and over: Mix one packet in 6 oz. of your favorite juice. Stir briskly for at least 15 seconds. Drink promptly. May repeat every 4 hours, not to exceed 4 doses in 24 hours. Do not give to children under 12.

INACTIVE INGREDIENTS
Hydroxypropyl Methylcellulose, Povidone, Silica, Starch, Stearic Acid, Sucrose, Tricalcium Phosphate.

HOW SUPPLIED
In packages containing 1 (trial size), 5 or 10 individual use packets.
Patent Pending
Shown in Product Identification Section, page 435.

Maximum Strength DRISTAN® COLD   OTC
MULTI-SYMPTOM FORMULA
Nasal Decongestant/Antihistamine/Analgesic
Gel Caplets

[See table on preceding page.]
DESCRIPTION
Each gel caplet contains: Acetaminophen 500mg, Pseudoephedrine HCl 30mg, and Brompheniramine Maleate 2mg.

INDICATIONS
MAXIMUM STRENGTH DRISTAN® COLD GEL CAPLETS contain a **decongestant** to temporarily relieve nasal congestion, sinus pressure and reduce swollen nasal passages; an **antihistamine** to temporarily relieve sneezing, runny nose, and watery eyes; and an **analgesic** to temporarily relieve headache, body aches, minor sore throat pain, and reduce fever.

ACTIONS
Acetaminophen is an analgesic and antipyretic. Pseudoephedrine HCl is an oral nasal decongestant. Brompheniramine Maleate is an antihistamine.

WARNINGS
Avoid alcoholic beverages and driving a motor vehicle or operating heavy machinery while taking this product. Do not take this product if you are taking sedatives or tranquilizers, without first consulting your doctor. May cause drowsiness or excitability especially in children. Persons with asthma, glaucoma, diabetes, heart or thyroid disease, or difficulty in urination due to an enlarged prostate gland, should use only as directed by a physican. *Drug Interaction Precaution:* Do not take this product if you are presently taking a prescription drug for high blood pressure or depression unless directed by a doctor. Do not exceed recommended dosage because at higher doses nervousness, dizziness, or sleeplessness may occur. If symptoms do not improve within 7 days or are accompanied by high fever, discontinue use and see a physician. If sore throat is severe, persists for more than 2 days, is accompanied by fever, headache, rash, nausea or vomiting, consult a doctor promptly. As with any drug, if you are pregnant or nursing a baby, seek the advice of a health professional before using this product. Do not give to children under 12. Keep this and all drugs out of the reach of children. In case of accidental overdose, seek professional assistance or contact a poison control center immediately. Prompt medical attention is critical for adults as well as for children even if you do not notice any signs or symptoms.

DIRECTIONS
Adults and children 12 years of age and over: 2 gel caplets every 6 hours, not to exceed 8 gel caplets in any 24 hour period. Do not give to children under 12 years of age.

INACTIVE INGREDIENTS
Calcium Stearate, Croscarmellose Sodium, D&C Red #30 Lake, EDTA, FD&C Blue #1 Lake, FD&C Red #40 Lake, Gelatin, Glycerin, Hydrogenated Vegetable Oil, Hydroxypropyl Methylcellulose, Iron Oxide, Lecithin, Microcrystalline Cellulose, Pharmaceutical Glaze, Polyethylene Glycol, Povidone, Simethicone, Starch, Stearic Acid, Titanium Dioxide, Triacetin.

HOW SUPPLIED
In packages of 4s (trial size), 16s and 36s.
Shown in Product Identification Section, page 435.

DRISTAN® SALINE SPRAY   OTC
Non-Medicated Nasal Moisturizer

DESCRIPTION
Dristan Saline Spray is a non-medicated moisturizer for dry, irritated nasal membranes. It is safe to use with oral cold, allergy and sinus medications.

INDICATIONS
For prompt, soothing relief of dry, irritated nasal membranes due to colds, allergies, low humidity, or other nasal irritations.

WARNINGS
Keep this and all drugs out of the reach of children. The use of this dispenser by more than one person may spread infection.

DIRECTIONS
Use as often as needed. **For Adults:** With head upright, insert nozzle in nostril and spray quickly and firmly. Spray 2 or 3 times as often as needed or as directed by a physician. **For Infants and Children:** With head back, turn bottle upside down and squeeze 2 to 3 drops in each nostril as often as needed or as directed by a physician. Wipe nozzle clean after use.

INGREDIENTS
Water, Sodium Chloride, Benzyl Alcohol, Hydroxypropyl Methylcellulose, Sodium Phosphate, Disodium Phosphate, Benzalkonium Chloride, Disodium EDTA.

HOW SUPPLIED
In ½ Fl. oz. (15 mL) plastic squeeze bottles.
Shown in Product Identification Section, page 435

DRISTAN®SINUS Caplets   OTC
Ibuprofen/Pseudoephedrine Caplets*
Pain Reliever/Nasal Decongestant
*Oval-shaped tablets

WARNING: ASPIRIN-SENSITIVE PATIENTS. Do not take this product if you have had a severe allergic reaction to aspirin, eg—asthma, swelling, shock or hives, because even though this product contains no aspirin or salicylates, cross-reactions may occur in patients allergic to aspirin. Use other Dristan formulas.

INDICATIONS
For temporary relief of symptoms associated with the common cold, sinusitis or flu including nasal congestion, headache, fever, body aches, and pains.

DIRECTIONS
Adults: Take 1 caplet every 4 to 6 hours while symptoms persist. If symptoms do not respond to 1 caplet, 2 caplets may be used, but do not exceed 6 caplets in 24 hours unless directed by a doctor. The smallest effective dose should be used. Take with food or milk if occasional and mild heartburn, upset stomach, or stomach pain occurs with use. Consult a doctor if these symptoms are more than mild or if they persist. *Children:* Do not give this product to children under 12 years of age except under the advice and supervision of a doctor.

WARNINGS
Do not take for colds for more than 7 days or for fever for more than 3 days unless directed by a doctor. If the cold or fever persists or gets worse, or if new symptoms occur, consult a doctor. These could be signs of serious illness. As with aspirin and acetaminophen, if you have any condition which requires you to take prescription drugs or if you have had any problems or serious side effects from taking any nonprescription pain reliever, do not take this product without first discussing it with your doctor.
IF YOU EXPERIENCE ANY SYMPTOMS WHICH ARE UNUSUAL OR SEEM UNRELATED TO THE CONDITION FOR WHICH YOU TOOK THIS PRODUCT, CONSULT A DOCTOR BEFORE TAKING ANY MORE OF IT. If you are under a doctor's care for any serious condition, consult a doctor before taking this product.
Do not exceed recommended dosage because at higher doses nervousness, dizziness or sleeplessness may occur. Do not take this product if you have high blood pressure, heart disease, diabetes, thyroid disease or difficulty in urination due to enlargement of the prostate gland, except under the advice and supervision of a doctor.

DRUG INTERACTION PRECAUTION
Do not take this product if you are presently taking a prescription drug for high blood pressure or depression without first consulting your doctor. Do not combine this product with other nonprescription pain relievers. Do not combine this product with any other ibuprofen-containing product. As with any drug, if you are pregnant or nursing a baby, seek the advice of a health professional before using this product. IT IS ESPECIALLY IMPORTANT NOT TO USE THIS PRODUCT DURING THE LAST 3 MONTHS OF PREGNANCY UNLESS SPECIFICALLY DIRECTED TO DO SO BY A DOCTOR BECAUSE IT MAY CAUSE PROBLEMS IN THE UNBORN CHILD OR COMPLICATIONS DURING DELIVERY. Keep this and all drugs out of the reach of children. In case of accidental overdose, seek professional assistance or contact a poison control center immediately. Store at room temperature; avoid excessive heat (40°C, 104°F).

ACTIVE INGREDIENTS
Each caplet contains Ibuprofen 200 mg and Pseudoephedrine HCl 30 mg.

INACTIVE INGREDIENTS
Carnauba or Equivalent Wax, Croscarmellose Sodium, Iron Oxide, Methylparaben, Microcrystalline Cellulose, Propylparaben, Silicon Dioxide, Sodium Benzoate, Sodium Lauryl Sulfate, Starch, Stearic Acid, Sucrose, Titanium Dioxide.

HOW SUPPLIED
Dristan Sinus is an oval-shaped white-colored caplet supplied in consumer blister packs of 20 and bottles of 40.
Shown on Product Identification Section, page 436

Continued on next page

Whitehall Laboratories—Cont.

Maximum Strength DRISTAN® COLD   OTC
NO DROWSINESS FORMULA
Nasal Decongestant/Analgesic Coated Caplets

[See table on page 2532.]

DESCRIPTION
Each Maximum Strength Dristan Cold Coated Caplet contains: Acetaminophen 500 mg and Pseudoephedrine HCl 30 mg.

ACTIONS
Acetaminophen is both an analgesic and an antipyretic. This maximum strength non-aspirin pain reliever effectively reduces elevated body temperature, headache pain and body aches associated with a cold. Pseudoephedrine HCl is an oral nasal decongestant and is effective in reducing nasal/sinus congestion, sinus pressure, and swollen nasal passages.

INDICATIONS
Maximum Strength Dristan Cold is indicated for effective relief without drowsiness from nasal congestion, headache, fever and minor aches and pains associated with colds, sinusitis, flu and upper respiratory allergies.

WARNINGS
Persons with asthma, glaucoma, high blood pressure, heart disease, diabetes, thyroid disease, difficulty in urination due to an enlarged prostate gland, or taking an antidepressant drug should use only as directed by a physician. Do not exceed recommended dosage because at higher doses nervousness, dizziness, or sleeplessness may occur. If symptoms do not improve within 7 days, or are accompanied by high fever, discontinue use and see a physician. Do not give to children under 12. As with any drug, if you are pregnant or nursing a baby, seek the advice of a health professional before using this product. Keep this and all drugs out of the reach of children. In case of accidental overdose, seek professional assistance or contact a poison control center immediately.

DOSAGE AND ADMINISTRATION
Adults and children over 12: Two caplets every 6 hours, not to exceed 8 caplets in any 24-hour period. Children under 12 should use only as directed by a physician.

INACTIVE INGREDIENTS
Calcium Stearate, Croscarmellose Sodium, D&C Red #7 Lake, D&C Yellow #10 Lake, FD&C Yellow #6 Lake, Hydrogenated Vegetable Oil, Hydroxypropyl Methylcellulose, Microcrystalline Cellulose, Pharmaceutical Glaze, Polyethylene Glycol, Povidone, Starch, Stearic Acid, Titanium Dioxide.

HOW SUPPLIED
Yellow coated caplets in blister packages of 20 and bottles of 40.

Shown in Product Identification Section, page 435

POSTURE®   OTC
[pos'tūr]
600 mg
High Potency Calcium Supplement
Micro-thin Coated for Easy Swallowing, No Gas Distress
No Calories • No Sugar • No Starch • No Preservatives

DESCRIPTION
Each film-coated tablet of POSTURE® contains Tribasic Calcium Phosphate 1565.2 mg which provides 600 mg of elemental calcium. POSTURE® is specially formulated not to produce gas.

	For Adults—	
Two tablets contain:		% U.S. RDA*
Elemental Calcium	1200 mg	120%
(as calcium phosphate)		

*Percentage of U.S. Recommended Daily Allowance

INDICATION
POSTURE® Tablets provide a daily source of calcium to help maintain healthy bones or to supplement dietary calcium intake when directed by a physician. Keep out of children.

DIRECTIONS FOR USE
One or two tablets daily, or as recommended by a physician.

INACTIVE INGREDIENTS
Croscarmellose Sodium, Ethylcellulose, Magnesium Stearate, Microcrystalline Cellulose, Polyethylene Glycol, Povidone, Sodium Lauryl Sulfate.

HOW SUPPLIED
In bottles of 60 scored tablets. Store at room temperature.

POSTURE®–D   OTC
[pos'tūr d]
600 mg
High Potency Calcium Supplement with Vitamin D
Micro-thin Coated for Easy Swallowing
No Calories • No Sugar • No Starch • No Preservatives

DESCRIPTION
Each film-coated tablet of POSTURE®–D contains Tribasic Calcium Phosphate 1565.2 mg which provides 600 mg of elemental calcium and 125 IU of Vitamin D. POSTURE®–D is specially formulated not to produce gas.

	For Adults—	
Two tablets contain:		% U.S. RDA*
Elemental Calcium	1200 mg	120%
(as calcium phosphate)		
Vitamin D	250 IU	63%

*Percentage of U.S. Recommended Daily Allowance.

INDICATION
POSTURE®-D Tablets provide a daily source of calcium and Vitamin D to help maintain healthy bones or to supplement dietary calcium and Vitamin D intake when directed by a physician.

DIRECTIONS FOR USE
One or two tablets daily, or as recommended by a physician. Keep out of reach of children.

INACTIVE INGREDIENTS
Croscarmellose Sodium, Ethylcellulose, Magnesium Stearate, Microcrystalline Cellulose, Polyethylene Glycol, Povidone, Sodium Lauryl Sulfate.

HOW SUPPLIED
In bottles of 60 scored tablets. Store at room temperature.

PREPARATION H®   OTC
[prep-e'rā-shen āch]
Hemorrhoidal Ointment and Cream
PREPARATION H®   OTC
Hemorrhoidal Suppositories

DESCRIPTION
Preparation H is available in ointment, cream, and suppository product forms.
The <u>Ointment</u> contains Live Yeast Cell Derivative supplying 2,000 units Skin Respiratory Factor per ounce of Ointment and Shark Liver Oil 3.0% in a specially prepared Rectal Petrolatum Base.
The <u>Cream</u> contains Live Yeast Cell Derivative supplying 2000 units Skin Respiratory Factor per ounce of cream and shark liver oil 3.0% in a specially prepared Rectal Cream Base containing Petrolatum.
The <u>Suppositories</u> contain Live Yeast Cell Derivative supplying 2,000 units Skin Respiratory Factor per ounce of Cocoa Butter Suppository Base and Shark Liver Oil 3.0%.

INDICATIONS
Preparation H helps shrink swelling of hemorrhoidal tissues caused by inflammation and gives prompt, temporary relief in many cases from pain and itching in tissues.

PRECAUTIONS
In case of bleeding, or if your condition persists, see your physician. Keep this and all drugs out of reach of children. In case of accidental ingestion, seek professional assistance or contact a poison control center immediately.

DOSAGE AND ADMINISTRATION
<u>Ointment/Cream:</u> Before applying, remove protective cover from applicator. Lubricate applicator before each application and thoroughly cleanse after use. It is recommended that Preparation H Hemorrhoidal ointment/cream be applied freely to the affected rectal area whenever symptoms occur, from three to five times per day, especially at night, in the morning and after each bowel movement. Frequent application with Preparation H ointment/cream provides continual therapy which leads to more rapid improvement of rectal conditions. <u>Suppositories:</u> Whenever symptoms occur, remove wrapper, insert one suppository rectally from three to five times per day, especially at night, in the morning and after each bowel movement. Frequent application with Preparation H suppositories provides continual therapy which leads to more rapid improvement of rectal conditions.
Inactive Ingredients: <u>Ointment</u>—Beeswax, Glycerin, Lanolin, Lanolin Alcohol, Mineral Oil, Paraffin, Phenylmercuric Nitrate (1:10,000 as a preservative), Thyme Oil.
<u>Cream</u>—BHA, Cellulose Gum, Cetyl Alcohol, Citric Acid, Disodium EDTA, Glycerin, Glyceryl Stearate, Lanolin, Methylparaben, Phenylmercuric Nitrate, 1:10,000 (as a preservative), Propyl Gallate, Propylene Glycol, Propylparaben, Simethicone, Sodium Lauryl Sulfate, Stearyl Alcohol, Wa-

ter, Xanthan Gum. May also contain Glyceryl Oleate and/or Polysorbate 80.
<u>Suppositories</u>—Beeswax, Glycerin, Phenylmercuric Nitrate 1:10,000 (as a preservative), Polyethylene Glycol 600 Dilaurate.

HOW SUPPLIED
Ointment: Net Wt. 1 oz. and 2 oz.
Cream: Net Wt. 0.9 oz. and 1.8 oz.
Suppositories: 12's, 24's, 36's, and 48's.
Store at controlled room temperature in cool place but not over 80°F.

Shown in Product Identification Section, page 436

PREPARATION H® HYDROCORTISONE 1%   OTC
[prep-e'ra-shen-ach]
Anti-Itch Cream

DESCRIPTION
Preparation H® Hydrocortisone 1% is an antipruritic external analgesic cream containing 1% Hydrocortisone.

INDICATIONS
For the temporary relief of external anal itch and itching associated with minor skin irritations and rashes. Other uses of this product should be only under the advice and supervision of a doctor.

WARNINGS
For external use only. Avoid contact with the eyes. If condition worsens, or if symptoms persist for more than 7 days or clear up and occur again within a few days, stop use of this product and do not begin use of any other hydrocortisone product unless you have consulted a doctor. Do not exceed the recommended daily dosage unless directed by a doctor. In case of bleeding, consult a doctor promptly. Do not put this product into the rectum by using fingers or any mechanical device or applicator. Do not use for the treatment of diaper rash. Keep this and all drugs out of the reach of children. In case of accidental ingestion, seek professional assistance or contact a Poison Control Center immediately.

DIRECTIONS
Adults: When practical, cleanse the affected area by patting or blotting with an appropiate cleansing tissue, such as Preparation H Cleansing Tissues. Gently dry by patting or blotting with toilet tissue or soft cloth before application of this product. Apply to affected area not more than 3 to 4 times daily.
Children under 12: consult a doctor.

INACTIVE INGREDIENTS
BHA, Cellulose Gum, Cetyl Alcohol, Citric Acid, Disodium EDTA, Glycerin, Glyceryl Oleate, Glyceryl Stearate, Lanolin, Methylparaben, Petrolatum, Propyl Gallate, Propylene Glycol, Propylparaben, Simethicone, Sodium Benzoate, Sodium Lauryl Sulfate, Stearyl Alcohol, Water, Xanthan Gum.

HOW SUPPLIED
Available in Net Wt. 0.9 oz. tube. Store at room temperature or in cool place not over 80°F.

Shown in Product Identification Section, page 436

PRIMATENE®   OTC
[prīm'a-tēn]
Mist
(Epinephrine Inhalation Aerosol)
Bronchodilator

DESCRIPTION
Primatene Mist contains Epinephrine 5.5 mg/mL.

ACTION
Epinephrine is a sympathomimetic agent which relaxes bronchial smooth muscle during an acute asthmatic attack.

INDICATIONS
Primatene Mist is indicated for temporary relief of shortness of breath, tightness of chest, and wheezing due to bronchial asthma. Eases breathing for asthma patients by reducing spasms of bronchial muscles.

DOSAGE AND ADMINISTRATION
Inhalation dosage for adults and children 4 years of age and older: Start with one inhalation, then wait at least 1 minute. If not relieved, use once more. Do not use again for at least 3 hours. The use of this product by children should be supervised by an adult. Children under 4 years of age: Consult a physician. Each inhalation delivers 0.22 mg of epinephrine.

WARNINGS
Do not use this product unless a diagnosis of asthma has been made by a physician. Do not use this product if you have heart disease, high blood pressure, thyroid disease, diabetes, or difficulty in urination due to enlargement of the prostate gland unless directed by a physician. As with any drug, if you

are pregnant or nursing a baby, seek the advice of a health professional before using this product. Do not use this product if you have ever been hospitalized for asthma or if you are taking any prescription drug for asthma unless directed by a physician.

Keep this and all drugs out of the reach of children. In case of accidental overdose, seek professional assistance or contact a poison control center immediately.

DO NOT CONTINUE TO USE THIS PRODUCT, BUT SEEK MEDICAL ASSISTANCE IMMEDIATELY IF SYMPTOMS ARE NOT RELIEVED WITHIN 20 MINUTES OR BECOME WORSE. DO NOT USE THIS PRODUCT MORE FREQUENTLY OR AT HIGHER DOSES THAN RECOMMENDED UNLESS DIRECTED BY A PHYSICIAN. EXCESSIVE USE MAY CAUSE NERVOUSNESS AND RAPID HEART BEAT AND POSSIBLY, ADVERSE EFFECTS ON THE HEART.

DRUG INTERACTION PRECAUTION: Do not use this product if you are presently taking a prescription drug for high blood pressure or depression, without first consulting your physician.

PRECAUTIONS

Contents under pressure. Do not puncture or throw container into incinerator. Using or storing near open flame or heating above 120° F (49° C) may cause bursting. Store at room temperature 59° F–86° F (15°C–30°C).

DIRECTIONS FOR USE OF THE MOUTHPIECE

The Primatene Mist mouthpiece, which is enclosed in the Primatene Mist 15mL size (not the refill size), should be used for inhalation only with Primatene Mist.

1. Take plastic cap off mouthpiece. (For refills, use mouthpiece from previous purchase.)
2. Take plastic mouthpiece off bottle.
3. Place other end of mouthpiece on bottle.
4. Turn bottle upside down. Place thumb on bottom of mouthpiece over circular button and forefinger on top of vial. Empty the lungs as completely as possible by exhaling.
5. Place mouthpiece in mouth with lips closed around opening. Inhale deeply while squeezing mouthpiece and bottle together. Release immediately and remove unit from mouth, then complete taking the deep breath, drawing medication into your lungs, holding breath as long as comfortable.
6. Then exhale slowly keeping the lips nearly closed. This distributes the medication in the lungs.
7. Replace plastic cap on mouthpiece.
8. The Primatene Mist mouthpiece should be washed once daily with soap and hot water, and rinsed thoroughly. Then it should be dried with a clean, lint-free cloth.

INACTIVE INGREDIENTS

Alcohol 34%, Ascorbic Acid, Fluorocarbons (Propellant), Water. Contains no Sulfites.

HOW SUPPLIED

½ Fl. oz. (15 mL) With Mouthpiece.
½ Fl. oz. (15 mL) Refill
¾ Fl. oz. (22.5 mL) Refill
Shown in Product Identification Section, page 436

PRIMATENE®　　OTC
[prīm 'a-tēn]
Mist Suspension
(Epinephrine Bitartrate Inhalation Aerosol Bronchodilator)

DESCRIPTION

Primatene Mist Suspension contains Epinephrine Bitartrate 7.0 mg/mL.

ACTION

Epinephrine is a sympathomimetic agent which relaxes bronchial smooth muscle and thereby eases breathing during an acute asthmatic attack.

INDICATIONS

Primatene Mist Suspension is indicated for temporary relief of shortness of breath, tightness of chest, and wheezing due to bronchial asthma. Eases breathing for asthma patients by reducing spasms of bronchial muscles.

DOSAGE AND ADMINISTRATION

Shake before using.
Inhalation dosage for adults and children 4 years of age and older: Start with one inhalation, then wait at least 1 minute. If not relieved, use once more. Do not use again for at least 3 hours. The use of this product by children should be supervised by an adult. Children under 4 years of age: Consult a physician. Each inhalation delivers 0.3 mg Epinephrine Bitartrate equivalent to 0.16 mg Epinephrine Base.

WARNINGS

Do not use this product unless a diagnosis of asthma has been made by a physician. Do not use this product if you have

heart disease, high blood pressure, thyroid disease, diabetes, or difficulty in urination due to enlargement of the prostate gland unless directed by a physician. As with any drug, if you are pregnant or nursing a baby, seek the advice of a health professional before using this product. Do not use this product if you have ever been hospitalized for asthma or if you are taking any prescription drug for asthma unless directed by a physician.

Keep this and all drugs out of the reach of children. In case of accidental overdose, seek professional assistance or contact a poison control center immediately.

DO NOT CONTINUE TO USE THIS PRODUCT, BUT SEEK MEDICAL ASSISTANCE IMMEDIATELY IF SYMPTOMS ARE NOT RELIEVED WITHIN 20 MINUTES OR BECOME WORSE. DO NOT USE THIS PRODUCT MORE FREQUENTLY OR AT HIGHER DOSES THAN RECOMMENDED UNLESS DIRECTED BY A PHYSICIAN. EXCESSIVE USE MAY CAUSE NERVOUSNESS AND RAPID HEART BEAT AND POSSIBLY, ADVERSE EFFECTS ON THE HEART.

DRUG INTERACTION PRECAUTION: Do not use this product if you are presently taking a prescription drug for high blood pressure or depression, without first consulting your physician.

PRECAUTIONS

Contents under pressure. Do not puncture or throw container into incinerator. Using or storing near open flame or heating above 120° F (49° C) may cause bursting. Store at room temperature 59° F–86° F (15° C–30° C).

DIRECTIONS FOR USE OF THE INHALER

1. SHAKE WELL BEFORE USING.
2. HOLD INHALER WITH NOZZLE DOWN WHILE USING. Empty the lungs as completely as possible by exhaling.
3. Purse the lips, as in saying "O" and hold the nozzle up to the lips keeping the tongue flat. As you start to take a deep breath, squeeze nozzle and can together, releasing one full application. Complete taking a deep breath, drawing medication into your lungs.
4. Hold breath for as long as comfortable. Then exhale slowly keeping the lips nearly closed. This distributes the medication in the lungs.
5. The Primatene Mist Suspension nozzle should be washed once daily. After removing the nozzle from the vial, wash it with soap and hot water, and rinse thoroughly. Then it should be dried with a clean, lint-free cloth.

INACTIVE INGREDIENTS

Fluorocarbons (Propellant), Sorbitan Trioleate. Contains No Sulfites.

HOW SUPPLIED

⅓ Fl. oz. (10 mL) pocket-size aerosol inhaler.

PRIMATENE®　　OTC
[prīm 'a-tēn]
Tablets

DESCRIPTION

Depending upon the state (see HOW SUPPLIED), Primatene Tablets are available in 3 formulations:
(regular formula): Theophylline Anhydrous 130 mg, Ephedrine Hydrochloride 24 mg.
P Formula: Theophylline Hydrous 130 mg, Ephedrine Hydrochloride 24 mg, Phenobarbital 8 mg (⅛ gr.) per tablet. (Warning: May be habit forming.)
M Formula: Theophylline Hydrous 130 mg, Ephedrine Hydrochloride 24 mg, Pyrilamine Maleate 16.6 mg per tablet.

INDICATIONS

Primatene Tablets are indicated for relief and control of attacks of bronchial asthma.

ACTIONS

Primatene Tablets contain two bronchodilators, theophylline, a methylxanthine, and ephedrine, a sympathomimetic amine. The pharmacologic action of theophylline may be mediated through inhibition of phosphodiesterase with a resulting increase in intracellular cyclic AMP. The β-adrenergic ephedrine acts by a different mechanism to produce cyclic AMP. The combination of a xanthine and a sympathomimetic appears to produce more smooth muscle relaxation than when either drug is used alone. Phenobarbital (present in the P formula) counteracts the possible stimulation produced by ephedrine and acts as a mild sedative. Pyrilamine maleate (present in the M Formula) is an antihistamine with mild sedating action.

WARNINGS

If symptoms persist, consult your physician. Some people are sensitive to ephedrine and, in such cases, temporary sleeplessness and nervousness may occur. These reactions will disappear if the use of the medication is discontinued. Do not exceed recommended dosage.

People who have heart disease, high blood pressure, diabetes, thyroid trouble, or difficulty in urination due to enlarged prostate gland, should take this preparation only on the advice of a physician. Both "M" and "P" formula may cause drowsiness. People taking the "M" or "P" formula should not drive or operate machinery.

As with any drug, if you are pregnant or nursing a baby, seek the advice of a health professional before using this product. Keep this and all medicines out of reach of children. In case of accidental overdose, seek professional assistance or contact a poison control center immediately.

DOSAGE AND ADMINISTRATION

Adults: 1 or 2 tablets initially and then one every 4 hours, as needed, not to exceed 6 tablets in 24 hours. Children (6–12): One half adult dose. For children under 6, consult a physician.

INACTIVE INGREDIENTS

(Regular Formula): Croscarmellose Sodium, D&C Yellow No. 10 Lake, FD&C Yellow No. 6 Lake, Magnesium Stearate, Microcrystalline Cellulose, Silica, Starch, Stearic Acid.
P Formula (Phenobarbital): Colloidal Silicon Dioxide, D&C Yellow No. 10, FD&C Yellow No. 6, Magnesium Stearate, Sodium Starch Glycolate, Starch, Surfactant.
M Formula (Pyrilamine Maleate): D&C Yellow No. 10 Lake, FD&C Yellow No. 6 Lake, Hydrogenated Vegetable Oil, Magnesium Stearate, Microcrystalline Cellulose, Sodium Starch Glycolate, Surfactant, Talc.
Contains No Sulfites.

HOW SUPPLIED

Available in three forms (regular) Primatene Tablets, "M" Formula, and "P" Formula. In those states where Phenobarbital is Rx only, "M" Formula, containing pyrilamine maleate, is available.
"P" Formula, containing phenobarbital, is available in other states.
Both "M" and "P" formulas are supplied in glass bottles of 24 and 60 tablets. (Regular) Primatene Tablets are supplied in 24 and 60 tablet thermoform blister cartons.
Shown in Product Identification Section, page 436

RIOPAN®　　OTC
[rī 'o pan]
magaldrate
Antacid

DESCRIPTION

RIOPAN is a buffer antacid containing the unique chemical entity Magaldrate. Each teaspoonful (5 mL) of suspension contains Magaldrate, 540 mg. RIOPAN is considered dietetically sodium-free [containing not more than 0.013 mEq. (0.3 mg.) sodium per teaspoonful.]

ACTIONS

The active ingredient in RIOPAN, Magaldrate demonstrates a rapid and uniform buffering action. The acid-neutralizing capacity of RIOPAN is 15.0 mEq per 5mL. RIOPAN does not produce acid rebound or alkalinization.

INDICATIONS

RIOPAN is indicated for the relief of heartburn, sour stomach and acid indigestion. For symptomatic relief of hyperacidity associated with the diagnosis of peptic ulcer, gastritis, peptic esophagitis, gastric hyperacidity, hiatal hernia and postoperative gas pain.

DOSAGE AND ADMINISTRATION

Take one or two teaspoonfuls, between meals and at bedtime, or as directed by the physician.

WARNINGS

Patients should not take more than 18 teaspoonfuls in a 24-hour period or use the maximum dosage for more than two weeks, or use if they have kidney disease, except under the advice and supervision of a physician. Keep this and all drugs out of the reach of children.

DRUG INTERACTION PRECAUTION

Do not use in patients presently taking a prescription antibiotic drug containing any form of tetracycline.

INACTIVE INGREDIENTS

Flavor, Glycerin, Potassium Citrate, Saccharin, Sorbitol, Xanthan Gum, Water.

HOW SUPPLIED

In 12 fl oz (355 mL) plastic bottles. Individual Cups, 1 fl oz (30 mL) ea., tray of 10—10 trays per packer. Store at room temperature (approximately 25°C or 77°F). Avoid freezing.
Shown in Product Identification Section, page 436

Continued on next page

Whitehall Laboratories—Cont.

RIOPAN PLUS®   OTC
[rī'opan]
magaldrate and simethicone
Antacid Plus Anti-Gas

DESCRIPTION
Riopan Plus is a buffer antacid plus anti-gas combination product containing the unique chemical entity Magaldrate. Each teaspoonful (5mL) of suspension contains Magaldrate, 540 mg and Simethicone, 40 mg. Riopan Plus is considered dietetically sodium-free [containing not more than 0.013 mEq. (0.3 mg.) sodium per teaspoonful.]

ACTIONS
The active antacid ingredient in Riopan Plus, Magaldrate, provides a rapid and uniform buffering action. The acid-neutralizing capacity of Riopan Plus is 15.0 mEq per 5mL. Riopan Plus does not produce acid rebound or alkalinization. Simethicone reduces the surface tension of gas bubbles so that the gas is more easily eliminated.

INDICATIONS
RIOPAN Plus is indicated for the relief of heartburn, sour stomach and acid indigestion accompanied by the symptoms of gas. For symptomatic relief of hyperacidity associated with the diagnosis of peptic ulcer, gastritis, peptic esophagitis, gastric hyperacidity, hiatal hernia, and postoperative gas pain.

DOSAGE AND ADMINISTRATION
Take one or two teaspoonfuls between meals and at bedtime, or as directed by the physician.

WARNINGS
Patients should not take more than 12 teaspoonfuls, in a 24-hour period or use the maximum dosage for more than two weeks, or use if they have kidney disease, except under the advice and supervision of a physician. Keep this and all drugs out of the reach of children.

DRUG INTERACTION PRECAUTION
Do not use in patients presently taking a prescription antibiotic drug containing any form of tetracycline.

INACTIVE INGREDIENTS
Flavor, Glycerin, PEG-8 Stearate, Potassium Citrate, Saccharin, Sorbitan Stearate, Sorbitol, Xanthan Gum, Water.

HOW SUPPLIED
In 12 fl oz (355 mL) plastic bottles. Individual Cups, 1 fl oz (30 mL) ea., tray of 10—10 trays per packer.
Store at room temperature (approximately 25℃ or 77°F). Avoid freezing.
Shown in Product Identification Section, page 436

RIOPAN PLUS® 2   OTC
[rī'opan plus 2]
magaldrate and simethicone Double Strength Antacid plus Anti-Gas
Mint and Cherry Flavors

DESCRIPTION
Riopan Plus 2 is a double strength buffer antacid plus anti-gas combination product containing the unique chemical entity Magaldrate. Each teaspoonful (5 mL) of suspension contains Magaldrate, 1080 mg and Simethicone, 40 mg. Riopan Plus 2 is considered dietetically sodium-free [containing not more than 0.013 mEq, (0.3) mg sodium per teaspoonful.]

ACTIONS
Magaldrate, the active antacid ingredient in Riopan Plus 2, provides a rapid and uniform buffering action. The acid-neutralizing capacity of Double Strength Riopan Plus 2 is 30 mEq per 5mL. Riopan Plus 2 does not produce acid rebound or alkalinization. Simethicone reduces the surface tension of gas bubbles so that the gas is more easily eliminated.

INDICATIONS
RIOPAN PLUS 2 is indicated for the relief of heartburn, sour stomach and acid indigestion accompanied by the symptoms of gas. For symptomatic relief of hyperacidity associated with the diagnosis of peptic ulcer, gastritis, peptic esophagitis, gastric hyperacidity, hiatal hernia, and postoperative gas pain.

DOSAGE AND ADMINISTRATION
Take one or two teaspoonfuls between meals and at bedtime, or as directed by the physician.

WARNINGS
Patients should not take more than 12 teaspoonfuls in a 24-hour period, or use the maximum dosage for more than two weeks, or use if they have kidney disease, except under the advice and supervision of a physician. Keep this and all drugs out of the reach of children.

DRUG INTERACTION PRECAUTION
Do not use in patients presently taking a prescription antibiotic drug containing any form of tetracycline.

INACTIVE INGREDIENTS
Flavor, Glycerin, PEG-8 Stearate, Potassium Citrate, Saccharin, Sorbitan Stearate, Sorbitol, Xanthan Gum, Water.

HOW SUPPLIED
In 12 fl oz (355 mL) plastic bottles and 6 fl oz (176 mL) plastic bottles. Available in mint and cherry flavors.
Store at room temperature (approximately 25℃ or 77°F). Avoid freezing.
Shown in Product Identification Section, page 436

SEMICID   OTC
[sěm'ē-sĭd]
Vaginal Contraceptive Inserts

See PDR For Nonprescription Drugs.
Shown in Product Identification Section, page 436

TODAY®   OTC
[tü-dā]
Vaginal Contraceptive Sponge

DESCRIPTION
Today Vaginal Contraceptive Sponge is a soft polyurethane foam sponge containing nonoxynol-9, a spermicide used by millions of women for over 25 years.
Today Sponge is Effective, Safe, and Convenient. Today Sponge provides 24-hour contraceptive protection without hormones, allowing spontaneity. Today Sponge is easy to use, non-messy, and disposable.

ACTIVE INGREDIENT
Each Today Sponge contains nonoxynol-9, one gram.

INACTIVE INGREDIENTS
Benzoic acid, citric acid, sodium dihydrogen citrate, sodium metabisulfite, sorbic acid, water in a polyurethane foam sponge.

INDICATION
For the prevention of pregnancy.

ACTIONS
Used as directed, Today Vaginal Contraceptive Sponge prevents pregnancy in three ways: 1) the spermicide nonoxynol-9 kills sperm before they can reach the egg; 2) Today Sponge traps and absorbs sperm; 3) Today Sponge blocks the cervix so that sperm cannot enter.
Today Sponge is designed for easy insertion into the vagina. It is positioned against the cervix, and while in place provides protection against pregnancy for 24 hours. The soft polyurethane foam sponge is formulated to feel like normal vaginal tissue and has a specially-designed ribbon loop attached to an interior web for maximum strength.
In clinical trials of Today Sponge in over 1,800 women worldwide who completed over 12,000 cycles of use, the method-effectiveness, i.e., the level of effectiveness seen in women who followed the printed instructions exactly and who used Today Sponge every time that they had intercourse, was 89 to 91%. In women who did not use Today Sponge consistently and properly, the effectiveness was 84–87%.

INSTRUCTIONS
Remove one Today Sponge from airtight inner pack, wet thoroughly with clean tap water, and squeeze gently several times until it becomes very sudsy. The water activates the spermicide. Fold the sides of Today Sponge upward until it looks long and narrow and then insert it deeply into the vagina with the string loop dangling below. Protection begins immediately and continues for 24 hours. It is not necessary to add creams, jellies, foams, or any other additional spermicide as long as Today Sponge is in place, no matter how many acts of intercourse may occur during a 24-hour period. Always wait 6 hours after your last act of intercourse before removing Today Sponge. If you have intercourse when Today Sponge has been in place for 24 hours, it must be left in place an additional 6 hours after intercourse before removing it. To remove Today Sponge, place a finger in the vagina and reach up and back to find the string loop. Hook a finger around the loop. Slowly and gently pull the Sponge out. Some women, especially first-time users, may have difficulty removing the Sponge. This situation may be due to tension or unusually strong muscular pressure. Simple relaxation of the vaginal muscles and bearing down should make it possible to remove the Sponge without difficulty. See User Instruction Booklet (Section 7) for details on removing Today Sponge or call the Today TalkLine 1-800-223-2329.

WARNINGS
Some cases of Toxic Shock Syndrome (TSS) have been reported in women using barrier contraceptives including the diaphragm, cervical cap and Today® Sponge. Although the occurrence of TSS is uncommon, some studies indicate that there is an increased risk of non-menstrual TSS with the use of barrier contraceptives, including the diaphragm, cervical cap and Today Sponge. Today Sponge should not be left in place for more than 30 hours after insertion. If you experience two or more of the warning signs of TSS including fever, vomiting, diarrhea, muscular pain, dizziness, and rash similar to sunburn, consult your physician or clinic immediately. If you have difficulty removing the sponge from your vagina or you remove only a portion of the sponge, contact the Today TalkLine or consult your physician or clinic immediately. Today Sponge should not be used during the menstrual period. After childbirth, miscarriage or other termination of pregnancy, it is important to consult your physician or clinic before using this product. If you have ever had Toxic Shock Syndrome do not use Today Sponge.
A small number of men and women may be sensitive to the spermicide in this product (nonoxynol-9) and should not use this product if irritation occurs and persists. If you or your partner have ever experienced an allergic reaction to the spermicide used in this product, it is best to consult a physician before using Today Vaginal Contraceptive Sponge. If either you or your partner develops burning or itching in the genital area, stop using this product and contact your physician.
A higher degree of protection against pregnancy will be afforded by using another method of contraception in addition to a spermicidal contraceptive. This is especially true during the first few months, until you become familiar with the method. In our clinical studies, approximately one-half of all accidental pregnancies occurred during the first three months of use. Where avoidance of pregnancy is essential, the choice of contraceptive should be made in consultation with a doctor or a family planning clinic. Any delay in your menstrual period may be an early sign of pregnancy. If this happens, consult your physician or clinic as soon as possible. Keep this and all drugs out of reach of children. In case of accidental ingestion of Today Sponge, call a poison control center, emergency medical facility or doctor (For most people ingestation of small quantities of spermicide alone should not be harmful.) As with any drug, if you are pregnant or nursing a baby, seek professional advice before using this product.

HOW TO STORE
Store at normal room temperature.

HOW SUPPLIED
Packages of 1s, 2s, 3s, 6s, and 12s.
Shown in Product Identification Section, page 436

EDUCATIONAL MATERIAL

Videos
Today Sponge Instructional Videotape for Patients available to physicians, pharmacists, and patients.
Books—Booklets—Brochures
Today Sponge patient pamphlet available to physicians, pharmacists, and patients.
Pictures—Charts
8½× 11 laminated Today Sponge Instructions for Use chart available to physicians.
Write to: TalkLine, Whitehall Laboratories, 685 Third Ave., New York, NY 10017, or call toll-free 1-800-223-2329.

Important Notice
Before prescribing or administering
any product described in
PHYSICIANS' DESK REFERENCE
always consult the PDR Supplement for
possible new or revised information.

Winthrop Pharmaceuticals
90 PARK AVENUE
NEW YORK, NY 10016

Winthrop Pharmaceuticals' products are now distributed by Sanofi Winthrop Pharmaceuticals.

Wyeth-Ayerst Laboratories
Division of American Home
Products Corporation
P.O. BOX 8299
PHILADELPHIA, PA 19101

For prescribing information for products of Elkins-Sinn Incorporated, see page 984 of the 1993 PDR, and page 1939 for products of A.H. Robins Company. Information for these products can also be obtained by writing to Professional Service, Wyeth-Ayerst Laboratories, P.O. Box 8299, Philadelphia, PA 19101, or by contacting your local Wyeth-Ayerst representative.

Product Identification Codes
The following is a numerical list of National Drug Code (NDC) numbers with their corresponding product names for all oral solid dosage forms manufactured by Wyeth-Ayerst Laboratories.

Numerical Listing
Wyeth-Labeled Products

Product Ident. Code	Product	
1	Equanil® (meprobamate) Tablet 400 mg.	℞IV
2	Equanil® (meprobamate) Tablet 200 mg.	℞IV
6	Serax® (oxazepam) Capsule 15 mg.	℞IV
13	Amphojel® [dried aluminum hydroxide gel (hydrated alumina)] Tablet 0.6 Gm. (10 gr.)	
19	Phenergan® (promethazine HCl) Tablet 12.5 mg.	
27	Phenergan® (promethazine HCl) Tablet 25 mg.	
28	Sparine® (promazine HCl) Tablet 50 mg.	
29	Sparine® (promazine HCl) Tablet 25 mg.	
51	Serax® (oxazepam) Capsule 10 mg.	℞IV
52	Serax® (oxazepam) Capsule 30 mg.	℞IV
53	Omnipen® (ampicillin) Capsule 250 mg.	
56	Ovral® (each tablet contains 0.5 mg. norgestrel with 0.05 mg. ethinyl estradiol) Tablet, white	
57	Unipen® [(nafcillin sodium) as the monohydrate] Capsule 250 mg.	
59	Pen·Vee® K (penicillin V potassium) Tablet 250 mg. (400,000 units)	
62	Ovrette® (norgestrel) Tablet	
64	Ativan® (lorazepam) Tablet 1 mg.	℞IV
65	Ativan® (lorazepam) Tablet 2 mg.	℞IV
71	Mazanor® (mazindol) Tablet 1 mg.	℞IV
73	Wytensin® (guanabenz acetate) Tablet 4 mg.	
74	Wytensin® (guanabenz acetate) Tablet 8 mg.	
75	Nordette-21® (each tablet contains 0.15 mg. levonorgestrel with 0.03 mg. ethinyl estradiol) Tablet	
78	Lo/Ovral® (each tablet contains 0.3 mg. norgestrel with 0.03 mg. ethinyl estradiol) Tablet, white	
81	Ativan® (lorazepam) Tablet 0.5 mg.	℞IV
85	Wygesic® (each tablet contains 65 mg. propoxyphene HCl, U.S.P., and 650 mg. acetaminophen, U.S.P.) Tablet	℞IV
91	Equagesic® (meprobamate with aspirin) Tablet	
119	Amphojel® [dried aluminum hydroxide gel (hydrated alumina)] Tablet 0.3 Gm. (5 gr.)	
200	Sparine® (promazine HCl) Tablet 100 mg.	
227	Phenergan® (promethazine HCl) Tablet 50 mg.	
261	Mepergan® Fortis (meperidine HCl and promethazine HCl) Capsule	℞II
308	Meperidine HCl Tablet USP 50 mg.	℞II
309	Omnipen® (ampicillin) Capsule 500 mg.	
317	Serax® (oxazepam) Tablet 15 mg.	℞IV
360	Pathocil® (dicloxacillin sodium monohydrate) Capsule 250 mg.	
390	Pen·Vee® K (penicillin V potassium) Tablet 500 mg. (800,000 units)	
445	Ovral®-28 pink inert tablet	
464	Unipen® [(nafcillin sodium) as the monohydrate] Tablet 500 mg.	
472	Basaljel® (dried basic aluminum carbonate gel) Capsule	
473	Basaljel® (dried basic aluminum carbonate gel) Tablet	
486	Nordette®-28, Lo/Ovral®-28 pink inert tablet	
559	Wymox® (amoxicillin) Capsule 250 mg.	
560	Wymox® (amoxicillin) Capsule 500 mg.	
576	Wyamycin®S (erythromycin stearate) Tablet, film coated, 250 mg.	
578	Wyamycin®S (erythromycin stearate) Tablet, film coated, 500 mg.	
593	Pathocil® (dicloxacillin sodium monohydrate) Capsule 500 mg	
771	Ismo™ (isosorbide dinitrate) Tablet 20 mg.	
2511	Ovral®-28 Pilpak® (21 white tablets each containing 0.5 mg. norgestrel with 0.05 mg. ethinyl estradiol and 7 pink inert tablets)	
2514	Lo/Ovral®-28 Pilpak® (21 white tablets each containing 0.3 mg. norgestrel with 0.03 mg. ethinyl estradiol and 7 pink inert tablets)	
2533	Nordette®-28 Pilpak® (21 light-orange tablets each containing 0.15 mg. levonorgestrel with 0.03 mg ethinyl estradiol and 7 pink inert tablets)	
2535	Triphasil®-21 Tablets (levonorgestrel and ethinyl estradiol tablets—triphasic regimen)	
2536	Triphasil®-28 Tablets (levonorgestrel and ethinyl estradiol tablets—triphasic regimen)	
4124	Cyclospasmol® (cyclandelate) Capsule 200 mg	
4125	Isordil® Tembids® Tablet 40 mg	
4126	Isordil® Sublingual Tablet 5 mg	
4130	Trecator®-SC (ethionamide) Tablet 250 mg	
4132	Surmontil® (trimipramine) Capsule 25 mg	
4133	Surmontil® (trimipramine) Capsule 50 mg	
4139	Isordil® (isosorbide dinitrate) Sublingual Tablet 2.5 mg	
4140	Isordil® (isosorbide dinitrate) Tembids Capsule 40 mg	
4148	Cyclospasmol® (cyclandelate) Capsule 400 mg	
4152	Isordil® (isosorbide dinitrate) 5 Titradose Tablet 5 mg	
4153	Isordil® (isosorbide dinitrate) 10 Titradose Tablet 10 mg	
4154	Isordil® (isosorbide dinitrate) 20 Titradose Tablet 20 mg	
4158	Surmontil® (trimipramine) Capsule 100 mg	
4159	Isordil® (isosorbide dinitrate) 30 Titradose Tablet 30 mg	
4161	Isordil® (isosorbide dinitrate) Sublingual Tablet 10 mg	
4177	Sectral® (acebutolol) Capsule 200 mg	
4179	Sectral® (acebutolol) Capsule 400 mg	
4181	Orudis® (ketoprofen) Capsule 50 mg	
4186	Orudis® (ketoprofen) Capsule 25 mg	
4187	Orudis® (ketoprofen) Capsule 75 mg	
4188	Cordarone® (amiodarone) Tablet 200 mg	
4191	Synalgos®-DC (each capsule contains 16 mg. dihydrocodeine bitartrate, 356.4 mg. aspirin, and 30 mg. caffeine) Capsule	
4192	Isordil® (isosorbide dinitrate) 40 Titradose Tablet 40 mg	

Ayerst-Labeled Products

243	Atromid-S® (clofibrate) Capsule 500 mg.	
421	Inderal® (propranolol HCl) Tablet 10 mg.	
422	Inderal® (propranolol HCl) Tablet 20 mg.	
424	Inderal® (propranolol HCl) Tablet 40 mg.	
426	Inderal® (propranolol HCl) Tablet 60 mg.	
428	Inderal® (propranolol HCl) Tablet 80 mg.	
430	Mysoline® (primidone) Tablet 250 mg.	
431	Mysoline® (primidone) Tablet 50 mg.	
435	Grisactin® Ultra (griseofulvin, ultramicrosize) Tablet 250 mg.	
437	Grisactin® Ultra (griseofulvin, ultramicrosize) Tablet 330 mg.	
443	Grisactin® 250 (griseofulvin, microsize) Capsule 250 mg.	
444	Grisactin® 500 (griseofulvin, microsize) Tablet 500 mg.	
455	Inderide® LA (each capsule contains 80 mg. Inderal® LA [propranolol HCl] and 50 mg. hydrochlorothiazide) Capsule	
457	Inderide® LA (each capsule contains 120 mg. Inderal® LA [propranolol HCl] and 50 mg. hydrochlorothiazide) Capsule	
459	Inderide® LA (each capsule contains 160 mg. Inderal® LA [propranolol HCl] and 50 mg. hydrochlorothiazide) Capsule	
470	Inderal® LA (propranolol HCl) Capsule 60 mg.	
471	Inderal® LA (propranolol HCl) Capsule 80 mg.	
473	Inderal® LA (propranolol HCl) Capsule 120 mg.	
479	Inderal® LA (propranolol HCl) Capsule 160 mg.	
484	Inderide® (each tablet contains 40 mg. Inderal® [propranolol HCl] and 25 mg. hydrochlorothiazide) Tablet	
488	Inderide® (each tablet contains 80 mg. Inderal® [propranolol HCl] and 25 mg. hydrochlorothiazide) Tablet	
702	Diucardin® (hydroflumethiazide) Tablet 50 mg.	
738	Lodine® (etodolac) Capsule 200 mg.	
739	Lodine® (etodolac) Capsule 300 mg.	
755	Plegine® (phendimetrazine tartrate) Tablet 35 mg.	℞III
786	Thiosulfil® Forte (sulfamethizole) Tablet 500 mg.	
809	Antabuse® (disulfiram) Tablet 250 mg.	
810	Antabuse® (disulfiram) Tablet 500 mg.	
864	Premarin® (conjugated estrogens tablets, USP) Tablet 0.9 mg.	
865	Premarin® (conjugated estrogens tablets, USP) Tablet 2.5 mg.	
866	Premarin® (conjugated estrogens tablets, USP) Tablet 1.25 mg.	
867	Premarin® (conjugated estrogens tablets, USP) Tablet 0.625 mg.	
868	Premarin® (conjugated estrogens tablets, USP) Tablet 0.3 mg.	
878	Premarin® with Methyltestosterone (each tablet contains 0.625 mg. Premarin® [conjugated estrogens, USP] and 5 mg. methyltestosterone) Tablet	
879	Premarin® with Methyltestosterone (each tablet contains 1.25 mg. Premarin® [conjugated estrogens, USP] and 10 mg. methyltestosterone) Tablet	
880	PMB® 200 (each tablet contains 0.45 mg. Premarin® [conjugated estrogens, USP] and 200 mg. meprobamate) Tablet	
881	PMB® 400 (each tablet contains 0.45 mg. Premarin® [conjugated estrogens, USP] and 400 mg. meprobamate) Tablet	
894	Aygestin® (norethindrone acetate, USP) Tablet 5 mg.	
896	Cycrin® (medroxyprogesterone acetate, USP) Tablet 10 mg.	

CHILDREN'S ADVIL® SUSPENSION   ℞
(ibuprofen) 100mg/5mL

SHAKE WELL BEFORE USE

DESCRIPTION
CHILDREN'S ADVIL® SUSPENSION contains ibuprofen which is $(\pm)$-2-(p-isobutylphenyl)-propionic acid. Ibuprofen is a white powder with a melting point of 74°–77°C and is very slightly soluble in water (< 1 mg/mL) and readily soluble in organic solvents such as ethanol and acetone.
Ibuprofen's structural formula is:

CHILDREN'S ADVIL® SUSPENSION is a nonsteroidal anti-inflammatory agent. It is available for oral administration as a sucrose-sweetened, fruit-flavored liquid suspension containing 100mg of ibuprofen per 5mL.
Inactive Ingredients: Cellulose Gum, Citric Acid, Disodium EDTA, FD&C Red No. 40, Flavors, Glycerin, Microcrystalline Cellulose, Polysorbate 80, Sodium Benzoate, Sorbitol, Sucrose, Water, Xanthan Gum.

CLINICAL PHARMACOLOGY
CHILDREN'S ADVIL® SUSPENSION is a nonsteroidal anti-inflammatory agent that possesses analgesic and antipyretic activities. Its mode of action, like that of other nonsteroidal anti-inflammatory agents, is not completely understood, but may be related to prostaglandin synthetase inhibition.
In clinical studies in adult patients with rheumatoid arthritis and osteoarthritis, ibuprofen has been shown to be comparable to aspirin in controlling pain and inflammation and to be associated with a statistically significant reduction in the milder gastrointestinal side effects (see **ADVERSE REACTIONS**). CHILDREN'S ADVIL® SUSPENSION may be well tolerated in some patients who have had gastrointestinal side effects with aspirin, but these patients, when treated with CHILDREN'S ADVIL® SUSPENSION, should be carefully followed for signs and symptoms of gastrointestinal ulceration and bleeding.
Although it is not definitely known whether ibuprofen causes less peptic ulceration than aspirin, in one study involving 885 adult patients with rheumatoid arthritis treated for up to one year, there were no reports of gastric ulceration with ibuprofen whereas frank ulceration was reported in 13 patients in the aspirin group (statistically significant $p < .001$). Gastroscopic studies at varying doses show an increased tendency toward gastric irritation at higher doses. However, at comparable doses, gastric irritation is approximately half that seen with aspirin. Studies using ^{51}Cr-tagged

Continued on next page

Wyeth-Ayerst Laboratories—Cont.

red cells indicate that fecal blood loss associated with ibuprofen in doses up to 2400mg daily did not exceed the normal range, and was significantly less than that seen in aspirin-treated patients.

In clinical studies in patients with rheumatoid arthritis, ibuprofen has been shown to be comparable to indomethacin in controlling the signs and symptoms of disease activity and to be associated with a statistically significant reduction of the milder gastrointestinal (see **ADVERSE REACTIONS**), and CNS side effects.

CHILDREN'S ADVIL® SUSPENSION may be used in combination with gold salts and/or corticosteroids.

In clinical studies in patients aged 2 to 15 with juvenile arthritis, CHILDREN'S ADVIL® SUSPENSION in doses of 20 to 50 mg/kg/day divided into 3 or 4 daily doses, has been shown to be similar to aspirin in controlling the signs and symptoms of their disease. In these trials, there was a significantly lower incidence of liver test abnormalities associated with CHILDREN'S ADVIL® SUSPENSION than with aspirin. Although ibuprofen may be better tolerated in terms of liver test abnormalities in children treated with CHILDREN'S ADVIL® SUSPENSION, they should be carefully followed for signs and symptoms suggesting liver dysfunction particularly with doses above 30mg/kg/day, or if abnormal liver tests have occurred with previous NSAID treatment (see **PRECAUTIONS**).

Controlled studies in adults have demonstrated that ibuprofen is a more effective analgesic than propoxyphene for the relief of episiotomy pain, pain following dental extraction procedures, and for the relief of the symptoms of primary dysmenorrhea.

In patients with primary dysmenorrhea, ibuprofen has been shown to reduce elevated levels of prostaglandin activity in the menstrual fluid and to reduce resting and active intrauterine pressure, as well as the frequency of uterine contractions. The probable mechanism of action is to inhibit prostaglandin synthesis rather than simply to provide analgesia.

Controlled clinical trials comparing doses of 5 and 10mg/kg ibuprofen and 10–15 mg/kg of acetaminophen have been conducted in children 6 months to 12 years of age with fever primarily due to viral illnesses. In these studies there were no differences between treatments in fever reduction for the first hour and maximum fever reduction occurred between 2 and 4 hours. Response after 1 hour was dependent on both the level of temperature elevation as well as the treatment. In children with baseline temperatures at or below 102.5°F, both ibuprofen doses and acetaminophen were equally effective in their maximum effect. In those children with temperatures above 102.5°F, the ibuprofen 10mg/kg dose was more effective. By 6 hours children treated with ibuprofen 5mg/kg tended to have recurrence of fever, whereas children treated with ibuprofen 10 mg/kg still had significant fever reduction at 8 hours. In control groups treated with 10mg/kg acetaminophen, fever reduction resembled that seen in children treated with 5mg/kg of ibuprofen, with the exception that temperature elevation tended to return 1–2 hours earlier. In other trials, the antipyretic effect of CHILDREN'S ADVIL® SUSPENSION at 10 mg/kg was similar to that of acetaminophen at 15 mg/kg.

Pharmacokinetics: Ibuprofen is rapidly absorbed when administered orally. As is true with most tablet and suspension formulations, CHILDREN'S ADVIL® SUSPENSION is absorbed somewhat faster than the tablet with a time to peak serum level generally within one hour. Peak serum ibuprofen levels are generally attained one to two hours after administration of ibuprofen tablets and within about 1 hour after the suspension. With single, oral, solid doses up to 800mg in adults, a linear relationship exists between the amount of drug administered and the integrated area under the serum drug concentration vs. time curve. Above 800mg, however, the area under the curve increase is less than proportional to the increase in dose. There is no evidence of age-dependent kinetics in patients 2 to 11 years old. With single doses of CHILDREN'S ADVIL® SUSPENSION ranging up to 10mg/kg, a dose/response relationship exists between the amount of drug administered to febrile children and the serum concentration vs. time curve. There is also a correlation between reduction of fever and drug concentration over time, although the peak reduction in fever occurs 2–4 hours after dosing.

No absorption differences are noticeable when ibuprofen tablets or suspension are given under fasting conditions or immediately before meals. When either product is taken with food, however, the peak levels are somewhat lower (up to 30%) and the time to reach peak levels is slightly prolonged (up to 30 min.) although the extent of absorption is unchanged. A bioavailability study has shown that there was no interference with the absorption of ibuprofen when given in conjunction with an antacid containing both aluminum hydroxide and magnesium hydroxide.

Ibuprofen is rapidly metabolized and eliminated in the urine. The excretion of ibuprofen is virtually complete 24 hours after the last dose. The serum half-life of ibuprofen is 1.8 to 2.0 hours.

Studies have shown that following ingestion of the drug, 45% to 79% of the dose was recovered in the urine within 24 hours as metabolite A (25%), (+)-2-4'-(2-hydroxy-2-methylpropyl)- phenylpropionic acid and metabolite B (37%), (+)-2-4'-(2-carboxypropyl)-phenyl propionic acid; the percentages of free and conjugated ibuprofen were approximately 1% and 14%, respectively.

INDICATIONS AND USAGE

CHILDREN'S ADVIL® SUSPENSION is indicated for relief of the signs and symptoms of juvenile arthritis, rheumatoid arthritis and osteoarthritis.

CHILDREN'S ADVIL® SUSPENSION is indicated for relief of mild to moderate pain in adults and of primary dysmenorrhea.

CHILDREN'S ADVIL® SUSPENSION is also indicated for the reduction of fever in patients ages 6 months and older. Since there have been no controlled trials to demonstrate whether there is any beneficial effect or harmful interaction with the use of ibuprofen in conjunction with aspirin, the combination cannot be recommended (see **Drug Interactions**).

CONTRAINDICATIONS

CHILDREN'S ADVIL® SUSPENSION should not be used in patients who have previously exhibited hypersensitivity to ibuprofen, or in individuals with all or part of the syndrome of nasal polyps, angioedema and bronchospastic reactivity to aspirin or other nonsteroidal anti-inflammatory agents. Anaphylactoid reactions have occurred in such patients.

WARNINGS

Risk of GI Ulceration, Bleeding and Perforation with NSAID Therapy.

Serious gastrointestinal toxicity such as bleeding, ulceration, and perforation, can occur at any time, with or without warning symptoms, in patients treated chronically with NSAID therapy. Although minor upper gastrointestinal problems, such as dyspepsia, are common, usually developing early in therapy, physicians should remain alert for ulceration and bleeding in patients treated chronically with NSAIDs even in the absence of previous GI tract symptoms. In patients observed in clinical trials of several months to two years duration, symptomatic upper GI ulcers, gross bleeding or perforation appear to occur in approximately 1% of patients treated for 3–6 months, and in about 2–4% of patients treated for one year. Physicians should inform patients about the signs and/or symptoms of serious GI toxicity and what steps to take if they occur. Studies to date have not identified any subset of patients not at risk of developing peptic ulceration and bleeding. Except for a prior history of serious GI events and other risk factors known to be associated with peptic ulcer disease, such as alcoholism, smoking, etc., no risk factors (e.g., age, sex) have been associated with increased risk. Elderly or debilitated patients seem to tolerate ulceration or bleeding less well than other individuals and most spontaneous reports of fatal GI events are in this population. Studies to date are inconclusive concerning the relative risk of various NSAIDs in causing such reactions. High doses of any NSAID probably carry a greater risk of these reactions, although controlled clinical trials showing this do not exist in most cases. In considering the use of relatively large doses (within the recommended dosage range), sufficient benefit should be anticipated to offset the potential increased risk of GI toxicity.

PRECAUTIONS

General:

Blurred and/or diminished vision, scotomata, and/or changes in color vision have been reported. If a patient develops such complaints while receiving CHILDREN'S ADVIL® SUSPENSION (ibuprofen), the drug should be discontinued and the patient should have an ophthalmologic examination which includes central visual fields and color vision testing. Fluid retention and edema have been reported in association with ibuprofen, therefore, the drug should be used with caution in patients with a history of cardiac decompensation or hypertension.

Ibuprofen, like other nonsteroidal anti-inflammatory agents, can inhibit platelet aggregation, but the effect is quantitatively less and of shorter duration than that seen with aspirin. Ibuprofen has been shown to prolong bleeding time (but within the normal range), in normal subjects. Because this prolonged bleeding effect may be exaggerated in patients with underlying hemostatic defects, CHILDREN'S ADVIL® SUSPENSION should be used with caution in persons with intrinsic coagulation defects and those on anticoagulant therapy. Patients on ibuprofen should report to their physicians signs or symptoms of gastrointestinal ulceration or bleeding, blurred vision or other eye symptoms, skin rash, weight gain, or edema.

In order to avoid exacerbation of disease or adrenal insufficiency, patients who have been on prolonged corticosteroid therapy should have their therapy tapered slowly rather than discontinued abruptly when ibuprofen is added to the treatment program.

The antipyretic and anti-inflammatory activity of ibuprofen may reduce fever and inflammation, thus diminishing their utility as diagnostic signs in detecting complications of presumed noninfectious, noninflammatory painful conditions.

Liver Effects: As with other nonsteroidal anti-inflammatory drugs, borderline elevations of one or more liver function tests may occur in up to 15% of patients. These abnormalities may progress, may remain essentially unchanged, or may be transient with continued therapy. The SGPT (ALT) test is probably the most sensitive indicator of liver dysfunction. Meaningful (3 times the upper limit of normal) elevations of SGPT or SGOT (AST) occurred in controlled clinical trials in less than 1% of patients. A patient with symptoms and/or signs suggesting liver dysfunction, or in whom an abnormal liver test has occurred, should be evaluated for evidence of the development of more severe hepatic reactions while on therapy with ibuprofen. Severe hepatic reactions, including jaundice and cases of fatal hepatitis, have been reported with ibuprofen as with other nonsteroidal anti-inflammatory drugs. Although such reactions are rare, if abnormal liver tests persist or worsen, if clinical signs and symptoms consistent with liver disease develop, or if systemic manifestations occur (e.g., eosinophilia, rash, etc.), CHILDREN'S ADVIL® SUSPENSION should be discontinued.

Hemoglobin Levels: In cross-study comparisons with doses ranging from 1200mg to 3200mg daily for several weeks, a slight dose-response decrease in hemoglobin/hematocrit was noted. This has been observed with other nonsteroidal anti-inflammatory drugs; the mechanism is unknown. However, even with daily doses of 3200mg, the total decrease in hemoglobin usually does not exceed 1 gram; if there are no signs of bleeding, it is probably not clinically important.

In two postmarketing clinical studies with ibuprofen the incidence of a decreased hemoglobin level was greater than previously reported. Decrease in hemoglobin of 1 gram or more was observed in 17.1% of 193 patients on 1600mg ibuprofen daily (osteoarthritis), and in 22.8% of 189 patients taking 2400mg of ibuprofen daily (rheumatoid arthritis). Positive stool occult blood tests and elevated serum creatinine levels were also observed in these studies.

Aseptic Meningitis: Aseptic meningitis with fever and coma has been observed on rare occasions in patients on ibuprofen therapy. Although it is probably more likely to occur in patients with systemic lupus erythematosus and related connective tissue diseases, it has been reported in patients who do not have an underlying chronic disease. If signs or symptoms of meningitis develop in a patient on CHILDREN'S ADVIL® SUSPENSION, the possibility of its being related to ibuprofen should be considered.

Renal Effects: As with other nonsteroidal anti-inflammatory drugs, long-term administration of ibuprofen to animals has resulted in renal papillary necrosis and other abnormal renal pathology. In humans, there have been reports of acute interstitial nephritis with hematuria, proteinuria, and occasionally nephrotic syndrome.

A second form of renal toxicity has been seen in patients with prerenal conditions leading to a reduction in renal blood flow or blood volume, where the renal prostaglandins have a supportive role in the maintenance of renal perfusion. In these patients administration of a nonsteroidal anti-inflammatory drug may cause a dose dependent reduction in prostaglandin formation and may precipitate overt renal decompensation.

Patients at greatest risk of this reaction are those with impaired renal function, heart failure, liver dysfunction, those taking diuretics and the elderly. Discontinuation of nonsteroidal anti-inflammatory drug therapy is typically followed by recovery to the pretreatment state.

Those patients at high risk who chronically take ibuprofen should have renal function monitored if they have signs or symptoms which may be consistent with mild azotemia, such as malaise, fatigue, loss of appetite, etc. Occasional patients may develop some elevation of serum creatinine and BUN levels without signs or symptoms.

Since ibuprofen is eliminated primarily by the kidneys, patients with significantly impaired renal function should be closely monitored and a reduction in dosage should be anticipated to avoid drug accumulation. Prospective studies on the safety of ibuprofen in patients with chronic renal failure have not been conducted.

Information for Patients: Ibuprofen, like other drugs of its class, is not free of side effects. The side effects of these drugs can cause discomfort and rarely, there are more serious side effects, such as gastrointestinal bleeding, which may result in hospitalization and even fatal outcomes. NSAIDs (Nonsteroidal Anti-Inflammatory Drugs) are often essential agents in the management of arthritis and have a major role in the treatment of pain, but they also may be commonly employed for conditions which are less serious. Physicians may wish to discuss with their patients the potential risks (see **WARNINGS, PRECAUTIONS,** and **ADVERSE REACTIONS**) and likely benefits of NSAID treatment, particularly when the drugs are used for less serious conditions where treat-

Children's Advil® (ibuprofen) Suspension Incidence Greater than 1% (but less than 3%) Probable Causal Relationship	Precise Incidence Unknown (but less than 1%) Probable Causal Relationship**	Precise Incidence Unknown (but less than 1%) Causal Relationship Unknown**
GASTROINTESTINAL Nausea*, epigastric pain*, heartburn*, diarrhea, abdominal distress, nausea and vomiting, indigestion, constipation, abdominal cramps or pain, fullness of GI tract (bloating and flatulence)	Gastric or duodenal ulcer with bleeding and/or perforation, gastrointestinal hemorrhage, melena, gastritis, hepatitis, jaundice, abnormal liver function tests; pancreatitis	
CENTRAL NERVOUS SYSTEM Dizziness*, headache, nervousness	Depression, insomnia, confusion, emotional lability, somnolence, aseptic meningitis with fever and coma	Paresthesias, hallucinations, dream abnormalities, pseudotumor cerebri
DERMATOLOGIC Rash* (including maculopapular type), pruritus	Vesiculobullous eruptions, urticaria, erythema multiforme, Stevens-Johnson syndrome, alopecia	Toxic epidermal necrolysis, photoallergic skin reactions
SPECIAL SENSES Tinnitus	Hearing loss, amblyopia (blurred and/or diminished vision, scotomata and/or changes in color vision) (see PRECAUTIONS)	Conjunctivitis, diplopia, optic neuritis, cataracts
HEMATOLOGIC	Neutropenia, agranulocytosis, aplastic anemia, hemolytic anemia (sometimes Coombs positive), thrombocytopenia with or without purpura, eosinophilia, decreases in hemoglobin and hematocrit (see PRECAUTIONS)	Bleeding episodes (e.g. epistaxis, menorrhagia)
METABOLIC/ENDOCRINE Decreased appetite		Gynecomastia, hypoglycemic reaction, acidosis
CARDIOVASCULAR Edema, fluid retention (generally responds promptly to drug discontinuation; see PRECAUTIONS)	Congestive heart failure in patients with marginal cardiac function, elevated blood pressure, palpitations	Arrhythmias (sinus tachycardia, sinus bradycardia)
ALLERGIC	Syndrome of abdominal pain, fever, chills, nausea and vomiting; anaphylaxis; bronchospasm (see CONTRAINDICATIONS)	Serum sickness, lupus erythematosus syndrome, Henoch-Schönlein vasculitis, angioedema
RENAL	Acute renal failure (see PRECAUTIONS), decreased creatinine clearance, polyuria, azotemia, cystitis, hematuria	Renal papillary necrosis
MISCELLANEOUS	Dry eyes and mouth, gingival ulcer, rhinitis	

*Reactions occurring in 3% to 9% of adult patients treated with ibuprofen. (Those reactions occurring in less than 3% of the patients are unmarked).
**Reactions are classified under "*Probable Causal Relationship (PCR)*" if there has been one positive rechallenge or if three or more cases occur which might be causally related. Reactions are classified under "*Causal Relationship Unknown*" if seven or more events have been reported but the criteria for PCR have not been met.

ment without NSAIDs may represent an acceptable alternative to both the patient and physician.
Laboratory Tests: Because serious GI tract ulceration and bleeding can occur without warning symptoms, physicians should follow chronically treated patients for the signs and symptoms of ulceration and bleeding and should inform them of the importance of this follow-up (see **WARNINGS**).
Drug Interactions: Coumarin-type anticoagulants. Several short-term controlled studies failed to show that ibuprofen significantly affected prothrombin times or a variety of other clotting factors when administered to individuals on coumarin-type anticoagulants.
However, because bleeding has been reported when ibuprofen and other nonsteroidal anti-inflammatory agents have been administered to patients on coumarin-type anticoagulants, the physician should be cautious when administering CHILDREN'S ADVIL® SUSPENSION to patients on anticoagulants.
Aspirin: Animal studies show that aspirin given with nonsteroidal anti-inflammatory agents, including ibuprofen, yields a net decrease in anti-inflammatory activity with lowered blood levels of the non-aspirin drug. Single dose bioavailability studies in normal volunteers have failed to show an effect of aspirin on ibuprofen blood levels. Correlative clinical studies have not been performed.
Methotrexate: Ibuprofen, as well as other nonsteroidal anti-inflammatory drugs, has been reported to competitively inhibit methotrexate accumulation in rabbit kidney slices. This may indicate that ibuprofen could enhance the toxicity of methotrexate. Caution should be used if CHILDREN'S ADVIL® SUSPENSION is administered concomitantly with methotrexate.
H₂ Antagonists: In studies with human volunteers, coadministration of cimetidine or ranitidine with ibuprofen had no substantive effect on ibuprofen serum concentrations.
Furosemide: Clinical studies, as well as random observations, have shown that ibuprofen can reduce the natriuretic effect of furosemide and thiazides in some patients. This response has been attributed to inhibition of renal prostaglan-

din synthesis. During concomitant therapy with ibuprofen, patients should be observed closely for signs of renal failure (See **PRECAUTIONS, Renal Effects**), as well as to assure diuretic efficacy.
Lithium: Ibuprofen produced an elevation of plasma lithium levels and a reduction in renal lithium clearance in a study of eleven normal volunteers. The mean minimum lithium concentration increased 15% and the renal clearance of lithium was decreased by 19% during this period of concomitant drug administration. This effect has been attributed to inhibition of renal prostaglandin synthesis by ibuprofen. Thus, when ibuprofen and aluminum are administered concurrently, patients should be observed carefully for signs of lithium toxicity. (Read package insert for lithium preparation before use of such concurrent therapy.)
Diabetes: Each 5mL of CHILDREN'S ADVIL® SUSPENSION contains approximately 2.5 grams of sucrose, which should be taken into consideration when treating patients with impaired glucose tolerance. It also contains 350mg of sorbitol per 5mL. Although in clinical trials CHILDREN'S ADVIL® SUSPENSION was not associated with more diarrhea than control treatments, should a patient develop diarrhea, the physician may wish to review the patient's dietary intake of sorbitol from other sources.
Pregnancy: Reproductive studies conducted in rats and rabbits at doses somewhat less than the maximal adult clinical dose did not demonstrate evidence of developmental abnormalities. However, animal reproduction studies are not always predictive of human response. As there are no adequate and well-controlled studies in pregnant women, this drug should be used during pregnancy only if clearly needed. Because of the known effects of nonsteroidal anti-inflammatory drugs on the fetal cardiovascular system (closure of ductus arteriosus), use during late pregnancy should be avoided. As with other drugs known to inhibit prostaglandin synthesis, an increased incidence of dystocia and delayed parturition occurred in rats. Administration of CHILDREN'S ADVIL® SUSPENSION is not recommended during pregnancy.
Nursing Mothers: In limited studies, an assay capable of detecting 1mcg/mL did not demonstrate ibuprofen in the milk of lactating mothers. However, because of the limited

nature of the studies and the possible adverse effects of prostaglandin-inhibiting drugs on neonates, CHILDREN'S ADVIL® SUSPENSION is not recommended for use by nursing mothers.
Infants: Safety and efficacy of CHILDREN'S ADVIL® SUSPENSION in children below the age of 6 months has not been established.

ADVERSE REACTIONS
The most frequent type of adverse reaction occurring with ibuprofen is gastrointestinal. In controlled clinical trials, the percentage of adult patients reporting one or more gastrointestinal complaints ranged from 4% to 16%.
In controlled studies in adults when ibuprofen was compared to aspirin and indomethacin in equally effective doses, the overall incidence of gastrointestinal complaints was about half that seen in either the aspirin- or indomethacin-treated patients.
In a 12-week comparison of CHILDREN'S ADVIL® SUSPENSION (n=45) and aspirin (n=47) in children with juvenile arthritis, the most common adverse experiences were also gastrointestinal in nature, usually of mild severity. Abdominal pain of possible drug relationship was reported in about 25% of patients on ibuprofen and/or aspirin; other possibly drug-related effects associated with the digestive system were reported in 42% of the children taking ibuprofen and in 70% of those taking aspirin.
Adverse reactions observed during controlled clinical trials in adults at an incidence greater than 1% are listed in the table. Those reactions listed in column one encompass observations in approximately 3,000 adult patients. More than 500 of these patients were treated for periods of at least 54 weeks.
Still other reactions occurring less frequently than 1 in 100 were reported in controlled clinical trials and from marketing experience. These reactions have been divided into two categories: column two of the table lists reactions with therapy with ibuprofen where the probability of a causal rela-

Continued on next page

Wyeth-Ayerst Laboratories—Cont.

tionship exists; for the reactions in column three, a causal relationship with ibuprofen has not been established.

Reported side effects were higher at doses of 3200mg/day than at doses of 2400mg or less per day in clinical trials of adults patients with rheumatoid arthritis. The increases in incidence were slight and still within the ranges reported in the table below. [See table on preceding page.]

OVERDOSAGE

Approximately 1½ hours after the reported ingestion of from 7 to 10 ibuprofen tablets (400mg), a 19-month-old child weighing 12 kg was seen in the hospital emergency room, apneic and cyanotic, responding only to painful stimuli. This type of stimulus, however, was sufficient to induce respiration. Oxygen and parenteral fluids were given; a greenish-yellow fluid was aspirated from the stomach with no evidence to indicate the presence of ibuprofen. Two hours after ingestion the child's condition seemed stable; she still responded only to painful stimuli and continued to have periods of apnea lasting from 5 to 10 seconds. She was admitted to intensive care and sodium bicarbonate was administered as well as infusions of dextrose and normal saline. By four hours post-ingestion she could be aroused easily, sit by herself and respond to spoken commands. Blood level of ibuprofen was 102.9 mcg/mL approximately 8½ hours after accidental ingestion. At 12 hours she appeared to be completely recovered.

In two other reported cases where children (each weighing approximately 10kg) accidentally, acutely ingested approximately 120mg/kg, there were no signs of acute intoxication or late sequelae. Blood level in one child 90 minutes after ingestion was 700 mcg/mL, about 10 times the peak levels seen in absorption-excretion studies.

A 19-year-old male who had taken 8,000mg of ibuprofen over a period of a few hours complained of dizziness, and nystagmus was noted. After hospitalization, parenteral hydration and three days' bed rest, he recovered with no reported sequelae.

In cases of acute overdosage, the stomach should be emptied by vomiting or lavage, though little drug will likely be recovered if more than an hour has elapsed since ingestion. Because the drug is acidic and is excreted in the urine, it is theoretically beneficial to administer alkali and induce diuresis. In addition to supportive measures, the use of oral activated charcoal may help to reduce the absorption and reabsorption of ibuprofen.

DOSAGE AND ADMINISTRATION

Shake well prior to administration.

Do not exceed 3200mg total daily dose. If gastrointestinal complaints occur, administer ibuprofen with meals or milk.

Juvenile Arthritis: The usual dose is 30 to 40mg/kg/day divided into 3 or 4 doses. Patients with milder disease may be adequately treated with 20mg/kg/day.

Doses above 50mg/kg/day are not recommended because they have not been studied and because side effects appear to be dose related.

Therapeutic response may require from a few days to several weeks to be achieved. Once a clinical response is obtained, dosage can be lowered to the smallest dose of CHILDREN'S ADVIL® SUSPENSION needed to maintain adequate control of disease.

Rheumatoid arthritis and osteoarthritis, including flare-ups of chronic disease: Suggested Adult Dosage: 1200–3200mg daily (300mg q.i.d., or 400mg, 600mg or 800mg t.i.d. or q.i.d.). Individual patients may show a better response to 3200mg daily, as compared with 2400mg, although in well-controlled clinical trials patients on 3200mg did not show a better mean response in terms of efficacy. Therefore, when treating patients with 3200mg/day, the physician should observe sufficient increased clinical benefits to offset potential increased risk.

The dose of CHILDREN'S ADVIL® SUSPENSION should be tailored to each patient, and may be lowered or raised from the suggested doses depending on the severity of symptoms either at the time of initiating drug therapy or as the patient responds or fails to respond.

In general, patients with rheumatoid arthritis seem to require higher doses of ibuprofen than do patients with osteoarthritis.

The smallest dose of CHILDREN'S ADVIL® SUSPENSION that yields acceptable control should be employed. A linear blood level dose-response relationship exists with single doses up to 800mg (see **CLINICAL PHARMACOLOGY, Pharmacokinetics** for effects of food on rate of absorption).

In chronic conditions, a therapeutic response to ibuprofen therapy is sometimes seen in a few days to a week but most often is observed by two weeks. After a satisfactory response has been achieved, the patient's dose should be reviewed and adjusted as required.

Mild to moderate pain: 400mg every 4 to 6 hours as necessary for relief of pain in adults.

In controlled analgesic clinical trials, doses of ibuprofen greater than 400mg were no more effective than the 400mg dose.

Dysmenorrhea: For the treatment of dysmenorrhea, beginning with the earliest onset of such pain, CHILDREN'S ADVIL® SUSPENSION should be given in a dose of 400mg every 4 hours as necessary for the relief of pain.

FEVER REDUCTION IN CHILDREN 6 months to 12 years of age: Dosage should be adjusted on the basis of the initial temperature level (see **CLINICAL PHARMACOLOGY** for a description of the controlled clinical trial results). The recommended dose is 5mg/kg if the baseline temperature is 102.5°F or below or 10mg/kg if the baseline temperature is greater than 102.5°F. The duration of fever reduction is generally 6–8 hours and is longer with the higher dose. The recommended maximum daily dose is 40mg/kg.

		5mg/kg (Fever ≤102.5°F)		10mg/kg (Fever >102.5°F)	
Age	Weight (lb)	(mg)	(tsp)	(mg)	(tsp)
6–11 mos	13–17	25	¼	50	½
12–23 mos	18–23	50	½	100	1
2–3 yrs	24–35	75	¾	150	1½
4–5 yrs	36–47	100	1	200	2
6–8 yrs	48–59	125	1¼	250	2½
9–10 yrs	60–71	150	1½	300	3
11–12 yrs	72–95	200	2	400	4

FEVER REDUCTION IN ADULTS:
400mg every 4–6 hours as necessary.

HOW SUPPLIED

CHILDREN'S ADVIL® SUSPENSION is supplied as a sucrose-sweetened, fruit-flavored, aqueous suspension of ibuprofen 100mg/5mL in 4 and 16-ounce (119 and 473mL) bottles.

4 Ounce Bottles NDC 0008-0800-01
16 Ounce Bottles NDC 0008-0800-03

CHILDREN'S ADVIL® SUSPENSION should be stored at room temperature; 15°C to 30°C (59°F to 86°F).

Shake well before use. Keep container tightly closed.

Caution: Federal law prohibits dispensing without prescription.

Shown in Product Identification Section, page 436

ALUDROX® OTC

[*al'u-drox*]
(alumina and magnesia)
ORAL SUSPENSION

COMPOSITION

Nonconstipating, noncathartic, effective and palatable antacid containing, in each 5 ml. teaspoonful of suspension, 307 mg. of aluminum hydroxide as a gel, and 103 mg. of magnesium hydroxide. The inactive ingredients present are artificial and natural flavors, benzoic acid, butylparaben, glycerin, hydroxypropyl methylcellulose, methylparaben, propylparaben, saccharin, simethicone, sorbitol solution, and water.

INDICATIONS

For the symptomatic relief of hyperacidity associated with the diagnosis of peptic ulcer, gastritis, peptic esophagitis, gastric hyperacidity, and hiatal hernia.

DOSAGE AND ADMINISTRATION

Two teaspoonfuls (10 ml.) of suspension every four hours, or as required. Suspension may be followed by a sip of water if desired. Ten ml. of ALUDROX suspension have the capacity to neutralize 24 mEq of acid.

WARNINGS

Patients are advised not to take more than 12 teaspoonfuls (60 ml) in a 24-hour period or use this maximum dosage for more than two weeks except under the advice and supervision of a physician. Prolonged use of aluminum-containing antacids in patients with renal failure may result in or worsen dialysis osteomalacia. Elevated tissue aluminum levels contribute to the development of dialysis encephalopathy and osteomalacia syndromes. Also, a number of cases of dialysis encephalopathy have been associated with elevated aluminum levels in the dialysate water. Small amounts of aluminum are absorbed from the gastrointestinal tract and renal excretion of aluminum is impaired in renal failure. Prolonged use of aluminum-containing antacids in such patients may contribute to increased plasma levels of aluminum. Aluminum is not well removed by dialysis because it is bound to albumin and transferrin, which do not cross dialysis membranes. As a result, aluminum is deposited in bone, and dialysis osteomalacia may develop when large amounts of aluminum are ingested orally by patients with impaired renal function. Pregnant women and nursing mothers are advised to seek the advice of a health professional before using this product.

DRUG INTERACTION PRECAUTIONS

This product must not be taken if the patient is presently taking a prescription antibiotic drug containing any form of tetracycline.

HOW SUPPLIED

Oral Suspension, bottles of 12 fluidounces.

AMPHOJEL® OTC

[*am'fo-jel*]
(aluminum hydroxide gel)
SUSPENSION • TABLETS

COMPOSITION

Suspension—Each 5 ml. teaspoonful contains 320 mg. of aluminum hydroxide as a gel, and not more than 0.10 mEq of sodium. The inactive ingredients present are butylparaben, calcium benzoate, glycerin, hydroxypropyl methylcellulose, methylparaben, propylparaben, saccharin, simethicone, sorbitol solution, and water. *Tablets* contain a dried gel. The 0.3 Gm. (5 grain) strength is equivalent to about 1 teaspoonful of the suspension and the 0.6 Gm. (10 grain) strength is equivalent to about 2 teaspoonfuls. Each 0.3 Gm tablet contains 0.08 mEq of sodium and each 0.6 Gm tablet contains 0.13 mEq of sodium.

INDICATIONS

For the symptomatic relief of hyperacidity associated with the diagnosis of peptic ulcer, gastritis, peptic esophagitis, gastric hyperacidity, and hiatal hernia.

DOSAGE

Suspension—two teaspoonfuls followed by a sip of water if desired, five or six times daily, between meals and at bedtime. Two teaspoonfuls have the capacity to neutralize 20 mEq of acid. *Tablets*—Two tablets of the 0.3 Gm. strength, or one tablet of the 0.6 Gm. strength, five or six times daily between meals and at bedtime. Two tablets have the capacity to neutralize 16 mEq of acid.

WARNINGS

Patients are advised not to take more than 12 teaspoonfuls (60 ml) or twelve (12) 0.3 Gm tablets or six (6) 0.6 Gm tablets in a 24-hour period or use this maximum dosage for more than two weeks except under the advice and supervision of a physician. Prolonged use of aluminum-containing antacids in patients with renal failure may result in or worsen dialysis osteomalacia. Elevated tissue aluminum levels contribute to the development of dialysis encephalopathy and osteomalacia syndromes. Also, a number of cases of dialysis encephalopathy have been associated with elevated aluminum levels in the dialysate water. Small amounts of aluminum are absorbed from the gastrointestinal tract and reneal excretion of aluminum is impaired in renal failure. Prolonged use of aluminum-containing antacids in such patients may contribute to increased plasma levels of aluminum. Aluminum is not well removed by dialysis because it is bound to albumin and transferrin, which do not cross dialysis membranes. As a result, aluminum is deposited in bone, and dialysis osteomalacia may develop when large amounts of aluminum are ingested orally by patients with impaired renal function. Pregnant women and nursing mothers are advised to seek the advice of a health professional before using this product.

PRECAUTION

May cause constipation.

DRUG INTERACTION PRECAUTIONS

This product must not be taken if the patient is presently taking a prescription antibiotic drug containing any form of tetracycline.

HOW SUPPLIED

Suspension—Peppermint flavored; without flavor—bottles of 12 fluidounces. *Tablets*—a convenient auxiliary dosage form—0.3 Gm. (5 gr.), bottles of 100; 0.6 Gm. (10 gr.), boxes of 100.

ANTABUSE® ℞

[*an'tah-būse*]
(disulfiram)
In Alcoholism

Caution: Federal law prohibits dispensing without prescription.

> **WARNING**
> ANTABUSE should never be administered to a patient when he is in a state of alcohol intoxication, or without his full knowledge.
> The physician should instruct relatives accordingly.

DESCRIPTION
CHEMICAL NAME: bis(diethylthiocarbamoyl) disulfide
STRUCTURAL FORMULA:

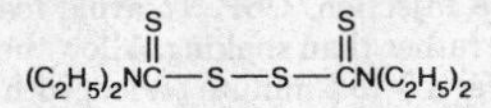

Antabuse occurs as a white to off-white, odorless, and almost tasteless powder, soluble in water to the extent of about 20 mg in 100 mL, and in alcohol to the extent of about 3.8 g in 100 mL.
Antabuse contains these inactive ingredients:
magnesium aluminum silicate;
magnesium stearate, NF.
povidone, USP;
starch, NF.

ACTION
Antabuse produces a sensitivity to alcohol which results in a highly unpleasant reaction when the patient under treatment ingests even small amounts of alcohol.
Antabuse blocks the oxidation of alcohol at the acetaldehyde stage. During alcohol metabolism following Antabuse intake, the concentration of acetaldehyde occurring in the blood may be 5- to 10-times higher than that found during metabolism of the same amount of alcohol alone.
Accumulation of acetaldehyde in the blood produces a complex of highly unpleasant symptoms referred to hereinafter as the Antabase-alcohol reaction. This reaction, which is proportional to the dosage of both Antabuse and alcohol, will persist as long as alcohol is being metabolized. Antabuse does not appear to influence the rate of alcohol elimination from the body.
Antabuse is absorbed slowly from the gastrointestinal tract and eliminated slowly from the body. One (or even two) weeks after a patient has taken his last dose of Antabuse, ingestion of alcohol may produce unpleasant symptoms.
Prolonged administration of Antabuse does not produce tolerance; the longer a patient remains on therapy, the more exquisitely sensitive he becomes to alcohol.

INDICATION
Antabuse is an aid in the management of selected chronic alcoholic patients who want to remain in a state of enforced sobriety so that supportive and psychotherapeutic treatment may be applied to best advantage. (Used alone, without proper motivation and supportive therapy, Antabuse is not a cure for alcoholism, and it is unlikely that it will have more than a brief effect on the drinking pattern of the chronic alcoholic.)

CONTRAINDICATIONS
Patients who are receiving or have recently received metronidazole, paraldehyde, alcohol, or alcohol-containing preparations, *e.g.*, cough syrups, tonics and the like, should not be given Antabuse.
Antabuse is contraindicated in the presence of severe myocardial disease or coronary occlusion, psychoses, and hypersensitivity to disulfiram or to other thiuram derivatives used in pesticides and rubber vulcanization.

WARNINGS

> ANTABUSE should never be administered to a patient when he is in a state of alcohol intoxication, or without his full knowledge.
> The physician should instruct relatives accordingly.

The patient must be fully informed of the Antabuse-alcohol reaction. He must be strongly cautioned against surreptitious drinking while taking the drug, and he must be fully aware of possible consequences. He should be warned to avoid alcohol in disguised form, *i.e.*, in sauces, vinegars, cough mixtures, and even aftershave lotions and back rubs. He should also be warned that reactions may occur with alcohol up to 14 days after ingesting Antabuse.
The ANTABUSE-ALCOHOL REACTION:
Antabuse plus alcohol, even small amounts, produces flushing, throbbing in head and neck, throbbing headache, respiratory difficulty, nausea, copious vomiting, sweating, thirst, chest pain, palpitation, dyspnea, hyperventilation, tachycardia, hypotension, syncope, marked uneasiness, weakness, vertigo, blurred vision, and confusion. In severe reactions there may be respiratory depression, cardiovascular collapse, arrhythmias, myocardial infarction, acute congestive heart failure, unconsciousness, convulsions, and death.
The intensity of the reaction varies with each individual but is generally proportional to the amounts of Antabuse and alcohol ingested. Mild reactions may occur in the sensitive individual when the blood alcohol concentration is increased to as little as 5 to 10 mg per 100 mL. Symptoms are fully developed at 50 mg per 100 mL and unconsciousness usually results when the blood alcohol level reaches 125 to 150 mg. The duration of the reaction varies from 30 to 60 minutes, to several hours in the more severe cases, or as long as there is alcohol in the blood.

DRUG INTERACTIONS:
Disulfiram appears to decrease the rate at which certain drugs are metabolized and therefore may increase the blood levels and the possibility of clinical toxicity of drugs given concomitantly.

DISULFIRAM SHOULD BE USED WITH CAUTION IN THOSE PATIENTS RECEIVING PHENYTOIN AND ITS CONGENERS, SINCE THE CONCOMITANT ADMINISTRATION OF THESE TWO DRUGS CAN LEAD TO PHENYTOIN INTOXICATION. PRIOR TO ADMINISTERING DISULFIRAM TO A PATIENT ON PHENYTOIN THERAPY, A BASELINE PHENYTOIN SERUM LEVEL SHOULD BE OBTAINED. SUBSEQUENT TO INITIATION OF DISULFIRAM THERAPY, SERUM LEVELS ON PHENYTOIN SHOULD BE DETERMINED ON DIFFERENT DAYS FOR EVIDENCE OF AN INCREASE OR FOR A CONTINUING RISE IN LEVELS. INCREASED PHENYTOIN LEVELS SHOULD BE TREATED WITH APPROPRIATE DOSAGE ADJUSTMENT.
It may be necessary to adjust the dosage of oral anticoagulants upon beginning or stopping disulfiram, since disulfiram may prolong prothrombin time.
Patients taking isoniazid when disulfiram is given should be observed for the appearance of unsteady gait or marked changes in mental status; the disulfiram should be discontinued if such signs appear.
In rats, simultaneous ingestion of disulfiram and nitrite in the diet for 78 weeks has been reported to cause tumors, and it has been suggested that disulfiram may react with nitrites in the rat stomach to form a nitrosamine, which is tumorigenic. Disulfiram alone in the rats' diet did not lead to such tumors. The relevance of this finding to humans is not known at this time.
CONCOMITANT CONDITIONS:
Because of the possibility of an accidental Antabuse-alcohol reaction, Antabuse should be used with extreme caution in patients with any of the following conditions: diabetes mellitus, hypothyroidism, epilepsy, cerebral damage, chronic and acute nephritis, hepatic cirrhosis or insufficiency.
USAGE IN PREGNANCY:
The safe use of this drug in pregnancy has not been established. Therefore, Antabuse should be used during pregnancy only when, in the judgment of the physician, the probable benefits outweigh the possible risks.

PRECAUTIONS
Patients with a history of rubber contact dermatitis should be evaluated for hypersensitivity to thiuram derivatives before receiving Antabuse (see **CONTRAINDICATIONS**).
It is suggested that every patient under treatment carry an Identification Card, stating that he is receiving Antabuse and describing the symptoms most likely to occur as a result of the Antabuse-alcohol reaction. In addition, this card should indicate the physician or institution to be contacted in emergency. (Cards may be obtained from Wyeth-Ayerst Laboratories upon request.)
Alcoholism may accompany or be followed by dependence on narcotics or sedatives. Barbiturates and Antabuse have been administered concurrently without untoward effects; the possibility of initiating a new abuse should be considered.
Baseline and follow-up transaminase tests (10 to 14 days) are suggested to detect any hepatic dysfunction that may result with Antabuse therapy. In addition, a complete blood count and a sequential multiple analysis-12 (SMA-12) test should be made every six months.
Patients taking Antabuse Tablets should not be exposed to ethylene dibromide or its vapors. This precaution is based on preliminary results of animal research currently in progress that suggest a toxic interaction between inhaled ethylene dibromide and ingested disulfiram resulting in a higher incidence of tumors and mortality in rats. A correlation between this finding and humans, however, has not been demonstrated.

ADVERSE REACTIONS
(See **CONTRAINDICATIONS, WARNINGS,** and **PRECAUTIONS.**)
OPTIC NEURITIS, PERIPHERAL NEURITIS, AND POLYNEURITIS MAY OCCUR FOLLOWING ADMINISTRATION OF ANTABUSE.
Multiple cases of both cholestatic and fulminant hepatitis have been reported to be associated with administration of Antabuse.
Occasional skin eruptions are, as a rule, readily controlled by concomitant administration of an antihistaminic drug.
In a small number of patients, a transient mild drowsiness, fatigability, impotence, headache, acneform eruptions, allergic dermatitis, or a metallic or garlic-like aftertaste may be experienced during the first two weeks of therapy. These complaints usually disappear spontaneously with the continuation of therapy, or with reduced dosage.
Psychotic reactions have been noted, attributable in most cases to high dosage, combined toxicity (with metronidazole or isoniazid), or to the unmasking of underlying psychoses in patients stressed by the withdrawal of alcohol.

DOSAGE AND ADMINISTRATION
Antabuse should never be administered until the patient has abstained from alcohol for at least 12 hours.
INITIAL DOSAGE SCHEDULE:
In the first phase of treatment, a maximum of 500 mg daily is given in a single dose for one to two weeks. Although usually taken in the morning, Antabuse may be taken on retiring by patients who experience a sedative effect. Alternatively, to minimize, or eliminate, the sedative effect, dosage may be adjusted downward.
MAINTENANCE REGIMEN:
The average maintenance dose is 250 mg daily (range, 125 to 500 mg); it should not exceed 500 mg daily.
NOTE: Occasionally patients, while seemingly on adequate maintenance doses of Antabuse, report that they are able to drink alcoholic beverages with impunity and without any symptomatology. All appearances to the contrary, such patients must be presumed to be disposing of their tablets in some manner without actually taking them. Until such patients have been observed reliably taking their daily Antabuse tablets (preferably crushed and well mixed with liquid), it cannot be concluded that Antabuse is ineffective.
DURATION OF THERAPY:
The daily, uninterrupted administration of Antabuse must be continued until the patient is fully recovered socially and a basis for permanent self-control is established. Depending on the individual patient, maintenance therapy may be required for months, or even years.
TRIAL WITH ALCOHOL:
During early experience with Antabuse, it was thought advisable for each patient to have at least one supervised alcohol-drug reaction. More recently, the test reaction has been largely abandoned. Furthermore, such a test reaction should never be administered to a patient over 50 years of age. A clear, detailed, and convincing description of the reaction is felt to be sufficient in most cases.
However, where a test reaction is deemed necessary, the suggested procedure is as follows:
After the first one to two weeks' therapy with 500 mg daily, a drink of 15 mL (½ oz) of 100 proof whiskey, or equivalent, is taken slowly. This test dose of alcoholic beverage may be repeated once only, so that the total dose does not exceed 30 mL (1 oz) of whiskey. Once a reaction develops, no more alcohol should be consumed. Such tests should be carried out only when the patient is hospitalized, or comparable supervision and facilities, including oxygen, are available.
MANAGEMENT OF ANTABUSE-ALCOHOL REACTION:
In severe reactions, whether caused by an excessive test dose or by the patient's unsupervised ingestion of alcohol, supportive measures to restore blood pressure and treat shock should be instituted. Other recommendations include: oxygen, carbogen (95% oxygen and 5% carbon dioxide), vitamin C intravenously in massive doses (1 g), and ephedrine sulfate. Antihistamines have also been used intravenously. Potassium levels should be monitored, particularly in patients on digitalis, since hypokalemia has been reported.

HOW SUPPLIED
Antabuse® (disulfiram) Tablets are available in the following dosage strengths:
250 mg, NDC 0046-0809-81, white-to-off-white, octagonal-shaped, scored, compressed tablet, embossed with a stylized "A" on one side and imprinted with "ANTABUSE" and "250" on the scored reverse side, in bottles of 100 tablets.
500 mg, NDC 0046-0810-50, white-to-off-white, octagonal-shaped, scored compressed tablet, embossed with a stylized "A" on one side and imprinted with "ANTABUSE" and "500" on the scored reverse side, in bottles of 50 tablets.
Shown in Product Identification Section, page 436

ANTIVENIN **(CROTALIDAE)** ℞
[*an"te ven'in*]
POLYVALENT
(equine origin)

IMPORTANT
Pit viper bites may cause severe tissue damage or fatal envenomation, or both. The physician responsible for treatment of an envenomated patient should be familiar with the contents of this brochure and the pertinent medical literature concerning current concepts of first-aid and general supportive therapy as presented in the references listed at the end of this pamphlet.

Continued on next page

Wyeth-Ayerst Laboratories—Cont.

COMPOSITION

Antivenin (Crotalidae) Polyvalent, Wyeth, is a refined and concentrated preparation of serum globulins obtained by fractionating blood from healthy horses immunized with the following venoms: *Crotalus adamanteus* (Eastern diamond rattlesnake), *C. atrox* (Western diamond rattlesnake), *C. durissus terrificus* (tropical rattlesnake, Cascabel), and *Bothrops atrox* ("Fer-de-lance"). Phenol, 0.25%, and thimerosal, 0.005%, are added as preservatives. The product is standardized by its ability to neutralize the lethal action of standard venoms by intravenous injection in mice.[1] Dried from the frozen state, the lyophilized serum has a moisture content of less than 1% and is soluble on addition of the diluent contained in each package (Bacteriostatic Water for Injection, USP, with preservative: 0.001% phenylmercuric nitrate).

Antivenin (Crotalidae) Polyvalent, Wyeth (hereinafter referred to as Antivenin) contains protective substances capable of neutralizing the toxic effects of venoms of crotalids (pit vipers) native to North, Central, and South America, including rattlesnakes *(Crotalus, Sistrurus)*; copperhead and cottonmouth moccasins *(Agkistrodon)*, including *A. halys* of Korea and Japan; the Fer-de-lance and other species of *Bothrops*; the tropical rattler (*Crotalus durissus* and similar species); the Cantil *(A. bilineatus)*; and bushmaster *(Lachesis mutus)* of South and Central America.

INDICATION

Antivenin is indicated only for the treatment of envenomation caused by bites of those crotalids (pit vipers) specified in the immediately preceding paragraph.

PIT VIPER BITES AND ENVENOMATION

The symptoms, signs, and severity of snake-venom poisoning resulting from pit viper bites depend on many factors, including, but not limited to, the following variables: species, age, and size of the biting snake; the number and location of bite(s); the depth of venom deposit by the snake's fangs; the condition of the snake's fangs and venom glands; the length of time the snake "hangs on"; the age, general health, and size of the victim; the type and efficacy of any first-aid treatment rendered in an attempt to remove venom and how soon such treatment was applied. In any venomous snake bite, the actual amount of venom introduced into the victim is always an unknown. Even the type of clothing or leg-footwear through which the snake's fangs pass may affect the amount of venom delivered by the bite. Although most North American pit vipers tend to bite and introduce venom superficially, their fangs may get hung-up in the subcutaneous tissues during the biting act and can penetrate deeper tissues during the attempt to release the bitten part. In some bites the fangs may penetrate into muscle. In such cases, the usual local superficial manifestations of envenomation may not appear early in the course of poisoning. In bites by some species, systemic evidence of envenomation may be present in the absence of significant local manifestations. It may be difficult to determine the severity of envenomation during the first several hours after a pit viper bite and estimates of severity may need to be revised as poisoning progresses. It must be remembered, too, that not all pit viper bites result in envenomation. In approximately 20% of rattlesnake bites, the snake may not inject any venom. The local and systemic symptoms and signs of envenomation include the following:

LOCAL:

Fang puncture(s).

Swelling—edema is usually seen around the site of bite within five minutes. It may progress rapidly and involve the entire extremity within an hour. More than 95% of all snakebites are inflicted on extremities.[2] Generally, however, edema spreads more slowly, usually over a period of 8 or more hours. Swelling is usually most severe following envenomation by the Eastern diamondback; less severe after bites by the Western diamondback, prairie, timber, red, Pacific, Mojave, and blacktailed rattlers, the sidewinder and cottonmouth moccasins; least severe after bites by copperheads, massasaugas, and pygmy rattlers.

Ecchymosis and discoloration of the skin—often appear in the area of the bite within a few hours. Vesicules may form within a few hours and are usually present at 24 hours. Hemorrhagic blebs and petechiae are common. Necrosis may develop, necessitating amputation of an extremity or a portion thereof.

Pain—frequently a complaint of the victim beginning shortly after the bite by most pit vipers. Pain may be absent after bites by Mojave rattlers.

SYSTEMIC:

Weakness; faintness; nausea; sweating; numbness or tingling around the mouth, tongue, scalp, fingers, toes, site of bite; muscle fasciculations; hypotension; prolongation of bleeding and clotting times; hemoconcentration, early followed by a decrease in erythrocytes; thrombocytopenia; hematuria; proteinuria; vomiting, including hematemesis; melena; hemoptysis; epistaxis. In fatal poisoning, a frequent cause of death is associated with destruction of erythrocytes and changes in capillary permeability, especially of the pulmonary vascular system, leading to pulmonary edema; hemoconcentration usually occurs early, probably as a result of plasma loss secondary to vascular permeability; the hemoglobin may fall, and bleeding may occur throughout the body as early as 6 hours after the bite. Renal involvement is not uncommon. Mojave rattler venom may cause neuromuscular changes leading to respiratory failure.

An estimate of the severity of envenomation should be made as soon as possible and before any Antivenin is administered. The amount (volume) of the first dose of Antivenin is determined on this estimate of severity. Every symptom, sign, laboratory-test result, and any other pertinent information should be considered in estimating severity—local manifestations; systemic manifestations, including abnormal laboratory findings; species and size of the biting snake, if known; number and location of bite(s); size and health of the patient; type of first-aid treatment rendered; and interval between bite and arrival for treatment. Russell et al,[3] and Wingert and Wainschel[4] grade severity as follows:

No envenomation—no local or systemic manifestations.

Minimal envenomation—local swelling and other local changes; no systemic manifestations; normal laboratory findings.

Moderate envenomation—swelling progressing beyond the site of bite and one or more systemic manifestations; abnormal laboratory findings, for example, a fall in hematocrit or platelets.

Severe envenomation—marked local response, severe systemic manifestations and significant alteration in laboratory findings.

Parrish and Hayes,[5] McCollough and Gennaro,[6] and Watt and Gennaro[7] have used a Grade 0 (no envenomation) through Grade IV (very severe) classification of severity which was developed for the most part in treatment of envenomation by the Eastern diamondback and timber rattlers. This classification is more dependent on local manifestations, or the absence thereof, as the venoms of these species seem to be more consistent in inducing local tissue damage.

Any suspected envenomation should be treated as a medical emergency, and until careful observation provides clear evidence that envenomation has not occurred or is minimal, the following procedures are recommended:

Monitor vital signs at frequent intervals: Blood pressure, pulse, respiration.

Draw sufficient blood as soon as possible for baseline laboratory studies, including type and cross-match, CBC, hematocrit, platelet count, prothrombin time, clot retraction, bleeding and coagulation times, BUN, electrolytes, bilirubin. Some of these studies may need to be repeated at daily intervals, or less, depending on the severity of envenomation and the response to treatment. During the first 4 or 5 days of severe envenomations, hemoglobin, hematocrit, and platelet counts should be carried out several times a day.

Obtain urine samples at frequent intervals for analysis, with special attention to microscopic examination for presence of erythrocytes.

Chart fluid intake and urine output.

Measure and record the circumference of the bitten extremity just proximal to the bite and at one or more additional points each several inches closer to the trunk. Repeat measurements every 15-30 minutes to obtain information about progression of edema.

Have available and ready for immediate use: oxygen, resuscitation equipment including airway, tourniquet, epinephrine, injectable antihistaminic agents and corticosteroids.

Start an intravenous infusion in one or two extremities: one line to be used for supportive therapy, if needed, such as whole blood, plasma, packed red cells, specific clotting factors, platelet transfusion, plasma expanders; the other line to be used for administration of Antivenin and electrolytes.

Carry out and interpret a skin test for horse-serum sensitivity. (See "Precautions" section below.)

DOSAGE AND ADMINISTRATION

Before administration, read "Precautions" and "Systemic Reactions" sections below. Since the possibility of a severe immediate reaction (anaphylaxis) exists whenever a horse-serum-containing product is administered, appropriate therapeutic agents, including a tourniquet, airway, oxygen, epinephrine, an injectable pressor amine, and corticosteroid, must be available and ready for immediate use. Constant attendance and observation of the patient for untoward reactions are mandatory when Antivenin is administered. Should any systemic reaction occur, administration should be discontinued immediately and appropriate treatment initiated.

The intravenous route of administration is preferred, and probably should always be used for moderate or severe envenomation. Intravenous administration is mandatory if venom-induced shock is present. To be most effective, Antivenin should be administered within 4 hours of the bite; it is less effective when given after 8 hours and may be of questionable value after 12 hours. However, it is recommended that Antivenin therapy be given in severe poisonings, even if 24 hours have elapsed since the time of the bite. It should be kept in mind that maximum blood levels of Antivenin may not be obtained for 8 or more hours after intramuscular administration.

For intravenous-drip use, prepare a 1:1 to 1:10 dilution of reconstituted Antivenin in Sodium Chloride Injection, USP, or 5% Dextrose Injection, USP. To avoid foaming, mix by gently swirling rather than shaking. Allow the initial 5 to 10 mL to infuse over a 3- to 5-minute period, with careful observation of the patient for evidence of untoward reaction. If no symptoms or signs of an immediate systemic reaction appear, continue the infusion with delivery at the maximum safe rate for intravenous fluid administration. The dilution of Antivenin to be used, the type of electrolyte solution used for dilution, and the rate of intravenous delivery of the diluted Antivenin must take into consideration the age, weight, and cardiac status of the patient; the severity of envenomation; the total amount and type of parenteral fluids it is anticipated will be given or are needed; and the interval between bite and initiation of specific therapy.

It is important to give as soon as possible the entire initial dose of Antivenin as based on the best estimate of the severity of envenomation at the time treatment is begun. The following initial doses are recommended:[3,4,8]

no envenomation—none

minimal envenomation—20-40 mL (contents of 2 to 4 vials)

moderate envenomation—50-90 mL (contents of 5 to 9 vials)

severe envenomation—100-150 mL or more (contents of 10 to 15 or more vials)

These recommended initial-dosage volumes are in general accord with those of others.[5-7,9]

The need for additional Antivenin must be based on the clinical response to the initial dose and continuing assessment of the severity of poisoning. If swelling continues to progress or if systemic symptoms or signs of envenomation increase in severity or if new manifestations appear, for example, fall in hematocrit or hypotension, administer an additional 10 to 50 mL (contents of 1 to 5 vials) intravenously.

Envenomation by large snakes in children or small adults requires larger doses of Antivenin. The amount administered to a child is not based on weight.

If Antivenin is given intramuscularly, it should be given into a large muscle mass, preferably the gluteal area, with care to avoid nerve trunks. Antivenin should never be injected into a finger or toe.

The effectiveness of corticosteroids in treatment of envenomation per se or venom shock is not resolved. Russell[3] and others[9,10] believe corticosteroids may mask the seriousness of hypovolemia in moderate or severe poisoning and have little, if any, effect on the local-tissue response to rattler venoms. Corticosteroids should not be given simultaneously with Antivenin on a routine basis or during the acute state of envenomation; however, their use may be necessary to treat immediate allergic reactions to Antivenin, and corticosteroids are the agents of choice for treating serious delayed reactions to Antivenin.

Snakes' mouths do not harbor *Clostridium tetani.* However, appropriate tetanus prophylaxis is indicated, since tetanus spores may be carried into the fang puncture wounds by dirt present on skin at time of bite or by nonsterile first-aid procedures.

A broad-spectrum antibiotic in adequate dosage is indicated if local tissue damage is evident.

Shock following envenomation is treated like shock resulting from hypovolemia from any cause, including administration of whole blood, plasma, albumin, or other plasma expanders, as indicated.

Aspirin or codeine is usually adequate for relieving pain. Sedation with phenobarbital or mild tranquilizers may be used if indicated, but not in the presence of respiratory failure.

The bitten extremity should not be packed in ice, and so-called "cryotherapy" is contraindicated.

Compartment syndromes may complicate pit viper envenomations, especially those caused by bites on the lower extremities. Prompt surgical consultation is indicated whenever a closed-compartment syndrome is suspected.[3,12]

Defibrination and disseminated intravascular coagulation (DIC) syndromes have been associated with envenomation caused by some pit vipers native to the United States, and appropriate therapy may be indicated.[3,9,10,13-17]

TECHNIC FOR RECONSTITUTING THE DRIED ANTIVENIN

Pry off the small metal disc in the cap over the diaphragms of the vials of Antivenin and diluent. Swab the exposed surface of the rubber diaphragms of both vials with an appropriate germicide. With a sterile 10 mL syringe and needle, withdraw the diluent (Bacteriostatic Water for Injection, USP, containing phenylmercuric nitrate 1:100,000) from the vial of diluent and inject it into the vial of Antivenin. Gentle agitation will hasten complete dissolution of the lyophilized Antivenin.

PRECAUTIONS

Before administration of any product prepared from horse serum, appropriate measures must be taken in an effort to

detect the presence of dangerous sensitivity: (1) A careful review of the patient's history, including any report of (a) asthma, hay fever, urticaria, or other allergic manifestations; (b) allergic reactions upon exposure to horses; and (c) prior injections of horse serum. (2) A suitable test for detection of sensitivity. A skin test should be performed in every patient prior to administration, regardless of clinical history.

Skin test—Inject intracutaneously 0.02 to 0.03 mL of a 1:10 dilution of Normal Horse Serum or Antivenin. A control test on the opposite extremity, using Sodium Chloride Injection, USP, facilitates interpretation. Use of larger amounts for the skin-test dose increases the likelihood of false-positive reactions, and in the exquisitely sensitive patient, increases the risk of a systemic reaction from the skin-test dose. A 1:100 or greater dilution should be used for preliminary skin testing if the history suggests sensitivity. A positive reaction to a skin test occurs within five to thirty minutes and is manifested by a wheal with or without pseudopodia and surrounding erythema. In general, the shorter the interval between injection and the beginning of the skin reaction, the greater the sensitivity.

If the history is negative for allergy and the result of a skin test is negative, proceed with administration of Antivenin as outlined above. If the history is positive and a skin test is strongly positive, administration may be dangerous, especially if the positive sensitivity test is accompanied by systemic allergic manifestations. In such instances, the risk of administering Antivenin must be weighed against the risk of withholding it, keeping in mind that severe envenomation can be fatal. (See last paragraph of this section.)

A negative allergic history and absence of reaction to a properly applied skin test do not rule out the possibility of an immediate reaction. Also, a negative skin test has no bearing on whether or not delayed serum reactions (serum sickness) will occur after administration of the full dose.

If the history is negative, and the skin test is mildly or questionably positive, administer as follows to reduce the risk of a severe immediate systemic reaction: (a) Prepare, in separate sterile vials or syringes, 1:100 and 1:10 dilutions of Antivenin. (b) Allow at least 15 minutes between injections and proceed with the next dose if no reaction follows the previous dose. (c) Inject subcutaneously, using a tuberculin-type syringe, 0.1, 0.2, and 0.5 mL of the 1:100 dilution at 15-minute intervals; repeat with the 1:10 dilution, and finally undiluted Antivenin. (d) If a systemic reaction occurs after any injection, place a tourniquet proximal to the site of injections and administer an appropriate dose of epinephrine, 1:1000, proximal to the tourniquet or into another extremity. Wait at least 30 minutes before injecting another dose. The amount of the next dose should be the same as the last that did not evoke a reaction. (e) If no reaction occurs after 0.5 mL of undiluted Antivenin has been administered, switch to the intramuscular route and continue doubling the dose at 15-minute intervals until the entire dose has been injected intramuscularly or proceed to the intravenous route as described above under "Dosage and Administration."

Obviously, if the just-described schedule is used, 3 to 5 or more hours would be required to administer the initial dose suggested for a moderate or severe envenomation, and time is an important factor in neutralization of venom in a critically ill patient. Wingert and Wainschel[4] have described a procedure based on the experience of their group which they have used in some severely envenomated patients who have positive sensitivity tests: 50 to 100 mg of diphenhydramine hydrochloride is given intravenously, followed by slow intravenous infusion of diluted Antivenin for 15 to 20 minutes while carefully observing the patient for symptoms and signs of anaphylaxis; if anaphylaxis does not occur, Antivenin is continued, maintaining close observation of the patient. Patients who require Antivenin but develop signs of impending anaphylaxis in spite of this or the procedure described earlier present a difficult problem, and consultation should be sought.

SYSTEMIC REACTIONS

A. The immediate reaction (shock, anaphylaxis) usually occurs within 30 minutes. Symptoms and signs may develop before the needle is withdrawn and may include apprehension, flushing, itching, urticaria; edema of the face, tongue, and throat; cough, dyspnea, cyanosis, vomiting, and collapse.

B. Serum sickness usually occurs 5 to 24 days after administration. The incubation period may be less than 5 days, especially in those who have received horse-serum-containing preparations in the past. The usual symptoms and signs are malaise, fever, urticaria, lymphadenopathy, edema, arthralgia, nausea, and vomiting. Occasionally, neurological manifestations develop, such as meningismus or peripheral neuritis. Peripheral neuritis usually involves the shoulders and arms. Pain and muscle weakness are frequently present, and permanent atrophy may develop.

REFERENCES

1. GINGRICH, W. & HOHENADEL, J.: Standardization of polyvalent antivenin. "Venoms", edited by E. Buckley and N. Porges. Publication No. 44, Amer. Assoc. for the Advancement of Science, Washington, D.C., 1956, Pages 337–80.
2. PARRISH, H.: Incidence of treated snakebite in the United States. Pub. Hlth. Rep. *81*:269, 1966.
3. RUSSELL, F., et al.: Snake venom poisoning in the United States. Experiences with 550 cases. JAMA *233*:341, 1975. RUSSELL, F.: Venomous bites and stings: Poisonous snakes. In The Merck Manual of Diagnosis and Therapy, pp. 2450–2456, 14th Ed., 1982.
4. WINGERT, W. and WAINSCHEL, J.: Diagnosis and management of envenomation by poisonous snakes. South. Med. J. *68*:1015, 1975.
5. PARRISH, H. & HAYES, R.: Hospital management of pit viper venenations. Clinical Toxicol. *3*:501, 1970.
6. McCOLLOUGH, N. & GENNARO, J.: Diagnosis, symptoms, treatment and sequelae of envenomation by *Crotalus adamanteus* and Genus *Agkistrodon*. J. Florida Med. Assoc. *55*:327, 1968.
7. WATT, C. & GENNARO, J.: Pit viper bites in South Georgia and North Florida. Tr. South. Surg. Assoc. *77*:378, 1966.
8. MINTON, S.: Venom Diseases: Snakebite. In Textbook of Medicine, P. Beeson and W. McDermott (Eds.), pp. 88–92; Saunders, Philadelphia, 1975.
9. VAN MIEROP, L.: Snakebite symposium. J. Florida Med. Assoc. *63*:101, 1976.
10. ARNOLD, R.: Treatment of snakebite. JAMA *236*:1843, 1976; Controversies and hazards in the treatment of pit viper bites. South Med. J. *72*:902, 1979.
11. Poisonous Snakes of the World. U.S. Government Printing Office, Washington, D.C., NAVMED, 1965.
12. GARFIN, S. et al.: Rattlesnake bites: Current concepts. Clin. Orthop. *140*:50, 1979; Role of surgical decompression in treatment of rattlesnake bites. Surg. Forum *30*:502, 1979.
13. VAN MIEROP, L. & KITCHENS, C.: Defibrination syndrome following bites by the Eastern diamondback rattlesnake. J. Florida Med. Assoc. *67*:21, 1980.
14. HASIBA, U. et al.: DIC-like syndrome after envenomation by the snake, *Crotalus horridus horridus*. New Eng. J. Med. *292*:505, 1975.
15. WEISS, H. et al.: Afibrinogenemia in man following the bite of a rattlesnake *(Crotalus adamanteus)*. Am. J. Med. *47*:625, 1969.
16. SIVAPRASAD, R. & CANTINI, E.: Western diamondback rattlesnake *(Crotalus atrox)* poisoning. Postgrad. Med. *71*:223, 1982.
17. SABBACK, M. et al.: A study of the treatment of pit viper envenomization in 45 patients. J. Trauma *17*:569, 1977.

HOW SUPPLIED

Each combination package contains one vacuum vial to yield 10 mL of serum—to be used immediately after reconstitution—(with preservatives: phenol 0.25% and thimerosal [mercury derivative] 0.005%). One vial containing 10 mL of Bacteriostatic Water for Injection, USP (with preservative: phenylmercuric nitrate 0.001%). One 1 mL vial of normal horse serum (diluted 1:10) as sensitivity testing material with preservatives: thimerosal (mercury derivative) 0.005% and phenol 0.35%. Not returnable.

ANTIVENIN (Micrurus fulvius) ℞

[an"te ven'in]
(equine origin)
North American Coral Snake Antivenin

COMPOSITION

Each combination package contains one vial of lyophilized Antivenin (Micrurus fulvius) with 0.25% phenol and 0.005% thimerosal (mercury derivative) as preservatives (before lyophilization); one vial of diluent containing 10 ml. of Bacteriostatic Water for Injection, U.S.P., with phenylmercuric nitrate (1:100,000) as preservative.

HOW SUPPLIED

Combination packages as described (not returnable).

For prescribing information write to Professional Service, Wyeth-Ayerst Laboratories, P.O. Box 8299, Philadelphia, PA 19101, or contact your local Wyeth-Ayerst representative.

A.P.L.® ℞

(chorionic gonadotropin for injection, USP)
For Intramuscular Injection Only

CAUTION: Federal law prohibits dispensing without prescription.

DESCRIPTION

Human chorionic gonadotropin (HCG), a polypeptide hormone produced by the human placenta, is composed of an alpha and a beta subunit. The alpha subunit is essentially identical to the alpha subunits of the human pituitary gonadotropins, luteinizing hormone (LH) and follicle-stimulating hormone (FSH), as well as to the alpha subunit of human thyroid stimulating hormone (TSH). The beta subunits of these hormones differ in amino acid sequence.

A.P.L. (chorionic gonadotropin, USP) is a gonad-stimulating principle obtained from the urine of pregnant women. It is a sterile, amorphous powder prepared by cryodesiccation, and is freely soluble in water.

When reconstituted with the accompanying 10 mL of sterile diluent water, each SECULE® vial contains:

5,000 USP units of chorionic gonadotropin, 2.0% benzyl alcohol, 0.9% lactose, and not more than 0.2% phenol;
10,000 USP units of chorionic gonadotropin, 2.0% benzyl alcohol, 1.8% lactose, and not more than 0.2% phenol;
20,000 USP units of chorionic gonadotropin, 2.0% benzyl alcohol, 3.6% lactose, and not more than 0.2% phenol.

The pH is adjusted with sodium hydroxide or hydrochloric acid.

After reconstitution, store refrigerated and use within 30 days.

THIS PRODUCT IS FOR INTRAMUSCULAR INJECTION ONLY.

CLINICAL PHARMACOLOGY

The action of HCG is virtually identical to that of pituitary LH, although HCG appears to have a small degree of FSH activity as well. It stimulates production of gonadal steroid hormones by stimulating the interstitial cells (Leydig cells) of the testis to produce androgens and the corpus luteum of the ovary to produce progesterone. Androgen stimulation in the male leads to the development of secondary sex characteristics and may stimulate testicular descent when no anatomical impediment to descent is present. This descent is usually reversible when HCG is discontinued. During the normal menstrual cycle, LH participates with FSH in the development and maturation of the normal ovarian follicle, and the midcycle LH surge triggers ovulation. HCG can substitute for LH in this function.

During a normal pregnancy, HCG secreted by the placenta maintains the corpus luteum after LH secretion decreases, supporting continued secretion of estrogen and progesterone, and preventing menstruation. HCG HAS NO KNOWN EFFECT ON FAT MOBILIZATION, APPETITE OR SENSE OF HUNGER, OR BODY FAT DISTRIBUTION.

Following intramuscular injection, a detectable rise in serum HCG levels is seen in 2 hours; peak levels are reached in 6 hours and remain at this level for 36 hours. HCG levels begin to decline at 48 hours and approach baseline (undetectable) levels at 72 hours.

INDICATIONS AND USAGE

HCG HAS NOT BEEN DEMONSTRATED TO BE EFFECTIVE ADJUNCTIVE THERAPY IN THE TREATMENT OF OBESITY. THERE IS NO SUBSTANTIAL EVIDENCE THAT IT INCREASES WEIGHT LOSS BEYOND THAT RESULTING FROM CALORIC RESTRICTION, THAT IT CAUSES A MORE ATTRACTIVE OR "NORMAL" DISTRIBUTION OF FAT, OR THAT IT DECREASES THE HUNGER AND DISCOMFORT ASSOCIATED WITH CALORIE RESTRICTED DIETS.

1. Cryptorchidism not due to anatomic obstruction. In general, A.P.L. is thought to induce testicular descent in situations when descent would have occurred at puberty. A.P.L. thus may help to predict whether or not orchiopexy will be needed in the future. Although, in some cases, descent following A.P.L. administration is permanent, in most cases the response is temporary. Therapy is usually instituted between the ages of 4 and 9.
2. Selected cases of male hypogonadism secondary to pituitary failure.
3. Induction of ovulation and pregnancy in the anovulatory, infertile woman in whom the cause of anovulation is secondary and not due to ovarian failure, and who has been appropriately pretreated with human menotropins.

CONTRAINDICATIONS

Precocious puberty.

Prostatic carcinoma or other androgen-dependent neoplasia.

Prior allergic reaction to chorionic gonadotropin.

Pregnancy. A.P.L. may cause fetal harm when administered to a pregnant woman. Combined HCG/PMS (pregnant mare's serum) therapy has been noted to induce high incidences of external congenital anomalies in the offspring of mice, in a dose-dependent manner. The potential extrapolation to humans has not been determined.

WARNINGS

HCG should be used in conjunction with human menopausal gonadotropins only by physicians experienced with infertility problems who are familiar with the criteria for patient selection, contraindications, warnings, precautions, and adverse reactions described in the package insert for menotropins. The principal serious adverse reactions during this use are: (1) ovarian hyperstimulation, a syndrome of sudden ovarian enlargement, ascites with or without pain, and/or

Continued on next page

Wyeth-Ayerst Laboratories—Cont.

pleural effusion; (2) enlargement of preexisiting ovarian cysts or rupture of ovarian cysts with resultant hemoperitoneum; (3) multiple births; and (4) arterial thromboembolism secondary to hyperestrogenism.

PRECAUTIONS

GENERAL: Induction of androgen secretion by chorionic gonadotropin may induce phallic enlargement; testicular enlargement and redness; development of pubic hair; aggressive behavior. These changes are reversible within four weeks of the last injection.

Since androgens may cause fluid retention, chorionic gonadotropin should be used with caution in patients with epilepsy, migraine, asthma, cardiac or renal disease.

LABORATORY TESTS: In adult males and females, the following hormone levels may be monitored depending on the nature of the diagnostic and therapeutic purpose: testosterone, dihydrotestosterone, 17β-estradiol, 17β-hydroxyprogesterone, progesterone, androstenedione. In prepubertal males, testosterone and dihydrotestosterone should be followed.

DRUG/LABORATORY TEST INTERACTIONS: HCG can crossreact in the radioimmunoassay of gonadotropins, especially luteinizing hormone. Each individual laboratory should establish the degree of crossreactivity with their gonadotropin assay. Physicians should make the laboratory aware of patients on HCG if gonadotropin levels are requested.

CARCINOGENESIS, MUTAGENESIS, IMPAIRMENT OF FERTILITY: There have been sporadic reports of testicular tumors in otherwise healthy young men receiving HCG for secondary infertility. A causative relationship between HCG and tumor development in these men has not been established.

Defects of forelimbs and of the central nervous system, as well as alterations in sex ratio, have been reported in mice on combined gonadotropin and HCG regimens. The dose of gonadotropin used was intended to induce superovulation. No mutagenic effect has been clearly established in humans. Fertility—see "Indications and Usage."

PREGNANCY: Teratogenic effects—Category X. See "Contraindications" section. Combined HCG/PMS (pregnant mare's serum) therapy has been noted to induce high incidences of external congenital anomalies in the offspring of mice, in a dose-dependent manner. The potential extrapolation to humans has not bee determined.

NURSING MOTHERS: It is not known whether this drug is excreted in human milk. Because many drugs are excreted in human milk, caution should be exercised when HCG is administered to a nursing woman.

PEDIATRIC USE: Safety and effectiveness in children below the age of 4 have not been established.

ADVERSE REACTIONS

Central Nervous System: Headache, Irritability, Restlessness, Depression, Tiredness, Aggressive behavior.

Body as a Whole: Edema.

Urogenital: Precocious puberty, Gynecomastia, Ovarian hyperstimulation syndrome, Enlargement of preexisting ovarian cysts and possible rupture, Phallic or testicular enlargement, Growth of pubic hair, Signs or symptoms of androgen excess.

Cardiovascular: Arterial thromboembolism.

Other: Pain at site of injection.

OVERDOSAGE

There is no experience to date with deliberate overdosage of A.P.L.

Treatment must be symptomatic and supportive.

DOSAGE AND ADMINISTRATION

Parenteral drug products should be inspected visually for particulate matter and discoloration prior to administration, whenever solution and container permit.

(Intramuscular Use Only): the dosage regimen to be used will depend upon the indication for use, the age and weight of the patient, and the physician's preference. The following regimens have been advocated by various authorities.

Cryptorchidism: (Therapy is usually instituted between the ages of 4 and 9.)

(1) 4,000 USP Units three times weekly for three weeks.

(2) 5,000 USP Units every second day for four injections.

(3) 15 injections of 500 to 1,000 USP Units over a period of six weeks.

(4) 500 USP Units three times weekly for four to six weeks. If this course of treatment is not successful, another is begun one month later, giving 1,000 USP Units per injection.

Selected cases of male hypogonadism secondary to pituitary failure:

(1) 500 to 1,000 USP Units three times a week for three weeks, followed by the same dose twice a week for three weeks.

(2) 1,000 to 2,000 USP Units three times weekly.

(3) 4,000 USP Units three times weekly for six to nine months, following which the dosage may be reduced to 2,000 USP Units three times weekly for an additional three months.

Induction of ovulation and pregnancy in the anovulatory, infertile woman in whom the cause of anovulation is not due to primary ovarian failure and who has been appropriately pretreated with human menotropins: (See prescribing information for menotropin dosage and administration of that drug product.)

5,000 to 10,000 USP units one day following the last dose of menotropins. (A dosage of 10,000 USP units is recommended in the labeling for menotropins.)

IMPORTANT: STORE IN REFRIGERATOR (APPROXIMATELY 4° C) PRIOR TO RECONSTITUTION. AFTER RECONSTITUTION, KEEP REFRIGERATED AND USE WITHIN 30 DAYS.

HOW SUPPLIED

A.P.L. (Chorionic Gonadotropin for Injection, USP)

NDC 0046-0970-10 — Each package provides:

(1) One vial containing 5,000 USP Units chorionic gonadotropin in dry form, and

(2) One 10 mL ampul sterile diluent.

NDC 0046-0971-10 — Each package provides:

(1) One vial containing 10,000 USP Units chorionic gonadotropin in dry form, and

(2) One 10 mL ampul sterile diluent.

NDC 0046-0972-10 — Each package provides:

(1) One vial containing 20,000 USP Units chorionic gonadotropin in dry form, and

(2) One 10 mL ampul sterile diluent.

The product is assayed in accord with USP method; USP potency units are defined in terms of the USP Chorionic Gonadotropin Reference Standard.

When reconstituted with 10 mL of accompanying sterile diluent, the resulting solutions also contain 2.0% benzyl alcohol, not more than 0.2% phenol, and the following concentrations of lactose: No. 970, 0.9%; No. 971, 1.8%; No. 972, 3.6%. The pH is adjusted with sodium hydroxide or hydrochloric acid.

DIRECTIONS FOR RECONSTITUTION

Withdraw sterile air from lyophilized vial and inject into sterile diluent vial. Remove 10 mL from diluent vial and add to lyophilized vial; agitate gently until powder is completely dissolved.

MAY BE STORED FOR 30 DAYS IN A REFRIGERATOR AFTER RECONSTITUTION.

ATIVAN® ℂ ℞

[at 'i-van]
(lorazepam)
Injection

DESCRIPTION

Ativan (lorazepam) Injection, a benzodiazepine with antianxiety and sedative effects, is intended for intramuscular or intravenous route of administration. It has the chemical formula: 7-chloro-5-(*o*-chlorophenyl)-1,3-dihydro-3-hydroxy-2*H*-1,4-benzodiazepin-2-one. The molecular weight is 321.2, and the C.A.S. No. is [846-49-1].

Lorazepam is a nearly white powder almost insoluble in water. Each mL of sterile injection contains either 2.0 or 4.0 mg of lorazepam, 0.18 mL polyethylene glycol 400 in propylene glycol with 2.0% benzyl alcohol as preservative.

CLINICAL PHARMACOLOGY

Intravenous or intramuscular administration of the recommended dose of 2 to 4 mg of Ativan (lorazepam) Injection to adult patients is followed by dose-related effects of sedation (sleepiness or drowsiness), relief of preoperative anxiety, and lack of recall of events related to the day of surgery in the majority of patients. The clinical sedation (sleepiness or drowsiness) thus noted is such that the majority of patients are able to respond to simple instructions whether they give the appearance of being awake or asleep. The lack of recall is relative rather than absolute, as determined under conditions of careful patient questioning and testing, using props designed to enhance recall. The majority of patients under these reinforced conditions had difficulty recalling perioperative events or recognizing props from before surgery. The lack of recall and recognition was optimum within 2 hours following intramuscular administration and 15 to 20 minutes after intravenous injection.

The intended effects of the recommended adult dose of lorazepam injection usually last 6 to 8 hours. In rare instances and where patients received greater than the recommended dose, excessive sleepiness and prolonged lack of recall were noted. As with other benzodiazepines, unsteadiness, enhanced sensitivity to CNS-depressant effects of ethyl alcohol and other drugs were noted in isolated and rare cases for greater than 24 hours.

Studies in healthy adult volunteers reveal that intravenous lorazepam in doses up to 3.5 mg/70 kg does not alter sensitivity to the respiratory stimulating effect of carbon dioxide and does not enhance the respiratory depressant effects of doses of meperidine up to 100 mg/70 kg (also determined by carbon dioxide challenge) as long as patients remain sufficiently awake to undergo testing. Upper airway obstruction has been observed in rare instances where the patient received greater than the recommended dose and was excessively sleepy and difficult to arouse. (See "Warnings" and "Adverse Reactions".)

Clinically employed doses of lorazepam injectable do not greatly affect the circulatory system in the supine position or employing a 70-degree tilt test. Doses of 8 mg to 10 mg of intravenous lorazepam (2 to 2½ times the maximum recommended dosage) will produce loss of lid reflexes within 15 minutes.

Studies in six (6) healthy young adults who received lorazepam injection and no other drugs revealed that visual tracking (the ability to keep a moving line centered) was impaired for a mean of eight (8) hours following administration of 4 mg of intramuscular lorazepam and four (4) hours following administration of 2 mg intramuscularly with considerable subject variation. Similar findings were noted with pentobarbital, 150 and 75 mg. Although this study showed that both lorazepam and pentobarbital interfered with eye-hand coordination, the data are insufficient to predict when it would be safe to operate a motor vehicle or engage in a hazardous occupation or sport.

PHARMACOKINETICS

Injectable Ativan (lorazepam) is readily absorbed when given intramuscularly. Peak plasma concentrations occur approximately 60 to 90 minutes following administration and appear to be dose-related, e.g., a 2.0 mg dose provides a level of approximately 20 ng/mL and a 4.0 mg dose approximately 40 ng/mL in plasma. The mean half-life of lorazepam is about 16 hours when given intravenously or intramuscularly. Ativan (lorazepam) is rapidly conjugated at the 3-hydroxyl group into its major metabolite, lorazepam glucuronide, which is then excreted in the urine. Lorazepam glucuronide has no demonstrable CNS activity in animals. When 5 mg of intravenous lorazepam was administered to volunteers once a day for four consecutive days, a steady state of free lorazepam was achieved by the second day (approximately 52 ng/mL of plasma three hours after the first dose and approximately 62 ng/mL three hours after each subsequent dose, one day apart). At clinically relevant concentrations, lorazepam is bound 85% to plasma proteins.

INDICATIONS AND USAGE

Ativan (lorazepam) Injection is indicated in adult patients for preanesthetic medication, producing sedation (sleepiness or drowsiness), relief of anxiety, and a decreased ability to recall events related to the day of surgery. It is most useful in those patients who are anxious about their surgical procedure and who would prefer to have diminished recall of the events of the day of surgery (see "Information for Patients").

CONTRAINDICATIONS

Ativan (lorazepam) Injection is contraindicated in patients with a known sensitivity to benzodiazepines or its vehicle (polyethylene glycol, propylene glycol, and benzyl alcohol) and in patients with acute narrow-angle glaucoma. The use of Ativan (lorazepam) Injection intra-arterially is contraindicated because, as with other injectable benzodiazepines, inadvertent intra-arterial injection may produce arteriospasm resulting in gangrene which may require amputation (see "Warnings").

WARNINGS

PRIOR TO INTRAVENOUS USE, ATIVAN INJECTION MUST BE DILUTED WITH AN EQUAL AMOUNT OF COMPATIBLE DILUENT (SEE "DOSAGE AND ADMINISTRATION"). INTRAVENOUS INJECTION SHOULD BE MADE SLOWLY AND WITH REPEATED ASPIRATION. CARE SHOULD BE TAKEN TO DETERMINE THAT ANY INJECTION WILL NOT BE INTRA-ARTERIAL AND THAT PERIVASCULAR EXTRAVASATION WILL NOT TAKE PLACE.

PARTIAL AIRWAY OBSTRUCTION MAY OCCUR IN HEAVILY SEDATED PATIENTS. INTRAVENOUS LORAZEPAM, WHEN GIVEN ALONE IN GREATER THAN THE RECOMMENDED DOSE, OR AT THE RECOMMENDED DOSE AND ACCOMPANIED BY OTHER DRUGS USED DURING THE ADMINISTRATION OF ANESTHESIA, MAY PRODUCE HEAVY SEDATION; THEREFORE, EQUIPMENT NECESSARY TO MAINTAIN A PATENT AIRWAY AND TO SUPPORT RESPIRATION/VENTILATION SHOULD BE AVAILABLE.

There is no evidence to support the use of lorazepam injection in coma, shock, or acute alcohol intoxication at this time. Since the liver is the most likely site of conjugation of lorazepam and since excretion of conjugated lorazepam (glucuronide) is a renal function, this drug is not recommended for use in patients with hepatic and/or renal *failure.* This does not preclude use of the drug in patients with mild-to-moderate hepatic or renal disease. When injectable

lorazepam is selected for use in patients with mild-to-moderate hepatic or renal disease, the lowest effective dose should be considered since drug effect may be prolonged. Experience with other benzodiazepines and limited experience with parenteral lorazepam has demonstrated that tolerance to alcoholic beverages and other central-nervous-system depressants is diminished when used concomitantly.

As is true of similar CNS-acting drugs, patients receiving injectable lorazepam should not operate machinery or engage in hazardous occupations or drive a motor vehicle for a period of 24 to 48 hours. Impairment of performance may persist for greater intervals because of extremes of age, concomitant use of other drugs, stress of surgery, or the general condition of the patient.

Clinical trials have shown that patients over the age of 50 years may have a more profound and prolonged sedation with intravenous lorazepam. Ordinarily, an initial dose of 2 mg may be adequate unless a greater degree of lack of recall is desired.

As with all central-nervous-system depressant drugs, care should be exercised in patients given injectable lorazepam that premature ambulation may result in injury from falling.

There is no added beneficial effect to the addition of scopolamine to injectable lorazepam, and their combined effect may result in an increased incidence of sedation, hallucination, and irrational behavior.

PREGNANCY
ATIVAN (LORAZEPAM) MAY CAUSE FETAL DAMAGE WHEN ADMINISTERED TO PREGNANT WOMEN. An increased risk of congenital malformations associated with the use of minor tranquilizers (chlordiazepoxide, diazepam, and meprobamate) during the first trimester of pregnancy has been suggested in several studies. In humans, blood levels obtained from umbilical cord blood indicate placental transfer of lorazepam and lorazepam glucuronide.

Ativan Injection should not be used during pregnancy. There are insufficient data regarding obstetrical safety of parenteral lorazepam, including use in cesarean section. Such use, therefore, is not recommended.

Reproductive studies in animals were performed in mice, rats, and two strains of rabbits. Occasional anomalies (reduction of tarsals, tibia, metatarsals, malrotated limbs, gastroschisis, malformed skull, and microphthalmia) were seen in drug-treated rabbits without relationship to dosage. Although all of these anomalies were not present in the concurrent control group, they have been reported to occur randomly in historical controls. At doses of 40 mg/kg orally or 4 mg/kg intravenously and higher, there was evidence of fetal resorption and increased fetal loss in rabbits which was not seen at lower doses.

ENDOSCOPIC PROCEDURES
There are insufficient data to support the use of Ativan (lorazepam) Injection for outpatient endoscopic procedures. Inpatient endoscopic procedures require adequate recovery room observations.

Pharyngeal reflexes are not impaired when Ativan Injection is used for peroral endoscopic procedures; therefore, adequate topical or regional anesthesia is recommended to minimize reflex activity associated with such procedures.

PRECAUTIONS
GENERAL
The additive central-nervous-system effects of other drugs such as phenothiazines, narcotic analgesics, barbiturates, antidepressants, scopolamine, and monoamine-oxidase inhibitors, should be borne in mind when these other drugs are used concomitantly with or during the period of recovery from Ativan (lorazepam) Injection. (See "Clinical Pharmacology" and "Warnings".)

Extreme care must be used in administering Ativan Injection to elderly patients, very ill patients, and to patients with limited pulmonary reserve because of the possibility that underventilation and/or hypoxic cardiac arrest may occur. Resuscitative equipment for ventilatory support should be readily available. (See "Warnings" and "Dosage and Administration".)

When lorazepam injection is used IV as the premedicant prior to regional or local anesthesia, the possibility of excessive sleepiness or drowsiness may interfere with patient cooperation to determine levels of anesthesia. This is most likely to occur when greater than 0.05 mg/kg is given and when narcotic analgesics are used concomitantly with the recommended dose. (See "Adverse Reactions".)

INFORMATION FOR PATIENTS
As appropriate, the patient should be informed of the pharmacological effects of the drug, such as sedation, relief of anxiety, and lack of recall, and the duration of these effects (about 8 hours), so that they may adequately perceive the risks as well as the benefits to be derived from its use.

Patients who receive Ativan Injection as a premedicant should be cautioned that driving an automobile or operating hazardous machinery, or engaging in a hazardous sport, should be delayed for 24 to 48 hours following the injection. Sedatives, tranquilizers, and narcotic analgesics may produce a more prolonged and profound effect when adminis-

tered along with injectable Ativan. This effect may take the form of excessive sleepiness or drowsiness and, on rare occasions, interfere with recall and recognition of events of the day of surgery and the day after.

Getting out of bed unassisted may result in falling and injury if undertaken within 8 hours of receiving lorazepam injection. Alcoholic beverages should not be consumed for at least 24 to 48 hours after receiving lorazepam injectable due to the additive effects on central-nervous-system depression seen with benzodiazepines in general. Elderly patients should be told that Ativan (lorazepam) Injection may make them very sleepy for a period longer than six (6) to eight (8) hours following surgery.

LABORATORY TESTS
In clinical trials no laboratory test abnormalities were identified with either single or multiple doses of Ativan (lorazepam) Injection. These tests included: CBC, urinalysis, SGOT, SGPT, bilirubin, alkaline phosphatase, LDH, cholesterol, uric acid, BUN, glucose, calcium, phosphorus, and total proteins.

DRUG INTERACTIONS
Ativan (lorazepam) Injection, like other injectable benzodiazepines, produces depression of the central nervous system when administered with ethyl alcohol, phenothiazines, barbiturates, MAO inhibitors, and other antidepressants. When scopolamine is used concomitantly with injectable lorazepam, an increased incidence of sedation, hallucinations, and irrational behavior has been observed.

DRUG/LABORATORY TEST INTERACTIONS
No laboratory test abnormalities were identified when lorazepam was given alone or concomitantly with another drug, such as narcotic analgesics, inhalation anesthetics, scopolamine, atropine, and a variety of tranquilizing agents.

CARCINOGENESIS, MUTAGENESIS, IMPAIRMENT OF FERTILITY
No evidence of carcinogenic potential emerged in rats and mice during an 18-month study with oral lorazepam. No studies regarding mutagenesis have been performed. Preimplantation study in rats was performed with oral lorazepam at a 20 mg/kg dose and showed no impairment of fertility.

PREGNANCY
Pregnancy Category D; See "Warnings."

LABOR AND DELIVERY
There are insufficient data to support the use of Ativan (lorazepam) Injection during labor and delivery, including cesarean section; therefore, its use in this situation is not recommended.

NURSING MOTHERS
Injectable lorazepam should not be administered to nursing mothers, because like other benzodiazepines, the possibility exists that lorazepam may be excreted in human milk and sedate the infant.

PEDIATRIC USE
There are insufficient data to support efficacy or make dosage recommendations for injectable lorazepam in patients less than 18 years of age; therefore, such use is not recommended.

ADVERSE REACTIONS
CENTRAL NERVOUS SYSTEM
The most frequent adverse effects seen with injectable lorazepam are an extension of the central-nervous-system depressant effects of the drug. The incidence varied from one study to another, depending on the dosage, route of administration, use of other central-nervous-system depressants, and the investigator's opinion concerning the degree and duration of desired sedation. Excessive sleepiness and drowsiness were the main side effects. This interfered with patient cooperation in approximately 6% (25/446) of patients undergoing regional anesthesia in that they were unable to assess levels of anesthesia in regional blocks or with caudal anesthesia. Patients over 50 years of age had a higher incidence of excessive sleepiness or drowsiness when compared with those under 50 (21/106 vs 24/245) when lorazepam was given intravenously (see "Dosage and Administration"). On rare occasion (3/1580) the patient was unable to give personal identification in the operating room on arrival, and one patient fell when attempting premature ambulation in the postoperative period.

Symptoms such as restlessness, confusion, depression, crying, sobbing, and delirium occurred in about 1.3% (20/1580). One patient injured himself by picking at his incision during the immediate postoperative period.

Hallucinations were present in about 1% (14/1580) of patients and were visual and self-limiting.

An occasional patient complained of dizziness, diplopia, and/or blurred vision. Depressed hearing was infrequently reported during the peak-effect period.

An occasional patient had a prolonged recovery room stay, either because of excessive sleepiness or because of some form of inappropriate behavior. The latter was seen most commonly when scopolamine was given concomitantly as a premedicant.

Limited information derived from patients who were discharged the day after receiving injectable lorazepam showed

one patient complained of some unsteadiness of gait and a reduced ability to perform complex mental functions. Enhanced sensitivity to alcoholic beverages has been reported more than 24 hours after receiving injectable lorazepam, similar to experience with other benzodiazepines.

LOCAL EFFECTS
Intramuscular injection of lorazepam has resulted in pain at the injection site, a sensation of burning, or observed redness in the same area in a very variable incidence from one study to another. The overall incidence of pain and burning was about 17% (146/859) in the immediate postinjection period, and about 1.4% (12/859) at the 24-hour observation time. Reactions at the injection site (redness) occurred in approximately 2% (17/859) in the immediate postinjection period and were present 24 hours later in about 0.8% (7/859).

Intravenous administration of lorazepam resulted in painful responses in 13/771 patients or approximately 1.6% in the immediate postinjection period, and 24 hours later 4/771 patients or about 0.5% still complained of pain. Redness did not occur immediately following intravenous injection but was noted in 19/771 patients at the 24-hour observation period. This incidence is similar to that observed with an intravenous infusion before lorazepam is given.

CARDIOVASCULAR SYSTEM
Hypertension (0.1%) and hypotension (0.1%) have occasionally been observed after patients have received injectable lorazepam.

RESPIRATORY SYSTEM
Five patients (5/446) who underwent regional anesthesia were observed to have partial airway obstruction. This was believed due to excessive sleepiness at the time of the procedure and resulted in temporary underventilation. Immediate attention to the airway, employing the usual countermeasures, will usually suffice to manage this condition (see also "Clinical Pharmacology," "Warnings," and "Precautions").

OTHER ADVERSE EXPERIENCES
Skin rash, nausea, and vomiting have occasionally been noted in patients who have received injectable lorazepam combined with other drugs during anesthesia and surgery.

DRUG ABUSE AND DEPENDENCE
As with other benzodiazepines, Ativan (lorazepam) Injection has a low potential for abuse and may lead to limited dependence. Although there are no clinical data available for injectable lorazepam in this respect, physicians should be aware that repeated doses over a prolonged period of time may result in limited physical and psychological dependence.

OVERDOSAGE
Overdosage of benzodiazepines is usually manifested by varying degrees of central-nervous-system depression, ranging from drowsiness to coma. In mild cases symptoms include drowsiness, mental confusion, and lethargy. In more serious examples, symptoms may include ataxia, hypotonia, hypotension, hypnosis, stages one (1) to three (3) coma, and very rarely death.

Treatment of overdosage is mainly supportive until the drug is eliminated from the body. Vital signs and fluid balance should be carefully monitored. An adequate airway should be maintained and assisted respiration used as needed. With normally functioning kidneys, forced diuresis with intravenous fluids and electrolytes may accelerate elimination of benzodiazepines from the body. In addition, osmotic diuretics, such as mannitol, may be effective as adjunctive measures. In more critical situations, renal dialysis and exchange blood transfusions may be indicated.

DOSAGE AND ADMINISTRATION
INTRAMUSCULAR INJECTION
For the designated indications as a premedicant, the usual recommended dose of lorazepam for intramuscular injection is 0.05 mg/kg up to a maximum of 4 mg. As with all premedicant drugs, the dose should be individualized. (See also "Clinical Pharmacology," "Warnings," "Precautions," and "Adverse Reactions.") Doses of other central-nervous-system depressant drugs should be ordinarily reduced. (See "Precautions.") *For optimum effect, measured as lack of recall, intramuscular lorazepam should be administered at least 2 hours before the anticipated operative procedure.* Narcotic analgesics should be administered at their usual preoperative time. There are insufficient data to support efficacy to make dosage recommendations for intramuscular lorazepam in patients less than 18 years of age; therefore, such use is not recommended.

INTRAVENOUS INJECTION
For the primary purpose of sedation and relief of anxiety, the usual recommended initial dose of lorazepam for intravenous injection is 2 mg total, or 0.02 mg/lb (0.044 mg/kg), whichever is smaller. This dose will suffice for sedating most adult patients, and should not ordinarily be exceeded in patients over 50 years of age. In those patients in whom a greater likelihood of lack of recall for perioperative events would be beneficial, larger doses as high as 0.05 mg/kg up to

Continued on next page

Wyeth-Ayerst Laboratories—Cont.

a total of 4 mg may be administered. (See "Clinical Pharmacology," "Warnings," "Precautions," and "Adverse Reactions.") Doses of other injectable central-nervous-system depressant drugs should ordinarily be reduced (see "Precautions"). *For optimum effect, measured as lack of recall, intravenous lorazepam should be administered 15 to 20 minutes before the anticipated operative procedure.*

EQUIPMENT NECESSARY TO MAINTAIN A PATENT AIRWAY SHOULD BE IMMEDIATELY AVAILABLE PRIOR TO INTRAVENOUS ADMINISTRATION OF LORAZEPAM (see "Warnings").

There are insufficient data to support efficacy or make dosage recommendations for intravenous lorazepam in patients less than 18 years of age; therefore, such use is not recommended.

ADMINISTRATION

When given intramuscularly, Ativan Injection, undiluted, should be injected deep in the muscle mass.

Injectable Ativan (lorazepam) can be used with atropine sulfate, narcotic analgesics, other parenterally used analgesics, commonly used anesthetics, and muscle relaxants.

Immediately prior to intravenous use, Ativan (lorazepam) Injection must be diluted with an equal volume of compatible solution. When properly diluted the drug may be injected directly into a vein or into the tubing of an existing intravenous infusion. The rate of injection should not exceed 2.0 mg per minute.

Parenteral drug products should be inspected visually for particulate matter and discoloration prior to administration, whenever solution and container permit. Do not use if solution is discolored or contains a precipitate.

Ativan (lorazepam) Injection is compatible for dilution purposes with the following solutions: Sterile Water for Injection, USP; Sodium Chloride Injection, USP; 5% Dextrose Injection, USP.

HOW SUPPLIED

Ativan® (lorazepam) Injection is available in the following dosage strengths in TUBEX® Sterile Cartridge-Needle Units (22 gauge × 1¼ inch needle), packaged in boxes of 10 TUBEX TAMP-R-TEL® tamper-resistant packages:

2 mg per mL, NDC 0008-0581-06, 1 mL fill in 2 mL size.
4 mg per mL, NDC 0008-0570-05, 1 mL fill in 2 mL size.

For IM or IV injection.
Protect from light.
Store in a refrigerator.
Use carton to protect contents from light.

ALSO AVAILABLE

TUBEX® Sterile Cartridge-Needle Units (22 gauge × 1¼ inch needle), in boxes of 10 TUBEX in the following dosage strengths:

2 mg per mL, NDC 0008-0581-02, 1 mL fill in 2 mL size
4 mg per mL, NDC 0008-0570-04, 1 mL fill in 2 mL size

Single-dose and multiple-dose vials are available as follows:
2 mg per mL, NDC 0008-0581-04, 1 mL vial and NDC 0008-0581-01, 10 mL vial
4 mg per mL, NDC 0008-0570-04, 1 mL and NDC 0008-0570-01, 10 mL vial

DIRECTIONS FOR DILUTION FOR IV USE

To dilute, adhere to the following procedure:

For TUBEX—

1. Extrude the entire amount of air in the half-filled TUBEX.
2. Slowly aspirate the desired volume of diluent.
3. Pull back slightly on the plunger to provide additional mixing space.
4. Immediately mix contents thoroughly by gently inverting TUBEX repeatedly until a homogenous solution results. Do not shake vigorously, as this will result in air entrapment.

For Vial—

Aspirate the desired amount of Ativan Injection into the syringe. Then proceed as described under TUBEX.

ATIVAN® Ⓒ℞
[at 'i-van]
(lorazepam)
Tablets

DESCRIPTION

Ativan (lorazepam), an antianxiety agent, has the chemical formula, 7-chloro-5-(*o*-chlorophenyl)-1,3-dihydro-3-hydroxy-2*H*-1,4-benzodiazepin-2-one.

It is a nearly white powder almost insoluble in water. Each Ativan (lorazepam) tablet, to be taken orally, contains 0.5 mg, 1 mg, or 2 mg of lorazepam. The inactive ingredients present are lactose and other ingredients.

CLINICAL PHARMACOLOGY

Studies in healthy volunteers show that in single high doses Ativan (lorazepam) has a tranquilizing action on the central nervous system with no appreciable effect on the respiratory or cardiovascular systems.

Ativan (lorazepam) is readily absorbed with an absolute bioavailability of 90 percent. Peak concentrations in plasma occur approximately 2 hours following administration. The peak plasma level of lorazepam from a 2 mg dose is approximately 20 ng/mL.

The mean half-life of unconjugated lorazepam in human plasma is about 12 hours and for its major metabolite, lorazepam glucuronide, about 18 hours. At clinically relevant concentrations, lorazepam is approximately 85% bound to plasma proteins. Ativan (lorazepam) is rapidly conjugated at its 3-hydroxy group into lorazepam glucuronide which is then excreted in the urine. Lorazepam glucuronide has no demonstrable CNS activity in animals.

The plasma levels of lorazepam are proportional to the dose given. There is no evidence of accumulation of lorazepam on administration up to six months.

Studies comparing young and elderly subjects have shown that the pharmacokinetics of lorazepam remain unaltered with advancing age.

INDICATIONS AND USAGE

Ativan (lorazepam) is indicated for the management of anxiety disorders or for the short-term relief of the symptoms of anxiety or anxiety associated with depressive symptoms. Anxiety or tension associated with the stress of everyday life usually does not require treatment with an anxiolytic.

The effectiveness of Ativan (lorazepam) in long-term use, that is, more than 4 months, has not been assessed by systematic clinical studies. The physician should periodically reassess the usefulness of the drug for the individual patient.

CONTRAINDICATIONS

Ativan (lorazepam) is contraindicated in patients with known sensitivity to the benzodiazepines or with acute narrow-angle glaucoma.

WARNINGS

Ativan (lorazepam) is not recommended for use in patients with a primary depressive disorder or psychosis. As with all patients on CNS-acting drugs, patients receiving lorazepam should be warned not to operate dangerous machinery or motor vehicles and that their tolerance for alcohol and other CNS depressants will be diminished.

PHYSICAL AND PSYCHOLOGICAL DEPENDENCE

Withdrawal symptoms, similar in character to those noted with barbiturates and alcohol (convulsions, tremor, abdominal and muscle cramps, vomiting, and sweating), have occurred following abrupt discontinuance of lorazepam. The more severe withdrawal symptoms have usually been limited to those patients who received excessive doses over an extended period of time. Generally milder withdrawal symptoms (e.g., dysphoria and insomnia) have been reported following abrupt discontinuance of benzodiazepines taken continuously at therapeutic levels for several months. Consequently, after extended therapy, abrupt discontinuation should generally be avoided and a gradual dosage-tapering schedule followed. Addiction-prone individuals (such as drug addicts or alcoholics) should be under careful surveillance when receiving lorazepam or other psychotropic agents because of the predisposition of such patients to habituation and dependence.

PRECAUTIONS

In patients with depression accompanying anxiety, a possibility for suicide should be borne in mind.

For elderly or debilitated patients, the initial daily dosage should not exceed 2 mg in order to avoid oversedation.

The usual precautions for treating patients with impaired renal or hepatic function should be observed.

In patients where gastrointestinal or cardiovascular disorders coexist with anxiety, it should be noted that lorazepam has not been shown to be of significant benefit in treating the gastrointestinal or cardiovascular component.

Esophageal dilation occurred in rats treated with lorazepam for more than one year at 6 mg/kg/day. The no-effect dose was 1.25 mg/kg/day (approximately 6 times the maximum human therapeutic dose of 10 mg per day). The effect was reversible only when the treatment was withdrawn within two months of first observation of the phenomenon. The clinical significance of this is unknown. However, use of lorazepam for prolonged periods and in geriatric patients requires caution, and there should be frequent monitoring for symptoms of upper G.I. disease.

Safety and effectiveness of Ativan (lorazepam) in children of less than 12 years have not been established.

INFORMATION FOR PATIENTS

To assure the safe and effective use of Ativan (lorazepam), patients should be informed that, since benzodiazepines may produce psychological and physical dependence, it is advisable that they consult with their physician before either increasing the dose or abruptly discontinuing this drug.

ESSENTIAL LABORATORY TESTS: Some patients on Ativan (lorazepam) have developed leukopenia, and some have had elevations of LDH. As with other benzodiazepines, periodic blood counts and liver-function tests are recommended for patients on long-term therapy.

CLINICALLY SIGNIFICANT DRUG INTERACTIONS: The benzodiazepines, including Ativan (lorazepam), produce CNS depressant effects when administered with such medications as barbiturates or alcohol.

CARCINOGENESIS AND MUTAGENESIS: No evidence of carcinogenic potential emerged in rats during an 18-month study with Ativan (lorazepam). No studies regarding mutagenesis have been performed.

PREGNANCY: Reproductive studies in animals were performed in mice, rats, and two strains of rabbits. Occasional anomalies (reduction of tarsals, tibia, metatarsals, malrotated limbs, gastroschisis, malformed skull, and microphthalmia) were seen in drug-treated rabbits without relationship to dosage. Although all of these anomalies were not present in the concurrent control group, they have been reported to occur randomly in historical controls. At doses of 40 mg/kg and higher, there was evidence of fetal resorption and increased fetal loss in rabbits which was not seen at lower doses.

The clinical significance of the above findings is not known. However, an increased risk of congenital malformations associated with the use of minor tranquilizers (chlordiazepoxide, diazepam, and meprobamate) during the first trimester of pregnancy has been suggested in several studies. Because the use of these drugs is rarely a matter of urgency, the use of lorazepam during this period should almost always be avoided. The possibility that a woman of childbearing potential may be pregnant at the time of institution of therapy should be considered. Patients should be advised that if they become pregnant, they should communicate with their physician about the desirability of discontinuing the drug.

In humans, blood levels obtained from umbilical cord blood indicate placental transfer of lorazepam and lorazepam glucuronide.

NURSING MOTHERS: It is not known whether oral lorazepam is excreted in human milk like the other benzodiazepine tranquilizers. As a general rule, nursing should not be undertaken while a patient is on a drug, since many drugs are excreted in human milk.

ADVERSE REACTIONS

Adverse reactions, if they occur, are usually observed at the beginning of therapy and generally disappear on continued medication or upon decreasing the dose. In a sample of about 3,500 anxious patients, the most frequent adverse reaction to Ativan (lorazepam) is sedation (15.9%), followed by dizziness (6.9%), weakness (4.2%), and unsteadiness (3.4%). Less frequent adverse reactions are disorientation, depression, nausea, change in appetite, headache, sleep disturbance, agitation, dermatological symptoms, eye function disturbance, together with various gastrointestinal symptoms and autonomic manifestations. The incidence of sedation and unsteadiness increased with age.

Small decreases in blood pressure have been noted but are not clinically significant, probably being related to the relief of anxiety produced by Ativan (lorazepam).

Transient amnesia or memory impairment has been reported in association with the use of benzodiazepines.

OVERDOSAGE

In the management of overdosage with any drug, it should be borne in mind that multiple agents may have been taken.

Manifestations of Ativan (lorazepam) overdosage include somnolence, confusion, and coma. Induced vomiting and/or gastric lavage should be undertaken, followed by general supportive care, monitoring of vital signs, and close observation of the patient. Hypotension, though unlikely, usually may be controlled with Levarterenol Bitartrate Injection, USP. The usefulness of dialysis has not been determined.

DOSAGE AND ADMINISTRATION

Ativan (lorazepam) is administered orally. For optimal results, dose, frequency of administration, and duration of therapy should be individualized according to patient response. To facilitate this, 0.5 mg, 1 mg, and 2 mg tablets are available.

The usual range is 2 to 6 mg/day given in divided doses, the largest dose being taken before bedtime, but the daily dosage may vary from 1 to 10 mg/day.

For anxiety, most patients require an initial dose of 2 to 3 mg/day given b.i.d. or t.i.d.

For insomnia due to anxiety or transient situational stress, a single daily dose of 2 to 4 mg may be given, usually at bedtime.

For elderly or debilitated patients, an initial dosage of 1 to 2 mg/day in divided doses is recommended, to be adjusted as needed and tolerated.

The dosage of Ativan (lorazepam) should be increased gradually when needed to help avoid adverse effects. When higher dosage is indicated, the evening dose should be increased before the daytime doses.

HOW SUPPLIED

Ativan® (lorazepam) Tablets, Wyeth®, are available in the following dosage strengths:
0.5 mg, NDC 0008-0081, white, five-sided tablet with a raised "A" on one side and "WYETH" and "81" on reverse side, in bottles of 100 and 500 tablets, in Redipak® cartons of 250 tablets (10 blister folders of 25), and in Redipak cartons of 100 tablets (10 blister strips of 10).
1 mg, NDC 0008-0064, white, five-sided tablet with a raised "A" on one side and "WYETH" and "64" on scored reverse side, in bottles of 100, 500, and 1000 tablets, in Redipak® cartons of 250 tablets (10 blister folders of 25), and in Redipak cartons of 100 tablets (10 blister strips of 10).
2 mg, NDC 0008-0065, white, five-sided tablet with a raised "A" on one side and "WYETH" and "65" on scored reverse side, in bottles of 100, 500, and 1000 tablets, in Redipak® cartons of 250 tablets (10 blister folders of 25), and in Redipak cartons of 100 tablets (10 blister strips of 10).
Store at controlled room temperature.
Keep bottles tightly closed.
Dispense in tight container.
The appearance of ATIVAN tablets is a registered trademark of Wyeth-Ayerst Laboratories.

Shown in Product Identification Section, page 436

ATROMID-S® ℞

[*ă'trō-mid*]
(clofibrate capsules)
Antilipidemic agent for reduction of elevated serum lipids

CAUTION: Federal law prohibits dispensing without prescription.

DESCRIPTION

ATROMID-S Capsules (clofibrate capsules) is ethyl 2-(p-chlorophenoxy)-2-methyl-propionate, an antilipidemic agent.

structural formula

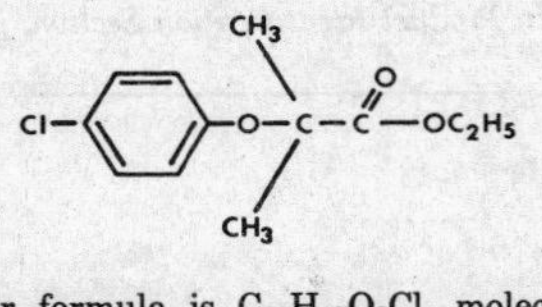

Its molecular formula is $C_{12}H_{15}O_3Cl$, molecular weight 242.7, and boiling point 148°–150°C at 25 mm Hg. It is a stable, colorless to pale-yellow liquid with a faint odor and characteristic taste, soluble in common solvents but not in water. Each ATROMID-S Capsule contains 500 mg clofibrate for oral administration.
ATROMID-S Capsules contain the following inactive ingredients: D&C Red No. 28, D&C Red No. 30, D&C Yellow No. 10, FD&C Blue No. 1, FD&C Red No. 3, FD&C Yellow No. 6, gelatin.

CLINICAL PHARMACOLOGY

ATROMID-S is an antilipidemic agent. It acts to lower elevated serum lipids by reducing the very low-density lipoprotein fraction (S_f20– 400) rich in triglycerides. Serum cholesterol may be decreased, particularly in those patients whose cholesterol elevation is due to the presence of IDL as a result of Type III hyperlipoproteinemia.
The mechanism of action has not been established definitively. Clofibrate may inhibit the hepatic release of lipoproteins (particularly VLDL), potentiate the action of lipoprotein lipase, and increase the fecal excretion of neutral sterols.
Between 95% and 99% of an oral dose of clofibrate is excreted in the urine as free and conjugated clofibric acid, thus, the absorption of clofibrate is virtually complete. The half-life of clofibric acid in normal volunteers averages 18 to 22 hours (range 14 to 35 hours) but can vary by up to 7 hours in the same subject at different times. Clofibric acid is highly protein-bound (95% to 97%). In subjects undergoing continuous clofibrate treatment, 1 g q12h, plasma concentrations of clofibric acid range from 120 to 125 mcg/mL to an approximate peak of 200 mcg/mL.
Several investigators have observed in their studies that clofibrate may produce a decrease in cholesterol linoleate but an increase in palmitoleate and oleate, the latter being considered atherogenic in experimental animals. The significance of this finding is unknown at this time.
Reduction of triglycerides in some patients treated with clofibrate or certain of its chemically and clinically similar analogs may be associated with an increase in LDL cholesterol. Increase in LDL cholesterol has been observed in patients whose cholesterol is initially normal.
Animal studies suggest that clofibrate interrupts cholesterol biosynthesis prior to mevalonate formation.

INDICATIONS AND USAGE

The initial treatment of choice for hyperlipidemia is dietary therapy specific for the type of hyperlipidemia.[1] Excess body weight and alcoholic intake may be important factors in hypertriglyceridemia and should be addressed prior to any drug therapy. Physical exercise can be an important ancillary measure. Estrogen therapy, some beta-blockers, and thiazide diuretics may also be associated with increases in plasma triglycerides. Discontinuation of such products may obviate the need for specific antilipidemic therapy. Contributory diseases such as hypothyroidism or diabetes mellitus should be looked for and adequately treated. The use of drugs should be considered only when reasonable attempts have been made to obtain satisfactory results with non-drug methods. If the decision ultimately is to use drugs, the patient should be instructed that this does not reduce the importance of adhering to diet.
Because ATROMID-S is associated with certain serious adverse findings reported in two large clinical trials (see WARNINGS), agents other than clofibrate may be more suitable for a particular patient.
ATROMID-S is indicated for Primary Dysbetalipoproteinemia (Type III hyperlipidemia) that does not respond adequately to diet.
ATROMID-S may be considered for the treatment of adult patients with very high serum-triglyceride levels (Types IV and V hyperlipidemia) who present a risk of abdominal pain and pancreatitis and who do not respond adequately to a determined dietary effort to control them. Patients who present such risk typically have serum triglycerides over 2000 mg/dl and have elevations of VLDL-cholesterol as well as fasting chylomicrons (Type V hyperlipidemia). Subjects who consistently have total serum or plasma triglycerides below 1000 mg/dl are unlikely to present a risk of pancreatitis. Atromid-S therapy may be considered for those subjects with triglyceride elevations between 1000 and 2000 mg/dl who have a history of pancreatitis or of recurrent abdominal pain typical of pancreatitis. It is recognized that some Type IV patients with triglycerides under 1000 mg/dl may, through dietary or alcoholic indiscretion, convert to a Type V pattern with massive triglyceride elevations accompanying fasting chylomicronemia, but the influence of Atromid-S therapy on the risk of pancreatitis in such situations has not been adequately studied.
Atromid-S is not useful for the hypertriglyceridemia of Type I hyperlipidemia, where elevations of chylomicrons and plasma triglycerides are accompanied by normal levels of very low-density lipoprotein (VLDL). Inspection of plasma refrigerated for 12 to 14 hours is helpful in distinguishing Types I, IV, and V hyperlipoproteinemia.[2]
ATROMID-S has not been shown to be effective for prevention of coronary heart disease.
The biochemical response to ATROMID-S is variable, and it is not always possible to predict from the lipoprotein type or other factors which patients will obtain favorable results. LDL cholesterol, as well as triglycerides, should be rechecked during the first several months of therapy in order to detect rises in LDL cholesterol that often accompany fibric-acid-type drug-induced reductions in elevated triglycerides. It is essential that lipid levels be reassessed periodically and that the drug be discontinued in any patient in whom lipids do not show significant improvement.

CONTRAINDICATIONS

Clofibrate is contraindicated in pregnant women. While teratogenic studies have not demonstrated any effect attributable to clofibrate, it is known that serum of the rabbit fetus accumulates a higher concentration of clofibrate than that found in maternal serum, and it is possible that the fetus may not have developed the enzyme system required for the excretion of clofibrate.
It is contraindicated in patients with clinically significant hepatic or renal dysfunction. Rhabdomyolysis and severe hyperkalemia have been reported in association with preexisting renal insufficiency.
It is contraindicated in patients with primary biliary cirrhosis since it may raise the already elevated cholesterol in these cases.
It is contraindicated in patients with a known hypersensitivity to clofibrate.
It is contraindicated in nursing women (see PRECAUTIONS).

WARNINGS

In a large prospective study involving 5,000 patients in a clofibrate-treated group and 5,000 in a placebo-treated group followed for an average of five years on drug or placebo and one year beyond (the WHO study), there was a statistically significant 36% higher mortality due to noncardiovascular causes in the clofibrate-treated group than in a comparable placebo group. Half of this difference was due to malignancy; other causes of death included postcholecystectomy complications and pancreatitis.[3] In another prospective study involving 1,000 clofibrate- and 3,000 placebo-treated patients followed for an average of six years on drug or placebo (the Coronary Drug Project study), the noncardiovascular mortality rate, including that of malignancy, was not significantly different in the clofibrate- and placebo-treated groups.[4] This should not be interpreted to mean that clofibrate is not associated with an increased risk of noncardiovascular death, because the patients in the Coronary Drug Project were much older than those in the WHO study and they all had had a previous myocardial infarction, so that the deaths in the Coronary Drug Project were overwhelmingly due to cardiovascular causes, and it would have been very difficult to discern a clofibrate-associated risk of death due to noncardiovascular causes if it existed. Both studies demonstrated that clofibrate users have twice the risk of developing cholelithiasis and cholecystitis requiring surgery as do nonusers.

A potential benefit of clofibrate was, however, reported in the WHO study which involved patients with hypercholesterolemia and no history of myocardial infarction or angina pectoris. In this study, there was a statistically significant 25% decrease in subsequent nonfatal myocardial infarctions in the clofibrate-treated group when compared with the placebo group. There was no difference in incidence of fatal myocardial infarction in the two groups. In the Coronary Drug Project study, which involved patients with or without hypercholesterolemia and/or hypertriglyceridemia and with a history of previous myocardial infarction, there was no significant difference in incidence of either nonfatal or fatal myocardial infarction between the clofibrate- and placebo-treated groups.[3]

As a result of these and other studies, the following can be stated:

1. Clofibrate, in general, causes a relatively modest reduction of serum cholesterol and a somewhat greater reduction of serum triglycerides. In Type III hyperlipidemia, however, substantial reductions of both cholesterol and triglycerides can occur with clofibrate use.
2. No study to date has shown a convincing reduction in incidence of *fatal* myocardial infarction.
3. A significantly increased incidence of cholelithiasis has been demonstrated consistently in clofibrate-treated groups, and an increase in morbidity from this complication and mortality from cholecystectomy must be anticipated during clofibrate treatment.
4. Several types of other undesirable events have been associated in a statistically significant way with clofibrate administration in the WHO and the Coronary Drug Project studies. There was an increase in incidence of noncardiovascular deaths reported in the WHO study. There was an increase in cardiac arrhythmias, intermittent claudication, and definite or suspected thromboembolic events, and angina reported in the Coronary Drug Project, which was not, however, reported in the WHO study.
5. Administration of clofibrate to mice and rats in long-term studies at eight times the human dose, and to rats at five times the human dose, resulted in a higher incidence of benign and malignant liver tumors than in controls. Lower doses were not included in these studies.
An increase in benign Leydig-cell tumors in male rats treated at 400 mg/kg (10 times the estimated human dose) was observed in a single study with clofibrate; similar increases were not observed in other studies conducted with clofibrate although they have been observed with other fibric-acid derivatives.
6. Administration of clofibrate to male monkeys at dosages of 2 to 6 times the human dose resulted in increases in mortality of 2- to 5-fold. As in the case of men in the WHO study, no single cause of death was identified.

BECAUSE OF THE TUMORIGENICITY OF CLOFIBRATE IN RODENTS AND THE POSSIBLE INCREASED RISK OF MALIGNANCY ASSOCIATED WITH CLOFIBRATE IN THE HUMAN, AS WELL AS THE INCREASED RISK OF CHOLELITHIASIS, AND BECAUSE THERE IS NOT, TO DATE, SUBSTANTIAL EVIDENCE OF A BENEFICIAL EFFECT ON CARDIOVASCULAR MORTALITY FROM CLOFIBRATE, THIS DRUG SHOULD BE UTILIZED ONLY FOR THOSE PATIENTS DESCRIBED IN THE "INDICATIONS AND USAGE" SECTION, AND SHOULD BE DISCONTINUED IF SIGNIFICANT LIPID RESPONSE IS NOT OBTAINED.

CONCOMITANT ANTICOAGULANTS
CAUTION SHOULD BE EXERCISED WHEN ANTICOAGULANTS ARE GIVEN IN CONJUNCTION WITH ATROMID-S. THE DOSAGE OF THE ANTICOAGULANT SHOULD BE REDUCED USUALLY BY ONE-HALF (DEPENDING ON THE INDIVIDUAL CASE) TO MAINTAIN

Continued on next page

Wyeth-Ayerst Laboratories—Cont.

THE PROTHROMBIN TIME AT THE DESIRED LEVEL TO PREVENT BLEEDING COMPLICATIONS. FREQUENT PROTHROMBIN DETERMINATIONS ARE ADVISABLE UNTIL IT HAS BEEN DEFINITELY DETERMINED THAT THE PROTHROMBIN LEVEL HAS BEEN STABILIZED.

SKELETAL MUSCLE
Myalgia, myositis, myopathy, and rhabdomyolysis with or without elevation of CPK have been associated with ATRO-MID-S therapy. Consideration should be given to withholding or discontinuing drug therapy in any patient with a risk factor predisposing to the development of renal failure secondary to rhabdomyolysis, including: severe acute infection; hypotension; major surgery; trauma; severe metabolic, endocrine, or electrolyte disorders; and uncontrolled seizures. ATROMID-S therapy should be discontinued if markedly elevated CPK levels occur or myositis is diagnosed.

AVOIDANCE OF PREGNANCY
Strict birth control procedures must be exercised by women of child-bearing potential. In patients who plan to become pregnant, clofibrate should be withdrawn several months before conception. Because of the possibility of pregnancy occurring despite birth control precautions in patients taking clofibrate, the possible benefits of the drug to the patient must be weighed against possible hazards to the fetus. (See Pregnancy section.)

PRECAUTIONS
GENERAL
Before instituting therapy with clofibrate, attempts should be made to control serum lipids with appropriate dietary regimens, weight loss in obese patients, control of diabetes mellitus, etc.

Because of the long-term administration of a drug of this nature, adequate baseline studies should be performed to determine that the patient has significantly elevated serum lipid levels. Frequent determinations of serum lipids should be obtained during the first few months of ATROMID-S administration, and periodic determinations thereafter. The drug should be withdrawn after three months if response is inadequate. However, in the case of xanthoma tuberosum, the drug should be employed for longer periods (even up to one year) provided that there is a reduction in the size and/or number of the xanthomata.

Since cholelithiasis is a possible side effect of clofibrate therapy, appropriate diagnostic procedures should be performed if signs and symptoms related to disease of the biliary system should occur.

Clofibrate may produce "flu-like" symptoms (muscular aching, soreness, cramping) associated with increased creatine kinase levels. The physician should differentiate this from actual viral and/or bacterial disease.

Use with caution in patients with peptic ulcer since reactivation has been reported. Whether this is drug related is unknown.

Various cardiac arrhythmias have been reported with the use of clofibrate.

LABORATORY TESTS
Subsequent serum lipid determinations should be done to detect a paradoxical rise in serum cholesterol or triglyceride levels. Clofibrate will not alter the seasonal variations of serum cholesterol: peak elevations in midwinter and late summer and decreases in fall and spring. If the drug is discontinued, the patient should be continued on an appropriate hypolipidemic diet, and serum lipids should be monitored until stabilized, as a rise in these values to or above the original baseline may occur.

During clofibrate therapy, frequent serum-transaminase determinations and other liver-function tests should be performed, since the drug may produce abnormalities in these parameters. These effects are usually reversible when the drug is discontinued. Hepatic biopsies are usually within normal limits. If the hepatic-function tests steadily rise or show excessive abnormalities, the drug should be withdrawn. Therefore, use with caution in those patients with a past history of jaundice or hepatic disease.

Complete blood counts should be done periodically since anemia, and more frequently, leukopenia have been reported in patients who have been taking clofibrate.

DRUG INTERACTIONS
Caution should be exercised when anticoagulants are given in conjunction with ATROMID-S. Usually, the dosage of the anticoagulant should be reduced by one-half (depending on the individual case) to maintain the prothrombin time at the desired level to prevent bleeding complications. Frequent prothrombin determinations are advisable until it has been determined definitely that the prothrombin level has been stabilized.

ATROMID-S may displace acidic drugs such as phenytoin or tolbutamide from their binding sites. Caution should be exercised when treating patients with either of these drugs or other highly protein-bound drugs and ATROMID-S. The hypoglycemic effect of tolbutamide has been reported to increase when ATROMID-S is given concurrently.

Fulminant rhabdomyolysis has been seen as early as three weeks after initiation of combined therapy with another fibrate and lovastatin but may be seen after several months. For these reasons, it is felt that, in most subjects who have had an unsatisfactory lipid response to either drug alone, the possible benefits of combined therapy with lovastatin and a fibrate do not outweigh the risks of severe myopathy, rhabdomyolysis, and acute renal failure. While it is not known whether this interaction occurs with fibrates other than gemfibrozil, myopathy and rhabdomyolysis has occasionally been associated with the use of fibrates alone, including clofibrate. Therefore, the combined use of lovastatin with fibrates should generally be avoided.

CARCINOGENESIS, MUTAGENESIS, IMPAIRMENT OF FERTILITY
See WARNINGS section for information on carcinogenesis and mutagenesis.

Arrest of spermatogenesis has been seen in both dogs and monkeys at doses approximately 4 to 6 times the human therapeutic dose.

PREGNANCY
Teratogenic effects
Pregnancy Category C. Animal reproduction studies have not been conducted with ATROMID-S. It is also not known whether ATROMID-S can cause fetal harm when administered to a pregnant woman or can affect reproductive capacity. However, animal reproduction studies with clofibrate plus androsterone showed increases in neonatal deaths and pup mortality during lactation.

NURSING MOTHERS
ATROMID-S is contraindicated in lactating women, since an active metabolite (CPIB) has been measured in breast milk.

PEDIATRIC USE
Safety and efficacy in children have not been established.

ADVERSE REACTIONS
The most common is nausea. Less frequently encountered gastrointestinal reactions are vomiting, loose stools, dyspepsia, flatulence, and abdominal distress. Reactions reported less often than gastrointestinal ones are headache, dizziness, and fatigue; muscle cramping, aching, and weakness; skin rash, urticaria, and pruritus; dry brittle hair, and alopecia. The following reported adverse reactions are listed alphabetically by systems:

CARDIOVASCULAR
Increased or decreased angina
Cardiac arrhythmias
Both swelling and phlebitis at site of xanthomas

DERMATOLOGIC
Allergic reactions including urticaria
Skin rash
Pruritus
Dry skin and dry, brittle hair
Alopecia
Toxic epidermal necrolysis

GASTROINTESTINAL
Gallstones
Nausea
Vomiting
Diarrhea
Gastrointestinal upset (bloating, flatulence, abdominal distress)
Hepatomegaly (not associated with hepatotoxicity)
Stomatitis and gastritis

GENITOURINARY
Findings consistent with renal dysfunction as evidenced by dysuria, hematuria, proteinuria, decreased urine output. One patient's renal biopsy suggested "allergic reaction."
Impotence and decreased libido

HEMATOLOGIC
Leukopenia
Potentiation of anticoagulant effect
Anemia
Eosinophilia
Agranulocytosis

MUSCULOSKELETAL
Myalgia (muscle cramping, aching, weakness)
"Flu-like" symptoms
Myositis
Myopathy
Rhabdomyolysis in the setting of preexisting renal insufficiency
Arthralgia

NEUROLOGIC
Fatigue, weakness, drowsiness
Dizziness
Headache

MISCELLANEOUS
Weight gain
Polyphagia

LABORATORY FINDINGS
Abnormal liver-function tests as evidenced by increased transaminase (SGOT and SGPT), BSP retention, and increased thymol turbidity

Proteinuria
Increased creatine phosphokinase
Hyperkalemia in association with renal insufficiency and continuous ambulatory peritoneal dialysis treatment

Reported adverse reactions whose direct relationship with the drug has not been established: peptic ulcer, gastrointestinal hemorrhage, rheumatoid arthritis, tremors, increased perspiration, systemic lupus erythematosus, blurred vision, gynecomastia, thrombocytopenic purpura.

OVERDOSAGE
While there has been no reported case of overdosage, should it occur, symptomatic supportive measures should be taken.

DOSAGE AND ADMINISTRATION
INITIAL: The recommended dosage for adults is 2 g daily in divided doses. Some patients may respond to a lower dosage.
MAINTENANCE: Same as for initial dosage.

HOW SUPPLIED
ATROMID-S CAPSULES (clofibrate capsules)—Each orange, oblong, soft gelatin capsule contains 500 mg clofibrate, in bottles of 100 (NDC 0046-0243-81).

The appearance of these orange, oblong, soft-gelatin capsules is a trademark of Ayerst Laboratories.

Store at room temperature (approximately 25° C). Avoid freezing and excessive heat.

REFERENCES
1. Coronary Risk Handbook (1973). American Heart Association.
2. Nikkila, E.A.: Familial lipoprotein lipase deficiency and related disorders of chylomicron metabolism. In Stanbury J.B. et al (eds): The Metabolic Basis of Inherited Disease, 5th ed., McGraw-Hill, 1983, Chap. 30 p.622–642.
3. Report from the Committee of Principal Investigators: A cooperative trial in the primary prevention of ischaemic heart disease using clofibrate. Br Heart J 40 :1069, 1978.
4. The Coronary Drug Project Research Group: Clofibrate and niacin in coronary heart disease. JAMA 231 :360, 1975.

Shown in Product Identification Section, page 436

AURALGAN®   ℞
[aw-răl 'gan]
Otic Solution

CAUTION: Federal law prohibits dispensing without prescription.

DESCRIPTION
Each mL contains:

Antipyrine .... 54.0 mg
Benzocaine .... 14.0 mg
Glycerin dehydrated q.s. to .... 1.0 mL
(contains not more than 0.6% moisture)
(also contains oxyquinoline sulfate)

TOPICAL DECONGESTANT AND ANALGESIC
AURALGAN is an otic solution containing antipyrine, benzocaine, and dehydrated glycerin. The solution congeals at 0° C (32° F), but returns to normal consistency, unchanged, at room temperature.

The structures of the components are:

antipyrine   benzocaine   glycerin

CLINICAL PHARMACOLOGY
AURALGAN combines the hygroscopic property of dehydrated glycerin with the analgesic action of antipyrine and benzocaine to relieve pressure, reduce inflammation and congestion, and alleviate pain and discomfort in acute otitis media.

AURALGAN does not blanch the tympanic membrane or mask the landmarks and, therefore, does not distort the otoscopic picture.

INDICATIONS AND USAGE
Acute otitis media of various etiologies
— prompt relief of pain and reduction of inflammation in the congestive and serous stages
— adjuvant therapy during systemic antibiotic administration for resolution of the infection
Because of the close anatomical relationship of the eustachian tube to the nasal cavity, otitis media is a frequent problem, especially in children in whom the tube is shorter, wider, and more horizontal than in adults.

Removal of cerumen
—facilitates the removal of excessive or impacted cerumen

CONTRAINDICATIONS

Hypersensitivity to any of the components or substances related to them.
Perforated tympanic membrane is considered a contraindication to the use of any medication in the external ear canal.

WARNINGS

Discontinue promptly if sensitization or irritation occurs.

PRECAUTIONS

Carcinogenesis, Mutagenesis, Impairment of Fertility:
No long-term studies in animals or humans have been conducted
Pregnancy Category C: Animal reproduction studies have not been conducted with AURALGAN. It is also not known whether AURALGAN can cause fetal harm when administered to a pregnant woman, or can affect reproduction capacity. AURALGAN should be given to a pregnant woman only if clearly needed.
Nursing Mothers: It is not known whether this drug is excreted in human milk. Because many drugs are excreted in human milk, caution should be exercised when AURALGAN is administered to a nursing woman.

DOSAGE AND ADMINISTRATION

Acute otitis media: Instill AURALGAN permitting the solution to run along the wall of the canal until it is filled. Avoid touching the ear with dropper. Then moisten a cotton pledget with AURALGAN and insert into meatus. Repeat every one to two hours until pain and congestion are relieved.
Removal of cerumen
Before: Instill AURALGAN three times daily for two or three days to help detach cerumen from wall of canal and facilitate removal.
After: AURALGAN is useful for drying out the canal or relieving discomfort.
Before and after removal of cerumen, a cotton pledget moistened with AURALGAN should be inserted into the meatus following instillation.
NOTE: Do not rinse dropper after use. Replace dropper in bottle after each use. Hold dropper assembly by screw cap and, without compressing the rubber bulb, insert into drug container and screw down tightly.
Protect the solution from light and heat, and do not use if it is brown or contains a precipitate.
DISCARD THIS PRODUCT SIX MONTHS AFTER DROPPER IS FIRST PLACED IN THE DRUG SOLUTION.

HOW SUPPLIED

AURALGAN® Otic Solution, in package containing 10 mL bottle with separate dropper-screw cap attachment (NDC 0046-1000-10).
Store at room temperature (approximately 25° C).

AYGESTIN®   ℞
[ā-jĕs 'tĭn]
(norethindrone acetate tablets, USP)

CAUTION: Federal law prohibits dispensing without prescription.

> **WARNING:**
> THE USE OF Aygestin® DURING THE FIRST FOUR MONTHS OF PREGNANCY IS NOT RECOMMENDED.
> Progestational agents have been used beginning with the first trimester of pregnancy in an attempt to prevent habitual abortion. There is no adequate evidence that such use is effective when such drugs are given during the first four months of pregnancy. Furthermore, in the vast majority of women, the cause of abortion is a defective ovum, which progestational agents could not be expected to influence. In addition, the use of progestational agents, with their uterine-relaxant properties, in patients with fertilized defective ova may cause a delay in spontaneous abortion. Therefore, the use of such drugs during the first four months of pregnancy is not recommended.
> Several reports suggest an association between intrauterine exposure to progestational drugs in the first trimester of pregnancy and genital abnormalities in male and female fetuses. The risk of hypospadias, 5 to 8 per 1,000 male births in the general population, may be approximately doubled with exposure to these drugs. There are insufficient data to quantify the risk to exposed female fetuses, but insofar as some of these drugs induce mild virilization of the external genitalia of the female fetus, and because of the increased association of hypospadias in the male fetus, it is prudent to avoid the use of these drugs during the first trimester of pregnancy.

If the patient is exposed to Aygestin® (norethindrone acetate tablets, USP) during the first four months of pregnancy or if she becomes pregnant while taking this drug, she should be apprised of the potential risks to the fetus.

DESCRIPTION

Aygestin® (norethindrone acetate tablets, USP)—
5 mg oral tablets
Aygestin, (17-hydroxy-19-nor-17α-pregn-4-en-20-yn-3-one acetate), a synthetic, orally active progestin, is the acetic acid ester of norethindrone. It is a white, or creamy white, crystalline powder.

Aygestin Tablets contain the following inactive ingredients: lactose, magnesium stearate, and microcrystalline cellulose.

CLINICAL PHARMACOLOGY

Norethindrone acetate induces secretory changes in an estrogen-primed endometrium. It acts to inhibit the secretion of pituitary gonadotropins which, in turn, prevent follicular maturation and ovulation. On a weight basis, it is twice as potent as norethindrone.

INDICATIONS AND USAGE

Aygestin is indicated for the treatment of secondary amenorrhea, endometriosis, and abnormal uterine bleeding due to hormonal imbalance in the absence of organic pathology, such as submucous fibroids or uterine cancer.

CONTRAINDICATIONS

Thrombophlebitis, thromboembolic disorders, cerebral apoplexy, or a past history of these conditions.
Markedly impaired liver function or liver disease.
Known or suspected carcinoma of the breast.
Undiagnosed vaginal bleeding.
Missed abortion.
As a diagnostic test for pregnancy.

WARNINGS

1. Discontinue medication pending examination if there is a sudden partial or complete loss of vision or if there is sudden onset of proptosis, diplopia, or migraine. If examination reveals papilledema or retinal vascular lesions, medication should be withdrawn.
2. Because of the occasional occurrence of thrombophlebitis and pulmonary embolism in patients taking progestogens, the physician should be alert to the earliest manifestations of the disease.
3. Masculinization of the female fetus has occurred when progestogens have been used in pregnant women.

PRECAUTIONS

A. GENERAL PRECAUTIONS.
1. The pretreatment physical examination should include special reference to breasts and pelvic organs, as well as a Papanicolaou smear.
2. Because this drug may cause some degree of fluid retention, conditions which might be influenced by this factor, such as epilepsy, migraine, asthma, cardiac or renal dysfunctions, require careful observation.
3. In cases of breakthrough bleeding, as in all cases of irregular bleeding per vaginam, nonfunctional causes should be borne in mind. In cases of undiagnosed vaginal bleeding, adequate diagnostic measures are indicated.
4. Patients who have a history of psychic depression should be carefully observed and the drug discontinued if the depression recurs to a serious degree.
5. Any possible influence of prolonged progestogen therapy on pituitary, ovarian, adrenal, hepatic, or uterine functions awaits further study.
6. Concomitant Use in Estrogen Replacement Therapy: In postmenopausal estrogen replacement therapy, studies of the addition of a progestin for 7 or more days of a cycle of estrogen administration have reported a lowered incidence of endometrial hyperplasia. Morphological and biochemical studies of the endometrium suggest that 10 to 13 days of progestin are needed to provide maximal maturation of the endometrium and to eliminate any hyperplastic changes. Whether this will provide protection from endometrial carcinoma has not been clearly established. There are possible additional risks which may be associated with the inclusion of progestin in estrogen replacement regimens. Progestin therapy may have an adverse effect on lipid metabolism.
7. A decrease in glucose tolerance has been observed in a small percentage of patients on estrogen-progestogen combination drugs. The mechanism of this decrease is obscure. For

this reason, diabetic patients should be carefully observed while receiving progestogen therapy.
8. The age of the patient constitutes no absolute limiting factor, although treatment with progestogens may mask the onset of the climacteric.
9. The pathologist should be advised of progestogen therapy when relevant specimens are submitted.
B. INFORMATION FOR THE PATIENT.
See text which appears at the end of this insert.
C. CARCINOGENESIS, MUTAGENESIS, AND IMPAIRMENT OF FERTILITY.
Some beagle dogs treated with medroxyprogesterone acetate developed mammary nodules. Although nodules occasionally appeared in control animals, they were intermittent in nature, whereas nodules in treated animals were larger and more numerous, and persisted. There is no general agreement as to whether the nodules are benign or malignant. Their significance with respect to humans has not been established.
D. PREGNANCY CATEGORY X.
See Boxed Warning.
E. NURSING MOTHERS.
Detectable amounts of progestogens have been identified in the milk of mothers receiving them. The effect of this on the nursing infant has not been determined.
F. PEDIATRIC USE.
Safety and effectiveness in children have not been established.

ADVERSE REACTIONS

The following adverse reactions have been observed in women taking progestins:
Breakthrough bleeding.
Spotting.
Change in menstrual flow.
Amenorrhea.
Edema.
Changes in weight (decreases, increases).
Changes in cervical erosion and cervical secretions.
Cholestatic jaundice.
Rash (allergic) with and without pruritus.
Melasma or chloasma.
Mental depression.
Progestins may alter the result of pregnanediol determinations. The following laboratory results may be altered by the concomitant use of estrogens with progestins:
Hepatic function.
Coagulation tests—increase in prothrombin, factors VII, VIII, IX, and X.
Increase in PBI, BEI, and a decrease in T^3 uptake.
Reduced response to metyrapone test.
A statistically significant association has been demonstrated between use of estrogen-progestogen combination drugs and the following serious adverse reactions: thrombophlebitis, pulmonary embolism, and cerebral thrombosis and embolism. For this reason, patients on progestogen therapy should be carefully observed. Although available evidence is suggestive of an association, such a relationship has been neither confirmed nor refuted for the following serious adverse reactions:
Neuro-ocular lesions, *e.g.*, retinal thrombosis and optic neuritis.
The following adverse reactions have been observed in patients receiving estrogen-progestogen combination drugs:
1.   Rise in blood pressure in susceptible individuals.
2.   Premenstrual-like syndrome.
3.   Changes in libido.
4.   Changes in appetite.
5.   Cystitis-like syndrome.
6.   Headache.
7.   Nervousness.
8.   Dizziness.
9.   Fatigue.
10.   Backache.
11.   Hirsutism.
12.   Loss of scalp hair.
13.   Erythema multiforme.
14.   Erythema nodosum.
15.   Hemorrhagic eruption.
16.   Itching.
In view of these observations, patients on progestogen therapy should be carefully observed.

DOSAGE AND ADMINISTRATION

Therapy with Aygestin® must be adapted to the specific indications and therapeutic response of the individual patient. This dosage schedule assumes the interval between menses to be 28 days.
Secondary amenorrhea, abnormal uterine bleeding due to hormonal imbalance in the absence of organic pathology: 2.5 to 10 mg Aygestin may be given daily for 5 to 10 days during the second half of the theoretical menstrual cycle to produce an optimum secretory transformation of an endometrium that

Continued on next page

Wyeth-Ayerst Laboratories—Cont.

has been adequately primed with either endogenous or exogenous estrogen.
Progestin withdrawal bleeding usually occurs within three to seven days after discontinuing Aygestin therapy. Patients with a past history of recurrent episodes of abnormal uterine bleeding may benefit from planned menstrual cycling with Aygestin.
Endometriosis:
Initial daily dosage of 5 mg Aygestin for two weeks. Dosage should be increased by 2.5 mg per day every two weeks until 15 mg per day of Aygestin is reached. Therapy may be held at this level for six to nine months or until annoying breakthrough bleeding demands temporary termination.

HOW SUPPLIED

Each scored Aygestin Tablet contains 5 mg norethindrone acetate, USP, in bottles of 50 (NDC 0046-0894-50).
Store at room temperature (approximately 25° C).
Dispense in a well-closed container as defined in the USP.

INFORMATION FOR THE PATIENT

Your doctor has prescribed Aygestin® (norethindrone acetate tablets, USP), a progestin, for you. Aygestin is similar to the progesterone hormones naturally produced by the body. Progestins are used to treat menstrual disorders and to test if the body is producing certain hormones.

Warning

Progesterone or progesterone-like drugs have been used to prevent miscarriage in the first few months of pregnancy. No adequate evidence is available to show that they are effective for this purpose. Furthermore, most cases of early miscarriage are due to causes which could not be helped by these drugs. There is an increased risk of minor birth defects in children whose mothers take this drug during the first four months of pregnancy. Several reports suggest an association between mothers who take these drugs in the first trimester of pregnancy and genital abnormalities in male and female babies. The risk to the male baby is the possibility of being born with a condition in which the opening of the penis is on the underside rather than the tip of the penis (hypospadias). Hypospadias occurs in about 5 to 8 per 1,000 male births and is about doubled with exposure to these drugs. There is not enough information to quantify the risk to exposed female fetuses, but enlargement of the clitoris and fusion of the labia may occur, although rarely.
Therefore, since drugs of this type may induce mild masculinization of the external genitalia of the female fetus, as well as hypospadias in the male fetus, it is wise to avoid using the drug during the first trimester of pregnancy.
These drugs have been used as a test for pregnancy but such use is no longer considered safe because of possible damage to a developing baby. Also, more rapid methods for testing for pregnancy are now available.
If you take Aygestin (norethindrone acetate tablets, USP) and later find you were pregnant when you took it, be sure to discuss this with your doctor as soon as possible.

HOW SUPPLIED

Aygestin® (norethindrone acetate tablets, USP)—scored 5 mg tablets, in bottles of 50, for oral administration.
Store at room temperature (approximately 25°C).
Shown in Product Identification Section, page 436

BASALJEL® OTC

[bā 'sel-jel]
(basic aluminum carbonate gel)
SUSPENSION • CAPSULES • TABLETS

COMPOSITION

Suspension—each 5 mL teaspoonful contains basic aluminum carbonate gel equivalent to 400 mg aluminum hydroxide. Inactive ingredients are artificial and natural flavors, butylparaben, calcium benzoate, glycerin, hydroxypropyl methylcellulose, methylparaben, mineral oil, propylparaben, saccharin, simethicone, sorbitol solution, and water.
Capsule contains dried basic aluminum carbonate gel equivalent to 608 mg of dried aluminum hydroxide gel or 500 mg aluminum hydroxide. Inactive ingredients are D&C Yellow 10, FD&C Blue 1, FD&C Red 40, FD&C Yellow 6, gelatin, polacrilin potassium, polyethylene glycol, talc, and titanium dioxide. Tablet contains dried basic aluminum carbonate gel equivalent to 608 mg of dried aluminum hydroxide gel or 500 mg aluminum hydroxide. Inactive ingredients are cellulose, hydrogenated vegetable oil, magnesium stearate, polacrilin potassium, starch, and talc.

INDICATIONS

Symptomatic relief of hyperacidity associated with peptic ulcer, gastritis, peptic esophagitis, gastric hyperacidity, and hiatal hernia. For the treatment, control, or management of hyperphosphatemia, or for use with a low phosphate diet to prevent formation of phosphate urinary stones, through the reduction of phosphates in the serum and urine.

WARNINGS

No more than 24 tablets/capsules/teaspoonfuls of BASALJEL should be taken in a 24-hour period. Aluminum forms insoluble complexes with phosphate in the gastrointestinal tract, thus decreasing phosphate absorption. Prolonged use of aluminum-containing antacids by normophosphatemic patients may result in hypophosphatemia if phosphate intake is not adequate. In its more severe forms, hypophosphatemia can lead to anorexia, malaise, muscle weakness, and osteomalacia. A usually transient hypercalciuria of mild degree may be associated with the early weeks of therapy. Prolonged use of aluminum-containing antacids in patients with renal failure may result in or worsen dialysis osteomalacia. Elevated tissue aluminum levels contribute to the development of dialysis encephalopathy and osteomalacia syndromes. Also, a number of cases of dialysis encephalopathy have been associated with elevated aluminum levels in the dialysate water. Small amounts of aluminum are absorbed from the gastrointestinal tract and renal excretion of aluminum is impaired in renal failure. Prolonged use of aluminum-containing antacids in such patients may contribute to increased plasma levels of aluminum. Aluminum is not well removed by dialysis because it is bound to albumin and transferrin, which do not cross dialysis membranes. As a result, aluminum is deposited in bone, and dialysis osteomalacia may develop when large amounts of aluminum are ingested orally by patients with impaired renal function. Pregnant women and nursing mothers are advised to seek the advice of a health professional before using this product.

PRECAUTIONS

May cause constipation. Adequate fluid intake should be maintained in addition to the specific medical or surgical management indicated by the patient's condition.

DRUG INTERACTIONS

Alumina-containing antacids should not be used concomitantly with any form of tetracycline therapy.

DOSAGE AND ADMINISTRATION

Suspension—2 teaspoonfuls (10 mL) in water or fruit juice taken as often as every 2 hours up to 12 times daily. Two teaspoonfuls have the capacity to neutralize 23 mEq of acid. Capsules—2 capsules as often as every 2 hours up to 12 times daily. Two capsules have the capacity to neutralize 24 mEq of acid. Tablets—2 tablets as often as every 2 hours up to 12 times daily. Two tablets have the capacity to neutralize 25 mEq of acid.
Hyperphosphatemia: An initial dose of Basaljel equivalent to 1.0 gm aluminum hydroxide—2 capsules, 2 tablets, or 2.5 teaspoonfuls (12 mL) suspension—taken 3 to 4 times per day with meals (total daily dose 3–4 gm) is recommended. After therapy is initiated, Basaljel dosage should be adjusted to the minimum required amount by carefully monitoring dietary phosphate intake (patients should be instructed on maintaining a low phosphate diet) and measurement of serum phosphorus levels on a regular basis. Sodium content is: 0.13 mEq/5 mL for the suspension, 0.12 mEq per capsule, and 0.12 mEq per tablet.

HOW SUPPLIED

Suspension—bottles of 12 fluidounces; Capsules—bottles of 100 and 500; Tablets (scored)—bottles of 100.

BICILLIN® C-R ℞

[bī-sil 'in]
(penicillin G benzathine and penicillin G procaine suspension)
INJECTION

FOR DEEP INTRAMUSCULAR INJECTION ONLY

DESCRIPTION

Bicillin C-R (penicillin G benzathine and penicillin G procaine suspension), Wyeth, contains equal amounts of the benzathine and procaine salts of penicillin G. It is available for deep intramuscular injection.
Penicillin G benzathine is prepared by the reaction of dibenzylethylene diamine with two molecules of penicillin G. It is chemically designated as 3,3-dimethyl-7-oxo-6-(2-phenylacetamido)-4-thia-1-azabicyclo [3.2.0] heptane-2-carboxylic acid compound with *N,N'* -dibenzylethylenediamine (2:1), tetrahydrate. It occurs as a white, crystalline powder and is very slightly soluble in water and sparingly soluble in alcohol.
Penicillin G procaine, 3,3-dimethyl-7-oxo-6-(2-phenylacetamido)-4-thia-1-azabicyclo [3.2.0] heptane-2-carboxylic acid 2-(diethylamino)ethyl p-aminobenzoate compound(1:1) monohydrate, is an equimolar salt of procaine and penicillin G. It occurs as white crystals or a white, microcrystalline powder and is slightly soluble in water.
Bicillin C-R (penicillin G benzathine and penicillin G procaine suspension) contains in each mL the equivalent of 150,000 units of penicillin G as the benzathine salt and 150,000 units of penicillin G as the procaine salt in a stabilized aqueous suspension with sodium citrate buffer; and as w/v, approximately 0.5% lecithin, 0.55% carboxymethylcellulose, 0.55% povidone, 0.1% methylparaben, and 0.01% propylparaben.
Each disposable syringe (2 mL size) contains the equivalent of 1,200,000 units of penicillin G comprising: the equivalent of 600,000 units penicillin G as the benzathine salt and the equivalent of 600,000 units penicillin G as the procaine salt in a stabilized aqueous suspension with sodium citrate buffer; and as w/v, approximately 0.5% lecithin, 0.55% carboxymethylcellulose, 0.55% povidone, 0.1% methylparaben, and 0.01% propylparaben.
Each disposable syringe (4 mL size) contains the equivalent of 2,400,000 units of penicillin G comprising: the equivalent of 1,200,000 units of penicillin G as the benzathine salt and the equivalent of 1,200,000 units of penicillin G as the procaine salt in a stabilized aqueous suspension with sodium citrate buffer; and as w/v, approximately 0.5% lecithin, 0.55% carboxymethylcellulose, 0.55% povidone, 0.1% methylparaben, and 0.01% propylparaben.
Each TUBEX cartridge (1 mL size) contains the equivalent of 600,000 units of penicillin G comprising: the equivalent of 300,000 units penicillin G as the benzathine salt and the equivalent of 300,000 units penicillin G as the procaine salt in a stabilized aqueous suspension with sodium citrate buffer; and as w/v, approximately 0.5% lecithin, 0.55% carboxymethylcellulose, 0.55% povidone, 0.1% methylparaben, and 0.01% propylparaben.
Each TUBEX cartridge (2 mL size) contains the equivalent of 1,200,000 units of penicillin G comprising: the equivalent of 600,000 units of penicillin G as the benzathine salt and the equivalent of 600,000 units of penicillin G as the procaine salt in a stabilized aqueous suspension with sodium citrate buffer; and as w/v, approximately 0.5% lecithin, 0.55% carboxymethylcellulose, 0.55% povidone, 0.1% methylparaben, and 0.01% propylparaben.
Bicillin C-R suspension in the multiple-dose-vial formulation, disposable-syringe formulation, and the TUBEX formulation is viscous and opaque. Read "Contraindications," "Warnings," "Precautions," and "Dosage and Administration" sections prior to use.

CLINICAL PHARMACOLOGY

GENERAL

Penicillin G benzathine and penicillin G procaine have a low solubility and, thus, the drugs are slowly released from intramuscular injection sites. The drugs are hydrolyzed to penicillin G. This combination of hydrolysis and slow absorption results in blood serum levels much lower but more prolonged than other parenteral penicillins. Intramuscular administration of 600,000 units of Bicillin C-R in adults usually produces peak blood levels of 1.0 to 1.3 units per mL within 3 hours; this level falls to an average concentration of 0.32 units per mL at 12 hours, 0.19 units per mL at 24 hours, and 0.03 units per mL at seven days.
Intramuscular administration of 1,200,000 units of Bicillin C-R in adults usually produces peak blood levels of 2.1 to 2.6 units per mL within 3 hours; this level falls to an average concentration of 0.75 units per mL at 12 hours, 0.28 units per mL at 24 hours, and 0.04 units per mL at seven days.
Approximately 60% of penicillin G is bound to serum protein. The drug is distributed throughout the body tissues in widely varying amounts. Highest levels are found in the kidneys with lesser amounts in the liver, skin, and intestines. Penicillin G penetrates into all other tissues and the spinal fluid to a lesser degree. With normal kidney function, the drug is excreted rapidly by tubuler excretion. In neonates and young infants and in individuals with impaired kidney function, excretion is considerably delayed.

MICROBIOLOGY

Penicillin G exerts a bactericidal action against penicillin-susceptible microorganisms during the stage of active multiplication. It acts through the inhibition of biosynthesis of cell-wall mucopeptide. It is not active against the penicillinase-producing bacteria, which include many strains of staphylococci. The following *in-vitro* data are available, but their clinical significance is unknown. Penicillin G exerts high *in-vitro* activity against staphylococci (except penicillinase-producing strains), streptococci (Groups A, C, G, H, L, and M), and pneumococci. Other organisms susceptible to penicillin G are *Neisseria gonorrhoeae, Corynebacterium diphtheriae, Bacillus anthracis,* Clostridia species, *Actinomyces bovis, Streptobacillus moniliformis, Listeria monocytogenes,* and Leptospira species. *Treponema pallidum* is extremely susceptible to the bactericidal action of penicillin G.
Susceptibility Test: If the Kirby-Bauer method of disc susceptibility is used, a 10-unit penicillin disc should give a zone greater than 28 mm when tested against a penicillin-sensitive bacterial strain.

INDICATIONS AND USAGE

This drug is indicated in the treatment of moderately severe infections due to penicillin-G-susceptible microorganisms that are susceptible to serum levels common to this particular dosage form. Therapy should be guided by bacteriological studies (including susceptibility testing) and by clinical response.

Bicillin C-R is indicated in the treatment of the following in children of all ages:

Moderately severe to severe infections of the upper-respiratory tract, scarlet fever, erysipelas, and skin and soft-tissue infections due to susceptible streptococci.

Note: Streptococci in Groups A, C, G, H, L, and M are very sensitive to penicillin G. Other groups, including Group D (enterococci), are resistant. Penicillin G sodium or potassium is recommended for streptococcal infections with bacteremia.

Moderately severe pneumonia and otitis media due to susceptible pneumococci.

Note: Severe pneumonia, empyema, bacteremia, pericarditis, meningitis, peritonitis, and arthritis of pneumococcal etiology are better treated with penicillin G sodium or potassium during the acute stage.

When high, sustained serum levels are required, penicillin G sodium or potassium, either IM or IV, should be used. This drug should not be used in the treatment of venereal diseases, including syphilis, gonorrhea, yaws, bejel, and pinta.

CONTRAINDICATIONS

A previous hypersensitivity reaction to any penicillin or to procaine is a contraindication.

Do not inject into or near an artery or nerve.

WARNINGS

The combination of penicillin G benzathine and penicillin G procaine should only be prescribed for the indications listed in this insert.

Serious and occasionally fatal hypersensitivity (anaphylactoid) reactions have been reported in patients on penicillin therapy. Although anaphylaxis is more frequent following parenteral therapy, it has occurred in patients on oral penicillins. These reactions are more apt to occur in individuals with a history of sensitivity to multiple allergens.

There are reports of patients with a history of penicillin hypersensitivity reactions who experienced severe hypersensitivity reactions when treated with a cephalosporin. Before therapy with a penicillin, careful inquiry should be made about previous hypersensitivity reactions to penicillins, cephalosporins, and other allergens. If an allergic reaction occurs, the drug should be discontinued and appropriate therapy should be instituted. Serious anaphylactoid reactions require immediate emergency treatment with epinephrine. Oxygen, intravenous steroids, airway management, including intubation, should also be administered as indicated.

Inadvertent intravascular administration, including inadvertent direct intraarterial injection or injection immediately adjacent to arteries, of Bicillin C-R and other penicillin preparations has resulted in severe neurovascular damage, including transverse myelitis with permanent paralysis, gangrene requiring amputation of digits and more proximal portions of extremities, and necrosis and sloughing at and surrounding the injection site. Such severe effects have been reported following injections into the buttock, thigh, and deltoid areas. Other serious complications of suspected intravascular administration which have been reported include immediate pallor, mottling or cyanosis of the extremity both distal and proximal to the injection site followed by bleb formation; severe edema requiring anterior and/or posterior compartment fasciotomy in the lower extremity. The above-described severe effects and complications have most often occurred in infants and small children. Prompt consultation with an appropriate specialist is indicated if any evidence of compromise of the blood supply occurs at, proximal to, or distal to the site of injection.[1–9] See "Contraindications," "Precautions," and "Dosage and Administration" sections.

Quadriceps femoris fibrosis and atrophy have been reported following repeated intramuscular injections of penicillin preparations into the anterolateral thigh.

Injection into or near a nerve may result in permanent neurological damage.

PRECAUTIONS

GENERAL

Penicillin should be used with caution in individuals with histories of significant allergies and/or asthma.

Care should be taken to avoid intravenous or intraarterial administration, or injection into or near major peripheral nerves or blood vessels, since such injections may produce neurovascular damage. See "Contraindications," "Warnings," and "Dosage and Administration" sections.

A small percentage of patients are sensitive to procaine. If there is a history of sensitivity make the usual test: Inject intradermally 0.1 mL of a 1 to 2 percent procaine solution. Development of an erythema, wheal, flare, or eruption indicates procaine sensitivity. Sensitivity should be treated by the usual methods, including barbiturates, and procaine penicillin preparations should not be used. Antihistaminics appear beneficial in treatment of procaine reactions.

The use of antibiotics may result in overgrowth of nonsusceptible organisms. Constant observation of the patient is essential. If new infections due to bacteria or fungi appear during therapy, the drug should be discontinued and appropriate measures taken.

Whenever allergic reactions occur, penicillin should be withdrawn unless, in the opinion of the physician, the condition being treated is life-threatening and amenable only to penicillin therapy.

In prolonged therapy with penicillin, and particularly with high-dosage schedules, periodic evaluation of the renal and hematopoietic systems is recommended.

LABORATORY TESTS

In streptococcal infections, therapy must be sufficient to eliminate the organism; otherwise, the sequelae of streptococcal disease may occur. Cultures should be taken following completion of treatment to determine whether streptococci have been eradicated.

DRUG INTERACTIONS

Tetracycline, a bacteriostatic antibiotic, may antagonize the bactericidal effect of penicillin, and concurrent use of these drugs should be avoided.

Concurrent administration of penicillin and probenecid increases and prolongs serum penicillin levels by decreasing the apparent volume of distribution and slowing the rate of excretion by competitively inhibiting renal tubular secretion of penicillin.

PREGNANCY CATEGORY B

Reproduction studies performed in the mouse, rat, and rabbit have revealed no evidence of impaired fertility or harm to the fetus due to penicillin G. Human experience with the penicillins during pregnancy has not shown any positive evidence of adverse effects on the fetus. There are, however, no adequate and well-controlled studies in pregnant women showing conclusively that harmful effects of these drugs on the fetus can be excluded. Because animal reproduction studies are not always predictive of human response, this drug should be used during pregnancy only if clearly needed.

NURSING MOTHERS

Soluble penicillin G is excreted in breast milk. Caution should be exercised when penicillin G benzathine and penicillin G procaine are administered to a nursing woman.

CARCINOGENESIS, MUTAGENESIS, IMPAIRMENT OF FERTILITY

No long-term animal studies have been conducted with these drugs.

PEDIATRIC USE

See "Indications and Usage" and "Dosage and Administration."

ADVERSE REACTIONS

As with other penicillins, untoward reactions of the sensitivity phenomena are likely to occur, particularly in individuals who have previously demonstrated hypersensitivity to penicillins or in those with a hstory of allergy, asthma, hay fever, or urticaria.

The following have been reported with parenteral penicillin G:

General: Hypersensitivity reactions including the following: skin eruptions (maculopapular to exfoliative dermatitis), urticaria, laryngeal edema, fever, eosinophilia; other serum-sicknesslike reactions (including chills, fever, edema, arthralgia, and prostration); anaphylaxis. Note: Urticaria, other skin rashes, and serum-sicknesslike reactions may be controlled with antihistamines and, if necessary, systemic corticosteriods. Whenever such reactions occur, penicillin G should be discontinued unless, in the opinion of the physician, the condition being treated is life-threatening and amenable only to therapy with penicillin G. Serious anaphylactic reactions require the immediate use of epinephrine, oxygen, and intravenous steroids.

Hematologic: Hemolytic anemia, leukopenia, thrombocytopenia.

Neurologic: Neuropathy.

Urogenital: Nephropathy.

OVERDOSAGE

Penicillin in overdosage has the potential to cause neuromuscular hyperirritability or convulsive seizures.

DOSAGE AND ADMINISTRATION

Shake multiple-dose vial vigorously before withdrawing the desired dose.

Administer by DEEP, INTRAMUSCULAR INJECTION in the upper, outer quadrant of the buttock. In infants and small children, the midlateral aspect of the thigh may be preferable. When doses are repeated, vary the injection site.

When using the multiple-dose vial:

After selection of the proper site and insertion of the needle into the selected muscle, aspirate by pulling back on the plunger. While maintaining negative pressure for 2–3 seconds, carefully observe the neck of the syringe immediately proximal to the needle hub for appearance of blood or any discoloration. Blood or "typical blood color" may *not* be seen if a blood vessel has been entered—only a mixture of blood and Bicillin C-R. The appearance of any discoloration is reason to withdraw the needle and discard the syringe. If it is elected to inject at another site, a new syringe and needle should be used. If no blood or discoloration appears, inject the contents of the syringe slowly. Discontinue delivery of the dose if the subject complains of severe immediate pain at the injection site or if in infants and young children symptoms or signs occur suggesting onset of severe pain.

When using the TUBEX cartridge:

The Wyeth TUBEX cartridge for this product incorporates several features that are designed to facilitate the visualization of blood on aspiration if a blood vessel is inadvertently entered.

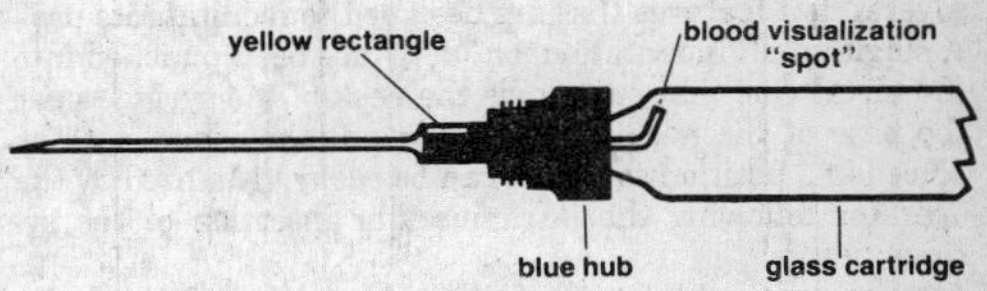

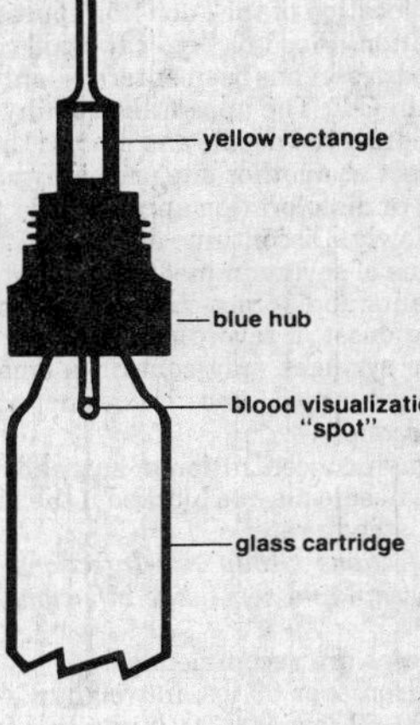

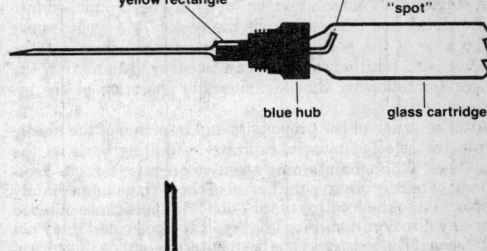

The design of this cartridge is such that blood which enters its needle will be quickly visualized as a red or dark-colored "spot." This "spot" will appear on the barrel of the glass cartridge immediately proximal to the blue hub. Prior to injection, in order to determine where this "spot" can be seen, the operator should first insert and secure the cartridge in the TUBEX syringe/injector in the usual fashion. The needle cover should then be partially removed to reveal a small yellow rectangle and the cartridge and syringe/injector held in one hand with the needle pointing away from the operator. If the 2 mL metal or plastic syringe is used, the glass cartridge should be rotated by turning the plunger of the syringe clockwise until the yellow rectangle is visualized. An imaginary straight line, drawn to extend the yellow rectangle to the shoulder of the glass cartridge, will point to the area on the cartridge where the "spot" can be visualized. If the 1 mL metal syringe is used, it will not be possible to continue to rotate the glass cartridge clockwise once it is properly engaged and fully threaded; it can, however, then be rotated counterclockwise as far as necessary to properly orient the yellow rectangle and locate the observation area. (In this same area in some cartridges, a dark spot may sometimes be visualized prior to injection. This is the proximal end of the needle and does not represent a foreign body in, or other abnormality of, the suspension.)

Thus, before the needle is inserted into the selected muscle, it is important for the operator to orient the yellow rectangle so that any blood which may enter after needle insertion and during aspiration can be visualized in the area on the cartridge where it will appear and not be obscured by any obstructions.

After selection of the proper site and insertion of the needle into the selected muscle, aspirate by pulling back on the plunger. While maintaining negative pressure for 2 to 3 seconds, carefully observe the barrel of the cartridge in the area

Continued on next page

Wyeth-Ayerst Laboratories—Cont.

previously identified (see above) for the appearance of a red or dark-colored "spot."

Blood or "typical blood color" may *not* be seen if a blood vessel has been entered—only a mixture of blood and Bicillin C-R. The appearance of *any* discoloration is reason to withdraw the needle and discard the glass TUBEX cartridge. If it is elected to inject at another site, a new cartridge should be used. If no blood or discoloration appears, inject the contents of the cartridge slowly. Discontinue delivery of the dose if the subject complains of severe immediate pain at the injection site or if, especially in infants and young children, symptoms or signs occur suggesting onset of severe pain.

Some TUBEX cartridges may contain a small air bubble which may be disregarded since it does not affect administration of the product. Because of the high concentration of suspended material in this product, the needle may be blocked if the injection is not made at a slow, steady rate.

When using the disposable syringe:

The Wyeth disposable syringe for this product incorporates several new features that are designed to facilitate its use. A single small indentation, or "dot," has been punched into the metal ring that surrounds the neck of the syringe near the base of the needle. It is important that this "dot" be placed in a position so that it can be easily visualized by the operator following the intramuscular insertion of the syringe needle.

After selection of the proper site and insertion of the needle into the selected muscle, aspirate by pulling back on the plunger. While maintaining negative pressure for 2 to 3 seconds, carefully observe the barrel of the syringe immediately proximal to the location of the "dot" for appearance of blood or any discoloration. Blood or "typical blood color" may *not* be seen if a blood vessel has been entered—only a mixture of blood and Bicillin C-R. The appearance of any discoloration is reason to withdraw the needle and discard the syringe. If it is elected to inject at another site, a new syringe should be used. If no blood or discoloration appears, inject the contents of the syringe slowly. Discontinue delivery of the dose if the subject complains of severe immediate pain at the injection site or if in infants and young children symptoms or signs occur suggesting onset of severe pain.

Some disposable syringes may contain a small air bubble which may be disregarded, since it does not affect administration of the product.

Because of the high concentration of suspended material in this product, the needle may be blocked if the injection is not made at a slow, steady rate.

Streptococcal infections Group A—Infections of the upper-respiratory tract, skin and soft-tissue infections, scarlet fever, and erysipelas.

The following doses are recommended:

Adults and children over 60 lbs. in weight: 2,400,000 units.
Children from 30–60 lbs.: 900,000 units to 1,200,000 units.
Infants and children under 30 lbs.: 600,000 units.

NOTE: Treatment with the recommended dosage is usually given at a single session using multiple IM sites when indicated. An alternative dosage schedule may be used, giving one-half ($\frac{1}{2}$) the total dose on day 1 and one-half ($\frac{1}{2}$) on day 3. This will also insure the penicillinemia required over a 10-day period; however, this alternate schedule should be used only when the physician can be assured of the patient's cooperation.

Pneumococcal infections (except pneumococcal meningitis): 600,000 units in children and 1,200,000 units in adults, repeated every 2 or 3 days until the temperature is normal for 48 hours. Other forms of penicillin may be necessary for severe cases.

Parenteral drug products should be inspected visually for particulate matter and discoloration prior to administration whenever solution and container permit.

HOW SUPPLIED

300,000 units per mL—multiple-dose vials of 10 mL, NDC 0008-0176-01. *600,000 units per mL*—1 mL TUBEX® Sterile Cartridge-Needle Units (20 gauge × 1$\frac{1}{4}$ inch needle) packages of 10, NDC 0008-0026-17; 2 mL TUBEX Sterile Cartridge-Needle Units (20 gauge × 1$\frac{1}{4}$ inch needle) (1,200,000 units per TUBEX), packages of 10, NDC 0008-0026-16; 4 mL single-dose (2,400,000 units) disposable syringes (18 gauge × 2 inch needle), packages of 10, NDC 0008-0026-22.

Store in a refrigerator.
Keep from freezing.
Shake multiple-dose vials well before using.

REFERENCES

1. SHAW, E.: Transverse myelitis from injection of penicillin. *Am. J. Dis. Child.*, 111 :548, 1966.
2. KNOWLES, J.: Accidental intra-arterial injection of penicillin. *Am. J. Dis. Child.*, 111 :552, 1966.
3. DARBY, C., et al: Ischemia following an intragluteal injection of benzathine-procaine penicillin G mixture in a one-year-old boy. *Clin. Pediatrics*, 12 :485, 1973.
4. BROWN, L. & NELSON, A.: Postinfectious intravascular thrombosis with gangrene. *Arch. Surg.*, 94 :652, 1967.
5. BORENSTINE, J.: Transverse myelitis and penicillin (Correspondence). *Am. J. Dis. Child.*, 112 :166, 1966.
6. ATKINSON, J.: Transverse myelopathy secondary to penicillin injection. *J. Pediatrics*, 75 :867, 1969.
7. TALBERT, J. et al: Gangrene of the foot following intramuscular injection in the lateral thigh: A case report with recommendations for prevention. *J. Pediatrics*, 70 :110, 1967.
8. FISHER, T.: Medicolegal affairs. *Canad. Med. Assoc. J.*, 112 :395, 1975.
9. SCHANZER, H. et al: Accidental intraarterial injection of penicillin G. *JAMA*, 242 :1289, 1979.

BICILLIN® C-R 900/300   ℞
[bī-sil'in]
(penicillin G benzathine and penicillin G procaine suspension)
INJECTION

FOR DEEP INTRAMUSCULAR INJECTION ONLY

DESCRIPTION

Bicillin C-R 900/300 (penicillin G benzathine and penicillin G procaine suspension), Wyeth, contains the equivalent of 900,000 units of penicillin G as the benzathine and 300,000 units of penicillin G as the procaine salts. It is available for deep, intramuscular injection.

Penicillin G benzathine is prepared by the reaction of dibenzylethylene diamine with two molecules of penicillin G. It is chemically designated as 3,3-dimethyl-7-oxo-6-(2-phenylacetamido)-4-thia-1-azabicyclo [3.2.0] heptane-2-carboxylic acid compound with *N,N'*-dibenzylethylenediamine (2:1), tetrahydrate. It occurs as a white, crystalline powder and is very slightly soluble in water and sparingly soluble in alcohol.

Penicillin G procaine, 3,3-dimethyl-7-oxo-6-(2-phenylacetamido)-4-thia-1-azabicyclo [3.2.0] heptane-2- carboxylic acid compound with 2-(diethylamino)ethyl *p*-aminobenzoate compound (1:1) monohydrate, is an equimolar salt of procaine and penicillin G. It occurs as white crystals or a white, microcrystalline powder and is slightly soluble in water.

Each TUBEX® cartridge (2 mL size) contains the equivalent to 1,200,000 units of penicillin G as follows: penicillin G benzathine equivalent to 900,000 units of penicillin G and penicillin G procaine equivalent to 300,000 units of penicillin G in a stabilized aqueous suspension with sodium citrate buffer; and as w/v, approximately 0.5% lecithin, 0.55% carboxymethylcellulose, 0.55% povidone, 0.1% methylparaben, and 0.01% propylparaben.

Bicillin C-R 900/300 suspension in the TUBEX formulation is viscous and opaque. Read "Contraindications," "Warnings," "Precautions," and "Dosage and Administration" sections prior to use.

CLINICAL PHARMACOLOGY
GENERAL

Penicillin G benzathine and penicillin G procaine have a low solubility and, thus, the drugs are slowly released from intramuscular injection sites. The drugs are hydrolyzed to penicillin G. This combination of hydrolysis and slow absorption results in blood serum levels much lower but more prolonged than other parenteral penicillins. Intramuscular administration of 1,200,000 units of Bicillin C-R 900/300 in patients weighing 100 to 140 lbs. usually produces average blood levels of 0.24 units/mL at 24 hours, 0.039 units/mL at 7 days, and 0.024 units/mL at 10 days.

Approximately 60% of penicillin G is bound to serum protein. The drug is distributed throughout the body tissues in widely varying amounts. Highest levels are found in the kidneys with lesser amounts in the liver, skin, and intestines. Penicillin G penetrates into all other tissues and the spinal fluid to a lesser degree. With normal kidney function, the drug is excreted rapidly by tubular excretion. In neonates and young infants and in individuals with impaired kidney function, excretion is considerably delayed.

MICROBIOLOGY

Penicillin G exerts a bactericidal action against penicillin-susceptible microorganisms during the stage of active multiplication. It acts through the inhibition of biosynthesis of cell-wall mucopeptide. It is not active against the penicillinase-producing bacteria, which include many strains of staphylococci.

The following *in-vitro* data are available, but their clinical significance is unknown. Penicillin G exerts high *in-vitro* activity against staphylococci (except penicillinase-producing strains), streptococci (Groups A, C, G, H, L, and M), and pneumococci. Other organisms susceptible to penicillin G are *Neisseria gonorrhoeae, Corynebacterium diphtheriae, Bacillus anthracis,* Clostridia species, *Actinomyces bovis, Streptobacillus moniliformis, Listeria monocytogenes,* and Leptospira species. *Treponema pallidum* is extremely susceptible to the bactericidal action of penicillin G.

Susceptibility Test: If the Kirby-Bauer method of disc susceptibility is used, a 10-unit penicillin disc should give a zone greater than 28 mm when tested against a penicillin-susceptible bacterial strain.

INDICATIONS AND USAGE

Bicillin C-R 900/300 is indicated in the treatment of infections as described below that are susceptible to serum levels characteristic of this particular dosage form. Therapy should be guided by bacteriological studies (including susceptibility testing) and by clinical response.

Bicillin C-R 900/300 is indicated in the treatment of the following in children of all ages:

Moderately severe to severe infections of the upper-respiratory tract, scarlet fever, erysipelas, and skin and soft-tissue infections due to susceptible streptococci.

Note: Streptococci in Groups A, C, G, H, L, and M are very susceptible to penicillin G. Other groups, including Group D (enterococci), are resistant. Penicillin G sodium or potassium is recommended for streptococcal infections with bacteremia.

Moderately severe pneumonia and otitis media due to susceptible pneumococci.

NOTE: Severe pneumonia, empyema, bacteremia, pericarditis, meningitis, peritonitis, and arthritis of pneumococcal etiology are better treated with penicillin G sodium or potassium during the acute stage.

When high, sustained serum levels are required, penicillin G sodium or potassium, either IM or IV, should be used. This drug should *not* be used in the treatment of venereal diseases, including syphilis, gonorrhea, yaws, bejel, and pinta.

CONTRAINDICATIONS

A previous hypersensitivity reaction to any penicillin or to procaine is a contraindication.

Do not inject into or near an artery or nerve.

WARNINGS

The combination of penicillin G benzathine and penicillin G procaine should only be prescribed for the indications listed in this insert.

Serious and occasionally fatal hypersensitivity (anaphylactoid) reactions have been reported in patients on penicillin therapy. Although anaphylaxis is more frequent following parenteral therapy, it has occurred in patients on oral penicillins. These reactions are more apt to occur in individuals with a history of sensitivity to multiple allergens.

There are reports of patients with a history of penicillin hypersensitivity reactions who experienced severe hypersensitivity reactions when treated with a cephalosporin. Before therapy with a penicillin, careful inquiry should be made about previous hypersensitivity reactions to penicillins, cephalosporins, and other allergens. If an allergic reaction occurs, the drug should be discontinued and appropriate therapy should be instituted. Serious anaphylactoid reactions require immediate emergency treatment with epinephrine. Oxygen, intravenous steroids, airway management, including intubation, should also be administered as indicated.

Inadvertent intravascular administration, including inadvertent direct intraarterial injection or injection immediately adjacent to arteries, of Bicillin C-R 900/300 and other penicillin preparations has resulted in severe neurovascular damage, including transverse myelitis with permanent paralysis, gangrene requiring amputation of digits and more proximal portions of extremities, and necrosis and sloughing at and surrounding the injection site. Such severe effects have been reported following injections into the buttock, thigh, and deltoid areas. Other serious complications of suspected intravascular administration which have been reported include immediate pallor, mottling or cyanosis of the extremity both distal and proximal to the injection site followed by bleb formation; severe edema requiring anterior and/or posterior compartment fasciotomy in the lower extremity. The above-described severe effects and complications have most often occurred in infants and small children. Prompt consultation with an appropriate specialist is indicated if any evidence of compromise of the blood supply occurs at, proximal to, or distal to the site of injection.[1-9] See "Contraindications," "Precautions," and "Dosage and Administration" sections.

Quadriceps femoris fibrosis and atrophy have been reported following repeated intramuscular injections of penicillin preparations into the anterolateral thigh.

Injection into or near a nerve may result in permanent neurological damage.

PRECAUTIONS
GENERAL

Penicillin should be used with caution in individuals with histories of significant allergies and/or asthma.

Care should be taken to avoid intravenous or intraarterial administration, or injection into or near major peripheral nerves or blood vessels, since such injections may produce neurovascular damage. See "Contraindications," "Warnings," and "Dosage and Administration" sections.

A small percentage of patients are sensitive to procaine. If there is a history of sensitivity make the usual test: Inject intradermally 0.1 mL of a 1 to 2 percent procaine solution.

Development of an erythema, wheal, flare, or eruption indicates procaine sensitivity. Sensitivity should be treated by the usual methods, including barbiturates, and procaine penicillin preparations should not be used. Antihistaminics appear beneficial in treatment of procaine reactions.

The use of antibiotics may result in overgrowth of nonsusceptible organisms. Constant observation of the patient is essential. If new infections due to bacteria or fungi appear during therapy, the drug should be discontinued and appropriate measures taken.

Whenever allergic reactions occur, penicillin should be withdrawn unless, in the opinion of the physician, the condition being treated is life-threatening and amenable only to penicillin therapy.

In prolonged therapy with penicillin, and particularly with high-dosage schedules, periodic evaluation of the renal and hematopoietic systems is recommended.

LABORATORY TESTS

In streptococcal infections, therapy must be sufficient to eliminate the organism; otherwise, the sequelae of streptococcal disease may occur. Cultures should be taken following completion of treatment to determine whether streptococci have been eradicated.

DRUG INTERACTIONS

Tetracycline, a bacteriostatic antibiotic, may antagonize the bactericidal effect of penicillin, and concurrent use of these drugs should be avoided.

Concurrent administration of penicillin and probenecid increases and prolongs serum penicillin levels by decreasing the apparent volume of distribution and slowing the rate of excretion by competitively inhibiting renal tubular secretion of penicillin.

PREGNANCY CATEGORY B

Reproduction studies performed in the mouse, rat, and rabbit have revealed no evidence of impaired fertility or harm to the fetus due to penicillin G. Human experience with the penicillins during pregnancy has not shown any positive evidence of adverse effects on the fetus. There are, however, no adequate and well-controlled studies in pregnant women showing conclusively that harmful effects of these drugs on the fetus can be excluded. Because animal reproduction studies are not always predictive of human response, this drug should be used during pregnancy only if clearly needed.

NURSING MOTHERS

Soluble penicillin G is excreted in breast milk. Caution should be exercised when penicillin G benzathine and penicillin G procaine are administered to a nursing woman.

CARCINOGENESES, MUTAGENESIS, IMPAIRMENT OF FERTILITY

No long-term animal studies have been conducted with these drugs.

PEDIATRIC USE

See "Indications and Usage" and "Dosage and Administration."

ADVERSE REACTIONS

As with other penicillins, untoward reactions of the sensitivity phenomena are likely to occur, particularly in individuals who have previously demonstrated hypersensitivity to penicillins or in those with a history of allergy, asthma, hay fever, or urticaria.

The following have been reported with parenteral penicillin G:

General: Hypersensitivity reactions including the following: skin eruptions (maculopapular to exfoliative dermatitis), urticaria, laryngeal edema, fever, eosinophilia; other serum-sicknesslike reactions (including chills, fever, edema, arthralgia, and prostration); anaphylaxis. Note: Urticaria, other skin rashes, and serum-sicknesslike reactions may be controlled with antihistamines and, if necessary, systemic corticosteroids.

Whenever such reactions occur, penicillin G should be discontinued unless, in the opinion of the physician, the condition being treated is life-threatening and amenable only to therapy with penicillin G. Serious anaphylactic reactions require the immediate use of epinephrine, oxygen, and intravenous steroids.

Hematologic: Hemolytic anemia, leukopenia, thrombocytopenia.

Neurologic: Neuropathy.

Urogenital: Nephropathy.

OVERDOSAGE

Penicillin in overdosage has the potential to cause neuromuscular hyperirritability or convulsive seizures.

DOSAGE AND ADMINISTRATION

Administer by DEEP, INTRAMUSCULAR INJECTION in the upper, outer quadrant of the buttock. In infants and small children, the midlateral aspect of the thigh may be preferable. When doses are repeated, vary the injection site. The Wyeth TUBEX cartridge for this product incorporates several features that are designed to facilitate the visualization of blood on aspiration if a blood vessel is inadvertently entered.

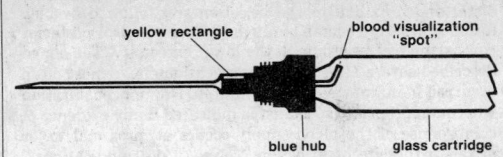

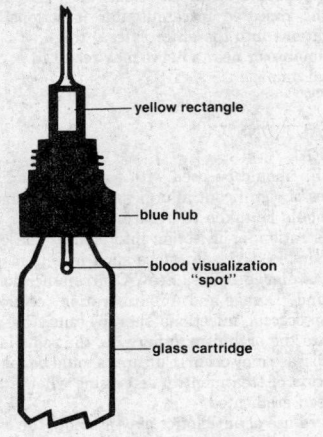

The design of this cartridge is such that blood which enters its needle will be quickly visualized as a red or dark-colored "spot." This "spot" will appear on the barrel of the glass cartridge immediately proximal to the blue hub. Prior to injection, in order to determine where this "spot" can be seen, the operator should first insert and secure the cartridge in the TUBEX syringe/injector in the usual fashion. The needle cover should then be partially removed to reveal a small yellow rectangle and the cartridge and syringe/injector held in one hand with the needle pointing away from the operator. If the 2 mL metal or plastic syringe is used, the glass cartridge should be rotated by turning the plunger of the syringe clockwise until the yellow rectangle is visualized. An imaginary straight line, drawn to extend the yellow rectangle to the shoulder of the glass cartridge, will point to the area on the cartridge where the "spot" can be visualized. If the 1 mL metal syringe is used, it will not be possible to continue to rotate the glass cartridge clockwise once it is properly engaged and fully threaded; it can, however, then be rotated counterclockwise as far as necessary to properly orient the yellow rectangle and locate the observation area. (In this same area in some cartridges, a dark spot may sometimes be visualized prior to injection. This is the proximal end of the needle and does not represent a foreign body in, or other abnormality of, the suspension.)

Thus, before the needle is inserted into the selected muscle, it is important for the operator to orient the yellow rectangle so that any blood which may enter after needle insertion and during aspiration can be visualized in the area on the cartridge where it will appear and not be obscured by any obstructions.

After selection of the proper site and insertion of the needle into the selected muscle, aspirate by pulling back on the plunger. While maintaining negative pressure for 2 to 3 seconds, carefully observe the neck of the glass TUBEX cartridge immediately proximal to the blue plastic needle hub for appearance of blood or any discoloration.

Blood or "typical blood color" may not be seen if a blood vessel has been entered—only a mixture of blood and Bicillin C-R 900/300. The appearance of *any* discoloration is reason to withdraw the needle and discard the TUBEX. If it is elected to inject at another site, a new TUBEX cartridge should be used. If no blood or discoloration appears, inject the contents of the TUBEX slowly. Discontinue delivery of the dose if the subject complains of severe immediate pain at the injection site or if in infants and young children symptoms or signs occur suggesting onset of severe pain.

Some TUBEX cartridges may contain a small air bubble which may be disregarded since it does not affect administration of the product. Because of the high concentration of suspended material in this product, the needle may be blocked if the injection is not made at a slow, steady rate.

STREPTOCOCCAL INFECTIONS—Group A Infections of the upper respiratory tract, skin and soft-tissue infections, scarlet fever, and erysipelas:

A single injection of Bicillin C-R 900/300 is usually sufficient for the treatment of Group A streptococcal infections in children of all ages.

PNEUMOCOCCAL INFECTIONS (except pneumococcal meningitis): One TUBEX Bicillin C-R 900/300 repeated at 2- or 3-day intervals until the temperature is normal for 48 hours. Other forms of penicillin may be necessary for severe cases. Parenteral drug products should be inspected visually for particulate matter and discoloration prior to administration, whenever solution and container permit.

HOW SUPPLIED

Bicillin® C-R 900/300 (penicillin G benzathine and penicillin G procaine suspension), Wyeth®, is supplied in 2 mL size TUBEX® Sterile Cartridge-Needle Units (20 gauge × 1¼ inch needle) in packages of 10 TUBEX, as follows: 1,200,000 units per TUBEX, NDC 0008-0079-01.

Store in a refrigerator.
Keep from freezing.

REFERENCES

1. SHAW, E.: Transverse myelitis from injection of penicillin. *Am. J. Dis. Child.,* 111: 548, 1966.
2. KNOWLES, J.: Accidental intra-arterial injection of penicillin. *Am. J. Dis. Child.,* 111: 552, 1966.
3. DARBY, C., et al: Ischemia following an intragluteal injection of benzathine-procaine penicillin G mixture in a one-year-old boy. *Clin. Pediatrics,* 12: 485, 1973.
4. BROWN, L. & NELSON, A.: Postinfectious intravascular thrombosis with gangrene. *Arch. Surg.,* 94: 652, 1967.
5. BORENSTINE, J.: Transverse myelitis and penicillin (Correspondence). *Am. J. Dis. Child.,* 112: 166, 1966.
6. ATKINSON, J.: Transverse myelopathy secondary to penicillin injection. *J. Pediatrics,* 75: 867, 1969.
7. TALBERT, J. et al: Gangrene of the foot following intramuscular injection in the lateral thigh: A case report with recommendations for prevention. *J. Pediatrics,* 70: 110, 1967.
8. FISHER, T.: Medicolegal affairs. *Canad. Med. Assoc. J.,* 112: 395, 1975.
9. SCHANZER, H. et al: Accidental intra-arterial injection of penicillin G. *JAMA,* 242: 1289, 1979.

BICILLIN® L-A   ℞
[bī-sil'in]
(sterile penicillin G benzathine suspension)
INJECTION
FOR DEEP INTRAMUSCULAR INJECTION ONLY

DESCRIPTION

Bicillin L-A (sterile penicillin G benzathine suspension), Wyeth, is prepared by the reaction of dibenzylethylene diamine with two molecules of penicillin G. It is chemically designated as 3,3-dimethyl-7-oxo-6-(2-phenylacetamido)-4-thia-1-azabicyclo[3.2.0]heptane-2-carboxylic acid compound with N,N'-dibenzylethylenediamine (2:1), tetrahydrate.

It is available for deep intramuscular injection. It contains sterile penicillin G benzathine in aqueous suspension with sodium citrate buffer and, as w/v, approximately 0.5% lecithin, 0.6% carboxymethylcellulose, 0.6% povidone, 0.1% methylparaben, and 0.01% propylparaben. It occurs as a white, crystalline powder and is very slightly soluble in water and sparingly soluble in alcohol.

Bicillin L-A suspension in the multiple-dose vial formulation, disposable syringe formulation and TUBEX formulation is viscous and opaque. The multiple-dose vial formulation contains the equivalent of 300,000 units per mL of penicillin G as the benzathine salt. The disposable syringe formulation is available in a 4 mL size containing the equivalent of 2,400,000 units of penicillin G as the benzathine salt. The TUBEX formulation is available in 1 mL and 2 mL TUBEX Sterile Cartridge-Needle Units containing the equivalent of 600,000 units and 1,200,000 units, respectively, of penicillin G as the benzathine salt. Read "Contraindications," "Warnings," "Precautions," and "Dosage and Administration" sections prior to use.

CLINICAL PHARMACOLOGY

GENERAL

Penicillin G benzathine has an extremely low solubility and, thus, the drug is slowly released from intramuscular injection sites. The drug is hydrolyzed to penicillin G. This combination of hydrolysis and slow absorption results in blood serum levels much lower but much more prolonged than other parenteral penicillins.

Intramuscular administration of 300,000 units of penicillin G benzathine in adults results in blood levels of 0.03 to 0.05 units per mL, which are maintained for 4 to 5 days. Similar blood levels may persist for 10 days following administration

Continued on next page

Wyeth-Ayerst Laboratories—Cont.

of 600,000 units and for 14 days following administration of 1,200,000 units. Blood concentrations of 0.003 units per mL may still be detectable 4 weeks following administration of 1,200,000 units.

Approximately 60% of penicillin G is bound to serum protein. The drug is distributed throughout the body tissues in widely varying amounts. Highest levels are found in the kidneys with lesser amounts in the liver, skin, and intestines. Penicillin G penetrates into all other tissues and the spinal fluid to a lesser degree. With normal kidney function, the drug is excreted rapidly by tubular excretion. In neonates and young infants and in individuals with impaired kidney function, excretion is considerably delayed.

MICROBIOLOGY

Penicillin G exerts a bactericidal action against penicillin-susceptible microorganisms during the stage of active multiplication. It acts through the inhibition of biosynthesis of cell-wall mucopeptide. It is not active against the penicillinase-producing bacteria, which include many strains of staphylococci.

The following *in-vitro* data are available, but their clinical significance is unknown. Penicillin G exerts high *in-vitro* activity against staphylococci (except penicillinase-producing strains), streptococci (Groups A, C, G, H, L, and M), and pneumococci. Other organisms susceptible to penicillin G are *Neisseria gonorrhoeae, Corynebacterium diphtheriae, Bacillus anthracis,* Clostridia species, *Actinomyces bovis, Streptobacillus moniliformis, Listeria monocytogenes,* and Leptospira species. *Treponema pallidum* is extremely susceptible to the bactericidal action of penicillin G.

Susceptibility Test: If the Kirby-Bauer method of disc susceptibility is used, a 20-unit penicillin disc should give a zone greater than 28 mm when tested against a penicillin-susceptible bacterial strain.

INDICATIONS AND USAGE

Intramuscular penicillin G benzathine is indicated in the treatment of infections due to penicillin-G-sensitive microorganisms that are susceptible to the low and very prolonged serum levels common to this particular dosage form. Therapy should be guided by bacteriological studies (including sensitivity tests) and by clinical response.

The following infections will usually respond to adequate dosage of intramuscular penicillin G benzathine:

Mild-to-moderate infections of the upper respiratory tract due to susceptible streptococci.

Venereal infections—Syphilis, yaws, bejel, and pinta.

Medical Conditions in Which Penicillin G Benzathine Therapy Is Indicated as Prophylaxis: Rheumatic fever and/or chorea—Prophylaxis with penicillin G benzathine has proven effective in preventing recurrence of these conditions. It has also been used as follow-up prophylactic therapy for rheumatic heart disease and acute glomerulonephritis.

CONTRAINDICATIONS

A history of a previous hypersensitivity reaction to any of the penicillins is a contraindication.

Do not inject into or near an artery or nerve.

WARNINGS

Penicillin G benzathine should only be prescribed for the indications listed in this insert.

Serious and occasionally fatal hypersensitivity (anaphylactoid) reactions have been reported in patients on penicillin therapy. Although anaphylaxis is more frequent following parenteral therapy, it has occurred in patients on oral penicillins. These reactions are more apt to occur in individuals with a history of sensitivity to multiple allergens.

There are reports of patients with a history of penicillin hypersensitivity reactions who experienced severe hypersensitivity reactions when treated with a cephalosporin. Before therapy with a penicillin, careful inquiry should be made about previous hypersensitivity reactions to penicillins, cephalosporins, and other allergens. If an allergic reaction occurs, the drug should be discontinued and appropriate therapy should be instituted. Serious anaphylactoid reactions require immediate emergency treatment with epinephrine. Oxygen, intravenous steroids, airway management, including intubation, should also be administered as indicated.

Inadvertent intravascular administration, including inadvertent direct intraarterial injection or injection immediately adjacent to arteries, of Bicillin L-A and other penicillin preparations has resulted in severe neurovascular damage, including transverse myelitis with permanent paralysis, gangrene requiring amputation of digits and more proximal portions of extremities, and necrosis and sloughing at and surrounding the injection site. Such severe effects have been reported following injections into the buttock, thigh, and deltoid areas. Other serious complications of suspected intravascular administration which have been reported include immediate pallor, mottling or cyanosis of the extremity both distal and proximal to the injection site followed by bleb formation; severe edema requiring anterior and/or posterior compartment fasciotomy in the lower extremity. The above-described severe effects and complications have most often occurred in infants and small children. Prompt consultation with an appropriate specialist is indicated if any evidence of compromise of the blood supply occurs at, proximal to, or distal to the site of injection.[1–9] See "Contraindications," "Precautions," and "Dosage and Administration" sections.

Quadriceps femoris fibrosis and atrophy have been reported following repeated intramuscular injections of penicillin preparations into the anterolateral thigh.

Injection into or near a nerve may result in permanent neurological damage.

PRECAUTIONS

GENERAL

Penicillin should be used with caution in individuals with histories of significant allergies and/or asthma.

Care should be taken to avoid intravenous or intraarterial administration, or injection into or near major peripheral nerves or blood vessels, since such injection may produce neurovascular damage. See "Contraindications," "Warnings," and "Dosage and Administration" sections.

In streptococcal infections therapy must be sufficient to eliminate the organism; otherwise, the sequelae of streptococcal disease may occur. Cultures should be taken following completion of treatment to determine whether streptococci have been eradicated.

Prolonged use of antibiotics may promote the overgrowth of nonsusceptible organisms, including fungi. Should superinfection occur, appropriate measures should be taken.

LABORATORY TESTS

In streptococcal infections, therapy must be sufficient to eliminate the organism; otherwise, the sequelae of streptococcal disease may occur. Cultures should be taken following completion of treatment to determine whether streptococci have been eradicated.

DRUG INTERACTIONS

Tetracycline, a bacteriostatic antibiotic, may antagonize the bactericidal effect of penicillin, and concurrent use of these drugs should be avoided.

Concurrent administration of penicillin and probenecid increases and prolongs serum penicillin levels by decreasing the apparent volume of distribution and slowing the rate of excretion by competitively inhibiting renal tubular secretion of penicillin.

PREGNANCY CATEGORY B

Reproduction studies performed in the mouse, rat, and rabbit have revealed no evidence of impaired fertility or harm to the fetus due to penicillin G. Human experience with the penicillins during pregnancy has not shown any positive evidence of adverse effects on the fetus. There are, however, no adequate and well-controlled studies in pregnant women showing conclusively that harmful effects of these drugs on the fetus can be excluded. Because animal reproduction studies are not always predictive of human response, this drug should be used during pregnancy only if clearly needed.

NURSING MOTHERS

Soluble penicillin G is excreted in breast milk. Caution should be exercised when penicillin G benzathine is administered to a nursing woman.

CARCINOGENESIS, MUTAGENESIS, IMPAIRMENT OF FERTILITY

No long-term animal studies have been conducted with this drug.

PEDIATRIC USE

See "Indications and Usage" and "Dosage and Administration."

ADVERSE REACTIONS

As with other penicillins, untoward reactions of the sensitivity phenomena are likely to occur, particularly in individuals who have previously demonstrated hypersensitivity to penicillins or in those with a history of allergy, asthma, hay fever, or urticaria.

As with other treatments for syphilis, the Jarisch-Herxheimer reaction has been reported.

The following have been reported with parenteral penicillin G:

General: Hypersensitivity reactions including the following: skin eruptions (maculopapular to exfoliative dermatitis), urticaria, laryngeal edema, fever, eosinophilia; other serum-sicknesslike reactions (including chills, fever, edema, arthralgia, and prostration); anaphylaxis. Note: Urticaria, other skin rashes, and serum-sicknesslike reactions may be controlled with antihistamines and, if necessary, systemic corticosteroids.

Whenever such reactions occur, penicillin G should be discontinued unless, in the opinion of the physician, the condition being treated is life-threatening and amenable only to therapy with penicillin G.

Serious anaphylactic reactions require the immediate use of epinephrine, oxygen, and intravenous steroids.

Hematologic: Hemolytic anemia, leukopenia, thrombocytopenia.

Neurologic: Neuropathy.

Urogenital: Nephropathy.

OVERDOSAGE

Penicillin in overdosage has the potential to cause neuromuscular hyperirritability or convulsive seizures.

DOSAGE AND ADMINISTRATION

Administer by DEEP INTRAMUSCULAR INJECTION in the upper, outer quadrant of the buttock. In infants and small children, the midlateral aspect of the thigh may be preferable. When doses are repeated, vary the injection site.

When using the multiple-dose vial:

Shake multiple-dose vial vigorously before withdrawing the desired dose.

After selection of the proper site and insertion of the needle into the selected muscle, aspirate by pulling back on the plunger. While maintaining negative pressure for 2–3 seconds, carefully observe the barrel of the syringe immediately proximal to the needle hub for appearance of blood or any discoloration. Blood or "typical blood color" may *not* be seen if a blood vessel has been entered—only a mixture of blood and Bicillin L-A. The appearance of any discoloration is reason to withdraw the needle and discard the syringe. If it is elected to inject at another site, a new syringe and needle should be used. If no blood or discoloration appears, inject the contents of the syringe slowly. Discontinue delivery of the dose if the subject complains of severe immediate pain at the injection site or if in infants and young children symptoms or signs occur suggesting onset of severe pain.

When using the TUBEX cartridge:

The Wyeth TUBEX® cartridge for this product incorporates several features that are designed to facilitate the visualization of blood on aspiration if a blood vessel is inadvertently entered.

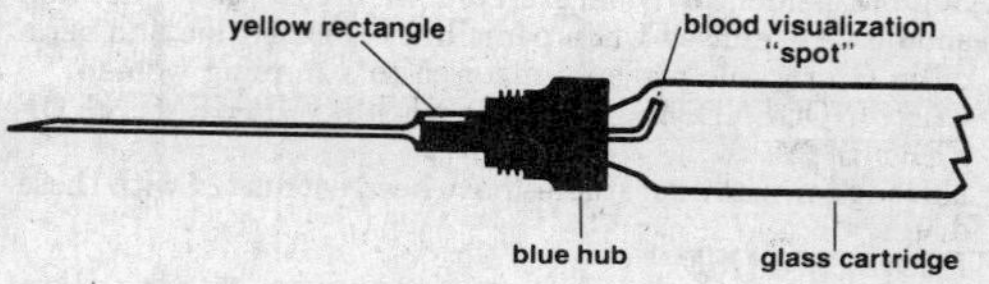

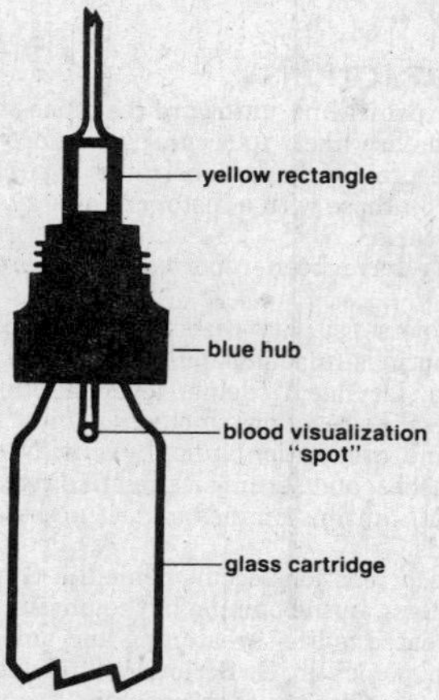

The design of this cartridge is such that blood which enters its needle will be quickly visualized as a red or dark-colored "spot." This "spot" will appear on the barrel of the glass cartridge immediately proximal to the blue hub. Prior to injection, in order to determine where this "spot" can be seen, the operator should first insert and secure the cartridge in the TUBEX syringe/injector in the usual fashion. The needle cover should then be partially removed to reveal a small yellow rectangle and the cartridge and syringe/injector held in one hand with the needle pointing away from the operator. If the 2 mL metal or plastic syringe is used, the glass cartridge should be rotated by turning the plunger of the syringe clockwise until the yellow rectangle is visualized. An imaginary straight line, drawn to extend the yellow rectangle to the shoulder of the glass cartridge, will point to the area on the cartridge where the "spot" can be visualized. If the 1 mL metal syringe is used, it will not be possible to continue to rotate the glass cartridge clockwise once it is prop-

erly engaged and fully threaded; it can, however, then be rotated counterclockwise as far as necessary to properly orient the yellow rectangle and locate the observation area. (In this same area in some cartridges, a dark spot may sometimes be visualized prior to injection. This is the proximal end of the needle and does not represent a foreign body in, or other abnormality of, the suspension.)

Thus, before the needle is inserted into the selected muscle, it is important for the operator to orient the yellow rectangle so that any blood which may enter after needle insertion and during aspiration can be visualized in the area on the cartridge where it will appear and not be obscured by any obstructions.

After selection of the proper site and insertion of the needle into the selected muscle, aspirate by pulling back on the plunger. While maintaining negative pressure for 2–3 seconds, carefully observe the barrel of the cartridge in the area previously identified (see above) for the appearance of a red or dark-colored "spot."

Blood or "typical blood color" may *not* be seen if a blood vessel has been entered—only a mixture of blood and Bicillin L-A. The appearance of *any* discoloration is reason to withdraw the needle and discard the glass TUBEX cartridge. If it is elected to inject at another site, a new cartridge should be used. If no blood or discoloration appears, inject the contents of the cartridge slowly. Discontinue delivery of the dose if the subject complains of severe immediate pain at the injection site or if, especially in infants and young children, symptoms or signs occur suggesting onset of severe pain.

Some TUBEX cartridges may contain a small air bubble which may be disregarded since it does not affect administration of the product.

Because of the high concentration of suspended material in this product, the needle may be blocked if the injection is not made at a slow, steady rate.

When using the disposable syringe:

The Wyeth disposable syringe for this product incorporates several new features that are designed to facilitate its use.

A single small indentation, or "dot," has been punched into the metal or plastic ring that surrounds the neck of the syringe near the base of the needle. It is important that this "dot" be placed in a position so that it can be easily visualized by the operator following the intramuscular insertion of the syringe needle.

After selection of the proper site and insertion of the needle into the selected muscle, aspirate by pulling back on the plunger. While maintaining negative pressure for 2–3 seconds, carefully observe the barrel of the syringe immediately proximal to the location of the "dot" for appearance of blood or any discoloration. Blood or "typical blood color" may *not* be seen if a blood vessel has been entered—only a mixture of blood and Bicillin L-A. The appearance of any discoloration is reason to withdraw the needle and discard the syringe. If it is elected to inject at another site, a new syringe should be used. If no blood or discoloration appears, inject the contents of the syringe slowly. Discontinue delivery of the dose if the subject complains of severe immediate pain at the injection site or if in infants and young children symptoms or signs occur suggesting onset of severe pain.

STREPTOCOCCAL (GROUP A) UPPER-RESPIRATORY INFECTIONS (for example, pharyngitis)

Adults—a single injection of 1,200,000 units; older children—a single injection of 900,000 units; infants and children (under 60 lbs.)—300,000 to 600,000 units.

SYPHILIS

Primary, secondary, and latent—2,400,000 (1 dose). Late (tertiary and neurosyphilis)—2,400,000 at 7-day intervals for three doses.

Congenital—under 2 years of age: 50,000 units/kg/body weight; ages 2–12 years: adjust dosage based on adult dosage schedule.

YAWS, BEJEL, and PINTA—1,200,000 (1 injection).

PROPHYLAXIS—for rheumatic fever and glomerulonephritis.

Following an acute attack, penicillin G benzathine (parenteral) may be given in doses of 1,200,000 units once a month or 600,000 units every 2 weeks.

Some disposable syringes may contain a small air bubble which may be disregarded, since it does not affect administration of the product.

Because of the high concentration of suspended material in this product, the needle may be blocked if the injection is not made at a slow, steady rate.

Parenteral drug products should be inspected visually for particulate matter and discoloration prior to administration whenever solution and container permit.

HOW SUPPLIED

BICILLIN® L-A (sterile penicillin G benzathine suspension) Injection: *300,000 units per ml*—multiple-dose vials of 10 ml (0008-0163-01); *600,000 units per 1 ml* TUBEX® sterile cartridge-needle unit, packages of 10 (0008-0021-08); *1,200,000 units per 2 ml* TUBEX, packages of 10 (0008-0021-07); *2,400,000 units per 4 ml* disposable syringe, packages of 10 (0008-0021-12).

Store in a refrigerator. Keep from freezing.
Shake disposable syringe well before using.

REFERENCES

1. SHAW, E.: Transverse myelitis from injection of penicillin. *Am. J. Dis. Child., 111:* 548, 1966.
2. KNOWLES, J.: Accidental intra-arterial injection of penicillin. *Am. J. Dis. Child., 111:* 552, 1966.
3. DARBY, C., et al: Ischemia following an intragluteal injection of benzathine-procaine penicillin G mixture in a one-year-old boy. *Clin. Pediatrics, 12:* 485, 1973.
4. BROWN, L. & NELSON, A.: Postinfectious intravascular thrombosis with gangrene. *Arch. Surg., 94:* 652, 1967.
5. BORENSTINE, J.: Transverse myelitis and penicillin (Correspondence). *Am. J. Dis. Child., 112:* 166, 1966.
6. ATKINSON, J.: Transverse myelopathy secondary to penicillin injection. *J. Pediatrics, 75:* 867, 1969.
7. TALBERT, J. et al: Gangrene of the foot following intramuscular injection in the lateral thigh: A case report with recommendations for prevention. *J. Pediatrics, 70:* 110, 1967.
8. FISHER, T.: Medicolegal affairs. *Canad. Med. Assoc. J., 112:* 395, 1975.
9. SCHANZER, H. et al: Accidental intra-arterial injection of penicillin G. *JAMA, 242:* 1289, 1979.

BIOLOGICALS

Each of Wyeth-Ayerst's biological products is listed separately in alphabetical order in Wyeth-Ayerst's Product Information Section.

For prescribing information on the products listed—and for which information is not provided—write to Professional Service, Wyeth-Ayerst Laboratories, P.O. Box 8299, Philadelphia, PA 19101, or contact your local Wyeth-Ayerst representative.

CEROSE–DM® OTC

[se-rōs' DM]
Antihistamine/Nasal Decongestant/Cough Suppressant

DESCRIPTION

Each teaspoonful (5 mL) contains 15 mg dextromethorphan hydrobromide, 4 mg chlorpheniramine maleate, and 10 mg phenylephrine hydrochloride. Alcohol 2.4%. The inactive ingredients present are artificial flavors, citric acid, edetate disodium, FD&C Yellow 6, glycerin, saccharin sodium, sodium benzoate, sodium citrate, sodium propionate, and water.

INDICATIONS

For the temporary relief of cough due to minor throat and bronchial irritation as may occur with the common cold or with inhaled irritants. Temporarily relieves nasal congestion, runny nose and sneezing due to the common cold, hay fever, or other upper respiratory allergies.

WARNINGS

May cause marked drowsiness; alcohol may increase the drowsiness effect. Avoid alcoholic beverages while taking this product. Use caution when driving a motor vehicle or operating machinery. Do not take this product if you have heart disease, high blood pressure, thyroid disease, diabetes, asthma, glaucoma, emphysema, chronic pulmonary disease, shortness of breath, difficulty in breathing, or difficulty in urination due to enlargement of the prostate gland unless directed by a doctor. This product may cause excitability especially in children. Do not exceed recommended dosage because at higher doses, nervousness, dizziness, or sleeplessness may occur. Do not take this product for more than 7 days. A persistent cough may be a sign of a serious condition. If symptoms persist for more than one week, tend to recur or are accompanied by fever, rash, or persistent headache, consult a doctor. Do not take this product for persistent or chronic cough such as occurs with smoking, or if cough is accompanied by excessive phlegm (mucus) unless directed by a doctor. As with any drug, if you are pregnant or nursing a baby, seek the advice of a health professional before using this product. Keep this and all drugs out of the reach of children. In case of accidental overdose, seek professional assistance or contact a Poison Control Center immediately.

DRUG INTERACTION PRECAUTION

Do not take this product if you are presently taking a prescription drug for high blood pressure or depression, without first consulting your doctor.

DIRECTIONS

Adults and children 12 years and over: One teaspoonful every four hours as needed. Children 6 to under 12 years of age: One-half teaspoonful every four hours as needed. Do not exceed six doses in a 24 hour period. For children under 6 years, consult a doctor.

HOW SUPPLIED

Cerose-DM® is available in bottles of 4 fl. oz., cases of 12 bottles; and bottles of 1 pint.

Keep tightly closed Store below 77°F (25°C)

CERUBIDINE® ℞

[sĭ-rew"bĭ'dēan]
(daunorubicin hydrochloride)
for Injection

WARNINGS

1. Cerubidine must be given into a rapidly flowing intravenous infusion. It must *never* be given by the intramuscular or subcutaneous route. Severe local tissue necrosis will occur if there is extravasation during administration.
2. Myocardial toxicity manifested in its most severe form by potentially fatal congestive heart failure may occur either during therapy or months to years after termination of therapy. The incidence of myocardial toxicity increases after a total cumulative dose exceeding 400–550 mg/m^2 in adults, 300 mg/m^2 in children more than 2 years of age, or 10 mg/kg in children less than 2 years of age.
3. Severe myelosuppression occurs when used in therapeutic doses.
4. It is recommended that Cerubidine be administered only by physicians who are experienced in leukemia chemotherapy and in facilities with laboratory and supportive resources adequate to monitor drug tolerance and protect and maintain a patient compromised by drug toxicity. The physician and institution must be capable of responding rapidly and completely to severe hemorrhagic conditions and/or overwhelming infection.
5. Dosage should be reduced in patients with impaired hepatic or renal function.

DESCRIPTION

Cerubidine (daunorubicin hydrochloride) is the hydrochloride salt of an anthracycline cytotoxic antibiotic produced by a strain of *Streptomyces coeruleorubidus*. It is provided as a sterile reddish lyophilized powder in vials for intravenous administration only. Each vial contains 20 mg of base activity (21.4 mg as the hydrochloride salt) and 100 mg of mannitol. It is soluble in water when adequately agitated and produces a reddish solution. It has the following structural formula which may be described with the chemical name of 7-(3-amino-2, 3, 6-trideoxy-L-lyxohexosyloxy) -9-acetyl-7, 8, 9, 10-tetrahydro-6,9,11-trihydroxy-4-methoxy-5, 12-naphthacenequinone hydrochloride. Its empirical formula is $C_{27}H_{29}NO_{10}HCl$ with a molecular weight of 563.99. It is a hygroscopic crystalline powder. The pH of a 5 mg/mL aqueous solution is 4.5 to 6.5.

STRUCTURAL FORMULA

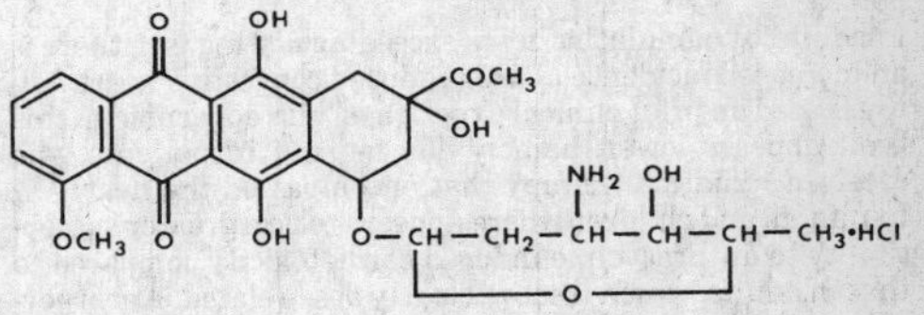

ACTION

Cerubidine inhibits the synthesis of nucleic acids; its effect on deoxyribonucleic acid is particularly rapid and marked. Cerubidine has antimitotic and cytotoxic activity although the precise mode of action is unknown. Cerubidine displays an immunosuppressive effect. It has been shown to inhibit the production of heterohemagglutinins in mice. *In vitro*, it inhibits blast-cell transformation of canine lymphocytes at 0.01 mcg/mL.

Cerubidine possesses a potent antitumor effect against a wide spectrum of animal tumors either grafted or spontaneous.

CLINICAL PHARMACOLOGY

Following intravenous injection of Cerubidine, plasma levels of daunorubicin decline rapidly, indicating rapid tissue uptake and concentration. Thereafter, plasma levels decline slowly with a half-life of 18.5 hours. By one hour after drug administration, the predominant plasma species is daunorubicinol, an active metabolite, which disappears with a half-life of 26.7 hours. Further metabolism via reduction cleavage of the glycosidic bond, 4-0 demethylation, and conjugation with both sulfate and glucuronide have been demonstrated. Simple glycosidic cleavage of daunorubicin or

Continued on next page

Wyeth-Ayerst Laboratories—Cont.

daunorubicinol is not a significant metabolic pathway in man. Twenty-five percent of an administered dose of Cerubidine is eliminated in an active form by urinary excretion and an estimated 40% by biliary excretion.

There is no evidence that Cerubidine crosses the blood-brain barrier.

In the treatment of adult acute nonlymphocytic leukemia, Cerubidine, used as a single agent, has produced complete remission rates of 40 to 50%, and in combination with cytarabine, has produced complete remission rates of 53 to 65%.

The addition of Cerubidine to the two-drug induction regimen of vincristine-prednisone in the treatment of childhood acute lymphocytic leukemia does not increase the rate of complete remission. In children receiving identical CNS prophylaxis and maintenance therapy (without consolidation), there is prolongation of complete remission duration (statistically significant, $p < 0.02$) in those children induced with the three-drug (Cerubidine-vincristine-prednisone) regimen as compared to two drugs. There is no evidence of any impact of Cerubidine on the duration of complete remission when a consolidation (intensification) phase is employed as part of a total treatment program.

In adult acute lymphocytic leukemia, in contrast to childhood acute lymphocytic leukemia, Cerubidine during induction significantly increases the rate of complete remission, but not remission duration, compared to that obtained with vincristine, prednisone, and L-asparaginase alone. The use of Cerubidine in combination with vincristine, prednisone, and L-asparaginase has produced complete remission rates of 83% in contrast to a 47% remission in patients not receiving Cerubidine.

INDICATIONS AND USAGE

Cerubidine in combination with other approved anticancer drugs is indicated for remission induction in acute nonlymphocytic leukemia (myelogenous, monocytic, erythroid) of adults and for remission induction in acute lymphocytic leukemia of children and adults.

WARNINGS

BONE MARROW—Cerubidine is a potent bone marrow suppressant. Suppression will occur in all patients given a therapeutic dose of this drug. Therapy with Cerubidine should not be started in patients with preexisting drug-induced bone-marrow suppression unless the benefit from such treatment warrants the risk.

CARDIAC EFFECTS—Special attention must be given to the potential cardiac toxicity of Cerubidine, particularly in infants and children. Preexisting heart disease and previous therapy with doxorubicin are co-factors of increased risk of Cerubidine-induced cardiac toxicity and the benefit-to-risk ratio of Cerubidine therapy in such patients should be weighed before starting Cerubidine. In adults, at total cumulative doses less than 550 mg/m^2, acute congestive heart failure is seldom encountered. However, rare instances of pericarditis-myocarditis, not dose-related, have been reported.

In adults, at cumulative doses exceeding 550 mg/m^2, there is an increased incidence of drug-induced congestive heart failure. Based on prior clinical experience with doxorubicin, this limit appears lower, namely 400 mg/m^2, in patients who received radiation therapy that encompassed the heart.[1]

In infants and children, there appears to be a greater susceptibility to anthracycline-induced cardiotoxicity compared to that in adults, which is more clearly dose-related. Anthracycline therapy (including daunorubicin) in pediatric patients has been reported to produce impaired left ventricular systolic performance, reduced contractility, congestive heart failure or death. These conditions may occur months to years following cessation of chemotherapy. This appears to be dose-dependent and aggravated by thoracic irradiation. Long-term periodic evaluation of cardiac function in such patients should, thus, be performed.[2–7] In both children and adults, the total dose of Cerubidine administered should also take into account any previous or concomitant therapy with other potentially cardiotoxic agents or related compounds such as doxorubicin.

There is no absolutely reliable method of predicting the patients in whom acute congestive heart failure will develop as a result of the cardiac toxic effect of Cerubidine. However, certain changes in the electrocardiogram and a decrease in the systolic ejection fraction from pretreatment baseline may help to recognize those patients at greatest risk to develop congestive heart failure. On the basis of the electrocardiogram, a decrease equal to or greater than 30% in limb lead QRS voltage has been associated with a significant risk of drug-induced cardiomyopathy. Therefore, an electrocardiogram and/or determination of systolic ejection fraction should be performed before each course of Cerubidine. In the event that one or the other of these predictive parameters should occur, the benefit of continued therapy must be weighed against the risk of producing cardiac damage.

Early clinical diagnosis of drug-induced congestive heart failure appears to be essential for successful treatment with digitalis, diuretics, sodium restriction, and bed rest.

EVALUATION OF HEPATIC AND RENAL FUNCTION—Significant hepatic or renal impairment can enhance the toxicity of the recommended doses of Cerubidine; therefore, prior to administration, evaluation of hepatic function and renal function using conventional clinical laboratory tests is recommended (see "Dosage and Administration").

PREGNANCY—Cerubidine may cause fetal harm when administered to a pregnant woman because of its teratogenic potential. An increased incidence of fetal abnormalities (parieto-occipital cranioschisis, umbilical hernias, or rachischisis) and abortions was reported in rabbits. Decreases in fetal birth weight and postdelivery growth rate were observed in mice. There are no adequate and well-controlled studies in pregnant women. If this drug is used during pregnancy, or if the patient becomes pregnant while taking this drug, the patient should be apprised of the potential hazard to the fetus. Women of childbearing potential should be advised to avoid becoming pregnant.

EXTRAVASATION AT INJECTION SITE—Extravasation of Cerubidine at the site of intravenous administration can cause severe local tissue necrosis.

PRECAUTIONS

Therapy with Cerubidine requires close patient observation and frequent complete blood-count determinations. Cardiac, renal, and hepatic function should be evaluated prior to each course of treatment.

Cerubidine may induce hyperuricemia secondary to rapid lysis of leukemic cells. As a precaution, allopurinol administration is usually begun prior to initiating antileukemic therapy. Blood uric acid levels should be monitored and appropriate therapy initiated in the event that hyperuricemia develops.

Appropriate measures must be taken to control any systemic infection before beginning therapy with Cerubidine.

Cerubidine may transiently impart a red coloration to the urine after administration, and patients should be advised to expect this.

CARCINOGENESIS, MUTAGENESIS, IMPAIRMENT OF FERTILITY

Cerubidine, when injected subcutaneously into mice, causes fibrosarcomas to develop at the injection site. When administered to mice orally or intraperitoneally, no carcinogenic effect was noted after 22 months of observation.

In male dogs at a daily dose of 0.25 mg/kg administered intravenously, testicular atrophy was noted at autopsy. Histologic examination revealed total aplasia of the spermatocyte series in the seminiferous tubules with complete aspermatogenesis.

PREGNANCY CATEGORY D. See "Warnings" section.

ADVERSE REACTIONS

Dose-limiting toxicity includes myelosuppression and cardiotoxicity (see Warnings). Other reactions include:

CUTANEOUS—Reversible alopecia occurs in most patients.

GASTROINTESTINAL—Acute nausea and vomiting occur but are usually mild. Antiemetic therapy may be of some help. Mucositis may occur three to seven days after administration. Diarrhea has occasionally been reported.

LOCAL—If extravasation occurs during administration, tissue necrosis can result at the site.

ACUTE REACTIONS—Rarely, anaphylactoid reaction, fever, chills, and skin rash can occur.

DOSAGE AND ADMINISTRATION

Parenteral drug products should be inspected visually for particulate matter and discoloration prior to administration, whenever solution and container permit.

PRINCIPLES—In order to eradicate the leukemic cells and induce a complete remission, a profound suppression of the bone marrow is usually required. Evaluation of both the peripheral blood and bone marrow are mandatory in the formulation of appropriate treatment plans.

It is recommended that the dosage of Cerubidine be reduced in instances of hepatic or renal impairment. For example, using serum bilirubin and serum creatinine as indicators of liver and kidney function, the following dose modifications are recommended:

Serum Bilirubin	Serum Creatinine	Recommended Dose
1.2 to 3.0 mg%		3/4 normal dose
> 3 mg%	> 3 mg%	1/2 normal dose

REPRESENTATIVE DOSE SCHEDULES AND COMBINATION FOR THE APPROVED INDICATION OF REMISSION INDUCTION IN ADULT ACUTE NONLYMPHOCYTIC LEUKEMIA:

IN COMBINATION[8,9]—For patients under age 60, Cerubidine 45 mg/m^2/day IV on days 1, 2, 3 of the first course and on days 1, 2 of subsequent courses AND cytosine arabinoside 100 mg/m^2/day IV infusion daily for 7 days for the first course and for 5 days for subsequent courses.

For patients 60 years of age and above, Cerubidine 30 mg/m^2/day IV on days 1, 2, 3 of the first course and on days 1, 2 of subsequent courses AND cytosine arabinoside 100 mg/m^2/day IV infusion daily for 7 days for the first course and for 5 days for subsequent courses.[9] This Cerubidine dose-reduction is based on a single study and may not be appropriate if optimal supportive care is available.

The attainment of a normal-appearing bone marrow may require up to three courses of induction therapy. Evaluation of the bone marrow following recovery from the previous course of induction therapy determines whether a further course of induction treatment is required.

REPRESENTATIVE DOSE SCHEDULE AND COMBINATION FOR THE APPROVED INDICATION OF REMISSION INDUCTION IN PEDIATRIC ACUTE LYMPHOCYTIC LEUKEMIA:

IN COMBINATION—Cerubidine 25 mg/m^2 IV on day 1 every week, vincristine 1.5 mg/m^2 IV on day 1 every week, prednisone 40 mg/m^2 PO daily. Generally, a complete remission will be obtained within four such courses of therapy; however, if after four courses the patient is in partial remission, an additional one or, if necessary, two courses may be given in an effort to obtain a complete remission.

In children less than 2 years of age or below 0.5 m^2 body surface area, it has been recommended that the Cerubidine dosage calculation should be based on weight (1.0 mg/kg) instead of body surface area.[17]

REPRESENTATIVE DOSE SCHEDULES AND COMBINATION FOR THE APPROVED INDICATION OF REMISSION INDUCTION IN ADULT ACUTE LYMPHOCYTIC LEUKEMIA:

IN COMBINATION[10]—Cerubidine 45 mg/m^2/day IV on days 1, 2, and 3 AND vincristine 2 mg IV on days 1, 8, and 15; prednisone 40 mg/m^2/day PO on days 1 thru 22, then tapered between days 22 to 29; L-asparaginase 500 IU/kg/day × 10 days IV on days 22 thru 32.

The contents of a vial should be reconstituted with 4 mL of Sterile Water for Injection, USP, and agitated gently until the material has completely dissolved. The withdrawable vial contents provide 20 mg of daunorubicin activity, with 5 mg of daunorubicin activity per mL. The desired dose is withdrawn into a syringe containing 10 mL to 15 mL of normal saline and then injected into the tubing or sidearm of a rapidly flowing IV infusion of 5 percent glucose or normal saline solution. Cerubidine should not be administered mixed with other drugs or heparin. The reconstituted solution is stable for 24 hours at room temperature and 48 hours under refrigeration. It should be protected from exposure to sunlight.

Procedures for proper handling and disposal of anticancer drugs should be considered. Several guidelines on this subject have been published.[11–16] There is no general agreement that all of the procedures recommended in the guidelines are necessary or appropriate.

HOW SUPPLIED

Cerubidine® (daunorubicin hydrochloride) for Injection, is available in butyl-rubber-stoppered vials, each containing 20 mg of base activity (21.4 mg as the hydrochloride salt) and 100 mg of mannitol, as a sterile reddish lyophilized powder. When reconstituted with 4 mL of Sterile Water for Injection, USP, each mL contains 5 mg of daunorubicin activity. Each package contains 10 vials. NDC 0008-4155-01.

STORAGE

(+15° to +25° C).

REFERENCES

1. Gilladoga AC, Manuel C, Tan CTC, et al: The cardiotoxicity of Adriamycin and daunomycin in children. Cancer *37:* 1070–1078, 1976.
2. Bleyer WA; Delayed toxicities of chemotherapy on childhood tissues. Front Radiat. Ther Onc *16:* 40–54, 1982.
3. Isner JM, Ferrans VJ, Cohen SR, et al: Clinical and morphological cardiac findings after anthracycline chemotherapy. Am J Cardiol *51:* 1167–1174, 1983.
4. Rhoden WE, Jenny M, Beton DC, et al: Long term effects on left ventricular function of treatment for childhood malignancy. Br Heart J *66:* 59, 1991.
5. Steinherz LJ, Steinherz PG, Tan CTC, et al: Cardiac toxicity 4 to 20 years after completing anthracycline therapy. JAMA *266:* 1672–1677, 1991.
6. Lipshultz SE, Colan SD, Gelber RD, et al: Late cardiac effects of doxorubicin therapy for acute lymphoblastic leukemia in childhood. N Engl J Med *324:* 808–815, 1991.
7. Steinherz L, Steinherz P: Delayed cardiac toxicity from anthracycline therapy. Pediatrician *18:* 49–52, 1991.
8. Rai KR, Holland JF, Glidewell O, et al: Treatment of acute myelocyctic leukemia: a study by Cancer and Leukemia Group B. Blood *58:* 1203–1212, 1981.
9. Yates J, Glidewell O, Wiernik P, et al: Cytosine arabinoside with daunorubicin or Adriamycin for therapy of acute myelocytic leukemia: a CALGB study. Blood *60:* 454–462, 1982.
10. Gottlieb AJ, Weinberg V, Ellison RR: Efficacy of daunorubicin in the therapy of adult acute lymphocytic

leukemia: a prospective randomized trial by Cancer and Leukemia Group B. Blood 64: 267–274, 1984.

11. Recommendations for the Safe Handling of Parenteral Antineoplastic Drugs. NIH Publication No. 83-2621. For sale by the Superintendent of Documents, U.S. Government Printing Office, Washington, D.C. 20402.

12. AMA Council Report. Guidelines for Handling Parenteral Antineoplastics. JAMA, March 15, 1985.

13. National Study Commission on Cytotoxic Exposure—Recommendations for Handling Cytotoxic Agents. Available from Louis P. Jeffrey, Sc. D., Director of Pharmacy Services, Rhode Island Hospital, 593 Eddy Street, Providence, Rhode Island 02902.

14. Clinical Oncological Society of Australia: Guidelines and recommendations for safe handling of antineoplastic agents. Med J Australia 1:426–428, 1983.

15. Jones RB, et al: Safe handling of chemotherapeutic agents: A report from the Mount Sinai Medical Center, Ca-A Cancer Journal for Clinicians Sept/Oct, 258–263, 1983.

16. American Society of Hospital Pharmacists technical assistance bulletin on handling cytotoxic drugs in hospitals. Am J Hosp Pharm 42:131–137, 1985.

17. Sallan SE: Personal Communication, 1981.

Manufactured by RPS PROPHARM, France
by arrangement with RHONE-POULENC France
Distributed by WYETH-AYERST LABORATORIES INC.,
Philadelphia, PA 19101.

CHOLERA VACCINE   ℞
USP

DESCRIPTION
CHOLERA VACCINE, USP, Wyeth, is a sterile suspension of equal parts of Ogawa and Inaba serotypes of killed *Vibrio cholerae (V. comma)* in buffered sodium chloride injection. The Inaba and Ogawa strains of *V. cholerae* are grown on trypticase soy agar medium, removed from the medium with buffered sodium chloride injection and killed by the addition of 0.5 percent phenol. Phenol in a concentration of 0.5 percent is also used as the preservative in the finished vaccine. The vaccine contains 8 units of each serotype antigen (Ogawa and Inaba) per milliliter.
Cholera vaccine may be injected intracutaneously (intradermally), subcutaneously or intramuscularly.

CLINICAL PHARMACOLOGY
Cholera vaccine is used for active immunization against cholera. Field studies carried out in endemic cholera areas have shown cholera vaccines to be approximately 50% effective in reducing incidence of disease and for only 3 to 6 months. Use of cholera vaccine does not prevent transmission of infection.

INDICATION AND USAGE
Active immunization against cholera is indicated only for individuals traveling to or residing in countries where cholera is endemic or epidemic.

CONTRAINDICATIONS
Use of cholera vaccine should be postponed in the presence of any acute illness.
A history of severe systemic reaction or allergic response following a prior dose of cholera vaccine is a contraindication to further use.

WARNINGS
DO NOT INJECT INTRAVENOUSLY.
Cholera vaccine should not be administered intramuscularly to persons with thrombocytopenia or any coagulation disorder that would contraindicate intramuscular injection.

PRECAUTIONS
GENERAL
A separate, sterilized syringe and needle should be used for each patient to prevent transmission of hepatitis B virus and other infectious agents from one person to another.
Before delivering the dose intramuscularly or subcutaneously, aspirate to help avoid inadvertent injection into a blood vessel.
Before the injection of any biological, the physician should take all precautions known for prevention of allergic or other side reactions. This should include: a review of the patient's history regarding possible sensitivity; and a knowledge of the recent literature pertaining to the use of the biological concerned.
Epinephrine (1:1000) should be available for immediate use when this product is injected.
Some data suggest that administration of cholera and yellow fever vaccines within three weeks of each other may result in decreased levels of antibody response to both vaccines as compared with administration at longer intervals. However, there is no evidence that protection to either disease is diminished following simultaneous administration.[1] It is currently recommended that, when feasible, cholera and yellow fever vaccines should be administered at a minimal interval

of three weeks, unless time constraints preclude this. If the vaccines cannot be administered at least three weeks apart, they should be given simultaneously.[2]

PREGNANCY
PREGNANCY CATEGORY C. Animal reproduction studies have not been conducted with cholera vaccine. It is also not known whether cholera vaccine can cause fetal harm when administered to a pregnant woman or can affect reproductive capacity. However, as with other inactivated bacterial vaccines, its use is not contraindicated during pregnancy unless the intended recipient has manifested significant systemic or allergic reaction following administration of prior doses. Use of cholera vaccine during pregnancy should be individualized to reflect actual need.[1,3]

ADVERSE REACTIONS
Local reactions manifested by erythema, induration, pain, and tenderness at the site of injection occur in most recipients, and such local reactions may persist for a few days. Recipients frequently develop malaise, headache, and mild-to-moderate temperature elevations which may persist for 1 to 2 days.[1,4]

DOSAGE AND ADMINISTRATION
Shake vial vigorously before withdrawing each dose.
Parenteral drug products should be inspected visually for presence of particulate matter and discoloration prior to use. The primary immunizing course consists of two doses administered one week to one month or more apart. The table below summarizes the recommended doses for both primary and booster immunizations by age, volume (mL), and route of administration.[3,5] The intracutaneous (intradermal) route is satisfactory for persons 5 years of age and older, but higher levels of antibody may be achieved in children less than 5 years old by the subcutaneous or intramuscular routes.

Dose number	Intradermal	Subcutaneous or Intramuscular		
	5 years and over	6 mos-4 years	5–10 years	Over 10 years
1 & 2	0.2 mL	0.2 mL	0.3 mL	0.5 mL
Booster	0.2 mL	0.2 mL	0.3 mL	0.5 mL

In areas where cholera is epidemic or endemic, booster doses should be given every six months.
The primary immunizing series need never be repeated for booster doses to be effective.
Before injection, the rubber diaphragm of the vial and the skin over the site to be injected should be cleansed and prepared with a suitable germicide.

HOW SUPPLIED
Cholera Vaccine, USP, is supplied as 1.5 and 20 mL vials.

STORAGE
Keep between 2 and 8°C (35 and 46°F).
Keep from freezing.

REFERENCES
1. Recommendation of the Immunization Practices Advisory Committee (ACIP). General recommendations on immunization. MMWR 32(1):1, 1983.
2. Recommendations of the Immunization Practices Advisory Committee (ACIP). Yellow fever vaccine. MMWR 32(52):679, 1984.
3. Recommendation of the Public Health Service Advisory Committee on Immunization Practices—Cholera Vaccine. MMWR 27(20):173, 1978.
4. GANGAROSA, E. and FAICH, G.: Cholera: The risk to American travelers. Ann. Int. Med. 74:412, 1971.
5. Report of the Committee on Infectious Diseases, American Academy of Pediatrics, 1982 (Red Book).

COLLYRIUM for FRESH EYES   OTC
[ko-lir′e-um]
A neutral borate solution
EYE WASH

DESCRIPTION
Soothing Collyrium Eye Wash for Fresh Eyes is specially formulated to soothe, refresh, and cleanse irritated eyes. Collyrium Eye Wash is a neutral borate solution that contains boric acid, sodium borate, benzalkonium chloride as a preservative and water.

INDICATIONS
Patients are advised of the following. Use Collyrium Eye Wash to cleanse the eye, loosen foreign material, air pollutants or chlorinated water.

RECOMMENDED USES
Home—For emergency flushing of foreign bodies or whenever a soothing eye rinse is necessary.

Hospitals, dispensaries and clinics—For emergency flushing of chemicals or foreign bodies from the eye.

DOSAGE AND ADMINISTRATION
Patients are advised of the following. Puncture bottle by twisting clear cap fully down onto bottle; then remove clear cap from bottle and discard. Remove the eyecup from plastic bag. Rinse blue eyecup with clear water immediately before and after each use. Avoid contamination of rim and interior surfaces of eyecup. Fill blue eyecup one-half full with Collyrium Eye Wash. Apply cup tightly to the affected eye to prevent the escape of the liquid and tilt head backward. Open eyelid wide and rotate eyeball to thoroughly wash eye. Recap by twisting blue eyecup fully onto bottle for storage and subsequent use.

WARNINGS
Patients are advised of the following. Do not use if solution changes color or becomes cloudy, or with a wetting solution for contact lenses or other eye care products containing polyvinyl alcohol.
To avoid contamination do not touch tip of container to any surface. Replace cap after using. If you experience eye pain, changes in vision, continued redness, irritation of the eye, or if the condition worsens or persists, consult a doctor. Obtain immediate medical treatment for all open wounds in or near the eyes.
The COLLYRIUM for FRESH EYES bottle is sealed for your protection. Prior to first use, remove cap and squeeze bottle. If bottle leaks, do not use.
Keep this and all medication out of the reach of children.
Keep bottle tightly closed at Room Temperature, Approx. 77° F (25° C).

HOW SUPPLIED
Bottles of 4 FL. OZ. (118 mL) with eyecup.

COLLYRIUM FRESH™   OTC
[ko-lir′e-um]
Sterile Eye Drops
Lubricant ● Redness Reliever

DESCRIPTION
Collyrium Fresh is a specially formulated sterile eye drop which can be used, up to 4 times daily, to relieve redness and discomfort due to minor eye irritations caused by dust, smoke, smog, swimming, or sun glare.
The active ingredients are tetrahydrozoline HCl (0.05%) and glycerin (1.0%). Other ingredients include benzalkonium chloride (0.01%) and edetate disodium (0.1%) as preservatives, boric acid, hydrochloric acid and sodium borate.

INDICATIONS
Patients are advised of the following. For the temporary relief of redness due to minor eye irritations or discomfort due to burning or exposure to wind or sun.

DOSAGE AND ADMINISTRATION
Patients are advised of the following. Tilt head back and squeeze 1 to 2 drops into each eye up to 4 times daily, or as directed by a physician.

WARNINGS
Patients are advised of the following. Do not use if solution changes color or becomes cloudy. Remove contact lenses before using. If you have glaucoma, do not use this product except under the advice and supervision of a physician. Overuse of this product may produce increased redness of the eye. To avoid contamination, do not touch tip of container to any surface. Replace cap after using. If you experience eye pain, changes in vision, continued redness or irritation of the eye, or if the condition worsens or persists for more than 72 hours, discontinue use and consult a physician.
Keep this and all medication out of the reach of children. The product's carton should be retained for complete product information.
Keep bottle tightly closed at Room Temperature, Approx. 77° F (25° C).

HOW SUPPLIED
Bottles of 0.5 FL. OZ. (15 mL) with built-in eye dropper.

CORDARONE®   ℞
[kŏr′dă-rōn]
(amiodarone HCl)
Tablets

DESCRIPTION
Cordarone is a member of a new class of antiarrhythmic drugs with predominantly Class III (Vaughan Williams classification) effects, available for oral administration as white, scored tablets containing 200 mg of amiodarone hydrochloride. The inactive ingredients present are colloidal silicon

Continued on next page

Wyeth-Ayerst Laboratories—Cont.

dioxide, lactose, magnesium stearate, povidone, starch, and FD&C Red 40. Cordarone is a benzofuran derivative: 2-butyl-3-benzofuranyl 4-[2-(diethylamino)-ethoxy]-3-5-diiodophenyl ketone, hydrochloride. It is not chemically related to any other available antiarrhythmic drug.
The structural formula is as follows:

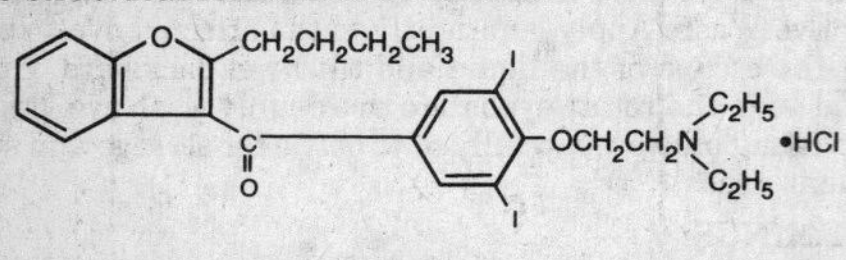

$C_{25}H_{29}I_2NO_3 \cdot HCl$ Molecular Weight: 681.8

Amiodarone HCl is a white to cream-colored crystalline powder. It is slightly soluble in water, soluble in alcohol, and freely soluble in chloroform. It contains 37.3% iodine by weight.

CLINICAL PHARMACOLOGY

ELECTROPHYSIOLOGY/MECHANISMS OF ACTION

In animals, Cordarone is effective in the prevention or suppression of experimentally induced arrhythmias. The antiarrhythmic effect of Cordarone may be due to at least two major properties: 1) a prolongation of the myocardial cell-action potential duration and refractory period and 2) noncompetitive alpha- and beta-adrenergic inhibition.

Cordarone prolongs the duration of the action potential of all cardiac fibers while causing minimal reduction of dV/dt (maximal upstroke velocity of the action potential). The refractory period is prolonged in all cardiac tissues. Cordarone increases the cardiac refractory period without influencing resting membrane potential, except in automatic cells where the slope of the prepotential is reduced, generally reducing automaticity. These electrophysiologic effects are reflected in a decreased sinus rate of 15 to 20%, increased PR and QT intervals of about 10%, the development of U-waves, and changes in T-wave contour. These changes should not require discontinuation of Cordarone as they are evidence of its pharmacological action, although Cordarone can cause marked sinus bradycardia or sinus arrest and heart block. On rare occasions, QT prolongation has been associated with worsening of arrhythmia (see "Warnings").

HEMODYNAMICS

In animal studies and after intravenous administration in man, Cordarone relaxes vascular smooth muscle, reduces peripheral vascular resistance (afterload), and slightly increases cardiac index. After oral dosing, however, Cordarone produces no significant change in left ventricular ejection fraction (LVEF), even in patients with depressed LVEF. After acute intravenous dosing in man, Cordarone may have a mild negative inotropic effect.

PHARMACOKINETICS

Following oral administration in man, Cordarone is slowly and variably absorbed. The bioavailability of Cordarone is approximately 50%, but has varied between 35 and 65% in various studies. Maximum plasma concentrations are attained 3 to 7 hours after a single dose. Despite this, the onset of action may occur in 2 to 3 days, but more commonly takes 1 to 3 weeks, even with loading doses. Plasma concentrations with chronic dosing at 100 to 600 mg/day are approximately dose proportional, with a mean 0.5 mg/L increase for each 100 mg/day. These means, however, include considerable individual variability.

Cordarone has a very large but variable volume of distribution, averaging about 60 L/kg because of extensive accumulation in various sites, especially adipose tissue and highly perfused organs, such as the liver, lung, and spleen. One major metabolite of Cordarone, desethylamiodarone, has been identified in man; it accumulates to an even greater extent in almost all tissues. The pharmacological activity of this metabolite, however, is not known. During chronic treatment, the plasma ratio of metabolite to parent compound is approximately one.

The main route of elimination is via hepatic excretion into bile, and some enterohepatic recirculation may occur. However, its kinetics in patients with hepatic insufficiency have not been elucidated. Cordarone has a very low plasma clearance with negligible renal excretion, so that it does not appear necessary to modify the dose in patients with renal failure. In patients with renal impairment, the plasma concentration of Cordarone is not elevated. Neither Cordarone nor its metabolite is dialyzable.

In patients, following discontinuation of chronic oral therapy, Cordarone has been shown to have a biphasic elimination with an initial one-half reduction of plasma levels after 2.5 to 10 days. A much slower terminal plasma-elimination phase shows a half-life of the parent compound ranging from 26 to 107 days, with a mean of approximately 53 days and most patients in the 40- to 55-day range. In the absence of a loading-dose period, steady-state plasma concentrations, at constant oral dosing, would therefore be reached between 130 and 535 days, with an average of 265 days. For the metabolite, the mean plasma-elimination half-life was approximately 61 days. These data probably reflect an initial elimination of the drug from well-perfused tissue (the 2.5- to 10-day half-life phase), followed by a terminal phase representing extremely slow elimination from poorly perfused tissue compartments such as fat.

The considerable intersubject variation in both phases of elimination, as well as uncertainty as to what compartment is critical to drug effect, requires attention to individual responses once arrhythmia control is achieved with loading doses because the correct maintenance dose is determined, in part, by the elimination rates. Daily maintenance doses of Cordarone should be based on individual patient requirements (see "Dosage and Administration").

Cordarone and its metabolite have a limited transplacental transfer of approximately 10 to 50%. The parent drug and its metabolite have been detected in breast milk.

Cordarone is highly protein-bound (approximately 96%).

Although electrophysiologic effects, such as prolongation of QTc, can be seen within hours after a parenteral dose of Cordarone, effects on abnormal rhythms are not seen before 2 to 3 days and usually require 1 to 3 weeks, even when a loading dose is used. There may be a continued increase in effect for longer periods still. There is evidence that the time to effect is shorter when a loading-dose regimen is used.

Consistent with the slow rate of elimination, antiarrhythmic effects persist for weeks or months after Cordarone is discontinued, but the time of recurrence is variable and unpredictable. In general, when the drug is resumed after recurrence of the arrhythmia, control is established relatively rapidly compared to the initial response, presumably because tissue stores were not wholly depleted at the time of recurrence.

PHARMACODYNAMICS

There is no well-established relationship of plasma concentration to effectiveness, but it does appear that concentrations much below 1 mg/L are often ineffective and that levels above 2.5 mg/L are generally not needed. Within individuals dose reductions and ensuing decreased plasma concentrations can result in loss of arrhythmia control. Plasma-concentration measurements can be used to identify patients whose levels are unusually low, and who might benefit from a dose increase, or unusually high, and who might have dosage reduction in the hope of minimizing side effects. Some observations have suggested a plasma concentration, dose, or dose/duration relationship for side effects such as pulmonary fibrosis, liver-enzyme elevations, corneal deposits and facial pigmentation, peripheral neuropathy, gastrointestinal and central nervous system effects.

MONITORING EFFECTIVENESS

Predicting the effectiveness of any antiarrhythmic agent in long-term prevention of recurrent ventricular tachycardia and ventricular fibrillation is difficult and controversial, with highly qualified investigators recommending use of ambulatory monitoring, programmed electrical stimulation with various stimulation regimens, or a combination of these, to assess response. There is no present consensus on many aspects of how best to assess effectiveness, but there is a reasonable consensus on some aspects:

1. If a patient with a history of cardiac arrest does not manifest a hemodynamically unstable arrhythmia during electrocardiographic monitoring prior to treatment, assessment of the effectiveness of Cordarone requires some provocative approach, either exercise or programmed electrical stimulation (PES).
2. Whether provocation is also needed in patients who do manifest their life-threatening arrhythmia spontaneously is not settled, but there are reasons to consider PES or other provocation in such patients. In the fraction of patients whose PES-inducible arrhythmia can be made noninducible by Cordarone (a fraction that has varied widely in various series from less than 10% to almost 40%, perhaps due to different stimulation criteria), the prognosis has been almost uniformly excellent, with very low recurrence (ventricular tachycardia or sudden death) rates. More controversial is the meaning of continued inducibility. There has been an impression that continued inducibility in Cordarone patients may not foretell a poor prognosis but, in fact, many observers have found greater recurrence rates in patients who remain inducible than in those who do not. A number of criteria have been proposed, however, for identifying patients who remain inducible but who seem likely nonetheless to do well on Cordarone. These criteria include increased difficulty of Induction (more stimuli or more rapid stimuli), which has been reported to predict a lower rate of recurrence, and ability to tolerate the induced ventricular tachycardia without severe symptoms, a finding that has been reported to correlate with better survival but not with lower recurrence rates. While these criteria require confirmation and further study in general, *easier* inducibility or *poorer* tolerance of the induced arrhythmia should suggest consideration of a need to revise treatment.

Several predictors of success not based on PES have also been suggested, including complete elimination of all nonsustained ventricular tachycardia on ambulatory monitoring and very low premature ventricular-beat rates (less than 1 VPB/1,000 normal beats).

While these issues remain unsettled for Cordarone, as for other agents, the prescriber of Cordarone should have access to (direct or through referral), and familiarity with, the full range of evaluatory procedures used in the care of patients with life-threatening arrhythmias.

It is difficult to describe the effectiveness rates of Cordarone, as these depend on the specific arrhythmia treated, the success criteria used, the underlying cardiac disease of the patient, the number of drugs tried before resorting to Cordarone, the duration of follow-up, the dose of Cordarone, the use of additional antiarrhythmic agents, and many other factors. As Cordarone has been studied principally in patients with refractory life-threatening ventricular arrhythmias, in whom drug therapy must be selected on the basis of response and cannot be assigned arbitrarily, randomized comparisons with other agents or placebo have not been possible. Reports of series of treated patients with a history of cardiac arrest and mean follow-up of one year or more have given mortality (due to arrhythmia) rates that were highly variable, ranging from less than 5% to over 30%, with most series in the range of 10 to 15%. Overall arrhythmia-recurrence rates (fatal and nonfatal) also were highly variable (and, as noted above, depended on response to PES and other measures), and depend on whether patients who do not seem to respond initially are included. In most cases, considering only patients who seemed to respond well enough to be placed on long-term treatment, recurrence rates have ranged from 20 to 40% in series with a mean follow-up of a year or more.

INDICATIONS AND USAGE

Because of its life-threatening side effects and the substantial management difficulties associated with its use (see "Warnings" below), Cordarone is indicated only for the treatment of the following documented, life-threatening recurrent ventricular arrhythmias when these have not responded to documented adequate doses of other available antiarrhythmics or when alternative agents could not be tolerated.

1. Recurrent ventricular fibrillation.
2. Recurrent hemodynamically unstable ventricular tachycardia.

As is the case for other antiarrhythmic agents, there is no evidence from controlled trials that the use of Cordarone favorably affects survival.

Cordarone should be used only by physicians familiar with and with access to (directly or through referral) the use of all available modalities for treating recurrent life-threatening ventricular arrhythmias, and who have access to appropriate monitoring facilities, including in-hospital and ambulatory continuous electrocardiographic monitoring and electrophysiologic techniques. Because of the life-threatening nature of the arrhythmias treated, potential interactions with prior therapy, and potential exacerbation of the arrhythmia, initiation of therapy with Cordarone should be carried out in the hospital.

CONTRAINDICATIONS

Cordarone is contraindicated in severe sinus-node dysfunction, causing marked sinus bradycardia; second- and third-degree atrioventricular block; and when episodes of bradycardia have caused syncope (except when used in conjunction with a pacemaker).

Cordarone is contraindicated in patients with a known hypersensitivity to the drug.

WARNINGS

Cordarone is intended for use only in patients with the indicated life-threatening arrhythmias because its use is accompanied by substantial toxicity.

Cordarone has several potentially fatal toxicities, the most important of which is pulmonary toxicity (hypersensitivity pneumonitis or interstitial/alveolar pneumonitis) that has resulted in clinically manifest disease at rates as high as 10 to 17% in some series of patients with ventricular arrhythmias given doses around 400 mg/day, and as abnormal diffusion capacity without symptoms in a much higher percentage of patients. Pulmonary toxicity has been fatal about 10% of the time. Liver injury is common with Cordarone, but is usually mild and evidenced only by abnormal liver enzymes. Overt liver disease can occur, however, and has been fatal in a few cases. Like other antiarrhythmics, Cordarone can exacerbate the arrhythmia, e.g., by making the arrhythmia less well tolerated or more difficult to reverse. This has occurred in 2 to 5% of patients in various series, and significant heart block or sinus bradycardia has been seen in 2 to 5%. All of these events should be manageable in the proper clinical setting in most cases. Although the frequency of such proarrhythmic events does not appear greater with Cordarone than with many other agents used in this population, the effects are prolonged when they occur.

Even in patients at high risk of arrhythmic death, in whom the toxicity of Cordarone is an acceptable risk, Cordarone poses major management problems that could be life-threatening in a population at risk of sudden death, so that every effort should be made to utilize alternative agents first.

The difficulty of using Cordarone effectively and safely itself poses a significant risk to patients. Patients with the indicated arrhythmias must be hospitalized while the loading dose of Cordarone is given, and a response generally requires at least one week, usually two or more. Because absorption and elimination are variable, maintenance-dose selection is difficult, and it is not unusual to require dosage decrease or discontinuation of treatment. In a retrospective survey of 192 patients with ventricular tachyarrhythmias, 84 required dose reduction and 18 required at least temporary discontinuation because of adverse effects, and several series have reported 15 to 20% overall frequencies of discontinuation due to adverse reactions. The time at which a previously controlled life-threatening arrhythmia will recur after discontinuation or dose adjustment is unpredictable, ranging from weeks to months. The patient is obviously at great risk during this time and may need prolonged hospitalization. Attempts to substitute other antiarrhythmic agents when Cordarone must be stopped will be made difficult by the gradually, but unpredictably, changing amiodarone body burden. A similar problem exists when Cordarone is not effective; it still poses the risk of an interaction with whatever subsequent treatment is tried.

PULMONARY TOXICITY

Cordarone may cause a clinical syndrome of cough and progressive dyspnea accompanied by functional, radiographic, gallium-scan, and pathological data consistent with pulmonary toxicity, the frequency of which varies from 2 to 7% in most published reports, but is as high as 10 to 17% in some reports. Therefore, when Cordarone therapy is initiated, a baseline chest X-ray and pulmonary-function tests, including diffusion capacity, should be performed. The patient should return for a history, physical exam, and chest X-ray every 3 to 6 months.

Preexisting pulmonary disease does not appear to increase the risk of developing pulmonary toxicity; however, these patients have a poorer prognosis if pulmonary toxicity does develop.

Pulmonary toxicity secondary to Cordarone seems to result from either indirect or direct toxicity as represented by hypersensitivity pneumonitis or interstitial/alveolar pneumonitis, respectively.

Hypersensitivity pneumonitis usually appears earlier in the course of therapy, and rechallenging these patients with Cordarone results in a more rapid recurrence of greater severity. Bronchoalveolar lavage is the procedure of choice to confirm this diagnosis, which can be made when a T suppressor/cytotoxic (CD8-positive) lymphocytosis is noted. Steroid therapy should be instituted and Cordarone therapy discontinued in these patients.

Interstitial/alveolar pneumonitis may result from the release of oxygen radicals and/or phospholipidosis and is characterized by findings of diffuse alveolar damage, interstitial pneumonitis or fibrosis in lung biopsy specimens. Phospholipidosis (foamy cells, foamy macrophages), due to inhibition of phospholipase, will be present in most cases of Cordarone-induced pulmonary toxicity; however, these changes also are present in approximately 50% of all patients on Cordarone therapy. These cells should be used as markers of therapy, but not as evidence of toxicity. A diagnosis of Cordarone-induced interstitial/alveolar pneumonitis should lead, at a minimum, to dose reduction or, preferably, to withdrawal of the Cordarone to establish reversibility, especially if other acceptable antiarrhythmic therapies are available. Where these measures have been instituted, a reduction in symptoms of amiodarone-induced pulmonary toxicity was usually noted within the first week, and a clinical improvement was greatest in the first two to three weeks. Chest X-ray changes usually resolve within two to four months. According to some experts, steroids may prove beneficial. Prednisone in doses of 40 to 60 mg/day or equivalent doses of other steroids have been given and tapered over the course of several weeks depending upon the condition of the patient. In some cases rechallenge with Cordarone at a lower dose has not resulted in return of toxicity. Recent reports suggest that the use of lower loading and maintenance doses of Cordarone are associated with a decreased incidence of Cordarone-induced pulmonary toxicity.

In a patient receiving Cordarone, any new respiratory symptoms should suggest the possibility of pulmonary toxicity, and the history, physical exam, chest X-ray, and pulmonary-function tests (with diffusion capacity) should be repeated and evaluated. A 15% decrease in diffusion capacity has a high sensitivity but only a moderate specificity for pulmonary toxicity; as the decrease in diffusion capacity approaches 30%, the sensitivity decreases but the specificity increases. A gallium scan also may be performed as part of the diagnostic workup.

Fatalities, secondary to pulmonary toxicity, have occurred in approximately 10% of cases. However, in patients with life-threatening arrhythmias, discontinuation of Cordarone therapy due to suspected drug-induced pulmonary toxicity should be undertaken with caution, as the most common cause of death in these patients is sudden cardiac death. Therefore, every effort should be made to rule out other causes of respiratory impairment (i.e., congestive heart failure with Swan-Ganz catheterization if necessary, respiratory infection, pulmonary embolism, malignancy, etc.) before discontinuing Cordarone in these patients. In addition, bronchoalveolar lavage, transbronchial lung biopsy, and/or open lung biopsy may be necessary to confirm the diagnosis, especially in those cases where no acceptable alternative therapy is available.

If a diagnosis of Cordarone-induced hypersensitivity pneumonitis is made, Cordarone should be discontinued, and treatment with steroids should be instituted. If a diagnosis of Cordarone-induced interstitial/alveolar pneumonitis is made, steroid therapy should be instituted and, preferably, Cordarone discontinued or, at a minimum, reduced in dosage. Some cases of Cordarone-induced interstitial/alveolar pneumonitis may resolve following a reduction in Cordarone dosage in conjunction with the administration of steroids. In some patients, rechallenge at a lower dose has not resulted in return of interstitial/alveolar pneumonitis; however, in some patients (perhaps because of severe alveolar damage) the pulmonary lesions have not been reversible.

WORSENED ARRHYTHMIA

Cordarone, like other antiarrhythmics, can cause serious exacerbation of the presenting arrhythmia, a risk that may be enhanced by the presence of concomitant antiarrhythmics. Exacerbation has been reported in about 2 to 5% in most series, and has included new ventricular fibrillation, incessant ventricular tachycardia, increased resistance to cardioversion, and polymorphic ventricular tachycardia associated with QT prolongation (Torsade de Pointes).

In addition, Cordarone has caused symptomatic bradycardia or sinus arrest with suppression of escape foci in 2 to 4% of patients.

LIVER INJURY

Elevations of hepatic enzyme levels are seen frequently in patients exposed to Cordarone and in most cases are asymptomatic. If the increase exceeds three times normal, or doubles in a patient with an elevated baseline, discontinuation of Cordarone or dosage reduction should be considered. In a few cases in which biopsy has been done, the histology has resembled that of alcoholic hepatitis or cirrhosis. Hepatic failure has been a rare cause of death in patients treated with Cordarone.

PREGNANCY: PREGNANCY CATEGORY D

Cordarone has been shown to be embryotoxic (increased fetal resorption and growth retardation) in the rat when given orally at a dose of 200 mg/kg/day (18 times the maximum recommended maintenance dose). Similar findings have been noted in one strain of mice at a dose of 5 mg/kg/day (approximately ½ the maximum recommended maintenance dose) and higher, but not in a second strain nor in the rabbit at doses up to 100 mg/kg/day (9 times the maximum recommended maintenance dose).

Neonatal hypo- or hyperthyroidism

Cordarone can cause fetal harm when administered to a pregnant woman. Although Cordarone use during pregnancy is uncommon, there have been a small number of published reports of congential goiter/hypothyroidism and hyperthyroidism. If Cordarone is used during pregnancy, or if the patient becomes pregnant while taking Cordarone, the patient should be apprised of the potential hazard to the fetus.

In general, Cordarone should be used during pregnancy only if the potential benefit to the mother justifies the unknown risk to the fetus.

PRECAUTIONS

CORNEAL MICRODEPOSITS; IMPAIRMENT OF VISION

Corneal microdeposits appear in the majority of adults treated with Cordarone. They are usually discernible only by slit-lamp examination, but give rise to symptoms such as visual halos or blurred vision in as many as 10% of patients. Corneal microdeposits are reversible upon reduction of dose or termination of treatment. Asymptomatic microdeposits are not a reason to reduce dose or discontinue treatment.

PHOTOSENSITIVITY

Cordarone has induced photosensitization in about 10% of patients; some protection may be afforded by the use of sun-barrier creams or protective clothing. During long-term treatment, a blue-gray discoloration of the exposed skin may occur. The risk may be increased in patients of fair complexion or those with excessive sun exposure, and may be related to cumulative dose and duration of therapy.

THYROID ABNORMALITIES

Cordarone inhibits peripheral conversion of thyroxine (T_4) to triiodothyronine (T_3) and may cause increased thyroxine levels, decreased T_3 levels, and increased levels of inactive reverse T_3 (rT_3) in clinically euthyroid patients. It is also a potential source of large amounts of inorganic iodine. Because of its release of inorganic iodine, or perhaps for other reasons, Cordarone can cause either hypothyroidism or hyperthyroidism. Thyroid function should be monitored prior to treatment and periodically thereafter, particularly in elderly patients, and in any patient with a history of thyroid nodules, goiter, or other thyroid dysfunction. Because of the slow elimination of Cordarone and its metabolites, high plasma iodide levels, altered thyroid function, and abnormal thyroid function tests may persist for several weeks or even months following Cordarone withdrawal.

Hypothyroidism has been reported in 2 to 4% of patients in most series, but in 8 to 10% in some series. This condition may be identified by relevant clinical symptoms and particularly by elevated serum TSH levels. In some clinically hypothyroid amiodarone-treated patients, free thyroxine index values may be normal. Hypothyroidism is best managed by Cordarone dose reduction and/or thyroid hormone supplement. However, therapy must be individualized, and it may be necessary to discontinue Cordarone in some patients. Hyperthyroidism occurs in about 2% of patients receiving Cordarone, but the incidence may be higher among patients with prior inadequate dietary iodine intake. Cordarone-induced hyperthyroidism usually poses a greater hazard to the patient than hypothyroidism because of the possibility of arrhythmia breakthrough or aggravation. In fact, IF ANY NEW SIGNS OF ARRHYTHMIA APPEAR, THE POSSIBILITY OF HYPERTHYROIDISM SHOULD BE CONSIDERED. Hyperthyroidism is best identified by relevant clinical symptoms and signs, accompanied usually by abnormally elevated levels of serum T_3 RIA, and further elevations of serum T_4, and a subnormal serum TSH level (using a sufficiently sensitive TSH assay). The finding of a flat TSH response to TRH is confirmatory of hyperthyroidism and may be sought in equivocal cases. Since arrhythmia breakthroughs may accompany Cordarone-induced hyperthyroidism, aggressive medical treatment is indicated, including, if possible, dose reduction or withdrawal of Cordarone. The institution of antithyroid drugs, beta-adrenergic blockers and/or temporary corticosteroid therapy may be necessary. The action of antithyroid drugs may be especially delayed in amiodarone-induced thyrotoxicosis because of substantial quantities of preformed thyroid hormones stored in the gland. Radioactive iodine therapy is contraindicated because of the low radioiodine uptake associated with amiodarone-induced hyperthyroidism. Experience with thyroid surgery in this setting is extremely limited, and this form of therapy runs the theoretical risk of inducing thyroid storm. Cordarone-induced hyperthyroidism may be followed by a transient period of hypothyroidism.

SURGERY

HYPOTENSION POSTBYPASS

Rare occurrences of hypotension upon discontinuation of cardiopulmonary bypass during open-heart surgery in patients receiving Cordarone have been reported. The relationship of this event to Cordarone therapy is unknown.

Adult Respiratory Distress Syndrome (ARDS): Postoperatively, rare occurrences of ARDS have been reported in patients receiving Cordarone therapy who have undergone either cardiac or noncardiac surgery. Although patients usually respond well to vigorous respiratory therapy, in rare instances the outcome has been fatal. One possible mechanism of this deleterious effect may be the generation of superoxide radicals during oxygenation; therefore, the operative FiO_2 should be kept as close to room air as possible.

LABORATORY TESTS

Elevations in liver enzymes (SGOT and SGPT) can occur. Liver enzymes in patients on relatively high maintenance doses should be monitored on a regular basis. Persistent significant elevations in the liver enzymes or hepatomegaly should alert the physician to consider reducing the maintenance dose of Cordarone or discontinuing therapy.

Cordarone alters the results of thyroid-function tests, causing an increase in serum T_4 and serum reverse T_3, and a decline in serum T_3 levels. Despite these biochemical changes, most patients remain clinically euthyroid.

DRUG INTERACTIONS

Although only a small number of drug-drug interactions with Cordarone have been explored formally, most of these have shown such an interaction. The potential for other interactions should be anticipated, particularly for drugs with potentially serious toxicity, such as other antiarrhythmics. If such drugs are needed, their dose should be reassessed and, where appropriate, plasma concentration measured.

In view of the long and variable half-life of Cordarone, potential for drug interactions exists not only with concomitant medication but also with drugs administered after discontinuation of Cordarone.

Digitalis

Administration of Cordarone to patients receiving digoxin therapy regularly results in an increase in the serum digoxin concentration that may reach toxic levels with resultant

Continued on next page

Wyeth-Ayerst Laboratories—Cont.

clinical toxicity. **On initiation of Cordarone, the need for digitalis therapy should be reviewed and the dose reduced by approximately 50% or discontinued.** If digitalis treatment is continued, serum levels should be closely monitored and patients observed for clinical evidence of toxicity. These precautions probably should apply to digitoxin administration as well.

Anticoagulants

Potentiation of warfarin-type anticoagulant response is almost always seen in patients receiving Cordarone and can result in serious or fatal bleeding. **The dose of the anticoagulant should be reduced by one-third to one-half, and prothrombin times should be monitored closely.**

Antiarrhythmic Agents

Other antiarrhythmic drugs, such as quinidine, procainamide, disopyramide, and phenytoin, have been used concurrently with Cordarone.

There have been case reports of increased steady-state levels of quinidine, procainamide, and phenytoin during concomitant therapy with Cordarone. In general, any added antiarrhythmic drug should be initiated at a lower than usual dose with careful monitoring.

In general, combination of Cordarone with other antiarrhythmic therapy should be reserved for patients with life-threatening ventricular arrhythmias who are incompletely responsive to a single agent or incompletely responsive to Cordarone. During transfer to Cordarone the dose levels of previously administered agents should be reduced by 30 to 50% several days after the addition of Cordarone, when arrhythmia suppression should be beginning. The continued need for the other antiarrhythmic agent should be reviewed after the effects of Cordarone have been established, and discontinuation ordinarily should be attempted. If the treatment is continued, these patients should be particularly carefully monitored for adverse effects, especially conduction disturbances and exacerbation of tachyarrhythmias, as Cordarone is continued. In Cordarone-treated patients who require additional antiarrhythmic therapy, the initial dose of such agents should be approximately half of the usual recommended dose.

Cordarone should be used with caution in patients receiving beta-blocking agents or calcium antagonists because of the possible potentiation of bradycardia, sinus arrest, and AV block; if necessary, Cordarone can continue to be used after insertion of a pacemaker in patients with severe bradycardia or sinus arrest. [See table above.]

ELECTROLYTE DISTURBANCES

Since antiarrhythmic drugs may be ineffective or may be arrhythmogenic in patients with hypokalemia, any potassium or magnesium deficiency should be corrected before instituting Cordarone therapy.

CARCINOGENESIS, MUTAGENESIS, IMPAIRMENT OF FERTILITY

Cordarone reduced fertility of male and female rats at a dose level of 90 mg/kg/day (8 × highest recommended human maintenance dose). Cordarone caused a statistically significant, dose-related increase in the incidence of thyroid tumors (follicular adenoma and/or carcinoma) in rats. The incidence of thyroid tumors was greater than control even at the lowest dose level of Cordarone tested, i.e., 5 mg/kg/day or approximately equal to ½ the highest recommended human maintenance dose. Mutagenicity studies (Ames, micronucleus, and lysogenic tests) with Cordarone were negative.

PREGNANCY: PREGNANCY CATEGORY D

See "Warnings."

LABOR AND DELIVERY

It is not known whether the use of Cordarone during labor or delivery has any immediate or delayed adverse effects. Preclinical studies in rodents have not shown any effect of Cordarone on the duration of gestation or on parturition.

NURSING MOTHERS

Cordarone is excreted in human milk, suggesting that breast-feeding could expose the nursing infant to a significant dose of the drug. Nursing offspring of lactating rats administered Cordarone have been shown to be less viable and have reduced body-weight gains. Therefore, when Cordarone therapy is indicated, the mother should be advised to discontinue nursing.

PEDIATRIC USE

The safety and effectiveness of Cordarone in children have not been established.

ADVERSE REACTIONS

Adverse reactions have been very common in virtually all series of patients treated with Cordarone for ventricular arrhythmias, with relatively large doses of drug (400 mg/day and above) occurring in about three-fourths of all patients and causing discontinuation in 7 to 18%. The most serious reactions are pulmonary toxicity, exacerbation of arrhythmia, and rare serious liver injury (see "Warnings"), but other adverse effects constitute important problems. They are often reversible with dose reduction and virtually always reversible with cessation of Cordarone treatment. Most of the adverse effects appear to become more frequent with continued treatment beyond six months, although rates appear to remain relatively constant beyond one year. The time and dose relationships of adverse effects are under continued study.

Neurologic problems are extremely common, occurring in 20 to 40% of patients and including malaise and fatigue, tremor and involuntary movements, poor coordination and gait, and peripheral neuropathy; they are rarely a reason to stop therapy and may respond to dose reductions.

Gastrointestinal complaints, most commonly nausea, vomiting, constipation, and anorexia, occur in about 25% of patients but rarely require discontinuation of drug. These commonly occur during high-dose administration (i.e., loading dose) and usually respond to dose reduction or divided doses.

Asymptomatic corneal microdeposits are present in virtually all adult patients who have been on drug for more than 6 months. Some patients develop eye symptoms of halos, photophobia, and dry eyes. Vision is rarely affected and drug discontinuation is rarely needed.

Dermatological adverse reactions occur in about 15% of patients, with photosensitivity being most common (about 10%). Sunscreen and protection from sun exposure may be helpful, and drug discontinuation is not usually necessary. Prolonged exposure to Cordarone occasionally results in a blue-gray pigmentation. This is slowly and occasionally incompletely reversible on discontinuation of drug but is of cosmetic importance only.

Cardiovascular adverse reactions, other than exacerbation of the arrhythmias, include the uncommon occurrence of congestive heart failure (3%) and bradycardia. Bradycardia usually responds to dosage reduction but may require a pacemaker for control. CHF rarely requires drug discontinuation. Cardiac conduction abnormalities occur infrequently and are reversible on discontinuation of drug.

The following side-effect rates are based on a retrospective study of 241 patients treated for 2 to 1,515 days (mean 441.3 days).

The following side effects were reported in 10 to 33% of patients:

Gastrointestinal: Nausea and vomiting.

The following side effects were each reported in 4 to 9% of patients:

Dermatologic: Solar dermatitis/photosensitivity.

Neurologic: Malaise and fatigue, tremor/abnormal involuntary movements, lack of coordination, abnormal gait/ataxia, dizziness, paresthesias.

Gastrointestinal: Constipation, anorexia.

Ophthalmologic: Visual disturbances.

Hepatic: Abnormal liver-function tests.

Respiratory: Pulmonary inflammation or fibrosis.

The following side effects were each reported in 1 to 3% of patients:

Thyroid: Hypothyroidism, hyperthyroidism.

Neurologic: Decreased libido, insomnia, headache, sleep disturbances.

Cardiovascular: Congestive heart failure, cardiac arrhythmias, SA node dysfunction.

Gastrointestinal: Abdominal pain.

Hepatic: Nonspecific hepatic disorders.

Other: Flushing, abnormal taste and smell, edema, abnormal salivation, coagulation abnormalities.

The following side effects were each reported in less than 1% of patients:

Blue skin discoloration, rash, spontaneous ecchymosis, alopecia, hypotension, and cardiac conduction abnormalities.

Rare occurrences of hepatitis, cholestatic hepatitis, cirrhosis, optic neuritis, epididymitis, vasculitis, pseudotumor cerebri, and thrombocytopenia have been reported in patients receiving Cordarone.

In surveys of almost 5,000 patients treated in open U.S. studies and in published reports of treatment with Cordarone, the adverse reactions most frequently requiring discontinuation of Cordarone included pulmonary infiltrates or fibrosis, paroxysmal ventricular tachycardia, congestive heart failure, and elevation of liver enzymes. Other symptoms causing discontinuations less often included visual disturbances, solar dermatitis, blue skin discoloration, hyperthyroidism and hypothyroidism.

SUMMARY OF DRUG INTERACTIONS WITH CORDARONE

Concomitant Drug	Interaction: Onset (days)	Interaction: Magnitude	Recommended Dose Reduction of Concomitant Drug
Warfarin	3 to 4	Increases prothrombin time by 100%	↓ ⅓ to ½
Digoxin	1	Increases serum concentration by 70%	↓ ½
Quinidine	2	Increases serum concentration by 33%	↓ ⅓ to ½ (or discontinue)
Procainamide	<7	Increases plasma concentration by 55%, NAPA* concentration by 33%	↓ ⅓ (or discontinue)

*NAPA = n-acetyl procainamide.

OVERDOSAGE

There have been a few reported cases of Cordarone overdose in which 3 to 8 grams were taken. There were no deaths or permanent sequelae. Animal studies indicate that Cordarone has a high oral LD_{50} (>3,000 mg/kg).

In addition to general supportive measures, the patient's cardiac rhythm and blood pressure should be monitored, and if bradycardia ensues, a β-adrenergic agonist or a pacemaker may be used. Hypotension with inadequate tissue perfusion should be treated with positive inotropic and/or vasopressor agents. Neither Cordarone nor its metabolite is dialyzable.

DOSAGE AND ADMINISTRATION

BECAUSE OF THE UNIQUE PHARMACOKINETIC PROPERTIES, DIFFICULT DOSING SCHEDULE, AND SEVERITY OF THE SIDE EFFECTS IF PATIENTS ARE IMPROPERLY MONITORED, CORDARONE SHOULD BE ADMINISTERED ONLY BY PHYSICIANS WHO ARE EXPERIENCED IN THE TREATMENT OF LIFE-THREATENING ARRHYTHMIAS, WHO ARE THOROUGHLY FAMILIAR WITH THE RISKS AND BENEFITS OF CORDARONE THERAPY, AND WHO HAVE ACCESS TO LABORATORY FACILITIES CAPABLE OF ADEQUATELY MONITORING THE EFFECTIVENESS AND SIDE EFFECTS OF TREATMENT.

In order to insure that an antiarrhythmic effect will be observed without waiting several months, loading doses are required. A uniform, optimal dosage schedule for administration of Cordarone has not been determined. Individual patient titration is suggested according to the following guidelines.

For life-threatening ventricular arrhythmias, such as ventricular fibrillation or hemodynamically unstable ventricular tachycardia: Close monitoring of the patients is indicated during the loading phase, particularly until risk of recurrent ventricular tachycardia or fibrillation has abated. Because of the serious nature of the arrhythmia and the lack of predictable time course of effect, loading should be performed in a hospital setting. Loading doses of 800 to 1,600 mg/day are required for 1 to 3 weeks (occasionally longer) until initial therapeutic response occurs. (Administration of Cordarone in divided doses with meals is suggested for total daily doses of 1,000 mg or higher, or when gastrointestinal intolerance occurs.) If side effects become excessive, the dose should be reduced. Elimination of recurrence of ventricular fibrillation and tachycardia usually occurs within 1 to 3 weeks, along with reduction in complex and total ventricular ectopic beats.

Upon starting Cordarone therapy, an attempt should be made to gradually discontinue prior antiarrhythmic drugs (see section on "Drug Interactions"). When adequate arrhythmia control is achieved, or if side effects become prominent, Cordarone dose should be reduced to 600 to 800 mg/day for one month and then to the maintenance dose, usually 400 mg/day (see "Clinical Pharmacology"—"Monitoring Effectiveness"). Some patients may require larger maintenance doses, up to 600 mg/day, and some can be controlled on lower doses. Cordarone may be administered as a single daily dose, or in patients with severe gastrointestinal intolerance, as a b.i.d. dose. In each patient, the chronic maintenance dose should be determined according to antiarrhythmic effect as assessed by symptoms, Holter recordings, and/or programmed electrical stimulation and by patient tolerance. Plasma concentrations may be helpful in evaluating nonresponsiveness or unexpectedly severe toxicity (see "Clinical Pharmacology").

	Loading Dose (Daily)	Adjustment and Maintenance Dose (Daily)	
Ventricular Arrhythmias	1 to 3 weeks	~1 month	usual maintenance
	800 to 1,600 mg	600 to 800 mg	400 mg

The lowest effective dose should be used to prevent the occurrence of side effects. In all instances, the physician must be guided by the severity of the individual patient's arrhythmia and response to therapy. When dosage adjustments are necessary, the patient should be closely monitored for an extended period of time because of the long and variable half-life of Cordarone and the difficulty in predicting the time required to attain a new steady-state level of drug. Dosage suggestions are summarized [in table at bottom of preceding page].

HOW SUPPLIED

Cordarone® (amiodarone HCl) Tablets are available in bottles of 60 tablets and in Redipak® cartons containing 100 tablets (10 blister strips of 10) as follows:

200 mg, NDC 0008-4188, round, convex-faced, pink tablets with a raised "C" and marked "200" on one side, with reverse side scored and marked "Wyeth" and "4188."

Keep tightly closed.

Store at Room Temperature, Approx. 25° C (77° F).

Protect from light

Caution: Federal law prohibits dispensing without prescription.

Manufactured for
Wyeth-Ayerst Laboratories, Inc., Philadelphia, PA 19101
by **Sanofi, S.A.**, Paris, France, by arrangement with
Sanofi Pharmaceuticals, Inc.

Shown in Product Identification Section, page 436

CYCRIN® ℞

[*sīc 'crin*]

(medroxyprogesterone acetate tablets, USP)

> **WARNING**
> THE USE OF CYCRIN DURING THE FIRST FOUR MONTHS OF PREGNANCY IS NOT RECOMMENDED.
> Progestational agents have been used, beginning with the first trimester of pregnancy, in an attempt to prevent habitual abortion. There is no adequate evidence that such use is effective when such drugs are given during the first 4 months of pregnancy. Furthermore, in the vast majority of women, the cause of abortion is a defective ovum, which progestational agents could not be expected to influence. In addition, the use of progestational agents with their uterine-relaxant properties, in patients with fertilized defective ova, may cause a delay in spontaneous abortion. Therefore, the use of such drugs during the first 4 months of pregnancy is not recommended.
> Several reports suggest an association between intrauterine exposure to progestational drugs in the first trimester of pregnancy and genital abnormalities in male and female fetuses. The risk of hypospadias, 5 to 8 per 1,000 male births in the general population, may be approximately doubled with exposure to these drugs. There are insufficient data to quantify the risk to exposed female fetuses, but insofar as some of these drugs induce mild virilization of the external genitalia of the female fetus, and because of the increased association of hypospadias in the male fetus, it is prudent to avoid the use of these drugs during the first trimester of pregnancy.
> If the patient is exposed to Cycrin (medroxyprogesterone acetate) during the first 4 months of pregnancy, or if she becomes pregnant while taking this drug, she should be apprised of the potential risks to the fetus.

DESCRIPTION

Cycrin tablets contain medroxyprogesterone acetate, which is a derivative of progesterone. It is a white to off-white, odorless, crystalline powder, stable in air, melting between 200°C and 210°C. It is freely soluble in chloroform, soluble in acetone and in dioxane, sparingly soluble in alcohol and in methanol, slightly soluble in ether, and insoluble in water.

The chemical name for medroxyprogesterone acetate is pregn-4-ene-3,20-dione, 17-(acetyloxy)-6-methyl-, (6α)-.

Its structural formula is:

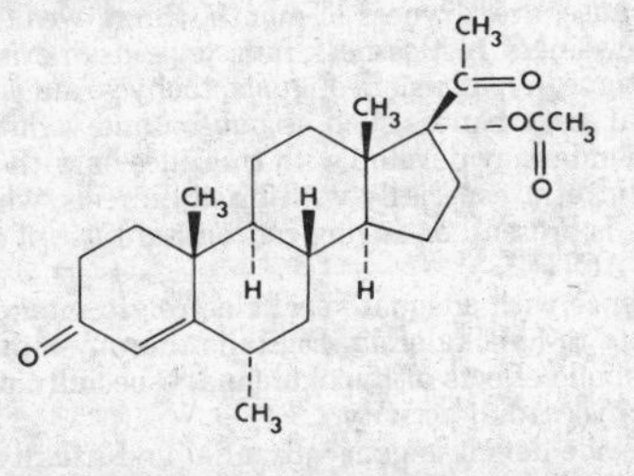

CYCRIN is available in tablet form for oral administration. Each tablet contains 10 mg of medroxyprogesterone acetate and the following inactive ingredients: lactose, magnesium stearate, methylcellulose, microcrystalline cellulose, D&C Red No. 30, and D&C Yellow No. 10.

CLINICAL PHARMACOLOGY

Medroxyprogesterone acetate, administered orally or parenterally in the recommended doses to women with adequate endogenous estrogen, transforms proliferative into secretory endometrium. Androgenic and anabolic effects have been noted, but the drug is apparently devoid of significant estrogenic activity. While parenterally administered medroxyprogesterone acetate inhibits gonadotropin production, which in turn prevents follicular maturation and ovulation, available data indicate that this does not occur when the usually recommended oral dosage is given as single daily doses.

INDICATIONS AND USAGE

Secondary amenorrhea; abnormal uterine bleeding due to hormonal imbalance in the absence of organic pathology, such as fibroids or uterine cancer.

CONTRAINDICATIONS

1. Thrombophlebitis, thromboembolic disorders, cerebral apoplexy, or patients with a past history of these conditions.
2. Liver dysfunction or disease.
3. Known or suspected malignancy of breast or genital organs.
4. Undiagnosed vaginal bleeding.
5. Missed abortion.
6. As a diagnostic test for pregnancy.
7. Known sensitivity to medroxyprogesterone acetate.

WARNINGS

1. The physician should be alert to the earliest manifestations of thrombotic disorders (thrombophlebitis, cerebrovascular disorders, pulmonary embolism, and retinal thrombosis). Should any of these occur or be suspected, the drug should be discontinued immediately.
2. Beagle dogs treated with medroxyprogesterone acetate developed mammary nodules, some of which were malignant. Although nodules occasionally appeared in control animals, they were intermittent in nature, whereas the nodules in the drug-treated animals were larger, more numerous, persistent, and there were some breast malignancies with metastases. Their significance with respect to humans has not been established.
3. Discontinue medication pending examination if there is sudden partial or complete loss of vision, or if there is a sudden onset of proptosis, diplopia, or migraine. If examination reveals papilledema or retinal vascular lesions, medication should be withdrawn.
4. Detectable amounts of progestin have been identified in the milk of mothers receiving the drug. The effect of this on the nursing infant has not been determined.
5. Usage in pregnancy is not recommended (see Boxed Warning).
6. Retrospective studies of morbidity and mortality in Great Britain and studies of morbidity in the United States have shown a statistically significant association between thrombophlebitis, pulmonary embolism, and cerebral thrombosis and embolism and the use of oral contraceptives.[1-4] The estimate of the relative risk of thromboembolism in the study by Vessey and Doll[3] was about sevenfold, while Sartwell and associates[4] in the United States found a relative risk of 4.4, meaning that the users are several times as likely to undergo thromboembolic disease without evident cause as nonusers. The American study also indicated that the risk did not persist after discontinuation of administration, and that it was not enhanced by long, continued administration. The American study was not designed to evaluate a difference between products.

PRECAUTIONS

1. The pretreatment physical examination should include special reference to breasts and pelvic organs, as well as Papanicolaou smear.
2. Because progestogens may cause some degree of fluid retention, conditions which might be influenced by this factor, such as epilepsy, migraine, asthma, cardiac or renal dysfunction, require careful observation.
3. In cases of breakthrough bleeding, as in all cases of irregular bleeding per vaginum, nonfunctional causes should be borne in mind. In cases of undiagnosed vaginal bleeding, adequate diagnostic measures are indicated.
4. Patients who have a history of psychic depression should be carefully observed and the drug discontinued if the depression recurs to a serious degree.
5. Any possible influence of prolonged progestin therapy on pituitary, ovarian, adrenal, hepatic, or uterine functions awaits further study.
6. A decrease in glucose tolerance has been observed in a small percentage of patients on estrogen-progestin combination drugs. The mechanism of this decrease is obscure. For this reason, diabetic patients should be carefully observed while receiving progestin therapy.
7. The age of the patient constitutes no absolute limiting factor, although treatment with progestins may mask the onset of the climacteric.
8. The pathologist should be advised of progestin therapy when relevant specimens are submitted.
9. Because of the occasional occurrence of thrombotic disorders (thrombophlebitis, pulmonary embolism, retinal thrombosis, and cerebrovascular disorders) in patients taking estrogen-progestin combinations, and since the mechanism is obscure, the physician should be alert to the earliest manifestation of these disorders.
10. CONCOMITANT USE IN ESTROGEN REPLACEMENT THERAPY: Studies of the addition of a progestin product to an estrogen replacement regimen for 7 or more days of a cycle of estrogen administration have reported a lowered incidence of endometrial hyperplasia. Morphological and biochemical studies of the endometrium suggest that 10 to 13 days of progestin are needed to provide maximal maturation of the endometrium and to eliminate any hyperplastic changes. Whether this will provide protection from endometrial carcinoma has not been clearly established. There are possible additional risks which may be associated with the inclusion of progestin in estrogen replacement regimens. The potential risks include adverse effects on carbohydrate and lipid metabolism. The dosage used may be important in minimizing these adverse effects.
11. Aminoglutethimide administered concomitantly with Cycrin may significantly depress the bioavailability of Cycrin.

CARCINOGENESIS, MUTAGENESIS, IMPAIRMENT OF FERTILITY

Long-term intramuscular administration of medroxyprogesterone acetate has been shown to produce mammary tumors in beagle dogs (see "Warnings" above). There was no evidence of a carcinogenic effect associated with the oral administration of medroxyprogesterone acetate to rats and mice. Medroxyprogesterone acetate was not mutagenic in a battery of *in vitro* or *in vivo* genetic toxicity assays. Medroxyprogesterone acetate at high doses is an antifertility drug and high doses would be expected to impair fertility until the cessation of treatment.

Information for the Patient

See Patient Information at the end of insert.

ADVERSE REACTIONS

PREGNANCY: (See Boxed Warning for possible adverse effects on the fetus.)

BREAST: Breast tenderness or galactorrhea has been reported rarely.

SKIN: Sensitivity reactions consisting of urticaria, pruritus, edema, and generalized rash have occurred in an occasional patient. Acne, alopecia, and hirsutism have been reported in a few cases.

THROMBOEMBOLIC PHENOMENA: Thromboembolic phenomena, including thrombophlebitis and pulmonary embolism, have been reported.

The following adverse reactions have been observed in women taking progestins, including Cycrin (medroxyprogesterone acetate tablets):

- breakthrough bleeding
- spotting
- change in menstrual flow
- amenorrhea
- edema
- change in weight (increase or decrease)
- change in cervical erosion and cervical secretions
- cholestatic jaundice
- anaphylactoid reactions and anaphylaxis
- rash (allergic) with and without pruritus
- mental depression
- pyrexia
- insomnia
- nausea
- somnolence

A statistically significant association has been demonstrated between use of estrogen-progestin combination drugs and the following serious adverse reactions: thrombophlebitis; pulmonary embolism; and cerebral thrombosis and embolism. For this reason patients on progestin therapy should be carefully observed.

Although available evidence is suggestive of an association, such a relationship has been neither confirmed nor refuted for the following serious adverse reactions:

- neuro-ocular lesions, e.g., retinal thrombosis, and optic neuritis.

The following adverse reactions have been observed in patients receiving estrogen-progestin combination drugs:

- rise in blood pressure in susceptible individuals
- premenstrual-like syndrome
- changes in libido
- changes in appetite

Continued on next page

Wyeth-Ayerst Laboratories—Cont.

cystitis-like syndrome
headache
nervousness
dizziness
fatigue
backache
hirsutism
loss of scalp hair
erythema multiforme
erythema nodosum
hemorrhagic eruption
itching

In view of these observations, patients on progestin therapy should be carefully observed.
The following laboratory results may be altered by the use of estrogen-progestin combination drugs:
Increased sulfobromophthalein retention and other hepatic-function tests.
Coagulation tests: increase in prothrombin factors VII, VIII, IX, and X.
Metyrapone test.
Pregnanediol determination
Thyroid function: increase in PBI, and butanol extractable protein bound iodine and decrease in T^3 uptake values.

DOSAGE AND ADMINISTRATION

SECONDARY AMENORRHEA—Cycrin (medroxyprogesterone acetate tablets) may be given in dosages of 5 mg to 10 mg daily for from 5 to 10 days. A dose for inducing an optimum secretory transformation of an endometrium that has been adequately primed with either endogenous or exogenous estrogen is 10 mg of Cycrin daily for 10 days. In cases of secondary amenorrhea, therapy may be started at any time. Progestin withdrawal bleeding usually occurs within 3 to 7 days after discontinuing Cycrin therapy.
ABNORMAL UTERINE BLEEDING DUE TO HORMONAL IMBALANCE IN THE ABSENCE OF ORGANIC PATHOLOGY—Beginning on the calculated 16th or 21st day of the menstrual cycle, 5 to 10 mg of medroxyprogesterone acetate may be given daily for from 5 to 10 days. To produce an optimum secretory transformation of an endometrium that has been adequately primed with either endogenous or exogenous estrogen, 10 mg of medroxyprogesterone acetate daily for 10 days beginning on the 16th day of the cycle is suggested. Progestin withdrawal bleeding usually occurs within three to seven days after discontinuing therapy with Cycrin. Patients with a past history of recurrent episodes of abnormal uterine bleeding may benefit from planned menstrual cycling with Cycrin.

HOW SUPPLIED

CYCRIN® (medroxyprogesterone acetate tablets, USP) is available for oral administration in the following dosage strength: 10 mg, peach, oval tablet with "CYCRIN" and a score debossed on one side and opposing "C"s debossed on the reverse, in bottles of 100 (NDC 0046-0896-81), and in Cycle Packs of 10 (NDC 0046-0896-10).
The appearance of these tablets is a registered trademark of Wyeth-Ayerst Laboratories.
Store at controlled room temperature, 15° C–30° C (59° F–86° F).
Dispense in a well-closed container as defined in the USP.
CAUTION: Federal law prohibits dispensing without prescription.

REFERENCES

1. Royal College of General Practitioners: Oral contraception and thromboembolic disease. *J Coll Gen Pract* 1967; 13:267-279.
2. Inman WHW, Vessey MP: Investigation of deaths from pulmonary, coronary, and cerebral thrombosis and embolism in women of childbearing age. *Br Med J* 1968; 2:193-199.
3. Vessey MP, Doll R: Investigation of relation between use of oral contraceptives and thromboembolic disease. A further report. *Br Med J* 1969; 2:651-657.
4. Sartwell PE, Masi AT, Arthes FG, et al: Thromboembolism and oral contraceptives: An epidemiological case-control study. *Am J Epidemiol* 1969; 90:365-380.

PATIENT INFORMATION

Cycrin tablets contain medroxyprogesterone acetate, a progesterone. The information below is that which the U.S. Food and Drug Administration requires be provided for all patients taking progesterones. The information below relates only to the risk to the unborn child associated with the use of progesterones during pregnancy. For further information on the use, side effects, and other risks associated with this product, ask your doctor.

WARNING FOR WOMEN

Progesterone or progesterone-like drugs have been used to prevent miscarriage in the first few months of pregnancy. No adequate evidence is available to show that they are effective for this purpose. Furthermore, most cases of early miscarriage are due to causes which could not be helped by these drugs.
There is an increased risk of minor birth defects in children whose mothers take this drug during the first four months of pregnancy. Several reports suggest an association between mothers who take these drugs in the first trimester of pregnancy and genital abnormalities in male and female babies. The risk to the male baby is the possibility of being born with a condition in which the opening of the penis is on the underside rather than the tip of the penis (hypospadias). Hypospadias occurs in about 5 to 8 per 1,000 male births and is about doubled with exposure to these drugs. There is not enough information to quantify the risk to exposed female fetuses, but enlargement of the clitoris and fusion of the labia may occur, although rarely.
Therefore, since drugs of this type may induce mild masculinization of the external genitalia of the female fetus, as well as hypospadias in the male fetus, it is wise to avoid using the drug during the first trimester of pregnancy.
These drugs have been used as a test for pregnancy, but such use is no longer considered safe because of possible damage to a developing baby. Also, more rapid methods of testing for pregnancy are now available.
If you take Cycrin (medroxyprogesterone acetate tablets, USP) and later find you were pregnant when you took it, be sure to discuss this with your doctor as soon as possible.
Shown in Product Identification Section, page 436

DIPHTHERIA AND TETANUS TOXOIDS ADSORBED ℞

[*dif-the're-ah and tet'ah-nus tok'soids*]
aluminum phosphate adsorbed
ULTRAFINED®
PEDIATRIC

DESCRIPTION

The diphtheria toxoid component is prepared by cultivating a suitable strain of *Corynebacterium diphtheriae* on a modified Mueller's casein hydrolysate medium (J. Immunology 37:103, 1939). The tetanus toxoid component is prepared by cultivating a suitable strain of *Clostridium tetani* on a protein-free semisynthetic medium (Appl. Microbiol. *10:* 146, 1962). Formaldehyde is used as the toxoiding (detoxifying) agent for both diphtheria and tetanus toxins. The final product contains no more than 0.02 percent free formaldehyde and contains 0.01 percent thimerosal (mercury derivative) as preservative.
The aluminum content of the final product does not exceed 0.85 mg per 0.5 mL dose.
During processing, hydrochloric acid and sodium hydroxide are used to adjust the pH. Sodium chloride is added to the finished product to control isotonicity.

HOW SUPPLIED

Vials of 5 mL., 0008-0338-02, and 0.5 mL TUBEX® Sterile Cartridge-Needle Units (25 gauge × 5/8 inch needle), packages of 10, 0008-0338-01.
For prescribing information write to Professional Service, Wyeth-Ayerst Laboratories, P.O. Box 8299, Philadelphia, PA 19101, or contact your local Wyeth-Ayerst representative.

DIUCARDIN® ℞

[*dī"ū-car'din*]
(hydroflumethiazide tablets, USP)

DESCRIPTION

Diucardin (hydroflumethiazide) is an oral thiazide (benzothiadiazide) diuretic-antihypertensive agent.
Diucardin is available as 50 mg tablets for oral administration.
Chemical name: 3,4-Dihydro-6-(trifluoromethyl)-2H-1,2,4-benzothiadiazine-7-sulfonamide 1,1-dioxide.
Structural formula:

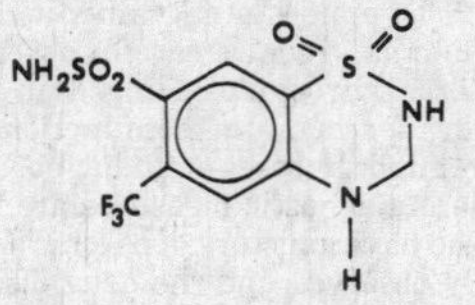

Hydroflumethiazide is an odorless white to cream-colored, finely divided, crystalline powder. It has a melting point between 270° and 275° C. Hydroflumethiazide is freely soluble in acetone, soluble in alcohol, and very slightly soluble in water.
The inactive ingredients contained in Diucardin Tablets are: lactose, magnesium stearate, microcrystalline cellulose, povidone, and starch.

CLINICAL PHARMACOLOGY

Hydroflumethiazide is incompletely but fairly rapidly absorbed from the gastrointestinal tract. It appears to have a biphasic biological half-life with an estimated alpha-phase of about 2 hours and an estimated beta-phase of about 17 hours; it has a metabolite with a longer half-life, which is extensively bound to the red blood cells. Hydroflumethiazide is excreted in the urine; its metabolite has also been detected in the urine.
The mechanism of action results in an interference with the renal tubular mechanism of electrolyte reabsorption. At maximal therapeutic dosage, all thiazides are approximately equal in their diuretic potency. The mechanism whereby thiazides function in the control of hypertension is unknown.

INDICATIONS AND USAGE

Diucardin is indicated as adjunctive therapy in edema associated with congestive heart failure, hepatic cirrhosis, and corticosteroid and estrogen therapy.
Diucardin has also been found useful in edema due to various forms of renal dysfunction such as: nephrotic syndrome; acute glomerulonephritis; and chronic renal failure.
Diucardin is indicated in the management of hypertension either as the sole therapeutic agent or to enhance the effect of other antihypertensive drugs in the more severe forms of hypertension.

USAGE IN PREGNANCY

The routine use of diuretics in an otherwise healthy woman is inappropriate and exposes mother and fetus to unnecessary hazard. Diuretics do not prevent development of toxemia of pregnancy, and there is no satisfactory evidence that they are useful in the treatment of developed toxemia.

Edema during pregnancy may arise from pathological causes or from the physiologic and mechanical consequences of pregnancy. Thiazides are indicated in pregnancy when edema is due to pathologic causes just as they are in the absence of pregnancy (however, see "Precautions—PREGNANCY," below). Dependent edema in pregnancy, resulting from restriction of venous return by the expanded uterus, is properly treated through elevation of the lower extremities and use of support hose. Use of diuretics to lower intravascular volume in this case is illogical and unnecessary. There is hypervolemia during normal pregnancy which is harmful to neither the fetus nor the mother (in absence of cardiovascular disease), but which is associated with edema, including generalized edema, in the majority of pregnant women. If this edema produces discomfort, increased recumbency will often provide relief. In rare instances, this edema may cause extreme discomfort which is not relieved by rest. In these cases, a short course of diuretics may provide relief and may be appropriate.

CONTRAINDICATIONS

Anuria.
Hypersensitivity to this or other sulfonamide-derived drugs.

WARNINGS

Diucardin should be used with caution in severe renal disease. In patients with renal disease, thiazides may precipitate azotemia. Cumulative effects of the drug may develop in patients with impaired renal function.
Thiazides should be used with caution in patients with impaired hepatic function or progressive liver disease, since minor alterations of fluid and electrolyte balance may precipitate hepatic coma.
Thiazides may add to or potentiate the action of other antihypertensive drugs. Potentiation occurs with ganglionic or peripheral adrenergic blocking drugs.
Sensitivity reactions may occur in patients with a history of allergy or bronchial asthma.
The possibility of exacerbation or activation of systemic lupus erythematosus has been reported.

PRECAUTIONS

GENERAL

All patients receiving thiazide therapy should be observed for clinical signs of fluid or electrolyte imbalance: namely, hyponatremia, hypochloremic alkalosis, and hypokalemia. Serum and urine electrolyte determinations are particularly important when the patient is vomiting excessively or receiving parenteral fluids. Medication such as digitalis may also influence serum electrolytes. Warning signs, irrespective of cause, are: dryness of mouth, thirst, weakness, lethargy, drowsiness, restlessness, muscle pains or cramps, muscular fatigue, hypotension, oliguria, tachycardia, and gastrointestinal disturbances such as nausea and vomiting.
Hypokalemia may develop with thiazides as with any other potent diuretic, especially with brisk diuresis, when severe cirrhosis is present, or during concomitant use of corticosteroids or ACTH.
Interference with adequate oral electrolyte intake will also contribute to hypokalemia. Digitalis therapy may exaggerate metabolic effects of hypokalemia, especially with reference to myocardial activity.
Any chloride deficit is generally mild and usually does not require specific treatment except under extraordinary circumstances (as in liver disease or renal disease). Dilutional

hyponatremia may occur in edematous patients in hot weather; appropriate therapy is water restriction, rather than administration of salt, except in rare instances when the hyponatremia is life-threatening. In actual salt depletion, appropriate replacement is the therapy of choice.
Hyperuricemia may occur or frank gout may be precipitated in certain patients receiving thiazide therapy.
Insulin requirements in diabetic patients may be increased, decreased, or unchanged. Latent diabetes mellitus may become manifested during thiazide administration.
The antihypertensive effects of the drug may be enhanced in the postsympathectomy patient.
If progressive renal impairment becomes evident, as indicated by a rising creatinine or blood urea nitrogen, a careful reappraisal of therapy is necessary with consideration given to withholding or discontinuing diuretic therapy.
Thiazides may decrease serum PBI levels without signs of thyroid disturbance.
Lithium generally should not be given with diuretics because they reduce its renal clearance and increase the risk of lithium toxicity. Read circulars for lithium preparations before use of such concomitant therapy with Diucardin.
Thiazides have been shown to increase the urinary excretion of magnesium; this may result in hypomagnesemia.
Calcium excretion is decreased by thiazides. Pathological changes in the parathyroid gland with hypercalcemia and hypophosphatemia have been observed in a few patients on prolonged thiazide therapy. The common complications of hyperparathyroidism, such as renal lithiasis, bone resorption, and peptic ulceration, have not been seen.

LABORATORY TESTS
Periodic determination of serum electrolytes to detect possible electrolyte imbalance should be performed at appropriate intervals.

DRUG INTERACTIONS
Anticoagulants, oral
(Effects may be decreased when used concurrently with thiazide diuretics; dosage adjustments may be necessary.)
Antigout medications
(Thiazide diuretics may raise the level of blood uric acid; dosage adjustment of antigout medications may be necessary to control hyperuricemia and gout.)
Antihypertensive medications, other, especially diazoxide, or preanesthetic and anesthetic agents used in surgery or skeletal-muscle relaxants, nondepolarizing, used in surgery
(Effects may be potentiated when used concurrently with thiazide diuretics; dosage adjustments may be necessary.)
Amphotericin B or Corticosteroids or Corticotropin (ACTH)
(Concurrent use with thiazide diuretics may intensify electrolyte imbalance, particularly hypokalemia.)
Cardiac glycosides
(Concurrent use with thiazide diuretics may enhance the possibility of digitalis toxicity associated with hypokalemia.)
Colestipol
(May inhibit gastrointestinal absorption of the thiazide diuretics; administration 1 hour before or 4 hours after colestipol is recommended.)
Hypoglycemics
(Thiazide diuretics may raise blood glucose levels; for adult-onset diabetics, dosage adjustment of hypoglycemic medications may be necessary during and after thiazide diuretic therapy; insulin requirements may be increased, decreased, or unchanged.)
Lithium salts
(Concurrent use with thiazide diuretics is not recommended, as they may provoke lithium toxicity because of reduced renal clearance.)
Methenamine
(Effectiveness may be decreased when used concurrently with thiazide diuretics because of alkalinization of the urine.)
Nonsteroidal anti-inflammatory agents
(In some patients, the steroidal anti-inflammatory agent can reduce the diuretic, natriuretic, and antihypertensive effects of loop, potassium sparing, and thiazide diuretics. Therefore, when hydroflumethiazide and nonsteroidal anti-inflammatory agents are used concomitantly, the patient should be observed closely to determine if the desired effect of the diuretic is obtained.)
Norepinephrine
(Thiazides may decrease arterial responsiveness to norepinephrine. This diminution is not sufficient to preclude effectiveness of the pressor agent for therapeutic use.)
Tubocurarine
(Thiazide drugs may increase the responsiveness to tubocurarine.)

DIAGNOSTIC INTERFERENCE—With expected physiologic effects
Blood and urine glucose levels (usually only in patients with a predisposition for glucose intolerance) and
Serum bilirubin levels (by displacement from albumin binding) and
Serum calcium levels (thiazide diuretics should be discontinued before parathyroid-function tests are carried out) and
Serum uric acid levels (may be increased)
Serum magnesium, potassium, and sodium levels (may be decreased; serum magnesium levels may increase in uremic patients)
Serum protein-bound iodine (PBI) levels (may be decreased)
Thiazides should be discontinued before carrying out tests for parathyroid function (see "Precautions—GENERAL, Calcium excretion").

CARCINOGENESIS, MUTAGENESIS, IMPAIRMENT OF FERTILITY
No studies have been performed to evaluate carcinogenic or mutagenic potential of Diucardin or the potential of Diucardin to impair fertility.

PREGNANCY
Teratogenic Effects—Pregnancy Category C
Animal reproduction studies have not been conducted with Diucardin. It is also not known whether Diucardin can cause fetal harm when administered to a pregnant woman or can affect reproduction capacity. Diucardin should be given to a pregnant woman only if clearly needed.
Nonteratogenic Effects
Fetal or neonatal jaundice, thrombocytopenia, and possibly other adverse reactions which have occurred in the adult.

NURSING MOTHERS
Thiazides appear in breast milk. If use of the drug is deemed essential, the patient may consider stopping nursing.

PEDIATRIC USE
Safety and effectiveness in children have not been established.

ADVERSE REACTIONS

The following adverse reactions have been observed, but there is not enough systematic collection of data to support an estimate of their frequency.

GASTROINTESTINAL SYSTEMS
Anorexia, gastric irritation, nausea, vomiting, cramping, diarrhea, constipation, jaundice (intrahepatic cholestatic jaundice), pancreatitis, sialadenitis.

CENTRAL NERVOUS SYSTEM
Dizziness, vertigo, paresthesias, headache, xanthopsia.

HEMATOLOGIC
Leukopenia, agranulocytosis, thrombocytopenia, aplastic anemia, hemolytic anemia.

CARDIOVASCULAR
Orthostatic hypotension (may be aggravated by alcohol, barbiturates, or narcotics).

DERMATOLOGIC—HYPERSENSITIVITY
Purpura, photosensitivity, rash, urticaria, necrotizing angiitis (vasculitis, cutaneous vasculitis), fever, respiratory distress including pneumonitis, anaphylactic reactions.

OTHER
Hyperglycemia, glycosuria, hyperuricemia, muscle spasm, weakness, restlessness, transient blurred vision.
Whenever adverse reactions are moderate or severe, thiazide dosage should be reduced or therapy withdrawn.

OVERDOSAGE

SIGNS AND SYMPTOMS
Diuresis, lethargy progressing to coma, with minimal cardiorespiratory depression and with or without significant serum electrolyte changes or dehydration; GI irritation; hypermotility; transient elevation in BUN level.

TREATMENT
Empty stomach by gastric lavage, taking care to avoid aspiration. Monitor serum electrolyte levels and renal function, and institute supportive measures, as required to maintain hydration, electrolyte balance, respiration, and cardiovascular and renal function. Treat GI effects symptomatically.

DOSAGE AND ADMINISTRATION

The average adult dose is 25 to 200 mg per day. The average adult antihypertensive dose is 50 to 100 mg per day.
Therapy should be individualized according to patient response. This therapy should be titrated to gain maximal response as well as the minimal dose possible to maintain that therapeutic response.

HOW SUPPLIED

Diucardin®—Each scored, white oval compressed tablet, inscribed "Diucardin 50," contains 50 mg hydroflumethiazide, in bottles of 100 (NDC 0046-0702-81).
Store at room temperature (approximately 25° C).
CAUTION: Federal law prohibits dispensing without prescription.

Shown in Product Identification Section, page 436

EQUAGESIC® Ⓒ ℞

[ek"wa-je'zik]
(meprobamate with aspirin)

DESCRIPTION

Each tablet of Equagesic contains 200 mg meprobamate and 325 mg aspirin. The inactive ingredients present are cellulose, D&C Yellow 10, FD&C Red 40, FD&C Yellow 6, hydrogenated vegetable oil, magnesium stearate, polacrilin potassium, and starch.

ACTIONS

Meprobamate is a carbamate derivative which has been shown (in animal and/or human studies) to have effects at multiple sites in the central nervous system, including the thalamus and limbic system.
Aspirin, acetylsalicylic acid, is a nonnarcotic analgesic with antipyretic and antiinflammatory properties.

INDICATIONS

As an adjunct in the short-term treatment of pain accompanied by tension and/or anxiety in patients with musculoskeletal disease. Clinical trials have demonstrated that in these situations relief of pain is somewhat greater than with aspirin alone.
The effectiveness of Equagesic in long-term use, that is, more than 4 months, has not been assessed by systematic clinical studies. The physician should periodically reassess the usefulness of the drug for the individual patient.

CONTRAINDICATIONS

ASPIRIN
Allergic or idiosyncratic reactions to aspirin or related compounds.

MEPROBAMATE
Acute intermittent porphyria and allergic or idiosyncratic reactions to meprobamate or related compounds, such as carisoprodol, mebutamate, or carbromal.

WARNINGS

ASPIRIN
Salicylates should be used with extreme caution in patients with peptic ulcer, asthma, coagulation abnormalities, hypoprothrombinemia, vitamin K deficiency, or in those on anticoagulant therapy.
In rare instances, the use of aspirin in persons allergic to salicylates may result in life-threatening allergic episodes.

MEPROBAMATE
DRUG DEPENDENCE: Physical dependence, psychological dependence, and abuse have occurred. Chronic intoxication from prolonged ingestion of, usually, greater-than-recommended doses is manifested by ataxia, slurred speech, and vertigo. Therefore, careful supervision of dose and amounts prescribed is advised, as well as avoidance of prolonged administration, especially for alcoholics and other patients with a known propensity for taking excessive quantities of drugs.
Sudden withdrawal of the drug after prolonged and excessive use may precipitate recurrence of preexisting symptoms such as anxiety, anorexia, or insomnia, or withdrawal reactions such as vomiting, ataxia, tremors, muscle twitching, confusional states, hallucinosis, and, rarely, convulsive seizures. Such seizures are more likely to occur in persons with central-nervous-system damage or preexistent or latent convulsive disorders. Onset of withdrawal symptoms occurs usually within 12 to 48 hours after discontinuation of meprobamate; symptoms usually cease within the next 12- to 48-hour period.
When excessive dosage has continued for weeks or months, dosage should be reduced gradually over a period of 1 to 2 weeks rather than abruptly stopped. Alternatively, a short-acting barbiturate may be substituted, then gradually withdrawn.
POTENTIALLY HAZARDOUS TASKS: Patients should be warned that meprobamate may impair the mental or physical abilities required for performance of potentially hazardous tasks, such as driving or operating machinery.
ADDITIVE EFFECTS: Since CNS-suppressant effects of meprobamate and alcohol or meprobamate and other psychotropic drugs may be additive, appropriate caution should be exercised with patients who take more than one of these agents simultaneously.

USAGE IN PREGNANCY AND LACTATION

An increased risk of congenital malformations associated with the use of minor tranquilizers (meprobamate, chlordiazepoxide, and diazepam) during the first trimester of pregnancy has been suggested in several studies. Because use of these drugs is rarely a matter of urgency, their use during this period should almost always be avoided. The possibility that a woman of childbearing potential may be pregnant at the time of institution of therapy should be considered. Patients should be advised that if they become pregnant during therapy or intend to become pregnant they should communicate with their physicians about the desirability of discontinuing the drug.
Meprobamate passes the placental barrier. It is present both in umbilical-cord blood at or near maternal plasma levels and in breast milk of lactating mothers at concentrations two to four times that of maternal plasma. When use of meprobamate is contemplated in breast-feeding patients, the drug's higher concentrations in breast milk as compared to maternal plasma levels should be considered.

Continued on next page

Wyeth-Ayerst Laboratories—Cont.

USAGE IN CHILDREN: Preparations containing aspirin should be kept out of the reach of children. Equagesic is not recommended for patients 12 years of age and under.

PRECAUTIONS

ASPIRIN
Salicylates antagonize the uricosuric activity of probenecid and sulfinpyrazone. Salicylates are reported to enhance the hypoglycemic effect of the sulfonylurea antidiabetic drugs.
MEPROBAMATE
The lowest effective dose should be administered, particularly to elderly and/or debilitated patients, in order to preclude oversedation.
Meprobamate is metabolized in the liver and excreted by the kidney; to avoid its excess accumulation, caution should be exercised in the administration to patients with compromised liver or kidney function.
Meprobamate occasionally may precipitate seizures in epileptic patients.
The drug should be prescribed cautiously and in small quantities to patients with suicidal tendencies.

ADVERSE REACTIONS

ASPIRIN
Aspirin may cause epigastric discomfort, nausea, and vomiting. Hypersensitivity reactions, including urticaria, angioneurotic edema, purpura, asthma, and anaphylaxis, may rarely occur.
Patients receiving large doses of salicylates may develop tinnitus.
MEPROBAMATE
CENTRAL NERVOUS SYSTEM: Drowsiness, ataxia, dizziness, slurred speech, headache, vertigo, weakness, paresthesias, impairment of visual accommodation, euphoria, overstimulation, paradoxical excitement, fast EEG activity.
GASTROINTESTINAL: Nausea, vomiting, diarrhea.
CARDIOVASCULAR: Palpitation, tachycardia, various forms of arrhythmia, transient ECG changes, syncope, hypotensive crisis.
ALLERGIC OR IDIOSYNCRATIC: Milder reactions are characterized by an itchy, urticarial, or erythematous maculopapular rash which may be generalized or confined to the groin.
Other reactions have included leukopenia, acute nonthrombocytopenic purpura, petechiae, ecchymoses, eosinophilia, peripheral edema, adenopathy, fever, fixed drug eruption with cross-reaction to carisoprodol, and cross-sensitivity between meprobamate/mebutamate and meprobamate/carbromal.
More severe hypersensitivity reactions, rarely reported, include hyperpyrexia, chills, angioneurotic edema, bronchospasm, oliguria, and anuria. Also, anaphylaxis, exfoliative dermatitis, stomatitis, and proctitis. Stevens-Johnson syndrome and bullous dermatitis have occurred.
HEMATOLOGIC (SEE ALSO "ALLERGIC OR IDIOSYNCRATIC"): Agranulocytosis, aplastic anemia have been reported, although no causal relationship has been established, and thrombocytopenic purpura.
OTHER: Exacerbation of porphyric symptoms.

DOSAGE AND ADMINISTRATION

The usual dosage of Equagesic is one or two tablets, each tablet containing meprobamate, 200 mg, and aspirin, 325 mg, orally 3 to 4 times daily as needed for the relief of pain when tension or anxiety is present.
Equagesic is not recommended for patients 12 years of age and under.

OVERDOSAGE

Treatment of overdose with Equagesic is essentially symptomatic and supportive. Any drug remaining in the stomach should be removed. Induction of vomiting or gastric lavage may be indicated. Activated charcoal may reduce absorption of both aspirin and meprobamate.
Overdosage with aspirin produces the usual symptoms and signs of salicylate intoxication. Observation and treatment should include management of hyperthermia, specific parenteral electrolyte therapy for ketoacidosis and dehydration, watching for evidence of hemorrhagic manifestations due to hypoprothrombinemia which, if it occurs, usually requires whole-blood transfusions.
Suicidal attempts with meprobamate have resulted in drowsiness, lethargy, stupor, ataxia, coma, shock, vasomotor and respiratory collapse. Some suicidal attempts have been fatal.
The following data have been reported in the literature and from other sources. These data are not expected to correlate with each case (considering factors such as individual susceptibility and length of time from ingestion to treatment), but represent the usual ranges reported.
Acute simple overdose (meprobamate alone): Death has been reported with ingestion of as little as 12 grams meprobamate and survival with as much as 40 grams.
BLOOD LEVELS
0.5 to 2.0 mg percent represents the usual blood-level range of meprobamate after therapeutic doses. The level may occasionally be as high as 3.0 mg percent.
3 to 10 mg percent usually corresponds to findings of mild-to-moderate symptoms of overdosage, such as stupor or light coma.
10 to 20 mg percent usually corresponds to deeper coma, requiring more intensive treatment. Some fatalities occur.
At levels greater than 20 mg percent, more fatalities than survivals can be expected.
Acute combined overdose (meprobamate with other psychotropic drugs or alcohol): Since effects can be additive, a history of ingestion of a low dose of meprobamate plus any of these compounds (or of a relatively low blood or tissue level) cannot be used as a prognostic indicator.
In cases where excessive doses have been taken, sleep ensues rapidly and blood pressure, pulse, and respiratory rates are reduced to basal levels. Any drug remaining in the stomach should be removed and symptomatic treatment given. Should respiration or blood pressure become compromised, respiratory assistance, central-nervous-system stimulants, and pressor agents should be administered cautiously as indicated. Diuresis, osmotic (mannitol) diuresis, peritoneal dialysis, and hemodialysis have been used successfully in removing both aspirin and meprobamate. Alkalinization of the urine increases the excretion of salicylates. Careful monitoring of urinary output is necessary, and caution should be taken to avoid overhydration. Relapse and death, after initial recovery, have been attributed to incomplete gastric emptying and delayed absorption.

HOW SUPPLIED

Equagesic® (meprobamate with aspirin) Tablets, 200 mg meprobamate and 325 mg aspirin, are available as follows:
NDC 0008-0091, pink and yellow, double-layer, round, scored tablet marked "WYETH" and "91", in bottles of 100 tablets.
Keep tightly closed.
Protect from light.
Dispense in light-resistant, tight container.
The appearance of EQUAGESIC tablets is a registered trademark of Wyeth-Ayerst Laboratories.

Shown in Product Identification Section, page 436

EQUANIL® Ⓒ ℞

[*ek 'wah-nil*]
(meprobamate)
Tablets

DESCRIPTION

Meprobamate is a white powder with a characteristic odor and a bitter taste. It is slightly soluble in water, freely soluble in acetone and alcohol, and sparingly soluble in ether.
Equanil tablets contain 200 mg or 400 mg meprobamate. The inactive ingredients present are lactose, methylcellulose, polacrilin potassium, and stearic acid.

HOW SUPPLIED

Equanil® (meprobamate) Tablets, Wyeth®, are available in the following dosage strengths:
200 mg, NDC 0008-0002, white, five-sided tablet marked "WYETH" and "2", in bottles of 100 tablets.
400 mg, NDC 0008-0001, white, round, scored tablet marked "WYETH" and "1", in bottles of 100 and 500 tablets.
Store at room temperature, approximately 25°C (77°F).
For prescribing information write to Professional Service, Wyeth-Ayerst Laboratories, P.O. Box 8299, Philadelphia, PA 19101, or contact your local Wyeth-Ayerst representative.

Shown in Product Identification Section, page 436

ESTRADURIN® ℞

[*ĕs "tra-dū 'rin*]
(polyestradiol phosphate)
For Intramuscular Injection Only

CAUTION: Federal law prohibits dispensing without prescription.

DESCRIPTION

ESTRADURIN is a water-soluble, high molecular weight polyester of phosphoric acid and 17β-estradiol.
It is provided in a SECULE® containing 40 mg polyestradiol phosphate, 0.022 mg phenylmercuric nitrate, and 5.2 mg sodium phosphate. As solubilizing agents for the active ingredient, 25 mg niacinamide and 4 mg propylene glycol are also present. The pH is adjusted with sodium hydroxide.
One 2 mL ampul of sterile diluent is also provided.

CLINICAL PHARMACOLOGY

Estrogens are important in the development and maintenance of the female reproductive system. In responsive tissues estrogens enter the cell and are transported into the nucleus.
In the male patient with androgenic hormone-dependent conditions, such as metastatic carcinoma of the prostate gland, the feedback mechanism of estrogens on the hypothalamus and the pituitary decreases FSH and LH which results in a decrease in testosterone. As a result of treatment with estrogens, metastatic lesions in the bone may also show improvement.
Biologically active estradiol units are gradually split off from the large parent molecule, thus providing a continuous level of active estrogen over a prolonged period. The liberated estradiol is metabolized by the body in the same manner as the endogenous hormone. There is no depot effect at the site of injection—90 percent of injected dose leaves the bloodstream within 24 hours. Passive storage occurs in the reticuloendothelial system. As circulating levels of estradiol drop, more returns to the bloodstream from the site of storage for an even, continuous therapeutic effect. Increasing the dose acts to prolong the duration of pharmacologic action rather than to increase blood levels.
Metabolism and inactivation occur primarily in the liver. Some estrogens are excreted into the bile; however they are reabsorbed from the intestine and returned to the liver through the portal venous system. Water-soluble estrogen conjugates are strongly acidic and are ionized in body fluids, which favor excretion through the kidneys since tubular reabsorption is minimal.

INDICATION

ESTRADURIN (polyestradiol phosphate) is indicated in the treatment of prostatic carcinoma—palliative therapy of advanced disease.

CONTRAINDICATIONS

Estrogens should not be used in men with any of the following conditions:

1. Known or suspected cancer of the breast except in appropriately selected patients being treated for metastatic disease.
2. Known or suspected estrogen-dependent neoplasia.
3. Active thrombophlebitis or thromboembolic disorders.

WARNINGS

1. *Induction of malignant neoplasms.* Long-term continuous administration of natural and synthetic estrogens in certain animal species increases the frequency of carcinomas of the breast, cervix, vagina, and liver.
2. *Gallbladder disease.* A recent study has reported a 2- to 3-fold increase in the risk of surgically confirmed gallbladder disease in women receiving postmenopausal estrogens,[1] similar to the 2-fold increase previously noted in users of oral contraceptives.[2,7a]
3. *Effects similar to those caused by estrogen-progestogen oral contraceptives.* There are several serious adverse effects of oral contraceptives. It has been shown that there is an increased risk of thrombosis in men receiving estrogens for prostatic cancer and women for postpartum breast engorgement.[3–6]

a. *Thromboembolic disease.* It is now well established that users of oral contraceptives have an increased risk of various thromboembolic and thrombotic vascular diseases, such as thrombophlebitis, pulmonary embolism, stroke, and myocardial infarction.[7–14] Cases of retinal thrombosis, mesenteric thrombosis, and optic neuritis have been reported in oral-contraceptive users. There is evidence that the risk of several of these adverse reactions is related to the dose of the drug.[15,16] An increased risk of postsurgery thromboembolic complications has also been reported in users of oral contraceptives.[17,18] If feasible, estrogen should be discontinued at least 4 weeks before surgery of the type associated with an increased risk of thromboembolism, or during periods of prolonged immobilization.
Estrogens should not be used in persons with active thrombophlebitis or thromboembolic disorders. They should be used with caution in patients with cerebral vascular or coronary artery disease and only for those in whom estrogens are clearly indicated.
Large doses of estrogen (5 mg conjugated estrogens per day), comparable to those used to treat cancer of the prostate, have been shown in a large prospective clinical trial in men[19] to increase the risk of nonfatal myocardial infarction, pulmonary embolism, and thrombophlebitis. When estrogen doses of this size are used, any of the thromboembolic and thrombotic adverse effects associated with oral-contraceptive use should be considered a clear risk.
b. *Hepatic adenoma.* Benign hepatic adenomas appear to be associated with the use of oral contraceptives.[20–22] Although benign, and rare, these may rupture and may cause death through intra-abdominal hemorrhage. Such lesions have not yet been reported in association with other estrogen or progestogen preparations but should be considered in estrogen users having abdominal pain and tenderness, abdominal mass, or hypovolemic shock. Hepatocellular carcinoma has also been reported in women taking estrogen-containing oral contraceptives.[21] The relationship of this malignancy to these drugs is not known at this time.
c. *Elevated blood pressure.* Women using oral contraceptives sometimes experience increased blood pressure which,

in most cases, returns to normal on discontinuing the drug. There is now a report that this may occur with use of estrogens in the menopause[23] and blood pressure should be monitored with estrogen use, especially if high doses are used.

d. *Glucose tolerance.* A worsening of glucose tolerance has been observed in a significant percentage of patients on estrogen-containing oral contraceptives. For this reason, diabetic patients should be carefully observed while receiving estrogen.

4. *Hypercalcemia.* Administration of estrogens may lead to severe hypercalcemia in patients with breast cancer and bone metastases. If this occurs, the drug should be stopped and appropriate measures taken to reduce the serum calcium level.

PRECAUTIONS

1. A complete medical and family history should be taken prior to the initiation of any estrogen therapy. The pretreatment and periodic physical examinations should include special reference to blood pressure, breasts, abdomen, and pelvic organs. As a general rule, estrogen should not be prescribed for longer than one year without another physical examination being performed.

2. Fluid retention—Because estrogens may cause some degree of fluid retention, conditions which might be influenced by this factor such as asthma, epilepsy, migraine, and cardiac or renal dysfunction, require careful observation.

3. Certain patients may develop undesirable manifestations of excessive estrogenic stimulation, such as gynecomastia.

4. Oral contraceptives appear to be associated with an increased incidence of mental depression.[7a] Although it is not clear whether this is due to the estrogenic or progestogenic component of the contraceptive, patients with a history of depression should be carefully observed.

5. The pathologist should be advised of estrogen therapy when relevant specimens are submitted.

6. If jaundice develops in any patient receiving estrogen, the medication should be discontinued while the cause is investigated.

7. Estrogens may be poorly metabolized in patients with impaired liver function, and they should be administered with caution in such patients.

8. Because estrogens influence the metabolism of calcium and phosphorus, they should be used with caution in patients with metabolic bone diseases that are associated with hypercalcemia or in patients with renal insufficiency.

9. Because of the effects of estrogens on epiphyseal closure, they should be used judiciously in young patients in whom bone growth is not complete.

10. Certain endocrine and liver-function tests may be affected by estrogen-containing oral contraceptives. The following similar changes may be expected with larger doses of estrogen:

a. Increased sulfobromophthalein retention.

b. Increased prothrombin and factors VII, VIII, IX, and X; decreased antithrombin 3; increased norepinephrine-induced platelet aggregability.

c. Increased thyroid-binding globulin (TBG) leading to increased circulating total thyroid hormone, as measured by PBI, T4 by column, or T4 by radioimmunoassay. Free T3 resin uptake is decreased, reflecting the elevated TBG; free T4 concentration is unaltered.

d. Impaired glucose tolerance.

e. Reduced response to metyrapone test.

f. Reduced serum folate concentration.

g. Increased serum triglyceride and phospholipid concentration.

ADVERSE REACTIONS

(See Warnings regarding induction of neoplasia, increased incidence of gallbladder disease, and adverse effects similar to those of oral contraceptives, including thromboembolism.) The following additional adverse reactions have been reported with estrogenic therapy, including oral contraceptives:

1. *Breasts:* Tenderness, enlargement, secretion.

2. *Gastrointestinal:* Nausea, vomiting; abdominal cramps, bloating; cholestatic jaundice.

3. *Skin:* Chloasma or melasma which may persist when drug is discontinued; erythema multiforme; erythema nodosum; hemorrhagic eruption; loss of scalp hair; hirsutism.

4. *Eyes:* Steepening of corneal curvature; intolerance to contact lenses.

5. *CNS:* Headache, migraine, dizziness; mental depression; chorea.

6. *Miscellaneous:* Increase or decrease in weight; reduced carbohydrate tolerance; aggravation of porphyria; edema; changes in libido.

ACUTE OVERDOSAGE

Numerous reports of ingestion of large doses of estrogen-containing oral contraceptives by young children indicate that acute serious ill effects do not occur. Overdosage of estrogen may cause nausea, and withdrawal bleeding may occur in females.

DOSAGE AND ADMINISTRATION

Inoperable progressing prostatic cancer:

40 mg intramuscularly every two to four weeks or less frequently, depending on clinical response of the patient. If the response is not satisfactory, doses up to 80 mg may be used. Experimental evidence indicates that increasing the dose primarily prolongs the duration of action, but the amount of estrogen available at any one time is not significantly increased. The dosage should be adjusted as indicated by careful observation of the patient.

Deep intramuscular injection only is recommended. (Initially, some patients may experience a burning sensation at site of injection. This is transitory, and it may not recur with subsequent injections, or may be obviated by concomitant administration of a local anesthetic.)

If a response to estrogen therapy is going to occur, it will be apparent within three months of the beginning of therapy. If it does occur, the hormone should be continued until the disease is again progressive. The hormone should then be stopped, and the patient may obtain another period of improvement known as "rebound regression." This occurs in 30% of the patients who show objective improvement on estrogens.

DIRECTIONS FOR USE

Reconstitution for use:

1. Introduce sterile diluent into SECULE, preferably with a 20-gauge needle affixed to a 5 mL syringe.

2. Swirl gently until a solution is effected. (DO NOT AGITATE VIOLENTLY.)

Stability: After reconstitution, if storage is desired, the solution should be kept at room temperature and away from direct light. Under these conditions the solution is stable for about 10 days, so long as cloudiness or evidence of a precipitate has not occurred.

HOW SUPPLIED

NDC 0046-0754-02—Each package provides:

1. One SECULE® containing 40 mg polyestradiol phosphate, 0.022 mg phenylmercuric nitrate, and 5.2 mg sodium phosphate. As solubilizing agents for the active ingredient, 25 mg niacinamide and 4 mg propylene glycol are also present. The pH is adjusted with sodium hydroxide.

2. One 2 mL ampul of sterile diluent.

ESTRADURIN (polyestradiol phosphate) is prepared by cryodesiccation.

PHYSICIAN REFERENCES

1. Boston Collaborative Drug Surveillance Program: N. Engl. J. Med. *290*:15–19, 1974.
2. Boston Collaborative Drug Surveillance Program: Lancet *1*:1399–1404, 1973.
3. Daniel, D. G., *et al.*: Lancet *2*:287–289, 1967.
4. The Veterans Administration Cooperative Urological Research Group: J. Urol. *98*:516–522, 1967.
5. Bailar, J. C.: Lancet *2*:560, 1967.
6. Blackard, C., *et al.*: Cancer *26*:249–256, 1970.
7. Royal College of General Practitioners: J. R. Coll. Gen. Pract. *13*:267–279, 1967.
7a. Royal College of General Practitioners: Oral Contraceptives and Health, New York, Pitman Corp., 1974.
8. Inman, W. H. W., *et al.*: Br. Med. J. *2*:193–199, 1968.
9. Vessey, M. P., *et al.*: Br. Med. J. *2*:651–657, 1969.
10. Sartwell, P. E., *et al.*: Am. J. Epidemiol. *90*:365–380, 1969.
11. Collaborative Group for the Study of Stroke in Young Women: N. Engl. J. Med. *288*:871–878, 1973.
12. Collaborative Group for the Study of Stroke in Young Women: J.A.M.A. *231*:718–722, 1975.
13. Mann, J. I., *et al.*: Br. Med. J. *2*:245–248, 1975.
14. Mann, J. I., *et al.*: Br. Med. J. *2*:241–245, 1975.
15. Inman, W. H. W., *et al.*: Br. Med. J. *2*:203–209, 1970.
16. Stolley, P. D., *et al.*: Am. J. Epidemiol. *102*:197–208, 1975.
17. Vessey, M. P., *et al.*: Br. Med. J. *3*:123–126, 1970.
18. Greene, G. R., *et al.*: Am. J. Public Health *62*:680–685, 1972.
19. Coronary Drug Project Research Group: J.A.M.A. *214*:1303–1313, 1970.
20. Baum, J., *et al.*: Lancet *2*:926–928, 1973.
21. Mays, E. T., *et al.*: J.A.M.A. *235*:730–732, 1976.
22. Edmondson, H. A., *et al.*: N. Engl. J. Med. *294*:470–472, 1976.
23. Pfeffer, R. I., *et al.*: Am. J. Epidemiol. *103*:445–456, 1976.

SECULE®—Trademark to designate a special vial containing an injectable preparation in dry form.

FACTREL®   ℞
[făc-trĕl']
(gonadorelin hydrochloride)
Synthetic Luteinizing Hormone Releasing Hormone (LH-RH)
DIAGNOSTIC USE ONLY

HOW SUPPLIED

LYOPHILIZED POWDER
in single-dose SECULE® vials containing 100 mcg (NDC 0046-0507-05) and 500 mcg (NDC 0046-0509-05) gonadorelin as the hydrochloride with 100 mg lactose, USP. Each SECULE® vial is accompanied by one ampul containing 2 mL sterile diluent of 2% benzyl alcohol in sterile water. SECULE®—Registered trademark to designate a vial containing an injectable preparation in dry form.

For full prescribing information turn to the Diagnostic Product Information section of this edition of the PDR.

Shown in Product Identification Section, page 436

FLUOTHANE®   ℞
[flū'o-thān]
(halothane, USP)
Inhalation

CAUTION: Federal law prohibits dispensing without prescription.

DESCRIPTION

Fluothane (halothane, USP) is supplied as a liquid and is vaporized for use as an inhalation anesthetic. It is 2-bromo-2-chloro-1, 1, 1-trifluoro-ethane and has the following structural formula:

$$\begin{array}{ccc} & Br & F \\ & | & | \\ H - & C - & C - F \\ & | & | \\ & Cl & F \end{array}$$

$$C_2HBrClF_3$$

The molecular weight is 197.38. The drug substance halothane molecule has an asymmetric carbon atom; the commercial product is a racemic mixture. Resolution of the mixture has not been reported.*

Halothane is miscible with alcohol, chloroform, ether, and other fat solvents.

The specific gravity is 1.872–1.877 at 20°C, and the boiling point (range) is 49°C–51°C at 760 mm Hg. The vapor pressure is 243 mm Hg at 20°C. The blood/gas coefficient is 2.5 at 37°C, and the olive oil/water coefficient is 220 at 37°C. Vapor concentrations within anesthetic range are nonirritating and have a pleasant odor. Fluothane is nonflammable, and its vapors mixed with oxygen in proportions from 0.5 to 50% (v/v) are not explosive.

Fluothane does not decompose in contact with warm soda lime. When moisture is present, the vapor attacks aluminum, brass, and lead, but not copper. Rubber, some plastics, and similar materials are soluble in Fluothane; such materials will deteriorate rapidly in contact with Fluothane vapor or liquid. Stability of Fluothane is maintained by the addition of 0.01% thymol (w/w), up to 0.00025% ammonia (w/w).

CLINICAL PHARMACOLOGY

Fluothane is an inhalation anesthetic. Induction and recovery are rapid, and depth of anesthesia can be rapidly altered. Fluothane progressively depresses respiration. There may be tachypnea with reduced tidal volume and alveolar ventilation. Fluothane is not an irritant to the respiratory tract, and no increase in salivary or bronchial secretions ordinarily occurs. Pharyngeal and laryngeal reflexes are rapidly obtunded. It causes bronchodilation. Hypoxia, acidosis, or apnea may develop during deep anesthesia.

Fluothane reduces the blood pressure and frequently decreases the pulse rate. The greater the concentration of the drug, the more evident these changes become. Atropine may reverse the bradycardia. Fluothane does not cause the release of catecholamines from adrenergic stores. Fluothane also causes dilation of the vessels of the skin and skeletal muscles.

Cardiac arrhythmias may occur during Fluothane anesthesia. These include nodal rhythm, AV dissociation, ventricular extrasystoles and asystole. Fluothane sensitizes the myocardial conduction system to the action of epinephrine and norepinephrine, and the combination may cause serious cardiac arrhythmias. Fluothane increases cerebrospinal-fluid pressure. Fluothane produces moderate muscular relaxation. Muscle relaxants are used as adjuncts in order to maintain lighter levels of anesthesia. Fluothane augments the action of nondepolarizing relaxants and ganglionic-blocking agents. Fluothane is a potent uterine relaxant.

*Klaus Florey, editor, Analytical Profiles of Drug Substances, Vol. 1, page 127, (1972).

Continued on next page

Wyeth-Ayerst Laboratories—Cont.

The mechanism(s) whereby Fluothane and other substances induce general anesthesia is unknown. Fluothane is a very potent anesthetic in humans, with a minimum alveolar concentration (MAC) determined to be 0.64%. The MAC has been found to decrease with age (see MAC table in DOSAGE AND ADMINISTRATION).

INDICATIONS AND USAGE
Fluothane (halothane, USP) is indicated for the induction and maintenance of general anesthesia.

CONTRAINDICATIONS
Fluothane is not recommended for obstetrical anesthesia except when uterine relaxation is required.

WARNINGS
When previous exposure to Fluothane was followed by unexplained hepatic dysfunction and/or jaundice, consideration should be given to the use of other agents.

PRECAUTIONS
GENERAL
Fluothane should be used in vaporizers that permit a reasonable approximation of output, and preferably of the calibrated type. The vaporizer should be placed out of circuit in closed-circuit rebreathing systems, otherwise overdosage is difficult to avoid. The patient should be closely observed for signs of overdosage, i.e., depression of blood pressure, pulse rate, and ventilation, particularly during assisted or controlled ventilation.

Fluothane increases cerebrospinal-fluid pressure. Therefore, in patients with markedly raised intracranial pressure, if Fluothane is indicated, administration should be preceded by measures ordinarily used to reduce cerebrospinal-fluid pressure. Ventilation should be carefully assessed, and it may be necessary to assist or control ventilation to ensure adequate oxygenation and carbon dioxide removal.

In susceptible individuals, halothane anesthesia may trigger a skeletal-muscle hypermetabolic state leading to a high oxygen demand and the clinical syndrome known as malignant hyperthermia. The syndrome includes nonspecific features such as muscle rigidity, tachycardia, tachypnea, cyanosis, arrhythmias, and unstable blood pressure. (It should also be noted that many of these nonspecific signs may appear with light anesthesia, acute hypoxia, etc.) An increase in overall metabolism may be reflected in an elevated temperature (which may rise rapidly early, or late in the case, but usually is not the first sign of augmented metabolism) and an increased usage of the CO_2 absorption system (hot canister). PaO_2 and pH may decrease, and hyperkalemia and a base deficit may appear. Treatment includes discontinuance of triggering agents (e.g., halothane), administration of intravenous dantrolene, and application of supportive therapy. Such therapy includes vigorous efforts to restore body temperature to normal, respiratory and circulatory support as indicated, and management of electrolyte-fluid-acid-base derangements. Renal failure may appear later, and urine flow should be sustained if possible. It should be noted that the syndrome of malignant hyperthermia secondary to halothane appears to be rare.

INFORMATION FOR PATIENTS
When appropriate, as in some cases where discharge is anticipated soon after general anesthesia, patients should be cautioned not to drive automobiles, operate hazardous machinery, or engage in hazardous sports for 24 hours or more (depending on the total dose of Fluothane, condition of the patient, and consideration given to other drugs administered after anesthesia).

DRUG INTERACTIONS
Epinephrine or norepinephrine should be employed cautiously, if at all, during Fluothane (halothane, USP) anesthesia since their simultaneous use may induce ventricular tachycardia or fibrillation.

Nondepolarizing relaxants and ganglionic-blocking agents should be administered cautiously, since their actions are augmented by Fluothane (halothane, USP).

Clinical experience and animal experiments suggest that pancuronium should be given with caution to patients receiving chronic tricyclic antidepressant therapy who are anesthetized with halothane because severe ventricular arrhythmias may result from such usage.

CARCINOGENESIS, MUTAGENESIS, IMPAIRMENT OF FERTILITY
An 18-month inhalational carcinogenicity study of halothane at 0.05% in the mouse revealed no evidence of anesthetic-related carcinogenicity. This concentration is equivalent to 24 hours of 1% halothane.

Mutagenesis testing of halothane revealed both positive and negative results. In the rat, one-year exposure to trace concentrations of halothane (1 and 10 ppm) and nitrous oxide produced chromosomal damage to spermatogonia cells and bone marrow cells. Negative mutagenesis tests included: Ames bacterial assay, Chinese hamster lung fibroblast as-

say, sister chromatid exchange in Chinese hamster ovary cells, and human leukocyte culture assay.

Reproduction studies of halothane (10 ppm) and nitrous oxide in the rat caused decreased fertility. This trace concentration corresponds to 1/1000 the human maintenance dose.

PREGNANCY
Teratogenic Effects; Pregnancy Category C. Some studies have shown Fluothane to be teratogenic, embryotoxic, and fetotoxic in the mouse, rat, hamster, and rabbit at subanesthetic and/or anesthetic concentrations. There are no adequate and well-controlled studies in pregnant women. Fluothane should be used during pregnancy only if the potential benefit justifies the potential risk to the fetus.

LABOR AND DELIVERY
The uterine relaxation obtained with Fluothane, unless carefully controlled, may fail to respond to ergot derivatives and oxytocic posterior pituitary extract.

NURSING MOTHERS
It is not known whether this drug is excreted in human milk. Because many drugs are excreted in human milk, caution should be exercised when Fluothane is administered to a nursing woman.

PEDIATRIC USE
Extensive clinical experience reveals that maintenance concentrations of halothane are generally higher in infants and children, and that maintenance requirements decrease with age. See MAC table, based upon age, in DOSAGE AND ADMINISTRATION.

ADVERSE REACTIONS
The following adverse reactions have been reported: mild, moderate, and severe hepatic dysfunction (including hepatic necrosis); cardiac arrest; hypotension; respiratory arrest; cardiac arrhythmias; hyperpyrexia; shivering; nausea; and emesis.

OVERDOSAGE
In the event of overdosage, or what may appear to be overdosage, drug administration should be stopped, and assisted or controlled ventilation with pure oxygen initiated.

DOSAGE AND ADMINISTRATION
Fluothane may be administered by the nonrebreathing technique, partial rebreathing, or closed technique. The induction dose varies from patient to patient but is usually within the range of 0.5% to 3%. The maintenance dose varies from 0.5% to 1.5%.

Fluothane may be administered with either oxygen or a mixture of oxygen and nitrous oxide.

Fluothane should not be kept indefinitely in vaporizer bottles not specifically designed for its use. Thymol does not volatilize along with Fluothane, and, therefore, accumulates in the vaporizer, and may, in time, impart a yellow color to the remaining liquid or to wicks in vaporizers. The development of such discoloration may be used as an indicator that the vaporizer should be drained and cleaned, and the discolored Fluothane (halothane, USP) discarded. Accumulation of thymol may be removed by washing with diethyl ether. After cleaning a wick or vaporizer, make certain all the diethyl ether has been removed before reusing the equipment to avoid introducing ether into the system.

Because of the more rapid uptake of Fluothane and the increased blood concentration required for anesthesia in younger patients, the minimum alveolar concentration (MAC)[1] values will decrease with age as follows:

Age	MAC %
Infants	1.08
3 yrs.	0.91
10 yrs.	0.87
15 yrs.	0.92
24 yrs.	0.84
42 yrs.	0.76
81 yrs.	0.64

HOW SUPPLIED
Fluothane® (halothane, USP) is available in unit packages of 125 mL (NDC 0046-3125-81) and 250 mL (NDC 0046-3125-82) of halothane, USP, stabilized with 0.01% thymol (w/w) and up to 0.00025% ammonia (w/w).

HANDLING AND STORAGE
Store at room temperature (approximately 25°C) in a tight, closed container.
Protect from light.

PHYSICIAN REFERENCE
1. Gregory, GA et al: *Anesthesiology* 1969; *30*(5):488–491.

GRISACTIN®

[grĭz-ăc′tĭn]
(griseofulvin) microsize

CAUTION: Federal law prohibits dispensing without prescription.

DESCRIPTION
Griseofulvin is an oral fungistatic antibiotic for the treatment of superficial mycoses. It is derived from a species of *Penicillium.*

Grisactin is produced by a special process that fractures griseofulvin particles into minute crystals of irregular shape offering a greater and more effective surface area for increased gastrointestinal absorption.

Grisactin Capsules and Tablets contain the following inactive ingredients:
—250 mg capsules: black iron oxide, D&C Yellow No. 10, FD&C Blue No. 2, FD&C Red No. 40, FD&C Yellow No. 6, gelatin, lactose, magnesium stearate, titanium dioxide, water.
—500 mg tablets: calcium carboxymethylcellulose, D&C Red No. 36, gelatin, magnesium stearate, starch.

ACTION
Griseofulvin is fungistatic with *in vitro* activity against various species of *Microsporum, Epidermophyton,* and *Trichophyton.* It has no effect on bacteria or on other genera of fungi. Griseofulvin is deposited in the keratin precursor cells and has a greater affinity for diseased tissue. The drug is tightly bound to the new keratin which becomes highly resistant to fungal invasions.

Griseofulvin absorption from the gastrointestinal tract varies considerably among individuals mainly because of insolubility of the drug in aqueous media of the upper G.I. tract. The peak serum level found in fasting adults given 0.5 g occurs at about four hours and ranges between 0.5 to 2.0 mcg/mL. The serum level may be increased by giving the drug with a meal with a high fat content.

INDICATIONS
Griseofulvin is indicated for the treatment of ringworm infections of the skin, hair, and nails, namely:
Tinea corporis
Tinea pedis
Tinea cruris
Tinea barbae
Tinea capitis
Tinea unguium (onychomycosis) when caused by one or more of the following genera of fungi:
Trichophyton rubrum
Trichophyton tonsurans
Trichophyton mentagrophytes
Trichophyton interdigitalis
Trichophyton verrucosum
Trichophyton megnini
Trichophyton gallinae
Trichophyton crateriform
Trichophyton sulphureum
Trichophyton schoenleini
Microsporum audouini
Microsporum canis
Microsporum gypseum
Epidermophyton floccosum
NOTE: Prior to therapy, the type of fungi responsible for the infection should be identified.

The use of this drug is not justified in minor or trivial infections which will respond to topical agents alone.
Griseofulvin is *not* effective in the following:
Bacterial infections
Candidiasis (Moniliasis)
Histoplasmosis
Actinomycosis
Sporotrichosis
Chromoblastomycosis
Coccidioidomycosis
North American Blastomycosis
Cryptococcosis (Torulosis)
Tinea versicolor
Nocardiosis

CONTRAINDICATIONS
This drug is contraindicated in patients with porphyria, hepatocellular failure, and in individuals with a history of hypersensitivity to griseofulvin.

WARNINGS
PROPHYLACTIC USAGE
Safety and efficacy of griseofulvin for prophylaxis of fungal infections has not been established.
ANIMAL TOXICOLOGY
Chronic feeding of griseofulvin, at levels ranging from 0.5-2.5% of the diet, resulted in the development of liver tumors in several strains of mice, particularly males. Smaller particle sizes result in an enhanced effect. Lower-oral dosage levels have not been tested. Subcutaneous administration of relatively small doses of griseofulvin, once a week, during the first three weeks of life has also been reported to induce hepatomata in mice. Although studies in other animal species have not yielded evidence of tumorigenicity, these studies were not of adequate design to form a basis for conclusions in this regard.

In subacute toxicity studies, orally administered griseofulvin produced hepatocellular necrosis in mice, but this has not

been seen in other species. Disturbances in porphyrin metabolism have been reported in griseofulvin-treated laboratory animals. Griseofulvin has been reported to have a colchicine-like effect on mitosis and cocarcinogenicity with methylcholanthrene in cutaneous tumor induction in laboratory animals.

USAGE IN PREGNANCY

The safety of this drug during pregnancy has not been established.

ANIMAL REPRODUCTION STUDIES

It has been reported in the literature that griseofulvin was found to be embryotoxic and teratogenic on oral administration to pregnant rats. Pups with abnormalities have been reported in the litters of a few bitches treated with griseofulvin. Additional animal reproduction studies are in progress. Suppression of spermatogenesis has been reported to occur in rats, but investigation in man failed to confirm this.

PRECAUTIONS

Patients on prolonged therapy with any potent medication should be under close observation. Periodic monitoring of organ-system function, including renal, hepatic, and hematopoietic, should be done.

Since griseofulvin is derived from species of *Penicillium*, the possibility of cross-sensitivity with penicillin exists; however, known penicillin-sensitive patients have been treated without difficulty.

Since a photosensitivity reaction is occasionally associated with griseofulvin therapy, patients should be warned to avoid exposure to intense natural or artificial sunlight. Lupus erythematosus, lupus-like syndromes, or exacerbation of existing lupus erythematosus have been reported in patients receiving griseofulvin.

Griseofulvin decreases the activity of warfarin-type anticoagulants, so that patients receiving these drugs concomitantly may require dosage adjustment of the anticoagulant during and after griseofulvin therapy.

Barbiturates usually depress griseofulvin activity and concomitant administration may require a dosage adjustment of the antifungal agent.

The effect of alcohol may be potentiated by griseofulvin, producing such effects as tachycardia and flush.

ADVERSE REACTIONS

When adverse reactions occur, they are most commonly of the hypersensitivity type such as skin rashes, urticaria, and rarely, angioneurotic edema, and may necessitate withdrawal of therapy and appropriate countermeasures. Paresthesias of the hands and feet have been reported rarely after extended therapy. Other side effects reported occasionally are oral thrush, nausea, vomiting, epigastric distress, diarrhea, headache, fatigue, dizziness, insomnia, mental confusion, and impairment of performance of routine activities. Proteinuria and leukopenia have been reported rarely. Administration of the drug should be discontinued if granulocytopenia occurs.

When rare, serious reactions occur with griseofulvin, they are usually associated with high dosages, long periods of therapy, or both.

DOSAGE AND ADMINISTRATION

Accurate diagnosis of the infecting organism is essential. Identification should be made either by direct microscopic examination of a mounting of infected tissue in a solution of potassium hydroxide or by culture on an appropriate medium.

Medication must be continued until the infecting organism is completely eradicated as indicated by appropriate clinical or laboratory examination. Representative treatment periods are—*tinea capitis*, 4 to 6 weeks; *tinea corporis*, 2 to 4 weeks; *tinea pedis*, 4 to 8 weeks; *tinea unguium*—depending on rate of growth—fingernails, at least 4 months; toenails, at least 6 months.

General measures in regard to hygiene should be observed to control sources of infection or reinfection. Concomitant use of appropriate topical agents is usually required, particularly in treatment of *tinea pedis*. In some forms of athlete's foot, yeasts and bacteria may be involved as well as fungi. Griseofulvin will not eradicate the bacterial or monilial infection.

ADULTS: 0.5 g daily (125 mg q.i.d., 250 mg b.i.d., or 500 mg/day). Patients with less severe or extensive infections may require less, whereas those with widespread lesions may require a starting dose of 0.75 g to 1.0 g a day. This may be reduced gradually to 0.5 g or less after a response has been noted. In all cases, the dosage should be individualized.

CHILDREN: A dosage of 10 mg/kg daily is usually adequate (children from 30 to 50 lb, 125 mg to 250 mg daily; children over 50 lb, 250 mg to 500 mg daily, in divided doses). Dosage should be individualized, as with adults.

Clinical relapse will occur if the medication is not continued until the infecting organism is eradicated.

HOW SUPPLIED

GRISACTIN (griseofulvin) microsize—
GRISACTIN 250, each capsule contains 250 mg, in bottles of 100 (NDC 0046-0443-81) and 500 (NDC 0046-0443-85).

GRISACTIN 500, each tablet (scored) contains 500 mg, in bottles of 60 (NDC 0046-0444-60).
Store at room temperature (approximately 25°C).
Shown in Product Identification Section, page 436

GRISACTIN® Ultra   ℞
[grĭz-ăc'tĭn]
(griseofulvin ultramicrosize)

CAUTION: Federal law prohibits dispensing without prescription.

DESCRIPTION

Griseofulvin is an oral fungistatic antibiotic for the treatment of superficial mycoses. It is derived from a species of *Penicillium*.

GRISACTIN Ultra tablets contain griseofulvin ultramicrosize in the following dosage strengths: 250 mg and 330 mg. GRISACTIN Ultra tablets contain the following inactive ingredients: lactose, magnesium stearate, microcrystalline cellulose, sodium starch glycolate.

ACTION

Griseofulvin is fungistatic with *in vitro* activity against various species of *Microsporum, Epidermophyton*, and *Trichophyton*. It has no effect on bacteria or on other genera of fungi.

Human Pharmacology: Following oral administration, griseofulvin is deposited in the keratin precursor cells and has a greater affinity for diseased tissue. The drug is tightly bound to the new keratin which becomes highly resistant to fungal invasions.

The efficiency of gastrointestinal absorption of ultramicrocrystalline griseofulvin is approximately one and one-half times that of the conventional microsize griseofulvin. This factor permits the oral intake of two-thirds as much ultramicrocrystalline griseofulvin as the microsize form. However, there is currently no evidence that this lower dose confers any significant clinical difference with regard to safety and/or efficacy.

INDICATIONS

Griseofulvin is indicated for the treatment of ringworm infections of the skin, hair, and nails, namely:

Tinea corporis
Tinea pedis
Tinea cruris
Tinea barbae
Tinea capitis
Tinea unguium (onychomycosis) when caused by one or more of the following genera of fungi:

Trichophyton rubrum
Trichophyton tonsurans
Trichophyton mentagrophytes
Trichophyton interdigitalis
Trichophyton verrucosum
Trichophyton megnini
Trichophyton gallinae
Trichophyton crateriform
Trichophyton sulphureum
Trichophyton schoenleini
Microsporum audouini
Microsporum canis
Microsporum gypseum
Epidermophyton floccosum

NOTE: Prior to therapy, the type of fungi responsible for the infection should be identified.

The use of this drug is not justified in minor or trivial infections which will respond to topical agents alone.

Griseofulvin is *not* effective in the following:

Bacterial infections
Candidiasis (Moniliasis)
Histoplasmosis
Actinomycosis
Sporotrichosis
Chromoblastomycosis
Coccidioidomycosis
North American Blastomycosis
Cryptococcosis (Torulosis)
Tinea versicolor
Nocardiosis

CONTRAINDICATIONS

This drug is contraindicated in patients with porphyria, hepatocellular failure, and in individuals with a history of hypersensitivity to griseofulvin.

WARNINGS

Prophylactic Usage
Safety and efficacy of griseofulvin for prophylaxis of fungal infections has not been established.

Animal Toxicology
Chronic feeding of griseofulvin, at levels ranging from 0.5–2.5% of the diet, resulted in the development of liver tumors in several strains of mice, particularly males. Smaller particle sizes result in an enhanced effect. Lower

oral dosage levels have not been tested. Subcutaneous administration of relatively small doses of griseofulvin, once a week, during the first three weeks of life has also been reported to induce hepatomata in mice. Although studies in other animal species have not yielded evidence of tumorigenicity, these studies were not of adequate design to form a basis for conclusions in this regard.

In subacute toxicity studies, orally administered griseofulvin produced hepatocellular necrosis in mice, but this has not been seen in other species. Disturbances in porphyrin metabolism have been reported in griseofulvin-treated laboratory animals. Griseofulvin has been reported to have a colchicine-like effect on mitosis and cocarcinogenicity with methylcholanthrene in cutaneous tumor induction in laboratory animals.

Usage in Pregnancy
The safety of this drug during pregnancy has not been established.

Animal Reproduction Studies
It has been reported in the literature that griseofulvin was found to be embryotoxic and teratogenic on oral administration to pregnant rats. Pups with abnormalities have been reported in the litters of a few bitches treated with griseofulvin. Additional animal reproduction studies are in progress. Suppression of spermatogenesis has been reported to occur in rats, but investigation in man failed to confirm this.

PRECAUTIONS

Patients on prolonged therapy with any potent medication should be under close observation. Periodic monitoring of organ system function, including renal, hepatic, and hematopoietic, should be done.

Since griseofulvin is derived from species of *Penicillium*, the possibility of cross-sensitivity with penicillin exists; however, known penicillin-sensitive patients have been treated without difficulty.

Since a photosensitivity reaction is occasionally associated with griseofulvin therapy, patients should be warned to avoid exposure to intense natural or artificial sunlight. Lupus erythematosus, lupus-like syndromes, or exacerbation of existing lupus erythematosus have been reported in patients receiving griseofulvin.

Griseofulvin decreases the activity of warfarin-type anticoagulants so that patients receiving these drugs concomitantly may require dosage adjustment of the anticoagulant during and after griseofulvin therapy.

Barbiturates usually depress griseofulvin activity and concomitant administration may require a dosage adjustment of the antifungal agent.

The effect of alcohol may be potentiated by griseofulvin, producing such effects as tachycardia and flush.

ADVERSE REACTIONS

When adverse reactions occur, they are most commonly of the hypersensitivity type such as skin rashes, urticaria, and rarely, angioneurotic edema, and may necessitate withdrawal of therapy and appropriate countermeasures. Paresthesias of the hands and feet have been reported rarely after extended therapy. Other side effects reported occasionally are oral thrush, nausea, vomiting, epigastric distress, diarrhea, headache, fatigue, dizziness, insomnia, mental confusion, and impairment of performance of routine activities. Proteinuria and leukopenia have been reported rarely. Administration of the drug should be discontinued if granulocytopenia occurs.

When rare, serious reactions occur with griseofulvin, they are usually associated with high dosages, long periods of therapy, or both.

DOSAGE AND ADMINISTRATION

Accurate diagnosis of the infecting organism is essential. Identification should be made either by direct microscopic examination of a mounting of infected tissue in a solution of potassium hydroxide or by culture on an appropriate medium.

Medication must be continued until the infecting organism is completely eradicated as indicated by appropriate clinical or laboratory examination. Representative treatment periods are—*tinea capitis*, 4 to 6 weeks; *tinea corporis*, 2 to 4 weeks; *tinea pedis*, 4 to 8 weeks; *tinea unguium*—depending on rate of growth—fingernails, at least 4 months; toenails, at least 6 months.

General measures in regard to hygiene should be observed to control sources of infection or reinfection. Concomitant use of appropriate topical agents is usually required, particularly in treatment of *tinea pedis*. In some forms of athlete's foot, yeasts and bacteria may be involved as well as fungi. Griseofulvin will not eradicate the bacterial or monilial infection.

Adults: Daily administration of 330 mg (as a single dose or in divided doses) will give a satisfactory response in most patients with *tinea corporis, tinea cruris*, and *tinea capitis*. For those fungal infections more difficult to eradicate such as *tinea pedis* and *tinea unguium*, a divided dose of 660 mg is recommended.

Continued on next page

Wyeth-Ayerst Laboratories—Cont.

Children: Approximately 3.3 mg per pound of body weight per day of ultramicrosize griseofulvin is an effective dose for most children. On this basis the following dosage schedules are suggested:

Children weighing 35 to 50 lbs: 125 to 165 mg
Children weighing 50 to 75 lbs: 165 to 250 mg
Children weighing 75 lbs and over: 250 to 330 mg
Children 2 years of age and younger: dosage has not been established.

Clinical experience with griseofulvin in children with *tinea capitis* indicates that a single daily dose is effective. Clinical relapse will occur if the medication is not continued until the infecting organism is eradicated.

HOW SUPPLIED

GRISACTIN® Ultra tablets, 250 mg: white, square shaped compressed tablets impressed with the trade name and dosage strength, in bottles of 100 (NDC 0046-0435-81).
GRISACTIN® Ultra tablets, 330 mg: scored, white, wide-oval shaped, compressed tablets impressed with the trade name and dosage strength, in bottles of 100 (NDC 0046-0437-81).
Store at room temperature (approximately 25° C).
Shown in Product Identification Section, page 436

HEPARIN ℞
[*hep 'ah-rin*]
Lock Flush Solution, USP
Heparin Flush Kits

Heparin Lock Flush Solution is intended for maintenance of patency of intravenous injection devices only, and is not to be used for anticoagulant therapy.

DESCRIPTION

Wyeth's TUBEX® Heparin Lock Flush Solution, USP, is a sterile solution. Each mL contains either 10 or 100 USP units heparin sodium derived from porcine intestinal mucosa (standardized for use as an anticoagulant) in normal saline solution, and not more than 10 mg benzyl alcohol as a preservative.

The potency is determined by biological assay, using a USP reference standard based upon units of heparin activity per milligram. The pH range is 5.0 to 7.5.

Heparin is a heterogenous group of straight-chain anionic mucopolysaccharides, called glycosaminoglycans, having anticoagulant properties. Although others may be present, the main sugars occurring in heparin are: (1) α-L-iduronic acid 2-sulfate, (2) 2-deoxy-2-sulfamino-α-D-glucose 6-sulfate, (3) β-D-glucuronic acid, (4) 2-acetamido-2-deoxy-α-D-glucose, and (5) α-L-iduronic acid. These sugars are present in decreasing amounts, usually in the order (2) > (1) > (4) > (3) > (5), and are joined by glycosidic linkages, forming polymers of varying sizes. Heparin is strongly acidic because of its content of covalently linked sulfate and carboxylic acid groups. In heparin sodium, the acidic protons of the sulfate units are partially replaced by sodium ions.

STRUCTURE OF HEPARIN SODIUM (representative subunits):

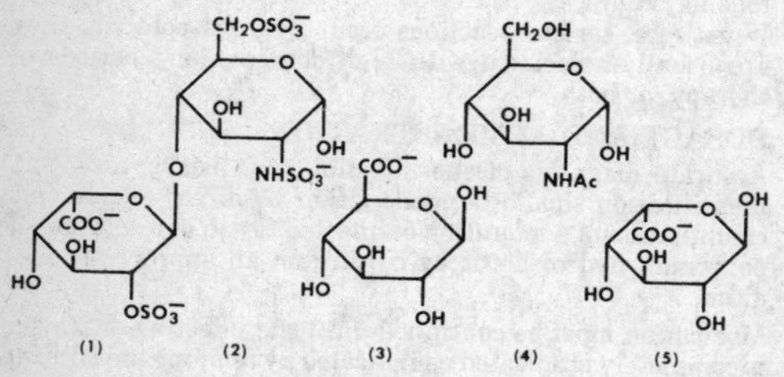

(1) (2) (3) (4) (5)

CLINICAL PHARMACOLOGY

Heparin inhibits reactions that lead to the clotting of blood and the formation of fibrin clots both *in vitro* and *in vivo.* Heparin acts at multiple sites in the normal coagulation system. Small amounts of heparin in combination with antithrombin III (heparin cofactor) can inhibit thrombosis by inactivating activated Factor X and inhibiting the conversion of prothrombin to thrombin. Once active thrombosis has developed, larger amounts of heparin can inhibit further coagulation by inactivating thrombin and preventing the conversion of fibrinogen to fibrin. Heparin also prevents the formation of a stable fibrin clot by inhibiting the activation of the fibrin stabilizing factor.

Bleeding time is usually unaffected by heparin. Clotting time is prolonged by full therapeutic doses of heparin; in most cases, it is not measurably affected by low doses of heparin. Peak plasma levels of heparin are achieved 2 to 4 hours following subcutaneous administration, although there are considerable individual variations. Loglinear plots of heparin plasma concentrations with time, for a wide range of dose levels, are linear which suggests the absence of zero order processes. Liver and the reticulo-endothelial system are the sites of biotransformation. The biphasic elimination curve, a rapidly declining alpha phase ($t_{1/2}$ = 10 min.), and after the age of 40 a slower beta phase, indicates uptake in organs. The absence of a relationship between anticoagulant half-life and concentration half-life may reflect factors such as protein binding of heparin.

Heparin does not have fibrinolytic activity; therefore, it will not lyse existing clots.

INDICATIONS AND USAGE

Heparin Lock Flush Solution, USP, is intended to maintain patency of an indwelling venipuncture device designed for intermittent injection or infusion therapy, or blood sampling. Heparin Lock Flush Solution, USP, may be used following initial placement of the device in the vein, after each injection of a medication, or after withdrawal of blood for laboratory tests.

Heparin Lock Flush Solution, USP, is not to be used for anticoagulant therapy.

CONTRAINDICATIONS

Heparin sodium should not be used in patients with the following conditions:
Severe thrombocytopenia;
An uncontrollable active bleeding state (see "Warnings"), except when this is due to disseminated intravascular coagulation.

WARNINGS

Heparin is not intended for intramuscular use.

HYPERSENSITIVITY
Patients with documented hypersensitivity to heparin should be given the drug only in clearly life-threatening situations.

HEMORRHAGE
Hemorrhage can occur at virtually any site in patients receiving heparin. An unexplained fall in hematocrit, fall in blood pressure, or any other unexplained symptom should lead to serious consideration of a hemorrhagic event.

Heparin sodium should be used with extreme caution in disease states in which there is increased danger of hemorrhage. Some of the conditions in which increased danger of hemorrhage exists are:

Cardiovascular—Subacute bacterial endocarditis. Severe hypertension.
Surgical—During and immediately following (a) spinal tap or spinal anesthesia or (b) major surgery, especially involving the brain, spinal cord, or eye.
Hematologic—Conditions associated with increased bleeding tendencies, such as hemophilia, thrombocytopenia, and some vascular purpuras.
Gastrointestinal—Ulcerative lesions and continuous tube drainage of the stomach or small intestine.
Other—Menstruation, liver disease with impaired hemostasis.

THROMBOCYTOPENIA
Thrombocytopenia has been reported to occur in patients receiving heparin with a reported incidence of 0 to 30%. Mild thrombocytopenia (count greater than 100,000/mm^3) may remain stable or reverse even if heparin is continued. However, thrombocytopenia of any degree should be monitored closely. If the count falls below 100,000/mm^3 or if recurrent thrombosis develops (see "White-clot Syndrome," "Precautions"), the heparin product should be discontinued. If continued heparin therapy is essential, administration of heparin from a different organ source can be reinstituted with caution.

MISCELLANEOUS
This product contains benzyl alcohol as preservative. Benzyl alcohol has been reported to be associated with a fatal "Gasping Syndrome" in premature infants.

PRECAUTIONS

GENERAL
White-clot Syndrome
It has been reported that patients on heparin may develop new thrombus formation in association with thrombocytopenia, resulting from irreversible aggregation of platelets induced by heparin, the so-called "white-clot syndrome." The process may lead to severe thromboembolic complications like skin necrosis, gangrene of the extremities that may lead to amputation, myocardial infarction, pulmonary embolism, stroke, and possibly death. Therefore, heparin administration should be promptly discontinued if a patient develops new thrombosis in association with thrombocytopenia.

Heparin Resistance
Increased resistance to heparin is frequently encountered in fever, thrombosis, thrombophlebitis, infections with thrombosing tendencies, myocardial infarction, cancer, and in postsurgical patients.

Increased Risk in Older Women
A higher incidence of bleeding has been reported in women over 60 years of age.

LABORATORY TESTS
Periodic platelet counts, hematocrits, and tests for occult blood in stool are recommended during the entire course of heparin therapy, regardless of the route of administration (see "Dosage and Administration").

DRUG INTERACTIONS
Platelet Inhibitors
Drugs such as acetylsalicylic acid, dextran, phenylbutazone, ibuprofen, indomethacin, dipyridamole, hydroxychloroquine, and others that interfere with platelet-aggregation reactions (the main hemostatic defense of heparinized patients) may induce bleeding and should be used with caution in patients receiving heparin sodium.

Other Interactions
Digitalis, tetracyclines, nicotine, or antihistamines may partially counteract the anticoagulant action of heparin sodium.

CARCINOGENESIS, MUTAGENESIS, IMPAIRMENT OF FERTILITY
No long-term studies in animals have been performed to evaluate carcinogenic potential of heparin. Also, no reproduction studies in animals have been performed concerning mutagenesis or impairment of fertility.

PREGNANCY
Teratogenic Effects —Pregnancy Category C
Animal reproduction studies have not been conducted with heparin sodium. It is also not known whether heparin sodium can cause fetal harm when administered to a pregnant woman or can affect reproduction capacity. Heparin sodium should be given to a pregnant woman only if clearly needed.

Nonteratogenic Effects
Heparin does not cross the placental barrier.

NURSING MOTHERS
Heparin is not excreted in human milk.

ADVERSE REACTIONS

HEMORRHAGE
Hemorrhage is the chief complication that may result from heparin therapy (see "Warnings"). An overly prolonged clotting time or minor bleeding during therapy can usually be controlled by withdrawing the drug (see "Overdosage"). It should be appreciated that gastrointestinal- or urinary-tract bleeding during anticoagulant therapy may indicate the presence of an underlying occult lesion. Bleeding can occur at any site but certain specific hemorrhagic complications may be difficult to detect:

a. Adrenal hemorrhage, with resultant acute adrenal insufficiency, has occurred during anticoagulant therapy. Therefore, such treatment should be discontinued in patients who develop signs and symptoms of acute adrenal hemorrhage and insufficiency. Initiation of corrective therapy should not depend on laboratory confirmation of the diagnosis, since any delay in an acute situation may result in the patient's death.
b. Ovarian (corpus luteum) hemorrhage developed in a number of women of reproductive age receiving short- or long-term anticoagulant therapy. This complication, if unrecognized, may be fatal.
c. Retroperitoneal hemorrhage.

LOCAL IRRITATION
Local irritation, erythema, mild pain, hematoma, or ulceration may follow deep, subcutaneous (intrafat) injection of heparin sodium. These complications are much more common after intramuscular use, and such use is not recommended.

HYPERSENSITIVITY
Generalized hypersensitivity reactions have been reported, with chills, fever, and urticaria as the most usual manifestations, and asthma, rhinitis, lacrimation, headache, nausea and vomiting, and anaphylactoid reactions, including shock, occurring more rarely. Itching and burning, especially on the plantar side of the feet, may occur.

Thrombocytopenia has been reported to occur in patients receiving heparin with a reported incidence of 0 to 30%. While often mild and of no obvious clinical significance, such thrombocytopenia can be accompanied by severe thromboembolic complications, such as skin necrosis, gangrene of the extremities that may lead to amputation, myocardial infarction, pulmonary embolism, stroke, and possibly death. (See "Warnings," "Precautions.")

Certain episodes of painful, ischemic and cyanosed limbs have in the past been attributed to allergic vasospastic reactions. Whether these are, in fact, identical to the thrombocytopenia-associated complications remains to be determined.

MISCELLANEOUS
Osteoporosis following long-term administration of high doses of heparin, cutaneous necrosis after systemic administration, suppression of aldosterone synthesis, delayed transient alopecia, priapism, and rebound hyperlipemia on discontinuation of heparin sodium have also been reported.

Significant elevations of aminotransferase (SGOT [S-AST] and SGPT [S-ALT]) levels have occurred in a high percentage of patients (and healthy subjects) who have received heparin.

OVERDOSAGE
SYMPTOMS
Bleeding is the chief sign of heparin overdosage. Nosebleeds, blood in urine, or tarry stools may be noted as the first sign of bleeding. Easy bruising or petechial formations may precede frank bleeding.
TREATMENT—Neutralization of Heparin Effect
When clinical circumstances (bleeding) require reversal of heparinization, protamine sulfate (1% solution) by slow infusion will neutralize heparin sodium. No more than 50 mg should be administered, very slowly, in any 10-minute period. Each mg of protamine sulfate neutralizes approximately 100 USP heparin units. The amount of protamine required decreases over time as heparin is metabolized. Although the metabolism of heparin is complex, it may, for the purpose of choosing a protamine dose, be assumed to have a half-life of about $\frac{1}{2}$ hour after intravenous injection.
Administration of protamine sulfate can cause severe hypotensive and anaphylactoid reactions. Because fatal reactions, often resembling anaphylaxis, have been reported, the drug should be given only when resuscitation techniques and treatment of anaphylactoid shock are readily available.
For additional information consult the labeling of Protamine Sulfate Injection, USP, products.

DOSAGE AND ADMINISTRATION
Parenteral drug products should be inspected visually for particulate matter and discoloration prior to administration, whenever solution and container permit. Slight discoloration does not alter potency.
MAINTENANCE OF PATENCY OF INTRAVENOUS DEVICES
To prevent clot formation in a heparin lock set or central venous catheter following its proper insertion, Heparin Lock Flush Solution, USP, is injected via the injection hub in a quantity sufficient to fill the entire device. This solution should be replaced each time the device is used. Aspirate before administering any solution via the device in order to confirm patency and location of needle or catheter tip. If the drug to be administered is incompatible with heparin, the entire device should be flushed with normal saline before and after the medication is administered; following the second saline flush, Heparin Lock Flush Solution, USP, may be reinstilled into the device. The device manufacturer's instructions should be consulted for specifics concerning its use. Usually this dilute heparin solution will maintain anticoagulation within the device for up to 4 hours.
NOTE: Since repeated injections of small doses of heparin can alter tests for activated partial thromboplastin time (APTT), a baseline value for APTT should be obtained prior to insertion of an intravenous device.
WITHDRAWAL OF BLOOD SAMPLES
Heparin Lock Flush Solution, USP, may also be used after each withdrawal of blood for laboratory tests. When heparin (or sodium chloride) would interfere with or alter the results of blood tests, the heparin solution should be cleared from the device by aspirating and discarding it before withdrawing the blood sample.

HOW SUPPLIED
Heparin Lock Flush Solution, USP, is supplied in TUBEX Sterile Cartridge-Needle Units which include 25 gauge × $\frac{5}{8}$ inch needles.
Each 1 mL size TUBEX contains one of the following concentrations of heparin sodium, in packages of 50 TUBEX:
10 USP units per mL, NDC 0008-0523-01.
100 USP Units per mL, NDC 0008-0487-01.
Each 2.5 mL size TUBEX contains one of the following concentrations of heparin sodium, in packages of 50 TUBEX:
25 USP Units per TUBEX or 10 USP Units per mL, NDC 0008-0523-02.
250 USP Units per TUBEX or 100 USP Units per mL, NDC 0008-0487-03.
Store at room temperature, 15°–25°C (59°–77°F).
Do not freeze
HEPARIN FLUSH KITS
NOTE: There are two package inserts associated with the use of Heparin Flush Kits (Heparin Lock Flush Solution, USP, and Bacteriostatic Sodium Chloride Injection, USP).
All TUBEX® Sterile Cartridge-Needle Units in the following packages include 25 gauge × $\frac{5}{8}$ inch needles.
10 USP UNITS HEPARIN SODIUM PER ML
Each Unit of Use Kit contains:
NDC 0008-2528-01; one TUBEX (1 mL) Heparin Lock Flush Solution, USP; two TUBEX (2.5 mL each) Bacteriostatic Sodium Chloride Injection, USP; in packages of 50 Kits.
NDC 0008-2528-02; one TUBEX (2.5 mL) Heparin Lock Flush Solution, USP (25 USP Units heparin sodium per TUBEX); two TUBEX (2.5 mL each) Bacteriostatic Sodium Chloride Injection, USP; in packages of 30 Kits.
NDC 0008-2528-03; one TUBEX (1 mL) Heparin Lock Flush Solution, USP; two TUBEX (1 mL each) Bacteriostatic Sodium Chloride Injection, USP; in packages of 50 Kits.
100 USP UNITS HEPARIN SODIUM PER ML
Each Unit of Use Kit contains:
NDC 0008-2529-01; one TUBEX (1 mL) Heparin Lock Flush Solution, USP; two TUBEX (2.5 mL each) Bacteriostatic Sodium Chloride Injection, USP; in packages of 50 Kits.
NDC 0008-2529-02; one TUBEX (2.5 mL) Heparin Lock Flush Solution, USP (250 USP Units heparin sodium per TUBEX); two TUBEX (2.5 mL each) Bacteriostatic Sodium Chloride Injection, USP; in packages of 30 Kits.
NDC 0008-2529-03; one TUBEX (1 mL) Heparin Lock Flush Solution, USP; two TUBEX (1 mL each) Bacteriostatic Sodium Chloride Injection, USP; in packages of 50 Kits.
Store at room temperature, 15°–25°C (59°–77°F).
Do not freeze

HEPARIN ℞
[*hep 'ah-rin*]
Sodium Injection, USP

DESCRIPTION
Wyeth's TUBEX® Heparin Sodium Injection, USP, is a sterile solution. Each mL contains 1,000, 2,500, 5,000, 7,500, 10,000, 15,000, or 20,000 USP units heparin sodium, derived from porcine intestinal mucosa (standardized for use as an anticoagulant), in water for injection, and not more than 10 mg benzyl alcohol as a preservative.
The potency is determined by biological assay, using a USP reference standard based upon units of heparin activity per milligram. The pH range is 5.0 to 7.5.
Heparin is a heterogenous group of straight-chain anionic mucopolysaccharides, called glycosaminoglycans, having anticoagulant properties. Although others may be present, the main sugars occurring in heparin are: (1) α-L-iduronic acid 2-sulfate, (2) 2-deoxy-2-sulfamino-α-D-glucose 6-sulfate, (3) β-D-glucuronic acid, (4) 2-acetamido-2-deoxy-α-D-glucose, and (5) α-L-iduronic acid. These sugars are present in decreasing amounts, usually in the order (2) > (1) > (4) > (3) > (5), and are joined by glycosidic linkages, forming polymers of varying sizes. Heparin is strongly acidic because of its content of covalently linked sulfate and carboxylic acid groups. In heparin sodium, the acidic protons of the sulfate units are partially replaced by sodium ions.
STRUCTURE OF HEPARIN SODIUM (representative subunits):

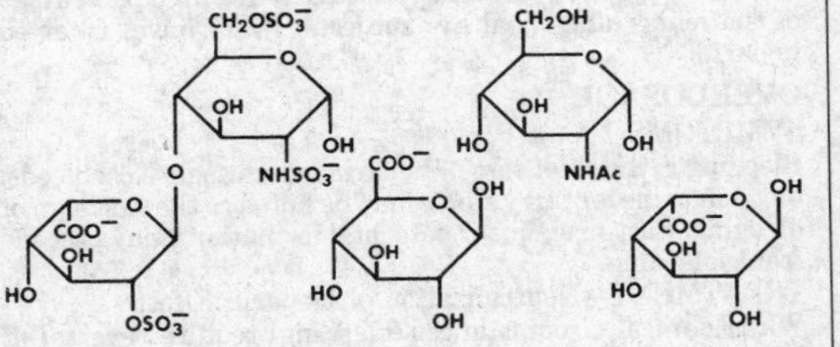

(1) (2) (3) (4) (5)

CLINICAL PHARMACOLOGY
Heparin inhibits reactions that lead to the clotting of blood and the formation of fibrin clots both *in vitro* and *in vivo.* Heparin acts at multiple sites in the normal coagulation system. Small amounts of heparin in combination with antithrombin III (heparin cofactor) can inhibit thrombosis by inactivating activated Factor X and inhibiting the conversion of prothrombin to thrombin. Once active thrombosis has developed, larger amounts of heparin can inhibit further coagulation by inactivating thrombin and preventing the conversion of fibrinogen to fibrin. Heparin also prevents the formation of a stable fibrin clot by inhibiting the activation of the fibrin stabilizing factor.
Bleeding time is usually unaffected by heparin. Clotting time is prolonged by full therapeutic doses of heparin; in most cases it is not measurably affected by low doses of heparin.
Peak plasma levels of heparin are achieved 2 to 4 hours following subcutaneous administration, although there are considerable individual variations. Loglinear plots of heparin plasma concentrations with time, for a wide range of dose levels, are linear which suggests the absence of zero order processes. Liver and the reticulo-endothelial system are the sites of biotransformation. The biphasic elimination curve, a rapidly declining alpha phase ($t_{1/2}$ = 10 min.), and after the age of 40 a slower beta phase, indicates uptake in organs. The absence of a relationship between anticoagulant half-life and concentration half-life may reflect factors such as protein binding of heparin.
Heparin does not have fibrinolytic activity; therefore, it will not lyse existing clots.

INDICATIONS AND USAGE
Heparin sodium injection is indicated for anticoagulant therapy in prophylaxis and treatment of venous thrombosis and its extension; in low-dose regimen for prevention of postoperative deep venous thrombosis and pulmonary embolism in patients undergoing major abdominothoracic surgery who are at risk of developing thromboembolic disease (see "Dosage and Administration"); for prophylaxis and treatment of pulmonary embolism; in atrial fibrillation with embolization; for diagnosis and treatment of acute and chronic consumptive coagulopathies (disseminated intravascular coagulation); for prevention of clotting in arterial and cardiac surgery; and for prophylaxis and treatment of peripheral arterial embolism.
Heparin may also be employed as an anticoagulant in blood transfusions, extracorporeal circulation, dialysis procedures, and in blood samples for laboratory purposes.

CONTRAINDICATIONS
Heparin sodium should not be used in patients:
with severe thrombocytopenia;
in whom suitable blood-coagulation tests—e.g., the whole-blood clotting time, partial thromboplastin time, etc.—cannot be performed at appropriate intervals (this contraindication refers to full-dose heparin; there is usually no need to monitor coagulation parameters in patients receiving low-dose heparin);
with an uncontrollable active bleeding state (see "Warnings"), except when this is due to disseminated intravascular coagulation.

WARNINGS
Heparin is not intended for intramuscular use.
HYPERSENSITIVITY
Patients with documented hypersensitivity to heparin should be given the drug only in clearly life-threatening situations.
HEMORRHAGE
Hemorrhage can occur at virtually any site in patients receiving heparin. An unexplained fall in hematocrit, fall in blood pressure, or any other unexplained symptom should lead to serious consideration of a hemorrhagic event.
Heparin sodium should be used with extreme caution in disease states in which there is increased danger of hemorrhage. Some of the conditions in which increased danger of hemorrhage exists are:
Cardiovascular—Subacute bacterial endocarditis. Severe hypertension.
Surgical—During and immediately following (a) spinal tap or spinal anesthesia or (b) major surgery, especially involving the brain, spinal cord, or eye.
Hematologic—Conditions associated with increased bleeding tendencies, such as hemophilia, thrombocytopenia, and some vascular purpuras.
Gastrointestinal—Ulcerative lesions and continuous tube drainage of the stomach or small intestine.
Other—Menstruation, liver disease with impaired hemostasis.
COAGULATION TESTING
When heparin sodium is administered in therapeutic amounts, its dosage should be regulated by frequent blood coagulation tests. If the coagulation test is unduly prolonged or if hemorrhage occurs, heparin sodium should be discontinued promptly (see "Overdosage").
THROMBOCYTOPENIA
Thrombocytopenia has been reported to occur in patients receiving heparin with a reported incidence of 0 to 30%. Mild thrombocytopenia (count greater than 100,000/mm^3) may remain stable or reverse even if heparin is continued. However, thrombocytopenia of any degree should be monitored closely. If the count falls below 100,000/mm^3 or if recurrent thrombosis develops (see "White-clot Syndrome," "Precautions"), the heparin product should be discontinued. If continued heparin therapy is essential, admistration of heparin from a different organ source can be reinstituted with caution.
MISCELLANEOUS
This product contains benzyl alcohol as preservative. Benzyl alcohol has been reported to be associated with a fatal "Gasping Syndrome" in premature infants.

PRECAUTIONS
GENERAL
White-clot Syndrome
It has been reported that patients on heparin may develop new thrombus formation in association with thrombocytopenia, resulting from irreversible aggregation of platelets induced by heparin, the so-called "white-clot syndrome." The process may lead to severe thromboembolic complications like skin necrosis, gangrene of the extremities that may lead to amputation, myocardial infarction, pulmonary embolism, stroke, and possibly death. Therefore, heparin administration should be promptly discontinued if a patient develops new thrombosis in association with thrombocytopenia.
Heparin Resistance
Increased resistance to heparin is frequently encountered in fever, thrombosis, thrombophlebitis, infections with thrombosing tendencies, myocardial infarction, cancer, and in postsurgical patients.

Continued on next page

Wyeth-Ayerst Laboratories—Cont.

Increased Risk in Older Women
A higher incidence of bleeding has been reported in women over 60 years of age.
LABORATORY TESTS
Periodic platelet counts, hematocrits, and tests for occult blood in stool are recommended during the entire course of heparin therapy, regardless of the route of administration (see "Dosage and Administration").
DRUG INTERACTIONS
Oral Anticoagulants
Heparin sodium may prolong the one-stage prothrombin time. Therefore, when heparin sodium is given with dicumarol or warfarin sodium, a period of at least 5 hours after the last intravenous dose or 24 hours after the last subcutaneous dose should elapse before blood is drawn if a valid prothrombin time is to be obtained.
Platelet Inhibitors
Drugs such as acetylsalicylic acid, dextran, phenylbutazone, ibuprofen, indomethacin, dipyridamole, hydroxychloroquine, and others that interfere with platelet-aggregation reactions (the main hemostatic defense of heparinized patients) may induce bleeding and should be used with caution in patients receiving heparin sodium.
Other Interactions
Digitalis, tetracyclines, nicotine, or antihistamines may partially counteract the anticoagulant action of heparin sodium.
DRUG/LABORATORY TEST INTERACTIONS
Hyperaminotransferasemia
Significant elevations of aminotransferase (SGOT [S-AST] and SGPT [S-ALT]) levels have occurred in a high percentage of patients (and healthy subjects) who have received heparin. Since aminotransferase determinations are important in the differential diagnosis of myocardial infarction, liver disease, and pulmonary emboli, rises that might be caused by drugs (like heparin) should be interpreted with caution.
CARCINOGENESIS, MUTAGENESIS, IMPAIRMENT OF FERTILITY
No long-term studies in animals have been performed to evaluate carcinogenic potential of heparin. Also, no reproduction studies in animals have been performed concerning mutagenesis or impairment of fertility.
PREGNANCY
Teratogenic Effects—Pregnancy Category C
Animal reproduction studies have not been conducted with heparin sodium. It is also not known whether heparin sodium can cause fetal harm when administered to a pregnant woman or can affect reproduction capacity. Heparin sodium should be given to a pregnant woman only if clearly needed.
Nonteratogenic Effects
Heparin does not cross the placental barrier.
NURSING MOTHERS
Heparin is not excreted in human milk.
PEDIATRIC USE
See "Dosage and Administration."

ADVERSE REACTIONS

HEMORRHAGE
Hemorrhage is the chief complication that may result from heparin therapy (see "Warnings").
An overly prolonged clotting time or minor bleeding during therapy can usually be controlled by withdrawing the drug (see "Overdosage"). It should be appreciated that gastrointestinal- or urinary-tract bleeding during anticoagulant therapy may indicate the presence of an underlying occult lesion. Bleeding can occur at any site but certain specific hemorrhagic complications may be difficult to detect:

a. Adrenal hemorrhage, with resultant acute adrenal insufficiency, has occurred during anticoagulant therapy. Therefore, such treatment should be discontinued in patients who develop signs and symptoms of acute adrenal hemorrhage and insufficiency. Initiation of corrective therapy should not depend on laboratory confirmation of the diagnosis, since any delay in an acute situation may result in the patient's death.
b. Ovarian (corpus luteum) hemorrhage developed in a number of women of reproductive age receiving short- or long-term anticoagulant therapy. This complication, if unrecognized, may be fatal.
c. Retroperitoneal hemorrhage.

LOCAL IRRITATION
Local irritation, erythema, mild pain, hematoma, or ulceration may follow deep, subcutaneous (intrafat) injection of heparin sodium. These complications are much more common after intramuscular use, and such use is not recommended.
HYPERSENSITIVITY
Generalized hypersensitivity reactions have been reported, with chills, fever, and urticaria as the most usual manifestations, and asthma, rhinitis, lacrimation, headache, nausea and vomiting, and anaphylactoid reactions, including shock, occurring more rarely. Itching and burning, especially on the plantar side of the feet, may occur.
Thrombocytopenia has been reported to occur in patients receiving heparin with a reported incidence of 0 to 30%. While often mild and of no obvious clinical significance, such thrombocytopenia can be accompanied by severe thromboembolic complications, such as skin necrosis, gangrene of the extremities that may lead to amputation, myocardial infarction, pulmonary embolism, stroke, and possibly death. (See "Warnings," "Precautions.")
Certain episodes of painful, ischemic and cyanosed limbs have in the past been attributed to allergic vasospastic reactions. Whether these are, in fact, identical to the thrombocytopenia-associated complications remains to be determined.
MISCELLANEOUS
Osteoporosis following long-term administration of high doses of heparin, cutaneous necrosis after systemic administration, suppression of aldosterone synthesis, delayed transient alopecia, priapism, and rebound hyperlipemia on discontinuation of heparin sodium have also been reported.
Significant elevations of aminotransferase (SGOT [S-AST] and SGPT [S-ALT]) levels have occurred in a high percentage of patients (and healthy subjects) who have received heparin.

OVERDOSAGE

SYMPTOMS
Bleeding is the chief sign of heparin overdosage. Nosebleeds, blood in urine, or tarry stools may be noted as the first sign of bleeding. Easy bruising or petechial formations may precede frank bleeding.
TREATMENT—Neutralization of Heparin Effect
When clinical circumstances (bleeding) require reversal of heparinization, protamine sulfate (1% solution) by slow infusion will neutralize heparin sodium. No more than 50 mg should be administered, very slowly, in any 10-minute period. Each mg of protamine sulfate neutralizes approximately 100 USP heparin units. The amount of protamine required decreases over time as heparin is metabolized. Although the metabolism of heparin is complex, it may, for the purpose of choosing a protamine dose, be assumed to have a half-life of about ½ hour after intravenous injection.
Administration of protamine sulfate can cause severe hypotensive and anaphylactoid reactions. Because fatal reactions, often resembling anaphylaxis, have been reported, the drug should be given only when resuscitation techniques and treatment of anaphylactoid shock are readily available.
For additional information consult the labeling of Protamine Sulfate Injection, USP, products.

DOSAGE AND ADMINISTRATION

Parenteral drug products should be inspected visually for particulate matter and discoloration prior to administration, whenever solution and container permit. Slight discoloration does not alter potency.
When heparin is added to an infusion solution for continuous intravenous administration, the container should be inverted at least six times to insure adequate mixing and prevent pooling of the heparin in the solution.
Heparin sodium is not effective by oral administration and should be given by intermittent intravenous injection, intravenous infusion, or deep, subcutaneous (intrafat, i.e., above the iliac crest or abdominal fat layer) injection. *The intramuscular route of administration should be avoided because of the frequent occurrence of hematoma at the injection site.*
The dosage of heparin sodium should be adjusted according to the patient's coagulation-test results. When heparin is given by continuous intravenous infusion, the coagulation time should be determined approximately every 4 hours in the early stages of treatment. When the drug is administered intermittently by intravenous injection, coagulation tests should be performed before each injection during the early stages of treatment and at appropriate intervals thereafter. Dosage is considered adequate when the activated partial thromboplastin time (APTT) is 1.5 to 2 times normal or when the whole-blood clotting time is elevated approximately 2.5 to 3 times the control value. After deep subcutaneous (intrafat) injections, tests for adequacy of dosage are best performed on samples drawn 4 to 6 hours after the injections.
Periodic platelet counts, hematocrits, and tests for occult blood in stool are recommended during the entire course of heparin therapy, regardless of the route of administration.
CONVERTING TO ORAL ANTICOAGULANT
When an oral anticoagulant of the coumarin or similar type is to be begun in patients already receiving heparin sodium, baseline and subsequent tests of prothrombin activity must be determined at a time when heparin activity is too low to affect the prothrombin time. This is about 5 hours after the last IV bolus and 24 hours after the last subcutaneous dose. If continuous IV heparin infusion is used, prothrombin time can usually be measured at any time.
In converting from heparin to an oral anticoagulant, the dose of the oral anticoagulant should be the usual initial amount, and thereafter prothrombin time should be determined at the usual intervals. To ensure continuous anticoagulation, it is advisable to continue full heparin therapy for several days after the prothrombin time has reached the therapeutic range. Heparin therapy may then be discontinued without tapering.
THERAPEUTIC ANTICOAGULANT EFFECT WITH FULL-DOSE HEPARIN
Although dosage must be adjusted for the individual patient according to the results of suitable laboratory tests, the following dosage schedules may be used as guidelines:
[See table below.]

Method of Administration	Frequency	Recommended Dose [based on 150 lb (68 kg) patient]
Deep, Subcutaneous (Intrafat) Injection	Initial Dose	5,000 units by IV injection followed by 10,000–20,000 units of a concentrated solution, subcutaneously
A different site should be used for each injection to prevent the development of massive hematoma.	Every 8 hours	8,000–10,000 units of a concentrated solution
	(or) Every 12 hours	15,000–20,000 units of a concentrated solution
Intermittent, Intravenous Injection	Initial Dose	10,000 units, either undiluted or in 50–100 ml isotonic sodium chloride injection
	Every 4 to 6 hours	5,000–10,000 units, either undiluted or in 50–100 mL isotonic sodium chloride injection
Intravenous Infusion	Initial Dose	5,000 units by IV injection
	Continuous	20,000–40,000 units in 1,000 mL of isotonic sodium chloride solution for infusion/day

PEDIATRIC USE
Follow recommendations of appropriate pediatric reference texts. In general, the following dosage schedule may be used as a guideline.
Initial Dose: 50 units/kg (IV, drip).
Maintenance Dose: 100 units/kg (IV, drip) every four hours, or 20,000 units/M^2/24 hours continuously.
SURGERY OF THE HEART AND BLOOD VESSELS
Patients undergoing total body perfusion for open-heart surgery should receive an initial dose of not less than 150 units of heparin sodium per kilogram of body weight. Frequently, a dose of 300 units of heparin sodium per kilogram of body weight is used for procedures estimated to last less than 60 minutes; or 400 units per kilogram for those estimated to last longer than 60 minutes.
LOW-DOSE PROPHYLAXIS OF POSTOPERATIVE THROMBOEMBOLISM
A number of well-controlled clinical trials have demonstrated that low-dose heparin prophylaxis, given just prior to and after surgery, will reduce the incidence of postoperative deep-vein thrombosis in the legs, as measured by the I-125 fibrinogen technique and venography, and of clinical pulmonary embolism. The most widely used dosage has been 5,000 units 2 hours before surgery and 5,000 units every 8 to 12 hours thereafter for 7 days or until the patient is fully ambulatory, whichever is longer. The heparin is given by deep, subcutaneous injection in the arm or abdomen with a fine needle (25 to 26 gauge) to minimize tissue trauma. A concentrated solution of heparin sodium is recommended. Such prophylaxis should be reserved for patients over 40 undergoing major surgery. Patients with bleeding disorders, those having neurosurgery, spinal anesthesia, eye surgery, or potentially sanguineous operations should be excluded, as well as patients receiving oral anticoagulants or platelet-active drugs (see "Warnings"). The value of such prophylaxis in hip surgery has not been established. The possibility of increased

bleeding during surgery or postoperatively should be borne in mind. If such bleeding occurs, discontinuance of heparin and neutralization with protamine sulfate is advisable. If clinical evidence of thromboembolism develops despite low-dose prophylaxis, full therapeutic doses of anticoagulants should be given unless contraindicated. All patients should be screened prior to heparinization to rule out bleeding disorders, and monitoring should be performed with appropriate coagulation tests just prior to surgery. Coagulation-test values should be normal or only slightly elevated. There is usually no need for daily monitoring of the effect of low-dose heparin in patients with normal coagulation parameters.

EXTRACORPOREAL DIALYSIS USE

Follow equipment manufacturer's operating directions carefully.

BLOOD TRANSFUSION

Addition of 400 to 600 USP units per 100 ml of whole blood. Usually, 7,500 USP units of heparin sodium are added to 100 mL of Sterile Sodium Chloride Injection (or 75,000 USP units per 1,000 mL of Sterile Sodium Chloride Injection) and mixed, and from this sterile solution, 6 to 8 mL is added per 100 mL of whole blood.

LABORATORY SAMPLES

Addition of 70 to 150 units of heparin sodium per 10 to 20 mL sample of whole blood is usually employed to prevent coagulation of the sample. Leukocyte counts should be performed on heparinized blood within two hours after addition of the heparin. Heparinized blood should not be used for isoagglutinin, complement, erythrocyte fragility tests, or platelet counts.

HOW SUPPLIED

Heparin Sodium Injection, USP, is supplied in TUBEX® Sterile Cartridge-Needle Units.

Each 1 mL size TUBEX contains one of the following concentrations of heparin sodium:

1,000 USP Units per mL (22 gauge × 1¼ inch needle), NDC 0008-0275-01, in packages of 10 TUBEX.

2,500 USP Units per mL (25 gauge × ⅝ inch needle), NDC 0008-0482-01, in packages of 10 TUBEX.

5,000 USP Units per 0.5 mL (10,000 USP Units per mL) (25 gauge × ⅝ inch needle), NDC 0008-0277-02, in packages of 10 TUBEX.

5,000 USP Units per 0.5 mL (10,000 USP Units per mL) (25 gauge × ⅝ inch needle), NDC 0008-0277-03, in packages of 50 TUBEX.

5,000 USP Units per mL (25 gauge × ⅝ inch needle), NDC 0008-0278-02, in packages of 10 TUBEX.

7,500 USP Units per mL (25 gauge × ⅝ inch needle), NDC 0008-0293-01, in packages of 10 TUBEX.

10,000 USP Units per mL (25 gauge × ⅝ inch needle), NDC 0008-0277-01, in packages of 10 TUBEX.

20,000 USP Units per mL (25 gauge × ⅝ inch needle), NDC 0008-0276-01, in packages of 10 TUBEX.

Store at room temperature, 15°–25°C (59°–77°F).

Do not freeze

INDERAL® ℞

[in 'der-al]

(propranolol hydrochloride)

TABLETS

CAUTION: Federal law prohibits dispensing without prescription.

DESCRIPTION

Inderal (propranolol hydrochloride) is a synthetic beta-adrenergic receptor blocking agent chemically described as 1-(Isopropylamino)-3-(1-naphthyloxy)-2-propanol hydrochloride. Its structural formula is

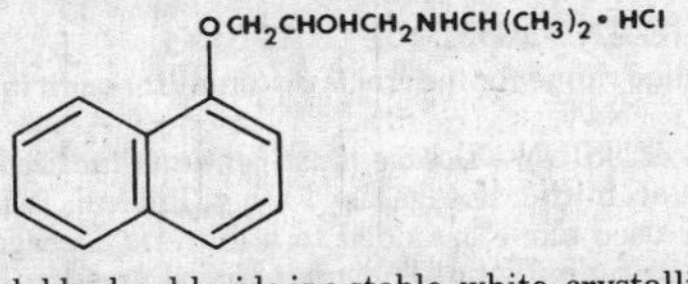
O CH2CHOHCH2NHCH(CH3)2 • HCl

Propranolol hydrochloride is a stable, white, crystalline solid which is readily soluble in water and ethanol. Its molecular weight is 295.81.

Inderal is available as 10 mg, 20 mg, 40 mg, 60 mg, and 80 mg tablets for oral administration and as a 1 mg/mL sterile injectable solution for intravenous administration.

The inactive ingredients contained in Inderal Tablets are: lactose, magnesium stearate, microcrystalline cellulose, and stearic acid. In addition, Inderal 10 mg and 80 mg Tablets contain FD&C Yellow No. 6 and D&C Yellow No. 10; Inderal 20 mg Tablets contain FD&C Blue No. 1; Inderal 40 mg Tablets contain FD&C Blue No. 1, FD&C Yellow No. 6 and D&C Yellow No. 10; Inderal 60 mg Tablets contain D&C Red No. 30.

CLINICAL PHARMACOLOGY

Inderal is a nonselective beta-adrenergic receptor blocking agent possessing no other autonomic nervous system activity. It specifically competes with beta-adrenergic receptor stimulating agents for available receptor sites. When access to beta-receptor sites is blocked by Inderal, the chronotropic, inotropic, and vasodilator responses to beta-adrenergic stimulation are decreased proportionately.

Propranolol is almost completely absorbed from the gastrointestinal tract, but a portion is immediately bound by the liver. Peak effect occurs in one to one and one-half hours. The biologic half-life is approximately four hours.

There is no simple correlation between dose or plasma level and therapeutic effect, and the dose-sensitivity range as observed in clinical practice is wide. The principal reason for this is that sympathetic tone varies widely between individuals. Since there is no reliable test to estimate sympathetic tone or to determine whether total beta blockade has been achieved, proper dosage requires titration.

The mechanism of the antihypertensive effect of Inderal has not been established. Among the factors that may be involved in contributing to the antihypertensive action are (1) decreased cardiac output, (2) inhibition of renin release by the kidneys, and (3) diminution of tonic sympathetic nerve outflow from vasomotor centers in the brain. Although total peripheral resistance may increase initially, it readjusts to or below the pretreatment level with chronic use. Effects on plasma volume appear to be minor and somewhat variable. Inderal has been shown to cause a small increase in serum potassium concentration when used in the treatment of hypertensive patients.

In angina pectoris, propranolol generally reduces the oxygen requirement of the heart at any given level of effort by blocking the catecholamine-induced increases in the heart rate, systolic blood pressure, and the velocity and extent of myocardial contraction. Propranolol may increase oxygen requirements by increasing left ventricular fiber length, end diastolic pressure, and systolic ejection period. The net physiologic effect of beta-adrenergic blockade is usually advantageous and is manifested during exercise by delayed onset of pain and increased work capacity.

Propranolol exerts its antiarrhythmic effects in concentrations associated with beta-adrenergic blockade and this appears to be its principal antiarrhythmic mechanism of action. In dosages greater than required for beta blockade, Inderal also exerts a quinidine-like or anesthetic-like membrane action, which affects the cardiac action potential. The significance of the membrane action in the treatment of arrhythmias is uncertain.

The mechanism of the antimigraine effect of propranolol has not been established. Beta-adrenergic receptors have been demonstrated in the pial vessels of the brain.

The specific mechanism of Inderal's antitremor effects has not been established, but beta-2 (noncardiac) receptors may be involved. A central effect is also possible. Clinical studies have demonstrated that Inderal is of benefit in exaggerated physiological and essential (familial) tremor.

Beta-receptor blockade can be useful in conditions in which, because of pathologic or functional changes, sympathetic activity is detrimental to the patient. But there are also situations in which sympathetic stimulation is vital. For example, in patients with severely damaged hearts, adequate ventricular function is maintained by virtue of sympathetic drive, which should be preserved. In the presence of AV block greater than first degree, beta blockade may prevent the necessary facilitating effect of sympathetic activity on conduction. Beta blockade results in bronchial constriction by interfering with adrenergic bronchodilator activity, which should be preserved in patients subject to bronchospasm.

Propranolol is not significantly dialyzable.

The Beta-Blocker Heart Attack Trial (BHAT) was a National Heart, Lung and Blood Institute-sponsored multicenter, randomized, double-blind, placebo-controlled trial conducted in 31 U.S. centers (plus one in Canada) in 3,837 persons without history of severe congestive heart failure or presence of recent heart failure; certain conduction defects; angina since infarction, who had survived the acute phase of myocardial infarction. Propranolol was administered at either 60 or 80 mg t.i.d. based on blood levels achieved during an initial trial of 40 mg t.i.d. Therapy with Inderal, begun 5-21 days following infarction, was shown to reduce overall mortality up to 39 months, the longest period of follow-up. This was primarily attributable to a reduction in cardiovascular mortality. The protective effect of Inderal was consistent regardless of age, sex, or site of infarction. Compared with placebo, total mortality was reduced 39% at 12 months and 26% over an average follow-up period of 25 months. The Norwegian Multicenter Trial in which propranolol was administered at 40 mg q.i.d. gave overall results which support the findings in the BHAT.

Although the clinical trials used either t.i.d. or q.i.d. dosing, clinical, pharmacologic, and pharmacokinetic data provide a reasonable basis for concluding that b.i.d. dosing with propranolol should be adequate in the treatment of post-infarction patients.

CLINICAL: In the BHAT, patients on Inderal were prescribed either 180 mg/day (82% of patients) or 240 mg/day (18% of patients). Patients were instructed to take the medication 3 times a day at mealtimes. This dosing schedule would result in an overnight dosing interval of 12 to 14 hours which is similar to the dosing interval for a b.i.d regimen. In addition, blood samples were drawn at various times and analyzed for propranolol. When the patients were grouped into tertiles based on the blood levels observed and the mortality in the upper and lower tertiles was compared, there was no evidence that blood levels affected mortality.

PHARMACOLOGIC: Studies in normal volunteers have shown that a 90 mg b.i.d. regimen maintains beta blockade at, or above, the minimum for 60 mg t.i.d. dosing for 24 hours even though differences occurred at two time intervals. At 10–12 hours after the first dose of the day, t.i.d. dosing gave more beta blockade than b.i.d. dosing; at 20–24 hours the trend of the relationship was reversed. These relationships were similar in direction to those observed for plasma propranolol levels. (See Pharmacokinetic.)

PHARMACOKINETIC: A bioavailability study in normal volunteers showed that the blood levels produced by 180 mg/day given b.i.d. are below those provided by the same daily dosage given t.i.d. at 10–12 hours after the first dose of the day, but above those of a t.i.d. regimen at 20–24 hours. However, the blood levels produced by b.i.d. dosing were always equivalent to or above the minimum for t.i.d. dosing throughout the 24 hours. In addition, the mean AUC on the fourth day for the b.i.d. regimen was about 17% greater than for the t.i.d. regimen (1,194 *vs.* 1,024 ng/mL·hr).

INDICATIONS AND USAGE

HYPERTENSION

Inderal is indicated in the management of hypertension. It may be used alone or used in combination with other antihypertensive agents, particularly a thiazide diuretic. Inderal is not indicated in the management of hypertensive emergencies.

ANGINA PECTORIS DUE TO CORONARY ATHEROSCLEROSIS

Inderal is indicated for the long-term management of patients with angina pectoris.

CARDIAC ARRHYTHMIAS

1.) Supraventricular arrhythmias

a) Paroxysmal atrial tachycardias, particularly those arrhythmias induced by catecholamines or digitalis or associated with the Wolff-Parkinson-White syndrome. (See W-P-W under WARNINGS.)

b) Persistent sinus tachycardia which is noncompensatory and impairs the well-being of the patient.

c) Tachycardias and arrhythmias due to thyrotoxicosis when causing distress or increased hazard and when immediate effect is necessary as adjunctive, short-term (2–4 weeks) therapy.

May be used with, but not in place of, specific therapy. (See THYROTOXICOSIS under WARNINGS.)

d) Persistent atrial extrasystoles which impair the well-being of the patient and do not respond to conventional measures.

e) Atrial flutter and fibrillation when ventricular rate cannot be controlled by digitalis alone, or when digitalis is contraindicated.

2.) Ventricular tachycardias

Ventricular arrhythmias do not respond to propranolol as predictably as do the supraventricular arrhythmias.

a) Ventricular tachycardias

With the exception of those induced by catecholamines or digitalis, Inderal is not the drug of first choice. In critical situations when cardioversion techniques or other drugs are not indicated or are not effective, Inderal may be considered. If, after consideration of the risks involved, Inderal is used, it should be given intravenously in low dosage and very slowly. (See DOSAGE AND ADMINISTRATION.) *Care in the administration of* Inderal *with constant electrocardiographic monitoring is essential as the failing heart requires some sympathetic drive for maintenance of myocardial tone.*

b) Persistent premature ventricular extrasystoles which do not respond to conventional measures and impair the well-being of the patient.

3.) Tachyarrhythmias of digitalis intoxication

If digitalis-induced tachyarrhythmias persist following discontinuance of digitalis and correction of electrolyte abnormalities, they are usually reversible with *oral* Inderal. Severe bradycardia may occur. (See OVERDOSAGE.)

Intravenous propranolol hydrochloride is reserved for life-threatening arrhythmias. Temporary maintenance with oral therapy may be indicated. (See DOSAGE AND ADMINISTRATION.)

4.) Resistant tachyarrhythmias due to excessive catecholamine action during anesthesia

Tachyarrhythmias due to excessive catecholamine action during anesthesia may sometimes arise because of release of endogenous catecholamines or administration of catecholamines. When usual measures fail in such arrhythmias, Inderal may be given intravenously to abolish them. All general inhalation anesthetics produce some degree of myocardial depression. Therefore, when Ind-

Continued on next page

Wyeth-Ayerst Laboratories—Cont.

eral is used to treat arrhythmias during anesthesia, it should be used with extreme caution and constant ECG and central venous pressure monitoring. (See WARNINGS.)

MYOCARDIAL INFARCTION

Inderal is indicated to reduce cardiovascular mortality in patients who have survived the acute phase of myocardial infarction and are clinically stable.

MIGRAINE

Inderal is indicated for the prophylaxis of common migraine headache. The efficacy of propranolol in the treatment of a migraine attack that has started has not been established, and propranolol is not indicated for such use.

ESSENTIAL TREMOR

Inderal is indicated in the management of familial or hereditary essential tremor. Familial or essential tremor consists of involuntary, rhythmic, oscillatory movements, usually limited to the upper limbs. It is absent at rest but occurs when the limb is held in a fixed posture or position against gravity and during active movement. Inderal causes a reduction in the tremor amplitude but not in the tremor frequency. Inderal is not indicated for the treatment of tremor associated with Parkinsonism.

HYPERTROPHIC SUBAORTIC STENOSIS

Inderal is useful in the management of hypertrophic subaortic stenosis, especially for treatment of exertional or other stress-induced angina, palpitations, and syncope. Inderal also improves exercise performance. The effectiveness of propranolol hydrochloride in this disease appears to be due to a reduction of the elevated outflow pressure gradient, which is exacerbated by beta-receptor stimulation. Clinical improvement may be temporary.

PHEOCHROMOCYTOMA

After primary treatment with an alpha-adrenergic blocking agent has been instituted, Inderal may be useful as *adjunctive* therapy if the control of tachycardia becomes necessary before or during surgery.

It is hazardous to use Inderal unless alpha-adrenergic blocking drugs are already in use, since this would predispose to serious blood pressure elevation. Blocking only the peripheral dilator (beta) action of epinephrine leaves its constrictor (alpha) action unopposed.

In the event of hemorrhage or shock, there is a disadvantage in having both beta and alpha blockade since the combination prevents the increase in heart rate and peripheral vasoconstriction needed to maintain blood pressure.

With inoperable or metastatic pheochromocytoma, Inderal may be useful as an adjunct to the management of symptoms due to excessive beta-receptor stimulation.

CONTRAINDICATIONS

Inderal is contraindicated in 1) cardiogenic shock, 2) sinus bradycardia and greater than first degree block, 3) bronchial asthma, 4) congestive heart failure (see WARNINGS) unless the failure is secondary to a tachyarrhythmia treatable with Inderal.

WARNINGS

CARDIAC FAILURE: Sympathetic stimulation may be a vital component supporting circulatory function in patients with congestive heart failure, and its inhibition by beta blockade may precipitate more severe failure. Although beta blockers should be avoided in overt congestive heart failure, if necessary, they can be used with close follow-up in patients with a history of failure who are well compensated and are receiving digitalis and diuretics. Beta-adrenergic blocking agents do not abolish the inotropic action of digitalis on heart muscle.

IN PATIENTS WITHOUT A HISTORY OF HEART FAILURE, continued use of beta blockers can, in some cases, lead to cardiac failure. Therefore, at the first sign or symptom of heart failure, the patient should be digitalized and/or treated with diuretics, and the response observed closely, or Inderal should be discontinued (gradually, if possible).

IN PATIENTS WITH ANGINA PECTORIS, there have been reports of exacerbation of angina and, in some cases, myocardial infarction, following *abrupt* discontinuance of Inderal therapy. Therefore, when discontinuance of Inderal is planned, the dosage should be gradually reduced over at least a few weeks and the patient should be cautioned against interruption or cessation of therapy without the physician's advice. If Inderal therapy is interrupted and exacerbation of angina occurs, it usually is advisable to reinstitute Inderal therapy and take other measures appropriate for the management of unstable angina pectoris. Since coronary artery disease may be unrecognized, it may be prudent to follow the above advice in patients considered at risk of having occult atherosclerotic heart disease who are given propranolol for other indications.

Nonallergic Bronchospasm (e.g., chronic bronchitis, emphysema)—PATIENTS WITH BRONCHOSPASTIC DISEASES SHOULD IN GENERAL NOT RECEIVE BETA BLOCKERS. Inderal should be administered with caution since it may block bronchodilation produced by endogenous and exogenous catecholamine stimulation of beta receptors.

MAJOR SURGERY: The necessity or desirability of withdrawal of beta-blocking therapy prior to major surgery is controversial. It should be noted, however, that the impaired ability of the heart to respond to reflex adrenergic stimuli may augment the risks of general anesthesia and surgical procedures.

Inderal, like other beta blockers, is a competitive inhibitor of beta-receptor agonists and its effects can be reversed by administration of such agents, e.g., dobutamine or isoproterenol. However, such patients may be subject to protracted severe hypotension. Difficulty in starting and maintaining the heartbeat has also been reported with beta blockers.

DIABETES AND HYPOGLYCEMIA: Beta blockers should be used with caution in diabetic patients if a beta-blocking agent is required. Beta blockers may mask tachycardia occurring with hypoglycemia, but other manifestations such as dizziness and sweating may not be significantly affected. Following insulin-induced hypoglycemia, propranolol may cause a delay in the recovery of blood glucose to normal levels.

THYROTOXICOSIS: Beta blockade may mask certain clinical signs of hyperthyroidism. Therefore, abrupt withdrawal of propranolol may be followed by an exacerbation of symptoms of hyperthyroidism, including thyroid storm. Propranolol may change thyroid-function tests, increasing T_4 and reverse T_3 and decreasing T_3.

IN PATIENTS WITH WOLFF-PARKINSON-WHITE SYNDROME, several cases have been reported in which, after propranolol, the tachycardia was replaced by a severe bradycardia requiring a demand pacemaker. In one case this resulted after an initial dose of 5 mg propranolol.

PRECAUTIONS

GENERAL: Propranolol should be used with caution in patients with impaired hepatic or renal function. Inderal is not indicated for the treatment of hypertensive emergencies. Beta-adrenoreceptor blockade can cause reduction of intraocular pressure. Patients should be told that Inderal may interfere with the glaucoma screening test. Withdrawal may lead to a return of increased intraocular pressure.

CLINICAL LABORATORY TESTS: Elevated blood urea levels in patients with severe heart disease, elevated serum transaminase, alkaline phosphatase, lactate dehydrogenase.

DRUG INTERACTIONS: Patients receiving catecholamine-depleting drugs such as reserpine should be closely observed if Inderal is administered. The added catecholamine-blocking action may produce an excessive reduction of resting sympathetic nervous activity, which may result in hypotension, marked bradycardia, vertigo, syncopal attacks, or orthostatic hypotension.

Caution should be exercised when patients receiving a beta blocker are administered a calcium-channel blocking drug, especially intravenous verapamil, for both agents may depress myocardial contractility or atrioventricular conduction. On rare occasions, the concomitant intravenous use of a beta blocker and verapamil has resulted in serious adverse reactions, especially in patients with severe cardiomyopathy, congestive heart failure or recent myocardial infarction. Blunting of the antihypertensive effect of beta-adrenoceptor blocking agents by nonsteroidal anti-inflammatory drugs has been reported.

Hypotension and cardiac arrest have been reported with the concomitant use of propranolol and haloperidol.

Aluminum hydroxide gel greatly reduces intestinal absorption of propranolol.

Ethanol slows the rate of absorption of propranolol.

Phenytoin, phenobarbitone, and *rifampin* accelerate propranolol clearance.

Chlorpromazine, when used concomitantly with propranolol, results in increased plasma levels of both drugs.

Antipyrine and *lidocaine* have reduced clearance when used concomitantly with propranolol.

Thyroxine may result in a lower than expected T_3 concentration when used concomitantly with propranolol.

Cimetidine decreases the hepatic metabolism of propranolol, delaying elimination and increasing blood levels.

Theophylline clearance is reduced when used concomitantly with propranolol.

CARCINOGENESIS, MUTAGENESIS, IMPAIRMENT OF FERTILITY: Long-term studies in animals have been conducted to evaluate toxic effects and carcinogenic potential. In 18-month studies, in both rats and mice, employing doses up to 150 mg/kg/day, there was no evidence of significant drug-induced toxicity. There were no drug-related tumorigenic effects at any of the dosage levels. Reproductive studies in animals did not show any impairment of fertility that was attributable to the drug.

PREGNANCY: Pregnancy Category C: Inderal has been shown to be embryotoxic in animal studies at doses about 10 times greater than the maximum recommended human dose.

There are no adequate and well-controlled studies in pregnant women. Inderal should be used during pregnancy only if the potential benefit justifies the potential risk to the fetus.

NURSING MOTHERS: Inderal is excreted in human milk. Caution should be exercised when Inderal is administered to a nursing woman.

PEDIATRIC USE: High serum propranolol levels have been noted in patients with Down's syndrome (trisomy 21), suggesting that the bioavailability of propranolol may be increased in patients with this condition.

Evaluation of the effects of propranolol in children, relative to the drug's efficacy and safety, has not been as systematically performed as in adults. Information is available in the medical literature to allow fair estimates, and specific dosing information has been reasonably studied.

Cardiovascular diseases that are common to adults and children are generally as responsive to propranolol intervention in children as they are in adults. Adverse reactions are also similar; for example, bronchospasm and congestive heart failure related to propranolol therapy have been reported in children and occur through the same mechanisms as previously described in adults.

The normal echocardiogram evolves through a series of changes as the heart matures during growth and development in children. Should echocardiography be used to monitor propranolol therapy in children, the age-related changes in the echocardiogram need to be borne in mind.

ADVERSE REACTIONS

Most adverse effects have been mild and transient and have rarely required the withdrawal of therapy.

Cardiovascular: Bradycardia; congestive heart failure; intensification of AV block; hypotension; paresthesia of hands; thrombocytopenic purpura; arterial insufficiency, usually of the Raynaud type.

Central Nervous System: Light-headedness; mental depression manifested by insomnia, lassitude, weakness, fatigue; reversible mental depression progressing to catatonia; visual disturbances; hallucinations, vivid dreams, an acute reversible syndrome characterized by disorientation for time and place, short-term memory loss, emotional lability, slightly clouded sensorium, and decreased performance on neuropsychometrics. Total daily doses above 160 mg (when administered as divided doses of greater than 80 mg each) may be associated with an increased incidence of fatigue, lethargy, and vivid dreams.

Gastrointestinal: Nausea, vomiting, epigastric distress, abdominal cramping, diarrhea, constipation, mesenteric arterial thrombosis, ischemic colitis.

Allergic: Pharyngitis and agranulocytosis, erythematous rash, fever combined with aching and sore throat, laryngospasm, and respiratory distress.

Respiratory: Bronchospasm.

Hematologic: Agranulocytosis, nonthrombocytopenic purpura, thrombocytopenic purpura.

Autoimmune: In extremely rare instances, systemic lupus erythematosus has been reported.

Miscellaneous: Alopecia, LE-like reactions, psoriasiform rashes, dry eyes, male impotence, and Peyronie's disease have been reported rarely. Oculomucocutaneous reactions involving the skin, serous membranes and conjunctivae reported for a beta blocker (practolol) have not been associated with propranolol.

DOSAGE AND ADMINISTRATION

The dosage range for Inderal is different for each indication.

ORAL

HYPERTENSION—*Dosage must be individualized.*

The usual initial dosage is 40 mg Inderal twice daily, whether used alone or added to a diuretic. Dosage may be increased gradually until adequate blood pressure control is achieved. The usual maintenance dosage is 120 mg to 240 mg per day. In some instances a dosage of 640 mg a day may be required. The time needed for full antihypertensive response to a given dosage is variable and may range from a few days to several weeks.

While twice-daily dosing is effective and can maintain a reduction in blood pressure throughout the day, some patients, especially when lower doses are used, may experience a modest rise in blood pressure toward the end of the 12-hour dosing interval. This can be evaluated by measuring blood pressure near the end of the dosing interval to determine whether satisfactory control is being maintained throughout the day. If control is not adequate, a larger dose, or 3-times-daily therapy may achieve better control.

ANGINA PECTORIS—*Dosage must be individualized.*

Total daily doses of 80 mg to 320 mg, when administered orally, twice a day, three times a day, or four times a day, have been shown to increase exercise tolerance and to reduce ischemic changes in the ECG.

If treatment is to be discontinued, reduce dosage gradually over a period of several weeks. (See WARNINGS.)
ARRHYTHMIAS—10 mg to 30 mg three or four times daily, before meals and at bedtime.
MYOCARDIAL INFARCTION—The recommended daily dosage is 180 mg to 240 mg per day in divided doses. Although a t.i.d. regimen was used in the Beta-Blocker Heart Attack Trial and a q.i.d. regimen in the Norwegian Multicenter Trial, there is a reasonable basis for the use of either a t.i.d. or b.i.d. regimen (see CLINICAL PHARMACOLOGY). The effectiveness and safety of daily dosages greater than 240 mg for prevention of cardiac mortality have not been established. However, higher dosages may be needed to effectively treat coexisting diseases such as angina or hypertension (see above).
MIGRAINE—*Dosage must be individualized.*
The initial oral dose is 80 mg Inderal daily in divided doses. The usual effective dose range is 160 mg to 240 mg per day. The dosage may be increased gradually to achieve optimum migraine prophylaxis.
If a satisfactory response is not obtained within four to six weeks after reaching the maximum dose, Inderal therapy should be discontinued. It may be advisable to withdraw the drug gradually over a period of several weeks.
ESSENTIAL TREMOR—*Dosage must be individualized.*
The initial dosage is 40 mg Inderal twice daily. Optimum reduction of essential tremor is usually achieved with a dose of 120 mg per day. Occasionally, it may be necessary to administer 240 mg to 320 mg per day.
HYPERTROPHIC SUBAORTIC STENOSIS—20 mg to 40 mg three or four times daily, before meals and at bedtime.
PHEOCHROMOCYTOMA—*Preoperatively*—60 mg daily in divided doses for three days prior to surgery, concomitantly with an alpha-adrenergic blocking agent.
—*Management of inoperable tumor*—30 mg daily in divided doses.
USE IN CHILDREN: Intravenous administration of Inderal is not recommended in children. Oral dosage for treating hypertension requires individual titration, beginning with a 1.0 mg per kg (body weight) per day dosage regimen (i.e., 0.5 mg per kg b.i.d.).
The usual pediatric dosage range is 2 mg to 4 mg per kg per day in two equally divided doses (i.e., 1.0 mg per kg b.i.d. to 2.0 mg per kg b.i.d.). Pediatric dosage calculated by weight (recommended) generally produces propranolol plasma levels in a therapeutic range similar to that in adults. On the other hand, pediatric doses calculated on the basis of body surface area (*not* recommended) usually result in plasma levels above the mean adult therapeutic range. Doses above 16 mg per kg per day should not be used in children.
If treatment with Inderal is to be discontinued, a gradually decreasing dose titration over a 7- to 14-day period is necessary.
INTRAVENOUS
Parenteral drug products should be inspected visually for particulate matter and discoloration prior to administration, whenever solution and container permit.
Intravenous administration is reserved for life-threatening arrhythmias or those occurring under anesthesia. The usual dose is from 1 mg to 3 mg administered under careful monitoring, e.g., electrocardiographic, central venous pressure. The rate of administration should not exceed 1 mg (1 mL) per minute to diminish the possibility of lowering blood pressure and causing cardiac standstill. Sufficient time should be allowed for the drug to reach the site of action even when a slow circulation is present. If necessary, a second dose may be given after two minutes. Thereafter, additional drug should not be given in less than four hours. Additional Inderal should not be given when the desired alteration in rate and/or rhythm is achieved.
Transference to oral therapy should be made as soon as possible.
The intravenous administration of Inderal has not been evaluated adequately in the management of hypertensive emergencies.
OVERDOSAGE
Inderal is not significantly dialyzable. In the event of overdosage or exaggerated response, the following measures should be employed:
General—If ingestion is or may have been recent, evacuate gastric contents, taking care to prevent pulmonary aspiration.
BRADYCARDIA—ADMINISTER ATROPINE (0.25 mg to 1.0 mg); IF THERE IS NO RESPONSE TO VAGAL BLOCKADE, ADMINISTER ISOPROTERENOL CAUTIOUSLY.
CARDIAC FAILURE—DIGITALIZATION AND DIURETICS.
HYPOTENSION—VASOPRESSORS, e.g., LEVARTERENOL OR EPINEPHRINE (THERE IS EVIDENCE THAT EPINEPHRINE IS THE DRUG OF CHOICE).
BRONCHOSPASM — ADMINISTER ISOPROTERENOL AND AMINOPHYLLINE.

HOW SUPPLIED

Inderal®
(propranolol hydrochloride)
TABLETS

INDERAL 10—Each hexagonal-shaped, orange, scored tablet, embossed with an "I" and imprinted with "Inderal 10," contains 10 mg propranolol hydrochloride, in bottles of 100 (NDC 0046-0421-81); 1,000 (NDC 0046-0421-91); and 5,000 (NDC 0046-0421-95). Also in Unit Dose packages of 100 (NDC 0046-0421-99).

INDERAL 20—Each hexagonal-shaped, blue, scored tablet, embossed with an "I" and imprinted with "Inderal 20", contains 20 mg propranolol hydrochloride, in bottles of 100 (NDC 0046-0422-81); 1,000 (NDC 0046-0422-91); and 5,000 (NDC 0046-0422-95). Also in Unit Dose packages of 100 (NDC 0046-0422-99).

INDERAL 40—Each hexagonal-shaped, green, scored tablet, embossed with an "I" and imprinted with "Inderal 40," contains 40 mg propranolol hydrochloride, in bottles of 100 (NDC 0046-0424-81); 1,000 (NDC 0046-0424-91); and 5,000 (NDC 0046-0424-95). Also in Unit Dose packages of 100 (NDC 0046-0424-99).

INDERAL 60—Each hexagonal-shaped, pink, scored tablet, embossed with an "I" and imprinted with "Inderal 60," contains 60 mg propranolol hydrochloride, in bottles of 100 (NDC 0046-0426-81) and 1,000 (NDC 0046-0426-91).

INDERAL 80—Each hexagonal-shaped, yellow, scored tablet, embossed with an "I" and imprinted with "Inderal 80", contains 80 mg propranolol hydrochloride, in bottles of 100 (NDC 0046-0428-81); 1,000 (NDC 0046-0428-91); and 5,000 (NDC 0046-0428-95). Also in Unit Dose packages of 100 (NDC 0046-0428-99).

The appearance of these tablets is a registered trademark of Wyeth-Ayerst Laboratories.
Store at room temperature (approximately 25°C).
Dispense in well-closed, light-resistant containers.
INJECTABLE
—Each mL contains 1 mg of propranolol hydrochloride in Water for Injection. The pH is adjusted with citric acid. Supplied as: 1 mL ampuls in boxes of 10 (NDC 0046-3265-10).
Store at room temperature (approximately 25°C).
Shown in Product Identification Section, page 436

INDERAL® LA ℞

[*ĭn 'der-al*]
(propranolol hydrochloride)
Long-Acting Capsules

CAUTION: Federal law prohibits dispensing without prescription.

DESCRIPTION

Inderal (propranolol hydrochloride) is a synthetic beta-adrenergic receptor-blocking agent chemically described as 1-(Isopropylamino)-3-(1-naphthyloxy)-2-propanol hydrochloride. Its structural formula is

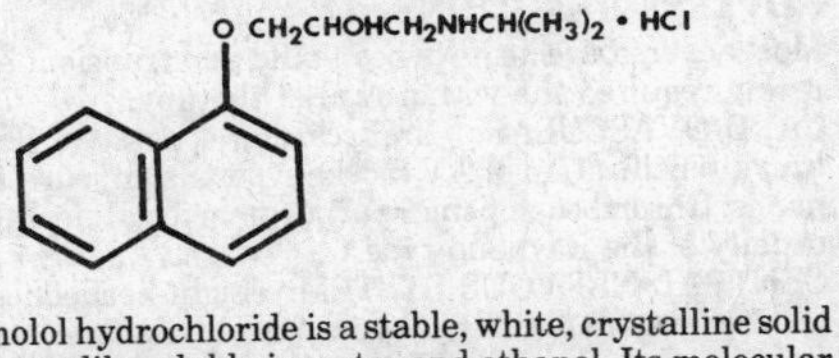
O CH2CHOHCH2NHCH(CH3)2 • HCl

Propranolol hydrochloride is a stable, white, crystalline solid which is readily soluble in water and ethanol. Its molecular weight is 295.81.
Inderal LA is formulated to provide a sustained release of propranolol hydrochloride. Inderal LA is available as 60 mg, 80 mg, 120 mg, and 160 mg capsules.
Inderal LA Capsules contain the following inactive ingredients: cellulose, ethylcellulose, gelatin capsules, hydroxypropyl methylcellulose, and titanium dioxide. In addition, Inderal LA 60 mg, 80 mg, and 120 mg capsules contain D&C Red No. 28 and FD&C Blue No. 1; Inderal LA 160 mg capsules contain FD&C Blue No. 1.
These capsules comply with USP Drug Release Test 1.

CLINICAL PHARMACOLOGY

Inderal is a nonselective, beta-adrenergic receptor-blocking agent possessing no other autonomic nervous system activity. It specifically competes with beta-adrenergic receptor-stimulating agents for available receptor sites. When access to beta-receptor sites is blocked by INDERAL, the chronotropic, inotropic, and vasodilator responses to beta-adrenergic stimulation are decreased proportionately.
INDERAL LA Capsules (60, 80, 120, and 160 mg) release propranolol HCl at a controlled and predictable rate. Peak blood levels following dosing with INDERAL LA occur at about 6 hours, and the apparent plasma half-life is about 10 hours. When measured at steady state over a 24-hour period the areas under the propranolol plasma concentration-time curve (AUCs) for the capsules are approximately 60% to 65% of the AUCs for a comparable divided daily dose of INDERAL Tablets. The lower AUCs for the capsules are due to greater hepatic metabolism of propranolol, resulting from the slower rate of absorption of propranolol. Over a twenty-four (24) hour period, blood levels are fairly constant for about twelve (12) hours, then decline exponentially.
INDERAL LA should not be considered a simple mg-for-mg substitute for conventional propranolol and the blood levels achieved do not match (are lower than) those of two to four times daily dosing with the same dose. When changing to INDERAL LA from conventional propranolol, a possible need for retitration upwards should be considered, especially to maintain effectiveness at the end of the dosing interval. In most clinical settings, however, such as hypertension or angina where there is little correlation between plasma levels and clinical effect, Inderal LA has been therapeutically equivalent to the same mg dose of conventional Inderal as assessed by 24-hour effects on blood pressure and on 24-hour exercise responses of heart rate, systolic pressure, and rate pressure product. Inderal LA can provide effective beta blockade for a 24-hour period.
The mechanism of the antihypertensive effect of Inderal has not been established. Among the factors that may be involved in contributing to the antihypertensive action are: (1) decreased cardiac output, (2) inhibition of renin release by the kidneys, and (3) diminution of tonic sympathetic nerve outflow from vasomotor centers in the brain. Although total peripheral resistance may increase initially, it readjusts to or below the pretreatment level with chronic use. Effects on plasma volume appear to be minor and somewhat variable. Inderal has been shown to cause a small increase in serum potassium concentration when used in the treatment of hypertensive patients.
In angina pectoris, propranolol generally reduces the oxygen requirement of the heart at any given level of effort by blocking the catecholamine-induced increases in the heart rate, systolic blood pressure, and the velocity and extent of myocardial contraction. Propranolol may increase oxygen requirements by increasing left ventricular fiber length, end diastolic pressure, and systolic ejection period. The net physiologic effect of beta-adrenergic blockade is usually advantageous and is manifested during exercise by delayed onset of pain and increased work capacity.
In dosages greater than required for beta blockade, Inderal also exerts a quinidine-like or anesthetic-like membrane action which affects the cardiac action potential. The significance of the membrane action in the treatment of arrhythmias is uncertain.
The mechanism of the antimigraine effect of propranolol has not been established. Beta-adrenergic receptors have been demonstrated in the pial vessels of the brain.
Beta-receptor blockade can be useful in conditions in which, because of pathologic or functional changes, sympathetic activity is detrimental to the patient. But there are also situations in which sympathetic stimulation is vital. For example, in patients with severely damaged hearts, adequate ventricular function is maintained by virtue of sympathetic drive, which should be preserved. In the presence of AV block, greater than first degree, beta blockade may prevent the necessary facilitating effect of sympathetic activity on conduction. Beta blockade results in bronchial constriction by interfering with adrenergic bronchodilator activity, which should be preserved in patients subject to bronchospasm.
Propranolol is not significantly dialyzable.

INDICATIONS AND USAGE

HYPERTENSION
Inderal LA is indicated in the management of hypertension; it may be used alone or used in combination with other antihypertensive agents, particularly a thiazide diuretic. Inderal LA is not indicated in the management of hypertensive emergencies.
ANGINA PECTORIS DUE TO CORONARY ATHEROSCLEROSIS
Inderal LA is indicated for the long-term management of patients with angina pectoris.
MIGRAINE
Inderal LA is indicated for the prophylaxis of common migraine headache. The efficacy of propranolol in the treatment of a migraine attack that has started has not been established and propranolol is not indicated for such use.
HYPERTROPHIC SUBAORTIC STENOSIS
Inderal LA is useful in the management of hypertrophic subaortic stenosis, especially for treatment of exertional or other stress-induced angina, palpitations, and syncope. Inderal LA also improves exercise performance. The effectiveness of propranolol hydrochloride in this disease appears to be due to a reduction of the elevated outflow pressure gradient which is exacerbated by beta-receptor stimulation. Clinical improvement may be temporary.

Continued on next page

Wyeth-Ayerst Laboratories—Cont.

CONTRAINDICATIONS

Inderal is contraindicated in 1) cardiogenic shock; 2) sinus bradycardia and greater than first-degree block; 3) bronchial asthma; 4) congestive heart failure (see WARNINGS), unless the failure is secondary to a tachyarrhythmia treatable with Inderal.

WARNINGS

CARDIAC FAILURE: Sympathetic stimulation may be a vital component supporting circulatory function in patients with congestive heart failure, and its inhibition by beta blockade may precipitate more severe failure. Although beta blockers should be avoided in overt congestive heart failure, if necessary, they can be used with close follow-up in patients with a history of failure who are well compensated and are receiving digitalis and diuretics. Beta-adrenergic blocking agents do not abolish the inotropic action of digitalis on heart muscle.

IN PATIENTS WITHOUT A HISTORY OF HEART FAILURE, continued use of beta blockers can, in some cases, lead to cardiac failure. Therefore, at the first sign or symptom of heart failure, the patient should be digitalized and/or treated with diuretics, and the response observed closely, or Inderal should be discontinued (gradually, if possible).

> IN PATIENTS WITH ANGINA PECTORIS, there have been reports of exacerbation of angina and, in some cases, myocardial infarction, following *abrupt* discontinuance of Inderal therapy. Therefore, when discontinuance of Inderal is planned, the dosage should be gradually reduced over at least a few weeks, and the patient should be cautioned against interruption or cessation of therapy without the physician's advice. If Inderal therapy is interrupted and exacerbation of angina occurs, it usually is advisable to reinstitute Inderal therapy and take other measures appropriate for the management of unstable angina pectoris. Since coronary artery disease may be unrecognized, it may be prudent to follow the above advice in patients considered at risk of having occult atherosclerotic heart disease who are given propranolol for other indications.

NONALLERGIC BRONCHOSPASM (e.g., CHRONIC BRONCHITIS, EMPHYSEMA)—PATIENTS WITH BRONCHOSPASTIC DISEASES SHOULD IN GENERAL NOT RECEIVE BETA BLOCKERS. INDERAL should be administered with caution since it may block bronchodilation produced by endogenous and exogenous catecholamine stimulation of beta receptors.

MAJOR SURGERY: The necessity or desirability of withdrawal of beta-blocking therapy prior to major surgery is controversial. It should be noted, however, that the impaired ability of the heart to respond to reflex adrenergic stimuli may augment the risks of general anesthesia and surgical procedures.

INDERAL, like other beta blockers, is a competitive inhibitor of beta-receptor agonists and its effects can be reversed by administration of such agents, e.g., dobutamine or isoproterenol. However, such patients may be subject to protracted severe hypotension. Difficulty in starting and maintaining the heartbeat has also been reported with beta blockers.

DIABETES AND HYPOGLYCEMIA: Beta blockers should be used with caution in diabetic patients if a beta-blocking agent is required. Beta blockers may mask tachycardia occurring with hypoglycemia, but other manifestations such as dizziness and sweating may not be significantly affected. Following insulin-induced hypoglycemia, propranolol may cause a delay in the recovery of blood glucose to normal levels.

THYROTOXICOSIS: Beta blockade may mask certain clinical signs of hyperthyroidism. Therefore, abrupt withdrawal of propranolol may be followed by an exacerbation of symptoms of hyperthyroidism, including thyroid storm. Propranolol may change thyroid-function tests, increasing T_4 and reverse T_3, and decreasing T_3.

IN PATIENTS WITH WOLFF-PARKINSON-WHITE SYNDROME, several cases have been reported in which, after propranolol, the tachycardia was replaced by a severe bradycardia requiring a demand pacemaker. In one case this resulted after an initial dose of 5 mg propranolol.

PRECAUTIONS

GENERAL

Propranolol should be used with caution in patients with impaired hepatic or renal function. Inderal is not indicated for the treatment of hypertensive emergencies.

Beta-adrenoreceptor blockade can cause reduction of intraocular pressure. Patients should be told that Inderal may interfere with the glaucoma screening test. Withdrawal may lead to a return of increased intraocular pressure.

CLINICAL LABORATORY TESTS

Elevated blood urea levels in patients with severe heart disease, elevated serum transaminase, alkaline phosphatase, lactate dehydrogenase.

DRUG INTERACTIONS

Patients receiving catecholamine-depleting drugs such as reserpine should be closely observed if INDERAL is administered. The added catecholamine-blocking action may produce an excessive reduction of resting sympathetic nervous activity, which may result in hypotension, marked bradycardia, vertigo, syncopal attacks, or orthostatic hypotension. Caution should be exercised when patients receiving a beta blocker are administered a calcium-channel-blocking drug, especially intravenous verapamil, for both agents may depress myocardial contractility or atrioventricular conduction. On rare occasions, the concomitant intravenous use of a beta blocker and verapamil has resulted in serious adverse reactions, especially in patients with severe cardiomyopathy, congestive heart failure or recent myocardial infarction.

Aluminum hydroxide gel greatly reduces intestinal absorption of propranolol.

Ethanol slows the rate of absorption of propranolol.

Phenytoin, phenobarbitone, and *rifampin* accelerate propranolol clearance.

Chlorpromazine, when used concomitantly with propranolol, results in increased plasma levels of both drugs.

Antipyrine and *lidocaine* have reduced clearance when used concomitantly with propranolol.

Thyroxine may result in a lower than expected T_3 concentration when used concomitantly with propranolol.

Cimetidine decreases the hepatic metabolism of propranolol, delaying elimination and increasing blood levels.

Theophylline clearance is reduced when used concomitantly with propranolol.

CARCINOGENESIS, MUTAGENESIS, IMPAIRMENT OF FERTILITY

Long-term studies in animals have been conducted to evaluate toxic effects and carcinogenic potential. In 18-month studies, in both rats and mice, employing doses up to 150 mg/kg/day, there was no evidence of significant drug-induced toxicity. There were no drug-related tumorigenic effects at any of the dosage levels. Reproductive studies in animals did not show any impairment of fertility that was attributable to the drug.

PREGNANCY: PREGNANCY CATEGORY C

Inderal has been shown to be embryotoxic in animal studies at doses about 10 times greater than the maximal recommended human dose.

There are no adequate and well-controlled studies in pregnant women. Inderal should be used during pregnancy only if the potential benefit justifies the potential risk to the fetus.

NURSING MOTHERS

Inderal is excreted in human milk. Caution should be exercised when Inderal is administered to a nursing woman.

PEDIATRIC USE

Safety and effectiveness in children have not been established.

ADVERSE REACTIONS

Most adverse effects have been mild and transient and have rarely required the withdrawal of therapy.

CARDIOVASCULAR: Bradycardia; congestive heart failure; intensification of AV block; hypotension; paresthesia of hands; thrombocytopenic purpura; arterial insufficiency, usually of the Raynaud type.

CENTRAL NERVOUS SYSTEM: Light-headedness, mental depression manifested by insomnia, lassitude, weakness, fatigue; reversible mental depression progressing to catatonia; visual disturbances; hallucinations; vivid dreams; an acute reversible syndrome characterized by disorientation for time and place, short-term memory loss, emotional lability, slightly clouded sensorium, and decreased performance on neuropsychometrics. For immediate formulations, fatigue, lethargy, and vivid dreams appear dose related.

GASTROINTESTINAL: Nausea; vomiting; epigastric distress; abdominal cramping; diarrhea; constipation; mesenteric arterial thrombosis; ischemic colitis.

ALLERGIC: Pharyngitis and agranulocytosis; erythematous rash; fever combined with aching and sore throat; laryngospasm, and respiratory distress.

RESPIRATORY: Bronchospasm.

HEMATOLOGIC: Agranulocytosis, nonthrombocytopenic purpura, thrombocytopenic purpura.

AUTOIMMUNE: In extremely rare instances, systemic lupus erythematosus has been reported.

MISCELLANEOUS: Alopecia; LE-like reactions; psoriasiform rashes; dry eyes; male impotence; and Peyronie's disease have been reported rarely. Oculomucocutaneous reactions involving the skin, serous membranes and conjunctivae reported for a beta blocker (practolol) have not been associated with propranolol.

DOSAGE AND ADMINISTRATION

Inderal LA provides propranolol hydrochloride in a sustained-release capsule for administration once daily. If pa-

tients are switched from Inderal Tablets to Inderal LA Capsules, care should be taken to assure that the desired therapeutic effect is maintained. Inderal LA should not be considered a simple mg-for-mg substitute for Inderal. Inderal LA has different kinetics and produces lower blood levels. Retitration may be necessary, especially to maintain effectiveness at the end of the 24-hour dosing interval.

HYPERTENSION

Dosage must be individualized. The usual initial dosage is 80 mg INDERAL LA once daily, whether used alone or added to a diuretic. The dosage may be increased to 120 mg once daily or higher until adequate blood pressure control is achieved. The usual maintenance dosage is 120 to 160 mg once daily. In some instances a dosage of 640 mg may be required. The time needed for full hypertensive response to a given dosage is variable and may range from a few days to several weeks.

ANGINA PECTORIS

Dosage must be individualized. Starting with 80 mg INDERAL LA once daily, dosage should be gradually increased at three- to seven-day intervals until optimal response is obtained. Although individual patients may respond at any dosage level, the average optimal dosage appears to be 160 mg once daily. In angina pectoris, the value and safety of dosage exceeding 320 mg per day have not been established.

If treatment is to be discontinued, reduce dosage gradually over a period of a few weeks (see WARNINGS).

MIGRAINE

Dosage must be individualized. The initial oral dose is 80 mg Inderal LA once daily. The usual effective dose range is 160 to 240 mg once daily. The dosage may be increased gradually to achieve optimal migraine prophylaxis. If a satisfactory response is not obtained within four to six weeks after reaching the maximal dose, Inderal LA therapy should be discontinued. It may be advisable to withdraw the drug gradually over a period of several weeks.

HYPERTROPHIC SUBAORTIC STENOSIS

80 to 160 mg Inderal LA once daily.

PEDIATRIC DOSAGE

At this time the data on the use of the drug in this age group are too limited to permit adequate directions for use.

OVERDOSAGE

Inderal is not significantly dialyzable. In the event of overdosage or exaggerated response, the following measures should be employed:

GENERAL

If ingestion is, or may have been, recent, evacuate gastric contents, taking care to prevent pulmonary aspiration.

BRADYCARDIA

ADMINISTER ATROPINE (0.25 to 1.0 mg); IF THERE IS NO RESPONSE TO VAGAL BLOCKADE, ADMINISTER ISOPROTERENOL CAUTIOUSLY.

CARDIAC FAILURE

DIGITALIZATION AND DIURETICS.

HYPOTENSION

VASOPRESSORS, e.g., LEVARTERENOL OR EPINEPHRINE (THERE IS EVIDENCE THAT EPINEPHRINE IS THE DRUG OF CHOICE).

BRONCHOSPASM

ADMINISTER ISOPROTERENOL AND AMINOPHYLLINE.

HOW SUPPLIED

INDERAL® LA CAPSULES (propranolol hydrochloride) Each white/light-blue capsule, identified by 3 narrow bands, 1 wide band, and "INDERAL LA 60," contains 60 mg of propranolol hydrochloride in bottles of 100 (NDC 0046-0470-81) and in bottles of 1,000 (NDC 0046-0470-91).

Each light-blue capsule, identified by 3 narrow bands, 1 wide band, and "INDERAL LA 80," contains 80 mg of propranolol hydrochloride in bottles of 100 (NDC 0046-0471-81) and in bottles of 1,000 (NDC 0046-0471-91). Also available in a Unit Dose package of 100 (NDC 0046-0471-99).

Each light-blue/dark-blue capsule, identified by 3 narrow bands, 1 wide band, and "INDERAL LA 120," contains 120 mg of propranolol hydrochloride in bottles of 100 (NDC 0046-0473-81) and in bottles of 1,000 (NDC 0046-0473-91). Also available in a Unit Dose package of 100 (NDC 0046-0473-99).

Each dark-blue capsule, identified by 3 narrow bands, 1 wide band, and "INDERAL LA 160," contains 160 mg of propranolol hydrochloride in bottles of 100 (NDC 0046-0479-81) and in bottles of 1,000 (NDC 0046-0479-91). Also available in a Unit Dose package of 100 (NDC 0046-0479-99).

The appearance of these capsules is a registered trademark of Wyeth-Ayerst Laboratories.

Store at room temperature (approximately 25° C). Protect from light, moisture, freezing, and excessive heat.

Dispense in a tight, light-resistant container as defined in the USP.

Use carton to protect contents from light.

Shown in Product Identification Section, page 436

INDERIDE® ℞

[ĭn 'de-rīde]
(propranolol hydrochloride [INDERAL®] and hydrochlorothiazide)

CAUTION: Federal law prohibits dispensing without prescription.

DESCRIPTION

INDERIDE Tablets for oral administration combine two antihypertensive agents: INDERAL (propranolol hydrochloride), a beta-adrenergic blocking agent, and hydrochlorothiazide, a thiazide diuretic-antihypertensive. INDERIDE 40/25 Tablets contain 40 mg propranolol hydrochloride and 25 mg hydrochlorothiazide; INDERIDE 80/25 Tablets contain 80 mg propranolol hydrochloride and 25 mg hydrochlorothiazide.

INDERAL (propranolol hydrochloride) is a synthetic beta-adrenergic receptor-blocking agent chemically described as 1-(Isopropylamino)-3-(1-naphthyloxy)-2-propanol hydrochloride. Its structural formula is:

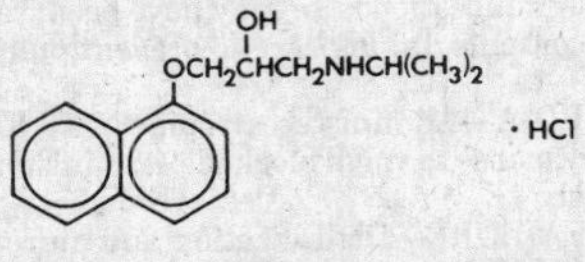
OH
OCH2CHCH2NHCH(CH3)2
· HCl

Propranolol hydrochloride is a stable, white, crystalline solid which is readily soluble in water and ethanol. Its molecular weight is 295.81.

Hydrochlorothiazide is a white, or practically white, practically odorless, crystalline powder. It is slightly soluble in water freely soluble in sodum hydroxide solution; sparingly soluble in methanol; insoluble in ether, chloroform, benzene, and dilute mineral acids. Its chemical name is: 6-Chloro-3,4-dihydro-2H-1,2,4-benzothiadiazine-7-sulfonamide 1,1-dioxide. Its structural formula is:

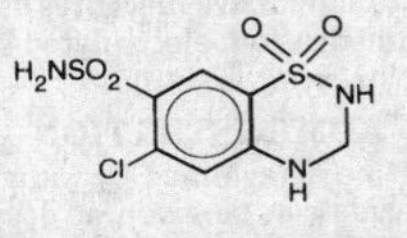
H2NSO2
O O
S
NH
Cl
N
H

The inactive ingredients contained in INDERIDE Tablets are lactose, magnesium stearate, microcrystalline cellulose, stearic acid, and yellow ferric oxide.

CLINICAL PHARMACOLOGY

Propranolol hydrochloride (INDERAL®):

Propranolol hydrochloride is a nonselective beta-adrenergic receptor blocking agent possessing no other autonomic nervous system activity. It specifically competes with beta-adrenergic receptor stimulating agents for available receptor sites. When access to beta-receptor sites is blocked by propranolol, the chronotropic, inotropic, and vasodilator responses to beta-adrenergic stimulation are decreased proportionately.

Propranolol is almost completely absorbed from the gastrointestinal tract, but a portion is immediately metabolized by the liver on its first pass through the portal circulation.

Peak effect occurs in one to one-and-one-half hours. The biologic half-life is approximately four hours. Propranolol is not significantly dialyzable. There is no simple correlation between dose or plasma level and therapeutic effect, and the dose-sensitivity range, as observed in clinical practice, is wide. The principal reason for this is that sympathetic tone varies widely between individuals. Since there is no reliable test to estimate sympathetic tone or to determine whether total beta blockade has been achieved, proper dosage requires titration.

The mechanism of the antihypertensive effects of propranolol has not been established. Among the factors that may be involved are (1) decreased cardiac output, (2) inhibition of renin release by the kidneys, and (3) diminution of tonic sympathetic nerve outflow from vasomotor centers in the brain. Although total peripheral resistance may increase initially, it readjusts to, or below, the pretreatment level with chronic usage. Effects on plasma volume appear to be minor and somewhat variable. Propranolol has been shown to cause a small increase in serum potassium concentration when used in the treatment of hypertensive patients. Propranolol hydrochloride decreases heart rate, cardiac output, and blood pressure.

Beta-receptor blockade can be useful in conditions in which, because of pathologic or functional changes, sympathetic activity is detrimental to the patient. But there are also situations in which sympathetic stimulation is vital. For example, in patients with severely damaged hearts, adequate ventricular function is maintained by virtue of sympathetic drive, which should be preserved. In the presence of AV block greater than first degree, beta blockade may prevent the necessary facilitating effect of sympathetic activity on conduction. Beta blockade results in bronchial constriction by interfering with adrenergic bronchodilator activity, which should be preserved in patients subject to bronchospasm.

The proper objective of beta-blockade therapy is to decrease adverse sympathetic stimulation, but not to the degree that may impair necessary sympathetic support.

Hydrochlorothiazide:

Hydrochlorothiazide is a benzothiadiazine (thiazide) diuretic closely related to chlorothiazide. The mechanism of the antihypertensive effect of the thiazides is unknown. Thiazides do not affect normal blood pressure.

Thiazides affect the renal tubular mechanism of electrolyte reabsorption. At maximal therapeutic dosage, all thiazides are approximately equal in their diuretic potency.

Thiazides increase excretion of sodium and chloride in approximately equivalent amounts. Natriuresis causes a secondary loss of potassium and bicarbonate. Onset of diuretic action of hydrochlorothiazide occurs in 2 hours, and the peak effect in about 4 hours. Its action persists for approximately 6 to 12 hours. Thiazides are eliminated rapidly by the kidney.

INDICATIONS AND USAGE

INDERIDE is indicated in the management of hypertension. **This fixed combination is not indicated for initial therapy of hypertension. Hypertension requires therapy titrated to the individual patient. If the fixed combination represents the dosage so determined, its use may be more convenient in patient management.**

CONTRAINDICATIONS

Propranolol hydrochloride (INDERAL®):

Propranolol is contraindicated in: 1) cardiogenic shock; 2) sinus bradycardia and greater than first-degree block; 3) bronchial asthma; 4) congestive heart failure (see WARNINGS) unless the failure is secondary to a tachyarrhythmia with propranolol.

Hydrochlorothiazide:

Hydrochlorothiazide is contraindicated in patients with anuria or hypersensitivity to this or other sulfonamide-derived drugs.

WARNINGS

Propranolol hydrochloride (INDERAL®):

CARDIAC FAILURE: Sympathetic stimulation is a vital component supporting circulatory function in congestive heart failure, and inhibition with beta blockade always carries the potential hazard of further depressing myocardial contractility and precipitating cardiac failure. Propranolol acts selectively without abolishing the inotropic action of digitalis on the heart muscle (i.e., that of supporting the strength of myocardial contractions). In patients already receiving digitalis, the positive inotropic action of digitalis may be reduced by propranolol's negative inotropic effect. The effects of propranolol and digitalis are additive in depressing AV conduction.

PATIENTS WITHOUT A HISTORY OF HEART FAILURE: Continued depression of the myocardium over a period of time can, in some cases, lead to cardiac failure. In rare instances, this has been observed during propranolol therapy. Therefore, at the first sign or symptom of impending cardiac failure, patients should be fully digitalized and/or given additional diuretic, and the response observed closely: a) if cardiac failure continues, despite adequate digitalization and diuretic therapy, propranolol therapy should be withdrawn (gradually, if possible); b) if tachyarrhythmia is being controlled, patients should be maintained on combined therapy and the patient closely followed until threat of cardiac failure is over.

> ANGINA PECTORIS: There have been reports of exacerbation of angina and, in some cases, myocardial infarction following *abrupt* discontinuation of propranolol therapy. Therefore, when discontinuance of propranolol is planned, the dosage should be gradually reduced and the patient should be carefully monitored. In addition, when propranolol is prescribed for angina pectoris, the patient should be cautioned against interruption or cessation of therapy without the physician's advice. If propranolol therapy is interrupted and exacerbation of angina occurs, it usually is advisable to reinstitute propranolol therapy and take other measures appropriate for the management of unstable angina pectoris. Since coronary artery disease may be unrecognized, it may be prudent to follow the above advice in patients considered at risk of having occult atherosclerotic heart disease, who are given propranolol for other indications.

NONALLERGIC BRONCHOSPASM (e.g., chronic bronchitis, emphysema): PATIENTS WITH BRONCHOSPASTIC DISEASES SHOULD, IN GENERAL, NOT RECEIVE BETA BLOCKERS. Propranolol should be administered with caution since it may block bronchodilation produced by endogenous and exogenous catecholamine stimulation of beta receptors.

MAJOR SURGERY: The necessity or desirability of withdrawal of beta-blocking therapy prior to major surgery is controversial. It should be noted, however, that the impaired ability of the heart to respond to reflex adrenergic stimuli may augment the risks of general anesthesia and surgical procedures.

Propranolol, like other beta blockers, is a competitive inhibitor of beta-receptor agonists, and its effects can be reversed by administration of such agents, e.g., dobutamine or isoproterenol. However, such patients may be subject to protracted severe hypotension. Difficulty in starting and maintaining the heartbeat has also been reported with beta blockers.

DIABETES AND HYPOGLYCEMIA: Beta blockers should be used with caution in diabetic patients if a beta-blocking agent is required. Beta blockers may mask tachycardia occurring with hypoglycemia, but other manifestations such as dizziness and sweating may not be significantly affected. Following insulin-induced hypoglycemia, propranolol may cause a delay in the recovery of blood glucose to normal levels.

THYROTOXICOSIS: Beta blockade may mask certain clinical signs of hyperthyroidism. Therefore, abrupt withdrawal of propranolol may be followed by an exacerbation of symptoms of hyperthyroidism, including thyroid storm. Propranolol may change thyroid-function tests, increasing T_4 and reverse T_3, and decreasing T_3.

WOLFF-PARKINSON-WHITE SYNDROME: Several cases have been reported in which, after propranolol, the tachycardia was replaced by a severe bradycardia requiring a demand pacemaker. In one case this resulted after an initial dose of 5 mg propranolol.

Hydrochlorothiazide:

Thiazides should be used with caution in severe renal disease. In patients with renal disease, thiazides may precipitate azotemia. In patients with impaired renal function, cumulative effects of the drug may develop.

Thiazides should also be used with caution in patients with impaired hepatic function or progressive liver disease, since minor alterations of fluid and electrolyte balance may precipitate hepatic coma.

Thiazides may add to or potentiate the action of other antihypertensive drugs. Potentiation occurs with ganglionic or peripheral adrenergic-blocking drugs.

Sensitivity reactions may occur in patients with a history of allergy or bronchial asthma. The possibility of exacerbation or activation of systemic lupus erythematosus has been reported.

PRECAUTIONS

GENERAL

Propranolol hydrochloride (INDERAL®):

Propranolol should be used with caution in patients with impaired hepatic or renal function. INDERIDE is not indicated for the treatment of hypertensive emergencies.

Hydrochlorothiazide:

All patients receiving thiazide therapy should be observed for clinical signs of fluid or electrolyte imbalance, namely hyponatremia, hypochloremic alkalosis, and hypokalemia. Serum and urine electrolyte determinations are particularly important when the patient is vomiting excessively or receiving parenteral fluids. Medication such as digitalis may also influence serum electrolytes. Warning signs, irrespective of cause, are: dryness of mouth, thirst, weakness, lethargy, drowsiness, restlessness, muscle pains or cramps, muscular fatigue, hypotension, oliguria, tachycardia, and gastrointestinal disturbances such as nausea and vomiting.

Hypokalemia may develop, especially with brisk diuresis or when severe cirrhosis is present.

Interference with adequate oral electrolyte intake will also contribute to hypokalemia. Hypokalemia can sensitize or exaggerate the response of the heart to the toxic effects of digitalis (e.g., increased ventricular irritability).

Hypokalemia may be avoided or treated by use of potassium supplements or foods with a high potassium content.

Any chloride deficit is generally mild, and usually does not require specific treatment except under extraordinary circumstances (as in liver or renal disease). Dilutional hyponatremia may occur in edematous patients in hot weather; appropriate therapy is water restriction rather than administration of salt, except in rare instances when the hyponatremia is life-threatening. In actual salt depletion, appropriate replacement is the therapy of choice.

Hyperuricemia may occur or frank gout may be precipitated in certain patients receiving thiazide therapy.

Diabetes mellitus which has been latent may become manifest during thiazide administration.

The antihypertensive effects of the drug may be enhanced in the postsympathectomy patient.

If progressive renal impairment becomes evident, consider withholding or discontinuing diuretic therapy.

Calcium excretion is decreased by thiazides. Pathologic changes in the parathyroid gland with hypercalcemia and hypophosphatemia have been observed in a few patients on prolonged thiazide therapy. The common complications of hyperparathyroidism, such as renal lithiasis, bone resorption, and peptic ulceration, have not been seen.

Continued on next page

Wyeth-Ayerst Laboratories—Cont.

INFORMATION FOR PATIENTS
Beta-adrenoreceptor blockade can cause reduction of intraocular pressure. Patients should be told that propranolol may interfere with the glaucoma screening test. Withdrawal may lead to a return of increased intraocular pressure.
LABORATORY TESTS
Propranolol hydrochloride (INDERAL®):
Elevated blood urea levels in patients with severe heart disease, elevated serum transaminase, alkaline phosphatase, lactate dehydrogenase.
Hydrochlorothiazide:
Periodic determination of serum electrolytes to detect possible electrolyte imbalance should be performed at appropriate intervals.
DRUG/DRUG INTERACTIONS
Propranolol hydrochloride (INDERAL®):
Patients receiving catecholamine-depleting drugs such as reserpine should be closely observed if INDERIDE is administered. The added catecholamine-blocking action may produce an excessive reduction of resting sympathetic nervous activity, which may result in hypotension, marked bradycardia, vertigo, syncopal attacks, or orthostatic hypotension.
Caution should be exercised when patients receiving a beta blocker are administered a calcium-channel blocking drug, especially intravenous verapamil, for both agents may depress myocardial contractility or atrioventricular conduction. On rare occasions, the concomitant intravenous use of a beta blocker and verapamil has resulted in serious adverse reactions, especially in patients with severe cardiomyopathy, congestive heart failure, or recent myocardial infarction.
Blunting of the antihypertensive effect of beta-adrenoceptor blocking agents by nonsteroidal anti-inflammatory drugs has been reported.
Hypotension and coronary arrest have been reported with the concomitant use of propranolol and haloperidol.
Aluminum hydroxide gel greatly reduces intestinal absorption of propranolol.
Ethanol slows the rate of absorption of propranolol.
Phenytoin, phenobarbitone, and rifampin accelerate propranolol clearance.
Chlorpromazine, when used concomitantly with propranolol, results in increased plasma levels of both drugs.
Antipyrine and *lidocaine* have reduced clearance when used concomitantly with propranolol.
Thyroxine may result in a lower than expected T_3 concentration when used concomitantly with propranolol.
Cimetidine decreases the hepatic metabolism of propranolol, delaying elimination and increasing blood levels.
Theophylline clearance is reduced when used concomitantly with propranolol.
Hydrochlorothiazide:
Thiazide drugs may increase the responsiveness to tubocurarine.
Thiazides may decrease arterial responsiveness to norepinephrine. This diminution is not sufficient to preclude effectiveness of the pressor agent for therapeutic use.
Insulin requirements in diabetic patients may be increased, decreased, or unchanged.
Hypokalemia may develop during concomitant use of corticosteroids or ACTH.
DRUG/LABORATORY TEST INTERACTIONS
Hydrochlorothiazide:
Thiazides may decrease serum PBI levels without signs of thyroid disturbance.
Thiazides should be discontinued before carrying out tests for parathyroid function (see PRECAUTIONS—General).
CARCINOGENESIS, MUTAGENESIS, IMPAIRMENT OF FERTILITY
Propranolol hydrochloride (INDERAL®):
Long-term studies in animals have been conducted to evaluate toxic effects and carcinogenic potential. In 18-month studies in both rats and mice, employing doses up to 150 mg/kg/day, there was no evidence of significant drug-induced toxicity. There were no drug-related tumorigenic effects at any of the dosage levels. Reproductive studies in animals did not show any impairment of fertility that was attributable to the drug. Long-term studies in animals have not been conducted to evaluate the toxic effects and carcinogenic potential of INDERIDE.
Hydrochlorothiazide:
Hydrochlorothiazide is presently under study for carcinogenesis in rats and mice in the National Toxicology Research and Testing Program.
Hydrochlorothiazide was not mutagenic in *in vitro* Ames mutagenicity assays of *Salmonella typhimurium* strains TA 98, TA 100, TA 1535, TA 1537, and TA 1538 or in *in vivo* mutagenicity assays of mouse germinal-cell chromosomes and Chinese hamster bone-marrow-cell chromosomes. It was, however, mutagenic in inducing nondisjunction (96% frequency) in diploid strains of *Aspergillus nidulans.* Hydrochlorothiazide had no adverse effects on fertility in rats at a dose equivalent to the recommended maximum human dose and in mice at a dose equivalent to 25 times the recommended maximum human dose (4 mg/kg, assumed body weight of 50 kg).
PREGNANCY: Pregnancy Category C
Propranolol hydrochloride (INDERAL®):
Propranolol has been shown to be embryotoxic in animal studies at doses about 10 times greater than the maximum recommended human dose. There are no adequate and well-controlled studies in pregnant women. Propranolol should be used during pregnancy only if the potential benefit justifies the potential risk to the fetus.
Hydrochlorothiazide:
Thiazides cross the placental barrier and appear in cord blood. The use of thiazides in pregnant women requires that the anticipated benefit be weighed against possible hazards to the fetus. These hazards include fetal or neonatal jaundice, thrombocytopenia, and possibly other adverse reactions which have occurred in the adult.
Available information indicates that hydrochlorothiazide at doses as high as 330 times the recommended maximum human dose was not teratogenic in pregnant rats.
NURSING MOTHERS
Propranolol hydrochloride (INDERAL®):
Propranolol is excreted in human milk. Caution should be exercised when INDERIDE is administered to a nursing woman.
Hydrochlorothiazide:
Thiazides appear in breast milk. If the use of drug is deemed essential, the patient should stop nursing.
PEDIATRIC USE
Safety and effectiveness in children have not been established.

ADVERSE REACTIONS

The following adverse reactions have been observed, but there is not enough systematic collection of data to support an estimate of their frequency. Within each category, adverse reactions are listed in decreasing order of severity. Although many side effects are mild and transient, some require discontinuation of therapy.
Propranolol hydrochloride (INDERAL®):
Cardiovascular: Congestive heart failure; hypotension; intensification of AV block; bradycardia; thrombocytopenic purpura; arterial insufficiency, usually of the Raynaud type; paresthesia of hands.
Central Nervous System: Reversible mental depression progressing to catatonia; mental depression manifested by insomnia, lassitude, weakness, fatigue; an acute reversible syndrome characterized by disorientation for time and place, short-term memory loss, emotional lability, slightly clouded sensorium, decreased performance on neuropsychometrics; hallucinations; visual disturbances; vivid dreams; lightheadedness. Total daily doses above 160 mg (when administered as divided doses of greater than 80 mg each) may be associated with an increased incidence of fatigue, lethargy, and vivid dreams.
Gastrointestinal: Mesenteric arterial thrombosis; ischemic colitis; nausea, vomiting, epigastric distress, abdominal cramping, diarrhea, constipation.
Allergic: Laryngospasm and respiratory distress; pharyngitis and agranulocytosis; fever combined with aching and sore throat; erythematous rash.
Respiratory: Bronchospasm.
Hematologic: Agranulcytosis; nonthrombocytopenic purpura; thrombocytopenic purpura.
Autoimmune: In extremely rare instances, systemic lupus erythematosus has been reported.
Miscellaneous: Male impotence. Alopecia, LE-like reactions, psoriasiform rashes, dry eyes, and Peyronie's disease have been reported rarely. Oculomucocutaneous reactions involving the skin, serous membranes, and conjunctivae reported for a beta blocker (practolol) have not been associated with propranolol.
Hydrochlorothiazide:
Cardiovascular: Orthostatic hypotension (may be aggravated by alcohol, barbiturates or narcotics).
Central Nervous System: Dizziness, vertigo, headache, xanthopsia, paresthesias.
Gastrointestinal: Pancreatitis; jaundice (intrahepatic cholestatic jaundice); sialadenitis; anorexia, nausea, vomiting, gastric irritation, cramping, diarrhea, constipation.
Hypersensitivity: Anaphylactic reactions; necrotizing angiitis (vasculitis, cutaneous vasculitis); respiratory distress including pneumonitis; fever; urticaria, rash, purpura, photosensitivity.
Hematologic: Aplastic anemia, agranulocytosis, leukopenia, thrombocytopenia.
Miscellaneous: Hyperglycemia, glycosuria; hyperuricemia; muscle spasm; weakness; restlessness; transient blurred vision.
Whenever adverse reactions are moderate or severe, thiazide dosage should be reduced or therapy withdrawn.

OVERDOSAGE

The propranolol hydrochloride component may cause bradycardia, cardiac failure, hypotension, or bronchospasm. Propranolol is not significantly dialyzable.
The hydrochlorothiazide component can be expected to cause diuresis. Lethargy of varying degree may appear and may progress to coma within a few hours, with minimal depression of respiration and cardiovascular function, and in the absence of significant serum electrolyte changes or dehydration. The mechanism of central nervous system depression with thiazide overdosage is unknown. Gastrointestinal irritation and hypermotility can occur, temporary elevation of BUN has been reported, and serum electrolyte changes could occur, especially in patients with impairment of renal function.
The oral LD_{50} dosages in rats and mice for propranolol, hydrochlorothiazide, and combined propranolol/hydrochlorothiazide (40/25, 80/25) are 364 to 533 mg/kg, greater than 2,750 to 5,000 mg/kg, and 538 to 845 mg/kg, respectively.
TREATMENT
The following measures should be employed:
GENERAL—If ingestion is, or may have been, recent, evacuate gastric contents, taking care to prevent pulmonary aspiration.
BRADYCARDIA—Administer atropine (0.25 to 1.0 mg). If there is no response to vagal blockade, administer isoproterenol cautiously.
CARDIAC FAILURE—Digitalization and diuretics.
HYPOTENSION—Vasopressors, e.g., levarterenol or epinephrine.
BRONCHOSPASM—Administer isoproterenol and aminophylline.
STUPOR OR COMA—Administer supportive therapy as clinically warranted.
GASTROINTESTINAL EFFECTS—Though usually of short duration, these may require symptomatic treatment.
ABNORMALITIES IN BUN AND/OR SERUM ELECTROLYTES—Monitor serum electrolyte levels and renal function; institute supportive measures as required individually to maintain hydration, electrolyte balance, respiration, and cardiovascular-renal function.

DOSAGE AND ADMINISTRATION

The dosage must be determined by individual titration.
Hydrochlorothiazide can be given at doses of 25 to 100 mg per day when used alone, but in most patients, 50 mg exerts a maximal effect. The initial dose of propranolol is 80 mg daily, and it may be increased gradually until optimal blood pressure control is achieved. The usual effective dose when used alone is 160 to 480 mg per day.
One INDERIDE Tablet twice daily can be used to administer up to 160 mg of propranolol and 50 mg of hydrochlorothiazide. For doses of propranolol greater than 160 mg the combination products are not appropriate, because their use would lead to an excessive dose of the thiazide component.
When necessary, another antihypertensive agent may be added gradually beginning with 50 percent of the usual recommended starting dose to avoid an excessive fall in blood pressure.

HOW SUPPLIED

INDERIDE 40/25
—Each hexagonal-shaped, off-white, scored tablet, embossed with an "I" and imprinted with "INDERIDE 40/25," contains 40 mg propranolol hydrochloride (INDERAL®) and 25 mg hydrochlorothiazide, in bottles of 100 (NDC 0046-0484-81) and 1,000 (NDC 0046-0484-91). Also in Unit Dose packages of 100 (NDC 0046-0484-99).
INDERIDE 80/25
—Each hexagonal-shaped, off-white, scored tablet, embossed with an "I" and imprinted with "INDERIDE 80/25," contains 80 mg propranolol hydrochloride (INDERAL®) and 25 mg hydrochlorothiazide, in bottles of 100 (NDC 0046-0488-81).
The appearance of these tablets is a registered trademark of Wyeth-Ayerst Laboratories.
Store at room temperature (approximately 25° C).
Dispense in well-closed, light-resistant containers.
Protect from moisture, freezing, and excessive heat.
Shown in Product Identification Section, page 436

INDERIDE® LA ℞

[ĭn 'de-rīde]
(propranolol hydrochloride and hydrochlorothiazide)
Long-Acting Capsules

No. 455—Each Inderide® LA 80/50 Capsule contains:
Propranolol hydrochloride
(Inderal® LA) .... 80 mg
Hydrochlorothiazide .... 50 mg
No. 457—Each Inderide® LA 120/50
Capsule contains:
Propranolol hydrochloride
(Inderal® LA) .... 120 mg
Hydrochlorothiazide .... 50 mg

No. 459—Each Inderide® LA 160/50
Capsule contains:
Propranolol hydrochloride
(Inderal® LA) .... 160 mg
Hydrochlorothiazide .... 50 mg
CAUTION: Federal law prohibits dispensing without prescription.

DESCRIPTION

Inderide LA is indicated in the once-daily management of hypertension.
Inderide LA combines two antihypertensive agents: Inderal (propranolol hydrochloride), a beta-adrenergic receptor-blocking agent, and hydrochlorothiazide, a thiazide diuretic-antihypertensive. Inderide LA is formulated to provide a sustained release of propranolol hydrochloride. Hydrochlorothiazide in Inderide LA exists in a conventional (not sustained-release) formulation.
Inderal (propranolol hydrochloride) is a synthetic beta-adrenergic receptor-blocking agent chemically described as 1-(Isopropylamino)-3-(1-naphthyloxy)-2-propanol hydrochloride. Its structural formula is:

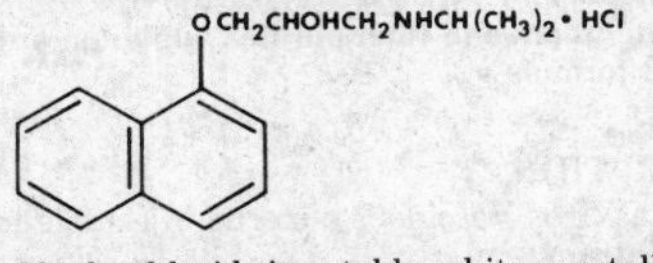

Propranolol hydrochloride is a stable, white, crystalline solid which is readily soluble in water and ethanol. Its molecular weight is 295.81.
Hydrochlorothiazide is a white, or practically white, practically odorless, crystalline powder. It is slightly soluble in water; freely soluble in sodium hydroxide solution; sparingly soluble in methanol; insoluble in ether, chloroform, benzene, and dilute mineral acids. Its chemical name is 6-Chloro-3,4-dihydro-2H-1,2,4-benzothiadiazine-7-sulfonamide 1,1-dioxide. Its structural formula is:

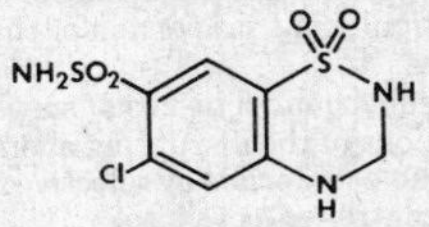

Inderide LA contains the following inactive ingredients: calcium carbonate, ethylcellulose, gelatin capsules, hydroxypropyl methylcellulose, lactose, magnesium stearate, microcrystalline cellulose, sodium lauryl sulfate, sodium starch glycolate, titanium dioxide, and D&C Yellow No. 10. In addition, Inderide LA 80/50 mg and 120/50 mg Capsules contain D&C Red No. 33; Inderide LA 120/50 mg and 160/50 mg Capsules contain FD&C Blue No. 1 and FD&C Red No. 40.

CLINICAL PHARMACOLOGY

PROPRANOLOL HYDROCHLORIDE (INDERAL®)
Inderal is a nonselective, beta-adrenergic receptor-blocking agent possessing no other autonomic nervous system activity. It specifically competes with beta-adrenergic receptor-stimulating agents for available receptor sites. When access to beta-receptor sites is blocked by Inderal, the chronotropic, inotropic, and vasodilator responses to beta-adrenergic stimulation are decreased proportionately.
Inderide LA Capsules (80/50, 120/50, and 160/50 mg) release propranolol hydrochloride at a controlled and predictable rate. Peak propranolol blood levels following dosing with Inderide LA occur at about 6 hours, and the apparent plasma half-life is about 10 hours. Over a 24-hour period, propranolol blood levels are fairly constant for about 12 hours, then decline exponentially. When measured at steady state over a 24-hour period, the areas under the propranolol plasma concentration-time curve (AUCs) for the capsules are approximately 60% to 65% of the AUCs for a comparable divided daily dose of Inderal Tablets. The lower AUCs for the capsules are due to greater hepatic metabolism of propranolol resulting from the slower rate of absorption of propranolol. Inderide LA should not be considered a simple mg-for-mg substitute for conventional Inderide Tablets, and the propranolol blood levels achieved do not match (are lower than) those of twice-daily dosing of Inderide Tablets with the same dose. When changing to Inderide LA from conventional Inderide Tablets, a possible need for retitration upwards should be considered.
The mechanism of the antihypertensive effect of propranolol has not been established. Among the factors that may be involved in contributing to the antihypertensive action are: (1) decreased cardiac output, (2) inhibition of renin release by the kidneys, and (3) diminution of tonic sympathetic nerve outflow from vasomotor centers in the brain.
Propranolol hydrochloride decreases heart rate, cardiac output, and blood pressure. Although total peripheral vascular resistance may increase initially, it readjusts to or below the pretreatment level with chronic usage. Effects on plasma volume appear to be minor and somewhat variable. Inderal has been shown to cause a small increase in serum potassium concentration when used in the treatment of hypertensive patients.
Beta-receptor blockade is useful in conditions in which, because of pathologic or functional changes, sympathetic activity is excessive or inappropriate, and detrimental to the patient. But there are also situations in which sympathetic stimulation is vital. For example, in patients with severely damaged hearts, adequate ventricular function is maintained by virtue of sympathetic drive, which should be preserved. In the presence of AV block, beta blockade may prevent the necessary facilitating effect of sympathetic activity on conduction. Beta blockade results in bronchial constriction by interfering with adrenergic bronchodilator activity, which should be preserved in patients subject to bronchospasm.
The proper objective of beta-blockade therapy is to decrease adverse sympathetic stimulation, but not to the degree that may impair necessary sympathetic support.
HYDROCHLOROTHIAZIDE
Hydrochlorothiazide is a benzothiadiazine (thiazide) diuretic closely related to chlorothiazide. The mechanism of the antihypertensive effect of the thiazides is unknown. Thiazides usually do not affect normal blood pressure.
Thiazides affect the renal tubular mechanism of electrolyte reabsorption. At maximal therapeutic dosage, all thiazides are approximately equal in their diuretic efficacy.
Thiazides increase excretion of sodium and chloride in approximately equivalent amounts. Natriuresis causes a secondary loss of potassium and bicarbonate.
Onset of diuretic action of thiazides occurs in 2 hours, and the peak effect in about 4 hours. Its action persists for approximately 6 to 12 hours. Thiazides are eliminated rapidly by the kidney. The hydrochlorothiazide in Inderide LA is a conventional (not sustained-release) formulation.

INDICATIONS AND USAGE

Inderide LA is indicated in the management of hypertension.
This fixed-combination drug is not indicated for initial therapy of hypertension. Hypertension requires therapy titrated to the individual patient. If the fixed combination represents the dosage so determined, its use may be more convenient in patient management. The treatment of hypertension is not static, but must be reevaluated as conditions in each patient warrant.

CONTRAINDICATIONS

PROPRANOLOL HYDROCHLORIDE (INDERAL®)
Propranolol is contraindicated in: 1) cardiogenic shock; 2) sinus bradycardia and greater than first-degree block; 3) bronchial asthma; 4) congestive heart failure (see WARNINGS), unless the failure is secondary to a tachyarrhythmia treatable with propranolol.
HYDROCHLOROTHIAZIDE
Hydrochlorothiazide is contraindicated in patients with anuria or hypersensitivity to this or other sulfonamide-derived drugs.

WARNINGS

PROPRANOLOL HYDROCHLORIDE (INDERAL®)
Cardiac Failure: Sympathetic stimulation may be a vital component supporting circulatory function in patients with congestive heart failure, and its inhibition by beta blockade may precipitate more severe failure. Although beta blockers should be avoided in overt congestive heart failure, if necessary, they can be used with close follow-up in patients with a history of failure who are well compensated and are receiving digitalis and diuretics. Beta-adrenergic blocking agents do not abolish the inotropic action of digitalis on heart muscle.
In Patients Without a History of Heart Failure, continued use of beta blockers can, in some cases, lead to cardiac failure. Therefore, at the first sign or symptom of heart failure, the patient should be digitalized and/or treated with diuretics, and the response observed closely, or propranolol should be discontinued (gradually, if possible).

In Patients with Angina Pectoris, there have been reports of exacerbation of angina and, in some cases, myocardial infarction, following *abrupt* discontinuance of propranolol therapy. Therefore, when discontinuance of propranolol is planned, the dosage should be gradually reduced and the patient carefully monitored. In addition, when propranolol is prescribed for angina pectoris, the patient should be cautioned against interruption or cessation of therapy without the physician's advice. If propranolol therapy is interrupted and exacerbation of angina occurs, it usually is advisable to reinstitute propranolol therapy and take other measures appropriate for the management of unstable angina pectoris. Since coronary artery disease may be unrecognized, it may be prudent to follow the above advice in patients considered at risk of having occult atherosclerotic heart disease who are given propranolol for other indications.

Thyrotoxicosis: Beta blockade may mask certain clinical signs of hyperthyroidism. Therefore, abrupt withdrawal of propranolol may be followed by an exacerbation of symptoms of hyperthyroidism, including thyroid storm. Propranolol does not distort thyroid function tests.
In Patients With Wolff-Parkinson-White Syndrome, several cases have been reported in which, after propranolol, the tachycardia was replaced by a severe bradycardia requiring a demand pacemaker. In one case this resulted after an initial dose of 5 mg propranolol.
Major Surgery: The necessity or desirability of withdrawal of beta-blocking therapy prior to major surgery is controversial. It should be noted, however, that the impaired ability of the heart to respond to reflex adrenergic stimuli may augment the risks of general anesthesia and surgical procedures.
Nonallergic Bronchospasm (e.g., chronic bronchitis, emphysema): PATIENTS WITH BRONCHOSPASTIC DISEASES SHOULD, IN GENERAL, NOT RECEIVE BETA BLOCKERS. INDERAL should be administered with caution since it may block bronchodilation produced by endogenous and exogenous catecholamine stimulation of beta receptors.
Diabetes and Hypoglycemia: Beta-adrenergic blockade may prevent the appearance of certain premonitory signs and symptoms (pulse rate and pressure changes) of acute hypoglycemia in labile insulin-dependent diabetes. In these patients, it may be more difficult to adjust the dosage of insulin. Hypoglycemic attacks may be accompanied by a precipitous elevation of blood pressure.
HYDROCHLOROTHIAZIDE

Thiazides should be used with caution in severe renal disease. In patients with renal disease, thiazides may precipitate azotemia. In patients with impaired renal function, cumulative effects of the drug may develop.
Thiazides should also be used with caution in patients with impaired hepatic function or progressive liver disease, since minor alterations of fluid and electrolyte balance may precipitate hepatic coma.
Thiazides may add to or potentiate the action of other antihypertensive drugs. Potentiation occurs with ganglionic or peripheral adrenergic-blocking drugs.
Sensitivity reactions may occur in patients with a history of allergy or bronchial asthma. The possibility of exacerbation or activation of systemic lupus erythematosus has been reported.

PRECAUTIONS

PROPRANOLOL HYDROCHLORIDE (INDERAL®)

General: Propranolol should be used with caution in patients with impaired hepatic or renal function. Propranolol is not indicated for the treatment of hypertensive emergencies.
Beta-adrenoreceptor blockade can cause reduction of intraocular pressure. Patients should be told that propranolol may interfere with the glaucoma screening test. Withdrawal may lead to a return of increased intraocular pressure.
Clinical Laboratory Tests: Elevated blood urea levels in patients with severe heart disease, elevated serum transaminase, alkaline phosphatase, lactate dehydrogenase.
Drug Interactions: Patients receiving catecholamine-depleting drugs, such as reserpine, should be closely observed if propranolol is administered. The added catecholamine-blocking action may produce an excessive reduction of resting sympathetic nervous activity, which may result in hypotension, marked bradycardia, vertigo, syncopal attacks, or orthostatic hypotension.
Carcinogenesis, Mutagenesis, Impairment of Fertility: Long-term studies in animals have been conducted to evaluate toxic effects and carcinogenic potential. In 18-month studies, in both rats and mice, employing doses up to 150 mg/kg/day there was no evidence of significant drug-induced toxicity. There were no drug-related tumorigenic effects at any of the dosage levels. Reproductive studies in animals did not show any impairment of fertility that was attributable to the drug.
Pregnancy: Pregnancy Category C. Propranolol has been shown to be embryotoxic in animal studies at doses about 10 times greater than the maximal recommended human dose. There are no adequate and well-controlled studies in pregnant women. Propranolol should be used during pregnancy only if the potential benefit justifies the potential risk to the fetus.
Nursing Mothers: Propranolol is excreted in human milk. Caution should be exercised when propranolol is administered to a nursing mother.
Pediatric Use: Safety and effectiveness in children have not been established.
HYDROCHLOROTHIAZIDE

General: Periodic determination of serum electrolytes to detect possible electrolyte imbalance should be performed at appropriate intervals.

Continued on next page

Wyeth-Ayerst Laboratories—Cont.

All patients receiving thiazide therapy should be observed for clinical signs of fluid or electrolyte imbalance, namely: hyponatremia, hypochloremic alkalosis, and hypokalemia. Serum and urine electrolyte determinations are particularly important when the patient is vomiting excessively or receiving parenteral fluids. Medication such as digitalis may also influence serum electrolytes. Warning signs irrespective of cause are: Dryness of mouth, thirst, weakness, lethargy, drowsiness, restlessness, muscle pains or cramps, muscular fatigue, hypotension, oliguria, tachycardia, and gastrointestinal disturbances such as nausea and vomiting.

Hypokalemia may develop, especially with brisk diuresis, when severe cirrhosis is present or during concomitant use of corticosteroids or ACTH.

Interference with adequate oral electrolyte intake will also contribute to hypokalemia. Hypokalemia can sensitize or exaggerate the response of the heart to the toxic effect of digitalis (e.g., increased ventricular irritability). Hypokalemia may be avoided or treated by use of potassium supplements, such as foods with a high potassium content.

Any chloride deficit is generally mild and usually does not require specific treatment, except under extraordinary circumstances (as in liver or renal disease). Dilutional hyponatremia may occur in edematous patients in hot weather; appropriate therapy is water restriction, rather than administration of salt, except in rare instances when the hyponatremia is life-threatening. In actual salt depletion, appropriate replacement is the therapy of choice.

Hyperuricemia may occur or frank gout may be precipitated in certain patients receiving thiazide therapy.

Insulin requirements in diabetic patients may be increased, decreased, or unchanged. Diabetes mellitus which has been latent may become manifest during thiazide administration.

If progressive renal impairment becomes evident, consider withholding or discontinuing diuretic therapy.

Thiazides may decrease serum PBI levels without signs of thyroid disturbance.

Calcium excretion is decreased by thiazides. Pathologic changes in the parathyroid gland with hypercalcemia and hypophosphatemia have been observed in a few patients on prolonged thiazide therapy. The common complications of hyperparathyroidism, such as renal lithiasis, bone resorption, and peptic ulceration have not been seen. Thiazides should be discontinued before carrying out tests for parathyroid function.

Drug Interactions: Thiazide drugs may increase the responsiveness to tubocurarine.

The antihypertensive effects of thiazides may be enhanced in the postsympathectomy patient. Thiazides may decrease arterial responsiveness to norepinephrine. This diminution is not sufficient to preclude effectiveness of the pressor agent for therapeutic use.

Pregnancy: Pregnancy Category C. Thiazides cross the placental barrier and appear in cord blood. The use of thiazides in pregnancy requires that the anticipated benefit be weighed against possible hazards to the fetus. These hazards include fetal or neonatal jaundice, thrombocytopenia, and possibly other adverse reactions which have occurred in the adult.

Nursing Mothers: Thiazides appear in human milk. If use of the drug is deemed essential, the patient should stop nursing.

Pediatric Use: Safety and effectivenss in children have not been established.

ADVERSE REACTIONS

PROPRANOLOL HYDROCHLORIDE (INDERAL®)

Most adverse effects have been mild and transient and have rarely required the withdrawal of therapy.

Cardiovascular: Bradycardia; congestive heart failure; intensification of AV block; hypotension; paresthesia of hands; thrombocytopenic purpura; arterial insufficiency, usually of the Raynaud type.

Central Nervous System: Light-headedness; mental depression manifested by insomnia, lassitude, weakness, fatigue; reversible mental depression progressing to catatonia; visual disturbances; hallucinations; an acute reversible syndrome characterized by disorientation for time and place, short-term memory loss, emotional lability, slightly clouded sensorium, and decreased performance on neuropsychometrics.

Gastrointestinal: Nausea, vomiting, epigastric distress, abdominal cramping, diarrhea, constipation, mesenteric arterial thrombosis, ischemic colitis.

Allergic: Pharyngitis and agranulocytosis; erythematous rash; fever combined with aching and sore throat; laryngospasm and respiratory distress.

Respiratory: Bronchospasm.

Hematologic: Agranulocytosis; nonthrombocytopenic purpura, thrombocytopenic purpura.

Autoimmune: In extremely rare instances, systemic lupus erythematosus has been reported.

Miscellaneous: Alopecia; LE-like reactions; psoriasiform rashes; dry eyes; male impotence; and Peyronie's disease

have been reported rarely. Oculomucocutaneous reactions involving the skin, serous membranes, and conjunctivae reported for a beta blocker (practolol) have not been associated with propranolol.

HYDROCHLOROTHIAZIDE

Gastrointestinal: Anorexia; gastric irritation, nausea, vomiting, cramping; diarrhea; constipation; jaundice (intrahepatic cholestatic jaundice); pancreatitis; sialadenitis.

Central Nervous System: Dizziness, vertigo; paresthesias; headache; xanthopsia.

Hematologic: Leukopenia; agranulocytosis; thrombocytopenia; aplastic anemia.

Cardiovascular: Orthostatic hypotension (may be aggravated by alcohol, barbiturates, or narcotics).

Hypersensitivity: Purpura; photosensitivity; rash; urticaria; necrotizing angiitis (vasculitis, cutaneous vasculitis); fever; respiratory distress, including pneumonitis; anaphylactic reactions.

Other: Hyperglycemia; glycosuria; hyperuricemia; muscle spasm; weakness; restlessness; transient blurred vision.

Whenever adverse reactions are moderate or severe, thiazide dosage should be reduced or therapy withdrawn.

DOSAGE AND ADMINISTRATION

The dosage must be determined by individual titration. Hydrochlorothiazide can be given at doses of 25 to 100 mg per day when used alone, but in most patients, 50 mg exerts a maximal effect. The initial dose of propranolol is 80 mg daily, and it may be increased gradually until optimal blood pressure control is achieved. The usual effective dose, when used alone, is 160 to 480 mg per day.

One INDERIDE LA Capsule once-a-day can be used to administer up to 160 mg of propranolol and 50 mg of hydrochlorothiazide. For doses of propranolol greater than 160 mg, the combination products are not appropriate because their use would lead to an excessive dose of the thiazide component. INDERIDE LA provides propranolol hydrochloride in a sustained-release form and hydrochlorothiazide in conventional formulation, for once-daily administration. If patients are switched from INDERIDE Tablets (or INDERAL plus hydrochlorothiazide) to INDERIDE LA, care should be taken to ensure that the desired therapeutic effect is maintained. INDERIDE LA should not be considered a mg-for-mg substitute for INDERIDE or INDERAL plus hydrochlorothiazide. INDERIDE LA has different kinetics and produces lower blood levels. Retitration may be necessary, especially to maintain effectiveness at the end of the 24-hour dosing interval.

When necessary, another antihypertensive agent may be added gradually, beginning with 50% of the usual recommended starting dose, to avoid an excessive fall in blood pressure.

OVERDOSAGE OR EXAGGERATED RESPONSE

The propranolol hydrochloride (INDERAL) component may cause bradycardia, cardiac failure, hypotension, or bronchospasm.

The hydrochlorothiazide component can be expected to cause diuresis. Lethargy of varying degree may appear and may progress to coma within a few hours, with minimal depression of respiration and cardiovascular function, and in the absence of significant serum electrolyte changes or dehydration. The mechanism of central nervous system depression with thiazide overdosage is unknown. Gastrointestinal irritation and hypermotility can occur; temporary elevation of BUN has been reported and serum electrolyte changes could occur, especially in patients with impairment of renal function.

TREATMENT

The following measures should be employed:

General: If ingestion is, or may have been, recent, evacuate gastric contents, taking care to prevent pulmonary aspiration.

Bradycardia: Administer atropine (0.25 to 1.0 mg). If there is no response to vagal blockade, administer isoproterenol cautiously.

Cardiac Failure: Digitalization and diuretics.

Hypotension: Vasopressors, e.g., levarterenol or epinephrine.

Bronchospasm: Administer isoproterenol and aminophylline.

Stupor or Coma: Administer supportive therapy as clinically warranted.

Gastrointestinal Effects: Though usually of short duration, these may require symptomatic treatment.

Abnormalities in BUN and/or Serum Electrolytes: Monitor serum electrolyte levels and renal function; institute supportive measures, as required individually, to maintain hydration, electrolyte balance, respiration, and cardiovascular function.

HOW SUPPLIED

Each beige capsule, identified by one wide band and 3 narrow bands, all in gold, and "INDERIDE LA 80/50," contains 80 mg of propranolol hydrochloride (INDERAL® LA) and 50 mg of hydrochlorothiazide, in bottles of 100 (NDC 0046-0455-81).

Each beige/brown capsule, identified by one wide band and 3 narrow bands, all in gold, and "INDERIDE LA 120/50," contains 120 mg of propranolol hydrochloride (INDERAL® LA) and 50 mg of hydrochlorothiazide, in bottles of 100 (NDC 0046-0457-81).

Each brown capsule, identified by one wide band and 3 narrow bands, all in gold, and "INDERIDE LA 160/50, contains 160 mg of propranolol hydrochloride (INDERAL® LA) and 50 mg of hydrochlorothiazide, in bottles of 100 (NDC 0046-0459-81).

Store at room temperature (approximately 25° C).
Protect from light, moisture, freezing, and excessive heat.
Dispense in a tight, light-resistant container as defined in the USP.
Use carton to protect contents from light.

The appearance of these capsules is a registered trademark of Wyeth-Ayerst Laboratories.

Shown in Product Identification Section, page 436

INFLUENZA VIRUS VACCINE, TRIVALENT, TYPES A AND B   ℞
(chromatograph- and filter-purified subvirion antigen)
1992-93 formula

DESCRIPTION

Influenza Virus Vaccine is a sterile injectable for administration intramuscularly.

Influenza Virus Vaccine is prepared from the allantoic fluids of chick embryos inoculated with a specific type of influenza virus. During processing, not more than 5 μg of gentamicin sulfate per mL is added. The harvested virus is inactivated with formaldehyde and is concentrated and purified.

Influenza Virus Vaccine, Trivalent (chromatograph- and filter-purified subvirion antigen), is concentrated and refined by a column-chromatographic procedure. At the same time, addition of tri(n)butylphosphate and Polysorbate 80, USP, to the column-eluting fluids effects disruption and inactivation of a significant proportion of the virus to smaller subunit particles.

The recovered subvirion (split-virus) suspension is freed of substantial portions of the disrupting agents by dialysis and of other undesirable materials by selective filtration through membranes of controlled pore size.

The viral antigen content has been standardized by immuno-diffusion tests, according to current U.S. Public Health Service requirements. Each dose (0.5 mL) contains the proportions and not less than the microgram amounts of hemagglutinin antigens (μg HA) representative of the specific components recommended for the 1992-1993 season: 15 μg HA of A/Texas/36/91 (H1N1), 15 μg HA of A/Beijing/353/89 (H3N2), and 15 μg HA of B/Panama/45/90. This is a split-virus suspension.

The vaccine contains 1:10,000 thimerosal (mercury derivative) as a preservative. Gentamicin sulfate is used during manufacturing but is not detectable in the final product by current assay procedures.

ISMO™   ℞
[ĭs 'mō]
(isosorbide mononitrate)
20 mg tablets

DESCRIPTION

Isosorbide mononitrate is 1,4:3,6-dianhydro-D-glucitol,5-nitrate, an organic nitrate whose structural formula is

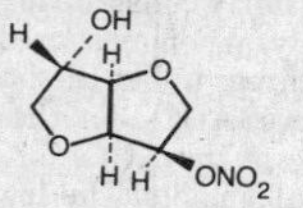

and whose molecular weight is 191.14. The organic nitrates are vasodilators, active on both arteries and veins. Each Ismo tablet contains 20 mg of isosorbide mononitrate. The inactive ingredients in each tablet are D&C Yellow 10 Aluminum Lake, FD&C Yellow 6 Aluminum Lake, hydroxypropyl methylcellulose, lactose, magnesium stearate, microcrystalline cellulose, polyethylene glycol, polysorbate 20, povidone, silicon dioxide, sodium starch glycolate, titanium dioxide and hydroxypropyl cellulose.

CLINICAL PHARMACOLOGY

Isosorbide mononitrate is the major active metabolite of isosorbide dinitrate (ISDN), and most of the clinical activity of the dinitrate is attributable to the mononitrate.

The principal pharmacological action of isosorbide mononitrate is relaxation of vascular smooth muscle and consequent dilatation of peripheral arteries and veins, especially the latter. Dilation of the veins promotes peripheral pooling of blood and decreases venous return to the heart, thereby reducing left ventricular end-diastolic pressure and pulmonary capillary wedge pressure (preload). Arteriolar relax-

ation reduces systemic vascular resistance, systolic arterial pressure, and mean arterial pressure (afterload). Dilatation of the coronary arteries also occurs. The relative importance of preload reduction, afterload reduction, and coronary dilatation remains undefined.

PHARMACODYNAMICS

Dosing regimens for most chronically used drugs are designed to provide plasma concentrations that are continuously greater than a minimally effective concentration. This strategy is inappropriate for organic nitrates. Several well-controlled clinical trials have used exercise testing to assess the antianginal efficacy of continuously-delivered nitrates. In the large majority of these trials, active agents were indistinguishable from placebo after 24 hours (or less) of continuous therapy. Attempts to overcome tolerance by dose escalation, even to doses far in excess of those used acutely, have consistently failed. Only after nitrates have been absent from the body for several hours has their antianginal efficacy been restored.

The drug-free interval sufficient to avoid tolerance to isosorbide mononitrate has not been completely defined. In the only regimen of twice-daily isosorbide mononitrate that has been shown to avoid development of tolerance, the two doses of Ismo tablets are given 7 hours apart, so there is a gap of 17 hours between the second dose of each day and the first dose of the next day. Taking account of the relatively long half-life of isosorbide mononitrate this result is consistent with those obtained for other organic nitrates.

The same twice-daily regimen of Ismo tablets successfully avoided significant rebound/withdrawal effects. The incidence and magnitude of such phenomena have appeared, in studies of other nitrates, to be highly dependent upon the schedule of nitrate administration.

PHARMACOKINETICS

In humans, isosorbide mononitrate is not subject to first pass metabolism in the liver. The absolute bioavailability of isosorbide mononitrate from Ismo tablets is nearly 100%. Maximum serum concentrations of isosorbide mononitrate are achieved 30 to 60 minutes after ingestion of Ismo.

The volume of distribution of isosorbide mononitrate is approximately 0.6 L/Kg, and less than 4% is bound to plasma proteins. It is cleared from the serum by denitration to isosorbide; glucuronidation to the mononitrate glucuronide; and denitration/hydration to sorbitol. None of these metabolites is vasoactive. Less than 1% of administered isosorbide mononitrate is eliminated in the urine.

The overall elimination half-life of isosorbide mononitrate is about 5 hours; the rate of clearance is the same in healthy young adults, in patients with various degrees of renal, hepatic, or cardiac dysfunction, and in the elderly. In a single-dose study, the pharmacokinetics of isosorbide mononitrate were dose-proportional up to at least 60 mg.

CLINICAL TRIALS

Controlled trials of single doses of Ismo tablets have demonstrated that antianginal activity is present about 1 hour after dosing, with peak effect seen from 1–4 hours after dosing. In placebo-controlled trials lasting 2–3 weeks, Ismo tablets were administered twice daily, in asymmetric regimens (with interdosing intervals of 7 and 17 hours) designed to avoid tolerance. One trial tested doses of 10 mg and 20 mg; one trial tested doses of 20 mg, 40 mg, and 60 mg; and three trials tested only doses of 20 mg. In each trial, the subjects were persons with known chronic stable angina, and the primary measure of efficacy was exercise tolerance on a standardized treadmill test. After initial dosing and for at least three weeks, exercise tolerance in patients treated with Ismo 20 mg tablets was significantly greater than that seen in patients treated with placebo, although there was some attenuation of effect with time. Treatment with Ismo tablets was superior to placebo for at least 12 hours after the first dose (i.e., 5 hours after the second dose) of each day. Significant tolerance and rebound phenomena were not observed.

The 10-mg dose was not unequivocally superior to placebo, while the effect of the 40-mg dose was similar to that of the 20-mg dose. The 60-mg dose appeared to be less effective, and it was associated with a rebound phenomenon (early-morning worsening).

INDICATIONS AND USAGE

Ismo tablets are indicated for the prevention of angina pectoris due to coronary artery disease. The onset of action of oral isosorbide mononitrate is not sufficiently rapid for this product to be useful in aborting an acute anginal episode.

CONTRAINDICATIONS

Allergic reactions to organic nitrates are extremely rare, but they do occur. Isosorbide mononitrate is contraindicated in patients who are allergic to it.

WARNINGS

The benefits of isosorbide mononitrate in patients with acute myocardial infarction or congestive heart failure have not been established. Because the effects of isosorbide mononitrate are difficult to terminate rapidly, this drug is not recommended in these settings.

If isosorbide mononitrate is used in these conditions, careful clinical or hemodynamic monitoring must be used to avoid the hazards of hypotension and tachycardia.

PRECAUTIONS

GENERAL

Severe hypotension, particularly with upright posture, may occur with even small doses of isosorbide mononitrate. This drug should therefore be used with caution in patients who may be volume depleted or who, for whatever reason, are already hypotensive. Hypotension induced by isosorbide mononitrate may be accompanied by paradoxical bradycardia and increased angina pectoris.

Nitrate therapy may aggravate the angina caused by hypertrophic cardiomyopathy.

In industrial workers who have had long-term exposure to unknown (presumably high) doses of organic nitrates, tolerance clearly occurs. Chest pain, acute myocardial infarction, and even sudden death have occurred during temporary withdrawal of nitrates from these workers, demonstrating the existence of true physical dependence. The importance of these observations to the routine, clinical use of oral isosorbide mononitrate is not known.

INFORMATION FOR PATIENTS

Patients should be told that the antianginal efficacy of Ismo tablets can be maintained by carefully following the prescribed schedule of dosing (two doses taken seven hours apart). For most patients, this can be accomplished by taking the first dose on awakening and the second dose 7 hours later.

As with other nitrates, daily headaches sometimes accompany treatment with isosorbide mononitrate. In patients who get these headaches, the headaches are a marker of the activity of the drug. Patients should resist the temptation to avoid headaches by altering the schedule of their treatment with isosorbide mononitrate, since loss of headache may be associated with simultaneous loss of antianginal efficacy. Aspirin and/or acetaminophen, on the other hand, often successfully relieve isosorbide mononitrate-induced headaches with no deleterious effect on isosorbide mononitrate's anti-anginal efficacy.

Treatment with isosorbide mononitrate may be associated with light-headedness on standing, especially just after rising from a recumbent or seated position. This effect may be more frequent in patients who have also consumed alcohol.

DRUG INTERACTIONS

The vasodilating effects of isosorbide mononitrate may be additive with those of other vasodilators. Alcohol, in particular, has been found to exhibit additive effects of this variety. Marked symptomatic orthostatic hypotension has been reported when calcium channel blockers and organic nitrates were used in combination. Dose adjustments of either class of agents may be necessary.

CARCINOGENESIS, MUTAGENESIS, AND IMPAIRMENT OF FERTILITY

No carcinogenic effects were observed in mice exposed to oral isosorbide mononitrate for 104 weeks at doses of up to 900 mg/kg/day (102 × the human exposure comparing body surface area). Rats treated with 900 mg/kg/day for 26 weeks (225 × the human exposure comparing body surface area) and 500 mg/kg/day for the remaining 95–111 weeks (males and females, respectively) showed no evidence of tumors.

No mutagenic activity was seen in a variety of *in vitro* and *in vivo* assays.

No adverse effects on fertility were observed when isosorbide mononitrate was administered to male and female rats at doses up to 500 mg/kg/day (125 × the human exposure comparing body surface area).

PREGNANCY CATEGORY C

Isosorbide mononitrate has been shown to be associated with stillbirths and neonatal death in rats receiving 500 mg/kg/day of isosorbide mononitrate (125 × the human exposure comparing body surface area). At 250 mg/kg/day, no adverse effects on reproduction and development were reported.

In rats and rabbits receiving isosorbide mononitrate at up to 250 mg/kg/day, no developmental abnormalities, fetal abnormalities, or other effects upon reproductive performance were detected; these doses are larger than the maximum recommended human dose by factors between 70 (body-surface-area basis in rabbits) and 310 (body-weight basis, either species). In rats receiving 500 mg/kg/day, there were small but statistically significant increases in the rates of prolonged gestation, prolonged parturition, stillbirth, and neonatal death; and there were small but statistically significant decreases in birth weight, live litter size, and pup survival.

There are no adequate and well-controlled studies in pregnant women. Isosorbide mononitrate should be used during pregnancy only if the potential benefit justifies the potential risk to the fetus.

NURSING MOTHERS

It is not known whether isosorbide mononitrate is excreted in human milk. Because many drugs are excreted in human milk, caution should be exercised when isosorbide mononitrate is administered to a nursing woman.

PEDIATRIC USE

Safety and effectiveness of isosorbide mononitrate in children have not been established.

ADVERSE REACTIONS

The table below shows the frequencies of the adverse reactions observed in more than 1% of the subjects (a) in 6 placebo-controlled domestic studies in which patients in the active-treatment arm received 20 mg of isosorbide mononitrate twice daily, and (b) in all studies in which patients received isosorbide mononitrate in a variety of regimens. In parentheses, the same table shows the frequencies with which these adverse reactions led to discontinuation of treatment. Overall, eleven percent of the patients who received isosorbide mononitrate in the six controlled U.S. studies discontinued treatment because of adverse reactions. Most of these discontinued because of headache. "Dizziness" and nausea were also frequently associated with withdrawal from these studies.

Frequency and Adverse Reactions (Discontinuations)*

	6 Controlled Studies		92 Clinical Studies
Dose	Placebo	20 mg	(varied)
Patients	204	219	3344
Headache	9% (0%)	38% (9%)	19% (4.3%)
Dizziness	1% (0%)	5% (1%)	3% (0.2%)
Nausea, Vomiting	<1% (0%)	4% (3%)	2% (0.2%)

* Some individuals discontinued for multiple reasons.

Other adverse reactions, each reported by fewer than 1% of exposed patients, and in many cases of uncertain relation to drug treatment, were:

Cardiovascular: angina pectoris, arrhythmias, atrial fibrillation, hypotension, palpitations, postural hypotension, premature ventricular contractions, supraventricular tachycardia, syncope.

Dermatologic: pruritus, rash.

Gastrointestinal: abdominal pain, diarrhea, dyspepsia, tenesmus, tooth disorder, vomiting.

Genitourinary: dysuria, impotence, urinary frequency.

Miscellaneous: asthenia, blurred vision, cold sweat, diplopia, edema, malaise, neck stiffness, rigors.

Musculoskeletal: arthralgia.

Neurologic: agitation, anxiety, confusion, dyscoordination, hypoesthesia, hypokinesia, increased appetite, insomnia, nervousness, nightmares.

Respiratory: bronchitis, pneumonia, upper respiratory tract infection.

Extremely rarely, ordinary doses of organic nitrates have caused methemoglobinemia in normal-seeming patients; for further discussion of its diagnosis and treatment see under **OVERDOSAGE.**

OVERDOSAGE

HEMODYNAMIC EFFECTS

The ill effects of isosorbide mononitrate overdose are generally the results of isosorbide mononitrate's capacity to induce vasodilatation, venous pooling, reduced cardiac output, and hypotension. These hemodynamic changes may have protean manifestations, including increased intracranial pressure, with any or all of persistent throbbing headache, confusion, and moderate fever; vertigo; palpitations; visual disturbances; nausea and vomiting (possibly with colic and even bloody diarrhea); syncope (especially in the upright posture); air hunger and dyspnea, later followed by reduced ventilatory effort; diaphoresis, with the skin either flushed or cold and clammy; heart block and bradycardia; paralysis; coma; seizures and death.

Laboratory determinations of serum levels of isosorbide mononitrate and its metabolites are not widely available, and such determinations have, in any event, no established role in the management of isosorbide mononitrate overdose.

There are no data suggesting what dose of isosorbide mononitrate is likely to be life-threatening in humans. In rats and mice, there is significant lethality at doses of 2000 mg/kg and 3000 mg/kg, respectively.

No data are available to suggest physiological maneuvers (e.g., maneuvers to change the pH of the urine) that might accelerate elimination of isosorbide mononitrate. In particular, dialysis is known to be ineffective in removing isosorbide mononitrate from the body.

No specific antagonist to the vasodilator effects of isosorbide mononitrate is known, and no intervention has been subject to controlled study as a therapy of isosorbide mononitrate overdose. Because the hypotension associated with isosorbide mononitrate overdose is the result of venodilatation and arterial hypovolemia, prudent therapy in this situation should be directed toward an increase in central fluid vol-

Continued on next page

Wyeth-Ayerst Laboratories—Cont.

ume. Passive elevation of the patient's legs may be sufficient, but intravenous infusion of normal saline or similar fluid may also be necessary.
The use of epinephrine or other arterial vasoconstrictors in this setting is likely to do more harm than good.
In patients with renal disease or congestive heart failure, therapy resulting in central volume expansion is not without hazard. Treatment of isosorbide mononitrate overdose in these patients may be subtle and difficult, and invasive monitoring may be required.

METHEMOGLOBINEMIA

Methemoglobinemia has been reported in patients receiving other organic nitrates, and it probably could also occur as a side effect of isosorbide mononitrate. Certainly nitrate ions liberated during metabolism of isosorbide mononitrate can oxidize hemoglobin into methemoglobin. Even in patients totally without cytochrome b_5 reductase activity, however, and even assuming that the nitrate moiety of isosorbide mononitrate is quantitatively applied to oxidation of hemoglobin, about 2 mg/kg of isosorbide mononitrate should be required before any of these patients manifests clinically significant ($\geq$ 10%) methemoglobinemia. In patients with normal reductase function, significant production of methemoglobin should require even larger doses of isosorbide mononitrate. In one study in which 36 patients received 2–4 weeks of continuous nitroglycerin therapy at 3.1 to 4.4 mg/hr (equivalent, in total administered dose of nitrate ions, to 7.8–11.1 mg of isosorbide mononitrate per hour), the average methemoglobin level measured was 0.2%; this was comparable to that observed in parallel patients who received placebo.
Notwithstanding these observations, there are case reports of significant methemoglobinemia in association with moderate overdoses of organic nitrates. None of the affected patients had been thought to be unusually susceptible.
Methemoglobin levels are available from most clinical laboratories. The diagnosis should be suspected in patients who exhibit signs of impaired oxygen delivery despite adequate cardiac output and adequate arterial pO_2. Classically, methemoglobinemic blood is described as chocolate brown, without color change on exposure to air.
When methemoglobinemia is diagnosed, the treatment of choice is methylene blue, 1–2 mg/kg intravenously.

DOSAGE AND ADMINISTRATION

The recommended regimen of Ismo tablets is 20 mg (one tablet) twice daily, with the two doses given seven hours apart. For most patients, this can be accomplished by taking the first dose on awakening and the second dose 7 hours later. Dosage adjustments are not necessary for elderly patients or patients with altered renal or hepatic function.
As noted above (**CLINICAL PHARMACOLOGY**), multiple studies of organic nitrates have shown that maintenance of continuous 24-hour plasma levels results in refractory tolerance. The dosing regimen for Ismo tablets provides a daily nitrate-free interval to avoid the development of this tolerance.
As also noted under **CLINICAL PHARMACOLOGY,** well-controlled studies have shown that tolerance to Ismo tablets is avoided when using the twice-daily regimen in which the two doses are given seven hours apart. This regimen has been shown to have antianginal efficacy beginning one hour after the first dose and lasting at least five hours after the second dose. The duration (if any) of antianginal activity beyond twelve hours has not been studied; large controlled studies with other nitrates suggest that no dosing regimen should be expected to provide more than about twelve hours of continuous antianginal efficacy per day.
In clinical trials, Ismo tablets have been administered in a variety of regimens. Single doses less than 20 mg have not been adequately studied, while single doses greater than 20 mg have demonstrated no greater efficacy than doses of 20 mg.

HOW SUPPLIED

Ismo (isosorbide mononitrate) tablets, 20 mg, are available in bottles of 100 (NDC 0008-0771-01) and in unit dose packages of 10 blister strips of 10 tablets (NDC 0008-0771-02). Each orange, round, film-coated tablet is engraved "ISMO 20" on one side and "W" on the reverse side.
Store at controlled room temperature between 15°C and 30°C (59°F and 86°F).
Dispense in tight container.

Shown in Product Identification Section, page 436

ISORDIL® ℞

[ī'sore"dĭl]
(isosorbide dinitrate)
(1,4,3,6-dianhydro-sorbitol-2,5-dinitrate)

DESCRIPTION

Isosorbide dinitrate, an organic nitrate, is a vasodilator with effects on both arteries and veins. Isordil is available as 2.5 mg, 5 mg, and 10 mg Sublingual tablets; 5 mg, 10 mg, 20 mg, 30 mg, and 40 mg standard oral Titradose® tablets; and 40 mg controlled-release oral Tembids® capsules and tablets.
Isordil Sublingual tablets contain 2.5 mg, 5 mg, or 10 mg isosorbide dinitrate. The inactive ingredients present are cellulose, lactose, magnesium stearate, and starch. The 2.5 mg dosage strength also contains D&C Yellow 10 and FD&C Yellow 6, and the 5 mg dosage strength also contains FD&C Red 40.
Isordil Titradose tablets contain 5 mg, 10 mg, 20 mg, 30 mg, or 40 mg isosorbide dinitrate. The inactive ingredients present are lactose, magnesium stearate, and other ingredients. The 5 mg, 20 mg, 30 mg, and 40 mg dosage strengths also contain the following: 5 mg—FD&C Red 40; 20 mg and 40 mg—D&C Yellow 10, FD&C Blue 1, and FD&C Yellow 6; 30 mg—FD&C Blue 1.
Isordil Tembids capsules contain 40 mg isosorbide dinitrate. The inactive ingredients present are confectioners sugar, starch, gelatin capsule, and other ingredients.
Isordil Tembids tablets contain 40 mg isosorbide dinitrate. The inactive ingredients present are D&C Yellow 10, FD&C Blue 1, FD&C Yellow 6, lactose, magnesium stearate, sodium silicoaluminate, talc, and other ingredients.
The chemical name for isosorbide dinitrate is 1,4,3,6-dianhydro-sorbitol-2,5-dinitrate, and compound has the following structural formula:

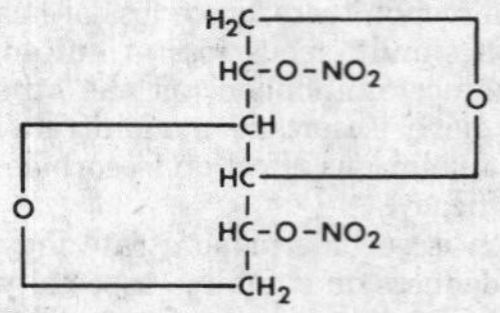

Molecular Weight 236.14

Isosorbide dinitrate is a white, crystalline, odorless compound which is stable in air and in solution, has a melting point of 70° C and has an optical rotation of +134° (c = 1.0, alcohol, 20° C). Isosorbide dinitrate is freely soluble in organic solvents such as acetone, alcohol, and ether, but is only sparingly soluble in water.

CLINICAL PHARMACOLOGY

The principal pharmacological action of Isordil is relaxation of vascular smooth muscle, producing a vasodilatory effect on both peripheral arteries and veins, with predominant effects on the latter. Dilation of the postcapillary vessels, including large veins, promotes peripheral pooling of blood and decreases venous return to the heart, thereby reducing left-ventricular end-diastolic pressure (preload). Arteriolar relaxation reduces systemic vascular resistance and arterial pressure (afterload).
The mechanism by which Isordil relieves angina pectoris is not fully understood. Myocardial oxygen consumption or demand (as measured by the pressure-rate product, tension-time index, and stroke-work index) is decreased by both the arterial and venous effects of Isordil, and, presumably, a more favorable supply-demand ratio is achieved. While the large epicardial coronary arteries are also dilated by Isordil, the extent to which this contributes to relief of exertional angina is unclear.
Therapeutic doses of Isordil may reduce systolic, diastolic, and mean arterial blood pressures, especially in the upright posture. Effective coronary perfusion is usually maintained. The decrease in systemic blood pressure may result in reflex tachycardia, an effect which could unfavorably influence myocardial oxygen demand. Hemodynamic studies indicate that Isordil may reduce the abnormally elevated left ventricular end-diastolic and pulmonary capillary wedge pressures that occur during an acute episode of angina pectoris.
Isordil is metabolized by enzymatic denitration to the intermediate products, isosorbide-2-mononitrate and isosorbide-5-mononitrate. Both metabolites have biological activity, especially the 5-mononitrate which is also the principal metabolite. The liver is a principal site of metabolism, and oral isosorbide dinitrate is subject to a large first pass effect. The systemic clearance of the drug following intravenous infusion is about 3.4 liters/min. Since the clearance exceeds hepatic blood flow, considerable extrahepatic metabolism must also occur.
The average bioavailability of Isordil is 59 and 22 percent following sublingual and oral administration, respectively. The terminal half-life is about 20 minutes, 60 minutes, and 4 hours following IV, sublingual, and oral administration, respectively. The dependence of half-life on the route of administration is not understood. Over limited ranges of IV dosing, the pharmacokinetics of isosorbide dinitrate appear linear. However, both the 2- and 5-mononitrate metabolites have been shown to decrease the rate of disappearance of the dinitrate from the blood. The half-lives of isosorbide-5-mononitrate and isosorbide-2-mononitrate range from 4.0 to 5.6 and 1.5 to 3.1 hours, respectively.
The pharmacokinetics and/or bioavailability of isosorbide dinitrate during multiple dosing have not been well studied. Because the metabolites influence the clearance of isosorbide dinitrate, prediction of blood levels of parent compound or metabolites from single-dose studies is uncertain.

INDICATIONS AND USAGE

Isordil is indicated for the treatment and prevention of angina pectoris. Controlled clinical trials have demonstrated that the sublingual, immediate release, and controlled-release oral dosage forms of Isordil are effective in improving exercise tolerance in patients with angina pectoris. When single sublingual doses (5 mg) of isosorbide dinitrate were administered prophylactically to patients with angina pectoris in various clinical studies, duration of exercise until chest pain or fatigue was significantly improved for at least 45 minutes (and as long as 2 hours in some studies) following dosing. Similar studies after single oral (15 to 120 mg) and oral controlled-release (40 to 80 mg) doses of isosorbide dinitrate have shown significant improvement in exercise tolerance for up to 8 hours following dosing. The exercise electrocardiographic evidence suggests that improved exercise tolerance with Isordil is not at the expense of greater myocardial ischemia. All dosage forms of Isordil may therefore be used prophylactically to decrease frequency and severity of anginal attacks and can be expected to decrease the need for sublingual nitroglycerin.
The sublingual form of the drug is indicated for acute prophylaxis of angina pectoris when taken a few minutes before situations likely to provoke anginal attacks. Because of a slower onset of effect, the oral forms of Isordil are not indicated for acute prophylaxis.
In controlled clinical trials, sublingual isosorbide dinitrate was effective in relieving an acute attack of angina pectoris. Relief occurred with a mean time of 3.4 minutes compared to relief of angina with a mean time of 1.9 minutes following sublingual nitroglycerin. Because of the more rapid relief of chest pain with sublingual nitroglycerin, the use of sublingual isosorbide dinitrate for aborting an acute anginal attack should be limited to patients intolerant or unresponsive to sublingual nitroglycerin.

CONTRAINDICATIONS

Isosorbide dinitrate is contraindicated in patients who have shown purported hypersensitivity or idiosyncrasy to it or other nitrates or nitrites.

WARNINGS

The benefits of isosorbide dinitrate during the early days of an acute myocardial infarction have not been established. If one elects to use organic nitrates in early infarction, hemodynamic monitoring and frequent clinical assessment should be used because of the potential deleterious effects of hypotension.

PRECAUTIONS

GENERAL

Severe hypotensive response, particularly with upright posture, may occur with even small doses of isosorbide dinitrate. The drug should therefore be used with caution in subjects who may have blood volume depletion from diuretic therapy or in subjects who have low systolic blood pressure (e.g., below 90 mm Hg). Paradoxical bradycardia and increased angina pectoris may accompany nitrate-induced hypotension.
Nitrate therapy may aggravate the angina caused by hypertrophic cardiomyopathy. Tolerance to this drug and cross-tolerance to other nitrates and nitrites may occur.
Marked symptomatic, orthostatic hypotension has been reported when calcium channel blockers and organic nitrates were used in combination. Dose adjustment of either class of agents may be necessary.
Tolerance to the vascular and antianginal effects of isosorbide dinitrate or nitroglycerin has been demonstrated in clinical trials, experience through occupational exposure, and in isolated tissue experiments in the laboratory. The importance of tolerance to the appropriate use of isosorbide dinitrate in the management of patients with angina pectoris has not been determined. However, one clinical trial using treadmill exercise tolerance (as an endpoint) found an 8-hour duration of action of oral isosorbide dinitrate following the first dose (after a 2-week placebo washout) and only a 2-hour duration of effect of the same dose after 1 week of repetitive dosing at conventional dosing intervals. On the other hand, several trials have been able to differentiate isosorbide dinitrate from placebo after 4 weeks of therapy, and in open trials an effect seems detectable for as long as several months.
Tolerance clearly occurs in industrial workers continuously exposed to nitroglycerin. Moreover, physical dependence also occurs, since chest pain, acute myocardial infarction,

and even sudden death have occurred during temporary withdrawal of nitroglycerin from the workers. In clinical trials in angina patients, there are reports of anginal attacks being more easily provoked and of rebound in the hemodynamic effects soon after nitrate withdrawal. The relative importance of these observations to the routine, clinical use of isosorbide dinitrate is not known. However, it seems prudent to gradually withdraw patients from isosorbide dinitrate when the therapy is being terminated, rather than stopping the drug abruptly.

INFORMATION FOR PATIENTS

Headache may occur during initial therapy with isosorbide dinitrate. Headache is usually relieved by the use of standard headache remedies, or by lowering the dose, and tends to disappear after the first week or two of use.

DRUG INTERACTIONS

Alcohol may enhance any marked sensitivity to the hypotensive effect of nitrates.

Isosorbide dinitrate acts directly on vascular smooth muscle; therefore, any other agent that depends on vascular smooth muscle as the final common path can be expected to have decreased or increased effect, depending on the agent.

CARCINOGENESIS, MUTAGENESIS, IMPAIRMENT OF FERTILITY

No long-term studies in animals have been performed to evaluate the carcinogenic potential of this drug. A modified two-litter reproduction study in rats fed isosorbide dinitrate at 25 or 100 mg/kg/day did not reveal any effects on fertility or gestation or any remarkable growth pathology in any parent or offspring fed isosorbide dinitrate as compared with rats fed a basal-controlled diet.

PREGNANCY CATEGORY C

Isosorbide dinitrate has been shown to cause a dose-related increase in embryotoxicity (increase in mummified pups) in rabbits at oral doses 35 and 150 times the maximum recommended human daily dose. There are no adequate and well-controlled studies in pregnant women. Isosorbide dinitrate should be used during pregnancy only if the potential benefit justifies the potential risk to the fetus.

NURSING MOTHERS

It is not known whether this drug is excreted in human milk. Because many drugs are excreted in human milk, caution should be exercised when isosorbide dinitrate is administered to a nursing woman.

PEDIATRIC USE

The safety and effectiveness of isosorbide dinitrate in children have not been established.

ADVERSE REACTIONS

Adverse reactions, particularly headache and hypotension, are dose-related. In clinical trials at various doses, the following have been observed.

Headache is the most common adverse reaction and may be severe and persistent; reported incidence varies widely, apparently being dose-related, with an average occurrence of about 25%.

Cutaneous vasodilation with flushing may occur.

Transient episodes of dizziness and weakness, as well as other signs of cerebral ischemia associated with postural hypotension, may occasionally develop (the incidence of reported symptomatic hypotension ranges from 2% to 36%).

An occasional individual will exhibit marked sensitivity to the hypotensive effects of nitrates, and severe responses (nausea, vomiting, weakness, restlessness, pallor, perspiration, and collapse) may occur even with the usual therapeutic dose. Drug rash and/or exfoliative dermatitis may occasionally occur. Nausea and vomiting appear to be uncommon.

OVERDOSAGE

SIGNS AND SYMPTOMS

These may include the following: a prompt fall in blood pressure, persistent and throbbing headache, vertigo, palpitation, visual disturbances, flushed and perspiring skin (later becoming cold and cyanotic), nausea and vomiting (possibly with colic and even bloody diarrhea), syncope (especially in the upright position), methemoglobinemia with cyanosis and anoxia, initial hyperpnea, dyspnea and slow breathing, slow pulse (dicrotic and intermittent), heart block, increased intracranial pressure with cerebral symptoms of confusion and moderate fever, paralysis and coma followed by clonic convulsions and possibly death due to circulatory collapse.

It is not known what dose of the drug is associated with symptoms of overdosing or what dose of the drug would be life-threatening. The acute oral LD50 of isosorbide dinitrate in rats was found to be approximately 1100 mg/kg of body weight. These animal experiments indicate that approximately 500 times the usual therapeutic dose would be required to produce such toxic symptoms in humans. It is not known whether the drug is dialyzable.

TREATMENT OF OVERDOSAGE

Prompt removal of the ingested material by gastric lavage is reasonable but not documented to be useful. Keep the patient recumbent in a shock position and comfortably warm. Passive movements of the extremities may aid venous return. Administer oxygen and artificial respiration if necessary. If methemoglobinemia is present, administer methylene blue (1% solution), 1 to 2 mg/kg intravenously.

METHEMOGLOBIN

Case reports of clinically significant methemoglobinemia are rare at conventional doses of organic nitrates. The formation of methemoglobin is dose-related, and in the case of genetic abnormalities of hemoglobin that favor methemoglobin formation, even conventional doses of organic nitrate could produce harmful concentrations of methemoglobin.

WARNING: Epinephrine is ineffective in reversing the severe hypotensive events associated with overdose. It and related compounds are contraindicated in this situation.

DOSAGE AND ADMINISTRATION

For the treatment of angina pectoris, the usual starting dose of sublingual Isordil is 2.5 to 5 mg.

Isordil should be titrated upward until angina is relieved or side effects limit the dose. In ambulatory patients, the magnitude of the incremental dose increase should be guided by measurements of standing blood pressure.

The initial dosage of sublingual Isordil for acute prophylactic therapy in angina pectoris patients is generally 5 or 10 mg every 2 to 3 hours. Adequate, controlled clinical studies demonstrating the effectiveness of chronic maintenance therapy with these dosage forms have not been reported.

For the treatment of chronic stable angina pectoris, the usual starting dose for immediate-release (swallowed) tablets is 5 to 20 mg; and for controlled release forms, 40 mg. For maintenance therapy, oral doses of 10 to 40 mg given every 6 hours or oral controlled-release doses of 40 to 80 mg given every 8 to 12 hours are generally recommended. The extent to which development of tolerance should modify the dosage program has not been defined. The oral controlled-release forms of Isordil should not be chewed.

HOW SUPPLIED

Isordil® (isosorbide dinitrate) Tablets, Wyeth®, are available as follows:

Sublingual, 2.5 mg, yellow tablets:
NDC 0008-4139-01, bottles of 100.
NDC 0008-4139-03, bottles of 500.
Sublingual, 5 mg, pink tablets:
NDC 0008-4126-01, bottles of 100.
NDC 0008-4126-03, bottles of 500.
Sublingual, 10 mg, white tablets:
NDC 0008-4161-01, bottles of 100.
Oral Titradose®, 5 mg, scored pink tablets:
NDC 0008-4152-01, bottles of 100.
NDC 0008-4152-02, bottles of 500.
NDC 0008-4152-03, bottles of 1000.
Oral Titradose, 10 mg, scored white tablets:
NDC 0008-4153-01, bottles of 100.
NDC 0008-4153-02, bottles of 500.
NDC 0008-4153-03, bottles of 1000.
Oral Titradose, 20 mg, scored green tablets:
NDC 0008-4154-01, bottles of 100.
NDC 0008-4154-02, bottles of 500.
Oral Titradose, 30 mg, scored blue tablets:
NDC 0008-4159-01, bottles of 100.
NDC 0008-4159-02, bottles of 500.
Oral Titradose, 40 mg, scored light-green tablets:
NDC 0008-4192-01, bottles of 100.
Tembids®, 40 mg, scored green controlled-release tablets:
NDC 0008-4125-01, bottles of 100.
NDC 0008-4125-02, bottles of 500.
NDC 0008-4125-03, bottles of 1000.

Keep bottles tightly closed.

Store at Room Temperature, Approx. 25° C (77° F).

ALSO AVAILABLE

Redipak® cartons of 100 tablets (10 blister strips of 10) as follows:
Sublingual, 2.5 mg, NDC 0008-4139-05.
Sublingual, 5 mg, NDC 0008-4126-07.
Oral Titradose, 5 mg, NDC 0008-4152-05.
Oral Titradose, 10 mg, NDC 0008-4153-05.
Oral Titradose, 20 mg, NDC 0008-4154-05.
Oral Titradose, 30 mg, NDC 0008-4159-04.
Oral Titradose, 40 mg, NDC 0008-4192-04.

Store at Room Temperature, Approx. 25° C (77° F).

Isordil® (isosorbide dinitrate) Tembids® Capsules, Wyeth®, are available in 40 mg, controlled-release capsules (opaque, blue cap and colorless, transparent body):
NDC 0008-4140-01, bottles of 100.
NDC 0008-4140-02, bottles of 500.

Keep bottles tightly closed.

Store at Room Temperature, Approx. 25° C (77° F).

US Pat. No. Re 29077 (Titradose®)

The appearances of Titradose® tablets and Tembids® tablets and capsules are trademarks of Wyeth-Ayerst Laboratories.

Shown in Product Identification Section, pages 436 and 437

LODINE® ℞

[*lō′deen*]
(etodolac)
Capsules

DESCRIPTION

Lodine (etodolac) is a pyranocarboxylic acid chemically designated as (±) 1,8-diethyl-1,3,4,9-tetrahydropyrano-[3,4-b]indole-1-acetic acid. The structural formula for etodolac is shown below:

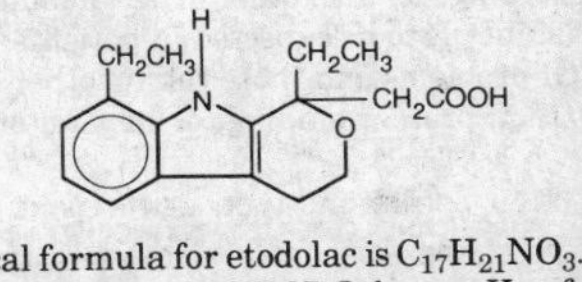

The empirical formula for etodolac is $C_{17}H_{21}NO_3$. The molecular weight of the base is 287.37. It has a pKa of 4.65 and an n-octanol:water partition coefficient of 11.4 at pH 7.4. Etodolac is a white crystalline compound, insoluble in water but soluble in alcohols, chloroform, dimethyl sulfoxide, and aqueous polyethylene glycol.

The inactive ingredients present are cellulose, gelatin, iron oxides, lactose, magnesium stearate, povidone, sodium lauryl sulfate, sodium starch glycolate, talc, and titanium dioxide.

Lodine is available in 200 and 300 mg capsules for oral administration.

CLINICAL PHARMACOLOGY

PHARMACOLOGY

Etodolac is a nonsteroidal anti-inflammatory drug (NSAID) that exhibits anti-inflammatory, analgesic and antipyretic activities in animal models. The mechanism of action of etodolac, like that of other NSAIDs, is not known but is believed to be associated with the inhibition of prostaglandin biosynthesis.

Lodine is a racemic mixture of R- and S-etodolac. As with other NSAIDs, it has been demonstrated in animals that the S-form is biologically active and the R-form is not. Both enantiomers are stable and there is no R-to-S conversion *in vivo.*

PHARMACODYNAMICS

Analgesia was demonstrable by ½ hour following single doses of 200 to 400 mg Lodine, with the peak effect occurring in 1 to 2 hours. The analgesic effect generally lasts for 4 to 6 hours (with some patients maintaining analgesia up to 8 to 12 hours; see "Analgesia" and "Osteoarthritis" sections under "CLINICAL TRIALS" below).

PHARMACOKINETICS

The pharmacokinetics of etodolac have been evaluated in 267 normal subjects, 44 elderly patients (> 65 years old), 19 patients with renal failure (creatinine clearance 37 to 88 mL/min), 9 patients on hemodialysis, and 10 patients with compensated hepatic cirrhosis. Lodine is well absorbed and had a relative bioavailability of 100% when 200 mg capsules were compared with a solution of etodolac. Based on mass balance studies, the systemic availability of Lodine is at least 80%, and etodolac does not undergo significant first-pass metabolism following oral administration. The dose-proportionality based on AUC (the area under the plasma concentration-time curve) is linear following doses up to 600 mg every 12 hours. Peak concentrations are dose-proportional for both total and free etodolac following doses up to 400 mg every 12 hours, but following a 600 mg dose, the peak is about 20% higher than predicted on the basis of lower doses. As shown on the graphs below, etodolac plasma concentrations, after multiple-dose administration, are slightly higher than after single doses, as predicted, indicating no change in pharmacokinetics with multiple dose use. Etodolac is more than 99% bound to plasma proteins. The free fraction is less than 1% and is independent of etodolac total concentration over the dose range studied.

Etodolac, when administered orally, exhibits characteristics which are well described by a two-compartment model with first-order absorption. Mean (± 1 SD) peak plasma concentrations range from approximately 14±4 to 37±9 μg/mL after 200 to 600 mg single doses and are reached in 80±30 minutes. The mean plasma clearance of etodolac is 47 (± 16) mL/h/kg, and terminal disposition half-life is 7.3 (± 4.0) hours (see Table for Summary of Pharmacokinetic Parameters [on next page]).

As with many drugs which are hepatically metabolized and not dosed on a mg/kg basis, the intersubject variability of etodolac plasma levels, achieved after recommended doses, is substantial. The graph of simulated curves demonstrates the range of plasma concentrations that would be expected for 95% of the patients following 200 or 400 mg single doses on the top and on t.i.d. regimens on the bottom (at steady-state). The cross-hatched area represents the overlap in plasma levels following 200 or 400 mg of Lodine orally as single or multiple doses. The area above the upper 95% C.L. lines represents blood levels which would be achieved by larger doses or in individuals with decreased clearance in

Continued on next page

Wyeth-Ayerst Laboratories—Cont.

whom one should anticipate increased adverse reactions. The area below the 95% C.L. lines represents blood levels following lower doses or in individuals with high clearance of etodolac, and one would expect less effectiveness in such patients. The data used to produce these simulations were derived from the mean ± 2 SD of the plasma concentrations at each time point from a total of 267 normal subjects following multiple dosing. As with other drugs, including NSAIDs, greater variability is to be expected in patients, particularly those with GI problems and those taking other drugs affecting the GI tract, protein binding, or hepatic or renal function.

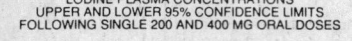

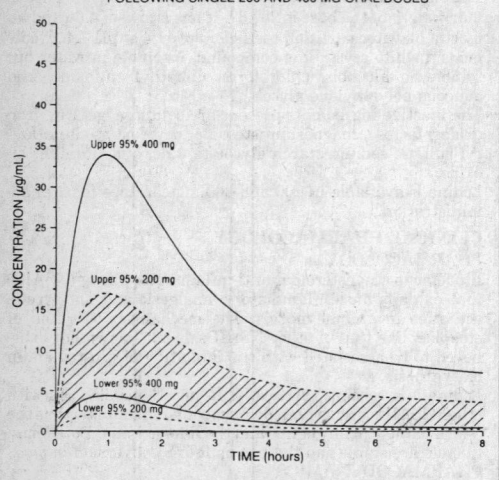

LODINE PLASMA CONCENTRATIONS
UPPER AND LOWER 95% CONFIDENCE LIMITS
FOLLOWING SINGLE 200 AND 400 MG ORAL DOSES

LODINE PLASMA CONCENTRATIONS
UPPER AND LOWER 95% CONFIDENCE LIMITS
FOLLOWING 200 AND 400 MG T.I.D. ORAL DOSES

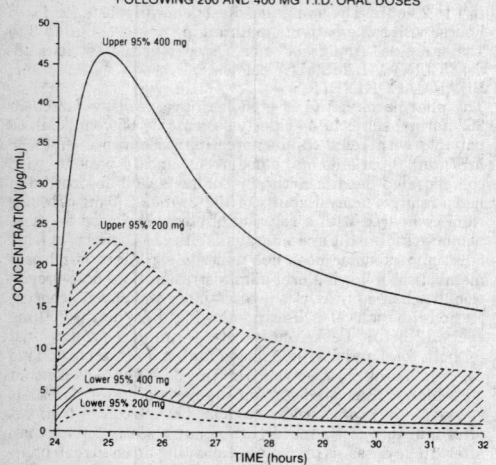

[See table below.]
Etodolac is extensively metabolized in the liver, with renal elimination of etodolac and its metabolites being the primary route of excretion. Approximately 72% of the adminis-

tered dose is recovered in the urine as the following, indicated as % of the administered dose:

—etodolac, unchanged	1%
—etodolac glucuronide	13%
—hydroxylated metabolites (6-, 7- and 8-OH)	5%
—hydroxylated metabolite glucuronides	20%
—unidentified metabolites	33%

Fecal excretion accounted for 16% of the dose. Therefore, enterohepatic circulation, if present, is not extensive.
The extent of absorption of etodolac is not affected when Lodine is administered after a meal or with an antacid. Food intake, however, reduces the peak concentration reached by approximately one half, and increases the time-to-peak concentration by 1.4 to 3.8 hours. Coadministration with antacid decreases the peak concentration reached by about 15 to 20%, with no measurable effect on time-to-peak.
In studies in the elderly, age was found to have no effect on etodolac $t_{1/2}$ or protein binding, and there was no drug accumulation. Etodolac clearance was reduced by about 15%. Because the reduction in clearance is small, no dosage adjustment is generally necessary in the elderly on the basis of pharmacokinetics. The elderly may need dosage adjustment, however, on the basis of body size (see GERIATRIC POPULATION), and they may be more sensitive to antiprostaglandin effects than younger patients (see PRECAUTIONS).
In studies of the effects of mild-to-moderate renal impairment, no significant differences in the disposition of total and free etodolac were observed. In patients undergoing hemodialysis, there was a 50% greater apparent clearance of total etodolac, due to a 50% greater unbound fraction. Free etodolac clearance was not altered, indicating the importance of protein binding in etodolac's disposition. Nevertheless etodolac is not dialyzable. No dosage adjustment of Lodine is generally required in patients with mild-to-moderate renal impairment; however, etodolac should be used with caution in such patients because, as with other NSAIDs, it may further decrease renal function in some patients with impaired renal function (see **PRECAUTIONS**).
In patients with compensated hepatic cirrhosis, the disposition of total and free etodolac is not altered. Although no dosage adjustment is generally required in this patient population, etodolac clearance is dependent on hepatic function and could be reduced in patients with severe hepatic failure.
SPECIAL STUDIES
Lodine was compared with other NSAIDs in inducing gastrointestinal (GI) microbleeding. Lodine 1200 mg/day caused less GI blood loss than ibuprofen 2400 mg/day, indomethacin 200 mg/day, or naproxen 750 mg/day. Lodine was also compared with piroxicam 20 mg/day in two studies; piroxicam caused more blood loss than Lodine in one of these studies but not the other.
Lodine was also compared to other NSAIDs in GI endoscopic studies. Endoscopic scores in studies of 12 healthy subjects following 1 week of Lodine 1200 mg/day showed significantly fewer GI mucosal erosions with Lodine than with aspirin 3900 mg/day. In another study performed in healthy males 18 to 41 years of age, 12 subjects treated with Lodine 1000 mg/day for one week had lower endoscopic scores than 12 subjects treated with indomethacin 200 mg/day, naproxen 1000 mg/day, or ibuprofen 2400 mg/day. Another endoscopic study comparing effects of Lodine 1000 mg/day with piroxicam 20 mg/day, each administered to 12 normal volunteers for one month, yielded equivocal results, with both treatments showing higher scores than the 12-subject placebo-treated group.
The clinical significance of these findings is unknown.

CLINICAL TRIALS
Analgesia
Controlled clinical trials in analgesia were single-dose, randomized, double-blind, parallel studies in 3 pain models (dental extractions, post-general surgery, and post-episiotomy pain). In these studies there were patients treated with placebo, 2 or more doses of etodolac, and varying combinations of aspirin, acetaminophen with codeine (oral surgery only), or zomepirac. The analgesic effective dose for Lodine established in these acute pain models was 200 to 400 mg. The onset of analgesia occurred approximately 30 minutes after oral administration and was comparable for Lodine (200 to 400 mg), aspirin (650 mg), acetaminophen with codeine (600 mg + 60 mg), and zomepirac (100 mg). The peak analgesic effect was between 1 to 2 hours. Duration of relief averaged 4 to 5 hours for 200 mg of Lodine and 5 to 6 hours for 400 mg of Lodine as measured by when approximately half of the patients required remedication. However, in some studies there were still statistically significant differences between the degree of pain relief experienced by patients treated with 200 and 400 mg of Lodine and placebo-treated patients at 8 hours.

Osteoarthritis
The use of Lodine in managing the signs and symptoms of osteoarthritis of the hip or knee was assessed in double-blind, randomized, controlled clinical trials in 341 patients. In patients with osteoarthritis of the knee, Lodine in doses of 600 to 1000 mg/day was better than placebo in 2 studies. The clinical trials in osteoarthritis used b.i.d. dosage regimens. The initial dosing recommendation for Lodine in patients with osteoarthritis is t.i.d. administration, due to etodolac's pharmacokinetic profile (See PHARMACOKINETICS and INDIVIDUALIZATION OF DOSAGE).

Rheumatoid Arthritis
Lodine is not recommended for the treatment of patients with rheumatoid arthritis because in controlled clinical trials, although Lodine treatment was sometimes better than placebo treatment, it was generally not as effective as treatment with other marketed NSAIDs.
INDIVIDUALIZATION OF DOSAGE
Lodine, like other NSAIDs, shows considerable interindividual variation in response. Consequently, the recommended strategy for initiating therapy is to use a starting dose likely to be effective for the majority of patients and to adjust dosage thereafter based on observations of Lodine's beneficial and adverse effects.
The effectiveness of Lodine in otherwise healthy, young to middle-aged adults in acute pain models showed symptom relief to last approximately 5 to 6 hours following single 400 mg doses and 4 to 5 hours following 200 mg doses as judged by the time by which approximately half of the patients needed remediation. In dental extraction studies, hourly comparisons were made of the number of placebo-treated patients versus the number of Lodine-treated patients who needed to be remediated. In these studies, the 200 mg Lodine group had significantly fewer patients who needed remediation up to 6 hours than the placebo group, while the 400 mg Lodine group had significantly fewer patients who required remediation for up to 12 hours.
These results suggest an initial Lodine dose of 400 mg for acute pain followed by doses of 200 to 400 mg every 6 to 8 hours, as needed, not to exceed a maximum total daily dose of 1200 mg. If a patient taking 400 mg doses has adequate pain relief that does not last 8 hours, then 300 mg every 6 hours (q.i.d.) is a reasonable schedule to try. As with all NSAIDs, if symptoms are still not adequately controlled by recommended doses, another analgesic should be tried.
In osteoarthritis, the recommended starting dose of Lodine is 800 to 1200 mg/day in divided doses: 400 mg t.i.d. or b.i.d. or 300 mg q.i.d. or t.i.d. which is derived from pharmacokinetic and single-dose analgesic trial data. In controlled clinical trials in patients with osteoarthritis, total daily doses of 600 to 1000 mg of Lodine were successfully given on a b.i.d. schedule. In one study some patients were apparently adequately treated with as little as 200 mg Lodine b.i.d. The pharmacokinetic profile of Lodine and the results of single-dose analgesia studies suggest, however, that the drug may provide greater benefit when given on a t.i.d. schedule. As with other NSAIDs, the lowest dose and longest dosing interval should be sought for each patient. Therefore, after observing the response to initial therapy with Lodine, the dose and frequency should be adjusted to suit individual patient's needs.
The recommended total daily dose of Lodine is 600 to 1200 mg/day given in divided doses: 400 mg t.i.d. or b.i.d.; 300 mg q.i.d., t.i.d. or b.i.d.; 200 mg q.i.d. or t.i.d..
Total daily doses of Lodine above 20 mg/kg/day have not been studied. Therefore, in patients weighing less than 60 kg (132 lbs), or where the severity of the disease, concomitant medications, or other diseases warrant, the maximum recommended total daily dose of 1200 mg should be reduced. (See **Precautions**)

Table of Etodolac Steady-State Pharmacokinetic Parameters (n=267)

Kinetic Parameters	Scientific Notation (units)	Mean±SD
Extent of oral absorption (bioavailability)	F (%)	≥ 80
Peak concentration time	t_{max} (h)	1.7 ± 1.3
Oral-dose clearance	CL/F (mL/h/kg)	47 ± 16
Central compartment volume	V_c/F (mL/kg)	132 ± 47
Steady-state volume	V_{ss}/F (mL/kg)	362 ± 129
Distribution half-life	$t_{1/2,\alpha}$ (h)	0.71 ± 0.50
Terminal half-life	$t_{1/2,\beta}$ (h)	7.3 ± 4.0

INDICATIONS AND USAGE

Lodine is indicated for acute and long-term use in the management of signs and symptoms of osteoarthritis. Lodine is also indicated for the management of pain.

CONTRAINDICATIONS

Lodine is contraindicated in patients who have previously shown hypersensitivity to it. Lodine should not be given to patients in whom Lodine, aspirin, or ther NSAIDs induce asthma, rhinitis, urticaria, or other allergic reactions. Fatal asthmatic reactions have been reported in such patients receiving NSAIDs.

WARNINGS

RISK OF GASTROINTESTINAL (GI) ULCERATION, BLEEDING, AND PERFORATION WITH NONSTEROIDAL ANTI-INFLAMMATORY DRUG THERAPY

Serious GI toxicity, such as bleeding, ulceration, and perforation, can occur at any time, with or without warning symptoms, in patients treated chronically with NSAIDs. Although minor upper GI problems, such as dyspepsia, are common, usually developing early in therapy, physicians should remain alert for ulceration and bleeding in patients treated chronically with NSAIDs even in the absence of previous GI-tract symptoms. In patients observed in clinical trials of such agents for several months to 2 years' duration, symptomatic upper GI ulcers, gross bleeding, or perforation appear to occur in approximately 1% of patients treated for 3 to 6 months and in about 2% to 4% of patients treated for 1 year. Physicians should inform patients about the signs and/or symptoms of serious GI toxicity and what steps to take if they occur.

Studies to date have not identified any subset of patients not at risk of developing peptic ulceration and bleeding. Except for a prior history of serious GI events and other risk factors known to be associated with peptic ulcer disease, such as alcoholism, smoking, etc., no risk factors (e.g., age, sex) have been associated with increased risk. Elderly or debilitated patients seem to tolerate ulceration or bleeding less well than other individuals, and most spontaneous reports of fatal GI events are in this population. Studies to date are inconclusive concerning the relative risk of various NSAIDs in causing such reactions. High doses of any NSAID probably carry a greater risk of these reactions, although controlled clinical trials showing this do not exist in most cases. In considering the use of relatively large doses (within the recommended dosage range), sufficient benefit should be anticipated to offset the potential increased risk of GI toxicity.

PRECAUTIONS

GENERAL PRECAUTIONS

Renal Effects

As with other NSAIDs, long-term administration of etodolac to rats has resulted in renal papillary necrosis and other renal medullary changes. Renal pelvic transitional epithelial hyperplasia, a spontaneous change occurring with variable frequency, was observed with increased frequency in treated male rats in a 2-year chronic study. The cause-effect relationship to etodolac has not been established.

A second form of renal toxicity encountered with Lodine, as with other NSAIDs, is seen in patients with conditions in which renal prostaglandins have a supportive role in the maintenance of renal perfusion. In these patients, administration of a nonsteroidal anti-inflammatory drug may cause a dose-dependent reduction in prostaglandin formation and, secondarily, in renal blood flow, which may precipitate overt renal decompensation. Patients at greatest risk of this reaction are those with impaired renal function, heart failure, liver dysfunction, those taking diuretics, and the elderly. Discontinuation of nonsteroidal anti-inflammatory drug therapy is usually followed by recovery to the pretreatment state.

Etodolac metabolites are eliminated primarily by the kidneys. The extent to which the inactive glucuronide metabolites may accumulate in patients with renal failure has not been studied. As with other drugs whose metabolites are excreted by the kidney, the possibility that adverse reactions (not listed in **ADVERSE REACTIONS**) may be attributable to these metabolites should be considered.

Hepatic Effects

As with all NSAIDs, borderline elevations of one or more liver tests may occur in up to 15% of patients. These abnormalities may disappear, remain essentially unchanged, or progress with continued therapy. Meaningful elevations of ALT or AST (approximately three or more times the upper limit of normal) have been reported in approxiamtely 1% of patients in clinical trials with Lodine. A patient with symptoms and/or signs suggesting liver dysfunction, or in whom an abnormal liver test has occurred, should be evaluated for evidence of the development of a more severe hepatic reaction while on therapy with Lodine. Although such reactions are rare, if abnormal liver tests persist or worsen, if clinical signs and symptoms consistent with liver disease develop, or if systemic manifestations occur (e.g., eosinophilia, rash, etc.), Lodine should be discontinued.

Hematological Effect

Anemia is sometimes seen in patients receiving Lodine or other NSAIDs. This may be due to fluid retention, gastrointestinal blood loss, or an incompletely described effect upon erythropoiesis. Patients on long-term treatment with NSAIDs, including Lodine, should have their hemoglobin or hematocrit checked if they develop signs or symptoms of anemia.

All drugs which inhibit the biosynthesis of prostaglandins may interfere to some extent with platelet function and vascular responses to bleeding. Patients receiving Lodine who may be adversely affected by such actions should be carefully observed.

Fluid Retention and Edema

Fluid retention and edema have been observed in some patients taking Lodine. Therefore, as with other NSAIDs, Lodine should be used with caution in patients with fluid retention, hypertension, or heart failure.

Information for Patients

Lodine, like other NSAIDs (Nonsteroidal Anti-inflammatory Drugs), is not free of side effects. The side effects of these drugs can cause discomfort and, rarely, there may be serious side effects, such as GI bleeding, that may result in hospitalization and even fatal outcomes.

NSAIDs are often essential agents in the management of arthritis and have a major role in the treatment of pain, but they also may be commonly employed for conditions that are less serious.

Physicians may wish to discuss with their patients the potential risks (see **WARNINGS, PRECAUTIONS,** and **ADVERSE REACTIONS** sections) and likely benefits of Lodine treatment, particularly when it may be used for less serious conditions in which treatment without Lodine may represent an acceptable alternative to both the patient and physician.

LABORATORY TESTS

Because serious GI-tract ulceration and bleeding can occur without warning symptoms, physicians should observe chronically treated patients for the signs and symptoms of ulceration and bleeding and should inform them of the importance of this follow-up (see "RISK OF GI ULCERATIONS, BLEEDING, AND PERFORATION WITH NSAID THERAPY").

DRUG INTERACTIONS

Antacids

The concomitant administration of antacids has no apparent effect on the extent of absorption of Lodine. However, antacids can decrease the peak concentration reached by 15 to 20% but have no detectable effect on the time-to-peak.

Aspirin

When Lodine is administered with aspirin, its protein binding is reduced, although the clearance of free etodolac is not altered. The clinical significance of this interaction is not known; however, as with other NSAIDs, concomitant administration of Lodine and aspirin is not generally recommended because of the potential of increased adverse effects.

Warfarin

Concomitant administration of warfarin and Lodine results in reduced protein binding warfarin, but there is no change in the clearance of free warfarin. There is no significant difference in the pharmacodynamic effect of warfarin administered alone and warfarin administered with Lodine as measured by prothrombin time. Thus, concomitant therapy with warfarin and Lodine should not require dosage adjustment of either drug. Caution should be exercised, nevertheless, because interactions have been seen with other NSAIDs.

Phenytoin

Lodine has no apparent pharmacokinetic interaction when administered with phenytoin.

Glyburide

Lodine has no apparent pharmacokinetic or pharmacodynamic interaction when administered with glyburide.

Diuretics

Lodine has no apparent pharmacokinetic interaction when administered with furosemide or hydrochlorothiazide; nor does Lodine attenuate the diuretic response of either of these drugs in normal volunteers. Lodine, and other NSAIDs, nevertheless, should be used with caution in patients receiving diuretics, who have cardiac, renal, or hepatic failure (see *Renal Effects*).

Cyclosporine, Digoxin, Lithium, Methotrexate

Lodine, like other NSAIDs, through effects on renal prostaglandins, may cause changes in the elimination of these drugs leading to elevated serum levels of digoxin, lithium, and methotrexate and increased toxicity. Nephrotoxicity associated with cyclosporine may also be enhanced. Patients receiving these drugs who are given Lodine, or any other NSAID, and particularly those patients with altered renal function, should be observed for the development of the specific toxicities of these drugs.

Protein Binding

Data from *in vitro* studies, using peak serum concentrations at reported therapeutic doses in humans, show that the etodolac free fraction is not significantly altered by acetaminophen, ibuprofen, indomethacin, naproxen, piroxicam, chlorpropamide, glipizide, glyburide, phenytoin, and probenecid. In contrast, phenylbutazone causes an increase (by about 80%) in the free fraction of etodolac. Although *in vivo* studies have not been done to see if etodolac clearance is changed by coadministration of phenylbutazone, it is not recommended that they be coadministered.

DRUG/LABORATORY TEST INTERACTIONS

The urine of patients who take Lodine can give a false-positive reaction for urinary bilirubin (urobilin) due to the presence of phenolic metabolites of etodolac.

Diagnostic dip-stick methodology, used to detect ketone bodies in urine, has resulted in false-positive findings in some patients treated with Lodine. Generally, this phenomenon has not been associated with other clinically significant events. No dose-relationship has been observed.

Lodine treatment is associated with a small decrease in serum uric acid levels. In clinical trials, mean decreases of 1–2 mg/dL were observed in arthritic patients receiving etodolac (600 mg to 1000 mg/day) after 4 weeks of therapy. These levels then remained stable for up to one year of therapy.

CARCINOGENESIS, MUTAGENESIS, AND IMPAIRMENT OF FERTILITY

No carcinogenic effect of etodolac was observed in mice or rats receiving oral doses of 15 mg/kg/day (45 to 89 mg/m^2, respectively) or less for periods of 2 years or 18 months, respectively. Etodolac was not mutagenic in *in vitro* tests performed with *S.* typhimurium and mouse lymphoma cells as well as in an *in vivo* mouse micronucleus test. However, data from the *in vitro* human peripheral lymphocyte test showed an increase ($p = 0.06$) in the number of gaps (3.0 to 5.3% unstained regions in the chromatid without dislocation) among the Lodine-treated cultures (50 to 200 μg/mL) compared to negative controls (2.0%); no other difference was noted between the controls and drug-treated groups. Etodolac showed no impairment of fertility in male and female rats up to oral doses of 16 mg/kg (94 mg/m^2). However, reduced implantation of fertilized eggs occurred in the 8 mg/kg group.

TERATOGENIC EFFECTS: PREGNANCY CATEGORY C

In teratology studies, isolated occurrences of alterations in limb development were found and included polydactyly, oligodactyly, syndactyly, and unossified phalanges in rats and oligodactyly and synostosis of metatarsals in rabbits. These were observed at dose levels (2 to 14 mg/kg/day) close to human clinical doses. However, the frequency and the dosage group distribution of these findings in initial or repeated studies did not establish a clear drug or dose-response relationship.

There are no adequate or well-controlled studies in pregnant women. Lodine should be used during pregnancy only if the potential benefits justifies the potential risk of the fetus. Because of the known effects of NSAIDs on parturition and on the human fetal cardiovascular system with respect to closure of the ductus arteriosus, use during late pregnancy should be avoided.

LABOR AND DELIVERY

In rat studies with etodolac, as with other drugs known to inhibit prostaglandin synthesis, an increased incidence of dystocia, delayed parturition, and decreased pup survival occurred. The effects of Lodine on labor and delivery in pregnant women are unknown.

NURSING MOTHERS

Caution should be exercised if Lodine is administered to a nursing woman, because many drugs are excreted in human milk. It is not known whether etodolac is excreted in human milk.

PEDIATRIC USE

Safety and effectiveness in children have not been established.

GERIATRIC POPULATION

In patients 65 years and older, no substantial differences in the pharmacokinetics or the side-effect profile of Lodine were seen compared with the general population. Therefore, no dosage adjustment is generally necessary in the elderly. As with any NSAID, however, caution should be exercised in treating the elderly, and when individualizing their dosage, extra care should be taken when increasing the dose because the elderly seem to tolerate NSAID side effects less well than younger patients. (See PHARMACOKINETICS)

ADVERSE REACTIONS

Adverse-reaction information for Lodine was derived from 2,629 arthritic patients treated with Lodine in double-blind and open-label clinical trials of 4 to 320 weeks in duration and worldwide postmarketing surveillance studies in approximately 60,000 patients.

In clinical trials, most adverse reactions were mild and transient. The discontinuation rate in controlled clinical trials, because of adverse events, was 9% for patients treated with Lodine.

New patient complaints (with an incidence greater than or equal to 1%) are listed below by body system. The incidences were determined from clinical trials involving 465 patients

Continued on next page

Wyeth-Ayerst Laboratories—Cont.

with osteoarthritis treated with 300 to 500 mg of Lodine b.i.d. (i.e., 600 to 1000 mg per day).

INCIDENCE GREATER THAN OR EQUAL TO 1%—PROBABLY CAUSALLY RELATED.

Body as a whole—Chills and fever.

Digestive system—Dyspepsia (10%), abdominal pain*, diarrhea*, flatulence*, nausea*, constipation, gastritis, melena, vomiting.

Nervous system—Asthenia/malaise*, dizziness*, depression, nervousness.

Skin and appendages—Pruritus, rash.

Special senses—Blurred vision, tinnitus.

Urogenital system—Dysuria, urinary frequency.

INCIDENCE LESS THAN 1%—PROBABLY CAUSALLY RELATED (Adverse reactions reported only in worldwide postmarketing experience, not seen in clinical trials, are considered rarer and are italicized.):

Cardiovascular system—Hypertension, congestive heart failure, flushing, palpitations, syncope.

Digestive system—Thirst, dry mouth, ulcerative stomatitis, anorexia, eructation, elevated liver enzymes, hepatitis, *jaundice*, PUB, i.e., peptic ulcer with or without bleeding and/or perforation.

Hemic and lymphatic system—Ecchymosis, anemia, thrombocytopenia, bleeding time increased.

Metabolic and nutritional—Edema, serum creatinine increase.

Nervous system—Insomnia, somnolence.

Respiratory system—Asthma.

Skin and appendages—Angioedema, sweating, urticaria, vesiculobullous rash, *cutaneous vasculitis with purpura, Stevens-Johnson Syndrome,* hyperpigmentation.

Special senses—Photophobia, transient visual disturbances.

INCIDENCE LESS THAN 1%—CAUSAL RELATIONSHIP UNKNOWN (Medical events occurring under circumstances where causal relationship to Lodine is uncertain. These reactions are listed as alerting information for physicians):

Body as a whole—Infection.

Cardiovascular system—Arrhythmias, myocardial infarction.

Digestive system—Esophagitis with or without stricture or cardiospasm, colitis.

Hemic and lympathic system—Leukopenia.

Metabolic and nutritional—Change in weight.

Nervous system—Paresthesia, confusion.

Respiratory system—Bronchitis, dyspnea, pharyngitis, rhinitis, sinusitis.

Skin and appendages—Maculopapular rash, alopecia, skin peeling, photosensitivity.

Special senses—Conjunctivitis, deafness, taste perversion.

Urogenital system—Cystitis, hematuria, leukorrhea, renal calculus, interstitial nephritis, uterine bleeding irregularities.

DRUG ABUSE AND DEPENDENCE

Lodine is a non-narcotic drug. Several predictive animal studies indicated that Lodine has no addiction potential in humans.

OVERDOSAGE

Symptoms following acute NSAID overdose are usually limited to lethargy, drowsiness, nausea, vomiting, and epigastric pain which are generally reversible with supportive care. Gastrointestinal bleeding can occur and coma has occurred following massive ibuprofen or mefenamic-acid overdose. Hypertension, acute renal failure, and respiratory depression may occur but are rare. Anaphylactoid reactions have been reported with therapeutic ingestion of NSAIDs, and may occur following overdose.

Patients should be managed by symptomatic and supportive care following an NSAID overdose. There are no specific antidotes. Gut decontamination may be indicated in patients seen within 4 hours of ingestion with symptoms or following a large overdose (5 to 10 times the usual dose). This should be accomplished via emesis and/or activated charcoal (60 to 100 g in adults, 1 to 2 g/kg in children) with an osmotic cathartic. Forced diuresis, alkalinization of the urine, hemodialysis or hemoperfusion would probably not be useful due to etodolac's high protein binding.

One case of intentional etodolac overdosage has been reported (Human Toxicol. 1988; 7:203–4). This 53-year-old female ingested from 15 to 46 two-hundred mg etodolac capsules (3 to 8.6 grams). Plasma etodolac concentrations were measured frequently over the next 4 days. At 5 hours after ingestion (3 hours after gastric lavage) the plasma etodolac level was 22 μg/mL. These plasma levels and her subsequent recovery with no signs or symptoms of etodolac toxicity were consistent with systemic absorption of 600 to 800 mg. Her laboratory tests on admission showed a prolonged prothrombin time and a false-positive urine bilirubin (attributed to the phenolic etodolac metabolites).

*Drug-related patient complaints occurring in 3 to 9% of patients treated with Lodine. Drug-related patient complaints occurring in fewer than 3%, but more than 1%, are unmarked.

DOSAGE AND ADMINISTRATION

ANALGESIA

The recommended dose of Lodine for acute pain is 200 to 400 mg every 6 to 8 hours, as needed, not to exceed a total daily dose of 1200 mg. For patients weighing 60 kg or less, the total daily dose of Lodine should not exceed 20 mg/kg. For more details see INDIVIDUALIZATION OF DOSAGE.

OSTEOARTHRITIS

The recommended dose of Lodine for the management of the signs and symptoms of osteoarthritis is initially 800 to 1200 mg/day in divided doses, followed by dosage adjustment within the range of 600 to 1200 mg/day given in divided doses: 400 mg t.i.d. or b.i.d.; 300 mg q.i.d., t.i.d., or b.i.d.; 200 mg q.i.d. or t.i.d.. The total daily dose of Lodine should not exceed 1200 mg. For patients weighing 60 kg or less, the total daily dose of Lodine should not exceed 20 mg/kg. For more details see INDIVIDUALIZATION OF DOSAGE.

HOW SUPPLIED

Lodine (etodolac) is available as:

LODINE® (etodolac) Capsules:

200 mg capsules (light gray with one wide red band with LODINE 200/dark gray with two narrow red bands)

—in bottles of 100, NDC 0046-0738-81

—in unit-dose packages of 100, NDC 0046-0738-99

300 mg capsules (light gray with one wide red band with LODINE 300/light gray with two narrow red bands)

—in bottles of 100, NDC 0046-0739-81

—in unit-dose packages of 100, NDC 0046-0739-99

CAPSULES IN BOTTLES

Store at 15°–30°C (59°–86°F), protected from moisture.

CAPSULES IN UNIT-DOSE PACKAGES

Store at 15°–25°C (59°–77°F), protected from moisture. For institutional use only.

The appearance of these capsules is a trademark of WYETH-AYERST LABORATORIES, Philadelphia, PA.

Caution: Federal law prohibits dispensing without a prescription.

Shown in Product Identification Section, page 437

LO/OVRAL® ℞

[lōh-ōh 'vral]

Tablets

(norgestrel and ethinyl estradiol tablets)

DESCRIPTION

Each LO/OVRAL tablet contains 0.3 mg of norgestrel (*dl* -13-beta-ethyl -17- alpha-ethinyl -17- beta-hydroxygon- 4- en-3-one), a totally synthetic progestogen, and 0.03 mg of ethinyl estradiol (19-nor-17α-pregna-1,3,5 (10)-trien-20-yne-3,17-diol). The inactive ingredients present are cellulose, lactose, magnesium stearate, and polacrilin potassium.

CLINICAL PHARMACOLOGY

Combination oral contraceptives act by suppression of gonadotropins. Although the primary mechanism of this action is inhibition of ovulation, other alterations include changes in the cervical mucus (which increase the difficulty of sperm entry into the uterus) and the endometrium (which reduce the likelihood of implantation).

INDICATIONS AND USAGE

Oral contraceptives are indicated for the prevention of pregnancy in women who elect to use this product as a method of contraception.

Oral contraceptives are highly effective. Table I lists the typical accidental pregnancy rates for users of combination oral contraceptives and other methods of contraception. The efficacy of these contraceptive methods, except sterilization and the IUD, depends upon the reliability with which they are used. Correct and consistent use of methods can result in lower failure rates.

CONTRAINDICATIONS

Oral contraceptives should not be used in women with any of the following conditions:

Thrombophlebitis or thromboembolic disorders

A past history of deep-vein thrombophlebitis or thromboembolic disorders

Cerebral-vascular or coronary-artery disease

Known or suspected carcinoma of the breast

Carcinoma of the endometrium or other known or suspected estrogen-dependent neoplasia

Undiagnosed abnormal genital bleeding

Cholestatic jaundice of pregnancy or jaundice with prior pill use

Hepatic adenomas or carcinomas

Known or suspected pregnancy

WARNINGS

Cigarette smoking increases the risk of serious cardiovascular side effects from oral-contraceptive use. This risk increases with age and with heavy smoking (15 or more cigarettes per day) and is quite marked in women over 35 years of age. Women who use oral contraceptives should be strongly advised not to smoke.

The use of oral contraceptives is associated with increased risks of several serious conditions including myocardial infarction, thromboembolism, stroke, hepatic neoplasia, gallbladder disease, and hypertension, although the risk of serious morbidity or mortality is very small in healthy women without underlying factors. The risk of morbidity and mortality increases significantly in the presence of other underlying risk factors such as hypertension, hyperlipidemias, obesity, and diabetes.

Practitioners prescribing oral contraceptives should be familiar with the following information relating to these risks.

The information contained in this package insert is based principally on studies carried out in patients who used oral contraceptives with higher formulations of estrogens and progestogens than those in common use today. The effect of long-term use of the oral contraceptives with lower formulations of both estrogens and progestogens remains to be determined.

Throughout this labeling, epidemiological studies reported are of two types: retrospective or case control studies and prospective or cohort studies. Case control studies provide a measure of the relative risk of disease, namely, a ratio of the incidence of a disease among oral-contraceptive users to that among nonusers. The relative risk does not provide information on the actual clinical occurrence of a disease. Cohort studies provide a measure of attributable risk, which is the difference in the incidence of disease between oral-contraceptive users and nonusers. The attributable risk does provide information about the actual occurrence of a disease in the population. For further information, the reader is referred to a text on epidemiological methods.

1. THROMBOEMBOLIC DISORDERS AND OTHER VASCULAR PROBLEMS

a. *Myocardial Infarction*

An increased risk of myocardial infarction has been attributed to oral-contraceptive use. This risk is primarily in smokers or women with other underlying risk factors for coronary-artery disease such as hypertension, hypercholesterolemia, morbid obesity, and diabetes. The relative risk of heart attack for current oral-contraceptive users has been estimated to be two to six. The risk is very low under the age of 30.

TABLE I: LOWEST EXPECTED AND TYPICAL FAILURE RATES DURING THE FIRST YEAR OF CONTINUOUS USE OF A METHOD

% of Women Experiencing an Accidental Pregnancy in the First Year of Continuous Use

Method	Lowest Expected*	Typical**
(No Contraception)	(89)	(89)
Oral contraceptives		3
combined	0.1	N/A***
progestin only	0.5	N/A***
Diaphragm with spermicidal cream or jelly	3	18
Spermicides alone (foam, creams, jellies and vaginal suppositories)	3	21
Vaginal Sponge		
nulliparous	5	18
multiparous	>8	>28
IUD (medicated)	1	6#
Condom without spermicides	2	12
Periodic abstinence (all methods)	2–10	20
Female sterilization	0.2	0.4
Male sterilization	0.1	0.15

Adapted from J. Trussell and K. Kost, Table 11, Studies in Family Planning, 18(5), Sept.–Oct. 1987.

* The authors' best guess of the percentage of women expected to experience an accidental pregnancy among couples who initiate a method (not necessarily for the first time) and who use it consistently and correctly during the first year if they do not stop for any other reason.

** This term represents "typical" couples who initiate use of a method (not necessarily for the first time), who experience an accidental pregnancy during the first year if they do not stop use for any other reason.

*** N/A—Data not available.

\# Combined typical rate for both medicated and non-medicated IUD. The rate for medicated IUD alone is not available.

Smoking in combination with oral contraceptive use has been shown to contribute substantially to the incidence of myocardial infarctions in women in their mid-thirties or older with smoking accounting for the majority of excess cases. Mortality rates associated with circulatory disease have been shown to increase substantially in smokers over the age of 35 and nonsmokers over the age of 40 (Table II) among women who use oral contraceptives.

CIRCULATORY DISEASE MORTALITY RATES PER 100,000 WOMAN YEARS BY AGE, SMOKING STATUS AND ORAL-CONTRACEPTIVE USE

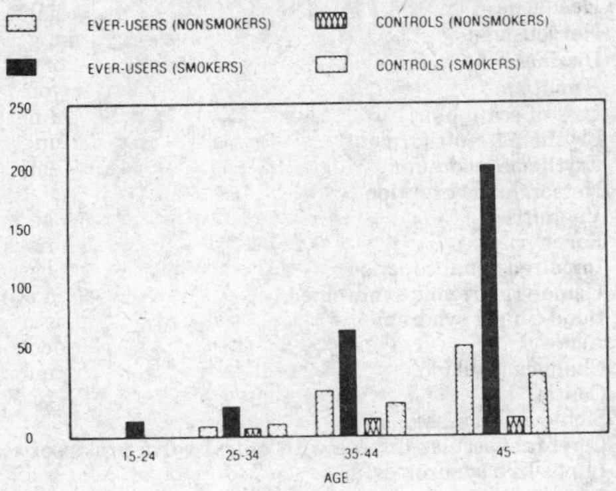

TABLE II. (Adapted from P.M. Layde and V. Beral, Lancet. 1:541–546, 1981.)

Oral contraceptives may compound the effects of well-known risk factors, such as hypertension, diabetes, hyperlipidemias, age, and obesity. In particular, some progestogens are known to decrease HDL cholesterol and cause glucose intolerance, while estrogens may create a state of hyperinsulinism. Oral contraceptives have been shown to increase blood pressure among users (see section 9 in Warnings). Similar effects on risk factors have been associated with an increased risk of heart disease. Oral contraceptives must be used with caution in women with cardiovascular disease risk factors.

b. *Thromboembolism*

An increased risk of thromboembolic and thrombotic disease associated with the use of oral contraceptives is well established. Case control studies have found the relative risk of users compared to nonusers to be 3 for the first episode of superficial venous thrombosis, 4 to 11 for deep vein thrombosis or pulmonary embolism, and 1.5 to 6 for women with predisposing conditions for venous thromboembolic disease. Cohort studies have shown the relative risk to be somewhat lower, about 3 for new cases and about 4.5 for new cases requiring hospitalization. The risk of thromboembolic disease due to oral contraceptives is not related to length of use and disappears after pill use is stopped.

A two- to four-fold increase in relative risk of postoperative thromboembolic complications has been reported with the use of oral contraceptives. The relative risk of venous thrombosis in women who have predisposing conditions is twice that of women without such medical conditions. If feasible, oral contraceptives should be discontinued at least four weeks prior to and for two weeks after elective surgery of a type associated with an increase in risk of thromboembolism and during and following prolonged immobilization. Since the immediate postpartum period is also associated with an increased risk of thromboembolism, oral contraceptives should be started no earlier than four to six weeks after delivery in women who elect not to breast-feed, or a midtrimester pregnancy termination.

c. *Cerebrovascular diseases*

Oral contraceptives have been shown to increase both the relative and attributable risks of cerebrovascular events (thrombotic and hemorrhagic strokes), although, in general, the risk is greatest among older (>35 years), hypertensive women who also smoke. Hypertension was found to be a risk factor for both users and nonusers, for both types of strokes, while smoking interacted to increase the risk for hemorrhagic strokes.

In a large study, the relative risk of thrombotic strokes has been shown to range from 3 for normotensive users to 14 for users with severe hypertension. The relative risk of hemorrhagic stroke is reported to be 1.2 for nonsmokers who used oral contraceptives, 2.6 for smokers who did not use oral contraceptives, 7.6 for smokers who used oral contraceptives, 1.8 for normotensive users, and 25.7 for users with severe hypertension. The attributable risk is also greater in older women.

d. *Dose-related risk of vascular disease from oral contraceptives*

A positive association has been observed between the amount of estrogen and progestogen in oral contraceptives and the risk of vascular disease. A decline in serum high-density lipoproteins (HDL) has been reported with many progestational agents. A decline in serum high-density lipoproteins has been associated with an increased incidence of ischemic heart disease. Because estrogens increase HDL cholesterol, the net effect of an oral contraceptive depends on a balance achieved between doses of estrogen and progestogen and the nature and absolute amount of progestogen used in the contraceptive. The amount of both hormones should be considered in the choice of an oral contraceptive.

Minimizing exposure to estrogen and progestogen is in keeping with good principles of therapeutics. For any particular estrogen/progestogen combination, the dosage regimen prescribed should be one which contains the least amount of estrogen and progestogen that is compatible with a low failure rate and the needs of the individual patient. New acceptors of oral-contraceptive agents should be started on preparations containing less than 50 mcg of estrogen.

e. *Persistence of risk of vascular disease*

There are two studies which have shown persistence of risk of vascular disease for ever-users of oral contraceptives. In a study in the United States, the risk of developing myocardial infarction after discontinuing oral contraceptives persists for at least 9 years for women 40 to 49 years who had used oral contraceptives for five or more years, but this increased risk was not demonstrated in other age groups. In another study in Great Britain, the risk of developing cerebrovascular disease persisted for at least 6 years after discontinuation of oral contraceptives, although excess risk was very small. However, both studies were performed with oral-contraceptive formulations containing 50 micrograms or higher of estrogens.

TABLE III—ANNUAL NUMBER OF BIRTH-RELATED OR METHOD-RELATED DEATHS ASSOCIATED WITH CONTROL OF FERTILITY PER 100,000 NONSTERILE WOMEN, BY FERTILITY-CONTROL METHOD ACCORDING TO AGE

Method of control and outcome	15–19	20–24	25–29	30–34	35–39	40–44
No fertility-control methods*	7.0	7.4	9.1	14.8	25.7	28.2
Oral contraceptives non-smoker**	0.3	0.5	0.9	1.9	13.8	31.6
Oral contraceptives smoker**	2.2	3.4	6.6	13.5	51.1	117.2
IUD**	0.8	0.8	1.0	1.0	1.4	1.4
Condom*	1.1	1.6	0.7	0.2	0.3	0.4
Diaphragm/spermicide*	1.9	1.2	1.2	1.3	2.2	2.8
Periodic abstinence*	2.5	1.6	1.6	1.7	2.9	3.6

* Deaths are birth related
** Deaths are method related

Adapted from H.W. Ory, Family Planning Perspectives, 15:57–63, 1983.

2. ESTIMATES OF MORTALITY FROM CONTRACEPTIVE USE

One study gathered data from a variety of sources which have estimated the mortality rate associated with different methods of contraception at different ages (Table III). These estimates include the combined risk of death associated with contraceptive methods plus the risk attributable to pregnancy in the event of method failure. Each method of contraception has its specific benefits and risks. The study concluded that with the exception of oral-contraceptive users 35 and older who smoke and 40 and older who do not smoke, mortality associated with all methods of birth control is less than that associated with childbirth. The observation of a possible increase in risk of mortality with age for oral-contraceptive users is based on data gathered in the 1970's—but not reported until 1983. However, current clinical practice involves the use of lower estrogen dose formulations combined with careful restriction of oral contraceptive use to women who do not have the various risk factors listed in this labeling.

Because of these changes in practice and, also, because of some limited new data which suggest that the risk of cardiovascular disease with the use of oral contraceptives may now be less than previously observed, the Fertility and Maternal Health Drugs Advisory Committee was asked to review the topic in 1989. The Committee concluded that although cardiovascular disease risks may be increased with oral-contraceptive use after age 40 in healthy nonsmoking women (even with the newer low-dose formulations), there are greater potential health risks associated with pregnancy in older women and with the alternative surgical and medical procedures which may be necessary if such women do not have access to effective and acceptable means of contraception.

Therefore, the Committee recommended that the benefits of oral-contraceptive use by healthy nonsmoking women over 40 may outweigh the possible risks. Of course, older women, as all women who take oral contraceptives, should take the lowest possible dose formulation that is effective.

3. CARCINOMA OF THE REPRODUCTIVE ORGANS

Numerous epidemiological studies have been performed on the incidence of breast, endometrial, ovarian, and cervical cancer in women using oral contraceptives. The overwhelming evidence in the literature suggests that use of oral contraceptives is not associated with an increase in the risk of developing breast cancer, regardless of the age and parity of first use or with most of the marketed brands and doses. The Cancer amd Steroid Hormone (CASH) study also showed no latent effect on the risk of breast cancer for at least a decade following long-term use. A few studies have shown a slightly increased relative risk of developong breast cancer, although the methodology of these studies, which included differences in examination of users and nonusers and differences in age at start of use, has been questioned.

Some studies suggest that oral-contraceptive use has been associated with an increase in the risk of cervical intraepithelial neoplasia in some populations of women. However, there continues to be controversy about the extent to which such findings may be due to differences in sexual behavior and other factors.

In spite of many studies of the relationship between oral-contraceptive use and breast and cervical cancers, a cause-and-effect relationship has not been established.

4. HEPATIC NEOPLASIA

Benign hepatic adenomas are associated with oral-contraceptive use, although the incidence of benign tumors is rare in the United States. Indirect calculations have estimated the attributable risk to be in the range of 3.3 cases/100,000 for users, a risk that increases after four or more years of use. Rupture of rare, benign, hepatic adenomas may cause death through intra-abdominal hemorrhage.

Studies from Britain have shown an increased risk of developing hepatocellular carcinoma in long-term (>8 years) oral-contraceptive users. However, these cancers are extremely rare in the U.S., and the attributable risk (the excess incidence) of liver cancers in oral contraceptive users approaches less than one per million users.

5. OCULAR LESIONS

There have been clincial case reports of retinal thrombosis associated with the use of oral contraceptives. Oral contraceptives should be discontinued if there is unexplained partial or complete loss of vision; onset of proptosis or diplopia; papilledema; or retinal vascular lesions. Appropriate diagnostic and therapeutic measures should be undertaken immediately.

6. ORAL-CONTRACEPTIVE USE BEFORE OR DURING EARLY PREGNANCY

Extensive epidemiological studies have revealed no increased risk of birth defects in women who have used oral contraceptives prior to pregnancy. Studies also do not suggest a teratogenic effect, particularly insofar as cardiac anomalies and limb reduction defects are concerned, when taken inadvertently during early pregnancy.

The administration of oral contraceptives to induce withdrawal bleeding should not be used as a test for pregnancy. Oral contraceptives should not be used during pregnancy to treat threatened or habitual abortion.

It is recommended that for any patient who has missed two consecutive periods, pregnancy should be ruled out before continuing oral contraceptive use. If the patient has not adhered to the prescribed schedule, the possibility of pregnancy should be considered at the time of the first missed period. Oral contraceptive use should be discontinued if pregnancy is confirmed.

7. GALLBLADDER DISEASE

Earlier studies have reported an increased lifetime relative risk of gallbladder surgery in users of oral contraceptives and estrogens. More recent studies, however, have shown that the relative risk of developing gallbladder disease among oral-contraceptive users may be minimal. The recent findings of minimal risk may be related to the use of oral-contraceptive formulations containing lower hormonal doses of estrogens and progestogens.

Continued on next page

Wyeth-Ayerst Laboratories—Cont.

8. CARBOHYDRATE AND LIPID METABOLIC EFFECTS

Oral contraceptives have been shown to cause glucose intolerance in a significant percentage of users. Oral contraceptives containing greater than 75 micrograms of estrogens cause hyperinsulinism, while lower doses of estrogen cause less glucose intolerance. Progestogens increase insulin secretion and create insulin resistance, this effect varying with different progestational agents. However, in the nondiabetic woman, oral contraceptives appear to have no effect on fasting blood glucose. Because of these demonstrated effects, prediabetic and diabetic women should be carefully observed while taking oral contraceptives.

A small proportion of women will have persistent hypertriglyceridemia while on the pill. As discussed earlier (see Warnings, 1a and 1d), changes in serum triglycerides and lipoprotein levels have been reported in oral-contraceptive users.

9. ELEVATED BLOOD PRESSURE

An increase in blood pressure has been reported in women taking oral contraceptives, and this increase is more likely in older oral-contraceptive users and with continued use. Data from the Royal College of General Practitioners and subsequent randomized trials have shown that the incidence of hypertension increases with increasing quantities of progestogens.

Women with a history of hypertension or hypertension-related diseases, or renal disease, should be encouraged to use another method of contraception. If women with hypertension elect to use oral contraceptives, they should be monitored closely, and if significant elevation of blood pressure occurs, oral contraceptives should be discontinued. For most women, elevated blood pressure will return to normal after stopping oral contraceptives, and there is no difference in the occurrence of hypertension among ever- and never-users.

10. HEADACHE

The onset or exacerbation of migraine or development of headache with a new pattern that is recurrent, persistent, or severe requires discontinuation of oral contraceptives and evaluation of the cause.

11. BLEEDING IRREGULARITIES

Breakthrough bleeding and spotting are sometimes encountered in patients on oral contraceptives, especially during the first three months of use. The type and dose of progestogen may be important. Non-hormonal causes should be considered and adequate diagnostic measures taken to rule out malignancy or pregnancy in the event of breakthrough bleeding, as in the case of any abnormal vaginal bleeding. If pathology has been excluded, time or a change to another formulation may solve the problem. In the event of amenorrhea, pregnancy should be ruled out.

Some women may encounter post-pill amenorrhea or oligomenorrhea, especially when such a condition was preexistent.

PRECAUTIONS

1. PHYSICAL EXAMINATION AND FOLLOW-UP

A complete medical history and physical examination should be taken prior to the initiation or reinstitution of oral contraceptives and at least annually during use of oral contraceptives. These physical examinations should include special reference to blood pressure, breasts, abdomen and pelvic organs, including cervical cytology, and relevant laboratory tests. In case of undiagnosed, persistent or recurrent abnormal vaginal bleeding, appropriate diagnostic measures should be conducted to rule out malignancy. Women with a strong family history of breast cancer or who have breast nodules should be monitored with particular care.

2. LIPID DISORDERS

Women who are being treated for hyperlipidemias should be followed closely if they elect to use oral contraceptives. Some progestogens may elevate LDL levels and may render the control of hyperlipidemias more difficult. (See Warnings, 1d.).

3. LIVER FUNCTION

If jaundice develops in any woman receiving such drugs, the medication should be discontinued. Steroid hormones may be poorly metabolized in patients with impaired liver function.

4. FLUID RETENTION

Oral contraceptives may cause some degree of fluid retention. They should be prescribed with caution, and only with careful monitoring, in patients with conditions which might be aggravated by fluid retention.

5. EMOTIONAL DISORDERS

Patients becoming significantly depressed while taking oral contraceptives should stop the medication and use an alternate method of contraception in an attempt to determine whether the symptom is drug related. Women with a history of depression should be carefully observed and the drug discontinued if depression recurs to a serious degree.

6. CONTACT LENSES

Contact lens wearers who develop visual changes or changes in lens tolerance should be assessed by an ophthalmologist.

7. DRUG INTERACTIONS

Reduced efficacy and increased incidence of breakthrough bleeding and menstrual irregularities have been associated with concomitant use of rifampin. A similar association, though less marked, has been suggested with barbiturates, phenylbutazone, phenytoin sodium, and possibly with griseofulvin, ampicillin, and tetracyclines.

8. INTERACTIONS WITH LABORATORY TESTS

Certain endocrine- and liver-function tests and blood components may be affected by oral contraceptives:

a. Increased prothrombin and factors VII, VIII, IX, and X; decreased antithrombin 3; increased norepinephrine-induced platelet aggregability.

b. Increased thyroid-binding globulin (TBG) leading to increased circulating total thyroid hormone, as measured by protein-bound iodine (PBI), T4 by column or by radioimmunoassay. Free T3 resin uptake is decreased, reflecting the elevated TBG; free T4 concentration is unaltered.

c. Other binding proteins may be elevated in serum.

d. Sex-binding globulins are increased and result in elevated levels of total circulating sex steroids and corticoids; however, free or biologically active levels remain unchanged.

e. Triglycerides may be increased.

f. Glucose tolerance may be decreased.

g. Serum folate levels may be depressed by oral-contraceptive therapy. This may be of clinical significance if a woman becomes pregnant shortly after discontinuing oral contraceptives.

9. CARCINOGENESIS

See "Warnings" section.

10. PREGNANCY

Pregnancy Category X. See "Contraindications" and "Warnings" sections.

11. NURSING MOTHERS

Small amounts of oral-contraceptive steroids have been identified in the milk of nursing mothers, and a few adverse effects on the child have been reported, including jaundice and breast enlargement. In addition, oral contraceptives given in the postpartum period may interfere with lactation by decreasing the quantity and quality of breast milk. If possible, the nursing mother should be advised not to use oral contraceptives but to use other forms of contraception until she has completely weaned her child.

INFORMATION FOR THE PATIENT

See Patient Labeling Printed Below.

ADVERSE REACTIONS

An increased risk of the following serious adverse reactions has been associated with the use of oral contraceptives (see "Warnings"section):

Thrombophlebitis.
Arterial thromboembolism.
Pulmonary embolism.
Myocardial infarction.
Cerebral hemorrhage.
Cerebral thrombosis.
Hypertension.
Gallbladder disease.
Hepatic adenomas or benign liver tumors.

There is evidence of an association between the following conditions and the use of oral contraceptives, although additional confirmatory studies are needed:

Mesenteric thrombosis.
Retinal thrombosis.

The following adverse reactions have been reported in patients receiving oral contraceptives and are believed to be drug related:

Nausea.
Vomiting.
Gastrointestinal symptoms (such as abdominal cramps and bloating).
Breakthrough bleeding.
Spotting.
Change in menstrual flow.
Amenorrhea.
Temporary infertility after discontinuation of treatment.
Edema.
Melasma which may persist.
Breast changes: tenderness, enlargement, secretion.
Change in weight (increase or decrease).
Change in cervical erosion and secretion.
Diminution in lactation when given immediately postpartum.
Cholestatic jaundice.
Migraine.
Rash (allergic).
Mental depression.
Reduced tolerance to carbohydrates.
Vaginal candidiasis.

Change in corneal curvature (steepening).
Intolerance to contact lenses.

The following adverse reactions have been reported in users of oral contraceptives, and the association has been neither confirmed nor refuted:

Congenital anomalies.
Premenstrual syndrome.
Cataracts.
Optic neuritis.
Changes in appetite.
Cystitis-like syndrome.
Headache.
Nervousness.
Dizziness.
Hirsutism.
Loss of scalp hair.
Erythema multiforme.
Erythema nodosum.
Hemorrhagic eruption.
Vaginitis.
Porphyria.
Impaired renal function.
Hemolytic uremic syndrome.
Budd-Chiari syndrome.
Acne.
Changes in libido.
Colitis.
Sickle cell disease.
Cerebral-vascular disease with mitral valve prolapse.
Lupus-like syndromes.

OVERDOSAGE

Serious ill effects have not been reported following acute ingestion of large doses of oral contraceptives by young children. Overdosage may cause nausea, and withdrawal bleeding may occur in females.

NONCONTRACEPTIVE HEALTH BENEFITS

The following noncontraceptive health benefits related to the use of oral contraceptives are supported by epidemiological studies which largely utilized oral contraceptive formulations containing doses exceeding 0.035 mg of ethinyl estradiol or 0.05 mg of mestranol.

Effects on menses:
Increased menstrual cycle regularity.
Decreased blood loss and decreased incidence of iron- deficiency anemia.
Decreased incidence of dysmenorrhea.

Effects related to inhibition of ovulation:
Decreased incidence of functional ovarian cysts.
Decreased incidence of ectopic pregnancies.

Effects from long-term use:
Decreased incidence of fibroadenomas and fibrocystic disease of the breast.
Decreased incidence of acute pelvic inflammatory disease.
Decreased incidence of endometrial cancer.
Decreased incidence of ovarian cancer.

DOSAGE AND ADMINISTRATION

To achieve maximum contraceptive effectiveness, LO/OVRAL must be taken exactly as directed and at intervals not exceeding 24 hours.

The dosage of LO/OVRAL is one tablet daily for 21 consecutive days per menstrual cycle according to prescribed schedule. Tablets are then discontinued for 7 days (three weeks on, one week off).

It is recommended that LO/OVRAL tablets be taken at the same time each day, preferably after the evening meal or at bedtime.

During the first cycle of medication, the patient is instructed to take one LO/OVRAL tablet daily for twenty-one consecutive days, beginning on day five of her menstrual cycle. (The first day of menstruation is day one.) The tablets are then discontinued for one week (7 days). Withdrawal bleeding should usually occur within 3 days following discontinuation of LO/OVRAL. (If LO/OVRAL is first taken later than the fifth day of the first menstrual cycle of medication or postpartum, contraceptive reliance should not be placed on LO/OVRAL until after the first seven consecutive days of administration. The possibility of ovulation and conception prior to initiation of medication should be considered.) The patient begins her next and all subsequent 21-day courses of LO/OVRAL tablets on the same day of the week that she began her first course, following the same schedule: 21 days on—7 days off. She begins taking her tablets on the 8th day after discontinuance, regardless of whether or not a menstrual period has occurred or is still in progress. Any time a new cycle of LO/OVRAL is started later than the 8th day, the patient should be protected by another means of contraception until she has taken a tablet daily for seven consecutive days.

If spotting or breakthrough bleeding occurs, the patient is instructed to continue on the same regimen. This type of bleeding is usually transient and without significance; however, if the bleeding is persistent or prolonged, the patient is advised to consult her physician. Although the occurrence of pregnancy is highly unlikely if LO/OVRAL is taken accord-

ing to directions, if withdrawal bleeding does not occur, the possibility of pregnancy must be considered. If the patient has not adhered to the prescribed schedule (missed one or more tablets or started taking them on a day later than she should have), the probability of pregnancy should be considered at the time of the first missed period and appropriate diagnostic measures taken before the medication is resumed. If the patient has adhered to the prescribed regimen and misses two consecutive periods, pregnancy should be ruled out before continuing the contraceptive regimen.

The patient should be instructed to take a missed tablet as soon as it is remembered. If two consecutive tablets are missed, they should both be taken as soon as remembered. The next tablet should be taken at the usual time.

Any time the patient misses one or two tablets, she should also use another method of contraception until she has taken a tablet daily for seven consecutive days. If breakthrough bleeding occurs following missed tablets, it will usually be transient and of no consequence. While there is little likelihood of ovulation occurring if only one or two tablets are missed, the possibility of ovulation increases with each successive day that scheduled tablets are missed. If three consecutive tablets are missed, all medication should be discontinued and the remainder of the package discarded. A new tablet cycle should be started on the 8th day after the last tablet was taken, and an alternate means of contraception should be prescribed during the seven days without tablets and until the patient has taken a tablet daily for seven consecutive days.

In the nonlactating mother, LO/OVRAL may be initiated postpartum, for contraception. When the tablets are administered in the postpartum period, the increased risk of thromboembolic disease associated with the postpartum period must be considered (see "Contraindications," "Warnings," and "Precautions" concerning thromboembolic disease). It is to be noted that early resumption of ovulation may occur if Parlodel® (bromocriptine mesylate) has been used for the prevention of lactation.

HOW SUPPLIED

LO/OVRAL® tablets (0.3 mg norgestrel and 0.03 mg ethinyl estradiol), Wyeth®, are available in packages of 6 PIL-PAK® dispensers with 21 tablets each as follows: NDC 0008-0078, white, round tablet marked "WYETH" and "78".

ALSO AVAILABLE

LO/OVRAL®-28 tablets in containers of 28 tablets, consisting of 21 white LO/OVRAL® tablets (0.3 mg norgestrel and 0.03 mg ethinyl estradiol) and 7 pink inert tablets.

REFERENCES

Available Upon Request.

Brief Summary Patient Package Insert

Oral contraceptives, also known as "birth-control pills" or "the pill," are taken to prevent pregnancy, and when taken correctly, have a failure rate of less than 1.0% per year when used without missing any pills. The typical failure rate of large numbers of pill users is less than 3.0% per year when women who miss pills are included. For most women oral contraceptives are also free of serious or unpleasant side effects. However, forgetting to take pills considerably increases the chances of pregnancy.

For the majority of women, oral contraceptives can be taken safely. But there are some women who are at high risk of developing certain serious diseases that can be life-threatening or may cause temporary or permanent disability or death. The risks associated with taking oral contraceptives increase significantly if you:

- smoke
- have high blood pressure, diabetes, high cholesterol
- have or have had clotting disorders, heart attack, stroke, angina pectoris, cancer of the breast or sex organs, jaundice, or malignant or benign liver tumors.

You should not take the pill if you suspect you are pregnant or have unexplained vaginal bleeding.

> Cigarette smoking increases the risk of serious cardiovascular side effects on the heart and blood vessels from oral contraceptive use. This risk increases with age and with heavy smoking (15 or more cigarettes per day) and is quite marked in women over 35 years of age. Women who use oral contraceptives should not smoke.

Most side effects of the pill are not serious. The most common such effects are nausea, vomiting, bleeding between menstrual periods, weight gain, breast tenderness, and difficulty wearing contact lenses. These side effects, especially nausea and vomiting, may subside within the first three months of use.

The serious side effects of the pill occur very infrequently, especially if you are in good health and do not smoke. However, you should know that the following medical conditions have been associated with or made worse by the pill:

1. Blood clots in the legs (thrombophlebitis), lungs (pulmonary embolism), stoppage or rupture of a blood vessel in the brain (stroke), blockage of blood vessels in the heart (heart attack or angina pectoris) or other organs of the body. As mentioned above, smoking increases the risk of heart attacks and strokes and subsequent serious medical consequences.

2. Liver tumors, which may rupture and cause severe bleeding. A possible but not definite association has been found with the pill and liver cancer. However, liver cancers are extremely rare. The chance of developing liver cancer from using the pill is thus even rarer.

3. High blood pressure, although blood pressure usually returns to normal when the pill is stopped.

The symptoms associated with these serious side effects are discussed in the detailed leaflet given to you with your supply of pills. Notify your doctor or health-care provider if you notice any unusual physical disturbances while taking the pill. In addition, drugs such as rifampin, as well as some anticonvulsants and some antibiotics, may decrease oral contraceptive effectiveness.

Studies to date of women taking the pill have not shown an increase in the incidence of cancer of the breast or cervix. There is, however, insufficient evidence to rule out the possibility that pills may cause such cancers.

Taking the pill provides some important noncontraceptive benefits. These include less painful menstruation, less menstrual blood loss and anemia, fewer pelvic infections, and fewer cancers of the ovary and the lining of the uterus.

Be sure to discuss any medical condition you may have with your health-care provider. Your health-care provider will take a medical and family history before prescribing oral contraceptives and will examine you. You should be reexamined at least once a year while taking oral contraceptives. The detailed patient information leaflet gives you further information which you should read and discuss with your health-care provider.

DETAILED PATIENT LABELING
INTRODUCTION

Any woman who considers using oral contraceptives (the birth-control pill or the pill) should understand the benefits and risks of using this form of birth control. This leaflet will give you much of the information you will need to make this decision and will also help you determine if you are at risk of developing any of the serious side effects of the pill. It will tell you how to use the pill properly so that it will be as effective as possible. However, this leaflet is not a replacement for a careful discussion between you and your health-care provider. You should discuss the information provided in this leaflet with him or her, both when you first start taking the pill and during your revisits. You should also follow your health-care provider's advice with regard to regular checkups while you are on the pill.

EFFECTIVENESS OF ORAL CONTRACEPTIVES

Oral contraceptives or "birth-control pills" or "the pill" are used to prevent pregnancy and are more effective than other nonsurgical methods of birth control. When they are taken correctly, the chance of becoming pregnant is less than 1.0% when used perfectly, without missing any pills. Typical failure rates are less than 3.0% per year. The chance of becoming pregnant increases with each missed pill during the menstrual cycle.

In comparison, typical failure rates for other nonsurgical methods of birth control during the first year of use are as follows:

IUD: 6%
Diaphragm with spermicides: 18%
Spermicides alone: 21%
Vaginal sponge: 18% to 30%
Condom alone: 12%
Periodic abstinence: 20%
No methods: 89%

WHO SHOULD NOT TAKE ORAL CONTRACEPTIVES

> Cigarette smoking increases the risk of serious adverse effects on the heart and blood vessels from oral contraceptive use. The risk increases with age and with heavy smoking (15 or more cigarettes per day) and is quite marked in women over 35 years of age. Women who use oral contraceptives should not smoke.

Some women should not use the pill. For example, you should not take the pill if you are pregnant or think you may be pregnant. You should also not use the pill if you have had any of the following conditions:

- Heart attack or stroke
- Blood clots in the legs (thrombophlebitis), lungs (pulmonary embolism), or eyes
- Blood clots in the deep veins of your legs
- Known or suspected breast cancer or cancer of the lining of the uterus, cervix, or vagina
- Liver tumor (benign or cancerous)

Or, if you have any of the following:

- Chest pain (angina pectoris)
- Unexplained vaginal bleeding (until a diagnosis is reached by your doctor)

- Yellowing of the whites of the eyes or of the skin (jaundice) during pregnancy or during previous use of the pill
- Known or suspected pregnancy

Tell your health-care provider if you have ever had any of these conditions. Your health-care provider can recommend another method of birth control.

OTHER CONSIDERATIONS BEFORE TAKING ORAL CONTRACEPTIVES

Tell your health-care provider if you or any family member has ever had:

- Breast nodules, fibrocystic disease of the breast, an abnormal breast X-ray or mammogram
- Diabetes
- Elevated cholesterol or triglycerides
- High blood pressure
- Migraine or other headaches or epilepsy
- Mental depression
- Gallbladder, heart, or kidney disease
- History of scanty or irregular menstrual periods

Women with any of these conditions should be checked often by their health-care provider if they choose to use oral contraceptives. Also, be sure to inform your doctor or health-care provider if you smoke or are on any medications.

RISKS OF TAKING ORAL CONTRACEPTIVES

1. Risk of developing blood clots

Blood clots and blockage of blood vessels are the most serious side effects of taking oral contraceptives and can be fatal. In particular, a clot in the legs can cause thrombophlebitis and a clot that travels to the lungs can cause a sudden blocking of the vessel carrying blood to the lungs. Rarely, clots occur in the blood vessels of the eye and may cause blindness, double vision, or impaired vision.

If you take oral contraceptives and need elective surgery, need to stay in bed for a prolonged illness, or have recently delivered a baby, you may be at risk of developing blood clots. You should consult your doctor about stopping oral contraceptives three to four weeks before surgery and not taking oral contraceptives for two weeks after surgery or during bed rest. You should also not take oral contraceptives soon after delivery of a baby or a midtrimester pregnancy termination. It is advisable to wait for at least four weeks after delivery if you are not breast-feeding. If you are breast-feeding, you should wait until you have weaned your child before using the pill. (See also the section on breast-feeding in General Precautions.)

2. Heart attacks and strokes

Oral contraceptives may increase the tendency to develop strokes (stoppage or rupture of blood vessels in the brain) and angina pectoris and heart attacks (blockage of blood vessels in the heart). Any of these conditions can cause death or serious disability.

Smoking greatly increases the possibility of suffering heart attacks and strokes. Furthermore, smoking and the use of oral contraceptives greatly increase the chances of developing and dying of heart disease.

3. Gallbladder disease

Oral-contraceptive users probably have a greater risk than nonusers of having gallbladder disease, although this risk may be related to pills containing high doses of estrogens.

4. Liver tumors

In rare cases, oral contraceptives can cause benign but dangerous liver tumors. These benign liver tumors can rupture and cause fatal internal bleeding. In addition, a possible but not definite association has been found with the pill and liver cancers in two studies in which a few women who developed these very rare cancers were found to have used oral contraceptives for long periods. However, liver cancers are extremely rare. The chance of developing liver cancer from using the pill is thus even rarer.

5. Cancer of the reproductive organs

There is, at present, no confirmed evidence that oral contraceptives increase the risk of cancer of the reproductive organs in human studies. Several studies have found no overall increase in the risk of developing breast cancer. However, women who use oral contraceptives and have a strong family history of breast cancer or who have breast nodules or abnormal mammograms should be closely followed by their doctors.

Some studies have found an increase in the incidence of cancer of the cervix in women who use oral contraceptives. However, this finding may be related to factors other than the use of oral contraceptives.

ESTIMATED RISK OF DEATH FROM A BIRTH-CONTROL METHOD OR PREGNANCY

All methods of birth control and pregnancy are associated with a risk of developing certain diseases which may lead to disability or death. An estimate of the number of deaths associated with different methods of birth control and pregnancy has been calculated and is shown in the following table. [See table on next page.]

In the above table, the risk of death from any birth control method is less than the risk of childbirth, except for oral-contraceptive users over the age of 35 who smoke and pill

Continued on next page

Wyeth-Ayerst Laboratories—Cont.

users over the age of 40 even if they do not smoke. It can be seen in the table that for women aged 15 to 39, the risk of death was highest with pregnancy (7–26 deaths per 100,000 women, depending on age). Among pill users who do not smoke, the risk of death was always lower than that associated with pregnancy for any age group, except for those women over the age of 40, when the risk increases to 32 deaths per 100,000 women, compared to 28 associated with pregnancy at that age. However, for pill users who smoke and are over the age of 35, the estimated number of deaths exceeds those for other methods of birth control. If a woman is over the age of 40 and smokes, her estimated risk of death is four times higher (117/100,000 women) than the estimated risk associated with pregnancy (28/100,000 women) in that age group.

The suggestion that women over 40 who don't smoke should not take oral contraceptives is based on information from older high-dose pills and on less-selective use of pills than is practiced today. An Advisory Committee of the FDA discussed this issue in 1989 and recommended that the benefits of oral-contraceptive use by healthy, nonsmoking women over 40 years of age may outweigh the possible risks. However, all women, especially older women, are cautioned to use the lowest dose pill that is effective.

WARNING SIGNALS

If any of these adverse effects occur while you are taking oral contraceptives, call your doctor immediately:

- Sharp chest pain, coughing of blood, or sudden shortness of breath (indicating a possible clot in the lung)
- Pain in the calf (indicating a possible clot in the leg)
- Crushing chest pain or heaviness in the chest (indicating a possible heart attack)
- Sudden severe headache or vomiting, dizziness or fainting, disturbances of vision or speech, weakness, or numbness in an arm or leg (indicating a possible stroke)
- Sudden partial or complete loss of vision (indicating a possible clot in the eye)
- Breast lumps (indicating possible breast cancer or fibrocystic disease of the breast; ask your doctor or health-care provider to show you how to examine your breasts)
- Severe pain or tenderness in the stomach area (indicating a possibly ruptured liver tumor)
- Difficulty in sleeping, weakness, lack of energy, fatigue, or change in mood (possibly indicating severe depression)
- Jaundice or a yellowing of the skin or eyeballs, accompanied frequently by fever, fatigue, loss of appetite, dark colored urine, or light-colored bowel movements (indicating possible liver problems)

SIDE EFFECTS OF ORAL CONTRACEPTIVES

1. Vaginal bleeding

Irregular vaginal bleeding or spotting may occur while you are taking the pills. Irregular bleeding may vary from slight staining between menstrual periods to breakthrough bleeding which is a flow much like a regular period. Irregular bleeding occurs most often during the first few months of oral-contraceptive use, but may also occur after you have been taking the pill for some time. Such bleeding may be temporary and usually does not indicate any serious problems. It is important to continue taking your pills on schedule. If the bleeding occurs in more than one cycle or lasts for more than a few days, talk to your doctor or health-care provider.

2. Contact lenses

If you wear contact lenses and notice a change in vision or an inability to wear your lenses, contact your doctor or health-care provider.

3. Fluid retention

Oral contraceptives may cause edema (fluid retention) with swelling of the fingers or ankles and may raise your blood pressure. If you experience fluid retention, contact your doctor or health-care provider.

4. Melasma

A spotty darkening of the skin is possible, particularly of the face.

5. Other side effects

Other side effects may include change in appetite, headache, nervousness, depression, dizziness, loss of scalp hair, rash, and vaginal infections.

If any of these side effects bother you, call your doctor or health-care provider.

GENERAL PRECAUTIONS

1. Missed periods and use of oral contraceptives before or during early pregnancy

There may be times when you may not menstruate regularly after you have completed taking a cycle of pills. If you have taken your pills regularly and miss one menstrual period, continue taking your pills for the next cycle but be sure to inform your health care provider before doing so. If you have not taken the pills daily as instructed and missed a menstrual period, or if you missed two consecutive menstrual periods, you may be pregnant. Check with your health care provider immediately to determine whether you are pregnant. Do not continue to take oral contraceptives until you are sure you are not pregnant, but continue to use another method of contraception.

There is no conclusive evidence that oral-contraceptive use is associated with an increase in birth defects, when taken inadvertently during early pregnancy. Previously, a few studies had reported that oral contraceptives might be associated with birth defects, but these findings have not been confirmed. Nevertheless, oral contraceptives or any other drugs should not be used during pregnancy unless clearly necessary and prescribed by your doctor. You should check with your doctor about risks to your unborn child of any medication taken during pregnancy.

2. While breast-feeding

If you are breast-feeding, consult your doctor before starting oral contraceptives. Some of the drug will be passed on to the child in the milk. A few adverse effects on the child have been reported, including yellowing of the skin (jaundice) and breast enlargement. In addition, oral contraceptives may decrease the amount and quality of your milk. If possible, do not use oral contraceptives while breast-feeding. You should use another method of contraception since breast-feeding provides only partial protection from becoming pregnant, and this partial protection decreases significantly as you breast-feed for longer periods of time. You should consider starting oral contraceptives only after you have weaned your child completely.

3. Laboratory tests

If you are scheduled for any laboratory tests, tell your doctor you are taking birth-control pills. Certain blood tests may be affected by birth-control pills.

4. Drug interactions

Certain drugs may interact with birth control pills to make them less effective in preventing pregnancy or cause an increase in breakthrough bleeding. Such drugs include rifampin, drugs used for epilepsy such as barbiturates (for example, phenobarbital) and phenytoin (Dilantin is one brand of this drug), phenylbutazone (Butazolidin is one brand) and possibly certain antibiotics. You may need to use an additional method of contraception during any cycle in which you take drugs that can make oral contraceptives less effective.

HOW TO TAKE ORAL CONTRACEPTIVES

1. General Instructions

You must take your pill every day according to the instructions. Oral contraceptives are most effective if taken no more than 24 hours apart. Take your pill at the same time every day so that you are less likely to forget to take it. You will then maintain an effective dose of the oral contraceptive in your body.

If your doctor has scheduled you for surgery, or you need prolonged bed rest, he or she may suggest that you stop taking the pill four weeks before surgery to avoid an increased

risk of blood clots. It is also advisable not to start oral contraceptives sooner than four weeks after delivery of a baby or a midtrimester pregnancy termination.

NORDETTE®-21, OVRAL®, LO/OVRAL®

The dosage of Nordette-21, Ovral and Lo/Ovral is one tablet daily for 21 days in a row per menstrual cycle. Tablets are then discontinued for 7 days. The basic schedule is 21 days on—7 days off.

During the first month, you should begin taking Nordette-21, Ovral or Lo/Ovral on Day 5 of your menstrual cycle whether or not you still have your period. (Day 1 is the first day of menstruation, even if it is almost midnight when you start.) Note: During your first month on Nordette-21, Ovral, or Lo/Ovral, if you start taking tablets later than Day 5 of your menstrual cycle, you should protect yourself by also using another method of birth control until you have taken a tablet daily for seven consecutive days. Thereafter, if you follow directions carefully, you will obtain the full contraceptive benefit. If you begin taking tablets later than the proper day, the possibility of ovulation and pregnancy occurring before beginning medication should be considered.

Take one tablet every day until you finish all 21 tablets. No tablets are then taken for one week (7 days). Your period will usually begin about three days after you take the last tablet. Don't be alarmed if the amount of bleeding is not the same as before. On the 8th day, start a new Pilpak®, even if you still have your period. If, for example, you took Nordette-21, Ovral, or Lo/Ovral for the first time on a Tuesday, the 8th day will also be a Tuesday. Thus, you will always begin a new cycle on the same day of the week as long as you do not interrupt your original schedule. If you start taking tablets later than the 8th day, you should protect yourself by also using another method of birth control until you have taken a tablet daily for seven days in a row.

NORDETTE®-28, OVRAL®-28, LO/OVRAL®-28

The dosage of Nordette-28, Ovral-28, and Lo/Ovral-28 is one white or light-orange active tablet daily for 21 consecutive days followed by one pink inactive tablet daily for 7 consecutive days. The basic schedule is 21 days on white or light-orange active tablets—7 days on pink inactive tablets. Always take all 21 white or light-orange tablets in each Pilpak before taking the pink tablets.

You should begin taking Nordette-28, Ovral-28, or Lo/Ovral-28 on the first Sunday after your menstrual period begins, whether or not you are still bleeding. If your period begins on a Sunday, take your first tablet that very same day. Your first white or light-orange tablet is marked with a large arrow and the word "Start". Note: During your first month on Nordette-28, Ovral-28, or Lo/Ovral-28, you should protect yourself by also using another method of birth control until you have taken a white or light-orange tablet daily for seven consecutive days. Thereafter, if you follow directions carefully, you will obtain the full contraceptive benefit. If you begin taking tablets later than the proper day, the possibility of ovulation and pregnancy occurring before beginning medication should be considered. Take one tablet every day until you finish all 21 white or light-orange tablets in a Pilpak, followed by all 7 pink tablets. Your period will usually begin about three days after you take the last white or light-orange tablet, which will be during the time you are taking the pink tablets. Don't be alarmed if the amount of bleeding is not the same as before. The day after you have taken your last pink tablet, begin a new Pilpak of tablets (taking all 21 white or light-orange tablets first, just as you did before) so that you will take a tablet every day without interruption. The starting day for each new Pilpak will always be Sunday. If in any cycle you start tablets later than the proper day, you should also use another method of birth control until you have taken a white or light-orange tablet daily for 7 days in a row.

SPOTTING OR BREAKTHROUGH BLEEDING:

Spotting is slight staining between menstrual periods which may not even require a pad. Breakthrough bleeding is a flow much like a regular period, requiring sanitary protection. Spotting is more common than breakthrough bleeding, and both occur more often in the first few cycles than in later cycles. These types of bleeding are usually temporary and without significance. It is important to continue taking your pills on schedule. If the bleeding persists for more than a few days, consult your doctor.

2. If you forget to take your pill

If you miss only one pill in a cycle, the chance of becoming pregnant is small. Take the missed pill as soon as you realize that you have forgotten it. Since the risk of pregnancy increases with each additional pill you skip, it is very important that you take one pill a day.

Nordette-21, Ovral and Lo/Ovral each contain 21 active white or light-orange tablets per Pilpak. Nordette-28, Ovral-28 and Lo/Ovral-28 each contain 21 active white or light-orange tablets plus 7 pink inactive tablets per Pilpak.

The chance of becoming pregnant is quite small if you miss only one white or light-orange tablet in a cycle. Of course, with each additional one you skip, the chance increases. If you miss one or more pink tablets (Nordette-28, Ovral-28, Lo/Ovral-28) you are still protected against pregnancy as

ANNUAL NUMBER OF BIRTH-RELATED OR METHOD-RELATED DEATHS ASSOCIATED WITH CONTROL OF FERTILITY PER 100,000 NONSTERILE WOMEN, BY FERTILITY CONTROL METHOD ACCORDING TO AGE

Method of control and outcome	15–19	20–24	25–29	30–34	35–39	40–44
No fertility control methods*	7.0	7.4	9.1	14.8	25.7	28.2
Oral contraceptives nonsmoker**	0.3	0.5	0.9	1.9	13.8	31.6
Oral contraceptives smoker**	2.2	3.4	6.6	13.5	51.1	117.2
IUD**	0.8	0.8	1.0	1.0	1.4	1.4
Condom*	1.1	1.6	0.7	0.2	0.3	0.4
Diaphragm/ spermicide*	1.9	1.2	1.2	1.3	2.2	2.8
Periodic abstinence*	2.5	1.6	1.6	1.7	2.9	3.6

* Deaths are birth-related
** Deaths are method-related

long as you begin taking your next white or light-orange tablet on the proper day.

It is important to take a missed white or light-orange tablet as soon as it is remembered. If two consecutive white or light-orange tablets are missed, they should both be taken as soon as remembered. The next tablet should then be taken at the usual time. Any time you miss one or two white or light-orange tablets, or begin a new Pilpak after the proper starting day, you should also use another method of birth control until you have taken a white or light-orange tablet daily for seven consecutive days. If breakthrough bleeding occurs following missed tablets, it will usually be temporary and of no consequence. While there is little likelihood of pregnancy occurring if only one or two white or light-orange tablets are missed, the possibility of pregnancy increases with each successive day that scheduled white or light-orange tablets are missed.

If you are taking Nordette-21, Ovral, or Lo/Ovral and forget to take three white or light-orange tablets in a row, do not take them when you remember. Wait four more days—which makes a whole week without tablets. Then begin a new Pilpak on the 8th day after the last tablet was taken. During the seven days without tablets, and until you have taken a white or light-orange tablet daily for seven consecutive days, you should protect yourself from pregnancy by also using another method of birth control.

If you are taking Nordette-28, Ovral-28, or Lo/Ovral-28 and forget to take three white or light-orange tablets in a row, do not take them when you remember. Stop taking all medication until the first Sunday following the last missed tablet. Then, whether or not you have had your period, and even if you are still bleeding, start a new Pilpak. During the days without tablets, and until you have taken a white or light-orange tablet daily for seven consecutive days, you should protect yourself from pregnancy by also using another method of birth control.

OVRETTE®

Ovrette is administered on a continuous daily dosage schedule, one tablet each day, every day of the year. Take the first tablet on the first day of your menstrual period. Tablets should be taken at the same time every day, without interruption, whether bleeding occurs or not. If bleeding is prolonged (more than 8 days) or unusually heavy, you should contact your doctor.

Forgotten Pills

The risk of pregnancy increases with each tablet missed. Therefore, it is very important that you take one tablet daily as directed. If you miss one tablet, take it as soon as you remember and also take your next tablet at the regular time. If you miss two tablets, take one of the missed tablets as soon as you remember, as well as your regular tablet for that day at the proper time. Furthermore, you should use another method of birth control in addition to taking Ovrette until you have taken fourteen days (2 weeks) of medication.

If more than two tablets have been missed, Ovrette should be discontinued immediately and another method of birth control used until the start of your next menstrual period. Then you may resume taking Ovrette.

At times there may be no menstrual period after a cycle of pills. Therefore, if you miss one menstrual period but have taken the pills **exactly as you were supposed to,** continue as usual into the next cycle. If you have not taken the pills correctly and miss a menstrual period, or if you are taking mini-pills and it is 45 days or more from the start of your last menstrual period, you may be pregnant and should stop taking oral contraceptives until your doctor determines whether or not you are pregnant. Until you can get to your doctor, use another form of nonhormonal contraception. If two consecutive menstrual periods are missed, you should stop taking pills until it is determined by a physician whether you are pregnant.

If you do become pregnant while using oral contraceptives, the risk to the fetus is small, on the order of no more than one per thousand. You should, however, discuss the risks to the developing child with your doctor.

3. *Pregnancy due to pill failure*

The incidence of pill failure resulting in pregnancy is approximately less than 1.0% if taken every day as directed, but more typical failure rates are less than 3.0%. If failure does occur, the risk to the fetus is minimal.

4. *Pregnancy after stopping the pill*

There may be some delay in becoming pregnant after you stop using oral contraceptives, especially if you had irregular menstrual cycles before you used oral contraceptives. It may be advisable to postpone conception until you begin menstruating regularly once you have stopped taking the pill and desire pregnancy.

There does not appear to be any increase in birth defects in newborn babies when pregnancy occurs soon after stopping the pill.

5. *Overdosage*

Serious ill effects have not been reported following ingestion of large doses of oral contraceptives by young children. Overdosage may cause nausea and withdrawal bleeding in females. In case of overdosage, contact your health-care provider or pharmacist.

6. *Other information*

Your health-care provider will take a medical and family history before prescribing oral contraceptives and will examine you. You should be reexamined at least once a year. Be sure to inform your health-care provider if there is a family history of any of the conditions listed previously in this leaflet. Be sure to keep all appointments with your health-care provider, because this is a time to determine if there are early signs of side effects of oral-contraceptive use.

Do not use the drug for any condition other than the one for which it was prescribed. This drug has been prescribed specifically for you; do not give it to others who may want birth-control pills.

HEALTH BENEFITS FROM ORAL CONTRACEPTIVES

In addition to preventing pregnancy, use of oral contraceptives may provide certain benefits. They are:

- Menstrual cycles may become more regular
- Blood flow during menstruation may be lighter, and less iron may be lost. Therefore, anemia due to iron deficiency is less likely to occur.
- Pain or other symptoms during menstruation may be encountered less frequently
- Ovarian cysts may occur less frequently
- Ectopic (tubal) pregnancy may occur less frequently
- Noncancerous cysts or lumps in the breast may occur less frequently
- Acute pelvic inflammatory disease may occur less frequently
- Oral contraceptive use may provide some protection against developing two forms of cancer: cancer of the ovaries and cancer of the lining of the uterus.

If you want more information about birth-control pills, ask your doctor or pharmacist. They have a more technical leaflet called the Professional Labeling which you may wish to read.

Shown in Product Identification Section, page 437

LO/OVRAL®-28 ℞

[*lōh-oh 'vral-28*]

Tablets

(norgestrel and ethinyl estradiol tablets)

DESCRIPTION

21 white LO/OVRAL® tablets, each containing 0.3 mg of norgestrel (*dl*-13-beta-ethyl-17-alpha-ethinyl-17-beta-hydroxygon-4-en-3-one), a totally synthetic progestogen, and 0.03 mg of ethinyl estradiol (19-nor-17α-pregna-1,3,5(10)-trien-20-yne-3,17-diol), and 7 pink inert tablets. The inactive ingredients present are cellulose, D&C Red 30, lactose, magnesium stearate, and polacrilin potassium.

CLINICAL PHARMACOLOGY

See LO/OVRAL®.

INDICATIONS AND USAGE

See LO/OVRAL.

CONTRAINDICATIONS

See LO/OVRAL.

WARNINGS

See LO/OVRAL.

PRECAUTIONS

See LO/OVRAL.

Drug Interactions: See LO/OVRAL.
Carcinogenesis: See LO/OVRAL.
Pregnancy: See LO/OVRAL.
Nursing Mothers: See LO/OVRAL.
Information for the Patient: See LO/OVRAL.

ADVERSE REACTIONS

See LO/OVRAL.

OVERDOSAGE

See LO/OVRAL.

NONCONTRACEPTIVE HEALTH BENEFITS

See LO/OVRAL.

DOSAGE AND ADMINISTRATION

To achieve maximum contraceptive effectiveness, LO/OVRAL-28 must be taken exactly as directed and at intervals not exceeding 24 hours.

The dosage of LO/OVRAL-28 is one white tablet daily for 21 consecutive days followed by one pink inert tablet daily for 7 consecutive days according to prescribed schedule. It is recommended that tablets be taken at the same time each day, preferably after the evening meal or at bedtime.

During the first cycle of medication, the patient is instructed to begin taking LO/OVRAL-28 on the first Sunday after the onset of menstruation. If menstruation begins on a Sunday, the first tablet (white) is taken that day. One white tablet should be taken daily for 21 consecutive days followed by one pink inert tablet daily for 7 consecutive days. Withdrawal bleeding should usually occur within three days following discontinuation of white tablets. During the first cycle, contraceptive reliance should not be placed on LO/OVRAL-28 until a white tablet has been taken daily for 7 consecutive days. The possibility of ovulation and conception prior to initiation of medication should be considered.

The patient begins her next and all subsequent 28-day courses of tablets on the same day of the week (Sunday) on which she began her first course, following the same schedule: 21 days on white tablets—7 days on pink inert tablets. If in any cycle the patient starts tablets later than the proper day, she should protect herself by using another method of birth control until she has taken a white tablet daily for 7 consecutive days.

If spotting or breakthrough bleeding occurs, the patient is instructed to continue on the same regimen. This type of bleeding is usually transient and without significance; however, if the bleeding is persistent or prolonged the patient is advised to consult her physician. Although the occurrence of pregnancy is highly unlikely if LO/OVRAL-28 is taken according to directions, if withdrawal bleeding does not occur, the possibility of pregnancy must be considered. If the patient has not adhered to the prescribed schedule (missed one or more tablets or started taking them on a day later than she should have), the probability of pregnancy should be considered at the time of the first missed period and appropriate diagnostic measures taken before the medication is resumed. If the patient has adhered to the prescribed regimen and misses two consecutive periods, pregnancy should be ruled out before continuing the contraceptive regimen.

The patient should be instructed to take a missed white tablet as soon as it is remembered. If two consecutive white tablets are missed, they should both be taken as soon as remembered. The next tablet should be taken at the usual time.

Any time the patient misses one or two white tablets, she should also use another method of contraception until she has taken a white tablet daily for seven consecutive days. If the patient misses one or more pink tablets she is still protected against pregnancy **provided** she begins taking white tablets again on the proper day.

If breakthrough bleeding occurs following missed white tablets, it will usually be transient and of no consequence. While there is little likelihood of ovulation occurring if only one or two white tablets are missed, the possibility of ovulation increases with each successive day that scheduled white tablets are missed. If three consecutive white LO/OVRAL tablets are missed, all medication should be discontinued and the remainder of the 28-day package discarded. A new tablet cycle should be started on the first Sunday following the last missed tablet, and an alternate means of contraception should be prescribed during the days without tablets and until the patient has taken a white tablet daily for 7 consecutive days.

In the nonlactating mother, LO/OVRAL-28 may be initiated postpartum, for contraception. When the tablets are administered in the postpartum period, the increased risk of thromboembolic disease associated with the postpartum period must be considered (see Contraindications, Warnings, and Precautions concerning thromboembolic disease). It is to be noted that early resumption of ovulation may occur if Parlodel® (bromocriptine mesylate) has been used for the prevention of lactation.

HOW SUPPLIED

LO/OVRAL®-28 Tablets (0.3 mg norgestrel and 0.03 mg ethinyl estradiol), Wyeth®, are available in packages of 6 PILPAK® dispensers, each containing 28 tablets as follows:
21 active tablets, NDC 0008-0078, white, round tablet marked "WYETH" and "78".
7 inert tablets, NDC 0008-0486, pink, round tablet marked "WYETH" and "486".

References available upon request.

Brief Summary Patient Package Insert: See LO/OVRAL.
DETAILED PATIENT LABELING: See LO/OVRAL.

Shown in Product Identification Section, page 437

MAXAQUIN® ℞

[*măx 'ah-kwĭn*]

(lomefloxacin hydrochloride)

Film-coated Tablets

DESCRIPTION

Maxaquin (lomefloxacin HCl) is a synthetic broad-spectrum antimicrobial agent for oral administration. Lomefloxacin HCl, a difluoroquinolone, is the monohydrochloride salt of (±)-1-ethyl-6,8-difluoro-1,4-dihydro-7-(3-methyl-1-piperazinyl)-4-oxo-3-quinolinecarboxylic acid. Its empirical formula is $C_{17}H_{19}F_2N_3O_3 \cdot HCl$, and its structural formula is:

[See chemical structure at top of next column.]

Lomefloxacin HCl is a white to pale yellow powder with a molecular weight of 387.8. It is slightly soluble in water and practically insoluble in alcohol. Lomefloxacin HCl is stable

Continued on next page

Wyeth-Ayerst Laboratories—Cont.

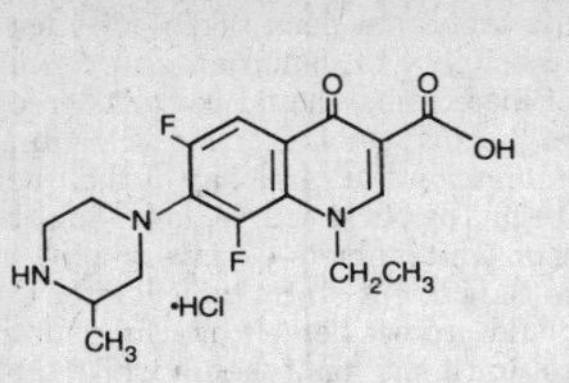

to heat and moisture but is sensitive to light in dilute aqueous solution.

Maxaquin is available as a film-coated tablet formulation containing 400 mg of lomefloxacin base, present as the hydrochloride salt. The base content of the hydrochloride salt is 90.6%. The inactive ingredients are carboxymethylcellulose calcium, hydroxypropyl cellulose, hydroxypropyl methylcellulose, lactose, magnesium stearate, polyethylene glycol, polyoxyl 40 stearate, and titanium dioxide.

CLINICAL PHARMACOLOGY

Pharmacokinetics in Healthy Volunteers: In 6 fasting healthy male volunteers, approximately 95% to 98% of a single oral dose of lomefloxacin was absorbed. Absorption was rapid following single doses of 200 and 400 mg (T_{max} 0.8 to 1.4 hours). Mean plasma concentration increased proportionally between 100 and 400 mg as shown below.

Dose (mg)	Mean Plasma Concentration (μg/mL)	Area Under Curve (AUC) (μg·h/mL)
100	0.8	5.6
200	1.4	10.9
400	3.2	26.1

In 6 healthy male volunteers administered 400 mg of lomefloxacin on an empty stomach q.d. for 7 days, the following mean pharmacokinetic parameter values were obtained:

C_{max}	2.8 μg/mL
C_{min}	0.27 μg/mL
$AUC_{0-24\ h}$	25.9 μg·h/mL
T_{max}	1.5 h
$t_{1/2}$	7.75 h

The elimination half-life in 8 subjects with normal renal function was approximately 8 hours. At 24 hours post dose, subjects with normal renal function receiving single doses of 200 or 400 mg had mean plasma lomefloxacin concentrations of 0.10 and 0.24 μg/mL, respectively. Steady-state concentrations were achieved within 48 hours of initiating therapy with once-a-day dosing. There was no drug accumulation with single daily dosing in patients with normal renal function.

Approximately 65% of an orally administered dose was excreted in the urine as unchanged drug in patients with normal renal function. Following a 400-mg dose of lomefloxacin administered q.d. for 7 days, the mean urine concentration was in excess of 300 μg/mL 4 hours post dose. The mean urine concentration exceeded 35 μg/mL for at least 24 hours after dosing.

Following a single 400-mg dose, lomefloxacin's solubility in urine usually exceeded its peak urinary concentration 2 to 6 fold. In this study, urine pH affected the solubility of lomefloxacin with solubilities ranging from 7.8 mg/mL at pH 5.2, to 2.4 mg/mL at pH 6.5, and 3.03 mg/mL at pH 8.12.

The urinary excretion of lomefloxacin was virtually complete within 72 hours after cessation of dosing, with approximately 65% of the dose being recovered as parent drug and 9% as its glucuronide metabolite. The mean renal clearance was 145 mL/min in subjects with normal renal function (GFR = 120 mL/min). This may indicate tubular secretion.

Food effect: When lomefloxacin and food were administered concomitantly, the rate of drug absorption was delayed [T_{max} increased to 2 hours (delayed by 41%), C_{max} decreased by 18%], and the extent of absorption (AUC) was decreased by 12%.

Pharmacokinetics in the Geriatric Population: In 16 healthy elderly volunteers (61 to 76 years of age) with normal renal function for their age, lomefloxacin's half-life (mean of 8 hours) and peak plasma concentration (mean of 4.2 μg/mL) following a single 400-mg dose were similar to those in 8 younger subjects dosed with a single 400-mg dose. Thus, drug absorption appears unaffected in the elderly. Plasma clearance was, however, reduced in this elderly population by approximately 25%, and the AUC was increased by approximately 33%. This slower elimination most likely reflects the decreased renal function normally observed in the geriatric population.

Pharmacokinetics in the Renally Impaired Patients: In 8 patients with creatinine clearance (Cl_{Cr}) between 10 and 40 mL/min/1.73 m^2, the mean AUC after a single 400-mg dose of lomefloxacin increased 335% over the AUC demonstrated in patients with a Cl_{Cr} > 80 mL/min/1.73 m^2. Also, in these patients, the mean $t_{1/2}$ increased to 21 hours. In 8 patients with Cl_{Cr} < 10 mL/min/1.73 m^2, the mean AUC after a single 400-mg dose of lomefloxacin increased 700% over the AUC demonstrated in patients with a Cl_{Cr} > 80 mL/min/1.73 m^2. In these patients with Cl_{Cr} < 10 mL/min/1.73 m^2, the mean $t_{1/2}$ increased to 45 hours. The plasma clearance of lomefloxacin was closely correlated with creatinine clearance, ranging from 31 mL/min/1.73 m^2 when creatinine clearance was zero to 271 mL/min/1.73 m^2 at a normal creatinine clearance of 110 mL/min/1.73 m^2. Peak lomefloxacin concentrations were not affected by the degree of renal function when single doses of lomefloxacin were administered. Adjustment of dosage schedules for patients with such decreases in renal function is warranted. (See **Dosage and Administration.**)

Pharmacokinetics in Patients with Cirrhosis: In 12 patients with histologically confirmed cirrhosis, no significant changes in rate or extent of lomefloxacin exposure (C_{max}, T_{max}, $t_{1/2}$ or AUC) were observed when they were administered 400 mg of lomefloxacin as a single dose. No data are available in cirrhotic patients treated with multiple doses of lomefloxacin. Cirrhosis does not appear to reduce the nonrenal clearance of lomefloxacin. There does not appear to be a need for a dosage reduction in cirrhotic patients, provided adequate renal function is present.

Metabolism and Pharmacodynamics of Lomefloxacin: Lomefloxacin is minimally metabolized although 5 metabolites have been identified in human urine. The glucuronide metabolite is found in the highest concentration and accounts for approximately 9% of the administered dose. The other 4 metabolites together account for less than 0.5% of the dose.

Approximately 10% of an oral dose was recovered as unchanged drug in the feces.

Serum protein binding of lomefloxacin is approximately 10%.

The following are mean tissue or fluid to plasma ratios of lomefloxacin following oral administration. Studies have not been conducted to assess the penetration of lomefloxacin into human cerebrospinal fluid.

Tissue or Body Fluid	Mean Tissue or Fluid to Plasma Ratio
Bronchial mucosa	2.1
Bronchial secretions	0.6
Prostatic tissue	2
Sputum	1.3
Urine	140.0

Microbiology: Lomefloxacin is a bactericidal agent with *in vitro* activity against a wide range of gram-negative and gram-positive organisms. The bactericidal action of lomefloxacin results from interference with the activity of the bacterial enzyme DNA gyrase, which is needed for the transcription and replication of bacterial DNA. The minimum bactericidal concentration (MBC) generally does not exceed the minimum inhibitory concentration (MIC) by more than a factor of 2, except for staphylococci, which usually have MBC's 2 to 4 times the MIC.

Lomefloxacin has been shown to be active against most strains of the following organisms both *in vitro* and in clinical infections: (See **Indications and Usage.**)

Gram-positive aerobes

Staphylococcus saprophyticus

Gram-negative aerobes

Citrobacter diversus
Enterobacter cloacae
Escherichia coli
Haemophilus influenzae
Klebsiella pneumoniae
Moraxella (Branhamella) catarrhalis
Proteus mirabilis
Pseudomonas aeruginosa (urinary tract only—See **Indications and Usage** and **Warnings**)

The following *in vitro* data are available; however, their clinical significance is unknown.

Lomefloxacin exhibits *in vitro* MIC's of 2 μg/mL or less against most strains of the following organisms; however, the safety and effectiveness of lomefloxacin in treating clinical infections due to these organisms have not been established in adequate and well-controlled trials:

Gram-positive aerobes

Staphylococcus aureus (including methicillin-resistant strains)
Staphylococcus epidermidis (including methicillin-resistant strains)

Gram-negative aerobes

Aeromonas hydrophila
Citrobacter freundii
Enterobacter aerogenes
Enterobacter agglomerans
Haemophilus parainfluenzae
Hafnia alvei
Klebsiella oxytoca
Klebsiella ozaenae
Morganella morganii
Proteus vulgaris
Providencia alcalifaciens
Providencia rettgeri
Serratia liquefaciens
Serratia marcescens

Other organisms:

Legionella pneumophila

Beta-lactamase production should have no effect on the *in vitro* activity of lomefloxacin.

Most group A, B, D, and G streptococci, *Streptococcus pneumoniae, Pseudomonas cepacia, Ureaplasma urealyticum, Mycoplasma hominis,* and anaerobic bacteria are resistant to lomefloxacin.

Lomefloxacin appears slightly less active *in vitro* when tested at acidic pH. An increase in inoculum size has little effect on the *in vitro* activity of lomefloxacin. *In vitro* resistance to lomefloxacin develops slowly (multiple-step mutation). Rapid one-step development of resistance occurs only rarely ($<10^{-9}$) *in vitro.*

Cross-resistance between lomefloxacin and other quinolone-class antimicrobial agents has been reported; however, cross-resistance between lomefloxacin and members of other classes of antimicrobial agents, such as aminoglycosides, penicillins, tetracyclines, cephalosporins, or sulfonamides has not yet been reported. Lomefloxacin is active *in vitro* against some strains of cephalosporin- and aminoglycoside-resistant gram-negative bacteria.

Susceptibility tests

Diffusion techniques: Quantitative methods that require measurement of zone diameters give the most precise estimate of the susceptibility of bacteria to antimicrobial agents. One such standardized procedure[1] that has been recommended for use with disks to test the susceptibility of organisms to lomefloxacin uses the 10-μg lomefloxacin disk. Interpretation involves correlation of the diameter obtained in the disk test with the MIC for lomefloxacin.

Reports from the laboratory giving results of the standard single-disk susceptibility test with a 10-μg lomefloxacin disk should be interpreted according to the following criteria:

Zone Diameter (mm)	Interpretation
≥22	Susceptible (S)
19–21	Intermediate (I)
≤18	Resistant (R)

A report of "Susceptible" indicates that the pathogen is likely to be inhibited by generally achievable drug concentrations. A report of "Intermediate" indicates that the result should be considered equivocal, and, if the organism is not fully susceptible to alternative clinically feasible drugs, the test should be repeated. This category provides a buffer zone that prevents small uncontrolled technical factors from causing major discrepancies in interpretation. A report of "Resistant" indicates that achievable drug concentrations are unlikely to be inhibitory, and other therapy should be selected.

Standardized susceptibility test procedures require the use of laboratory control organisms. The 10-μg lomefloxacin disk should give the following zone diameters:

Organism	Zone Diameter (mm)
S. aureus (ATCC 25923)	23–29
E. coli (ATCC 25922)	27–33
P. aeruginosa (ATCC 27853)	22–28

Dilution techniques: Use a standardized dilution method[2] (broth, agar, or microdilution) or equivalent with lomefloxacin powder. The MIC values obtained should be interpreted according to the following criteria:

MIC (μg/mL)	Interpretation
≤2	Susceptible (S)
4	Intermediate (I)
≥8	Resistant (R)

As with standard diffusion techniques, dilution methods require the use of laboratory control organisms. Standard lomefloxacin powder should provide the following MIC values:

Organism	MIC (μg/mL)
S. aureus (ATCC 29213)	0.25–2.0
E. coli (ATCC 25922)	0.03–0.12
P. aeruginosa (ATCC 27853)	1.0–4.0

INDICATIONS AND USAGE

TREATMENT:

Maxaquin (lomefloxacin HCl) film-coated tablets are indicated for the treatment of adults with mild to moderate infections caused by susceptible strains of the designated microorganisms in the conditions listed below: (See **Dosage and Administration** for specific dosing recommendations.)

LOWER RESPIRATORY TRACT

Acute Bacterial Exacerbation of Chronic Bronchitis caused by *Haemophilus influenzae* or *Moraxella (Branhamella) catarrhalis**.

NOTE: MAXAQUIN IS NOT INDICATED FOR THE EMPIRIC TREATMENT OF ACUTE BACTERIAL EXACERBATION OF CHRONIC BRONCHITIS WHEN IT IS PROBABLE THAT *S. PNEUMONIAE* IS A CAUSATIVE PATHOGEN. *S. PNEUMONIAE* EXHIBITS *IN VITRO* RESISTANCE TO LOMEFLOXACIN, AND THE SAFETY AND EFFICACY OF LOMEFLOXACIN IN THE TREATMENT OF PATIENTS WITH ACUTE BACTERIAL EXACERBATION OF CHRONIC BRONCHITIS CAUSED BY *S. PNEUMONIAE* HAVE NOT BEEN DEMONSTRATED. IF LOMEFLOXACIN IS TO BE PRESCRIBED FOR GRAM-STAIN GUIDED EMPIRIC THERAPY OF ACUTE BACTERIAL EXACERBATION OF CHRONIC BRONCHITIS, IT SHOULD BE USED ONLY IF SPUTUM GRAM STAIN DEMONSTRATES AN ADEQUATE QUALITY OF SPECIMEN (>25 PMN'S/LPF) AND THERE IS BOTH A PREDOMINANCE OF GRAM NEGATIVE ORGANISMS AND NOT A PREDOMINANCE OF GRAM POSITIVE ORGANISMS.

URINARY TRACT

Uncomplicated Urinary Tract Infections (cystitis) caused by *Escherichia coli, Klebsiella pneumoniae, Proteus mirabilis,* or *Staphylococcus saprophyticus.*

Complicated Urinary Tract Infections caused by *Escherichia coli, Klebsiella pneumoniae, Proteus mirabilis, Pseudomonas aeruginosa, Citrobacter diversus**, or *Enterobacter cloacae**.

NOTE: In clinical trials of complicated urinary tract infections due to *P. aeruginosa,* 12 of 16 patients had the organism eradicated from the urine after therapy with lomefloxacin. No patients had concomitant bacteremia. Serum levels of lomefloxacin do not reliably exceed the MIC of *Pseudomonas* isolates. THE SAFETY AND EFFICACY OF LOMEFLOXACIN IN TREATING PATIENTS WITH *PSEUDOMONAS* BACTEREMIA HAS NOT BEEN ESTABLISHED.

Appropriate culture and susceptibility tests should be performed before antimicrobial treatment in order to isolate and identify organisms causing infection and to determine their susceptibility to lomefloxacin. In patients with urinary tract infections, therapy with Maxaquin film-coated tablets may be initiated before results of these tests are known; once these results become available, appropriate therapy should be continued. In patients with an acute bacterial exacerbation of chronic bronchitis, therapy should not be started empirically with lomefloxacin when there is a probability the causative pathogen is *S. pneumoniae.*

Beta-lactamase production should have no effect on lomefloxacin activity.

PROPHYLAXIS:

Maxaquin (lomefloxacin HCl) film-coated tablets are indicated pre-operatively to reduce the incidence of urinary tract infections in the early post-operative period (3–5 days post-surgery) in patients undergoing transurethral surgical procedures. Efficacy in decreasing the incidence of infections other than urinary tract infections in the early post-operative period has not been established. Maxaquin, like all drugs for prophylaxis of transurethral surgical procedures, usually should not be used in minor urologic procedures for which prophylaxis is not indicated (e.g., simple cystoscopy or retrograde pyelography).

CONTRAINDICATIONS

Lomefloxacin is contraindicated in patients with a history of hypersensitivity to lomefloxacin or to any of the quinolone group of antimicrobial agents.

WARNINGS

THE SAFETY AND EFFICACY OF LOMEFLOXACIN IN CHILDREN, ADOLESCENTS (UNDER THE AGE OF 18 YEARS), PREGNANT WOMEN, AND LACTATING WOMEN HAVE NOT BEEN ESTABLISHED. (See PRECAUTIONS—***Pregnancy; Nursing Mothers;* and *Pediatric Use.***) The oral administration of multiple doses of lomefloxacin to juvenile dogs at 0.3 and to rats at 5.4 times the recommended adult human dose based on mg/m^2 (0.6 and 34 times the recommended adult human dose based on mg/kg, respectively) caused arthropathy and lameness. Histopathological examination of the weight-bearing joints of these animals revealed permanent lesions of the cartilage. Other quinolones also produce erosions of cartilage of weight-bearing joints and other signs of arthropathy in juvenile animals of various species. (See **Animal Pharmacology.**)

The safety and efficacy of lomefloxacin in the treatment of acute bacterial exacerbation of chronic bronchitis due to *S. pneumoniae* have not been demonstrated. This product should not be used empirically in the treatment of acute bacterial exacerbation of chronic bronchitis when it is probable that *S. pneumoniae* is a causative pathogen.

In clinical trials of complicated urinary tract infections due to *P. aeruginosa,* 12 of 16 patients had the organism eradicated from the urine after therapy with lomefloxacin. No patients had concomitant bacteremia. Serum levels of lomefloxacin do not reliably exceed the MIC of *Pseudomonas* isolates. THE SAFETY AND EFFICACY OF LOMEFLOXACIN IN TREATING PATIENTS WITH *PSEUDOMONAS* BACTEREMIA HAS NOT BEEN ESTABLISHED.

Serious and occasionally fatal hypersensitivity (anaphylactoid or anaphylactic) reactions, some following the first dose, have been reported in patients receiving quinolone therapy. Some reactions were accompanied by cardiovascular collapse, loss of consciousness, tingling, pharyngeal or facial edema, dyspnea, urticaria, or itching. Only a few of these patients had a history of previous hypersensitivity reactions. Serious hypersensitivity reactions have also been reported following treatment with lomefloxacin. If an allergic reaction to lomefloxacin occurs, discontinue the drug. Serious acute hypersensitivity reactions may require immediate emergency treatment with epinephrine. Oxygen, intravenous fluids, antihistamines, corticosteroids, pressor amines, and airway management, including intubation, should be administered as indicated.

Convulsions have been reported in patients receiving lomefloxacin. Whether the convulsions were directly related to lomefloxacin administration has not yet been established. However, convulsions, increased intracranial pressure, and toxic psychoses have been reported in patients receiving other quinolones. Quinolones may also cause central nervous system stimulation, which may lead to tremors, restlessness, lightheadedness, confusion, and hallucinations. If any of these reactions occurs in patients receiving lomefloxacin, the drug should be discontinued and appropriate measures instituted. No evidence of an effect of lomefloxacin on the electrical activity of the brain has been demonstrated. Lomefloxacin does not alter cerebral blood flow or cerebral glucose uptake in the central nervous system based on positron emission tomography. However, until more information becomes available, lomefloxacin, like all other quinolones, should be used with caution in patients with known or suspected central nervous system disorders, such as severe cerebral arteriosclerosis, epilepsy, or other factors that predispose to seizures. (See **Adverse Reactions.**)

Pseudomembranous colitis has been reported with nearly all antibacterial agents, including quinolones, and may range from mild to life-threatening in severity. Therefore, it is important to consider this diagnosis in patients who present with diarrhea subsequent to the administration of antibacterial agents. Treatment with broad-spectrum antibiotics alters the normal flora of the colon and may permit overgrowth of clostridia. Studies indicate that a toxin produced by *Clostridium difficile* is a primary cause of "antibiotic-associated colitis." After the diagnosis of pseudomembranous colitis has been established, therapeutic measures should be initiated. Mild cases of pseudomembranous colitis usually respond to discontinuation of drug alone. In moderate to severe cases, consideration should be given to management with fluid and electrolytes, protein supplementation, and treatment with an antibacterial drug clinically effective against *C. difficile* colitis.

PRECAUTIONS

General:

Alteration of the dosage regimen is recommended for patients with impairment of renal function (Cl_{Cr} < 40 mL/min/1.73 m^2). (See **Dosage and Administration.**)

Moderate to severe phototoxicity reactions have been observed in patients exposed to excessive sunlight or artificial ultraviolet light while receiving lomefloxacin or some other quinolones. Excessive sunlight and artificial ultraviolet light should be avoided while taking lomefloxacin. Lomefloxacin therapy should be discontinued if phototoxicity occurs.

Information for patients:

Patients should be advised

- to drink fluids liberally,
- that lomefloxacin can be taken without regard to meals,
- that mineral supplements or vitamins with iron or minerals should not be taken within the 2-hour period before or after taking lomefloxacin (see **Drug Interactions**),
- that sucralfate or antacids containing magnesium or aluminum should not be taken within 4 hours before or 2 hours after taking lomefloxacin (see **Drug Interactions**),
- that lomefloxacin can cause dizziness and lightheadedness and, therefore, patients should know how they react to lomefloxacin before they operate an automobile or machinery or engage in activities requiring mental alertness and coordination,
- that lomefloxacin may be associated with hypersensitivity reactions, even following the first dose, and to discontinue the drug at the first sign of a skin rash or other allergic reaction, and
- to avoid excessive sunlight and artificial ultraviolet light while receiving lomefloxacin and to discontinue therapy if phototoxicity occurs.

Drug interactions:

Theophylline: In 3 pharmacokinetic studies including 46 normal, healthy subjects, theophylline clearance and concentration were not significantly altered by the addition of lomefloxacin. In clinical studies where patients were on chronic theophylline therapy, lomefloxacin had no measurable effect on the mean distribution of theophylline concentrations or the mean estimates of theophylline clearance. Though individual theophylline levels fluctuated, there were no clinically significant symptoms of drug interaction.

Antacids and sucralfate: Sucralfate and antacids containing magnesium or aluminum form chelation complexes with lomefloxacin and interfere with its bioavailability. Sucralfate administered 2 hours before lomefloxacin resulted in a slower rate of absorption (mean C_{max} decreased by 30% and mean T_{max} increased by 1 hour) and a lesser extent of absorption (mean AUC decreased by approximately 25%). Magnesium- and aluminum-containing antacids, administered concomitantly with lomefloxacin, significantly decreased the bioavailability (48%) of lomefloxacin. Separating the doses of antacid and lomefloxacin minimizes this decrease in bioavailability; therefore, administration of these agents should precede lomefloxacin dosing by 4 hours or follow lomefloxacin dosing by at least 2 hours.

Caffeine: One hundred mg of caffeine (equivalent to 1 to 3 cups of American coffee) was administered to 16 normal, healthy volunteers who had achieved steady-state blood concentrations of lomefloxacin after being dosed at 400 mg q.d. This did not result in any statistically or clinically relevant changes in the pharmacokinetic parameters of either caffeine or lomefloxacin. No data are available on potential interactions in individuals who consume greater than 100 mg of caffeine per day or in those, such as the geriatric population, who are generally believed to be more susceptible to the development of drug-induced central nervous system-related adverse effects. Other quinolones have demonstrated moderate to marked interference with the metabolism of caffeine, resulting in a reduced clearance, a prolongation of plasma half-life, and an increase in symptoms that accompany high levels of caffeine.

Cimetidine: Cimetidine has been demonstrated to interfere with the elimination of other quinolones. This interference has resulted in significant increases in half-life and AUC. Interaction between lomefloxacin and cimetidine has not been studied.

Cyclosporine: Elevated serum levels of cyclosporine have been reported with concomitant use of cyclosporine with other members of the quinolone class. Interaction between lomefloxacin and cyclosporine has not been studied.

Non-steroidal anti-inflammatory drugs (NSAID's): Concomitant administration of the NSAID, fenbufen, with some quinolones has been reported to increase the risk of CNS stimulation and convulsive seizures.

There was an increase in the incidence of seizures in mice treated with fenbufen, when fenbufen was administered to mice that had been concomitantly treated with a dose of lomefloxacin equivalent to the recommended human dose on a mg/m^2 basis (10 times the recommended human dose on a mg/kg basis). Fenbufen is not presently an approved drug in the United States. (See **Animal Pharmacology**).

Probenecid: Probenecid slows the renal elimination of lomefloxacin. An increase of 63% in the mean AUC and increases of 50% and 4%, respectively, in the mean T_{max} and mean C_{max} were noted in 1 study of 6 individuals.

Warfarin: Quinolones may enhance the effects of the oral anticoagulant, warfarin, or its derivatives. When these products are administered concomitantly, prothrombin or other suitable coagulation test should be monitored closely.

Carcinogenesis, mutagenesis, impairment of fertility:

Carcinogenesis: Long-term carcinogenicity studies of lomefloxacin in animals have not been performed.

Mutagenesis: One *in vitro* mutagenicity test (CHO/HGPRT assay) was weakly positive at lomefloxacin concentrations of 226 μg/mL and greater and negative at concentrations less than 226 μg/mL. Two other *in vitro* mutagenicity tests (chromosomal aberrations in Chinese hamster ovary cells, chromosomal aberrations in human lymphocytes) and two *in vivo* mouse micronucleus mutagenicity tests were all negative.

Impairment of Fertility: Lomefloxacin did not affect the fertility of male and female rats at oral doses up to 8 times the recommended human dose based on mg/m^2 (34 times the recommended human dose based on mg/kg).

Continued on next page

* = Although treatment of infections due to this organism in this organ system demonstrated a clinically acceptable overall outcome, efficacy was studied in fewer than 10 infections.

Wyeth-Ayerst Laboratories—Cont.

Pregnancy: Teratogenic Effects. Pregnancy Category C. Reproductive function studies have been performed in rats at doses up to 8 times the recommended human dose based on mg/m^2 (34 times the recommended human dose based on mg/kg), and no impaired fertility or harm to the fetus was reported due to lomefloxacin. Increased incidence of fetal loss in monkeys has been observed at approximately 3 to 6 times the recommended human dose based on mg/m^2 (6 to 12 times the recommended human dose based on mg/kg). No teratogenicity has been observed in rats and monkeys at up to 16 times the recommended human dose exposure. In the rabbit, maternal toxicity and associated fetotoxicity, decreased placental weight, and variations of the coccygeal vertebrae occurred at doses 2 times the recommended human exposure based on mg/m^2. There are, however, no adequate and well-controlled studies in pregnant women. Lomefloxacin should be used during pregnancy only if the potential benefit justifies the potential risk to the fetus.

Nursing mothers:
It is not known whether lomefloxacin is excreted in human milk. However, it is known that other drugs of this class are excreted in human milk and that lomefloxacin is excreted in the milk of lactating rats. Because of the potential for serious adverse reactions from lomefloxacin in nursing infants, a decision should be made whether to discontinue nursing or to discontinue the drug, taking into account the importance of the drug to the mother.

Pediatric use:
The safety and effectiveness of lomefloxacin in children and adolescents below the age of 18 years have not been established. Lomefloxacin causes arthropathy in juvenile animals of several species. (See **Warnings** and **Animal Pharmacology.**)

Geriatric use:
Of the total number of patients in clinical studies of lomefloxacin, 26% were ≥ 65 years of age. No overall differences in effectiveness or safety were observed between these patients and younger patients. (See **Clinical Pharmacology**—Pharmacokinetics in the Geriatric Population.)

ADVERSE REACTIONS

In clinical trials, most of the adverse events reported were mild to moderate in severity and transient in nature. During these clinical investigations, 2869 patients received Maxaquin. In 2.6% of the patients, lomefloxacin was discontinued because of adverse events, primarily involving the gastrointestinal system (0.7%), skin (1.0%), or central nervous system (0.5%).

Adverse Clinical Events: The events with the highest incidence (≥ 1%) in patients, regardless of relationship to drug, were nausea (3.7%), headache (3.2%), photosensitivity (2.4%), dizziness (2.3%), and diarrhea (1.4%).

Additional clinical events reported in less than 1% of patients treated with Maxaquin, regardless of relationship to drug, are listed below:

Autonomic: dry mouth, flushing, increased sweating.
Body as a Whole: fatigue, back pain, malaise, asthenia, chest pain, chills, allergic reaction, face edema, influenza-like symptoms, decreased heat tolerance.
Cardiovascular: hypotension, hypertension, edema, syncope, tachycardia, bradycardia, arrhythmia, extrasystoles, cyanosis, cardiac failure, angina pectoris, myocardial infarction, pulmonary embolism, cerebrovascular disorder, cardiomyopathy, phlebitis.
Central Nervous System: convulsions, coma, hyperkinesia, tremor, vertigo, paresthesias.
Gastrointestinal: abdominal pain, dyspepsia, vomiting, flatulence, constipation, gastrointestinal inflammation, dysphagia, gastrointestinal bleeding, tongue discoloration.
Hearing: earache, tinnitus.
Hematologic: thrombocytopenia, thrombocythemia, purpura, lymphadenopathy, increased fibrinolysis.
Metabolic: thirst, gout, hypoglycemia.
Musculoskeletal: leg cramps, arthralgia, myalgia.
Ophthalmologic: abnormal vision, conjunctivitis, eye pain.
Psychiatric: somnolence, insomnia, nervousness, anorexia, confusion, anxiety, depression, agitation, increased appetite, depersonalization, paroniria.
Reproductive System: Female: vaginitis, leukorrhea, intermenstrual bleeding, perineal pain, vaginal moniliasis. Male: orchitis, epididymitis.
Respiratory: dyspnea, respiratory infection, epistaxis, respiratory disorder, bronchospasm, cough, increased sputum, stridor.
Skin/Allergic: pruritus, rash, urticaria, eczema, skin exfoliation, skin disorder.
Special Senses: taste perversion.
Urinary: dysuria, hematuria, strangury, micturition disorder, anuria.

Adverse Laboratory Events: Changes in laboratory parameters, listed as adverse events, without regard to drug relationship include:
Hepatic: elevations of ALT (SGPT) (0.4%), AST (SGOT) (0.3%), bilirubin (0.1%), alkaline phosphatase (0.1%).
Hematologic: monocytosis (0.3%), elevated ESR (0.1%).
Renal: elevated BUN (0.1%), decreased potassium (0.1%).

Additional laboratory changes occurring in ≤0.1% in the clinical studies included: elevation of serum gamma glutamyl transferase, decrease in total protein or albumin, prolongation of prothrombin time, anemia, decrease in hemoglobin, leukopenia, eosinophilia, thrombocytopenia, abnormalities of urine specific gravity or serum electrolytes, decrease in blood glucose.

Quinolone-class Adverse Events: Although not reported in completed clinical studies with Maxaquin, a variety of adverse events have been reported with other quinolones.
Clinical adverse events include: anaphylactoid reactions, erythema nodosum, Stevens-Johnson syndrome, exfoliative dermatitis, toxic epidermal necrolysis, hepatic necrosis, possible exacerbation of myasthenia gravis, dysphasia, nystagmus, pseudomembranous colitis, painful oral mucosa, intestinal perforation, hallucinations, manic reaction, ataxia, phobia, hyperpigmentation, diplopia, interstitial nephritis, renal failure, renal calculi, polyuria, urinary retention, acidosis, cardiopulmonary arrest, cerebral thrombosis, laryngeal or pulmonary edema, hiccough, dysgeusia, and photophobia.
Laboratory adverse events include: agranulocytosis, elevation of serum triglycerides, elevation of serum cholesterol, elevation of blood glucose, elevation of serum potassium, albuminuria, candiduria, and crystalluria.

OVERDOSAGE

Information on overdosage in humans is limited. In the event of acute overdosage, the stomach should be emptied by inducing vomiting or by gastric lavage, and the patient should be carefully observed and given supportive treatment. Adequate hydration must be maintained. Hemodialysis or peritoneal dialysis is unlikely to aid in the removal of lomefloxacin as less than 3% is removed by these modalities.

Clinical signs of acute toxicity in rodents progressed from salivation to tremors, decreased activity, dyspnea, and clonic convulsions prior to death. These signs were noted in rats and mice as lomefloxacin doses were increased.

DOSAGE AND ADMINISTRATION

Maxaquin (lomefloxacin HCl) may be taken without regard to meals. (See **Clinical Pharmacology.**)
See **Indications and Usage** for information on appropriate pathogens and patient populations.

TREATMENT:
Patients with Normal Renal Function: The recommended daily dose of Maxaquin is described in the following chart: [See table below.]
Elderly Patients: No dosage adjustment is needed for elderly patients with normal renal function (Cl_{cr} ≥ 40 mL/min/1.73 m^2).
Patients with Impaired Renal Function: Lomefloxacin is primarily eliminated by renal excretion. (See *Clinical Pharmacology.*) Modification of dosage is recommended in patients with renal dysfunction. In patients with a creatinine clearance greater than 10 but less than 40 mL/min/1.73 m^2, the recommended dosage is an initial loading dose of 400 mg followed by daily maintenance doses of 200 mg (½ tablet) once daily for the duration of treatment. It is suggested that serial determinations of lomefloxacin levels be performed to determine any necessary alteration in the appropriate next dosing interval.

Body System	Infection	Unit Dose	Frequency	Duration	Daily Dose
Lower respiratory tract	Acute bacterial exacerbation of chronic bronchitis	400 mg	q.d.	10 days	400 mg
Urinary tract	Cystitis	400 mg	q.d.	10 days	400 mg
	Complicated Urinary Tract Infections	400 mg	q.d.	14 days	400 mg

If only the serum creatinine is known, the following formula may be used to estimate creatinine clearance.

$$\text{Men: } \frac{(\text{weight in kg}) \times (140 - \text{age})}{(72) \times \text{serum creatinine (mg/dL)}}$$

Women: (0.85) × (calculated value for men)

Dialysis patients: Hemodialysis removes only a negligible amount of lomefloxacin (3% in 4 hours). Hermodialysis patients should receive an initial loading dose of 400 mg followed by daily maintenance doses of 200 mg (½ tablet) once daily for the duration of treatment.
Patients with Cirrhosis: Cirrhosis does not reduce the nonrenal clearance of lomefloxacin. The need for a dosage reduction in this population should be based on the degree of renal function of the patient and on the plasma concentrations. (See **Clinical Pharmacology** and **Dosage and Administration**—Impaired Renal Function.)

PROPHYLAXIS

A single dose of 400 mg of Maxaquin should be administered orally 2 to 6 hours prior to surgery when oral pre-operative prophylaxis for transurethral surgical procedures is considered appropriate.

HOW SUPPLIED

Maxaquin (lomefloxacin HCl) is supplied as a scored, film-coated tablet containing the equivalent of 400 mg of lomefloxacin base present as the hydrochloride. The tablet is oval, white, and film-coated with "MAXAQUIN 400" debossed on one side and scored on the other side and is supplied in:

NDC Number	Size
0025-1651-20	bottle of 20
0025-1651-34	carton of 100 unit dose

Store at 59° to 86°F (15° to 30°C).

Caution: Federal law prohibits dispensing without prescription.

ANIMAL PHARMACOLOGY

Lomefloxacin and other quinolones have been shown to cause arthropathy in juvenile animals. Arthropathy, involving multiple diarthrodial joints, was observed in juvenile dogs administered lomefloxacin at doses as low as 4.5 mg/kg for 7 to 8 days (0.3 times the recommended human dose based on mg/m^2 or 0.6 times the recommended human dose based on mg/kg). In juvenile rats, no changes were observed in the joints with doses up to 91 mg/kg for 7 days (2 times the recommended human dose based on mg/m^2 or 11 times the recommended human dose based on mg/kg). (See **Warnings.**)

In a 13-week oral rat study, gamma globulin decreased when lomefloxacin was administered at less than the recommended human exposure. Beta globulin decreased when lomefloxacin was administered at 0.6 to 2 times the recommended human dose based on mg/m^2. The A/G ratio increased when lomefloxacin was administered at 6 to 20 times the human dose. Following a 4-week recovery period, beta globulins in the females and A/G ratios in the females returned to control values. Gamma globulin values in the females and beta and gamma globulins and A/G ratios in the males were still statistically significantly different from control values. No effects on globulins were seen in oral studies in dogs or monkeys in the limited number of specimens collected.

Twenty-seven NSAID's, administered concomitantly with lomefloxacin, were tested for seizure induction in mice at approximately 2 times the recommended human dose based on mg/m^2. At a dose of lomefloxacin equivalent to the recommended human exposure based on mg/m^2 (10 times the human dose based on mg/kg), only fenbufen, when co-administered, produced an increase in seizures.

Crystalluria and ocular toxicity, seen with some related quinolones, were not observed in any lomefloxacin-treated animals, either in studies designed to look for these effects specifically or in subchronic and chronic toxicity studies in rats, dogs, and monkeys.

Long-term, high-dose systemic use of other quinolones in experimental animals has caused lenticular opacities; however, this finding was not observed with lomefloxacin.

REFERENCES

1. National Committee for Clinical Laboratory Standards, *Performance Standards for Antimicrobial Disk Susceptibility Tests*—Fourth Edition. Approved Standard NCCLS Document M2-A4, Vol. 10, No. 7, NCCLS, Villanova, PA, 1990. **2.** National Committee for Clinical Laboratory Standards, *Methods for Dilution Antimicrobial Susceptibility Tests for Bacteria that Grow Aerobically*—Second Edition. Approved Standard NCCLS Document M7-A2, Vol. 10, No. 8, NCCLS, Villanova, PA, 1990.

3/2/92 • A05215

MAZANOR® C R

[*maz'a-nor*]

(mazindol)

DESCRIPTION

Mazanor (mazindol) is an imidazoisoindole anorectic agent. It is chemically designated as 5-p-chloro-phenyl-5-hydroxy-2,3-dihydro-5H-imidazo (2,1-a) isoindole, a tautomeric form of 2-[2'-(p-chlorobenzoyl) phenyl]-2-imidazoline. Mazanor tablets contain 1 mg mazindol. The inactive ingredients present are calcium sulfate, cellulose, lactose, magnesium stearate, povidone, and talc.

HOW SUPPLIED

Mazanor® (mazindol) Tablets, Wyeth®, are available in the following dosage strength in bottles of 30 tablets:

1 mg, NDC 0008-0071, white, round, scored tablet marked "WYETH" and "71".

Keep tightly closed.

Store below 25° C (77° F).

Dispense in tight container.

For prescribing information, write to Professional Service, Wyeth-Ayerst Laboratories, P.O. Box 8299, Philadelphia, PA 19101, or contact your local Wyeth-Ayerst representative.

Shown in Product Identification Section, page 437

MEPERGAN® CII R

[*mep'er-gan*]

(meperidine HCl and promethazine HCl) Injection

DESCRIPTION

This product is available in concentration providing 25 mg each of meperidine hydrochloride and promethazine hydrochloride per mL with 0.1 mg edetate disodium, 0.04 mg calcium chloride, and not more than 0.75 mg sodium formaldehyde sulfoxylate, 0.25 mg sodium metabisulfite, and 5 mg phenol with sodium acetate buffer.

ACTIONS

Meperidine hydrochloride is a narcotic analgesic with multiple actions qualitatively similar to those of morphine. Phenergan® (promethazine HCl) is a phenothiazine derivative that has several different pharmacologic properties including antihistaminic, sedative, and antiemetic actions.

INDICATIONS

As a preanesthetic medication when analgesia and sedation are indicated. As an adjunct to local and general anesthesia.

CONTRAINDICATIONS

Hypersensitivity to meperidine or promethazine.

Under no circumstances should Mepergan be given by intra-arterial injection, due to the likelihood of severe arteriospasm and the possibility of resultant gangrene (see "Warnings").

Mepergan should not be given by the subcutaneous route; evidence of chemical irritation has been noted, and necrotic lesions have resulted on rare occasions following subcutaneous injection. The preferred parenteral route of administration is by deep, intramuscular injection.

Meperidine is contraindicated in patients who are receiving monoamine-oxidase inhibitors (MAOI) or those who have received such agents within 14 days.

Therapeutic doses of meperidine have inconsistently precipitated unpredictable, severe, and occasionally fatal reactions in patients who have received such agents within 14 days. The mechanism of these reactions is unclear. Some have been characterized by coma, severe respiratory depression, cyanosis, and hypotension and have resembled the syndrome of acute narcotic overdose. In other reactions the predominant manifestations have been hyperexcitability, convulsions, tachycardia, hyperpyrexia, and hypertension. Although it is not known that other narcotics are free of the risk of such reactions, virtually all of the reported reactions have occurred with meperidine. If a narcotic is needed in such patients, a sensitivity test should be performed in which repeated, small, incremental doses of morphine are administered over the course of several hours while the patient's condition and vital signs are under careful observation. (Intravenous hydrocortisone or prednisolone have been used to treat severe reactions, with the addition of intravenous chlorpromazine in those cases exhibiting hypertension and hyperpyrexia. The usefulness and safety of narcotic antagonists in the treatment of these reactions is unknown.)

WARNINGS

Mepergan Injection contains sodium metabisulfite, a sulfite that may cause allergic-type reactions, including anaphylactic symptoms and life-threatening or less severe asthmatic episodes, in certain susceptible people. The overall prevalence of sulfite sensitivity in the general population is unknown and probably low. Sulfite sensitivity is seen more frequently in asthmatic than in nonasthmatic people.

Tolerance and Addiction Liability

Warning—may be habit forming

DRUG DEPENDENCE: Meperidine can produce drug dependence of the morphine type and therefore has the potential for being abused. Psychic dependence, physical dependence, and tolerance may develop upon repeated administration of meperidine, and it should be prescribed and administered with the same degree of caution appropriate to the use of morphine. Like other narcotics, meperidine is subject to the provisions of the Federal narcotic laws.

INTERACTION WITH OTHER CENTRAL NERVOUS SYSTEM DEPRESSANTS: Meperidine should be used with great caution and in reduced dosage in patients who are concurrently receiving other narcotic analgesics, general anesthetics, phenothiazines, other tranquilizers, sedative-hypnotics, tricyclic antidepressants, and other CNS depressants (including alcohol). Respiratory depression, hypotension, and profound sedation or coma may result.

The sedative action of promethazine hydrochloride is additive to the sedative effects of central nervous system depressants; therefore, agents such as alcohol, barbiturates, and narcotic analgesics should either be eliminated or given in reduced dosage in the presence of promethazine hydrochloride. When given concomitantly with promethazine hydrochloride, the dose of barbiturates should be reduced by at least one-half and the dose of analgesic depressants, such as morphine or meperidine, should be reduced by one-quarter to one-half.

HEAD INJURY AND INCREASED INTRACRANIAL PRESSURE: The respiratory-depressant effects of meperidine and its capacity to elevate cerebrospinal-fluid pressure may be markedly exaggerated in the presence of head injury, other intracranial lesions, or a preexisting increase in intracranial pressure. Furthermore, narcotics produce adverse reactions which may obscure the clinical course of patients with head injuries. In such patients, meperidine must be used with extreme caution and only if its use is deemed essential.

INADVERTENT INTRA-ARTERIAL INJECTION: Due to the close proximity of arteries and veins in the areas most commonly used for intravenous injection, extreme care should be exercised to avoid perivascular extravasation or inadvertent intra-arterial injection of Mepergan. Reports compatible with inadvertent intra-arterial injection suggest that pain, severe chemical irritation, severe spasm of distal vessels, and resultant gangrene requiring amputation is likely under such circumstances. Intravenous injection was intended in all the cases reported, but perivascular extravasation or arterial placement of the needle is now suspect. There is no proven successful management of this condition after it occurs, although sympathetic block and heparinization are commonly employed during the acute management because of the results of animal experiments with other known arteriolar irritants. Aspiration of dark blood does not preclude intra-arterial needle placement, because blood is discolored upon contact with promethazine. Use of syringes with rigid plungers or of small bore needles might obscure typical arterial backflow if this is relied upon alone.

INTRAVENOUS USE: If necessary, meperidine may be given intravenously, but the injection should be given very slowly, preferably in the form of a diluted solution. Rapid intravenous injection of narcotic analgesics, including meperidine, increases the incidence of adverse reactions; severe respiratory depression, apnea, hypotension, peripheral circulatory collapse, and cardiac arrest have occurred. Meperidine should not be administered intravenously unless a narcotic antagonist and the facilities for assisted or controlled respiration are immediately available. When meperidine is given parenterally, especially intravenously, the patient should be lying down.

When used intravenously, Mepergan should be given at a rate not to exceed 1 mL (25 mg of each component) per minute. When administering any irritant drug intravenously, it is usually preferable to inject it through the tubing of an intravenous infusion set that is known to be functioning satisfactorily. In the event that a patient complains of pain during intended intravenous injection of Mepergan, the injection should immediately be stopped to provide for evaluation of possible arterial placement or perivascular extravasation.

ASTHMA AND OTHER RESPIRATORY CONDITIONS: Meperidine should be used with extreme caution in patients having an acute asthmatic attack, patients with chronic obstructive pulmonary disease or cor pulmonale, patients having a substantially decreased respiratory reserve, and patients with preexisting respiratory depression, hypoxia, or hypercapnia. In such patients, even usual therapeutic doses of narcotics may decrease respiratory drive while simultaneously increasing airway resistance to the point of apnea.

HYPOTENSIVE EFFECT: The administration of meperidine may result in severe hypotension in an individual whose ability to maintain his blood pressure has already been compromised by a depleted blood volume or concurrent administration of drugs such as the phenothiazines or certain anesthetics.

USAGE IN AMBULATORY PATIENTS: Meperidine may impair the mental and/or physical abilities required for the performance of potentially hazardous tasks, such as driving a car or operating machinery. The patient should be cautioned accordingly.

Meperidine, like other narcotics, may produce orthostatic hypotension in ambulatory patients.

USAGE IN PREGNANCY AND LACTATION: Meperidine should not be used in pregnant women prior to the labor period, unless in the judgment of the physician the potential benefits outweigh the possible hazards, because safe use in pregnancy prior to labor has not been established relative to possible adverse effects on fetal development.

When used as an obstetrical analgesic, meperidine crosses the placental barrier and can produce respiratory depression in the newborn; resuscitation may be required (see "Overdosage").

Meperidine appears in the milk of nursing mothers receiving the drug.

PRECAUTIONS

SUPRAVENTRICULAR TACHYCARDIAS: Meperidine should be used with caution in patients with atrial flutter and other supraventricular tachycardias because of a possible vagolytic action which may produce a significant increase in the ventricular response rate.

CONVULSIONS: Meperidine may aggravate preexisting convulsions in patients with convulsive disorders. If dosage is escalated substantially above recommended levels because of tolerance development, convulsions may occur in individuals without a history of convulsive disorders.

ACUTE ABDOMINAL CONDITIONS: The administration of meperidine or other narcotics may obscure the diagnosis or clinical course in patients with acute abdominal conditions.

SPECIAL-RISK PATIENTS: Meperidine should be given with caution, and the initial dose should be reduced in certain patients, such as the elderly or debilitated, and those with severe impairment of hepatic or renal function, hypothyroidism, Addison's disease, and prostatic hypertrophy or urethral stricture.

Antiemetics may mask the symptoms of an unrecognized disease and thereby interfere with diagnosis.

Patients in pain who have received inadequate or no analgesia have been noted to develop "athetoidlike" movements of the upper extremities following the parenteral administration of promethazine. These symptoms usually disappear upon adequate control of the pain.

Ambulatory patients should be cautioned against driving automobiles or operating dangerous machinery until it is known that they do not become drowsy or dizzy from promethazine hydrochloride therapy.

ADVERSE REACTIONS

The major hazards of meperidine, as with other narcotic analgesics, are respiratory depression and, to a lesser degree, circulatory depression; respiratory arrest, shock, and cardiac arrest have occurred.

The most frequently observed adverse reactions include light-headedness, dizziness, sedation, nausea, vomiting, and sweating. These effects seem to be more prominent in ambulatory patients and in those who are not experiencing severe pain. In such individuals, lower doses are advisable. Some adverse reactions in ambulatory patients may be alleviated if the patient lies down.

Other adverse reactions include:

CENTRAL NERVOUS SYSTEM: Euphoria, dysphoria, weakness, headache, agitation, tremor, uncoordinated muscle movements, transient hallucinations and disorientation, visual disturbances and, rarely, extrapyramidal reactions.

GASTROINTESTINAL: Dry mouth, constipation, biliary-tract spasm.

CARDIOVASCULAR: Flushing of the face, tachycardia, bradycardia, palpitation, faintness, syncope.

Cardiovascular effects from promethazine have been rare. Minor increases in blood pressure and occasional mild hypotension have been reported. Venous thrombosis at the injection site has been reported. Intra-arterial injection of Mepergan may result in gangrene of the affected extremity (see "Warnings").

GENITOURINARY: Urinary retention.

ALLERGIC: Pruritus, urticaria, other skin rashes, wheal and flare over the vein with IV injection.

Photosensitivity, although extremely rare, has been reported. Occurrence of photosensitivity may be a contraindication to further treatment with promethazine or related drugs.

OTHER: Pain at injection site; local tissue irritation, induration, and possible tissue necrosis, particularly when injection is repeated at same site; antidiuretic effect.

Patients may occasionally complain of autonomic reactions, such as dryness of the mouth, blurring of vision and, rarely, dizziness following the use of promethazine.

Very rare cases have been reported where patients receiving promethazine have developed leukopenia. In one instance agranulocytosis has been reported. In nearly every instance

Continued on next page

Wyeth-Ayerst Laboratories—Cont.

reported, other toxic agents known to have caused these conditions have been associated with the administration of promethazine.

DOSAGE AND ADMINISTRATION

Parenteral drug products should be inspected visually for particulate matter and discoloration prior to administration, whenever solution and container permit.

WARNING—BARBITURATES ARE NOT CHEMICALLY COMPATIBLE IN SOLUTION WITH MEPERGAN (MEPERIDINE HYDROCHLORIDE AND PROMETHAZINE HYDROCHLORIDE) AND SHOULD NOT BE MIXED IN THE SAME SYRINGE.

The TUBEX® Sterile Cartridge-Needle Unit is designed for single-dose use. VIALS should be used when required doses are fractions of a milliliter, as indicated below.

Mepergan is usually administered intramuscularly. However, in certain specific situations, the intravenous route may be employed. INADVERTENT INTRA-ARTERIAL INJECTION CAN RESULT IN GANGRENE OF THE AFFECTED EXTREMITY (see "Warnings"). SUBCUTANEOUS ADMINISTRATION IS CONTRAINDICATED, AS IT MAY RESULT IN TISSUE NECROSIS (see "Contraindications"). INJECTION INTO OR NEAR PERIPHERAL NERVES MAY RESULT IN PERMANENT NEUROLOGICAL DEFICIT.

When used intravenously, the rate should not be greater than 1 mL of Mepergan (25 mg of each component) per minute; it is preferable to inject through the tubing of an intravenous infusion set that is known to be functioning satisfactorily.

ADULT DOSE: 1 to 2 mL (25 to 50 mg of each component) per single injection, which can be repeated every 3 to 4 hours.

CHILDREN 12 YEARS OF AGE AND UNDER: 0.5 mg of each component per pound of body weight. The dosage may be repeated every 3 to 4 hours as necessary. For preanesthetic medication the usual adult dose is 2 mL (50 mg of each component) intramuscularly with or without appropriate atropinelike drug. Atropine sulfate, 0.3 to 0.4 mg, or scopolamine hydrobromide, 0.25 to 0.4 mg, in sterile solution may be mixed in the same syringe with Mepergan. Repeat doses of 50 mg or less of both promethazine and meperidine may be administered by either route at 3- to 4-hour intervals, as necessary. As an adjunct to local or general anesthesia, the usual dose is 2 mL (50 mg each of meperidine and promethazine).

OVERDOSAGE

SYMPTOMS: Serious overdose with meperidine is characterized by respiratory depression (a decrease in respiratory rate and/or tidal volume, Cheyne-Stokes respiration, cyanosis), extreme somnolence progressing to stupor or coma, skeletal muscle flaccidity, cold and clammy skin, and sometimes bradycardia and hypotension. In severe overdosage, particularly by the intravenous route, apnea, circulatory collapse, cardiac arrest, and death may occur.

TREATMENT: Primary attention should be given to the reestablishment of adequate respiratory exchange through provision of a patent airway and institution of assisted or controlled ventilation. The narcotic antagonist, naloxone hydrochloride, is a specific antidote against respiratory depression which may result from overdosage or unusual sensitivity to narcotics, including meperidine. The usual initial adult dose of naloxone is 0.4 to 2.0 mg, administered intravenously. If the desired degree of counteraction and improvement in respiratory functions is not obtained, this dosage can be repeated at two- to three-minute intervals while resuscitation efforts continue. If 10 mg of naloxone have been administered without an improvement in the clinical situation, the diagnosis of MEPERGAN overdose should be questioned.

An antagonist should not be administered in absence of clinically significant respiratory or cardiovascular depression. Oxygen, intravenous fluids, vasopressors, and other supportive measures should be employed as indicated.

NOTE: In an individual physically dependent on narcotics, the administration of the usual dose of a narcotic antagonist will precipitate an acute withdrawal syndrome. The severity of this syndrome will depend on the degree of physical dependence and the dose of antagonist administered. The use of narcotic antagonists in such individuals should be avoided if possible. If a narcotic antagonist must be used to treat serious respiratory depression in the physically dependent patient, the antagonist should be administered with extreme care and only one-tenth to one-fifth the usual initial dose administered.

Attempted suicides with promethazine have resulted in deep sedation, coma, rarely convulsions and cardiorespiratory symptoms compatible with the depth of sedation present. Extrapyramidal reactions may be treated with anticholinergic antiparkinson agents, diphenhydramine, or barbiturates.

If severe hypotension occurs, levarterenol or phenylephrine may be indicated. Epinephrine is probably best avoided, since it has been suggested that promethazine overdosage could produce a partial alpha-adrenergic blockade.

A paradoxical reaction, characterized by hyperexcitability and nightmares, has been reported in children receiving large single doses of promethazine.

HOW SUPPLIED

Mepergan® (meperidine HCl and promethazine HCl) Injection, Wyeth®, is supplied as follows:

NDC 0008-0234-01, in 10 mL vials, as single vials.

NDC 0008-0235-01, in TAMP-R-TEL® Tamper-Resistant packages of 10 TUBEX® Sterile Cartridge-Needle Units, 2 mL size (22 gauge × 1¼ inch needle).

Protect from light

MYSOLINE® ℞

[mī'sō-lēn]

(primidone)

Anticonvulsant

CAUTION: Federal law prohibits dispensing without prescription.

DESCRIPTION

Chemical name: 5-ethyldihydro-5-phenyl-4,6 (1H, 5H) pyrimidinedione.

Structural formula:

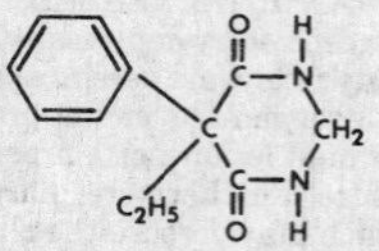

Mysoline is a white, crystalline, highly stable substance, M.P. 279–284°C. It is poorly soluble in water (60 mg per 100 mL at 37°C) and in most organic solvents. It possesses no acidic properties, in contrast to its barbiturate analog.

Mysoline 50 mg and 250 mg tablets contain the following inactive ingredients: Microcrystalline Cellulose, NF; Lactose, USP; Methylcellulose, USP; Sodium Starch Glycolate, NF; Talc, USP; Sodium Lauryl Sulfate, NF; Magnesium Stearate, NF; Water, USP, Purified.

Mysoline 250 mg tablets also contain Yellow Iron Oxide, NF.

Mysoline suspension contains these inactive ingredients: Ammonia Solution, Diluted; Citric Acid, USP; D&C Yellow No. 10; FD&C Yellow No. 6; Magnesium Aluminum Silicate; Methylparaben, NF; Propylparaben, NF; Saccharin Sodium, NF; Sodium Alginate; Sodium Citrate; Sodium Hypochlorite Solution, USP; Sorbic Acid, NF; Sorbitan Monolaurate; Water, USP, Purified; Flavors.

ACTIONS

Mysoline raises electro- or chemoshock seizure thresholds or alters seizure patterns in experimental animals. The mechanism(s) of primidone's antiepileptic action is not known.

Primidone *per se* has anticonvulsant activity as do its two metabolites, phenobarbital and phenylethylmalonamide (PEMA). In addition to its anticonvulsant activity, PEMA potentiates the anticonvulsant activity of phenobarbital in experimental animals.

INDICATIONS

Mysoline, used alone or concomitantly with other anticonvulsants, is indicated in the control of grand mal, psychomotor, and focal epileptic seizures. It may control grand mal seizures refractory to other anticonvulsant therapy.

CONTRAINDICATIONS

Primidone is contraindicated in: 1) patients with porphyria and 2) patients who are hypersensitive to phenobarbital (see ACTIONS).

WARNINGS

The abrupt withdrawal of antiepileptic medication may precipitate status epilepticus.

The therapeutic efficacy of a dosage regimen takes several weeks before it can be assessed.

USAGE IN PREGNANCY

The effects of Mysoline in human pregnancy and nursing infants are unknown.

Recent reports suggest an association between the use of anticonvulsant drugs by women with epilepsy and an elevated incidence of birth defects in children born to these women. Data are more extensive with respect to diphenylhydantoin and phenobarbital, but these are also the most commonly prescribed anticonvulsants; less systematic or anecdotal reports suggest a possible similar association with the use of all known anticonvulsant drugs.

The reports suggesting an elevated incidence of birth defects in children of drug-treated epileptic women cannot be regarded as adequate to prove a definite cause and effect relationship. There are intrinsic methodologic problems in obtaining adequate data on drug teratogenicity in humans; the possibility also exists that other factors leading to birth defects, *e.g.,* genetic factors or the epileptic condition itself, may be more important than drug therapy. The majority of mothers on anticonvulsant medication deliver normal infants. It is important to note that anticonvulsant drugs should not be discontinued in patients in whom the drug is administered to prevent major seizures because of the strong possibility of precipitating status epilepticus with attendant hypoxia and threat to life. In individual cases where the severity and frequency of the seizure disorders are such that the removal of medication does not pose a serious threat to the patient, discontinuation of the drug may be considered prior to and during pregnancy, although it cannot be said with any confidence that even minor seizures do not pose some hazard to the developing embryo or fetus.

The prescribing physician will wish to weigh these considerations in treating or counseling epileptic women of childbearing potential.

Neonatal hemorrhage, with a coagulation defect resembling vitamin K deficiency, has been described in newborns whose mothers were taking primidone and other anticonvulsants. Pregnant women under anticonvulsant therapy should receive prophylactic vitamin K_1 therapy for one month prior to, and during, delivery.

PRECAUTIONS

The total daily dosage should not exceed 2 g. Since Mysoline therapy generally extends over prolonged periods, a complete blood count and a sequential multiple analysis-12 (SMA-12) test should be made every six months.

IN NURSING MOTHERS

There is evidence that in mothers treated with primidone, the drug appears in the milk in substantial quantities. Since tests for the presence of primidone in biological fluids are too complex to be carried out in the average clinical laboratory, it is suggested that the presence of undue somnolence and drowsiness in nursing newborns of Mysoline-treated mothers be taken as an indication that nursing should be discontinued.

ADVERSE REACTIONS

The most frequently occurring early side effects are ataxia and vertigo. These tend to disappear with continued therapy, or with reduction of initial dosage. Occasionally, the following have been reported: nausea, anorexia, vomiting, fatigue, hyperirritability, emotional disturbances, sexual impotency, diplopia, nystagmus, drowsiness, and morbilliform skin eruptions. Granulocytopenia, and red-cell hypoplasia and aplasia, have been reported rarely. These and, occasionally, other persistent or severe side effects may necessitate withdrawal of the drug. Megaloblastic anemia may occur as a rare idiosyncrasy to Mysoline and to other anticonvulsants. The anemia responds to folic acid without necessity of discontinuing medication.

DOSAGE AND ADMINISTRATION

ADULT DOSAGE

Patients 8 years of age and older who have received no previous treatment may be started on Mysoline according to the following regimen using either 50 mg or scored 250 mg Mysoline tablets.

Days 1 to 3: 100 to 125 mg at bedtime
Days 4 to 6: 100 to 125 mg b.i.d.
Days 7 to 9: 100 to 125 mg t.i.d.
Day 10 to maintenance: 250 mg t.i.d.

For most adults and children 8 years of age and over, the usual maintenance dosage is three to four 250 mg Mysoline tablets daily in divided doses (250 mg t.i.d. or q.i.d.). If required, an increase to five or six 250 mg tablets daily may be made but daily doses should not exceed 500 mg q.i.d.

INITIAL: ADULTS AND CHILDREN OVER 8

KEY: · = 50 mg tablet ● = 250 mg tablet

DAY	1	2	3	4	5	6
AM				··	··	··
NOON						
PM	··	··	··	··	··	··

DAY	7	8	9	10	11	12
AM	··	··	··	●		
NOON	··	··	··	●	Adjust to Maintenance	
PM	··	··	··	●		

Dosage should be individualized to provide maximum benefit. In some cases, serum blood level determinations of primidone may be necessary for optimal dosage adjustment. The clinically effective serum level for primidone is between 5 to 12 μg/mL.

IN PATIENTS ALREADY RECEIVING OTHER ANTICONVULSANTS

Mysoline should be started at 100 to 125 mg at bedtime and gradually increased to maintenance level as the other drug is gradually decreased. This regimen should be continued until satisfactory dosage level is achieved for the combination, or

the other medication is completely withdrawn. When therapy with Mysoline alone is the objective, the transition from concomitant therapy should not be completed in less than two weeks.

PEDIATRIC DOSAGE

For children under 8 years of age, the following regimen may be used:

Days 1 to 3:   50 mg at bedtime
Days 4 to 6:   50 mg b.i.d.
Days 7 to 9:   100 mg b.i.d.
Day 10 to maintenance: 125 mg t.i.d. to 250 mg t.i.d.

For children under 8 years of age, the usual maintenance dosage is 125 to 250 mg three times daily or, 10 to 25 mg/kg/day in divided doses.

HOW SUPPLIED

MYSOLINE TABLETS

Each square-shaped, scored, yellow tablet, identified by "MYSOLINE 250" and an embossed *M*, contains 250 mg of primidone, in bottles of 100 (NDC 0046-0430-81) and 1,000 (NDC 0046-0430-91).

Also available in a unit-dose package of 100 (NDC 0046-0430-99).

Each square-shaped, scored, white tablet, identified by "MYSOLINE 50 " and an embossed *M*, contains 50 mg of primidone, in bottles of 100 (NDC 0046-0431-81) and 500 (NDC 0046-0431-85).

The appearance of these tablets is a trademark of Wyeth-Ayerst Laboratories.

MYSOLINE SUSPENSION

Each 5 mL (teaspoonful) contains 250 mg of primidone, in bottles of 8 fluid ounces (NDC 0046-3850-08).

Store at room temperature, approximately 25° C (77° F).
Dispense in a tight, light-resistant container as defined in the U.S.P.

Shown in Product Identification Section, page 437

NORDETTE®–21   ℞
[*nor-det'-21*]
TABLETS
(levonorgestrel and ethinyl estradiol tablets)

DESCRIPTION

ORAL CONTRACEPTIVE

Each Nordette tablet contains 0.15 mg of levonorgestrel (*d* (-)-13 beta-ethyl-17-alpha-ethinyl-17-beta-hydroxygon-4-en-3-one), a totally synthetic progestogen, and 0.03 mg of ethinyl estradiol (19-nor-17α-pregna-1,3,5 (10)-trien-20-yne-3,17-diol). The inactive ingredients present are cellulose, FD&C Yellow 6, lactose, magnesium stearate, and polacrilin potassium.

CLINICAL PHARMACOLOGY

Combination oral contraceptives act by suppression of gonadotropins. Although the primary mechanism of this action is inhibition of ovulation, other alterations include changes in the cervical mucus (which increase the difficulty of sperm entry into the uterus) and the endometrium (which reduce the likelihood of implantation).

INDICATIONS AND USAGE

Oral contraceptives are indicated for the prevention of pregnancy in women who elect to use this product as a method of contraception.

Oral contraceptives are highly effective. Table I lists the typical accidental pregnancy rates for users of combination oral contraceptives and other methods of contraception. The efficacy of these contraceptive methods, except sterilization and the IUD, depends upon the reliability with which they are used. Correct and consistent use of methods can result in lower failure rates.

CONTRAINDICATIONS

Oral contraceptives should not be used in women with any of the following conditions:

Thrombophlebitis or thromboembolic disorders
A past history of deep-vein thrombophlebitis or thromboembolic disorders
Cerebral-vascular or coronary-artery disease
Known or suspected carcinoma of the breast
Carcinoma of the endometrium or other known or suspected estrogen-dependent neoplasia
Undiagnosed abnormal genital bleeding
Cholestatic jaundice of pregnancy or jaundice with prior pill use
Hepatic adenomas or carcinomas
Known or suspected pregnancy

WARNINGS

Cigarette smoking increases the risk of serious cardiovascular side effects from oral-contraceptive use. This risk increases with age and with heavy smoking (15 or more cigarettes per day) and is quite marked in women over 35 years of age. Women who use oral contraceptives should be strongly advised not to smoke.

The use of oral contraceptives is associated with increased risks of several serious conditions including myocardial infarction, thromboembolism, stroke, hepatic neoplasia, gallbladder disease, and hypertension, although the risk of serious morbidity or mortality is very small in healthy women without underlying risk factors. The risk of morbidity and mortality increases significantly in the presence of other underlying risk factors such as hypertension, hyperlipidemias, obesity, and diabetes.

Practitioners prescribing oral contraceptives should be familiar with the following information relating to these risks. The information contained in this package insert is based principally on studies carried out in patients who used oral contraceptives with higher formulations of estrogens and progestogens than those in common use today. The effect of long-term use of the oral contraceptives with lower formulations of both estrogens and progestogens remains to be determined.

Throughout this labeling, epidemiological studies reported are of two types: retrospective or case control studies and prospective or cohort studies. Case control studies provide a measure of the relative risk of disease, namely, a ratio of the incidence of a disease among oral-contraceptive users to that among nonusers. The relative risk does not provide information on the actual clinical occurrence of a disease. Cohort studies provide a measure of attributable risk, which is the difference in the incidence of disease between oral-contraceptive users and nonusers. The attributable risk does provide information about the actual occurrence of a disease in the population. For further information, the reader is referred to a text on epidemiological methods.

1. THROMBOEMBOLIC DISORDERS AND OTHER VASCULAR PROBLEMS

a. *Myocardial Infarction*

An increased risk of myocardial infarction has been attributed to oral-contraceptive use. This risk is primarily in smokers or women with other underlying risk factors for coronary-artery disease such as hypertension, hypercholesterolemia, morbid obesity, and diabetes. The relative risk of heart attack for current oral-contraceptive users has been estimated to be two to six. The risk is very low under the age of 30.

Smoking in combination with oral-contraceptive use has been shown to contribute substantially to the incidence of myocardial infarctions in women in their mid-thirties or older with smoking accounting for the majority of excess cases. Mortality rates associated with circulatory disease have been shown to increase substantially in smokers over

TABLE I: LOWEST EXPECTED AND TYPICAL FAILURE RATES DURING THE FIRST YEAR OF CONTINUOUS USE OF A METHOD

% of Women Experiencing an Accidental Pregnancy in the First Year of Continuous Use

Method	Lowest Expected*	Typical**
(No Contraception)	(89)	(89)
Oral contraceptives		3
combined	0.1	N/A***
progestin only	0.5	N/A***
Diaphragm with spermicidal cream or jelly	3	18
Spermicides alone (foam, creams, jellies and vaginal suppositories)	3	21
Vaginal Sponge		
nulliparous	5	18
multiparous	>8	>28
IUD (medicated)	1	6#
Condom without spermicides	2	12
Periodic abstinence (all methods)	2–10	20
Female sterilization	0.2	0.4
Male sterilization	0.1	0.15

Adapted from J. Trussell and K. Kost, Table 11, Studies in Family Planning, 18(5), Sept.–Oct. 1987.

---

* The authors' best guess of the percentage of women expected to experience an accidental pregnancy among couples who initiate a method (not necessarily for the first time) and who use it consistently and correctly during the first year if they do not stop for any other reason.

** This term represents "typical" couples who initiate use of a method (not necessarily for the first time), who experience an accidental pregnancy during the first year if they do not stop use for any other reason.

*** N/A—Data not available

\# Combined typical rate for both medicated and non-medicated IUD. The rate for medicated IUD alone is not available.

---

the age of 35 and nonsmokers over the age of 40 (Table II) among women who use oral contraceptives.

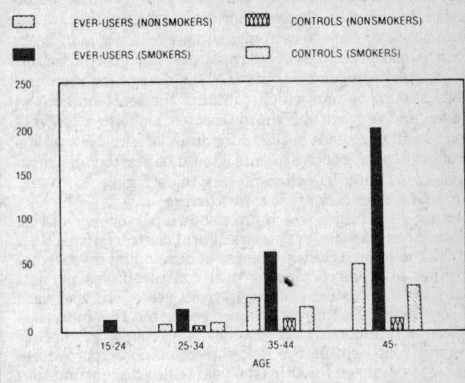

CIRCULATORY DISEASE MORTALITY RATES PER 100,000 WOMAN YEARS BY AGE, SMOKING STATUS AND ORAL-CONTRACEPTIVE USE

EVER-USERS (NONSMOKERS)   CONTROLS (NONSMOKERS)
EVER-USERS (SMOKERS)   CONTROLS (SMOKERS)

TABLE II.   (Adapted from P.M. Layde and V. Beral, Lancet. 1:541–546, 1981.)

Oral contraceptives may compound the effects of well-known risk factors, such as hypertension, diabetes, hyperlipidemias, age, and obesity. In particular, some progestogens are known to decrease HDL cholesterol and cause glucose intolerance, while estrogens may create a state of hyperinsulinism. Oral contraceptives have been shown to increase blood pressure among users (see section 9 in "Warnings"). Similar effects on risk factors have been associated with an increased risk of heart disease. Oral contraceptives must be used with caution in women with cardiovascular disease risk factors.

b. *Thromboembolism*

An increased risk of thromboembolic and thrombotic disease associated with the use of oral contraceptives is well established. Case control studies have found the relative risk of users compared to nonusers to be 3 for the first episode of superficial venous thrombosis, 4 to 11 for deep vein thrombosis or pulmonary embolism, and 1.5 to 6 for women with predisposing conditions for venous thromboembolic disease. Cohort studies have shown the relative risk to be somewhat lower, about 3 for new cases and about 4.5 for new cases requiring hospitalization. The risk of thromboembolic disease due to oral contraceptives is not related to length of use and disappears after pill use is stopped.

A two- to four-fold increase in relative risk of postoperative thromboembolic complications has been reported with the use of oral contraceptives. The relative risk of venous thrombosis in women who have predisposing conditions is twice that of women without such medical conditions. If feasible, oral contraceptives should be discontinued at least four weeks prior to and for two weeks after elective surgery of a type associated with an increase in risk of thromboembolism and during and following prolonged immobilization. Since the immediate postpartum period is also associated with an increased risk of thromboembolism, oral contraceptives should be started no earlier than four to six weeks after delivery in women who elect not to breast feed, or a midtrimester pregnancy termination.

c. *Cerebrovascular diseases*

Oral contraceptives have been shown to increase both the relative and attributable risks of cerebrovascular events (thrombotic and hemorrhagic strokes), although, in general, the risk is greatest among older (> 35 years), hypertensive women who also smoke. Hypertension was found to be a risk factor for both users and nonusers, for both types of strokes, while smoking interacted to increase the risk for hemorrhagic strokes.

In a large study, the relative risk of thrombotic strokes has been shown to range from 3 for normotensive users to 14 for users with severe hypertension. The relative risk of hemorrhagic stroke is reported to be 1.2 for nonsmokers who used oral contraceptives, 2.6 for smokers who did not use oral contraceptives, 7.6 for smokers who used oral contraceptives, 1.8 for normotensive users and 25.7 for users with severe hypertension. The attributable risk is also greater in older women.

d. *Dose-related risk of vascular disease from oral contraceptives*

A positive association has been observed between the amount of estrogen and progestogen in oral contraceptives and the risk of vascular disease. A decline in serum high-density lipoproteins (HDL) has been reported with many progestational agents. A decline in serum high-density lipoproteins has been associated with an increased incidence of ischemic heart disease. Because estrogens increase HDL cholesterol, the net effect of an oral contraceptive depends on a balance achieved between doses of estrogen and progesto-

Continued on next page

Wyeth-Ayerst Laboratories—Cont.

gen and the nature and absolute amount of progestogen used in the contraceptive. The amount of both hormones should be considered in the choice of an oral contraceptive.

Minimizing exposure to estrogen and progestogen is in keeping with good principles of therapeutics. For any particular estrogen/progestogen combination, the dosage regimen prescribed should be one which contains the least amount of estrogen and progestogen that is compatible with a low failure rate and the needs of the individual patient. New acceptors of oral-contraceptive agents should be started on preparations containing less than 50 mcg of estrogen.

e. *Persistence of risk of vascular disease*

There are two studies which have shown persistence of risk of vascular disease for ever-users of oral contraceptives. In a study in the United States, the risk of developing myocardial infarction after discontinuing oral contraceptives persists for at least 9 years for women 40 to 49 years who had used oral contraceptives for five or more years, but this increased risk was not demonstrated in other age groups. In another study in Great Britain, the risk of developing cerebrovascular disease persisted for at least 6 years after discontinuation of oral contraceptives, although excess risk was very small. However, both studies were performed with oral contraceptive formulations containing 50 micrograms or higher of estrogens.

2. ESTIMATES OF MORTALITY FROM CONTRACEPTIVE USE

One study gathered data from a variety of sources which have estimated the mortality rate associated with different methods of contraception at different ages (Table III). These estimates include the combined risk of death associated with contraceptive methods plus the risk attributable to pregnancy in the event of method failure. Each method of contraception has its specific benefits and risks. The study concluded that with the exception of oral-contraceptive users 35 and older who smoke and 40 and older who do not smoke, mortality associated with all methods of birth control is less than that associated with childbirth. The observation of a possible increase in risk of mortality with age for oral-contraceptive users is based on data gathered in the 1970's—but not reported until 1983. However, current clinical practice involves the use of lower estrogen dose formulations combined with careful restriction of oral-contraceptive use to women who do not have the various risk factors listed in this labeling.

Because of these changes in practice and, also, because of some limited new data which suggest that the risk of cardiovascular disease with the use of oral contraceptives may now be less than previously observed, the Fertility and Maternal Health Drugs Advisory Committee was asked to review the topic in 1989. The Committee concluded that although cardiovascular-disease risks may be incraesed with oral-contraceptive use after age 40 in healthy nonsmoking women (even with the newer low-dose formulations), there are greater potential health risks associated with pregnancy in older women and with the alternative surgical and medical procedures which may be necessary if such women do not have access to effective and acceptable means of contraception. Therefore, the Committee recommended that the benefits of oral-contraceptive use by healthy nonsmoking women over 40 may outweigh the possible risks. Of course, older women, as all women who take oral contraceptives, should take the lowest possible dose formulation that is effective.

3. CARCINOMA OF THE REPRODUCTIVE ORGANS

Numerous epidemiological studies have been performed on the incidence of breast, endometrial, ovarian, and cervical cancer in women using oral contraceptives. The overwhelming evidence in the literature suggests that the use of oral contraceptives is not associated with an increase in the risk of developing breast cancer, regardless of the age and parity of first use or with most of the marketed brands and doses. The Cancer and Steroid Hormone (CASH) study also showed no latent effect on the risk of breast cancer for at least a decade following long-term use. A few studies have shown a slightly increased relative risk of developing breast cancer, although the methodology of these studies, which included differences in examination of users and nonusers and differences in age at start of use, has been questioned.

Some studies suggest that oral-contraceptive use has been associated with an increase in the risk of cervical intraepithelial neoplasia in some populations of women. However, there continues to be controversy about the extent to which such findings may be due to differences in sexual behavior and other factors.

In spite of many studies of the relationship between oral-contraceptive use and breast and cervical cancers, a cause-and-effect relationship has not been established.

4. HEPATIC NEOPLASIA

Benign hepatic adenomas are associated with oral-contraceptive use, although the incidence of benign tumors is rare in the United States. Indirect calculations have estimated the attributable risk to be in the range of 3.3 cases/100,000 for users, a risk that increases after four or more years of use. Rupture of rare, benign, hepatic adenomas may cause death through intra-abdominal hemorrhage.

Studies from Britain have shown an increased risk of developing hepatocellular carcinoma in long-term (>8 years) oral-contraceptive users. However, these cancers are extremely rare in the U.S. and the attributable risk (the excess incidence) of liver cancers in oral-contraceptive users approaches less than one per million users.

5. OCULAR LESIONS

There have been clincial case reports of retinal thrombosis associated with the use of oral contraceptives. Oral contraceptives should be discontinued if there is unexplained partial or complete loss of vision; onset of proptosis or diplopia; papilledema; or retinal vascular lesions. Appropriate diagnostic and therapeutic measures should be undertaken immediately.

6. ORAL-CONTRACEPTIVE USE BEFORE OR DURING EARLY PREGNANCY

Extensive epidemiological studies have revealed no increased risk of birth defects in women who have used oral contraceptives prior to pregnancy. Studies also do not suggest a teratogenic effect, particularly insofar as cardiac anomalies and limb-reduction defects are concerned, when taken inadvertently during early pregnancy.

The administration of oral contraceptives to induce withdrawal bleeding should not be used as a test for pregnancy. Oral contraceptives should not be used during pregnancy to treat threatened or habitual abortion.

It is recommended that for any patient who has missed two consecutive periods, pregnancy should be ruled out before continuing oral-contraceptive use. If the patient has not adhered to the prescribed schedule, the possibility of pregnancy should be considered at the time of the first missed period. Oral-contraceptive use should be discontinued until pregnancy is confirmed.

7. GALLBLADDER DISEASE

Earlier studies have reported an increased lifetime relative risk of gallbladder surgery in users of oral contraceptives and estrogens. More recent studies, however, have shown that the relative risk of developing gallbladder disease among oral-contraceptive users may be minimal. The recent findings of minimal risk may be related to the use of oral-contraceptive formulations containing lower hormonal doses of estrogens and progestogens.

TABLE III—ANNUAL NUMBER OF BIRTH-RELATED OR METHOD-RELATED DEATHS ASSOCIATED WITH CONTROL OF FERTILITY PER 100,000 NONSTERILE WOMEN, BY FERTILITY-CONTROL METHOD ACCORDING TO AGE

Method of control and outcome	15–19	20–24	25–29	30–34	35–39	40–44
No fertility-control methods*	7.0	7.4	9.1	14.8	25.7	28.2
Oral contraceptives nonsmoker**	0.3	0.5	0.9	1.9	13.8	31.6
Oral contraceptives smoker**	2.2	3.4	6.6	13.5	51.1	117.2
IUD**	0.8	0.8	1.0	1.0	1.4	1.4
Condom*	1.1	1.6	0.7	0.2	0.3	0.4
Diaphragm/spermicide*	1.9	1.2	1.2	1.3	2.2	2.8
Periodic abstinence*	2.5	1.6	1.6	1.7	2.9	3.6

* Deaths are birth related
** Deaths are method related

Adapted from H.W. Ory, Family Planning Perspectives, 15:57–63, 1983.

8. CARBOHYDRATE AND LIPID METABOLIC EFFECTS

Oral contraceptives have been shown to cause glucose intolerance in a significant percentage of users. Oral contraceptives containing greater than 75 micrograms of estrogens cause hyperinsulinism, while lower doses of estrogen cause less glucose intolerance. Progestogens increase insulin secretion and create insulin resistance, this effect varying with different progestational agents. However, in the nondiabetic woman, oral contraceptives appear to have no effect on fasting blood glucose. Because of these demonstrated effects, prediabetic and diabetic women should be carefully observed while taking oral contraceptives.

A small proportion of women will have persistent hypertriglyceridemia while on the pill. As discussed earlier (see Warnings 1a and 1d), changes in serum triglycerides and lipoprotein levels have been reported in oral-contraceptive users.

9. ELEVATED BLOOD PRESSURE

An increase in blood pressure has been reported in women taking oral contraceptives, and this increase is more likely in older oral-contraceptive users and with continued use. Data from the Royal College of General Practitioners and subsequent randomized trials have shown that the incidence of hypertension increases with increasing quantities of progestogens.

Women with a history of hypertension or hypertension-related diseases, or renal disease should be encouraged to use another method of contraception. If women with hypertension elect to use oral contraceptives, they should be monitored closely, and if significant elevation of blood pressure occurs, oral contraceptives should be discontinued. For most women, elevated blood pressure will return to normal after stopping oral contraceptives, and there is no difference in the occurrence of hypertension among ever- and never-users.

10. HEADACHE

The onset or exacerbation of migraine or development of headache with a new pattern that is recurrent, persistent, or severe requires discontinuation of oral contraceptives and evaluation of the cause.

11. BLEEDING IRREGULARITIES

Breakthrough bleeding and spotting are sometimes encountered in patients on oral contraceptives, especially during the first three months of use. The type and dose of progestogen may be important. Non-hormonal causes should be considered and adequate diagnostic measures taken to rule out malignancy or pregnancy in the event of breakthrough bleeding, as in the case of any abnormal vaginal bleeding. If pathology has been excluded, time or a change to another formulation may solve the problem. In the event of amenorrhea, pregnancy should be ruled out.

Some women may encounter post-pill amenorrhea or oligomenorrhea, especially when such a condition was preexistent.

PRECAUTIONS

1. PHYSICAL EXAMINATION AND FOLLOW-UP

A complete medical history and physical examination should be taken prior to the initiation or reinstitution of oral contraceptives and at least annually during use of oral contraceptives. These physical examinations should include special reference to blood pressure, breasts, abdomen and pelvic organs, including cervical cytology, and relevant laboratory tests. In case of undiagnosed, persistent or recurrent abnormal vaginal bleeding, appropriate diagnostic measures should be conducted to rule out malignancy. Women with a strong family history of breast cancer or who have breast nodules should be monitored with particular care.

2. LIPID DISORDERS

Women who are being treated for hyperlipidemias should be followed closely if they elect to use oral contraceptives. Some progestogens may elevate LDL levels and may render the control of hyperlipidemias more difficult. (See "Warnings," 1d.).

3. LIVER FUNCTION

If jaundice develops in any woman receiving such drugs, the medication should be discontinued. Steroid hormones may be poorly metabolized in patients with impaired liver function.

4. FLUID RETENTION

Oral contraceptives may cause some degree of fluid retention. They should be prescribed with caution, and only with careful monitoring, in patients with conditions which might be aggravated by fluid retention.

5. EMOTIONAL DISORDERS

Patients becoming significantly depressed while taking oral contraceptives should stop the medication and use an alternate method of contraception in an attempt to determine whether the symptom is drug related. Women with a history of depression should be carefully observed and the drug discontinued if depression recurs to a serious degree.

6. CONTACT LENSES

Contact lens wearers who develop visual changes or changes in lens tolerance should be assessed by an ophthalmologist.

7. DRUG INTERACTIONS

Reduced efficacy and increased incidence of breakthrough bleeding and menstrual irregularities have been associated with concomitant use of rifampin. A similar assocation, though less marked, has been suggested with barbiturates, phenylbutazone, phenytoin sodium, and possibly with griseofulvin, ampicillin and tetracyclines.

8. INTERACTIONS WITH LABORATORY TESTS

Certain endocrine- and liver-function tests and blood components may be affected by oral contraceptives:

a. Increased prothrombin and factors VII, VIII, IX, and X; decreased antithrombin 3; increased norepinephrine-induced platelet aggregability.
b. Increased thyroid-binding globulin (TBG) leading to increased circulating total thyroid hormone, as measured by protein-bound iodine (PBI), T4 by column or by radioimmunoassay. Free T3 resin uptake is decreased, reflecting the elevated TBG; free T4 concentration is unaltered.
c. Other binding proteins may be elevated in serum.
d. Sex-binding globulins are increased and result in elevated levels of total circulating sex steroids and corticoids; however, free or biologically active levels remain unchanged.
e. Triglycerides may be increased.
f. Glucose tolerance may be decreased.
g. Serum folate levels may be depressed by oral contraceptive therapy. This may be of clinical significance if a woman becomes pregnant shortly after discontinuing oral contraceptives.

9. CARCINOGENESIS
See "Warnings" section.

10. PREGNANCY
Pregnancy Category X. See Contraindications and Warnings sections.

11. NURSING MOTHERS
Small amounts of oral-contraceptive steroids have been identified in the milk of nursing mothers, and a few adverse effects on the child have been reported, including jaundice and breast enlargement. In addition, oral contraceptives given in the postpartum period may interfere with lactation by decreasing the quantity and quality of breast milk. If possible, the nursing mother should be advised not to use oral contraceptives but to use other forms of contraception until she has completely weaned her child.

INFORMATION FOR THE PATIENT
See Patient Labeling Printed Below.

ADVERSE REACTIONS

An increased risk of the following serious adverse reactions has been associated with the use of oral contraceptives (see "Warnings" section):

Thrombophlebitis.
Arterial thromboembolism.
Pulmonary embolism.
Myocardial infarction.
Cerebral hemorrhage.
Cerebral thrombosis.
Hypertension.
Gallbladder disease.
Hepatic adenomas or benign liver tumors.

There is evidence of an association between the following conditions and the use of oral contraceptives, although additional confirmatory studies are needed:

Mesenteric thrombosis.
Retinal thrombosis.

The following adverse reactions have been reported in patients receiving oral contraceptives and are believed to be drug-related:

Nausea.
Vomiting.
Gastrointestinal symptoms (such as abdominal cramps and bloating).
Breakthrough bleeding.
Spotting.
Change in menstrual flow.
Amenorrhea.
Temporary infertility after discontinuation of treatment.
Edema.
Melasma which may persist.
Breast changes: tenderness, enlargement, secretion.
Change in weight (increase or decrease).
Change in cervical erosion and secretion.
Diminution in lactation when given immediately postpartum.
Cholestatic jaundice.
Migraine.
Rash (allergic).
Mental depression.
Reduced tolerance to carbohydrates.
Vaginal candidiasis.
Change in corneal curvature (steepening).
Intolerance to contact lenses.

The following adverse reactions have been reported in users of oral contraceptives, and the association has been neither confirmed nor refuted:

Congenital anomalies.
Premenstrual syndrome.
Cataracts.
Optic neuritis.
Changes in appetite.
Cystitis-like syndrome.
Headache.
Nervousness.
Dizziness.
Hirsutism.
Loss of scalp hair.
Erythema multiforme.
Erythema nodosum.
Hemorrhagic eruption.
Vaginitis.
Porphyria.
Impaired renal function.
Hemolytic uremic syndrome.
Budd-Chiari syndrome.
Acne.
Changes in libido.
Colitis.
Sickle-cell disease.
Cerebral-vascular disease with mitral valve prolapse.
Lupus-like syndromes.

OVERDOSAGE

Serious ill effects have not been reported following acute ingestion of large doses of oral contraceptives by young children. Overdosage may cause nausea, and withdrawal bleeding may occur in females.

NONCONTRACEPTIVE HEALTH BENEFITS

The following noncontraceptive health benefits related to the use of oral contraceptives are supported by epidemiological studies which largely utilized oral-contraceptive formulations containing doses exceeding 0.035 mg of ethinyl estradiol or 0.05 mg of mestranol.

Effects on menses:
Increased menstrual cycle regularity
Decreased blood loss and decreased incidence of iron deficiency anemia
Decreased incidence of dysmenorrhea
Effects related to inhibition of ovulation:
Decreased incidence of functional ovarian cysts
Decreased incidence of ectopic pregnancies
Effects from long-term use:
Decreased incidence of fibroadenomas and fibrocystic disease of the breast
Decreased incidence of acute pelvic inflammatory disease
Decreased incidence of endometrial cancer
Decreased incidence of ovarian cancer

DOSAGE AND ADMINISTRATION

To achieve maximum contraceptive effectiveness, Nordette-21 must be taken exactly as directed and at intervals not exceeding 24 hours. The dosage of Nordette-21 is one tablet daily for 21 consecutive days per menstrual cycle according to prescribed schedule. Tablets are then discontinued for 7 days (three weeks on, one week off).

It is recommended that Nordette-21 tablets be taken at the same time each day, preferably after the evening meal or at bedtime. During the first cycle of medication, the patient is instructed to take one Nordette-21 tablet daily for twenty-one consecutive days beginning on day five of her menstrual cycle. (The first day of menstruation is day one.) The tablets are then discontinued for one week (7 days). Withdrawal bleeding should usually occur within three days following discontinuation of Nordette-21.

(If Nordette-21 is first taken later than the fifth day of the first menstrual cycle of medication or postpartum, contraceptive reliance should not be placed on Nordette-21 until after the first seven consecutive days of administration. The possibility of ovulation and conception prior to initiation of medication should be considered.)

The patient begins her next and all subsequent 21-day courses of Nordette-21 tablets on the same day of the week that she began her first course, following the same schedule: 21 days on—7 days off. She begins taking her tablets on the 8th day after discontinuance regardless of whether or not a menstrual period has occurred or is still in progress. Any time a new cycle of Nordette-21 is started later than the 8th day, the patient should be protected by another means of contraception until she has taken a tablet daily for seven consecutive days.

If spotting or breakthrough bleeding occurs, the patient is instructed to continue on the same regimen. This type of bleeding is usually transient and without significance; however, if the bleeding is persistent or prolonged the patient is advised to consult her physician. Although the occurrence of pregnancy is highly unlikely if Nordette-21 is taken according to directions, if withdrawal bleeding does not occur, the possibility of pregnancy must be considered. If the patient has not adhered to the prescribed schedule (missed one or more tablets or started taking them on a day later than she should have) the probability of pregnancy should be considered at the time of the first missed period and appropriate

diagnostic measures taken before the medication is resumed. If the patient has adhered to the prescribed regimen and misses two consecutive periods, pregnancy should be ruled out before continuing the contraceptive regimen.

The patient should be instructed to take a missed tablet as soon as it is remembered. If two consecutive tablets are missed, they should both be taken as soon as remembered. The next tablet should be taken at the usual time.

Any time the patient misses one or two tablets she should also use another method of contraception until she has taken a tablet daily for seven consecutive days. If breakthrough bleeding occurs following missed tablets it will usually be transient and of no consequence. While there is little likelihood of ovulation occurring if only one or two tablets are missed, the possibility of ovulation increases with each successive day that scheduled tablets are missed. If three consecutive tablets are missed, all medication should be discontinued and the remainder of the package discarded. A new tablet cycle should be started on the 8th day after the last tablet was taken, and an alternate means of contraception should be prescribed during the seven days without tablets and until the patient has taken a tablet daily for seven consecutive days.

In the nonlactating mother, Nordette-21 may be initiated postpartum, for contraception. When the tablets are administered in the postpartum period, the increased risk of thromboembolic disease associated with the postpartum period must be considered (see "Contraindications," "Warnings," and "Precautions" concerning thromboembolic disease). It is to be noted that early resumption of ovulation may occur if Parlodel® (bromocriptine mesylate) has been used for the prevention of lactation.

HOW SUPPLIED

Nordette®-21 Tablets (0.15 mg levonorgestrel and 0.03 mg ethinyl estradiol), Wyeth®, are available in 6 PILPAK® dispensers of 21 tablets each as follows: NDC 0008-0075, light-orange, round tablet marked "WYETH" and "75".

References available upon request.
Brief Summary Patient Package Insert: See Lo/Ovral.
DETAILED PATIENT LABELING: See Lo/Ovral.
Shown in Product Identification Section, page 437

NORDETTE®-28   ℞
[nor-det '-28]
TABLETS
(levonorgestrel and ethinyl estradiol tablets)

DESCRIPTION

21 light-orange Nordette tablets, each containing 0.15 mg of levonorgestrel (d (-)-13 beta-ethyl -17-alpha-ethinyl-17-beta-hydroxygon-4-en-3-one), a totally synthetic progestogen, and 0.03 mg of ethinyl estradiol (19-nor-17α-pregna-1,3,5 (10)-trien-20-yne-3,17-diol), and 7 pink inert tablets. The inactive ingredients present are cellulose, D&C Red 30, FD&C Yellow 6, lactose, magnesium stearate, and polacrilin potassium.

CLINICAL PHARMACOLOGY
See NORDETTE®-21

INDICATIONS AND USAGE
See NORDETTE-21

CONTRAINDICATIONS
See NORDETTE-21

WARNINGS
See NORDETTE-21

PRECAUTIONS
See NORDETTE-21
Drug Interactions: See NORDETTE-21
Carcinogenesis: See NORDETTE-21
Nursing Mothers: See NORDETTE-21
Information for the Patient: See NORDETTE-21

ADVERSE REACTIONS
See NORDETTE-21

OVERDOSAGE
See NORDETTE-21

NONCONTRACEPTIVE HEALTH BENEFITS
See NORDETTE-21

DOSAGE AND ADMINISTRATION
To achieve maximum contraceptive effectiveness, Nordette-28 must be taken exactly as directed and at intervals not exceeding 24 hours.
The dosage of Nordette-28 is one light-orange tablet daily for 21 consecutive days, followed by one pink inert tablet daily for 7 consecutive days, according to prescribed schedule. It is recommended that tablets be taken at the same time each day, preferably after the evening meal or at bedtime.

Continued on next page

Wyeth-Ayerst Laboratories—Cont.

During the first cycle of medication, the patient is instructed to begin taking Nordette-28 on the first Sunday after the onset of menstruation. If menstruation begins on a Sunday, the first tablet (light-orange) is taken that day. One light-orange tablet should be taken daily for 21 consecutive days, followed by one pink inert tablet daily for 7 consecutive days. Withdrawal bleeding should usually occur within three days following discontinuation of light-orange tablets.
During the first cycle, contraceptive reliance should not be placed on Nordette-28 until a light-orange tablet has been taken daily for 7 consecutive days. The possibility of ovulation and conception prior to initiation of medication should be considered.
The patient begins her next and all subsequent 28-day courses of tablets on the same day of the week (Sunday) on which she began her first course, following the same schedule: 21 days on light-orange tablets—7 days on pink inert tablets. If in any cycle the patient starts tablets later than the proper day, she should protect herself by using another method of birth control until she has taken a light-orange tablet daily for 7 consecutive days.
If spotting or breakthrough bleeding occurs, the patient is instructed to continue on the same regimen. This type of bleeding is usually transient and without significance; however, if the bleeding is persistent or prolonged, the patient is advised to consult her physician. Although the occurrence of pregnancy is highly unlikely if Nordette-28 is taken according to directions, if withdrawal bleeding does not occur, the possibility of pregnancy must be considered. If the patient has not adhered to the prescribed schedule (missed one or more tablets or started taking them on a day later than she should have), the probability of pregnancy should be considered at the time of the first missed period and appropriate diagnostic measures taken before the medication is resumed. If the patient has adhered to the prescribed regimen and misses two consecutive periods, pregnancy should be ruled out before continuing the contraceptive regimen.
The patient should be instructed to take a missed light-orange tablet as soon as it is remembered. If two consecutive light-orange tablets are missed, they should both be taken as soon as remembered. The next tablet should be taken at the usual time.
Any time the patient misses one or two light-orange tablets, she should also use another method of contraception until she has taken a light-orange tablet daily for seven consecutive days. If the patient misses one or more pink tablets, she is still protected against pregnancy **provided** she begins taking light-orange tablets again on the proper day.
If breakthrough bleeding occurs following missed light-orange tablets, it will usually be transient and of no consequence. While there is little likelihood of ovulation occurring if only one or two light-orange tablets are missed, the possibility of ovulation increases with each successive day that scheduled light-orange tablets are missed. If three consecutive light-orange Nordette tablets are missed, all medication should be discontinued and the remainder of the 28-day package discarded. A new tablet cycle should be started on the first Sunday following the last missed tablet, and an alternate means of contraception should be prescribed during the days without tablets and until the patient has taken a light-orange tablet daily for 7 consecutive days.
In the nonlactating mother, Nordette-28 may be initiated postpartum, for contraception. When the tablets are administered in the postpartum period, the increased risk of thromboembolic disease associated with the postpartum period must be considered (see Contraindications, Warnings, and Precautions concerning thromboembolic disease). It is to be noted that early resumption of ovulation may occur if Parlodel® (bromocriptine mesylate) has been used for the prevention of lactation.

HOW SUPPLIED

Nordette®-28 Tablets (0.15 mg levonorgestrel and 0.03 mg ethinyl estradiol), Wyeth®, are available in 6 PILPAK® dispensers, each containing 28 tablets as follows:
21 active tablets, NDC 0008-2533, light-orange, round tablet marked "WYETH" and "75".
7 inert tablets, NDC 0008-0486, pink, round tablet marked "WYETH" and "486".

References available upon request.
Brief Summary Patient Package Insert: See LO/OVRAL.
DETAILED PATIENT LABELING: See LO/OVRAL.
Shown in Product Identification Section, page 437

NORPLANT® SYSTEM ℞
(levonorgestrel implants)

DESCRIPTION

The NORPLANT SYSTEM kit contains levonorgestrel implants, a set of six flexible closed capsules made of Silastic®

TABLE 1
Annual and Five-Year Cumulative Pregnancy Rates
Per 100 Users by Weight Class

Weight class	year 1	year 2	year 3	year 4	year 5	Cumulative
<50 kg (<110 lbs)	0.2	0	0	0	0	0.2
50–59 kg (110–130 lbs)	0.2	0.5	0.4	2.0	0.4	3.4
60–69 kg (131–153 lbs)	0.4	0.5	1.6	1.7	0.8	5.0
≥70 kg (≥154 lbs)	0	1.1	5.1	2.5	0	8.5
All	0.2	0.5	1.2	1.6	0.4	3.9

(dimethylsiloxane/methylvinylsiloxane copolymer), each containing 36 mg of the progestin levonorgestrel contained in an insertion kit to facilitate implantation. The capsules are sealed with Silastic (polydimethylsiloxane) adhesive and sterilized. Each capsule is 2.4 mm in diameter and 34 mm in length. The capsules are inserted in a superficial plane beneath the skin of the upper arm.
Information contained herewith regarding safety and efficacy was derived from studies which used two slightly different Silastic tubing formulations. The formulation being used in the NORPLANT SYSTEM has slightly higher release rates of levonorgestrel and at least comparable efficacy.
Evidence indicates that the dose of levonorgestrel provided by the NORPLANT SYSTEM is initially about 85 mcg/day followed by a decline to about 50 mcg/day by 9 months and to about 35 mcg/day by 18 months with a further decline thereafter to about 30 mcg/day. The NORPLANT SYSTEM is a progestin-only product and does not contain estrogen.
Levonorgestrel, (d(-)-13-beta-ethyl-17-alpha-ethinyl-17-beta-hydroxygon-4-en-3-one), the active ingredient in the NORPLANT SYSTEM, has a molecular weight of 312.46 and the following structural formula:

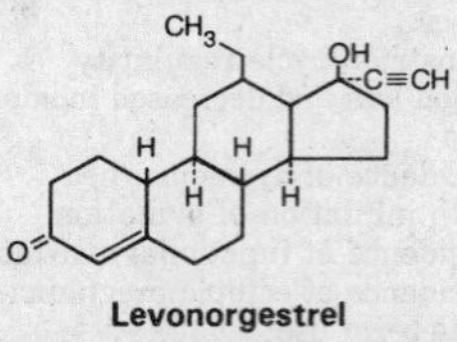

Levonorgestrel

CLINICAL PHARMACOLOGY

Levonorgestrel is a totally synthetic and biologically active progestin which exhibits no significant estrogenic activity and is highly progestational. The absolute configuration conforms to that of D-natural steroids. Levonorgestrel is not subjected to a "first-pass" effect and is virtually 100% bioavailable. Plasma concentrations average approximately 0.30 ng/mL over 5 years but are highly variable as a function of individual metabolism and body weight.
Diffusion of levonorgestrel through the wall of each capsule provides a continuous low dose of the progestin. Resulting blood levels are substantially below those generally observed among users of combination oral contraceptives containing the progestins norgestrel or levonorgestrel. Because of the range of variability in blood levels and variation in individual response, blood levels alone are not predictive of the risk of pregnancy in an individual woman.
At least two mechanisms are active in preventing pregnancy: ovulation inhibition and thickening of the cervical mucus. Other mechanisms may add to these contraceptive effects.
Levonorgestrel concentrations among women show considerable variation depending on individual clearance rates, body weight, and possibly other factors. Levonorgestrel concentrations reach a maximum, or near maximum, within 24 hours after placement with mean values of 1600 ± 1100 pg/mL. They decline rapidly over the first month partially due to a circulating protein, SHBG, that binds levonorgestrel and which is depressed by the presence of levonorgestrel. At 3 months, mean levels decline to values of around 400 pg/mL while concentrations normalized to a 60 kg body weight were 327 ± 119 (SD) pg/mL at 12 months with further decline by 1.4 pg/mL/month to reach 258 ± 95 (SD) pg/mL at 60 months.
Concentrations decreased with increasing body weight by a mean of 3.3 pg/mL/kg. After capsule removal, mean concentrations drop to below 100 pg/mL by 96 hours and to below assay sensitivity (50 pg/mL) by 5 to 14 days. Fertility rates return to levels comparable to those seen in the general population of women using no method of contraception. Circulating concentrations can be used to forecast the risk of pregnancy only in a general statistical sense. Mean concentrations associated with pregnancy have been 210 ± 60 (SD) pg/mL. However, in clinical studies, 20 percent of women had one or more values below 200 pg/mL but an average annual gross pregnancy rate of less than 1.0 per 100 women through 5 years.
Although lipoprotein levels were altered in several clinical studies with the NORPLANT SYSTEM, the long-term clinical effects of these changes have not been determined. A decrease in total cholesterol levels has been reported in all lipoprotein studies and reached statistical significance in several. Both increases and decreases in high-density lipoprotein (HDL) levels have been reported in clinical trials. No statistically significant increases have been reported in the ratio of total cholesterol to HDL-cholesterol. Low-density lipoprotein (LDL) levels decreased during NORPLANT SYSTEM use. Triglyceride levels also decreased from pretreatment values.

INDICATIONS AND USAGE

The NORPLANT SYSTEM is indicated for the prevention of pregnancy and is a long-term (up to 5 years) reversible contraceptive system. The capsules should be removed by the end of the 5th year. New capsules may be inserted at that time if continuing contraceptive protection is desired.
In multicenter trials with the NORPLANT SYSTEM, involving 2470 women, the relationship between body weight and efficacy was investigated. Tabulated below is the pregnancy experience as a function of body weight. Because NORPLANT SYSTEM is a long-term method of contraception, this is reported over five years of use. [See Table 1.]
Typically, pregnancy rates with contraceptive methods are reported for only the first year of use as shown below. The efficacy of these contraceptive methods, except the IUD and sterilization, depends in part on the reliability of use. The efficacy of the NORPLANT SYSTEM does not depend on patient compliance.

TABLE 2
Lowest Expected and Typical Failure Rates (%)
During the First Year of Use of a Contraceptive Method

Method	Lowest Expected	Typical
Male Sterilization	0.1	0.15
NORPLANT SYSTEM	0.2	0.2
Female Sterilization	0.2	0.4
Oral contraceptives		3
Combined	0.1	N/A
Progestin only	0.5	N/A
IUD	<1	3
Condom without spermicide	2	12
Cervical Cap	6	18
Diaphragm with spermicide cream or jelly	6	18
Vaginal sponge		
nulliparous	6	18
parous	9	28
Spermicides alone (foam, creams, jellies, and vaginal suppositories)	3	21
Periodic abstinence (all methods)	1–9	20
No contraception (planned pregnancy)	85	85

N/A—not available

NORPLANT SYSTEM gross annual discontinuation and continuation rates are summarized in Table 3.
[See table on next page.]

CONTRAINDICATIONS

1. Active thrombophlebitis or thromboembolic disorders.
2. Undiagnosed abnormal genital bleeding.
3. Known or suspected pregnancy.
4. Acute liver disease; benign or malignant liver tumors.
5. Known or suspected carcinoma of the breast.

WARNINGS

A. WARNINGS BASED ON EXPERIENCE WITH THE NORPLANT SYSTEM

1. *Bleeding Irregularities*

Most women can expect some variation in menstrual bleeding patterns. Irregular menstrual bleeding, intermenstrual spotting, prolonged episodes of bleeding and spotting, and amenorrhea occur in some women. Irregular bleeding patterns associated with the NORPLANT SYSTEM could mask symptoms of cervical or endometrial cancer. Overall, these irregularities diminish with continuing use. Since some NORPLANT SYSTEM users experience periods of amenorrhea, missed menstrual periods cannot serve as the only

means of identifying early pregnancy. Pregnancy tests should be performed whenever a pregnancy is suspected. Six (6) weeks or more of amenorrhea after a pattern of regular menses may signal pregnancy. If pregnancy occurs, the capsules must be removed.

Although bleeding irregularities have occurred in clinical trials, proportionately more women had increases rather than decreases in hemoglobin concentrations, a difference that was highly statistically significant. This finding generally indicates that reduced menstrual blood loss is associated with the use of the NORPLANT SYSTEM. In rare instances, blood loss did result in hemoglobin values consistent with anemia.

2. *Delayed Follicular Atresia*

If follicular development occurs with the NORPLANT SYSTEM, atresia of the follicle is sometimes delayed, and the follicle may continue to grow beyond the size it would attain in a normal cycle. These enlarged follicles cannot be distinguished clinically from ovarian cysts. In the majority of women, enlarged follicles will spontaneously disappear and should not require surgery. Rarely, they may twist or rupture, sometimes causing abdominal pain, and surgical intervention may be required.

3. *Ectopic Pregnancies*

Ectopic pregnancies have occurred among NORPLANT SYSTEM users, although clinical studies have shown no increase in the rate of ectopic pregnancies per year among NORPLANT SYSTEM users as compared with users of no method or of IUDs. The incidence among NORPLANT SYSTEM users was 1.3 per 1000 woman-years, a rate significantly below the rate that has been estimated for noncontraceptive users in the United States (2.7 to 3.0 per 1000 woman-years). The risk of ectopic pregnancy may increase with the duration of NORPLANT SYSTEM use and possibly with increased weight of the user. Physicians should be alert to the possibility of an ectopic pregnancy among women using the NORPLANT SYSTEM who become pregnant or complain of lower-abdominal pain. Any patient who presents with lower-abdominal pain must be evaluated to rule out ectopic pregnancy.

4. *Breast-feeding*

Steroids are not considered the contraceptives of first choice for lactating women. Levonorgestrel has been identified in the breast milk of lactating women. No significant effects were observed on the growth or health of infants whose mothers used the NORPLANT SYSTEM beginning 6 weeks after parturition in comparative studies with mothers using IUDs or barrier methods. Eighty (80) infants were monitored for three years. No information is available beyond that time. No data are available on use in breast-feeding mothers earlier than 6 weeks after parturition.

5. *Foreign-body Carcinogenesis*

Rarely, cancers have occurred at the site of foreign-body intrusions or old scars. None has been reported in NORPLANT SYSTEM clinical trials. In rodents, which are highly susceptible to such cancers, the incidence decreases with decreasing size of the foreign body. Because of the resistance of human beings to these cancers and because of the small size of the capsules, the risk to users of the NORPLANT SYSTEM is judged to be minimal.

6. *Thromboembolic Disorders*

Patients who develop active thrombophlebitis or thromboembolic disease should have the NORPLANT SYSTEM capsules removed. Removal should also be considered in women who will be subjected to prolonged immobilization due to surgery or other illnesses.

B. WARNINGS BASED ON EXPERIENCE WITH COMBINATION (PROGESTIN PLUS ESTROGEN) ORAL CONTRACEPTIVES

1. *Cigarette Smoking*

Cigarette smoking increases the risk of serious cardiovascular side effects from the use of combination oral contraceptives. This risk increases with age and with heavy smoking (15 or more cigarettes per day) and is quite marked in women over 35 years old. While this is believed to be an estrogen-related effect, it is not known whether a similar risk exists with progestin-only methods such as the NORPLANT SYSTEM; however, women who use the NORPLANT SYSTEM should be advised not to smoke.

2. *Elevated Blood Pressure*

Increased blood pressure has been reported in users of combination oral contraceptives. The prevalence of elevated blood pressure increases with long exposure. Although there were no statistically significant trends among NORPLANT SYSTEM users in clinical trials, physicians should be aware of the possibility of elevated blood pressure with the NORPLANT SYSTEM.

3. *Thromboembolic Disorders and Other Vascular Problems*

An increased risk of thromboembolic and thrombotic disease (pulmonary embolism, superficial venous thrombosis, and deep-vein thrombosis) has been found to be associated with the use of combination oral contraceptives. The relative risk has been estimated to be 4- to 11-fold higher for users than for nonusers. While there is evidence of an association between the estrogen content of combination oral contraceptives and thromboembolic risk, the association of the NORPLANT SYSTEM progestin-only method to this risk is not known.

TABLE 3
Annual and Five-Year Cumulative Rates
per 100 Users

	year 1	year 2	year 3	year 4	year 5	Cumulative
Pregnancy	0.2	0.5	1.2	1.6	0.4	3.9
Bleeding Irregularities	9.1	7.9	4.9	3.3	2.9	25.1
Medical (excl. bleeding irreg.)	6.0	5.6	4.1	4.0	5.1	22.4
Personal	4.6	7.7	11.7	10.7	11.7	38.7
Continuation	81.0	77.4	79.2	76.7	77.6	29.5

Cerebrovascular Disorders: Combination oral contraceptives have been shown to increase both the relative and attributable risks of cerebrovascular events (thrombotic and hemorrhagic strokes), although, in general, the risk is greatest among older (>35 years) hypertensive women who also smoke. Hypertension was found to be a risk factor for both users and nonusers for both types of strokes, while smoking interacted to increase the risk for hemorrhagic strokes. The association of the NORPLANT SYSTEM progestin-only method to this risk is not known.

Myocardial Infarction: An increased risk of myocardial infarction has been attributed to combination oral-contraceptive use. This is thought to be primarily thrombotic in origin and is related to the estrogen component of combination oral contraceptives. This increased risk occurs primarily in smokers or in women with other underlying risk factors for coronary-artery disease, such as family history of coronary-artery disease, hypertension, hypercholesterolemia, morbid obesity, and diabetes. The current relative risk of heart attack for combination oral-contraceptive users has been estimated as 2 to 6 times the risk for nonusers. The absolute risk is very low for women under 30 years of age.

Studies indicate a significant trend toward higher rates of myocardial infarctions and strokes with increasing doses of progestin in combination oral contraceptives. However, a recent study showed no increased risk of myocardial infarction associated with the past use of levonorgestrel-containing combination oral contraceptives. The association of the NORPLANT SYSTEM progestin-only method with the risk of cardiovascular diseases is not known.

4. *Carcinoma*

Numerous epidemiological studies have been performed to determine the incidence of breast, endometrial, ovarian, and cervical cancer in women using combination oral contraceptives. Recent evidence in the literature suggests that use of combination oral contraceptives is not associated with an increased risk of developing breast cancer in the overall population of users. The Cancer and Steroid Hormone (CASH) study also showed no latent effect on the risk of breast cancer for at least a decade following long-term use. However, some of these same recent studies have shown an increased relative risk of breast cancer in certain subgroups of combination oral-contraceptive users, although no consistent pattern of findings has been identified. This information should be considered when prescribing the NORPLANT SYSTEM.

Some studies suggest that combination oral-contraceptive use has been associated with an increase in the risk of cervical intraepithelial neoplasia in some populations of women. However, there continues to be controversy about the extent to which such findings may be due to differences in sexual behavior and other factors. In spite of many studies of the relationship between combination oral-contraceptive use and breast and cervical cancers, a cause-and-effect relationship has not been established.

Evidence indicates that combination oral contraceptives may decrease the risk of ovarian and endometrial cancer. Irregular bleeding patterns associated with the NORPLANT SYSTEM could mask symptoms of cervical or endometrial cancer.

5. *Hepatic Tumors*

Hepatic adenomas have been found to be associated with the use of combination oral contraceptives with an estimated incidence of about 3 occurrences per 100,000 users per year, a risk that increases after 4 or more years of use. Although benign, hepatic adenomas may rupture and cause death through intra-abdominal hemorrhage. The contribution of the progestin component of oral contraceptives to the development of hepatic adenomas is not known.

6. *Ocular Lesions*

There have been clinical case reports of retinal thrombosis associated with the use of oral contraceptives. Although it is believed that this adverse reaction is related to the estrogen component of oral contraceptives, the NORPLANT SYSTEM capsules should be removed if there is unexplained partial or complete loss of vision; onset of proptosis or diplopia; papilledema; or retinal vascular lesions. Appropriate diagnostic and therapeutic measures should be undertaken immediately.

7. *Use Before or During Early Pregnancy*

Extensive epidemiological studies have revealed no increased risk of birth defects in women who have used oral contraceptives prior to pregnancy. Studies also do not suggest a teratogenic effect, particularly insofar as cardiac anomalies and limb-reduction defects are concerned, when taken inadvertently during early pregnancy. There is no evidence suggesting that the risk associated with NORPLANT SYSTEM use is different.

8. *Gallbladder Disease*

Earlier studies have reported an increased lifetime relative risk of gallbladder surgery in users of oral contraceptives and estrogens. More recent studies, however, have shown that the relative risk of developing gallbladder disease among oral-contraceptive users may be minimal. The recent findings of minimal risk may be related to the use of oral-contraceptive formulations containing lower hormonal doses of estrogens and progestins. The association of this risk with use of the NORPLANT SYSTEM progestin-only method is not known.

PRECAUTIONS

GENERAL

1. *Physical Examination and Follow-Up*

A complete medical history and physical examination should be taken prior to the implantation or reimplantation of NORPLANT SYSTEM capsules and at least annually during its use. These physical examinations should include special reference to the implant site, blood pressure, breasts, abdomen and pelvic organs, including cervical cytology and relevant laboratory tests. In case of undiagnosed, persistent or recurrent abnormal vaginal bleeding, appropriate diagnostic measures should be conducted to rule out malignancy. Women with a strong family history of breast cancer or who have breast nodules should be monitored with particular care.

2. *Carbohydrate Metabolism*

An altered glucose tolerance characterized by decreased insulin sensitivity following glucose loading has been found in some users of combination and progestin-only oral contraceptives. The effects of the NORPLANT SYSTEM on carbohydrate metabolism appear to be minimal. In a study in which pretreatment serum-glucose levels were compared with levels after 1 and 2 years of NORPLANT SYSTEM use, no statistically significant differences in mean serum-glucose levels were evident 2 hours after glucose loading. The clinical significance of these findings is unknown, but diabetic and prediabetic patients should be carefully observed while using the NORPLANT SYSTEM.

Women who are being treated for hyperlipidemias should be followed closely if they elect to use the NORPLANT SYSTEM. Some progestins may elevate LDL levels and may render the control of hyperlipidemias more difficult. (See "Warnings," B.3.)

3. *Liver Function*

If jaundice develops in any women while using the NORPLANT SYSTEM, consideration should be given to removing the capsules. Steroid hormones may be poorly metabolized in patients with impaired liver function.

4. *Fluid Retention*

Steroid contraceptives may cause some degree of fluid retention. They should be prescribed with caution, and only with careful monitoring, in patients with conditions which might be aggravated by fluid retention.

5. *Emotional Disorders*

Consideration should be given to removing NORPLANT SYSTEM capsules in women who become significantly depressed since the symptom may be drug-related. Women with a history of depression should be carefully observed and removal considered if depression recurs to a serious degree.

6. *Contact Lenses*

Contact-lens wearers who develop visual changes or changes in lens tolerance should be assessed by an ophthalmologist.

7. *Insertion and Removal*

To be sure that the woman is not pregnant at the time of capsule placement and to assure contraceptive effectiveness during the first cycle of use, it is advisable that insertion be done during the first 7 days of the cycle or immediately following an abortion. Insertion is not recommended before 6 weeks post-partum in breast-feeding women.

Continued on next page

Wyeth-Ayerst Laboratories—Cont.

Insertion and removal are not difficult procedures but instructions must be followed closely. It is strongly advised that all health-care professionals who insert and remove NORPLANT SYSTEM capsules be instructed in the procedures before they attempt them. A proper insertion just under the skin will facilitate removals. Proper NORPLANT SYSTEM insertion and removal should result in minimal scarring. If the capsules are placed too deeply, they can be harder to remove. If all capsules cannot be removed at the first attempt, removal should be attempted later when the site has healed. Bruising may occur at the implant site during insertion or removal. In some women, hyperpigmentation occurs over the implantation site but is usually reversible following removal. See detailed Insertion and Removal Instructions below.

8. *Infections*
Infection at the implant site has been uncommon (0.7%) Attention to aseptic technique and proper insertion and removal of the NORPLANT SYSTEM capsules reduces the possibility of infection. If infection occurs, suitable treatment should be instituted. If infection persists, the capsules should be removed.

9. *Expulsion*
Expulsion of capsules was uncommon. It occurred more frequently when placement of the capsules was extremely shallow, too close to the incision, or when infection was present. Replacement of an expelled capsule must be accomplished using a new sterile capsule. If infection is present, it should be treated and cured before replacement. Contraceptive efficacy may be inadequate with fewer than 6 capsules.

10. *Provisions for Removal*
Women should be advised that the capsules will be removed at any time for any reason. The removal should be done on such request or at the end of 5 years of usage by personnel instructed in the removal technique.
Upon removal, NORPLANT SYSTEM capsules should be disposed of in accordance with Center for Disease Control Guidelines for the handling of biohazardous waste.

DRUG INTERACTIONS
Reduced efficacy (pregnancy) has been reported for NORPLANT SYSTEM users taking phenytoin and carbamazepine. NORPLANT SYSTEM users should be warned of the possibility of decreased efficacy with use of any related drugs.

DRUG/LABORATORY TEST INTERACTIONS
Certain endocrine tests may be affected by NORPLANT SYSTEM use:
1. Sex-hormone-binding globulin concentrations are decreased.
2. Thyroxine concentrations may be slightly decreased and triiodothyronine uptake increased.

CARCINOGENESIS
See "Warnings" section.

PREGNANCY
Pregnancy Category X. See "Warnings" section.

NURSING MOTHERS
See "Warnings" section.

INFORMATION FOR THE PATIENT
See Patient Labeling.
Two copies of the Patient Labeling are included to help describe the characteristics of the NORPLANT SYSTEM to the patient. One copy should be provided to the patient. Patients should also be advised that the Prescribing Information is available to them at their request. It is recommended that propective users be fully informed about the risks and benefits associated with use of the NORPLANT SYSTEM, with other forms of contraception, and with no contraception at all. It is also recommended that prospective users be fully informed about the insertion and removal procedures. Health-care providers may wish to obtain informed consent from all patients in light of the techniques involved with insertion and removal.

ADVERSE REACTIONS
The following adverse reactions have been associated with the NORPLANT SYSTEM during the first year of use. They include:

Many bleeding days or prolonged bleeding	27.6%
Spotting	17.1%
Amenorrhea	9.4%
Irregular (onsets of) bleeding	7.6%
Frequent bleeding onsets	7.0%
Scanty bleeding	5.2%
Pain or itching near implant site (usually transient)	3.7%
Infection at implant site	0.7%
Removal difficulties affecting subject (based on 849 removals)	6.2%

Controlled clinical studies suggest that the following adverse reactions occurring during the first year are probably associated with NORPLANT SYSTEM use:

Headache
Nervousness
Nausea
Dizziness
Adnexal enlargement
Dermatitis
Acne
Change of appetite
Mastalgia
Weight gain
Hirsutism, hypertrichosis, and scalp-hair loss
In addition, the following adverse reactions have been reported with a frequency of 5% or greater during the first year and possibly may be related to NORPLANT SYSTEM use:
Breast discharge
Cervicitis
Musculoskeletal pain
Abdominal discomfort
Leukorrhea
Vaginitis

OVERDOSAGE
Overdosage can result if more than six capsules of the NORPLANT SYSTEM are in situ. All implanted NORPLANT SYSTEM capsules should be removed before inserting a new set of NORPLANT SYSTEM capsules. Overdosage may cause fluid retention with its associated effects and uterine bleeding irregularities.

DOSAGE AND ADMINISTRATION
The NORPLANT SYSTEM consists of six Silastic capsules, each containing 36 mg of the progestin, levonorgestrel. The total administered (implanted) dose is 216 mg. Implantation of all six capsules should be performed during the first 7 days of the onset of menses by a health-care professional instructed in the NORPLANT SYSTEM insertion technique. Insertion is subdermal in the midportion of the upper arm about 8 to 10 cm above the elbow crease. Distribution should be in a fanlike pattern, about 15 degrees apart, for a total of 75 degrees. Proper insertion will facilitate later removal. (See section on Insertion/Removal.)

HOW SUPPLIED
The NORPLANT SYSTEM Kit includes the following items:
1 NORPLANT SYSTEM (levonorgestrel implants), a set of six implants (capsules)
1 NORPLANT SYSTEM trocar
1 Scalpel
1 Forceps
1 Syringe
2 Syringe needles
1 Package of skin closures
3 Packages of gauze sponges
1 Stretch bandage
1 Surgical drape (fenestrated)
2 Surgical drapes
Store at room temperature away from excess heat and moisture.
NDC 0008-2564-01
References available upon request.

INSTRUCTIONS FOR INSERTION AND REMOVAL
The NORPLANT SYSTEM consists of six levonorgestrel-releasing capsules that are inserted subdermally in the medial aspect of the upper arm.
The NORPLANT SYSTEM provides up to 5 years of effective contraceptive protection.
The basis for successful use and subsequent removal of NORPLANT SYSTEM capsules is a correct and carefully performed subdermal insertion of the six capsules. It is recommended that health-care professionals performing insertions or removals of NORPLANT SYSTEM capsules avail themselves of instruction and supervision in the proper technique prior to attempting these procedures. During insertion, special attention should be given to the following:
—asepsis.
—correct subdermal placement of the capsules.
—careful technique to minimize tissue trauma.
This will help to avoid infections and excessive scarring at the insertion area and will help keep the capsules from being inserted too deeply in the tissue. If the capsules are placed too deeply, they will be more difficult to remove than correctly placed subdermal capsules.

INSERTION PROCEDURE
Insertion should be performed within seven days from the onset of menses. However, NORPLANT SYSTEM capsules may be inserted at any time during the cycle provided pregnancy has been excluded and a nonhormonal contraceptive method is used for the remainder of the cycle. A gynecological examination should be performed before the insertion of NORPLANT SYSTEM capsules, as would be the case before initiating any hormonal contraception. Determine if the subject has any allergies to the antiseptic or anesthetic to be used or contraindications to progestin-only contraception. If none are found, the capsules are inserted using the procedure outlined below.

One NORPLANT SYSTEM set consists of six capsules in a sterile pouch. The insertion is performed under aseptic conditions using a trocar to place the capsules under the skin.

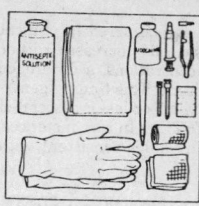
Figure 1: The following equipment is recommended for the insertion:
—an examining table for the patient to lie on.
—sterile surgical drapes, sterile gloves (free of talc), antiseptic solution.
—local anesthetic, needles, and syringe.
—#11 scalpel, #10 trocar, forceps.
—skin closure, sterile gauze, and compresses.

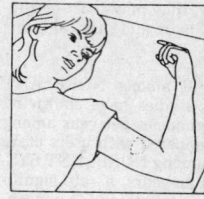
Figure 2: Have the patient lie on her back on the examination table with her left arm (if the patient is left-handed, the right arm) flexed at the elbow and externally rotated so that her hand is lying by her head. The capsules will be inserted subdermally through a small 2-mm incision and positioned in a fanlike manner with the fan opening towards the shoulder.

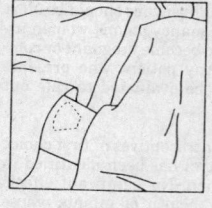
Figure 3: Prep the patient's upper arm with antiseptic solution; cover the arm above and below the insertion area with a sterile cloth. The optimal insertion area is in the inside of the upper arm about 8 to 10 cm above the elbow crease.

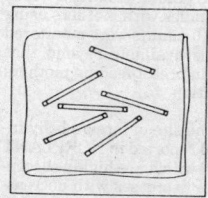
Figure 4: Open the sterile NORPLANT SYSTEM package carefully by pulling apart the sheets of the pouch, allowing the capsules to fall onto a sterile cloth. Count the six capsules.

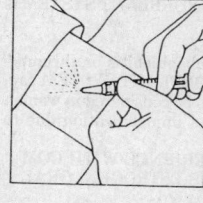
Figure 5: After determining the absence of known allergies to the anesthetic agent or related drugs, fill a 5-mL syringe with the local anesthetic. Anesthetize the insertion area by first inserting the needle under the skin and releasing a small amount of anesthetic. Then anesthetize six areas about 4 to 4.5 cm long, to mimic the fanlike position of the implanted capsules.

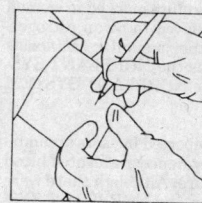
Figure 6: Use the scalpel to make a small, shallow incision (about 2 mm) through the skin.

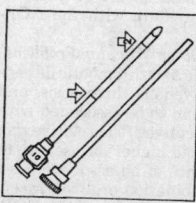
Figure 7: The trocar has two marks on it. The first mark is closer to the hub and indicates how far the trocar should be introduced under the skin before the loading of each capsule. The second mark is close to the tip and indicates how much of the trocar should remain under the skin following the insertion of each implant.

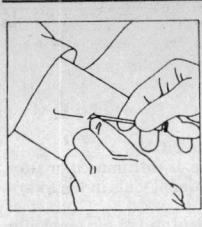

Figure 8: Insert the tip of the trocar through the incision beneath the skin at a shallow angle. Once the trocar is inserted, it should be oriented with the the bevel up toward the skin to keep the capsules in a superficial plane. It is important to keep the trocar subdermal by tenting the skin with the trocar, as failure to do so may result in deep placement of the capsules and could make removal more difficult.

Advance the trocar gently under the skin to the first mark near the hub of the trocar. The tip of the trocar is now at a distance of about 4 to 4.5 cm from the incision.

Do not force the trocar, and if resistance is felt, try another direction.

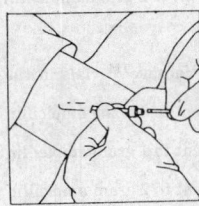

Figure 9: When the trocar has been inserted the appropriate distance, remove the obturator and load the first capsule into the trocar using the thumb and forefinger.

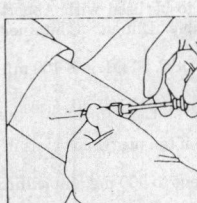

Figure 10: Gently advance the capsule with the obturator towards the tip of the trocar until you feel resistance. Never force the obturator.

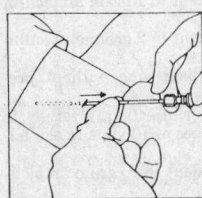

Figure 11: Hold the obturator steady, and bring the trocar back until it touches the handle of the obturator.

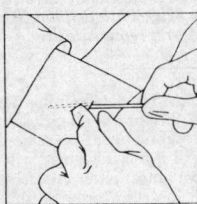

Figure 12: The capsule should have been released under the skin when the mark close to the tip of the trocar is visible in the incision. Release of the capsule can be checked by palpation. It is important to keep the obturator steady and not to push the capsule into the tissue.

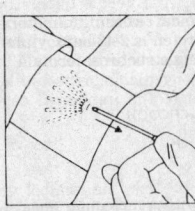

Figure 13: Do not remove the trocar from the incision until all capsules have been inserted. The trocar is withdrawn only to the mark close to its tip. Each succeeding capsule is always inserted next to the previous one, to form a fanlike shape. Fix the position of the previous capsule with the forefinger and and middle finger of the free hand, and advance the trocar along the tips of the fingers. This will ensure a suitable distance of about 15 degrees between capsules and keep the trocar from puncturing any of the previously inserted capsules.

Leave a distance of about 5 mm between the incision and the tips of the capsules. This will help avoid spontaneous expulsions. The correct position of the capsules can be ensured by feeling them with the fingers after the insertion has been completed.

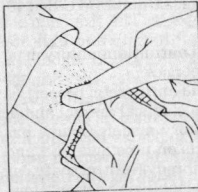

Figure 14: After the insertion of the sixth capsule, palpate the capsules to make sure that all six have been inserted.

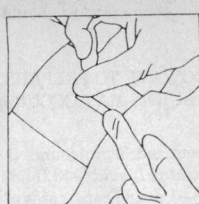

Figure 15: Press the edges of the incision together, and close the incision with a skin closure. Suturing the incision should not be necessary.

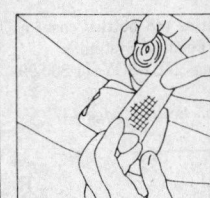

Figure 16: Cover the insertion area with a dry compress, and wrap gauze around the arm to ensure hemostasis.

Observe the patient for a few minutes for signs of syncope or bleeding from the incision before she is discharged.

Advise the patient to keep the insertion area dry for 2 to 3 days. The gauze may be removed after 1 day, and the butterfly bandage as soon as the incision has healed, i.e., normally in 3 days.

REMOVAL PROCEDURE

It is recommended that removals be prescheduled so that preparations for carrying out the procedure can be facilitated.

Removal of the capsules should be performed very gently and will take more time than insertion. Capsules are sometimes nicked or cut during removal. The incidence of overall removal difficulties, including damage to capsules, has been 13.2 percent. Less than half of these removal difficulties have caused inconvenience to the patient. If the removal of some of the capsules proves difficult, have the patient return for a second visit. The remaining capsule(s) will be easier to remove after the area is healed. If contraception is still desired, a barrier method should be advised until all capsules are removed.

The position of the patient and the asepsis are the same as for insertion.

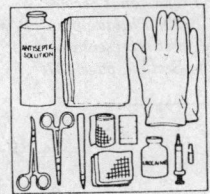

Figure 17: The following equipment is needed for the removal:
—an examining table for the patient to lie on.
—sterile surgical drapes, sterile gloves (free of talc), antiseptic solution.
—local anesthetic, needles, and syringe.
—#11 scalpel, forceps (straight and curved mosquito).
—skin closure, sterile gauze, and compresses.

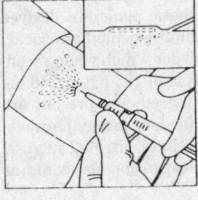

Figure 18: Locate the implanted capsules by palpation, possibly marking their position with a sterile skin marker. Apply a small amount of local anesthetic *under* the capsule ends nearest the original incision site. This will serve to raise the ends of the capsules. Anesthetic injected over the capsules will obscure them and make removal more difficult.

Additional small amounts of the anesthetic can be used for the removal of each of the capsules, if required.

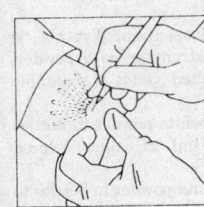

Figure 19: Make a 4-mm incision with the scalpel close to the ends of the capsules. Do not make a large incision.

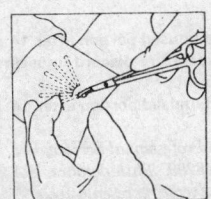

Figure 20: Push each capsule gently towards the incision with the fingers. When the tip is visible or near to the incision, grasp it with a mosquito forceps.

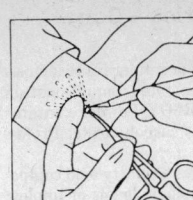

Figure 21: Use the scalpel very gently to open the tissue sheath that has formed around the capsule.

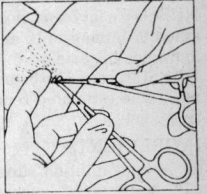

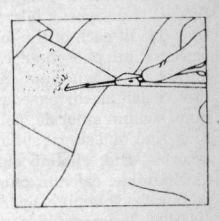

Figures 22 and 23: Remove the capsule from the incision with the second forceps.

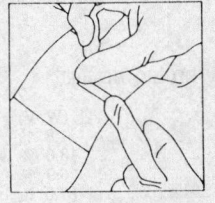

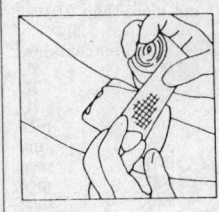

Figures 24 and 25: After the procedure is completed, the incision is closed and bandaged as with insertion. The upper arm should be kept dry for a few days.

Following removal, a return to the previous level of fertility is usually prompt, and a pregnancy may occur at any time. If the patient wishes to continue using the method, a new set of NORPLANT SYSTEM capsules can be inserted through the same incision in the same or opposite direction.

HINTS
Insertion
—Counselling of the patient on the benefits and side effects of the method prior to insertion will greatly increase patient satisfaction.
—Correct subdermal placement of the capsules will facilitate removal.
—Before insertion, apply the anesthetic just beneath the skin so as to raise the dermis above the underlying tissue.
—Never force the trocar.
—To ensure subdermal placement, the trocar with bevel up should be supported by the index finger and should visibly raise the skin at all times during insertion.
—To avoid damaging the previous implanted capsule, stabilize the capsule with your forefinger and middle finger and advance the trocar alongside the finger tips at an angle of 15 degrees.
—After insertion, make a drawing for the patient's file showing the location of the 6 capsules and describe any variations in placement. This will greatly aid removal.

Removal
—The removal of the implanted capsules will take a little more time than the insertion.
—Before removal, apply the anesthetic *under* the capsule ends nearest the original incision site.
—If the removal of some of the capsules proves difficult, interrupt the procedure and have the patient return for a second visit. The remaining capsule(s) will be easier to remove after the area is healed.

Shown in Product Identification Section, page 437

NURSOY®
[*nur-soy*]
Soy protein formula
READY-TO-FEED
CONCENTRATED LIQUID
POWDER

NURSOY® milk free formula is intended to meet the nutritional needs of infants and children who are not breast-fed

Continued on next page

Wyeth-Ayerst Laboratories—Cont.

and are allergic to cow's milk protein or intolerant to lactose. NURSOY Ready-to-Feed and Concentrated Liquid contain sucrose as their carbohydrate. NURSOY Powder contains corn syrup solids and sucrose as its carbohydrate. Professional advice should be followed.

NURSOY's fat blend closely resembles the fatty acid composition of human milk and has physiologic levels of linoleic and linolenic acid.

NURSOY contains beta carotene, a component of human milk. The estimated renal solute load of NURSOY is relatively low.

INGREDIENTS

(in normal dilution supplying 20 calories per fluidounce): 87% water; 6.7% sucrose; 3.4% oleo, coconut, oleic (safflower) and soybean oils; 2.0% soy protein isolate; and less than 1% of each of the following: potassium citrate; monobasic sodium phosphate; calcium carbonate; dibasic calcium phosphate; magnesium chloride; calcium chloride; soy lecithin; calcium carrageenan; calcium hydroxide; L-methionine; sodium chloride; potassium bicarbonate; taurine; ferrous, zinc, and cupric sulfates; L-carnitine; potassium iodide; ascorbic acid; choline chloride; alpha-tocopheryl acetate; niacinamide; calcium pantothenate; riboflavin; vitamin A palmitate; thiamine hydrochloride; pyridoxine hydrochloride; beta-carotene; phytonadione; folic acid; biotin; cholecalciferol; cyanocobalamin.

PROXIMATE ANALYSIS

at 20 calories per fluidounce
READY-TO-FEED, CONCENTRATED LIQUID and POWDER

	(W/V)	
Protein	1.8	%
Fat	3.6	%
Carbohydrate	6.9	%
Water	87.0	%
Crude fiber	not more than 0.01%	
Calories/fl. oz.	20	

Vitamins, Minerals: In normal dilution, each liter contains:

A	2,000	IU
D$_3$	400	IU
E	9.5	IU
K$_1$	100	mcg
C (ascorbic acid)	55	mg
B$_1$ (thiamine)	670	mcg
B$_2$ (riboflavin)	1000	mcg
B$_6$	420	mcg
B$_{12}$	2	mcg
Niacin	5000	mcg
Pantothenic acid	3000	mcg
Folic acid (folacin)	50	mcg
Choline	85	mg
Inositol	27	mg
Biotin	35	mcg
Calcium	600	mg
Phosphorus	420	mg
Sodium	200	mg
Potassium	700	mg
Chloride	375	mg
Magnesium	67	mg
Manganese	200	mcg
Iron	12.0	mg
Copper	470	mcg
Zinc	5	mg
Iodine	60	mcg

PREPARATION

Ready-to-Feed (32 fl. oz. cans of 20 calories per fluidounce formula)—shake can, open and pour into previously sterilized nursing bottle; attach nipple and feed. Cover opened can and immediately store in refrigerator. Use contents of can within 48 hours of opening.

Prolonged storage of can at excessive temperatures should be avoided.

Expiration date is on top of can.

WARNING: DO NOT USE A MICROWAVE TO PREPARE OR WARM FORMULA. SERIOUS BURNS MAY OCCUR.

Concentrated Liquid—For normal dilution supplying 20 calories per fluidounce, use equal amounts of Nursoy® liquid and cooled, previously boiled water. *Note: Prepared formula should be used within 24 hours.*

Prolonged storage of can at excessive temperatures should be avoided.

Expiration date is on top of can.

WARNING: DO NOT USE A MICROWAVE TO PREPARE OR WARM FORMULA. SERIOUS BURNS MAY OCCUR.

Powder—For normal dilution supplying 20 calories per fluidounce, add 1 scoop (8.9 grams or 1 standard tablespoonful) of NURSOY POWDER, packed and leveled, to 2 fluidounces of water. For larger amounts of formula, add ¼ standard measuring cup of powder (35.5 grams), packed and leveled, to 8 fluidounces (1 standard measuring cup) of water.

Prolonged storage of can at excessive temperatures should be avoided.

Expiration date is on bottom of can.

WARNING: DO NOT USE A MICROWAVE TO PREPARE OR WARM FORMULA. SERIOUS BURNS MAY OCCUR.

HOW SUPPLIED

Ready-to-Feed—presterilized and premixed, 32 fluidounce (1 quart) cans, cases of 6 cans; *Concentrated Liquid*—13 fluidounce cans, cases of 12 cans; *Powder*—1 pound cans, cases of 6 cans.

Also available to hospitals only:

Ready-to-Feed 4 oz. disposable bottles (48 bottles/case) as part of the Wyeth Hospital Infant Feeding System.

Questions or Comments regarding NURSOY: 1-800-99-WYETH.

Shown in Product Identification Section, page 437

OMNIPEN®   ℞
[om ′nĭ-pen]
(ampicillin)
CAPSULES

DESCRIPTION

Omnipen (ampicillin) is a semisynthetic penicillin derived from the basic penicillin nucleus, 6-amino-penicillanic acid. Omnipen capsules contain 250 mg or 500 mg ampicillin. The inactive ingredients present are D&C Red 22, D&C Red 28, FD&C Blue 1, gelatin, lactose, methylcellulose, stearic acid, and titanium dioxide.

HOW SUPPLIED

Omnipen® (ampicillin) Capsules, Wyeth®, contain 250 mg or 500 mg ampicillin anhydrous and are available as follows: 250 mg, NDC 0008-0053, violet and pink capsule marked "WYETH" and "53", in bottles of 500 capsules.

500 mg, NDC 0008-0309, violet and pink capsule marked "WYETH" and "309", in bottles of 100 and 500 capsules.

For prescribing information write to Professional Service, Wyeth-Ayerst Laboratories, P.O. Box 8299, Philadelphia, PA 19101, or contact your local Wyeth-Ayerst representative.

Shown in Product Identification Section, page 437

OMNIPEN®   ℞
[om ′nĭ-pen]
(ampicillin)
ORAL SUSPENSION

DESCRIPTION

Omnipen (ampicillin) is a semisynthetic penicillin derived from the basic penicillin nucleus, 6-amino-penicillanic acid. Omnipen for oral suspension is a powder which when reconstituted as directed yields a suspension of 125 mg or 250 mg ampicillin per 5 mL. The inactive ingredients present are artificial flavors, colloidal silicon dioxide, methylparaben, propylparaben, sodium benzoate, sodium citrate, sucrose, and water. Each dosage strength of suspension also contains the following:

125 mg per 5 mL—carboxymethylcellulose sodium FD&C Blue 1, FD&C Red 40, FD&C Yellow 6, and natural flavors; 250 mg per 5 mL—D&C Red 28.

HOW SUPPLIED

Omnipen® (ampicillin) for Oral Suspension, Wyeth®, is available in the following dosage strengths as a powder, which when reconstituted as directed yields a palatable suspension:

125 mg per 5 mL, NDC 0008-0054, white powder in bottles to make 100 mL, 150 mL, or 200 mL of salmon-colored suspension.

250 mg per 5 mL, NDC 0008-0055, pink powder in bottles to make 100 mL, 150 mL, or 200 mL of pink suspension.

Shake well before using.

Keep tightly closed.

When stored in refrigerator discard unused portion after 14 days, or when stored at room temperature discard unused portion after 7 days (250 mg per 5 mL).

When stored in refrigerator discard unused portion after 14 days (125 mg per 5 mL).

For prescribing information write to Professional Service, Wyeth-Ayerst Laboratories, P.O. Box 8299, Philadelphia, PA 19101, or contact your local Wyeth-Ayerst representative.

OMNIPEN®-N   ℞
[om ′nĭ-pen-N]
(ampicillin sodium)
INJECTION

HOW SUPPLIED

FOR PARENTERAL ADMINISTRATION

Conventional Vials (for intravenous or intramuscular use)

Supplied in packages of ten conventional vials in the following dosage strengths:

125 mg, NDC 0008-0315-07, equivalent to 125 mg ampicillin per vial.

250 mg, NDC 0008-0315-05, equivalent to 250 mg ampicillin per vial.

500 mg, NDC 0008-0315-06, equivalent to 500 mg ampicillin per vial.

1 gram, NDC 0008-0315-08, equivalent to 1 gram ampicillin per vial.

2 gram, NDC 0008-0315-10, equivalent to 2 gram ampicillin per vial.

FOR INTRAVENOUS USE ONLY

ADD-Vantage™ Vials

Supplied in packages of ten ADD-Vantage™ vials in the following dosage strengths:

500 mg, NDC 0008-0315-38, equivalent to 500 mg ampicillin per vial.

1 gram, NDC 0008-0315-40, equivalent to 1 gram ampicillin per vial.

2 gram, NDC 0008-0315-42, equivalent to 2 gram ampicillin per vial.

The ADD-Vantage Vials are only to be used with Abbott Laboratories' ADD-Vantage Flexible Diluent Container containing:

   0.9% Sodium Chloride Injection, USP, 50 mL and 100 mL sizes.

   5% Dextrose Injection, USP, 50 mL and 100 mL sizes.

Piggyback Vials

Supplied as single units in packages of ten piggyback vials in the following dosage strengths:

500 mg, NDC 0008-0315-28, equivalent to 500 mg ampicillin per vial.

1 gram, NDC 0008-0315-24, equivalent to 1 gram ampicillin per vial.

2 gram, NDC 0008-0315-26, equivalent to 2 gram ampicillin per vial.

Caution: Federal law prohibits dispensing without prescription.

Omnipen®-N (ampicillin sodium) for Injection, Wyeth®, is available in Pharmacy Bulk Packages of 10 vials in the following dosage strength:

10 gram, NDC 0008-0315-43, equivalent to 10 gram ampicillin per vial.

For prescribing information write to Professional Service, Wyeth-Ayerst Laboratories, P.O. Box 8299, Philadelphia, PA 19101, or contact your local Wyeth-Ayerst representative.

ORUDIS®   ℞
[ō″roo′dĭs]
(ketoprofen)
Capsules

DESCRIPTION

Orudis (ketoprofen) is a nonsteroidal antiinflammatory drug. The chemical name for ketoprofen is 2-(3-benzoylphenyl)-propionic acid with the following structural formula:

Its empirical formula is $C_{16}H_{14}O_3$, with a molecular weight of 254.29.

Ketoprofen is a white or off-white, odorless, nonhygroscopic, fine to granular powder, melting at about 95℃. It is freely soluble in ethanol, chloroform, acetone, and ether; soluble in benzene and strong alkali, but practically insoluble in water at 20℃.

Orudis capsules contain 25 mg, 50 mg, or 75 mg of ketoprofen for oral administration. The inactive ingredients present are D&C Yellow 10, FD&C Blue 1, FD&C Yellow 6, gelatin, lactose, magnesium stearate, and titanium dioxide. The 25 mg dosage strength also contains D&C Red 28 and FD&C Red 40.

CLINICAL PHARMACOLOGY

Orudis (ketoprofen) is a nonsteroidal antiinflammatory drug with analgesic and antipyretic properties.

The antiinflammatory, analgesic, and antipyretic properties of Orudis have been demonstrated in classical animal and *in vitro* test systems. In antiinflammatory models Orudis has been shown to have inhibitory effects on prostaglandin and leukotriene synthesis, to have antibradykinin activity, as well as to have lysosomal membrane-stabilizing action. How-

ever, its mode of action, like that of other nonsteroidal antiinflammatory drugs, is not fully understood.

Orudis is rapidly and completely absorbed from the gastrointestinal tract. Mean Orudis peak plasma levels are reached in 0.5 to 2 hours. The total absolute bioavailability of Orudis, as demonstrated by area under the plasma concentration-time curve (AUC), is approximately 90% for capsule formulations tested when compared to IV administration and is linear for 75 to 200 mg single doses. The plasma clearance of ketoprofen is approximately 0.08 L/kg/hr with a V_d of 0.1 L/kg after IV administration. The mean plasma elimination half-life of Orudis ranged from 2 to 4 hours in 14 pharmacokinetic studies which included 6 to 24 normal volunteers. Following absorption, Orudis can be detected in plasma as the unchanged compound, hydroxylated metabolites and their respective glucuronides. There are no known active metabolites of Orudis. The drug is 99% bound to plasma proteins, mainly to the albumin fraction. Approximately 60% of an administered dose of Orudis is excreted in the urine primarily as the glucuronide metabolite in the first 24 hours. Enterohepatic recirculation of the drug has been postulated to account for the other 40% of the absorbed ketoprofen, although biliary levels have never been measured to confirm this.

Orudis has been shown to not induce drug-metabolizing enzymes.

Steady-state concentrations of Orudis are attained within 24 hours after commencing treatment.

When ketoprofen is administered with food, its total bioavailability (AUC) is not altered; however, the rate of absorption is slowed, resulting in delayed and reduced peak concentrations (C_{max}). Following a single 50 mg dose of Orudis while fasting, the mean C_{max} is 4.1 mg/L (at 1.1 hours); when administered after food, it decreases to 2.4 mg/L (at 2.0 hours).

To date, studies of the effects of age and renal-function impairment have been small, generally involving 5 to 8 subjects per group, but they indicate modest decrease in clearance in the elderly and in patients with impaired renal function. In normal elderly volunteers (mean age 73 years), the plasma and renal clearance and protein-binding were reduced while the V_d increased when compared to a younger normal population (mean age 27 years). (Plasma clearance and V_d were 0.05 L/kg/hr and 0.4 L/kg in elderly and 0.06 L/kg/hr and 0.3 L/kg in young subjects, respectively.) The mean half-life of Orudis in this normal geriatric population, as well as in a rheumatoid elderly population (mean age 64 years), was about 5 hours as compared to 3 hours in the younger population.

Patients with impaired renal function (mean age 44 years) also demonstrate decreases in plasma clearance (0.04 L/kg/hr) of drug, with the mean half-life increasing to about 3.5 hours.

For patients with alcoholic cirrhosis, no significant changes in the kinetic disposition of Orudis were observed relative to age-matched normal subjects; the plasma clearance of drug was 0.07 L/kg/hr) in both groups (N = 8 for each group) and total bioavailability was comparable. However, the protein unbound (biologically active) fraction was increased from 0.85% to 1.15%, probably due to hypoalbuminemia, and high variability was observed in the pharmacokinetics in cirrhotic patients. Therefore, these patients should be carefully monitored and daily doses kept at the minimum levels providing the desired therapeutic effect.

In healthy men, the average blood loss in stool, measured over a one-week period during administration of 200 mg per day of Orudis, was 50% lower than that resulting from administration of 3,900 mg per day of aspirin. In addition, a double-blind crossover trial using gastroscopy in 13 normal volunteers demonstrated fewer mucosal lesions with Orudis than aspirin.

The efficacy of Orudis has been demonstrated in patients with rheumatoid arthritis and osteoarthritis. Using standard assessment of therapeutic response, Orudis demonstrated effectiveness comparable to aspirin, ibuprofen, and indomethacin.

In studies in patients with rheumatoid arthritis, Orudis was administered in combination with gold salts, antimalarials, and/or corticosteroids with results comparable to those seen with the control nonsteroidal drugs.

The effectiveness of Orudis as a general purpose analgesic has been studied in standard pain models which have shown the effectiveness of doses of 25 to 150 mg. Doses of 25 mg were superior to placebo. Larger doses than 25 mg generally could not be shown significantly more effective but there was a tendency toward faster onset and greater duration of action with 50 mg and, in the case of dysmenorrhea, a significantly greater effect overall with 75 mg. Doses greater than 50 to 75 mg did not have increased analgesic effect.

INDICATIONS AND USAGE

Orudis is indicated for the acute or long-term treatment of the signs and symptoms of rheumatoid arthritis and osteoarthritis.

Orudis is indicated for the relief of mild-to-moderate pain. Orudis is also indicated for treatment of primary dysmenorrhea.

CONTRAINDICATIONS

Orudis is contraindicated in patients who have shown hypersensitivity to it. Orudis should not be given to patients in whom aspirin or other nonsteroidal antiinflammatory drugs induce asthma, urticaria, or other allergic-type reactions, because severe, rarely fatal, anaphylactic reactions to Orudis have been reported in such patients.

WARNINGS

RISK OF GI ULCERATION, BLEEDING, AND PERFORATION WITH NSAID THERAPY:

Serious gastrointestinal toxicity, such as bleeding, ulceration, and perforation, can occur at any time, with or without warning symptoms, in patients treated chronically with NSAID therapy. Although minor upper-gastrointestinal problems, such as dyspepsia, are common, usually developing early in therapy, physicians should remain alert for ulceration and bleeding in patients treated chronically with NSAIDs even in the absence of previous GI-tract symptoms. In patients observed in clinical trials of several months to two years duration, symptomatic upper-GI ulcers, gross bleeding, or perforation appear to occur in approximately 1% of patients treated for 3 to 6 months, and in about 2–4% of patients treated for one year. Physicians should inform patients about the signs and/or symptoms of serious GI toxicity and what steps to take if they occur.

Studies to date have not identified any subset of patients not at risk of developing peptic ulceration and bleeding. Except for a prior history of serious GI events and other risk factors known to be associated with peptic ulcer disease, such as alcoholism, smoking, etc., no risk factors (e.g., age, sex) have been associated with increased risk. Elderly or debilitated patients seem to tolerate ulceration or bleeding less well than other individuals, and most spontaneous reports of fatal GI events are in this population. Studies to date are inconclusive concerning the relative risk of various NSAIDs in causing such reactions. High doses of any NSAID probably carry a greater risk of these reactions, although controlled clinical trials showing this do not exist in most cases. In considering the use of relatively large doses (within the recommended dosage range), sufficient benefit should be anticipated to offset the potential increased risk of GI toxicity.

GENERAL PRECAUTIONS

Orudis and other nonsteroidal antiinflammatory drugs cause nephritis in mice and rats associated with chronic administration. Cases of interstitial nephritis and nephrotic syndrome have been reported with Orudis since it has been marketed abroad.

A second form of renal toxicity has been seen in patients with conditions leading to a reduction in renal blood flow or blood volume, where renal prostaglandins have a supportive role in the maintenance of renal blood flow. In these patients administration of a nonsteroidal antiinflammatory drug results in a dose-dependent decrease in prostaglandin synthesis and, secondarily, in renal blood flow which may precipitate overt renal failure. Patients at greatest risk of this reaction are those with impaired renal function, heart failure, liver dysfunction, those taking diuretics, and the elderly. Discontinuation of nonsteroidal antiinflammatory drug therapy is typically followed by recovery to the pretreatment state.

Since ketoprofen is primarily eliminated by the kidneys and its pharmacokinetics are altered by renal failure (see "Clinical Pharmacology"), patients with significantly impaired renal function should be closely monitored, and a reduction of dosage should be anticipated to avoid accumulation of ketoprofen and/or its metabolites.

As with other nonsteroidal antiinflammatory drugs, borderline elevations of one or more liver-function tests may occur in up to 15% of patients. These abnormalities may progress, may remain essentially unchanged, or may disappear with continued therapy. The SGPT (ALT) test is probably the most sensitive indicator of liver dysfunction. Meaningful (3 times the upper limit of normal) elevations of SGPT or SGOT (AST) occurred in controlled clinical trials in less than 1% of patients. A patient with symptoms and/or signs suggesting liver dysfunction, or in whom an abnormal liver test has occurred, should be evaluated for evidence of the development of a more severe hepatic reaction while on therapy with ketoprofen. Serious hepatic reactions, including jaundice, have been reported from postmarketing experience with ketoprofen as well as with other nonsteroidal antiinflammatory drugs.

If steroid dosage is reduced or eliminated during therapy, it should be reduced slowly and the patients observed closely for any evidence of adverse effects, including adrenal insufficiency and exacerbation of symptoms of arthritis.

Anemia is commonly observed in rheumatoid arthritis and is sometimes aggravated by nonsteroidal antiinflammatory drugs, which may produce fluid retention or minor gastrointestinal blood loss in some patients. Therefore, patients with initial hemoglobin values of 10 g/dL or less who are to re-

ceive long-term therapy should have hemoglobin values determined frequently.

Peripheral edema has been observed in approximately 2% of patients taking ketoprofen. Therefore, as with other nonsteroidal antiinflammatory drugs, ketoprofen should be used with caution in patients with fluid retention, hypertension, or heart failure.

INFORMATION FOR PATIENTS

Orudis, like other drugs of its class, is not free of side effects. The side effects of these drugs can cause discomfort and, rarely, there are more serious side effects, such as gastrointestinal bleeding, which may result in hospitalization and even fatal outcomes.

NSAIDs (Nonsteroidal Anti-Inflammatory Drugs) are often essential agents in the management of arthritis and have a major role in the treatment of pain, but they also may be commonly employed for conditions which are less serious. Physicians may wish to discuss with their patients the potential risks (see "Warnings," "Precautions," and "Adverse Reactions" sections) and likely benefits of NSAID treatment, particularly when the drugs are used for less serious conditions where treatment without NSAIDs may represent an acceptable alternative to both the patient and physician.

Because aspirin causes an increase in the level of unbound ketoprofen, patients should be advised not to take aspirin while taking Orudis (see "Drug Interactions"). It is possible that minor adverse symptoms of gastric intolerance may be prevented by administering Orudis with antacids, food, or milk. Because antacids do not affect bioavailability (see "Drug Interactions") but food and milk do affect the rate but not the extent of absorption (see "Clinical Pharmacology"), physicians may want to make specific recommendations to patients about when they should take Orudis in relation to food and/or what patients should do if they experience minor GI symptoms associated with Orudis therapy.

LABORATORY TESTS

Because serious GI-tract ulceration and bleeding can occur without warning symptoms, physicians should follow chronically treated patients for the signs and symptoms of ulceration and bleeding and should inform them of the importance of this follow-up (see "Risk of GI Ulceration, Bleeding, and Perforation with NSAID Therapy").

DRUG INTERACTIONS

The following drug interactions were studied with Orudis doses of 200 mg per day (50 mg q.i.d.). The possibility of increased interaction should be kept in mind when Orudis doses greater than 50 mg as a single dose or 200 mg per day are used concomitantly with highly bound drugs.

1. Antacids
Concomitant administration of magnesium hydroxide and aluminum hydroxide does not interfere with the rate or extent of the absorption of ketoprofen.

2. Aspirin
Orudis does not alter aspirin absorption; however, in a study of 12 normal subjects, concurrent administration of aspirin decreased ketoprofen protein-binding and increased ketoprofen plasma clearance from 0.07 L/kg/hr without aspirin to 0.11 L/kg/hr with aspirin. The clinical significance of these changes has not been adequately studied. Therefore, concurrent use of aspirin and ketoprofen is not recommended.

3. Diuretic
Hydrochlorothiazide, given concomitantly with Orudis, produces a reduction in urinary potassium and chloride excretion compared to hydrochlorothiazide alone. Patients taking diuretics are at greater risk of developing renal failure secondary to a decrease in renal blood flow caused by prostaglandin inhibition (see "General Precautions").

4. Digoxin
In a study in 12 patients with congestive heart failure where Orudis and digoxin were concomitantly administered, Orudis did not alter the serum levels of digoxin.

5. Warfarin
In a short-term controlled study in 14 normal volunteers, Orudis did not significantly interfere with the effect of warfarin on prothrombin time. Bleeding from a number of sites may be a complication of warfarin treatment and GI bleeding a complication of Orudis treatment. Because prostaglandins play an important role in hemostasis and ketoprofen has an effect on platelet function as well (see "Blood Coagulation"), concurrent therapy with Orudis and warfarin requires close monitoring of patients on both drugs.

6. Probenecid
Probenecid increases both free and bound ketoprofen by reducing the plasma clearance of ketoprofen to about one-third, as well as decreasing its protein-binding. Therefore, the combination of Orudis and probenecid is not recommended.

7. Methotrexate
The coadministration of Orudis and methotrexate should be avoided because increased toxicity due to displacement of protein-bound methoxtrexate has been reported to occur

Continued on next page

Wyeth-Ayerst Laboratories—Cont.

when nonsteroidal antiinflammatory agents are administered simultaneously with methotrexate.

8. *Lithium*

Nonsteroidal antiinflammatory agents have been reported to increase steady-state plasma lithium levels. It is recommended that plasma lithium levels be monitored when Orudis is coadministered with lithium.

DRUG/LABORATORY TEST INTERACTIONS:
EFFECT ON BLOOD COAGULATION

Orudis decreases platelet adhesion and aggregation. Therefore, it can prolong bleeding time by approximately 3 to 4 minutes from baseline values. There is no significant change in platelet count, prothrombin time, partial thromboplastin time, or thrombin time.

CARCINOGENESIS, MUTAGENESIS, IMPAIRMENT OF FERTILITY

Chronic oral toxicity studies in mice (up to 32 mg/kg/day) did not indicate a carcinogenic potential for Orudis (maximum recommended human therapeutic dose for a 50 kg man is 6 mg/kg/day). A chronic oral toxicity study was also performed in rats (up to 12.5 mg/kg/day) with no statistically significant increase in any tumor type; however, this study was unacceptable because of poor survival. Orudis did not show mutagenic potential in the Ames Test. Orudis administered to male rats (up to 9 mg/kg/day) had no significant effect on reproductive performance or fertility. In female rats administered 6 or 9 mg/kg/day, a decrease in the number of implantation sites has been noted.

Abnormal spermatogenesis or inhibition of spermatogenesis developed in rats and dogs at high doses, and a decrease in the weight of the testes occurred in dogs and baboons at high doses.

TERATOGENIC EFFECTS: PREGNANCY CATEGORY B

In teratology studies Orudis administered to mice at doses up to 12 mg/kg/day and rats at doses up to 9 mg/kg/day, the approximate equivalent of 1.5 times the maximum recommended therapeutic dose in (a 50 kg) man, showed no teratogenic or embryotoxic effects. In separate studies in rabbits, maternally toxic doses were associated with embryotoxicity but not teratogenicity.

There are no adequate and well-controlled studies in pregnant women. Because animal teratology studies are not always predictive of the human response, Orudis should be used during pregnancy only if the potential benefit justifies the risk.

LABOR AND DELIVERY

The effects of Orudis on labor and delivery in pregnant women are unknown. Studies in rats have shown Orudis at doses of 6 mg/kg (approximately equal to the maximum recommended human dose) prolong pregnancy when given before the onset of labor. Because of the known effects of prostaglandin-inhibiting drugs on the fetal cardiovascular system (closure of ductus arteriosus), use of Orudis during late pregnancy should be avoided.

NURSING MOTHERS

In rats, Orudis at doses of 9 mg/kg (approximately 1.5 times the maximum human therapeutic dose) did not affect perinatal development. Upon administration to lactating dogs, the milk concentration of Orudis was found to be 4 to 5% of the plasma drug level. Data on secretion in human milk after ingestion of ketoprofen do not exist. As with other drugs that are excreted in milk, Orudis is not recommended for use in nursing mothers.

PEDIATRIC USE

Orudis is not recommended for use in children, because its safety and effectiveness have not been studied in children.

ADVERSE REACTIONS

The incidence of common adverse reactions (above 1%) was obtained from a population of 835 ketoprofen-treated patients in double-blind trials lasting from 4 to 54 weeks.

Minor gastrointestinal side effects predominated; upper gastrointestinal symptoms were more common than lower gastrointestinal symptoms. Peptic ulcer or GI bleeding occurred in controlled clinical trials in less than 1% of 1,076 patients; however, in open label continuation studies in 1,292 patients the rate was greater than 2%. The incidence of peptic ulceration in patients on NSAIDs is dependent on many risk factors including age, sex, smoking, alcohol use, diet, stress, concomitant drugs such as aspirin and corticoids, as well as the dose and duration of treatment with NSAIDs (see "Warnings"). These were followed in frequency by central nervous system side effects, such as headache, dizziness, or drowsiness. The incidence of some adverse reactions appears to be dose-related (see "Dosage and Administration").

Those rare adverse reactions (incidence less than 1%) were collected from foreign reports to manufacturers and regulatory agencies, publications, and U.S. clinical trials.

In double-blind trials, 233 ketoprofen-treated patients had fewer minor gastrointestinal complaints, tinnitus and hearing impairment, fluid retention, and minor abnormalities in liver-function tests than 228 aspirin-treated patients.

INCIDENCE GREATER THAN 1%
(PROBABLE CAUSAL RELATIONSHIP)

Digestive: Dyspepsia (11.5%), nausea*, abdominal pain*, diarrhea*, constipation*, flatulence*, anorexia, vomiting, stomatitis.

Central Nervous System: Headache*, dizziness, CNS inhibition (i.e., pooled reports of somnolence, malaise, depression, etc.) or excitation (i.e., insomnia, nervousness, dreams, etc.).*

Special Senses: Tinnitus, visual disturbance.

Skin and Appendages: Rash.

Urogenital: Impairment of renal function (edema, increased BUN)*, signs or symptoms of urinary-tract irritation.

INCIDENCE LESS THAN 1%
(PROBABLE CAUSAL RELATIONSHIP)

Digestive: Appetite increased, dry mouth, eructation, gastritis, rectal hemorrhage, melena, fecal occult blood, salivation, peptic ulcer, gastrointestinal perforation, hematemesis, intestinal ulceration.

Central Nervous System: Amnesia, confusion, impotence, migraine, paresthesia, vertigo.

Special Senses: Conjunctivitis, conjunctivitis sicca, eye pain, hearing impairment, retinal hemorrhage and pigmentation change, taste perversion.

Skin and Appendages: Alopecia, eczema, pruritus, purpuric rash, sweating, urticaria, bullous rash, exfoliative dermatitis, photosensitivity, skin discoloration, onycholysis.

Body as a Whole: Chills, facial edema, infection, pain, allergic reaction, anaphylaxis.

Cardiovascular: Hypertension, palpitation, tachycardia, congestive heart failure, peripheral vascular disease, vasodilation.

Hemic: Hypocoagulability, agranulocytosis, anemia, hemolysis, purpura, thrombocytopenia.

Metabolic and Nutritional: Thirst, weight gain, weight loss, hepatic dysfunction, hyponatremia.

Musculoskeletal: Myalgia.

Respiratory: Dyspnea, hemoptysis, epistaxis, pharyngitis, rhinitis, bronchospasm, laryngeal edema.

Urogenital: Menometrorrhagia, hematuria, renal failure, interstitial nephritis, nephrotic syndrome.

INCIDENCE LESS THAN 1%
(CAUSAL RELATIONSHIP UNKNOWN)

The following rare adverse reactions, whose causal relationship to ketoprofen is uncertain, are being listed to serve as alerting information to the physician.

Digestive: Buccal necrosis, ulcerative colitis.

Central Nervous System: Dysphoria, hallucination, libido disturbance, nightmares, personality disorder.

Body as a Whole: Septicemia, shock.

Cardiovascular: Arrhythmias, myocardial infarction.

Endocrine: Diabetes mellitus (aggravated).

Metabolic and Nutritional: Jaundice.

Urogenital: Acute tubulopathy, gynecomastia.

OVERDOSAGE

The reports of overdosage with Orudis are rare. Of the 20 subjects reported in Great Britain (5 children, 14 adolescents or young adults, and 1 man 80-years-old), only 4 had mild symptoms (vomiting in 3, drowsiness in 1 child). The highest reported dose was 5,000 mg in the elderly man who displayed no symptoms.

Tonic-clonic seizures and metabolic acidosis were reported in a 12-year-old female who attempted suicide by ingestion of an unknown quantity of ketoprofen, hydrocodone, and acetaminophen. The patient recovered within 18 hours of ingestion.

Should a patient ingest a large number of capsules, the stomach should be emptied by gastric lavage or induction of vomiting and usual supportive measures employed. The drug is dialyzable; therefore, hemodialysis may be useful to remove circulating drug and to assist in case of renal failure.

DOSAGE AND ADMINISTRATION

RHEUMATOID ARTHRITIS AND OSTEOARTHRITIS

The recommended daily dose of Orudis is 150 to 300 mg, divided in three or four doses. The recommended starting dose is 75 mg three times or 50 mg four times a day. If minor side effects appear, they may disappear at a lower dose which may still have an adequate therapeutic effect. If well tolerated but not optimally effective, the dosage may be increased. Individual patients may show a better response to 300 mg daily as compared to 200 mg, although in well-controlled clinical trials patients on 300 mg did not show greater mean effectiveness. They did, however, show an increased frequency of upper- and lower-GI distress and headaches. It is of interest that women also had an increased frequency of these adverse effects compared to men. When treating patients with 300 mg a day, the physician should observe sufficient increased clinical benefit to offset potential increased risk. Dosages higher than 300 mg per day are not recommended because they have not been adequately studied. Relatively small people may need smaller doses.

Orudis is eliminated primarily by renal excretion; therefore, initial dosage should be reduced by $\frac{1}{2}$ to $\frac{1}{3}$ in patients with impaired renal function, including the elderly who normally have decreased renal function even with normal serum creatinine and/or BUN, because the lean body weight of older patients results in less creatinine formation.

Because hypoalbuminemia and reduced renal function both increase the fraction of free drug (biologically active form), patients who have both conditions may be at greater risk of adverse effects. Therefore, it is recommended that such patients also be started on lower doses and closely monitored.

As with other nonsteroidal antiinflammatory drugs, the predominant adverse effects of ketoprofen are gastrointestinal. To attempt to minimize these effects, physicians may wish to prescribe that Orudis be taken with antacids, food, or milk. Although food affects the bioavailability of Orudis (see "Clinical Pharmacology"), in most of the clinical trials Orudis was taken with food or milk.

MILD-TO-MODERATE PAIN AND DYSMENORRHEA

The usual dose of Orudis recommended for mild-to-moderate pain and dysmenorrhea is 25 to 50 mg every 6 to 8 hours as necessary. A smaller dose should be utilized initially in small individuals, in debilitated or elderly patients, or in patients with renal or liver disease (see "Precautions"). A larger dose may be tried if the patient's response to a previous dose was less than satisfactory, but doses above 75 mg have not been shown to give added analgesia. Daily doses above 300 mg are not recommended because they have not been adequately studied. Because of its typical nonsteroidal antiinflammatory drug-side-effect profile, including as its principal adverse effect GI side effects (see "Warnings" and "Adverse Reactions"), higher doses of Orudis should be used with caution and patients receiving them observed carefully.

*Side effects with incidence greater than 3%.

HOW SUPPLIED

Orudis® (ketoprofen) Capsules, Wyeth®, are available as follows:

25 mg, NDC 0008-4186, dark-green and red capsule marked "WYETH 4186" on one side and "ORUDIS 25" on the reverse side, in bottles of 100 capsules.

50 mg, NDC 0008-4181, dark-green and light-green capsule marked "WYETH 4181" on one side and "ORUDIS 50" on the reverse side, in bottles of 100 capsules.

75 mg, NDC 0008-4187, dark-green and white capsule marked "WYETH 4187" on one side and "ORUDIS 75" on the reverse side, in bottles of 100 and 500 capsules, and in Redipak® cartons each containing 10 blister strips of 10 capsules.

Keep tightly closed.
Dispense in tight container.
Store at room temperature, approx. 25° C (77° F).

The appearance of these capsules is a trademark of Wyeth-Ayerst Laboratories.

Shown in Product Identification Section, page 437

OVRAL® ℞
[oh 'vral]
TABLETS
(norgestrel and ethinyl estradiol tablets)

DESCRIPTION

Each Ovral tablet contains 0.5 mg of norgestrel (*dl* -13-beta-ethyl-17-alpha-ethinyl -17- beta-hydroxygon -4- en -3- one), a totally synthetic progestogen, and 0.05 mg of ethinyl estradiol (19-nor-17α-pregna-1,3,5 (10)-trien-20-yne-3,17-diol). The inactive ingredients present are cellulose, lactose, magnesium stearate, and polacrilin potassium.

CLINICAL PHARMACOLOGY

See LO/OVRAL®.

INDICATIONS AND USAGE

Oral contraceptives are indicated for the prevention of pregnancy in women who elect to use this product as a method of contraception.

Oral contraceptives are highly effective. Table I lists the typical accidental pregnancy rates for users of combination oral contraceptives and other methods of contraception. The efficacy of these contraceptive methods, except sterilization and the IUD, depends upon the reliability with which they are used. Correct and consistent use of methods can result in lower failure rates. [See table on next page.]

CONTRAINDICATIONS

See LO/OVRAL.

WARNINGS

See LO/OVRAL.

PRECAUTIONS

See LO/OVRAL.

Drug Interactions: See LO/OVRAL

Carcinogenesis: See LO/OVRAL

Pregnancy: See LO/OVRAL

Nursing Mothers: See LO/OVRAL

Information For The Patient: See LO/OVRAL.

TABLE I: LOWEST EXPECTED AND TYPICAL FAILURE RATES DURING THE FIRST YEAR OF CONTINUOUS USE OF A METHOD

% of Women Experiencing an Accidental Pregnancy in the First Year of Continuous Use

Method	Lowest Expected*	Typical**
(No Contraception)	(89)	(89)
Oral contraceptives		3
combined	0.1	N/A***
progestin only	0.5	N/A***
Diaphragm with spermicidal cream or jelly	3	18
Spermicides alone (foam, creams, jellies and vaginal suppositories)	3	21
Vaginal Sponge		
nulliparous	5	18
multiparous	>8	>28
IUD (medicated)	1	6#
Condom without spermicides	2	12
Periodic abstinence (all methods)	2–10	20
Female sterilization	0.2	0.4
Male sterilization	0.1	0.15

Adapted from J. Trussell and K. Kost, Table 11, Studies in Family Planning, 18(5), Sept.–Oct. 1987.

* The authors' best guess of the percentage of women expected to experience an accidental pregnancy among couples who initiate a method (not necessarily for the first time) and who use it consistently and correctly during the first year if they do not stop for any other reason.

** This term represents "typical" couples who initiate use of a method (not necessarily for the first time), who experience an accidental pregnancy during the first year if they do not stop use for any other reason.

*** N/A—Data not available

\# Combined typical rate for both medicated and non-medicated IUD. The rate for medicated IUD alone is not available.

ADVERSE REACTIONS
See LO/OVRAL.

OVERDOSAGE
See LO/OVRAL.

NONCONTRACEPTIVE HEALTH BENEFITS
See LO/OVRAL.

DOSAGE AND ADMINISTRATION
To achieve maximum contraceptive effectiveness, Ovral must be taken exactly as directed and at intervals not exceeding 24 hours.

The dosage of Ovral is one tablet daily for 21 consecutive days per menstrual cycle according to prescribed schedule. Tablets are then discontinued for 7 days (three weeks on, one week off).

It is recommended that Ovral tablets be taken at the same time each day, preferably after the evening meal or at bedtime.

During the first cycle of medication, the patient is instructed to take one Ovral tablet daily for twenty-one consecutive days beginning on day five of her menstrual cycle. (The first day of menstruation is day one.) The tablets are then discontinued for one week (7 days). Withdrawal bleeding should usually occur within three days following discontinuation of Ovral. (If Ovral is first taken later than the fifth day of the first menstrual cycle of medication or postpartum, contraceptive reliance should not be placed on Ovral until after the first seven consecutive days of administration. The possibility of ovulation and conception prior to initiation of medication should be considered.) The patient begins her next and all subsequent 21-day courses of Ovral tablets on the same day of the week that she began her first course, following the same schedule: 21 days on—7 days off. She begins taking her tablets on the 8th day after discontinuance regardless of whether or not a menstrual period has occurred or is still in progress. Any time a new cycle of Ovral is started later than the 8th day, the patient should be protected by another means of contraception until she has taken a tablet daily for seven consecutive days.

If spotting or breakthrough bleeding occurs, the patient is instructed to continue on the same regimen. This type of bleeding is usually transient and without significance; however, if the bleeding is persistent or prolonged, the patient is advised to consult her physician. Although the occurrence of pregnancy is highly unlikely if Ovral is taken according to directions, if withdrawal bleeding does not occur, the possibility of pregnancy must be considered. If the patient has not adhered to the prescribed schedule (missed one or more tablets or started taking them on a day later than she should

have), the probability of pregnancy should be considered at the time of the first missed period and appropriate diagnostic measures taken before the medication is resumed. If the patient has adhered to the prescribed regimen and misses two consecutive periods, pregnancy should be ruled out before continuing the contraceptive regimen.

The patient should be instructed to take a missed tablet as soon as it is remembered. If two consecutive tablets are missed, they should both be taken as soon as remembered. The next tablet should be taken at the usual time.

Any time the patient misses one or two tablets, she should also use another method of contraception until she has taken a tablet daily for seven consecutive days. If breakthrough bleeding occurs following missed tablets, it will usually be transient and of no consequence. While there is little likelihood of ovulation occurring if only one or two tablets are missed, the possibility of ovulation increases with each successive day that scheduled tablets are missed. If three consecutive tablets are missed, all medication should be discontinued and the remainder of the package discarded. A new tablet cycle should be started on the 8th day after the last tablet was taken, and an alternate means of contraception should be prescribed during the seven days without tablets and until the patient has taken a tablet daily for seven consecutive days.

In the nonlactating mother, Ovral may be initiated postpartum, for contraception. When the tablets are administered in the postpartum period, the increased risk of thromboembolic disease associated with the postpartum period must be considered (see Contraindications, Warnings, and Precautions concerning thromboembolic disease). It is to be noted that early resumption of ovulation may occur if Parlodel® (bromocriptine mesylate) has been used for the prevention of lactation.

HOW SUPPLIED
Ovral® Tablets (0.5 mg norgestrel and 0.05 mg ethinyl estradiol), Wyeth®, are available in packages of 6 PILPAK® dispensers with 21 tablets each as follows: NDC 0008-0056, white, round tablet marked "WYETH" and "56".

References available upon request.

Brief Summary Patient Package Insert: See LO/OVRAL.
DETAILED PATIENT LABELING: See LO/OVRAL.

Shown in Product Identification Section, page 437

OVRAL®-28   ℞
[oh'vral-28]
Tablets
(norgestrel and ethinyl estradiol tablets)

DESCRIPTION
21 white Ovral tablets, each containing 0.5 mg of norgestrel (*dl* -13-beta-ethyl-17-alpha-ethinyl-17-beta-hydroxygon-4-en-3-one), a totally synthetic progestogen, and 0.05 mg of ethinyl estradiol (19-nor-17α-pregna-1,3,5 (10)-trien-20-yne-3,17-diol), and 7 pink inert tablets. The inactive ingredients present are cellulose, D&C Red 30, lactose, magnesium stearate, and polacrilin potassium.

CLINICAL PHARMACOLOGY
See LO/OVRAL®.

INDICATIONS AND USAGE
See OVRAL®.

CONTRAINDICATIONS
See LO/OVRAL.

WARNINGS
See LO/OVRAL.

PRECAUTIONS
See LO/OVRAL.
Drug Interactions: See LO/OVRAL.
Carcinogenesis: See LO/OVRAL.
Pregnancy: See LO/OVRAL.
Nursing Mothers: See LO/OVRAL.
Information for the Patient:10 See LO/OVRAL.

ADVERSE REACTIONS
See LO/OVRAL.

OVERDOSAGE
See LO/OVRAL.

NONCONTRACEPTIVE HEALTH BENEFITS
See LO/OVRAL

DOSAGE AND ADMINISTRATION
To achieve maximum contraceptive effectiveness, Ovral-28 must be taken exactly as directed and at intervals not exceeding 24 hours.

The dosage of Ovral-28 is one white tablet daily for 21 consecutive days followed by one pink inert tablet daily for 7 consecutive days according to prescribed schedule. It is recommended that OVRAL-28 tablets be taken at the same time each day, preferably after the evening meal or at bedtime. During the first cycle of medication, the patient is instructed

to begin taking Ovral-28 on the first Sunday after the onset of menstruation. If menstruation begins on a Sunday, the first tablet (white) is taken that day. One white tablet should be taken daily for 21 consecutive days followed by one pink inert tablet daily for 7 consecutive days. Withdrawal bleeding should usually occur within three days following discontinuation of white tablets. During the first cycle, contraceptive reliance should not be placed on Ovral-28 until a white tablet has been taken daily for 7 consecutive days. The possibility of ovulation and conception prior to initiation of medication should be considered.

The patient begins her next and all subsequent 28-day courses of tablets on the same day of the week (Sunday) on which she began her first course, following the same schedule: 21 days on white tablets—7 days on pink inert tablets. If in any cycle the patient starts tablets later than the proper day, she should protect herself by using another method of birth control until she has taken a white tablet daily for 7 consecutive days.

If spotting or breakthrough bleeding occurs, the patient is instructed to continue on the same regimen. This type of bleeding is usually transient and without significance; however, if the bleeding is persistent or prolonged, the patient is advised to consult her physician. Although the occurrence of pregnancy is highly unlikely if Ovral-28 is taken according to directions, if withdrawal bleeding does not occur, the possibility of pregnancy must be considered. If the patient has not adhered to the prescribed schedule (missed one or more tablets or started taking them on a day later than she should have), the probability of pregnancy should be considered at the time of the first missed period and appropriate diagnostic measures taken before the medication is resumed. If the patient has adhered to the prescribed regimen and misses two consecutive periods, pregnancy should be ruled out before continuing the contraceptive regimen.

The patient should be instructed to take a missed white tablet as soon as it is remembered. If two consecutive white tablets are missed they should both be taken as soon as remembered. The next tablet should be taken at the usual time.

Any time the patient misses one or two white tablets she should also use another method of contraception until she has taken a white tablet daily for seven consecutive days. If the patient misses one or more pink tablets she is still protected against pregnancy **provided** she begins taking white tablets again on the proper day.

If breakthrough bleeding occurs following missed white tablets, it will usually be transient and of no consequence. While there is little likelihood of ovulation occurring if only one or two white tablets are missed, the possibility of ovulation increases with each successive day that scheduled white tablets are missed. If three consecutive white Ovral tablets are missed, all medication should be discontinued and the remainder of the 28-day package discarded. A new tablet cycle should be started on the first Sunday following the last missed tablet, and an alternate means of contraception should be prescribed during the days without tablets and until the patient has taken a white tablet daily for 7 consecutive days.

In the nonlactating mother, Ovral-28 may be initiated postpartum, for contraception. When the tablets are administered in the postpartum period, the increased risk of thromboembolic disease associated with the postpartum period must be considered (see Contraindications, Warnings, and Precautions concerning thromboembolic disease). It is to be noted that early resumption of ovulation may occur if Parlodel® (bromocriptine mesylate) has been used for the prevention of lactation.

HOW SUPPLIED
Ovral®-28 Tablets (0.5 mg norgestrel and 0.05 mg ethinyl estradiol), Wyeth®, are available in packages of 6 PILPAK® dispensers, each containing 28 tablets as follows: 21 active tablets, NDC 0008-0056, white, round tablet marked "WYETH" and "56".
7 inert tablets, NDC 0008-0445, pink, round tablet marked "WYETH" and "445".

References available upon request.

Brief Summary Patient Package Insert: See LO/OVRAL.
DETAILED PATIENT LABELING: See LO/OVRAL.

Shown in Product Identification Section, page 437

OVRETTE®   ℞
[oh-vret']
Tablets
(norgestrel tablets)

Each OVRETTE® tablet contains 0.075 mg of norgestrel (*dl* -13-beta-ethyl-17-alpha-ethinyl-17-beta-hydroxygon-4-en-3-one). The inactive ingredients present are cellulose, FD&C Yellow 5, lactose, magnesium stearate, and polacrilin potassium.

Continued on next page

Wyeth-Ayerst Laboratories—Cont.

DESCRIPTION

Each OVRETTE tablet contains 0.075 mg of a single active steroid ingredient, norgestrel, a totally synthetic progestogen. The available data suggest that the d (-)enantiomeric form of norgestrel is the biologically active portion. This form amounts to 0.0375 mg per OVRETTE tablet.

CLINICAL PHARMACOLOGY

The primary mechanism through which OVRETTE prevents conception is not known, but progestogen-only contraceptives are known to alter the cervical mucus, exert a progestational effect on the endometrium, interfering with implantation, and, in some patients, suppress ovulation.

INDICATIONS AND USAGE

OVRETTE is indicated for the prevention of pregnancy in women who elect to use oral contraceptives as a method of contraception. Oral contraceptives are highly effective. The pregnancy rate in women using conventional combination oral contraceptives (containing 35 mcg or more of ethinyl estradiol or 50 mcg or more of mestranol) is generally reported as less than one pregnancy per 100 women-years of use. Slightly higher rates (somewhat more than 1 pregnancy per 100 woman-years of use) are reported for some combination products containing 35 mcg or less of ethinyl estradiol, and rates on the order of 3 pregnancies per 100 woman-years are reported for the progestogen-only oral contraceptives. These rates are derived from separate studies conducted by different investigators in several population groups and cannot be compared precisely. Furthermore, pregnancy rates tend to be lower as clinical studies are continued, possibly due to selective retention in the longer studies of those patients who accept the treatment regimen and do not discontinue as a result of adverse reactions, pregnancy, or other reasons.

In clinical trials with OVRETTE, 2.752 patients completed 38.245 cycles, and a total of 78 pregnancies were reported. This represents a pregnancy rate of 2.45 per 100 woman-years. Approximately one-half of the pregnancies reported in these trials were due to method failure, and the other half were due to patient failure.

Table 1 gives ranges of pregnancy rates reported in the literature[1] for other means of contraception. The efficacy of these means of contraception (except the IUD) depends upon the degree of adherence to the method.

TABLE 1
PREGNANCIES PER 100 WOMAN-YEARS
IUD, less than 1-6; Diaphragm with spermicidal products (creams or jellies), 2-20; Condom, 3-36; Aerosol foams, 2-29; Jellies and creams, 4-36;
Periodic abstinence (rhythm) all types, less than 1-47:
1. Calendar method, 14-47;
2. Temperature method, 1-20;
3. Temperature method—intercourse only in postovulatory phase, less that 1-7;
4. Mucus method, 1-25;
No contraception, 60-80.
Dose-Related Risk of Thromboembolism from Oral Contraceptives: See LO/OVRAL®.

CONTRAINDICATIONS
See LO/OVRAL.

WARNINGS
See LO/OVRAL.

PRECAUTIONS
See LO/OVRAL.

INFORMATION FOR THE PATIENT
See LO/OVRAL.

DRUG INTERACTIONS
See LO/OVRAL.

CARCINOGENESIS
See LO/OVRAL.

PREGNANCY
See LO/OVRAL.

NURSING MOTHERS
See LO/OVRAL.

ADVERSE REACTIONS
See LO/OVRAL.

OVERDOSAGE
See LO/OVRAL.

DOSAGE AND ADMINISTRATION

To achieve maximum contraceptive effectiveness, OVRETTE (norgestrel) must be taken exactly as directed and at intervals not exceeding 24 hours. OVRETTE is administered on a continuous daily dosage regimen starting on the first day of menstruation, i.e., one tablet each day, every day of the year.

Tablets should be taken at the same time each day and continued daily, without interruption, whether bleeding occurs or not. The patient should be advised that, if prolonged bleeding occurs, she should consult her physician. In the non-nursing mother, OVRETTE may be prescribed in the postpartum period either immediately or at the first postpartum examination whether or not menstruation has resumed.

The risk of pregnancy increases with each tablet missed. If the patient misses one tablet, she should be instructed to take it as soon as she remembers and to also take her next tablet at the regular time. If she misses two tablets, she should take one of the missed tablets as soon as she remembers, as well as taking her regular tablet for that day at the proper time. Furthermore, she should use a method of nonhormonal contraception in addition to taking OVRETTE until fourteen tablets have been taken. If more than 2 tablets have been missed, OVRETTE should be discontinued immediately and a method of nonhormonal contraception should be used until menses has appeared or pregnancy has been excluded. If menses does not appear within 45 days from the last period, a method of nonhormonal contraception should be substituted until the start of the next menstrual period or an appropriate diagnostic procedure is performed to rule out pregnancy.

HOW SUPPLIED

OVRETTE® tablets (0.075 mg norgestrel), Wyeth®, are available in packages of 6 PILPAK® dispensers with 28 tablets each as follows: NDC 0008-0062, yellow, round tablet marked "WYETH" and "62".

REFERENCES

Available upon request.
Brief Summary Patient Package Insert: See LO/OVRAL
DETAILED PATIENT LABELING: See LO/OVRAL.

OXYTOCIN   ℞
[ok "se-to 'sin]
Injection, USP
(synthetic)

DESCRIPTION

Each mL of TUBEX® Oxytocin Injection sterile solution contains an oxytocic activity equivalent to 10 USP Posterior Pituitary Units, chlorobutanol (a chloroform derivative), 0.5%, as a preservative, and acetic acid to adjust pH (2.5 to 4.5). Wyeth Oxytocin is intended for IM or IV use. Oxytocin is a synthetic polypeptide; it occurs as a white powder and is soluble in water.

CLINICAL PHARMACOLOGY

The pharmacologic and clinical properties of oxytocin are identical with those of the naturally occurring oxytocin principle of the posterior lobe of the pituitary. Oxytocin exerts a selective action on the smooth musculature of the uterus, particularly toward the end of pregnancy, during labor, and immediately following delivery. Oxytocin stimulates rhythmic contractions of the uterus, increases the frequency of existing contractions, and raises the tone of the uterine musculature.

When given in appropriate doses during pregnancy, oxytocin is capable of eliciting graded increases in uterine motility from a moderate increase in the rate and force of spontaneous motor activity to sustained tetanic contraction. The sensitivity of the uterus to oxytocic activity increases progressively throughout pregnancy until term when it is maximal. Oxytocin is distributed throughout the extracellular fluid. Small amounts of this drug probably reach the fetal circulation. Oxytocin has a plasma half-life of about 3 to 5 minutes. Following parenteral administration, uterine response occurs within 3 to 5 minutes and persists for 2 to 3 hours. Its rapid removal from plasma is accomplished largely by the kidney and the liver. Only small amounts of oxytocin are excreted in the urine unchanged.

INDICATIONS AND USAGE

> **IMPORTANT NOTICE**
>
> Oxytocin is indicated for the medical rather than the elective induction of labor. Available data and information are inadequate to define the benefits-to-risks considerations in the use of the drug product for elective induction. Elective induction of labor is defined as the initiation of labor for convenience in an individual with a term pregnancy who is free of medical indications.

ANTEPARTUM: Oxytocin is indicated for the initiation or improvement of uterine contractions, where this is desirable and considered suitable for reasons of fetal or maternal concern, in order to achieve early vaginal delivery. It is indicated for (1) induction of labor in patients with a medical indication for the initiation of labor, such as Rh problems, maternal diabetes, preeclampsia at or near term, when delivery is in the best interest of mother and fetus or when membranes are prematurely ruptured and delivery is indicated;

(2) stimulation or reinforcement of labor, as in selected cases of uterine inertia; (3) as adjunctive therapy in the management of incomplete or inevitable abortion. In the first trimester, curettage is generally considered primary therapy. In second trimester abortion, oxytocin infusion will often be successful in emptying the uterus. Other means of therapy, however, may be required in such cases.
POSTPARTUM: Oxytocin is indicated to produce uterine contractions during the third stage of labor and to control postpartum bleeding or hemorrhage.

CONTRAINDICATIONS

Oxytocin is contraindicated in any of the following conditions:
significant cephalopelvic disproportion;
unfavorable fetal positions or presentations which are undeliverable without conversion prior to delivery, e.g., transverse lies;
in obstetrical emergencies where the benefit-to-risk ratio for either the fetus or the mother favors surgical intervention;
in cases of fetal distress where delivery is not imminent;
hypertonic uterine patterns;
hypersensitivity to the drug.
Prolonged use in uterine inertia or severe toxemia is contraindicated.
Oxytocin should not be used in cases where vaginal delivery is not indicated, such as cord presentation or prolapse, total placenta previa, and vasa previa.

WARNINGS

Oxytocin, when given for induction or stimulation of labor, must be administered only by intravenous infusion (drip method) and with adequate medical supervision in a hospital.

PRECAUTIONS

GENERAL:
1. All patients receiving intravenous infusions of oxytocin must be under continuous observation by trained personnel with a thorough knowledge of the drug and qualified to identify complications. A physician qualified to manage any complications should be immediately available.
2. When properly administered, oxytocin should stimulate uterine contractions similar to those seen in normal labor. Overstimulation of the uterus by improper administration can be hazardous to both mother and fetus. Even with proper administration and adequate supervision, hypertonic contractions can occur in patients whose uteri are hypersensitive to oxytocin.
3. Except in unusual circumstances, oxytocin should not be administered in the following conditions: prematurity, borderline cephalopelvic disproportion, previous major surgery on the cervix or uterus, including cesarean section, overdistention of the uterus, grand multiparity, or invasive cervical carcinoma. Because of the variability of the combinations of factors which may be present in the conditions listed above, the definition of "unusual circumstances" must be left to the judgment of the physician. The decision can only be made by carefully weighing the potential benefits which oxytocin can provide in a given case against the rare occurrence of hypertonicity or tetanic spasm with this drug.
4. Maternal deaths due to hypertensive episodes, subarachnoid hemorrhage, rupture of the uterus, fetal deaths and permanent CNS or brain damage of the infant due to various causes have been reported to be associated with the use of parenteral oxytocic drugs for induction of labor or for augmentation in the first and second stages of labor.
5. Oxytocin has been shown to have an intrinsic antidiuretic effect, acting to increase water reabsorption from the glomerular filtrate. Consideration should, therefore, be given to the possibility of water intoxication, particularly when oxytocin is administered continuously by infusion and the patient is receiving fluids by mouth.
6. Oxytocin should be considered for use only in patients who have been carefully selected. Pelvic adequacy must be considered and maternal and fetal conditions thoroughly evaluated before use of the drug.
DRUG INTERACTIONS
Severe hypertension has been reported when oxytocin was given 3 to 4 hours following prophylactic administration of a vasoconstrictor in conjunction with caudal-block anesthesia. Cyclopropane anesthesia may modify oxytocin's cardiovascular effects, so as to produce unexpected results such as hypotension. Maternal sinus bradycardia with abnormal atrioventricular rhythms has also been noted when oxytocin was used concomitantly with cyclopropane anesthesia.
CARCINOGENESIS, MUTAGENESIS, IMPAIRMENT OF FERTILITY
There are no animal or human studies on the carcinogenicity and mutagenicity of this drug, nor is there any information on its effect on fertility.
PREGNANCY
See "Indications and Usage."
Teratogenic Effects
Animal reproduction studies have not been conducted with oxytocin. There are no known indications for use in the first trimester of pregnancy other than in relation to spontaneous

or induced abortion. Based on the wide experience with this drug and its chemical structure and pharmacological properties, it would not be expected to present a risk of fetal abnormalities when used as indicated.

Nonteratogenic Effects

See "Adverse Reactions" in the fetus or infant.

LABOR AND DELIVERY

See "Indications and Usage."

ADVERSE REACTIONS

The following adverse reactions have been reported in the mother:

Anaphylactic reaction

Postpartum hemorrhage

Cardiac arrhythmia

Fatal afibrinogenemia

Nausea

Vomiting

Premature ventricular contractions

Pelvic hematoma

Excessive dosage or hypersensitivity to the drug may result in uterine hypertonicity, spasm, tetanic contraction, or rupture of the uterus.

The possibility of increased blood loss and afibrinogenemia should be kept in mind when administering the drug.

Severe water intoxication with convulsions and coma has occurred, associated with a slow oxytocin infusion over a 24-hour period. Maternal death due to oxytocin-induced water intoxication has been reported.

The following adverse reactions have been reported in the fetus or infant:

(Due to induced uterine motility)

Bradycardia

Premature ventricular contractions and other arrhythmias

Permanent CNS or brain damage

Fetal death

(Due to use of oxytocin in the mother)

Low Apgar scores at five minutes

Neonatal jaundice

Neonatal retinal hemorrhage

OVERDOSAGE

Overdosage with oxytocin depends essentially on uterine hyperactivity whether or not due to hypersensitivity to this agent. Hyperstimulation with strong (hypertonic) or prolonged (tetanic) contractions, or a resting tone of 15 to 20 mmH$_2$O or more between contractions can lead to tumultuous labor, uterine rupture, cervical and vaginal lacerations, postpartum hemorrhage, utero-placental hypoperfusion, and variable deceleration of fetal heart, fetal hypoxia, hypercapnia, or death. Water intoxication with convulsions, which is caused by the inherent antidiuretic effect of oxytocin, is a serious complication that may occur if large doses (40 to 50 milliunits/minute) are infused for long periods. Management consists of immediate discontinuation of oxytocin, and symptomatic and supportive therapy.

DOSAGE AND ADMINISTRATION

Parenteral drug products should be inspected visually for particulate matter and discoloration prior to administration, whenever solution and container permit.

Dosage of oxytocin is determined by uterine response. The following dosage information is based upon the various regimens and indications in general use.

A. INDUCTION OR STIMULATION OF LABOR

Intravenous infusion (drip method) is the only acceptable method of administration for the induction or stimulation of labor.

Accurate control of the rate of infusion flow is essential. An infusion pump or other such device and frequent monitoring of strength of contractions and fetal heart rate are necessary for the safe administration of oxytocin for the induction or stimulation of labor. If uterine contractions become too powerful, the infusion can be abruptly stopped, and oxytocic stimulation of the uterine musculature will soon wane.

1. An intravenous infusion of nonoxytocin-containing solution should be started. Physiologic electrolyte solution should be used except under unusual circumstances.

2. To prepare the usual solution for infusion, the contents of one 1-mL TUBEX® (10 units) is combined aseptically with 1,000 mL of nonhydrating diluent (physiologic electrolyte solution). The combined solution, rotated in the infusion bottle to insure thorough mixing, contains 10 mU/mL. Add the container with dilute oxytocic solution to the system through use of a constant infusion pump or other such device, to control accurately the rate of infusion.

3. The initial dose should be no more than 1 to 2 mU/min. The dose may be gradually increased in increments of no more than 1 to 2 mU/min. until a contraction pattern has been established which is similar to normal labor.

4. The fetal heart rate, resting uterine tone, and the frequency, duration, and force of contractions should be monitored.

5. The oxytocin infusion should be discontinued immediately in the event of uterine hyperactivity or fetal distress.

Oxygen should be administered to the mother. The mother and the fetus must be evaluated by the responsible physician.

B. CONTROL OF POSTPARTUM UTERINE BLEEDING

1. Intravenous Infusion (Drip Method):

To control postpartum bleeding, 10 to 40 units of oxytocin may be added to 1,000 mL of a nonhydrating diluent (physiologic electrolyte solution) and run at a rate necessary to control uterine atony.

2. Intramuscular Administration:

1 mL (10 units) of oxytocin can be given after delivery of the placenta.

C. TREATMENT OF INCOMPLETE OR INEVITABLE ABORTION

Intravenous infusion with physiologic saline solution, 500 mL, or 5% dextrose in physiologic saline solution to which 10 units of oxytocin have been added should be infused at a rate of 20 to 40 drops per minute.

HOW SUPPLIED

Oxytocin Injection, USP (synthetic), 10 USP units in 1 mL TUBEX® Sterile Cartridge-Needle Unit (22 gauge × 1¼ inch needle), is supplied as follows:

NDC 0008-0406-01, package of 10 TUBEX.

Store in a refrigerator; do not freeze.

When stored out of refrigeration at temperatures of up to 26° C (79° F), this product has exhibited acceptable data for a period not exceeding three (3) months.

PATHOCIL®   ℞

[*path 'o-sil*]

(dicloxacillin sodium monohydrate)

CAPSULES • ORAL SUSPENSION

DESCRIPTION

Dicloxacillin sodium monohydrate is an isoxazolyl penicillin which resists destruction by the enzyme penicillinase (betalactamase). It is the monohydrate sodium salt of 6-[3-(2, 6-Dichlorophenyl)-5-methyl-4-isoxazolecarboxamido]-3,3-dimethyl -7- oxo -4- thia-1-azabicyclo-[3.2.0] heptane-2-carboxylic acid.

Pathocil capsules contain dicloxacillin sodium monohydrate equivalent to 250 mg or 500 mg dicloxacillin. The inactive ingredients present are D&C Red 28, FD&C Blue 1, FD&C Red 40, gelatin, lactose, stearic acid, talc, and titanium dioxide.

Pathocil oral suspension is a powder which when reconstituted as directed yields a suspension of dicloxacillin sodium monohydrate equivalent to 62.5 mg dicloxacillin per 5 mL. The inactive ingredients present are artificial and natural flavors, carboxymethylcellulose sodium, citric acid, colloidal silicon dioxide, D&C Red 28, edetate disodium, saccharin sodium, sodium benzoate, sodium citrate, sucrose, and water.

HOW SUPPLIED

Pathocil® (dicloxacillin sodium monohydrate) Capsules, Wyeth®, contain dicloxacillin sodium monohydrate equivalent to 250 mg or 500 mg dicloxacillin and are supplied as follows:

250 mg, NDC 0008-0360-02, purple and white capsule marked "WYETH" and "360", in bottles of 100 capsules.

500 mg, NDC 0008-0593-01, purple and white capsule marked "WYETH" and "593", in bottles of 50 capsules.

Keep tightly closed.

Dispense in tight container.

Pathocil® (dicloxacillin sodium monohydrate) for Oral Suspension, Wyeth®, is available as a white to light-pink powder which when reconstituted as directed yields a palatable, pink suspension of dicloxacillin sodium monohydrate equivalent to 62.5 mg dicloxacillin per 5 mL and is supplied as follows:

62.5 mg per 5 mL, NDC 0008-0361-03, in bottles to make 100 mL.

Shake well before using.

Keep tightly closed.

After reconstitution store in refrigerator. Discard any unused portion after two weeks.

Bibliography: A bibliography is available upon request.

For prescribing information write to Professional Service, Wyeth-Ayerst Laboratories, P.O. Box 8299, Philadelphia, PA 19101, or contact your local Wyeth-Ayerst representative.

Shown in Product Identification Section, page 437

PEN•VEE® K   ℞

[*pen-vee-kay*]

(penicillin V potassium)

TABLETS • FOR ORAL SOLUTION

DESCRIPTION

Penicillin V is the phenoxymethyl analog of penicillin G. Penicillin V potassium is the potassium salt of penicillin V. Pen•Vee K tablets contain penicillin V potassium equivalent to 250 mg (400,000 units) or 500 mg (800,000 units) peni-

cillin V. The inactive ingredients present are carboxymethylcellulose sodium, magnesium stearate, and stearic acid. The 250 mg dosage strength also contains lactose.

Pen•Vee K for oral solution is a powder which when reconstituted as directed yields a suspension of penicillin V potassium equivalent to 125 mg (200,000 units) or 250 mg (400,000 units) penicillin V per 5 mL. The inactive ingredients present are artificial and natural flavors, citric acid, FD&C Red 40, saccharin sodium, sodium benzoate, sodium citrate, sodium propionate, sucrose, and water. The 250 mg per 5 mL dosage strength also contains edetate disodium and FD&C Yellow 6.

HOW SUPPLIED

Pen•Vee® K (penicillin V potassium) Tablets contain penicillin V potassium equivalent to 250 mg (400,000 units) or 500 mg (800,000 units) penicillin V. They are white, round, scored tablets supplied as follows:

250 mg (400,000 units), NDC 0008-0059, marked "WYETH" and "59", in bottles of 100 or 500 tablets, and in Redipak® cartons of 100 individually wrapped tablets.

500 mg (800,000 units), NDC 0008-0390, marked "WYETH" and "390", in bottles of 100 or 500 tablets, and in Redipak cartons of 100 individually wrapped tablets.

Keep tightly closed.

Dispense in tight container.

Pen•Vee® K (penicillin V potassium) for Oral Suspension is available as a powder which when reconstituted as directed yields a palatable suspension of penicillin V potassium equivalent to 125 mg (200,000 units) or 250 mg (400,000 units) penicillin V per 5 mL and is supplied as follows:

125 mg (200,000 units) per 5 mL, NDC 0008-0004, faint pink powder, in bottles to make 100 mL or 200 mL of red solution.

250 mg (400,000 units) per 5 mL, NDC 0008-0036, light peach-colored powder, in bottles to make 100 mL, 150 mL, or 200 mL of light-orange solution.

Keep tightly closed.

After reconstitution, solution must be stored in a refrigerator.

Discard any unused portion after 14 days.

For prescribing information write to Professional Service, Wyeth-Ayerst Laboratories, P.O. Box 8299, Philadelphia, PA 19101, or contact your local Wyeth-Ayerst representative.

Shown in Product Identification Section, page 437

PEPTAVLON®   ℞

[*pĕp-tăv 'lon*]

Brand of

pentagastrin

for subcutaneous injection

HOW SUPPLIED

PEPTAVLON (pentagastrin) is available in 2 mL ampuls. Each mL contains 0.25 mg (250 micrograms) pentagastrin. Cartons of 10 ampules (NDC 0046-3290-10).

REFRIGERATE, 2°C to 8°C (36°F to 46°F), AND PROTECT FROM LIGHT.

DO NOT USE IF DISCOLORED.

For full prescribing information turn to the Diagnostic Product Information section of this edition of the PDR.

PHENERGAN®   ℞

[*fen 'er-gan*]

(promethazine HCl)

INJECTION

DESCRIPTION

Promethazine HCl (10*H*-phenothiazine-10-ethanamine, *N*, *N*,α-trimethyl-, monohydrochloride).

Each mL of ampul contains either 25 mg or 50 mg promethazine hydrochloride with 0.1 mg edetate disodium, 0.04 mg calcium chloride, not more than 0.25 mg sodium metabisulfite and 5 mg phenol with sodium acetate-acetic acid buffer. Sealed under nitrogen.

Each mL of TUBEX® Sterile Cartridge-Needle Unit contains either 25 or 50 mg promethazine hydrochloride with 0.1 mg edetate disodium, 0.04 mg calcium chloride, not more than 5 mg monothioglycerol and 5 mg phenol with sodium acetate-acetic acid buffer.

ACTIONS

Promethazine hydrochloride, a phenothiazine derivative, possesses antihistaminic, sedative, antimotion-sickness, antiemetic, and anticholinergic effects. The duration of action is generally from four to six hours. The major side reaction of this drug is sedation. As an antihistamine, it acts by competitive antagonism but does not block the release of histamine. It antagonizes in varying degrees most but not all of the pharmacological effects of histamine.

Continued on next page

INDICATIONS

The injectable form of promethazine hydrochloride is indicated for the following conditions:

1. Amelioration of allergic reactions to blood or plasma.
2. In anaphylaxis as an adjunct to epinephrine and other standard measures after the acute symptoms have been controlled.
3. For other uncomplicated allergic conditions of the immediate type when oral therapy is impossible or contraindicated.
4. Active treatment of motion sickness.
5. Preoperative, postoperative, and obstetric (during labor) sedation.
6. Prevention and control of nausea and vomiting associated with certain types of anesthesia and surgery.
7. As an adjunct to analgesics for the control of postoperative pain.
8. For sedation and relief of apprehension and to produce light sleep from which the patient can be easily aroused.
9. Intravenously in special surgical situations, such as repeated bronchoscopy, ophthalmic surgery, and poor-risk patients, with reduced amounts of meperidine or other narcotic analgesic as an adjunct to anesthesia and analgesia.

CONTRAINDICATIONS

Promethazine is contraindicated in comatose states, in patients who have received large amounts of central-nervous-system depressants (alcohol, sedative hypnotics, including barbiturates, general anesthetics, narcotics, narcotic analgesics, tranquilizers, etc.), and in patients who have demonstrated an idiosyncrasy or hypersensitivity to promethazine. Under no circumstances should promethazine be given by intra-arterial injection due to the likelihood of severe arteriospasm and the possibility of resultant gangrene (see "Warnings").

Phenergan Injection should not be given by the subcutaneous route; evidence of chemical irritation has been noted, and necrotic lesions have resulted on rare occasions following subcutaneous injection. The preferred parenteral route of administration is by deep, intramuscular injection.

WARNINGS

Phenergan Injection (ampuls only) contains sodium metabisulfite, a sulfite that may cause allergic-type reactions, including anaphylactic symptoms and life-threatening or less severe asthmatic episodes, in certain susceptible people. The overall prevalence of sulfite sensitivity in the general population is unknown and probably low. Sulfite sensitivity is seen more frequently in asthmatic than in nonasthmatic people.

Promethazine may impair the mental and/or physical abilities required for the performance of potentially hazardous tasks, such as driving a vehicle or operating machinery. The concomitant use of alcohol, sedative hypnotics (including barbiturates), general anesthetics, narcotics, narcotic analgesics, tranquilizers or other central-nervous-system depressants may have an additive sedative effect. Patients should be warned accordingly.

USAGE IN PREGNANCY

The safe use of promethazine has not been established with respect to the possible adverse effects upon fetal development. Therefore, the need for the use of this drug during pregnancy should be weighed against the possible but unknown hazards to the developing fetus.

USE IN CHILDREN

Excessively large dosages of antihistamines, including promethazine, in children may cause hallucinations, convulsions, and sudden death. In children who are acutely ill associated with dehydration, there is an increased susceptibility to dystonias with the use of promethazine hydrochloride injection.

CAUTION SHOULD BE EXERCISED WHEN ADMINISTERING PHENERGAN TO CHILDREN. ANTIEMETICS ARE NOT RECOMMENDED FOR TREATMENT OF UNCOMPLICATED VOMITING IN CHILDREN, AND THEIR USE SHOULD BE LIMITED TO PROLONGED VOMITING OF KNOWN ETIOLOGY. THE EXTRAPYRAMIDAL SYMPTOMS WHICH CAN OCCUR SECONDARY TO PHENERGAN ADMINISTRATION MAY BE CONFUSED WITH THE CNS SIGNS OF UNDIAGNOSED PRIMARY DISEASE, e.g., ENCEPHALOPATHY OR REYE'S SYNDROME. THE USE OF PHENERGAN SHOULD BE AVOIDED IN CHILDREN WHOSE SIGNS AND SYMPTOMS MAY SUGGEST REYE'S SYNDROME OR OTHER HEPATIC DISEASES.

USE IN THE ELDERLY (APPROXIMATELY 60 YEARS OR OLDER)

Since therapeutic requirements for sedative drugs tend to be less in elderly patients, the dosage of Phenergan should be reduced for these patients.

OTHER CONSIDERATIONS

Drugs having anticholinergic properties should be used with caution in patients with asthmatic attack, narrow-angle glaucoma, prostatic hypertrophy, stenosing peptic ulcer, pyloroduodenal obstruction, and bladder-neck obstruction. Phenergan should be used with caution in patients with bone-marrow depression. Leukopenia and agranulocytosis have been reported, usually when Phenergan has been used in association with other known toxic agents.

INADVERTENT INTRA-ARTERIAL INJECTION

Due to the close proximity of arteries and veins in the areas most commonly used for intravenous injection, extreme care should be exercised to avoid perivascular extravasation or inadvertent intra-arterial injection. Reports compatible with inadvertent intra-arterial injection of promethazine, usually in conjunction with other drugs intended for intravenous use, suggest that pain, severe chemical irritation, severe spasm of distal vessels, and resultant gangrene requiring amputation are likely under such circumstances. Intravenous injection was intended in all the cases reported but perivascular extravasation or arterial placement of the needle is now suspect. There is no proven successful management of this condition after it occurs, although sympathetic block and heparinization are commonly employed during the acute management because of the results of animal experiments with other known arteriolar irritants. Aspiration of dark blood does not preclude intra-arterial needle placement, because blood is discolored upon contact with promethazine. Use of syringes with rigid plungers or of small bore needles might obscure typical arterial backflow if this is relied upon alone.

When used intravenously, promethazine hydrochloride should be given in a concentration no greater than 25 mg per mL and at a rate not to exceed 25 mg per minute. When administering any irritant drug intravenously, it is usually preferable to inject it through the tubing of an intravenous infusion set that is known to be functioning satisfactorily. In the event that a patient complains of pain during intended intravenous injection of promethazine, the injection should immediately be stopped to provide for evaluation of possible arterial placement or perivascular extravasation.

PRECAUTIONS

Promethazine may significantly affect the actions of other drugs. It may increase, prolong, or intensify the sedative action of central-nervous-system depressants, such as alcohol, sedative hypnotics (including barbiturates), general anesthetics, narcotics, narcotic analgesics, tranquilizers, etc. When given concomitantly with promethazine hydrochloride, the dose of barbiturates should be reduced by at least one-half, and the dose of narcotics should be reduced by one-quarter to one-half. Dosage must be individualized. Excessive amounts of promethazine relative to a narcotic may lead to restlessness and motor hyperactivity in the patient with pain; these symptoms usually disappear with adequate control of the pain. Promethazine should be used cautiously in persons with cardiovascular disease or impairment of liver function.

Although reversal of the vasopressor effect of epinephrine has not been reported with promethazine, the possibility should be considered in case of promethazine overdose.

ADVERSE REACTIONS

CNS EFFECTS

Drowsiness is the most prominent CNS effect of this drug. Extrapyramidal reactions may occur with high doses; this is almost always responsive to a reduction in dosage. Other reported reactions include dizziness, lassitude, tinnitus, incoordination, fatigue, blurred vision, euphoria, diplopia, nervousness, insomnia, tremors, convulsive seizures, oculogyric crises, excitation, catatoniclike states, and hysteria.

CARDIOVASCULAR EFFECTS

Tachycardia, bradycardia, faintness, dizziness, and increases and decreases in blood pressure have been reported following the use of promethazine hydrochloride injection. Venous thrombosis at the injection site has been reported. INTRA-ARTERIAL INJECTION MAY RESULT IN GANGRENE OF THE AFFECTED EXTREMITY ("see Warnings").

GASTROINTESTINAL

Nausea and vomiting have been reported, usually in association with surgical procedures and combination drug therapy.

ALLERGIC REACTIONS

These include urticaria, dermatitis, asthma, and photosensitivity. Angioneurotic edema has been reported.

OTHER REPORTED REACTIONS

Leukopenia and agranulocytosis, usually when Phenergan has been used in association with other known toxic agents, have been reported. Thrombocytopenic purpura and jaundice of the obstructive type have been associated with the use of promethazine. The jaundice is usually reversible on discontinuation of the drug. Subcutaneous injection has resulted in tissue necrosis. Nasal stuffiness may occur. Dry mouth has been reported.

LABORATORY TESTS

The following laboratory tests may be affected in patients who are receiving therapy with promethazine hydrochloride:

Pregnancy Tests—Diagnostic pregnancy tests based on immunological reactions between HCG and anti-HCG may result in false-negative or false-positive interpretations.

Glucose Tolerance Test—An increase in glucose tolerance has been reported in patients receiving promethazine hydrochloride.

PARADOXICAL REACTIONS (OVERDOSAGE)

Hyperexcitability and abnormal movements, which have been reported in children following a single administration of promethazine, may be manifestations of relative overdosage, in which case, consideration should be given to the discontinuation of the promethazine and to the use of other drugs. Respiratory depression, nightmares, delirium, and agitated behavior have also been reported in some of these patients.

DRUG INTERACTIONS

NARCOTICS AND BARBITURATES

The CNS-depressant effects of narcotics and barbiturates are additive with promethazine hydrochloride.

MONOAMINE OXIDASE INHIBITORS (MAOI)

Drug interactions, including an increased incidence of extrapyramidal effects, have been reported when some MAOI and phenothiazines are used concomitantly. Although such a reaction has not been reported with promethazine, the possibility should be considered.

DOSAGE AND ADMINISTRATION

The preferred parenteral route of administration for promethazine hydrochloride is by deep, intramuscular injection. The proper intravenous administration of this product is well tolerated, but use of this route is not without some hazard.

INADVERTENT INTRA-ARTERIAL INJECTION CAN RESULT IN GANGRENE OF THE AFFECTED EXTREMITY (see "Warnings"). SUBCUTANEOUS INJECTION IS CONTRAINDICATED, AS IT MAY RESULT IN TISSUE NECROSIS (see "Contraindications"). When used intravenously, promethazine hydrochloride should be given in concentration no greater than 25 mg/mL at a rate not to exceed 25 mg per minute; it is preferable to inject through the tubing of an intravenous infusion set that is known to be functioning satisfactorily.

ALLERGIC CONDITIONS

The average adult dose is 25 mg. This dose may be repeated within two hours if necessary, but continued therapy, if indicated, should be via the oral route as soon as existing circumstances permit. After initiation of treatment, dosage should be adjusted to the smallest amount adequate to relieve symptoms. The average adult dose for amelioration of allergic reactions to blood or plasma is 25 mg.

SEDATION

In hospitalized adult patients, nighttime sedation may be achieved by a dose of 25 to 50 mg of promethazine hydrochloride.

PRE- AND POSTOPERATIVE USE

As an adjunct to pre- or postoperative medication, 25 to 50 mg of promethazine hydrochloride in adults may be combined with appropriately reduced doses of analgesics and atropinelike drugs as desired. Dosage of concomitant analgesic or hypnotic medication should be reduced accordingly.

NAUSEA AND VOMITING

For control of nausea and vomiting, the usual adult dose is 12.5 to 25 mg, not to be repeated more frequently than every four hours. When used for control of postoperative nausea and vomiting, the medication may be administered either intramuscularly or intravenously and dosage of analgesics and barbiturates reduced accordingly.

OBSTETRICS

Phenergan in doses of 50 mg will provide sedation and relieve apprehension in the early stages of labor. When labor is definitely established, 25 to 75 mg (average dose, 50 mg) promethazine hydrochloride may be given intramuscularly or intravenously with an appropriately reduced dose of any desired narcotic. Amnesic agents may be administered as necessary. If necessary, Phenergan with a reduced dose of analgesic may be repeated once or twice at four-hour intervals in the course of a normal labor. A maximum total dose of 100 mg of Phenergan may be administered during a 24-hour period to patients in labor.

CHILDREN

In children under the age of 12 years, the dosage should not exceed half that of the suggested adult dose. As an adjunct to premedication, the suggested dose is 0.5 mg per lb. of body weight in combination with an equal dose of narcotic or barbiturate and the appropriate dose of an atropinelike drug. Antiemetics should not be used in vomiting of unknown etiology in children.

Parenteral drug products should be inspected visually for particulate matter and discoloration prior to administration, whenever solution and container permit.

MANAGEMENT OF OVERDOSAGE

Signs and symptoms of overdosage range from mild depression of the central nervous system and cardiovascular system to profound hypotension, respiratory depression, and unconsciousness. Stimulation may be evident, especially in

children and geriatric patients. Atropinelike signs and symptoms—dry mouth, fixed, dilated pupils, flushing, etc., as well as gastrointestinal symptoms, may occur. The treatment of overdosage is essentially symptomatic and supportive. Early gastric lavage may be beneficial if promethazine has been taken orally. Centrally acting emetics are of little use.

Avoid analeptics, which may cause convulsions. Severe hypotension usually responds to the administration of levarterenol or phenylephrine. EPINEPHRINE SHOULD NOT BE USED, since its use in a patient with partial adrenergic blockade may further lower the blood pressure. Extrapyramidal reactions may be treated with anticholinergic antiparkinson agents, diphenhydramine, or barbiturates. Additional measures include oxygen and intravenous fluids. Limited experience with dialysis indicates that it is not helpful.

HOW SUPPLIED

Phenergan® (promethazine HCl) Injection, is available in packages of 25 ampules of 1 mL as follows:
25 mg per mL, NDC 0008-0063.
50 mg per mL, NDC 0008-0746.

Store at Room Temperature between 15°C-25°C (59°F-77°F). Protect from light.

Do not use if soluton is discolored or contains a precipitate.

ALSO AVAILABLE

Phenergan® (promethazine HCl) Injection, Wyeth®, is also available in TUBEX® Sterile Cartridge-Needle Units, (22 gauge × 1¼ inch needle) in packages of 10 TUBEX (1 mL size), as follows:
25 mg per mL, NDC 0008-0416.
50 mg per mL, NDC 0008-0417.

Store at Room Temperature, between 15°C-25°C (59°F-77°F). Protect from light.

PHENERGAN® ℞

[fen 'er-gan]
(promethazine hydrochloride)
Syrup Plain and

PHENERGAN® ℞

(promethazine hydrochloride)
Syrup Fortis

DESCRIPTION

Each teaspoon (5 mL) of Phenergan Syrup Plain contains 6.25 mg promethazine hydrochloride in a flavored syrup base with a pH between 4.7 and 5.2. Alcohol 7%. The inactive ingredients present are artificial and natural flavors, citric acid, D&C Red 33, D&C Yellow 10, FD&C Blue 1, FD&C Yellow 6, glycerin, saccharin sodium, sodium benzoate, sodium citrate, sodium propionate, water, and other ingredients.

Each teaspoon (5 mL) of Phenergan Syrup Fortis contains 25 mg promethazine hydrochloride in a flavored syrup base with a pH between 5.0 and 5.5. Alcohol 1.5%. The inactive ingredients present are artificial and natural flavors, citric acid, saccharin sodium, sodium benzoate, sodium propionate, water, and other ingredients.

Promethazine hydrochloride is a racemic compound; the empirical formula is $C_{17}H_{20}N_2S \cdot HCl$ and its molecular weight is 320.88.

Promethazine hydrochloride, a phenothiazine derivative, is designated chemically as N,N,α-trimethyl-10*H*-phenothiazine-10-ethanamine monohydrochloride with the following structural formula:

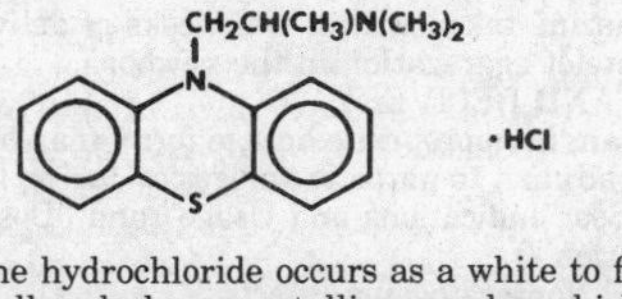
CH2CH(CH3)N(CH3)2
N
S
•HCl

Promethazine hydrochloride occurs as a white to faint yellow, practically odorless, crystalline powder which slowly oxidizes and turns blue on prolonged exposure to air. It is soluble in water and freely soluble in alcohol.

CLINICAL PHARMACOLOGY

Promethazine is a phenothiazine derivative which differs structurally from the antipsychotic phenothiazines by the presence of a branched side chain and no ring substitution. It is thought that this configuration is responsible for its relative lack (1/10 that of chlorpromazine) of dopaminergic (CNS) action.

Promethazine is an H_1 receptor blocking agent. In addition to its antihistaminic action, it provides clinically useful sedative and antiemetic effects. In therapeutic dosage, promethazine produces no significant effects on the cardiovascular system.

Promethazine is well absorbed from the gastrointestinal tract. Clinical effects are apparent within 20 minutes after oral administration and generally last four to six hours, although they may persist as long as 12 hours. Promethazine is metabolized by the liver to a variety of compounds; the sulfoxides of promethazine and N-demethylpromethazine are the predominant metabolites appearing in the urine.

INDICATIONS AND USAGE

Phenergan is useful for:
Perennial and seasonal allergic rhinitis.
Vasomotor rhinitis.
Allergic conjunctivitis due to inhalant allergens and foods.
Mild, uncomplicated allergic skin manifestations of urticaria and angioedema.
Amelioration of allergic reactions to blood or plasma.
Dermographism.
Anaphylactic reactions, as adjunctive therapy to epinephrine and other standard measures, after the acute manifestations have been controlled.
Preoperative, postoperative, or obstetric sedation.
Prevention and control of nausea and vomiting associated with certain types of anesthesia and surgery.
Therapy adjunctive to meperidine or other analgesics for control of postoperative pain.
Sedation in both children and adults, as well as relief of apprehension and production of light sleep from which the patient can be easily aroused.
Active and prophylactic treatment of motion sickness.
Antiemetic therapy in postoperative patients.

CONTRAINDICATIONS

Promethazine is contraindicated in individuals known to be hypersensitive or to have had an idiosyncratic reaction to promethazine or to other phenothiazines.

Antihistamines are contraindicated for use in the treatment of lower respiratory tract symptoms including asthma.

WARNINGS

Promethazine may cause marked drowsiness. Ambulatory patients should be cautioned against such activities as driving or operating dangerous machinery until it is known that they do not become drowsy or dizzy from promethazine therapy.

The sedative action of promethazine hydrochloride is additive to the sedative effects of central nervous system depressants; therefore, agents such as alcohol, narcotic analgesics, sedatives, hypnotics, and tranquilizers should either be eliminated or given in reduced dosage in the presence of promethazine hydrochloride. When given concomitantly with promethazine hydrochloride, the dose of barbiturates should be reduced by at least one-half, and the dose of analgesic depressants, such as morphine or meperidine, should be reduced by one-quarter to one-half.

Promethazine may lower seizure threshold. This should be taken into consideration when administering to persons with known seizure disorders or when giving in combination with narcotics or local anesthetics which may also affect seizure threshold.

Sedative drugs or CNS depressants should be avoided in patients with a history of sleep apnea.

Antihistamines should be used with caution in patients with narrow-angle glaucoma, stenosing peptic ulcer, pyloroduodenal obstruction, and urinary bladder obstruction due to symptomatic prostatic hypertrophy and narrowing of the bladder neck.

Administration of promethazine has been associated with reported cholestatic jaundice.

PRECAUTIONS

GENERAL

Promethazine should be used cautiously in persons with cardiovascular disease or with impairment of liver function.

INFORMATION FOR PATIENTS

Phenergan may cause marked drowsiness or impair the mental and/or physical abilities required for the performance of potentially hazardous tasks, such as driving a vehicle or operating machinery. Ambulatory patients should be told to avoid engaging in such activities until it is known that they do not become drowsy or dizzy from Phenergan therapy. Children should be supervised to avoid potential harm in bike riding or in other hazardous activities.

The concomitant use of alcohol or other central nervous system depressants, including narcotic analgesics, sedatives, hypnotics, and tranquilizers, may have an additive effect and should be avoided or their dosage reduced.

Patients should be advised to report any involuntary muscle movements or unusual sensitivity to sunlight.

DRUG INTERACTIONS

The sedative action of promethazine is additive to the sedative effects of other central nervous system depressants, including alcohol, narcotic analgesics, sedatives, hypnotics, tricyclic antidepressants, and tranquilizers; therefore, these agents should be avoided or administered in reduced dosage to patients receiving promethazine.

DRUG/LABORATORY TEST INTERACTIONS

The following laboratory tests may be affected in patients who are receiving therapy with promethazine hydrochloride:

Pregnancy Tests

Diagnostic pregnancy tests based on immunological reactions between HCG and anti-HCG may result in false-negative or false-positive interpretations.

Glucose Tolerance Test

An increase in blood glucose has been reported in patients receiving promethazine.

CARCINOGENESIS, MUTAGENESIS, IMPAIRMENT OF FERTILITY

Long-term animal studies have not been performed to assess the carcinogenic potential of promethazine, nor are there other animal or human data concerning carcinogenicity, mutagenicity, or impairment of fertility with this drug. Promethazine was nonmutagenic in the *Salmonella* test system of Ames.

PREGNANCY

Teratogenic Effects —Pregnancy Category C

Teratogenic effects have not been demonstrated in rat-feeding studies at doses of 6.25 and 12.5 mg/kg of promethazine. These doses are from approximately 2.1 to 4.2 times the maximum recommended total daily dose of promethazine for a 50-kg subject, depending upon the indication for which the drug is prescribed. Specific studies to test the action of the drug on parturition, lactation, and development of the animal neonate were not done, but a general preliminary study in rats indicated no effect on these parameters. Although antihistamines, including promethazine, have been found to produce fetal mortality in rodents, the pharmacological effects of histamine in the rodent do not parallel those in man. There are no adequate and well-controlled studies of promethazine in pregnant women. Phenergan should be used during pregnancy only if the potential benefit justifies the potential risk to the fetus.

Nonteratogenic Effects

Promethazine taken within two weeks of delivery may inhibit platelet aggregation in the newborn.

LABOR AND DELIVERY

Phenergan, in appropriate dosage form, may be used alone or as an adjunct to narcotic analgesics during labor and delivery. (See "Indications and Usage" and "Dosage and Administration.")

See also "Nonteratogenic Effects."

NURSING MOTHERS

It is not known whether promethazine is excreted in human milk. Caution should be exercised when promethazine is administered to a nursing woman.

PEDIATRIC USE

This product should not be used in children under 2 years of age because safety for such use has not been established.

ADVERSE REACTIONS

Nervous System —Sedation, sleepiness, occasional blurred vision, dryness of mouth, dizziness; rarely confusion, disorientation, and extrapyramidal symptoms such as oculogyric crisis, torticollis, and tongue protrusion (usually in association with parenteral injection or excessive dosage).
Cardiovascular —Increased or decreased blood pressure.
Dermatologic —Rash, rarely photosensitivity.
Hematologic —Rarely leukopenia, thrombocytopenia; agranulocytosis (1 case).
Gastrointestinal —Nausea and vomiting.

OVERDOSAGE

Signs and symptoms of overdosage with promethazine range from mild depression of the central nervous system and cardiovascular system to profound hypotension, respiratory depression, and unconsciousness.

Stimulation may be evident, especially in children and geriatric patients. Convulsions may rarely occur. A paradoxical reaction has been reported in children receiving single doses of 75 mg to 125 mg orally, characterized by hyperexcitability and nightmares.

Atropinelike signs and symptoms—dry mouth, fixed, dilated pupils, flushing, as well as gastrointestinal symptoms, may occur.

TREATMENT

Treatment of overdosage is essentially symptomatic and supportive. Only in cases of extreme overdosage or individual sensitivity do vital signs including respiration, pulse, blood pressure, temperature, and EKG need to be monitored. Activated charcoal orally or by lavage may be given, or sodium or magnesium sulfate orally as a cathartic. Attention should be given to the reestablishment of adequate respiratory exchange through provision of a patent airway and institution of assisted or controlled ventilation. Diazepam may be used to control convulsions. Acidosis and electrolyte losses should be corrected. Note that any depressant effects of promethazine are not reversed by naloxone. Avoid analeptics which may cause convulsions.

Severe hypotension usually responds to the administration of norepinephrine or phenylephrine. EPINEPHRINE SHOULD NOT BE USED, since its use in patients with partial adrenergic blockade may further lower the blood pressure.

Limited experience with dialysis indicates that it is not helpful.

Continued on next page

Wyeth-Ayerst Laboratories—Cont.

DOSAGE AND ADMINISTRATION
ALLERGY
The average oral dose is 25 mg taken before retiring; however, 12.5 mg may be taken before meals and on retiring, if necessary. Children tolerate this product well. Single 25-mg doses at bedtime or 6.25 to 12.5 mg taken three times daily will usually suffice. After initiation of treatment in children or adults, dosage should be adjusted to the smallest amount adequate to relieve symptoms.

Phenergan Rectal Suppositories may be used if the oral route is not feasible, but oral therapy should be resumed as soon as possible if continued therapy is indicated.

The administration of promethazine hydrochloride in 25-mg doses will control minor transfusion reactions of an allergic nature.

MOTION SICKNESS
The average adult dose is 25 mg taken twice daily. The initial dose should be taken one-half to one hour before anticipated travel and be repeated 8 to 12 hours later, if necessary. On succeeding days of travel, it is recommended that 25 mg be given on arising and again before the evening meal. For children, Phenergan Tablets, Syrup, or Rectal Suppositories, 12.5 to 25 mg, twice daily, may be administered.

NAUSEA AND VOMITING
The average effective dose of Phenergan for the active therapy of nausea and vomiting in children or adults is 25 mg. When oral medication cannot be tolerated, the dose should be given parenterally (cf. Phenergan Injection) or by rectal suppository. 12.5- to 25-mg doses may be repeated, as necessary, at 4- to 6-hour intervals.

For nausea and vomiting in children, the usual dose is 0.5 mg per pound of body weight, and the dose should be adjusted to the age and weight of the patient and the severity of the condition being treated.

For prophylaxis of nausea and vomiting, as during surgery and the postoperative period, the average dose is 25 mg repeated at 4- to 6-hour intervals, as necessary.

SEDATION
This product relieves apprehension and induces a quiet sleep from which the patient can be easily aroused. Administration of 12.5 to 25 mg Phenergan by the oral route or by rectal suppository at bedtime will provide sedation in children. Adults usually require 25 to 50 mg for nighttime, presurgical, or obstetrical sedation.

PRE- AND POSTOPERATIVE USE
Phenergan in 12.5- to 25-mg doses for children and 50-mg doses for adults the night before surgery relieves apprehension and produces a quiet sleep.

For preoperative medication children require doses of 0.5 mg per pound of body weight in combination with an equal dose of meperidine and the appropriate dose of an atropinelike drug.

Usual adult dosage is 50 mg Phenergan with an equal amount of meperidine and the required amount of a belladonna alkaloid.

Postoperative sedation and adjunctive use with analgesics may be obtained by the administration of 12.5 to 25 mg in children and 25- to 50-mg doses in adults.

Phenergan Syrup Plain and Phenergan Syrup Fortis are not recommended for children under 2 years of age.

HOW SUPPLIED
Phenergan® (Promethazine Hydrochloride) Syrup Plain is a clear, green solution supplied as follows:
NDC 0008-0549-02, case of 24 bottles of 4 fl. oz. (118 mL).
NDC 0008-0549-03, bottle of 1 pint (473 mL).
Phenergan® (Promethazine Hydrochloride) Syrup Fortis is a clear, light straw-colored solution supplied as follows:
NDC 0008-0231-01, bottle of 1 pint (473 mL).
Keep bottles tightly closed.
Store at Room Temperature, between 15° C and 25° C (59° F and 77° F).
Protect from light.
Dispense in light-resistant, glass, tight containers.

PHENERGAN®   ℞
[fen´er-gan]
(promethazine HCl)
TABLETS •
SUPPOSITORIES

DESCRIPTION
Each tablet of Phenergan contains 12.5 mg, 25 mg, or 50 mg promethazine hydrochloride. The inactive ingredients present are lactose, magnesium stearate, and methylcellulose. Each dosage strength also contains the following:

12.5 mg—FD&C Yellow 6 and saccharin sodium;
25 mg—saccharin sodium;
50 mg—FD&C Red 40.
Each rectal suppository of Phenergan contains 12.5 mg, 25 mg, or 50 mg promethazine hydrochloride with ascorbyl palmitate, silicon dioxide, white wax, and cocoa butter.
Promethazine hydrochloride is a racemic compound; the empirical formula is $C_{17}H_{20}N_2S\cdot HCl$ and its molecular weight is 320.88.
Promethazine hydrochloride, a phenothiazine derivative, is designated chemically as N,N,α-trimethyl-10H-phenothiazine-10-ethanamine monohydrochloride.
Promethazine hydrochloride occurs as a white to faint yellow, practically odorless, crystalline powder which slowly oxidizes and turns blue on prolonged exposure to air. It is soluble in water and freely soluble in alcohol.

CLINICAL PHARMACOLOGY
Promethazine is a phenothiazine derivative which differs structurally from the antipsychotic phenothiazines by the presence of a branched side chain and no ring substitution. It is thought that this configuration is responsible for its relative lack ($\frac{1}{10}$ that of chlorpromazine) of dopaminergic (CNS) action.
Promethazine is an H_1 receptor blocking agent. In addition to its antihistaminic action, it provides clinically useful sedative and antiemetic effects. In therapeutic dosage, promethazine produces no significant effects on the cardiovascular system.
Promethazine is well absorbed from the gastrointestinal tract. Clinical effects are apparent within 20 minutes after oral administration and generally last four to six hours, although they may persist as long as 12 hours. Promethazine is metabolized by the liver to a variety of compounds; the sulfoxides of promethazine and N-demethylpromethazine are the predominant metabolites appearing in the urine.

INDICATIONS AND USAGE
Phenergan, either orally or by suppository, is useful for:
Perennial and seasonal allergic rhinitis.
Vasomotor rhinitis.
Allergic conjunctivitis due to inhalant allergens and foods.
Mild, uncomplicated allergic skin manifestations of urticaria and angioedema.
Amelioration of allergic reactions to blood or plasma.
Dermographism.
Anaphylactic reactions, as adjunctive therapy to epinephrine and other standard measures, after the acute manifestations have been controlled.
Preoperative, postoperative, or obstetric sedation.
Prevention and control of nausea and vomiting associated with certain types of anesthesia and surgery.
Therapy adjunctive to meperidine or other analgesics for control of postoperative pain.
Sedation in both children and adults, as well as relief of apprehension and production of light sleep from which the patient can be easily aroused.
Active and prophylactic treatment of motion sickness.
Antiemetic therapy in postoperative patients.

CONTRAINDICATIONS
Promethazine is contraindicated in individuals known to be hypersensitive or to have had an idiosyncratic reaction to promethazine or to other phenothiazines.
Antihistamines are contraindicated for use in the treatment of lower respiratory tract symptoms including asthma.

WARNINGS
Promethazine may cause marked drowsiness. Ambulatory patients should be cautioned against such activities as driving or operating dangerous machinery until it is known that they do not become drowsy or dizzy from promethazine therapy.
The sedative action of promethazine hydrochloride is additive to the sedative effects of central nervous system depressants; therefore, agents such as alcohol, narcotic analgesics, sedatives, hypnotics, and tranquilizers should either be eliminated or given in reduced dosage in the presence of promethazine hydrochloride. When given concomitantly with promethazine hydrochloride, the dose of barbiturates should be reduced by at least one-half, and the dose of analgesic depressants, such as morphine or meperidine, should be reduced by one-quarter to one-half.
Promethazine may lower seizure threshold. This should be taken into consideration when administering to persons with known seizure disorders or when giving in combination with narcotics and local anesthetics which may also affect seizure threshold.
Sedative drugs or CNS depressants should be avoided in patients with a history of sleep apnea.
Antihistamines should be used with caution in patients with narrow-angle glaucoma, stenosing peptic ulcer, pyloroduodenal obstruction, and urinary bladder obstruction due to symptomatic prostatic hypertrophy and narrowing of the bladder neck.
Administration of promethazine has been associated with reported cholestatic jaundice.

PRECAUTIONS
GENERAL
Promethazine should be used cautiously in persons with cardiovascular disease or with impairment of liver function.
INFORMATION FOR PATIENTS
Phenergan may cause marked drowsiness or impair the mental and/or physical abilities required for the performance of potentially hazardous tasks, such as driving a vehicle or operating machinery. Ambulatory patients should be told to avoid engaging in such activities until it is known that they do not become drowsy or dizzy from Phenergan therapy. Children should be supervised to avoid potential harm in bike riding or in other hazardous activities.
The concomitant use of alcohol or other central nervous system depressants, including narcotic analgesics, sedatives, hypnotics, and tranquilizers, may have an additive effect and should be avoided or their dosage reduced.
Patients should be advised to report any involuntary muscle movements or unusual sensitivity to sunlight.
DRUG INTERACTIONS
The sedative action of promethazine is additive to the sedative effects of other central nervous system depressants, including alcohol, narcotic analgesics, sedatives, hypnotics, tricyclic antidepressants, and tranquilizers; therefore, these agents should be avoided or administered in reduced dosage to patients receiving promethazine.
DRUG/LABORATORY TEST INTERACTIONS
The following laboratory tests may be affected in patients who are receiving therapy with promethazine hydrochloride:
Pregnancy Tests
Diagnostic pregnancy tests based on immunological reactions between HCG and anti-HCG may result in false-negative or false-positive interpretations.
Glucose Tolerance Test
An increase in blood glucose has been reported in patients receiving promethazine.
CARCINOGENESIS, MUTAGENESIS, IMPAIRMENT OF FERTILITY
Long-term animal studies have not been performed to assess the carcinogenic potential of promethazine, nor are there other animal or human data concerning carcinogenicity, mutagenicity, or impairment of fertility with this drug. Promethazine was nonmutagenic in the *Salmonella* test system of Ames.
PREGNANCY
Teratogenic Effects—Pregnancy Category C
Teratogenic effects have not been demonstrated in rat-feeding studies at doses of 6.25 and 12.5 mg/kg of promethazine. These doses are from approximately 2.1 to 4.2 times the maximum recommended total daily dose of promethazine for a 50-kg subject, depending upon the indication for which the drug is prescribed. Specific studies to test the action of the drug on parturition, lactation, and development of the animal neonate were not done, but a general preliminary study in rats indicated no effect on these parameters. Although antihistamines, including promethazine, have been found to produce fetal mortality in rodents, the pharmacological effects of histamine in the rodent do not parallel those in man. There are no adequate and well-controlled studies of promethazine in pregnant women. Phenergan should be used during pregnancy only if the potential benefit justifies the potential risk to the fetus.
Nonteratogenic Effects
Promethazine taken within two weeks of delivery may inhibit platelet aggregation in the newborn.
LABOR AND DELIVERY
Phenergan, in appropriate dosage form, may be used alone or as an adjunct to narcotic analgesics during labor and delivery. (See "Indications and Usage" and "Dosage and Administration.")
See also "Nonteratogenic Effects."
NURSING MOTHERS
It is not known whether promethazine is excreted in human milk. Caution should be exercised when promethazine is administered to a nursing woman.
PEDIATRIC USE
This product should not be used in children under 2 years of age because safety for such use has not been established.

ADVERSE REACTIONS
Nervous System —Sedation, sleepiness, occasional blurred vision, dryness of mouth, dizziness; rarely confusion, disorientation, and extrapyramidal symptoms such as oculogyric crisis, torticollis, and tongue protrusion (usually in association with parenteral injection or excessive dosage).
Cardiovascular —Increased or decreased blood pressure.
Dermatologic —Rash, rarely photosensitivity.
Hematologic —Rarely leukopenia, thrombocytopenia; agranulocytosis (1 case).
Gastrointestinal —Nausea and vomiting.

OVERDOSAGE
Signs and symptoms of overdosage with promethazine range from mild depression of the central nervous system and car-

diovascular system to profound hypotension, respiratory depression, and unconsciousness.

Stimulation may be evident, especially in children and geriatric patients. Convulsions may rarely occur. A paradoxical reaction has been reported in children receiving single doses of 75 mg to 125 mg orally, characterized by hyperexcitability and nightmares.

Atropinelike signs and symptoms—dry mouth, fixed, dilated pupils, flushing, as well as gastrointestinal symptoms, may occur.

TREATMENT

Treatment of overdosage is essentially symptomatic and supportive. Only in cases of extreme overdosage or individual sensitivity do vital signs, including respiration, pulse, blood pressure, temperature, and EKG, need to be monitored. Activated charcoal orally or by lavage may be given, or sodium or magnesium sulfate orally as a cathartic. Attention should be given to the reestablishment of adequate respiratory exchange through provision of a patent airway and institution of assisted or controlled ventilation. Diazepam may be used to control convulsions. Acidosis and electrolyte losses should be corrected. Note that any depressant effects of promethazine are not reversed by naloxone. Avoid analeptics which may cause convulsions.

Severe hypotension usually responds to the administration of norepinephrine or phenylephrine. EPINEPHRINE SHOULD NOT BE USED, since its use in patients with partial adrenergic blockade may further lower the blood pressure.

Limited experience with dialysis indicates that it is not helpful.

DOSAGE AND ADMINISTRATION

Allergy: The average oral dose is 25 mg taken before retiring; however, 12.5 mg may be taken before meals and on retiring, if necessary. Children tolerate this product well. Single 25-mg doses at bedtime or 6.25 to 12.5 mg taken three times daily will usually suffice. After initiation of treatment in children or adults, dosage should be adjusted to the smallest amount adequate to relieve symptoms. The administration of promethazine hydrochloride in 25-mg doses will control minor transfusion reactions of an allergic nature.

Motion Sickness: The average adult dose is 25 mg taken twice daily. The initial dose should be taken one-half to one hour before anticipated travel and be repeated 8 to 12 hours later, if necessary. On succeeding days of travel, it is recommended that 25 mg be given on arising and again before the evening meal. For children, Phenergan Tablets, Syrup, or Rectal Suppositories, 12.5 to 25 mg, twice daily, may be administered.

Nausea and Vomiting: The average effective dose of Phenergan for the active therapy of nausea and vomiting in children or adults is 25 mg. When oral medication cannot be tolerated, the dose should be given parenterally (cf. Phenergan Injection) or by rectal suppository. 12.5- to 25-mg doses may be repeated as necessary at 4- to 6-hour intervals.

For nausea and vomiting in children, the usual dose is 0.5 mg per pound of body weight, and the dose should be adjusted to the age and weight of the patient and the severity of the condition being treated.

For prophylaxis of nausea and vomiting, as during surgery and the postoperative period, the average dose is 25 mg repeated at 4- to 6-hour intervals, as necessary.

Sedation: This product relieves apprehension and induces a quiet sleep from which the patient can be easily aroused. Administration of 12.5 to 25 mg Phenergan by the oral route or by rectal suppository at bedtime will provide sedation in children. Adults usually require 25 to 50 mg for nighttime, presurgical, or obstetrical sedation.

Pre- and Postoperative Use: Phenergan in 12.5- to 25-mg doses for children and 50-mg doses for adults the night before surgery relieves apprehension and produces a quiet sleep.

For preoperative medication children require doses of 0.5 mg per pound of body weight in combination with an equal dose of meperidine and the appropriate dose of an atropinelike drug.

Usual adult dosage is 50 mg Phenergan with an equal amount of meperidine and the required amount of a belladonna alkaloid.

Postoperative sedation and adjunctive use with analgesics may be obtained by the administration of 12.5 to 25 mg in children and 25- to 50-mg doses in adults.

Phenergan tablets and Phenergan suppositories are not recommended for children under 2 years of age.

HOW SUPPLIED

Phenergan® (promethazine HCl) Tablets are available as follows:

12.5 mg, orange tablet with "WYETH" on one side and "19" on the scored reverse side.

NDC 0008-0019-01, bottle of 100 tablets.

25 mg, white tablet with "WYETH" and "27" on one side and scored on the reverse side.

NDC 0008-0027-02, bottle of 100 tablets.

NDC 0008-0027-07, Redipak® carton of 100 tablets (10 blister strips of 10).

50 mg, pink tablet with "WYETH" on one side and "227" on the other side.

NDC 0008-0227-01, bottle of 100 tablets.

Keep tablets in tightly closed bottles.

Store at Room Temperature, between 15°C and 25°C (59°F and 77°F).

Protect from light.

Dispense in light-resistant, tight container.

Phenergan® (promethazine HCl) Suppositories are available in boxes of 12 as follows:

12.5 mg, ivory, cone-shaped suppository wrapped in copper-colored foil, NDC 0008-0498-01.

25 mg, ivory, cone-shaped suppository wrapped in light-green foil, NDC 0008-0212-01.

50 mg, ivory, torpedo-shaped suppository wrapped in light-green foil, NDC 0008-0229-01.

Store refrigerated 2°–8°C (36°–46°F).

Dispense in well-closed container.

Shown in Product Identification Section, page 437

PHENERGAN® ℭ ℞

[fen 'er-gan]

with codeine

(Promethazine Hydrochloride and Codeine Phosphate) Syrup

DESCRIPTION

Each teaspoon (5 mL) of Phenergan with codeine contains 10 mg (1/6 grain) codeine phosphate (Warning—may be habit-forming) and 6.25 mg promethazine hydrochloride in a flavored syrup base with a pH between 4.7 and 5.2. Alcohol 7%. The inactive ingredients present are artificial and natural flavors, citric acid, D&C Red 33, FD&C Blue 1, FD&C Yellow 6, glycerine, saccharin sodium, sodium benzoate, sodium citrate, sodium propionate, water, and other ingredients.

Codeine is one of the naturally occurring phenanthrene alkaloids of opium derived from the opium poppy; it is classified pharmacologically as a narcotic analgesic. Codeine phosphate may be chemically named as (5α,6α)-7, 8-didehydro-4, 5-epoxy-3-methoxy-17-methylmorphinan-6-ol phosphate (1:1) (salt) hemihydrate with the following structural formula:

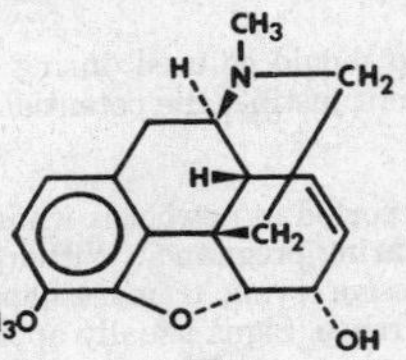

• H_3PO_4 • $\frac{1}{2}H_2O$

The phosphate salt of codeine occurs as white, needle-shaped crystals or white crystalline powder. Codeine phosphate is freely soluble in water and slightly soluble in alcohol, with a molecular weight of 406.37. The empirical formula is $C_{18}H_{21}NO_3 \cdot H_3PO_4 \cdot \frac{1}{2}H_2O$, and the stereochemistry is 5α, 6α isomer as indicated in the structure.

Promethazine hydrochloride is a racemic compound; the empirical formula is $C_{17}H_{20}N_2S \cdot HCl$ and its molecular weight is 320.88.

Promethazine hydrochloride, a phenothiazine derivative, is designated chemically as N,N,α-trimethyl-10*H*-phenothiazine-10-ethanamine monohydrochloride with the following structural formula:

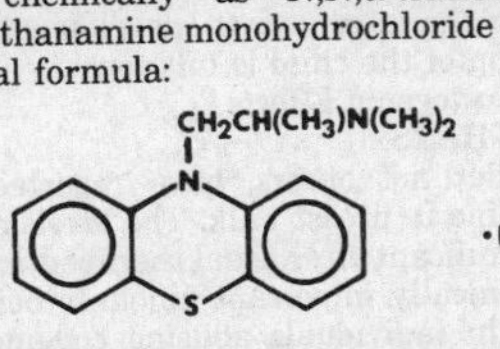

• HCl

Promethazine hydrochloride occurs as a white to faint yellow, practically odorless, crystalline powder which slowly oxidizes and turns blue on prolonged exposure to air. It is soluble in water and freely soluble in alcohol.

CLINICAL PHARMACOLOGY

CODEINE

Narcotic analgesics, including codeine, exert their primary effects on the central nervous system and gastrointestinal tract. The analgesic effects of codeine are due to its central action; however, the precise sites of action have not been determined, and the mechanisms involved appear to be quite complex. Codeine resembles morphine both structurally and pharmacologically, but its actions at the doses of codeine used therapeutically are milder, with less sedation, respiratory depression, and gastrointestinal, urinary, and pupillary effects. Codeine produces an increase in biliary tract pressure, but less than morphine or meperidine. Codeine is less constipating than morphine.

Codeine has good antitussive activity, although less than that of morphine at equal doses. It is used in preference to morphine, because side effects are infrequent at the usual antitussive dose of codeine.

Codeine in oral therapeutic dosage does not usually exert major effects on the cardiovascular system.

Narcotic analgesics may cause nausea and vomiting by stimulating the chemoreceptor trigger zone (CTZ); however, they also depress the vomiting center, so that subsequent doses are unlikely to produce vomiting. Nausea is minimal after usual oral doses of codeine.

Narcotic analgesics cause histamine release, which appears to be responsible for wheals or urticaria sometimes seen at the site of injection on parenteral administration. Histamine release may also produce dilation of cutaneous blood vessels, with resultant flushing of the face and neck, pruritus, and sweating.

Codeine and its salts are well absorbed following both oral and parenteral administration. Codeine is about 2/3 as effective orally as parenterally. Codeine is metabolized primarily in the liver by enzymes of the endoplasmic reticulum, where it undergoes O-demethylation, N-demethylation, and partial conjugation with glucuronic acid. The drug is excreted primarily in the urine, largely as inactive metabolites and small amounts of free and conjugated morphine. Negligible amounts of codeine and its metabolites are found in the feces.

Following oral or subcutaneous administration of codeine, the onset of analgesia occurs within 15 to 30 minutes and lasts for four to six hours.

The cough-depressing action, in animal studies, was observed to occur 15 minutes after oral administration of codeine, peak action at 45 to 60 minutes after ingestion. The duration of action, which is dose-dependent, usually did not exceed 3 hours.

PROMETHAZINE

Promethazine is a phenothiazine derivative which differs structurally from the antipsychotic phenothiazines by the presence of a branched side chain and no ring substitution. It is thought that this configuration is responsible for its lack (1/10 that of chlorpromazine) of dopaminergic (CNS) action.

Promethazine is an H_1 receptor blocking agent. In addition to its antihistaminic action, it provides clinically useful sedative and antiemetic effects. In therapeutic dosages, promethazine produces no significant effects on the cardiovascular system.

Promethazine is well absorbed from the gastrointestinal tract. Clinical effects are apparent within 20 minutes after oral administration and generally last four to six hours, although they may persist as long as 12 hours. Promethazine is metabolized by the liver to a variety of compounds; the sulfoxides of promethazine and N-demethylpromethazine are the predominant metabolites appearing in the urine.

INDICATIONS AND USAGE

Phenergan with codeine is indicated for the temporary relief of coughs and upper respiratory symptoms associated with allergy or the common cold.

CONTRAINDICATIONS

Codeine is contraindicated in patients with a known hypersensitivity to the drug.

Promethazine is contraindicated in individuals known to be hypersensitive or to have had an idiosyncratic reaction to promethazine or to other phenothiazines.

Antihistamines and codeine are both contraindicated for use in the treatment of lower respiratory tract symptoms, including asthma.

WARNINGS

CODEINE

Dosage of codeine SHOULD NOT BE INCREASED if cough fails to respond; an unresponsive cough should be reevaluated in 5 days or sooner for possible underlying pathology, such as foreign body or lower respiratory tract disease.

Codeine may cause or aggravate constipation.

Respiratory depression leading to arrest, coma, and death has occurred with the use of codeine antitussives in young children, particularly in the under-one-year infants whose ability to deactivate the drug is not fully developed.

Administration of codeine may be accompanied by histamine release and should be used with caution in atopic children.

Head Injury and Increased Intracranial Pressure

The respiratory-depressant effects of narcotic analgesics and their capacity to elevate cerebrospinal fluid pressure may be markedly exaggerated in the presence of head injury, intracranial lesions, or a preexisting increase in intracranial pressure. Narcotics may produce adverse reactions which may obscure the clinical course of patients with head injuries.

Asthma and Other Respiratory Conditions

Narcotic analgesics or cough suppressants, including codeine, should not be used in asthmatic patients (see "Contraindications"). Nor should they be used in acute febrile illness associated with productive cough or in chronic respiratory disease where interference with ability to clear the tracheobronchial tree of secretions would have a deleterious effect on the patient's respiratory function.

Continued on next page

Wyeth-Ayerst Laboratories—Cont.

Hypotensive Effect

Codeine may produce orthostatic hypotension in ambulatory patients.

PROMETHAZINE

Promethazine may cause marked drowsiness. Ambulatory patients should be cautioned against such activities as driving or operating dangerous machinery until it is known that they do not become drowsy or dizzy from promethazine therapy.

The sedative action of promethazine hydrochloride is additive to the sedative effects of central nervous system depressants; therefore, agents such as alcohol, narcotic analgesics, sedatives, hypnotics, and tranquilizers should either be eliminated or given in reduced dosage in the presence of promethazine hydrochloride. When given concomitantly with promethazine hydrochloride, the dose of barbiturates should be reduced by at least one-half, and the dose of analgesic depressants, such as morphine or meperidine, should be reduced by one-quarter to one-half.

Promethazine may lower seizure threshold. This should be taken into consideration when administering to persons with known seizure disorders or when giving in combination with narcotics or local anesthetics which may also affect seizure threshold.

Sedative drugs or CNS depressants should be avoided in patients with a history of sleep apnea.

Antihistamines should be used with caution in patients with narrow-angle glaucoma, stenosing peptic ulcer, pyloroduodenal obstruction, and urinary bladder obstruction due to symptomatic prostatic hypertrophy and narrowing of the bladder neck.

Administration of promethazine has been associated with reported cholestatic jaundice.

PRECAUTIONS

Animal reproduction studies have not been conducted with the drug combination—promethazine and codeine. It is not known whether this drug combination can cause fetal harm when administered to a pregnant woman or can affect reproduction capacity. Phenergan with codeine should be given to a pregnant woman only if clearly needed.

GENERAL

Narcotic analgesics, including codeine, should be administered with caution and the initial dose reduced in patients with acute abdominal conditions, convulsive disorders, significant hepatic or renal impairment, fever, hypothyroidism, Addison's disease, ulcerative colitis, prostatic hypertrophy, in patients with recent gastrointestinal or urinary tract surgery, and in the very young or elderly or debilitated patients. Promethazine should be used cautiously in persons with cardiovascular disease or with impairment of liver function.

INFORMATION FOR PATIENTS

Phenergan with codeine may cause marked drowsiness or may impair the mental and/or physical abilities required for the performance of potentially hazardous tasks, such as driving a vehicle or operating machinery. Ambulatory patients should be told to avoid engaging in such activities until it is known that they do not become drowsy or dizzy from Phenergan with codeine therapy. Children should be supervised to avoid potential harm in bike riding or in other hazardous activities.

The concomitant use of alcohol or other central nervous system depressants, including narcotic analgesics, sedatives, hypnotics, and tranquilizers, may have an additive effect and should be avoided or their dosage reduced.

Patients should be advised to report any involuntary muscle movements or unusual sensitivity to sunlight.

Codeine, like other narcotic analgesics, may produce orthostatic hypotension in some ambulatory patients. Patients should be cautioned accordingly.

DRUG INTERACTIONS

CODEINE

In patients receiving MAO inhibitors, an initial small test dose is advisable to allow observation of any excessive narcotic effects or MAOI interaction.

PROMETHAZINE

The sedative action of promethazine is additive to the effects of other central nervous system depressants, including alcohol, narcotic analgesics, sedatives, hypnotics, tricyclic antidepressants, and tranquilizers; therefore, these agents should be avoided or administered in reduced dosage to patients receiving promethazine.

DRUG/LABORATORY TEST INTERACTIONS

Because narcotic analgesics may increase biliary tract pressure, with resultant increases in plasma amylase or lipase levels, determination of these enzyme levels may be unreliable for 24 hours after a narcotic analgesic has been given. The following laboratory tests may be affected in patients who are receiving therapy with promethazine hydrochloride:

Pregnancy Tests

Diagnostic pregnancy tests based on immunological reactions between HCG and anti-HCG may result in false-negative or false-positive interpretations.

Glucose Tolerance Test

An increase in blood glucose has been reported in patients receiving promethazine.

CARCINOGENESIS, MUTAGENESIS, IMPAIRMENT OF FERTILITY

Long-term animal studies have not been performed to assess the carcinogenic potential of codeine or of promethazine, nor are there other animal or human data concerning carcinogenicity, mutagenicity, or impairment of fertility with these agents. Codeine has been reported to show no evidence of carcinogenicity or mutagenicity in a variety of test systems, including the micronucleus and sperm abnormality assays and the *Salmonella* assay. Promethazine was nonmutagenic in the *Salmonella* test system of Ames.

PREGNANCY

Teratogenic Effects—Pregnancy Category C

CODEINE

A study in rats and rabbits reported no teratogenic effect of codeine administered during the period of organogenesis in doses ranging from 5 to 120 mg/kg. In the rat, doses at the 120-mg/kg level, in the toxic range for the adult animal, were associated with an increase in embryo resorption at the time of implantation. In another study a single 100-mg/kg dose of codeine administered to pregnant mice reportedly resulted in delayed ossification in the offspring.

There are no studies in humans, and the significance of these findings to humans, if any, is not known.

PROMETHAZINE

Teratogenic effects have not been demonstrated in rat-feeding studies at doses of 6.25 and 12.5 mg/kg of promethazine. These doses are 8.3 and 16.7 times the maximum recommended total daily dose of promethazine for a 50-kg subject. Specific studies to test the action of the drug on parturition, lactation, and development of the animal neonate were not done, but a general preliminary study in rats indicated no effect on these parameters. Although antihistamines, including promethazine, have been found to produce fetal mortality in rodents, the pharmacological effects of histamine in the rodent do not parallel those in man. There are no adequate and well-controlled studies of promethazine in pregnant women.

Phenergan with codeine should be used during pregnancy only if the potential benefit justifies the potential risk to the fetus.

Nonteratogenic Effects

Dependence has been reported in newborns whose mothers took opiates regularly during pregnancy. Withdrawal signs include irritability, excessive crying, tremors, hyperreflexia, fever, vomiting, and diarrhea. Signs usually appear during the first few days of life.

Promethazine taken within two weeks of delivery may inhibit platelet aggregation in the newborn.

LABOR AND DELIVERY

Narcotic analgesics cross the placental barrier. The closer to delivery and the larger the dose used, the greater the possibility of respiratory depression in the newborn. Narcotic analgesics should be avoided during labor if delivery of a premature infant is anticipated. If the mother has received narcotic analgesics during labor, newborn infants should be observed closely for signs of respiratory depression. Resuscitation may be required (see "Overdosage"). The effect of codeine, if any, on the later growth, development, and functional maturation of the child is unknown.

See also "Nonteratogenic Effects."

NURSING MOTHERS

Some studies, but not others, have reported detectable amounts of codeine in breast milk. The levels are probably not clinically significant after usual therapeutic dosage. The possibility of clinically important amounts being excreted in breast milk in individuals abusing codeine should be considered.

It is not known whether promethazine is excreted in human milk.

Caution should be exercised when Phenergan with codeine is administered to a nursing woman.

PEDIATRIC USE

This product should not be used in children under 2 years of age because safety for such use has not been established.

ADVERSE REACTIONS

CODEINE

Nervous System—CNS depression, particularly respiratory depression, and to a lesser extent circulatory depression; light-headedness, dizziness, sedation, euphoria, dysphoria, headache, transient hallucination, disorientation, visual disturbances, and convulsions.

Cardiovascular—Tachycardia, bradycardia, palpitation, faintness, syncope, orthostatic hypotension (common to narcotic analgesics).

Gastrointestinal—Nausea, vomiting, constipation, and biliary tract spasm. Patients with chronic ulcerative colitis may

experience increased colonic motility; in patients with acute ulcerative colitis, toxic dilation has been reported.

Genitourinary—Oliguria, urinary retention; antidiuretic effect has been reported (common to narcotic analgesics).

Allergic—Infrequent pruritus, giant urticaria, angioneurotic edema, and laryngeal edema.

Other—Flushing of the face, sweating and pruritus (due to opiate-induced histamine release); weakness.

PROMETHAZINE

Nervous System—Sedation, sleepiness, occasional blurred vision, dryness of mouth, dizziness; rarely confusion, disorientation, and extrapyramidal symptoms such as oculogyric crisis, torticollis, and tongue protrusion (usually in association with parenteral injection or excessive dosage).

Cardiovascular—Increased or decreased blood pressure.

Dermatologic—Rash, rarely photosensitivity.

Hematologic—Rarely leukopenia, thrombocytopenia; agranulocytosis (1 case).

Gastrointestinal—Nausea and vomiting.

DRUG ABUSE AND DEPENDENCE

CONTROLLED SUBSTANCE

Phenergan with codeine is a Schedule V Controlled Substance.

ABUSE

Codeine is known to be subject to abuse; however, the abuse potential of oral codeine appears to be quite low. Even parenteral codeine does not appear to offer the psychic effects sought by addicts to the same degree as heroin or morphine. However, codeine must be administered only under close supervision to patients with a history of drug abuse or dependence.

DEPENDENCE

Psychological dependence, physical dependence, and tolerance are known to occur with codeine.

OVERDOSAGE

CODEINE

Serious overdose with codeine is characterized by respiratory depression (a decrease in respiratory rate and/or tidal volume, Cheyne-Stokes respiration, cyanosis), extreme somnolence progressing to stupor or coma, skeletal muscle flaccidity, cold and clammy skin, and sometimes bradycardia and hypotension. The triad of coma, pinpoint pupils, and respiratory depression is strongly suggestive of opiate poisoning. In severe overdosage, particularly by the intravenous route, apnea, circulatory collapse, cardiac arrest, and death may occur. Promethazine is additive to the depressant effects of codeine.

It is difficult to determine what constitutes a standard toxic or lethal dose. However, the lethal oral dose of codeine in an adult is reported to be in the range of 0.5 to 1.0 gram. Infants and children are believed to be relatively more sensitive to opiates on a body-weight basis. Elderly patients are also comparatively intolerant to opiates.

PROMETHAZINE

Signs and symptoms of overdosage with promethazine range from mild depression of the central nervous system and cardiovascular system to profound hypotension, respiratory depression, and unconsciousness.

Stimulation may be evident, especially in children and geriatric patients. Convulsions may rarely occur. A paradoxical reaction has been reported in children receiving single doses of 75 mg to 125 mg orally, characterized by hyperexcitability and nightmares.

Atropine-like signs and symptoms—dry mouth, fixed, dilated pupils, flushing, as well as gastrointestinal symptoms, may occur.

TREATMENT

The treatment of overdosage with Phenergan with codeine is essentially symptomatic and supportive. Only in cases of extreme overdosage or individual sensitivity do vital signs including respiration, pulse, blood pressure, temperature, and EKG need to be monitored. Activated charcoal orally or by lavage may be given, or sodium or magnesium sulfate orally as a cathartic. Attention should be given to the reestablishment of adequate respiratory exchange through provision of a patent airway and institution of assisted or controlled ventilation. The narcotic antagonist, naloxone hydrochloride, may be administered when significant respiratory depression occurs with Phenergan with codeine; any depressant effects of promethazine are not reversed with naloxone. Diazepam may be used to control convulsions. Avoid analeptics, which may cause convulsions. Acidosis and electrolyte losses should be corrected. A rise in temperature or pulmonary complications may signal the need for institution of antibiotic therapy.

Severe hypotension usually responds to the administration of norepinephrine or phenylephrine. EPINEPHRINE SHOULD NOT BE USED, since its use in a patient with partial adrenergic blockade may further lower the blood pressure.

Limited experience with dialysis indicates that it is not helpful.

PHENERGAN WITH CODEINE

Adults	1 teaspoon (5 mL) every 4 to 6 hours, not to exceed 30.0 mL in 24 hours.
Children 6 years to under 12 years	$\frac{1}{2}$ to 1 teaspoon (2.5 to 5 mL) every 4 to 6 hours, not to exceed 30.0 mL in 24 hours.
Children under 6 years (weight: 18 kg or 40 lbs)	$\frac{1}{4}$ to $\frac{1}{2}$ teaspoon (1.25 to 2.5 mL) every 4 to 6 hours, not to exceed 9.0 mL in 24 hours.
Children under 6 years (weight: 16 kg or 35 lbs)	$\frac{1}{4}$ to $\frac{1}{2}$ teaspoon (1.25 to 2.5 mL) every 4 to 6 hours, not to exceed 8.0 mL in 24 hours.
Children under 6 years (weight: 14 kg or 30 lbs)	$\frac{1}{4}$ to $\frac{1}{2}$ teaspoon (1.25 to 2.5 mL) every 4 to 6 hours, not to exceed 7.0 mL in 24 hours.
Children under 6 years (weight: 12 kg or 25 lbs)	$\frac{1}{4}$ to $\frac{1}{2}$ teaspoon (1.25 to 2.5 mL) every 4 to 6 hours, not to exceed 6.0 mL in 24 hours.

Phenergan with codeine is not recommended for children under 2 years of age.

DOSAGE AND ADMINISTRATION
The average effective dose is given in the table above:

HOW SUPPLIED
Phenergan® with codeine is a clear, purple solution supplied as follows:
NDC 0008-0550-02, case of 24 bottles of 4 fl. oz. (118 mL).
NDC 0008-0550-03, bottle of 1 pint (473 mL).
Keep bottles tightly closed—Store at Room Temperature, between 15° C and 25° C (59° F and 77° F).
Protect from light.
Dispense in light-resistant, glass, tight containers.

PHENERGAN®   ℞
[fen 'er-gan]
with dextromethorphan
(Promethazine Hydrochloride and Dextromethorphan Hydrobromide)
Syrup

DESCRIPTION
Each teaspoon (5 mL) of Phenergan with dextromethorphan contains 6.25 mg promethazine hydrochloride and 15 mg dextromethorphan hydrobromide in a flavored syrup base with a pH between 4.7 and 5.2. Alcohol 7%. The inactive ingredients present are artificial and natural flavors, citric acid, D&C Yellow 10, FD&C Yellow 6, glycerin, saccharin sodium, sodium benzoate, sodium citrate, sodium propionate, water, and other ingredients.

Promethazine hydrochloride is a racemic compound; the empirical formula is $C_{17}H_{20}N_2S \cdot HCl$ and its molecular weight is 320.88.

Promethazine hydrochloride, a phenothiazine derivative, is designated chemically as N,N,α-trimethyl-10H -phenothiazine-10-ethanamine monohydrochloride with the following structural formula:

CH$_2$CH(CH$_3$)N(CH$_3$)$_2$

· HCl

Promethazine hydrochloride occurs as a white to faint yellow, practically odorless, crystalline powder which slowly oxidizes and turns blue on prolonged exposure to air. It is soluble in water and freely soluble in alcohol.

Dextromethorphan hydrobromide is a salt of the methyl ether of the dextrorotatory isomer of levorphanol, a narcotic analgesic. It is chemically named as 3-methoxy-17-methyl-9α, 13α, 14α-morphinan hydrobromide monohydrate with the following structural formula:

· HBr · H$_2$O

Dextromethorphan hydrobromide monohydrate occurs as white crystals, is sparingly soluble in water, and is freely soluble in alcohol. The empirical formula is $C_{18}H_{25}NO \cdot HBr \cdot H_2O$, and the molecular weight of the monohydrate is 370.33. Dextromethorphan HBr monohydrate is dextrorotatory with a specific rotation of +27.6 degrees in water (20 degrees C, sodium D-line).

CLINICAL PHARMACOLOGY
PROMETHAZINE
Promethazine is a phenothiazine derivative which differs structurally from the antipsychotic phenothiazines by the presence of a branched side chain and no ring substitution. It is thought that this configuration is responsible for its rela-

tive lack (1/10 that of chlorpromazine) of dopaminergic (CNS) action.

Promethazine is an H$_1$ receptor blocking agent. In addition to its antihistaminic action, it provides clinically useful sedative and antiemetic effects. In therapeutic dosages, promethazine produces no significant effects on the cardiovascular system.

Promethazine is well absorbed from the gastrointestinal tract. Clinical effects are apparent within 20 minutes after oral administration and generally last four to six hours, although they may persist as long as 12 hours. Promethazine is metabolized by the liver to a variety of compounds; the sulfoxides of promethazine and N-demethylpromethazine are the predominant metabolites appearing in the urine.

DEXTROMETHORPHAN
Dextromethorphan is an antitussive agent and, unlike the isomeric levorphanol, it has no analgesic or addictive properties.

The drug acts centrally and elevates the threshold for coughing. It is about equal to codeine in depressing the cough reflex. In therapeutic dosage dextromethorphan does not inhibit ciliary activity.

Dextromethorphan is rapidly absorbed from the gastrointestinal tract and exerts its effect in 15 to 30 minutes. The duration of action after oral administration is approximately three to six hours. Dextromethorphan is metabolized primarily by liver enzymes undergoing O-demethylation, N-demethylation, and partial conjugation with glucuronic acid and sulfate. In humans, (+)-3-hydroxy-N-methylmorphinan, (+)-3-hydroxymorphinan, and traces of unmetabolized drug were found in urine after oral administration.

INDICATIONS AND USAGE
Phenergan with dextromethorphan is indicated for the temporary relief of coughs and upper respiratory symptoms associated with allergy or the common cold.

CONTRAINDICATIONS
Promethazine is contraindicated in individuals known to be hypersensitive or to have had an idiosyncratic reaction to promethazine or to other phenothiazines.

Antihistamines are contraindicated for use in the treatment of lower respiratory tract symptoms, including asthma.

Dextromethorphan should not be used in patients receiving a monoamine oxidase inhibitor (MAOl).

WARNINGS
PROMETHAZINE
Promethazine may cause marked drowsiness. Ambulatory patients should be cautioned against such activities as driving or operating dangerous machinery until it is known that they do not become drowsy or dizzy from promethazine therapy.

The sedative action of promethazine hydrochloride is additive to the sedative effects of central nervous system depressants; therefore, agents such as alcohol, narcotic analgesics, sedatives, hypnotics, and tranquilizers should either be eliminated or given in reduced dosage in the presence of promethazine hydrochloride. When given concomitantly with promethazine hydrochloride, the dose of barbiturates should be reduced by at least one-half, and the dose of analgesic depressants, such as morphine or meperidine, should be reduced by one-quarter to one-half.

Promethazine may lower seizure threshold. This should be taken into consideration when administering to persons with known seizure disorders or when giving in combination with narcotics or local anesthetics which may also affect seizure threshold.

Sedative drugs or CNS depressants should be avoided in patients with a history of sleep apnea.

Antihistamines should be used with caution in patients with narrow-angle glaucoma, stenosing peptic ulcer, pyloroduodenal obstruction, and urinary bladder obstruction due to symptomatic prostatic hypertrophy and narrowing of the bladder neck.

Administration of promethazine has been associated with reported cholestatic jaundice.

DEXTROMETHORPHAN
Administration of dextromethorphan may be accompanied by histamine release and should be used with caution in atopic children.

PRECAUTIONS
Animal reproduction studies have not been conducted with the drug combination—promethazine and dextromethorphan. It is not known whether this drug combination can cause fetal harm when administered to a pregnant woman or can affect reproduction capacity. Phenergan with dextromethorphan should be given to a pregnant woman only if clearly needed.

GENERAL
Promethazine should be used cautiously in persons with cardiovascular disease or with impairment of liver function. Dextromethorphan should be used with caution in sedated patients, in the debilitated, and in patients confined to the supine position.

INFORMATION FOR PATIENTS
Phenergan with dextromethorphan may cause marked drowsiness or impair the mental and/or physical abilities required for the performance of potentially hazardous tasks, such as driving a vehicle or operating machinery. Ambulatory patients should be told to avoid engaging in such activities until it is known that they do not become drowsy or dizzy from Phenergan with dextromethorphan therapy. Children should be supervised to avoid potential harm in bike riding or in other hazardous activities.

The concomitant use of alcohol or other central nervous system depressants, including narcotic analgesics, sedatives, hypnotics, and tranquilizers, may have an additive effect and should be avoided or their dosage reduced.

Patients should be advised to report any involuntary muscle movements or unusual sensitivity to sunlight.

DRUG INTERACTIONS
The sedative action of promethazine is additive to the sedative effects of other central nervous system depressants, including alcohol, narcotic analgesics, sedatives, hypnotics, tricyclic antidepressants, and tranquilizers; therefore, these agents should be avoided or administered in reduced dosage to patients receiving promethazine.

DRUG/LABORATORY TEST INTERACTIONS
The following laboratory tests may be affected in patients who are receiving therapy with promethazine hydrochloride:
Pregnancy Tests
Diagnostic pregnancy tests based on immunological reactions between HCG and anti-HCG may result in false-negative or false-positive interpretations.
Glucose Tolerance Test
An increase in blood glucose has been reported in patients receiving promethazine.

CARCINOGENESIS, MUTAGENESIS, IMPAIRMENT OF FERTILITY
Long-term animal studies have not been performed to assess the carcinogenic potential of promethazine or of dextromethorphan. There are no animal or human data concerning the carcinogenicity, mutagenicity, or impairment of fertility with these drugs. Promethazine was nonmutagenic in the *Salmonella* test system of Ames.

PREGNANCY
Teratogenic Effects —Pregnancy Category C
Teratogenic effects have not been demonstrated in rat-feeding studies at doses of 6.25 and 12.5 mg/kg of promethazine. These doses are 8.3 and 16.7 times the maximum recommended total daily dose for a 50-kg subject. Specific studies to test the action of the drug on parturition, lactation, and development of the animal neonate were not done, but a general preliminary study in rats indicated no effect on these parameters. Although antihistamines, including promethazine, have been found to produce fetal mortality in rodents, the pharmacological effects of histamine in the rodent do not parallel those in man. There are no adequate and well-controlled studies of promethazine in pregnant women.

Phenergan with dextromethorphan should be used during pregnancy only if the potential benefit justifies the potential risk to the fetus.

Nonteratogenic Effects
Promethazine taken within two weeks of delivery may inhibit platelet aggregation in the newborn.

LABOR AND DELIVERY
See "Nonteratogenic Effects."

NURSING MOTHERS
It is not known whether promethazine or dextromethorphan is excreted in human milk. Caution should be exercised when Phenergan with dextromethorphan is administered to a nursing woman.

PEDIATRIC USE
This product should not be used in children under 2 years of age because safety for that use has not been established.

ADVERSE REACTIONS
PROMETHAZINE
Nervous System —Sedation, sleepiness, occasional blurred vision, dryness of mouth, dizziness; rarely confusion, disorientation, and extrapyramidal symptoms such as oculogyric

Continued on next page

Wyeth-Ayerst Laboratories—Cont.

crisis, torticollis, and tongue protrusion (usually in association with parenteral injection or excessive dosage).
Cardiovascular—Increased or decreased blood pressure.
Dermatologic—Rash, rarely photosensitivity.
Hematologic—Rarely leukopenia, thrombocytopenia; agranulocytosis (1 case).
Gastrointestinal—Nausea and vomiting.
DEXTROMETHORPHAN
Dextromethorphan hydrobromide occasionally causes slight drowsiness, dizziness, and gastrointestinal disturbances.

DRUG ABUSE AND DEPENDENCE

According to the WHO Expert Committee on Drug Dependence, dextromethorphan could produce very slight psychic dependence but no physical dependence.

OVERDOSAGE

PROMETHAZINE
Signs and symptoms of overdosage with promethazine range from mild depression of the central nervous system and cardiovascular system to profound hypotension, respiratory depression, and unconsciousness.
Stimulation may be evident, especially in children and geriatric patients. Convulsions may rarely occur. A paradoxical reaction has been reported in children receiving single doses of 75 mg to 125 mg orally, characterized by hyperexcitability and nightmares.
Atropine-like signs and symptoms—dry mouth, fixed, dilated pupils, flushing, as well as gastrointestinal symptoms, may occur.
DEXTROMETHORPHAN
Dextromethorphan may produce central excitement and mental confusion. Very high doses may produce respiratory depression. One case of toxic psychosis (hyperactivity, marked visual and auditory hallucinations) after ingestion of a single dose of 20 tablets (300 mg) of dextromethorphan has been reported.
TREATMENT
Treatment of overdosage with Phenergan with dextromethorphan is essentially symptomatic and supportive. Only in cases of extreme overdosage or individual sensitivity do vital signs including respiration, pulse, blood pressure, temperature, and EKG need to be monitored. Activated charcoal orally or by lavage may be given, or sodium or magnesium sulfate orally as a cathartic. Attention should be given to the reestablishment of adequate respiratory exchange through provision of a patent airway and institution of assisted or controlled ventilation. Diazepam may be used to control convulsions. Acidosis and electrolyte losses should be corrected. The antidotal efficacy of narcotic antagonists to dextromethorphan has not been established; note that any of the depressant effects of promethazine are not reversed by naloxone. Avoid analeptics, which may cause convulsions.
Severe hypotension usually responds to the administration of norepinephrine or phenylephrine. EPINEPHRINE SHOULD NOT BE USED, since its use in a patient with partial adrenergic blockade may further lower the blood pressure.
Limited experience with dialysis indicates that it is not helpful.

DOSAGE AND ADMINISTRATION

The average effective dose for adults is one teaspoon (5 mL) every 4 to 6 hours, not to exceed 30.0 mL in 24 hours. For children 6 years to under 12 years of age, the dose is one-half to one teaspoon (2.5 to 5.0 mL) every 4 to 6 hours, not to exceed 20.0 mL in 24 hours. For children 2 years to under 6 years of age, the dose is one-quarter to one-half teaspoon (1.25 to 2.5 mL) every 4 to 6 hours, not to exceed 10.0 mL in 24 hours.
Phenergan with dextromethorphan is not recommended for children under 2 years of age.

HOW SUPPLIED

Phenergan® with dextromethorphan (Promethazine Hydrochloride and Dextromethorphan Hydrobromide) Syrup is a clear, yellow solution supplied as follows:
NDC 0008-0548-02, case of 24 bottles of 4 fl. oz. (118 mL).
NDC 0008-0548-03, bottle of 1 pint (473 mL).
Keep bottles tightly closed and store at room temperature between 15° and 25°C (59° and 77°F).
Protect from light.
Dispense in light-resistant, glass, tight containers.

PHENERGAN® VC ℞

[fen 'er-gan]
(Promethazine Hydrochloride and Phenylephrine Hydrochloride) Syrup

DESCRIPTION

Each teaspoon (5 mL) of Phenergan VC contains 6.25 mg promethazine hydrochloride and 5 mg phenylephrine hydrochloride in a flavored syrup base with a pH between 4.7 and 5.2. Alcohol 7%. The inactive ingredients present are artificial and natural flavors, citric acid, FD&C Yellow 6, glycerin, saccharin sodium, sodium benzoate, sodium citrate, sodium propionate, water, and other ingredients.
Promethazine hydrochloride is a racemic compound; the empirical formula is $C_{17}H_{20}N_2S \cdot HCl$ and its molecular weight is 320.88.
Promethazine hydrochloride, a phenothiazine derivative, is designated chemically as N,N,α-trimethyl-10*H*-phenothiazine-10-ethanamine monohydrochloride with the following structural formula:

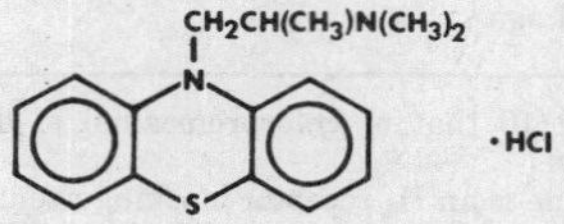
CH₂CH(CH₃)N(CH₃)₂
N
S
·HCl

Promethazine hydrochloride occurs as white to faint yellow, practically odorless, crystalline powder which slowly oxidizes and turns blue on prolonged exposure to air. It is soluble in water and freely soluble in alcohol.
Phenylephrine hydrochloride is a sympathomimetic amine salt. It may be chemically named as 3-hydroxy-α-[(methylamino)methyl]-benzenemethanol hydrochloride and has the following chemical formula:

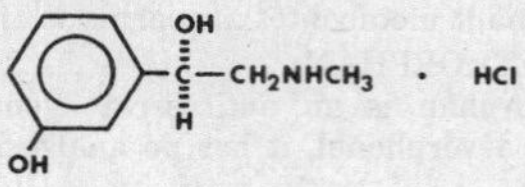
OH
C—CH₂NHCH₃ · HCl
H
OH

Phenylephrine hydrochloride occurs as white or nearly white crystals, having a bitter taste. It is freely soluble in water and alcohol, with a molecular weight of 203.67. The empirical formula is $C_9H_{13}NO_2 \cdot HCl$, and the stereochemistry is R-isomer as indicated in the structure; Specific Rotation—between −42° and −47.5°. Phenylephrine hydrochloride is subject to oxidation and must be protected from light and air.

CLINICAL PHARMACOLOGY

PROMETHAZINE
Promethazine is a phenothiazine derivative which differs structurally from the antipsychotic phenothiazines by the presence of a branched side chain and no ring substitution. It is thought that this configuration is responsible for its relative lack (1/10 that of chlorpromazine) of dopaminergic (CNS) action.
Promethazine is an H_1 receptor blocking agent. In addition to its antihistaminic action, it provides clinically useful sedative and antiemetic effects. In therapeutic dosages, promethazine produces no significant effects on the cardiovascular system.
Promethazine is well absorbed from the gastrointestinal tract. Clinical effects are apparent within 20 minutes after oral administration and generally last four to six hours, although they may persist as long as 12 hours. Promethazine is metabolized by the liver to a variety of compounds; the sulfoxides of promethazine and N-demethylpromethazine are the predominant metabolites appearing in the urine.
PHENYLEPHRINE
Phenylephrine is a potent postsynaptic α-receptor agonist with little effect on β receptors of the heart. Phenylephrine has no effect on β-adrenergic receptors of the bronchi or peripheral blood vessels. A direct action at receptors accounts for the greater part of its effects, only a small part being due to its ability to release norepinephrine.
Therapeutic doses of phenylephrine mainly cause vasoconstriction. Phenylephrine increases resistance and, to a lesser extent, decreases capacitance of blood vessels. Total peripheral resistance is increased, resulting in increased systolic and diastolic blood pressure. Pulmonary arterial pressure is usually increased, and renal blood flow is usually decreased. Local vasoconstriction and hemostasis occur following topical application or infiltration of phenylephrine into tissues.
The main effect of phenylephrine on the heart is bradycardia; it produces a positive inotropic effect on the myocardium in doses greater than those usually used therapeutically. Rarely, the drug may increase the irritability of the heart, causing arrhythmias. Cardiac output is decreased slightly. Phenylephrine increases the work of the heart by increasing peripheral arterial resistance.
Phenylephrine has a mild central stimulant effect.
Following oral administration or topical application of phenylephrine to the mucosa, constriction of blood vessels in the nasal mucosa relieves nasal congestion associated with allergy or head colds. Following oral administration, nasal decongestion may occur within 15 or 20 minutes and may persist for up to 4 hours.
Phenylephrine is irregularly absorbed from and readily metabolized in the gastrointestinal tract. Phenylephrine is metabolized in the liver and intestine by monoamine oxidase. The metabolites and their route and rate of excretion have not been identified. The pharmacologic action of phenylephrine is terminated at least partially by uptake of the drug into tissues.

INDICATIONS AND USAGE

Phenergan VC is indicated for the temporary relief of upper respiratory symptoms, including nasal congestion, associated with allergy or the common cold.

CONTRAINDICATIONS

Promethazine is contraindicated in individuals known to be hypersensitive or to have had an idiosyncratic reaction to promethazine or to other phenothiazines.
Antihistamines are contraindicated for use in the treatment of lower respiratory tract symptoms or asthma.
Phenylephrine is contraindicated in patients with hypertension or with peripheral vascular insufficiency (ischemia may result with risk of gangrene or thrombosis of compromised vascular beds). Phenylephrine should not be used in patients known to be hypersensitive to the drug or in those receiving a monoamine oxidase inhibitor (MAOI).

WARNINGS

PROMETHAZINE
Promethazine may cause marked drowsiness. Ambulatory patients should be cautioned against such activities as driving or operating dangerous machinery until it is known that they do not become drowsy or dizzy from promethazine therapy.
The sedative action of promethazine hydrochloride is additive to the sedative effects of central nervous system depressants; therefore, agents such as alcohol, narcotic analgesics, sedatives, hypnotics, and tranquilizers should either be eliminated or given in reduced dosage in the presence of promethazine hydrochloride. When given concomitantly with promethazine hydrochloride, the dose of barbiturates should be reduced by at least one-half, and the dose of analgesic depressants, such as morphine or meperidine, should be reduced by one-quarter to one-half.
Promethazine may lower seizure threshold. This should be taken into consideration when administering to persons with known seizure disorders or when giving in combination with narcotics or local anesthetics which may also affect seizure threshold.
Sedative drugs or CNS depressants should be avoided in patients with a history of sleep apnea.
Antihistamines should be used with caution in patients with narrow-angle glaucoma, stenosing peptic ulcer, pyloroduodenal obstruction, and urinary bladder obstruction due to symptomatic prostatic hypertrophy and narrowing of the bladder neck.
Administration of promethazine has been associated with reported cholestatic jaundice.
PHENYLEPHRINE
Because phenylephrine is an adrenergic agent, it should be given with caution to patients with thyroid diseases, diabetes mellitus, and heart diseases or those receiving tricyclic antidepressants.
Men with symptomatic, benign prostatic hypertrophy can experience urinary retention when given oral nasal decongestants.
Phenylephrine can cause a decrease in cardiac output, and extreme caution should be used when administering the drug, parenterally or orally, to patients with arteriosclerosis, to elderly individuals, and/or to patients with initially poor cerebral or coronary circulation.
Phenylephrine should be used with caution in patients taking diet preparations, such as amphetamines or phenylpropanolamine, because synergistic adrenergic effects could result in serious hypertensive response and possible stroke.

PRECAUTIONS

Animal reproduction studies have not been conducted with the drug combination—promethazine and phenylephrine. It is not known whether this drug combination can cause fetal harm when administered to a pregnant woman or can affect reproduction capacity. Phenergan VC should be given to a pregnant woman only if clearly needed.
GENERAL
Promethazine should be used cautiously in persons with cardiovascular disease or impairment of liver function.
Phenylephrine should be used with caution in patients with cardiovascular disease, particularly hypertension.
INFORMATION FOR PATIENTS
Phenergan VC may cause marked drowsiness or impair the mental and/or physical abilities required for the performance of potentially hazardous tasks, such as driving a vehicle or operating machinery. Ambulatory patients should be told to avoid engaging in such activities until it is known that they do not become drowsy or dizzy from Phenergan VC therapy. Children should be supervised to avoid potential harm in bike riding or other hazardous activities.
The concomitant use of alcohol or other central nervous system depressants, including narcotic analgesics, sedatives, hypnotics, and tranquilizers, may have an additive effect and should be avoided or their dosage reduced.

Patients should be advised to report any involuntary muscle movements or unusual sensitivity to sunlight.

DRUG INTERACTIONS
PROMETHAZINE
The sedative action of promethazine is additive to the sedative effects of other central nervous system depressants, including alcohol, narcotic analgesics, sedatives, hypnotics, tricyclic antidepressants, and tranquilizers; therefore, these agents should be avoided or administered in reduced dosage to patients receiving promethazine. [See table at right.]

DRUG/LABORATORY TEST INTERACTIONS
The following laboratory tests may be affected in patients who are receiving therapy with promethazine hydrochloride:

Pregnancy Tests
Diagnostic pregnancy tests based on immunological reactions between HCG and anti-HCG may result in false-negative or false-positive interpretations.

Glucose Tolerance Test
An increase in blood glucose has been reported in patients receiving promethazine.

CARCINOGENESIS, MUTAGENESIS, IMPAIRMENT OF FERTILITY
PROMETHAZINE
Long-term animal studies have not been performed to assess the carcinogenic potential of promethazine, nor are there other animal or human data concerning carcinogenicity, mutagenicity, or impairment of fertility with this drug. Promethazine was nonmutagenic in the *Salmonella* test system of Ames.

PHENYLEPHRINE
A study which followed the development of cancer in 143,574 patients over a four-year period indicated that in 11,981 patients who received phenylephrine (systemic or topical), there was no statistically significant association between the drug and cancer at any or all sites.

Long-term animal studies have not been performed to assess the carcinogenic potential of phenylephrine, nor are there other animal or human data concerning mutagenicity.

A study of the effects of adrenergic drugs on ovum transport in rabbits indicated that treatment with phenylephrine did not alter incidence of pregnancy; the number of implantations was significantly reduced when high doses of the drug were used.

PREGNANCY
Teratogenic Effects —Pregnancy Category C
PROMETHAZINE
Teratogenic effects have not been demonstrated in rat-feeding studies at doses of 6.25 and 12.5 mg/ kg of promethazine. These doses are 8.3 and 16.7 times the maximum recommended total daily dose of promethazine for a 50-kg subject. Specific studies to test the action of the drug on parturition, lactation, and development of the animal neonate were not done, but a general preliminary study in rats indicated no effect on these parameters. Although antihistamines, including promethazine, have been found to produce fetal mortality in rodents, the pharmacological effects of histamine in the rodent do not parallel those in man. There are no adequate and well-controlled studies of promethazine in pregnant women.

PHENYLEPHRINE
A study in rabbits indicated that continued moderate overexposure to phenylephrine (3 mg/ day) during the second half of pregnancy (22nd day of gestation to delivery) may contribute to perinatal wastage, prematurity, premature labor, and possibly fetal anomalies; when phenylephrine (3 mg/day) was given to rabbits during the first half of pregnancy (3rd day after mating for seven days), a significant number gave birth to litters of low birth weight. Another study showed that phenylephrine was associated with anomalies of aortic arch and with ventricular septal defect in the chick embryo. Phenergan VC should be used during pregnancy only if the potential benefit justifies the potential risk to the fetus.

Nonteratogenic Effects
Promethazine taken within two weeks of delivery may inhibit platelet aggregation in the newborn.

LABOR AND DELIVERY
Administration of phenylephrine to patients in late pregnancy or labor may cause fetal anoxia or bradycardia by increasing contractility of the uterus and decreasing uterine blood flow.
See also "Nonteratogenic Effects."

NURSING MOTHERS
It is not known whether promethazine or phenylephrine is excreted in human milk.
Caution should be exercised when Phenergan VC is administered to a nursing woman.

PEDIATRIC USE
This product should not be used in children under 2 years of age because safety for such use has not been established.

ADVERSE REACTIONS
PROMETHAZINE
Nervous System —Sedation, sleepiness, occasional blurred vision, dryness of mouth, dizziness; rarely confusion, disori-

---

PHENYLEPHRINE Drug	Effect
Phenylephrine with prior administration of monoamine oxidase inhibitors (MAOI).	Cardiac pressor response potentiated. May cause acute hypertensive crisis.
Phenylephrine with tricyclic antidepressants.	Pressor response increased.
Phenylephrine with ergot alkaloids.	Excessive rise in blood pressure.
Phenylephrine with bronchodilator sympathomimetic agents and with epinephrine or other sympathomimetics.	Tachycardia or other arrhythmias may occur.
Phenylephrine with prior administration of propranolol or other β-adrenergic blockers.	Cardiostimulating effects blocked.
Phenylephrine with atropine sulfate.	Reflex bradycardia blocked; pressor response enhanced.
Phenylephrine with prior administration of phentolamine or other α-adrenergic blockers.	Pressor response decreased.
Phenylephrine with diet preparations, such as amphetamines or phenylpropanolamine.	Synergistic adrenergic response.

entation, and extrapyramidal symptoms such as oculogyric crisis, torticollis, and tongue protrusion (usually in association with parenteral injection or excessive dosage).
Cardiovascular —Increased or decreased blood pressure.
Dermatologic —Rash, rarely photosensitivity.
Hematologic —Rarely leukopenia, thrombocytopenia; agranulocytosis (1 case).
Gastrointestinal —Nausea and vomiting.

PHENYLEPHRINE
Nervous System —Restlessness, anxiety, nervousness, and dizziness.
Cardiovascular —Hypertension (see "Warnings").
Other —Precordial pain, respiratory distress, tremor, and weakness.

OVERDOSAGE
PROMETHAZINE
Signs and symptoms of overdosage with promethazine range from mild depression of the central nervous system and cardiovascular system to profound hypotension, respiratory depression, and unconsciousness.
Stimulation may be evident, especially in children and geriatric patients. Convulsions may rarely occur. A paradoxical reaction has been reported in children receiving single doses of 75 mg to 125 mg orally, characterized by hyperexcitability and nightmares.
Atropine-like signs and symptoms—dry mouth, fixed, dilated pupils, flushing, as well as gastrointestinal symptoms, may occur.

PHENYLEPHRINE
Signs and symptoms of overdosage with phenylephrine include hypertension, headache, convulsions, cerebral hemorrhage, and vomiting. Ventricular premature beats and short paroxysms of ventricular tachycardia may also occur. Headache may be a symptom of hypertension. Bradycardia may also be seen early in phenylephrine overdosage through stimulation of baroreceptors.

TREATMENT
Treatment of overdosage with Phenergan VC is essentially symptomatic and supportive. Only in cases of extreme overdosage or individual sensitivity do vital signs including respiration, pulse, blood pressure, temperature, and EKG need to be monitored. Activated charcoal orally or by lavage may be given, or sodium or magnesium sulfate orally as a cathartic. Attention should be given to the reestablishment of adequate respiratory exchange through provision of a patent airway and institution of assisted or controlled ventilation. Diazepam may be used to control convulsions. Acidosis and electrolyte losses should be corrected. Note that any depressant effects of promethazine are not reversed by naloxone. Avoid analeptics which may cause convulsions. Severe hypotension usually responds to the administration of norepinephrine or phenylephrine. EPINEPHRINE SHOULD NOT BE USED, since its use in patients with partial adrenergic blockade may further lower the blood pressure.
Limited experience with dialysis indicates that it is not helpful.

DOSAGE AND ADMINISTRATION
The recommended adult dose is one teaspoon (5 mL) every 4 to 6 hours, not to exceed 30.0 mL in 24 hours. For children 6 years to under 12 years of age, the dose is one-half to one teaspoon (2.5 to 5.0 mL) repeated at 4- to 6-hour intervals, not to exceed 30.0 mL in 24 hours. For children 2 years to under 6 years of age, the dose is one-quarter to one-half teaspoon (1.25 to 2.5 mL) every 4 to 6 hours.
Phenergan VC is not recommended for children under 2 years of age.

HOW SUPPLIED
Phenergan® VC (Promethazine Hydrochloride and Phenylephrine Hydrochloride) Syrup, is a clear, orange-yellow solution supplied as follows:
NDC 0008-0551-02, case of 24 bottles of 4 fl. oz. (118 mL).
NDC 0008-0551-03, bottle of 1 pint (473 mL).
Keep bottles tightly closed and store at room temperature between 15° and 25°C (59° and 77°F).
Protect from light.
Dispense in light-resistant, glass, tight containers.

PHENERGAN® VC   © ℞
[fen 'er-gan]
with codeine
(Promethazine Hydrochloride,
Phenylephrine Hydrochloride, and
Codeine Phosphate) Syrup

DESCRIPTION
Each teaspoon (5 mL) of Phenergan VC with codeine contains 10 mg ($\frac{1}{6}$ grain) codeine phosphate (Warning—may be habit-forming), 6.25 mg promethazine hydrochloride, and 5 mg phenylephrine hydrochloride in a flavored syrup base with a pH between 4.7 and 5.2. Alcohol 7%. The inactive ingredients present are artificial and natural flavors, citric acid, D&C Red 33, FD&C Yellow 6, glycerin, saccharin sodium, sodium benzoate, sodium citrate, sodium propionate, water, and other ingredients.
Codeine is one of the naturally occurring phenanthrene alkaloids of opium derived from the opium poppy; it is classified pharmacologically as a narcotic analgesic. Codeine phosphate may be chemically named as (5α,6α)–7,8–didehydro–4,5–epoxy–3–methoxy–17–methylmorphinan–6–ol phosphate (1:1) (salt) hemihydrate with the following structural formula:

$$\cdot \, H_3PO_4 \cdot \tfrac{1}{2}H_2O$$

The phosphate salt of codeine occurs as white, needle-shaped crystals or white crystalline powder. Codeine phosphate is freely soluble in water and slightly soluble in alcohol, with a molecular weight of 406.37. The empirical formula is $C_{18}H_{21}NO_3 \cdot H_3PO_4 \cdot \tfrac{1}{2}H_2O$, and the stereochemistry is 5α, 6α isomer as indicated in the structure.
Promethazine hydrochloride is a racemic compound; the empirical formula is $C_{17}H_{20}N_2S \cdot HCl$ and its molecular weight is 320.88.
Promethazine hydrochloride, a phenothiazine derivative, is designated chemically as N,N,α-trimethyl-10*H* -phenothiazine-10-ethanamine monohydrochloride with the following structural formula:
[See chemical structure at top of next page.]
Promethazine hydrochloride occurs as a white to faint yellow, practically odorless, crystalline powder which slowly oxidizes and turns blue on prolonged exposure to air. It is soluble in water and freely soluble in alcohol.

Continued on next page

Wyeth-Ayerst Laboratories—Cont.

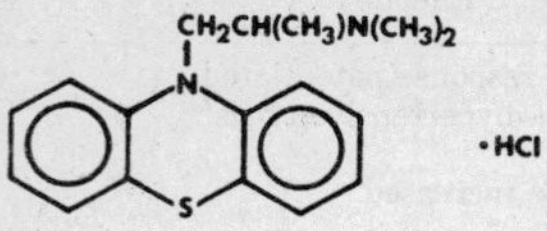

Phenylephrine hydrochloride is a sympathomimetic amine salt. It may be chemically named as 3-hydroxy-α-[(methylamino)methyl]-benzenemethanol hydrochloride and has the following chemical formula:

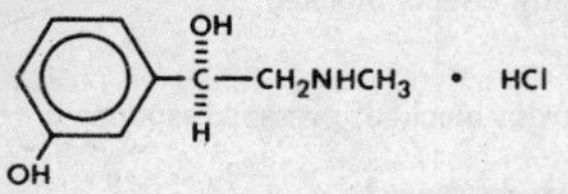

Phenylephrine hydrochloride occurs as white or nearly white crystals, having a bitter taste. It is freely soluble in water and alcohol, with a molecular weight of 203.67. The empirical formula is $C_9H_{13}NO_2 \cdot HCl$, and the stereochemistry is R-isomer as indicated in the structure; Specific Rotation—between −42° and −47.5°. Phenylephrine hydrochloride is subject to oxidation and must be protected from light and air.

CLINICAL PHARMACOLOGY

CODEINE: Narcotic analgesics, including codeine, exert their primary effects on the central nervous system and gastrointestinal tract. The analgesic effects of codeine are due to its central action; however, the precise sites of action have not been determined, and the mechanisms involved appear to be quite complex. Codeine resembles morphine both structurally and pharmacologically, but its actions at the doses of codeine used therapeutically are milder, with less sedation, respiratory depression, and gastrointestinal, urinary, and pupillary effects. Codeine produces an increase in biliary tract pressure, but less than morphine or meperidine. Codeine is less constipating than morphine.

Codeine has good antitussive activity, although less than that of morphine at equal doses. It is used in preference to morphine, because side effects are infrequent at the usual antitussive dose of codeine.

Codeine in oral therapeutic dosage does not usually exert major effects on the cardiovascular system.

Narcotic analgesics may cause nausea and vomiting by stimulating the chemoreceptor trigger zone (CTZ); however, they also depress the vomiting center, so that subsequent doses are unlikely to produce vomiting. Nausea is minimal after usual oral doses of codeine.

Narcotic analgesics cause histamine release, which appears to be responsible for wheals or urticaria sometimes seen at the site of injection on parenteral administration. Histamine release may also produce dilation of cutaneous blood vessels, with resultant flushing of the face and neck, pruritus, and sweating.

Codeine and its salts are well absorbed following both oral and parenteral administration. Codeine is about ⅔ as effective orally as parenterally. Codeine is metabolized primarily in the liver by enzymes of the endoplasmic reticulum, where it undergoes O-demethylation, N-demethylation, and partial conjugation with glucuronic acid. The drug is excreted primarily in the urine, largely as inactive metabolites and small amounts of free and conjugated morphine. Negligible amounts of codeine and its metabolites are found in the feces. Following oral or subcutaneous administration of codeine, the onset of analgesia occurs within 15 to 30 minutes and lasts for four to six hours.

The cough-depressing action, in animal studies, was observed to occur 15 minutes after oral administration of codeine, peak action at 45 to 60 minutes after ingestion. The duration of action, which is dose-dependent, usually did not exceed 3 hours.

PROMETHAZINE: Promethazine is a phenothiazine derivative which differs structurally from the antipsychotic phenothiazines by the presence of a branched side chain and no ring substitution. It is thought that this configuration is responsible for its relative lack (1/10 that of chlorpromazine) of dopaminergic (CNS) action.

Promethazine is an H_1 receptor blocking agent. In addition to its antihistaminic action, it provides clinically useful sedative and antiemetic effects. In therapeutic dosages, promethazine produces no significant effects on the cardiovascular system.

Promethazine is well absorbed from the gastrointestinal tract. Clinical effects are apparent within 20 minutes after oral adminstration and generally last four to six hours, although they may persist as long as 12 hours. Promethazine is metabolized by the liver to a variety of compounds; the sulfoxides of promethazine and N-demethylpromethazine are the predominant metabolites appearing in the urine.

PHENYLEPHRINE: Phenylephrine is a potent postsynaptic α-receptor agonist with little effect on β receptors of the heart. Phenylephrine has no effect on β-adrenergic receptors of the bronchi or peripheral blood vessels. A direct action at receptors accounts for the greater part of its effects, only a small part being due to its ability to release norepinephrine.

Therapeutic doses of phenylephrine mainly cause vasoconstriction. Phenylephrine increases resistance and, to a lesser extent, decreases capacitance of blood vessels. Total peripheral resistance is increased, resulting in increased systolic and diastolic blood pressure. Pulmonary arterial pressure is usually increased, and renal blood flow is usually decreased. Local vasoconstriction and hemostasis occur following topical application or infiltration of phenylephrine into tissues.

The main effect of phenylephrine on the heart is bradycardia; it produces a positive inotropic effect on the myocardium in doses greater than those usually used therapeutically. Rarely, the drug may increase the irritability of the heart, causing arrhythmias. Cardiac output is decreased slightly. Phenylephrine increases the work of the heart by increasing peripheral arterial resistance.

Phenylephrine has a mild central stimulant effect.

Following oral administration or topical application of phenylephrine to the mucosa, constriction of blood vessels in the nasal mucosa relieves nasal congestion associated with allergy or head colds. Following oral administration, nasal decongestion may occur within 15 or 20 minutes and may persist for up to 4 hours.

Phenylephrine is irregularly absorbed from and readily metabolized in the gastrointestinal tract. Phenylephrine is metabolized in the liver and intestine by monoamine oxidase. The metabolites and their route and rate of excretion have not been identified. The pharmacologic action of phenylephrine is terminated at least partially by uptake of the drug into tissues.

INDICATIONS AND USAGE

Phenergan VC with codeine is indicated for the temporary relief of coughs and upper respiratory symptoms, including nasal congestion, associated with allergy or the common cold.

CONTRAINDICATIONS

Codeine is contraindicated in patients with a known hypersensitivity to the drug.

Promethazine is contraindicated in individuals known to be hypersensitive or to have had an idiosyncratic reaction to promethazine or to other phenothiazines.

Phenylephrine is contraindicated in patients with hypertension or with peripheral vascular insufficiency (ischemia may result with risk of gangrene or thrombosis of compromised vascular beds). Phenylephrine should not be used in patients known to be hypersensitive to the drug or in those receiving a monoamine oxidase inhibitor (MAOI).

Antihistamines and codeine are both contraindicated for use in the treatment of lower respiratory tract symptoms, including asthma.

WARNINGS

CODEINE: Dosage of codeine SHOULD NOT BE INCREASED if cough fails to respond; an unresponsive cough should be reevaluated in 5 days or sooner for possible underlying pathology, such as foreign body or lower respiratory tract disease.

Codeine may cause or aggravate constipation.

Respiratory depression leading to arrest, coma, and death has occurred with the use of codeine antitussives in young children, particularly in the under-one-year infants whose ability to deactivate the drug is not fully developed.

Administration of codeine may be accompanied by histamine release and should be used with caution in atopic children.

Head Injury and Increased Intracranial Pressure

The respiratory-depressant effects of narcotic analgesics and their capacity to elevate cerebrospinal fluid pressure may be markedly exaggerated in the presence of head injury, intracranial lesions, or a preexisting increase in intracranial pressure. Narcotics may produce adverse reactions which may obscure the clinical course of patients with head injuries.

Asthma and Other Respiratory Conditions

Narcotic analgesics or cough suppressants, including codeine, should not be used in asthmatic patients (see "Contraindications"). Nor should they be used in acute febrile illness associated with productive cough or in chronic respiratory disease where interference with ability to clear the tracheobronchial tree of secretions would have a deleterious effect on the patient's respiratory function.

Hypotensive Effect

Codeine may produce orthostatic hypotension in ambulatory patients.

PROMETHAZINE: Promethazine may cause marked drowsiness. Ambulatory patients should be cautioned against such activities as driving or operating dangerous machinery until it is known that they do not become drowsy or dizzy from promethazine therapy.

The sedative action of promethazine hydrochloride is additive to the sedative effects of central nervous system depressants; therefore, agents such as alcohol, narcotic analgesics, sedatives, hypnotics, and tranquilizers should either be eliminated or given in reduced dosage in the presence of promethazine hydrochloride. When given concomitantly with promethazine hydrochloride, the dose of barbiturates should be reduced by at least one-half, and the dose of analgesic depressants, such as morphine or meperidine, should be reduced by one-quarter to one-half.

Promethazine may lower seizure threshold. This should be taken into consideration when administering to persons with known seizure disorders or when giving in combination with narcotics or local anesthetics which may also affect seizure threshold.

Sedative drugs or CNS depressants should be avoided in patients with a history of sleep apnea. Antihistamines should be used with caution in patients with narrow-angle glaucoma, stenosing peptic ulcer, pyloroduodenal obstruction, and urinary bladder obstruction due to symptomatic prostatic hypertrophy and narrowing of the bladder neck.

Administration of promethazine has been associated with reported cholestatic jaundice.

PHENYLEPHRINE: Because phenylephrine is an adrenergic agent, it should be given with caution to patients with thyroid diseases, diabetes mellitus, and heart diseases or those receiving tricyclic antidepressants.

Men with symptomatic, benign prostatic hypertrophy can experience urinary retention when given oral nasal decongestants.

Phenylephrine can cause a decrease in cardiac output, and extreme caution should be used when administering the drug, parenterally or orally, to patients with arteriosclerosis, to elderly individuals, and/or to patients with initially poor cerebral or coronary circulation.

Phenylephrine should be used with caution in patients taking diet preparations, such as amphetamines or phenylpropanolamine, because synergistic adrenergic effects could result in serious hypertensive response and possible stroke.

PRECAUTIONS

Animal reproduction studies have not been conducted with the drug combination—promethazine, phenylephrine, and codeine. It is not known whether this drug combination can cause fetal harm when administered to a pregnant woman or can affect reproduction capacity. Phenergan VC with codeine should be given to a pregnant woman only if clearly needed.

GENERAL

Narcotic analgesics, including codeine, should be administered with caution and the initial dose reduced in patients with acute abdominal conditions, convulsive disorders, significant hepatic or renal impairment, fever, hypothyroidism, Addison's disease, ulcerative colitis, prostatic hypertrophy, in patients with recent gastrointestinal or urinary tract surgery, and in the very young or elderly or debilitated patients.

Promethazine should be used cautiously in persons with cardiovascular disease or with impairment of liver function.

Phenylephrine should be used with caution in patients with cardiovascular disease, particularly hypertension.

INFORMATION FOR PATIENTS

Phenergan VC with codeine may cause marked drowsiness or impair the mental and/or physical abilities required for the performance of potentially hazardous tasks, such as driving a vehicle or operating machinery. Ambulatory patients should be told to avoid engaging in such activities until it is known that they do not become drowsy or dizzy from Phenergan VC with codeine therapy. Children should be supervised to avoid potential harm in bike riding or in other hazardous activities.

The concomitant use of alcohol or other central nervous system depressants, including narcotic analgesics, sedatives, hypnotics, and tranquilizers, may have an additive effect and should be avoided or their dosage reduced.

Patients should be advised to report any involuntary muscle movements or unusual sensitivity to sunlight.

Codeine, like other narcotic analgesics, may produce orthostatic hypotension in some ambulatory patients. Patients should be cautioned accordingly.

DRUG INTERACTIONS

CODEINE: In patients receiving MAO inhibitors, an initial small test dose is advisable to allow observation of any excessive narcotic effects or MAOI interaction.

PROMETHAZINE: The sedative action of promethazine is additive to the effects of other central nervous system depressants, including alcohol, narcotic analgesics, sedatives, hypnotics, tricyclic antidepressants, and tranquilizers; therefore, these agents should be avoided or administered in reduced dosage to patients receiving promethazine.

[See table on next page.]

DRUG/LABORATORY TEST INTERACTIONS

Because narcotic analgesics may increase biliary tract pressure, with resultant increases in plasma amylase or lipase levels, determination of these enzyme levels may be unreliable for 24 hours after a narcotic analgesic has been given.

The following laboratory tests may be affected in patients who are receiving therapy with promethazine hydrochloride:

PHENERGAN VC WITH CODEINE

PHENYLEPHRINE

Drug	Effect
Phenylephrine with prior administration of monoamine oxidase inhibitors (MAOI).	Cardiac pressor response potentiated. May cause acute hypertensive crisis.
Phenylephrine with tricyclic antidepressants.	Pressor response increased.
Phenylephrine with ergot alkaloids.	Excessive rise in blood pressure.
Phenylephrine with bronchodilator sympathomimetic agents and with epinephrine or other sympathomimetics.	Tachycardia or other arrhythmias may occur.
Phenylephrine with prior administration of propranolol or other β-adrenergic blockers.	Cardiostimulating effects blocked.
Phenylephrine with atropine sulfate.	Reflex bradycardia blocked; pressor response enhanced.
Phenylephrine with prior administration of phentolamine or other α-adrenergic blockers.	Pressor response decreased.
Phenylephrine with diet preparations, such as amphetamines or phenylpropanolamine.	Synergistic adrenergic response.

Pregnancy Tests

Diagnostic pregnancy tests based on immunological reactions between HCG and anti-HCG may result in false-negative or false-positive interpretations.

Glucose Tolerance Test

An increase in blood glucose has been reported in patients receiving promethazine.

CARCINOGENESIS, MUTAGENESIS, IMPAIRMENT OF FERTILITY

CODEINE AND PROMETHAZINE

Long-term animal studies have not been performed to assess the carcinogenic potential of codeine or of promethazine, nor are there other animal or human data concerning carcinogenicity, mutagenicity, or impairment of fertility with these agents. Codeine has been reported to show no evidence of carcinogenicity or mutagenicity in a variety of test systems, including the micronucleus and sperm abnormality assays and the *Salmonella* assay. Promethazine was nonmutagenic in the *Salmonella* test system of Ames.

PHENYLEPHRINE

A study which followed the development of cancer in 143,574 patients over a four-year period indicated that in 11,981 patients who received phenylephrine (systemic or topical), there was no statistically significant association between the drug and cancer at any or all sites.

Long-term animal studies have not been performed to assess the carcinogenic potential of phenylephrine, nor are there other animal or human data concerning mutagenicity.

A study of the effects of adrenergic drugs on ovum transport in rabbits indicated that treatment with phenylephrine did not alter incidence of pregnancy; the number of implantations was significantly reduced when high doses of the drug were used.

PREGNANCY

Teratogenic Effects—Pregnancy Category C

CODEINE: A study in rats and rabbits reported no teratogenic effect of codeine administered during the period of organogenesis in doses ranging from 5 to 120 mg/kg. In the rat, doses at the 120-mg/kg level, in the toxic range for the adult animal, were associated with an increase in embryo resorption at the time of implantation. In another study a single 100-mg/kg dose of codeine administered to pregnant mice reportedly resulted in delayed ossification in the offspring.

There are no studies in humans, and the significance of these findings to humans, if any, is not known.

PROMETHAZINE: Teratogenic effects have not been demonstrated in rat-feeding studies at doses of 6.25 and 12.5 mg/kg of promethazine. These doses are 8.3 and 16.7 times the maximum recommended total daily dose for a 50-kg subject. Specific studies to test the action of the drug on parturition, lactation, and development of the animal neonate were not done, but a general preliminary study in rats indicated no effect on these parameters. Although antihistamines, including promethazine, have been found to produce fetal mortality in rodents, the pharmacological effects of histamine in the rodent do not parallel those in man. There are no adequate and well-controlled studies of promethazine in pregnant women.

PHENYLEPHRINE: A study in rabbits indicated that continued moderate overexposure to phenylephrine (3 mg/day) during the second half of pregnancy (22nd day of gestation to delivery) may contribute to perinatal wastage, prematurity, premature labor, and possibly fetal anomalies; when phenylephrine (3 mg/day) was given to rabbits during the first half of pregnancy (3rd day after mating for seven days), a significant number gave birth to litters of low birth weight. Another study showed that phenylephrine was associated with anomalies of aortic arch and with ventricular septal defect in the chick embryo.

Phenergan VC with codeine should be used during pregnancy only if the potential benefit justifies the potential risk to the fetus.

Nonteratogenic Effects

Dependence has been reported in newborns whose mothers took opiates regularly during pregnancy. Withdrawal signs include irritability, excessive crying, tremors, hyperreflexia, fever, vomiting, and diarrhea. Signs usually appear during the first few days of life.

Promethazine taken within two weeks of delivery may inhibit platelet aggregation in the newborn.

LABOR AND DELIVERY

Narcotic analgesics cross the placental barrier. The closer to delivery and the larger the dose used, the greater the possibility of respiratory depression in the newborn. Narcotic analgesics should be avoided during labor if delivery of a premature infant is anticipated. If the mother has received narcotic analgesics during labor, newborn infants should be observed closely for signs of respiratory depression. Resuscitation may be required (see "Overdosage"). The effect of codeine, if any, on the later growth, development, and functional maturation of the child is unknown.

Administration of phenylephrine to patients in late pregnancy or labor may cause fetal anoxia or bradycardia by increasing contractility of the uterus and decreasing uterine blood flow.

See also "Nonteratogenic Effects."

NURSING MOTHERS

Some studies, but not others, have reported detectable amounts of codeine in breast milk. The levels are probably not clinically significant after usual therapeutic dosage. The possibility of clinically important amounts being excreted in breast milk in individuals abusing codeine should be considered.

It is not known whether either phenylephrine or promethazine is excreted in human milk.

Caution should be exercised when Phenergan VC with codeine is administered to a nursing woman.

PEDIATRIC USE

This product should not be used in children under 2 years of age because safety for such use has not been established.

ADVERSE REACTIONS

CODEINE

Nervous System—CNS depression, particularly respiratory depression, and to a lesser extent circulatory depression; light-headedness, dizziness, sedation, euphoria, dysphoria, headache, transient hallucination, disorientation, visual disturbances, and convulsions.

Cardiovascular—Tachycardia, bradycardia, palpitation, faintness, syncope, orthostatic hypotension (common to narcotic analgesics).

Gastrointestinal—Nausea, vomiting, constipation, and biliary tract spasm. Patients with chronic ulcerative colitis may experience increased colonic motility; in patients with acute ulcerative colitis, toxic dilation has been reported.

Genitourinary—Oliguria, urinary retention; antidiuretic effect has been reported (common to narcotic analgesics).

Allergic—Infrequent pruritus, giant urticaria, angioneurotic edema, and laryngeal edema.

Other—Flushing of the face, sweating and pruritus (due to opiate-induced histamine release); weakness.

PROMETHAZINE

Nervous System—Sedation, sleepiness, occasional blurred vision, dryness of mouth, dizziness; rarely confusion, disorientation, and extrapyramidal symptoms such as oculogyric crisis, torticollis, and tongue protrusion (usually in association with parenteral injection or excessive dosage).

Cardiovascular—Increased or decreased blood pressure.

Dermatologic—Rash, rarely photosensitivity.

Hematologic—Rarely leukopenia, thrombocytopenia; agranulocytosis (1 case).

Gastrointestinal—Nausea and vomiting.

PHENYLEPHRINE

Nervous System—Restlessness, anxiety, nervousness, and dizziness.

Cardiovascular—Hypertension (see "Warnings").

Other—Precordial pain, respiratory distress, tremor, and weakness.

DRUG ABUSE AND DEPENDENCE

CONTROLLED SUBSTANCE

Phenergan VC with codeine is a Schedule V Controlled Substance.

ABUSE

Codeine is known to be subject to abuse; however, the abuse potential of oral codeine appears to be quite low. Even parenteral codeine does not appear to offer the psychic effects sought by addicts to the same degree as heroin or morphine. However, codeine must be administered only under close supervision to patients with a history of drug abuse or dependence.

DEPENDENCE

Psychological dependence, physical dependence, and tolerance are known to occur with codeine.

OVERDOSAGE

CODEINE: Serious overdose with codeine is characterized by respiratory depression (a decrease in respiratory rate and/or tidal volume, Cheyne-Stokes respiration, cyanosis), extreme somnolence progressing to stupor or coma, skeletal muscle flaccidity, cold and clammy skin, and sometimes bradycardia and hypotension. The triad of coma, pinpoint pupils, and respiratory depression is strongly suggestive of opiate poisoning. In severe overdosage, particularly by the intravenous route, apnea, circulatory collapse, cardiac arrest, and death may occur. Promethazine is additive to the depressant effects of codeine.

It is difficult to determine what constitutes a standard toxic or lethal dose. However, the lethal oral dose of codeine in an adult is reported to be in the range of 0.5 to 1.0 gram. Infants and children are believed to be relatively more sensitive to opiates on a body-weight basis. Elderly patients are also comparatively intolerant to opiates.

PROMETHAZINE: Signs and symptoms of overdosage with promethazine range from mild depression of the central nervous system and cardiovascular system to profound hypotension, respiratory depression, and unconsciousness.

Stimulation may be evident, especially in children and geriatric patients. Convulsions may rarely occur. A paradoxical reaction has been reported in children receiving single doses of 75 mg to 125 mg orally, characterized by hyperexcitability and nightmares.

Atropine-like signs and symptoms—dry mouth, fixed, dilated pupils, flushing, as well as gastrointestinal symptoms, may occur.

PHENYLEPHRINE: Signs and symptoms of overdosage with phenylephrine include hypertension, headache, convulsions, cerebral hemorrhage, and vomiting. Ventricular premature beats and short paroxysms of ventricular tachycardia may also occur. Headache may be a symptom of hypertension. Bradycardia may also be seen early in phenylephrine overdosage through stimulation of baroreceptors.

TREATMENT

Treatment of overdosage with Phenergan VC with codeine is essentially symptomatic and supportive. Only in cases of extreme overdosage or individual sensitivity do vital signs including respiration, pulse, blood pressure, temperature, and EKG need to be monitored. Activated charcoal orally or by lavage may be given, or sodium or magnesium sulfate orally as a cathartic. Attention should be given to the reestablishment of adequate respiratory exchange through provision of a patent airway and institution of assisted or controlled ventilation. The narcotic antagonist, naloxone hydrochloride, may be administered when significant respiratory depression occurs with Phenergan VC with codeine; any depressant effects of promethazine are not reversed by naloxone. Diazepam may be used to control convulsions. Avoid analeptics, which may cause convulsions. Acidosis and electrolyte losses should be corrected. A rise in temperature or pulmonary complications may signal the need for institution of antibiotic therapy.

Severe hypotension usually responds to the administration of norepinephrine or phenylephrine. EPINEPHRINE SHOULD NOT BE USED, since its use in a patient with partial adrenergic blockade may further lower the blood pressure.

Limited experience with dialysis indicates that it is not helpful.

Continued on next page

Wyeth-Ayerst Laboratories—Cont.

DOSAGE AND ADMINISTRATION
The average effective dose is given in the following table:
[See table at right.]

HOW SUPPLIED
Phenergan® VC with codeine is a clear, reddish-orange solution supplied as follows:
NDC 0008-0552-02, case of 24 bottles of 4 fl. oz. (118 mL).
NDC 0008-0552-03, bottle of 1 pint (473 mL).
Keep bottles tightly closed—Stored at Room Temperature, between 15° C and 25° C (59° F and 77° F).
Protect from light.
Dispense in light-resistant, glass, tight containers.

PHOSPHOLINE IODIDE®   ℞
[fŏs 'fo-lĭn ī 'o-dīd]
(echothiophate iodide for ophthalmic solution)

HOW SUPPLIED
Each package contains sterile PHOSPHOLINE IODIDE (echothiophate iodide), sterile diluent, and dropper for dispensing 5 mL eyedrops of the strength indicated on the label. Four potencies are available:
NDC 0046-1062-05 .... 1.5 mg package
for 0.03%

White amorphous deposit on bottle walls. Aluminum crimp seal is blue.

NDC 0046-1064-05 .... 3.0 mg package
for 0.06%

White amorphous deposit on bottle walls. Aluminum crimp seal is red.

NDC 0046-1065-05 .... 6.25 mg package
for 0.125%

White amorphous deposit on bottle walls. Aluminum crimp seal is green.

NDC 0046-1066-05 .... 12.5 mg package
for 0.25%

White amorphous deposit on bottle walls. Aluminum crimp seal is yellow.

Handling and Storage:
Store at room temperature (approximately 25°C).
After reconstitution, keep eyedrops in refrigerator to obtain maximum useful life of 6 months. Room temperature is acceptable if drops will be used within a month.
Full prescribing information for this product appears in the PHYSICIANS' DESK REFERENCE FOR OPHTHALMOLOGY. Please refer to this book or, for prescribing information write to Professional Service, Wyeth-Ayerst Laboratories, P.O. Box 8299, Philadelphia, PA 19101, or contact your local Wyeth-Ayerst representative.

PLEGINE®   Ⓒ ℞
[plĕj-ēn ']
(phendimetrazine tartrate tablets)
Anorexiant

CAUTION: Federal law prohibits dispensing without prescription.

DESCRIPTION
Chemical name: (+)-3,4-Dimethyl-2-phenylmorpholine Tartrate
Structural formula:

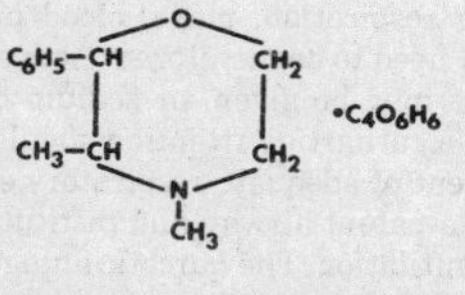

Plegine is the dextro isomer of phendimetrazine tartrate. Phendimetrazine tartrate is a white, odorless powder with a bitter taste. It is soluble in water, methanol, and ethanol. Plegine contains these inactive ingredients: D&C Yellow No. 10; FD&C Yellow No. 6; Lactose, NF; Magnesium Stearate, NF; Polyethylene Glycol 8000, NF.

ACTIONS
Plegine is a phenylalkylamine sympathomimetic with pharmacologic activity similar to the prototype drugs of this class used in obesity, the amphetamines. Actions include central nervous system (CNS) stimulation and elevation of blood pressure. Tachyphylaxis and tolerance have been demonstrated with all drugs of this class in which these phenomena have been looked for.
Drugs of this class used in obesity are commonly known as "anorectics" or "anorexigenics." It has not been established,

---

PHENERGAN VC WITH CODEINE

Adults	1 teaspoon (5 mL) every 4 to 6 hours, not to exceed 30.0 mL in 24 hours.
Children 6 years to under 12 years	½ to 1 teaspoon (2.5 to 5 mL) every 4 to 6 hours, not to exceed 30.0 mL in 24 hours.
Children under 6 years (weight: 18 kg or 40 lbs)	¼ to ½ teaspoon (1.25 to 2.5 mL) every 4 to 6 hours, not to exceed 9.0 mL in 24 hours.
Children under 6 years (weight: 16 kg or 35 lbs)	¼ to ½ teaspoon (1.25 to 2.5 mL) every 4 to 6 hours, not to exceed 8.0 mL in 24 hours.
Children under 6 years (weight: 14 kg or 30 lbs)	¼ to ½ teaspoon (1.25 to 2.5 mL) every 4 to 6 hours, not to exceed 7.0 mL in 24 hours.
Children under 6 years (weight: 12 kg or 25 lbs)	¼ to ½ teaspoon (1.25 to 2.5 mL) every 4 to 6 hours, not to exceed 6.0 mL in 24 hours.

Phenergan VC with codeine is not recommended for children under 2 years of age.

---

however, that the action of such drugs in treating obesity is primarily one of appetite suppression. Other CNS actions, or metabolic effects, may be involved.
Adult obese subjects instructed in dietary management and treated with "anorectic" drugs, lose more weight on the average than those treated with placebo and diet, as determined in relatively short-term clinical trials.

The magnitude of increased weight loss of drug-treated patients over placebo-treated patients is only a fraction of a pound a week. The rate of weight loss is greatest in the first weeks of therapy for both drug and placebo subjects and tends to decrease in succeeding weeks. The possible origins of the increased weight loss due to the various drug effects are not established. The amount of weight loss associated with use of an "anorectic" drug varies from trial to trial, and the increased weight loss appears to be related, in part, to variables other than the drug prescribed, such as the physician-investigator, the population treated, and the diet prescribed. Studies do not permit conclusions as to the relative importance of the drug and non-drug factors on weight loss.
The natural history of obesity is measured in years, whereas the studies cited are restricted to a few weeks' duration; thus, the total impact of drug-induced weight loss over that of diet alone must be considered clinically limited.

INDICATIONS
Plegine is indicated in the management of exogenous obesity as a short-term adjunct (a few weeks) in a regimen of weight reduction based on caloric restriction. The limited usefulness of agents of this class should be measured against possible risk factors inherent in their use (see ACTIONS).

CONTRAINDICATIONS
Known hypersensitivity or idiosyncratic reactions to sympathomimetics.

Advanced arteriosclerosis, symptomatic cardiovascular disease, moderate and severe hypertension, hyperthyroidism, glaucoma.

Highly nervous or agitated patients.

Patients with a history of drug abuse.

Patients taking other CNS stimulants, including monamine oxidase inhibitors.

WARNINGS
DRUG DEPENDENCE
Plegine is related chemically and pharmacologically to the amphetamines. Amphetamines and related stimulant drugs have been abused extensively, and the possibility of Plegine abuse should be kept in mind when evaluating the desirability of including a drug as part of a weight reduction program. Abuse of amphetamines and related drugs may be associated with intense psychological dependence and severe social dysfunction. There are reports of patients who have increased the dosage to many times that recommended. Abrupt cessation following prolonged high-dosage administration results in extreme fatigue and mental depression; changes are also noted on the sleep EEG. Manifestations of chronic intoxication with anorectic drugs include severe dermatoses, marked insomnia, irritability, hyperactivity, and personality changes. The most severe manifestation of chronic intoxication is psychosis, often indistinguishable clinically from schizophrenia.
Tolerance to the anorectic effect of Plegine develops within a few weeks. When this occurs, its use should be discontinued; the maximum recommended dose should not be exceeded. Use of Plegine within 14 days following the administration of monamine oxidase inhibitors may result in a hypertensive crisis.
Abrupt cessation of administration following prolonged high dosage results in extreme fatigue and depression. Because of the effect on the central nervous system Plegine may impair the patient's ability to engage in potentially hazardous activities such as operating machinery or driving a motor vehicle; the patient should therefore be cautioned accordingly.
USAGE IN PREGNANCY
Safe use in pregnancy has not been established. Until more information is available, phendimetrazine tartrate should not be taken by women who are, or may become, pregnant unless, in the opinion of the physician, the potential benefits outweigh the possible hazards.

USAGE IN CHILDREN
Plegine is not recommended for use in children under 12 years of age.
PRECAUTIONS
Caution is to be exercised in prescribing Plegine for patients with even mild hypertension.
Insulin requirements in diabetes mellitus may be altered in association with the use of Plegine and the concomitant dietary regimen.
Plegine may decrease the hypotensive effect of guanethidine.
The least amount feasible should be prescribed or dispensed at one time in order to minimize the possibility of overdosage.
ADVERSE REACTIONS
CENTRAL NERVOUS SYSTEM
Overstimulation, restlessness, insomnia, agitation, flushing, tremor, sweating, dizziness, headache, psychotic states, blurring of vision.
CARDIOVASCULAR
Palpitation, tachycardia, elevated blood pressure.
GASTROINTESTINAL
Mouth dryness, nausea, diarrhea, constipation, stomach pain.
GENITOURINARY
Urinary frequency, dysuria, changes in libido.
DOSAGE AND ADMINISTRATION
USUAL ADULT DOSAGE
1 tablet (35 mg) b.i.d. or t.i.d., one hour before meals. Dosage should be individualized to obtain an adequate response with the lowest effective dosage. In some cases, ½ tablet per dose may be adequate; dosage should not exceed 2 tablets t.i.d.
OVERDOSAGE
Acute overdosage of phendimetrazine tartrate may manifest itself by the following signs and symptoms: unusual restlessness, confusion, belligerence, hallucinations, and panic states. Fatigue and depression usually follow the central stimulation. Cardiovascular effects include arrhythmias, hypertension or hypotension, and circulatory collapse. Gastrointestinal symptoms include nausea, vomiting, diarrhea, and abdominal cramps. Poisoning may result in convulsions, coma, and death.

The management of overdosage is largely symptomatic. It includes sedation with a barbiturate. If hypertension is marked, the use of a nitrate or rapid-acting alpha receptor-blocking agent should be considered. Experience with hemodialysis or peritoneal dialysis is inadequate to permit recommendations for its use.

HOW SUPPLIED
Plegine—Each scored tablet contains 35 mg phendimetrazine tartrate, in bottles of 100 (NDC 0046-0755-81).
Store at room temperature, approximately 25°C.
Shown in Product Identification Section, page 437

PMB® 200   ℞

Each tablet contains:
Premarin® (conjugated
estrogens, USP) .... 0.45 mg
Meprobamate .... 200.0 mg

PMB® 400

Each tablet contains:
Premarin® (conjugated
estrogens, USP) .... 0.45 mg
Meprobamate .... 400.0 mg

CAUTION: Federal law prohibits dispensing without prescription.

---

1. ESTROGENS HAVE BEEN REPORTED TO INCREASE THE RISK OF ENDOMETRIAL CARCINOMA.

Three independent, case-controlled studies have reported an increased risk of endometrial cancer in post-

menopausal women exposed to exogenous estrogens for more than one year.[1–3] This risk was independent of the other known risk factors for endometrial cancer. These studies are further supported by the finding that incidence rates of endometrial cancer have increased sharply since 1969 in eight different areas of the United States with population-based cancer reporting systems, an increase which may be related to the rapidly expanding use of estrogens during the last decade.[4]

The three case-controlled studies reported that the risk of endometrial cancer in estrogen users was about 4.5 to 13.9 times greater than in nonusers. The risk appears to depend on both duration of treatment[1] and on estrogen dose.[3] In view of these findings, when estrogens are used for the treatment of menopausal symptoms, the lowest dose that will control symptoms should be utilized and medication should be discontinued as soon as possible. When prolonged treatment is medically indicated, the patient should be reassessed, on at least a semi-annual basis to determine the need for continued therapy. Although the evidence must be considered preliminary, one study suggests that cyclic administration of low doses of estrogen may carry less risk than continuous administration.[3] It therefore appears prudent to utilize such a regimen.

Close clinical surveillance of all women taking estrogens is important. In all cases of undiagnosed persistent or recurring abnormal vaginal bleeding, adequate diagnostic measures should be undertaken to rule out malignancy.

There is no evidence at present that "natural" estrogens are more or less hazardous than "synthetic" estrogens at equi-estrogenic doses.

2. ESTROGENS SHOULD NOT BE USED DURING PREGNANCY.

The use of female sex hormones, both estrogens and progestogens, during early pregnancy may seriously damage the offspring. It has been shown that females exposed in utero to diethylstilbestrol, a nonsteroidal estrogen, have an increased risk of developing, in later life, a form of vaginal or cervical cancer that is ordinarily extremely rare.[5,6] This risk has been estimated as not greater than 4 per 1,000 exposures.[7] Furthermore, a high percentage of such exposed women (from 30% to 90%) have been found to have vaginal adenosis,[8–12] epithelial changes of the vagina and cervix. Although these changes are histologically benign, it is not known whether they are precursors of malignancy. Although similar data are not available with the use of other estrogens, it cannot be presumed they would not induce similar changes.

Several reports suggest an association between intrauterine exposure to female sex hormones and congenital anomalies, including congenital heart defects and limb-reduction defects.[13–16] One case-controlled study[16] estimated a 4.7-fold increased risk of limb-reduction defects in infants exposed in utero to sex hormones (oral contraceptives, hormone withdrawal tests for pregnancy, or attempted treatment for threatened abortion). Some of these exposures were very short and involved only a few days of treatment. The data suggest that the risk of limb-reduction defects in exposed fetuses is somewhat less than 1 per 1,000.

In the past, female sex hormones have been used during pregnancy in an attempt to treat threatened or habitual abortion. There is considerable evidence that estrogens are ineffective for these indications, and there is no evidence from well-controlled studies that progestogens are effective for these uses.

If PMB is used during pregnancy, or if the patient becomes pregnant while taking this drug, she should be apprised of the potential risks to the fetus, and the advisability of pregnancy continuation.

3. THIS FIXED-COMBINATION DRUG IS NOT INDICATED FOR INITIAL THERAPY.

In cases where estrogen given alone has not alleviated anxiety and tension existing as part of the menopausal symptom complex, therapy may then consist of separate administration of estrogen and meprobamate in order to determine the appropriate dosage of each drug for the patient. If this fixed combination represents the dosage so determined, its use may be more convenient in patient management. The treatment of such patients is not static, but must be re-evaluated as conditions in each patient warrant.

DESCRIPTION

PMB is a combination of PREMARIN® (conjugated estrogens, USP) and meprobamate, a tranquilizing agent, in tablet form for oral administration.

PREMARIN (conjugated estrogens, USP) is a mixture of estrogens, obtained exclusively from natural sources, occurring as the sodium salts of water-soluble estrogen sulfates blended to represent the average composition of material derived from pregnant mares' urine. It contains estrone, equilin, and 17α-dihydroequilin, together with smaller amounts of 17α-estradiol, equilenin, and 17 α-dihydroequilenin as salts of their sulfate esters.

Meprobamate, USP, is the dicarbamic acid ester of 2-methyl-2-*n*-propyl-1,3-propanediol.

PMB 200: Each tablet contains 0.45 mg of PREMARIN® (conjugated estrogens, USP) and 200 mg Meprobamate, USP.

PMB 400: Each tablet contains 0.45 mg of PREMARIN® (conjugated estrogens, USP) and 400 mg Meprobamate, USP.

PMB Tablets contain the following inactive ingredients: calcium phosphate, calcium sulfate, carnauba wax, cellulose, lactose, magnesium stearate, methylcellulose, pharmaceutical glaze, sucrose, talc, titanium dioxide.

—PMB 200 Tablets also contain: D&C Yellow No. 10, FD&C Blue No. 1, FD&C Yellow No. 6.

—PMB 400 Tablets also contain: FD&C Blue No. 2, D&C Red No. 7, D&C Red No. 27.

CLINICAL PHARMACOLOGY

Estrogens are important in the development and maintenance of the female reproductive system and secondary sex characteristics. They promote growth and development of the vagina, uterus, and fallopian tubes, and enlargement of the breasts. Indirectly, they contribute to the shaping of the skeleton, maintenance of tone and elasticity of urogenital structures, changes in the epiphyses of the long bones that allow for the pubertal growth spurt and its termination, growth of axillary and pubic hair, and pigmentation of the nipples and genitals. Decline of estrogenic activity at the end of the menstrual cycle can bring on menstruation, although the cessation of progesterone secretion is the most important factor in the mature ovulatory cycle. However, in the preovulatory or nonovulatory cycle, estrogen is the primary determinant in the onset of menstruation. Estrogens also affect the release of pituitary gonadotropins.

The pharmacologic effects of conjugated estrogens are similar to those of endogenous estrogens. They are soluble in water and are well absorbed from the gastrointestinal tract.

In responsive tissues (female genital organs, breasts, hypothalamus, pituitary) estrogens enter the cell and are transported into the nucleus. As a result of estrogen action, specific RNA and protein synthesis occurs.

Metabolism and inactivation occur primarily in the liver. Some estrogens are excreted into the bile; however, they are reabsorbed from the intestine and returned to the liver through the portal venous system. Water-soluble estrogen conjugates are strongly acidic and are ionized in body fluids, which favor excretion through the kidneys since tubular reabsorption is minimal.

Meprobamate is used clinically for the reduction of anxiety and tension. The precise mechanism(s) of its action is not known. It is well absorbed from the gastrointestinal tract and has a physiological half-life of about 10 hours. It is excreted in the urine primarily as hydroxymeprobamate and as a glucuronide.

The combination of PREMARIN with meprobamate as provided in PMB relieves the underlying estrogen deficiency and affords tranquilizing activity to ameliorate the anxiety and tension not due to estrogen deficiency.

INDICATIONS AND USAGE

For the treatment of moderate-to-severe vasomotor symptoms of the menopause when anxiety and tension are part of the symptom complex and only in those cases in which the use of estrogens alone has not resulted in alleviation of such symptoms.

PMB HAS NOT BEEN SHOWN TO BE EFFECTIVE FOR ANY PURPOSE DURING PREGNANCY AND ITS USE MAY CAUSE SEVERE HARM TO THE FETUS (SEE BOXED WARNING).

CONTRAINDICATIONS

Estrogens should not be used in women with any of the following conditions:

1. Known or suspected cancer of the breast except in appropriately selected patients being treated for metastatic disease.
2. Known or suspected estrogen-dependent neoplasia.
3. Known or suspected pregnancy (see Boxed Warning).
4. Undiagnosed abnormal genital bleeding.
5. Active thrombophlebitis or thromboembolic disorders.
6. A past history of thrombophlebitis, thrombosis, or thromboembolic disorders associated with previous estrogen use.

Meprobamate should not be used in patients with the following conditions:

1. A history of allergic or idiosyncratic reactions to meprobamate or related compounds such as carisoprodol, mebutamate, tybamate, or carbromal.
2. Acute intermittent porphyria.

WARNINGS

USAGE IN PREGNANCY AND LACTATION.

An increased risk of congenital malformations associated with the use of minor tranquilizers (meprobamate, chlordiazepoxide, and diazepam) during the first trimester of pregnancy has been suggested in several studies. Because use of these drugs is rarely a matter of urgency, their use during this period should almost always be avoided. The possibility that a woman of childbearing potential may be pregnant at the time of institution of therapy should be considered. Patients should be advised that if they become pregnant during therapy or intend to become pregnant they should communicate with their physicians about the desirability of discontinuing the drug.

Meprobamate passes the placental barrier. It is present both in umbilical cord blood at or near maternal plasma levels and in breast milk of lactating mothers at concentrations two to four times that of maternal plasma. When use of meprobamate is contemplated in breast-feeding patients, the drug's higher concentrations in breast milk as compared to maternal plasma levels should be considered.

Usage in Children—PMB is not intended for use in children.

Associated with Estrogen Administration:

1. *Induction of malignant neoplasms.* Estrogens have been reported to increase the risk of endometrial carcinoma. (See Boxed Warning.) However, a recent, large, case-controlled study indicated no increase in risk of breast cancer in postmenopausal women.[18]

2. *Gallbladder disease.* A recent study has reported a 2- to 3-fold increase in the risk of surgically confirmed gallbladder disease in women receiving postmenopausal estrogens,[17] similar to the 2-fold increase previously noted in users of oral contraceptives.[19,24a]

3. *Effects similar to those caused by estrogen-progestogen oral contraceptives.* There are several serious adverse effects of oral contraceptives, most of which have not, up to now, been documented as consequences of postmenopausal estrogen therapy. This may reflect the comparatively low doses of estrogen used in postmenopausal women. It would be expected that the larger doses of estrogen used to treat prostatic or breast cancer, or postpartum breast engorgement, are more likely to result in these adverse effects, and, in fact, it has been shown that there is an increased risk of thrombosis in men receiving estrogens for prostatic cancer and women for postpartum breast engorgement.[20–23]

a. *Thromboembolic disease.* It is now well established that users of oral contraceptives have an increased risk of various thromboembolic and thrombotic vascular diseases, such as thrombophlebitis, pulmonary embolism, stroke, and myocardial infarction.[24–31] Cases of retinal thrombosis, mesenteric thrombosis, and optic neuritis have been reported in oral-contraceptive users. There is evidence that the risk of several of these adverse reactions is related to the dose of the drug.[32,33] An increased risk of postsurgery thromboembolic complications has also been reported in users of oral-contraceptives.[34,35] If feasible, estrogen should be discontinued at least 4 weeks before surgery of the type associated with an increased risk of thromboembolism, or during periods of prolonged immobilization.

While an increased rate of thromboembolic and thrombotic disease in postmenopausal users of estrogens has not been found,[17–24,25–36] this does not rule out the possibility that such an increase may be present or that subgroups of women who have underlying risk factors or who are receiving relatively large doses of estrogens may have increased risk. Therefore estrogens should not be used in persons with active thrombophlebitis or thromboembolic disorders, and they should not be used (except in treatment of malignancy) in persons with a history of such disorders in association with estrogen use. They should be used with caution in patients with cerebral vascular or coronary artery disease and only for those in whom estrogens are clearly needed.

Large doses of estrogen (5 mg conjugated estrogens per day), comparable to those used to treat cancer of the prostate and breast, have been shown in a large prospective clinical trial in men[37] to increase the risk of nonfatal myocardial infarction, pulmonary embolism, and thrombophlebitis. When estrogen doses of this size are used, any of the thromboembolic and thrombotic adverse effects associated with oral contraceptive use should be considered a clear risk.

b. *Hepatic adenoma.* Benign hepatic adenomas appear to be associated with the use of oral contraceptives.[38–40] Although benign, and rare, these may rupture and may cause death through intra-abdominal hemorrhage. Such lesions have not yet been reported in association with other estrogen or progestogen preparations but should be considered in estrogen users having abdominal pain and tenderness, abdominal mass, or hypovolemic shock. Hepatocellular carcinoma has also been reported in women taking estrogen-containing oral contraceptives.[39] The relationship of this malignancy to these drugs is not known at this time.

Continued on next page

Wyeth-Ayerst Laboratories—Cont.

c. *Elevated blood pressure.* Women using oral contraceptives sometimes experience increased blood pressure which, in most cases, returns to normal on discontinuing the drug. There is now a report that this may occur with use of estrogens in the menopause[41] and blood pressure should be monitored with estrogen use, especially if high doses are used.

d. *Glucose tolerance.* A worsening of glucose tolerance has been observed in a significant percentage of patients on estrogen-containing oral contraceptives. For this reason, diabetic patients should be carefully observed while receiving estrogen.

4. *Hypercalcemia.* Administration of estrogens may lead to severe hypercalcemia in patients with breast cancer and bone metastases. If this occurs, the drug should be stopped and appropriate measures taken to reduce the serum calcium level.

Associated with Meprobamate Administration:

1. *Drug Dependence*—Physical dependence, psychological dependence, and abuse have occurred. When chronic intoxication from prolonged use occurs, it usually involves ingestion of greater than recommended doses and is manifested by ataxia, slurred speech, and vertigo. Therefore, careful supervision of dose and amounts prescribed is advised, as well as avoidance of prolonged administration, especially for alcoholics and other patients with a known propensity for taking excessive quantities of drugs.

Sudden withdrawal of the drug after prolonged and excessive use may precipitate recurrence of pre-existing symptoms, such as anxiety, anorexia, or insomnia, or withdrawal reactions, such as vomiting, ataxia, tremors, muscle twitching, confusional states, hallucinosis, and, rarely, convulsive seizures. Such seizures are more likely to occur in persons with central nervous system damage or pre-existent or latent convulsive disorders. Onset of withdrawal symptoms occurs usually within 12 to 48 hours after discontinuation of meprobamate; symptoms usually cease within the next 12 to 48 hours.

When excessive dosage has continued for weeks or months, dosage should be reduced gradually over a period of one or two weeks rather than abruptly stopped. Alternatively, a short-acting barbiturate may be substituted, then gradually withdrawn.

2. *Potentially Hazardous Tasks*—Patients should be warned that this drug may impair the mental and/or physical abilities required for the performance of potentially hazardous tasks such as driving a motor vehicle or operating machinery.

3. *Additive Effects*—Since the effects of meprobamate and alcohol or meprobamate and other CNS depressants or psychotropic drugs may be additive, appropriate caution should be exercised with patients who take more than one of these agents simultaneously.

PRECAUTIONS

A. General Precautions.

Associated with Estrogen:

1. A complete medical and family history should be taken prior to the initiation of any estrogen therapy. The pretreatment and periodic physical examinations should include special reference to blood pressure, breasts, abdomen, and pelvic organs, and should include a Papanicolaou smear. As a general rule, estrogen should not be prescribed for longer than one year without another physical examination being performed.

2. *Fluid retention*—Because estrogens may cause some degree of fluid retention, conditions which might be influenced by this factor such as asthma, epilepsy, migraine, and cardiac or renal dysfunction, require careful observation.

3. Certain patients may develop undesirable manifestations of excessive estrogenic stimulation, such as abnormal or excessive uterine bleeding, mastodynia, etc.

4. Prolonged administration of unopposed estrogen therapy has been reported to increase the risk of endometrial hyperplasia in some patients.

5. Oral contraceptives appear to be associated with an increased incidence of mental depression.[24a] Although it is not clear whether this is due to the estrogenic or progestogenic component of the contraceptive, patients with a history of depression should be carefully observed.

6. Pre-existing uterine leiomyomata may increase in size during estrogen use.

7. The pathologist should be advised of estrogen therapy when relevant specimens are submitted.

8. Patients with a past history of jaundice during pregnancy have an increased risk of recurrence of jaundice while receiving estrogen-containing oral contraceptive therapy. If jaundice develops in any patient receiving estrogen, the medication should be discontinued while the cause is investigated.

9. Estrogens may be poorly metabolized in patients with impaired liver function and should be administered with caution in such patients.

10. Because estrogens influence the metabolism of calcium and phosphorus, they should be used with caution in patients with metabolic bone diseases that are associated with hypercalcemia or in patients with renal insufficiency.

11. Because of the effects of estrogens on epiphyseal closure, they should be used judiciously in young patients in whom bone growth is not complete.

Concomitant Progestin Use: The lowest effective dose appropriate for the specific indication should be utilized. Studies of the addition of a progestin for 7 or more days of a cycle of estrogen administration have reported a lowered incidence of endometrial hyperplasia. Morphological and biochemical studies of the endometrium suggest that 10 to 13 days of progestin are needed to provide maximal maturation of the endometrium and to eliminate any hyperplastic changes. Whether this will provide protection from endometrial carcinoma has not been clearly established. There are possible additional risks which may be associated with the inclusion of progestin in estrogen replacement regimens. If concomitant progestin therapy is used, potential risks may include adverse effects on carbohydrate and lipid metabolism. The choice of progestin and dosage may be important in minimizing these adverse effects.

Associated with Meprobamate:

1. The lowest effective dose should be administered, particularly to debilitated patients, in order to preclude oversedation.

2. The possibility of suicide attempts should be considered and the least amount of drug feasible should be dispensed at any one time.

3. Meprobamate is metabolized in the liver and excreted by the kidney; to avoid its excess accumulation, caution should be exercised in administration to patients with compromised liver or kidney function.

4. Meprobamate occasionally may precipitate seizures in epileptic patients.

B. Information for Patients. (See text which appears after the PHYSICIAN REFERENCES.)

C. Drug/Laboratory Test Interactions: Certain endocrine and liver function tests may be affected by estrogen-containing oral contraceptives. The following similar changes may be expected with larger doses of estrogen.

a. Increased sulfobromophthalein retention.

b. Increased prothrombin and factors VII, VIII, IX, and X; decreased antithrombin 3; increased norepinephrine-induced platelet aggregability.

c. Increased thyroid binding globulin (TBG) leading to increased circulating total thyroid hormone, as measured by PBI, T_4 by column, or T_4 by radioimmunoassay. Free T_3 resin uptake is decreased, reflecting the elevated TBG; free T_4 concentration is unaltered.

d. Impaired glucose tolerance.

e. Decreased pregnanediol excretion.

f. Reduced response to metyrapone test.

g. Reduced serum folate concentration.

h. Increased serum triglyceride and phospholipid concentration.

D. Mutagenesis and Carcinogenesis. Long-term, continuous administration of natural and synthetic estrogens in certain animal species increases the frequency of carcinomas of the breast, cervix, vagina, and liver. However, in a recent, large, case-controlled study of postmenopausal women, there was no increase in risk of breast cancer with use of conjugated estrogens.[18]

E. Pregnancy Category X. (See CONTRAINDICATIONS and Boxed Warning.)

F. Nursing Mothers. Because of the potential for serious adverse reactions in nursing infants from PMB, a decision should be made whether to discontinue nursing or to discontinue the drugs, taking into account the importance of the drug to the mother. (See WARNINGS section for information on use in pregnancy and lactation.)

G. Pediatric Use. Safety and effectiveness in children have not been established.

ADVERSE REACTIONS

Associated with Estrogen Administration

(See WARNINGS regarding induction of neoplasia, adverse effects on the fetus, increased incidence of gallbladder disease, and adverse effects similar to those of oral contraceptives, including thromboembolism.) The following additional adverse reactions have been reported with estrogenic therapy, including oral contraceptives:

1. *Genitourinary system:* Breakthrough bleeding, spotting, change in menstrual flow; dysmenorrhea; premenstrual-like syndrome; amenorrhea during and after treatment; increase in size of uterine fibromyomata; vaginal candidiasis; change in cervical erosion and in degree of cervical secretion; cystitis-like syndrome.

2. *Breasts:* Tenderness, enlargement, secretion.

3. *Gastrointestinal:* Nausea, vomiting; abdominal cramps, bloating; cholestatic jaundice.

4. *Skin:* Chloasma or melasma which may persist when drug is discontinued; erythema multiforme; erythema nodosum; hemorrhagic eruption; loss of scalp hair; hirsutism.

5. *Eyes:* Steepening of corneal curvature; intolerance to contact lenses.

6. *CNS:* Headache, migraine, dizziness; mental depression; chorea.

7. *Miscellaneous:* Increase or decrease in weight; reduced carbohydrate tolerance; aggravation of porphyria; edema; changes in libido.

The following have been reported with meprobamate therapy:

1. *Central Nervous System*—Drowsiness, ataxia, dizziness, slurred speech, headache, vertigo, weakness, paresthesias, impairment of visual accommodation, euphoria, overstimulation, paradoxical excitement, fast EEG activity.

2. *Gastrointestinal*—Nausea, vomiting, diarrhea.

3. *Cardiovascular*—Palpitations, tachycardia, various forms of arrhythmia, transient ECG changes, syncope; also, hypotensive crises (including one fatal case).

4. *Allergic or Idiosyncratic*—Allergic or idiosyncratic reactions are usually seen within the period of the first to fourth dose in patients having had no previous contact with the drug. Milder reactions are characterized by an itchy, urticarial, or erythematous maculopapular rash which may be generalized or confined to the groin. Other reactions have included leukopenia, acute nonthrombocytopenic purpura, petechiae, ecchymoses, eosinophilia, peripheral edema, adenopathy, fever, fixed drug eruption with cross reaction to carisoprodol, and cross sensitivity between meprobamate/mebutamate and meprobamate/carbromal.

More severe hypersensitivity reactions, rarely reported, include hyperpyrexia, chills, angioneurotic edema, bronchospasm, oliguria, and anuria. Also, anaphylaxis, erythema multiforme, exfoliative dermatitis, stomatitis, proctitis, Stevens-Johnson syndrome, and bullous dermatitis, including one fatal case of the latter, following administration of meprobamate in combination with prednisolone.

In case of allergic or idiosyncratic reactions to meprobamate, discontinue the drug and initiate appropriate symptomatic therapy, which may include epinephrine, antihistamines, and in severe cases corticosteroids. In evaluating possible allergic reactions, also consider allergy to excipients (information on excipients is available to physicians on request).

5. *Hematologic* (See also *Allergic or Idiosyncratic.*)—Agranulocytosis and aplastic anemia have been reported, although no causal relationship has been established. These cases rarely were fatal. Rare cases of thrombocytopenic purpura have been reported.

6. *Other*—Exacerbation of porphyric symptoms.

OVERDOSAGE

Acute overdosage (estrogen alone):

Numerous reports of ingestion of large doses of estrogen-containing oral contraceptives by young children indicate that acute serious ill effects do not occur. Overdosage of estrogen may cause nausea, and withdrawal bleeding may occur in females.

Acute simple overdosage (meprobamate alone): Death has been reported with ingestion of as little as 12 grams meprobamate and survival with as much as 40 grams.

Blood levels: 0.5—2.0 mg% represents the usual blood level range of meprobamate after therapeutic doses. The level may occasionally be as high as 3.0 mg%.

3—10 mg% usually corresponds to findings of mild-to-moderate symptoms of overdosage, such as stupor or light coma.

10—20 mg% usually corresponds to deeper coma, requiring more intensive treatment. Some fatalities occur.

At levels greater than 20 mg%, more fatalities than survivals can be expected.

Acute combined (alcohol or other CNS depressants or psychotropic drugs) Overdosage: Since effects can be additive, a history of ingestion of a low dose of meprobamate plus any of these compounds (or of a relatively low blood or tissue level) cannot be used as a prognostic indicator.

In cases where excessive doses have been taken, sleep ensues rapidly and blood pressure, pulse, and respiratory rates are reduced to basal levels. Any drug remaining in the stomach should be removed and symptomatic therapy given. Should respiration or blood pressure become compromised, respiratory assistance, central nervous system stimulants, and pressor agents should be administered cautiously as indicated. Meprobamate is metabolized in the liver and excreted by the kidney. Diuresis, osmotic (mannitol) diuresis, peritoneal dialysis, and hemodialysis have been used successfully. Careful monitoring of urinary output is necessary and caution should be taken to avoid overhydration. Relapse and death, after initial recovery, have been attributed to incomplete gastric emptying and delayed absorption. Meprobamate can be measured in biological fluids by two methods: colorimetric[42] and gas chromatographic.[43]

DOSAGE AND ADMINISTRATION

Given cyclically for short-term use only:

For the treatment of moderate-to-severe vasomotor symptoms of the menopause when anxiety and tension are part of the symptom complex and only in those cases in which the use of estrogens alone has not resulted in alleviation of such symptoms.

The lowest dose that will control symptoms should be chosen and medication should be discontinued as promptly as possible. The usual dosage of conjugated estrogen is 1.25 milligrams daily. The usual dosage of meprobamate is 1,200 to 1,600 milligrams daily.

Administration should be cyclic (eg, three weeks on and one week off).

Attempts to discontinue or taper medication should be made at three- to six-month intervals.

PMB® 200 & PMB® 400: The usual dosage is one tablet of either strength three times daily administered cyclically. Use of meprobamate during the rest period should be considered for those patients who may require continuing medication with tranquilizer. After the first few cycles of therapy, the patient's need for continuing the use of the meprobamate component should be re-evaluated.

Daily dosage should be adjusted to individual requirements. The daily dosage should not exceed 6 tablets of PMB 200 per day or 4 tablets of PMB 400 per day.

Treated patients with an intact uterus should be monitored closely for signs of endometrial cancer and appropriate diagnostic measures should be taken to rule out malignancy in the event of persistent or recurring abnormal vaginal bleeding.

HOW SUPPLIED

PMB® 200 [PREMARIN (conjugated estrogens, USP) with Meprobamate, USP] Tablets

Each oblong *green* tablet contains 0.45 mg PREMARIN and 200 mg meprobamate, in bottles of 60 (NDC 0046-0880-60).

PMB® 400 [PREMARIN (conjugated estrogens, USP) with Meprobamate, USP] Tablets

Each oblong *pink* tablet contains 0.45 mg PREMARIN and 400 mg meprobamate, in bottles of 60 (NDC 0046-0881-60).

The appearance of these tablets is a trademark of Wyeth-Ayerst Laboratories.

Store at room temperature (approximately 25°C).

PHYSICIAN REFERENCES

1. Ziel, H. K., *et al.*: N. Engl. J. Med. *293*:1167–1170, 1975.
2. Smith, D. C., *et al.*: N. Engl. J. Med. *293*:1164–1167, 1975.
3. Mack, T. M., *et al.*: N. Engl. J. Med. *294*:1262–1267, 1976.
4. Weiss, N. S., *et al.*: N. Engl. J. Med. *294*:1259–1262, 1976.
5. Herbst, A. L., *et al.*: N. Engl. J. Med. *284*:878–881, 1971.
6. Greenwald, P., *et al.*: N. Engl. J. Med. *285*:390–392, 1971.
7. Lanier, A., *et al.*: Mayo Clin. Proc. *48*:793–799, 1973.
8. Herbst, A., *et al.*: Obstet. Gynecol. *40*:287–298, 1972.
9. Herbst, A., *et al.*: Am. J. Obstet. Gynecol. *118*:607–615, 1974.
10. Herbst, A., *et al.*: N. Engl. J. Med. *292*:334–339, 1975.
11. Stafl, A., *et al.*: Obstet. Gynecol. *43*:118–128, 1974.
12. Sherman, A. I., *et al.*: Obstet. Gynecol. *44*:531–545, 1974.
13. Gal, I., *et al.*: Nature *216*:83, 1967.
14. Levy, E. P., *et al.*: Lancet *1*:611, 1973.
15. Nora, J., *et al.*: Lancet *1*:941–942, 1973.
16. Janerich, D. T., *et al.*: N. Engl. J. Med. *291*:697–700, 1974.
17. Boston Collaborative Drug Surveillance Program: N. Engl. J. Med. *290*:15–19, 1974.
18. Kaufman, D.W., *et al.*: J.A.M.A. 252:63–67, 1984.
19. Boston Collaborative Drug Surveillance Program: Lancet *1*:1399–1404, 1973.
20. Daniel, D. G., *et al.*: Lancet *2*:287–289, 1967.
21. The Veterans Administration Cooperative Urological Research Group: J. Urol. *98*:516–522, 1967.
22. Bailar, J. C.: Lancet *2*:560, 1967.
23. Blackard, C., *et al.*: Cancer *26*:249–256, 1970.
24. Royal College of General Practitioners: J. R. Coll. Gen. Pract. *13*:267–279, 1967.

24a. Royal College of General Practitioners: Oral Contraceptives and Health, New York, Pitman Corp., 1974.

25. Inman, W. H. W., *et al.*: Br. Med. J. *2*:193–199, 1968.
26. Vessey, M. P., *et al.*: Br. Med. J. *2*:651–657, 1969.
27. Sartwell, P. E., *et al.*: Am. J. Epidemiol. *90*:365–380, 1969.
28. Collaborative Group for the Study of Stroke in Young Women: N. Engl. J. Med. *288*:871–878, 1973.
29. Collaborative Group for the Study of Stroke in Young Women: J.A.M.A. *231*:718–722, 1975.
30. Mann, J. I., *et al.*: Br. Med. J. *2*:245–248, 1975.
31. Mann, J. I., *et al.*: Br. Med. J. *2*:241–245, 1975.
32. Inman, W. H. W., *et al.*: Br. Med. J. *2*:203–209, 1970.
33. Stolley, P. D., *et al.*: Am. J. Epidemiol. *102*:197–208, 1975.
34. Vessey, M. P., *et al.*: Br. Med. J. *3*:123–126, 1970.
35. Greene, G. R., *et al.*: Am. J. Public Health *62*:680–685, 1972.
36. Rosenberg, L., *et al.*: N. Engl. J. Med. *294*:1256–1259, 1976.
37. Coronary Drug Project Research Group: J.A.M.A. *214*:1303–1313, 1970.
38. Baum, J., *et al.*: Lancet *2*:926–928, 1973.
39. Mays, E. T., *et al.*: J.A.M.A. *235*:730–732, 1976.
40. Edmondson, H. A., *et al.*: N. Engl. J. Med. *294*:470–472, 1976.
41. Pfeffer, R. I., *et al.*: Am. J. Epidemiol. *103*:445–456, 1976.
42. Hoffman, A. J., *et al.*: J. Am. Pharm. Assoc. *48*:740, 1959.
43. Douglas, J. F., *et al.*: Anal. Chem. *39*:956, 1967.

INFORMATION FOR THE PATIENT

WHAT YOU SHOULD KNOW ABOUT ESTROGENS

Estrogens are female hormones produced by the ovaries. The ovaries make several different kinds of estrogens. In addition, scientists have been able to make a variety of synthetic estrogens. As far as we know, all these estrogens have similar properties and, therefore, much the same usefulness, side effects, and risks. This leaflet is intended to help you understand what estrogens are used for, the risks involved in their use, and how to use them as safely as possible.

This leaflet includes the most important information about estrogens, but not all the information. If you want to know more, you should ask your doctor for more information, or you can ask your doctor or pharmacist to let you read the package insert prepared for the doctor.

USES OF ESTROGEN

THERE IS NO PROPER USE OF ESTROGENS IN A PREGNANT WOMAN

Estrogens are prescribed by doctors for a number of purposes, including:

1. To provide estrogen during a period of adjustment when a woman's ovaries stop producing a majority of her estrogens, in order to prevent certain uncomfortable symptoms of estrogen deficiency. (With the menopause, which generally occurs between the ages of 45 and 55, women produce a much smaller amount of estrogens.)
2. To prevent symptoms of estrogen deficiency when a woman's ovaries have been removed surgically before the natural menopause.
3. To prevent pregnancy. (Estrogens are given along with a progestogen, another female hormone; these combinations are called oral contraceptives, or birth control pills. Patient labeling is available to women taking oral contraceptives and they will not be discussed in this leaflet.)
4. To treat certain cancers in women and men.
5. To prevent painful swelling of the breasts after pregnancy in women who choose not to nurse their babies.

ESTROGENS IN THE MENOPAUSE

In the natural course of their lives, all women eventually experience a decrease in estrogen production. This usually occurs between ages 45 and 55, but may occur earlier or later. Sometimes the ovaries may need to be removed before natural menopause by an operation, producing a "surgical menopause."

When the amount of estrogen in the blood begins to decrease, many women may develop typical symptoms: feelings of warmth in the face, neck, and chest or sudden intense episodes of heat and sweating throughout the body (called "hot flashes" or "hot flushes"). These symptoms are sometimes very uncomfortable. Some women may also develop changes in the vagina (called "atrophic vaginitis") that cause discomfort, especially during and after intercourse.

Estrogens can be prescribed to treat these symptoms of the menopause. It is estimated that considerably more than half of all women undergoing the menopause have only mild symptoms or no symptoms at all and therefore do not need estrogens. Other women may need estrogens for a few months, while their bodies adjust to lower estrogen levels. Sometimes the need will be for periods longer than six months. In an attempt to avoid overstimulation of the uterus (womb), estrogens are usually given cyclically during each month of use, such as three weeks of pills followed by one week without pills.

Sometimes women experience nervous symptoms or depression during menopause. There is no evidence that estrogens are effective for such symptoms without associated vasomotor symptoms. In the absence of vasomotor symptoms, estrogens should not be used to treat nervous symptoms, although other treatment may be needed.

You may have heard that taking estrogens for long periods (years) after the menopause will keep your skin soft and supple and keep you feeling young. There is no evidence that this is so, however, and such long-term treatment carries important risks.

ESTROGENS TO PREVENT SWELLING OF THE BREASTS AFTER PREGNANCY

If you do not breast-feed your baby after delivery, your breasts may fill up with milk and become painful and engorged. This usually begins about 3 to 4 days after delivery and may last for a few days to up to a week or more. Sometimes the discomfort is severe, but usually it is not and can be controlled by pain-relieving drugs such as aspirin and by binding the breasts up tightly. Estrogens can be used to try to prevent the breasts from filling up. While this treatment is sometimes successful, in many cases the breasts fill up to some degree in spite of treatment. The dose of estrogens needed to prevent pain and swelling of the breasts is much larger than the dose needed to treat symptoms of the menopause and this may increase your chances of developing blood clots in the legs or lungs (see below). Therefore, it is important that you discuss the benefits and the risks of estrogen use with your doctor if you have decided not to breast-feed your baby.

THE DANGERS OF ESTROGENS

1. *Endometrial cancer.* There are reports that if estrogens are used in the postmenopausal period for more than a year, there is an increased risk of *endometrial cancer* (cancer of the lining of the uterus). Women taking estrogens have roughly 5- to 10-times as great a chance of getting this cancer as women who take no estrogens. To put this another way, while a postmenopausal woman not taking estrogens has 1 chance in 1,000 each year of getting endometrial cancer, a woman taking estrogens has 5 to 10 chances in 1,000 each year. For this reason *it is important to take estrogens only when they are really needed.*

The risk of this cancer is greater the longer estrogens are used and when larger doses are taken. Therefore, you should not take more estrogen than your doctor prescribes. *It is important to take the lowest dose of estrogen that will control symptoms and to take it only as long as it is needed.* If estrogens are needed for longer periods of time, your doctor will want to re-evaluate your need for estrogens at least every six months.

Women using estrogens should report any vaginal bleeding to their doctors; such bleeding may be of no importance, but it can be an early warning of endometrial cancer. If you have undiagnosed vaginal bleeding, you should not use estrogens until a diagnosis is made and you are certain there is no endometrial cancer.

NOTE: If you have had your uterus removed (total hysterectomy), there is no danger of developing endometrial cancer.

2. *Other possible cancers.* Estrogens can cause development of other tumors in animals, such as tumors of the breast, cervix, vagina, or liver, when given for a long time. At present there is no good evidence that women using estrogen in the menopause have an increased risk of such tumors, but there is no way yet to be sure they do not; and one study raises the possibility that use of estrogens in the menopause may increase the risk of breast cancer many years later. This is a further reason to use estrogens only when clearly needed. While you are taking estrogens, it is important that you go to your doctor at least once a year for a physical examination. Also, if members of your family have had breast cancer or if you have breast nodules or abnormal mammograms (breast x-rays), your doctor may wish to carry out more frequent examinations of your breasts.

3. *Gallbladder disease.* Women who use estrogens after menopause are more likely to develop gallbladder disease needing surgery then women who do not use estrogens. Birth control pills have a similar effect.

4. *Abnormal blood clotting.* Oral contraceptives increase the risk of blood clotting in various parts of the body. This can result in a stroke (if the clot is in the brain), a heart attack (clot in a blood vessel of the heart), or a pulmonary embolus (a clot which forms in the legs or pelvis, then breaks off and travels to the lungs). Any of these can be fatal.

At this time, use of estrogens in the menopause is not known to cause such blood clotting, but this has not been fully studied and there could still prove to be such a risk. It is recommended that if you have had clotting in the legs or lungs, or a heart attack or stroke while you were using estrogens or birth control pills, you should not use estrogens (unless they are being used to treat cancer of the breast or prostate). If you have had a stroke or heart attack, or if you have angina pectoris, estrogens should be used with great caution and only if clearly needed (for example, if you have severe symptoms of the menopause).

The larger doses of estrogen used to prevent swelling of the breasts after pregnancy have been reported to cause clotting in the legs and lungs.

SPECIAL WARNING ABOUT PREGNANCY

You should not receive estrogen if you are pregnant. If this should occur, there is a greater than usual chance that the developing child will be born with a birth defect, although the possibility remains fairly small. A female child may have an increased risk of developing cancer of the vagina or cervix later in life (in the teens or twenties). Every possible effort should be made to avoid exposure to estrogens during pregnancy. If exposure occurs, see your doctor.

OTHER EFFECTS OF ESTROGENS

In addition to the serious known risks of estrogens described above, estrogens have the following side effects and potential risks:

1. *Nausea and vomiting.* The most common side effect of estrogen therapy is nausea. Vomiting is less common.

Continued on next page

Wyeth-Ayerst Laboratories—Cont.

2. *Effects on breasts.* Estrogens may cause breast tenderness or enlargement and may cause the breasts to secrete a liquid. These effects are not dangerous.

3. *Effects on the uterus.* Estrogens may cause benign fibroid tumors of the uterus to get larger.

4. *Effects on liver.* Women taking oral contraceptives develop, on rare occasions, a tumor of the liver which can rupture and bleed into the abdomen and may cause death. So far, these tumors have not been reported in women using estrogens in the menopause, but you should report any swelling or unusual pain or tenderness in the abdomen to your doctor immediately.

Women with a past history of jaundice (yellowing of the skin and white parts of the eyes) may get jaundice again during estrogen use. If this occurs, stop taking estrogens and see your doctor.

5. *Other effects.* Estrogens may cause excess fluids to be retained in the body. This may make some conditions worse, such as asthma, epilepsy, migraine, heart disease, or kidney disease.

SUMMARY

Estrogens have important uses, but they have serious risks as well. You must decide, with your doctor, whether the risks are acceptable to you in view of the benefits of treatment. Except where your doctor has prescribed estrogens for use in special cases of cancer of the breast or prostate, you should not use estrogens if you have cancer of the breast or uterus, are pregnant, have undiagnosed abnormal vaginal bleeding, clotting in the legs or lungs, or have had a stroke, heart attack or angina, or clotting in the legs or lungs in the past while you were taking estrogens.

You can use estrogens as safely as possible by understanding that your doctor will require regular physical examinations while you are taking them and will try to discontinue the drug as soon as possible and use the smallest dose possible. Be alert for signs of trouble including:

1. Abnormal bleeding from the vagina.
2. Pains in the calves or chest or sudden shortness of breath, or coughing blood.
3. Severe headache, dizziness, faintness, or changes in vision.
4. Breast lumps (you should ask your doctor how to examine your own breasts).
5. Jaundice (yellowing of the skin).
6. Mental depression.

Your doctor has prescribed this drug for you and you alone. Do not give the drug to anyone else.

Shown in Product Identification Section, page 437

PREMARIN® INTRAVENOUS　　　℞

[prĕm 'a-rĭn]
(conjugated estrogens, USP)
for Injection
Specially prepared for Intravenous &
Intramuscular use

CAUTION: Federal law prohibits dispensing without prescription.

1. ESTROGENS HAVE BEEN REPORTED TO INCREASE THE RISK OF ENDOMETRIAL CARCINOMA.

Three independent, case-controlled studies have reported an increased risk of endometrial cancer in postmenopausal women exposed to exogenous estrogens for more than one year.[1-3] This risk was independent of the other known risk factors for endometrial cancer. These studies are further supported by the finding that incidence rates of endometrial cancer have increased sharply since 1969 in eight different areas of the United States with population-based cancer-reporting systems, an increase which may be related to the rapidly expanding use of estrogens during the last decade.[4]

The three case-controlled studies reported that the risk of endometrial cancer in estrogen users was about 4.5 to 13.9 times greater than in nonusers. The risk appears to depend on both duration of treatment[1] and on estrogen dose.[3] In view of these findings, when estrogens are used for the treatment of menopausal symptoms, the lowest dose that will control symptoms should be utilized and medication should be discontinued as soon as possible. When prolonged treatment is medically indicated, the patient should be reassessed, on at least a semi-annual basis, to determine the need for continued therapy. Although the evidence must be considered preliminary, one study suggests that cyclic administration of low doses of estrogen may carry less risk than continuous administration.[3] It therefore appears prudent to utilize such a regimen.

Close clinical surveillance of all women taking estrogens is important. In all cases of undiagnosed persistent or recurring abnormal vaginal bleeding, adequate diagnostic measures should be undertaken to rule out malignancy.

There is no evidence at present that "natural" estrogens are more or less hazardous than "synthetic" estrogens at equi-estrogenic doses.

2. ESTROGENS SHOULD NOT BE USED DURING PREGNANCY.

The use of female sex hormones, both estrogens and progestogens, during early pregnancy may seriously damage the offspring. It has been shown that females exposed *in utero* to diethylstilbestrol, a nonsteroidal estrogen, have an increased risk of developing, in later life, a form of vaginal or cervical cancer that is ordinarily extremely rare.[5,6] This risk has been estimated as not greater than 4 per 1,000 exposures.[7] Furthermore, a high percentage of such exposed women (from 30% to 90%) have been found to have vaginal adenosis,[8-12] epithelial changes of the vagina and cervix. Although these changes are histologically benign, it is not known whether they are precursors of malignancy. Although similar data are not available with the use of other estrogens, it cannot be presumed they would not induce similar changes.

Several reports suggest an association between intrauterine exposure to female sex hormones and congenital anomalies, including congenital heart defects and limb-reduction defects.[13-16] One case-controlled study[16] estimated a 4.7-fold increased risk of limb-reduction defects in infants exposed *in utero* to sex hormones (oral contraceptives, hormone withdrawal tests for pregnancy, or attempted treatment for threatened abortion). Some of these exposures were very short and involved only a few days of treatment. The data suggest that the risk of limb-reduction defects in exposed fetuses is somewhat less than 1 per 1,000.

In the past, female sex hormones have been used during pregnancy in an attempt to treat threatened or habitual abortion. There is considerable evidence that estrogens are ineffective for these indications, and there is no evidence from well-controlled studies that progestogens are effective for these uses.

If PREMARIN Intravenous (conjugated estrogens, USP) for injection is used during pregnancy, or if the patient becomes pregnant while taking this drug, she should be apprised of the potential risks to the fetus, and the advisability of pregnancy continuation.

DESCRIPTION

Each Secule® vial contains 25 mg of conjugated estrogens, USP, in a sterile lyophilized cake which also contains lactose 200 mg, sodium citrate 12.2 mg and simethicone 0.2 mg. The pH is adjusted with sodium hydroxide or hydrochloric acid. A sterile diluent (5 mL) containing 2% benzyl alcohol in sterile water is provided for reconstitution. The reconstituted solution is suitable for intravenous or intramuscular injection.

PREMARIN (conjugated estrogens, USP) is a mixture of estrogens obtained exclusively from natural sources, occurring as the sodium salts of water-soluble estrogen sulfates blended to represent the average composition of material derived from pregnant mares' urine. It contains estrone, equilin, and 17 α-dihydroequilin, together with smaller amounts of 17 α-estradiol, equilenin, and 17 α-dihydroequilenin as salts of their sulfate esters.

CLINICAL PHARMACOLOGY

Estrogens are important in the development and maintenance of the female reproductive system and secondary sex characteristics. They promote growth and development of the vagina, uterus, and fallopian tubes, and enlargement of the breasts. Indirectly, they contribute to: the shaping of the skeleton; maintenance of tone and elasticity of urogenital structures; changes in the epiphyses of the long bones that allow for the pubertal growth spurt and its termination; growth of axillary and pubic hair; and pigmentation of the nipples and genitals. Decline of estrogenic activity at the end of the menstrual cycle can bring on menstruation, although the cessation of progesterone secretion is the most important factor in the mature ovulatory cycle. However, in the preovulatory or nonovulatory cycle, estrogen is the primary determinant in the onset of menstruation. Estrogens also affect the release of pituitary gonadotropins.

The pharmacologic effects of conjugated estrogens are similar to those of endogenous estrogens. They are soluble in water and may be administered by intravenous or intramuscular injection.

In responsive tissues (female genital organs, breasts, hypothalamus, pituitary) estrogens enter the cell and are transported into the nucleus. As a result of estrogen action, specific RNA and protein synthesis occurs.

Metabolism and inactivation occur primarily in the liver. Some estrogens are excreted into the bile; however, they are reabsorbed from the intestine and returned to the liver through the portal venous system. Water-soluble estrogen conjugates are strongly acidic and, therefore, ionized in body fluids, which favor excretion through the kidneys since tubular reabsorption is minimal.

INDICATION

PREMARIN Intravenous (conjugated estrogens, USP, for injection) is indicated in the treatment of abnormal uterine bleeding due to hormonal imbalance in the absence of organic pathology.

CONTRAINDICATIONS

Estrogens should not be used in women with any of the following conditions:
1. Known or suspected cancer of the breast, except in appropriately selected patients being treated for metastatic disease.
2. Known or suspected estrogen-dependent neoplasia.
3. Known or suspected pregnancy (see Boxed Warning).
4. Undiagnosed abnormal genital bleeding.
5. Active thrombophlebitis or thromboembolic disorders.
6. A past history of thrombophlebitis, thrombosis, or thromboembolic disorders associated with previous estrogen use (except when used in treatment of breast malignancy).

WARNINGS

1. *Induction of malignant neoplasms.* Long-term, continuous administration of natural and synthetic estrogens in certain animal species increases the frequency of carcinomas of the breast, cervix, vagina, and liver. There are now reports that estrogens increase the risk of carcinoma of the endometrium in humans (see Boxed Warning).

At the present time there is no satisfactory evidence that estrogens given to postmenopausal women increase the risk of cancer of the breast,[17] although a recent long-term follow-up of a single physician's practice has raised this possibility.[18] Because of the animal data, there is a need for caution in prescribing estrogens for women with a strong family history of breast cancer, or who have breast nodules, fibrocystic disease, or abnormal mammograms.

2. *Gallbladder disease.* A recent study has reported a 2- to 3-fold increase in the risk of surgically confirmed gallbladder disease in women receiving postmenopausal estrogens,[17] similar to the 2-fold increase previously noted in users of oral contraceptives.[19,24a]

3. *Effects similar to those caused by estrogen-progestogen oral contraceptives.* There are several serious adverse effects of oral contraceptives, most of which have not, up to now, been documented as consequences of postmenopausal estrogen therapy. This may reflect the comparatively low doses of estrogen used in postmenopausal women. It would be expected that the larger doses of estrogen used to treat prostatic or breast cancer are more likely to result in these adverse effects, and, in fact, it has been shown that there is an increased risk of thrombosis in men receiving estrogens for prostatic cancer.[20-23]

a. *Thromboembolic disease.* It is now well established that users of oral contraceptives have an increased risk of various thromboembolic and thrombotic vascular diseases, such as thrombophlebitis, pulmonary embolism, stroke, and myocardial infarction.[24-31] Cases of retinal thrombosis, mesenteric thrombosis, and optic neuritis have been reported in oral-contraceptive users. There is evidence that the risk of several of these adverse reactions is related to the dose of the drug.[32,33] An increased risk of postsurgery thromboembolic complications has also been reported in users of oral contraceptives.[34,35] If feasible, estrogen should be discontinued at least 4 weeks before surgery of the type associated with an increased risk of thromboembolism, or during periods of prolonged immobilization.

While an increased rate of thromboembolic and thrombotic disease in postmenopausal users of estrogens has not been found,[17-24,25-36] this does not rule out the possibility that such an increase may be present, or that subgroups of women who have underlying risk factors, or who are receiving relatively large doses of estrogens, may have increased risk. Therefore estrogens should not be used in persons with active thrombophlebitis or thromboembolic disorders, and they should not be used (except in treatment of malignancy) in persons with a history of such disorders in association with estrogen use. They should be used with caution in patients with cerebral vascular or coronary artery disease and only for those in whom estrogens are clearly needed.

Large doses of estrogen (5 mg conjugated estrogens per day), comparable to those used to treat cancer of the prostate and breast, have been shown in a large prospective clinical trial in men[37] to increase the risk of nonfatal myocardial infarction, pulmonary embolism, and thrombophlebitis. When estrogen doses of this size are used, any of the thromboembolic and thrombotic adverse effects associated with oral-contraceptive use should be considered a clear risk.

b. *Hepatic adenoma.* Benign hepatic adenomas appear to be associated with the use of oral contraceptives.[38-40] Although benign, and rare, these may rupture and may cause death through intra-abdominal hemorrhage. Such lesions have not yet been reported in association with other estrogen or progestogen preparations but should be considered in estrogen users having abdominal pain and tenderness, abdomi-

nal mass, or hypovolemic shock. Hepatocellular carcinoma has also been reported in women taking estrogen-containing oral contraceptives.[39] The relationship of this malignancy to these drugs is not known at this time.

c. *Elevated blood pressure.* Women using oral contraceptives sometimes experience increased blood pressure which, in most cases, returns to normal on discontinuing the drug. There is now a report that this may occur with use of estrogens in the menopause[41] and blood pressure should be monitored with estrogen use, especially if high doses are used.

d. *Glucose tolerance.* A worsening of glucose tolerance has been observed in a significant percentage of patients on estrogen-containing oral contraceptives. For this reason, diabetic patients should be carefully observed while receiving estrogen.

4. *Hypercalcemia.* Administration of estrogens may lead to severe hypercalcemia in patients with breast cancer and bone metastases. If this occurs, the drug should be stopped and appropriate measures taken to reduce the serum calcium level.

PRECAUTIONS

A. General Precautions.

1. A complete medical and family history should be taken prior to the initiation of any estrogen therapy. The pretreatment and periodic physical examinations should include special reference to blood pressure, breasts, abdomen, and pelvic organs, and should include a Papanicolaou smear. As a general rule, estrogen should not be prescribed for longer than one year without another physical examination being performed.

2. Fluid retention—Because estrogens may cause some degree of fluid retention, conditions which might be influenced by this factor such as asthma, epilepsy, migraine, and cardiac or renal dysfunction, require careful observation.

3. Certain patients may develop undesirable manifestations of excessive estrogenic stimulation, such as abnormal or excessive uterine bleeding, mastodynia, etc.

4. Oral contraceptives appear to be associated with an increased incidence of mental depression.[24a] Although it is not clear whether this is due to the estrogenic or progestogenic component of the contraceptive, patients with a history of depression should be carefully observed.

5. Pre-existing uterine leiomyomata may increase in size during estrogen use.

6. The pathologist should be advised of estrogen therapy when relevant specimens are submitted.

7. Patients with a past history of jaundice during pregnancy have an increased risk of recurrence of jaundice while receiving estrogen-containing oral contraceptive therapy. If jaundice develops in any patient receiving estrogen, the medication should be discontinued while the cause is investigated.

8. Estrogens may be poorly metabolized in patients with impaired liver function and they should be administered with caution in such patients.

9. Because estrogens influence the metabolism of calcium and phosphorus, they should be used with caution in patients with metabolic bone diseases that are associated with hypercalcemia or in patients with renal insufficiency.

10. Because of the effects of estrogens on epiphyseal closure, they should be used judiciously in young patients in whom bone growth is not yet complete.

11. Certain endocrine and liver function tests may be affected by estrogen-containing oral contraceptives. The following similar changes may be expected with larger doses of estrogen:

a. Increased sulfobromophthalein retention.

b. Increased prothrombin and factors VII, VIII, IX, and X; decreased antithrombin 3; increased norepinephrine-induced platelet aggregability.

c. Increased thyroid binding globulin (TBG) leading to increased circulating total thyroid hormone, as measured by PBI, T4 by column, or T4 by radioimmunoassay. Free T3 resin uptake is decreased, reflecting the elevated TBG; free T4 concentration is unaltered.

d. Impaired glucose tolerance.

e. Decreased pregnanediol excretion.

f. Reduced response to metyrapone test.

g. Reduced serum folate concentration.

h. Increased serum triglyceride and phospholipid concentration.

B. Information for the Patient. (See text which appears after the PHYSICIAN REFERENCES.)

C. Pregnancy Category X. (See CONTRAINDICATIONS and Boxed Warning.)

D. Nursing Mothers. As a general principle, the administration of any drug to nursing mothers should be done only when clearly necessary, since many drugs are excreted in human milk.

ADVERSE REACTIONS

(See WARNINGS regarding induction of neoplasia, adverse effects on the fetus, increased incidence of gallbladder disease, and adverse effects similar to those of oral contraceptives, including thromboembolism.) The following additional adverse reactions have been reported with estrogenic therapy, including oral contraceptives:

1. *Genitourinary system:* Breakthrough bleeding, spotting, change in menstrual flow; dysmenorrhea; premenstrual-like syndrome; amenorrhea during and after treatment; increase in size of uterine fibromyomata; vaginal candidiasis; change in cervical erosion and in degree of cervical secretion; cystitis-like syndrome.

2. *Breasts:* Tenderness, enlargement, secretion.

3. *Gastrointestinal:* Nausea, vomiting; abdominal cramps, bloating; cholestatic jaundice.

4. *Skin:* Chloasma or melasma which may persist when drug is discontinued; erythema multiforme; erythema nodosum; hemorrhagic eruption; loss of scalp hair; hirsutism.

5. *Eyes:* Steepening of corneal curvature; intolerance to contact lenses.

6. *CNS:* Headache, migraine, dizziness; mental depression; chorea.

7. *Miscellaneous:* Increase or decrease in weight; reduced carbohydrate tolerance; aggravation of porphyria; edema; changes in libido.

ACUTE OVERDOSAGE

Numerous reports of ingestion of large doses of estrogen-containing oral contraceptives by young children indicate that acute serious ill effects do not occur. Overdosage of estrogen may cause nausea, and withdrawal bleeding may occur in females.

DOSAGE AND ADMINISTRATION

Abnormal uterine bleeding due to hormonal imbalance: One 25 mg injection, intravenously or intramuscularly. Intravenous use is preferred since more rapid response can be expected from this mode of administration.

Repeat in 6 to 12 hours if necessary. The use of PREMARIN Intravenous (conjugated estrogens, USP) for injection does not preclude the advisability of other appropriate measures. The usual precautionary measures governing intravenous administration should be adhered to. Injection should be made SLOWLY to obviate the occurrence of flushes.

Infusion of PREMARIN Intravenous (conjugated estrogens, USP) for injection with other agents is not generally recommended. In emergencies, however, when an infusion has already been started it may be expedient to make the injection into the tubing just distal to the infusion needle. If so used, compatibility of solutions must be considered.

Compatibility of solutions: PREMARIN Intravenous is compatible with normal saline, dextrose, and invert sugar solutions. IT IS NOT COMPATIBLE WITH PROTEIN HYDROLYSATE, ASCORBIC ACID, OR ANY SOLUTION WITH AN ACID pH.

Treated patients with an intact uterus should be monitored closely for signs of endometrial cancer, and appropriate diagnostic measures should be taken to rule out malignancy in the event of persistent or recurring abnormal vaginal bleeding.

DIRECTIONS FOR STORAGE AND RECONSTITUTION:

Storage before reconstitution: Store package in refrigerator, 2°–8°C (36°–46°F).

To reconstitute: First withdraw air from Secule® vial so as to facilitate introduction of sterile diluent. Then, flow the sterile diluent slowly against side of Secule® vial and agitate gently. DO NOT SHAKE VIOLENTLY.

Storage after reconstitution: It is common practice to utilize the reconstituted solution within a few hours. If it is necessary to keep the reconstituted solution for more than a few hours, store the reconstituted solution under refrigeration (2°–8°C). Under these conditions, the solution is stable for 60 days, and is suitable for use unless darkening or precipitation occurs.

HOW SUPPLIED

NDC 0046-0749-05—Each package provides: (1) One Secule® vial containing 25 mg of conjugated estrogens, USP, for injection (also lactose 200 mg, sodium citrate 12.2 mg, and simethicone 0.2 mg). The pH is adjusted with sodium hydroxide or hydrochloric acid. (2) One 5 mL ampul sterile diluent with 2% benzyl alcohol in sterile water. PREMARIN Intravenous (conjugated estrogens, USP) for injection is prepared by cryodesiccation.

Secule®—Registered trademark to designate a vial containing an injectable preparation in dry form.

PHYSICIAN REFERENCES

1. Ziel, H. K., et al.: N. Engl. J. Med. *293* :1167–1170, 1975.
2. Smith, D. C., et al.: N. Engl. J. Med. *293* :1164–1167, 1975.
3. Mack, T. M., et al.: N. Engl. J. Med. *294* :1262–1267, 1976.
4. Weiss, N. S., et al.: N. Engl. J. Med. *294* :1259–1262, 1976.
5. Herbst, A. L., et al.: N. Engl. J. Med. *284* :878–881, 1971.
6. Greenwald, P., et al.: N. Engl. J. Med. *285* :390–392, 1971.
7. Lanier, A., et al.: Mayo Clin. Proc. *48* :793–799, 1973.
8. Herbst, A., et al.: Obstet. Gynecol. *40* :287–298, 1972.
9. Herbst, A., et al.: Am. J. Obstet. Gynecol. *118* :607–615, 1974.
10. Herbst, A., et al.: N. Engl. J. Med. *292* :334–339, 1975.
11. Stafl, A., et al.: Obstet. Gynecol. *43* :118–128, 1974.
12. Sherman, A. I., et al.: Obstet. Gynecol. *44* :531–545, 1974.
13. Gal, I., et al.: Nature *216* :83, 1967.
14. Levy, E. P., et al.: Lancet *1* :611, 1973.
15. Nora, J., et al.: Lancet *1* :941–942, 1973.
16. Janerich, D. T., et al.: N. Engl. J. Med. *291* :697–700, 1974.
17. Boston Collaborative Drug Surveillance Program: N. Engl. J. Med. *290* :15–19, 1974.
18. Hoover, R., et al.: N. Engl. J. Med. *295* :401–405, 1976.
19. Boston Collaborative Drug Surveillance Program: Lancet *1* :1399–1404, 1973.
20. Daniel, D. G., et al.: Lancet *2* :287–289, 1967.
21. The Veterans Administration Cooperative Urological Research Group: J. Urol. *98* :516–522, 1967.
22. Bailar, J. C.: Lancet *2* :560, 1967.
23. Blackard, C., et al.: Cancer *26* :249–256, 1970.
24. Royal College of General Practitioners: J. R. Coll. Gen. Pract. *13* :267–279, 1967.
24a. Royal College of General Practitioners: Oral Contraceptives and Health, New York, Pitman Corp., 1974.
25. Inman, W. H. W., et al.: Br. Med. J. *2* :193–199, 1968.
26. Vessey, M. P., et al.: Br. Med. J. *2* :651–657, 1969.
27. Sartwell, P. E., et al.: Am. J. Epidemiol. *90* :365–380, 1969.
28. Collaborative Group for the Study of Stroke in Young Women: N. Engl. J. Med. *288* :871–878, 1973.
29. Collaborative Group for the Study of Stroke in Young Women: J.A.M.A. *231* :718–722, 1975.
30. Mann, J. I., et al.: Br. Med. J. *2* :245–248, 1975.
31. Mann, J. I., et al.: Br. Med. J. *2* :241–245, 1975.
32. Inman, W. H. W., et al.: Br. Med. J. *2* :203–209, 1970.
33. Stolley, P. D., et al.: Am. J. Epidemiol. *102* :197–208, 1975.
34. Vessey, M. P., et al.: Br. Med. J. *3* :123–126, 1970.
35. Greene, G. R., et al.: Am. J. Public Health *62* :680–685, 1972.
36. Rosenberg, L., et al.: N. Engl. J. Med. *294* :1256–1259, 1976.
37. Coronary Drug Project Research Group: J.A.M.A. *214* :1303–1313, 1970.
38. Baum, J., et al.: Lancet *2* :926–928, 1973.
39. Mays, E. T., et al.: J.A.M.A. *235* :730–732, 1976.
40. Edmondson, H. A., et al.: N. Engl. J. Med. *294* :470–472, 1976.
41. Pfeffer, R. I., et al.: Am. J. Epidemiol. *103* :445–456, 1976.

INFORMATION FOR THE PATIENT

WHAT YOU SHOULD KNOW ABOUT ESTROGENS

Estrogens are female hormones produced by the ovaries. The ovaries make several different kinds of estrogens. In addition, scientists have been able to make a variety of synthetic estrogens. As far as we know, all these estrogens have similar properties and, therefore, much the same usefulness, side effects, and risks. This leaflet is intended to help you understand what estrogens are used for, the risks involved in their use, and how to use them as safely as possible.

This leaflet includes the most important information about estrogens, but not all the information. If you want to know more, you should ask your doctor for more information, or you can ask your doctor or pharmacist to let you read the package insert prepared for the doctor.

USES OF ESTROGEN

THERE IS NO PROPER USE OF ESTROGENS IN A PREGNANT WOMAN.

Estrogens are prescribed by doctors for a number of purposes, including:

1. To provide estrogen during a period of adjustment when a woman's ovaries stop producing a majority of her estrogens, in order to prevent certain uncomfortable symptoms of estrogen deficiency. (With the menopause, which generally occurs between the ages of 45 and 55, women produce a much smaller amount of estrogens.)

2. To prevent symptoms of estrogen deficiency when a woman's ovaries have been removed surgically before the natural menopause.

3. To prevent pregnancy. (Estrogens are given along with a progestogen, another female hormone; these combinations are called oral contraceptives, or birth control pills. Patient labeling is available to women taking oral contraceptives and they will not be discussed in this leaflet.)

4. To treat certain cancers in women and men.

ESTROGENS IN THE MENOPAUSE

In the natural course of their lives, all women eventually experience a decrease in estrogen production. This usually

Continued on next page

Wyeth-Ayerst Laboratories—Cont.

occurs between ages 45 and 55, but may occur earlier or later. Sometimes the ovaries may need to be removed before natural menopause by an operation, producing a "surgical menopause."

When the amount of estrogen in the blood begins to decrease, many women may develop typical symptoms: feelings of warmth in the face, neck, and chest, or sudden intense episodes of heat and sweating throughout the body (called "hot flashes" or "hot flushes"). These symptoms are sometimes very uncomfortable. Some women may also develop changes in the vagina (called "atrophic vaginitis") that cause discomfort, especially during and after intercourse.

Estrogens can be prescribed to treat these symptoms of the menopause. It is estimated that considerably more than half of all women undergoing the menopause have only mild symptoms or no symptoms at all and, therefore, do not need estrogens. Other women may need estrogens for a few months, while their bodies adjust to lower estrogen levels. Sometimes the need will be for periods longer than six months. In an attempt to avoid overstimulation of the uterus (womb), estrogens are usually given cyclically during each month of use, such as three weeks of pills followed by one week without pills.

Sometimes women experience nervous symptoms or depression during menopause. There is no evidence that estrogens are effective for such symptoms without associated vasomotor symptoms. In the absence of vasomotor symptoms, estrogens should not be used to treat nervous symptoms, although other treatment may be needed.

You may have heard that taking estrogens for long periods (years) after the menopause will keep your skin soft and supple and keep you feeling young. There is no evidence that this is so, however, and such long-term treatment carries important risks.

THE DANGERS OF ESTROGENS

1. *Endometrial cancer.* There are reports that if estrogens are used in the postmenopausal period for more than a year, there is an increased risk of *endometrial cancer* (cancer of the lining of the uterus). Women taking estrogens have roughly 5- to 10-times as great a chance of getting this cancer as women who take no estrogens. To put this another way, while a postmenopausal woman not taking estrogens has 1 chance in 1,000 each year of getting endometrial cancer, a woman taking estrogens has 5 to 10 chances in 1,000 each year. For this reason *it is important to take estrogens only when they are really needed.*

The risk of this cancer is greater the longer estrogens are used and when larger doses are taken. Therefore, you should not take more estrogen than your doctor prescribes. *It is important to take the lowest dose of estrogen that will control symptoms and to take it only as long as it is needed.* If estrogens are needed for longer periods of time, your doctor will want to reevaluate your need for estrogens at least every six months.

Women using estrogens should report any vaginal bleeding to their doctors; such bleeding may be of no importance, but it can be an early warning of endometrial cancer. If you have undiagnosed vaginal bleeding, you should not use estrogens until a diagnosis is made and you are certain there is no endometrial cancer.

NOTE: If you have had your uterus removed (total hysterectomy), there is no danger of developing endometrial cancer.

2. *Other possible cancers.* Estrogens can cause development of other tumors in animals, such as tumors of the breast, cervix, vagina, or liver, when given for a long time. At present there is no good evidence that women using estrogen in the menopause have an increased risk of such tumors, but there is no way yet to be sure they do not; and one study raises the possibility that use of estrogens in the menopause may increase the risk of breast cancer many years later. This is a further reason to use estrogens only when clearly needed. While you are taking estrogens, it is important that you go to your doctor at least once a year for a physical examination. Also, if members of your family have had breast cancers, or if you have breast nodules, or abnormal mammograms (breast Xrays), your doctor may wish to carry out more frequent examinations of your breasts.

3. *Gallbladder disease.* Women who use estrogens after menopause are more likely to develop gallbladder disease needing surgery than women who do not use estrogens. Birth-control pills have a similar effect.

4. *Abnormal blood clotting.* Oral contraceptives increase the risk of blood clotting in various parts of the body. This can result in a stroke (if the clot is in the brain), a heart attack (a clot in a blood vessel of the heart), or a pulmonary embolus (a clot which forms in the legs or pelvis, then breaks off and travels to the lungs). Any of these can be fatal. At this time, use of estrogens in the menopause is not known to cause such blood clotting, but this has not been fully studied and there could still prove to be such a risk. It is recommended that if you have had clotting in the legs or lungs, or a

heart attack or stroke, while you were using estrogens or birth control pills, you should not use estrogens (unless they are being used to treat cancer of the breast or prostate). If you have had a stroke or heart attack, or if you have angina pectoris, estrogens should be used with great caution and only if clearly needed (for example, if you have severe symptoms of the menopause).

SPECIAL WARNING ABOUT PREGNANCY

You should not receive estrogen if you are pregnant. If this should occur, there is a greater than usual chance that the developing child will be born with a birth defect, although the possibility remains fairly small. A female child may have an increased risk of developing cancer of the vagina or cervix later in life (in the teens or twenties). Every possible effort should be made to avoid exposure to estrogens during pregnancy. If exposure occurs, see your doctor.

OTHER EFFECTS OF ESTROGENS

In addition to the serious known risks of estrogens described above, estrogens have the following side effects and potential risks:

1. *Nausea and vomiting.* The most common side effect of estrogen therapy is nausea. Vomiting is less common.
2. *Effects on breasts.* Estrogens may cause breast tenderness or enlargement and may cause the breasts to secrete a liquid. These effects are not dangerous.
3. *Effects on the uterus.* Estrogens may cause benign fibroid tumors of the uterus to get larger.
4. *Effects on liver.* Women taking oral contraceptives develop, on rare occasions, a tumor of the liver which can rupture and bleed into the abdomen and may cause death. So far, these tumors have not been reported in women using estrogens in the menopause, but you should report any swelling or unusual pain or tenderness in the abdomen to your doctor immediately.

Women with a past history of jaundice (yellowing of the skin and white parts of the eyes) may get jaundice again during estrogen use. If this occurs, stop taking estrogens and see your doctor.

5. *Other effects.* Estrogens may cause excess fluid to be retained in the body. This may make some conditions worse, such as asthma, epilepsy, migraine, heart disease, or kidney disease.

SUMMARY

Estrogens have important uses, but they have serious risks as well. You must decide, with your doctor, whether the risks are acceptable to you in view of the benefits of treatment. Except where your doctor has prescribed estrogens for use in special cases of cancer of the breast or prostate, you should not use estrogens if you have cancer of the breast or uterus, are pregnant, have undiagnosed abnormal vaginal bleeding, clotting in the legs or lungs, or have had a stroke, heart attack or angina, or clotting in the legs or lungs in the past while you were taking estrogens.

You can use estrogens as safely as possible by understanding that your doctor will require regular physical examinations while you are taking them, will try to discontinue the drug as soon as possible, and use the smallest dose possible. Be alert for signs of trouble including:

1. Abnormal bleeding from the vagina.
2. Pains in the calves or chest, or sudden shortness of breath, or coughing blood.
3. Severe headache, dizziness, faintness, or changes in vision.
4. Breast lumps (you should ask your doctor how to examine your own breasts).
5. Jaundice (yellowing of the skin).
6. Mental depression.

Your doctor has prescribed this drug for you and you alone. Do not give the drug to anyone else.

HOW SUPPLIED

PREMARIN® (conjugated estrogens tablets, USP) tablets for oral administration.

PREMARIN® VAGINAL CREAM—PREMARIN® in a nonliquefying base, designed for vaginal use.

PREMARIN® with METHYLTESTOSTERONE—a combination of PREMARIN® and methyltestosterone (an androgen) in tablet form for oral administration.

PMB® 200, 400—a combination of PREMARIN® and meprobamate (a tranquilizing agent) in tablet form for oral administration.

PREMARIN® INTRAVENOUS—PREMARIN® specially prepared for intravenous and intramuscular use.

ESTROGENIC SUBSTANCE (estrone) in Aqueous Suspension—a sterile aqueous suspension of estrone, a short-acting estrogen, for intramuscular injection only.

PREMARIN®   ℞

[prĕm 'a-rĭn]
(conjugated estrogens tablets, USP)

CAUTION: Federal law prohibits dispensing without prescription.

> 1. ESTROGENS HAVE BEEN REPORTED TO INCREASE THE RISK OF ENDOMETRIAL CARCINOMA IN POSTMENOPAUSAL WOMEN.
> Close clinical surveillance of all women taking estrogens is important. Adequate diagnostic measures, including endometrial sampling when indicated, should be undertaken to rule out malignancy in all cases of undiagnosed persistent or recurring abnormal vaginal bleeding. There is currently no evidence that "natural" estrogens are more or less hazardous than "synthetic" estrogens at equiestrogenic doses.
> 2. ESTROGENS SHOULD NOT BE USED DURING PREGNANCY.
> Estrogen therapy during pregnancy is associated with an increased risk of congenital defects in the reproductive organs of the male and female fetus, an increased risk of vaginal adenosis, squamous-cell dysplasia of the uterine cervix, and vaginal cancer in the female later in life. The 1985 DES Task Force concluded that women who used DES during their pregnancies may subsequently experience an increased risk of breast cancer. However, a causal relationship is still unproven, and the observed level of risk is similar to that for a number of other breast-cancer risk factors.
> There is no indication for estrogen therapy during pregnancy. Estrogens are ineffective for the prevention or treatment of threatened or habitual abortion.

DESCRIPTION

PREMARIN (conjugated estrogens tablets, USP) for oral administration contains a mixture of estrogens obtained exclusively from natural sources, occurring as the sodium salts of water-soluble estrogen sulfates blended to represent the average composition of material derived from pregnant mares' urine. It contains estrone, equilin, and 17 α-dihydroequilin, together with smaller amounts of 17 α-estradiol, equilenin, and 17 α-dihydroequilenin as salts of their sulfate esters. Tablets for oral administration are available in 0.3 mg, 0.625 mg, 0.9 mg, 1.25 mg, and 2.5 mg strengths of conjugated estrogens.

PREMARIN Tablets contain the following inactive ingredients: calcium phosphate tribasic, calcium sulfate anhydrous, carnauba wax, glyceryl mono-oleate, lactose, magnesium stearate, methylcellulose, microcrystalline cellulose, pharmaceutical glaze, polyethylene glycol, stearic acid, sucrose, talc, titanium dioxide.

—0.3 mg tablets also contain: D&C Yellow No. 10, FD&C Blue No. 1, FD&C Yellow No. 6;
—0.625 mg tablets also contain: FD&C Blue No. 2, D&C Red No. 27, FD&C Red No. 40;
—0.9 mg tablets also contain: D&C Red No. 6, D&C Red No. 7, polysorbate 20;
—1.25 mg tablets also contain: black iron oxide, D&C Yellow No. 10, FD&C Yellow No. 6;
—2.5 mg tablets also contain: FD&C Blue No. 2, D&C Red No. 7.

CLINICAL PHARMACOLOGY

Estrogens are important in the development and maintenance of the female reproductive system and secondary sex characteristics. They promote growth and development of the vagina, uterus, and fallopian tubes, and enlargement of the breasts. Indirectly, they contribute to the shaping of the skeleton, maintenance of tone and elasticity of urogenital structures, changes in the epiphyses of the long bones that allow for the pubertal growth spurt and its termination, growth of axillary and pubic hair, and pigmentation of the nipples and genitals. Decline of estrogenic activity at the end of the menstrual cycle can bring on menstruation, although the cessation of progesterone secretion is the most important factor in the mature ovulatory cycle. However, in the preovulatory or nonovulatory cycle, estrogen is the primary determinant in the onset of menstruation. Estrogens also affect the release of pituitary gonadotropins.

The pharmacologic effects of conjugated estrogens are similar to those of endogenous estrogens. They are soluble in water and are well absorbed from the gastrointestinal tract. In responsive tissues (female genital organs, breasts, hypothalamus, pituitary) estrogens enter the cell and are transported into the nucleus. As a result of estrogen action, specific RNA and protein synthesis occurs.

Metabolism and inactivation occur primarily in the liver. Some estrogens are excreted into the bile; however, they are reabsorbed from the intestine and returned to the liver through the portal venous system. Water-soluble estrogen conjugates are strongly acidic and are ionized in body fluids,

which favor excretion through the kidneys since tubular reabsorption is minimal.

INDICATIONS AND USAGE

PREMARIN (conjugated estrogens tablets, USP) is indicated in the treatment of:

1. Moderate to severe vasomotor symptoms associated with the menopause. There is no adequate evidence that estrogens are effective for nervous symptoms or depression which might occur during menopause and they should not be used to treat these conditions.
2. Atrophic vaginitis.
3. Atrophic urethritis.
4. Osteoporosis (loss of bone mass). The mainstays of prevention and management of osteoporosis are estrogen and calcium; exercise and nutrition may be important adjuncts. Estrogen replacement therapy is the most effective single modality for the prevention of osteoporosis in women. Estrogen reduces bone resorption and retards or halts postmenopausal bone loss. Case-controlled studies have shown an approximately 60-percent reduction in hip and wrist fractures in women whose estrogen replacement was begun within a few years of menopause. Studies also suggest that estrogen reduces the rate of vertebral fractures. Even when started as late as 6 years after menopause, estrogen prevents further loss of bone mass but does not restore it to premenopausal levels. The lowest effective dose for prevention and treatment of osteoporosis should be utilized. (See DOSAGE AND ADMINISTRATION.)

Woman are at higher risk than men because they have less bone mass, and for several years following natural or induced menopause, the rate of bone mass decline is accelerated. Early menopause is one of the strongest predictors for the development of osteoporosis. White women are at higher risk than black women, and white men are at higher risk than black men. Women who are underweight also have osteoporosis more often than overweight women. Cigarette smoking may be an additional factor in increasing risk. Calcium deficiency has been implicated in the pathogenesis of the disease. Therefore, when not contraindicated, it is recommended that postmenopausal women receive an elemental calcium intake of 1000 to 1500 mg/day.

Immobilization and prolonged bed rest produce rapid bone loss, while weight-bearing exercise has been shown both to reduce bone loss and to increase bone mass. The optimal type and amount of physical activity that would prevent osteoporosis have not been established.

5. Hypoestrogenism due to hypogonadism, castration, or primary ovarian failure.
6. Breast cancer (for palliation only) in appropriately selected women and men with metastatic disease.
7. Advanced androgen-dependent carcinoma of the prostate (for palliation only).

CONTRAINDICATIONS

Estrogens should not be used in women (or men) with any of the following conditions:

1. Known or suspected pregnancy (see Boxed Warning). Estrogen may cause fetal harm when administered to a pregnant woman.
2. Known or suspected cancer of the breast except in appropriately selected patients being treated for metastatic disease.
3. Known or suspected estrogen-dependent neoplasia.
4. Undiagnosed abnormal genital bleeding.
5. Active thrombophlebitis or thromboembolic disorders.
6. Women on estrogen replacement therapy have not been reported to have an increased risk of thrombophlebitis and/or thromboembolic disease. However, there is insufficient information regarding women who have had previous thromboembolic disease.

PREMARIN Tablets should not be used in patients hypersensitive to their ingredients.

WARNINGS

1. *Induction of malignant neoplasms.* Some studies have suggested a possible increased incidence of breast cancer in those women on estrogen therapy taking higher doses for prolonged periods of time. The majority of studies, however, have not shown an association with the usual doses used for estrogen replacement therapy. Women on this therapy should have regular breast examinations and should be instructed in breast self-examination. The reported endometrial cancer risk among estrogen users was about 4-fold or greater than in nonusers and appears dependent on duration of treatment and on estrogen dose. There is no significant increased risk associated with the use of estrogens for less than one year. The greatest risk appears associated with prolonged use—five years or more. In one study, persistence of risk was demonstrated for 10 years after cessation of estrogen treatment. In another study, a significant decrease in the incidence of endometrial cancer occurred six months after estrogen withdrawal.

Estrogen therapy during pregnancy is associated with an increased risk of fetal congenital reproductive-tract disorders. In females there is an increased risk of vaginal adenosis, squamous-cell dysplasia of the cervix, and cancer later in

life; in the male, urogenital abnormalities. Although some of these changes are benign, it is not known whether they are precursors of malignancy.

2. *Gallbladder disease.* A recent study has reported a 2.5-fold increase in the risk of surgically confirmed gallbladder disease in women receiving postmenopausal estrogens.
3. *Cardiovascular disease.* Large doses of estrogen (5 mg conjugated estrogens per day), comparable to those used to treat cancer of the prostate and breast, have been shown in a large prospective clinical trial in men to increase the risk of nonfatal myocardial infarction, pulmonary embolism, and thrombophlebitis. It cannot necessarily be extrapolated from men to women. However, to avoid the theoretical cardiovascular risk caused by high estrogen doses, the doses for estrogen replacement therapy should not exceed the recommended dose.
4. *Elevated blood pressure.* There is no evidence that this may occur with use of estrogens in the menopause. However, blood pressure should be monitored with estrogen use, especially if high doses are used.
5. *Hypercalcemia.* Administration of estrogen may lead to severe hypercalcemia in patients with breast cancer and bone metastases. If this occurs, the drug should be stopped and appropriate measures taken to reduce the serum calcium level.

PRECAUTIONS

A. General.

1. *Addition of a progestin.* Studies of the addition of a progestin for seven or more days of a cycle of estrogen administration have reported a lowered incidence of endometrial hyperplasia. Morphological and biochemical studies of endometrium suggest that 10 to 13 days of progestin are needed to provide maximal maturation of the endometrium and to eliminate any hyperplastic changes. Whether this will provide protection from endometrial carcinoma has not been clearly established. There are possible additional risks which may be associated with the inclusion of progestin in estrogen replacement regimens. The potential risks include adverse effects on carbohydrate and lipid metabolism. The choice of progestin and dosage may be important in minimizing these adverse effects.
2. *Physical examination.* A complete medical and family history should be taken prior to the initiation of any estrogen therapy. The pretreatment and periodic physical examinations should include special reference to blood pressure, breasts, abdomen, and pelvic organs, and should include a Papanicolaou smear. As a general rule, estrogen should not be prescribed for longer than one year without another physical examination being performed.
3. *Fluid retention.* Because estrogens may cause some degree of fluid retention, conditions which might be influenced by this factor, such as asthma, epilepsy, migraine, and cardiac or renal dysfunction, require careful observation.
4. *Uterine bleeding and mastodynia.* Certain patients may develop undesirable manifestations of estrogenic stimulation, such as abnormal uterine bleeding and mastodynia.
5. *Uterine fibroids.* Preexisting uterine leiomyomata may increase in size during prolonged high-dose estrogen use.
6. *Impaired liver function.* Estrogens may be poorly metabolized in patients with impaired liver function and should be administered with caution.
7. *Hypercalcemia and renal insufficiency.* Prolonged use of estrogens can alter the metabolism of calcium and phosphorus. Estrogens should be used with caution in patients with metabolic bone disease.

B. Information for the Patient.

See text of Patient Package Insert which appears after the HOW SUPPLIED section.

C. Laboratory Tests.

Clinical response at the smallest dose should generally be the guide to estrogen administration for relief of symptoms for those indications in which symptoms are observable. However, for prevention and treatment of osteoporosis see DOSAGE AND ADMINISTRATION section. Tests used to measure adequacy of estrogen replacement therapy include serum estrone and estradiol levels and suppression of serum gonadotrophin levels.

D. Drug/Laboratory Test Interactions.

Some of these drug/laboratory test interactions have been observed only with estrogen-progestin combinations (oral contraceptives):

1. Increased prothrombin and factors VII, VIII, IX and X; decreased antithrombin 3; increased norepinephrine-induced platelet aggregability, decreased fibrinolysis.
2. Increased thyroid-binding globulin (TBG) leading to increased circulating total thyroid hormone, as measured by T4 levels determined either by column or by radioimmunoassay. Free T3 resin uptake is decreased, reflecting the elevated TBG; free T4 concentration is unaltered.

3. Impaired glucose tolerance.
4. Reduced response to metyrapone test.
5. Reduced serum folate concentration.

E. Mutagenesis and Carcinogenesis.

Long-term, continuous administration of natural and synthetic estrogens in certain animal species increases the frequency of carcinomas of the breast, cervix, vagina, and liver.

F. Pregnancy Category X.

Estrogens should not be used during pregnancy. See CONTRAINDICATIONS and Boxed Warning.

G. Nursing Mothers.

As a general principle, the administration of any drug to nursing mothers should be done only when clearly necessary since many drugs are excreted in human milk.

ADVERSE REACTIONS

(See WARNINGS regarding induction of neoplasia, adverse effects on the fetus, increased incidence of gallbladder disease.) The following additional adverse reactions have been reported with estrogenic therapy.

1. *Genitourinary system.* Changes in vaginal bleeding pattern and abnormal withdrawal bleeding or flow. Breakthrough bleeding, spotting. Increase in size of uterine fibromyomata. Vaginal candidiasis. Change in amount of cervical secretion.
2. *Breasts.* Tenderness, enlargement.
3. *Gastrointestinal.* Nausea, vomiting; abdominal cramps, bloating; cholestatic jaundice.
4. *Skin.* Chloasma or melasma that may persist when drug is discontinued; erythema multiforme; erythema nodosum; hemorrhagic eruption; loss of scalp hair; hirsutism.
5. *Eyes.* Steepening of corneal curvature; intolerance of contact lenses.
6. *CNS.* Headache, migraine, dizziness; mental depression; chorea.
7. *Miscellaneous.* Increase or decrease in weight; reduced carbohydrate tolerance; aggravation of porphyria; edema; changes in libido.

ACUTE OVERDOSAGE

Numerous reports of ingestion of large doses of estrogen-containing oral contraceptives by young children indicate that acute serious ill effects do not occur. Overdosage of estrogen may cause nausea and vomiting.

DOSAGE AND ADMINISTRATION

1. For treatment of moderate to severe vasomotor symptoms, atrophic vaginitis, and atrophic urethritis associated with the menopause. The lowest dose that will control symptoms should be chosen, and medication should be discontinued as promptly as possible.

Attempts to discontinue or taper medication should be made at 3-month to 6-month intervals.

Usual dosage ranges:

Vasomotor symptoms—1.25 mg daily. If the patient has not menstruated within the last two months or more, cyclic administration is started arbitrarily. If the patient is menstruating, cyclic (e.g., three weeks on and one week off) administration is started on day 5 of bleeding.

Atrophic vaginitis and Atrophic urethritis—0.3 mg to 1.25 mg or more daily, depending upon the tissue response of the individual patient. Administer cyclically.

2. Hypoestrogenism due to:
a. Female hypogonadism—2.5 mg to 7.5 mg daily, in divided doses for 20 days, followed by a rest period of 10 days' duration. If bleeding does not occur by the end of this period, the same dosage schedule is repeated. The number of courses of estrogen therapy necessary to produce bleeding may vary depending on the responsiveness of the endometrium.

If bleeding occurs before the end of the 10-day period, begin a 20-day estrogen-progestin cyclic regimen with PREMARIN, 2.5 mg to 7.5 mg daily in divided doses, for 20 days. During the last five days of estrogen therapy, give an oral progestin. If bleeding occurs before this regimen is concluded, therapy is discontinued and may be resumed on the fifth day of bleeding.

b. Female castration or primary ovarian failure— 1.25 mg daily, cyclically. Adjust dosage, upward or downward, according to severity of symptoms and response of the patient. For maintenance, adjust dosage to lowest level that will provide effective control.

3. Osteoporosis (loss of bone mass)—0.625 mg daily. Administration should be cyclic (e.g., three weeks on and one week off).

4. Advanced androgen-dependent carcinoma of the prostate, for palliation only—1.25 mg to 2.5 mg three times daily. The effectiveness of therapy can be judged by phosphatase determinations as well as by symptomatic improvement of the patient.

5. Breast cancer (for palliation only) in appropriately selected women and men with metastatic disease. Suggested dosage is 10 mg three times daily for a period of at least three months.

Treated patients with an intact uterus should be monitored closely for signs of endometrial cancer, and appropriate diag-

Continued on next page

Wyeth-Ayerst Laboratories—Cont.

nostic measures should be taken to rule out malignancy in the event of persistent or recurring abnormal vaginal bleeding.

HOW SUPPLIED

PREMARIN® (conjugated estrogens tablets, USP)
—Each oval purple tablet contains 2.5 mg, in bottles of 100 (NDC 0046-0865-81) and 1,000 (NDC 0046-0865-91).
—Each oval yellow tablet contains 1.25 mg, in bottles of 100 (NDC 0046-0866-81); 1,000 (NDC 0046-0866-91); 5,000 (NDC 0046-0866-95); and Unit-Dose packages of 100 (NDC 0046-0866-99).
—Each oval white tablet contains 0.9 mg, in bottles of 100 (NDC 0046-0864-81).
—Each oval maroon tablet contains 0.625 mg, in bottles of 100 (NDC 0046-0867-81); 1,000 (NDC 0046-0867-91); 5,000 (NDC 0046-0867-95); and Unit-Dose packages of 100 (NDC 0046-0867-99).
—Each oval green tablet contains 0.3 mg, in bottles of 100 (NDC 0046-0868-81) and 1,000 (NDC 0046-0868-91).
The appearance of these tablets is a trademark of Wyeth-Ayerst Laboratories.
Store at room temperature (approximately 25° C).

INFORMATION FOR THE PATIENT

This leaflet describes when and how to use estrogens and the risks of estrogen treatment.

ESTROGEN DRUGS

Estrogens have several important uses but also some risks. You must decide, with your doctor, whether the risks of estrogens are acceptable in view of their benefits. If you decide to start taking estrogens, check with your doctor to make sure you are using the lowest possible effective dose. The length of treatment with estrogens will depend upon the reason for use. This should also be discussed with your doctor.

USES OF ESTROGEN

To reduce menopausal symptoms. Estrogens are hormones produced by the ovaries. The decrease in the amount of estrogen that occurs in all women, usually between ages 45 and 55, causes the menopause. Sometimes the ovaries are removed by an operation, causing "surgical menopause." When the amount of estrogen begins to decrease, some women develop very uncomfortable symptoms, such as feelings of warmth in the face, neck and chest or sudden intense episodes of heat and sweating ("hot flashes"). The use of drugs containing estrogens can help the body adjust to lower estrogen levels.
Most women have none or only mild menopausal symptoms and do not need estrogens. Other women may need estrogens for a few months while their bodies adjust to lower estrogen levels. The majority of women do not need estrogen replacement for longer than six months for these symptoms.
To prevent brittle bones. After age 40, and especially after menopause, some women develop osteoporosis. This is a thinning of the bones that makes them weaker and more likely to break, often leading to fractures of vertebrae, hip, and wrist bones. Taking estrogens after the menopause slows down bone loss and may prevent bones from breaking. Eating foods that are high in calcium (such as milk products) or taking calcium supplements (1,000 to 1,500 milligrams per day) and certain types of exercise may also help prevent osteoporosis. Since estrogen use is associated with some risk, its use in the prevention of osteoporosis should be confined to women who appear to be susceptible to this condition. The following characteristics are often present in women who are likely to develop osteoporosis: white race, thinness, and cigarette smoking.
Women who had their menopause by the surgical removal of their ovaries at a relatively young age are good candidates for estrogen replacement therapy to prevent osteoporosis.
To treat certain types of abnormal uterine bleeding due to hormonal imbalance.
To treat atrophic vaginitis (itching, burning, dryness in or around the vagina) and *atrophic urethritis* (which may cause difficulty or burning on urination).
To treat certain cancers.

WHEN ESTROGENS SHOULD NOT BE USED

Estrogens should not be used:
During pregnancy. Although the possibility is fairly small, there is a greater risk of having a child born with a birth defect if you take estrogens during pregnancy. A male child may have an increased risk of developing abnormalities of the urinary system and sex organs. A female child may have an increased risk of developing cancer of the vagina or cervix in her teens or twenties. Estrogen is not effective in preventing miscarriage (abortion).
If you have had any heart or circulation problems. Estrogen therapy should be used only after consultation with your physician and only in recommended doses. Patients with a tendency for abnormal blood clotting should avoid estrogen use (see [next column]).

If you have had cancer. Since estrogens increase the risk of certain cancers, you should not take estrogens if you have ever had cancer of the breast or uterus. In certain situations, your doctor may choose to use estrogen in the treatment of breast cancer.
When they are ineffective. Sometimes women experience nervous symptoms or depression during menopause. There is no evidence that estrogens are effective for such symptoms. You may have heard that taking estrogens for long periods (years) after menopause will keep your skin soft and supple and keep you feeling young. There is no evidence that this is so and such long-term treatment may carry serious risks.

DANGERS OF ESTROGENS

Cancer of the uterus. The risk of cancer of the uterus increases the longer estrogens are used and when larger doses are taken. One study showed that when estrogens are discontinued, this increased risk of cancer seems to fall off quickly. In another study, the persistence of risk was demonstrated for 10 years after stopping estrogen treatment. Because of this risk, *it is important to take the lowest dose of estrogen that will control your symptoms and to take it only as long as you need it.* There is a higher risk of cancer of the uterus if you are overweight, diabetic, or have high blood pressure.
If you have had your uterus removed (total hysterectomy), there is no danger of developing cancer of the uterus.
Cancer of the breast. The majority of studies have shown no association with the usual doses used for estrogen replacement therapy and breast cancer. Some studies have suggested a possible increased incidence of breast cancer in those women taking estrogens for prolonged periods of time and especially if higher doses are used.
Regular breast examinations by a health professional and self-examination are recommended for women receiving estrogen therapy, as they are for all women.
Gallbladder disease. Women who use estrogens after menopause are more likely to develop gallbladder disease needing surgery than women who do not use estrogens.
Abnormal blood clotting. Taking estrogens may increase the risk of blood clots. These clots can cause a stroke, heart attack or pulmonary embolus, any of which may be fatal.

SIDE EFFECTS

In addition to the risk listed above, the following side effects have been reported with estrogen use:
● Nausea and vomiting.
● Breast tenderness or enlargement.
● Enlargement of benign tumors of the uterus.
● Retention of excess fluid. This may make some conditions worsen, such as asthma, epilepsy, migraine, heart disease, or kidney disease.
● A spotty darkening of the skin, particularly on the face.

REDUCING RISK OF ESTROGEN USE

If you decide to take estrogens, you can reduce your risks by carefully monitoring your treatment.
See your doctor regularly. While you are taking estrogens, it is important that you visit your doctor at least once a year for a physical examination. If members of your family have had breast cancer or if you have ever had breast nodules or an abnormal mammogram (breast Xray), you may need to have more frequent breast examinations.
Reevaluate your need for estrogens. You and your doctor should reevaluate your need for estrogens at least every six months.
Be alert for signs of trouble. Report these or any other unusual side effects to your doctor immediately:
● Abnormal bleeding from the vagina.
● Pains in the calves or chest, a sudden shortness of breath or coughing blood (indicating possible clots in the legs, heart, or lungs).
● Severe headache, dizziness, faintness, or changes in vision, indicating possible clots in the brain or eye.
● Breast lumps.
● Yellowing of the skin.
● Pain, swelling, or tenderness in the abdomen.

OTHER INFORMATION

Some physicians may choose to prescribe another hormonal drug to be used in association with estrogen treatment. These drugs, progestins, have been reported to lower the frequency of occurrence of a possible precancerous condition of the uterine lining. Whether this will provide protection from uterine cancer has not been clearly established. There are possible additional risks that may be associated with the inclusion of a progestin in estrogen treatment. The possible risks include unfavorable effects on blood fats and sugars. The choice of progestin and its dosage may be important in minimizing these effects.
Your doctor has prescribed this drug for you and you alone. Do not give the drug to anyone else.
If you will be taking calcium supplements as part of the treatment to help prevent osteoporosis, check with your doctor about the amounts recommended.
Keep this and all drugs out of the reach of children. In case of overdose, call your doctor, hospital, or poison control center immediately.

This leaflet provides the most important information about estrogens. If you want to read more, ask your doctor or pharmacist to let you read the professional labeling.

HOW SUPPLIED

PREMARIN® (conjugated estrogens tablets, USP)—tablets for oral administration.
　　Each oval purple tablet contains 2.5 mg.
　　Each oval yellow tablet contains 1.25 mg.
　　Each oval white tablet contains 0.9 mg.
　　Each oval maroon tablet contains 0.625 mg.
　　Each oval green tablet contains 0.3 mg.
The appearance of these tablets is a trademark of Wyeth-Ayerst Laboratories.
Shown in Product Identification Section, page 437

PREMARIN®　　　　　　　　　　　　　　　　　　　　　℞
[*prĕm'a-rin*]
(conjugated estrogens)
VAGINAL CREAM
in a nonliquefying base

CAUTION: Federal law prohibits dispensing without prescription.

---

1. ESTROGENS HAVE BEEN REPORTED TO INCREASE THE RISK OF ENDOMETRIAL CARCINOMA.
Three independent, case-controlled studies have reported an increased risk of endometrial cancer in postmenopausal women exposed to exogenous estrogens for more than one year.[1–3] This risk was independent of the other known risk factors for endometrial cancer. These studies are further supported by the finding that incidence rates of endometrial cancer have increased sharply since 1969 in eight different areas of the United States with population-based cancer reporting systems, an increase which may be related to the rapidly expanding use of estrogens during the last decade.[4]
The three case-controlled studies reported that the risk of endometrial cancer in estrogen users was about 4.5 to 13.9 times greater than in nonusers. The risk appears to depend on both duration of treatment[1] and on estrogen dose.[3] In view of these findings, when estrogens are used for the treatment of menopausal symptoms, the lowest dose that will control symptoms should be utilized and medication should be discontinued as soon as possible. When prolonged treatment is medically indicated, the patient should be reassessed, on at least a semi-annual basis, to determine the need for continued therapy. Although the evidence must be considered preliminary, one study suggests that cyclic administration of low doses of estrogen may carry less risk than continuous administration.[3] It therefore appears prudent to utilize such a regimen.
Close clinical surveillance of all women taking estrogens is important. In all cases of undiagnosed persistent or recurring abnormal vaginal bleeding, adequate diagnostic measures should be undertaken to rule out malignancy.
There is no evidence at present that "natural" estrogens are more or less hazardous than "synthetic" estrogens at equi-estrogenic doses.
2. ESTROGENS SHOULD NOT BE USED DURING PREGNANCY.
The use of female sex hormones, both estrogens and progestogens, during early pregnancy may seriously damage the offspring. It has been shown that females exposed in utero to diethylstilbestrol, a nonsteroidal estrogen, have an increased risk of developing, in later life, a form of vaginal or cervical cancer that is ordinarily extremely rare.[5,6] This risk has been estimated as not greater than 4 per 1,000 exposures.[7] Furthermore, a high percentage of such exposed women (from 30% to 90%) have been found to have vaginal adenosis,[8–12] epithelial changes of the vagina and cervix. Although these changes are histologically benign, it is not known whether they are precursors of malignancy. Although similar data are not available with the use of other estrogens, it cannot be presumed they would not induce similar changes.
Several reports suggest an association between intrauterine exposure to female sex hormones and congenital anomalies, including congenital heart defects and limb reduction defects.[13–16] One case-controlled study[16] estimated a 4.7-fold increased risk of limb-reduction defects in infants exposed *in utero* to sex hormones (oral contraceptives, hormone withdrawal tests for pregnancy, or attempted treatment for threatened abortion). Some of these exposures were very short and involved only a few days of treatment. The data suggest that the risk of limb-reduction defects in exposed fetuses is somewhat less than 1 per 1,000.
In the past, female sex hormones have been used during pregnancy in an attempt to treat threatened or habitual

abortion. There is considerable evidence that estrogens are ineffective for these indications, and there is no evidence from well-controlled studies that progestogens are effective for these uses.

If PREMARIN (conjugated estrogens) Vaginal Cream is used during pregnancy, or if the patient becomes pregnant while taking this drug, she should be apprised of the potential risks to the fetus, and the advisability of pregnancy continuation.

DESCRIPTION

Each gram of PREMARIN (conjugated estrogens) Vaginal Cream contains 0.625 mg conjugated estrogens. USP, in a nonliquefying base containing cetyl esters wax, cetyl alcohol, white wax, glyceryl monostearate, propylene glycol monostearate, methyl stearate, phenylethyl alcohol, sodium lauryl sulfate, glycerin, and mineral oil. PREMARIN Vaginal Cream is applied intravaginally.

PREMARIN (conjugated estrogens) is a mixture of estrogens obtained exclusively from natural sources, occurring as the sodium salts of water-soluble estrogen sulfates blended to represent the average composition of material derived from pregnant mares' urine. It contains estrone, equilin, and 17 α-dihydroequilin, together with smaller amounts of 17 α-estradiol, equilenin, and 17 α-dihydroequilenin as salts of their sulfate esters.

CLINICAL PHARMACOLOGY

Estrogens are important in the development and maintenance of the female reproductive system and secondary sex characteristics. They promote growth and development of the vagina, uterus, and fallopian tubes, and enlargement of the breasts. Indirectly, they contribute to the shaping of the skeleton, maintenance of tone and elasticity of urogenital structures, changes in the epiphyses of the long bones that allow for the pubertal growth spurt and its termination, growth of axillary and pubic hair, and pigmentation of the nipples and genitals. Decline of estrogenic activity at the end of the menstrual cycle can bring on menstruation, although the cessation of progesterone secretion is the most important factor in the mature ovulatory cycle. However, in the preovulatory or nonovulatory cycle, estrogen is the primary determinant in the onset of menstruation. Estrogens also affect the release of pituitary gonadotropins.

The pharmacologic effects of conjugated estrogens are similar to those of endogenous estrogens. They are soluble in water and may be absorbed from mucosal surfaces after local administration.

In responsive tissues (female genital organs, breasts, hypothalamus, pituitary) estrogens enter the cell and are transported into the nucleus. As a result of estrogen action, specific RNA and protein synthesis occurs.

Metabolism and inactivation occur primarily in the liver. Some estrogens are excreted into the bile; however, they are reabsorbed from the intestine and returned to the liver through the portal venous system. Water-soluble estrogen conjugates are strongly acidic and, therefore, ionized in body fluids, which favor excretion through the kidneys since tubular reabsorption is minimal.

INDICATIONS AND USAGE

PREMARIN (conjugated estrogens) Vaginal Cream is indicated in the treatment of atrophic vaginitis and kraurosis vulvae.

PREMARIN Vaginal Cream HAS NOT BEEN SHOWN TO BE EFFECTIVE FOR ANY PURPOSE DURING PREGNANCY AND ITS USE MAY CAUSE SEVERE HARM TO THE FETUS (SEE BOXED WARNING).

CONTRAINDICATIONS

Estrogens should not be used in women with any of the following conditions:

1. Known or suspected cancer of the breast except in appropriately selected patients being treated for metastatic disease.
2. Known or suspected estrogen-dependent neoplasia.
3. Known or suspected pregnancy (see Boxed Warning).
4. Undiagnosed abnormal genital bleeding.
5. Active thrombophlebitis or thromboembolic disorders.
6. A past history of thrombophlebitis, thrombosis, or thromboembolic disorders associated with previous estrogen use (except when used in treatment of breast malignancy).

PREMARIN Vaginal Cream should not be used in patients hypersensitive to its ingredients.

WARNINGS

1. *Induction of malignant neoplasms.* Long-term continuous administration of natural and synthetic estrogens in certain animal species increases the frequency of carcinomas of the breast, cervix, vagina, and liver. There are now reports that estrogens increase the risk of carcinoma of the endometrium in humans (see Boxed Warning).

At the present time there is no satisfactory evidence that estrogens given to postmenopausal women increase the risk of cancer of the breast,[17] although a recent long-term follow-up of a single physician's practice has raised this possibility.[18] Because of the animal data, there is a need for caution in prescribing estrogens for women with a strong family history of breast cancer or who have breast nodules, fibrocystic disease, or abnormal mammograms.

2. *Gallbladder disease.* A recent study has reported a 2- to 3-fold increase in the risk of surgically confirmed gallbladder disease in women receiving postmenopausal estrogens,[17] similar to the 2-fold increase previously noted in users of oral contraceptives.[19,24a]

3. *Effects similar to those caused by estrogen-progestogen oral contraceptives.* There are several serious adverse effects of oral contraceptives, most of which have not, up to now, been documented as consequences of postmenopausal estrogen therapy. This may reflect the comparatively low doses of estrogen used in postmenopausal women. It would be expected that the larger doses of estrogen used to treat prostatic or breast cancer, or postpartum breast engorgement, are more likely to result in these adverse effects, and, in fact, it has been shown that there is an increased risk of thrombosis in men receiving estrogens for prostatic cancer and women for postpartum breast engorgement.[20–23]

a. *Thromboembolic disease.* It is now well established that users of oral contraceptives have an increased risk of various thromboembolic and thrombotic vascular diseases, such as thrombophlebitis, pulmonary embolism, stroke, and myocardial infarction.[24–31] Cases of retinal thrombosis, mesenteric thrombosis, and optic neuritis have been reported in oral-contraceptive users. There is evidence that the risk of several of these adverse reactions is related to the dose of the drug.[32,33] An increased risk of postsurgery thromboembolic complications has also been reported in users of oral contraceptives.[34,35] If feasible, estrogen should be discontinued at least 4 weeks before surgery of the type associated with an increased risk of thromboembolism, or during periods of prolonged immobilization.

While an increased rate of thromboembolic and thrombotic disease in postmenopausal users of estrogens has not been found,[17–24,25–36] this does not rule out the possibility that such an increase may be present or that subgroups of women who have underlying risk factors or who are receiving relatively large doses of estrogens may have increased risk. Therefore estrogens should not be used in persons with active thrombophlebitis or thromboembolic disorders, and they should not be used (except in treatment of malignancy) in persons with a history of such disorders in association with estrogen use. They should be used with caution in patients with cerebral vascular or coronary artery disease and only for those in whom estrogens are clearly needed.

Large doses of estrogen (5 mg conjugated estrogens per day), comparable to those used to treat cancer of the prostate and breast, have been shown in a large prospective clinical trial in men[37] to increase the risk of nonfatal myocardial infarction, pulmonary embolism, and thrombophlebitis. When estrogen doses of this size are used, any of the thromboembolic and thrombotic adverse effects associated with oral contraceptive use should be considered a clear risk.

b. *Hepatic adenoma.* Benign hepatic adenomas appear to be associated with the use of oral contraceptives.[38–40] Although benign and rare, these may rupture and may cause death through intra-abdominal hemorrhage. Such lesions have not yet been reported in association with other estrogen or progestogen preparations but should be considered in estrogen users having abdominal pain and tenderness, abdominal mass, or hypovolemic shock. Hepatocellular carcinoma has also been reported in women taking estrogen-containing oral contraceptives.[39] The relationship of this malignancy to these drugs is not known at this time.

c. *Elevated blood pressure.* Women using oral contraceptives sometimes experience increased blood pressure which, in most cases, returns to normal on discontinuing the drug. There is now a report that this may occur with use of estrogens in the menopause[41] and blood pressure should be monitored with estrogen use, especially if high doses are used.

d. *Glucose tolerance.* A worsening of glucose tolerance has been observed in a significant percentage of patients on estrogen-containing oral contraceptives. For this reason, diabetic patients should be carefully observed while receiving estrogen.

4. *Hypercalcemia.* Administration of estrogens may lead to severe hypercalcemia in patients with breast cancer and bone metastases. If this occurs, the drug should be stopped and appropriate measures taken to reduce the serum calcium level.

PRECAUTIONS

A. GENERAL PRECAUTIONS.

1. A complete medical and family history should be taken prior to the initiation of any estrogen therapy. The pretreatment and periodic physical examinations should include special reference to blood pressure, breasts, abdomen, and pelvic organs, and should include a Papanicolaou smear. As a general rule, estrogen should not be prescribed for longer than one year without another physical examination being performed.
2. Fluid retention—Because estrogens may cause some degree of fluid retention, conditions which might be influenced by this factor such as asthma, epilepsy, migraine, and cardiac or renal dysfunction, require careful observation.
3. Certain patients may develop undesirable manifestations of excessive estrogenic stimulation, such as abnormal or excessive uterine bleeding, mastodynia, etc.
4. Prolonged administration of unopposed estrogen therapy has been reported to increase the risk of endometrial hyperplasia in some patients.
5. Oral contraceptives appear to be associated with an increased incidence of mental depression.[24a] Although it is not clear whether this is due to the estrogenic or progestogenic component of the contraceptive, patients with a history of depression should be carefully observed.
6. Preexisting uterine leiomyomata may increase in size during estrogen use.
7. The pathologist should be advised of estrogen therapy when relevant specimens are submitted.
8. Patients with a past history of jaundice during pregnancy have an increased risk of recurrence of jaundice while receiving estrogen-containing oral contraceptive therapy. If jaundice develops in any patient receiving estrogen, the medication should be discontinued while the cause is investigated.
9. Estrogens may be poorly metabolized in patients with impaired liver function and they should be administered with caution in such patients.
10. Because estrogens influence the metabolism of calcium and phosphorus, they should be used with caution in patients with metabolic bone diseases that are associated with hypercalcemia or in patients with renal insufficiency.
11. Because of the effects of estrogens on epiphyseal closure, they should be used judiciously in young patients in whom bone growth is not complete.

CONCOMITANT PROGESTIN USE: The lowest effective dose appropriate for the specific indication should be utilized. Studies of the addition of a progestin for 7 or more days of a cycle of estrogen administration have reported a lowered incidence of endometrial hyperplasia. Morphological and biochemical studies of the endometrium suggest that 10 to 13 days of progestin are needed to provide maximal maturation of the endometrium and to eliminate any hyperplastic changes. Whether this will provide protection from endometrial carcinoma has not been clearly established. There are possible additional risks which may be associated with the inclusion of progestin in estrogen replacement regimens. If concomitant progestin therapy is used, potential risks may include adverse effects on carbohydrate and lipid metabolism. The choice of progestin and dosage may be important in minimizing these adverse effects.

B. Information for Patients. (See text which appears after the PHYSICIAN REFERENCES.)

C. Drug/Laboratory Test Interactions. Certain endocrine and liver function tests may be affected by estrogen-containing oral contraceptives. The following similar changes may be expected with larger doses of estrogen:

a. Increased sulfobromophthalein retention.
b. Increased prothrombin and factors VII, VIII, IX, and X; decreased antithrombin 3; increased norepinephrine-induced platelet aggregability.
c. Increased thyroid binding globulin (TBG) leading to increased circulating total thyroid hormone, as measured by PBI, T4 by column, or T4 by radioimmunoassay. Free T3 resin uptake is decreased, reflecting the elevated TBG; free T4 concentration is unaltered.
d. Impaired glucose tolerance.
e. Decreased pregnanediol excretion.
f. Reduced response to metyrapone test.
g. Reduced serum folate concentration.
h. Increased serum triglyceride and phospholipid concentration.

D. Carcinogenesis, Mutagenesis, Impairment of Fertility. (See WARNINGS section for information on carcinogenesis.)

E. Pregnancy Category X. (See CONTRAINDICATIONS and Boxed Warning.)

F. Nursing Mothers. It is not known whether this drug is excreted in human milk. Because many drugs are excreted in human milk and because of the potential for serious adverse reactions in nursing infants from estrogens, a decision should be made whether to discontinue nursing or to discontinue the drug, taking into account the importance of the drug to the mother.

G. Pediatric Use. Safety and effectiveness in children have not been established.

ADVERSE REACTIONS

(See WARNINGS regarding induction of neoplasia, adverse effects on the fetus, increased incidence of gallbladder disease, and adverse effects similar to those of oral contraceptives, including thromboembolism.) The following additional adverse reactions have been reported with estrogenic therapy, including oral contraceptives:

1. *Genitourinary system:* Breakthrough bleeding, spotting, change in menstrual flow; dysmenorrhea; premenstrual-like

Continued on next page

Wyeth-Ayerst Laboratories—Cont.

syndrome; amenorrhea during and after treatment; increase in size of uterine fibromyomata; vaginal candidiasis; change in cervical erosion and in degree of cervical secretion; cystitis-like syndrome.

2. *Breasts:* Tenderness, enlargement, secretion.
3. *Gastrointestinal:* Nausea, vomiting; abdominal cramps, bloating; cholestatic jaundice.
4. *Skin:* Chloasma or melasma which may persist when drug is discontinued; erythema multiforme; erythema nodosum; hemorrhagic eruption; loss of scalp hair; hirsutism.
5. *Eyes:* Steepening of corneal curvature; intolerance to contact lenses.
6. *CNS:* Headache, migraine, dizziness; mental depression; chorea.
7. *Miscellaneous:* Increase or decrease in weight; reduced carbohydrate tolerance; aggravation of porphyria; edema; changes in libido.

OVERDOSAGE

Numerous reports of ingestion of large doses of estrogen-containing oral contraceptives by young children indicate that acute serious ill effects do not occur. Overdosage of estrogens may cause nausea, and withdrawal bleeding may occur in females.

DOSAGE AND ADMINISTRATION

Given cyclically for short-term use only:
For treatment of atrophic vaginitis, or kraurosis vulvae.
The lowest dose that will control symptoms should be chosen and medication should be discontinued as promptly as possible.
Administration should be cyclic (e.g., three weeks on and one week off).
Attempts to discontinue or taper medication should be made at three- to six-month intervals.

USUAL DOSAGE RANGE:

2 to 4 g (½ applicatorful to 1 applicatorful) daily, intravaginally, depending on the severity of the condition.
Treated patients with an intact uterus should be monitored closely for signs of endometrial cancer, and appropriate diagnostic measures should be taken to rule out malignancy in the event of persistent or recurring abnormal vaginal bleeding.

INSTRUCTIONS FOR USE OF APPLICATOR:

1. Remove cap from tube.
2. Screw nozzle end of applicator onto tube.
3. *Gently* squeeze tube from the *bottom* to force sufficient cream into the barrel to provide the prescribed dose.
4. Unscrew applicator from tube.
5. Lie on back with knees drawn up. To deliver medication, gently insert applicator deeply into vagina and press plunger downward to its original position.
TO CLEANSE: Pull plunger out from barrel. Wash with mild soap and warm water.
DO NOT BOIL OR USE HOT WATER.

HOW SUPPLIED

PREMARIN (conjugated estrogens) Vaginal Cream—Each gram contains 0.625 mg conjugated estrogens, USP. (Also contains cetyl esters wax, cetyl alcohol, white wax, glyceryl monostearate, propylene glycol monostearate, methyl stearate, phenylethyl alcohol, sodium lauryl sulfate, glycerin, and mineral oil.)
Combination package: Each contains Net Wt. 1½ oz (42.5 g) tube with one plastic applicator calibrated in 1 g increments to a maximum of 4 g (NDC 0046-0872-93).
Also Available—Refill package: Each contains Net Wt. 1½ oz (42.5 g) tube (NDC 0046-0872-01).
Store at room temperature (approximately 25° C).

PHYSICIAN REFERENCES

1. Ziel, H. K., *et al.*: N. Engl. J. Med. *293* :1167–1170, 1975.
2. Smith, D. C., *et al.*: N. Engl. J. Med. *293* :1164–1167, 1975.
3. Mack, T. M., *et al.*: N. Engl. J. Med *294* :1262–1267, 1976.
4. Weiss, N. S., *et al.*: N. Engl. J. Med. *294* :1259–1262, 1976.
5. Herbst, A. L., *et al.*: N. Engl. J. Med. *284* :878–881, 1971.
6. Greenwald, P., *et al.*: N. Engl. J. Med. *285* :390–392, 1971.
7. Lanier, A., *et al.*: Mayo Clin. Proc. *48* :793–799, 1973.
8. Herbst, A., *et al.*: Obstet. Gynecol. *40* :287–298, 1972.
9. Herbst, A., *et al.*: Am. J. Obstet. Gynecol. *118* :607–615, 1974.
10. Herbst, A., *et al.*: N. Engl. J. Med. *292* :334–339, 1975.
11. Stafl, A., *et al.*: Obstet. Gynecol. *43* :118–128, 1974.
12. Sherman, A. I., *et al.*: Obstet. Gynecol. *44* :531–545, 1974.
13. Gal, I., *et al.*: Nature *216* :83, 1967.
14. Levy, E. P., *et al.*: Lancet *1* :611, 1973.
15. Nora, J., *et al.*: Lancet *1* :941–942, 1973.
16. Janerich, D. T., *et al.*: N. Engl. J. Med. *291* :697–700, 1974.
17. Boston Collaborative Drug Surveillance Program: N. Engl. J. Med. *290* :15–19, 1974.
18. Hoover, R., *et al.*: N. Engl. J. Med. *295* :401–405, 1976.
19. Boston Collaborative Drug Surveillance Program: Lancet *1* :1399–1404, 1973.
20. Daniel, D. G., *et al.*: Lancet *2* :287–289, 1967.
21. The Veterans Administration Cooperative Urological Research Group: J. Urol. *98* :516–522, 1967.
22. Bailar, J. C.: Lancet *2* :560, 1967.
23. Blackard, C., *et al.*: Cancer *26* :249–256, 1970.
24. Royal College of General Practitioners: J. R. Coll. Gen. Pract. *13* :267–279, 1967.
24a. Royal College of General Practitioners: Oral Contraceptives and Health, New York, Pitman Corp., 1974.
25. Inman, W. H. W., *et al.*: Br. Med. J. *2* :193–199, 1968.
26. Vessey, M. P., *et al.*: Br. Med. J. *2* :651–657, 1969.
27. Sartwell, P. E., *et al.*: Am. J. Epidemiol. *90* :365–380, 1969.
28. Collaborative Group for the Study of Stroke in Young Women: N. Engl. J. Med. *288* :871–878, 1973.
29. Collaborative Group for the Study of Stroke in Young Women: J.A.M.A. *231* :718–722, 1975.
30. Mann, J. I., *et al.*: Br. Med. J. *2* :245–248, 1975.
31. Mann, J. I., *et al.*: Br. Med. J. *2* :241–245, 1975.
32. Inman, W. H. W., *et al.*: Br. Med. J. *2* :203–209, 1970.
33. Stolley, P. D., *et al.*: Am. J. Epidemiol. *102* :197–208, 1975.
34. Vessey, M. P., *et al.*: Br. Med. J. *3* :123–126, 1970.
35. Greene, G. R., *et al.*: Am. J. Public Health *62* :680–685, 1972.
36. Rosenberg, L., *et al.*: N. Engl. J. Med. *294* :1256–1259, 1976.
37. Coronary Drug Project Research Group: J.A.M.A. *214* :1303–1313, 1970.
38. Baum, J., *et al.*: Lancet *2* :926–928, 1973.
39. Mays, E. T., *et al.*: J.A.M.A. *235* :730–732, 1976.
40. Edmondson, H. A., *et al.*: N. Engl. J. Med. *294* :470–472, 1976.
41. Pfeffer, R. I., *et al.*: Am. J. Epidemiol. *103* :445–456, 1976.

INFORMATION FOR THE PATIENT

WHAT YOU SHOULD KNOW ABOUT ESTROGENS

Estrogens are female hormones produced by the ovaries. The ovaries make several different kinds of estrogens. In addition, scientists have been able to make a variety of synthetic estrogens. As far as we know, all these estrogens have similar properties and, therefore, much the same usefulness, side effects, and risks. This leaflet is intended to help you understand what estrogens are used for, the risks involved in their use, and how to use them as safely as possible.
This leaflet includes the most important information about estrogens, but not all the information. If you want to know more, you should ask your doctor for more information or you can ask your doctor or pharmacist to let you read the package insert prepared for the doctor.

USES OF ESTROGEN

THERE IS NO PROPER USE OF ESTROGENS IN A PREGNANT WOMAN.
Estrogens are prescribed by doctors for a number of purposes, including:
1. To provide estrogen during a period of adjustment when a woman's ovaries stop producing a majority of her estrogens, in order to prevent certain uncomfortable symptoms of estrogen deficiency. (With the menopause, which generally occurs between the ages of 45 and 55, women produce a much smaller amount of estrogens.)
2. To prevent symptoms of estrogen deficiency when a woman's ovaries have been removed surgically before the natural menopause.
3. To prevent pregnancy. (Estrogens are given along with a progestogen, another female hormone; these combinations are called oral contraceptives or birth control pills. Patient labeling is available to women taking oral contraceptives and they will not be discussed in this leaflet.)
4. To treat certain cancers in women and men.

ESTROGENS IN THE MENOPAUSE

In the natural course of their lives, all women eventually experience a decrease in estrogen production. This usually occurs between ages 45 and 55 but may occur earlier or later. Sometimes the ovaries may need to be removed before natural menopause by an operation, producing a "surgical menopause."
When the amount of estrogen in the blood begins to decrease, many women may develop typical symptoms: feelings of warmth in the face, neck, and chest or sudden intense episodes of heat and sweating throughout the body (called "hot flashes" or "hot flushes"). These symptoms are sometimes very uncomfortable. Some women may also develop changes in the vagina (called "atrophic vaginitis") which cause discomfort, especially during and after intercourse.
Estrogens can be prescribed to treat these symptoms of the menopause. It is estimated that considerably more than half of all women undergoing the menopause have only mild symptoms or no symptoms at all and therefore do not need

estrogens. Other women may need estrogens for a few months, while their bodies adjust to lower estrogen levels. Sometimes the need will be for periods longer than six months. In an attempt to avoid overstimulation of the uterus (womb), estrogens are usually given cyclically during each month of use, such as three weeks of pills followed by one week without pills.
Sometimes women experience nervous symptoms or depression during menopause. There is no evidence that estrogens are effective for such symptoms without associated vasomotor symptoms. In the absence of vasomotor symptoms, estrogens should not be used to treat nervous symptoms, although other treatment may be needed.
You may have heard that taking estrogens for long periods (years) after the menopause will keep your skin soft and supple and keep you feeling young. There is no evidence that this is so, however, and such long-term treatment carries important risks.

THE DANGERS OF ESTROGENS

1. *Endometrial cancer.* There are reports that if estrogens are used in the postmenopausal period for more than a year, there is an increased risk of *endometrial cancer* (cancer of the lining of the uterus). Women taking estrogens have roughly 5 to 10 times as great a chance of getting this cancer as women who take no estrogens. To put this another way, while a postmenopausal woman not taking estrogens has 1 chance in 1,000 each year of getting endometrial cancer, a woman taking estrogens has 5 to 10 chances in 1,000 each year. For this reason, *it is important to take estrogens only when they are really needed.*
The risk of this cancer is greater the longer estrogens are used and when larger doses are taken. Therefore, you should not take more estrogen than your doctor prescribes. *It is important to take the lowest dose of estrogen that will control symptoms and to take it only as long as it is needed.* If estrogens are needed for longer periods of time, your doctor will want to re-evaluate your need for estrogens at least every six months.
Women using estrogens should report any vaginal bleeding to their doctors; such bleeding may be of no importance, but it can be an early warning of endometrial cancer. If you have undiagnosed vaginal bleeding, you should not use estrogens until a diagnosis is made and you are certain there is no endometrial cancer.
NOTE: If you have had your uterus removed (total hysterectomy), there is no danger of developing endometrial cancer.
2. *Other possible cancers.* Estrogens can cause development of other tumors in animals, such as tumors of the breast, cervix, vagina, or liver, when given for a long time. At present there is no good evidence that women using estrogen in the menopause have an increased risk of such tumors, but there is no way yet to be sure they do not; and one study raises the possibility that use of estrogens in the menopause may increase the risk of breast cancer many years later. This is a further reason to use estrogens only when clearly needed. While you are taking estrogens, it is important that you go to your doctor at least once a year for a physical examination. Also, if members of your family have had breast cancer or if you have breast nodules or abnormal mammograms (breast x-rays), your doctor may wish to carry out more frequent examinations of your breasts.
3. *Gallbladder disease.* Women who use estrogens after menopause are more likely to develop gallbladder disease needing surgery than women who do not use estrogens. Birth control pills have a similar effect.
4. *Abnormal blood clotting.* Oral contraceptives increase the risk of blood clotting in various parts of the body. This can result in a stroke (if the clot is in the brain), a heart attack (a clot in a blood vessel of the heart), or a pulmonary embolus (a clot which forms in the legs or pelvis, then breaks off and travels to the lungs). Any of these can be fatal.
At this time use of estrogens in the menopause is not known to cause such blood clotting, but this has not been fully studied and there could still prove to be such a risk. It is recommended that if you have had clotting in the legs or lungs or a heart attack or stroke while you were using estrogens or birth control pills, you should not use estrogens (unless they are being used to treat cancer of the breast or prostate). If you have had a stroke or heart attack or if you have angina pectoris, estrogens should be used with great caution and only if clearly needed (for example, if you have severe symptoms of the menopause).

SPECIAL WARNING ABOUT PREGNANCY

You should not receive estrogen if you are pregnant. If this should occur, there is a greater than usual chance that the developing child will be born with a birth defect, although the possibility remains fairly small. A female child may have an increased risk of developing cancer of the vagina or cervix later in life (in the teens or twenties). Every possible effort should be made to avoid exposure to estrogens during pregnancy. If exposure occurs, see your doctor.

OTHER EFFECTS OF ESTROGENS

In addition to the serious known risks of estrogens described above, estrogens have the following side effects and potential risks:

1. *Nausea and vomiting.* The most common side effect of estrogen therapy is nausea. Vomiting is less common.
2. *Effects on breasts.* Estrogens may cause breast tenderness or enlargement and may cause the breasts to secrete a liquid. These effects are not dangerous.
3. *Effects on the uterus.* Estrogens may cause benign fibroid tumors of the uterus to get larger.
4. *Effects on liver.* Women taking oral contraceptives develop, on rare occasions, a tumor of the liver which can rupture and bleed into the abdomen and may cause death. So far, these tumors have not been reported in women using estrogens in the menopause, but you should report any swelling or unusual pain or tenderness in the abdomen to your doctor immediately.

Women with a past history of jaundice (yellowing of the skin and white parts of the eyes) may get jaundice again during estrogen use. If this occurs, stop taking estrogens and see your doctor.

5. *Other effects.* Estrogens may cause excess fluid to be retained in the body. This may make some conditions worse, such as asthma, epilepsy, migraine, heart disease, or kidney disease.

SUMMARY

Estrogens have important uses, but they have serious risks as well. You must decide, with your doctor, whether the risks are acceptable to you in view of the benefits of treatment. Except where your doctor has prescribed estrogens for use in special cases of cancer of the breast or prostate, you should not use estrogens if you have cancer of the breast or uterus, are pregnant, have undiagnosed abnormal vaginal bleeding, clotting in the legs or lungs, or have had a stroke, heart attack or angina, or clotting in the legs or lungs in the past while you were taking estrogens.

You can use estrogens as safely as possible by understanding that your doctor will require regular physical examinations while you are taking them, will try to discontinue the drug as soon as possible, and use the smallest dose possible. Be alert for signs of trouble including:

1. Abnormal bleeding from the vagina.
2. Pains in the calves or chest, sudden shortness of breath, or coughing blood.
3. Severe headache, dizziness, faintness, or changes in vision.
4. Breast lumps (you should ask your doctor how to examine your own breasts).
5. Jaundice (yellowing of the skin).
6. Mental depression.

Your doctor has prescribed this drug for you and you alone. Do not give the drug to anyone else.

HOW SUPPLIED

PREMARIN (conjugated estrogens) Vaginal Cream—Each gram contains 0.625 mg conjugated estrogens, USP. (Also contains cetyl esters wax, cetyl alcohol, white wax, glyceryl monostearate, propylene glycol monostearate, methyl stearate, phenylethyl alcohol, sodium lauryl sulfate, glycerin, and mineral oil.)

Combination package: Each contains Net Wt. 1½ oz (42.5 g) tube with one plastic applicator calibrated in 1 g increments to a maximum of 4 g (NDC 0046-0872-93).

Also Available —Refill package: Each contains Net Wt. 1½ oz (42.5 g) tube (NDC 0046-0872-01).

Store at room temperature (approximately 25° C).

INSTRUCTIONS FOR USE OF PREMARIN®
(conjugated estrogens)
VAGINAL CREAM APPLICATOR:

1. Remove cap from tube.
2. Screw nozzle end of applicator onto tube.
3. *Gently* squeeze tube from the *bottom* to force sufficient cream into the barrel to provide the prescribed dose.
4. Unscrew applicator from tube.
5. Lie on back with knees drawn up. To deliver medication, gently insert applicator deeply into vagina and press plunger downward to its original position.

TO CLEANSE: Pull plunger out from barrel. Wash with mild soap and warm water.

DO NOT BOIL OR USE HOT WATER.

Shown in Product Identification Section, page 437

PREMARIN® ℞

[*prem 'a-rin with meth "yl-tĕs-tŏs 'ta-rōn*]

(conjugated estrogens)
with METHYLTESTOSTERONE

No. 879—Each *yellow* tablet contains:

Premarin® (conjugated estrogens, USP)	1.25 mg
Methyltestosterone	10.0 mg

No. 878—Each *white* tablet contains:

Premarin® (conjugated estrogens, USP)	0.625 mg
Methyltestosterone	5.0 mg

CAUTION: Federal law prohibits dispensing without prescription.

1. ESTROGENS HAVE BEEN REPORTED TO INCREASE THE RISK OF ENDOMETRIAL CARCINOMA.

Three independent, case-controlled studies have reported an increased risk of endometrial cancer in postmenopausal women exposed to exogenous estrogens for more than one year.[1–3] This risk was independent of the other known risk factors for endometrial cancer. These studies are further supported by the finding that incidence rates of endometrial cancer have increased sharply since 1969 in eight different areas of the United States with population-based cancer reporting systems, an increase which may be related to the rapidly expanding use of estrogens during the last decade.[4]

The three case-controlled studies reported that the risk of endometrial cancer in estrogen users was about 4.5 to 13.9 times greater than in nonusers. The risk appears to depend on both duration of treatment[1] and on estrogen dose.[3] In view of these findings, when estrogens are used for the treatment of menopausal symptoms, the lowest dose that will control symptoms should be utilized and medication should be discontinued as soon as possible. When prolonged treatment is medically indicated, the patient should be reassessed on at least a semi-annual basis to determine the need for continued therapy. Although the evidence must be considered preliminary, one study suggests that cyclic administration of low doses of estrogen may carry less risk than continuous administration.[3] It, therefore, appears prudent to utilize such a regimen.

Close clinical surveillance of all women taking estrogens is important. In all cases of undiagnosed persistent or recurring abnormal vaginal bleeding, adequate diagnostic measures should be undertaken to rule out malignancy.

There is no evidence at present that "natural" estrogens are more or less hazardous than "synthetic" estrogens at equi-estrogenic doses.

2. ESTROGENS SHOULD NOT BE USED DURING PREGNANCY.

The use of female sex hormones, both estrogens and progestogens, during early pregnancy may seriously damage the offspring. It has been shown that females exposed *in utero* to diethylstilbestrol, a nonsteroidal estrogen, have an increased risk of developing, in later life, a form of vaginal or cervical cancer that is ordinarily extremely rare.[5,6] This risk has been estimated as not greater than 4 per 1,000 exposures.[7] Furthermore, a high percentage of such exposed women (from 30% to 90%) have been found to have vaginal adenosis,[8–12] epithelial changes of the vagina and cervix. Although these changes are histologically benign, it is not known whether they are precursors of malignancy. Although similar data are not available with the use of other estrogens, it cannot be presumed they would not induce similar changes.

Several reports suggest an association between intrauterine exposure to female sex hormones and congenital anomalies, including congenital heart defects and limb-reduction defects.[13–16] One case-controlled study[16] estimated a 4.7-fold increased risk of limb reduction defects in infants exposed *in utero* to sex hormones (oral contraceptives, hormone withdrawal tests for pregnancy, or attempted treatment for threatened abortion). Some of these exposures were very short and involved only a few days of treatment. The data suggest that the risk of limb-reduction defects in exposed fetuses is somewhat less than 1 per 1,000.

In the past, female sex hormones have been used during pregnancy in an attempt to treat threatened or habitual abortion. There is considerable evidence that estrogens are ineffective for these indications, and there is no evidence from well-controlled studies that progestogens are effective for these uses.

If Premarin with Methyltestosterone is used during pregnancy, or if the patient becomes pregnant while taking this drug, she should be apprised of the potential risks to the fetus, and the advisability of pregnancy continuation.

DESCRIPTION

Premarin with Methyltestosterone is provided in tablets for oral administration.

Premarin (conjugated estrogens, USP) is a mixture of estrogens, obtained exclusively from natural sources, occurring as the sodium salts of water-soluble estrogen sulfates blended to represent the average composition of material derived from pregnant mares' urine. It contains estrone, equilin, and 17 α-dihydroequilin, together with smaller amounts of 17 α-estradiol, equilenin, and 17 α-dihydroequilenin as salts of their sulfate esters.

Methyltestosterone is an androgen.

Androgens are derivatives of cyclopentano-perhydrophenanthrene. Endogenous androgens are C-19 steroids with a side chain at C-17, and with two angular methyl groups. Testosterone is the primary endogenous androgen. Fluoxymesterone and methyltestosterone are synthetic derivatives of testosterone.

Methyltestosterone is a white to light-yellow crystalline substance that is virtually insoluble in water but soluble in organic solvents. It is stable in air but decomposes in light.

Premarin with Methyltestosterone Tablets contain the following inactive ingredients: calcium phosphate tribasic, calcium sulfate carnauba wax, cellulose, glyceryl monooleate, guar gum, lactose, magnesium stearate, methylcellulose, pharmaceutical glaze, polyethylene glycol, stearic acid, sucrose, talc, titanium dioxide.

—1.25 mg Premarin with 10.0 mg methyltestosterone tablets also contain: D&C Yellow #10, FD&C Yellow #6.

CLINICAL PHARMACOLOGY

ESTROGENS

Estrogens are important in the development and maintenance of the female reproductive system and secondary sex characteristics. They promote growth and development of the vagina, uterus, and fallopian tubes, and enlargement of the breasts. Indirectly, they contribute to the shaping of the skeleton, maintenance of tone and elasticity of urogenital structures, changes in the epiphyses of the long bones that allow for the pubertal growth spurt and its termination, growth of axillary and pubic hair, and pigmentation of the nipples and genitals. Decline of estrogenic activity at the end of the menstrual cycle can bring on menstruation, although the cessation of progesterone secretion is the most important factor in the mature ovulatory cycle. However, in the preovulatory or nonovulatory cycle, estrogen is the primary determinant in the onset of menstruation. Estrogens also affect the release of pituitary gonadotropins.

The pharmacologic effects of conjugated estrogens are similar to those of endogenous estrogens. They are soluble in water and are well absorbed from the gastrointestinal tract. In responsive tissues (female genital organs, breasts, hypothalamus, pituitary) estrogens enter the cell and are transported into the nucleus. As a result of estrogen action, specific RNA and protein synthesis occurs.

Estrogen Pharmacokinetics

Metabolism and inactivation occur primarily in the liver. Some estrogens are excreted into the bile; however, they are reabsorbed from the intestine and returned to the liver through the portal venous system. Water-soluble estrogen conjugates are strongly acidic and are ionized in body fluids, which favor excretion through the kidneys since tubular reabsorption is minimal.

ANDROGENS

Endogenous androgens are responsible for the normal growth and development of the male sex organs and for maintenance of secondary sex characteristics. These effects include the growth and maturation of prostate, seminal vesicles, penis, and scrotum; the development of male hair distribution, such as beard, pubic, chest, and axillary hair, laryngeal enlargement, vocal chord thickening, alterations in body musculature, and fat distribution. Drugs in this class also cause retention of nitrogen, sodium, potassium, phosphorus, and decreased urinary excretion of calcium. Androgens have been reported to increase protein anabolism and decrease protein catabolism. Nitrogen balance is improved only when there is sufficient intake of calories and protein.

Androgens are responsible for the growth spurt of adolescence and for the eventual termination of linear growth which is brought about by fusion of the epiphyseal growth centers. In children, exogenous androgens accelerate linear growth rates but may cause a disproportionate advancement in bone maturation. Use over long periods may result in fusion of the epiphyseal growth centers and termination of growth process. Androgens have been reported to stimulate the production of red blood cells by enhancing the production of erythropoietic stimulating factor.

Androgen Pharmacokinetics

Testosterone given orally is metabolized by the gut and 44% is cleared by the liver in the first pass. Oral doses as high as 400 mg per day are needed to achieve clinically effective blood levels for full replacement therapy. The synthetic androgens (methyltestosterone and fluoxymesterone) are less extensively metabolized by the liver and have longer half-lives. They are more suitable than testosterone for oral administration. Testosterone in plasma is 98% bound to a specific testosterone-estradiol binding globulin, and about 2% is free. Generally, the amount of this sex-hormone-binding globulin in the plasma will determine the distribution of testosterone between free and bound forms, and the free testosterone concentration will determine its half-life.

About 90% of a dose of testosterone is excreted in the urine as glucuronic and sulfuric acid conjugates of testosterone

Continued on next page

Wyeth-Ayerst Laboratories—Cont.

and its metabolites; about 6% of a dose is excreted in the feces, mostly in the unconjugated form. Inactivation of testosterone occurs primarily in the liver. Testosterone is metabolized to various 17-keto steroids through two different pathways. There are considerable variations of the half-life of testosterone as reported in the literature, ranging from 10 to 100 minutes.

In many tissues the activity of testosterone appears to depend on reduction to dihydrotestosterone, which binds to cytosol receptor proteins. The steroid-receptor complex is transported to the nucleus where it initiates transcription events and cellular changes related to androgen action.

INDICATIONS

Premarin (conjugated estrogens, USP) with Methyltestosterone is indicated in the treatment of:

Moderate to severe *vasomotor* symptoms associated with the menopause in those patients not improved by estrogens alone. (There is no evidence that estrogens are effective for nervous symptoms or depression without associated vasomotor symptoms, and they should not be used to treat such conditions.)

PREMARIN with METHYLTESTOSTERONE HAS NOT BEEN SHOWN TO BE EFFECTIVE FOR ANY PURPOSE DURING PREGNANCY, AND ITS USE MAY CAUSE SEVERE HARM TO THE FETUS (SEE BOXED WARNING).

CONTRAINDICATIONS

Estrogens should not be used in women with any of the following conditions:

1. Known or suspected cancer of the breast, except in appropriately selected patients being treated for metastatic disease.
2. Known or suspected estrogen-dependent neoplasia.
3. Known or suspected pregnancy (see Boxed Warning).
4. Undiagnosed abnormal genital bleeding.
5. Active thrombophlebitis or thromboembolic disorders.
6. A past history of thrombophlebitis, thrombosis, or thromboembolic disorders associated with previous estrogen use (except when used in treatment of breast malignancy). Methyltestosterone should not be used in:
1. The presence of severe liver damage.
2. Pregnancy and in breast-feeding mothers because of the possibility of masculinization of the female fetus or breast-fed infant.

WARNINGS

ASSOCIATED WITH ESTROGENS

1. *Induction of malignant neoplasms.* Long-term continuous administration of natural and synthetic estrogens in certain animal species increases the frequency of carcinomas of the breast, cervix, vagina, and liver. There are now reports that estrogens increase the risk of carcinoma of the endometrium in humans. (See Boxed Warning.)

At the present time there is no satisfactory evidence that estrogens given to postmenopausal women increase the risk of cancer of the breast,[17] although a recent, long-term follow-up of a single physician's practice has raised this possibility.[18] Because of the animal data, there is a need for caution in prescribing estrogens for women with a strong family history of breast cancer or who have breast nodules, fibrocystic disease, or abnormal mammograms.

2. *Gallbladder disease.* A recent study has reported a 2- to 3-fold increase in the risk of surgically confirmed gallbladder disease in women receiving postmenopausal estrogens,[17] similar to the 2-fold increase previously noted in users of oral contraceptives.[19,24a]

3. *Effects similar to those caused by estrogen-progestogen oral contraceptives.* There are several serious adverse effects of oral contraceptives, most of which have not, up to now, been documented as consequences of postmenopausal estrogen therapy. This may reflect the comparatively low doses of estrogen used in postmenopausal women. It would be expected that the larger doses of estrogen used to treat prostatic or breast cancer are more likely to result in these adverse effects, and, in fact, it has been shown that there is an increased risk of thrombosis in men receiving estrogens for prostatic cancer.[20–23]

a. *Thromboembolic disease.* It is now well established that users of oral contraceptives have an increased risk of various thromboembolic and thrombotic vascular diseases, such as thrombophlebitis, pulmonary embolism, stroke, and myocardial infarction.[24–31] Cases of retinal thrombosis, mesenteric thrombosis, and optic neuritis have been reported in oral-contraceptive users. There is evidence that the risk of several of these adverse reactions is related to the dose of the drug.[32,33] An increased risk of postsurgery thromboembolic complications has also been reported in users of oral contraceptives.[34,35] If feasible, estrogen should be discontinued at least 4 weeks before surgery of the type associated with an increased risk of thromboembolism, or during periods of prolonged immobilization.

While an increased rate of thromboembolic and thrombotic disease in postmenopausal users of estrogens has not been found,[17–24,25–36] this does not rule out the possibility that such an increase may be present or that subgroups of women who have underlying risk factors or who are receiving relatively large doses of estrogens may have increased risk. Therefore estrogens should not be used in persons with active thrombophlebitis or thromboembolic disorders, and they should not be used (except in treatment of malignancy) in persons with a history of such disorders in association with estrogen use. They should be used with caution in patients with cerebral-vascular or coronary-artery disease and only for those in whom estrogens are clearly needed.

Large doses of estrogen (5 mg conjugated estrogens per day), comparable to those used to treat cancer of the prostate and breast, have been shown in a large prospective clinical trial in men[37] to increase the risk of nonfatal myocardial infarction, pulmonary embolism, and thrombophlebitis. When estrogen doses of this size are used, any of the thromboembolic and thrombotic adverse effects associated with oral-contraceptive use should be considered a clear risk.

b. *Hepatic adenoma.* Benign hepatic adenomas appear to be associated with the use of oral contraceptives.[38–40] Although benign, and rare, these may rupture and may cause death through intra-abdominal hemorrhage. Such lesions have not yet been reported in association with other estrogen or progestogen preparations but should be considered in estrogen users having abdominal pain and tenderness, abdominal mass, or hypovolemic shock. Hepatocellular carcinoma has also been reported in women taking estrogen-containing oral contraceptives.[39] The relationship of this malignancy to these drugs is not known at this time.

c. *Elevated blood pressure.* Women using oral contraceptives sometimes experience increased blood pressure which, in most cases, returns to normal on discontinuing the drug. There is now a report that this may occur with use of estrogens in the menopause,[41] and blood pressure should be monitored with estrogen use, especially if high doses are used.

d. *Glucose tolerance.* A worsening of glucose tolerance has been observed in a significant percentage of patients on estrogen-containing oral contraceptives. For this reason, diabetic patients should be carefully observed while receiving estrogens.

4. *Hypercalcemia.* Administration of estrogens may lead to severe hypercalcemia in patients with breast cancer and bone metastases. If this occurs, the drug should be stopped and appropriate measures taken to reduce the serum calcium level.

ASSOCIATED WITH METHYLTESTOSTERONE

In patients with breast cancer, androgen therapy may cause hypercalcemia by stimulating osteolysis. In this case, the drug should be discontinued.

Prolonged use of high doses of androgens has been associated with the development of peliosis hepatis and hepatic neoplasms including hepatocellular carcinoma. (See PRECAUTIONS—*Carcinogenesis*). Peliosis hepatis can be a life-threatening or fatal complication.

Cholestatic hepatitis and jaundice occur with 17-alpha-alkylandrogens at a relatively low dose. If cholestatic hepatitis with jaundice appears, or if liver function tests become abnormal, the androgen should be discontinued and the etiology should be determined. Drug-induced jaundice is reversible when the medication is discontinued.

Edema with or without heart failure may be a serious complication in patients with pre-existing cardiac, renal, or hepatic disease. In addition to discontinuation of the drug, diuretic therapy may be required.

PRECAUTIONS

ASSOCIATED WITH ESTROGENS

A. General.

1. Addition of a progestin—Studies of the addition of a progestin for 7 or more days of a cycle of estrogen administration have reported a lowered incidence of endometrial hyperplasia. Morphological and biochemical studies of the endometrium suggest that 10 to 13 days of progestin are needed to provide maximal maturation of the endometrium and to eliminate any hyperplastic changes. Whether this will provide protection from endometrial carcinoma has not been clearly established. There are possible additional risks which may be associated with the inclusion of progestin in estrogen-replacement regimens. The potential risks include adverse effects on carbohydrate and lipid metabolism. The choice of progestin and dosage may be important in minimizing these adverse effects.

2. Physical examination—A complete medical and family history should be taken prior to the initiation of any estrogen therapy. The pretreatment and periodic physical examinations should include special reference to blood pressure, breasts, abdomen, and pelvic organs, and should include a Papanicolaou smear. As a general rule, estrogen should not be prescribed for longer than one year without another physical examination being performed.

3. Fluid retention—Because estrogens may cause some degree of fluid retention, conditions which might be influenced by this factor such as asthma, epilepsy, migraine, and cardiac or renal dysfunction, require careful observation.

4. Certain patients may develop undesirable manifestations of excessive estrogenic stimulation, such as abnormal or excessive uterine bleeding, mastodynia, etc.

5. Prolonged administration of unopposed estrogen therapy has been reported to increase the risk of endometrial hyperplasia in some patients.

6. Oral contraceptives appear to be associated with an increased incidence of mental depression.[24a] Although it is not clear whether this is due to the estrogenic or progestogenic component of the contraceptive, patients with a history of depression should be carefully observed.

7. Preexisting uterine leiomyomata may increase in size during estrogen use.

8. The pathologist should be advised of estrogen therapy when relevant specimens are submitted.

9. Patients with a past history of jaundice during pregnancy have an increased risk of recurrence of jaundice while receiving estrogen-containing oral contraceptive therapy. If jaundice develops in any patient receiving estrogen, the medication should be discontinued while the cause is investigated.

10. Estrogens may be poorly metabolized in patients with impaired liver function and should be administered with caution in such patients.

11. Because estrogens influence the metabolism of calcium and phosphorus, they should be used with caution in patients with metabolic bone diseases that are associated with hypercalcemia or in patients with renal insufficiency.

12. Because of the effects of estrogens on epiphyseal closure, they should be used judiciously in young patients in whom bone growth is not yet complete.

13. Certain endocrine and liver function tests may be affected by estrogen-containing oral contraceptives. The following similar changes may be expected with larger doses of estrogen.

a. Increased sulfobromophthalein retention.

b. Increased prothrombin and factors VII, VIII, IX, and X; decreased antithrombin 3; increased norepinephrine-induced platelet aggregability.

c. Increased thyroid binding globulin (TBG) leading to increased circulating total thyroid hormone, as measured by PBI, T_4 by column, or T_4 by radioimmunoassay. Free T_3 resin uptake is decreased, reflecting the elevated TBG; free T_4 concentration is unaltered.

d. Impaired glucose tolerance.

e. Decreased pregnanediol excretion.

f. Reduced response to metyrapone test.

g. Reduced serum folate concentration.

h. Increased serum triglyceride and phospholipid concentration.

B. Information for the Patient. (See text which appears after the PHYSICIAN REFERENCES.)

C. Pregnancy Category X. See CONTRAINDICATIONS and Boxed Warning.

D. Nursing Mothers. As a general principle, the administration of any drug to nursing mothers should be done only when clearly necessary since many drugs are excreted in human milk.

ASSOCIATED WITH METHYLTESTOSTERONE

A. General Precautions

1. Women should be observed for signs of virilization (deepening of the voice, hirsutism, acne, clitoromegaly, and menstrual irregularities). Discontinuation of drug therapy at the time of evidence of mild virilism is necessary to prevent irreversible virilization. Such virilization is usual following androgen use at high doses.

2. Prolonged dosage of androgen may result in sodium and fluid retention. This may present a problem, especially in patients with compromised cardiac reserve or renal disease.

3. Hypersensitivity may occur rarely.

4. PBI may be decreased in patients taking androgens.

5. Hypercalcemia may occur. If this does occur, the drug should be discontinued.

B. Information for the Patient

The physician should instruct patients to report any of the following side effects of androgens:

Women: Hoarseness, acne, changes in menstrual periods, or more hair on the face.

All Patients: Any nausea, vomiting, changes in skin color or ankle swelling.

C. Laboratory Tests

1. Women with disseminated breast carcinoma should have frequent determination of urine and serum calcium levels during the course of androgen therapy (See WARNINGS).

2. Because of the hepatotoxicity associated with the use of 17-alpha-alkylated androgens, liver-function tests should be obtained periodically.

3. Hemoglobin and hematocrit should be checked periodically for polycythemia in patients who are receiving high doses of androgens.

D. Drug Interactions

1. *Anticoagulants.* C-17 substituted derivatives of testosterone, such as methandrostenolone, have been reported to

decrease the anticoagulant requirements of patients receiving oral anticoagulants. Patients receiving oral anticoagulant therapy require close monitoring, especially when androgens are started or stopped.

2. *Oxyphenbutazone.* Concurrent administration of oxyphenbutazone and androgens may result in elevated serum levels of oxyphenbutazone.

3. *Insulin.* In diabetic patients the metabolic effects of androgens may decrease blood glucose and insulin requirements.

E. Drug/Laboratory Test Interferences

Androgens may decrease levels of thyroxine-binding globulin, resulting in decreased T_4 serum levels and increased resin uptake of T_3 and T_4. Free thyroid hormone levels remain unchanged, however, and there is no clinical evidence of thyroid dysfunction.

F. Carcinogenesis

Animal Data. Testosterone has been tested by subcutaneous injection and implantation in mice and rats. The implant induced cervical-uterine tumors in mice, which metastasized in some cases. There is suggestive evidence that injection of testosterone into some strains of female mice increases their susceptibility to hepatoma. Testosterone is also known to increase the number of tumors and decrease the degree of differentiation of chemically induced carcinomas of the liver in rats.

Human Data. There are rare reports of hepatocellular carcinoma in patients receiving long-term therapy with androgens in high doses. Withdrawal of the drugs did not lead to regression of the tumors in all cases.

Geriatric patients treated with androgens may be at an increased risk for the development of prostatic hypertrophy and prostatic carcinoma.

G. Pregnancy

Teratogenic Effects. Pregnancy Category X (see CONTRAINDICATIONS).

H. Nursing Mothers

It is not known whether androgens are excreted in human milk. Because many drugs are excreted in human milk and because of the potential for serious adverse reactions in nursing infants from estrogens, a decision should be made whether to discontinue nursing or to discontinue the drug, taking into account the importance of the drug to the mother.

ADVERSE REACTIONS

ASSOCIATED WITH ESTROGENS

(See WARNINGS regarding induction of neoplasia, adverse effects on the fetus, increased incidence of gallbladder disease, and adverse effects similar to those of oral contraceptives, including thromboembolism.) The following additional adverse reactions have been reported with estrogenic therapy, including oral contraceptives:

1. *Genitourinary system:* Breakthrough bleeding, spotting, change in menstrual flow; dysmenorrhea; premenstrual-like syndrome; amenorrhea during and after treatment; increase in size of uterine fibromyomata; vaginal candidiasis; change in cervical erosion and in degree of cervical secretion; cystitis-like syndrome.

2. *Breasts:* Tenderness, enlargement, secretion.

3. *Gastrointestinal:* Nausea, vomiting; abdominal cramps, bloating; cholestatic jaundice.

4. *Skin:* Chloasma or melasma which may persist when drug is discontinued; erythema multiforme; erythema nodosum; hemorrhagic eruption; loss of scalp hair; hirsutism.

5. *Eyes:* Steepening of corneal curvature; intolerance to contact lenses.

6. *CNS:* Headache, migraine, dizziness; mental depression; chorea.

7. *Miscellaneous:* Increase or decrease in weight; reduced carbohydrate tolerance; aggravation of porphyria; edema; changes in libido.

ASSOCIATED WITH METHYLTESTOSTERONE

A. Endocrine and Urogenital

1. *Female:* The most common side effects of androgen therapy are amenorrhea and other menstrual irregularities, inhibition of gonadotropin secretion, and virilization, including deepening of the voice and clitoral enlargement. The latter usually is not reversible after androgens are discontinued. When administered to a pregnant woman androgens cause virilization of external genitalia of the female fetus.

2. *Skin and Appendages:* Hirsutism, male pattern of baldness, and acne.

3. *Fluid and Electrolyte Disturbances:* Retention of sodium, chloride, water, potassium, calcium, and inorganic phosphates.

4. *Gastrointestinal:* Nausea, cholestatic jaundice, alterations in liver-function tests, rarely hepatocellular neoplasms, and peliosis hepatis (see WARNINGS).

5. *Hematologic:* Suppression of clotting factors II, V, VII, and X, bleeding in patients on concomitant anticoagulant therapy, and polycythemia.

6. *Nervous System:* Increased or decreased libido, headache, anxiety, depression, and generalized paresthesia.

7. *Metabolic:* Increased serum cholesterol.

8. *Miscellaneous:* Inflammation and pain at the site of intramuscular injection or subcutaneous implantation of testosterone-containing pellets, stomatitis with buccal preparations, and rarely anaphylactoid reactions.

ACUTE OVERDOSAGE

Numerous reports of ingestion of large doses of estrogen-containing oral contraceptives by young children indicate that acute serious ill effects do not occur. Overdosage of estrogens may cause nausea, and withdrawal bleeding may occur in females.

There have been no reports of acute overdosage with the androgens.

DOSAGE AND ADMINISTRATION

GIVEN CYCLICALLY FOR SHORT-TERM USE ONLY:

For treatment of moderate-to-severe *vasomotor* symptoms associated with the menopause in patients not improved by estrogen alone.

The lowest dose that will control symptoms should be chosen and medication should be discontinued as promptly as possible.

Administration should be cyclic (eg, three weeks on and one week off).

Attempts to discontinue or taper medication should be made at 3- to 6-month intervals.

USUAL DOSAGE RANGE:

1.25 mg Conjugated Estrogens, USP, and 10.0 mg Methyltestosterone (1 yellow tablet, No. 879, or 2 white tablets, No. 878), daily and cyclically.

Treated patients with an intact uterus should be monitored closely for signs of endometrial cancer and appropriate diagnostic measures should be taken to rule out malignancy in the event of persistent or recurring abnormal vaginal bleeding.

HOW SUPPLIED

Premarin (conjugated estrogens, USP) with Methyltestosterone Tablets

—Each round *yellow* tablet contains 1.25 mg Premarin and 10.0 mg Methyltestosterone, in bottles of 100 (NDC 0046-0879-81).

—Each round *white* tablet contains 0.625 mg Premarin and 5.0 mg Methyltestosterone, in bottles of 100 (NDC 0046-0878-81).

Store at room temperature (approximately 25° C).

The appearance of these tablets is a trademark of Wyeth-Ayerst Laboratories.

PHYSICIAN REFERENCES

1. Ziel, H. K., *et al.*: N. Engl. J. Med. *293* :1167–1170, 1975.
2. Smith, D. C., *et al.*: N. Engl. J. Med. *293* :1164–1167, 1975.
3. Mack, T. M., *et al.*: N. Engl. J. Med. *294* :1262–1267, 1976.
4. Weiss, N. S., *et al.*: N. Engl. J. Med. *294* :1259–1262, 1976.
5. Herbst, A. L., *et al.*: N. Engl. J. Med. *284* :878–881, 1971.
6. Greenwald, P., *et al.*: N. Engl. J. Med. *285* :390–392, 1971.
7. Lanier, A., *et al.*: Mayo Clin. Proc. *48* :793–799, 1973.
8. Herbst, A., *et al.*: Obstet. Gynecol. *40* :287–298, 1972.
9. Herbst, A., *et al.*: Am. J. Obstet. Gynecol. *118* :607–615, 1974.
10. Herbst, A., *et al.*: N. Engl. J. Med. *292* :334–339, 1975.
11. Stafl, A., *et al.*: Obstet. Gynecol. *43* :118–128, 1974.
12. Sherman, A. I., *et al.*: Obstet. Gynecol. *44* :531–545, 1974.
13. Gal, I., *et al.*: Nature *216* :83, 1967.
14. Levy, E. P., *et al.*: Lancet *1* :611, 1973.
15. Nora, J., *et al.*: Lancet *1* :941–942, 1973.
16. Janerich, D. T., *et al.*: N. Engl. J. Med. *291* :697–700, 1974.
17. Boston Collaborative Drug Surveillance Program: N. Engl. J. Med. *290* :15–19, 1974.
18. Hoover, R., *et al.*: N. Engl. J. Med. *295* : 401–405, 1976.
19. Boston Collaborative Drug Surveillance Program: Lancet *1* :1399–1404, 1973.
20. Daniel, D. G., *et al.*: Lancet *2* :287–289, 1967.
21. The Veterans Administration Cooperative Urological Research Group: J. Urol. *98* :516–522, 1967.
22. Bailar, J. C.: Lancet *2* :560, 1967.
23. Blackard, C., *et al.*: Cancer *26* :249–256, 1970.
24. Royal College of General Practitioners: J. R. Coll. Gen. Pract. *13* :267–279, 1967.
24a. Royal College of General Practitioners: Oral Contraceptives and Health, New York, Pitman Corp., 1974.
25. Inman, W. H. W., *et al.*: Br. Med. J. *2* :193–199, 1968.
26. Vessey, M. P., *et al.*: Br. Med. J. *2* :651–657, 1969.
27. Sartwell, P. E., *et al.*: Am. J. Epidemiol. *90* :365–380, 1969.
28. Collaborative Group for the Study of Stroke in Young Women: N. Engl. J. Med. *288* :871–878, 1973.
29. Collaborative Group for the Study of Stroke in Young Women: J.A.M.A. *231* : 718–722, 1975.
30. Mann, J. I., *et al.*: Br. Med. J. *2* :245–248, 1975.
31. Mann, J. I., *et al.*: Br. Med. J. *2* :241–245, 1975.
32. Inman, W. H. W., *et al.*: Br. Med. J. *2* :203–209, 1970.
33. Stolley, P. D., *et al.*: Am. J. Epidemiol. *102* :197–208, 1975.
34. Vessey, M. P., *et al.*: Br. Med. J. *3* :123–126, 1970.
35. Greene, G. R., *et al.*: Am. J. Public Health *62* :680–685, 1972.
36. Rosenberg, L., *et al.*: N. Engl. J. Med. *294* : 1256–1259, 1976.
37. Coronary Drug Project Research Group: J.A.M.A. *214* :1303–1313, 1970.
38. Baum, J., *et al.*: Lancet *2* :926–928, 1973.
39. Mays, E. T., *et al.*: J.A.M.A. *235* :730–732, 1976.
40. Edmondson, H. A., *et al.*: N. Engl. J. Med. *294* :470–472, 1976.
41. Pfeffer, R. I., *et al.*: Am. J. Epidemiol. *103* :445–456, 1976.

Androgen references available upon request.

INFORMATION FOR THE PATIENT

What You Should Know About Estrogens

Estrogens are female hormones produced by the ovaries. The ovaries make several different kinds of estrogens. In addition, scientists have been able to make a variety of synthetic estrogens. As far as we know, all these estrogens have similar properties and, therefore, much the same usefulness, side effects, and risks. This leaflet is intended to help you understand what estrogens are used for, the risks involved in their use, and how to use them as safely as possible.

This leaflet includes the most important information about estrogens, but not all the information. If you want to know more, you should ask your doctor for more information or you can ask your doctor or pharmacist to let you read the package insert prepared for the doctor.

Uses of Estrogen

THERE IS NO PROPER USE OF ESTROGENS IN A PREGNANT WOMAN.

Estrogens are prescribed by doctors for a number of purposes, including:

1. To provide estrogen during a period of adjustment when a woman's ovaries stop producing a majority of her estrogens, in order to prevent certain uncomfortable symptoms of estrogen deficiency. (With the menopause, which generally occurs between the ages of 45 and 55, women produce a much smaller amount of estrogens.)

2. To prevent symptoms of estrogen deficiency when a woman's ovaries have been removed surgically before the natural menopause.

3. To prevent pregnancy. (Estrogens are given along with a progestogen, another female hormone; these combinations are called oral contraceptives or birth-control pills. Patient labeling is available to women taking oral contraceptives and they will not be discussed in this leaflet.)

4. To treat certain cancers in women and men.

Estrogens in the Menopause

In the natural course of their lives, all women eventually experience a decrease in estrogen production. This usually occurs between ages 45 and 55, but may occur earlier or later. Sometimes the ovaries may need to be removed before natural menopause by an operation, producing a "surgical menopause."

When the amount of estrogen in the blood begins to decrease, many women may develop typical symptoms: feelings of warmth in the face, neck, and chest, or sudden intense episodes of heat and sweating throughout the body (called "hot flashes" or "hot flushes"). These symptoms are sometimes very uncomfortable. Some women may also develop changes in the vagina (called "atrophic vaginitis") that cause discomfort, especially during and after intercourse.

Estrogens can be prescribed to treat these symptoms of the menopause. It is estimated that considerably more than half of all women undergoing the menopause have only mild symptoms or no symptoms at all and, therefore, do not need estrogens. Other women may need estrogens for a few months, while their bodies adjust to lower estrogen levels. Sometimes the need will be for periods longer than six months. In an attempt to avoid overstimulation of the uterus (womb), estrogens are usually given cyclically during each month of use, such as three weeks of pills followed by one week without pills.

Sometimes women experience nervous symptoms or depression during menopause. There is no evidence that estrogens are effective for such symptoms without associated vasomotor symptoms. In the absence of vasomotor symptoms, estrogens should not be used to treat nervous symptoms, although other treatment may be needed.

You may have heard that taking estrogens for long periods (years) after the menopause will keep your skin soft and supple and keep you feeling young. There is no evidence that this is so, however, and such long-term treatment carries important risks.

Continued on next page

Wyeth-Ayerst Laboratories—Cont.

The Dangers of Estrogens

1. *Endometrial cancer.* There are reports that if estrogens are used in the postmenopausal period for more than a year, there is an increased risk of *endometrial cancer* (cancer of the lining of the uterus). Women taking estrogens have roughly 5- to 10-times as great a chance of getting this cancer as women who take no estrogens. To put this another way, while a postmenopausal woman not taking estrogens has 1 chance in 1,000 each year of getting endometrial cancer, a woman taking estrogens has 5 to 10 chances in 1,000 each year. For this reason *it is important to take estrogens only when they are really needed.*

The risk of this cancer is greater the longer estrogens are used and when larger doses are taken. Therefore you should not take more estrogen than your doctor prescribes. *It is important to take the lowest dose of estrogen that will control symptoms and to take it only as long as it is needed.* If estrogens are needed for longer periods of time, your doctor will want to reevaluate your need for estrogens at least every six months.

Women using estrogens should report any vaginal bleeding to their doctors; such bleeding may be of no importance, but it can be an early warning of endometrial cancer. If you have undiagnosed vaginal bleeding, you should not use estrogens until a diagnosis is made and you are certain there is no endometrial cancer.

NOTE: If you have had your uterus removed (total hysterectomy), there is no danger of developing endometrial cancer.

2. *Other possible cancers.* Estrogens can cause development of other tumors in animals, such as tumors of the breast, cervix, vagina, or liver, when given for a long time. At present there is no good evidence that women using estrogen in the menopause have an increased risk of such tumors, but there is no way yet to be sure they do not; and one study raises the possibility that use of estrogens in the menopause may increase the risk of breast cancer many years later. This is a further reason to use estrogens only when clearly needed. While you are taking estrogens, it is important that you go to your doctor at least once a year for a physical examination. Also, if members of your family have had breast cancer or if you have breast nodules or abnormal mammograms (breast x-rays), your doctor may wish to carry out more frequent examinations of your breasts.

3. *Gallbladder disease.* Women who use estrogens after menopause are more likely to develop gallbladder disease needing surgery than women who do not use estrogens. Birth-control pills have a similar effect.

4. *Abnormal blood clotting.* Oral contraceptives increase the risk of blood clotting in various parts of the body. This can result in a stroke (if the clot is in the brain), a heart attack (a clot in a blood vessel of the heart), or a pulmonary embolus (a clot which forms in the legs or pelvis, then breaks off and travels to the lungs). Any of these can be fatal.

At this time, use of estrogens in the menopause is not known to cause such blood clotting, but this has not been fully studied and there could still prove to be such a risk. It is recommended that if you have had clotting in the legs or lungs or a heart attack or stroke while you were using estrogens or birth control pills, you should not use estrogens (unless they are being used to treat cancer of the breast or prostate). If you have had a stroke or heart attack, or if you have angina pectoris, estrogens should be used with great caution and only if clearly needed (for example, if you have severe symptoms of the menopause).

Special Warning About Pregnancy

You should not receive estrogen if you are pregnant. If this should occur, there is a greater than usual chance that the developing child will be born with a birth defect, although the possibility remains fairly small. A female child may have an increased risk of developing cancer of the vagina or cervix later in life (in the teens or twenties). Every possible effort should be made to avoid exposure to estrogens during pregnancy. If exposure occurs, see your doctor.

Other Effects of Estrogens

In addition to the serious known risks of estrogens described above, estrogens have the following side effects and potential risks:

1. *Nausea and vomiting.* The most common side effect of estrogen therapy is nausea. Vomiting is less common.
2. *Effects on breasts.* Estrogens may cause breast tenderness or enlargement and may cause the breasts to secrete a liquid. These effects are not dangerous.
3. *Effects on the uterus.* Estrogens may cause benign fibroid tumors of the uterus to get larger.
4. *Effects on liver.* Women taking oral contraceptives develop, on rare occasions, a tumor of the liver which can rupture and bleed into the abdomen and may cause death. So far, these tumors have not been reported in women using estrogens in the menopause, but you should report any swelling or unusual pain or tenderness in the abdomen to your doctor immediately.

Women with a past history of jaundice (yellowing of the skin and white parts of the eyes) may get jaundice again during estrogen use. If this occurs, stop taking estrogens and see your doctor.

5. *Other effects.* Estrogens may cause excess fluid to be retained in the body. This may make some conditions worse, such as asthma, epilepsy, migraine, heart disease, or kidney disease.

Summary

Estrogens have important uses, but they have serious risks as well. You must decide, with your doctor, whether the risks are acceptable to you in view of the benefits of treatment. Except where your doctor has prescribed estrogens for use in special cases of cancer of the breast or prostate, you should not use estrogens if you have cancer of the breast or uterus, are pregnant, have undiagnosed abnormal vaginal bleeding, clotting in the legs or lungs, or have had a stroke, heart attack or angina, or clotting in the legs or lungs in the past while you were taking estrogens.

You can use estrogens as safely as possible by understanding that your doctor will require physical examinations while you are taking them and will try to discontinue the drug as soon as possible and use the smallest dose possible. Be alert for signs of trouble including:

1. Abnormal bleeding from the vagina.
2. Pains in the calves or chest or sudden shortness of breath, or coughing blood.
3. Severe headache, dizziness, faintness, or changes in vision.
4. Breast lumps (you should ask your doctor how to examine your own breasts).
5. Jaundice (yellowing of the skin).
6. Mental depression.

Your doctor has prescribed this drug for you and you alone. Do not give the drug to anyone else.

HOW SUPPLIED

Premarin® with Methyltestosterone—a combination of Premarin and methyltestosterone (an androgen) in tablet form for oral administration.

Each round *yellow* tablet contains 1.25 mg Premarin and 10.0 mg methyltestosterone

Each round *white* tablet contains 0.625 mg Premarin and 5 mg methyltestosterone

Shown in Product Identification Section, page 437

PROTOPAM® CHLORIDE ℞

(pralidoxime chloride)
Lyophilized Powder for Injection

CAUTION: Federal law prohibits dispensing without prescription.

DESCRIPTION

Chemical name: 2-formyl-1-methylpyridinium chloride oxime. Available in the United States as Protopam Chloride, pralidoxime chloride is frequently referred to as 2-PAM Chloride.

Structural formula:

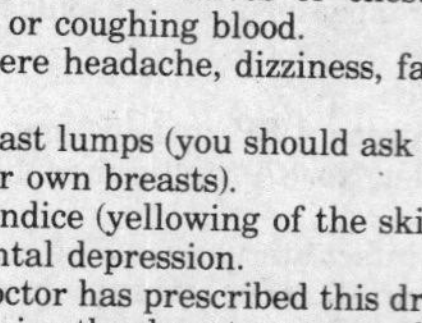

$C_7H_9ClN_2O$

Pralidoxime chloride occurs as an odorless, white, nonhygroscopic, crystalline powder which is soluble in water to the extent of 1 g in less than 1 mL. Stable in air, it melts between 215° and 225°C, with decomposition.

The specific activity of the drug resides in the 2-formyl-1-methylpyridinium ion and is independent of the particular salt employed. The chloride is preferred because of physiologic compatibility, excellent water solubility at all temperatures, and high potency per gram, due to its low (173) molecular weight.

Pralidoxime chloride is a cholinesterase reactivator.

Protopam Chloride for intravenous injection or infusion is prepared by cryodesiccation. Each vial contains 1 g of sterile pralidoxime chloride, and NaOH to adjust pH, to be reconstituted with 20 mL of Sterile Water for Injection, USP. The pH of the reconstituted solution is 3.5 to 4.5. Intramuscular or subcutaneous injection may be used when intravenous injection is not feasible.

CLINICAL PHARMACOLOGY

The principal action of pralidoxime is to reactivate cholinesterase (mainly outside of the central nervous system) which has been inactivated by phosphorylation due to an organophosphate pesticide or related compound. The destruction of accumulated acetylcholine can then proceed, and neuromuscular junctions will again function normally. Pralidoxime also slows the process of "aging" of phosphorylated cholinesterase to a nonreactivatable form, and detoxifies certain organophosphates by direct chemical reaction. The drug has its most critical effect in relieving paralysis of the muscles of respiration. Because pralidoxime is less effective in relieving depression of the respiratory center, atropine is always required concomitantly to block the effect of accumulated acetylcholine at this site. Pralidoxime relieves muscarinic signs and symptoms, salivation, bronchospasm, etc., but this action is relatively unimportant since atropine is adequate for this purpose.

Pralidoxime is distributed throughout the extracellular water; it is not bound to plasma protein. The drug is rapidly excreted in the urine partly unchanged, and partly as a metabolite produced by the liver. Consequently, pralidoxime is relatively short acting, and repeated doses may be needed, especially where there is any evidence of continuing absorption of the poison.

The minimum therapeutic concentration of pralidoxime in plasma is 4 μg/mL; this level is reached in about 16 minutes after a single injection of 600 mg Protopam Chloride. The apparent half-life of Protopam Chloride is 74 to 77 minutes.

It has been reported[1] that the supplemental use of oxime cholinesterase reactivators (such as pralidoxime) reduces the incidence and severity of developmental defects in chick embryos exposed to such known teratogens as parathion, bidrin, carbachol, and neostigmine. This protective effect of the oximes was shown to be dose related.

INDICATIONS AND USAGE

Protopam is indicated as an antidote: (1) in the treatment of poisoning due to those pesticides and chemicals of the organophosphate class which have anticholinesterase activity and (2) in the control of overdosage by anticholinesterase drugs used in the treatment of myasthenia gravis.

The principal indications for the use of pralidoxime are muscle weakness and respiratory depression. In severe poisoning, respiratory depression may be due to muscle weakness.

CONTRAINDICATIONS

There are no known absolute contraindications for the use of Protopam. Relative contraindications include known hypersensitivity to the drug and other situations in which the risk of its use clearly outweighs possible benefit (see "Precautions").

WARNINGS

Protopam is not effective in the treatment of poisoning due to phosphorus, inorganic phosphates, or organophosphates not having anticholinesterase activity

Protopam is **not** indicated as an antidote for intoxication by pesticides of the carbamate class since it may increase the toxicity of carbaryl.

PRECAUTIONS

GENERAL

Pralidoxime has been very well tolerated in most cases, but it must be remembered that the desperate condition of the organophosphate-poisoned patient will generally mask such minor signs and symptoms as have been noted in normal subjects.

Intravenous administration of Protopam should be carried out slowly and, preferably, by infusion, since certain side effects, such as tachycardia, laryngospasm, and muscle rigidity, have been attributed in a few cases to a too-rapid rate of injection. (See "Dosage and Administration".)

Protopam should be used with great caution in treating organophosphate overdosage in cases of myasthenia gravis since it may precipitate a myasthenic crisis.

Because pralidoxime is excreted in the urine, a decrease in renal function will result in increased blood levels of the drug. Thus, the dosage of pralidoxime should be reduced in the presence of renal insufficiency.

LABORATORY TESTS

Treatment of organophosphate poisoning should be instituted without waiting for the results of laboratory tests. Red blood cell, plasma cholinesterase, and urinary paranitrophenol measurements (in the case of parathion exposure) may be helpful in confirming the diagnosis and following the course of the illness. A reduction in red blood cell cholinesterase concentration to below 50% of normal has been seen only with organophosphate ester poisoning.

DRUG INTERACTIONS

When atropine and pralidoxime are used together, the signs of atropinization (flushing, mydriasis, tachycardia, dryness of the mouth and nose) may occur earlier than might be expected when atropine is used alone. This is especially true if the total dose of atropine has been large and the administration of pralidoxime has been delayed.[2–4]

The following precautions should be kept in mind in the treatment of anticholinesterase poisoning, although they do not bear directly on the use of pralidoxime: since barbiturates are potentiated by the anticholinesterases, they should be used cautiously in the treatment of convulsions; morphine, theophylline, aminophylline, succinylcholine, reserpine, and phenothiazine-type tranquilizers should be avoided in patients with organophosphate poisoning.

CARCINOGENESIS, MUTAGENESIS, IMPAIRMENT OF FERTILITY

Since pralidoxime chloride is indicated for short-term emergency use only, no investigations of its potential for carcinogenesis, mutagenesis, or impairment of fertility have been conducted by the manufacturer, or reported in the literature.

PREGNANCY

Teratogenic Effects —Pregnancy Category C:
Animal reproduction studies have not been conducted with pralidoxime. It is also not known whether pralidoxime can cause fetal harm when administered to a pregnant woman or can affect reproduction capacity. Pralidoxime should be given to a pregnant woman only if clearly needed.

NURSING MOTHERS

It is not known whether this drug is excreted in human milk. Because many drugs are excreted in human milk, caution should be exercised when pralidoxime is administered to a nursing woman.

PEDIATRIC USE

Safety and effectiveness in children have not been established.

ADVERSE REACTIONS

Forty to 60 minutes after intramuscular injection, mild to moderate pain may be experienced at the site of injection. Pralidoxime may cause blurred vision, diplopia and impaired accommodation, dizziness, headache, drowsiness, nausea, tachycardia, increased systolic and diastolic blood pressure, hyperventilation, and muscular weakness when given parenterally to normal volunteers who have not been exposed to anticholinesterase poisons. In patients, it is very difficult to differentiate the toxic effects produced by atropine or the organophosphate compounds from those of the drug.

Elevations in SGOT and/or SGPT enzyme levels were observed in 1 of 6 normal volunteers given 1200 mg of pralidoxime chloride intramuscularly, and in 4 of 6 volunteers given 1800 mg intramuscularly. Levels returned to normal in about 2 weeks. Transient elevations in creatine phosphokinase were observed in all normal volunteers given the drug. A single intramuscular injection of 330 mg in 1 mL in rabbits caused myonecrosis, inflammation, and hemorrhage.

When atropine and pralidoxime are used together, the signs of atropinization may occur earlier than might be expected when atropine is used alone. This is especially true if the total dose of atropine has been large and the administration of pralidoxime has been delayed.[2-4] Excitement and manic behavior immediately following recovery of consciousness have been reported in several cases. However, similar behavior has occurred in cases of organophosphate poisoning that were not treated with pralidoxime.[3,5,6]

DRUG ABUSE AND DEPENDENCE

Pralidoxime chloride is not subject to abuse and possesses no known potential for dependence.

OVERDOSAGE

MANIFESTATIONS OF OVERDOSAGE

Observed in normal subjects only: dizziness, blurred vision, diplopia, headache, impaired accommodation, nausea, slight tachycardia. In therapy it has been difficult to differentiate side effects due to the drug from those due to the effects of the poison.

TREATMENT OF OVERDOSAGE

Artificial respiration and other supportive therapy should be administered as needed.

ACUTE TOXICITY

IV—man TDLo: 14 mg/kg (toxic effects: CNS)
IV—rat LD50: 96 mg/kg
IM—rat LD50: 150 mg/kg
ORAL—mouse LD50: 4100 mg/kg
IP—mouse LD50: 155 mg/kg
IV—mouse LD50: 90 mg/kg
IM—mouse LD50: 180 mg/kg
IV—rabbit LD50: 95 mg/kg
IM—guinea pig LD50: 168 mg/kg

DOSAGE AND ADMINISTRATION

ORGANOPHOSPHATE POISONING

"Pralidoxime is most effective if administered immediately after poisoning. Generally, little is accomplished if the drug is given more than 36 hours after termination of exposure. When the poison has been ingested, however, exposure may continue for some time due to slow absorption from the lower bowel, and fatal relapses have been reported after initial improvement. Continued administration for several days may be useful in such patients. Close supervision of the patient is indicated for at least 48 to 72 hours. If dermal exposure has occurred, clothing should be removed and the hair and skin washed thoroughly with sodium bicarbonate or alcohol as soon as possible. Diazepam may be given cautiously if convulsions are not controlled by atropine."[7] Severe poisoning (coma, cyanosis, respiratory depression) requires intensive management. This includes the removal of secretions, airway management, the correction of acidosis, and hypoxemia.

AAT—see PARATHION

AFLIX®—see FORMOTHION

ALKRON®—See PARATHION

AMERICAN CYANAMID 3422—see PARATHION

AMITON—diethyl-S-(2-diethylaminoethyl)phosphorothiolate

ANTHIO®—see FORMOTHION

APHAMITE—see PARATHION

ARMIN—ethyl-4-nitrophenylethylphosphonate

AZINPHOS-METHYL—dimethyl-S-(4-oxo-1,2,3,-benzotriazin-3 (4H)-ylmethyl) phosphorodithioate

MORPHOTHION—dimethyl-S-2-keto-2-(N-morpholyl)ethyl-phosphorodithioate

NEGUVON®—see TRICHLOROFON

NIRAN®—see PARATHION

NITROSTIGMINE—see PARATHION

O,O-DIETHYL-O-p-NITROPHENYL PHOSPHOROTHIOATE—see PARATHION

O,O-DIETHYL-O-p-NITROPHENYLTHIO PHOSPHATE—see PARATHION

OR 1191—see PHOSPHAMIDON

OS 1836—see VINYLPHOS

OXYDEMETONMETHYL—dimethyl-S-2-(ethylsulfinyl) ethyl phosphorothiolate

PARAOXON-diethyl (4-nitrophenyl) phosphate

PARATHION—diethyl (4-nitrophenyl) phosphorothionate

PENPHOS—see PARATHION

PHENCAPTON—diethyl-S-(2,5-dichlorophenylmercaptomethyl) phosphorodithioate

---

Atropine should be given as soon as possible after hypoxemia is improved. Atropine should not be given in the presence of significant hypoxia due to the risk of atropine-induced ventricular fibrillation. In adults, atropine may be given intravenously in doses of 2 to 4 mg. This should be repeated at 5- to 10-minute intervals until full atropinization (secretions are inhibited) or signs of atropine toxicity appear (delirium, hyperthermia, muscle twitching).

The dosage of atropine for children, 0.05 to 0.10 mg/kg, should be given on a similar schedule.

Some degree of atropinization should be maintained for at least 48 hours, and until any depressed blood cholinesterase activity is reversed.

Morphine, theophylline, aminophylline, and succinylcholine are contraindicated. Tranquilizers of the reserpine or phenothiazine type are to be avoided.

After the effects of atropine become apparent, Protopam may be administered.

PROTOPAM CHLORIDE INJECTION

Parenteral drug products should be inspected visually for particulate matter and discoloration prior to administration, whenever solution and container permit.

Discard unused solution after a dose has been withdrawn.

In adults, inject an initial dose of 1 to 2 g of Protopam, preferably as an infusion in 100 mL of saline, over a 15- to 30-minute period. If this is not practical or if pulmonary edema is present, the dose should be given slowly by intravenous injection as a 5 percent solution in water over not less than five minutes. After about an hour, a second dose of 1 to 2 g will be indicated if muscle weakness has been relieved. Additional doses may be given cautiously if muscle weakness persists. Too-rapid administration may result in temporary worsening of cholinergic manifestations. Injection rate should not exceed 200 mg/minute. If intravenous administration is not feasible, intramuscular or subcutaneous injection should be used.

In children, the dose should be 20 to 40 mg/kg body weight using the same procedure.

In severe cases, especially after ingestion of the poison, it may be desirable to monitor the effect of therapy electrocardiographically because of the possibility of heart block due to the anticholinesterase. Where the poison has been ingested, it is particularly important to take into account the likeli-

---

PHOSDRIN®—see MEVINPHOS

PHOS-KIL—see PARATHION

PHOSPHAMIDON—1-chloro-1-diethylcarbamoyl-1-propen-2-yl-dimethylphosphate

PHOSPHOLINE IODIDE®—see echothiophate iodide

PHOSPHOROTHIOIC ACID, O,O-DIETHYL-O-p-NITROPHENYL ESTER—see PARATHION

PLANTHION—see PARATHION

QUELETOX—see FENTHION

RHODIATOX®—see PARATHION

RUELENE®—4-tert-butyl-2-chlorophenylmethyl-N-methylphosphoroamidate

SARIN—isopropyl-methylphosphonofluoridate

SHELL OS 1836—see VINYLPHOS

SHELL 2046—see MEVINPHOS

SNP—see PARATHION

SOMAN—pinacolyl-methylphosphonofluoridate

SYSTOX®—diethyl-(2-ethylmercaptoethyl) phosphorothionate

TEP—see TEPP

TEPP—tetraethylpyro phosphate

THIOPHOS®—see PARATHION

TIGUVON—see FENTHION

TRICHLOROFON—dimethyl-1-hydroxy-2,2,2-trichloroethylphosphonate

VAPONA®—see DICHLORVOS

VAPOPHOS—see PARATHION

VINYLPHOS—diethyl-2-chloro-vinylphosphate

---

hood of continuing absorption from the lower bowel since this constitutes new exposure. In such cases, additional doses of Protopam (pralidoxime) may be needed every three to eight hours. In effect, the patient should be "titrated" with Protopam as long as signs of poisoning recur. As in all cases of organophosphate poisoning, care should be taken to keep the patient under observation for at least 24 hours.

If convulsions interfere with respiration, they may be controlled by the slow intravenous injection of diazepam, up to 20 mg in adults and at 0.1 to 0.2 mg/kg in children.

ANTICHOLINESTERASE OVERDOSAGE

As an antagonist to such anticholinesterases as neostigmine, pyridostigmine, and ambenonium, which are used in the treatment of myasthenia gravis, Protopam may be given in a dosage of 1 to 2 g intravenously followed by increments of 250 mg every five minutes.

HOW SUPPLIED

NDC 0046-0374-06—*Hospital Package:* This contains six 20 mL vials of 1 g each of sterile Protopam Chloride (pralidoxime chloride) white to off-white porous cake*, without diluent or syringe. Solution may be prepared by adding 20 mL of Sterile Water for Injection, USP. These are single-dose vials for intravenous injection or for intravenous infusion after further dilution with physiologic saline. Intramuscular or subcutaneous injection may be used when intravenous injection is not feasible.

Store at room temperature (approximately 25°C).

ANIMAL PHARMACOLOGY AND TOXICOLOGY

The above table lists chemical and trade or generic names of pesticides, chemicals, and drugs against which Protopam (usually administered in conjunction with atropine) has been found to have antidotal activity on the basis of animal experiments. All compounds listed are organophosphates having anticholinesterase activity. A great many additional substances are in industrial use but have been omitted because of lack of special information.

PROTOPAM appears to be ineffective, or marginally effective, against poisoning by:

*When necessary, sodium hydroxide is added during processing to adjust the pH.

Continued on next page

Wyeth-Ayerst Laboratories—Cont.

CIODRIN® (alpha-methylbenzyl-3[dimethoxyphosphinyloxy]-ciscrotonate)
DIMEFOX (tetramethylphosphorodiamidic fluoride)
DIMETHOATE (dimethyl-S-[N-methylcarbamoylmethyl]-phosphorodithioate)
METHYL DIAZINON (dimethyl-[2-isopropyl-4-methyl-pyrimidyl]-phosphorothionate)
METHYL PHENCAPTON (dimethyl-S-[2,5-dichlorophenyl-mercaptomethyl]phosphorodithioate)
PHORATE (diethyl-S-ethylmercaptomethylphosphorodithioate)
SCHRADAN (octamethylpyrophosphoramide)
WEPSYN® (5-amino-1-[bis-(dimethylamino) phosphinyl]-3-phenyl-1,2,4-triazole).

The use of Protopam should, nevertheless, be considered in any life-threatening situation resulting from poisoning by these compounds, since the limited and arbitrary conditions of pharmacologic screening do not always accurately reflect the usefulness of Protopam in the clinical situation.

CLINICAL STUDIES

The use of Protopam (pralidoxime) has been reported in the treatment of human cases of poisoning by the following substances:

Azodrin	Methyldemeton
Diazinon	Methylparathion
Dichlorvos (DDVP) with chlordane	Mevinphos
	Parathion
Disulfoton	Parathion and Mevinphos
EPN	Phosphamidon
Isoflurophate	Sarin
Malathion	Systox®
Metasystox I® and Fenthion	TEPP

Of these cases, over 100 were due to parathion, about a dozen each to malathion, diazinon, and mevinphos, and a few to each of the other compounds.

REFERENCES

1. LANDAUER, W.: Cholinomimetic teratogens. V. The effect of oximes and related cholinesterase reactivators, *Teratology 15*:33 (Feb) 1977.
2. MOLLER, K.O., JENSEN-HOLM, J., and LAUSEN, H.H.: *Ugeskr. Laeg. 123*:501, 1961.
3. NAMBA, T., NOLTE, C.T., JACKREL, J. and GROB, D.: Poisoning due to organophosphate insecticides. Acute and chronic manifestations, *Amer. J. Med. 50*:475 (Apr), 1971.
4. ARENA, J.M.: Poisoning, Toxicology Symptoms, Treatments, ed. 4, Springfield, IL, Charles C. Thomas, 1979, p. 133.
5. BRACHFELD, J., and ZAVON, M.R.: Organic phosphate (Phosdrin®) intoxication. Report of a case and the results of treatment with 2-PAM, *Arch. Environ. Health 11*:859, 1965.
6. HAYES, W.J., Jr.: Toxicology of Pesticides, Baltimore, The Williams & Wilkins Company, 1975, p. 416.
7. AMA Department of Drugs: AMA Drug Evaluations, ed. 4, Chicago, American Medical Association, 1980, p. 1455.

SECTRAL® ℞

[sek 'tral]
(acebutolol hydrochloride)
Capsules

DESCRIPTION

Sectral® (acebutolol HCl) is a selective, hydrophilic beta-adrenoreceptor blocking agent with mild intrinsic sympathomimetic activity for use in treating patients with hypertension and ventricular arrhythmias. It is marketed in capsule form for oral administration. Sectral capsules are provided in two dosage strengths which contain 200 or 400 mg of acebutolol as the hydrochloride salt. The inactive ingredients present are D&C Red 22, FD&C Blue 1, FD&C Yellow 6, gelatin, povidone, starch, stearic acid, and titanium dioxide. The 200 mg dosage strength also contains D&C Red 28 and the 400 mg dosage strength also contains FD&C Red 40.

Acebutolol HCl has the following structural formula:

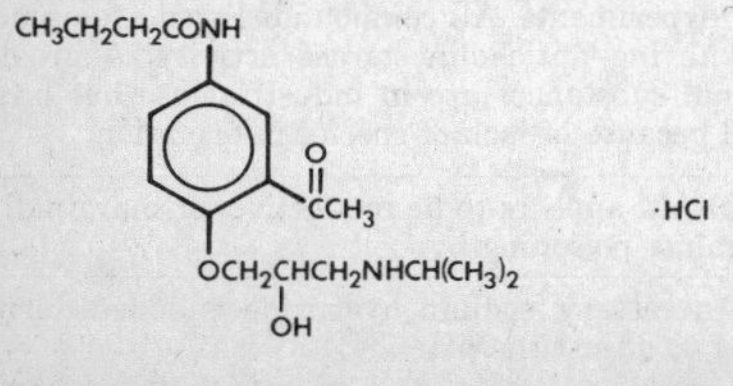

$C_{18}H_{28}N_2O_4 \cdot HCl$ M.W. 372.9

Acebutolol HCl is a white or slightly off-white powder freely soluble in water, and less soluble in alcohol. Chemically it is defined as Butanamide, N-[3-acetyl-4-[2-hydroxy-3-[(1-methylethyl)amino]propoxy]phenyl]-, (±)- or (±)-3'-Acetyl-4'-[2-hydroxy -3- (isopropylamino) propoxy] butyranilide.

CLINICAL PHARMACOLOGY

Sectral is a cardioselective, β-adrenoreceptor blocking agent, which possesses mild intrinsic sympathomimetic activity (ISA) in its therapeutically effective dose range.

PHARMACODYNAMICS

β_1-cardioselectivity has been demonstrated in experimental animal studies. In anesthetized dogs and cats, Sectral is more potent in antagonizing isoproterenol-induced tachycardia (β_1) than in antagonizing isoproterenol-induced vasodilatation (β_2). In guinea pigs and cats, it is more potent in antagonizing this tachycardia than in antagonizing isoproterenol-induced bronchodilatation (β_2). ISA of Sectral has been demonstrated in catecholamine-depleted rats by tachycardia induced by intravenous administration of this agent. A membrane-stabilizing effect has been detected in animals, but only with high concentrations of Sectral.

Clinical studies have demonstrated β_1-blocking activity at the recommended doses by: a) reduction in the resting heart rate and decrease in exercise-induced tachycardia; b) reduction in cardiac output at rest and after exercise; c) reduction of systolic and diastolic blood pressures at rest and postexercise; d) inhibition of isoproterenol-induced tachycardia.

The β_1-selectivity of Sectral has also been demonstrated on the basis of the following vascular and bronchial effects:

Vascular Effects: Sectral has less antagonistic effects on peripheral vascular β_2-receptors at rest and after epinephrine stimulation than nonselective β-antagonists.

Bronchial Effects: In single-dose studies in asthmatics examining effects of various beta-blockers on pulmonary function, low doses of acebutolol produce less evidence of bronchoconstriction and less reduction of beta$_2$ agonist, bronchodilating effects, than nonselective agents like propranolol but more than atenolol.

ISA has been observed with Sectral in man, as shown by a slightly smaller (about 3 beats per minute) decrease in resting heart rate when compared to equivalent β-blocking doses of propranolol, metoprolol or atenolol. Chronic therapy with Sectral induced no significant alteration in the blood lipid profile.

Sectral has been shown to delay AV conduction time and to increase the refractoriness of the AV node without significantly affecting sinus node recovery time, atrial refractory period, or the HV conduction time. The membrane-stabilizing effect of Sectral is not manifest at the doses used clinically.

Significant reductions in resting and exercise heart rates and systolic blood pressures have been observed 1.5 hours after Sectral administration with maximal effects occurring between 3 and 8 hours postdosing in normal volunteers. Sectral has demonstrated a significant effect on exercise-induced tachycardia 24 to 30 hours after drug administration.

There are significant correlations between plasma levels of acebutolol and both the reduction in resting heart rate and the percent of β-blockade of exercise-induced tachycardia.

The antihypertensive effect of Sectral has been shown in double-blind controlled studies to be superior to placebo and similar to propranolol and hydrochlorothiazide. In addition, patients responding to Sectral administered twice daily had a similar response whether the dosage regimen was changed to once daily administration or continued on a b.i.d. regimen. Most patients responded to 400 to 800 mg per day in divided doses.

The antiarrhythmic effect of Sectral was compared with placebo, propranolol, and quinidine. Compared with placebo, Sectral significantly reduced mean total ventricular ectopic beats (VEB), paired VEB, multiform VEB, R-on-T beats, and ventricular tachycardia (VT). Both Sectral and propranolol significantly reduced mean total and paired VEB and VT. Sectral and quinidine significantly reduced resting total and complex VEB; the antiarrhythmic efficacy of Sectral was also observed during exercise.

PHARMACOKINETICS AND METABOLISM

Sectral is well absorbed from the GI tract. It is subject to extensive first-pass hepatic biotransformation, with an absolute bioavailability of approximately 40% for the parent compound. The major metabolite, an N-acetyl derivative (diacetolol), is pharmacologically active. This metabolite is equipotent to Sectral and in cats is more cardioselective than Sectral; therefore, this first-pass phenomenon does not attenuate the therapeutic effect of Sectral. Food intake does not have a significant effect on the area under the plasma concentration-time curve (AUC) of Sectral although the rate of absorption and peak concentration decreased slightly.

The plasma elimination half-life of Sectral is approximately 3 to 4 hours, while that of its metabolite, diacetolol, is 8 to 13 hours. The time to reach peak concentration for Sectral is 2.5 hours and for diacetolol, after oral administration of Sectral, 3.5 hours.

Within the single oral dose range of 200 to 400 mg, the kinetics are dose proportional. However, this linearity is not seen at higher doses, probably due to saturation of hepatic biotransformation sites. In addition, after multiple dosing the lack of linearity is also seen by AUC increases of approximately 100% as compared to single oral dosing. Elimination via renal excretion is approximately 30% to 40% and by nonrenal mechanisms 50% to 60%, which includes excretion into the bile and direct passage through the intestinal wall.

Sectral has a low binding affinity for plasma proteins (about 26%). Sectral and its metabolite, diacetolol, are relatively hydrophilic and, therefore, only minimal quantities have been detected in the cerebrospinal fluid (CSF).

Drug interaction studies with tolbutamide and warfarin indicated no influence on the therapeutic effects of these compounds. Digoxin and hydrochlorothiazide plasma levels were not affected by concomitant Sectral administration. The kinetics of Sectral were not significantly altered by concomitant administration of hydrochlorothiazide, hydralazine, sulfinpyrazone, or oral contraceptives.

In patients with renal impairment, there is no effect on the elimination half-life of Sectral, but there is decreased elimination of the metabolite, diacetolol, resulting in a two- to three-fold increase in its half-life. For this reason, the drug should be administered with caution in patients with renal insufficiency (see "Precautions"). Sectral and its major metabolite are dialyzable.

Sectral crosses the placental barrier and is secreted in breast milk.

In geriatric patients, the bioavailability of Sectral and its metabolite is increased, approximately two-fold, probably due to decreases in the first-pass metabolism and renal function in the elderly.

INDICATIONS AND USAGE

HYPERTENSION: Sectral is indicated for the management of hypertension in adults. It may be used alone or in combination with other antihypertensive agents, especially thiazide-type diuretics.

VENTRICULAR ARRHYTHMIAS: Sectral is indicated in the management of ventricular premature beats; it reduces the total number of premature beats, as well as the number of paired and multiform ventricular ectopic beats, and R-on-T beats.

CONTRAINDICATIONS

Sectral is contraindicated in: 1) persistently severe bradycardia; 2) second- and third-degree heart block; 3) overt cardiac failure; and 4) cardiogenic shock. (See "WARNINGS.")

WARNINGS

CARDIAC FAILURE: Sympathetic stimulation may be essential for support of the circulation in individuals with diminished myocardial contractility, and its inhibition by β-adrenergic receptor blockade may precipitate more severe failure. Although β-blockers should be avoided in overt cardiac failure, Sectral can be used with caution in patients with a history of heart failure who are controlled with digitalis and/or diuretics. Both digitalis and Sectral impair AV conduction. If cardiac failure persists, therapy with Sectral should be withdrawn.

IN PATIENTS WITHOUT A HISTORY OF CARDIAC FAILURE: In patients with aortic or mitral valve disease or compromised left ventricular function, continued depression of the myocardium with β-blocking agents over a period of time may lead to cardiac failure. At the first signs of failure, patients should be digitalized and/or be given a diuretic and the response observed closely. If cardiac failure continues despite adequate digitalization and/or diuretic, Sectral therapy should be withdrawn.

EXACERBATION OF ISCHEMIC HEART DISEASE FOLLOWING ABRUPT WITHDRAWAL: Following abrupt cessation of therapy with certain β-blocking agents in patients with coronary artery disease, exacerbation of angina pectoris and, in some cases, myocardial infarction and death have been reported. Therefore, such patients should be cautioned against interruption of therapy without a physician's advice. Even in the absence of overt ischemic heart disease, when discontinuation of Sectral is planned, the patient should be carefully observed, and should be advised to limit physical activity to a minimum while Sectral is gradually withdrawn over a period of about two weeks. (If therapy with an alternative β-blocker is desired, the patient may be transferred directly to comparable doses of another agent without interruption of β-blocking therapy.) If an exacerbation of angina pectoris occurs, antianginal therapy should be restarted immediately in full doses and the patient hospitalized until his condition stabilizes.

PERIPHERAL VASCULAR DISEASE: Treatment with β-antagonists reduces cardiac output and can precipitate or aggravate the symptoms of arterial insufficiency in patients with peripheral or mesenteric vascular disease. Caution should be exercised with such patients, and they should be observed closely for evidence of progression of arterial obstruction.

BRONCHOSPASTIC DISEASES: PATIENTS WITH BRONCHOSPASTIC DISEASE SHOULD, IN GENERAL, NOT RECEIVE A β-BLOCKER. Because of its relative β_1-selectivity, however, low doses of Sectral may be used with caution in patients with bronchospastic disease who do not respond to, or who cannot tolerate, alternative treatment. Since β_1-selectivity is not absolute and is dose-dependent, the lowest possible dose of Sectral should be used initially, preferably in divided doses to avoid the higher plasma levels associated with the longer dose-interval. A bronchodilator, such as a theophylline or a β_2-stimulant, should be made available in advance with instructions concerning its use.

ANESTHESIA AND MAJOR SURGERY: The necessity, or desirability, of withdrawal of a β-blocking therapy prior to major surgery is controversial. β-adrenergic receptor blockade impairs the ability of the heart to respond to β-adrenergically mediated reflex stimuli. While this might be of benefit in preventing arrhythmic response, the risk of excessive myocardial depression during general anesthesia may be enhanced and difficulty in restarting and maintaining the heart beat has been reported with beta-blockers. If treatment is continued, particular care should be taken when using anesthetic agents which depress the myocardium, such as ether, cyclopropane and trichlorethylene, and it is prudent to use the lowest possible dose of Sectral. Sectral, like other β-blockers, is a competitive inhibitor of β-receptor agonists, and its effect on the heart can be reversed by cautious administration of such agents (e.g., dobutamine or isoproterenol—see "Overdose").

Manifestations of excessive vagal tone (e.g., profound bradycardia, hypotension) may be corrected with atropine 1 to 3 mg IV in divided doses.

DIABETES AND HYPOGLYCEMIA: β-blockers may potentiate insulin-induced hypoglycemia and mask some of its manifestations such as tachycardia; however, dizziness and sweating are usually not significantly affected. Diabetic patients should be warned of the possibility of masked hypoglycemia.

THYROTOXICOSIS: β-adrenergic blockade may mask certain clinical signs (tachycardia) of hyperthyroidism. Abrupt withdrawal of β-blockade may precipitate a thyroid storm; therefore, patients suspected of developing thyrotoxicosis from whom Sectral therapy is to be withdrawn should be monitored closely.

PRECAUTIONS

IMPAIRED RENAL OR HEPATIC FUNCTION: Studies on the effect of acebutolol in patients with renal insufficiency have not been performed in the U.S. Foreign published experience shows that acebutolol has been used successfully in chronic renal insufficiency. Acebutolol is excreted through the G.I. tract, but the active metabolite, diacetolol, is eliminated predominantly by the kidney. There is a linear relationship between renal clearance of diacetolol and creatinine clearance. Therefore, the daily dose of acebutolol should be reduced by 50% when the creatinine clearance is less than 50 mL/min and by 75% when it is less than 25 mL/min. Sectral should be used cautiously in patients with impaired hepatic function.

Sectral has been used successfully and without problems in elderly patients in the U.S. clinical trials without specific adjustment of dosage. However, elderly patients may require lower maintenance doses because the bioavailability of both Sectral and its metabolite are approximately doubled in this age group.

INFORMATION FOR PATIENTS: Patients, especially those with evidence of coronary artery disease, should be warned against interruption or discontinuation of Sectral therapy without a physician's supervision. Although cardiac failure rarely occurs in properly selected patients, those being treated with β-adrenergic blocking agents should be advised to consult a physician if they develop signs or symptoms suggestive of impending CHF, or unexplained respiratory symptoms.

Patients should also be warned of possible severe hypertensive reactions from concomitant use of α-adrenergic stimulants, such as the nasal decongestants commonly used in OTC cold preparations and nasal drops.

CLINICAL LABORATORY FINDINGS: Sectral, like other β-blockers, has been associated with the development of antinuclear antibodies (ANA). In prospective clinical trials, patients receiving Sectral had a dose-dependent increase in the development of positive ANA titers and the overall incidence was higher than that observed with propranolol. Symptoms (generally persistent arthralgias and myalgias) related to this laboratory abnormality were infrequent (less than 1% with both drugs). Symptoms and ANA titers were reversible upon discontinuation of treatment.

DRUG INTERACTIONS: Catecholamine-depleting drugs, such as reserpine, may have an additive effect when given with β-blocking agents. Patients treated with Sectral plus catecholamine depletors should, therefore, be observed closely for evidence of marked bradycardia or hypotension which may present as vertigo, syncope/presyncope, or orthostatic changes in blood pressure without compensatory tachycardia. Exaggerated hypertensive responses have been reported from the combined use of β-adrenergic antagonists and α-adrenergic stimulants, including those contained in proprietary cold remedies and vasoconstrictive nasal drops. Patients receiving β-blockers should be warned of this potential hazard.

Blunting of the antihypertensive effect of beta-adrenoceptor blocking agents by nonsteroidal anti-inflammatory drugs has been reported.

No significant interactions with digoxin, hydrochlorothiazide, hydralazine, sulfinpyrazone, oral contraceptives, tolbutamide, or warfarin have been observed.

CARCINOGENESIS, MUTAGENESIS, IMPAIRMENT OF FERTILITY: Chronic oral toxicity studies in rats and mice, employing dose levels as high as 300 mg/kg/day, which is equivalent to 15 times the maximum recommended (60 kg) human dose, did not indicate a carcinogenic potential for Sectral. Diacetolol, the major metabolite of Sectral in man, was without carcinogenic potential in rats when tested at doses as high as 1800 mg/kg/day. Sectral and diacetolol were also shown to be devoid of mutagenic potential in the Ames Test. Sectral, administered orally to two generations of male and female rats at doses of up to 240 mg/kg/day (equivalent to 12 times the maximum recommended therapeutic dose in a 60-kg human) and diacetolol, administered to two generations of male and female rats at doses of up to 1000 mg/kg/day, had no significant impact on reproductive performance or fertility.

PREGNANCY

Teratogenic Effects:

Pregnancy Category B: Reproduction studies have been performed with Sectral in rats (up to 630 mg/kg/day) and rabbits (up to 135 mg/kg/day). These doses are equivalent to approximately 31.5 and 6.8 times the maximum recommended therapeutic dose in a 60-kg human, respectively. The compound was not teratogenic in either species. In the rabbit, however, doses of 135 mg/kg/day caused slight fetal growth retardation; this effect was considered to be a result of maternal toxicity, as evidenced by reduced food intake, a lowered rate of body weight gain, and mortality. Studies have also been performed in these species with diacetolol (at doses of up to 450 mg/kg/day in rabbits and up to 1800 mg/kg/day in rats.) Other than a significant elevation in postimplantation loss with 450 mg/kg/day diacetolol, a level at which food consumption and body weight gain were reduced in rabbit dams and a nonstatistically significant increase in incidence of bilateral cataract in rat fetuses from dams treated with 1800 mg/kg/day diacetolol, there was no evidence of harm to the fetus. There are no adequate and well-controlled trials in pregnant women. Because animal teratology studies are not always predictive of the human response, Sectral should be used during pregnancy only if the potential benefit justifies the risk to the fetus.

Nonteratogenic Effects:

Studies in humans have shown that both acebutolol and diacetolol cross the placenta. Neonates of mothers who have received acebutolol during pregnancy have reduced birth weight, decreased blood pressure, and decreased heart rate. In the newborn the elimination half-life of acebutolol was 6 to 14 hours, while the half-life of diacetolol was 24 to 30 hours for the first 24 hours after birth, followed by a half-life of 12 to 16 hours. Adequate facilities for monitoring these infants at birth should be available.

LABOR AND DELIVERY: The effect of Sectral on labor and delivery in pregnant women is unknown. Studies in animals have not shown any effect of Sectral on the usual course of labor and delivery.

NURSING MOTHERS: Acebutolol and diacetolol also appear in breast milk with a milk:plasma ratio of 7.1 and 12.2, respectively. Use in nursing mothers is not recommended.

PEDIATRIC USE: Safety and effectiveness in children have not been established.

ADVERSE REACTIONS

Sectral is well tolerated in properly selected patients. Most adverse reactions have been mild, not required discontinuation of therapy, and tended to decrease as duration of treatment increases.

The following table shows the frequency of treatment-related side effects derived from controlled clinical trials in patients with hypertension, angina pectoris, and arrhythmia. These patients received Sectral, propranolol, or hydrochlorothiazide as monotherapy, or placebo.

[See table above.]

TOTAL VOLUNTEERED AND ELICITED (U.S. STUDIES)

Body System/ Adverse Reaction	SECTRAL (N = 1002) %	Propranolol (N = 424) %	Hydrochlorothiazide (N = 178) %	Placebo (N = 314) %
Cardiovascular				
Chest Pain	2	4	4	1
Edema	2	2	4	1
Central Nervous System				
Depression	2	1	3	1
Dizziness	6	7	12	2
Fatigue	11	17	10	4
Headache	6	9	13	4
Insomnia	3	6	5	1
Abnormal dreams	2	3	0	1
Dermatologic				
Rash	2	2	4	1
Gastrointestinal				
Constipation	4	2	7	0
Diarrhea	4	5	5	1
Dyspepsia	4	6	3	1
Flatulence	3	4	7	1
Nausea	4	6	3	0
Genitourinary				
Micturition (frequency)	3	1	9	<1
Musculoskeletal				
Arthralgia	2	1	3	2
Myalgia	2	1	4	0
Respiratory				
Cough	1	1	2	0
Dyspnea	4	6	4	2
Rhinitis	2	1	4	<1
Special Senses				
Abnormal Vision	2	2	3	0

The following selected (potentially important) side effects were seen in up to 2% of Sectral patients:

Cardiovascular: hypotension, bradycardia, heart failure.

Central Nervous System: anxiety, hyper/hypoesthesia, impotence.

Dermatological: pruritus.

Gastrointestinal: vomiting, abdominal pain.

Genitourinary: dysuria, nocturia.

Liver and Biliary System: A small number of cases of liver abnormalities (increased SGOT, SGPT, LDH) have been reported in association with acebutolol therapy. In some cases increased bilirubin or alkaline phosphatase, fever, malaise, dark urine, anorexia, nausea, headache, and/or other symptoms have been reported. In some of the reported cases, the symptoms and signs were confirmed by rechallenge with acebutolol. The abnormalities were reversible upon cessation of acebutolol therapy.

Musculoskeletal: back pain, joint pain.

Respiratory: pharyngitis, wheezing.

Special Senses: conjunctivitis, dry eye, eye pain.

Autoimmune: In extremely rare instances, systemic lupus erythematosus has been reported.

The incidence of drug-related adverse effects (volunteered and solicited) according to Sectral dose is shown below. (Data from 266 hypertensive patients treated for 3 months on a constant dose.)

[See table at top of next page.]

POTENTIAL ADVERSE EFFECTS

In addition, certain adverse effects not listed above have been reported with other β-blocking agents and should also be considered as potential adverse effects of Sectral.

Central Nervous System: Reversible mental depression progressing to catatonia (an acute syndrome characterized by

Continued on next page

Wyeth-Ayerst Laboratories—Cont.

Body System	400 mg/day (N = 132)	800 mg/day (N = 63)	1200 mg/day (N = 71)
Cardiovascular	5%	2%	1%
Gastrointestinal	3%	3%	7%
Musculoskeletal	2%	3%	4%
Central Nervous System	9%	13%	17%
Respiratory	1%	5%	6%
Skin	1%	2%	1%
Special Senses	2%	2%	6%
Genitourinary	2%	3%	1%

disorientation for time and place), short-term memory loss, emotional lability, slightly clouded sensorium, and decreased performance (neuropsychometrics).
Cardiovascular: Intensification of AV block (see "Contraindications").
Allergic: Erythematous rash, fever combined with aching and sore throat, laryngospasm, and respiratory distress.
Hematologic: Agranulocytosis, nonthrombocytopenic, and thrombocytopenic purpura.
Gastrointestinal: Mesenteric arterial thrombosis and ischemic colitis.
Miscellaneous: Reversible alopecia and Peyronie's disease.
The oculomucocutaneous syndrome associated with the β-blocker practolol has not been reported with Sectral during investigational use and extensive foreign clinical experience.

OVERDOSAGE

No specific information on emergency treatment of overdosage is available for Sectral. However, overdosage with other β-blocking agents has been accompanied by extreme bradycardia, advanced atrioventricular block, intraventricular conduction defects, hypotension, severe congestive heart failure, seizures, and in susceptible patients, bronchospasm and hypoglycemia. Although specific information on the emergency treatment of Sectral overdose is not available, on the basis of the pharmacological actions and the observations in treating overdoses with other β-blockers, the following general measures should be considered:

1. Empty stomach by emesis or lavage.
2. Bradycardia: IV atropine (1 to 3 mg in divided doses). If antivagal response is inadequate, administer isoproterenol cautiously since larger than usual doses of isoproterenol may be required.
3. Persistent hypotension in spite of correction of bradycardia: Administer vasopressor (e.g., epinephrine, levarterenol, dopamine, or dobutamine) with frequent monitoring of blood pressure and pulse rate.
4. Bronchospasm: A theophylline derivative, such as aminophylline and/or parenteral β_2-stimulant, such as terbutaline.
5. Cardiac failure: Digitalize the patient and/or administer a diuretic. It has been reported that glucagon is useful in this situation.

Sectral is dialyzable.

DOSAGE AND ADMINISTRATION

HYPERTENSION: The initial dosage of Sectral in uncomplicated mild-to-moderate hypertension is 400 mg. This can be given as a single daily dose, but in occasional patients twice daily dosing may be required for adequate 24-hour blood-pressure control. An optimal response is usually achieved with dosages of 400 to 800 mg per day, although some patients have been maintained on as little as 200 mg per day. Patients with more severe hypertension or who have demonstrated inadequate control may respond to a total of 1200 mg daily (administered b.i.d.), or to the addition of a second antihypertensive agent. Beta-1 selectivity diminishes as dosage is increased.
VENTRICULAR ARRHYTHMIA: The usual initial dose of Sectral is 400 mg daily given as 200 mg b.i.d. Dosage should be increased gradually until an optimal clinical response is obtained, generally at 600 to 1200 mg per day. If treatment is to be discontinued, the dosage should be reduced gradually over a period of about two weeks.
USE IN OLDER PATIENTS: Older patients have an approximately 2-fold increase in bioavailability and may require lower maintenance doses. Doses above 800 mg/day should be avoided in the elderly.

HOW SUPPLIED

Sectral® (acebutolol HCl), Wyeth®, is available in the following dosage strengths:
200 mg, opaque purple and orange capsule marked "WYETH 4177" and "Sectral 200"
NDC 0008-4177-01, in bottles of 100 capsules.
NDC 0008-4177-04, in Redipak® cartons of 100 capsules (10 blister strips of 10).
400 mg, opaque brown and orange capsule marked "WYETH 4179" and "Sectral 400"
NDC 0008-4179-01, in bottles of 100 capsules.
Keep at Room Temperature, Approx. 25° C (77° F).
The appearance of these capsules is a trademark of Wyeth-Ayerst Laboratories.
by arrangement with RHÔNE-POULENC France
Shown in Product Identification Section, page 437

SERAX® Ⓒ℞

[ser'aks]
(oxazepam)
CAPSULES • TABLETS

DESCRIPTION

Serax is the first of a chemically new series of compounds, the 3-hydroxybenzodiazepinones. A new therapeutic agent providing versatility and flexibility in control of common emotional disturbances, this product exerts prompt action in a wide variety of disorders associated with anxiety, tension, agitation, and irritability, and anxiety associated with depression. In tolerance and toxicity studies on several animal species, this product reveals significantly greater safety factors than related compounds (chlordiazepoxide and diazepam) and manifests a wide separation of effective doses and doses inducing side effects.
Serax capsules contain 10 mg, 15 mg, or 30 mg oxazepam. The inactive ingredients present are gelatin, lactose, titanium dioxide, and other ingredients. Each dosage strength also contains the following:
10 mg—D&C Red 22, D&C Red 28, and FD&C Blue 1;
15 mg—FD&C Red 40 and FD&C Yellow 6;
30 mg—D&C Red 28, FD&C Red 40, and FD&C Blue 1.
Serax tablets contain 15 mg oxazepam. The inactive ingredients present are FD&C Yellow 5, lactose, magnesium stearate, methylcellulose, and polacrilin potassium.
Serax is 7 chloro-1,3,-dihydro-3-hydroxy-5-phenyl-2*H*-1,4-benzodiazepin-2-one, a white crystalline powder with a molecular weight of 286.7.

CLINICAL PHARMACOLOGY

Pharmacokinetic testing in twelve volunteers demonstrated that when given as a single 30 mg dose, the capsule, tablet, and suspension were equivalent in extent of absorption. For the capsule and tablet, peak plasma levels averaged 450 ng/mL and were observed to occur about 3 hours after dosing. The mean elimination half-life for oxazepam was approximately 8.2 hours (range 5.7 to 10.9 hours).
This product has a single, major inactive metabolite in man, a glucuronide excreted in the urine.

ANIMAL PHARMACOLOGY AND TOXICOLOGY

In mice, Serax exerts an anticonvulsant (anti-Metrazol®) activity at 50-percent-effective doses of about 0.6 mg/kg orally. (Such anticonvulsant activity of benzodiazepines correlates with their tranquilizing properties.) To produce ataxia (rotabar test) and sedation (abolition of spontaneous motor activity), the 50 percent effective doses of this product are greater than 5 mg/kg orally. Thus, about ten times the therapeutic (anticonvulsant) dose must be given before ataxia ensues, indicating a wide separation of effective doses and doses inducing side effects.
In evaluation of antianxiety activity of compounds, conflict behavioral tests in rats differentiate continuous response for food in the presence of anxiety-provoking stress (shock) from drug-induced motor incoordination. This product shows significant separation of doses required to relieve anxiety and doses producing sedation or ataxia. Ataxia-producing doses exceed those of related CNS-acting drugs.
Acute oral LD_{50} in mice is greater than 5000 mg/kg, compared to 800 mg/kg for a related compound (chlordiazepoxide).
Subacute toxicity studies in dogs for four weeks at 480 mg/kg daily showed no specific changes; at 960 mg/kg two out of eight died with evidence of circulatory collapse. This wide margin of safety is significant compared to chlordiazepoxide HCl, which showed nonspecific changes in six dogs at 80 mg/kg. On chlordiazepoxide, two out of six died with evidence of circulatory collapse at 127 mg/kg, and six out of six died at 200 mg/kg daily. Chronic toxicity studies of Serax in dogs at 120 mg/kg/day for 52 weeks produced no toxic manifestation.
Fatty metamorphosis of the liver has been noted in six-week toxicity studies in rats given this product at 0.5% of the diet. Such accumulations of fat are considered reversible as there is no liver necrosis or fibrosis.
Breeding studies in rats through two successive litters did not produce fetal abnormality.
Oxazepam has not been adequately evaluated for mutagenic activity.
In a carcinogenicity study, oxazepam was administered with diet to rats for two years. Male rats receiving 30 times the maximum human dose showed a statistical increase, when compared to controls, in benign thyroid follicular cell tumors, testicular interstitial cell adenomas, and prostatic adenomas. An earlier published study reported that mice fed dietary dosages of 35 or 100 times the human daily dose of oxazepam for 9 months developed a dose-related increase in liver adenomas.[1] In an independent analysis of some of the microscopic slides from this mouse study several of these tumors were classified as liver carcinomas. At this time, there is no evidence that clinical use of oxazepam is associated with tumors.

INDICATIONS

Serax (oxazepam) is indicated for the management of anxiety disorders or for the short-term relief of the symptoms of anxiety. Anxiety or tension associated with the stress of everyday life usually does not require treatment with an anxiolytic.
Anxiety associated with depression is also responsive to Serax therapy.
This product has been found particularly useful in the management of anxiety, tension, agitation, and irritability in older patients.
Alcoholics with acute tremulousness, inebriation, or with anxiety associated with alcohol withdrawal are responsive to therapy.
The effectiveness of Serax in long-term use, that is, more than 4 months, has not been assessed by systematic clinical studies. The physician should reassess periodically the usefulness of the drug for the individual patient.

CONTRAINDICATIONS

History of previous hypersensitivity reaction to oxazepam.
Oxazepam is not indicated in psychoses.

WARNINGS

As with other CNS-acting drugs, patients should be cautioned against driving automobiles or operating dangerous machinery until it is known that they do not become drowsy or dizzy on oxazepam therapy.
Patients should be warned that the effects of alcohol or other CNS-depressant drugs may be additive to those of Serax, possibly requiring adjustment of dosage or elimination of such agents.
PHYSICAL AND PSYCHOLOGICAL DEPENDENCE
Withdrawal symptoms, similar in character to those noted with barbiturates and alcohol (convulsions, tremor, abdominal and muscle cramps, vomiting, and sweating), have occurred following abrupt discontinuance of oxazepam. The more severe withdrawal symptoms have usually been limited to those patients who received excessive doses over an extended period of time. Generally milder withdrawal symptoms (e.g., dysphoria and insomnia) have been reported following abrupt discontinuance of benzodiazepines taken continuously at therapeutic levels for several months. Consequently, after extended therapy, abrupt discontinuation should generally be avoided and a gradual dosage-tapering schedule followed. Addiction-prone individuals (such as drug addicts or alcoholics) should be under careful surveillance when receiving oxazepam or other psychotropic agents because of the predisposition of such patients to habituation and dependence.

SERAX (oxazepam)
USUAL DOSE

Mild-to-moderate anxiety, with associated tension, irritability, agitation, or related symptoms of functional origin or secondary to organic disease.	10 to 15 mg, 3 or 4 times daily
Severe anxiety syndromes, agitation, or anxiety associated with depression.	15 to 30 mg, 3 or 4 times daily
Older patients with anxiety, tension, irritability, and agitation.	Initial dosage: 10 mg, 3 times daily. If necessary, increase cautiously to 15 mg, 3 or 4 times daily
Alcoholics with acute inebriation, tremulousness, or anxiety on withdrawal.	15 to 30 mg, 3 or 4 times daily

USE IN PREGNANCY

An increased risk of congenital malformations associated with the use of minor tranquilizers (chlordiazepoxide, diazepam, and meprobamate) during the first trimester of pregnancy has been suggested in several studies. Serax, a benzodiazepine derivative, has not been studied adequately to determine whether it, too, may be associated with an increased risk of fetal abnormality. Because use of these drugs is rarely a matter of urgency, their use during this period should almost always be avoided. The possibility that a woman of childbearing potential may be pregnant at the time of institution of therapy should be considered. Patients should be advised that if they become pregnant during therapy or intend to become pregnant they should communicate with their physician about the desirability of discontinuing the drug.

PRECAUTIONS

Although hypotension has occurred only rarely, oxazepam should be administered with caution to patients in whom a drop in blood pressure might lead to cardiac complications. This is particularly true in the elderly patient.

Serax 15 mg tablets, *but none of the other available dosage forms of this product,* contain FD&C Yellow 5 (tartrazine) which may cause allergic-type reactions (including bronchial asthma) in certain susceptible individuals. Although the overall incidence of FD&C Yellow 5 (tartrazine) sensitivity in the general population is low, it is frequently seen in patients who also have aspirin hypersensitivity.

INFORMATION FOR PATIENTS

To assure the safe and effective use of Serax (oxazepam), patients should be informed that, since benzodiazepines may produce psychological and physical dependence, it is advisable that they consult with their physician before either increasing the dose or abruptly discontinuing this drug.

ADVERSE REACTIONS

The necessity for discontinuation of therapy due to undesirable effects has been rare. Transient mild drowsiness is commonly seen in the first few days of therapy. If it persists, the dosage should be reduced. In few instances, dizziness, vertigo, headache, and rarely syncope have occurred either alone or together with drowsiness. Mild paradoxical reactions, i.e., excitement, stimulation of affect, have been reported in psychiatric patients; these reactions may be secondary to relief of anxiety and usually appear in the first two weeks of therapy.

Other side effects occurring during oxazepam therapy include rare instances of minor diffuse skin rashes—morbilliform, urticarial and maculopapular—nausea, lethargy, edema, slurred speech, tremor, and altered libido. Such side effects have been infrequent and are generally controlled with reduction of dosage.

Although rare, leukopenia and hepatic dysfunction including jaundice have been reported during therapy. Periodic blood counts and liver-function tests are advisable.

Ataxia with oxazepam has been reported in rare instances and does not appear to be specifically related to dose or age.

Although the following side reactions have not as yet been reported with oxazepam, they have occurred with related compounds (chlordiazepoxide and diazepam): paradoxical excitation with severe rage reactions, hallucinations, menstrual irregularities, change in EEG pattern, blood dyscrasias including agranulocytosis, blurred vision, diplopia, incontinence, stupor, disorientation, fever, and euphoria. Transient amnesia or memory impairment has been reported in association with the use of benzodiazepines.

DOSAGE AND ADMINISTRATION

Because of the flexibility of this product and the range of emotional disturbances responsive to it, dosage should be individualized for maximum beneficial effects.

[See table at bottom of preceding page.]

This product is not indicated in children under 6 years of age. Absolute dosage for children 6 to 12 years of age is not established.

HOW SUPPLIED

Serax® (oxazepam) Capsules and Tablets, Wyeth® are available in the following dosage strengths:

10 mg, NDC 0008-0051, white and pink capsule banded with Wyeth logo and marked "SERAX", "10", and "51", in bottles of 100 and 500 capsules, and in Redipak cartons of 25 capsules.

15 mg, NDC 0008-0006, white and red capsule banded with Wyeth logo and marked "SERAX", "15", and "6", in bottles of 100 and 500 capsules, and in Redipak® cartons of 25 capsules.

30 mg, NDC 0008-0052, white and maroon capsule banded with Wyeth logo and marked "SERAX", "30", and "52", in bottles of 100 and 500 capsules, and in Redipak® cartons of 25 capsules.

15 mg, NDC 0008-0317, yellow, five-sided tablet with a raised "S" and a "15" on one side and "WYETH" and "317" on reverse side, in bottles of 100 tablets.

The appearance of SERAX capsules and tablets is a trademark of Wyeth-Ayerst Laboratories.

Keep bottles tightly closed. Dispense in tight container.

REFERENCE

1. FOX, KA.; LAHCEN, R.B.: Liver-cell Adenomas and Peliosis Hepatis in Mice Associated with Oxazepam. Res. Commun. Chem. Pathol. Pharmacol. 8 :481–488, 1974.
Shown in Product Identification Section, page 437

SMA®
[ess-em-ay]
Iron fortified
infant formula
READY–TO–FEED
CONCENTRATED LIQUID
POWDER

Breast milk is the preferred feeding for newborns. Infant formula is intended to replace or supplement breast milk when breast feeding is not possible or is insufficient, or when mothers elect not to breast feed.

Good maternal nutrition is important for the preparation and maintenance of breast feeding. Extensive or prolonged use of partial bottle feeding, before breast feeding has been well established, could make breast feeding difficult to maintain. A decision not to breast feed could be difficult to reverse.

Professional advice should be followed on all matters of infant feeding. Infant formula should always be prepared and used as directed. Unnecessary or improper use of infant formula could present a health hazard. Social and financial implications should be considered when selecting the method of infant feeding.

SMA is close in overall nutrient composition to human milk with its physiologic fat blend, whey-dominated protein composition, and inclusion of beta-carotene and nucleotides.

SMA, utilizing a hybridized safflower (oleic) oil, became the first infant formula offering fat and calcium absorption closest to that of human milk, with physiologic levels of linoleic acid and linolenic acid. Thus, the fat blend in SMA provides a ready source of energy, helps protect infants against neonatal tetany and produces a ratio of vitamin E to polyunsaturated fatty acids (linoleic acid) more than adequate to prevent hemolytic anemia and yields a serum lipid profile close to that of the breast fed infant.

By combining reduced minerals whey with skimmed cow's milk, SMA reduces the protein content to fall within the range of human milk, adjusts the whey-protein to casein ratio to that of human milk, and subsequently reduces the mineral content to a physiologic level.

The resultant 60:40 whey-protein to casein ratio provides protein nutrition superior to a casein-dominated formula. In addition, the essential amino acids, including cystine, are present in amounts close to those of human milk. So the protein in SMA is of high biologic value.

Five nucleotides found in higher amounts in human milk compared to infant formula have been added to SMA at levels found in breast milk.

The physiologic mineral content makes possible a low renal solute load which helps protect the functionally immature infant kidney, increases expendable water reserves and helps protect against dehydration.

Use of lactose as the carbohydrate results in a physiologic stool flora and a low stool pH, decreasing the incidence of perianal dermatitis.

INGREDIENTS

SMA® Concentrated Liquid or Ready-to-Feed. WATER; NONFAT MILK; REDUCED MINERALS WHEY; OLEO, COCONUT, OLEIC (SAFFLOWER OR SUNFLOWER), AND SOYBEAN OILS; LACTOSE; SOY LECITHIN; TAURINE; CYTIDINE-5'-MONOPHOSPHATE; CALCIUM CARRAGEENAN; ADENOSINE-5'-MONOPHOSPHATE; DISODIUM URIDINE-5'-MONOPHOSPHATE; DISODIUM INOSINE-5'MONOPHOSPHATE; DISODIUM GUANOSINE-5'-MONOPHOSPHATE. **MINERALS:** POTASSIUM BICARBONATE AND CHLORIDE; CALCIUM CHLORIDE AND CITRATE; SODIUM BICARBONATE AND CITRATE; FERROUS, ZINC, CUPRIC, AND MANGANESE SULFATES. **VITAMINS:** ASCORBIC ACID, ALPHA TOCOPHERYL ACETATE, NIACINAMIDE, VITAMIN A PALMITATE, CALCIUM PANTOTHENATE, THIAMINE HYDROCHLORIDE, RIBOFLAVIN, PYRIDOXINE HYDROCHLORIDE, BETA-CAROTENE, FOLIC ACID, PHYTONADIONE, BIOTIN, CHOLECALCIFEROL, CYANOCOBALAMIN. **SMA® Powder:** LACTOSE; OLEO, COCONUT, OLEIC (SAFFLOWER OR SUNFLOWER), AND SOYBEAN OILS; NONFAT MILK; WHEY PROTEIN CONCENTRATE; SOY LECITHIN; TAURINE; CYTIDINE-5'-MONOPHOSPHATE; ADENOSINE-5'-MONOPHOSPHATE; DISODIUM URIDINE-5'-MONOPHOSPHATE; DISODIUM INOSINE-5'MONOPHOSPHATE; DISODIUM GUANOSINE-5'-MONOPHOSPHATE. **MINERALS:** POTASSIUM PHOSPHATE; CALCIUM HYDROXIDE; MAGNESIUM CHLORIDE; CALCIUM CHLORIDE; SODIUM BICARBONATE; FERROUS SULFATE; POTASSIUM HYDROXIDE; POTASSIUM BICARBONATE; ZINC, CUPRIC, AND MANGANESE SULFATES; POTASSIUM IODIDE. **VITAMINS:** ASCORBIC ACID, CHOLINE CHLORIDE, INOSITOL, ALPHA TOCOPHERYL ACETATE, NIACINAMIDE, CALCIUM PANTOTHENATE, VITAMIN A PALMITATE, RIBOFLAVIN, THIAMINE HYDROCHLORIDE, PYRIDOXINE HYDROCHLORIDE, BETA-CAROTENE, FOLIC ACID, PHYTONADIONE, BIOTIN, CHOLECALCIFEROL, CYANOCOBALAMIN.

PROXIMATE ANALYSIS

at 20 calories per fluidounce
READY-TO-FEED, POWDER, and CONCENTRATED LIQUID:

	(w/v)
Fat	3.6%
Carbohydrate	7.2%
Protein	1.5%
60% Lactalbumin (whey protein)	0.9%
40% Casein	0.6%
Crude Fiber	None
Total Solids	12.6%
Calories/fl. oz.	20

Vitamins, Minerals: In normal dilution, each liter contains:

A	2000 IU
D_3	400 IU
E	9.5 IU
K_1	55 mcg
C (ascorbic acid)	55 mg
B_1 (thiamine)	670 mcg
B_2 (riboflavin)	1000 mcg
B_6 (pyroxidine hydrochloride)	420 mcg
B_{12}	1.3 mcg
Niacin	5000 mcg
Pantothenic Acid	2100 mcg
Folic Acid (folacin)	50 mcg
Choline	100 mg
Biotin	15 mcg
Calcium	420 mg
Phosphorus	280 mg
Sodium	150 mg
Potassium	560 mg
Chloride	375 mg
Magnesium	45 mg
Manganese	100 mcg
Iron	12 mg
Copper	470 mcg
Zinc	5 mg
Iodine	60 mcg

PREPARATION

Ready-to-Feed (8 and 32 fl. oz. cans of 20 calories per fluidounce formula)—shake can, open and pour into previously sterilized nursing bottle; attach nipple and feed. Cover opened can and immediately store in refrigerator. Use contents of can within 48 hours of opening.

Prolonged storage of can at excessive temperatures should be avoided.

Expiration date is on top of can.

WARNING: DO NOT USE A MICROWAVE TO PREPARE OR WARM FORMULA. SERIOUS BURNS MAY OCCUR.

Powder—(1 pound can)—For normal dilution supplying 20 calories per fluidounce, use 1 level measuring scoop to 2 fluidounces of cooled, previously boiled water.

Prolonged storage of can at excessive temperatures should be avoided.

Expiration date is on bottom of can.

WARNING: DO NOT USE A MICROWAVE TO PREPARE OR WARM FORMULA. SERIOUS BURNS MAY OCCUR.

Concentrated Liquid —For normal dilution supplying 20 calories per fluidounce, use equal amounts of SMA liquid and cooled, previously boiled water.

Prolonged storage of can at excessive temperatures should be avoided.

Expiration date is on top of can.

WARNING: DO NOT USE A MICROWAVE TO PREPARE OR WARM FORMULA. SERIOUS BURNS MAY OCCUR.

Note: Prepared formula should be used within 24 hours.

HOW SUPPLIED

Ready-to-Feed —presterilized and premixed, 32 fluidounce (1 quart) cans, cases of 6 cans; 8 fluidounce cans, cases of 24 (4 carriers of 6 cans). *Powder*—1 pound cans with measuring scoop, cases of 6 cans. *Concentrated Liquid* — 13 fluidounce cans, cases of 24 cans.

For Hospital Nursery Use —an infant feeding system which provides premixed, presterilized, ready-to-feed items, thus saving space, time and equipment. It eliminates washing, measuring, mixing, sterilizing, refrigerating and heating.

The system is offered in a choice of two forms:

1. Prefilled and presterilized 4 oz. glass bottles for which sterile nipple assemblies are available, to be attached before feeding. These units may be used again after resterilizing or may be discarded, as desired.

Continued on next page

Wyeth-Ayerst Laboratories—Cont.

The following items are supplied in both the forms described above:

SMA® Ready-to-Feed	
13 calories/oz.	48 bottles of 4 fl. oz.
20 calories/oz.	48 bottles of 4 fl. oz.
24 calories/oz.	48 bottles of 4 fl. oz.
27 calories/oz.	48 bottles of 4 fl. oz.
SMA® lo-iron Ready-to-Feed	
13 calories/oz.	48 bottles of 4 fl. oz.
20 calories/oz.	48 bottles of 4 fl. oz.
24 calories/oz.	48 bottles of 4 fl. oz.
"preemie" SMA® Ready-to-Feed	
24 calories/oz.	48 bottles of 4 fl. oz.
Distilled Water	48 bottles of 4 fl. oz.
Glucose, 5% in Distilled Water, 6 calories/oz.	48 bottles of 4 fl. oz.
Glucose, 10% in Distilled Water, 12 calories/oz.	48 bottles of 4 fl. oz.
NURSOY® (soy protein formula)	
20 calories/oz.	48 bottles of 4 fl. oz.

Supplied in 8 oz. bottles, to which sterile nipple assemblies must be attached before feeding, are the following:

SMA® Ready-to-Feed	
20 calories/oz.	24 bottles of 8 fl. oz.
Oral Electrolyte Solution	24 bottles of 8 fl. oz.
Distilled Water	24 bottles of 8 fl. oz.

NIPPLE ASSEMBLIES—presterilized, for both premature and term infants, single-hole and suitable for use with all ready-to-feed products requiring them, cartons of 288 nipple units. Single-hole and orthodontic nipples.

ACCUFEED™, Wyeth Graduated Nursers—presterilized, disposable nursers (60 ml capacity) for accurately measured feedings, packages of 200.

Also Available: SMA® lo-iron. Those who appreciate the particular advantages of SMA® infant formula close in nutrient composition to mother's milk, sometimes need or wish to recommend a formula that does not contain a high level of iron. SMA lo-iron has all the benefits of regular SMA but with a reduced level of iron of 1.4 mg per quart. Infants should receive supplemental dietary iron from an outside source to meet daily requirements.

Concentrated Liquid, 13 fl. oz. cans, cases of 12 cans. Powder, 1 pound cans with measuring scoop, cases of 6 cans. Ready-to-Feed, 32 fl. oz. cans, cases of 6 cans.

Preparation of the standard 20 calories per fluidounce formula of SMA lo-iron is the same as SMA iron fortified given above.

Questions or Comments regarding SMA: 1-800-99-WYETH.

Shown in Product Identification Section, page 437

SURMONTIL® ℞

[*sir 'mon "til*]

(trimipramine maleate)

DESCRIPTION

Surmontil (trimipramine maleate) is 5-(3-dimethylamino-2-methylpropyl)-10,11-dihydro-5H-dibenz (b,f) azepine acid maleate (racemic form).

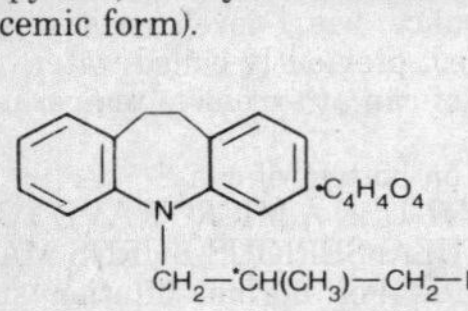

MOLECULAR FORMULA: $C_{20}H_{26}N_2 \cdot C_4H_4O_4$

MOLECULAR WEIGHT: 410.5

Surmontil capsules contain trimipramine maleate equivalent to 25 mg, 50 mg, or 100 mg of trimipramine as the base. The inactive ingredients present are FD&C Blue 1, gelatin, lactose, magnesium stearate, and titanium dioxide. The 25 mg dosage strength also contains D&C Yellow 10 and FD&C Yellow 6; the 50 mg dosage strength also contains D&C Red 28, FD&C Red 40, and FD&C Yellow 6.

Trimipramine maleate is prepared as a racemic mixture which can be resolved into levorotatory and dextrorotatory isomers. The asymmetric center responsible for optical isomerism is marked in the formula by an asterisk. Trimipramine maleate is an almost odorless, white or slightly cream-colored, crystalline substance, melting at 140–144°C. It is very slightly soluble in ether and water, is slightly soluble in ethyl alcohol and acetone, and freely soluble in chloroform and methanol at 20°C.

CLINICAL PHARMACOLOGY

Surmontil is an antidepressant with an anxiety-reducing sedative component to its action. The mode of action of Surmontil on the central nervous system is not known. However, unlike amphetamine-type compounds it does not act primarily by stimulation of the central nervous system. It does not act by inhibition of the monoamine oxidase system.

INDICATIONS

Surmontil is indicated for the relief of symptoms of depression. Endogenous depression is more likely to be alleviated than other depressive states. In studies with neurotic outpatients, the drug appeared to be equivalent to amitriptyline in the less-depressed patients but somewhat less effective than amitriptyline in the more severely depressed patients. In hospitalized depressed patients, trimipramine and imipramine were equally effective in relieving depression.

CONTRAINDICATIONS

Surmontil is contraindicated in cases of known hypersensitivity to the drug. The possibility of cross-sensitivity to other dibenzazepine compounds should be kept in mind. Surmontil should not be given in conjunction with drugs of the monoamine oxidase inhibitor class (e.g., tranylcypromine, isocarboxazid or phenelzine sulfate). The concomitant use of monoamine oxidase inhibitors (MAOI) and tricyclic compounds similar to Surmontil has caused severe hyperpyretic reactions, convulsive crises, and death in some patients. At least two weeks should elapse after cessation of therapy with MAOI before instituting therapy with Surmontil. Initial dosage should be low and increased gradually with caution and careful observation of the patient. The drug is contraindicated during the acute recovery period after a myocardial infarction.

WARNINGS

USE IN CHILDREN

This drug is not recommended for use in children, since safety and effectiveness in the pediatric age group have not been established.

GENERAL CONSIDERATION FOR USE

Extreme caution should be used when this drug is given to patients with any evidence of cardiovascular disease because of the possibility of conduction defects, arrhythmias, myocardial infarction, strokes, and tachycardia.

Caution is advised in patients with increased intraocular pressure, history of urinary retention, or history of narrow-angle glaucoma because of the drug's anticholinergic properties; hyperthyroid patients or those on thyroid medication because of the possibility of cardiovascular toxicity; patients with a history of seizure disorder, because this drug has been shown to lower the seizure threshold; patients receiving guanethidine or similar agents, since Surmontil may block the pharmacologic effects of these drugs.

Since the drug may impair the mental and/or physical abilities required for the performance of potentially hazardous tasks, such as operating an automobile or machinery, the patient should be cautioned accordingly.

PRECAUTIONS

The possibility of suicide is inherent in any severely depressed patient and persists until a significant remission occurs. When a patient with a serious suicidal potential is not hospitalized, the prescription should be for the smallest amount feasible.

In schizophrenic patients activation of the psychosis may occur and require reduction of dosage or the addition of a major tranquilizer to the therapeutic regime.

Manic or hypomanic episodes may occur in some patients, in particular those with cyclic-type disorders. In some cases therapy with Surmontil must be discontinued until the episode is relieved, after which therapy may be reinstituted at lower dosages if still required.

Concurrent administration of Surmontil and electroshock therapy may increase the hazards of therapy. Such treatment should be limited to those patients for whom it is essential. When possible, discontinue the drug for several days prior to elective surgery.

There is evidence that cimetidine inhibits the elimination of tricyclic antidepressants. Downward adjustment of Surmontil dosage may be required if cimetidine therapy is initiated: upward adjustment if cimetidine therapy is discontinued.

Patients should be warned that the concomitant use of alcoholic beverages may be associated with exaggerated effects.

It has been reported that tricyclic antidepressants can potentiate the effects of catecholamines. Similarly, atropinelike effects may be more pronounced in patients receiving anticholinergic therapy. Therefore, particular care should be exercised when it is necessary to administer tricyclic antidepressants with sympathomimetic amines, local decongestants, local anesthetics containing epinephrine, atropine or drugs with an anticholinergic effect. In resistant cases of depression in adults, a dose of 2.5 mg/kg/day may have to be exceeded. If a higher dose is needed, ECG monitoring should be maintained during the initiation of therapy and at appropriate intervals during stabilization of dose.

USAGE IN PREGNANCY

Pregnancy Category C

Surmontil has shown evidence of embryo-toxicity and/or increased incidence of major anomalies in rats or rabbits at doses 20 times the human dose. There are no adequate and well-controlled studies in pregnant women. Surmontil should be used during pregnancy only if the potential benefit justifies the potential risk to the fetus.

Semen studies in man (four schizophrenics and nine normal volunteers) revealed no significant changes in sperm morphology. It is recognized that drugs having a parasympathetic effect, including tricyclic antidepressants, may alter the ejaculatory response.

Chronic animal studies showed occasional evidence of degeneration of seminiferous tubules at the highest dose of 60 mg/kg/day.

Surmontil should be used with caution in patients with impaired liver function.

Chronic animal studies showed occasional occurrence of hepatic congestion, fatty infiltration, or increased serum liver enzymes at the highest dose of 60 mg/kg/day.

Both elevation and lowering of blood sugar have been reported with tricyclic antidepressants.

ADVERSE REACTIONS

Note: The pharmacological similarities among the tricyclic antidepressants require that each of the reactions be considered when Surmontil is administered. Some of the adverse reactions included in this listing have not in fact been reported with Surmontil.

CARDIOVASCULAR

Hypotension, hypertension, tachycardia, palpitation, myocardial infarction, arrhythmias, heart block, stroke.

PSYCHIATRIC

Confusional states (especially the elderly) with hallucinations, disorientation, delusions; anxiety, restlessness, agitation; insomnia and nightmares; hypomania; exacerbation of psychosis.

NEUROLOGICAL

Numbness, tingling, paresthesias of extremities; incoordination, ataxia, tremors, peripheral neuropathy; extrapyramidal symptoms; seizures, alterations in EEG patterns; tinnitus; syndrome of inappropriate ADH (antidiuretic hormone) secretion.

ANTICHOLINERGIC

Dry mouth and, rarely, associated sublingual adenitis; blurred vision, disturbances of accommodation, mydriasis, constipation, paralytic ileus; urinary retention, delayed micturition, dilation of the urinary tract.

ALLERGIC

Skin rash, petechiae, urticaria, itching, photosensitization, edema of face and tongue.

HEMATOLOGIC

Bone-marrow depression including agranulocytosis, eosinophilia; purpura; thrombocytopenia. Leukocyte and differential counts should be performed in any patient who develops fever and sore throat during therapy; the drug should be discontinued if there is evidence of pathological neutrophil depression.

GASTROINTESTINAL

Nausea and vomiting, anorexia, epigastric distress, diarrhea, peculiar taste, stomatitis, abdominal cramps, black tongue.

ENDOCRINE

Gynecomastia in the male; breast enlargement and galactorrhea in the female; increased or decreased libido, impotence; testicular swelling; elevation or depression of blood-sugar levels.

OTHER

Jaundice (simulating obstructive); altered liver function; weight gain or loss; perspiration; flushing; urinary frequency; drowsiness, dizziness, weakness, and fatigue; headache; parotid swelling; alopecia.

WITHDRAWAL SYMPTOMS

Though not indicative of addiction, abrupt cessation of treatment after prolonged therapy may produce nausea, headache, and malaise.

DOSAGE AND ADMINISTRATION

Dosage should be initiated at a low level and increased gradually, noting carefully the clinical response and any evidence of intolerance.

Lower dosages are recommended for elderly patients and adolescents. Lower dosages are also recommended for outpatients as compared to hospitalized patients who will be under close supervision. It is not possible to prescribe a single dosage schedule of Surmontil that will be therapeutically effective in all patients. The physical psychodynamic factors contributing to depressive symptomatology are very complex; spontaneous remissions or exacerbations of depressive symptoms may occur with or without drug therapy. Consequently, the recommended dosage regimens are furnished as a guide which may be modified by factors such as the age of the patient, chronicity and severity of the disease, medical condition of the patient, and degree of psychotherapeutic support.

Most antidepressant drugs have a lag period of ten days to four weeks before a therapeutic response is noted. Increasing the dose will not shorten this period but rather increase the incidence of adverse reactions.

USUAL ADULT DOSE

Outpatients and Office Patients—Initially, 75 mg/day in divided doses, increased to 150 mg/day. Dosages over 200 mg/

day are not recommended. Maintenance therapy is in the range of 50 to 150 mg/day. For convenient therapy and to facilitate patient compliance, the total dosage requirement may be given at bedtime.

Hospitalized Patients—Initially, 100 mg/day in divided doses. This may be increased gradually in a few days to 200 mg/day, depending upon individual response and tolerance. If improvement does not occur in 2 to 3 weeks, the dose may be increased to the maximum recommended dose of 250 to 300 mg/day.

Adolescent and Geriatric Patients—Initially, a dose of 50 mg/day is recommended, with gradual increments up to 100 mg/day, depending upon patient response and tolerance.

Maintenance—Following remission, maintenance medication may be required for a longer period of time, at the lowest dose that will maintain remission. Maintenance therapy is preferably administered as a single dose at bedtime. To minimize relapse, maintenance therapy should be continued for about three months.

OVERDOSAGE

SIGNS AND SYMPTOMS

The response of the patient to toxic overdosage of tricyclic antidepressants may vary in severity and is conditioned by factors such as age, amount ingested, amount absorbed, interval between ingestion and start of treatment. Surmontil is not recommended for infants or young children. Should accidental ingestion occur in any amount, it should be regarded as serious and potentially fatal.

CNS abnormalities may include drowsiness, stupor, coma, ataxia, restlessness, agitation, hyperactive reflexes, muscle rigidity, athetoid and choreiform movements, and convulsions. Cardiac abnormalities may include arrhythmia, tachycardia, ECG evidence of impaired conduction, and signs of congestive failure. Other symptoms may include respiratory depression, cyanosis, hypotension, shock, vomiting, hyperpyrexia, mydriasis, and diaphoresis.

Treatment is supportive and symptomatic as no specific antidote is known. Depending upon need the following measures can be considered:

1. Surmontil is not recommended for use in infants and children. Hospitalization with continuous cardiac monitoring for up to 4 days is recommended for children who have ingested Surmontil in any amount. This is based on the reported greater sensitivity of children to acute overdosage with tricyclic antidepressants.
2. Blood and urine levels may not reflect the severity of the poisoning and are mostly of diagnostic value.
3. CNS involvement, respiratory depression, or cardiac arrhythmia can occur suddenly; hospitalization and close observation are necessary, even when the amount ingested is thought to be small or initial toxicity appears slight. Patients with any alteration of ECG should have continuous cardiac monitoring for at least 72 hours and be observed until well after the cardiac status has returned to normal; relapses may occur after apparent recovery.
4. The slow intravenous administration of physostigmine salicylate has been reported to reverse most of the cardiovascular and CNS effects of overdosage with tricyclic antidepressants. In adults, 1 to 3 mg has been reported to be effective. In children, start with 0.5 mg and repeat at 5-minute intervals to determine the minimum effective dose; do not exceed 2.0 mg. Avoid rapid injection, to reduce the possibility of physostigmine-induced convulsions. Because of the short duration of action of physostigmine, it may be necessary to repeat doses at 30- to 60-minute intervals as necessary.
5. In the alert patient, empty the stomach rapidly by induced emesis, followed by lavage. In the obtunded patient, secure the airway with a cuffed endotracheal tube before beginning lavage (do not induce emesis). Instillation of activated-charcoal slurry may help reduce absorption of trimipramine.
6. Minimize external stimulation to reduce the tendency to convulsions. If anticonvulsants are necessary, diazepam, short-acting barbiturates, paraldehyde, or methocarbamol may be useful. Do not use barbiturates if MAO inhibitors have been taken recently.
7. Maintain adequate respiratory exchange. Do not use respiratory stimulants.
8. Shock should be treated with supportive measures, such as intravenous fluids, oxygen, and corticosteroids. Digitalis may increase conduction abnormalities and further irritate an already sensitized myocardium. If congestive heart failure necessitates rapid digitalization, particular care must be exercised.
9. Hyperpyrexia should be controlled by whatever external means available, including ice packs and cooling sponge baths if necessary.
10. Hemodialysis, peritoneal dialysis, exchange transfusions, and forced diuresis have been generally reported as ineffective in tricyclic poisoning.

HOW SUPPLIED

Surmontil® (trimipramine maleate) Capsules, Wyeth®, are available in the following dosage strengths:

25 mg, NDC 0008-4132, opaque blue and yellow capsule marked "WYETH" and "4132", in bottles of 100 capsules.

50 mg, NDC 0008-4133, opaque blue and orange capsule marked "WYETH" and "4133", in bottles of 100 capsules and in Redipak cartons of 100 capsules (10 blister strips of 10).

100 mg, NDC 0008-4158, opaque blue and white capsule marked "WYETH" and "4158", in bottles of 100 capsules.

Keep bottles tightly closed.

Dispense in tight container.

Protect capsules packaged in blister strips from moisture.

The appearance of these capsules is a trademark of Wyeth-Ayerst Laboratories.

by arrangement with RHONE-POULENC France

Shown in Product Identification Section, page 438

SYNALGOS®-DC ℞

[*sĭn 'al "gōs*]

Capsules

DESCRIPTION

Each Synalgos-DC capsule contains 16 mg drocode (dihydrocodeine) bitartrate (Warning—may be habit-forming), 356.4 mg aspirin, and 30 mg caffeine.

The inactive ingredients present are alginic acid, cellulose, D&C Red 28, FD&C Blue 1, gelatin, iron oxides, stearic acid, and titanium dioxide.

ACTIONS

Dihydrocodeine is a semisynthetic narcotic analgesic, related to codeine, with multiple actions qualitatively similar to those of codeine; the most prominent of these involve the central nervous system and organs with smooth-muscle components. The principal action of therapeutic value is analgesia.

Synalgos-DC also contains the non-narcotic antipyretic-analgesic, aspirin.

INDICATIONS

For the relief of moderate to moderately severe pain.

CONTRAINDICATIONS

Hypersensitivity to dihydrocodeine, codeine, or aspirin.

WARNINGS

Salicylates should be used with extreme caution in the presence of peptic ulcer or coagulation abnormalities.

DRUG DEPENDENCE

Dihydrocodeine can produce drug dependence of the codeine type and therefore has the potential of being abused. Psychic dependence, physical dependence, and tolerance may develop upon repeated administration of dihydrocodeine, and it should be prescribed and administered with the same degree of caution appropriate to the use of other oral narcotic-containing medications.

Like other narcotic-containing medications, dihydrocodeine is subject to the provisions of the Federal Controlled Substances Act.

USAGE IN AMBULATORY PATIENTS

Dihydrocodeine may impair the mental and/or physical abilities required for the performance of potentially hazardous tasks, such as driving a car or operating machinery. The patient using Synalgos-DC should be cautioned accordingly.

INTERACTIONS WITH OTHER CENTRAL NERVOUS SYSTEM DEPRESSANTS

Patients receiving other narcotic analgesics, general anesthetics, tranquilizers, sedative-hypnotics, or other CNS depressants (including alcohol) concomitantly with Synalgos-DC may exhibit an additive CNS depression. When such combined therapy is contemplated, the dose of one or both agents should be reduced.

USAGE IN PREGNANCY

Reproduction studies have not been performed in animals. There is no adequate information on whether this drug may affect fertility in human males and females or has a teratogenic potential or other adverse effect on the fetus.

USAGE IN CHILDREN

Preparations containing aspirin should be kept out of the reach of children. Synalgos-DC is not recommended for patients 12 years of age and under. Since there is no experience in children who have received this drug, safety and efficacy in children have not been established.

PRECAUTIONS

Synalgos-DC should be given with caution to certain patients, such as the elderly or debilitated.

ADVERSE REACTIONS

The most frequently observed reactions include light-headedness, dizziness, drowsiness, sedation, nausea, vomiting, constipation, pruritus, and skin reactions.

DOSAGE AND ADMINISTRATION

Dosage should be adjusted according to the severity of the pain and the response of the patient. Synalgos-DC is given orally. The usual adult dose is two capsules every 4 hours as needed for pain.

DRUG INTERACTIONS

The CNS-depressant effects of Synalgos-DC may be additive with that of other CNS depressants.

See "Warnings."

Aspirin may enhance the effects of anticoagulants and inhibit the uricosuric effects of uricosuric agents.

HOW SUPPLIED

Synalgos®-DC Capsules, Wyeth®, are supplied in bottles of 100 and 500 capsules as follows:

NDC 0008-4191, blue and gray capsule marked "WYETH" and "4191".

Store below 25°C (77°F).

Keep tightly closed.

Dispense in tight container.

Shown in Product Identification Section, page 438

TETANUS AND DIPHTHERIA TOXOIDS ADSORBED for Adult Use ℞

[*tet 'ah-nus and dif-the 're-ah tok 'soids*]

aluminum phosphate adsorbed

ULTRAFINED®

DESCRIPTION

The diphtheria toxoid component is prepared by cultivating a suitable strain of *Corynebacterium diphtheriae* on a modified Mueller's casein hydrolysate medium (J. Immunology *37:* 103, 1939). The tetanus toxoid component is prepared by cultivating a suitable strain of *Clostridium tetani* on a protein-free semisynthetic medium (Appl. Microbiol. *10:* 146, 1962). Formaldehyde is used as the toxoiding (detoxifying) agent for both diphtheria and tetanus toxins. The final product is sterile and contains no more than 0.02 percent free formaldehyde and contains 0.01 percent thimerosal (mercury derivative) as preservative. Each dose (0.5 mL) for intramuscular use contains the same amount of purified tetanus toxoid that is in an individual dose of Tetanus Toxoid Adsorbed, Aluminum Phosphate Adsorbed, Ultrafined, Wyeth. In addition, each dose contains no more than 2 Lf of purified diphtheria toxoid. The aluminum content of the final product does not exceed 0.85 mg per 0.5 mL dose. During processing hydrochloric acid and sodium hydroxide are used to adjust the pH. Sodium chloride is added to the finished product to control isotonicity.

HOW SUPPLIED

Tetanus and Diphtheria Toxoids Adsorbed **for Adult Use**, Aluminum Phosphate Adsorbed, Ultrafined®, is available in vials of 5 mL (0008-0341-02) and 0.5 mL TUBEX® Sterile Cartridge-Needle Units (25 gauge × 5/8 inch needle) packaged in cartons of 10 TUBEX, NDC 0008-0341-01.

Store between 2° and 8° C (35° and 46°F)

Do not freeze

Shake the vial vigorously before withdrawing each dose

For prescribing information write to Professional Service, Wyeth-Ayerst Laboratories, P.O. Box 8299, Philadelphia, PA 19101, or contact your local Wyeth-Ayerst representative.

TETANUS TOXOID ℞

[*tet 'ahnus tok 'soid*]

fluid, purified

ULTRAFINED®

DESCRIPTION

Tetanus Toxoid, fluid, is prepared by growing a suitable strain of *Clostridium tetani* on a protein-free semisynthetic medium (Appl. Microbiol. *10:* 146, 1962). Formaldehyde is used as the toxoiding (detoxifying) agent for tetanus toxin. The final product contains no more than 0.02% free formaldehyde and contains 0.01% thimerosal (mercury derivative) as preservative.

Tetanus toxoid is refined by methods perfected in the Wyeth Institute for Medical Research. These methods eliminate at least 97% of the nontoxoid nitrogen. During processing, hydrochloric acid and sodium hydroxide are used to adjust the pH. Sodium chloride is added to the finished product to control isotonicity.

HOW SUPPLIED

Tetanus Toxoid, fluid, purified, Ultrafined®, Wyeth®, is available in vials of 7.5 mL (0008-0340-02) and in 0.5 mL TUBEX® Sterile Cartridge-Needle Units (25 gauge × 5/8 inch needle), packaged in boxes of 10 TUBEX (0008-0340-01).

Continued on next page

Wyeth-Ayerst Laboratories—Cont.

Keep between 2° and 8°C (35° and 46°F)
Keep from freezing
For prescribing information write to Professional Service, Wyeth-Ayerst Laboratories, P.O. Box 8299, Philadelphia, PA 19101, or contact your local Wyeth-Ayerst representative.

TETANUS TOXOID ADSORBED ℞
[tet'ah-nus tok'soid]
aluminum phosphate adsorbed,
ULTRAFINED®

DESCRIPTION
TETANUS TOXOID ADSORBED, Aluminum Phosphate Adsorbed, Wyeth, is prepared by growing a suitable strain of Cl. tetani on a protein-free, semisynthetic medium (Appl. Microbiol. *10:* 146, 1962). Formaldehyde is used as the toxoiding (detoxifying) agent for tetanus toxin. The final product contains no more than 0.02% free formaldehyde and contains 0.01% thimerosal (mercury derivative) as preservative.
TETANUS TOXOID ADSORBED, Wyeth, is refined by methods which eliminate at least 97% of the nontoxoid nitrogen. Adsorption of purified antigens on an optimal quantity of aluminum phosphate, a mineral adjuvant, prolongs and enhances the antigenic properties by retarding the rate of absorption. The alumium content of the final product does not exceed 0.85 mg per 0.5 mL dose. During processing, hydrochloric acid and sodium hydroxide are used to adjust the pH. Sodium chloride is added to the finished product to control isotonicity.

HOW SUPPLIED
Vials of 5 mL. (0008-0339-03); and 0.5-mL. TUBEX ® Sterile Cartridge-Needle Units, packages of 10 (0008-0339-01).
Keep between 2° and 8°C (35° and 46°F)
Do not freeze
Shake well
For prescribing information write to Professional Service, Wyeth-Ayerst Laboratories, P.O. Box 8299, Philadelphia, PA 19101, or contact your local Wyeth-Ayerst representative.

THIOSULFIL® Forte ℞
[thī"o-sul'fil fawrta]
(sulfamethizole 500 mg)

CAUTION: Federal law prohibits dispensing without prescription.

DESCRIPTION
Thiosulfil Forte is an antibacterial sulfonamide available in tablet form for oral administration.
Chemical name: N′-(5-methyl-1,3,4-thiadiazol-2-yl) sulfanilamide.
Structural formula:

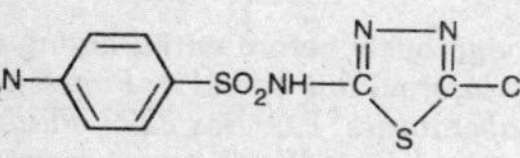

Sulfamethizole is a 5-membered heterocyclic sulfanilamide, occurring as a white or light buff-colored crystalline powder. Solubility in water is dependent upon the pH (1 g/5 mL at pH 7.5; 1 g/4000 mL at pH 6.5). It is soluble in alcohol, and practically insoluble in benzene.
Thiosulfil Forte Tablets contain the following inactive ingredients: gelatin, magnesium stearate, microcrystalline cellulose, starch.

CLINICAL PHARMACOLOGY
MECHANISM OF SULFONAMIDE BACTERIOSTATIC ACTION
The primary mechanism of bacteriostatic action by Thiosulfil Forte is the same as that of most sulfonamides. By competing with the precursor para-aminobenzoic acid, sulfonamides inhibit bacterial synthesis of folic (pteroylglutamic) acid which is required for bacterial growth. Resistant strains are capable of utilizing folic acid precursors or preformed folic acid.
ANTIBACTERIAL SPECTRUM
The antibacterial spectrum of all sulfonamides is similar. *In vitro* sensitivity of bacteria to sulfonamides does not always reflect *in vivo* sensitivity. Therefore, efficacy must be carefully evaluated with bacteriologic and clinical responses in the individual patient. (See WARNINGS.)
FACTORS DETERMINING EFFICACY
Efficacy of antimicrobial therapy is dependent upon a number of factors including the *in vivo* sensitivity of the involved organisms, the concentration of the drug required for bacteriostasis, and the achievable concentration of the sulfonamide at the desired site of action.
Because of the very rapid renal clearance of sulfamethizole, the blood levels attained are low, and accumulation of the drug in tissues outside the urinary tract is very limited. Therefore, sulfamethizole is not appropriate for treatment of systemic infections such as nocardiosis or for local lesions outside the urinary tract such as chancroid and trachoma. However, its low degree of acetylation and its rapid renal clearance permit high concentrations of active sulfamethizole to occur in the urinary tract, making it especially applicable for the treatment of infections of this tract. In addition, the possibility of crystalluria is minimized because of the high solubility of the drug in urine.
Approximately 95% of a given dose of sulfamethizole is not metabolized; less than 5% is acetylated. As a consequence, almost all of a given dose of Thiosulfil Forte is present in its active form in the body.
Approximately 80% of an administered dose is recoverable within eight hours; approximately 98% is cleared within 15 to 24 hours. Sulfamethizole is cleared by the kidney at a rate only 10 to 20% lower than that for creatinine.
BLOOD CONCENTRATIONS
Following a single 2 g dose of sulfamethizole, peak total drug levels in whole blood are in the range of 6 mg %, the levels fall to about 50% in four hours, and are negligible at eight hours. Approximately the same concentrations are found in children following a single dose of 100 mg/kg.
URINE CONCENTRATIONS
The following average values of free drug in mg/mL were found after a single 4 g dose of sulfamethizole:

0 to 2 hours—	7.01
2 to 4 " —	10.97
4 to 6 " —	5.93
6 to 10 " —	1.09
10 to 24 " —	0.31

Following a single 2 g dose, the following average concentrations of total drug in mg/mL of urine were found:

0 to 4 hours—	5.15
4 to 8 " —	1.8
8 to 12 " —	0.4
16 to 24 " —	0.1

Following a single 1 g dose of sulfamethizole, the average concentration of total drug during the first 3.5 hours was 2.9 mg/mL.
SOLUBILITY IN URINE
Sulfamethizole is highly soluble in urine. The solubilities of free and acetylated drug in buffered urine at 37° C at various pH's, in mg/mL, are given below:

pH	*free*	*acetylated*
4.5	108	33
5.3	220	.....
5.6	480	278
6.0	729	310
6.5	5,650	380
7.0	8,250	1,500
7.5	54,000	.....

INDICATIONS AND USAGE
Thiosulfil Forte is indicated in the treatment of urinary tract infections (primarily pyelonephritis, pyelitis, and cystitis) in the absence of obstructive uropathy or foreign bodies, when these infections are caused by susceptible strains of the following organisms: *Escherichia coli, Klebsiella-Enterobacter, Staphylococcus aureus, Proteus mirabilis,* and *Proteus vulgaris.*
IMPORTANT NOTE: In In vitro sulfonamide sensitivity tests are not always reliable. The test must be carefully coordinated with bacteriologic and clinical reponse. When the patient is already taking sulfonamides, follow-up cultures should have aminobenzoic acid added to the culture media.
Currently, the increasing frequency of resistant organisms is a limitation of the usefulness of antibacterial agents, including the sulfonamides, especially in the treatment of recurrent and complicated urinary tract infections.

Wide variation in blood levels may result with identical doses. Blood levels should be measured in patients receiving sulfonamides for serious infections. Free sulfonamide blood levels of 5–15 mg per 100 mL may be considered therapeutically effective for most infections, with blood levels of 12–15 mg per 100 mL optimal for serious infections; 20 mg per 100 mL should be the maximum total sulfonamide level, as adverse reactions occur more frequently above this level.

CONTRAINDICATIONS
Sulfonamides should not be used in patients hypersensitive to sulfa drugs. They should not be used in infants less than two months of age, in pregnancy at term, and during the nursing period because sulfonamides cross the placenta and are excreted in breast milk and may cause kernicterus.

WARNINGS
Deaths associated with the administration of sulfonamides have been reported from hypersensitivity reactions, agranulocytosis, aplastic anemia, and other blood dyscrasias. The occurrence of sore throat, fever, pallor, purpura, or jaundice during sulfonamide administration may be an early indication of serious blood dyscrasias.

PRECAUTIONS
GENERAL
The usual precautions used in sulfonamide therapy should be observed, including the maintenance of an adequate fluid intake. Sulfonamides should be used with caution in patients with impairment of hepatic or renal function, severe allergy or bronchial asthma, and in patients with glucose-6-phosphate dehydrogenase deficiency since sulfas may cause hemolysis in this latter group.
Information for the Patient: Adequate fluid intake should be maintained while taking Thiosulfil Forte. Patients should drink a full 8 oz. glass of water with each dose of Thiosulfil Forte and drink additional fluids at frequent intervals throughout the day. Patients should immediately report any adverse side effects to their physician.
LABORATORY TESTS
Frequent blood counts and renal function tests should be carried out during sulfonamide treatment, especially during prolonged administration. Microscopic urinalyses should be done once a week when a patient is treated for longer than two weeks. Urine cultures should be made to confirm eradication of bacteriuria.
DRUG INTERACTIONS
The most important interactions between the sulfonamides and other drugs involve those with oral anticoagulants, the sulfonylurea hypoglycemic agents, and the hydantoin anticonvulsants. In each case, sulfonamides can potentiate the effects of the other drug. Dosage adjustments may have to be made when these drugs are given concomitantly. Cross sensitivity may exist with these agents. PABA and certain local anesthetics such as procaine that are esters of PABA, antagonize the effects of sulfonamides and therefore decrease their effectiveness.
An insoluble precipitate may form in acidic urine when sulfamethizole is used concomitantly with methenamine mandelate.
Tolbutamide, diphenylhydantoin, phenytoin, and warfarin may have prolonged half-lives when administered with sulfamethizole.
CARCINOGENESIS, MUTAGENESIS, IMPAIRMENT OF FERTILITY
Rats appear to be especially susceptible to the goitrogenic effects of sulfonamides, and long-term administration has produced thyroid malignancies in the species.
No long-term fertility or mutagenicity studies have been conducted in animals or humans.
Pregnancy: Teratogenic Effects, Pregnancy Category C.
USAGE IN PREGNANCY
The safe use of sulfonamides in pregnancy has not been established. The teratogenicity potential of most sulfonamides has not been thoroughly investigated in either animals or humans. However, a significant increase in the incidence of cleft palate and other bony abnormalities of offspring has been observed when certain sulfonamides of the short-, intermediate-, and long-acting types were given to pregnant rats and mice at high oral doses (7 to 25 times the human dose).
Thiosulfil Forte should be used during pregnancy only if the potential benefit justifies the potential risk to the fetus.
NURSING MOTHERS
Thiosulfil Forte is contraindicated in pregnant women and nursing mothers. Sulfonamides cross the placenta and are excreted in breast milk to a significant degree. Because of the potential for serious adverse reactions in nursing infants from sulfonamides, a decision should be made whether to discontinue nursing or to discontinue the drug, taking into account the importance of the drug to the mother. See CONTRAINDICATIONS.
PEDIATRIC USE
Sulfamethizole is not indicated for use in infants less than two months old. See CONTRAINDICATIONS and DOSAGE AND ADMINISTRATION.

ADVERSE REACTIONS
BLOOD DYSCRASIAS
Agranulocytosis, aplastic anemia, thrombocytopenia, leukopenia, hemolytic anemia, purpura, hypoprothrombinemia, and methemoglobinemia.
ALLERGIC REACTIONS
Drug fever, erythema multiforme (Stevens-Johnson syndrome), generalized skin eruptions, epidermal necrolysis, urticaria, serum sickness, pruritus, exfoliative dermatitis, anaphylactoid reactions, periorbital edema, conjunctival and scleral injection, photosensitization, arthralgia, and allergic myocarditis.
GASTROINTESTINAL REACTIONS
Nausea, emesis, abdominal pains, hepatitis, diarrhea, anorexia, pancreatitis, and stomatitis.
CNS REACTIONS
Headache, peripheral neuritis, mental depression, convulsions, ataxia, hallucinations, tinnitus, vertigo, and insomnia.

RENAL

Crystalluria, toxic nephrosis with oliguria and anuria.

MISCELLANEOUS REACTIONS

Chills, periarteritis nodosum, and LE phenomenon.

The sulfonamides bear certain chemical similarities to some goitrogens, diuretics (acetazolamide and the thiazides), and oral hypoglycemic agents. Goiter production, diuresis, and hypoglycemia have occurred rarely in patients receiving sulfonamides. Cross-sensitivity may exist with these agents. (See PRECAUTIONS: Carcinogenesis, Mutagenesis, Impairment of Fertility.)

OVERDOSAGE

The maximum tolerated single dose of sulfa drug has not been established. Sulfamethoxazole has been given in single doses up to 2000 mg. The acute signs and symptoms associated with sulfonamide overdose include anorexia, nausea, colicky abdominal pain, vertigo, headache, drowsiness and unconsciousness. Pyrexia, hematuria and crystalluria have been reported. Blood dyscrasias and jaundice are late manifestations of overdosing.

General treatment of overdose for sulfonamides includes induction of emesis and gastric lavage. Urine output should be maintained by either oral or I.V. fluid administration in patients with normal renal function. Renal function with appropriate blood chemistries including electrolytes should be monitored closely in the acute period. Hematologic parameters should be followed over the next 10 days to two weeks after the overdose ingestion. Methemoglobinuria can be acutely reversed with intravenous 1% methylene blue. Sulfamethizole is only minimally dialyzable by hemodialysis and is not dialyzable by peritoneal dialysis. Other supportive measures should be instituted appropriate to signs and symptoms.

DOSAGE AND ADMINISTRATION

USUAL DOSAGE

Adults: 500 mg to 1 g, three or four times daily.

Children and infants (over 2 months of age): 30 to 45 mg/kg/24 hours, divided into 4 doses.

HOW SUPPLIED

Thiosulfil Forte—Each white, biconvex, scored, oval tablet contains sulfamethizole 500 mg (scored), in bottles of 100 (NDC 0046-0786-81).

Store at room temperature (approximately 25° C.)

Shown in Product Identification Section, page 438

TRECATOR®-SC   ℞

[trek "ā'tōre]

(ethionamide)

Sugar-Coated Tablets

DESCRIPTION

Trecator-SC (ethionamide) is used in the treatment of tuberculosis. The chemical name for ethionamide is 2-ethyl-thioisonicotinamide with the following structural formula:

Ethionamide is a yellow, crystalline, nonhygroscopic compound with a faint-to-moderate sulfide odor. It is practically insoluble in water and ether but soluble in methanol and ethanol. It melts at about 162°C and is stable at ordinary temperatures and humidities.

Trecator-SC tablets contain 250 mg of ethionamide. The inactive ingredients present are acacia, calcium carbonate, carnauba wax, confectioners sugar, FD&C Yellow 6, gelatin, lactose, magnesium stearate, methylcellulose, pharmaceutical glaze, polacrilin potassium, povidone, sodium benzoate, sucrose, talc, titanium dioxide, and white wax.

ACTION

Bacteriostatic against *Mycobacterium tuberculosis.*

INDICATIONS

Failure after adequate treatment with primary drugs (i.e., isoniazid, streptomycin, aminosalicylic acid) in any form of active tuberculosis. Ethionamide should only be given with other effective antituberculous agents.

CONTRAINDICATIONS

Severe hypersensitivity.

Severe hepatic damage.

WARNING

USE IN PREGNANCY

Teratogenic effects have been demonstrated in animals (rabbits, rats) receiving doses in excess of those recommended in humans. Use of the drug should be avoided during pregnancy or in women of childbearing potential unless the benefits outweigh its possible hazard.

USE IN CHILDREN

Optimum dosage for children has not been established. This, however, does not preclude use of the drug when its use is crucial to therapy.

PRECAUTIONS

Pretreatment examinations should include *in vitro* susceptibility tests of recent cultures of *M. tuberculosis* from the patient as measured against ethionamide and the usual primary antituberculous drugs.

Determinations of serum transaminase (SGOT, SGPT) should be made prior to and every 2 to 4 weeks during therapy.

In patients with diabetes mellitus, management may be more difficult and hepatitis occurs more frequently.

Ethionamide may intensify the adverse effects of the other antituberculous drugs administered concomitantly. Convulsions have been reported, and special care should be taken, particularly when ethionamide is administered with cycloserine.

ADVERSE REACTIONS

The most common side effect is gastrointestinal intolerance. Other adverse effects similar to those seen with isoniazid have been reported: peripheral neuritis, optic neuritis, psychic disturbances (including mental depression), postural hypotension, skin rashes, thrombocytopenia, pellagralike syndrome, jaundice and/or hepatitis, increased difficulty in management of diabetes mellitus, stomatitis, gynecomastia, and impotence.

DOSAGE AND ADMINISTRATION

Ethionamide should be administered with at least one other effective antituberculous drug.

Average Adult Dose: 0.5 gram to 1.0 gram/day in divided doses.

Concomitant administration of pyridoxine is recommended.

HOW SUPPLIED

Trecator®-SC (ethionamide) Tablets are supplied in bottles of 100 tablets as follows:

250 mg, NDC 0008-4130, orange, sugar-coated tablet marked "WYETH" and "4130".

Keep tightly closed

Dispense in tight container.

TRIPHASIL®-21   ℞

[tri-fa'sil]

Tablets

(levonorgestrel and ethinyl estradiol tablets—triphasic regimen)

DESCRIPTION

Each Triphasil cycle of 21 tablets consists of three different drug phases as follows: Phase 1 comprised of 6 brown tablets, each containing 0.050 mg of levonorgestrel (d(-)-13 beta-ethyl-17-alpha-ethinyl-17-beta-hydroxygon-4-en-3-one), a totally synthetic progestogen, and 0.030 mg of ethinyl estradiol (19-nor-17α-pregna-1,3,5(10)-trien-20-yne-3,17-diol); phase 2 comprised of 5 white tablets, each containing 0.075 mg levonorgestrel and 0.040 mg ethinyl estradiol; and phase 3 comprised of 10 light-yellow tablets, each containing 0.125 mg levonorgestrel and 0.030 mg ethinyl estradiol. The inactive ingredients present are calcium carbonate, glycerin, iron oxides, lactose, magnesium stearate, methylparaben, polyethylene glycol, povidone, propylparaben, sodium benzoate, starch, sucrose, talc, and titanium dioxide.

Levonorgestrel

Ethinyl Estradiol

CLINICAL PHARMACOLOGY

Combination oral contraceptives act by suppression of gonadotropins. Although the primary mechanism of this action is inhibition of ovulation, other alterations include changes in the cervical mucus (which increase the difficulty of sperm entry into the uterus) and the endometrium (which reduce the likelihood of implantation).

INDICATIONS AND USAGE

Oral contraceptives are indicated for the prevention of pregnancy in women who elect to use this product as a method of contraception.

Oral contraceptives are highly effective. Table I lists the typical accidental pregnancy rates for users of combination oral contraceptives and other methods of contraception. The efficacy of these contraceptive methods, except sterilization and the IUD, depends upon the reliability with which they are used. Correct and consistent use of methods can result in lower failure rates.

TABLE I: LOWEST EXPECTED AND TYPICAL FAILURE RATES DURING THE FIRST YEAR OF CONTINUOUS USE OF A METHOD

% of Women Experiencing an Accidental Pregnancy in the First Year of Continuous Use

Method	Lowest Expected*	Typical**
(No Contraception)	(89)	(89)
Oral contraceptives		3
combined	0.1	N/A***
progestin only	0.5	N/A***
Diaphragm with spermicidal cream or jelly	3	18
Spermicides alone (foam, creams, jellies and vaginal suppositories)	3	21
Vaginal Sponge		
nulliparous	5	18
multiparous	>8	>28
IUD (medicated)	1	6#
Condom without spermicides	2	12
Periodic abstinence (all methods)	2–10	20
Female sterilization	0.2	0.4
Male sterilization	0.1	0.15

Adapted from J. Trussell and K. Kost, Table 11, Studies in Family Planning, 18(5), Sept.–Oct. 1987.

---

* The authors' best guess of the percentage of women expected to experience an accidental pregnancy among couples who initiate a method (not necessarily for the first time) and who use it consistently and correctly during the first year if they do not stop for any other reason.

** This term represents "typical" couples who initiate use of a method (not necessarily for the first time), who experience an accidental pregnancy during the first year if they do not stop use for any other reason.

*** N/A—Data not available.

\# Combined typical rate for both medicated and non-medicated IUD. The rate for medicated IUD alone is not available.

CONTRAINDICATIONS

Oral contraceptives should not be used in women with any of the following conditions:

Thrombophlebitis or thromboembolic disorders

A past history of deep-vein thrombophlebitis or thromboembolic disorders

Cerebral-vascular or coronary-artery disease

Known or suspected carcinoma of the breast

Carcinoma of the endometrium or other known or suspected estrogen-dependent neoplasia

Undiagnosed abnormal genital bleeding

Cholestatic jaundice of pregnancy or jaundice with prior pill use

Hepatic adenomas or carcinomas

Known or suspected pregnancy

WARNINGS

> **Cigarette smoking increases the risk of serious cardiovascular side effects from oral-contraceptive use. This risk increases with age and with heavy smoking (15 or more cigarettes per day) and is quite marked in women over 35 years of age. Women who use oral contraceptives should be strongly advised not to smoke.**

The use of oral contraceptives is associated with increased risks of several serious conditions including myocardial infarction, thromboembolism, stroke, hepatic neoplasia, gallbladder disease, and hypertension, although the risk of serious morbidity or mortality is very small in healthy women without underlying factors. The risk of morbidity and mortality increases significantly in the presence of other underlying risk factors such as hypertension, hyperlipidemias, obesity, and diabetes.

Continued on next page

Wyeth-Ayerst Laboratories—Cont.

Practitioners prescribing oral contraceptives should be familiar with the following information relating to these risks.
The information contained in this package insert is based principally on studies carried out in patients who used oral contraceptives with higher formulations of estrogens and progestogens than those in common use today. The effect of long-term use of the oral contraceptives with lower formulations of both estrogens and progestogens remains to be determined.
Throughout this labeling, epidemiological studies reported are of two types: retrospective or case control studies and prospective or cohort studies. Case control studies provide a measure of the relative risk of disease, namely, a ratio of the incidence of a disease among oral-contraceptive users to that among nonusers. The relative risk does not provide information on the actual clinical occurrence of a disease. Cohort studies provide a measure of attributable risk, which is the difference in the incidence of disease between oral-contraceptive users and nonusers. The attributable risk does provide information about the actual occurrence of a disease in the population. For further information, the reader is referred to a text on epidemiological methods.

1. THROMBOEMBOLIC DISORDERS AND OTHER VASCULAR PROBLEMS

a. *Myocardial Infarction*
An increased risk of myocardial infarction has been attributed to oral-contraceptive use. This risk is primarily in smokers or women with other underlying risk factors for coronary-artery disease such as hypertension, hypercholesterolemia, morbid obesity, and diabetes. The relative risk of heart attack for current oral-contraceptive users has been estimated to be two to six. The risk is very low under the age of 30.
Smoking in combination with oral-contraceptive use has been shown to contribute substantially to the incidence of myocardial infarctions in women in their mid-thirties or older with smoking accounting for the majority of excess cases. Mortality rates associated with circulatory disease have been shown to increase substantially in smokers over the age of 35 and nonsmokers over the age of 40 (Table II) among women who use oral contraceptives.

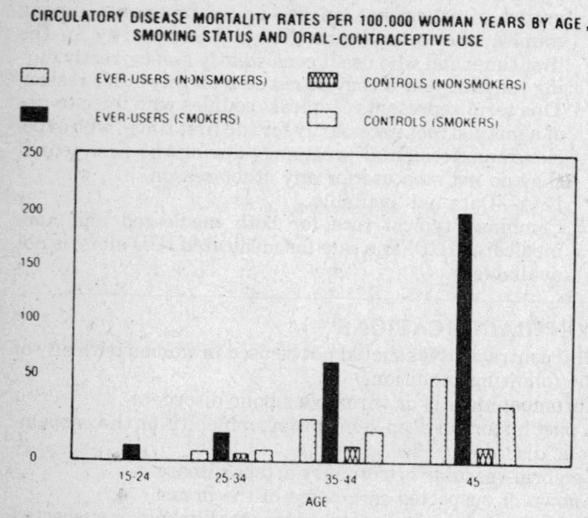

TABLE II. (Adapted from P.M. Layde and V. Beral, Lancet, 1:541–546, 1981.)

Oral contraceptives may compound the effects of well-known risk factors, such as hypertension, diabetes, hyperlipidemias, age, and obesity. In particular, some progestogens are known to decrease HDL cholesterol and cause glucose intolerance, while estrogens may create a state of hyperinsulinism. Oral contraceptives have been shown to increase blood pressure among users (see section 9 in Warnings). Similar effects on risk factors have been associated with an increased risk of heart disease. Oral contraceptives must be used with caution in women with cardiovascular disease risk factors.

b. *Thromboembolism*
An increased risk of thromboembolic and thrombotic disease associated with the use of oral contraceptives is well established. Case control studies have found the relative risk of users compared to nonusers to be 3 for the first episode of superficial venous thrombosis, 4 to 11 for deep vein thrombosis or pulmonary embolism, and 1.5 to 6 for women with predisposing conditions for venous thromboembolic disease. Cohort studies have shown the relative risk to be somewhat lower, about 3 for new cases and about 4.5 for new cases requiring hospitalization. The risk of thromboembolic disease due to oral contraceptives is not related to length of use and disappears after pill use is stopped.
A two- to four-fold increase in relative risk of postoperative thromboembolic complications has been reported with the use of oral contraceptives. The relative risk of venous thrombosis in women who have predisposing conditions is twice that of women without such medical conditions. If feasible, oral contraceptives should be discontinued at least four weeks prior to and for two weeks after elective surgery of a type associated with an increase in risk of thromboembolism and during and following prolonged immobilization. Since the immediate postpartum period is also associated with an increased risk of thromboembolism, oral contraceptives should be started no earlier than four to six weeks after delivery in women who elect not to breast-feed, or a midtrimester pregnancy termination.

c. *Cerebrovascular diseases*
Oral contraceptives have been shown to increase both the relative and attributable risks of cerebrovascular events (thrombotic and hemorrhagic strokes), although, in general, the risk is greatest among older (>35 years), hypertensive women who also smoke. Hypertension was found to be a risk factor for both users and nonusers, for both types of strokes, while smoking interacted to increase the risk for hemorrhagic strokes.
In a large study, the relative risk of thrombotic strokes has been shown to range from 3 for normotensive users to 14 for users with severe hypertension. The relative risk of hemorrhagic stroke is reported to be 1.2 for nonsmokers who used oral contraceptives, 2.6 for smokers who did not use oral contraceptives, 7.6 for smokers who used oral contraceptives, 1.8 for normotensive users, and 25.7 for users with severe hypertension. The attributable risk is also greater in older women.

d. *Dose-related risk of vascular disease from oral contraceptives*
A positive association has been observed between the amount of estrogen and progestogen in oral contraceptives and the risk of vascular disease. A decline in serum high-density lipoproteins (HDL) has been reported with many progestational agents. A decline in serum high-density lipoproteins has been associated with an increased incidence of ischemic heart disease. Because estrogens increase HDL cholesterol, the net effect of an oral contraceptive depends on a balance achieved between doses of estrogen and progestogen and the nature and absolute amount of progestogen used in the contraceptive. The amount of both hormones should be considered in the choice of an oral contraceptive.
Minimizing exposure to estrogen and progestogen is in keeping with good principles of therapeutics. For any particular estrogen/progestogen combination, the dosage regimen prescribed should be one which contains the least amount of estrogen and progestogen that is compatible with a low failure rate and the needs of the individual patient. New acceptors of oral-contraceptive agents should be started on preparations containing less than 50 mcg of estrogen.

e. *Persistence of risk of vascular disease*
There are two studies which have shown persistence of risk of vascular disease for ever-users of oral contraceptives. In a study in the United States, the risk of developing myocardial infarction after discontinuing oral contraceptives persists for at least 9 years for women 40 to 49 years who had used oral contraceptives for five or more years, but this increased risk was not demonstrated in other age groups. In another study in Great Britain, the risk of developing cerebrovascular disease persisted for at least 6 years after discontinuation of oral contraceptives, although excess risk was very small. However, both studies were performed with oral- contraceptive formulations containing 50 micrograms or higher of estrogens.

2. ESTIMATES OF MORTALITY FROM CONTRACEPTIVE USE
One study gathered data from a variety of sources which have estimated the mortality rate associated with different methods of contraception at different ages (Table III). These estimates include the combined risk of death associated with contraceptive methods plus the risk attributable to pregnancy in the event of method failure. Each method of contraception has its specific benefits and risks. The study concluded that with the exception of oral-contraceptive users 35 and older who smoke and 40 and older who do not smoke, mortality associated with all methods of birth control is less than that associated with childbirth. The observation of a possible increase in risk of mortality with age for oral-contraceptive users is based on data gathered in the 1970's—but not reported until 1983. However, current clinical practice involves the use of lower estrogen dose formulations combined with careful restriction of oral-contraceptive use to women who do not have the various risk factors listed in this labeling.
Because of these changes in practice and, also, because of some limited new data which suggest that the risk of cardiovascular disease with the use of oral contraceptives may now be less than previously observed, the Fertility and Maternal Health Drugs Advisory Committee was asked to review the topic in 1989. The Committee concluded that although cardiovascular-disease risks may be increased with oral-contraceptive use after age 40 in healthy nonsmoking women (even with the newer low-dose formulations), there are greater potential health risks associated with pregnancy in older women and with the alternative surgical and medical procedures which may be necessary if such women do not have access to effective and acceptable means of contraception. Therefore, the Committee recommended that the benefits of oral-contraceptive use by healthy nonsmoking women over 40 may outweigh the possible risks. Of course, older women, as all women who take oral contraceptives, should take the lowest possible dose formulation that is effective.

3. CARCINOMA OF THE REPRODUCTIVE ORGANS
Numerous epidemiological studies have been performed on the incidence of breast, endometrial, ovarian, and cervical cancer in women using oral contraceptives. The overwhelming evidence in the literature suggests that the use of oral contraceptives is not associated with an increase in the risk of developing breast cancer, regardless of the age and parity of first use or with most of the marketed brands and doses. The Cancer and Steroid Hormone (CASH) study also showed no latent effect on the risk of breast cancer for at least a decade following long-term use. A few studies have shown a slightly increased relative risk of developing breast cancer, although the methodology of these studies, which included differences in examination of users and nonusers and differences in age at start of use, has been questioned.
Some studies suggest that oral-contraceptive use has been associated with an increase in the risk of cervical intraepithelial neoplasia in some populations of women. However, there continues to be controversy about the extent to which such findings may be due to differences in sexual behavior and other factors.
In spite of many studies of the relationship between oral-contraceptive use and breast and cervical cancers, a cause-and-effect relationship has not been established.

4. HEPATIC NEOPLASIA
Benign hepatic adenomas are associated with oral-contraceptive use, although the incidence of benign tumors is rare in the United States. Indirect calculations have estimated the attributable risk to be in the range of 3.3 cases/100,000 for users, a risk that increases after four or more years of use. Rupture of rare, benign, hepatic adenomas may cause death through intra-abdominal hemorrhage.
Studies from Britain have shown an increased risk of developing hepatocellular carcinoma in long-term (>8 years) oral-contraceptive users. However, these cancers are extremely rare in the U.S., and the attributable risk (the excess incidence) of liver cancers in oral-contraceptive users approaches less than one per million users.

TABLE III—ANNUAL NUMBER OF BIRTH-RELATED OR METHOD-RELATED DEATHS ASSOCIATED WITH CONTROL OF FERTILITY PER 100,000 NONSTERILE WOMEN, BY FERTILITY-CONTROL METHOD ACCORDING TO AGE

Method of control and outcome	15–19	20–24	25–29	30–34	35–39	40–44
No fertility-control methods*	7.0	7.4	9.1	14.8	25.7	28.2
Oral contraceptives nonsmoker**	0.3	0.5	0.9	1.9	13.8	31.6
Oral contraceptives smoker**	2.2	3.4	6.6	13.5	51.1	117.2
IUD**	0.8	0.8	1.0	1.0	1.4	1.4
Condom*	1.1	1.6	0.7	0.2	0.3	0.4
Diaphragm/spermicide*	1.9	1.2	1.2	1.3	2.2	2.8
Periodic abstinence*	2.5	1.6	1.6	1.7	2.9	3.6

* Deaths are birth related
** Deaths are method related

Adapted from H.W. Ory, Family Planning Perspectives, 15:57–63, 1983.

5. OCULAR LESIONS

There have been clincial case reports of retinal thrombosis associated with the use of oral contraceptives. Oral contraceptives should be discontinued if there is unexplained partial or complete loss of vision; onset of proptosis or diplopia; papilledema; or retinal vascular lesions. Appropriate diagnostic and therapeutic measures should be undertaken immediately.

6. ORAL-CONTRACEPTIVE USE BEFORE OR DURING EARLY PREGNANCY

Extensive epidemiological studies have revealed no increased risk of birth defects in women who have used oral contraceptives prior to pregnancy. Studies also do not suggest a teratogenic effect, particularly insofar as cardiac anomalies and limb-reduction defects are concerned, when taken inadvertently during early pregnancy.

The administration of oral contraceptives to induce withdrawal bleeding should not be used as a test for pregnancy. Oral contraceptives should not be used during pregnancy to treat threatened or habitual abortion.

It is recommended that for any patient who has missed two consecutive periods, pregnancy should be ruled out before continuing oral-contraceptive use. If the patient has not adhered to the prescribed schedule, the possibility of pregnancy should be considered at the time of the first missed period. Oral-contraceptive use should be discontinued if pregnancy is confirmed.

7. GALLBLADDER DISEASE

Earlier studies have reported an increased lifetime relative risk of gallbladder surgery in users of oral contraceptives and estrogens. More recent studies, however, have shown that the relative risk of developing gallbladder disease among oral-contraceptive users may be minimal. The recent findings of minimal risk may be related to the use of oral-contraceptive formulations containing lower hormonal doses of estrogens and progestogens.

8. CARBOHYDRATE AND LIPID METABOLIC EFFECTS

Oral contraceptives have been shown to cause glucose intolerance in a significant percentage of users. Oral contraceptives containing greater than 75 micrograms of estrogens cause hyperinsulinism, while lower doses of estrogen cause less glucose intolerance. Progestogens increase insulin secretion and create insulin resistance, this effect varying with different progestational agents. However, in the non-diabetic woman, oral contraceptives appear to have no effect on fasting blood glucose. Because of these demonstrated effects, prediabetic and diabetic women should be carefully observed while taking oral contraceptives.

A small proportion of women will have persistent hypertriglyceridemia while on the pill. As discussed earlier (see "WARNINGS" 1a. and 1d.), changes in serum triglycerides and lipoprotein levels have been reported in oral-contraceptive users.

9. ELEVATED BLOOD PRESSURE

An increase in blood pressure has been reported in women taking oral contraceptives, and this increase is more likely in older oral-contraceptive users and with continued use. Data from the Royal College of General Practitioners and subsequent randomized trials have shown that the incidence of hypertension increases with increasing quantities of progestations.

Women with a history of hypertension or hypertension-related diseases, or renal disease, should be encouraged to use another method of contraception. If women with hypertension elect to use oral contraceptives, they should be monitored closely, and if significant elevation of blood pressure occurs, oral contraceptives should be discontinued. For most women, elevated blood pressure will return to normal after stopping oral contraceptives, and there is no difference in the occurrence of hypertension between ever- and never-users.

10. HEADACHE

The onset or exacerbation of migraine or development of headache with a new pattern that is recurrent, persistent, or severe requires discontinuation of oral contraceptives and evaluation of the cause.

11. BLEEDING IRREGULARITIES

Breakthrough bleeding and spotting are sometimes encountered in patients on oral contraceptives, especially during the first three months of use. The type and dose of progestogen may be important. Non-hormonal causes should be considered and adequate diagnostic measures taken to rule out malignancy or pregnancy in the event of breakthrough bleeding, as in the case of any abnormal vaginal bleeding. If pathology has been excluded, time or a change to another formulation may solve the problem. In the event of amenorrhea, pregnancy should be ruled out.

Some women may encounter post-pill amenorrhea or oligomenorrhea, especially when such a condition was preexistent.

PRECAUTIONS

1. PHYSICAL EXAMINATION AND FOLLOW-UP

A complete medical history and physical examination should be taken prior to the initiation or reinstitution of oral contraceptives and at least annually during use of oral contraceptives. These physical examinations should include special reference to blood pressure, breasts, abdomen and pelvic organs, including cervical cytology, and relevant laboratory tests. In case of undiagnosed, persistent or recurrent abnormal vaginal bleeding, appropriate diagnostic measures should be conducted to rule out malignancy. Women with a strong family history of breast cancer or who have breast nodules should be monitored with particular care.

2. LIPID DISORDERS

Women who are being treated for hyperlipidemias should be followed closely if they elect to use oral contraceptives. Some progestogens may elevate LDL levels and may render the control of hyperlipidemias more difficult. (See "Warnings," 1d.)

3. LIVER FUNCTION

If jaundice develops in any woman receiving such drugs, the medication should be discontinued. Steroid hormones may be poorly metabolized in patients with impaired liver function.

4. FLUID RETENTION

Oral contraceptives may cause some degree of fluid retention. They should be prescribed with caution, and only with careful monitoring, in patients with conditions which might be aggravated by fluid retention.

5. EMOTIONAL DISORDERS

Patients becoming significantly depressed while taking oral contraceptives should stop the medication and use an alternate method of contraception in an attempt to determine whether the symptom is drug related. Women with a history of depression should be carefully observed and the drug discontinued if depression recurs to a serious degree.

6. CONTACT LENSES

Contact lens wearers who develop visual changes or changes in lens tolerance should be assessed by an ophthalmologist.

7. DRUG INTERACTIONS

Reduced efficacy and increased incidence of breakthrough bleeding and menstrual irregularities have been associated with concomitant use of rifampin. A similar association, though less marked, has been suggested with barbiturates, phenylbutazone, phenytoin sodium, and possibly with griseofulvin, ampicillin, and tetracyclines.

8. INTERACTIONS WITH LABORATORY TESTS

Certain endocrine- and liver-function tests and blood components may be affected by oral contraceptives:

a. Increased prothrombin and factors VII, VIII, IX, and X; decreased antithrombin 3; increased norepinephrine-induced platelet aggregability.

b. Increased thyroid-binding globulin (TBG) leading to increased circulating total thyroid hormone, as measured by protein-bound iodine (PBI), T4 by column or by radioimmunoassay. Free T3 resin uptake is decreased, reflecting the elevated TBG; free T4 concentration is unaltered.

c. Other binding proteins may be elevated in serum.

d. Sex-binding globulins are increased and result in elevated levels of total circulating sex steroids and corticoids; however, free or biologically active levels remain unchanged.

e. Triglycerides may be increased.

f. Glucose tolerance may be decreased.

g. Serum folate levels may be depressed by oral-contraceptive therapy. This may be of clinical significance if a woman becomes pregnant shortly after discontinuing oral contraceptives.

9. CARCINOGENESIS

See "Warnings" section.

10. PREGNANCY

Pregnancy Category X. See "Contraindications" and "Warnings" sections.

11. NURSING MOTHERS

Small amounts of oral-contraceptive steroids have been identified in the milk of nursing mothers, and a few adverse effects on the child have been reported, including jaundice and breast enlargement. In addition, oral contraceptives given in the postpartum period may interfere with lactation by decreasing the quantity and quality of breast milk. If possible, the nursing mother should be advised not to use oral contraceptives but to use other forms of contraception until she has completely weaned her child.

INFORMATION FOR THE PATIENT

See Patient Labeling Printed Below.

ADVERSE REACTIONS

An increased risk of the following serious adverse reactions has been associated with the use of oral contraceptives (see "Warnings" section):

Thrombophlebitis.
Arterial thromboembolism.
Pulmonary embolism.
Myocardial infarction.
Cerebral hemorrhage.
Cerebral thrombosis.
Hypertension.

Gallbladder disease.
Hepatic adenomas or benign liver tumors.

There is evidence of an association between the following conditions and the use of oral contraceptives, although additional confirmatory studies are needed:

Mesenteric thrombosis.
Retinal thrombosis.

The following adverse reactions have been reported in patients receiving oral contraceptives and are believed to be drug-related:

Nausea
Vomiting
Gastrointestinal symptoms (such as abdominal cramps and bloating).
Breakthrough bleeding.
Spotting.
Change in menstrual flow.
Amenorrhea.
Temporary infertility after discontinuation of treatment.
Edema.
Melasma which may persist.
Breast changes: tenderness, enlargement, secretion.
Change in weight (increase or decrease).
Change in cervical erosion and cervical secretion.
Diminution in lactation when given immediately postpartum.
Cholestatic jaundice.
Migraine.
Rash (allergic).
Mental depression.
Reduced tolerance to carbohydrates.
Vaginal candidiasis.
Change in corneal curvature (steepening).
Intolerance to contact lenses.

The following adverse reactions have been reported in users of oral contraceptives, and the association has been neither confirmed nor refuted:

Congenital anomalies.
Premenstrual syndrome.
Cataracts.
Optic neuritis.
Changes in appetite.
Cystitis-like syndrome.
Headache.
Nervousness.
Dizziness.
Hirsutism.
Loss of scalp hair.
Erythema multiforme.
Erythema nodosum.
Hemorrhagic eruption.
Vaginitis.
Porphyria.
Impaired renal function.
Hemolytic uremic syndrome.
Budd-Chiari syndrome.
Acne.
Changes in libido.
Colitis.
Sickle-cell disease.
Cerebral-vascular disease with mitral valve prolapse.
Lupus-like syndromes.

OVERDOSAGE

Serious ill effects have not been reported following acute ingestion of large doses of oral contraceptives by young children. Overdosage may cause nausea, and withdrawal bleeding may occur in females.

NONCONTRACEPTIVE HEALTH BENEFITS

The following noncontraceptive health benefits related to the use of combination oral contraceptives are supported by epidemiological studies which largely utilized oral-contraceptive formulations containing doses exceeding 0.035 mg of ethinyl estradiol or 0.05 mg of mestranol.

Effects on menses:
Increased menstrual cycle regularity
Decreased blood loss and decreased incidence of iron deficiency anemia
Decreased incidence of dysmenorrhea
Effects related to inhibition of ovulation:
Decreased incidence of functional ovarian cysts
Decreased incidence of ectopic pregnancies
Effects from long-term use:
Decreased incidence of fibroadenomas and fibrocystic disease of the breast
Decreased incidence of acute pelvic inflammatory disease
Decreased incidence of endometrial cancer
Decreased incidence of ovarian cancer

DOSAGE AND ADMINISTRATION

To achieve maximum contraceptive effectiveness, Triphasil-21 Tablets (levonorgestrel and ethinyl estradiol tablets—triphasic regimen) must be taken exactly as directed and at intervals not exceeding 24 hours.

Continued on next page

Wyeth-Ayerst Laboratories—Cont.

Triphasil-21 Tablets are a three-phase preparation. The dosage of Triphasil-21 Tablets is one tablet daily for 21 consecutive days per menstrual cycle in the following order: 6 brown tablets (phase 1), followed by 5 white tablets (phase 2), and then followed by the last 10 light-yellow tablets (phase 3), according to the prescribed schedule. Tablets are then discontinued for 7 days (three weeks on, one week off). It is recommended that Triphasil-21 Tablets be taken at the same time each day, preferably after the evening meal or at bedtime. During the first cycle of medication, the patient should be instructed to take one Triphasil-21 Tablet daily in the order of 6 brown, 5 white and, finally, 10 light-yellow tablets for twenty-one (21) consecutive days, beginning on day one (1) of her menstrual cycle. (The first day of menstruation is day one.) The tablets are then discontinued for one week (7 days). Withdrawal bleeding usually occurs within 3 days following discontinuation of Triphasil-21 Tablets. (If Triphasil-21 Tablets are first taken later than the first day of the first menstrual cycle of medication or postpartum, contraceptive reliance should not be placed on Triphasil-21 Tablets until after the first 7 consecutive days of administration. The possibility of ovulation and conception prior to initiation of medication should be considered.)

When switching from another oral contraceptive, Triphasil-21 Tablets should be started on the first day of bleeding following the last tablet taken of the previous oral contraceptive.

The patient begins her next and all subsequent 21-day courses of Triphasil-21 Tablets on the same day of the week that she began her first course, following the same schedule: 21 days on—7 days off. She begins taking her brown tablets on the 8th day after discontinuance regardless of whether or not a menstrual period has occurred or is still in progress. Any time the next cycle of Triphasil-21 Tablets is started later than the 8th day, the patient should be protected by another means of contraception until she has taken a tablet daily for seven consecutive days.

If spotting or breakthrough bleeding occurs, the patient is instructed to continue on the same regimen. This type of bleeding is usually transient and without significance; however, if the bleeding is persistent or prolonged, the patient is advised to consult her physician. Although the occurrence of pregnancy is highly unlikely if Triphasil-21 Tablets are taken according to directions, if withdrawal bleeding does not occur, the possibility of pregnancy must be considered. If the patient has not adhered to the prescribed schedule (missed one or more tablets or started taking them on a day later than she should have), the probability of pregnancy should be considered at the time of the first missed period and appropriate diagnostic measures taken before the medication is resumed. If the patient has adhered to the prescribed regimen and misses two consecutive periods, pregnancy should be ruled out before continuing the contraceptive regimen.

The risk of pregnancy increases with each tablet missed. If the patient misses one tablet, she should be instructed to take it as soon as she remembers, and also to take her next tablet at the regular time, which means that she will be taking two tablets on that day. If she misses two tablets consecutively, she should take the second missed tablet as soon as she remembers, discard the first missed tablet and take her regular tablet for that day at the proper time. Furthermore, she should use an additional method of birth control in addition to Triphasil®-21 until menses has appeared or pregnancy has been excluded. If breakthrough bleeding occurs following missed tablets, it will usually be transient and of no consequence. If three consecutive tablets are missed, all medication should be discontinued and the remainder of the package discarded. A new package of Triphasil-21 Tablets should be started on the first day of the patient's next bleed after the last tablet was taken. An alternate means of birth control should be prescribed during the days without tablets and continued until the patient has taken a tablet daily for seven consecutive days (six brown, and one white).

In the nonlactating mother, Triphasil-21 may be initiated postpartum, for contraception. When the tablets are administered in the postpartum period, the increased risk of thromboembolic disease associated with the postpartum period must be considered (See Contraindications, Warnings, and Precautions concerning thromboembolic disease). It is to be noted that early resumption of ovulation may occur if Parlodel® (bromocriptine mesylate) has been used for the prevention of lactation.

HOW SUPPLIED

Triphasil®-21 Tablets (levonorgestrel and ethinyl estradiol tablets—triphasic regimen), Wyeth®, NDC 0008-2535, are available in packages of 3 compacts, and in packages of 6 compact refills. Each cycle contains 21 round coated tablets as follows:

NDC 0008-0641, six brown tablets marked "WYETH" and "641", each containing 0.050 mg levonorgestrel and 0.030 mg ethinyl estradiol;

NDC 0008-0642, five white to off-white tablets marked "WYETH" and "642", each containing 0.075 mg levonorgestrel and 0.040 mg ethinyl estradiol; and

NDC 0008-0643, ten light-yellow tablets marked "WYETH" and "643", each containing 0.125 mg levonorgestrel and 0.030 mg ethinyl estradiol.

References available upon request.

Brief Summary Patient Package Insert

Oral contraceptives, also known as "birth control pills" or "the pill," are taken to prevent pregnancy, and when taken correctly, have a failure rate of less than 1.0% per year when used without missing any pills. The typical failure rate of large numbers of pill users is less than 3.0% per year when women who miss pills are included. For most women oral contraceptives are also free of serious or unpleasant side effects. However, forgetting to take pills considerably increases the chances of pregnancy.

For the majority of women, oral contraceptives can be taken safely. But there are some women who are at high risk of developing certain serious diseases that can be life-threatening or may cause temporary or permanent disability or death. The risks associated with taking oral contraceptives increase significantly if you:

- smoke
- have high blood pressure, diabetes, high cholesterol
- have or have had clotting disorders, heart attack, stroke, angina pectoris, cancer of the breast or sex organs, jaundice or malignant or benign liver tumors

You should not take the pill if you suspect you are pregnant or have unexplained vaginal bleeding.

Cigarette smoking increases the risk of serious adverse effects on the heart and blood vessels from oral-contraceptive use. This risk increases with age and with heavy smoking (15 or more cigarettes per day) and is quite marked in women over 35 years of age. Women who use oral contraceptives should not smoke.

Most side effects of the pill are not serious. The most common such effects are nausea, vomiting, bleeding between menstrual periods, weight gain, breast tenderness, and difficulty wearing contact lenses. These side effects, especially nausea and vomiting, may subside within the first three months of use.

The serious side effects of the pill occur very infrequently, especially if you are in good health and do not smoke. However, you should know that the following medical conditions have been associated with or made worse by the pill:

1. Blood clots in the legs (thrombophlebitis), lungs (pulmonary embolism), stoppage or rupture of a blood vessel in the brain (stroke), blockage of blood vessels in the heart (heart attack and angina pectoris) or other organs of the body. As mentioned above, smoking increases the risk of heart attacks and strokes and subsequent serious medical consequences.
2. Liver tumors, which may rupture and cause severe bleeding. A possible but not definite association has been found with the pill and liver cancer. However, liver cancers are extremely rare. The chance of developing liver cancer from using the pill is thus even rarer.
3. High blood pressure, although blood pressure usually returns to normal when the pill is stopped.

The symptoms associated with these serious side effects are discussed in the detailed leaflet given to you with your supply of pills. Notify your doctor or health-care provider if you notice any unusual physical disturbances while taking the pill. In addition, drugs such as rifampin, as well as some anticonvulsants and some antibiotics, may decrease oral-contraceptive effectiveness.

Studies to date of women taking the pill have not shown an increase in the incidence of cancer of the breast or cervix. There is, however, insufficient evidence to rule out the possibility that pills may cause such cancers.

Taking the pill provides some important noncontraceptive benefits. These include less painful menstruation, less menstrual blood loss and anemia, fewer pelvic infections, and fewer cancers of the ovary and the lining of the uterus.

Be sure to discuss any medical condition you may have with your health care provider. Your health-care provider will take a medical and family history before prescribing oral contraceptives and will examine you. You should be reexamined at least once a year while taking oral contraceptives. The detailed patient information leaflet gives you further information which you should read and discuss with your health-care provider.

DETAILED PATIENT LABELING

INTRODUCTION

Any woman who considers using oral contraceptives (the birth control pill or the pill) should understand the benefits and risks of using this form of birth control. This leaflet will give you much of the information you will need to make this decision and will also help you determine if you are at risk of developing any of the serious side effects of the pill. It will tell you how to use the pill properly so that it will be as effective as possible. However, this leaflet is not a replacement for a careful discussion between you and your health-care provider. You should discuss the information provided in this leaflet with him or her, both when you first start taking the pill and during your revisits. You should also follow your health-care provider's advice with regard to regular check-ups while you are on the pill.

EFFECTIVENESS OF ORAL CONTRACEPTIVES

Oral contraceptives or "birth-control pills" or "the pill" are used to prevent pregnancy and are more effective than other nonsurgical methods of birth control. When they are taken correctly, the chance of becoming pregnant is less than 1.0% when used perfectly, without missing any pills. Typical failure rates are actually 3.0% per year. The chance of becoming pregnant increases with each missed pill during the menstrual cycle.

In comparison, typical failure rates for other nonsurgical methods of birth control during the first year of use are as follows:

IUD: 6%
Diaphragm with spermicides: 18%
Spermicides alone: 21%
Vaginal sponge: 18 to 30%
Condom alone: 12%
Periodic abstinence: 20%
No methods: 89%

WHO SHOULD NOT TAKE ORAL CONTRACEPTIVES

Cigarette smoking increases the risk of serious adverse effects on the heart and blood vessels from oral-contraceptive use. This risk increases with age and with heavy smoking (15 or more cigarettes per day) and is quite marked in women over 35 years of age. Women who use oral contraceptives should not smoke.

Some women should not use the pill. For example, you should not take the pill if you are pregnant or think you may be pregnant. You should also not use the pill if you have any of the following conditions:

- Heart attack or stroke
- Blood clots in the legs (thrombophlebitis), lungs (pulmonary embolism), or eyes
- Blood clots in the deep veins of your legs
- Known or suspected breast cancer or cancer of the lining of the uterus, cervix, or vagina
- Liver tumor (benign or cancerous)

Or, if you have any oif the following:

- Chest pain (angina pectoris)
- Unexplained vaginal bleeding (until a diagnosis is reached by your doctor)
- Yellowing of the whites of the eyes or of the skin (jaundice) during pregnancy or during previous use of the pill
- Known or suspected pregnancy

Tell your health-care provider if you have ever had any of these conditions. Your health-care provider can recommend another method of birth control.

OTHER CONSIDERATIONS BEFORE TAKING ORAL CONTRACEPTIVES

Tell your health-care provider if you or any family member has ever had:

- Breast nodules, fibrocystic disease of the breast, an abnormal breast x-ray or mammogram
- Diabetes
- Elevated cholesterol or triglycerides
- High blood pressure
- Migraine or other headaches or epilepsy
- Mental depression
- Gallbladder, heart or kidney disease
- History of scanty or irregular menstrual periods

Women with any of these conditions should be checked often by their health-care provider if they choose to use oral contraceptives. Also, be sure to inform your doctor or health-care provider if you smoke or are on any medications.

RISKS OF TAKING ORAL CONTRACEPTIVES

1. *Risk of developing blood clots*

Blood clots and blockage of blood vessels are the most serious side effects of taking oral contraceptives and can be fatal. In particular, a clot in the legs can cause thrombophlebitis and a clot that travels to the lungs can cause a sudden blocking of the vessel carrying blood to the lungs. Rarely, clots occur in the blood vessels of the eye and may cause blindness, double vision, or impaired vision.

If you take oral contraceptives and need elective surgery, need to stay in bed for a prolonged illness, or have recently delivered a baby, you may be at risk of developing blood clots. You should consult your doctor about stopping oral contraceptives three to four weeks before surgery and not taking oral contraceptives for two weeks after surgery or during bed rest. You should also not take oral contraceptives soon after delivery of a baby or a midtrimester pregnancy termination. It is advisable to wait for at least four weeks after delivery if you are not breast feeding. If you are breast-feeding, you should wait until you have weaned your child before using

the pill. (See also the section on breast-feeding in General Precautions.)

2. Heart attacks and strokes
Oral-contraceptives may increase the tendency to develop strokes (stoppage or rupture of blood vessels in the brain) and angina pectoris and heart attacks (blockage of blood vessels in the heart). Any of these conditions can cause death or serious disability.

Smoking greatly increases the possibility of suffering heart attacks and strokes. Furthermore, smoking and the use of oral contraceptives greatly increase the chances of developing and dying of heart disease.

3. Gallbladder disease
Oral contraceptive users probably have a greater risk than nonusers of having gallbladder disease, although this risk may be related to pills containing high doses of estrogens.

4. Liver tumors
In rare cases, oral contraceptives can cause benign but dangerous liver tumors. These benign liver tumors can rupture and cause fatal internal bleeding. In addition, a possible but not definite association has been found with the pill and liver cancers in two studies in which a few women who developed these very rare cancers were found to have used oral contraceptives for long periods. However, liver cancers are extremely rare. The chance of developing liver cancer from using the pill is thus even rarer.

5. Cancer of the reproductive organs
There is, at present, no confirmed evidence that oral contraceptives increase in the risk of cancer of the reproductive organs in human studies. Several studies have found no overall increase in the risk of developing breast cancer. However, women who use oral contraceptives and have a strong family history of breast cancer or who have breast nodules or abnormal mammograms should be closely followed by their doctors.

Some studies have found an increase in the incidence of cancer of the cervix in women who use oral contraceptives. However, this finding may be related to factors other than the use of oral contraceptives.

ESTIMATED RISK OF DEATH FROM A BIRTH-CONTROL METHOD OR PREGNANCY

All methods of birth control and pregnancy are associated with a risk of developing certain diseases which may lead to disability or death. An estimate of the number of deaths associated with different methods of birth control and pregnancy has been calculated and is shown in the following table.

[See table above.]

In the above table, the risk of death from any birth-control method is less than the risk of childbirth, except for oral contraceptive users over the age of 35 who smoke and pill users over the age of 40 even if they do not smoke. It can be seen in the table that for women aged 15 to 39, the risk of death was highest with pregnancy (7 to 26 deaths per 100,000 women, depending on age). Among pill users who do not smoke, the risk of death was always lower than that associated with pregnancy for any age group, except for those over the age of 40, when the risk increases to 32 deaths per 100,000 women, compared to 28 associated with pregnancy at that age. However, for pill users who smoke and are over the age of 35, the estimated number of deaths exceeds those for other methods of birth control. If a woman is over the age of 40 and smokes, her estimated risk of death is four times higher (117/100,000 women) than the estimated risk associated with pregnancy (28/100,000 women) in that age group.

The suggestion that women over 40 who don't smoke should not take oral contraceptives is based on information from older high-dose pills and on less-selective use of pills than is practiced today. An Advisory Committee of the FDA discussed this issue in 1989 and recommended that the benefits of oral-contraceptive use by healthy, nonsmoking women over 40 years of age may outweigh the possible risks. However, all women, especially older women, are cautioned to use the lowest-dose pill that is effective.

WARNING SIGNALS

If any of these adverse effects occur while you are taking oral contraceptives, call your doctor immediately:

- Sharp chest pain, coughing of blood, or sudden shortness of breath (indicating a possible clot in the lung)
- Pain in the calf (indicating a possible clot in the leg)
- Crushing chest pain or heaviness in the chest (indicating a possible heart attack)
- Sudden severe headache or vomiting, dizziness or fainting, disturbances of vision or speech, weakness, or numbness in an arm or leg (indicating a possible stroke)
- Sudden partial or complete loss of vision (indicating a possible clot in the eye)
- Breast lumps (indicating possible breast cancer or fibrocystic disease of the breast; ask your doctor or health care provider to show you how to examine your breasts)
- Severe pain or tenderness in the stomach area (indicating a possibly ruptured liver tumor)
- Difficulty in sleeping, weakness, lack of energy, fatigue, or change in mood (possibly indicating severe depression)
- Jaundice or a yellowing of the skin or eyeballs, accompanied frequently by fever, fatigue, loss of appetite, dark colored urine, or light-colored bowel movements (indicating possible liver problems)

ANNUAL NUMBER OF BIRTH-RELATED OR METHOD-RELATED DEATHS ASSOCIATED WITH CONTROL OF FERTILITY PER 100,000 NONSTERILE WOMEN, BY FERTILITY-CONTROL METHOD ACCORDING TO AGE

Method of control and outcome	15–19	20–24	25–29	30–34	35–39	40–44
No fertility-control methods*	7.0	7.4	9.1	14.8	25.7	28.2
Oral contraceptives nonsmoker**	0.3	0.5	0.9	1.9	13.8	31.6
Oral contraceptives smoker**	2.2	3.4	6.6	13.5	51.1	117.2
IUD**	0.8	0.8	1.0	1.0	1.4	1.4
Condom*	1.1	1.6	0.7	0.2	0.3	0.4
Diaphragm/spermicide*	1.9	1.2	1.2	1.3	2.2	2.8
Periodic abstinence*	2.5	1.6	1.6	1.7	2.9	3.6

* Deaths are birth related
** Deaths are method related

SIDE EFFECTS OF ORAL CONTRACEPTIVES

1. Vaginal bleeding
Irregular vaginal bleeding or spotting may occur while you are taking the pills. Irregular bleeding may vary from slight staining between menstrual periods to breakthrough bleeding which is a flow much like a regular period. Irregular bleeding occurs most often during the first few months of oral contraceptive use, but may also occur after you have been taking the pill for some time. Such bleeding may be temporary and usually does not indicate any serious problems. It is important to continue taking your pills on schedule. If the bleeding occurs in more than one cycle or lasts for more than a few days, talk to your doctor or health-care provider.

2. Contact lenses
If you wear contact lenses and notice a change in vision or an inability to wear your lenses, contact your doctor or health care provider.

3. Fluid retention
Oral contraceptives may cause edema (fluid retention) with swelling of the fingers or ankles and may raise your blood pressure. If you experience fluid retention, contact your doctor or health care provider.

4. Melasma
A spotty darkening of the skin is possible, particularly of the face.

5. Other side effects
Other side effects may include change in appetite, headache, nervousness, depression, dizziness, loss of scalp hair, rash, and vaginal infections.

If any of these side effects bother you, call your doctor or health care provider.

GENERAL PRECAUTIONS

1. Missed periods and use of oral contraceptives before or during early pregnancy
There may be times when you may not menstruate regularly after you have completed taking a cycle of pills. If you have taken your pills regularly and miss one menstrual period, continue taking your pills for the next cycle but be sure to inform your health care provider before doing so. If you have not taken the pills daily as instructed and missed a menstrual period, or if you missed two consecutive menstrual periods, you may be pregnant. Check with your health care provider immediately to determine whether you are pregnant. Do not continue to take oral contraceptives until you are sure you are not pregnant, but continue to use another method of contraception.

There is no conclusive evidence that oral-contraceptive use is associated with an increase in birth defects when taken inadvertently during early pregnancy. Previously, a few studies had reported that oral contraceptives might be associated with birth defects, but these studies have not been confirmed. Nevertheless, oral contraceptives or any other drugs should not be used during pregnancy unless clearly necessary and prescribed by your doctor. You should check with your doctor about risks to your unborn child of any medication taken during pregnancy.

2. While breast-feeding
If you are breast-feeding, consult your doctor before starting oral contraceptives. Some of the drug will be passed on to the child in the milk. A few adverse effects on the child have been reported, including yellowing of the skin (jaundice) and breast enlargement. In addition, oral contraceptives may decrease the amount and quality of your milk. If possible, do not use oral contraceptives while breast-feeding. You should use another method of contraception since breast-feeding provides only partial protection from becoming pregnant and this partial protection decreases significantly as you breast-feed for longer periods of time. You should consider starting oral contraceptives only after you have weaned your child completely.

3. Laboratory tests
If you are scheduled for any laboratory tests, tell your doctor you are taking birth control pills. Certain blood tests may be affected by birth control pills.

4. Drug interactions
Certain drugs may interact with birth-control pills to make them less effective in preventing pregnancy or cause an increase in breakthrough bleeding. Such drugs include rifampin, drugs used for epilepsy such as barbiturates (for example, phenobarbital) and phenytoin (Dilantin is one brand of this drug), phenylbutazone (Butazolidin is one brand) and possibly certain antibiotics. You may need to use an additional method of contraception during any cycle in which you take drugs that can make oral contraceptives less effective.

HOW TO TAKE ORAL CONTRACEPTIVES

1. General Instructions
You must take your pill every day according to the instructions. Oral contraceptives are most effective if taken no more than 24 hours apart. Take your pill at the same time every day so that you are less likely to forget to take it. You will then maintain an effective dose of the oral contraceptive in your body.

If your doctor has scheduled you for surgery, or you need prolonged bed rest, he or she may suggest that you stop taking the pill four weeks before surgery to avoid increased risk of blood clots. It is also advisable not to start oral contraceptives sooner than four weeks after delivery of a baby or a midtrimester pregnancy termination.

TRIPHASIL®-21 TABLETS (levonorgestrel and ethinyl estradiol tablets—triphasic regimen)

Triphasil is a three-phased contraceptive, different from the usual same-dose-every-day combination oral contraceptive. Triphasil-21 Tablets contain 21 active pills divided among 6 brown pills, 5 white pills, and 10 light-yellow pills in each package.

The dosage of Triphasil-21 Tablets is **one pill daily** for 21 days in a row in your menstrual cycle beginning with the first brown pill, continuing through the white pills, and finishing the cycle with the light-yellow pills, **in that order.** Pills are then discontinued for 7 days. The basic schedule is 21 days on—7 days off.

In the first month, you should begin taking Triphasil-21 Tablets on day one (1) of your menstrual cycle, which is the first day of your menstruation regardless of the amount of bleeding or spotting. (Day 1 is the first day of menstruation, even if it is almost midnight when you start.) NOTE: During the first month of Triphasil-21 Tablets, if you start taking pills later than day 1 of your menstrual cycle, you should protect yourself by also using another method of birth control until you have taken a pill daily for seven days in a row (6 brown pills followed by 1 white pill). Thereafter, if you follow directions carefully, you should obtain the full contraceptive benefit. If you begin taking pills later than the proper day, the possibility of ovulation and pregnancy occurring before or during the taking of the brown pills should be considered.

Take one pill every day until you finish all 21 pills. No pills are then taken for one week (7 days). Your period will usually begin about three days after you take the last light-yellow pill. Don't be alarmed if the amount of bleeding is not the same as before. On the 8th day, start with a brown pill from a new package, even if you still have your period. If, for example, you took Triphasil-21 Tablets for the first time on a Tuesday, the 8th day will also be a Tuesday. **If you have taken the pills as directed,** you will begin the next cycle on the same day of the week. If you start taking pills later than the 8th day, you should protect yourself by also using another method of birth control until you have taken a pill daily for seven days in a row.

Continued on next page

Wyeth-Ayerst Laboratories—Cont.

When switching from another oral contraceptive, Triphasil®-21 Tablets should be started on the first day of bleeding following the last active pill taken of the previous oral contraceptive.

TRIPHASIL®-28 TABLETS (levonorgestrel and ethinyl estradiol tablets—triphasic regimen)

Triphasil is a three-phased contraceptive, different from the usual same-dose-every-day combination oral contraceptive.

Triphasil-28 Tablets contain 21 active pills divided among 6 brown pills, 5 white pills, and 10 light-yellow pills plus 7 light-green inactive pills per package.

The dosage of Triphasil-28 Tablets is one active pill daily for 21 days in a row beginning with the 6 brown pills, followed by the 5 white pills, followed by the 10 light-yellow pills, and then one of the 7 light-green inactive pills daily for the next 7 days, **in that order,** for a total of 28 days or 4 weeks. The basic schedule is 21 days on active pills (brown, white, and light-yellow)—7 days on light-green inactive pills. Always take all of the 21 active pills (brown, white, and light-yellow) in each package before taking the light-green pills.

When you start your **first** cycle of Triphasil-28 Tablets, you should begin taking your pills on the **first** day of your next menstrual period, regardless of the day of the week or the amount of the bleeding or spotting. NOTE: During the first month on Triphasil-28 Tablets, if you start taking pills later than day 1 of your menstrual cycle, you should protect yourself by also using another method of birth control until you have taken a pill daily for seven days in a row (6 brown pills followed by 1 white pill). Thereafter, if you follow directions carefully you should obtain the full contraceptive benefit. If you begin taking pills later than the proper day, the possibility of ovulation and pregnancy occurring before or during the taking of the brown pills should be considered. Take one pill every day until you finish all 6 brown, 5 white, and 10 light-yellow pills in a package followed by all 7 light-green pills. Your period will usually begin about three days after you take the last light-yellow pill, which will be during the time you are taking the light-green pills. Don't be alarmed if the amount of bleeding is not the same as before.

The day after you have taken your last light-green pill, begin a new package of pills (first taking the 6 brown, then the 5 white, and then the 10 light-yellow pills, one a day just as you did before) so that you will take a pill every day without interruption. **If you have taken the pills as directed,** the starting day for each new package will always be the same day as in the previous cycle. When switching from another oral contraceptive, Triphasil-28 Tablets should be started on the first day of bleeding following the last active pill taken of the previous oral contraceptive.

SPOTTING OR BREAKTHROUGH BLEEDING:

Spotting is slight staining between menstrual periods which may not even require a pad. Breakthrough bleeding is a flow much like a regular period, requiring sanitary protection. Spotting is more common than breakthrough bleeding, and both occur more often in the first few cycles than in later cycles. These types of bleeding are usually temporary and without significance. It is important to continue taking your pills on schedule. If the bleeding persists for more than a few days, consult your doctor.

2. If You Forget to Take Your Pill

If you miss only one pill in a cycle, the chance of becoming pregnant is small. Take the missed pill as soon as you realize that you have forgotten it. Since the risk of pregnancy increases with each additional pill you skip, it is very important that you take one pill a day.

There is a chance of becoming pregnant if you miss one brown, white, or light-yellow pill, and that chance increases with each additional brown, white, or light-yellow pill missed. If you miss any one of these pills, it is important that it be taken as soon as remembered, and also take your next pill at the regular time, which means that you will be taking two pills on that day. If you miss any two of these pills consecutively, it is important that you take the second missed pill as soon as you remember, discard the first missed pill, and take your regular pill that day at the proper time (which means you will be taking two pills on that day). Furthermore, you should use an additional method of birth control for the remainder of the cycle in addition to taking your pills as directed above. If breakthrough occurs following missed pills, it will usually be temporary and of no consequence. If you miss three or more of any of the brown, white, or light-yellow pills in succession, discontinue the medication and discard the pill card. Then start a new refill card beginning with the first brown pill on the first day of bleeding of your next period. During the days without pills and until you have taken a pill daily for seven consecutive days (six brown and one white), you should also use another means of birth control. If you miss one or more light-green inactive pills (Triphasil-28 Tablets only), you are still protected against pregnancy **provided** you begin taking your next brown pill on the proper day.

At times there may be no menstrual period after a cycle of pills. Therefore, if you miss one menstrual period but have taken the pills **exactly as you were supposed to,** continue as usual into the next cycle. If you have not taken the pills correctly and miss a menstrual period, you may be pregnant and should stop taking oral contraceptives until your doctor determines whether or not you are pregnant. Until you can get to your doctor, use another form of nonhormonal contraception. If two consecutive menstrual periods are missed, you should stop taking pills until it is determined by a physician whether you are pregnant.

If you do become pregnant while using oral contraceptives, the risk to the fetus is small, on the order of no more than one per thousand. You should, however, discuss the risks to the developing child with your doctor.

3. Pregnancy Due to Pill Failure

The incidence of pill failure resulting in pregnancy is approximately less than 1.0% if taken every day as directed, but more typical failure rates are less than 3.0%. If failure does occur, the risk to the fetus is minimal.

4. Pregnancy After Stopping the Pill

There may be some delay in becoming pregnant after you stop using oral contraceptives, especially if you had irregular menstrual cycles before you used oral contraceptives. It may be advisable to postpone conception until you begin menstruating regularly once you have stopped taking the pill and desire pregnancy.

There does not appear to be any increase in birth defects in newborn babies when pregnancy occurs soon after stopping the pill.

5. Overdosage

Serious ill effects have not been reported following ingestion of large doses of oral contraceptives by young children. Overdosage may cause nausea and withdrawal bleeding in females. In case of overdosage, contact your health-care provider or pharmacist.

6. Other Information

Your health-care provider will take a medical and family history before prescribing oral contraceptives and will examine you. You should be reexamined at least once a year. Be sure to inform your health-care provider if there is a family history of any of the conditions listed previously in this leaflet. Be sure to keep all appointments with your health care provider, because this is a time to determine if there are early signs of side effects of oral-contraceptive use.

Do not use the drug for any condition other than the one for which it was prescribed. This drug has been prescribed specifically for you; do not give it to others who may want birth control pills.

HEALTH BENEFITS FROM ORAL CONTRACEPTIVES

In addition to preventing pregnancy, use of oral contraceptives may provide certain benefits. They are:

- Menstrual cycles may become more regular
- Blood flow during menstruation may be lighter and less iron may be lost. Therefore, anemia due to iron deficiency is less likely to occur.
- Pain or other symptoms during menstruation may be encountered less frequently
- Ovarian cysts may occur less frequently
- Ectopic (tubal) pregnancy may occur less frequently
- Noncancerous cysts or lumps in the breast may occur less frequently
- Acute pelvic inflammatory disease may occur less frequently
- Oral contraceptive use may provide some protection against developing two forms of cancer: cancer of the ovaries and cancer of the lining of the uterus.

If you want more information about birth control pills, ask your doctor or pharmacist. They have a more technical leaflet called the Professional Labeling which you may wish to read.

Shown in Product Identification Section, page 438

TRIPHASIL®-28 ℞

[tri-fa 'sil]

Tablets

(levonorgestrel and ethinyl estradiol tablets—triphasic regimen)

DESCRIPTION

Each Triphasil cycle of 28 tablets consists of three different drug phases as follows: Phase 1 comprised of 6 brown tablets, each containing 0.050 mg of levonorgestrel (d(-)-13-beta-ethyl-17-alpha-ethinyl-17-beta-hydroxygon-4-en-3-one), a totally synthetic progestogen, and 0.030 mg of ethinyl estradiol (19-nor-17α-pregna-1,3,5(10)-trien-20-yne-3,17-diol); phase 2 comprised of 5 white tablets, each containing 0.075 mg levonorgestrel and 0.040 mg ethinyl estradiol; and phase 3 comprised of 10 light-yellow tablets, each containing 0.125 mg levonorgestrel and 0.030 mg ethinyl estradiol; then followed by 7 light-green inert tablets. The inactive ingredients present are calcium carbonate, cellulose, FD&C Blue 1, glycerin, iron oxides, lactose, magnesium stearate, methylparaben, polyethylene glycol, povidone, propylparaben, sodium benzoate, starch, sucrose, talc, and titanium dioxide.

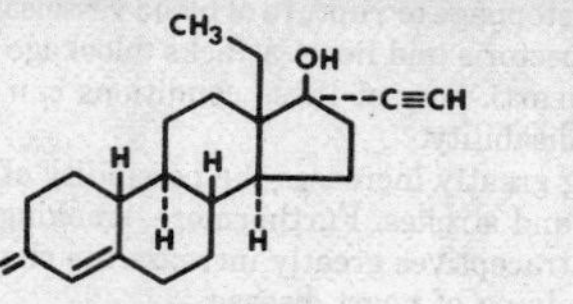

Levonorgestrel

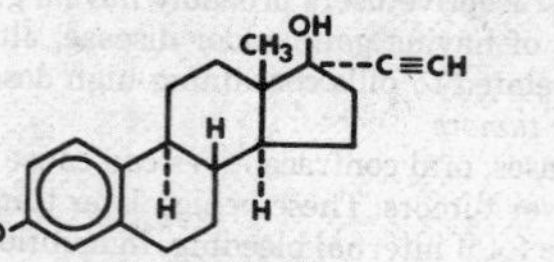

Ethinyl Estradiol

CLINICAL PHARMACOLOGY

See Triphasil®-21.

INDICATIONS AND USAGE

See Triphasil-21.

CONTRAINDICATIONS

See Triphasil-21.

WARNINGS

See Triphasil-21.

PRECAUTIONS

See Triphasil-21.

DRUG INTERACTIONS

See Triphasil-21.

CARCINOGENESIS

See Triphasil-21.

PREGNANCY

See Triphasil-21.

NURSING MOTHERS

See Triphasil-21.

INFORMATION FOR THE PATIENT

See Triphasil-21.

ADVERSE REACTIONS

See Triphasil-21.

OVERDOSAGE

See Triphasil-21.

NONCONTRACEPTIVE HEALTH BENEFITS

See Triphasil-21.

DOSAGE AND ADMINISTRATION

To achieve maximum contraceptive effectiveness, Triphasil-28 Tablets (Levonorgestrel and Ethinyl Estradiol Tablets—Triphasic Regimen) must be taken exactly as directed and at intervals not exceeding 24 hours.

Triphasil-28 Tablets are a three-phase preparation plus 7 inert tablets. The dosage of Triphasil-28 Tablets is **one tablet daily** for 28 consecutive days per menstrual cycle in the following order: 6 brown tablets (phase 1), followed by 5 white tablets (phase 2), followed by 10 light-yellow tablets (phase 3), plus 7 light-green inert tablets, according to the prescribed schedule.

It is recommended that Triphasil-28 Tablets be taken at the same time each day, preferably after the evening meal or at bedtime. During the first cycle of medication, the patient should be instructed to take one Triphasil-28 Tablet daily in the order of 6 brown, 5 white, 10 light-yellow tablets, and then 7 light-green inert tablets for twenty-eight (28) consecutive days, beginning on day one (1) of her menstrual cycle. (The first day of menstruation is day one.) Withdrawal bleeding usually occurs within 3 days following the last light-yellow tablet. (If Triphasil-28 Tablets are first taken later than the first day of the first menstrual cycle of medication or postpartum, contraceptive reliance should not be placed on Triphasil-28 Tablets until after the first 7 consecutive days of administration. The possibility of ovulation and conception prior to initiation of medication should be considered.)

When switching from another oral contraceptive, Triphasil-28 Tablets should be started on the first day of bleeding following the last active tablet taken of the previous oral contraceptive.

The patient begins her next and all subsequent 28-day courses of Triphasil-28 Tablets on the same day of the week that she began her first course, following the same schedule. She begins taking her brown tablets on the next day after ingestion of the last light-green tablet, regardless of whether or not a menstrual period has occurred or is still in progress. Any time a subsequent cycle of Triphasil-28 Tablets is started later than the next day, the patient should be pro-

tected by another means of contraception until she has taken a tablet daily for seven consecutive days.

If spotting or breakthrough bleeding occurs, the patient is instructed to continue on the same regimen. This type of bleeding is usually transient and without significance; however, if the bleeding is persistent or prolonged, the patient is advised to consult her physician. Although the occurrence of pregnancy is highly unlikely if Triphasil-28 Tablets are taken according to directions, if withdrawal bleeding does not occur, the possibility of pregnancy must be considered. If the patient has not adhered to the prescribed schedule (missed one or more tablets or started taking them on a day later than she should have), the probability of pregnancy should be considered at the time of the first missed period and appropriate diagnostic measures taken before the medication is resumed. If the patient has adhered to the prescribed regimen and misses two consecutive periods, pregnancy should be ruled out before continuing the contraceptive regimen.

The risk of pregnancy increases with each active (brown, white, or light-yellow) tablet missed. If the patient misses one active tablet, she should be instructed to take it as soon as she remembers, and also to take her next tablet at the regular time, which means that she will be taking two tablets on that day. If she misses two active tablets consecutively, she should take the second missed tablet as soon as she remembers, discard the first missed tablet and take her regular tablet for that day at the proper time. Furthermore, she should use an additional method of birth control in addition to taking Triphasil®-28 until menses has appeared or pregnancy has been excluded. If breakthrough bleeding occurs following missed active tablets, it will usually be transient and of no consequence. If three consecutive active tablets are missed, all medication should be discontinued and the remainder of the package discarded. A new package of Triphasil®-28 Tablets should be started on the first day of the patient's next bleed after the last tablet was taken. An alternate means of birth control should be prescribed during the days without tablets and continued until the patient has taken a tablet daily for seven consecutive days (six brown, and one white). If the patient misses one or more light-green tablets, she is still protected against pregnancy **provided** she begins taking brown tablets again on the proper day.

In the nonlactating mother, Triphasil®-28 may be initiated postpartum, for contraception. When the tablets are administered in the postpartum period, the increased risk of thromboembolic disease associated with the postpartum period must be considered (See Contraindications, Warnings, and Precautions concerning thromboembolic disease). It is to be noted that early resumption of ovulation may occur if Parlodel® (bromocriptine mesylate) has been used for the prevention of lactation.

HOW SUPPLIED

Triphasil®-28 Tablets (Levonorgestrel and Ethinyl Estradiol Tablets—Triphasic Regimen), Wyeth®, NDC 0008-2536, are available in packages of 3 compacts, and in packages of 6 compact refills; packages of 12 Pilpak® dispensers are also available for clinic use only. Each cycle contains 28 round, coated tablets as follows:

NDC 0008-0641, six brown tablets marked "WYETH" and "641", each containing 0.050 mg levonorgestrel and 0.030 mg ethinyl estradiol;

NDC 0008-0642, five white to off-white tablets marked "WYETH" and "642", each containing 0.075 mg levonorgestrel and 0.040 mg ethinyl estradiol;

NDC 0008-0643, ten light-yellow tablets marked "WYETH" and "643", each containing 0.125 mg levonorgestrel and 0.030 mg ethinyl estradiol; and

NDC 0008-0650, seven light-green inert tablets marked "WYETH" and "650".

REFERENCES

Available upon request.

Brief Summary Patient Package Insert: See Triphasil-21.

DETAILED PATIENT LABELING: See Triphasil-21.

Shown in Product Identification Section, page 438

TUBEX® Closed Injection System
[tū'beks]

The TUBEX® closed injection system delivers injectable medication in accurately machine-measured doses with each sterile, prefilled cartridge-needle unit permanently identified up to the moment of injection. Precisely calibrated single-use cartridge-needle units eliminate cross contamination and minimize dosage errors. Super-sharp, siliconized needles minimize penetration pressure. Medication is easily delivered via the TUBEX Injector.

TUBEX sterile cartridge-needle units are ready for instant use, fit easily into the physician's bag, and are readily stored and inventoried in the office.

TAMP-R-TEL® (tamper-resistant package) — a clear, sturdy plastic package for all TUBEX narcotics and barbiturates — adds a new dimension to the handling and record keeping of

these controlled drugs. In TAMP-R-TEL, each TUBEX sterile cartridge-needle unit is locked into an individual slot within the package by its own end-lock tab, which is easily broken to release the unit for use. Once the end-lock tab is broken, it is almost impossible to replace it. TAMP-R-TEL thus enhances package integrity, discourages pilferage and facilitates "at a glance" drug count.

The following products are currently available in TUBEX closed injection system. *For prescribing information on products listed, write to Professional Service, Wyeth-Ayerst Laboratories, P.O. Box 8299, Philadelphia, PA 19101, or contact your local Wyeth-Ayerst representative.*

Product and Needle Size Units Per Pkg	NDC 0008-

NARCOTICS in TAMP-R-TEL®
(tamper-resistant package)

CODEINE PHOSPHATE, USP Ⓒ●
30 mg (½ gr.) (25 G × ⅝″)
  10—1 mL   0728-01

60 mg (1 gr.) (25 G × ⅝″)
  10—1 mL   0729-01

HYDROMORPHONE HYDROCHLORIDE, USP Ⓒ●
1 mg (1/60 gr.) (22 G × 1¼″)
  10—1 mL fill in 2 mL   0387-03

2 mg (1/30 gr.) (22 G × 1¼″)
  10—1 mL fill in 2 mL   0295-01

4 mg (1/15 gr.) (22 G × 1¼″)
  10—1 mL fill in 2 mL   0296-01

MEPERGAN® (Meperidine HCl and Promethazine HCl) 25 mg each/mL Ⓒ●
(22 G × 1¼″)
  10—2 mL   0235-01

MEPERIDINE HYDROCHLORIDE, USP Ⓒ●
25 mg (22 G × 1¼″)
  10—1 mL fill in 2 mL   0601-02

50 mg (22 G × 1¼″)
  10—1 mL fill in 2 mL   0602-02

75 mg (22 G × 1¼″)
  10—1 mL fill in 2 mL   0605-02

100 mg (22 G × 1¼″)
  10—1 mL fill in 2 mL   0613-02

MORPHINE SULFATE, USP Ⓒ●
2 mg (¹⁄₃₀ gr.) (25 G × ⅝″)
  10—1 mL   0649-01

4 mg (¹⁄₁₅ gr.) (25 G × ⅝″)
  10—1 mL   0653-01

8 mg (1/8 gr.) (25 G × ⅝″)
  10—1 mL fill in 2 mL   0655-01

8 mg (1/8 gr.) (22 G × 1¼″)
  10—1 mL fill in 2 mL   0655-03

10 mg (1/6 gr.) (25 G × ⅝″)
  10—1 mL fill in 2 mL   0656-02

10 mg (1/6 gr.) (22 G × 1¼″)
  10—1 mL fill in 2 mL   0656-01

15 mg (¼ gr.) (25 G × ⅝″)
  10—1 mL fill in 2 mL   0657-02

15 mg (¼ gr.) (22 G × 1¼″)
  10—1 mL fill in 2 mL   0657-01

BARBITURATES in TAMP-R-TEL®
PENTOBARBITAL SODIUM, USP Ⓒ●
100 mg (1½ gr.) (22 G × 1¼″)
  10—2 mL   0303-02

PHENOBARBITAL SODIUM, USP Ⓒ
30 mg (½ gr.) (22 G × 1¼″)
  10—1 mL   0499-01

60 mg (1 gr.) (22 G × 1¼″)
  10—1 mL   0747-01

130 mg (2 gr.) (22 G × 1¼″)
  10—1 mL   0304-01

SECOBARBITAL SODIUM, USP Ⓒ●
100 mg (1½ gr.) (22 G × 1¼″)
  10—2 mL   0305-02

● Narcotic order blank required.

ANTIBIOTICS
BICILLIN® C-R (Penicillin G Benzathine and Penicillin G Procaine Suspension) 300,000 U each/mL
600,000 U (20 G × 1¼″)
  10—1 mL   0026-17

1,200,000 U (20 G × 1¼″)
  10—2 mL   0026-16

2,400,000 U (18 G × 2″)
  10—4 mL   0026-22
(disposable syringe)

BICILLIN C-R 900/300
(900,000 units Penicillin G Benzathine and 300,000 units Penicillin G Procaine in suspension)
1,200,000 U (20 G × 1¼″)
  10—2 mL   0079-01

BICILLIN LONG-ACTING (Sterile Penicillin G Benzathine Suspension)
600,000 U (20 G × 1¼″)
  10—1 mL   0021-08

1,200,000 U (20 G × 1¼″)
  10—2 mL   0021-07

2,400,000 U (18 G × 2″)
  10—4 mL   0021-12
(disposable syringe)

WYCILLIN® (Sterile Penicillin G Procaine Suspension)
600,000 U (20 G × 1¼″)
  10—1 mL   0018-10

1,200,000 U (20 G × 1¼″)
  10—2 mL   0018-08

2,400,000 U (18 G × 2″)
  10—4 mL   0018-12
(disposable syringe)

WYCILLIN Injection and PROBENECID Tablets
(Sterile Penicillin G Procaine Suspension and Probenecid Tablets)
2,400,000 U (18 G × 2″)
4 mL   2517-01
(package contains two disposable syringes and two 0.5 gram Probenecid tablets, USP)

BIOLOGICALS
DIPHTHERIA and TETANUS TOXOIDS ADSORBED (PEDIATRIC)
(25 G × ⅝″)
  10—0.5 mL   0338-01

INFLUENZA VIRUS VACCINE
(purified subvirion)
1992-1993 Formula
(25 G × ⅝″)
  10—0.5 mL   0815-02

TETANUS and DIPHTHERIA TOXOIDS ADSORBED for Adult Use
(25 G × ⅝″)
  10—0.5 mL   0341-01

TETANUS TOXOID ADSORBED
(25 G × ⅝″)
  10—0.5 mL   0339-01

TETANUS TOXOID FLUID
(25 G × ⅝″)
  10—0.5 mL   0340-01

VITAMINS
CYANOCOBALAMIN, USP
100 mcg (22 G × 1¼″)
  10—1 mL   0265-01

1,000 mcg (25 G × ⅝″)
  10—1 mL   0264-03

1,000 mcg (22 G × 1¼″)
  10—1 mL   0264-01

Continued on next page

Wyeth-Ayerst Laboratories—Cont.

THIAMINE HYDROCHLORIDE, USP
100 mg (22 G × 1¼")
10—1 mL fill in 2 mL   0302-01

CARDIOVASCULAR AGENTS

DIGOXIN, USP
0.25 mg (22 G × 1¼")
10—1 mL   0480-02

0.5 mg (22 G × 1¼")
10—2 mL   0480-01

EPINEPHRINE, USP (1:1000)
(25 G × ⅝")
10—1 mL   0263-01

HEPARIN SODIUM, USP
1,000 USP units (22 G × 1¼")
10—1 mL   0275-01

2,500 USP units (25 G × ⅝")
10—1 mL   0482-01

5,000 USP units (25 G × ⅝")
10—0.5 mL   0277-02

5,000 USP units (25 G × ⅝")
50—0.5 mL   0277-03

5,000 USP units (25 G × ⅝")
10—1.0 mL   0278-02

7,500 USP units (25 G × ⅝")
10—1 mL   0293-01

10,000 USP units (25 G × ⅝")
10—1 mL   0277-01

20,000 USP units (25 G × ⅝")
10—1 mL   0276-01

SPECIAL AGENTS

ATIVAN® (Lorazepam) ℃
2 mg/mL (22 G × 1¼")
10—1 mL fill in 2 mL   0581-02

2 mg/mL (22 G × 1¼")
10—1 mL fill in 2 mL
in TAMP-R-TEL   0581-06

4 mg/mL (22 G × 1¼")
10—1 mL fill in 2 mL   0570-02

4 mg/mL (22 G × 1¼")
10—1mL fill in 2 mL
in TAMP-R-TEL   0570-05

DIMENHYDRINATE, USP
50 mg (22 G × 1¼")
10—1 mL   0485-01

DIPHENHYDRAMINE HYDROCHLORIDE, USP
50 mg (22 G × 1¼")
10—1 mL   0485-01

CVC HEPARIN FLUSH KITS
25 USP units
(25 G × ⅝")
30 Kits   2528-02
Each Unit of Use Kit contains:
One 2.5 mL size (25 G × ⅝") TUBEX Heparin Lock Flush Solution, USP, 10 USP units per mL and two 2.5 mL size (25 G × ⅝") TUBEX Bacteriostatic Sodium Chloride Injection, USP.

250 USP units
(25 G × ⅝")
30 Kits   2529-02
Each Unit of Use Kit contains:
One 2.5 mL size (25 G × ⅝") TUBEX Heparin Lock Flush Solution, USP, 100 USP units per mL and two 2.5 mL size (25 G × ⅝") TUBEX Bacteriostatic Sodium Chloride Injection, USP.

HEPARIN FLUSH KITS
10 USP units
(25 G × ⅝")
50 Kits   2528-01
Each Unit of Use Kit contains:
One 1 mL size (25 G × ⅝") TUBEX Heparin Lock Flush Solution, USP, 10 USP units per mL and two 2.5 mL size (25 G × ⅝") TUBEX Bacteriostatic Sodium Chloride Injection, USP.

100 USP units
(25 G × ⅝")
50 Kits   2529-01
Each Unit of Use Kit contains:
One 1 mL size (25 G × ⅝") TUBEX Heparin Lock Flush Solution, USP, 100 USP units per mL and two 2.5 mL size (25 G × ⅝") TUBEX Bacteriostatic Sodium Chloride Injection, USP.

HEPARIN FLUSH 1 mL KITS
10 USP units
(25 G × ⅝")
50 Kits   2528-03
Each Unit of Use Kit contains:
One 1 mL size (25 G × ⅝") TUBEX Heparin Lock Flush Solution, USP, 10 USP units per mL and two 1 mL size (25 G × ⅝") TUBEX Bacteriostatic Sodium Chloride Injection, USP.

100 USP units
(25 G × ⅝")
50 Kits   2529-03
Each Unit of Use Kit contains:
One 1 mL size (25 G × ⅝") TUBEX Heparin Lock Flush Solution, USP, 100 USP units per mL and two 1 mL size (25 G × ⅝") TUBEX Bacteriostatic Sodium Chloride Injection, USP.

HEPARIN LOCK FLUSH Solution, USP
10 USP units per mL (25 G × ⅝")
50—1 mL   0523-01

100 USP units per mL (25 G × ⅝")
50—1 mL   0487-01

10 USP units per mL—25 USP units per TUBEX
(25 G × ⅝")
50—2.5 mL   0523-02

100 USP units per mL—250 USP units per TUBEX
(25 G × ⅝")
50—2.5 mL   0487-03

OXYTOCIN, USP (Synthetic)
10 USP units (22 G × 1¼")
10—1 mL   0406-01

PHENERGAN® (Promethazine HCl)
25 mg (22 G × 1¼")
10—1 mL   0416-01

50 mg (22 G × 1¼")
10—1 mL   0417-01

PROCHLORPERAZINE EDISYLATE, USP
5 mg (22 G × 1¼")
10—1 mL   0542-01

10 mg (22 G × 1¼")
10—2 mL   0542-02

SODIUM CHLORIDE, USP (Bacteriostatic)
(25 G × ⅝")
50—1 mL   0333-08

(22 G × 1¼")
50—2.5 mL   0333-05

(25 G × ⅝")
50—2.5 mL   0333-02

Wyeth®
PLEASE NOTE: THE WYETH-AYERST METAL TUBEX HYPODERMIC SYRINGE AND TUBEX FAST-TRAK SYRINGE HAVE BEEN DISCONTINUED AND REPLACED BY THE TUBEX INJECTOR. EXCHANGE OF THESE DISCONTINUED SYRINGES IS AVAILABLE, FREE OF CHARGE, FROM YOUR WYETH-AYERST AND/OR ELKINS-SINN SALES REPRESENTATIVE, OR FROM WYETH-AYERST DIRECTLY. FOR LOADING AND UNLOADING INFORMATION OF THESE DISCONTINUED SYRINGES, CONTACT THE MEDICAL AFFAIRS DEPARTMENT, AT WYETH-AYERST LABORATORIES, P.O. BOX 8299, PHILADELPHIA, PA 19101.

TUBEX® Injector
NOTE: The TUBEX® Injector is reusable; do not discard.

DIRECTIONS FOR USE

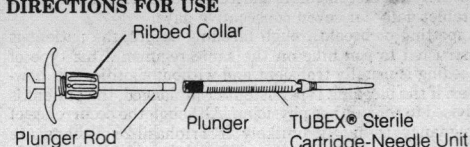

Ribbed Collar   Plunger   TUBEX® Sterile Cartridge-Needle Unit
Plunger Rod

To load a TUBEX® Sterile Cartridge-Needle Unit into the TUBEX® Injector
1. Turn the ribbed collar to the "OPEN" position until it stops.

CLOSE   OPEN

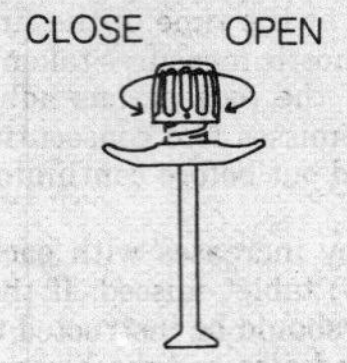

2. Hold the Injector with the open end up and fully insert the TUBEX® Sterile Cartridge-Needle Unit.
Firmly tighten the ribbed collar in the direction of the "CLOSE" arrow.

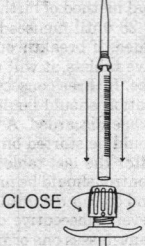

CLOSE

3. Thread the plunger rod into the plunger of the TUBEX® Sterile Cartridge-Needle Unit until slight resistance is felt.

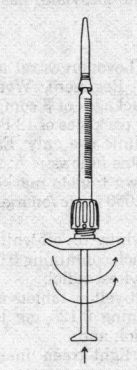

The Injector is now ready for use in the usual manner.

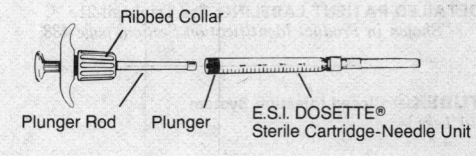

Ribbed Collar
Plunger Rod   Plunger   E.S.I. DOSETTE® Sterile Cartridge-Needle Unit

CLOSE   OPEN

To load an E.S.I. DOSETTE® Sterile Cartridge-Needle Unit into the TUBEX® Injector
1. Turn the ribbed collar to the "OPEN" position until it stops.

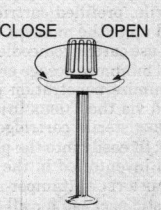

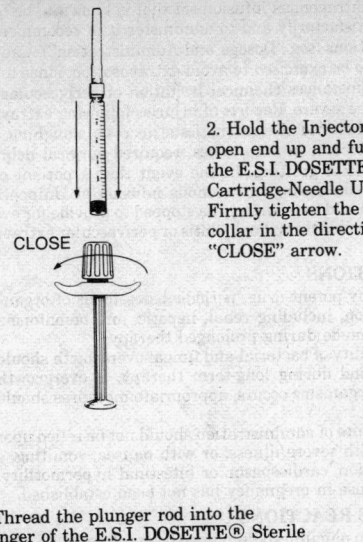

CLOSE

2. Hold the Injector with the open end up and fully insert the E.S.I. DOSETTE® Sterile Cartridge-Needle Unit. Firmly tighten the ribbed collar in the direction of the "CLOSE" arrow.

3. Thread the plunger rod into the plunger of the E.S.I. DOSETTE® Sterile Cartridge-Needle Unit until slight resistance is felt.

4. Engage the needle-cap assembly by pulling the cap down over the silver cartridge hub. The needle is fully engaged when the silver hub is completely covered.
The Injector is now ready for use in the usual manner.

To administer
Method of administration is the same as with conventional syringe. Remove needle cover by grasping it securely; twist and pull. Introduce needle into patient, aspirate by pulling back slightly on the plunger, and inject.

To remove the empty TUBEX® or DOSETTE® Cartridge- Needle Unit and dispose into a vertical needle disposal container

1. Do not recap the needle.
Disengage the plunger rod.

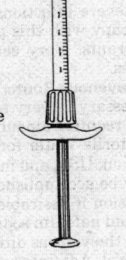

2. Hold the Injector, needle down, over a verticle needle disposal container and loosen the ribbed collar. TUBEX® or DOSETTE® Cartridge-Needle Unit will drop into the container.

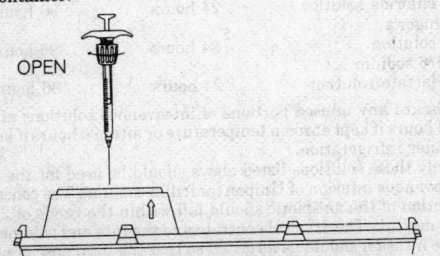

OPEN

---

3. Discard the needle cover.
To remove the empty TUBEX® or DOSETTE® Cartridge-Needle Unit and dispose into a horizontal (mailbox) needle disposal container

1. Do not recap the needle. Disengage the plunger rod.
2. Open the horizontal (mailbox) needle disposal container. Insert TUBEX® or DOSETTE® Cartridge-Needle Unit, needle pointing down, halfway into container. Close the container lid on cartridge. Loosen ribbed collar; TUBEX® or DOSETTE® Cartridge-Needle Unit will drop into the container.

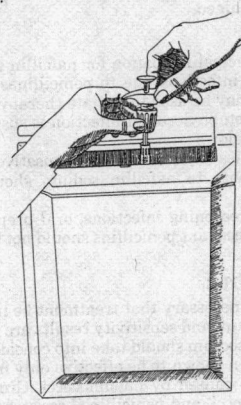

3. Discard the needle cover.
The TUBEX® Injector is reusable and should not be discarded.
Used TUBEX® or DOSETTE® Cartridge-Needle Units should not be employed for successive injections or as multiple-dose containers. They are intended to be used only once and discarded.

NOTE: Any graduated markings on TUBEX® or DOSETTE® Sterile Cartridge-Needle Units are to be used only as a guide in mixing, withdrawing, or administering measured doses.

Wyeth-Ayerst does not recommend and will not accept responsibility for the use of any cartridge-needle unit other than TUBEX® or E.S.I. DOSETTE® Cartridge-Needle Units in the TUBEX® Injector.

Shown in Product Identification Section, page 438

TYPHOID VACCINE   ℞
USP

DESCRIPTION
Typhoid Vaccine, USP, Wyeth, is a saline suspension containing not more than 1000 million Salmonella typhosa (Ty-2-strain) organisms per mL. After growing on veal infusion agar (containing 0.5 percent sodium chloride, 2 percent peptone, and 5 percent agar), the bacteria are washed off the medium, suspended in buffered sodium chloride injection, and killed by a combination of phenol and heat. Phenol (0.5 percent) is added to the final vaccine as preservative. Typhoid Vaccine, USP, Wyeth, is tested for safety, potency, and purity and standardized according to F.D.A. Additional Standards for Bacterial Vaccines, 21 C.F.R. 620.10-620.15.

INDICATIONS
Typhoid Vaccine, USP, Wyeth, is indicated for active immunization against typhoid fever. Based on data obtained from field studies, it has been estimated that typhoid vaccine is 70% or more effective in preventing typhoid fever, depending in part on the degree of exposure.
Routine immunization against typhoid is no longer recommended for persons residing in the United States. Selective immunization is indicated in the following situations:
1. Intimate exposure to a known typhoid carrier, as would occur with continued household contact.
2. Foreign travel to areas where typhoid fever is endemic. Although at one time typhoid immunization was suggested for persons attending summer camps or for residents of areas where flooding has occurred, there are no data to support continuation of such practices.[1,2]

CONTRAINDICATIONS
Administration should be postponed in the presence of acute respiratory or other active infection.
A severe systemic or allergic reaction following a prior dose is a contraindication to further use.[3]

PRECAUTIONS
A sterile syringe and needle should be used for each patient to prevent transmission of hepatitis B virus and other infectious agents from one person to another.
Specific information concerning use of typhoid vaccine during pregnancy is not available. However, as with other inactivated bacterial vaccines, its use is not contraindicated during pregnancy unless the intended recipient has manifested significant systemic or allergic reactions following administration of prior doses. Use of typhoid vaccine during pregnancy should be individualized to reflect actual need. Before the injection of any biological, the physician should take all precautions known for prevention of allergic or any other side reactions. This should include: A review of the patient's history regarding possible sensitivity; the ready availability of epinephrine 1:1000 and other appropriate agents used for control of immediate allergic reactions; and a knowledge of the recent literature pertaining to use of the biological concerned.

REACTIONS
Most recipients of typhoid vaccine experience some degree of local and systemic response, usually beginning within 24 hours of administration and persisting for one or two days. Local reactions are usually manifested by erythema, induration, and tenderness and should be expected in all those injected intracutaneously.
Systemic manifestations may include malaise, headache, myalgia, and elevated temperature.

DOSAGE
PRIMARY IMMUNIZATION
1. Adults and children over 10 years of age:
Two doses of 0.5 mL each, administered subcutaneously, at an interval of four or more weeks.
2. Children less than 10 years of age:
Two doses of 0.25 mL, each administered subcutaneously, at an interval of four or more weeks.
In instances where there is insufficient time for two doses administered at the specified intervals, three doses of the appropriate volume may be given at weekly intervals.
BOOSTER DOSES
1. Adults and children over 10 years of age:
0.5 mL, administered subcutaneously, or 0.1 mL, injected intracutaneously (intradermally).
2. Children 6 months to 10 years of age:
0.25 mL, administered subcutaneously, or 0.1 mL, intracutaneously (intradermally)
Under conditions of continued or repeated exposure, a booster dose should be given at least every three years. In instances where an interval of more than three years has elapsed since primary immunization or the last booster dose, a single booster dose is considered sufficient; it is not necessary to repeat the primary immunizing series.

ADMINISTRATION
Shake vial vigorously before withdrawing each dose.
Before injection, the rubber diaphragm of the vial and the skin over the site to be injected should be cleansed and prepared with a suitable germicide.
After insertion of the needle, aspirate to help avoid inadvertent injection into a blood vessel.

HOW SUPPLIED
Typhoid Vaccine, USP, Wyeth, is supplied in vials of 5 mL and 10 mL, each containing 8 units per mL.

REFERENCES
1. Recommendations of the Public Health Service Advisory Committee on Immunization Practices—Typhoid Vaccine. Morbidity and Mortality Weekly Report 27 (No. 27): 231, 1978.
2. Report of the Committee on Infectious Diseases, American Academy of Pediatrics, 1982 (Red Book).
3. Recommendations of the Public Health Service Advisory Committee on Immunization Practices—General Recommendations on Immunization. Morbidity and Mortality Weekly Report (No.7): 76, 1980.

UNIPEN®   ℞
[ū′ni-pen]
(nafcillin sodium) as the monohydrate
**INJECTION • CAPSULES • POWDER
FOR ORAL SOLUTION • TABLETS**

DESCRIPTION
Unipen is a semisynthetic penicillin developed by Wyeth research. Although primarily designed as an antistaphylococcal penicillin, in limited clinical trials it has been shown to be effective in the treatment of infections caused by pneumococci and Group A beta-hemolytic streptococci. Because of this wide gram-positive spectrum, this product is particularly suitable for *Initial Therapy* in severe or poten-

Continued on next page

Wyeth-Ayerst Laboratories—Cont.

tially severe infections before definitive culture results are known and in which staphylococci are suspected.

This product is readily soluble and can be conveniently administered in both oral and parenteral dosage forms. It is resistant to inactivation by staphylococcal penicillinase. Following intramuscular administration in humans, it rapidly appears in the plasma, penetrates body tissues in high concentration, and diffuses well into pleural, pericardial, and synovial fluids.

Unipen capsules contain nafcillin sodium as the monohydrate equivalent to 250 mg nafcillin. The inactive ingredients present are calcium carbonate, D&C Yellow 10, FD&C Blue 1, FD&C Yellow 6, gelatin, mineral oil, and titanium dioxide.

Unipen tablets contain nafcillin sodium as the monohydrate equivalent to 500 mg nafcillin. The inactive ingredients present are calcium carbonate, cellulose, hydroxypropyl methylcellulose, lactose, magnesium stearate, polacrilin potassium, starch, and talc.

Unipen for oral solution is a powder which when reconstituted as directed yields a solution of nafcillin sodium as the monohydrate equivalent to 250 mg nafcillin per 5 mL. The inactive ingredients present are artificial and natural flavors, citric acid, edetate disodium, FD&C Red 40, FD&C Yellow 6, saccharin sodium, sodium benzoate, sodium citrate, sodium propionate, sucrose, and water.

Unipen (nafcillin sodium) as the monohydrate is available for parenteral administration in vials of 500 mg, 1 gram, or 2 grams nafcillin. When reconstituted as directed, each vial contains, respectively, 2 mL, 4 mL, or 8 mL of solution.

Each mL contains nafcillin sodium equivalent to 250 mg nafcillin buffered with 10 mg sodium citrate.

NOTE: Unipen contains 2.9 milliequivalents of sodium per gram of nafcillin as the sodium salt.

MICROBIOLOGY

Unipen is a bactericidal penicillin which has shown activity *in vitro* against both penicillin-G-sensitive and penicillin-G-resistant strains of *Staphylococcus aureus* as well as against pneumococcus, beta-hemolytic streptococcus, and alpha streptococcus (viridans).

In experimental mouse infections induced with pneumococci, beta-hemolytic streptococci, and both penicillin-G-susceptible and penicillin-G-resistant strains of *Staph. aureus,* nafcillin sodium was compared with methicillin and oxacillin. Regardless of the route of drug administration (intramuscular or oral), nafcillin sodium was consistently and significantly more effective than the other two penicillins.

The fate of a penicillin-G-resistant strain of *Staph. aureus* was determined in the kidneys of mice treated with penicillin G, methicillin, and nafcillin sodium. Animals injected with the nafcillin sodium showed negative cultures after the fourteenth day, whereas positive kidney cultures were obtained during the entire 28-day period from mice treated with penicillin G and methicillin.

PHARMACOLOGY

Unipen is relatively nontoxic for animals. The acute LD50 of this product by oral administration in rats and mice was greater than 5 g/kg; by intramuscular administration in rats, 2800 mg/kg; by intraperitoneal administration in rats, 1240 mg/kg; and by intravenous administration in mice, 1140 mg/kg. The intraperitoneal LD50 in dogs is 600 mg/kg.

Animal studies indicated that local tissue responses following intramuscular administration of 25% solutions were minimal and resembled those of penicillin G rather than methicillin.

Animal studies indicate that antibacterial amounts are concentrated in the bile, kidney, lung, heart, spleen, and liver. Eighty-four percent of an intravenously administered dose can be recovered by biliary cannulation and 13 percent by renal excretion in 24 hours. High and prolonged tissue levels can be demonstrated by both biological activity assays and C^{14} distribution patterns.

At comparable dosage, intramuscular absorption of this product is nearly equivalent to that of intramuscular methicillin, and oral absorption to that of oral oxacillin. Blood concentrations may be tripled by the concurrent use of probenecid. Clinical studies with nafcillin sodium monohydrate in infants under three days of age and prematures have revealed higher blood levels and slower rates of urinary excretion than in older children and adults.

Studies of the effect of this product on reproduction in rats and rabbits have been completed and reveal no fetal or maternal abnormalities. These studies include the observation of the effects of administration of the drug before conception and continuously through weaning (one generation).

Disc Susceptibility Tests: Quantitative methods that require measurement of zone diameters give the most precise estimates of antibiotic susceptibility. One such procedure* has been recommended for use with discs for testing susceptibility to penicillinase-resistant penicillin-class antibiotics. Interpretations correlate diameters on the disc test with MIC values for penicillinase-resistant penicillins. With this procedure, a report from the laboratory of "susceptible" indicates that the infecting organism is likely to respond to therapy. A report of "resistant" indicates that the infecting organism is not likely to respond to therapy. A report of "intermediate susceptibility" suggests that the organism would be susceptible if high dosage is used, or if the infection is confined to tissues and fluids (e.g., urine) in which high antibiotic levels are attained.

INDICATIONS

Although the principal indication for nafcillin sodium is in the treatment of infections due to penicillinase-producing staphylococci, it may be used to initiate therapy in such patients in whom a staphylococcal infection is suspected. (See Important Note below.)

Bacteriologic studies to determine the causative organisms and their sensitivity to nafcillin sodium should be performed.

In serious, life-threatening infections, oral preparations of the penicillinase-resistant penicillins should not be relied on for initial therapy.

IMPORTANT NOTE

When it is judged necessary that treatment be initiated before definitive culture and sensitivity results are known, the choice of nafcillin sodium should take into consideration the fact that it has been shown to be effective only in the treatment of infections caused by pneumococci, Group A beta-hemolytic streptococci, and penicillin-G-resistant and penicillin-G-sensitive staphylococci. If the bacteriology report later indicates the infection is due to an organism other than a penicillin-G-resistant staphylococcus sensitive to nafcillin sodium, the physician is advised to continue therapy with a drug other than nafcillin sodium or any other penicillinase-resistant, semisynthetic penicillin.

Recent studies have reported that the percentage of staphylococcal isolates resistant to penicillin G outside the hospital is increasing, approximating the high percentage of resistant staphylococcal isolates found in the hospital. For this reason, it is recommended that a penicillinase-resistant penicillin be used as initial therapy for any suspected staphylococcal infection until culture and sensitivity results are known.

Methicillin is a compound that acts through a mechanism similar to that of nafcillin sodium against penicillin-G-resistant staphylococci. Strains of staphylococci resistant to methicillin have existed in nature, and it is known that the number of these strains reported has been increasing. Such strains of staphylococci have been capable of producing serious disease, in some instances resulting in fatality. Because of this there is concern that widespread use of the penicillinase-resistant penicillins may result in the appearance of an increasing number of staphylococcal strains which are resistant to these penicillins.

Methicillin-resistant strains are almost always resistant to all other penicillinase-resistant penicillins (cross-resistance with cephalosporin derivatives also occurs frequently). Resistance to any penicillinase-resistant penicillin should be interpreted as evidence of clinical resistance to all, in spite of the fact that minor variations in *in vitro* sensitivity may be encountered when more than one penicillinase-resistant penicillin is tested against the same strain of staphylococcus.

CONTRAINDICATIONS

A history of allergic reaction to any of the penicillins is a contraindication.

WARNINGS

Serious and occasionally fatal hypersensitivity (anaphylactoid) reactions have been reported in patients on penicillin therapy. Although anaphylaxis is more frequent following parenteral therapy, it has occurred in patients on oral penicillins. These reactions are more apt to occur in individuals with a history of sensitivity to multiple allergens.

There have been reports of individuals with a history of penicillin hypersensitivity reactions who have experienced severe hypersensitivity reactions when treated with a cephalosporin. Before therapy with a penicillin, careful inquiry should be made concerning previous hypersensitivity reactions to penicillins, cephalosporins, and other allergens. If an allergic reaction occurs, appropriate therapy should be instituted, and discontinuation of nafcillin therapy considered. The usual agents (antihistamines, pressor amines, corticosteroids) should be readily available.

Unipen injection should be used with caution when administered by the intravenous route because of the possibility of thrombophlebitis. To help minimize the risk of thrombophlebitis, it is important to administer Unipen through the tubing of an intravenous infusion set that is known to be functioning satisfactorily and to administer it in recommended concentrations (see "Dosage and Administration"). Caution should also be exercised to avoid extravasation, since under such circumstances chemical irritation of perivascular tissues may be severe. Reports of injuries following extravasation have included ulceration, tissue necrosis, sloughing, and gangrene which, in some cases, required surgical debridement and skin grafting. In the event that a patient complains of pain during intravenous infusion of Unipen, the infusion should immediately be stopped to provide for evaluation of possible thrombophlebitis or perivascular extravasation.

PRECAUTIONS

As with any potent drug, periodic assessment of organ-system function, including renal, hepatic, and hematopoietic, should be made during prolonged therapy.

The possibility of bacterial and fungal overgrowth should be kept in mind during long-term therapy. If overgrowth of resistant organisms occurs, appropriate measures should be taken.

The oral route of administration should not be relied upon in patients with severe illness, or with nausea, vomiting, gastric dilatation, cardiospasm, or intestinal hypermotility.

Safety for use in pregnancy has not been established.

ADVERSE REACTIONS

Reactions to nafcillin sodium have been infrequent and mild in nature. As with other penicillins, the possibility of an anaphylactic reaction or serum-sickness like reactions should be considered. A careful history should be taken. Patients with histories of hay fever, asthma, urticaria, or previous sensitivity to penicillin are more likely to react adversely.

Transient leukopenia, neutropenia with evidence of granulocytopenia or thrombocytopenia are infrequent and usually associated with prolonged therapy with high doses of penicillin. These alterations have been noted to return to normal after cessation of therapy.

The few reactions associated with the intramuscular use of nafcillin sodium have been skin rash, pruritus, and possible drug fever. As with other penicillins, reactions from oral use of the drug have included nausea, vomiting, diarrhea, urticaria, and pruritus.

DOSAGE AND ADMINISTRATION

Parenteral drug products should be inspected visually for particulate matter and discoloration prior to administration, whenever solution and container permit.

It is recommended that parenteral therapy be used initially in severe infections. The patient should be placed on oral therapy with this product as soon as the clinical condition warrants. Very severe infections may require very high doses.

Intravenous Route: 500 mg every 4 hours; double the dose if necessary in very severe infections.

The required amount of drug should be diluted in 15 to 30 mL of Sterile Water for Injection, USP, or Sodium Chloride Injection, USP, and injected over a 5- to 10-minute period. This may be accomplished through the tubing of an intravenous infusion if desirable.

To add nafcillin sodium to an intravenous solution, reconstitute the vials as directed under "How Supplied"—"For Parenteral Administration." Add the reconstituted vial contents immediately to the intravenous solution or within 8 hours following reconstitution if the vials are kept at room temperature (25° C) or within 48 hours following reconstitution if the vials are kept at refrigeration (2°-8° C).

Stability studies on nafcillin sodium at concentrations of 2 mg/mL to 40 mg/mL in the following intravenous solutions indicate the drug will lose less than 10% activity at room temperature (70° F) or, if kept under refrigeration, during the time period stipulated:

STABILITY OF	ROOM TEMPERATURE	REFRIGERATED
Sterile Water for Injection	24 hours	96 hours
Isotonic sodium chloride	24 hours	96 hours
5% dextrose in water	24 hours	96 hours
5% dextrose in 0.4% sodium chloride solution	24 hours	96 hours
Ringer's solution	24 hours	96 hours
M/6 sodium lactate solution	24 hours	96 hours

Discard any unused portions of intravenous solutions after 24 hours if kept at room temperature or after 96 hours if kept under refrigeration.

Only those solutions listed above should be used for the intravenous infusion of Unipen (nafcillin sodium). The concentration of the antibiotic should fall within the range of 2 to 40 mg/mL. The drug concentrate and the rate and volume of the infusion should be adjusted so that the total dose of naf-

*Bauer, A.W., Kirby, W.M.M., Sherris, J.C., and Turck, M.: Antibiotic Testing by a Standardized Single-Discs Method, Am. J. Clin. Pathol., *45*:493, 1966; Standardized Disc Susceptibility Test, FEDERAL REGISTER *37*:20527–29, 1972.

cillin is administered before the drug loses its stability in the solution in use.

There is no clinical experience available on the use of this agent in neonates or infants for this route of administration.

This route of administration should be used for relatively short-term therapy (24 to 48 hours) because of the occasional occurrence of thrombophlebitis, particularly in elderly patients.

This route of administration requires care be taken not to allow perivascular extravasation (see "Warnings").

PIGGYBACK UNITS (for Intravenous Drip Use)

As diluents, use the following solutions: Sterile Water for Injection, Isotonic Sodium Chloride, 5% dextrose in water, 5% dextrose in 0.4% sodium chloride solution, Ringer's solution, or M/6 sodium lactate solution.

1-GRAM BOTTLE:

Add a minimum of 49 mL diluent and shake well. If lower concentrations are desired, the solution could be further diluted with up to a total of 99 mL of diluent.

Amount of Diluent	Concentration of Solution
49 mL	20 mg/mL
99 mL	10 mg/mL

2-GRAM BOTTLE:

Add a minimum of 49 mL diluent and shake well. If lower concentrations are desired, the solution could be further diluted with up to a total of 99 mL of diluent.

Amount of Diluent	Concentration of Solution
49 mL	40 mg/mL
99 mL	20 mg/mL

The resulting solutions may then be administered alone or with the intravenous solutions listed above. Discard unused solution after 24 hours at room temperature (70°F) or 96 hours if kept under refrigeration. Administer piggyback through an IV tubing very slowly (at least 30 to 60 minutes) to avoid vein irritation.

At times it may be desired to use the contents of the piggyback bottles for addition to large-volume IV fluids. In this case the entire vial contents should be dissolved in not less than 25 mL of Sterile Water for Injection. Use the resulting concentration within 24 hours when kept at room temperature or within 96 hours when kept under refrigeration.

TEN-GRAM BOTTLE

Add 94 mL Sterile Water for Injection, USP, or Sodium Chloride Injection, USP, and shake well. For ease of reconstitution, the amount of diluent should be added in two portions; the first portion should not exceed 25 mL. Shake gently after each addition and before using. The final concentration will be approximately 100 mg/mL. After reconstitution, use within 8 hours if kept at room temperature or within 48 hours if kept under refrigeration.

The closure shall be penetrated only one time after reconstitution with a suitable sterile transfer device or dispensing set which allows measured dispensing of the contents. The Pharmacy Bulk Package is to be used only in a suitable work area, such as a laminar flow hood (or an equivalent clean-air compounding area).

IV INFUSION

The recommended dosage should be withdrawn from the stock solution and further diluted with water or saline to a maximum concentration of 40 mg/mL or less. The solution thus diluted will remain stable for 24 hours at room temperature or 96 hours under refrigeration. Any unused portion of the above-mentioned solutions must be discarded after the time periods specified above.

Caution: Administer slowly by intravenous route over a period of at least 30 to 60 minutes to avoid vein irritation.

ADD-Vantage™ VIALS—500 mg, 1 gram, and 2 gram. Unipen® (nafcillin sodium) in the ADD-Vantage system is intended as a single dose for intravenous administration after dilution with the ADD-Vantage Flexible Diluent Container containing 50 mL or 100 mL of 0.9% Sodium Chloride Injection, USP, or 5% Dextrose, USP. See "Instructions for Use of the Add-Vantage Vial."

Stability studies on reconstituted Unipen at concentrations of 5 mg/mL to 40 mg/mL in the ADD-Vantage system's various intravenous solutions indicate that the drug will lose less than 10% activity at room temperature (70°F) during the time period stated:

Intravenous Solutions	Room Temperature
0.9% Sodium Chloride Inj.	24 hours
5% Dextrose Inj.	24 hours

CAUTION: Administer slowly by intravenous route over a period of at least 20 minutes. More rapid administration may result in convulsive seizures.

CONVENTIONAL VIALS—500 mg, 1 gram, and 2 gram.

Intramuscular Route: 500 mg every 6 hours in adults; decrease the interval to 4 hours if necessary in severe infections. In infants and children, a dose of 25 mg/kg (about 12 mg/lb) twice daily is usually adequate.

For neonates, 10 mg/kg is recommended twice daily.

To reconstitute see directions and table below.

The clear solution should be administered by deep intragluteal injection immediately after reconstitution. After reconstitution, keep refrigerated (2°–8° C) and use within 7 days, keep at room temperature (25° C) and use within 3 days, or keep frozen (−20° C) for up to 3 months.

Oral Route: In adults a dose of 250 to 500 mg every 4 to 6 hours is sufficient for mild-to-moderate infections. In severe infections 1 gram every 4 to 6 hours may be necessary.

In children, streptococcal pharyngitis cases have responded to a dosage of 250 mg t.i.d. Beta-hemolytic streptococcal infections should be treated for at least ten days to prevent development of acute rheumatic fever or glomerulonephritis.

Children and infants with scarlet fever and pneumonia should receive 25 mg/kg/day in four divided doses. For staphylococcal infections, 50 mg/kg/day in four divided doses is recommended. For neonates, 10 mg/kg three to four times daily is recommended. If inadequate, resort to parenteral UNIPEN® (nafcillin sodium, Wyeth).

To reconstitute the powder for oral solution, add the water in two separate portions. Shake well after each addition. After reconstitution the solution must be refrigerated. Discard any unused portion after 7 days.

HOW SUPPLIED

FOR ORAL ADMINISTRATION

Capsules

Supplied as capsules containing nafcillin sodium, as the monohydrate, equivalent to 250 mg nafcillin buffered with calcium carbonate as follows:

NDC 0008-0057, green and yellow capsule marked "WYETH" and "57", in bottles of 100 capsules.

Keep tightly closed.

Dispense in tight container.

The appearance of these capsules is a trademark of Wyeth-Ayerst Laboratories.

Tablets

Supplied as tablets containing nafcillin sodium as the monohydrate, equivalent to 500 mg nafcillin buffered with calcium carbonate, as follows:

NDC 0008-0464, white, capsule-shaped, scored, film-coated tablet marked "WYETH" and "464", in bottles of 50 tablets.

Keep tightly closed.

Protect from light.

Dispense in light-resistant, tight container.

FOR PARENTERAL ADMINISTRATION

Conventional Vials (for intravenous or intramuscular use)

Supplied in vials of nafcillin sodium as the monohydrate equivalent to 500 mg, 1 gram, or 2 grams nafcillin per vial, buffered with 40 mg sodium citrate per gram, as follows:

NDC 0008-0751, in packages of 10 vials.

When reconstituted as recommended (see table below) with Sterile Water for Injection, USP, Sodium Chloride Injection, USP, Bacteriostatic Water for Injection, USP (TUBEX®), or Bacteriostatic Water for Injection, USP, with parabens or with benzyl alcohol, each vial contains, respectively, 2 mL, 4 mL, or 8 mL of solution. Each mL contains nafcillin sodium equivalent to 250 mg nafcillin, buffered with 10 mg sodium citrate.

Vial Size	Amount of Diluent	Nafcillin Sodium Solution
500 mg	1.7 mL	2 mL
1 gram	3.4 mL	4 mL
2 gram	6.8 mL	8 mL

FOR INTRAVENOUS USE ONLY

ADD-Vantage™ Vials

Supplied in vials of nafcillin sodium as the monohydrate equivalent to 500 mg, 1 gram, or 2 grams nafcillin per vial, buffered with 40 mg sodium citrate per gram, as follows:

NDC 0008-0751, in packages of 10 ADD-Vantage Vials.

The ADD-Vantage Vials are only to be used with Abbott Laboratories' ADD-Vantage Flexible Diluent Container containing:

0.9% Sodium Chloride Injection, USP, 50 mL and 100 mL sizes.

5% Dextrose Injection, USP, 50 mL and 100 mL sizes.

Piggyback Units

Supplied in single units of nafcillin sodium as the monohydrate equivalent to 1 gram or 2 grams nafcillin per unit, buffered with 40 mg sodium citrate per gram, as follows:

NDC 0008-0751, in packages of 10 PIGGYBACK vials.

Bulk Vial (for IV stock solution only)

Supplied in vials of nafcillin sodium as the monohydrate equivalent to 10 grams nafcillin per vial, buffered with 40 mg sodium citrate per gram, as follows:

NDC 0008-0751, in packages of 10 vials.

Shake vial well after adding diluent and before using.

Use solution within 8 hours if kept at room temperature or 48 hours if kept under refrigeration.

Caution: Federal law prohibits dispensing without prescription.

BIBLIOGRAPHY

A bibliography is available upon request.

Shown in Product Identification Section, page 438

VERELAN® ℞

(Verapamil HCl)

Sustained-Release Pellet-Filled Capsules

DESCRIPTION

VERELAN (verapamil hydrochloride capsules) is a calcium influx inhibitor (slow channel blocker or calcium ion antagonist). VERELAN is available for oral administration as a 240 mg hard gelatin capsule (blue cap/yellow body) and a 120 mg hard gelatin capsule (yellow cap/yellow body). These pellet-filled capsules provide a sustained-release of the drug in the gastrointestinal tract.

Chemical name: Benzeneacetonitrile, α-[3-[[2-(3,4-dimethoxyphenyl)-ethyl] methylamino]propyl]-3,4-dimethoxy-α-(1-methylethyl) monohydrochloride.

Verapamil HCl is an almost white, crystalline powder, practically free of odor, with a bitter taste. It is soluble in water, chloroform and methanol. Verapamil HCl is not structurally related to other cardioactive drugs.

In addition to verapamil HCl the VERELAN capsule contains the following inactive ingredients: fumaric acid, talc, sugar spheres, povidone, shellac, gelatin, FD&C red #40, yellow iron oxide, titanium dioxide, methylparaben, propylparaben, silicon dioxide, and sodium lauryl sulfate; in addition the VERELAN 240 mg capsule contains FD&C blue #1 and D&C red #28.

CLINICAL PHARMACOLOGY

VERELAN is a calcium ion influx inhibitor (slow channel blocker or calcium ion antagonist) which exerts its pharmacologic effects by modulating the influx of ionic calcium across the cell membrane of the arterial smooth muscle as well as in conductile and contractile myocardial cells.

Normal sinus rhythm is usually not affected by verapamil HCl. However in patients with sick sinus syndrome, verapamil HCl may interfere with sinus node impulse generation and may induce sinus arrest or sinoatrial block. Atrioventricular block can occur in patients without preexisting condition defects (see **WARNINGS**). Verapamil HCl does not alter the normal atrial action potential or intraventricular conduction time, but depresses amplitude, velocity of depolarization and conduction in depressed atrial fibers. Verapamil HCl may shorten the antegrade effective refractory period of accessory bypass tracts. Acceleration of ventricular rate and/or ventricular fibrillation has been reported in patients with atrial flutter or atrial fibrillation and a coexisting accessory AV pathway following administration of verapamil (see **WARNINGS**).

Verapamil HCl has a local anesthetic action that is 1.6 times that of procaine on an equimolar basis. It is not known whether this action is important at the doses used in man.

Mechanism of Action

Essential Hypertension

Verapamil HCl exerts antihypertensive effects by decreasing systemic vascular resistance, usually without orthostatic decreases in blood pressure or reflex tachycardia; bradycardia (rate less than 50 beats/minute) is uncommon. Verapamil HCl regularly reduces arterial pressure at rest and at a given level of exercise by dilating peripheral arterioles and reducing the total peripheral resistance (afterload) against which the heart works.

Pharmacokinetics and Metabolism

With the immediate release formulations, more than 90% of the orally administered dose is absorbed, and peak plasma concentrations of verapamil are observed 1 to 2 hours after dosing. Because of rapid biotransformation of verapamil during its first pass through the portal circulation, the absolute bioavailability ranges from 20% to 35%. Chronic oral administration of the highest recommended dose (120 mg every 6 hours) resulted in plasma verapamil levels ranging from 125 to 400 ng/mL with higher values reported occasionally. A nonlinear correlation between the verapamil HCl dose administered and verapamil plasma levels does exist. During initial dose titration with verapamil a relationship exists between verapamil plasma concentrations and the prolongation of the PR interval. However, during chronic administration this relationship may disappear.

In a multiple dose pharmacokinetic study, peak concentrations for a single daily dose of VERELAN 240 mg were approximately 65% of those obtained with an 80 mg tid dose of the conventional immediate release tablets, and the 24 hour post-dose concentrations were approximately 30% higher. At a total daily dose of 240 mg, VERELAN was shown to have a similar extent of verapamil bioavailability based on the AUC-24 as that obtained with the conventional immediate release tablets. In this same study VERELAN doses of 120 mg, 240 mg, and 360 mg once daily were compared after multiple doses. The ratios of the verapamil and norverapamil AUCs for the VERELAN 120 mg, 240 mg, and 360 mg once daily doses are 1 (565 ng·hr/ mL):3 (1660 ng·hr/mL):5 (2729 ng·hr/mL) and 1 (621 ng·hr/mL):3 (1614 ng·hr/mL):4 (2535 ng·hr/mL), respectively, indicating that the AUC increased non-proportionately with increasing doses.

Continued on next page

Wyeth-Ayerst Laboratories—Cont.

Food does not affect the extent or rate of the controlled absorption of verapamil from the VERELAN capsule. The VERELAN 240 mg capsule when administered with food had a ^{C}max of 77 ng/mL which occurred 9.0 hours after dosing, and an AUC(O-inf) of 1387 ng·hr/mL. VERELAN 240 mg under fasting conditions had a ^{C}max of 77 ng/mL which occurred 9.8 hours after dosing, and an AUC(O-inf) of 1541 ng·hr/mL.

The time to reach maximum verapamil concentrations (T_{max}) with VERELAN has been found to be approximately 7 to 9 hours in each of the single dose (fasting), single dose (fed), the multiple dose (steady state) studies, and dose proportionality pharmacokinetic studies. Similarly the apparent half-life ($t_{1/2}$) has been found to be approximately 12 hours independent of dose. Aging may affect the pharmacokinetics of verapamil. Elimination half-life may be prolonged in the elderly.

In healthy man, orally administered verapamil HCl undergoes extensive metabolism in the liver. Twelve metabolites have been identified in plasma; all except norverapamil are present in trace amounts only. Norverapamil can reach steady-state plasma concentrations approximately equal to those of verapamil itself. The biologic activity of norverapamil appears to be approximately 20% that of verapamil.

Approximately 70% of an administered dose of verapamil HCl is excreted as metabolites in the urine and 16% or more in the feces within 5 days. About 3% to 4% is excreted in the urine as unchanged drug. Approximately 90% is bound to plasma proteins. In patients with hepatic insufficiency, metabolism is delayed and elimination half-life prolonged up to 14 to 16 hours (see **PRECAUTIONS**), the volume of distribution is increased, and plasma clearance reduced to about 30% of normal. Verapamil clearance values suggest that patients with liver dysfunction may attain therapeutic verapamil plasma concentrations with one third of the oral daily dose required for patients with normal liver function.

After 4 weeks of oral dosing (120 mg qid), verapamil and norverapamil levels were noted in the cerebrospinal fluid with estimated partition coefficient of 0.06 for verapamil and 0.04 for norverapamil.

Hemodynamics and Myocardial Metabolism

Verapamil HCl reduces afterload and myocardial contractility. Improved left ventricular diastolic function in patients with IHSS and those with coronary heart disease has also been observed with verapamil HCl therapy. In most patients, including those with organic cardiac disease, the negative inotropic action of verapamil HCl is countered by reduction of afterload and cardiac index is usually not reduced. In patients with severe left ventricular dysfuntion however (e.g., pulmonary wedge pressure above 20 mmHg or ejection fraction lower than 30%), or in patients on beta-adrenergic blocking agents or other cardiodepressant drugs, deterioration of ventricular function may occur (see **DRUG INTERACTIONS**).

Pulmonary Function

Verapamil HCl does not induce broncho-constriction and hence, does not impair ventilatory function.

INDICATIONS AND USAGE

VERELAN (verapamil HCl) is indicated for the management of essential hypertension.

CONTRAINDICATIONS

Verapamil HCl is contraindicated in:

1. Severe left ventricular dysfunction (see **WARNINGS**).
2. Hypotension (less than 90 mmHg systolic pressure) or cardiogenic shock.
3. Sick sinus syndrome (except in patients with a functioning artificial ventricular pacemaker).
4. Second- or third-degree AV block (except in patients with a functioning artificial ventricular pacemaker).
5. Patients with atrial flutter or atrial fibrillation and an accessory bypass tract (e.g., Wolff-Parkinson-White, Lown- Ganong-Levine syndromes) (see **WARNINGS**).
6. Patients with known hypersensitivity to verapamil HCl.

WARNINGS

Heart Failure

Verapamil has a negative inotropic effect which, in most patients, is compensated by its afterload reduction (decreased systemic vascular resistance) properties without a net impairment of ventricular performance. In clinical experience with 4,954 patients, 87 (1.8%) developed congestive heart failure or pulmonary edema. Verapamil should be avoided in patients with severe left ventricular dysfunction (eg, ejection fraction less than 30% or moderate to severe symptoms of cardiac failure) and in patients with any degree of ventricular dysfunction if they are receiving a beta-adrenergic blocker (see **DRUG INTERACTIONS**). Patients with milder ventricular dysfunction should, if possible, be controlled with optimum doses of digitalis and/or diuretics before verapamil treatment (note interactions with digoxin under **PRECAUTIONS**).

Hypotension

Occasionally, the pharmacologic action of verapamil may produce a decrease in blood pressure below normal levels which may result in dizziness or symptomatic hypotension. The incidence of hypotension observed in 4,954 patients enrolled in clinical trials was 2.5%. In hypertensive patients, decreases in blood pressure below normal are unusual. Tilt table testing (60 degrees) was not able to induce orthostatic hypotension.

Elevated Liver Enzymes

Elevations of transaminases with and without concomitant elevations in alkaline phosphatase and bilirubin have been reported. Such elevations have sometimes been transient and may disappear even in the face of continued verapamil treatment. Several cases of hepatocellular injury related to verapamil have been proven by rechallenge; half of these had clinical symptoms (malaise, fever, and/or right upper quadrant pain) in addition to elevations of SGOT, SGPT, and alkaline phosphatase. Periodic monitoring of liver function in patients receiving verapamil is therefore prudent.

Accessory Bypass Tract (Wolff-Parkinson-White or Lown-Ganong-Levine)

Some patients with paroxysmal and/or chronic atrial flutter or atrial fibrillation and a coexisting accessory AV pathway have developed increased antegrade conduction across the accessory pathway bypassing the AV node, producing a very rapid ventricular response or ventricular fibrillation after receiving intravenous verapamil (or digitalis). Although a risk of this occurring with oral verapamil has not been established, such patients receiving oral verapamil may be at risk and its use in these patients is contraindicated (see **CONTRAINDICATIONS**).

Treatment is usually DC-cardioversion. Cardioversion has been used safely and effectively after oral verapamil.

Atrioventricular Block

The effect of verapamil on AV conduction and the SA node may lead to asymptomatic first-degree AV block and transient bradycardia, sometimes accompanied by nodal escape rhythms. PR interval prolongation is correlated with verapamil plasma concentrations, especially during the early titration phase of therapy. Higher degrees of AV block, however, were infrequently (0.8%) observed.

Marked first-degree block or progressive development to second- or third-degree AV block requires a reduction in dosage or, in rare instances, discontinuation of verapamil HCl and institution of appropriate therapy depending upon the clinical situation.

Patients with Hypertrophic Cardiomyopathy (IHSS)

In 120 patients with hypertrophic cardiomyopathy (most of them refractory or intolerant to propranolol) who received therapy with verapamil at doses up to 720 mg/day, a variety of serious adverse effects were seen. Three patients died in pulmonary edema; all had severe left ventricular outflow obstruction and a past history of left ventricular dysfunction. Eight other patients had pulmonary edema and/or severe hypotension; abnormally high (over 20 mmHg) capillary wedge pressure and a marked left ventricular outflow obstruction were present in most of these patients. Concomitant administration of quinidine (see **DRUG INTERACTIONS**) preceded the severe hypotension in 3 of the 8 patients (2 of whom developed pulmonary edema). Sinus bradycardia occurred in 11% of the patients, second-degree AV block in 4% and sinus arrest in 2%. It must be appreciated that this group of patients had a serious disease with a high mortality rate. Most adverse effects responded well to dose reduction and only rarely did verapamil have to be discontinued.

PRECAUTIONS

General

Use in Patients with Impaired Hepatic Function

Since verapamil is highly metabolized by the liver, it should be administered cautiously to patients with impaired hepatic function. Severe liver dysfunction prolongs the elimination half-life of immediate release verapamil to about 14 to 16 hours; hence, approximately 30% of the dose given to patients with normal liver function should be administered to these patients. Careful monitoring for abnormal prolongation of the PR interval or other signs of excessive pharmacologic effects (see **OVERDOSAGE**) should be carried out.

Use in Patients with Attenuated (Decreased) Neuromuscular Transmission

It has been reported that verapamil decreases neuromuscular transmission in patients with Duchenne's muscular dystrophy, and that verapamil prolongs recovery from the neuromuscular blocking agent vecuronium. It may be necessary to decrease the dosage of verapamil when it is administered to patients with attenuated neuromuscular transmission.

Use in Patients with Impaired Renal Function

About 70% of an administered dose of verapamil is excreted as metabolites in the urine. Until further data are available, verapamil should be administered cautiously to patients with impaired renal function. These patients should be carefully monitored for abnormal prolongation of the PR interval or other signs of overdosage (see **OVERDOSAGE**).

Drug Interactions

Beta Blockers

Concomitant therapy with beta-adrenergic blockers and verapamil may result in additive negative effects on heart rate, atrioventricular conduction, and/or cardiac contractility. The combination of sustained-release verapamil and beta-adrenergic blocking agents has not been studied. However, there have been reports of excess bradycardia and AV block, including complete heart block, when the combination has been used for the treatment of hypertension. For hypertensive patients, the risk of combined therapy may outweigh the potential benefits. The combination should be used only with caution and close monitoring.

Asymptomatic bradycardia (36 beats/min) with a wandering atrial pacemaker has been observed in a patient receiving concomitant timolol (a beta-adrenergic blocker) eyedrops and oral verapamil.

A decrease in metoprolol clearance has been reported when verapamil and metoprolol were administered together. A similar effect has not been observed when verapamil and atenolol are given together.

Digitalis

Clinical use of verapamil in digitalized patients has shown the combination to be well tolerated if digoxin doses are properly adjusted. Chronic verapamil treatment can increase serum digoxin levels by 50% to 75% during the first week of therapy, and this can result in digitalis toxicity. In patients with hepatic cirrhosis the influence of verapamil on digoxin kinetics is magnified. Maintenance digitalis doses should be reduced when verapamil is administered, and the patient should be carefully monitored to avoid over- or underdigitalization. Whenever overdigitalization is suspected, the daily dose of digoxin should be reduced or temporarily discontinued. Upon discontinuation of verapamil HCl, the patient should be reassessed to avoid underdigitalization.

Antihypertensive Agents

Verapamil administered concomitantly with oral antihypertensive agents (eg, vasodilators, angiotensin-converting enzyme inhibitors, diuretics, beta blockers) will usually have an additive effect on lowering blood pressure. Patients receiving these combinations should be appropriately monitored. Concomitant use of agents that attenuate alpha-adrenergic function with verapamil may result in reduction in blood pressure that is excessive in some patients. Such an effect was observed in one study following the concomitant administration of verapamil and prazosin.

Antiarrhythmic Agents

Disopyramide: Until data on possible interactions between verapamil and disopyramide phosphate are obtained, disopyramide should not be administered within 48 hours before or 24 hours after verapamil administration.

Flecainide: A study in healthy volunteers showed that the concomitant administration of flecainide and verapamil may have additive effects on myocardial contractility, AV conduction, and repolarization. Concomitant therapy with flecainide and verapamil may result in additive negative inotropic effect and prolongation of atrioventricular conduction.

Quinidine: In a small number of patients with hypertrophic cardiomyopathy (IHSS), concomitant use of verapamil and quinidine resulted in significant hypotension. Until further data are obtained, combined therapy of verapamil and quinidine in patients with hypertrophic cardiomyopathy should probably be avoided.

The electrophysiological effects of quinidine and verapamil on AV conduction were studied in 8 patients. Verapamil significantly counteracted the effects of quinidine on AV conduction. There has been a report of increased quinidine levels during verapamil therapy.

Nitrates: Verapamil has been given concomitantly with short- and long-acting nitrates without any undesirable drug interactions. The pharmacologic profile of both drugs and the clinical experience suggest beneficial interactions.

Other

Cimetidine: The interaction between cimetidine and chronically administered verapamil has not been studied. Variable results on clearance have been obtained in acute studies of healthy volunteers; clearance of verapamil was either reduced or unchanged.

Lithium: Pharmacokinetic and pharmacodynamic interactions between oral verapamil and lithium have been reported. The former may result in a lowering of serum lithium levels in patients receiving chronic stable oral lithium therapy. The latter may result in an increased sensitivity to the effects of lithium. Patients receiving both drugs must be monitored carefully.

Carbamazepine: Verapamil therapy may increase carbamazepine concentrations during combined therapy. This may produce carbamazepine side effects such as diplopia, headache, ataxia, or dizziness.

Rifampin: Therapy with rifampin may markedly reduce oral verapamil bioavailability.

Phenobarbital: Phenobarbital therapy may increase verapamil clearance.

Cyclosporine: Verapamil therapy may increase serum levels of cyclosporine.

Inhalation Anesthetics: Animal experiments have shown that inhalation anesthetics depress cardiovascular activity by decreasing the inward movement of calcium ions. When used concomitantly, inhalation anesthetics and calcium antagonists, such as verapamil, should be titrated carefully to avoid excessive cardiovascular depression.
Neuromuscular Blocking Agents: Clinical data and animal studies suggest that verapamil may potentiate the activity of neuromuscular blocking agents (curare-like and depolarizing). It may be necessary to decrease the dose of verapamil and/or the dose of the neuromuscular blocking agent when the drugs are used concomitantly.

Carcinogenesis, Mutagenesis, Impairment of Fertility
An 18-month toxicity study in rats, at a low multiple (sixfold) of the maximum recommended human dose, and not the maximum tolerated dose, did not suggest a tumorigenic potential. There was no evidence of a carcinogenic potential of verapamil administered in the diet of rats for 2 years at doses of 10, 35, and 120 mg/kg per day or approximately 1x, 3.5x, and 12x, respectively, the maximum recommended human daily dose (480 mg per day or 9.6 mg/kg/day.
Verapamil was not mutagenic in the Ames test in five test strains at 3 mg per plate, with or without metabolic activation.
Studies in female rats at daily dietary doses up to 5.5 times (55 mg/kg/day) the maximum recommended human dose did not show impaired fertility. Effects on male fertility have not been determined.

Pregnancy
Pregnancy Category C: Reproduction studies have been performed in rabbits and rats at oral doses up to 1.5 (15 mg/kg/day) and 6 (60 mg/kg/day) times the maximum recommended human daily dose, respectively, and have revealed no evidence of teratogenicity. In the rat, however, this multiple of the human dose was embryocidal and retarded fetal growth and development, probably because of adverse maternal effects reflected in reduced weight gains of the dams. This oral dose has also been shown to cause hypotension in rats. There are no adequate and well-controlled studies in pregnant women. Because animal reproduction studies are not always predictive of human response, this drug should be used during pregnancy only if clearly needed. Verapamil crosses the placental barrier and can be detected in umbilical vein blood at delivery.

Labor and Delivery
It is not known whether the use of verapamil during labor or delivery has immediate or delayed adverse effects on the fetus, or whether it prolongs the duration of labor or increases the need for forceps delivery or other obstetric intervention. Such adverse experiences have not been reported in the literature, despite a long history of use of verapamil HCl in Europe in the treatment of cardiac side effects of beta-adrenergic agonist agents used to treat premature labor.

Nursing Mothers
Verapamil is excreted in human milk. Because of the potential for adverse reactions in nursing infants from verapamil, nursing should be discontinued while verapamil is administered.

Pediatric Use
Safety and efficacy of verapamil in children below the age of 18 years have not been established.

Animal Pharmacology and/or Animal Toxicology
In chronic animal toxicology studies verapamil causes lenticular and/or suture line changes at 30mg/kg/day or greater and frank cataracts at 62.5 mg/kg/day or greater in the beagle dog but not the rat. Development of cataracts due to verapamil has not been reported in man.

ADVERSE REACTIONS

Serious adverse reactions are uncommon when verapamil HCl therapy is initiated with upward dose titration within the recommended single and total daily dose. See **WARNINGS** for discussion of heart failure, hypotension, elevated liver enzymes, AV block, and rapid ventricular response.
In clinical trials involving 285 hypertensive patients on VERELAN for greater than 1 week the following adverse reactions were reported in greater than 1.0% of the patients:

Constipation	7.4%
Headache	5.3%
Dizziness	4.2%
Lethargy	3.2%
Dyspepsia	2.5%
Rash	1.4%
Ankle Edema	1.4%
Sleep Disturbance	1.4%
Myalgia	1.1%

In clinical trials of other formulations of verapamil HCl (N=4,954) the following reactions have occurred at rates greater than 1.0%: [See table at top of next column.]

Constipation	7.3%
Dizziness	3.3%
Nausea	2.7%
Hypotension	2.5%
Edema	1.9%
Headache	2.2%
CHF/Pulmonary Edema	1.8%
Fatigue	1.7%
Bradycardia (HR <50/min)	1.4%
AV block-total	
1°, 2°, 3°	1.2%
2°and 3°	0.8%
Flushing	0.6%
Elevated Liver Enzymes (see **WARNINGS.**)	

In clinical trials related to the control of ventricular response in digitalized patients who had atrial fibrillation or atrial flutter, ventricular rate below 50/min at rest occurred in 15% of patients and asymptomatic hypotension occurred in 5% of patients.
The following reactions, reported in 1.0% or less of patients, occurred under conditions (open trials, marketing experience) where a causal relationship is uncertain; they are listed to alert the physician to a possible relationship:
Cardiovascular: angina pectoris, atrioventricular dissociation, chest pain, claudication, myocardial infarction, palpitations, purpura (vasculitis), syncope.
Digestive System: diarrhea, dry mouth, gastrointestinal distress, gingival hyperplasia.
Hemic and Lymphatic: ecchymosis or bruising.
Nervous System: cerebrovascular accident, confusion, equilibrium disorders, insomnia, muscle cramps, paresthesia, psychotic symptoms, shakiness, somnolence.
Respiratory: dyspnea.
Skin: arthralgia and rash, exanthema, hair loss, hyperkeratosis, maculae, sweating, urticaria, Stevens-Johnson syndrome, erythema multiforme.
Special Senses: blurred vision.
Urogenital: gynecomastia, impotence, increased urination, spotty menstruation.

Treatment of Acute Cardiovascular Adverse Reactions
The frequency of cardiovascular adverse reactions which require therapy is rare; hence, experience with their treatment is limited. Whenever severe hypotension or complete AV block occur following oral administration of verapamil, the appropriate emergency measures should be applied immediately, eg, intravenously administered isoproterenol HCl, levarterenol bitartrate, atropine (all in the usual doses), or calcium gluconate (10% solution). In patients with hypertrophic cardiomyopathy (IHSS), alpha-adrenergic agents (phenylephrine, metaraminol bitartrate or methoxamine) should be used to maintain blood pressure, and isoproterenol and levarterenol should be avoided. If further support is necessary, inotropic agents (dopamine or dobutamine) may be administered. Actual treatment and dosage should depend on the severity and the clinical situation and the judgment and experience of the treating physician.

OVERDOSAGE

Treatment of overdosage should be supportive. Beta-adrenergic stimulation or parenteral administration of calcium solutions may increase calcium ion flux across the slow channel, and have been used effectively in treatment of deliberate overdosage with verapamil. Verapamil cannot be removed by hemodialysis. Clinically significant hypotensive reactions or high degree AV block should be treated with vasopressor agents or cardiac pacing, respectively. Asystole should be handled by the usual measures including cardiopulmonary resuscitation.

DOSAGE AND ADMINISTRATION

Essential Hypertension
The dose of VERELAN should be individualized by titration. The usual daily dose of sustained-release verapamil, VERELAN, in clinical trials has been 240 mg given by mouth once daily in the morning. However, initial doses of 120 mg a day may be warranted in patients who may have an increased response to verapamil (eg, elderly, small people, etc). Upward titration should be based on therapeutic efficacy and safety evaluated approximately 24 hours after dosing. The antihypertensive effects of VERELAN are evident within the first week of therapy.
If adequate response is not obtained with 120 mg of VERELAN, the dose may be titrated upward in the following manner: (a) 240 mg in the morning, (b) 360 mg in the morning, (c) 480 mg in the morning. VERELAN sustained-release capsules are for once-a-day administration. When switching from immediate-release verapamil to VERELAN capsules, the same total daily dose of VERELAN capsules can be used.
As with immediate-release verapamil, dosages of VERELAN capsules should be individualized and titration may be needed in some patients.

HOW SUPPLIED

VERELAN *verapamil HCl* capsules are supplied in two dosage strengths:
120 mg—Two-piece, size 2 hard gelatin capsule (yellow cap/yellow body), printed with Lederle over V8 on one side and VERELAN *verapamil HCl* over 120 mg on the other in black ink, supplied as follows:
NDC 0005-2490-23—Bottle of 100
240 mg—Two-piece, size 0 hard gelatin capsule (blue cap/yellow body), printed with Lederle over V9 on one side and VERELAN over 240 mg on the other in black ink, supplied as follows:
NDC 0005-2491-23—Bottle of 100
STORE AT CONTROLLED ROOM TEMPERATURE 15°-30°C (59°-86°F), PROTECTED FROM MOISTURE.
Dispense in tight, light-resistant container as defined in USP.

Manufactured for
LEDERLE LABORATORIES DIVISION
American Cyanamid Company
Pearl River, NY 10965
by
ELAN PHARMACEUTICAL RESEARCH CORP.
Gainesville, GA 30501

Shown in Product Identification Section, page 416

WYAMYCIN® S ℞
[*wi-a-mi 'sin*]
Film-coated Tablets
(erythromycin stearate)

DESCRIPTION

Wyamycin S (erythromycin stearate) is produced by a strain of *Streptomyces erythraeus* and belongs to the macrolide group of antibiotics. It is basic and readily forms salts with acids. The base, the stearate salt, and the esters are poorly soluble in water and are suitable for oral administration.
Each film-coated tablet contains 250 mg or 500 mg erythromycin as erythromycin stearate, USP. The inactive ingredients present are acetylated monoglycerides, D&C Yellow 10, ethylcellulose, FD&C Blue 2, FD&C Yellow 6, hydroxypropyl methylcellulose, magnesium stearate, povidone, sodium citrate, sodium starch glycolate and titanium dioxide.

HOW SUPPLIED

Wyamycin® S (erythromycin stearate) Tablets, Wyeth®, containing the equivalent of 250 mg or 500 mg erythromycin, are available as follows:
250 mg, NDC 0008-0576, yellow, round, film-coated tablet marked "WYETH" and "576", in bottles of 500 tablets.
500 mg, NDC 0008-0578, yellow, elliptical, film-coated tablet marked "WYETH" and "578", in bottles of 100 tablets.
Keep tightly closed.
Protect from light and moisture.
Dispense in light-resistant, tight container.
For prescribing information write to Professional Service, Wyeth-Ayerst Laboratories, P.O. Box 8299, Philadelphia, PA 19101, or contact your local Wyeth-Ayerst representative.

Shown in Product Identification Section, page 438

WYANOIDS® Relief Factor OTC
[*wi 'a-noids*]
Hemorrhoidal Suppositories

DESCRIPTION

Active ingredients: Live Yeast Cell Derivative, Supplying 2,000 units Skin Respiratory Factor Per Ounce of Cocoa Butter Suppository Base and Shark Liver Oil 3%. Inactive Ingredients: Beeswax Glycerin, Phenylmercuric Nitrate 1:10,000 (as a preservative), Polyethylene Glycol 600 Dilaurate.

INDICATIONS

To help shrink swelling of hemorrhoidal tissues and provide prompt, temporary relief from pain and itching.

USUAL DOSAGE

Patients are advised to use one suppository up to five times daily, especially in the morning, at night, and after bowel movements, or as directed by a physician.

DIRECTIONS

Remove wrapper and insert one suppository rectally using gentle pressure. Frequent application and lubrication with Wyanoids® Relief Factor provide continual therapy which will lead to more rapid improvement of rectal conditions.

CAUTION

In case of bleeding or if the condition persists, the patient should consult a physician. Keep this and all medications out of the reach of children. Do not store above 80° F.

HOW SUPPLIED

Boxes of 12 and 24.
Shown in Product Identification Section, page 438

Continued on next page

Wyeth-Ayerst Laboratories—Cont.

WYCILLIN®   ℞

[*wi-sil'in*]
(sterile penicillin G procaine suspension)
INJECTION

FOR DEEP INTRAMUSCULAR INJECTION ONLY

DESCRIPTION

This product is designed to provide a stable aqueous suspension of sterile penicillin G procaine, ready for immediate use. This eliminates the necessity for addition of any diluent, required for the usual dry formulation of injectable penicillin.

Each TUBEX® Sterile Cartridge-Needle Unit, Wyeth, 1,200,000 units (2 mL size) or 600,000 units (1 mL size) or disposable syringe, 2,400,000 units (4 mL size), contains penicillin G procaine in a stabilized aqueous suspension with sodium citrate buffer; and as w/v, approximately 0.5% lecithin, 0.5% carboxymethylcellulose, 0.5% povidone, 0.1% methylparaben, and 0.01% propylparaben.

Each TUBEX, 300,000 units (1 mL size), contains penicillin G procaine in a stabilized aqueous suspension with sodium citrate buffer; and as w/v, approximately 0.3% lecithin, 0.9% carboxymethylcellulose, 0.9% povidone, 0.14% methylparaben, and 0.015% propylparaben.

Each syringe, 2,400,000 units (4 mL size), contains penicillin G procaine in a stabilized aqueous suspension with sodium citrate buffer; and as w/v, approximately 0.5% lecithin, 0.5% carboxymethylcellulose, 0.5% povidone, 0.1% methylparaben, and 0.01% propylparaben.

Wycillin must be stored in a refrigerator. Keep from freezing. This will prevent deterioration and assure that no significant loss of potency occurs within the expiration date.

Wycillin suspension in the TUBEX and disposable syringe formulations is viscous and opaque. Read "Contraindications," "Warnings," "Precautions," and "Dosage and Administration" sections prior to use.

ACTIONS AND PHARMACOLOGY

Penicillin G exerts a bactericidal action against penicillin-sensitive microorganisms during the stage of active multiplication. It acts through the inhibition of biosynthesis of cell-wall mucopeptide. It is not active against the penicillinase-producing bacteria, which include many strains of staphylococci. Penicillin G exerts high *in vitro* activity against staphylococci (except penicillinase-producing strains), streptococci (Groups A, C, G, H, L, and M), and pneumococci. Other organisms sensitive to penicillin G are *Neisseria gonorrhoeae, Corynebacterium diphtheriae, Bacillus anthracis,* Clostridia, *Actinomyces bovis, Streptobacillus moniliformis, Listeria monocytogenes,* and Leptospira. *Treponema pallidum* is extremely sensitive to the bactericidal action of penicillin G.

Sensitivity Plate Testing: If the Kirby-Bauer method of disc sensitivity is used, a 10-unit penicillin disc should give a zone greater than 28 mm when tested against a penicillin-sensitive bacterial strain.

Penicillin G procaine is an equimolecular compound of procaine and penicillin G, administered intramuscularly as a suspension. It dissolves slowly at the site of injection, giving a plateau type of blood level at about 4 hours which falls slowly over a period of the next 15 to 20 hours.

Approximately 60% of penicillin G is bound to serum protein. The drug is distributed throughout the body tissues in widely varying amounts. Highest levels are found in the kidneys with lesser amounts in the liver, skin, and intestines. Penicillin G penetrates into all other tissues to a lesser degree with a very small level found in the cerebrospinal fluid. With normal kidney function, the drug is excreted rapidly by tubular excretion. In neonates and young infants and in individuals with impaired kidney functions, excretion is considerably delayed. Approximately 60 to 90 percent of a dose of parenteral penicillin G is excreted in the urine within 24 to 36 hours.

INDICATIONS

Penicillin G procaine is indicated in the treatment of moderately severe infections due to penicillin-G-sensitive microorganisms that are sensitive to the low and persistent serum levels common to this particular dosage form. Therapy should be guided by bacteriological studies (including sensitivity tests) and by clinical response.

NOTE: When high, sustained serum levels are required, aqueous penicillin G, either IM or IV, should be used.

The following infections will usually respond to adequate dosages of intramuscular penicillin G procaine:

Streptococcal infections (Group A—without bacteremia). Moderately severe to severe infections of the upper respiratory tract, skin and soft-tissue infections, scarlet fever, and erysipelas.

NOTE: Streptococci in Groups A, C, G, H, L, and M are very sensitive to penicillin G. Other groups, including Group D (enterococcus), are resistant. Aqueous penicillin is recommended for streptococcal infections with bacteremia.

Pneumococcal infections. Moderately severe infections of the respiratory tract.

NOTE: Severe pneumonia, empyema, bacteremia, pericarditis, meningitis, peritonitis, and arthritis of pneumococcal etiology are better treated with aqueous penicillin G during the acute stage.

Staphylococcal infections—penicillin-G-sensitive. Moderately severe infections of the skin and soft tissues.

NOTE: Reports indicate an increasing number of strains of staphylococci resistant to penicillin G, emphasizing the need for culture and sensitivity studies in treating suspected staphylococcal infections.

Indicated surgical procedures should be performed.

Fusospirochetosis (Vincent's gingivitis and pharyngitis). Moderately severe infections of the oropharynx respond to therapy with penicillin G procaine.

NOTE: Necessary dental care should be accomplished in infections involving the gum tissue.

Treponema pallidum (syphilis); all stages.

N. gonorrhoeae; acute and chronic (without bacteremia).

Yaws, Bejel, Pinta.

C. diphtheriae —penicillin G procaine as an adjunct to antitoxin for prevention of the carrier stage.

Anthrax.

Streptobacillus moniliformis and *Spirillum minus* infections (rat-bite fever).

Erysipeloid.

Subacute bacterial endocarditis (Group A streptococcus), only in extremely sensitive infections.

Although no controlled clinical efficacy studies have been conducted, aqueous crystalline penicillin G for injection and penicillin G procaine suspension have been suggested by the American Heart Association and the American Dental Association for use as part of a combined parenteral-oral regimen for prophylaxis against bacterial endocarditis in patients who have congenital heart disease or rheumatic or other acquired valvular heart disease when they undergo dental procedures and surgical procedures of the upper respiratory tract.[1]

Since it may happen that *alpha* -hemolytic streptococci relatively resistant to penicillin may be found when patients are receiving continuous oral penicillin for secondary prevention of rheumatic fever, prophylactic agents other than penicillin may be chosen for these patients and prescribed in addition to their continuous rheumatic fever prophylactic regimen.

NOTE: When selecting antibiotics for the prevention of bacterial endocarditis, the physician or dentist should read the full joint statement of the American Heart Association and the American Dental Association.[1]

CONTRAINDICATIONS

A previous hypersensitivity reaction to any penicillin is a contraindication.

Do not inject into or near an artery or nerve.

WARNINGS

Serious and occasionally fatal hypersensitivity (anaphylactoid) reactions have been reported in patients on penicillin therapy.

Serious anaphylactoid reactions require immediate emergency treatment with epinephrine. Oxygen and intravenous corticosteroids should also be administered as indicated.

Although anaphylaxis is more frequent following parenteral therapy, it has occurred in patients on oral penicillins. These reactions are more apt to occur in individuals with a history of sensitivity to multiple allergens.

There have been well-documented reports of individuals with a history of penicillin hypersensitivity reactions who have experienced severe hypersensitivity reactions when treated with a cephalosporin. Before therapy with a penicillin, careful inquiry should be made concerning previous hypersensitivity reactions to penicillins, cephalosporins, and other allergens. If an allergic reaction occurs, the drug should be discontinued and the patient treated with the usual agents, e.g., pressor amines, antihistamines, and corticosteroids.

Immediate toxic reactions to procaine may occur in some individuals, particularly when a large single dose is administered in the treatment of gonorrhea (4.8 million units). These reactions may be manifested by mental disturbances, including anxiety, confusion, agitation, depression, weakness, seizures, hallucinations, combativeness, and expressed "fear of impending death." The reactions noted in carefully controlled studies occurred in approximately one in 500 patients treated for gonorrhea. Reactions are transient, lasting from 15 to 30 minutes.

Inadvertent intravascular administration, including inadvertent direct intra-arterial injection or injection immediately adjacent to arteries, of Wycillin and other penicillin preparations has resulted in severe neurovascular damage, including transverse myelitis with permanent paralysis, gangrene requiring amputation of digits and more proximal portions of extremities, and necrosis and sloughing at and surrounding the injection site. Such severe effects have been reported following injections into the buttock, thigh, and deltoid areas. Other serious complications of suspected intravascular administration which have been reported include immediate pallor, mottling or cyanosis of the extremity both distal and proximal to the injection site followed by bleb formation; severe edema requiring anterior and/or posterior compartment fasciotomy in the lower extremity. The above described severe effects and complications have most often occurred in infants and small children. Prompt consultation with an appropriate specialist is indicated if any evidence of compromise of the blood supply occurs at, proximal to, or distal to the site of injection.[2-10] See "Contraindications," "Precautions," and "Dosage and Administration" sections. Quadriceps femoris fibrosis and atrophy have been reported following repeated intramuscular injections of penicillin preparations into the anterolateral thigh.

Injection into or near a nerve may result in permanent neurological damage.

PRECAUTIONS

Penicillin should be used with caution in individuals with histories of significant allergies and/or asthma.

Care should be taken to avoid intravenous or intraarterial administration, or injection into or near major peripheral nerves or blood vessels, since such injections may produce neurovascular damage. See "Contraindications," "Warnings," and "Dosage and Administration" sections.

In suspected staphylococcal infections, proper laboratory studies, including sensitivity tests, should be performed.

A small percentage of patients are sensitive to procaine. If there is a history of sensitivity, make the usual test: Inject intradermally 0.1 mL of a 1 to 2 percent procaine solution. Development of an erythema, wheal, flare, or eruption indicates procaine sensitivity. Sensitivity should be treated by the usual methods, including barbiturates, and procaine penicillin preparations should not be used. Antihistaminics appear beneficial in treatment of procaine reactions.

The use of antibiotics may result in overgrowth of nonsusceptible organisms. Constant observation of the patient is essential. If new infections due to bacteria or fungi appear during therapy, the drug should be discontinued and appropriate measures taken.

Whenever allergic reactions occur, penicillin should be withdrawn unless, in the opinion of the physician, the condition being treated is life-threatening and amenable only to penicillin therapy.

In prolonged therapy with penicillin, and particularly with high-dosage schedules, periodic evaluation of the renal and hematopoietic systems is recommended.

When treating gonococcal infections in which primary or secondary syphilis may be suspected, proper diagnostic procedures, including dark-field examinations, should be done. In all cases in which concomitant syphilis is suspected, monthly serological tests should be made for at least four months.

ADVERSE REACTIONS

Penicillin is a substance of low toxicity but does possess a significant index of sensitization. The following hypersensitivity reactions associated with use of penicillin have been reported: Skin rashes, ranging from maculopapular eruptions to exfoliative dermatitis; urticaria; serum-sicknesslike reactions, including chills, fever, edema, arthralgia, and prostration. Severe and often fatal anaphylaxis has been reported (see "Warnings"). As with other treatments for syphilis, the Jarisch-Herxheimer reaction has been reported. Procaine toxicity manifestations have been reported (see "Warnings"). Although procaine hypersensitivity reactions have not been reported with this drug, there are patients who are sensitive to procaine (see "Precautions").

DOSAGE AND ADMINISTRATION

Parenteral drug products should be inspected visually for particulate matter and discoloration prior to administration, whenever solution and container permit.

Penicillin G procaine (aqueous) is for intramuscular injection only.

Administer by DEEP, INTRAMUSCULAR INJECTION in the upper, outer quadrant of the buttock. In infants and small children, the midlateral aspect of the thigh may be preferable. When doses are repeated, vary the injection site.

When using the TUBEX cartridge:

The Wyeth TUBEX cartridge for this product incorporates several features that are designed to facilitate the visualization of blood on aspiration if a blood vessel is inadvertently entered.

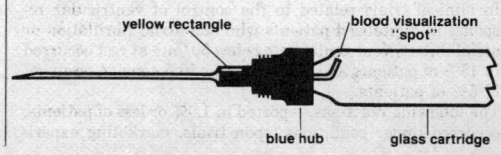

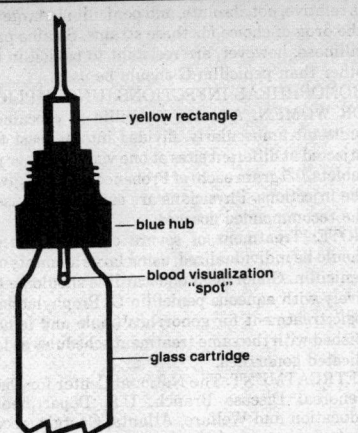

yellow rectangle

blue hub

blood visualization "spot"

glass cartridge

The design of this cartridge is such that blood which enters its needle will be quickly visualized as a red or dark-colored "spot." This "spot" will appear on the barrel of the glass cartridge immediately proximal to the blue hub. Prior to injection, in order to determine where this "spot" can be seen, the operator should first insert and secure the cartridge in the TUBEX syringe/injector in the usual fashion. The needle cover should then be partially removed to reveal a small yellow rectangle and the cartridge and syringe/injector held in one hand with the needle pointing away from the operator. If the 2 mL metal or plastic syringe is used, the glass cartridge should be rotated by turning the plunger of the syringe clockwise until the yellow rectangle is visualized. An imaginary straight line, drawn to extend the yellow rectangle to the shoulder of the glass cartridge, will point to the area on the cartridge where the "spot" can be visualized. If the 1 mL metal syringe is used, it will not be possible to continue to rotate the glass cartridge clockwise once it is properly engaged and fully threaded; it can, however, then be rotated counterclockwise as far as necessary to properly orient the yellow rectangle and locate the observation area. (In this same area in some cartridges, a dark spot may sometimes be visualized prior to injection. This is the proximal end of the needle and does not represent a foreign body in, or other abnormality of, the suspension.)

Thus, before the needle is inserted into the selected muscle, it is important for the operator to orient the yellow rectangle so that any blood which may enter after needle insertion and during aspiration can be visualized in the area on the cartridge where it will appear and not be obscured by any obstructions.

After selection of the proper site and insertion of the needle into the selected muscle, aspirate by pulling back on the plunger. While maintaining negative pressure for 2 to 3 seconds, carefully observe the barrel of the cartridge in the area previously identified (see above) for the appearance of a red or dark-colored "spot."

Blood or "typical blood color" may not be seen if a blood vessel has been entered—only a mixture of blood and Wycillin. The appearance of any discoloration is reason to withdraw the needle and discard the glass TUBEX cartridge. If it is elected to inject at another site, a new cartridge should be used. If no blood or discoloration appears, inject the contents of the cartridge slowly. Discontinue delivery of the dose if the subject complains of severe immediate pain at the injection site or if, especially in infants and young children, symptoms or signs occur suggesting onset of severe pain.

Some TUBEX cartridges may contain a small air bubble which may be disregarded, since it does not affect administration of the product.

Because of the high concentration of suspended material in this product, the needle may be blocked if the injection is not made at a slow, steady rate.

When using the disposable syringe:
The Wyeth disposable syringe for this product incorporates several features that are designed to facilitate its use.
A single small indentation, or "dot", has been punched into the metal ring that surrounds the neck of the syringe near the base of the needle. It is important that this "dot" be placed in a position so that it can be easily visualized by the operator following the intramuscular insertion of the syringe needle.

After selection of the proper site and insertion of the needle into the selected muscle, aspirate by pulling back on the plunger. While maintaining negative pressure for 2 to 3 seconds, carefully observe the barrel of the syringe immediately proximal to the location of the "dot" for appearance of blood or any discoloration. Blood or "typical blood color" may *not* be seen if a blood vessel has been entered—only a mixture of blood and Wycillin. The appearance of any discoloration is reason to withdraw the needle and discard the syringe. If it is elected to inject at another site, a new syringe should be used. If no blood or discoloration appears, inject the contents

of the syringe slowly. Discontinue delivery of the dose if the subject complains of severe immediate pain at the injection site or if in infants and young children symptoms or signs occur suggesting onset of severe pain.

Pneumonia (pneumococcal), moderately severe (uncomplicated): 600,000–1,000,000 units daily.

Streptococcal infections (Group A), moderately severe to severe tonsillitis, erysipelas, scarlet fever, upper respiratory tract, skin and soft tissue: 600,000–1,000,000 units daily for 10-day minimum.

Staphylococcal infections, moderately severe to severe: 600,000–1,000,000 units daily.

In pneumonia, streptococcal (Group A) and staphylococcal infections in children under 60 pounds: 300,000 units daily.

Bacterial endocarditis (Group A streptococci) only in extremely sensitive infections: 600,000–1,000,000 units daily.

For prophylaxis against bacterial endocarditis[1] in patients with congenital heart disease or rheumatic or other acquired valvular heart disease when undergoing dental procedures or surgical procedures of the upper respiratory tract, use a combined parenteral-oral regimen. One million units of aqueous crystalline penicillin G (30,000 units/kg in children) intramuscularly mixed with 600,000 units penicillin G procaine (600,000 units for children) should be given one-half to one hour before the procedure. Oral penicillin V (phenoxymethyl penicillin), 500 mg for adults or 250 mg for children less than 60 lbs., should be given every 6 hours for 8 doses. Doses for children should not exceed recommendations for adults for a single dose or for a 24-hour period.

Syphilis—
Primary, secondary, and latent with a negative spinal fluid in adults and children over 12 years of age: 600,000 units daily for 8 days—total 4,800,000 units.

Late (tertiary, neurosyphilis, and latent syphilis with positive spinal-fluid examination or no spinal-fluid examination): 600,000 units daily for 10 to 15 days—total 6 to 9 million units.

Congenital syphilis under 70-lb. body weight: 10,000 units/ kg/day for 10 days.

Yaws, Bejel, and Pinta: Treatment as syphilis in corresponding stage of disease.

Although some isolates of *Neisseria gonorrhoeae* have decreased susceptibility to penicillin, this inherent resistance is relative, not absolute, and penicillin in large doses remains the drug of choice for these strains. Strains producing penicillinase, however, are resistant to penicillin G, and a drug other than penicillin G should be used. Physicians are cautioned not to use less than the recommended doses.

GONORRHEAL INFECTIONS (UNCOMPLICATED)—
MEN OR WOMEN: Aqueous penicillin G procaine, 4.8 million units intramuscularly, divided into at least two doses and injected at different sites at one visit, together with 1 gram of oral probenecid, preferably given just before the injection.

NOTE: Treatment of severe complications of gonorrhea should be individualized, using large amounts of short-acting penicillin. Gonorrheal endocarditis should be treated intensively with aqueous penicillin G. Prophylactic or epidemiologic treatment for gonorrhea (male and female) is accomplished with the same treatment schedules as for the uncomplicated gonorrhea.

Retreatment
The National Center for Disease Control, Venereal Disease Branch, U.S. Department of Health, Education and Welfare, Atlanta, Georgia, recommends:
Test of cure procedures at approximately 7 to 14 days after therapy. In the male, a gram-stained smear is adequate if positive; otherwise, a culture specimen should be obtained from the anterior urethra. In the female, culture specimens should be obtained from both the endocervical and anal canal sites.

Retreatment in the male is indicated if the urethral discharge persists for three or more days following initial therapy and the smear or culture remains positive. Follow-up treatment consists of 4,800,000 units of aqueous penicillin G procaine intramuscularly, divided in two injection sites at a single visit.

In uncomplicated gonorrhea in the female, retreatment is indicated if follow-up cervical or rectal cultures remain positive for *N. gonorrhoeae*. Follow-up treatment consists of 4,800,000 units of aqueous penicillin G procaine daily on two successive days.

SYPHILIS: All gonorrhea patients should have a serologic test for syphilis at the time of diagnosis. Patients with gonorrhea who also have syphilis should be given additional treatment appropriate to the stage of syphilis.

Diphtheria — adjunctive therapy with antitoxin: 300,000 to 600,000 units daily.

Diphtheria carrier state: 300,000 units daily for 10 days.

Anthrax-cutaneous: 600,000 to 1,000,000 units/day.

Vincent's infection (fusospirochetosis): 600,000 to 1,000,000 units/day.

Erysipeloid: 600,000 to 1,000,000 units/day.

Streptobacillus moniliformis and *Spirillum minus* (rat-bite fever): 600,000 to 1,000,000 units/day.

HOW SUPPLIED
Wycillin® (sterile penicillin G procaine suspension), Wyeth®, is available in packages of 10 TUBEX Sterile Cartridge-Needle Units (20 gauge × 1¼ inch needle), NDC 0008-0018, as follows: 1 mL size, 600,000 units per TUBEX; and 2 mL size, 1,200,000 units per TUBEX; and in 4 mL size single-dose disposable syringe (18 gauge × 2 inch needle), 2,400,000 units, in packages of 10 disposable syringes.
Store in a refrigerator.
Keep from freezing.

REFERENCES
1. American Heart Association: Prevention of bacterial endocarditis. *Circulation,* 56: 139A-143A, 1977.
2. SHAW, E.: Transverse myelitis from injection of penicillin. *Am. J. Dis. Child.,* 11: 548, 1966.
3. KNOWLES, J.: Accidental intra-arterial injection of penicillin. *Am. J. Dis. Child.,* 111: 552, 1966.
4. DARBY, C., et al: Ischemia following an intragluteal injection of benzathine-procaine penicillin G mixture in a one-year-old boy. *Clin. Pediatrics,* 12: 485, 1973.
5. BROWN, L. & NELSON, A.: Postinfectious intravascular thrombosis with gangrene. *Arch. Surg.,* 94: 652, 1967.
6. BORENSTINE, J.: Transverse myelitis and penicillin (Correspondence). *Am. J. Dis. Child.,* 112: 166, 1966.
7. ATKINSON, J.: Transverse myelopathy secondary to penicillin injection. *J. Pediatrics,* 75: 867, 1969.
8. TALBERT, J. et al: Gangrene of the foot following intramuscular injection in the lateral thigh: A case report with recommendations for prevention. *J. Pediatrics,* 70: 110, 1967.
9. FISHER, T.: Medicolegal affairs. *Canad. Med. Assoc. J.,* 112: 395, 1975.
10. SCHANZER, H. et al: Accidental intra-arterial injection of penicillin G. *JAMA,* 242: 1289, 1979.

WYCILLIN® and PROBENECID   ℞
[*wi-sil'in and pro-ben'is-id*]
(sterile penicillin G procaine suspension and probenecid tablets)
Disposable Syringe and Tablets
Wycillin is for deep IM injection only.

DESCRIPTION
The Wycillin disposable syringe is designed to provide a stable aqueous suspension of sterile penicillin G procaine, ready for immediate use. This eliminates the necessity for addition of any diluent, required for the usual dry formulation of injectable penicillin.

Each syringe, 2,400,000 units (4 mL size), contains penicillin G procaine in a stabilized aqueous suspension with sodium citrate buffer; and as w/v, approximately 0.5% lecithin, 0.5% carboxymethylcellulose, 0.5% povidone, 0.1% methylparaben, and 0.01% propylparaben.

Wycillin must be stored in a refrigerator. Keep from freezing. This will prevent deterioration and assure that no significant loss of potency occurs within the expiration date.

Probenecid is a uricosuric and renal tubular-blocking agent. Probenecid tablets contain 0.5 gram probenecid. The inactive ingredients present are calcium stearate, D&C Yellow 10, gelatin, hydroxypropyl methylcellulose, iron oxide, magnesium carbonate, polyethylene glycol, starch, talc, and titanium dioxide.

Wycillin suspension in the disposable syringe formulation is viscous and opaque. Read "Contraindications," "Warnings," "Precautions," and "Dosage and Administration" sections prior to use.

ACTIONS AND PHARMACOLOGY
Penicillin G exerts a bactericidal action against penicillin-sensitive microorganisms during the stage of active multiplication. It acts through the inhibition of biosynthesis of cell-wall mucopeptide. It is not active against the penicillinase-producing bacteria, which include many strains of staphylococci. *Neisseria gonorrhoeae* are included among the various organisms which are sensitive to penicillin G. Penicillin G procaine is an equimolecular salt of procaine and penicillin G, administered intramuscularly as a suspension. It dissolves slowly at the site of injection, giving a plateau type of blood level at about 4 hours which falls slowly over a period of the next 15 to 20 hours. Approximately 60% to 90% of a dose of penicillin G is excreted in the urine within 24 to 36 hours.

Approximately 60% of penicillin G is bound to serum protein. The drug is distributed throughout the body tissues in widely varying amounts, with highest levels found in the kidneys and lesser amounts in the liver, skin, and intestines. Penicillin G penetrates into all other tissues to a lesser degree, with a very small level found in the cerebrospinal fluid. With normal kidney function the drug is excreted rapidly by tubular excretion. In neonates and young infants and in individuals with impaired kidney function, excretion is considerably delayed.

Continued on next page

Wyeth-Ayerst Laboratories—Cont.

Probenecid inhibits the tubular reabsorption of urate, thus increasing the urinary excretion of uric acid and decreasing serum uric acid levels. It also inhibits the tubular excretion of penicillin and usually increases penicillin plasma levels, regardless of the route by which the antibiotic is given. A 2-fold to 4-fold elevation has been demonstrated for various penicillins. Probenecid does not influence plasma concentrations of salicylates, nor the excretion of streptomycin, chloramphenicol, chlortetracycline, oxytetracycline, or neomycin.

INDICATIONS

Wycillin and Probenecid is indicated for the single-dose treatment of uncomplicated (without bacteremia) urethral, cervical, rectal, or pharyngeal infections caused by *Neisseria gonorrhoeae* (gonorrhea) in men and women.
Susceptibility studies should be performed when recurrent infections or resistant strains are encountered. Urethritis and the presence of gram-negative diplococci in urethral smears are strong presumptive evidence of gonorrhea. Culture or fluorescent antibody studies will confirm the diagnosis. Therapy may be instituted prior to obtaining results of susceptibility testing.

CONTRAINDICATIONS

A history of a previous hypersensitivity reaction to any of the penicillins or to Probenecid is a contraindication.
Probenecid is not recommended in persons with known blood dyscrasias or uric acid kidney stones or during an acute attack of gout. It is not recommended in conjunction with penicillin G procaine suspension in the presence of known renal impairment.
Do not inject into or near an artery or nerve.

WARNINGS

PENICILLIN G PROCAINE: Serious and occasionally fatal hypersensitivity (anaphylactoid) reactions have been reported in patients on penicillin therapy. Serious anaphylactoid reactions require immediate emergency treatment with epinephrine. Oxygen and intravenous corticosteroids should also be administered as indicated. Although anaphylaxis is more frequent following parenteral therapy, it has occurred in patients on oral penicillins. These reactions are more apt to occur in individuals with a history of sensitivity to multiple allergens.

There have been well-documented reports of individuals with a history of penicillin-hypersensitivity reactions who have experienced severe hypersensitivity reactions when treated with a cephalosporin. Before therapy with a penicillin, careful inquiry should be made concerning previous hypersensitivity reactions to penicillins, cephalosporins, and other allergens. If an allergic reaction occurs, the drug should be discontinued and the patient treated with the usual agents, e.g., pressor amines, antihistamines, and corticosteroids.

Immediate toxic reactions to procaine may occur in some individuals, particularly when a large single dose is administered in the treatment of gonorrhea (4.8 million units). These reactions may be manifested by mental disturbances, including anxiety, confusion, agitation, depression, weakness, seizures, hallucinations, combativeness, and expressed "fear of impending death." The reactions noted in carefully controlled studies occurred in approximately one in 500 patients treated for gonorrhea. Reactions are transient, lasting from 15 to 30 minutes.

Inadvertent intravascular administration, including inadvertent direct intraarterial injection or injection immediately adjacent to arteries, of Wycillin and other penicillin preparations has resulted in severe neurovascular damage, including transverse myelitis with permanent paralysis, gangrene requiring amputation of digits and more proximal portions of extremities, and necrosis and sloughing at and surrounding the injection site. Such severe effects have been reported following injections into the buttock, thigh, and deltoid areas. Other serious complications of suspected intravascular administration which have been reported include immediate pallor, mottling or cyanosis of the extremity both distal and proximal to the injection site followed by bleb formation; severe edema requiring anterior and/or posterior compartment fasciotomy in the lower extremity. The above-described severe effects and complications have most often occurred in infants and small children. Prompt consultation with an appropriate specialist is indicated if any evidence of compromise of the blood supply occurs at, proximal to, or distal to the site of injection.[1-9] See "Contraindications," "Precautions," and "Dosage and Administration" sections.
Quadriceps femoris fibrosis and atrophy have been reported following repeated intramuscular injections of penicillin preparations into the anterolateral thigh.
Injection into or near a nerve may result in permanent neurological damage.
PROBENECID: Exacerbation of gout following therapy with Probenecid may occur; in such cases colchicine therapy is advisable.

In patients on Probenecid, the use of salicylates in either small or large doses is not recommended because it antagonizes the uricosuric action of Probenecid. Patients on Probenecid who require a mild analgesic agent should receive acetaminophen rather than salicylates, even in small doses.
USAGE IN PREGNANCY: The safety of these drugs for use in pregnancy has not been established.

PRECAUTIONS

PENICILLIN G PROCAINE: When treating gonococcal infections in which primary or secondary syphilis may be suspected, proper diagnostic procedures, including dark-field examinations, should be done. In all cases in which concomitant syphilis is suspected, monthly serological tests should be made for at least four months. Patients with gonorrhea, who also have syphilis, should be given additional appropriate parenteral penicillin treatment.
Penicillin should be used with caution in individuals with histories of significant allergies and/or asthma. When administering Wycillin, care should be taken to avoid intravenous or intra-arterial administration, or injection into or near major peripheral nerves or blood vessels, since such injections may produce neurovascular damage. See "Contraindications," "Warnings," and "Dosage and Administration" sections.
A small percentage of patients are sensitive to procaine. If there is a history of sensitivity, make the usual test: Inject intradermally 0.1 mL of a 1- to 2-percent procaine solution. Development of an erythema, wheal, flare, or eruption indicates procaine sensitivity. Sensitivity should be treated by the usual methods, including barbiturates, and procaine penicillin preparations should not be used. Antihistaminics appear beneficial in treatment of procaine reactions.
PROBENECID: Use Probenecid with caution in patients with a history of peptic ulcer. A reducing substance may appear in the urine of patients receiving Probenecid. Although this disappears with discontinuance of therapy, a false diagnosis of glycosuria may be made because of a false-positive Benedict's test.

ADVERSE REACTIONS

WYCILLIN: Penicillin is a substance of low toxicity but does possess a significant index of sensitization. The following hypersensitivity reactions associated with use of penicillin have been reported: skin rashes, ranging from maculopapular eruptions to exfoliative dermatitis; urticaria; serum-sickness like reactions, including chills, fever, edema, arthralgia, and prostration. Severe and often fatal anaphylaxis has been reported (see "Warnings"). As with other treatments for syphilis, the Jarisch-Herxheimer reaction has been reported.
Procaine toxicity manifestations have been reported (see "Warnings"). Although procaine hypersensitivity reactions have not been reported with this drug, there are patients who are sensitive to procaine (see "Precautions").
PROBENECID: The following are the principal adverse reactions which have been reported as associated with the use of Probenecid, generally with more prolonged or repeated administration: Hypersensitivity reactions (including anaphylaxis), nephrotic syndrome, hepatic necrosis, aplastic anemia; also other anemias, including hemolytic anemia related to genetic deficiency of glucose-6-phosphate dehydrogenase.

DOSAGE AND ADMINISTRATION

Parenteral drug products should be inspected visually for particulate matter and discoloration prior to administration, whenever solution and container permit.
Penicillin G procaine (aqueous) is for intramuscular injection only.
Administer by DEEP INTRAMUSCULAR INJECTION in the upper, outer quadrant of the buttock. When doses are repeated, vary the injection site.
The Wyeth disposable syringe for this product incorporates several new features that are designed to facilitate its use. A single small indentation, or "dot", has been punched into the metal ring that surrounds the neck of the syringe near the base of the needle. It is important that this "dot" be placed in a position so that it can be easily visualized by the operator following the intramuscular insertion of the syringe needle.
After selection of the proper site and insertion of the needle into the selected muscle, aspirate by pulling back on the plunger. While maintaining negative pressure for 2 to 3 seconds, carefully observe the barrel of the syringe immediately proximal to the location of the "dot" for appearance of blood or any discoloration. Blood or "typical blood color" may *not* be seen if a blood vessel has been entered—only a mixture of blood and Wycillin. The appearance of any discoloration is reason to withdraw the needle and discard the syringe. If it is elected to inject at another site, a new syringe should be used. If no blood or discoloration appears, inject the contents of the syringe slowly. Discontinue delivery of the dose if the subject complains of severe immediate pain at the injection site or if in infants and young children symptoms or signs occur suggesting onset of severe pain.
Although some isolates of *Neisseria gonorrhoeae* have decreased susceptibility to penicillin, this inherent resistance

is relative, not absolute, and penicillin in large doses remains the drug of choice for these strains. Strains producing penicillinase, however, are resistant to penicillin G, and a drug other than penicillin G should be used.
GONORRHEAL INFECTIONS (UNCOMPLICATED) MEN OR WOMEN: Aqueous penicillin G procaine, 4.8 million units intramuscularly, divided into at least two doses and injected at different sites at one visit, together with 1 gram (2 tablets, 0.5 gram each) of Probenecid orally, given just before the injections. Physicians are cautioned to use no less than the recommended dosages.
NOTE: Treatment of severe complications of gonorrhea should be individualized, using large amounts of short-acting penicillin. Gonorrheal endocarditis should be treated intensively with aqueous penicillin G. Prophylactic or epidemiologic treatment for gonorrhea (male and female) is accomplished with the same treatment schedules as for the uncomplicated gonorrhea.
RETREATMENT: The National Center for Disease Control, Venereal Disease Branch, U.S. Department of Health, Education and Welfare, Atlanta, Georgia, recommends:
Test of cure procedures at approximately 7 to 14 days after therapy. In the male, a gram-stained smear is adequate if positive; otherwise, a culture specimen should be obtained from the anterior urethra. In the female, culture specimens should be obtained from both the endocervical and anal canal sites.
Retreatment in the male is indicated if the urethral discharge persists for three or more days following initial therapy and the smear or culture remains positive. Follow-up treatment consists of 4,800,000 units of aqueous penicillin G procaine, intramuscular, divided in two injection sites at a single visit.
In uncomplicated gonorrhea in the female, retreatment is indicated if follow-up cervical or rectal cultures remain positive for *N. gonorrhoeae*. Follow-up treatment consists of 4,800,000 units of aqueous penicillin G procaine daily on two successive days.
SYPHILIS: All gonorrhea patients should have a serologic test for syphilis at the time of diagnosis. Patients with gonorrhea who also have syphilis should be given additional treatment appropriate to the stage of syphilis.

HOW SUPPLIED

Wycillin® (sterile penicillin G procaine suspension) Injection and Probenecid Tablets is supplied as a combination package, NDC 0008-2517, containing the following:
Two disposable syringes of Wycillin (2,400,000 units each), 4 mL size (18 gauge × 2 inch needle), and
Two tablets Probenecid, Benemid® (0.5 gram each).
Store in a refrigerator—Keep from freezing.
Wycillin® Disposable Syringes manufactured by **Wyeth-Ayerst Laboratories Inc.**, Philadelphia, PA 19101
Probenecid Tablets (Benemid®) manufactured by **Merck, Sharp and Dohme,** Division of Merck & Co., West Point, PA 19486

REFERENCES

1. SHAW, E.: Transverse myelitis from injection of penicillin. *Am. J. Dis. Child.,* 111: 548, 1966.
2. KNOWLES, J.: Accidental intra-arterial injection of penicillin. *Am. J. Dis. Child.,* 111: 552, 1966.
3. DARBY, C., et al: Ischemia following an intragluteal injection of benzathine-procaine penicillin G mixture in a one-year-old boy. *Clin. Pediatrics,* 12: 485, 1973.
4. BROWN, L. & NELSON, A.: Postinfectious intravascular thrombosis with gangrene. *Arch. Surg.,* 94: 652, 1967.
5. BORENSTINE, J.: Transverse myelitis and penicillin (Correspondence). *Am. J. Dis. Child.,* 112: 166, 1966.
6. ATKINSON, J.: Transverse myelopathy secondary to penicillin injection. *J. Pediatrics,* 75: 867, 1969.
7. TALBERT, J. et al: Gangrene of the foot following intramuscular injection in the lateral thigh: A case report with recommendations for prevention. *J. Pediatrics,* 70: 110, 1967.
8. FISHER, T.: Medicolegal affairs. *Canad. Med. Assoc. J.,* 112: 395, 1975.
9. SCHANZER, H. et al: Accidental intra-arterial injection of penicillin G. *JAMA,* 242: 1289, 1979.

WYDASE®   ℞
[wi-dās]
(hyaluronidase)

DESCRIPTION

Wydase, a protein enzyme, is a preparation of highly purified bovine testicular hyaluronidase. The exact chemical structure of this enzyme is unknown. Wydase is available in two dosage forms:
WYDASE LYOPHILIZED
Hyaluronidase, dehydrated in the frozen state under high vacuum, with lactose and thimerosal (mercury derivative), is supplied as a sterile, white, odorless, amorphous solid and is to be reconstituted with Sodium Chloride Injection, USP,

before use, usually in the proportion of one mL per 150 USP units of hyaluronidase (Wydase Lyophilized).

Each vial of 1,500 USP units contains 1.0 mg thimerosal (mercury derivative), added as a preservative, and 13.3 mg lactose. Each vial of 150 USP units contains 0.075 mg thimerosal (mercury derivative), added as a preservative, and 2.66 mg lactose.

WYDASE STABILIZED SOLUTION

A hyaluronidase injection solution ready for use, colorless and odorless, containing 150 USP units of hyaluronidase per mL with 8.5 mg sodium chloride, 1 mg edetate disodium, 0.4 mg calcium chloride, monobasic sodium phosphate buffer, and not more than 0.1 mg thimerosal (mercury derivative).

The USP and the NF hyaluronidase units are the equivalent to the turbidity-reducing (TR) unit and to the International Unit.

HOW SUPPLIED

Wydase®, Lyophilized, Wyeth®, is supplied as follows:

150 USP (TR) units of hyaluronidase

NDC 0008-0121-01, 1 mL vial, as single vials.

Not Recommended for IV Use.

Store at controlled room temperature in a dry place. Store sterile reconstituted solution below 30°C (86°F). Use within 24 hours.

1,500 USP (TR) units of hyaluronidase

NDC 0008-0149-01, 10 mL vial, as single vials.

Not Recommended for IV Use.

Store at controlled room temperature in a dry place. Store sterile reconstituted solution below 30°C (86°F). Use within 14 days.

Wydase®, Stabilized Solution, Wyeth®, is supplied as follows:

150 USP (TR) units of hyaluronidase per mL

NDC 0008-0170-01, 1 mL vial, as single vials.

NDC 0008-0170-02, 10 mL vial, as single vials.

Not Recommended for IV Use.

Must be refrigerated.

Do not use if solution is discolored or contains a precipitate.
For prescribing information write to Professional Service, Wyeth-Ayerst Laboratories, P.O. Box 8299, Philadelphia, PA 19101, or contact your local Wyeth-Ayerst representative.

WYGESIC®
[wi-je'zik]
(propoxyphene HCl and acetaminophen)
Tablets

Ⓒ℞

DESCRIPTION

Wygesic tablets contain 65 mg propoxyphene HCl and 650 mg acetaminophen. The inactive ingredients present are cellulose, D&C Yellow 10, FD&C Blue 1, FD&C Yellow 6, hydrogenated vegetable oil, hydroxypropyl methylcellulose, methylcellulose, polacrilin potassium, and titanium dioxide. Propoxyphene hydrochloride is an odorless white crystalline powder with a bitter taste. It is freely soluble in water. Chemically, it is [S-(R*,S*)]-α[2-(dimethylamino)-1-methylethyl]-α-phenylbenzeneethanol, propanoate (ester), hydrochloride, which can be represented by the following structural formula:

$$(CH_3)_2NCH_2-\underset{\underset{H}{|}}{\overset{\overset{CH_3}{|}}{C}}-\underset{C_6H_5}{\overset{\overset{O}{\overset{||}{OCC_2H_5}}}{C}}-CH_2-C_6H_5 \cdot HCl$$

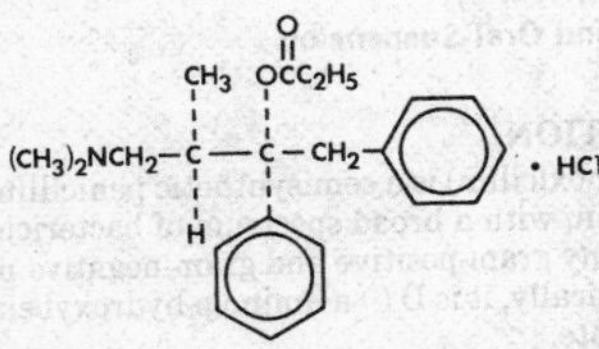

Acetaminophen is a white, crystalline powder, possessing a slightly bitter taste. It is soluble in boiling water and freely soluble in alcohol. Chemically, it is N-Acetyl-p-aminophenol, which can be presented by the following structural formula:

$$HO-C_6H_4-NHCOCH_3$$

CLINICAL PHARMACOLOGY

Propoxyphene is a centrally acting narcotic analgesic agent. Equimolar doses of propoxyphene hydrochloride provide similar plasma concentrations. Following administration of 65, 130, or 195 mg of propoxyphene hydrochloride, the bioavailability of propoxyphene is equivalent to that of 100, 200, or 300 mg respectively of propoxyphene napsylate. Peak plasma concentrations of propoxyphene are reached in 2 to 2½ hours. After a 65 mg oral dose of propoxyphene hydrochloride, peak plasma levels of 0.05 to 0.1 mcg/mL are achieved.

Repeated doses of propoxyphene at 6-hour intervals lead to increasing plasma concentrations, with a plateau after the ninth dose at 48 hours.

Propoxyphene is metabolized in the liver to yield norpropoxyphene. Propoxyphene has a half-life of 6 to 12 hours, whereas that of norpropoxyphene is 30 to 36 hours.

Norpropoxyphene has substantially less central nervous system depressant effect than propoxyphene, but a greater local anesthetic effect, which is similar to that of amitriptyline and antiarrhythmic agents, such as lidocaine and quinidine.

In animal studies in which propoxyphene and norpropoxyphene were continuously infused in large amounts, intracardiac conduction time (P-R and QRS intervals) was prolonged. Any intracardiac conduction delay attributable to high concentrations of norpropoxyphene may be of relatively long duration.

ACTIONS

Propoxyphene is a mild narcotic analgesic structurally related to methadone. The potency of propoxyphene hydrochloride is from two-thirds to equal that of codeine.

Propoxyphene hydrochloride and acetaminophen provide the analgesic activity of propoxyphene napsylate and the antipyretic-analgesic activity of acetaminophen.

The combination of propoxyphene and acetaminophen produces greater analgesia than that produced by either propoxyphene or acetaminophen alone.

INDICATIONS

Wygesic is indicated for the relief of mild-to-moderate pain, either when pain is present alone or when it is accompanied by fever.

CONTRAINDICATIONS

Hypersensitivity to propoxyphene or to acetaminophen.

WARNINGS

Do not prescribe propoxyphene for patients who are suicidal or addiction-prone.

Prescribe propoxyphene with caution for patients taking tranquilizers or antidepressant drugs and patients who use alcohol in excess.

Tell your patients not to exceed the recommended dose and to limit their intake of alcohol.

Propoxyphene products in excessive doses, either alone or in combination with other CNS depressants, including alcohol, are a major cause of drug-related deaths. Fatalities within the first hour of overdosage are not uncommon. In a survey of deaths due to overdosage conducted in 1975, in approximately 20% of the fatal cases, death occurred within the first hour (5% occurred within 15 minutes). Propoxyphene should not be taken in doses higher than those recommended by the physician. The judicious prescribing of propoxyphene is essential to the safe use of this drug. With patients who are depressed or suicidal, consideration should be given to the use of nonnarcotic analgesics. Patients should be cautioned about the concomitant use of propoxyphene products and alcohol because of potentially serious CNS-additive effects of these agents. Because of its added depressant effects, propoxyphene should be prescribed with caution for those patients whose medical condition requires the concomitant administration of sedatives, tranquilizers, muscle relaxants, antidepressants, or other CNS-depressant drugs. Patients should be advised of the additive depressant effects of these combinations.

Many of the propoxyphene-related deaths have occurred in patients with previous histories of emotional disturbances or suicidal ideation or attempts as well as histories of misuse of tranquilizers, alcohol, and other CNS-active drugs. Some deaths have occurred as a consequence of the accidental ingestion of excessive quantities of propoxyphene alone or in combination with other drugs. Patients taking propoxyphene should be warned not to exceed the dosage recommended by the physician.

DRUG DEPENDENCE:

Propoxyphene, when taken in higher-than-recommended doses over long periods of time, can produce drug dependence characterized by psychic dependence and, less frequently, physical dependence and tolerance. Propoxyphene will only partially suppress the withdrawal syndrome in individuals physically dependent on morphine or other narcotics. The abuse liability of propoxyphene is qualitatively similar to that of codeine although quantitatively less, and propoxyphene should be prescribed with the same degree of caution appropriate to the use of codeine.

USAGE IN AMBULATORY PATIENTS:

Propoxyphene may impair the mental and/or physical abilities required for the performance of potentially hazardous tasks, such as driving a car or operating machinery. The patient should be cautioned accordingly.

PRECAUTIONS

GENERAL:

Propoxyphene should be administered with caution to patients with hepatic or renal impairment since higher serum concentrations or delayed elimination may occur.

DRUG INTERACTIONS:

The CNS-depressant effect of propoxyphene is additive with that of other CNS depressants, including alcohol.

As is the case with many medicinal agents, propoxyphene may slow the metabolism of a concomitantly administered drug. Should this occur, the higher serum concentrations of that drug may result in increased pharmacologic or adverse effects of that drug. Such occurrences have been reported when propoxyphene was administered to patients on antidepressants, anticonvulsants, or warfarin-like drugs.

USAGE IN PREGNANCY:

Safe use in pregnancy has not been established relative to possible adverse effects on fetal development. Instances of withdrawal symptoms in the neonate have been reported following usage during pregnancy. Therefore, propoxyphene should not be used in pregnant women unless, in the judgment of the physician, the potential benefits outweigh the possible hazards.

USAGE IN NURSING MOTHERS:

Low levels of propoxyphene have been detected in human milk. In postpartum studies involving nursing mothers who were given propoxyphene, no adverse effects were noted in infants receiving mother's milk.

USAGE IN CHILDREN:

Propoxyphene is not recommended for use in children, because documented clinical experience has been insufficient to establish safety and a suitable dosage regimen in the pediatric age group.

A Patient Information Sheet is available for this product. See text following "How Supplied" section below.

ADVERSE REACTIONS

In a survey conducted in hospitalized patients, less than 1% of patients taking propoxyphene hydrochloride at recommended doses experienced side effects. The most frequently reported have been dizziness, sedation, nausea, and vomiting. Some of these adverse reactions may be alleviated if the patient lies down.

Other adverse reactions include constipation, abdominal pain, skin rashes, light-headedness, headache, weakness, euphoria, dysphoria, and minor visual disturbances.

Liver dysfunction has been reported in association with both active components of propoxyphene and acetaminophen tablets.

Propoxyphene therapy has been associated with abnormal liver-function tests and, more rarely, with instances of reversible jaundice.

Hepatic necrosis may result from acute overdoses of acetaminophen (see Management of Overdosage). In chronic ethanol abusers, this has been reported rarely with short-term use of acetaminophen doses of 2.5 to 10 g/day. Fatalities have occurred.

MANAGEMENT OF OVERDOSAGE

In all cases of suspected overdosage, call your regional Poison Control Center to obtain the most up-to-date information about the treatment of overdosage. This recommendation is made because, in general, information regarding the treatment of overdosage may change more rapidly than do package inserts.

Initial consideration should be given to the management of the CNS effects of propoxyphene overdosage. Resuscitative measures should be initiated promptly.

SYMPTOMS OF PROPOXYPHENE OVERDOSAGE:

The manifestations of acute overdosage with propoxyphene are those of narcotic overdosage. The patient is usually somnolent, but may be stuporous or comatose and convulsing. Respiratory depression is characteristic. The ventilatory rate and/or tidal volume is decreased, which results in cyanosis and hypoxia. Pupils, initially pinpoint, may become dilated as hypoxia increases. Cheyne-Stokes respiration and apnea may occur. Blood pressure and heart rate are usually normal initially, but blood pressure falls and cardiac performance deteriorates, which ultimately results in pulmonary edema and circulatory collapse unless the respiratory depression is corrected and adequate ventilation is restored promptly. Cardiac arrhythmias and conduction delay may be present. A combined respiratory-metabolic acidosis occurs, owing to retained CO_2 (hypercapnea) and to lactic acid formed during anaerobic glycolysis. Acidosis may be severe if large amounts of salicylates have also been ingested. Death may occur.

TREATMENT OF PROPOXYPHENE OVERDOSAGE:

Attention should be directed first to establishing a patent airway and to restoring ventilation. Mechanically assisted ventilation, with or without oxygen, may be required, and positive-pressure respiration may be desirable if pulmonary edema is present.

Continued on next page

Wyeth-Ayerst Laboratories—Cont.

The narcotic antagonist naloxone hydrochloride will markedly reduce the degree of respiratory depression, and 0.4 to 2 mg should be administered promptly, preferably intravenously. If the desired degree of counteraction with improvement in respiratory function is not obtained, naloxone should be repeated at 2- to 3-minute intervals. The duration of action of the antagonist may be brief. If no response is observed after 10 mg of naloxone have been administered, the diagnosis of propoxyphene toxicity should be questioned. Naloxone hydrochloride may also be administered by continuous intravenous infusion.

TREATMENT OF PROPOXYPHENE OVERDOSAGE IN CHILDREN:
The usual initial dose of naloxone in children is 0.01 mg/kg body weight given intravenously. If this dose does not result in the desired degree of clinical improvement, a subsequent increased dose of 0.1 mg/kg body weight may be administered. If an IV route of administration is not available, naloxone may be administered IM or subcutaneously in divided doses. If necessary, naloxone can be diluted with sterile water for injection.

Blood gases, pH, and electrolytes should be monitored in order that acidosis and any electrolyte disturbance present may be corrected promptly. Acidosis, hypoxia, and generalized CNS depression predispose to the development of cardiac arrhythmias. Ventricular fibrillation or cardiac arrest may occur and necessitate the full complement of cardiopulmonary resuscitation (CPR) measures. Respiratory acidosis rapidly subsides as ventilation is restored and hypercapnea eliminated, but lactic acidosis may require intravenous bicarbonate for prompt correction.

Electrocardiographic monitoring is essential. Prompt correction of hypoxia, acidosis, and electrolyte disturbance (when present) will help prevent these cardiac complications and will increase the effectiveness of agents administered to restore normal cardiac function.

In addition to the use of a narcotic antagonist, the patient may require careful titration with an anticonvulsant to control convulsions. Analeptic drugs (for example, caffeine or amphetamine) should not be used because of their tendency to precipitate convulsions.

General supportive measures, in addition to oxygen, include, when necessary, intravenous fluids, vasopressor-inotropic compounds, and, when infection is likely, anti-infective agents. Gastric lavage may be useful, and activated charcoal can adsorb a significant amount of ingested propoxyphene. Dialysis is of little value in poisoning due to propoxyphene. Efforts should be made to determine whether other agents, such as alcohol, barbiturates, tranquilizers, or other CNS depressants, were also ingested, since these increase CNS depression as well as cause specific toxic effects.

SYMPTOMS OF ACETAMINOPHEN OVERDOSAGE:
Shortly after oral ingestion of an overdosage of acetaminophen and for the next 24 hours, anorexia, nausea, vomiting, and abdominal pain have been noted. The patient may then present no symptoms, but evidence of liver dysfunction may be apparent during the next 24 to 48 hours, with elevated serum transaminase and lactic dehydrogenase levels, an increase in serum bilirubin concentrations, and a prolonged prothrombin time. Death from hepatic failure may result 3 to 7 days after overdosage.

Acute renal failure may accompany the hepatic dysfunction and has been noted in patients who do not exhibit signs of fulminant hepatic failure. Typically, renal impairment is more apparent 6 to 9 days after ingestion of the overdose.

TREATMENT OF ACETAMINOPHEN OVERDOSAGE:
Acetaminophen in massive overdosage may cause hepatic toxicity in some patients. In all cases of suspected overdose, you may wish to call your regional poison center for assistance in diagnosis and for directions in the use of N-acetylcysteine as an antidote.

In adults, hepatic toxicity has rarely been reported with acute overdoses of less than 10 g and fatalities with less than 15 g. Importantly, young children seem to be more resistant than adults to the hepatotoxic effect of an acetaminophen overdose. Despite this, the measures outlined below should be initiated in any adult or child suspected of having ingested an acetaminophen overdose. Clinical and laboratory evidence of hepatic toxicity may not be apparent until 48 to 72 hours postingestion. Early symptoms following a potentially hepatotoxic overdose may include: nausea, vomiting, diaphoresis, and general malaise.

The stomach should be emptied promptly by lavage or by induction of emesis with syrup of ipecac. Patients' estimates of the quantity of a drug ingested are notoriously unreliable. Therefore, if an acetaminophen overdose is suspected, a serum acetaminophen assay should be obtained as early as possible, but no sooner than four hours following ingestion. Liver-function studies should be obtained initially and repeated at 24-hour intervals.

The antidote, N-acetylcysteine, should be administered as early as possible, preferably within 16 hours of the overdose

ingestion for optimal results, but in any case, within 24 hours. Following recovery, there are no residual, structural or functional hepatic abnormalities.

ANIMAL TOXICOLOGY:
The acute lethal doses of the hydrochloride and napsylate salts of propoxyphene were determined in 4 species. The results shown in Figure 1 indicate that on a molar basis, the napsylate salt is less toxic than the hydrochloride. This may be due to the relative insolubility and retarded absorption of propoxyphene napsylate.

FIGURE 1
ACUTE ORAL TOXICITY OF PROPOXYPHENE
LD50 (mg/kg)=SE
LD50 (mMole/kg)

Species	Propoxyphene Hydrochloride	Propoxyphene Napsylate
Mouse	282 ± 39	915 ± 163
	0.75	1.62
Rat	230 ± 44	647 ± 95
	0.61	1.14
Rabbit	ca. 82	>183
	0.22	>0.32
Dog	ca. 100	>183
	0.27	>0.32

Some indication of the relative insolubility and retarded absorption of propoxyphene napsylate was obtained by measuring plasma propoxyphene levels in 2 groups of 4 dogs following oral administration of equimolar doses of the 2 salts. Although none of the animals in this experiment died, 3 of the 4 dogs given propoxyphene hydrochloride exhibited convulsive seizures during the time interval corresponding to the peak plasma levels. The 4 animals receiving the napsylate salt were ataxic but not acutely ill.

DOSAGE AND ADMINISTRATION
The product is given orally. The usual dose is 65 mg propoxyphene HCl and 650 mg acetaminophen every 4 hours as needed for pain. The maximum recommended dose of propoxyphene HCl is 390 mg per day.
Consideration should be given to a reduced total daily dosage in patients with hepatic or renal impairment.

HOW SUPPLIED
Wygesic® (propoxyphene HCl and acetaminophen) Tablets, Wyeth®, 65 mg propoxyphene and 650 mg acetaminophen, are available as follows:
NDC 0008-0085, green, capsule-shaped, scored, film-coated tablet marked "WYETH" and "85", in bottles of 100 and 500 tablets, and in REDIPAK® cartons of 100 tablets (10 blister strips of 10).
Keep tightly closed.
Protect from light.
Store at controlled room temperature, 15°–30°C (59°–86°F).
Dispense in light-resistant, tight container as defined in the USP.

PATIENT INFORMATION
Summary
Products containing propoxyphene are used to relieve pain. LIMIT YOUR INTAKE OF ALCOHOL WHILE TAKING THIS DRUG. Make sure your doctor knows if you are taking tranquilizers, sleep aids, antidepressants, antihistamines, or any other drugs that make you sleepy. Combining propoxyphene with alcohol or these drugs in excessive doses is dangerous.
Use care while driving a car or using machines until you see how the drug affects you, because propoxyphene can make you sleepy. Do not take more of the drug than your doctor prescribed. Dependence has occurred when patients have taken propoxyphene for a long period of time at doses greater than recommended.
The rest of this leaflet gives you more information about propoxyphene. Please read it and keep it for further use.
Uses for Propoxyphene
Products containing propoxyphene are used for the relief of mild to moderate pain. Products which contain propoxyphene plus acetaminophen are prescribed for the relief of pain or pain associated with fever.
Before taking Propoxyphene
Make sure your doctor knows if you have ever had an allergic reaction to propoxyphene or acetaminophen.
The effect of propoxyphene in children under 12 has not been studied. Therefore, use of the drug in this age group is not recommended.
How to take Propoxyphene
Follow your doctor's directions exactly. Do not increase the amount you take without your doctor's approval. If you miss a dose of the drug, do not take twice as much the next time.
Pregnancy
Do not take propoxyphene during pregnancy unless your doctor knows you are pregnant and specifically recommends its use. Cases of temporary dependence in the newborn have occurred when the mother has taken propoxyphene consistently in the weeks before delivery. As a general principle, no drug should be taken during pregnancy unless it is clearly necessary.

General Caution
Heavy use of alcohol with propoxyphene is hazardous and may lead to overdosage symptoms (see "Overdosage" below); THEREFORE, LIMIT YOUR INTAKE OF ALCOHOL WHILE TAKING PROPOXYPHENE.
Combinations of excessive doses of propoxyphene, alcohol, and tranquilizers are dangerous. Make sure your doctor knows if you are taking tranquilizers, sleep aids, antidepressant drugs, antihistamines, or any other drugs that make you sleepy. The use of these drugs with propoxyphene increases their sedative effects and may lead to overdosage symptoms, including death (see "Overdosage" below).
Propoxyphene may cause drowsiness or impair your mental and/or physical abilities; therefore, use caution when driving a vehicle or operating dangerous machinery. DO NOT perform any hazardous task until you have seen your response to this drug.
Propoxyphene may increase the concentration in the body of medications such as anticoagulants ("blood thinners"), antidepressants, or drugs used for epilepsy. The result may be excessive or adverse effects of these medications. Make sure your doctor knows if you are taking any of these medications.
Dependence
You can become dependent on propoxyphene if you take it in higher than recommended doses over a long period of time. Dependence is a feeling of need for the drug and a feeling that you cannot perform normally without it.
Overdosage
An overdosage of propoxyphene, alone or in combination with other drugs, including alcohol, may cause weakness, difficulty in breathing, confusion, anxiety, and more severe drowsiness and dizziness. Extreme overdosage may lead to unconsciousness and death.
If the propoxyphene product contains acetaminophen, the overdosage symptoms include nausea, vomiting, lack of appetite, and abdominal pain. Liver damage may occur.
In any suspected overdosage situation, contact your doctor or nearest hospital emergency room. GET EMERGENCY HELP IMMEDIATELY. KEEP THIS AND ALL DRUGS OUT OF THE REACH OF CHILDREN.
Possible Side Effects
When propoxyphene is taken as directed, side effects are infrequent. Among those reported are drowsiness, dizziness, nausea, and vomiting. If these effects occur, it may help if you lie down and rest.
Less frequently reported side effects are constipation, abdominal pain, skin rashes, light-headedness, headache, weakness, minor visual disturbances, and feelings of elation or discomfort.
If side effects occur and concern you, contact your doctor.
Other Information
The safe and effective use of propoxyphene depends on your taking it exactly as directed. This drug has been prescribed specifically for you and your present condition. Do not give this drug to others who may have similar symptoms. Do not use it for any other reason.
If you would like more information about propoxyphene, ask your doctor or pharmacist. They have a more technical leaflet (professional labeling) you may read.
Shown in Product Identification Section, page 438

WYMOX®   **℞**
[wi 'moks]
(amoxicillin)
Capsules and Oral Suspension

DESCRIPTION
Wymox (amoxicillin) is a semisynthetic penicillin, an analog of ampicillin, with a broad spectrum of bactericidal activity against many gram-positive and gram-negative microorganisms. Chemically, it is D-(-)-a-amino-p-hydroxybenzyl penicillin trihydrate.
Wymox capsules contain amoxicillin as the trihydrate equivalent to 250 mg or 500 mg amoxicillin. The inactive ingredients present are colloidal silicon dioxide, D&C Yellow 10, FD&C Blue 1, gelatin, iron oxide, magnesium stearate, sodium lauryl sulfate, and titanium dioxide.
Wymox oral suspension is a powder which when reconstituted as directed yields a suspension of amoxicillin trihydrate equivalent to 125 mg or 250 mg amoxicillin per 5 mL. The inactive ingredients present are artificial flavors, carboxymethylcellulose sodium, cellulose, citric acid, D&C Red 28; FD&C Red 40, mannitol, sodium citrate, sucrose, and water.

HOW SUPPLIED
Wymox® (amoxicillin) Capsules contain amoxicillin as the trihydrate equivalent to 250 mg or 500 mg amoxicillin and are supplied as follows:
250 mg, NDC 0008-0559, grey and green capsule marked "WYETH" and "559", in bottles of 100 and 500 capsules.
500 mg, NDC 0008-0560, grey and green capsule marked "WYETH" and "560", in bottles of 50 and 500 capsules.

Store at room temperature, approx. 25°C (77°F).
Keep tightly closed.
Protect from light.
Dispense in light-resistant, tight container.
Wymox® (amoxicillin) Oral Suspension is available as a pink powder which when reconstituted as directed yields a palatable, pink suspension of amoxicillin trihydrate equivalent to 125 mg or 250 mg amoxicillin per 5 mL and is supplied as follows:
125 mg per 5 mL, NDC 0008-0557, in bottles to make 100 mL or 150 mL.
250 mg per 5 mL, NDC 0008-0558, in bottles to make 80 mL, 100 mL, or 150 mL.
Store at room temperature, [approx. 25°C (77°F)] before reconstitution.
Keep tightly closed.
Shake well before using.
Store under refrigeration. Discard any unused portion after 14 days.
For prescribing information write to Professional Service, Wyeth-Ayerst Laboratories, P.O. Box 8299, Philadelphia, PA 19101, or contact your local Wyeth-Ayerst representative.
Shown in Product Identification Section, page 438

WYTENSIN® ℞
[wi-ten 'sin]
(guanabenz acetate)

DESCRIPTION
Wytensin (guanabenz acetate), an antihypertensive agent for oral administration, is an aminoguanidine derivative, 2,6-dichlorobenzylideneaminoguanidine acetate, and its structural formula is:

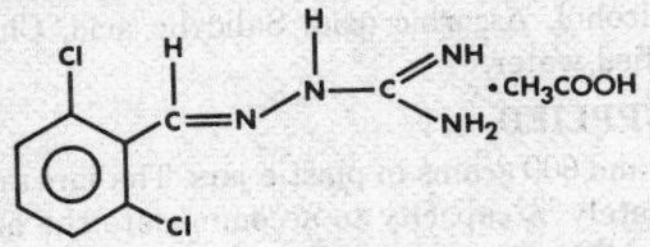

It is an odorless, white to off-white, crystalline substance, sparingly soluble in water and soluble in alcohol, with a molecular weight of 291.14. Each tablet of Wytensin is equivalent to 4 mg or 8 mg of free guanabenz base. The inactive ingredients present are cellulose, iron oxide, lactose, and magnesium stearate. The 8 mg dosage strength also contains FD&C Blue 2.
Wytensin is available as 4 mg or 8 mg tablets for oral administration.

CLINICAL PHARMACOLOGY
Wytensin is an orally active central alpha-2 adrenergic agonist. Its antihypertensive action appears to be mediated via stimulation of central alpha adrenergic receptors, resulting in a decrease of sympathetic outflow from the brain at the bulbar level to the peripheral circulatory system.
PHARMACOKINETICS
In human studies, about 75% of an orally administered dose of Wytensin is absorbed and metabolized with less than 1% of unchanged drug recovered from the urine. Peak plasma concentrations of unchanged drug occur between two and five hours after a single oral dose. The average half-life for Wytensin is about 6 hours. The site or sites of metabolism of Wytensin have not been determined. The effect of meals on the absorption of Wytensin has not been studied.
PHARMACODYNAMICS
The onset of the antihypertensive action of Wytensin begins within 60 minutes after a single oral dose and reaches a peak effect within two to four hours. The effect of an acute single dose is reduced appreciably six to eight hours after administration, and blood pressure approaches baseline values within 12 hours of administration.
The acute antihypertensive effect of Wytensin occurs without major changes in peripheral resistance, but its chronic effect appears to be a decrease in peripheral resistance. A decrease in blood pressure is seen in both the supine and standing positions without alterations of normal postural mechanisms, so that postural hypotension has not been observed. Wytensin decreases pulse rate by about 5 beats per minute. Cardiac output and left ventricular ejection fraction are unchanged during long-term therapy.
In clinical trials, Wytensin, given orally to hypertensive patients, effectively controlled blood pressure without any significant effect on glomerular filtration rate, renal blood flow, body fluid volume or body weight. Wytensin given parenterally to dogs has produced a natriuresis. Similarly, hypertensive subjects, 24 hours after salt loading, have shown a decrease in blood pressure and a natriuresis (5% to 240% increase in sodium excretion) following a single oral dose of Wytensin. After seven consecutive days of administration and effective blood-pressure control, no significant change on glomerular filtration rate, renal blood flow, or body weight was observed. However, in clinical trials of six to thirty months duration, hypertensive patients with effective blood-pressure control by Wytensin lost one to four pounds of body weight. The mechanism of this weight loss has not been established. Tolerance to the antihypertensive effect of Wytensin has not been observed.
During long-term administration of Wytensin, there is a small decrease in serum cholesterol and total triglycerides without any change in the high-density lipoprotein fraction. Plasma norepinephrine, serum dopamine beta-hydroxylase and plasma renin activity are decreased during chronic administration of Wytensin. No changes in serum electrolytes, uric acid, blood-urea nitrogen, calcium, or glucose have been observed.
Wytensin and hydrochlorothiazide have been shown to have at least partially additive effects in patients not responding adequately to either drug alone.

INDICATIONS AND USAGE
Wytensin (guanabenz acetate) is indicated in the treatment of hypertension. It may be employed alone or in combination with a thiazide diuretic.

CONTRAINDICATION
Wytensin is contraindicated in patients with a known sensitivity to the drug.

PRECAUTIONS
1. Sedation: Wytensin causes sedation or drowsiness in a large fraction of patients. When Wytensin is used with centrally active depressants, such as phenothiazines, barbiturates, and benzodiazepines, the potential for additive sedative effects should be considered.
2. Patients with vascular insufficiency: Wytensin, like other antihypertensive agents, should be used with caution in patients with severe coronary insufficiency, recent myocardial infarction, cerebrovascular disease, or severe hepatic or renal failure.
3. Rebound: Sudden cessation of therapy with central alpha agonists like Wytensin may rarely result in "overshoot" hypertension and more commonly produces an increase in serum catecholamines and subjective symptomatology.
4. Patients with hepatic impairment: The disposition of orally administered Wytensin is altered in patients with alcohol-induced liver disease. Mean plasma concentrations of Wytensin were higher in these patients than in healthy subjects. The clinical significance of this finding is unknown. However, careful monitoring of blood pressure is suggested when Wytensin is administered to patients with hypertension and coexisting chronic hepatic dysfunction.
5. Patients with renal impairment: The disposition of orally administered Wytensin is altered modestly in patients with renal impairment. Wytensin's half-life is prolonged and clearance decreased, more so in patients on hemodialysis. The clinical significance of these findings is unknown. Careful monitoring of blood pressure during Wytensin dose titration is suggested in patients with coexisting hypertension and renal impairment.

INFORMATION FOR PATIENTS
Patients who receive Wytensin should be advised to exercise caution when operating dangerous machinery or driving motor vehicles until it is determined that they do not become drowsy or dizzy from the medication. Patients should be warned that their tolerance for alcohol and other CNS depressants may be diminished. Patients should be advised not to discontinue therapy abruptly.
LABORATORY TESTS
In clinical trials, no clinically significant laboratory-test abnormalities were identified during either acute or chronic therapy with Wytensin. Tests carried out included CBC, urinalysis, electrolytes, SGOT, bilirubin, alkaline phosphatase, uric acid, BUN, creatinine, glucose, calcium, phosphorus, total protein, and Coombs' test. During long-term administration of Wytensin, there was a small decrease in serum cholesterol and total triglycerides without any change in the high-density lipoprotein fraction. In rare instances an occasional nonprogressive increase in liver enzymes has been observed. However, no clinical evidence of hepatic disease has been found.
DRUG INTERACTIONS
Wytensin has not been demonstrated to cause any drug interactions when administered with other drugs, such as digitalis, diuretics, analgesics, anxiolytics, and antiinflammatory or antiinfective agents, in clinical trials. However, the potential for increased sedation when Wytensin is administered concomitantly with CNS-depressant drugs should be noted.
DRUG/LABORATORY TEST INTERACTIONS
No laboratory-test abnormalities were identified with the use of Wytensin.
CARCINOGENESIS, MUTAGENESIS, IMPAIRMENT OF FERTILITY
No evidence of carcinogenic potential emerged in rats during a two-year oral study with Wytensin at doses up to 9.5 mg/kg/day, i.e., about 10 times the maximum recommended human dose. In the Salmonella microsome mutagenicity (Ames) test system, Wytensin at 200 to 500 mcg per plate or at 30 to 50 mcg/mL in suspension gave dose-related increases in the number of mutants in one (TA 1537) of five *Salmonella typhimurium* strains with or without inclusion of rat liver microsomes. No mutagenic activity was seen at doses up to those which inhibit growth in the eukaryotic microorganism, *Schizosaccharomyces pombe*, or in Chinese hamster ovary cells at doses up to those which were lethal to the cells in culture. In another eukaryotic system, *Saccharomyces cerevisiae*, Wytensin produced no activity in an assay measuring induction of repairable DNA damage. Reproductive studies showed a decreased pregnancy rate in rats administered high oral doses (9.6 mg/kg) of Wytensin, suggesting an impairment of fertility. The fertility of treated males (9.6 mg/kg) may also have been affected, as suggested by the decreased pregnancy rate of their mates, even though the females received Wytensin only during the last third of pregnancy.
PREGNANCY
Pregnancy Category C
WYTENSIN MAY HAVE ADVERSE EFFECTS ON THE FETUS WHEN ADMINISTERED TO PREGNANT WOMEN. A teratology study in mice has indicated a possible increase in skeletal abnormalities when Wytensin is given orally at doses of 3 to 6 times the maximum recommended human dose of 1.0 mg/kg. These abnormalities, principally costal and vertebral, were not noted in similar studies in rats and rabbits. However, increased fetal loss has been observed after oral Wytensin administration to pregnant rats (14 mg/kg) and rabbits (20 mg/kg). Reproductive studies of Wytensin in rats have shown slightly decreased live-birth indices, decreased fetal survival rate, and decreased pup body weight at oral doses of 6.4 and 9.6 mg/kg. There are no adequate, well-controlled studies in pregnant women. Wytensin should be used during pregnancy only if the potential benefit justifies the potential risk to the fetus.
NURSING MOTHERS
Because no information is available on the excretion of Wytensin in human milk, it should not be administered to nursing mothers.
PEDIATRIC USE
The safety and effectiveness of Wytensin in children less than 12 years of age have not been demonstrated. Therefore, its use in this age group cannot be recommended at this time.

ADVERSE REACTIONS
The incidence of adverse effects has been ascertained from controlled clinical studies conducted in the United States and is based on data from 859 patients who received Wytensin for up to 3 years. There is some evidence that the side effects are dose-related.
The following table shows the incidence of adverse effects occurring in at least 5% of patients in a study comparing Wytensin (guanabenz acetate) to placebo, at a starting dose of 8 mg b.i.d.

Adverse Effect	Placebo (%) n=102	Wytensin (%) n=109
Dry mouth	7	28
Drowsiness or sedation	12	39
Dizziness	7	17
Weakness	7	10
Headache	6	5

In other controlled clinical trials at the starting dose of 16 mg/day in 476 patients, the incidence of dry mouth was slightly higher (38%) and that of dizziness was slightly lower (12%), but the incidence of the most frequent adverse effects was similar to the placebo-controlled trial. Although these side effects were not serious, they led to discontinuation of treatment about 15% of the time. In more recent studies using an initial dose of 8 mg/day in 274 patients, the incidence of drowsiness or sedation was lower, about 20%.
Other adverse effects were reported during clinical trials with Wytensin but are not clearly distinguishable from placebo effects and occurred with a frequency of 3% or less:
Cardiovascular — chest pain, edema, arrhythmias, palpitations.
Gastrointestinal—nausea, epigastric pain, diarrhea, vomiting, constipation, abdominal discomfort.
Central nervous system—anxiety, ataxia, depression, sleep disturbances.
ENT disorders—nasal congestion.
Eye disorders—blurring of vision.
Musculoskeletal—aches in extremities, muscle aches.
Respiratory—dyspnea.
Dermatologic—rash, pruritus.
Urogenital—urinary frequency, disturbances of sexual function (decreased libido, impotence).
Other—gynecomastia, taste disorders.
In very rare instances atrioventricular dysfunction, up to and including complete AV block, has been caused by Wytensin.

Continued on next page

Wyeth-Ayerst Laboratories—Cont.

DRUG ABUSE AND DEPENDENCE
No reported dependence or abuse has been associated with the administration of Wytensin.

OVERDOSAGE
Accidental ingestion of Wytensin caused hypotension, somnolence, lethargy, irritability, miosis, and bradycardia in two children aged one and three years. Gastric lavage and administration of pressor substances, fluids, and oral activated charcoal resulted in complete and uneventful recovery within 12 hours in both patients.

Since experience with accidental overdosage is limited, the suggested treatment is mainly supportive while the drug is being eliminated from the body and until the patient is no longer symptomatic. Vital signs and fluid balance should be carefully monitored. An adequate airway should be maintained and, if indicated, assisted respiration instituted. There are no data available on the dialyzability of Wytensin.

DOSAGE AND ADMINISTRATION
Dosage with Wytensin should be individualized. A starting dose of 4 mg twice a day is recommended, whether Wytensin is used alone or with a thiazide diuretic. Dosage may be increased in increments of 4 to 8 mg per day every one to two weeks, depending on the patient's response. The maximum dose studied to date has been 32 mg twice daily, but doses as high as this are rarely needed.

HOW SUPPLIED
Wytensin® (guanabenz acetate) Tablets, Wyeth®, are available in the following dosage strengths:

4 mg, NDC 0008-0073, orange, five-sided tablet with a raised "W"and a "4"under the "W" on one side and "WYETH 73" on reverse side, in bottles of 100 and 500 tablets and in Redipak® cartons of 100 tablets (10 blister strips of 10).

8 mg, NDC 0008-0074, gray, five-sided tablet with a raised "W" and an "8" under the "W" on one side and "WYETH 74" on scored reverse side, in bottles of 100 tablets.

The appearance of these tablets is a trademark of Wyeth-Ayerst Laboratories.

Keep tightly closed.
Dispense in tight container.
Protect from light.

Shown in Product Identification Section, page 438

ZOVIRAX® Capsules　　　　　　　　　　　　℞
ZOVIRAX® Tablets　　　　　　　　　　　　　℞
ZOVIRAX® Suspension　　　　　　　　　　　℞
[zō"vī'răx]
(Acyclovir)

For full prescribing information for ZOVIRAX® Capsules, Tablets, and Suspension, see page 844 of the Burroughs-Wellcome section of this *PDR*.

Shown in Product Identification Section, page 407

> ### EDUCATIONAL MATERIAL

Films—Slides—Videos
The Wyeth-Ayerst Audiovisual Catalog, listing films, audiovisual, and slide programs available through the Wyeth-Ayerst Film Library or on loan through the local Wyeth-Ayerst representative, can be obtained by writing Professional Service, Wyeth-Ayerst Laboratories, P.O. Box 8299, Philadelphia, PA 19101.

Young Pharmaceuticals Inc.
1840 BERLIN TURNPIKE
WETHERSFIELD, CT 06109

BLEMERASE™　　　　　　　　　　　　　　　℞
10% Benzoyl peroxide Acne Masking Lotion

DESCRIPTION
Contains 10% Benzoyl peroxide in a unique blemish-masking lotion consisting of Chrome oxides, Iron oxides, Methylparaben, Mg Al silicate, Povidone, Propylene glycol, Purified water, Sodium polynaphthalene sulfonate, Talc, Titanium dioxide and Xanthan gum.

HOW SUPPLIED
10 grams in plastic bottles with controlled-drop dispensing tip in Fair (NDC 52185-250-10), Medium (NDC 52185-251-10) and Deep (NDC 52185-252-10) complexion shades.
Each bottle contains a mixing ball to insure lotion uniformity.

CURASTAIN™　　　　　　　　　　　　　　OTC
Dermatologic Stain Reducing Spray

DESCRIPTION
Contains Water, Triethanolamine, Benzyl alcohol, Glycerin, Hydroxypropyl cellulose, Allantoin, Imidurea and Polyoxyethylene lauryl ether. US and foreign patents pending.

HOW SUPPLIED
4 Fl. ozs. in a plastic bottle with spray pump closure.

PHARMACREME™　　　　　　　　　　　　　OTC
Emollient Topical Vehicle

DESCRIPTION
Contains White Petrolatum, Sodium lauryl sulfate, Cetostearyl alcohol, Ascorbic acid, Salicylic acid, Chlorocresol and Purified water.

HOW SUPPLIED
30 grams and 600 grams in plastic jars. The jars are filled to approximately ⅔ capacity to accommodate the addition of selected additives.

For additional information, call Young Pharmaceuticals Inc. Professional Services Department toll-free at 1-800-874-9686. In Connecticut, call (203) 529-7919 collect.

Discontinued Products

Listed below are products that pharmaceutical companies have removed from the market during the past year. Please consult the Product Name Index to determine if another company is now marketing a particular pharmaceutical.

Allen & Hanburys

Trandate HCT Tablets

Astra Pharmaceutical Products, Inc.

Calcium Gluconate 10% Injection

Biocraft Laboratories, Inc.

Amoxicillin Pediatric Drops
Cyclacillin Tablets 250 mg
Cyclacillin Tablets 500 mg

Central Pharmaceuticals, Inc.

Adronaq-50 Sterile Suspension
Adronaq-LA Injectable
Codimal Expectorant
Estronol Aqueous Sterile Suspension
Neocyten Injection
Synophylate-GG Tablets

Cetus Oncology Corporation

Fluorouracil Injection 1 g

CIBA Pharmaceutical Company

Apresoline-Esidrix
Metandren
Serpasil
Serpasil-Apresoline
Serpasil-Esidrix

GEIGY Pharmaceuticals

Butazolidin

Johnson & Johnson o MERCK Consumer Pharmaceuticals Co.

Orexin Softab Tablets

3M Pharmaceuticals

Medihaler Ergotamine
Tepanil 25 mg Tablets
Tepanil Ten-Tab 75 mg Tablets

**Miles Inc.
Consumer Healthcare Products**

Alka-Seltzer Advanced Formula

Ortho Pharmaceutical Corporation

Ortho-Cyclen

Par Pharmaceutical, Inc.

Doxylamine Succinate Tablets 25 mg
Meprobamate and Aspirin Tablets
   200 mg/325 mg
Thioridazine HCl Tablets 150 mg
Thioridazine HCl Tablets 200 mg
Trichlormethiazide Tablets 2 mg

Procter & Gamble Pharmaceuticals, Inc. (Norwich Eaton Pharmaceuticals, Inc.)

Dopar Capsules
Macrodantin MACPAC

Reed & Carnrick

Alphosyl Lotion/Cream

Rhone-Poulenc Rorer Pharmaceuticals, Inc.

Arlidin Tablets 6 mg
Arlidin Tablets 12 mg

Sanofi Winthrop Pharmaceuticals

Aralen Phosphate with Primaquine
   Phosphate
Demerol APAP
Tornalate

Schering Corporation

Diprolene Cream 0.05%
Normozide Tablets
Rela Tablets
Tindal Tablets

Schiapparelli Searle

Diulo
Haloperidol Tablets

**Schwarz Pharma
Kremers Urban Company**

Nitrocine Timecaps 2.5 mg
Nitrocine Timecaps 6.5 mg
Nitrocine Timecaps 9 mg
Nitrocine Transdermal System
   0.6 mg/hr

G.D. Searle & Co.

Aminophyllin Tablets
Theo-24

SmithKline Beecham Pharmaceuticals

Darbid
Daricon
Dasin

Solvay Pharmaceuticals

Cin-Quin
Vio-Bec
Vio-Bec Forte

Upsher-Smith Laboratories, Inc.

Acetaminophen Uniserts Suppositories

SECTION 7
Diagnostic Product Information

Products described in PHYSICIANS' DESK REFERENCE® which have official package circulars must be in full compliance with Food & Drug Administration regulations pertaining to labeling for prescription drugs. These regulations require that for PDR® copy, "indications, effects, dosages, routes, methods, and frequency and duration of administration, and any relevant warnings, hazards, contraindications, side effects, and precautions" must be the "*same in language and emphasis*" as the approved labeling for the product. FDA regards the words "*same in language and emphasis*" as requiring VERBATIM use of the approved labeling providing such information. Furthermore, information in the approved labeling that is emphasized by the use of type set in a box or in capitals, bold face, or italics must also be given the same emphasis in PDR. For products which do not have official package circulars, the Publisher emphasized to manufacturers the necessity of describing such products comprehensively so that physicians would have access to all information essential for intelligent and informed prescribing. In organizing and presenting the material in PHYSICIANS' DESK REFERENCE, the Publisher is providing all the information made available to PDR by manufacturers.

This edition of PHYSICIANS' DESK REFERENCE contains the latest product information available at press-time. During the year, however, new and revised information about the products described herein may be furnished us. This information will be published in the PDR Supplement. Therefore, before prescribing or administering any product described in the following pages, you should first consult the PDR Supplement.

In presenting the following material to the medical profession, the Publisher is not necessarily advocating the use of any product listed.

Connaught Laboratories, Inc.
A Pasteur Mérieux Company
SWIFTWATER, PA 18370

MULTITEST CMI®   ℞
[mul'tĭ-test]
(Skin Test Antigens for Cellular Hypersensitivity)

NDC 50361-780-80

DESCRIPTION
Skin Test Antigens for Cellular Hypersensitivity, MULTI-TEST CMI® is a disposable, plastic applicator consisting of eight sterile test heads preloaded with the following seven delayed hypersensitivity skin test antigens and glycerin negative control for precutaneous administration: Tetanus Toxoid Antigen, Diphtheria Toxoid Antigen, Streptococcus Antigen, Old Tuberculin, Candida Antigen, Trichophyton Antigen, and Proteus Antigen.

MULTITEST CMI® provides a quick, convenient and uniform procedure for delayed cutaneous hypersensitivity testing.

Supplied in box of 10 individual cartons containing one pre-loaded MULTITEST CMI® per carton.

TUBERCULIN, MONO-VACC®   ℞
TEST (O.T.)
[tu-ber'ku-lin mon'ō-vak]
(old tuberculin)
Multiple Puncture Device

NDC 50361-770-40   25 tests per box
Supplied in plastic tamper proof box of 25 tests per box; test reading cards in English, Spanish, Vietnamese and Chinese are also available.

Ferring Laboratories, Inc.
400 RELLA BLVD, SUITE 201
SUFFERN, NY 10901

RELEFACT® TRH   ℞
(protirelin)
Injection
FOR INTRAVENOUS ADMINISTRATION

DESCRIPTION
Chemically, Relefact TRH (protirelin) is identified as 5-oxo-L-prolyl-L-histidyl-L-proline amide. It is a synthetic tripeptide which is believed to be structurally identical with the naturally-occurring thyrotropin-releasing hormone produced by the hypothalamus. The CAS Registry Number is 24305-27-9. The structural formula is:

Relefact TRH is supplied as 1 mL ampuls. Each ampul contains 500 µg protirelin in a sterile non-pyrogenic isotonic saline solution having a pH of approximately 6.5. In addition, each ampul contains sodium chloride 9.0 mg, Water for Injection, hydrochloric acid and sodium hydroxide as needed to adjust pH. Relefact TRH is intended for intravenous administration.

CLINICAL PHARMACOLOGY
Pharmacologically, Relefact TRH increases the release of the thyroid stimulating hormone (TSH) from the anterior pituitary. Prolactin release is also increased. It has recently been observed that approximately 65% of acromegalic patients tested respond with a rise in circulating growth hormone levels; the clinical significance is as yet not clear. Following intravenous administration, the mean plasma half-life of protirelin in normal subjects is approximately five minutes. TSH levels rise rapidly and reach a peak at 20 to 30 minutes. The decline in TSH levels takes place more slowly, approaching baseline levels after approximately three hours.

INDICATIONS AND USAGE
Relefact TRH is indicated as an adjunctive agent in the diagnostic assessment of thyroid function. As an adjunct to other diagnostic procedures, testing Relefact TRH (protirelin) may yield useful information in patients with pituitary or hypothalamic dysfunction.

Relefact TRH is indicated as an adjunct to evaluate the effectiveness of thyrotropin suppression with a particular dose of T4 in patients with nodular or diffuse goitre. A normal TSH baseline value and a minimal difference between the 30 minute and baseline response to Relefact TRH injection would indicate adequate suppression of the pituitary secretion of TSH. Relefact TRH may be used, adjunctively, for adjustment of thyroid hormone dosage given to patients with primary hypothyroidism. A normal or slightly blunted TSH response, thirty minutes following Relefact TRH injection, would indicate adequate replacement therapy.

CONTRAINDICATIONS
Relefact TRH (protirelin) is contraindicated in patients with a known hypersensitivity to the drug.

WARNINGS
Transient changes in blood pressure, either increases or decreases, frequently occur immediately following administration of Relefact TRH. Blood pressure should therefore be measured before Relefact TRH is administered and at frequent intervals during the first 15 minutes after its administration.

Increases in systolic pressure (usually less than 30 mm Hg) and/or increases in diastolic pressure (usually less than 20 mm Hg) have been observed more frequently than decreases in pressure. These changes have not ordinarily persisted for more than 15 minutes nor have they required therapy. More severe degrees of hypertension or hypotension with or without syncope have been reported in a few patients. To minimize the incidence and/or severity of hypotension, the patient should be supine before, during, and after Relefact TRH administration. If a clinically important change in blood pressure occurs, monitoring of blood pressure should be continued until it returns to baseline levels. Relefact TRH should not be administered to patients in whom marked, rapid changes in blood pressure would be dangerous unless the potential benefit clearly outweighs the potential risk.

PRECAUTIONS
Thyroid hormones reduce the TSH response to Relefact TRH. Accordingly, patients in whom Relefact TRH (protirelin) is to be used diagnostically should be taken off liothyronine (T3) approximately seven days prior to testing and should be taken off thyroid medications containing levothyroxine (T4), e.g., desiccated thyroid, thyroglobulin, or liotrix, at least 14 days before testing. Hormone therapy is NOT to be discontinued when the test is used to evaluate the effectiveness of thyroid suppression with a particular dose of T4 in patients with nodular or diffuse goitre, or for adjustment of thyroid hormone dosage given to patients with primary hypothyroidism.

Chronic administration of levodopa has been reported to inhibit the TSH response to Relefact TRH.

It is not advisable to withdraw maintenance doses of adrenocortical drugs used in the therapy of known hypopituitarism. Several published reports have shown that prolonged treatment with glucocorticoids at physiologic doses has no significant effect on the TSH response to thyrotropin releasing hormone, but that the administration of pharmacologic doses of steroids reduces the TSH response. Therapeutic doses of acetylsalicylic acid (2 to 3.6 g/day) have been reported to inhibit the TSH response to protirelin. The ingestion of acetylsalicylic acid caused the peak level of TSH to decrease approximately 30% as compared to values obtained without acetylsalicylic acid administration. In both cases, the TSH peak occurred 30 minutes post-administration of protirelin.

Carcinogenesis, Mutagenesis, Impairment of Fertility
Long-term animal studies have not been performed to evaluate the carcinogenic potential of protirelin. Studies to determine potential effects concerning mutagenesis or impairment of fertility have also not been performed.

Pregnancy (Category C)
Protirelin has been shown to increase the number of resorptions in rabbits, but not in rats, when given in doses 1½ and 6 times the human dose. There are no adequate and well-controlled studies in pregnant women. Relefact TRH (protirelin) should be used during pregnancy only if the potential benefit justifies the potential risk to the fetus.

Nursing Mothers
It is not known whether this drug is excreted in human milk. Because many drugs are excreted in human milk, caution should be exercised when Relefact TRH is administered to a nursing woman.

ADVERSE REACTIONS
Side effects have been reported in about 50% of the patients tested with Relefact TRH. Generally, the side effects are minor, have occurred promptly, and have persisted for only a few minutes following injection.

Cardiovascular reactions:
Marked changes in blood pressure, including both hypertension and hypotension with or without syncope, have been reported in a small number of patients.

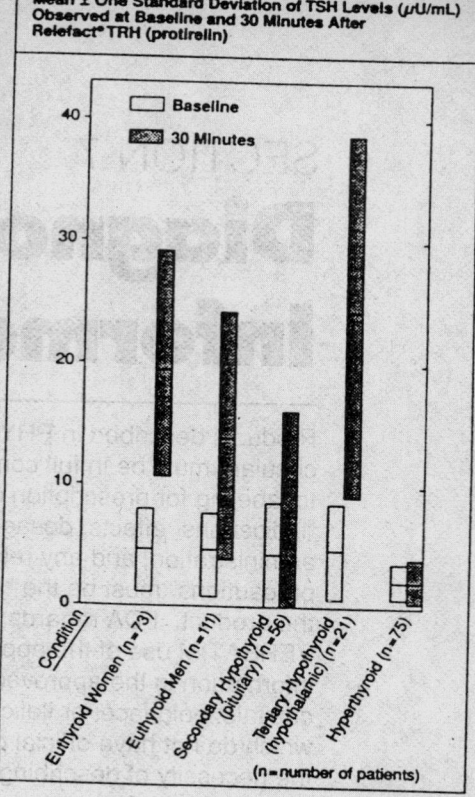

Figure 1

Mean ± One Standard Deviation of TSH Levels (µU/mL) Observed at Baseline and 30 Minutes After Relefact® TRH (protirelin)

(n = number of patients)

Endocrine reaction:
Breast enlargement and leakage in lactating women for up to two or three days.

Other reactions:
Headaches, sometimes severe,, and transient amaurosis in patients with pituitary tumors. Rarely, convulsions may occur in patients with predisposing conditions, e.g. epilepsy, brain damage. Nausea; urge to urinate; flushed sensation; lightheadedness; bad taste; abdominal discomfort; and dry mouth. Less fequently reported were: anxiety; sweating; tightness in the throat; pressure in the chest; tingling sensation; drowsiness; and allergic reactions.

Pituitary apoplexy requiring acute neurosurgical intervention has been reported infrequently for patients with pituitary macroadenomas following the acute administration of protirelin (TRH) injection in the setting of combined anterior pituitary function testing in conjunction with LHRH and insulin.

DOSAGE AND ADMINISTRATION
Relefact TRH is intended for intravenous administration with the patient in the supine position. The drug is administered as a bolus over a period of 15 to 30 seconds, with the patient remaining supine until all scheduled postinjection blood samples have been taken. Blood pressure should be measured before Relefact TRH (protirelin) is administered and at frequent intervals during the first 15 minutes thereafter (see WARNINGS). Have the patient urinate before injecting Relefact TRH.

Dosage:
Adults: 500 µg. Doses between 200 and 500 µg have been used. 500 µg is considered the optimum dose to give the maximum response in the greatest number of patients. Doses greater than 500 µg are unlikely to elicit a greater TSH response.

Children age 6 to 16 years: 7 µg/kg body weight up to a dose of 500 µg.

Infants and children up to 6 years: Experience is limited in this age group; doses of 7 µg/kg have been administered. One blood sample for TSH assay should be drawn immediately prior to the injection of Relefact TRH, and a second sample should be obtained 30 minutes after injection. The TSH response to Relefact TRH is reduced by repetitive administration of the drug. Accordingly, if the Relefact TRH test is repeated, an interval of seven days before testing is recommended. Elevated serum lipids may interfere with the TSH assay. Thus, fasting (except in patients with hypopituitarism) or a low-fat meal is recommended prior to the test.

for possible revisions

INTERPRETATION OF TEST RESULTS

Interpretation of the TSH response to Relefact TRH requires an understanding of thyroid-pituitary-hypothalamic physiology and knowledge of the clinical status of the individual patient.

Because the TSH test results may vary with the laboratory, the physician should be familiar with the TSH assay method used and the normal range for the laboratory performing the assay. TSH response 30 minutes after Relefact TRH administration in normal subjects and in patients with hyperthyroidism and hypothyroidism are presented in Figure 1. The diagnoses were established prior to the administration of Relefact TRH on the basis of the clinical history, physical examination, and the results of other thyroid and/or pituitary function tests. [See Figure 1 on preceding page.]

Among the normal euthyroid subjects, women and children were found to have higher levels of TSH at 30 minutes than men. Among the patients with hyperthyroidism or primary (thyroidal), secondary (pituitary), or tertiary (hypothalamic) hypothyroidism, no significant differences in TSH levels by age or sex were found.

Normal: Baseline TSH levels of less than 10 microunits/mL (μU/mL) were observed in 97% of euthyroid normal subjects tested. Thirty minutes after Relefact TRH, the serum TSH increased by 2.0 μU/mL or more in 95% of euthyroid subjects.

Hyperthyroidism: All hyperthyroid patients tested had baseline TSH levels of less than 10 μU/mL and a rise of less than 2 μU/mL 30 minutes after Relefact TRH (protirelin). Primary (thyroidal) hypothyroidism: The diagnosis of primary hypothyroidism is frequently supported by finding clearly elevated baseline TSH levels; 93% of patients tested had levels above 10 μU/mL. Relefact TRH administration to these patients generally would not be expected to yield additional useful information. Ninety-four percent of patients with primary hypothyroidism given Relefact TRH in clinical trials responded with a rise in TSH of 2.0 μU/mL or greater, since this response is also found in normal subjects. Relefact TRH testing does not differentiate primary hypothyroidism from normal.

Table 1

Characterization Based on Serum TSH Levels at Baseline and 30 Minutes after Relefact TRH

	Baseline (Serum TSH μU/mL)	Change of Serum TSH (μU/mL) at 30 minutes
Euthyroidism (normal thyroid function)	10 or less (usually 6 or less; 20% have <1.5 μU/mL)	2 or more (usually 6 to 30)
Hyperthyroidism	10 or less (usually 4 or less)	less than 2
Primary Hypothyroidism (thyroidal)	more than 10 (usually 15 to 100)	2 or more (usually 20 or more)
Secondary Hypothyroidism (pituitary)	10 or less (usually 6 or less)	less than 2 (59%) 2 to 50 (41%)
Tertiary Hypothyroidism (hypothalamic)	10 or less (often less than 2)	2 or more

Secondary (pituitary) and tertiary (hypothalamic) hypothyroidism: In the presence of clinical and other laboratory evidence of hypothyroidism, the finding of a baseline TSH level less than 10 μU/mL should suggest secondary or tertiary hypothyroidism. In this situation, a response to Relefact TRH (protirelin) of less than 2 μU/mL suggests secondary hypothyroidism since this response was observed in about 60% of patients with secondary hypothyroidism and only approximately 5% of patients with tertiary hypothyroidism. A TSH response to Relefact TRH greater than 2 μU/mL is not helpful in differentiating between secondary and tertiary hypothyroidism since this response was noted in about 40% of the former and about 95% in the latter. Establishing the diagnosis of secondary or tertiary hypothyroidism requires a careful history and physical examination along with appropriate test of anterior pituitary and/or target gland function. The Relefact TRH test should not be used as the only laboratory determinant for establishing these diagnoses.

HOW SUPPLIED

As 1 mL ampuls – boxes of 5 (NDC 55566-0081-5). Each mL contains Relefact TRH 0.50 mg (500 μg), sodium chloride 9.0 mg for isotonicity, hydrochloric acid and sodium hydroxide as needed to adjust pH.

Store at controlled room temperature (59 – 86°F).

Caution: Federal law prohibits dispensing without a prescription.

Manufacturer for:
FERRING LABORATORIES, INC.
Suffern, NY 10901
By: Taylor Pharmacal Co.
Decatur, IL 62525
RELEFACT REG TM HOECHST AG
0081-5-DC-115   (6/92)

Shown in Product Identification Section, page 409

SECRETIN–FERRING   ℞
[si-krē'tin]
secretin
For diagnostic use in pancreatic dysfunction and gastrinoma (Zollinger-Ellison syndrome)

DESCRIPTION

Secretin is a gastrointestinal peptide hormone that was first extracted from porcine duodenum by Jorpes & Mutt (1961). The heptacosa-peptide was subsequently sequenced and synthesized by Mutt, Bodansky and their co-workers at the Karolinska Institute. Secretin-Ferring is a highly purified naturally occurring porcine hormone with a potency of not less than 3000 clinical units (CU) per mg peptide. Secretin is chemically defined as follows:

Mol.Wt. 3055.5
Empirical Formula: $C_{130}H_{220}N_{44}O_{41}$
Structural Formula: H-His-Ser-Asp-Gly-Thr-Phe-Thr-Ser-Glu-Leu-Ser-Arg-Leu-Arg-Asp-Ser-Ala-Arg-Leu-Gln-Arg-Leu-Leu-Gln-Gly-Leu-Val-NH$_2$

Secretin-Ferring contains 75 CU of lyophilized, sterile purified secretin, 1 mg of L-cysteine hydrochloride, and 20 mg of mannitol per vial. When reconstituted in 7.5 ml of Sodium Chloride Injection USP, each ml of solution contains 10 CU secretin for intravenous use. The pH of the reconstituted solution has a range of 2.5-5.0.

CLINICAL PHARMACOLOGY

The primary action of secretin is to increase the volume and bicarbonate content of secreted pancreatic juices. The standard unit of activity used for Secretin-Ferring is the clinical unit defined by Jorpes & Mutt in 1966. In a study of 6 healthy subjects the t(½) for secretin approximated 4 minutes with a clearance rate of 540 ml/min (Kolts and McGuigan, 1977). Normal ranges for pancreatic secretory response to intravenous secretin in patients with defined pancreatic diseases have been shown to vary. The variation is related to the secretin product used as well as inter-investigator differences in operative technique. However, it has been demonstrated that properly performed tests with secretin will identify pancreatic disease (Gutierrez and Baron, 1972, Lagerlöf et al., 1967).

The pancreatic secretory responses to secretin in normal subjects and patients with well-documented pancreatitis are shown in Table 1 (Gutierrez and Baron, 1972).

The values obtained for Table 1 are derived from a single study by investigators skilled in performing the secretin test and are to be taken only as guidelines. These results should not be generalized to results of secretin testing conducted in other laboratories. However, a volume response of less than 2.0 ml/kg/hr, bicarbonate concentration of less than 90 mEq/liter and bicarbonate output of less than 0.2 mEq/kg/hr are consistent with impaired pancreatic function. A physician or institution planning to perform secretin testing for diagnosis of pancreatic disease should begin by assessing enough normal subjects (≥ 5) to develop proficiency in proper technique and to generate normal response ranges for the three commonly assessed parameters of pancreatic exocrine response to Secretin-Ferring.

Proper technique for carrying out the secretin test of pancreatic function is described in DOSAGE AND ADMINISTRATION.

Secretin-Ferring administered intravenously stimulates gastrin release in patients with gastrinoma (Zollinger-Ellison syndrome), whereas no or only small changes in serum gastrin concentrations occur in normal subjects. Secretin-Ferring may produce a small decrease in serum gastrin levels in patients with duodenal ulcer disease. This gastrin response is the basis for the use of Secretin-Ferring as a provocative test in the evaluation of patients in whom gastrinoma is a diagnostic consideration. Accepted technique for carrying out the secretin provocation test is detailed in DOSAGE AND ADMINISTRATION.

INDICATIONS AND USAGE

Secretin-Ferring (secretin) is indicated for:
(1) Diagnosis of pancreatic exocrine disease.
(2) As an adjunct in obtaining desquamated pancreatic cells for cytopathologic examination.
(3) Diagnosis of gastrinoma (Zollinger-Ellison syndrome).

CONTRAINDICATIONS

Patients suffering from actue pancreatitis should not receive Secretin-Ferring until the attack has subsided.

WARNING

Because of a potential allergic reaction to secretin, patients should receive an initial intravenous test dose of 0.1-1.0 CU. If no allergic reaction is noted after one minute the recommended dose may be injected slowly over 1 minute. A test dose is especially important in patients with a history of atopic allergy and/or asthma. Appropriate measures for the treatment of acute hypersensitivity reactions should be immediately available.

PRECAUTIONS

GENERAL: Patients who have undergone vagotomy, or are receiving anticholinergics at the time of secretin testing, or who have inflammatory bowel disease may be hyporesponsive to secretin stimulation. This response does not indicate pancreatic disease. A greater than normal volume response to secretin stimulation, which can mask coexisting pancreatic disease, is occasionally encountered in patients with alcoholic or other liver disease.

DRUG/LABORATORY TEST INTERACTION: The concomitant use of anticholinergic agents may make patients hyporesponsive (false positive).

CARCINOGENSIS, MUTAGENESIS, IMPAIRMENT OF FERTILITY:
Long-term studies in animals have not been performed to evaluate the carcinogenic, mutagenic potential or possible impairment of fertility effects of secretin.

PREGNANCY CATEGORY C: Animal reproduction studies have not been conducted with Secretin-Ferring. It is also not known whether Secretin-Ferring can cause fetal harm when administered to a pregnant woman or can affect reproductive capacity. Secretin-Ferring should be given to a pregnant woman for diagnosis of gastrinoma (Zollinger-Ellison syndrome) only if clearly needed. Insofar as fluoroscopic guidance is usually necessary to position the double-lumen tube used in the pancreatic function test, this test should be postponed until after delivery.

NURSING MOTHERS: It is not known whether secretin is excreted in human milk. Because many drugs are excreted in human milk, caution is advised when Secretin-Ferring is administered to a nursing woman. Further, normal values for pancreatic secretory response to Secretin-Ferring and for serum gastrin response have not been established for nursing women.

PEDIATRIC USE: Safety and effectiveness in children have not been established.

ADVERSE REACTIONS

No adverse reactions to Secretin-Ferring have been reported.

DOSAGE AND ADMINISTRATION

Secretin-Ferring should be prepared immediately prior to use. The contents of a vial are dissolved in 7.5 ml of Sodium Chloride Injection USP, to yield a concentration of 10 CU per ml. Avoid vigorous shaking. Discard any unused portion after reconstitution.

Continued on next page

Table 1

	Normal male subjects (10)[a]		Chronic Pancreatitis (5)
Volume secreted (ml/kg/hr)	3.6 ± 0.8[b]		1.1 ± 0.6
HCO$_3$ content (mEq/l)	114 ± 20		71 ± 33
HCO$_3$ output (mEq/kg/hr)	0.436 ± 0.141		0.105 ± 0.093

[a] number of subjects.
[b] $\overline{x}\pm$S.D.

Ferring—Cont.

The reconstituted drug product should be inspected visually prior to administration. If particulate matter or discoloration are seen, the product should be discarded.

DOSAGE

PANCREATIC FUNCTION TESTING AND PROCEDURE FOR OBTAINING DESQUAMATED PANCREATIC CELLS FOR CYTOPATHOLOGY: 1 CU per kg body weight by slow intravenous injection over 1 minute.

DIAGNOSIS OF GASTRINOMA (Zollinger-Ellison syndrome): 2 CU per kg body weight by slow intravenous injection over 1 minute.

ADMINISTRATION

1. PANCREATIC FUNCTION TESTING: A Dreiling type, radioopaque, double-lumen tube is passed through the mouth following a 12-15 hour fast. The proximal lumen of the tube is placed in the gastric antrum and the distal lumen just beyond the pailla of Vater with the aid of fluoroscopic guidance. The positioning of the tube must be confirmed and the tube secured prior to secretin testing. A negative pressure of 25-40 mm Hg is applied to both lumens and maintained throughout the test. Interruption of suction at 1 minute intervals improves the reliability of fluid collections. When uncontaminated duodenal contents are obtained - i.e., when these secretions are clear, although possibly bile stained, and have a pH of ≥6.0 - a baseline sample of duodenal fluids is collected for 2 consecutive 10 minute periods. Subsequent to the baseline collections, Secretin-Ferring at a dose of 1 CU/kg of body weight is injected intravenously in approximately 1 minute. Duodenal fluid is then collected for 60 minutes after secretin administration. The aspirate is fractioned into four collection periods, the first two at 10 minute intervals, and the last two at 20 minute intervals. The duodenal lumen of the tube is cleared with an injection of air after collection of each fraction. Wide variations in volume of the aspirate will be indicative of incomplete aspiration or contamination. Each fraction of duodenal fluid is to be chilled and subsequently analyzed for volume and bicarbonate concentration.
2. PROCEDURE FOR OBTAINING DESQUAMATED PANCREATIC CELLS FOR CYTOPATHOLOGY: A duodenal aspirate obtained as under Pancreatic Function Testing is submitted for cytopathological examination.
3. SECRETIN TESTING FOR GASTRINOMA (Zollinger-Ellison syndrome). The patient should have fasted for at least 12 hours prior to beginning the test. Prior to injection of Secretin-Ferring, two blood samples are drawn for determination of fasting serum gastrin levels (baseline values). Subsequently, 2 CU of Secretin-Ferring per kg of body weight are administered intravenously over 1 minute; post-injection blood samples are collected after 1,2,5,10 and 30 minutes for determination of serum gastrin concentrations.

Gastrinoma is strongly indicated in patients with elevated fasting serum gastrin concentrations in the 120-500 pg/ml range (determined by RIA using an antibody to gastrin similar to that prepared by Rehfeld) and in patients who show an increase in serum gastrin concentration of more than 110 pg per ml over basal level.

HOW SUPPLIED

Secretin-Ferring is supplied as a lyophilized sterile powder in 10 ml vials (NDC 55566-1075-1) containing 75 CU. The unreconstituted product should be stored at −20°C (freezer). However, the biological activity of Secretin-Ferring will not be significantly decreased by storage at temperatures up to 25°C for up to 3 weeks. Expiration date is marked on the label.

Caution: Federal (USA) law prohibits dispensing without prescription.

REFERENCES

Jorpes, E., and Mutt, V.
On the biological activity and amino acid composition of secretin.
Acta Chem Scand 15 (1961) 1790–1791.
Jorpes, E., and Mutt V.
On the biological assay of secretin. The reference standard.
Acta Physiol Scand 66 (1966) 316–325.
Kolts, B.E. and Mc Guigan, J.E.
Radioimmunoassay Measurement of Secretin Half-Life in Man.
Gastroenterol. 72 (1977) 55–60.
Lagerlöf, H.O., et al.
A secretin test with high doses of secretin and correction for incomplete recovery of duodenal juice.
Gastroenterol 52 (1967) 67–77.
Gutierrez, L.V., and Baron, J.H.
A comparison of Boots and GIH secretin as stimuli of pancreatic secretin in human subjects with or without chronic pancreatitis.
Gut 13 (1972) 721–725.

Manufactured by Ferring AB, Malmö, Sweden, for
FERRING LABORATORIES, INC.
Suffern, N.Y. 10901
Revision date May '92

Shown in Product Identification Section, page

Lederle Laboratories

A Division of American Cyanamid Co.
ONE CYANAMID PLAZA
WAYNE, NJ 07470

PPD TINE TEST® ℞

[*tine tĕst*]
Tuberculin, Purified Protein Derivative

DESCRIPTION

The Tuberculin, Purified Protein Derivative (PPD) TINE TEST is a simple, multiple-puncture, disposable intradermal test device for the detection of tuberculin reactivity. These convenient devices are especially useful in mass tuberculosis screening programs.

Each test unit consists of a stainless steel disc attached to a light blue plastic handle. Projecting from the disc are four triangular-shaped prongs (tines) which are 2 mm long and approximately 4 mm apart. The tines have been mechanically dipped into a concentrated solution of PPD. The PPD concentrate is prepared by the Seibert Process[1,2] and is stabilized with 7% acacia (gum arabic), 30% dextrose, and 5% glycerol. The glycerol also acts as a humectant preventing the film on the tines from becoming brittle-dry. The final PPD concentrate is standardized against U.S. Standard PPD. Following dipping, the tines are capped and sterilized with ethylene oxide. No preservative has been added. The unit is disposable, and there is no need for syringes, needles, and other equipment necessary for the standard intradermal tests.

PPD TINE TEST units have been standardized by clinical evaluation in human subjects to give reactions equivalent to or more potent than 5 TU (US tuberculin units) of standard PPD administered intradermally in the Mantoux test. However, all multiple puncture-type devices must be regarded as screening tools and other appropriate diagnostic procedures such as the Mantoux test should be utilized for retesting individuals with positive reactions.

CLINICAL PHARMACOLOGY

Tuberculin deposited in the skin of tuberculin reactive individuals reacts with sensitized lymphocytes to effect the release of mediators of cellular hypersensitivity. Some of these mediators (eg, skin reactive factor) induce an inflammatory response in the skin causing the induration and erythema characteristic of a "positive" reaction.[3,4]

INDICATIONS AND USAGE

Tuberculin, Purified Protein Derivative (PPD) TINE TEST is indicated to detect tuberculin-sensitive individuals. PPD TINE TEST units are also useful in programs to determine priorities for additional testing (eg, chest X-rays) and in epidemiological surveys to identify those areas having high levels of infection.

Data obtained from clinical studies with a total of 3,062 volunteer subjects (males and females), ranging in age from 4 to 96 years, of which 47.5% (1,443) were Mantoux positive, clearly demonstrates that PPD TINE TEST, when used as a screening test to determine tuberculin reactivity is associated with very little, if any, adverse reactivity. Other than the skin test reaction itself, slight vesiculation and slight ulceration were the only adverse experiences reported. The slight to mild vesiculation was equally divided between the two tests (TINE TEST, 54/3062, 1.78%, and PPD-T Mantoux, 55/3062, 1.81%). The slight ulceration observed with one subject at 72 hours was associated with the TINE TEST site. Of the subjects classified as positive or intermediate by PPD-T Mantoux, 93.8% were classified similarly with the TINE TEST. The results of the clinical trials revealed a 72-hour false positive rate of 10.9% and a false negative rate of 6.2%. In clinical studies of more than 1,800 PPD-S Mantoux positive subjects, only 6.3% gave negative PPD TINE TEST reactions at 72 hours; of more than 1,900 PPD TINE TEST positive tests, less than 11% gave negative Mantoux results.

The frequency of repeated tuberculin tests depends on risk of exposure of the individual and on the prevalence of tuberculosis in the population group. The repeated testing of uninfected individuals does not sensitize to tuberculin. Among individuals with waning sensitivity to homologous or heterologous mycobacterial antigens, however, the stimulus of a tuberculin test may "boost" or increase the size of the reaction to a second test, even causing an apparent development of sensitivity in some cases.[3]

Tuberculin testing should be done with caution in individuals with active tuberculosis. (See **PRECAUTIONS**.)

CONTRAINDICATIONS

There are no known contraindications for use of Tuberculin, Purified Protein Derivative (PPD) TINE TEST. See **PRECAUTIONS** for information regarding special care to be exercised for safe and effective use.

WARNINGS

There are no known serious adverse reactions or potential safety hazards associated with the use of Tuberculin, Purified Protein Derivative (PPD) TINE TEST. However, as with the use of any biological product, the possibility of anaphylactic reaction should be considered. See **PRECAUTIONS** for information regarding special care to be exercised for safe and effective use.

PRECAUTIONS

Tuberculin testing should be done with caution in individuals with active tuberculosis. Although activation of quiescent lesions is rare, if a patient has a history of occurrence of vesiculation and necrosis with a previous tuberculin test by any method, tuberculin testing should be avoided.

Although clinical allergy to acacia is very rare, this product contains some acacia as stabilizer and should be used with caution in patients with known allergy to this component. In these instances remedial measures for anaphylactoid reactions, including epinephrine injection (1:1000), must be available for immediate use.

Reactivity to the test may be suppressed in patients who are receiving corticosteroids or immunosuppressive agents, or those who have recently been immunized with live virus vaccines such as measles, mumps, rubella, polio. If tuberculin skin testing is indicated it should be done preceding, or at the time of such immunization, and read 48 to 72 hours later. If the test is not administered in the time suggested, an interval of 4 to 6 weeks should be allowed between tuberculin skin testing and immunization with live virus vaccines to prevent suppression of tuberculin reactivity.[5]

With a positive reaction further diagnostic procedures must be considered. These may include X-ray of the chest, microbiological examinations of sputa and other specimens, and confirmation of the positive TINE TEST reaction (except vesiculation reactions) using the Mantoux method. In general, the TINE TEST does not need to be repeated.

Antituberculous chemotherapy should not be instituted solely on the basis of a single positive TINE TEST.

When vesiculation occurs, the reaction is to be interpreted as strongly positive and a repeat test by the Mantoux method must not be attempted. Similar or more severe vesiculation with or without necrosis is likely to occur.

Pregnancy Category C: Animal reproduction studies have not been conducted with Tuberculin, Purified Protein Derivative (PPD) TINE TEST. It is also not known whether PPD TINE TEST can cause fetal harm when administered to a pregnant woman or affect reproduction capacity. Tuberculin, Purified Protein Derivative (PPD) TINE TEST should be given to a pregnant woman only if clearly needed. During pregnancy, known positive reactors may demonstrate a negative response to a PPD TINE TEST.

Tuberculin, Purified Protein Derivative (PPD) TINE TEST units must never be reused.

ADVERSE REACTIONS

Vesiculation (positive reaction), ulceration, or necrosis may occur at the test site in highly sensitive persons. Pain, pruritus, and discomfort at the test site may be relieved by cold packs or by topical glucocorticoid ointment or cream. Transient bleeding may be observed at a puncture site and is of no significance.

DOSAGE AND ADMINISTRATION

PPD TINE TEST units have been standardized by clinical evaluation in human subjects to give reactions equivalent to or more potent than 5 TU (US tuberculin units) of standard PPD administered intradermally in the Mantoux test. However, all multiple puncture-type devices must be regarded as screening tools and other appropriate diagnostic procedures such as the Mantoux test should be utilized for retesting reactors.

The volar surface of the upper one-third of the forearm, over a muscle belly, is the preferred site. Hairy areas, and areas without adequate subcutaneous tissue, eg, concavities over a tendon or bone should be avoided.

Alcohol, acetone, ether, or soap and water may be used to cleanse the skin. The area must be clean and thoroughly dry before application of the PPD TINE TEST.

Expose the four coated tines by removing the protective cap while holding the plastic handle. Grasp the patient's forearm firmly, since the sharp momentary sting may cause the patient to jerk his or her arm, resulting in scratching. Stretch the skin of the forearm tightly and apply the disc with the other hand. **Hold at least one second.** Release tension grip on forearm. Withdraw tine unit.

Sufficient pressure should be exerted so that the four puncture sites, and circular depression of the skin from the plastic base are visible.

After administration of the test, local care of the skin is not necessary.

Tuberculin, Purified Protein Derivative (PPD) TINE TEST units **must never be reused.**

Reading Reactions: Tests should be read at 48 to 72 hours. Vesiculation or the extent of induration are the determining factors; erythema without induration is of no significance. Readings should be made in good light with the forearm slightly flexed. The size of the induration in millimeters should be determined by inspection, measuring, and palpation with gentle finger stroking. Identification of the application site is usually easy because of the distinct four-point pattern. The diameter of the largest single reaction around one of the puncture sites should be measured. With pronounced reactions, the areas of induration around the puncture sites may coalesce.

INTERPRETATION

Positive Reactions:

A. **Vesiculation.** If vesiculation is present the test may be interpreted as positive, in which case the management of the patient is the same as that for one classified as positive to the Mantoux test.[3]

B. **Induration, 2 mm or greater.** The test may be interpreted as positive but further diagnostic procedures must be considered. These may include X-ray of the chest, microbiological examination of sputa and other specimens, and confirmation of the positive TINE TEST reaction using the Mantoux method.

Negative Reaction:

Induration less than 2 mm. With a negative reaction there is no need for retesting unless the person is a contact of a patient with tuberculosis or there is clinical evidence suggestive of the disease.[3]

Induration indicator cards illustrating typical reactions are enclosed.

HOW SUPPLIED

Tuberculin, Purified Protein Derivative (PPD) TINE TEST is supplied as follows:
NDC 0005-2720–25   25 individual tests
NDC 0005-2720–28   100 individual tests

STORAGE

STORE AT CONTROLLED ROOM TEMPERATURE 15°C–30°C (59°F–86°F). DO NOT REFRIGERATE.

REFERENCES

1. Seibert FB. Isolation and properties of purified protein derivative of tuberculin. *Am Rev Tuberc.* 1934;30:713.
2. Seibert FB, Glenn JF. Tuberculin purified protein derivative—preparation and analysis of a large quantity for standard. *Am Rev Tuberc.* 1941;44:9.
3. Comstock CW, et al. The tuberculin skin test. *Am Rev Respir Dis.* 1981;124:356–363.
4. Freeman BA. *Burrows Textbook of Microbiology.* 22nd ed. Philadelphia, Pa: W. B. Saunders Company; 1985: 295–299.
5. *Report of the Committee on Infectious Diseases.* 21st ed. Elk Grove Village, Ill: American Academy of Pediatrics. 1988:429–447.

LEDERLE LABORATORIES DIVISION
American Cyanamid Company
Pearl River, NY 10965   Rev. 7/89
                                  22796

Shown in Product Identification Section, page 416

TUBERCULIN, OLD, TINE TEST®   ℞
[*to-ber-cu-lĭn*]

DESCRIPTION

The Tuberculin, Old, TINE TEST is a sterile, simple, multiple-puncture, disposable intradermal test device for the detection of tuberculin reactivity. These convenient devices are especially useful in mass tuberculosis screening programs. Each test unit consists of a stainless steel disc attached to a white plastic handle. Projecting from the disc are four triangular-shaped prongs (tines) which are 2 mm long and approximately 4 mm apart. The tines have been mechanically dipped into a solution of Old Tuberculin, containing 7% acacia (gum arabic) and 8.5% lactose as stabilizers, and then dried. The entire unit has been sterilized by Cobalt 60 irradiation. No preservative has been added. The unit is disposable and there is no need for syringes, needles, and other equipment necessary for the standard intradermal tests.

Tuberculin, Old, TINE TEST units have been standardized by clinical evaluation in human subjects to give reactions equivalent to or more potent than 5 TU (US tuberculin units) of standard Old Tuberculin administered intradermally in the Mantoux test. However, all multiple puncture-type devices must be regarded as screening tools, and other appropriate diagnostic procedures, such as the Mantoux test, should be utilized for retesting individuals with positive reactions.

CLINICAL PHARMACOLOGY

Tuberculin deposited in the skin of tuberculin reactive individuals reacts with sensitized lymphocytes to effect the release of mediators of cellular hypersensitivity. Some of these mediators (eg, skin reactive factor) induce an inflammatory response in the skin causing the induration and erythema characteristic of a "positive" reaction.[1,2]

INDICATIONS AND USAGE

Tuberculin, Old, TINE TEST is indicated to detect tuberculin-sensitive individuals. Tuberculin, Old, TINE TEST units are also useful in programs to determine priorities for additional testing (eg, chest X-rays) and in epidemiological surveys to identify those areas having high levels of infection. In clinical studies covering various geographical areas of the US and all age groups, with a total of 30,588 test subjects, there were 911 (4%) false positive reactors among 26,236 subjects who were Mantoux negative, and 342 (8%) false negative reactors among 4,352 subjects who were Mantoux positive.

The frequency of repeated tuberculin tests depends on risk of exposure of the individual and on the prevalence of tuberculosis in the population group. The repeated testing of uninfected individuals does not sensitize to tuberculin. Among individuals with waning sensitivity to homologous or heterologous mycobacterial antigens, however, the stimulus of a tuberculin test may "boost" or increase the size of the reaction to a second test, even causing an apparent development of sensitivity in some cases.[1]

Tuberculin testing should be done with caution in individuals with active tuberculosis (see **PRECAUTIONS**).

CONTRAINDICATIONS

There are no known contraindications for use of Tuberculin, Old, TINE TEST. See **PRECAUTIONS** for information regarding special care to be exercised for safe and effective use.

WARNINGS

There are no known serious adverse reactions or potential safety hazards associated with the use of Tuberculin, Old, TINE TEST. However, as with the use of any biological product, the possibility of anaphylactic reaction should be considered. See **PRECAUTIONS** for information regarding special care to be exercised for safe and effective use.

PRECAUTIONS

Tuberculin testing should be done with caution in individuals with active tuberculosis. Although activation of quiescent lesions is rare, if a patient has a history of occurrence of vesiculation and necrosis with a previous tuberculin test by any method, tuberculin testing should be avoided.

Although clinical allergy to acacia is very rare, this product contains some acacia as stabilizer and should be used with caution in patients with known allergy to this component. In these instances, remedial measures for anaphylactoid reactions, including epinephrine injection (1:1000), must be available for immediate use.

Reactivity to the test may be suppressed in patients who are receiving corticosteroids or immunosuppressive agents, or those who have recently been immunized with live virus vaccines such as measles, mumps, rubella, polio. If tuberculin skin testing is indicated it should be done preceding, or at the time of such immunization, and read 48 to 72 hours later. If the test is not administered in the time suggested, an interval of 4 to 6 weeks should be allowed between tuberculin skin testing and immunization with live virus vaccines to prevent suppression of tuberculin reactivity.[3]

With a positive reaction further diagnostic procedures must be considered. These may include X-ray of the chest, microbiological examinations of sputa and other specimens, and confirmation of the positive TINE TEST reaction (except vesiculation reactions) using the Mantoux method. In general, the TINE TEST does not need to be repeated.

Antituberculous chemotherapy should not be instituted solely on the basis of a single positive TINE TEST.

When vesiculation occurs, the reaction is to be interpreted as strongly positive and a repeat test by the Mantoux method must not be attempted. Similar or more severe vesiculation with or without necrosis is likely to occur.

Pregnancy Category C: Animal reproduction studies have not been conducted with Tuberculin, Old, TINE TEST. It is also not known whether Tuberculin, Old, TINE TEST can cause fetal harm when administered to a pregnant woman or affect reproduction capacity. Tuberculin, Old, TINE TEST should be given to a pregnant woman only if clearly needed. During pregnancy, known positive reactors may demonstrate a negative response to a Tuberculin, Old, TINE TEST. Tuberculin, Old, TINE TEST units must never be reused.

ADVERSE REACTIONS

Vesiculation (positive reaction), ulceration, or necrosis may occur at the test site in highly sensitive persons. Pain, pruritus, and discomfort at the test site may be relieved by cold packs or by topical glucocorticoid ointment or cream. Transient bleeding may be observed at a puncture site and is of no significance.

DOSAGE AND ADMINISTRATION

Tuberculin, Old, TINE TEST units have been standardized by clinical evaluation in human subjects to give reactions equivalent to or more potent than 5 TU (US tuberculin units) of standard Old Tuberculin administered intradermally in the Mantoux test. However, all multiple puncture-type devices must be regarded as screening tools and other appropriate diagnostic procedures, such as the Mantoux test, should be utilized for retesting reactors.

The volar surface of the upper one-third of the forearm, over a muscle belly, is the preferred site. Hairy areas, and areas without adequate subcutaneous tissue, eg, concavities over a tendon or bone, should be avoided.

Alcohol, acetone, ether, or soap and water may be used to cleanse the skin. The area must be clean and thoroughly dry before application of the Tuberculin, Old, TINE TEST.

Expose the four coated tines by removing the protective cap while holding the plastic handle. Grasp the patient's forearm firmly, since the sharp momentary sting may cause the patient to jerk his or her arm, resulting in scratching. Stretch the skin of the forearm tightly and apply the disc with the other hand. **Hold at least one second.** Release tension grip on forearm. Withdraw tine unit.

Sufficient pressure should be exerted so that the four puncture sites, and circular depression of the skin from the plastic base are visible.

After administration of the test, local care of the skin is not necessary.

Tuberculin, Old, TINE TEST units **must never be reused.**

Reading Reactions: Tests should be read at 48 to 72 hours. Vesiculation or the extent of induration are the determining factors; erythema without induration is of no significance. Readings should be made in good light with the forearm slightly flexed. The size of the induration in millimeters should be determined by inspection, measuring, and palpation with gentle finger stroking. Identification of the application site is usually easy because of the distinct four-point pattern. The diameter of the largest single reaction around one of the puncture sites should be measured. With pronounced reactions, the areas of induration around the puncture sites may coalesce.

INTERPRETATION

Positive Reactions:

A. **Vesiculation.** If vesiculation is present, the test may be interpreted as positive, in which case the management of the patient is the same as that for one classified as positive to the Mantoux test.[1]

B. **Induration, 2 mm or greater.** The test may be interpreted as positive but further diagnostic procedures must be considered. These may include X-ray of the chest, microbiological examination of sputa and other specimens, and confirmation of the positive TINE TEST reaction using the Mantoux method.

Negative Reaction:

Induration less than 2 mm. With a negative reaction there is no need for retesting unless the person is a contact of a patient with tuberculosis or there is clinical evidence suggestive of the disease.[1]

Induration indicator cards illustrating typical reactions are enclosed.

HOW SUPPLIED

Tuberculin, Old, TINE TEST is supplied as follows:
NDC 0005-2722-25 25 individual tests
NDC 0005-2722-28 100 individual tests
NDC 0005-2722-34 250 individual tests

Military Depots:
NSN 6505-00-890-1534 25 tests

STORE AT CONTROLLED ROOM TEMPERATURE 15°C–30°C (59°F–86°F). DO NOT REFRIGERATE.

REFERENCES

1. Comstock CW, et al: The tuberculin skin test. *Am Rev Respir Dis.* 1981;124:356–363.
2. Freeman BA: *Burrows Textbook of Microbiology,* 22nd ed. Philadelphia, Pa: W. B. Saunders Company; 1985: 295–299.
3. Report of the Committee on Infectious Diseases. American Academy of Pediatrics. 21st ed. Elk Grove Village, Ill; 1988: 429–447.

LEDERLE LABORATORIES DIVISION
American Cyanamid Company
Pearl River, NY 10965   Rev. 7/89
                                  22795

Shown in Product Identification Section, page 416

Information on Lederle products listed on these pages is the full prescribing information from product literature or package inserts effective in August 1992. Information concerning all Lederle products may be obtained from the Professional Services Department, Lederle Laboratories, Pearl River, New York, 10965.

LifeScan Inc.
a Johnson & Johnson Company
1000 GIBRALTAR DR.
MILPITAS, CA 95035-6312

ONE TOUCH® II
BLOOD GLUCOSE MONITORING SYSTEM

DESCRIPTION

The ONE TOUCH® II System provides very accurate blood glucose results for your patients with diabetes through a simple three-step procedure which requires no user timing, wiping, or blotting. Simply press power and insert test strip, apply blood sample, accurate results in 45 seconds. Memory stores the most recent 250 results with date and time. Automatically averages last 14 days of blood glucose values excluding Check Strip and Control results. Signals when the Meter must be cleaned, and detects and notifies patients of most errors in blood sample size and application. In clinical studies, patients using the ONE TOUCH II Meter achieved results that were 99% clinically accurate, compared to the YSI reference standard.[1]

HOW SUPPLIED

ONE TOUCH II Blood Glucose Monitoring Kit—Each Complete Kit contains everything your patient needs to begin blood glucose monitoring:
ONE TOUCH II Blood Glucose Meter
—with 250-Test Memory with date and time
—Display prompts in eight languages, including Spanish
25 ONE TOUCH Test Strips
Carry Case
PENLET® II Automatic Blood Sampler
25 Lancets
ONE TOUCH Normal Glucose Control Solution
Instructional Audio Cassette
Owner's Booklet
Logbook
Size J Battery

For a ONE TOUCH II System demonstration and a complete review of clinical data, contact your LifeScan Professional Representative. For the name of your local representative, call toll free:

In the United States:	1 800 227-8862
In Canada:	1 800 663-5521

1. Clinical accuracy is defined as test results within 20% of reference method. Data on file, available upon request.

Eli Lilly and Company
LILLY CORPORATE CENTER
INDIANAPOLIS, IN 46285

TES-TAPE® OTC
[tĕs ′tāp]
(glucose enzymatic test strip)
USP

For In Vitro Diagnostic Use in Testing for the Presence and Semiquantitative Measurement of Glucose in Human Urine

Tes-Tape® (Glucose Enzymatic Test Strip, Lilly) has been used since 1956, when Dr. A. S. Keston described the novel idea of using 2 enzymes simultaneously to test for glucose and Dr. J. P. Comer published data on the specificity and accuracy of Tes-Tape for the semiquantitative analysis of urine glucose.

During the development and testing of this urine test method, Tes-Tape was found to be an accurate and reliable semiquantitative method for determining urine glucose. To date, relatively few instances of faulty results have occurred with the use of Tes-Tape. Problems associated with the product are usually due to improper techniques, exposure of the tape to adverse conditions, or drugs that have an inhibitory effect on the enzyme reaction. Considerable data may be found in the published scientific documents.

Tes-Tape is impregnated with the enzymes glucose oxidase and peroxidase and an oxidizable substrate, orthotolidine. When the tape is dipped into urine containing glucose, the glucose oxidase catalyzes the reaction of the glucose in the urine with oxygen from the air to form gluconic acid and hydrogen peroxide. The enzyme peroxidase (from horseradish) then catalyzes the reaction of hydrogen peroxide and orthotolidine, forming a blue color. With the addition of a yellow dye (FDC Yellow No. 5) to the paper, the possible color range of the test is extended from yellow to light green to deep blue. If no glucose is present, the tape maintains its yellow color.

Reactive Ingredient	Approximate Amount per 1.5 Inches of Tape
Glucose oxidase	3.78 units
Horseradish peroxidase	2.82 PZ units
O-tolidine	0.136 mg

Nonreactive ingredients include filter paper, FDC Yellow No. 5 coloring, buffers, stabilizers, and wetting agents.

For in vitro diagnostic use. Store below 86°F (30°C). Protect from high humidity and light.

Do not use if the tape becomes dark yellow or yellowish-brown or if a 2% reading is not obtained when the reliability is tested, as described under the heading *Important*.

The urine should be collected in a container free of chemicals and glucose.

If the freshly voided specimen is not to be tested within 4 hours, it should be refrigerated.

Drugs that are known to have an inhibitory effect on the enzyme reactions include ascorbic acid (vitamin C), dipyrone, gentisic acid (a metabolite of aspirin), homogentisic acid (present in alkaptonuria), levodopa, meralluride injection, and methyldopa. The inhibiting effect is notable on the dipped part of the tape, but accurate readings may be obtained by observing the narrow band of color at the junction of the dry and wet portions. A separation of glucose from the inhibitory substances occurs as the urine travels along the dry portion of the tape. Ingestion of more than 1.5 g of ascorbic acid may produce urine with inhibitory action on Tes-Tape due to acidity.

Specimens for storage or shipment should be refrigerated or preserved with up to 0.37% formaldehyde.

All materials are provided for the test; these include dispenser, tape, and color chart.

Results on the color chart are expressed in percent of glucose (urine sugar) and by a corresponding arbitrary system of 0, +, + +, + + +, + + + +, representing 0, $\frac{1}{10}$, $\frac{1}{4}$, $\frac{1}{2}$, 2 (or more) % of glucose respectively.

When testing, do not place the tape on the lavatory or on paper or allow moistened portion to contact fingers. Contamination of the tape by glucose from other sources (eg, perspiration, tears, and saliva) or with a residue of chlorine from lavatory cleansing agents can cause false-positive results.

Patients who are receiving high doses of ascorbic acid or whose urine contains dipyrone, meralluride, homogentisic acid, gentisic acid, levodopa, or methyldopa should read only the very narrow band of color in the moist portion of the tape above the level to which it was dipped into the specimen.

Very high doses of ascorbic acid may cause a false-negative test despite taking the above precaution. (Urinary levels of ascorbic acid in excess of 0.1% are necessary to block the test completely. This concentration is most likely to appear within 3 to 7 hours after a single dose of 1.5 g or more.) Penicillin, cephalosporin, and aminoglycoside antibiotics have not been shown to adversely influence Tes-Tape accuracy in measuring urine glucose levels.

Normal urine should test 0% with Tes-Tape. Persons using Tes-Tape for a screening test should report all values above 0% to their physician. Diabetic urine values in the range of the color chart should also be recorded and reported to the patient's physician. Measured values of 2% should be reported as 2% or more.

The overall semiquantitative accuracy of Tes-Tape originally reported in 1956 on 1,000 determinations was 96%. This was confirmed in 1973 on 14,000 determinations over a 2-year period. These data were obtained by taking urine samples containing concentrations of glucose at each measurable increment on the color chart. The color chart provided is based on the average color perception of many observers. Patients who have difficulty in differentiating color should seek the advice of their physician before using Tes-Tape.

Numerous other clinical and laboratory studies have shown that Tes-Tape is accurate in qualitative and semiquantitative determinations of urine sugar. Tes-Tape is specific for glucose in urine sugar testing. Contamination of the tape or urine receptacle with glucose from other sources (eg, perspiration, tears, and saliva) or with a residue of chlorine from cleansing agents, have produced false-positive results for glucose. False high values can also be obtained if Tes-Tape is exposed to peroxide-containing detergents. When Tes-Tape is exposed to these detergents (ie, inadequately rinsed urine specimen containers cleansed with these detergents), the peroxides in the detergent can oxidize the dye in the enzyme strip, producing a false-positive reaction. Except for the instances mentioned above, there are no known clinical situations in which a false-positive test for glucose occurs with Tes-Tape. The sensitivity of Tes-Tape is such that it will react with concentrations of 0.05% glucose or more. Trace reactions, shown by the development of a very light yellow-green color, may be observed with less than this amount of glucose.

After opening plastic wrapper, use tape within 4 months. It must be used prior to expiration date.

IMPORTANT

The reliability of a roll of Tes-Tape may easily be checked by dipping a piece into a properly prepared glucose solution.* The tape should be removed immediately, as one would when testing a urine specimen. After 2 minutes have elapsed, the reading obtained when the tape is compared with the color chart should be approximately + + + + (2%). If such a reading is not obtained, the tape has apparently deteriorated and should not be used.

Measurements for the amount of glucose present (semiquantitative) should not be made after 2 minutes because the colors gradually change as the tape dries. Screening tests for the presence of glucose (qualitative) in urine may be made for several hours after the tape has dried.

The patient should consult the package insert in regard to Procedure, What to Do If Tape Breaks, and a record chart for urine sugar tests with Tes-Tape.

*If a properly prepared glucose solution is not available, any nationally known *sugar (glucose)-containing* beverage from a freshly opened bottle or can is satisfactory. (Diet beverages would not be satisfactory.) DO NOT INGEST GLUCOSE SOLUTION OR BEVERAGE AFTER USING FOR A GLUCOSE TEST.

HOW SUPPLIED

M-73, Tes-Tape® (Glucose Enzymatic Test Strip, USP), dispenser package, approximately 100 tests, in single packages. (NDC 0002-2344-41) [043090]

Parke-Davis
Division of Warner-Lambert Company
201 TABOR ROAD
MORRIS PLAINS, NEW JERSEY 07950

APLISOL® ℞
[ă ′plĭ-sŏl ″]
(Tuberculin Purified Protein Derivative, Diluted [Stabilized Solution])

DESCRIPTION

Aplisol (tuberculin PPD, diluted) is a sterile aqueous solution of a purified protein fraction for intradermal administration as an aid in the diagnosis of tuberculosis. The solution is stabilized with polysorbate (Tween) 80, buffered with potassium and sodium phosphates and contains approximately 0.35% phenol as a preservative.

The product is clinically equivalent in potency to the standard PPD-S* (5 TU** per 0.1 ml) of the U.S. Public Health Service, National Center for Disease Control, and is ready for immediate use without further dilution. This product meets all applicable standards.

CLINICAL PHARMACOLOGY

The purified protein fraction is isolated from culture filtrates of human type strains of *Mycobacterium tuberculosis* by the method of F.B. Seibert.[1,2] This product is made from a single master lot (No. 924994) to eliminate lot to lot variation inherent in manufacturing.

The 5 TU dose of Tuberculin PPD intradermally (Mantoux) is recommended as the standard tuberculin test, and Tuberculin PPD is recommended by the American Lung Association as an aid in the detection of infection with *Mycobacterium tuberculosis.*

Reactions to the Mantoux test are interpreted on the basis of a quantitative measurement of the response to a specific dose (5 TU PPD-S or equivalent) of Tuberculin PPD. Other dosages are regarded as having no demonstrable usefulness in ordinary practice.[3] Accordingly, Aplisol is available in only one potency (5 TU equivalent) and the use of this potency only is recommended. The selection of 5 TU as the test dose is based upon data indicating that (1) the 5 TU dose gives measurable reactions in over 95 percent of the known tuberculous infected; (2) doses larger than 5 TU might elicit reactions not caused by tuberculosis infection; and (3) nonreactors to doses considerably less than 5 TU are not accepted as negative but are retested with a stronger dose.[3]

INDICATIONS AND USAGE

Tuberculin PPD is recommended by the American Lung Association as an aid in the detection of infection with *Mycobacterium tuberculosis.* The standard tuberculin test recommended employs the intradermal (Mantoux) test using a 5 TU dose of tuberculin PPD.[3] The 0.1 ml test dose of Aplisol (tuberculin PPD, diluted) is equivalent to the 5 TU dose recommended as clinically established and standardized with PPD-S.

CONTRAINDICATIONS

None known.

WARNINGS

Tuberculin should not be administered to known tuberculin-positive reactors because of the severity of reactions (e.g.,

*PPD-S (No. 49608) World Health Organization International PPD-Tuberculin Standard (PPD-S is a dried powder from which WHO and U.S. Standard tuberculin solutions are made.)

**U.S. Tuberculin Unit

vesiculation, ulceration or necrosis) that may occur at the test site in very highly sensitive individuals.
Avoid injecting tuberculin subcutaneously. If this occurs, no local reaction develops, but a general febrile reaction and/or acute inflammation around old tuberculous lesions may occur in highly sensitive individuals.

PRECAUTIONS

General
A separate heat sterilized syringe and needle, or a sterile disposable unit, should be used for each individual patient to prevent possible transmission of homologous serum hepatitis virus and other infectious agents from one person to another.
Syringes that have previously been used with histoplasmin, blastomycin and other antigens should not be used for tuberculin.
As with any biological product, epinephrine should be immediately available in case an anaphylactoid or acute hypersensitivity reaction occurs.

Pregnancy
Teratogenic effects: Pregnancy Category C. Animal reproduction studies have not been conducted with Aplisol. It is also not known whether Aplisol can cause fetal harm when administered to a pregnant woman or can affect the reproduction capacity. Aplisol should be given to a pregnant woman only if clearly needed.
However, the risk of unrecognized tuberculosis and the close postpartum contact between a mother with active disease and an infant leaves the infant in grave danger of tuberculosis and complications such as tuberculous meningitis. Although there have been not been reported any adverse effects upon the fetus recognized as being due to tuberculosis skin testing, the prescribing physician will want to consider if the potential benefits outweigh the possible risks for performing the tuberculin test on a pregnant woman or woman of childbearing age, particularly in certain high risk populations.

ADVERSE REACTIONS

In highly sensitive individuals, strongly positive reactions including vesiculation, ulceration or necrosis may occur at the test site. Cold packs or topical steroid preparations may be employed for symptomatic relief of the associated pain, pruritus, and discomfort.
Strongly positive test reactions may result in scarring at the test site.
Immediate erythematous or other reactions may occur at the injection site. The reason(s) for these infrequent occurrences are presently unknown.

DOSAGE AND ADMINISTRATION

Standard Method (Mantoux Test)
The Mantoux test is performed by intradermally injecting with a syringe and needle exactly 0.1 ml of tuberculin PPD, diluted. The result is read 48 to 72 hours later and induration only is considered in interpreting the test. The standard test is performed as follows:

1. The site of the test is usually the flexor or dorsal surface of the forearm about 4″ below the elbow. Other skin sites may be used, but the flexor surface of the forearm is preferred.
2. The skin at the injection site is cleansed with 70% alcohol and allowed to dry.
3. The test material is administered with a tuberculin syringe (0.5 or 1.0 ml) fitted with a short (½″) 26 or 27 gauge needle.
4. The syringe and needle should be of a sterile disposable, single use type or should have been sterilized by autoclaving, boiling or by the use of dry heat. A separate sterile unit should be used for each person tested.
5. The diaphragm of the vial-stopper should be wiped with 70% alcohol.
6. The needle is inserted through the stopper diaphragm of the inverted vial. Exactly 0.1 ml is filled into the syringe, with care being taken to exclude air bubbles and to maintain the lumen of the needle filled.
7. The point of the needle is inserted into the most superficial layers of the skin with the needle bevel pointing upward. As the tuberculin solution is injected, a pale bleb 6 to 10 mm in size (⅜″) will rise over the point of the needle. This is quickly absorbed and no dressing is required.

In the event the injection is delivered subcutaneously (ie, no bleb will form), or if a significant part of the dose leaks from the injection site, the test should be repeated immediately at another site at least 5 cm (2″) removed.
Aplisol vials should be inspected visually for particulate matter and discoloration prior to administration.
The Mantoux test is the standard of comparison for all other tuberculin tests.
Aplisol is a stabilized solution of Tuberculin PPD. Data indicate that Aplisol is stable when prefilled into syringes and stored in a refrigerator for up to 30 days.
However, the practice of storing such prefilled syringes is not recommended as good practice because of the increased potential for contamination.

Interpretation of Tuberculin Reaction
Readings of Mantoux reactions should be made during the period from 48 to 72 hours after the injection. Induration only should be considered in interpreting the test. The diameter of induration should be measured transversely to the long axis of the forearm and recorded in millimeters. Erythema of less than 10 mm should be disregarded. If the area of erythema is greater than 10 mm and induration is absent the injection may have been made too deeply and retesting is indicated.
Reactions should be interpreted as follows:
Positive—Induration measuring 10 mm or more. This indicates hypersensitivity to tuberculoprotein and should be interpreted as positive for past or present infection with *M. tuberculosis.*
Doubtful—Induration measuring 5 to 9 mm. Retesting is indicated using a different site of injection. Evaluation to rule out cross-reaction from other mycobacterial infection should be considered.
Negative—Induration of less than 5 mm. This indicates a lack of hypersensitivity to tuberculoprotein and tuberculous infection is highly unlikely.
It should be noted that reactivity to tuberculin may be depressed or suppressed for as long as four weeks by viral infections, live virus vaccines (i.e., measles, smallpox, polio, rubella and mumps), or by the administration of corticosteroids. Malnutrition may also have a similar effect. When of diagnostic importance, a negative test should be accepted as proof that hypersensitivity is absent only after normal reactivity to nonspecific irritants has been demonstrated. A primary injection of tuberculin may possibly have a boosting effect on subsequent tuberculin reactions.
A child who is known to have been exposed to a tuberculous adult must not be adjudged free of infection until he has a negative tuberculin reaction at least ten weeks after contact with the tuberculous person has ceased.[4]
A positive tuberculin reaction does not necessarily signify the presence of active disease. Further diagnostic procedures should be carried out before a diagnosis of tuberculosis is made. A small percentage of responders may not have been infected with *M. tuberculosis* but by some other mycobacterium.

HOW SUPPLIED

N 0071-4525-03 (Bio. 1525)
1 ml (10 tests)—rubber-diaphragm-capped vial
N 0071-4525-08 (Bio. 1607)
5 ml (50 tests)—rubber-diaphragm-capped vial
This product should be stored at 2° to 8°C (36° to 46°F), and protected from light.

REFERENCES

1. Seibert, F.B.: Am. Rev. Tuberc. 30:713, 1934.
2. Seibert, F.B., and Glenn, J.T.: Am. Rev. Tuberc. 44:9, 1941.
3. Diagnostic Standards and Classification of Tuberculosis and Other Mycobacterial Diseases, American Lung Association, New York, 1974.
4. Sewell, E.M., O'Hare, D., and Kendig, E.L., Jr.: The Tuberculin Test, Pediatrics, Vol. 54, No. 5, Nov. 1974.

4525G033

APLITEST® ℞

[ă ′plĭ-tĕst″]
Tuberculin Purified Protein Derivative
Multiple-Puncture Device

DESCRIPTION

Aplitest (tuberculin PPD) is a sterile, single-use, multiple-puncture type device for percutaneous administration for use in determining the tuberculin sensitivity status of individuals. Aplitest, a diagnostic aid, has been clinically compared with 5 US Tuberculin Units of PPD-S administered intradermally.
These disposable devices are useful in mass tuberculosis screening programs. The product packaging facilitates the use of Aplitest units for testing of individual patients in office, ward, or clinic settings.
Each Aplitest unit consists of a cylindrical plastic holder bearing four equally spaced stainless steel tines at one end. The tines have been coated by dipping in a solution of tuberculin PPD and dried. The tuberculin solution applied to the tines is buffered with potassium and sodium phosphates and contains approximately 0.5% phenol as a preservative. The narrow (tine-bearing) end of each unit fits into a protective cap to protect the tines and maintain their sterility.
The purified tuberculin protein fraction is isolated from culture filtrates of human-type strains of *Mycobacterium tuberculosis* by the method of F.B. Seibert.[1,2] Purified tuberculin protein solution is prepared from a single master lot (No. 975302) to eliminate lot to lot variation.

CLINICAL PHARMACOLOGY

Tuberculin deposited in the skin of tuberculin-reactive individuals reacts with sensitized lymphocytes to effect the release of mediators of cellular hypersensitivity. Some of these mediators, eg, skin reactive factor, induce an inflammatory response to the skin, causing the induration characteristic of a "positive" or "significant" reaction.
Aplitest has been standardized by clinical studies in human subjects against 5 TU* of PPD-S administered intradermally by the Mantoux test, and guidelines relating response to the two treatments have been formulated. (See "Interpretation of Response" section.)

INDICATIONS AND USAGE

Aplitest is indicated to detect tuberculin-sensitive individuals. Aplitest units are also useful in programs to establish priorities for additional testing (ie, chest x-rays) and in epidemiological surveys to identify areas with high levels of infection.
All multiple-puncture type devices should be regarded as screening tools, and appropriate diagnostic procedures (eg, Mantoux test with tuberculin PPD diluted, Aplisol®) should be employed for retesting "doubtful" reactors.
Regular periodic (annual or biennial)[3] testing of tuberculin-negative persons is recommended and is especially valuable because the conversion of an individual from negative to positive is highly indicative of recent tuberculosis infection. Repeated testing of the uninfected individual does not sensitize to tuberculin. In persons with waning sensitivity to homologous or heterologous mycobacterial antigens, however, the stimulus of a tuberculin test may "boost" or increase the size of reaction to a second test, even causing an apparent development of sensitivity in some instances.

CONTRAINDICATIONS

None known.

WARNINGS

Tuberculin should not be administered to known tuberculin-positive reactors because of the severity of reactions (eg, vesiculation, ulceration or necrosis) that may occur at the test site in very highly sensitive individuals.
As with any biological product, epinephrine should be immediately available in case an anaphylactoid or acute hypersensitivity reaction occurs.

PRECAUTIONS

General: A separate, sterile unit must be used for each individual patient and disposed of after use.
Sensitivity may decrease or disappear temporarily during or immediately following severe febrile illness, measles, and other exanthemas, live virus vaccination, sarcoidosis, overwhelming miliary or pulmonary tuberculosis, and the administration of corticosteroids or immunosuppressive drugs. Severe malnutrition may also have a similar effect.
A positive tuberculin reaction does not necessarily signify the presence of active disease. Further diagnostic procedures should be carried out before a diagnosis of tuberculosis is made.
Simultaneous application of two or more multiple-puncture devices is not recommended. The response of an individual to a single multiple-puncture device may be altered by the simultaneous administration of additional tuberculin tests (multiple-puncture or Mantoux).[4]
Pregnancy: Teratogenic effects: Pregnancy Category C. Animal reproduction studies have not been conducted with Aplitest. It is also not known whether Aplitest can cause fetal harm when administered to a pregnant woman or can affect reproduction capacity. Aplitest should be given to a pregnant woman only if clearly needed.
However, the risk of unrecognized tuberculosis and the close postpartum contact between a mother with active disease and an infant leaves the infant in grave danger of tuberculosis and complications such as tuberculous meningitis. Although there have not been reported any adverse effects upon the fetus recognized as being due to tuberculosis skin testing, the prescribing physician will want to consider if the potential benefits outweigh the possible risks for performing the tuberculin test on a pregnant woman or a woman of childbearing age, particularly in certain high risk populations.

ADVERSE REACTIONS

In highly sensitive individuals, strongly positive reactions including vesiculation, ulceration or necrosis, may occur at the test site. Cold packs or topical steroid preparations may be employed for symptomatic relief of the associated pain pruritus and discomfort.

*U.S. (International) tuberculin units.

Continued on next page

This product information was prepared in August, 1992. On these and other Parke-Davis Products, information may be obtained by addressing PARKE-DAVIS, Division of Warner-Lambert Company, Morris Plains, New Jersey 07950.

Parke-Davis—Cont.

Strongly positive test reactions may result in scarring at the test site.
Minimal bleeding may be experienced at a puncture site. This occurs infrequently and does not affect the interpretation of the test.

DOSAGE AND ADMINISTRATION

Each Aplitest unit provides for the intradermal administration of one test-dose of tuberculin PPD.

Method of Application

1. The preferred site of the test is the flexor surface of the forearm about 4 inches below the elbow. Other suitable skin sites, such as the dorsal surface of the forearm, may be used. Areas without adequate subcutaneous tissue, such as over a tendon, should be avoided.
2. The skin at the test site should be cleaned with 70% alcohol, or other suitable agent, and allowed to dry thoroughly.
3. To expose the four impregnated tines, grasp the device and twist to break the perforated label seal.
4. Grasp the patient's forearm firmly to stretch the skin taut at the test site and to prevent any jerking motion of the arm that could cause scratching with the tines.
5. Apply the Aplitest unit firmly and without twisting to the test area for approximately one second. Sufficient pressure should be exerted to assure that all four tines have penetrated the skin of the test area.
6. Dispose of used units in a manner to avoid accidents. Do not reuse.

Interpretation of Response

Selection of the appropriate criteria for interpretation of response to the tuberculin PPD Aplitest should be made in accordance with the objectives of the specific testing program and with consideration of the history and clinical status of the individuals.
Reading of reactions should be made during the period from 48 to 72 hours after application of Aplitest and should be conducted under good lighting conditions. Induration only should be considered in interpreting the test. Erythema should be disregarded. The diameter of the induration of the greatest response at any of the four puncture points should be determined by visual inspection and palpation. If there is coalescence of reaction, the largest diameter of coalescent induration should be measured and recorded.
The American Thoracic Society recommends that all multiple-puncture tuberculin skin test devices be interpreted as follows: If vesiculation is present, the test may be interpreted as positive. If vesiculation is not present, induration of 2 mm or more is considered as a doubtful reaction and a Mantoux test for diagnostic evaluation should be given. Decisions concerning management should be based on the reaction to the Mantoux test and relevant diagnostic criteria. Induration of less than 2 mm and/or erythema of any size is a negative test and there is no need for retesting.[5]
In clinical studies with Aplitest, it has been determined that coalescence of the induration around two or more puncture sites corresponds more than 90% of the time to 10 mm or more of induration in the same individual tested by Mantoux test at the 5 TU level with PPD-S.†
Thus, the following criteria of interpretation have been established.

1. Vesiculation—Positive Reaction
The test should be interpreted as positive and the management of the subject is the same as that for one classified as positive by Mantoux test.

2. Coalescence of induration from two or more puncture points—Doubtful Reaction
A subject with a coalescent reaction may be considered for Mantoux retest. However, more than 90% of the time this reaction was equivalent to a reaction of 10 mm or more of induration with PPD-S (5 TU) administered by Mantoux test.[6] Other criteria, such as contact with tuberculosis patients and case history, should be considered to determine the likelihood that such a reaction is considered positive.

3. 2 mm or more of induration without coalescence—Doubtful Reaction
Reactions of this size range reflect sensitivity that can result from infection with either atypical mycobacteria or *M tuberculosis;* hence, they are classified as doubtful.
A standard Mantoux test should be done on all subjects in this group. Management should be based on the reaction to the Mantoux test, as well as other clinical considerations.

4. Less than 2 mm of induration—Negative Reaction
There is no need for retesting unless the individual is in contact with a case of tuberculosis or there is clinical evidence suggestive of the disease.

†Purified Protein Derivative (Seibert). Lot No. 49608, the standard adopted by the World Health Organization in 1952 as International PPD Tuberculin and used to prepare the official U.S. Public Health Service 5 TU solution of tuberculin for skin testing known as PPD-S.

HOW SUPPLIED

N 0071-4589-13 (Bio. 1590) 25-test package. Twenty-five individually capped Aplitest units in a dispensing package.
Aplitest (tuberculin PPD, multiple-puncture device) units should be stored at no warmer than 30°C (86°F).

REFERENCES

1. Seibert, F.B.: Am. Rev. Tuberc. 30:713, 1934.
2. Seibert, F.B., and Glenn J.T.: Am. Rev. Tuberc. 44:9, 1941.
3. Report of the Committee on Infectious Diseases, American Academy of Pediatrics, 1982.
4. Rosenthal, S.R., and Libby, J.E.P.: Bull. Wld. Hlth. Org. 23:689, 1960.
5. Diagnostic Standards and Classification of Tuberculosis and Other Mycobacterial Diseases, American Lung Association, 1974.
6. Unpublished data from Warner-Lambert Co. available upon request.

4589G022

Sanofi Winthrop Pharmaceuticals
90 PARK AVENUE
NEW YORK, NY 10016

OMNIPAQUE® 140 180 210 240 300 350 ℞

INJECTION (IOHEXOL)
Section I—Intrathecal
Section II—Intravascular
Section III—Oral/Body Cavity Use

DESCRIPTION

Iohexol, *N,N'*-Bis(2,3-dihydroxypropyl)-5-[*N*-(2,3-dihydroxypropyl)-acetamido]-2,4,6-triiodoisophthalamide, is a nonionic, water-soluble radiographic contrast medium with a molecular weight of 821.14 (iodine content 46.36%). In aqueous solution each triiodinated molecule remains undissociated.
OMNIPAQUE is provided as a sterile, pyrogen-free, colorless to pale yellow solution, in the following iodine concentrations: 140, 180, 210, 240, 300, and 350 mgI/mL. OMNIPAQUE 140 contains 302 mg of iohexol equivalent to 140 mg of organic iodine per mL; OMNIPAQUE 180 contains 388 mg of iohexol equivalent to 180 mg of organic iodine per mL; OMNIPAQUE 210 contains 453 mg of iohexol equivalent to 210 mg of organic iodine per mL; OMNIPAQUE 240 contains 518 mg of iohexol equivalent to 240 mg of organic iodine per mL; OMNIPAQUE 300 contains 647 mg of iohexol equivalent to 300 mg of organic iodine per mL; and OMNIPAQUE 350 contains 755 mg of iohexol equivalent to 350 mg of organic iodine per mL. Each milliliter of iohexol solution contains 1.21 mg tromethamine and 0.1 mg edetate calcium disodium with the pH adjusted between 6.8 and 7.7 with hydrochloric acid or sodium hydroxide. All solutions are sterilized by autoclaving and contain no preservatives. Unused portions must be discarded. Iohexol solution is sensitive to light and therefore should be protected from exposure.
The available concentrations have the following physical properties: [See table below.]

OMNIPAQUE 140, OMNIPAQUE 180, OMNIPAQUE 210, OMNIPAQUE 240, OMNIPAQUE 300, and OMNIPAQUE 350 have osmolalities from approximately 1.1 to 3.0 times that of plasma (285 mOsm/kg water) or cerebrospinal fluid (301 mOsm/kg water) as shown in the table below and are hypertonic under conditions of use.

SECTION I

CLINICAL PHARMACOLOGY—Intrathecal

Iohexol is absorbed from cerebrospinal fluid (CSF) into the bloodstream and is eliminated by renal excretion. No significant metabolism, deiodination, or biotransformation occurs.
In five adult patients receiving 16 to 18 milliliters of iohexol (180 mgI/mL) by lumbar intrathecal injection, approximately 88 (73.1–98.2) percent of the injected dose was excreted in the urine within the first 24 hours after administration. The renal and body clearances were 99 (47–137) milliliters per minute and 109 (52–138) milliliters per minute. The mean maximal plasma concentration was 119 (72–177) micrograms of iohexol per milliliter and occurred after 3.8 (2–6) hours. The volume of distribution was 557 (350–849) milliliters per kilogram. In one patient with a large spinal cord tumor, excretion was delayed (67 percent of the dose appeared in the urine within the first 24 hours) with no difference in the total overall recovery in the urine after 48 hours. The delay in excretion appeared to be related to a decrease in the rate of transfer of iohexol from the cerebrospinal fluid to the blood (plasma maximal concentration was approximately 30 micrograms/mL).
The initial concentration and volume of the medium, in conjunction with appropriate patient manipulation and the volume of CSF into which the medium is placed, will determine the extent of the diagnostic contrast that can be achieved.
Following intrathecal injection in conventional radiography, OMNIPAQUE 180, OMNIPAQUE 210, OMNIPAQUE 240, and OMNIPAQUE 300 will continue to provide good diagnostic contrast for at least 30 minutes. Slow diffusion of iohexol takes place throughout the CSF with subsequent absorption into the bloodstream. Once in the systemic circulation, iohexol displays little tendency to bind to serum or plasma proteins. At approximately 1 hour following injection, contrast of diagnostic quality will no longer be available for conventional myelography. If computerized tomographic (CT) myelography is to follow, consideration should be given to a delay of several hours to allow the degree of contrast to decrease.
After administration into the lumbar subarachnoid space, computerized tomography shows the presence of contrast medium in the thoracic region in about 1 hour, in the cervical region in about 2 hours, and in the basal cisterns in 3 to 4 hours.
In patients with renal impairment, depending on the degree of impairment, prolonged plasma iohexol levels may be anticipated due to decreased renal elimination.

INDICATIONS AND USAGE—Intrathecal

OMNIPAQUE 180, OMNIPAQUE 240, and OMNIPAQUE 300 are indicated for intrathecal administration in adults including myelography (lumbar, thoracic, cervical, total columnar) and in contrast enhancement for computerized tomography (myelography, cisternography, ventriculography).
OMNIPAQUE 180 and OMNIPAQUE 210 are indicated for intrathecal administration in children including myelography (lumbar, thoracic, cervical, total columnar) and in contrast enhancement for computerized tomography (myelography, cisternography).

CONTRAINDICATIONS—Intrathecal

OMNIPAQUE should not be administered to patients with a known hypersensitivity to iohexol.
Myelography should not be performed in the presence of significant local or systemic infection where bacteremia is likely.
Intrathecal administration of corticosteroids with OMNIPAQUE (iohexol) is contraindicated.
Because of the possibility of overdosage, immediate repeat myelography in the event of technical failure is contraindicated (see DOSAGE AND ADMINISTRATION).

WARNINGS—General

If grossly bloody CSF is encountered, the possible benefits of a myelographic procedure should be considered in terms of the risk to the patient.
Caution is advised in patients with a history of epilepsy, severe cardiovascular disease, chronic alcoholism, or multiple sclerosis.
Elderly patients may present a greater risk following myelography. The need for the procedure in these patients should be evaluated carefully. Special attention must be paid to dose and concentration of the medium, hydration, and technique used.
Patients who are receiving anticonvulsants should be maintained on this therapy. Should a seizure occur, intravenous diazepam or phenobarbital sodium is recommended. In patients with a history of seizure activity who are not on anticonvulsant therapy, premedication with barbiturates should be considered.

Concentration (mgI/mL)	Osmolality* (mOsm/kg water)	Osmolarity (mOsm/L)	Absolute Viscosity (cp) 20°C	Absolute Viscosity (cp) 37°C	Specific Gravity 37°C
140	322	273	2.3	1.5	1.164
180	408	331	3.1	2.0	1.209
210	460	362	4.2	2.5	1.244
240	520	391	5.8	3.4	1.280
300	672	465	11.8	6.3	1.349
350	844	541	20.4	10.4	1.406

*By vapor-pressure osmometry.

Prophylactic anticonvulsant treatment with barbiturates should be considered in patients with evidence of inadvertent intracranial entry of a large or concentrated bolus of the contrast medium since there may be an increased risk of seizure in such cases.

Drugs which lower the seizure threshold, especially phenothiazine derivatives, including those used for their antihistamine properties, are not recommended for use with OMNIPAQUE (iohexol). Others include MAO inhibitors, tricyclic antidepressants, CNS stimulants, and psychoactive drugs described as analeptics, major tranquilizers, or antipsychotic drugs. While the contributory role of these medications has not been established, the use of such drugs should be based on physician evaluation of potential benefits and potential risks. Physicians have discontinued these agents at least 48 hours before and for at least 24 hours postprocedure.

Care is required in patient management to prevent inadvertent intracranial entry of a large dose or concentrated bolus of the medium. Also, effort should be directed to avoid rapid dispersion of the medium causing inadvertent rise to intracranial levels (eg, by active patient movement). Direct intracisternal or ventricular administration for standard radiography (not CT) is not recommended.

In most reported cases of major motor seizures with nonionic myelographic media, one or more of the following factors were present. Therefore avoid:

- Deviations from recommended procedure or in myelographic management.
- Use in patients with a history of epilepsy.
- Overdosage.
- Intracranial entry of a bolus or premature diffusion of a high concentration of the medium.
- Medication with neuroleptic drugs or phenothiazine antinauseants.
- Failure to maintain elevation of the head during the procedure, on the stretcher, or in bed.
- Excessive and particularly active patient movement or straining.

PRECAUTIONS—General

Diagnostic procedures which involve the use of radiopaque diagnostic agents should be carried out under the direction of personnel with the prerequisite training and with a thorough knowledge of the particular procedure to be performed. Appropriate facilities should be available for coping with any complication of the procedure, as well as for emergency treatment of severe reactions to the contrast agent itself. After parenteral administration of a radiopaque agent, competent personnel and emergency facilities should be available for at least 30 to 60 minutes since severe delayed reactions have occurred. (See ADVERSE REACTIONS.)

Preparatory dehydration is dangerous and may contribute to acute renal failure in patients with advanced vascular disease, diabetic patients, and in susceptible nondiabetic patients (often elderly with preexisting renal disease). Dehydration in these patients seems to be enhanced by the osmotic diuretic action of contrast agents. *Patients should be well hydrated prior to and following administration of any contrast medium, including iohexol.*

The possibility of a reaction, including serious, life-threatening, fatal, anaphylactoid, cardiovascular or central nervous system reactions, should always be considered (see ADVERSE REACTIONS). Therefore, it is of utmost importance that a course of action be carefully planned in advance for the immediate treatment of serious reactions, and that adequate and appropriate facilities and personnel be readily available in case of any reaction.

The possibility of an idiosyncratic reaction in susceptible patients should always be considered (see ADVERSE REACTIONS). The susceptible population includes, but is not limited to, patients with a history of a previous reaction to contrast media, patients with a known sensitivity to iodine per se, and patients with a known clinical hypersensitivity: bronchial asthma, hay fever, and food allergies.

The occurrence of severe idiosyncratic reactions has prompted the use of several pretesting methods. However, pretesting cannot be relied upon to predict severe reactions and may itself be hazardous for the patient. It is suggested that a thorough medical history with emphasis on allergy and hypersensitivity, prior to the injection of any contrast media, may be more accurate than pretesting in predicting potential adverse reactions.

A positive history of allergies or hypersensitivity does not arbitrarily contraindicate the use of a contrast agent where a diagnostic procedure is thought essential, but caution should be exercised (see ADVERSE REACTIONS). Premedication with antihistamines or corticosteroids to avoid or minimize possible allergic reactions in such patients should be considered. Recent reports indicate that such pretreatment does not prevent serious life-threatening reactions, but may reduce both their incidence and severity.

In patients with severe renal insufficiency or failure, compensatory biliary excretion of the drug is anticipated to occur, with a slow clearance into the bile. Patients with hepatorenal insufficiency should not be examined unless the possibility of benefit clearly outweighs the additional risk.

Administration of contrast media should be performed by qualified personnel familiar with the procedure and appropriate patient management (see PATIENT MANAGEMENT). Sterile technique must be used with any spinal puncture.

When OMNIPAQUE (iohexol) is to be injected using plastic disposable syringes, the contrast medium should be drawn into the syringe and used immediately.

If nondisposable equipment is used, scrupulous care should be taken to prevent residual contamination with traces of cleansing agents.

Parenteral products should be inspected visually for particulate matter and discoloration prior to administration. If particulate matter or discoloration is present, do not use.

Repeat Procedures: If in the clinical judgment of the physician sequential or repeat examinations are required, a suitable interval of time between administrations should be observed to allow for normal clearance of the drug from the body (see DOSAGE AND ADMINISTRATION and CLINICAL PHARMACOLOGY).

Information for Patients (or if applicable, children)

Patients receiving injectable radiopaque diagnostic agents should be instructed to:

1. Inform your physician if you are pregnant (see CLINICAL PHARMACOLOGY).
2. Inform your physician if you are diabetic or if you have multiple myeloma, pheochromocytoma, homozygous sickle cell disease or known thyroid disorder (see WARNINGS).
3. Inform your physician if you are allergic to any drugs, food, or if you had any reactions to previous injections of dyes used for x-ray procedures (see PRECAUTIONS—General).
4. Inform your physician about any other medications you are currently taking, including nonprescription drugs, before you are administered this drug.

Drug Interactions

Drugs which lower seizure threshold, especially phenothiazine derivatives including those used for their antihistaminic or antinauseant properties, are not recommended for use with OMNIPAQUE. Others include monoamine oxidase (MAO) inhibitors, tricyclic antidepressants, CNS stimulants, psychoactive drugs described as analeptics, major tranquilizers, or antipsychotic drugs. Such medications should be discontinued at least 48 hours before myelography, should not be used for the control of nausea or vomiting during or after myelography, and should not be resumed for at least 24 hours postprocedure. In nonelective procedures in patients on these drugs, consider prophylactic use of anticonvulsants.

Carcinogenesis, Mutagenesis, Impairment of Fertility

No long-term animal studies have been performed to evaluate carcinogenic potential, mutagenesis, or whether OMNIPAQUE (iohexol) can affect fertility in men or women.

Pregnancy Category B

Reproduction studies have been performed in rats and rabbits with up to 100 times the recommended human dose. No evidence of impaired fertility or harm to the fetus has been demonstrated due to OMNIPAQUE. There are, however, no studies in pregnant women. Because animal reproduction studies are not always predictive of human response, this drug should be used during pregnancy only if clearly needed.

Nursing Mothers

It is not known to what extent iohexol is excreted in human milk. However, many injectable contrast agents are excreted unchanged in human milk. Although it has not been established that serious adverse reactions occur in nursing infants, caution should be exercised when intravascular contrast media are administered to nursing women. Bottle feedings may be substituted for breast feedings for 24 hours following administration of OMNIPAQUE.

Pediatric Use

Pediatric patients at higher risk of experiencing adverse events during contrast medium administration may include those having asthma, a sensitivity to medication and/or allergens, congestive heart failure, a serum creatinine greater than 1.5 mg/dL or those less than 12 months of age.

ADVERSE REACTIONS—Intrathecal

The most frequently reported adverse reactions with OMNIPAQUE are headache, mild to moderate pain including backache, neckache and stiffness, nausea, and vomiting. These reactions usually occur 1 to 10 hours after injection, and almost all occur within 24 hours. They are usually mild to moderate in degree, lasting for a few hours, and usually disappearing within 24 hours. Rarely, headaches may be severe or persist for days. Headache is often accompanied by nausea and vomiting and tends to be more frequent and persistent in patients not optimally hydrated.

Transient alterations in vital signs may occur and their significance must be assessed on an individual basis. Those reactions reported in clinical studies with OMNIPAQUE are listed below in decreasing order of occurrence, based on clinical studies of 1531 patients.

Headaches: The most frequently occurring adverse reaction following myelography has been headache, with an incidence of approximately 18%. Headache may be caused by either a direct effect of the contrast medium or by CSF leakage at the dural puncture site. However, in managing the patient, it is considered more important to minimize intracranial entry of contrast medium by postural management than attempting to control possible CSF leakage (see PATIENT MANAGEMENT).

Pain: Mild to moderate pain including backache, neckache and stiffness, and neuralgia occurred following injection with an incidence of about 8%.

Nausea and Vomiting: Nausea was reported with an incidence of about 6%, and vomiting about 3% (see PATIENT MANAGEMENT). Maintaining normal hydration is very important. The use of phenothiazine antinauseants is not recommended. (See WARNINGS —General.) Reassurance to the patient that the nausea will clear usually is all that is required.

Dizziness: Transient dizziness was reported in about 2% of the patients.

Other Reactions: Other reactions occurring with an individual incidence of less than 0.1% included: feeling of heaviness, hypotension, hypertonia, sensation of heat, sweating, vertigo, loss of appetite, drowsiness, hypertension, photophobia, tinnitus, neuralgia, paresthesia, difficulty in micturition, and neurological changes. All were transient and mild with no clinical sequelae.

Pediatrics

In controlled clinical trials involving 152 patients for pediatric myelography by lumbar puncture, adverse events following the use of OMNIPAQUE 180 and OMNIPAQUE 210 were generally less frequent than with adults.

Headache: 9%
Vomiting: 6%
Backache: 1.3%

Other Reactions: Other reactions occurring with an individual incidence of less than 0.7% included: fever, hives, stomachache, visual hallucination, and neurological changes. All were transient and mild with no clinical sequelae.

General Adverse Reactions to Contrast Media

Physicians should remain alert for the occurrence of adverse effects in addition to those discussed above, particularly the following reactions which have been reported in the literature for other nonionic, water-soluble myelographic media, and rarely with iohexol. These have included, but are not limited to, convulsion, aseptic and bacterial meningitis, and CNS and other neurological disturbances.

An aseptic meningitis syndrome has been reported rarely (less than 0.01%). It was usually preceded by pronounced headaches, nausea and vomiting. Onset usually occurred about 12 to 18 hours postprocedure. Prominent features were meningismus, fever, sometimes with oculomotor signs and mental confusion. Lumbar puncture revealed a high white cell count, high protein content often with a low glucose level and with absence of organisms. The condition usually started to clear spontaneously about 10 hours after onset, with complete recovery over 2 to 3 days.

Allergy or Idiosyncrasy: Chills, fever, profuse diaphoresis, pruritus, urticaria, nasal congestion, dyspnea, and a case of Guillain-Barré syndrome.

CNS Irritation: Mild and transitory perceptual aberrations such as hallucinations, depersonalization, amnesia, hostility, amblyopia, diplopia, photophobia, psychosis, insomnia, anxiety, depression, hyperesthesia, visual or auditory or speech disturbances, confusion and disorientation. In addition, malaise, weakness, convulsion, EEG changes, meningismus, hyperreflexia or areflexia, hypertonia or flaccidity, hemiplegia, paralysis, quadriplegia, restlessness, tremor, echoacousia, echolalia, asterixis, cerebral hemorrhage, and dysphasia have occurred.

Profound mental disturbances have also rarely been reported. They have usually consisted of various forms and degrees of aphasia, mental confusion, or disorientation. The onset is usually at 8 to 10 hours and lasts for about 24 hours, without aftereffects. However, occasionally they have been manifest as apprehension, agitation, or progressive withdrawal in several instances to the point of somnolence, stupor, and coma. In a few cases these have been accompanied by transitory hearing loss or other auditory symptoms and visual disturbances (believed subjective or delusional), including unilateral or bilateral loss of vision which may last for hours. In one case, persistent cortical loss of vision has been reported in association with convulsions. Ventricular block has been reported; amnesia of varying degrees may be present for the reaction event.

Rarely, persistent though transitory weakness in the leg or ocular muscles has been reported.

Continued on next page

This product information was prepared in August 1992. On these and other products of Sanofi Winthrop Pharmaceuticals, detailed information may be obtained on a current basis by direct inquiry to Product Information Services, 90 Park Avenue, New York, NY 10016 (toll free 1-800-446-6267).

Sanofi Winthrop—Cont.

Peripheral neuropathies have been rare and transitory. They include sensory and/or motor or nerve root disturbances, myelitis, persistent leg muscle pain or weakness, 6th nerve palsy, or cauda equina syndrome. Muscle cramps, fasciculation or myoclonia, spinal convulsion, or spasticity is unusual and has responded promptly to a small intravenous dose of diazepam.

In general, the reactions which are known to occur upon parenteral administration of iodinated contrast agents are possible with any nonionic agent. Approximately 95 percent of adverse reactions accompanying the use of water-soluble contrast agents are mild to moderate in degree. However, severe, life-threatening, anaphylactoid and fatal reactions, mostly of cardiovascular origin and central nervous system origin, have occurred.

Adverse reactions to injectable contrast media fall into two categories: chemotoxic reactions and idiosyncratic reactions. Chemotoxic reactions result from the physicochemical properties of the contrast media, the dose, and speed of injection. All hemodynamic disturbances and injuries to organs or vessels perfused by the contrast medium are included in this category.

Idiosyncratic reactions include all other reactions. They occur more frequently in patients 20 to 40 years old. Idiosyncratic reactions may or may not be dependent on the amount of dose injected, the speed of injection, and the radiographic procedure. Idiosyncratic reactions are subdivided into minor, intermediate, and severe. The minor reactions are self-limited and of short duration; the severe reactions are life-threatening and treatment is urgent and mandatory.

The reported incidence of adverse reactions to contrast media in patients with a history of allergy is twice that of the general population. Patients with a history of previous reactions to a contrast medium are three times more susceptible than other patients. However, sensitivity to contrast media does not appear to increase with repeated examinations.

Most adverse reactions to injectable contrast media appear within 1 to 3 minutes after the start of injection, but delayed reactions may occur.

OVERDOSAGE

Clinical consequences of overdosage with OMNIPAQUE (iohexol) have not been reported. However, based on experience with other nonionic myelographic media, physicians should be alert to a potential increase in frequency and severity of CNS-mediated reactions. Even use of a recommended dose can produce effects tantamount to overdosage, if incorrect management of the patient during or immediately following the procedure permits inadvertent early intracranial entry of a large portion of the medium.

The intracisternal LD_{50} value of OMNIPAQUE (in grams of iodine per kilogram body weight) is greater than 2.0 in mice.

DOSAGE AND ADMINISTRATION—Intrathecal

The volume and concentration of OMNIPAQUE 180, OMNIPAQUE 210, OMNIPAQUE 240, or OMNIPAQUE 300 to be administered will depend on the degree and extent of contrast required in the area(s) under examination and on the equipment and technique employed.

OMNIPAQUE 180 at a concentration of 180 mgI/mL, OMNIPAQUE 240 at a concentration of 240 mgI/mL, or OMNIPAQUE 300 at a concentration of 300 mgI/mL is recommended for the examination of the lumbar, thoracic, and cervical regions in adults by lumbar or direct cervical injection and is slightly hypertonic to CSF.

OMNIPAQUE 180 at a concentration of 180 mgI/mL or OMNIPAQUE 210 at a concentration of 210 mgI/mL is recommended for the examination of the lumbar, thoracic, and cervical regions in children by lumbar injection and is slightly hypertonic to CSF.

A total dose of 3060 mg iodine or a concentration of 300 mgI/mL should not be exceeded in adults and a total dose of 2940 mg iodine or a concentration of 210 mgI/mL should not be exceeded in children in a single myelographic examination. This is based on clinical trial evaluation to date. As in all diagnostic procedures, the minimum volume and dose to produce adequate visualization should be used. Most procedures do not require either maximum dose or concentration. Anesthesia is not necessary. Premedication sedatives or tranquilizers are usually not needed (see PRECAUTIONS). Patients should be well hydrated prior to and following contrast administration. Seizure-prone patients should be maintained on anticonvulsant medication.

Many radiopaque contrast agents are incompatible in vitro with some antihistamines and many other drugs; therefore, concurrent drugs should not be physically admixed with contrast agents.

Rate of Injection: To avoid excessive mixing with CSF and consequent dilution of contrast, injection should be made slowly over 1 to 2 minutes.

Depending on the estimated volume of contrast medium which may be required for the procedure a small amount of

Procedure	Formulations	Concentration (mgI/mL)	Volume (mL)	Dose (gI)
Lumbar Myelography (via lumbar injection)	OMNIPAQUE 180 OMNIPAQUE 240	180 240	10–17 7–12.5	1.8–3.06 1.7–3.0
Thoracic Myelography (via lumbar or cervical injection)	OMNIPAQUE 240 OMNIPAQUE 300	240 300	6–12.5 6–10	1.7–3.0 1.8–3.0
Cervical Myelography (via lumbar injection)	OMNIPAQUE 240 OMNIPAQUE 300	240 300	6–12.5 6–10	1.4–3.0 1.8–3.0
Cervical Myelography (via C1-2 injection)	OMNIPAQUE 180 OMNIPAQUE 240 OMNIPAQUE 300	180 240 300	7–10 6–12.5 4–10	1.3–1.8 1.4–3.0 1.2–3.0
Total Columnar Myelography (via lumbar injection)	OMNIPAQUE 240 OMNIPAQUE 300	240 300	6–12.5 6–10	1.4–3.0 1.8–3.0

CSF may be removed to minimize distention of the subarachnoid spaces.

The lumbar or cervical puncture needle may be removed immediately following injection since it is not necessary to remove OMNIPAQUE (iohexol) after injection into the subarachnoid space.

Adults: The usual recommended total doses for use in lumbar, thoracic, cervical, and total columnar myelography in adults are 1.2 gI to 3.06 gI as follows: [See table above.]

Pediatrics: The usual recommended total doses for lumbar, thoracic, cervical, and/or total columnar myelography by lumbar puncture in children are 0.36 gI to 2.94 gI (see table below). Actual volumes administered depend largely on patient age and the following guidelines are recommended.

Age	Conc. (mgI/mL)	Volume (mL)	Dose (gI)
0 to < 3 mos.	180 210	2–4 2–3	0.36–0.72 0.42–0.63
3 to < 36 mos.	180 210	4–8 3–6	0.72–1.44 0.63–1.26
3 to < 7 yrs.	180 210	5–10 5–8	0.9–1.8 1.05–1.68
7 to < 13 yrs.	180 210	5–12 5–10	0.9–2.16 1.05–2.1
13 to 18 yrs.	180 210	6–15 6–14	1.08–2.7 1.26–2.94

Withdrawal of contrast agents from their containers should be accomplished under aseptic conditions with sterile syringes. Spinal puncture must always be performed under sterile conditions.

Parenteral products should be inspected visually for particulate matter or discoloration prior to administration. If particulate matter or discoloration is present, do not use.

Repeat Procedures: If in the clinical judgment of the physician sequential or repeat examinations are required, a suitable interval of time between administrations should be observed to allow for normal clearance of the drug from the body. An interval of at least 48 hours should be allowed before repeat examination; however, whenever possible, 5 to 7 days is recommended.

PATIENT MANAGEMENT—Intrathecal

Suggestions for Usual Patient Management

Good patient management should be exercised at all times to minimize the potential for procedurally related complications.

Preprocedure
- Discontinuance of neuroleptic drugs (including phenothiazines, eg, chlorpromazine, prochlorperazine, and promethazine) at least 48 hours beforehand should be considered.
- Maintain normal diet up to 2 hours before procedure.
- Ensure hydration—fluids up to procedure.

During Procedure
- Use minimum dose and concentration required for satisfactory contrast (see DOSAGE AND ADMINISTRATION).
- In all positioning techniques keep the patient's head elevated above highest level of spine.
- Do not lower head of table more than 15° in moving contrast medium cranially.
- In patients with excessive lordosis, consider lateral position for injection and movement of the medium cephalad.
- Inject slowly (over 1 to 2 minutes) to avoid excessive mixing.
- To maintain as a bolus, move medium to distal area very slowly. Use fluoroscopic monitoring.

- Avoid intracranial entry of a bolus.
- Avoid early and high cephalad dispersion of the medium.
- Avoid abrupt or active patient movement to minimize excessive mixing of medium with CSF. Instruct patient to remain passive. Move patient slowly and only as necessary.

Postprocedure
- Raise head of stretcher to at least 30° before moving patient onto it.
- Movement onto and off the stretcher should be done slowly with the patient completely passive, maintaining head-up position.
- Before moving patient onto bed, raise head of bed 30° to 45°.
- Advise patient to remain still in bed, in a sitting or semisitting position, especially in the first few hours.
- Maintain close observation for at least 12 hours after myelogram.
- Obtain visitors' cooperation in keeping the patient quiet and in head-up position, especially in first few hours.
- Encourage oral fluids. Diet as tolerated.
- If nausea or vomiting occurs, do not use phenothiazine antinauseants. Persistent nausea and vomiting will result in dehydration. Therefore, prompt consideration of replacement by intravenous fluids is recommended.

Alternative Postprocedure Method
- Recent evidence with nonionic, water-soluble contrast media suggests that maintaining the patient postmyelography in an upright position (via wheelchair or ambulation) may help minimize adverse effects. The upright position may help to delay upward dispersion of the medium and to maximize the spinal arachnoid absorption.

HOW SUPPLIED

OMNIPAQUE 180
Vials of 10 mL, 180 mgI/mL, boxes of 10 (NDC 0024-1411-10)
Vials of 20 mL, 180 mgI/mL, boxes of 10 (NDC 0024-1411-20)
OMNIPAQUE 210
Vials of 15 mL, 210 mgI/mL, boxes of 10 (NDC 0024-1402-15)
OMNIPAQUE 240
Vials of 10 mL, 240 mgI/mL, boxes of 10 (NDC 0024-1412-10)
Vials of 20 mL, 240 mgI/mL, boxes of 10 (NDC 0024-1412-20)
OMNIPAQUE 300
Vials of 10 mL, 300 mgI/mL, boxes of 10 (NDC 0024-1413-10)
MYELO-KIT® containing: One 10 mL sterile vial of OMNIPAQUE 180, 180 mgI/mL, in REDI-UNIT™, and one sterile myelogram tray, boxes of 5 (NDC 0024-1415-05)
MYELO-KIT containing: One 20 mL sterile vial of OMNIPAQUE 180, 180 mgI/mL, in REDI-UNIT, and one sterile myelogram tray, boxes of 5 (NDC 0024-1415-06)
MYELO-KIT containing: One 10 mL sterile vial of OMNIPAQUE 240, 240 mgI/mL, in REDI-UNIT and one sterile myelogram tray, boxes of 5 (NDC 0024-1416-05)
REDI-UNIT containing: One sterile 10 mL vial of OMNIPAQUE 180, 180 mgI/mL, boxes of 5 (NDC 0024-1411-07)
REDI-UNIT containing: One sterile 20 mL vial of OMNIPAQUE 180, 180 mgI/mL, boxes of 5 (NDC 0024-1411-08)
REDI-UNIT containing: One sterile 10 mL vial of OMNIPAQUE 240, 240 mgI/mL, boxes of 5 (NDC 0024-1412-07)
Storage: Protect vials of OMNIPAQUE from strong daylight and direct exposure to sunlight. Do not freeze. Store at 59°F to 86°F (15°C to 30°C).

SECTION II

CLINICAL PHARMACOLOGY—Intravascular

Following intravascular injection, iohexol is distributed in the extracellular fluid compartment and is excreted un-

changed by glomerular filtration. It will opacify those vessels in the path of flow of the contrast medium permitting radiographic visualization of the internal structures until significant hemodilution occurs.

Approximately 90% or more of the injected dose is excreted within the first 24 hours, with the peak urine concentrations occurring in the first hour after administration. Plasma and urine iohexol levels indicate that the iohexol body clearance is due primarily to renal clearance. An increase in the dose from 500 mgI/kg to 1500 mgI/kg does not significantly alter the clearance of the drug. The following pharmacokinetic values were observed following the intravenous administration of iohexol (between 500 mgI/kg to 1500 mgI/kg) to 16 adult human subjects: renal clearance—120 (86-162) mL/min; total body clearance—131 (98-165) mL/min; and volume of distribution—165 (108-219) mL/kg.

Renal accumulation is sufficiently rapid that the period of maximal opacification of the renal passages may begin as early as 1 minute after intravenous injection. Urograms become apparent in about 1 to 3 minutes with optimal contrast occurring between 5 to 15 minutes. In nephropathic conditions, particularly when excretory capacity has been altered, the rate of excretion may vary unpredictably, and opacification may be delayed after injection. Severe renal impairment may result in a lack of diagnostic opacification of the collecting system and, depending on the degree of renal impairment, prolonged plasma iohexol levels may be anticipated. In these patients, as well as in infants with immature kidneys, the route of excretion through the gallbladder and into the small intestine may increase.

Iohexol displays a low affinity for serum or plasma proteins and is poorly bound to serum albumin. No significant metabolism, deiodination or biotransformation occurs.

OMNIPAQUE (iohexol) probably crosses the placental barrier in humans by simple diffusion. It is not known to what extent iohexol is excreted in human milk.

Animal studies indicate that iohexol does not cross an intact blood-brain barrier to any significant extent following intravascular administration.

OMNIPAQUE enhances computed tomographic imaging through augmentation of radiographic efficiency. The degree of density enhancement is directly related to the iodine content in an administered dose; peak iodine blood levels occur immediately following rapid intravenous injection. Blood levels fall rapidly within 5 to 10 minutes and the vascular compartment half-life is approximately 20 minutes. This can be accounted for by the dilution in the vascular and extravascular fluid compartments which causes an initial sharp fall in plasma concentration. Equilibration with the extracellular compartments is reached in about ten minutes; thereafter, the fall becomes exponential.

The pharmacokinetics of iohexol in both normal and abnormal tissue have been shown to be variable. Contrast enhancement appears to be greatest immediately after bolus administration (15 seconds to 120 seconds). Thus, greatest enhancement may be detected by a series of consecutive two-to-three second scans performed within 30 to 90 seconds after injection (ie, dynamic computed tomographic imaging). Utilization of a continuous scanning technique (ie, dynamic CT scanning) may improve enhancement and diagnostic assessment of tumor and other lesions such as abscess, occasionally revealing unsuspected or more extensive disease. For example, a cyst may be distinguished from a vascularized solid lesion when precontrast and enhanced scans are compared; the nonperfused mass shows unchanged x-ray absorption (CT number). A vascularized lesion is characterized by an increase in CT number in the few minutes after a bolus of intravascular contrast agent; it may be malignant, benign, or normal tissue, but would probably not be a cyst, hematoma, or other nonvascular lesion.

Because unenhanced scanning may provide adequate diagnostic information in the individual patient, the decision to employ contrast enhancement, which may be associated with risk and increased radiation exposure, should be based upon a careful evaluation of clinical, other radiological, and unenhanced CT findings.

CT SCANNING OF THE HEAD
In contrast enhanced computed tomographic head imaging, OMNIPAQUE does not accumulate in normal brain tissue due to the presence of the normal blood-brain barrier. The increase in x-ray absorption in normal brain is due to the presence of contrast agent within the blood pool. A break in the blood-brain barrier such as occurs in malignant tumors of the brain allows for the accumulation of contrast medium within the interstitial tissue of the tumor. Adjacent normal brain tissue does not contain the contrast medium.

Maximum contrast enhancement in tissue frequently occurs after peak blood iodine levels are reached. A delay in maximum contrast enhancement can occur. Diagnostic contrast enhanced images of the brain have been obtained up to 1 hour after intravenous bolus administration. This delay suggests that radiographic contrast enhancement is at least in part dependent on the accumulation of iodine containing medium within the lesion and outside the blood pool, al-

though the mechanism by which this occurs is not clear. The radiographic enhancement of nontumoral lesions, such as arteriovenous malformations and aneurysms, is probably dependent on the iodine content of the circulating blood pool. In patients where the blood-brain barrier is known or suspected to be disrupted, the use of any radiographic contrast medium must be assessed on an individual risk to benefit basis. However, compared to ionic media, nonionic media are less toxic to the central nervous system.

CT SCANNING OF THE BODY
In contrast enhanced computed tomographic body imaging (nonneural tissue), OMNIPAQUE diffuses rapidly from the vascular into the extravascular space. Increase in x-ray absorption is related to blood flow, concentration of the contrast medium, and extraction of the contrast medium by interstitial tissue of tumors since no barrier exists. Contrast enhancement is thus due to the relative differences in extravascular diffusion between normal and abnormal tissue, quite different from that in the brain.

INDICATIONS AND USAGE, General—Intravascular
OMNIPAQUE 350 is indicated in adults for angiocardiography (ventriculography, selective coronary arteriography), aortography including studies of the aortic root, aortic arch, ascending aorta, abdominal aorta and its branches, contrast enhancement for computed tomographic head and body imaging, intravenous digital subtraction angiography of the head, neck, abdominal, renal and peripheral vessels, peripheral arteriography, and excretory urography.

OMNIPAQUE 350 is indicated in children for angiocardiography (ventriculography, pulmonary arteriography, and venography; studies of the collateral arteries and aortography, including the aortic root, aortic arch, ascending and descending aorta).

OMNIPAQUE 300 is indicated in adults for aortography including studies of the aortic arch, abdominal aorta and its branches, contrast enhancement for computed tomographic head and body imaging, cerebral arteriography, peripheral venography (phlebography), and excretory urography.

OMNIPAQUE 300 is indicated in children for angiocardiography (ventriculography), excretory urography, and contrast enhancement for computed tomographic head imaging.

OMNIPAQUE 240 is indicated in adults for contrast enhancement for computed tomographic head imaging and peripheral venography (phlebography).

OMNIPAQUE 140 is indicated in adults for intra-arterial digital subtraction angiography of the head, neck, abdominal, renal and peripheral vessels.

OMNIPAQUE 240 is indicated in children for contrast enhancement for computed tomographic head imaging.

CONTRAINDICATIONS
OMNIPAQUE (iohexol) should not be administered to patients with a known hypersensitivity to iohexol.

WARNINGS—General
Nonionic iodinated contrast media inhibit blood coagulation, in vitro, less than ionic contrast media. Clotting has been reported when blood remains in contact with syringes containing nonionic contrast media.

Serious, rarely fatal, thromboembolic events causing myocardial infarction and stroke have been reported during angiographic procedures with both ionic and nonionic contrast media. Therefore, meticulous intravascular administration technique is necessary, particularly during angiographic procedures, to minimize thromboembolic events. Numerous factors, including length of procedure, catheter and syringe material, underlying disease state, and concomitant medications may contribute to the development of thromboembolic events. For these reasons, meticulous angiographic techniques are recommended including close attention to guidewire and catheter manipulation, use of manifold systems and/or three-way stopcocks, frequent catheter flushing with heparinized saline solutions and minimizing the length of the procedure. The use of plastic syringes in place of glass syringes has been reported to decrease but not eliminate the likelihood of in vitro clotting.

OMNIPAQUE should be used with extreme care in patients with severe functional disturbances of the liver and kidneys, severe thyrotoxicosis, or myelomatosis. Diabetics with a serum creatinine level above 3 mg/dL should not be examined unless the possible benefits of the examination clearly outweigh the additional risk. OMNIPAQUE (iohexol) is not recommended for use in patients with anuria.

Radiopaque contrast agents are potentially hazardous in patients with multiple myeloma or other paraproteinemia, particularly in those with therapeutically resistant anuria. Although neither the contrast agent nor dehydration has separately proven to be the cause of anuria in myeloma, it has been speculated that the combination of both may be causative factors. The risk in myelomatous patients is not a contraindication; however, special precautions are necessary. Partial dehydration in the preparation of these patients prior to injection is not recommended since this may

predispose the patient to precipitation of the myeloma protein in the renal tubules. No form of therapy, including dialysis, has been successful in reversing the effect. Myeloma, which occurs most commonly in persons over age 40, should be considered before instituting intravascular administration of contrast agents.

Ionic contrast media, when injected intravenously or intra-arterially, may promote sickling in individuals who are homozygous for sickle cell disease.

Administration of radiopaque materials to patients known or suspected of having pheochromocytoma should be performed with extreme caution. If, in the opinion of the physician, the possible benefits of such procedures outweigh the considered risks, the procedures may be performed; however, the amount of radiopaque medium injected should be kept to an absolute minimum. The patient's blood pressure should be assessed throughout the procedure and measures for the treatment of hypertensive crisis should be readily available.

Reports of thyroid storm following the use of iodinated, ionic radiopaque contrast media in patients with hyperthyroidism or with an autonomously functioning thyroid nodule suggest that this additional risk be evaluated in such patients before use of any contrast medium.

Urography should be performed with caution in patients with severely impaired renal function and patients with combined renal and hepatic disease.

PRECAUTIONS—General
Diagnostic procedures which involve the use of radiopaque diagnostic agents should be carried out under the direction of personnel with the prerequisite training and with a thorough knowledge of the particular procedure to be performed. Appropriate facilities should be available for coping with any complication of the procedure, as well as for emergency treatment of severe reactions to the contrast agent itself. After parenteral administration of a radiopaque agent, competent personnel and emergency facilities should be available for at least 30 to 60 minutes since severe delayed reactions have occurred (see ADVERSE REACTIONS: Intravascular—General).

Preparatory dehydration is dangerous and may contribute to acute renal failure in patients with advanced vascular disease, diabetic patients, and in susceptible nondiabetic patients (often elderly with preexisting renal disease), infants and small children. Dehydration in these patients seems to be enhanced by the osmotic diuretic action of urographic agents. It is believed that overnight fluid restriction prior to excretory urography generally does not provide better visualization in normal patients. *Patients should be well hydrated prior to and following administration of any contrast medium, including iohexol.*

Acute renal failure has been reported in diabetic patients with diabetic nephropathy and in susceptible nondiabetic patients (often elderly with preexisting renal disease) following excretory urography. Therefore, careful consideration of the potential risks should be given before performing this radiographic procedure in these patients.

Immediately following surgery, excretory urography should be used with caution in renal transplant recipients.

The possibility of a reaction, including serious, life-threatening, fatal, anaphylactoid or cardiovascular reactions should always be considered (see ADVERSE REACTIONS: Intravascular—General). It is of utmost importance that a course of action be carefully planned in advance for immediate treatment of serious reactions, and that adequate and appropriate personnel be readily available in case of any reaction.

The possibility of an idiosyncratic reaction in susceptible patients should always be considered (see ADVERSE REACTIONS: Intravascular—General). The susceptible population includes, but is not limited to, patients with a history of a previous reaction to contrast media, patients with a known sensitivity to iodine per se, and patients with a known clinical hypersensitivity: bronchial asthma, hay fever, and food allergies.

The occurrence of severe idiosyncratic reactions has prompted the use of several pretesting methods. However, pretesting cannot be relied upon to predict severe reactions and may itself be hazardous for the patient. It is suggested that a thorough medical history with emphasis on allergy and hypersensitivity, prior to the injection of any contrast media, may be more accurate than pretesting in predicting potential adverse reactions.

A positive history of allergies or hypersensitivity does not arbitrarily contraindicate the use of a contrast agent where a diagnostic procedure is thought essential, but caution

Continued on next page

This product information was prepared in August 1992. On these and other products of Sanofi Winthrop Pharmaceuticals, detailed information may be obtained on a current basis by direct inquiry to Product Information Services, 90 Park Avenue, New York, NY 10016 (toll free 1-800-446-6267).

Sanofi Winthrop—Cont.

should be exercised (see ADVERSE REACTIONS: Intravascular—General). Premedication with antihistamines or corticosteroids to avoid or minimize possible allergic reactions in such patients should be considered and administered using separate syringes. Recent reports indicate that such pretreatment does not prevent serious life-threatening reactions, but may reduce both their incidence and severity.

Even though the osmolality of OMNIPAQUE is low compared to diatrizoate- or iothalamate-based ionic agents of comparable iodine concentration, the potential transitory increase in the circulatory osmotic load in patients with congestive heart failure requires caution during injection. These patients should be observed for several hours following the procedure to detect delayed hemodynamic disturbances.

General anesthesia may be indicated in the performance of some procedures in selected adult patients; however, a higher incidence of adverse reactions has been reported in these patients, and may be attributable to the inability of the patient to identify untoward symptoms, or to the hypotensive effect of anesthesia which can reduce cardiac output and increase the duration of exposure to the contrast agent.

Angiography should be avoided whenever possible in patients with homocystinuria, because of the risk of inducing thrombosis and embolism.

In angiographic procedures, the possibility of dislodging plaques or damaging or perforating the vessel wall should be borne in mind during the catheter manipulations and contrast medium injection. Test injections to ensure proper catheter placement are recommended.

Selective coronary arteriography should be performed only in those patients in whom the expected benefits outweigh the potential risk. The inherent risks of angiocardiography in patients with chronic pulmonary emphysema must be weighed against the necessity for performing this procedure.

When OMNIPAQUE (iohexol) is to be injected using plastic disposable syringes, the contrast medium should be drawn into the syringe and used immediately.

If nondisposable equipment is used, scrupulous care should be taken to prevent residual contamination with traces of cleansing agents.

Parenteral products should be inspected visually for particulate matter and discoloration prior to administration. If particulate matter or discoloration is present, do not use.

Information for Patients
Patients receiving injectable radiopaque diagnostic agents should be instructed to:

1. Inform your physician if you are pregnant (see CLINICAL PHARMACOLOGY—Intravascular).
2. Inform your physician if you are diabetic or if you have multiple myeloma, pheochromocytoma, homozygous sickle cell disease, or known thyroid disorder (see WARNINGS).
3. Inform your physician if you are allergic to any drugs, food, or if you had any reactions to previous injections of dyes used for x-ray procedures (see PRECAUTIONS—General).
4. Inform your physician about any other medications you are currently taking, including nonprescription drugs, before you are administered this drug.

Drug/Laboratory Test Interaction
If iodine-containing isotopes are to be administered for the diagnosis of thyroid disease, the iodine-binding capacity of thyroid tissue may be reduced for up to 2 weeks after contrast medium administration. Thyroid function tests which do not depend on iodine estimation, eg, T_3 resin uptake or direct thyroxine assays, are not affected.

Many radiopaque contrast agents are incompatible in vitro with some antihistamines and many other drugs; therefore, no other pharmaceuticals should be admixed with contrast agents.

Carcinogenesis, Mutagenesis, Impairment of Fertility
No long-term animal studies have been performed to evaluate carcinogenic potential, mutagenesis, or whether OMNIPAQUE (iohexol) can affect fertility in men or women.

Pregnancy Category B
Reproduction studies have been performed in rats and rabbits with up to 100 times the recommended human dose. No evidence of impaired fertility or harm to the fetus has been demonstrated due to OMNIPAQUE. There are, however, no studies in pregnant women. Because animal reproduction studies are not always predictive of human response, this drug should be used during pregnancy only if clearly needed.

Nursing Mothers
It is not known to what extent iohexol is excreted in human milk. However, many injectable contrast agents are excreted unchanged in human milk. Although it has not been established that serious adverse reactions occur in nursing infants, caution should be exercised when intravascular contrast media are administered to nursing women. Bottle feedings may be substituted for breast feedings for 24 hours following administration of OMNIPAQUE.

Pediatric Use
Pediatric patients at higher risk of experiencing adverse events during contrast medium administration may include those having asthma, a sensitivity to medication and/or allergens, congestive heart failure, a serum creatinine greater than 1.5 mg/dL or those less than 12 months of age.

ADVERSE REACTIONS

Intravascular—General
Adverse reactions following the use of OMNIPAQUE 140, OMNIPAQUE 240, OMNIPAQUE 300, and OMNIPAQUE 350 are usually of mild to moderate severity. However, serious, life-threatening and fatal reactions, mostly of cardiovascular origin, have been associated with the administration of iodine-containing contrast media, including OMNIPAQUE. The injection of contrast media is frequently associated with the sensation of warmth and pain, especially in peripheral angiography; pain and warmth are less frequent and less severe with OMNIPAQUE than with many contrast media.

Cardiovascular System: Arrhythmias including PVCs and PACs (2%), angina/chest pain (1%), and hypotension (0.7%). Others including cardiac failure, asystole, bradycardia, tachycardia, and vasovagal reaction were reported with an individual incidence of 0.3% or less. In controlled clinical trials involving 1485 patients, one fatality occurred. A cause and effect relationship between this death and iohexol has not been established.

Nervous System: Vertigo (including dizziness and lightheadedness) (0.5%), pain (3%), vision abnormalities (including blurred vision and photomas) (2%), headache (2%), and taste perversion (1%). Others including anxiety, fever, motor and speech dysfunction, convulsion, paresthesia, somnolence, stiff neck, hemiparesis, syncope, shivering, transient ischemic attack, cerebral infarction, and nystagmus were reported, with an individual incidence of 0.3% or less.

Respiratory System: Dyspnea, rhinitis, coughing, and laryngitis, with an individual incidence of 0.2% or less.

Gastrointestinal System: Nausea (2%) and vomiting (0.7%). Others including diarrhea, dyspepsia, cramp, and dry mouth were reported, with an individual incidence of less than 0.1%.

Skin and Appendages: Urticaria (0.3%), purpura (0.1%), abscess (0.1%), and pruritus (0.1%).

Individual adverse reactions which occurred to a significantly greater extent for a specific procedure are listed under that indication.

Pediatrics
In controlled clinical trials involving 391 patients for pediatric angiocardiography, urography, and contrast enhanced computed tomographic head imaging, adverse reactions following the use of OMNIPAQUE (iohexol) 240, OMNIPAQUE 300, and OMNIPAQUE 350 were generally less frequent than with adults.

Cardiovascular System: Ventricular tachycardia (0.5%), 2:1 heart block (0.5%), hypertension (0.3%), and anemia (0.3%).

Nervous System: Pain (0.8%), fever (0.5%), taste abnormality (0.5%), and convulsion (0.3%).

Respiratory System: Congestion (0.3%) and apnea (0.3%).

Gastrointestinal System: Nausea (1%), hypoglycemia (0.3%), and vomiting (2%).

Skin and Appendages: Rash (0.3%).

General Adverse Reactions to Contrast Media
Physicians should remain alert for the occurrence of adverse effects in addition to those discussed above.

The following reactions have been reported after administration of other intravascular iodinated contrast media, and rarely with iohexol. *Reactions due to technique:* hematomas and ecchymoses. *Hemodynamic reactions:* vein cramp and thrombophlebitis following intravenous injection. *Cardiovascular reactions:* rare cases of cardiac arrhythmias, reflex tachycardia, chest pain, cyanosis, hypertension, hypotension, peripheral vasodilatation, shock, and cardiac arrest. *Renal reactions:* occasionally, transient proteinuria, and rarely, oliguria or anuria. *Allergic reactions:* asthmatic attacks, nasal and conjunctival symptoms, dermal reactions such as urticaria with or without pruritus, as well as pleomorphic rashes, sneezing and lacrimation and, rarely, anaphylactic reactions. Rare fatalities have occurred, due to this or unknown causes. *Signs and symptoms related to the respiratory system:* pulmonary or laryngeal edema, bronchospasm, dyspnea; *or to the nervous system:* restlessness, tremors, convulsions. *Other reactions:* flushing, pain, warmth, metallic taste, nausea, vomiting, anxiety, headache, confusion, pallor, weakness, sweating, localized areas of edema, especially facial cramps, neutropenia, and dizziness. Rarely, immediate or delayed rigors can occur, sometimes accompanied by hyperpyrexia. Infrequently, "iodism" (salivary gland swelling) from organic iodinated compounds appears two days after exposure and subsides by the sixth day.

In general, the reactions which are known to occur upon parenteral administration of iodinated contrast agents are possible with any nonionic agent. Approximately 95 percent of adverse reactions accompanying the use of water-soluble intravascularly administered contrast agents are mild to moderate in degree. However, severe, life-threatening anaphylactoid reactions, mostly of cardiovascular origin, have occurred. Reported incidences of death range from 6.6 per 1 million (0.00066 percent) to 1 in 10 000 (0.01 percent). Most deaths occur during injection or 5 to 10 minutes later; the main feature being cardiac arrest with cardiovascular disease as the main aggravating factor. Isolated reports of hypotensive collapse and shock are found in the literature. The incidence of shock is estimated to be 1 out of 20 000 (0.005 percent) patients.

Adverse reactions to injectable contrast media fall into two categories: chemotoxic reactions and idiosyncratic reactions. Chemotoxic reactions result from the physicochemical properties of the contrast media, the dose, and speed of injection. All hemodynamic disturbances and injuries to organs or vessels perfused by the contrast medium are included in this category.

Idiosyncratic reactions include all other reactions. They occur more frequently in patients 20 to 40 years old. Idiosyncratic reactions may or may not be dependent on the amount of dose injected, the speed of injection, and the radiographic procedure. Idiosyncratic reactions are subdivided into minor, intermediate, and severe. The minor reactions are self-limited and of short duration; the severe reactions are life-threatening and treatment is urgent and mandatory.

The reported incidence of adverse reactions to contrast media in patients with a history of allergy are twice that of the general population. Patients with a history of previous reactions to a contrast medium are three times more susceptible than other patients. However, sensitivity to contrast media does not appear to increase with repeated examinations. Most adverse reactions to injectable contrast media appear within 1 to 3 minutes after the start of injection, but delayed reactions may occur.

Regardless of the contrast agent employed, the overall estimated incidence of serious adverse reactions is higher with angiocardiography than with other procedures. Cardiac decompensation, serious arrhythmias, angina pectoris, or myocardial ischemia or infarction may occur during angiocardiography and left ventriculography. Electrocardiographic and hemodynamic abnormalities occur less frequently with OMNIPAQUE than with diatrizoate meglumine and diatrizoate sodium injection.

OVERDOSAGE
Overdosage may occur. The adverse effects of overdosage are life-threatening and affect mainly the pulmonary and cardiovascular systems. The symptoms included: cyanosis, bradycardia, acidosis, pulmonary hemorrhage, convulsions, coma, and cardiac arrest. Treatment of an overdosage is directed toward the support of all vital functions, and prompt institution of symptomatic therapy.

The intravenous LD_{50} values of OMNIPAQUE (iohexol) (in grams of iodine per kilogram body weight) are 24.2 in mice and 15.0 in rats.

DOSAGE AND ADMINISTRATION—General
As with all radiopaque contrast agents, the lowest dose of OMNIPAQUE necessary to obtain adequate visualization should be used. A lower dose may reduce the possibility of an adverse reaction. Most procedures do not require use of either the maximum volume or the highest concentration of OMNIPAQUE. The combination of volume and concentration of OMNIPAQUE (iohexol) to be used should be carefully individualized accounting for factors such as age, body weight, size of the vessel and the rate of blood flow within the vessel. Other factors such as anticipated pathology, degree and extent of opacification required, structure(s) or area to be examined, disease processes affecting the patient, and equipment and technique to be employed should be considered.

Sterile technique must be used in all vascular injections involving contrast media.

Withdrawal of contrast agents from their containers should be accomplished under aseptic conditions with sterile equipment. Sterile techniques must be used with any invasive procedure.

If nondisposable equipment is used, scrupulous care should be taken to prevent residual contamination with traces of cleansing agents.

It may be desirable that solutions of radiopaque diagnostic agents be used at body temperature when injected.

Parenteral products should be inspected visually for particulate matter and discoloration prior to administration whenever solution and container permit. Solutions of OMNIPAQUE should be used only if clear and within the normal colorless to pale yellow range. If particulate matter or discoloration is present, do not use.

INDIVIDUAL INDICATIONS AND USAGE
ANGIOCARDIOGRAPHY
Pharmacology—Hemodynamic Changes
OMNIPAQUE 350 at a concentration of 350 mgI/mL is indicated in adults for angiocardiography (ventriculography, aortic root injections, and selective coronary arteriography). OMNIPAQUE 350 at a concentration of 350 mgI/mL is indicated in children for angiocardiography (ventriculography, pulmonary arteriography, and venography, and studies of the collateral arteries).

OMNIPAQUE 300 at a concentration of 300 mgI/mL is indicated in children for angiocardiography (ventriculography). After both ventricular and coronary injection, decreases in systolic pressure were less pronounced and returned to baseline values earlier with OMNIPAQUE 350 than with diatrizoate meglumine and diatrizoate sodium injection. OMNIPAQUE 350 produced less Q–T interval prolongation than seen with diatrizoate meglumine and diatrizoate sodium injection.

In children, after injection of all sites, but particularly following ventricular and pulmonary artery injections, decreases in both systolic and diastolic intravascular pressure were significantly less pronounced with OMNIPAQUE 350 than with diatrizoate meglumine and diatrizoate sodium injection. In children, OMNIPAQUE 350 produced significantly less shortening of the R-R interval than seen with diatrizoate meglumine and diatrizoate sodium injection.

If repeat injections are made in rapid succession, all these changes are likely to be more pronounced. (See DOSAGE AND ADMINISTRATION.)

Precautions: During administration of large doses of OMNIPAQUE 350, continuous monitoring of vital signs is desirable. Caution is advised in the administration of large volumes to patients with incipient heart failure because of the possibility of aggravating the preexisting condition. Hypotension should be corrected promptly since it may induce serious arrhythmias.

Special care regarding dosage should be observed in patients with right ventricular failure, pulmonary hypertension, or stenotic pulmonary vascular beds because of the hemodynamic changes which may occur after injection into the right heart outflow tract. (See PRECAUTIONS—General.) Pediatric patients at higher risk of experiencing adverse events during contrast medium administration may include those having asthma, a sensitivity to medication and/or allergens, congestive heart failure, a serum creatinine greater than 1.5 mg/dL or those less than 12 months of age.

Adverse Reactions: Cardiovascular system reactions in angiocardiography included angina (8%), hypotension (2.5%), bradycardia (1.0%), and tachycardia (1.0%). (See ADVERSE REACTIONS: Intravascular—General.)

Dosage and Administration: The individual dose or volume is determined by the size of the structure to be visualized, the anticipated degree of hemodilution, and valvular competence. Weight is a minor consideration in adults, but must be considered in infants and young children. The volume of each individual injection is a more important consideration than the total dosage used. When large individual volumes are administered, as in ventriculography and aortography, it has been suggested that several minutes be permitted to elapse between each injection to allow for subsidence of possible hemodynamic disturbances.

The recommended single injection volume of OMNIPAQUE 350 for angiocardiographic procedures in adults and the recommended single injection volumes of OMNIPAQUE 350 and OMNIPAQUE 300 for angiographic procedures in children are as follows:

Ventriculography
Adults: The usual adult volume for a single injection is 40 mL with a range of 30 mL to 60 mL. This may be repeated as necessary. When combined with selective coronary arteriography, the total administered volume should not exceed 250 mL (87.5 gI).
Pediatrics: The usual single injection dose of OMNIPAQUE 350 is 1.25 mL/kg of body weight with a range of 1.0 mL/kg to 1.5 mL/kg. For OMNIPAQUE 300 the usual single injection dose is 1.75 mL/kg with a range of 1.5 mL/kg to 2.0 mL/kg. When multiple injections are given, the total administered dose should not exceed 5 mL/kg up to a total volume of 250 mL of OMNIPAQUE 350 or up to a total volume of 291 mL of OMNIPAQUE 300.

Selective Coronary Arteriography
The usual adult volume for right or left coronary arteriography is 5 mL (range 3 mL to 14 mL) per injection.

Aortic Root and Arch Study When Used Alone
The usual adult single injection volume is 50 mL, with a range of 20 mL to 75 mL.

Pulmonary Angiography
Pediatrics: The usual single injection dose is 1.0 mL/kg of OMNIPAQUE (iohexol) 350.

Combined Angiocardiographic Procedures
Multiple Procedures
Adults: The visualization of multiple vascular systems and target organs is possible during a single radiographic examination of the patient.
Large doses of OMNIPAQUE 350 were well tolerated in angiographic procedures requiring multiple injections.
The maximum total volume for multiple procedures should not exceed 250 mL of 350 mgI/mL (87.5 gI).
Pediatrics: Visualization of multiple vascular systems and target organs is possible during a single radiographic examination of the patient.
The maximum total dose for multiple injection procedures should not exceed 5.0 mL/kg up to a total volume of 250 mL of OMNIPAQUE 350 or 6.0 mL/kg up to a total volume of 291 mL of OMNIPAQUE 300.

AORTOGRAPHY AND SELECTIVE VISCERAL ARTERIOGRAPHY

OMNIPAQUE 300 at a concentration of 300 mgI/mL and OMNIPAQUE (iohexol) 350 at a concentration of 350 mgI/mL are indicated in adults for use in aortography and selective visceral arteriography including studies of the aortic arch, ascending aorta, and abdominal aorta and its branches (celiac, mesenteric, renal, hepatic and splenic arteries).

OMNIPAQUE 350 at a concentration of 350 mgI/mL is indicated in children for use in aortography including studies of the aortic root, aortic arch, ascending and descending aorta.

Precautions: Under conditions of slowed aortic circulation there is an increased likelihood for aortography to cause muscle spasm. Occasional serious neurologic complications, including paraplegia, have also been reported in patients with aortoiliac obstruction, femoral artery obstruction, abdominal compression, hypotension, hypertension, spinal anesthesia, and injection of vasopressors to increase contrast. In these patients the concentration, volume, and number of repeat injections of the medium should be maintained at a minimum with appropriate intervals between injections. The position of the patient and catheter tip should be carefully monitored.

Entry of a large aortic dose into the renal artery may cause, even in the absence of symptoms, albuminuria, hematuria, and an elevated creatinine and urea nitrogen. Rapid and complete return of function usually follows. (See PRECAUTIONS—General.)

Adverse Reactions: See ADVERSE REACTIONS: Intravascular—General and ADVERSE REACTIONS—ANGIOCARDIOGRAPHY.

Dosage and Administration:
Adults: The usual adult volume as a single injection is 50 mL to 80 mL for the aorta, 30 mL to 60 mL for major branches including celiac and mesenteric arteries, and 5 mL to 15 mL for renal arteries. Repeated injections may be performed if indicated, but the total volume should not exceed 291 mL of OMNIPAQUE 300 or 250 mL of OMNIPAQUE 350 (87.5 gI/mL).
Pediatrics: The usual single injection dose is 1.0 mL/kg of OMNIPAQUE 350 and should not exceed 5.0 mL/kg up to a total volume of 250 mL of OMNIPAQUE 350.

CEREBRAL ARTERIOGRAPHY

OMNIPAQUE 300 at a concentration of 300 mgI/mL is indicated in adults for use in cerebral arteriography.

The degree of pain and flushing as the result of the use of OMNIPAQUE 300 in cerebral arteriography is less than that seen with comparable injections of many contrast media.

In cerebral arteriography, patients should be appropriately prepared consistent with existing or suspected disease states.

Precautions: Cerebral arteriography should be undertaken with extreme care with special caution in elderly patients, patients in poor clinical condition, advanced arteriosclerosis, severe arterial hypertension, recent cerebral embolism or thrombosis, and cardiac decompensation.

Since the contrast medium is given by rapid injection, the patient should be monitored for possible untoward reactions. (See PRECAUTIONS—General.)

Adverse Reactions: Cerebral arteriography with water-soluble contrast media has been associated with temporary neurologic complications including seizures, drowsiness, transient paresis, and mild disturbances in vision such as photomas of 1-second or less duration.

Central nervous system reactions in cerebral arteriography included photomas (15%), headache (5.5%), and pain (4.5%). (See ADVERSE REACTIONS: Intravascular—General.)

Dosage and Administration: OMNIPAQUE 300 is recommended for cerebral arteriography at the following volumes: common carotid artery (6 mL to 12 mL), internal carotid artery (8 mL to 10 mL), external carotid artery (6 mL to 9 mL), and vertebral artery (6 mL to 10 mL).

CONTRAST ENHANCED COMPUTED TOMOGRAPHY

OMNIPAQUE 240 at a concentration of 240 mgI/mL, OMNIPAQUE 300 at a concentration of 300 mgI/mL, and OMNIPAQUE 350 at a concentration of 350 mgI/mL are indicated in adults for use in intravenous contrast enhanced computed tomographic head and body imaging by rapid injection or infusion technique.

OMNIPAQUE 240 at a concentration of 240 mgI/mL and OMNIPAQUE 300 at a concentration of 300 mgI/mL are indicated in children for use in intravenous contrast enhanced computed tomographic head imaging by rapid bolus injection.

CT SCANNING OF THE HEAD

OMNIPAQUE may be used to redefine diagnostic precision in areas of the brain which may not otherwise have been satisfactorily visualized.

Tumors
OMNIPAQUE (iohexol) may be useful to investigate the presence and extent of certain malignancies such as: gliomas including malignant gliomas, glioblastomas, astrocytomas,

oligodendrogliomas and gangliomas, ependymomas, medulloblastomas, meningiomas, neuromas, pinealomas, pituitary adenomas, carniopharyngiomas, germinomas, and metastatic lesions. The usefulness of contrast enhancement for the investigation of the retrobulbar space and in cases of low grade or infiltrative glioma has not been demonstrated. In calcified lesions, there is less likelihood of enhancement. Following therapy, tumors may show decreased or no enhancement. The opacification of the inferior vermis following contrast media administration has resulted in false-positive diagnosis in a number of otherwise normal studies.

Nonneoplastic Conditions
OMNIPAQUE may be beneficial in the image enhancement of nonneoplastic lesions. Cerebral infarctions of recent onset may be better visualized with contrast enhancement, while some infarctions are obscured if contrast medium is used. The use of iodinated contrast media results in enhancement in about 60 percent of cerebral infarctions studied from one to four weeks from the onset of symptoms.

Sites of active infection may also be enhanced following contrast medium administration.

Arteriovenous malformations and aneurysms will show contrast enhancement. For these vascular lesions the enhancement is probably dependent on the iodine content of the circulating blood pool. Hematomas and intraparenchymal bleeders seldom demonstrate contrast enhancement. However, in cases of intraparenchymal clot, for which there is no obvious clinical explanation, contrast media administration may be helpful in ruling out the possibility of associated arteriovenous malformation.

CT SCANNING OF THE BODY

OMNIPAQUE (iohexol) may be useful for enhancement of computed tomographic images for detection and evaluation of lesions in the liver, pancreas, kidneys, aorta, mediastinum, pelvis, abdominal cavity, and retroperitoneal space. Enhancement of computed tomography with OMNIPAQUE may be of benefit in establishing diagnoses of certain lesions in these sites with greater assurance than is possible with CT alone. In other cases, the contrast agent may allow visualization of lesions not seen with CT alone (ie, tumor extension) or may help to define suspicious lesions seen with unenhanced CT (ie, pancreatic cyst).

For information regarding the use of dilute oral plus intravenous OMNIPAQUE in CT of the abdomen, see INDIVIDUAL INDICATIONS AND USAGE—Oral Use.

Precautions: See PRECAUTIONS—General.
Adverse Reactions: Immediately following intravascular injection of contrast medium, a transient sensation of mild warmth is not unusual. Warmth is less frequent with OMNIPAQUE than with ionic media. (See ADVERSE REACTIONS: Intravascular—General.)

Dosage and Administration: The concentration and volume required will depend on the equipment and imaging technique used.

OMNIPAQUE Injection (Iohexol)
The dosage recommended for use in adults for contrast enhanced computed tomography is as follows:

Head Imaging by Injection:	70 mL to 150 mL (21 gI to 45 gI) of OMNIPAQUE 300 (300 mgI/mL) 80 mL (28 gI) of OMNIPAQUE 350 (350 mgI/mL)
Head Imaging by Infusion:	120 mL to 250 mL (29 gI to 60 gI) of OMNIPAQUE 240 (240 mgI/mL)
Body Imaging by Injection:	50 mL to 200 mL (15 gI to 60 gI) of OMNIPAQUE 300 (300 mgI/mL) 60 mL to 100 mL (21 gI to 35 gI) of OMNIPAQUE 350 (350 mgI/mL)

The dosage recommended for use in children for contrast enhanced computed tomographic head imaging is 1.0 mL/kg to 2.0 mL/kg for OMNIPAQUE 240 or OMNIPAQUE 300. It should not be necessary to exceed a maximum dose of 28 gI with OMNIPAQUE 240 or 35 gI with OMNIPAQUE 300.

DIGITAL SUBTRACTION ANGIOGRAPHY

Intravenous Administration
OMNIPAQUE 350 at a concentration of 350 mgI/mL is indicated in adults for use in intravenous digital subtraction angiography (I.V. DSA) of the vessels of the head, neck, and abdominal, renal and peripheral vessels.

Arteriograms of diagnostic quality can be obtained following the intravenous administration of contrast media employing

Continued on next page

This product information was prepared in August 1992. On these and other products of Sanofi Winthrop Pharmaceuticals, detailed information may be obtained on a current basis by direct inquiry to Product Information Services, 90 Park Avenue, New York, NY 10016 (toll free 1-800-446-6267).

Sanofi Winthrop—Cont.

digital subtraction and computer imaging enhancement techniques. The intravenous route of administration using these techniques has the advantage of being less invasive than the corresponding selective catheter placement of medium. The dose is administered into a peripheral vein, the superior vena cava or right atrium, usually by mechanical injection although sometimes by rapid manual injection. The technique has been used to visualize the ventricles, aorta and most of its larger branches, including the carotids, cerebrals, vertebrals, renal, celiac, mesenterics, and the major peripheral vessels of the limbs. Radiographic visualization of these structures is possible until significant hemodilution occurs.

OMNIPAQUE 350 can be injected intravenously as a rapid bolus to provide arterial visualization using digital subtraction radiography. Preprocedural medications are not considered necessary. OMNIPAQUE 350 has provided diagnostic arterial radiographs in about 95% of patients. In some cases, poor arterial visualization has been attributed to patient movement. OMNIPAQUE (iohexol) 350 is very well tolerated in the vascular system. Patient discomfort (general sensation of heat and/or pain) following injection is less than with various other contrast media.

Precautions: Since the contrast medium is usually administered mechanically under high pressure, rupture of smaller peripheral veins can occur. It has been suggested that this can be avoided by using an intravenous catheter threaded proximally beyond larger tributaries or, in the case of the antecubital vein, into the superior vena cava. Sometimes the femoral vein is used. (See PRECAUTIONS—General.)

Adverse Reactions: Cardiovascular system reactions in digital arteriography included transient PVCs (16%) and PACs (6.5%). (See ADVERSE REACTIONS: Intravascular—General.)

Dosage and Administration: The usual injection volume of OMNIPAQUE 350 for the intravenous digital technique is 30 mL to 50 mL of a 350 mgI/mL solution. This is administered as a bolus at 7.5 to 30 mL/second using a pressure injector. The volume and rate of injection will depend primarily on the type of equipment and technique used.

Frequently three or more injections may be required, up to a total volume not to exceed 250 mL (87.5 gI).

Intra-arterial Administration

OMNIPAQUE 140 at a concentration of 140 mgI/mL is indicated for use in intra-arterial digital subtraction angiography of head, neck, abdominal, renal and peripheral vessels. The intra-arterial route of administration has the advantages of allowing a lower total dose of contrast agent since there is less hemodilution than with the intravenous route of administration. Patients with poor cardiac output would be expected to have better contrast enhancement following intra-arterial administration as compared with intravenous administration. A higher concentration of contrast agent may be needed to facilitate catheter placement under fluoroscopic control.

Precautions: High pressure intra-arterial injections may cause the rupture of smaller peripheral arteries. (See PRECAUTIONS—General.)

Adverse Reactions: Central nervous system reactions in intra-arterial digital angiography include transient ischemia attacks (1.6%) and cerebral infarctions (1.6%). These occurred in high risk patients having a cerebral examination and the relationship to the contrast medium was uncertain. (See ADVERSE REACTIONS—General.) Headache occurred in 6.3% of the patients, all of whom were having cerebral examinations.

Dosage and Administration: Mechanical or hand injection can be used to administer one or more bolus intra-arterial injections of OMNIPAQUE 140. The volume and rate of injection will depend on the type of equipment, technique used, and the vascular area to be visualized. The following volumes and rates of injection have been used with OMNIPAQUE 140.

Arteries	Volume/ Injection (mL)	Rate of Injection (mL/sec)
Aorta	20–45	8–20
Carotid	5–10	3–6
Femoral	9–20	3–6
Vertebral	4–10	2–8
Renal	6–12	3–6
Other Branches of the Aorta (includes subclavian, axillary, innominate and iliac)	8–25	3–10

PERIPHERAL ANGIOGRAPHY

OMNIPAQUE (iohexol) 300 at a concentration of 300 mgI/mL or OMNIPAQUE 350 at a concentration of 350 mgI/mL is indicated in adults for use in peripheral arteriography. OMNIPAQUE 240 at a concentration of 240 mgI/mL or OMNIPAQUE 300 at a concentration of 300 mgI/mL is indicated in adults for use in peripheral venography.

Sedative medication may be employed prior to use. Anesthesia is not considered necessary.

Patient discomfort during and immediately following injection is substantially less than that following injection of various other contrast media. Moderate to severe discomfort is very unusual.

Precautions: Pulsation should be present in the artery to be injected. In thromboangiitis obliterans, or ascending infection associated with severe ischemia, angiography should be performed with extreme caution, if at all. (See PRECAUTIONS—General.)

Adverse Reactions: A transient sensation of mild warmth is usual, immediately following injection. This has not interfered with the procedure.

In phlebography the incidence of leg pain was 21%. This usually was mild and lasted a short time after injection. (See ADVERSE REACTIONS: Intravascular—General.)

Dosage and Administration: The volume required will depend on the size, flow rate, and disease state of the injected vessel and on the size and condition of the patient, as well as the imaging technique used.

The dosage recommended for use in peripheral angiography is as follows:

Aortofemoral runoffs:
20 mL to 70 mL of OMNIPAQUE 350 (350 mgI/mL)
30 mL to 90 mL of OMNIPAQUE 300 (300 mgI/mL)

Selective arteriograms (femoral/iliac):
10 mL to 30 mL of OMNIPAQUE 350 (350 mgI/mL)
10 mL to 60 mL of OMNIPAQUE 300 (300 mgI/mL)

Venography (per leg):
20 mL to 150 mL of OMNIPAQUE 240 (240 mgI/mL)
40 mL to 100 mL of OMNIPAQUE 300 (300 mgI/mL)

EXCRETORY UROGRAPHY

OMNIPAQUE (iohexol) 300 at a concentration of 300 mgI/mL or OMNIPAQUE 350 at a concentration of 350 mgI/mL is indicated for use in adults in excretory urography to provide diagnostic contrast of the urinary tract.

OMNIPAQUE 300 at a concentration of 300 mgI/mL is indicated in children for excretory urography. (See Section III for information on voiding cystourethrography.)

For pharmacokinetics of excretion in adults, see CLINICAL PHARMACOLOGY—Intravascular.

Precautions: Preparatory dehydration is not recommended in the elderly, infants, young children, diabetic or azotemic patients, or in patients with suspected myelomatosis.

Pediatric patients at higher risk of experiencing adverse events during contrast medium administration may include those having asthma, a sensitivity to medication and/or allergens, congestive heart failure, a serum creatinine greater than 1.5 mg/dL or those less than 12 months of age.

Since there is a possibility of temporary suppression of urine formation, it is recommended that a suitable interval elapse before excretory urography is repeated, especially in patients with unilateral or bilateral reduction in renal function. (See PRECAUTIONS—General.)

Adverse Reactions: See ADVERSE REACTIONS: Intravascular—General.

Dosage and Administration: *Adults:* OMNIPAQUE 300 and OMNIPAQUE 350 at dosages from 200 mgI/kg body weight to 350 mgI/kg body weight have produced diagnostic opacification of the excretory system in patients with normal renal function.

Pediatrics

Excretory Urography

OMNIPAQUE 300 at doses of 0.5 mL/kg to 3.0 mL/kg of body weight has produced diagnostic opacification of the excretory tract. The usual dose for children is 1.0 mL/kg to 1.5 mL/kg. Dosage for infants and children should be administered in proportion to age and body weight. The total administered dose should not exceed 3 mL/kg.

SECTION III

CLINICAL PHARMACOLOGY—Oral/Body Cavity Use

For most body cavities, the injected iohexol is absorbed into the surrounding tissue and eliminated by the kidneys and bowel as previously described in SECTION II, CLINICAL PHARMACOLOGY—Intravascular. Examinations of the uterus (hysterosalpingography) and bladder (voiding cystourethrography) involve the almost immediate drainage of contrast medium from the cavity upon conclusion of the radiographic procedure.

Orally administered iohexol is very poorly absorbed from the normal gastrointestinal tract. Only 0.1 to 0.5 percent of the oral dose was excreted by the kidneys. This amount may increase in the presence of bowel perforation or bowel obstruction. Iohexol is well tolerated and readily absorbed if leakage into the peritoneal cavity occurs.

Visualization of the joint spaces, uterus, fallopian tubes, peritoneal herniations, pancreatic and bile ducts, and bladder can be accomplished by direct injection of contrast medium into the region to be studied. The use of appropriate iodine concentrations assures diagnostic density.

Orally administered OMNIPAQUE produces good visualization of the gastrointestinal tract. OMNIPAQUE is particularly useful when barium sulfate is contraindicated as in patients with suspected bowel perforation or those where aspiration of contrast medium is a possibility.

INDICATIONS AND USAGE

General—Oral/Body Cavity Use

OMNIPAQUE 210, OMNIPAQUE 240, OMNIPAQUE 300, and OMNIPAQUE 350 have osmolalities from approximately 1.6 to 3.0 times that of plasma (285 mOsm/kg water) and are hypertonic under conditions of use.

Adults: OMNIPAQUE 350 is indicated in adults for arthrography and oral pass-thru examination of the gastrointestinal tract.

OMNIPAQUE 300 is indicated in adults for arthrography and hysterosalpingography.

OMNIPAQUE 240 is indicated in adults for arthrography, endoscopic retrograde pancreatography and cholangiopancreatography, herniography, and hysterosalpingography.

OMNIPAQUE 210 is indicated in adults for arthrography.

OMNIPAQUE diluted to concentrations from 6 mgI/mL to 9 mgI/mL administered orally in conjunction with OMNIPAQUE 300 at a concentration of 300 mgI/mL administered intravenously is indicated in adults for contrast enhanced computed tomography of the abdomen.

Children: OMNIPAQUE diluted to concentrations from 50 mgI/mL to 100 mgI/mL is indicated in children for voiding cystourethrography.

OMNIPAQUE (iohexol) diluted to concentrations from 9 mgI/mL to 21 mgI/mL administered orally in conjunction with OMNIPAQUE 240 at a concentration of 240 mgI/mL or OMNIPAQUE 300 at a concentration of 300 mgI/mL administered intravenously are indicated in children for use in contrast enhanced computed tomography of the abdomen.

CONTRAINDICATIONS

OMNIPAQUE should not be administered to patients with a known hypersensitivity to iohexol.

WARNINGS—General

See SECTION II, WARNINGS—General.

PRECAUTIONS—General

See SECTION II, PRECAUTIONS—General.

Orally administered hypertonic contrast media draw fluid into the intestines which, if severe enough, could result in hypovolemia. Plasma fluid loss in elderly cachectic patients may be sufficient to cause a shock-like state which, if untreated, could be dangerous. It is advisable to correct any electrolyte disturbances before using hypertonic contrast media and promptly correct any hypovolemic episodes caused by the media.

Bronchial entry of hypertonic contrast medium causes osmotic effusion and should be avoided.

ADVERSE REACTIONS: Oral/Body Cavity Use—General

Body Cavities

In controlled clinical trials involving 285 adult patients for various body cavity examinations using OMNIPAQUE 210, 240, 300, and 350, the following adverse reactions were reported.

Cardiovascular System
Incidence > 1%: None
Incidence ≤ 1%: Hypertension

Nervous System
Incidence > 1%: Pain (26%)
Incidence ≤ 1%: Headache, somnolence, fever, muscle weakness, burning, unwell feeling, tremors, lightheadedness, syncope

Respiratory System
None

Gastrointestinal System
Incidence > 1%: None
Incidence ≤ 1%: Flatulence, diarrhea, nausea, vomiting, abdominal pressure

Skin and Appendages
Incidence > 1%: Swelling (22%), heat (7%)
Incidence ≤ 1%: Hematoma at injection site

The most frequent reactions, pain and swelling, were almost exclusively reported after arthrography and were generally related to the procedure rather than the contrast medium. Gastrointestinal reactions were almost exclusively reported after oral pass-thru examinations. For additional information on adverse reactions that may be expected with specific procedures, see INDIVIDUAL INDICATIONS AND USAGE. For information on general adverse reactions to contrast media, see SECTION II, ADVERSE REACTIONS: Intravascular—General.

No adverse reactions associated with the use of OMNIPAQUE (iohexol) for VCU procedures were reported in 51 pediatric patients studied.

Oral Use

See INDIVIDUAL INDICATIONS AND USAGE; Oral Use—Adverse Reactions.

To Achieve	Add		To
One Liter of Contrast Medium at A Final Concentration (mgI/mL) of	Stock Concentration of OMNIPAQUE (mgI/mL)	Volume (mL)	Water, Carbonated Beverage, Milk, or Juice (mL)
6	240	25	975
	300	20	980
	350	17	983
9	240	38	962
	300	30	970
	350	26	974
12	240	50	950
	300	40	960
	350	35	965
15	240	63	937
	300	50	950
	350	43	957
18	240	75	925
	300	60	940
	350	52	948
21	240	88	912
	300	70	930
	350	60	940

OVERDOSAGE

See also SECTION II, OVERDOSAGE.

The recommended dose of OMNIPAQUE 350 at a concentration of 350 mgI/mL for adult oral pass-thru examination of the gastrointestinal tract is 50 mL to 100 mL. In a Phase I study, 150 mL of OMNIPAQUE 350 was administered orally to 11 healthy male subjects. The incidence of diarrhea was 91% (10 of 11) and abdominal cramping was 27% (3 of 11). Despite all of these events being mild and transient the occurrences were more than double that seen at the recommended doses. It is apparent from this finding that larger volumes of hypertonic contrast media, like OMNIPAQUE, increase the osmotic load in the bowel which may result in greater fluid shifts.

DOSAGE AND ADMINISTRATION—General

See SECTION II, DOSAGE AND ADMINISTRATION—General.

INDIVIDUAL INDICATIONS AND USAGE

Oral Use

Adults: OMNIPAQUE 350 at a concentration of 350 mgI/mL is indicated in adults for use in oral pass-thru examination of the gastrointestinal tract.

OMNIPAQUE diluted to concentrations from 6 mgI/mL to 9 mgI/mL administered orally in conjunction with OMNIPAQUE 300 at a concentration of 300 mgI/mL administered intravenously are indicated in adults for use in contrast enhanced computed tomography of the abdomen. Dilute oral plus intravenous OMNIPAQUE may be useful when unenhanced imaging does not provide sufficient delineation between normal loops of the bowel and adjacent organs or areas of suspected pathology.

Children: OMNIPAQUE diluted to concentrations from 9 mgI/mL to 21 mgI/mL administered orally in conjunction with OMNIPAQUE 240 at a concentration of 240 mgI/mL or OMNIPAQUE 300 at a concentration of 300 mgI/mL administered intravenously are indicated in children for use in contrast enhanced computed tomography of the abdomen.

Precautions: See PRECAUTIONS—General.

Adverse Reactions: Oral administration of OMNIPAQUE is most often associated with mild, transient diarrhea especially when high concentrations and large volumes are administered. Nausea, vomiting, and moderate diarrhea have also been reported following orally administered OMNIPAQUE, but much less frequently. For CT examinations using dilute oral plus intravenous contrast medium, adverse events are more likely to be associated with the intravenous injection than the hypotonic oral solution. It should be noted that serious or anaphylactoid reactions that may occur with intravascular iodinated media are possible following administration by other routes.

In controlled clinical trials involving 54 adult patients for oral pass-thru examination of the gastrointestinal tract using OMNIPAQUE 350, the following adverse reactions were reported: diarrhea (42%), nausea (15%), vomiting (11%), abdominal pain (7%), flatulence (2%), and headache (2%).

In controlled clinical studies involving 44 adult patients for dilute oral plus intravenous CT examination of the gastrointestinal tract using OMNIPAQUE 300, adverse reactions were limited to a single report of vomiting (2%).

In controlled clinical studies involving 69 pediatric patients for dilute oral plus intravenous CT examination of the gastrointestinal tract using OMNIPAQUE 240 and OMNIPAQUE 300, adverse reactions were limited to a single report of vomiting (1.4%).

Dosage and Administration: *Adults:* The recommended dosage of OMNIPAQUE 350 at a concentration of 350 mgI/mL for oral pass-thru examination of the gastrointestinal tract in adults is 50 mL to 100 mL depending on the nature of the examination and the size of the patient.

The recommended oral dosage of OMNIPAQUE diluted to concentrations of 6 mgI/mL to 9 mgI/mL for contrast enhanced computed tomography of the abdomen in adults is 500 mL to 1000 mL. Smaller administered volumes are needed as the concentration of the final solution is increased (see Table above). In conjunction with dilute oral administration, the recommended dosage of OMNIPAQUE 300 administered intravenously is 100 mL to 150 mL. The oral dose is administered about 20 to 40 minutes prior to the intravenous dose and image acquisition.

Children: The recommended oral dosage of OMNIPAQUE diluted to concentrations of 9 mgI/mL to 21 mgI/mL for contrast enhanced computed tomography of the abdomen in children is 180 mL to 750 mL. Smaller administered volumes are needed as the concentration of the final solution is increased (see Table below). The total oral dose in grams of iodine should generally not exceed 5 gI for children under 3 years of age and 10 gI for children from 3 to 18 years of age. The oral dosage may be given all at once or over a period of 30 to 45 minutes if there is difficulty in consuming the required volume.

In conjunction with dilute oral administration the recommended dosage of OMNIPAQUE 240 and OMNIPAQUE 300 is 2.0 mL/kg when administered intravenously with a range of 1.0 mL/kg to 2.0 mL/kg. Dosage for infants and children should be administered in proportion to age and body weight. The total intravenously administered dose should not exceed 3 mL/kg. The oral dose is administered about 30 to 60 minutes prior to the intravenous dose and image acquisition.

OMNIPAQUE may be diluted with water or beverage as follows:

[See table above.]

Dilutions of OMNIPAQUE should be prepared just prior to use and any unused portion discarded after the procedure.

VOIDING CYSTOURETHROGRAPHY (VCU)

OMNIPAQUE (iohexol) diluted to concentrations from 50 mgI/mL to 100 mgI/mL is indicated in children for voiding cystourethrography. VCUs are often performed in conjunction with excretory urography.

Precautions: See PRECAUTIONS—General.

Since the VCU procedure requires instrumentation, special precautions should be observed in those patients known to have an acute urinary tract infection. Filling of the bladder should be done at a steady rate, exercising caution to avoid excessive pressure. Sterile procedures are essential.

Adverse Reactions: See ADVERSE REACTIONS—General.

Dosage and Administration: OMNIPAQUE may be diluted, utilizing aseptic technique, with Sterile Water for Injection to a concentration of 50 mgI/mL to 100 mgI/mL for voiding cystourethrography. The concentration may vary depending upon the patient's size and age and also with the technique and equipment used. Sufficient volume of contrast medium should be administered to adequately fill the bladder. The usual volume ranges from 50 mL to 300 mL of OMNIPAQUE at a concentration of 100 mgI/mL and 50 mL to 600 mL of OMNIPAQUE at a concentration of 50 mgI/mL. OMNIPAQUE may be diluted with Sterile Water for Injection as indicated in the table below:

Dilutions of OMNIPAQUE should be prepared just prior to use and any unused portion discarded after the procedure.

ARTHROGRAPHY

OMNIPAQUE 240 at a concentration of 240 mgI/mL or OMNIPAQUE 300 at a concentration of 300 mgI/mL or OMNIPAQUE 350 at a concentration of 350 mgI/mL is indicated in radiography of the knee joint in adults, and OMNIPAQUE 210 at a concentration of 210 mgI/mL or OMNIPAQUE 240 at a concentration of 240 mgI/mL or OMNIPAQUE 300 at a concentration of 300 mgI/mL is indicated in radiography of the shoulder joint in adults, and OMNIPAQUE 300 at a concentration of 300 mgI/mL is indicated in radiography of the temporomandibular joint in adults. Arthrography may be helpful in the diagnosis of post-traumatic or degenerative joint diseases, synovial rupture, the visualization of communicating bursae or cysts, and in meniscography.

Precautions: See PRECAUTIONS—General.

Strict aseptic technique is required to prevent infection. Fluoroscopic control should be used to ensure proper needle placement, prevent extracapsular injection, and prevent dilution of contrast medium. Undue pressure should not be exerted during injection.

Adverse Reactions: Injection of OMNIPAQUE into the joint is associated with transient discomfort, ie, pain, swelling. However, delayed, severe or persistent discomfort may occur occasionally. Severe pain may often result from undue use of pressure or the injection of large volumes. Joint swelling after injection is less with OMNIPAQUE than with high osmolar ionic contrast medium. These types of reactions are generally procedurally dependent and of greater frequency when double-contrast technique is employed.

Nervous system: Swelling sensation (42%), pain (29%), heat sensation (13%), and muscle weakness (0.7%).

Skin and appendages: Hematoma at injection site (0.7%).

Dosage and Administration: Arthrography is usually performed under local anesthesia. The amount of OMNIPAQUE (iohexol) injected is dependent on the size of the joint to be examined and the technique employed. Lower volumes of contrast medium are usually injected for knee and shoulder arthrography when double-contrast examinations using 15 mL to 100 mL of air are performed.

The following concentrations and volumes are recommended for normal adult knee, shoulder, and temporomandibular joints but should serve as guidelines since joints may require more or less contrast medium for optimal visualization.

KNEE		
OMNIPAQUE 240	5 mL to 15 mL	
OMNIPAQUE 300	5 mL to 15 mL	Lower volumes
OMNIPAQUE 350	5 mL to 10 mL	recommended for
SHOULDER		double-contrast
OMNIPAQUE 300	10 mL	examinations;
OMNIPAQUE 240	3 mL	higher volumes
OMNIPAQUE 210	3 mL	recommended
TEMPOROMANDIBULAR		for single-contrast
OMNIPAQUE 300	0.5 mL to 1.0 mL	examinations.

Passive or active manipulation is used to disperse the medium throughout the joint space.

ENDOSCOPIC RETROGRADE PANCREATOGRAPHY (ERP)/ENDOSCOPIC RETROGRADE CHOLANGIOPANCREATOGRAPHY (ERCP)

OMNIPAQUE 240 at a concentration of 240 mgI/mL is indicated in adults for use in ERP/ERCP.

Precautions: See PRECAUTIONS—General.

Continued on next page

This product information was prepared in August 1992. On these and other products of Sanofi Winthrop Pharmaceuticals, detailed information may be obtained on a current basis by direct inquiry to Product Information Services, 90 Park Avenue, New York, NY 10016 (toll free 1-800-446-6267).

To Achieve	Add to		
A Final Concentration	Each 100 mL of OMNIPAQUE Sterile Water for Injection, USP (mL)		
(mgI/mL) of	OMNIPAQUE 240	OMNIPAQUE 300	OMNIPAQUE 350
100	140	200	250
90	167	233	289
80	200	275	338
70	243	330	400
60	300	400	483
50	380	500	600

Sanofi Winthrop—Cont.

Adverse Reactions: Injection of OMNIPAQUE (iohexol) in ERP/ERCP is associated with transient pain. However, delayed, severe or persistent pain may occur and can persist for 24 hours. The cause of the pain may be due as much to the procedure itself as to the contrast medium injected, therefore, attention should be paid to the injection pressure and total volume injected to minimize disruptive distention of the ducts examined.

Cardiovascular system: Hypertension (1%).

Nervous system: Pain (17%), somnolence (1%), and burning (1%).

Gastrointestinal system: Vomiting, diarrhea, and pressure, each with an individual incidence of 1%.

Dosage and Administration: The recommended dose of OMNIPAQUE 240 at a concentration of 240 mgI/mL is 10 mL to 50 mL but may vary depending on individual anatomy and/or disease state.

HYSTEROSALPINGOGRAPHY

OMNIPAQUE 240 at a concentration of 240 mgI/mL or OMNIPAQUE 300 at a concentration of 300 mgI/mL is indicated in radiography of the internal group of adult female reproductive organs; ovaries, fallopian tubes, uterus, and vagina. Hysterosalpingography is utilized as a diagnostic and therapeutic modality in the treatment of infertility and other abnormal gynecological conditions.

Contraindications: The procedure should not be performed during the menstrual period or when menstrual flow is imminent, nor should it be performed when infection is present in any portion of the genital tract, including the external genitalia. The procedure is also contraindicated for pregnant women or for those in whom pregnancy is suspected. Its use is not advised for 6 months after termination of pregnancy or 30 days after conization or curettage.

Precautions: In patients with carcinoma or in those in whom the condition is suspected, caution should be exercised to avoid possible spreading of the lesion by the procedure.

Adverse Reactions: Injection of OMNIPAQUE in hysterosalpingography is associated with immediate but transient pain. The cause of the pain may be due as much to the procedure itself as to the contrast medium injected, therefore attention should be paid to the injection pressure and volume instilled to avoid disruptive distention of the uterus and fallopian tubes. Fluoroscopic monitoring is recommended.

Nervous system: Pain (49%), somnolence and fever each with an individual incidence of 3%.

Gastrointestinal system: Nausea (3%).

Dosage and Administration: The recommended dosage of OMNIPAQUE 240 is 15 mL to 20 mL and of OMNIPAQUE 300 is 15 mL to 20 mL but will vary depending on individual anatomy and/or disease state.

HERNIOGRAPHY

OMNIPAQUE 240 at a concentration of 240 mgI/mL is indicated in adults for use in herniography.

Precautions: See PRECAUTIONS—General.

Adverse Reactions: Nervous system: Pain (7%), headache (3%), and unwell feeling (3%).

Gastrointestinal system: Diarrhea (3%) and flatulence (10%).

Dosage and Administration: The recommended dosage of OMNIPAQUE 240 is 50 mL but may vary depending on individual anatomy and/or disease state.

DO NOT USE FLEXIBLE CONTAINER IN SERIES CONNECTIONS.

HOW SUPPLIED

OMNIPAQUE 140
Vials of 50 mL, 140 mgI/mL, boxes of 10
(NDC 0024-1401-50)
50 mL bottle with hanger, 140 mgI/mL, boxes of 10
(NDC 0024-1401-51)

OMNIPAQUE 210
Vials of 15 mL, 210 mgI/mL, boxes of 10
(NDC 0024-1402-15)

OMNIPAQUE 240
Vials of 10 mL, 240 mgI/mL, boxes of 10
(NDC 0024-1412-10)
Vials of 20 mL, 240 mgI/mL, boxes of 10
(NDC 0024-1412-20)
Vials of 50 mL, 240 mgI/mL, boxes of 10
(NDC 0024-1412-50)
50 mL bottle with hanger, 240 mgI/mL, boxes of 10
(NDC 0024-1412-51)
100 mL fill in 100 mL bottle with hanger, 240 mgI/mL, boxes of 10
(NDC 0024-1412-60)
150 mL fill in 200 mL bottle with hanger, 240 mgI/mL, boxes of 10
(NDC 0024-1412-49)
200 mL fill in 200 mL bottle with hanger, 240 mgI/mL, boxes of 10
(NDC 0024-1412-17)

100 mL flexible container, 240 mgI/mL, boxes of 10
(NDC 0024-1412-70)
150 mL flexible container, 240 mgI/mL, boxes of 10
(NDC 0024-1412-75)
200 mL flexible container, 240 mgI/mL, boxes of 10
(NDC 0024-1412-72)

OMNIPAQUE 300
Vials of 10 mL, 300 mgI/mL, boxes of 10
(NDC 0024-1413-10)
Vials of 30 mL, 300 mgI/mL, boxes of 10
(NDC 0024-1413-30)
Vials of 50 mL, 300 mgI/mL, boxes of 10
(NDC 0024-1413-50)
50 mL bottle with hanger, 300 mgI/mL, boxes of 10
(NDC 0024-1413-51)
100 mL fill in 100 mL bottle with hanger, 300 mgI/mL, boxes of 10
(NDC 0024-1413-60)
150 mL fill in 200 mL bottle with hanger, 300 mgI/mL, boxes of 10
(NDC 0024-1413-90)
100 mL flexible container, 300 mgI/mL, boxes of 10
(NDC 0024-1413-80)
150 mL flexible container, 300 mgI/mL, boxes of 10
(NDC 0024-1413-85)

OMNIPAQUE 350
Vials of 50 mL, 350 mgI/mL, boxes of 10
(NDC 0024-1414-50)
50 mL bottle with hanger, 350 mgI/mL, boxes of 10
(NDC 0024-1414-51)
75 mL fill in 100 mL bottle with hanger, 350 mgI/mL, boxes of 10
(NDC 0024-1414-75)
100 mL fill in 100 mL bottle with hanger, 350 mgI/mL, boxes of 10
(NDC 0024-1414-60)
125 mL fill in 200 mL bottle with hanger, 350 mgI/mL, boxes of 10
(NDC 0024-1414-76)
150 mL fill in 200 mL bottle with hanger, 350 mgI/mL, boxes of 10
(NDC 0024-1414-03)
175 mL fill in 200 mL bottle with hanger, 350 mgI/mL, boxes of 10
(NDC 0024-1414-77)
200 mL fill in 200 mL bottle with hanger, 350 mgI/mL, boxes of 10
(NDC 0024-1414-04)
100 mL flexible container, 350 mgI/mL, boxes of 10
(NDC 0024-1414-61)
150 mL flexible container, 350 mgI/mL, boxes of 10
(NDC 0024-1414-65)
200 mL flexible container, 350 mgI/mL, boxes of 10
(NDC 0024-1414-62)

Storage: Protect vials, bottles, and flexible containers of OMNIPAQUE (iohexol) from strong daylight and direct exposure to sunlight. Do not freeze. Store at controlled room temperature 59°F to 86°F (15°C to 30°C).

Caution: Federal law prohibits dispensing without prescription.

OSW-1

Manufactured by Sterling Pharmaceuticals Inc.
Barceloneta, Puerto Rico 00617

Savage Laboratories
a division of Altana Inc.
60 BAYLIS ROAD
MELVILLE, NY 11747

ETHIODOL®   ℞
[ĕ-thī'ō'dŏl]
(brand of ethiodized oil injection)

DESCRIPTION

Ethiodol®, brand of ethiodized oil, is a sterile injectable radio-opaque diagnostic agent for use in hysterosalpingography and lymphography. It contains 37% iodine (475 mg/ml) organically combined with ethyl esters of fatty acids (primarily as ethyl monoiodostearate and ethyl diiodostearate) of poppyseed oil. Stabilized with poppyseed oil, 1%. The precise structure of Ethiodol® is unknown at this time. Ethiodol® is a straw to amber colored, oil fluid, which because of simplified molecular structure, possesses a greatly reduced viscosity (1.280 specific gravity at 15°C yields viscosity of 0.5 to 1.0 poise). This high fluidity provides a new flexibility for radiographic exploration.

HOW SUPPLIED

Ethiodol® (brand of ethiodized oil for injection) is supplied in a box of two 10 ml ampules, NDC 0281-7062-37.

Serono Laboratories, Inc.
100 LONGWATER CIRCLE
NORWELL, MA 02061

GEREF®   ℞
(sermorelin acetate for injection)
For intravenous injection only
FOR DIAGNOSTIC USE ONLY

DESCRIPTION

Geref® (sermorelin acetate for injection) is a sterile, non-pyrogenic, lyophilized preparation containing 50 mcg sermorelin (as the acetate), 5 mg mannitol, 0.66 mg monobasic sodium phosphate, and 0.04 mg dibasic sodium phosphate. Geref® may contain up to 1% albumin (human), which is used during Geref® manufacturing. Sermorelin acetate is an acetate salt of a synthetic, 29-amino acid polypeptide that is the amino-terminal segment of the naturally occurring human growth hormone-releasing hormone (GHRH or GRH) consisting of 44 amino acid residues. The structural formula for sermorelin acetate is presented below:

Tyr-Ala-Asp-Ala-Ile-Phe-Thr-Asn-Ser-Tyr-
Arg-Lys-Val-Leu-Gly-Gln-Leu-Ser-Ala-Arg-
Lys-Leu-Leu-Gln-Asp-Ile-Met-Ser-Arg-$NH_2 \cdot (C_2H_4O_2)_{3-6}$

The free base of sermorelin has the empirical formula $C_{149}H_{246}N_{44}O_{42}S_1$ and a molecular weight of 3,358 daltons. Sermorelin appears to be equivalent to GRH (1-44) in its ability to stimulate growth hormone secretion in humans. It has also been called GRH (1-29) and GHRH (1-29).

CLINICAL PHARMACOLOGY

Sermorelin increases plasma growth hormone (GH) concentrations by direct stimulation of the pituitary gland to release GH.

Because baseline GH levels are generally very low (< 4 ng/mL), provocative tests may be useful in determining the functional GH-secreting capability of the pituitary somatotroph. Adults and children with normal responses to standard provocative tests of GH secretion were used to define the range of normal plasma GH-level responses to Geref.® It was found that the absolute peak GH level following Geref® infusion and the time elapsed from infusion to that peak are appropriate measures to evaluate the response to GH infusion. Doses of Geref® used in children and adults in these studies ranged from 0.3 to 6.06 mcg/kg with a majority of patients receiving 1 mcg/kg. Based on these studies and published reports, 1 mcg/kg was chosen as the recommended dose for diagnostic purposes.

A total of 71 Geref® injection tests were performed on 47 boys and 24 girls who showed normal responses to standard, indirect provocative tests such as clonidine, L-dopa, and arginine. The GH peak plasma response to Geref® was 28 ± 15 ng/mL (average $\pm$ S.D.) and the time to this peak was 30 ± 27 minutes (average $\pm$ S.D.).

Of all children who had GH responses of > 7 ng/mL to standard provocative tests, 96% also had responses to Geref® of > 7 ng/mL. In 77 patients who failed to respond to standard provocative tests, mean GH peak responses to Geref® were significantly lower compared to the mean GH peak response of normal control children. However, 53% of the children who failed to respond to standard tests had a GH response to Geref® of more than 7 ng/mL, suggesting that clinical GH deficiency is frequently not due to somatotroph failure.

The following figure shows the time course of average plasma GH-level responses to Geref® injection in normal children and those with subnormal responses to standard provocative tests, i.e., growth hormone-deficient (GHD) children.

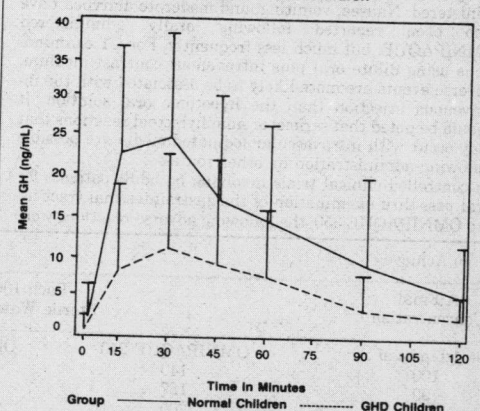

**Mean (& SD) of GH Response to Geref®
in Normal and GHD Children**

Group   —— Normal Children   ------ GHD Children

In 14 published reports that utilized different forms of GRH including GRH (1-44), GRH (1-40), and formulations of GRH

(1-29) other than Geref,® 167 normal young adults of both sexes, 19 to 40 years old, were tested with approximately 1 mcg/kg GRH peptide. The data derived from pooling these results are similar to the results obtained from 14 normal male adults, 19 to 30 years old tested with Geref®:

ADULT VOLUNTEERS

Source	N	Age Range	Range of Mean Peak GH (ng/mL)	Mean Peak GH (ng/mL)
14 Studies	167	19–40	10–41	22
Geref®	14	19–30	—	24

In adults, time to peak GH response to Geref® was 35 ± 29 minutes (average $\pm$ S.D.).
Preliminary studies have demonstrated a decline in GH responsiveness to GRH with age in persons over 40 years old, but the normal range of GH response to Geref® in older adults has not been established.

INDICATIONS AND USAGE
Geref® as a single intravenous injection is indicated for evaluating the ability of the somatotroph of the pituitary gland to secrete growth hormone (GH). A normal plasma GH response to Geref® demonstrates that the somatotroph is intact. However, a normal response does not exclude GH deficiency because this deficiency is frequently the result of hypothalamic dysfunction in the presence of an intact somatotroph. The Geref® stimulation test is most easily interpreted when there is a subnormal response to conventional provocative testing and a normal response to Geref.® Such findings suggest that hypothalamic dysfunction is the cause for the growth hormone deficiency. When both conventional and Geref® testing result in subnormal GH responses, the site of dysfunction cannot be determined with certainty because some patients with GH deficiency due to hypothalamic dysfunction require repeated Geref® administration before demonstrating a normal response.
The Geref® test has not been found useful in the diagnosis of acromegaly.

CONTRAINDICATIONS
Geref® is contraindicated in patients hypersensitive to sermorelin acetate or any of the excipients.

WARNINGS
Although hypersensitivity reactions have been observed with other polypeptide hormones, to date no such reactions have been reported following the administration of a single dose of Geref.® Antibody formation has been reported in humans after chronic subcutaneous administration of large doses of sermorelin (see Adverse Reactions section).

PRECAUTIONS
Drug Interactions: The Geref® test should not be conducted in the presence of drugs that directly affect the pituitary secretion of somatotropin. These include preparations that contain or release somatostatin, insulin, glucocorticoids, or cyclooxygenase inhibitors such as aspirin or indomethacin. Somatotropin levels may be transiently elevated by clonidine, levodopa, and insulin-induced hypoglycemia. Response to Geref® may be blunted in patients who are receiving muscarinic antagonists (atropine) or who are hypothyroid or being treated with antithyroid medications such as propylthiouracil. Obesity, hyperglycemia, and elevated plasma fatty acids generally are associated with subnormal GH responses to Geref.® Exogenous growth hormone therapy should be discontinued at least one week before administering the Geref® test.
Carcinogensis, Mutagenesis, Impairment of Fertility: There have been no long-term studies performed in animals to assess the carcinogenic potential of Geref.® Geref® was not mutagenic in *in vitro* or *in vivo* genetic toxicology studies.
Pregnancy Category C: Sermorelin acetate has been shown to produce minor variations in fetuses of rats and rabbits when given in subcutaneous doses of 50, 150, and 500 mcg/kg. In the rat teratology study, external malformations (thin tail) were observed in the higher dose groups, and there was an increase in minor skeletal variants at the high dose. Some visceral malformations (hydroureter) were observed in all treatment groups, with the incidence greatest in the high-dose group. In rabbits, minor skeletal anomalies were significantly greater in the treated animals than in the controls. There are no adequate and well-controlled studies in pregnant women. Geref® should be used during pregnancy only if the potential benefit justifies the potential risk to the fetus.
Nursing Mothers: It is not known whether this drug is excreted in human milk. Because many drugs are excreted in human milk, caution should be exercised when Geref® is administered to a nursing woman.

ADVERSE REACTIONS
The following adverse reactions, in decreasing order of frequency, have been reported following sermorelin administration:

Transient warmth and/or flushing of the face
Injection site pain
Redness and/or swelling at injection site
Nausea
Headache
Vomiting
Strange taste in the mouth
Paleness
Tightness in the chest
Approximately one in four patients given repeated doses of one or more of the three forms of GRH (1-29, 1-40, and 1-44) has developed antibodies to GRH. The clinical significance of these antibodies is unknown. One patient who developed antibodies to GRH (1-44) also experienced an allergic reaction described as severe redness, swelling, and urticaria at the injection sites. No long-lasting effects from this reaction were reported. No symptomatic allergic reactions to GRH (1-29) have been reported.

OVERDOSAGE
Changes of heart rate and blood pressure have been reported with the various GRH peptides in intravenous doses exceeding 10 mcg/kg. Cardiovascular collapse is a conceivable, but as of yet, unreported, complication of overdosage with GRH (1-29).

DOSAGE AND ADMINISTRATION
Geref® dosage should be individualized for each patient according to his/her weight. It is recommended that Geref® be administered in a single intravenous dose of 1.0 mcg/kg body weight in the morning following an overnight fast.
DIRECTIONS
Children (or subjects less than 50 kg)
1) Reconstitute the contents of one 50 mcg ampule of Geref® with a minimum of 0.5 mL of the accompanying sterile diluent.
2) Venous blood samples for growth hormone determinations should be drawn 15 minutes before and immediately prior to Geref® administration.
3) Administer a bolus of 1 mcg/kg body weight Geref® intravenously followed by a 3 mL normal saline flush.
4) Draw venous blood samples for growth hormone determinations at 15, 30, 45, and 60 minutes after Geref® administration.
Adults (or subjects over 50 kg)
1) Determine the number of ampules needed, based on a dose of 1 mcg/kg body weight.
2) Reconstitute the contents of each ampule with a minimum of 0.5 mL of the accompanying sterile diluent.
3) Follow steps 2–4 above.
Parenteral drug products should be inspected visually for particulate matter and discoloration prior to administration, whenever solution and container permit. The drug should be discarded if not dissolved or if the reconstituted solution is cloudy or discolored.

HOW SUPPLIED
Geref® is supplied in sterile, nonpyrogenic, lyophilized form in ampules containing 50 mcg sermorelin (as the acetate). The following package combination is available:
NDC 44087-4050-1
1 ampule containing 50 mcg sermorelin (as the acetate) and 1 vial containing 2 mL 0.9% Sodium Chloride Injection, USP
The lyophilized product must be stored refrigerated (2°–8°C/36°–46°F). Use immediately after reconstitution. Discard unused material.
Caution: Federal law prohibits dispensing without prescription.
References available on request.
Manufactured for:
SERONO LABORATORIES, INC.
Randolph, MA 02368 USA
by: Laboratoires Serono, SA
Aubonne, Switzerland
© SERONO LABORATORIES, INC. 1991

Winthrop Pharmaceuticals
90 PARK AVENUE
NEW YORK, NY 10016

Winthrop Pharmaceuticals' products are now distributed by Sanofi Winthrop Pharmaceuticals.

Wyeth-Ayerst Laboratories
Division of American Home
Products Corporation
P.O. BOX 8299
PHILADELPHIA, PA 19101

FACTREL®   ℞
[fắc'trel]
(gonadorelin hydrochloride)
Synthetic Luteinizing Hormone Releasing
Hormone (LH-RH)
DIAGNOSTIC USE ONLY

CAUTION: Federal law prohibits dispensing without prescription.

DESCRIPTION
An agent for use in evaluating hypothalamic-pituitary gonadotropic function. FACTREL (gonadorelin hydrochloride) injectable is available as a sterile lyophilized powder for reconstitution and administration by subcutaneous or intravenous routes.
Chemical Name: 5-oxo-L-prolyl-L-histidyl-L-tryptophyl-L-seryl -L- tyrosyl-glycyl -L- leucyl-L-arginyl-L-prolyl glycinamide hydrochloride
[See structural formula below.]

FACTREL is $C_{55}H_{75}N_{17}O_{13}HCl$, as the mono- or dihydrochloride, or their mixture. The gonadorelin base has a molecular weight of 1182.33. It is a white powder, soluble in alcohol and water, hygroscopic and moisture-sensitive, and stable at room temperature. The synthetic decapeptide, FACTREL, has a chemical composition and structure identical to the natural hormone, identified from porcine or ovine hypothalami.
Each SECULE® vial of FACTREL contains 100 or 500 mcg gonadorelin as the hydrochloride, with 100 mg lactose, USP. Each ampul of sterile diluent contains 2% benzyl alcohol in sterile water.

CLINICAL PHARMACOLOGY
FACTREL has been shown to have gonadotropin-releasing effects upon the anterior pituitary. The range for normal baseline LH levels, as determined from the literature, is 5–25 mIU/mL in postpubertal males, and postpubertal and premenopausal females. The standard used is the Second International Reference Preparation—HMC. This range may not correspond in each laboratory performing the assay since the concentration of LH in normal individuals varies with different assay methods. The normal responses to FACTREL analyzed from the results of clinical studies included:
(1) LH peak (mIU/mL)
   (highest LH value post-FACTREL administration)
(2) Maximum LH increase (mIU/mL)
   (peak LH value—LH baseline value)
(3) LH percent response
$$\frac{peak\ LH - baseline\ LH}{baseline\ LH} \times 100\%$$
(4) Time to peak (minutes)
   (time required to reach LH peak value)
Normal adult subjects were shown to have these LH responses following FACTREL administration by subcutaneous or intravenous routes.

FACTREL®   Structural Formula:

Continued on next page

Wyeth-Ayerst—Cont.

I. MALE ADULTS:

A) Subcutaneous Administration

The results are based on 18 tests in males between the ages of 18–42 years, inclusive:
(1) LH peak: mean 60.3 ± 26.2 mIU/mL
   100% ≥ 24.0 mIU/mL
   90% ≥ 32.8 mIU/mL
(2) Maximum LH increase: mean 46.7 ± 20.8 mIU/mL
   100% ≥ 12.3 mIU/mL
   90% ≥ 20.9 mIU/mL
(3) LH percent response: mean 437 ± 243%
   range: 66–1853%
   90% ≥ 188%
(4) Time to peak: mean 34 ± 13 min

B) Intravenous Administration

The results are based on 26 tests in males between the ages of 19–58 years, inclusive:
(1) LH peak: mean 63.8 ± 40.3 mIU/mL
   100% ≥ 12.6 mIU/mL
   90% ≥ 26.0 mIU/mL
(2) Maximum LH increase: mean 51.3 ± 35.2 mIU/mL
   100% ≥ 7.4 mIU/mL
   90% ≥ 14.8 mIU/mL
(3) LH percent response: mean 481 ± 184%
   range: 67–2139%
   90% ≥ 142%
(4) Time to peak: mean 27 ± 14 min

In males older than 50 years, the LH baseline and peak levels tend to be higher; however, the maximum LH increases do not differ in regard to age.

II. FEMALE ADULTS:

A) Subcutaneous Administration

The results are based on 38 tests in females between the ages of 19–36 years, inclusive:
(1) LH peak: mean 67.9 ± 27.5 mIU/mL
   100% ≥ 12.5 mIU/mL
   90% ≥ 39.0 mIU/mL
(2) Maximum LH increase: mean 52.8 ± 26.4 mIU/mL
   100% ≥ 7.5 mIU/mL
   90% ≥ 23.8 mIU/mL
(3) LH percent response: mean 374 ± 221%
   range: 108–981%
   90% ≥ 185%
(4) Time to peak: mean 71.5 ± 49.6 min

B) Intravenous Administration

The results are based on 31 tests in females between the ages of 20–35 years inclusive:
(1) LH peak: mean 57.6 ± 36.7 mIU/mL
   100% ≥ 20.0 mIU/mL
   90% ≥ 24.6 mIU/mL
(2) Maximum LH increase: mean 44.5 ± 31.8 mIU/mL
   100% ≥ 7.5 mIU/mL
   90% ≥ 16.2 mIU/mL
(3) LH percent response: mean 356 ± 282%
   range: 60–1300%
   90% ≥ 142%
(4) Time to peak: mean 36 ± 24 min

The FACTREL tests on which the normal female responses are based were performed in the early follicular phase of the menstrual cycle (Days 1–7).

In menopausal and postmenopausal females, the baseline LH levels are elevated and the maximum LH increases are exaggerated when compared with the premenopausal levels. Patients with clinically diagnosed or suspected pituitary and/or hypothalamic dysfunction were often shown to have subnormal or no LH responses following FACTREL administration. For example, in clinical studies of 6 patients with known postpubertal panhypopituitarism, and 11 patients with Prader-Willi syndrome, 100% showed subnormal responses or no rise in LH. Subnormal responses to the FACTREL test also were observed in 21 (95%) of 22 patients with prepubertal panhypopituitarism. In 19 patients with Sheehan's syndrome, 16 (84%) had a subnormal response. In the FACTREL test in 44 patients with Kallmann's syndrome, 33 (77%) had subnormal LH responses.

INDICATIONS AND USAGE

FACTREL as a single injection is indicated for evaluating the functional capacity and response of the gonadotropes of the anterior pituitary. This single-injection test does not measure pituitary gonadotropic reserve, for which more prolonged or repeated administration may be required. The LH response is useful in testing patients with suspected gonadotropin deficiency, whether due to the hypothalamus alone or in combination with anterior pituitary failure. FACTREL is also indicated for evaluating residual gonadotropic function of the pituitary following removal of a pituitary tumor by surgery and/or irradiation. In clinical studies to date, however, the single-injection test has not been useful in

differentiating pituitary disorders from hypothalamic disorders. The FACTREL test can be performed concomitantly with other post-treatment evaluations. The results of the FACTREL test complement the clinical examination and other laboratory tests used to confirm or substantiate hypogonadotropic hypogonadism.

In cases where there is a normal response, it indicates the presence of functional pituitary gonadotropes. The single-injection test does not measure pituitary gonadotropic reserve.

CONTRAINDICATIONS

Hypersensitivity to gonadorelin hydrochloride or any of the components.

PRECAUTIONS

Although allergic and hypersensitivity reactions have been observed with other polypeptide hormones, and rarely with multiple doses of FACTREL, to date no such reactions have been reported following the administration of a single 100 mcg dose of FACTREL.

Antibody formation has been reported rarely after chronic administration of large doses of FACTREL.

The FACTREL test should be conducted in the absence of other drugs which directly affect the pituitary secretion of the gonadotropins. These would include a variety of preparations which contain androgens, estrogens, progestins, or glucocorticoids. The gonadotropin levels may be transiently elevated by spironolactone, minimally elevated by levodopa, and suppressed by oral contraceptives and digoxin. The response to FACTREL may be blunted by phenothiazines and dopamine antagonists which cause a rise in prolactin.

Pregnancy Category B. Reproduction studies have been performed in mice, rats, and rabbits at doses up to 50 times the human dose, and have revealed no evidence of harm to the fetus due to FACTREL. There are, however, no adequate and well-controlled studies in pregnant women. Because animal reproduction studies are not always predictive of human response, this drug should be used during pregnancy only if clearly needed.

Appropriate precautions should be taken because the effects of LH-RH on the fetus and developing offspring have not been adequately evaluated. Repetitive, high doses of FACTREL may cause luteolysis and inhibition of spermatogenesis.

ADVERSE REACTIONS

Systemic complaints such as headaches, nausea, light-headedness, abdominal discomfort, and flushing have been reported rarely following administration of 100 mcg of FACTREL. Local swelling, occasionally with pain and pruritus, at the injection site may occur if FACTREL is administered subcutaneously. Local and generalized skin rash have been noted after chronic subcutaneous administration.

Rare instances of hypersensitivity reaction (bronchospasm, tachycardia, flushing, urticaria, induration at injection site) and anaphylactic reactions have been reported following multiple-dose administration.

OVERDOSAGE

FACTREL has been administered parenterally in doses up to 3 mg bid for 28 days without any signs or symptoms of overdosage. In case of overdosage or idiosyncrasy, symptomatic treatment should be administered as required.

DOSAGE AND ADMINISTRATION

Parenteral drug products should be inspected visually for particulate matter and discoloration prior to administration, whenever solution and container permit.

Adults: 100 mcg dose, subcutaneously or intravenously. In females for whom the phase of the menstrual cycle can be established, the test should be performed in the early follicular phase (Days 1–7).

TEST METHODOLOGY

To determine the status of the gonadotropin secretory capacity of the anterior pituitary, a test procedure requiring seven venous blood samples for LH is recommended.

PROCEDURE:

1. Venous blood samples should be drawn at -15 minutes and immediately prior to FACTREL administration. The LH baseline is obtained by averaging the LH values of the two samples.
2. Administer a bolus of 100 mcg of FACTREL subcutaneously or intravenously.
3. Draw venous blood samples at 15, 30, 45, 60, and 120 minutes after administration.
4. Blood samples should be handled as recommended by the laboratory that will determine the LH content. It must be emphasized that the reliability of the test is directly related to the inter-assay and intra-assay reliability of the laboratory performing the assay.

INTERPRETATION OF TEST RESULTS

Interpretation of the LH response to FACTREL requires an understanding of the hypothalamic-pituitary physiology, knowledge of the clinical status of the individual patient, and familiarity with the normal ranges and the standards used in the laboratory performing the LH assays.

Figures 1 through 4 represent the LH response curves after FACTREL administration in normal subjects. The normal LH response curves were established between the 10th percentile (B line) and 90th percentile (A line) of all LH responses in normal subjects analyzed from the results of clinical studies. LH values are reported in units of mIU/mL and time is displayed in minutes. Individual patient responses should be plotted on the appropriate curve. A subnormal response in patients is defined as three or more LH values which fall below the B line of the normal LH response curve. In cases where there is a blunted or borderline response, the FACTREL test should be repeated.

Fig. 1

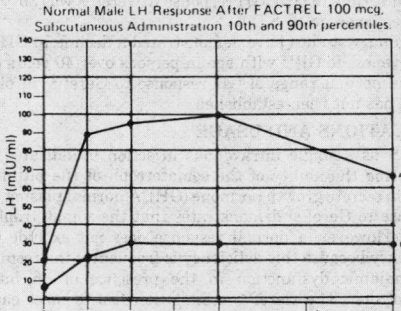

Normal Male LH Response After FACTREL 100 mcg, Subcutaneous Administration 10th and 90th percentiles

Fig. 2

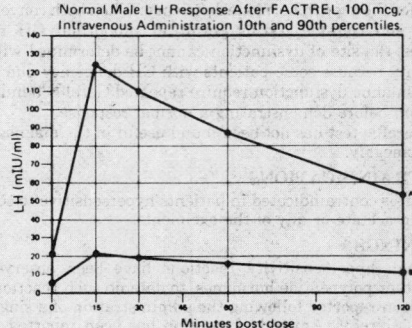

Normal Male LH Response After FACTREL 100 mcg, Intravenous Administration 10th and 90th percentiles

Fig. 3

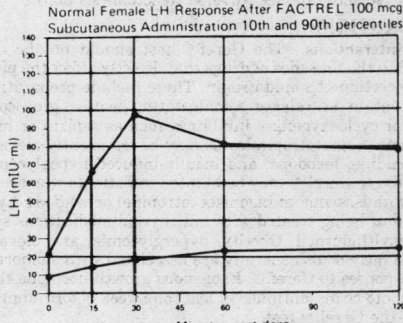

Normal Female LH Response After FACTREL 100 mcg, Subcutaneous Administration 10th and 90th percentiles

Fig. 4

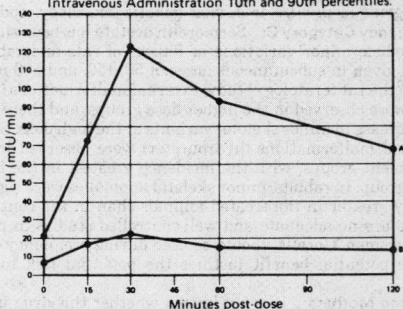

Normal Female LH Response After FACTREL 100 mcg, Intravenous Administration 10th and 90th percentiles

The FACTREL test complements the clinical assessment of patients with a variety of endocrine disorders involving the hypothalamic-pituitary axis. In cases where there is a normal response, it indicates the presence of functional pituitary gonadotropes. The single-injection test does not determine the pathophysiological cause for the subnormal response and does not measure pituitary gonadotropic reserve.

HOW SUPPLIED

LYOPHILIZED POWDER—
in single-dose SECULE® vials containing 100 mcg (NDC 0046-0507-05) and 500 mcg (NDC 0046-0509-05) gonadorelin as the hydrochloride with 100 mg lactose, USP. Each SECULE® vial is accompanied by one ampul containing 2 mL sterile diluent of 2% benzyl alcohol in sterile water.

DIRECTIONS

Store at room temperature (approximately 25°C).
Reconstitute <u>100</u> mcg SECULE® vial with <u>1.0</u> mL of the accompanying sterile diluent.
Reconstitute <u>500</u> mcg SECULE® vial with <u>2.0</u> mL of the accompanying sterile diluent.
Prepare solution immediately before use.
After reconstitution, store at room temperature and use within 1 day.
Discard unused reconstituted solution and diluent.
Diagnostic Method of Use Patent 3,947,569
SECULE®—Registered trademark to designate a vial containing an injectable preparation in dry form.
Shown in Product Identification Section, page 436

PEPTAVLON®   ℞

[pĕp-tăv′lon]
(pentagastrin)
for subcutaneous injection

CAUTION: Federal law prohibits dispensing without prescription.

DESCRIPTION

Peptavlon (pentagastrin) is a diagnostic agent for evaluation of gastric acid secretory function.
Chemical name: N-t-butyloxycarbonyl-B-alanyl-L-tryptophyl-L-methionyl-L-aspartyl-L-phenylalanyl amide.
Structural formula:

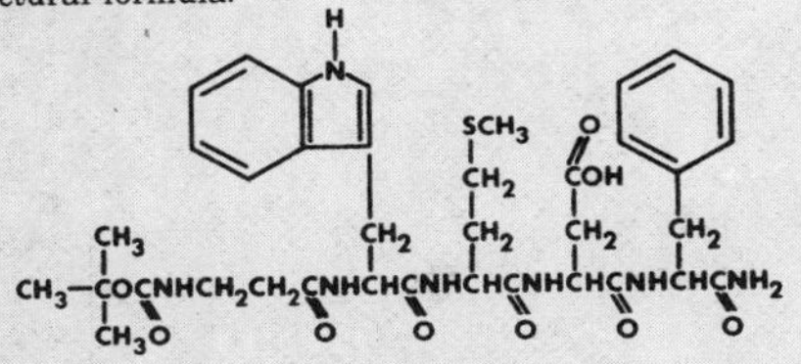

Pentagastrin is a synthetic pentapeptide containing the carboxyl terminal tetrapeptide, the active portion found in all natural gastrins. Pentagastrin is a colorless crystalline solid. It is soluble in dimethylformamide and dimethylsulfoxide; it is almost insoluble in water, ethanol, ether, benzene, chloroform, and ethyl acetate.
Pentagastrin is sterile and nonpyrogenic.
Each mL of injection contains 0.25 mg (250 mcg) pentagastrin. Peptavlon also contains 8.8 mg sodium chloride and Water for Injection, USP. The pH is adjusted with ammonium hydroxide and/or hydrochloric acid.
Peptavlon is available in 2 mL ampules for subcutaneous administration.

CLINICAL PHARMACOLOGY

PEPTAVLON (pentagastrin) contains the C-terminal tetrapeptide responsible for the actions of the natural gastrins and, therefore, acts as a physiologic gastric acid secretagogue. The recommended dose of 6 mcg/kg subcutaneously produces a peak acid output which is reproducible when used in the same individual.
PEPTAVLON stimulates gastric acid secretion approximately ten minutes after subcutaneous injection, with peak responses occurring in most cases twenty to thirty minutes after administration. Duration of activity is usually between sixty and eighty minutes.
In amounts in excess of recommended dose, pentagastrin may cause inhibition of gastric acid secretion.
In clinical studies of gastric acid secretion, peak gastric output in mEq/hr resulting from the subcutaneous injection of 6 mcg/kg pentagastrin does not differ significantly from that caused by the standard subcutaneous injection of the histamine acid phosphate dose used in the augmented histamine test (40 mcg/kg). For example, in 25 normal volunteers, pentagastrin produced an average peak acid output of 28.4 mEq/hr, compared with 24.7 mEq/hr by histamine. In 45 patients with duodenal ulcer, or suspected duodenal ulcer, pentagastrin produced an average peak gastric acid output of 39.7 mEq/hr, compared with 33.7 mEq/hr by histamine.
In 18 patients with gastric ulcer, or suspected gastric ulcer, pentagastrin produced an average peak acid output of 17.4 mEq/hr, compared with 19.4 mEq/hr by histamine. The overall mean for peak acid secretion by pentagastrin was 24.8 mEq/hr, compared with 22.6 mEq/hr by histamine. No biochemical abnormality which might indicate specific organ toxicity has been encountered following the administration of pentagastrin.

INDICATIONS AND USAGE

PEPTAVLON is used as a diagnostic agent to evaluate gastric acid secretory function. It is useful in testing for:
Anacidity:—as a diagnostic aid in patients with suspected pernicious anemia, atrophic gastritis, or gastric carcinoma.
Hypersecretion:—as a diagnostic aid in patients with suspected duodenal ulcer or postoperative stomal ulcer, and for the diagnosis of Zollinger-Ellison tumor.
PEPTAVLON (pentagastrin) is also useful in determining the adequacy of acid-reducing operations for peptic ulcer.

CONTRAINDICATIONS

Hypersensitivity or idiosyncrasy to pentagastrin.

WARNINGS

In amounts in excess of the recommended dose, pentagastrin may cause inhibition of gastric acid secretion.

PRECAUTIONS

Use with caution in patients with pancreatic, hepatic, or biliary disease. Like gastrin, pentagastrin could, in some cases, have the physiologic effect of stimulating pancreatic enzyme and bicarbonate secretion, as well as biliary flow.
CARCINOGENESIS, MUTAGENESIS, IMPAIRMENT OF FERTILITY
Long-term studies in animals to evaluate carcinogenic potential and studies to evaluate the mutagenic potential or effect on fertility have not been conducted.

PREGNANCY: TERATOGENIC EFFECTS

Pregnancy Category C—Animal reproduction studies have not been conducted with Peptavlon. It is also not known whether Peptavlon can cause fetal harm when administered to a pregnant woman or can affect reproduction capacity. Peptavlon should be given to a pregnant woman only if clearly needed.
NURSING MOTHERS
It is not known whether this drug is excreted in human milk. Because many drugs are excreted in human milk, caution should be exercised when Peptavlon is administered to a nursing woman.
PEDIATRIC USE Safety and effectiveness in children have not been established.

ADVERSE REACTIONS

Pentagastrin causes fewer and less severe cardiovascular and other adverse reactions than histamine or betazole. The majority of reactions to pentagastrin are related to the gastrointestinal tract.
The following reactions associated with the use of pentagastrin have been reported.
Gastrointestinal: Abdominal pain, desire to defecate, nausea, vomiting, borborygmi, blood-tinged mucus
Cardiovascular: Flushing, tachycardia
Central Nervous System: Dizziness, faintness or light-headedness, drowsiness, sinking feeling, transient blurring of vision, tiredness, headache
Allergic and Hypersensitivity Reactions: May occur in some patients.
Miscellaneous: Shortness of breath, heavy sensation in arms and legs, tingling in fingers, chills, sweating, generalized burning sensation, warmth, pain at site of injection, bile in collected specimens

OVERDOSAGE

In case of overdosage or idiosyncrasy, symptomatic treatment should be administered as required.

DOSAGE AND ADMINISTRATION

Adults: 6 mcg/kg subcutaneously. Effect begins in about ten minutes; peak response usually occurs in twenty to thirty minutes. (For discussion of the test and explicit directions, consult Baron, JH: Gastric Function Tests, in Wastell, C: *Chronic Duodenal Ulcer,* New York, Appleton-Century-Crofts, 1972, pp 82–114.)
Parenteral drug products should be inspected visually for particulate matter and discoloration prior to administration, whenever solution and container permit.

HOW SUPPLIED

PEPTAVLON (pentagastrin) is available in 2 mL ampuls. Each mL contains 0.25 mg (250 micrograms) pentagastrin. Cartons of 10 ampules (NDC 0046-3290-10).
REFRIGERATE, 2°C to 8°C (36°F to 46°F), AND PROTECT FROM LIGHT.
DO NOT USE IF DISCOLORED.

Certified Poison Control Centers

The poison control centers in the following list are certified by the American Association of Poison Control Centers. To receive certification, each center must meet certain criteria. It must, for example, serve a large geographic area; it must be open 24 hours a day and provide direct-dialing or toll-free access; it must be supervised by a medical director; and it must have registered pharmacists or nurses available to answer questions from the public.

Staff members of these centers are trained to resolve toxic situations in the home of the caller, but, in some instances, hospital referrals are given.

The centers have a wide variety of toxicology resources, including a computer capability covering some 350,000 substances that are updated quarterly. They also offer a range of educational services to the public as well as to the health care professional. In some states, these large centers exist side by side with smaller poison control centers that provide more limited information.

AMERICAN ASSOCIATION OF POISON CONTROL CENTERS

ALABAMA

Regional Poison Control Center
The Children's Hospital of Alabama
1600 Seventh Ave. S.
Birmingham, AL 35233-1711
Emergency Numbers:
(205) 939-9201
(205) 933-4050
(800) 292-6678 (Alabama only)

ARIZONA

Arizona Poison and Drug
Information Center
Arizona Health Sciences Center
Room 3204-K
1501 N. Campbell Ave.
Tucson, AZ 85724
Emergency Numbers:
(602) 626-6016
(800) 362-0101 (Arizona only)

Samaritan Regional Poison Center
Good Samaritan Regional
Medical Center
1130 E. McDowell, Suite A-5
Phoenix, AZ 85006
Emergency Number:
(602) 253-3334

CALIFORNIA

Fresno Regional Poison Control Center
of Fresno Community Hospital
and Medical Center
2823 Fresno St.
Fresno, CA 93721
Emergency Numbers:
(209) 445-1222
(800) 346-5922 (California only)

San Diego Regional Poison Center
UCSD Medical Center
225 Dickinson St.
San Diego, CA 92103-8925
Emergency Numbers:
(619) 543-6000
(800) 876-4766 (619 area code only)

San Francisco Bay Area Regional
Poison Control Center
San Francisco General Hospital
1001 Potrero Ave., Bldg. 80., Room 230
San Francisco, CA 94122
Emergency Number:
(415) 476-6600

Santa Clara Valley Medical Center
Regional Poison Center
751 S. Bascom Ave.
San Jose, CA 95128
Emergency Numbers:
(408) 299-5112
(800) 662-9886 (California only)

University of California, Davis,
Medical Center
Regional Poison Control Center
2315 Stockton Blvd.
Sacramento, CA 95817
Emergency Numbers:
(916) 734-3692
(800) 342-9293 (Northern California only)

UCI Regional Poison Center
UCI Medical Center
101 The City Dr.
Route 78
Orange, CA 92668-3298
Emergency Numbers:
(714) 634-5988
(800) 544-4404 (Southern California only)

COLORADO

**Rocky Mountain Poison and
Drug Center**
645 Bannock St.
Denver, CO 80204
Emergency Number:
(303) 629-1123

DISTRICT OF COLUMBIA

National Capital Poison Center
Georgetown University Hospital
3800 Reservoir Rd., N.W.
Washington, DC 20007
Emergency Numbers:
(202) 625-3333
(202) 784-4660 (TTY*)

FLORIDA

**The Florida Poison Information Center
at Tampa General Hospital**
P.O. Box 1289
Tampa, FL 33601
Emergency Numbers:
(813) 253-4444
(800) 282-3171 (Florida only)

GEORGIA

Georgia Poison Center
Grady Memorial Hospital
80 Butler St., S.E.
P.O. Box 26066
Atlanta, GA 30335-3801
Emergency Numbers:
(404) 589-4400
(800) 282-5846 (Georgia only)

INDIANA

Indiana Poison Center
Methodist Hospital of Indiana
1701 N. Senate Blvd.
P.O. Box 1367
Indianapolis, IN 46206-1367
Emergency Numbers:
(317) 929-2323
(800) 382-9097 (Indiana only)

KENTUCKY

**Kentucky Regional Poison Center
of Kosair Children's Hospital**
315 E. Broadway
P.O. Box 35070
Louisville, KY 40232
Emergency Numbers:
(502) 629-7275
(800) 722-5725 (Kentucky only)

MARYLAND

Maryland Poison Center
20 N. Pine St.
Baltimore, MD 21201
Emergency Numbers:
(410) 528-7701
(800) 492-2414 (Maryland only)

**National Capital Poison Center
(D.C. suburbs only)**
Georgetown University Hospital
3800 Reservoir Rd., N.W.
Washington, DC 20007
Emergency Numbers:
(202) 625-3333
(202) 784-4660 (TTY*)

MASSACHUSETTS

Massachusetts Poison Control System
300 Longwood Ave.
Boston, MA 02115
Emergency Numbers:
(617) 232-2120
(800) 682-9211

MICHIGAN

Blodgett Regional Poison Center
1840 Wealthy S.E.
Grand Rapids, MI 49506-2968
Emergency Numbers:
(800) 632-2727 (Michigan only)
(800) 356-3232 (TTY*)

Poison Control Center
Children's Hospital of Michigan
3901 Beaubien Blvd.
Detroit, MI 48201
Emergency Number:
(313) 745-5711

MINNESOTA

Hennepin Regional Poison Center
Hennepin County Medical Center
701 Park Ave.
Minneapolis, MN 55415
Emergency Numbers:
(612) 347-3141
(612) 337-7474 (TDD†)
Petline (612) 337-7387

Minnesota Regional Poison Center
St. Paul-Ramsey Medical Center
640 Jackson St.
St. Paul, MN 55101
Emergency Number:
(612) 221-2113

---

*TTY = teletype (for hearing-impaired individuals).
†TDD = telecommunication device for the deaf.

MISSOURI

Cardinal Glennon Children's Hospital Regional Poison Center
1465 S. Grand Blvd.
St. Louis, MO 63104
Emergency Numbers:
(314) 772-5200
(800) 366-8888

MONTANA

Rocky Mountain Poison and Drug Center
645 Bannock St.
Denver, CO 80204
Emergency Number:
(303) 629-1123

NEBRASKA

The Poison Center
8301 Dodge St.
Omaha, NE 68114
Emergency Numbers:
(402) 390-5555 (Omaha)
(800) 955-9119 (Nebraska only)

NEW JERSEY

New Jersey Poison Information and Education System
201 Lyons Ave.
Newark, NJ 07112
Emergency Number:
(800) 962-1253

NEW MEXICO

New Mexico Poison and Drug Information Center
University of New Mexico
Albuquerque, NM 87131-1076
Emergency Numbers:
(505) 843-2551
(800) 432-6866 (New Mexico only)

NEW YORK

Long Island Regional Poison Control Center
Nassau County Medical Center
2201 Hempstead Turnpike
East Meadow, NY 11554
Emergency Numbers:
(516) 542-2323, 2324, 2325, 3813

New York City Poison Control Center
N.Y.C. Department of Health
455 First Ave., Room 123
New York, NY 10016
Emergency Numbers:
(212) 340-4494
(212) POISONS
(212) 689-9014 (TDD†)

OHIO

Central Ohio Poison Center
700 Children's Drive
Columbus, OH 43205-2696
Emergency Numbers:
(614) 228-1323
(614) 461-2012
(800) 682-7625
(614) 228-2272 (TTY*)

Cincinnati Drug and Poison Information Center and Regional Poison Control System
231 Bethesda Ave.
M.L. 144
Cincinnati, OH 45267-0144
Emergency Numbers:
(513) 558-5111
(800) 872-5111 (Ohio only)

OREGON

Oregon Poison Center
Oregon Health Sciences University
3181 S.W. Sam Jackson Park Rd.
Portland, OR 97201
Emergency Numbers:
(503) 494-8968
(800) 452-7165 (Oregon only)

PENNSYLVANIA

Central Pennsylvania Poison Center
University Hospital
Milton S. Hershey Medical Center
Hershey, PA 17033
Emergency Number:
(800) 521-6110

The Poison Control Center serving the greater Philadelphia metropolitan area
One Children's Center
Philadelphia, PA 19104-4303
Emergency Number:
(215) 386-2100

Pittsburgh Poison Center
3705 Fifth Ave. at DeSoto St.
Pittsburgh, PA 15213
Emergency Number:
(412) 681-6669

RHODE ISLAND

Rhode Island Poison Center
593 Eddy St.
Providence, RI 02903
Emergency Number:
(401) 277-5727

TEXAS

North Texas Poison Center
5201 Harry Hines Blvd.
P.O. Box 35926
Dallas, TX 75235
Emergency Numbers:
(214) 590-5000
(800) 441-0040 (Texas WATS)

*TTY = teletype (for hearing-impaired individuals).
†TDD = telecommunication device for the deaf.

UTAH

**Intermountain Regional Poison
Control Center**
50 N. Medical Dr.
Bldg. 428
Salt Lake City, UT 84132
Emergency Numbers:
(801) 581-2151
(800) 456-7707 (Utah only)

VIRGINIA

Blue Ridge Poison Center
Box 67
Blue Ridge Hospital
Charlottesville, VA 22901
Emergency Numbers:
(804) 925-5543
(800) 451-1428

**National Capital Poison Center
(Northern Virginia only)**
Georgetown University Hospital
3800 Reservoir Rd., N.W.
Washington, DC 20007
Emergency Numbers:
(202) 625-3333
(202) 784-4660 (TTY*)

WEST VIRGINIA

West Virginia Poison Center
3110 MacCorkle Ave., S.E.
Charleston, WV 25304
Emergency Numbers:
(304) 348-4211
(800) 642-3625 (West Virginia only)

WYOMING

The Poison Center
8301 Dodge St.
Omaha, NE 68114
Emergency Numbers:
(402) 390-5555 (Omaha)
(800) 955-9119 (Nebraska only)

---

*TTY = teletype (for hearing-impaired individuals).

Key to Controlled Substances Categories

Products listed with the symbols shown below are subject to the Controlled Substances Act of 1970. These drugs are categorized according to their potential for abuse. The greater the potential, the more severe the limitations on their prescription.

CATEGORY   INTERPRETATION

Ⓒ II   **High potential for abuse.** Use may lead to severe physical or psychological dependence. Prescriptions must be written in ink, or typewritten and signed by the practitioner. Verbal prescriptions must be confirmed in writing within 72 hours, and may be given only in a genuine emergency. No renewals are permitted.

Ⓒ III   **Some potential for abuse.** Use may lead to low-to-moderate physical dependence or high psychological dependence. Prescriptions may be oral or written. Up to 5 renewals are permitted within 6 months.

Ⓒ IV   **Low potential for abuse.** Use may lead to limited physical or psychological dependence. Prescriptions may be oral or written. Up to 5 renewals are permitted within 6 months.

Ⓒ V   **Subject to state and local regulation.** Abuse potential is low; a prescription may not be required.

Key to FDA Use-in-pregnancy Ratings

The Food and Drug Administration's Pregnancy Categories are based on the degree to which available information has ruled out risk to the fetus, balanced against the drug's potential benefits to the patient. Ratings range from "A," for drugs that have been tested for teratogenicity under controlled conditions without showing evidence of damage to the fetus, to "D" and "X" for drugs that are definitely teratogenic. The "D" rating is generally reserved for drugs with no safer alternatives. The "X" rating means there is absolutely no reason to risk using the drug in pregnancy.

CATEGORY   INTERPRETATION

A   **Controlled studies show no risk.** Adequate, well-controlled studies in pregnant women have failed to demonstrate risk to the fetus.

B   **No evidence of risk in humans.** Either animal findings show risk, but human findings do not; or, if no adequate human studies have been done, animal findings are negative.

C   **Risk cannot be ruled out.** Human studies are lacking, and animal studies are either positive for fetal risk, or lacking as well. However, potential benefits may justify the potential risk.

D   **Positive evidence of risk.** Investigational or post-marketing data show risk to the fetus. Nevertheless potential benefits may outweigh the potential risk.

X   **Contraindicated in pregnancy.** Studies in animals or human, or investigational or post-marketing reports have shown fetal risk which clearly outweighs any possible benefit to the patient.

Key to Controlled Substances Categories

Products listed with the symbols shown below are subject to the Controlled Substances Act of 1970. These drugs are categorized according to their potential for abuse. The greater the potential, the more severe the limitations on their prescription.

CATEGORY   INTERPRETATION

① High potential for abuse. Use may lead to severe physical or psychological dependence. Prescriptions must be written in ink, or typewritten and signed by the practitioner. Verbal prescriptions must be confirmed in writing within 72 hours, and may be given only in a genuine emergency. No renewals are permitted.

② Some potential for abuse. Use may lead to low-to-moderate physical dependence or high psychological dependence. Prescriptions may be oral or written. Up to 5 renewals are permitted within 6 months.

④ Low potential for abuse. Use may lead to limited physical or psychological dependence. Prescriptions may be oral or written. Up to 5 renewals are permitted within 6 months.

⑤ Subject to State and local regulation. Abuse potential is low; a prescription may not be required.

Key to FDA Use-in-pregnancy Ratings

The Food and Drug Administration's Pregnancy Categories are based on the degree to which available information has ruled out risk to the fetus, balanced against the drug's potential benefits to the patient. Ratings range from "A," for drugs that have been tested for teratogenicity under controlled conditions with no showing evidence of damage to the fetus, to "D" and "X" for drugs that are definitely teratogenic. The "D" rating is generally reserved for drugs with no safer alternatives. The "X" rating means there is absolutely no reason to risk using the drug in pregnancy.

CATEGORY   INTERPRETATION

A. Controlled studies show no risk. Adequate, well-controlled studies in pregnant women have failed to demonstrate risk to the fetus.

B. No evidence of risk in humans. Either animal findings show risk, but human findings do not; or, if no adequate human studies have been done, animal findings are negative.

C. Risk cannot be ruled out. Human studies are lacking, and animal studies are either positive for fetal risk, or lacking as well. However, potential benefits may justify the potential risk.

D. Positive evidence of risk. Investigational or post-marketing data show risk to the fetus. Nevertheless, potential benefits may outweigh the potential risk.

X. Contraindicated in pregnancy. Studies in animals or humans, or investigational or post-marketing reports, have shown fetal risk which clearly outweighs any possible benefit to the patient.

Vaccine Adverse Event Reporting System

Health care providers and manufacturers are required by law (42 USC 300aa-25) to report reactions to vaccines listed in the Vaccine Injury Table. Reports for reactions to other vaccines are voluntary except when required as a condition of immunization grant awards.

The form appears overleaf and may be photocopied for submission.

DIRECTIONS FOR COMPLETING FORM
(Additional pages may be attached if more space is needed.)

GENERAL

- Use a separate form for each patient. Complete the form to the best of your abilities. Items 3, 4, 7, 8, 10, 11, and 13 are considered essential and should be completed whenever possible. Parents/Guardians may need to consult the facility where the vaccine was administered for some of the information (such as manufacturer, lot number or laboratory data.)
- Refer to the Vaccine Injury Table (VIT) for events mandated for reporting by law. Reporting for other serious events felt to be related but not on the VIT is encouraged.
- Health care providers other than the vaccine administrator (VA) treating a patient for a suspected adverse event should notify the VA and provide the information about the adverse event to allow the VA to complete the form to meet the VA's legal responsibility.
- These data will be used to increase understanding of adverse events following vaccination and will become part of CDC Privacy Act System 09-20-0136, "Epidemiologic Studies and Surveillance of Disease Problems". Information identifying the person who received the vaccine or that person's legal representative will not be made available to the public, but may be available to the vaccinee or legal representative.
- Postage will be paid by addressee. Forms may be photocopied (must be front & back on same sheet).

SPECIFIC INSTRUCTIONS

Form Completed By: To be used by parents/guardians, vaccine manufacturers/distributors, vaccine administrators, and/or the person completing the form on behalf of the patient or the health professional who administered the vaccine.

Item 7:   Describe the suspected adverse event. Such things as temperature, local and general signs and symptoms, time course, duration of symptoms diagnosis, treatment and recovery should be noted.

Item 9:   Check "YES" if the patient's health condition is the same as it was prior to the vaccine, "NO" if the patient has not returned to the pre-vaccination state of health, or "UNKNOWN" if the patient's condition is not known.

Item 10:   Give dates and times as specifically as you can remember. If you do not know the exact time, please
and 11:   indicate "AM" or "PM" when possible if this information is known. If more than one adverse event, give the onset date and time for the most serious event.

Item 12:   Include "negative" or "normal" results of any relevant tests performed as well as abnormal findings.

Item 13:   List ONLY those vaccines given on the day listed in Item 10.

Item 14:   List ANY OTHER vaccines the patient received within four weeks of the date listed in Item 10.

Item 16:   This section refers to how the person who gave the vaccine purchased it, not to the patient's insurance.

Item 17:   List any prescription or non-prescription medications the patient was taking when the vaccine(s) was given.

Item 18:   List any short term illnesses the patient had on the date the vaccine(s) was given (i.e., cold, flu, ear infection).

Item 19:   List any pre-existing physician-diagnosed allergies, birth defects, medical conditions (including developmental and/or neurologic disorders) the patient has.

Item 21:   List any suspected adverse events the patient, or the patient's brothers or sisters, may have had to previous vaccinations. If more than one brother or sister, or if the patient has reacted to more than one prior vaccine, use additional pages to explain completely. For the onset age of a patient, provide the age in months if less than two years old.

Item 26:   This space is for manufacturers' use only.

VACCINE ADVERSE EVENT REPORTING SYSTEM
24 Hour Toll-free information line 1-800-822-7967
P.O. Box 1100, Rockville, MD 20849-1100
PATIENT IDENTITY KEPT CONFIDENTIAL

VAERS

Patient Name:

_____
Last   First   M.I.

Address

_____

_____

City   State   Zip

Telephone no. (_____) _____

Vaccine administered by (Name):

Responsible
Physician _____

Facility Name/Address

_____

_____

City   State   Zip

Telephone no. (_____) _____

Form completed by (Name):

Relation   Vaccine Provider   Patient/Parent
to Patient   Manufacturer   Other

Address (if different from patient or provider)

_____

_____

City   State   Zip

Telephone no. (_____) _____

1. State	2. County where administered	3. Date of birth / / mm dd yy	4. Patient age	5. Sex M F	6. Date form completed / / mm dd yy

7. Describe adverse event(s) (symptoms, signs, time course) and treatment, if any

8. Check all appropriate:
Patient died   (date ____ / ____ / ____)
Life threatening illness   mm   dd   yy
Required emergency room/doctor visit
Required hospitalization (_____days)
Resulted in prolongation of hospitalization
Resulted in permanent disability
None of the above

9. Patient recovered   YES   NO   UNKNOWN

12. Relevant diagnostic tests/laboratory data

10. Date of vaccination / / mm dd yy   Time _____ AM PM

11. Adverse event onset / / mm dd yy   Time _____ AM PM

13. Enter all vaccines given on date listed in no. 10

	Vaccine (type)	Manufacturer	Lot number	Route/Site	No. Previous doses
a.					
b.					
c.					
d.					

14. Any other vaccinations within 4 weeks of date listed in no. 10

	Vaccine (type)	Manufacturer	Lot number	Route/Site	No. Previous doses	Date given
a.						
b.						

15. Vaccinated at:
Private doctor's office/hospital   Military clinic/hospital
Public health clinic/hospital   Other/unknown

16. Vaccine purchased with:
Private funds   Military funds
Public funds   Other /unknown

17. Other medications

18. Illness at time of vaccination (specify)

19. Pre-existing physician-diagnosed allergies, birth defects, medical conditions (specify)

20. Have you reported this adverse event previously?
No   To health department
To doctor   To manufacturer

Only for children 5 and under

22. Birth weight _____ lb. _____ oz.

23. No. of brothers and sisters

21. Adverse event following prior vaccination (check all applicable, specify)

	Adverse Event	Onset Age	Type Vaccine	Dose no. in series
In patient				
In brother or sister				

Only for reports submitted by manufacturer/immunization project

24. Mfr. / imm. proj. report no.

25. Date received by mfr. / imm. proj.

26. 15 day report?   Yes   No

27. Report type   Initial   Follow-Up

Health care providers and manufacturers are required by law (42 USC 300aa-25) to report reactions to vaccines listed in the Vaccine Injury Table.
Reports for reactions to other vaccines are voluntary except when required as a condition of immunization grant awards.

Form VAERS -1

Adverse Reaction Report

INSTRUCTIONS FOR COMPLETING FORM FDA - 1639

REPORTING ADVERSE REACTIONS TO FDA

All health care providers who observe *suspect* reactions to drugs or biologics are encouraged to report these to FDA. Serious reactions, observations of events not described in the package insert, and reactions to newly marketed products are of particular importance.

The form appears overleaf and may be photocopied for submission.

GENERAL
- Use a separate Form FDA-1639 for each patient.
- Additional pages may be attached if space provided on the Form FDA-1639 is inadequate.
- For questions call: 301-443-4580
- Patient and initial reporter identification is held in confidence by the FDA.

SPECIFIC INSTRUCTIONS
I. Reaction Information
    Item 2.   Age—For children under 5 years of age, also write date of birth (DOB) in Item 1. For congenital malformations, give the age and sex of the infant (even though the mother was exposed).
    Item 7.   Describe Reaction(s)—Give signs and/or symptoms, diagnoses, course, etc.
    Item 13. Relevant Tests/Laboratory Data—Both pre- and post-drug values should be provided if known.
II. Suspect Drug Information
    Item 14. Suspect Drug—The trade name is preferred. If a generically produced product is involved, the manufacturer should be identified.
    Item 15. Dose—For pediatric patients, also give body weights.
    Item 20 and 21. NA—is defined as nonapplicable *(e.g. when only one dose given or outcome was irreversible).*
V. Initial Reporter
    Item 26c. Have you also reported this reaction to the manufacturer? Your answer facilitates identification of duplicates in the central adverse reaction file. FDA encourages direct reporting even if a report has been submitted to the manufacturer.

NOTE TO MANUFACTURERS *(Refer to 21 CFR 314.80 and 21 CFR 310.305).* Detailed instructions are contained in the "Guideline for Postmarketing Reporting of Adverse Drug Reactions."

Public reporting burden for this collection of information is estimated to average 5 hours per response, including the time for review instructions, searching existing data sources, gathering and maintaining the data needed, and completing and reviewing the collection of information. Send comments regarding this burden estimate or any other aspect of this collection of information, including suggestions for reducing this burden to:

Reports Clearance Officer, PHS
Hubert H. Humphrey Building, Room 721-B
200 Independence Avenue, S.W.
Washington, DC 20201
Attn: PRA

and to:

Office of Management and Budget
Paperwork Reduction Project (0910-0230)
Washington, DC 20503

Please DO NOT RETURN your questionnaire to either of these addresses
After completing the form, please mail to the following address:

Food and Drug Administration
Division of Epidemiology and Surveillance (HFD-730)
Public Health Service
5600 Fishers Lane
Rockville, MD 20852-9787

DEPARTMENT OF HEALTH AND HUMAN SERVICES
PUBLIC HEALTH SERVICE
FOOD AND DRUG ADMINISTRATION (HFD-730)
ROCKVILLE, MD 20857

Form Approved: OMB No. 0910-0230
See OMB Statement on the Reverse

FDA CONTROL NO.

ADVERSE REACTION REPORT
(Drugs and Biologics)

ACCESSION NO.

I. REACTION INFORMATION

1. PATIENT ID / INITIALS (In.Confidence)	2. AGE YRS.	3. SEX	4 -6. REACTION ONSET			8 -12. CHECK ALL APPROPRIATE
			MO.	DA.	YR.	

8-12. CHECK ALL APPROPRIATE
- ☐ PATIENT DIED
- ☐ REACTION TREATED WITH R$_x$ DRUG
- ☐ RESULTED IN, OR PROLONGED, INPATIENT HOSPITALIZATION
- ☐ RESULTED IN PERMANENT DISABILITY
- ☐ NONE OF THE ABOVE

7. DESCRIBE REACTION(S)

13. RELEVANT TESTS/LABORATORY DATA

II. SUSPECT DRUG(S) INFORMATION

14. SUSPECT DRUG(S) (Give manufacturer and lot no. for vaccines/biologics)

20. DID REACTION ABATE AFTER STOPPING DRUG?
☐ YES   ☐ NO   ☐ NA

15. DAILY DOSE	16. ROUTE OF ADMINISTRATION

21. DID REACTION REAPPEAR AFTER REINTRODUCTION?

17. INDICATION(S) FOR USE

18. DATES OF ADMINISTRATION (From/To)	19. DURATION OF ADMINISTRATION

☐ YES   ☐ NO   ☐ NA

III. CONCOMITANT DRUGS AND HISTORY

22. CONCOMITANT DRUGS AND DATES OF ADMINISTRATION (Exclude those used to treat reaction)

23. OTHER RELEVANT HISTORY (e.g. diagnoses, allergies, pregnancy with LMP, etc.)

IV. ONLY FOR REPORTS SUBMITTED BY MANUFACTURER	V. INITIAL REPORTER (In confidence)
24. NAME AND ADDRESS OF MANUFACTURER (Include Zip Code)	26.-26a. NAME AND ADDRESS OF REPORTER (Include Zip Code)

24a. IND/NDA NO. FOR SUSPECT DRUG	24b. MFR CONTROL NO.	26b. TELEPHONE NO. (Include area code)

24c. DATE RECEIVED BY MANUFACTURER	24d. REPORT SOURCE (Check all that apply)	26c. HAVE YOU ALSO REPORTED THIS REACTION TO THE MANUFACTURER?
	☐ FOREIGN ☐ STUDY ☐ LITERATURE ☐ HEALTH PROFESSIONAL ☐ CONSUMER	☐ YES ☐ NO

25. 15 DAY REPORT?	25a. REPORT TYPE	26d. ARE YOU A HEALTH PROFESSIONAL?	
☐ YES ☐ NO	☐ INITIAL ☐ FOLLOWUP	☐ YES ☐ NO	Submission of a report does not necessarily constitute an admission that the drug caused the adverse reaction.

NOTE: Required of manufacturers by 21 CFR 314.80

FORM FDA 1639 (12/91)   PREVIOUS EDITION MAY BE USED